11th Edition

Davis-Christopher

TEXTBOOK
OF
SURGERY

The Biological Basis of
Modern Surgical Practice

Edited by

DAVID C. SABISTON, Jr., M.D.

James B. Duke Professor and Chairman, Department
of Surgery, Duke University Medical Center,
Durham, North Carolina

W. B. SAUNDERS COMPANY / **Philadelphia** / **London** / **Toronto**

W. B. Saunders Company: West Washington Square
                          Philadelphia, PA   19105

                          1 St. Anne's Road
                          Eastbourne, East Sussex BN21 3UN, England

                          1 Goldthorne Avenue
                          Toronto, Ontario M8Z 5T9, Canada

Listed here is the latest translated edition of this book together with
the language of the translation and the publisher.

Portuguese (9th Edition) — Editora Guanabara Koogan, Rio de Janeiro, Brazil
Spanish (9th Edition) — Editorial Interamericana, Mexico
Japanese (10th Edition) — Igaku Shoin Ltd., Tokyo, Japan

Davis-Christopher TEXTBOOK OF SURGERY   Single Volume   0-7216-7868-8
                                                    Volume 1   0-7216-7869-6
                                                    Volume 2   0-7216-7870-X

Last digit is the print number: 9   8   7   6   5   4   3

DEDICATION

To medical students and residents, who
through their commitment, innovative thinking, and searching minds
continuously stimulate the entire profession to make
improvements in the diagnosis and management of the sick.

PREFACE

In the eleventh edition of this text, continuing emphasis is placed upon the *biological* derangements which form the basis of disease. The fundamental roles of physiology, biochemistry, immunology, pharmacology, and pathology form the foundation for discussion in relation to the pathogenesis, clinical manifestations, diagnosis, and management of each disorder. While such an approach has obvious merit of its own, it is perhaps even more significant that the contemporary student with complete justification insists that these fundamental biological features form the basis of a modern text.

Recognizing the fact that readers clearly prefer contributors of recognized authority, this policy has been continued in the present edition such that the subject and author may be clearly identified. The annotated bibliography, introduced in the last edition, has been expanded with concise descriptions of the most important references in the literature. Renewed emphasis has also been placed upon *illustrations,* with the best of those available in the current literature being selected for reproduction.

A number of new chapters and subjects have been added, including surgical problems associated with diabetes mellitus; the acute care unit — monitoring of the surgical patient; medullary carcinoma of the thyroid and multiple endocrine neoplasias; the diagnosis and management of massive gastrointestinal bleeding by arteriography and vasoconstrictors; hemobilia; intestinal bypass for hypercholesterolemia and morbid obesity; and plastic procedures for augmentation and reduction of the breast. Dr. J. Leonard Goldner and associates have prepared new sections on the musculoskeletal system, including fractures and dislocations, amputations, infections and neoplasms of bone, and the hand. The coronary circulation has received additional emphasis in view of the large number of surgical procedures being performed for myocardial ischemia. A new section on pathological changes occurring in venous autografts has been added, and all aspects of the text have been thoroughly revised and updated. The chapter on "Fluid and Electrolyte Balance in Surgical Patients" has been rewritten in an exemplary manner by Shires, as has the chapter on "Principles of Preoperative Preparation of the Surgical Patient" by Polk.

Finally, it has been necessary in this edition to make a major policy decision in order that it continue both as a definitive textbook of surgery and as a reference source to meet the needs of medical students, residents, practicing surgeons, and teachers of surgery. This decision was clearly necessary in order to include the many advances which characterize modern scientific surgery.

DAVID C. SABISTON, JR.

CONTRIBUTORS

PAUL C. ADKINS, M.D.
: Professor and Chairman, Department of Surgery, George Washington University School of Medicine, Washington, D.C.
Tumors of the Esophagus

J. WESLEY ALEXANDER, M.D., Sc.D.
: Professor of Surgery, University of Cincinnati College of Medicine. Attending Surgeon, Cincinnati General Hospital, Christian R. Holmes Hospital, Christ Hospital, and Shriners Burns Hospital, Cincinnati, Ohio.
Surgical Infections and Choice of Antibiotics

WILLIAM A. ALTEMEIER, M.D.
: Christian R. Holmes Professor of Surgery and Chairman of the Department, University of Cincinnati College of Medicine. Director, Surgical Services, Cincinnati General Hospital; Surgeon in Chief, Children's Hospital and Christian R. Holmes Hospital, Cincinnati, Ohio.
Surgical Infections and Choice of Antibiotics

D. BERNARD AMOS, M.D.
: James B. Duke Professor of Immunology and Experimental Surgery, Duke University School of Medicine. Chief, Division of Immunology, Duke University Medical Center, Durham, North Carolina.
Transplantation Antigens; Immune Mechanisms and Allograft Destruction

ROBERT W. ANDERSON, M.D.
: Associate Professor of Surgery, University of Minnesota Medical School, Minneapolis, Minnesota.
Bronchoscopy

WILLIAM G. ANLYAN, M.D.
: Professor of Surgery, Duke University School of Medicine. Vice President for Health Affairs, Duke University, Durham, North Carolina.
Carcinoid Tumors and the Carcinoid Syndrome

CURTIS P. ARTZ, M.D.
: Professor of Surgery and Chairman of the Department, Medical University of South Carolina. Chief of Surgery, Medical University Hospital; Chief Surgical Consultant, Veterans Administration Hospital and Charleston County Hospital, Charleston, South Carolina.
Burns: Including Cold, Chemical, and Electrical Injuries

J. BRADLEY AUST, M.D., Ph.D.
: Professor and Chairman, Department of Surgery, The University of Texas Health Science Center at San Antonio—Medical School. Chief of Surgery, Bexar County Teaching Hospitals, San Antonio, Texas.
Pyogenic Liver Abscess

W. GERALD AUSTEN, M.D.

Edward D. Churchill Professor of Surgery, Harvard Medical School. Chief of Surgical Services, Massachusetts General Hospital, Boston, Massachusetts.

Lung Function: Physiologic Considerations Applicable to Surgery; Acquired Mitral and Tricuspid Valvular Disease

HENRY T. BAHNSON, M.D.

George V. Foster Professor and Chairman, Department of Surgery, University of Pittsburgh School of Medicine. Chief of Surgery, Presbyterian-University Hospital; Attending Surgeon, Children's Hospital of Pittsburgh, Montefiore Hospital, and Veterans Administration Hospital, Pittsburgh, Pennsylvania.

Patent Ductus Arteriosus, Coarctation of the Aorta, Aortic Vascular Ring, and Interruption of the Aortic Arch

WALTER F. BALLINGER, M.D.

Bixby Professor of Surgery and Chairman of the Department, Washington University School of Medicine. Surgeon in Chief, The Barnes Group of Hospitals, St. Louis, Missouri.

The Spleen

HENDRICK B. BARNER, M.D.

Professor of Vascular Surgery, St. Louis University School of Medicine. Attending Surgeon, Firmin Desloge Hospital, St. Louis, Missouri.

Carotid Occlusive Disease

FRANK H. BASSETT, III, M.D.

Professor of Orthopaedic Surgery and Assistant Professor of Anatomy, Duke University School of Medicine. Attending Surgeon, Durham County General Hospital, Lenox Baker Cerebral Palsy and Crippled Children's Hospital of North Carolina, and Veterans Administration Hospital, Durham, North Carolina.

Fractures of the Tibia, Fibula, Ankle, and Foot

ARTHUR E. BAUE, M.D.

Professor and Chairman of Surgery, Yale University School of Medicine. Chief of Surgery, Yale-New Haven Hospital, New Haven, Connecticut.

The Rationale and Scientific Basis of Current Examinations in Surgery

STEPHEN B. BAYLIN, M.D.

Assistant Professor of Medicine and Assistant Professor of Oncology, The Johns Hopkins University School of Medicine. Attending Physician, Johns Hopkins Hospital, Baltimore, Maryland.

The Multiple Endocrine Neoplasias

JOHN M. BEAL, M.D.

Professor and Chairman, Department of Surgery, Northwestern University Medical School. Chairman, Department of Surgery, Northwestern Memorial Hospital, Chicago, Illinois.

The Acute Abdomen

FOLKERT O. BELZER, M.D.

Professor of Surgery, University of Wisconsin Medical School. Chairman, Department of Surgery, Division of General Surgery, and Section of Transplant Surgery, University Hospitals, Madison, Wisconsin.

Preservation of the Kidney

HARVEY W. BENDER, JR., M.D.

Professor of Surgery, Vanderbilt University School of Medicine. Chairman, Department of Cardiac and Thoracic Surgery, Vanderbilt University Hospital, Nashville, Tennessee.

Tricuspid Atresia

JOHN J. BERGAN, M.D.
  Magerstadt Professor of Surgery and Director, Vascular Training Program, North-western University Medical School. Attending Surgeon, Northwestern Memorial Hospital and Lake Side Veterans Administration Hospital, Chicago, Illinois.
Visceral Ischemic Syndrome

RICHARD J. BING, M.D.
  Professor of Medicine, University of Southern California School of Medicine, Los Angeles. Director of Cardiology and Intramural Medicine, Huntington Memorial Hospital, Pasadena, California.
Cardiac Catheterization

WILLIAM S. BLAKEMORE, M.D.
  Professor and Chairman, Department of Surgery, Medical College of Ohio at Toledo. Attending Surgeon, Medical College of Ohio Hospital, Toledo, Ohio.
Angiography in Diagnosis and Treatment of Gastrointestinal Bleeding

C. THOMAS BOMBECK, M.D.
  Associate Professor of Surgery, The Abraham Lincoln School of Medicine of the University of Illinois College of Medicine. Chief, Division of Gastroenterological Surgery, University of Illinois Hospital, Chicago, Illinois.
Hernias

EDWARD L. BRADLEY, III, M.D.
  Associate Professor of Surgery, Emory University School of Medicine. Attending Surgeon, Emory University Hospital; Director, Elective Surgical Service, Grady Memorial Hospital; Consultant, Veterans Administration Hospital, Atlanta, Georgia.
The Pancreas

ROBERT K. BRAWLEY, M.D.
  Associate Professor of Surgery, The Johns Hopkins University School of Medicine. Attending Surgeon, Johns Hopkins Hospital; Consultant Surgeon, Veterans Administration Hospital, Baltimore City Hospitals, and U.S. Public Health Service Hospital, Baltimore, Maryland.
Double Outlet Right Ventricle

GERT H. BRIEGER, M.D., Ph.D.
  Professor and Chairman, Department of History of the Health Sciences, University of California, San Francisco, School of Medicine, San Francisco, California.
The Development of Surgery

DONALD S. BRIGHT, M.D.
  Assistant Professor of Orthopaedic Surgery, Duke University School of Medicine. Attending Surgeon, Duke University Medical Center, Veterans Administration Hospital, Durham, and Cabarrus Memorial Hospital, Concord, North Carolina.
Fractures and Dislocations of the Shoulder

EDWARD A. BRUNNER, M.D.
  Professor and Chairman, Department of Anesthesia, Northwestern University Medical School, Chicago, Illinois.
Anesthesia

HENRY BUCHWALD, M.D., Ph.D.
  Associate Professor of Surgery, University of Minnesota Medical School. Attending Surgeon, University of Minnesota Hospitals, Minneapolis, Minnesota.
Intestinal Bypass for Hyperlipidemia and Morbid Obesity

FRED T. CALDWELL, M.D.
  Professor of Surgery, University of Arkansas School of Medicine, Little Rock, Arkansas.
Fever

GILBERT S. CAMPBELL, M.D., Ph.D.
    Chairman and Professor of Surgery, University of Arkansas School of Medicine,
    Little Rock, Arkansas.
Bronchiectasis

PETER C. CANIZARO, M.D.
    Associate Professor, Cornell University Medical College. Attending Physician, The
    New York Hospital, New York, New York.
Fluid and Electrolyte Management of the Surgical Patient

LARRY C. CAREY, M.D.
    Professor and Chairman of the Department of Surgery, Ohio State University College
    of Medicine. Attending Surgeon, Ohio State University Hospitals, Columbus, Ohio.
Acute Cholecystitis

PHILIP W. CATALANO, M.D.
    Clinical Instructor in Surgery, Ohio State University College of Medicine. Resident
    Staff, Ohio State University Hospitals, Columbus, Ohio.
Acute Cholecystitis

WILLIAM M. CHARDACK, M.D.
    Associate Professor of Surgery, State University of New York at Buffalo School of
    Medicine. Thoracic Surgeon, Veterans Administration Hospital, Buffalo, New York.
Cardiac Pacemakers

FRANK W. CLIPPINGER, JR., M.D.
    Professor of Orthopaedic Surgery, Duke University School of Medicine. Attending
    Surgeon, Duke University Medical Center and Lenox Baker Cerebral Palsy and
    Crippled Children's Hospital of North Carolina, Durham; Consultant, McCain
    Hospital, McCain, North Carolina.
Amputations and Limb Substitutions

ISIDORE COHN, JR., M.D., M.Sc.(Med.), D.Sc.(Med.)
    Professor and Chairman, Department of Surgery, Louisiana State University School
    of Medicine. Senior Visiting Surgeon and Surgeon in Chief, Louisiana State Uni-
    versity Hospital and Charity Hospital of Louisiana, New Orleans, Louisiana.
The Colon and Rectum

JACK W. COLE, M.D.
    Ensign Professor of Surgery, Yale University School of Medicine. Director, Division
    of Oncology and Yale Comprehensive Cancer Center; Attending Surgeon, Yale-New
    Haven Hospital, New Haven, Connecticut.
Polyps of the Colon and Rectum

ROBERT E. CONDON, M.D.
    Professor of Surgery, The Medical College of Wisconsin. Chief of Surgical Services,
    Wood Veterans Administration Hospital; Consultant or Attending Surgeon, Mil-
    waukee County General Hospital, Columbia Hospital, and Deaconess Hospital,
    Milwaukee, Wisconsin.
Appendicitis

REX B. CONN, M.D.
    Professor of Laboratory Medicine, The Johns Hopkins University School of Medi-
    cine. Director, Department of Laboratory Medicine, The Johns Hopkins Hospital,
    Baltimore, Maryland.
Normal Laboratory Values of Clinical Importance

JOHN E. CONNOLLY, M.D.
    Professor and Chairman, Department of Surgery, University of California, Irvine,
    California College of Medicine, Irvine, California. Consultant, Long Beach

Veterans Administration Hospital and Long Beach Naval Hospitals, Long Beach, California.
Assisted Circulation

WILLARD M. DAGGETT, M.D.
Associate Professor of Surgery, Harvard Medical School. Associate Visiting Surgeon, Massachusetts General Hospital, Boston, Massachusetts.
Pharmacology of the Cardiovascular System in the Surgical Patient

JOHN H. DAVIS, M.D.
Professor and Chairman, Department of Surgery, University of Vermont College of Medicine. Surgeon-in-Chief, Medical Center Hospital of Vermont, Burlington, Vermont.
Surgical Aspects of Diabetes Mellitus

JEROME J. DeCOSSE, M.D., Ph.D.
Professor and Chairman of Surgery, Medical College of Wisconsin. Director of Surgery, Milwaukee County General Hospital, Milwaukee, Wisconsin.
Radiation Injury to the Intestinal Tract

MARCUS L. DILLON, JR., M.D.
Professor of Surgery, University of Kentucky College of Medicine. Chief, Cardio-thoracic Surgery, Veterans Administration Hospital, Lexington, Kentucky.
Benign Tumors of the Trachea and Bronchi

ARTHUR J. DONOVAN, M.D.
Professor and Chairman, Department of Surgery, University of South Alabama, Mobile, Alabama.
Benign Tumors of the Stomach

THEODORE DRAPANAS, M.D.†
Trauma

WILLIAM R. DRUCKER, M.D.
Dean and Professor of Surgery, University of Virginia School of Medicine. Chief of Staff, University of Virginia Hospital, Charlottesville, Virginia.
Regional Enteritis

STANLEY J. DUDRICK, M.D.
Chairman, Department of Surgery, The University of Texas Health Science Center at Houston – Medical School. Chief of Surgical Services, The Hermann Hospital; Consultant in Surgery, The University of Texas System Cancer Center, M.D. Anderson Hospital and Tumor Institute, Houston, Texas.
Metabolism in Surgical Patients

PAUL A. EBERT, M.D.
Professor and Chairman, Department of Surgery, University of California, San Francisco, School of Medicine, San Francisco, California.
Thoracic Trauma; The Pericardium; Transposition of the Great Arteries

JAMES E. ECKENHOFF, M.D.
Dean and Professor of Anesthesia, Northwestern University Medical School, Chicago, Illinois.
Anesthesia

MILTON T. EDGERTON, M.D.
Professor and Chairman, Department of Plastic Surgery, University of Virginia School of Medicine. Plastic Surgeon in Chief, University of Virginia Hospital,

---

†Deceased

Charlottesville, Virginia; Consultant Plastic Surgeon, Clinical Center, National Institutes of Health, Bethesda, Maryland, and Veterans Administration Hospital, Salem, Virginia.
The Mouth, Tongue, Jaws, and Salivary Glands

W. STERLING EDWARDS, M.D.

Professor and Chairman, Department of Surgery, University of New Mexico School of Medicine, Albuquerque, New Mexico.
Aneurysms of the Sinus of Valsalva

F. HENRY ELLIS, JR., M.D., Ph.D.

Associate Clinical Professor of Surgery, Harvard Medical School. Chief of Thoracic and Cardiovascular Surgery, Lahey Clinic Foundation and New England Deaconess Hospital, Boston, Massachusetts.
The Esophagus

ANTHONY J. FEDERICO, M.D.

Assistant Clinical Professor of Surgery, State University of New York at Buffalo School of Medicine. Chief, Cardio-Thoracic Service, Sisters of Charity Hospital, Buffalo, New York.
Cardiac Pacemakers

WILLIAM T. FITTS, JR., M.D.

Professor of Surgery, University of Pennsylvania School of Medicine. Associate Chief of Surgery, Hospital of the University of Pennsylvania, Philadelphia, Pennsylvania.
Polycythemia Vera

THOMAS J. FOGARTY, M.D.

Cardiovascular Surgeon, Stanford University Hospital, Stanford, California.
Acute Arterial Occlusion

JOHN E. FOKER, M.D., Ph.D.

Assistant Professor of Surgery, University of Minnesota Medical School. Attending Surgeon, University of Minnesota Health Science Center, St. Paul-Ramsey Hospital, and Hennepin County General Hospital, Minneapolis, Minnesota.
Principles of Immunosuppression

MORRIS E. FRANKLIN, JR., M.D.

Assistant Professor of Surgery, University of Texas Health Science Center at San Antonio — Medical School. Attending Surgeon, Bexar County Hospital, Baptist Memorial Hospital, and Santa Rosa Memorial Hospital, San Antonio, Texas, and Penrose Hospital and St. Francis Hospital, Colorado Springs, Colorado.
Pyogenic Liver Abscess

ROBERT J. FREEARK, M.D.

Professor and Chairman, Department of Surgery, Loyola University of Chicago Stritch School of Medicine, Chicago. Surgeon in Chief, Foster G. McGaw Hospital of Loyola University, Maywood; Consultant, Hines Veterans Administration Hospital, Hines, Illinois.
Arterial Injuries

HARRY FRIEDMAN, B.S., M.D.

Instructor in Neurosurgery, University of Tennessee College of Medicine. Associate Staff, Baptist Memorial Hospital; Consulting Staff, Le Bonheur Children's Hospital and St. Joseph Hospital, Memphis, Tennessee.
Neurosurgical Relief of Pain

WILLIAM J. FRY, M.D.

Professor and Chairman, Department of Surgery, University of Texas Health Science Center at Dallas — Southwestern Medical School. Senior Attending Staff, General

Surgery and Peripheral Vascular Surgery, University of Texas Health Science Center and Parkland Memorial Hospital, Dallas, Texas.
Femoral and Popliteal Artery Aneurysms

JAMES C. A. FUCHS, M.D.
Burroughs Wellcome Associate Professor of Surgery and Assistant Professor of Pharmacology, Duke University School of Medicine. Attending Physician, Duke University Medical Center, Durham, North Carolina.
Pathologic Changes Occurring in Venous Autografts

ANDREW A. GAGE, M.D.
Professor of Surgery, State University of New York at Buffalo School of Medicine. Chief, Surgical Service and Chief of Staff, Veterans Administration Hospital, Buffalo, New York.
Cardiac Pacemakers

SUNILENDU N. GANGULY, M.D.
Assistant Professor of Medicine, Wayne State University School of Medicine. Chief, Section of Cardiology, Hutzel Hospital, Detroit, Michigan.
Cardiac Catheterization

WILLIAM A. GAY, JR., M.D.
Associate Professor of Surgery, Cornell University Medical Center. Associate Attending Surgeon, The New York Hospital, New York, New York.
Ventricular Aneurysm

NICHOLAS G. GEORGIADE, M.D.
Professor of Plastic, Maxillofacial, and Reconstructive Surgery, Duke University School of Medicine. Chief, Division of Plastic, Maxillofacial, and Reconstructive Surgery, Duke University Medical Center, Durham, North Carolina.
Reconstructive Surgery of the Breast

JAMES F. GLENN, M.D.
Professor of Urology, Duke University School of Medicine. Chief, Division of Urology, Duke University Medical Center, Durham, North Carolina.
The Male Genital System

J. LEONARD GOLDNER, M.D.
Professor of Orthopaedic Surgery, Duke University School of Medicine. Chief, Division of Orthopaedic Surgery, Duke University Medical Center, Durham, North Carolina.
Fractures of the Carpal Bones; Fractures and Dislocations of the Hand; The Hand

HARRY S. GOLDSMITH, M.D.
Samuel D. Gross Professor of Surgery and Chairman, Department of Surgery, Jefferson Medical College of Thomas Jefferson University. Surgeon in Chief, Thomas Jefferson University Hospital, Philadelphia, Pennsylvania.
Disorders of the Lymphatic System

JOHN T. GRAYHACK, M.D.
Professor and Chairman, Department of Urology, Northwestern University Medical School. Attending Physician and Chairman of Urology, Northwestern Memorial Hospital; Consultant, Lake Side Veterans Administration Hospital, Chicago, Illinois.
The Urinary System

LAZAR J. GREENFIELD, M.D.
Stuart McGuire Professor and Chairman, Department of Surgery, Medical College of Virginia of Virginia Commonwealth University. Chief of Surgery, Medical College of Virginia Hospitals, Richmond, Virginia.
Cardiac Arrest

RANDALL B. GRIEPP, M.D.
Professor of Surgery, State University of New York, Downstate Medical Center,

College of Medicine. Chief, Division of Cardiothoracic Surgery, State University Hospital, Brooklyn, New York.
Cardiac Homotransplants

WARD O. GRIFFEN, JR., M.D., Ph.D.
Professor and Chairman, Department of Surgery, University of Kentucky College of Medicine. Chief of Surgery, University Hospital; Consultant Surgeon, Veterans Administration Hospital; Attending Surgeon, Central Baptist Hospital, St. Joseph Hospital, and Good Samaritan Hospital, Lexington, Kentucky.
Meckel's Diverticulum

HERMES C. GRILLO, M.D.
Professor of Surgery, Harvard Medical School. Chief of General Thoracic Surgery, Massachusetts General Hospital, Boston, Massachusetts.
Tracheostomy and Its Complications

J. CAULIE GUNNELLS, JR., M.D.
Professor of Medicine, Duke University School of Medicine, Durham, North Carolina.
Surgical Management of Renovascular Hypertension

CHARLES B. HAMMOND, M.D.
Associate Professor of Obstetrics and Gynecology, Duke University School of Medicine. Director, Division of Reproductive Endocrinology, Department of Obstetrics and Gynecology, Duke University Medical Center, Durham, North Carolina.
Gynecology

JAMES D. HARDY, M.D.
Professor and Chairman, Department of Surgery, University of Mississippi School of Medicine. Surgeon in Chief, University Hospital; Surgical Consultant, Veterans Administration Hospital, Jackson, Mississippi.
Surgical Complications

JOHN M. HARRELSON, M.D.
Assistant Professor of Orthopaedic Surgery and Associate in Pathology, Duke University School of Medicine, Durham, North Carolina.
Fractures and Dislocations: General Principles; Infections and Neoplasms of Bone

TIMOTHY S. HARRISON, M.D.
Professor of Surgery and Physiology, Pennsylvania State University College of Medicine. Attending Surgeon, Milton S. Hershey Medical Center, Hershey, Pennsylvania.
The Thyroid Gland

BRACK G. HATTLER, JR., M.D., Ph.D.
Associate Professor of Surgery, University of Arizona Medical Center. Attending Surgeon, Veterans Administration Hospital and Porter Memorial Hospital, Denver, and Swedish Medical Center, Englewood, Colorado.
Cardiac Neoplasms

DAVID B. HINSHAW, M.D.
Professor and Chairman, Department of Surgery, Loma Linda University School of Medicine, Loma Linda, California.
Acute Suppurative Cholangitis

THOMAS M. HOLDER, M.D.
Clinical Professor of Surgery, University of Missouri—Kansas City School of Medicine. Chief, Thoracic and Cardiovascular Surgery, Children's Mercy Hospital, Kansas City, Missouri.
Pediatric Surgery

THOMAS W. HOYT, M.D.
Assistant Professor, University of New Mexico School of Medicine. Attending Surgeon, Presbyterian Hospital and Bernalillo County Hospital, Albuquerque, New Mexico.
Aneurysms of the Sinus of Valsalva

LOREN J. HUMPHREY, M.D., Ph.D.
Professor and Chairman, Department of Surgery, University of Kansas School of Medicine, Kansas City, Kansas.
Malignant Melanoma

ADOLPH M. HUTTER, JR., M.D.
Associate Professor of Medicine, Harvard Medical School. Assistant Physician, Massachusetts General Hospital, Boston, Massachusetts.
Acquired Mitral and Tricuspid Valvular Disease

GLYN G. JAMIESON, M.B., B.S., F.R.A.C.S.
Senior Lecturer in Surgery, University of Adelaide. Visiting Surgeon, Royal Adelaide Hospital; Consultant in Surgery, Queen Elizabeth Hospital; Associate in Vascular Surgery, Adelaide Children's Hospital, Adelaide, South Australia.
Disorders of Systemic Veins

R. SCOTT JONES, M.D.
Professor of Surgery, Duke University School of Medicine. Attending Physician, Duke University Hospital and Veterans Administration Hospital, Durham, North Carolina.
The Small Intestine

ROBERT H. JONES, M.D.
Assistant Professor of Surgery, Duke University School of Medicine. Attending Surgeon, Duke University Medical Center, Durham, North Carolina.
Radioisotope Techniques for Diagnosis of Surgical Disorders

GEORGE L. JORDAN, JR., M.D., M.S.(Surgery)
Professor of Surgery, Baylor College of Medicine. Chief of Staff, Harris County Hospital District; Senior Attending Physician, The Methodist Hospital; Consultant, Veterans Administration Hospital, St. Luke's Episcopal Hospital, and Texas Children's Hospital, Houston, Texas.
Neoplasms of the Liver

RICHARD C. KARL, M.D.
Professor and Chairman, Department of Surgery, Dartmouth Medical School. Chairman, Department of Surgery, Mary Hitchcock Memorial Hospital, Hanover, New Hampshire; Consultant in Surgery, Veterans Administration Hospital, White River Junction, Vermont.
Lymphomas of the Stomach

J. MICHAEL KELLY, M.D.
Professor and Chief, Division of Plastic Surgery, University of Oklahoma College of Medicine. Chief of Plastic Surgery, Oklahoma University Health Sciences Center, Veterans Administration Hospital, and Oklahoma Children's Memorial Hospital, Oklahoma City, Oklahoma.
Replantation of the Extremities

JOHN M. KINNEY, M.D.
Professor of Surgery, Columbia University College of Physicians and Surgeons. Attending Surgeon, Presbyterian Hospital, New York, New York.
Fever

JOHN W. KIRKLIN, M.D.
Fay Fletcher Kerner Professor and Chairman, Department of Surgery, University

of Alabama School of Medicine. Surgeon in Chief, University of Alabama Hospitals, Birmingham, Alabama.
Ventricular Septal Defects

NICHOLAS T. KOUCHOUKOS, M.D.
    Professor of Surgery, University of Alabama School of Medicine. Attending Surgeon, University of Alabama Hospitals and Veterans Administration Hospital, Birmingham, Alabama.
Ventricular Septal Defects

SAMUEL L. KOUNTZ, M.D.
    Professor of Surgery, State University of New York, Downstate Medical Center, College of Medicine. Attending Surgeon, State University Hospital, Brooklyn, New York.
Autotransplantation

WILLIAM W. KRIPPAEHNE, M.D.
    Professor and Chairman, Department of Surgery, University of Oregon Medical School, Portland, Oregon.
Arterial Substitutes

FRANK T. KURZWEG, M.D., M.S.(Surgery)
    Professor and Head, Department of Surgery, Louisiana State University School of Medicine in Shreveport. Chief, Surgical Service, Confederate Memorial Medical Center and Veterans Administration Hospital, Shreveport, Louisiana.
Mesenteric Cysts

HIRAM T. LANGSTON, M.D.
    Professor of Surgery, Abraham Lincoln School of Medicine of the University of Illinois College of Medicine. Thoracic Surgeon, St. Joseph Hospital, Grant Hospital, and Cook County Hospital, Chicago, Illinois.
The Development of Thoracic Surgery

ALLAN M. LANSING, M.D., Ph.D.
    Clinical Professor of Surgery, University of Louisville School of Medicine. Chief of Cardiovascular Surgery, Jewish Hospital; Chief of Pediatric Cardiac Surgery, Norton-Children's Hospitals; Attending Staff, Methodist Evangelical Hospital and St. Joseph Infirmary, Louisville, Kentucky.
Traumatic Aneurysms of the Aorta

DEMETRIOS G. LAPPAS, M.D.
    Assistant Professor of Anesthesia, Harvard Medical School. Assistant Anesthetist, Massachusetts General Hospital, Boston, Massachusetts.
Pharmacology of the Cardiovascular System in the Surgical Patient

MYRON B. LAVER, M.D.
    Professor of Anesthesia, Harvard Medical School. Anesthetist, Massachusetts General Hospital, Boston, Massachusetts.
Lung Function: Physiologic Considerations Applicable to Surgery

LUCIAN L. LEAPE, M.D.
    Professor of Surgery, Tufts University School of Medicine. Chief of Pediatric Surgery, New England Medical Center Hospital, Boston, Massachusetts.
Pediatric Surgery

LaSALLE D. LEFFALL, JR., M.D.
    Professor and Chairman, Department of Surgery, Howard University College of Medicine. Chief, Department of Surgery, Howard University Hospital, Washington, D.C.
Soft Tissue Sarcomas

MARTIN S. LITWIN, M.D.
  Professor of Surgery, Tulane University School of Medicine. Visiting Surgeon, Charity Hospital of Louisiana; Medical Director, Tulane Clinical Care Center, New Orleans, Louisiana.
Trauma

WILLIAM P. LONGMIRE JR., M.D.
  Professor of Surgery, UCLA School of Medicine. Surgeon in Chief, UCLA Hospital, Los Angeles, California.
Carcinoma of the Stomach

JOHN LUDBROOK, M.D., Ch.M., B.Med.Sc., F.R.C.S., F.R.A.C.S.
  Dorothy Mortlock Professor of Surgery, University of Adelaide. Visiting Surgeon, Royal Adelaide Hospital; Consultant in Surgery, Queen Elizabeth Hospital and Adelaide Children's Hospital, Adelaide, South Australia.
Disorders of Systemic Veins

ROBERT A. MACBETH, M.D., M.Sc.
  Associate Dean and Professor of Surgery, Dalhousie University, Halifax, Nova Scotia. Director of Postgraduate Medical Education (New Brunswick); Active Staff, Saint John General Hospital, Saint John, New Brunswick, Canada.
The Abdominal Wall, Umbilicus, Peritoneum, Mesenteries, and Retroperitoneum

JAMES W. MacKENZIE, M.D.
  Professor and Chairman, Department of Surgery, College of Medicine and Dentistry of New Jersey—Rutgers Medical School, Piscataway. Attending Surgeon, Raritan Valley Hospital, Green Brook, and Medical Center at Princeton, Princeton, New Jersey.
Diagnostic Thoracoscopy

LLOYD D. MacLEAN, M.D.
  Professor of Surgery, McGill University. Surgeon in Chief, Royal Victoria Hospital, Montreal, Quebec, Canada.
Shock

JOHN W. MADDEN, M.D.
  Director, The Hand Rehabilitation Center, Inc., Tucson. Staff Surgeon, St. Joseph's Hospital and Tucson Medical Center, Tucson, Arizona.
Wound Healing

M. STEPHEN MAHALEY, JR., M.D., Ph.D.
  Professor and Chief, Division of Neurosurgery, University of North Carolina School of Medicine. Chief of Neurosurgery, North Carolina Memorial Hospital, Chapel Hill, North Carolina.
Diagnostic Studies in Neurosurgery; Intracranial Tumors; Spinal Tumors; Congenital Neurosurgical Abnormalities

DEV R. MANHAS, M.D., M.S.(Surgery)
  Clinical Assistant Professor of Surgery, University of Washington School of Medicine. Consultant, Veterans Administration Hospital; Active Staff, Providence Medical Center and Swedish Hospital Medical Center, Seattle, Washington.
Disorders of Pulmonary Venous Return

JOHN A. MANNICK, M.D.
  Moseley Professor of Surgery, Harvard Medical School. Surgeon in Chief, Peter Bent Brigham Hospital, Boston, Massachusetts.
Subclavian Steal Syndrome

ARLIE R. MANSBERGER, JR., M.D., Sc.D.
  Professor and Chairman, Department of Surgery, Medical College of Georgia School

of Medicine. Consultant in Surgery, Forest Hills Veterans Administration Hospital, Augusta, Georgia.
Vascular Compression of the Duodenum

G. ROBERT MASON, M.D., Ph.D.
Professor and Chairman, Department of Surgery, University of Maryland School of Medicine, Baltimore, Maryland.
Tumors of the Duodenum and Small Intestine

DONALD E. McCOLLUM, M.D.
Professor of Orthopaedic Surgery, Duke University School of Medicine, Durham, North Carolina.
Fractures of the Pelvis, Femur, and Knee

ARTHUR S. McFEE, M.D., Ph.D.
Professor of Surgery, University of Texas Health Science Center at San Antonio—Medical School. Staff Physician, Bexar County Hospital and Veterans Administration Hospital; Consultant, Santa Rosa Medical Center and Methodist Hospital, San Antonio, Texas.
Pyogenic Liver Abscess

EMMANUEL G. MELISSINOS, M.D.
Instructor in Surgery, University of Pennsylvania School of Medicine. Attending Surgeon, Veterans Administration Hospital and Hospital of the University of Pennsylvania, Philadelphia, Pennsylvania.
Polycythemia Vera

K. ALVIN MERENDINO, M.D., Ph.D.
Professor of Surgery, University of Washington School of Medicine. Active Medical Staff, General, Thoracic, and Cardiovascular Surgery, Harborview Medical Center; Consultant in Surgery, Veterans Administration Hospital and Children's Orthopedic Hospital, Seattle, Washington. Chairman, Department of Surgery, King Faisal's Specialist Hospital and Research Center, Riyadh, Saudi Arabia.
Disorders of Pulmonary Venous Return

FRANK G. MOODY, M.D.
Professor and Chairman, Department of Surgery, University of Utah College of Medicine. Attending Surgeon, University of Utah Medical Center, Salt Lake City, Utah.
Ulcerative Colitis

GORDON F. MOOR, M.D.
Attending Surgeon, Watson Clinic. Chief, Thoracic and Cardiovascular Section, Lakeland General Hospital, Lakeland, Florida.
Surgical Treatment of Pulmonary Tuberculosis

FRANCIS D. MOORE, M.D.
Moseley Professor Emeritus of Surgery, Harvard Medical School. Surgeon in Chief Emeritus, Peter Bent Brigham Hospital, Boston, Massachusetts.
Homeostasis: Bodily Changes in Trauma and Surgery

RICHARD B. MOORE, M.D.
Assistant Professor of Medicine, University of Minnesota Medical School. Attending Surgeon, University of Minnesota Hospitals, Minneapolis, Minnesota.
Intestinal Bypass for Hyperlipidemia and Morbid Obesity

DONALD L. MORTON, M.D.
Professor of Surgery, UCLA School of Medicine. Chief, Division of Surgical Oncology, Department of Surgery, UCLA Hospital, Los Angeles; Chief, Oncology Section, Surgical Service, Veterans Administration Hospital, Sepulveda, California.
Immunobiology and Immunotherapy of Neoplastic Disease

JOSEPH A. MOYLAN, M.D.
> Associate Professor of Surgery, Duke University School of Medicine. Chief, Trauma Service, and Surgeon in Charge, Emergency Department, Duke University Medical Center, Durham, North Carolina.

Fat Embolism Syndrome

WILLIAM H. MULLER, JR., M.D.
> Stephen H. Watts Professor and Chairman, Department of Surgery, Vice-President for Medical Affairs, University of Virginia School of Medicine. Surgeon in Chief, University of Virginia Medical Center, Charlottesville, Virginia.

Acquired Disorders of the Aortic Valve

RICHARD T. MYERS, M.D.
> Professor and Chairman, Department of Surgery, Bowman Gray School of Medicine of Wake Forest University. Chief of Surgery, North Carolina Baptist Hospital, Winston-Salem, North Carolina.

Carcinoma of the Gallbladder

HASSAN NAJAFI, M.S., M.D.
> Professor of Surgery, Rush Medical College. Chairman, Department of Cardiovascular-Thoracic Surgery, Rush-Presbyterian-St. Luke's Medical Center, Chicago, Illinois.

Ebstein's Anomaly

JOHN S. NAJARIAN, M.D.
> Professor and Chairman, Department of Surgery, University of Minnesota Medical School, Minneapolis, Minnesota.

Principles of Immunosuppression

FRANCIS C. NANCE, M.S.(Physiology), M.D.
> Professor of Surgery and Physiology, Louisiana State University School of Medicine in New Orleans. Visiting Surgeon, Charity Hospital of Louisiana, New Orleans, Louisiana.

The Colon and Rectum

BLAINE S. NASHOLD, JR., M.D.
> Professor of Neurosurgery, Duke University School of Medicine, Durham, North Carolina.

Neurosurgical Relief of Pain; Neurosurgical Treatment of Epilepsy; Stereotactic Neurosurgery

RUSSELL M. NELSON, M.D., Ph.D.
> Research Professor of Surgery, University of Utah College of Medicine. Division of Thoracic Surgery, Latter-Day Saints Hospital; Director, Thoracic Surgical Residency, University of Utah Affiliated Hospitals, Salt Lake City, Utah.

Extracorporeal Circulation

STANTON P. NOLAN, M.D., M.S.
> Professor of Surgery, Division of Thoracic Cardiovascular Surgery, University of Virginia School of Medicine. Surgeon in Charge, Division of Thoracic Cardiovascular Surgery, University of Virginia Medical Center, Charlottesville, Virginia.

Acquired Disorders of the Aortic Valve

LLOYD M. NYHUS, M.D.
> Warren H. Cole Professor and Head, Department of Surgery, The Abraham Lincoln School of Medicine of the University of Illinois College of Medicine. Surgeon in Chief, University of Illinois Hospital, Chicago, Illinois.

Hernias

GUY L. ODOM, M.D.
> Professor of Neurological Surgery, Duke University School of Medicine. Attending

Surgeon, Duke University Medical Center and Veterans Administration Hospital, Durham, North Carolina.
Neurosurgery; Craniocerebral Injuries; Cervical Disc Lesions

H. NEWLAND OLDHAM, JR., M.D.
Professor of Surgery, Duke University School of Medicine, Durham, North Carolina.
The Mediastinum; Congenital Aortic Stenosis

MARSHALL J. ORLOFF, M.D.
Professor and Chairman, Department of Surgery, University of California, San Diego, School of Medicine. Surgeon in Chief, University of California Medical Center, San Diego, California.
The Liver; The Biliary System

FREDERICK B. PARKER, JR., M.D.
Associate Professor and Director, Division of Thoracic Surgery, State University of New York, Upstate Medical Center, College of Medicine. Attending Surgeon, State University Hospital, Crouse-Irving Memorial Hospital, Veterans Administration Hospital, and St. Joseph's Hospital Health Center, Syracuse, New York.
Aneurysms of the Thoracic Aorta

ALAN G. PARKS, M.D.
Teacher in Surgery, The London Hospital Medical College. Consultant Surgeon, The London Hospital and St. Mark's Hospital, London, England.
The Rectum and Anal Canal

JAMES W. PATE, M.D.
Professor and Chairman of Surgery, University of Tennessee College of Medicine. Chief of Surgery, City of Memphis Hospital; Consultant, Veterans Administration Hospital, U.S. Naval Hospital, Baptist Memorial Hospital, Methodist Hospital, St. Joseph Hospital, St. Jude Children's Research Hospital, West Tennessee Chest Disease Hospital, Tennessee Psychiatric Hospital and Institute, and Le Bonheur Children's Hospital, Memphis, Tennessee.
Bronchial Adenoma

GORDON W. PHILPOTT, M.D.
Associate Professor of Surgery, Washington University School of Medicine. Hospital Staff, The Barnes Group of Hospitals; Visiting Surgeon, St. Louis City Hospital, St. Louis, Missouri.
The Spleen

KENNETH L. PICKRELL, M.D.
Professor of Plastic Surgery, Duke University School of Medicine. Attending Plastic Surgeon, Duke University Medical Center, Durham; Consultant Plastic Surgeon, Veterans Administration Hospitals, Durham and Fayetteville, and Womack Army Hospital, Fort Bragg, North Carolina.
Surgical Disorders of the Skin

HIRAM C. POLK, JR., M.D.
Professor and Chairman, Department of Surgery, The University of Louisville School of Medicine, Louisville, Kentucky.
Principles of Preoperative Preparation of the Surgical Patient

JOHN M. PORTER, M.D.
Associate Professor of Surgery and Head, Division of Vascular Surgery, University of Oregon Medical School, Portland, Oregon.
Arterial Substitutes; Raynaud's Syndrome

RAYMOND W. POSTLETHWAIT, M.D.
Professor of Surgery, Duke University School of Medicine. Chief of Surgery, Veterans Administration Hospital, Durham, North Carolina.
Principles of Operative Surgery

W. JOHN POWELL, JR., M.D.
Associate Professor of Medicine, Harvard Medical School. Assistant Physician, Massachusetts General Hospital, Boston, Massachusetts.
Pharmacology of the Cardiovascular System in the Surgical Patient

SAMUEL R. POWERS, JR., M.D.
Professor and Chairman, Department of Surgery, Albany Medical College of Union University. Surgeon in Chief, Albany Medical Center Hospital; Attending Surgeon, Veterans Administration Hospital, Albany, New York.
Acute Postoperative Renal Failure

CHARLES W. PUTNAM, M.D.
Assistant Professor of Surgery, University of Colorado School of Medicine. Attending Surgeon, Colorado General Hospital and Veterans Administration Hospital, Denver, Colorado.
Liver Homotransplantation

KENNETH P. RAMMING, M.D.
Assistant Professor of Surgery, Divisions of Oncology and Thoracic Surgery, Department of Surgery, UCLA School of Medicine. Attending Surgeon, UCLA Hospital, Los Angeles, and Veterans Administration Hospital, Sepulveda, California.
Bites and Stings

MARK M. RAVITCH, M.D.
Professor of Surgery, University of Pittsburgh. Surgeon in Chief, Montefiore Hospital; Attending Surgeon, Presbyterian-University Hospital and Children's Hospital of Pittsburgh; Consultant, Veterans Administration Hospital, Pittsburgh, Pennsylvania.
Disorders of the Chest Wall

KEITH REEMTSMA, M.D.
Professor and Chairman, Department of Surgery, Columbia University College of Physicians and Surgeons. Attending Surgeon and Director of Surgical Service, Presbyterian Hospital, New York, New York.
Lung Transplantation; Pancreas and Pancreatic Islet Transplantation

FREDERICK A. REICHLE, M.D.
Professor of Surgery, Temple University School of Medicine. Attending Surgeon, Temple University Hospital; Associate Attending Surgeon, Episcopal Hospital, St. Mary's Hospital, and St. Christopher's Hospital for Children, Philadelphia; Consultant, Veterans Administration Hospital, Wilkes Barre, Pennsylvania.
Femoropopliteal and Femorotibial Bypass

JONATHAN E. RHOADS, M.D., D.Sc.(Med.)
Professor of Surgery, The University of Pennsylvania School of Medicine. Surgical Staff, Hospital of the University of Pennsylvania; Consultant, Germantown Dispensary and Hospital, Children's Hospital of Philadelphia, Pennsylvania Hospital, and Veterans Administration Hospital, Philadelphia; Bryn Mawr Hospital, Bryn Mawr, Pennsylvania; and Monmouth Medical Center, Long Branch, New Jersey.
Metabolism in Surgical Patients

ERWIN ROBIN, M.D.
Clinical Associate Professor of Medicine, Loyola University of Chicago Stritch School of Medicine, Chicago. Attending Cardiologist, Hines Veterans Administration Hospital, Maywood, and Sherman Hospital and St. Joseph Hospital, Elgin, Illinois.
Cardiac Catheterization

BRADLEY M. RODGERS, M.D.
Assistant Professor of Surgery and Pediatrics, University of Florida College of Medicine, Gainesville, Florida.
Esophagoscopy

FRANCIS E. ROSATO, M.D.
Professor and Chairman, Department of Surgery, Eastern Virginia Medical School.

Director of Surgery, Norfolk General Hospital; Attending Surgeon, De Paul Hospital, Norfolk; Consultant in Surgery, U.S. Naval Hospital, Portsmouth, Virginia.
Gallstone Ileus and Fistula

LEONARD ROSOFF, SR., M.D.
Professor and Chairman, Department of Surgery, University of Southern California School of Medicine. Director of Surgery, Los Angeles County-University of Southern California Medical Center; Affiliating Staff, Hospital of the Good Samaritan; Consultant, Cedars-Sinai Medical Center and Children's Hospital, Los Angeles; and Huntington Memorial Hospital, Pasadena, California.
Amebic Abscess of the Liver

DAVID C. SABISTON, JR., M.D.
James B. Duke Professor and Chairman, Department of Surgery, Duke University School of Medicine. Chief of Staff, Duke University Hospital, Durham, North Carolina.
Pulmonary Embolism; Anatomy of the Arterial System; Aneurysms of the Subclavian Artery, Visceral Arteries, and Abdominal Aorta; Thrombo-obliterative Disease of the Aorta and Its Branches; Arteriovenous Fistula; Surgical Management of Renovascular Hypertension; Carcinoma of the Lung; The Mediastinum; Tetralogy of Fallot; The Coronary Circulation; Cardiac Neoplasms

WORTHINGTON G. SCHENK, JR., M.D.
Professor and Chairman, Department of Surgery, State University of New York at Buffalo School of Medicine. Director of Surgery, Edward J. Meyer Memorial Hospital, Buffalo, New York.
The Surgical Acute Care Unit

WILLIAM R. SCHILLER, M.D.
Associate Professor of Surgery, Medical College of Ohio at Toledo. Attending Surgeon, Medical College of Ohio Hospital, Toledo, Ohio.
Angiography in Diagnosis and Treatment of Gastrointestinal Bleeding

H. WILLIAM SCOTT, JR., M.D.
Professor and Chairman, Department of Surgery, Vanderbilt University School of Medicine; Professor of Clinical Surgery, Meharry Medical School. Surgeon in Chief, Vanderbilt University Hospital; Consultant in Surgery, Veterans Administration Hospital, Nashville General Hospital, and St. Thomas Hospital, Nashville, Tennessee.
The Pituitary and Adrenals

WILL C. SEALY, M.D.
Professor of Thoracic Surgery, Duke University School of Medicine. Duke University Hospital, Durham, North Carolina.
Surgical Treatment of Supraventricular Tachyarrhythmias Associated with the Wolff-Parkinson-White Syndrome

H. F. SEIGLER, M.D.
Professor of Surgery and Immunology, Duke University School of Medicine. Attending Surgeon, Veterans Administration Hospital. Consulting Surgeon, Durham County General Hospital, Durham, and Cabarrus Memorial Hospital, Concord, North Carolina.
Historical Aspects of Transplantation; Renal Allografts

WILLIAM W. SHINGLETON, M.D.
Professor of Surgery, Duke University School of Medicine. Attending Surgeon, Duke University Hospital, Durham, North Carolina.
Malabsorption Syndromes

G. THOMAS SHIRES, M.D.
Professor and Chairman, Department of Surgery, Cornell University Medical College. Chairman, Department of Surgery, The New York Hospital-Cornell Medical Center, New York, New York.
Fluid and Electrolyte Management of the Surgical Patient

NORMAN E. SHUMWAY, M.D., Ph.D.
The Frances and Charles D. Field Professor and Chairman, Department of Cardiovascular Surgery, Stanford University School of Medicine, Stanford, California.
Cardiac Homotransplants

JOHN H. SIEGEL, M.D.
Professor of Surgery and Research Professor of Biophysical Sciences, State University of New York at Buffalo School of Medicine. Chief, Department of Surgery, Buffalo General Hospital, Buffalo, New York.
Computers and Mathematical Techniques in Surgery

DONALD SILVER, M.D.
Professor of Surgery and Chairman of the Department, University of Missouri—Columbia School of Medicine. Attending Surgeon, Veterans Administration Hospital, Columbia, Missouri.
Blood Transfusions and Disorders of Surgical Bleeding; Circulatory Problems of the Upper Extremity; Thoracic Outlet Syndrome

RICHARD L. SIMMONS, M.D.
Professor, Department of Surgery, University of Minnesota Medical School, Minneapolis, Minnesota.
Principles of Immunosuppression

DAVID B. SKINNER, M.D.
Dallas B. Phemister Professor of Surgery, University of Chicago Pritzker School of Medicine. Chairman, Department of Surgery, University of Chicago Hospitals and Clinics, Chicago, Illinois.
Perforation of the Esophagus

JAMES B. SNOW, JR., M.D.
Professor and Chairman, Department of Otorhinolaryngology and Human Communication, University of Pennsylvania School of Medicine. Chairman, Department of Otorhinolaryngology, Hospital of the University of Pennsylvania; Chief, Section of Otolaryngology, Veterans Administration Hospital; Senior Surgeon, Children's Hospital of Philadelphia, Graduate Hospital of the University of Pennsylvania, and Pennsylvania Hospital, Philadelphia, Pennsylvania.
Surgical Disorders of the Ears, Nose, Paranasal Sinuses, Pharynx, and Larynx

HENRY M. SPOTNITZ, M.D.
Assistant Professor of Surgery, Columbia University College of Physicians and Surgeons. Attending Surgeon, Presbyterian Hospital, New York, New York.
Lung Transplantation

THOMAS E. STARZL, M.D., Ph.D.
Professor and Chairman of Surgery, University of Colorado School of Medicine. Attending Surgeon, Colorado General Hospital and Veterans Administration Hospital, Denver, Colorado.
Liver Homotransplantation

DELFORD L. STICKEL, M.D.
Professor of Surgery, Duke University School of Medicine, Durham, North Carolina.
Historical Aspects of Transplantation; Renal Allografts

TIMOTHY TAKARO, M.D., M.S.(Surgery)
Associate Clinical Professor of Surgery, Duke University School of Medicine, Durham. Chief, Surgical Service, Veterans Administration Hospital, Asheville, North Carolina.
Lung Abscess and Fungal Infections; The Pleura and Empyema

JAMES L. TALBERT, M.D.
Professor of Surgery and Pediatrics and Chief, Division of Pediatric Surgery, University of Florida College of Medicine. Chief, Division of Pediatric Surgery, Shands Teaching Hospital; Consultant in Surgery, Veterans Administration Hospital, Gainesville, and University Hospital of Jacksonville, Jacksonville, Florida.
Corrosive Strictures of the Esophagus

COLIN G. THOMAS, JR., M.D.
     Professor and Chairman, Department of Surgery, University of North Carolina
     School of Medicine. Chief of Surgery, North Carolina Memorial Hospital, Chapel
     Hill, North Carolina.
Nodular Goiter and Neoplasms of the Thyroid

JAMES C. THOMPSON, M.D.
     Professor, Department of Surgery, University of Texas Medical Branch at Galveston
     — Medical School. Chief of Surgery, The University of Texas Hospitals at Galveston,
     Galveston, Texas.
The Stomach

JESSE E. THOMPSON, M.D.
     Clinical Professor of Surgery, University of Texas Southwestern Medical School.
     Attending Surgeon, Baylor University Medical Center, Dallas, Texas.
Aneurysms of the Carotid Artery; Carotid Body Tumors

JAMES P. S. THOMSON, M.S., F.R.C.S.
     Consultant Surgeon, St. Mark's Hospital, London, England.
The Rectum and Anal Canal

G. FRANK O. TYERS, M.D., F.R.C.S.(C)
     Associate Professor of Surgery, Pennsylvania State University College of Medicine.
     Attending Surgeon, The Milton S. Hershey Medical Center, Hershey, Pennsylvania.
Atrial Septal Defects, Ostium Primum Defects, and Atrioventricular Canals

JAMES R. URBANIAK, M.D.
     Professor of Orthopaedic Surgery, Duke University School of Medicine, Durham,
     North Carolina.
Fractures of the Spine

RICHARD L. VARCO, M.D., Ph.D.
     Professor of Surgery, University of Minnesota Medical School. Attending Surgeon,
     University of Minnesota Hospitals, Minneapolis, Minnesota.
Intestinal Bypass for Hyperlipidemia and Morbid Obesity

JOHN A. WALDHAUSEN, M.D.
     Professor and Chairman, Department of Surgery, Pennsylvania State University
     College of Medicine. Attending Surgeon, The Milton S. Hershey Medical Center,
     Hershey, Pennsylvania.
Atrial Septal Defects, Ostium Primum Defects, and Atrioventricular Canals

ROBERT B. WALLACE, M.D.
     Professor, Mayo Medical School. Chairman, Department of Surgery, The Mayo
     Clinic and its Affiliated Hospitals, Rochester, Minnesota.
Truncus Arteriosus

ALEXANDER J. WALT, M.B., Ch.B.
     Penberthy Professor and Chairman, Department of Surgery, Wayne State Uni-
     versity School of Medicine. Chief of Surgery, Harper-Grace Hospital and Detroit
     General Hospital; Consultant in Surgery, Hutzel Hospital and Veterans Administra-
     tion Hospital, Detroit, Michigan.
Erosive Gastritis

W. DEAN WARREN, M.D.
     Joseph B. Whitehead Professor and Chairman, Department of Surgery, Emory
     University School of Medicine. Chief of Surgery, Grady Memorial Hospital, Veterans
     Administration Hospital, Henrietta Egleston Hospital for Children, and Emory
     University Hospitals, Atlanta, Georgia.
The Pancreas

ALVIN L. WATNE, M.D.
Professor of Surgery, West Virginia University School of Medicine, Morgantown, West Virginia.
Gardner's Syndrome

WATTS R. WEBB, M.D.
Professor and Chairman, Department of Surgery, Tulane University School of Medicine, New Orleans, Louisiana.
Aneurysms of the Thoracic Aorta

COLLIN J. WEBER, M.D.
Visiting Clinical Fellow, Columbia University College of Physicians and Surgeons. Assistant Resident, Department of Surgery, Presbyterian Hospital, New York, New York.
Pancreas and Pancreatic Islet Transplantation

ANDREW S. WECHSLER, M.D.
Associate Professor of Surgery and Assistant Professor of Physiology and Pharmacology, Duke University School of Medicine. Chief, Cardiac Surgery, Veterans Administration Hospital, and Clinical Investigator, Veterans Administration, Durham, North Carolina.
Physiology of the Arterial System

SAMUEL A. WELLS, JR., M.D.
Professor of Surgery and Assistant Professor of Immunology, Duke University School of Medicine. Attending Surgeon, Duke University Medical Center and Veterans Administration Hospital, Durham, North Carolina.
Immunobiology and Immunotherapy of Neoplastic Disease; The Multiple Endocrine Neoplasias; The Parathyroid Glands

MYRON W. WHEAT, JR., M.D.
Chairman, Department of Surgery, Diagnostic Clinic, Largo, Florida; Staff, Bayfront Medical Center, St. Petersburg, Florida.
Dissecting Aneurysms of the Aorta

H. BROWNELL WHEELER, M.D.
Professor and Chairman, Department of Surgery, University of Massachusetts Medical School. Surgeon in Chief, University of Massachusetts Hospital, Worcester, Massachusetts.
Buerger's Disease

THOMAS J. WHELAN, JR., M.D.
Professor and Chairman, Department of Surgery, University of Hawaii School of Medicine. Attending Surgeon, Queen's Hospital, St. Francis Hospital, Kuakini Hospital, Kauikeolani Children's Hospital, Kapiolani Hospital, and Straub Hospital, Honolulu, and Castle Hospital, Kailua, Hawaii.
Hemobilia

ROBERT H. WILKINS, M.D.
Professor of Neurosurgery, Duke University School of Medicine, Chief, Division of Neurosurgery, Duke University Medical Center, Durham, North Carolina.
Historical Aspects of Neurosurgery; Spontaneous Intracranial Hemorrhage; Intracranial Infections

GAYLORD S. WILLIAMS, M.D., M.S.(Surgery)
Associate Professor of Plastic Surgery, University of Virginia School of Medicine. Plastic Surgeon, University of Virginia Medical Center, Charlottesville; Consultant, Veterans Administration Hospital, Salem, Virginia.
The Mouth, Tongue, Jaws, and Salivary Glands

G. RAINEY WILLIAMS, M.D.
  Professor and Chairman, Department of Surgery, University of Oklahoma College
  of Medicine. Attending Surgeon, General and Thoracic/Cardiovascular Surgery,
  University Hospital and Clinics, Veterans Administration Hospital, and Oklahoma
  Children's Memorial Hospital; Associate Medical Staff, Presbyterian Hospital,
  Oklahoma City, Oklahoma.
Replantation of the Extremities

VALLEE L. WILLMAN, M.D.
  Professor and Chairman, Department of Surgery, St. Louis University School of
  Medicine, St. Louis, Missouri.
Carotid Occlusive Disease

RICHARD E. WILSON, M.D.
  Professor of Surgery, Harvard Medical School. Chief, Surgical Oncology, Peter Bent
  Brigham Hospital and Sidney Farber Cancer Center, Boston, Massachusetts.
The Breast

WALTER G. WOLFE, M.D.
  Associate Professor of Surgery, Duke University School of Medicine, Durham,
  North Carolina.
Anatomy of the Lungs, Pleura, and Chest Wall

BARNES WOODHALL, M.D.
  James B. Duke Professor Emeritus of Neurosurgery, Duke University School of
  Medicine. Distinguished Physician, Veterans Administration Hospital, Durham,
  North Carolina.
Rupture of Lumbar Intervertebral Discs; Peripheral Nerve Injuries

EDWARD R. WOODWARD, M.D.
  Professor and Chairman, University of Florida College of Medicine. Chief of Surgery,
  Shands Teaching Hospital and Clinics; Consultant in Surgery, Veterans Adminis-
  tration Hospitals, Lake City and Gainesville, Florida.
Hiatus Hernia

JAMES S. T. YAO, M.D., Ph.D.
  Associate Professor of Surgery, Northwestern University Medical School. Attend-
  ing Surgeon and Director, Blood Flow Laboratory, Northwestern Memorial Hos-
  pital; Visiting Surgeon, Lake Side Veterans Administration Hospital; Consultant,
  Rehabilitation Institute of Chicago, Chicago, Illinois.
Visceral Ischemic Syndromes

DABNEY R. YARBROUGH, III, M.D.
  Associate Professor of Surgery, Medical University of South Carolina College of
  Medicine. Attending Surgeon, Medical University Hospital and Veterans Adminis-
  tration Hospital, Charleston, South Carolina.
Burns: Including Cold, Chemical, and Electrical Injuries

W. GLENN YOUNG, JR., M.D.
  Professor of Surgery, Duke University School of Medicine. Consulting Thoracic
  Surgeon, McCain Hospital, McCain, and Eastern North Carolina Hospital, Wilson,
  North Carolina.
Surgical Treatment of Pulmonary Tuberculosis

ROBERT ZEPPA, M.D.
  Professor and Chairman, Department of Surgery, University of Miami School of
  Medicine. Attending Surgeon, National Children's Cardiac Hospital, Jackson
  Memorial Hospital, and Veterans Administration Hospital, Miami, Florida.
The Pancreas

ACKNOWLEDGMENTS

The current text is the result of contributions by a number of authorities in surgery. Each has worked diligently to produce a section based upon an appropriate combination of basic and clinical science. Particular appreciation is due the contributors for attention to detail in the preparation of all sections, including a review of the stepwise development of our understanding of the various surgical disorders as well as for the quality of the illustrations and the choice of annotated references.

Special thanks are due Mr. Robert B. Rowan of the W. B. Saunders Company for his continuing advice and assistance in all phases of the extensive revisions required in the present text. The editorial assistance of Miss Elizabeth J. Taylor and Ms. Donna K. Musser, both of the Saunders staff, has been invaluable and much appreciation is expressed to them for their tireless efforts in establishing the high standards of editing which characterize the eleventh edition.

Many thanks are due Mr. Herbert J. Powell, Jr., and his associates in the Production Department of Saunders. They have made possible the printing of this exceptionally large volume in an amazingly brief period of time, and simultaneously they have maintained the highest standards of accuracy and attractiveness.

Finally, deep appreciation is expressed to Mrs. Kathryn Slaughter for the remarkable personal interest she has continued in the eleventh edition. Her careful review of each contribution and attention to even the smallest detail are fully recognized. She has served as a stimulus to many others in achieving editorial perfection and is clearly due much credit for many hours of work dedicated to this text. Her loyalty and enthusiasm for the entire venture are gratefully acknowledged.

DAVID C. SABISTON, JR.

CONTENTS

55

56

57

59

THE DEVELOPMENT OF SURGERY

Historical Aspects Important in the Origin and Development of Modern Surgical Science

Gert H. Brieger, M.D.

Those who cannot remember the past are condemned to repeat it.

— Santayana

There is a long and honorable tradition for inclusion of the history of surgery in the major surgical texts of the last hundred years. In fact, some of these chapters have been among the most frequently cited sources of surgical history.[8] This in itself is not a cause for congratulation, for a new historical approach to the development of modern surgery is needed. It is no longer sufficient to list the great surgeons and their contributions, or to focus only on the great operations, which is merely a variation of the old approach, since quite naturally the great advances in technique were made by great men. This is not to say that much useful history of surgery has not already been written. Throughout this chapter some of these earlier writings will be cited as references that are intended as guides for those who wish to pursue further various aspects of the history of surgery.

This chapter will follow the thinking of recent historians who have directed more attention to the proper integration of the history of surgery with the history of medicine as a whole. In addition, much research and thought have been devoted to the parts played by surgery and surgeons in effecting nonscientific changes in medical care, and to the influence of surgery upon the society in which it is practiced, and in turn the influence of various social, cultural, and economic institutions upon surgery. These aspects also will be stressed in this chapter.

Every field has its great men and each of us has his heroes. A history of surgery without Paré, Vesalius, Hunter, Lister, and Halsted would be a strange history indeed; the magnitude of the achievements of these men warrants discussion of their lives and work. Nevertheless, many justly famous names will be missing. The emphasis will be placed on the *recent* past, *especially the last hundred years*, although the reader should keep in mind always that surgery's history is as old as man's on earth.

The history of disease is at least as old as the history of man. One can assume that surgical disease, or the surgical response to disease, is of similar antiquity. The basic forms of disease—tumors, infections, trauma, and congenital abnormalities—have existed unchanged.[51] Today's surgeon obviously manages them in different fashion than did his colleague of prehistoric time, yet some aspects of the surgeon's work are timeless. Ackerknecht, who has written extensively on primitive medicine, has emphasized that surgery was not defined as a special field by the primitives,[1] yet much of their medical treatment would be termed *surgical.* They treated wounds and tried to stop hemorrhage, and they trephined for injury to the head as well as for ritual reasons, such as the release of demons.

The single most important factor limiting the work of these early surgeons was their lack of knowledge of anatomy. It is true that evidence has been found of very successful bone-setting for fractures in some tribes, but these good results may have been due to chance. The study of the anthropologist Adolph Schultz has shown that the efficacy of medical men cannot simply be assumed. Nature, too, as the ancients well knew, is a powerful healer in its own right. In 1939 Schultz reported finding healed fractures in wild apes; in one series of 118 wild adult gibbons, 42, or 36 per cent, had well-healed fractures.[77] Since these animals obviously did not have the benefit of surgical assistance, one must take pause, then, before too quickly assigning credit for cures.

Ancient Egypt, long a fascinating subject for historians and archeologists, provides examples of some of the earliest known medical writings. The papyri that have been found deal with medicine, surgery, obstetrics and gynecology, and veterinary problems. The Edwin Smith Papyrus, of greatest interest to surgeons, is one of the oldest. It was written about 1600 B.C. but probably was copied from a still older version. It consists of 48 cases, mostly wounds, arranged in the order that later was to become the traditional one, *a capite ad calcem*.[78]

Egyptian medicine had both a rational-empirical element and a magical-religious one. To ascribe any great knowledge of anatomy to the Egyptian physicians would be to claim too much. The mummification procedure included a crude evisceration and was performed by lower class men who were not interested in the study of medicine. Though knowledge of human anatomy was minimal, the writer of the Smith Papyrus obviously had observed enough to prescribe clearly and effectively in many of the cases.

Ancient India also has a rich medical legacy, all too often ignored by Western writers. Susruta described more than 100 surgical instruments, including scalpels, bistouries, lancets, scarifiers, saws, bone nippers, trocars, and needles. The Indian surgeons are best known for their great skill in plastic surgery, especially the restoration of noses and ears.

In Greek and Roman antiquity the surgeon existed as a specialist, but only when diet and drugs were of no effect did doctors resort to surgery. In cases of injury, of course, the surgeon might be called upon immediately. In the great Greek medical works that are ascribed to Hippocrates, but certainly not all written by him, there are books on fractures, dislocations, and other surgical disorders. One of the most interesting is simply entitled *On the Surgery*. Here the author described what it was the surgeon should know, how he should proceed with the treatment, and the general qualifications he should possess. Much of the work relates to bandaging of various types of injuries. "The things relating to surgery are," the Hippocratic author wrote around 400 B.C., "the patient; the operator; the assistants; the instruments; the light; where and how; how many things, and how; where the body, and the instruments; the time; the manner; the place."

Besides the 70 books of the Hippocratic works, one of our best authorities for Greek medicine is the Roman encyclopedist of the early first century A.D., Aulus Cornelius Celsus. His *De medicina,* in several volumes, reflects much learning, though its author was himself probably not a medical practitioner. This book was one of the earliest medical books to be printed (1478) after the invention of movable type. Of interest to surgeons is the classic description Celsus left us of inflammation: "Now the characteristics of inflammation are four: redness and swelling, with heat and pain" (Book III). Of more direct interest, though, is what he had to say about surgery. He went into great detail regarding some surgical remedies, but his general comments found in the *Prooemium* of Book VII are timeless and bear repeating:

The third part of the Art of Medicine is that which cures by the hand. . . . It does not omit medicaments and regulated diets [the other two parts of medicine], but does most by hand. The effects of this treatment are more obvious than any other kind; in as much as in diseases since luck helps much, and the same things are often salutary, often of no use at all, it may be doubted whether recovery has been due to medicine or a sound body or good luck. . . . But in that part of medicine which cures by hand, it is obvious that all improvement comes chiefly from this, even if it be assisted somewhat in other ways. This branch, although very ancient, was more practiced by Hippocrates, the father of all medical art, than by his forerunners. . . .

Now a surgeon should be youthful or at any rate nearer youth than age; with a strong and steady hand which never trembles, and ready to use the left hand as well as the right; with vision sharp and clear, and spirit undaunted; filled with pity, so that he wishes to cure his patient, yet is not moved by his cries, to go too fast, or cut less than is necessary; but he does everything just as if the cries of pain cause him no emotion.

It is usually said that medicine in the Middle Ages slavishly followed the doctrines of Galen of the second century A.D., and that because of adherence to his humoral concept of disease, which he in turn took over and elaborated from the Hippocratic writers of five centuries earlier, no advances were made. Only in a general sense is this true. The sins of the followers of Galen should not be attributed to Galen himself, but this is beyond the scope of this discussion. Of importance, however, is that if one holds that disease is caused by the humors—yellow bile, black bile, blood, and phlegm—being either in excess or in the wrong location within the body, then surgery cannot be of much use. How can one operate on the humors? If the humoral excess should manifest itself as a pus-filled swelling it might be incised and drained, but the chances for operative intervention were generally few under this system or theory of pathology.

The surgery of the early Middle Ages has been described by Bishop as merely meddlesome. Itinerant surgeons operated for stone, cataract, and hernia. Since these procedures were likely to be associated with complications, the operators often hit and ran. Surgeons also cared for wounds and injuries, and later all skin diseases, especially syphilis, came within their province.

In the later Middle Ages, when medicine was in a stagnant state except for the contributions of the Arabs, surgery was the branch that began again to show progress. Surgery was separated from medicine during the time of Galen or before, and the two branches of medicine took quite different paths in the following 1500 years. There were probably many reasons why the surgeons were accorded less prestige and became a much less learned group than their medical colleagues, but the separation of surgery from medicine was not decreed by the church, as history books said for years. What misled historians of surgery was the phrase *Ecclesia abhorret a sanguine* (the Church abhors blood). This is not to be found in the text of the Council of Tours (1163), as was commonly claimed, or in any papal decree, although certainly the idea that the church wished its monks to spend more time on matters of religion and less on such secular things as medicine and surgery seems reasonable enough. It was Quesnay, the eighteenth century French historian of surgery, who disseminated the mistaken notion that the church actually forbade surgery, and the phrase and his interpretation were repeated over and over again.[81]

By the thirteenth and fourteenth centuries surgery was looked down upon and avoided by physicians, who had received their education in the universities that were now arising all over Europe. Along with theology and law, medicine was usually one of the basic faculties. Surgeons, on the other hand, were often unlettered, lower-class men who were scorned in clerical circles. The surgeons were taught the ways of their craft by apprenticeship. But, as Sir Clifford Allbutt has written, "by the expulsion of surgery from the liberal arts medicine herself was eviscerated."[3]

That surgery had also declined there is no doubt. The Salernitan surgeons of the twelfth century, when the rebirth of medicine and surgery may be said to occur, believed that surgery's decadence could be ascribed to two causes: its division from medicine and the neglect of anatomy. It was not long thereafter, however, that two major developments greatly affected the future course of surgery. One was the invention of gunpowder and its use in human warfare beginning in the fourteenth century; the other was the beginning of a renewed interest in the study of anatomy about the same time. Thus with greater call for their services and with the beginnings of greater fundamental knowledge from which advance could be made, the surgeons can be credited with having carried medicine forward from the time of the fourteenth century. The texts of Guy de Chauliac, who unfortunately favored suppuration in healing, and the works of Theodoric and Henri de Mondeville, whom we like to honor because they stressed clean wounds, reflected great credit upon the whole of medicine.

Guy de Chauliac, in his fourteenth century book on surgery, carried on the custom begun by Celsus of including a history of surgery within his text. Moreover, he identified five different surgical schools existing at the time, and differentiated one from the other on the basis of their treatment of wounds. The followers of Galen, who applied salves to promote pus formation, he called the orthodox school. A second group followed the teachings of Theodoric, who stressed clean wounds and healing by first intention. A third group deviated slightly by applying mild substances to the wound. A fourth group relied on charms and incantations to help them heal wounds, and the fifth were called the "women and silly folk." They depended on nature or God.

From 1200 on there is little doubt that surgeons existed as separate practitioners. They were especially to be found in the newly rising cities, where they joined guilds. Earlier, they had sometimes been admitted to the universities, where they could even lecture. But as time passed they were excluded and thus formed their own colleges, such as the Collège de St. Côme in Paris.[76] Along with these surgeons of the long robe, who were often clerics, arose the barbers, the even less learned surgeons. The physicians usually favored the barbers because, being simpler men, they were more likely to be willing to be at the beck and call of the learned doctors.

The barbers and surgeons of England had belonged to separate guilds since the fourteenth century. In 1540 a compromise as to the rights and duties of each was achieved, and a single company of Barbers and Surgeons was formed. Surgeons agreed to do no barbering and the barbers restricted their surgery to dentistry. The union lasted 200 years. In 1745 it was dissolved and the surgeons' company again existed

independently, jealously guarding its prerogatives and protecting its interests. In 1800 George III chartered the Royal College of Surgeons of London, which by charter from Queen Victoria in 1843 became the Royal College of Surgeons of England.

The works of many surgeons of the fourteenth to the seventeenth century were important, but there is little point in reviewing them here. For greater detail the reader should see the references by Billings,[8] Bishop,[11] Graham,[42] Zimmerman and Veith,[90] and Malgaigne.[59] Suffice it to say that the surgeon of four centuries ago had the same aims as his counterpart today, though his methods and results were severely limited. Witness, for instance, what the British surgeon Peter Lowe (1550–1613) had to say in his *A Discourse of the Whole Art of Chirurgerie* (1597), the first real textbook of surgery written in English. Lowe asks: "What is chirurgerie?" The answer is as true today as four centuries ago: "It is a science or Arte that sheweth the manner howe to work on man's body, exercising all manuall operations necessary to heal man, or as much as is possible by using of most expedient medicines." Lowe's textbook, incidentally, is arranged under five headings, also used by Paré: (1) to take away; (2) to help and add; (3) to put in place that which is out; (4) to separate; and (5) to join what is separated.[28]

These early surgeons also had a clear conception of what kind of man the surgeon should be. Who can improve upon the qualifications set forth by Thomas Vicary, mid-sixteenth century surgeon and author?

Now then to know what properties and conditions this man must have before he be a perfect chirurgien. I doe note foure things most specially that every chirurgien ought so to have: the first, that he be learned; the second, that he be expert; the third, that he be ingenious; the fourth, that he be well mannered.[83]

Some physicians in the Renaissance saw clearly that medicine and surgery, united in ancient times, must be brought together again. During the Renaissance surgery did slowly begin to attain a higher social position once again. No longer primarily in the hands of barbers, surgery was taught and practiced by some of the most illustrious physicians and anatomists. Vesalius and Fabricius of Aquapendente, the teacher of William Harvey, were but two of many.

Paracelsus, the sixteenth century rebel against the dead hand of the past, whom some have called the Luther of Medicine, called for a reunion of medicine and surgery:

How can ye establish it as another faculty and profession? Ye wood doctor and fool! . . . In *judicando* ye are a physician, in *curando* a surgeon. The patient asks for cure – surgery – and not for theory – medicine – it is the doctor who needs the latter. That is: there can be no surgeon who is not also a physician; the latter begets the surgeon and the surgeon tests the physician by the result of his work. Where the physician is not also a surgeon, he is an idol that is nothing but a painted monkey.[70]

In this hurried survey we must pause at least long enough to recognize Ambrose Paré (1510–1590). Few men in the history of medicine have been more popular than this sixteenth century French surgeon. There

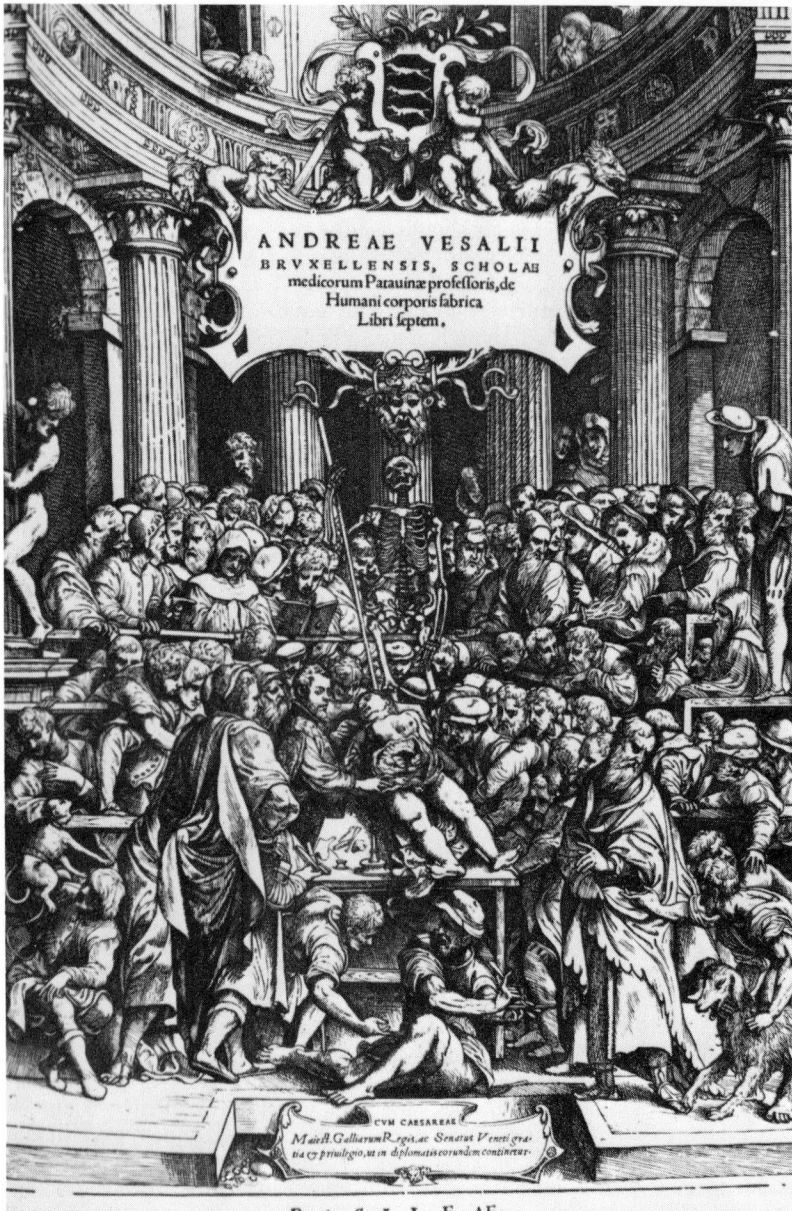

Figure 1. Frontispiece from Vesalius's *Fabrica*, published in 1543.

are many reasons for his high standing. His superb work, his pleasing personality, his humility, and, not least, the loving study made of his life and work by the nineteenth century surgeon Joseph Malgaigne all help to account for Paré's place in the history of surgery.

Born of humble parents in the province of Maine in 1510, Paré received his medical training as an apprentice barber-surgeon and then went to Paris, where he was appointed a house surgeon at the Hôtel-Dieu, already a famous charity hospital. Here he learned anatomy and surgery and began to develop the superb manual dexterity and sound general knowledge of medicine of his time that led to his success. He served four successive kings of France as a military surgeon and

wrote books in his own tongue instead of Latin, in which he and his fellow barber-surgeons were not schooled. Thus, in his writing as well as in his surgical treatment, Paré's achievement was a victory of experience over tradition.

The use of a digestive solution of egg yolk, rose oil, and turpentine to dress gunshot wounds was a discovery Paré made when the hot oil usually used to cauterize wounds ran out during the war between Francis I and Charles V. Those men treated with Paré's improvised methods, he tells us, did much better, and he resolved to treat all gunshot wounds without boiling oil in the future.[71] Remarkable as were his results, of equal note is that Paré here knowingly challenged authority. The text of Giovanni da Vigo on wounds was widely followed by all the famous surgeons from whom Paré had learned and whom he was following and copying in battle. That he realized the meaning of his little chance experiment is no less wondrous then.

One can readily see in Paré's approach a great similarity to our own, doubtless still another reason why he should be so attractive to us today. He stressed, for instance, the importance of anatomy, which in his time was beginning to come out of its doldrums.

Anatomy

Anatomy, so avidly pursued in the school of Alexandria in Hellenistic times, became detached from the medical curriculum. Its revival in the sixteenth century is closely related to several outside or nonmedical influences. One was the interest in the human form expressed by artists, such as Leonardo da Vinci, Raphael, Donatello, and Michelangelo; the other was the invention of printing with movable type, making books readily available. Even more important, illustrations, so necessary to anatomic study, could be faithfully reproduced and distributed. One need only look at the magnificent book by Vesalius to realize immediately the impact that illustration could have.

The origins of anatomy are veiled in obscurity, but early wound surgeons and those who butchered animals must have had some notions of structure. The Greeks pursued animal anatomy, and one must keep in mind that ancient anatomy, except for the school of Alexandria in the time of Herophilus and Erasistratus in the third century B.C., was largely animal anatomy. It was one of the great accomplishments of the Renaissance to rediscover the fine structure of the body and to impress upon the medical world the essential knowledge of anatomy that underlies all medical knowledge.

Anatomic dissection began to be more common again at the end of the thirteenth century. With the first manual for dissection written by Mondino de Luzzi in 1316, students had some guide. The early dissections were still often confined to the bodies of animals and sometimes were really autopsies performed to ascertain the cause of death, especially if foul play was suspected. These dissections were usually the responsibility of the surgeon. Only by the

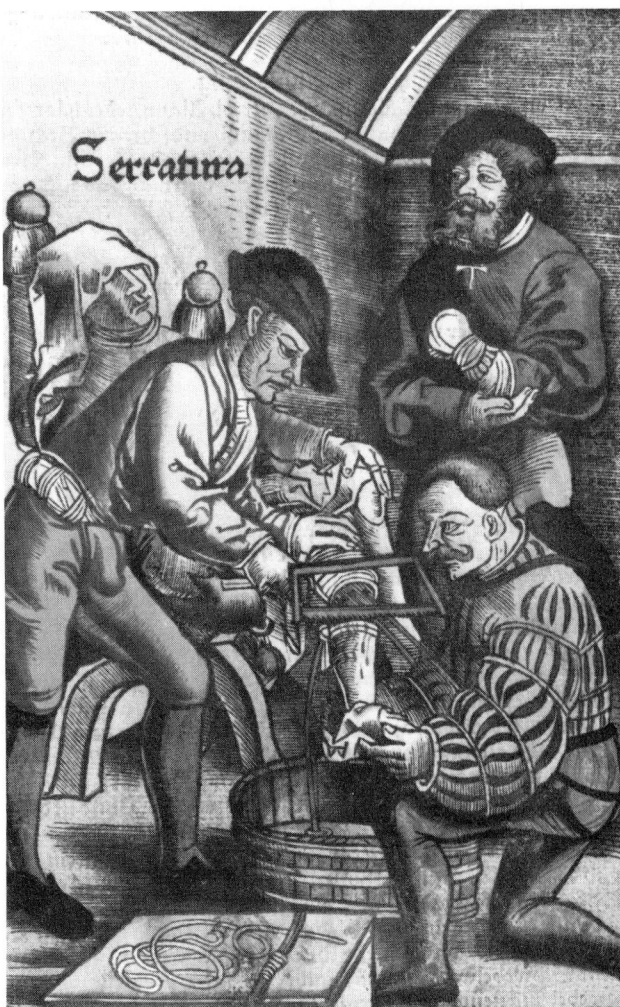

Figure 2. Illustration of an early amputation of the leg from Hans von Gersdorf's *Feldtbuch der Wundt Artzney*, Frankfort, 1551. (Trent Collection, Duke University Medical Center Library.)

middle of the fifteenth century did anatomic dissection become common enough that a special theater for it was built in Padua.

A basic requirement of any descriptive science is the ability to make pictures that can be readily duplicated so that men in many centers can use them for instruction and for learning. Woodcuts with pictures began to be made in Europe probably late in the fourteenth century, mainly as a labor-saving device for turning out sacred images. It was some time before biologists took up the idea, but by the end of the fifteenth and early in the sixteenth century occasional illustrated medical works began to appear. Johannes de Ketham's *Fasiculus medicinae,* Venice, 1491, and Berengario da Carpi's *Commentari... Super Anatomia Mundini...* are two of the best known. Others appeared, but the best and most lasting proved to be the *De humani corporis fabrica* of Andreas Vesalius. The publication of the *Fabrica* in 1543 coincided with the publication of another great book in the history of science, the *De revolutionibus orbium coelestium* of Nicolaus Copernicus. Thus in a single year, the modern understanding of both microscosm and macrocosm was set under way, and man's place in the world took on new dimensions.

The disputed points in Vesalian history, such as the identity of the artist, the magnitude of Vesalius' own work, and his originality, need not concern us here. Certainly his was neither the first nor the last great anatomic book, but the important point is that by his work and example he set forth a program. The famous frontispiece depicting Vesalius at the dissecting table, knife in hand, is itself programmatic. This young man, born into a family of physicians in Louvain in 1514, educated in Brussels and Paris, went to Padua to finish his medical study. At the age of 23, upon receiving his degree, he was appointed professor of anatomy and surgery, an important academic combination for centuries to come. Vesalius was certainly not alone in his attack upon the ancients, particularly the anatomic and physiologic system of Galen. Yet his great achievement set a tone. One must also remember that in the same year as the *Fabrica* Vesalius also published the *Epitome,* a shorter book intended to serve as a guide for students. The great rarity of original editions of the *Epitome* probably attests to its heavy use.[69]

The relationship of Vesalius and his study of anatomy to the field of surgery was self-evident to him, yet he speaks of it in the preface of the *Fabrica.* "At Padua, in that most famous university of the whole world... I gave the lectures on surgical medicine, and because anatomy is related to this, I devoted myself to the investigation of man's structure."

The surgeon-anatomists, Vesalius being one of their number, played an increasingly important role as time went on and knowledge of anatomy advanced. Thomas Vicary in his anatomy text quoted Galen's saying that it is as possible for a surgeon not knowing anatomy to work in man's body without error as it is for a blind man to carve an image and make it perfect. The tradition of teaching both surgery and anatomy was carried on by the professors of surgery in medical schools until the early twentieth century.

William Cheselden, the eighteenth century British surgeon, wrote a textbook of anatomy that was standard for nearly a hundred years.[18, 21] Henry Gray, who in 1859, the year of Darwin's *Origin of Species,* introduced the first edition of his *Anatomy,* not only was a surgeon but gave his book the title *Anatomy, Descriptive and Surgical.*[41]

Pathology and Experimental Surgery

The eighteenth century has often been called the century of systems in the history of medicine. The work of William Cullen, John Brown, and Benjamin Rush affords some proof for such an assertion, but in the history of surgery the eighteenth century saw the development of modern pathology and experimental surgery, all associated with the name of John Hunter. To him as much as to any single individual must go credit for ushering in the modern medicine of the nineteenth century. Again, because this essay is not a general history of medicine or a monograph on the history of surgery, we see a greatly simplified and thereby somewhat distorted view of things.

One of the great medical events of the eighteenth century was the publication of *On the Seats and Causes of Disease Investigated by Anatomy (De sedibus et causus morborum . . .)* by Giovanni Battista Morgagni, Padua's gifted professor of anatomy for nearly 60 years, in 1761 when the author was 79 years old. It represented a lifetime of work and stands as one of the great classics of medicine. Morgagni insisted that clinical observations be correlated with postmortem findings. He intended his book to be a useful one; he dealt with common diseases faced by physicians, not the rare and unusual ones usually written about by previous authors. Morgagni wrote his book as a series of 70 letters, composed in elegant Latin. Not until 1793 did Matthew Baillie, a nephew of the Hunters, write a book on morbid anatomy in English. In the tradition of Morgagni, then, John Hunter was to bring pathologic study to surgery.

John Hunter, born in Scotland in 1728, was the youngest son in a large family.[29, 55] He was a poor student and was little interested in his studies except those having to do with natural history. At age 20 he was apprenticed to his brother William, 10 years his senior, who earlier that year had begun giving private anatomic lessons for surgeons in London. Such anatomic schools became legal in England in 1745 with the dissolution of the Barber-Surgeons' Company, and their founding ushered in the great era of body snatching.[4]

John Hunter had been a poor student, but he took to dissection immediately, and his brother quickly recognized his talents. This was the beginning of a long, illustrious career that was to find John Hunter as a naturalist who collected a large museum of specimens, as an anatomist and experimental surgeon, and as a teacher of great influence. That he should have been the preceptor of so many pupils who later became famous in their own right is the more remarkable when one considers that he was a poor lecturer and an obtuse writer. Nevertheless, his precepts were stimulating and his writings widely read. His work on venereal disease confused syphilis and gonorrhea, but

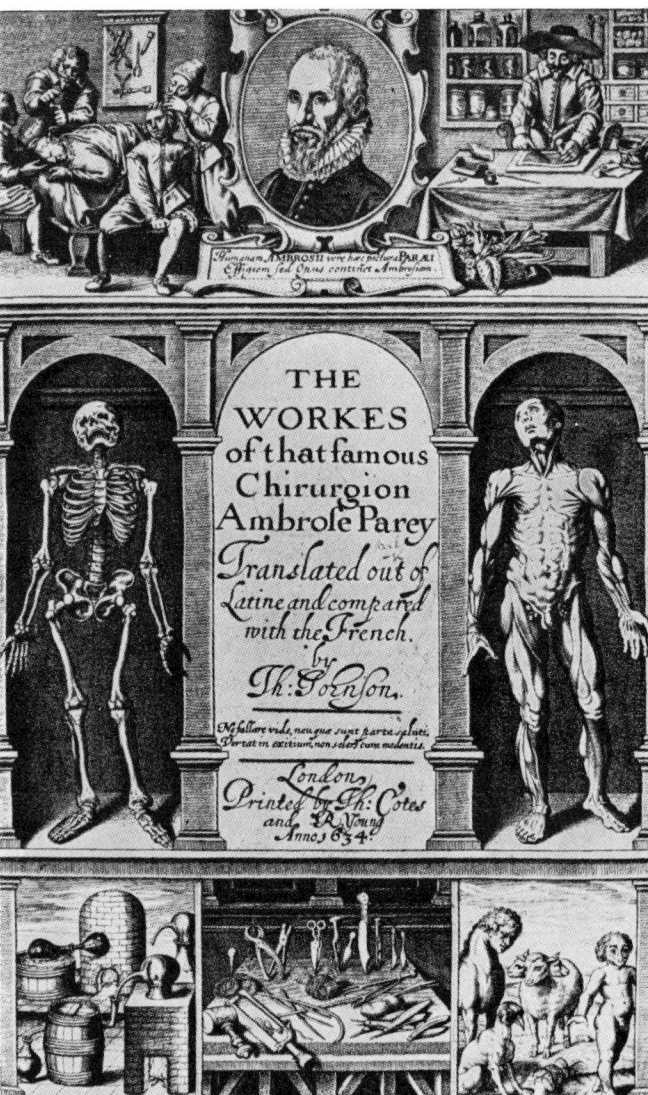

Figure 3. The title page of the first English edition of the works of Ambroise Paré (London, 1634).

was a major study of the subject. In 1794, a year after Hunter's death, his *Treatise on the Blood, Inflammation and Gun-Shot Wounds* appeared. Here one finds ample reason why Hunter's lectures on surgery, physiology, and pathology, often a combination of the three, were so successful. Hunter believed that "inflammation is not only occasionally the cause of disease, but it is often a mode of cure...." Inflammation thus became "the first principle in surgery."

Equally well known was his study of ligation of arterial vessels in cases of aneurysm. By supposed experimental study on the antlers of deer, Hunter realized that collateral circulation would probably suffice if the vessel involved by aneurysm were ligated in its healthy part.[80] By this means, amputation, if the aneurysm was in the femoral or popliteal arteries, for instance, could be avoided. This was a major advance in surgical therapy, and was the real beginning of what came to prominence in the nineteenth century as

conservative surgery. Thus Hunter amply earned the epitaph given him by the medical historian Fielding H. Garrison when he said, "With the advent of John Hunter, surgery ceased to be regarded as a mere technical mode of treatment, and began to take its place as a branch of scientific medicine, firmly grounded in physiology and pathology."[37]

The influence of John Hunter was still keenly felt in the first half of the nineteenth century. Many of the leading surgeons of Britain and America had been his pupils, and since any great man must give credit to those who taught and influenced him, Hunter's accomplishments stand out sharply. He made certain that all his students received thorough grounding in anatomy, physiology, and surgical pathology. And so medicine, surgery included, began gradually to take on a more scientific character.

Sir Astley Cooper, perhaps the most popular London surgeon of the first part of the nineteenth century, was

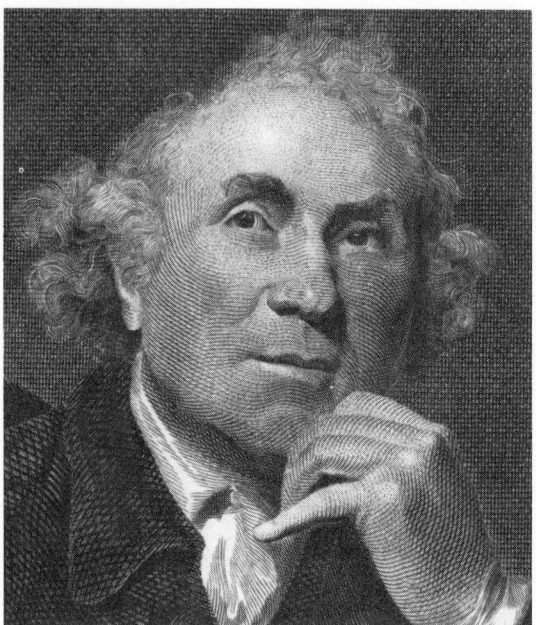

Figure 4. John Hunter (1728–1793), the father of experimental surgery and a superb anatomist and teacher.

a pupil of Hunter and a very fine operator. Part of his secret, no doubt, was his devotion to anatomic study, which he practiced and taught in his private dissecting room. "If I laid my head upon my pillow at night," Cooper said, "without having dissected something in the day, I should think that I had lost that day."[14]

Anesthesia and Antisepsis

Surgery of the twentieth century has been characterized by "a lifting of the eyes from the local lesion and the operation designed to deal with it to regard the more general aspects of surgical disorders," according to Churchill.[20] While this approach is certainly a hallmark of our time, we did not invent it. The institutes of surgery, as they were called in previous times, "are its settled principles," Henry J. Bigelow told his students in 1849.[7] Although the principles were still excessively general, discussion of constitution and disease was not entirely neglected by the surgeons. But in the field of operative surgery, Bigelow confessed, "we occupy more directly what is popularly considered to be the province of the surgeon. The surgeon, with the public, is associated with surgical operations; and his notoriety is in measure with the belief which the world may entertain of the number of or magnitude of the operations he may perform."[7] The public may be impressed, warned Bigelow, and the surgeon should guard against much of the exaggerated sense of worth and of drama.

Both Bigelow and his Boston colleague, J. Mason Warren, wrote about the all-too-frequent sepsis that appeared after the drama in the amphitheater had run its course. Primary healing, Warren wrote in 1864, "is seldom attained in city practice."[86] Union by first intention had been rare for 20 years, he claimed. Part of the blame, Warren believed, could be laid at the doors

of the city fathers who were responsible for the unhygienic conditions then prevailing. Thus some surgeons looked well beyond the local lesion, but they were usually powerless to make change.

The surgeons of the nineteenth century, incidentally, played an honorable part in the movement for sanitary reform. Edmund Parke and John Simon in England, and Stephen Smith and Willard Parker in New York, for instance, were both surgeons and sanitarians. The French surgeon, E. Doyen, in his *Surgical Therapeutics and Operative Technique* of the early twentieth century, entitled one chapter "Parallelism of the Evolution of Surgical Asepsis and the Progress of Public Hygiene." "We may readily admit," wrote Doyen, "that while the discovery of antisepsis proved the starting point for the improvement of public hygiene, the subsequent progress of the latter may be credited with advancement of surgical practice." The principles of antisepsis were carried over into the public hygiene, and the early resistance to Lister's ideas was due in part, Doyen believed, to the fact that the surgeons "had been brought up in a period in which personal cleanliness was generally neglected."

In the early nineteenth century surgical operations were still infrequent. Many hospitals in England and America had their weekly operating days on which one or two procedures might be performed. In many major hospitals there were fewer operations in 1 year than are performed in 2 days in one of our modern busy surgical services. The surgery of tuberculosis, especially its bony complications, accounted for a significant proportion of operations; accidents, strangu-

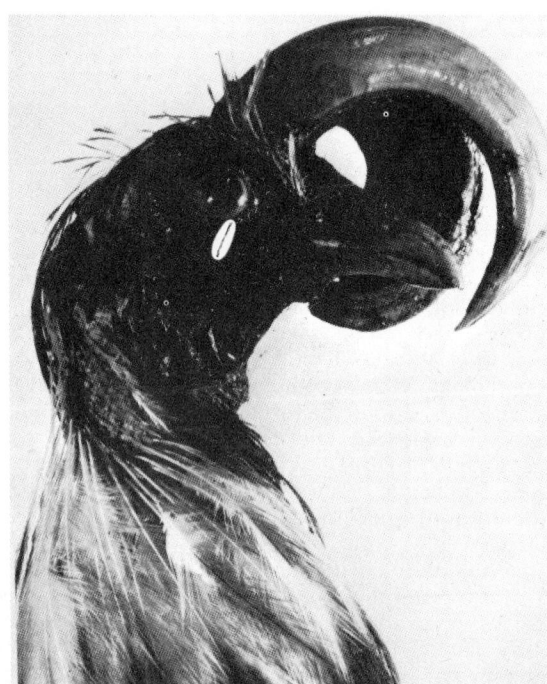

Figure 5. Photograph of a specimen from the Royal College of Surgeons of England of a spur that grew after being transplanted to the cock's comb by John Hunter (example of tissue transplantation).

lated hernias, abscesses, and aneurysms accounted for most of the rest. Mortality varied from hospital to hospital and differed in different countries.[79] It was generally highest on the Continent, amounting to 40 to 60 per cent, depending on the operative procedure.

There were numerous obstacles blocking the advance of surgery. Pain, infection, hemorrhage, and shock were four of the most difficult to overcome. As each was dealt with, the bounds of surgery enlarged. As the limits of surgery extended, the field of the individual surgeons seems to have become more and more restricted.

Since the fundamental aim of all medical art and science has always been to alleviate human pain and suffering, the development of anesthesia for use during surgical operations ranks as one of the most dramatic discoveries in the annals of medicine. The use of alcohol, mandrake root, opium, and even bleeding or reduction of blood flow to the brain to reduce sensibility was known to the ancients in a crude sense, but the really effective use of general anesthesia can be very precisely dated to the 1840s. In 1842 a rural Georgia practitioner, Crawford W. Long, used ether to remove small skin tumors, but he did not report his results until 3 years after William Morton successfully etherized a patient for John Collins Warren on October 16, 1846, at the Massachusetts General Hospital. James Young Simpson of Edinburgh introduced chloroform in the next year, and a new age in surgery was born. Speed of operation would now no longer be the hallmark of the great surgeons.

The history of anesthesia, like that of most medical accomplishments, is quite long.[54] To pass over it in a simple paragraph does it an injustice, but the story, with its technical details and tragic priority conflicts, has been well told so often that it need not be repeated here. What should be stressed is that the development of anesthesia and its very rapid acceptance after its introduction may be seen as part of a larger movement of humanitarianism. Reforms of prisons, public health, schools, almshouses, and mental hospitals, the crusades against the evils of drinking, and, in this country especially, the abolitionist movement all had at root a genuine concern for human life and dignity. Also noteworthy in the story of anesthesia, especially in the twentieth century development of intratracheal and intravenous routes of administration, as well as conduction or nerve block methods, is that physiology and surgery here became inseparably combined.

Although the mid-nineteenth century English physician John Snow, famous for his writing about cholera and the Broad Street pump, was one of the first to call himself an anesthesiologist, not until the years just before World War II did the specialty of anesthesiology really begin to develop. No longer was it sufficient for a surgical house officer or even a medical student to be delegated the task of administering the anesthetic and monitoring the patient, who often was neglected as the student eagerly watched the surgeon operate.

Several associations and meetings devoted to anesthesia began in the 1920s. Not until 1941 did the American Medical Association include a section on

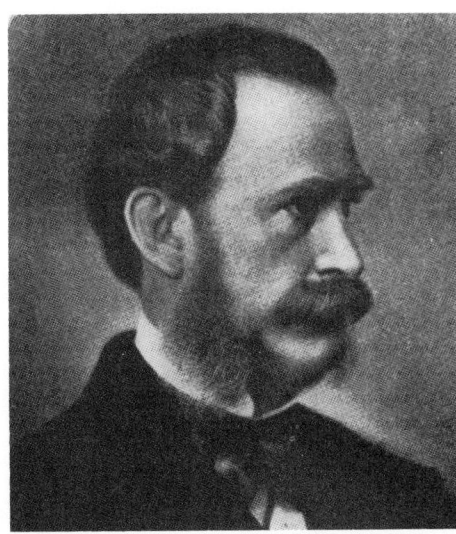

Figure 6. William T. G. Morton (1819–1868), a Boston dentist whose successful demonstration of ether anesthesia on October 16, 1846, at the Massachusetts General Hospital was a landmark in the history of surgery.

Anesthesia at its annual meeting, and not until after World War II did the specialty begin to grow and to train men and women seriously for full-time work in anesthesiology.

Anesthesia found speedy acceptance. The same, unfortunately, cannot be said for the attempts to control infection. Wound healing in the days before Lister was a confused and depressing aspect of surgery. Wounding, either accidental or done by the surgeon, was often followed by what was called irritative fever, usually lasting a few days and resulting in accumulation of pus in the wound. Sometimes the pus was creamy white; this thick exudate was often called "laudable pus." If the patient was fortunate, he then went through a slow healing process to recovery. This was the state of surgery seen from the patient's view, and it had existed for centuries.

The problem of surgical dressings was one of trial and error.[10] Surgeons in the early nineteenth century were still using dressing materials that were as old as recorded surgical history. Some, of course, acted very beneficially, but even with the most ingenious technique, the most agile and skilled operator all too often found that his work went for nought because his patient succumbed to postoperative infection. The term hospitalism was used by surgeons to describe the postsurgical infections so commonly found in surgical wards: erysipelas, pyemia, septicemia, and hospital gangrene.[53, 56] While the cause of these infections may have been guessed by some shrewd surgeons of the prebacteriologic era, by and large most surgeons felt helpless in the wake of them. Sir James Simpson, the Scottish surgeon who introduced chloroform, strongly urged his colleagues to do their operating on kitchen tables or in small cottage hospitals, for here the patients stood much less chance of becoming infected.

The history of the idea of so-called "laudable pus" is very difficult to trace. Some ancient writers mention pus formation as a normal part of healing, but the mere presence of pus does not yet make it laudable. What is certain, however, is that only within the last 100 years have surgeons been able to deal with the problem effectively. The comments of Sir Clifford Allbutt about his experiences in the years just before antisepsis was introduced are typical of what may be found in the literature.

> ... in the third quarter of the nineteenth century, in my callow days as a physician, the apothecary of a large hospital showed me a row of amputations, with stumps pouring out pus in cataracts upon the cushions, and exclaimed—"That, Sir, is what I like to see; nothing so wholesome in a wound as a good discharge of laudable pus." As a university graduate, for as universities were then we knew nothing of surgery,—I assented in superior ignorance."[3]

Joseph Lister was faced with these problems and watched the wretched patients in his surgical wards with increasing frustration and concern. Although he was not alone, he was the first to combat this major surgical obstacle successfully. The Hungarian obstetrician Ignaz Semmelweis and the American anatomist and writer Oliver Wendell Holmes had clearly shown in the 1840s that puerperal fever was carried to parturient women on the hands of their doctors. Simple washing in chlorinated lime solutions was extremely successful in Semmelweis's wards, but his Viennese colleagues and the world paid scant heed. Thus it was left to Lister doggedly to convince the world that wound infection was evil, not laudable, and that it could be effectively prevented.

Joseph Lister was born in Essex in 1827.[40] He was imbued with a love for science early in life by his father, Joseph Jackson Lister, a wine merchant who soon after his son's birth reported an important advance in microscopy to the Royal Society. An amateur scientist in the best tradition, the elder Lister perfected an achromatic lens that lessened the artifacts that had plagued the users of the earlier microscopes.

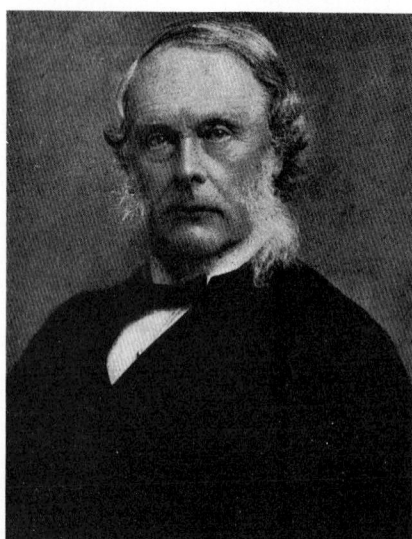

Figure 7. Joseph Lister (1827–1912), the originator of antiseptic surgery.

Young Lister attended University College, London, the common school for dissenters such as the Quaker Listers. He was graduated in 1847 and received his medical degree in 1852. In the following year he journeyed to Edinburgh to work and study with James Syme, one of the outstanding surgeons and surgical teachers of the midcentury. Syme was a leader in the movement toward a conservative surgery, one that tried to conserve limbs by exsection of parts of bone, with preservation of the limb as a whole. Lister remained in Edinburgh and became a member of the surgical staff of the Royal Infirmary, and he married Syme's eldest daughter, Agnes. In 1861 Lister moved to the chair of surgery at the Royal Infirmary in Glasgow, and it was during 8 fruitful years there that he began to develop his principles and practice of antisepsis. In 1869 he was called back to Edinburgh to fill Syme's chair, and in 1877 he moved to King's College Hospital in London. In 1897 he became the first medical man elevated to the peerage.

In his earlier Edinburgh and Glasgow years Lister investigated a number of problems closely related to surgery, such as inflammation, wound healing, and the role of blood coagulation in both. His approach to the problems of surgery was distinctly modern, in the sense that it was scientific and physiologic. Despite Lister's attempts to clean up his wards and to perform surgery as cleanly as possible, there was still an appalling rate of the common surgical complications of hospital gangrene, pyemia, and erysipelas among his patients.

In the years just prior to 1865 the French scientist Louis Pasteur slowly worked out what came to be a germ theory of disease. He clearly showed that fermentation and putrefaction, observed since ancient days, were caused by living, multiplying matter. He reasoned that pus formation and wound infection and some fevers must also be caused by minute organisms from the environment.[30]

It has never been entirely clear how Lister became aware of Pasteur's work. That he gave him specific credit there is no doubt. Rickman Godlee, Lister's surgical pupil, nephew, and biographer, claimed that it was a Glasgow colleague, the professor of chemistry, who suggested the practical implications of Pasteur's work to Lister and also suggested the use of carbolic acid. There is another possibility, however, that though not provable without more information, seems very plausible.

In the latter part of 1864, the year before Lister began to use carbolic acid on wounds, T. Spencer Wells, the eminent British surgeon, published a paper in the *British Medical Journal* entitled "Some Causes of Excessive Mortality After Surgical Operations." Wells described the work of Pasteur and said that it might well have an "important bearing upon the development of purulent infection and the whole class of diseases most fatal in hospitals and other overcrowded places."[88] Wells further suggested that germs might find their appropriate medium in wounds, causing pus and subsequent septicemia. Though clearly set forth, Well's argument seems to have borne little fruit, unless, of course, Lister was indeed stimulated by it.

Lister's first papers describing his method and its

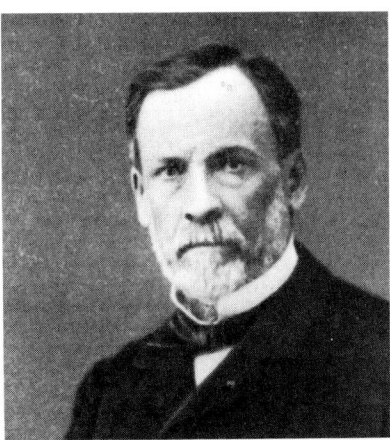

Figure 8. Louis Pasteur (1822–1895), the originator of the germ theory of disease.

success appeared in 1867. In the following years he changed the technical details of his method, added the steam-powered spray for the operating environment, and continued to fight for his idea in many publications. As the years went by he was able to perform safely operations that previously no capable surgeon would have dared attempt. The successful wiring of a fractured patella in 1877, thereby converting a closed fracture to an open one, brought much scorn upon him, but patience, doggedness, and scrupulous attention to detail led eventually to complete success. Lister admitted in the 1880s that the spray was not necessary, and indeed may have been harmful to operators and patients alike. He gracefully accepted the development of aseptic surgery by the Germans and acknowledged that it was but a step beyond his own work and a logical extension of it.

The acceptance of listerism, as I have already indicated, was uneven and, in our eyes, with the advantage of retrospective view, quite slow. There were many reasons for this, most of them not tied to simple conservatism or resistance to change. Lister's method was complicated; the carbolic acid was an unpleasant nuisance and could be actually harmful, and the method was time-consuming and expensive and required assistance. Some surgeons and medical men believed the germ theory to be mere speculation; hence the underlying theory or the rationale for Lister's technique was also slow of acceptance.[13] Also one must remember that many leading surgeons simply could not duplicate Lister's good results, hard as they might try. Theodor Billroth was one who tried the method, wanted to accept it, but found it somewhat frustrating. By the late 1870s he had adopted listerism fully, but not without much discouragement.[91]

Other surgeons reported that they used Lister's techniques but that their results were not much improved. In reading case reports in medical journals of the period one must evaluate carefully such phrases as "listerism used" or "Lister's technique followed throughout." In the case of President James Garfield in 1881, for instance, the extensive medical bulletins

issued during his 2-month lingering battle with an abdominal gunshot wound inflicted through the back, often reported, "Lister's dressings used." Yet we know, too, that fingers and instruments probed the wound from the first day on. Little real understanding of the germ theory can be ascribed to surgeons who carefully soaked their instruments in carbolic acid, but then reused them without resoaking after they had dropped on the floor, or, even more commonly used them after they had been wiped on the operator's nonsterile apron or held between his teeth. Thus the full realization by Lister of the meaning of Pasteur's work is perhaps his greatest achievement.

Rudolph Matas, one of the young American surgeons of the first generation of Lister disciples, has emphasized that certain features of the typical Lister dressing routine were more readily adopted than parts of the doctrine itself. Carbolic acid was accepted as the preferred antiseptic; Chassaignac's rubber drainage tubes again came into wider use, and the ligatures, soaked in carbolic solution, were cut short. "But even this marvelous improvement in technique was slow in coming, for, in 1878 and 1879, I saw a number of amputation stumps from which long ligatures dangled, waiting to ripen in pus to drop off."[48, 61]

In the 1880s, Matas recalled, the head, chest, and abdomen were still sanctuaries not to be opened, unless by accident.[61] It has frequently been stressed that the development of anesthesia and antisepsis greatly increased the numbers of operations performed, but a look at the statistics reveals that the increase was very slow. Halsted in 1904 showed that in the decade following the fairly wide acceptance of antisepsis in this country (1878–1888) the numbers of operations performed increased only slightly.[44] This decade, we must remember, was the second after Lister's first enunciation of his principles in 1867. Matas gave the figures for the Charity Hospital in New

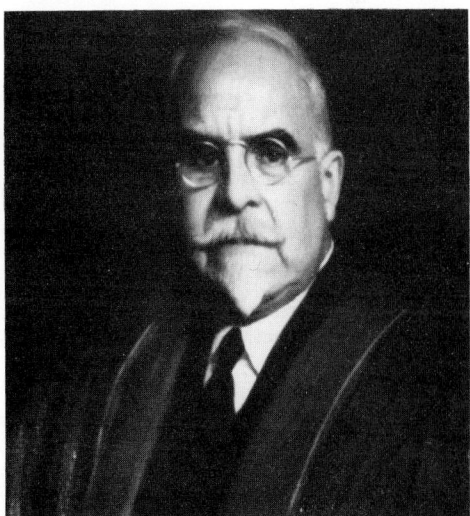

Figure 9. Rudolph Matas (1860–1957), Professor of Surgery at Tulane University in Louisiana and a pioneer in vascular surgery. He introduced the technique of endoaneurysmorrhaphy in the treatment of arterial aneurysm.

Orleans, where in 1881 only 172 operations were done among 5300 admissions, or about 3.2 per cent. In 1890, the Charity Hospital admitted 6083 patients, but only 291, or 4.7 per cent, had major surgical procedures. By 1939, about 40 per cent of admissions were surgical.[61]

In the decade after Lister's momentous papers on the efficacy of antisepsis, there was still much reticence, as has already been indicated, about accepting the method as well as its theoretical foundation, the germ theory of disease. There was also some reluctance to hope for much more improvement in the art of surgery. After the Napoleonic wars at the beginning of the century, the French surgeon and author of surgical texts, Alexis Boyer, is supposed to have said, "Surgery seems to have attained the highest degree of perfection of which it is capable."[72] Despite anesthesia and the development of many new techniques, and despite the promise of antisepsis, John Eric Erichsen, one of the most perceptive and influential surgeons of latter nineteenth century Britain, came to similar conclusions in 1873:

That there must be a final limit to development in this department of our profession there can be no doubt. . . . Like every other art, be it manipulative, plastic, or imitative, it can only be carried to a certain definite point of excellence. An art may be modified, it may be varied, but it cannot be perfected beyond certain attainable limits. . . . There cannot always be fresh fields for conquest by the knife; there must be portions of the human frame that will ever remain sacred from intrusion, at least in the surgeon's hands. That we have nearly, if not quite, reached these final limits there can be little question.[72]

The story of the last hundred years has proved Erichsen a poor prophet, yet most of those engaged in medicine have at one time or another shared his feelings. What Erichsen and his contemporaries could not foresee was that within two decades medicine (including surgery now) would join hands with biology as a whole and thereby be able to expand its horizon in ways previously unthought of. Chemotherapy, cardiac surgery, and transplantation are but a few examples of significant teamwork between basic scientists and surgeons.

Abdominal Surgery

Among the many difficult technical problems faced by nineteenth century surgeons was that of reconnecting the divided ends of hollow tubes, especially blood vessels and intestine. The story of the former is part of the history of transplantation, and it will be discussed in that context. Intestinal suture is part of the story of abdominal surgery, an important epoch in surgical history.

Just as cardiovascular surgery has captured both public and professional attention in the past two decades, 80 to 90 years ago it was abdominal surgery that played the same role. The successful removal of an inflamed appendix prior to rupture, the Billroth operations for esophageal and gastric cancer causing obstruction, the improved hernia operations of Bassini and Halsted, and abdominal operations for such other reasons as diseases of the ovary all caused great ex-

citement in the medical world of the late nineteenth century.

The problem of intestinal obstruction faced surgeons long before the 1880s. Strangulated hernia, for instance, was not uncommon. Before the introduction of antisepsis, laparotomy was not usually performed. Ephraim McDowell, the Kentucky physician who successfully removed a huge ovarian tumor from Mrs. Jane Todd Crawford in 1809, was skilled, to be sure, but also very lucky. An indication of how his townsmen felt is that they gathered in large numbers around his house on that Christmas Day in Danville, Kentucky, with a rope slung over a tree, ready for use if the doctor should fail in the butchery they were convinced he was committing. They might well have hanged him had his patient died.[34]

The basic principle of intestinal suture, that the serous coats must be brought into contact, was not discovered until early in the nineteenth century, and not put into use until some decades later. The British surgeon Benjamin Travers in 1812 published *An Inquiry Into the Process of Nature in Preparing Injuries of Intestines.* About the same time, Guillaume Dupuytren, one of the best trained and ablest surgeons of France, whose approach to surgery was much like John Hunter's in the use of experimental physiology and pathology, also concerned himself with intestinal suture. Although apparently quite a mean and unscrupulous man, he was a great teacher and surgical innovator. Unfortunately his name is associated today mainly with an uncommon malady of the hand caused by contraction of the palmar fascia. Dupuytren's student, Antoine Lembert, is known for his suture, which resulted from the observation that careful approximation of the peritoneal coats of divided intestine would result in good healing. Not until the German and German-trained surgeons (including Swiss and Austrians) began putting antiseptic and aseptic principles to work did the techniques of abdominal surgery find their way into common practice.

In America, one of the important contributions to the advance of surgery stemmed from the work of a pathologist, Reginald Heber Fitz of Boston, and the surgeons Charles McBurney and Henry B. Sands of New York and John B. Murphy of Chicago. Fitz in 1886 published his classic paper on appendicitis, a term he coined.[32] Known for centuries under a variety of names such as perityphlitis and iliac passion, acute inflammation of the *vermiform* appendix was a surgical disease according to Fitz. "The vital importance of the early recognition of perforating appendix is unmistakable," Fitz concluded. "Its diagnosis, in most cases, is comparatively easy. Its eventual treatment by laparotomy is generally indispensable." Fritz analyzed 257 cases with careful preoperative and postmortem correlation.

Charles McBurney, professor of surgery at the College of Physicians and Surgeons, working mainly at Roosevelt Hospital in New York, described in 1889 the point of maximal tenderness now bearing his name, and 5 years later proposed a new incision for appendectomy.[62, 63] J. B. Murphy in this country and Lord Moynihan of Leeds in England and others at the turn of the century led the vigorous campaign for withholding purgatives and for resorting to prompt surgery. It should be noted that the understanding of this common disease and the operative concept for it were worked out by the cooperative efforts of medical men of several specialities.

This use for surgery, self-evident to us today, took some years to become assimilated into standard medical practice. In 1900 abdominal surgery was not yet something undertaken lightly by most doctors and patients. The successful drainage of an appendiceal abscess of King Edward VII of England, forcing the delay of his coronation in 1902, helped make appendicitis a fashionable disease, and also helped break down further the resistance to surgery.

Another important contribution in the epoch of abdominal surgery of the last decades of the nineteenth century stemmed from work in pathologic physiology, especially in the various German medical centers. It was in these years that the German physiologist Heidenhain devised his pouches for the study of gastric physiology and Nickolai Eck, a Russian, his anastomosis of vena cava and portal vein. This latter experimental surgical procedure, devised in 1877, was then widely utilized by Mering, Minkowski, and other physiologists and internists in their study of digestion and liver function.

During these decades after 1860 the German clinics made numerous advances in scientific medicine. The concept of organ insufficiency put forward by Ottomar Rosenbach, for instance, had led to more frequent diagnosis of functional entities such as hyperactivity or hypersecretion and less frequent diagnosis of specific disorders such as gastric or duodenal ulcer. It was surgeons, with their new freedom to explore the abdomen, who redirected the attention of the medical world to the importance of anatomic diagnosis.[31]

Physiology and Surgery

The alliance of surgery with physiology, although not as long-standing as that with anatomy, still has quite a history. The mid-eighteenth century Swiss, Albrecht von Haller, was professor of both surgery and physiology in Göttingen. Trained by the most famous medical teacher of his day, Hermann Boerhaave of Leyden, Haller wanted to teach medicine as a science in Göttingen as his master had done in Holland. To Haller must go the credit for animating anatomy and for stressing the importance of a systematic study of function. It must be admitted that although Haller taught the subject of surgery, he probably never took knife in hand except for anatomic dissection or physiologic experiment.

Many of the nineteenth century physiologists became superb experimental surgeons. François Magendie and Claude Bernard in France and Rudolph Heidenhain in Germany are good examples. Bernard joined Charles Huette in writing a manual of operative surgery. Similarly, some men who were primarily surgeons became well known for their contributions to physiology. Benjamin Collins Brodie, sergeant-surgeon to two kings of England, did important work on the effects of alcohol and curare as well as on the relationship of heat and respiration.

To William Beaumont's surgical skills and wound

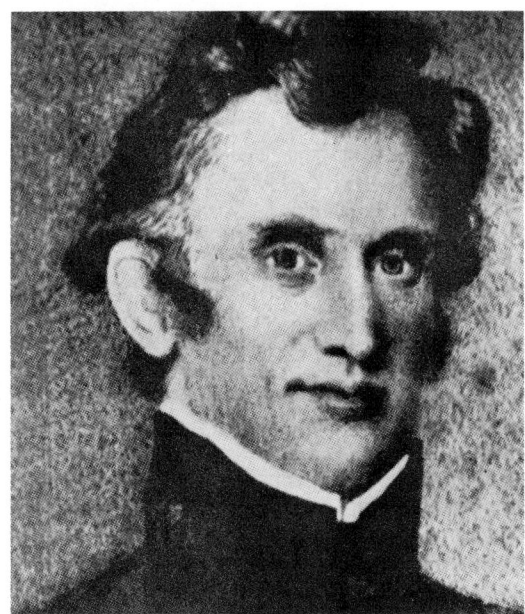

Figure 10. William Beaumont (1785–1853), an Army surgeon who performed pioneer studies in gastric physiology on the post-traumatic gastric fistula of Alexis St. Martin.

dressing is ascribed the fact that his patient, Alexis St. Martin, survived to become the most famous human experimental subject in the nineteenth century. St. Martin was wounded in the left lower chest by a musket shot at close range in 1822. Only after 3 years of constant and careful tending of the wounded area did Beaumont begin the famous investigations of gastric function.[5]

It was in the twentieth century, however, that surgeons began to deal consistently with a variety of physiologic problems almost every time they operated. Early in this century pain and infection were under control, but shock and the problem of maintaining respiration when the pleura was entered remained to be solved.

Training of the Surgeon

Much has been written in the last hundred years about the training of the surgeon, his proper qualifications, and what it means to be a surgeon. Between the simple apprenticeship or even the transfer of knowledge from father to son that held sway until the nineteenth century and the thorough grounding in pathology, research, and operative and postoperative management required of today's surgeon, much surgical history has passed.[38, 75]

The subject of surgical training in America invariably brings to mind the name of William S. Halsted, no doubt partly because of his famous address entitled "The Training of the Surgeon" delivered at Yale in 1904.[44] Halsted, who was born in New York City in 1852 and died in Baltimore 70 years later, made numerous important contributions to surgical technique and teaching.[50] After graduation from the Col-

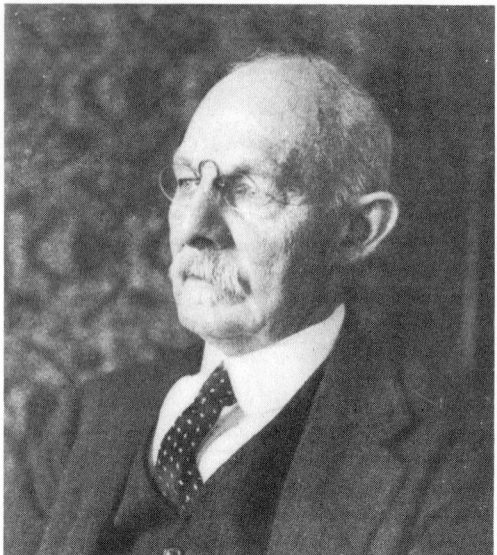

Figure 11. William S. Halsted (1852–1922), prominent American surgeon who introduced the German system of residency training to the United States. He also made fundamental contributions to the surgery of the thyroid, breast, and blood vessels, and to the surgical treatment of hernia.

lege of Physicians and Surgeons and a trip to Europe, he quickly established himself as an energetic researcher, gifted operator, and popular young teacher in New York. While working with cocaine for nerve block anesthesia, he and some of his associates became addicted. Only after hospitalization and prolonged convalescence, and with the faithful help of his friend, William H. Welch, who invited him to Baltimore in 1886, did Halsted recover. Historians are still working at unraveling the circumstances of further addiction during his later and very productive years.

When the Johns Hopkins Hospital opened in 1889, Halsted was appointed acting surgeon and head of the outpatient clinic. He became professor of surgery in 1892, the year before admission of the first medical school class. Halsted developed improved methods for operating on hernias and cancer of the breast; he introduced the use of rubber gloves in surgery, and he constantly stressed the relationship of surgery to physiology. Careful handling of tissues and minimizing blood loss were concepts he passed on to the many fine surgeons he trained during 30 years. Justifiable as has been his fame, Halsted was not solely responsible for establishing the surgical residency system as we know it. He himself would have been the first to note that the great German teachers of surgery, especially von Langenbeck and his pupils, including Billroth, were his models. Furthermore, Halsted's colleague William Osler deserves equal credit for instituting the system at Hopkins.

Why was it in Germany that the surgeons first adopted antisepsis, Halsted asked in his Yale lecture. The answer lay, he believed, "in the character of the scientific and practical training of surgeons in Germany." The assistants or "residents" in these programs enjoyed good research facilities, ample clinical

material, and excellent instruction, and this is what Halsted successfully duplicated in Baltimore. "We need a system," he said at Yale in 1904, "and we shall surely have it, which will produce not only surgeons but surgeons of the highest type, men who will stimulate the first youths of our country to study surgery and to devote their energies and their lives to raising the standard of surgical science."[44] Reforms, Halsted stressed, had to come from both hospital and university, and the medical school should control a hospital of its own.

Halsted's German model was based mainly on the system founded by Bernhard Rudolf Konrad von Langenbeck (1810–1887), one of Germany's most distinguished nineteenth century surgeons. He took his degree in Göttingen in 1835, 7 years later became professor of surgery at Kiel, and in 1847 moved to Berlin, where he assumed what was probably the most prestigious chair in Germany, succeeding the illustrious Johann Friedrich Dieffenbach, who had done much to make orthopedic surgery and plastic surgery successful modes of treatment. Langenbeck thus followed in the footsteps of a superb operator, an imaginative innovator, and a highly popular teacher, but he was superbly equal to the task.

In 1861 Langenbeck, along with two of his pupils, Theodor Billroth, who became equally prominent, and Ernst Gurlt, the historian of surgery, founded the *Archive für klinische Chirurgie*. Langenbeck's editorial contributions and surgical improvements alone would assure him a very high rank in the history of

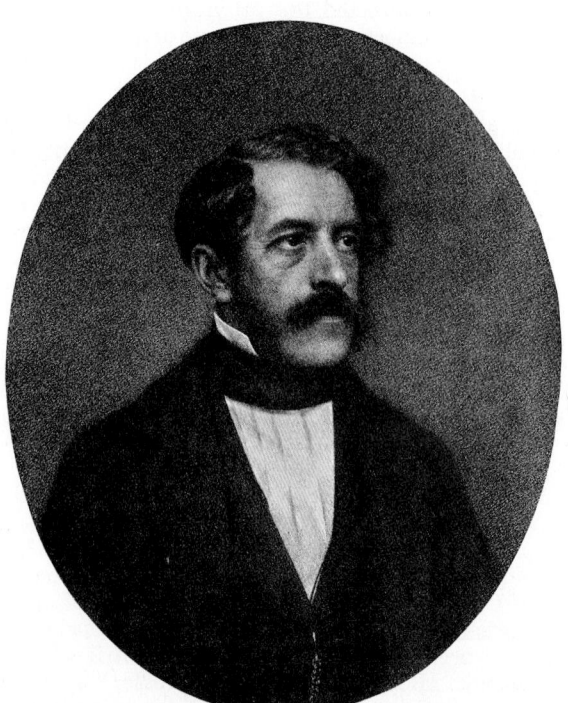

Figure 12. Bernhard von Langenbeck (1810–1887), master German surgeon who is acknowledged by many to be the father of the modern residency system in surgery. His students included Billroth and Kocher.

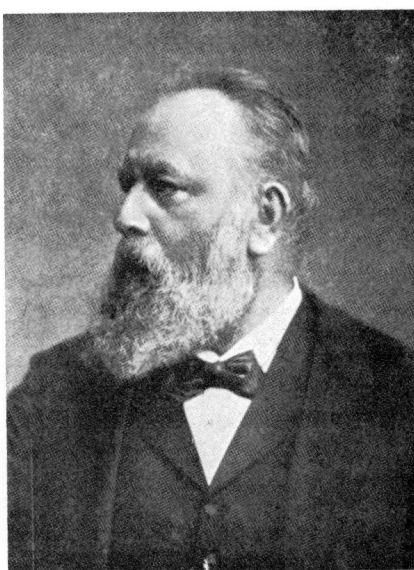

Figure 13. Theodor Billroth (1829–1894), Professor of Surgery at the University of Vienna and pioneer abdominal surgeon. Billroth was one of the most influential teachers of his time.

surgery, but perhaps his greatest contribution was his stress on a systematic way of training young surgeons. In general, this is what we now know as the surgical residency system.[9]

Halsted spent 2 years studying surgery, histology, and pathology in various German centers. He watched the work of Bergmann, Volkmann, Billroth, Esmarch, and Mikulicz in their surgical clinics. He was thus favorably inclined to the use of antisepsis, and the German thoroughness and insistence on knowledge of the basic sciences as a foundation for surgery were to be the hallmarks of his own career as well. Halsted's 17 residents and more than 50 assistant residents carried this "German method" to many teaching centers in the United States. The second and third generations from this "Johns Hopkins school" are still to be seen in American academic centers.

William Halsted was a keen judge of surgical talent, among both his peers and his students. That he considered Theodor Kocher of Berne perhaps the greatest surgeon of his time was one reason why Kocher was very popular with American students. He was known for his work on the brain and spinal cord and especially for his careful techniques and study of the thyroid gland. His surgical treatment of goiter, a particularly severe disease in his native Switzerland, earned Kocher the Nobel Prize in 1909, the first time it was awarded to a surgeon.[57]

Kocher was born in Berne in 1841, and was trained in several European centers, although he considered himself a pupil of Theodor Billroth, the great surgical teacher of Vienna. Kocher was professor of surgery at the University of Berne and headed its surgical clinic for 45 years. Among his students were Harvey Cushing and many other Americans.

In his work on the surgical relief of goiter, Kocher not only developed the surgical technique necessary for removal of the thyroid but also added immeasurably to the understanding of its role in the body's metabolism. In his early thyroidectomy patients, if removal was complete, myxedema developed, accompanied by all its unpleasant and stunting side effects. When his colleagues pointed out this tragic aftereffect, Kocher took positive steps to learn from his mistake instead of engaging in scientific polemics, so common for his age.

Neurosurgery and Thoracic Surgery

It should be clear that the latter decades of the nineteenth century gave rise to numerous developments in surgery and that these developments clearly set the stage for advances in our own century. Changing concepts in pathology during the nineteenth century greatly influenced surgery. Especially important was the idea that disease was localized, and hence remediable by surgical attack. In addition to his many other talents, the pathologist Rudolph Virchow, who in 1858 published his *Cellular Pathology,* was also a superb historian. He spoke in his essays about the "anatomical idea," the progressive localization of life and disease in the body. The "anatomical idea" originated in the mid-eighteenth century with Morgagni, who believed disease had its seat within the organs of the body. At the beginning of the nineteenth century the French surgeon Xavier Bichat claimed that it was to the tissues that one must look.[2] He identified 21 kinds, such as muscle, bone, and nerve, and pointed out that when epithelium became inflamed, the reaction was similar no matter where in the body it might occur. Virchow took the last step and localized disease

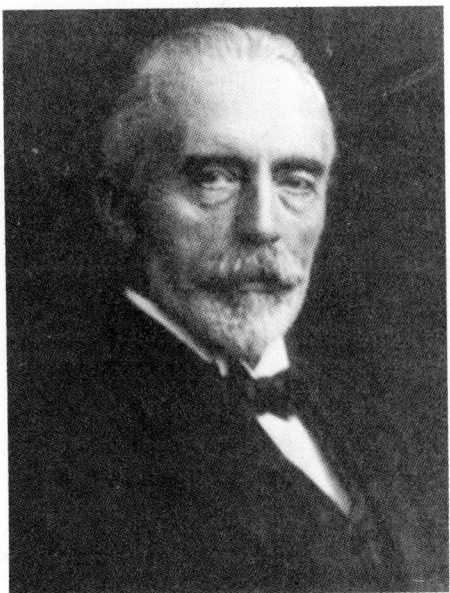

Figure 14. Theodor Kocher (1841–1917), Professor of Surgery at the University of Berne and pioneer in the development of surgery of the thyroid. He received the Nobel Prize in 1909.

processes within the cell. This view has held sway
since, though today we also discuss disease on the molecular or even the submolecular level.[82]

Some aspects of the surgical approach to disease
that the student of the 1970s may take for granted
have, actually, quite a short history. The twentieth
century is the century especially of neurosurgery,
thoracic surgery, and the whole field of transplantation.

The field of neurosurgery, so much of it brought to
its modern state by the work of Harvey Cushing,
Walter Dandy, and others, is similar in its historical
development to general surgery in a variety of ways.
The operation of trephination of the skull is one of the
oldest in the annals of surgery but since it was done
only to release evil spirts, to relieve pressure from injuries, or for the treatment of epilepsy, it hardly
qualifies for pride of place as neurosurgery. Not until
work on cerebral localization was done in the latter
nineteenth century could the surgeon really begin to
attack effectively lesions within the cranium. As in
other branches of surgery, diagnostic means had to be
developed, along with safe and efficient operative
measures.

Harvey Cushing, like all neurosurgeons until fairly
recent times (after World War II), was trained in general surgery.[35] He was William Halsted's resident,
though emotionally and personally he felt much closer
to the professor of medicine at Hopkins, William
Osler. While still a medical student at Harvard, Cushing devised a chart for continuous recording of respiration and blood pressure by the anesthetist and some
years later brought to American operating rooms the
practice of sphygmomanometry. While at Hopkins he
helped found the "Hunterian" surgical laboratory,
where the modern practice of experimental surgery in
dogs for medical students began.[24]

In thoracic surgery, the story is much the same.
Basic cardiac and pulmonary physiology had to be understood before surgical therapy could be contemplated.
The problems of operating on a beating heart were as
hard to overcome as was the difficulty of maintaining
pressure relationships within the chest. It was not
until the 1890s that direct wounds of the heart were
successfully sutured. Before this time chest surgery
consisted primarily of evacuation of empyema or
drainage of a pericardial sac filled with fluid or blood.

The story of the surgical treatment of cardiac lesions, traumatic, congenital, degenerative, or postin-
fective, has been told in some detail in recent books by
Meade,[64] Richardson,[74] and Johnson.[52] There is no
need to repeat the story here except to point out certain interesting aspects. In the first place, it is almost
entirely a twentieth century story. Historians, particularly thoracic surgeons, have taken some measure of
pride from disproving the statement of Stephen Paget
in *The Surgery of the Chest* in 1896:

Surgery of the heart has probably reached the limits set by
Nature to all surgery: no new method, and no new discovery,
can overcome the natural difficulties that attend a wound of
the heart. It is true that "heart suture" has been vaguely
proposed as a possible procedure, and has been done on
animals: but I cannot find that it has ever been attempted in
practice.

In the same year that Paget's book was published,
Ludwig Rehn of Frankfort became the first surgeon to
suture successfully a human heart laceration.

The history of valvular surgery has been one of
steady progress since the operations were reintroduced
in the late 1940s. The progress relates not only to
direct improvements in operative approach and technique, but also, as is the case in most thoracic surgery,
to technical developments by which physiologic conditions can be made suitable for surgery. There is an interesting connection between surgeons and internists
in the story of the surgical alleviation of valvular
disease. As has been true throughout the history of
medicine, the underlying theory regarding causation
of disease has been closely intertwined with the therapy made available. In the case of mitral valve disease, for instance, a great English clinician, the London cardiologist Sir Lauder Brunton, suggested in
1902 that animal experiments showed the feasibility
of a surgical approach to the disease. This suggestion
was not well received, and no surgeon seems to have
acted upon it until a London colleague, Henry Souttar,
operated on a woman in 1925. Souttar, instead of inserting an instrument into the ventricle to reach the
valve, used his finger to push through the valve from
the atrium. The patient, a 19-year-old girl, lived in
fair health for 5 years and died of a cerebral embolus.

New theories and innovations should not be accepted uncritically. The medical profession has been
accused of being too conservative, but for the sake of
our patients this is a necessary trait. Other aspects of
the resistance to change are not so defensible, as the
story of listerism has shown. Once again, in the
story of mitral valve surgery, a major theoretical
hurdle had to be overcome before real progress could
be made. James MacKenzie, who was Britain's leading
cardiologist and a respected teacher, hastened to con-
demn Souttar's attempted treatment, basing his objections on the belief that the abnormality of mitral
stenosis was in the myocardium, not in the valve.
With this theory, as with that of a basically humoral
pathology, surgical therapy made little sense. Theory
must affect practice; one cannot be divorced from the
other, as this example clearly illustrates.

By 1928 Elliot Cutler and Claude Beck could summarize only 12 known cases of valvular surgery, and
the results were discouraging. Mortality was 83 per
cent. The truly remarkable changes that have occurred in the years since 1955 are now known to all
students of surgery.

Experimental cardiac surgery began nearly 100
years ago. M. H. Block, a German surgeon, published
a report on wounds of the heart in 1882 in which he
described successful suture of rabbit hearts, and he
strongly urged that the procedure be used in man. In
the best surgical circles of the time, however, resistance to his innovation was strong. Billroth is reported
to have said a year later, "A surgeon who would attempt such an operation should lose the respect of his
colleagues." Here, too, the exact anatomic and functional relationships of various forms of heart disease
had to be clearly understood before surgical intervention could be contemplated. In addition, there were
technical problems of pressure relationships in the

chest, stilling the heart, and maintaining the circulation during surgery that had to be mastered before practical application was possible. Claude Beck was perfectly correct in 1926 when he predicted, "These technical problems should be capable of solution, as were problems in the past, by methods, instruments, and gentleness."[6]

One of the very basic physiologic obstacles that had already been overcome was the problem of negative pressure within the pleural cavity. Ferdinand Sauerbruch, working in the clinic of his teacher, Mikulicz, in Breslau, devised an apparatus in which negative pressure for the open thorax could be maintained. These experiments in 1903 and 1904 led to the construction of a large chamber in the next years, and the technical difficulties involved were soon alleviated by the introduction of endotracheal or insufflation anesthesia around 1910. Not until the late 1930s was a reliable apparatus available that would give good control of the respiration.

Hypothermia and the heart-lung machine are even more recent developments. Hypothermia had been used in the treatment of cancer and other medical problems when it was adapted for surgery by groups in Philadelphia, Minneapolis, and Denver in the 1950s. Many of the same surgeons also did much to develop a safe and efficient means of extracorporeal circulation. Dr. John H. Gibbon began to work on this problem before World War II.[39] He and others, especially C. Walton Lillehei and Clarence Dennis and their co-workers, made the possibility of extensive cardiac surgery an everyday reality in large hospital surgical services.

The problem of shock is important for all surgery, especially in times of war. Major surgical texts of the late nineteenth century rarely devoted more than a

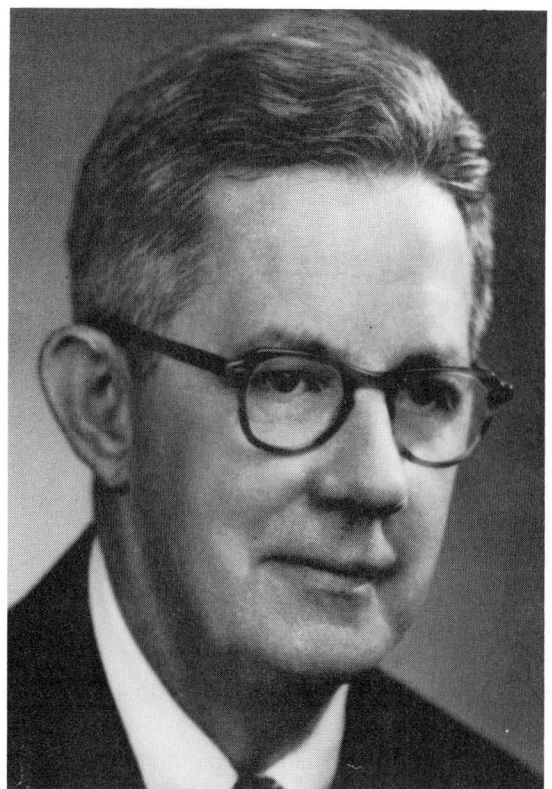

Figure 16. Alfred Blalock (1889–1964), noted investigator and clinical surgeon who made basic contributions to the understanding of the pathogenesis of shock. He also was a pioneer and innovator in the field of cardiac surgery.

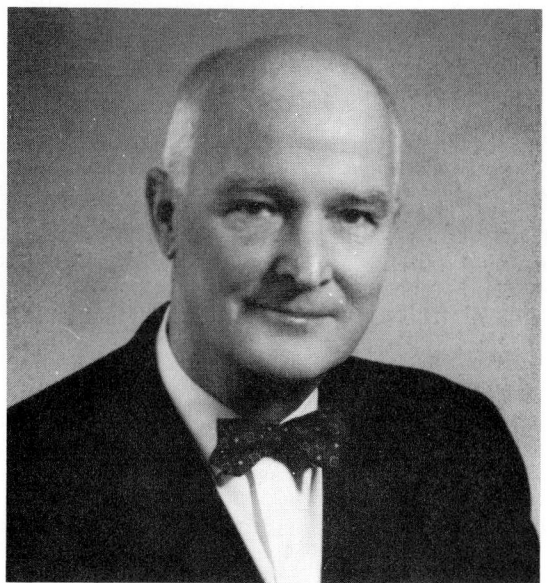

Figure 15. John H. Gibbon (1903–1973), pioneer cardiothoracic surgeon who developed extracorporeal circulation.

page to the subject. Loss of blood was known to be a cause, but beyond that not much more was known, nor could much have been done to counteract the effects. The list of credit for unraveling the story is a long one, but certainly two American surgeons, George Crile and Alfred Blalock, deserve special mention.[23]

Blalock, while he was at Vanderbilt University in the late 1920s and the 1930s, published significant papers on the cause and treatment of shock. The prevailing theory of the time was that the most likely cause for shock was release of a toxin, very possibly histamine. In studies of shock produced by muscle injury, Blalock and his co-workers found a large accumulation of blood at the site of trauma, be it in an extremity or the intestinal tract. In 1964, shortly before his death, Blalock summarized his work and added, "After thirty-four years have elapsed there still is much to be learned about shock."[12]

The contributions of surgical teachers and investigators such as Alfred Blalock, to single out just one among many, also illustrate the importance and influence of the scientific and academic environment upon the man. In Blalock's case, he was fortunate in having gone to Vanderbilt, a new medical center with many young men ambitious to do research. His former Hopkins roommate, Tinsley Harrison, was a resident in medicine at Vanderbilt when Blalock was a resident in surgery, and Harrison's influence, though hard to measure exactly, was doubtless important. After returning to Johns Hopkins in the early 1940s, Blalock worked in one of the finest medical research centers in any academic institution. His cooperation with the pediatrics department, particularly with Dr. Edwards A. Park and Dr. Helen Taussig, resulted in the discovery of a successful method of surgical treatment of tetralogy of Fallot. This in no way detracts from what Blalock or any other single individual may have contributed. It merely illustrates that an important change in scientific medicine has come about since the time when Claude Bernard or Louis Pasteur worked in inadequate quarters with a handful of students and assistants. Science today is, more than ever before, a great cooperative venture. To conduct such a venture successfully, academic and scientific leadership of high quality is required. Perhaps it is for this kind of leadership, for the stimulus provided to a whole school of research, rather than for individual surgical feats, that the recent great teachers such as Blalock and Owen Wangensteen will be best remembered. "My principle role," Dr. Wangensteen has said, "has been essentially that of trying to create an atmosphere friendly to learning."[58]

Electrolyte and Fluid Balance, Chemotherapy, and Radiology

Just as surgery has had profound effects on many aspects of health, disease, and the practice of medicine, numerous medical and biologic advances have greatly altered the work and the results of the surgeon. These nonsurgical developments are most obvious in such fields as cardiac surgery, as already discussed. Three further examples might be cited here, because modern surgery has been so dependent upon

them. Today surgeons, and, for that matter, all physicians, take for granted that proper electrolyte and fluid balance, chemotherapy, and x-ray studies are part of the medical regimen, if indicated. Each of these fields has an interesting history that is far too involved to describe in a few words, but it would be misleading not to include any part of the story here.

The concept of balance is an ancient one. The Greeks strove for a golden mean in life, and one of the pre-Socratic philosophers, Alcamaeon of Crotona, believed that the body's health depended on an equal combination of the four elements, earth, air, fire, and water. When this was achieved, there was *isonomia,* but when one element dominated a *monarchia* resulted.

Not until the 1850s and the work of Claude Bernard was a definition of the role of the blood and the body fluids clearly enunciated. In his *Liquids of the Organism,* a series of lectures published in 1859, Bernard first used the word *milieu* to express the internal environment. In the following years he elaborated his concept of the *milieu intérieur,* the physiologic state that allows the organism to exist independently.[68] In our own century these earlier ideas of Bernard were taken over by many, including Walter Cannon of Harvard, who coined the term homeostasis, and by Lawrence J. Henderson, also of Harvard, who wrote much on the mechanism of acid-base balance,[15, 49] and whose name is familiar to all medical students who have mastered the Henderson-Hasselbalch equation, at least for biochemistry examinations.

Neither Cannon nor Henderson was a surgeon, and although both were medically trained, neither practiced. Another Harvard physician, the Moseley Professor of Surgery, Francis D. Moore, early in his career became interested in the metabolic problems of surgical patients. The Coconut Grove fire in 1942 was a sad stimulus to learning for many. Moore continued to learn and to write and in 1952 published *Metabolic Response to Surgery,*[66] a surgical landmark. He greatly expanded his ideas in *Metabolic Care of the Surgical Patient,*[65] which has been a standard work since it was published in 1959. Moore's definition of the boundaries of surgery is of interest to the historian as well, because it sets his task.

> The fundamental act of medical care is assumption of responsibility. Surgery has assumed responsibility for the cure of a large section of human illness: a segment of disease which is largely acute, focal, or traumatic. This is responsibility for the care of the entire range of injuries and wounds, local infections, benign and malignant tumors, as well as a large fraction of those various pathologic processes and anomalies which are localized in the organs of the body. The study of surgery is a study of these diseases, the conditions and details of their care.[65]

What should also be noted here is that the techniques and the outcome that a patient and his surgeon can reasonably expect have drastically changed over time, though the basic disease processes confronting the surgeon have changed very little.

The story of modern chemotherapy began with the successful use of the arsenical salvarsan or "606" introduced by Paul Ehrlich and his co-worker Sahachiro Hata in 1910. Actually, as Ehrlich described his ap-

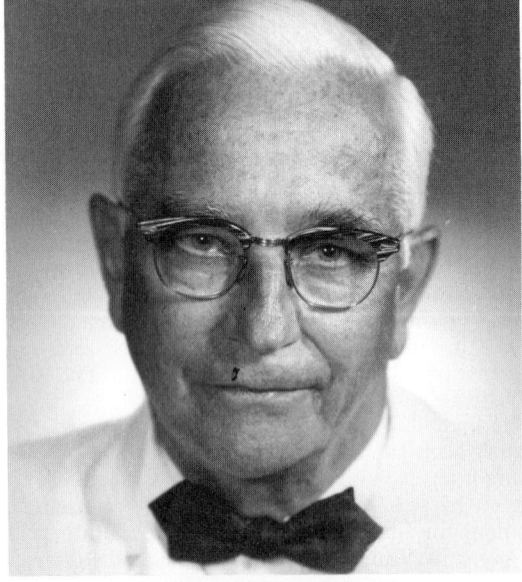

Figure 17. Owen H. Wangensteen, who for more than half a century has been a leading teacher of surgeons at the University of Minnesota.

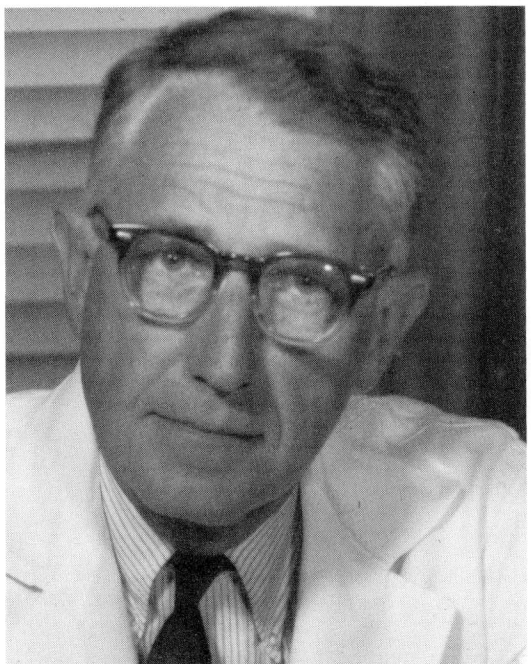

Figure 18. Francis D. Moore, leading investigative surgeon who defined objective aspects of metabolism in surgical patients.

proach to research, the idea began to evolve several decades earlier in his work on the development of tissue stains. The story continues with the work of the British pathologist Sir Alexander Fleming, who said in his Nobel Lecture, "To my generation of bacteriologists the inhibition of one microbe by another was commonplace. We were all taught about these inhibi-

tions and indeed it is seldom that an observant clinical bacteriologist can pass a week without seeing ... very definite instances of antibacterial antagonism."[33]

In 1921 Fleming described and isolated such an inhibiting agent, and called it lysozyme. Unfortunately, the bacteria inhibited by this natural enzyme are not those harmful to man. But the lysozyme work alerted him to be on the lookout for other suitable antagonistic candidates. In the fall of 1928 Fleming noted that some of his plates of staphylococcal cultures contaminated by laboratory air grew a mold that inhibited growth of the bacteria.

Fleming's observation, so often ascribed to chance, was actually made in the course of careful laboratory investigation. Part of Fleming's goal was to find just such a substance. What did prove to be extremely fortuitous was that the product of the contaminating mold, penicillin, was a powerful antibacterial substance, effective against some of the common pathogens of man, yet remarkably free of toxicity for man. Why Fleming's important discovery was not commercially produced until the war years is not entirely clear. Fleming himself claimed that medical men became interested in the possibility of antibiotics only after the demonstrated usefulness of the sulfonamide drugs introduced by Gerhard Domagk in 1935. Not until several American manufacturing plants entered the picture in the early 1940s was there enough penicillin for a clinical trial.

If Fleming fully recognized the momentous nature of his discovery, and every indication points to the fact that he did, the question still remains why he and others did not push harder for earlier penicillin synthesis or isolation.

Another development that deserves emphasis is the discovery of x-rays by Röntgen in 1895. This was a discovery that, although part of a general physical investigation, was accidental. Moreover, it was the first modern scientific discovery to receive banner headlines in the papers. The public was fascinated and

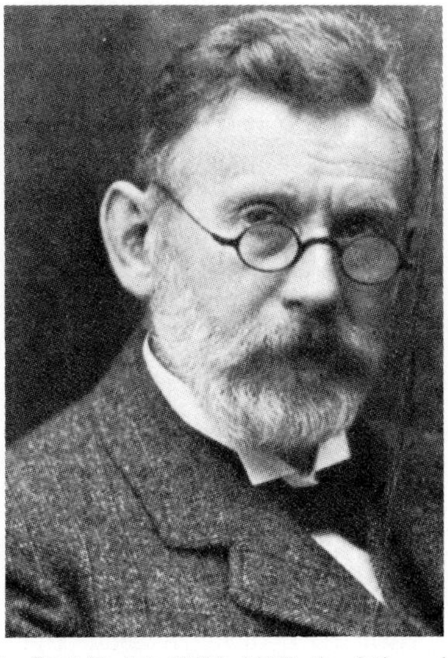

Figure 19. Paul Ehrlich (1854–1915), the father of modern chemotherapy, who introduced the use of the arsenicals (salvarsan) in 1910 for the treatment of syphilis.

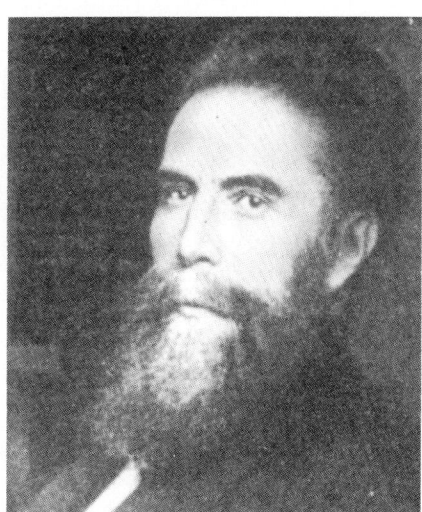

Figure 20. Wilhelm K. Röntgen (1845–1923), who discovered x-rays in 1895.

frightened. "Old ladies," Derek Price tells us, "went into their baths fully clothed, being convinced that the scientists now had mystery rays that could look through brick walls and round corners."[73] It was only a matter of months after the discovery that Frau Röntgen's hand and wrist bones could be clearly visualized that clinical application of the finding was made. Within a few years the use of the rays was expanded to include physiologic studies such as that of swallowing and intestinal motion. Walter B. Cannon used fluoroscopy for this purpose while he was still a medical student in 1901.

The daily use of x-rays for complex diagnostic and therapeutic reasons is now accepted procedure. Orthopedics, neurosurgery, cardiovascular surgery, and gastrointestinal surgery all have advanced rapidly because of the use of x-rays before and during surgery. It should be noted, too, that the need for complicated, expensive, and bulky equipment for radiologic studies helped establish the hospital as the primary locus for medical, especially surgical, care.

Organ Transplantation

Probably no recent development in surgery has so captured the public interest as has organ transplantation. Like some other recent aspects of medicine, transplantation has a long history.[89] An integral part of the story of transplantation is to be found in the annals of plastic surgery. The ancient Hindus were adept at transplanting skin from the buttocks area to refashion noses and ears. Even more common was the forehead flap method that was given wide publicity with a picture in *The Gentleman's Magazine* in 1794. This can be traced back to much earlier times.

In the sixteenth century the Italian surgeon Gasparo Tagliacozzi gained fame for his method of rhinoplasty. One sees in the history of plastic surgery a close connection between social customs and civilization as a whole and the surgeon's responses to the resultant needs. During the Renaissance and beyond, frequent street brawls, the cutting off of the nose or ears as punishment for thievery and adultery, and the devastating effects of leprosy, syphilis, and mercury treatment all made the need for a method to rebuild the face very evident. The history of plastic surgery can be seen in terms of man's increasing facility with transplanting skin.

Another aspect of transplantation that has direct bearing on surgery is tissue and cell culture, more properly called explantation. Here medicine and biology met and joined forces in the early twentieth century. What happened in this one field is thus a typical case study for the development of twentieth century medicine and surgery generally. To understand the story of tissue culture and cell culture, one must go back into the history of botany, especially the history of plant grafting, and also into the history of experimental embryology, because it was the embryologists at the end of the last century who made extensive use of explantation of embryos to observe their subsequent growth and development. The history of tissue culture is really one of the more recent episodes in the history of medicine. It began with the work of Ross G. Harrison in the first decade of this century. Born in Ger-

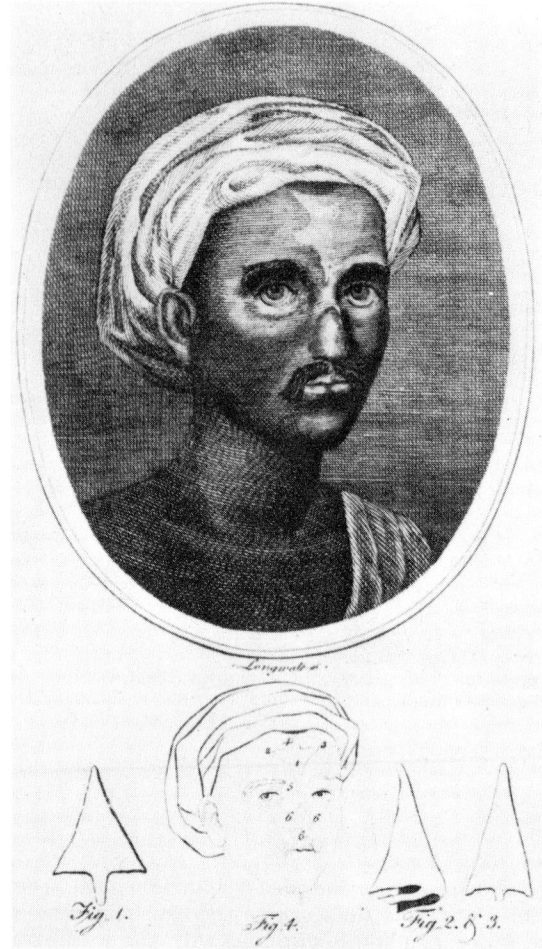

Figure 21. The forehead flap method for plastic reconstruction employing transplant of skin from the buttocks to refashion the nose and ears. (From The Gentleman's Magazine, 1794).

mantown near Philadelphia in 1870, Harrison was among many illustrious students in the early years of The Johns Hopkins University, where he received his undergraduate degree in biology in 1889. After further study, including medical education, Harrison went to Yale in 1907, and in the same year published the paper that is generally considered to contain the rudiments of the method of modern tissue culture so widely used today.[46, 47]

Harrison hoped to settle the controversy then being aired in the scientific journals over the growth of the nerve cell. Was its long process an outgrowth of the cell or was it an independent unit, growing toward the cell body? By means of a hanging-drop preparation, Harrison was able to observe under direct vision the growth of frog embryo nervous tissue in clotted lymph. Soon after Harrison moved to New Haven, Montrose Burrows came from the newly established Rockefeller Institute in New York to learn about the method of independent cell growth.[22]

Burrows suggested improvements in the medium

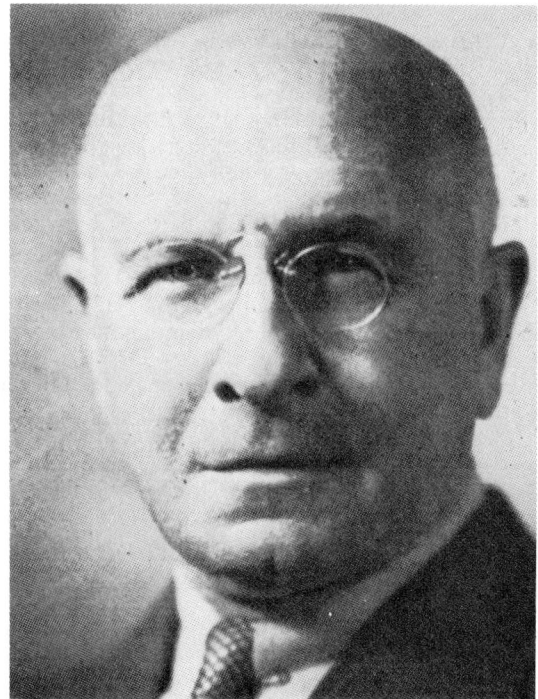

Figure 22. Alexis Carrel (1873–1944), an experimental surgeon interested in wound healing, tissue culture, organ transplantation, and blood vessel anastomosis. He was awarded the Nobel Prize in 1912.

and, incidentally, probably also deserves credit for suggesting the term tissue culture. He returned to New York to report his findings to the man who had sent him to New Haven, the French-born surgeon Alexis Carrel.

Carrel, born in Lyon in 1873, was one of the most colorful and most interesting figures in the medicine of the first half of the century. He was trained in France and became a skilled and imaginative experimental surgeon who developed the finest of techniques. Carrel was much interested in Harrison's work because he saw its potential for his own work on wound healing and tissue proliferation. These problems could be much better studied if they were isolated from the body as a whole. Carrel and Burrows

did indeed manage to grow tissues in flasks. The next step was to grow entire organs. Carrel had already been involved in extensive transplantation of organs in the decade 1902–1912.

Here, in the work of this one man, there is a close connection between surgery and transplantation of organs and the growth of cells and tissues. What Carrel accomplished with the delicate instruments he devised was to suture blood vessels, end to end, without leaving tissue hanging into the lumen that could then act as a focus for clot formation. Previous attempts to transplant organs and to re-establish their blood supply had met with failure because of infection and thrombosis. Carrel first reported his technique in 1902, when he was not yet 30 and only 2 years after

Figure 23. Joining blood vessels by suture anastomosis. Adapted from the line drawing by Alexis Carrel published in *Lyon Medical* in 1902. The walls of the two blood vessels (here drawn as about 5 mm. in diameter) are held together by three holding sutures. Another is then used to sew over and over, with very fine needles ("aiguilles extrêmement fines"). This method of suture anastomosis, demonstrated initially by Carrel, is still used throughout surgery, and particularly in the transplantation of organs.

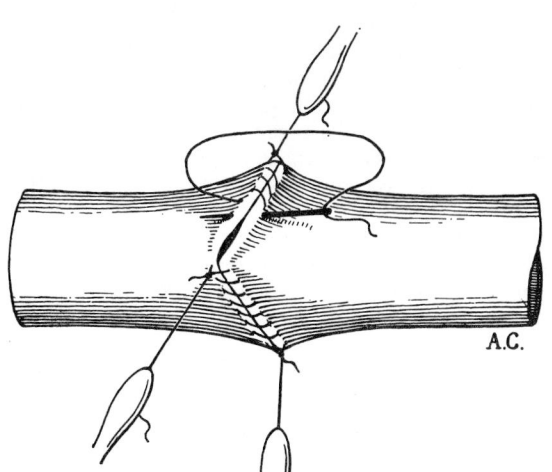

he had obtained his M.D. degree. His method was to use three retaining sutures, thereby converting a round hole to a triangular one, which could then be easily sutured, a simple but lasting technique for which he was awarded the Nobel Prize in 1912.[16]

Carrel came to the United States in 1905 and that summer worked with Charles Claude Guthrie at the Hull Physiological Laboratory at the University of Chicago. Guthrie, medically trained but a physiologist most of his career, is the unsung hero in the story of vascular suture and hence organ transplantation. Guthrie suggested improvements to Carrel's technique and the two men collaborated in numerous experiments and papers. Guthrie urged Carrel to include all layers of the vessel wall, even the endothelium, in the suture to prevent wrinkling.[45, 87]

In 1906 Carrel presented the results of the work he and Guthrie had done on organ transplantation and discussed the clinical implications for cure of aneurysm and other conditions. Carrel said, in words that have a very timely ring,

> The question of the transplantation of organs in man is a very serious one and difficult, for will the transplanted organ remain and function normally after a long period of time? Another difficulty would be that of finding organs suitable for transplantation into man. A process of immunization would no doubt be necessary before the organs of animals would be suitable for transplantation into man. Organs from a person killed by accident would no doubt be suitable.[17]

William Halsted, commenting on this paper in 1906, said, "There is work here for an army of investigators." Forty years were to pass before the army began its work. One reason why rapid strides in both experimental surgery and tissue culture were delayed until after World War II was that antibiotics were not readily available until then.

One of the prime contributors to the field of cardiovascular surgery has been Michael E. DeBakey of Houston. In 1934 he first described the occlusive roller pump, which has been widely used throughout the world in extracorporeal circulation. Following this basic contribution, he became a leader in the field of direct surgery for the treatment of thoracic and abdominal aneurysms, including complicated resections of lesions of the aortic arch. Moreover, he and his associates dedicated much time and effort to the development of plastic prosthetic arterial substitutes, which have been widely adopted and highly successful. He was the first to perform a successful carotid endarterectomy in 1953 and, in addition, he and his colleagues were also the first to report the successful use of a saphenous vein bypass graft for coronary arterial occlusion, a procedure which they accomplished in 1964.

In addition to his important surgical contributions, Dr. DeBakey has for more than 25 years been an influential member of an advisory group that has been important in shaping biomedical research. His influence on Mary and Albert Lasker and on members of Congress has been instrumental in the evolution of support for research and for health care.

To go further in describing recent events in surgery would be futile in a short space and surely foolish

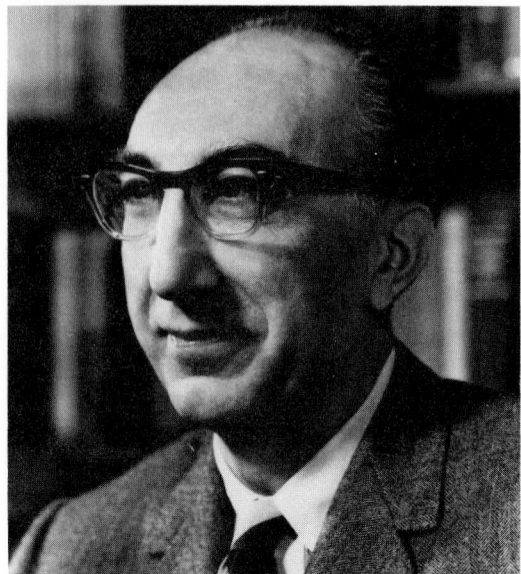

Figure 24. Michael E. DeBakey, American pioneer in cardiovascular surgery who has been a leading spokesman of medicine and medical research.

boldness for a medical historian. One need only compare the table of contents of any recent issue of any surgical journal with one from a decade or two ago to note differences in emphasis. How lasting or productive one approach will be compared to another is for the prophet to predict.

In looking back over the history of surgery one of the themes that stand out is progress. Though uneven over the years, and certainly not a straight line of advance after advance, the progress of man's ability to contribute to the well-being of his fellow man by means of surgery seems impressive indeed.

Intimately related to this progress has been the increasing specialization in medicine as a whole and within the field of surgery itself. Surgery as a specialty began with the wound surgeons of early antiquity. From later antiquity to the early twentieth century, surgeons for the most part did not confine themselves to operative therapy; they were also charged with care for a variety of dermatologic disorders, especially syphilis. It is no accident that Sir Jonathan Hutchinson (1828–1913), a surgeon, described the triad of congenital syphilis: deformed incisor teeth, interstitial keratitis, and deafness. It was not until the great advances made by surgery in the nineteenth century that surgeons as a group began to regain prestige, which they did for themselves as well as for the medical profession as a whole.

In America, most historians have pointed out, no definite separation of medicine and surgery ever existed, despite the early attempts of John Morgan to have university-educated medical men desist from the work of the apothecary and the surgeon. The most widely known statement regarding the lack of separation comes from a long review article by Samuel D.

Gross on the achievements of surgery in the first hundred years of the country:

Although this paper is designed to record the achievements of American surgeons, there are, strange to say, as a separate and distinct class, no such persons among us. It is safe to affirm that there is not a medical man on this continent who devotes himself exclusively to the practice of surgery. On the other hand, there are few physicians, even in our larger cities, who do not treat the more common surgical diseases and injuries.... In short, American medical men are general practitioners, ready for the most part, if well-educated, to meet any and every emergency, whether in medicine, surgery or midwifery.[43]

Interestingly, a few years later, Gross welcomed the newly founded American Surgical Association to its inaugural meeting in 1882. He justifies the existence of the new society by pointing out that there were in the United States about 60,000 medical men, large numbers being surgeons.

In a general sense, surgeons doubtless practiced family medicine or the like, but there is evidence that they did exist as a distinct specialty even at the time of Gross and before. According to the *Seventh Census of the United States*, 1850, the State of New York, for instance, is credited with 5060 physicians for a population of 3,097,394. In addition, listed separately among the occupations are 54 surgeons. Five years later, in a census of New York State, the City of New York claimed 1252 physicians and 19 surgeons. More and more, as the nineteenth century progressed, surgery was performed by those who called themselves surgeons. This became true especially in the urban areas and for the increasingly complex operations within the abdomen after the introduction of antisepsis. In rural areas there was less reluctance to do surgery among those not specifically trained. This is still true of the general practitioner today.

The founding of the American Surgical Association in 1880, the American College of Surgeons in 1913, and the American Board of Surgery in 1937 has played an important part in setting and maintaining high professional standards and providing a forum for communication among men with similar scientific interests. Like their European predecessors, these surgical organizations have thus aided the process of professionalization by insisting on standards for both surgeons and hospitals.[25, 60]

In conclusion, a few comments concerning the development of this textbook are appropriate. Dr. Frederick Christopher was Associate Professor of Surgery at Northwestern University when he originally assumed the gigantic task of coordinating the writings of nearly 200 leaders of American surgery between the covers of one book. Christopher was born in Cincinnati in 1889. He received a bachelor's degree from Northwestern University in 1911, and the M.D. degree in 1915 from the Johns Hopkins Medical School. Christopher then returned to Evanston, where he spent the rest of his illustrious professional career. He retired to Seattle and died there in 1967 at the age of 77.[19]

In the mid 1920s Christopher began work on his *Minor Surgery,* which was published in 1929. Stimu-

lated by its success, and by that of the multiple-author *Textbook of Medicine* edited by Russell Cecil, the W. B. Saunders Company prevailed upon him in 1934 to begin work on a similar text in surgery. The result was the first edition of what has, since its publication in 1936, been referred to by several generations of medical students and surgeons as "Christopher's Surgery."

The mid-1930s was an exciting period in medical science. Insulin had become available, sulfonamide drugs were just appearing, and the scent of progress was again in the air. Since the bacteriologic discoveries of Pasteur, Koch, and others, and their practical application by Lister, Bergmann, and Schimmelbusch, to name but a few, surgery had assumed an increasingly important role. It must be remembered, however, that this period was not the best time to launch a new and expensive publishing venture. The book's success, despite the Depression, is indicative of its merit.

Perhaps the most concise summary of the overall needs and conditions of surgery in the mid-1930s was made by Alton Ochsner and Owen Wangensteen, the editors of *Surgery,* founded in 1937, about the time the first edition of Christopher appeared. In their editorial announcement, the two surgeons wrote:

There can be no longer a sharp distinction between that which is medical and that which is surgical. The borders between medicine and surgery are not fixed, but are constantly changing. There is a continual striving to find means of treating surgical diseases which are refractory to medical management; at the same time an uninterrupted search is always in progress for conservative agents which may adequately replace satisfactory, but more energetic, operative methods. The sole anxiety of surgery is no longer concerned with the treatment of wounds. Surgery has emerged from a handicraft to occupy an important position in the treatment of disease. Its influence has been felt in every branch of medical science and practice.[67]

Surgery, like all medicine at the time, was rapidly becoming far too complex for one author to handle competently. Of even greater importance in the history of this book, only a team approach could ensure that it would continue to be current in subsequent editions. This was a point not lost upon the reviewers, who praised Christopher, and then his successor, Loyal Davis, who assumed the editorship with the sixth edition in 1956, for the broad updating of each new edition. "The dominant plan of this textbook," Christopher's first sentence read in 1936, "is to give the student a concise presentation of surgery which is characterized by the maximum authority." The list of authors reads like a who's who of surgery, and has continued to do so.

One could, with some justification and accuracy, write the history of surgery of the 40 years between the first and eleventh editions of this book by using each edition as a primary source for material. A simple comparison of the tables of contents of the first and present editions is revealing.

The 1936 edition began with a section on inflammation and repair, followed by a widely prized chapter on the bacteriology of surgery by Frank L. Meleney. Then came sections on anthrax, fungus disease, tularemia, and thermal, chemical, and electrical injuries, and on page 64 the discussion of the various systems or regions of the body began. After final sections on aseptic technique and anesthesia, fewer than 30 pages were devoted to preoperative and postoperative care.

The chapter titles in the present edition reflect the sounder physiologic basis of surgery of more recent years, and presumably better surgical management. Full chapters are devoted to discussion of surgical metabolism, shock, and preoperative and postoperative care.

The book reviews of each of the ten editions have been uniformly warm in their praise of the scope and modernity of the book. The readers must have been satisfied, because the sales figures show quite an astounding success. The last edition of the text was published in English, Japanese, and Spanish.

SELECTED REFERENCES

Bishop, W. J.: The Early History of Surgery. London, Robert Hale, 1960.
As suggested by the title, the history of surgery through the seventeenth century comprises two thirds of the book. It provides a general, not overly detailed history of premodern surgery and its role in the history of medicine.

Cartwright, F. F.: The Development of Modern Surgery. New York, Thomas Y. Crowell Company, 1968.
This text stresses the last 100 years and is rich in detail and interpretation.

Cope, Z.: A History of the Acute Abdomen. New York, Oxford University Press, 1965.
The author gives an excellent description of the evolution of surgical methods of treatment of abdominal emergencies.

Dale, W. A.: The beginnings of vascular surgery. Surgery, 76:849, 1974.
A fine review of an important aspect of twentieth century surgery, with many references.

Earle, A. S.: Surgery in America: From the Colonial Era to the Twentieth Century. Philadelphia, W. B. Saunders Company, 1965.
Long excerpts from original papers in the American medical literature provide ready access to some of the best in surgical writing.

Forssmann, W.: Experiments on Myself, Memoirs of a Surgeon in Germany. Trans. H. Davies. New York, St. Martin's Press, Inc., 1974.
The autobiographical account of the Nobel prize-winning surgeon, including the fascinating story of contrast radiography and catheterization of the heart.

Gnudi, M. T., and Webster, J. P.: The Life and Times of Gasparo Tagliacozzi, Surgeon of Bologna 1545–1599. New York, Herbert Reichner, 1950.
The main emphasis of this book is on the accomplishments of Tagliacozzi in the field of plastic surgery. Other superb chapters deal with the history of plastic surgery before and after Tagliacozzi, and student life and the teaching of surgery in his time. There are many illustrations of sixteenth century medicine, particularly surgery.

Graham, H.: The Story of Surgery. New York, Doubleday & Company, 1939.
This is a well written, informative general history of surgery, though lacking in a bibliography and weak in the twentieth century part of the story.

Johnson, S. L.: The History of Cardiac Surgery 1896–1955. Baltimore, The Johns Hopkins Press, 1970.
This short but superior book describes the advances in physiology and technology that necessarily preceded or accompanied the development of cardiac surgery. The illustrations help make the story more readily understandable for those who are not specialists in thoracic surgery.

Majno, G.: The Healing Hand, Man and Wound in the Ancient World. Boston, Harvard University Press, 1975.
A superbly illustrated book describing wound care and the treatment of inflammation in the ancient cultures of Mesopotamia, Egypt, Arabia, China, India, and Greece.

Malgaigne, J. F.: Surgery and Ambroise Paré. Trans. W. B. Hamby. Norman, University of Oklahoma Press, 1965.
In 1840 Malgaigne brought out a large, three-volume Oeuvres de Paré. The first volume included a "History of Western Surgery from the Sixth to the Sixteenth Century," "Surgery During the First Half of the Sixteenth Century," and a long biographic sketch of Paré. These are now here available in English for the first time. Although it is now over 135 years old, Malgaigne's is still a very useful history of early surgery.

Meade, R. H.: A History of Thoracic Surgery. Springfield, Ill., Charles C Thomas, Publisher, 1960.
This large book deals with the increasing complexity of thoracic surgery from antiquity to the 1950s, with an extensive bibliography.

Meade, R. H.: An Introduction to the History of General Surgery. Philadelphia, W. B. Saunders Company, 1968.
This is the most ambitious attempt in recent years to cover the entire history of surgery. The 30 chapters are organized by individual organs or parts of the body, and each has an extensive list of references, with emphasis on the literature of the past 25 years.

Moore, F. D.: Give and Take, The Biology of Tissue Transplantation. Philadelphia, W. B. Saunders Company, 1964.
This is an excellent, concise description of the development of renal transplants and the surgical and biologic problems encountered by the pioneering group at Peter Bent Brigham Hospital.

Richardson, R. G.: Surgery: Old and New Frontiers. New York, Charles Scribner's Sons, 1969.
This revised edition of Surgeon's Tale is a very satisfactory book for a general understanding of the historical background of the recent trends in surgery.

Richardson, R. G.: The Scalpel and the Heart. New York, Charles Scribner's Sons, 1970.
This book covers much the same ground as Johnson's, but has the added advantage of bringing the story to very recent times, including many of the events since 1955.

Shryock, R. H.: The Development of Modern Medicine. New York, Alfred A. Knopf, 1947.
In spite of its age, this is still the most satisfactory single volume on the history of medicine. The role of surgery in the development of medicine as a whole is well described.

Zimmerman, L. M., and Veith, I.: Great Ideas in the History of Surgery. Baltimore, Williams & Wilkins Company, 1961; 2nd ed. New York, Dover Publications, 1967.
Because of its availability in a paperback edition, its judicious combination of readings from the great surgeons of antiquity to the early twentieth century with a well-written narrative by the authors, and the inclusion of many useful references, this book is highly recommended for further reading.

REFERENCES

1. Ackerknecht, E. H.: Primitive surgery. Am. Anthropol., *49*:25, 1947.
2. Ackerknecht, E. H.: Medicine at the Paris Hospital 1794–1848. Baltimore, The Johns Hopkins Press, 1967.
3. Allbutt, T. C.: The Historical Relations of Medicine and Surgery to the End of the Sixteenth Century. London, Macmillan & Company, 1905.
4. Ball, J. M.: The Sack-em Up Men; an Account of the Rise and Fall of the Modern Resurrectionists. Edinburgh, Oliver & Boyd, 1928.
5. Beaumont, W.: Experiments and Observations on the Gastric Juice and the Physiology of Digestion, 1833. New York, Dover Publications, 1959.
6. Beck, C. S.: The operative story of the heart. Ann. Med. Hist., *8*:224, 1926.
7. Bigelow, H. J.: Introductory Lecture. Boston, Mussey, 1850.
8. Billings, J. S.: The history and literature of surgery. *In* Dennis, F.

(Ed.): System of Surgery. Philadelphia, Lea, 1895, Volume 1, pp. 17–144.

9. Billroth, T.: The Medical Sciences in the German Universities New York, The Macmillan Company, 1924.

10. Bishop, W. J.: A History of Surgical Dressings. Chesterfield, Robinson & Sons, 1959.

11. Bishop, W. J.: The Early History of Surgery. London, Robert Hale, 1960.

12. Blalock, A.: Reminiscence: Shock after thirty-four years. In Ravitch, M. (Ed.): The Papers of Alfred Blalock. Baltimore, The Johns Hopkins Press, 1966, Volume 1, pp. 16–19.

13. Brieger, G. H.: American surgery and the germ theory of disease. Bull. Hist. Med., 40:135, 1966.

14. Brock, R. C.: The Life and Work of Astley Cooper. Edinburgh, E. & S. Livingstone, 1952.

15. Cannon, W. B.: The Wisdom of the Body. New York, W. W. Norton, 1932.

16. Carrel, A.: La technique opératoire des anastomoses vasculaires et la transplantation des viscères. Lyon Med., 98:859, 1902.

17. Carrel, A.: Surgery of the blood vessels and its application to changes in circulation and transplantation of organs. Bull. Johns Hopkins Hosp., 17:236, 1906.

18. Cheselden, W.: The Anatomy of the Humane Body. London, 1713; 13th ed., 1792.

19. Christopher, F.: One Surgeon's Practice. Philadelphia, W. B. Saunders Company, 1957.

20. Churchill, E. D.: Surgery in the twentieth century. In Nardi, G. L., and Zuidema, G. D. (Eds.): Surgery, A Concise Guide to Clinical Practice, 2nd ed. Boston, Little, Brown and Company, 1965, pp. 1–8.

21. Cope, Z.: William Cheselden 1688–1752. Edinburgh, E. & S. Livingstone, 1953.

22. Corner, G. W.: A History of the Rockefeller Institute 1901–1953. New York, Rockefeller Institute Press, 1964.

23. Crile, G. W.: An Autobiography. Crile, G. (Ed.): 2 vols. Philadelphia, J. B. Lippincott Company, 1947.

24. Cushing, H.: Instruction in operative medicine with the description of a course given in the Hunterian Laboratory of experimental medicine. Bull. Johns Hopkins Hosp., 17:123, 1906.

25. Davis, L.: Fellowship of Surgeons, A History of the American College of Surgeons. Springfield, Ill., Charles C Thomas, 1960.

26. DeBakey, M. E.: A simple continuous-flow blood transfusion instrument. New Orleans Med. Surg. J., 87:383, 1934.

27. DeBakey, M. E.: Successful carotid endarterectomy for cerebrovascular insufficiency. Nineteen-year follow-up. J.A.M.A., 233:1083, 1975.

28. Dobson, J.: The training of a surgeon. Ann. R. Coll. Surg. Engl., 34:1, 1964.

29. Dobson, J.: John Hunter. Edinburgh, E. & S. Livingstone, 1969.

30. Dubos, R.: Louis Pasteur: Free Lance of Science. Boston, Little, Brown and Company, 1950.

31. Faber, K.: Nosography in Modern Internal Medicine. New York, Paul B. Hoeber, 1923.

32. Fitz, R. H.: Perforating inflammation of the vermiform appendix; with special reference to its early diagnosis and treatment. Trans. Assoc. Am. Physicians, 1:107, 1886.

33. Fleming, A.: Penicillin. In Nobel Lectures, Physiology-Medicine. Vol. 3, 1942–1962. New York, American Elsevier Publishing Company, 1964, pp. 77–95.

34. Flexner, J. T.: Doctors on Horseback. New York, Dover Publications, 1969.

35. Fulton, J. F.: Harvey Cushing: A Biography. Springfield, Ill., Charles C Thomas, 1946.

36. Garrett, H. E., Dennis, E. W., and DeBakey, M. E.: Aortocoronary bypass with saphenous vein graft. Seven-year follow-up. J.A.M.A., 223:792, 1973.

37. Garrison, F. H.: History of Medicine, 4th ed. Philadelphia, W. B. Saunders Company, 1960.

38. Gelfand, T.: Empiricism and eighteenth century French surgery. Bull. Hist. Med., 44:40, 1970.

39. Gibbon, J. H.: Development of the artificial heart and lung extracorporeal blood circuit. J.A.M.A., 206:1983, 1968.

40. Godlee, R. J.: Lord Lister. London, Macmillan & Company, 1917.

41. Goss, C. M.: A Brief Account of Henry Gray, F.R.S., and his Anatomy, Descriptive and Surgical. Philadelphia, Lea & Febiger, 1959.

42. Graham, H.: The Story of Surgery. New York, Doubleday & Company, 1939.

43. Gross, S. D.: A century of American medicine, 1776–1876. II. Surgery. Am. J. Med. Sci., 71:431, 1876.

44. Halsted, W. S.: The training of the surgeon. Bull. Johns Hopkins Hosp., 15:267, 1904.

45. Harbison, S. P.: Origins of vascular surgery: The Carrel-Guthrie letters. Surgery, 52:406, 1962.

46. Harrison, R. G.: Observations on the living developing nerve fiber. Anat. Rec., 1:116, 1907.

47. Harrison, R. G.: On the status and significance of tissue culture. Arch. Exp. Zellforsch., 6:4, 1928.

48. Harvey, S. C.: The history of hemostasis. Ann. Med. Hist., 1:127, 1929.

49. Henderson, L. J.: Blood; A Study in General Physiology. New Haven, Yale University Press, 1928.

50. Heuer, G. W.: Dr. Halsted. Bull. Johns Hopkins Hosp. (Suppl.), 90:1, 1952.

51. Janssens, P. A.: Palaeopathology; Diseases and Injuries of Prehistoric Man. London, John Baker Publishers, 1970.

52. Johnson, S. L.: The History of Cardiac Surgery 1896–1955. Baltimore, The Johns Hopkins Press, 1970.

53. Jones, J.: Notes upon the history of hospital gangrene. Southern Med. Surg. J., 1:55, 1866–67.

54. Keys, T. E.: The History of Surgical Anesthesia. New York, Dover Publications, 1963.

55. Kobler, J.: The Reluctant Surgeon. A Biography of John Hunter. Garden City, Doubleday & Company, 1960.

56. Koch, R.: Investigations into the Etiology of Traumatic Infective Diseases. Trans. W. W. Cheyne. London, New Sydenham Society, 1880.

57. Kocher, E. T.: Concerning pathological manifestations in low-grade thyroid diseases. In Nobel Lectures, Physiology-Medicine. Vol. 1, 1901–1921. New York, American Elsevier Publishing Company, 1967, pp. 327–386.

58. Leonard, A. S.: Reflections of the Retiring Chief, Minneapolis, University of Minnesota Press, 1967.

59. Malgaigne, J. F.: Surgery and Ambroise Paré. Trans. W. B. Hamby. Norman, University of Oklahoma Press, 1965.

60. Martin, F. H.: Fifty Years of Medicine and Surgery, An Autobiographical sketch. Chicago, The Surgical Publishing Company, 1934.

61. Matas, R.: Surgical operations fifty years ago. Am. J. Surg., 82:111, 1951.

62. McBurney, C.: Experience with early operative interference in cases of disease of the vermiform appendix. N. Y. Med. J., 50:676, 1889.

63. McBurney, C.: The incision made in the abdominal wall in cases of appendicitis, with a description of a new method of operating. Ann. Surg., 20:38, 1894.

64. Meade, R. H.: A History of Thoracic Surgery. Springfield, Ill., Charles C Thomas, 1960.

65. Moore, F. D.: Metabolic Care of the Surgical Patient. Philadelphia, W. B. Saunders Company, 1959.

66. Moore, F. D., and Ball, M. R.: Metabolic Response to Surgery. Springfield, Ill., Charles C Thomas, 1952.

67. Ochsner, A., and Wangensteen, O.: Editorial announcement. Surgery, 1:4, 1937.

68. Olmsted, J. M. D., and Olmsted, E. H.: Claude Bernard and The Experimental Method. New York, Henry Schuman Publishers, 1952.

69. O'Malley, C. D.: Andreas Vesalius of Brussels 1514–1564. Berkeley, University of California Press, 1965.

70. Pagel, W., and Rattansi, P.: Vesalius and Paracelsus. Med. Hist., 8:309, 1964.

71. Paré, A.: The Apologie and Treatise of Ambroise Paré. G. Keynes (Ed.). New York, Dover Publications, 1968.

72. Poland, J.: A Retrospect of Surgery During the Past Century. London, Smith, Elder, 1901.

73. Price, D. J. D.: Science Since Babylon. New Haven, Yale University Press, 1961.

74. Richardson, R. G.: The Scalpel and the Heart. New York, Charles Scribner's Sons, 1970.

75. Sabiston, D. C., Jr.: A continuum in surgical education. Surgery, 66:1, 1969.

76. Schecter, D. C.: Role of the confraternity of St. Cosmas in the evolution of French Surgery. Surgery, 64:1002, 1968.

77. Schultz, A. H.: Notes on diseases and healed fractures of wild apes and their bearing on the antiquity of pathological conditions in man. Bull. Hist. Med., 7:571, 1939.

78. Sigerist, H. E.: A History of Medicine. Volume 1. Primitive and Archaic Medicine. New York, Oxford University Press, 1951.

79. Smith, S.: The comparative results of operations in Bellevue Hospital. Med. Rec., 28:427, 1885.

80. Stevenson, L. G.: The stag of Richmond Park: A note on John Hunter's most famous animal experiment. Bull. Hist. Med., *22*:467, 1948.
81. Talbot, C. H.: Medicine in Medieval England. New York, American Elsevier Publishing Company, 1967.
82. Temkin, O.: The role of surgery in the rise of modern medical thought. Bull. Hist. Med., *25*:248, 1951.
83. Vicary, T.: The English-Man's Treasure. With the True Anatomie of Man's Body. London, 1633.
84. Wangensteen, O.: Reflections on the Blalock Papers. Bull. Hist. Med., *42*:357, 1968.
85. Wangensteen, O. H., Smith, J., and Wangensteen, S. D.: Some highlights in the history of amputation reflecting lessons in wound healing. Bull. Hist. Med., *41*:97, 1967.
86. Warren, J. M.: Recent Progress in Surgery. Boston, Clapp, 1864.
87. Watts, S. H.: The suture of blood vessels. Implantation and transplantation of vessels and organs. An historical and experimental study. Bull. Johns Hopkins Hosp., *18*:153, 1907.
88. Wells, T. S.: Some causes of excessive mortality after surgical operations. Br. Med. J., *2*:384, 1864.
89. Woodruff, M. F. A.: The Transplantation of Tissues and Organs. Springfield, Ill., Charles C Thomas, 1960.
90. Zimmerman, L. M., and Veith, I.: Great Ideas in the History of Surgery. Baltimore, Williams & Wilkins, 1961.
91. Zimmerman, L. M., and Veith, I.: Billroth's troubles with listerian antisepsis. Mod. Med., March 10, 1969, pp. 213–215.

2

HOMEOSTASIS: BODILY CHANGES IN TRAUMA AND SURGERY

The Responses to Injury in Man as the Basis for Clinical Management

Francis D. Moore, M.D.

I. INTRODUCTION: THE JOINING OF TWO STREAMS OF KNOWLEDGE

Our current awareness of an integral endocrine and metabolic response to injury may be traced to two streams of thought, which are now confluent in a single river of knowledge and practice.

One of these streams is based on the biologic adaptation of the species to conditions of external stress (such as injury and starvation) through the survival of the fittest. This provides an understanding of mammalian survival mechanisms: biochemical, nutritional, and endocrine. These have evolved by the process of natural selection acting on favorable mutants, through the struggle for existence. This is the Darwinian stream.

The second stream of knowledge is that of constancy in the internal environment after its distortion by external stresses. This is an understanding of the *milieu intérieur* of Bernard and its autoregulation toward normal after disorders that threaten life acutely: the *homeostasis* of Cannon. The former term was coined by Bernard to signify the composition of body fluids that constitute the environment of all body cells. The latter term was invented by Cannon to indicate the totality of physiologic responses that return the internal environment to a normal steady state after an acute challenge such as injury.

In the past 30 years these two streams of thought have joined. Metabolic adaptations to injury and starvation (such as the mobilization of amino acids for gluconeogenesis) go far beyond any information that Darwin had on the adjustment of the higher vertebrates to the survival hazards of their environment. Likewise, the Bernard-Cannon concept of homeostasis in the milieu intérieur has been decorated by a whole variety of mechanisms beyond the chemistry or physiology of adrenal medullary stimulation with which these pioneers were familiar.

The joining of these two streams of knowledge is nowhere better epitomized than by the demonstration that simple blood loss, isotonic volume reduction, is a challenge that elicits many mechanisms of both types: metabolic adaptations and acute autoregulatory homeostatic responses. After a brisk hemorrhage there is an increased secretion of epinephrine and norepinephrine, arising in the adrenal medulla and in nerve synapses. Among other actions, epinephrine inhibits the production of insulin, while it stimulates glycogenolysis and the hydrolysis of depot fat to free fatty acids. This insulin inhibition favors the release of amino acids from muscle, some of which pass through a 3-carbon step to glucose, other components appearing as increased nitrogen excretion in the urine. At the same time, there is a decreased perfusion of the juxtaglomerular apparatus of the kidney, which stimulates the production of renin, angiotensin, and aldosterone, supporting the blood pressure and conserving sodium, and with it the interstitial fluid and plasma volume. A mild stimulus to the pituitary, this produces an increase in blood glucocorticoids that has a permissive action for the intensification of the foregoing changes. This particular example of the response to a brisk hemorrhage merely demonstrates the integrated response to one challenge met by every patient who is injured or operated upon.

There follow a few biographic notes on some of the scientists who established the basis for our understanding of survival responses in surgical patients.

Charles Darwin (1809–1882), an English biologist, was 22 years of age when he shipped as a junior scientist-observer on the geographic explorations of the "Beagle." Coasting southward along the South American littoral, then through the Straits of Magel-

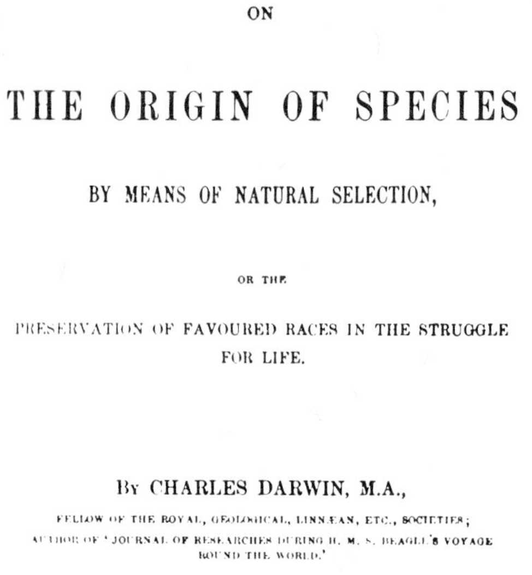

ON

THE ORIGIN OF SPECIES

BY MEANS OF NATURAL SELECTION,

OR THE

PRESERVATION OF FAVOURED RACES IN THE STRUGGLE
FOR LIFE.

By CHARLES DARWIN, M.A.,

FELLOW OF THE ROYAL, GEOLOGICAL, LINNÆAN, ETC., SOCIETIES;
AUTHOR OF 'JOURNAL OF RESEARCHES DURING H. M. S. BEAGLE'S VOYAGE
ROUND THE WORLD.'

LONDON:
JOHN MURRAY, ALBEMARLE STREET.
1859.

Figure 1. Title sheet of Darwin's book in which he first set forth a new concept: that animals have inheritable body features, varying between members of the same species, some of which have superior survival value in the struggle for existence. The transmission of these features by heredity produced a constant improvement and finally led to differentiation of species that Darwin likened to the improvement of domestic animals through a selection process imposed by their breeders. He conceived of the struggle for existence largely in terms of competition for a limited food supply or by the process of sexual selection. Writing in 1859, about the time of Claude Bernard, Darwin did not think in terms of physiologic mechanisms, although he perceived that such variations would also have survival value. Much of surgical physiology, metabolism, endocrinology, and wound healing represents the expression, in man, of inheritable responses with survival value, of the type first described in *The Origin of Species.*

lan to the Galápagos Islands, he observed living forms with great care. He later stated that his greatest insight came in the Galápagos Islands, where he perceived that the tremendous variety of living forms might have a unifying basis in a process for the origin of species that we now call "evolution." He conceived of the process of natural selection as acting on minor variants through the struggle for existence and the survival of the fittest individuals. Although the term "gene" had not yet been coined, he clearly understood that what we would now call an isolated gene pool (i.e., an interbreeding subspecies sharing the same nucleic acid configurations) was essential to this process and would most likely be observed on islands.

Such isolated species would achieve adaptation to a newer challenging environment by the survival and reproduction of those members of the group in whom mutations — many of them very minor — favored survival. Isolation, in turn, was essential so that the genetic configurations achieved by the new interbreeding and stressed mutants would not continuously be diluted back to the ancestral type through contact with a larger unchallenged stem population.

Although Darwin himself never studied survival mechanisms following physical injury, hemorrhage, starvation, burns, or cold, it is evident that the evolution of strong protective mechanisms against all of these agencies must arise through the operation of environmental challenge on mutant forms over the millennia of evolution. The obvious survival value of many adaptive mechanisms in the surgical patient indicates their significance as the products of evolution in the terms of Darwin: *survival of the fittest in the struggle for existence.*

Claude Bernard (1813–1878), a Frenchman, was the first physiologist. He was an "antivitalist," meaning that he regarded all living processes as due to analyzable chemical reactions, could we but understand the detailed chemistry involved. His major contributions were elucidation of the chemistry of pancreatic enzymatic digestion of foods, the formation of sugars from glycogen substrates in the liver, the carbohydrate changes in diabetes, and the delineation of vasoconstrictor and vasodilator nerves by experimental nerve section and electrical stimulation. In his *Introduction to the Study of Experimental Medicine,* Bernard described the basic methods needed to elucidate natural phenomena in precise scientific terms. His methods laid the foundation for the work of a whole generation of physiologists, including Walter Cannon. An interesting critique of Bernard's work will be found in Henderson's book on *Blood.* Claude Bernard first used the term *milieu intérieur* to mean the chemical composition of the body, and clearly perceived that its constancy was one of the remarkable features of animal life.

Walter Cannon (1871–1945) was an American physiologist, born in Wisconsin, who did most of his work at the Harvard Medical School. He is best known for his detailed study of the autonomic nervous system, evolving the concept of a sympathetic and parasympathetic system, one devoted to the circulation, and the other to vegetative functions. He worked in many other fields of physiology and medicine as well. He invented the term *homeostasis* for the tendency of the organism to maintain constancy of the internal environment but more especially to include the autoregulatory adjustments that maintain this constancy.

Lawrence J. Henderson (1878–1942) was Professor of Biological Chemistry at Harvard during the years just before, during, and after World War I. Working with A. V. Bock and D. B. Dill, he established precise chemical investigation of man as a scientific method. He was truly the first clinical investigator. He studied man himself by the methods that Bernard had thought of as applicable largely to animals: controlled clinical experiment. Henderson's major work was on blood, and his book of that name remains a classic. In

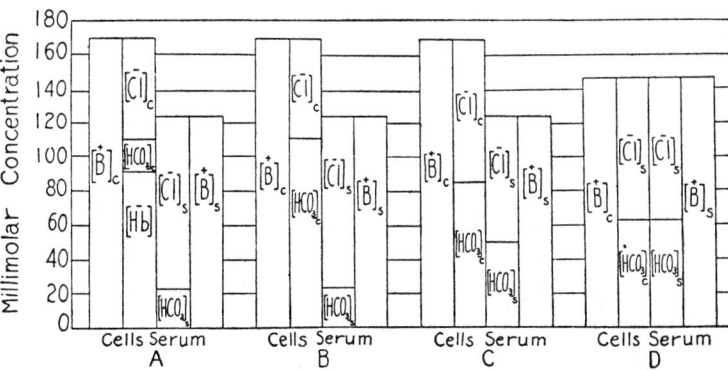

Figure 2. Illustration from Lawrence Henderson's book, *Blood*, published in 1928. Henderson was known as a mathematician and as a superb planner of experimental design. Most of the actual work was performed by Bock and Dill. This was the first clinical investigation in normal subjects designed to cast light on the compensations in blood to the stresses of exercise and acidosis. Here are shown changes in ionic equilibrium between cells and serum. Bar graphs of this type relating to millimolar concentrations were later used extensively by Gamble in his book, *The Chemical Anatomy of the Extracellular Fluid*.

performing these studies, he sampled his own blood and that of co-workers under conditions of rest and exercise and applied to this blood the precise quantitative analyses that were becoming available at that time.

The present era is notable for the broad concern of many scientists about social ills. Both Cannon and

BODILY CHANGES IN PAIN, HUNGER, FEAR AND RAGE

AN ACCOUNT OF RECENT RESEARCHES INTO THE FUNCTION OF EMOTIONAL EXCITEMENT

BY

WALTER B. CANNON

GEORGE HIGGINSON PROFESSOR OF PHYSIOLOGY IN HARVARD UNIVERSITY

NEW YORK AND LONDON
D. APPLETON AND COMPANY
1915

Figure 3. Title sheet of Walter Cannon's book, *Bodily Changes in Pain, Hunger, Fear and Rage*. This book was a review of work done by Cannon over a number of years, describing autonomic reactions to physical and emotional stresses, making use of the isolated cat heart as a built-in bioassay for blood catecholamines. Cannon, like Benedict and Henderson, was looking at complex physiologic adaptations to stress, adaptations that have survival value in Darwinian terms and that provide the basis for the patient's response to injury and surgery.

Henderson, 50 years ago, were similarly concerned. Cannon became involved in social change and hoped that some of the wisdom of the body might be manifested in social organisms. In his later years, Henderson became a Professor of Sociology, with a particular interest in economic theory.

The contributions of the *chemists* after World War I were vitally essential to the foundations of clinical investigation, and Henderson and Cannon acknowledged their debt to these men, including *Donald D. Van Slyke,* who worked with Henderson and later at the Rockefeller Institute, and *John Peters*, who worked with Van Slyke and later was Professor of Medicine at Yale. Peters and Van Slyke together published an epoch-making two-volume work entitled *Quantitative Clinical Chemistry* in 1935. These volumes were the laboratory bible for all hospital and research laboratories until the most modern era of flame photometry and isotope quantification. *Otto Folin*, Professor of Biological Chemistry at Harvard after Henderson, was also a pioneer in developing quantitative clinical methods. *James L. Gamble* was particularly interested in the biochemistry of the extracellular fluid. His small monograph on *The Anatomy of the Extracellular Fluid*, published in 1938, had almost as much impact as the Peters-Van Slyke volumes because it assumed their methods and built a precise interpretive framework still used in the daily care of the sick.

Francis G. Benedict (1870–1957) was a nutritionist at the Carnegie Institute and Carnegie Laboratories, and later at the Harvard Medical School. He was one of the first to study what would now be called "metabolism"; he measured the basal metabolic rate and invented an apparatus for so doing. Most important, he described prolonged starvation in a volunteer human subject in a book (published in 1915) that is so strikingly modern that its charts are still being replotted, reinterpreted, and published anew over 60 years later.

Harvey Cushing (1869–1939), renowned in surgery for his work in cerebrospinal fluid physiology and brain tumors, was also America's first great endocrinologist. His book on the pituitary gland, published in 1912, described syndromes, pictured pathologic characteristics, and elucidated relationships between the pituitary and the target glands. His description of the syndrome that bears his name was based on studies on patients he had seen at the Johns Hopkins during the period 1905 to 1912, and was later to provide one of the early insights into the pathophysiology of injury itself. He influenced several generations of neurosurgeons by his personal example of excellence in surgery; physiologists and endocrinologists have spent half a century working out in detail the endocrine mechanisms that he described in broad clinical outline.

David Cuthbertson (b. 1900) is a Scots nutritionist. Working in an agricultural laboratory, he first described, in accurate biochemical terms, the negative nitrogen balance that follows injury. This work was published in 1930, and was based on the study of fractures in rats. Prior workers had described similar changes in infection and typhoid fever; Cuthbertson related them to trauma. The balance between catabolism and anabolism after injury has occupied surgical investigators ever since that time. It remains a sort of barometer as to whether the patient is still undergo-

ing tissue lysis as a response to injury or has commenced to anabolize *en route* to the completion of convalescence. While this field of work has gradually enlarged to include study of hormone interrelationships and body fuel utilization, Cuthbertson's contribution remains basic, and he himself continues active investigation.

Fuller Albright (1900–1970) was a clinical investigator who traced his own work directly back to that of Bernard, Henderson, and Cannon. Before his work was cut short by Parkinson's disease, and in the short space of his active career in internal medicine (about 15 years), Albright perceived many features of surgical metabolism. Among the most important was his observation that prolonged illness and tissue injury appeared to resemble prolonged stimulation of the adrenal cortex, as seen in Cushing's syndrome, a

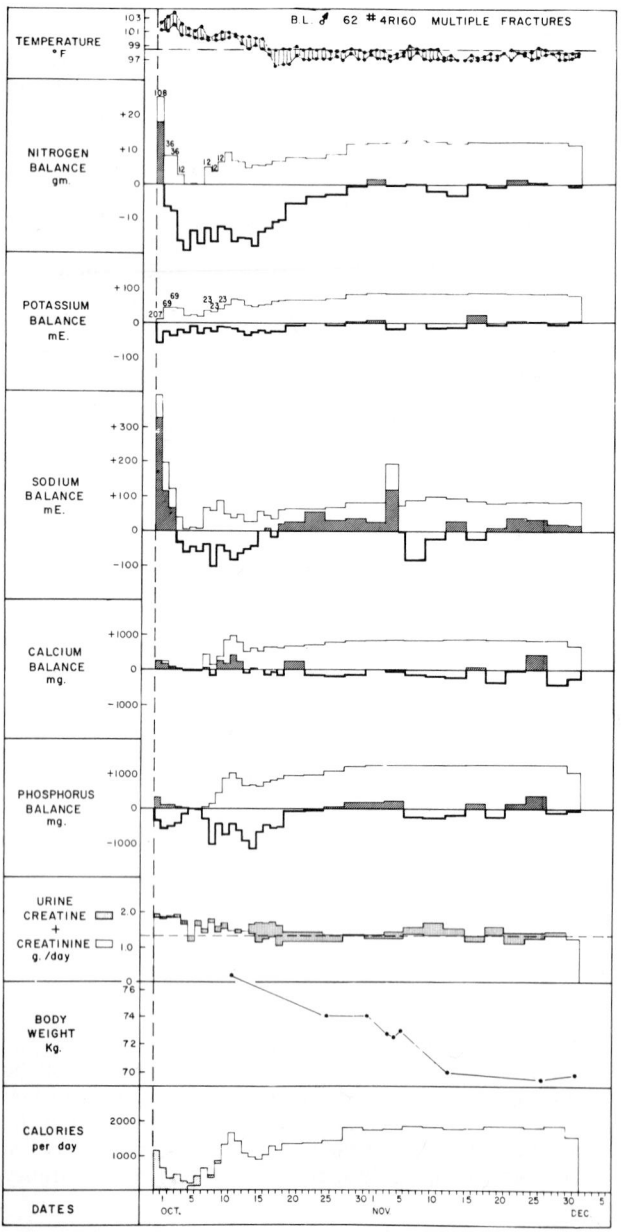

Figure 4. Patient B.L.—Multiple fractures. Here is shown a surgical metabolic chart of the type commonly employed to demonstrate the intake and output of certain elements as shown on the vertical coordinate. The overall metabolic balance of an element tells of the daily flux but does not indicate details of intermediary metabolism. Since body nitrogen exists almost wholly as protein, the nitrogen balance is in most circumstances a linear function of net protein degradation or synthesis.

Intake is measured upward from the baseline, and *output* is measured downward from the top of the intake line. If the patient eats more than he excretes, the balance is positive and is shown as a shaded area above the zero line. If he loses more than he takes in, the balance is negative, and is shown by a heavily enclosed or white area below the zero line. Because hundreds of metabolic measurements have been made in surgical patients, many charts can now be reduced to "typical" or "theoretical" reconstructions as shown in Figures 6, 21, and 22.

Here are shown actual data from a patient recently studied after an automobile accident, demonstrating the daily variability and some of the fascinating problems in interpretation. This patient lost about 17 pounds in his acute catabolism. The loss of nitrogen was extremely brisk, running as high as 20 gm. per day even with modest caloric supply during the first week. Sodium balance was strongly positive during the period of wound edema and aldosterone increase. Urinary creatinine shows an early increase, suggesting that muscle is the source of most of the nitrogen. Calcium balance departs inconsequentially from zero, and there is marked calcium economy during an early period of zero intake. The phosphorus balance parallels the nitrogen balance, suggesting that most of the urinary phosphorus comes from soft tissue rather than bone.

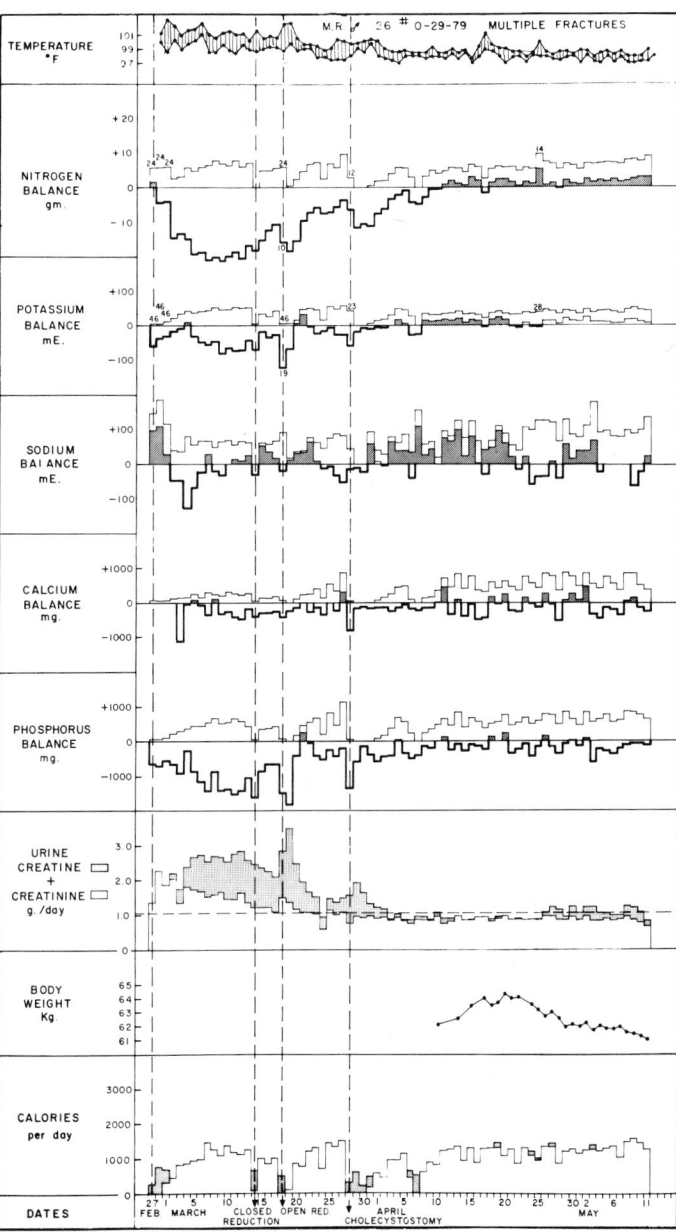

Figure 5. Metabolic balance chart from a patient with multiple fractures. Many features are rather similar to those shown in Figure 4, although potassium losses were more marked here, as were calcium losses. Again, the loss of phosphorus correlates much more closely with that of nitrogen than with that of calcium, and the urinary creatine shows the remarkable phenomenon of large increases in excretion during the first 2 weeks, and then a return to an almost zero value, normal for the adult male. Creatinine is also increased at this time, the sum of the two indicating in an approximate way the mass of muscle protoplasm undergoing lysis during catabolism.

It is interesting that open reduction and cholecystostomy both were followed by an increased tendency to catabolism even on a second and third stress in a previously healty and vigorous young man. In older persons, repeated injuries do not usually summon an additional catabolism of significance, the changes being merely those of starvation. The secondary increases in excretion of creatine, phosphorus, nitrogen, and potassium all suggest that this young man (despite the brisk catabolic loss of the principal injury) was still capable of mobilizing additional soft tissue in response to his later operations.

theory Albright elaborated in his Harvey Lecture in 1943. This lecture of Albright's influenced many persons, and his methods of metabolic balance study represented an advance over those used by prior workers. Both of these inspired the author of this chapter while he was an intern and resident in surgery. Our own work in this field began about that time, using metabolic methods to describe the phenomena of electrolyte and nitrogen balance in surgical patients. To this we added endocrine concepts borrowed from Albright's work, and the application of radioactive and stable isotopes to elaborate the body compositional changes in the surgical patient. For this biophysical component of our work, we owe a particular debt to *Joseph C. Aub,* who was himself a contemporary and collaborator of Albright and a pioneer in the application of radioactive isotopes to human metabolism.

Hans Selye (b. 1907), a French-Canadian experimental biologist working in Montreal, attempted to form a unified theory of "stress" by which, through a variety of endocrine mechanisms, all of the stresses of life were thought to produce a variety of disease processes, especially arthritis, chronic vascular disease, and hypertension. He popularized the term "alarm reaction," published a journal called *Stress,* and included tissue injury in this concept. Some of the confusion that surrounds the term "shock" relates to Selye's terminology in the "alarm reaction," in which the first injury is referred to as "shock" and the response thereto as "counter-shock," even though no reduction in tissue perfusion or blood flow, in the true sense of surgical shock, is involved.

George W. Thorn (b. 1904), Hersey Professor of Medicine at Harvard during the years 1941 to 1972, occupied about 20 years of his active scientific career with de-

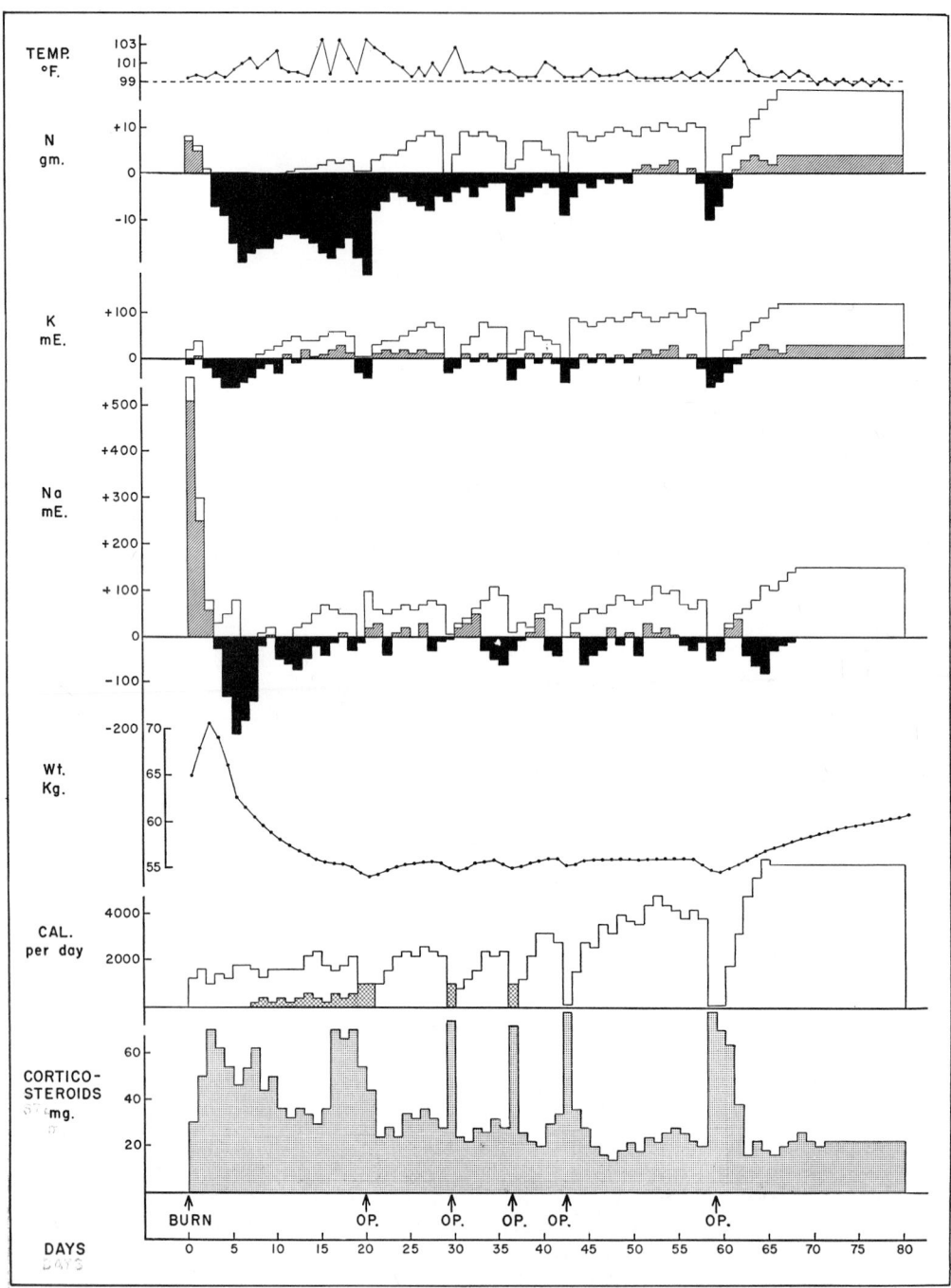

Figure 6. Metabolism after burn. Here, in a "theoretical" or "typical" chart the metabolic findings in burn patients have been gathered and typified. There are many differences from the changes seen in Figures 4 and 5. The negative balance of nitrogen (shown here in black rather than a dark enclosed line) proceeds with few interruptions for almost 2 months until the wound starts to close completely. The initial positive balance of sodium is of spectacular extent and far exceeds that seen in a fracture. It is associated with weight gain during the period of early fluid therapy, such fluid therapy being essential to maintain the circulation while at the same time satisfying the demand of the burn edema, thus producing a positive sodium balance and gain in weight. Caloric intake is here shown as being maintained quite well for a burned patient. Urinary steroid excretion is high throughout and shows repeated peaks with multiple grafting operations. This long-continued adrenal stimulation produces the adrenal hyperplasia so commonly seen in burn patients at autopsy, and is likewise associated, in some cases, with acid-peptic ulceration.

These metabolic charts (Figures 4, 5, and 6) show but one aspect of endocrine and biochemical survival responses of the injured human patient—modified by the conditions of care itself, by the administration of drugs, anesthetics, and transfusions, and by infection.

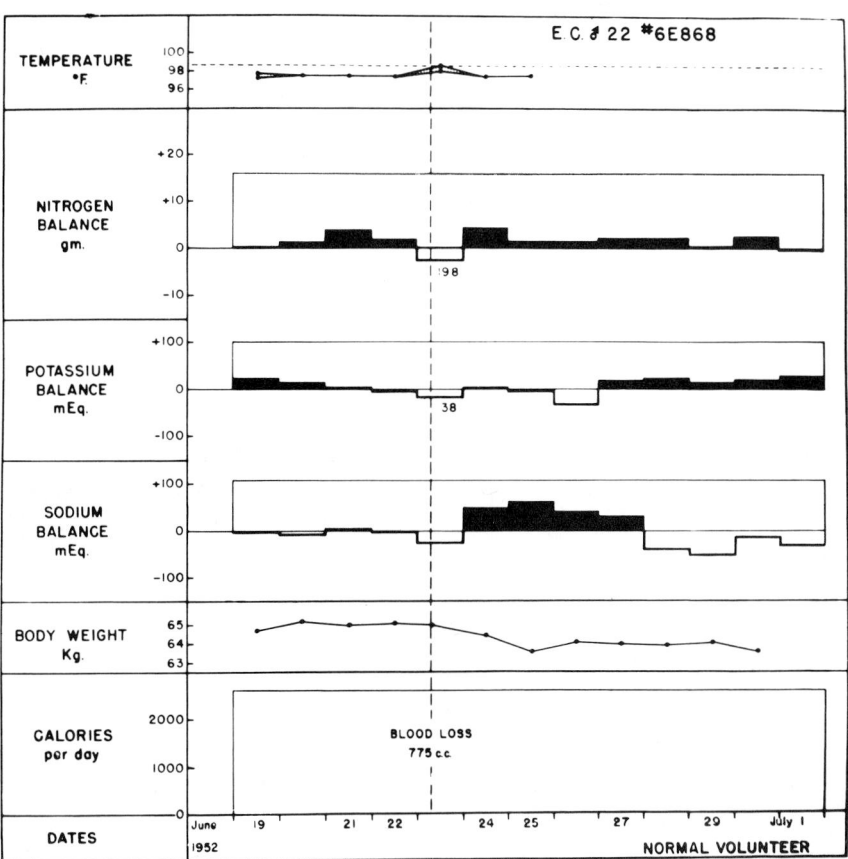

Figure 7. Balance studies after hemorrhage in a normal, young, male volunteer. This study was of historic interest from the point of view of our laboratories. Done in 1952, prior to the isolation or description of aldosterone, it demonstrates a strongly positive sodium balance and a weakly but statistically significant negative potassium balance, after hemorrhage alone. This is an example of a gross external change in ion flux in response to isotonic volume reduction due, at least in part, to alterations in endocrine activity. This is an adaptation in man, the main thrust of which is the maintenance intact of extracellular fluid volume to support the transcapillary refilling of the plasma volume and thus the maintenance of the circulation after bleeding.

tailed studies on the activation of the adrenal cortex. In this interest he was joined by a generation of investigators including such persons as *Edward Kendall* of the Mayo Clinic, who isolated cortisol (leading to its synthesis), and a number of surgical and physiologic researchers of the pituitary-ACTH-adrenal cortical axis. Among these workers were *David Hume* of Boston and Richmond, *Francis Ganong* of Boston and San Francisco, and *Richard Egdahl* of Minneapolis and Boston. The work of these men joined to elucidate the pathway by which physical injury, such as a burn, fracture, or surgical incision, communicates a message via the nervous system to the basal ganglia of the brain, and thence to the pituitary gland, finally stimulating the adrenal cortex to produce a variety of corticosteroid hormones. Thorn should be credited with the first clinical investigations that provided quantitative measures of adrenal function, particularly through his early use of ACTH testing, the study of the eosinophil, and blood steroid measurements.

John Kinney of Boston and New York was among the first to recognize the fundamental problems of energetics in trauma: the changeover in energy source from exogenous diet to endogenous fat oxidation, the partition of energy expenditure, and the partition of energy source among the components of weight loss after injury. Dr. Kinney devised a continuous gas-flow method for studying energy exchange even in critically ill surgical patients, which has been widely used in similar studies at other universities.

Starting at the time of World War II, many of these surgical laboratories, including ours, became involved with quantitative studies of the systemic changes following injury and surgery. References to this recent and sometimes current work will be found in the bibliography. From this work have emerged two basic messages for the surgeons: first, that his patient is exhibiting a biologic response to physical injury which is deeply ingrained in the species, and valuable to survival, healing, and ultimate return to social usefulness; and, second, that the practical daily steps devoted to the care of that patient can be most effective if they are carried out with a full understanding of the patient's own bodily changes.

It is the purpose of this chapter to review briefly the homeostatic and adaptive responses of the patient to injury, and then to identify as nearly as we can the contributions to that response of specific stimuli such as the wound, volume reduction, low flow states, starvation, and infection. Activating endocrine mediators that translate the message of peripheral injury into systemic and visceral changes will be described. Discussion of the phases of convalescence through which the surgical patient normally passes will close the chapter.

The Contents of this chapter are arranged as follows:
    I. Introduction
   II. Acute Injury: Changes in Biochemistry, Metabolism, and Visceral Function
  III. Acute Injury: Endocrine Changes

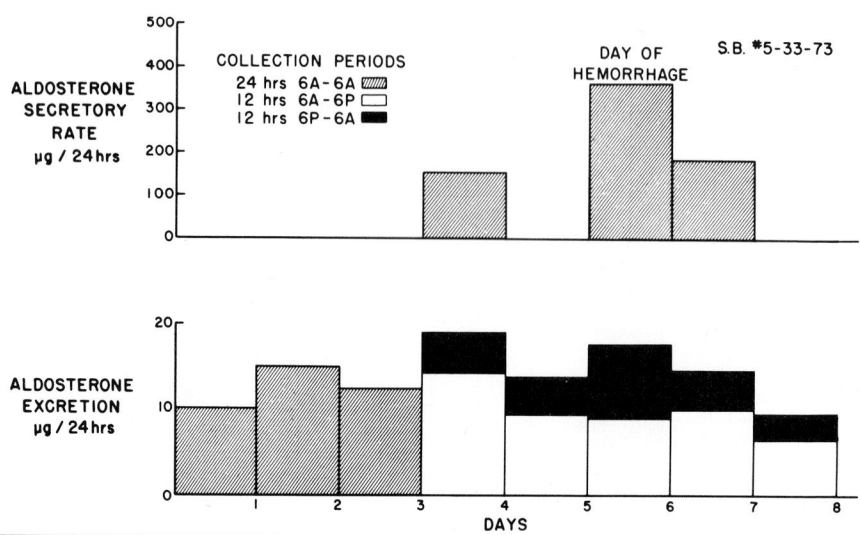

Figure 8. These data represent 20 years of advance in study of human adaptive responses to hemorrhage as they bear on maintenance of interstitial fluid volume; to be contrasted with Figure 7.

Here are shown data on the aldosterone secretory rate based on a double isotope dilution technique, and, below, the gross aldosterone excretion in the urine of a normal, healthy, male volunteer bled on the day shown. The increase in aldosterone secretory rate is highly significant. Total urinary aldosterone excretion is not grossly increased, but that component excreted at night, following the hemorrhage, is increased. This increase in aldosterone activity produced by isotonic volume reduction is responsible for restricted excretion of sodium bicarbonate, an acid urine containing increased amounts of potassium, a strong tendency toward the buildup of positive sodium balances, and the maintenance intact of interstitial fluid volume for plasma volume refilling. This example is used in this chapter to typify the complex integrative activity of the neural-endocrine-compositional system in response to a single component of surgical injury, in this case hemorrhage. Not shown in this chart are data likewise reported by Skillman et al. from our laboratories, showing that renin and angiotensin are appropriately elevated following this challenge.

The type of injury to be considered here consists of major trauma *without* a low flow state or "shock." We are examining the effects of an injury of the type associated with military or civilian trauma (fractures, burns), or major operations involving widespread dissection or visceral removal. Although changes in distribution of blood flow and some degree of volume reduction are universal in patients with such injuries, we are not here considering the effects of prolonged hypoperfusion of tissues or low flow states *per se*. The contributions of flow deficiency to the metabolism of trauma are considered later as a specific variant superimposing severe tissue hypoxia on the normal response to the injury itself.

The compositional metabolism of acute injury may be considered under four headings: (1) loss of body cell mass, (2) conservation of extracellular fluid, (3) change in energy source, and (4) alterations in neutrality regulation.

II. ACUTE INJURY: CHANGES IN BIOCHEMISTRY, METABOLISM, AND VISCERAL FUNCTION*

1. Loss of Body Cell Mass

The basic transaction between the body cell mass and the extracellular fluid after injury is the lysis of cellular protoplasm and conservation of extracellular fluid volume. The products of this cellular lysis are released into the extracellular fluid, some compounds are converted to glucose and burned through the carbohydrate-oxidative pathway, and most of the nitrogen is excreted in the urine as urea. The tissue most prominently involved is skeletal muscle; this is demonstrated by the increased amount of creatine and creatinine in blood and urine, and by the evident rapid decrease in the bulk of palpable muscles. Transient immobiliza-

*Background reading on biochemical, metabolic, and visceral changes will be found in the Bibliography, references 10, 11, 14, 20, 21, 24, 25, 41, 43, 45, and 46.

TABLE 1. Normal Adult Body Composition (Age 40)

	Male 70 kg.		Female 60 kg.	
	Absolute	*Relative*	*Absolute*	*Relative*
A. Intravascular Phase				
Hematocrit (LVH)	0.43		0.40	
Plasma volume (PV)	3150 ml.	4.5% b.wt.	2630 ml.	4.4% b.wt.
Red cell volume (RV)	1930 ml.	2.8% b.wt.	1400 ml.	2.3% b.wt.
Blood volume (BV)	5080 ml.	7.3% b.wt.	4030 ml.	6.7% b.wt.
RV/BV (WBH)	0.38		0.35	
WBH/LVH	0.87		0.87	
PV/IF	0.22		0.23	
B. Body Water and Extracellular Phase				
Total body water (TBW)	39.4 l.	56.3% b.wt.	29.5 l.	49.2% b.wt.
Extracellular water (ECW)	17.3 l.	24.7% b.wt.	14.0 l.	23.3% b.wt.
Interstitial water (IF)	14.3 l.	20.4% b.wt.	11.4 l.	19.0% b.wt.
Total exchangeable sodium (Na_e)	2980 mEq.	42.6 mEq./kg.	2360 mEq.	39.3 mEq./kg.
C. Intracellular Phase				
Intracellular water (ICW)	22.1 l.	31.6% b.wt.	15.5 l.	25.8% b.wt.
Total exchangeable potassium (K_e)	3380 mEq.	48.3 mEq./kg.	2380 mEq.	39.7 mEq./kg.
Average intracellular potassium concentration	150 mEq./l.		150 mEq./l.	
ICW/TBW	0.56		0.52	
D. Derived Values				
Total body solids (TBS)	30.6 kg.	43.7% b.wt.	30.5 kg.	50.8% b.wt.
Total body fat (TBF)	16.2 kg.	23.1% b.wt.	19.7 kg.	32.8% b.wt.
Total body cell mass (BCM)	30.9 kg.	44.1% b.wt.	21.7 kg.	36.2% b.wt.
Estimated skeletal weight	4.5 kg.	6.4% b.wt.	3.4 kg.	5.7% b.wt.

tion and starvation add to this impost on the skeletal muscle mass.

This release of the products of cellular protoplasm to the extracellular fluid (and their subsequent excretion) accounts for several events: the *negative nitrogen balance* (largely as urinary urea), the appearance of *new glucose* from noncarbohydrate sources, the relative *inability of the body to synthesize new muscle protein* immediately after injury, and the *loss of intracellular electrolytes* (particularly potassium, phosphate, and sulfate) into the extracellular fluid and thence to the urine via the kidneys, as well as the *appearance in the urine of increased amounts of xanthines* found in muscle (creatine, creatinine, uric acid).

Normal values for body composition in the resting normal person, together with constants and coefficients for metabolic calculation, are shown in Tables 1 through 4.

There is little evidence that this type of post-traumatic catabolism has much impact on the total cell mass of visceral organs such as brain, heart, lungs, kidneys, gastrointestinal tract, and liver. The fact that muscle recovers completely without any evidence of residual weakness suggests that each muscle cell is maintained intact with its neuromuscular apparatus despite the severity of a draft on its nitrogen and protoplasm that may at times amount to 50 or 60 per cent of the muscle mass (as in very severe injury with infection).

An appreciation of the significance of cellular reaction after injury requires some appreciation of normal basic body composition. Body compositional methods for the measurement of red cell and plasma volume, extracellular fluid volume, total body water, and total body electrolyte have been made available by the widespread use of stable and radioactive isotopes. Though rarely needed in daily bedside care, they have provided a valuable framework for the clinical management of surgical patients.

The normal draft on muscle cells after medium-grade injury in the adult amounts to about 30 gm. of nitrogen, corresponding to about 220 gm. of protein, and approximately 1 kg. of wet lean tissue. This is about 5 per cent of the fat-free body mass. There is a concomitant loss of body fat (see p. 39). There is no evidence from either animals or man that this transient post-traumatic draft on muscle cells and fat has any adverse effect on the healing of wounds or fractures, the formation of albumin or hemoglobin, or the subsequent achievement of anabolism. Within this range of severity the post-traumatic cellular catabolism appears to be a species adaptation analogous, in a sense, to the bodily changes of pregnancy: a new set of metabolic conditions imposed by new demands placed

TABLE 2. Equivalents and Calculations
Constants Useful in Estimating Metabolic Change

---

1. Lean Tissue

     Protein = nitrogen $\times$ 6.25
     Wet lean tissue = nitrogen $\times$ 30
     Wet lean tissue = protein $\times$ 4.75
     Wet cellular tissue = 73% water, 27% protein; whole wet muscle = approx. 79% water, 21% protein.
   Muscle tissue
     Extracellular potassium concentration = 3.8–4.3 mEq./l.
     Intracellular potassium concentration = 148–155 mEq./l.
     Potassium content = 100 mEq./kg. wet weight
     Body cell mass (kg.) estimated as $\left(K_e \text{ (mEq.)} \times \dfrac{9.14}{1000} \right)$

2. Extracellular Fluids and Urine

     Sodium balance $\div$ plasma sodium concentration = change in isotonic extracellular fluid volume
     Hydration of lean tissue = 0.73 (range 0.68–0.82)
     Plasma volume $\div$ interstitial fluid volume = 0.23 (range 0.18–0.27)
     Glomerular filtration rate = 80–120 ml./min.
     Plasma sodium concentration is proportional to $\dfrac{Na_e + K_e}{TBW}$
     Sodium concentration in plasma water = $([Na]_p = 1.1 \times \dfrac{Na_e + K_e}{TBW} - 26)$
     Total body water is proportional to sum of exchangeable cations ($Na_e + K_e$)
     $(Na_e + K_e) = 163\,[TBW] - 70$

3. Energy Sources

     Total body fat = body weight $- \dfrac{(TBW)}{(0.73)}$
      As first approximation — very thin man — 10% fat
                        — normally built man — 20% fat
                        — normally built woman — 30% fat
                        — obese woman — 40% fat
                        — very obese man or woman — 50% fat
   Caloric equivalents
     (gm.) Glucose $\times$ 4 = calories
     (gm.) Triglycerides or neutral fat $\times$ 9 = calories
     (gm.) Protein $\times$ 4 = calories
     (gm.) Alcohol $\times$ 7 = calories
   Respiratory quotient (CO_2/O_2)

Carbohydrate oxidation	1.00
Fat oxidation	0.70
Carbohydrate to fat conversion	>1.00
Mixed diet	0.75–0.85

   Metabolic rate = 1800 cal./day
   Oxygen consumption = 250 ml./min.
   Carbohydrate consumption = 400 cal./day (100 gm.)
   Fat = 1160 cal./day (130 gm.)
   Protein = 240 cal./day (60 gm.)
     Total = 1800 cal./day
   Plasma free fatty acids = 300–600 μEq./l.

---

upon the organism. As will be described in greater detail later, most wounds heal to tensile integrity during the catabolic phase; nitrogen anabolism of the whole body is not required for healing of a local wound; abolition of nitrogen and fat loss during this period by forced feeding has no demonstrable effect upon convalescence. By sharp contrast, *prolonged* post-traumatic starvation has extremely adverse effects upon all aspects of the bodily economy and is most favorably affected by increased intakes by mouth or vein.

2. Conservation of Extracellular Fluid

While the body cell mass is being reduced by lysis of protoplasm, the organism is devoting several active mechanisms to the conservation of extracellular fluid and thus to the maintenance of plasma and blood volume.

The tendency to conserve extracellular fluid after trauma is manifested by a decreased absolute sodium excretion rate, a decreased sodium concentration in the urine, inability to excrete sodium bicarbonate, a tendency toward aciduria, and decreased sodium content of saliva and sweat. There is some evidence that the distal small bowel also participates in this regulation with increased reabsorption of sodium from distal ileum.

There is now good evidence from both man and experimental animals that in the injured vertebrate conservation of the volume of extracellular fluid has a higher biologic priority than the maintenance of its exact chemical composition. These volume-conserving mechanisms consist primarily in the reduction of sodium loss in urine, saliva, and sweat, and a reduction in water loss in all these body fluids, including gas-

TABLE 3. Equivalents and Calculations
Constants Useful in Estimating Blood Volumes

Blood Volume Formulations

Normal blood volume in males	$= \pm 7.0\%$ b.wt.
Normal blood volume in females	$= \pm 6.5\%$ b.wt.
Normal red cell volume in males	$= \pm 3.0\%$ b.wt.
Normal red cell volume in females	$= \pm 2.8\%$ b.wt.
Normal plasma volume in males	$= \pm 4.0\%$ b.wt.
Normal plasma volume in females	$= \pm 3.7\%$ b.wt.

Expression for *plasma volume requirement* with rising hematocrit, plasma loss, but no red cell loss (as in early burns or peritonitis):

$$\text{PV deficit} = BV_1 - \frac{(BV_1 \times LVH_1)}{LVH_2}$$

Where:
PV deficit = plasma volume deficit at time of observation
BV_1 = normal blood volume for that individual
LVH_1 = normal large vessel hematocrit for that individual
LVH_2 = observed large vessel hematocrit at time of study

Expression for *red cell deficit* with low hematocrit and normal blood volume (as in a stabilized posthemorrhagic fully hemodiluted anemia):

$$\text{RV deficit} = RV_1 - (BV_1 \times LVH_2)$$

Where:
RV deficit = red cell deficit at time of observation
RV_1 = starting normal red cell volume for that individual
LVH_2 = observed large vessel hematocrit at time of study

---

trointestinal juice. The significance of sodium conservation after injury lies in the fact that the total osmolality of extracellular fluid (and therefore its total volume) is largely determined by the sodium content. Sodium is the water-holding ion of extracellular fluid. The total exchangeable or "available" sodium determines the volume of the extracellular fluid; the sum of the total exchangeable sodium and potassium of the body together determines, within extremely tight limits, the volume of total body water. Because the interstitial component of the extracellular fluid (i.e., that fraction outside cells and likewise outside the plasma) supports the plasma volume after hemorrhage by transcapillary refilling, the total extracellular sodium and its degree of hydration may be considered as measures of the volume reserves of the body that can be called upon to replace losses by hemorrhage. The sodium area of the body consists of the plasma volume,

TABLE 4. Equivalents and Calculations
Constants Useful in Estimating Respiratory, Pulmonary, and Oxygen Changes

1. Arterial Blood Gases

Variable	Abbreviation	Normal Value
O_2 saturation	S_aO_2	97.0%
O_2 tension	P_aO_2	95 mm.Hg
CO_2 tension	P_aCO_2	40 mm.Hg
pH		7.4
Alveolar-arterial PO_2 diff. (on room air)	A-a DO_2	9 mm.Hg
Alveolar-arterial PCO_2 diff. (on room air)	A-a DCO_2	0
Alveolar-arterial PO_2 diff. (on 100% O_2)	A-a DO_2	35–150 mm.Hg

Note: By usual clinical methods of measurement any arterial oxygen tension of 500 mm.Hg or above can be considered normal for the 100% O_2 test.

2. Pulmonary Circulation

Variable	Abbreviation	Normal Value
Pulmonary artery pressure	PAP	25/8 mm.Hg
Pulmonary capillary blood pressure (wedge)	PCW	7 mm.Hg
Pulmonary capillary blood flow	$\dot{Q}c$	5400 ml./min.
Pulmonary capillary blood volume	Qc	90 ml.
Pulmonary extravascular water volume	PEWV	194 ml. H_2O

3. Oxygen Consumption (males)

Formula: O_2 consumption $= S \times$ body surface area (ml./min.)

1. 0–5% b.wt. as fat	$S = 141.2$
2. 5–10% b.wt. as fat	$S = 139.4$
3. 10–15% b.wt. as fat	$S = 134.9$
4. >15% b.wt. as fat	$S = 130.5$

extracellular fluid in tissue spaces and lymph, special transcellular fluids such as joint fluid and gastrointestinal fluid, and the sodium of the skeleton (slowly available and to only a minor extent for the restoration of sodium losses). This contrasts with the distribution of body potassium, which is almost wholly within body cells, is entirely ionized, and therefore is wholly exchangeable in isotopic equilibrium.

In many post-traumatic states, there is a trade-off or ion pair effect between sodium and either potassium or hydrogen ion. When sodium is retained, potassium and hydrogen ions are lost, or move into cells, and there is a tendency toward extracellular alkalosis. By contrast, when sodium is lost, potassium and hydrogen ions are retained (or move out of the cell), and there is a tendency toward extracellular acidosis and hyperkalemia. The plasma concentrations of sodium and potassium characteristically move in opposite directions and at similar proportional rates.

The administration of large loads of sodium-containing fluids after operation or injury will give the illusion of overcoming a tendency toward sodium conservation because sodium excretion is increased thereby. But retention still occurs, and the ease with which positive sodium balances are achieved after trauma demonstrates that renal salt conservation is still present. Following injury, patients are much more easily swamped with sodium and water loads than they are in the normal state. A dilutional hypoproteinemia with a tendency toward tissue edema, particularly of lungs, brain, and peripheral areas, ensues. This contrasts with the finding in a normal uninjured person who, with a healthy heart, liver, and kidneys, will excrete an administered load of sodium quantitatively.

Retention of the sodium ion in the body tends to maintain the volume of extracellular fluid, as mentioned before. After injury, another fluid-conserving mechanism also comes into play in the form of a sharp restriction in the excretion of free water, or anti-diuresis.

The tendency to conserve body water (antidiuresis) is demonstrated by a rising urine osmolality due to distal tubular water reabsorption. With the urine sodium content markedly reduced, the increased urine osmolality must be due to the presence of other substances at increased concentrations. These are chiefly phosphate, potassium, and urea.

Large water loads given to postoperative patients will increase water excretion and thus (as with the case of sodium) give the superficial appearance to the uncritical observer of overcoming the water-conserving mechanism. Actually, the postoperative or post-traumatic patient is much more apt to retain this water than is the normal patient and will develop a dilutional hyponatremia with much greater ease.

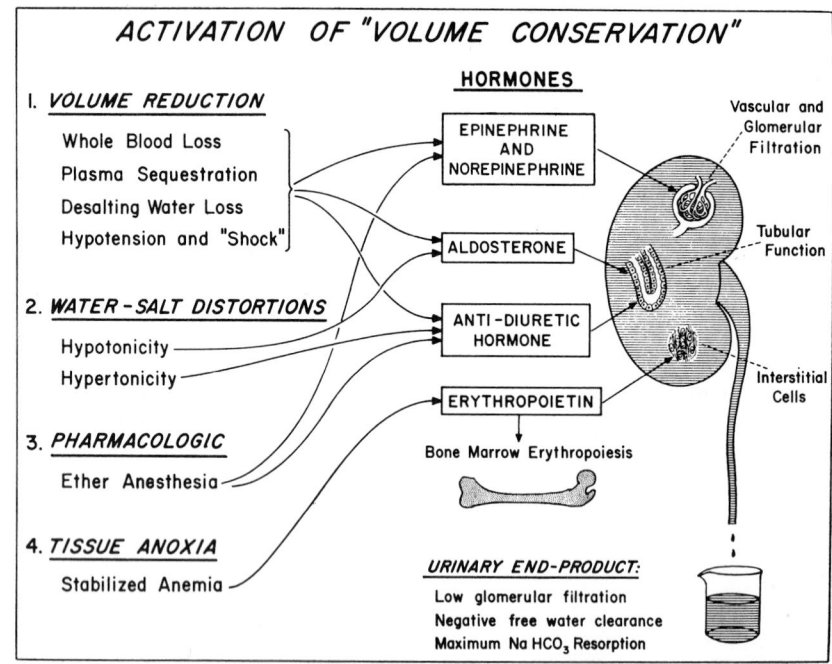

Figure 9. This chart demonstrates some of the activation mechanisms that conserve effective volume of body water, plasma, and interstitial fluid in man. Most of these activations are noted after simple hemorrhage without a low flow state. Others are observed as distortions of water and salt metabolism or after pharmacologic or respiratory stimulus as noted to the left.

Possibly most noteworthy are the effects of the catecholamines. While one may think of the pituitary as the "master gland" of the endocrine system, the catecholamines are the "front-runner" hormones in the response to injury. In addition to these local effects on the kidney their widespread effects on the circulatory system conserve blood flow for critical areas. Moreover, they demonstrate, as described in the text, significant effects on the intermediary metabolism of fat, nitrogen, and carbohydrate. Catecholamine effects—first described by Cannon—are common denominators of the neuroendocrine response to injury.

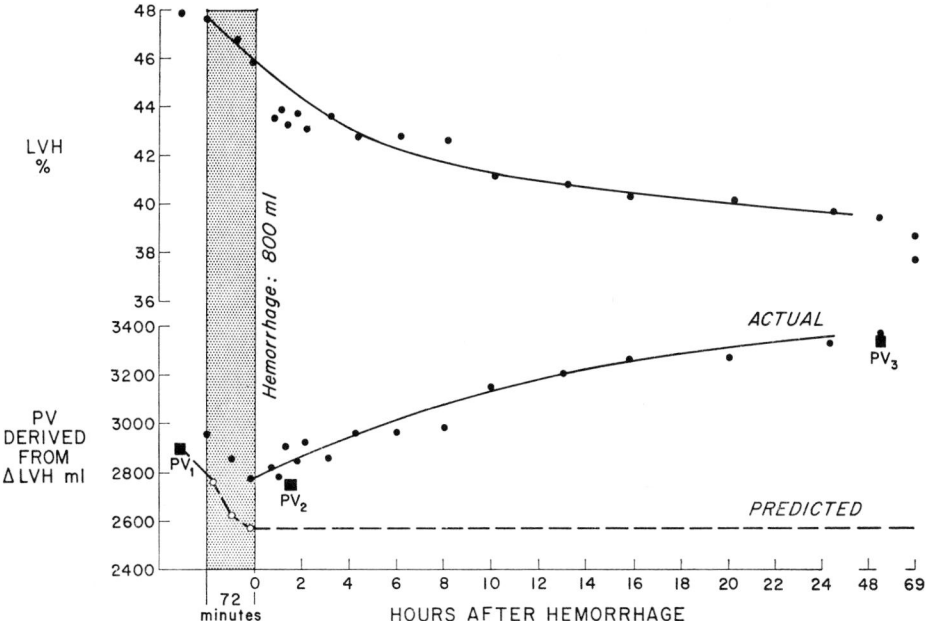

Figure 10. Transcapillary refilling of blood volume after hemorrhage. In this experiment a normal young man was bled by slow arterial hemorrhage of 825 ml., corresponding to approximately 15 per cent of his blood volume. Above is shown the gradual fall in hematocrit resulting from the entry of interstitial fluid across the capillary into the bloodstream, finally producing a stabilized, fully hemodiluted posthemorrhagic anemia with a hematocrit of 40, to be contrasted with the initial hematocrit of 52. Below are shown the plasma volume data in which the solid squares represent actual measurements of the plasma volume and demonstrate the increase in plasma volume, which is responsible for the fall in hematocrit after bleeding. The multiple small points indicate the plasma volume increases as calculated from the hematocrit, and are contrasted with the lower straight line marked "predicted," which merely indicates what the plasma volume would have been had no further change occurred following hemorrhage.

It is evident that in this case almost 1000 ml. of fluid was added to the circulation by this endogenous plasma transfusion occurring across the capillary. Transcapillary refilling was 104 per cent complete in 24 hours. During the 108 minutes occupied by the hemorrhage itself almost 200 ml. of plasma entered the circulation. The volume of plasma entering the circulation after hemorrhage equals *the sum of cells and plasma lost.* It is the total blood volume that is restored to normal, with an associated fall in peripheral concentration of erythrocytes as measured by hematocrit, red count, or hemoglobin concentration.

Although our evidence would suggest that this response is not driven by hormones alone, the aldosterone-sodium mechanism maintains intact the volume of refill fluid that enables this response to occur. (From Skillman, J. J., et al.: Surg. Gynecol. Obstet., *125*:983, 1967. Used by permission of Surgery, Gynecology & Obstetrics.)

This tendency is so regular that some degree of dilutional hyponatremia may be regarded as a normal feature of the effects of trauma on plasma chemistry.

Moderation must therefore be used in the administration of water and sodium after trauma; the administration of an amount required to maintain intact extracellular and circulating blood volume with normal renal function is advantageous; any excess will produce hypoproteinemia* and hyponatremia. This is a classic example of the need for the surgeon to understand the patient's own reaction in order to adapt therapy to his needs.

---

*The term "hypoproteinemia" means a low concentration of protein in the blood. This should not be equated with either starvation or specific protein starvation. Most hypoproteinemia is due to *dilution* of plasma protein during a period of water and salt retention. The hepatic synthesis of albumin has a very high priority in the human; if the liver is not primarily diseased, and if water and salt loading are avoided, plasma protein concentrations are maintained near normal until very late in human starvation. Gross alterations in nitrogen balance occur daily in surgical patients with little reflection in plasma albumin concentrations.

3. Change in Energy Source

In addition to this loss of muscle protoplasm and conservation of extracellular fluid, the severely injured vertebrate is faced with another inevitable condition of his wound: acute starvation.

The third fundamental characteristic of the posttraumatic patient is therefore his shift in energy source from a mixed *exogenous* diet to *endogenous* fat oxidation. Although body glycogen supplies some carbohydrate energy in the first few hours after injury (often at an increased rate and associated with hyperglycemia), and although the mobilization of muscle protein provides some energy by the ultimate oxidation of its carbon moieties, it is fat that provides most of the patient's energy requirements during a period of zero or negligible food intake. This fat is mobilized from depot fat by its hydrolysis to free fatty acids and glycerol. These compounds are circulated to the tissues, certain of which (largely muscle) can burn the fatty acids directly; in other instances they are degraded to 2-carbon fragments in the liver prior to utilization in other tissues. Each kilogram of fat thus mobilized yields about 1 liter of water of oxidation.

This change in energy source is signified by a rise in plasma free fatty acids, a fall in the respiratory quotient toward that of fat oxidation (0.7), and a small and persistent rise in blood sugar unaccompanied by an appropriate rise in plasma immunoreactive insulin. As will be described, this combination of events suggests the preferential oxidation of fat, the inhibition of insulin production from the pancreas, the mobilization of muscle protein to produce alanine for gluconeogenesis, and a transient pseudodiabetic state. Many factors enter into this endocrine sequence, among the most important being an increased production of epinephrine and norepinephrine from the adrenal medulla and at nerve synapses.

4. Neutrality Regulation*

The fourth feature of the post-traumatic state is an alteration in neutrality regulation. Initially, this change favors the development of extracellular alkalosis. If visceral failure or low flow state supervenes, this mild alkalosis is quickly overwhelmed by a mixed metabolic and respiratory acidosis, involving all phases of body water.

The most important early effect of trauma (without a low flow state) is a strong trend toward alkalosis, as mentioned above. Post-traumatic alkalosis results from the interaction of four components: (1) post-traumatic aldosteronism stimulated by volume reduction: inability to excrete sodium bicarbonate in an alkaline urine; (2) the oxidation of transfused citrate: a sodium bicarbonate load; (3) the removal of gastric juice by nasogastric tube: loss of hydrogen ion; and (4) hyperventilation: respiratory removal of carbon dioxide and with it a loss of hydrogen ion in water.

This mixed metabolic and respiratory alkalosis

---

*Information relating to neutrality regulation, fluid metabolism in surgical patients, and body composition will be found in references 29, 31, 35, 37, 38, and 41.

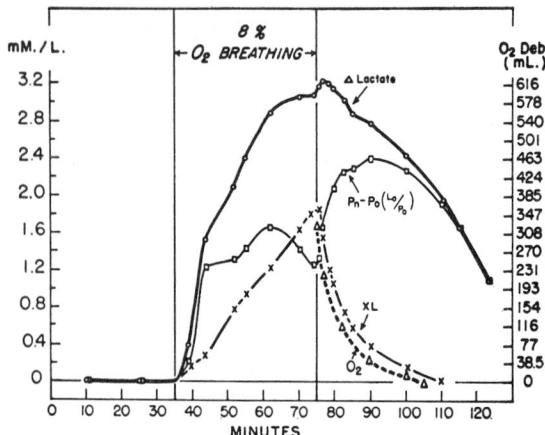

Figure 12. In this experiment, analogous to that shown in Figure 11, the accumulation of lactate during ventilatory anoxia is shown, together with the extent of oxygen debt. Below the upper line, which demonstrates change in total lactate, is a line (hollow squares) showing the lactate:pyruvate ratio and a solid line (connected by x) showing the excess lactate accumulation. The curve of oxygen utilization, as shown by the dotted lines in the triangles, returns toward normal much as in Figure 11. Excess lactate returns to normal at about the same kinetic rate that oxygen debt is repaid.

In surgical patients or in animals in low flow experiments, decreased tissue perfusion is a much more abundant stimulus to lactic acid production than is ventilatory anoxia, the stimulus used in these experiments. (From Huckabee, W. E.: J. Clin. Invest., 37:264, 1958. With permission.)

quite regularly reaches pH levels of 7.50 to 7.60. In severe cases when all of these four factors become accumulated over time, blood pH may reach 7.65 or higher.

Mild transient alkalosis is a normal response to trauma and has no severe significance. When it is marked or prolonged, however, it has several adverse effects, as follows: (1) left-shifted oxyhemoglobin dissociation curve with impaired tissue oxygen delivery; (2) increased impost on cardiac output; (3) hypokalemia; (4) cardiac arrhythmias; (5) digitalis toxicity in the digitalized patient; and (6) cerebral vasoconstriction.

The left-shifted oxyhemoglobin dissociation curve that results from alkalosis produces an anomalous increase in venous oxygen saturation, which may masquerade as peripheral shunting. This decrease in tissue oxygenation results in a slight buildup of lactate to levels of 2 to 4 mM. per liter.

Post-traumatic alkalosis might be thought of as the normal acid-base change of the surgical patient, particularly with volume reduction and blood transfusion. When a pathologic low flow state supervenes, with prolonged deficiency of blood flow in skeletal muscle, there is an accumulation of lactic acid. The initial alkalotic trend is overwhelmed by a severe metabolic acidosis. This results largely from hypoperfusion of muscle, although lactate can be produced in almost any tissue of the body that is inadequately perfused with blood. It is notable that ventilatory anoxemia is but a mild stimulus to lactic acidosis (severe anoxia of a transient sort will produce lactate levels of 3 to 5 mM. per liter, for example). In sharp contrast, even

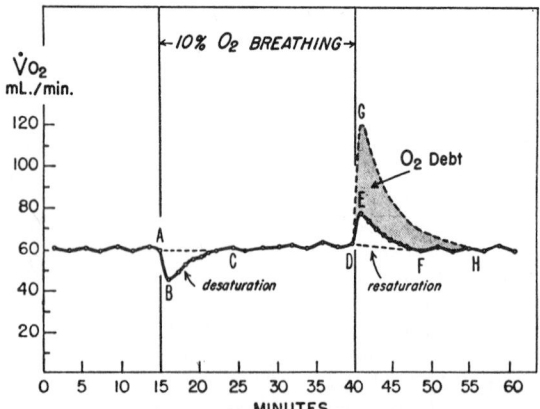

Figure 11. This, and Figure 12, are taken from the work of Huckabee. In this chart is shown the meaning of the term "oxygen debt" as indicated by change in oxygen consumption ($\dot{V}o_2$) in a period of rebreathing after anoxia. This work was done in the dog, and demonstrates doubling (for a few minutes) of oxygen consumption as the debt is "repaid," largely by lactate oxidation. (From Huckabee, W. E.: J. Clin. Invest., 37:264, 1958. With permission.)

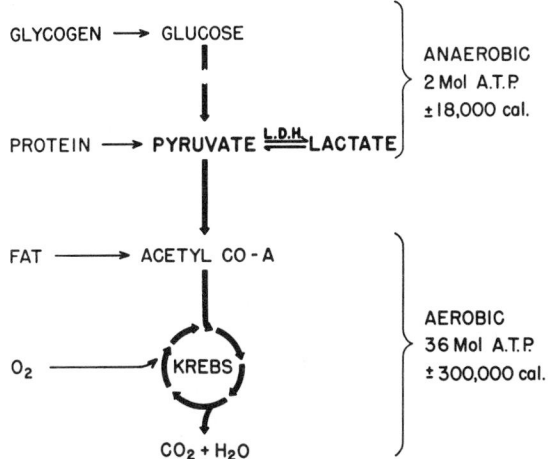

Figure 13. The degradation of 1 mol of glucose. This chart demonstrates that the anaerobic degradation of glucose by glycolytic metabolism yields only a small amount of energy as high-energy phosphate (adenosine triphosphate or ATP), and if anaerobic metabolism is maintained, produces a 3-carbon compound, lactic acid. This arises within the cell, and donates hydrogen ions to the cell. These hydrogen ions leak through the cell membrane, and the result is the production of a diffuse acidosis starting in the cell and later buffered by extracellular means.

When aerobic metabolism is restored, the 3-carbon compound passes via pyruvate to the 2-carbon compounds of the Krebs cycle, finally yielding CO_2 and H_2O with the release of 18 times as much energy.

It is thus clear that tissue anaerobiosis resulting from a low flow state not only yields acid but likewise deprives the body of the energy that should be gained from full aerobic oxidation of glucose. (From Lyons, J. H., Jr., and Moore, F. D. *In* Lewis-Walter's Practice of Surgery. New York, Hoeber Medical Division, Harper & Row, 1969, Volume 1, pp. 1–82. With permission.)

short periods of hypoperfusion will yield very high levels of blood lactate, as high as 25 to 30 mM. per liter. This lactate is produced at a far higher rate than pyruvate, when hypoperfusion is its cause. The lactate is therefore referred to as excess lactate or as lactate at a high lactate-pyruvate ratio. In such instances the reduction in standard bicarbonate is quantitatively related to the lactate level.

It must be emphasized that the lactate ion itself is quite nontoxic. It is a normal intermediary 3-carbon step in glycolysis. Its importance in surgical patients is its value as a barometer of the amount of new hydrogen ion produced in the cells of anoxic tissue. The lactate level observed at any moment is the net result of the rate of lactic acid production in anoxic tissue, the rate of lactate excretion, and the ability of other tissues to cause combustion of lactate in an aerobic environment. The lactic acid of low flow acidosis arises in the cells themselves. The cellular buffers are therefore taken up first, and the change in buffer base in the plasma represents an end stage. This must be considered as a uniquely intracellular acidosis, and it cannot be reproduced by the intravenous infusion of lactic acid.

5. Cardiac Output

In the post-traumatic patient (the individual resuscitated after injury or operation, or following a low

flow state), elevated cardiac output is the norm. This results from the effects of catecholamines on resting cardiac function, and from the increased demands of tissues for blood flow when the oxyhemoglobin dissociation curve is shifted "to the left" (a reduction in the P_{50} or oxygen tension required for 50 per cent saturation). The normal P_{50} for human hemoglobin is about 27 mm. Hg. With post-traumatic alkalosis this value may be shifted to the vicinity of 20 to 22 mm. Hg. Diphosphoglycerate deficiency also shifts this curve to the left, lowering the P_{50} value. Alkalosis and DPG deficiency are additive in their effects, as observed in the severely injured patient who has received massive blood transfusions. These factors therefore combine to force an increase in cardiac output. Counteracting this effect is the fact that the left-shifted oxyhemoglobin will pick up oxygen more readily in the lungs, and peripheral tissue acidosis in a low flow state will tend to normalize the curve by a right shift as the blood passes through tissue. In addition to this complex interaction there are many other factors that decrease oxygen supply to tissues in special cases. These include mild carbon monoxide poisoning in burns, and minor blood group incompatibility. Increased demand for cardiac output also arises from shivering in the

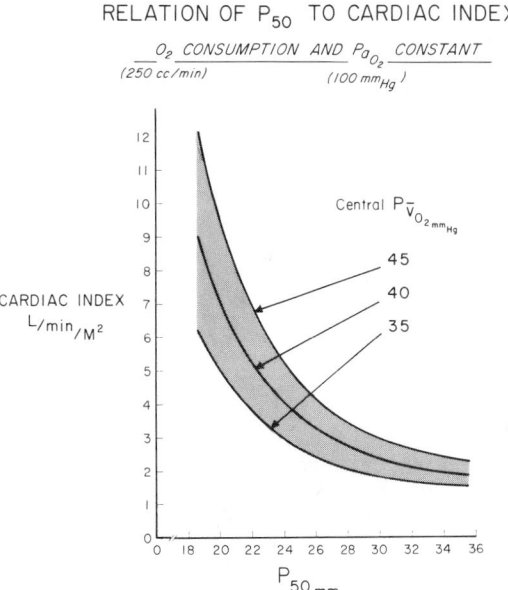

Figure 14. Effect of the oxyhemoglobin dissociation curve on cardiac index. In this theoretical diagram, based on constancy of oxygen consumption and oxygen tensions, it is demonstrated that with a left shift of the oxyhemoglobin dissociation curve (i.e., a reduction in the P_{50} value), cardiac output must increase to maintain oxygen supply normal to the tissues. This is because of decreased oxygen extraction from each quantum of blood passing through the tissues. This type of left-shifted oxyhemoglobin curve places an added impost on cardiac output, and is a typical result of post-traumatic alkalosis. In addition, a deficiency of 2,3-DPG in the erythrocytes (usually due to transfusion of banked blood) produces the same effect. The two causes are additive, as stimuli to a left-shifted curve. This finding appears to explain, for the first time, the markedly elevated cardiac output seen in many severely injured surgical patients who have been successfully resuscitated.

cold, muscular exercise in the restless or disoriented patient, increased work of breathing, increased temperature, and sepsis.

Some controversy has revolved around the interpretation of this increased cardiac output so often observed after injury. It seems clear that in the previously healthy young person whose heart can respond to this load, the increased cardiac output merely represents a central circulatory response to a disorder of oxygen transport. If the demand is constant, output must rise to compensate for decreased extraction. In persons with heart disease who cannot support an increased cardiac output (or in older individuals with chronic coronary insufficiency), four types of undesirable changes can result from this challenge: (1) acute congestive heart failure, (2) an acute cardiac arrhythmia, (3) peripheral tissue anoxia with lactic acidosis, and (4) outright visceral failure (brain or kidneys). For reasons not well understood by the cardiologist, sudden exertion, placing a demand on the heart unaccustomed to it, is associated with acute myocardial infarction or arrhythmias. This is the sort of phenomenon seen in older men with sudden exertion followed by sudden fatality, as in running, snow shoveling, or sexual intercourse. This mechanism is apparently operative in some older persons after injury or operation, when there is a sudden increase in demand for cardiac output but the heart is unable to respond.

6. Renal Function*

Detailed effects of trauma on renal function have already been described. An early tendency to hypoperfusion of the kidneys ("differential renal vasoconstriction") is a response to any volume or flow challenge. This is coupled with shunting of blood away from the renal cortex, decreased filtration fraction of renal blood flow, and a maximal tubular resorptive stimulus by aldosterone and antidiuretic hormone. When glomerular filtration rate falls below 20 ml. per minute, the kidney under these influences becomes extremely vulnerable to nephrotic damage from porphyrin pigments, drugs, or exogenous chemical poisons. It is this combination of factors that results in post-traumatic renal insufficiency.

The maintenance of adequate hydration and an osmotic load (as either mannitol, glucose, or salts) serves to maintain well-filled renal tubular lumina and high glomerular filtration rates. These are among the chief mechanisms by which adequate hydration and solute loading are protective for the kidney.

The kidney is thus the target organ for the interplay of a very wide variety of influences after trauma; the precise weighting of these various factors determines the renal response. The risk of severe renal damage is greatly increased if there is some degree of renal disease prior to injury, as in an elderly person with nephrosclerosis or in a younger person with chronic nephritis.

7. Gastrointestinal Tract

After severe injury anywhere in the body, the absorptive and propulsive effect of the gastrointestinal tract is reduced; if this injury involves the peritoneal cavity itself, the reduction in gastrointestinal function is much more profound and prolonged. Efforts to feed the patient during this early period result in abdominal distention, decreased diaphragmatic excursions, severe peristaltic abdominal pain, vomiting, and the threat of aspiration of vomitus.

As the patient recovers from this initial inhibition, and if the stress of tissue injury is long-continued (burns, myocardial infarction, pulmonary insufficiency, or rapidly growing cancer especially around the head and neck), acid-peptic autodigestion of the stomach and duodenum becomes commonplace and stress ulcer results. The acid-peptic mechanism (altered gastric barrier function) that permits stress ulcer to develop can also result in a diffuse hemorrhagic gastritis with multiple small erosions or reactivation of duodenal ulcer. The isolated punched-out deep gastric ulcer is much more characteristic of cortisone administration than it is of surgical stress itself. Massive hemorrhage from the upper gastrointestinal tract is the terminal mechanism in many patients with acute infection after injury, as in burns or bacteremia, and in patients with post-traumatic pulmonary insufficiency.

When gastrointestinal propulsive and absorptive activity has been returned but the total surface of available gastrointestinal tract is inadequate for ordinary diet, the use of elemental diets has made a notable contribution to the anabolic and synthetic period of surgical convalescence.

8. Lungs*

A variety of mechanisms after trauma combine to threaten the integrity of the lungs. These adverse influences may be thought of as arriving at the lungs either by the airway, by the bloodstream, or by direct trauma, as follows:

Airway
>   Aspiration of gastric contents
>   Prolonged exposure to high oxygen tensions
>   Inhalation of smoke chronically (heavy smoking history) or acutely (burns)
>   Prolonged mechanical ventilation
>   Disorders of ventilation-perfusion ratios due to posture (i.e., prolonged immobilization in one position)

Bloodstream
>   Fluid overload with oncotic dilution and pulmonary edema
>   Heart failure often due in part to fluid overload
>   Multiple small platelet emboli from the area of trauma
>   Multiple "debris emboli" from banked blood
>   Microorganisms from peripheral infection
>   Vasoactive substances affecting pulmonary perfu-

---

*Because of the increasing importance of diuretics in surgical care, the few references in this small bibliography dealing with renal function relate to the use of diuretics; see references 16, 28, and 35.

---

*See reference 40 for a review of post-traumatic pulmonary insufficiency; references 12, 26, and 52 deal with infection.

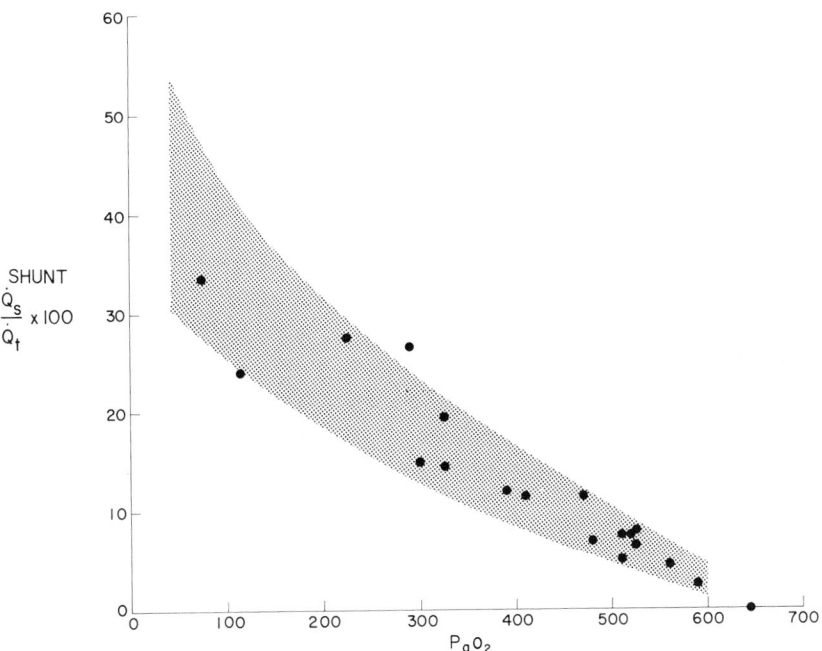

Figure 15. Nomogram for estimating the shunt fraction in pulmonary insufficiency, as based on observation of the arterial oxygen tension after a test inhalation of 100 per cent oxygen for 20 to 30 minutes.

The observed arterial oxygen tension after the test period of inhalation is read upward from the bottom line of the chart. The intercept through the shaded area from the vertical coordinate shows the approximate fraction of blood passing through the lungs without oxygenation $\frac{(\dot{Q}_s)}{(\dot{Q}_t)}$. The black dots are observed points from work in our laboratories. The shaded area shows the general order of magnitude. It is evident that in a patient acutely ill with post-traumatic pulmonary insufficiency whose arterial oxygen tension can be raised only to 100 mm. Hg after one-half hour of inhaling 100 per cent oxygen, 30 to 50 per cent of the blood volume is moving through the lungs without ventilation or oxygenation. This type of greatly increased pulmonary shunting is characteristic of post-traumatic pulmonary insufficiency and is a characteristic cause of lethal anoxia in such patients. (From Moore, F. D., et al.: Post-traumatic Pulmonary Insufficiency. Philadelphia, W. B. Saunders Company, 1969. With permission.)

sion, especially serotonin, the catecholamines, and the kinins

Direct Trauma to the Chest and Lungs

Unstable rib cage, fractures, crushed chest

Solid blow to chest or abdomen, traumatic wet lung

Prolonged open chest with collapsed or underperfused lung tissue

Explosive compression or decompression

Post-traumatic pulmonary insufficiency results when the net vector of these forces is greater than the tolerance of that patient's lungs. A heavy smoking history, chronic asthma, emphysema, and bronchiectasis are the most common conditions predisposing to pulmonary insufficiency. Loss of compliance, possibly due to loss of surfactants, is a universal result.

The characteristic physiological disorder detected in the periphery is shunting, i.e., the appearance of abnormally large amounts of venous blood containing reduced hemoglobin in the arterial output from the left heart. This is revealed, or quantified, by a test period of inhalation of 100 per cent oxygen when the expected normal response to an arterial oxygen tension of 450 mm. Hg, or higher, is not achieved. The extent of shunting can be estimated from a nomogram. The precise amount of oxygen required to satisfy the patient's needs can be gauged thereby, and prolonged exposure to inappropriate and unnecessarily high oxygen tensions can be avoided.

Anoxemia resulting from pulmonary shunting is associated with increased efforts at ventilation that result in overventilation of the remaining portions of lung. Therefore the characteristic carbon dioxide tension is below normal, often far below normal. Hyperventilation, with hypocarbia, a respiratory alkalosis, and prolonged anoxemia insensitive to increased oxygen tensions in the airway, are characteristic of post-traumatic pulmonary insufficiency.

9. Brain

When fixed vessel disease is present (as in older people), cerebral function is very sensitive to perfusion and oxygenation. The left-shifted oxyhemoglobin dissociation curve of alkalosis reduces cerebral function, with resulting disorientation, hallucination, extreme restlessness, or coma. Much that is termed metabolic encephalopathy represents inadequate perfusion or oxygenation of the brain.

Hypocarbia or alkalosis (or both) reduces cerebral perfusion by producing cerebral vasoconstriction. The effects on consciousness and respiratory drive are additive. There is no more ominous sign in the surgical patient than loss of consciousness and with it the ability to cooperate. Repairing these deficiencies by mechanical ventilation and mechanical restraints is no substitute for a proper understanding of the need of the patient's brain for adequate perfusion with well-oxygenated blood and a normal supply of glucose.

Although the brain acutely requires glucose as its obligate metabolic substrate, this is rarely in short supply in the post-traumatic patient unless blood supply itself is unable to transport the substrate to the tissue. Oxygen and perfusion are the limiting factors.

10. Endocrine Glands

Two of the glands most extensively concerned with the response to trauma—the pituitary and adrenals—may become either hyperemic or infarcted in severe injury or prolonged low flow states. This is observed in Sheehan's syndrome after obstetric hemorrhage. This is the syndrome of pituitary infarction during a low flow state associated with parturition. Hemorrhage into the adrenal is occasionally seen as "adrenal apoplexy" after burns and severe injury. These post-traumatic losses of pituitary-adrenal function, occurring after specific injury, are very rare. But the fact that they can occur constitutes an indication for the test infusion of glucocorticoids intravenously in any patient whose circulation is not supported by ordinary measures after severe injury, burns, or a low flow state. Adrenal failure also results from hemorrhage into the adrenal cortex, in patients being given anticoagulants, or from the cortical localization of bacteria from the bloodstream. Prolonged administration of corticosteroids produces atrophy of the adrenal cortex which may not be noticeable in the stresses of everyday life, but which will be associated with poor blood pressure maintenance if the patient is injured or operated upon. Additional corticosteroid administration is mandatory in such patients.

III. ACUTE INJURY: ENDOCRINE CHANGES

Accompanying the biochemical, metabolic, and visceral changes are a series of endocrine alterations, many of which were initially inferred from the associated chemical abnormalities. During the past decade, as precise methods of endocrine assay have become available for almost all of the pituitary and target-gland hormones, it has become possible to assign numerical values to the hormone changes in blood, urine, and glandular secretory rate. In this section will be reviewed briefly the endocrine changes that are involved in surgical convalescence.

1. Glucocorticoids*

A rise in the level of blood cortisol is characteristic after trauma. This is a rise in the level of both free and conjugated steroids of the Porter-Silber reacting variety (i.e., 17-hydroxycorticosteroids). This output of hormone is followed by increased hepatic reduction in ring A (to tetrahydro compounds) and an excretion of representative compounds of all of these groups of cortisone metabolites in the urine. When the injury is

*Bibliographic references on neuroendocrine activation and hormone changes are to be found in references 6, 17, 19, 22, 23, 29, 32, 33, 34, 47, 48, 50, 54, 56, 57, and 60.

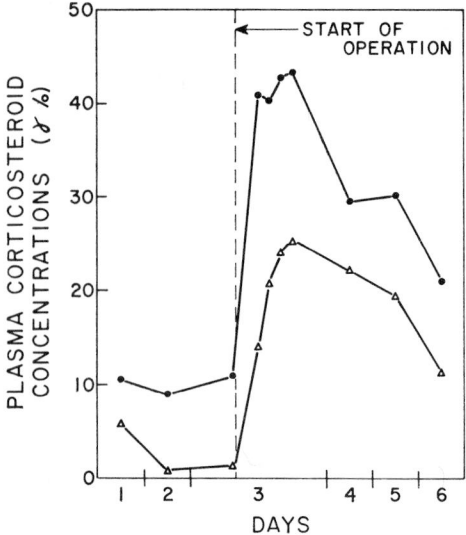

Figure 16. Rise in free and conjugated steroids after subtotal gastrectomy. This demonstrates the rise of plasma corticosteroids after an operation. The free steroids are shown by black dots, and the conjugated steroids by small triangles. In such a patient the steroid values return toward normal by the third postoperative day. The presence of surgical complications produces a higher level for a longer time. (From Smith, L. L., et al.: J. Clin. Endocr., 20:919, 1960. With permission.)

self-limited, as in the typical elective clean civilian surgical operation, these hormone values quickly fall to normal. When the trauma is long-continued (as in the transportation of a military casualty), or when infection supervenes and maintains the traumatic status for a long time (as in burns), the free and conjugated blood steroids remain at high levels for many weeks and even months.

The result of prolonged stimulation of the production of glucocorticoids from the adrenal cortex is hypertrophy of the adrenal cortex. This is regularly found after prolonged or recurrent injury. The concept of "adrenal exhaustion" has little basis in post-traumatic adrenal physiology. When there has been hemorrhage into the adrenal (particularly in patients given anticoagulants), or the localization of bacteria from the bloodstream (during invasive infection with bacteremia), then adrenal failure can occur. This is a rarity even after severe injury. In a patient with adrenal atrophy prior to operation (as with Addison's disease or following prolonged use of corticosteroids), the expected post-traumatic rise in adrenal cortical function does not occur. Such patients exhibit very poor maintenance of blood pressure, pass into a low flow state, and will die rapidly if not treated with cortisone.

This increase in the secretion, concentration, and excretion of glucocorticoids results from ACTH stimulation of the adrenal cortex. Trauma stimulates the pituitary by a variety of pathways, including the peripheral nerves and the catecholamines. The neuroendocrine activation of the pituitary-adrenal axis involves medullary extensions of the spinal tracts, the supraoptic nuclei of the hypothalamus, and the release there of humoral substances, as yet unidentified, which stimulate the pituitary. Increased ACTH concentrations in the blood are regularly observed. Only

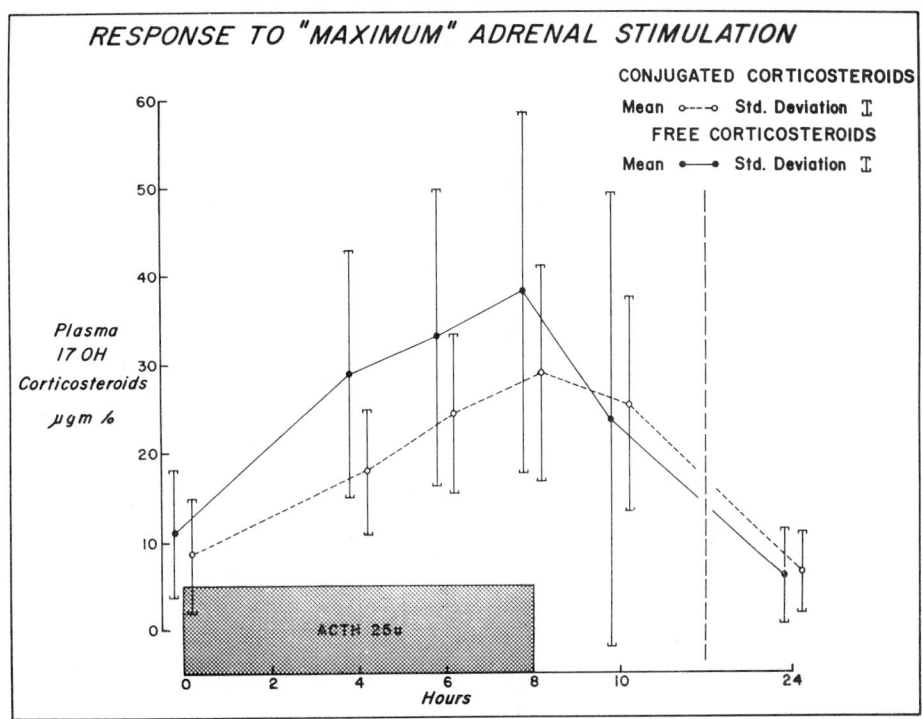

Figure 17. Effects of ACTH on blood steroids. Here, to contrast with the data in Figures 16 and 18 are shown the effects of maximal ACTH stimulation on free and conjugated blood corticosteroids. (From Steenburg, R. W., et al.: J. Clin. Endocr. *21*:39, 1961. With permission.)

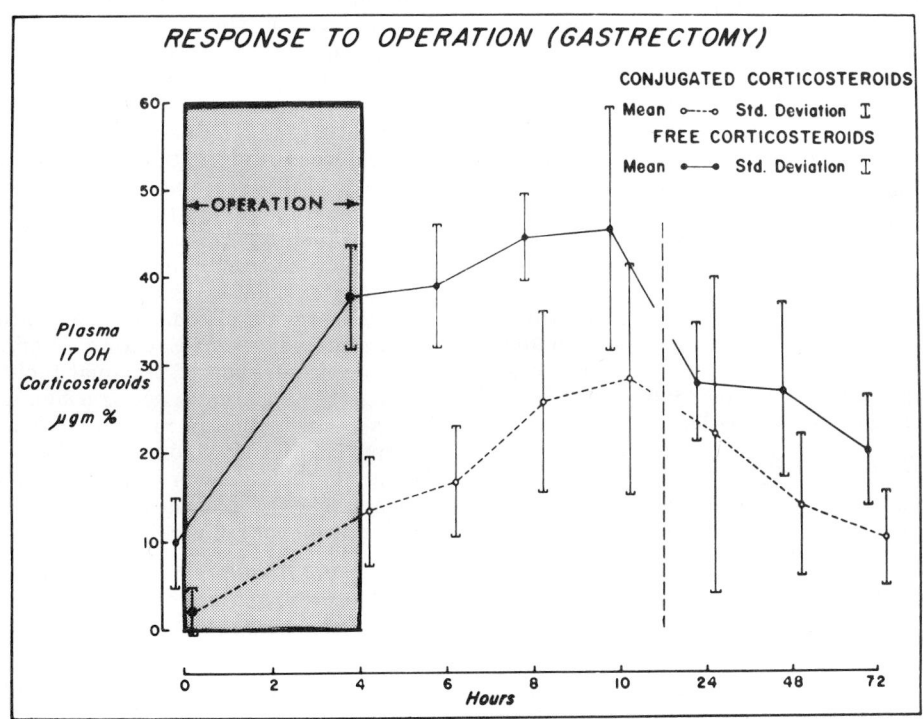

Figure 18. Response to operation in a group of eight patients undergoing gastrectomy plotted as in Figure 17. These data are to be compared with those of ACTH stimulation. They indicate that, with operation, a higher level of free steroid was attained than with maximal ACTH stimulation, and that conjugation of steroids was not quite as marked. Other data not shown here suggest that this fault in conjugation may be due to minor alterations in liver function due to the operation itself, changes in liver blood flow, or the anesthetic agent.

when the pituitary has been directly damaged, or inhibited by prolonged administration of steroids, does this expected rise in ACTH fail to occur. If the patient is in a profound low flow state, with prolonged hypotension and hypoperfusion of all tissues, including the adrenal cortex, this normal adrenal response to the ACTH stimulus is blunted. As soon as tissue flow is restored so that the adrenal can function again, the expected rise in blood cortisol metabolites is seen.

2. Aldosterone[1, 16, 22, 36, 39, 51]

Isotonic volume reduction (as in simple blood loss) is one of the most potent stimuli to aldosterone secretion in man. This is detected by an increased concentration of aldosterone in adrenal vein blood and an increase in aldosterone secretory and excretory rate. The hormone is active in such tiny concentrations that its measurement is difficult, and it is best detected by measurement of alterations in the aldosterone secretory rate by isotope dilution.

There is good evidence that this stimulus to aldosterone production after blood loss is activated through the secretion of renin by the juxtaglomerular apparatus of the kidney in response to decreased renal blood flow. This in turn stimulates the production of angiotensin, which directly stimulates the adrenal cortex to produce aldosterone. In addition, ACTH itself is a potent stimulator of the adrenal production of aldosterone. Other metabolic events that stimulate this change include a decrease in sodium concentration in the plasma, a decrease in extracellular volume, and an increase in potassium concentration in the plasma. Simple restriction of water and salt will, over the course of a few hours, stimulate the production of aldosterone.

The characteristic renal effects of aldosterone are decreased renal excretion of sodium bicarbonate in an acid urine containing increased amounts of potassium. This is characteristic of the post-traumatic state. These effects of aldosterone support the circulation in several ways; the net vector is pressor in character. Chronic administration or oversecretion of aldosterone results in hypertension. Although the most obvious pressor effect of aldosterone in surgical trauma is the support of the plasma volume by sodium conservation and thus maintenance of interstitial fluid volume, there may be other more subtle pressor effects of aldosterone bearing directly on ion exchange in heart muscle and vascular smooth muscle.

3. Antidiuretic Hormone[16, 22, 50]

The production of vasopressin from the supraoptic tract and its release from the posterior pituitary is likewise stimulated by loss of blood volume even though the plasma remains isotonic. It appears that trauma itself stimulates the production of antidiuretic hormone. If the plasma becomes hypertonic for any reason, the secretion of antidiuretic hormone is further accentuated. For all these reasons, the postoperative patient demonstrates decreased free water clearance for many hours or days after injury (as previously mentioned) and hyponatremia will develop if he is treated with an excess of sodium-free water.

The mild hypertonicity of water deprivation stimu-lates the production of antidiuretic hormone. This appropriate antidiuresis ceases promptly (with the renewed excretion of free water) when water is taken by mouth and the plasma hypertonicity restored to normal. By contrast, the antidiuresis that follows surgery is in a sense inappropriate, since it is activated by tissue trauma and isotonic volume reduction. Water administration therefore produces hyponatremia and hypotonicity rather than merely shutting off the antidiuretic hormone production.

4. Sensors for Volume Regulation

Peripheral tissue injury appears to activate the pituitary-adrenal axis by central nervous pathways to the brain and thence by a mixed neuroendocrine activation of the anterior pituitary. Negative feedback is provided by the plasma free cortisol level, which in turn tends to inhibit ACTH production.

A sensing mechanism or "volume receptor" is needed to explain the variety of mechanisms activated after injury that help to support the circulation.

The right and left atria appear to be sensing agencies regulating production of aldosterone and antidiuretic hormone secretion, respectively. Certainly there is good evidence that in a normal person a low central venous pressure (as exhibited, for example, after hemorrhage) is a stimulus to the production of both aldosterone and antidiuretic hormone. By the same token, a rise in atrial pressure appears to be associated with a cutoff in these secretory rates and an increased urinary sodium excretion. When there is a cutoff in the secretory rate of aldosterone or antidiuretic hormone, there is a free diuresis of water and salt. This accounts for the diuresis observed when anemic patients are treated by blood transfusion. It also accounts for the free diuresis exhibited by the convalescent burned patient when reabsorption of burn edema occurs through the recovering capillary wall.

Special renal sensors that regulate aldosterone production via the renin-angiotensin mechanism have been located in the juxtaglomerular apparatus of the kidney, which appears to be very sensitive to minor changes in arteriolar inflow pressures to the glomerulus. Immediately adjacent is the macula densa, a specialized region of renal tubular epithelium which, it is postulated, is sensitive to small alterations in the sodium concentration of proximal tubular urine. The two together apparently act as a fine regulator of aldosterone production in response either to changes in effective circulating volume as reflected by arteriolar pressure in the kidney or to alterations in sodium concentration in the plasma as reflected in the sodium content or tonicity of proximal tubular urine.

5. Body Fuel Regulators and the Energy Cycle — Insulin, Its Cooperators, and Antagonists — Amino Acid Changes*

Any rise in blood sugar in a normal person stimulates the pancreatic islet cells to increased insulin

---

*Suggested reading in the field of starvation endocrinology, energy metabolism, and hormone interrelationships regulating the utilization of body fuels will be found in references 10, 11, 24, 25, 30, 47, and 48.

production. This endogenous influence favors the oxidation of carbohydrate through an alteration in cellular permeability, and has the additional effect of inhibiting the release of amino acids from muscle and the hydrolysis of depot fat to free fatty acids. One might paraphrase this by stating that insulin secretion not only is activated by the presence of glucose, but also favors the preferential combustion of glucose as the primary fuel, inhibiting the mobilization and oxidation of other fuel sources. Contrariwise, when blood glucose concentrations are low and insulin secretion therefore inhibited, the body releases amino acids

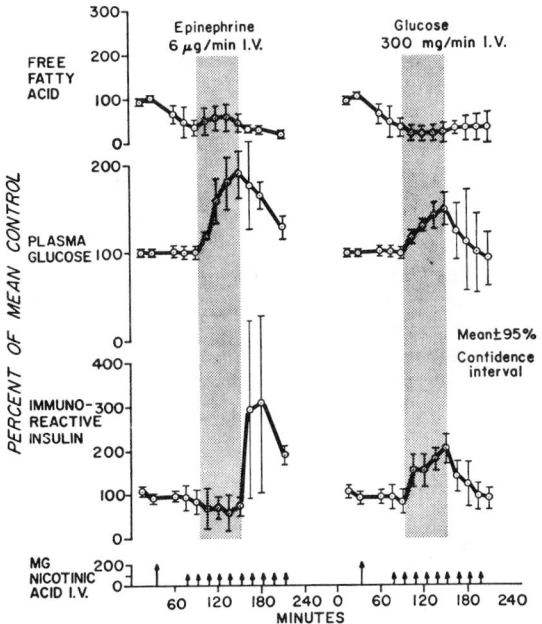

Figure 19. The inhibition of insulin output by epinephrine. The data shown above are the classic findings upon which is based the concept that catecholamine output after injury inhibits the output of insulin, producing a transient pseudodiabetic state. More important, the inhibition of insulin production permits an expanded leak of amino acids from muscle; the mobilization of free fatty acids from adipose tissue is favored; insulin effects that favor the combustion of glucose are also antagonized in the periphery by epinephrine.

In this experiment, the animal was prepared by nicotinic acid injection to prevent fatty acid mobilization. The animal was then given intravenous glucose with the rise in plasma glucose as shown. In the left-hand chart, this was accompanied by epinephrine infusion, which completely inhibited the production of insulin in response to hyperglycemia until the epinephrine was stopped. At that time insulin reacted smartly to the glucose challenge. On the right, epinephrine was not given with the glucose and a typical insulin rise was observed.

As described in the text, these data demonstrating a profound effect of catecholamines on the intermediary metabolism of carbohydrate, fat, and protein (mediated at least in part by insulin inhibition) constitute an important link between the emergency endocrine adjustments to blood loss or low flow states on the one hand, and the more slowly reacting metabolic consequences of injury, on the other. Many aspects of both types of bodily adjustment are thus paced by the catecholamine levels and are most marked in severe low flow states or sepsis. (From Porte, D.: J. Clin. Invest., 46:86, 1967. With permission.)

from muscle. These are converted into glucose largely through interconversion to alanine, its deamination, and therefrom the synthesis of 6-carbon sugars, some of which are polymerized to glycogen. At the same time, depot fat is hydrolyzed, the level of free fatty acids rises, and fat becomes the major caloric source. Insulin is therefore a prime regulator of many of the intermediary metabolic changes of the post-traumatic state. The brain is an obligate glucose burner, at least over the short term, and certain of the acute changes after both starvation and trauma suggest a bodily adjustment favoring increased availability of glucose.

The appearance and biochemistry of recently injured patients suggest a reduction in available insulin. There is a blood sugar level that is slightly elevated for several days; accompanying this blood sugar level is a concentration of serum immunoreactive insulin that is significantly lower than one would expect for the observed glucose level. In states of relative hypoinsulinism the glucose-insulin ratio is elevated. This is the case following trauma. In addition, there is a gradually rising concentration of glucagon in the blood that may reach its peak as long as five days after the injury. The interpretation has been offered that these two changes both result from catecholamine secretion. There is an inhibition of insulin production and of peripheral insulin effect; there is a gradual rise in glucagon. All of these changes are produced by catecholamine secretion. In addition there is an increased rate of mobilization of body fat indicated by an increased level of free fatty acids in the plasma, likewise an effect of catecholamine stimulation.

Growth hormone antagonizes the effect of insulin in the periphery, and therefore has a diabetogenic action. In addition, it diverts small molecular weight nitrogen compounds toward protein synthesis with a resultant enlargement in muscle and bone mass. Growth hormone and similar molecules favor the synthesis of milk protein in lactating animals.

In the past few years there has been increased interest and a wealth of new data on the intermediary metabolism of amino acids in muscle, and a beginning flow of information on the changes in this system imposed by injury and starvation. These data will profoundly affect the mixture of nutrients that the surgeon finds best adapted to the needs of the injured and starving individual. A few of these findings can be mentioned here. First, the inappropriately low level of circulating insulin favors a leak of amino acids from muscle. Second, alanine appears to have a shunt function recirculating between muscle and liver, carrying amino groups from muscle to liver and returning to muscle as a carbohydrate. This may account for its anomalous high concentration in the starving patient given glucose. Third, the branched-chain amino acids (leucine, isoleucine, and valine) appear to have a particular metabolic property: once they have been lost from muscle they are irreversibly deaminated and disappear from the nitrogen pool. Recent evidence suggests that their provision has a special nitrogen-sparing affect. Of these amino acids, leucine may be the most important. There is suggestive evidence that providing leucine in excess prevents loss of other nitrogen compounds from muscle. Finally, it has been nicely shown in isolated muscle preparations that exercise or even passive stretch prevents the loss of nitrogen from muscle. This is a laboratory finding that corroborates the common clinical precept that exercise prevents muscle wasting. This may have a particular message in the resting immobilized surgical patient: the muscles that show the greatest wasting are the peripheral muscles that are immobilized. The heart, intercostal muscles, and diaphragm (which must continue to exercise) show much less evidence of loss of tissue. In patients on prolonged respiratory assistance, some of the difficulty in "weaning" may be due to actual loss of muscular mass from the diaphragm owing to prolonged rest. Early mobilization, exercise, and physiotherapy thus have metabolic effects far more profound than previously suspected. Bibliographic references on this new and interesting field of endocrinology and metabolism are found in the bibliography, references 3, 4, 5, 9, 14, 15, 18, 49, 55, and 58.

The level of thyroglobulins circulating in the blood determines the basal requirement of peripheral tissues for oxygen. There is no evidence for any systematic change after trauma despite conflicting reports in the literature for many years. Measurements of oxygen consumption after injury demonstrate that the relationship of oxygen consumption to body temperature and exercise is perfectly normal. Only when infection is superimposed, or with large open wounds and excessive water loss from the body, imposing a thermal load, is there an increased caloric turnover. Such changes can occur in otherwise normal individuals with changes in body temperature, without presupposing any change in thyroid hormone production.

6. The Adrenal Medulla and Catecholamines[19, 56, 57]

As mentioned in the historical introduction to this chapter, Cannon was the first to demonstrate a systematic endocrine change after injury: increased secretion of "adrenalin" (i.e., epinephrine plus norepinephrine). It could well be that these two hormones, the first to be described, are also among the most basic of post-traumatic hormonal responses in the surgical patient because of their manifold and widespread activities both in circulation and in metabolism, their effect on the activity of other hormones, and their stimulation by almost all of the components of trauma.

The adrenal medulla is the sole source in the body of epinephrine. Epinephrine is the prototype beta-receptor stimulant of the catecholamine group. Its peripheral metabolic activities are chiefly those of hepatic glycogenolysis with increase in blood glucose formation, inhibition of insulin production leading in turn to amino acid release from muscle, and, finally, direct stimulation of the hydrolysis of fat and release of free fatty acids. Increased levels of epinephrine are readily demonstrable in the experimental animal after hemorrhage, minor reductions in circulating blood or plasma volume, or tissue injury. The metabolic effects are all seen regularly after severe injury. In addition, epinephrine is a vasodilator in certain vascular beds; in other circumstances, or at different concentrations, it is a mild vasoconstrictor.

Possibly the most enigmatic feature of epinephrine activity after injury is that bilateral adrenalectomy, which effectively removes epinephrine entirely and permanently from body fluids, is not followed by any severe metabolic disorder so long as corticosteroids are provided. This may be because of the fact that norepinephrine has weak epinephrine-like effects, or that intermediary metabolites substitute for epinephrine in its peripheral metabolic activities when glucocorticoids are in slight excess. The peripheral vasomotor activity of both epinephrine and norepinephrine requires the basal presence of glucocorticoids in order that tissues may exhibit a vasomotor response.

Norepinephrine is produced throughout the body at nerve synapses. Bilateral total adrenalectomy has no effect whatsoever on blood or urine norepinephrine levels. The intermediary metabolic effects of norepinephrine are not marked although it is active as a fat mobilizer; its principal activity is as the prototype stimulator of alpha receptors in peripheral vascular smooth muscle with a resultant vasomotor effect that is vasoconstrictor throughout the body save for the myocardium.

Increased catecholamine secretion might be considered the primal endocrine response to trauma, not only because of their widespread effects, but also because they are stimulators of the pituitary, producing ACTH and therefore glucocorticoids and aldosterone. In addition, they are produced by a large variety of characteristic traumatic stimuli, including excitement, fear, apprehension, anger, cross-sectional tissue injury, fractures, burns, and volume reduction.

The teleologic interpretation of catecholamine responses to injury is most appealing as long as the response is transient. These hormones have an extremely short biologic half-life. They may well be thought of as emergency mechanisms. If, because of the conditions of continuing trauma, or through the error of overadministration by the surgeon, catecholamine levels remain high for a prolonged period of time, then the metabolic effects and prolonged vasoconstriction becomes deleterious to the organism through exhaustion of energy stores and ischemia of cellular tissues.

7. Gonadal Steroids

Starvation, subnormal nutrition, the winter season in northern nonhibernating mammals, and prolonged illness all result in a decreased urinary excretion of 17-ketosteroids. These ketogenic steroids are excreted in the urine as the end product of metabolism of a variety of precursors, particularly adrenal and testicular androgens and to a minor extent, glucocorticoids. After trauma or with prolonged severe illness, there is decreased libido in the male and cessation of menses in the female. These changes suggest that reproductive potential drops and that gonadal steroid activity is decreased after injury. There have been few systematic studies of blood and urine levels of gonadal steroids, measured either directly or by bioassay, to give us any concept of the regularity or metabolic significance of this change.

Androgens, of both adrenal and testicular origin, are anabolic in character, sharing with growth hormone the property of diverting nitrogen compounds toward protein synthesis. Androgenic growth in the male at puberty is largely the growth of skeletal muscle, which is thus ε secondary sex character of the male. Since it is this tissue that suffers most in the catabolism of trauma, it is attrative to assume that a decreased androgenicity characterizes the post-traumatic state. Although the weight of evidence favors such an interpretation, there is a paucity of quantitative data on the point.

The administration of androgens such as testosorone immediately after injury has little effect on nitrogen metabolism. Within a few days it can be demonstrated that androgen administration favors protein synthesis. It is unknown whether or not this helps the patient clinically. The exogenous administration of androgens inhibits the patient's own pituitary production of gonadotropins and will, in the long run, result in gonadal atrophy.

As regards the female, the cessation of menses in chronically ill patients has long been observed. The usual teleologic interpretation given is that a female must be in good health and good nutrition in order to ovulate and be fertile. This is obviously in the best interest of the species. Whatever the interpretation, one would expect amenorrhea to be associated with a decreased level of pituitary gonadotropins or of ovarian steroid hormones (estradiol or progesterone). If a woman is in the premenstrual period at the time of operation or injury, she will frequently have a bloody vaginal discharge after the operation. This is often interpreted as menstruation, when in point of fact it is merely the discharge of an early secretory endometrium when its progesterone support is withdrawn.

8. The Calcium Regulators: Skeletal-Salt Hormones

Parathyroid hormone and calcitonin act in antagonism to maintain a normal serum calcium concentration, the normal renal excretion of phosphate, and the mass of calcified bone matrix. There is no direct evidence at present that trauma itself alters the activity or concentration of these hormones, although methods are now at hand to make possible such observations. Parathyroid hormone raises the serum calcium concentration and lowers the phosphate concentration by decreasing renal tubular phosphate absorption, mobilizing calcium from bone, and increasing the kinetic transport of calcium across the gastrointestinal mucous membrane. Calcitonin—a product of the interstitial cells of the thyroid—acts to lower the serum calcium concentration by direct action in depositing calcium in bone. It would be attractive to postulate that the repair of fractures, or the prevention of osteoporosis during prolonged immobilization, elicits a response of these two balancing hormones so as to favor the repair or maintenance of skeletal integrity. Up to this time there are no data as yet available to settle the question of systematic alterations in these hormones after injury. It has recently been demonstrated that the administration of intravenous nourishment, including glucose and amino acids, lowers the serum phosphate concentration to very low

values, in some cases. Gastrin, by contrast, stimulates calcitonin production, while hypercalcemia stimulates gastrin production and gastric hydrochloric acid secretion. When to this is added the fact that skeletal salt mobilization increases body buffers and is a response to acidosis, we glimpse a new set of interrelationships between the stomach, the parathyroids, and the skeleton that bear not only on calcification and gastric digestion, but also on neutrality regulation.

9. Other Endocrine Mechanisms: the Liver and Cyclic AMP*

In patients with pre-existent liver disease, or after prolonged low flow conditions, liver function is impaired by injury. In such cases one might expect that the activity of hormones predominantly conjugated or inactivated in the liver would be accentuated. This is especially true of aldosterone, antidiuretic hormone, and estrogens. In certain surgical patients, therefore, inability to excrete salt and water and decreased androgenic appearances may both be assigned, at least

---

*See reference 29 for a recent review of cyclic adenosine monophosphate metabolism.

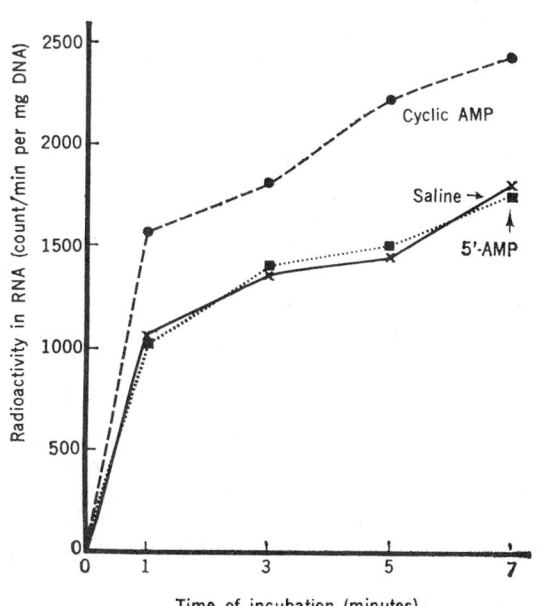

Figure 20. This chart demonstrates experimental data illustrating the mechanism by which cyclic AMP may act in the cell. In this experiment cyclic AMP has been injected into rats prior to analysis of liver nuclei for RNA synthesis. It is evident that in those animals given cyclic AMP the compound has resulted in an increased synthesis of RNA. In those animals given saline as a control, or an analogous compound, 5'-AMP, there has been no comparable rise. The authors conclude that cyclic AMP hastens the induction of enzyme synthesis, and thus of cellular activity, through an increased rate of gene transcription at the DNA-RNA step.

Although suggestive changes in AMP activity after injury have been reported, and although several of the hormones activated by trauma stimulate this "second messenger," it is premature at this time to indicate which tissues show increased gene transcription, activated by cyclic AMP, after injury. (From Dokas, D. F., and Kleinsmith, L. J.: Science, 172:1237, 1971. With permission.)

in part, to alterations in liver function, as well as to intrinsic changes in the secretion of water- and salt-conserving hormones and androgens.

Many hormones are low molecular weight polypeptides or small proteins (including insulin, ACTH, parathyroid hormone, thyrocalcitonin, thyroglobulin, and glucagon). These apparently act on the cell through a common effector mechanism involving a stimulus to the production of cyclic adenosine monophosphate (AMP) within the cell. Although the catecholamines and glucocorticoids are not protein hormones, they also affect the levels of cyclic AMP in cells. It is of interest that catecholamine stimulation of the alpha type decreases cellular AMP, while beta stimulation increases cellular AMP.

Cyclic AMP stimulates the cell to perform synthetic or metabolic functions at an increased rate. This mechanism has been of interest to cellular biologists as an example of a "second messenger system" or a final common pathway for endocrine actions. It suggests a possible mechanism for overlap of various hormone actions (e.g., aldosterone and deoxycorticosterones, growth hormone, and lactogenic hormone; epinephrine and norepinephine), and for the "permissive action" of other hormones. By the latter term is meant that a basal level of activity must be present (possibly providing substrates in the cell) before other hormones can act. An outstanding example of this effect is the basal requirement for the presence of glucocorticoids to enable appropriate actions of the catecholamines, insulin, or the lactogenic hormones. It remains to be seen whether severe injury, low flow states, or starvation materially alters the level of adenyl cyclase or cyclic AMP.

IV. COMPONENTS OF ACUTE INJURY*

Here, and in the subsequent four sections, will be examined briefly those particular features of injury that contribute to the endocrine and metabolic response. Both in clinical management and in research on the biology of trauma, it is of the greatest importance to distinguish between these various components and to avoid lumping them all together under the heading of "trauma."

1. The Tissue Wound

Some degree of tissue damage, a *wound*, is a common denominator in all surgical injury. This wound affects the organism in many ways, including local loss of blood and fluid, direct pain with efferent neural stimuli to the brain and endocrine organs, and release of cellular products to the circulation. A wound initiates catabolism, and a continuously open wound inhibits anabolism. A number of other aspects of local tissue trauma are mentioned here because of their particular bearing on the biochemistry and metabolism of the patient after injury. A detailed discussion of wound healing itself is presented in Chapter 12.

---

*Suggested background reading on injury components — the wound, volume reduction, starvation, and infection — will be found in bibliographic references 1, 27, 29, 31, 35, 38, 39, 44, and 53.

Most wounds heal to tensile integrity during the period of negative nitrogen balance. By "tensile integrity" is meant the restoration of sufficient tensile strength in the tissue itself so that artificial supports can be withdrawn. This can be noted by the removal of sutures from skin, in the function of gastrointestinal anastomoses, and in the healing of blood vessels or visceral suture lines. The restoration of nitrogen metabolism to the anabolic state — protein synthesis — is far more important for resumption of muscular strength and vigor than it is for wound healing *per se*. Virtually the only nutritional substance needed from outside of the body for the healing of the wound is ascorbic acid. Even here, storage mechanisms are such that deprivation of this substance for up to a month has no effect on wound healing if the subject has normal stores to begin with.

Hematomas and blood in the tissues are a common result of injury or surgical operations; such blood undergoes hemolysis, presenting the body with a load of porphyrin pigments for metabolism and excretion. If liver function is compromised, a mild increase in indirect-reacting bilirubin is observed. If renal function is compromised by maximal endocrine activity or low flow states, or both, the presentation of these pigments as hemoglobin, methemoglobin, myoglobin, or related compounds is nephrotoxic and plays a role in the production of acute renal failure. Blood in the tissues also provides increased urinary nitrogen excretion in an otherwise normal convalescent patient. One must make corrections for this in assigning the loss of nitrogen in the urine to muscle catabolism after injury.

Fractures initiate a series of wound healing changes that pursue a very long course. The restoration of tensile integrity requires many months, especially in major midshaft long bone fractures. Fractures often impose a greater need for strict immobilization. Fractures are therefore associated with larger alterations in calcium and phosphate metabolism than are other sorts of trauma; it has yet to be proved that this is due to any particular sensing mechanism on the part of the body that mobilizes calcium from one place to favor calcification in another. The early healing of a fracture does not involve calcification of collagen, and calcium changes in the fracture itself, after a period of acute bone resorption, are not observable for many weeks. In fractures, the final restoration to tensile integrity and weight-bearing strength occurs during the anabolic phase of convalescence. This is likewise the period of calcification of osteoid matrix, an event which, in a linear fracture, involves only a tiny amount of calcium as compared either with the total amount of calcium in the skeleton as a whole or with the negative calcium balance associated with either immobilization or parathyroid hormone stimulation.

In all wounds there is a continuous metabolic alteration in progress for many weeks, months, or even years after the healing process has reached tensile integrity. In a normal person these late changes occur during nitrogen positivity. The wound has a high priority in its demand on biologic substrates. It is notable that even in patients with late cancer undergoing palliative surgery, and in whom weight loss and negative balance of all nutrients (including negative calorie balance) persist up to the time of death, one commonly observes strong healing, and at autopsy a firmly cicatrized healing process. Conversely, the primary failure of wound healing identified as "wound dehiscence," in which almost no fibroplasia whatsoever is observed, is as apt to occur in the previously normal and healthy person undergoing surgery as it is in the nutritionally depleted patient.

These comments should not be taken to negate the value of increased feedings by mouth or vein in surgical patients in whom starvation is present either before or after the injury. At the same time, one must be realistic in the evaluation of such measures. The early achievement of positive nitrogen balance has never been proved to have any effect on wound healing per se. Certain laboratory animals, particularly the rat, are extremely vulnerable to total starvation, and show alterations after only a week or two of food deprivation that are of an entirely different magnitude than those observed in man after a similar time. As repeatedly emphasized in this chapter, the early loss of nitrogen after injury occurs from striated muscle and its restoration has to do with the resumption of muscular strength and work potential. It should again be emphasized that although the oncotic pressure of the plasma is almost wholly traceable to its albumin concentration, there is no systematic reduction in this concentration as the result of post-traumatic muscle catabolism and negative nitrogen balance unless, at the same time, the patient is treated with an overload of water and salt.

Burns constitute a prototype for wounds that cannot be closed for many weeks or months; they are chronically colonized and infected. So long as they remain open and uncovered, it is a rarity for the patient to pass into nitrogen anabolism.

We can therefore identify a further principle of surgical metabolism in relation to wound healing: *a continuously open wound inhibits protein anabolism and the resumption of convalescent growth.* Burns demonstrate this phenomenon very clearly. So long as the burn wound is open, discharging exudate, infected, and painful, the patient remains systemically ill with a tendency toward negative nitrogen balance. The negativity of nitrogen balance cannot be appreciated unless the nitrogen loss in the exudate is measured directly. When the wound is then healed by grafting or closure, a marked change occurs which is evident clinically, and which is associated with an increased readiness to assume nitrogen anabolism on relatively low calorie-nitrogen ratios by mouth or vein.*

---

*The concept of the "hypermature burn wound" came from observations that some patients with very late unhealed burns (up to a year or 18 months after the original injury) appeared to have grown fat and passed into an anabolic stage without healing the wound. It seemed as though the normal balance between an open wound and catabolic mobilization of substrates had been lost. The biologic priority of the wound had been dropped. The patient had progressed to a systemic state usually unassociated with a wound, that of muscle and fat anabolism. The organism was not diverting substrates for other purposes. In a few such instances the administration of ACTH, accompanied by a short period of starvation (to mimic the early trauma phase), has favored wound healing and skin coverage.

The early wound accumulates a protein-rich slurry of mucopolysaccharides, plasma albumin, and globulin. This is then changed to procollagen, and with the invasion of fibroblasts, collagen is formed and tensile strength gradually is resumed. In most soft tissue injury followed by normal healing without sepsis, tensile integrity is resumed some time between the seventh and the fifteenth day. Sufficient tensile strength has then been restored to permit resumption of function independent of sutures. This phenomenon is associated with a brisk nitrogen catabolism in the body as a whole; the early and most significant phases of wound healing are completed during the nitrogen-negative, calorie-poor phase. The provision of macronutrient cannot be demonstrated to hasten the normal curve of wound healing; it remains to be seen whether energy-rich phosphate compounds such as AMP (see earlier) will have any effect on the healing of clean or infected wounds.

The transmission of the message from the wound to the organism remains at once both obvious and subtle. The post-traumatic neuroendocrine and metabolic response appears to favor wound healing. Afferent nervous stimuli, blood loss, and infection all join to inform the rest of the organism that a wound or an incision has occurred, and initiate the appropriate systemic changes. Injuries in which nerve impulses are impaired, as in a denervated extremity or in diabetic neuropathy (or below the level of transection of the spinal cord), are notable for a lack of systemic neuroendocrine and metabolic response. Such wounds are notoriously slow to heal and the organism shows few changes of the post-traumatic metabolism.

2. Volume Reduction, Hypoperfusion, and the Low Flow State*

The confusion of injury with shock is a major point of difficulty in many writings on trauma. This major distinction is absolutely essential in consideration of the biology of trauma. Acute volume reduction of the type associated with ordinary injury is a nonlethal stimulus to which the body has normal and effective responses; changes in blood flow or tissue perfusion are minor and transient. By contrast, the state of prolonged hypoperfusion of tissue—"shock"—is a severe pathologic state. This is a prolonged deficiency of blood flow, or low flow state, which leads to gradual destruction of body cells, death of tissues through loss of substrate supply and oxygen during a period of continued demand, and ultimately death of the organs and of the organism.

The surgeon must therefore distinguish sharply between hemorrhage or fluid loss as a metabolic and endocrine stimulus incident to injury, and prolonged low flow states.

Some of the historic confusion between ordinary injury and low flow states arose from the employment by Selye of the term "shock" as mentioned in the historical introduction; he meant to use the term merely to indicate the sudden collapse to the organism of whatever type. Confusion also arose from the tremendous variety of animal shock models used in the laboratory,

---

*Suggested reading on low flow physiology and lacticacidosis includes references 20, 21, 26, and 52.

some of them far removed from anything seen in ordinary injury. Finally, confusion on this point arose from work with small laboratory rodents by some investigators who were quite unaware of the clear differences in man between simple compensated hemorrhage, or fluid loss, and a prolonged deficiency of blood flow or low flow state. The difference between the two is not easy to see in an injured mouse or hamster; it is quite obvious in man.

Because of this historic intermingling and confusion, we prefer to avoid the term "shock" altogether, and to distinguish between volume reduction as a normal traumatic stimulus and the low flow situation as a severely pathologic state.

The term *volume reduction* signifies reduction in the effective circulating volume of blood. This alters the renal handling of water and sodium, activates aldosterone and antidiuretic hormone, and initiates mass transport of fluid inward across the capillary toward the plasma volume. Even in cases of traumatic edema there may be inward traffic or fluid transport from the interstitial fluid to the plasma volume in uninjured areas. Because effective circulating blood volume can be reduced by so many different mechanisms, the term "volume reduction" is intentionally indefinite, requiring in the next phrase a specific definition of the mechanism.

The simplest and most frequent form of volume reduction is *simple hemorrhage*. Here there is no initial change in plasma total osmolality or tonicity; the serum sodium concentration is initially unchanged. It is therefore referred to as "isotonic volume reduction." The mass transport of fluid is across the capillary into the bloodstream: transcapillary refilling of the blood volume. This is associated with a drop in the peripheral concentration of red cells (as measured by hematocrit, hemoglobin, and red count), and a slight dilution of serum protein concentration. With loss of 1000 ml. of blood in an adult, the transcapillary refill requires about 24 hours.

Volume reduction can also arise from *acute desalting water loss*, as in vomiting, diarrhea, pancreatic fistula, uncontrolled ileostomy losses, intestinal obstruction, and so forth. Here there are changes in tonicity that result from the mobilization of cell water relatively free of sodium; in the initial phases of acute gastrointestinal fluid loss (as in cholera, for example), there is no change in sodium concentration, but within minutes or hours the sodium concentration falls. Osmolality changes are prominent and the biochemical changes are distinct from those of isotonic volume reduction due to hemorrhage or plasma loss.

Finally, the fluid loss may involve all the tissues of the body as in *desiccation-dehydration* (with hypertonicity) seen in excessive water losses from skin or lungs, in which virtually pure water is lost proportionally from all components of body composition. In desiccation-dehydration, hypertonicity is inevitable. Hypertonic syndromes can also result from the continued loss of large volumes of dilute urine in a continuous solute diuresis as seen in the tube feeding syndrome, untreated diabetic acidosis, or the provision of hypercaloric feedings by vein in a person with inadequate insulin coverage from his own pancreas.

By sharp contrast, the *low flow state* is defined as a situation in which hypoperfusion of tissues passes the boundaries of physiologic compensation, with alterations in the metabolism of all tissue cells as a result of anoxia. *Volume reduction of any type, if severe and prolonged, leads to a low flow state.*

The body as a whole, as well as the individual tissues, may be thought of as existing in a balance between perfusional supply of substrate with oxygen and metabolic demand determined by temperature and exercise. *This supply-demand ratio is the perfusion-metabolism ratio.* In a low flow state the perfusion-metabolism ratio is markedly reduced and deterioration of tissues is inevitable.

The key differentiation between simple volume reduction and a low flow state lies in the occurrence of cellular deterioration. This can be measured in many ways: by the deterioration of specific organs such as the brain or kidneys whose function is obvious; by the accumulation of intracellular electrolytes and enzymes in the blood and their excretion in the urine, or by the accumulation of abnormal pigments; by the patient's temperature and pulse rate; and by the blood level of catecholamines, all of which are far more elevated in a low flow state than they are in simple volume reduction. The production of prolonged severe tissue acidosis is characteristic of a low flow state. This is due to the intracellular accumulation of lactic acid. A rising lacticacidemia is therefore characteristic of the low flow state; any value over 5 mM. per liter may be considered as pathognomonic of a significant hypoperfusion of tissue somewhere in the body. Values for lactate that are elevated, but below this high level, may be produced by simple alteration of the oxyhemoglobin dissociation curve or by alkalosis, either respiratory or metabolic.

Low flow pathology involves a parallelogram of forces, each of the four corners being represented by one prime cause of tissue hypoperfusion, as follows:

1. *Volume reduction*—reduction in effective circulating blood volume: hypovolemia.
2. *Tissue injury*—traumatic or ischemic injury to tissue with direct killing of cells.
3. *Pump failure*—failure of the heart to maintain a forward output adequate for peripheral perfusion of tissues.
4. *Infection*—local cellular damage plus the release to the organism of the toxic products of bacterial growth.

An alteration in the weighting of any corner of this parallelogram will distort balance in the other three corners. If blood volume reduction is very severe, cardiac output falls, tissue deterioration begins (as evidenced by release of lactic acid), and infection, especially anaerobic infection, is much more apt to occur.

As a stimulus to post-traumatic changes in endocrinology and metabolism, prolonged deficiency of blood flow exceeds in intensity all of the other components of acute injury considered in this chapter. All of the endocrine and metabolic changes that form the body of this chapter are immensely exaggerated if the initial injury is sufficiently severe that a low flow state is produced. The treatment of "shock" is described in Chapter 3.

3. Starvation*

As mentioned in the introductory section, the studies of Benedict introduced to science an analysis of the metabolic kinetics of starvation. He laid the basis for many of our modern views of starvation. Investigators since that time have been concerned not only with the kinetics and endocrinology of starvation, but likewise with an attempt to compare the effects of starvation with the effects of surgical injury alone. If the surgical trauma is rather minor and followed by starvation of but short duration, as in an uneventful clean cholecystectomy or a simple gastrectomy without hemorrhage or infection, then the differences between starvation alone and the post-traumatic catabolism are minor.

Any person abruptly starved shows alterations in intermediary metabolism of protein, carbohydrate, and fat. There is an elaborate interaction between available glucose and the demands of the brain for 6-carbon sugars as its obligate and sole source of energy. There is mobilization of amino acids from skeletal muscle to provide building blocks for those sugars via gluconeogenesis, the mobilization of free fatty acids from depot fat (with recycling of glycerol), and the gradual (over several weeks) shiftover of the brain to an adaptive combustion of ketones. After several weeks almost all the urinary nitrogen is present as ammonia rather than urea.

These changes and their understanding are of central importance to surgery because all surgical patients who have undergone trauma of any magnitude are starving for at least a short time after the injury. In many cases, especially in cancer of the gastrointestinal tract, patients have been starving for many weeks or months prior to the operation.

Post-traumatic catabolism (as observed in a previously normal person, severely injured) has a number of striking differences from simple starvation. There is no more need to confuse the two than there is to confuse any two biologic processes involving similar metabolic systems. Examples of these types of distinction are found in the differentiation between postprandial hyperglycemia and diabetes, the differentiation between simple volume reduction and the low flow state, as just discussed, or the differentiation between convalescent anabolism and normal growth.

A list of the most pronounced differences between post-traumatic catabolism, as observed in a previously healthy person undergoing a severe trauma, and simple starvation is as follows:

1. *Rate of proteolysis and nitrogen loss* — in simple starvation the peak rate is about 5 to 7 gm. of nitrogen per 70 kg. per day; in post-traumatic catabolism similar rates may reach 15 to 25 gm. of nitrogen per 70 kg. per day.

2. *Changes in blood sugar and insulin* — in simple starvation the blood sugar falls and remains low throughout; after severe trauma it rises and has a pseudodiabetic curve for several hours or days, depending upon the nature and severity of the injury. In starvation the administration of glucose produces an immediate rise of blood insulin; while blood epinephrine levels are still high following injury, an elevation of blood sugar is unaccompanied by a rise in insulin concentration.

3. *Blood urea nitrogen* — in simple starvation blood urea nitrogen falls to very low levels (e.g., 3 to 5 mg. per 100 ml.), whereas after major injury the value is normal or elevated in all cases.

4. *Xanthine metabolism* — in simple starvation there is no change in the urinary excretion of creatinine save for a very gradual reduction as the body cell mass falls; there is an initial reduction in creatine excretion in the female. After severe injury there is a sharp rise in urinary excretion of both creatine and creatinine in both sexes; it appears for the first time in the urine in the male and disappears again in about 4 days. These changes in xanthines apparently have to do with muscle catabolism and are never seen in simple starvation.

5. *Calorie-nitrogen ratio* — in feeding after simple starvation the optimal calorie-nitrogen ratio for tissue synthesis is probably close to 100 calories per gram of nitrogen; after severe trauma the figure is much higher (the absolute level is unknown) and this elevation is one manifestation of the increased energy required for protein anabolism following injury.

6. *Endocrinology* — in simple starvation acute elevations of catecholamines, renin, angiotensin, aldosterone, antidiuretic hormone, and free blood cortisol are not observed. With prolonged starvation there is an evident renal conservation of sodium, starting at the second or third week (nicely shown in Benedict's charts), which we might assume was associated with aldosterone secretion even though this has not been sought or demonstrated. In trauma, the sudden sharp rise of all these endocrine values is a distinct point of differentiation from simple starvation. Differences in glucose and insulin have already been mentioned.

7. *Reversal* — of all these differences between the post-traumatic metabolism and starvation, the most striking difference is that revealed by efforts to reverse the process. Simple starvation is readily and immediately reversed by feeding; if food cannot be taken by mouth, a balanced intravenous infusion providing vitamins, amino acids, and an energy source such as glucose or fat will easily reverse the process. By contrast, after severe injury the ingestion of macronutrients by any route is accompanied by a markedly increased wastage in the urine, particularly of nitrogenous substrates. It is possible to administer them so fast that a positive nitrogen balance is achieved, but only at the expense of large nitrogen excretions in the urine which in themselves bespeak a most important contrast with starvation wherein refeeding is accompanied by improved nitrogen economy, and the ready achievement of zero or positive balance.

Despite these clear differences, starvation contributes an important component to the post-traumatic metabolism, especially when it is continued more than 2 to 5 days after the injury or operation. The present

---

*A review of energy requirements in surgery is found in reference 24; references 8 and 13 deal with oral and intravenous feedings, respectively. Studies of hormone interrelationships, insulin inhibition, and so forth, will be found in references 10, 11, 46, 47, and 48.

availability of "predigested" foods for oral administration when there is gastrointestinal disability and of balanced intravenous feeding mixtures represents a practical contribution of major importance in damping out the starvation component in the post-traumatic period. This is especially important in chronically ill patients with intestinal diseases, wounds, burns, or chronic sepsis.

4. Infection

Any consideration of the surgical patient must differentiate sharply between the *presence of microorganisms* (positive culture), *colonization* (the growth of these organisms over time), and *invasive infection* (tissue destruction with systemic response).

Humans are colonized throughout their skin, respiratory tract, and gastrointestinal tract (as well as the lower female reproductive tract) with a normal mix of microorganisms, including bacteria, fungi, and viruses. The same organisms introduced by continuous leak into a new area, such as the peritoneal cavity or the subcutaneous tissues, can produce local infection, abscess, and bloodstream invasion. This heightens the virulence of the organisms, by a process identified by bacteriologists as the effect of animal passage. When organisms of heightened virulence from one person are transferred to another, this is nosocomial infection even though the organism involved (for example, Staphylococcus or Pseudomonas) may be a normal inhabitant of persons without disease. By contrast, many pathogenic organisms are not normal inhabitants of the human body. These include the tubercle bacillus, meningococcus, gonococcus, and the spirochete of syphilis.

Any patient with an open wound will have colonization of that wound with the normal human flora. Even in clean incised surgical incisions of the type associated with orthopedic operations or herniorrhaphy, organisms are readily detected by positive cultures from the wound at the time of its closure in a high percentage of cases. Infection is rare.

In patients with burns, colonization of the burn wound with a healthy mix of normal skin and intestinal flora does not seem to be associated with clinical burn wound sepsis. When, as a result of cross infection or prolonged antibiotic therapy, this normal healthy mix of organisms is changed to monocolonization with any one organism of this same group, its virulence heightened by animal passage, a sinister alteration has occurred, invasive infection becomes inevitable, and outlook for survival is ominous.

The foregoing may seem out of place in a chapter on endocrinology and metabolism in surgery. It serves to emphasize the fact that colonization with microorganisms has almost no metabolic effect save for the synthesis of certain vitamins in the gastrointestinal tract and the maintenance of the normal odor of the skin and intestinal discharges. By contrast, invasive infection has profound effects on biochemistry and metabolism. Increased virulence and altered immunity play a role in the pathogenesis of invasive infection; the presence of organisms alone is not enough.

The local metabolic effects of infection are due to tissue destruction with cell death and the accumulation of a protein-rich exudate of leukocytes, immunoglobulins, and plasma, viewed externally as pus. These local effects can be quantitatively small in very severe infections that have marked systemic effects. In other cases, local systemic effects can be quantitatively massive, as for example in large infected wounds or burns, where the total nitrogen loss from the wound itself may equal or exceed that excreted in the urine, and the loss of whole protein may necessitate the repeated administration of plasma, albumin, or whole blood.

The systemic effects of infection greatly exaggerate the metabolic response to injury and when severe invasive infection is the primary event, the metabolic effects are almost indistinguishable from those of injury itself. In some instances the infection alone involves minimal tissue mass. Examples are urinary or gynecologic sepsis arising from instrumentation, infection from an intravenous catheter, or other cases of bloodstream inoculation. Here, the infection activates all the characteristic and metabolic alterations of trauma itself. Especially prominent are the catecholamine stimuli, with tachycardia, increased cardiac output, changes in peripheral resistance, and greatly increased catabolic lysis of muscle tissue. The muscle wasting of severe infection equals and often exceeds that of uninfected injury.

When severe injury is closely followed by invasive infection (as in septic fractures, visceral perforation with peritonitis, anaerobic infection in wounds, or early invasive infection of burns), the catabolic result is more severe than any other seen in surgery. This may reach levels of a kilogram of tissue per day, of which about two thirds is muscle tissue (approximately 73 per cent water) and one third is fat (accounting for about 2700 calories).

It has already been mentioned that the closure of an open wound is associated with return of the patient toward anabolism on progressively lower calorie-nitrogen ratios. The same gratifying change toward metabolic recovery occurs with the drainage of pus under pressure or with sudden defervescence following control of a bloodstream infection by surgical means (such as drainage or amputation) or by the use of antibiotics.

Severe and prolonged low flow states resulting from gram-negative infection have become loosely referred to as "endotoxemia" despite conflicting evidence on the actual or measurable amounts of endotoxin present. Bloodstream infection with any organism can cause hypoperfusion in tissues. The coliform organisms are especially prone to do this because their capsular lipopolysaccharides have marked vasoactive properties. In any event the organism should be accurately identified by culture, the infection should be treated, and undrained sepsis should be exteriorized. Until this is done, the catabolism of trauma will be greatly exaggerated and the anabolism of convalescence forestalled.

5. Drugs, Transfusion, and Emotional Stress

An injured vertebrate in the primordial environment either survives his injury or dies as its result, on the basis of his own protective responses. By contrast, the injured human being is without treatment for only short periods of time, and even in the military, self-injection of morphine or antibiotics may modify the patient's internal environment before he reaches the first casualty clearing station. Some understanding of the pharmacologic response to the various treatment modalities that we employ in injury and operation is therefore basic to an understanding of endocrinology and metabolism after injury. In this section, necessarily very brief, only a few of these chirurgenic factors will be listed.

a. Anesthetic Agents

This book is published during a period of wide swings of enthusiasm for various anesthetic agents. In the 1950s the use of intravenous barbiturates with muscle relaxants and endotracheal intubation replaced the widespread use of ether and other gaseous fat-soluble inhalation agents. This modality was then replaced by the use of halogenated hydrocarbons. Early evidence suggested liver damage from these, but a national study of "halothane" based on a search for lethal cases produced a negative result that proved, in retrospect, to be misleading. Had the investigators looked instead for mild cases of liver damage, they would have found a wealth of evidence. This was later found, and the use of such anesthetics became less widespread. These agents in turn have been replaced by a whole variety of agents, many of which are more hazardous (especially in inexperienced hands) than agents with which the physician has long been familiar, such as ether (the diethyl variety), intravenous barbiturates, nitrous oxide, and subarachnoid block with cocaine derivatives.

Because of this polypharmacy of his anesthesiologic colleague, it has become impossible for the surgeon to characterize in any simple terms the endocrine and metabolic changes in his patient due to the anesthetic itself. In general, they fall into three classifications:

1. *Specific endocrine effects*—examples are the stimulation of the adrenal medulla by ether, the stimulation of antidiuretic hormone by morphine, and the blocking out of afferent impulses from the area of trauma to the midbrain (with sustained diuresis until the anesthetic wears off) by spinal anesthesia.

2. *Specific organ damage*—examples here are the hypersensitivity lesions observed in the liver in certain persons repeatedly exposed to halothane; the effects on the heart of cyclopropane; the severe and continuing anomalous water loss in the urine (renal diabetes insipidus) produced by Penthrane; and the occasional epidural abscess or exacerbation of central nervous system disease produced by spinal anesthesia.

3. *Autonomic changes, blockade, or stimulation*—the effects here are too numerous even to give reasonable examples. Curare and the curare-like agents interfere with cholinergic activity at neuromuscular synapses throughout the body, and therefore interfere with venous return to the heart. The use of autonomic blockade to produce hypotension or of autonomic stimulus to produce vasoconstriction or support blood pressure has become a commonplace practice of the anesthesiologist. High spinal anesthesia interferes with all vasomotion below the level of the lowermost thoracodorsal input affected by that particular level of anesthesia. There can be disastrous falls in perfusion pressure at the glomerulus, the coronary ostia, or the circle of Willis despite the fact that cardiac output is maintained and the periphery is pink and vasodilated. Although pink vasodilated hypotension is far to be preferred to the vasoconstriction of a low flow state, the total perfusion of brain, myocardium, and kidneys is very sensitive to arterial inflow pressure in elderly persons in whom there is fixed vessel disease and significant luminal encroachment by atherosclerotic plaques. It is in this type of patient that unexpected hypotension under anesthesia—even if "vasodilated"—is followed by renal failure, myocardial infarction, and infarction of the brain.

In the words of Emerson, "In Nature nothing is given, all things are sold." The patient pays a price for insensibility to pain. The carping critic might explain the current tendency of anesthesiologists to experiment with multiple agents merely as failure to keep track of this physiologic price of anesthesia. The surgeon must also share responsibility for the desire to achieve speed of induction, ease of maintenance, rapid arousal, or some other highly specific clinical objective attained at an unexpectedly high pharmacologic price.

Drugs other than anesthetics must also be counted in the endocrine and metabolic mix. Large amounts of potassium penicillin salts can cause hyperkalemia and renal failure; morphine and most of its substitutes are markedly antidiuretic; with a fixed dose and fixed blood level of digitalis alkaloids, the effects upon the heart are profoundly altered by changes in certain ion pairs. It is quite a challenge for the surgeon of the present day to evaluate the totality of influences that bear upon his patient. A conscientious attempt to do so, even if it fails to consider every variable and every unknown, will nonetheless contribute to the patient's welfare.

A wide variety of mild sedatives and tranquilizers have become available. There can be little question that they are overused by the practicing physician in this country and prescribed for a whole variety of organic and psychologic ills. Some of them are remarkably treacherous in the surgical patient, in whom there are so many other acute metabolic events. An example is to be found in the prolonged administration of Valium (diazepam). If it is withdrawn for operation, a delirium tremens-like state can result, which is most baffling when observed about the fourth postoperative day in a person who has never consumed alcohol. Another example is acetylsalicylic acid, so useful in certain cases of arthritis or hypercoagulability, but associated with a bleeding tendency due to alterations in the adherence of platelets to collagen.

b. Blood Transfusion[29, 31, 35]

Blood transfusion is an abundant source of metabolic change. Two commonplace effects of blood transfusion are as follows:

1. Bank blood over 4 days old alters *oxygen transport*.[2, 7] This old blood is deficient in 2,3-diphosphoglycerate, adenosine triphosphate, and glucose, with excessively high levels of potassium in the plasma. Infusions of large amounts of this blood, therefore, tend to produce a left-shifted oxyhemoglobin

curve, with deficient delivery to tissues and an obligatory increase in cardiac output; hyperkalemia and hyperkaliuria can also result.

2. Aged blood is likewise rich in small aggregates of platelets and cellular debris large enough to produce *multiple small pulmonary emboli,* even when routine filtration methods are used. This contributes to the pulmonary insufficiency so notable following massive transfusion. While aged blood is undesirable in this regard, very fresh blood (i.e., freshly collected in plastic containers and administered within an hour) contains many immunologically competent lymphocytes that will mount a graft-versus-host reaction in the first tissue whose capillaries they pass. This tissue is the lung. The importance of this allograft histocompatibility phenomenon in blood transfusion is still poorly understood. It is evident that its severity will depend upon prior sensitization of the donor with antigens shared by the transfusion recipient.

The very rapid infusion of large amounts of *cold* citrated blood is in itself dangerous and sometimes lethal. The pathologic changes induced by sudden rapid infusion of massive amounts of cold citrated blood may be listed as follows:

1. *Hypothermia*—with a marked reduction in hepatic and renal function, loss of coagulation effectiveness, and a left-shifted oxyhemoglobin dissociation curve.

2. *Citrate toxicity*—with acute acidosis, calcium-binding tetany, and electrocardiographic changes of hypocalcemia progressing toward diastolic arrest. If this is tolerated and the citrate is oxidized, severe sodium bicarbonate loads result, with an increased tendency to post-traumatic alkalosis and cardiac arrhythmias.

3. *Thrombocytopenia*—the usual transient dilutional thrombocytopenia of banked blood (eventually platelet-free) is readily overcome. When the blood transfusion amounts to several exchanges in a short period of time, the bone marrow cannot keep pace and a dangerous thrombocytopenia results. This is differentiated from a consumptive coagulopathy by the absence of fibrin split products in the blood in the latter.

4. *Hyperkalemia and acute phosphoglycerate deficiency*—as already described.

5. *Multiple small pulmonary emboli or immunologic activity in the lungs*—as already described.

The incidence of severe pulmonary insufficiency can be arranged in an approximately linear relationship to the number of transfusions given. Such a finding is ambivalent as to interpretation: it is, after all, the severely injured person who needs the transfusion. Nonetheless the occurrence of severe pulmonary insufficiency after massive blood transfusions for bleeding ulcer or varices indicates that tissue trauma may be minimal and lung damage severe if blood transfusions are multiple and closely spaced.

Hepatitis is transmitted by blood transfusion. The virus, whether or not of the Australia antigen type, resides in the plasma. The use of washed red cell suspensions markedly decreases the hazard of hepatitis transmission.

c. Antibiotics

The systemic effects of antibiotics are poorly understood at this time, but they must be included as an almost universal accompaniment of surgical management in severe injury, infection, burns, and extensive operations.

There is evidence that *antibiotics are immunosuppressive.* This is traceable to two drug actions: first, by rapidly killing sensitive flora the antibiotics prevent the immune apparatus of the patient from "seeing" or making effective molecular contact with specific bacterial antigens. Secondly, certain of the antibiotics (particularly chloramphenicol) can specifically inhibit protein synthesis and produce leukopenia.

Antibiotics produce a selective change in flora. This is in part due to obliteration of sensitive strains, enabling the overgrowth of others. In other instances antibiotics favor the growth of resistant mutants and a molecular change in some organisms associated with the transfer of resistance to others of similar strains, formerly sensitive. Widespread severe infections with such organisms as *Candida, Proteus,* and *Pseudomonas* are in part due to the widespread and sometimes careless use of antibiotics.

Antibiotics can cause disorders of water and salt metabolism. This is most commonly due to continuous intravenous administration of antibiotics resulting in excessive water loads; some antibiotics are given as sodium and potassium salts and carry an unusual or unexpected salt load.

Antibiotics can cause specific tissue and visceral damage. These well-known reactions will not be listed here, since they would be more appropriate in a section on the treatment of infection. Ototoxicity, liver damage, kidney damage, and severe ulcerating colitis have all been recorded as dose-related responses to antibiotics, causing life-endangering or crippling damage. Leukopenia, blindness, and peripheral neuropathy, often on the basis of hypersensitivity, have been reported.

Finally, antibiotics may cause a surgeon to overlook significant local infection. The metabolic significance of this is inestimable. Undrained pus is one of the strongest stimuli to the lysis of lean tissue and the deterioration of the patient's visceral and muscular function. When antibiotics are mistakenly given instead of the needed surgical drainage, a severe impost is made on the patient's survival mechanisms.

As is evident from even such a brief enumeration, the biochemical, metabolic, and visceral effects of antibiotics must always be considered in evaluating the total response of the surgical patient to his injury and treatment. Antibiotics should be used with the greatest of care and, when properly used, are often life-saving. Nevertheless, it is difficult to avoid the conclusion that in the past 30 years, since the discovery of penicillin, they have been overused in surgical practice and have been responsible for many adverse reactions.

d. Psychologic Stress

Pain, fear of pain, and fear of disease play a role in activating adrenal medullary responses in many surgical patients. These factors can be minimized under the care of an understanding team of doctors and nurses, by staying with the patient or talking to him. There are many other psychologic factors that enter into surgical care today, often neglected by the surgeon or his assistants. These include the following:

1. *Fear of malignancy*—it is estimated that 30 per cent of patients having exploratory operations assume that malignancy has been found unless they are specifically told otherwise; this is true despite the fact that the finding of malignancy may have been the furthest thing from the surgeon's mind in undertaking the operation in the first place.

2. *Isolation from a normal ambience*—this is the "intensive care unit" syndrome. The playing of sweet Muzak in the distance is no substitute for normal persons, conversation, a diurnal variation of light and temperature, and, preferably, an outside view. If the patient is unconscious, these features lose importance.

3. *Lack of sleep*—this is particularly notable under the intensive care environment and with burned patients. It has been demonstrated that severe chronic autonomic stimulation becomes manifest if patients go for many hours without sleep. In badly burned patients the intentional induction of general anesthesia with intravenous barbiturates is sometimes required to give the patient some sleep. The rewards therefrom can be quite remarkable in lowered pulse rate, as one sign of subsiding autonomic activity.

4. *Cultural isolation and rejection*—many older people have lost contact with family, friends, and any meaningful social environment. Language difficulties and racist fears are commonplace. The lack of desire to cooperate or even to live often results in suicidal thoughts arising from this cultural isolation. Intelligent understanding of this problem can be of major assistance in avoiding such unhappy disorders in a hospitalized patient.

5. *Desire for death*—if a palliative period has come to an end in late malignant diseases, or if no palliation is possible for intelligent persons still possessed of their faculties, they will frequently adopt an attitude that hastens their demise. The mechanism of death here remains unknown, and has attracted the attention of both pathologists and mystics for generations. Its importance lies in the fact that if nothing further can be offered the patient, he certainly should be permitted this demise without disturbance.* Even if cardiac arrest or pulmonary embolism is the terminal event, attempts at resuscitation or stimulatory medication are inhumane.

---

*There has recently grown up a clerical subculture of theologians who exclaim against the habit of doctors—especially surgeons—of prolonging the death agonies of their patients, keeping patients unnecessarily alive, or "machine living." Clearly, a day-to-day decision is needed for each patient to decide whether or not continued treatment is merciful as well as feasible. It is my conviction that needless or unnecessary prolongation of the patient's life is far less common now than it was 25 years ago. Death in any form is not pleasant for either the patient or the family, and patients left alone die neither with dignity nor with a beatific expression on their faces. Nonetheless the avoidance of meddlesome interference and the use of large doses of simple medication can help both the patient and the family through this most difficult of all of life's experiences.

V. SEQUELAE OF INJURY: THE FOUR PHASES OF CONVALESCENCE*

Thus far we have been considering *acute* injury, its various components, and some of its visceral sequelae. In this section there will be summarized briefly the long-range dynamic course of the surgical patient through several identifiable phases of convalescence on to complete rehabilitation.

Recovery from injury is a dynamic process in which the patient rapidly changes and progresses, presenting each day a different clinical appearance and physiologic balance. An important component in the skill and experience of the surgeon comes in his understanding of the changing face of recovery from day to day. This is a wisdom often gained by years of experience. The expectation of dynamic recovery permits the surgeon to sense those important occasions in which complications or difficulties are signaled, not so much by any deterioration as by failure to progress or failure to thrive. Dividing the steady march of normal convalescence after severe injury into four phases is merely a convenient device for describing some of these dynamic appearances.

1. Acute Injury Phase

The many components of human biology and pathophysiology entering into the first phase of acute injury have already been described in detail in the foregoing pages.

Clinically, the patient tends to have a rapid pulse (often associated with the elevated cardiac output referred to earlier), feels ill or listless, often desires to sleep excessive lengths of time, if in pain requires medication, does not wish to be disturbed, often avoids strong lights, and, once he finds a comfortable position, will wish to remain immobile and undisturbed.

As in so many features of normal convalescence, it is difficult here to sort out the normal from the abnormal. There is no question that a smoothly done operation reduces the magnitude and duration of pathologic disorders in this first phase. With a minimum of tissue trauma there is minimal bleeding or hematoma left in tissue planes. Accurate restoration of body fluid volumes to normal, careful placement of strong sutures in soft tissue incisions, and adequate immobilization in bone injury all join to minimize pain, endocrine response, and total stimulus of injury. *The purpose of excellence in surgical technique is to diminish the depth and duration of the injury components in surgical operations;* excellence in surgical care diminishes the magnitude and duration of the endocrine and metabolic changes and reduces the likelihood of local or systemic complications.

In clean elective civilian surgery the operation initiates the injury. If surgical technique is meticulous and effective, the first phase of injury is minimized. After operations of the magnitude of colectomy, pneumonec-

---

*Additional background reading on the four phases of convalescence and some of the late rehabilitative changes will be found in the bibliography, references 8, 13, 30, 36, and 37.

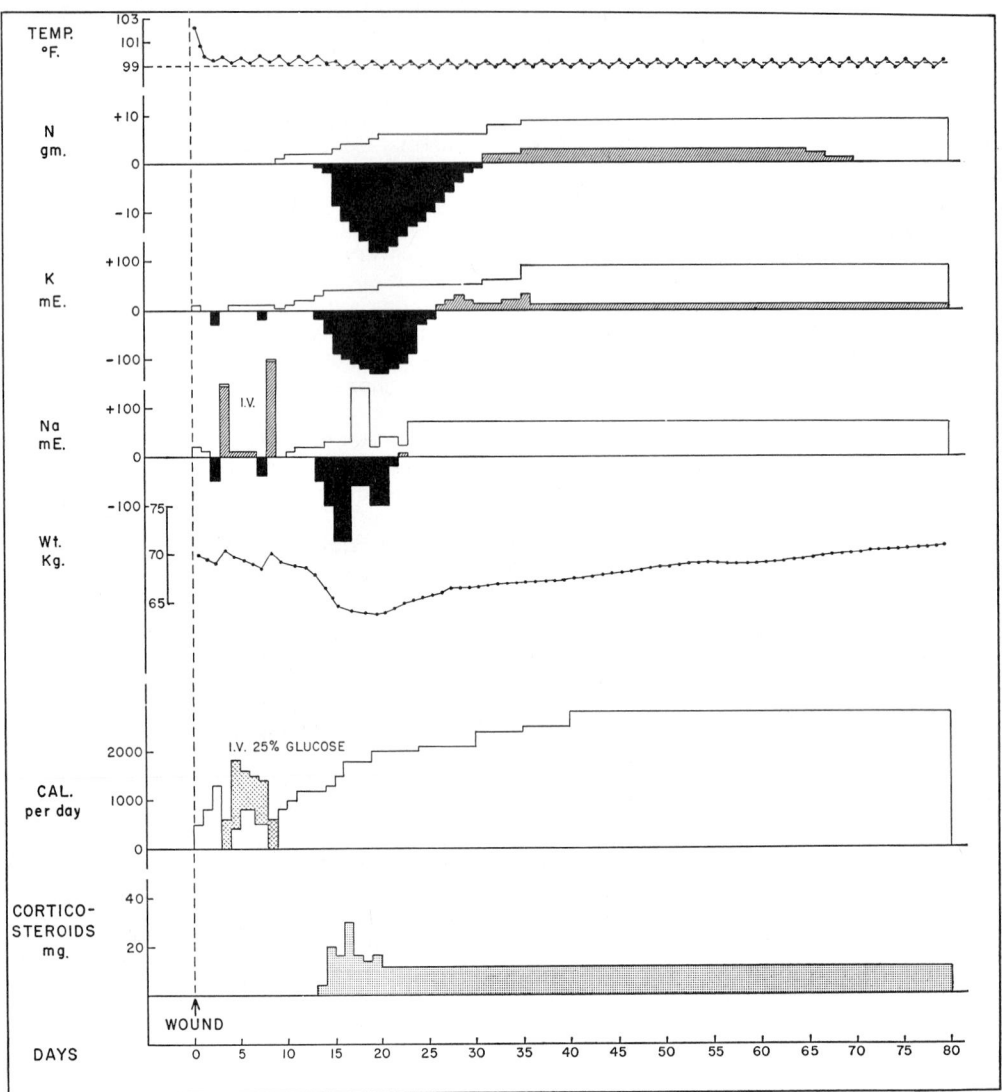

Figure 21. Metabolic chart in post-traumatic renal insufficiency. This chart, like that in Figure 6, is a normalized or "theoretical" metabolic chart of a patient with post-traumatic renal insufficiency, representing the average of many findings in a variety of patients.

It will be noted that during the anuric phase the patient loses weight but slowly, and positive sodium balances are readily attained. As urine output begins again (here shown on the eleventh day), nitrogen excretion begins and becomes very marked as the load of unexcreted catabolic nitrogen, represented only in small part by the blood urea nitrogen level, is excreted. With this nitrogen a load of potassium is also excreted, and there is a brisk sodium diuresis with loss of weight. This diuretic phase is shown here as lasting approximately 2 weeks, after which anabolism and normal salt excretions return. (From Moore, F. D.: Metabolic Care of the Surgical Patient. Philadelphia, W. B. Saunders Company, 1959. With permission.)

tomy, heart valve replacement, gastrectomy, pancreatectomy, or major limb amputations this first phase of injury lasts 2 to 5 days.

By contrast, in civilian accidents or military casualties, the injury initiates and the definitive surgical operation limits the duration of the injury phase. In military casualties and civilian trauma the purpose of operation is to permit convalescence to commence. The many steps of traumatic or military surgery include immobilization of injured parts, exteriorization of holed hollow viscera, control of hemorrhage, amputation of mangled extremities, débridement of large soft tissue wounds, adequate drainage, relief of pneumo-

thorax, and tracheostomy in injuries of the head and neck. These are merely examples of the many steps that enable the patient to be returned to the recovery room with the acute challenge mended, blood volume restored, and infection drained or obviated, so that the dynamic phases of convalescence can begin.

Body temperature is usually elevated after injury. Excellence of surgical and anesthesia technique reduces this fever to a minimum, with maintenance of perfect ventilation of all pulmonary segments. Most early postoperative fever over 100° F. is due to blood in the tissues or to small areas of pulmonary atelectasis—that is, presuming the absence of invasive infection. In 2 to 5 days (depending upon the nature of the trauma and the accuracy of volume restoration), the injury phase begins to draw to a close as the patient looks brighter, pulse rate and temperature are reduced, and he enters the turning point. Catecholamine responses have ceased.

2. The Turning Point Phase

This is possibly the most spectacular of the dynamic phases of convalescence observed after injury. It is characterized by a return of peristalsis, of expulsion of flatus, of appetite, and of a strong desire for food, diuresis, a renewed interest in surroundings, and a desire to see visitors, to read, and to "return to living."

While these clinical and external appearances are often quite spectacular, there is a metabolic change that is the most eloquent biochemical evidence of the turning point: a spontaneous reduction in urinary nitrogen excretion without change in intake. If the patient is being maintained on either constant or zero nitrogen intake, it will be noted during these few days that the amount of urinary nitrogen loss is sharply reduced. This is interpreted as meaning a reduction in glucagon activity, restoration of insulin to normal levels, and decrease of the catecholamine components; there is a decline in both the clinical and endocrinologic stress factors. Now, if the patient is given food either by mouth or by vein he will assimilate it in an avid way, reminiscent of simple starvation. The turning point is therefore associated with a dramatic alteration in the metabolic set of the patient, changing in a few days from the post-traumatic rejection of substrate, to the normal avidity for food and nourishment that characterizes the unstressed starving patient. Now is the time that the gastrointestinal tract as well as the appetite of the patient are ready for nourishment; muscle protein resynthesis will occur with great rapidity as the anabolic phase begins.

Like all aspects of convalescence, this clinical event has many causes and several effects. The lowering of pulse, sitting up, and moving around in bed, and increased interest in surroundings and food result also from the diminution in incisional pain that comes at about the third to fifth day. The final restoration of body fluid volumes to normal with the cessation of aldosterone secretion and the occurrence of a free diuresis is characteristic. The clinical appearances are unmistakable. The young woman who now seeks to restore her cosmetics has given rise to the term "positive lipstick sign" to indicate that the patient is rounding the bend and starting recovery normally; the man only asks for a newspaper, though he may think more tenderly of his wife or girl friend.

3. The Anabolic Phase

While the phase of acute injury has yielded the most metabolic and endocrine data, and the turning point is the most obvious and spectacular, this phase of positive anabolism is the most important in terms of the social, psychologic, sexual, and economic rehabilitation of the patient. It is for this reason that in the writings of the physiotherapist (and in much of the literature on "convalescence and rehabilitation") this is the only phase that is thought of as "convalescence,"

when in point of fact the two preceding phases set the stage for its occurrence.

The anabolic phase of convalescence is characterized by increasing strength, appetite, and food intake, normal absorption, and the occurrence of a prolonged positive nitrogen balance which is maintained until the initial nitrogen losses have been restored. Normal nitrogen anabolism occurs at the rate of 3 to 5 gm. of nitrogen per 70 kg. per day; it is possible, therefore, to predict the duration of this phase once the initial losses are known. When there has been a very massive injury, as, for example, in a civilian accident with multiple fractures and a ruptured spleen, the total nitrogen lost during the first phase may be as much as 75 gm. It is thus clear that the anabolic phase must take at least 15 days, and usually somewhat longer, since the maximal anabolism is not always attained early or maintained throughout.

The calorie-nitrogen ratio of intake required in the anabolic phase of convalescence is about 150 calories per gram of nitrogen.

It is during this period that the patient begins to regain muscular strength and vigor. Patients universally observe that their muscular strength and achievement, as in walking or climbing stairs or even riding in an automobile, are not as great as their anticipation or ambition. It is during the nitrogen anabolic phase that performance starts to meet expectation, and most patients are returned home.

Sutures are usually removed from elective clean soft tissue incisions during the turning point phase or immediately thereafter. As already noted, the attainment of positive nitrogen balance is not necessary for the healing per primam of ordinary wounds or incisions. Despite this reservation, there is a healing aspect of the anabolic phase, since large tissue defects and abdominal wall defects of the type associated with fistulas progress toward closure better during anabolism, with disposition of subcutaneous fat.

Little is known about the endocrinology of the anabolic phase in convalescent recovery. From current constructs of the interplay of hormones in the metabolism of body fuels, we would consider this to be a period during which both growth hormone and insulin are active, restoring nitrogen compounds to the synthesis of actin and myosin in muscle, maintaining normal blood sugar levels despite large intakes, and turning nitrogen compounds toward protein synthesis with a minimal urinary spill of urea.

Many surgical complications and disease processes inhibit normal nitrogen anabolism. If these are present or long-continued, anabolism will not occur and the patient cannot recover his social role. The commonest causes of this arrested anabolism are prolonged wound sepsis, unhealed wounds or burns, osteomyelitis, septic fractures, intestinal fistulas, chronic bronchopleural sepsis, and the continued rapid growth of cancer. In all such cases the patient does not recover; he does not convalesce. He must remain hospitalized or be discharged from the hospital to remain in bed at home or in a nursing home. *Positive nitrogen balance after injury, while not required for the healing of the wound per primam, is absolutely essential for the social rehabilitation of the patient.*

The amount of nitrogen laid down in muscle is determined by the genetic body composition of the patient, as well as his exercise requirements. If for some reason excessive exercise comes too soon—as in a person returning to work too soon after an operation—then nitrogen anabolism is slowed down by the diversion of calories to other purposes.

Weight gain during the anabolic phase is not spectacular. During the early days of the anabolic phase of convalescence the patient may actually still be losing some weight because of the diuresis of water and salt. As a general rule, about 30 gm. of lean wet muscle tissue is synthesized per gram of nitrogen retained for anabolism. It is thus evident that in a person with a maximal positive nitrogen anabolism of 5 gm. of nitrogen per 70 kg. per day, the weight gain will be only about 150 gm. per day, which would mean that it would take him about a week to gain a kilogram. This slow rate of gain is measured carefully. If the patient is doing well in all other regards, one must not be disappointed by the slowness of weight gain during this period. It is the gain in muscle protein and in strength that counts. During this time menses return; reproductive function is restored in both sexes.

4. The Fat Gain Phase

Following the return of nitrogen metabolism to zero balance (indicating that muscle mass has been restored and nitrogen retention is reduced to only that required to replace wear-and-tear losses), the patient continues to gain weight and remains in positive caloric balance if his work impost is not too great. He now gains fat almost exclusively. When there have been very large losses of weight, as in extensive multivisceral cancer operations, massive multisystem trauma, and military casualties, this fat gain phase may go on for several weeks or months as the normal stores of body fat are regained. It has been body fat that has provided the endogenous source of calories required for maintenance during the early post-traumatic period, and this fat is now restored. The provision of high caloric sources by vein (glucose or fat) in large amounts during the early injury phase has as one of its chief effects the reduction in the

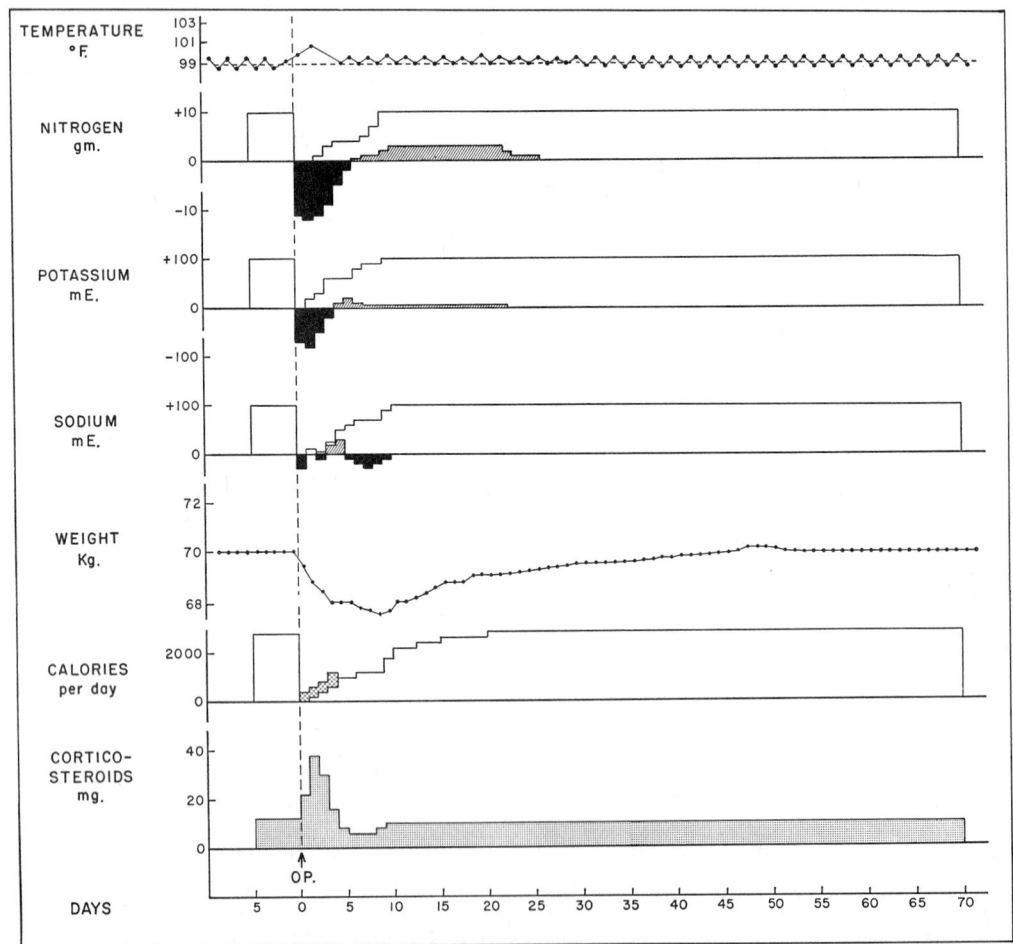

Figure 22. Illustration of the metabolic response to trauma of moderate severity. Transient loss of nitrogen at a rate slightly higher than that observed in starvation alone, a minor loss of potassium, and a transient positive sodium balance followed by a diuresis are the most striking features. After the twenty-fifth day, nitrogen anabolism has been completed, and the continued gain of weight is due to the redeposition of body fat. (From Moore, F. D.: Metabolic Care of the Surgical Patient. Philadelphia, W. B. Saunders Company, 1959. With permission.)

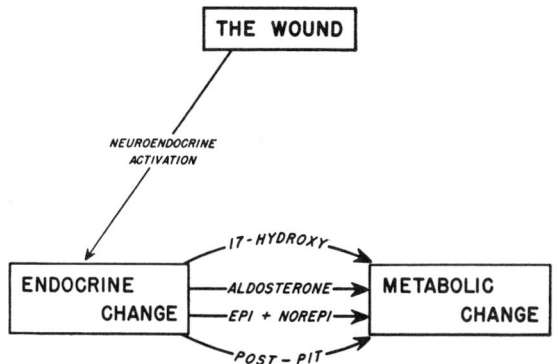

Figure 23. This diagram shows the presumed interaction between the wound, endocrine change, and metabolic change. The various aspects of this triangular relationship have been described in detail in the text. (From Moore, F. D.: Harvey Lect., *52*:74, 1958. With permission.)

obligate call on body fat stores for calories, and weight loss is minimized.

This tendency to regain weight after injury is most clearly perceived by the patient. For several months after his operation his clothing does not fit him even though he is back to normal activities and back to work. Then, over the course of several months he gains weight through fat accumulation and his clothes again fit normally.

If for some reason the patient passes into the fat gain phase but is denied adequate exercise, he may become overweight or even obese as this strong tendency to late post-traumatic fat gain expresses itself. This is especially seen in persons who are paralyzed, as with paraplegia or poliomyelitis, or immobilized because of multiple fractures or burns. Here we frequently see patients who become quite obese during their late post-traumatic period. Such obesity is un-

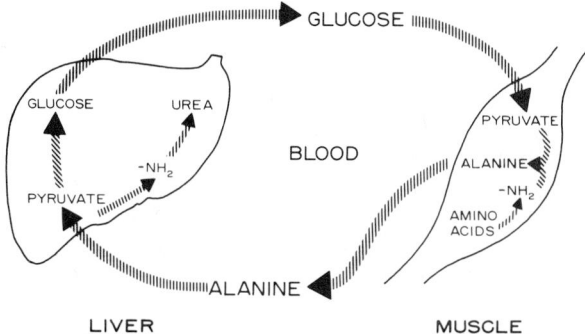

Figure 24. *The alanine shunt.* This diagram demonstrates the concept, supported by recent evidence from in vitro laboratory experiments, that alanine, a straight-chain three-carbon amino acid, acts as a carrier of amino groups from muscle to liver. This provides one of the mechanisms by which amino acids or other compounds are transaminated in muscle itself. Alanine provides a substrate from which urea is synthesized in the liver, and a recirculation mechanism by which energy-rich carbon fragments can return to muscle either for resynthesis into glycogen or protein, or for oxidation. In trauma, intravenous feeding, and starvation, this cycle is altered in rate according to the nature of the injury and the substrate provided. A small fraction of the nitrogen lost from muscle after injury occurs by this route. (From Moore, F. D., and Brennan, M. B.: Surgical injury. *In* Ballinger, W. F. (Ed.): Manual of Surgical Nutrition. Philadelphia, W. B. Saunders Company, 1974. With permission.)

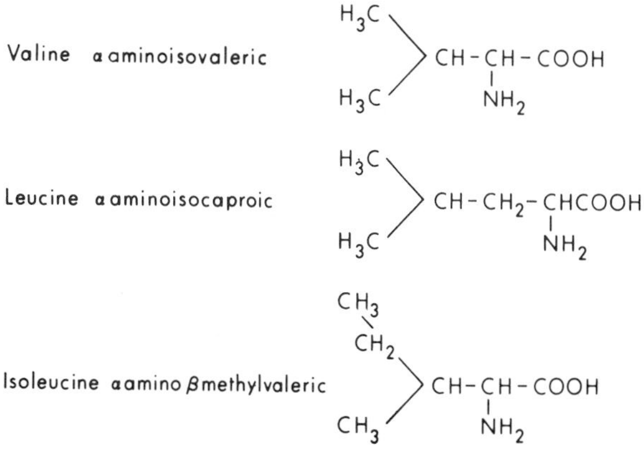

Figure 25. *The branched-chain amino acids.* Leucine, isoleucine, and valine are shown here. It has been known for many years that the shape of the carbon skeleton of amino acids is more important in determining their metabolic fate (as well as their utility in protein synthesis) than is the nature or position of their nitrogen-containing amino groups. The three branched-chain amino acids are of particular importance in surgical metabolism because they are lost abundantly from muscle in the stress phase after injury. Once lost they are irreversibly deaminated, oxidized, and excreted. When provided in the diet they appear to have a special protein-sparing effect. (From Moore, F. D., and Brennan, M. B.: Surgical injury. *In* Ballinger, W. F. (Ed.): Manual of Surgical Nutrition. Philadelphia, W. B. Saunders Company, 1974. With permission.)

desirable for the patient from the point of view not only of appearance, but also of ventilation, lipoprotein levels in the blood, and degenerative vascular disease. Some degree of dietary restraint should be imposed if normal work and exercise cannot be undertaken after post-traumatic anabolism is complete.

VI. SUMMARY

Although the interlocking events of surgical biology are complicated, they are also fascinating. They evidence the evolutionary adaptations postulated by Charles Darwin, the constancy of the *milieu intérieur* as conceived by Claude Bernard, and the autoregulation or homeostasis of bodily processes through the activity of the neuroendocrine system as pictured by Walter Cannon.

The surgeon is privileged to witness, at times to assist, and but rarely to modify these deeply ingrained responses of higher vertebrates such as his patients. At best the surgeon appreciates these processes and assists them, and at the very least he must understand them if he is to be competent in his service to the sick. If his operative technique is clean and effective, it will impose a minimal catabolic change in the patient's body composition.

As his reward, there is no more gratifying experience in all of medicine than for the surgeon to see a critically ill patient pass through the deep valley of challenge and catabolism, finally to emerge, climb the mountain of anabolic gain, and return to the peak of normal living with his wound healed, and his body composition restored so that he may fulfill the role in society offered to him by his genes, his schooling, and his motivation.

SELECTED HISTORICAL REFERENCES

Albright, F.: Cushing's syndrome. Its pathologic physiology, its relationship to the adreno-genital syndrome, and its connection with the problem of the reaction of the body to injurious agents ("alarm reaction" of Selye). Harvey Lect., *28*:123, 1942–43.

Albright knew from metabolic study that certain types of adrenal stimulation produced nitrogen loss, gluconeogenesis from amino acids, a diabetes-like state, and, given sufficient oral intake, an accumulation of excess body fat. Adrenal hormones could be measured in the urine, but not in the blood. Cortisone and aldosterone had been neither isolated, identified, nor synthesized. In this lecture he postulates that acute injury produces the transient state of hyperadrenocorticism resembling, at least for a few days, the metabolic abnormality of Cushing's syndrome. This lecture inspired many laboratories, including our own, to pursue this subject further.

Benedict, F. G.: A Study of Prolonged Fasting. Washington, D. C., The Carnegie Institute of Washington, 1915.

Benedict, long interested in metabolism, and a pioneer in the development of apparatus for the measurement of oxygen consumption and carbon dioxide production, perceived that in responding to the stress of fasting without thirsting, the human body would unmask and demonstrate many physiologic mechanisms important to survival, and of key interest in the interconversion of protein, fat, and carbohydrate. He had devised the first practical apparatus for the measurement of "basal metabolic rate" and by combining these gasometric measurements with biochemical studies in blood and urine, this book revealed data on the bodily economy of protein, fat, and carbohydrate that are an important basis for the understanding of problems of surgical patients, most of whom undergo a period of starvation during their illness. Like the work of Henderson, the studies of Benedict were so carefully done that half a century later they can still be profitably reanalyzed using the original numbers themselves in the light of modern body-fuel endocrinology.

Bernard, C.: An Introduction to the Study of Experimental Medicine. Translated by H. C. Greene. Introduction by L. J. Henderson. New York, The Macmillan Company, 1927.

Bernard's work, originally published in 1865, stamped a template for the physiologic study of whole organ systems, the whole organism, and chemical reactions within that body. Sixty years later, Henderson's book on Blood established a prototype for quantitative clinical investigation based on mathematical analysis of physicochemical systems. In his Introduction to the edition of Bernard's Introduction referred to here, Henderson described the influence of Bernard on himself and on a whole generation of physiologists. Bernard was born in 1813, and Henderson in 1878. It took 50 or 60 years for Bernard's teaching to reach fruition, whereas with the faster pace of modern clinical investigation, the effect of Henderson's book was much more rapid though equally profound. As mentioned in the text, the acceptance of modern quantitative chemistry and biology into the mainstream of surgery occurred as a result of the work of Bernard, Henderson, and Cannon, and then of their more modern offspring, including Van Slyke, Peters, Hastings, Gamble, and Albright.

Cannon, W. B.: The isolated heart as an indicator of adrenal secretion induced by pain, asphyxia, and excitement. Am. J. Physiol., *50*:3959, 1919.

Cannon, W. B.: Bodily Changes in Pain, Hunger, Fear and Rage, 2nd ed. New York, D. Appleton & Company, 1929.

Cannon, W. B.: The Wisdom of the Body. New York, W. W. Norton & Company, 1939.

Walter Cannon was responsible for many advances of interest in surgery, including the use of contrast meals for the study of anatomy and physiology of the gastrointestinal tract, and many other types of physiologic observations now made regularly on patients. He was also interested in the patient's record and several aspects of hospital routine. His main work was on the autonomic nervous system, and he viewed this as an autoregulatory mechanism for the achievement of homeostasis in the internal environment, originally conceived by Bernard as the milieu intérieur. Cannon was interested in stresses of both a physiologic and psychologic nature. He used the isolated cat heart as a built-in bioassay for catecholamines in the blood. He perceived that there were two basic types of autonomic response in the sympathetic side, somewhat analogous to those we would now identify as alpha and beta receptors; he also perceived the differences between sympathetic and parasympathetic responses. Later in his life he transferred these concepts of "the wisdom of the body" (as he entitled one of his later rather philosophic books) to the body politic, believing that people and nations should also have ways of internal regulation without strife.

Cushing, H.: The Pituitary Body and Its Disorders; Clinical States Produced by Disorders of the Hypophysis Cerebri. Philadelphia, J. B. Lippincott & Company, 1912.

This book was an amplification of Cushing's Harvey Lecture of 1910. In it he described many patients he had seen, their pituitary pathologic changes, and their neurologic, physiologic, and psychologic abnormalities. The syndrome later referred to as "Cushing's syndrome" was clearly delineated, and considered to be primarily a basophilic disorder of the pituitary. Cushing was America's first endocrinologist, and he was the leading pituitary endocrinologist of the world. Our later understanding of the role of the pituitary in activating the target glands, whether in starvation or in physical injury, and of the effect on bodily processes of pituitary hormones of all three lobes, must be traced to work of Harvey Cushing. Many physicians and endocrinologists have spent the subsequent 60 years elucidating the details of Cushing's syndrome, and from his analysis of the syndrome, Dr. Fuller Albright formed his theory on the endocrinology of physical injury.

Cuthbertson, D. P.: The disturbance of metabolism produced by bony and non-bony injury, with notes on certain abnormal conditions of bone. Biochem. J., *24*:1244, 1930.

Cuthbertson, D. P.: Observations on the disturbance of metabolism produced by injury to the limbs. Q. J. Med. n.s., *1*:233, 1932.

The work of David Cuthbertson, a Scots veterinarian nutritionist, is an example of the high level of scientific achievement that the British veterinary research establishment has achieved in their desire to improve agriculture in a small island, heavily populated. Cuthbertson described a brisk loss of nitrogen in rats after fracture. From this initial description grew 30 years of quantitative study, in man, of nitrogen metabolism after injury, and now, in the past 5 years, an elucidation of the mechanism of this loss through the effects of catecholamines on insulin production and the peripheral action of insulin.

Darwin, C.: On the Origin or the Species by Means of Natural Selection, or, the Preservation of Favoured Races in the Struggle for Life, London, John Murray, 1859.

In this book Darwin set forth his concept of the struggle for existence, and on the origin of species by the survival of the fittest members of that species, their fitness often being manifested by minor variations in bodily structure on which the process of natural selection could act. He also indicated the action of sexual selection on minor variations, resulting in marked sexual dimorphism in some species (i.e., the males and females having very different bodily habitus, skin, fur, or feather configuration). He considered the minor variations as being transmitted by heredity, and understood the meaning of an isolated gene pool though not in modern terms. He perceived that the struggle for existence included, necessarily, physical, thermal, nutritional, and combative injury, and that certain members would, by minor variations, be better able to survive such injury, thus passing the survival responses along to their offspring.

Gamble, J. L.: Chemical anatomy, Physiology and Pathology of Extracellular Fluid. Cambridge, Mass., Harvard University Press, 1952.

Gamble was a pediatric investigator who first systematized a way of analyzing the biochemical changes in extracellular fluid which results when the milieu intérieur of Bernard has not yet been restored to normal by the homeostatic mechanisms of Cannon. His clear and systematic way of dealing with this, including his particular illustrative way of diagraming the balance of anions and cations and his popularization of the milliequivalent unit of weight so as to make it possible to think of various ions in equivalent terms, helped to spread the working knowledge of extracellular chemistry from the laboratory to the hospitals of the country, and from the minds of the investigator to the awareness of all practitioners of medicine.

Henderson, L. J.: Blood. A study in General Physiology. New Haven, Yale University Press, 1928.

This book comprises the Silliman Lectures that Henderson, Professor of Biological Chemistry at Harvard, gave at Yale College in New Haven in 1927–1928. Henderson's predecessors in the Silliman Lectureship were Haldane and Krogh. He acknowledged his debt also to Barcroft, Warburg, and Van Slyke. He had worked in collaboration with Van Slyke and indicated his great indebtedness to Bock and Dill. In the Introduction to his book Henderson states, "The subject of this book is the red blood of vertebrates. We shall study this substance as a physical-chemical system and as a tissue, seeking in its properties the exemplification of some of the general characteristics of protoplasm. In its physiologic function and interrelation with other parts of the body, we shall look for an illustration of organic integration and adaptation. We shall also study it comparatively from species to species, in rest and activity, in health and disease. So far as possible these studies will be quantitative and mathematical."

This book was a milestone, being the first modern clinical investigation dealing with the living physical-chemical system in man on a quantitative mathematical basis. At the end of the book Henderson wrote, "The elementary conditions of the phenomena of life is a particular kind of physical-chemical system." In Henderson's book will be found quantitative data on blood chemistry which are still, 50 years later, being further elucidated by experienced investigators, or painfully relearned by the neophyte.

Moore, F. D., and Ball, M. R.: The Metabolic Response to Surgery. Springfield, Ill. Charles C Thomas, 1952.

This was the first publication from our laboratories delineating in man the changes described in animals by Cuthbertson, and adding to them a variety of measurements of fluid and eletrolyte change. We also tried to mimic the operative metabolism by adding a course of ACTH treatment to starvation in the normal human volunteer. This improved the resemblance to injury, suggesting that the latter metabolism was a combination of adrenal stimulation plus starvation. Had we further added an infusion of catecholamines to inhibit insulin production, increasing amino acid mobilization from muscle as well as fat mobilization, we might have come somewhat closer to the true "artificial production of post-traumatic metabolism." A method of charting metabolism after surgery was perfected which we and others have used since that time.

REFERENCES

1. Bartter, F. C., Liddle, G. W., Duncan, L. E., and Delea, C.: Role of extracellular fluid volume in control of aldosterone secretion in man. J. Clin. Invest., 35:688, 1956.
2. Benesch, R., and Benesch, R. E.: Intracellular organic phosphates as regulators of oxygen release by hemoglobin. Nature, 221:618, 1969.
3. Bergstrom, J., Furst, P., Noree, L. O., and Vinnars, E.: Intracellular free amino acid concentration in human muscle tissue. J. Appl. Physiol., 36:693, 1974.
4. Blackburn, G. L., Flatt, J. P., Clowes, G. H. A., and O'Donnell, T. F.: Peripheral intravenous feeding with isotonic amino acid solutions. Am. J. Surg., 125:447, 1973.
5. Brennan, M. F., Aoki, T. T., and Cahill, G. F., Jr.: The effect of insulin on glutamate uptake in the forearm muscles of postabsorptive man. Surg. Forum, 23:64, 1972.
6. Brennan, M. F., Aoki, T. T., Muller, W. A., and Cahill, G. F., Jr.: The effect of insulin on glutamate catabolic hormone. Surg. Forum, 25:72, 1974.
7. Bunn, H. F., and Jandl, J. H.: Control of hemoglobin function within the red cell. N. Engl. J. Med., 25:1414, 1970.
8. Bury, K. D., Stephens, R. V., and Randall, H. T.: Use of a chemically defined liquid elemental diet for nutritional management of fistulas of the alimentary tract. Am. J. Surg., 121:174, 1971.
9. Buse, M. G., and Reid, S. S.: Leucine a possible regulator of protein turnover in muscle. J. Clin. Invest., 56:1250–1261, 1975.
10. Cahill, G. F., Jr.: Body fuels and their metabolism. Bull. Am. Coll. Surg., Nov., 1970, pp. 12–18.
11. Cahill, G. F., Jr., and Owen, O. E.: Some observations on carbohydrate metabolism in man. In Dickens, F., Randle, P. J., and Whelan, W. J. (Eds.): Carbohydrate Metabolism and Its Disorders. London, Academic Press, 1958, pp. 497–522.
12. Clowes, G. H. A., O'Donnell, T. F., Ryan, N. T., and Blackburn, G. L.: Energy metabolism in sepsis. Ann. Surg., 179:684, 1974.
13. Dudrick, S. J., Wilmore, D. W., Vars, H. M., and Rhoads, J. E.: Long term total parenteral nutrition with growth development and positive nitrogen balance. Surgery, 64:134, 1968.
14. Duke, J. H., Jr., Jorgensen, S. B., Broell, J. R., Long, C. L., and Kinney, J. M.: Contribution of protein to caloric expenditure following injury. Surgery, 68:168, 1970.
15. Felig, P.: The glucose-alanine cycle. Metabolism, 22:179, 1973.
16. Ganong, W. F.: Functions of the nervous system. In Ganong, W. F. (Ed.): Review of Medical Physiology. Los Altos, Calif., Lange Medical Publications, 1963.
17. Gold, N. I., Smith, L. L., and Moore, F. D.: Cortisol metabolism in man: Observations of pathways, pool sizes of metabolites and rates of formation of metabolites. J. Clin. Invest. 38:2238, 1959.
18. Goldberg, A. L., and Odessey, R.: Oxidation of amino acids by diaphragms from fed and fasted rats. Am. J. Physiol., 6:1384, 1972.
19. Hammond, W. G., Aronow, L., and Moore, F. D.: Studies in surgical endocrinology. III. Plasma concentrations of epinephrine and norepinephrine in anesthesia, trauma and surgery, as measured by a modification of the method of Weil-Malherbe and Bone. Ann. Surg., 144:715, 1956.
20. Huckabee, W. E.: Relationships of pyruvate and lactate during anaerobic metabolism. I. Effects of infusion of pyruvate or glucose and of hyperventilation. J. Clin. Invest. 37:244, 1958.
21. Huckabee, W. E.: Relationships of pyruvate and lactate during anaerobic metabolism. II. Exercise and formation of O_2-debt. J. Clin. Invest., 37:255, 1958.
22. Hume, D. M.: The neuro-endocrine response to injury: Present status of the problem. Ann. Surg., 138:548, 1953.
23. Hume, D. M., and Egdahl, R. H.: The importance of the brain to injury in the endocrine response. Ann. Surg., 150:697, 1959.
24. Kinney, J. M.: A consideration of energy exchange in human trauma. Bull. N. Y. Acad. Med., 36:617, 1960.
25. Kinney, J. M.: A consideration of energy exchange in human trauma. Bull. N. Y. Acad. Med., 36:617, 1960.
26. Levin, J., Poore, T. E., Zauber, N. P., and Oser, R. S.: Detection of endotoxin in blood of patients with sepsis due to gram negative bacteria. N. Engl. J. Med., 283:1313, 1970.
27. Levin, N. W.: Furosemide and ethacrynic acid in renal insufficiency. Med. Clin. North Am., 55:107, 1971.
28. Liddle, G. W., and Hardman, J. G.: Cyclic adenosine monophosphate as a mediator of hormone action. N. Engl. J. Med., 285:560, 1971.
29. Litwin, M. S., Smith, L. L., and Moore, F. D.: Metabolic alkalosis following massive transfusion. Surgery, 45:805, 1959.
30. Long, C. L., Zikria, B. A., Kinney, J. M., and Geiger, J. W.: Comparison of fibrin hydrolysates and crystalline amino acid solutions in parenteral nutrition. Am. J. Clin. Nutr., 27:163, 1974.
31. Lyons, J. H., Jr., and Moore, F. D.: Posttraumatic alkalosis: Incidence and pathophysiology of alkalosis in surgery. Surgery, 60:93, 1966.
32. Meguid, M. M., Brennan, M. F., Aoki, T. T., Muller, W. A., Ball, M. R., and Moore, F. D.: Hormone substrate relationships following trauma. Arch. Surg., 109:176, 1974.
33. Meguid, M. M., Brennan, M. F., Muller, W. A., and Aoki, T. T.: Glucagon after trauma. Lancet, 2:1145, 1972.
34. Meguid, M. M., Moore-Ede, M. C., Fitzpatrick, G. F., and Moore, F. D.: Norepinephrine-induced insulin and substrate changes in normal man; incomplete reversal by phentolamine. J. Surg. Res., 18:365, 1975.
35. Miller, R. D., Tong, M. J., and Robinson, T. O.: Effects of massive transfusion of blood on acid-base balance. J.A.M.A., 216:1762, 1971.
36. Moore, F. D.: Metabolism in trauma. The meaning of definitive surgery. The wound, the endocrine glands, and metabolism. Harvey Lect., 52:745, 1958.
37. Moore, F. D.: Metabolic Care of the Surgical Patient. Philadelphia, W. B. Saunders Company, 1959.
38. Moore, F. D.: Volume and tonicity in body water (Baxter Lecture). Surg. Gynecol. Obstet., 114:276, 1962.
39. Moore, F. D.: The effect of hemorrhage on body composition. N. Engl. J. Med., 273:563, 1965.
40. Moore, F. D., Lyons, J. H., Jr., Pierce, E. C., Jr., Morgan, A. P., Jr., Drinker, P. A., MacArthur, J. D., and Dammin, G. J.: Posttraumatic Pulmonary Insufficiency. Philadelphia, W. B. Saunders Company, 1969.
41. Moore, F. D., Olesen, K. H., McMurrey, J. D., Parker, H. V., Ball, M. R., and Boyden, C. M.: The Body Cell Mass and its Supporting Environment: Body Composition in Health and Disease. Philadelphia, W. B. Saunders Company, 1963.
42. Moore, F. D., Steenburg, R. W., Ball, M. R., Wilson, G. W., and Myrden, J. A.: Studies in surgical endocrinology. I. The urinary excretion of 17-hydroxycorticoids and associated metabolic changes in cases of soft tissue trauma of varying severity and in bone trauma. Ann. Surg., 141:145, 1955.

43. Moore, F. D., and Brennan, M. F.: Surgical injury: Body composition; protein metabolism, and neuroendocrinology: Nitrogen flux and the effects of substrate provision; changing priorities of muscle and wound; anabolic convalescence. *In* American College of Surgeons Manual of Surgical Nutrition. Philadelphia, W. B. Saunders Company, 1975, p. 169.

44. Mueller, C. B.: Use of solute diuresis in the prevention of acute renal failure. Am. J. Surg., *114*:695, 1967.

45. O'Connell, R. C., Morgan, A. P., Aoki, T. T., Ball, M. R., and Moore, F. D.: Nitrogen conservation in starvation: Graded response to intravenous glucose. J. Clin. Endocrinol. Metab., *39*:555, 1974.

46. Owen, O. E., Morgan, A. P., Kemp, H. G., Sullivan, J. M., Herrera, M. G., and Cahill, G. F., Jr.: Brain metabolism during fasting. J. Clin. Invest., *46*:1589, 1967.

47. Porte, D.: A receptor mechanism for the inhibition of insulin release by epinephrine in man. J. Clin. Invest., *46*:86, 1967.

48. Ross, H., Johnston, I. D. A., Welbourn, T. A., and Wright, A. D.: Effect of abdominal operations on glucose tolerance and serum levels of insulin growth hormone and hydrocortisone. Lancet, *2*:563, 1966.

49. Schloerb, P. R.: Essential L-amino acid administration in uremia. Am. J. Med. Sci., *252*:650, 1966.

50. Shu'ayb, W. A., Moran, W. H., Jr., and Zimmermann, B.: Studies of the mechanism of antidiuretic hormone secretion and the post-commissurotomy dilutional syndrome. Ann. Surg., *162*:690, 1965.

51. Skillman, J. J., Lauler, D. P., Hickler, R. B., Lyons, J. H., Olson, J. E., Ball, M. R., and Moore, F. D.: Hemorrhage in normal man: Effect on renin, cortisol, aldosterone, and urine composition. Ann. Surg., *166*:865, 1967.

52. Smith, L. L., and Moore, F. D.: Refractory hypotension in man—is this irreversible shock? N. Engl. J. Med., *267*:733, 1962.

53. Stahl, W. M., and Stone, A. M.: Prophylactic diuresis with ethacrynic acid for prevention of postoperative renal failure. Ann. Surg., *172*:361, 1970.

54. Steenburg, R. W., Smith, L. L., and Moore, F. D.: Conjugated 17-hydroxycorticosteroids in plasma: Measurement and significance in relation to surgical trauma. J. Clin. Endocrinol., *21*:39, 1961.

55. Vinnars, E., Bergston, J., and Furst, P.: Influence of the postoperative state on the intracellular free amino acids in human muscle tissue. Ann. Surg., *182*:665, 1975.

56. Walker, W. F., Reutter, F. W., Zileli, M. S., Friend, D., and Moore, F. D.: Effects of infusion of norepinephrine on blood hormone levels, electrolytes and water excretion in man. J. Surg. Res., *1*:272, 1961.

57. Walker, W. F., Zileli, M. S., Reutter, F. W., Shoemaker, W. C., Friend, D., and Moore, F. D.: Adrenal medullary secretion in hemorrhagic shock. Am. J. Physiol., *197*:773, 1959.

58. Walser, M., Lund, P., Ruderman, N. B., and Coulter, A. W.: Synthesis of essential amino acids from their alpha ketoanalogues, by perfused rat liver and muscle. J. Clin. Invest., *52*:2865, 1973.

59. Wilmore, D. W., Lindsey, C. A., Moylan, J. A., and Pruitt, B.: Hypergluconemia after burns. Lancet, *1*:73, 1974.

60. Wilmore, D. W., Long, J. M., Mason, A. D., Skreen, R. W., and Pruitt, B. A.: Catecholamines: Mediator of the hypermetabolic response to thermal injury. Ann. Surg., *180*:653, 1974.

3

SHOCK: CAUSES AND MANAGEMENT OF CIRCULATORY COLLAPSE

Lloyd D. MacLean, M.D.

HISTORICAL ASPECTS

The word "shock," first used medically in 1743 by the unnamed English translator of Henri François Le Dran's *A Treatise of Reflections Drawn from Experience with Gunshot Wounds*, has been used for more than two centuries in all clinical disciplines to describe a progressive but gradual collapse of vital organ functions after injury or surgery. The initiating injuries seemed disproportionately small when compared with the effect on vital processes. Pathologic findings failed to supply a reasonable cause of death.

At the end of the nineteeth century surgeons recognized shock when they saw it. The definition at that time was descriptive and usually referred to post-traumatic or secondary shock. The observations of John Collins Warren,[81] Professor of Surgery, Harvard University, in 1895 are representative:

A patient is brought into the hospital with a compound comminuted fracture..., where the bleeding has been slight. As the litter is gently deposited on the floor he makes no effort to move or look about him. He lies staring at the surgeon with an expression of complete indifference as to his condition. There is no movement of the muscles of the face; the eyes, which are deeply sunken in their sockets, have a weird, uncanny look. The features are pinched and the face shrunken. A cold, clammy sweat exudes from the pores of the skin, which has an appearance of profound anaemia. The lips are bloodless and the fingers and nails are blue. The pulse is almost imperceptible; a weak, thread-like stream may, however, be detected in the radial artery. The thermometer, placed in the rectum, registers 96° or 97° F. The muscles are not paralyzed anywhere, but the patient seems disinclined to make any muscular effort. Even respiratory movements seem for the time to be reduced to a minimum. Occasionally the patient may feebly throw about one of his limbs and give vent to a hoarse, weak groan. There is no insensibility..., but he is strangely apathetic, and seems to realize but imperfectly the full meaning of the questions put to him. It is of no use to attempt an operation until appropriate remedies have brought about a reaction. The pulse, however, does not respond; it grows feebler and finally disappears, and "this

momentary pause in the act of death" is soon followed by the grim reality. A post-mortem examination reveals no visible changes in the internal organs.

The progressively deleterious effects of hypovolemia were not fully recognized by clinicians or even investigated at that time.

In 1899 George W. Crile[18] published the first extensive *experimental* study devoted principally to the solution of the problem of shock. These pioneering experiments were the basis for much of our understanding of traumatic and hypovolemic shock today. Crile noted that the animal in shock responded to intravenous administration of warm saline. He correlated this favorable response with an increased venous pressure, which in turn filled the heart. The heart beat more vigorously, and pumped larger quantities of blood, which, he reasoned, nourished the exhausted and starving vital centers, and improved oxygenation within the lungs. Crile should be credited with observing for the first time the most important characteristics of hypovolemic shock, i.e., failure of venous return, low central venous pressure, and the favorable response of the venous pressure to infusion, accompanied in turn by an increased cardiac output. He ascribed failure of this treatment, which occurred in many of his animals, to exhaustion of the vasomotor center.

During the first two decades of this century, the two principal theories to explain the phenomenon of shock were *vasomotor exhaustion* (which was believed to cause pooling of the blood in the great veins with failure of venous return) and *vasoconstriction* (with failure of blood flow to vital organs). In treating war casualties, surgeons had noted the pallor of tissues of patients in shock, the disappearance of peripheral pulses at a time when the femoral and carotid pulses were palpable, and the constriction of peripheral veins, which supported the latter concept.

The birth of the team approach for investigation and treatment of patients in shock occurred during World

War I, when American and British physiologists, as well as clinicians, led by Cannon and Bayliss[14] provided the opportunity to collect clinical descriptions by front-line medical officers, and to measure physiologic and biochemical phenomena in patients in shock. Parallel studies in animals were conducted at the same time. The data collected were interpreted and published in a classic monograph on traumatic shock in 1923.[14] While a wealth of information of great value exists in this volume, the final conclusion that a toxemia, possibly involving a histamine-like substance, was produced in the wound was misleading. The observations of Keith[37] and of Robertson and Bock,[66] which related the presence or absence and the severity of shock to deficits in circulating blood volume, were recognized but unfortunately believed at the time to be of secondary importance.

A most important observation by Cannon in 1918 was the correlation between *low blood pressure* and arterial blood *acidosis*. He postulated that the fall in alkali reserve was due to the accumulation of fixed acids, such as lactic acid, as a result of impaired oxygen transport. He noted improvement in patients in shock after the administration of sodium bicarbonate.[13]

It was known at the time that the blood volume was reduced in both clinical and experimental shock, without any indication of external hemorrhage. This observed fact raised the question, "Where in the body is the blood which is out of currency?" The shock team at Béthune in World War I noted a high capillary red cell count in patients in shock from trauma without notable hemorrhage. Of a series of 27 patients classified as having severe traumatic shock, all but one had a capillary red count of 6 million or higher, and in eight it was more than 7 million. It was not certain at the time whether the increased concentration of red cells was due to transudation of plasma or to slowing of the circulation from a diminished arterial blood pressure.[14]

Members of these early shock teams recognized a difference between blood flow and blood pressure in shock. In 1917 Archibald and McLean[4] noted that "while a low blood pressure is one of the most constant signs of shock, it is not the essential thing, let alone the cause of it. We have focused our attention far too much on blood pressure."

Cannon believed that the problem of shock still required the demonstration of some factor, naturally related to the onset of shock, which might so operate in the body that when hemorrhage and infection were ruled out, the persistent low blood pressure characteristics of the shock state would become gradually established. While working with Bayliss in London in 1918, Cannon[13] investigated the question of whether the acid known to be developed in injured tissue might be a contributory factor in the production of shock seen in man. They first showed that acid production was not an essential factor in the complex, and in order to establish in lower animals trauma similar to that giving rise to shock in man, the thigh muscles in the anesthetized cat were repeatedly struck with a blunt, wedge-shaped hammer, or crushed by compression. The trauma usually failed to break the skin, so

that infection from without was unlikely. The course of events was followed by observations of the pulse, respiration, alkali reserve, and corpuscular volume. After about 20 minutes (and still longer in the dog) the blood pressure began to fall, and a condition resembling post-traumatic shock in man ensued. It was known at the time that Dale and Laidlaw had been able, in 1910, to induce hypotension by the injection of extremely minute amounts (1 to 2 mg. per kilogram in the anesthetized animal) of histamine.[20] The view was taken that secondary shock was due to the action of toxins arising in injured tissues, and histamine was considered the specific offender.

Blalock,[8] and separately Phemister and Parsons,[61] challenged the theory of *toxemia* as a mechanism of traumatic shock, and, utilizing a model similar to that of Cannon and Bayliss, demonstrated that the shock observed after trauma to a dog's leg was due clearly to the accumulation of blood and plasma in and around the wound and throughout the tissue spaces far beyond the area of local injury. It was found that trauma of sufficient severity to cause low blood pressure produced extravasation of blood not only into the tissues of the thigh, but also into the loose tissues of the groin and flank. Therefore, amputation at the upper part of the thigh to demonstrate the difference in weight between the injured and uninjured legs as had been done by Cannon and Bayliss was shown to be inadequate. A wider dissection that permitted weighing the two halves of the lower body demonstrated that the blood and plasma lost into the traumatized side could easily explain the shock observed.[8, 61]

Blalock noticed that transfusion of blood from one dog, in which a low blood pressure had been produced by trauma to an extremity, to another dog, in which a low blood pressure had been produced by loss of blood either outside the body or into the tissues of the body, resulted in all instances in an elevation of blood pressure in the recipient rather than a fall. The intravenous injection of histamine caused definite alteration in the gallbladder. Trauma to an extremity did not produce these changes, further suggesting that histamine release was not a factor in traumatic shock.

During World War II several units were established to study battle casualties and air raid victims. Notable among these was a board headed by Beecher, which concluded that the major cause of shock was *hemorrhage and fluid loss*, which in turn led to metabolic acidosis when the condition was severe and protracted.[7] Table 1 summarizes some of the historical landmarks in our understanding of shock.

Definitions of Shock

The earliest definitions of shock were a clinical description of injury, a typical appearance, and if death followed, no suitable explanation at autopsy. During World War I, blood pressure was measured in battle casualties and shock and hypotension were equated.

During the 1960s, following the earlier clinical investigations of Cournand and Richards,[17] cardiac output was commonly measured in seriously ill or injured patients. A suitable definition of shock then was "decreased blood flow to vital organs." It became obvious

TABLE 1.   Some Historical Landmarks in Shock

1743   *Henri Francois Le Dran*—Shock is progressive deterioration following injury.

1831   *Thomas Latta*—First use of intravenous saline for hypovolemic shock.

1895   *John Collins Warren*—Shock is an adaptive response to life-threatening injury.

1899   *George W. Crile*—First extensive experimental studies of shock; defined dangers of hemorrhage, hypothermia, anesthesia, and fluid loss in surgical shock; noted value of measurement of central venous pressure in hypovolemic shock.

1908   *Yandell Henderson*—"Venous pressure is . . . the fulcrum of the circulation. Shock as surgeons use the word is failure of the fulcrum."

1917   *Edward Archibald and W. S. McLean*—"While a low blood pressure is one of the most constant signs of shock, it is not the essential thing, let alone the cause of it . . . we have focused our attention far too much on blood pressure, so much so as unconsciously to have come to regard it as almost causal."

1917   *W. B. Cannon*—Noted correlation between hypotension and reduction in alkali reserve. Postulated accumulation of fixed acids (lactic acid) due to impaired oxygen transport.

1919   *N. M. Keith*—The severity of shock is correlated with the magnitude of decrease in blood volume.

1923   *W. B. Cannon and W. M. Bayliss*—Organizers and leaders of first shock team. Best clinical descriptions and first battlefield measurements of physiologic and biochemical phenomena in patients in shock.

1930   *A. Blalock and D. B. Phemister*—Demonstrated conclusively that traumatic shock is due to hypovolemia. There was no suggestion of a toxic factor such as histamine as a causal factor in their well planned studies.

1943   *A. Cournand and D. W. Richards*—First measurements of cardiac output in patients in shock.

that one could have severely decreased blood flow with normal blood pressure. It was possible to follow patients who survived who had a very low blood pressure but a normal or elevated cardiac output.

During the 1970s, the definition of shock has again been altered because hemodynamic measurements on patients in shock due to sepsis frequently reveal a high cardiac output and low peripheral resistance.[9, 47, 74] These patients have many characteristics of shock, including elevated arterial blood lactate, hypotension, and oliguria, but differ from patients with hypovolemic or traumatic shock in that they frequently have warm, dry extremities and severe respiratory alkalosis from hyperventilation. They appear to have sufficient blood flow to the cells of vital organs but these cells fail to perform normally. Even oxygen uptake may be entirely normal despite vital organ failure.

A current *definition* to include all these possibilities is "inadequate blood flow to vital organs or the inability of the body cell mass to metabolize nutrients normally."

CLASSIFICATION OF SHOCK

A classification of shock based on our most recent understanding appears in Table 2. The purpose of any classification is to facilitate recognition and to promote correct and specific therapy as quickly as possible. This classification suggests that a hemodynamic diagnosis should be made as soon as possible, and treatment based on this started before a clinical diagnosis is necessarily established. The ultimate welfare of the patient will depend also upon excellent medical and surgical care directed to the clinical diagnosis. For example, it would be important to repair surgically a perforated duodenal ulcer in a patient in shock, but the recognition beforehand that hypovolemia is the cause of the shock and correction of it is of equal importance.

Aphorisms:

Never leave a hypovolemic patient in shock. Start restoration of volume before hematocrit.

Assessment of Patients in Shock

Eight measurements are extremely useful in the initial assessment and follow-up on all patients in shock (Table 3). Seven of the eight are readily measured in most hospitals. Only cardiac output is difficult to measure accurately. Fortunately, in most instances the information provided by the other measurements alone establishes a hemodynamic diagnosis.

The Important Relationship of Oxygen Saturation, Hemoglobin Concentration and Cardiac Output in Shock

The central problem in shock is the impairment and eventual failure of cellular metabolism. As will be emphasized later, it is believed that in hypovolemic and cardiogenic shock, cellular damage follows the development of a tissue oxygen debt due to low tissue perfusion.[45] In contrast, in shock due to a cellular defect,

TABLE 2.   Classification of Shock

I. Hypovolemic
 1. Blood loss
 2. Plasma loss
 3. Water loss
II. Cardiogenic
 1. Myocardial infarction
 2. Arrhythmia
 3. Tamponade
 4. Late hypovolemia
 5. Epidural and general anesthesia
 6. Pulmonary embolism
III. Peripheral Pooling
 1. Loss of tone in resistance vessels—spinal anesthesia
 2. Trapping in capacitance vessels—endotoxin shock in the dog
IV. Septic
 Failure of cells of vital organs to perform normal metabolic function despite availability of oxygen

TABLE 3. The Critical Hemodynamic and Metabolic Measurements in Shock

Primary Measurements	Normal Values	Secondary Measurements	Normal Values in Adult Man
Arterial blood pressure (B.P.)	120/80 mm. Hg	Pulse pressure Position change	40 mm. Hg 0 mm. Hg
Pulse rate	70/min.	EKG	Sinus rhythm
Central venous pressure (CVP)	5 ± 2 cm. saline	Pulmonary artery wedge pressure (PAWP)	5 ± 2 cm. saline
Cardiac index (C.I.)	3.20 ± 0.20 L./min./M.²	Stroke index	46.0 ± 5.0 ml./M.²
		Systemic vascular resistance	2100 ± 200 dyne-sec./cm.⁵/M.²
		Left ventricular stroke work index (LVSWI)	56.0 ± 6.0 gm. meters/M²
		Starling performance curves	
Urine flow	50 ml./hour	Specific gravity	1.003–1.030
		Urine to plasma creatinine ratio	> 20
		Urine sodium concentration	< 20 mEq./L.

Arterial blood pO_2
    pCO_2
    pH
	100 torr
	40 torr
	7.4
		Arterial oxygen content	19.0 ± 1.0 ml./100 ml.

		Arteriovenous oxygen content difference	4.60 ± 0.40 ml./100 ml.
		Oxygen consumption	140.0 ± 25.0 ml./min./M.²
		Alveolar-arterial oxygen content difference	< 100 torr
Arterial blood lactate	1 mM./L.		
Hematocrit	35–45%	P_{50}	27 ± 1.5 mm. Hg

as seen in many patients with sepsis, a primary cellular defect occurs that is often characterized by low oxygen utilization. The hyperdynamic circulation seen in many patients with septic shock is then a compensatory mechanism.

Nunn and Freeman[59] have quantitated the available oxygen in hypovolemic shock in the following way: Available oxygen = Cardiac output × Arterial O_2 saturation × Hemoglobin concentration × 1.34, which becomes

$$\underset{\text{ml./min.}}{1000} = \underset{\text{ml./min.}}{5250} \times \frac{95}{100} \times \underset{\text{gm./ml.}}{\frac{15}{100}} \times \underset{\text{ml./min.}}{1.34}$$

The body utilizes oxygen at approximately 250 ml. per minute in the resting state; this might at first glance suggest a large reserve. More specifically, the formula suggests that if normally 5 volumes per cent of oxygen is extracted from arterial blood containing 20 volumes per cent, a reserve of 15 volumes per cent remains. This supposition must be modified in two ways:

1. A certain partial pressure gradient is needed for transfer of oxygen from capillary to tissue, and below a critical partial pressure of oxygen in capillary blood

tissue hypoxia will result. The critical value may vary from tissue to tissue and, of course, with pH and temperature, but a reasonable range is approximately 20 to 30 mm. Hg. This corresponds to an oxygen saturation of 35 to 55 per cent. This in turn means that of the 20 volumes per cent oxygen normally carried in arterial blood, approximately 7 to 11 volumes per cent is unavailable to the tissues. Of the original 1000 ml. per minute of oxygen potentially available, only about 600 to 700 ml. per minute is actually available to the tissues when circumstances are ideal.

2. There is also a variation in oxygen uptake and requirements by different tissues of the body. While the overall oxygen uptake per 100 ml. of blood is approximately 5 volumes per cent, the chemoreceptors of the body have no measurable oxygen uptake, the kidney 1.5 volumes per cent, and the heart approximately 11.5 volumes per cent with little or no oxygen reserve.[59] Only a selective increase in coronary blood flow can prevent the heart from being the first organ to suffer in general hypoxia. This offers an explanation of why cardiac failure (inadequate cardiac output with high filling pressure) may supervene in certain pa-

tients with hypovolemia who have at first inadequate volume replacement, followed later by large volumes because of persistent or recurrent hypotension. Vigorous and quick volume replacement in the beginning would likely avoid the secondary form of shock, which is, from the hemodynamic viewpoint, cardiogenic.

Having established that available oxygen has a limited reserve and is dependent upon cardiac output, arterial O_2 saturation, and hemoglobin concentration, let us follow the calculations of Nunn and Freeman[59] for specific deficits. If any one of the three variables is reduced, the available oxygen is reduced proportionately. Therefore, if saturation and hemoglobin remain constant, a halving of cardiac output will halve the available oxygen and a small margin of safety still exists.

If two of the variables are lowered at the same time, the effect on available oxygen will equal the product of the individual changes. Thus, if cardiac output and hemoglobin are both one half of normal, the available oxygen will be reduced to one quarter, or 250 ml. per minute. This is a most dangerous level in critically ill patients and is compatible with life only for short periods.

If all three factors are moderately reduced, the effect on available oxygen will be great, since this will reduce available oxygen by a factor equal to the product of the three individual changes. Thus, if cardiac output, hemoglobin, and saturation are each reduced by one third, the available oxygen will be only 300 ml., a level that is rapidly fatal. For example,[5, 9] Available oxygen = Carbon dioxide × Oxygen saturation × Hemoglobin concentration × 1.34.

$$\frac{3500}{\text{ml./min.}} \times \frac{64}{100} \times \frac{10}{100} \times 1.34 = 300 \text{ ml.}$$

In this circumstance, none of the values is particularly alarming and all are seen individually with great frequency during shock and anesthesia. All three should be observed carefully and corrected in seriously ill patients before irreversible damage has occurred.

HYPOVOLEMIC SHOCK

(Low blood pressure, low cardiac output with low central venous pressure)

J. J., a college student aged 21 years, was run over one morning by a truck, and both legs were severely crushed. He became temporarily unconscious but was able to talk on the way to the hospital. Three broken bones were easily set; there was no visible bleeding, and after taking a sedative he felt well enough to smile and appeared to be on the road to recovery. In the afternoon, however, he became restless; his face showed an anxious expression, with pallor; his pulse became weak and rapid, his skin cold and clammy and his breathing labored and shallow; he sank into coma despite a 500 ml. blood transfusion and, toward evening, died.[32]

This boy, seen over 25 years ago and reported by Rhoads and Harkins, died of hypovolemic shock. In no form of shock has our ability to save life shown greater progress than in hypovolemic or post-traumatic shock.

To Archibald and McLean[4] in World War I, the clinical picture of shock was equally sharp: "a low tension pulse, usually rapid, shallow breathing, pallor, sometimes going on into a light cyanosis, lack of apparent suffering, carelessness as to one's surroundings, preservation of a clear though lethargic mind up to the very last." None of 17 patients admitted to a casualty clearing station in France with a systolic blood pressure below 75 mm. Hg survived. Saline, gelatin with saline, and, in three patients, 16 to 20 ounces of blood were given by Archibald and McLean for volume replacement at that time. In contrast, in Korea and in Vietnam, Howard and Brown[33] report that "pre-operative irreversible shock is not recognized, for, without exception, the blood pressure can be returned to normal in the pre-operative period if bleeding can be controlled. . . . Continued hypotension means continued bleeding or inadequate transfusion."

The course of an elderly patient seen in civilian practice with a crushing injury of both legs, with fractures of both femora and both tibiae and fibulae, is shown in Figure 1. The patient required 8000 ml. of blood over a 7-hour period to stabilize his vital signs. There was no external blood loss. The frequent use of chest auscultation was the only means available to avoid overtransfusion in this elderly, vulnerable patient. The need for a quick, easy method for guidance in blood volume replacement was obvious. Measurements of central venous pressure now make replacement of blood volume in hypovolemic shock rapid, easier, and safer.

Central Venous Pressure

Central venous pressure (CVP) is the function of four measurable and independent forces: the volume of blood in the central veins; the distensibility and contractility of the right heart chambers; venomotor activity in the central veins; and intrathoracic pressure. If one can rule out abnormal causes of elevated intrathoracic pressure, e.g., hemothorax, the CVP reflects principally the volume of blood returning to the heart and the ability of both the right and left ventricles to propel it. One is impressed with the great value of serial measurements of the CVP and the advantages of this over individual or serial measurements of blood volume. Figure 2 summarizes a comparison in 16 patients of the normal blood volume and the effective blood volume after treatment for hypovolemic shock at a time when blood pressure, urine flow, and tissue perfusion had returned to normal. The effective blood volume exceeded the normal blood volume in all these patients soon after the correction of hypovolemic shock. The CVP at that time was between 10 and 20 cm. H_2O in all patients and between 10 and 15 cm. H_2O in 15 of the 16 patients. In some, the data suggest that the measurement of blood volume would persuade one not to transfuse at a time when the patient required a greater volume and thereby would be misleading rather than helpful.

The late recognition of hypovolemic shock or inadequate volume replacement can lead to another syndrome even in young adults without a history of cardiac disease. Hypovolemic shock, seen early, is characterized by a low CVP, low blood pressure, low cardiac output, and high peripheral resistance, all of which respond favorably to adequate and rapid volume

77 YR. W.M. – Fx FEMORA, TIBIA & FIBULA – BILATERALLY

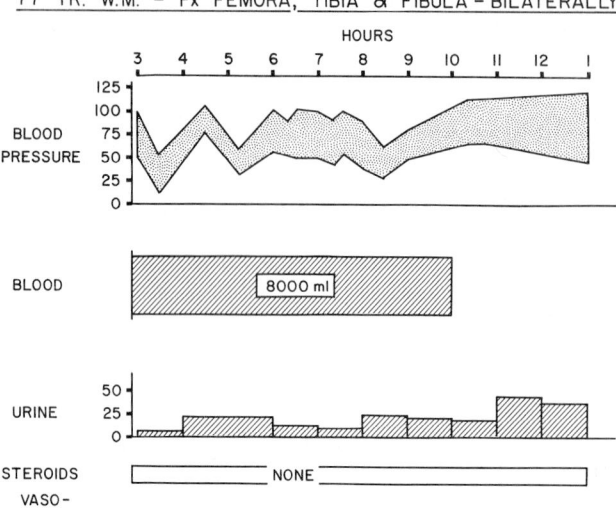

Figure 1. Favorable clinical response to 16 units of blood in an elderly patient in post-traumatic shock in whom there was no external blood loss. The amount of blood necessary to achieve hemodynamic stability frequently exceeds the anticipated amount. (From MacLean, L. D., et al.: Can. Med. Assoc. J., *105*:78, 1971.)

replacement. In contrast, inadequate volume replacement in the patient with hypovolemic shock can, when vigorous attempts are made to elevate blood pressure and promote urine output, result in a high CVP, low blood pressure, and persistently low cardiac output. At this point, the patient has cardiogenic shock (Fig. 3).

Pulmonary Arterial Wedge Pressure and Other Secondary Measurements in Shock

Although central venous pressure monitoring is of great importance, there are instances when the CVP does not reflect left atrial or left ventricular filling pressure. This discrepancy occurs most frequently in patients with a history of cardiopulmonary disease or with an unsuspected myocardial infarct.

Measurement of left-sided heart pressure is a better guide to volume replacement because the volume and distensibility on the left are less (Fig. 4). In patients being closely monitored we found a greater change in pulmonary artery wedge pressure (PAWP) than in CVP after a 500-ml. injection of saline over a 30- to 60-minute period. It has also been shown that the PAWP coincides very closely with the left atrial pressure when these two have been compared in patients in whom a catheter was placed directly into the left atrium at the time of surgery. The Swan-Ganz[77] flow-guided catheter serves admirably to obtain PAWP and in addition provides a means to sample true mixed venous blood and thereby to measure cardiac output by the direct Fick technique. The simpler technique of measuring cardiac output by thermodilution[82] is currently favored and is extremely useful. In the intensive care unit, a major goal of treatment for the critically ill is frequently the improvement of myocardial function. This technique is easier than previous methods and can be repeated at freqent intervals to assess therapy.

From the measurements of cardiac index and arterial blood pressure one can calculate systemic resistance. By knowing the pulse rate, the stroke index, and the PAWP, one can calculate the left ventricular

stroke work index (LVSWI). With the information assembled from repeated measurements of PAWP and LVSWI, one can plot a Starling curve of left heart performance as it responds to volume expansion, to intra-aortic balloon pumping, to inotropic agents, to the mixture of glucose, insulin, and potassium, or to any therapy designed to maximize myocardial performance. Using these techniques Weisel et al.[2] showed a marked difference in myocardial performance between

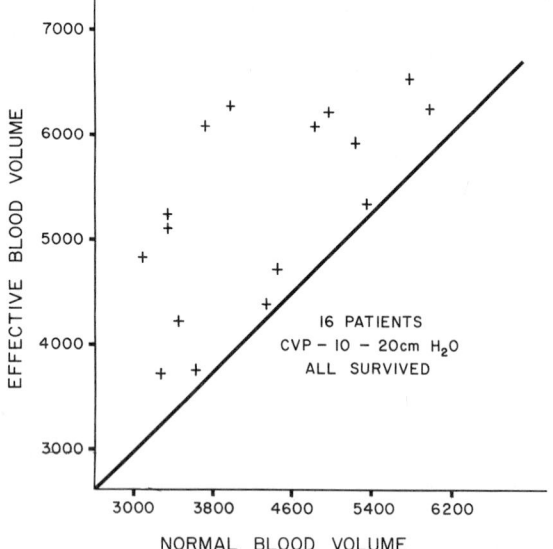

Figure 2. "Effective blood volume," or that volume which restored arterial blood pressure, urine output, and tissue perfusion, exceeds the "normal blood volume" for each of these patients in hypovolemic shock. The CVP is an excellent guide for replacement of effective blood volume, whereas the measurement of the blood volume can be quite misleading. With "normal blood volume" many patients will remain in shock with a low CVP. (From MacLean, L. D., et al.: Surg. Gynecol. Obstet., *120*:1, 1965.)

Figure 3. Patient E. C. presented for surgery with a low CVP, low cardiac index, high peripheral resistance, and normal blood pressure suggesting hypovolemia. With induction of anesthesia there was a marked drop in blood pressure and flow. Following the operation and after transfusion of three units of blood, the blood pressure was normal but the CVP was elevated, the cardiac index was very low, and the arterial blood lactate was elevated, all suggestive of cardiogenic shock. The patient had a cardiac arrest the following day, but she recovered. There was no evidence of myocardial infarction. Improperly treated hypovolemia became cardiogenic shock in this patient.

(Mrs. E.C., 75)	CARCINOMA OF CECUM				
• TIME	11:00 am	1:35 pm	1:37 pm	4:00 pm	
• TREATMENT	PRE-OP	PENTOTHAL ANECTINE CURARE	TRENDELENBURG POSITION	BLOOD ×3	CARDIAC ARREST (Next day)
• BP (mm Hg)	100/45	57/30	75/35	125/75	
• CVP (cm H$_2$O)	0.5	2.5	–	15	
• CO (l/min)	3.3	1.9	2.4	2.14	
• CI (l/min/M^2)	2.2	1.2	1.5	1.4	
• PR (dynes/sec×cm^{-5})	1475	1400	–	2950	
• LACTATE (mg%)	8.4	–	–	23	

patients with sepsis and patients recovering from open-heart surgery. In the former group, volume infusions induced a rapid rise in stroke work, which reached a peak at a low PAWP (10 ± 3 mm. Hg). In contrast, the heart patients had a slow rise in stroke work after volume loading and reached a lower peak at a much higher wedge pressure (17 ± 6.5 mm. Hg). The implications for therapy are obvious, especially since respiratory failure is related to volume overloading, particularly in the septic group.

Other secondary measurements (summarized in Table 3) that help assess the patient and his response to therapy include the pulse pressure, which is a measure of flow and may be greater with a low systolic pressure than with a normal systolic pressure accompanied by intense vasoconstriction. Normally, there is no change in blood pressure with a change in position of the patient. A rise with elevation of the legs or a fall with sitting suggests hypovolemia.

Pulse monitoring is essential for all seriously ill patients and patients being treated for shock. Arrythmias occur suddenly, must be diagnosed quickly, and are amenable to therapy.

Secondary measurements that reflect the adequacy of ventilation and oxygen consumption include arterial oxygen content, arteriovenous oxygen content dif-

ference, oxygen consumption, and alveolar–arterial oxygen difference. The treatment of shock is designed to deliver oxygen to the tissues that may require an increase in flow rate and oxygen content by increasing hematocrit or pulmonary transport. Despite all these steps, oxygen uptake in the periphery may not respond. Measurements of oxygen consumption can now be made with accuracy to document this abnormality.

Arterial Blood Lactate

Cannon in 1918[13] recorded a rough correlation between the severity or duration of hypotension and the decrease in carbon dioxide–combining power of the blood. Peretz et al.[62] in 1964 were the first to show, in man in shock, a close correlation between arterial blood lactate levels and survival. Their observations suggested that inadequate perfusion of tissues results in partial arrest of glycolysis at the anaerobic phase, with accumulation of lactate and other ions as a consequence of decreased tissue pO$_2$. Crowell and Guyton[19] showed that death occurs inevitably in dogs subjected to hemorrhagic shock when an oxygen debit of 150 ml. of oxygen per kilogram occurs, regardless of the measures taken.

There is no advantage in shock studies to measure "excess lactate," i.e., the disproportionate elevation of the level of lactate in relation to that of pyruvate. There is no correlation between blood pressure and lactate elevation, but there is a close correlation between the lactate level when the patient is first seen and the prognosis, as shown in Figure 5. Serial measurements of arterial blood lactate are of even greater prognostic importance and represent a valuable measurement to follow the adequacy of treatment.[73]

Some investigators have questioned the cause-and-effect relationship between lactate rise and tissue hypoxia or oxygen debt, and it is known that nonhypoxic hyperventilation will cause a marked elevation of blood lactate.[87]

We were surprised to find, in a recent study in dogs with shock induced by hemorrhage, cardiac tamponade, or endotoxin, that the elevation of lactate did not correlate with oxygen lack or decreased carbon dioxide production.[21] This study included measurements of lactate production and utilization, not just concentration, as well as oxygen uptake and carbon dioxide production. The conclusions, which must be confirmed in man in shock, were (1) there is an increased utiliza-

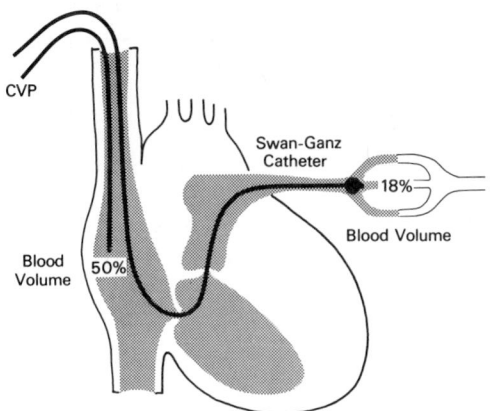

Figure 4. The central venous catheter in the right atrium "sees" 50 per cent of the blood volume. It follows that a greater change in volume will be necessary to effect a change in pressure than at the pulmonary artery wedge position. The latter catheter "sees" only 18 per cent of the blood volume.

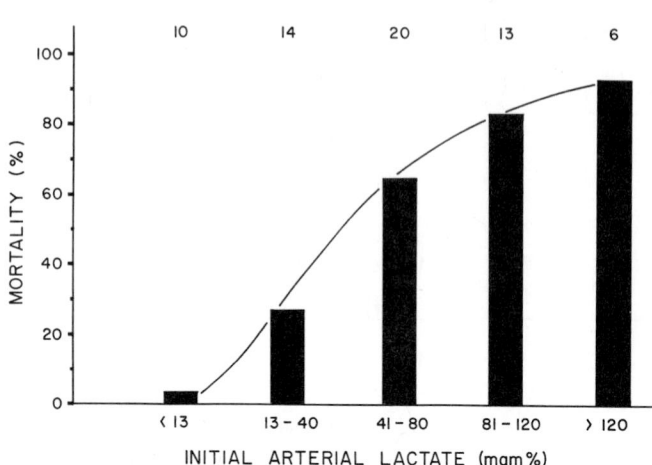

NUMBER OF PATIENTS = 63

Figure 5. Mortality rate and initial value for arterial blood lactate concentration in 63 patients in shock. There is a close correlation between the lactate level and prognosis. There was no correlation between blood pressure when the patient was initially seen and prognosis. (From MacLean, L. D., et al.: Can. Med. Assoc. J., *105*:78, 1971.)

tion and production of lactate in shock, even though both oxygen uptake and carbon dioxide production are normal; (2) there is decreased metabolic clearance of lactate; (3) there is abnormal substrate utilization, i.e., decrease in oxidation of fatty acids and increased metabolic breakdown and oxidation of liver and muscle glycogen and amino acids (Fig. 6). While an excellent guide to therapy, it is quite possible that in man the elevated arterial blood lactate may not reflect oxygen debt but a change in substrate utilization by the body. The body utilizes substrates (carbohydrates and amino acids) that pass through lactate and pyruvate to enter the Krebs cycle, and for this reason lactate is elevated. These data also suggest that specific nutritional support of the patient in shock may become of greater importance than was formerly believed.

Summary

Most patients with hypovolemic shock have a low blood pressure (under 90 mm. Hg systolic), rapid pulse (over 100), low CVP (under 2 cm. H_2O), low cardiac index (under 2.5 liters per minute per square meter), low urine flow (under 20 ml. per hour), near-normal arterial pO_2, increased arteriovenous oxygen difference, and a moderately elevated arterial blood lactate (20 to 30 mg. per 100 ml.) (Fig. 7). There is a dramatic response to rapid volume replacement, first with normal saline, Ringer's lactate, or buffered saline (44 mEq. of sodium bicarbonate in each liter of saline), followed by the fluid lost, which is usually blood or plasma. If bleeding can be arrested, and the replacement is prompt (the patient has normal vital signs within 1 to 2 hours of onset), the prognosis is excellent, even in the elderly. A comparison of these hemodynamic and metabolic phenomena with those in other forms of shock appears in Table 4.

The hematocrit is useful as a guide of what intravenous replacement to give rather than when to give it. Therefore, plasma and saline should be given for a patient with hypovolemic shock due to pancreatitis who might have a hematocrit of 60. This patient will improve, as evidenced by an increased cardiac output, urine flow, and blood pressure, and decreased pulse

rate, if the hematocrit is promptly lowered from 60 to 35 by saline alone. Conversely, the patient in shock with a bleeding duodenal ulcer who has a hematocrit of 20 will require blood. Maximal oxygen-carrying capacity is achieved with a hematocrit between 35 and 45.

In experimental animals the resistance to hypovolemic shock, produced by bleeding to a mean blood pressure of 30 mm. Hg, has been found to be greatest if the animal started with a hematocrit of 42 per cent.[6] The available oxygen reached its highest values at the same hematocrit. Resistance to hemorrhage and available oxygen both fell with higher or lower values.[6]

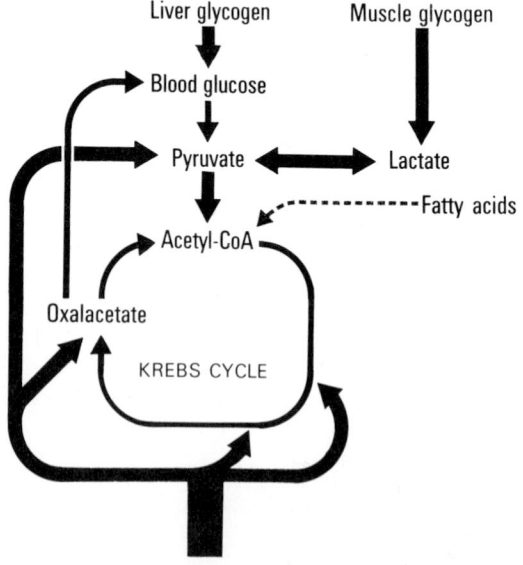

Figure 6. Probable metabolic pathways in shock which account for the elevated arterial blood lactate. The body utilizes substrates that pass through lactate and pyruvate to enter the Krebs cycle. Fatty acids are not utilized.

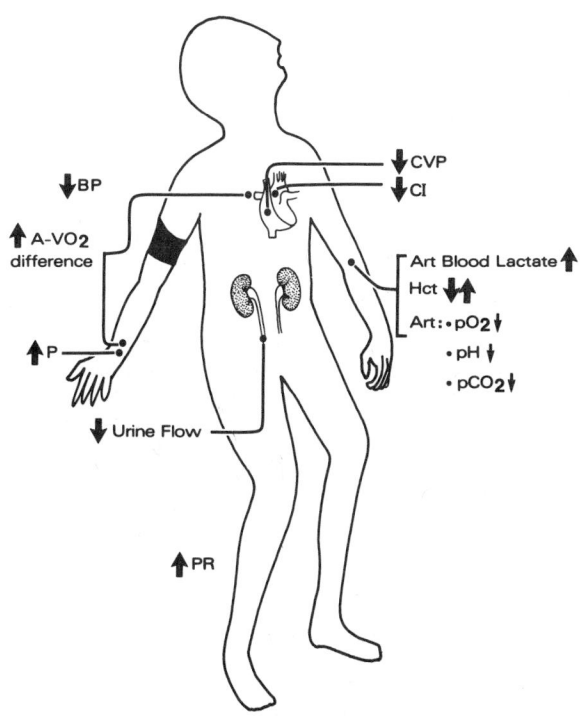

Figure 7. The principal hemodynamic and metabolic abnormalities seen in hypovolemic or traumatic shock.

A decrease in peripheral resistance is achieved by volume replacement alone in hypovolemic shock. The use of vasodilators for this purpose does not seem justified. The lowering of blood pressure induced by phenoxybenzamine in a hypovolemic patient will promote rapid volume replacement but does not seem necessary.

Aphorism:

Increased peripheral resistance is the result, not the cause, of shock.

PATHOPHYSIOLOGY OF HYPOVOLEMIC SHOCK

CARDIOVASCULAR RESPONSES

With the clinical characteristics of hypovolemic shock clearly in mind, the known and postulated un- derlying mechanisms should be reviewed. The cardio- vascular system is continuously regulated by the vaso- motor center in the medulla. This center is supplied with information via the ninth and tenth cranial nerves from stretch receptors monitoring pressure in the carotid sinus and aortic arch. A fall in arterial blood pressure produces a response predominantly through the sympathetic nervous system, which in- creases peripheral resistance by arteriolar constriction and cardiac output by augmenting the rate and force of cardiac contraction. The effective blood volume is enhanced by increased venomotor tone, which squeezes blood from large venous reservoirs into the central circulation. The sympathetic responses seen in shock divert blood from the extremities, bowel, and kidney to the more vital areas of heart and brain, the vessels of which constrict little under intense sympa- thetic stimulation.

Transcapillary Refilling

In the microcirculation, when capillary pressure falls there is a net movement of extracellular fluid into the capillary, restoring plasma volume. This phe- nomenon of transcapillary refilling is seen after mod- erate blood loss (up to 1500 ml. in the adult). Moore[41] has measured refilling at the rate of 50 to 120 ml. per hour until plasma volume is restored. Normal trans- capillary refilling does not produce hypoalbuminemia. With infusion of salt solution there is a simultaneous movement of salt and water out of the circulation and a net movement of albumin into the circulation. In severe shock, postcapillary venous pressure rises to the point where net capillary influx ceases. Both nor- epinephrine and angiotensin, known to elevate capil- lary venous pressure, also interfere with capillary refilling after hemorrhage. In experimental studies on cats, Mellander and Lewis found that postcapillary ve- nous sphincters maintained their state of vasoconstric- tion long after precapillary sphincters failed to re- spond to sympathetic stimulation. When capillary hydrostatic pressure exceeds plasma colloid pressure, there is a net loss of fluid from the vascular space into the interstitial space. This loss, in the experiments of Mellander and Lewis, occurred approximately 2 hours after continuous hypotension. Anomalous movement of water into cells is not required to explain the decreased plasma and extracellular water volumes after hypovolemia and trauma.

TABLE 4.   Hemodynamic and Metabolic Differences in Various Types of Shock*

	Blood Pressure	Pulse Rate	CVP	Cardiac Index	Urine Flow	Response to Volume Load	Arterial pO_2	Arteriove- nous O_2 Difference	Arterial Blood Lactate
Hypovolemic shock	↓	↑	↓	↓	↓	↑	↓	↑	↑
Cardiogenic shock	↓	↑ or ↓	↑	↓	↓	↓	↓	↑	↑
Peripheral pooling	↓	↑	↓	↓	↓	↓	↓	↑	↑
Septic shock (hyperdynamic)	↓	↑	↑	↑	↓	↓	↓	↓	↑

* ↑ increased; ↓ decreased.

ENDOCRINE RESPONSES

Shock and severe injury cause three main endocrine responses to maintain flow to vital organs and to retain volume.

1. Catecholamine discharge occurs from the adrenal medulla and from nerve endings throughout the autonomic nervous system. Catecholamine release is an important part of the primary reaction to injury, which assists man to maintain blood flow to the heart and brain. The best known hemodynamic effects are related to inotropic and chronotropic stimulation of the heart, constriction of the arterioles in skin, kidney, and viscera, a dilatation of arteries in striated muscle and the myocardium, and constriction of most veins. In addition to their vasoactive effects, catecholamines stimulate the production of glucagon, inhibit both the central production and peripheral action of insulin and accelerate muscle and liver glycogenolysis, and stimulate the production of ACTH from the pituitary. Catecholamines do not cause lipolysis in shock as in other forms of stress.

Insulin, "the banker hormone," which promotes storage of metabolic fuels, is inhibited during times of stress. Glucagon, "the spender," has actions diametrically opposed to insulin. Glucagon enhances production of glucose by the liver through breakdown of glycogen and gluconeogenesis. The lowered serum insulin or its decreased peripheral effect promotes amino acid mobilization from muscle and increases hepatic gluconeogenesis from amino acids.

Sharp reduction in blood volume is the prime stimulus to the production of norepinephrine from nerve endings; acidosis, hypercarbia, sepsis, and prolonged low-flow states are very strong stimuli for the production of both epinephrine and norepinephrine, which initiate the above-mentioned chain of hormonal events[70, 80] so important in fuel control.

2. Pituitary-adrenal-renal stimulation: Hypovolemia is a potent stimulus to aldosterone production by the adrenals. There are two mechanisms. ACTH is itself a potent stimulator of the adrenal production of aldosterone. The second mechanism is due to decreased renal blood flow, with a decreased pulse pressure that activates the secretion of renin by the juxtaglomerular apparatus. This stimulates the production of angiotensin, which directly promotes the elaboration of aldosterone by the adrenal. This has a pressor effect by conserving sodium bicarbonate and promoting the excretion of potassium.

3. Posterior pituitary stimulation: The restoration of plasma volume by retention of water is augmented further by antidiuretic hormone (ADH), which is released by increased baroreceptor firing due to hypotension, changes in plasma osmolality, and reduced left atrial filling pressure.

VISCOSITY

A good measure of circulatory adequacy is generally agreed to be the quantity of blood flow to the tissues of vital organs. Most emphasis has been placed on total blood flow, even though a large literature on the rheologic behavior of blood exists.

Replogle et al.[65] have described the interrelationships of viscosity, shear stress, and shear rate in a readily understandable manner. Newtonian fluids, such as water or saline, are those for which there is a constant relationship between flow and pressure (viscosity) regardless of the pressure or flow rate at which the measurement is made. In contrast, for colloidal suspensions such as blood, the viscosity varies with the flow (shear rate) at which it is measured. For this reason, at very slow flow rates the viscosity of normal blood in small vessels can increase 40 times over blood flowing rapidly in the aorta. If whole blood is defibrinated or if washed red cells are suspended in saline or Ringer's solution, Newtonian behavior is restored. When fibrinogen is added to these suspensions, they again demonstrate non-Newtonian characteristics. It is apparent then that it is fibrinogen and its effect on red cells that are largely responsible for the anomalous rheologic behavior of whole blood.

While it is apparent that slow flow and hemoconcentration will increase viscosity, and therefore decrease tissue blood flow, is there anything we can do at this time to render blood more Newtonian by means other than changing the hematocrit? Despite the abundant literature describing red cell aggregation in the microcirculation as a disease or a symptom of disease, it seems clear that the extent of "blood sludging" is a function of red cell–fibrinogen interaction and the extent of this interaction is dependent upon the concentrations of each. As the concentration of red cells increases, the contribution by direct red cell-to-red cell interaction becomes increasingly important. The combination of polycythemia and hyperfibrinogenemia is the worst possible rheologic combination.

The thesis that red cell aggregation and rouleaux formation depend, in fact, upon the net charge on the red cell is no longer tenable. Those treatments designed to alter red cell charge are likewise suspect. The extensive studies of Gelin[28, 29] demonstrated that intravascular red cell aggregation and blood viscosity were increased after various types of trauma. Gelin observed that the adverse rheologic effects of trauma could be reversed by the infusion of low molecular weight dextran (LMWD). There is undoubtedly dramatic improvement in circulation in various types of shock following the infusion of LMWD, but it should be noted that this effect is associated with hemodilution as well as fibrinogen dilution. If hemodilution is avoided by infusing the LMWD into a suspension of packed red blood cells, keeping the hematocrit constant, no effect on blood flow during hemorrhagic hypertension is observed. Further support for the idea that viscosity is directly related to red cell and fibrinogen concentrations is offered by the investigations of Branemark. This worker implanted transparent chambers into the skin of human volunteers under circumstances of a skin tube pedicle. Under these normal conditions there was no tendency for erythrocytes to adhere. When blood flow was reduced by compression of the pedicle, however, erythrocyte aggregation was seen in rouleaux formation. When flow was reestablished these rouleaux were quickly broken apart and washed away. Even when flow had been reduced for 3 hours there was aggregation but no tendency for agglutination. Under these conditions, elevated hema-

(Mr. J.F., 53)	PERFORATED DUODENAL ULCER		
• TREATMENT	PHLEBOTOMY	SALINE	
• TIME	10 pm	3pm	4pm
• BP (mmHg)	130/70	140/50	120/65
• CVP (cm H_2O)	20	14	5
• CI (l/min/M^2)	1.7	2.3	2.6
• PR (dynes/sec cm^{-5})	2050	1393	1300
• HEART RATE(beats/min)	100	120	110
• Hct.	73	–	59
• LACTATE (mg%)	27	–	20
• URINE FLOW (ml/hr)	0	10	83
• BLOOD VOL. (ml)	+1500	–	+800

Figure 8. Clinical and laboratory data from a patient who received a large quantity of blood despite a rising hematocrit, which resulted in a very low cardiac output, high peripheral resistance, and elevated arterial blood lactate. Phlebotomy alone was beneficial, but over a period of 7 hours the use of saline resulted in a significant rise in cardiac output, a fall in arterial blood lactate, and increased urine flow.

tocrit together with low flow, red cell aggregates appeared to plug capillaries and venules. Again, restoration of flow readily initiated breakup of the erythrocyte mass. Replogle[65] concludes that intravascular aggregation should at the moment be viewed as a result of diminished flow rather than its cause. This does not suggest that correction of a high hematocrit is not extremely important in the treatment of shock. The ideal range still appears to be between 35 and 45 per cent. The decreases in blood flow above this range and the increases below it are due to the effects of viscosity, and not due to vasoconstriction and vasodilation (Fig. 8).

RENAL RESPONSES

In hypovolemic shock, cardiac output falls, renal vascular resistance usually increases, and there is a reduction of renal blood flow. The decrease in renal plasma flow may persist for several days after cardiac output has returned to normal.[67] The striking finding is usually oliguria. If this is due to a diminished effective plasma volume, there will be a diminished glomerular filtration rate but increased renal tubular transport of salt and creatinine. This will result in a low urinary concentration of sodium and a high urine creatinine to plasma creatinine ratio.

In contrast, if the oliguria is associated with renal parenchymal destruction, the diminished glomerular filtration rate will exist with evidence of impaired tubular function as well. The urine to plasma concentration ratios for creatinine will be low, frequently less than 20, and the urinary concentration of sodium in excess of 20 mEq. per liter.

A common finding after major operations and trauma is an impaired ability of the kidney to concentrate the urine to more than 600 mOsm. per liter. Furthermore, a large volume is required in sepsis and trauma to excrete the increased osmolar load. Azo-

temia can result for this reason unless urine volumes are at least 1000 ml. per day in patients with sepsis and trauma.

Acute renal failure is the result of several concurrent factors: (1) a period of decreased rate of urine flow sets the stage for renal injury; (2) obstruction of tubules may result from precipitation of casts from a concentrated urine; and (3) trauma and sepsis are frequently associated.

High-output renal failure (large volume, high sodium, low U/P ratio for creatine) is frequently observed with sepsis. This may be related to the generalized vasodilation and increased blood flow seen in sepsis.[44]

INCREASED ARTERIOVENOUS OXYGEN DIFFERENCE

Cournand's pioneering hemodynamic studies in shock patients stressed a decrease in cardiac output associated with peripheral vasoconstriction.[17] Oxygen consumption was maintained in the face of decreased blood flow by greater than normal oxygen extraction, as judged by an increase in the arteriovenous oxygen difference. These findings also apply to exercise, in which condition it is known that oxygen saturation of mixed venous blood falls as soon as exercise is started, and that increased oxygen extraction enables the body to double the amount of oxygen available to the tissues without any increase in cardiac output. The extraction percentage for oxygen has been shown to increase approximately threefold in exercising subjects, and slightly more than twofold in patients with hemorrhagic shock.[31] Death in experimental animals in hemorrhagic shock has been correlated with total oxygen debt. This concept has not been confirmed in man. In septic shock in man there is frequently a wide discrepancy between the high cardiac output and low oxygen uptake, with a narrow arteriovenous oxygen difference.

TREATMENT OF HYPOVOLEMIC SHOCK

The eight measurements listed in Table 3 and the observed response to therapy present an organized approach to the supervision of patients in hypovolemic shock. If prompt infusion of 2000 ml. of crystalloid solution and 1000 ml. of blood in 4 hours to a patient with a fractured pelvis restores blood pressure and pulse to normal, elevates CVP from 0 to 5 cm. H_2O, the cardiac index from 2 to 5 liters per minute per square meter, lowers the arterial blood lactate from 40 to 15 mg. per 100 ml., the urine flow from 10 to 70 ml. per hour, the hematocrit from 25 to 35 per cent, the arterial pO_2 from 60 to 90 mm. Hg and the pCO_2 from 20 to 35, and the arterial pH from 7.21 to 7.35, the problem is under good initial control. Failure to accomplish hemodynamic and metabolic stability promptly has several hazards. The chronic low-flow state promotes vital organ failure of the kidney, liver, and heart in particular. While not proved in man, susceptibility to infection and cellular breakdown, with a greater obligatory fluid deficit and a refractory state, all probably supervene as a direct result of "too little, too late."

Aphorism:

Prompt treatment with adequate volume replacement based on hemodynamic and metabolic monitoring is the keystone to uncomplicated survival from hypovolemic shock.

If the patient does not respond to this therapy, then some or all of the secondary measurements may be required (Table 3). Failure of response of urine flow demands immediate monitoring of specific gravity, U/P ratio of creatinine or urea concentration, and knowledge of urine sodium concentration. Likewise, the onset of pulmonary edema, with a persistently low cardiac output, requires the placement of a Swan-Ganz catheter to measure PAWP and the other guides to cardiac function.

The differences in treatment now, compared to 20 years ago, are the larger volumes administered and the use of 8 to 10 meaurements of vital organ function rather than 1 or 2 to follow the patients. There are at least three reasons to use crystalloid in addition to blood in trauma associated with hypovolemia. Shires and colleagues have demonstrated by direct measurement a change in active transport of sodium and potassium in living muscle cells. Shock encourages the intracellular accumulation of sodium and water and loss of potassium to the extracellular fluid. There is also the possibility of loss of fluid into the operated, injured, or inflamed area. A third reason to give fluid is to decrease hematocrit and fibrinogen concentration in small vessels to decrease viscosity and thereby promote flow in nutrient vessels. Patients in shock will achieve better oxygen transport at the capillary level with an hematocrit of 30 per cent rather than 50 per cent.

Arterial blood pressure remains a good guide to therapy; in seriously ill or injured patients, accurate and constant monitoring demands intra-arterial recording via a plastic catheter placed percutaneously into the radial artery.* A prompt rise in pressure with elevation of the legs (an internal transfusion) or a prompt fall when the patient assumes the sitting position assists one in confirming the presence of hypovolemia and its severity. In the average patient, the blood volume must be reduced by 15 to 25 per cent before systolic blood pressure begins to fall below 80 to 90 mm. Hg. The margin between the onset of hypotension and death may be only 20 per cent of the blood volume or about 1.0 liter in a 70-kg. adult male. Even when the systolic blood pressure is restored to normal, there may still be a reduction of 15 to 25 per cent in the blood volume. If the patient is alert, with a normal EKG, and urine flow of 50 ml. per hour, the systolic pressure is probably adequate even if it is only 80 mm. Hg.

Pulse rate usually elevates with hypovolemia and returns to under 100 beats per minute when normovolemia is approached but is much less reliable than blood pressure as a guide to volume replacement. The

---

*We favor a 20-gauge Argyle Medicut catheter available from Aloe Medical, St. Louis, Mo. 63103. An automatic, disposable flushing device, "Intraflo," available from Sorenson Research Co., Salt Lake City, Utah, keeps the connection to the strain gauge clear.

pulse pressure can be helpful. The diastolic pressure determines the degree of arteriolar constriction and pulse pressure reflects the stroke volume. A blood pressure of 80/40 mm. Hg is frequently preferable to one of 120/100 mm. Hg. The higher diastolic pressure is usually due to severe arteriolar vasoconstriction and poor tissue perfusion.

Anxiety, fright, or pain may cause the pulse rate to exceed 120 to 130 beats per minute even if the blood flow is adequate. Continuous EKG monitoring of the seriously ill or injured patient is important to detect arrythmias. If the pulse rate remains low despite obvious hypovolemia and hypotension, isoproterenol is useful to restore cardiac output.

Fluid Administration

Crystalloids. The all-purpose fluid begun on most patients in shock or with trauma is 5 per cent glucose in Ringer's lactate. Equally effective and also readily available is 5 per cent glucose in normal saline with two ampules (90 mEq.) of sodium bicarbonate added to each liter to buffer the solution to pH 7.4. After two to three liters of crystalloid are given, additional fluid should consist roughly of half crystalloid and half fresh frozen plasma, albumin, or whole blood.

Colloids. Albumin — 25 to 50 gm. in each liter of normal saline or Ringer's lactate — has been recommended by Wilson et al.[83] Plasma or fresh frozen plasma that contains clotting factors is useful. The controversy concerning the relative value of albumin or protein-free fluids in the control of transcapillary fluid exchange is not resolved. Oncotic pressure, circulating protein, and their interrelationships vary greatly in ill patients. Furthermore, the interstitial pool of albumin is twice the size of the intravascular pool, and intravenously infused albumin rapidly equilibriates with the interstitial pool, which has the potential to aggravate edema rather than help it.[48] Type-specific blood can usually be available in an emergency in 5 to 15 minutes. A saline crossmatch requires an additional 5 to 10 minutes. Blood that has been completely crossmatched should be used whenever possible but requires at least one hour. The rate of crystalloid and colloid administration depends upon the response to the eight key measurements.

In conditions in which there is excessive loss of plasma proteins, as in acute pancreatitis, peritonitis, or burns, the use of plasma or electrolyte solutions to which albumin is added is of great value.

Plasmanate is a sterile solution of human plasma proteins obtained by cold ethanol fractionation. No blood coagulating factors or immune globulins are included. The solution has the advantage of being heat-treated as 60° C to reduce the likelihood of hepatitis.

Commercial dextran (molecular weight 70,000) is a better volume expander than low-molecular-weight dextran (molecular weight 40,000) because it leaves the vascular space less readily. Both dextrans have been used to prevent thrombosis or sludging in small vessels, but a unique value for the dextran in shock has not been established. Use of either dextran in volumes over two liters carries the hazard of abnormal bleeding.

Ventilation. All patients in shock should receive oxygen by mask. Respiratory failure may require further measures (see discussion of shock lung below).

Diuretics. If hypovolemia has been corrected, i.e., the CVP has responded briskly to a further volume load, the blood pressure and cardiac output have returned to normal but oliguria (< 25 ml. per hour) persists, diuretics are indicated. Urinary output should be monitored hourly with an indwelling catheter. The three diuretics in common use are mannitol, ethacrynic acid, and furosemide. The osmotic diuretic mannitol is given as 25 gm. in 100 to 500 ml. of 5 per cent glucose in water over a 15- to 30-minute period. If there is a response, the dose may be repeated, up to 100 gm. of mannitol in any 24-hour period, in order to maintain a urine output of 50 ml. per hour. The CVP and, in a patient with borderline cardiopulmonary status, the pulmonary artery wedge pressure must be closely monitored because of the increase in intravascular volume.

Ethacrynic acid and furosemide are very effective in preventing as well as in treating acute renal failure. Furosemide is administered intravenously in a dose of 40 mg. If an adequate response is not obtained, the dose is doubled every half hour until a total of 2 gm. has been given. Occasionally, 50 to 100 mg. of ethacrynic acid intravenously will produce a diuresis. If not, the diagnosis of acute renal failure is established and limitation of fluid administration, careful monitoring of serum electrolytes, particularly potassium, and hemodialysis may all be indicated.

Furosemide is a powerful diuretic that inhibits the active reabsorption of sodium in the proximal tubule, in the ascending loop of Henle, and possibly in the distal tubule. Sodium concentration in the distal tubule is an important factor in the control of glomerular filtration rate (G.F.R.), especially following a period of hypotension. The decrease in blood pressure results in a decreased filtration into the tubule and a fall in the sodium load. Tubular urine that has passed through the loop of Henle arrives with a very low sodium concentration, which, by means not established, promotes further reduction of G.F.R. in these nephrons to conserve volume. If the sodium is artificially increased in the distal tubule, the central mechanisms will maintain G.F.R. This is done using either an osmotic diuretic (mannitol) or one of the loop diuretics (furosemide or ethacrynic acid). These agents protect the kidney from damage. If the urine sodium remains below 20 mEq. and the urine to plasma ratio for creatinine remains above 20 or is moving in the appropriate direction with diuresis, further confirmatory evidence of the value of therapy is established.

Acid-Base Correction

Treatment of metabolic acidosis in shock is accomplished best by restoring tissue perfusion, not simply by loading with buffer. In severe metabolic acidosis, especially with an arterial blood pH under 7.1, sodium bicarbonate is indicated. At this level cardiac function is adversely affected by the acidosis per se. A 50-ml. ampule of 7 per cent sodium bicarbonate contains approximately 45 mEq. of bicarbonate in water and is available containing 595 mEq. of sodium and an equal

concentration of bicarbonate. The dosage may be roughly determined by the following formula:

Dosage of sodium bicarbonate in milliequivalents = 0.2 × body weight in kg. × 27 mEq. per liter − sodium bicarbonate in mEq. per liter in the patient's serum.

In severe acidosis, half the calculated dose is given initially and the dose is then adjusted according to pH determinations.

Although normal patients can readily tolerate and buffer the acidity in banked blood, the patient with poor tissue perfusion has an impaired ability to maintain a normal pH. When massive blood transfusions are given to patients in severe shock, an ampule of sodium bicarbonate should probably be given with every 2 to 3 units of whole blood.

Vasoactive Drugs Used in the Treatment of Shock

Methoxamine. Methoxamine (Vasoxyl) is a pure alpha-adrenergic receptor stimulating agent. It is a potent vasopressor with little, if any, direct effect on the heart. This agent causes a rise in arterial blood pressure at the expense of peripheral perfusion and cardiac output. The reduced cardiac output results from a reflex bradycardia and negative inotropic effects of the vagus on the heart. Blood flow to most organs, with the exception of the heart and brain, is decreased.

Norepinephrine. Norepinephrine (levarterenol) is the chemical transmittor at the postganglionic sympathetic nerve endings. This agent has a primary alpha-adrenergic receptor stimulating effect on the peripheral circulation but has, in addition, beta-adrenergic activity on the heart and metabolism. The overall effect of this agent is an increase in total peripheral resistance and arterial blood pressure with a reflex bradycardia that can be blocked by atropine. Cardiac output is usually decreased with the administration of this agent in man. When used with an alpha-adrenergic blocking agent, norepinephrine has been shown to increase cardiac output in man and in the dog. In large concentrations it increases pulmonary artery pressures as a result of an increase in left atrial pressure. There is a rise in venous tone and a shift of blood centrally to the lungs in the dog and possibly in man.

Metaraminol. Metaraminol (Aramine) is a potent vasopressor and functions to deplete norepinephrine at the postganglionic sympathetic nerve endings. These actions are almost identical to those of norepinephrine with the exception that metaraminol appears not to reduce renal blood flow as much as norepinephrine does in man.

Epinephrine. Epinephrine is one of the oldest known adrenergic stimulants. It is predominantly a beta-adrenergic stimulant at low doses, although it does possess potent alpha-mimetic effects in high doses. When infused intravenously, epinephrine causes an increase in heart rate, which is due to the direct action of this agent on the sinoatrial node. In a standard normotensive preparation, stroke volume increases as the result of the direct action of epinephrine on the force of myocardial contractility, and cardiac output increases as a result of the increased stroke volume and heart rate. Total peripheral resistance falls with physiologic doses only, although systolic pressure increases and diastolic pressure remains unchanged or increases slightly, causing a moderate increase in mean blood pressure. Coronary, cerebral, splanchnic, and skeletal muscle blood flows increase, whereas renal blood flow and blood flow through skin and mucous membranes decrease.

The use of these potent vasoconstrictors may be useful for short periods of time if the heart beat is strong but the patient remains hypotensive. Unless the systolic blood pressure is raised above 50 mm. Hg, cerebral and coronary blood flow may be inadequate. The usual dose of norepinephrine is 4 ampules (16 milligrams in 500 ml. of 5 per cent glucose in water). The addition of 2 ampules, 10 mg., of phentolamine (Regitine) to the same bottle reduces the toxicity of the norepinephrine and decreases the chance of its causing a skin slough if it extravasates. The intravenous drip is controlled to keep the blood pressure above 80 mm. Hg systolic or at the level needed to maintain adequate cerebral, cardiac, and renal function. The indications for metaraminol are similar. Mild degrees of hypotension may be controlled with a slow intravenous infusion of a solution containing 20 to 100 mg. of metaraminol in 500 ml. of intravenous solution.

Vasoconstrictors may be especially valuable in patients who have been on antihypertensive drugs and in those with significant atherosclerosis, in contrast to young patients with little or no vascular disease, who can often tolerate hypotension well. Older patients with significant narrowing of coronary or cerebral vessels may require increased blood pressure to maintain an adequate flow to these vital organs. If the arterial blood pressure falls below the critical closing pressure of an important part of the coronary or cerebral circulation, a myocardial or cerebral infarct may result.

Digitalis. Digitalis is extremely useful in patients with any history or evidence of congestive heart failure and an abnormally elevated central venous pressure or a severe persistent atrial tachycardia (above 130 to 140), especially in the older age groups. The usual intravenous digitalizing dose of digoxin is 1.25 to 1.75 mg. The dose required to obtain an optimal effect when shock is present is variable because of acid-base abnormalities, electrolyte imbalance, and altered cellular metabolism. A useful dose schedule is immediate infusion of 0.5 to 0.75 mg. of digoxin intravenously, followed by 0.25 mg. every two hours for two doses, then 0.125 mg. every two hours for four doses until there is evidence of a digitalis effect. An EKG is taken before each dose is given. If there is evidence of digitalis effect or toxicity, no further drug is administered until the maintenance doses are required.

Dopamine. Dopamine is one of the intermediates in the synthesis of norepinephrine and epinephrine. In intact animals both norepinephrine and dopamine cause vasoconstriction in the skeletal muscle, the kidney, and the splanchnic organs. Dopamine may be an effective agent in increasing myocardial contractility without excessive peripheral vasoconstrictive effects and can often produce a dramatic improvement in cardiac output and blood pressure. It is administered with a slow intravenous infusion of a solution containing 200 mg. of dopamine in 250 ml. of 5 per cent glucose in water and may be increased as required.

Isoproterenol. Isoproterenol (Isuprel) is a pure beta-adrenergic receptor stimulating agent. The drug increases both the rate of firing of the sinoatrial node and the rate of atrioventricular node conduction and reduces the refractory period of cardiac muscle. This results in a tachycardia, i.e., increased myocardial contactility. Cardiac output is increased while mean blood pressure decreases. The reduction in total peripheral resistance is due to the active vasodilation induced by this agent. Blood flow to all organs is increased, with the exception, perhaps, of the brain. Isoproterenol can be extremely useful if the pulse rate is slow (below 80 beats per minute) with a high cardiac filling pressure and low output. The usual intravenous infusion rate is 1 to 5 micrograms per minute (0.25 to 1.25 ml. per minute of a solution containing 2 mg. of isoproterenol in 500 ml. of intravenous fluid).

Phenoxybenzamine. Phenoxybenzamine (Dibenzyline) is an alpha-adrenergic receptor blocking agent. This agent, when given intravenously to healthy, recumbent, normovolemic patients or animals, causes minor changes in systolic blood pressure, although diastolic pressure usually decreases. A reflex tachycardia results from the mild hypotension and decreased baroreceptor activity on the vasomotor center. Cardiac output usually increases owing to the tachycardia and the effects of endogenous catecholamines on the heart not inhibited by the baroreceptor reflex. The effects of phenoxybenzamine differ greatly in the upright individual or in a patient with hypovolemia or excess sympathetic activity from stress or other factors. Orthostatic hypotension is common and may exist for 24 hours or more after administration of this drug. Administration to a hypovolemic patient results in mild tachycardia, hypotension, and variable changes in cardiac output. This hypotension can be reversed only with large volumes of fluid or administration of a vasoconstrictor.

Predominantly vasoconstrictor agents, such as methoxamine, metaraminol, and norepinephrine, have detrimental effects when used as primary treatment for hypovolemia. The advanced type of hypovolemic shock associated with cardiac failure, low cardiac output, increased peripheral resistance, and high venous pressure is the prime indication for the use of isoproterenol, dopamine, glucagon, and possibly phenoxybenzamine in selected patients. The clinical use of phenoxybenzamine in shock is predicated on the prior demonstration of an adequate or increased filling pressure but persistently poor tissue perfusion. Questions that have not been answered concerning this drug are: (1) What precisely are the microcirculatory pathways opened up after adrenergic receptor blockade? and (2) Are these channels nutritive in vital organs or elsewhere?

CARDIOGENIC SHOCK

Cardiogenic shock may be defined as "inadequate blood flow to vital organs due to inadequate cardiac output despite a normal cardiac filling pressure." Although it is classically associated with myocardial infarction, this form of shock occurs in many patients with surgical problems.

Previously, the term "cardiogenic shock" pointed to the heart as the culprit, but this is no longer true. Neither mechanism nor therapy is specified. Since different causes require different treatment, precision in diagnosis is not an academic luxury.

Once the heart is recognized, or suspected, as the cause of the shock state, a crucial diagnostic question must always be posed. Is the shock due to generalized depression of myocardial function or is it due, entirely or in part, to a mechanical lesion? Such lesions often require specific treatment and a systematic search for their presence should be made. Cardiac tamponade due to pericardial effusion, tight mitral or aortic stenosis, acute mitral or aortic insufficiency, ventricular septal rupture, and aortic dissection all produce reasonably characteristic signs on physical examination. Chest x-rays and electrocardiograms are often helpful, and the echocardiogram is now a powerful tool to confirm many of these diagnoses.[24] It is important to note that the hemodynamic assessment of shock that will be outlined will not make these diagnoses. Once made, however (and confirmed if necessary by cardiac catheterization), therapy may often be directed at the specific hemodynamic abnormality. For example, relieving tamponade due to pericardial effusion by pericardiocentesis and, if required, by pericardiectomy will usually dramatically improve the patient's clinical state.

Frequently, cardiogenic shock reflects desperately poor ventricular function following myocardial infarction. The cardinal hemodynamic abnormalities characterizing this state are low blood pressure (80 mm. Hg or less), low cardiac output (2.0 liters per minute per square meter), and peripheral vascular resistance that is usually normal but often raised. The objectives of therapy are (1) to raise cardiac output, (2) to reduce cardiac work, and (3) to maintain coronary blood flow.

Cardiac output is the product of heart rate times stroke volume (where stroke volume is the amount of blood ejected from the left ventricle with each beat). Stroke volume is determined by preload, afterload, myocardial contractility, and heart rate.[68] Attempts to improve stroke volume depend on influencing these determinants of ventricular performance.

Preload. The amount the myocardial fiber is stretched before stimulation determines, in part, the force and velocity of contraction. By increasing stretch (preload) and optimizing the potential interaction between contractile proteins, more force is developed. In the intact heart, a greater stroke volume results (Frank-Starling mechanism). Even in the abnormal heart, stroke volume will be maximal at an ideal preload. Clinically, preload is measured as the pressure in the left ventricle at the end of diastole (normal LVEDP is 12 mm. Hg). This pressure is generally the same as mean left atrial pressure, which in turn is usually the same as the pulmonary artery wedge pressure (PAWP). The introduction of the flow-directed balloon-tipped catheter allows relatively facile measurement of both the wedge pressure and cardiac out-

put (generally by thermodilution) in the acutely ill patient with only minimal risk. For the patient in shock with a low wedge pressure (low preload), a trial of fluid therapy is reasonable.[69] When between 12 and 20 mm. Hg, although abnormal, the wedge pressure may still not be optimal for left ventricular performance. This is frequently seen in the postcardiac surgical patient and often following myocardial infarction. In such patients, in the absence of pulmonary edema, a cautious trial of volume expansion may still be attempted. With a wedge pressure greater than 24 mm. Hg, pulmonary edema is usually present or imminent, and little benefit but considerable hazard accrues from such therapy.

Contractility. At a given length (preload) and given afterload (see below), the force developed by a myocardial fiber is dependent on contractility. Increasing contractility is the major effect of low doses of norepinephrine, metaraminol, or epinephrine. Cardiac output rises, as does aortic pressure, thus maintaining coronary perfusion. Higher doses cause an inordinate increase in peripheral resistance, which, as will be shown, both increases myocardial oxygen needs and diminishes ventricular performance.

Recently, favorable experience has been gained with dopamine,[30] which combines the myocardial stimulant properties with a greater preservation of renal blood flow. The greater tachycardia following isoproterenol, coupled with a drop in aortic pressure due to skeletal muscle vasodilation, has diminished enthusiasm for its use. Nevertheless, occasional patients, particularly those with high peripheral resistance, still respond well. With such agents, the mortality of cardiogenic shock due to myocardial infarction has been reduced from 90 to perhaps 75 per cent, but not beyond.

Afterload. Afterload is the tension developed by the left ventricle in opening the aortic valve and is related to aortic pressure and the radius of the left ventricular cavity. By increasing aortic diastolic pressure and left ventricular cavity size, afterload is increased. If preload and contractility are kept constant, stroke volume is inversely related to afterload. Thus, a decrease in aortic pressure or left ventricular volume will increase stroke volume. As well, we should note that myocardial oxygen consumption is directly related to heart rate, preload, contractility, and afterload. A diminution in afterload should improve cardiac performance and reduce myocardial oxygen needs. Such considerations form the basis for use of vasodilators such as sodium nitroprusside. Indeed, studies demonstrate that following nitroprusside, there is often a drop in wedge pressure, a drop in afterload, and an increase in cardiac output.[26] More importantly, the mortality may be reduced,[15] although further trials are required to confirm this observation.

All of these effects are favorable, but they occur at the risk of diminishing coronary perfusion. The major portion of coronary flow occurs in diastole, and in the normal heart is reasonably independent of aortic diastolic pressure (between 60 and 120 mm. Hg). As perfusion pressure in this range diminishes, so does coronary resistance, and thus flow is maintained. Beyond this range of pressures, flow is pressure-dependent. With obstructive atheromas, the driving pressure across the heart is no longer the aortic diastolic pressure but the lesser pressure distal to the obstruction. Thus, a difficult therapeutic problem arises. By increasing aortic pressure, coronary perfusion is increased but so is myocardial oxygen demand, which may cause further ischemia and necrosis. On the other hand, decreasing afterload reduces myocardial work but at the risk of diminishing coronary flow. This sequence may also cause further ischemia and ultimately necrosis. This dilemma is neatly resolved (at least theoretically) by circulatory support devices such as the intra-aortic balloon pump.[76] Systolic pressure (and thus, to a degree, afterload) is reduced while diastolic pressure is raised, thus increasing coronary perfusion. Happily, ventricular performance is often improved with such devices. In a minority of patients, this is sufficient, but for the majority, successful counterpulsation provides only temporary stabilization.[40] Pharmacologic therapy may be a valuable adjunct to counterpulsation.

The cause of cardiogenic shock has become clear from pathologic studies. A fatal outcome is associated with necrosis of 40 per cent or more of the left ventricle.[60] Austen and his colleagues have acted on two important hypotheses. First, although myocardial infarction causes shock, the abnormal hemodynamics produce a vicious cycle of further ischemia and ventricular necrosis that continues until death is inevitable. Secondly, this cycle may be interrupted by emergency aortic coronary bypass, which, if performed in time, may improve myocardial performance because of the increased coronary perfusion. Cardiac catheterization performed with the intra-aortic balloon pump in place will outline coronary anatomy and the degree of left ventricular dysfunction. A surprising number, up to 40 per cent, of patients with shock due to infarction have recovered.[71]

Heart Rate and Rhythm. Cardiac output may be reduced if the rate is either too slow (< 60 beats per minute) or too rapid (> 150). In sinus rhythm, atrial and ventricular contraction are coordinated. In some patients, particularly those with valvular disease or cardiomyopathy, the onset of atrial fibrillation may result in acute cardiac decompensation. Both direct current countershock and drug therapy may be used to terminate tachyarrhythmias. Specific therapy depends on the arrhythmia, its cause, and the patient's clinical state.

The diagnosis and management of cardiogenic shock is complex even in the coronary care unit. This complexity may be multiplied in the surgical patient in whom cardiac dysfunction may be only one of the abnormalities affecting the circulation. Nevertheless, the same priniciples of diagnosis and therapy may be applied.

Output after Recovery of Rate and Rhythm

Agents with positive inotropy can restore circulation in those cirumstances which frequently follow cardiac arrest. Calcium chloride, isoproterenol, dopamine, and glucagon all increase myocardial contractility. In normotensive man dopamine in doses of 2 to 6 μg. per kilogram per minute has been reported to produce fewer arrhythmias and chronotropic effects than isoproterenol in doses of 0.01 to 0.06 μg. per kilogram per minute. Further studies of dopamine during shock are needed, particularly with larger doses (10 to 20 μg. per kilogram per minute). Glucagon may also be a useful agent. Its mode of action in producing increased contractility is unknown, but it is independent of that of digitalis. The dose used is 5 mg. per kilogram repeated every 30 minutes, or 100 mg. per minute as a continuous fusion.

The Poor-Risk Patient

Age, obesity, specific organ failure, chronic illness, and infection are all well-known causes of increased operative risk. Many of these factors cannot be corrected, but optimal hemodynamic status can be evaluated conveniently preoperatively by measuring the eight factors used to assess patients in shock (see Table 3).

An example of the possible use of this technique to evaluate the "risk status" of a patient has already been described (Fig. 3). In this patient shock and subsequent cardiac arrest probably would not have developed if at the time of operation the CVP had been brought to between 5 and 10 cm. H$_2$O and the cardiac index raised to more than 3.2 liters per minute per square meter.

Cardiopulmonary resuscitation for cardiac arrest has been most useful. At present, 30 per cent of patients in the hospital are resuscitated and 19 per cent leave the hospital. The survival at 1 year in a group of 230 patients discharged from the hospital after resuscitation from cardiac arrest was 74 per cent, at the end of 2 years 59 per cent, and at the end of 3 years 41 per cent.[38] It is also clear that in most patients who survive, the reason for resuscitation was myocardial infarction or reversible pulmonary failure. Cardiac arrest associated with complicated surgical problems is best treated by prevention (see Fig. 3). In many cases, cardiac arrest in the surgical patient could be avoided if careful attention were paid to the eight measurements outlined in Table 3 and the patient's state corrected or partially corrected accordingly.

Epidural and General Anesthesia

Most general anesthetics decrease cardiac output with no change or an actual rise in the CVP, indicating a compromise of cardiac function. Profound and prolonged declines in blood pressure and cardiac output with induction of anesthesia are best treated by correction of venous return as assessed by CVP, blood gases and pH, hematocrit, and urine flow before the operation rather than by emergency measures after the fall in arterial pressure.

It is not generally realized that epidural anesthesia or high spinal blockade can result in cardiac sympathetic block, which causes a decrease in the cardiac index with an elevated CVP. The cardiac deficit occurs mainly through loss of rate control, resulting in bradycardia as well as further loss of performance through decreased myocardial contractility despite adequate filling.

Epidural anesthesia or analgesia offers excellent relaxation for abdominal surgery, and has been very successful in relieving pain associated with thoracic trauma and pancreatitis. However, the fact that in several instances hepatorenal failure after epidural and spinal blockade was not prevented by the use of vasoconstrictors suggests that cardiogenic shock was the cause. Restoration of cardiac output to normal is easily accomplished with isoproterenol. Norepinephrine, on the other hand, failed to restore cardiac performance to control levels.[51] It is likely that cardiac sympathectomy occurs even when the analgesic is administered in the lumbar region. Total epidural block adds peripheral dilatation and pooling to the cardiac effect and further decreases output by decreasing venous return. A vasoconstrictor is useful for this abnormality.

Pulmonary Embolus

Dyspnea is the commonest symptom in pulmonary embolus. The classic findings of hemoptysis, pleural friction rub, gallop rhythm, cyanosis, and splinting of the chest are found in only about one quarter of patients with proved pulmonary embolus. Only one third have phlebitis that is clinically recognized at the time of embolus. The patient with pulmonary embolus who presents with shock usually has an elevated CVP or even obvious jugular venous distention and jugular hepatic reflux. The chest film and electrocardiogram are of little value at this time in differentiating embolism from myocardial infarction or even from septic shock.

A bedside scanning technique is available that is quick and safe and does not require moving the patient. Macroaggregates of radioiodinated serum albumin (RISA), 1 μc. per pound of body weight, are injected via a brachial vein and, with a handheld scintillation counter, radioactivity over the anterior, posterior, and lateral aspects of the chest is recorded within 5 to 10 minutes of injection. An area of decreased activity is suspect unless there is an obvious pleural effusion or other space-occupying lesion to explain it. If the scan is negative, one can pursue other lines of investigation with considerable assurance that massive pulmonary embolus does not exist. If the scan is positive one can initiate intravenous heparin therapy, or, if the patient is seriously ill or in shock, obtain pulmonary artery angiograms. At the time the catheter is advanced for pulmonary angiography, pressure recordings in the right ventricle and pulmonary artery are useful to determine outcome. If the mean pressure in the right ventricle is over 25 mm. Hg, it is safer to operate on the patient and perform embolectomy. If the patient has a lower pressure than 25 mm. Hg, we have found it better to give heparin every four hours intravenously to keep the partial thromboplastin time two to three times normal one hour before the next dose. Clotting times must be measured daily to maintain adequate protection and avoid bleeding complications.

When this scanning procedure was used with 104 patients suspected of having pulmonary embolus, the scan was negative in 51, and no subsequent diagnosis of pulmonary embolus was made in these patients, including eight who died and underwent autopsy examination. False negatives were for this reason considered unlikely, making the test ideal as a screening procedure. Of the 53 patients in whom bedside scan was positive, 47 were treated with heparin alone. There were eight deaths in this group, three from pulmonary embolus and five from unrelated causes. The other six patients were in severe shock and all survived after treatment with isoproterenol and either pulmonary embolectomy and inferior vena caval plication, or with vena caval plication alone. Vena caval plication alone was performed in patients in shock but with a mean pressure in the right ventricle of less than 25 mm. Hg.

Prophylactic administration of heparin or coumadin is recommended for high-risk patients, for example, patients over 45 years of age with lower extremity fractures. Lower doses than those used therapeutically may be effective prophylactically. Dextran has also been suggested and may be effective, with a lower risk of bleeding from operative sites. Routine prophylactic measures to prevent pulmonary embolus should be considered for every patient in the intensive care unit. Rapid resolution of demonstrated pulmonary emboli is the rule in man. Direct injection of thrombolytic substances via catheter into the pulmonary artery may hasten this resolution with a more rapid return of normal pressures in the right heart. Inferior vena cava interruption is reserved for patients who cannot be managed with heparin, or who have had several emboli not controlled by heparin, and for certain patients with septic emboli.

In summary, cardiogenic shock is seen in a wide variety of surgical patients and may be due to (1) myocardial infarction, (2) arrhythmias, (3) cardiac tamponade, (4) delayed and inadequate volume replacement in hypovolemia, (5) inappropriate volume replacement in hypovolemia with the creation of a high hematocrit, (6) epidural anesthesia with resultant cardiac sympathectomy, (7) adrenal insufficiency, and (8) pulmonary embolism. The patient usually presents with a lowered arterial pressure, a slow or rapid pulse, an elevated CVP, decreased urine flow, decreased cardiac index, lowered arterial pO_2, moderately elevated lactate (15 to 30 mg. per 100 ml.), and increased arterial-mixed venous difference (Fig. 9, Table 4).

Peripheral Pooling

This hemodynamic abnormality is classically seen in experimental hemorrhage or endotoxin shock in the dog. The syndrome is characterized by a low blood pressure, rapid pulse, low CVP despite massive volume replacement, low cardiac index owing to failure of venous return, low arterial pO_2, but increased arteriovenous oxygen difference owing to increased oxygen extraction. Many studies have revealed that in the dog the area of trapping is principally the liver and splanchnic bed. *This syndrome is not characteristic of hypovolemic or septic shock in man, but it may be observed in patients with hypotension due to spinal anesthesia.*

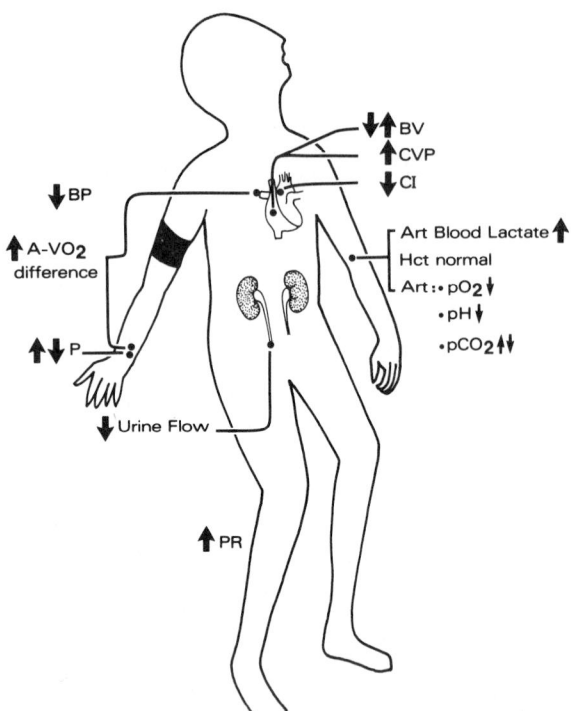

Figure 9. The principal hemodynamic and metabolic abnormalities seen in cardiogenic shock.

SEPTIC SHOCK

Septic shock in man is the principal cause of a primary cellular defect in shock. Evidence will be presented in this section that sepsis causes a cellular defect that inhibits oxygen utilization and that this occurs before the hemodynamic changes. Not all patients with septic shock present with a cellular defect; hypovolemia and even cardiogenic shock are occasionally seen as a consequence of sepsis.

Septic shock has emerged as the *primary unsolved problem in shock* both in understanding the mechanisms involved and in successful therapy. It is now common practice to resuscitate *successfully* patients with devastating injuries and associated hypovolemic shock. Many of these patients, however, succumb days or weeks later from septic shock.

There are several factors that predispose to sepsis in medical and surgical patients, including underlying neoplastic disease, diabetes mellitus, old age, hypovolemia, steroid therapy, immunosuppressive therapy, indwelling urinary or intravenous catheters, indiscriminate use of prophylactic antibiotics, overconfidence in the effectiveness of antibiotic agents, cancer chemotherapy, cirrhosis of the liver, tracheostomy, and radiation therapy. Recognition of these predisposing factors is especially important on surgical services, where more complicated operations are being performed with increasing frequency on patients more likely to be affected by them.[3]

Origins of Knowledge of Septic Shock

Septicemia caused by coliform bacilli and other intestinal organisms has been recognized at least since the reports of Jacob in 1909[35] and Felty and Keefer in 1924.[25] However, bacteremic shock as a clinical entity was first described only in 1951 by Waisbren.[79] Over the subsequent 10 years many experimental studies were conducted using the cell walls of gram-negative organisms, i.e., endotoxin, in dogs. These hemodynamic studies showed that endotoxin given in appropriate doses to the dog produced hypotension, a rise in portal pressure with a simultaneous constriction of hepatic veins, and great increase in the weight of the liver. This reaction was usually transitory and after approximately 1 hour the animal partially recovered, at which time the liver weight and portal pressure returned to normal. The animals frequently died in shock several hours later when the site of pooling was predominantly in the intestine. A hemorrhagic gut was the predominant lesion at autopsy. This form of shock was always characterized by a failure of venous return, and massive transfusions were never ameliorating. Hemorrhagic shock in the dog is characterized by the same intestinal lesion and has been a subject of interest to Gurd and his colleagues,[10] who showed that despite restoration of flow to the mesenteric artery after shock, mucosal flow remained deficient. They postulated that metabolic depression renders the mucosal cells susceptible to permeation by intraluminal proteolytic enzymes such as trypsin. The characteristic hemorrhagic enteritis could be prevented by inactivating the trypsin by means of the inhibitor Trasylol. It was further shown by these workers that the "shocked" intestine becomes permeable to curare and that this is related to a significant reduction in mucin production at the tips of the villi.[11] Protection to the intestine was afforded by feeding an "elemental" or predigested diet prior to injury.[12] This protection was believed to result from reduction of the burden of intracellular digestion by the cells of the intestinal epithelium while maintaining absorption and nutrition. It is possible that such preparation for colon surgery would decrease intraluminal toxic factors and leave the intestinal epithelium in a favorable metabolic state.

More recently, attention has been focused on the patient in septic shock, even though the opportunity to control the many variables that determine outcome is limited. Clinical studies of septic shock have established the following: the patient is usually over 45 years of age, the problem is increasing in frequency, the genitourinary and gastrointestinal tracts are the commonest sites of invasion, only 30 per cent of cases of this form of shock occur before admission to the hospital, shock persists for an average of 2.3 days in survivors, adrenal insufficiency is rarely, if ever, a feature, and shock develops in approximately 30 per cent of patients with gram-negative bacteremia.

Patterns of Septic Shock

Hyperdynamic or Warm Shock. These patients present with the syndrome summarized in Table 5 and are now recognized commonly.[47, 74] Hyperventilation is especially valuable as an early sign of septic shock. The true cause of hyperventilation may be overlooked, especially after operation when atelectasis, pneumonia, pulmonary embolism, or even myocardial infarc-

TABLE 5. Early Bacteremic Shock

Hyperventilation
High central venous pressure
High cardiac index
Alkalosis
Oliguria
Profound hypotension
Warm, dry extremities
Low peripheral resistance
Lacticacidosis

tion is likely to be thought of first. The clinical and laboratory data of a typical patient with the hyperdynamic type of septic shock are illustrated in Figure 10. This patient with septic abortion and *Escherichia coli* septicemia had hypotension, rapid pulse rate, high cardiac index, elevated arterial blood lactate, hypoxia, respiratory alkalosis, a high-normal CVP, and elevated plasma volume. After evacuation of the uterus the blood pressure remained low, the cardiac index dropped, and the arterial blood pH indicated progressive acidosis. This trend was reversed by raising the cardiac index with isoproterenol and additional blood and saline. The patient appeared to require a much higher cardiac index than normal, and when this was maintained she showed a favorable response with a decline of arterial blood lactate to near normal.

A summary of the hemodynamic findings before and after therapy, including the survival rate of 28 patients with hyperdynamic septic shock, appears in Figure 11. Salvage is related to maintaining a higher than normal flow rate, and to prompt and complete drainage or excision of the source of infection.

DISSEMINATED INTRAVASCULAR COAGULATION. The widespread clinical manifestations of the established disseminated intravascular coagulation (DIC) syndrome are unmistakable. Figure 12 summarizes the clinical findings of the patient with septic abortion whose course is shown in Figure 10. Many stimuli, including endotoxin, can initiate this abnormal acceleration of the clotting process. Even though the type of stimulus varies, the end result is the same: the formation of thrombin with the deposition of microthrombi

of different combinations of agglutinated platelets, fibrin, and red and white cells in the microcirculation, resulting in occlusion of small vessels. Local fibrinolysis almost invariably accompanies the clotting, but in some patients thrombosis with infarction and necrosis of tissue occurs with the syndrome (Fig. 12). Disseminated intravascular coagulation is an intermediary mechanism of disease. With massive coagulation a patient may die rapidly in irreversible shock. Minor clotting episodes usually result only in transient platelet agglutination, with a slight deposition of fibrin and mild reversible shock. With somewhat more severe stimuli, the patient may survive shock only to develop a bleeding diathesis due to the consumption of platelets, fibrinogen, and other clotting factors during the intravascular coagulation. This is called consumptive coagulopathy.

With any degree of DIC, *hemorrhage* usually occurs. It is most often manifested by bleeding where surgical or obstetric trauma has left an open wound, but it may occur from all mucous membranes in the severely affected patient. The bleeding may be produced by consumption of the coagulation proteins, or activated by the anticoagulant activity of fibrin split products that form from the activity of fibrinolytic substances such as plasmin and may not be cleared from the circulation for several hours. In acute situations, the following group of tests is helpful to determine the type of abnormality present:

1. Fibrinogen titer—this will be moderately to severely decreased in DIC.

2. Platelet count—platelets are decreased in the same proportions as fibrinogen.

3. Whole blood clotting and lysis—in DIC whole blood tends to clot in normal or near-normal time, and the clot retracts rapidly.

4. Prothrombin time—although nonspecific, the prothrombin time is usually slightly prolonged in DIC.

5. Activated partial thromboplastin time (APTT)—this test measures the time required for clotting by the intrinsic pathway. If the test is prolonged, it should be repeated with a mixture of the patient's plasma and an equal volume of normal plasma. Correction would indicate that the abnormal result was due to a deficiency of clotting factors rather than to

Figure 10. Clinical and laboratory findings in septic abortion in a 35-year-old female. Drainage of the abscess and administration of antibiotics alone did not solve the problem. There was a falling cardiac index, low blood pressure, and elevated arterial blood lactate. Stimulation of cardiac index to twice normal by means of isoproterenol, blood, and saline over a 2-day period resulted in a fall in arterial blood lactate, a rise in arterial blood pressure, and, ultimately, survival.

(Mrs. P.S., 35)	SEPTIC ABORTION (E. coli bacteremia)			
• TIME	1:30 am	SEPT 21 2:20 am	4:00 am	23 10:00 am
• TREATMENT	D&C ANTIBIOTICS		ISOPROTERENOL	
			SOLUCORTEF	BLOOD SALINE
• BP (mm Hg)	85/55	80/50	100/45	115/65
• PULSE	–	120	126*	–
• CVP (cm H2O)	19	16	11*	–
• CI (l/min/M2)	4.5	3.6*	6.5*	5.2
• PR (dynes/sec×cm-5)	609	774	452	780
• LACTATE (mg%)	70	–	–	16*
• pH	7.49	7.26	7.4	–

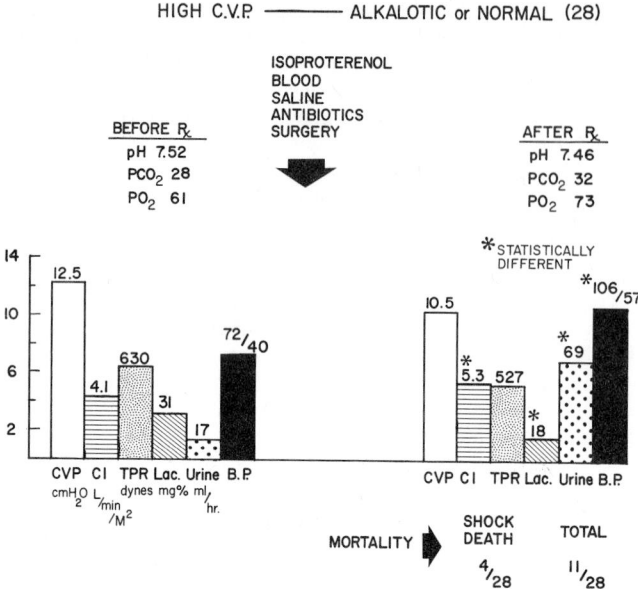

HIGH C.V.P. ———— ALKALOTIC or NORMAL (28)

ISOPROTERENOL
BLOOD
SALINE
ANTIBIOTICS
SURGERY

BEFORE Rx
pH 7.52
PCO₂ 28
PO₂ 61

AFTER Rx
pH 7.46
PCO₂ 32
PO₂ 73

* STATISTICALLY DIFFERENT

MORTALITY → SHOCK DEATH 4/28   TOTAL 11/28

Figure 11. A summary of the response to treatment in 28 patients with hyperdynamic septic shock. These patients presented with hypoxia, low pCO_2, and alkalosis. Central venous pressure and cardiac index were elevated, the peripheral resistance was lowered, the arterial blood lactate was elevated, and urine flow and blood pressure were markedly diminished. There was a favorable response to isoproterenol, blood, saline, and antibiotics, as well as surgical drainage when the patient was hemodynamically stable. (From MacLean, L. D., et al.: Ann. Surg., *166*:543, 1967.)

the anticoagulant effects of fibrin split products. It would also suggest that the patient's situation could be improved by giving blood or plasma.

6. Thrombin time—this test measures the time required for the clotting of plasma, after addition of extrinsic thrombin. It is influenced by the level of fibrinogen and fibrin split products.

7. Fibrin split products—these products are detected qualitatively in serum with the Fi test by reaction with an antifibrinogen serum in the presence of latex particles to produce agglutination.

In general, if the episode is minor no therapy should be instituted. If the patient is in clinical shock and massive hemorrhage is accompanied by a consumptive coagulopathy, the most immediate need is a restoration of tissue perfusion, preferably by the administration of whole fresh blood. If there is good evidence that the stimulus to clotting is still operating, intravenous heparin is the treatment of choice. Heparin inhibits the intravascular coagulation sufficiently to allow the gradual return to normal of depleted clotting factors. The dosage should be sufficient to double the clotting time, and is best given by a continuous intravenous drip using a motor-driven syringe. DIC accompanying septicemia with shock responds less well to heparin than other causes of DIC. The combination of dextran-70 and heparin may be better in this setting.

The antifibrinolytic agent epsilon-aminocaproic acid (EACA) should be used in those patients with exaggerated fibrinolysis. The possible situations include hemorrhage due to the activation of the fibrinolytic systems secondary to DIC, when the clotting has stopped and fibrinolysis has persisted; and hemorrhage associated with decrease in antifibrinolytic activity, as occurs in liver disease. The drug should never be given alone if there is even a suspicion of intravascular clotting, because of the danger of thrombosis leading to ischemic necrosis. However, when

heparin is used with EACA, this danger is reduced, suggesting that the combination of these two drugs may represent an effective way of treating patients with continuing clotting and exaggerated lysis. If increased clot lysis cannot be demonstrated in vivo as the primary abnormality, there is no indication for the isolated therapeutic use of this drug.

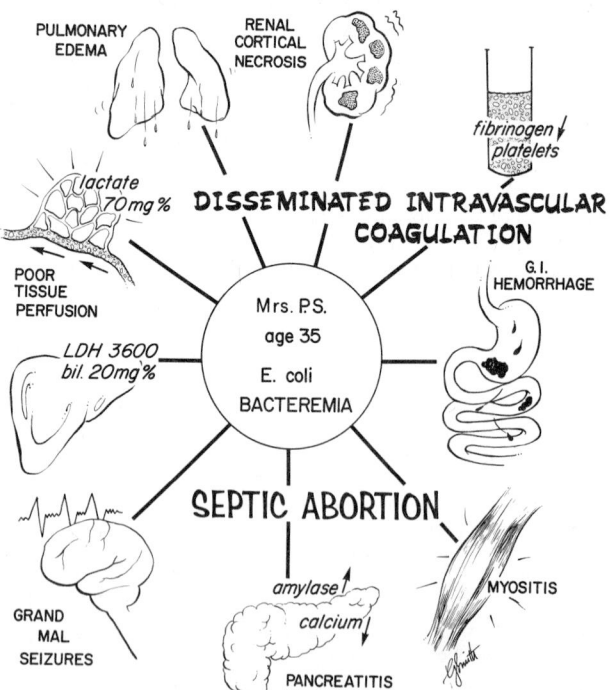

Figure 12. The clinical characteristics of disseminated intravascular coagulation in a patient with *Escherichia coli* septicemia and septic shock. The patient, the same one as in Figure 10, recovered.

Hypodynamic Septic Shock. In contrast to the hyperdynamic state, this form of septic shock is seen in patients with evidence of a "third space" loss prior to the septic process. Most have gangrenous intestinal obstruction, mesenteric thrombosis, or peritonitis. The clinical presentation suggests hypovolemic shock with a low CVP, hypotension, low cardiac output, increased peripheral resistance, elevated lactate, low urine output, and cold cyanotic extremities.

In both the hyperdynamic and hypodynamic types of septic shock, respiratory alkalosis is an early manifestation. Patients treated at this stage have a mortality rate lower than that of patients seen late when they are overwhelmed with severe metabolic acidosis and an elevated arterial blood lactate. An illustrative case history follows:

A 52-year-old female, who several years previously had received radiotherapy for carcinoma of the cervix, had abdominal distention and rigidity. Her blood pressure was 80/40, pulse 140, and CVP 0. Her extremities were cold, moist, and slightly cyanotic and there was no urine output. Arterial blood gas studies showed a pO_2 of 86 mm. Hg, pH of 7.42, pCO_2 of 25 mm. Hg, and base deficit of 6.5 mEq. per liter. Hemoglobin concentration was 10 gm. per 100 ml., hematocrit 34 per cent, and white blood count 16,000 per cubic millimeter. Prior to resuscitation, the cardiac index was 2.8 liters per minute per square meter. Preparation for surgery over a 4-hour period included administration of blood, saline, mannitol, and sodium bicarbonate, which brought the CVP to 6 cm. H_2O and the cardiac index to 3.1 liters per minute per square meter. At operation, massive small bowel infarction due to volvulus was found and extensive resection was carried out with a successful outcome. During operation, the CVP was maintained at 7 to 14 cm. H_2O by administering blood, and the patient remained normotensive. Postoperatively, blood pressure was 130/80 mm. Hg and the CVP was 6.5 cm. H_2O, yet, disturbingly, the cardiac index had declined to 2.7 liters per minute per square meter. Repeat hematocrit was 51 per cent, indicating hemoconcentration. With correction of this disorder, the cardiac index promptly rose to 5.4 liters per minute per square meter and there was a marked improvement in urine flow. Twelve hours later blood lactic acid had declined from the initial value when first seen of 61 mg. per 100 ml. to 15 mg. per 100 ml. The patient was discharged well 10 days later.

Preoperative preparation based on the eight key measurements can be quickly and easily accomplished in hypodynamic septic shock. There is a tendency to treat hypotension occurring during surgery, especially for gangrenous small bowel obstruction, with blood and this is effective. It is suggested that a hematocrit between 30 and 40 per cent be maintained. Massive quantities of Ringer's lactate that lower the hematocrit below 30 to 35 per cent would represent poor treatment.

Gram-Negative versus Gram-Positive Infections

Gram-negative organisms are by far the commonest cause of septic shock and are associated with both types of hemodynamic abnormality. Gram-positive organisms and fungi are associated with septic shock, which is usually hyperdynamic because "third space" losses are not as commonly due to these organisms as to the gram-negative group.

Defective Oxygen Consumption in Septic Shock

With accurate methods of collection and analysis of inspired and expired air, oxygen uptake has been shown to be decreased or normal in patients with septic shock who have a normal or increased cardiac output. Furthermore, these same patients have an elevated arterial blood lactate and an inappropriately low arterial–mixed venous oxygen difference.

In exercise, where the need for oxygen increases, there is an increased cardiac output and, at the same time, an increased oxygen extraction and increased arteriovenous difference (Fig. 13). In hypovolemic shock, cardiogenic shock, and endotoxic shock in the dog, there is a decreased cardiac output but an increased oxygen extraction and therefore a wide arteriovenous difference, which is an appropriate response. Patients with septic shock probably have a need for a larger than normal oxygen uptake (fever, rapid pulse, and infection) but have a normal or low uptake when related to flow. This might be due to a failure of oxygen transport in the lungs, failure of flow to the tissues of utilization, failure of oxygen release from hemoglobin in the tissues, arteriovenous shunting in the periphery, or failure of oxygen utilization by the cells of vital organs. While arterial oxygen content of arterial blood is decreased in most patients with sepsis, correction of arterial pO_2 does not improve oxygen uptake (Fig. 14), and large increases of arterial blood pO_2 as accomplished by hyperbaric oxygen therapy have been of no value.[47] The second possibility is a failure of flow, but we have already established that increased cardiac output is a characteristic of this form of shock.

The final two possibilities to account for the decreased oxygen uptake in septic shock are arteriovenous shunting and a primary cellular defect due to a direct effect of sepsis. Using the model of Clowes et al.[16] to produce hyperdynamic septic shock in dogs, Wright et al.[85] measured cardiac output, blood flow

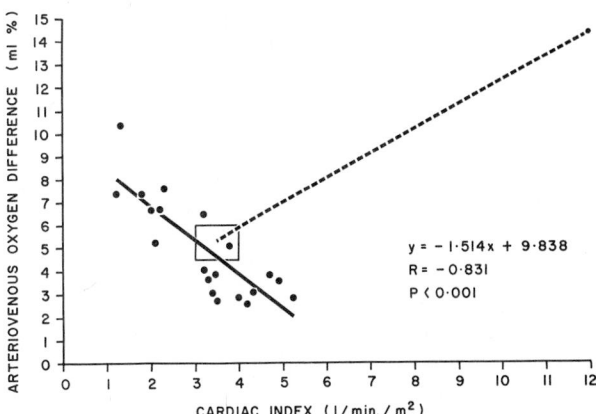

$$y = -1.514x + 9.838$$
$$R = -0.831$$
$$P < 0.001$$

Figure 13. The relationship between arteriovenous oxygen difference and cardiac index in a group of septic shock patients, represented by solid dots. It appears that as the arteriovenous oxygen difference drops, the cardiac index increases. In contrast, the interrupted line represents the known and appropriate response of cardiac index and arteriovenous oxygen difference related to exercise. In both situations, there are increased oxygen requirements. In sepsis the response is inappropriate.

PATIENTS WITH HYPOXEMIA

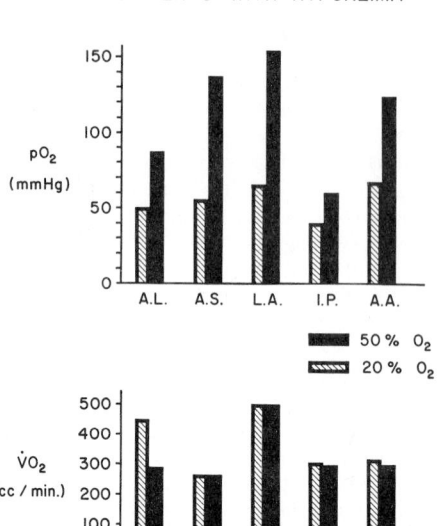

Figure 14. The response in six septic shock patients to breathing 20 per cent oxygen and 50 per cent oxygen. Although it is possible to increase arterial pO_2 in these patients, this does not result in increased oxygen uptake, indicating a peripheral failure of utilization rather than a limitation of oxygen availability due to a lung deficiency.

in skeletal muscle, oxygen uptake, and femoral and total arteriovenous oxygen differences. Muscle blood flow was determined by xenon-133 clearance, which measures only tissue capillary flow. There was a highly significant correlation between the rise in cardiac index and the increased muscle blood flow in animals with hyperdynamic sepsis, demonstrating that no capillary arteriovenous shunting was taking place but that the decreased oxygen uptake was likely due to a primary cellular defect. The hyperdynamic circulation is probably a compensatory mechanism to increase flow and oxygen supply to those deficient cells. This may be the direct result of persistent catecholamine stimulation.

Catabolism of Sepsis and Shock

A prominent feature of sepsis and septic shock is the rapid and excessive protein wasting. The precise mechanisms responsible for the proteolysis and gluconeogenesis, which far exceed those seen in starvation, are only now being clarified. Clinical observations of the cardiac output during uneventful convalescence from major operations suggest that a slight elevation above the patient's resting basal value is required to maintain normal metabolic conditions and to effect recovery. In the presence of severe infection, however, cardiac output twice or three times normal is commonly seen, and the ability to raise cardiac output has been suggested as a necessity for survival. Albrecht and Clowes[2] showed in dogs that survival after cecal ligation with abscess formation was related to a progressive and significant increase of the cardiac output. At the end of a week, this amounted to almost twice

the basal value observed in uninfected animals. The concept that a greater demand for circulation is occasioned by sepsis and gangrene was further substantiated by the dramatic reductions in cardiac output that occurred in animals in which the abscesses were drained.

The discrepancy documented in man now suggests that while sepsis calls upon the organism for greater flow and oxygen delivery there is not an appropriate response in extraction of oxygen at the tissue level.

The metabolic peculiarities of sepsis documented by Immaura et al.[34] suggest insulin resistance in the periphery, especially in muscle, as an initiating factor to account for the excessive proteolysis, which is not prevented by glucose infusion. They suggest that energy needs are met by oxidation of branched-chain amino acids. Other amino acids including alanine are also released into the blood stream. If the liver is functioning normally, alanine and lactate are converted to glucose to elevate this level in blood and tissue and thereby elevate blood insulin. There is a resultant suppression of lipolysis and a further fuel deficit in muscle, which causes further proteolysis.

If there is liver failure, which may occur frequently if shock supervenes in addition to sepsis, the conversion of lactate and alanine to glucose is impeded and very high serum levels of alanine and lactate occur with hypoglycemia and frequently death.

Phenylalanine, which is detoxified exclusively in the liver. and methionine, which is known to be elevated in liver failure, are both elevated in some patients with sepsis. Glucagon and insulin, which was found by Woolf et al.[86] to be elevated in one investigation on patients, would not be expected to elevate but rather to lower the serum concentration of these amino acids. This manifestation of abnormal liver function was not found in patients after uncomplicated surgery or trauma with fractures.

Successful therapy of septic shock in the future, in addition to the very important prophylactic measures, will probably alter metabolic functions of cells rather than increase blood flow to them.

In summary, the patient with *hyperdynamic septic shock* has hyperventilation, a low blood pressure, rapid pulse, high CVP, low urine flow, high cardiac index, low peripheral resistance, normal hematocrit, narrow arteriovenous oxygen difference, low oxygen uptake, mild lactic acidosis, and, if seen early, respiratory alkalosis, or later, when the prognosis is poor, uncompensated metabolic acidosis (Fig. 15). *Hypodynamic septic shock* presents as hypovolemic shock with the addition of narrow arteriovenous oxygen difference and subnormal oxygen uptake, indicating a cellular defect in addition to the consequences of hypovolemia.

THE LUNG LESION IN SHOCK

Interstitial or diffuse air space pulmonary edema can be the result of sepsis, fat embolism, cardiac failure, crystalloid overload, lung contusion, oxygen toxicity, aspiration of gastric contents, and microemboli contained in blood transfusions. The resulting acute

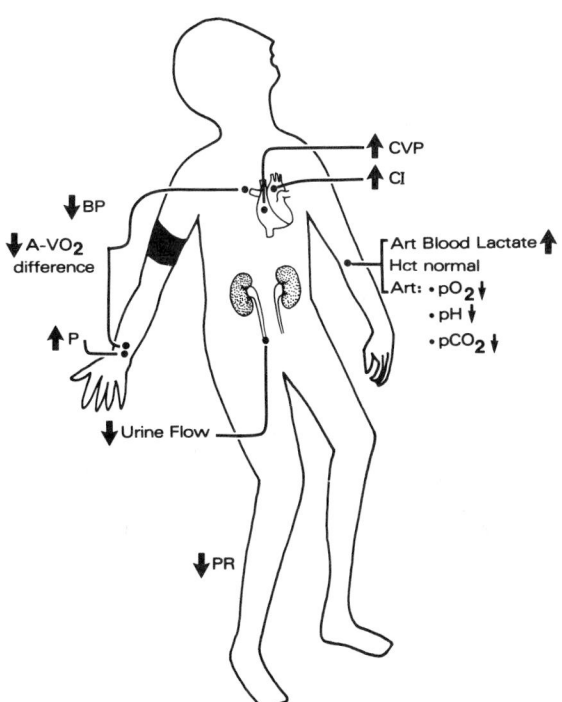

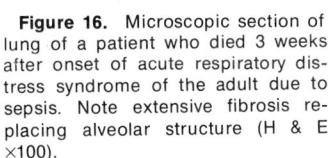

Figure 15. The principal hemodynamic and metabolic abnormalities seen in hyperdynamic septic shock.

respiratory failure (ARF) is a major cause of death in injured patients and patients receiving intensive care.[56] Most forms of respiratory failure start with edema. If this is due to cardiac failure the prognosis is good. Gas exchange returns to normal when the cardiac failure is treated. If the respiratory failure is as-sociated with sepsis, the problem is much more hazardous and the outlook is poor even if the infection is controlled.

What are the basic differences between the types of acute respiratory failure? In heart failure or simple crystalloid overload, fluid leaves the pulmonary capillary because of increased pressure or possibly decreased colloid osmotic pressure within the pulmonary capillary. In the dog, marked crystalloid overload causes only interstitial edema.[57] This does not alter gas exchange. With the addition of heart failure by inflating a balloon in the thoracic aorta, Muir et al. created alveolar edema, but again gas exchange was protected by reduction of blood flow to the dependent, most edematous, areas.[57] Great amounts of lung edema are also required in the goat to reduce arterial oxygen tension and is best explained, as by Barcroft in 1920, if blood flow is reduced to the edematous areas.[5] In contrast, in respiratory failure associated with sepsis, hypoxia is prominent and usually cannot be explained by elevated pulmonary capillary pressure or decreased colloid osmotic pressure.[50]

The hypoxia of ARF is resistant to breathing 100 per cent oxygen, which suggests that areas of lung that have no ventilation are being perfused, i.e., a true anatomic shunt rather than ventilation-perfusion admixture that will respond to breathing 100 per cent oxygen and is characteristic of simple pulmonary edema. Autopsy examinations of patients dying of ARF due to sepsis reveal air space edema early, frequently without pneumonia, later formation of hyaline membrane and diffuse fibrosis, and honeycombing of the lung in patients who survive for longer periods (Fig. 16). A reasonable postulate is that ARF due to sepsis destroys the Type 1 cells of the alveolus, which are responsible for gas exchange. If the lesion is severe

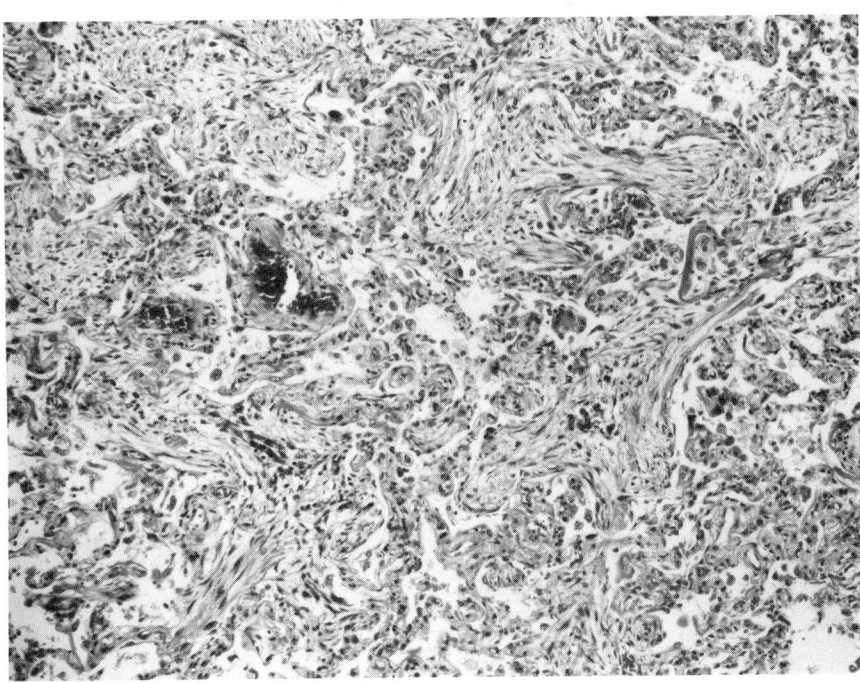

Figure 16. Microscopic section of lung of a patient who died 3 weeks after onset of acute respiratory distress syndrome of the adult due to sepsis. Note extensive fibrosis replacing alveolar structure (H & E ×100).

enough to damage capillaries and to permit passage of the large fibrinogen molecule, hyaline membranes may form. Healing may occur from the Type 2 cells of the alveolus (responsible for production of surfactant), or if destruction has been more severe, healing may occur by fibrosis of the lung,[1, 39] which may be incompatible with life. Late evaluation of pulmonary function in patients who have survived ARF associated with sepsis has not been reported to determine if a restriction of function characteristic of fibrosis persists.

Does hypovolemic shock produce abnormalities of lung function? Lowery et al.[42] originally noted hypoxemia in battle casualties in Vietnam. In an experimental model in the pig, they noted that the onset of hypoxemia coincided with the period of reinfusion and that at the same time moderate to very severe focal interstitial and alveolar edema and hemorrhage occurred. One possible explanation was an increase in alveolar-capillary permeability, which occurs during the period of hypoperfusion but manifests itself only after pulmonary perfusion is returned to normal.[43]

This concept is supported by the work of Todd et al.[78] and of Northrup and Humphrey.[58] Both these studies show that simple hemorrhagic shock causes increased permeability of the pulmonary capillary to protein. This increased permeability appears to be due to an increase in the capillary pore number rather than in the radius of the pores in the capillary membrane.[78] Similar studies which measure all forces and flows to and from the pulmonary capillary are not available for septic shock.

In summary, acute respiratory failure is well tolerated if simple edema is the cause. Compensation occurs through alteration in perfused areas of the lung to maximize oxygenation and the great ability of the pulmonary lymphatics to rid the lung of edema. It takes great crystalloid overload to increase the wet weight to dry weight ratio of the lung of experimental animals, which is an index of the capacity of pulmonary lymphatics. Damage to alveolar cells and the pulmonary capillaries, which can occur from sepsis, aspiration, oxygen, and other agents, is much less well tolerated because an active process of healing is required, which in itself may limit the capacity of the lung to exchange oxygen and carbon dioxide.

PREVENTION OR TREATMENT OF ACUTE RESPIRATORY FAILURE (ARF)

While the normal lung tolerates fluid overload very well, it is nevertheless clear that the accumulation of lung water is a constant feature of ARF. Prevention is aimed at avoiding positive water balance in patients who have a high risk of sepsis in particular. Many patients are in positive water balance in the hospital because of the vigorous measures currently and properly taken to restore blood flow to vital organs as promptly as possible when shock exists. Others are in positive sodium and water balance because of chronic or malignant disease states. The latter are malnourished and have an increased total body sodium to total body potassium ratio, i.e., there has been a loss of a body cell mass in relationship to the extracellular supporting structure of the body.

Careful calculation of water and sodium requirements, the use of diuretics, daily weighings, and total parenteral nutrition all may be necessary to avoid ARF. Frequent change of position to prevent fluid accumulation and air space closure in one area of the lung is extremely important. Correction of hypoxemia by increasing inspired oxygen concentration, or if not sufficient, artificial ventilation including positive end-expiratory pressure, should be used.

Relief of pain without central depression of respiration is an ideal not usually attained. The use of epidural anesthesia in the early postoperative period following upper abdominal surgery is particularly useful in the obese and for the first 24 to 48 hours when tidal volume may be below the closing volume in patients with a high diaphragm and an expanded functional residual capacity. The measurement of single-breath peak expiratory flow rates in patients before and after epidural anesthesia provides objective evidence that flows sufficient to initiate a cough (> 125 liters per minute) are possible only after adequate relief of pain.[54]

The value of a 40-micron filter in the system when several blood transfusions are given is strongly suggested by the randomized study of Jordan et al.[36] They had significantly less ARF when a mean of 10 units of blood was given if the filter was used.

Serial quantitative tracheal cultures for patients with endotracheal tubes are useful to differentiate between contamination that does not require antibiotic therapy and invasive infection that does. Polk[63] showed that bacterial concentrations that do not exceed 10,000 organisms per milliliter of aspirate are seldom if ever associated with respiratory infection. Patients with more than 100,000 organisms per ml. had respiratory infections regularly, which may have become obvious clinically or on roentgenogram only at a later time.

In established ARF, therapy is directed primarily toward correction of physiological abnormalities rather than toward the primary mechanism of injury. Guidelines for ventilatory support have been summarized by Wilson and Pontoppidan[84] and appear in Table 6. Positive end-expiratory pressure (PEEP) during mechanical ventilation is widely used to prevent and treat small airway closure with subsequent gas trapping and atelectasis, as well as alveolar collapse from other causes. Response in PaO_2 to various pressures is the usual method to determine adequacy of treatment, but measurement of all the variables in Table 6 may be necessary, as well as determination of the influence of continuous positive pressure on pulmonary capillary wedge pressure and cardiac output.

TREATMENT OF SEPTIC SHOCK

The treatment of septic shock is much more difficult than treatment of either hypovolemic or cardiogenic shock and must appear to us now as traumatic shock did to Archibald and McLean[3] in World War I.

Evaluation of Host Resistance

The status of host resistance to infection is only very generally assessed in patients at this time. Many fac-

TABLE 6. Guidelines for Ventilatory Support in Adults With Acute Respiratory Failure*

Parameter	Normal Range	Indication for Tracheal Intubation and Ventilation
Mechanics		
Respiratory rate	12–20	>35
Vital capacity (ml./kg. body weight)	65–75	<15
FEV_1 (ml./kg. body weight)	50–60	<10
Inspiratory force (cm. H_2O)	75–100	<25
Oxygenation		
PaO_2 (torr)	100–75	<70
	air	(on mask O_2)
PA-a DO_2 (torr)†	25–65	>450
Ventilation		
$PaCO_2$	35–45	>55‡
V_D/V_T	0.25–0.40	>60

The trend of values is important and the values are meant to be guides only and are not intended to be used to the exclusion of clinical judgment.

*Adapted from Pontoppidan, H., Geffin, B., Lowenstein, E.: N. Engl. J. Med., 287:743, 1972.

†After 10 min. of 100% oxygen

‡Except in patients with chronic hypercapnia

tors are known to influence the development of infection following surgery or injury. The relative importance of these is difficult to quantitate in any single patient. The five most important factors predisposing to infection of the surgical wound, according to Davidson et al.,[22] are (1) a potentially contaminated procedure arising as a result of division of the gastrointestinal or genitourinary tracts; (2) the presence of bacteria in the wound at the end of the operation; (3) the age of the patient; (4) the duration of the operation; and (5) the ward environment (an open ward increases the risk). Davidson's study is particularly valuable because 14 factors believed to be important were monitored in a prospective fashion in all 1000 patients studied. Linear regression analyses of these data permitted a prediction of the likelihood of wound infection in any given patient.

Using all factors, an 80.6 per cent correct incidence of the state of a wound could be predicted. Factors of borderline significance were glove punctures at the end of the operation, nasal carrier state of the patient, emergency procedures, and failure to use skin towels. Factors of no significance in the development of wound sepsis were type of skin preparation, drainage of the wound, skin carrier state, and poor skin preparation before disinfection. Surgical technique, while more difficult to measure, is obviously of great importance in preserving blood supply to healing edges, in eliminating dead spaces, in establishing hemostasis, and in excising devitalized tissue, all of which have the potential to influence infection rates.

It is also likely that host resistance to infection can determine the outcome; indeed, this may be the determining factor for increased infection rates in the elderly following a contaminated operation. It would be worthwhile knowing before operation to what degree a given patient has been compromised by age alone. Not all the elderly are poor risks. It also follows that host resistance is dependent upon more than the age of the patient.[52]

Host defense mechanisms may be subdivided into five components: (1) the inflammatory response; (2) the humoral (immunoglobin) system; (3) the phagocytic system (neutrophil and macrophages); (4) cell-mediated immunity; and (5) the complement system. The inflammatory response serves to deliver polymorphonuclear leukocytes (PMN) and plasma proteins (immunoglobulins, complement, and fibrinogen) to the pathogenic invading bacteria. After the first 24 hours, the monocyte replaces the neutrophil as the predominant phagocytic cell.

The crucial role of complement is to attract PMNs to the bacteria and, with IgG, to opsonize them for effective phagocytosis. In the absence of complement or immunoglobins, phagocytosis is substantially decreased. Fibrinogen facilitates localization of the infection. The processes by which the bacterium is prepared and destroyed appear in Figure 17. The burn injury is known to be associated with cyclic depression of intracellular killing of pathogenic bacteria after phagocytosis.

The second line of phagocytic response is the monocyte. The cells that take part in this activity may be bone marrow (B) lymphocytes or thymus-derived (T) lymphocytes. B cells produce specific antibodies and T cells produce specifically sensitized lymphocytes with a major role in protection against intracellular parasites, most notably Mycobacterium tuberculosis, Listeria monocytogenes, and viral and fungal infections. Delayed hypersensitivity is mediated through cell-mediated immunity (CMI), and failure to respond appropriately to skin antigens to which the patient has likely had previous exposure documents a depressed host resistance not only to intracellular parasites but also to more usual bacteria found in surgical patients.

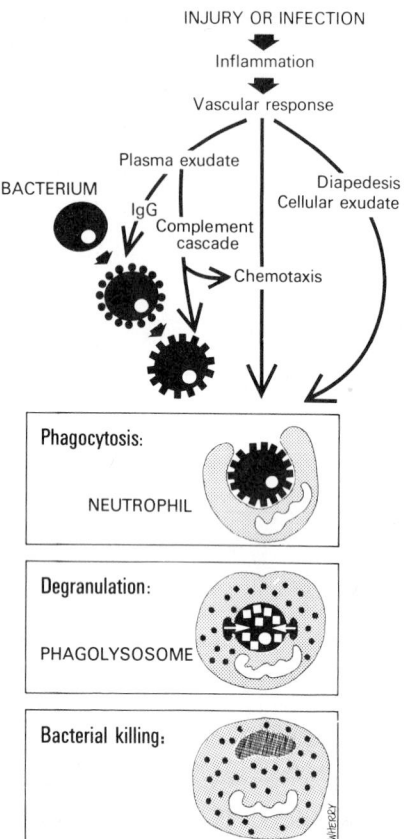

Figure 17. Initial response to injury or infection. The preparation and destruction of bacteria depend upon a vascular response, the opsonic preparation of complement, and phagocytosis.

The latter is based on data which showed an increased rate of infection, invasiveness of the infection, and mortality from infection in patients who did not possess CMI as measured by skin reactivity (anergy).[46]

Treatment of septic shock is properly based on prevention. The discovery of defects in host defense in surgical candidates might assist in their treatment. The laboratory evaluation of the status of host defense will probably enlarge in the future. The present status

is summarized in Table 7. Defects in CMI that are amenable to therapy occur with malnutrition, which does not have to be clinically obvious or profound. It is also possible that nonspecific stimulators of CMI such as levamisole may be useful in patients who demonstrate poor host resistance before or after surgery or injury.

Prophylaxis

Antibiotics. Antibiotic therapy has not reduced the incidence of infection with complicating septicemia. Furthermore, intensive or prolonged antibiotic therapy permits the emergence of antibiotic-resistant strains of gram-negative bacteria and their invasion of the blood stream.[2] Most studies of the use of prophylactic antibiotics in surgery are not definitive. One excellent, prospective, double-blind decisive study by Polk and Lopez-Mayor on patients undergoing elective surgery on the gastrointestinal tract strongly supports the use of prophylactic antibiotics.[64] These authors advise the prophylactic use of cephaloridine, 1 gm. intramuscularly, on call to surgery, and at 5 hours and 12 hours postoperatively. In their study this short course avoided toxicity, provided a high blood level at the time of risk, did not result in emergence of resistant strains, and greatly lowered the infection rate in clean contaminated cases. Prophylactic use of antibiotics is not bad; it is the regimens of use that have been faulty.

A reasonable approach to prevention of wound and intra-abdominal abscesses following surgery is the following: for clean cases, no antibiotics and primary wound closure; for clean contaminated cases (gastrointestinal or genitourinary tracts divided but no gross spillage), prophylactic antibiotics such as cefazolin, 1 gm. on call to surgery and at 5 hours and 12 hours postoperatively, with primary wound closure; for contaminated cases (same as clean contaminated but with gross spillage), prophylactic cefazolin but delayed primary wound closure; and for dirty cases (pus or perforation encountered), antibiotics and secondary wound closure.

Catheters. Intravenous, intra-arterial, and urinary catheters are frequent sources of infection and septicemia. The use of total parenteral alimentation has

TABLE 7.   Laboratory Investigation of Host Defense Against Infection

Host Defense Mechanism	Primary	Secondary
Inflammatory	Skin window	
Humoral	Immunoelectrophoresis Quantitation of IgG, IgA, and IgM	Complement Antibody response to specific antigens
Phagocytic	Neutrophil, monocytes: count and morphology	PMN Monocytes } bacterial function: Macrophages } motility, chemotaxis

Cell-mediated	Lymphocytes: count, morphology
	Skin tests: P. P. D., varidase,
	    mumps, trichophyton,
	    Candida
		D.N.C.B. sensitization
		Skin graft rejection
		Mixed lymphocyte culture
		Lymphokine quantitation

aggravated the problem because these solutions are good media for bacterial growth and one is reluctant to remove central venous lines if they are functioning. We favour "scalp vein" needles for routine intravenous fluid therapy and plastic catheters for patients who might require large volume replacements. These should be removed within 48 hours; central venous lines (subclavian or brachial) to be used for parenteral nutrition should be placed using operating room technique and dressed three times weekly using an occlusive dressing. This line must be used only for parenteral nutrition. The preparation of parenteral nutrition fluids should be done using a laminar flow hood in the hospital pharmacy.

Two techniques have been used to decrease septicemia from the urinary tract associated with catheterization. These are the use of a three-way catheter with antibiotic irrigation and the strict use of a constantly sealed drainage system. We favor the latter as being more effective and cheaper.

Many other diagnostic and therapeutic procedures provide a direct route for the introduction of gram-negative bacilli. Ventilatory equipment with nebulizers, a notorious source, must be cultured and cleaned and sterilized daily. Pump oxygenators and dialysis equipment are easily contaminated and must be monitored frequently.

Infection Control Committee. In hospitals where infections are a problem, an infection control committee, by evaluating procedures used, may effect a lowering of the infection rate.

Restoration and Maintenance of Nutrition. Many patients in whom septic complications develop following surgery have a negative nitrogen balance when first seen or may actually be in this state at the time of surgery because of a prolonged period of investigation. If a complication does develop postoperatively, the period of inadequate intake may easily reach 3 weeks, in which time a deficit of approximately 20,000 calories can easily develop. It is a widely held opinion since the establishment of hyperalimentation[23] that septic complications can be avoided and more successfully treated when present if nutritional deficits are vigorously corrected.

Treatment

Assessment of Results of Treatment of Septic Shock. The evaluation of treatment based on mortality rate is always hazardous in retrospective trials but is especially so in septic shock because of the great influence of underlying disease on the eventual outcome. McCabe and Jackson[49] have classified underlying diseases associated with sepsis as rapidly fatal, ultimately fatal, and nonfatal. Freid and Vosti[27] applying this classification to 270 patients with gram-negative bacteremia, of whom 34 per cent had shock, found an overall mortality rate of 36 per cent. However, for diseases that are "rapidly fatal," such as acute leukemia, postnecrotic cirrhosis, and bacterial endocarditis, the mortality was 86 per cent. In the "ultimately fatal" group, with diseases such as lymphoma, gastrointestinal neoplasms, gynecologic cancer, renal malignancy, and chronic leukemia, the mortality was 46 per cent. In the "nonfatal" category,

which included patients with anatomic defects and nonmalignant disease of the urinary and gastrointestinal tracts as well as prematurity and septic abortion, the mortality rate was 16 per cent. One must look skeptically at studies that claim benefit from a given treatment when the underlying disease process is not taken into account.

Early Recognition. The early signs of septic shock are listed in Table 5. Hyperventilation is a particularly valuable warning sign. Mortality is decreased when sepsis is recognized before the onset of shock.[3]

Appropriate Antibiotic. Altemeier et al.[3] have shown in a large series of patients a mortality rate of 54 per cent for sepsis when the patient was given an inappropriate antibiotic and 28 per cent when an appropriate antibiotic, chosen on the basis of culture sensitivities, was used.

The inadequate perfusion of tissues that can occur with shock precludes the use of oral or intramuscular administration of antibiotics. Antibiotics must be given intravenously. It is now apparent that appropriate antibiotic therapy given early will decrease the incidence of shock related to septicemia. Bactericidal or bacteriostatic agents are equally effective in gram-negative infections. The patterns of susceptibility vary widely from hospital to hospital, and familiarity with local factors is essential to appropriate initial treatment. Treatment is usually started with one of the aminoglycosides (kanamycin or gentamicin), but when cultures and susceptibility tests are available, a less toxic but effective drug should be substituted. If the infection is gram-positive and the organisms are cocci on smear, a synthetic penicillin should be used. In anaerobic infections such as necrotizing fasciitis, the smear frequently shows pleomorphic gram-negative bacilli (Bacteroides) and a mixture of aerobes and anaerobes. The treatment regimen is currently 10 to 20 million units of penicillin G, 600 mg. clindamycin, and 5 mg. per kilogram per day of gentamicin. If gram-positive rods are present, a clostridial infection is more likely, in which case penicillin only is required.

Restoration of Normal Hemodynamics. A higher than normal cardiac output with normal filling pressure and normal hematocrit should be sought. This may require administration of blood, saline, isoproterenol, or all three. Unfortunately, many patients die of a cellular defect despite this treatment. However, the survival rate does appear to be better in patients in whom the cardiac index can be elevated 1 liter per minute per square meter than in those in whom it cannot.

Abscess Drainage. Patients in whom the septic source is amenable to surgical treatment and who are treated surgically have a better prognosis than patients who do not satisfy these criteria. Adequate and continuous drainage of abscesses and fistulas of the gastrointestinal tract is best accomplished with continuous suction with air vent catheters.

Decompression of the small intestine via a long tube without enterostomy is important in small bowel obstruction to lower the incidence of peritonitis and sepsis due to spillage at the time of surgery.

Corticosteroids. This therapy, though not of proven

value, is widely used. The basis for the large doses used (50 to 150 mg. per kilogram of hydrocortisone in a single bolus) is threefold. First, clinical observations suggest benefit, in pulmonary and renal function particularly. Second, steroids stabilize cellular and subcellular membranes. The most important of the organelles are the lysosomes, which may release hydrolytic enzymes that adversely affect the mitochondria, which in inactivity prevent oxygen utilization. Third, corticosteroids stabilize the membranous portion of the microcirculation. A summary of the abundant literature on this subject, generally supporting the use of steroids, especially in septic shock, appears in a recent monograph.[72] There is no clinical proof that steroids alter the mortality rate in septic shock.

SELECTED REFERENCES

Altemeier, W. A.: Significance of infection in trauma. Bull. Am. Coll. Surg., 57:7, 1972.
A classic review of the profound increase in infection, which complicates care of surgical patients.

Ballinger, W. F., Collins, J. A., Drucker, W. R., Dudrick, S. J., and Zeppa, R.: Manual of Surgical Nutrition. Philadelphia, W. B. Saunders Company, 1975.
An excellent source of current thinking on nutritional requirements of the surgical patient. It contains many important guidelines for prevention of sepsis and septic shock and maintenance of host resistance.

Cannon, W. B.: Traumatic Shock. New York, D. Appleton and Company, 1923.
This scholarly monograph summarizes the field of shock through World War I, as well as the observations and experiments of the first "shock team." The importance of low blood volume and acidosis in traumatic shock is noted, but greatest emphasis is placed on toxemia as the cause of shock due to trauma.

Crile, G. W.: An Experimental Research into Surgical Shock. Philadelphia, J. B. Lippincott Company, 1899.
The experimental basis for the modern understanding of shock. The first experiments showing the value of the central venous pressure.

Gump, F. E., Price, J. B., Jr., and Kinney, J. M.: Whole body and splanchnic blood flow and oxygen consumption measurements in patients with intraperitoneal infection. Ann. Surg., 171:321, 1970.
In this study measurements of regional as well as whole-body flow and oxygen consumption were made. The authors noted that an increase in the splanchnic fraction of cardiac output was evident in those patients whose infections were associated with increased resting oxygen consumption. The methodology is particularly interesting and important.

MacLean, L. D., Duff, J. H., Scott, H. M., and Peretz, D. I.: Treatment of shock in man based on hemodynamic diagnosis. Surg. Gynecol. Obstet., 120:1, 1965.
This report presents detailed hemodynamic studies from 20 patients with various types of shock. Two patterns of shock were recognized: hypovolemic, with low cardiac output, low central venous pressure, low blood pressure, and elevated arterial blood lactate that responded to inotropic and chronotropic stimulation of the heart by isoproterenol; and septic shock. Emphasis is placed on establishing a hemodynamic diagnosis in all patients in shock before treatment is started.

Moore, F. D.: The effects of hemorrhage on body composition. N. Engl. J. Med., 273:567, 1965.
Classic description of changes in body composition with venous hemorrhage of 500 to 1000 ml. in man. Concepts and quantitation of plasma volume refill are introduced. Simultaneous movement of salt and water out of the circulation and albumin into the circulation in response to salt infusion is noted and its significance discussed in terms of the microcirculation and therapy.

Nickerson, M.: Vascular adjustments during the development of shock. Can. Med. Assoc. J., 103:853, 1970.
In this paper, Nickerson, who has greatly influenced and stimulated modern workers in shock, summarizes his concepts as they have developed over the past 15 years. His conclusion is that shock may be initiated by a variety of primary events but appears to have a common pattern of progressive hemodynamic deterioration characterized by excessive constriction of peripheral blood vessels.

Pontoppidan, H., Geffin, B., and Lowenstein, E.: Acute Respiratory Failure in the Adult. Boston, Little, Brown and Company, 1973.
This compact monograph, which appeared originally as a three-part New England Journal of Medicine Progress Report, presents the physiological basis and pathology of acute respiratory failure. Clinical applications are emphasized.

Powers, S. R.: The maintenance of renal function following massive trauma. J. Trauma, 10:554, 1970.
The experimental basis for understanding the abnormal intrarenal distribution of blood flow during shock and trauma together with the rationale for use of saline solution, mannitol, and ethacrynic acid in therapy.

Shires, G. T., Carrico, C. J., and Canizaro, P. C.: Shock. Philadelphia, W. B. Saunders Company, 1973.
This text summarizes the clinical manifestations of shock, the physiological responses, especially of fluid and electrolyte shifts, and pulmonary and kidney function. The cellular response to shock with direct measurements of changes in active transport of ions, which has been the basis for the use of larger quantities of crystalloid solution for resuscitation, is herein carefully documented.

Walt, A. J., and Wilson, R. F.: Management of Trauma: Pitfalls and Practice. Philadelphia, Lea and Febiger, 1975.
An excellent text which covers trauma management from the emergency room to the court room. The do's and don'ts of shock therapy are particularly interesting and based on extensive experience at the Detroit General Hospital.

REFERENCES

1. Adamson, I. Y. R., and Bowden, D. H.: The type 2 cell as progenitor of alveolar epithelial regeneration. Lab. Invest., 30:35, 1974.
2. Albrecht, M., and Clowes, G. H. A., Jr.: The increase of circulatory requirements in the presence of inflammation. Surgery, 56:158, 1964.
3. Altemeier, W. A., Todd, J. C., and Wellford, W. I.: Gram-negative septicemia: A growing threat. Ann. Surg., 166:530, 1967.
4. Archibald, E. W., and McLean, W. S.: Observations upon shock with particular reference to the condition as seen in war surgery. Ann Surg., 66:280, 1917.
5. Barcroft, J: Some problems of the circulation during gas poisoning. J. R. Army Med. Corp., 34:155, 1920.
6. Baue, A. E., Tragus, E. T., Wolfson, S. K., Cary, A. L., and Parkins, W. M.: Hemodynamic and metabolic effects of Ringer's lactate solution in hemorrhagic shock. Ann. Surg., 166:29, 1967.
7. Beecher, H. K. (Ed.): Medical Department of the Army in World War II: Surgery in World War II: Physiologic Effects of Wounds, by the Board for Study of Severely Wounded, North African and Mediterranean Theatre of Operation. Washington, D.C., Army Medical Service of the Defense Department, 1952.
8. Blalock, A.: Experimental shock, the cause of the low blood pressure produced by muscle injury. Arch. Surg., 20:959, 1930.
9. Border, J. R., Gallo, E., and Schenk, W. G., Jr.: Systemic arteriovenous shunts in patients under severe stress: A common cause of high output cardiac failure? Surgery, 60:225, 1966.
10. Bounous, G., Hampson, L. G., and Gurd, F. N.: Cellular nucleotides in hemorrhagic shock: Relationship of intestinal metabolic changes to hemorrhagic enteritis and the barrier function of intestinal mucosa. Ann. Surg., 160:650, 1964.
11. Bounous, G., McArdle, A. H., Hodges, D. M., Hampson, L. G., and Gurd, F. N.: Biosynthesis of intestinal mucin in shock: Relationship to tryptic hemorrhagic enteritis and permeability to curare. Ann. Surg., 164:13, 1966.

12. Bounous, G., Sutherland, N. G., McArdle, A. H., and Gurd, F. N.: The prophylactic use of an "elemental" diet in experimental hemorrhagic and intestinal ischemia. Ann. Surg., 166:312, 1967.

13. Cannon, W. B.: Acidosis in cases of shock, hemorrhage and gas infection. J.A.M.A., 70:531, 1918.

14. Cannon, W. B.: Traumatic Shock, New York, D. Appleton and Company, 1923.

15. Chatterjee, K., Parmley, W. W., Ganz, W., et al.: Hemodynamic and metabolic responses to vasodilator therapy in acute myocardial infarction. Circulation, 48:1183–1193, 1973.

16. Clowes, G. H., Jr., Zuschneid, W., Turner, M., Blackburn, G., Rubin, J., Toala, P., and Green, G.: Observations on the pathogenesis of the pneumonitis associated with severe infections in other parts of the body. Ann. Surg., 167:630, 1968.

17. Cournand, A., Riley, R. L., Bradley, S. E., Breed, E. D., Noble, R. P., Lauson, H. D., Gregersen, M. I., and Richards, D. W.: Studies of the circulation in clinical shock. Surgery, 13:964, 1943.

18. Crile, G. W.: An Experimental Research into Surgical Shock. Philadelphia, J. B. Lippincott Company, 1889.

19. Crowell, J. W., and Guyton, A. C.: Further evidence favoring a cardiac mechanism in irreversibile hemorrhagic shock. Am. J. Physiol., 203:248, 1962.

20. Dale, H. H., and Laidlaw, P. P.: The physiological action of B-iminazolythylamine. J. Physiol., 41:318, 1910.

21. Daniel, A., Pierce, C. H., MacLean, L. D., and Shizgal, H. M.: Lactate metabolism during canine shock from hemorrhage, cardiac tamponade, or endotoxin. In press.

22. Davidson, A. I. G., Clark, C., and Smith, G.: Postoperative wound infections: A computer analysis. Br. J. Surg., 58:333, 1971.

23. Dudrick, S. J., Wilmore, D. W., Vars, H. M., and Rhoads, J. E.: Long-term parenteral nutrition with growth, development, and positive nitrogen balance. Surgery, 64:134, 1968.

24. Feigenbaum, H.: Echocardiography. Philadelphia, Lea & Febiger, 1973.

25. Felty, A. R., and Keefer, C. S.: Bacillus coli sepsis: A clinical study of twenty-eight cases of blood stream infection by the colon bacillus. J.A.M.A., 82:1430, 1924.

26. Franciosa, J. A., Guiha, N. H., Limas, C. J., et al.: Improved left ventricular function during nitroprusside infusion in acute myocardial infarction. Lancet, 1:650–654, 1972.

27. Freid, M. A., and Vosti, K. L.: The importance of underlying disease in patients with gram-negative bacteremia. Arch. Intern. Med., 121:418, 1968.

28. Gelin, L. E.: Intravascular aggregation and capillary flow. Acta Chir. Scand., 113:463, 1957.

29. Gelin, L. E.: Disturbance of the flow properties of blood and its counteraction in surgery. Acta Chir. Scand., 122:287, 1961.

30. Goldberg, L. I.: Drug therapy: Dopamine – Uses of an endogenous catecholamine. N. Engl. J. Med., 291:707–710, 1974.

31. Gump, F. E., Kinney, J. M., and Price, J. B.: Energy metabolism in surgical patients: Oxygen consumption and blood flow. J. Surg. Res., 10:613, 1970.

32. Harkins, H. N., and Rhoads, J. E.: Shock. In Rhoads, J. E., Allen, J. G., Harkins, H. N., and Moyer, C. A. (Eds.): Surgery, Principles and Practice, 4th ed. Philadelphia, J. B. Lippincott Company, 1970, pp. 121–148.

33. Howard, J. M., and Brown, R. B.: Military surgery. In Rhoads, J. E., Allen, J. G., Harkins, H. N., and Moyer, C. A. (Eds.): Surgery, Principles and Practice, 4th ed. Philadelphia, J. B. Lippincott Company, 1970, pp. 599–648.

34. Imamura, M., Clowes, G. H. A., Jr., Blackburn, G. L., O'Donnell, T. F., Jr., Trerice, M., Bhimjee, Y., and Ryan, N. T.: Liver metabolism and glucogenesis in trauma and sepsis. Surgery, 77:868, 1975.

35. Jacob, L.: Uber Allgemeininfektion durch Bacterium coli commune. Deutsche Arch. Klin. Med., 97:303, 1909.

36. Jordan, G. L., Jr., Reul, G. J., Greenberg, S. D., Lefrak, E. A., McCollum, W. B., and Beall, A. C., Jr.: Prevention of post-traumatic pulmonary insufficiency. Arch. Surg., 106:386, 1973.

37. Keith, N. M.: Blood volume changes in wound shock and primary hemorrhage. Report No. IX of the Special Investigation Committee on Surgical Shock and Allied Conditions. Special Report Series No. 27. London, Great Britain Medical Research Council, 1919.

38. Lemire, J., and Johnson, A. L.: Is cardiac resuscitation worthwhile? A decade of experience. N. Engl. J. Med., 286:970, 1972.

39. Liebow, A. A.: Definition and classification of interstitial pneumonias in human pathology. Prog. Resp. Res., 8:1, 1975.

40. Liotta, D., Crawford, E. S., Cooley, D. A., DeBakey, M. E., DeUrguia, M., and Feldman, L.: Prolonged partial left ventricular bypass of means of an intrathoracic pump implanted in the left chest. Trans. Am. Soc. Artif. Intern. Organs, 8:90, 1962.

41. Lister, J., McNeill, I. F., Marshall, V. C., Plzak, L. F., Dagher, F. J., and Moore, F. D.: Transcapillary refilling and hemorrhage in normal man: Basal rates and volumes; effect of norepinephrine. Ann. Surg., 158:698, 1963.

42. Lowery, B. D., Cloutier, C. T., and Carey, L. C.: Blood gas determinations in the severely wounded in hemorrhagic shock. Arch. Surg., 99:330, 1969.

43. Lowery, B. D., Mulder, D. S., Joyal, E. M., and Palmer, W. H.: The effect of hemorrhagic shock on the lung of the pig. Surg. Forum, 21:21, 1970.

44. Lucas, C. E., Rector, F. E., Werner, M., and Rosenberg, I. K.: Altered renal homeostasis with acute sepsis. Arch. Surg., 106:444, 1973.

45. MacLean, L. D., Duff, J. H., Scott, H. M., and Peretz, D. I.: Treatment of shock in man based on hemodynamic diagnosis. Surg. Gynecol. Obstet., 120:1, 1965.

46. MacLean, L. D., Meakins, J. L., Taguchi, K., Duignan, J. P., Dhillon, K. S., and Gordon, J.: Host resistance in sepsis and trauma. Ann. Surg., 182:207, 1975.

47. MacLean, L. D., Mulligan, W. G., McLean, A. P. H., and Duff, J. H.: Patterns of septic shock in man – a detailed study of 56 patients. Ann Surg., 166:543, 1967.

48. Marty, A. T.: Hyperoncotic albumin therapy. Surg. Gynecol. Obstet., 139:105, 1974.

49. McCabe, W. R., and Jackson, G. G.: Gram-negative bacteremia. Arch. Intern. Med., 110:847, 1962.

50. McLean, A. P. H., Duff, J. H., and MacLean, L. D.: Lung lesions associated with septic shock. J. Trauma, 8:891, 1968.

51. McLean, A. P. H., Mulligan, G. W., Otton, P., and MacLean, L. D.: Hemodynamic alterations associated with epidural anaesthesia. Surgery, 62:79, 1967.

52. Meakins, J. L.: Host defense mechanisms: Evaluation and roles of acquired defects and immunotherapy. Can. J. Surg., 18:259, 1975.

53. Mellander, S., and Lewis, D. H.: Effect of hemorrhagic shock on the reactivity of resistance and capacitance vessels and on capillary filtration transfer in cat skeletal muscle. Circ. Res., 13:105, 1963.

54. Miller, L., Gertel, M., Fox, G. S., and MacLean, L. D.: A comparison of narcotic and epidural analgesia on post-operative respiratory function. Am. J. Surg., 131:291, 1976.

55. Moore, F. D., Dagher, F. J., Boyden, C. M., Lee, C. J., and Lyons, J. H.: Hemorrhage in normal man: I. Distribution and dispersal of saline infusion following acute blood loss: Clinical kinetics of blood volume support. Ann. Surg., 163:485, 1966.

56. Moore, F. D., Lyons, J. H., Jr., Pierce, E. C., Jr., Morgan, A. P., Jr., Drinker, P. A., MacArthur, J. D., and Dammin, G. J.: Post-traumatic Pulmonary Insufficiency; Pathophysiology of Respiratory Failure and Principles of Respiratory Care after Surgical Operations, Trauma, Hemorrhage, Burns and Shock. Philadelphia, W. B. Saunders Company, 1969.

57. Muir, A. L., Hall, D. L., Despas, P., and Hogg, J. C.: Distribution of blood flow in the lungs in acute pulmonary edema in dogs. J. Appl. Physiol., 33:763, 1972.

58. Northrup, W. F., III, and Humphrey, E. W.: Relationship of pulmonary capillary protein flux to irreversible hypotension following hemorrhagic shock and reinfusion. Surg. Forum, 26:13, 1975.

59. Nunn, J. F., and Freeman, J.: Problems of oxygenation and oxygen transport during hemorrhage. Anaesthesia, 19:206, 1964.

60. Page, D. L., Canfield, J. B., Kastor, J. A., and DeSanctis, R. W.: Myocardial changes associated with cardiogenic shock. N. Engl. J. Med., 285:133, 1971.

61. Parsons, E., and Phemister, D. B.: Hemorrhage and "shock" in traumatized limbs; an experimental study. Surg. Gynecol. Obstet., 51:196, 1930.

62. Peretz, D. I., McGregor, M., and Dosetor, J. B.: Lactic-acidosis: A clinically significant aspect of shock. Can. Med. Assoc. J., 90:673, 1964.

63. Polk, H. C., Jr.: Quantitative tracheal cultures in surgical patients requiring mechanical ventilatory assistance. Surgery, 78:485, 1975.

64. Polk, H. C., Jr., and Lopez-Mayor, J. F.: Post-operative wound infection: A prospective study of determinant factors and prevention. Surgery, 66:97, 1969.
65. Replogle, R. L., Meiselman, H. J., and Merrill, E. W.: Clinical implications of blood rheology studies. Circulation, 36:148, 1967.
66. Robertson, O. H., and Bock, A. V.: Memorandum on blood volume after hemorrhage. Report No. VI of the Special Investigation Committee on Surgical Shock and Allied Conditions. Special Report Series No. 25. London, Great Britain Medical Research Council, 1919, pp. 213–244.
67. Rosenberg, I. K.: Acute vasomotor nephropathy. In Walt, A. J., and Wilson, R. F.: Management of Trauma: Pitfalls and Practice. Philadelphia, Lea and Febiger, 1970, p. 485.
68. Ross, J., Jr., and Sobel, B. E.: Regulation of cardiac contraction. Ann. Rev. Physiol., 34:47, 1972.
69. Russell, R. O., Jr., Ruckley, C. E., Pumbo, J., Hunt, D., Potanin, C., and Dodge, H. T.: Effects of increasing left ventricular filling pressure in patients with acute myocardial infarction. J. Clin. Invest., 49:1539, 1970.
70. Russell, R. C. G., Walker, C., and Bloom, S. R.: Hyperglucagonemia in the surgical patient. Br. Med. J., 1:10, 1975.
71. Sanders, C. A., Buckley, M. J., Leinbach, R. C., Mundth, E. D., and Austen, W. G.: Mechanical circulatory assistance, current status and experience with combining circulatory assistance, emergency coronary angiography and acute myocardial revascularization. Circulation, 45:1292, 1972.
72. Schumer, W., and Nyhus, L. M. (Eds.): Corticosteroids in the Treatment of Shock. New York, Academic Press, 1968.
73. Shepro, D., and Fulton, G. P. (Eds.): Conference on Microcirculation as Related to Shock. New York, Academic Press, 1968.
74. Siegal, J. H., Greenspan, M., and Del Guercio, L. R. M.: Abnormal vascular tone, defective oxygen transport and myocardial failure in human septic shock. Ann. Surg., 165:504, 1967.
75. Skillman, J. J., Lauler, D. P., Hickler, R. B., Lyons, J. H., Olson, J. E., Ball, M. R., and Moore, F. D.: Hemorrhage in normal man: Effect on renin, cortisol, aldosterone and urine composition. Ann. Surg., 166:865, 1967.
76. Soroff, H. S., Levine, H. J., Sachs, B. F., Birtwell, W. C., and Deterling, R. A., Jr.: Assisted circulation. II. Effects of counterpulsation of left ventricular oxygen consumption and hemodynamics. Circulation, 27:722, 1963.
77. Swan, H. J. C., Ganz, W. F., Forrester, J., Marcus, H., Diamond, G., and Chonette, D.: Catheterization of the heart in man with use of a flow-directed balloon-tipped catheter. N. Engl. J. Med., 283:447, 1970.
78. Todd, T. R. J., Baile, E. M., and Hogg, J. C.: The effect of hemorrhagic shock on the pulmonary capillary membrane. Physiologist, 18:423, 1975.
79. Waisbren, B. A.: Bacteremia due to gram-negative bacilli other than the Salmonella. Arch. Intern. Med., 88:467, 1951.
80. Walker, W. E., Zileli, M. S., Reutter, F. W., Shoemaker, W. C., Friend, D., and Moore, F. D.: Adrenal medullary secretion in hemorrhagic shock. Am. J. Physiol., 197:773, 1959.
81. Warren, J. C.: Surgical Pathology and Therapeutics. Philadelphia, W. B. Saunders Company, 1895.
82. Weisel, R. D., Berger, R. L., and Hechtman, H. B.: Measurement of cardiac output by thermodilution. N. Engl. J. Med., 292:682, 1975.
83. Wilson, R. F., Leblanc, L. P., and Walt, A. J.: Shock due to Trauma in Management of Trauma: Pitfalls and Practice. Philadelphia, Lea and Febiger, 1975, p. 56.
84. Wilson, R. S., and Pontoppidan, H.: Acute respiratory failure: Diagnostic and therapeutic criteria. Crit. Care Med., 2:293, 1974.
85. Wright, C. J., Duff, J. H., McLean, A. P. H., and MacLean, L. D.: Regional capillary blood flow and oxygen uptake in severe sepsis. Surg. Gynecol. Obstet., 132:637, 1971.
86. Woolf, L. I., Groves, A. C., Moore, J. P., Duff, J. H., Finley, R. J., and Loomer, R. L.: Arterial plasma amino acids in patients with serious post-operative infection and in patients with major fractures. Surgery, in press.
87. Zborowska-Sluis, D. T., and Dossetor, J. B.: Hyperlactatemia of hyperventilation. J. Appl. Physiol., 22:746, 1967.

4

FLUID AND ELECTROLYTE MANAGEMENT OF THE SURGICAL PATIENT

G. Tom Shires, M.D.,
and Peter C. Canizaro, M.D.

Fluid and electrolyte management is an integral part of the care of surgical patients, and it may be a critical factor in certain patients. Many diseases, injuries, and operative trauma often impose a great impact on the physiology of fluids and electrolytes within the body, far greater than the changes associated with a simple lack of alimentation. Therefore, a thorough understanding of the metabolism of salt, water, and other electrolytes and of certain metabolic responses is essential to the care of surgical patients.

An attempt will be made in this chapter to define the anatomy of body fluid compartments and the physiologic principles relating to fluids and electrolytes. In addition to the normal functions, a classification of derangements will be developed so that therapy may be described.

ANATOMY OF BODY FLUIDS

A prerequisite to the understanding of fluid and electrolyte management is knowledge of the extent and composition of the various body fluid compartments. Early attempts to define these compartments were relatively accurate, but a more precise definition has been obtained by many investigators through the use of isotopic tracer techniques. The wide range of normal values is a function of body size, weight, and sex, but these compartments are relatively constant in size for the individual patient in the normal steady state. The figures used in this section are approximate and reported as a percentage of body weight.

TOTAL BODY WATER

Water constitutes between 50 and 70 per cent of total body weight. Using deuterium oxide or tritiated water for measurement of total body water (TBW), the average normal value for young adult males is 60 per cent of body weight, and 50 per cent for young adult females. A normal variation of ± 15 per cent applies to both groups. The actual figure for a healthy individual is remarkably constant and is a function of several variables, including lean body mass and age. Since fat contains little water, the lean individual has a greater proportion of water to total body weight than the obese person. Thus, an extremely obese individual may have 25 to 30 per cent less body water than a lean individual of the same weight. The lower percentage of total body water in females correlates with a relatively large amount of subcutaneous adipose tissue and small muscle mass. Moore et al. have shown that total body water, as a percentage of total body weight, decreases steadily and significantly with age to a low of 52 and 47 per cent in males and females respectively.[21] Conversely, the highest proportion of total body water is found in newborn infants, with a maximum of 75 to 80 per cent. During the first several months following birth there is a gradual "physiologic" loss of body water as the infant adjusts to his environment. At one year of age, the total body water averages approximately 65 per cent of the body weight and remains relatively constant throughout the remainder of infancy and childhood.

The water of the body is divided into three functional compartments (Fig. 1). The fluid within the body's diverse cell population, intracellular water, represents between 30 and 40 per cent of the body weight. The extracellular water represents approximately 20 per cent of the body weight and is divided between the intravascular fluid, or plasma (5 per cent of body weight), and the interstitial, or extravascular, extracellular fluid (15 per cent of body weight).

Intracellular Fluid

Measurement of intracellular fluid is determined indirectly by subtraction of the measured extracellular fluid from the measured total body water. The intracellular water is between 30 and 40 per cent of the body weight, with the largest proportion in the skeletal muscle mass. Because of the smaller muscle mass in the female, the percentage of intracellular water is lower than in the male.

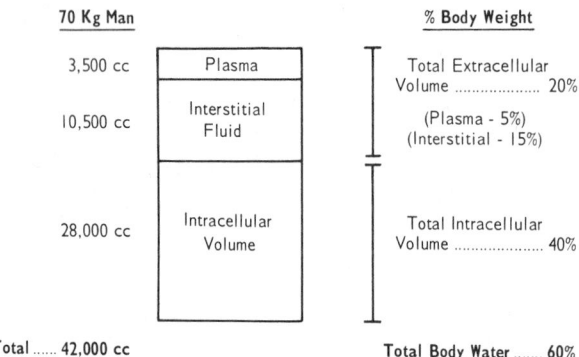

Figure 4–1. Functional compartments of body fluids.

The chemical composition of the intracellular fluid is shown in Figure 2, with potassium and magnesium the principal cations, and phosphates and proteins the principal anions. This is an approximation, since so few data concerning the intracellular fluid are available.

Extracellular Fluid

The total extracellular fluid volume represents approximately 20 per cent of the body weight. The extracellular fluid compartment has two major subdivisions. The plasma volume is approximately 5 per cent of the body weight in the normal adult. The intersti-

tial, or extravascular, extracellular fluid volume, obtained by subtracting the plasma volume from the measured total extracellular fluid volume, comprises approximately 15 per cent of the body weight.

The interstitial fluid is further complicated by having, normally, a rapidly equilibrating, or functional, component, as well as several more slowly equilibrating, or relatively nonfunctioning, components. The nonfunctioning components include connective tissue water as well as water that has been termed *transcellular,* which includes cerebrospinal and joint fluids. This nonfunctional component normally represents only 10 per cent of the interstitial fluid volume (1 to 2 per cent of body weight) and is not to be confused with the relatively nonfunctional extracellular fluid, often called a "third space," found in burns and soft tissue injuries.

The normal constituents of the extracellular fluid are shown in Figure 2, with sodium the principal cation and chloride and bicarbonate the principal anions. There are minor differences in ionic composition between the plasma and interstitial fluid occasioned by the difference in protein concentration. Because of the higher protein content (organic anions) of the plasma, the total concentration of cations is higher and the concentration of inorganic anions somewhat lower than in the interstitial fluid, as explained by the Gibbs-Donnan equilibrium equation.* For practical

---

*The product of the concentrations of any pair of diffusible cations and anions on one side of a semipermeable membrane will equal the product of the same pair of ions on the other side.

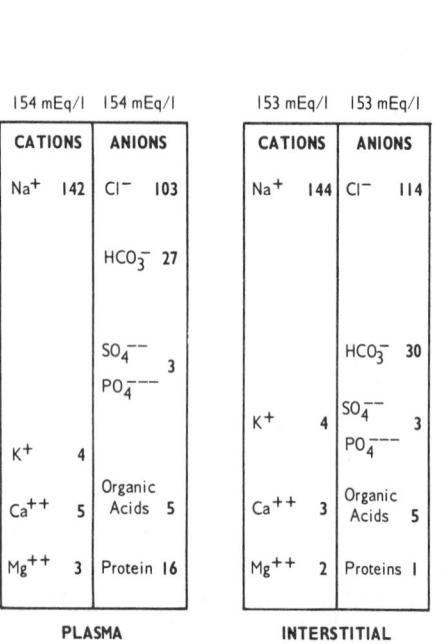
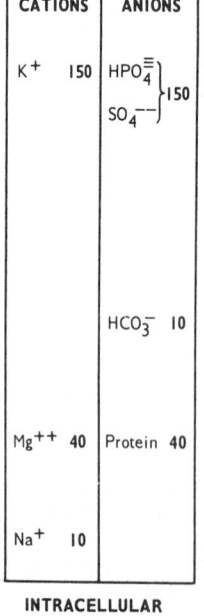

Figure 4–2. Chemical composition of body fluid compartments.

consideration, however, they may be considered equal. The total concentration of intracellular ions exceeds that of the extracellular compartment and would seem to violate the concept of osmolar equilibrium between the two compartments. This apparent discrepancy is due to the fact that the concentration of ions is expressed in milliequivalents (mEq.) without regard to osmotic activity. In addition, some of the intracellular cations probably exist in undissociated form.

Osmotic Pressure

Relevant to a discussion of the complicated interactions between the various body fluid compartments is the definition of commonly used terms: The physiologic and chemical activity of electrolytes depends on (1) the *number of particles* present per unit volume (moles or millimoles (mM.) per liter), (2) the *number of electric charges* per unit volume (equivalents or milliequivalents (mEq.) per liter), and (3) the *number of osmotically active particles,* or ions per unit volume (osmoles or milliosmoles (mOsm.) per liter). The use of the term *grams* or *milligrams per 100 milliliters* expresses the weight of the electrolytes per unit volume but does not allow a physiologic comparison of the solutes in a solution.

A mole of a substance is the molecular weight of that substance in grams, and a millimole is that figure expressed in milligrams. For example, a mole of sodium chloride is 58 grams (Na–23, Cl–35), and a millimole is 58 milligrams. This expression, however, gives no direct information as to the number of osmotically active ions in solution or the electrical charges that they carry.

The electrolytes of the body fluids then may be expressed in terms of chemical combining activity, or "equivalents." An equivalent of an ion is its atomic weight expressed in grams divided by the valence, whereas a milliequivalent of an ion is that figure expressed in milligrams. In the case of univalent ions, a milliequivalent is the same as a millimole. However, in the case of divalent ions, such as calcium or magnesium, one millimole equals two milliequivalents. The importance of this expression is that a milliequivalent of any substance will combine chemically with a milliequivalent of any other substance; in any given solution, the number of milliequivalents of cations present is balanced precisely by the same number of milliequivalents of anions.

When the osmotic pressure of a solution is considered, it is more descriptive to employ the terms osmole and milliosmole. These terms refer to the actual number of osmotically active particles present in solution, but are not dependent on the chemical combining capacities of the substances. Thus, a millimole of sodium chloride, which dissociates nearly completely into sodium and chloride, contributes two milliosmoles, and one millimole of sodium sulfate (Na_2SO_4), which dissociates into three particles, contributes three milliosmoles. One millimole of an un-ionized substance such as glucose is equal to one milliosmole of the substance.

The differences in ionic composition between intracellular and extracellular fluid are maintained by the cell wall, which functions as a semipermeable membrane. The total number of osmotically active particles is 290 to 310 mOsm. in each compartment. Although the osmotic pressure of a fluid is the sum of the partial pressures contributed by each of the solutes in that fluid, the *effective* osmotic pressure is dependent on those substances that fail to pass through the pores of the semipermeable membrane. The dissolved proteins in the plasma, therefore, are primarily responsible for effective osmotic pressure between the plasma and the interstitial fluid compartments. This is frequently referred to as the *colloid osmotic pressure.* The effective osmotic pressure between the extracellular and intracellular fluid compartments would be contributed to by any substance that does not traverse the cell membranes freely. Thus, sodium, which is the principal cation of the extracellular fluid, contributes a major portion of the osmotic pressure, but substances that fail to penetrate the cell membrane freely, such as glucose, also increase the effective osmotic pressure.

Since the cell membranes are completely permeable to water, the effective osmotic pressures in the two compartments are considered to be equal. Any condition that alters the effective osmotic pressure in either compartment will result in redistribution of water between the compartments. Thus, an increase in effective osmotic pressure in the extracellular fluid, which would occur most frequently as a result of increased sodium concentration, would cause a net transfer of water from the intracellular to the extracellular fluid compartment. This transfer of water would continue until the effective osmotic pressures in the two compartments were equal. Conversely, a decrease in the sodium concentration in the extracellular fluid will cause a transfer of water from the extracellular to the intracellular fluid compartment. However, depletion of the extracellular fluid volume without a change in the concentration of ions will not result in transfer of free water from the intracellular space.

Thus, the intracellular fluid shares in losses that involve a change in concentration or composition of the extracellular fluid but shares slowly in changes involving loss of isotonic volume alone. For practical consideration, most losses and gains of body fluid are directly from the extracellular compartment.

CLASSIFICATION OF BODY FLUID CHANGES

The disorders in fluid balance may be classified in three general categories: disturbances of (1) volume, (2) concentration, and (3) composition (Table 1). Of primary importance is the concept that although these disturbances are interrelated, each is a separate entity.

If an isotonic salt solution is added to or lost from the body fluids, only the volume of the extracellular fluid is changed. The acute loss of an isotonic extracellular solution, such as intestinal juice, is followed by a significant decrease in the extracellular fluid volume and little, if any, change in the intracellular fluid volume. Fluid will not be transferred from the intracellu-

Volume abnormalities
  Extracellular fluid deficit
  Extracellular fluid excess

Concentration abnormalities
  Hyponatremia
  Hypernatremia

Compositional abnormalities
  Acidosis-alkalosis
  Hypo-hyperkalemia
  Hypo-hypercalcemia
  Hypo-hypermagnesemia

lar space to refill the depleted extracellular space as long as the osmolarity remains the same in the two compartments.

If water alone is added to or lost from the extracellular fluid, the *concentration* of osmotically active particles will change. Sodium ions account for 90 per cent of the osmotically active particles in the extracellular fluid and generally reflect the tonicity of body fluid compartments. If the extracellular fluid is depleted of sodium, water will pass into the intracellular space until osmolarity is again equal in the two compartments.

The concentration of most other ions within the extracellular fluid compartment can be altered without significant change in the total number of osmotically active particles, thus producing only a *compositional* change. For instance, a rise of the serum potassium concentration from 4 to 8 mEq. per liter would have a significant effect on the myocardium, but it would not significantly change the effective osmotic pressure of the extracellular fluid compartment. Normally functioning kidneys minimize these changes considerably, particularly if the addition or loss of solute or water is gradual.

An internal loss of extracellular fluid into a nonfunctional space, such as the sequestration of isotonic fluid in a burn, peritonitis, ascites, or muscle trauma, is termed a *distributional* change. This transfer or functional loss of extracellular fluid internally may be extracellular (e.g., as in peritonitis) or intracellular (e.g., as in hemorrhagic shock).[29] In any event, all distributional shifts or losses result in a contraction of the *functional* extracellular fluid space.

VOLUME CHANGES

Volume deficit or excess generally must be diagnosed by clinical examination of the patient. There are no readily available laboratory tests of benefit in the acute phase except measurement of the plasma volume. Changes secondary to long-standing derangements in volume, however, may be discernible by laboratory tests. For example, the blood urea nitrogen (BUN) level slowly rises with a long-standing extracellular fluid deficit of sufficient magnitude to reduce glomerular filtration. The concentration of serum sodium is *not* related to the volume status of extracellular fluid; a severe volume deficit may exist with a normal, low, or high serum sodium level.

Volume Deficit. Extracellular fluid volume deficit is by far the most common fluid disorder in the surgical patient. The loss of fluid is not water alone, but water and electrolytes in approximately the same proportion as that in which they exist in normal extracellular fluid. The most common disorders leading to an extracellular fluid volume deficit include losses of gastrointestinal fluids due to vomiting, nasogastric suction, diarrhea, and fistular drainage. Other common causes include sequestration of fluid in soft tissue injuries and infections, intra-abdominal and retroperitoneal inflammatory processes, peritonitis, intestinal obstruction, and burns. The signs and symptoms of this state are easily recognized and are listed in Table 2. The central nervous system and cardiovascular signs occur early with acute rapid losses, whereas tissue signs may be absent until the deficit has existed for at least 24 hours. The central nervous system signs are similar to barbiturate intoxication and may be missed by the casual observer if the volume deficit is mild. The cardiovascular signs are secondary to a decrease in plasma volume and may be associated with varying degrees of hypotension in the patient with a severe extracellular fluid volume deficit. Skin turgor may be difficult to assess in the elderly patient or in the patient with recent weight loss and is not diagnostic in the absence of other confirmatory signs. The body temperature tends to vary with the environmental temperature. In a cool room, the patient may be slightly hypothermic, and the febrile response to an illness may be suppressed. The latter occurs frequently and can be very misleading during clinical evaluation of the septic patient. After partial correction of the volume deficit, the temperature will generally rise to the appropriate level.

Volume Excess. Extracellular fluid volume excess is generally iatrogenic or secondary to renal insufficiency. Both the plasma and interstitial fluid volumes are increased. In the healthy young adult, the signs are generally those of circulatory overload, manifested primarily in the pulmonary circulation, and of excessive fluid in other tissue (Table 2). In the elderly patient, congestive heart failure with pulmonary edema may develop rather quickly with a moderate volume excess.

CONCENTRATION CHANGES

Since the sodium ion is primarily responsible for the osmolarity of the extracellular fluid space, determination of the serum concentration of sodium generally indicates the tonicity of body fluids. Hyponatremia and hypernatremia can be diagnosed by clinical manifestations (Table 3), but discernible signs and symptoms are not generally present until the changes are severe. Changes in concentration should be noted early by appropriate laboratory tests and corrected promptly. Clinical signs of hyponatremia or hypernatremia tend to occur early and with greater severity if the rate of change in extracellular sodium concentration is very rapid.

TABLE 2. Extracellular Fluid Volume

| | Deficit | | Excess | |
	Moderate	Severe	Moderate	Severe
CNS	Sleepiness Apathy Slow responses Anorexia Cessation of usual activity	Decreased tendon reflexes Anesthesia of distal extremities Stupor Coma	None	None
Gastrointestinal	Progressive decrease in food consumption	Nausea, vomiting Refusal to eat Silent ileus and distention	*At Surgery:* Edema of stomach, colon, lesser and greater omenta, and small bowel mesentary	
Cardiovascular	Orthostatic hypotension Tachycardia Collapsed veins Collapsing pulse	Cutaneous lividity Hypotension Distant heart sounds Cold extremities Absent peripheral pulses	Elevated venous pressure Distension of peripheral veins Increased cardiac output Loud heart sounds Functional murmurs Bounding pulse High pulse pressure Increased pulmonary 2nd sound Gallop	Pulmonary edema
Tissue Signs	Soft, small tongue with longitudinal wrinkling Decreased skin turgor	Atonic muscles Sunken eyes	Subcutaneous pitting edema Basilar rales	Anasarca Moist rales Vomiting Diarrhea
Metabolism	Mild decrease of temperature 97–99° ℝ	Marked decrease of temperature 95–98° ℝ	None	None

Hyponatremia. Acute symptomatic hyponatremia (sodium generally less than 130 mEq. per liter) clinically is characterized by central nervous system signs of increased intracranial pressure and tissue signs of excessive intracellular water. There are no cardiovascular signs per se. The hypertension is probably induced by the rise in intracranial pressure, since the blood pressure generally returns to normal with the

TABLE 3. Acute Changes in Osmolar Concentration

| | Hyponatremia (Water Intoxication) | | Hypernatremia (Water Deficit) | |
	Moderate	Severe	Moderate	Severe
CNS	Muscle twitching Hyperactive tendon reflexes Increased intracranial pressure (compensated phase)	Convulsions Loss of reflexes Increased intracranial pressure (decompensated phase)	Restlessness Weakness	Delirium Maniacal behavior
Cardiovascular	Changes in blood pressure and pulse secondary to increased intracranial pressure		Tachycardia Hypotension (if severe)	
Tissue Signs	Salivation, lacrimation Watery diarrhea "Finger printing" of skin (sign of intracellular volume excess)		Decreased saliva and tears Dry and sticky mucous membranes Red, swollen tongue Skin flushed	
Renal	Oliguria progressing to anuria		Oliguria	
Metabolic	None		Fever	

administration of hypertonic solutions of sodium salts. Of importance with severe hyponatremia is the relatively rapid development of oliguric renal failure, which may not be reversible if therapy is delayed.

Many *hyponatremic* states are asymptomatic until the serum sodium level falls below 120 mEq. per liter. One important exception is the patient with increased cerebrospinal fluid pressure, as following closed head injury, where mild hyponatremia may be extremely deleterious, even fatal. This is due to the progressive increase in intracellular water as the extracellular fluid osmolarity falls.

Hypernatremia. Central nervous system tissue signs (listed in Table 3) characterize acute symptomatic hypernatremia. This is the only state in which dry, sticky mucous membranes are characteristic. This sign does not occur with pure extracellular fluid volume deficit alone and may be misleading in the patient who breathes through his mouth. Body temperature is generally elevated and may approach a lethal level, as in the patient with heatstroke. While volume changes occur frequently without a change in serum sodium, the reverse is not true. The disease states that cause a significant acute alteration in the serum sodium frequently produce a concomitant change in the extracellular fluid volume.

MIXED VOLUME AND CONCENTRATION ABNORMALITIES

Mixed volume and concentration abnormalities may develop as a consequence of the disease state or occasionally may result from inappropriate parenteral fluid therapy. Moyer noted that the clinical picture associated with a combination of fluid abnormalities will tend to be an algebraic composite of the signs and symptoms of each state.[22] Like signs produced by both abnormalities will be additive, and opposing signs will tend to nullify one another. For example, the tendency for the body temperature to fall with an extracellular volume deficit may be counteracted by the tendency for it to rise with severe hypernatremia.

One of the more common mixed abnormalities is an extracellular fluid deficit and hyponatremia. This state is readily produced in the patient who continues to drink water while losing large volumes of gastrointestinal fluids. It may also occur in the postoperative period when gastrointestinal losses are replaced with only 5 per cent dextrose in water or a hypotonic sodium solution. An extracellular volume deficit accompanied by hypernatremia may be produced by the loss of a large amount of hypotonic salt solution, such as sweat, in the absence of fluid intake.

The prolonged administration of excessive quantities of sodium salts with restricted water intake may result in an extracellular volume excess and hypernatremia. This may also occur when pure water losses (such as insensible loss of water from the skin and lungs) are replaced with sodium-containing solutions only. Similarly, the excessive administration of water or hypotonic salt solutions to the patient with oliguric renal failure may rapidly produce an extracellular volume excess and hyponatremia.

Normally functioning kidneys may minimize these changes to some extent and compensate for many of the errors associated with parenteral fluid administration. In contrast, the patient in anuric or oliguric renal failure is particularly prone to develop these mixed volume and osmolar concentration abnormalities. Fluid and electrolyte management in these patients, therefore, must be precise. Unfortunately, the fact that a patient with normal kidneys who develops a significant volume deficit may be in a state of "functional" renal failure is often not appreciated. As the volume deficit progresses, the glomerular filtration rate falls precipitously, and the kidneys' unique functions for maintaining fluid homeostasis are lost. These changes may occur with only a mild volume deficit in the elderly patient with borderline renal function. In these elderly patients, the blood urea nitrogen level may rise higher than 100 mg. per 100 ml. in response to the fluid deficit, with a concomitant rise in the serum creatinine level. Fortunately, these changes are usually reversible with early and adequate correction of the extracellular fluid volume deficit.

COMPOSITION CHANGES

Compositional abnormalities of importance include changes in acid-base balance and concentration changes of potassium, calcium, and magnesium.

Acid-Base Balance

The pH (the negative logarithm of the hydrogen ion concentration) of the body fluids is normally maintained within narrow limits in spite of the rather large load of acid produced endogenously as a by-product of body metabolism. The acids are neutralized efficiently by several buffer systems and subsequently excreted by the lungs and kidneys. The important buffers include proteins and phosphates, which play a primary role in maintaining intracellular pH, and the bicarbonate–carbonic acid system, which operates principally in the extracellular fluid space. The proteins and hemoglobin have only minor influence in the extracellular fluid space, but the latter is of prime significance as a buffer in the red cell.

A buffer system consists of a weak acid or base and the salt of that acid or base. The buffering effect is the result of the formation of an amount of weak acid or base equivalent to the amount of strong acid or base added to the system. The resultant change in pH is considerably less than if the substance were added to water alone. Thus, inorganic acids (e.g., hydrochloric, sulfuric, phosphoric) and organic acids (e.g., lactic, pyruvic, keto acids) combine with base bicarbonate, producing the sodium salt of the acid and carbonic acid:

$$(HCL + NaHCO_3 \rightarrow NaCl + H_2CO_3)$$

The carbonic acid formed is then excreted via the lungs as CO_2. The inorganic acid anions are excreted by the kidneys with hydrogen or as ammonium salts. The organic acid anions generally are metabolized as the underlying disorder is corrected, although some renal excretion may occur with high levels.

The functions of the buffer systems are expressed in the Henderson-Hasselbalch equation, which defines the pH in terms of the ratio of the salt and acid. The pH of the extracellular fluid is defined primarily by the ratio of the amount of base bicarbonate (majority as sodium bicarbonate) to the amount of carbonic acid (related to the CO_2 content of alveolar air) present in the blood:

$$\left(pH = pK + \log \frac{BHCO_3}{H_2CO_3} = \frac{27 \text{ mEq./L.}}{1.33 \text{ mEq./L.}} = \frac{20}{1} = 7.4 \right)$$

pK represents the dissociation constant of carbonic acid in the presence of base bicarbonate and by measurement is 6.1. At a body pH of 7.4, the ratio must be 20:1, as depicted. From a chemical standpoint, this is an inefficient buffer system, but the unusual property of CO_2 to behave as an acid or to change to a neutral gas subsequently excreted by the lungs makes it quite efficient biologically.

As long as the 20:1 ratio is maintained, regardless of the absolute values, the pH will remain at 7.4. When an acid is added to the system, the concentration of bicarbonate (the numerator in the Henderson-Hasselbalch equation) will decrease. Ventilation will immediately increase to eliminate larger quantities of CO_2 with a subsequent decrease in the carbonic acid (the denominator in the Henderson-Hasselbalch equation) until the 20:1 ratio is re-established. Slower, more complete compensation is effected by the kidneys with increased excretion of acid salts and retention of bicarbonate. The reverse will occur if an alkali is added to the system. Respiratory acidosis and alkalosis are produced by disturbances of ventilation, with

an increase or decrease in the denominator and a resultant change of the 20:1 ratio. Compensation is primarily renal, with a retention of bicarbonate and increased excretion of acid salts in respiratory acidosis and the reverse process in respiratory alkalosis.

The four types of acid-base disturbances are listed in Table 4. Use of the CO_2 combining power (approximates the plasma bicarbonate) or CO_2 content (includes bicarbonate, carbonic acid, and dissolved CO_2) and knowledge of the patient's disease may allow an accurate diagnosis in the uncomplicated case. However, use of the CO_2 content or CO_2 combining power alone is generally inadequate as an index of acid-base balance. Both these tests principally reflect the level of plasma bicarbonate, since dissolved CO_2 and carbonic acid contribute no more than a few millimoles under most circumstances. In the acute phase, therefore, respiratory acidosis or alkalosis may exist without any change in the CO_2 content; determinations of the pH and P_{CO_2} from a freshly drawn arterial blood sample are necessary for diagnosis. Thus, measurements of pH, bicarbonate concentration, and P_{CO_2} are required for a more complete understanding of the acid-base status in most patients (Table 5).

Unfortunately, more complex acid-base disturbances are frequently encountered. Combinations of respiratory and metabolic changes occur and may represent compensation for the initial acid-base disturbance or may indicate two or more coexisting primary disorders (e.g., a *primary* respiratory acidosis complicated by a *primary* metabolic acidosis or alkalosis).

Usually primary acid-base disturbances are compensated to some extent. A primary metabolic disturbance is initially compensated by changes in pulmonary

TABLE 4.   Acidosis-Alkalosis

	Defect	Common Causes	$\frac{BHCO_3}{H_2CO_3} = \frac{20}{1}$	Compensation
Respiratory acidosis	Retention of CO_2 (decreased alveolar ventilation)	Depression of respiratory center by morphine CNS injury Pulmonary disease— emphysema, pneumonia	↑ Denominator Ratio less than 20:1	Renal Retention of bicarbonate, excretion of acid salts, increased ammonia formation Chloride shift into red cells
Respiratory alkalosis	Excessive loss of CO_2 (increased alveolar ventilation)	Hyperventilation: emotional, severe pain, assisted ventilation, encephalitis	↓ Denominator Ratio greater than 20:1	Renal Excretion of bicarbonate, retention of acid salts, decreased ammonia formation
Metabolic acidosis	Retention of fixed acids or loss of base bicarbonate	Diabetes, azotemia, lactic acid accumulation, starvation Diarrhea, small bowel fistulae	↓ Numerator Ratio less than 20:1	Pulmonary (rapid): increased rate and depth of breathing Renal (slow): As in respiratory acidosis
Metabolic alkalosis	Loss of fixed acids Gain of base bicarbonate Potassium depletion	Vomiting or gastric suction with pyloric obstruction Excessive intake of bicarbonate Diuretics	↑ Numerator Ratio greater than 20:1	Pulmonary (rapid): Decreased rate and depth of breathing Renal (slow): As in respiratory alkalosis

TABLE 5. Respiratory and Metabolic Components of Acid-Base Disorders

	Acute (uncompensated)			Chronic (partially compensated)		
	pH	P_{CO_2} (respiratory component)	Plasma HCO_3^-* (metabolic component)	pH	P_{CO_2} (respiratory component)	Plasma HCO_3^-* (metabolic component)
Respiratory acidosis	↓↓	↑↑	N	↓	↑↑	↑
Respiratory alkalosis	↑↑	↓↓	N	↑	↓↓	↓
Metabolic acidosis	↓↓	N	↓↓	↓	↓	↓
Metabolic alkalosis	↑↑	N	↑↑	↑	↑?	↑

*Measured as standard bicarbonate, whole-blood buffer base, CO_2-content or CO_2-combining power. The *base excess value* is positive when the standard bicarbonate is above normal and negative when the standard bicarbonate is below normal.

ventilation, while respiratory disturbances are compensated by renal mechanisms. For example, the initial compensation for an acute metabolic acidosis is an increase in the rate and depth of breathing to lower the arterial P_{CO_2}. As pointed out by Astrup et al., the actual state of the acid-base disorder may be characterized by the degree of compensation—*not compensated* (early or compensatory mechanisms not functioning), *partially compensated* (pH has not returned to a normal value), *compensated,* or *overcompensated.*[3]

As previously noted, a knowledge of the pH, bicarbonate concentration, and P_{CO_2} will allow an accurate diagnosis of most acid-base disturbances. However, the clinical interpretation of these measurements is associated with some inherent problems. Although the arterial P_{CO_2} is considered an accurate index of primary respiratory disturbances, changes in the level may represent compensation for a primary metabolic alteration. Thus, a depressed P_{CO_2} (below 40 mm. Hg) is characteristic of respiratory alkalosis but also represents the normal compensatory response to a metabolic acidosis. Similarly, the level of plasma bicarbonate cannot be regarded exclusively as an index of metabolic disturbances. An elevated plasma bicarbonate level may indicate a primary metabolic alkalosis or a compensatory response to chronic respiratory acidosis.

In an effort to separate the respiratory and metabolic components of acid-base disorders, two other approaches have been introduced: In 1948 Singer and Hastings[30] introduced the concept of *whole blood buffer base,* and later Astrup and his colleagues proposed the use of the *standard bicarbonate* and *base excess* values.[2, 3, 18] The approach advocated by Astrup has been the more popular of the two, although both are attempts to quantify the metabolic, or nonrespiratory, component in an acid-base disturbance and separate it from the respiratory component.

The standard bicarbonate is defined as the concentration of bicarbonate in plasma, when whole blood with fully oxygenated hemoglobin has been equilibrated with CO_2 at a P_{CO_2} of 40 mm. Hg at a temperature of 38° C. This value may be rapidly and accurately determined using the Astrup technique by measuring pH values at two known levels of P_{CO_2} and reading the standard bicarbonate directly from a nomogram. The normal mean value for standard bicarbonate is 24.5 mEq. per liter of plasma. As a measure of bicarbonate concentration in plasma, the standard bicarbonate is probably superior to both the CO_2 content and CO_2 combining power values, since the latter two determinations vary with the actual P_{CO_2} and oxygen saturation. Unfortunately, the standard bicarbonate, unlike the whole blood buffer base, does not indicate the total amount of surplus acid or base present, since the bicarbonate–carbonic acid system does not account for the entire buffering capacity of the blood. This information can be obtained by expressing the base content of the blood as *base excess* or *base deficit.* Base excess (or deficit) directly expresses the amount, in milliequivalents, of fixed base (or fixed acid) added to each liter of blood. This value is obtained by multiplying the deviation of standard bicarbonate from the normal mean by a factor of 1.2. This factor corrects for the buffering capacity of the red cells and will vary slightly with changes in hemoglobin concentration.[3] To avoid calculations, the base excess may be read directly from a nomogram. When the term *base excess* is used exclusively, the *positive* values represent the excess of base, and the *negative* values reflect the deficit of base (or excess of acid).*

In an excellent review of the Singer-Hastings and the Astrup systems, Schwartz and Relman state that neither system offers any advantage over the classic approach for the diagnosis of acid-base disorders.[24] They question the validity of using an in vitro CO_2 titration curve as a measure of in vivo acid-base changes. Additionally, they note that the use of either of the two systems may be misleading in the analysis of chronic disorders. For example, a low pH with an elevated P_{CO_2}, a normal standard bicarbonate value, and a base excess value of zero are compatible with a diagnosis of primary uncompensated respiratory acidosis. After several hours or days, compensatory renal mechanisms would cause elevation of standard bicarbonate level above normal, resulting in a positive base

*The deficit or excess of base in the extracellular compartment can be estimated in milliequivalents by multiplying the negative or positive value for base excess, in milliequivalents per liter of blood, by 0.3 times the body weight in kilograms (Mellemgaard and Astrup).

excess value. This partially compensated respiratory acidosis, then, may be erroneously interpreted as a respiratory acidosis *plus* metabolic alkalosis as indicated by a significant base excess.

Despite these shortcomings, either approach may be useful when properly interpreted as a single laboratory test. Other systems have been recommended, some with ingeniously devised nomograms, but all are subject to misinterpretation. Unfortunately, there are no shortcuts. Regardless of the methods used, the proper analysis of complex acid-base disorders requires a thorough knowledge of the clinical situation, good judgment, and a sound understanding of acid-base physiology.

Respiratory Acidosis. This condition is associated with retention of CO_2 secondary to decreased alveolar ventilation. The more common causes are listed in Table 4. Initially, the arterial Pco_2 is elevated (usually above 50 mm. Hg), and the plasma bicarbonate concentration (measured as CO_2 combining power, CO_2 content, or standard bicarbonate) is normal. In the chronic form, the Pco_2 remains elevated, and the bicarbonate concentration rises as compensation occurs.

This problem may be particularly serious in the patient with chronic pulmonary disease in whom pre-existing respiratory acidosis may be accentuated in the postoperative period. A number of conditions resulting in inadequate ventilation—airway obstruction, atelectasis, pneumonia, pleural effusion, hypoventilation due to the pain of upper abdominal incisions, or abdominal distention limiting diaphragmatic excursion—may exist singly or in combination to produce respiratory acidosis. Although restlessness, hypertension, and tachycardia in the immediate postoperative period may be due to pain, similar signs indicate inadequate ventilation with hypercapnia. The use of narcotics in this situation will compound the problem by further depressing respiration.

Management involves prompt correction of the pulmonary defect, when feasible, and measures to ensure adequate ventilation. Endotracheal intubation and mechanical ventilation are occasionally necessary to achieve this objective. Strict attention to tracheobronchial hygiene during the postoperative period is an important preventive measure in all patients, particularly those with chronic pulmonary disease. Encouraging deep breathing and coughing, using humidified air to prevent inspissation of secretions, and avoiding oversedation are all indicated.

Respiratory Alkalosis. Respiratory alkalosis is a more common problem in the surgical patient than previously recognized. Hyperventilation due to apprehension, pain, hypoxia, central nervous system injury, and assisted ventilation are all common causes. Any of these conditions may cause a rapid depression of the arterial Pco_2 and elevation of the pH. The plasma bicarbonate concentration is normal in the acute phase but falls with compensation if the condition persists.

Mild respiratory alkalosis secondary to hyperventilation during the operative procedure frequently occurs. This is of little consequence in the majority of patients and generally requires no therapy. One important exception is the patient with impaired cerebral blood flow from obstructive arterial disease (or during performance of carotid endarterectomy), in whom modest hypocapnia with cerebral vasoconstriction may cause irreparable damage.

The majority of patients who require ventilatory support in the postoperative period will develop varying degrees of respiratory alkalosis. This may be inadvertent, owing to improper use of the mechanical respirator, or it may occur during attempts to raise the Po_2 in a hypoxic patient. Proper management of the patient on a mechanical ventilator requires frequent measurements of blood gases and appropriate corrections of the ventilatory pattern when indicated. The arterial Pco_2 should not be allowed to fall below 30 mm. Hg, as serious complications may occur, particularly in the presence of a complicating hypokalemia or metabolic alkalosis. Generally, the Pco_2 can be maintained at an acceptable level by proper adjustments of the ventilatory rate and volume. Increasing the pulmonary dead space is of doubtful benefit, while adding 5 per cent CO_2 to the inspired air is potentially dangerous and poorly tolerated by most patients.

The dangers of a severe respiratory alkalosis are those related to potassium depletion and include the development of ventricular arrhythmias and fibrillation, particularly in patients who are digitalized or have pre-existing hypokalemia. Other complications include a shift of the oxygen dissociation curve to the left, which limits the ability of hemoglobin to unload oxygen at the tissue level except at low intracellular Po_2, and the development of tetany and convulsions if the level of ionized calcium is significantly depressed. The development of hypokalemia may be quite sudden and is related to entry of potassium ions into the cells in exchange for hydrogen and an excessive urinary potassium loss in exchange for sodium. Severe and persistent respiratory alkalosis is often difficult to correct and may be associated with a poor prognosis because of the underlying cause of hyperventilation. Treatment is primarily directed toward preventing the condition by the proper use of mechanical respirators and correcting any pre-existing potassium deficits.

Metabolic Acidosis. Metabolic acidosis results from the retention or gain of fixed acids (diabetic acidosis, lactic acidosis, azotemia) or the loss of base bicarbonate (diarrhea, small bowel fistula, renal insufficiency with inability to resorb bicarbonate). The excess of hydrogen ion results in lower pH and plasma bicarbonate concentration. The initial compensation is pulmonary, with an increase of the rate and depth of breathing and depression of the arterial Pco_2.

Renal damage may interfere with the important role of the kidneys in the regulation of acid-base balance. The kidneys serve a vital function in this regard through the excretion of nitrogenous waste products and acid metabolites and the resorption of bicarbonates. If renal damage occurs and these functions are lost, metabolic acidosis develops rapidly and may be difficult to control.

With normal kidneys, metabolic acidosis may develop when the capacity of the kidneys for handling chlorides is exceeded. This is particularly common in patients who have excessive losses of alkaline gastrointestinal fluids (biliary, pancreatic, small bowel secretions) and are maintained on parenteral fluids for an extended period of time. Continued replacement of these losses with fluids having an inappropriate chloride/bicarbonate ratio, such as isotonic sodium chloride solution, will not correct the pH change; the use of a balanced salt solution, such as lactated Ringer's, is indicated.

One of the most common causes of severe metabolic acidosis in surgical patients is acute circulatory failure with accumulation of lactic acid. This is a reflection of tissue hypoxia due to inadequate perfusion, although it is only one of the manifestations of cellular dysfunction. Acute hemorrhagic shock may result in a rapid and profound drop in the pH, and attempts to raise the blood pressure with vasopressors will simply compound the problem. Similarly, attempts to correct the acidosis by the infusion of large quantities of sodium bicarbonate without restoration of flow are futile. Following restoration of adequate tissue perfusion by proper volume replacement, the lactic acid is quickly metabolized and the pH returned to normal. The use of lactated Ringer's solution to replace the extracellular fluid deficit incurred with hemorrhagic shock concomitant with administration of whole blood does not accentuate the lactic acidosis. Instead, there is a rapid decrease in the lactate level and return of pH toward normal, as opposed to the results when whole blood alone is used.[7, 17]

The indiscriminate use of sodium bicarbonate during the resuscitation of patients in hypovolemic shock is discouraged for several reasons. A mild metabolic acidosis is a common finding following resuscitation, in part due to the alkalinizing effects of blood transfusion and the administration of lactated Ringer's solution. After infusion (and partial restoration of hepatic blood flow), the citrate contained in the transfused blood and the lactate in lactated Ringer's solution are metabolized, and bicarbonate is formed. The organic acidosis (lactic acid) that developed during the shock episode is rapidly cleared once adequate tissue perfusion is restored. Lactic acid production ceases, the hydrogen ion load is buffered and excreted via the lungs as CO_2, and the organic anion, lactate, is metabolized by the liver. If excessive quantities of sodium bicarbonate were administered simultaneously, severe metabolic alkalosis could result. An alkaline pH may be highly undesirable in this situation, particularly in patients with hypoxia or low fixed cardiac outputs, because it shifts the oxygen dissociation curve to the left. Other factors that tend to shift the oxygen dissociation curve to the left in this situation include the depressed level of erythrocyte 2,3-diphosphoglycerate in the transfused blood, and the development of hypothermia. If the curve shifts far enough to the left, significant interference with oxygen unloading at the cellular level may occur.[8]

The treatment of metabolic acidosis, therefore, should be directed toward correction of the underlying disorder when possible. Bicarbonate therapy properly may be reserved for the treatment of severe metabolic acidosis, particularly following cardiac arrest, when partial correction of the pH may be essential to restore myocardial function. However, recent studies indicate that the acidosis accompanying cardiac arrest is well compensated for a significant period of time if the patient is well ventilated and not previously acidotic.[6]

In addition, the administration of bicarbonate in the usual recommended doses may induce an acute and severe hypernatremia and hyperosmolarity.[16] Thus, bicarbonate should be used judiciously during cardiac arrest. Mattar et al. recommended that the initial dose of bicarbonate not exceed 50 ml. of 7.5 per cent solution (45 mEq. $NaHCO_3$ containing 90 mOsm.), and the decision for additional doses be based on measurements of pH and Pco_2 when possible.[16] Similarly, pH correction of more protracted states of metabolic acidosis may be indicated but should be accomplished slowly. Frequent measurements of serum electrolytes and blood pH are the best guides to therapy, since a satisfactory formula to estimate the amount of alkali needed has not been devised.

Metabolic Alkalosis. Metabolic alkalosis results from the loss of fixed acids or the gain of base bicarbonate and is aggravated by any pre-existing potassium depletion. Both the pH and plasma bicarbonate concentration are elevated. Compensation for metabolic alkalosis is primarily by renal mechanisms, since respiratory compensation is generally small and cannot be detected in most patients. Rarely, hypercapnia may represent a compensatory response to metabolic alkalosis in patients without chronic pulmonary disease.[32] When this is suspected, rapid reduction in Pco_2 by mechanical ventilation should be avoided. Rather, the Pco_2 will fall as the metabolic alkalosis is corrected.

The majority of patients with metabolic alkalosis have some degree of hypokalemia. Depletion of cellular potassium results in entry of hydrogen and sodium ions into the cells with resultant lowering of intracellular pH and an extracellular alkalosis. Metabolic alkalosis, in turn, results in excessive urinary potassium loss in exchange for sodium, which further accentuates the alkalosis. The dangers of metabolic alkalosis are the same as discussed with respiratory alkalosis.

An interesting and not infrequent problem in the surgical patient is *hypochloremic, hypokalemic metabolic alkalosis* resulting from persistent vomiting or gastric suction in the patient with pyloric obstruction. Unlike vomiting with an open pylorus (involving a loss of gastric, pancreatic, biliary, and intestinal secretions), this entity results in loss of fluid with high chloride and hydrogen ion concentration in relation to sodium. The loss of chloride causes accelerated loss of sodium and bicarbonate in the urine and partial compensation of the alkalosis. In addition, the alkalosis itself causes increased renal excretion of potassium. As the volume deficit progresses, potassium and hydrogen ions are excreted into the urine in increasing quantities in an attempt to conserve sodium, resulting in an uncompensated alkalosis and hypokalemia. The initially alkaline urine becomes acid after a period of time owing to the hydrogen ion excretion ("paradoxic aciduria"). Proper management includes replacement of the extracellular fluid volume deficit with isotonic sodium chloride solution in addition to replacement of potassium. A severe potassium depletion is invariably present but may be overlooked owing to concentration of the serum potassium by a severe volume deficit. However, volume repletion should be started and a good urine output obtained before potassium is administered.

Rarely, severe hypokalemic metabolic alkalosis in a patient with pyloric outlet obstruction may be refractory to standard therapy. This occurs most often in patients who also have severe hypochloremia and several liters of nasogastric drainage daily. In the past, the infusion of ammonium chloride or arginine hydrochloride has been the usual method for increasing the level of nonvolatile acids. However, infusion of the former may produce ammonia toxicity, and the latter solution is no longer available commercially. Recently, the use of 0.1N to 0.2N hydrochloric acid has been shown to be safe and effective therapy for correction of severe, resistant metabolic alkalosis.[1, 13, 25] The technique for infusion of hydrochloric acid, as described by Abouna et al., involves the preparation of an isotonic solution by the addition of 150 ml. of *one normal* hydrochloric acid (300 mEq. of hydrogen and chloride) to one liter of sterile water. The hydrochloric acid can be added to a liter of isotonic saline or 5 per cent dextrose solution if desired. The infusion should be administered over a 6- to 24-hour period with measurements of pH, P_{CO_2} and serum electrolytes every 4 to 6 hours. Generally, one or two liters of solution over a period of 24 hours is sufficient, although one should not hesitate to infuse additional hydrochloric acid when the need is based on appropriate clinical and laboratory evidence. Temporary control of the alkalosis with this method is usually successful, but control of the underlying cause should be obtained as soon as possible.

A rough estimate of the initial dose of hydrochloric acid solution can be calculated from the estimated chloride or hydrogen ion deficit. The chloride deficit is calculated from the plasma chloride concentration and the chloride space (approximately 20 per cent of body weight). The hydrogen ion deficit can be calculated from the plasma base excess and the hydrogen ion space (approximately 60 per cent of total body weight).

As an example, for a 70-kg. patient with a metabolic alkalosis and a plasma chloride of 80 mEq. per liter, the initial dose of hydrochloric acid is calculated as follows:

Chloride deficit = (20% of body weight) × (normal plasma chloride − observed plasma chloride)
= (0.2 × 70 kg.) × (103 mEq./L. − 80 mEq./L.)
= 322 mEq.

This amount of chloride (as hydrochloric acid) would be contained in approximately 2 liters of the solution described above. It is emphasized that while calculations of this type are helpful, close monitoring of pH and serum electrolytes is essential.

Potassium Abnormalities

The normal dietary intake of potassium is approximately 50 to 100 mEq. daily, and in the absence of hypokalemia, the majority of this is excreted in the urine. Ninety-eight per cent of the potassium in the body is located within the intracellular compartment at a concentration of approximately 150 mEq. per liter, and it is the major cation of intracellular water. Although the total extracellular potassium in a 70-kg. male would approximate only 63 mEq. (4.5 mEq./L. × 14 L.), this small amount is critical to cardiac and neuromuscular function. In addition, the turnover rate in the extracellular fluid compartment may be extremely rapid.

The intracellular and extracellular distribution of potassium is influenced by many factors. Significant quantities of intracellular potassium are released into the extracellular space in response to severe injury or surgical stress, acidosis, and the catabolic state. A significant rise in serum potassium may occur in these states in the presence of oliguric or anuric renal failure, but dangerous hyperkalemia (greater than 6 mEq. per liter) is rarely encountered if renal function is normal. After severe trauma, however, normal or excessive urinary volumes may not reflect the ability of the kidney to clear solutes or to excrete potassium. (See the section High-Output Renal Failure.)

Hyperkalemia. The signs of a significant hyperkalemia are limited to the cardiovascular and gastrointestinal systems. The gastrointestinal symptoms include nausea, vomiting, intermittent intestinal colic, and diarrhea. The cardiovascular signs are apparent on the electrocardiogram initially, with high peaked T waves, widened QRS complex, and depressed ST segments. Disappearance of T waves, heart block, and diastolic cardiac arrest may develop with increasing levels of potassium.

Treatment of hyperkalemia consists of immediate measures to reduce the serum potassium level, withholding of exogenously administered potassium, and correction of the underlying cause if possible. Temporary suppression of the myocardial effects of a sudden rapid rise of potassium level can be accomplished by the intravenous administration of a solution containing 80 mEq. of sodium lactate, 100 ml. of calcium gluconate, and 100 ml. of 50 per cent dextrose in water. The administration of dextrose stimulates the synthesis of glycogen, resulting in an uptake of potassium. Insulin may also be given, but it should be limited to 1 unit per 5 gm. or more of glucose, since rebound hypoglycemia may occur. The sodium lactate raises the pH and shifts potassium intracellularly, and the calcium gluconate tends to counteract the myocardial effects of hyperkalemia. Administration of this solution over a 2-hour period allows time to prepare for definitive removal of the excess potassium by hemodialysis or peritoneal dialysis. A slow rise of potassium level (less than 1 mEq. per liter per day) can be controlled by the use of cation-exchange resins, preferably in the sodium cycle,* administered by rectum in doses of 24 gm. every 12 hours. To prevent rapid absorption of water from the colon, 200 ml. of 10 per cent dextrose in water is used as the vehicle.

Hypokalemia. The more common problem in the surgical patient is hypokalemia, which may occur as a

---

*Kayexalate

result of (1) excessive renal excretion, (2) movement of potassium into cells, (3) prolonged administration of potassium-free parenteral fluids with continued obligatory renal loss of potassium (20 mEq. per day or more), (4) parenteral hyperalimentation with inadequate potassium replacement, and (5) loss of gastrointestinal secretions.

Potassium plays an important role in the regulation of acid-base balance. Increased renal excretion occurs with both respiratory and metabolic alkalosis. Potassium is in competition with hydrogen ion for renal tubular excretion in exchange for sodium ion. Thus, in alkalosis, the increased potassium ion excretion in exchange for sodium ion permits hydrogen ion conservation. Hypokalemia itself may produce a metabolic alkalosis, since an increase in excretion of hydrogen ions occurs when the concentration of potassium in the tubular cell is low. In addition, movement of hydrogen ions into the cells as a consequence of potassium loss is partly responsible for the alkalosis. In metabolic acidosis the reverse process occurs, and the excess hydrogen ion exchanges for sodium with retention of greater amounts of potassium.

Renal tubular excretion of potassium ion is increased when large quantities of sodium are available for excretion. The more sodium ion available for resorption, the more potassium is exchanged for it in the lumen. Potassium requirements for prolonged or massive isotonic fluid volume replacement are increased, probably on this basis. The same mechanism may also explain the increased potassium ion excretion with steroid administration.

The renal excretion of potassium may be small when compared to the amount of potassium that may be lost in gastrointestinal secretions. The amount per liter in various types of gastrointestinal fluids is shown in Table 6. Although the average potassium concentration of some of these fluids is relatively low, significant hypokalemia will result if potassium-free fluids are used for replacement.

Hypokalemia also may be a serious problem in the patient maintained on intravenous hyperalimenta-tion. Large quantities of supplemental potassium generally are necessary to restore depleted intracellular stores and to meet the requirements for tissue synthesis during the anabolic phase.

In summary, most of the factors that tend to influence potassium metabolism result in excess excretion, and a tendency toward hypokalemia occurs frequently in the surgical patient except when shock or acidosis interferes with the normal renal handling of potassium.

The signs of potassium deficit are related to failure of normal contractility of skeletal, smooth, and cardiac muscle and include weakness that may progress to flaccid paralysis, diminished to absent tendon reflexes, and paralytic ileus. Sensitivity to digitalis with cardiac arrhythmias and electrocardiographic signs of low voltage, flattening of T waves, and depression of ST segments are characteristic. However, signs of potassium deficit may be masked by those of a severe extracellular fluid volume deficit. Repletion of the volume deficit may further aggravate the situation by lowering the serum potassium level secondary to dilution.

The treatment of hypokalemia involves, first, prevention of this state. In the replacement of gastrointestinal fluids, it is safe to replace the upper limits of loss, since an excess is readily handled by the patient with normal renal function. Potassium is available in 20-mEq. and 40-mEq. ampules for addition to intravenous fluids. No more than 40 mEq. should be added to a liter of intravenous fluid, and the rate of administration should not exceed 40 mEq. per hour unless the electrocardiogram is being monitored. In the absence of specific indications, potassium should not be given to the oliguric patient or during the first 24 hours following severe surgical stress or trauma.

Calcium Abnormalities

The majority of the 1000 to 1200 gm. of body calcium in the average-size adult is found in the bone in the form of phosphate and carbonate. Normal daily intake of calcium is between 1 and 3 gm. Most of this is

TABLE 6. Composition of Gastrointestinal Secretions

	Volume (ml./24 hr.)	Na (mEq./L.)	K (mEq./L.)	Cl (mEq./L.)	HCO₃ (mEq./L.)
Salivary	1500 (500–2000)	10 (2–10)	26 (20–30)	10 (8–18)	30
Stomach	1500 (100–4000)	60 (9–116)	10 (0–32)	130 (8–154)	
Duodenum	(100–2000)	140	5	80	
Ileum	3000 (100–9000)	140 (80–150)	5 (2–8)	104 (43–137)	30
Colon		60	30	40	
Pancreas	(100–800)	140 (113–185)	5 (3–7)	75 (54–95)	115
Bile	(50–800)	145 (131–164)	5 (3–12)	100 (89–180)	35

excreted via the gastrointestinal tract, and 200 mg. or less is excreted in the urine daily. The normal serum level is between 9 and 11 mg. per 100 ml. (depending on the individual laboratory's normal range), and approximately half of this is not ionized and is bound to plasma protein. An additional nonionized fraction (5 per cent) is bound to other substances in the plasma and interstitial fluid, whereas the remaining 45 per cent is the ionized portion that is responsible for neuromuscular stability. Determination of the plasma protein level, therefore, is essential for proper analysis of the serum calcium level. The ratio of ionized to nonionized calcium is also related to the pH; acidosis causes an increase in the ionized fraction, whereas alkalosis causes a decrease.

Disturbances of calcium metabolism generally are not a problem in the uncomplicated postoperative patient, with the exception of skeletal loss during prolonged immobilization. Routine administration of calcium to the surgical patient, therefore, is not needed in the absence of specific indications.

Hypocalcemia. The symptoms of hypocalcemia (serum level less than 8 mg. per 100 ml.) are numbness and tingling of the circumoral region and the tips of the fingers and toes. The signs are of neuromuscular origin and include hyperactive tendon reflexes, positive Chvostek's sign, muscle and abdominal cramps, tetany with carpopedal spasm, convulsions (with severe deficit), and prolongation of the Q-T interval on the electrocardiogram.

The common causes include acute pancreatitis, massive soft tissue infections (necrotizing fasciitis), acute and chronic renal failure, pancreatic and small intestinal fistulas, and hypoparathyroidism. Transient hypocalcemia is a frequent occurrence in the hyperparathyroid patient following removal of a parathyroid adenoma, owing to atrophy of the remaining glands. Asymptomatic hypocalcemia may occur with hypoproteinemia (normal ionized fraction), whereas symptoms may appear with a normal serum calcium level in a patient with severe alkalosis. The latter is due to a decrease in the physiologically active or ionized fraction of total serum calcium. Calcium levels also may fall with a severe depletion of magnesium.

Treatment is directed toward correction of the underlying cause with concomitant repletion of the deficit. Acute symptoms may be relieved by the intravenous administration of calcium gluconate or calcium chloride. Calcium lactate may be given orally, with or without supplemental vitamin D, in the patient requiring prolonged replacement.

The routine administration of calcium during massive transfusions of blood remains controversial and reflects a paucity of studies where calcium *ion* levels are measured. In the majority of studies, calcium ion concentrations have been estimated from measured *total* serum calcium levels. At present, available data indicated that the majority of patients receiving blood transfusions do not require calcium supplementation.[9, 10] The binding of ionized calcium by citrate is generally compensated for by the mobilization of calcium from body stores. For patients receiving blood as rapidly as 500 ml. every five to ten minutes, however, calcium administration is recommended. An appropri-

ate dose, obtained from the data of Moore, is 0.2 gm. of calcium chloride (2 ml. of 10 per cent calcium chloride solution) administered intravenously in a separate line, for every 500 ml. of blood transfused.[21] To avoid dangerous levels of hypercalcemia, this dose of calcium is recommended only while blood is being transfused at the rate noted above. Additionally, the total dose of calcium generally should not exceed 3 gm. unless there is objective evidence of hypocalcemia. Larger doses are rarely indicated, since there is some mobilization of calcium and citrate breakdown with release of calcium ion, even with shock and inadequate peripheral perfusion. During massive transfusions some attempt should be made to monitor the calcium level. A rough approximation of calcium ion concentration can be obtained by monitoring the Q-T interval on the electrocardiogram, although techniques for the rapid measurement of calcium ion concentration are now available.

Hypercalcemia. The symptoms of hypercalcemia are rather vague and of gastrointestinal, renal, musculoskeletal, and central nervous system origin. The early manifestations of hypercalcemia include easy fatigue, lassitude, weakness of varying degree, anorexia, nausea, vomiting, and weight loss. With higher serum calcium levels, lassitude gives way to somnambulism, stupor, and finally coma. Other symptoms include severe headaches, pains in the back and extremities, thirst, polydypsia, and polyuria. The critical level for serum calcium is between 16 and 20 mg. per 100 ml., and unless treatment is instituted promptly, the symptoms may rapidly progress to death. The two major causes of hypercalcemia are hyperparathyroidism and cancer with bony metastasis. The latter is most frequently seen in the patient with metastatic breast cancer who is receiving estrogen therapy.

The treatment of acute hypercalcemia is an emergency. Measures to lower the serum calcium level are instituted immediately while preparations are being made for more definitive treatment. Of particular importance is the rapid repletion of the associated extracellular fluid volume deficit, which will immediately lower the calcium level by dilution. Other measures that have been used and may be of temporary benefit include the use of a chelating agent (EDTA), steroids, sodium sulfate solution, and hemodialysis. Recently, intravenous mithromycin has been shown to reduce the serum calcium level in normocalcemic and hypercalcemic patients.[12] The definitive treatment of acute hypercalcemic crisis in patients with hyperparathyroidism is immediate surgery.[4]

Treatment of hypercalcemia in the patient with metastatic cancer is primarily that of prevention. The serum calcium level is checked frequently; if it is elevated, the patient is placed on a low-calcium diet, and measures to ensure adequate hydration are instituted.

Magnesium Abnormalities

The infrequent occurrence of magnesium deficiency and the previous lack of a rapid, precise technique for measurement of magnesium ion concentration account for the late appreciation of this entity. The total body content of magnesium in the average adult is approximately 2000 mEq., about half of which is incorporated in bone and only slowly exchangeable. The distribution of magnesium is similar to that of potassium, the major portion being intracellular. Plasma magnesium concentration normally ranges between 1.5 and 2.5 mEq. per liter. The normal dietary intake of magnesium is approximately 20 mEq. (240 mg.) daily. The larger part is excreted in the feces, and the remainder in the urine. The kidneys show a remarkable ability to conserve magnesium; on a magnesium-free diet, renal excretion of this ion may be less than 1 mEq. per day.

Magnesium Deficiency. Magnesium deficiency is known to occur with starvation, malabsorption syndromes, protracted losses of gastrointestinal fluid, prolonged parenteral fluid therapy with magnesium-free solutions, and parenteral hyperalimentation when inadequate quantities of magnesium have been added to the solution. Other causes include acute pancreatitis, diabetic acidosis during treatment, primary aldosteronism, chronic alcoholism, and burns (late stage).

The magnesium ion is essential for proper function of most enzyme systems, and depletion is characterized by neuromuscular and central nervous system hyperactivity. The signs and symptoms are quite similar to those of calcium deficiency, including hyperactive tendon reflexes, muscle tremors, and tetany with a positive Chvostek sign. Progression to delirium and convulsions may occur with a severe deficit. A concomitant calcium deficiency occasionally is noted, particularly in those with clinical signs of tetany.

The diagnosis of magnesium deficiency depends on an awareness of the syndrome and clinical recognition of the symptoms. Laboratory confirmation is available but not reliable, as the syndrome may exist in the presence of a normal serum magnesium level. The possibility of magnesium deficiency should always be considered in the surgical patient who exhibits disturbed neuromuscular or cerebral activity in the postoperative period. This is particularly important in patients who have had protracted dysfunction of the gastrointestinal tract with long-term maintenance on parenteral fluids and in patients on parenteral hyperalimentation. Routine administration of magnesium is always indicated in the management of these patients.

Treatment of magnesium deficiency is by the parenteral administration of magnesium sulfate or magnesium chloride solution. If renal function is normal, as much as 2 mEq. of magnesium per kilogram of body weight can be administered in a day in the face of a severe depletion. Magnesium sulfate (50 per cent solution contains approximately 4 mEq. of magnesium ion per milliliter) may be given intravenously or intramuscularly. The intravenous route is preferable for the initial treatment of a severe symptomatic deficit. This can be accomplished by the addition of 80 mEq. of magnesium sulfate (20 ml. of 50 per cent solution) to a liter of intravenous fluid administered over a four-hour period.[14] If the patient is not symptomatic, the infusion should be given over a longer period of time. The possibility of acute magnesium toxicity should be kept in mind when giving this ion intravenously. When large doses are given, the heart rate, blood pres-

sure, respiration, and electrocardiogram should be monitored closely for signs of magnesium toxicity, which could lead to cardiac arrest. It is advisable to have calcium chloride or calcium gluconate available to counteract any adverse effects of a rapidly rising plasma magnesium level.

Partial or complete relief of symptoms may follow this infusion as a result of increased concentration of magnesium ion in the extracellular fluid compartment, although continued replacement over a one- to three-week period is necessary to replenish the intracellular compartment. For this purpose and for the asymptomatic patient who is likely to have significant magnesium depletion, 10 to 20 mEq. of 50 per cent magnesium sulfate solution is given daily by the intramuscular route or in infusion fluids. When magnesium sulfate is used, it should be given in divided doses or at multiple sites, since the intramuscular injection of this salt is painful. Following complete repletion of intracellular magnesium and in the absence of abnormal loss, balance may be maintained by the administration of as little as 4 mEq. of magnesium ion daily. The amount of magnesium supplementation required for patients on parenteral hyperalimentation varies, but approximates 12 to 24 mEq. daily for the average patient.[11]

Magnesium ion should not be given to the oliguric patient or in the presence of severe volume deficit unless actual magnesium depletion is demonstrated. If given to a patient with renal insufficiency, considerably smaller doses are used, and the patient is carefully observed for signs or symptoms of toxicity.

Magnesium Excess. Symptomatic hypermagnesemia, although rare, is most commonly seen with severe renal insufficiency. Retention and accumulation of magnesium may occur in any patient with impaired glomerular or renal tubular function, and the presence of acidosis may rapidly compound the situation. Serum magnesium levels tend to parallel changes in potassium concentration in these cases. Therefore, magnesium levels should be carefully monitored in cases of acute and chronic renal failure and in selected patients with borderline renal function. Randall et al. have shown that in patients on ordinary dietary intakes of magnesium, increased serum concentrations of the ion do not occur until the glomerular filtration rate falls below 30 ml. per minute.[23] As noted by Henzel et al., however, magnesium-containing antacids and laxatives (milk of magnesia, epsom salts, Gelusil, Maalox) are commonly administered in quantities sufficient to produce toxic serum levels of magnesium where impaired renal function is present.[14] Other conditions that may be associated with symptomatic hypermagnesemia include early-stage burns, massive trauma or surgical stress, severe extracellular volume deficit, and severe acidosis.

The early signs and symptoms include lethargy and weakness with progressive loss of deep tendon reflexes. Interference with cardiac conduction occurs with increasing levels of magnesium, and changes in the electocardiogram (increased P-R interval, widened QRS complex, and elevated T waves) resemble those seen with hyperkalemia. Somnolence leading to coma and muscular paralysis occur in the later stages, and death is usually caused by respiratory or cardiac arrest.

Treatment consists of immediate measures to lower the serum magnesium level by correcting any acidosis, replenishing any pre-existing extracellular volume deficit, and withholding exogenously administered magnesium. Acute symptoms may be temporarily controlled by the slow intravenous administration of 5 to 10 mEq. of calcium chloride or calcium gluconate. If elevated levels or symptoms persist, peritoneal dialysis or hemodialysis is indicated.

NORMAL EXCHANGE OF FLUID AND ELECTROLYTES

Knowledge of the basic principles governing both the internal and external exchanges of water and salt is mandatory for care of the patient undergoing major operative surgery. The stable internal fluid environment, which is maintained by the kidneys, brain, lungs, skin, and gastrointestinal tract, may be compromised by severe surgical stress or direct damage to any of these organs.

WATER EXCHANGE

The normal individual consumes an average of 2000 to 2500 ml. water per day; approximately 1500 ml. water is taken by mouth, and the rest is extracted from solid food, either from the contents of the food or as the product of oxidation (Table 7). The daily water losses include 250 ml. in stools, 800 to 1500 ml. as urine, and approximately 600 to 900 ml. as insensible loss. A patient deprived of all external access to water must still excrete a minimum of 500 to 800 ml. of urine per day in order to excrete the products of catabolism, in addition to the mandatory insensible loss through the skin and lungs.

Insensible loss of water occurs through the skin (75 per cent) and the lungs (25 per cent) and is increased by hypermetabolism, hyperventilation, and fever. The insensible water loss through the skin is not from evaporation of water from sweat glands but from water vapor formed within the body and lost through the skin. With excessive heat production (or excessive environmental heat), the capacity for insensible loss through the skin is exceeded, and sweating occurs. These losses may, but seldom do, exceed 250 ml. per day per degree of fever. An unhumidified tracheostomy with hyperventilation increases the loss through the lungs and results in a total insensible loss up to 1.5 liters per day.

A frequently overlooked source of gain is the water of solution, which is the water that holds carbohydrates and proteins in solution in the cell. Normally, gain of water from this source is zero, but after four to five days without food intake, the postoperative patient may begin to gain significant quantities of water (maximum 500 ml. daily) from excessive cellular catabolism. The amount depends on the degree of trauma and the complications occurring postoperatively.

SALT GAIN AND LOSSES

In the normal individual, the salt intake per day varies between 50 and 90 mEq. (3 to 5 gm.) as sodium chloride (Table 8). Balance is maintained primarily by the normal kidneys that excrete the excess salt. Under conditions of reduced intake or extrarenal losses, the normal kidney can reduce sodium excretion to less than 1 mEq. per day within 24 hours after restriction. In the patient with salt-wasting kidneys, however, the loss may exceed 200 mEq. per liter of urine. Sweat represents a hypotonic loss of fluids with an average sodium concentration of 15 mEq. per liter in the acclimatized patient. In the unacclimatized individual,

TABLE 7. Water Exchange (60- to 80-kg. man)

H₂O Gain—Routes	Average Daily Volume (ml.)	Minimal (ml.)	Maximal (ml.)
Sensible			
Oral fluids	800–1500	0	1500/hr.
Solid foods	500– 700	0	1500
Insensible			
Water of oxidation	250	125	800
Water of solution	0	0	500
H₂O Loss—Routes			
Sensible			
Urine	800–1500	300	1400/hr. (diabetes insipidus)
Intestinal	0–250	0	2500/hr.
Sweat	0	0	4000/hr.
Insensible			
Lungs and skin	600–900	600–900	1500

TABLE 8.   Sodium (Salt) Exchange (60- to 80-kg. man)

Sodium Exchange	Average	Minimal	Maximal
Sodium gain			
Diet	50–90 mEq./day	0	75–100 mEq./hr. (oral)
Sodium loss			
Skin (sweat)	10–60 mEq./day*	0	300 mEq./hr.
Urine	10–80 mEq./day	<1 mEq./day†	110–200 mEq./L.‡
Intestines	0–20 mEq./day	0	300 mEq./hr.

*Depending on the degree of acclimatization of the individual.
†With normal renal function.
‡With renal salt wasting.

the sodium concentration in sweat may be 60 mEq. per liter or more. Insensible fluid lost from the skin and lungs, by definition, is pure water. For practical considerations, then, normal losses may be relatively free of salt in the healthy individual with normal renal function.

The volume and composition of various types of gastrointestinal secretions are shown in Table 6. Gastrointestinal losses are usually isotonic or slightly hypotonic, although there is considerable variation in the composition. These should be replaced by an essentially isotonic salt solution. It is also important to reiterate that distributional or sequestration losses of extracellular fluid at any point in the operative or postoperative course also represent isotonic losses of salt and water.

FLUID AND ELECTROLYTE THERAPY

PARENTERAL SOLUTIONS

The composition of various parenteral fluids available for administration is shown in Table 9. There is sufficient variety to satisfy the majority of fluid requirements in the surgical patient. The proper choice of parenteral fluid in a given situation will correct the abnormalities but impose minimal demands on the kidneys.

A good available isotonic salt solution for replacing gastrointestinal losses and repairing pre-existing volume deficits, in the absence of gross abnormalities of concentration and composition, is lactated Ringer's solution. This solution is "physiologic" and contains 130 mEq. sodium balanced by 109 mEq. chloride and 28 mEq. lactate. This fluid has minimal effects on normal body fluid composition and pH even when infused in large quantities. The chief disadvantage of lactated Ringer's solution is the slight hypo-osmolarity with respect to sodium. Each liter of lactated Ringer's solution furnishes approximately 100 to 150 ml. free water. This rarely presents a clinical problem if it is considered in calculating water replacement. The remainder of the solutions listed in Table 9 are used to correct specific defects. Choice of a particular fluid depends on the volume status of the patient and the type of concentration or compositional abnormality present.

Isotonic sodium chloride contains 154 mEq. sodium and 154 mEq. chloride per liter. The high concentration of chloride above the normal serum concentration of 103 mEq. per liter imposes on the kidneys an appreciable load of excess chloride that cannot be rapidly excreted. Thus, a dilutional acidosis may develop.* This solution is ideal, however, for the initial cor-

---

*Infusion of a large volume of isotonic sodium chloride solution may induce or aggravate a pre-existing acidosis by reducing the amount of base bicarbonate in the body relative to the carbonic acid content.[26]

TABLE 9.   Composition of Parenteral Fluids: Electrolyte Content (mEq./L.)

Solutions	Cations					Anions		
	Na	K	Ca	Mg	NH₄	Cl	HCO₃⁻	HPO₄⁻
Extracellular fluid	142	4	5	3	.3	103	27	3
Lactated Ringer's	130	4	2.7			109	28*	
0.9% sodium chloride (saline)	154					154		
M/6 sodium lactate	167						167*	
M (molar) sodium lactate	1000						1000*	
3% sodium chloride	513					513		
5% sodium chloride	855					855		
0.9% ammonium chloride					168	168		
21.4% ammonium chloride					400	400		

*Present in solution as lactate, which is converted to bicarbonate.

rection of an extracellular fluid volume deficit in the presence of hyponatremia, hypochloremia, and metabolic alkalosis. In a similar situation with moderate metabolic acidosis, M/6 sodium lactate (167 mEq. per liter each of sodium and lactate) may be given. Another solution for this purpose can be made by adding one ampule of sodium bicarbonate (40 ml. solution containing 40 mEq. each of sodium and bicarbonate) to 1000 ml. lactated Ringer's solution.

Molar sodium lactate solution or 3 or 5 per cent sodium chloride may be used to correct symptomatic hyponatremic states. The choice of anion (lactate or chloride) is determined by the accompanying acid-base derangement. Following the correction of concentration or compositional abnormalities using specific repair solutions, a balanced salt solution is used to replenish the remaining volume deficit.

PREOPERATIVE FLUID THERAPY

Preoperative evaluation and correction of existing fluid disorders is an integral part of surgical care. An orderly approach to these problems requires an understanding of the common fluid disturbances associated with surgical illness and adherence to a few simple guidelines. There are no shortcuts; close observation of the patient and frequent re-evaluation of the clinical situation is the most rewarding approach.

The analysis of a fluid disorder may be facilitated by categorizing the abnormalities into *volume, concentration,* and *compositional* changes. Although some disease states produce characteristic changes in fluid balance, much confusion may be avoided by regarding each disturbance as a separate entity. For example, volume changes cannot be accurately predicted from a knowledge of the level of serum sodium, since an extracellular fluid volume deficit or excess may exist with a normal, low, or high sodium concentration. Similarly, any of the four primary acid-base disturbances may be associated with any combination of volume and concentration abnormalities.

Correction of Volume Changes

Changes in the volume of extracellular fluid are the most frequent and important abnormalities encountered in the surgical patient. Depletion of the extracellular fluid compartment without changes in concentration or composition is a common problem. The diagnosis of volume changes is made almost entirely on clinical grounds. The signs that will be present in an individual patient depend not only on the relative or absolute quantity of extracellular fluid that has been lost but also on the rapidity with which it is lost and the presence or absence of signs of associated disease.

Volume deficits in the surgical patient may result from external loss of fluids or from an internal redistribution of extracellular fluid into a nonfunctional compartment. Generally, it involves a combination of the two, but the internal redistribution is frequently overlooked.

The phenomenon of internal redistribution or translocation of extracellular fluid is peculiar to many surgical diseases; in the individual patient, the loss may be quite large. Although the concept of a "third space" is not new, it is generally considered only in relation to patients with massive ascites, burns, or crush injuries. Of more importance, however, is the "third space" loss into the peritoneum, the bowel wall, and other tissues with inflammatory lesions of the intra-abdominal organs. The magnitude of these losses may not be fully appreciated without realization of the fact that the peritoneum alone has approximately 1 sq. meter of surface area. A slight increase in thickness from sequestration of fluid, which would not be appreciated on casual observation, may result in a functional loss of several liters of fluid. Swelling of the bowel wall and mesentery and secretion of fluid into the lumen of the bowel will cause even larger losses. Similar deficits may occur with massive infection of the subcutaneous tissues (necrotizing fasciitis) or with severe crush injury.

These "parasitic" losses remain a part of the extracellular fluid space and may be measured as a slowly equilibrating volume. The term *nonfunctional* is used because the fluid is no longer able to participate in the normal functions of the extracellular fluid compartment and may just as well have been lost externally. Any transfer of intracellular fluid to the extracellular compartment for replenishment of the loss is insignificant in the acute phase. The patient with ascites may have an enormous total extracellular fluid volume although the functional component is severely depleted. The same is true of extensive inflammatory or obstructive lesions of the gastrointestinal tract, although the loss is not as obvious. These losses will evoke the signs and symptoms of an extracellular fluid volume deficit with or without the concomitant external loss of fluids.

Exact quantification of these deficits is impossible and, at the present time, probably unnecessary. The defect can be estimated on the basis of the severity of the clinical signs. A mild deficit represents a loss of approximately 4 per cent of body weight, a moderate loss is 6 to 8 per cent of body weight, and a severe deficit is approximately 10 per cent of body weight. It is important to re-emphasize the fact that cardiovascular signs predominate when there is acute rapid loss of fluid from the extracellular fluid compartment with few or no tissue signs. In addition to the estimated deficit, fluids lost during the period of treatment must be replaced.

Fluid replacement should be started and changed according to the response of the patient noted on frequent clinical observation. Reliance on a formula or single clinical sign to determine adequacy of resuscitation is fraught with danger. Rather, reversal of the signs of the volume deficit, combined with stabilization of the blood pressure and pulse, and an hourly urine volume of 30 to 50 ml. are used as general guidelines. An adequate hourly urine output, although usually a reliable index of volume replacement, may be totally misleading. The excessive administration of glucose (over 50 gm. in a 2- to 3-hour period) may result in osmotic diuresis, while an osmotic agent such as mannitol tends to produce urine at the expense of the vascular volume. Patients with chronic renal disease or incipient acute renal damage from shock and injury also may have inappropriately high urinary volumes. In addition, the rapid administration of salt solutions may transiently expand the intravascular volume, increase the glomerular filtration rate, and result in an immediate outpouring of urine, although the total extracellular fluid space remains quite depleted.

The choice of the proper fluid for replacement depends on the existence of concomitant concentration or compositional abnormalities. With pure extracellular fluid volume loss or when only minimal concentration or compositional abnormalities are present, the use of a balanced salt solution, such as lactated Ringer's, is desirable.

Correction of Concentration Changes

If severe *symptomatic* hyponatremia or hypernatremia complicates the volume loss, prompt correction of the concentration abnormality to the extent that symptoms are relieved is necessary. Volume replenishment then should be accomplished with slower correction of the remaining concentration abnormality. For immediate correction of severe hyponatremia, a 5 per cent sodium chloride solution or molar sodium lactate solution is used, depending on the patient's acid-base status. In any case, the sodium deficit can be estimated by multiplying the decrease in serum sodium concentration below normal (in milliequivalents per liter) *times* the liters of total body water. Total body water averages 60 per cent of the body weight in young adult males and 50 per cent in young adult females. Initially, up to half of the calculated amount of sodium may be administered slowly, followed by clinical and chemical re-evaluation of the patient before any additional infusion of sodium salts.

Example: A 24-year-old female with symptomatic hyponatremia, weight = 60 kg., serum sodium = 120 mEq. per liter:

Total body water = 60 kg. × 0.50 = 30 liters
Sodium deficit = (140 − 120 mEq./L.) × 30 liters
= 600 mEq.

Half of this amount (300 mEq.) could be given by slowly infusing approximately 350 ml. of 5 per cent sodium chloride solution. Note that this estimate is based on total body water, since the effective osmotic pressure in the extracellular compartment cannot be increased without increasing this function proportionately in the intracellular compartment. Although absolute reliance on any formula is undesirable, proper use of this estimate will allow a safe quantitative approximation of the sodium deficit. Generally, only a portion of the total deficit is replaced initially to relieve acute symptoms. Further correction is facilitated when renal function is restored by correction of the volume deficit. If the total calculated deficit were given rapidly, symptomatic hypervolemia might occur, particularly in patients with limited cardiac reserve. In practice, the infusion of small, successive increments of hypertonic saline solution with frequent evaluation of the clinical response and serum sodium concentration is recommended.

In the treatment of moderate hyponatremia with an associated volume deficit, volume replacement can be started immediately with concomitant correction of the serum sodium deficit. Isotonic sodium chloride solution (normal saline) is used initially in the presence of metabolic alkalosis, whereas M/6 sodium lactate is used to correct an associated acidosis. Only a few liters of these solutions may be necessary to correct the serum sodium concentration; the remainder of the volume deficit may be repaired with lactated Ringer's solution.

Treatment of hyponatremia associated with volume excess is by restriction of water. In the presence of severe symptomatic hyponatremia, a small amount of hypertonic salt solution may be infused cautiously to alleviate symptoms. As this will cause additional volume expansion, it is contraindicated in patients with limited cardiac reserve; peritoneal dialysis or hemodialysis is preferred in this situation.

For the correction of severe, symptomatic hypernatremia with an associated volume deficit, 5 per cent dextrose in water may be infused slowly until symptoms are relieved. If the extracellular osmolarity is reduced too rapidly, however, convulsions and coma may result. For this reason, correction of hypernatremia concomitant with repletion of the volume deficit by half-strength sodium chloride or half-strength lactated Ringer's solution is safer in most cases. In the absence of a significant volume deficit, water should be administered cautiously, since dangerous hypervolemia may result; constant observation and frequent determinations of the serum sodium concentration are indicated. The problem is somewhat simplified once a sufficient quantity of fluid has been given to permit renal excretion of the solute load.

Rate of Fluid Administration. This varies considerably, depending on the severity and type of fluid disturbance, the presence of continuing losses, and the cardiac status. In general, the most severe volume deficits may be safely replaced initially with isotonic solutions at a rate of 2000 ml. per hour, reducing the rate as the fluid status improves. Constant observation by a physician is mandatory when the administration exceeds 1000 ml. per hour. At these rates, a significant portion may be lost as urinary output owing to a transient overexpansion of the plasma volume.

In elderly patients, associated cardiovascular disorders do not preclude correction of existing volume deficits, but they do require slower, more careful correction with constant monitoring of all functions including the central venous, pulmonary artery, or wedge pressure. Hypertonic salt solutions should be given under close supervision, and the rate of administration generally should not exceed 100 to 150 ml. per hour.

Composition and Miscellaneous Considerations

Correction of existing potassium deficits should be started *after* an adequate urine output is obtained, particularly in the patient with metabolic alkalosis, since this may be secondary to or aggravated by potassium depletion. Potassium chloride is available in 20-mEq. and 40-mEq. ampules for addition to intravenous fluids. A maximum of 40 mEq. of potassium chloride per hour may be safely administered to the adult of average size who is not severely depleted of extracellular fluid volume, in frank hypovolemic shock, or in established oliguric or high-output renal failure. The concentration of potassium chloride should not exceed 40 mEq. per liter of intravenous fluids, with rare exception, such as the treatment of digitalis intoxication during which the electrocardiogram must be constantly monitored. Calcium and magnesium rarely are needed during preoperative resuscitation, but should be given if any doubt exists, particularly to patients with massive subcutaneous infections, those with acute pancreatitis, and those who have been chronically starved.

Fluid abnormalities also must be suspected in the patient for whom an elective procedure is planned. Chronic illnesses frequently are associated with extracellular fluid volume deficits, and concentration and compositional changes are not uncommon. Correction of anemia and recognition of the fact that a contracted blood volume may exist in the chronically debilitated patient are of obvious importance. The choice of whole blood versus packed cells for correction of anemia depends on the volume status. If there is any question, one unit of packed cells may be given and the hemoglobin and hematocrit determined subsequently. The hemoglobin generally increases approximately 1.5 gm. per 100 ml. following the infusion of 250 ml. of packed cells into the adult of average size. The increase will be significantly greater than 1.5 gm. per 100 ml. in the patient with a contracted intravascular volume, indicating the probable need for whole blood transfusions. If available, measurement of the blood volume is obviously more accurate.

Of additional importance is the prevention of volume depletion during the preoperative period. Prolonged periods of fluid restriction in preparation for various diagnostic procedures, and the use of cathartics and enemas for preparation of the bowel, may cause a significant acute loss of extracellular fluid. Prompt recognition and treatment of these losses is necessary to prevent complications during the operative period.

INTRAOPERATIVE MANAGEMENT OF FLUIDS

If preoperative replacement of extracellular fluid volume has been incomplete, hypotension may develop promptly with the induction of anesthesia. This can be quite insidious, as the ability of the awake patient to compensate for mild volume deficit is revealed only when the compensatory mechanisms are abolished with anesthesia. This problem is prevented by maintaining baseline requirements and replacing abnormal losses of fluids and electrolytes by intravenous infusions in the preoperative period.

Blood lost during the operative procedure should be replaced steadily. It is usually unnecessary to replace blood loss of less than 500 ml., but after the loss has exceeded this, replacement should begin. The warnings against the use of a single transfusion during operation have been somewhat confusing. There may be a very definite need for a single-unit transfusion in the patient who loses between 500 and 1000 ml. of blood during operation.

In addition to blood losses during operation, there appear to be extracellular fluid losses during major operative procedures. Some of these, including edema from extensive dissection, collections within the lumen and wall of the small bowel, and accumulations of fluid in the peritoneal cavity, are clinically discernible and well recognized. They generally are felt to represent distributional shifts, in that the functional volume of extracellular fluid is reduced but not externally lost from the body. These functional losses are often referred to as "a parasitic loss of extracellular fluid," "a third space edema," or "a sequestration" of extracellular fluid. Another source of extracellular fluid loss during major operative trauma is the wound itself. This is a relatively smaller loss that is very difficult to quantify except in extensive and major operative procedures.

At the beginning of this century, surgeons became aware that many changes occurred in urinary output, blood volume, and fluid and electrolyte composition during and after surgery. Assessment of these changes, however, awaited the development of analytic techniques and their application to patient studies. In the following 25 years, saline solutions in varying combinations were given to patients undergoing operation, often in excessive amounts. Work in the late 1930s and early 1940s by Moyer and by many others indicated that during and after operative procedures, saline and water solutions should be withheld entirely because most of the fluid administered is retained.[19]

The possibility existed that the operative and postoperative retention of salt and water administered in relatively small amounts might simply be physiologic retention to replace a deficit of salt and water incurred by the operative procedure. Subsequent studies have revealed that functional extracellular fluid decreases with major abdominal operations, largely as sequestered loss into the operative site.[27, 28] This extracellular fluid volume deficit can be replaced during the operative procedure. These data have led to the conclusion that the need for an extracellular "mimic" in the form of balanced salt solution now can be clinically estimated. Intraoperative correction of the volume deficit with salt solution markedly reduces "postoperative salt intolerance" but is not intended to substitute for blood replacement. Rather, it is felt to be a physiologic supplement, or adjunct, to replace sequestered losses.

Thus, the pendulum has swung from indiscriminate use of salt solutions in the first quarter of this century to almost total withholding of fluid and electrolytes from surgical patients in the second quarter of the century; indications at present are that proper management lies somewhere between these two extremes. Some guidelines are necessary for the intraoperative administration of saline solutions as a "mimic" for the sequestered extracellular fluid. Since this varies from an almost imperceptible minimum to a high of approximately 3 liters during an uncomplicated procedure, quantification is extremely difficult with the currently available means of measuring functional extracellular fluid. Consequently, no accurate formula for intraoperative fluid administration can yet be derived. Some arbitrary but clinically useful guidelines are the following: (1) Blood should be replaced as lost, irrespective of any additional fluid and electrolyte therapy. (2) The replacement of extracellular fluid should begin during the operative procedure. (3) Balanced salt solution needed during operation is approximately 0.5 to 1 liter per hour, but only to a maximum of 2 to 3 liters during a four-hour major abdominal procedure, unless there are other measurable losses.

Using a similar fluid regimen, Thompson reported experiences in a series of 670 patients undergoing major aortoiliac reconstructive procedures.[31] In this group, the average amount of Ringer's lactate solution administered was 3555 ml., giving an average intraoperative replacement of salt solution of 677 ml. per hour of operative procedure. In the last six years of this study, there were only two deaths in 298 operations, an operative mortality of 0.67 per cent. Among the entire 670 patients, only two patients died of renal failure, an incidence of 0.3 per cent. No patient died of pulmonary insufficiency. This extremely low incidence of renal failure, even in the presence of extensive operative trauma, is similar to the authors' data for major abdominal operative procedures.

POSTOPERATIVE MANAGEMENT OF FLUIDS

Immediate Postoperative Period

Orders for postoperative fluids are not written until the patient is in the recovery room and the fluid status has been assessed. Evaluation at this point should include a review of preoperative fluid status, the amount of fluid loss and gain during operation, and clinical examination of the patient with assessment of the vital signs and urinary output. Initial fluid orders are written to correct any *existing* deficit, followed by maintenance fluids for the remainder of the day. For the patient with complications who has received or lost large amounts of fluid, it is frequently difficult to estimate the fluid requirements for the ensuing 24 hours. In this situation, intravenous fluids are ordered 1 liter at a time and the patient checked frequently until the situation is clarified. Proper replacement of fluids during this relatively short period will facilitate subsequent fluid management.

Immediately after operation, extracellular fluid volume depletion may occur as a result of continued losses of fluid at the site of injury or operative trauma—for example, into the wall or lumen of the small intestine. Several liters of extracellular fluid may be slowly deposited in such areas within a few hours or more during the first day or so from the time of the injury. Unrecognized deficits of extracellular fluid volume during the early postoperative period are manifest primarily as circulatory instability. The signs of volume deficiency in other organ systems may be delayed for several hours with this type of fluid loss. Postoperative hypotension and tachycardia require prompt investigation, followed by appropriate therapy. The generally accepted adequate blood pressure of 90/60 mm. Hg and a pulse of less than 120 in postoperative patients may not be sufficient to prevent

renal ischemia unless, in addition to lack of signs of shock, urine flow is adequate. Evaluation of the level of consciousness, pupillary size, airway patency, breathing patterns, pulse rate and volume, skin warmth, color, body temperature, and a 30- to 50-ml. hourly urine output, combined with critical review of the operative procedure and the operative fluid management, usually is rewarding. Since operative trauma frequently involves loss or transfer of significant quantities of whole blood, plasma, or extracellular fluid which can be only grossly estimated, circulatory instability is most commonly caused by underestimated initial losses or insidious, concealed continued losses. Operative blood loss is usually estimated by the operating surgeon to be 15 to 40 per cent less than the isotopically measured blood loss from the patient.[15] In addition, several liters of extravascular, extracellular fluid can be sequestered in areas of injury and manifested only by oliguria and mild depression of the blood pressure with a rapid pulse. For a patient with circulatory instability, further volume replacement of an additional 1000 ml. isotonic salt solution, while determining whether continuing losses or other causes are present, often resolves the problem. Contributing causes must be vigorously pursued with all diagnostic aids before excessive volumes of fluid have been administered.

It is unnecessary and probably unwise to administer potassium during the first 24 hours postoperatively, unless a definite potassium deficit exists. This is particularly important for the patient subjected to prolonged operative trauma involving one or more episodes of hypotension and for the post-traumatic patient with hemorrhagic hypotension. Oliguric renal failure or the more insidious high-output renal failure may develop, and the administration of even a small quantity of potassium may be quite detrimental.

Later Postoperative Period

The problem of volume management during the postoperative convalescent phase is one of accurate measurement and replacement of all losses. In the otherwise healthy individual, this involves the replacement of measured sensible losses, which are generally of gastrointestinal origin, and the estimation and replacement of insensible losses.

The insensible loss is usually relatively constant and will average 600 to 900 ml. daily. This may be increased by hypermetabolism, hyperventilation, and fever to a maximum of approximately 1500 ml. daily. The estimated insensible loss is replaced with 5 per cent dextrose in water. This loss may be partially offset by an insensible gain of water from excessive tissue catabolism in the complicated postoperative patient, particularly if associated with oliguric renal failure.

Approximately 1 liter of fluid should be given to replace that volume of urine required to excrete the catabolic end products of metabolism (800 to 1000 ml. per day). In the individual with normal renal function, this may be given as 5 per cent dextrose in water, since the kidneys are able to conserve sodium with excretion of less than 1 mEq. daily. It is probably unnecessary to stress the kidneys to this degree, however, and a small amount of salt solution may be given in addition to water to cover urinary loss. In the elderly patient with salt-losing kidneys or in patients with head injuries, an insidious hyponatremia may develop if urinary losses are replaced with water. Urinary sodium in these circumstances may exceed 100 mEq. per liter and result in a daily loss of significant amounts of sodium. Measurement of urinary sodium will facilitate accurate replacement.

Urine volume is not replaced on a milliliter-for-milliliter basis. A urinary output of 2000 to 3000 ml. on a given day may simply represent diuresis of fluids given during surgery or may represent excessive fluid administration. If these large losses are completely replaced, the urine output will progressively increase, and this may logically progress to a unique situation resembling diabetes insipidus with urinary output in excess of 10 liters daily.

Sensible losses, by definition, can be measured or, as in the case of sweating, the amount can be estimated. Gastrointestinal losses are usually isotonic or slightly hypotonic, and they are replaced with an essentially isotonic salt solution. When the estimated loss is slightly above or below isotonicity, appropriate corrections can be made in the daily water administration, while isotonic salt solutions are used to replace these losses volume for volume. Sweating is not usually a problem except with the febrile patient in whom losses may, but seldom do, exceed 250 ml. per day per degree of fever. Excessive sweating may, in addition, represent a considerable loss of sodium in the unacclimatized individual.

Determination of serum electrolyte levels is generally unnecessary in the patient with an uncomplicated postoperative course maintained on parenteral fluids for two to three days. A more prolonged period of parenteral replacement or one complicated by excessive fluid losses requires frequent determinations of the serum sodium, potassium, and chloride levels and carbon dioxide combining power. Adjustments then can be made with intravenous fluids of appropriate composition. For example, gastrointestinal losses should be replaced with isotonic sodium chloride solution in a patient with hyponatremia, hypochloremia, and mild metabolic alkalosis, and this should be continued until these abnormalities are corrected. In the hyponatremic patient with obvious overload, the amount of water given is restricted. In the presence of hyponatremia and mild metabolic acidosis, M/6 sodium lactate or lactated Ringer's solution with added sodium bicarbonate may be used. In this way, severe concentration and compositional changes can be avoided while an adequate extracellular fluid volume is maintained by appropriate maintenance fluids.

Maintenance fluids are administered at a steady rate over an 18- to 24-hour period as the losses are incurred. If given over a shorter period of time, renal excretion of the excess salt and water may occur while the normal losses continue over the full 24-hour period. For the same reason, fluids of different composition are alternated, and additives to intravenous fluids (e.g., potassium chloride and antibiotics) are evenly distributed in the total volume of fluid given.

In summary, daily fluid orders should begin with an assessment of the patient's volume status and a check for possible concentration or compositional disorders as reflected by proper laboratory determinations. All measured and insensible losses are replaced with fluids of appropriate composition, allowing for any pre-existing deficit or excess. The amount of potassium replacement is 40 mEq. daily for renal excretion of potassium, in addition to approximately 20 mEq. per liter for replacement of gastrointestinal losses. Inadequate replacement may prolong the usual postoperative ileus and contribute to the insidious development of a resistant metabolic alkalosis. Calcium and magnesium are replaced when needed, as previously discussed.

Special Consideration in the Postoperative Patient

Volume Excesses. The administration of isotonic salt solutions in excess of volume losses (external or internal) may result in overexpansion of the extracellular fluid space. The otherwise normal person in a postoperative state tolerates an acute overexpansion extremely well. Excesses administered over a period of several days, however, will soon exceed the kidneys' ability to excrete sodium; since water losses continue, hypernatremia will ensue. Therefore, it is important to determine as accurately as possible from intake and output records and serum sodium concentrations the actual needs of the patient managed over several postoperative days. Attention to the signs and symptoms of overload usually prevents this fluid abnormality. It arises most frequently with attempts to meet excessive volume losses that are not measurable, such as those occurring from incompletely controlled fistula drainage.

The earliest sign is a weight gain (when measurable) during the catabolic period, when the patient should be losing $1/4$ to $1/2$ pound per day. Heavy eyelids, hoarseness, or dyspnea on exertion may rapidly appear. Circulatory and pulmonary signs of overload appear late and represent a rather massive overload. Peripheral edema may be a sign, but it does not necessarily indicate volume excess. In the absence of additional evidence for volume overload, other causes for peripheral edema should be considered. Of particular importance is the fact that overexpansion of the *total* extracellular fluid may coexist with *depletion* of the functional extracellular fluid compartment. Central venous pressure measurements may be helpful during volume replacement but may be misleading, as a rapid rise may indicate an excessive rate of fluid administration or primary pump failure, but it does not accurately establish volume status.

Hyponatremia. Significant postoperative alterations in serum sodium concentration are not frequently observed if the fluid resuscitation during operation has included adequate volumes of isotonic salt solutions. The kidneys retain the ability to excrete moderate excesses of salt water administered in the early postoperative period if functional extracellular fluid has been adequately replaced during the operative or immediate postoperative period. Previous studies of sodium balance have revealed that patients do excrete sodium after the functional deficit incurred by the shift of extracellular fluid has been replaced. Wright and Gann have demonstrated normal capacity to excrete water postoperatively when isotonic salt solutions are administered prior to a challenge with a water load.[33] Thus, the commonly described hyponatremia associated with surgical procedures and traumatic injury is prevented by the replacement of extracellular fluid deficits. The daily maintenance of normal osmolarity is simplified by the replacement of observable losses of known sodium content.

Hyponatremia may easily occur when water is given to replace losses of sodium-containing fluids or when water administration consistently exceeds water losses. The latter may occur with oliguria or in association with decreased water loss through the skin and lungs, intracellular shifts of sodium, or the cellular release of excessive amounts of endogenous water. Severe or refractory hyponatremia, however, is difficult to produce if renal function remains normal.

REPLACEMENT OF SODIUM LOSSES WITH WATER. A common error is replacement of gastrointestinal and other salt losses with only water or a hypotonic solution. Patients with head injury or with pre-existing renal disease (loss of concentrating ability) may elaborate urine with a high salt concentration (50 to 200 mEq. per liter).

Progressive hyponatremia in the patient with head injury, despite adequate salt administration, is believed to be due to excessive secretion of antidiuretic hormone with consequent water retention. The loss of renal concentrating ability due to impairment of renal tubular function ("salt-wasting kidneys") is a common problem in elderly patients. This source of sodium loss is frequently not anticipated, since the blood urea nitrogen and creatinine levels usually fall within normal limits. Continued replacement of these urinary losses with water only eventually may result in symptomatic hyponatremia. The urine sodium concentration should be determined if the diagnosis is in doubt; with hyponatremia and normal renal function, the urine should be virtually free of sodium.

DECREASED URINARY VOLUME. Oliguria, from whatever cause (prerenal or renal), reduces the daily water requirements if not corrected. Cellular catabolism and the metabolic acidosis produced by the retention of nitrogenous waste products increases the cellular release of water. Therefore, the gain of endogenous water decreases the total water requirement beyond that expected when the urinary volume is low.

DECREASED INSENSIBLE LOSS. Cutaneous vasoconstriction from any cause decreases both insensible and evaporative water loss by this route. This condition most commonly accompanies generalized hypothermia.

ENDOGENOUS WATER RELEASE. The patient maintained on intravenous fluids without adequate caloric intake will, between the fifth and tenth days, gain significant quantities of water (maximum, 500 ml. daily) from excessive cellular catabolism, thus decreasing the quantity of exogenous water required per day.

INTRACELLULAR SHIFTS. Systemic bacterial sepsis is often accompanied by a precipitous drop in serum sodium concentration. This sudden change is poorly understood, but usually accompanies loss of extracellular fluid as either interstitial or intracellular sequestrations. This can be treated by withholding free water, restoring extracellular fluid volume, and initiating treatment of the sepsis.

Many hyponatremic states are asymptomatic until the serum sodium level falls below 120 mEq. per liter. This moderate asymptomatic hyponatremia, however, signifies inappropriate therapy or indicates the basic underlying condition. Symptomatic hyponatremia, or water intoxication, is difficult to produce if renal function is normal. Convulsions and apnea from uncorrected water excesses occur most often in children and elderly adults. Within the limits imposed by the circulatory apparatus, these deficits should be corrected by the administration of hypertonic salt solution to a serum sodium level above 130 mEq. per liter. Mild or moderate degrees of hyponatremia may be simply corrected by temporary restriction of water intake.

In the presence of hyperglycemia, determination of the glucose concentration is necessary to evaluate the significance of a depressed serum sodium level. Since glucose does not enter cells by passive diffusion, it exerts an osmotic force in the extracellular compartment. This contribution to osmotic pressure is normally small, but with an elevated glucose concentration, the increased osmotic pressure causes the transfer of cellular water into the extracellular compartment, resulting in a dilutional hyponatremia. Hyponatremia therefore may be observed when the total effective osmotic pressure in the extracellular compartment is normal or even above normal. In terms of tonicity, each 100 mg. per 100 ml. rise in the blood glucose *above normal* is roughly equivalent to a 3 mEq. per liter rise in the serum sodium concentration. Consider a patient with a serum sodium concentration of 125 mEq. per liter and a blood glucose level of 500 mg. per 100 ml. The glucose level is approximately 400 mg. per 100 ml. above normal, which is equivalent to a 12 mEq. per liter rise in the serum sodium level. Thus, 125 + 12 = 137 mEq. per liter; the tonicity is normal despite the marked reduction in sodium concentration. In this instance, therapy is directed toward lowering the blood glucose level. The sodium concentration will return toward normal as the excess water leaves the extracellular compartment. In practice, a true sodium deficit may be secondary to the underlying disorder and must be corrected.

Hypernatremia. Hypernatremia (serum sodium concentration above 150 mEq. per liter), although uncommon, is a dangerous abnormality. In contradistinction to decreased serum sodium concentration, hypernatremia is easily produced when renal function is normal. The extracellular fluid hyperosmolarity results in a shift of intracellular water from within the cell to the extracellular fluid compartment; in this situation, a high serum sodium level may indicate a significant deficit of total body water. In surgical patients hypernatremia arises most often from excessive or unexpected water losses, although it may result from use of salt-containing solutions to replace water losses. The following classification of water losses may be helpful in preventing and treating this abnormality.

EXCESSIVE EXTRARENAL WATER LOSSES. With increased metabolism from any cause, but particularly associated with fever, the water loss through evaporation of sweat may reach several liters daily. Patients with tracheostomies in dry environments can (with excessive minute volume air exchange) lose as much as 1 to 1.5 liters of water per day by this route. Increased water evaporation from a granulating surface is of significant magnitude in the thermally injured patient, and losses may be as great as 3 to 5 liters per day.[20]

INCREASED RENAL WATER LOSSES. Extremely large volumes of solute-poor urine may result from hypoxic damage to the distal tubules and collecting ducts or loss of antidiuretic hormone stimulation from damage to the central nervous system. In both instances, facultative water resorption is impaired. The former occurs in high-output renal failure; in our experience, this is the most common type of renal failure following severe injury or operative trauma. The latter occurs with extensive head injuries accompanied by temporary diabetes insipidus.

SOLUTE LOADING. High protein intake may produce an increased osmotic load of urea, which necessitates the excretion of large volumes of water. Hypernatremia, azotemia, and extracellular fluid volume deficits follow. In general, these can be prevented by an intake of 7 ml. of water per gram of dietary protein.

Excessive glucose administration results in the need for a large volume of water for excretion. Osmotic diuretics such as mannitol and urea also result in the obligatory excretion of a large volume of water as well as increasing urinary sodium losses. In addition, isotonic salt solutions, if used to replace pure water losses, rapidly produce hypernatremia.

High-Output Renal Failure. Acute renal insufficiency following trauma or surgical stress may be a lethal complication. The diagnosis is classically based on persistent oliguria and chemical evidence of uremia after stabilization of the circulation. The clinical course is characterized by oliguria lasting from several days to several weeks, followed by a progressive rise in daily urine volume until both the excretory and concentrating functions of the kidney are gradually restored.

Uremia, occurring without a period of oliguria and accompanied by a daily urine volume greater than 1000 to 1500 ml. per day, is a more frequent but less well recognized entity.[5] Clinical experience and laboratory experiments suggest that high-output renal failure represents the renal response to a less severe or modified episode of renal injury than that required to produce classic oliguric renal failure. Its importance lies in the fact that it is a milder form of renal insufficiency and that realization of its presence, by serial measurement of blood urea nitrogen and serum electrolytes, permits intelligent chemical and fluid volume management with a much greater latitude because of the daily urine volume excretion. Normal extracellular fluid volume and normal serum sodium concentration, therefore, are quite easily maintained when accurate daily outputs of each are obtained and replaced accordingly. The sodium-containing fluids may be administered as lactate to control the mild metabolic acidosis that occurs. Severe acidosis may develop if isotonic losses from the gastrointestinal tract or renal excretion of sodium are replaced with sodium chloride.

The chief dangers of high-output renal failure are failure to recognize its existence because of normal output, and the intravenous administration of potassium salts. Good urinary output and gastrointestinal involvement requiring suction usually indicate the need for daily potassium replacement. With this type of renal failure, however, potassium intoxication may be produced. As little as 20 mEq. of potassium chloride given intravenously may rapidly produce myocardial potassium intoxication requiring resin or hemodialysis treatment.

The typical course of high-output renal failure begins without a period of oliguria. The daily urine volumes are normal or greater than normal, often reaching levels of 3 to 5 liters per day while blood urea nitrogen is increasing. An attempt to decrease urine output by water restriction rapidly results in hypernatremia without a change in urine volume. On the average, urea nitrogen continues to increase for 8 to 12 days before a downward trend occurs. The blood/urine urea ratio is about 1:10 until a decrease occurs in the blood urea concentration.

Functionally, the lesion is characterized by a glomerular filtration rate of less than 20 per cent of normal and complete resistance to vasopressin for one to three weeks after the blood urea nitrogen has declined. During the next six to eight weeks, the glomerular filtration rate gradually rises, and the response to vasopressin becomes normal. The early recognition of high-output renal failure by serial blood determinations of blood urea nitrogen is important. Failure to recognize its presence may result in death from hyperkalemia, hypernatremia, or acidosis. As alluded to previously, it is unwise to administer potassium during the first 24 postoperative hours unless a definite potassium deficit exists. This is particularly important in the patient subjected to prolonged operative trauma involving one or more episodes of hypotension and in the patient with post-traumatic hemorrhagic hypotension.

REFERENCES

1. Abouna, G. M., Veazey, P. R., and Terry, D. B.: Intravenous infusion of hydrochloric acid for treatment of severe metabolic alkalosis. Surgery, 75:194, 1974.
2. Andersen, O. S., and Engel, K.: A new acid-based nomogram: An improved method for the calculation of the relevant blood acid-base data. Scand. J. Clin. Lab. Invest., 12:177, 1960.
3. Astrup, P., Jorgensen, K., Andersen, O. S., and Engel, K.: The acid-base metabolism: A new approach. Lancet, 1:1035, 1960.
4. Bartlett, W. C.: Acute hyperparathyroid crisis. Am. J. Surg., 114:796, 1967.
5. Baxter, C. R., Zedlitz, W. H., and Shires, G. T.: High-output acute renal failure complicating traumatic injury. J. Trauma, 4:467, 1964.
6. Bishop, R. L., and Weisfeldt, M. L.: Sodium bicarbonate administration during cardiac arrest: Effect on arterial pH, Pco₂ and osmolality, J.A.M.A., 235:506, 1976.
7. Canizaro, P. C., Prager, M. D., and Shires, G. T.: The infusion of Ringer's lactate solution during shock. Am. J. Surg., 122:494, 1971.
8. Canizaro, P. C., Nelson, J., and Hennessy, J.: Alterations in oxygen transport. In Shires, G. T., Carrico, C. J., and Canizaro, P. C. (Eds.): Shock. Philadelphia, W. B. Saunders Company, 1973.
9. Collins, J. A.: Problems associated with the massive transfusion of stored blood. Surgery, 75:274, 1974.

10. Cooper, N., Brazier, J. R., Hottenrott, C., Mulder, D. G., Maloney, J. V., and Buckberg, C. D.: Myocardial depression following citrated blood transfusion. Arch. Surg., 107:756, 1973.
11. Dudrick, S. J., et al.: General principles and techniques of intravenous hyperalimentation. In Cowan, G. S. M., and Schutz, W. L. (Eds.): Intravenous Hyperalimentation. Philadelphia, Lea and Febiger, 1972.
12. Elias, E. G., and Evans, J. T.: Hypercalcemic crisis in neoplastic diseases: Management with mithramycin. Surgery, 71:631, 1972.
13. Harken, A. H., Gabel, R. A., Fencl, V., and Moore, F. D.: Hydrochloric acid in the correction of metabolic acidosis. Arch. Surg., 110:819, 1975.
14. Henzel, J. H., DeWeese, M. S., and Ridenhour, G.: Significance of magnesium and zinc metabolism in the surgical patient. I. Magnesium. Arch. Surg., 95:974, 1967.
15. Jenkins, M. T., and Beck, G. P.: Differential diagnosis of hypotension occurring during anesthesia and surgery. Clin. Anesth., 3:106, 1963.
16. Mattar, J. A., Weil, M. H., Shubin, H., and Stein, L.: Cardiac arrest in the critically ill: II. Hyperosmolal states following cardiac arrest. Am. J. Med., 56:162, 1974.
17. McClelland, R. N., Shires, G. T., Baxter, C. R., Coln, C. D., and Carrico, C. J.: Balanced salt solution in the treatment of hemorrhagic shock studies in dogs. J.A.M.A., 199:830, 1967.
18. Mellemgaard, K., and Astrup, P.: The quantitative determination of surplus amounts of acid or base in the human body. Scand. J. Clin. Lab. Invest., 12:187, 1960.
19. Mengoli, L. R.: Experts from the history of postoperative fluid therapy. Am. J. Surg., 121:311, 1971.
20. Moncrief, J. A., and Mason, A. D.: Water vapor loss in the burned patient. Surg. Forum, 13:38, 1962.
21. Moore, F. D., Olesen, K. H., McMurrey, J. D., Parker, H. V., Ball, M. R., and Boyden, C. M.: The Body Cell Mass and Its Supporting Environment. Philadelphia, W. B. Saunders Company, 1963.
22. Moyer, C. A.: Fluid Balance. Chicago, Year Book Medical Publishers, Inc., 1954.
23. Randall, R. E., Jr., Cohen, M. D., Spray, C. C., Jr., and Rossmeisl, E. C.: Hypermagnesemia in renal failure: Etiology and toxic manifestations. Ann. Intern. Med., 61:73, 1964.
24. Schwarz, W. B., and Relman, A. S.: A critique of the parameters used in the evaluation of acid-base disorders. N. Engl. J. Med., 268:1382, 1963.
25. Shavelle, H. S., and Parke, R.: Postoperative alkalosis and acute renal failure: Rationale for the use of hydrochloric acid. Surgery, 78:439, 1975.
26. Shires, G. T., and Holman, V.: Dilutional acidosis. Ann. Intern. Med., 28:551, 1948.
27. Shires, T., Williams, J., and Brown, F.: Acute changes in extracellular fluids associated with major surgical procedures. Ann. Surg., 154:803, 1961.
28. Shires, T., and Jackson, D. E.: Postoperative salt tolerance. Arch. Surg., 84:703, 1962.
29. Shires, G. T., Cunningham, J. N., Baker, C. R. F., Reeder, S. F., Illner, H., Wagner, I. Y., and Maher, J.: Alterations in cellular membrane function during hemorrhagic shock in primates. Ann. Surg., 176:288, 1972.
30. Singer, R. B., and Hastings, A. B.: An improved clinical method for the estimation of disturbances of the acid-base balance of human blood. Medicine, 27:223, 1948.
31. Thompson, J. E., Vollman, R. W., Austin, D. J., and Kartchner, M. M.: Prevention of hypotensive and renal complications of aortic surgery using balanced salt solution. Ann. Surg., 167:767, 1968.
32. Tuller, M. A., and Mehdi, F.: Compensatory hypoventilation and hypercapnia in primary metabolic alkalosis. Am. J. Med., 50:281, 1971.
33. Wright, H. K., and Gann, D. S.: Correction of defect in free water excretion in postoperative patients by extracellular fluid volume expansion. Ann. Surg., 158:70, 1963.

5

PRINCIPLES OF PREOPERATIVE PREPARATION OF THE SURGICAL PATIENT

Hiram C. Polk, Jr., M.D.

No single development more aptly characterizes the transfer of the surgical disciplines from art to science than the preparation of the ill patient for surgical intervention. Indeed, surgery languished in a primitive state, properly associated with the barber-surgeons, until the latter half of the nineteenth century, when two sequential discoveries initiated the conversion of the art to the science of today. These were the development of *anesthesia* followed by introduction of the *antiseptic concepts* of Semmelweiss and Lister.

ASSESSMENT OF OPERATIVE RISK

Inherent in discussion of operative risk is the consideration each physician must make regarding the relative rewards and risks of treatment of a given illness. The surgeon is particularly fortunate that the dramatic nature of his method magnifies the significance of adverse results and allows clear perception of this expression of the therapeutic ratio. There are few more valuable parameters than the *natural history* of a given illness, that is, the course of the disease and its ultimate outcome if untreated. Classic examples are the study by Estes[10] on the natural history of untreated abdominal aortic aneurysms and the important report by Greenwood[13] on the course of untreated mammary carcinoma. Such data are of particular significance in an era of therapeutic chauvinism. One must further ascertain that the *stages* of disease being considered are *clinically* comparable.[11]

Special problems that influence operative risk are of major concern in the preoperative preparation of the patient. The first of these is the relative urgency of the operative procedure. The therapeutic ratio of appendectomy for *suspected* appendicitis is quite clearly in favor of intervention. The treatment of appendicitis by excision, even with a 20 per cent incidence of normal appendices, is much better than allowing a single appendix to perforate, in view of the exaggerated morbidity and geometric effect upon mortality if the latter occurs. Similarly, the urgency of a given procedure is once more a function of the relative risks and rewards. In suspected appendicitis, the rewards of treatment are very clear in controlling an inflamed focus or dealing with a systemic complication that will very likely be fatal if untreated. Another example is the treatment of a free perforation of a sigmoid colonic diverticulum. The benefits compared to results of nonoperative treatment point strongly toward operation, and a principal determinant of those benefits is the promptness with which contamination is terminated or otherwise treated. While the urgency of an operation may determine the period of time and indirectly limit the measures taken to prepare the patient, it is all the more important that these preparations be accomplished promptly. While one cannot correct chronic malnutrition in 2 to 3 hours, it is possible to initiate correction of certain concentrational and volume deficiencies in a similar period.

In addition to urgency, the nature of the illness being treated sharply influences outcome by virtue of only partially alterable secondary effects. For example, a patient with advanced neoplastic disease often presents with anemia, profound weight loss, and evidence of metastases that alter hepatic, pulmonary, or cerebral function. Once the decision is made for operation, each consideration becomes important in preparing the individual for definitive treatment. By contrast, the systemic effects of an inflammatory process that has led to contamination of the entire peritoneal cavity may be treated vigorously with parenteral fluids, antibiotics, and intestinal decompression, with full knowledge that operative correction of the offending focus, whether perforated appendix, duodenal ulcer, or sigmoid diverticulum, is definitive in eliminating the source of continuing contamination.

A very special problem in treatment of the elderly is the appropriate management of multiple-organ degenerative disease. When one disease produces a complication that can be controlled only by surgery, particular attention should be given to the often subtle but physiologically important alterations of the organs essential for life support. Among the specific considerations that markedly influence operative risk are cardiovascular disease, respiratory insufficiency, renal disease, and gastrointestinal disease. Significant impairment of more than one organ system profoundly influences operative risk. For example, Irvin and Zeppa[15] recently determined that an individual with severe respiratory disease plus major renal insufficiency bore only one chance in 50 of surviving definitive surgical treatment of a duodenal ulcer.

The capacity for sound clinical *judgment* is the ultimate tribute to a qualified physician. Yet the parameters involved in clinical decisions are frequently difficult to define, and it is clear that quantification of these factors is desirable both to assess the physician's initial professional judgment and also to provide the younger physician a means of more promptly acquiring professional excellence. Some have criticized a quantitative approach as unnecessary, because all good physicians are assumed to be capable of sound clinical judgment, but there is continuing evidence that more is required in this area. Linn and Linn,[20] Knutson and Watson,[18] and Irvin and Zeppa[15] have each provided clear examples of efforts to achieve additional objectivity in the crucial area of judgment. Linn and Linn[20] found that the presence of systemic and local disease is generally additive in determining the probability of death during hospitalization. In prospective and retrospective studies of peptic ulcer disease, Irvin and Zeppa[15] showed that the effects of multiple organ system disease may be so profound as to *eliminate* from surgical consideration some patients previously recognized as having an increased but tolerable risk.

In determining operative risk and factors requiring specific preoperative correction, a simple list should be made part of each physical examination, including (1) personal and familial history of any past bleeding tendency, with laboratory definition of its significance; (2) allergic responses to medication or prior treatments; (3) current list of medications (with awareness that patients may forget to list some drugs or to recognize that nonprescription products may contain active medicinal agents. Examples are the intermittent use of corticosteroids with the real possibility of adrenal insufficiency at the time of stress and the use of diuretics with induced hypokalemia and its obvious systemic effects at time of anesthesia and operation).

PERSONAL RELATIONSHIPS

When a surgical procedure is being considered, it is crucial that a genuine bond of communication and personal responsibility be established between the surgeon and the patient. The patient's confidence is inherent in the agreement when an operation is planned. This confidence is established upon genuine understanding, allowing the patient to participate, when appropriate, in judgments affecting risks, future life style, and the process of postoperative recovery.

Many have emphasized the infrequency, even rarity, of legal action taken by a patient when a genuinely careful effort has been made by the physician to achieve such understanding prior to operation. This relationship evolves with a carefully informed and accurate statement of the relative risks and rewards of the operation. Most patients today have an increasing insight regarding such matters and should be allowed to participate actively in the decisions. In achieving this goal, the physician should not convey a sense of hurry or inadequate time for explanations, no matter how small or seemingly unimportant the operation might be. Finally, there are occasions when a direct answer may not be possible, and it has been said that the measure of a physician is his capacity to say "I don't know."

Another attribute of the mature and capable physician is his desire to involve consultants who may have additional or parallel skills to contribute to diagnosis and treatment. From recriminations about unnecessary operations and other largely unfounded criticisms that have been directed at the profession, there has evolved a desire for and understanding of the value of a *second opinion* concerning the necessity of the operative procedure. If there is reasonable question on the part of a patient that an operation is indicated, the surgeon should be certain to obtain the independent view of another surgeon to reassure the patient of the necessity for an operation.

The patient in a teaching institution finds his illness and operation a focal point for the education of students at several levels. Properly conducted, this can be a tremendous asset for the patient psychologically, as most enjoy such attention, provided it is conducted to involve the patient personally and to consider the medical problems in a tactful manner. Most discussions can be done at the bedside and do much to reassure the patient as to the total understanding of the illness and of the projected treatment.

For the young surgeon, there are few issues less well understood than the concept of optimal relationships with referring physicians. In most situations patients are referred to surgeons by physicians in other disciplines; it is important to have an understanding of the wishes and views of the referring physician at the outset. On some occasions the referring physician will have made certain judgments that are at variance with those of the surgeon, differences that must be discussed with him and, if unresolved, with the patient. Further, it is very helpful to have a clear understanding of the projected course of treatment and the relative participation of the referring physician in the postoperative care.

The *specific permission* for conduct of an operative procedure is a focal point of medical, legal, and sociologic discussion. Local custom and recent legal practice will often determine which of these is most appropriate. The surest perception of true *informed consent* can be attained in a setting in which there is a full and frank discussion with the patient as well as a close relative and an appropriate professional witness. It is also wise to record a summary of this encounter in the hospital chart.

Some procedures have such major measurable risk

that the real possibility of death and disability must be discussed as part of the mutual decision-making process. It is usually sufficient to inform the patient that there are risks of both complications and death, no matter how well or carefully the operation is conducted. One must carefully consider the patient's options, and it is important to avoid arousal of fear.

GENERAL PREPARATION OF THE PATIENT

Although the basic principles of preparation of the patient for a major operative procedure can be readily enumerated, it is much more difficult to determine the rapidity with which such preparation must be accomplished. For example, time may be of minor importance when an operation is being planned for a patient with an intractable duodenal ulcer but is more often a matter of personal convenience for the patient, the family, and the surgeon. In contrast is the patient with a radiographically demonstrated carcinoma of the colon, who should undergo definitive operation within a short time in order to prevent extension of the lesion. In the patient suspected of having acute appendicitis, operation should be performed within a few hours. Moreover, in a patient with rupture of an abdominal aortic aneurysm or with shock and peritonitis following mesenteric vascular occlusion, the lethality of uncontrolled hemorrhage in the first and the rapid progression of intestinal gangrene in the second require surgical treatment immediately, with few if any factors sufficiently important to justify delay. Thus, there is a measurable *spectrum of urgency* that directly warrants the promptness, the speed, and the adequacy of preoperative preparation.

PSYCHOLOGICAL PREPARATION

A frank discussion, planned to be as optimistic as possible, of the possibilities ahead is of great value for the patient who is about to undergo a major surgical procedure. The preoperative steps should be enumerated, justified, and explained in detail. The experience of being in the operating room and in the recovery area should be thoughtfully reviewed. The use of drainage devices and various forms of intubation are better tolerated, both physiologically and psychologically, if their need has been previously explained. The patient then anticipates and understands the benefits and realizes that the period of discomfort is for an identifiable purpose.

A frank attitude should be the standard procedure in discussing possible disfiguring operations, such as upon the head and neck, the breast or genital organs, and most especially with respect to methods of urinary or fecal eliminations, as in the creation of an ileal bladder or a colostomy.

Plans and Projections for Certain Chronic Illnesses

When an illness is apt to have a clinically significant course beyond the duration of the hospitalization and early postoperative follow-up, it is often reassur-ing for the surgeon to outline this situation with care. This is particularly helpful for the patient with neoplastic disease, who may correctly or incorrectly perceive his life expectancy to be 6 months or less. The surgeon should make realistic projections about continuing office visits at progressively longer intervals as the patient continues to do well after treatment. The critical factor is not only the reassurance of anticipated longevity on the part of the patient, but the assurance that the physician will indeed be his partner in the long-term management of the disease or any complication that may arise from the treatment. In such a setting, the problem of honesty as to preoperative and postoperative diagnosis always arises.

Some well-intentioned members of the family may wish to shield the patient from unpleasant facts. This is generally unwise, and the surgeon should carefully consider the fact that his contract is with the patient. When the medical facts are unpleasant, it is wise to allow the patient an opportunity to recover from the immediate effects of the operation and to ascertain that he is alert before such information is provided. Often it is useful to see if the patient will ask about the status of his disease spontaneously. However, if this has not occurred within a period of several days, the surgeon should take the initiative and review with the patient the observations and the probable prognosis. Such honesty guarantees that the patient who reaches the more difficult stages of his illness will once again turn to his physician as a person who has been honest with him in his prospects. He likewise will once more expect that physician to be thoroughly honest about the treatments available in difficult circumstances. At the point of first information, the prognosis, if poor, should not be presented as a hopeless situation. Such would not only be unjustified biologically, but experience has shown that even a small degree of justifiable optimism will support a patient with a grim prognosis surprisingly well.

PHYSIOLOGIC PREPARATION

Fluid and Blood Volume

A variety of chronic disease processes are associated with anemia. In some instances, these represent visible, external losses, such as in carcinoma of the cecum. Other instances are far less clear and are associated with chronic infection or with chronic inflammatory processes of the bowel. These patients all fit a pattern in which there is substantial blood loss associated with reduction of red cell mass. Indeed, such patients have a normal total blood *volume* (Fig. 1). They have compensated for a significantly decreased red blood cell volume by expansion of the plasma volume to supernormal levels.[26] While *acute* intravascular volume deficiencies are manifested by an increased pulse rate or decreased blood pressure, these are poorly tolerated on a chronic basis. Such volume is restored by expanding the plasma volume, often at the expense of the extracellular fluid, to compensate for the loss of or nonproduction of red cell mass.

Before correcting these concentrational deficits prior to an elective operation, it must be appreciated that

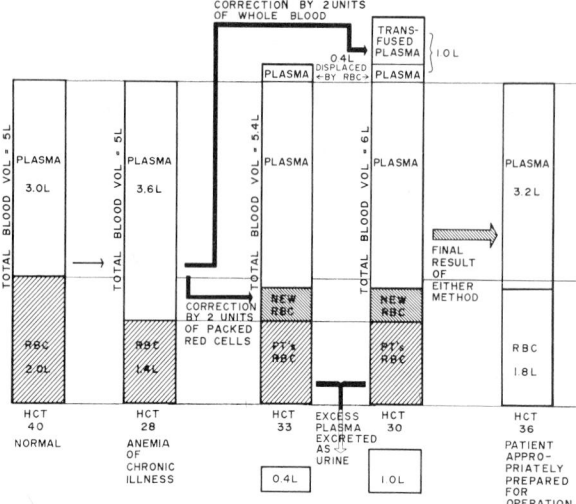

Figure 1. Schematic drawing illustrating anemia of chronic illness and the advantages of appropriate correction with packed red blood cells as compared to inefficient, and possibly dangerous, use of whole blood.

large deficits in red cell mass occurring over a long period are well tolerated. There are isolated but verified instances of a patient entering the hospital with a hemoglobin below 5 gm. per 100 ml. with no evidence of tachycardia or hypovolemia. Uniformly the red cell concentrational deficit has been sustained over an extended period and is of fundamental importance when considering general anesthesia. Although 10 gm. per 100 ml. of hemoglobin is regarded by many as minimal, what must be determined is the physiologic limits safe for tissue oxygen delivery. Enhanced oxygen delivery can be achieved in the following ways: (a) increase in heart rate, (b) increase in stroke volume, and (c) increase in oxygen extraction. This last way may be set almost unalterably, and to increase stroke volume or pulse rate places a definite physiologic stress upon the heart, which often is diseased itself in the elderly who acquire such chronic illnesses. Therefore, there is a reasonable limit to the hemoglobin concentrations that are likely to be safe for a major operation. Indeed, if one could ascertain that no unforeseen blood losses or inadvertent hypoxia would occur, a patient could with some safety expect to undergo an elective operation with a distinctly low hemoglobin concentration. However, the risk of one of these untoward events is greater than the hazard of the correction of this deficit. Thus, patients being prepared for operation with an anemia commonly associated with chronic disease should have replacement of the red cell mass up to nearly 10 gm. per 100 ml., or even more nearly normal when there is evidence of associated cardiovascular disease (e.g., prior myocardial infarct, congestive heart failure, etc.).

A useful rule when attempting physiologic correction of chronic anemia is to administer more than 1 unit of blood per day only rarely, thereby allowing time for excretion of excess plasma in an orderly fashion. A hemoglobin concentration deficit that has been acquired over months need not be corrected in a matter of hours. Whereas blood deficits are primarily con-

centrational, plasma and extracellular fluid deficits are significant in both volume and concentration in terms of the preparation of most patients preoperatively.

Special problems are presented when the volume deficiencies are pre-existing or concealed. For example, pre-existing losses may represent vomitus and/or diarrhea occurring for 3 to 4 days before hospitalization. It is quite difficult if not impossible for the patient to estimate the volume of such losses. While other losses occur rather visibly in a fracture of the femur or in a major third-degree burn of an extremity and are manifested by visible swelling, more often such fluid losses are concealed and thus inadequately estimated. A patient with intestinal obstruction may present with vomiting of 3 days' duration with signs of dry mucous membranes and tongue and complaining of thirst. Yet the patient has continued to vomit, although he has taken several hundred milliliters of liquid orally over each of the 3 days. His hemoglobin concentration might well be an index of dehydration, but this requires a recent known normal value for that patient. For example, if the hemoglobin is normal, one could postulate either that there had been very little volume loss or that there had been a major blood volume loss superimposed upon pre-existing anemia. Such occurs with a colonic carcinoma, which may produce significant red blood cell deficiency, and then leads to intestinal obstruction, which produces an extracellular fluid volume deficit. Together these losses produce a hemoglobin concentration that is in the normal range.

Objective determination of fluid deficits should be obtained, and one of the most useful is urinary output. Hourly urine output through an indwelling catheter can be followed as an objective measure of efficacy of replenishment. Other parameters such as hemoglobin concentration, appearance of the mucous membranes, and skin turgor assist in such a judgment. It should be emphasized that standard losses in these circumstances total approximately 3 liters a day or 125 ml. an hour in adults. Therefore, the rate of fluid resuscitation in a *deficit* situation should begin with at least 250 ml. an hour. The hourly urinary output should be assessed over a period of 3 to 4 hours for determination of volume deficiency and the rate at which replenishment should be continued.

The problem of concealed loss is particularly difficult. These "third space losses" in which blood, plasma, and/or extracellular fluid are extravasated are often associated with fractures, and it is only upon careful comparison of the fractured and unfractured limb for circumference that one can appreciate the magnitude of such losses.

A common error in quantitating concentrational deficits is to ascertain the serum concentration of a given electrolyte and, finding it normal, to postulate that there has been no loss. Isotonic losses of water, salt, chloride, and potassium may produce profound volume deficiencies with maintenance of normal concentrations of the commonly measured serum electrolytes. When concentrational abnormalities exist, they imply only that the loss of electrolyte concentration has been relatively greater than the loss of water or

TABLE 1. Conditions That Adversely Affect Nutritional Balance

I. Inadequate intake and inflow
  A. Anorexia
    1. Hepatic disease
    2. Chronic infectious disease
    3. Visceral colic (gastrocolic reflex in presence of lesion of colon)
    4. Senility
    5. Emotional disturbances
  B. Malfunction of gastrointestinal tract
    1. Ineffective mastication (inadequate dentures)
    2. Interference with swallowing
      a. Cerebrovascular disease
      b. Obstructing esophageal lesions
    3. Obstructing lesions of stomach and intestine
  C. Malabsorption
    1. Gastritis and/or prior extensive gastric resection
    2. Pancreatitis
    3. Enteritis and colitis (see also II. A. 3. below)
    4. Inadequate length of small bowel for effective absorption
II. Excessive outflow
  A. Intestinal losses (diarrhea)
    1. Internal enteric fistulas (gastrocolic, enterocolic, enteroenteral)
    2. External gastrointestinal fistulas
    3. Various forms of enteritis and colitis with excessive losses of proteins, fats, water, electrolytes, and vitamins (Zollinger-Ellison syndrome; villous adenoma of colon)
III. Metabolic demands and disturbances
  A. Endocrine effects on metabolic rate
    1. Thyrotoxicosis
    2. Diabetes
    3. Leukemia
  B. Burns and caloric loss
  C. Infections and fever
  D. Trauma and stress
    1. Severe fractures
    2. Operations

vice versa. Although administration of any fluid containing the electrolytes will ultimately be of value, it may be an inefficient approach, as, for example, replenishing sodium chloride and potassium deficits by administration of 5 per cent dextrose in half-normal (0.45 per cent) saline. Reasonably normal kidneys will conserve all sodium and chloride administered. However, to do so will be metabolically expensive because the kidney must excrete large amounts of free water. Ultimately, correction will be accomplished, but infusion of solutions proportionate to losses is much more precise and definitive. In the above example, the patient probably should be given normal saline.

Under what circumstances should hypertonic resuscitative solutions be used? Notwithstanding their apparent marginal benefit in the resuscitation of some forms of experimental hemorrhagic shock and some clinical usefulness in burn shock,[23] the method has relatively limited indications. A useful rule is to employ isotonic solutions unless cerebral abnormalities deemed attributable to concentrational deficits in sodium are present. In the presence of severe dysfunction attributed to hyponatremia (coma, etc.), the limited administration of hypertonic solution is therapeutically acceptable. Unless there is history of renal disease, potassium replenishment should proceed along with sodium infusion.

The urgency of the operation is the major determinant in the time available for correction of fluid and electrolyte balance. All volume and concentrational deficits need not be corrected before operation is undertaken, but a significant fraction of the total deficit should be corrected in order to enhance the safety of anesthesia and operation. For example, in a patient with nonstrangulating intestinal obstruction of 3 days' duration and normal electrolyte concentrations without signs of urinary or hemoconcentration, one may assume that there has been a significant isotonic loss of electrolytes and water. Resuscitation should be initiated with Ringer's lactate solution with added potassium at a rate of 500 ml. in the first hour. If the urinary response to such administration is only 10 ml., another 500 ml. should be infused during the next hour. Should urinary output increase to 20 ml. per hour, one might reasonably anticipate operation. Sufficient replenishment of extracellular fluid in such patients would require another 2 liters of fluid, for a total preparatory period of about 6 hours in a patient who has been ill for 3 days. In general, the longer a patient has been ill, the more time one can take to correct the deficiencies. In other words, the patient has adjusted physiologically to the deficiency induced by the illness; one must be certain that the rapid replenishment of those deficits does not impose a risk greater than the illness itself. The overly rapid correction of fluid deficits and induction of pulmonary edema, particularly in elderly patients with marginal cardiovascular compensation, may represent a risk that would not otherwise exist in the young patient with a normal cardiovascular system and acutely encountered disease.

The desired and usual preoperative state is one of abundant nutritional intake. A surgical procedure, together with the pharmacologic effects of preoperative drugs, the dietary restrictions, and sometimes the preliminary preparations, imposes metabolic stresses that must be met by the patient's normal physiologic reactions supported by appropriate therapy. Special postoperative problems include (1) depletion of stored glycogen such that emergency gluconeogenesis from this source is quickly exhausted; (2) inability of the heart to increase its output; (3) inability of the liver to produce adequate protein; (4) respiratory insufficiency such that the lungs cannot eliminate carbon dioxide and maintain HCO_3/H_2CO_3 ratio near 20; and (5) inability of kidneys to change selectively the glomerular filtrate to maintain normal composition of body fluids.

Insulin is an important determinant of protein breakdown and synthesis, and its role in the feedback mechanism responsible for glucose homeostasis and nitrogen metabolism is shown in Figure 1. Low levels of circulating insulin, as found in fasting after an operation and in other conditions of negative nutritional balance, enhance the release of fatty acids from neutral fat and of amino acids from muscle.

In times of abundance, when intake of energy-providing substances exceeds utilization, carbohydrate is stored largely as fat. Some is stored as glycogen, but

TABLE 2. Sources of Fuel*
Body Composition of 70-kg. Man

	Kilograms →	can yield → Calories
Body parenchyma		
Fat	15	141,000
Protein	6	24,000
Glycogen from muscle	0.15	600
Glycogen from liver	0.075	300
Extracellular fluid (ECF)		
Glucose from ECF	0.02	80
Free fatty acids from plasma	0.0003	3
Triglycerides from plasma	0.003	30
		166,013

*Modified from Cahill, G. F., Jr.: Starvation in man. N. Engl. J. Med., *282*:668, 1970.

for each gram of glycogen stored an equal weight of water enters the cells along with electrolytes to preserve normal intracellular osmotic relationships. This is an inefficient method for storing calories as carbohydrate, the yield upon demand being only 2 calories per gram instead of 4. Nor is protein economically stored as fuel. Proteins exist to perform specific functions: as enzymes, buffers, antibodies, and contractile elements in cardiac, smooth, and skeletal muscle. They have some oncotic functions in body fluids. The average 70-kg. man has 6 kg. of protein, of which as much as 20 per cent can be used for gluconeogenesis (Table 2). Theoretically, total destruction of body mass could provide 3000 calories per day for 55 days of survival. A patient so depleted, however, is not a good candidate for operation. Once the normal protein composition is attained, additional nitrogen intake is not stored but is metabolized to glucose and stored as fat.

Fat is the body's best fuel reservoir. It is stored with very little water: adipose tissue contains only 10 per cent water. The mechanisms that govern the utilization of carbohydrate, fat, and protein are not entirely understood, but insulin and the liver play vital regulatory functions in this aspect of energy metabolism.

Typical Problems

Brief Negative Caloric Balance. It is important to distinguish brief from prolonged periods of negative caloric balance.[2] With brief negative caloric balance, as in fasting, the sources of energy include the following:

1. Oxidation of glucose to carbon dioxide and water in the tricarboxylic acid cycle, which occurs almost entirely in the brain.

2. Glycolysis, with lactic acid as the end product, occurring largely in the formed elements of the blood, renal medulla, bone marrow, peripheral nerves, and skeletal muscles. The lactate is converted in the liver to glucose by way of the Cori cycle. Anaerobic glycolysis is a far less efficient source of energy than oxidative glucose metabolism.

3. Oxidation of free fatty acids and ketone bodies. The transformation of lactate into glucose requires energy, the source of which is mainly the oxidation of free fatty acids to ketone bodies.

Fasting results in the release of (a) free fatty acids from the triglycerides of depot fat to fulfill the caloric requirements of the body (except for the brain) and (b) amino acids from the body proteins for gluconeogenesis to provide dextrose for the brain and spinal cord. Unfortunately, in man this carbohydrate cannot be derived from amino acids obtained from hydrolysis of body proteins.

In a desirable nutritional state, body proteins are protected from such depletion. Enough nitrogen must be obtained to supply the body's requirement, but when malnutrition pre-exists, enough must be ingested to achieve a positive nitrogen balance and rebuild protein. Proteins are not present as stores with no other function than to wait to be used as fuel in times of need. Protein comprises the working elements of the body's composition of its "machinery." The loss of one third of the body's protein content is thought to be incompatible with life.

For many years it has been known that the administration of carbohydrate in relatively small amounts has a demonstrable protein-sparing effect. Presumably, the increased concentration of dextrose induces the secretion of insulin by pancreatic islet beta cells, and insulin inhibits the hydrolysis of protein to amino acids, thus saving the protein. Similarly, the need for the liver to derive energy from the oxidation of free fatty acids ceases and ketogenesis decreases. The administration of 2 liters of 5 per cent dextrose, or 1 liter of a 10 per cent solution, will protect 50 gm. of protein from hydrolysis. However, the protein-sparing action of these small amounts of carbohydrate is *not* increased by administering larger amounts. To maintain a positive nitrogen balance, building blocks from proteins must be provided. Deficits of caloric requirements are met by oxidation of free fatty acids derived from depots of neutral fat, which are readily available in the absence of chronic starvation.

In planning the nutritional preparation of the malnourished patient preoperatively, note that while nitrogen is necessary as amino acids to serve as protein building blocks, glucose must be provided to satisfy the caloric requirements of the brain, and the two sources of energy must be provided at the same time. Insufficient carbohydrate administration permits the obligatory gluconeogenesis from amino acids derived from the breakdown of body protein to continue.

Prolonged Negative Caloric Balance. In contrast to the patient whose imbalance before and after operation is brief, the patient who has been deficient for days or weeks before operation requires aggressive attention to nutritional balance to avoid loss of body protein, most of which comes from muscle. The loss of muscle mass at the rate of 50 to 75 gm. per day soon decreases body proteins to levels that are physiologically intolerable. Smooth and skeletal muscle, as well as cardiac muscle, would suffer a decrease in contractile protein elements to the point of interference with cardiovascular dynamics and ventilation. Recall that an operation often places a serious demand upon the heart to increase its output if morbidity and mortality are to be minimized.[4]

Some metabolic adaptation takes place with prolonged fasting. There is progressively less excretion of urea and more excretion of ammonia, while other nitrogenous urinary constituents remain unchanged.

With chronic fasting, the brain gradually stops demanding glucose for its source of energy and turns to keto acids for its needs.[25] Protein mobilization and catabolism decrease in proportion to the diminished demands for gluconeogenesis by the brain. Except for amino acids, which are diminished after prolonged fasting, these adaptations take place without significant alterations in the concentrations of substrates in the blood (glucose, free fatty acids, acetoacetate, beta-hydroxybutyrate, glycerol, lactate, and pyruvate.)

Gluconeogenesis by the liver decreases as adaptation of the brain to keto acid utilization increases. More than three fourths of the glucose produced by the liver comes from lactate, pyruvate, and glycerol and amounts to as much as 45 gm. per day. A nearly equal amount of glucose, approximately 40 gm. per day, is produced by the kidneys via gluconeogenesis from amino acids. The amine and amide groups are converted to ammonia, which combines with the keto acids for excretion by the kidneys, and thus also spares sodium.

Preoperative Correction of Caloric Deficit

The principle that the malnourished patient approaching surgical intervention is at serious disadvantage bears emphasis. Not only has he lost or greatly depleted his fuel stores, but his loss of muscle mass makes it difficult for him to move about because of weakness, and breathing itself becomes a tiring effort. Cough becomes ineffective for lack of muscle strength, a situation commonly seen among the elderly.

Nutritional deficits can be corrected either orally or parenterally. The choice between the two, or a combination of the two, is based upon the circumstances. If the patient can take the usual diet with supplements, there is no need for special diets, tube feedings, or parenteral administration. In the absence of sufficient gastrointestinal function, special diets can be designed that may be self-sufficient or may require only parenteral supplements. Occasionally, a complete parenteral alimentation is necessary.

Oral Nutrition. The oral administration of natural or specially prepared food, whenever possible, is by far the best way to correct malnutrition. When solid food cannot be swallowed because of dentitional problems or esophageal, gastric, or duodenal obstruction, a liquid diet may be administered by a small nasogastric tube passed into the stomach or duodenum in the patient with obstruction so severe as to cause difficulty in swallowing his own saliva. The passage of such a tube can permit administration of calories and needed

TABLE 4. Comparison of Basal Nutrient Requirements and Influence of Trauma and/or Sepsis*

	Basal State	Hypermetabolism in Trauma and/or Sepsis
Water	30 ml.	60 ml.
Calories	30 cal.	55 cal.
Protein	1.5 gm.	2.5 gm.
Carbohydrate	2 gm.	5 gm.
Fat	2 gm.	4 gm.

*Estimates per kilogram of body weight.

nutrient elements for several days or weeks before operation. Tube feeding is also useful when patients, particularly the elderly, refuse to eat for psychological reasons. Aspiration is an ever-present hazard with tube feeding.

Occasionally, obstructions are practically complete and food must be directed into the gastrointestinal tract by gastrostomy or jejunostomy. Except for special technical considerations, as in instances of carcinoma near the cardia in which reconstruction may require use of the stomach itself, gastrostomy is preferred to jejunostomy.

Before correcting deficiencies in caloric body composition, the daily energy requirements of the individual must be met (Table 3). To them must be added losses through abnormal avenues, as in severe ulcerative colitis, high intestinal fistulas, and extensive surface burns (Table 4). Added to these losses are relative deficits imposed by increased metabolic rate, as in thyrotoxicosis and fever (10 per cent increase in metabolic activity per degree centigrade). For the patient who can eat, a palatable diet containing essential requirements in twice the basal amounts is arranged. With encouragement, a daily intake of perhaps 6000 calories can be achieved. However, patients, especially the elderly, are often totally incapable of eating a diet so high in calories.

The administration of more nutrients than are required to meet basal needs plus losses through abnormal channels is referred to as hyperalimentation. The administration of carbohydrate, protein, and fat must be sufficient to spare protein, to replace obligatory protein breakdown, and to begin restoration of the essential and "reserve" protein mass.

Parenteral Alimentation. Until about three decades ago, parenteral alimentation was confined to the subcutaneous administration of isotonic solutions of dextrose and electrolytes to patients who could ingest food and water[9] in only insufficient amounts or not at all. Such injections were made into the subcutaneous compartment of the thighs or of the subpectoral region. Injections into the marrow spaces were occasionally used. Intravenous infusions were avoided because of the unacceptable frequency of pyrogenic and other reactions. In infants and children, intraperitoneal injections were commonly employed. These routes of fluid administration are now almost never used because convenient pyrogen-free solutions are available for intravenous administration.

The advent of convenient and safe solutions for in-

TABLE 3. Daily Energy Requirements*
(Basal: 70-kg. Man)

	Amount →	can yield →	Calories
Protein	75 gm.		300
Fat as triglycerides	160 gm.		1440
Carbohydrate as glucose	180 gm.		720
			2460

*Modified from Cahill, G. F., Jr.: Starvation in man. N. Engl. J. Med., *282*:668, 1970.

travenous administration led to the successful use of precisely constituted solutions for the treatment of dehydration and electrolyte imbalance. Dextrose solutions are useful for providing water and the relatively small amount of carbohydrates needed to spare proteins. The drastically hyperosmotic solutions necessary to meet the total caloric requirement in a reasonable volume of water made it impractical to use dextrose solutions for this purpose until techniques for delivering solutions into the large central veins proved practical. Dudrick and his associates[8] have achieved remarkable results with this approach to nutrition, and their method, which is discussed in a separate chapter, has been widely accepted.

Vitamins. The role of the vitamins in health and their therapeutic implementation bear emphasis. In this country it is rather uncommon to encounter a patient with a specific vitamin deficiency. The typical American example of chronic adult malnutrition is often complicated by a sociopathic state and/or acute and chronic alcoholism. Vitamin replenishment is warranted in such patients, as well as in those who have advanced chronic illnesses and are being prepared for operation. Administration of both water-soluble and fat-soluble vitamins should be included in preoperative preparation.

The utilization of vitamins in postoperative parenteral fluids is a common practice that is routinely unnecessary and rarely beneficial. Only the patient who is markedly malnourished before operation or who will be late into the postoperative period before he can resume normal nutrition will benefit from vitamin infusions. Clearly such treatment should be the exception rather than the rule.

PREVENTION OF INFECTION

Infection continues to be a major source of morbidity and a disconcerting source of mortality in the surgical patient. The patient who is badly injured or who undergoes a major operation and survives despite the development of secondary shock and electrolyte disturbances is a high-risk candidate for serious infection. Therefore, control of infection is a major consideration before, during, and after every operation. Only certain aspects of the problem of infection as it particularly pertains to the preoperative assessment of the patient are here reviewed.

The first consideration is to identify the *genuine* high-risk factors for infection. For example, diabetics have long been considered particularly prone to infection. As a matter of fact, this is correct, as long as one considers their well-known propensity to develop infection in the lower extremities related to small vessel arteriosclerosis and peripheral neuropathy. If these possibilities are eliminated, as in extensive cooperative studies, the diabetic patient is probably no more prone to infection than any other individual of similar age and illness.[24] Some other risk factors, however, are indeed genuine. Among the risks that do increase the likelihood of infection are extremes of obesity or malnutrition, evidence of remote infection elsewhere in the patient's body, the use of acute or chronic corticosteroid medicinal therapy, and several metabolic dis-

eases.[24] Data on the potentiation of infection under these circumstances are virtually unequivocal. Nevertheless, clinical compromises are sometimes inescapable. Termination of steroid medication must be considered carefully in view of the obvious risk of acute adrenal insufficiency in the intra- or postoperative patient who has been receiving exogenous steroids for a long period.

Furthermore, during preoperative evaluation, the patient should be protected from any patient with extramural or hospital-acquired infections. The proposed operative site should be washed with an appropriate antiseptic agent on several occasions before operation, and shaving should be done either as close to the time of operation as feasible or not at all, substituting either clipping or depilatory agents where removal of hair is mandated.[7]

Among other factors that should be considered in preparation of the patient are *antibiotics*. Despite their widespread use since 1948, only recently has evidence of the efficacy of preoperative intestinal preparation with antimicrobial agents been shown for colon operations.[38] Systemic antibiotics for alleged prophylaxis of operative wound infection acquired a poor reputation in the years after their introduction, largely because the patients so treated were already at greater risk of infection compared to those from whom antibiotics were withheld and because the antibiotics used were initiated in the recovery room *after* the operation was complete. Explicit laboratory studies[31] were confirmed by randomized clinical trials that showed systemic antibiotics highly effective when used just before, during, and immediately after an operation.[29] However, one must always balance the risk of an adverse effect of an antibiotic with its potential benefit. To date, most studies showing clearcut benefit from such antibiotic use have been in operations that bore an appreciable risk of infection, such as those on the gastrointestinal tract or on other contaminated foci.[1, 3, 19]

Urgency of operation, reflecting limited time for preparation and the nature of the illnesses requiring immediate intervention, is another major determinant. Furthermore, the type of operation in terms of contamination is substantially determinative of the probability of postoperative infection. If ideal preoperative preparation has been obtained, one can then consider those operative maneuvers that are likely to control infection. The elimination of unnecessary conversation and traffic in the operating room, as well as strict adherence to sterile technique, and the precise use of noninjurious methods of handling tissue are each critical in controlling infection. A recent report suggests that it is the combination of all these factors that leads to the lowest possible infection rate.[12] If contamination of the wound edges is likely, specific protective drapes[5] are available to minimize the dose of bacteria delivered to the subcutaneous fat, which with relatively poor blood supplies is the most common site of bacterial infection.

With regard to the prevention of wound infection, one may administer systemic antibiotics or choose topical antibiotics for the wound itself. This latter is controversial, but clinical data show a consistent value when contamination of the operative wound is likely to occur.[6] A method of wound management that has been efficacious for a very long time in badly contaminated cases is *delayed* primary closure of the wound.[35] The peritoneum and muscle layers are closed securely, and the subcutaneous fat and skin are left open and covered with gauze treated with either saline or an antimicrobial agent. At a suitable time postoperatively when the wounds are shown to be free of infection by inspection or by culture, the subcutaneous fat and skin are closed with tape or previously placed sutures. Although sometimes cumbersome, this method has been a standby for many years and should continue to be so.

No single technical complication is as frequently associated with infection as is the presence of a *hematoma*, implying poor hemostasis. Often thought to represent poor technique and to provide a medium for bacterial growth, there is increasing evidence that iron-binding proteins contribute directly to the nonspecific host defense response to bacteria, functioning very effectively when incompletely bound with iron and becoming ineffective when highly saturated with iron. A hematoma of the wound has the theoretical and probably practical capacity to abrogate the effect of this important defense mechanism.[30] Therefore, hematoma must be avoided by meticulous technique and by closed suction drainage at a distance from the wound where avoidance seems otherwise impossible.

SPECIFIC ORGANS AND SYSTEMS

CARDIOVASCULAR

Each patient scheduled for an operation should have careful evaluation of the cardiovascular system. In the young, previously overlooked congenital heart disease may be discovered. Arteriosclerosis affects an increasingly broad segment of the older population and is of considerable concern.[14] Although this is an identifiable adverse determinant of outcome, one must look for the lesson in the evolution of coronary artery surgery.

Several significant groups of patients with arteriosclerotic heart disease deserve specific mention:

1. *Previous myocardial infarction:* the patient who has undergone a documented myocardial infarct engenders optimal care at every level in the preoperative evaluation and can generally undergo major operations with an acceptable risk, especially those who are a functional Class I. These patients deserve and receive careful preoperative assessment with particular attention to oxygenation, hemoglobin concentration, and anesthetic and postoperative respiratory management. Patients with recent infarcts should be allowed a healing period of three months or so before an elective operation.

2. *Angina pectoris:* angina before operation is a serious problem. The presence of angina indicates significant coronary ischemia that could lead to ventricular fibrillation or intraoperative myocardial infarct, should hypoxia and/or hypotension supervene in the procedure itself. In the past, best management has consisted of accurate monitoring during and after operation. In some instances the patient with continuing angina requiring an elective operation should be evaluated for a coronary bypass before considering the planned operation.

3. The patient with *congestive* heart failure poses an absolutely prohibitive operative risk and should not undergo operation, except those known to be immediately and unequivocally lifesaving. One striking exception to this consideration is the patient whose congestive heart failure is unmasked only by profound anemia with its secondary demand for increased cardiac output. Once hemoglobin concentration returns to normal, these patients are readily converted from the congestive state and approach the risk of the patient with stable heart disease.

One of the most hazardous conditions is occult or unrecognized heart disease, such as a silent myocardial infarct, for which there may be no EKG or in which the EKG is misinterpreted.

Arrhythmias and/or treatment with digitalis are common considerations before operation. In general, atrial fibrillation, depending on underlying cause, is relatively well tolerated during anesthesia and operation and does not require specific treatment. Continuing digitalis during and after operative procedures is generally warranted. With respect to perioperative digitalis, the critical factor is to maintain a normal serum potassium level throughout the postoperative period for maximal synergistic effect. In every case, patients with arrhythmias benefit from continuing electrocardiographic monitoring during the intra- and early postoperative periods.

RESPIRATORY

Respiratory complications of operations fall into two major groups: first, the development of respiratory abnormalities secondary to the anesthetic agent and the operation in patients with grossly normal lungs; second, the increasing number of patients with measurable chronic lung disease who require operation, thus superimposing the problems of anesthesia and operation upon intrinsically diseased pulmonary tissue.

Patients with normal lung function sustain pulmonary complications more often after *upper* abdominal operations than *lower* ones. The complication rate is also higher in individuals who are cigarette smokers. Therefore, elimination of the use of tobacco for as long a period as possible, preferably at least 2 weeks before a major operation, has a measurable benefit upon the incidence and severity of postoperative complications.

Preoperative pulmonary insufficiency represents a critical problem. The crucial distinction between nonobstructive and obstructive pulmonary emphysema can be made with the standard tests of pulmonary function. In general, patients below the age of 40 who have no pulmonary signs or symptoms do not require special tests. In older patients and those with pre-existing disease, especially in lesions requiring upper abdominal operations, tests of pulmonary function can provide useful information. Abnormalities of the lungs and tracheobronchial tree are detected in some patients despite a history negative for pulmonary disease. What levels of pulmonary function are consistent with tolerating a major operation remains a subject of debate with respect to two categories of patients: those who will require excision of functioning or nonfunctioning lung tissue and those who undergo nonpulmonary operations. Although there are a variety of specific tests that delineate minimal function, careful evaluation by the physician, in consultation with pulmonary medicine, is usually indicated. It should be remembered that a simple, useful test is a brisk walk of the patient up a flight of stairs with observation of tolerance. One test of proven value in the diagnosis and management of patients with pulmonary insufficiency is documentation of the normal resting *arterial blood gases*. A preoperative base line study is especially valuable to the patient with respiratory disease.

RENAL

With appropriate hydration, renal complications of major surgical endeavors have become relatively uncommon. Of those that remain, most represent a failure to appreciate the renal status preoperatively. A normal level of blood urea nitrogen may be misleading. Surely, where there is the slightest suspicion of intrinsic renal disease, appropriate creatinine studies should be undertaken. However, perhaps the most inappropriate consideration in the surgical patient is the fear that renal disease exists. Renal disease is not nearly so frequent in the apparently asymptomatic population as are cardiovascular and respiratory diseases. With the screening procedures of the BUN, creatinine determination, and urinalysis, one may proceed to an operative procedure and subsequent fluid therapy reasonably confident that the patient will tolerate judiciously managed fluid loads with ease. The most common cause of oliguria on surgical services continues to be hypovolemia rather than incipient renal failure.

A special type of renal disease is that associated with obstruction in the lower urinary tract, especially prostatic hypertrophy in elderly men. If time permits, free drainage of the obstructed urinary tract and elimination of infection should be done before an elective procedure, allowing return of adequate function. A secondary operation for treatment of prostatic obstruction may later be necessary. If time does not permit, drainage by an indwelling catheter and sufficient fluid therapy to provide some indices of renal function should be accomplished.

HEPATIC

The signs and symptoms of significant liver impairment are detectable on a variety of standard examinations. The typical patient has obvious signs of advanced nutritional cirrhosis or widespread metastatic liver disease. In many instances, these abnormalities can be only marginally corrected before operation. With cirrhotic patients, a substantial preoperative period must be allowed if any recovery of function is to be achieved, again concentrating on nutrition and

TABLE 5. Relationship of Life Expectancy to Certain Evidence of Hepatic Metastases*

Characteristic	Estimated Median Survival After Diagnosis of Hepatic Metastases (Days)
Metastases	
Multiple in one lobe	95
Multiple in both lobes	70
Solitary	140
Ascites	
Present	30
Absent	100
Jaundice	
Present	30
Absent	80
BSP retention	
<10%	140
>11%	30
Alkaline phosphatase	
<5.0	140
5.1–15.0	70
>15.1	20

*Modified from Jaffe, B. M., Donegan, W. L., Watson, F., and Spratt, J. S.: Factors influencing survival in patients with untreated hepatic metastases. Surg. Gynecol. Obstet., *127*:1, 1968.

avoidance of hepatotoxins in any form. The effect of metastatic liver disease, such as from an intestinal neoplasm, has been characterized by Jaffe and associates.[16] The anticipated median survival for such patients, depending on clinical, laboratory, or operative findings, is depicted on Table 5. Such observations allow objectivity in the assessment of the standard therapeutic risk-reward balance and provide a measure of confidence in recommending palliative operations with evidence of potential duration of benefit.

NEUROLOGIC

One special aspect of cerebral function ever must stand first among preoperative considerations for the patient who is suspected to have cardiovascular disease. Significant carotid artery narrowing enhances the risk of stroke during any operation or anesthesia in which hypotension and/or hypoxia may occur. A specific history should be taken and the neck examined for bruits. Should a question arise, a neurologic consultation and perhaps carotid arteriography are warranted. Should carotid stenosis be documented, operative correction thereof should be considered, and if performed, one or two weeks or longer should elapse before the originally planned operation is undertaken. This policy is a function of both the very low risk and substantial efficacy of carotid endarterectomy in symptomatic patients.

TABLE 6.   A Sample Preoperative Check List

1. Operative permit—appropriately signed and witnessed
2. Dietary considerations
   A. For abdominal operation, liquid diet and laxatives to ensure clean collapsed bowel
   B. NPO at least 6 hours before operation
3. Review of life-support systems
   A. Vital signs recorded often enough to establish "normal"
   B. Pulmonary system—chest x-rays; other studies as indicated
   C. Cardiac function—electrocardiogram; other studies as indicated
   D. Renal function—urinalysis; BUN and creatinine determinations
4. Adequate hydration up to time of operation—especially to compensate for laxatives and fasting
5. Area of operation washed with appropriate germicidal detergent and shaved, dipped, or cleansed with depilatory agent
6. Blood transfusions prepared as anticipated
7. Order that patient should void on call to OR
8. Preoperative medications—vagolytic and sedative drugs
9. Special medications—digitalis, insulin, etc.

SPECIAL PROBLEMS

A variety of special problems demand preoperative correction. Foremost among these is incomplete cleansing of the alimentary tract. Pulmonary aspiration is a dreaded surgical complication, the treatment for which remains inadequate, whereas prevention is simple. There are almost no circumstances when general anesthesia should be induced without specific question as to evacuation of the patient's stomach, ascertained in any questionable case by the surgeon himself. So simple to prevent, aspiration remains one of the more common causes of surgical mortality. A useful checklist of preoperative considerations that should be reviewed at the time of writing preoperative hospital orders is depicted in Table 6.

SELECTED REFERENCES

Blalock, A.: Principles of Surgical Care, Shock and Other Problems. St. Louis, The C. V. Mosby Company, 1940.

Elman, R.: Surgical Care. A Practical Physiologic Guide. New York, Appleton-Century-Crofts, 1951.

These two monographs reflect the vision of far-sighted and imaginative surgeons of the entire process of the physiologic disturbances of the surgical patient. Blalock's chapter on shock is a classic, particularly when one views the time frame in which it was first offered. Elman's understanding of parenteral alimentation and its importance in the surgical setting is more apparent today than at any time in the past.

Feinstein, A. R.: Clinical Judgment. Baltimore, The Williams and Wilkins Company, 1967.

The process of assessing operative risk is discussed in detail in this rambling but enormously incisive monograph about a variety of considerations. Clinical examples are drawn to provide objectivity and specificity, and most apply to the surgical setting.

Moore, F. D.: Metabolic Care of the Surgical Patient. Philadelphia, W. B. Saunders Company, 1959.

Moore, F. D., Olesen, K. H., McMurrey, J. D., Parker, H. V., Ball, M. R., and Boyden, C. M.: The Body Cell Mass and Its Supporting Environment. Philadelphia, W. B. Saunders Company, 1963.

These contributions from Moore's productive and life-long inquiry into the metabolic process form the basis of modern perception of surgical physiology and contain the principles of preparation of the patient for operation. These careful and specific studies have unmasked many heretofore unappreciated or misunderstood entities, in terms of their routine prevention and/or correction in a very simple fashion.

Moyer, C. A.: The assessment of operative risk. *In* Rhoads, J. E., Allen, J. G., Harkins, H. N., and Moyer, C. A.: Surgery. Principles and Practice, 4th ed. Philadelphia, J. B. Lippincott Company, 1970, pp. 232–243.

The requisite process for evaluating factors that genuinely influence operative risk is explicitly reviewed and documented. Mechanisms by which future risk factors can be evaluated are also presented in detail.

REFERENCES

1. Bernard, H. R., and Cole, W. R.: Wound infection following potentially contaminated operations. The effect of delayed primary closure on the skin and subcutaneous tissue. J.A.M.A., *184*:290, 1963.
2. Cahill, G. F., Jr.: Starvation in man. N. Engl. J. Med., *282*:668, 1970.
3. Chetlin, S. H., and Elliott, D. W.: Preoperative antibiotics in biliary surgery. Arch. Surg., *107*:319, 1973.
4. Clowes, G. H. A., Jr., Del Guercio, L. R., and Barwinsky, J.: The cardiac output in response to surgical trauma. A comparision between patients who survived and those who died. Arch. Surg., *81*:212, 1960.
5. Cole, W. R., and Bernard, H. R.: Wound isolation in prevention of postoperative wound infection. Surg. Gynecol. Obstet., *125*:251, 1967.
6. Coller, F. A., and Valk, W. L.: The delayed closure of contaminated wounds: A preliminary report. Ann. Surg., *112*:256, 1940.
7. Cruse, P. J. E., and Foord, R. A.: A five-year prospective study of 23, 649 surgical wounds. Arch. Surg., *107*:206, 1973.
8. Dudrick, S. J., MacFadyen, B. V., Jr., Van Buren, C. T., Ruberg, R. L., and Maynard, A. T.: Parenteral hyperalimentation. Metabolic problems and solutions. Ann. Surg., *176*:259, 1972.
9. Elman, R.: Surgical Care. A Practical Physiologic Guide. New York, Appleton-Century-Crofts, 1951.
10. Estes, J. E., Jr.: Abdominal aortic aneurysms; a study of 102 cases. Circulation, *2*:258, 1950.
11. Feinstein, A. R.: Clinical Judgment. Baltimore, The Williams and Wilkins Company, 1967.
12. Fikri, E., and McAdams, A. J.: Wound infection in colonic surgery. Ann. Surg., *182*:724, 1975.
13. Greenwood, M.: A Report on the Natural Duration of Cancer. Ministry of Health Reports on Public Health and Medical Subjects, No. 33. London, Her Majesty's Stationery Office, 1926.
14. Hunter, P. R., Endrey-Walder, P., Bauer, G. E., and Stephens, F. O.: Myocardial infarction following surgical operations. Br. Med. J., *4*:725, 1968.
15. Irvin, G. L., III, and Zeppa, R.: Predicted survival in peptic ulcer patients based on computer analysis of preoperative variables. Ann. Surg., Vol. 183, 1976.
16. Jaffe, B. M., Donegan, W. L., Watson, F., and Spratt, J. S.: Factors influencing survival in patients with untreated hepatic metastases. Surg. Gynecol. Obstet., *127*:1, 1968.
17. Knutson, C. O., and Polk, H. C., Jr.: Decisions in the operative management of colon cancer—An objective determinant of quality surgical care. To be published.
18. Knutson, C. O., and Watson, F. R.: Preliminary results of a computer logic program for the operative management of colon cancer. Surgery, *76*:298, 1974.
19. Ledger, W. J., Sweet, R. L., and Headington, J. T.: The prophylactic use of cephaloridine in the prevention of pelvic infections in premenopausal women undergoing vaginal hysterectomy. Am. J. Obstet. Gynecol., *115*:766, 1973.
20. Linn, B. S., Linn, M. W., and Gurel, L.: Physical resistance and longevity. Gerontol. Clin., *11*:362, 1969.
21. McConnell, D. H., Maloney, J. V., Jr., and Buckberg, G. D.: Postoperative intermittent positive-pressure breathing treatments. Physiological considerations. J. Thorac. Cardiovasc. Surg., *68*:944, 1974.
22. Miles, A. A., Miles, E. M., and Burke, J.: The value and duration of defense reactions of the skin to the primary lodgement of bacteria. Br. J. Exp. Pathol., *38*:79, 1957.

23. Monafo, W. W.: Hypertonic sodium solutions for the treatment of burn shock. *In* Polk, H. C., Jr., and Stone, H. H. (Eds.): Contemporary Burn Management. Boston, Little, Brown and Company, 1971, pp. 33–42.

24. National Academy of Sciences – National Research Council: Postoperative wound infections: The influence of ultraviolet irradiation of the operating room and of various other factors. Ann. Surg., *160*(Suppl.):1, 1964.

25. Owen, O. E., Morgan, A. P., and Kemp, H. G.: Brain metabolism during fasting. J. Clin. Invest., *46*:1589, 1967.

26. Peden, J. E., Jr., Maxwell, M., Ohin, A., and Moyer, C. A.: A consideration of indications for preoperative transfusion based on analysis of blood volumes and circulating proteins in normal and malnourished patients with or without cancer. Ann. Surg., *151*:303, 1960.

27. Polk, H. C., Jr.: The surgical treatment of carcinoma of the colon and rectum: Its evolution in one university hospital. Arch. Surg., *91*:985, 1965.

28. Polk, H. C., Jr., Ahmad, W., and Knutson, C. O.: Carcinoma of the colon and rectum. Curr. Probl. Surg., January, 1973.

29. Polk, H. C., Jr., and Lopez-Mayor, J. F.: Postoperative wound infection: A prospective study of determinant factors and prevention. Surgery, *66*:97, 1969.

30. Polk, H. C., Jr., and Miles, A. A.: Enhancement of bacterial infection by ferric iron: Kinetics, mechanisms and surgical significance. Surgery, *70*:71, 1971.

31. Polk, H. C., Jr., and Miles, A. A.: The decisive period in the primary infection of muscle by *Escherichia coli*. Br. J. Exp. Pathol., *54*:99, 1973.

32. Poth, E. J.: The role of intestinal antisepsis in the preoperative preparation of the colon. Surgery, *47*:1018, 1960.

33. Simeone, F. A.: Principles of preoperative preparation of the surgical patient. *In* Sabiston, D. C., Jr. (Ed.): Davis-Christopher Textbook of Surgery, 10th ed. Philadelphia, W. B. Saunders Company, 1972, pp. 112–130.

34. Stein, M., and Cassara, E. L.: Preoperative pulmonary evaluation and therapy for surgical patients. J.A.M.A., *211*:787, 1970.

35. Stone, H. H., and Hester, T. R., Jr.: Incisional and peritoneal infection after emergency celiotomy. Ann. Surg., *177*:669, 1973.

36. Stone, H. H., Kolb, L. D., Currie, C. A., Geheber, C. E., and Cuzzell, J. Z.: Candida sepsis: Pathogenesis and principles of treatment. Ann. Surg., *179*:697, 1974.

37. Subcommittee on the National Halothane Study: Summary of the national halothane study. J.A.M.A., *197*:775, 1966.

38. Washington, J. A., II, Dearing, W. H., Judd, E. S., and Elveback, L. R.: Effect of preoperative antibiotic regimen on development of infection after intestinal surgery: Prospective, randomized, double-blind study. Ann. Surg., *180*:567, 1974.

6

BLOOD TRANSFUSIONS AND DISORDERS OF SURGICAL BLEEDING

Donald Silver, M.D.

BLOOD TRANSFUSIONS

Historical Aspects

Although blood letting and the use of blood as an oral or topical medication had been utilized from the earliest times, it was not until 1665 that Richard Lower demonstrated the feasibility of transfusing blood from one animal to another. In June, 1667, Jean Baptiste Denis and Emmerez successfully transfused sheep blood into a teenage boy and a 45-year-old man. These successes prompted three more animal-to-human transfusions. The death of two of these recipients and the exaggerated claims of the benefits of transfusion precipitated a lawsuit against Denis. Denis was acquitted, but an edict was issued prohibiting the practice of blood transfusion unless "approved by the physicians of the Faculty of Paris."[44] In 1818, James Blundell of St. Thomas and Guy's Hospital performed the first man-to-man transfusion.[49] Blood transfusions became popular in the second half of the nineteenth century, with William Stewart Halsted supporting the procedure. In 1881, Halsted transfused his sister with his own blood after she had a postpartum hemorrhage.[20]

A major advance in blood transfusion technology occurred in 1900 when Landsteiner observed the agglutination of human red blood cells by human sera. Thirty years later he received the Nobel Prize for his discovery of the ABO blood groups.[74] In 1926, Landsteiner and Levine discovered the MN and the P blood groups (which, though of genetic interest, usually have little influence on transfusion). In 1940, Landsteiner and Wiener discovered the Rh groups and in 1941 Levine and associates noted the relation of these groups to the hemolytic disease of the newborn.[55] Since 1940, the Ss, Lutheran, Kell, Lewis, Duffy, Kidd, Vel, and other blood group systems have been identified.

The recognition of these blood groups, the development of high-quality antisera for testing for these groups, and improved methods for collecting and storing blood have made blood transfusion a safe procedure.

Blood Bank

The problems associated with obtaining, preserving, storing, and administering blood prompted the development of central facilities to provide these services. The first "modern" blood bank was established in 1937 at the Cook County Hospital in Chicago by Bernard Fantus.[30] In 1938, Mount Sinai Hospital and Bellevue Hospital in New York opened blood banks and other institutions quickly followed.

The functions of a modern blood bank include (1) the procurement, testing, typing, labeling, storage, crossmatching, and disbursement of blood; (2) the preparation of blood products for specific needs, e.g., platelet transfusions for symptomatic thrombocytopenia, cryoprecipitate for hemophilia, packed cells for patients with low hemoglobin and borderline cardiac reserve; (3) the long-term storage of blood cells and blood products, e.g., frozen blood, fresh frozen plasma; and (4) the performance of those tests of coagulation-fibrinolysis which will help the clinician determine the etiology of nonmechanical bleeding[89] and select the proper blood product(s) or pharmacologic agents to treat the bleeding.

Crossmatching

All blood must be crossmatched prior to insuring its safeness for transfusion purposes. Crossmatching includes selecting blood of the same ABO and Rh type as the recipient's, and then (1) reacting the cells of the donor, suspended in saline, with the serum of the recipient at room temperature to detect complete agglutinins; (2) performing an indirect antiglobulin test (Coombs' test) at 37° C. to detect incomplete antibodies that do not produce agglutination during the first test; and (3) reacting the serum of the donor with recipient cells to detect incompatible donor antibodies.[98]

Patients who receive multiple transfusions may develop antibodies to the infused blood that could cause reactions during subsequent transfusions. Therefore, new recipient serum should be used for compatibility testing each day that repeat transfusions are given. Blood that was previously found to be compatible should be recrossmatched with the new serum.

Cold Agglutinins

Most humans have agglutinins that agglutinate their own red cells at low temperatures (0 to 20° C.). Cold agglutinins are increased in Raynaud's disease, paroxysmal hemoglobinuria, some hemolytic anemias, and many chronic diseases, e.g., cirrhosis. Cold agglutinins have two important effects on blood transfusions. First, if the serum for crossmatching is cold or the blood bank is cold, agglutination may occur because of the cold agglutinin and interfere with the crossmatch. Second, if cold blood is given to a patient with cold agglutinins, agglutination and a hemolytic reaction may occur. These adverse effects of the cold agglutinins may be obviated by warming serum prior to using it for crossmatching and warming the infused blood for patients with cold agglutinins.

Emergency Transfusion

Blood of the same ABO and Rh groups as the patient's should be transfused whenever possible. ABO compatibility must always be respected. Rh-negative blood, when otherwise compatible, may safely be given to Rh-positive recipients. Rh-positive blood may be given, during emergencies, to Rh-negative patients safely for a few days, but should not be given to Rh-negative women in the childbearing age, to sensitized Rh-negative patients, or to Rh-positive infants with hemolytic disease of the newborn who require exchange transfusion.

Many emergency situations arise because the blood loss is not anticipated and blood is not requested until needed. Most transfusion emergencies can be avoided by proper physician planning. If a situation arises during which there is an exsanguinating hemorrhage such that blood volume expanders will not suffice, the "universal" blood, type O, Rh-negative, may be administered while a crossmatch is being performed. However, harmful isoantibodies may occur in some type O plasmas. The effect of these antibodies may be reduced by using only O Rh-negative cells (removing the plasma) or by adding A and B antigens to the donor blood. If a nongroup O patient receives several units of type O blood, he will have significant levels of transfused antibodies in his plasma that may react with his own red cells. Consequently, it may be necessary to use type O blood until the antibody titer decreases.

Transfusion

Although blood transfusion is an accepted method for replacing lost blood, blood is frequently transfused when minor, clinically insignificant losses have occurred. It has been estimated that 35 to 50 per cent of all blood transfusions are unnecessary,[33, 47] and only about 1 per cent are given as lifesaving procedures.[24] If transfusions were innocuous, this unnecessary transfusion of blood might be condoned. However, each transfusion exposes the patient to several potential risks, and the indication for blood transfusion must be firmly understood by the clinician.[103]

The major indications for blood transfusion are to restore blood volume and/or to improve the oxygen-carrying capacity of the blood. Many agents function quite well as plasma volume expanders, e.g., plasma, plasma protein fractions, dextran, and crystalloids, but erythrocytes transport almost all of the oxygen to the tissues. Although precise data are not available, it has been accepted that a hematocrit of 30 per cent or a hemoglobin of 10 gm. per 100 ml. will insure an adequate tissue oxygen supply. However, recent studies have indicated that, in selected situations, significant hemodilution is safe and reduces blood bank requirements and the risk associated with homologous blood transfusion.[18, 36]

Autologous blood transfusions, during which patients receive their own previously donated blood, have been safely and effectively utilized in elective surgery,[54, 63] while mechanical autotransfusion is being evaluated as a means of reducing the needs for homologous blood during times of emergency and elective surgery.[11, 12, 75] Although mechanical autotransfusion may provide a lifesaving supply of blood,[77] its utilization should be limited to emergency situations until the effects of autotransfusion on the coagulation system and organ function can be determined.

Regardless of the type of blood administered, the single unit transfusion is almost never indicated, because volume and oxygen-carrying capacity can be compensated by other means.

Anticoagulants

The clotting of blood plagued all of the early transfusion attempts. In 1821, Prevost and Dumas[72] demonstrated that blood could be made incoagulable by defibrination. Arthus and Pages, in 1890, discovered that citrate and oxalate bound calcium and acted as anticoagulants.[7] In 1915, Lewisohn reported his experience with transfusions of citrated blood.[57] Further work of Lewisohn established citrate as a safe and useful anticoagulant.[58]

It has been found that red cells have better survival in slightly acid — pH 7 — storage solutions, and that the addition of dextrose as a source of energy will further improve cell viability. Consequently, a slightly acid anticoagulant solution containing dextrose was developed. Acid-citrate-dextrose (ACD, Table 1) has been the most popular anticoagulant storage medium until recently. ACD solutions and refrigeration at 4° C. permitted blood to be stored up to 21 days with approximately 70 per cent survival of the transfused red cells. In 1957, Gibson demonstrated the superiority of a citrate-phosphate anticoagulant over ACD solutions.[35] Subsequently, it has been shown that citrate-phosphate-dextrose (CPD, Table 1) maintains a higher pH, lower potassium concentration, and higher 2,3-diphosphoglycerate (2,3-DPG) level in stored blood than does ACD (Table 2).[34] The red cell survival in CPD is quite good,[88, 90] and the higher level of 2,3-DPG in CPD-stored blood means better oxygenation of tissues with transfused blood.[14] CPD is currently the most widely utilized anticoagulant-preservative.

Heparin interferes with the coagulation mechanism at multiple sites and may be used to anticoagulate donor blood. Blood is collected in heparin (see Table 1) only for special uses, e.g., extracorporeal circulation. Blood collected in heparin has an accelerated rate of glycolysis, deteriorates rapidly, and may be safely used for only 48 hours after collection. If blood collec-

TABLE 1. Anticoagulants*

ACD Solution "A"

Sodium citrate, hydrous, USP	2.20 gm.
Citric acid, anhydrous, USP	0.80 gm.
Dextrose, hydrous, USP	2.45 gm.
Water, USP	to vol. of 100 ml.
67.5 ml. for collection of 450 ml. blood	

CPD Solution

Sodium citrate, hydrous, USP	2.63 gm.
Citric acid, hydrous, USP	0.327 gm.
Monobasic sodium phosphate, monohydrate, USP	0.222 gm.
Dextrose, hydrous, USP	2.55 gm.
Water, USP	to vol. of 100 ml.
63 ml. for collection of 450 ml. of blood	

Heparin Solution

Heparin sodium, USP	2115 units
Sodium chloride, USP, 0.9%	28.2 ml.
Sodium citrate (buffer), USP	84.6 mg.
For collection of 470 ml. of blood	

*From Hospital Medicine, 6:63, June, 1970. © Hospital Publications, Inc., by permission.

tion in heparin is not used CPD solution may be added within 48 hours after collection and the blood's usefulness prolonged to 12 days. Heparin is not recommended for routine blood collection.

Blood obtained from patients experiencing sudden death may undergo spontaneous fibrinolysis and become incoagulable. In 1930, Yudin utilized 420 ml. of blood from a 60-year-old man who died after a basilar skull fracture to resuscitate a young engineer suicide victim. He was encouraged by the successful results and initiated the use of cadaver blood on a large scale. By 1937 he reported over 1000 "highly successful" cadaver transfusions.[104] More recently, Tarasov has emphasized the practical usefulness and safeness of cadaver blood transfusions.[96] He noted that approximately 24,000 transfusions of cadaver blood have been performed in the Moscow Sklifosovsky Institute during the past 30 years with "no danger where infection or toxicity is concerned." The erythrocytes of cadaver blood have a normal in vivo survival; however, the coagulation factors, platelets, and white cells are reduced. One should await the autopsy findings before utilizing the blood.

Frozen Blood

If the safe storage time for blood could be significantly prolonged, the supply of blood would be increased proportionately. Better storage solutions will help, but long-term storage requires stopping or markedly slowing the blood's metabolism. Techniques have been developed whereby blood may be frozen and stored for long periods at very low temperatures (−80 to −190° C.). The process includes adding glycerol to freshly collected blood after removing the plasma. The glycerolization protects the red cells during the freezing and thawing process.

Varying techniques for glycerolization, freezing, and thawing are being evaluated.[41, 48, 50, 100] Current methods utilize either a high concentration of glycerol (approximately 45 per cent weight per volume) and a slow freeze-thaw technique (−80° C. storage), or a low concentration of glycerol (approximately 18 per cent weight per volume) with a rapid freeze-thaw technique. Studies have shown that those frozen cells which are viable at 24 hours post transfusion have normal survival times.

Advantages of frozen blood include: the supply of red cells for transfusion purposes is significantly increased; rare blood types may be preserved in sufficient quantities to be useful clinically; blood may be collected and reserved for those patients who will accept only autotransfusions; thawed, washed, frozen blood is free of platelets and white cells and seems to be the ideal blood for transfusing transplantation recipients and for use during cardiopulmonary bypass; frozen blood seems to be free of viable hepatitis viruses. Disadvantages of frozen blood include: the need for special freezing, thawing, and storage facilities; limited post-thaw stability of red cells, and the absence of coagulation factors, platelets, and white cells in the thawed blood. Frozen blood should be ad-

TABLE 2. Changes in Stored ACD (CPD) Blood*

	Days Stored			
	0	7	14	21
pH	7.00 (7.20)	6.79 (7.00)	6.73 (6.89)	6.71 (6.84)
Hemoglobin	10 (4)	22 (10)	35 (21)	53 (30)
Potassium mEq./L.	10 (4)	20 (10)	29 (20)	35 (25)
Inorganic phosphate mM./L.	0.6 (3.6)	1.5 (3.6)	2.2 (4.2)	3.0 (4.9)
2,3-DPG μg./gm. Hgb	15 (12.5)	9 (12)	3.5 (7)	1.5 (3.7)
Ammonia mg./100 ml.	113 (95)	145 (160)	263 (255)	373 (330)
Dextrose mg./100 ml.	331 (333)	296 (267)	260 (260)	211 (191)
Viable RBC %†	100	98	85	70

*Data from Beutler et al.: Transfusion, 9:109, 1969; Epstein: Abbott Laboratories, Chicago. Verbal communication; Gibson et al;[34] and National Academy of Sciences: General Principles of Blood Transfusion. Philadelphia, J. B. Lippincott Co., 1963.

†Most studies indicate a greater than 70 per cent viability of red blood cells stored in CPD at 28 and, in some reports, 35 days.

ministered soon after it is thawed to obtain maximal survival of the red cells.

Many blood banks are freezing red cells and plasma components to increase their stocks of blood products and to stop the waste of blood dictated by routine storage methods.

Blood Components

Simple techniques have been developed that permit blood to be separated into its components (Table 3). Figure 1 illustrates the technique for preparing blood components by means of a plastic quadruple blood set. By utilizing double or triple blood-collecting sets, other combinations of components can be prepared.[51] The components from a single unit of blood may be used therapeutically in several patients and the effectiveness of donated blood may be greatly extended.

Transfusion of packed red cells is an excellent way to improve oxygenation ability without overloading the circulation.[78] Washed, packed red cell transfusions are preferred in patients with hepatic or renal insufficiency to reduce the amount of potassium, ammonia, excessive acid, etc., that is infused. Packed red cell transfusions may be safely utilized to replace operative blood loss, provided it is remembered that (1) approximately 55 to 60 per cent of the blood lost is plasma so that appropriate crystalloid (2 to 3 ml. for each milliliter of packed cells) or colloid (1 ml. for each milliliter of packed cell) solutions are also given; and (2) the coagulation factors are in the plasma, so that fresh frozen plasma, platelets, or other blood components are available if needed. However, most patients receiving multiple transfusions will not require fresh frozen plasma, fresh blood, or blood components to maintain an adequate coagulation profile. When large amounts of blood have been transfused, monitoring of the coagulation profile will alert the surgeon to the need for appropriate blood components.[83, 85]

Platelet transfusions may be required to control bleeding in patients with a deficient number of platelets, i.e., less then 30,000 per cu. mm. or with platelets that function improperly. Platelet concentrates enable one to increase the number of circulating platelets without expanding the circulating volume excessively. The platelet concentrate from a unit of blood can, unless platelet antibodies, hypersplenism, etc. are present, increase the circulating number of platelets by 10,000 to 15,000 per cu. mm. Because platelets cannot be stored, the need for platelets should be anticipated and appropriate platelet concentrates prepared.

Although "warm" fresh whole blood has been utilized to "correct" or "prevent" coagulopathies,[87] this practice is rarely indicated.[85] Appropriate component therapy, as determined by laboratory testing, will adequately correct the deficit without exposing the patient to the potential dangers inherent in transfusing blood before its serology or hepatitis antigen concentration has been determined.

It behooves all physicians to utilize only the specific blood components necessary for their patient's welfare so that the other components from donated units of blood can be available for other patients.

Complications of Blood Transfusions

The complications of blood transfusion include those of any intravenous fluid administration, i.e., volume overload, phlebitis, air embolism, and so forth, in addition to complications peculiar to the administration of blood. General principles of sterility, clean venipunctures, and monitored rates of infusion must be observed.

Hemolytic Reactions. A hemolytic tranfusion reaction, the most common of all severe transfusion reactions, occurs approximately once in 15,000 to 20,000 transfusions. Most often this reaction results when red cells are transfused into a patient who possesses antibodies against one or more of the antigens on the infused cells. Occasionally transfused plasma contains high titers of hemolytic antibodies that "attack" the recipient cells and produce a hemolytic reaction. Therefore, cells *and* serum of recipient and donor must be shown to be compatible prior to transfusion. The titer and potency of antibody and the amount of blood infused have significant effects on the outcome of the hemolytic reaction. As little as 25 to 50 ml. of the transfused blood may cause a significant reaction, or as much as 500 ml. may be transfused before the reaction can be detected.

The clinical manifestations of a transfusion reaction include fever, chills, flushing, headache, a tight constricting pain in the chest, breathlessness, nausea, and pain in the flanks. The first manifestations may be followed by further increases of temperature, vomiting or diarrhea, hypotension, hemoglobinuria, and unexplained bleeding. Most reactions occur during the early period of the transfusion, and therefore all blood recipients should be observed carefully for the first 20 to 30 minutes of their transfusion. All anesthetized or otherwise unconscious patients who receive blood must be carefully monitored during the transfusion period. The only manifestation of a transfusion reaction in an anesthetized patient may be tachycardia, hypotension, or the sudden increase of bleeding.

As soon as a transfusion reaction is suspected, the transfusion should be discontinued. The blood, transfusion set, and a fresh blood sample from the patient should be sent to the blood bank for repeat compatibility testing. The patient's blood should be examined for hemoglobinemia. Urine samples may become dark brown to black and contain hemoglobin, red cells, and casts. After a few hours, bilirubinemia, spherocytosis and fragments of red cells, and severe anemia may appear.

Management of a transfusion reaction includes stopping the transfusion and initiating measures to correct the hypotension, controlling the hemorrhagic state, if it is present, and preventing anuria. Although

---

TABLE 3.   Blood and Its Components

Whole blood
Packed red blood cells
Fresh plasma
Fresh frozen plasma
Platelet-rich plasma
Platelet concentrate
Cryoprecipitate
Reconstituted whole blood

PREPARATION OF FOUR BLOOD COMPONENTS UTILIZING A PREASSEMBLED PLASTIC CONTAINER WITH FOUR COMPARTMENTS (QUADRUPLE PACK)

The four products are packed red cells, platelet concentrate, cryoprecipitate, and single donor plasma

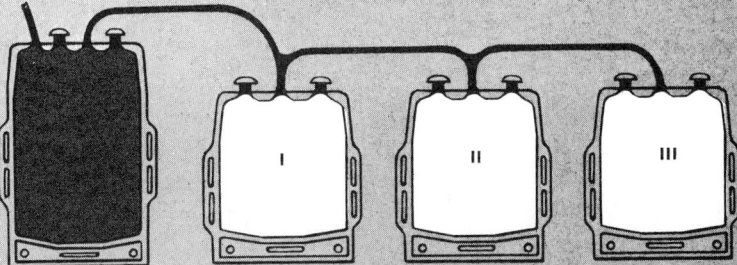

WHOLE BLOOD IN QUADRUPLE CONTAINER

Step 1: Whole blood is collected in the primary pouch of a preassembled quadruple container (primary plus three satellites).

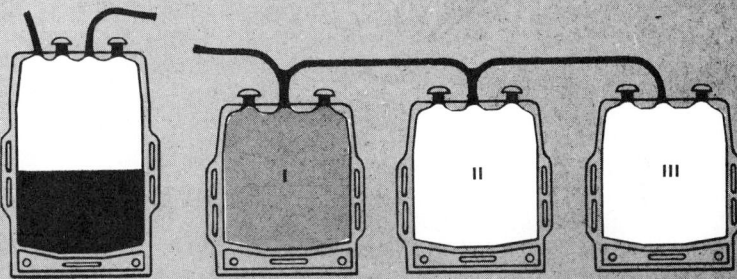

PLATELET-RICH PLASMA AND PACKED RED CELLS

Step 2: The container is centrifuged at a speed which produces packed red cells and platelet-rich plasma. The plasma is expressed into the first satellite container, and the satellite assembly is separated from the packed red cells in the primary container.

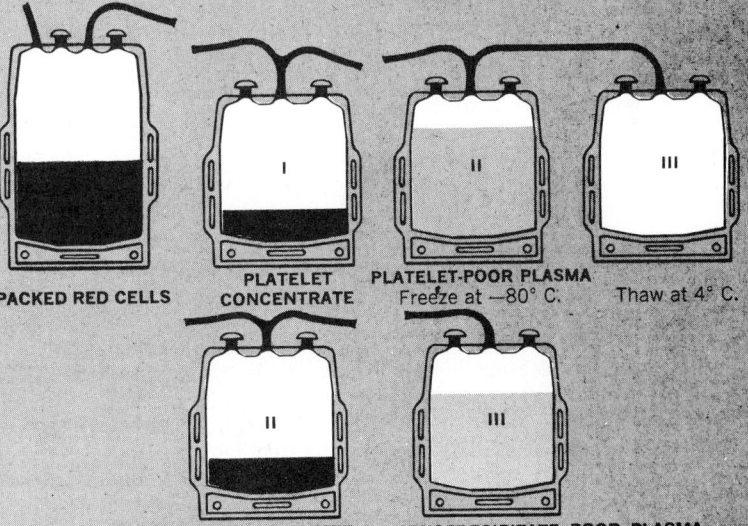

Step 3: To get platelet concentrate, the platelet-rich plasma is centrifuged at high speed and the supernatant is expressed into the second satellite container leaving the concentrate in the first satellite.

Step 4: To get cryoprecipitate, the platelet-poor plasma is quick frozen at −80° C. and then thawed at 4° C. Another high speed centrifugation separates the cold-precipitated material (cryoprecipitate) from the supernatant platelet-poor, cryoprecipitate-poor plasma (single donor plasma). Sterility is maintained in all products by making two seals in the connecting tubing and cutting between seals to separate the containers.

Figure 1. (From Kliman, A.: Hospital Medicine, *6*:63, June 1970. Copyright Hospital Publications, Inc., by permission.)

the transfusion must be discontinued, the needle or catheter should be left in the vein because circulatory collapse may impede the establishment of another intravenous route. Compatible blood may be carefully transfused. If a hemorrhagic state is present, blood should be obtained for coagulation and fibrinolytic studies and appropriate treatment instituted. Most often a profound thrombocytopenia will be present and frequently there will be other evidence of a consumptive coagulopathy. The hemorrhagic diathesis is usually self-limiting and stops when the hypotension and other symptoms are corrected.

Although attention is directed to supporting the patient's circulation and respiratory function, the insult to the kidneys requires prompt and vigorous therapy to prevent or minimize the tubular necrosis and anuria that frequently occur after major transfusion reactions.[56] Hypotension, acidosis, and free hemoglobin provide a severe insult to the kidneys during a transfusion reaction. The best way to treat acute tubular necrosis is to prevent it. This frequently can be accomplished by combating the hypotension with appropriate fluids, vasopressors, and so forth, by using bicarbonate or other buffers to maintain an alkaline urine pH, and by providing osmotic diuresis with mannitol or similar agents. If these measures are begun promptly after the transfusion reaction is detected, tubular necrosis and anuria are not likely to happen. If anuria does occur, then the patient must be treated for acute renal failure with limitation of fluid intake to 400 to 500 ml. plus his daily output, and careful monitoring of potassium, blood urea, creatinine, and so forth. Peritoneal dialysis or hemodialysis should be performed when indicated.

Post-transfusion jaundice may occur when a patient has been transfused with several units of older bank blood. The shorter survival of the red cells causes an increase in free hemoglobin and, later, bilirubinemia. Usually no treatment is required for this condition. Occasionally a patient will receive provocative blood antigens during a transfusion and will rapidly produce antibodies to the infused blood. The infused red cells are then destroyed over the next few days and hemoglobinemia, hyperbilirubinemia, and mild hemoglobinuria may occur. Usually this type of reaction does little, if any, harm to the patient; however, it should be detected by appropriate immunologic studies so that additional transfusions of similar incompatible blood can be avoided.

Nonhemolytic Reactions. Pyrexial reactions are the most common untoward consequences of blood transfusions. Reactions may vary from mild chilliness and transient rise in temperature to severe chills and high fever. The severe symptoms may be accompanied by headache, muscle pain, nausea, and vomiting. Symptoms are treated with antipyretic drugs and there are no known lasting ill effects. Since a pyrexial reaction cannot be distinguished from an early hemolytic reaction, the transfusion must be discontinued and blood samples sent to the blood bank for studies. Most often no incompatabilities can be detected and the cause of the reaction remains uncertain. The utilization of sterile disposable plastic tranfusion sets has reduced the incidence of the pyrogenic reactions by markedly reducing the possibility of bacterial contamination, and currently most pyrexial reactions are assumed to be reactions to some components of the donor's blood. White blood cells and platelets may cause such reactions, and it may be necessary to prepare transfusions of washed packed red cells for some patients to prevent pyrexial reactions.

Allergic reactions occur in 2 to 3 per cent of patients receiving transfusions.[37] The reaction is usually characterized by the appearance of hives, itching, and a diffuse rash. Rarely the reaction may be severe enough to produce laryngeal edema and collapse. The reactions are probably caused by the recipient's response to allergens in the donor's blood. Treatment consists of stopping the transfusion and treating the recipient with antihistaminic drugs. If the reaction is mild and the antihistamine effective, the transfusion may be completed. The antihistamine should be given to the patient and not added to the blood being infused. If the symptoms are severe or recur when the infusion is continued, blood should be returned to the blood bank for crossmatching and another unit of compatible blood from another donor used for transfusion purposes. Steroid preparations may be required in severe allergic reactions.

Contaminated blood may cause reactions in the recipient. Most of the reactions are produced by the endotoxin of gram-negative bacteria. Bacteria will survive but not multiply significantly in refrigerated blood. However, if the blood is allowed to warm, bacteria will grow. Therefore, blood transfusions should be completed within 2 hours after the blood is removed from the blood bank. For those patients who receive multiple transfusions during a short period of time, warming devices are available to warm the blood. This blood must be infused immediately after it is warmed. Warm blood should *not* be returned to the blood bank or given as a delayed transfusion.

The contaminated blood may produce chills, fever, general pain, hypotension, and shock. The transfusion must be stopped and the blood cultured. Prompt utilization of antibiotics, steroids, and fluid replacement may be lifesaving.

Microcirculation Blockade. Aggregates of platelets, fibrin, white cells, and other proteins which form in banked blood may accumulate in the lung at the arterial-arteriolar level and be a contributing factor in the acute respiratory insufficiency that occurs in patients with severe trauma or complex surgical procedures or in those requiring multiple blood transfusions.[27, 32] Micropore filters that remove most of the debris from stored blood have been developed and often reduce the frequency and intensity of the respiratory distress syndrome.[21, 27] The current policy at the University of Missouri–Columbia Medical Center is to utilize a 40-micron filter for each unit of blood transfused into all patients with multiple trauma or chronic obstructive pulmonary disease, or who are likely to require more than 4 units of blood.

Transmission of Disease. Blood obtained from an infected donor with a circulating causative organism may infect the recipient. Careful questioning and examination of donors will eliminate most of the acute febrile illnesses. If the donor becomes ill after giving the blood, the blood bank should be notified and the blood discarded. If the blood has been transfused, the recipient must be informed and proper precautions and treatment begun.

Although most infectious diseases are readily detected, there are three such processes that are difficult to detect and that are readily transmitted via transfusions. These diseases are malaria, syphilis, and hepatitis.

The travel habits of American citizens and the deployment of servicemen and civilians in tropical areas have once again established malaria as a problem for blood banks.[23] Several thousand servicemen contract malaria each year (approximately 6000 cases in 1966). The number of cases in this country is increasing, with 722 cases of malaria being recorded in the first 3½ months of 1967.[91] Donors who have had malaria or an unexplained febrile illness with jaundice, or who are from an endemic malaria area, are permanently rejected. Persons who remain well with no therapy for 6 months after traveling through an endemic area may serve as donors. Any patient who has an unexplained febrile illness or jaundice after receiving blood should, after the usual causes are excluded, be suspected of having malaria. If the malaria organism is found, an evaluation of the donor(s) should be undertaken. Therapy for the donor and the patient is mandatory. Malaria is transmitted only in the red cells and cannot be transmitted by those blood components which do not contain red cells.

Venereal disease continues to be a significant public health problem. Early stages of syphilis are difficult to detect and donors may not be aware of their infection. Serologic testing for syphilis must be performed on all blood before it is released for transfusion purposes. If fresh blood is given for an emergency, the serologic test must be performed afterwards. Any positive test must be called to the attention of the physician and the patient. Because spirochetes do not survive at blood bank temperatures for more than 4 days,[52] only relatively fresh blood can transmit syphilis. Blood with a positive serologic reaction should be discarded and the donor reported to appropriate public health authorities.

Hepatitis constitutes a serious and increasing risk of the administration of blood or blood products. Hepatitis occurs in 0.3 to 0.8 per cent of those persons receiving blood transfusions, and is accompanied by a mortality that varies from 1 or 2 to 20 or 30 per cent, according to the age, illness, general condition, and so forth, of the patient. Transfused blood causes at least 30,000 cases of overt hepatitis, with 1500 to 3000 deaths per year. If all of the subclinical cases of hepatitis were detected, the annual incidence might be as high as 150,000.[31, 84]

Serum hepatitis (SH) is transmitted by the parenteral route, while infectious hepatitis (IH) is transmitted parenterally or orally. The incubation period of IH is 15 to 40 days with an average of 25 days; the incubation period for SH ranges from 50 to 160 days. There is no known way to eliminate the hepatitis virus from whole blood, packed red cells, platelet preparations, fresh frozen plasma, fibrinogen, or antihemophilic globulin. Infusions of albumin that has been heated to 60° C. for 10 hours and of gamma glob-

ulin have not produced hepatitis. Virus activity deteriorates in plasma stored at room temperature, and plasma kept at room temperature for 6 months is considered to be virus-free.

The hepatitis problem is compounded by the asymptomatic carrier and the prolonged postinfection time (3 years or longer) that a person may transmit the disease. The increasing practice of experimental drug use will further increase the number of cases of hepatitis. Drug users frequently become blood donors to obtain money for drugs. The hepatitis infection rate in recipients of blood from paid blood donors is 3.3 times greater than in those who received blood only from volunteers.[95] All donors with a history of hepatitis or exposure to hepatitis should be excluded.

Two recent developments may reduce the magnitude of the hepatitis problem. Tullis and associates have demonstrated that high glycerolization and a slow freeze-thaw process for preserving red cells significantly reduces the incidence of post-transfusion hepatitis.[101] Secondly, a radioimmunoassay for the hepatitis antigen (HA) has been developed.[73] Current methods for testing will detect 75 to 85 per cent of infected donors. Testing for the HA antigen should be performed on each unit of blood obtained. It is to be hoped that the development of better serologic testing will permit the detection of all infected donors.

Other Complications. Many of the undesirable aspects of blood transfusion are caused by the metabolic changes that occur in the blood during storage (see Table 2). There is a progressive loss of potassium from the erythrocytes into the plasma. The plasma potassium concentration may reach 30 or 40 mEq. per liter in 3-week-old blood. The transfusion of several units of aged blood may produce cardiac arrhythmias and arrest from the hyperkalemia. The hyperkalemia is further compounded by decreased renal function so often found in patients requiring multiple transfusions. The renal insufficiency may be adversely affected by the low pH and high hemoglobin concentration in the old blood.

Excess citrate in transfused blood will bind some of the recipient's calcium. The reduced calcium augments the cardiac effects of hyperkalemia, and calcium gluconate infusions should be given whenever hyperkalemia and acidosis exist and whenever the adult patient receives more than two units of blood. Ten milliliters of 10 per cent calcium gluconate for each two units of blood received is usually given, through a vein other than that through which the blood is being infused.

The progressive increase in ammonia makes aged blood unsatisfactory for use in patients with hepatic insufficiency. The infusion of several units of aged blood into patients with cirrhosis may precipitate hepatic coma. Certainly all patients should receive the freshest blood possible. Careful control of a blood bank inventory should establish guidelines for supply and demand so that most blood is utilized before it is 7 to 10 days old.

Plasmapheresis

Plasmapheresis is the process of withdrawing blood from a donor to obtain plasma, plasma components, or nonerythrocytic blood elements and then reinfusing the red cells back into the donor. When the erythrocytes are reinfused, donors may give 500 to 1000 ml. of plasma every 1 to 4 weeks. One must be careful not to deplete the donor's protein stores by allowing him to donate too often.

White Blood Cells

White blood cell transfusions are being investigated. White cells have a very short survival time and there is no good evidence that white cell transfusions provide any lasting beneficial effects to the recipient.[38]

DISORDERS OF SURGICAL BLEEDING

This section will discuss those bleeding diatheses that result from insufficient, ineffective, or too much clotting; from excessive activity of the fibrinolytic system; from platelet abnormalities; and from excessive anticoagulation.

COAGULATION SYSTEM

Although man has been intrigued with blood coagulation since earliest times, it was not until 1771 that William Hewson noted that intravascular stagnation of blood resulted in clotting; blood always clotted when shed; cooling blood prolonged its clotting time; and the plasma contained the substance(s) responsible for coagulation.[42] In 1859 Denis[25] isolated the substance (fibrinogen) that Virchow in 1856 had postulated to be the precursor of fibrin. In 1861 Schmidt[82] extracted thrombin from serum and presented evidence for the presence of prothrombin. In 1875 the importance of calcium was discovered.[40]

In 1906, Morawitz[66] presented his classic theory that blood coagulation proceeded in three phases. The first was concerned with the production of thromboplastin; in the second the thromboplastin converted prothrombin to thrombin; and in the third phase thrombin stimulated the conversion of fibrinogen to fibrin.

Table 4 lists the known coagulation factors, their synonyms, and whether the factors may be found in therapeutic quantities in banked or fresh blood. Factor VI is probably the same as factor V. It should be noted that "banked" blood provides all the coagulation factors except IV (calcium is usually bound by the anticoagulant), V, and VIII. Fresh blood, fresh plasma, or fresh frozen plasma will provide all of the factors except calcium. Unless the patient receives excessive amounts of citrate, he will have sufficient calcium for coagulation purposes.

Blood coagulation may be initiated by intrinsic or extrinsic mechanisms. Once active thromboplastin is formed, it splits each prothrombin molecule into two molecules of thrombin. This reaction (second phase of coagulation) is accelerated by factors V and VII. In the third phase of coagulation, the proteolytic enzyme thrombin "breaks" fibrinogen into a fibrin monomer and two polypeptides. Factor XIII mediates this reaction. An outline of the coagulation scheme is presented in Figure 2. It should be noted that the autoactivation of the first two phases of coagulation enables a small initial stimulus to produce a large thrombus. Macfarlane has described this process as a "waterfall mechanism."[60]

Theoretically, once coagulation is initiated it could go to completion and produce massive intravenous thrombosis. However, several processes prevent this from occurring. Phase I proceeds relatively slowly; factor V is consumed during phases I and II; the presence of fibrin activates the fibrinolytic system, which digests fibrin; the "split" products of fibrin act as an-

TABLE 4. Names and Synonyms of Coagulation Factors

Roman Numeral	Name	Synonym	Source*
I	Fibrinogen		Banked blood
II	Prothrombin		Banked blood
III	Thromboplastin		
IV	Calcium		
V	Proaccelerin	Labile factor, Accelerator globulin (Ac-G)	Fresh blood
VI	Same as V (no longer used)		
VII	Proconvertin	Stable factor, Serum prothrombin conversion accelerator (SPCA)	Banked blood
VIII	Antihemophilic globulin (AHG)	Antihemophilic factor A	Fresh blood
IX	Plasma thromboplastin component (PTC)	Christmas factor, Antihemophilic factor B	Banked blood
X	Stuart-Prower factor	Thrombokinase, Autoprothrombin C	Banked blood
XI	Plasma thromboplastin antecedent (PTA)	Antihemophilic factor C	Banked blood
XII	Hageman factor	Contact factor, Glass factor	Banked blood
XIII	Fibrin stabilizing factor	Laki-Lorand factor, Fibrinase	

*The coagulation factors are in the plasma, and bank plasma or fresh plasma may be substituted for whole blood if the red cells are not required.

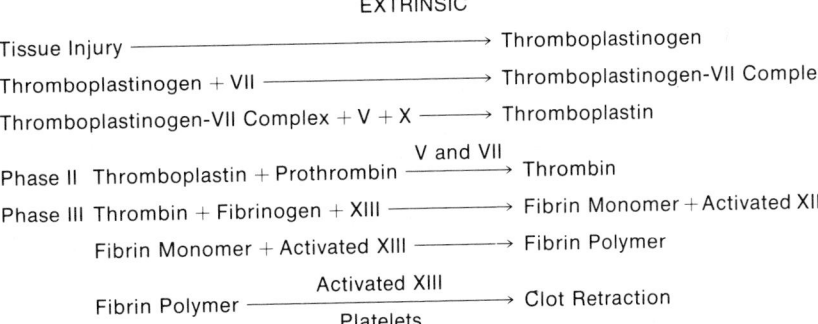

Phase I

INTRINSIC

Inactive XII $\xrightarrow{\text{Exposed collagen or foreign surface}}$ Active XII

Active XII + Inactive XI $\longrightarrow$ Active XI-XII Complex

Active XI-XII Complex + Inactive IX $\longrightarrow$ Active IX

Active IX + VIII + X $\xrightarrow{\text{Platelet factors}}$ Thromboplastinogen

Autoactivation of Thromboplastinogen + V $\longrightarrow$ Thromboplastin

Figure 2. Coagulation mechanism. Calcium is required in all of the stages and is not shown.

EXTRINSIC

Tissue Injury $\longrightarrow$ Thromboplastinogen

Thromboplastinogen + VII $\longrightarrow$ Thromboplastinogen-VII Complex

Thromboplastinogen-VII Complex + V + X $\longrightarrow$ Thromboplastin

Phase II Thromboplastin + Prothrombin $\xrightarrow{\text{V and VII}}$ Thrombin

Phase III Thrombin + Fibrinogen + XIII $\longrightarrow$ Fibrin Monomer + Activated XII

Fibrin Monomer + Activated XIII $\longrightarrow$ Fibrin Polymer

Fibrin Polymer $\xrightarrow[\text{Platelets}]{\text{Activated XIII}}$ Clot Retraction

ticoagulants, and natural antithrombins are present in blood. Fortunately, most often the coagulation mechanism rapidly and efficiently inhibits the excessive loss of blood and excessive coagulation does not occur. Occasionally, however, because of genetic errors or disease processes, the coagulation system does not function properly and excessive bleeding may occur.

Congenital Abnormalities of the Coagulation Mechanism

Hemophilia (Factor VIII Deficiency, AHG Deficiency, Hemophilia A). Hemophilia was described in 1803[68] and was well known in the royal houses of England, Russia, and Spain in the nineteenth century. It is the most common genetic bleeding disorder, occurring approximately once in 25,000 births. It is transmitted as a sex-linked recessive trait, with the male usually being the bleeder and the female the carrier. There are estimated to be 20,000 moderate and severe hemophiliacs in the United States, with a median age of 11.5 years.[93] Most hemophiliacs have sufficient quantities of factor VIII for daily consumption, but seem to be unable to replace the factor when it is consumed during the clotting that occurs after trauma or surgery.

Symptoms of hemophilia usually have their onset during the latter half of the first year of life. Although hemorrhage may occur at the time of circumcision, hemophilic babies appear to be protected, either by a protective immunity from their mother or by their protective environment, during the first few months of life. Mild hemophiliacs frequently note only prolonged bleeding after dental extractions or minor cuts. Moderate to severe hemophiliacs bleed into joints or muscles after minor trauma.

Hemophiliacs with abdominal pain present a diag-

nostic problem. The differential diagnosis usually is between retroperitoneal, mesenteric, or intramural hematomas of the bowel and an inflammatory disease of the bowel, especially acute appendicitis. The likelihood that the pain is related to the hemophilia increases in direct proportion to the severity of the bleeding disorder. In general, the more severe the hemophilia, the more conservative one should be in his decision regarding operative intervention. More hemophiliacs have died from unnecessary operations than from the complications of appendicitis.[15, 19, 67, 97]

Current management of hemophilia has reduced the risk of surgery, but the hemophiliac still represents an increased surgical risk and operations must be performed for definite reasons and expeditiously, with precise hemostasis and adequate replacement of factor VIII. Not infrequently, intestinal obstruction develops from intramural hematomas or retroperitoneal bleeds in hemophiliacs. Nonoperative management usually is very satisfactory for these patients.

The diagnosis of hemophilia is usually suspected from the history. Most often the diagnosis has been established in early childhood. Correction of the clotting deficiency with normal plasma, but not with hemophiliac plasma, establishes the diagnosis. The partial thromboplastin time (PTT) is an excellent diagnostic screening test. Careful manipulation of the PTT will permit diagnosis of hemophilia or the various hemophilioid disorders.[89] Routine bleeding and clotting times are not reliable and have little value in the preoperative assessment of the hemostatic mechanism of these patients. The clotting time may be normal when the patient's factor VIII concentration is less than 5 per cent of normal.

The PTT is a simple way to follow the effectiveness of replacement therapy. Normal PTT values range from 65 to 85 seconds. Hemophiliacs who are bleeding frequently have PTT values in excess of 250 to 300 seconds. Factor VIII–containing preparations are given in sufficient amounts to return the PTT to 120 seconds or less (factor VIII concentration of 30 per cent or more). Although the shortened PTT is an excellent index of successful replacement therapy, a "rule of thumb" for replacement therapy is that 1 ml. of fresh normal plasma per kilogram of patient's weight will raise the factor VIII level about 2 per cent.[1] The short half-life of factor VIII—6 to 8 hours—requires replacement of at least one half the required amount at these time intervals.

Frequently, large amounts of factor VIII are required for lengthy periods. If a patient were transfused only with fresh (or fresh frozen) plasma during this time, his cardiovascular volume might be exceeded and pulmonary edema, congestive heart failure, and so forth, might result. Fortunately, factor VIII has been concentrated by freezing plasma (cryoprecipitate) or by a freezing-glycine precipitation method. In order to provide the millions of equivalents of whole blood required by our hemophiliac population,[93] it is mandatory that virtually all donated blood be processed as components.

Cryoprecipitate may be easily prepared in most blood banks, is available in all fresh blood, and is the agent most often used for treating hemophiliacs. Cryoprecipitate contains 15 to 34 times the concentration of factor VIII that is found in the plasma and can raise the factor VIII concentration with minimal effects on the blood volume. Cryoprecipitate administration should be monitored by the PTT.

Five to 20 per cent of hemophiliacs develop antibody inhibitors to factor VIII during increasing exposure to transfusion of the antigen.[86] These patients may be treated with infusions of factor VIII in doses that overwhelm the inhibitors, immunosuppression and factor VIII,[39] or animal factor VIII.[81] The concomitant administration of epsilon-aminocaproic acid, a fibrinolytic inhibitor, to selected hemophiliac patients has reduced the patients' requirement of factor VIII.[1, 28]

Care of the hemophiliac patient includes meticulous attention to all aspects of his illness. Besides restoring the factor VIII level, infection should be treated promptly and vigorously with antibiotics, and drainage if indicated. Fractures or hematomas should be immobilized, intravenous catheters should be inserted carefully, and intratracheal intubations or suction must be done extremely carefully and only for definite indications. Prophylactic home and hospital treatment programs have been successful in reducing the amount of hospitalization time for hemophiliacs but not the yearly number of infusions of factor VIII.[1]

Hemophilioid Disorders. There are several congenital bleeding disorders that resemble hemophilia. These disorders are not as common as hemophilia, rarely are severe, and are more easily managed.

FACTOR IX DEFICIENCY (CHRISTMAS DISEASE, PTC DEFICIENCY, HEMOPHILIA B). Factor IX deficiency is a mild bleeding disorder that was described in 1952.[3] Its clinical manifestations are similar to but less severe than those of true hemophilia. The disease is transmitted as a sex-linked recessive trait and occurs in approximately one patient per 100,000 births. It is the second most common genetic bleeding disorder.

Spontaneous bleeding may occur in severely affected patients who have 1 per cent, or less, of factor IX. A factor IX level greater than 1 per cent seems to protect against spontaneous bleeding but not against bleeding from trauma or surgery. A factor IX level of 10 to 15 per cent appears to be necessary to provide adequate hemostasis during the time of surgery or trauma. Unlike factor VIII, factor IX is stable in both plasma and serum and loses little activity during storage. The circulating half-life of factor IX is 24 to 30 hours, and therefore replacement therapy can be done daily with banked blood or plasma. The PTT is a satisfactory test for factor IX replacement. Recently, new clotting factor concentrates, which contain factors II, VII, IX, and X, have become available for replacing factor IX.[10, 43, 53] The concentration of factor IX in the new concentrate is 10 to 20 times that found in plasma.

FACTOR XI DEFICIENCY (ROSENTHAL SYNDROME, PTA DEFICIENCY, HEMOPHILIA C). This bleeding disorder is very mild and is transmitted by a simple dominant gene that occurs in males and females with equal frequency. It was discovered in 1953. Spontaneous hemorrhages and hemarthroses rarely occur, but postpartum hemorrhage and bleeding after trauma may occur. Factor XI–deficient patients may have prolonged and delayed postoperative bleeding, which responds very well to fresh or banked plasma or blood. The bleeding is not likely to be of serious concern to the surgeon. Preoperative transfusion may prevent the bleeding. It has been suggested that transfusions may be required intermittently postoperatively for up to 5 days.[70]

FACTOR V DEFICIENCY (PARAHEMOPHILIA, OWREN'S DISEASE). This is a very rare, mild hemorrhagic disorder that was described in 1947.[69] It is transmitted as an autosomal recessive and affects both sexes equally.[45] The disorder manifests itself early in life by epistaxis or excessive bleeding from minor trauma or minor surgery. Factor V, like factor VIII, is moderately unstable and disappears during the coagulation process. Deficiencies of factor V can be corrected by transfusion of fresh blood or plasma and should be monitored (like all the other hemophiliac-like conditions, save for factor VII deficiency) with the PTT.

FACTOR VII DEFICIENCY (PROCONVERTIN DEFICIENCY, PSEUDOHEMOPHILIA). A mild hemorrhagic and purpuric condition due to the deficiency of factor VII was described in 1951.[4] It is transmitted as a recessive autosomal character and occurs about once in 500,000 births. Homozygotes vary from severe bleeders to nonbleeders. Severe bleeders frequently bleed in early childhood, so that the diagnosis is established prior to surgical procedures. Uncorrected factor VII deficiency may result in moderate to severe intraoperative and postoperative bleeding. These patients have a normal PTT and a prolonged one-stage prothrombin time. The deficiency is readily corrected by stored blood or plasma. Preoperative transfusion may be all that is necessary to insure adequate operative and postoperative hemostasis. The concentrate of factors II, VII, IX, and X will also correct hemostatic defects.

FACTOR X DEFICIENCY (CONGENITAL DEFICIENCY OF STUART-PROWER FACTOR). Factor X deficiency produces a mild hemorrhagic diathesis that was described in 1955.[26] The sexes are equally affected. Although the hemorrhagic diathesis is mild, mucosal bleeding, articular bleeding, and other spontaneous hemorrhages do occur. Factor X is stable in bank blood, which readily corrects any bleeding disorder. The PTT serves as an adequate guide of replacement therapy.

FACTOR XII DEFICIENCY (HAGEMAN TRAIT). Congenital absence of factor XII was discovered in 1965.[62] Absence of factor XII has no effect on clotting in vivo, but does markedly prolong blood clotting in vitro. Patients with this deficiency do not have a hemorrhagic tendency and do not bleed postoperatively. A prolonged clotting time in an otherwise healthy individual should be evaluated in terms of this defect.

VON WILLEBRAND'S DISEASE (VASCULAR HEMOPHILIA). This disorder is inherited as an autosomal dominant trait and is characterized by prolonged bleeding time, reduced platelet adhesiveness, deficiency of factor VIII coagulant activity, and an over-response of factor VIII to transfusions. It has a very mild hemorrhagic diathesis. Epistaxis, easy bruisability, and purpura appear as early diagnostic clues in childhood in approximately 75 per cent of the cases. Hemorrhages and deep intramuscular hemarthroses are rare but may occur. The bleeding times are usually prolonged, platelet adhesiveness to glass is reduced, factor VIII is reduced, and the ristocetin-Willebrand factor is decreased.[9] Other clotting studies usually are normal unless there is a significant deficiency of factor VIII or, on rare occasions, one of the other coagulation factors. Surgery rarely presents a problem in these patients. If bleeding does occur, fresh blood or plasma usually is effective in controlling the bleeding.

Other Congenital Deficiencies of Coagulation Factors

FACTOR I DEFICIENCY (FIBRINOGEN DEFICIENCY). Congenital deficiencies of factor I are quite rare. The severity of the clinical course is determined by the fibrinogen level. Persons with reduced fibrinogen levels may be asymptomatic, whereas afibrinogenemic children have a high incidence of serious and frequently fatal bleeding in the neonatal and infant period. Children with afibrinogenemia rarely survive, so that few adults with congenital afibrinogenemia are seen.

FACTOR II DEFICIENCY (PROTHROMBIN DEFICIENCY). This congenital condition is extremely rare and is unlikely to present a problem to the surgeon. Transfusion with bank blood or plasma will stop the hemorrhages that occur with this deficiency.

THE FIBRINOLYTIC SYSTEM

Although fibrinolysis had been observed for many years, it was not until the early part of the twentieth century that studies on induced and spontaneous fibrinolysis were begun. In 1933, Tillett and Gardner[99] demonstrated that cultures and filtrates of strains of beta hemolytic streptococci obtained from patients were capable of liquefying human fibrin clots. In 1941,

Milstone noted that a thermolabile nondialyzable factor present in the euglobulin fraction of normal human serum was needed before the streptococcal filtrate could exert its action on human fibrin.[65] In 1956–57, Cliffton and associates were able to induce systemic fibrinolytic activity in patients.[16] Subsequently, numerous investigations of induced fibrinolysis have been performed.[6, 17] Many of the recent studies on induced fibrinolysis are being conducted under the auspices of the Committee of Thrombolytic Agents of the National Heart and Lung Institute.[102]

Although the fibrinolytic system serves primarily as a "balance" for the coagulation system and acts to maintain vessel patency, pathologically significant hyperfibrinolytic activity may occur during or after major operations performed on poor-risk patients who have required multiple blood transfusions. These patients usually have experienced hypoxia, hypoperfusion, hypotension, and acidosis. Pathologic hypofibrinolysis has been reported in patients with carcinoma of the prostate,[5, 61] carcinoma of the pancreas,[76] hepatic cirrhosis,[29] polycythemia vera, sarcoidosis, leukemia, and other blood dyscrasias.[71]

Fibrinolytic Mechanism

The fibrinolytic mechanism is quite similar to, although not yet as well understood as, the coagulation mechanism (Fig. 3). Plasminogen, or profibrinolysin, is converted to plasmin (fibrinolysin) by activator(s). Plasmin produces fibrinolysis by enzymatically breaking fibrin into polypeptides (split products). Plasminogen has a strong affinity for fibrinogen and becomes incorporated into the fibrin gel during clotting. Thus, plasminogen is available in the circulation and in the thrombus for conversion to plasmin, and fibrinolysis may occur from within the thrombus or from without.

Although fibrinolytic activators are found in all tissues, the most important physiologic fibrinolytic activator is the intravascular activator found in the endothelium of veins, venules, and capillaries and in the vasa vasorum of arteries and arterioles. Except in the pulmonary vasculature, where the reverse is true, veins contain much more of the activator than do arteries. The intravascular fibrinolytic activator may be released into the circulation or may diffuse into adjacent thrombi and plays a major role in initiating in vivo thrombolysis.

Hyperfibrinolysis. Hyperfibrinolysis occurs whenever the amount of plasmin produced exceeds the quantity of naturally occurring plasmin inhibitors. Hyperfibrinolysis produces proteolysis with digestion of fibrin, fibrinogen, and other plasma proteins. During times of hyperfibrinolysis, protecting thrombi may be lysed and secondary bleeding may occur. New thrombi cannot form because of proteolysis of the coagulation proteins. Hyperfibrinolysis has little effect upon the intact vascular system; however, it frequently occurs during clinical situations that are associated with defects in vascular integrity, and bleeding occurs.

Hyperfibrinolysis may be produced by the infusion of plasminogen activators (urokinase, streptokinase, and so forth) or plasmin. However, this type of hyperfibrinolysis is readily treated by stopping the infusion,

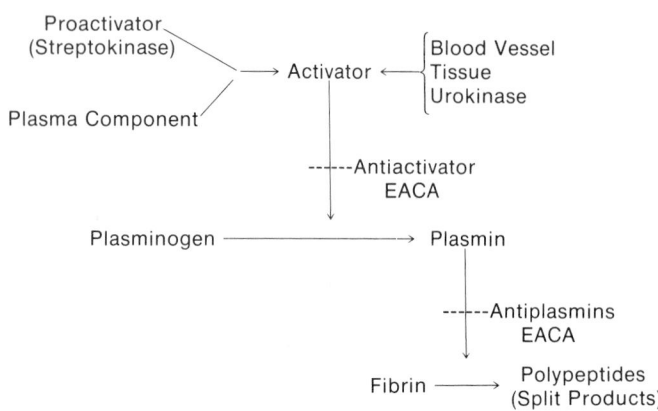

Figure 3. Fibrinolytic mechanism. Plasmin is a proteolytic enzyme with a special affinity for fibrin (and fibrinogen). During times of hyperplasminemia, a generalized proteolysis occurs and many of the coagulation proteins and other plasma proteins undergo digestion.

or by infusing fibrinolytic inhibitors. Spontaneous hyperfibrinolysis usually is unsuspected and is responsible for 1 per cent of the cases of nonmechanical surgical bleeding. Hyperfibrinolysis has occurred after sudden death from trauma or electric shock, after a massive hemorrhage, during times of profound hypoxia or shock, during and after cardiopulmonary bypass, in patients with carcinoma of the prostate or with cirrhosis, and in patients with blood dyscrasias.

Increased fibrinolytic activity usually accompanies all thrombotic processes. Occasionally it is difficult to determine whether the bleeding is produced from too much clotting with consumption of the coagulation factors[89] or from clotting with secondary lysis. It is likely that many of the so-called hyperfibrinolytic states are a type of consumption coagulopathy. Bleeding from hyperfibrinolysis occurs much *less* frequently than does bleeding from other causes.

Consumption Coagulopathy

In 1965 Rodriguez-Erdmann[80] introduced the term "consumption coagulopathy" to describe the common features of a variety of bleeding disorders, e.g., afibrinogenemia, defibrination syndrome, acquired hypofibrinogenemia, and purpura fulminans. Consumption coagulopathy is a hemorrhagic disorder that results when widespread activation of the clotting mechanism occurs and there is consumption of plasma clotting factors (especially factors I, II, V, and VIII, and platelets). Consumption coagulopathy may be thought of as an end stage of disseminated intravascular coagulation. It may be caused by a Shwartzman-like reaction, an infusion of thromboplastin, fat embolism, and the Kasabach-Merritt syndrome.[79]

Regardless of the initiating events, the excessive coagulation that occurs during this disorder results in consumption of many of the coagulation factors and a secondary hyperfibrinolysis. Laboratory studies reveal low platelet counts (20,000 to 60,000) and low values (10 to 30 per cent of normal range) of factors II, V, VII, and VIII. Increased fibrinolytic activity is usually present.

Management is directed primarily toward alleviating the precipitating cause of the syndrome. Shock, sepsis, acidosis, hypoxia, and so forth, are treated. If the consumptive coagulopathy continues, heparin, paradoxically, is the treatment of choice. Heparin inhibits

thrombin's action, slows the rate of thromboplastin production, and permits a gradual restoration of coagulation factors. The constant infusion of about one third to one half of an anticoagulating dose of heparin will usually restore the coagulation factors toward normal levels within 24 to 36 hours. Administration of blood, plasma, or fibrinogen to a patient with a consumption coagulopathy is dangerous because the large amounts of circulating thrombin will rapidly convert the infused fibrinogen to fibrin and major vessels may be occluded.

PLATELETS

Platelets have a major role in hemostasis. The ability of platelets to adhere to injured endothelium, especially to exposed collagen, and to form aggregates permits them to reduce hemorrhage by occluding the severed ends of small vessels. Platelets contain factors that accelerate or activate stages of the coagulation mechanism, interfere with the action of heparin or heparin-like substances, and are responsible for clot retraction. Platelets deserve their title as the keystone of the hemostatic arch.[92]

Bleeding may be caused by too few, too many, or physiologically inadequate platelets. The bleeding of thrombocytopenia is characterized by spontaneous capillary hemorrhages into the skin and mucous membranes, with resultant petechiae and ecchymoses. There is a marked reduction in the number of platelets, a prolonged bleeding time, and a positive tourniquet test. Although hematuria and gastrointestinal bleeding occur frequently, hemarthrosis and intramuscular bleeding rarely occur.

Thrombocytopenia may be primary or secondary. Primary (idiopathic) thrombocytopenia purpura is a condition in which the platelets are reduced, but the platelet precursors, the megakaryocytes, are normal or increased; the spleen is usually not enlarged.[22] Secondary thrombocytopenia occurs after viral infection, with hypersplenism, during anaphylactoid reactions, after incompatible blood transfusion, during disseminated intravascular coagulation, and after drug administration or irradiation. When the diagnosis is established platelet transfusions will, unless there are antibodies to the platelets, restore platelet levels to those adequate for hemostasis. Thirty to 40 thousand normal platelets per cu. mm. are sufficient for hemostatic purposes.

Too many platelets may cause bleeding by producing platelet plugs in multiple small vessels and secondary ischemic necrosis, by stimulating diffuse intravascular coagulation with a secondary consumption coagulopathy, or by being physiologically inadequate. Thrombocytosis, a temporary increase of platelets, occurs most often after splenectomy but is also seen after other surgical procedures, especially cardiopulmonary bypass. It occurs after inflammation, trauma, and parturition and with various disease states. Bleeding usually does not occur during these temporary increases of platelets. If bleeding does occur, it is usually managed with dextran or heparin to reduce the platelet plugging and secondary ulceration.

Thrombocythemia refers to a sustained increase in platelet count. Bleeding that occurs in association with thrombocythemia is called hemorrhagic thrombocythemia. The patients usually bleed from the mucous membranes and the gastrointestinal tract, and frequently have an enlarged spleen. Many patients with thrombocythemia have a myeloproliferative disorder. Treatment is directed at treating the thrombotic and bleeding process and then reducing the platelet count with appropriate chemotherapeutic agents.

Although disorders of platelet function may be inherited, e.g., Glanzmann's thrombasthenia,[13] Bernard-Soulier syndrome,[8] most disorders of platelet function are acquired. Occasionally platelets are coated with abnormal proteins, such as occurs during cryoglobulinemia, macroglobulinemia, and hyperglobulinemia, which interfere with platelet functions. Abnormal platelet function has also been described in patients with burns, congestive heart failure, scurvy, leukemia, cirrhosis, and some collagen disorders. Many drugs may inhibit platelet release and/or aggregation, e.g., aspirin, antihistamines, alcohol, barbiturates, dipyridamole, ethacrynic acid, indomethacin.[94] These patients have prolonged thrombin consumption times, prolonged bleeding times, and prolonged clotting times. Treatment of the basic disease process and platelet transfusions will help control the bleeding in most of these patients.

ANTICOAGULANTS

Heparin

Heparin is the most widely used and reliable anticoagulant. It was discovered by McLean, a second-year medical student, in 1916,[64] and given its name in 1918.[46] Heparin has a strong negative charge which allows it to interfere with most reactions involving proteins. It acts as an anticoagulant by its antithrombin effect, by its antithromboplastic effect (it interferes with factors IX, XI, XII, and activated factor X), and by interfering with platelet function. Although it is extracted from animal sources commercially, toxic or sensitivity reactions are quite rare.

The effectiveness of heparin is directly related to the amount given and the activity of the coagulation mechanism. The dose must be titrated for each patient. In general, the larger the patient or the more extensive the thrombosis, the greater the amount of heparin required to inhibit the coagulation process. The clotting time (CT) and partial thromboplastin time (PTT) or its modifications are utilized to monitor the effect of heparin. The CT should be 25 to 30 minutes and the PTT 120 seconds when there is a constant infusion of heparin. If the heparin is given intermittently, the heparin dosage should be regulated so that the above values are obtained when blood samples are drawn 30 minutes before the next dose is given.

If excessive amounts of heparin are given, coagulation will be completely inhibited and bleeding will ensue. Usually stopping the heparin will control the bleeding. However, if the bleeding persists the heparin can be "neutralized" with protamine sulfate, a basic amine.[2] The amount of protamine required can be estimated from the protamine titration test. Usually 50 to 75 per cent of the estimated amount is administered and another protamine titration test performed in 10 to 15 minutes. Additional amounts of protamine are given as indicated by the titration test. Protamine should be used with caution because it will act as an anticoagulant when given in excessive amounts and hypertension may result if it is infused rapidly.

Indirect Anticoagulants

The discovery of *Dicumarol* by Link in 1943[59] led to the development of a variety of indirect anticoagulants. Long-term therapy with oral anticoagulants is used for a variety of reasons, e.g., for stroke or myocardial infarction prophylaxis, to reduce the thromboembolism associated with artificial heart valves, or to prevent recurrence of pulmonary embolism. Taking this medicine may be part of a patient's daily routine and he may not voluntarily relate it when his history is taken.

The prothrombinopenic agents do not directly interfere with coagulation but decrease the production of some of the coagulation factors (especially factors II, VII, IX, and X). The reduction of these factors slows the rate and amount of thrombin produced. Most often the effect of the prothrombinopenic agents is monitored with periodic determinations of the prothrombin time. Beneficial interference with coagulation without bleeding occurs when a prothrombin time is maintained at 20 to 30 per cent of normal. Patients with prothrombin times greater than 30 per cent of the control (less than 19 seconds when the control is 13 seconds) will usually not bleed spontaneously or excessively during an operation. Only when the prothrombin time is less than 10 per cent of the control is spontaneous or excessive bleeding likely to occur.

Other medications should be prescribed carefully for patients taking a prothrombinopenic agent. Synergistic drugs such as salicylates, oral antibiotics (which alter the intestinal flora and reduce the amount of vitamin K produced), phenylbutazone, quinidine, clofibrate, and ethanol will potentiate the effects of the prothrombinopenic drugs and may induce bleeding in a previously stable patient. Other drugs such as barbiturates, chloral hydrate, oral contraceptives, and vitamin K preparations decrease the effectiveness of the prothrombinopenic drugs.

If bleeding occurs because of the excessive action of a prothrombinopenic agent, one should stop the agent and administer 25 to 50 mg. of vitamin K_1 intravenously. If liver failure is not present, the prothrombin time will return to normal in 24 to 48 hours and restoration of the coagulation mechanism will usually be sufficient to control bleeding in 4 to 6 hours. If the bleeding is excessive it can be stopped by the infusion of bank blood or plasma because the involved factors are relatively stable. Infusion of the factor II, VII, IX, and X concentrate will also control the bleeding. Vitamin K_1 is given simultaneously with transfusion.

SELECTED REFERENCES

Aledort, L. M. (Ed.): Recent Advances in Hemophilia. N.Y. Acad. Sci., 240: 1975.
> An excellent current review of the genetic, biochemical, psychosocial, diagnostic, and therapeutic aspects of hemophilia.

Hutchin, P.: History of blood transfusion: A tercentennial look. Surgery, 64:685, 1968.
> This is an excellent review of the history of blood transfusions. It includes reports of the earliest transfusion, transfusing devices, anticoagulants, blood banks, and the use of cadaver blood and should be included in the library of those interested in the history of medicine.

Owen, C. A., Bowie, E. J. W., and Thompson, J. H.: The Diagnosis of Bleeding Disorders, 2nd ed. Boston, Little, Brown and Company, 1975.
> This text reviews the mechanisms of coagulation and hemostasis. In addition to discussions of the congenital and acquired coagulation disorders, special emphasis is given to the intravascular coagulation syndrome, platelet diseases, and a clinical and laboratory investigation of the bleeding patient.

REFERENCES

1. Abildgaard, C. F.: Current concepts in the management of hemophilia. Sem. Hematol., 12:223, 1975.
2. Adkins, J. R., and Hardy, J. D.: Sodium heparin neutralization and the anticoagulant effects of protamine sulfate. Arch. Surg., 94:175, 1967.
3. Aggeler, P. M., White, S. G., Glendining, M. D., Page, E. W., Leake, T. B., and Bates, G.: Plasma thromboplastin component (PTC) deficiency: A new disease resembling hemophilia. Proc. Soc. Exper. Biol. Med., 79:692, 1952.
4. Alexander, B., Goldstein, R., Landwehr, G., and Cook, C. D.: Congenital SPCA deficiency: A hitherto unrecognized coagulation defect with hemorrhage rectified by serum and serum fractions. J. Clin. Invest., 30:596, 1951.
5. Andersson, L.: Fibrinolytic states in prostatic disease and their treatment with epsilon-amino-caproic acid. Acta Chir. Scand., 126:251, 1963.
6. Anlyan, W. G., Deaton, H. L., and Silver, D.: Experiences with fibrinolysin in peripheral vascular occlusive disease. Am. J. Cardiol., 6:507, 1960.
7. Arthus, M., and Pages, C.: Nouvelle théorie chimique de la coagulation du sang. Arch. Physiol. Norm. Pathol., 2:739, 1890 (cited in Hutchin, P.: History of blood transfusion: A tercentennial look. Surgery, 64:685, 1968.)
8. Bithell, T. C., Parekh, S. J., and Strong, R. R.: Platelet-function studies in the Bernard-Soulier syndrome. Ann. N.Y. Acad. Sci., 201:145, 1972.
9. Bowie, E. J. W., Fass, D. N., Olson, J. D., and Owen, C. A., Jr.: The spectrum of von Willebrand's disease revisited. Mayo Clin. Proc., 51:35, 1975.
10. Breen, F. A., and Tullis, J. L.: Prothrombin concentrates in treatment of Christmas disease and allied disorders. J.A.M.A., 208:1848, 1969.
11. Brener, B. J., Raines, J. K., and Darling, R. C.: Intraoperative autotransfusion in abdominal aortic resection. Arch. Surg., 107:78, 1973.
12. Buth, J., Raines, J. K., Kolodny, G. M., and Darling, R. C.: Effect of intraoperative autotransfusion on red cell mass and red cell survival. Surg. Forum, 26:276, 1975.
13. Caen, J.: Glanzmann thrombasthenia. Clin. Haematol., 1:383, 1972.
14. Chanutin, A., and Curnish, R. R.: Effect of organic and inorganic phosphates on the oxygen equilibrium of human erythrocytes. Arch. Biochem., 121:96, 1967.
15. Cheek, J. H., Aguillon, A., and Nafrawi, A.: Major surgery on the hemophilic patient. Surgery, 54:699, 1963.
16. Cliffton, E. E.: The use of plasmin in humans. Ann. N.Y. Acad. Sci., 68:209, 1957.
17. Cliffton, E. E.: Review of clinical experience with clot-lysing agents. Am. J. Cardiol., 6:476, 1960.
18. Cohn, L. H., Fosberg, A. M., Anderson, W. P., and Collins, J. J., Jr.: The effects of phlebotomy, hemodilutions, and autologous transfusion on systemic oxygenation and whole blood utilization in open heart surgery. Chest, 68:283, 1975.
19. Craddock, C. G., Jr., Fenninger, L. D., and Simmons, B.: Hemophilia. Problem of surgical intervention for accompanying diseases. Review of the literature and report of a case. Ann. Surg., 128:888, 1948.
20. Crowe, S. J.: Halsted of Johns Hopkins. The Man and His Men. Springfield, Ill., Charles C Thomas, Publisher, 1957.
21. Cullen, D. J., and Ferrara, L.: Comparative evaluation of blood filters: A study in vitro. Anesthesia, 41:568, 1974.
22. Dameshek, W.: "I.T.P." Tricky disease. Med. Clin. North Am., 46:1135, 1962.
23. Danziger, S. J.: Transfusion malaria (Letter to the Editor). Lancet, 2:312, 1970.
24. Davidsohn, I., and Stern, K.: Blood transfusion reactions: Their causes and identification. Med. Clin. North Am., 44:281, 1960.
25. Denis, P. S.: Memoires sur le sang, considéré quand il est fluide, pendant qu'il se coagule et lorsqu'il est coagulé. Paris, Bailliere et Fils, 1859 (cited in von Kaulla, K. N.: Chemistry of Thrombolysis: Human Fibrinolytic Enzymes. Springfield, Ill., Charles C Thomas, Publisher, 1963, pp. 9–20).
26. Duckert, F., Flückiger, P., Matter, M., and Koller, F.: Clotting factor X. Physiology and physico-chemical properties. Proc. Soc. Exper. Biol. Med., 90:17, 1955.
27. Dunbar, R. W., Price, K. A., and Cannarella, C. F.: Microaggregate blood filters: Effects on filtration time, plasma hemoglobin, and fresh blood platelet counts. Anesth. Analg., 53:577, 1974.
28. Duthie, R. B.: Reconstructive surgery in hemophilia. Ann. N.Y. Acad. Sci., 240:295, 1975.
29. Ende, N., and Auditore, J. V.: Circulating fibrinolytic activity and hemorrhagic diathesis. Ann. Surg., 158:117, 1963.
30. Fantus, B.: The therapy of the Cook County Hospital. J.A.M.A., 109:128, 1937.
31. Garrott, A. J., and Sayman, W. A.: Serum hepatitis from transfusions of blood. J.A.M.A., 180:1029, 1966.
32. Geelhoed, G. W., and Bennett, S. H.: "Shock lung" resulting from perfusion of canine lungs with stored bank blood. Am. Surg., 41:671, 1975.
33. Gibbs, C. E., and Misenhimer, H. R.: The use of blood transfusion in obstetrics. Am. J. Obstet. Gynecol., 93:26, 1965.
34. Gibson, J. G., Gregory, C. B., and Button, L. N.: Citrate-phosphate-dextrose solution for preservation of human blood: A further report. Transfusion, 1:280, 1961.
35. Gibson, J. G., Rees, S. B., McManus, T. J., and Scheitlin, W. A.: A citrate-phosphate-dextrose solution for the preservation of human blood. Am. J. Clin. Pathol., 28:569, 1957.
36. Gollub, S., Svigals, R., Bailey, C. P., Hirose, T., and Schaefer, C.: Electrolyte solution in surgical patients refusing transfusion. J.A.M.A., 215:2077, 1971.
37. Grant, J.: Complications of blood transfusion. Practitioner, 195:1796, 1965.
38. Graw, R. G., Jr., Herzig, G., Perry, S., and Henderson, E. S.: Normal granulocyte transfusion therapy: Treatment of septicemia due to gram-negative bacteria. N. Engl. J. Med., 287:367, 1972.
39. Green, D.: Factor VIII antibodies: Immunosuppressive therapy. Ann. N.Y. Acad. Sci., 240:389, 1975.
40. Hammarsten, O.: Quoted in Hougie, C.: Fundamentals of Blood Coagulation in Clinical Medicine. New York, McGraw-Hill Book Company, 1963.
41. Haynes, L., Tullis, J. L., Pyle, H. M., Sproul, M. T., Wallach, S., and Turville, W. C.: Clinical use of glycerolized frozen blood. J.A.M.A., 173:1657, 1960.

42. Hewson, W.: An experimental Inquiry into the Properties of the Blood, 2nd ed. London, T. Cadell, 1772.

43. Hoag, M. S., Johnson, F. F., Robinson, J. A., and Aggeler, P. M.: Treatment of hemophilia B with a new clotting-factor concentrate. N. Engl. J. Med., 280:581, 1969.

44. Hoff, H. E., and Guilemin, R.: The tercentenary transfusion in man. Cardiovasc. Res. Cent. Bull., 6:47, 1967.

45. Hougie, C.: Fundamentals of Blood Coagulation in Clinical Medicine. New York, McGraw-Hill Book Company, 1963.

46. Howell, W. H., and Holt, E.: Two new factors in blood coagulation—heparin and ago-antithrombin. Am. J. Physiol., 47:328, 1918.

47. Hoxworth, P. I., Haesler, W. E., Jr., and Smith, H., Jr.: The risk of hepatitis from whole blood and stored plasma. Surg. Gynecol. Obstet., 109:38, 1959.

48. Huggins, C. C.: Frozen blood. Ann. Surg., 160:643, 1964.

49. Hutchin, P.: History of blood tranfusion: A tercentennial look. Surgery, 64:685, 1968.

50. Ketchel, M. M., Tullis, J. L., Tinch, R. J., Driscoll, S. G., and Surgenor, D. M.: Use of biochemical equipment for the long-term preservation of erythrocytes. J.A.M.A., 168:404, 1958.

51. Kliman, A.: Modern blood component therapy. Hosp. Med., 6:59, 1970.

52. Kolmer, J. A., and Rule, A. M.: Survival of Treponema pallidum in preserved citrated human blood and plasma. Amer. J. Syph. Gonor. Ven. Dis., 26:156, 1942.

53. Kurczynski, E. M., and Penner, J. A.: Activated prothrombin concentrate for patients with factor VIII inhibitors. N. Engl. J. Med., 291:164, 1974.

54. Langston, H. T., Callaghan, R. S., and Mehl, R.: Blood for autologous transfusion. Bull. Soc. Intern. Chir., 6:514, 1972.

55. Levine, P., Katzin, E. M., and Burnham, L.: Isoimmunization in pregnancy. J.A.M.A., 116:825, 1941.

56. Lewers, D. T., Mathew, T. H., Maher, J. F., and Schreiner, G. E.: Long-term follow-up of renal function and histology after acute tubular necrosis. Ann. Intern. Med., 73:523, 1970.

57. Lewisohn, R.: New and greatly simplified method of blood transfusion. Med. Rec., 87:141, 1915.

58. Lewisohn, R.: Blood transfusion: 50 years ago and today. Surg. Gynecol. Obstet., 101:362, 1955.

59. Link, K. P.,: The anticoagulant from spoiled sweet clover hay. Harvey Lect., 34:162, 1943–1944.

60. Macfarlane, R. G.: A clotting scheme for 1964. Thromb. Diath. Haemorrh., 17(Suppl.):45, 1965.

61. Malcolm, D., and O'Connor, J. J.: Generalized fibrinolytic bleeding following cystoscopy in a patient with carcinoma of the prostate. J. Urol., 90:458, 1963.

62. Margolius, A., Jr., and Ratnoff, O. D.: Observations on the hereditary nature of Hageman trait. Blood, 11:565, 1956.

63. McKittrick, J. E.: Banked autologous blood in elective surgery. Am. J. Surg., 128:137, 1974.

64. McLean, J.: The thromboplastic action of cephalin. Am. J. Physiol., 41:250, 1916.

65. Milstone, H.: A factor in normal human blood which participates in streptococcal fibrinolysis. J. Immunol., 42:109, 1941.

66. Morawitz, P.: Uber einige postmortale Blutveranderungen. Beitr. Chem. Physiol. Pathol., 8:1, 1906.

67. Ochsner, A., and Johnston, J. H.: Appendiceal peritonitis. Surgery, 17:873, 1945.

68. Otto, J. C.: Account of an hemorrhagic disposition existing in certain families. Med. Repository, 6:1, 1803.

69. Owren, P. A.: Parahaemophilia—hemorrhagic diathesis due to the absence of a previously unknown clotting factor. Lancet, 1:446, 1947.

70. Phillips, L. L., Hyman, G. A., and Rosenthal, R. L.: Prolonged postoperative bleeding in a patient with factor XI (PTA) deficiency. Ann. Surg., 162:37, 1965.

71. Piscoitta, A. V., and Schulz, E. J.: Fibrinolytic purpura in acute leukemia. Am. J. Med., 19:824, 1955.

72. Prevost, J. L., and Dumas, J. B. A.: Examen du sang et de son action dans les divers phenomenes de la vie. Ann. Chim. (Phys.), 18:1, 1821 (cited in Hutchin, P.: History of blood transfusion: A tercentennial look. Surgery, 64:685, 1968).

73. Prince, A. M., Brotman, B., Jass, D., and Ikram, H.: Specificity of the direct solid phase radioimmunoassay for detection of hepatitis B antigen. Lancet, 1:1346, 1973.

74. Race, R. R., and Sanger, R.: Blood Groups in Man. Oxford, Blackwell Scientific Publications, 1958.

75. Rakower, S. R., and Worth, M. H., Jr.: Massive intraoperative autotransfusion of blood. Surg. Gynecol. Obstet., 137:633, 1973.

76. Ratnoff, O. D.: Studies on a proteolytic enzyme in human plasma. VII. A fatal hemorrhagic state associated with excessive plasma proteolytic activity in a patient undergoing surgery for carcinoma of the head of the pancreas. J. Clin. Invest., 31:521, 1952.

77. Reul, G. J., Jr., Solis, R. T., Greenberg, S. D., Mattox, K. L., and Whisennard, H. H.: Experience with autotransfusion in the surgical management of trauma. Surgery, 76:546, 1974.

78. Robertson, H. D., and Polk, H. C., Jr.: Blood transfusions in elective operations: Comparison of whole blood versus packed red cells. Ann. Surg., 181:778, 1975.

79. Rodriguez-Erdmann, F.: Studies on the pathogenesis of the generalized Shwartzman reaction. III. Trigger mechanism for activation of prothrombin molecule. Thromb. Diath. Haemorrh., 12:471, 1964.

80. Rodriguez-Erdmann, F.: Bleeding due to increased intravascular blood coagulation. Hemorrhagic syndromes caused by consumption of blood-clotting factors (consumption-coagulopathies). N. Engl. J. Med., 273:1370, 1965.

81. Rubin, H., Niemetz, J., and Estren, S.: Use of animal AHG concentrates (factor VIII) in the treatment of life-threatening hemorrhage in patients with factor VIII antibodies. Ann. N.Y. Acad. Sci., 240:362, 1975.

82. Schmidt, A.: Uber den Faserstoff und die Ursachen seiner Gerinnung. Arch. Anat. Physiol., 1861, p. 545 (cited by Biggs, R., and Macfarlane, R. G.: Human Blood Coagulation, 3rd ed. Oxford, Blackwell Scientific Publications, 1962).

83. Schorr, J. B., and Marx, G. F.: New trends in intraoperative blood replacement. Anesth. Analg., 49:646, 1970.

84. Screening for hepatitis made possible through NIH-licensed reagent. NIH Record, 23:8, 1971.

85. Shafer, A. W.: Use of blood and blood components. South. Med. J., 68:631, 1975.

86. Shapiro, S. S.: Characterization of factor VIII. Ann. N.Y. Acad. Sci., 240:350, 1975.

87. Sheldon, G. F., Lim, R. C., and Blaisdell, F. W.: The use of fresh blood in the treatment of critically injured patients. J. Trauma, 15:670, 1975.

88. Shields, C. E.: Comparison studies of whole blood stored in ACD and CPD with adenine. Transfusion, 8:1, 1968.

89. Silver, D.: Nonmechanical causes of surgical bleeding. Curr. Probl. Surg., Jan., 1970.

90. Simon, E. R., Chapman, R. G., and Finch, C. A.: Adenine in red cell preservation. J. Clin. Invest., 41:351, 1962.

91. Skrzypek, G., and Barrett, O.: The problem of vivax malaria in Vietnam returnees. Part II. Malaria chemoprophylaxis survey. Milit. Med., 133:449, 1968.

92. Spaet, T.: The platelet in hemostasis. Ann. N.Y. Acad., Sci., 115:31, 1964.

93. Stengle, J. M.: The hemophiliacs demand on blood resources: The magnitude of the problem. Ann. N.Y. Acad. Sci., 240:155, 1975.

94. Stuart, M. J.: Inherited defects of platelet function. Sem. Hematol., 12:233, 1975.

95. Survey data support link between hepatitis and Australia antigen. J.A.M.A., 214:1405, 1970.

96. Tarasov, M. M.: Cadaveric blood transfusion. Ann. N.Y. Acad. Sci., 87:512, 1960.

97. Tashiro, S., and Zinnenger, M. M.: Appendicitis. A review of nine hundred and thirty-six cases at the Cincinnati General Hospital. Arch. Surg., 53:545, 1946.

98. Technical Methods and Procedures of the American Association of Blood Banks, 4th ed. Chicago, American Associations of Blood Banks, 1966.

99. Tillett, W. S., and Gardner, R. H.: The fibrinolytic activity of hemolytic streptococci. J. Exp. Med., 58:485, 1933.

100. Tullis, J. L., and Lionetti, F. J.: The preservation of blood by freezing. Anesthesiology, 27:483, 1966.

101. Tullis, J. L., Hinman, J., Sproul, M. T., and Nickerson, R. J.: Incidence of posttransfusion hepatitis in previously frozen blood. J.A.M.A., 214:1405, 1970.

102. Urokinase Pulmonary Embolism Trial: A National Cooperative Study. Circulation, 47(Suppl. 2):4, 1973.

103. Young, L. E.: Complications of blood transfusion. Ann. Intern. Med., 61:136, 1964.

104. Yudin, S. S.: Transfusion of stored cadaver blood. Lancet, 2:361, 1937.

POLYCYTHEMIA VERA

William T. Fitts, Jr., M.D.,
and Emmanuel G. Melissinos, M.D.

Surgeons frequently are the first physicians to treat patients with polycythemia vera, but they may fail to recognize it. Polycythemia vera combines the elements that render a disease a challenge to any physician: it is an uncommon disorder (estimated incidence only five cases per million per year),[10] has protean manifestations, and carries an extremely high incidence of serious complications. It has been clearly shown that the high morbidity and mortality that accompany surgical procedures for coincidental or complicating disease can be considerably improved by establishing the diagnosis and properly preparing the polycythemic patient *preoperatively.*[4, 11] Polycythemia is only rarely discussed in surgical journals. Since many of the patients with polycythemia vera die paradoxically from either hemorrhage or thrombosis, surgeons are vitally concerned.

PATHOPHYSIOLOGY OF POLYCYTHEMIA VERA AND ITS PROGNOSIS

Polycythemia vera (erythremia, Vaquez-Osler disease) is considered one of the myeloproliferative disorders, a panmyelosis, in which the hematopoietic tissue produces an excess of erythrocytes and usually of leukocytes and thrombocytes. Its cause is unknown, despite the vast improvement in our understanding of the physiology of erythropoiesis since the disease was first described by Vaquez in 1892[9] and clarified by Osler (1903).[7] Recent evidence indicates that the elevated numbers of circulating cells in polycythemia vera result from the abnormal proliferation of an altered clone of the pluripotential hematopoietic precursor cell which escapes from the ordinary control of erythropoietin.[12] Recently a factor structurally similar to erythropoietin capable of stimulating erythropoiesis has been found in the serum of polycythemia vera patients. The site and mode of production, as well as the interrelation of this factor with erythropoietin, remain at present unclear, but its discovery indicates that at least erythrocyte production may be humorally controlled in this disease.[12]

The cytopathologic changes that occur during the early course of polycythemia vera are characterized by hyperactivity of the bone marrow cells (erythroblasts, granulocytes, megakaryoblasts, and fibroblasts), resulting in complete filling of the total marrow space and depletion of the marrow iron stores. In the peripheral blood an absolute increase in the red cell mass is detected, usually accompanied by leukocytosis, thrombocytosis, and immature red and white cells. Simultaneously, hematopoietic cells in extramedullary sites (liver, spleen) become active, and extraosseous hematopoiesis begins. With time, fibroblastic proliferation in the limited bone marrow space encroaches on the hematopoietic tissue, with diminution in erythrogenesis. The extramedullary sites become the major sites of erythropoiesis in the expanding parenchyma of the enlarging spleen and liver. Blood examination at this stage reveals anemia, morphologically bizarre red cells, leukocytosis, and thrombocytopenia or thrombocytosis (state of myelofibrosis). As myelofibrosis progresses, all blood formation may occur in extraosseous hematopoietic sites with tremendous hepatosplenomegaly accompanied by severe anemia, leukopenia, and thrombopenia (myeloid metaplasia). It should be emphasized that the cytopathologic picture may vary markedly in individual cases at any particular stage of the disease.[3, 10]

Polycythemia vera is not a benign disease but may be considered cancer of the mesenchymal tissues with only a moderately good prognosis. Death occurs from thrombosis, hemorrhage, congestive heart failure, or the development of chronic myelogenous leukemia or myelofibrosis. In a number of patients, death has resulted from acute leukemia. Recent reports indicate that only 50 per cent of the untreated patients survive for as long as 18 months, patients treated with phlebotomy alone have a 50 per cent survival of 3 to 9 years, and the ones treated with ^{32}P or alkylating agents have a median survival of 10 to 15 years.[10]

CLASSIFICATION OF THE POLYCYTHEMIAS AND THEIR DIFFERENTIATION (Table 1)

Polycythemia vera should be differentiated from (a) *secondary polycythemia* due to increased erythropoietin production caused by a distinct mechanism, physiologically appropriate or not, or genetically transmitted (see Table 1) and (b) *relative polycythemia* (also called stress or spurious polycythemia), in which the elevation of the hematocrit is due to reduced plasma volume, the total circulating red cell mass being normal. Some hematologists have estimated that they see as many as ten patients with relative polycythemia for every patient with polycythemia vera.[1]

The history may be helpful in differentiating the three types of polycythemia: (1) the age of onset is higher in polycythemia vera when compared with relative polycythemia (mean age of 60 in polycythemia vera in contrast to 52 in relative polycythemia); (2) the male to female ratio is much higher in relative polycythemia than in polycythemia vera (1.2:1 in polycythemia vera in contrast to about 5:1 or even 20:1,

TABLE 1. Types of Polycythemia*

I. Polycythemia vera
II. Secondary polycythemia (increased erythropoietin production)
  A. Physiologically appropriate (decreased blood oxygen saturation)
    1. High altitude
    2. Chronic obstructive pulmonary disease
    3. Postural hypoxemia
    4. Cardiovascular shunt (right to left)
    5. Pickwickian syndrome (massive obesity)
    6. High oxygen affinity hemoglobinopathy
    7. Congenital decreased red cell DPG
  B. Physiologically inappropriate increased erythropoietin production
    1. Tumor
      a. Renal carcinoma
      b. Cerebellar hemangioblastoma
      c. Hepatoma
      d. Uterine fibroid
      e. Adrenal cortical adenoma (and/or hyperplasia)
      f. Ovarian carcinoma
    2. Renal
      a. Cysts
      b. Hydronephrosis
      c. Bartter's syndrome
      d. Transplantation
    3. Cobalt
  C. Recessive familial polycythemia
III. Relative polycythemia (also called stress, spurious, pseudopolycythemia, Gaisbock's syndrome)

*From Berlin, N. I.: Diagnosis and classification of the polycythemias. Semin. Hematol., *12*:340, 1975. By permission of Grune & Stratton, Inc.

according to some reports, in relative polycythemia); and (3) each case of secondary polycythemia (see Table 1) is associated with a group of symptoms that characterize that particular entity.[1]

The detection of splenomegaly on physical examination is a very important differentiating sign as it is present in at least 70 per cent of patients with polycythemia vera and never accompanies secondary or relative polycythemia. Occasionally, though, a left upper quadrant mass representing an enlarged left kidney producing secondary polycythemia causes confusion.

The study of a patient who has been found to have an elevated hematocrit (above 50 per cent) can be accomplished in a methodical manner by following a suggested decision tree that will permit the classification of most cases[1] (see Table 2). To start, a measurement of the total red cell volume will separate the patients with absolute polycythemia (polycythemia vera or secondary polycythemia) from those with relative polycythemia. Following this, the determination of arterial oxygen saturation and the discovery of a reduced value will isolate a number of secondary polycythemias associated with specific causes. An intravenous pyelogram should be done next to investigate the presence of renal abnormalities that may be the cause of secondary polycythemia. If the intravenous pyelogram is normal, determination of hemoglobin $P_{50}O_2$ to rule out high oxygen affinity hemoglobinopathy should be obtained. Finally, whenever necessary, and if available, an erythropoietin assay of urine differentiates polycythemia vera patients, who

TABLE 2. Decision Tree for the Evaluation of an Elevated Hematocrit*

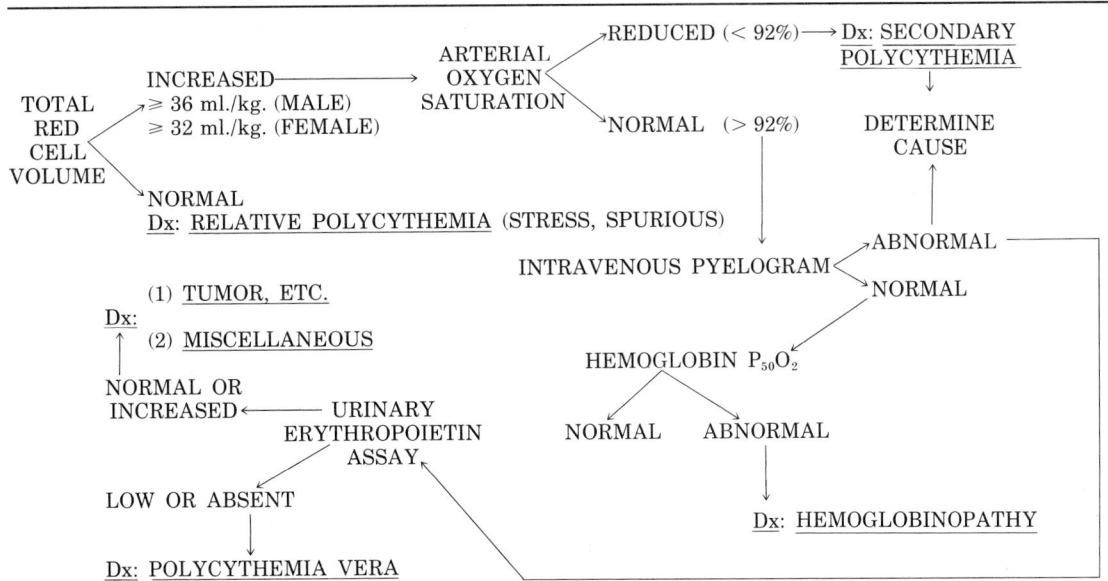

*From Berlin, N. I.: Diagnosis and classification of the polycythemias. Semin. Hematol., *12*:343, 1975. By permission of Grune & Stratton, Inc.

have low or absent amounts of erythropoietin, from those with secondary polycythemia, who have increased amounts in the urine.

SYMPTOMS AND SIGNS OF POLYCYTHEMIA VERA

The onset of polycythemia vera is often insidious. The disease may go unrecognized until the physician discovers splenomegaly or finds an elevated hematocrit value.

Early symptoms include nonspecific malaise, headaches, weakness, dizziness, visual disturbances, and paresthesias (Table 3). Circulatory disturbances of the brain probably account for the majority of the subjective symptoms.[5] They can also be partially related to the mild anemia that is sometimes present at the time of diagnosis. Pruritis, especially after a hot shower or bath, often adds to the patient's discomfort and is probably related to the increased histamine production by the myeloid cells. Splenic enlargement or infarction is frequently the cause of upper abdominal discomfort or pain and early satiety. Peptic ulcer disease is relatively common in polycythemia vera patients and probably is associated with the aforementioned hyperhistaminemia.[5] Secondary hyperuricemia due to increased catabolism of nucleated cells is the cause of gouty arthritis or renal colic in 5 to 20 per cent of patients.[6] Spontaneous purpura, epistaxis, and prolonged bleeding following minor injury are probably related to the abnormal structure and function (abnormal aggregation, adhesiveness, defective factor III release)[2] of the patient's platelets. Sluggish circulation of the highly viscous blood to the extremities is occasionally the cause of troublesome swelling and pain.

The physical findings are not very helpful. In addition to the previously mentioned splenomegaly, the most frequently observed signs, as reported by the Polycythemia Vera Study Group, are ruddy cyanosis (67 per cent of the patients), conjunctival plethora (59 per cent), engorgement of the veins of the fundus (46 per cent), and palpable liver (40 per cent).[1]

LABORATORY FINDINGS IN POLYCYTHEMIA VERA

Laboratory features as noted by the Polycythemia Vera Study Group include an increase in hematocrit, elevated white blood counts (above 12,000 in 43 per cent of the cases with presence of 5 to 10 per cent blasts), platelet count above 400,000 in 63 per cent, reticulocyte count greater than 1.5 per cent in 54 per cent of the patients, and leukocyte alkaline phosphatase score greater than 100 in 70 per cent. Blood viscosity is greatly increased, but conventional coagulation tests are usually normal. The principal radiologic finding is osteosclerosis, which tends to be symmetrical in distribution and is usually detected in the vertebral bodies, pelvis, ribs, clavicles, and metaphyseal portions of the femur and humerus.[6]

In untreated polycythemia vera, the bone marrow picture exhibits increases in marrow cellularity, in the number and size of megakaryocytes, in the number of eosinophils, in the amount of reticulin, and/or myelofibrosis and depletion of marrow iron stores.[3]

COMPLICATIONS OF POLYCYTHEMIA VERA

The most serious, life-threatening complications of the disease are related to abnormal hemostasis and paradoxically include both hemorrhagic and thromboembolic phenomena. These complications occur in about one third of polycythemia vera patients. The exact causes of the hemostatic disorders are still incompletely understood. In addition to the already mentioned intrinsic defects in platelet function, a large number of elements have been implicated, including increased viscosity of the blood, weakness of the vascular bed combined with reduced ability to react from stretching, and splenic pooling of the platelets.

In nontraumatized patients, thrombotic episodes are the most catastrophic complications, cerebral, coronary, and peripheral venous thrombosis being the most frequent causes of death. Occlusion of the hepatic veins (Budd-Chiari syndrome) and of the mesenteric, splenic, or portal veins has also been reported. Hemorrhagic episodes are usually mild in this category of patients, although they may be the cause of troublesome menometrorrhagia in menstruating females.[5]

The complication rate of 46 per cent and death rate of 16 per cent, following major surgery in patients with polycythemia vera, as reported in the classic study of Wasserman and Gilbert,[11] illustrate strikingly the risks accompanying operation on these patients. Of extreme significance is the observation that the incidence of complications was 79 per cent in patients whose hemoglobin and/or hematocrit were greater than normal before operation, whereas, in hematologically controlled patients, complications were significantly reduced (28 per cent). In the uncontrolled group of patients, the incidence of complications was increased threefold and the incidence of death sevenfold. Most importantly, the morbidity and mortality diminished strikingly (complication rate 5 per cent, no deaths) for patients treated properly for four or more months before operation. This also has

TABLE 3. Symptoms of Polycythemia*

Headache	48%
Weakness	47%
Pruritus	43%
Dizziness	43%
Sweating	33%
Visual disturbances	31%
Weight loss	29%
Paresthesias	29%
Dyspnea	26%
Joint symptoms	26%
Epigastric distress	24%

*From Berlin, N. I.: Diagnosis and classification of the polycythemias. Semin. Hematol., *12*:343, 1975. By permission of Grune & Stratton, Inc.

been our experience at the Hospital of the University of Pennsylvania. Comparison of the data published in the first report on the subject from our hospital[4] with the results of management over recent years reveals an impressive improvement that we attribute mainly to the increased awareness of the danger of operations in the untreated patient with polycythemia vera.

The majority of the complications occurring in surgical patients are hemorrhage (65 per cent), followed in frequency by thrombosis (arterial or venous) and infection. More than half of the hemorrhagic complications develop during the first 48 hours following operation.[3]

MANAGEMENT OF THE PATIENT WITH POLYCYTHEMIA VERA

From the foregoing, it seems clear that the patient with polycythemia vera represents an unusual surgical risk which should be weighed accordingly against the need for operation. All elective procedures must be preceded by therapy directed toward controlling the disease.[10]

There are a number of effective therapeutic maneuvers available today for managing polycythemia vera, but the argument as to which is the safest and most efficient mode of treatment continues. Most agree that the plan of treatment must be individualized, taking into consideration the stage of the disease, the hematologic picture, the marrow histology, and the magnitude of the problems caused by hepatosplenomegaly.[10] Phlebotomy is a long-used, important mode of treatment permitting the reduction of the blood volume by withdrawing 250 to 500 ml. of blood every second or third day until the hematocrit has been reduced to normal levels. A more gradual reduction is indicated in elderly patients. For a number of easily manageable patients having a benign course, an occasional phlebotomy is the only required therapy.[10] Although immediate relief from headaches, dizziness, and other symptoms related to the high viscosity of the blood follows this procedure, it does not offer any protection against the thrombotic complications to which patients with elevated platelet count are exposed. This type of polycythemia vera patient requires judiciously administered myelosuppressive therapy using ^{32}P and/or chemotherapy for patients above the age of 40. Radiation therapy is also a valuable mode of treatment, despite the known incidence of acute leukemia (10 to 15 per cent) that accompanies its use. Unfortunately, it appears now that a similar incidence of acute leukemia develops in patients treated with antimitotic drugs. Even patients with polycythemia vera treated with phlebotomy alone have been reported to develop this fatal complication. Females in the child-bearing age and young males should be treated with phlebotomies only, unless extreme need for supplementary treatment exists.

The problem of massive splenomegaly producing severe pressure symptoms may not be solved with radiotherapy or oral alkylating agents. If these measures are unsuccessful, the patient should be considered a candidate for splenectomy.

Before emergency operations, every attempt should be made to reduce the hematocrit to normal as rapidly as possible by frequent phlebotomies. This can be accomplished in a relatively short period of time, as the average patient with polycythemia vera can tolerate removal of 1000 to 1500 ml. of blood a day. It is wise to save the blood for subsequent reinfusion if bleeding ensues during or after operation. Early ambulation is understandably important following surgery.[4] Anticoagulants can be cautiously administered when thrombotic complications necessitate their use, heparin being the agent of choice because it can be counteracted promptly with protamine sulfate. If hemorrhage occurs, venesection, estrogens, transfusions with fresh frozen plasma or fresh blood, and the application of local pressure and ice may be helpful in the control of bleeding.[4]

SELECTED REFERENCES

Berlin, N. I.: Polycythemia. Semin. Hematol., *12*:4, 1975, and *13*:1, 1976.

This is an excellent, up-to-date summary of the present knowledge and the ongoing investigation of the disease. In the two seminars the initial results of the Polycythemia Vera Study Group are detailed.

Wasserman, L. R., and Gilbert, H. S.: Surgery in polycythemia vera. N. Engl. J. Med., *269*:1226, 1963.

This is a classic study, detailing the dangers of complications accompanying operations on patients with polycythemia vera.

REFERENCES

1. Berlin, N. I.: Diagnosis and classification of the polycythemias. Semin. Hematol., *12*:337, 1975.
2. Cardamone, J. M., Edson, J. R., McArthur, J. R., and Jacob, H. S.: Abnormalities of platelet function in the myeloproliferative disorders. J.A.M.A., *221*:270, 1972.
3. Ellis, J. T., Silver, R. T., Coleman, M., et al.: The bone marrow in polycythemia vera. Semin. Hematol., *12*:433, 1975.
4. Fitts, W. T., Jr., Erde, A., Peskin, G. W., and Frost, J. W.: Surgical implications of polycythemia vera. Ann. Surg., *151*:548, 1960.
5. Jacob, H. S.: The polycythemias and their relationship to erythropoietin. Disease-a-Month, August, 1974, p. 19.
6. Laszlo, J.: Myeloproliferative disorders. Semin. Hematol., *12*:409, 1975.
7. Osler, W.: Chronic cyanosis with polycythemia and enlarged spleen. A new clinical entity. Am. J. Med. Sci., *12*:187, 1903.
8. Silverstein, M. N.: The evolution into the treatment of late stage polycythemia vera. Semin. Hematol., *13*:79, 1976.
9. Vaquez, M. H.: Concerning a special form of cyanosis with accompanying excessive and persistent polycythemia. C. R. Soc. Biol., *49*:384, 1892.
10. Wasserman, L. R.: The treatment of polycythemia vera. Semin. Hematol., *13*:57, 1976.
11. Wasserman, L. R., and Gilbert, H. S.: Surgery in polycythemia vera. N. Engl. J. Med., *269*:1226, 1963.
12. Zanzani, E. D.: Hematopoietic factors in polycythemia vera. Semin. Hematol., *13*:1, 1976.

7

METABOLISM IN SURGICAL PATIENTS: PROTEIN, CARBOHYDRATE, AND FAT UTILIZATION BY ORAL AND PARENTERAL ROUTES

Stanley J. Dudrick, M.D., and Jonathan E. Rhoads, M.D.

The metabolic status of the patient has become the critical factor in an increasing number of surgical decisions. The health of the patient clearly exerts a major influence upon the ultimate outcome of a surgical procedure. It often determines whether a larger curative operation can be attempted safely as opposed to a smaller palliative operation, and, indeed, whether an operation can be undertaken at all.

Changes in blood volume are considered in detail in the chapter on shock. Alterations in electrolyte concentrations and composition of the various fluid compartments of the body are discussed in Chapter 4. This chapter will focus upon the nutrient requirements and nutritional status of the patient. The assessment of overall metabolic status, the disease factors that affect it, the operative factors that influence it, and the effects of nutritional deficits on the incidence of complications will be considered. With this information as a background, the several methods of preventing, correcting, or compensating for these deficits will be presented, with special emphasis on intravenous hyperalimentation.

Evaluation of Nutritional Status

Preoperative evaluation of the cardiovascular, pulmonary, hepatic, and renal functions, together with an assessment of the hematologic status and physiologic age, is performed routinely in the preparation of a patient for operation in order to minimize operative and postoperative risks. However, an equally critical, though sometimes disregarded, factor affecting surgical judgment is the nutritional condition of the patient. Nutritional status is very important in surgery because certain forms of malnutrition increase the morbidity and mortality of operations; because particular types of surgical procedures necessitate periods of relative or complete starvation preoperatively and/or

postoperatively; and because specific pathological conditions or lesions that have caused or contributed to the state of malnutrition often require operative therapy. Moreover, accidental or surgical trauma precipitates the catabolic response described by Cuthbertson and his associates in 1935,[5] promoting excessive nitrogen losses and accentuating any existing protein deficits.

Certain specific nutritional problems that occur less frequently in other disciplines of medicine often confront the surgeon. There may be prolonged periods of time during which patients cannot be fed by mouth or by intestinal tube because of bowel obstruction, primary gastrointestinal disease, peritonitis, or other alimentary tract conditions. Such patients usually require parenteral means of nourishment. Other patients may have sustained major burns, soft tissue trauma, or large metabolic losses. Protein-rich exudates from the mucosal surface of extensive areas of inflamed bowel or from indolent infected wounds can cause rapid and severe depletion of body stores of protein. Still other patients can be nutritionally depleted by the seemingly autonomous metabolic demands of malignant tumors and systemic infection.

An adequate understanding of the nutritional aspects of surgery requires a knowledge of the "normal" requirements for carbohydrate, fat, protein, electrolytes, and micronutrients such as vitamins and trace elements, together with some appreciation of the ways in which surgical diseases, trauma, operations, and complications alter the usual requirements for these nutrients.

Potential Dangers of Inadequate Nutrition

Although much emphasis of recent studies of nutrition has been placed on the primacy of proteins or their building blocks—the amino acids and peptides—the effects secondary to a deficiency of protein and the effects secondary to a deficiency of total calories in the diet cannot be easily separated under clinical conditions. Because both carbohydrate and fat can spare protein, they can significantly affect nitrogen balance. Although there have been many demonstrations of the high degree to which carbohydrates can spare protein, the degree to which fats are able to spare protein is significantly less, but remains incompletely defined. However, recent work in surgical patients fed intravenously has confirmed work done orally in rats more than three decades ago by showing again that calories added to a dietary regimen as fat do not significantly increase nitrogen retention above that which is achieved by the carbohydrate and amino acid components of the diet alone.

Jones and Eaton[15] were among the first to call attention to the frequent development of hypoproteinemia in postoperative patients and the sensitivity of such patients to large quantities of intravenous saline. Subsequently, Mecray, Barden, and Ravdin[16] defined an inverse relationship between the serum protein concentration and the gastric emptying time in dogs and in patients. Serial roentgenographic studies revealed that this effect was not limited to the stomach alone, but was also evident in the small intestine by the prolonged transit time of a barium meal from the pylorus to the cecum in hypoproteinemic subjects. During their studies on hypoproteinemic dogs, wound dehiscence was encountered quite frequently, and experiments directed toward the explanation of this phenomenon disclosed that the hypoproteinemic animals were disposed to disruption of abdominal wounds.[24] Histologic examination revealed a marked delay in fibroplasia with concomitant impaired wound healing in these animals. Restoration of serum proteins to normal levels on the day the test wound was made led to prompt wound healing and normal histologic appearance.

In experimental animals rendered hypoproteinemic by repeated plasmapheresis, a reduced blood volume will result, and it has been shown that these animals are predisposed to hemorrhagic shock. An average blood loss of only 26 ml. per kilogram body weight will produce a degree of shock comparable to that caused by the loss of 45 ml. of blood per kilogram body weight in normal animals.[19] The clinical counterpart of this observation has been noted frequently in man.

Interference with the appearance of calcified bone callus following experimental fractures of the ulnas of hypoproteinemic dogs has been verified by serial roentgenograms[22] and histologic examination. Other effects of hypoproteinemia include depression of bone marrow activity and atrophy of the spleen and lymphoid tissue, resulting in anemia and leukopenia.

Impaired antibody production[4] and possible decreased resistance to infection[28] have been shown to occur in the presence of hypoproteinemia. However, the interrelationships between host resistance to infection and hypoproteinemia are complex and poorly defined. Indeed, some investigators have accumulated data that indicate that under certain conditions, malnutrition appears to increase resistance to some forms of infection. It has been a clinical impression that the incidence and severity of infection are increased in malnourished patients, and studies are available that directly correlate infectious complications with hypoproteinemia in man.[21] However, these studies do not establish unequivocally which element was present first. It seems that hypoproteinemia is often an unfavorable factor as far as susceptibility to infection is concerned but that the host has considerable capacity to resist many pathologic organisms even in states of moderately advanced protein depletion. In ongoing clinical studies in our institutions, normal serum levels of immunoglobins A, G, and M were noted in adult patients with severe anorexia, weight loss, and hypoalbuminemia, but lymphocyte proliferative responses and delayed skin reactivity to primary and secondary antigens were depressed. Both responses improved significantly within 18 days of nutritional rehabilitation intravenously.

Protein malnutrition may result in a number of other adverse effects. The resistance of the liver to various toxic agents may be lowered,[20] and susceptibility to trauma may be increased. Reduction in several hepatic oxidative enzyme activities has been demonstrated in starvation, although the cytochrome oxidases tend to be fairly well preserved. An increased morbidity and delayed postoperative convalescence as well as an increased operative mortality rate are associated with lack of adequate protein intake. Decubitus ulcers in patients who are confined to bed and not turned frequently are most likely to develop in those who are undernourished. The poor nutritional status of such patients is aggravated by the negative nitrogen balance that is often associated with inactivity or immobilization. Urine output can be significantly reduced, and excessive water can be retained. Subjectively, protein depletion for even relatively short periods of time can cause weakness, lassitude, and an impaired feeling of well-being.

It has been evident clinically that starvation alone is rarely the sole cause for impaired wound healing, impaired fracture healing, impaired granulation tissue formation, or wound dehiscence. The vast majority of the failures of the healing process are related to either local wound complications, inadequate visceral decompression, other concomitant systemic diseases, vitamin deficiencies, or errors in technique. Conversely, protein anabolism is rarely achieved in the presence of an open or unhealed wound. The best examples of this are observed in the management of compound fractures or major burns. Conscientious attention to the wound and to the diet simultaneously will yield the best results.

It is not generally appreciated that prolonged protein depletion will have a rather profound adverse effect on pulmonary function and ventilatory capacity. Death from starvation is most often manifested as death from pneumonia. An explanation for this is that, except for the serum proteins and so-called labile proteins, there are no body depots of spare protein. Each molecule of proteins serves a purpose, e. g., as part of a contractile element in muscle, as an enzyme, or as part of the cell membrane or intracellular contents of all cells. Loss of protein, therefore, is necessarily accompanied by some loss of essential function.

Skeletal muscle, for example, which performs many important functions in the body, also is the chief source of protein lost in starvation. However, it is a poor source of fuel, yielding only 4 calories per gram of dry protein oxidized. The respiratory complications that occur in malnourished patients are often secondary to the loss of strength and function of the abdominal, intercostal, shoulder, and diaphragmatic muscles. As a result of muscle weakness, full ventilatory excursions are not maintained, the vigor and ability to expel mucus is lowered, and bronchial exudates accumulate excessively. Furthermore, the hypoproteinemia favors the development of both interstitial edema and bronchial secretions. It must be emphasized that just as the resumption of protein anabolism is necessary for muscular integrity, conversely, protein catabolism takes its toll in terms of muscular performance, and this decline of function is most critical in those muscles that surround the thorax.

Muscle protein constitutes by far the greatest mass of body protein. The total amount of muscle protein varies with the size of the individual, but in the average adult it accounts for approximately 30 per cent of the body weight. Inasmuch as 80 per cent of the weight of muscle is made up of water, the actual amount of anhydrous muscle protein present in an average man is approximately 4000 gm. This is in contrast to the 245 gm. of total plasma protein and 350 gm. of liver protein. During bed rest, skeletal muscle protein may be considered physiologically useless except as it is used for respiration. It can also be used as an excellent source of protein by the rest of the body whenever the dietary intake is inadequate. Although this concept is attractive and somewhat popular, deprivation of dietary protein is quickly followed not only by utilization of muscle protein, but by the concomitant consumption of other body proteins as well. All endogenous proteins seem to be susceptible to utilization in supplying the daily catabolic needs, including those that play important metabolic roles, such as the plasma proteins, digestive enzymes, and liver enzymes. During starvation there seems to be no selective use of muscle protein or other stores of protein except, perhaps, those in the liver and plasma. Muscular activity may increase neither the requirement for nor the breakdown of protein, and there is little if any, difference in the needs for protein nourishment whether the individual is active or at bed rest, provided that his energy requirements are met by fat and carbohydrate.[3] As a matter of fact, there is a considerable loss of muscle protein during bed rest, and especially during skeletal immobilization, because of the atrophy of disuse. It might be expected that this breakdown of muscle protein would yield amino acids or nitrogenous moieties of value in other areas of higher priority to the body. However, there is no sound evidence that such is the case, and apparently most of these catabolic metabolites are not utilized elsewhere but are lost in the urine primarily as urea.

Plasma contains a number of different proteins, many of which perform very important physiologic activities. As there is approximately 3500 ml. of plasma in the normal adult, and the total plasma protein concentration is about 7 gm. per 100 ml., the total amount of plasma protein can be readily calculated at 245 gm. From the standpoint of protein nutrition, the albumin fraction of plasma protein is of the greatest significance, primarily because in most surgical diseases, it is the fraction that is characteristically most adversely affected. Indeed, many of the clinical manifestations in both acute and chronic protein deficiency states occur secondarily to the decreased colloid osmotic pressure associated with hypoalbuminemia. The albumin fraction contributes approximately 85 per cent of the total colloidal osmotic pressure because its molecular weight is 70,000, in contrast to the much larger globulin molecules, and because its concentration is nearly twice that of globulin in normal plasma. The importance of albumin in delicately balancing capillary filtration pressure, thus maintaining the integrity of the microcirculation and controlling fluid interchange across the capillary wall in accordance with Starling's hypothesis, cannot be overemphasized.

The plasma globulins serve entirely different functions from albumin. For example, gamma globulin, which is probably synthesized in the reticuloendothelial system, is undoubtedly concerned with immunologic mechanisms and infection control. On the other hand, fibrinogen and prothrombin, which are synthesized in the liver like albumin, function in the coagulation mechanism. Further discussion of the other plasma proteins is beyond the scope of this chapter.

Although plasma proteins represent a small portion of the total body protein, a quantitative relationship is constantly maintained between plasma and body proteins in both health and disease. During protein starvation, the losses from plasma albumin and protein from the rest of the body have a relatively constant and definite relationship of approximately 1 to 30,[11] and this same partition of body protein occurs during the anabolism that occurs after protein alimentation. In other words, for each gram of plasma albumin lost or gained, 30 gm. of tissue protein is lost or gained, respectively, during protein starvation or feeding.

Inasmuch as the normal adult has approximately 7000 ml. of whole blood, which contains 15 gm. per 100 ml. of hemoglobin, more than 1000 gm. of body protein is in the form of hemoglobin. Unlike the extracellular circulating plasma proteins, hemoglobin is intracellular, and therefore undergoes metabolic degradation much more slowly. Thus, hemoglobin is depleted rather late in protein starvation, and apparently both iron and protein are conserved for the maintenance of red blood cells at a time when plasma proteins have become significantly depleted.

The relationship of the liver to protein metabolism is of paramount importance but is only partially understood. In the average adult, the liver normally weighs approximately 1500 to 2000 gm. and contains about 350 gm. of protein. However, the total protein content of the liver varies according to the type and quantity of dietary protein and greatly influences hepatic function. Whenever the supply of protein is inadequate in the diet, liver protein is not conserved, but is drawn upon from the very beginning of protein malnutrition. However, sublethal resection of the liver in rats results in anabolism in the liver at the expense of other body tissues. In animals, considerable histologic changes occur in the liver after even a short period of protein deprivation. In man, inadequate protein intake together with a high calorie-to-protein dietary ratio (>200:1) can result in extensive fatty metamorphosis and impaired function of the liver as manifested by kwashiorkor in children and as a complication of jejunoileal bypass procedures in some adults. The many functions of the liver accentuate the importance of protecting this master organ as much as possible by preventing protein depletion.

Mechanism of Protein Loss

Protein is lost from the body by one or more of several different routes, some of them normal, and others as a result of disease. The loss of body protein that occurs as the result of tissue catabolism can be measured readily by collecting the entire 24-hour urine, stool, and other output, and determining the nitrogen content of all of the excrement. A good reflection of the degree of protein catabolism can thus be derived because all body protein, when broken down, is excreted largely in the urine as simple nitrogenous compounds such as urea and ammonia. When there is no nitrogen intake in the diet, all of the nitrogen in the urine necessarily originates from tissue protein catabolism. Under ordinary dietary conditions, much of the nitrogen in the urine originates from the portion of dietary protein that was not utilized for the synthesis of tissue protein. Addition of protein to the diet is always followed by an increase in the nitrogen excretion in the urine. In order to estimate net tissue protein losses, it is necessary to subtract the nitrogen intake from the nitrogen output. It is obvious that if a patient's nitrogen output equals his nitrogen intake, he is in balance, and is not being depleted of protein. If nitrogen output exceeds nitrogen intake, the patient is in negative nitrogen balance, and the degree of negative nitrogen balance is a fairly accurate quantitative measurement of the amount of protein tissue that is being broken down and lost. Conversely, when nitrogen intake exceeds nitrogen output, the patient is in positive nitrogen balance, which is a good indication of the degree to which protein synthesis is occurring. To quantify the actual skeletal protein breakdown more precisely, 3-methyl histidine, a nonreutilizable product of muscle degradation, can be measured in the urine.

Most of the body proteins contain about 16 per cent nitrogen. By dividing 16 into 100, a constant (6.25) can be derived. By multiplying the total nitrogen gain or loss by 6.25, the actual weight of protein gain or loss can be simply calculated. To determine the equivalent weight of lean wet tissue, such as muscle, it is necessary to multiply 6.25×5, because muscle protein is bound to four volumes of water by weight.[11] Thus, a rough factor can be derived to equate 1 gm. of nitrogen to about 30 gm. of muscle tissue.

During the course of normal metabolism, the body is constantly building up and breaking down protein. When buildup exceeds breakdown, the body is in a state of anabolism, and when breakdown exceeds buildup, the body is in a state of catabolism. During the normal catabolic processes of the body, there is a loss of protein tissue that has been described as physiologic or endogenous. In the average adult, this tissue turnover amounts to approximately 4 gm. of nitrogen per day, or the equivalent of 120 gm. of wet muscle tissue.

Whenever an inadequate amount of carbohydrate is supplied in the diet, tissue protein will be broken down, apparently to provide substrates for gluconeogenesis. Such protein losses can be prevented almost entirely by the ingestion of adequate calories, preferably as carbohydrates, thus sparing the protein. The amount of protein lost in this manner varies under differing conditions, but even during complete starvation, only approximately 13 per cent of the calories is provided by catabolism of tissue protein.

Extensive tissue protein losses accompany the peculiar, poorly understood phenomenon known as the catabolic response. This inordinate destruction of tissue protein has been observed after major surgical operations and extensive trauma, especially burns and long bone fractures, and during sepsis. The magnitude of this protein loss may approach 30 gm. or more of nitrogen a day, or the equivalent of approximately 2 pounds of muscle tissue.

In addition to catabolic losses, protein can be lost directly as such in a wide variety of conditions, the simplest being hemorrhage. In addition to the erythrocyte protein, a liter of whole blood contains about 35 to 40 gm. of plasma protein. Extensive protein losses can also occur in conditions in which plasma or other protein-containing fluids escape. For example, in burns, large quantities of plasma protein are lost from the circulation into the injured tissues as well as from the weeping surfaces. Such wound losses have been quantitated in amounts as high as 50 gm. of protein a day. With intestinal obstruction or general peritonitis, large amounts of protein are lost into the wall of the bowel and from the extensive surface of peritoneum into the abdominal cavity. With pneumonia, large losses of protein occur into the alveoli and interstitium of the lungs and with empyema, into the pleural cavities. Major crush injuries to soft tissue result in losses of plasma protein into the traumatized areas. In extensive infections, considerable protein is lost in the exudate and pus.

Significant loss of nitrogen in the urine accompanies disuse atrophy of the skeletal structures, primarily bone and muscle. It is probable that this component of nitrogen loss cannot always be reversed by provision of adequate dietary protein alone, but must be combated by exercise of the involved muscle as well.

One or more of these mechanisms of protein loss are present to some extent in all surgical patients. Quantitatively, protein depletion can be tremendous, and as much as 40 gm. of nitrogen has been measured in the urine in the course of 24 hours. In a patient not receiving any dietary protein, this represents a daily loss of more than 250 gm. of protein or 1250 gm. of muscle tissue. In addition, there may be protein losses of 10 to 50 gm. as a result of hemorrhage and wound exudates. Thus, in critical surgical conditions, it is possible for a patient to lose more than 3 pounds of muscle tissue or its equivalent in the course of a day. It should not be surprising, therefore, that tremendous body wasting often occurs after major trauma or operation. It is obvious that daily protein requirements will vary greatly under different conditions in different people. Normally, a daily ration of about 10 gm. of nitrogen, equivalent to 62.5 gm. of protein, will promote positive nitrogen balance and prevent protein malnutrition. The normal protein requirement of a well-balanced diet is about 1 gm. per kilogram of body weight. This figure will vary slightly depending upon the quality or biologic value of the protein ingested. It has been shown that the body can assimilate as much as 10 gm. of protein per kilogram body weight per day, which would amount to about 700 gm. of protein equivalent and to more than 100 gm. of nitrogen in the average adult.[12] This probably represents the practical maximum of protein utilization by man.

Protein requirements differ from water and electrolyte requirements in that chronic deficiencies of protein are cumulative and may exist for long periods of time. Inadequate protein intake leads immediately and inevitably to tissue wasting, which appears to be fairly well tolerated by the body. This is probably the major reason why the importance of providing protein needs is so frequently overlooked by physicians.

In a chronically protein-depleted patient, it is not uncommon that body weight loss approximates 25 to 30 pounds in a few weeks. It is an unfortunate truth that many such cases develop while in the hospital during medical or surgical treatment. If one estimates that one third of a 15-kg. loss in body weight has been from muscle, and that 20 per cent of wet muscle is protein, the simple calculation of 0.2 × 5 kg. muscle would yield 1 kg. of protein.

Although it would be possible theoretically to replace the deficit of 1000 gm. of protein parenterally by the administration of 100 to 300 gm. of protein a day for a period of one or more weeks, it may well be that such complete replacement is not actually necessary. On the other hand, it should be emphasized that such deficits should be corrected as rapidly and as completely as possible by the administration of such protein nourishment as is convenient and feasible. Obviously, the improvement in the patient's nutritional status will be considerable even if only one fourth to one third of this deficit is corrected. As great as one half of the protein deficit may be corrected without inordinately prolonging the period of preoperative preparation. Extended deferment of operation is not justifiable in the presence of malignant disease because extirpation of neoplastic lesions should be accomplished as soon as possible. On the other hand, total parenteral nutrition may be given coincidentally with decompression of the stomach, chemotherapy, bowel preparation, or other indicated preoperative procedures that may necessarily delay operation anyway.

In order to regenerate cellular protoplasm, the importance of simultaneously providing adequate quantities of essential calories, electrolytes, trace minerals, and other micronutrients cannot be overlooked, and these requirements (Table 1) and their relationships to protein synthesis will be discussed in subsequent sections of this chapter.

Body Composition and Energy Stores

The ability of the patient to meet the energy requirements exacted by severe trauma, major

TABLE 1. Requirements of Basic Nutrients per Kilogram Body Weight

	Basal	Hypermetabolic (Trauma, Sepsis)
Water	25–35 ml.	50–70 ml.
Calories	25–30 Cal.	40–70 Cal.
Protein	0.9–1.9 gm.	1.5–3.5 gm.
Carbohydrate	2 gm.	4–6 gm.
Fat	2 gm.	3–5 gm.

surgery, sepsis, or starvation, alone or in combination, depends entirely upon the total body stores of potential energy and biochemically active substrates, the capacity of the patient to mobilize and to utilize these stores, and the extent to which exogenous essential nutrients can be provided, assimilated, and used to prevent depletion of body stores. Latent body sources of fuel are stored in a rather dormant form as neutral fat or glycogen, and in a dynamic form as protein. Fat in human adipose tissue is stored in essentially water-free form, yields approximately 9 calories per gram, and is available in abundant quantities in the majority of the American population. A limited amount of carbohydrate is stored in the body in the form of muscle and liver glycogen. In the average patient, approximately 200 gm. of glycogen is present in the body reserves, approximately two thirds in the muscle and one third in the liver, most of which is completely utilized within 18 to 24 hours of complete starvation. Although most carbohydrates yield approximately 4 calories per gram, each gram of glycogen, which is stored with 1 or 2 gm. of intracellular water and electrolytes, yields only 1 to 2 calories per gram, and is thus a relatively small source of energy. As emphasized earlier, protein is not stored as a static source of nitrogen or energy, but serves an essential function as a part of an enzyme, oncotic molecule, cell, or muscle. Pure animal protein, which yields 4.25 calories per gram, is stored in the body mostly in the form of skeletal muscle, which yields only 1 calorie per gram when oxidized.

According to a recent report by Cahill,[3] an average man in the resting state who normally consumes up to 1800 calories a day will break down about 75 gm. of protein, mostly from skeletal muscle, and about 160 gm. of triglyceride from adipose tissue, when fasting for 24 hours (Table 2). During this time, he will also excrete 12 to 15 gm. of nitrogen in his urine, mostly in the form of urea, and will lose approximately 500 gm. of body weight.[18] Glycogen stores will yield about 180 gm. of endogenous glucose, most of which will be utilized by the brain and central nervous system, and will be completely oxidized to carbon dioxide and water in the process. A small fraction of the glucose from glycogen catabolism will be used by other tissues such as the bone marrow, red blood cells, white blood cells, kidneys, and striated muscle. This portion of glucose is converted primarily to lactate and pyruvate, returned to the liver, and resynthesized into glucose

TABLE 2. Body Composition of "Normal Man"*
(70 kg.)

Kg.	Components	Caloric Equivalent
48.7	Water and minerals	0
15.0	Fat (adipose triglyceride)	141,000
6.0	Protein (mainly muscle)	24,000
0.150	Glycogen (muscle)	600
0.075	Glycogen (liver)	300
	Subtotal	165,900
0.020	Glucose (extracellular fluid)	80
0.0003	Free fatty acids (plasma)	3
0.003	Triglycerides (plasma)	30
~70.	Total	166,013

*Modified from Cahill, G. F.: N. Engl. J. Med., 282:669, 1970.

via the Cori cycle. The glycerol and the glucogenic amino acids are also converted into glucose by the liver, which uses fatty acids as its own primary energy source. The rest of the body tissues also use either fatty acids or partially oxidized fatty acids for energy. Because glucose cannot be synthesized from fatty acids directly, use of fatty acids and ketones by most of the body tissues in effect spares protein as a glucogenic precursor by reducing glucose requirements. In a well-nourished person during complete starvation, about 87 per cent of the caloric requirement is derived from tissue fat and about 13 per cent of the caloric need is derived from tissue protein. This amount of tissue protein is apparently the minimum required to provide glucose by neogenesis, without which metabolism of fat would produce ketosis. The body tends to utilize tissue fat and to conserve tissue protein as much as possible. A daily ration of about 100 to 150 gm. of glucose, providing 350 to 500 calories, will prevent ketosis, will spare the catabolism of tissue protein, and will reduce the average urinary nitrogen losses by about 50 per cent. It is of significance to note that even when exogenous calories are provided in quantities sufficient to effect maximal endogenous protein sparing, reducing daily nitrogen losses from an average of 12 to 15 gm. a day to as little as 4 gm. of nitrogen a day (equivalent to 25 gm. of protein or 150 gm. of muscle), death will result in most patients secondary to protein loss and muscle weakness before all of the adipose tissue stores are depleted.

CAUSES OF INADEQUATE NUTRITION

Preoperative Deficiencies

Currently, in this country, nutritional deficiencies are usually not secondary to lack of availability of foodstuff, but rather result from a variety of defects in individual patients. The most frequent causes of malnutrition today are related not only to inadequate quantity but also to inadequate quality of dietary nutrients. For example, unbalanced, incomplete diets are still encountered among exclusively milk-fed infants, food faddists, and persons on self-imposed, poorly conceived, weight-losing diets. Causes of deficient food intake in our increasingly enlarging geriatric population include lack of teeth, poor oral hygiene, poor dentures, and meager finances. Additional factors contributing to malnutrition include dietary idiosyncrasies, inactivity, drug addiction, alcoholism, and chronic illness with associated anorexia. Obstructing lesions of the alimentary tract such as pyloric stenosis, atresia, neoplasia, ulceration, or cicatrization can cause insufficient ingestion of nutrients directly or as a result of vomiting.

Endocrinologic diseases or disorders that result in hyperthyroidism, hyperparathyroidism, hypopituitarism, or hypoadrenalism impair nutritional status primarily by altering the metabolic rate or by causing anorexia, nausea, or vomiting. Fever secondary to acute infections and other causes also increases the metabolic rate, significantly increasing caloric requirements. Metabolism increases approximately 7 per cent per degree Fahrenheit, and in some febrile patients, it has been shown that it is necessary to exceed the theoretical caloric requirement by 50 to 110 per cent in order to bring the patient into nitrogen and weight equilibrium. Other factors such as pregnancy and lactation can also significantly alter basal caloric requirements by altering metabolic rate.

Interference with the normal digestive and absorptive processes of the gastrointestinal tract constitutes a major nutritional problem in surgical patients. Deficiencies of digestive enzymes may allow food to pass through the alimentary tract unabsorbed and be lost in the stool. Obstruction of the common bile duct by a calculus or neoplasm with the resultant absence of bile in the alimentary canal leads eventually to improper digestion and reduced absorption of fats and fat-soluble vitamins. Chronic pancreatitis, mucoviscidosis, and malignant disease may result in deficiencies of the pancreatic enzymes so essential for adequate hydrolysis of ingested carbohydrate, protein, and fat. Bowel hypermotility with diarrhea can cause enormous deficits, not only of water and electrolytes, but also of vitamins and other nutrients, by decreasing the transit time through the small intestine, where the major digestive and absorptive processes take place. Other examples of pathologic conditions that may be accompanied by malabsorption and that may eventually require surgical intervention are regional enteritis, ulcerative or granulomatous colitis, blind loops or diverticula, and parasitic infestations. Shunting of partially digested nutriment through external or internal fistulas can prevent proper nutrient absorption and assimilation with significant losses from the body despite even a very large oral intake. Vitamin deficiencies of the fat- and water-soluble type as well as secondary hypocalcemia and hypomagnesemia may attend any of these conditions.

Despite normal ingestion, digestion, and absorption, malnutrition can be manifest in diseases that interfere with proper utilization of foods. In patients with hepatic insufficiency secondary to hepatitis, hepatoma, cirrhosis, or other liver diseases, the metabolism of carbohydrates, fats, and proteins can be severely impaired. This is true also in glycogen storage disease and in untreated or decompensated diabetes mellitus.

Insidious loss of protein from the body is another important contributing factor to malnutrition. This may occur in patients with carcinoma of the alimentary tract, giant hypertrophic gastritis (Menetrier's disease), regional enteritis, and ulcerative colitis. Chronic overt or occult hemorrhage from the gastrointestinal or genitourinary tract may result in significant protein losses because each 100 ml. of blood is approximately equivalent to 3 gm. of nitrogen or to 19 gm. of protein. Massive albuminuria in nephrosis may severely deplete body protein stores rapidly. Chronic suppuration from draining sinus tracts, large open wounds, and oozing burn surfaces can also contribute significantly to protein malnutrition. Protein losses can also follow prolonged gastrointestinal suction, repeated paracentesis or thoracentesis, and, as previously mentioned, prolonged vomiting or diarrhea. A large, rapidly growing neoplasm can act like a parasite to deprive the body of exogenous and endogenous nutrient substrates, leading to hypoproteinemia. Some of the reported preoperative nitrogen losses in various surgical patients are partially quantitated in Table 3.

A patient who is a candidate for operation often has medical disorders that are related directly or indirectly to his surgical problem and either have required or will require preoperative therapeutic measures. Potassium depletion, sodium retention, and negative nitrogen balance characteristically attend the use of systemic corticosteroids. Water losses induced by diuretics may be accompanied by potassium and sodium deficits as well as losses of water-soluble vitamins. Use of broad-spectrum antibiotics for treatment for preoperative infections or for bowel preparation can alter or even destroy the normal intestinal flora, thereby interfering with the bacterial production of vitamin K in the intestine and the absorption of some of the B-complex vitamins. Anorexia, vomiting, and diarrhea are other complications of antibiotic therapy that can result in a substandard nutritional state.

Losses During Surgery

The most significant measurable protein loss that occurs during surgery is secondary to hemorrhage. Additional plasma protein losses occur in response to tissue trauma. Examples of the extent of nitrogen losses

TABLE 3. Nitrogen Losses in Various Conditions Before Operation

	Average Nitrogen Loss	Time Period
Small bowel obstruction	11.0 gm.	1 day
Major thermal burns	630.0 gm.	3 weeks
Surface exudate	7.8 gm.	1 day
Total nitrogen excretion	40.0 gm.	1 day
Bleeding peptic ulcer	90.7 gm.	5 days
Long bone fracture	137.0 gm.	10 days
Multiple fractures	190.0 gm.	2–3 weeks
Total starvation	56.0 gm.	4 days
	248.0 gm.	31 days

TABLE 4. Nitrogen Losses in Various Conditions During Operation*

	Nitrogen Loss in Grams			
	Minimum	Average	Maximum	Total Cases
Thyroidectomy	3	12	21	8
Abdomino-perineal resection	6	12	21	12
Complicated gastric operations	9	18	24	3
Thoracoplasty	12	23	60	10
Pneumonectomy	21	57	108	16
Radical mastectomy	15	24	32	4

*Assuming 3 gm. of nitrogen per 100 ml. blood

associated with various operative procedures are outlined in Table 4. Because the caloric requirement usually increases or decreases by 5 per cent for every 10° C change in environmental temperature, excessive caloric expenditure can occur during long operations in air-conditioned operating theaters, especially in infants and children. Water and electrolyte derangements that occur during lengthy operative procedures have been known to occur, but their effects on the nutritional status of the patient are generally transitory and easily corrected.

Losses After Injury and Operation

The pioneer work of Cuthbertson[5] first demonstrated the "catabolic response" to injury in man, although the phenomenon had been observed previously in laboratory animals by Whipple.[26] Subsequently, it has been shown that protein catabolism consistently occurs immediately after operation or injury, accompanied by markedly increased excretions of potassium and nitrogen in the urine. During this immediate post-trauma period, a negative balance may persist despite a large protein intake. Generally, this response lasts two to five days, but varies in intensity and duration with the type and extent of injury, and may last several weeks after major complicated surgical procedures. Postoperative nitrogen losses following various types of surgical procedures are given in Table 5. It has been a frequent observation that the amount of nitrogen loss in an undernourished patient is less than in a well-nourished patient after comparable degrees of trauma. Thus, it appears that the extent to which the body will mobilize nitrogen from protein stores depends in part upon the size of the endogenous protein mass.

The true significance of the catabolic response remains debatable. Some have regarded it teleologically as an attempt on the part of the body to rid itself of excess nitrogen at a time when its presence might in some way be harmful. They hold the view that this phenomenon neither requires nor is amenable to cor-

TABLE 5. Nitrogen Losses in Various Conditions after Operation

	Average Nitrogen Loss	Time Period
Radical mastectomy	15 gm.	10 days
Inguinal herniorrhaphy	18 gm.	10 days
Perforated appendicitis	49 gm.	10 days
Subtotal gastrectomy	54 gm.	5 days
Subtrochanteric osteotomy	65 gm.	2 weeks
Vagotomy and pyloroplasty	75 gm.	5 days
Cholecystectomy	114 gm.	10 days
Suture of perforated peptic ulcer	136 gm.	10 days
Gastrectomy	175 gm.	10 days

rection. Others believe that the catabolic response to injury, including the negative nitrogen balance in the immediate postoperative period, is a physiologic attempt to mobilize tissue nitrogen because of increased requirements for specific protein moieties. In support of this hypothesis are data that imply that the mobilization of protein stores is important after liver injury. There is histologic evidence available to show that injury to the livers of experimental animals subjected to toxic doses of chloroform was reduced if the animals were already in a catabolic state produced by inflammation resulting from hypodermic injections of sodium ricinoleate.[20] In this experiment, it appeared that the injured liver actually benefited as a result of the pre-existing state of protein catabolism. This led to the observation that diets high in protein and very high in carbohydrate protected the liver against noxious agents. If this is a general phenomenon and not peculiarly related to the liver, food nitrogen intake should be augmented after injury in order to provide the body with additional protein substrates. Still others believe that the protein is mobilized and oxidized in an attempt to satisfy increased caloric requirements following trauma. The energy produced by catabolism of endogenous protein stores under these conditions, however, is only a small fraction of total caloric expenditure, and this explanation seems inadequate to explain fully the phenomenon observed. The lysis and reabsorption of injured tissue such as torn muscle and extravasated blood about a fracture and the atrophy of disuse are other probable contributory factors to the catabolic response.

There has been general agreement that vigorous measures should be employed to induce positive nitrogen balance in the surgical patient after the severe catabolic phase of the immediate postoperative or post-trauma period is over. The authors believe that there is no reason to wait and that positive nitrogen balance frequently can be maintained in the face of injury of operation by means that will be described later in this chapter.

Massive small bowel resection following mesenteric venous or arterial occlusion, volvulus, or multiple operations for adhesions or granulomatous disease constitutes a particularly difficult nutritional handicap in that it not only inflicts a metabolic insult of great magnitude, but reduces vital areas for the absorption of food. It often requires meticulous attention, patience, and ingenuity in order to provide the patient with adequate nutrients to allow him to withstand this massive insult and to assist his residual short gut to compensate.

EVALUATION OF NUTRITIONAL STATUS

Evidence of malnutrition may not be apparent on casual clinical examination. However, an accurate evaluation of the nutritional status of the surgical patient can be obtained readily from a carefully directed history, physical examination, and series of laboratory studies. The data assembled may be very helpful in planning preoperative and postoperative nutritional regimens specifically for each patient.

History

An accurate determination of the dietary intake of the patient is most important in evaluating the nutritional status, especially as it relates to the degree and time course of weight loss. Other helpful points include the presence or absence of anorexia, diarrhea, dysphagia, nausea, vomiting, lethargy, loss of vitality, and decreased sense of well-being. A pointed systemic view and past medical history may elicit other signs, symptoms, or causes of malnutrition. An idea of the social and economic status of the patient is essential in determining the quality and quantity of food he may usually ingest. In some instances, the age of the patient is important in evaluating the dietary history, especially in the geriatric population.

Physical Examination

Although apparently well nourished, a patient may be in a state of negative nitrogen balance and relative malnutrition as a result of a recent or current catabolic pathologic process. Careful examination of a rather healthy-appearing person may reveal that his tissues are edematous as a result of hypoproteinemia. On the other hand, a severe case of malnutrition is easily recognized by the loose inelastic skin, loss of subcutaneous fat, atrophy of muscle mass, hepatomegaly, and massive peripheral edema. Diagnosis of specific vitamin or mineral deficiencies can often be made by recognition of characteristic signs on physical examination. Quite commonly, however, protein malnutrition is expressed very subtly, and specific deficiencies are masked. In such cases, clinical anthropometric measurements such as the triceps skin-fold thickness, mid upper arm circumference, mid upper arm muscle circumference, and height-creatinine index may be helpful in the clinical assessment of nutritional status.

Laboratory Examination

Biochemical and hematologic studies are usually helpful in accurately estimating the nutritional status of a patient. Determinations of the hemoglobin and hematocrit in correlation with deviations in hydration and body weight may be very useful, although both measurements can be misleading and inaccurate after recent blood loss. Routine urinalysis may reveal significant protein, sugar, or electrolyte losses. A fasting blood sugar or two-hour postprandial determination may indicate previously unsuspected diabetes mellitus. The blood urea nitrogen or nonprotein nitrogen may reflect a catabolic state or gastrointestinal bleeding in addition to helping assess the renal status. Detection of occult blood in the stool by guaiac or benzidine determinations may yield a clue to the etiology of a pathologic process that is adversely affecting nutritional status. Measurement of serum protein, albumin, and globulin levels should be obtained with the realization that these determinations can be misleading at times. The total serum protein level alone is of questionable value because a high serum globulin may mask a significant decrease in the serum albumin level. Electrophoretic fractionation of serum proteins provides more complete and reliable data than the traditional salting-out methods. Dehydration may mask hypoproteinemia to some extent by producing hemoconcentration, but a prompt fall in the serum protein level is usually observed after adequate replacement of existing water and electrolyte deficits. The critical levels of serum proteins, below which there is obligatory edema formation, have been defined as 5.5 gm. per 100 ml. for total serum proteins and 2.5 gm. per 100 ml. for albumin, the latter fraction being responsible for most of the colloid osmotic pressure of plasma. It must be appreciated, however, that there is no specific protein level below which edema fluid suddenly appears; the tendency to increase interstitial water occurs progressively as the serum protein concentrations fall over quite a broad range. There is poor correlation between serum protein levels and deviations in body weight, the serum protein levels being maintained for a considerable period after initial weight loss, and then suddenly decreasing in the latter stages of protein depletion.

Total circulating plasma protein is a more sensitive indication of protein deficiency than is the serum protein concentration. The total circulating plasma protein can be readily determined if the serum protein concentration and the plasma volume are known. Another rapidly responding index of protein nutrition can be obtained by measuring serial fasting plasma amino acid levels.[1] However, this rather tedious and expensive procedure is generally reserved for only the most complex nutritional problems.

In the presence of known or suspected hepatic disease, liver function studies should be performed because the patient with liver insufficiency is peculiarly unable to compensate well for the metabolic stresses of surgical procedures. In selected patients, it can be helpful to determine the serum lipid profile, specific individual serum vitamin levels, and serum levels of most of the biologically active electrolytes in addition to assessment of acid-base balance. Other indices which have gained increasing importance and application in the serial evaluation of nutritional status include the total lymphocyte count, serum transferrin (TIBC) level, and cellular immunity skin testing.

ROUTES OF ALIMENTATION

Other than restoring the plasma volume and red blood cell mass to normal levels, the preoperative replenishment of protein deficits is not feasible in some surgical patients because positive nitrogen balance often cannot be achieved until the required surgical procedure has been completed or because the operation cannot be safely postponed. Provided that the erythrocytes, plasma proteins, and water and electrolytes are in the proper proportion, moderate protein deficits are compatible with recovery from the stresses of major operations.

Common sense dictates that prevention of losses of body stores is equally important to providing adequate nutritional substrates. Prevention of blood loss from a gastrointestinal malignant lesion by early operation is much more sensible than attempting to reverse negative nitrogen balance in a few days with high-caloric and high-protein alimentation. Similarly, the early closure or grafting of large weeping wound or burn surfaces reduces the requirements for protein replacement. However, when protein deficiency exists in a patient with a benign lesion not requiring immediate operation, it is to his advantage to reverse his negative nitrogen balance by providing adequate nutrients enterally or parenterally or by both routes. This does not necessarily mean that his body weight or serum proteins must be restored completely to normal levels, because neither is a necessary prerequisite to achieving positive nitrogen balance. However, there are indications that morbidity and mortality rates are higher in patients whose serum albumin levels are below 3 gm. per 100 ml. In a severely depleted patient in whom a malignant neoplasm is present or suspected, attempts at preoperative restoration of positive nitrogen balance or normal body weight should not exceed a week or 10 days, for obvious reasons, if he is otherwise a satisfactory surgical candidate.

The routes available for providing nourishment are oral, rectal (nasogastric, esophagostomy, gastrostomy, jejunostomy), subcutaneous, intramedullary, intraperitoneal, intra-arterial, and intravenous.

Although it has been shown that glucose and certain protein derivatives can be absorbed from the colon, the quantities absorbed are too small to be of practical value. The rectal route for feeding has not been used extensively since the nineteenth century and is generally not recommended now.

The complications, discomfort, and limited usefulness of the subcutaneous, intraperitoneal, intramedullary, and intra-arterial routes make them impractical and undesirable avenues for nutrient administration. The other routes (oral, tube, intravenous) for providing nutrition will be discussed in some detail.

Oral Route

Fortunately, in the management of the average surgical patient who requires a major operative procedure, no significant nutritional problem exists other than providing the normal daily dietary intake. Even in patients with moderate nutritional deficiencies who may not be able to obtain nourishment orally for 5 to 7 days after operation, a complex nutritional regimen is not always required.

It must be emphasized that if alimentary tract function is normal or only moderately impaired, it is both the preferred and most effective route for supplying nutrients. Should anorexia or nausea interfere with oral food intake, such measures as physician encouragement, attentive nursing care, frequent small meals, supplementary, high-protein, interval feedings, and desirable foods served in an attractive manner can be very rewarding in improving the patient's attitude toward eating. Other measures include judicious use of ethanol-containing appetite stimulants, and the addition of desiccated bile, bile salts, or pancreatic enyzmes to the diets of patients whose endogenous supplies are inadequate. Antiemetics, tranquilizers, anticholinergics, testosterone or other anabolic agents, and therapeutic dosages of vitamins may exert a beneficial effect in selected patients. Consultation with a dietician regarding the particular dietary needs and preferences of the individual patient is frequently indicated and rewarding.

The use of chemically formulated diets of high biologic value for human nutrition is a relatively new clinical feeding technique that resulted from research efforts directed toward devising high-efficiency, bulk-free diets suitable for use in space by our astronauts. However, the use of chemically defined diets in rats has been studied extensively for many years, and these diets have been shown to support normal longevity, reproduction, growth, and lactation in these animals. The chemically formulated diets consist primarily of mixtures of purified L-amino acids derived from acid hydrolysis of casein (adjusted to restore normal amino acid profiles), carbohydrate in the form of glucose, sucrose, or a mixture of glucose and partially hydrolyzed starch, baseline requirements of electrolytes, water- and fat-soluble vitamins exclusive of vitamin K, and trace elements (Table 6). Various flavoring materials have been added to the diet to disguise the rather strong organic taste and odor inherent in amino acid mixtures. Although this is successfully accomplished at the low amino acid concentrations, the high-protein chemically formulated diets currently available are fairly unpalatable and must often be fed by tube.

The chemically formulated diets have several advantages over the usual high-calorie, high-protein supplements. They are completely bulk-free and virtually fat-free, and require minimal digestion, thus avoiding the need for most pancreatic and biliary secretions. Although stool volume is reduced because of lack of bulk, diarrhea sometimes occurs if the concentration or rate of administration is too high. The chemically formulated diets permit close physician control of caloric intake, water volume, and electrolytes. They obviate the risk of infection associated with intravenous infusions, but have the limitation of requiring at least a sufficient segment of functional small bowel to permit absorption of simple sugars and amino acids in adequate amounts.

Some complications of the elemental diet include nausea, vomiting, and diarrhea, all of which are related to the nutrient concentration and rate of ad-

TABLE 6. Comparison of Compositions of Chemically Formulated Diets

(per 1000 ml. of 25 per cent weight per volume)

		Codelid*	Vivonex High Nitrogen†	Vivonex 100†	Flexical‡
Calories	kcal.	1000	1000	1000	1000
Carbohydrate	gm.	198	203	212	155
Amino acids	gm.	37.6	45.5	19.2	28
Nitrogen	gm.	6.0	7.2	3.1	3.5
Fat	gm.	0	0.44	0.7	33.9
Sodium	mEq.	25	33.5	52.3	15.2
Potassium	mEq.	24	23	17.9	38.5
Chloride	mEq.	37	52.5	73.2	33.8
Magnesium	mEq.	7	4.3	6.6	14.4
Calcium	mEq.	24	13.3	20.7	25.0
Osmolality	mOsm.	1100	840	1000	805
Acidity	pH	5.4	4.3	5.5	6.0

*Codelid diet—Schwarz BioResearch, Mountain View Avenue, Orangeburg, New York 10962

†Vivonex diet—Eaton Laboratories, Norwich, New York 13815

‡Flexical diet—Mead Johnson Laboratories, Evansville, Indiana 47721

ministration. Aspiration of vomitus is a real risk in the elderly, weakened, or unconscious patient, but is usually preventable by elevating the head of the bed, by avoiding night feeding, and by careful attention to gastric retention. Hypertonic dehydration and hyperosmolar nonketotic coma may occur if the diets are used in too high amounts and concentrations or if inadequate water is provided. Hyperglycemia and glycosuria tend to occur in patients with diabetes, in severely stressed patients, and in the presence of sepsis. Hypoprothrombinemia may occur unless vitamin K is added, because there is no vitamin K present in currently available chemically formulated diets. By cautiously adjusting the concentration and administration rate of the diets and allowing time for increased tolerance, as many as 5200 calories have been given daily for prolonged periods of time. Randall and co-workers[2] have reported a series of surgical patients who were provided long-term total nutrition by means of chemically formulated diets in a variety of pathologic conditions.

Generally, these diets are prepared as 25 per cent weight per volume solutions, providing about 1000 calories per liter and 20 to 40 gm. of amino acids per liter. Because of their high osmolality (840 to 1100 milliosmols per liter), only about 100 to 150 ml. should be given per feeding, and no more than 2000 ml. can be administered per day in the average patient.

Chemically formulated diets currently represent an intermediate step in surgical nutrition between high-calorie, high-protein, total parenteral nutrition and the oral ingestion and digestion of regular food. They have their greatest value in the treatment of patients who require additional support and who have at least a part of their small intestine available for absorption, but who are unable to eat and digest enough whole protein and sufficient calories to meet their needs.

Tube Feeding

Occasionally, patients with severe anorexia, weakness, and malnutrition are refractory to oral feedings and can best be fed via a small rubber or plastic nasogastric tube to minimize the effort and discomfort of eating. In the special instance in which nutritional difficulties secondary to technical difficulties or anastomotic edema are anticipated in a patient undergoing gastric surgery, the orojejunal or gastrojejunal routes may be helpful. Esophagostomy with major head and neck tumors, gastrostomy with esophageal obstruction, and jejunostomy with pyloric obstruction have been recommended in patients prior to or at the time of major surgery.

Various commercially available powders and liquids are available that fulfill nutrient requirements and can be fed by tube. Indeed, there is a wide spectrum of formulas, each specifically tailored to satisfy individual needs, especially for pediatric patients. A simple and economic way to prepare gastrostomy feedings is to homogenize a normal house diet. In special instances, chemically formulated diets may be indicated and can be infused into the stomach or small bowel. The diet should be kept cold in a small reservoir and initially should be administered at a concentration of 12.5 to 15 per cent weight per volume at a rate of 40 to 50 ml. per hour through a nasogastric tube or gastrostomy. If this is well tolerated without nausea, vomiting, or gastric retention, the concentration can be increased to 25 per cent weight per volume in 24 to 48 hours. Daily total volume can then be progressively increased by increments of 500 ml. or more until the desired caloric and protein levels are achieved. If nausea or diarrhea occurs, administration of the diet should be slowed or stopped entirely for 12 to 24 hours, and then restarted more slowly. In elderly or unconscious patients, it is wise to elevate the head of the bed and to discontinue feeding at night in order to reduce the danger of aspiration, and to check the stomach for retention and dilatation at frequent intervals.

Chemically formulated diets can also be fed directly into the small bowel either through a long tube or a jejunostomy, provided that there are at least a few feet of bowel distal to the end of the tube. Initial feedings should be diluted to isotonicity at about 5 to 10 per cent weight per volume concentration and delivered at a rate of 40 to 60 ml. per hour. Gradually the concentration can be increased according to tolerance. Parenteral codeine in doses of 15 to 30 mg., given every 4 to 6 hours, can be quite helpful in controlling diarrhea. If excessive stool output persists, the infusion may have to be slowed or stopped, and restarted later at a slower rate.

Liquid vitamins and oral medications can be added to any of the tube feedings as desired. Addition of substances such as paregoric, kaolin-pectin mixtures, diphenoxylate (Lomotil), or belladonna alkaloids, or combinations of them, can be helpful in controlling hyperperistalsis, but in some patients diarrhea may persist in spite of these measures. In selected patients, the provision of essential fatty acids in the form of short- and medium-chain triglycerides or the provision of calcium, or both, can be valuable in maintaining homeostasis and controlling frequency and consistency of bowel movements.

Another troublesome complication of tube feeding is azotemia secondary to high nitrogen intake in the presence of inadequate hydration. In most instances, this can be prevented or corrected by supplementing the total ration with additional water by tube or by vein. Regular determinations of blood urea nitrogen are advisable in all patients on tube feeding, but particularly those with compromised renal function.

Parenteral Nutrition

When feeding via the gastrointestinal tract is inadequate, ill advised, impractical, or impossible, it is necessary to provide nutrients parenterally. Although parenteral implies by any other means than the alimentary tract, the only avenue by which total nutrition is currently feasible is the intravenous route. In addition to water, electrolytes, and vitamins, the nutrients available for intravenous alimentation include dextrose, fructose, invert sugar, ethyl alcohol, various protein hydrolysates and amino acid mixtures, human serum albumin, plasma protein fraction, and whole blood. In some countries, glycerol, gelatin, sorbitol, xylitol, and fat emulsions are also used, but not in the United States. These nutrient substrates are present in various concentrations and combinations for both peripheral and central venous administration.

Carbohydrates for Intravenous Administration. Dextrose is probably the most commonly employed parenteral nutrient. This should not be surprising in view of its essential role in metabolism, its normal presence in the blood, its availability, and its low cost. A 5 per cent dextrose solution is about isotonic with plasma, provides approximately 170 calories per liter, and is compatible with almost all other parenteral solutions. It is not generally realized that the USP dextrose used in intravenous solutions is not anhydrous, but monohydrated. Thus, a 5 per cent dextrose solution is really a 5 per cent dextrose monohydrate solution, the net effect being that only 91 per cent of the solute is calorigenic (Table 7).

Additionally, the caloric equivalent of dextrose is actually 3.75 calories per gram rather than the usual 4.1 calories per gram derived from carbohydrates in general.[25] Therefore, the true caloric potential of a liter of 5 per cent solution is $50 \times 0.91 \times 3.75 = 170$ calories, instead of the often stated theoretical 200 calories. In addition to the water infused with dextrose solutions, 0.6 ml. of water is produced within the body per gram of glucose oxidized. Although the basal functional caloric intake of about 25 calories per kilogram body weight per day for the average adult can be supplied by dextrose, much of the protein-sparing effect in fasting persons is achieved with the infusion of about 100 gm. of dextrose per day. The maximal speed of administration of glucose without exceeding metabolic capabilities and producing glycosuria is approximately 0.5 gm. per kilogram per hour for adults and about 1.2 gm. per kilogram per hour for full-term infants.[13] The rate of glucose utilization, however, will vary greatly among patients from premature infants to those in the geriatric age groups. It will also vary in an individual patient under different conditions. In

TABLE 7. Comparison of Caloric Values of Parenteral and Conventional Dietary Nutrients

	Quantity	Absolute Caloric Value	Conventional Caloric Value
Dextrose monohydrate	1 gm.	3.4	4
Dextrose anhydrous	1 gm.	3.75	4
Fructose (levulose)	1 gm.	3.75	4
Invert sugar	1 gm.	3.75	4
Lactate	1 gm.	3.6	4
Amino acids	1 gm.	3.5	4
Protein hydrolysates	1 gm.	3.5	4
Animal protein (albumin)	1 gm.	4.25	4
Ethyl alcohol— absolute	1 ml.	5.6	5.6
Ethyl alcohol— absolute	1 gm.	7	7
Lecithin	1 gm.	7.5	9
Cottonseed oil	1 gm.	9	9
Soybean oil	1 gm.	9	9

view of the fact that extreme variations of tolerance can occur, it is desirable to ascertain glucose utilization regularly in all patients fed by vein, as such information is deemed critical in order to assess the optimal caloric intake.

Unlike dextrose, fructose can be phosphorylated in the absence of insulin and can thus be advantageous in the parenteral nourishment of patients with diabetes mellitus. A liter of 5 per cent fructose (levulose) will yield 188 calories. Although there have been numerous reports in the literature attesting to the virtues of the use of fructose intravenously, our experience has indicated no practical advantage of fructose over dextrose. It is noteworthy that fructose metabolism raises blood lactate levels.

Invert sugar is a mixture of equal parts of dextrose and fructose that provides approximately 188 calories per liter of 5 per cent concentration in water. Here again, there is no practical advantage of invert sugar over dextrose alone.

According to Weisburg,[25] the administration of carbohydrate solutions by vein has served several functions: (1) Both the water of solution and the water of oxidation of the carbohydrate are used to supply the body requirements for replacement of insensible water losses and urine output. (2) Required calories are provided to meet the metabolic needs of the patient, especially for the synthesis of protein. (3) Excess protein catabolism and the resulting nitrogen losses from the body tissues are spared. (4) Depletion of glycogen and production by the liver of excess ketone bodies are prevented. (5) Losses of intracellular water are reduced. (6) Losses of intracellular electrolytes especially potassium, are reduced. (7) Losses of extracellular electrolytes, especially sodium, are decreased. (8)

The amount of water needed for renal excretory functions is decreased by reducing the quantities of ketone bodies, nitrogenous metabolites, and electrolytes that are presented to the kidneys.

Ethanol as an Energy Substrate. Absolute alcohol yields 5.6 calories per milliliter or 7.0 calories per gram. Therefore, a 5 per cent alcohol solution by volume will yield about 280 calories per liter. Although some of the calories derived from alcohol have the ability to spare nitrogen and can provide energy that would otherwise be produced necessarily from body reserves, daily metabolism of alcohol is limited to about 3 to 4.5 gm. per kilogram of body weight.[17] In addition to the fact that it is impossible to achieve positive nitrogen balance with the use of alcohol as the sole source of non-nitrogen calories, the side effects of intoxication, obtundity, and potential cellular damage have restricted its usefulness as a nutrient. The practical limit is not much more than 100 to 150 ml. a day for the average adult.

Protein Derivatives for Intravenous Administration. Intravenous protein hydrolysates are derived by the acid or enzymatic hydrolysis of casein or fibrin. Solutions of such substances contain approximately 50 to 60 per cent amino acids and 40 to 45 per cent dipeptides and tripeptides. Although the average caloric equivalency of 1 gm. of animal protein is 4.25 calories, the protein hydrolysates are approximately equal to 80 per cent whole protein. Thus, a 5 per cent solution of protein hydrolysates or amino acids can yield approximately 170 calories per liter. The true importance of protein hydrolysate or amino acid solutions, however, is not to provide calories, but to supply the amino acids and nitrogen that are essential for growth, cellular repair, and healing. Given an adequate caloric intake of about 125 to 200 calories per gram of nitrogen, intravenously administered amino acids and hydrolysates will be utilized most effectively for protein synthesis.

It has been held that little or nothing can be done to prevent the negative nitrogen balance and weight loss that occur postoperatively or after major trauma. Many physicians have felt that such losses are obligatory and have done nothing to prevent them. However, the most important factors responsible for this phenomenon are inadequate caloric and nitrogen intake. Nitrogen deficits simply cannot be corrected unless exogenous protein moieties are supplied to the patient and protected with ample quantities of protein-sparing foods (25 to 35 calories per gram of protein).

Fat Emulsions for Intravenous Administration. Because fat has a high caloric density of 9 calories per gram, attempts have been made to utilize fat emulsions for intravenous feeding in man. A 10 per cent fat emulsion contributes little to osmotic pressure and provides approximately 900 calories per liter. Its use can also provide essential fatty acids, allowing parenteral nutrition regimens to be formulated that could be truly complete. However, because of some difficulties with adverse reactions, with maintaining uniform particle size of the emulsion under various conditions, and with the deposition of fatty pigments in the liver, the cottonseed oil emulsion was withdrawn from clinical use in the United States by the Food and Drug Administration in 1966. The use of soybean oil emulsion has gained popularity in the last few years throughout Europe and other parts of the world, and clinical experience with this emulsion is currently being gained in the United States.

With the use of isotonic solutions in most routine intravenous feeding regimens, parenteral alimentation can provide only a small fraction of the nutritional requirements of a patient. Infusion of 5 per cent dextrose or other carbohydrate solutions within the limits of water tolerance of 2500 to 3500 ml. per day in the average human adult provides about 500 to 700 calories. In the average resting patient, basal caloric requirements are approximately three times this amount. Thus all of the peripherally infused nutrients will be metabolized for heat and energy rather than for tissue synthesis, and additional energy requirements must often be met by the catabolism of the body stores of glycogen, fat, and protein. If normal nutrient requirements are increased by pre-existing deficits, trauma, sepsis, hypermetabolic states, or other pathologic processes, the patient supported exclusively by the usual peripheral intravenous feeding is clearly subsisting on a starvation regimen.

There are several factors that impose limitations upon the provision of nourishment by vein, the most critical being that the tolerable water volume is limited to about three liters per day for the average sick adult. Larger amounts may overload the circulation and produce congestive heart failure or pulmonary edema. The concentrations of the nutrients dissolved in the water are limited to a total of approximately 5 to 10 per cent for peripheral infusion because higher concentrations lead to a significant incidence of inflammation of the intima, clotting, and occlusion of the veins.

Several approaches have been taken to increasing the efficacy of intravenous alimentation in the past, with limited clinical success. By infusing somewhat hypertonic (10 to 15 per cent) solutions of dextrose, fructose, or invert sugar, with or without additional ethyl alcohol or protein moities, 2000 to 2400 calories per day have been administered by peripheral vein within the limits of water tolerance. However, long-term parenteral nutrition by this technique is limited by a prohibitive incidence of thrombophlebitis. Several years ago, advantage was taken of the development of diuretics of high efficiency, and these potent medications were added intravenously to infusion volumes of 5 to 7 liters of isotonic or slightly hypertonic nutrient solutions, allowing the provision of up to 2600 calories per day while facilitating renal excretion of the extra vehicular water used to deliver the nutrients.[23] With this technique, nitrogen equilibrium and slightly positive nitrogen balance were achieved in animals and man. Its major disadvantage was that it required fairly constant attention to maintain the dynamic water and electrolyte equilibrium. The physician had to be assured that urine output had increased sufficiently as a result of the diuretic action before administering amounts of nutrient solutions beyond three liters, in order that the positive water balance never exceeded 2000 ml. per 24 hours. The risks of water overload, electrolyte imbalance, and cardiovas-

cular decompensation have restricted the widespread use of this technique. Ethyl alcohol and fat emulsions have limitations as energy sources, as mentioned earlier, and have fallen short of expectations. Thus, the only uniformly applicable approach to providing adequate nutrition parenterally was to concentrate the nutrients known to be safe and efficacious into the volume of water known to be safely tolerated and to infuse the resulting concentrated solution into a large venous channel such as the superior vena cava where it is immediately diluted.

In order to infuse nutrient solutions successfully by vein, several criteria must first be satisfied. The solution must not contain pyrogens or cause fever for any other reasons. It must exert at least sufficient total osmotic pressure to avoid injury to the cellular elements of the blood. The foodstuff must be in forms that normally travel in the circulatory system, such as glucose, fructose, amino acids, or peptides of very short chain length. It must preserve or permit the body to maintain normal concentrations of the various biologic ions such as sodium, potassium, chloride, calcium, phosphorous, magnesium, and bicarbonate, with a resultant pH in the normal range. The method must avoid the production of thrombosis and embolism and should not necessarily confine the patient to bed or other forms of inactivity. The technique of infusion must include stringent precautions against infection and must be sufficiently safe and stable that administration apparatus can be left in place and kept functioning for several days or weeks when required.

Parenteral Hyperalimentation

The primary aim of total parenteral nutrition is to provide suitable carbohydrates, protein moieties, and other essential nutrients exclusively by vein for prolonged periods of time in quantities substantially greater than the basal requirements for caloric and nitrogen equilibrium in order to achieve positive nitrogen balance and an anabolic state during conditions usually associated with a catabolic response. In infants, an additional goal is to maintain normal weight gain, growth, and development until adequate enteral feeding can be initiated or resumed. During the past few years, the development of the technique of intravenous hyperalimentation has allowed prolonged total parenteral nutrition to become practical. The basic principles leading to the success of this technique included the provision of all nutrients available in intravenous form, concentrated in a fluid volume equal to normal daily water requirements and infused into a high-flow, large-diameter central vein such as the superior vena cava. The infusion should be given at a constant rate over 24 hours a day to permit a maximal utilization and minimal renal excretion of the substrates.

The original experiments that established the safety, efficacy, and practicality of this technique were performed in dogs.[7, 9] A specially prepared complete parenteral diet was infused continuously into the superior venae cavae of beagle puppies for periods up to 256 days. During the course of total parenteral nutrition, the dogs showed normal growth and development for the first time in any animal species, exactly paral-

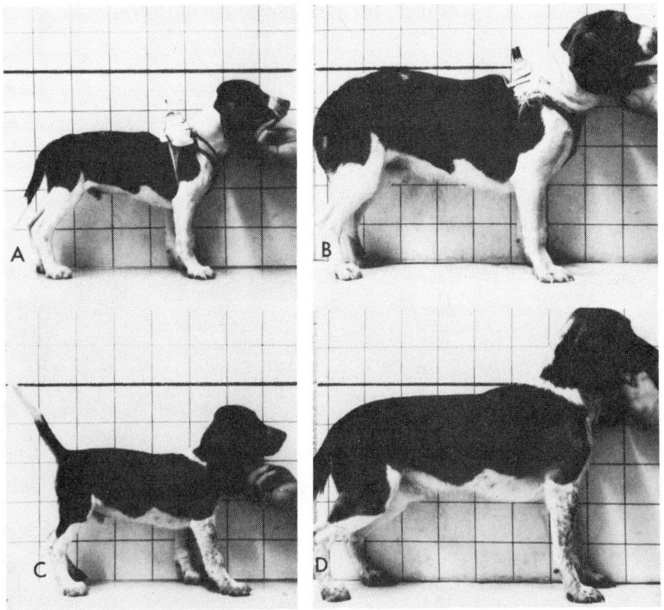

Figure 1. The growth and development of a puppy fed entirely by vein (A and B) was normal, comparable to that of a littermate (C and D) fed an optimal oral diet, during the study period, which began at 12 weeks of age (A and C) and was completed 235 days later (B and D).

leling that of their littermates fed isocalorically on a standard oral diet concurrently (Fig. 1). The technique and principles defined in the laboratory were then applied clinically to infant[27] and adult human patients.[10] The continuous infusion of the concentrated nutrients into the superior vena cava proved successful in achieving normal growth and development in newborn infants and positive nitrogen balance, weight gain, and wound healing in adults. Increased experience with the technique has led to modifications and refinements in methodology and to the application of intravenous hyperalimentation principles to an ever increasing number of clinical problems.

TECHNIQUE OF INTRAVENOUS HYPERALIMENTATION

Preparation of the Nutrient Solution

The basic nutrient mixture is a hypertonic solution about six times more concentrated than the blood, and consists of approximately 20 to 25 per cent dextrose and 4 to 5 per cent protein hydrolysates and crystalline amino acids. It provides about 5.25 to 6.0 gm. of nitrogen, equivalent to 32.5 to 37.5 gm. of protein, and approximately 900 to 1000 calories per liter. The base mixture can be formulated in bulk amounts from commercially available parenteral solutions by a manufacturing pharmacist or a specially trained technician, or in individual units by a physician, pharmacist, nurse, or technician, using strict aseptic mixing techniques. Hyperalimentation kits containing the basic solution components, transfer apparatus, and administration tubing are now marketed by intravenous solution manufacturers to increase the safety, availability, and facility of formulating the nutrient mixtures.

In the manufacturing pharmacy of the Hospital of the University of Pennsylvania, the bulk method of base solution preparation consists of dissolving anhydrous dextrose in one of several commercially available solutions of 5 per cent protein hydrolysate in 5 per cent dextrose in the ratio of 165 gm. of the former to 860 ml. of the latter (Table 8).

The resultant solution is sterilized immediately after mixing by passage through a 0.22 μ cellulose membrane filter 6 inches in diameter into sterile liter bottles. Sterilization of the concentrated solution is not possible by steam autoclaving because of the intense browning or Maillard reaction that occurs under these conditions. Several aliquots are taken from each lot of solution and are tested for the presence of bacteria, fungi, or pyrogens. Each lot is quarantined under refrigeration and is not released for clinical use until negative results of these tests have been received.

Individual units of the base solution can be prepared immediately prior to infusion from various commercially obtainable parenteral solutions. With strict aseptic mixing technique and, ideally, under a laminar-flow, filtered-air hood, 350 ml. of 50 per cent dextrose is added to 750 ml. of 5 per cent protein hydrolysate in 5 per cent dextrose. A unit of nutrient base solution prepared by this technique provides 100 ml. more water and slightly less nitrogen, dextrose, and calories than a liter of solution prepared by the bulk method. A safer and more convenient method of preparing a unit of base solution is by use of the hyperalimentation kits which contain a liter bottle half-filled with 40 to 50 per cent dextrose under vacuum, a half-liter bottle containing 8 to 10 per cent protein hydrolysate or crystalline amino acids, a transfer set for aseptically combining the two solutions, and an administration set for delivering the reconstituted solution to the patient. In our most recent experience, the best and safest technique for preparing, handling,

TABLE 8. Adult Hyperalimentation Solution Preparation*

Unit Preparation of Base Solution — Bulk Method (Pharmacy)
165 gm. anhydrous dextrose USP + 860 ml. 5% dextrose in 5% fibrin hydrolysate
Sterilization through 0.22 μ membrane filter under laminar-flow, filtered-air hood

Volume	1000 ml.
Calories	1000 Cal.
Dextrose	208 gm.
Hydrolysates	43 gm.
Nitrogen	6.0 gm.
Sodium	8 mEq.
Potassium	14 mEq.

Single Unit Method (Ward or Pharmacy)
350 ml. 50% dextrose + 750 ml. 5% dextrose in 5% fibrin hydrolysate
Aseptic mixing technique under laminar-flow, filtered-air hood

Volume	1100 ml.
Calories	1000 Cal.
Dextrose	212 gm.
Hydrolysates	37 gm.
Nitrogen	5.25 gm.
Sodium	7 mEq.
Potassium	13 mEq.

Additions to Each Unit of Base Solution (Average Adult)

Sodium (chloride and/or bicarbonate)	40–50 mEq.
Potassium (chloride or acid phosphate)	30–40 mEq.
Magnesium (sulfate)	4–8 mEq.

Additions to Only One Unit Daily (Average Adult)

Vitamin A	5000–10,000 USP units
Vitamin D	500–1000 USP units
Vitamin E	2.5–5.0 I.U.
Ascorbic acid	250–500 mg.
Thiamin hydrochloride	25–50 mg.
Riboflavin	5–10 mg.
Pyridoxine hydrochloride	7.5–15 mg.
Niacin	50–100 mg.
Pantothenic acid	12.5–25 mg.

Optional Additions to One Unit (as indicated by serum studies)

Phytonadione (vitamin K)	5–10 mg.
Cyanocobalamin (vitamin B_{12})	10–30 μg.
Folic acid	0.5–1.5 mg.
Iron (dextriferron)	2.0–3.0 mg.
Calcium (gluconate)	4.5–9 mEq.
Phosphate (potassium acid salt)	4–10 mEq.

*Micronutrients such as zinc, copper, manganese, cobalt, and iodine are present as contaminants in hydrolysate solutions, but may be given in plasma transfusion once or twice weekly if desired.

and administering the nutrient solutions involves the use of commercially available plastic bags and specially designed vacuum filling apparatus.

Although the base solution contains various quantities of some of the essential minerals, the composition and concentrations of which differ significantly from one product to another, electrolyte additives must be made immediately prior to infusion in order to satisfy the nutrient and metabolic requirements of most pa-

tients (Table 8). For the average adult patient with no significant renal, hepatic, or cardiovascular dysfunction, 40 to 50 mEq. of sodium as the chloride and/or acetate, bicarbonate, or lactate salt and 30 to 40 mEq. of potassium as the chloride and/or acetate, lactate, or acid phosphate salt are added to each liter of base solution. To base solutions prepared from crystalline amino acids, which may contain a combined total of 25 to 50 mEq. of chloride and/or hydrochloride per liter, sodium should be added as the acetate, bicarbonate, or lactate, and not the chloride salt, in order to avoid production or aggravation of hyperchloremic acidosis. Four to eight milliequivalents of magnesium sulfate is added to each liter of solution. Calcium in organic form, usually as the gluconate salt to avoid precipitation, is not administered routinely to all adults, but is added to the nutrient regimen as indicated by weekly determinations of the serum levels of calcium. Generally, 4 to 5 mEq. of calcium is added per liter of the base solution. However, phosphorus, a major intracellular ion, must be added in dosages of 18 to 25 mEq. per liter as the potassium acid phosphate salt, if significant hypophosphatemia and its attendant complications are to be avoided during anabolism. To only one bottle of solution daily is added an ampule of water- and fat-soluble vitamins in therapeutic dosages. Vitamin B_{12}, vitamin K, and folic acid, which are not present in intravenous vitamin mixtures, can be added to one bottle of the solution daily or given less frequently intravenously or intramuscularly as indicated in required dosages. Iron can be added to the solution daily or less frequently in appropriately calculated doses or given intramuscularly in depot form. In patients who are anemic, it is advisable to restore normal red cell volume by judicious transfusion of whole blood or packed erythrocytes upon initiation of intravenous hyperalimentation. Trace elements, such as cobalt, copper, iodine, manganese, molybdenum, and zinc, are present as contaminants in most parenteral solutions, particularly in protein hydrolysate solutions, and are therefore not added routinely to the hyperalimentation regimen. In newborn infants or in severely malnourished adults, trace elements may be infused intermittently as specially prepared additives, or alternatively provided by administration of 10 ml. of plasma or albumin per kilogram body weight per week.

To provide the requirements necessary for normal growth and development in newborn infants, who have no appreciable nutrient stores, more complete mixtures are required for daily infusion. Bulk or individual unit preparation of pediatric nutrient solutions is possible as outlined in Tables 9 and 10. Commercially available pediatric hyperalimentation kits can increase the ease and safety of solution formulation for infants. Moreover, the recent release of soybean oil emulsion for clinical use in this country has allowed complete parenteral nutrition by peripheral veins to become a practical reality in infants for limited periods of time.

Modifications of the standard adult formula are required for treatment of patients with congestive heart failure, liver disease, or massive nutritional edema, in whom sodium administration is reduced. In

TABLE 9. Bulk Preparation of Pediatric Hyperalimentation Solution

5% Dextrose in 5% protein hydrolysate	12,000 ml.
Anhydrous dextrose USP	2,200 ml.
10% Calcium gluconate	150 ml.
Multiple vitamin infusion	100 ml.
Potassium phosphate monobasic (2 mEq./ml.)	30 ml.
50% Magnesium sulfate	5 ml.
Phytonadione (10 mg./ml.)	2 ml.
Dextriferron (20 mg./ml.)	2 ml.
Cyanocobalamin (100 μ/ml.)	2 ml.
Folic acid (15 mg./ml.)	2 ml.
Trace elements (optional)	7 ml.
Total volume	14,500 ml.

Final pH of 5.2 to 5.5 may be adjusted to neutrality immediately prior to infusion with sodium bicarbonate or sodium hydroxide. Additional sodium, chloride, or other electrolytes may be added as indicated by metabolic studies.

TABLE 11. Renal Failure Solution Preparation

Preparation of Amino Acid Mixture		Preparation of Nutrient Solution†	
Essential Amino Acids*	Minimum Daily Requirement (gm.)		
L-Isoleucine	0.70	(750–1000 ml. 50–70% glucose)	
L-Leucine	1.10	+	
L-Lysine	0.80	100 ml. essential L-amino acids (6.35 gm.)	
L-Methionine	1.10	Volume	850–1100 ml.
L-Phenylalanine	1.10	Calories	1500–2500 Cal.
L-Threonine	0.50	Glucose	375–500 gm.
L-Tryptophan	0.25	Nitrogen	1.0 gm.
L-Valine	0.80		
Total	6.35		

*Crystalline amino acids are dissolved in 100 ml. sterile, pyrogen-free water and sterilized by passage through a 0.22 μ membrane filter. Amino acid mixture = 6.35 gm. per 100 ml.

†Final mixing is carried out under a laminar-flow, filtered-air hood with additions of vitamins and electrolytes as indicated.

elderly patients or in those with compromised renal function, potassium administration is reduced or temporarily omitted, and in patients with overt renal or hepatic dysfunction, protein hydrolysates or racemic mixtures of crystalline amino acids are restricted. Special solutions for the treatment of acute or chronic renal failure contain nitrogen of the highest biologic value in the form of essential L-amino acids in 50 to 70 per cent dextrose, thus restricting water administration, but providing adequate nutrition and promoting

reduction of blood urea nitrogen and ammonia[8] (Table 11).

Modifications of the solution are often necessary following the initiation of intravenous hyperalimentation, depending upon the patient's metabolic response to the disease, trauma, operation, infection, or other intercurrent conditions. It is essential for the physician to recognize that no single intravenous nutrient solution can be ideal for all conditions in all patients at all times, or for the same patient during the various phases of his pathologic process. Individual metabolic requirements may be satisfied by appropriate alterations in the solution formulas.

Administration of the Nutrient Solutions

The average daily ration of hypertonic nutrient solution contains about 25 to 30 per cent solute and should be infused continuously over 24 hours at a constant rate in order to allow maximal assimilation of the nutrients without exceeding the patient's capabilities for water, dextrose, amino acid, or mineral metabolism. Because the hypertonic solution is six times the osmolality of the blood, it must gain entry into the circulatory system through a large-diameter, high-flow blood vessel, preferably the superior vena cava. Starting at generally safe levels of water metabolism (2000 to 2500 ml. per day in adults or 100 ml. per kilogram per day in infants) and dextrose utilization (0.4 to 1.2 gm. per kilogram per hour), the daily intravenous nutrient ration is gradually increased as indicated or tolerated (3000 to 4000 ml. per day in adults or 130 to 150 ml. per kilogram per day in infants).

Basic guidelines for safe intravenous hyperalimentation include accurate determinations of: body weight daily; water balance every 4 to 8 hours; fractional urine sugar concentrations every 6 hours; serum electrolytes, blood sugar, and blood urea nitrogen daily until stable, then every 2 or 3 days thereafter; and complete blood count, serum proteins, calcium, phosphorous, and magnesium weekly. Hepatic and renal function tests should be evaluated initially and every 2 or 3 weeks during intravenous hyperalimentation.

TABLE 10. Pediatric Hyperalimentation Solution Preparation

Unit Composition of Base Solution

400 ml.	5% dextrose in 5% fibrin hydrolysate	160 Cal.	{ 20 gm. hydrolysate { 20 gm. dextrose
250 ml.	50% dextrose	500 Cal.	
650 ml.		660 Cal.	

Additions to Each Unit of Base Solution

Sodium	20 mEq.	Sodium chloride (2 mEq./ml.)	10	ml.
Potassium	25 mEq.	Potassium acid phosphate (2 mEq./ml.)	13	ml.
Phosphorus	25 mEq.			
Calcium	20 mEq.	Calcium gluconate 10% (0.45 mEq./ml.)	44	ml.
Magnesium	10 mEq.	Magnesium sulfate 50% (4 mEq./ml.)	2.4	ml.
Multiple vitamin infusion			4	ml.
Vitamin K Cyanocobalamin Folic acid Iron		Added to solution daily or weekly or given intramuscularly	1	ml.
Trace elements		Added to solution daily or given as 10 ml./kg. plasma twice weekly	1	ml.
			~75	ml.

Base solution 650 ml.
Additives 75 ml.

Final solution 725 ml. (Given at a rate of 145 ml./kg./day = 130 Cal./kg./day)

Intermittent measurements of serum osmolality and vitamin levels, and urine specific gravity, osmolality, and electrolytes, may be helpful in monitoring certain patients. Periodic determinations of arterial and central venous pressures, blood gases, and pH may also be indicated in the management of critically ill patients with significant cardiovascular, respiratory, or metabolic derangements, and in premature or full-term newborn infants.

Adjustments of water volume, sugar concentration, protein source, or electrolyte content in the nutrient solution may be necessary during the treatment of a critically ill or traumatized patient. Relative glucose intolerance is most likely to be manifest at the initiation of intravenous hyperalimentation, immediately following trauma, during operation, in the immediate postoperative period, in premature or newborn infants, in the aged, in patients with pancreatic disorders, or in the presence of shock or sepsis. To avoid excessive glycosuria, which may result in water and electrolyte imbalances, or hyperosmolar, hyperglycemic, nonketotic coma, the infusion is maintained at a rate that will not allow quantitative urinary glucose to exceed 1 gm. per 100 ml. (3+ nitroprusside reaction). Ideally, the patient will not excrete any sugar in his urine. However, trace amounts of glucose in the urine do not represent significant losses of the total sugar administered, and such small amounts of glycosuria will induce a mild diuresis which may actually be helpful in excreting any excess vehicular water, and in indicating that the limit of the patient's ability to metabolize glucose has been approached.

In all patients with diabetes mellitus, crystalline insulin is given routinely either subcutaneously in divided doses or equally distributed in the intravenous solution. At times in nondiabetic patients with relative glucose intolerance, crystalline insulin is added to nutrient solution in amounts of 5 to 50 units per 1000 calories. Addition of insulin is indicated in the presence of an elevated blood sugar in order to encourage more rapid and efficient glucose utilization and positive nutritional balance in elderly patients with dysfunction of the pancreas, in the early postoperative period, and in critically ill, nutritionally depleted patients whose survival appears to depend upon the expeditious achievement of positive caloric and nitrogen balance.

Albumin or blood is usually given early in the course of intravenous hyperalimentation to restore normal colloid osmotic pressure and red blood cell mass in patients with marked hypoproteinemia or anemia. In patients with borderline serum protein concentrations, administration of the nutrient solution alone is sufficient to correct the deficiencies.

Long-Term Central Venous Catheterization

The preferred method of infusion of the hypertonic nutrient solution at the Hermann Hospital – The University of Texas Medical School at Houston is via the subclavian route. It consists of the percutaneous introduction of an 8 inch long polyethylene, polyvinyl, or silicone rubber catheter, having an external diameter of 1 to 2 mm., into the superior vena cava via one of the subclavian veins (Fig. 2). The catheterization can be accomplished safely and effectively in 99 per cent of patients if the following principles are conscientiously

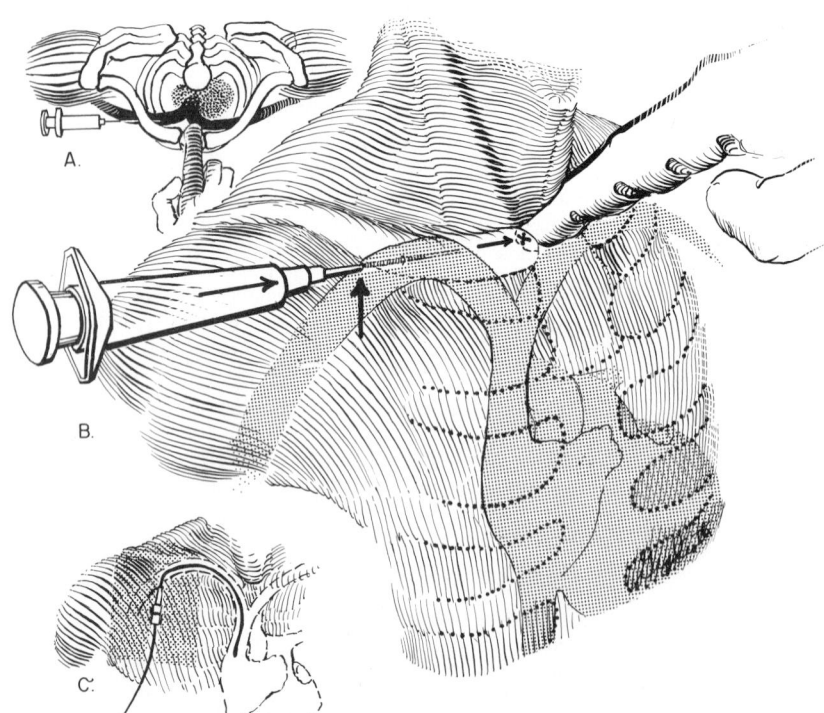

Figure 2. With the shoulders of the patient extended maximally, the deltoid prominence falls backward, allowing the syringe and needle to be aimed from the midpoint of the inferior margin of the clavicle, in a line parallel to the coronal plane of the patient *(A)*, to the tip of a finger placed firmly into the suprasternal notch *(B)*. After accurate subclavian venipuncture is accomplished, the catheter is advanced through the needle a distance of 5 to 6 inches, so that the tip of the catheter is positioned in the middle of the superior vena cava *(C)*.

observed. The patient is placed in bed on his back with his head 15 degrees lower than his feet, to allow maximal filling and dilatation of the subclavian vein to a diameter of 1 to 2 cm., thus making it a fairly large target. The shoulders are extended backward, and the head is turned to the opposite side, thus allowing the ipsilateral subclavian vein to become most easily accessible for percutaneous puncture. The skin of the lower neck, shoulder, and upper chest is shaved, cleansed with ether or acetone to remove skin oil, and prepared with tincture of USP in a manner identical to skin preparation prior to a major operation. With strict aseptic technique, including sterile gloves and surgical instruments, the prepared area of skin is draped with sterile towels, and local anesthetic solution is infiltrated into the skin, subcutaneous tissue, and periosteum at the inferior surface of the midpoint of the clavicle. A needle 2 inches long and 2.5 mm. in diameter, attached to a 2 ml. syringe, is inserted beneath the clavicle in a horizontal plane, with its tip aimed at the posterior aspect of the sternal notch. When the needle enters the subclavian vein, blood can easily be withdrawn from the vein into the syringe. The syringe is then disconnected from the needle, the bevel of which is directed caudally, and the catheter is introduced its full length into the subclavian vein and down into the superior vena cava. If any difficulty is encountered in advancing the catheter, both the needle and the catheter should be withdrawn together as a unit, and another venipuncture attempted. Withdrawal of the catheter alone with the needle in place may result in transection of the catheter and embolism of the distal segment. During the time that the needle is detached from the syringe, the patient is asked to hold his breath, or manual pressure is applied to his abdomen, to minimize the risk of air embolism. The needle is then withdrawn its full length, with approximately 5½ inches of catheter left within the central venous system, its tip lying in the midportion of the superior vena cava. The catheter is secured firmly with a suture, and broad-spectrum antibiotic-antifungal ointment or antiseptic ointment is applied around the catheter exit site from the skin. A sterile gauze dressing is then applied and fixed in place with tincture of benzoin and adhesive tape. Intravenous administration tubing is connected to the hub of the catheter, and an infusion is begun with an isotonic solution. After a roentgenogram has been obtained to confirm the desired position of the catheter, infusion of the concentrated nutrient solution can begin.

In infants who weigh less than 10 pounds, the relatively small subclavian vein and high position of the apex of the lung can render percutaneous subclavian vein puncture difficult and dangerous. Long-term central venous catheterization in these patients is achieved more safely and effectively by inserting a proportionally smaller catheter under direct vision into an external or internal jugular vein through a 1 cm. long incision made at the base of the neck.[6] After the catheter is secured in proper position in the vein, its proximal end is tunneled subcutaneously behind the ear to emerge through the parietal scalp. The skin exit site is thereby removed to a point distal from the neck incision, and the risks of infection and mechanical kinking of the catheter are reduced.

To accomplish safe, long-term intravenous catheterization, *meticulous* and *compulsive* care in the maintenance of the catheter is as important and necessary as proper catheter insertion. The intravenous administration tubing is replaced daily, while the patient is supine to minimize the risk of air embolism, and three times a week the dressing over the puncture site is changed. With aseptic techniques and sterile gloves, the skin area around the catheter is again prepared as it was at the time of catheterization. Antimicrobial or antiseptic ointment is reapplied, and a sterile gauze dressing is again secured over the site. Withdrawal or administration of blood through the catheter should be avoided because these practices significantly increase the possibility of contamination or clotting in the catheter. Extreme care should be exercised in adding medications or measuring central venous pressure through the catheter to prevent contamination of the solution or tubing. The catheter should be regarded by all in attendance of the patient as his lifeline, with the full realization that it must be given the care, respect, and considerations commensurate with its importance in maintaining the patient's life.

Infusion Apparatus for Intravenous Hyperalimentation

In ambulatory patients, standard intravenous solution bottles or plastic bags and infusion sets are used to deliver the nutrient solution at a constant rate of gravity drip. Rolling I.V. poles allow the mobility and exercise that are essential for optimal nutrition and rehabilitation of these patients. Use of closed, filtered infusion systems provides maximal safety against the ever-present airborne microorganisms which may gain entry into the solution or tubing. Portable lightweight AC-DC pumps, attached to the I.V. pole or directly to the patient, can be used to ensure a constant rate of infusion, while allowing considerable freedom of position and activity of the patient.

In newborn infants, nutrient solution can best be delivered continuously at a constant rate by means of a variable-speed pump, whose propelling mechanism is external to the tubing and solution. Syringe pumps must never be used to infuse nutrient solutions because the risk of contaminating the solution with such pumps is exceedingly great. A membrane filter 1 inch in diameter with 0.22 μ pores is attached to the infusion system between the pump tubing and the catheter. This in-line "final filter" prevents the transmission of micro-organisms and inert contaminants that may be introduced into the solution or tubing and prevents inadvertent air embolism, because air cannot pass through the pores after the filter has been moistened with the solution. These filters may also be used in adult patients, but a membrane of larger diameter or slightly larger pore size is necessary to permit satisfactory delivery of the greater volumes of solution required for adults. Work is currently in progress in several institutions to develop new apparatus and techniques to maximize the safety and efficacy of intravenous hyperalimentation while minimizing its risks and complications.

COMPLICATIONS OF INTRAVENOUS HYPERALIMENTATION

Prevention of *infection* or sepsis is of paramount importance to the success of long-term intravenous hyperalimentation. The occurrence of infection is very rare if the aseptic and antiseptic principles previously discussed are conscientiously observed in the insertion and maintenance of the central venous catheters. Because the nutrient solutions are good culture media for fungi and some species of bacteria, meticulous asepsis must also be maintained in preparing the base solution, making additives, and changing bottles and tubing. Should fever arise without an obvious cause, the solution and tubing are immediately replaced, and specimens of the blood and solution are sent promptly to the laboratory for microbiologic examination and culture. If the fever persists for more than a few hours after the solution and tubing are changed, the infusion is terminated. The central venous catheter is then removed, and its tip is immediately cultured for bacteria and fungi. Depending upon the clinical situation, either another catheter may be inserted into the contralateral subclavian vein, or administration of isotonic dextrose solution may be started via a peripheral vein to prevent rebound hypoglycemia. Antibiotics may not be required, but administration of broad-spectrum antimicrobial drugs is usually started if the temperature elevation persists and is modified appropriately when specific sensitivity testing is completed.

Fever or infection in a patient prior to the institution of intravenous hyperalimentation is not a contraindication to use of the technique. In a critically ill patient, infection actually accentuates the need for nutritional support. Antibiotic therapy may have already been instituted in many such patients, and although seeding of the indwelling catheter by circulating microorganisms in the blood is a real possibility, it has not been a frequent problem, and complete resolution of systemic infections has occurred frequently during the course of intravenous hyperalimentation. It is a cardinal rule that whenever a physician suspects that the infectious course of a patient might be caused or aggravated by the central venous catheter, it should be removed and cultured immediately.

Although intravenous *thrombosis* is a worrisome possibility with the long-term use of catheters and hypertonic solutions, clotting of the superior vena cava has not been observed clinically in the more than 4000 adult patients treated in our hospitals. The usual high blood flow in this vessel assures prompt dilution of the hypertonic fluid and, with maintenance of sterility, practically eliminates the threat of significant thrombosis. Rare instances of clotting have occurred, however, particularly in patients in whom the catheter tip was misdirected into an internal jugular, external jugular, internal mammary, or axillary vein.

Other complications such as *air embolism, catheter embolism, and clotting of the catheter* itself can be avoided readily by adherence to principles and techniques previously discussed. A thorough knowledge of anatomy, combined with common sense and strict adherence to the technique of percutaneous subclavian catheterization, should minimize the risk of accidental pneumothorax, hydrothorax, hemothorax, subclavian artery puncture, bleeding, or injury to the thoracic duct or brachial plexus.

Hyperosmolar coma can be precipitated acutely by too rapid infusion of the hypertonic solution, causing marked osmotic diuresis, serum and urine electrolyte aberrations, dehydration, and malfunction of the central nervous system. A chronic form of this syndrome can occur surreptitiously when impaired glucose tolerance is not recognized, particularly in the presence of diabetes mellitus, after some extensive burns or major trauma, or after intracranial operations or trauma. Hyperosmolar coma is seldom seen with blood sugar levels below 400 mg. per 100 ml., and in most instances the blood sugar concentration has been 600 mg. per 100 ml. or higher.

If blood and urine sugar levels are not conscientiously measured in such patients, hyperglycemia may occur with marked elevation of blood sugar, accompanied by weakness, listlessness, and coma. If the condition is not recognized and corrected promptly, permanent neurologic damage can ensue. Treatment of this syndrome consists of prompt infusion of isotonic or half-strength solutions of saline or glucose together with insulin, while frequent measurements of fluid losses, central venous pressure, electrolytes, and blood sugar are obtained. A thorough assessment and understanding of the patient's disease, his metabolic status, and the established principles of the technique of intravenous hyperalimentation will prevent the great majority of these complications.

SPECIFIC INDICATIONS FOR INTRAVENOUS HYPERALIMENTATION

A primary goal of intravenous hyperalimentation is to provide essential nutrients exclusively by vein for prolonged periods of time if necessary in quantities as high as two and one-half times the basal requirements. Thus, a state of anabolism can be achieved during conditions usually associated with a catabolic response. In infants requiring total intravenous feeding, an obvious goal is to promote normal weight gain, growth, and development until adequate feeding can be resumed via the alimentary tract. Intravenous hyperalimentation has proved efficacious in the treatment of more than 4000 adult patients and 300 infants for periods as long as one year in the former group and 22 months in the latter group at the Hospitals of The University of Pennsylvania and The University of Texas Medical School at Houston. Weight gain, wound healing, increased strength and activity, and an improved feeling of well-being have been observed in the vast majority of adults, and normal growth and development have been attained regularly in infants fed entirely by vein.

Enterocutaneous Fistulas

Patients with high enterocutaneous fistulas, resulting in losses of food and fluid from the alimentary tract through an abnormal opening in the skin, have been in the past extremely refractory to both nonoperative and operative treatment. With the advent of hyperalimentation, the fistulas have healed without operative intervention in more than 70 per cent of such patients, and in the remainder the nutritional status has improved sufficiently to lessen the risks of surgical correction.

Regional Enterocolitis and Ulcerative Colitis

Patients with severe inflammatory disease of the alimentary tract, such as regional enteritis, granulomatous colitis, or ulcerative colitis, often cannot tolerate food by mouth, both because the food cannot be absorbed properly by the diseased bowel and because administration of food orally seems to aggravate further the bowel symptoms. With hyperalimentation, such patients can be put on a regimen of nothing by mouth and still be given sufficient food by vein to gain weight and to synthesize body proteins. Moreover, they can be nourished into better condition to undergo surgical procedures, and, indeed, many of them have had spontaneous remissions of their disease on this regimen so that operation was postponed or obviated.

Renal Failure and Hepatic Decompensation

Patients with renal failure or impaired hepatic function have also been supported adequately by vein with the specially formulated solutions previously described, when feeding through the gastrointestinal tract was impossible or inadequate.

Burns

In patients with complicated major burns, in whom nutrient needs have been too great to be met by enteral feeding alone, as many as 6000 calories have been delivered by vein daily to supplement oral or tube feedings of 4000 to 5000 calories.

Short-Bowel Syndrome

Following massive small bowel resection, intravenous hyperalimentation has allowed provision of sufficient nutrient substrates and time for wound healing and bowel adaptation to occur, thus significantly reducing the ravages of the "short-gut syndrome."

Adjunctive to anticancer therapy in patients receiving chemotherapy for alimentary tract tumors, intravenous hyperalimentation and "bowel rest" have reduced gastrointestinal toxicity symptoms, thus allowing the delivery of two to three times the usual dose of chemotherapy medication. In patients receiving radiation therapy, particularly of the esophagus, this regimen has resulted in less pain, nausea, vomiting, diarrhea, and weight loss than in those fed by mouth or tube.

EFFECTS ON CONVALESCENCE

Many clinicians have the strong impression not only that more ill patients recover with the use of hyperalimentation, but that recovery is expedited for most patients who receive it. It is hoped that eventually data will be collected in sufficiently large numbers of patients to show that maintenance of the anabolic state in all patients requiring extensive operative procedures may allow a decreased incidence of complica-

tions and may achieve more rapid patient rehabilitation, thus reducing the duration and cost of hospitalization.

RESULTS OF INTRAVENOUS HYPERALIMENTATION

The following representative case reports may help to illustrate some specific spectacular results achieved with the use of intravenous hyperalimentation in the treatment of complicated conditions.

Case 1. Massive Intestinal Resection

The first infant to receive intravenous hyperalimentation underwent massive small bowel resection and transverse colon resection for congenital atresia.[22] Despite heroic attempts at conventional intravenous feeding by peripheral vein for 19 days after birth, body weight declined from 5 pounds 2 ounces to 4 pounds, and the child appeared moribund. After 45 days of intravenous hyperalimentation, her weight nearly doubled, to 7½ pounds, her body length increased by 2½ inches. This was the first association of long-term total intravenous feeding with normal growth and development in man (Fig. 3). At six months of age, she continued to grow and develop, having received 97 per cent of her nutrition by vein to this time. By one year of age, she had more than tripled her birth weight, and eventually achieved a maximal weight of 18½ pounds during her 22 months of intravenous hyperalimentation support.

Case 2. Congenital Gastrointestinal Tract Anomaly

A female infant was transferred to the Children's Hospital of Philadelphia shortly after birth for surgical correction of a ruptured omphalocele. The abdominal wall defect required temporary use of a large plastic patch to achieve complete coverage of the viscera.[10] After two weeks of intravenous hyperalimentation, the infant regained some function of the bowel and began taking small quantities of food by mouth. Within four weeks, the patient could ingest adequate amounts of formula, and the central venous catheter was removed. She had grown sufficiently during this time that the temporary patch could be removed, and the abdominal wall closed spontaneously (Fig. 4). She has continued to grow and develop normally without further difficulty for more than three years to date.

Case 3. Postoperative Enterocutaneous Fistula

A 46-year-old man with a 10-year history of regional enteritis was admitted to the hospital with severe abdominal pain, weight loss, and diarrhea. After one month of unsuccessful conservative medical management of this exacerbation of his inflammatory bowel disease, he underwent surgical resection of three feet of his intestine. Postoperatively, signs of bowel obstruction developed and he was operated upon a second time, less than two weeks after the first operation. Another 12 inches of diseased bowel was removed, and he initially recovered well after the operation.

Three weeks later, however, it was obvious that the sutures in the bowel had not held, and he began leaking 2 to 3 liters of fecal material daily through the wound and two drain sites in the abdomen. By this time, he had lost 30 pounds and appeared moribund. Roentgenographic examination confirmed that there was a large hole in the bowel at the site of the previous anastomosis (Fig. 5). Food by mouth was stopped, and the patient was started on a regimen of intravenous hyperalimentation and broad-spectrum antibiotics.

Text continued on page 173

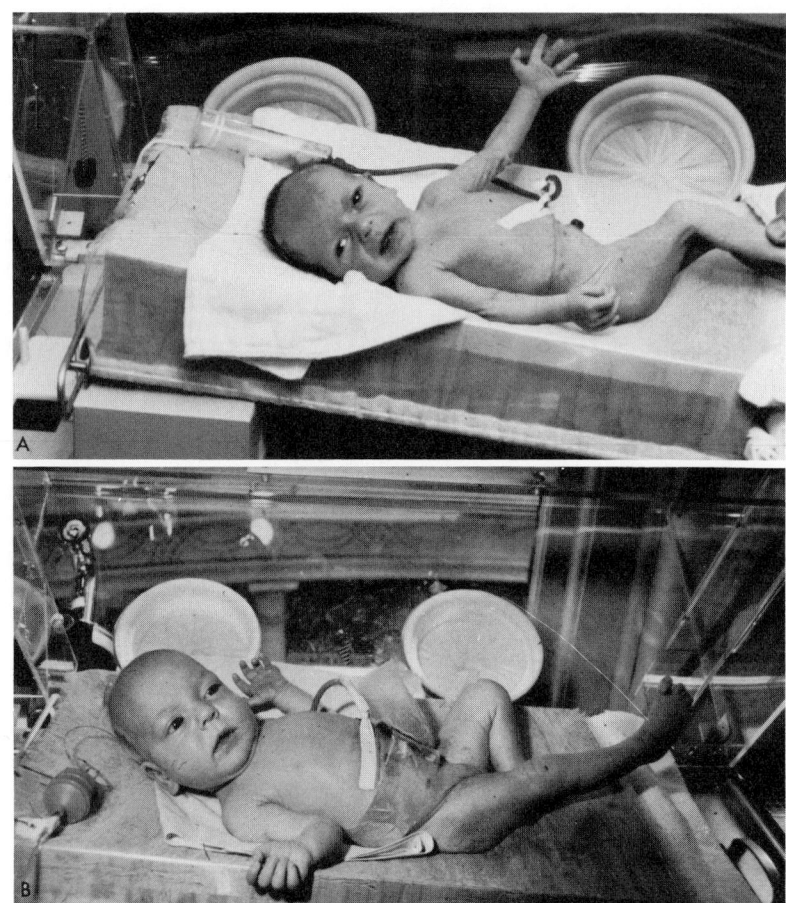

Figure 3.   During 45 days of intravenous hyperalimentation, this 19-day-old infant weighing 4 pounds (*A*) grew and developed normally, achieving a weight of 7½ pounds (*B*).

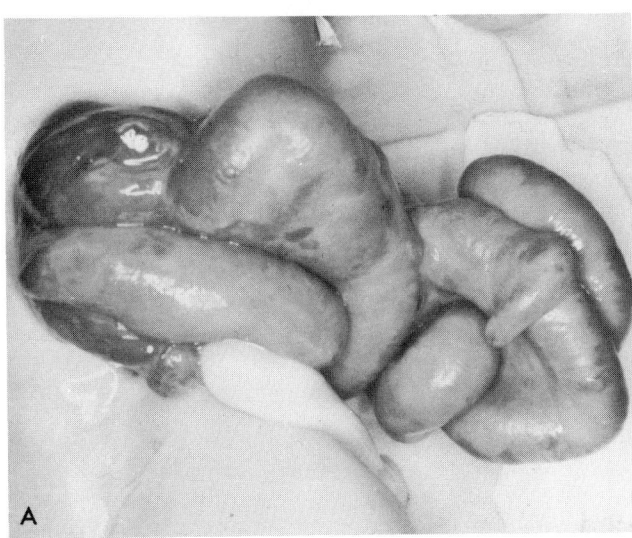

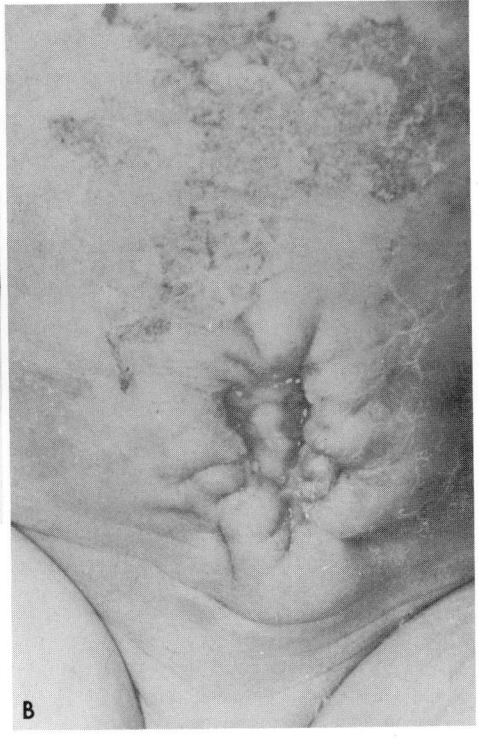

Figure 4. During four weeks of intravenous hyperalimentation and bowel rest, the abdominal cavity of this newborn infant with a ruptured omphalocele grew sufficiently to accommodate the extraperitoneal viscera *(A)*, and the fascial defect closed spontaneously *(B)*. Within nine additional days, epithelialization of the wound was complete.

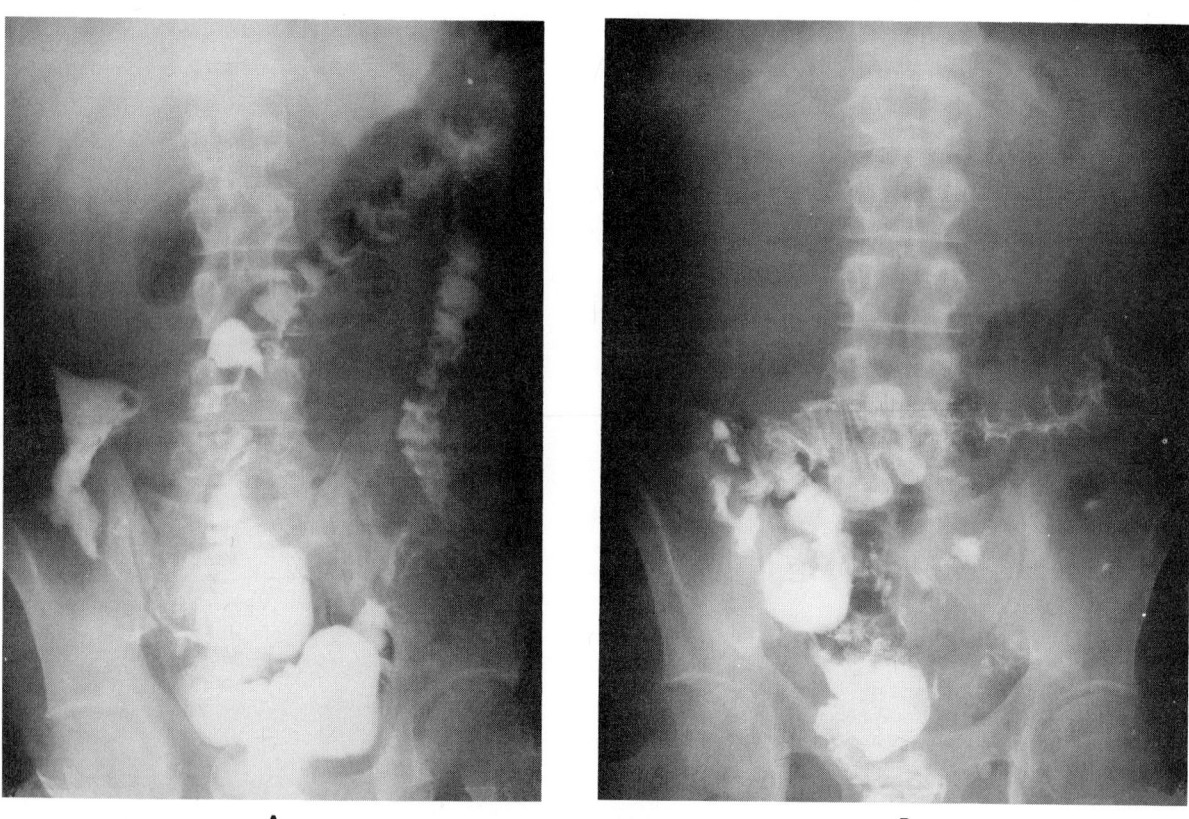

Figure 5.   Radiographic contrast medium can be seen emanating from the ileocolic anastomotic site on the left side of this roentgenogram (*A*). A similar study performed after six weeks of intravenous hyperalimentation and bowel rest showed no evidence of the previous enterocutaneous fistula (*B*).

Within 10 days, the fecal drainage ceased, the abdominal wall fistula closed spontaneously, and the patient began to gain weight. Within 40 days, repeat roentgenographic examination demonstrated complete healing of the bowel, and oral feedings were successfully reinstituted (Fig. 5). During this time, the patient had received a total of 176 liters of intravenous hyperalimentation solution and had gained 15 pounds of weight despite the total absence of oral feeding for 41 days (Fig. 6). Following discharge, he returned to his normal weight within three months and was able to resume his previous employment and activities.

Case 4. Inflammatory Disease of the Alimentary Tract

A 17-year-old-boy with a previous history of gastrointestinal dysfunction had abdominal pain, fever, anorexia, and weight loss from 205 pounds to 145 pounds over a three-month period. During this time, he was managed by conventional modes of medical therapy in the hospital without any signs of improvement in his condition. When first seen in consultation by the intravenous hyperalimentation team, his temperature was 102° F, and a 3 by 4 inch tender mass was felt in the right lower quadrant of the abdomen. Roentgenographic studies demonstrated severe regional enteritis of the terminal 2 feet of small bowel and cecum, and an associated inflammatory mass that produced complete obstruction of the right ureter. His therapeutic regimen consisted solely of nothing by mouth, antibiotics, and intravenous hyperalimentation. After only three days of bowel rest following institution of this therapy, the abdominal mass had regressed sufficiently to relieve the ureteral obstruction, and the patient's fever and pain disappeared. His nutrient intake was gradually increased to 5000 calories a day, entirely by vein. During seven weeks of intravenous hyperalimentation, he gained 12 pounds, and repeat roentgenographic examination revealed resolution of the granulomatous bowel disease. He was discharged on no therapy other than a low-roughage diet and tranquilizers, has returned to his original weight prior to his illness, and has been in good health for more than one year.

Case 5. Short-Gut Syndrome

Mesenteric venous thrombosis in a 44-year-old woman necessitated the resection of a length of the small intestine from the distal 2 inches of duodenum to the terminal 4 inches of ileum. Only 16 inches of small bowel remained for digestion and absorption of foodstuff (Fig. 7). Postoperatively, she was maintained on intravenous hyperalimentation for three months in order to allow her to recover from the massive insult of the surgical procedure and to permit bowel adaptation to occur. She was discharged at her normal weight, but within a month she lost about 20 pounds despite extensive dietary and pharmacologic therapeutic measures, and was hospitalized for another course of hyperalimentation. She required nine months of total and partial intravenous hyperalimenation support during the first year after operation.

During the second year, she was readmitted three times for three-week courses of supplementary intravenous feeding to restore body weight and strength, with increasing intervals of time between each admission. As a result of providing her with sufficient nutrient substrates and time, bowel adaptation gradually occurred with increased absorption, decreased motility, and cessation of diarrhea. Body weight stabilized at about 100 pounds, only 10 pounds below her usual weight. In addition to a low-fat, low-roughage, 3000 calorie diet, her therapeutic regimen currently includes multivitamins, iron, calcium, and anticholinergic-antiperistaltic medications orally; and vitamin B_{12} and folic acid intramuscularly. She has not required parenteral nutrition for more than six months to date, and it is hoped her intestinal absorptive capacities will continue to improve with time.

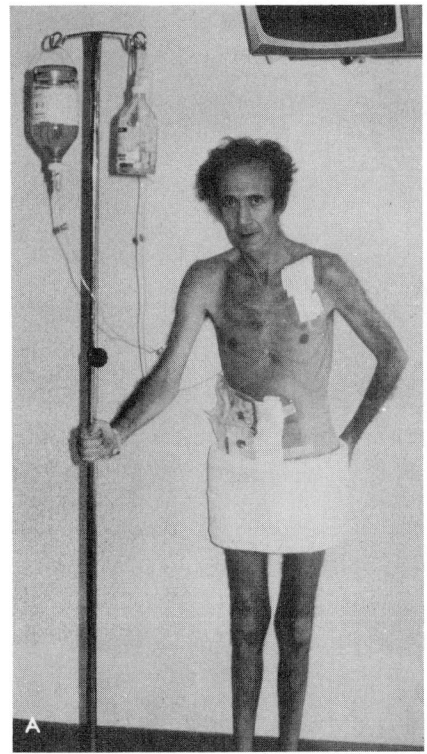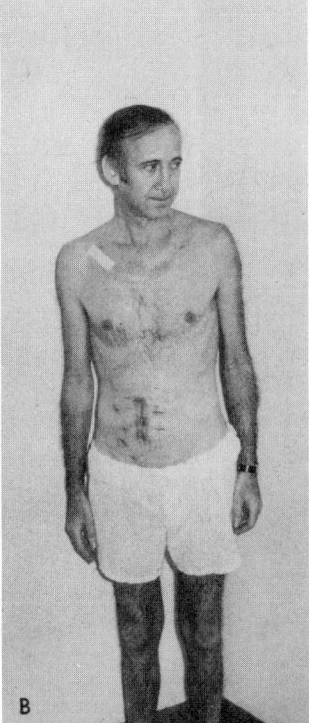

Figure 6. The large ileocolocutaneous fistula of this patient, who weighed 111½ pounds at the beginning of intravenous hyperalimentation therapy (A), healed without operation, and the patient gained 15 pounds in six weeks (B).

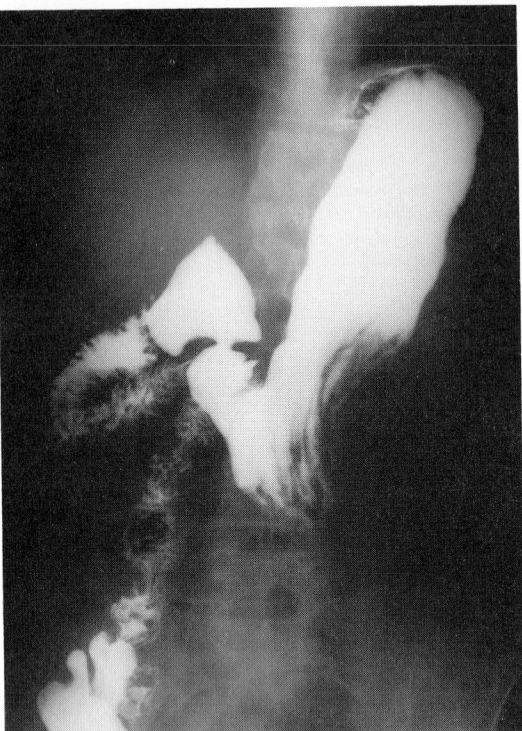

Figure 7. This roentgenogram of the gastrointestinal tract taken three years after massive small bowel resection shows the anastomosis of the third portion of the duodenum to the terminal four inches of the ileum.

Case 6. Acute Renal Failure

A previously healthy 42-year-old man sustained multiple injuries in an automobile collision and underwent celiotomy for drainage of a large retroperitoneal hematoma. The patient had a stormy septic course for three weeks, when another abdominal exploration was necessary to drain a large abscess. After the second operation, the patient became anuric and failed to respond to fluid and diuretic administration. He was transferred to the Hospital of the University of Pennsylvania for hemodialysis.

On admission he was hypothermic, hypotensive, hyponatremic, hypocalcemic, and hyperphosphatemic. His BUN was 80 mg. per 100 ml. and his creatinine was 8.9 mg. per 100 ml. Bile-stained purulent drainage emanated from a duodenal-cutaneous fistula at his right flank. He had lost 40 pounds since his accident. Because of persistent metabolic derangement, severe neuromuscular irritability, disorientation, and confusion, hemodialysis was performed.

Intravenous hyperalimentation with 50 to 70 per cent dextrose and essential L-amino acids infused via the subclavian vein was begun the day after dialysis.[8] Within 24 hours, urine output increased significantly. The dependent edema gradually disappeared, and over the next four weeks he gained 6 pounds, the duodenal fistula closed without further operation, and he resumed normal oral feedings (Fig. 8). From the fifth to the twenty-fifth day of total intravenous nutrition, positive nitrogen balance was maintained (Fig. 9) in the presence of positive potassium balance, normal water balance, and normal serum potassium levels. The BUN dropped to 26 mg. per 100 ml., and the serum creatinine fell to 1.8 mg. per 100 ml. Serum phosphorus and calcium levels returned to normal. Serum albumin increased from 2.5 to 3.2 gm. per 100 ml. without administration of exogenous plasma or albumin.

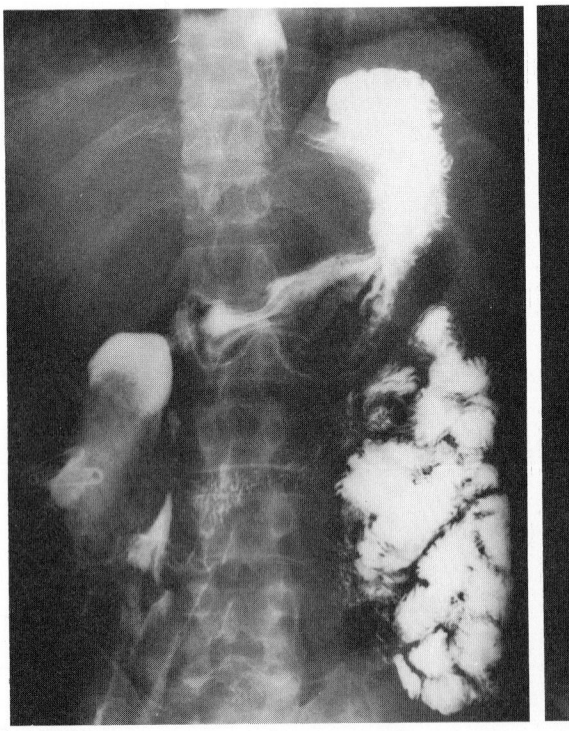

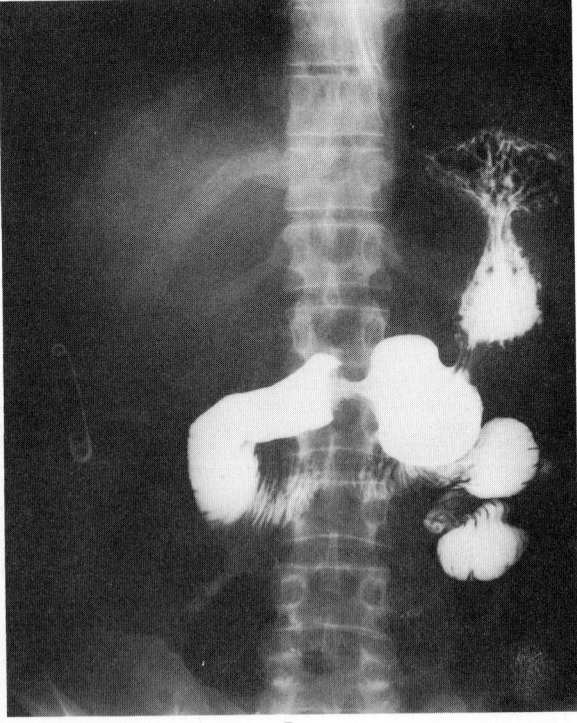

A　　　**B**

Figure 8. A large fistula following traumatic duodenal transection and unsuccessful operative repair is confirmed by the leak of contrast medium from the duodenal bulb toward the safety pin in the drain at the extreme left side of the roentgenogram (A). Complete healing of the duodenum is confirmed by follow-up roentgenography four weeks after intravenous hyperalimentation with renal failure solution (B).

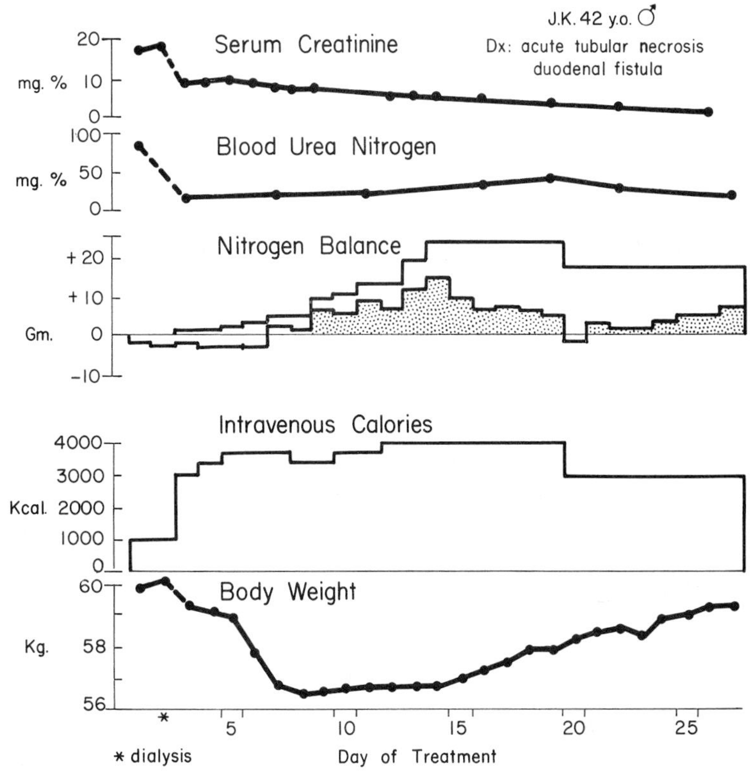

Figure 9. Metabolic data confirming the large amounts of nitrogen and calories that can be infused as essential L-amino acids and hypertonic dextrose without adversely affecting BUN and serum creatinine values in the presence of renal failure.

Two weeks after parenteral hyperalimentation was discontinued, he was discharged in good condition with normal renal function. Within two months, he attained his preaccident weight on an unrestricted diet and resumed his previous employment.

Therapeutic feeding has been progressively improved in each decade of the past century, but rarely until now has a prolonged, sustained, and meaningful state of anabolism been achieved exclusively by intravenous feedings, particularly under conditions ordinarily associated with a catabolic response. Critically ill patients require increased nutritional support for restoration of body tissues and normal metabolism. Superimposed on this need are the increased energy and nutrient requirements resulting from preoperative and intraoperative relative starvation, the postoperative catabolic response, and the accelerated metabolism associated with postoperative complications. With conscientious attention to established principles and techniques of intravenous hyperalimentation, long-term parenteral nutrition can be an effective and practical adjunct to the therapy of virtually every alimentary tract disease or disorder in which oral feeding is inadequate, ill advised, or impossible. Since there is virtually no pathologic process that can be treated better in a malnourished patient than in a well nourished patient, it no longer seems justifiable that critically ill patients be nutritionally deprived or subject to the ravages of starvation because they cannot obtain nourishment through the alimentary tract.

SELECTED REFERENCES

1. Albanese, A. A., Orto, L. A., and Zavatarro, D. N.: Biochemical significance of plasma amino nitrogen in man with a comparison of other criteria of protein metabolism. Metabolism, 7:256, 1958.
   Plasma amino nitrogen levels as indices of nutritional status were evaluated in 200 adults and correlated with body weight, nitrogen balance, exogenous protein load, and blood protein levels. The findings suggest that measurements of plasma amino nitrogen may provide a useful criterion of protein nutrition.

2. Bury, K. D., Stephens, R. V., and Randall, H. T.: Use of a chemically defined, liquid, elemental diet for nutritional management of fistulae of the alimentary tract. Am. J. Surg., 121:174, 1971.
   Thirteen patients with a variety of fistulas of the gastrointestinal tract were supported nutritionally with chemically defined liquid diets for 5 to 50 days. More than 50 per cent of the fistulas closed without operation, and the mortality rate was 15.4 per cent. Positive nitrogen, caloric, potassium, and magnesium balances were achieved in a significant number of patients.

3. Cahill, G. F.: Starvation in man. N. Engl. J. Med., 282:668, 1970.
   A series of metabolic adaptations that man undergoes during starvation in order to derive energy from adipose tissue and to conserve as efficiently as possible his protein reserves is discussed. The importance of insulin and other hormones in controlling fuel mobilization and homeostasis during starvation is outlined. The importance of fat and fat-derived fuels which are utilized preferentially and almost exclusively during starvation is elucidated and emphasized.

4. Cannon, P. R., Wissler, R. W., Woolridge, R. L., and Benditt, E. P.: Relationship of protein deficiency to surgical infection. Ann. Surg., 120:514, 1944.
   Attention is directed to the role of the blood and tissue globulins, especially gamma globulin fraction, in the mechanism of acquired resistance and to their origin from dietary amino acids. Evidence is presented that, to the extent that protein deficiency leads to

depression of the capacity of certain tissues to fabricate antibody globulin, the potential ability to elaborate specific antibodies is concomitantly impaired. The implications of protein depletion with respect to starvation, particularly in surgical patients, are discussed.

5. Cuthbertson, D. P.: Further observations on the disturbance of metabolism caused by injury, with particular reference to the dietary requirements of fracture cases. Br. J. Surg., 23:505, 1935.
The catabolic results and response to injury are classically described in this communication, together with the results of attempts to modify the marked loss of body protein that normally occurs under such circumstances. Countermeasures such as massage and manipulation, addition of meat extracts, gelatin, amino acids, protein hydrolysates to the diet, and use of diets of high caloric value are described and discussed. The importance of ingesting diets rich in first-class-protein and of high caloric value by patients sustaining long bone fractures from direct violence is emphasized.

6. Dudrick, S. J., Groff, D. B., and Wilmore, D. W.: Long-term venous catheterization in infants. Surg. Gynecol. Obstet., 129:805, 1969.
This paper describes in detail the technique for insertion and maintenance of long-term central venous catheters in infants requiring intravenous hyperalimentation.

7. Dudrick, S. J., Rhoads, J. E., and Vars, H. M.: Growth of puppies receiving all nutritional requirements by vein. In Fortschritte der parenteralen Ernährung. Lochham bei Munchen, West Germany, Pallas Verlag, 1967.
Results are reported on four puppies fed entirely intravenously for 72, 100, 200, and 255 days. This is the first demonstration of long-term intravenous feeding of sufficient quantity and quality to support growth and development in an immature animal of any species. The infusion techniques and diets utilized are described in detail.

8. Dudrick, S. J., Steiger, E., and Long, J. M.: Renal failure in surgical patients—treatment with intravenous essential amino acids and hypertonic glucose. Surgery, 68:180, 1970.
Solutions containing balanced quantities of essential L-amino acids, hypertonic dextrose, and other essential nutrients were administered by vein to 10 patients who had acute or chronic renal failure associated with or resulting from catastrophic complications precluding use of the gastrointestinal tract for alimentation. Weight gain, wound healing, and positive nitrogen balance occurred uniformly during periods of total intravenous nutrition, while blood urea nitrogen remained stable or decreased and the signs and symptoms of azotemia resolved. The data presented indicate that restoration of nutritional balance and achievement of protein synthesis is possible in patients who have renal failure and gastrointestinal dysfunction by the judicious administration of diets of high biologic value exclusively by vein.

9. Dudrick, S. J., Wilmore, D. W., Vars, H. M., and Rhoads, J. E.: Long-term total parenteral nutrition with growth, development and positive nitrogen balance. Surgery, 64:134, 1968.
The results of feeding six puppies entirely intravenously for 72 to 256 days are summarized. The successful application of the total intravenous technique developed in the animal laboratory to the first 30 surgical patients is reported, together with metabolic data on six of the patients. The results of intravenous hyperalimentation therapy of a newborn infant for 75 days are also presented.

10. Dudrick, S. J., Wilmore, D. W., Vars, H. M., and Rhoads, J. E.: Can intravenous feeding as the sole means of nutrition support growth in the child and restore weight loss in an adult? An affirmative answer. Ann. Surg., 169:974, 1969.
This paper outlines in detail the methods of total intravenous nutrition including catheter placement, catheter maintenance, infusion apparatus, and nutrient solution preparation and administration. Clinical application of intravenous hyperalimentation in the first 100 adult patients is tabulated, together with metabolic data in 11 patients. Spontaneous closure of enterocutaneous fistulas and results of intravenous hyperalimentation in the first nine newborn infants so treated are reported.

11. Elman, R.: Parenteral Alimentation in Surgery. New York, Paul B. Hoeber, 1947.
This primer is a most valuable compilation of the history of parenteral alimentation together with the results of the author's lifetime studies of parenteral amino acid and protein nutrition and its importance in surgical patients. All aspects of total intravenous feed-

12. Elman, R., Charnas, R., and Davey, H. W.: Ceiling of utilization of nitrogen. Arch. Surg., 47:216, 1943.
Positive nitrogen balance and regeneration of serum albumin were demonstrated in protein-depleted dogs given casein hydrolysate by vein. The importance of giving the total dose of nitrogen continuously during the 24 hours of the day if maximal utilization is to be achieved is emphasized. This study also established that the capacity of the body to assimilate protein was greater than the 1 gm. of protein per kilogram per day assumed as the maximum at that time.

13. Geyer, R. P.: Parenteral nutrition. Physiol. Rev., 40:150, 1960.
This is the most extensive and comprehensive review of the subject to the date of publication and is "must" reading for those interested in parenteral nutrition. An exhaustive search of the literature, which is brilliantly summarized and presented, forms the basis of this review. The properties, advantages, limitations, complications, and principles of administration of all of the basic parenteral nutrients are discussed succinctly.

14. Goldschmidt, S., Vars, H. M., and Ravdin, I. S.: Influence of foodstuffs upon the susceptibility of the liver to injury by chloroform, and the probable mechanism of their action. J. Clin. Invest., 18:277, 1939.
Studies in rats demonstrated that the incidence and severity of damage to hepatic cells 24 hours after 1 hour of chloroform anesthesia increased progressively with an increase in the lipid content of the liver. An adequate high-carbohydrate diet, by virtue of its effects in lowering hepatic lipids and sparing protein, decreased somewhat the incidence and severity of liver damage. A high-protein diet fed previous to chloroform anesthesia markedly reduced the incidence of hepatic cellular necrosis, even in livers with high lipid content. The importance of the relationship between starvation and the susceptibility of the liver to toxic agents is stressed.

15. Jones, C. M., and Eaton, F. B.: Post-operative nutritional edema. Arch. Surg., 27:159, 1933.
Data are presented from 34 surgical patients in whom critically low serum protein levels developed after routine surgical procedures. It is suggested that usually the low values for serum proteins and the consequent edema were the results of protein undernutrition before or after operation or both. The additional factors in production and treatment of these complications are discussed, and the possibility of nutritional edema of the intestinal wall as a cause of a poorly functioning gastroenterostomy was suggested.

16. Mecray, P. M., Barden, R. P., and Ravdin, I. S.: Nutritional edema: Its effect on gastric emptying time before and after gastric operations. Surgery, 1:53, 1937.
Data are presented from animals and man to demonstrate that gastric emptying time increases as the serum protein concentration decreases, whether the stomach is intact or whether it has been subjected to an operation. These findings were associated with edema of the gastric wall, and the implications of these relationships for the surgeon are discussed.

17. Newman, H. W., Wilson, R. H. L., and Newman, E. J.: Direct determinations of maximal daily metabolism of alcohol. Science, 116:328, 1952.
Administration of alcohol over several days to four subjects demonstrated a maximal metabolic capability of approximately 4.5 gm. of alcohol per kilogram body weight per day, equivalent to about 760 ml. of 100 proof liquor or 380 ml. of absolute alcohol. The data disregarded the fact that about 10 per cent of ingested alcohol is excreted, primarily via the lungs and kidneys. Increasing the blood alcohol concentration increased the rate of alcohol metabolism to only a minor degree.

18. Randall, H. T., and Dudrick, S. J.: Surgical nutrition: Parenteral and oral. In American College of Surgeons, Committee on Pre- and Postoperative Care: Manual of Preoperative and Postoperative Care, 2nd ed. Philadelphia, W. B. Saunders Company, 1971.
In this most up-to-date chapter are outlined the techniques and results of all of the currently possible means of providing adequate nutrition to surgical patients.

19. Ravdin, I. S., McNamee, H. G., Kamholz, J. H., and Rhoads, J. E.: Effect of hypoproteinemia on susceptibility to shock resulting from hemorrhage. Arch. Surg., 48:491, 1944.
Experiments in dogs demonstrated clearly for the first time the positive relationship between hypoproteinemia and increased sus-

ceptibility to hemorrhagic shock. Following plasmapheresis, the mean loss of blood necessary to produce a standard effect on the circulation in the normal animals was 67 per cent greater than the mean loss of blood required to produce the same effect in the hypoproteinemic animals.

20. Ravdin, I. S., Vars, H. M., and Goldschmidt, S.: The nonspecificity of suspensions of sodium xanthine in protecting the liver against injury by chloroform, and the probable cause of its action. J. Clin. Invest., 18:633, 1939.
    Irritating solutions of sodium xanthine or ricinoleate injected subcutaneously 24 hours before chloroform anesthesia protected the rat liver from injury. It is hypothesized that the inflammatory reaction aroused by these chemical agents afforded protection to the liver by increasing the protein split products made available to the body as a result of the increased protein catabolism incident to the inflammation.

21. Rhoads, J. E., and Alexander, C. E.: Nutritional problems of surgical patients. Ann. N.Y. Acad. Sci., 63:268, 1955.
    A rather broad review of the experimental and clinical evidence of the correlation between protein nutritional status and the responses of patients to surgical conditions is presented. The incidence of infectious and noninfectious complications is related to the serum protein concentration, and nitrogen losses before, during, and after various operations are compiled. The importance of finding ways to adequately nourish surgical patients by the simplest routes possible is emphasized.

22. Rhoads, J. E., and Kasinskas, W.: Influence of hypoproteinemia on the formation of callus in experimental fracture. Surgery, 11:38, 1942.
    Experimental data are presented to indicate that severe hypoproteinemia retards the formation of bony callus in fractures produced in dogs by section of the ulna with a saw.

23. Rhoads, J. E., Rawnsley, H. M., Vars, H. M., Crichlow, R. W., Nelson, H. M., Spagna, P. M., Dudrick, S. J., and Rhoads, J. E., Jr.: The use of diuretics as an adjunct in parenteral hyperalimentation for surgical patients with prolonged disability of the gastrointestinal tract. Bull. Int. Soc. Surg., 24:59, 1965.
    Surgical patients were maintained in a state of nitrogen equilibrium or positive nitrogen balance by infusing 5 to 7 liters of 10 to 15 per cent nutrient solutions by peripheral vein, together with sufficient intravenous chlorothiazide to promote diuresis of the extra vehicular water. Up to 150 gm. of protein equivalent was given in the form of fibrin hydrolysate daily, together with as much as 2400 calories in the form of slightly hypertonic dextrose. Frequent assessments of water and electrolyte balances were necessary to prevent untoward aberrations from normal.

24. Thompson, W. D., Ravdin, I. S., and Frank, I. L.: Effect of hypoproteinemia on wound disruption. Arch. Surg., 36:500, 1938.
    When every other factor that could be controlled was controlled, the incidence (72 per cent) of disruption of abdominal wounds in dogs was higher in animals with hypoproteinemia than in normal animals. Histologic evidence of decreased fibroplasia and tissue edema was present in the wounds of the hypoproteinemic animals.

25. Weisberg, H. F.: Water, Electrolyte, and Acid-Base Balance. Baltimore, Williams & Wilkins Company, 1962.
    This is a most handy and comprehensive reference manual, for both the novice and the expert, in fluid, electrolyte, and acid-base problems and their management. The author has a unique, thoughtful, and at times amusing technique of presenting and explaining complex problems and concepts in a simple, straightforward, and understandable manner.

26. Whipple, G. W.: Protein production and exchange in the body, including hemoglobin, plasma protein and cell protein. Am. J. Med. Sci., 196:609, 1938.
    This extensive summary of protein nutrition highlights the most significant experiments to that time and points out the primary importance of the liver in body protein metabolism. The production of hemoglobin, plasma proteins, and labile protein reserves and the exchange of protein materials within the body are described and discussed.

27. Wilmore, D. W., and Dudrick, S. J.: Growth and development of an infant receiving all nutrients exclusively by vein. J.A.M.A., 203:860, 1968.
    The techniques and solution used, together with the metabolic data and other results obtained, during the first 44 days in the first infant fed exclusively by vein with intravenous hyperalimentation are reported. Normal growth and development were achieved, as manifested by increases of 5.0 cm. in head circumference, 6.3 cm. in length, 8.9 cm. in chest circumference, and 1447 gm. in weight. The 30 per cent solution containing all required nitrogen, calories, and essential nutrients was infused continuously through a 0.22 μ membrane filter into the superior vena cava via a single catheter for the entire duration of the study.

28. Wohl, M. D., Reinholt, J. G., and Rose, S. B.: Antibody response in patients with hypoproteinemia. Arch. Intern. Med., 83:402, 1949.
    In an immunologic study of 102 patients, those with a disturbance of protein metabolism sufficient to cause low serum albumin showed an appreciable impairment of antibody production. Supplementation of the diets of these patients with lactalbumin or casein hydrolysate enhanced antibody formation but did not allow the antibody titer to rise to the same extent as in normal patients receiving the same antigenic stimulation.

8

SURGICAL ASPECTS OF DIABETES MELLITUS

John H. Davis, M.D.

Since diabetes mellitus may affect from 1 to 10 per cent of the general population, depending upon age, it is an ever present problem. The surgeon's interest in diabetes derives from the multiple ways in which it can affect the surgical patient. The following points are pertinent: (1) Diabetes is a major metabolic defect of carbohydrate and fat metabolism which may require therapy to successfully carry the patient through a surgical procedure. (2) This disorder may cause surgical conditions or complications such as infection, vascular disease, and neurological abnormalities that require surgical intervention. (3) Surgical intervention and general anesthesia alter normal glucose metabolism in normal patients, creating a state of mild diabetes and aggravating the diabetic state in the patient who already has diabetes mellitus. (4) Diabetes and hypoglycemia must always be considered as a cause of unconsciousness in any patient seen by the surgeon, particularly those who are seen following an injury.

HISTORY

The term "diabetes" was introduced by Aretaeus of Cappadocia and means to syphon or pass through. It was originally thought to be a weakness of the kidney because of the polyuria so commonly seen in the disease. Avicenna (about A.D. 1000) wrote a clinical description of this disease and noted many of the complications, including pyodermic infections and diabetic gangrene as well as the sweetness or honey-like substance found in the urine of the diabetic patients. Many other physicians associated a sweet urine with diabetes, but at the time specific tests for urine sugar were unknown. It was not until 1848 that the cupric oxide test for urinary sugar was developed by von Fehling.

In 1682, Brunner noted polyuria and polydipsia occurring in experimental animals following total pancreatectomy. He apparently did not associate this with diabetes, and it was not until 1778 that Cawley was the first to connect diabetes with the pancreas.

Claude Bernard was the first to demonstrate the presence of glycogen in the liver and to suggest the theory of glucose formation from glycogen. He believed that the high blood sugar level found in the patient with diabetes was due to an overproduction of sugar by the liver.

In 1869 the islets of the pancreas were discovered by Paul Langerhans and were subsequently named in his honor. Von Mering and Minkowski deserve the credit for demonstrating that the totally depancreatized dog develops hyperglycemia and glycosuria, followed by ketosis, coma, and death. While studying the role of the pancreas in fat digestion, pancreatectomy was performed, and it was noted that the dog passed large quantities of urine at irregular intervals. Minkowski tested the urine for sugar and connected the cause of the diabetic state with the removal of the pancreas. In this same year (1889) Brown-Sequard introduced the term "internal secretion," which later was applied to the secretion of the islet cells as well as other endocrine organs.

In 1920 an orthopedic surgeon, F. G. Banting, and a medical student, Charles H. Best, produced diabetes in dogs by total pancreatectomy and were the first to demonstrate a method of therapy. They isolated insulin from dog pancreas, fetal calf pancreas, and adult beef pancreas utilizing methods that protected the insulin from the action of the proteolytic enzymes of the pancreas. They were the first to recognize that any extraction process might allow the proteolytic enzymes of the pancreas to destroy material contained in the islets. Utilizing cold, acid, and alcohol as protective agents, they were able to extract from the islet cells a substance that was clear and sterile and contained from 12 to 16 international units of insulin per cubic centimeter. This purified extract was given to diabetic animals and to human beings and was found to produce a marked fall in the blood sugar and no local reaction at the injection site. Subsequent studies have led to purified insulin in its crystalline form, and a variety of compounds have been developed that permit a delayed release or utilization of the insulin when administered to the patient.

In summary, these studies show that the islets of the pancreas are responsible for insulin production and that insulin in some way controls glucose metabolism. Subsequent investigators have elucidated multiple chemical pathways of glucose production, release, and breakdown, as well as many aspects of insulin production and transport, plus a number of other factors such as glucagon which affect insulin action. With all of this increased knowledge, we are reasonably able to treat the patient with diabetes mellitus. As yet, however, we do not completely understand how insulin works. While insulin is involved in the control of glucose metabolism, a simple deficiency of insulin is not the entire picture of diabetes; it is merely one aspect of a major metabolic defect.[16]

PATHOPHYSIOLOGY

There are about 1.5 million islets in the pancreas with a total weight of about one gram. This small mass of tissue exercises control over much of the metabolic function of the body. The islets contain three types of cells—alpha, beta, and delta. The beta cells comprise about 75 per cent of the total cellular mass and are responsible for insulin production. The alpha cells secrete glucagon and the delta cells produce gastrin. It has been estimated that the adult pancreas contains about 200 units of insulin and secretes about 35 to 50 units per day. Insulin is released in the form of proinsulin, which is subsequently cleaved by trypsin-like enzymes.

Glucagon and insulin are interrelated but in exactly what manner is unknown. Glucagon is secreted by the alpha cells and is in excess of insulin by a factor of 100 in fetal pancreas. Glucagon reaches its highest level in fetal pancreas in the second trimester of pregnancy, and the alpha cells outnumber the beta cells from the tenth week to the fifth month of pregnancy. After this period the alpha cells progressively decline in number.[16]

We will next examine the data available about these compounds, their relationship, and their effect on the diabetic syndrome. Inadequate insulin leads to hyperglycemia, impaired transport of glucose into muscle and fat, release of glucose by the liver, and increased lipolysis. When insulin levels are insufficient and the blood sugar rises above 160 mg. per 100 ml., glycosuria develops. This creates an osmotic diuresis with loss of water, and an increase in serum osmolality, with the development of thirst. Sodium and potassium are also lost in the osmotic diuresis, and protein catabolism is increased. If this is allowed to continue, ketonemia develops secondary to increased lipolysis with a rise in serum fatty acids, mostly acetoacetic and beta-hydroxybutyric acid. These dissociate to release H^+, with a subsequent fall in the blood pH. When the pH drops below 7.2, respiratory compensation takes place with deep and prolonged respirations (Kussmaul respirations) and the loss of CO_2. This tends to correct the pH toward normal. If the process is allowed to continue, the pH continues to fall, further dehydration occurs, and compensation fails, leading to reduced cerebral function, coma, and death.

Glucagon secreted by the alpha cells of the islets has some equally potent effects on carbohydrate metabolism. Glucagon seems to have a reciprocal relationship to insulin; therefore, high plasma insulin suppresses glucagon and a low plasma insulin stimulates glucagon secretion. Hyperglucagonemia is associated with every known cause of hyperglycemia. When both glucagon and insulin are suppressed, there is no hyperglycemia unless the glucagon level is restored to normal. *Somatostatin* suppression of glucagon in diabetic animals restores the blood glucose levels to normal. (Somatostatin inhibits the release of somatotropin or growth hormone and its site of action appears to be the pancreas.[11]

Insulin appears to act by removing glucose from the blood and causing it to be stored in the liver, muscle, and adipose tissue. Glucagon, on the other hand, causes mobilization from storage deposits in the liver and makes it readily available for utilization by peripheral tissues, such as brain.[6]

Inadequate insulin causes a failure of removal of glucose from the blood into its storage areas, resulting in hyperglycemia, and too much glucagon causes excessive release of glucose with subsequent hyperglycemia. Whether this relationship is causative in the development of diabetes mellitus is not clear at present. Because the etiology of diabetes mellitus is still unclear, the investigation of its cause continues, and new evidence developed when Craighead demonstrated that a diabetes-like disease could be produced in mice by the encephalomyocarditis virus (EMC).[10] This picornavirus was first isolated from the heart of a pig dying of myocarditis. This virus replicates in the pancreas, parotid, and lacrimal glands as well as in the myocardium and central nervous system. One strain of the virus, known as the M variant, replicates exclusively in the islets of Langerhans. Immunofluorescent techniques have demonstrated that the viral antigens are found exclusively in the beta cells of the islets. Some of the damage may be the result of an autoimmune reaction because the islets are infiltrated by immunoreactive lymphocytes and macrophages. This experimental diabetes is worse in males than in females but lessened if the testicles of the male are removed prior to innoculation with the virus. The disease is also made worse if the animals are obese or if they have had pharmacologic doses of steroids. Renal lesions similar to those occurring in human diabetes are also found with the virus-produced disease.

The most important factor in the etiology of diabetes in man or animals appears to be a genetic trait. There is ample suggestion for this in man, and Craighead has shown a similar effect in mice. Two selected strains were given EMC virus: both developed infection of the pancreas, and both developed antibody to the same extent, but the majority of one strain developed diabetes whereas very few of the other strain developed the disease. Two other members of the picornavirus family, namely, Coxsackie B4 and the Venezuelan equine encephalomyelitis (VEE), have also been implicated as potential causes of diabetes. While these agents do not cause all of the pathologic changes seen in human diabetes, such as vascular lesions and blindness, they do provide a fundamental model for study. The added possibility of a viral etiology coupled with the generally accepted genetic basis for diabetes makes the role of these hormones in the pathogenesis of diabetes even more difficult to understand. However, further understanding of the relationship of these hormones should permit a clearer understanding of the biochemical process and lead to better methods of control. If we can eventually provide a more satisfactory control of the hyperglycemia, we may be able to prevent some of the complications that are so devastating to the patient.

PREOPERATIVE AND INTRAOPERATIVE MANAGEMENT OF THE DIABETIC PATIENT

Elective Surgery. It is an extremely rare situation in which the patient with known diabetes cannot be satisfactorily brought under control prior to elective surgery. It should be remembered that the diabetic who is normally controlled by diet alone may rapidly escape from balance under the stress of operation with its increased catabolism and often a large amount of glucose infusion. The diabetic who is controlled by insulin therapy may require larger amounts of insulin during the operative stress, but one must be careful that excessive amounts are not given so that a hypoglycemic state develops with its attendant serious complications. Finally, latent diabetes mellitus is not uncommon and every prospective patient must be screened by a urine examination and perhaps by a two-hour postprandial blood sugar determination as part of the initial evaluation.

The patient who is a known diabetic and on insulin control should be prepared for surgery by additional studies, which include serum electrolytes, blood urea nitrogen, or serum creatinine, as well as blood gases. These baseline data can be of great help in managing the patient preoperatively and bringing him into the best possible control, as well as serving as a guide for following the patient throughout the operative and immediate postoperative stress. The ideal management consists of keeping the patient slightly hyperglycemic with a mild glycosuria during this period. Hypoglycemia should be avoided at all times; the slight hyperglycemia and glycosuria are not harmful. The patient who has been on an oral hypoglycemia agent or on long-acting insulin may be easier to control if this is discontinued on the day prior to surgery and regular insulin substituted with doses given every four to six hours. The daily dose of regular insulin should be approximately equal to that of the long-acting insulin that the patient was taking prior to surgery.

On the day of operation, an intravenous infusion of 5 per cent glucose is started and about one half of the morning dose of regular insulin is given subcutaneously. It has been a common practice to add the regular insulin to the intravenous bottle, but there is some loss of the insulin activity in its contact with the glass. However, if one is aware of this and monitors the patient's urine and/or blood glucose, this method is satisfactory. Normally one uses about 10 units of regular insulin per liter of 5 per cent glucose. The glucose should be administered through a separate IV line so that continuous infusion is possible and is not interrupted by the administration of blood or other fluids. If blood or other fluids are administered during the operative period, they should be given through a separate intravenous line. If the surgical procedure is to be a long one, the patient's glucose should be monitored during the procedure and appropriate corrections made.

Postoperatively, a sliding scale may be used to provide the proper dose of insulin until the patient is back on an oral regimen. For the majority of patients the following schedule is satisfactory:

Urinalysis	Insulin
++++ sugar	15 units
+++	10 units
++	5 units
+	None

Most elective surgery will permit the patient to resume an oral intake by the third postoperative day, and then glucose infusions can be discontinued as the caloric intake is picked up via the oral route. Careful monitoring of the blood sugar and urine sugar is important throughout this period in order to prevent the extreme hyperglycemia that may result from excess glucose infusion or the hypoglycemia that may result from excess insulin administration.

Emergency Surgery. Occasionally a patient is admitted in severe diabetic acidosis or coma secondary to a problem demanding urgent surgical intervention. For example, a patient may have had his diabetes under good control until he developed a silent appendicitis with perforation and peritonitis. Such a patient may not realize his diabetes is getting out of control before his cerebral function becomes obtunded and he is admitted to the emergency room. The most immediate diagnostic steps to be taken include the determination of the serum acetone as well as electrolytes, blood sugar, and urinalysis. Immediate infusion of normal saline with the administration of regular insulin through the intravenous line should be initiated. Depending on the degree of ketosis, insulin administration may range from 50 to 300 units, with half being given intravenously and the remainder subcutaneously. (If the patient is in shock the entire dose of insulin should be given intravenously because of the poor absorption of medication by the patient in shock.) The patient is then carefully monitored with hourly blood glucose levels as well as frequent evaluation of the hypovolemic state, usually with the aid of a central venous catheter and an indwelling urinary catheter. As soon as the serum electrolytes are known, one can switch to Ringer's lactate solution to help correct the acidosis. Potassium which has also been lost through the osmotic diuresis that occurs in this state should be added to the intravenous solution as soon as an adequate urinary output has been obtained. (When the urine output approximates 30 ml. per hour, potassium replacement therapy should be started.) As soon as the acidosis is corrected or at least is well on its way to correction and the dehydration has been corrected, the patient may undergo the emergency surgical procedure for the original cause of the problem. The same therapy used to carry a diabetic patient through elective surgery may now be followed in carrying this patient through the emergency procedure.

COMPLICATIONS

Vascular. One of the most devastating aspects of diabetes mellitus is the pathologic changes that occur in both the large and small blood vessels. The large vessels begin to develop atherosclerosis at a much earlier age than that seen in the normal population. In addition to large vessel disease, there is a microangiopathy that occurs in the small blood vessels brought about by thickening of the basement membrane and resulting in a malfunction of these vessels.[14] The cause of these changes is unknown, but until recently it had not been believed to be dependent upon the control of glucose metabolism. Several studies in which comparisons of patients under so-called tight control of their glycosuria versus those not as adequately controlled did not appear to show any difference in the onset or severity of the vascular disease. One must bear in mind, however, that control of glucose metabolism by present methods is a relative thing. While insulin may be given in a variety of ways, the glucose level in the bloodstream may be fluctuating so that there are periods of hyperglycemia with mild glycosuria even though the total spillage for a 24-hour period is not great. Since the normal feedback mechanism, which occurs when the plasma glucose rises about 120 mg. per 100 ml. and mediates the release of insulin to bring it within normal limits, is not available to the diabetic, control by Depo-insulin that has been injected is much less responsive. Recent studies suggest that the hyperglycemia may play a role in the development of the pathologic changes in blood vessels as well as in some other organs.[13] It is known that in the rabbit aorta the polyol or sorbitol pathway may be utilized when insulin is not available and the glucose is converted to sorbitol and eventually to fructose.[1, 7] The sorbitol attracts water, causing edema in the area, and this may play a role in development of vascular disease. (This mechanism seems to be operative in the development of cataracts, as the sorbitol pathway is utilized in the lens of the eye.) These studies suggest, then, that the hyperglycemia results in significant alterations in the metabolism of the aortic intima and media.

The same sorbitol pathway is utilized by nerve cells, and it has been clearly demonstrated that swelling occurs in the Schwann cell. This may result in impaired nerve conduction and diabetic neuropathy. The sorbitol pathway in the diabetic nerve appears to be much more responsive to fluctuations in blood glucose than in the nondiabetic nerve. Diabetic neuropathy so often accompanies the vascular disease that they should be considered together when one is managing the vascular complications.

The alterations in basement membranes which affect the fine vessels of the kidney are not explained by the sorbitol mechanism. There seems to be an overproduction of basement membrane units, particularly those containing hydroxylysine and its glycosidically linked disaccharide unit. Recent studies suggest that while this thickened basement membrane is present in almost all adult diabetics, it is not present in all juvenile diabetics. However, the thickening is unrelated to the duration of the diabetes. This suggests that it is not affected by the duration of hyperglycemia but may well be independent of it. It may in fact be a primary lesion of the diabetic syndrome.[2, 3, 15]

Clinical Management of the Diabetic Foot. Every patient with known diabetes should have the peripheral circulation carefully evaluated with respect to the peripheral pulses, condition of the skin, and sensation in the foot. One of the most serious complications of diabetes mellitus is the early onset of atherosclerosis of both large and small vessels, particularly those involving the leg and foot. If the circulation appears to be normal and there is no evidence of neuropathy, the patient need have no further concern at present, but he should be cautioned about meticulous care of his feet and rechecked periodically for the premature onset of ischemic changes.

If there is evidence of diminished circulation, even though it is minimal as measured by the peripheral pulses, changes in skin sensation, or changes in the skin of the foot, the following measures should be instituted to prevent any damage to the skin which might lead to ulceration and gangrene. Of paramount importance is the wearing of well-fitted shoes so that corns and calluses or other trauma to the skin does not occur. This rather simple measure is often a difficult one, because many patients either are not interested or do not feel they can afford the type of shoe that is proper for their feet. The surgeon must emphasize the risk involved in possible loss of the extremity due to minor ulcerations; this will often encourage the patient to seek properly fitting shoes regardless of the cost. These patients should not be allowed to go barefoot at any time because of their increased susceptibility to skin breakdown from minor trauma. They must be warned about the difficulties that may be encountered if too much heat is applied to the foot or if the foot is allowed to get too cold. The normal foot responds to heat or cold by rapid dilatation or constriction of the peripheral circulation, but the patient with arteriosclerosis cannot respond in a normal manner. An all too common problem is the patient with diabetes and an impaired circulation, who allows his feet to become too cold while hunting or hiking and then believes that he will improve the situation by plunging them into hot water to restore the circulation. While tissue damage may have occurred from the cold itself, it more often occurs when extremely hot water is used to warm the feet. This is particularly true if there is any evidence of neuropathy, so that the patient's sensation is diminished and he does not realize that a burn of the foot may be occurring.

Meticulous care of the foot in the form of proper nail cutting, management of corns and calluses, and the prevention of dryness and fissuring of the skin is paramount. The extremities should have lanolin applied morning and evening to prevent the dry, flaking skin and fissures that often occur. The lanolin keeps the skin pliable and makes it more able to withstand the minor trauma that occurs from socks and shoes. The nails should be carefully trimmed by someone else if the patient's vision is impaired. The nails should be trimmed straight across and care must be taken not to allow the cutting instrument to dig into the surrounding skin. Corns and calluses should be managed by removing the pressure points that are causing them. Properly fitting shoes, metatarsal bars, and ring pads will often reduce these so that no further treatment is necessary.

If ulcers or gangrenous spots have already occurred on the foot or between the toes, a very urgent situation is present. The parts should be put at rest if at all possible, but if this is not practical because of the patient's need to work, very careful protection of the damaged area must be provided. The ulcerated area should be cleansed daily with tepid water and a mild soap, followed by the careful application of a dressing. A nonstick type of dressing should be applied, overlaid with cotton padding, and held in place by a loose-fitting bandage without tape. Cultures of the area should be taken; they will almost always be positive, but this does not demand immediate antibiotic therapy. If there is evidence of inflammation about the ulcer or if systemic signs of infection occur, systemic antibiotics should be started immediately. In most instances the bacteria cultured from such ulcers are surface contaminants and can be managed by the local means mentioned above.

The patient should sleep with his feet lowered approximately 5 degrees, usually accomplished by placing two bricks under each of the two headposts of the bed. This permits some relief of the pain if present and permits the patient to get a night's sleep without having the leg hang down and develop edema. Too often these patients find that they can relieve the pain by sitting up in a chair and allowing the feet to be dependent. Swelling then begins to occur, and a relentless cycle is initiated in which dependent edema develops, causing a further reduction in the circulation which often progresses to a wet gangrenous foot. If elevation of the head of the bed is not adequate to allow a night's sleep, analgesics must be used. Narcotics may be necessary to alleviate the ischemic pain and permit a night's sleep while the ulcer is healing. These conservative measures may result in the healing of a small ulcerated area, but unfortunately many will be progressive and no measure seems to be entirely satisfactory in preventing this.

Vascular reconstructive operations should be considered in patients with diabetic ischemia of the lower extremity, since many of them have large vessel occlusion in addition to small vessel disease. If the patient has evidence of ischemia, such as intermittent claudication or ulceration, and the pulses are diminished or absent, arteriography is indicated to determine whether or not surgical reconstruction is feasible. Some surgeons believe that these patients should have prophylactic arterial reconstruction when an occluded vessel is found, whether or not symptoms are present in the extremity. It is my belief that these patients are no different from any other patient with an arterial occlusion and arterial reconstruction should be performed only to relieve symptoms. Fortunately, successful arterial reconstruction will often result in the improvement of circulation in the foot, but the disease still may be rapidly progressive and the result is not as long-lasting as it may be in the nondiabetic. However, the points to be stressed are that the patient's diabetes does not mean that arterial reconstruction cannot be performed and that these patients should not be ignored by the surgeon, as has been the custom in the past. Too often no attempt at visualization of the arterial tree and possible reconstruction has been made because the patient has diabetes; the assumption has been made that small vessel disease is the cause and therefore surgical therapy is useless.

INFECTION

The patient with diabetes may or may not be more susceptible to infection, but treatment of an established infection must be viewed as a serious matter. It has long been thought that the diabetic is more susceptible to infection, but the evidence for this is not conclusive, with a few exceptions. There is reasonable evidence that they are definitely more susceptible to mucormycosis, for example. However, increased susceptibility to the ordinary bacterial and viral infections is not clear. The role of control of the diabetes and its effect on the patient's susceptibility to infection also remain unclear. We were able to show in the experimental laboratory that the alloxan diabetic rat is more susceptible to ascending pyelonephritis than the normal animal and that careful insulin control of the diabetes made no difference in this risk.[4, 5] We also demonstrated that a subcutaneous infection with *Staphylococcus aureus* was far more serious in the diabetic animal,[8] but this did not hold for a hematoma infected with *Eschericia coli.*[9]

Regardless of the risk of susceptibility to infection, there is little doubt that *the presence of an infection in the diabetic may have more serious consequences than if the patient were not diabetic.*

It is impossible to separate the role of vascular disease in infection. There is no doubt that, if the tissue is ischemic, what might be only surface contamination in the normal patient can become invasive infection in the diabetic patient. Since infection may be very serious in the young diabetic person or in the alloxan diabetic animal in which vascular changes have not yet occurred, it is a serious problem demanding attention and is worsened by the presence of vascular disease.

Diabetes is a major metabolic defect which affects almost all cells in the body and may interfere with their ability to respond to infectious agents in the normal way. It is known that the polymorphonuclear leukocyte of the diabetic has a normal phagocytic mechanism but appears to have a markedly decreased power to kill the engulfed bacteria. Thus, one of the body's major defense mechanisms becomes less efficient. Careful insulin control tends to ameliorate this problem. When infection occurs, it alters the insulin requirement of the diabetic and unless carefully monitored can rapidly lead to ketoacidosis. Thus, strenuous efforts should be made to prevent infection, but once it occurs equally strenuous therapy should be instituted.

Traumatic Wounds. Unless very small, these should be managed under medical supervision. The same principles apply to these wounds as to others. Careful inspection, irrigation, and débridement should be performed. If the wound is over 8 to 12 hours old, *delayed* closure should be planned; if less than this and otherwise clean, primary closure should be utilized. If the wound is heavily contaminated, or if it is in possibly ischemic tissue, broad spectrum prophylactic antibiotics should be instituted. We use penicillin and tetracycline until such time as culture data reveal the need for a more specific agent.

Elective Surgery. Patients undergoing an elective operation should have every effort made to clear up any existing infection unless this is the reason for operation. Patients often forget to tell the surgeon about some small infection that has been present for a few days, and it may very well be overlooked at the time of examination. There is a much higher incidence of wound infection in nondiabetics who undergo operative intervention with the presence of a remote infection. Since the diabetic responds in a more serious fashion, remote infection should be carefully searched for and eliminated prior to operation. If the infection cannot be eliminated, the patient should have antibiotic therapy started the morning of operation and continued for three to four days after surgery.

The role of prophylactic antibiotics in elective surgery is controversial and requires good judgment on the part of the surgeon. It seems wise to start intravenous antibiotics about one hour prior to surgery, in any diabetic patient who is to have a hollow viscus entered, or a foreign body, such as a vascular prosthesis, implanted.

When prophylactic antibiotics are used, a time limit order should be written so that they are not continued for prolonged periods of time. It is unlikely that they are required only for the day of operation, but most surgeons use them for about three to four days. By that time the wound is well sealed and its defenses should be able to manage any circulating or local bacteria, or if not, evidence of infection in spite of the prophylactic antibiotics will be seen and this requires culture data followed by the appropriate antibiotic plus surgical drainage.

Patients with diabetes who have undergone elective surgery and require postoperative ventilatory support are usually given prophylactic antibiotics. These are frequently patients who have had vascular procedures, open-heart procedures, or very major abdominal procedures. If continued ventilatory support is necessary, careful clinical and bacteriologic evaluation of the patient determines the need for additional antibiotic therapy.

NEUROLOGIC DISORDERS

Trauma: The Unconscious Patient. The surgeon who sees emergency cases, particularly trauma, must be wary of the unconscious or confused patient. While not common, an occasional patient has sustained the trauma because of ketoacidosis or hypoglycemia secondary to an insulin reaction. It should be routine procedure to obtain a blood sugar analysis of any patient admitted to the emergency department in a confused or unconscious state. Most of these patients will immediately have electrolyte solutions, such as Ringer's lactate, started upon admission and this will help to correct the acidosis if present. We ordinarily do not start a glucose solution unless it is known that the patient is a diabetic on insulin therapy. In addition to the injuries sustained in the accident, proper management of the diabetic state can prevent needless complications.

It is clear that we can reasonably manage the diabetic patient with exogenous hormones, but this approach does not cure the patient nor does it prevent complications. There is some expectation that a cure for diabetes may be developed, and three lines of investigation are under way that may provide the answer: (a) transplantation of healthy pancreas; (b)

transplantation of islet cells; and (c) implantation of an artificial pancreas.

There have been some 46 cadaver transplants of the pancreas attempted in 45 patients. Only one of these is alive at the end of 42 months. Technical problems as well as the problem of immunosuppression have impeded progress in this approach, but the effort continues.

The demonstration that rat islets could be isolated from the endocrine portion of the gland suggested another approach to therapy. The yield of islets has been low but is improving with new techniques. Because of the difficulty in obtaining adequate numbers of islet cells from adult organs, the isolation of islets from the fetus is being carefully studied. Islets from 2- to 3-day-old rats provide relatively the largest volume of cells, and these increase by 25-fold in tissue culture. Normoglycemia has been achieved in the adult diabetic rat using the islets from one or two rat fetuses. At the moment portal injection of the islets appears to be the best approach for a successful "take."

The use of an artificial pancreas was first tried in 1962, using a Technicon Auto-analyzer set to inject either insulin or glucose. This large, cumbersome, and slow device is not practical, but it did open this field of investigation. Computer control of the Auto-analyzer has been developed to automate the system. It has been shown that this system can maintain normoglycemia in man far more successfully than manual injection techniques. A production model of this instrument will soon be tested in several hospitals. Miniaturization of both sensors and pumps is under way, and a prototype of a battery-operated implantable device is ready for animal testing. One of these latter methods, if successful and practical, opens the possibility of cure.[12]

SELECTED REFERENCES

Beisswenger, P. J., and Spiro, R. G.: Studies on the human glomerular basement membrane: Composition, nature of the carbohydrate units and chemical changes in diabetes mellitus, Diabetes, 22:180, 1973.
  Studies of pooled, isolated, and purified human glomerular basement membrane were analyzed. The peptide portion was characterized by large amounts of glycine as well as by the occurrence of a substantial number of hydroxyproline, hydroxylysine, and cystine residues. The renal basement membranes of diabetic patients when compared to those from nondiabetetic patients indicated an increase in the basement membrane-like material in the diabetic. The studies suggest an overproduction of basement membrane, particularly those subunits that are rich in hydroxylysine and its glycosidally linked disaccharide unit. The authors postulate that inadequate insulin may lead to defective basement membrane synthesis owing to the overproduction and assembly of basement membrane subunits. This may be caused by an altered metabolism of the substrate glucose.

Gabbay, K. H.: The sorbitol pathway and the complications of diabetes. N. Engl. J. Med., 288:831, 1973.
  This article outlines the biochemistry of the sorbitol pathway. The mechanism of cataract formation, as well as the pathologic lesion in the peripheral nerve, is discussed. The experimental work which had laid the basis for this theory of tissue alteration in diabetes is explained in a lucid fashion. The author raises several important questions which must be answered in order to prove the theories that are outlined. There are good references listed in the article which allow the reader access to all of the material available on the subject.

Maugh, T. H.: Diabetes therapy: Can new techniques halt complications? Science, *190*:1281, 1975.

This author reports three techniques for the restoration of normoglycemia in the diabetic patient. These are transplantation of a cadaver pancreas, transplantation of the islets of Langerhans, and finally, the implantation of an artificial pancreas. The success rate with transplantation of the human cadaver pancreas is reviewed and the problems are discussed.

The use of isolated islets for transplantation has been worked out in the experimental animal and seems to offer a promise of success. The isolation of the islets is still not satisfactory in that the yields are low, but improving. Apparently the islets' "take" is best when they are injected into the portal vein, from which they take up residence in the sinusoids of the liver. Because they are antigenic, immunosuppressive therapy is required to maintain viability of the transplant.

The use of an artificial pancreas is discussed in some detail and the mechanical devices that are being utilized are set forth with respect to their advantages and disadvantages. This is a good review of some of the mechanical problems that exist and some of the methods that have been developed to circumvent these problems.

While none of these methods is entirely satisfactory for the management of the diabetic patient at this time, this review gives excellent insight into the problems and the progress being made.

Morrison, A. D., Clements, R. S., Jr., and Winegrad, A. I.: The effects of elevated glucose concentrations on the metabolism of the aortic wall. J. Clin. Invest., *51*:3114, 1972.

An experimental method that has been used to study vascular tissue with respect to changes brought about by hyperglycemia and diabetes is presented in this study. The aortic intima and media were separated from the adventitia and incubated with an elevated glucose concentration. This demonstrated an increased water content of the tissue and a decreased O_2 uptake, but no increase in the inulin space. The aortic intima and media from alloxan diabetic rabbits also exhibited an increased water content when incubated in an elevated ambient glucose concentration. These studies, while not proving that glucose excess is the cause of the vascular lesion, do suggest that exposure to elevated glucose concentration results in marked changes in the metabolism of aortic intima and media.

Raskin, P., Marks, J. F., Burns, H., Jr., Plumer, M. E., and Siperstein, M. D.: Capillary basement membrane width in diabetic children. Am. J. Med., *58*:365, 1975.

This interesting clinical study compares the capillary basement membrane of the quadriceps muscle of juvenile diabetics with adult diabetics as well as normal patients. Electron microscopic methods developed in their laboratory were utilized to evaluate the basement membrane. While there is almost constant thickening of the basement membrane in diabetic adults, this was found in only 40 per cent of children with diabetes mellitus. The basement membrane thickening appears to be unrelated to the duration of the diabetes in either adults or children. Of particular importance was the finding that the basement membrane hypertrophy was present at the time of onset of juvenile diabetes in 30 per cent of the children, indicating that the lesion occurs prior to the onset of

hyperglycemia. They conclude that diabetic microangiography is independent of the hyperglycemia and may well be the primary lesion of the diabetic syndrome.

Williams, R. H.: Etiologic, pathophysiologic and clinical interrelationships in diabetes. Johns Hopkins Med. J., *136*:25, 1975.

This excellent review by one of the outstanding authorities in the field of diabetes updates the reader on the theories of the etiology and pathology of diabetes. Various forms of insulin and their action are discussed in detail, providing a rational basis for understanding the action of insulin on the cell. This review is worth reading by anyone interested in the subject. An excellent bibliography is appended.

REFERENCES

1. Anderson, J. W.: Metabolic abnormalities contributing to diabetic complications. 1. Glucose metabolism in insulin-insensitive pathways. Am. J. Clin. Nutr., *28*:273, 1975.
2. Beisswenger, P. J.: Specificity of the chemical alteration in the diabetic glomerular basement membrane. Diabetes, *22*:744, 1973.
3. Beisswenger, P. J., and Spiro, R. G.: Studies on the human glomerular basement membrane: Composition, nature of the carbohydrate units and chemical changes in diabetes mellitus. Diabetes, *22*:180, 1973.
4. Coil, J. A., and Davis, J. H.: Altered host response to experimental pyelonephritis in alloxan diabetic rats. J. Surg. Res., *7*:26, 1967.
5. Davis, J. H., and Coil, J. A.: Studies of surgically induced pyelonephritis. Surgery, *50*:169, 1961.
6. Elbrink, J., and Bihler, I.: Membrane transport: Its relation to cellular metabolic rates. Science, *188*:1177, 1975.
7. Gabbay, K. H.: The sorbitol pathway and the complications of diabetes. N. Engl. J. Med., *288*:831, 1973.
8. Krizek, T. J., and Davis, J. H.: Experimental staphylococcal infection in the diabetic. Surg. Forum, *16*:394, 1965.
9. Krizek, T. J., and Davis, J. H.: Effect of diabetes on experimental infection. Surg. Forum, *15*:60, 1964.
10. Maugh, T. H.: Diabetes (II): Model systems indicate virus a cause. Science, *188*:436, 1975.
11. Maugh, T. H.: Diabetes (III): New hormones promise more effective therapy. Science, *188*:920, 1975.
12. Maugh, T. H.: Diabetic therapy: Can new techniques halt complications? Science, *190*:1281, 1975.
13. Morrison, A. D., Clements, R. S., Jr., and Winegrad, A. I.: The effects of elevated glucose concentrations on the metabolism of the aortic wall. J. Clin. Invest., *51*:3114, 1972.
14. Raskin, P., Marks, J. F., Burns, H., Jr., Plumer, M. E., and Siperstein, M. D.: Capillary basement membrane width in diabetic children. Am. J. Med., *58*:365, 1975.
15. Spiro, R. G., and Spiro, M. J.: Effect of diabetes on the biosynthesis of the renal glomerular basement membrane. Studies on glucosyltransferase. Diabetes, *20*:642, 1971.
16. Williams, R. H.: Etiologic, pathophysiologic and clinical interrelationships in diabetes. Johns Hopkins Med. J., *136*:25, 1975.

9

FEVER: ETIOLOGY, PHYSIOLOGIC AND METABOLIC EFFECTS, AND MANAGEMENT IN SURGICAL PATIENTS

John M. Kinney, M.D., and Fred T. Caldwell, Jr., M.D.

Concern with body temperature has been an important medical consideration since the days of Hippocrates. The earliest patients probably complained of "feeling hot" or "feeling cold" and were treated to add or subtract heat from the body. The symptom complex associated with "fever" was described in detail long before the advent of clinical thermometry. Only during the past century has fever come to mean a measured elevation of body temperature above a certain normal range.

The problem of fever is regarded by most clinicians in terms of infectious disease. The continued importance of surgical infections alone justifies attention to fever in a surgical textbook. However, there is also growing information about body temperature that has potential value in surgical care beyond its relation to infection, namely:

1. The ways in which surgical disease and injury may alter both heat production and heat loss.

2. The physiologic and metabolic significance of fever to the surgical patient.

3. An appreciation of the hazards of spontaneous hypothermia as well as the potential benefits of therapeutic hypothermia.

4. The alterations in central nervous system control of body temperature that may occur as a result of shock or injury.

Body Temperature and Body Heat Content. An extremely narrow range of body temperatures is one of the requirements for breadth and flexibility of behavior in normal man. However, different areas of the body differ in their intrinsic mechanisms for heat production and heat loss as well as their response to the temperature of the environment. The variation in temperature is greatest in the most exposed parts, such as skin of the extremities, and least in the interior of the body.

While the mouth reflects the internal temperature and is usually the most convenient site for measurement, oral readings are less constant than rectal, since the mouth is often exposed to heat loss or gain from food, liquids, or air temperature. In general, the normal range of oral temperature is from 36.5° C. (97.7° F.) to 37.5° C. (99.5° F.), with an average of 37.0° C. (98.6° F.); rectal temperature is approximately 1° F. higher and the axillary temperature 1 to 3° F. lower. In children, the normal range is more variable and tends to be 0.3 to 0.6° C. (0.5 to 1.0° F.) higher than corresponding temperatures in adults.

The measurement of body temperature is a reflection of body heat content. When the rate of heat loss to the environment is not balanced exactly by the rate of heat production, the difference is added to or removed from the body heat stores. A change in this heat content of the body can be calculated by multiplying the specific heat capacity of mammalian tissue by the body mass times the change in the mean body temperature. The specific heat of body tissue is approximately 0.83 kilocalories per kilogram per degree centigrade change in temperature. This relatively high value is due to the high water content of body tissue. The mean body temperature can be estimated roughly from a weighted average of skin and rectal temperatures. Under normal conditions the mean body temperature is considered to be 0.3 times the skin temperature plus 0.7 times the rectal temperature. Therefore a drop of 1° C. in the mean body temperature of a 70-kg. man would result in the loss of approximately 58 kilocalories, or the basal heat production of an average adult for about 1 hour. Because of the high heat capacity of the adult human body, heat production and loss may be unbalanced for up to several hours with only slight alteration in body temperature. This has the advantage of not requiring an immediate physiologic response to transient changes in the environmental temperature. It also provides an important lag period for the individual to escape from a thermally stressful situation in which adequate physiologic compensation would not be possible.

Heat Transfer Within the Body. Heat lost to the environment is transferred from the site of production to the body surface by combined conduction and circulatory convection. Conduction is a process of heat transfer through a material by transfer of thermal energy between adjacent atoms. Convective heat transfer occurs within the body with the bulk movement of body fluids. Of primary importance is forced convection via the circulatory system. The circulation is important to minimize temperature differences within the body and to control effective body insulation. The tissues of the body are relatively poor heat conductors. Thus if the heat exchange within the body were solely conductive, large internal temperature gradients would be necessary to conduct metabolic heat away. Compensation for changing internal and external thermal stress would be difficult since the thermal conductance of any particular tissue is constant.

Most of the metabolic heat is produced in the deep organs, the heart, viscera, and brain, except during vigorous exercise. For this heat to be lost, these organs must be warmer than the perfusing blood of the surrounding tissues.

For purposes of discussion, the human body may be regarded in two parts: an interior "core," which represents the viscera plus head where the primary heat-producing tissues are located; and the remainder of the body, including the surface, which is referred to as the "shell," which fluctuates at lower temperatures than the core of the body.[7] Those perfused tissues with temperatures within a few tenths of a degree of the rectal temperature are considered to be the body core. Thus the core comprises almost the entire body when cutaneous vasodilatation is maximal and the shell is reduced to the thickness of the skin. When heat must be conserved, vasoconstriction reduces circulation to the periphery, the central core contracts, and the thickness of the shell increases (Fig. 1). The vasoconstriction directly reduces the ease of heat transport to the surface and indirectly reduces heat loss to the environment by lowering the surface temperature.

Influence of Environmental Temperatures. Within the zone of thermal neutrality, man loses 25 per cent of his total heat

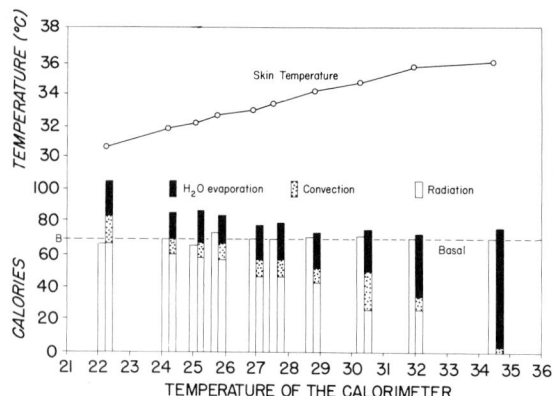

Figure 2. The rate of heat production and partitioned heat loss from seminude man over a wide range of environmental temperatures. (Modified from DuBois, E. F.: Trans. Assoc. Am. Physicians, *51*:252, 1936.)

loss by evaporation. One quarter of this is from water added to inspired air saturated with water vapor while in the respiratory tract, and three quarters is lost as water vapor passing through intact skin. It is important to note that there is no salt loss by either route. Neither route should be considered a regulatory physiologic function, since for the most part each process is passive and depends on physical vapor pressure gradients between the host and his environment. The remainder of the heat lost within the zone of thermal neutrality is by radiation (65 per cent) and conduction plus convection (10 per cent). Figure 2, taken from DuBois,[21] shows the pattern of heat loss for man over a wide range of environmental temperatures. Two things are readily apparent from this chart: one, vasoconstriction, represented as a fall in skin temperature, is not a very effective way to conserve heat (which is why man invented clothes); and two, above an ambient temperature of 36° C., man can lose heat only by evaporating sweat or applying water. The cooling effect of the evaporating sweat makes it impossible to increase skin temperature above 36° C., making further heat loss by radiation impossible.

Eventually, any decrease in environmental temperature below 27° C. will result in an increase in the rate of heat production, but it will not reach a point that will permit man to forgo clothing. Increasing the rate of heat production by chemical or metabolic means involves shivering, but shivering is severely limited in the maximal increases that can be sustained for any length of time. Man is far better equipped to withstand heat than cold without assistance. True cold acclimation has never been demonstrated for man. Nonshivering thermogenic and increased calorigenic effect from norepinephrine are probably not available without clothing.

Regulation of Body Temperature. Body temperature is regulated with the same degree of finesse as plasma pH, osmolality, or sodium concentration, and may be considered one of the characteristics of the milieu intérieur. The question of what is regulated—a temperature in a certain location, average body temperature, body heat content, or some other variable—has been the subject of much discussion and investigation. Current thermoregulatory theory suggests that the temperature to be regulated is the temperature of the anterior hypothalamus. Since the hypothalamic temperature changes little if at all when the host is subjected to a change in environmental temperature, an operational theory of thermoregulation must explain this fact. One plausible explanation has been offered by Hammel,[30] who has suggested that the output of the controlled system is fed back to the control-

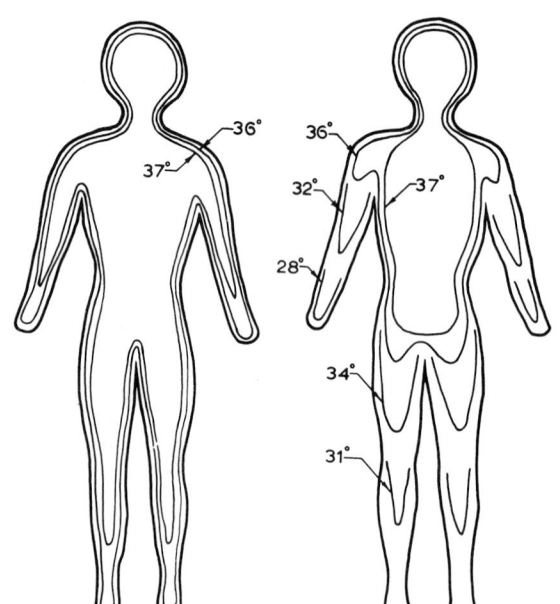

Figure 1. The influence of environmental temperature on blood flow and temperature of the body surface. The isotherms (surfaces connecting points of equal temperature) for a warm environment are shown on the left and for a cold environment on the right. (From Brengelmann, G., and Brown, A. C. *In* Ruch, T. C., and Patton, H. D. (Eds.): Physiology and Biophysics, 20th ed. Philadelphia, W. B. Saunders Company, 1973.)

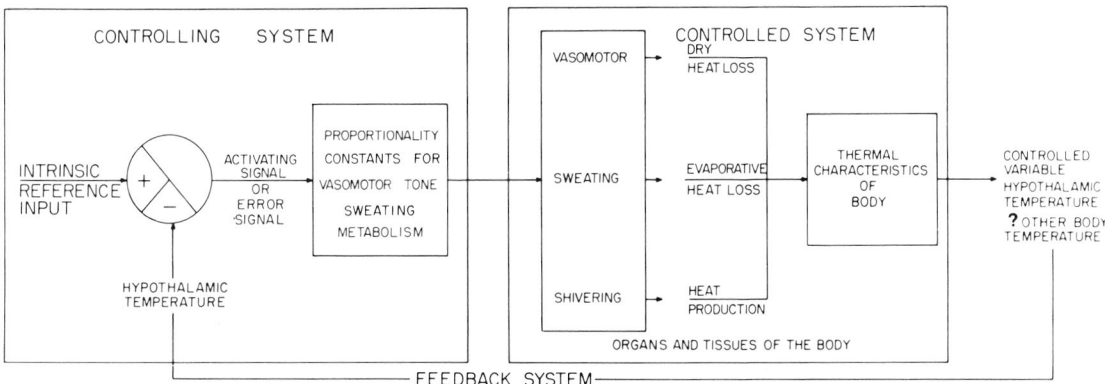

Figure 3. Block diagram for regulation of internal body temperature. (Modified from Hammel, H. T.: Ann. Rev. Physiol., *30*:641, 1968.)

ling system. In this case the output would be internal body temperature or only a special part of it, namely hypothalamic temperature. Central to this model is the stipulation that the controlling system must produce a reference signal, and thus the feed-back signal representing hypothalamic temperature may be continually compared with a reference signal or "set temperature." The difference is the error signal. A second essential feature of Hammel's model is that the set or reference temperature may shift, depending upon the neural input from skin, core, or muscle, or with the onset of sleep or exercise. As a result *the error signal may change with no change in the actual hypothalamic temperature.* The third essential feature of this model is that the threshold (or size of the error signal) for the various thermoregulatory responses, such as sweating, vasomotor tone, and shivering, changes with a change in environmental temperature. A block diagram of the model proposed by Hammel is shown in Figure 3. Thermal neutrality is a useful term to remember when making clinical use of thermoregulatory theory. Thermoneutrality is defined as the environmental temperature at which heat loss from the body is equal to the minimal heat production, with body heat content constant. For seminude man this occurs at an ambient temperature between 28 and 29° C. Above air temperatures of 30 to 32° C., sweating begins and increases by recruitment and increased secretory rate as the environmental temperature increases. Within the narrow temperature range of thermal neutrality, body temperature is regulated by small changes in vasomotor tone and the resulting small increases or decreases in heat loss by radiation. Below an ambient temperature of 28° C., vasoconstriction rapidly becomes maximal. Then shivering obtains as our only, not very effective, physiologic thermoregulatory response to a negative thermal load.

GENERAL ASPECTS OF FEVER

Pathogenesis of Fever

An increase in body temperature may occur alone for any of several reasons: infection, pyrogens, dehydration, increased heat production with extra muscle activity, acute endocrine stimulation, loss of the normal cooling mechanisms, or certain lesions in the anterior hypothalamus. Fever can be a manifestation of many diverse kinds of disease processes and the only obvious common factor in these circumstances appears to be tissue injury or inflammation. Most clinical observations of febrile conditions suggest that central thermal regulation has been altered and that the dis-

turbance of the brain centers is caused by the action of some product or products of tissue injury. Experimental work on the pathogenesis of fever has usually been carried out with bacterial pyrogens. These substances are endotoxins, or complex lipopolysaccharides of high molecular weight that form part of the cell wall of gram-negative bacteria. Such materials are extremely potent pharmacologic agents. In minute amounts they produce a wide variety of reactions including fever, leukopenia, and alterations in blood coagulation, and large doses can produce shock and death. There is a variable latent period of 15 to 30 minutes after intravenous inoculation before the onset of fever. During this period circulating granulocytes virtually disappear from the bloodstream. Therefore, it has been suggested that the fever following endotoxin administration arises from the release of an intermediary pyrogen from a tissue source within the body, presumably the white blood cell. Originally the polymorphonuclear leukocytes were thought to be the only source of this substance; however, more recent studies indicate that extracts of many normal tissues can produce pyrogens. A substance known as endogenous pyrogen with biologic properties similar to those of the leukocyte pyrogen appears in the blood of animals and man after intravenous endotoxin is given. Experimental studies indicate that a subtle balance probably exists between various activators and inhibitors of endogenous pyrogen in the body. When the balance is disturbed by certain influences, there is production and release of endogenous pyrogen into the bloodstream, which in turn causes fever.

The setpoint concept of temperature regulation is useful in understanding the mode of action of a bacterial pyrogen.[16] The host responds to a dose of bacterial pyrogen as if the thermoregulatory setpoint within the hypothalamus has been shifted upward (Fig. 4). A "chill" with shivering ensues, with a resulting rise in body temperature. When the hypothalamic temperature reaches the point of the new reference setpoint, the shivering stops and body temperature is now regulated around the "new" setpoint. Except for side effects such as headache or arthralgia associated with the fever, the host may be unaware that the body temperature is elevated.

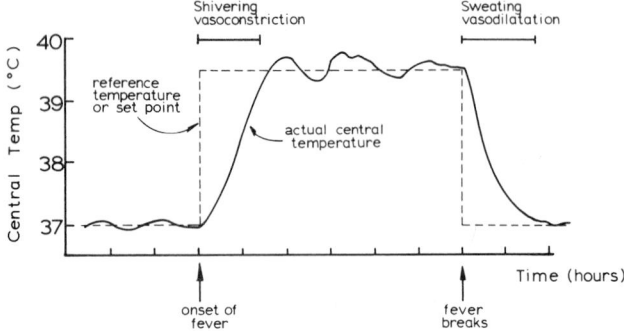

Figure 4. Time course of a typical febrile episode. The actual body temperature lags behind the rapid shifts in set point. (From Brengelmann, G., and Brown, A. C. In Ruch, T. C., and Patton, H. D. (Eds.): Physiology and Biophysics. 20th ed. Philadelpia, W. B. Saunders Company, 1973.)

The hypothalamus is essential for a response to a pyrogen. Figure 5A shows that in a dog displacement of the hypothalamic temperature upward prior to administration of a bacterial pyrogen will eliminate the febrile response. Figure 5B shows the reverse: cooling the hypothalamus before administration of a pyrogen will result in a "hyperfever." In the first example, the error signal is reduced or eliminated by artificially increasing the hypothalamic temperature by use of implanted thermodes. In the second example, the error signal is increased by decreasing the hypothalamic temperature, by circulating cold water through thermodes implanted in the hypothalamus.[3]

Temperature Regulation and Fever

The patient's body temperature, pulse, and respiratory rate are time-honored indices of disease and illness. With a multitude of new and complicated diagnostic and therapeutic procedures available today, there is a tendency for clinicians to attach less significance to these parameters. Yet within a hospital environment, abnormalities of body temperature almost invariably deserve investigation. The diurnal variation in body temperature of approximately 0.5° C. begins a cycle with the lowest temperature noted before the patient arises in the morning. In hospitalized patients, the body temperature slowly increases throughout the day and reaches a peak in the early evening before the patient retires. With the onset of sleep, there begins a fall in body temperature that may be associated with diaphoresis. This pattern suggests that the onset of sleep is associated with a shift downward in the thermoregulatory setpoint.

It has been commonly taught that the increase in resting metabolism of the body can be predicted from the degree of elevation in the body temperature. DuBois[21] studied a variety of medical conditions (Fig. 6) and found an approximate increase of 13 per cent for each degree rise in body temperature centigrade (7 per cent for each degree Fahrenheit). He expressed the opinion that the effects of fever on the metabolic rate corresponded to the principle of van't Hoff: that the velocity of chemical reactions is proportional to the temperature at which they occur. Therefore at a tempera-

ture of 40.5° C. (105° F.) the average human body would have an increase of approximately 50 per cent in resting metabolism. Comparison of the resting metabolic expenditure with body temperature in postoperative patients revealed that the 13 per cent relationship of DuBois provided only an approximate correlation for brief periods of low-grade fever.[36] This was in contrast with cases of major peritonitis and burns, in which the metabolic expenditure was increased well beyond the value predicted from the extent of fever.[48]

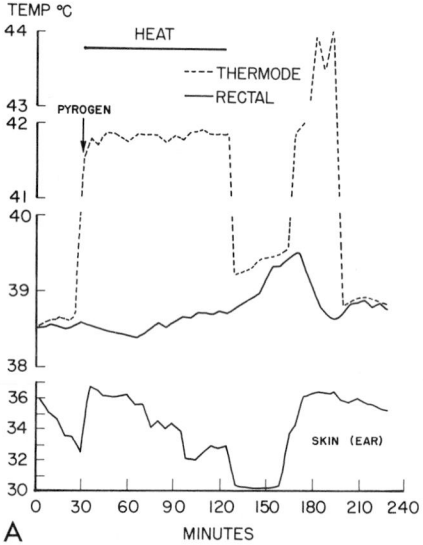

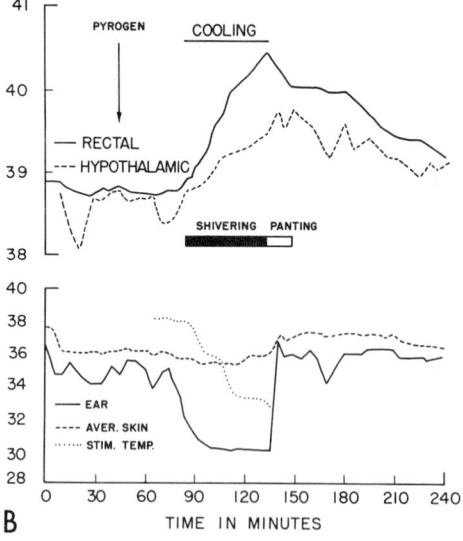

Figure 5. A, Modification of the febrile response in the dog to Pseudomonas polysaccharide by warming the anterior hypothalamus and inhibiting the production of fever. B, Cooling the hypothalamus results in a "hyperfever" since the error signal is increased in addition to the effect of the pyrogen. (From Andersen, H. T., Hammel, H. T., and Hardy, J. D. In American Institute of Physics: Temperature, Its Measurement and Control in Science and Industry. Volume 3, Part 3. New York, Reinhold Publishing Company, 1963.)

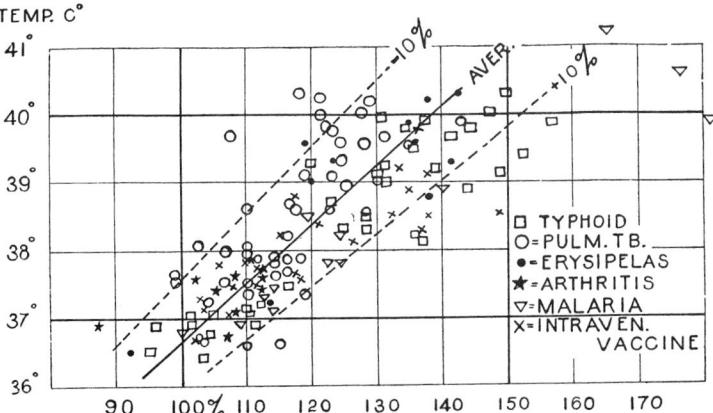

Figure 6. Relation of basal metabolism to body temperature in six different fevers. The dotted lines are drawn to represent 10 per cent above and below the average relationship. (From DuBois, E. F. *In* Basal Metabolism in Health and Disease. Philadelphia, Lea & Febiger, 1924.)

From an analysis of over 1700 temperature readings in 357 febrile patients, DuBois concluded that the temperature-regulating mechanism continued to function during fever, but at the "thermostatic level" set by the particular stage of the disease.[22] The sharp limitation of temperature elevation at the level of approximately 41.1° C. (106° F.) suggested to DuBois that an "emergency regulatory mechanism" must come into play during fever and protect the body from extreme hyperthermia.

Ventilatory changes during fever usually involve an increase in both respiratory rate and tidal volume. The alveolar ventilation is usually stimulated to a greater degree than minute ventilation, resulting in some decrease in carbon dioxide stores of the body and an associated respiratory alkalosis. The frequency of hyperventilation in the presence of clinical fever has prompted the suggestion that perhaps some of the circulating pyrogenic materials that influence the heat-regulating centers of the brain also stimulate the respiratory center.

Studies of experimental fever in man suggest that the increase in cardiac output is somewhat slower to appear than the increase in minute ventilation but that both rise in parallel with the increase in oxygen consumption.[40] This parallel rise is in contrast to the findings that are becoming evident in clinical sepsis, particularly when there is a large area of local inflammation. Clowes and co-workers[15] have emphasized that following appropriate therapy for shock, injury, or sepsis, the subsequent convalescence will often be characterized by a period of high cardiac output with a decreased total peripheral resistance. These workers have suggested that the decrease in peripheral resistance may be associated with arteriovenous shunting in the area of acute inflammation. Thal and Hermbeck[33] have shown in the dog that only about half of the increase in cardiac output in acute sepsis can be explained by increased flow in the area of the infection.

Water and Electrolyte Metabolism in Fever

When the body is faced with a rising environmental temperature, the capability for radiative heat loss is progressively decreased and the body's main compensation is to increase heat loss by means of evaporative cooling. Therefore at a specific setpoint, which is approximately 31° C. (87.8° F.), the body will begin to actively cool by means of sweating. Surgical patients with large areas of skin damage that have reduced their ability to sweat and patients with surgical dressings that do not allow for the transfer of water vapor may be unable to compensate for increased heat production or for an increase in heating from external sources, and thus may be unable to prevent a rise in body temperature.

The insensible water loss that occurs under normal conditions is electrolyte-free, whereas sweat contains all of the crystalloids of plasma in hypotonic concentrations. There is great variation in the concentration of sodium and chloride in human sweat, with reported values ranging from 5 to 100 mEq. per liter of each ion. Normal man performing daily work in a hot, dry environment acclimatizes himself so that the sodium chloride concentration steadily decreases to the point that daily balance is usually established to equal the level of intake of the ion.

Acute rises in sodium concentration of the extracellular fluid are associated with the development of fever and an increase in the rate of oxygen consumption. The development of hyponatremia is associated with a decrease in oxygen consumption and hypothermia.[27] The oxygen consumption of tissue slices is linearly related to the sodium concentration of the incubating media for the reason that the energy used, and heat produced secondary to operation of the sodium pump, is directly related to the sodium concentration outside the cells of the body.[45] In the intact body this effect is apparently peripheral, although recent work suggests that the central thermoregulatory centers are sensitive to the concentration ratios of several pairs of ions.[43]

There is little doubt that the adult patient who has experienced dehydration with rapid loss of both water and electrolytes from the gastrointestinal tract may have a temperature of 0.5 to 1.0° C. above normal, which responds to rehydration. Infants and small children are more prone to a variety of stimuli causing fever and demonstrate higher levels of fever than adults with comparable hydration. The frequency in clinical practice is not well established and the mechanism by which rehydration restores body temperature to normal is not known. For these reasons, the presence of fever in any patient should prompt a search for other explanations, and fever from dehydration should be a diagnosis by exclusion.

Protein Metabolism in Fever

At the normal body temperature the rate of destruction of cell proteins occurs so slowly that the normal concentration of a specific type of protein is readily maintained by synthesis. As the body temperature rises, both the synthetic repair process and the destruction of the protein increase, but at widely different rates, until a temperature level is reached at which the rate of destruction equals the rate of repair. Any further increment in temperature leads to a rate of protein destruction that rapidly exceeds that for repair because of the great disparity in the temperature coefficients of the opposing processes. Metabolic activity begins to fail unless the system is cooled, and the cell dies at a temperature only a few degrees above the temperature of balance between production and breakdown. The temperature at which death occurs for indefinitely long exposure is called the thermal death point. For skin, this temperature corresponds to the threshold temperature for burn injury.

There appear to be qualitative changes in intermediary metabolism in febrile conditions of certain types. It has long been recognized that patients with a variety of acute infections "use protein extravagantly."[35] This toxic destruction of protein cannot be overcome except by the administration of supranormal amounts of protein and calories. The phenomenon is not a specific reaction to infection but also occurs following severe injury or major surgical operation. The nitrogen loss cannot be attributed merely to accelerated energy expenditure, since protein can be conserved in both exercise and hyperthyroidism if caloric balance is maintained. The tendency to waste protein appears to be a reaction to injury that is most characteristic of previously healthy, well-nourished patients. Late in the convalescence after major infections, the nitrogen excretion is decreased and nitrogen equilibrium may be established more readily. In extremely depleted patients, the resting metabolic expenditure as well as the nitrogen excretion is usually decreased below normal and each will show only minimal, if any, elevation with the onset of fever.

Beisel and co-workers[4] conducted extensive metabolic studies in experimental infections in man. Their studies revealed that circulating amino acids began to drop for one or two days before the febrile period began. Further studies have gone on to demonstrate an endogenous mediator substance that is elaborated from polymorphonuclear leukocytes in the presence of various infective agents.[52] This material has been demonstrated during infections of both animals and man. Chemical characterization is not complete but has proceeded far enough to show that this substance is not endotoxin, as would be expected from gram-negative bacteria.[46] It is of particular interest that the assay for this material is based on the demonstration of more rapid uptake of amino acids and zinc from the circulating bloodstream to the liver cells. It has been further demonstrated that this amino acid uptake is not for gluconeogenesis but rather for protein synthesis, apparently for the synthesis of acute phase proteins as part of the metabolic response to infection. This is noteworthy, because the organ that is responsible for the majority of new glucose formation during catabolic states is the same organ that is involved in acute-phase protein synthesis, since all of the acute-phase proteins are glycoproteins. Stimulation of this process represents muscle protein breakdown that is in addition to the amount of breakdown that would be predicted by the extra urea excretion. Therefore, this may help to explain the observation that the most rapid and extreme muscle wasting in clinical conditions is observed in the well-muscled young adult male who is febrile as a result of injuries and secondary infection.

Splanchnic Metabolism and Surgical Fever

The increase in resting heat production associated with fever has never been clearly identified as to the tissues involved and the chemical reactions that are responsible. Studies on nonshivering thermogenesis in small animals emphasize increased peripheral utilization of fatty acids. Yet the hypermetabolism of clinical fever may not be equivalent to nonshivering thermogenesis induced by environmental changes.

The old observation of increased heat production following protein ingestion (specific dynamic action) has been linked to the deamination of certain amino acids. Cuthbertson and co-workers[9] have suggested that the increased heat production after skeletal injury in the rat might be due to an "endogenous specific dynamic action" that was underlying the increased nitrogen excretion. Since urea synthesis is increased in protein feeding, injury, and a variety of febrile conditions, and the liver is the sole organ to synthesize urea, is the hypermetabolism of clinical fever limited to the liver?

The gastrointestinal blood supply under normal resting conditions could conceivably determine hepatic function through its domination of the substrate supply. But, in fact, the hepatic blood supply appears to be adjusted to the metabolic requirements of the body as a whole. The hepatic blood flow has been shown to increase after a protein meal in proportion to the rise in cardiac output and blood flow to the entire body that occurs at the same time. Similar changes in systemic and hepatic circulation have been detected in man during febrile reactions to pyrogenic agents that increase total oxygen consumption. Liver temperature rises after protein feeding and during fever, presumably as a result of augmented hepatocellular metabolism. Myers[42] has confirmed that the relationship between cardiac output and arteriovenous oxygen difference for the whole body has a similar pattern to that which exists for the liver. This investigator found that the rapid intravenous injection of amino acids caused a prompt rise in the splanchnic oxygen consumption as a result of widening the arteriovenous oxygen difference without increasing hepatic blood flow. This pattern differs from that following the administration of an intravenous pyrogen to normal man, in which the arteriovenous oxygen difference remains essentially normal while the hepatic blood flow is promptly increased.

The extent of increase in splanchnic blood flow and oxygen consumption was studied by Gump and co-workers in 15 patients who were febrile as a result of intraperitoneal infection.[28] Whole-body and splanchnic blood flow were measured together with whole-body and splanchnic oxygen consumption. These studies revealed that approximately one third of the patients had no increase in oxygen consumption despite the presence of fever. Such patients had small increases in cardiac output with no significant change in the proportion of blood flow or oxygen consumption across the splanchnic bed. The patients with an increase in resting oxygen consumption always had an increased cardiac output and increased splanchnic blood flow. The increase in blood flow and oxygen consumption across the splanchnic viscera accounted for only 40 to 50 per cent of the total increase, establishing that the hypermetabolism of this form of surgical fever involved tissues other than the liver, and chemical reactions other than deamination and urea synthesis (Fig. 7). It is of interest that three burn patients studied in a similar fashion revealed much larger increases in resting oxygen consumption; however, the resting blood flow to the liver was of the same order of magnitude as that seen with intra-abdominal infection.[29] This is consistent with the fact that the fever and increase in nitrogen excretion of burn patients are of the same order of magnitude as those seen in cases of major peritoneal infection.

BODY TEMPERATURE AND THE SURGICAL PATIENT

Intraoperative Hypothermia

Shivering in the recovery room can be observed in one fourth to one half of all patients who have undergone general anesthesia, and some patients have increased skeletal muscle activity without gross shivering being observed. This shivering is related to a drop in body temperature during operation, which is usually unnoticed. Body temperature is seldom monitored as part of intraoperative management and is measured only sporadically in the recovery room. The range of normal body temperature in any large group of persons can vary as much as 1.5° C. Thus an isolated observation of body temperature in the recovery room may be assumed to be normal, yet actually be as much as a degree below what is normal for that patient and thus stimulate reflex responses that are undesirable at that time.

The normal response to a drop in body temperature is peripheral vasoconstriction, which decreases the transport of heat to the surface and hence preserves body heat. At the same time there is usually an increase in metabolism, primarily of the skeletal muscles, which increases heat production. General anesthesia modifies or prevents this normal response by restricting heat production at a time when body heat loss may be increased. There are other reasons for increased heat loss in surgical patients during an

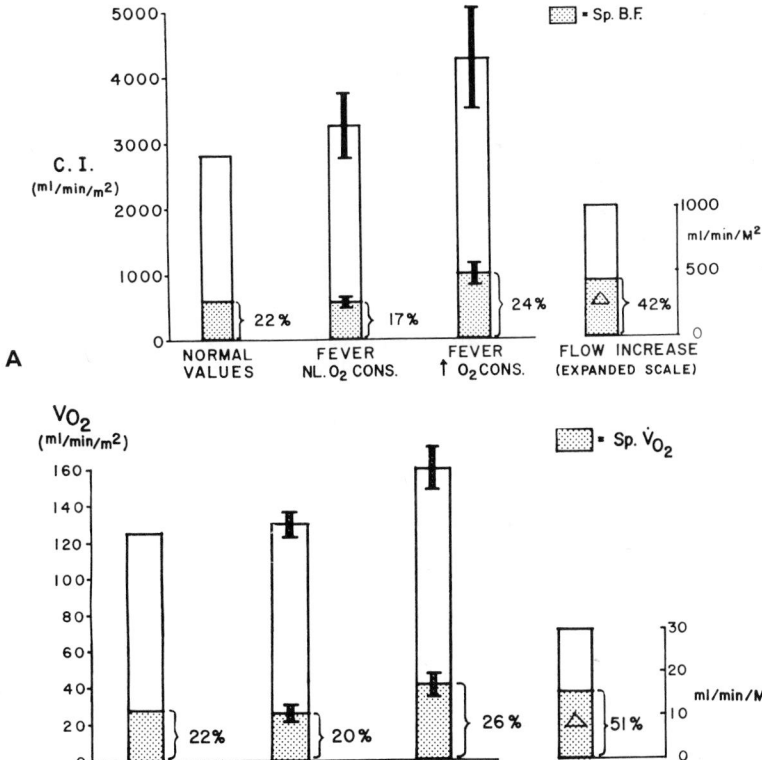

Figure 7. *A,* Splanchnic and total blood flow for 15 patients who were febrile with intraperitoneal infection. *B,* Corresponding values for splanchnic and total oxygen consumption. In the hypermetabolic patients, 40 to 50 per cent of the increased blood flow and oxygen consumption was associated with the splanchnic area. (From Gump, F. E., Price, J. B., Jr., and Kinney, J. M.: Ann. Surg., *171*:321, 1970.)

operation. Significant areas of skin are exposed to cool air and then prepared with volatile agents that rapidly evaporate and contribute vaporizational cooling. Certain operations, particularly in the abdomen and the chest, may leave large serous surfaces exposed, allowing continuous evaporative cooling at the expense of body water and body heat content. The administration of cool body fluids or blood transfusions can be additional causes of heat loss.

Goldberg and associates[24] reported that 78 per cent of adult surgical patients undergoing elective operation had some decrease in body temperature. The duration of the operation, the type of procedure, and the use of a muscle relaxant were important factors in whether the patient's temperature was decreased at the end of the operation. However, all these factors taken together were less important than the age of the patient. The older patients had the greatest decrease in body temperature, and measurements of oxygen consumption suggested that this was because their heat production was decreased more than that of the younger adults. Infants and young children have additional reasons for hypothermia. The infant undergoing operation has an increased heat loss because of a larger surface area for the body mass, a smaller body heat content, and sometimes a poorly developed temperature-regulating mechanism. For these reasons the body temperature of the pediatric patient can drop seriously during operation and requires careful monitoring throughout any operative procedure.

Wilson and co-workers[54] studied 90 burned children who were operated upon for late reconstructive procedures under standardized anesthesia technique and ambient conditions. Despite the usual measures to counteract unintentional hypothermia, they observed an unusual fall in body temperature that bore a linear relationship to the extent of scarring and the length of operation. The authors felt this was evidence of various thermoregulatory losses of the burn scar: decreased vasoactivity, loss of sweating and piloerection, loss of the thermal receptor activity, attenuated insulation properties, and loss of control by the sympathetic nervous system.

The postoperative treatment of spontaneous hypothermia is always more difficult than its prevention. Prevention is never possible without adequate monitoring. Current techniques are available for the continuous measurement of rectal temperature throughout an operation and this should become part of the anesthesia record. The temperature of the operating room plays a larger role than other factors in governing the rate of heat loss. It is now evident that the temperature and humidity of the operating room have been designed more for the comfort of the surgeon than for the physiologic or thermal stability of the patient. Morris[39] reported studies of patients undergoing elective abdominal operations in which he noted that when the operating room was kept at a temperature less than 21° C, all of the patients were hypothermic at the end of the procedure. In subsequent studies, when the temperature of the operating room was kept between 21 and 24° C., only a third of the patients became hypothermic.

The patient offers no resistance to body cooling during anesthesia because central thermoregulatory centers are inactive. As the patient awakens after the surgical procedure, function of the thermoregulatory center returns. With the return, a large "error signal" becomes apparent; i.e., the hypothalamic temperature is 1 to 1.5° C. (1.8 to 2.7° F.) or more below the reference setpoint of approximately 37° C. (98.6° F.). Shivering, sometimes violent, and peripheral vasoconstriction result in an effort to increase the rate of heat production, reduce heat loss, and thus increase body temperature. Shivering will continue until the patient's core temperature returns to normal. This situation may be serious if ventilation is compromised by the operation, surgical dressings, or retained secretions, together with the possibility of a marginal circulation from unreplaced blood loss. Roe and others[47] studied 24 patients following surgical procedures, and demonstrated an average fall in body temperature of 1.1° C. during the operative procedures and an average increase in maximal rate of heat production of 80 per cent during the first 4 hours following operation.

Why is postoperative shivering commonly tolerated? Surgeons have come to believe that hypothermia is beneficial because it reduces metabolic rate and therefore is a protective influence. This principle has been utilized effectively in open-heart surgery and other specialized procedures in which blood flow to vital organs has to be interrupted. However, spontaneous hypothermia carries a different connotation and sets the stage for potential problems. Any spontaneous drop in body temperature, even if less than a degree centigrade, should be regarded as a failure of a sensitive and highly developed thermoregulatory system. The cause for the drop in body temperature should be sought and efforts made to provide thermal support as well as to minimize excessive heat losses.

It is important that the hypothermic patient not be allowed to restore his own body heat by shivering. Shivering can be abolished by the use of medication such as promethazine (Phenergan) and meperidine (Demerol). Rewarming should proceed gently and slowly so that there is no excessive cutaneous vasodilatation, which might further lower peripheral vascular resistance and compromise a marginal circulation. Under special circumstances it is possible to use radiant heating with lamps placed at an appropriate distance so that the patient and bedclothes are gently warmed to prevent a net heat loss into the room.

Malignant Hyperpyrexia

Life-threatening hyperthermia is commonly considered to be a complication of unacclimated people living in hot climates. However, it has assumed surgical significance during the last few years with an increasing number of reports of "malignant hyperpyrexia," a condition occurring during or immediately at the conclusion of *general anesthesia*. This is a rare complication but one that is reported to be fatal in over 70 per cent of cases. In this condition the patients are usually young and healthy with a previously normal body temperature. There appears to be no sex predominance or any particular area of the body commonly associated with the complication. Some reports have emphasized the higher incidence of this complication when either succinylcholine or halothane was used. Temperature recording should be routinely used in all patients undergoing general anesthesia, since the present lack of understanding of the mechanisms in this condition makes early detection extremely important. The signs of impending difficulty are the rapid onset of diaphoresis, increased radiation of body heat, an increase in muscle tone, perhaps cardiovascular changes secondary to hypoxia, the appearance of dark blood despite adequate oxygenation with elevated oxygen concentration, and the terminal appearance of convulsions.

In each of the reported cases in the literature, the rapid rise in body temperature could not be attributed to thyrotoxicosis, the administration of fluids contaminated by bacterial pyrogens, environmental factors, or other well-established causes of fever in patients undergoing an operation. Uncoupling of oxidative phosphorylation within the mitochondria has been postulated as an etiologic possibility but has yet to be proved. The combination of unexplained hyperpyrexia and tonic contraction of muscles has led to the suggestion that the hyperthermia may be related to an undetected or subclinical genetic disorder of the neuromuscular system. Aldrete and co-workers[1] have reported high creatine phosphokinase and pyrophosphate levels in the serum of a surviving patient. Similar findings in a group of relatives led these authors to propose the tests as useful in predicting the patients in whom malignant hyperthermia might develop during anesthesia. Harrison and co-workers[31] have reported on a strain of pigs in which there is an "explosive thermal idiosyncrasy" to general anesthesia in 25 per cent of the animals. The syndrome is similar to that seen in human patients with malignant hyperpyrexia, and histologic investigation of muscle biopsies from the affected pigs showed an abnormal fall in adenosine triphosphate (ATP) content in response to incubation and also when exposed to certain anesthetic agents.

The rate of resting metabolism can be expected to approximately double, should the body temperature approach 43° C. (110° F.). Unfortunately there is a limit to the rate at which the body can lose heat even with maximal sweating. Furthermore, when the hypothalamus becomes excessively heated, its heat-regulating ability becomes greatly depressed and sweating diminishes. As a result, a vicious cycle develops: high temperature causes increased production of heat, which increases the body temperature still higher, causing still greater production of heat and still higher body temperature. Once the body temperature rises above 42° C., the heat-regulating mechanisms often can no longer dissipate the excessive heat being produced. Therefore the temperature may then rise abruptly until it causes death.

The signs of impending difficulty are unexplained increase in muscle tone, severe acidosis secondary to a rise in plasma lactate, the appearance of dark blood despite adequate oxygenation, and rapid rise in core temperature at a rate of 1° C. every 10 to 15 minutes. In Landrace pigs, which are subject to a syndrome very similar to that observed in man, there is a rise in the rate of oxygen consumption that corresponds to the amount predicted by the rise in body temperature; however, there is an inordinate increase in the rate of CO_2 production with an increase in RQ to above one. In these pigs halothane initiates massive and uncontrolled glycogenolysis with production of excess lactate and a rise in blood glucose.

A review of human data makes it clear that aerobic metabolism, even if totally uncoupled, cannot account for the heat needed to produce an increase in core temperature of 6° C. in one hour. An 80-kg. man has a thermal capacity of about 76 w per degree C. Thus, to increase the average body temperature 6° C. in one hour would require 456 w. This same man produces 46 w per M^2 or 92 w per hr. Oxidative phosphorylation is normally 40 to 50 per cent efficient in converting energy into a usable form (ATP). However, even if no ATP were found, this would account for only 20 per cent of the energy needed for the time rate of change in body heat content. Even if oxygen consumption doubled and the total energy converted to heat, it would not account for enough heat to produce observed rates of increase in body temperature.[5]

As with susceptible pigs, uncontrolled massive anaerobic glycogenolysis and severe acidosis support this hypothesis. The seriousness of this problem is compounded by the total absence of temperature regulation during anesthesia.

Malignant hyperpyrexia is transmitted as a genetic disease with a dominant gene. A careful family history is probably the most reliable way to detect high risk individuals. The metabolic defect is most likely in muscle, and although serum creatine phosphokinase is usually increased in susceptible individuals, this has not developed as a reliable screening test.[23]

One theory as to etiology places the essential defect in the inability of the sarcoplasmic reticulum membrane of muscle to accumulate calcium when exposed to halothane. The resulting high myoplasmic calcium activates phosphorylase kinase, thus accelerating glycolysis and myosin ATPase, which in turn accelerate hydrolysis of ATP to ADP, phosphate, and heat. Calcium is also taken up by mitochondria where it triggers secondary uncoupling of oxidative phosphorylation with a decrease in ATP formation and an increase in heat formation. Primary uncoupling of oxidative phosphorylation does not seem to be part of malignant hyperpyrexia.[8]

When the body temperature rises above approximately 41.5° C., the parenchyma of many cells usually begins to be damaged. When the body temperature exceeds approximately 42° C., the person usually has only a few hours to live unless his temperature can be immediately reduced by external means. The pathologic findings in a person who dies of hyperthermia are local hemorrhages and parenchymatous degeneration of cells throughout the entire body.

The treatment is first directed at decreasing the body temperature. This treatment must be aggressive, since surface cooling alone will often be inadequate. Cooling solutions can be introduced into the stomach or occasionally into the peritoneal or pleural cavity. While cooling the patient it is necessary to control shivering to avoid further increase in heat production. Hyperventilation and sodium bicarbonate may be needed to combat the severe acidosis that commonly occurs. Adequate oxygenation is critical to combat the hypoxia that is probably a combination of pulmonary shunting and increased peripheral utilization. Because of the high carbon dioxide levels that occur, there may be increased intracranial pressure. Therefore, in addition to hyperventilation, agents such as mannitol or urea may be employed. Hyperkalemia may be found on electrocardiographic monitoring and require treatment with intravenous calcium gluconate or peritoneal dialysis. The most important aspect of therapy is immediate cessation of the anesthetic and some form of body cooling. However, certain authors have recommended the administration of intravenous procainamide.[34]

In addition to malignant hyperpyrexia there is growing interest in the relationship between circulating endotoxin, its pyrogenic activity, and the possibility that it may occasionally contribute to fatal heat stroke. Graber and co-workers[26] have reported a case of an 18-year-old healthy male who collapsed during football practice on a hot day. There was rapid onset of tachycardia, hypotension, stupor, and convulsive movements of the extremities. On arrival at the hospital the patient's body temperature exceeded 44° C. and he died 4 days later following persistent coma, hyperkalemia, and acidosis. The authors present the possibility that unsuspected bacterial illness had produced the onset of this clinical picture with recurrent bacteremia and ultimately an endotoxemia. Measured levels of circulating endotoxin were extremely high and at the time of death there were widespread intravascular thrombi, pulmonary interstitial hemorrhage, and gastric ulceration. In view of the frequency with which critically ill surgical patients are faced with problems of fever, infection, and upper gastrointestinal hemorrhage, the possibility of circulating endotoxin must be borne in mind. This is particularly probable in patients in whom damage to the liver or other elements of the reticuloendothelial system would prevent clearance of circulating endotoxin.

Influence of Injury on Thermoregulation

The pioneering observations of Cuthbertson[18] on the metabolic response to injury were divided into the early events of the shock or "ebb" phase and the later events of the "flow" phase. The early or "ebb" phase can arbitrarily be considered to last for 12 to 36 hours following injury. If the animal or patient survives this period of depressed vitality, he then passes into the "flow" phase with resurgence of vitality (Fig. 8). Characteristic of the first phase is a normal or decreased level of heat production with some drop in core temperature. The later "flow" phase is characterized by an excessive protein breakdown, an increase in resting metabolic expenditure, and perhaps a rise in core temperature (sometimes called traumatic fever).

The initial or "ebb" phase after injury may influence heat metabolism by decreased circulation to heat-producing tissues and by decreased transport of heat to the body surface. In addition, the animal in shock has been reported to fail to shiver as the core temperature is falling.[41] Stoner has performed detailed studies of shivering in rats injured by bilateral hind limb ischemia.[51] When the core temperature fell in a cool

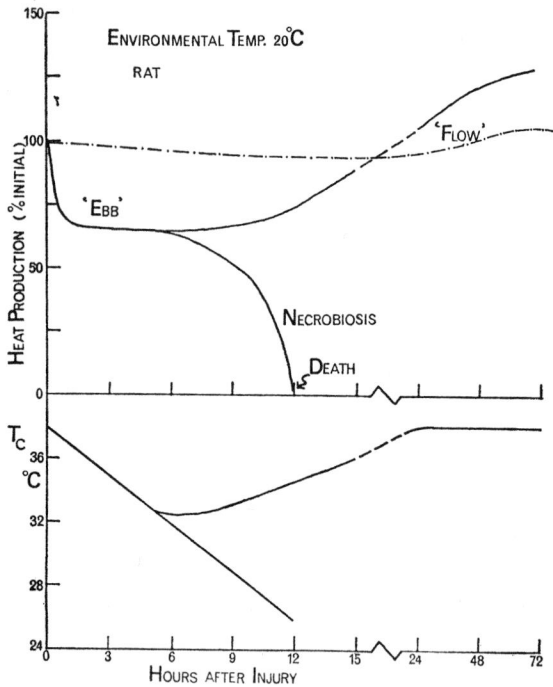

Figure 8. Changes in heat production and colon temperature (T_c) for rats injured by bilateral hind limb ischemia (70 to 80 per cent mortality) and 20 per cent burn (nonfatal) vs. heat production (broken line) after femoral fracture in the rat. (From Cuthbertson, D. P. *In* Porter, R., and Knight, J. (Eds.): Energy Metabolism in Trauma. London, J. & A. Churchill, 1970.)

environment to levels that provoked shivering in uninjured animals, no shivering was observed in those with limb ischemia. This was interpreted as a lowering of the "set point" for thermogenesis by the injury.

Kovach[37] has studied the central nervous system after hemorrhagic shock, with findings that may be relevant to the altered temperature control seen after injury. Blood flow is shown to be reduced to a greater degree in the hypothalamus than in the brain as a whole after hemorrhage. A progressive loss of peripheral circulatory changes following direct hypothalamic stimulation occurred during hypotension. These workers suggested that a similar loss of hypothalamic temperature control might also be occurring. The pO_2 of the hypothalamus was followed by means of platinum microelectrodes in the tissue, which indicated that the oxygen tension fell to less than 20 per cent of control values during hemorrhage. The observation that the pO_2 did not rise when the blood flow increased with reinfusion was interpreted as indicating that the oxygen consumption of the hypothalamus had increased as a result of the hemorrhage. Animals treated with phenoxybenzamine showed much less change in hypothalamic pO_2 during the hypotensive period and values returned to normal during reinfusion. The brain arteriovenous difference (carotid artery to saggital vein) increased in the untreated animals, but was unchanged in the pretreated animals. The protective effect of the drug appeared to be more than could be explained by changes in blood flow, perhaps indicating a local metabolic effect, such as a reversible inhibition of mitochondrial respiration.

Environmental Temperature and Experimental Injury

Environmental factors exert a profound effect on the response to injury in the rat and other small mammals. Qualitatively, similar changes can be expected to occur in larger mammals such as man, although the exploration of this area is just beginning. The growing interest in the relation of environmental conditions to convalescence after various forms of trauma in man justifies a brief review of current knowledge from small animal studies.

Various investigators have shown that the rat has an increased mortality and shortened survival time following various forms of injury, when the ambient temperature is raised significantly above control values anywhere in the range of 10 to 37° C. Increasing the temperature of the damaged part increases the severity of the tissue damage and consequent loss of fluid into the area. At a later stage, both burns and surgical wounds of the skin have been shown to heal faster at 30° C. than at 20° C., perhaps because of better circulation in the area of the wound.[19]

When rats are injured at an ordinary room temperature of about 20° C., the injury is rapidly followed by a fall in deep body or core temperature. Except in major hemorrhage this is not due, in the early stages, to a failure of oxygen transport to the heat-producing organs. This is in contrast to the later stages leading to death, in which the picture is dominated by a failure of oxygen transport. An optimal temperature for survival after various forms of injury has been reported from many laboratories for various species. This optimal temperature is always below the thermoneutral zone and is associated with a temporary decrease in core temperature. Stoner has observed, "From a teleological standpoint the optimum environmental temperature is one which allows the body temperature to fall at an optimum rate to a level which is not so low that unaided recovery is impossible yet which confers advantages by limiting the injury and husbanding the body's metabolic resources."[50]

Environmental Conditions and Human Injury

A reduction in post-traumatic nitrogen loss and a more normal plasma protein metabolism have recently been shown in the rat and in man following fracture of a long bone if convalescence was in an environment of 28 to 30° C. (82.4 to 86.0° F.) rather than 20 to 21° C. (68.0 to 69.8° F.).[19] The mechanism for this improvement is not clear and is the subject of active study. An ambient temperature below the thermoneutral zone in the patient area may cause an increased nitrogen loss as a result of a greater food requirement or of some unidentified neuroendocrine stimulus.

Advances in construction of buildings have included higher elevators, decreased window space, artificial lighting, and so forth, all of these things contributing to a separation of man from his natural environment. None of these architectural features have more physiologic significance than modern ventilation and air conditioning. The ease of manipulating temperature, humidity, and air flow in modern hospitals has outdistanced our knowledge of physiologic requirements and how they are altered in the critically ill patient. Too often the ventilation and air conditioning are regulated for the comfort of the professional staff rather than the physiologic needs of the patient.

One suggestion has been that the thermoneutral zone (28 to 30° C.) for seminude man should be the guide for the ambient temperature of hospital wards and particularly intensive care units. Perhaps in the hospital, graduated patient care from areas such as the recovery room and the intensive care unit to areas of intermediate care and to areas of limited care for late convalescence should be accompanied by changes in ambient temperature, from 25° C. (77° F.) for an area of intermediate care to conventional indoor temperature—21 to 22° C. (70 to 72° F.)—for late convalescence. Thus the transition in graduated medical care could have a parallel stepwise return toward the mild environmental stress associated with conditions of ordinary indoor living.

Temperature Regulation and Energy Metabolism Following Burn Injury

No injury results in greater changes in the host for a longer period of time than a thermal burn. Twenty-five years ago, burn cachexia was frequently observed but poorly understood. Patients with large burns lost weight progressively, and weeks after injury they became hypoalbuminemic and anemic. Frequently skin grafts failed to take, and the rate of dying was very high. Cope et al. in 1953 first reported that burned patients demonstrated a chronic increase in metabolic rate without any change in the circulating levels of thyroid hormone. This report also noted that the hypermetabolism persisted until wound closure.[17] Lieberman and Lansche[38] demonstrated an increase in evaporative heat loss and metabolic rate in burned rats and suggested that there was a causal relationship. They observed that both the evaporative heat loss and rate of heat production returned toward normal when such burn wounds were covered with a material impermeable to water. Caldwell et al. demonstrated that thyroid function was not necessary for the hypermetabolism in burned rats and that increasing the ambient temperature for such animals resulted in a return to near normal of the metabolic rate without affecting the increased evaporative heat loss.[14] With partitional calorimetry it was demonstrated that the decrease in metabolism effected by a warm ambient temperature was due to a decrease in heat loss by radiation, conduction, and convection.[10]

Caldwell et al. showed that burned rats housed at 30° C., with their total caloric intake fixed at preburned levels, were able to maintain positive nitrogen balance and gain body weight, whereas similarly burned and nourished animals housed at 20° C. lost weight rapidly and sustained a negative nitrogen balance for more than 40 days following the injury.[13] Thus, reduction of dry heat loss for burned rats through the medium of increased ambient temperature above thermal neutrality resulted in a great nutritional advantage.

Goodall et al. first recorded large increases in the rate of excretion of catecholamines in patients with large burns.[25] These authors noted that the major portion of the increase was noradrenaline and that the amount of increase roughly paralleled the size of the burn.

Harrison et al. showed a positive correlation between the metabolic rate and rate of catecholamine excretion for burned patients and postulated that an increased catecholamine excretion is responsible for the elevated metabolic rate seen in burned patients.[32]

Zawacki et al. studied 12 burned patients before and after their burn wounds had been covered for 12 hours with an impermeable material.[55] In these 12 patients (average burn size 40 per cent BSA, average day of study 14th PBD) with medium size burns studied in the early postburn period, covering the burn wound did not produce a fall in the rate of heat production and increased body temperature only an average of 0.5° F. If there was no associated decrease in the rate of heat production, covering the burn wound should have resulted in a rise in body temperature of one degree per hour in some of these patients. From these observations Zawacki challenged the idea that in man increased evaporative heat loss occurring through the burn wound was the primary drive for the hypermetabolism following thermal trauma.

In contrast to Zawacki, Neely et al. found a prompt decrease in the metabolic rate of five of six burned patients after their burn wounds were covered with a water-impermeable dressing. Metabolic rates remained elevated when the burn wounds were covered, but five of the six patients were febrile.[44]

Birke et al. studied burned man at environmental temperatures of 22° C. and 32° C. This group found a decrease in the rate of heat production and catecholamine excretion at 32° C. compared with 22° C., without a change in the rate of evaporative heat loss. Similarly, Barr et al. and Davis et al. showed that housing burned patients in a warm (32° C.), dry environment resulted in less loss of body weight, less excretion of urinary nitrogen, and a lower metabolic rate than keeping them at an ambient temperature of 22° C.[6, 20]

Wilmore et al. confirmed the findings of Birke and demonstrated further that the febrile burn patients showed increased tissue conduction and heat loss via radiation. This study also showed a lack of correlation between the rate of catecholamine excretion and metabolic rate when the metabolic rate was very high. Combined alpha and beta blockade of these patients produced a fall in metabolic rate, but 64 per cent of the original increase persisted.[53] Wilmore suggested that alterations in "hypothalamic function due to injury resulting in increased catecholamine elaboration would explain the metabolic response to thermal injury." This statement seems untenable in view of (a) the persistent hypermetabolic state of Wilmore's patients following alpha and beta blockade, and (b) the inability of even adrenaline to produce more than a 30 to 35 per cent increase in metabolic rate in man, while noradrenaline (which accounts for 90 per cent of the late increase in catecholamine in burned patients) can produce only a 21 ± 8 per cent increase in the met-

abolic rate in man.[49] Furthermore, burned rats with no adrenal medullary function are still hypermetabolic at ambient temperatures of 20° and 28° C., although they demonstrate chronic whole-body hypothermia when housed at 20° C.[12]

In summary, burned man demonstrates an increased metabolic rate that correlates very well with an increased evaporative heat loss. There is in addition a chronic febrile state with increased tissue conduction and dry heat loss as a result. Catecholamine turnover, principally of noradrenaline, is increased.

Elevating the ambient temperature for such patients results in a lowering of the metabolic rate, a decrease in the rate of excretion of catecholamines, a probable decrease in dry heat loss, and little or no change in the evaporative heat loss. Patients treated in this manner lose less body weight and excrete less urinary nitrogen.

These data indicate that the zone of thermal neutrality for the burned patient is increased (see page 192). Wilmore stated that the burned patient is internally warm but not externally cold. The evidence suggests that he is both internally warm and externally cold. The burned patient acts as though the regulatory setpoint for body temperature has been shifted upward. (Discussion of the metabolic effects of fever is presented elsewhere in this chapter.) Special consideration of the effects of fever should be given in the burned patient, for the fever persists for so long that the cumulative metabolic effect becomes more important. Efforts to explain the hypermetabolic state following thermal trauma must include the metabolic effects of fever.

What then is the primary drive and/or drives for the hypermetabolic state following thermal trauma? These authors interpret the data as supporting the idea that increased evaporative heat loss and chronic elevation of the body temperature are the primary etiological factors producing an increased metabolic rate. The possibility of interaction between these two factors is very real, for an increase in metabolic rate may produce fever, and fever definitely increases the metabolic rate following the van't Hoff law, as if the whole body had a Q_{10} of 2.3 to 2.5. Most of the data from both man and animals fit this area. The metabolic effect of fever is more subtle and has not been adequately studied. Even the basic cause of fever in burned patients is not understood. Increases in the excretion rates for catecholamines, principally noradrenaline, respond as if secondary to the chronic stress of hypermetabolism; increased release and turnover of catecholamines is a nonspecific response seen to some degree after all trauma and is not a very effective way to increase heat production. Most investigators agree that the burned patient should be cared for in a warm ambient environment.

The Meaning of Fever During the Postoperative Period

The idea that surgical convalescence is characterized by a low-grade fever most likely developed because of the high incidence of temperature elevation due to specific causes in the postoperative period. In the immediate postoperative period, most temperature elevations have their etiology in bacterial infections of the lung, urinary tract, or surgical wound. The surgeon should investigate by history and examination each patient in whom a fever of 38° C. (100.4° F.) or more develops. This arbitrary cutoff eliminates the majority of cases with temperature elevations falling within the range of normal variation. The history will reveal whether aspiration has occurred, whether the patient has been catheterized and now has dysuria, or whether he has pain in the area of the surgical wound. Physical examination will detect evidence of atelectasis or pneumonia within the chest, a tender, red, warm incision, or a red streak running along a vein leading from a vein puncture site. Treatment of each complication is beyond the scope of this chapter; however, the principle of *"no benign fever,"* with special investigation of each patient with postoperative fever, is stressed here. Core temperature is a tightly regulated characteristic of the body, and any variation should lead the clinician to seek an explanation.

Altemeier and associates[2] have reported on "third day surgical fever," a syndrome of sepsis arising on the third day after operation, trauma, or intensive care and caused by infection introduced through continuous intravenous devices which results in acute thrombophlebitis. The most frequent organisms cultured from the catheter tip and the bloodstream were Serratia, Klebsiella, Bacteroides, and Staphylococcus. Early recognition of the syndrome, prompt removal of the intravenous device, and administration of appropriate antibiotics are necessary to prevent secondary abscess formation.

Special Cases of Fever in Surgical Patients

Patients with thermal injury and neurosurgical patients who have had operative procedures about the base of the brain are two types of surgical patients who may show temperature elevation of a nonbacterial origin. The neurosurgical patient may demonstrate no thermoregulatory responses to a positive or negative thermal load. In such cases he may actually require treatment as if he were poikilothermic.

Burn patients are febrile before there is significant bacterial colonization of burn wound. The fever appears in 2 to 4 days and later becomes obscured by fever from secondary bacterial pyrogens originating in the burn wound. Although evidence is lacking, one possible explanation of the early fever seen with thermal injury is absorption of heat-modified protein fragments from the burn wound that have the capacity to act as pyrogens at a hypothalamic level.

TREATMENT OF FEVER

Fever in surgical patients commonly represents bacterial infection. Therefore the cornerstone of all treatment of febrile surgical patients is the location of any source of infection, identification of the infecting organisms, and appropriate local as well as systemic treatment. The surgical drainage of an abscess, or the relief of obstruction in an infected viscus such as a ureter or the common duct, must be done promptly in order that other therapy may be effective. In general, patients with intra-abdominal infections tend to have intermittent fever with moderate swings, marked leukocytosis, often with a shift to the left, shaking chills, and drenching sweats. The majority of these infections originate in the right upper quadrant in the form of subphrenic, subhepatic, or intrahepatic abscesses, cholangitis, or abscesses related to a perforated ulcer or appendix. Blood cultures may be positive and usually grow enteric bacilli, enterococci, or Salmonella. Laparotomy may be the only means of diagnosis of right upper quadrant infection. Liver biopsy will usually reveal only the changes of bile stasis or acute inflammation and will not be diagnostic.

The importance of antibacterial therapy in the treatment of surgical fever is obvious. However, this type of treatment requires more sophistication than in past years because of the increasing number of agents that are available, and the variation in sensitivity of a given strain to various antibiotics. The additional difficulty exists in some surgical conditions of delivering high antibiotic concentrations to the site of the infection because of local thrombosis of small vessels around the area of an abscess or previous radiation therapy. There is increasing evidence that diffuse coagulation abnormalities occur in the presence of certain forms of sepsis. The dissemination of microemboli added to some degree of intravascular coagulation may further complicate the administration of antibiotics.

In addition to antibiotic therapy and surgical drainage, the treatment of fever involves efforts to reduce the elevated body temperature. The salicylates are known for their effectiveness in lowering body temperature. This antipyretic action is usually rapid and effective in febrile patients, but no effect is demonstrable when the temperature is normal. The normal regulation of body temperature requires a delicate balance between heat production and heat loss. In fever, the balance between heat production and heat loss still persists, except that the hypothalamic "thermostat" is set at a higher level. The salicylates appear to act by resetting the hypothalamic "thermostat" toward a normal body temperature. Heat production is not inhibited, but heat dissipation is augmented by increased peripheral blood flow and sweating. Sweating is so prominently associated with the use of antipyretic drugs that it has come to be looked upon as a major response. Marked sweating, however, does not occur unless there is fever, and fever can be lowered with salicylates even if sweating is prevented by administration of atropine. In most febrile patients the metabolic rate is lowered by antipyretic drugs, consequent to the fall in temperature. It is not commonly appreciated that salicylates in moderate doses lower an elevated body temperature despite the fact that they increase oxygen consumption. Toxic doses can produce a febrile effect that results in sweating, thus enhancing the dehydration seen in salicylate intoxication.

The treatment of the febrile patient commonly includes measures to lower body temperature by various methods of body cooling. This is based on an effort to make the patient more comfortable because of subjective complaints of headache and aching of joints. With extreme levels of fever, lowering body temperature by increased cooling becomes an urgent matter to preserve the cells of vital organs, particularly the brain. Lowering body temperature by external cooling has the dual effect of protecting cells from direct thermal damage and also reducing the metabolic demands of cells by virtue of the "Q_{10} effect" on the enzyme reactions, which can be shown to be temperature-sensitive in the test tube. Hence a lower body temperature means less demand on the lungs, the heart, and the peripheral circulation to provide gas exchange for elevated levels of cellular metabolism.

External cooling can vary from simply reducing the bedclothes covering the patient to actually applying ice bags, turning a fan on the moistened body surface, or increasing evaporation with an alcohol solution applied to the body surface. The most effective cooling occurs by internal cooling of viscera such as the stomach, where heat can be rapidly removed without the peripheral vasoconstriction of surface cooling, which tends to limit heat loss from the body.

SELECTED REFERENCES

Carlson, L. D., and Hsieh, A. C. L.: Control of Energy Exchange. New York, The MacMillan Company, 1970.
An excellent little monograph in paperback that presents thermal physiology and temperature regulation as integral parts of overall energy exchange. A discussion of selected measurements and models of energy exchange is given in the appendix.

Hardy, J. D., Gagge, A. P., and Stolwijk, J. A. J. (Eds.): Physiological and Behavioral Temperature Regulation. Springfield, Ill., Charles C Thomas, Publisher, 1970.
The contributions to the First International Symposium on Temperature Regulation held in August, 1968, at the John B. Pierce Foundation Laboratory and Yale University School of Medicine. This book is recommended for the advanced student who wishes to explore areas of contemporary research and current controversy.

Newburgh, L. H. (Ed.): Physiology of Heat Regulation and the Science of Clothing. New York, Hafner Publishing Company, 1968.
The reprinting of a 1949 classic stimulated by the demands of the military in World War II to protect the fighting man from extremes of environmental temperature and humidity, when combat was taking place for the first time around the globe in every season and climate.

Roe, C. F.: Fever and energy metabolism in surgical disease. Monogr. Surg. Sci., 3:85, 1966.
A review of heat exchange, fever, and various clinical conditions that influence mechanisms of heat production and heat loss.

Wolstenholme, G. E. W., and Birch, J. (Eds.): Pyrogens and Fever: A Ciba Symposium. London, Churchill Livingstone, 1971.
This volume is a series of papers by leading authorities dealing with thermoregulation, pyrogenicity and antigenicity, and pyrogen production. The material provides extensive background with references and also highlights current areas of investigation.

REFERENCES

1. Aldrete, J. A., Padfield, A., Solomon, C. C., and Rubright, M. W.: Possible predictive tests for malignant hyperthermia during anesthesia. J.A.M.A., 215:1465, 1971.
2. Altemeier, W. A., McDonough, J. J., and Fullen, W. D.: Third day surgical fever. Arch. Surg., 103:158, 1971.
3. Anderson, H. T., Hammel, H. T., and Hardy, J. D.: Modifications of the febrile response to pyrogen by hypothalamic heating and cooling in the unanesthetized dog. In American Institute of Physics: Temperature, Its Measurement and Control in Science and Industry. Volume 3, Part 3. New York, Reinhold Publishing Company, 1963, pp. 597-601.
4. Beisel, W. R., Sawyer, E. D., Ryll, E. D., and Crozier, D.: Metabolic effects of intracellular infections in man. Ann. Intern. Med., 67:744-779, 1967.
5. Berman, M. C., Harrison, G. G., Bull, A. B., and Kench, J. E.: Changes underlying halothane-induced malignant hyperpyrexia in Landrace pigs. Nature, 225:653, 1970.

6. Birke, G., Carlson, L. A., von Euler, U. S., Liljedahl, S. O., and Plantin, L. O.: Studies on burns. XII. Lipid metabolism, catecholamine excretion, basal metabolic rate, and water loss during treatment of burns with warm dry air. Acta Chir. Scand., 138:321, 1972.
7. Brengelmann, G., and Brown, A. C.: Temperature regulation. In Ruch, T. C., and Patton, H. D.: Physiology and Biophysics. 20th ed. Philadelphia, W. B. Saunders Company, 1965.
8. Britt, B. A., Kalow, W., Gordon, A., Humphrey, J. G., and Rewcastle, N. B.: Malignant hyperthemia: An investigation of five patients. Can. Anaesth. Soc. J., 20:431, 1973.
9. Cairnie, A. B., Campbell, R. M., Pullar, J. D., and Cuthbertson, D. P.: The heat production consequent on injury. Br. J. Exp. Pathol., 38:504, 1957.
10. Caldwell, F. T., Hammel, H. D., and Dolan, F.: A calorimeter for simultaneous determination of heat production and heat loss in the rat. J. Appl. Physiol., 21:1655, 1966.
11. Caldwell, F. T., Smith, V., Bowser, B., Warren, L., and Baxter, G.: On the relationship of energy metabolism and adrenomedullary function in the rat following thermal burns. In preparation.
12. Caldwell, F. T.: Energy metabolism following thermal burns. Arch. Surg., in press.
13. Caldwell, F. T.: Metabolic response to thermal trauma: II. Nutritional studies with rats at two environmental temperatures. Ann. Surg., 115:119, 1962.
14. Caldwell, F. T., Osterholm, J. L., Sower, N. D., and Moyer, C. A.: Metabolic response to thermal trauma of normal and thyroprivic rats at three environmental temperatures. Ann. Surg., 150:976, 1959.
15. Clowes, G. H. A., Jr., Vucinic, M., and Weidner, M. G.: Circulatory and metabolic alterations associated with survival or death in peritonitis: Clinical analysis of 25 cases. Ann. Surg., 163:866, 1966.
16. Cooper, K. E., Cranston, W. I., and Snell, E. S.: Temperature regulation during fever in man. Clin. Sci., 27:345, 1964.
17. Cope, O., Nardi, G. L., Quijano, M., Rovit, R. L., Stanbury, J. B., and Wright, A.: Metabolic rate and thyroid function following acute thermal trauma in man. Ann. Surg., 137:165, 1953.
18. Cuthbertson, D. P.: Observations of the disturbance of metabolism produced by injury to the limbs. Q. J. Med., 1:233, 1932.
19. Cuthbertson, D., and Tilstone, W. J.: Metabolism during the postinjury period. In Sobotka, H., and Stewart, C. P. (Eds.): Advances in Clinical Chemistry. Volume 12. New York, Academic Press, 1969.
20. Davies, J. W. L., Liljedahl, S. O., and Birke, G.: Protein metabolism in burned patients treated in a warm (32° C.) or cool (22° C.) environment. Injury, 1:43, 1969.
21. DuBois, E. F.: Fever. In Basal Metabolism in Health and Disease. Philadelphia, Lea & Febiger, 1924, pp. 311-340.
22. DuBois, E. F.: Lane Medical Lectures: The Mechanism of Heat Loss and Temperature Regulation. Stanford, Calif., Stanford University Press, 1937.
23. Ellis, F. R., Keaney, N. P., Harriman, D. G. F., Sumner, D. W., Kyei-Mensah, K., Tyrrell, J. H., Hargreaves, J. B., Parikh, R. K., and Mulrooney, P. L.: Screening for malignant hyperpyrexia. Br. Med. J., 3:559, 1972.
24. Goldberg, M. J., and Roe, F.: Temperature changes during anesthesia and operations. Arch. Surg., 93:365, 1966.
25. Goodall, McC., Stone, C., and Haynes, B. W., Jr.: Urinary output of adrenaline and noradrenaline in severe thermal burns. Ann. Surg., 145:479, 1957.
26. Graber, C. D., Reinhold, R. B., Breman, J. G., Harley, R. A., and Hennigar, G. R.: Fatal heat stroke—circulating endotoxin and gram-negative sepsis as complications. J.A.M.A., 216:1195, 1971.
27. Grayson, T. L., White, J. E., and Moyer, C. A.: Oxygen consumptions: Concentrations of inorganic ions in urine, serum and duodenal fluid, hematocrits, urinary excretions; pulse rates and blood pressure during duodenal depletions of sodium salts in normal and alcoholic man. Ann. Surg., 158:840, 1963.
28. Gump, F. E., Price, J. B., Jr., and Kinney, J. M.: Whole body and splanchnic blood flow and oxygen consumption measurements in patients with intraperitoneal infection. Ann. Surg., 171:321, 1970.
29. Gump, F. E., Price, J. B., Jr., and Kinney, J. M.: Blood flow and oxygen consumption in patients with severe burns. Surg. Gynecol. Obstet., 130:641, 1970.
30. Hammel, H. T.: Regulation of internal body temperature. Ann. Rev. Physiol., 30:641, 1968.
31. Harrison, G. G., Saunders, S. J., et al.: Anaesthetic-induced

malignant hyperpyrexia and a method for its prediction. Br. J. Anaesth., 41:844, 1969.

32. Harrison, T. S., Seaton, J. F., and Feller, I.: Relationship of increased oxygen consumption to catecholamine excretion in thermal burns. Ann. Surg., 165:169, 1967.

33. Hermbeck, A. S., and Thal, H. P.: Mechanisms for the high circulatory requirements in sepsis and septic shock. Ann. Surg., 170:677, 1969.

34. Isaeas, H., and Barlow, M. B.: Malignant hyperpyrexia. J. Neurol., Neurosurg. Psychiatr., 36:228, 1973.

35. Kinney, J. M., Long, C. L., and Duke, J. H.: Carbohydrate and nitrogen metabolism after injury. In Porter, R., and Knight, J. (Eds.): Energy Metabolism in Trauma. London, J. & A. Churchill, 1970, pp. 103–126.

36. Kinney, J. M., and Roe, C. F.: Caloric equivalent of fever: I. Patterns of postoperative response. Ann. Surg., 156:610, 1962.

37. Kovach, A. G. B.: The function of the central nervous system after hemorrhage. J. Clin. Pathol., 23 (Suppl.), 4:202, 1970.

38. Lieberman, Z. H., and Lansche, J. M.: Effects of thermal injury on metabolic rate of insensible water loss in the rat. Surg. Forum, 7:83, 1957.

39. Morris, R. H.: Influence of ambient temperature on patient temperature during intraabdominal surgery. Ann. Surg., 173:230, 1971.

40. Moser, K. M., Perry, R. B., and Luchsinger, P. C.: Cardiopulmonary consequences of pyrogen-induced hyperpyrexia in man. J. Clin. Invest., 42:626, 1963.

41. Mott, J.: The effects of baroreceptor and chemoreceptor stimulation of shivering. J. Physiol., 166:563, 1963.

42. Myers, J. D.: The circulation in the splanchnic area. In Green, H. D. (Ed.): Shock and Circulatory Homeostasis. New York, Josiah Macy, Jr., Foundation, 1955, pp. 121–165.

43. Myers, R. D., and Veale, W. L.: Body temperature; possible ionic mechanism in the hypothalamus controlling the setpoint. Science, 170:95, 1970.

44. Neely, W. A., Petro, A. B., Holloman, G. H., Jr., Rushton, F. W.,

Turner, M. D., and Hardy, J. D.: Researchers on the cause of burn hypermetabolism. Ann. Surg., 179:291, 1974.

45. Nissan, S., et al.: Increased O_2 consumption of the rat diaphragm by elevated NaCl concentrations. Am. J. Physiol., 210:1222, 1966.

46. Pekarek, R., Wannemacher, R. W., Jr., Powandan, M. C., Abels, F., Mosher, D., Dinterman, R., and Beisel, W. R.: Further evidence that leukocytic endogenous mediator (LEM) is not endotoxin. Life Sci., 14:1765, 1974.

47. Roe, C. F., Goldberg, M. J., Blair, C. S., and Kinney, J. M.: The influence of body temperature on early postoperative oxygen consumption. Surgery, 60:85, 1966.

48. Roe, C. F., and Kinney, J. M.: The caloric equivalent of fever: II. Influence of major trauma. Ann. Surg., 161:140, 1965.

49. Steinberg, D., Nestel, P. J., Buskirk, E. R., and Thompson, R. H.: Calorigenic effect of norepinephrine correlated with plasma free fatty acid turnover and oxidation. J. Clin. Invest., 43:167, 1964.

50. Stoner, H. B.: The effect of environment on the response to injury in the rat. Postgrad. Med. J., 45:555, 1969.

51. Stoner, H. B.: Effect of injury on shivering thermogenesis in the rat. J. Physiol., 214:599, 1971.

52. Wannemacher, R. W., Jr., Dupont, H. L., Pekarek, R. S., Powanda, M. C., Schwartz, A., Hornick, R. B., and Beisel, W. R.: An endogenous mediator of depression of amino acids and trace metals in serum during typhoid fever. J. Infect. Dis., 126:77, 1972.

53. Wilmore, D. W., Long, J. M., Mason, A. D., Jr., Skreen, R. W., and Pruitt, B. A.: Catecholamines: Mediator of the hypermetabolic response to thermal injury. Ann. Surg., 180:653, 1974.

54. Wilson, R. D., Knapp, C., et al.: Thermoregulatory failure of the burn scar. J. Trauma, 2:518, 1971.

55. Zawacki, B. E., Spitzer, K. W., Mason, A. D., and Johns, L. A.: Does increased evaporative water loss cause hypermetabolism in burned patients? Ann. Surg., 171:236, 1970.

10

ANESTHESIA

Edward A. Brunner, M.D., and James E. Eckenhoff, M.D.

The analgesic properties of nitrous oxide were recognized by Sir Humphrey Davy as early as 1800, and he suggested its use for relief of the pain of surgery. It was not until 1844 that Horace Wells, a Hartford dentist who had employed nitrous oxide as an anesthetic for dentistry, tried to demonstrate its utility during surgical operation. His attempt was a failure. Michael Faraday, a student of Davy, after noting the effect of diethyl ether in animal experiments, suggested its use as an anesthetic in 1818. A quarter of a century later, ether was employed successfully for surgical anesthesia by two men working separately and independently. Crawford Long, a Georgia physician, used ether for surgical anesthesia as early as 1842, but did not publicize his discovery. W. T. G. Morton, on the other hand, gave a public demonstration of ether anesthesia at the Massachusetts General Hospital in 1846. A written account appeared in the Boston Medical and Surgical Journal, and within a few weeks this report was disseminated to England, where several physicians recognized its importance. John Snow adopted the use of ether and described the clinical signs of anesthetic depth. James Y. Simpson, having tried ether, abandoned it in favor of chloroform. His use of chloroform in childbirth for Queen Victoria led to widespread acceptance of anesthesia in both surgery and obstetrics. Carl Koller's clinical demonstration of the local anesthetic actions of cocaine in 1884 and its use by Halsted for infiltration and by Bier in 1899 for intrathecal injection led to the establishment of regional anesthesia. By 1900, the basic discoveries on which the clinical practice of anesthesia is based had been made.

The usual concept of anesthesiology relates primarily to the prevention of pain perception during an operation. Initially, such a concept was appropriate and perhaps for as long as six decades after the introduction of ether, this was the only concern of the anesthetist. Because the hazards associated with anesthesia became apparent early, the British entrusted the administration of ether or chloroform to physicians. The American philosophy of training nurses as anesthetists materialized during the late nineteenth century, and many years passed before physician anesthetists appeared in this country. It is likely that the early reliance of the British on the more dangerous chloroform and the preference of Americans for the safety of ether were responsible for this divergent development.

As surgical procedures became more complex, the demands upon anesthesia and anesthetists increased. The physiologic and pharmacologic effects of old and new anesthetic agents had to be thoroughly understood. Profound muscle relaxation had to be provided safely and because this often led to respiratory insufficiency, a background knowledge of pulmonary physiology and the control of ventilation became a necessity. As the critically ill and those at the extremes of life began to be operated upon, a sound foundation in medicine became mandatory to prepare these patients successfully for operation, and to care for them during the procedure. More recently, it became apparent that the expertise gained by the anesthetist should be utilized in the entire perioperative period; hence the modern participation of anesthetists in preoperative preparation of the surgical patient, in respiratory therapy, and in intensive care units.

General Considerations

A classification of the methods by which anesthesia may be provided should be preceded by an outline of the mechanisms by which a patient interacts with his environment, because anesthesia is a modification of such interaction. Sensory perception requires a stimulus to excite a receptor. This sets into motion events leading to awareness of the stimulus and ultimately to action by the organism. This is represented schematically in Figure 1. A stimulus excites a receptor *(a)*. The response of the receptor is to initiate a nerve impulse *(b)*, which is conducted to the central nervous system at the level of the spinal cord or brain stem *(c)*. In the spinal cord, the impulse may be transferred to motor pathways, which initiate an involuntary response *(i)*, thereby completing a reflex arc; or the impulse may be transmitted to higher centers in the central nervous system *(d)*, where perception of the sensation *(e)* combines with a psychologic reaction to that sensation *(f)* to produce knowledgeable awareness *(g)*, which may be stored in memory *(h)* subject to recall. Knowledgeable awareness may initiate a voluntary response *(i)*, thus completing the interaction of the organism and its environment.

The pathways outlined in this schema may be interrupted at different points to alter environmental interaction seemingly to provide the same result. For example, a blindfold placed over the eyes prevents light from exciting the retinal receptors and blocks visual awareness of the environment; injection of local anesthetic agents into the retrobulbar space blocks the transmission of the nerve action potential from the retina to the brain but just as surely blocks knowledgeable awareness of the environment; a neuromuscular blocking agent, on the other hand, leaves the receptors intact, transmission unimpeded, and perceptive areas of the brain active, but response to the stimulus becomes impossible. Following this pattern, one or more anesthetics, acting at known sites in the pathway, can be chosen to provide desirable and acceptable conditions for a surgical procedure, or for the relief of painful states.

Classification of Anesthetic Techniques

In a broad sense, all types of anesthesia may be classified as either regional or general. Regional anesthesia is more discrete in that the sensorium remains clear and pain relief follows a block of the sensory receptor or of peripheral nerve conduction. Sensory perception from unblocked areas remains intact, and sight, sound, taste, or smell may evoke an undesirable response during an operative procedure. General anesthesia is produced by agents that act primarily on the brain and interfere with normal neuronal activation,

sensory perception, or knowledgeable awareness. Some drugs can influence many pathways; for example, narcotic analgesics may alter reaction to pain as well as diminish perception of the stimulus. Pain may be perceived but it does not cause discomfort. Psychologic support from a physician, the family, or a religious counselor can mimic this effect.[15] Drugs such as scopolamine are capable of blocking memory and are sometimes employed for their amnesic qualities. The neuromuscular and ganglionic blocking agents and the belladonna alkaloids are examples of drugs that act at the terminal portions of nerve pathways to prevent activation of peripheral end organs.

REGIONAL ANESTHESIA

Regional anesthesia implies reversible blockade of pain perception or transmission by local anesthetic drugs, although physical agents such as cold or pressure can act similarly. In appropriate concentrations, these drugs prevent activation of pain receptors and block the transmission of nerve action potentials along all types of nerve fibers. The area influenced by the agent is governed by the anatomic site of application.

Regional anesthesia is classified into seven types on an anatomic basis. The first two types, topical anesthesia and local infiltration, involve principally sen-

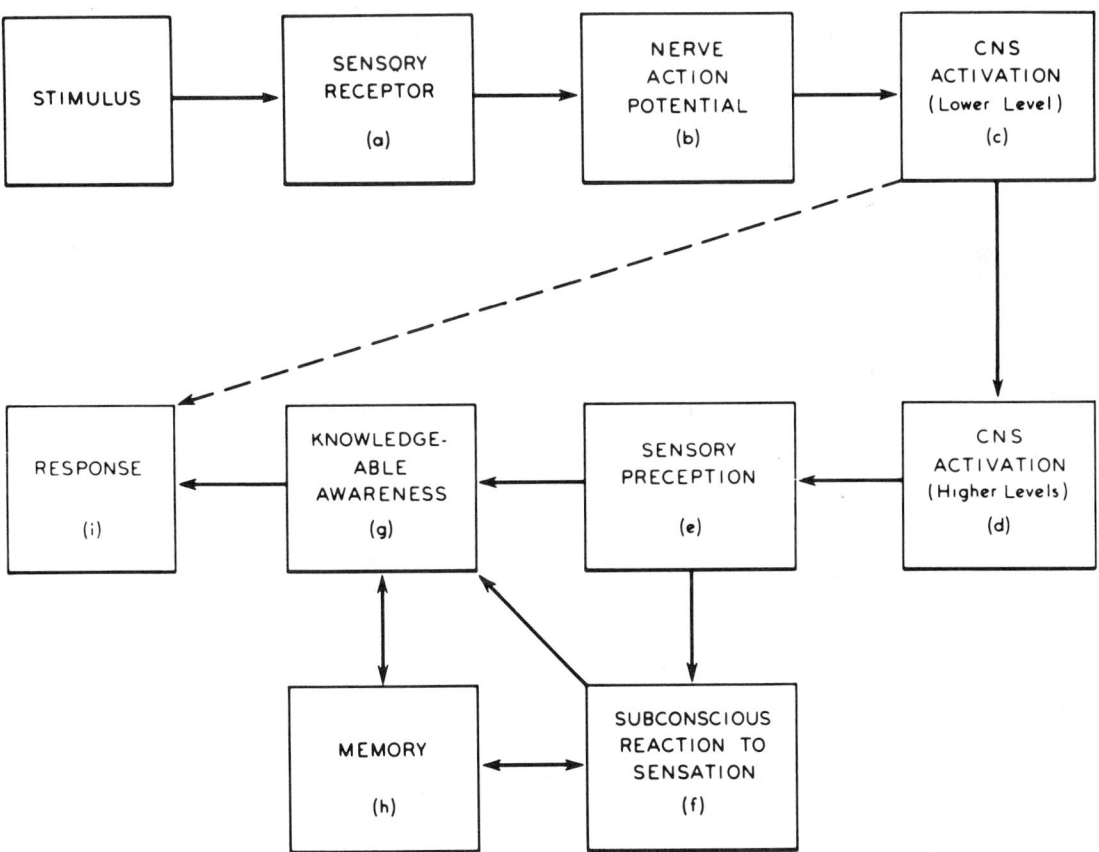

Figure 1. Schematic representation of the interaction of a patient and his environment.

sory receptors. The next four, field block, peripheral nerve block, epidural anesthesia, and spinal anesthesia, involve nerve conduction; hence the use of the term conduction anesthesia. The mechanism of action of the last type, intravenous regional anesthesia, is unclear.

Topical anesthesia results from the application of certain local anesthetics to skin or mucous membranes.[1] The technique is ineffective if the skin is intact and healthy, because aqueous solutions of the salts of local anesthetics lack penetrability of normal epidermis. When they are applied to inflamed or diseased skin, an anesthetic action will result. Ointments containing local anesthetic bases are effective on normal skin. Aqueous solutions of the salts of cocaine, lidocaine, or tetracaine will block the sensory receptors of mucous membranes. Good surface anesthesia of the conjunctiva and cornea, of oral, nasal, and pharyngeal cavities, of esophagus, larynx, and trachea, and of urethra and anus will result from application of these agents. Because the blood supply to mucous membranes is rich, absorption of the drug is rapid. The amount of local anesthetic used topically must be reduced to one fourth to one half of the maximum allowable by infiltration.

Local infiltration involves the injection of the anesthetic directly into the operative field so that the sensory receptors that would be stimulated by the surgical procedures are rendered insensitive. Obviously, some of the most distal segments of the conduction system will be blocked.

Field block is produced by circumscribing the operative field with a continuous wall of local anesthetic. Nerve fibers supplying the site of operation and traversing this barrier are blocked and the operative area is rendered insensitive. Large volumes of anesthetic agents are usually required so that most dilute effective concentrations must be injected to minimize the possibility of overdosage and toxic reactions.

Peripheral nerve block is performed by depositing a local anesthetic in proximity to major nerve trunks. Combinations of several nerve blocks, or injection of a nerve plexus, will render a large area of the body anesthetic. Nerve blocks may be combined with local infiltration to provide anesthesia for a particular surgical procedure. Examples include brachial plexus block to provide regional anesthesia for operations on the hand, forearm, or arm; femoral, sciatic, and obturator nerve block to anesthetize the entire lower extremity; and a combination of intercostal nerve blocks with celiac plexus block to provide anesthesia for laparotomy.

Epidural anesthesia follows the deposition of a local anesthetic agent into the extradural space within the vertebral canal. When anesthesia of caudal, sacral, or low lumbar dermatomes is indicated, the sacrococcygeal hiatus is a convenient approach to the epidural space. This is called caudal anesthesia, a technique particularly useful in perineal and rectal operations and for pain relief in the terminal stages of labor and delivery. The epidural space extends cephalad to the foramen magnum and may be penetrated at any level, although the lumbar area is most frequently used because of the ease of approach and the minimal

danger of trauma to the spinal cord. Thoracic and cervical epidural blocks are not used as often because the epidural space is narrow and the risk of injury to the cord is greater. The site of action of local anesthetics injected into the epidural space is in doubt but in all likelihood it is at the point where the nerves lose their dural sleeves at the intervertebral foramina. Some contend that the site of action is central to the pia arachnoid because an appreciable concentration of local anesthetic is detectable in cerebrospinal fluid after epidural block.

The injection into the epidural space of long-acting steroids combined with local anesthetic solutions has been advocated by some for treatment of the symptoms generally associated with herniation of an intervertebral disc. Long-term results of the treatment still need evaluation.

The physiologic changes associated with epidural anesthesia are similar to those observed with spinal anesthesia, since widespread sympathetic blockade is produced with both techniques. However, larger volumes of local anesthetic drugs are required for epidural anesthesia, and systemic reactions are more likely because the epidural space contains an extensive vascular network, making rapid uptake of injected substances possible. Systemic toxic effects of local anesthetic agents are not seen with spinal anesthesia, since the injected drug dosage is small. Catheters can be placed into the epidural space with relative ease, thus permitting the intermittent injection of local anesthetics for prolonged operations or for nonsurgical applications. The latter include control of pain due to operation, pancreatitis, or malignant disease; vasodilation of the lower extremities in acute vascular occlusion; sympathetic blockade to allow for the evaluation of effects of sympathectomy prior to operation; and use as a differential diagnostic measure in chronic pain states. The major advantage of the epidural technique compared to spinal anesthesia is that it produces extensive regional anesthesia without the hazards of dural puncture and injection of foreign substances into the cerebrospinal fluid. Heachache following epidural anesthesia is virtually nonexistent except when the dural sac is entered unintentionally.

Spinal anesthesia results from the injection of a local anesthetic into the cerebrospinal fluid so that the drug bathes the origin of the peripheral nerve roots. The term "saddle block" designates spinal anesthesia limited to the sacral and caudal dermatomes and is obtained by injection of a small volume of hyperbaric anesthetic solution, usually with the patient in the sitting position.

Puncture of the dural sac in the low lumbar area can be performed easily. In this area the sac is about 15 mm. in diameter, narrowing as it extends caudally to terminate at the level of the second lumbar vertebra. The area between L2 and L4 is nearly always chosen for lumbar puncture, since the spinal cord terminates between L1 and L2 vertebral bodies and the risk of cord puncture is negligible below this level.

The choice of drugs and technique depends upon the level and duration of anesthesia desired, the position and height of the patient, and the presence or absence of factors that modify cerebrospinal fluid dynamics.

The duration of anesthesia is largely determined by the local anesthetic used, although duration of block tends to be longer in the elderly. Procaine produces a block lasting less than an hour, tetracaine acts for $1\frac{1}{2}$ to 2 hours, and dibucaine about 3 hours. The addition of 0.3 to 0.5 mg. of epinephrine increases the average duration by 50 per cent or more. The level of sensory and motor block obtained is a function of the length of the dural sac and the volume and specific gravity of the drug mixture injected. As the volume becomes larger, the spread of the anesthetic increases and the level of anesthesia rises. In conditions associated with increased intra-abdominal pressure, the epidural venous plexus is usually engorged, constricting the dural sac and reducing the volume of spinal fluid. The volume of drug injected intrathecally should be reduced under these circumstances to prevent inordinately high levels of spinal anesthesia.

The specific gravity of cerebrospinal fluid is 1.006. Drug mixtures with greater specific gravity are called hyperbaric and tend to settle by gravity to the lowest point of the dural sac. Those which are lighter are hypobaric and rise in the cerebrospinal fluid; those of similar specific gravity are isobaric and are inclined to layer without rising or falling, unless influenced by extraneous factors that alter cerebrospinal fluid dynamics, such as coughing or straining. About 90 per cent of spinal anesthetic procedures in the United States are performed using hyperbaric techniques, with 10 per cent dextrose providing the greater specific gravity.

Local anesthetics injected into the subarachnoid space block autonomic preganglionic fibers as well as motor and sensory nerves. The sympathetic blockade results in peripheral arterial and venous dilation and pooling of blood in the peripheral vascular system. This normally reduces venous return to the heart. If the anesthesia extends high enough, sympathetic fibers innervating the heart may be blocked. Both factors usually combine to reduce cardiac output and blood pressure during spinal anesthesia. This can be overcome by rapid infusion of 500 to 1000 ml. of crystalloid solution or by the prophylactic intramuscular injection of sympathomimetic drugs five minutes before administration of a spinal anesthetic. An intravenous infusion of a pressor agent may be required in some patients.

Spinal anesthesia has advantages other than simplicity. Complete anesthesia is readily obtained for operations on the lower extremities, the perineal area, and the lower abdominal wall. Good conditions for intra-abdominal operations can be provided, accompanied by profound muscular relaxation, quiet breathing, constricted bowel, and lack of venous congestion. Spinal anesthesia is an excellent choice for patients who have eaten recently because the protective pharyngeal reflexes are intact in case vomiting should occur. It is also a good choice in the alcoholic, who might otherwise require large quantities of general anesthetics. There is no danger of systemic toxicity from local anesthetic agents, because little drug is needed for the desired effect.

The disadvantages of the technique include the lack of patient acceptance of a method that does not provide sleep, fear of permanent neurologic impairment, and its limitation to operations below the diaphragm. The incompleteness of autonomic blockade during operations in the abdominal cavity, particularly in the upper abdomen, may at times be bothersome because visceral traction may cause discomfort, nausea, or vomiting. Supplementation with light levels of general anesthesia may overcome some of these disadvantages. Despite impressions to the contrary, high spinal anesthesia has little effect upon pulmonary ventilation, presumably because the diaphragm compensates for the paralyzed abdominal and thoracic muscles.

The presence of disease of the central nervous system, whether neoplastic, infectious, traumatic, or degenerative, is a contraindication to the use of spinal anesthesia. Peripheral neuropathies, such as those associated with diabetes or syphilis, represent relative contraindications to subarachnoid block. A history of frequent severe headache warrants careful consideration before choosing the technique. Skin disease, or infection of the area chosen for lumbar puncture, and fear of spinal anesthesia will exclude some patients. The administration of spinal anesthesia to patients with marked hypovolemia will often result in precipitous hypotension. The technique should be avoided in this circumstance unless the volume deficit can be corrected.

Despite the ease with which it can be performed and the excellence of the operating conditions offered, spinal anesthesia has been associated with controversy and emotionalism. Reports of major neurologic sequelae have caused concern about the safety of the technique. A wide variation in the incidence of neurologic complications has been reported. Although one study reported six instances of residual paralysis following 1200 spinal anesthetics, several other studies of more than 10,000 patients each, in whom this technique was employed with careful follow-up, failed to uncover major neurologic sequelae.[12, 13]

Puncture of the dural sac and injection of foreign substances into the cerebrospinal fluid can be dangerous. Even without injection, lumbar puncture produces local trauma, changes cerebrospinal fluid dynamics, and may lead to the introduction of infection into the subarachnoid space. With attention to detail, the risk of lumbar puncture can be minimized. The injection of toxic substances into the intrathecal space must be avoided. In the past, carelessness in this respect has undoubtedly contributed to the complications reported. The availability of self-contained disposable sterile trays for spinal anesthesia has minimized risks previously arising from improper drug and equipment preparation and sterilization. By use of a meticulous technique, selection of drugs and equipment provided by reputable manufacturers, use of safe concentrations, and careful selection of patients, the risks associated with spinal anesthesia can be made comparable to those of general anesthesia. Minor neurologic sequelae related to spinal anesthesia may occur but are usually transient. These often relate to poor technique and improper positioning of the patient on the operating table. The mortality rate following spinal anesthesia is similar to that recorded in comparable series after general anesthesia.

The headache that may follow spinal anesthesia in some patients is thought to be caused by leakage of cerebrospinal fluid from the dural puncture site. This produces a decrease in cerebrospinal fluid pressure and when the patient assumes an upright position, the lack of fluid support for the intracranial contents produces tension on surrounding pain-sensitive structures. In severe cases diplopia and tinnitus may accompany headache in the upright position. Relief is obtained when the patient assumes the horizontal position. Systemic hydration and mild analgesics are effective in most cases, but more severe ones may require the injection of large volumes of saline into the epidural space to prevent further cerebrospinal fluid leakage. The injection of 10 ml. of autologous blood into the epidural space at the site of the dural puncture, to form a "blood patch," has been highly successful in treating spinal headache.[10]

Intravenous regional anesthesia follows the injection of a large volume of dilute local anesthetic solution into a vein of a bloodless extremity. The injected solution is confined to the extremity by a tourniquet. The anatomic site of action of the anesthetic is not clear. This technique may represent either a massive transvascular infiltration blockade of the extremity, or a conduction blockade resulting from the anesthetic agent leaking extravascularly near major nerve trunks.[8] Anesthesia obtained by this means is effective only as long as the tourniquet remains inflated. With deflation of the cuff, the blood level of the local anesthetic drug rises rapidly, creating the risk of systemic toxic reaction. This is a problem only if the operation requires less than 30 minutes. Intermittent release of the tourniquet minimizes this danger. Operations of or below the elbow require 25 to 40 ml. of 0.5 per cent procaine or lidocaine, whereas procedures below the knee require 40 to 60 ml. of solution. The technique is most suitable for superficial procedures.

USEFUL LOCAL ANESTHETICS

A variety of unrelated chemical compounds are capable of reversibly blocking neural transmission. To be clinically useful, an agent must be nonirritating, must not produce local tissue destruction in therapeutic concentrations, and must have low systemic toxicity in relation to nerve-blocking potency. Most of the currently used local anesthetics are relatively simple synthetic chemical compounds, but cocaine is a natural alkaloid. Procaine, the synthetic prototype, characterizes the fundamental chemical structure typical of drugs of this type (Fig. 2). The common components of this structure are a secondary or tertiary amino group (1); an aromatic group, often an acid (2); an aliphatic chain joining the two (3); and an ester, amide, or ether linkage (4). A large number of local anesthetics are modifications of this basic chemical structure (Table 1).

Cocaine is used exclusively as a topical anesthetic and is the only one to possess a prominent vasoconstrictor action. It must not be combined with epinephrine because of the potentiation of the cardiovascu-

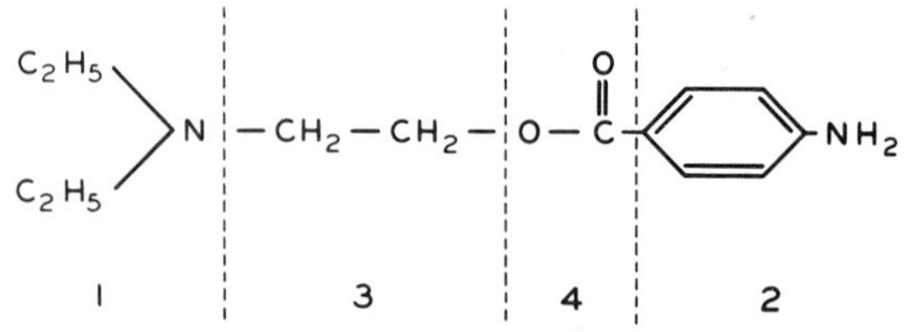

Figure 2. Chemical structure of procaine as a prototype of the synthetic local anesthetic agents, illustrating common features of chemical structure often found in these drugs.

lar effects of epinephrine by cocaine. It is particularly valuable for operations in the nasal cavity and is used in concentrations ranging from 4 to 10 per cent. The maximal safe dosage is 200 mg., although toxic effects from as little as 20 mg. have been witnessed. It may be applied by droplet, spray, pledget, or pack. At one time, it was used extensively in the eye but now has been almost abandoned in favor of safer agents. The ability of cocaine to produce mild central nervous system excitation has led to problems of addiction, so its use is controlled by federal narcotics regulations. Toxic symptoms from central nervous system stimulation may appear abruptly and run a rapid course. A high index of suspicion must be maintained because early manifestations are often mistaken for apprehension.

Procaine (Novocain) is an efficient local anesthetic that has had extensive clinical use since its introduction in 1905. It is not effective topically but has been used by all other methods. It is one fourth as toxic as cocaine and amounts of up to 1 gm. may be administered by infiltration in the average adult. Concentrations of 0.5 per cent are suitable for infiltration anesthesia, but 2 per cent may be needed for major nerve blocks. Procaine acts relatively rapidly but has a short duration of action. A congener, chloroprocaine (Nesacaine), is of equal potency but has a more rapid onset of action and a more evanescent effect. Vasoconstrictors are often added to slow absorption and prolong the duration of block with procaine. Plasma contains procaine esterase, which rapidly hydrolyzes the drug.

Lidocaine (Xylocaine) is a widely used drug, effective by topical application or by injection. Solutions of 2 to 4 per cent strength are used topically, 0.5 per cent for local infiltration, and 1 to 2 per cent for conduction anesthesia. A maximal injected dose of 500 mg. should not be exceeded in the average adult. The chemical structure of lidocaine is characterized by its amide linkage, which resists hydrolysis by plasma esterase. It produces a more prompt and longer lasting anesthesia than equal concentrations of procaine and appears to spread better in the tissues. Mild sedation often accompanies its use. It depresses the myocardium and the cardiac conduction system and can be used intravenously as an antiarrhythmic agent.

Mepivacaine (Carbocaine), like lidocaine, is an amide. Its onset of action is slightly more rapid, duration longer, and sedative effect less. The two drugs are similar in other respects.

Tetracaine (Pontocaine) is about 10 times more potent and toxic than procaine. It is effective by all methods of application and is widely used, especially for spinal anesthesia. Concentrations of 1 to 2 per cent produce adequate topical anesthesia for the respiratory tract and concentrations of 0.1 to 0.25 per cent are enough for infiltration and nerve block. For spinal anesthesia doses of 5 to 20 mg. are used, depending on the level of anesthesia sought. The maximal allowable dosage in any circumstance is about 75 mg. in the average adult. The chief disadvantage of tetracaine is its slow onset of action, although its duration of effect is twice that of procaine.

Benzocaine typifies the local anesthetics that are poorly soluble in water. It is effective when applied to mucous membranes or open wounds, and remains localized for long periods, which accounts for its sustained action and relatively low toxicity. It is the active ingredient in many analgesic ointments but is not useful for injection procedures.

Bupivacaine (Marcaine) is a long-lasting local anesthetic closely related to mepivacaine in its chemical structure. It is useful when prolonged sensory or sympathetic blockade is indicated. Its motor-blocking ability is inferior to that of other drugs. The interval required for onset of block and for the establishment of maximal sensory anesthesia is comparable to that required with lidocaine and shorter than with tetracaine. Duration of block is two to three times as long as with lidocaine and about 50 per cent longer than with tetracaine. Bupivacaine is used as a 0.1 per cent solution for infiltration, as a 0.25 to 0.75 per cent solution for epidural or caudal anesthesia, and in 0.25 to 0.50 per cent concentration for peripheral nerve block.

GENERAL RULES FOR USE OF LOCAL ANESTHETICS

Toxicity

The total dose should be limited to the smallest amount that will serve the purpose. Local anesthetics are toxic drugs that produce dangerous side effects on the cardiovascular and central nervous system.

Latency

There is a characteristic period of latency between application of drug and onset of block. It is essential to wait for the full effect before evaluating the response to the drug and before beginning the operation or administering additional drug.

Concentration

For each agent there is a minimal effective concentration below which adequate block will not appear. Higher concentrations often produce more rapid onset but also increase the possibility of toxic reactions. The concentration used should be appropriately selected and should be the least that will provide the desired effect.

Maximal Dose

A maximal dose for each local anesthetic is recommended in Table 1, but symptoms of toxicity may occur below that dose level if inadvertent intravascular injection occurs. Doses must be reduced by one half to one third when intravenous techniques are used or when the drug is applied topically in the respiratory tract.

TABLE 1. Commonly Used Local Anesthetic Agents

Technique	Local Anesthetic	Concentration Range	Duration of Action	Maximal Safe Dose*
Topical anesthesia (mucous membranes)	Lidocaine	2–4%	15 minutes	100 mg.
	Cocaine	4–10%	30 minutes	100–200 mg.
	Tetracaine	1–2%	45 minutes	40 mg.
	Benzocaine†	2–10%	Several hours	–
Local infiltration	Procaine	0.5%	1/4–1/2 hour	1000 mg.‡
	Lidocaine	0.5–1%	1/2–1 hour	500 mg.‡
	Mepivacaine	0.5–1%	1/2–1 hour	500 mg.‡
	Tetracaine	0.025–0.1%	2–3 hours	75 mg.‡
Major nerve block	Lidocaine	1–2%	1–2 hours	500 mg.‡
	Mepivacaine	1–2%	1–2 1/4 hours	500 mg.‡
	Tetracaine	0.1–0.25%	2–3 hours	75 mg.‡
Epidural anesthesia	Procaine	1–2%	1/2–1 hour	1000 mg.‡
	Lidocaine	1–2%	3/4–1 1/2 hours	500 mg.‡
	Mepivacaine	1–2%	1–2 1/4 hours	500 mg.‡
	Tetracaine	0.1–0.25%	2–3 hours	75 mg.‡
Spinal anesthesia	Procaine	5%	1/2–1 hour	–
	Lidocaine	5%	3/4–1 1/2 hours	–
	Tetracaine	0.5%	1–2 hours	–
Intravenous regional anesthesia	Lidocaine	0.25–0.5%	Varies	100–150 mg.

*The maximal safe dose listed is that dose most widely accepted as safe for administration to an average adult. Lower doses may produce toxic symptoms if inadvertent intravascular injection occurs. The safe dose must be reduced if disease, small patient size, and other factors might act to produce high blood levels of local anesthetic.

†As the base.

‡With epinephrine, 1:200,000, added.

Use of Vasoconstrictors

The addition of epinephrine to local anesthetic solutions produces vasoconstriction and slows absorption from the injection site, prolongs duration of anesthesia, and reduces the total dosage of drug required. The optimal concentration of epinephrine to be used in this manner is 1:200,000.[5] Stronger concentrations may lead to symptoms that mimic reactions to a local anesthetic. Its use with cocaine is contraindicated.

TOXIC REACTIONS TO LOCAL ANESTHETICS

Acute systemic toxicity from local anesthetics is caused by high blood levels of these agents acting on the central nervous, cardiovascular, and respiratory systems. Measures which minimize systemic uptake reduce toxicity. Premedication with diazepam (Valium) raises brain threshold to local anesthetics and is a useful prophylactic measure. Central nervous system stimulation occurs and is characterized by high voltage spike waves originating in the amygdaloid nuclei and radiating to the cortex. These are accompanied by grand mal seizures followed by postictal depression. Garrulousness sometimes precedes other symptoms and should be regarded as an early warning. Restlessness, anxiety, confusion, and twitching may also precede convulsions. Cardiovascular depression may be prominent. Arterial hypotension results from vasodilation and cardiac depression. Cardiac action may cease or become ineffective owing to depression of the myocardium or its conducting system. Inadequate ventilation occurs during the convulsion or following depression of the central respiratory center.

Therapy must support the cardiovascular and respiratory systems and control convulsions, if present.

Currently, there are two different therapeutic approaches to control convulsions. The first considers the increased electrical activity of the cortex during convulsions to be detrimental and attempts to abolish this with small doses of rapidly acting barbiturates. Thiopental is preferable because of its ability to penetrate brain tissue most rapidly, but some prefer to use diazepam. This method recognizes that postictal depression will occur and can summate with the barbiturate-induced depression. By the use of small doses of drug, prolonged depression is avoided. A second approach treats the peripheral manifestations of the convulsion. Succinylcholine is injected to suppress convulsive muscular motions, thereby permitting artificial ventilation of lungs.[22] With either therapy, the administration of oxygen, maintenance of adequate ventilation, and support of the cardiovascular system with intravenous fluids and pressor drugs are indicated.

GENERAL ANESTHESIA

General anesthesia is defined as a reversible state of insensibility with loss of consciousness. It can be produced by a variety of chemical agents that act on the brain. Neither the mechanism nor the exact site of action of the general anesthetic agents has been classified, probably because the structural and functional complexity of the central nervous system has escaped full definition. It is known, however, that there are two afferent systems that carry information to the brain (Table 2). The lateral ascending sensory pathways rapidly conduct afferent impulses to primary receiving areas in the brain by means of fibers that are specific with respect to modality and topography. The medial multisynaptic ascending pathways in the core of the

---

TABLE 2.   Ascending Pathways to the Brain

Long Ascending Sensory Pathways	Ascending Reticular Pathways
I. Somatotopical Organization (a) Point-for-point projection from periphery to thalamus to cortex (b) Modality-specific fiber pathways	I. No Somatotopical Organization (a) Single reticular unit responds to afferent stimulation from widely separated peripheral areas (b) Single unit responds to a variety of sensory modalities
II. Discrete, Well Defined Pathways Usually a three neuron pathway: neuron I with axon extending from sensory receptor to central nervous system, where synapse occurs with neuron II whose axon joins modality-specific fiber pathways to thalamus; neuron III projects from thalamus to specific area of cortex	II. Diffuse Pathways A multineuron pathway: input to ascending reticular system from (a) ascending sensory pathways of cord, (b) sensory nuclei of brain stem, (c) cerebral cortex, (d) cerebellum, (e) basal ganglia; neurons of medial reticular formation of brain stem are of small ($12\ \mu$) to large ($90\ \mu$) size, with short to long axons, ascending in direction; conduction in short or long steps with multiple collateral synapses; there is lack of modality-specific pathways; reticulofugal projections via thalamic relay or directly to widespread areas of cortex
III. Discrete Electrophysiologic Response Pattern A single peripheral stimulus produces a discrete response in the thalamus and a discrete projection to a specific location in the cortex	III. Widespread Response Pattern with Long Time Course Single peripheral stimulus evokes a bombardment of impulses over a considerable period of time in intralaminar nuclei of thalamus; this in turn projects to entire cortex by diffuse thalamocortical circuits to produce electrical desynchronization of resting EEG

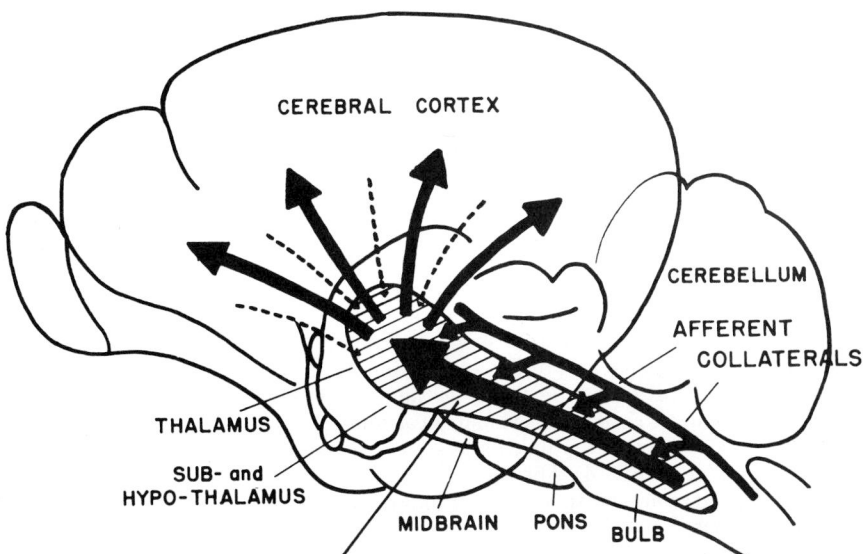

Figure 3. Outline of brain of cat showing extent of medially placed ascending reticular activating system of the brain stem (cross-lining) and distribution of collaterals to it from laterally situated long ascending sensory pathways. Diffuse projection to cortex from ascending reticular activating system is also shown. (From Starzl, T. E., et al.: J. Neurophysiol., 14:479, 1951.)

brain stem serve as a second and nonspecific sensory system which is important in the regulation of consciousness and is valuable in the integration of central nervous system function. Collaterals from the primary lateral pathways carry impulses to this system, called the ascending reticular activating system, in which conduction is slow and transmission diffuse. Peripheral and cortical impulses converge and interact and modalities lose their individuality. This system projects to wide areas of the cortex and promotes wakefulness and alertness[20] (Fig. 3). Experimental interruption of the ascending reticular activating system results in somnolence or unconsciousness, although sensory conduction via the classic sensory pathways remains intact. General anesthetic agents produce similar changes in a reversible manner. This has led Brazier to conclude that "it is the ascending activating influence of the brain stem reticular system on cortical excitability that is impaired by most anesthetics."[3]

The site of anesthetic action may be anywhere in the ascending reticular activating system between the peripheral afferents and the outflow to the cortex, with location differing among agents and dose. Stimulation of the anesthetized animal leads to recordable activity in the reticular formation; therefore, the collateral input from the primary sensory pathways is not blocked. Anesthetic agents do block synaptic transmission at lower concentrations than those which influence conduction in nerve fibers.[18] Comparison of the multisynaptic character of the reticular pathways with the paucisynaptic lateral pathways suggests greater susceptibility of the former to anesthetic depression and supports the concept that a primary mechanism of anesthetic action may be suppression of synaptic transmission in the ascending reticular activating system.

Anesthetic agents influence portions of the central nervous system other than the ascending reticular activating system. Primary sensory pathways can be depressed as anesthetic concentrations increase. Amnesia prior. to loss of consciousness may indicate synaptic blockade in the hippocampus by anesthetic agents at concentrations too low to affect the ascending reticular activating system. The analgesic effects of subanesthetic doses of some volatile liquid anesthetics and nitrous oxide may indicate a site of action in the limbic system or in the rhinencephalon at doses insufficient to affect the reticular system.

Body systems other than the central nervous system are also susceptible to the effects of general anesthetic agents. Before the introduction of curare into clinical medicine, muscular relaxation was produced by deep anesthesia, probably through a direct depression of muscle. Hypotension, cardiac arrhythmias, and prolonged postoperative ileus bear witness to other extraneural effects of anesthetics.

Neurophysiologic studies continue to disclose previously unrecognized effects of anesthetics upon the central nervous system; however, these studies are hampered by the imprecise methods available for measuring and controlling the depth of general anesthesia. The electroencephalograph has been disappointing as a clinically useful instrument to document varying levels of anesthesia, although it may be useful to detect cerebral hypoxia in the anesthetized patient. The depth of anesthesia in animals or man is as accurately determined by clinical signs as by any other means. This aspect of anesthesiology is much the same today as it was decades ago. In short, an agent known to produce unconsciousness, analgesia, and sometimes relaxation safely and reversibly is administered to a patient; its pharmacologic effects are evaluated on the basis of the anesthetist's experience; adjustments in concentration are made; and the patient is again observed. The cycle is repeated again and again. The practice of anesthesia, despite modern knowledge, is still an art.

Anesthetists have attempted to define a method for assessing the degree of anesthetic-induced depression ever since ether was introduced. Guedel's guide to the levels of ether anesthesia stands today as the classic. This requires assessment of muscle function, respiratory and eye motions, pupillary size, and presence or absence of certain reflexes, without consideration of the degree of surgical stimulation taking place. Despite its reliability, the system is little used today because ether has largely been replaced by modern anesthetic agents.

Current anesthetists use a more sophisticated approach than that proposed by Guedel by employing a fact recognized by all physicians: a patient is a living responsive organism in whom a graded set of stimuli will produce a graded set of responses. Anesthetics alter patient reactivity and allow application of stimuli of large magnitude while limiting the size of the resulting response. Three stages of surgical anesthesia are commonly accepted: too light, adequately anesthetized, and too deep (Fig. 4). The thoughtful anesthetist follows a specific method in making a judgment of his patient's status. First, he evaluates the afferent input to the patient's nervous system; next, those responses available are evaluated; finally, an estimate of the interaction of patient, stimulus, and drug is made and a judgment of level of surgical anesthesia is deduced. To evaluate fully the effect of an anesthetic drug, the anesthetist must evaluate both the stimulus and the resulting response.

Stimulus Assessment

Stimulus intensity is arbitrarily classified as strong, moderate, or weak (Table 3). Strong stimulation results from skin incision, raising a split thickness skin graft, anal dilation, periosteal stimulation, fracture manipulation, visceral traction, peritoneal stimulation, cervical dilation, diaphragmatic stimulation, manipulation of the cornea, excessive distension of the bladder or viscera, stimulation of the urethral mucosa, and stimulation of any inflamed structure. Moderate stimulation results from curettage of the uterine cavity, retroperitoneal dissection, wound débridement,

TABLE 3.   Stimulus Assessment

Strong
Skin cutting
Anal dilation
Peritoneal stimulation
Visceral traction
Periosteal stimulation
Fracture manipulation
Dilation of uterine cervix
Diaphragmatic stimulation
Nerve traction
Corneal manipulation
Excessive distension of bladder or viscera

Moderate
Curettage of uterine cavity
Retroperitoneal dissection
Wound débridement
Mild distension of bladder
Manipulation without traction of fascia, muscle, fat,
   or omentum

Weak
Brain dissection
Muscle dissection
Connective tissue dissection
Vascular cutting and suturing
Bowel cutting and suturing
Lung cutting and suturing

mild distension of the bladder and other viscera, and manipulations of fascia, muscle, or fat if done without traction. Weak stimulation occurs during surgical dissection of brain, muscle, and connective tissue, vascular cutting and suturing, bowel cutting and suturing, and lung resection and suturing.

The above listing gives examples of stimulus intensity commonly observed but is not complete nor rigid. Inflammation increases intensity of the stimulation arising on manipulation. Manipulation by a careful surgeon may produce less intense stimuli than cited. Other factors, i.e., an individual patient's pain threshold or age, may also be operative. One fact stands out: the anesthetist must continuously monitor surgical activity if he is to have the information required to perform his function in patient care adequately.

Response Evaluation

Patient responses are not as easily evaluated as when Guedel's scheme was employed. He cited a limited set of observations to be made. Modern anesthesia techniques invalidated many of them but have provided no obvious substitutes. The anesthetist is forced to make a large number of more subtle observations to compensate. Woodbridge[24] cites four components of the anesthetic state: sensory, motor, mental, and reflex functions. Table 4 attempts to classify intensity of responses that may be observed with reference to Woodbridge's four components. Note that observations made to evaluate depression in one component involve nearly all body systems. Moreover, a single response may relate to several components. For example, if a patient takes a deep breath, turns

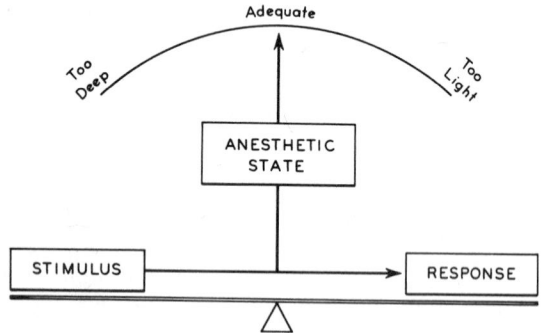

Figure 4.   The interaction of strength of surgical stimulation and patient response in determining depth of anesthesia. If response to stimulus is excessive, the pointer swings to the "Too Light" side. If the response is too small for the strength of stimulation, the pointer swings to the "Too Deep" side. The anesthetic state is modified to balance stimulus and resultant response at the "Just Right" point. This requires assessment of both stimulus and response.

TABLE 4. Signs of Depth of the Four Components of Anesthesia*

	Sensory	Motor	Mental	Reflex		
				Circulatory	Respiratory	Gastrointestinal
Insufficient depth of anesthesia	Breath holding Deep breathing Phonation Laryngospasm Tachycardia Rise or fall of blood pressure Movement with painful stimulus Coughing	Movement Insufficient muscle relaxation for surgical procedure	Motor response to stimulation Delirium Uninhibited speech or actions	Bradycardia and hypotension Tachycardia and hypertension Arrhythmias	Mucus Spasm: laryngeal bronchiolar chest wall Sucking	Nausea and retching Salivation Swallowing
Sufficient depth of anesthesia	Minimal response to painful stimulus followed by accommodation Stability of cardiovascular and respiratory systems	Quiet surgical field Adequate muscle relaxation when needed	Amnesia Ataraxia Sleep	Absence of troublesome reflexes from cardiovascular, respiratory, and gastrointestinal systems		
Excessive depth of anesthesia	No response	Muscular flaccidity Inability to reestablish normal ventilatory function at termination of anesthesia	Prolonged obtundation in pre- or postanesthetic period	Bradycardia or tachycardia Hypotension Arrhythmias Intolerance to change of position	Respiratory arrest†	Intestinal atony during surgery Postoperative ileus

*Adapted from Woodbridge, P. D.: Anesthesiology, *18*:536, 1957.
†In absence of muscle relaxants or hyperventilation.

his head, and develops tachycardia and hypertension when an abdominal incision is made, it is obvious that he has inadequate sensory depression. Whether he also has inadequate motor depression depends upon the site of surgery. Head motion is acceptable for abdominal but not for facial surgery. Most anesthetists avoid drug doses which produce responses associated with excessive depth of anesthesia. Utilization of this or a similar system allows logical evaluation of specific drug effects in each of Woodbridge's component areas.

Evaluation of Anesthetic Requirement

Comparison of strength of surgical stimulus and observation of intensity of response allows for evaluation of specific anesthetic requirements. If response is excessive in one of Woodbridge's component areas, then compensatory action is required. More inhalation anesthetic may be administered with the full recognition that this will increase depression in all four components; alternately, a specific drug, such as a muscle relaxant, may be chosen to correct a specific defect. Observations are made repeatedly and adjustments instituted when appropriate. Occasionally, the system will be disturbed by design to test the resulting response. The anesthetist may increase or reduce inhaled concentration of anesthetic in order to observe the effect. Inherent is the assumption that alterations are being made in a responsive system.

In many ways, this is merely a restatement of what the good clinician has always tried to do. The beginner will find, as his powers of observation and experience increase, that a combination of signs will provide a satisfactory guide to determination of anesthetic depth. It is well known, for example, that reactivity to stimuli diminishes with age and is always less marked in the desperately ill. Under these circumstances the careful observer can still detect useful signs of anesthetic requirements. He must be all the more alert and observant, however, because overdosage will result if he is unaware of the increased potency of these depressants.

GENERAL ANESTHETIC AGENTS

There are nearly 20 general anesthetic agents available for clinical use, but nitrous oxide, alone or in combination with other drugs, is chosen for most of the general anesthesias administered today. During the first half of the last decade, an increasing preference for halothane usage was clearly demonstrated.[7] By 1966, 70 per cent of patients who had general anesthesia in this country received halothane. Because of the danger of hepatotoxicity associated with the administration of halothane, this trend now has been clearly reversed. There has been a corresponding increase in this country in the use of nitrous oxide–narcotic–muscle relaxant combinations to fill the continual need for nonexplosive techniques of general anesthesia. Within the last five years extensive use of enflurane (Ethrane) has re-established the place of fluorinated hydrocarbons in modern anesthetic practice. The use of fluoroxene is limited because of its marginal explosiveness. Agents such as ethylene, chloroform, divinyl ether, and ethyl chloride are seldom used except by an occasional enthusiast. Ether and cyclopropane retain few proponents.

Recent investigative efforts have shown that anesthetic drugs have a much greater effect on cellular physiology and on biochemical mechanisms than was previously realized. The inhalation agents may depress the bone marrow, alter phagocytic activity of leukocytes, arrest cell division of rapidly multiplying cell lines, activate the microsomal drug-metabolizing enzyme system, and alter the body's normal response to treatment with drugs, radiation, and other therapeutic modalities. Similarly, it is now realized that most general inhalation anesthetic agents, previously thought to be excreted unchanged by the body, are in fact actively metabolized. The nephrotoxicity associated with methoxyflurane has been demonstrated to be caused by free fluoride ion formed during metabolic degradation of the drug. Changing patterns of anesthetic practice can be expected as this new knowledge is applied to patient care.

INHALATION AGENTS

Inhalation anesthetic agents may exist at room temperature either as gases or as volatile liquids that must be vaporized prior to administration. The gases are compressed and stored in metal cylinders which are painted characteristic colors to indicate their contents. Two color standards exist. In the United States, the National Bureau of Standards of the Department of Commerce has issued a color code. The remaining countries of the world follow a color code promulgated by the World Health Organization (Table 5).

Gases

Nitrous oxide was the first anesthetic gas described and today is probably the most widely used anesthetic agent. Many operating rooms have nitrous oxide as well as oxygen supplied to wall outlets from remote bulk storage areas. The gas comes in steel cylinders as a liquid under pressure and when released from the cylinder is colorless with a sweet odor. The possibility of contamination of nitrous oxide with toxic higher oxides of nitrogen has been noted recently. This is the least potent of the anesthetic gases and its effectiveness is further reduced by the necessity that it be administered with at least 20 per cent oxygen. Seldom

TABLE 5. National Bureau of Standards Color Markings for Anesthetic Gas Cylinders

Oxygen	green (white)*
Nitrous oxide	blue
Cyclopropane	orange
Ethylene	red (purple)*
Carbon dioxide	gray
Helium	brown

*The World Health Organization specifies that oxygen cylinders be painted white and ethylene cylinders be painted purple.

used alone because of its inability to produce surgical anesthesia, it is most often combined with a narcotic or barbiturate, a muscle relaxant, or a volatile agent such as halothane. In the absence of hypoxia, there is little effect on the circulation, respiration, liver, or kidney. It is nonexplosive and does not provide muscle relaxation. It is an analgesic and if inhaled in subanesthetic concentrations of 20 to 50 per cent, analgesia sufficient to allay the discomfort of uterine contractions during labor will result.

Cyclopropane is a potent, flammable anesthetic gas capable of producing deep anesthesia, muscle relaxation, and cardiovascular and respiratory depression. Ethylene is only slightly more potent than nitrous oxide, but like cyclopropane it also is explosive. Both of these drugs are seldom used today, having been replaced by the safer nonexplosive fluorinated hydrocarbon anesthetics.

Volatile Liquids

Halothane (Fluothane) is a potent, nonflammable, halogenated hydrocarbon with which anesthesia may be induced smoothly although relatively slowly. It is supplied in 125 to 250 ml. brown bottles and is usually given with 50 to 60 per cent nitrous oxide, although many use it with oxygen alone. With the latter technique, higher concentrations of the agent are required. Because of its potency, special vaporizers such as the Fluotec or Copper Kettle are usually indicated. Rapid recovery from anesthesia relates to the low (1 to 2 per cent) concentration usually inhaled and the short duration of administration. High concentrations or long periods of anesthesia will result in slow awakening. The incidence of nausea and vomiting with recovery is small.

Halothane causes depression of normal ventilatory responses to carbon dioxide, and respiratory acidosis develops if ventilation is not supported. Laryngeal and pharyngeal reflexes are obtunded early in the course of anesthesia. Respiratory tract secretions are minimal and bronchodilation occurs, making halothane the anesthetic of choice for patients with bronchial asthma. Halothane, like cyclopropane, is a cardiovascular depressant but does not cause stimulation of the sympathetic nervous system. The direct myocardial and vascular smooth muscle depressant effects of halothane are, therefore, unopposed and anesthesia is characterized by a decrease in both cardiac output and total peripheral resistance, resulting in hypotension. Arrhythmias are less common with halothane than with cyclopropane, although the myocardium is sensitized to catecholamines. The heart rate slows in deep levels of anesthesia. Some degree of muscle relaxation is characteristic with halothane, but supplemental relaxant drugs are usually required for abdominal operations.

The role of halothane in producing postoperative hepatic damage has been studied extensively after suspicion was raised that it was hazardous in this respect. Definitive findings have been elusive because of the difficulty in differentiating hepatitis of viral origin from that caused by halothane. It appears, however, that there is an etiologic relationship between halothane administration and some cases of postoperative liver dysfunction. The mechanism by which this occurs is not as yet clear. Repeated halothane exposure leading to hypersensitivity has been suggested as a possible cause and several persons with specific hypersensitivity to low concentrations of halothane have been identified. It has also been shown that halothane is an immunodepressant and the postulate that hepatitis following halothane may represent activation of a pre-existing latent viral hepatitis has been put forth. Finally, since halothane is in part metabolized, it has been suggested that a toxic metabolite may be formed in susceptible persons. The etiologic mechanisms remain to be solved. Halothane should be avoided in patients in whom eosinophilia, right upper quadrant tenderness, malaise, unexplained fever, or jaundice has occurred following prior halothane exposure. Some anesthesiologists consider a prior exposure to halothane a relative contraindication to its further use. It should be clearly recognized, however, that the risk of liver failure is only one factor in the total evaluation that must be made in the choice of an anesthetic agent. If the alternate choices offer risks that are significantly greater than the risk of liver failure following halothane, then obviously halothane may still be the agent of choice.

The smoothness of induction of anesthesia, ease of maintenance, lack of flammability, and pleasantness of recovery have led to wide acceptance of halothane.

Enflurane (Ethrane), first synthesized and introduced in clinical trials in 1963, was released for general use in 1972. It is a stable nonflammable liquid, somewhat less volatile than halothane, which produces rapid smooth induction of anesthesia, easy maintenance, and rapid recovery. Cardiac rhythm tends to be stable and there is only mild sensitization of the heart to epinephrine. Anesthesia with enflurane is accompanied in about 2 per cent of patients by signs of motor hyperactivity, such as twitching, of the muscles of the jaw, face, neck, or extremities. These are accompanied by EEG seizure patterns[6] and are more likely to appear at high concentrations of enflurane and at low levels of Pa_{CO_2}. Seizures are not associated with evidences of cerebral hypoxia and are not accompanied by permanent sequelae. Ventilatory depression parallels anesthetic depth. The decrease in slope of ventilatory response to CO_2 with enflurane is similar to that seen with comparable MAC equivalents of halothane. Control of ventilation at surgical depths of anesthesia is generally indicated. Cardiac output is well maintained and the cardiac responses to hypercarbia are similar to those seen in awake man (i.e., markedly increased cardiac output). Cardiac output is not altered by hypocarbia. These changes probably reflect an intact cardiac sympathetic control mechanism which is activated by CO_2. Enflurane depresses myocardial contractility in a dose-related and reversible manner. Arterial hypotension occurs with enflurane anesthesia, indicating a fall in peripheral resistance. Cardiovascular reflexes remain intact. Muscular relaxation occurs in a dose-related manner with surgical depths of anesthesia, and the relaxant properties of the curariform drugs are potentiated.[16] Generally, small doses of either curare or pancuronium are administered to allow lighter levels of enflurane

anesthesia to be employed. Enflurane is metabolized in the liver by defluorination to produce free fluoride, but serum fluoride levels are far less than seen with methoxyflurane. There is a relative contraindication to the use of enflurane in patients with renal disease or in those with decreased renal output.

Isoflurane (Forane), an isomer of enflurane, was synthesized in 1969, studied extensively, and eventually withdrawn from use because of a preliminary report suggesting that the drug may be a carcinogen. It causes neither central nervous system excitation nor seizures, as does enflurane. Cardiac performance is well maintained and arterial pressure falls because of a decrease in peripheral vascular resistance, but perfusion in all vascular beds is well maintained. It is a profound respiratory depressant and muscular relaxant. Competitive neuromuscular blocking drugs are markedly potentiated. This drug will be a useful anesthetic if it is not a carcinogen.

Diethyl ether is a highly volatile liquid with a pungent, flammable vapor capable of producing all depths of surgical anesthesia to respiratory arrest. Like other flammable anesthetics, its use is now markedly restricted in the United States, but it is still widely used in emerging countries.

Induction is prolonged, respiratory secretions are copious, and struggling and vomiting may occur before an adequate level of anesthesia is obtained. The signs of anesthetic depth are well demarcated, and muscle relaxation is present for most surgical procedures without the need for supplementary neuromuscular blocking drugs. Ether enhances the neuromuscular blocking effect of curare and if both drugs are used concomitantly, the dose of curare must be reduced. The irritation of ether vapor reflexly stimulates respiration, and respiratory alkalosis appears early, although this may be superseded subsequently with a metabolic acidosis. Blood pressure, pulse, and cardiac rhythm are normal in lighter levels, and hypotension may occur at deep stages. Direct myocardial depression by the anesthetic is counterbalanced by stimulation of the sympathetic nervous system, but the myocardium is not sensitized to catecholamines.

Methoxyflurane (Penthrane) is another potent, nonflammable, liquid ether with a low vapor pressure and high fat solubility. Azotemia associated with polyuria may follow anesthesia with methoxyflurane and has been attributed to renal tubular effects of free fluoride ion formed by metabolic degradation of the drug. Its use is relatively contraindicated in circumstances such as anesthesia of long duration, in obese patients, or at high inspired concentrations, all of which may lead to high blood fluoride levels. Recovery is slow and may be accompanied by prolonged analgesia. Nausea and vomiting are infrequent. This drug is rapidly disappearing from clinical use.

Other volatile anesthetics are available but are not widely used clinically. *Divinyl ether* and *ethyl chloride,* once used for the rapid induction of inhalation anesthesia by the open drop technique, are now seldom employed. *Trichloroethylene* is a halogenated hydrocarbon, nonflammable, and useful to supplement nitrous oxide for minor surgical procedures or manipulations, or for use alone as an inhalational analgesic.

However, it is not potent and reacts with soda lime in the presence of heat to form toxic products.

TECHNIQUES OF ADMINISTRATION OF INHALATION AGENTS

The original technique of administering volatile anesthetic agents was to pour them on a folded towel or gauze placed over the patient's nose and mouth. This provided a vaporizing surface and as air was breathed through the mask, the vapor was drawn into the lungs. There were disadvantages such as poorly controlled anesthetic concentration, inability to assist ventilation, and increased dead space leading to hypoxia and hypercarbia. Although this technique was popular in America for nearly a century, it has largely been abandoned in the operating room. It still proves useful in certain circumstances.

Current techniques employ sophisticated equipment to administer anesthesia. The equipment is relatively simple to understand and operate if one understands its basic components (Fig. 5).

Gas sources (A) of oxygen and other anesthetic gases are supplied in tanks as pressurized liquids or gases. Machines are equipped with a pin index system

to prevent improper placement of cylinders. Anesthetic machines often incorporate gauges so that the gas pressure in the tanks can be observed. Many modern machines are equipped with "fail-safe" devices or warning systems to alert the operator in the event of failure of the oxygen supply. Usually two tanks each of oxygen and nitrous oxide are available. These gases are sometimes supplied from remote sources to the anesthetic machine by high-pressure hoses.

Reducing valves (B) or pressure regulators are built into most anesthetic machines. Frequently pressure reduction is accomplished in several stages, so that the high pressures within the tanks are reduced to safe levels within the machines.

Metering devices (C) are calibrated, tapered glass tubes in which lightweight bobbins float in the flowing gas streams. The most common metering devices incorporated in modern anesthetic machines are Rotometers. The rate of gas flow is regulated by a needle valve at the bottom of the meter. As the aperture becomes wider, the flow of gas increases and the bobbin rises in the tube. Gas flow rates are read directly from the calibrated tube.

The mixing manifold (D) acts as a collecting and mixing space for the gases at the outflow end of the meter.

Vaporizers (E) of various designs may be included in the equipment. The simplest of these is the draw-over type, in which variable amounts of inspired air are drawn through a bottle containing a volatile anesthetic and in which a wick is placed to increase the volatilizing surface. More modern devices are flow- and temperature-compensated. Many factors govern the efficiency of a vaporizer, including ambient temperature and pressure, the liquid agent being used, the rate of gas flow through the vaporizer, and the surface area of the gas-liquid interface. Modern vaporizers are commonly constructed of copper because of the efficiency with which this metal conducts heat and keeps volatile anesthetic at a reasonably constant temperature.

A *reservoir bag (F)* is usually necessary so that the rate of gas flow demanded by the patient at any phase of respiration need not be matched throughout the respiratory cycle by that supplied from the meters. Respiratory gas flow in the patient's airway is intermittent and bidirectional. Anesthetic machines are available that provide intermittent gas flow on demand by the patient, but most modern machines provide for constant flow of anesthetic agents into a reservoir bag. With these machines the bag fills when the flow from the machine exceeds the inspiratory demands of the patient, and provides a ready supply of anesthetic gases at all times. In addition, the bag furnishes a means of applying pressure to the airway to assist or control ventilation. The reservoir is most often a part of the delivery apparatus.

The *delivery apparatus (G)* may be one of many arrangements to control the inspired atmosphere of the anesthetized patient and to provide for the elimination of expired carbon dioxide. These can be designated by two systems of nomenclature, one describing the pathway of respiratory gases in the anesthetic apparatus, the other the method of dealing with expired gases.[17] According to the latter, the apparatus is either

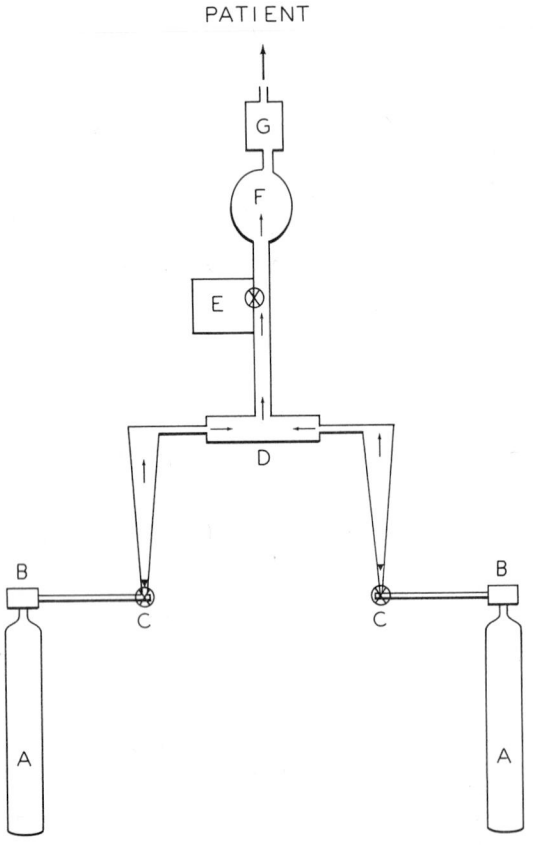

PATIENT

Figure 5. The components of an anesthetic machine. *A*, Source of anesthetic gases and oxygen. *B*, Reducing valves. *C*, Needle valves and flowmeters. *D*, Mixing manifold. *E*, Vaporizer for volatile anesthetic liquids. *F*, Reservoir bag. *G*, Delivery apparatus.

TABLE 6. Anesthetic Mortality Related to Physical Status*

Physical Status	Number of Patients	Number of Deaths	Ratio: Deaths/Patients
I	16,192	0	0/16,000
II	12,154	7	1/1740
III	4,070	11	1/370
IV	720	17	1/40
V	87	4	1/20

*Data from Dripps, R. D., Lamont, A., and Eckenhoff, J. E.: J.A.M.A., *178*:261, 1961.

open, semiopen, semiclosed, or closed. In an open system, expired gases are completely vented to the atmosphere and carbon dioxide is thus eliminated. In a closed system, expired gas is retained within the system and is rebreathed during subsequent respiratory cycles. This requires inclusion of a chemical method for the removal of carbon dioxide. Semiopen and semiclosed systems incorporate intermediate degrees of rebreathing.

The pathway of gas flow in nearly all anesthetic systems can be described by one of three terms: to and fro, nonrebreathing, or circle (Fig. 6). If the inspira-

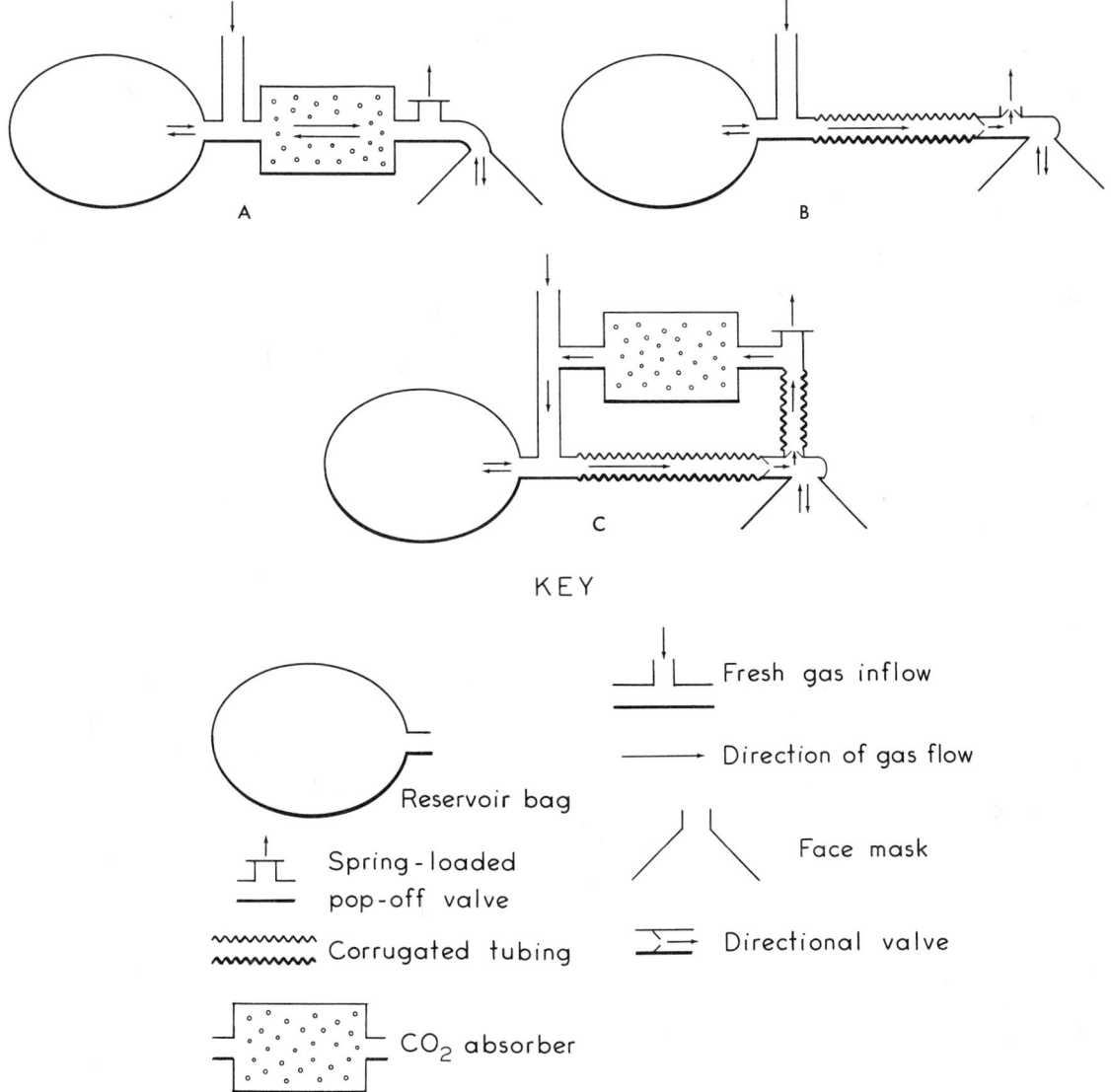

Figure 6. The to-and-fro (*A*), nonrebreathing (*B*), and circle (*C*) systems for delivering anesthesia. There is a common pathway for inspiratory and expiratory gases in the to-and-fro system, and a separation of these pathways by valves in the nonrebreathing and circle systems. The circle system provides for return of expired gas to the system by way of a carbon dioxide absorber.

tory and expiratory gases use a common pathway, the apparatus is named to and fro *(A)*. This does not require valves to direct gas flow, although a spring-loaded valve to allow venting of excess gas may be included. If directional valves separate inspiratory and expiratory pathways, the system is called either nonrebreathing or circle. In a nonrebreathing system *(B)* the inspiratory pathway is unidirectional, from the reservoir to the patient, and the expiratory pathway vents expired gases to the atmosphere. All nonrebreathing systems are open systems as well and demand a fresh gas supply in excess of the patient's respiratory minute volume. In circle systems *(C)*, which are commonly used in this country, valves direct expired gas completely or partially to a reservoir bag or to a spring-loaded vent, depending largely upon the rate of fresh gas flow being provided to the apparatus. Circle systems are either closed or semiclosed and usually depend on the chemical removal of carbon dioxide within the circuit.

All anesthetic apparatus must provide for the disposal of expired carbon dioxide. In open systems, because expired gases are vented to atmosphere, the patient inspires only fresh anesthetic mixtures. Systems in which both fresh and expired gases pass together into the reservoir usually include a carbon dioxide absorption canister charged with soda lime, which is a mixture of sodium hydroxide and calcium hydroxide, or Baralyme, a mixture of hydroxides of barium and calcium. Both mixtures contain sufficient moisture to allow formation of carbonic acid from exhaled carbon dioxide. The acid is then chemically neutralized. In this manner, expired carbon dioxide is eliminated. Alternately, if fresh gases are added to the system at a rate equal to twice the minute volume of ventilation, the expired carbon dioxide is usually flushed from the apparatus.

Each of these delivery systems has advantages and disadvantages that determine the selection for a particular clinical situation. Circle systems, because of the use of directional valves, add significantly to ventilatory resistance and the work of breathing but they are convenient to use. Respiratory resistance can be overcome by assisting or controlling ventilation. To-and-fro systems, on the other hand, incorporate the advantage of low respiratory resistance because directional valves are needed, but when used with soda lime canisters they are cumbersome. Open systems allow loss of heat and moisture from the respiratory tract, a factor of importance particularly in small children. Closed systems require the use of soda lime or Baralyme and, therefore, cannot be used with trichloroethylene, but they are particularly indicated when explosive agents are being administered. Circle systems represent considerable initial cost but offer the versatility of either high- or low-flow techniques. Open systems are relatively inexpensive but require high flows of anesthetic gases, adding to the cost of each procedure. The simple equipment used for a to-and-fro system is easily sterilized, making it an ideal choice in patients with a pulmonary infection. Increase in respiratory dead space and in resistance to respiration occurs with the best anesthetic equipment but is generally of little consequence in the adult. In children,

this consideration is important and special equipment is required.

UPTAKE AND DISTRIBUTION OF ANESTHETIC AGENTS

The depth of anesthesia produced by inhalation agents varies according to the partial pressure of the anesthetic in the brain. This can be controlled only indirectly. Altering the composition of the inspired atmosphere leads to successive pressure gradients from inspired atmosphere to alveolus, arterial blood, and brain. The partial pressure of agents in the brain always attempts to reach equilibrium with that in arterial blood. If blood gas tension is higher than that in the brain, anesthetic agents enter the brain and depth of anesthesia increases; if arterial tension is lower than that of brain, the reverse occurs. A similar relationship occurs in the lung, where alveolar tension determines the arterial tension. The uptake and transport of anesthetic agent from the external environment to its site of action in the brain is affected by inspired concentration of the agent; ventilatory factors, such as minute volume of ventilation, functional residual capacity, respiratory dead space, and distribution of inspired gas within the lung; circulatory factors, such as cardiac output and its distribution in lung and body tissues; physical factors, such as solubility of the agent in blood, partition of the agent between blood and body tissues, particularly brain, and partial pressure gradients of the agent within the body.

During induction of inhalation anesthesia, the higher the partial pressure of anesthetic inhaled, the faster the anesthetic tension rises in the lung and the faster the arterial tension rises. Large minute volumes of ventilation also hasten the buildup of anesthetic in the lung. When there is an abnormally great functional residual capacity, as in pulmonary emphysema, the rise in alveolar tension of the agent is slowed and induction prolonged.

If the anesthetic is highly soluble in blood, as is true, for example, of methoxyflurane or ether, it is removed from the lung rapidly. This impedes the rate at which the partial pressure in the lung approaches that in the inspired air. Similarly, a high cardiac output, such as is present in an apprehensive patient or one with hyperthyroidism, causes a fast removal of anesthetic agent from the lung and a slow rise of pulmonary partial pressure of the agent. On the other hand, nitrous oxide is of low solubility and is sparingly removed from the lung; the alveolar tension rapidly reflects the inspired tension. If abnormalities exist in the distribution of inspired gas within the lungs, or of pulmonary blood flow, or if ventilation-perfusion ratios are abnormal, then gradients in alveolar and arterial anesthetic tensions may occur and slow the rate of induction.

The delivery of anesthetic agent from the lung to tissues is dependent on the distribution of the cardiac output throughout the body. Hemorrhage, vascular shunts, or other factors that alter the proportion of cardiac output delivered to the brain may significantly influence the clinical management of an anesthetic.

The solubility of an anesthetic agent in body tissues influences its uptake. This is most often expressed as the blood-tissue partition coefficient and for most anesthetics and tissues is near 1.0, indicating that the agent is equally soluble in blood and tissue. Fat has a greater affinity for anesthetic agents, particularly for ether, halothane, and methoxyflurane, than do other body tissues. When anesthesia is prolonged, enough anesthetic agent may be sequestered in fat deposits to impede normal recovery significantly.

INTRAVENOUS ANESTHETIC AGENTS

Although a wide variety of drugs ranging from diethyl ether to a nonhormonal steroid have been administered intravenously to produce general anesthesia, only the ultra-short-acting barbiturates have gained wide support for use by this route until relatively recently. In the last two decades a variety of intravenously administered drugs or drug mixtures have been introduced into anesthetic practice but none approach the popularity of the thiobarbiturates or have gained widespread patient appeal for induction of anesthesia. In recent years some anesthesiologists have relied more heavily on intravenously administered mixtures of narcotics and tranquilizers in an attempt to avoid the use of halogenated hydrocarbon volatile anesthetics to supplement nitrous oxide and oxygen anesthesia.

Ultra-short-acting Barbiturates. The thiobarbiturates thiopental (Pentothal) and thiamylal (Surital) are administered intravenously in 2.5 per cent or more dilute solution, care being taken to avoid intra-arterial injection, which can lead to arterial occlusion, or subcutaneous injection, which may cause tissue slough. Methohexital (Brevital) as a 1 per cent solution is also used for induction of anesthesia. These drugs are useful because of two characteristics of the anesthetic state that they produce: rapid onset and short duration. Their high fat solubility allows them to penetrate all tissues of the body without delay, the tissue uptake being a function of local blood flow and arterial concentration of the drug. Because the brain receives a high proportion of the cardiac output, a large percentage of the injected dose reaches the brain rapidly and causes unconsciousness. Excitement is rare. The duration of the central depression is dependent upon the redistribution of the drug from the brain to viscera and other well-perfused body tissues.

After a single dose, the concentration of barbiturate at the neural site of action declines rapidly and progressively and central depression is reversed. The duration of the initial effect is dependent upon the size of the initial dose and the adequacy of the circulation. Anesthesia induced by these drugs is associated with respiratory depression or apnea if the dose given is large. Little analgesia or muscle relaxation is provided. Cardiovascular depression is dependent upon the dose but may be profound in hypovolemic or debilitated patients. By using fractional doses that are carefully administered, this can be avoided. Large amounts of the agent, even though injected over periods of several hours, slowly saturate fatty deposits, leading to sustained blood levels and to prolonged

unconsciousness. For this reason, the thiobarbiturates are seldom given as the sole anesthetic for other than very brief operations.

Ketamine is a parenterally administered phencyclidine derivative used to produce a state called "dissociative anesthesia." After the administration of 6 to 12 mg. per kilogram intramuscularly or of 1 to 3 mg. per kilogram intravenously, the patient rapidly becomes dissociated from his environment. Analgesia, amnesia, and lack of response to verbal stimuli develop. In this state, painful surgical procedures such as burn dressings and orthopedic manipulations can be carried out. Supplemental doses may be required at about 15 minute intervals. Spontaneous random muscular movements may occur. The technique is best suited for short procedures that involve "somatic" pain and less suitable for procedures involving "visceral" organs. Awakening from ketamine has been associated with a high incidence of visual hallucinations which may be of an unpleasant nature.

Innovar is a prepared mixture of fentanyl, a short-acting narcotic analgesic, and of droperidol, a butyrophenone tranquilizer, that has been used together with nitrous oxide to produce neuroleptanesthesia. The butyrophenone potentiates the central nervous system depressant effect of the other drugs and adds an antiemetic, an antiarrhythmic, and an alpha-adrenergic blocking effect. The result is an improvement over previous techniques of administration of nitrous oxide and oxygen potentiated by narcotic analgesics. The action of fentanyl is short-lived, and supplemental doses are often indicated after establishment of an initial stable anesthetic state.

NEUROMUSCULAR BLOCKING AGENTS

Prior to 1945, the muscle relaxation required for abdominal operations was provided either by deep general anesthesia or by spinal anesthesia. This was unsatisfactory because many patients were too ill to tolerate either technique and spinal anesthesia was often insufficient for extensive upper abdominal procedures. The introduction of muscle relaxants solved this problem and changed the concepts of general anesthesia.[21] Now deep general anesthesia is rarely required; only light planes of anesthesia need be provided and if relaxation is needed, the appropriate relaxant drug can be administered intravenously. Some have even advocated techniques that combine the minimal anesthesia of nitrous oxide with complete flaccidity provided by muscle relaxants. Classically, the action of muscle relaxants has been explained by a postsynaptic mechanism. Current investigations of neuromuscular pharmacology indicate involvement of the nerve terminal and imply a presynaptic site of action. The importance of the two sites in the clinical action of the muscle relaxants remains to be evaluated. The mechanism described here is based on the classic concept but soon may require modification. The muscle relaxants are divided into two classes according to their mode of action. The nondepolarizing competitive blocking agents prevent combination of normally liberated acetylcholine with the muscle endplate receptors, thereby blocking normal neuromuscular transmission. d-Tubocurarine, gallamine (Flaxedil) dimethyl tubocurarine (Metubine), and pancuronium (Pavulon) belong to this group. The depolarizing agents combine with the endplate receptor to cause an initial but prolonged depolarization of the postjunctional membrane, resulting in blockade of normal neuromuscular transmission. Succinylcholine (Anectine, Scoline, Quelicin) and decamethonium (Syncurine) belong to this group. There are other pharmacologic and pathologic causes of neuromuscular blockade.[19] Some diseases and drugs decrease the mobilization or release of acetylcholine upon nerve stimulation. These include magnesium ion excess, calcium ion deficit, botulinus toxin, antibiotics, quinine, and procaine. A postjunctional desensitization action has been described that explains, in part, the muscle relaxation caused by ether and halothane, as well as the otherwise ill-defined occasional persistent effect of depolarizing agents.[9]

The neuromuscular block produced by the competitive agents can be antagonized by substances that increase the concentration of acetylcholine at the motor endplate. An anticholinesterase drug, either pyridostigmine (Mestinon) or neostigmine (Prostigmin), is used for this purpose and is preceded by a large dose of atropine to block muscarinic actions such as excessive airway secretions and bradycardia. Antagonists to the action of depolarizing blocking agents are not available. The usefulness of the depolarizers is dependent upon dissipation of the pharmacologically induced paralysis which, with succinylcholine, usually occurs within five minutes. Prolonged blockade is occasionally seen after use of these drugs in two groups of patients. In the first, relative overdosage occurs because of the presence of an atypical plasma pseudocholinesterase. This enzyme normally metabolizes and inactivates succinylcholine. The atypical enzyme is unable to hydrolyze the drug in a normal manner, and succinylcholine remains in the plasma until slower nonenzymatic hydrolysis occurs, usually within an hour or two depending on the dose given. This condition can be recognized early and treated with respira-

tory support without risk to the patient. In the second group, prolonged paralysis results from a change in the character of the block produced by depolarizing agents.[9] When relaxation has been prolonged by repeated injections or infusions of depolarizing drugs, the blocking effect sometimes outlasts the depolarizing action. In this situation, there is a return of membrane potential toward normal but a persistence of blockade. This has been called "desensitization blockade." It is similar in some respects, but different in others, to the blockade produced by the competitive blocking agents. The treatment of prolonged paralysis in both these groups is maintenance of pulmonary ventilation until spontaneous respiration becomes adequate. Attempts at pharmacologic therapy under these circumstances may confuse the issue and prolong the block.

The muscle relaxants are usually given intravenously and the paralyzing effect follows promptly. There is a question as to whether or not the various muscle groups are affected equally, but it should be assumed that the respiratory muscles will be affected and that respiratory support will be required. These drugs should never be administered unless the means for artificial ventilation are immediately available and assembled for use. The dose of curare required to produce a given effect is dependent on many factors. These include physical fitness, muscular development, age, body temperature, concomitant diseases, anesthetic agent, and depth of general anesthesia. Some anesthesiologists apply a stimulator to a motor nerve in order to observe the normal motor response to supramaximal stimulation and the alteration of that response by curare. Patient susceptibility to curare is extremely variable (Fig. 7), but the response at low doses predicts the response at higher doses. It is always wise to give a small dose first, 0.1 mg. per kilogram, observe the effect, and repeat or increase the dose as indicated. When curare is being used with nitrous oxide and oxygen, the initial total dose required to provide adequate surgical relaxation is usually 0.3 or 0.4 mg. per kilogram. Doses of 0.5 mg. per kilogram

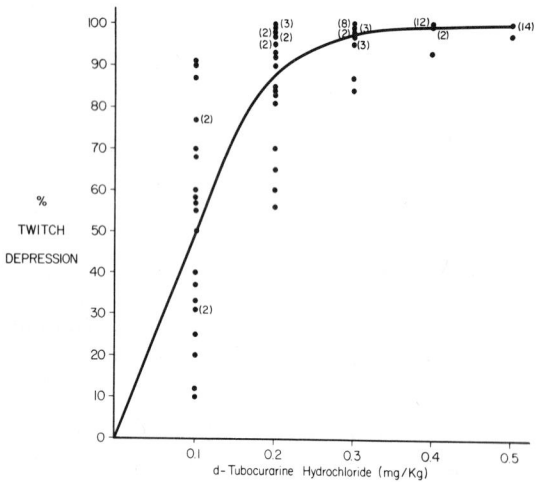

Figure 7. The cumulative dose response curve of curare, in man. This graph demonstrates the marked variability in response to various doses of curare in man: 0.1 mg. per kilogram results in twitch depression which varies from 10 to 90 per cent. Patients resistant to low doses retain resistance throughout the dose scale. Patients sensitive at low doses are sensitive throughout. (From Brunner, E. A.: Unpublished observations.)

need never be exceeded. Supplemental doses may be required for long surgical procedures.

The ease with which muscle relaxation can be produced with these agents has deluded many into believing their use is innocuous. Nothing could be further from the truth. Precipitous elevation of serum potassium levels may follow the administration of depolarizing muscle relaxants to patients with burns, massive trauma, and spinal cord injury. The changes in potassium levels may be great enough to produce cardiac arrest, and the depolarizing drugs should be avoided in the cited groups of patients.[23] Even in the healthy patient scheduled only for minor surgery, the administration of succinylcholine can cause muscle pain persisting for several days. Elevation of intraocular pressure, bradycardia, arrhythmia, and ganglionic blockade are all likely to occur at high dosage levels. Prolonged apnea may be associated with the use of drugs of either group. Incomplete antagonism of a curare block leaves a patient in a state akin to myasthenia gravis and susceptible to hypoventilation because of muscle weakness. Adequate respiratory reserve must be re-established prior to extubation of a patient who has received muscle relaxants during surgery. Occasionally, the use of a mechanical ventilator may be required for a period postoperatively before a patient can be allowed to breathe spontaneously.

THE PREANESTHETIC EVALUATION

The objectives of the preanesthetic evaluation are to identify abnormalities that are likely to affect the anesthetic and surgical risk,[4] to ensure that, when possible, action has been taken to correct or improve abnormalities; to help prepare the patient emotionally as well as physiologically for the stress of anesthesia and operation; to assess the need for special intraoperative monitoring devices or anesthetic techniques and to plan for special postoperative care; and to determine the patient's concurrent and past experience with drugs and anesthetics. It is well to determine the frequency with which alcohol or barbiturates are used because either may affect the tolerance to anesthetics. Many drugs may influence the course of an anesthetic. Included among these are antibiotics, digitalis, adrenal steroids, phenothiazines, rauwolfia, and monoamine oxidase inhibitors.

Ideally, all patients should be evaluated preoperatively by an anesthesiologist. This is not possible at present because of an acute shortage of physician anesthetists. Of necessity, therefore, a surgeon or internist sometimes assumes responsibility for preanesthetic evaluation and preparation. Because these physicians lack extensive experience with the physiologic changes that occur during anesthesia and with the pharmacologic idiosyncrasies of the anesthetized patient, this must be regarded as a temporary necessity that is less than ideal. If a physician anesthetist is available and fails to assume his responsibility in this respect, he is not giving his patients the care due them and he risks being considered a technician rather than a physician.

The examination, evaluation, and preoperative treatment of most surgical patients take place after their admission to the hospital. Before the anesthesiologist sees the patient, the results of the history and physical examination should be written on the chart, and a hemoglobin determination and a urinalysis report appended. If surgery is to be performed on an outpatient, the same information must be provided. The need for further laboratory information must relate to the history and physical examination. The Committee on Pre- and Postoperative Care of the American College of Surgeons suggests a routine chest x-ray for all preoperative patients, and for those over 50 years of age, an electrocardiogram and fasting blood sugar and blood urea nitrogen determinations. If a history of cardiovascular, pulmonary, renal, or hepatic disease exists, further evaluation may be necessary. Patients with heart disease should be classified as to type of disease, functional capacity of the heart, and evidence for or against decompensation. If this has not been done by the referring physician, it should be done by a cardiologist. Patients with pulmonary disease are especially prone to postoperative lung complications and deserve careful preoperative attention. Chest physiotherapy and intermittent positive-pressure treatments with bronchodilator and mucolytic agents are helpful in improving the ventilatory status. More extensive use of pulmonary function tests in evaluation of these patients is encouraged. Modern equipment allows preliminary tests to be performed at the bedside to identify those who may require more extensive pulmonary function studies. The availability of equipment for blood gas analysis and acid-base balance determinations leads to better preparation of surgical patients. It is unrealistic to believe that this type of preparation or these studies can be completed overnight.

In the case of an emergency operation, the same considerations apply but may be superseded by the urgency of the situation. Emergencies vary in degree, and fixed rules for rapid evaluation cannot be given. However, the patient must be examined by an anesthesiologist under even the most dire circumstances. In an emergency situation, each physician tends to view the patient in the light of his own specialty. For instance, recent food intake is often ignored in the patient with an acute surgical emergency, until an anesthesiologist's examination, although the risk of vomiting and aspiration is well known.

Physical Status

The preoperative status of the patient often dictates his response to anesthetic drugs. The risk[4] associated with anesthesia and operation is directly related to the patient's physical condition. Because of this the American Society of Anesthesiologists has adopted the following *Classification of Physical Status:*

Class I
> Patients with no organic, physiologic, biochemical, or psychologic disturbance. The pathologic process for which the operation is to be performed is localized and not related to a systemic

disturbance. Examples are the physically fit for elective inguinal herniorrhaphy or hysterectomy.

Class II
Patients with mild to moderate systemic disturbance caused by the condition to be treated surgically or by other pathophysiologic processes. Examples are patients with mild diabetes or mild hypertension.

Class III
Patients with systemic disturbance from whatever the cause even though it may not be possible to define the degree of disability with finality. Examples are patients with recent myocardial infarction or severe thyrotoxicosis.

Class IV
Patients with severe systemic disorder already life-threatening and not always correctable by the operative procedure. Examples are patients with cardiac insufficiency or advanced pulmonary disease.

Class V
Moribund patients with little chance for survival who are subject to operation in desperation. Examples are moribund patients with a ruptured aortic aneurysm or a mesenteric thrombosis.

The significance of the assignment of physical status to a patient should not be lost to the anesthesiologist or to the patient's surgeon and internist. Experience has shown that as the physical condition of the patient worsens, the possibility of mortality from anesthesia increases. In a study of the causes of death in 33,224 surgical patients, the figures reproduced in Table 5 were obtained.[11] Only those deaths thought definitely related to the anesthesia were included.

Preoperative Medication

Traditionally, preanesthetic drugs have been administered to allay apprehension, to provide a basal state of depression in preparation for anesthesia, to protect against undesirable reflexes, and to dry secretions in the respiratory tract. Belladonna drugs have generally been chosen for the latter two objectives, but the introduction of newer anesthetic agents that do not induce secretions has altered this approach. Atropine is often omitted from the preanesthetic orders and administered intravenously in the operating room on specific indication. The aim of premedication in modern anesthetic practice is to provide a patient who is comfortably sedated, free from apprehension, and able to cooperate in the preliminary preparations for anesthesia. The choice of preanesthetic medication should be left to the anesthesiologist, since the anesthesia really begins at the time the premedication is administered. Drugs may be chosen not only for their effect preoperatively but also for their effect during anesthesia. For instance, a narcotic analgesic is frequently chosen prior to administration of thiopental (Pentothal) and nitrous oxide to minimize the dose of thiopental required. Only the anesthesiologist can plan this integration of the actions of drugs administered in the preoperative and intraoperative periods. The confidence engendered in the patient by a preoperative visit with his anesthesiologist plays an important role in patient preparation, preoperatively. This confidence helps to develop a state of complacency which can be augmented by mild doses of depressant drugs to achieve the desired state of sedation.[14] Drugs are generally chosen from the barbiturate sedatives, the narcotic analgesics, or the tranquilizers. Intramuscular diazepam or hydroxyzine is often chosen today in preference to barbiturates for a sedative effect. Narcotics are frequently employed in low doses for their sedative and tranquilizing effects but are generally avoided in the elderly.

THE CHOICE OF ANESTHESIA

For nearly 90 years after the introduction of surgical anesthesia, a choice among anesthetic agents or techniques was negligible. During this period, interest lay only in providing oblivion and freedom from pain during operations. The last several decades have seen a change in this attitude. There is now available a wide variety of anesthetic agents and adjuvants with pharmacologic activities reasonably well defined. The wide scope of modern surgical procedures has also individualized anesthetic requirements. Choices do exist, but for the most part they are relative. Nonetheless, there are a few specific contraindications to agent or technique. Halothane is strictly contraindicated in a patient who has previously had signs of posthalothane hepatitis. Methoxyflurane is contraindicated in long operations or in obese patients or in patients with kidney disease. The patient with a family history of malignant hyperpyrexia presents a dilemma, since nearly all anesthetic techniques are contraindicated. Spinal anesthesia is contraindicated in the patient with pre-existing central nervous system disease, as is the use of muscle relaxants in patients with myasthenia gravis, and the administration of thiobarbiturates to patients with acute intermittent porphyria. An anesthetist skilled in a variety of anesthetic techniques can usually so apply them that a patient can be anesthetized in several ways. The final selection of agents and techniques is often a matter of individual preference or experience.

Although indications and contraindications are admittedly few, the skilled anesthetist has several ways of choosing agents and techniques for individual patients. The following are some guidelines:

Preoperative Disease

This can justify exclusion of certain agents or techniques. Some agents are poorly tolerated by patients with certain diseases, for example, muscle relaxants in postpoliomyelitis patients with thoracic muscle involvement. Similarly, fear of confusing the natural progress of disease with possible late postanesthetic complication may interdict the use of spinal anesthesia in patients with diabetic neuropathy or central nervous system syphilis.

Maintenance Medications

Many surgical patients receive maintenance drugs for concurrent medical disease. The anesthetist must consider possible effects of prior medication and either alter drug therapy or design an anesthetic management that will not threaten the patient's well-being because of drug interactions. Hypokalemia seen in patients maintained on diuretics contributes to the risk of arrhythmia during general anesthesia and should be corrected preoperatively. Antihypertensive drugs should be continued until the day of surgery, since the cardiovascular instability seen in hypertensive patients is more likely due to their disease than to their medication and in any case can be treated. Patients receiving doses of propranolol exceeding 240 mg. per day are subject to cardiovascular collapse during anesthesia, and the drug dose should be gradually reduced to below that level if time permits. Abrupt withdrawal is contraindicated. The resulting beta-adrenergic blockade can be antagonized by adequately large doses of isoproterenol in most cases. Patients receiving maintenance doses of steroids within the last six months may have secondary depression of adrenocortical function and should receive replacement doses of hydrocortisone on the day of surgery and in decreasing doses for several days thereafter. Patients with diabetes may be managed with either long-acting or crystalline insulin as long as tight control of the diabetic state and glucose load is maintained. There are many subtle interactions of anesthetics and other drugs: most anesthetics partially antagonize the effect of digitalis on the heart; quinidine and some of the antibiotics potentiate the competitive neuromuscular blockers; both the tricyclic antidepressants and the monoamine oxidase inhibitors interact with the narcotics. A well-informed anesthetist is aware of these interactions and takes every reasonable precaution to avoid adverse consequences.

The Bodily Habitus of the Patient

The asthenic, frail, elderly, or chronically ill generally require minimal amounts of anesthetics. They do best with inhalational agents. The robust often require larger concentrations of anesthetics and metabolize injected substances quickly. Weak anesthetics are ineffectual. The obese patient absorbs large amounts of volatile anesthetic and presents the problem of respiratory obstruction soon after induction of general anesthesia. Spinal anesthesia is often a better choice.

Preoperative Emotional State

The emotionally unstable and very apprehensive require heavy premedication and rapid induction of anesthesia. They do poorly with regional techniques or those which provide a slow induction of general anesthesia.

Requirements of the Surgeon

Important considerations that help dictate the choice of anesthetic agents and techniques include intended use of electrocautery, the need for muscle relaxation in an abdominal operation, the duration of the operation, and the position of the patient during the operation.

Requirements of the Recovery Period

The postanesthetic disposition of the patient may influence the choice of anesthesia. Rapid recovery of consciousness is important in outpatients or in those who do not receive recovery room care. If postoperative straining must be especially avoided, as in removal of cataract, agents associated with a high incidence of vomiting, such as ether or cyclopropane, are contraindicated.

The Experience of the Anesthetist

At times this may be a most important consideration. Physician specialists should be familiar with all agents and techniques, but even the busiest may not have enough personal experience to be expert with all. Nurse anesthetists have a more limited spectrum of experience which usually excludes regional techniques.

These judgements are best made by the anesthesiologist, not by the internist or the surgeon. Few internists or surgeons have made a study of anesthesia and its problems. Few have knowledge of the detailed pharmacology of anesthetic agents. Lacking such experience and training, they are not equipped to make a choice of anesthetics in the presence of a more qualified person, the anesthesiologist. As in other branches of medicine, the final decision should follow consideration and discussion and should not be accomplished by mandate.

ADMINISTRATION OF THE ANESTHETIC

Anesthesia begins with the administration of the premedication. After this has been given, the patient should be confined to bed. Ideally, after all has been prepared, the patient should be moved directly to the room where his operation will be performed, although modern operating suites have a holding area in which patients wait their turn for operation. These areas should be quiet, or have soft music. They should be apart from the sights and sounds of an operating room, and an attendant should be assigned to observe the occupants.

The patient should be moved from the transportation cart to the operating table with assistance because of the effects of the premedication. The table should be slightly flexed for the patient's comfort. At this point, the need for fluids is considered. When there is a possibility that a large blood loss may occur, it may be wise to provide several intravenous routes. A large reserve supply of blood serves little purpose if it cannot be given quickly when it is needed. For minor procedures in healthy patients an indwelling scalp vein needle may suffice, but in most cases a short plastic cannula is placed in a peripheral vein to insure that a patent intravenous route is available.

Monitoring Equipment

Equipment to monitor vital functions is now available. Periodic determinations of arterial blood pressure and heart rate are traditional. However, the practice of counting respiratory rate during anesthesia has lost its significance because of the employment of muscle relaxants as well as the use of assisted or controlled respiration. Little refuge can be taken in counting the rate of respiration, either spontaneous, assisted, or controlled, because it signifies so little in reference to pulmonary ventilation. Several ventilation meters are available but often are inaccurate, and may give false security. Improvement is needed in monitoring equipment in this area. Breath and heart sounds are often monitored continuously, either by affixing a stethoscope to the chest wall or by the use of an esophageal stethoscope. Auscultatory monitoring is especially common in pediatric patients. Temperature monitoring, especially in children, has become commonplace since the recognition of the syndrome of malignant hyperpyrexia.

Electroencephalographic monitors are available and are used extensively to observe the surgical patient. Although the electroencephalogram is seldom used today to assess depth of anesthetic, it is useful to detect cerebral hypoxia in specific circumstances, such as during extracorporeal circulation or during operations upon the carotid artery. Monitors for oxygen and carbon dioxide tensions of respired gases are available but are not yet adequately developed for wide clinical use. Monitors of neuromuscular function are gaining in popularity for diagnosing the cause of persistent neuromuscular blockade. Central venous pressure is frequently monitored in those operations in which blood loss may be excessive or hypovolemia is feared. The interpretation of the data requires careful standardization as well as an understanding of circulatory physiology. The use of flow-directed catheters has facilitated monitoring of the pulmonary wedge pressure and allows better evaluation of left ventricular function. The development of the thermal dilution technique for measurement of cardiac output brings to the operating room a measurement previously restricted to the cardiac catheterization laboratory. The proper choice of adequate monitoring devices to assist in observation of the patient is important because there is a danger that the anesthetist's attention may be centered on this type of device to the exclusion of an overall observation. The patient's condition may then be jeopardized.

Preparation for the Anesthetic

There is no substitute for prior planning in conducting an anesthesia. The anesthetic machine must be checked to see that it functions properly and is adequately supplied with gases, volatile agents, and drugs. This is true whether a general or regional technique is to be employed. Equipment must be available for supporting the patient's ventilation and for intubating the trachea. Fluids and drugs should be readily accessible for the support of the cardiovascular system and treatment of unexpected cardiac arrhythmias and arrest.

If a regional technique has been chosen, it should be performed in advance of the projected operating time to allow establishment of sensory anesthesia. If the patient is to remain awake during the operation, personnel should be instructed to speak quietly. Some patients may require heavy sedation or light general anesthesia for supplementation of regional blocks and preparation must be made for this. When local anesthetic agents are injected or applied topically, treatment of toxic reactions should be anticipated. When spinal anesthesia is chosen, hypotension or a total spinal paralysis may result. Preparation for treatment should be made before the intrathecal injection. Only in this way will these complications be readily and successfully treated.

When general anesthesia has been chosen, additional preparations are indicated. A functioning suction apparatus must be at hand to clear airway secretions and vomitus. Induction of anesthesia produces relaxation of the jaw and soft tissues and results in airway obstruction. Anesthesia must not be induced unless an adequate airway can be guaranteed. In most situations, extension of the head upon the neck, elevation of the jaw, or insertion of an oropharyngeal airway suffices to maintain airway patency. For most upper abdominal operations and all intracranial and intrathoracic procedures, endotracheal anesthesia and control of ventilation are indicated. In rare instances, the surgeon may be required to perform a tracheostomy under local anesthesia before general anesthesia is induced.

Tracheal Intubation

There are advantages to the intubation of the trachea. The airway is likely to remain patent. The respiratory dead space is reduced, and the removal of secretions is facilitated. Control of respiration is made easier and the danger of inflation of the stomach from pressure applied to a face mask is removed. By the use of cuffed tracheal tubes, the danger of aspirating gastric contents is minimized. The patient can be placed in any position, and the anesthetist can be situated away from the patient's face and yet retain control of ventilation. There are also disadvantages and these must always be weighed against the advantages. The trachea in some patients is difficult or impossible to intubate under any circumstances. A variety of technical difficulties can lead to trauma from the laryngoscope to the lips, teeth, gums, and oral or pharyngeal structures. The use of a tube of improper size may lead to increased resistance to respiration if too small, or to layngeal or tracheal damage if too large. The use of long tubes may result in bronchial intubation and contralateral pulmonary collapse. Contaminated equipment or mechanical trauma to the larynx may precipitate laryngeal edema in children. This is a valuable technique but it should not be taken lightly and should be used only if needed.

Maintenance

The anesthesiologist should observe the patient constantly throughout the anesthesia and operation, making frequent assessment of the vital signs and paying attention to the progress of the operation. He should stand to observe the surgical field or sit so that he can see over the screen. Among the things he should watch are the color of the blood, the degree of muscle relaxation, and the stage of the surgical procedure. An anesthetist unable or unwilling to watch the surgical field can be compared with a person driving a car in a fog and being unable to see the road clearly. Legible, accurate, and up-to-the-minute records should be kept during the anesthesia and operation. The medical reasons for this do not require amplification but the medicolegal reasons have assumed increasing importance in recent years. Most malpractice suits involving anesthesiologists are notable for the poor records kept by the defendant.

Termination of the Operation

By the end of the operation, the patient should be breathing spontaneously with a good respiratory exchange. He should have regained normal muscle tone as well as his protective airway reflexes. Little is gained, however, by having him wide awake before being moved from the operating table, particularly if the operation was a major one. Under these circumstances, the patient would as soon be oblivious to his surroundings for a few hours. The anesthetist must use good judgment in this matter. Transfer from the operating table to bed or litter must be made with care and at least four people should participate. The blood pressure should be checked immediately after the move because hypotension is common at this moment. Having satisfied himself that the blood pressure and respiration are satisfactory, the anesthesiologist may move the patient to the recovery room where he should remain with the patient until he has rechecked the vital signs and assigned supervision to another competent person.

If there is a reasonable risk that the patient may develop airway obstruction or respiratory inadequacy in the early postoperative period, the anesthetist may elect to leave the endotracheal tube in place or to support ventilation by mechanical ventilator in the recovery room. Generally, this is a safer course than attempting to withdraw support and monitor the patient who is then at risk. Many cardiovascular services electively ventilate postoperative cardiac bypass patients because of the reduced metabolic demand that accompanies mechanical ventilation.

THE RECOVERY ROOM

The purpose of the recovery room is to provide close observation and patient care during a period when normal protective mechanisms may be obtunded and the sensorium clouded.[2] The unit should be immediately adjacent to the operating rooms. Because the patients in this unit are usually under the influence of an anesthetic, it is logical for the anesthesiologist to continue his supervision. Because of the interaction of anesthetic agents with other drugs, therapy should not be administered in the recovery room without his express approval. He knows better than others what the patient has had in the way of depressants. He knows, for instance, that because of general anesthesia, narcotic analgesics must be injected in sharply reduced doses to avoid respiratory and circulatory catastrophe.

The heart of the recovery room is its professional staff. An anesthesiologist must always be available. Nursing personnel should be permanently assigned and specially trained for their work. Private duty nurses have no place either in a recovery room or in an intensive care unit. A supervisor, responsible to the chief of anesthesia, should be in charge during all hours the unit is open. A suggested ratio of one nurse to three patients with a minimum of two nurses always available in the unit is appropriate.

Maximal observation of unconscious patients is the primary consideration of a recovery room. It is essential that the room be well lighted and of open construction to allow for constant surveillance of the patients.

Each bed area should be provided with wall oxygen and suction, adequate electrical outlets, supports for intravenous solutions, and a supply of disposable suction and oxygen catheters, syringes, needles, and the like. In addition, emergency equipment must be available to provide for intubation of the trachea, treatment of cardiac arrest, cardiac defibrillation, mechanical ventilation, thoracentesis, and electrocardiographic monitoring. A supply of intravenous fluids, plasma expanders, and resuscitative and supportive drugs must be at hand. Ideally, type O, Rh-negative blood should be stored in a refrigerator and replaced if unused each week. Patients should not be discharged from the unit until an anesthesiologist has signed their release.

POSTOPERATIVE COMPLICATIONS

Those complications that are most likely to occur during the immediate postanesthetic period fall into two groups, respiratory and circulatory.

RESPIRATORY COMPLICATIONS

Aspiration

Vomiting may occur in any patient awakening from anesthesia, particularly in the patient whose abdomen has been opened. The inhalation of gastric contents into the tracheobronchial tract may be disastrous. Aspiration of large volumes, as may follow gastric dilation, can result in death from drowning; smaller volumes induce laryngospasm or bronchospasm and produce acute hypoxia. Aspiration of acid liquid gastric contents leads to chemical pneumonitis, whereas particulate matter can cause atelectasis, pneumonia, or lung abscess. Prophylaxis is best achieved by placing the patient in the lateral recumbent position with a pillow against the abdomen to prevent his rolling face downward. If regurgitation occurs, the head should be kept low and the mouth and pharynx cleared by suction. Once an airway has been obtained, ventilation and oxygenation are provided if necessary. If aspiration has occurred, treatment should consist of suctioning the trachea, washing it with 10 ml. volumes of saline, followed immediately by suctioning. Antibiotic therapy should be withheld until there is evidence of bacterial infection. The use of steroids is controversial, but ultrasonic mist may be helpful to keep secretions liquefied.

Airway Obstruction

This can sometimes be anticipated before the patient leaves the operating room and transportation delayed, an endotracheal tube left in place, or rarely a tracheostomy performed. Such patients require close supervision and should never be left in the care of the less experienced until the concern has subsided. The most common site of airway obstruction in the postanesthetic period is the upper airway. This is most easily treated by inserting an oropharyngeal airway if tolerated or by hyperextension of the head on the neck with elevation of the jaw. It may be necessary to free the airway of secretions by frequent use of a suction device. If a patent airway cannot be maintained by these simple procedures, an endotracheal tube can be reinserted. Airway obstruction may not be recognized in the obtunded patient and may lead to inadequate ventilation.

Hypoventilation

This may occur because of the action of anesthetics, narcotic analgesics, and muscle relaxants, along with or superimposed on underlying medical disease. Abdominal or thoracic incisions markedly reduce maximal breathing capacity, and many patients have some degree of hypoxia and hypercapnia after these procedures. Treatment of respiratory insufficiency, regardless of cause, requires two simple steps: establishment of a clear airway and maintenance of adequate pulmonary ventilation. The latter can be accomplished by mouth-to-mouth ventilation, use of a self-inflation bag and mask, manual compression of a breathing bag, or ventilation with a mechanical respirator. All recovery room personnel should be trained in the use of each of these methods. Even a brief period of hypoventilation can induce hypoxia sufficient to precipitate cardiac arrest. The administration of oxygen by a disposable face mask has much to recommend it during the early postanesthetic period.

CIRCULATORY COMPLICATIONS

Circulatory complications occur because of the effects of anesthesia, operation, or antecedent respiratory insufficiency. All patients in the recovery room should have blood pressure, pulse, and respiratory rate recorded at least every five minutes. At the same time, the patient should be evaluated for respiratory adequacy, changes in level of consciousness, and skin color. Moderate elevation or depression of blood pressure and pulse sometimes occurs because of awakening and perception of pain. Marked changes in blood pressure or pulse are not to be expected. Blood pressures below 90 mm. Hg and above 180 mm. Hg systolic in previously normotensive patients are to be viewed with concern. Pulse rates below 60 per minute or above 110 are likewise unusual in the recovery period. A persistent bradycardia from continuing action of drugs used during anesthesia may reduce cardiac output and cause hypotension. Atropine is sometimes helpful in this situation. Tachycardia may result from pain, apprehension, hypoventilation, or hypovolemia. If the tachycardia is caused by hypoxia, administration of oxygen by mask decreases the heart rate promptly by at least 20 beats per minute. If it is caused by hypercarbia, assisted ventilation is required. Hypotension with or without tachycardia may indicate hypovolemia, which must be appropriately treated. The use of Trendelenburg's position, which has been traditional in the treatment of hypovolemia, is no longer accepted because of associated diaphragmatic elevation and decreased vital capacity. Elevation of the legs mobilizes blood from the periphery but the body should remain horizontal. Occasionally, a severe hypertension may require small doses of short-acting vasodilating agents, such as sodium nitroprusside, for control. This must always be combined with respiratory support.

SURGEON-ANESTHETIST RELATIONSHIPS

Surgeons and anesthetists form a team of physicians striving for the welfare of the patient. The discipline of each is different but the common meeting ground is the patient. Each member of the team must recognize his own responsibilities and yet be aware of the difficulties faced by the other. The anesthetist must be aware of the patient's medical history, the proposed surgical procedure, and the risk involved from both the surgical and anesthetic points of view. He should confer with the surgeons, the internist, or other consultants about vague aspects of the patient's disease. He must keep the surgeon informed of the patient's condition during the operation by transmission of important details, and continue the care of the patient during the immediate postoperative period when the attention of the surgeon may be elsewhere.

The surgeon should inform the anesthetist of any unusual aspect of the patient's disease or of the surgical procedure. He should not insist upon one anesthetic agent or technique, although he should convey the patient's wishes. He should not promise the patient one anesthetic or another but leave this to the discretion of the anesthesiologist. Rapid induction, prompt awakening, or profound relaxation should not be demanded or expected with every procedure. It should be understood that anesthetists as well as surgeons sometimes have difficulties and complications.

At one time, the surgeon was medicolegally responsible for all that took place in the operating room. Today, each member of the surgical team, being specifically trained for his task, is likely to be responsible for his own acts, although the tendency is to name all physicians involved with a patient's care in case of suit. The surgeon should not assume that the ultimate responsibility for the anesthetic rests on his shoulders. This may be true if the anesthetic is administered by a technician but is unlikely if it is given by a physician.

The best relationships between anesthesiologists

and surgeons are based upon and promoted by mutual professional confidence, respect, and an awareness of each other's problems.

THE ANESTHESIOLOGIST OUTSIDE THE OPERATING ROOM

Daily experience in managing anesthetized patients under a variety of stressful situations has made the anesthesiologist a specialist in the care of critically ill and comatose patients.[13] Skill in supporting normal pulmonary and circulatory function, in managing fluid therapy, and in using vasopressors, narcotics, local anesthetics, antiarrhythmics, and other drugs is equally applicable to the nonanesthetized. This has led to the current participation of the anesthetist in surgical, cardiac, and respiratory intensive care units and in inhalation therapy. This interest is not confined to the postsurgical patient. It extends to the care of any critically ill patient, including those with strokes, shock, head injuries, drug intoxication, crushed chest, chronic cardiac or pulmonary failure, and certain advanced neurologic diseases. The anesthesiologist is also active in the resuscitation field and in many hospitals he directs the cardiopulmonary resuscitation team.

The anesthesiologist has also made significant contributions in the management of patients with acute or chronic pain. Proficiency in the application of spinal, epidural, and caudal anesthesia, regional nerve blocks, local anesthetics, and narcotic analgesics is useful in both diagnosis and treatment of pain. Work in this field may be useful in helping to establish a diagnosis to permit a more definitive surgical operation or to provide optimal conditions while a patient recovers from an operation such as continued sympathetic blockade after embolectomy or arterial graft. Therapy must also be directed toward the relief of acute pain, chronic pain, or intractable pain of terminal cancer. In some institutions, pain clinics have been established and are jointly managed by anesthesiologists, surgeons, neurosurgeons, neurologists, and psychiatrists. The current daily activities of the staff of an anesthesia department range beyond the confines of the operating room.

SELECTED REFERENCES

Dripps, R. D., Eckenhoff, J. E., and Vandam, L. D.: Introduction to Anesthesia, 5th ed. Philadelphia, W. B. Saunders Company, 1977.
The death of the senior author of this outstanding text has not detracted from the quality of the current edition, although its character has changed. The number of contributors has been expanded, but a strong editorial policy maintains a uniformity of presentation. This is still the best introductory text in the field.

Eger, E. I., II: Anesthetic Uptake and Action. Baltimore, Williams & Wilkins, 1974.
A clear and detailed presentation of the pharmacokinetics of drugs of importance in anesthesia. Mechanisms of general and local anesthetic action and of muscle relaxant action are discussed. Uptake and distribution of inhaled anesthetics and barbiturates are discussed in detail.

Greene, N. M.: Physiology of Spinal Anesthesia, 2nd ed. Baltimore, Williams & Wilkins, 1969.

This monograph has reached the status of a classic in its field. This is not a guide to the clinical technique of spinal anesthesia but rather a scholarly analysis of the process by which spinal anesthesia is accomplished and of the subsequent induced physiologic changes. An extensive bibliography is included.

Levin, R. M.: Pediatric Anesthesia Handbook. Flushing, Medical Examination Publishing Co., Inc., 1973.
A practical handbook for anesthetic care of the infant and child. The orientation is toward utility rather than theory.

Scurr, C., and Feldman, S. (Eds.): Scientific Foundations of Anesthesia. Philadelphia, F. A. Davis Co., 1970.
This multiauthor reference reviews the physical, physiologic, and pharmacologic basis of anesthetic practice. Principles underlying the functioning of flowmeters, pressure gauges, blood gas electrodes, temperature-measuring devices, transducers, and the like are explained. A review of pertinent cardiovascular and respiratory physiology includes a well-illustrated section on the microcirculation. The section on uptake and distribution of inhaled anesthetics by Eger is clearly and concisely written. The section on anesthetic apparatus may be useful for those interested in this subject.

Shapiro, B. A., Harrison, R. A., and Trout, C. A.: Clinical Application of Respiratory Care. Chicago, Year Book Medical Publishers, 1975.
The early chapters of this text review the basic principles of cardiopulmonary physiology. This establishes the basis for the subsequent discussions of the clinical uses of oxygen, humidity, physiotherapy, mechanical ventilation, and bronchial hygiene. Airway management and consideration of special problems complete the text.

REFERENCES

1. Adriani, J., Zepernick, R., Arens, J., and Authement, G.: The comparative potency and effectiveness of topical anesthetics in man. Clin. Pharmacol. Ther., 5:49, 1964.
2. Beal, J. M., and Eckenhoff, J. E. (Eds.): Intensive and Recovery Room Care. New York, The Macmillan Company, 1969.
3. Brazier, M. A.: Some effects of anaesthesia on the brain. Br. J. Anaesth., 33:194, 1961.
4. Brunner, E. A.: Factors related to anesthetic risk. Surg. Gynecol. Obstet., 141:761, 1975.
5. Burfoot, M. F., and Bromage, P. R.: The effect of epinephrine on mepivacaine absorption from the spinal epidural space. Anesthesiology, 35:488, 1971.
6. Clark, D. L., Hosick, E. C., and Rosner, B. S.: Neurophysiologic effects of different anesthetics in unconscious man. J. Appl. Physiol., 31:884, 1971.
7. Committee on Anesthesia, National Academy of Sciences, National Research Council: Summary of the national halothane study. J.A.M.A., 197:775, 1966.
8. Cotev, S., and Robin, G. C.: Experimental studies in intravenous regional anesthesia using radioactive lignocaine. Br. J. Anaesth., 38:936, 1966.
9. Crul, J. F., Long, G. J., Brunner, E. A., and Coolen, J. M.: The changing pattern of neuromuscular blockade caused by succinylcholine in man. Anesthesiology, 27:729, 1966.
10. DiGiovanni, A. J., Galbert, M. W., and Wahle, W. M.: Epidural injection of autologous blood for post-lumbar puncture headache. Anesth. Analg., 51:226, 1972.
11. Dripps, R. D., Lamont, A., and Eckenhoff, J. E.: The role of anesthesia in surgical mortality. J.A.M.A., 178:261, 1961.
12. Dripps, R. D., and Vandam, L. D.: Long term follow-up of patients who received 10,098 spinal anesthetics. I. Failure to discover major neurological sequelae. J.A.M.A., 156:1486, 1954.
13. Dripps, R. D., and Vandam, L. D.: Long term follow-up of patients who received 10,098 spinal anesthetics. II. Incidence and analysis of minor sensory neurological defects. Surgery, 38:463, 1955.
14. Egbert, L. D., Battit, G. E., Turndorf, H., and Beecher, H. K.: The value of the preoperative visit by the anesthetist. J.A.M.A., 185:553, 1963.
15. Egbert, L. D., Battit, G. E., Welch, C. F., and Bartlett, M. D.: Reduction of postoperative pain by encouragement and instruction of patients: Study of doctor-patient rapport. N. Engl. J. Med., 270:825, 1964.
16. Fogdall, R. P., and Miller, R. D.: Neuromuscular effects of enflurane. Anesthesiology, 42:173, 1975.

17. Hamilton, W. K.: Nomenclature of inhalation anesthetic systems. Anesthesiology, *25*:3, 1964.
18. Larabee, M. G., and Posternak, J. M.: Selective action of anesthetics on synapses and axons in mammalian sympathetic ganglia. J. Neurophysiol., *15*:91, 1952.
19. Linssen, A.: Curariform Drugs. Nijmegan, The Netherlands, Thoben, 1961.
20. Magoun, H. W.: Brain mechanisms for wakefulness. Br. J. Anaesth., *33*:183, 1961.
21. Mark, L. C., and Papper, E. M.: Advances in Anesthesiology: Muscle Relaxants. New York, Hoeber Medical Division, Harper & Row, 1967.
22. Moore, D. C., and Bridenbaugh, D.: Oxygen: The antidote for systemic toxic reaction from local anesthetic drugs. J.A.M.A., *174*:842, 1960.
23. Tobey, R. E.: Paraplegia, succinylcholine and cardiac arrest. Anesthesiology, *32*:359, 1970.
24. Woodbridge, P. D.: Changing concepts concerning depth of anesthesia. Anesthesiology, *18*:536, 1957.

11

THE SURGICAL ACUTE CARE UNIT

Worthington G. Schenk, Jr., M.D.

In the recent past, much progress has been made in the design and function of surgical acute care units. Some feeling for the newness of this concept can be appreciated by review of four surgical texts published between 1970 and 1972, in which there is no mention of such units. In two texts published in 1973, however, the subject is introduced.

Historically, the origin of such units appears to have begun with the military "shock" units devised for resuscitation during World War II. The first civilian application of such special care units for surgical patients was the anesthetic recovery room, which has now been in use for more than 20 years. As a matter of fact, many surgical special care units have been developed as outgrowths or merely extensions of anesthetic recovery rooms. It is probably the *special care* afforded by the recovery room units which, more than any other single experience, has convinced surgeons of the need for surgical special care units.

The next major contribution, the development of *coronary* care units, should be attributed to cardiologists. These units are perhaps better labeled *intensive observation units,* and they have clearly demonstrated the significant improvement in patient survival that can be attained in a specially designed unit with sophisticated monitoring and specially trained personnel for the management of specific cardiac conditions.

The advantages of a contemporary surgical intensive care unit are striking to the older surgeons, who often wonder how it was possible to manage without them. In the pre-World War II era, the patient needing special care postoperatively was often supplied with "special" nurses, who often did not have specialized training and were *special* only in that they were assigned to a single patient without other patient responsibilities.

A surgical acute care unit has three essential components. If any of these three is lacking, the unit will either not function at all or will function suboptimally. The first of these is a concept in *team care.* While the surgeon must always be in primary charge of his patient, it should be recognized that, for maximal effectiveness, such special care units should be staffed by a group of experts in respective areas of acute care.

The second requirement is that of *specially trained personnel.* While there are now special postgraduate courses for nurses who wish to enter any one of the special care fields, over the years most such nursing specialists have developed through extending their knowledge acquired either in the anesthetic recovery room or in emergency and trauma units. Whatever the method of training, it is essential that such nursing personnel be specially trained for this unique and critical professional position.

Third, a surgical intensive care unit represents a definite *physical location with specialized physical facilities, including appropriate laboratory support.* While the ideal architectural plan for such units is still in the process of evolution, the most effective units developed to date appear to be those in which the nursing personnel are stationed in the center of the unit and the patient cubicles are distributed around the periphery, enabling the nursing supervisor to maintain visual contact with all patients from the central location of the nursing station. Such units must be completely equipped with all currently available life support systems at each bed as well as provided with the generally accepted instruments for monitoring. Two of the most frequently used basic configurations are shown in Figure 1. The circular configuration has the advantage that all patients are equally distant from a central nursing station. Its disadvantages include the fact that it is difficult to construct such a unit in an existing rectangular building, and it results in somewhat more wasted space than the rectangular configuration. Moreover, it is difficult to expand. The rectangular configuration has the disadvantage that the most peripheral patients cannot be easily seen by the nurse in a central station, but its advantages are that it can be fitted into most existing buildings and can be more easily expanded if necessary.

Equipment

Fixed equipment at each patient unit should include the usual support systems, such as intravenous brackets, vacuum outlets, oxygen supply, and multiple electrical outlets. An emergency power source capable of providing adequate electrical power for portable x-rays, adequate lighting for performance of emergency procedures in the bed, and an efficient nurse call system should be available.

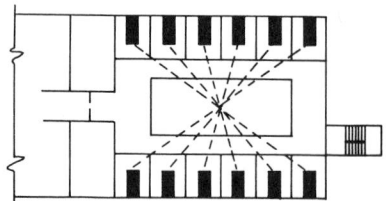

The central nursing station with beds on each side.

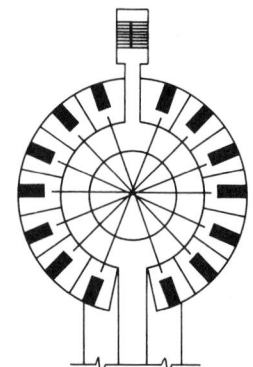

Circular pattern with all patients equidistant from the nurse.

Figure 1.   From Rourke, A. J. J.: Intensive Care Units. Functional Planning of General Hospitals. New York, McGraw-Hill, 1969.

Perhaps the single most widely used monitoring device is the *electrocardiogram*. While a wide variety of commercial units having a broad scope of optional features are available, most include the following features: (1) an audible signal or "beep" synchronous with each "R" wave, (2) a continuous display of the ECG on an oscilloscope at the patient's bedside, and (3) a remote oscilloscope that reproduces the ECG at the nursing station. Optional features include a cardiotachometer (a device which calculates heart rate and provides a direct numerical readout), and warning devices in the event that previously set limits are exceeded. For example, if the pulse rate falls below 60 or exceeds 120, an audible warning sounds. Other devices with an audible alarm can detect cardiac arrhythmias when certain preset limits are exceeded, as well as make permanent recordings of the abnormal cardiac rhythm.

Pressure Recording Devices.   The simplest and most used *pressure recording devices* are water manometers, usually used for determination of central venous pressure, and available in disposable plastic packs. For determination of arterial pressure, electronic transducers are in common use. These devices are compact and require that a needle or catheter be introduced into an artery (radial, brachial, femoral, etc.) and connected to the transducer. The transducer then converts the pressure changes to an electrical signal which is displayed on an oscilloscope, often a multichannel scope showing the ECG as well. This pressure information can be recorded either as the pulsatile trace showing the systolic and diastolic values or as a mean pressure. Accessories which sound an alarm if the pressure falls below or rises above preset limits are also available for such pressure recording systems.

While *central venous pressure* is a quantity interpreted somewhat differently by different authors, most surgeons now define it as the pressure recorded from the superior vena cava near the right atrium. The catheter used for recording this pressure is usually introduced through either the subclavian or the external jugular vein. Each of these routes has advantages; the subclavian route requires only a percutaneous needle puncture[5] but is associated with the risk of inducing a pneumothorax. Thus, after introduction of a catheter by this technique, a chest film should always be obtained to exclude the possibility of this complication. The external jugular approach usually requires a cutdown rather than a percutaneous puncture but does not have the same risk of pneumothorax.[1]

The central venous pressure usually yields information regarding cardiac filling pressure, which can be assumed to be representative of changes in the right atrium and to provide some evidence of left atrial pressure. There are a few notable exceptions, however, especially in mitral valve disease, severe lung disease, and recent cardiotomy or myocardial infarct, in which the central venous pressure may be quite misleading as a guide to the left atrial pressure. In these circumstances, it is well to consider the use of the Swan-Ganz catheter,[5] a soft, flexible catheter with a balloon near its tip (Fig. 2). It is usually introduced through an antecubital venous cutdown and advanced to the right ventricle. The balloon is then inflated and allowed to "float" into the pulmonary artery. In this location, pulsatile recording of pulmonary pressure can be observed, bearing in mind the fact that pulmonary diastolic pressure generally has a close relationship to mean left atrial pressure. The balloon can then be

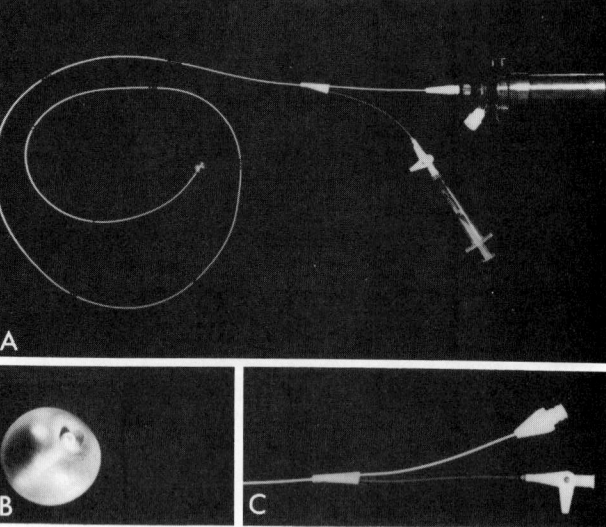

Figure 2.   *A,* Picture of the standard 5F balloon-tipped flow-directed catheter. The balloon is inflated and the stopcock of the inflation lumen closed. A pressure transducer is attached to the larger lumen. *B,* Close-up view of the inflated balloon protruding above the tip of the catheter. *C,* Close-up view of the proximal ends of the pressure lumen and of the inflation lumen in the stopcock. (Reproduced with permission from Swan, H. J. C., and Ganz, W.: Use of balloon flotation catheters in critically ill patients. Surg. Clin. North Am., *55:*501, 1975.)

deflated and the catheter advanced until it is "wedged" into a small pulmonary artery branch. In this "wedged" position, the pressure recorded is largely a reflection of left atrial pressure and can be most helpful in following function of the left side of the heart. Correlation between central venous pressure and left atrial pressure has been shown to be particularly poor following open-heart surgery,[2] while the pulmonary wedge pressure shows a much better, although not perfect, correlation with left atrial pressure.

Estimation of *cardiac output* is being more widely used in selected patients in acute care units, particularly those with known cardiac or circulatory disorders. The dye-dilution technique is usually employed, in which indocyanine green in measured amount is injected into the central venous line (ideally into the pulmonary artery), and a dye concentration-versus-time curve is recorded from an arterial sampling site. From this curve a cardiac output estimation can be made by plotting the area under a curve or more easily by automatic instrumentation with direct computation of cardiac output. There is evidence that the indocyanine green method may overestimate cardiac output in *high flow states*[3] and is considerably more reliable in normal or low flow states.

Increased attention is being given the thermodilution method of determining cardiac output. This technique requires the injection of a small quantity of cold solution into the central venous line (again ideally the pulmonary artery) following which a temperature-versus-time curve is plotted from a distal sampling site.[4] This is most often done using an inlying catheter having a thermistor at its tip. A more recent modification of this technique has been the addition of a thermistor probe to the Swan-Ganz catheter.[6] This device enables the estimation of cardiac output without the need for obtaining serial arterial thermal changes. At present, one basic difficulty with the interpretation of cardiac output is the fact that the ideal or "normal" cardiac output for critically ill patients is controversial. While it is generally higher than normal resting values for cardiac output, the volume of optimal increase has not been definitely established.

Urinary Output. Any patient ill enough to be in an intensive care unit will, with rare exception, be a candidate for an indwelling urethral catheter with continuous recording of urinary output. The urinary flow rate is indispensable in assessing the status of a patient's hydration, renal function, and cardiodynamic status.

Blood Gases. Highly important information concerning the patient's circulatory and respiratory status can be obtained from knowledge of arterial and central venous values of Po_2, Pco_2, and pH. Samples for such analysis are obtained by periodic collection of a small amount of blood from the arterial pressure line (or arterial puncture if such a line is not available) and from the central venous catheter which is usually in place. Several commercially available units enable the *rapid* determination of Po_2, Pco_2, and pH from less than 1 ml. of blood. The design and operational principles of these instruments are well described.[7] In most situations, the demand for blood gas

determinations is great enough to justify and indeed to require the establishment of a small laboratory directly adjacent to the intensive care unit, in which such studies are performed and are immediately available. Of the three values, Po_2, Pco_2, and pH, the single result which most often results in clinical decision making is the Po_2. The Po_2 is the partial pressure exerted by oxygen in blood, and the relationship between saturation of hemoglobin with oxygen and Po_2 is highly nonlinear. When the arterial Po_2 falls from 100 to 60 mm. Hg, the oxyhemoglobin saturation falls only from 100 to 88 per cent at normal pH (Fig. 3). However, when the Po_2 falls only 20 mm. Hg further, from 60 to 40 mm. Hg, the oxyhemoglobin saturation falls from 88 to 65 per cent. The manner in which the oxyhemoglobin dissociation curve is shifted by pH change is also shown in Figure 3. Acidosis produces a shift to the *right* so that oxyhemoglobin gives up its oxygen to the tissue more "easily" (i.e., at a higher Po_2 than at pH 7.4). Alkalosis, on the other hand, produces a shift to the *left* so that hemoglobin retains a greater affinity for oxygen and the Po_2 must fall to a lower value before giving up an equivalent amount of oxygen. As an exercise to demonstrate this point, the change can be calculated in oxyhemoglobin saturation as the Po_2 falls from 95 to 40 mm. Hg, with a pH of 7.3 as compared with 7.6. The significance of this difference is the amount of oxygen that can be delivered to the tissues with an arterial to venous Po_2 change from 95 to 40 mm. Hg in the *acidotic* versus the *alkalotic* patient.

For smaller hospitals in which it is impractical to employ biochemical technicians 24 hours daily, the direct reading oximeter is available. This instrument indicates per cent oxyhemoglobin saturation directly from a 1 ml. sample of blood and can be operated by the attending surgeon or a nurse.[2] Some clinical examples will probably serve best to illustrate the manner in which the information gathered by the above-described techniques is used in patient care.

Hypotension

The most common physiologic derangement requiring specific attention is the patient with *hypotension*. While a single blood pressure reading is difficult or

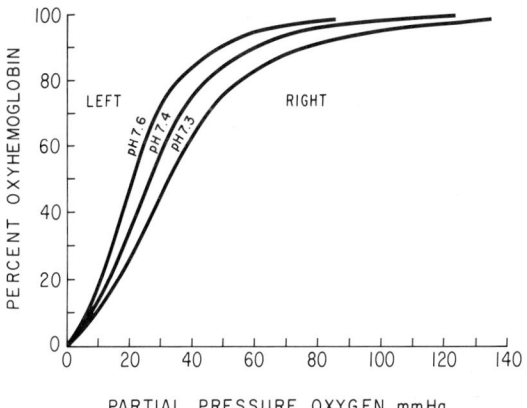

Figure 3. From Hill, R.: Proc. R. Soc. Biol., *120*:472, 1936.

impossible to interpret, previous blood pressures are available either from preoperative examinations, intraoperative charting, or recovery room notations. By comparison with previous values, a declining blood pressure is always a signal of concern. Whether or not a declining blood pressure indicates a clinically significant trend can usually be determined by two simple bedside observations. Significant hypotension is followed promptly by compensatory peripheral vasoconstriction. This is evidenced at the bedside by the typically *cold, clammy extremities*. The other simple observation is *urinary output*. A decrease in urinary output occurring simultaneously with a fall in blood pressure indicates *significant hypotension*. A reasonable figure to bear in mind is that a urinary output of 30 ml. per hour is a minimal amount for a 70 kg. adult.

Venous pressure is also a valuable factor to monitor. Normal pressure for the patient in the supine position is approximately +5 to +12 cm. of saline. A pressure in the zero or negative range, when accompanied by hypotension, is usually a sign of clinically significant *hypovolemia*.

Management of Hypotension. Once significant hypotension has been identified, with corroboration by peripheral vasoconstriction, decreased urinary output, or low central venous pressure, a rapid intravenous fluid infusion of a crystalloid solution such as a balanced salt solution should be started. This should be done through a large-bore needle, or preferably a large-bore inlying catheter, and if not already in place, a central venous catheter and urinary catheter should be inserted.

The series of events just described should be accomplished in 5 minutes or less, but it should be appreciated that this is only the beginning of the management problem. The initial therapy being instituted is based on *probability;* that is, hypotension is most often due to hypovolemia. Therefore, the physiologic derangement can be most quickly reversed by rapid infusion. However, after these initial steps have been accomplished, two additional things must be done promptly: (1) identify and treat the physiologic derangement, and (2) identify and correct the underlying pathologic defect producing the physiologic derangement. Several illustrative examples follow.

EXAMPLE 1. The patient has a blood pressure of 70/40 mm. Hg; the extremities are cold and clammy, and the central venous pressure is recorded at −1 cm. saline with a urinary output of 5 ml. in the last 20 minutes. The diagnosis is hypotension due to hypovolemia. *Question:* What is the basic pathologic defect? It must be appreciated that at this point it may be unknown and, if it remains unknown, is unlikely to be treated properly. Again, on the basis of probability, a frequent cause of hypovolemia in the surgical patient is hemorrhage, and all dressings and drain sites should be inspected for obvious blood loss as well as observation of any increase in girth of extremities or abdomen which might represent *sequestered* blood loss. If hemorrhage has been identified as the basic pathologic defect, whole blood should then be infused and the bleeding controlled by reoperation or whatever technical means necessary.

EXAMPLE 2. The patient's blood pressure is 70/40 mm. Hg; the extremities are cold and clammy; the urinary output is less than 5 ml. during the past 20 minutes, and the central venous pressure +20 cm. H_2O. The diagnosis is hypotension that is clinically significant but not in this instance due *solely* to hypovolemia, in view of the elevated central venous pressure. Rather, the high central venous pressure suggests primary cardiac failure or cardiac tamponade as a cause of the hypotension. The treatment should consist of immediate intravenous administration of one of the fast-acting cardiac glycosides in a full therapeutic dose (provided the patient has not been on cardiac glycosides previously) with very cautious continued fluid infusion. A search for the pathologic defect in this instance includes careful cardiac auscultation for valvar or pericardial disease as well as an electrocardiogram and enzyme studies for acute myocardial infarction. The lungs should be examined for possible pulmonary edema and a chest film obtained.

Hypoxia

Another common derangement requiring special attention is *hypoxia*. Only in recent years has the frequency with which arterial hypoxia occurs been appreciated, particularly the type present in the absence of obvious clinical signs. The appearance of the skin and mucous membranes or evidence of ventilatory distress are unreliable signs of the presence or absence of arterial hypoxia. It is now generally recommended that arterial blood samples be obtained at least as often as every four hours in any critically ill surgical patient. In addition, the Po_2 should be determined at any time any new physiologic derangement such as hypotension, abrupt change in central venous pressure, or change in urinary output occurs.

While an inlying radial artery catheter is often placed by the anesthesiologist both for continuous recording of arterial pressure and for easy collection of arterial samples during the course of anesthesia and in the recovery room, it is not always feasible to leave such catheters in for days at a time in the surgical intensive care unit. Therefore, arterial samples must then be obtained by direct puncture, with the radial, brachial, and common femoral being the most frequently used sites. It is well to bear in mind that the color of the blood obtained should not be used as a guide to whether it is arterial or venous blood; one can be sure that the sample is arterial only if the blood pulsates into the collecting syringe. The blood sample should be analyzed promptly.

EXAMPLE. The patient has dyspnea, tachycardia, and cyanosis. The blood gas values are: Po_2, 70 mm. Hg; Pco_2, 50 mm. Hg; and pH, 7.16, confirming arterial hypoxia. The treatment is immediate assisted ventilation with a bag and mask combination using a 40 per cent concentration of oxygen. After approximately 5 minutes of such manually assisted ventilation, a second series of arterial blood gas values should be obtained. These values in the normal range are: Pa_{O_2}, 85 to 110 mm. Hg (when breathing room air, and as high as twice these values when breathing a 40 per cent oxygen concentration); PCO_2, 35 to 45 mm. Hg; and pH, 7.36 to 7.44.

Should ventilatory insufficiency persist, the management should be assisted ventilation, probably with insertion of an endotracheal tube and connection to a volume-cycled ventilator with adjustment of the inspired oxygen concentration over a period of time to only that level required to maintain PaO_2 in the normal range. Approximately +5 cm. H_2O positive end-expiratory pressure (PEEP) should be added to help expand atelectatic portions of the lung of the patient and as future prophylaxis.

A relatively common variant of the above clinical manifestations of hypoxia is that in which ventilation is *difficult* when assisted with a mask and bag. When such difficult assisted ventilation is encountered, the cause must be sought and corrected. Most frequently this is found to be due to *upper airway obstruction* as a result of partial occlusion of the pharynx by the tongue or some degree of laryngeal obstruction from foreign bodies, mucus, or edema. The form of obstruction caused by the tongue may be corrected by the insertion of an oropharyngeal airway, while obstruction at the laryngeal level is usually best managed by direct laryngoscopy with removal of obstructing material and insertion of an endotracheal tube. If ventilation is easy following placement of the endotracheal tube, ventilatory assistance can be continued as described above. However, if ventilatory assistance is difficult through an endotracheal tube, an intrathoracic explanation for this difficulty must be sought. Marked atelectasis, pneumothorax (with or without hemothorax), and pulmonary edema should be considered. If a significant amount of air is present in the pleural cavity, a clinical diagnosis of pneumothorax can usually be made on physical examination of the chest. In a truly emergency situation, a chest needle or tube should be inserted on the affected side and connected to an underwater seal *without* waiting for a confirmatory x-ray when the clinical diagnosis is made. Provided the patient's condition permits, x-ray confirmation is clearly desirable, since errors can be made in the clinical diagnosis of pneumothorax. Both severe atelectasis and pulmonary edema will gradually improve with assisted ventilation provided positive end-expiratory pressure is added. PEEP is usually added at about 5 cm. H_2O pressure, but this may be increased, particularly in the presence of pulmonary edema.

Occult Hypoxia. It has become increasingly apparent since the start of routinely obtaining arterial blood gas studies in the critically ill that occult hypoxia is a *common* and not a rare condition. Between a third and a half of seriously ill patients in acute care units are hypoxic at the time of the first arterial blood sample if assisted ventilation has not been previously initiated. All too frequently these patients have few if any of the clinical signs of hypoxia but rather the most common clinical finding is *restlessness*. The hazard resulting from this observation in the past was the ordering of additional narcotic sedation, which, understandably, accentuated the hypoxia and probably has resulted in death. It must be emphasized that additional sedation should not be ordered for restlessness until the presence of hypoxia has been *excluded* by arterial blood gas values. Clearly, one may see patients with an arterial PO_2 in the range of 40 mm. Hg exhibiting no dyspnea or cyanosis.

In recent years, it has also become apparent that the arterial PO_2 is by far the most valuable of the three regularly obtained values, that is, PO_2, PCO_2, and pH. This is true because hypoxia cannot be tolerated except for very brief periods and, even in brief periods, initiates a chain of deleterious effects. Contrariwise, somewhat elevated PCO_2 values are not only well tolerated, but they may be persistently elevated in patients with chronic obstructive lung disease with no clinically apparent ill effect. Blood pH is so well buffered that it does not change acutely except in extreme states; even when changes are observed, they may be compensatory, which may be desirable rather than undesirable in view of their metabolic or respiratory origin. From the above, it then follows that a low arterial PO_2 must *always* be treated as an *acute emergency* and must be reversed immediately. Abnormal PCO_2 and pH values, however, require a somewhat less urgent evaluation, consultation, and decision as to whether to correct them or accept them as compensatory phenomena.

Renal Insufficiency

The suspected diagnosis of renal insufficiency begins with the observation that the urinary output is less than 5 ml. in a 15-minute period. This confirms that oliguria is present, and in order to interpret its significance, a prompt determination of the urinary specific gravity is required. If the specific gravity is 1.015 or above, the indication is that the patient has functioning renal parenchyma which is producing urinary concentration; therefore, in all probability, the physiologic defect is continued hypovolemia and the management will be to further increase the blood volume by increased intravenous infusion. If the specific gravity is low, approaching 1.010, this suggests the onset of oliguric renal insufficiency, but, again, the immediate management is to increase the fluid infusion, with close observation of the urinary volume output and specific gravity response.

If oliguria is observed after hydration and in the presence of normal arterial blood pressure, high or normal central venous pressure, and evidence of adequate peripheral perfusion, the diagnosis is clearly early oliguric failure. Management includes the immediate intravenous administration of 25 gm. of mannitol and 40 mg. of furosemide (Lasix). Urinary volume, specific gravity, and circulatory status are re-evaluated after 30 minutes. If the circulatory status remains good, while the urinary status is unchanged, an additional 80 mg. of furosemide is given intravenously. Contrariwise, if the circulatory status is good and the urinary status has improved, with an increase in urinary volume and a decrease in specific gravity, it will be apparent that the problem is being corrected.

Finally, if a very high urinary volume continues with a low specific gravity approaching 1.010, the diagnosis of a clinical syndrome designated as *high output renal failure* will be confirmed. In this instance, increased infusion must be administered to compensate for urinary losses. Such a patient may otherwise succumb to hypovolemia due to an excess urinary loss.

and the measurements of cardiac output with comparison by dye dilution techniques are of considerable significance.

SELECTED REFERENCES

Skillman, J. J.: Intensive Care. Boston, Little, Brown and Co., 1975.
This is an excellent monograph published under the editorship of an acknowledged and scholarly authority in the field. Detailed consideration is given each of the major aspects of appropriate management of an acute care unit, and the text is highly recommended as an updated source of the latest information presented both clearly and concisely.

Sørensen, M. B., Bille-Brahe, N. E., and Engell, H. C.: Cardiac output measurement by thermal dilution. Reproducibility and comparison with the dye-dilution technique. Ann. Surg., *183*:67, 1976.
This is a useful reference source in which a group of seriously ill surgical patients were monitored by use of a Swan-Ganz pulmonary artery thermodilution catheter before, during, and after major vascular surgery. The details of the usefulness of this technique

REFERENCES

1. Goldin, M. D.: Intensive care of the surgical patient. Chicago, Year Book Medical Publishers, 1971.
2. Lee, L. W.: Elementary Principles of Laboratory Instruments. St. Louis, The C. V. Mosby Co., 1974.
3. Merjang, J. P., Hahn, J. W., and Barner, H. B.: Comparison of thermodilution cardiac output and electromagnetic flowmeter. Surg. Forum, *25*:145, 1975.
4. Mills, A. B.: Intensive care units. *In* Functional Planning of General Hospitals. New York, McGraw-Hill, 1969.
5. Phillips, S. J.: Technique of percutaneous subclavian vein catheterization. Surg. Gynecol. Obstet., *127*:1079, 1968.
6. Skillman, J. J.: Intensive Care. Boston, Little, Brown and Co., 1975.
7. Subramanian, V. A., Hai, M. A., Sherman, M. M., and Berger, R. L.: Filling pressures of the heart following open heart surgery. Surg. Forum, *26*:236, 1975.

12

COMPUTERS AND MATHEMATICAL TECHNIQUES IN SURGERY

John H. Siegel, M.D.

Like a sluggish caterpillar which undergoes a gradual metamorphosis into a spectacular creature of great vitality, computer technology applied to surgical problems also has undergone a sophisticated maturation. The transformation of a pedestrian effort into a jet-engine flying machine is far from complete, but remarkable progress in the use of this technology has occurred in the field of surgery. This is largely a consequence of the heightened awareness of surgeons that they must rethink surgical problems in terms of the data to be obtained and must learn to formulate their questions prospectively in a manner which will allow computer analysis. An equally positive trend has been the mutual pragmatic recognition that the computer scientist and the statistician make good collaborators and colleagues of the academically oriented surgeon, and that working as a team more can be achieved by interaction than separately. The development of this mutual understanding and recognition of the limitations of their respective techniques have already produced some outstanding applications of computer technology to surgical problems, and it now seems evident that more impressive contributions are in the offing.

Computer-Based Patient Monitoring

A number of important efforts have centered about the acquisition of physiologic data in an on-line mode.[25, 34, 40, 56, 70, 74, 100] Most of these approaches have been directed primarily at obtaining an automated assessment of the cardiovascular[25, 70, 74, 100] or respiratory[34, 40, 56] systems, to obtain measurements and derive computations of the standard physiologic parameters of function.[25, 36, 41, 57, 73, 100] The initial assumptions underlying this approach were that if the well-studied physiologic interrelationships could be determined in an on-line basis, then trend analysis and early warning of dysfunction would be self-evident. In retrospect this seems naive, but the initial workers in this field had few means of comprehending the enormous magnitude that the task of reliable data acquisition presented. Furthermore, in spite of more than a quarter century of modern cardiorespiratory physiologic research, only a very small number of patients had been studied in a sufficiently similar manner to yield statistically significant data by which questions relevant to trend analysis in an abnormal population could be answered.

The result of these early failures was the realization by nearly all investigators that mere technologic expertise was not sufficient, but that studies had to be undertaken to define the relevant questions for analysis in terms that could be answered with the data available. These questions were related to delineation of the necessary set of primary measurements needed to define key physiologic functions, the required frequency of sampling of these data streams, and the types of analysis of these measurements that would be sufficient to provide a characterization of the patient's physiologic state and to serve as a predictor of the onset of a crisis situation.[3, 4, 20, 23, 36, 55, 63, 72, 77, 81] This latter requirement, related to the need to define a normal state of physiologic affairs in sick patients by which deleterious change can be quantified, has of necessity directed attention toward the establishment of data banks of patient information so that the nature and variety of physiologic patterns present in different types of critical illness can be understood.[25, 26]

One of the earliest approaches to the use of a computer for on-line physiologic measurements in the critically ill was made by Shubin and Weil,[73] who attempted to automate the data collection and computation of cardiovascular parameters in patients undergoing intensive care. These workers developed an efficient system for the derivation of cardiac output, using an algorithm that permitted the computation via the Stewart-Hamilton method of indicator dilution curve analysis. This system also allowed the extraction of systolic, diastolic, and mean blood pressures from a signal-processing technique applied to the arterial pressure pulse. In addition, their computer-transducer system permitted continuous monitoring of the

231

central venous pressure. Using these measurements, plus the heart rate obtained from either the electrocardiogram or the arterial pressure pulse, they computed the standard cardiovascular parameters of stroke work, total peripheral resistance, ejection rate, and so forth. An attempt was made to provide a graphic output of these data, as well as information about their time course, and to associate this information with other types of data, such as hourly urine output, in order to provide some kind of picture of the patient's clinical course and response to therapy.

In a similar but somewhat more imaginative approach, Warner and his colleagues[100] attempted to derive stroke volume, estimated from mathematic analysis of the central aortic pressure. Their aim was to obtain a measure of cardiac output that was not dependent upon analysis of the indicator dilution method, and that they felt would enable frequent sequential measures of changes in aortic flow. This method, which has considerable intellectual and mathematical sophistication, is based on an application of signal-processing techniques (Fig. 1) in which the computer is programed to recognize critical points on the arterial pressure pulse. Since the arterial bed has elements both of resistance and capacitance, only a portion of the blood ejected from the left ventricle during systole will leave the large vessels of the arterial system during systole. A considerable portion of the blood ejected from the heart is held within the elastic reservoir of the vascular bed and leaves large vessels during diastole. In Warner's analysis, the stroke volume (Sv) can therefore be divided into a systolic drainage (Sd) and the diastolic drainage (Dd); Sv = Sd + Dd, where Dd equals the change in arterial volume (Δv). In this analysis the difference in the volume (Δv) of the arterial bed has been assumed to be proportional to the square root of the change in pressure in the arterial bed (Pmd) at two points in time—the onset of systole and the end of systole. To approximate this change in pressure (Pmd), the pres-

sure was integrated to the point of systole (T2) from a point 80 milliseconds before the onset, (T1), since this would be the pressure at the other end of the arterial bed when systole begins. In the same way, the pressure at the end of systole averaged over the length of the arterial bed can be approximated by the integration of pressure to the dicrotic notch (T4) from a point 80 milliseconds earlier (T3). The difference in these two mean pressures is the mean distending pressure (Pmd). It is also assumed that flow (F) from the arterial bed during systole and during diastole is directly proportional to the pressure above 20 mm. Hg, $F = K_2$ (P − 20). This proportionality constant K_2 depends on peripheral resistance. However, it is Warner's contention that since only the ratio of systolic drainage to diastolic drainage is needed, K_2 is not necessary because this method is independent of peripheral resistance. Therefore, in his analysis, the final equation (see Fig. 1) involves only one constant (K_1), which relates pressure to volume in the aorta, and in practice is obtained for each individual by a single measurement of cardiac output by the indicator dilution technique.

Experimentally, Warner was able to show that this method had a considerable degree of reproducibility when compared to the standard indicator dilution method, even when peripheral vasoconstrictors or vasodilators were given. It also has been his contention that even if an absolute measurement of cardiac output cannot be obtained, this technique provides a method of detecting the change in the state of the patient by virtue of the relative change in cardiac output. In general, this ingenious technique appears to be a reasonable measure of cardiac output which can be obtained on a beat-by-beat basis in many clinical situations. However, it has recently been shown by the studies of Kouchoukos et al.[37] that major changes in the constant K_1, which relates pressure to volume, may occur in individual patients during their time course. Kirklin's group also noted that the disparity between actual flow and the derived measure may be as great as 30 per cent in patients immediately following cardiac surgery. In addition, the studies of Siegel et al.[83, 86] on vascular tone relations in the critically ill have shown that very major changes in the pressure-flow relationship can occur in patients with severe sepsis and septic shock, and in patients suffering from extensive cirrhotic liver disease. Other investigators have also confirmed the difficulties of using this method of estimating cardiac output without frequent recalibration by indicator dilution techniques.[25, 35, 92] Nevertheless, with the proper updating of the relevant constant (K_1), it remains an excellent means of reflecting changes in cardiovascular status from an on-line measurement.

Warner[100] and others[10, 11] have also attempted to apply a variety of signal-processing techniques to the analysis of electrocardiograms in order to obtain the heart rate and detect the presence of cardiac arrhythmias. Similar programs developed by Osborn and his colleagues[56, 57] have demonstrated that changes in rate and the development of ventricular ectopic beats are the most useful information in terms of developing alarms to be used in the monitoring of the critically ill

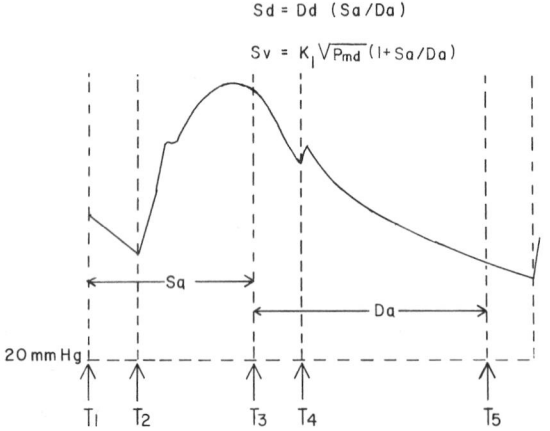

$$Sd = Dd \ (Sa/Da)$$

$$Sv = K_1 \sqrt{Pmd} \ (1 + Sa/Da)$$

Figure 1. Diagram of technique of stroke volume determination from arterial pressure pulse analysis. (Redrawn from Warner, H. R., et al.: Circulation (Suppl. 2), 37:68, 1968. By permission of American Heart Association, Inc.)

TABLE 1. Trend Display Summary*

Name	Displayed Component(s)	Signal Source	Continuous Sampling Rate (sam/sec)	Comments
1. Heart rate (HR)	(a) heart rate, and (b) ECG data loss	ECG Lead 1, 2, or 3	500	Derived from ECG PRIMITIVE processor output
2. Arterial pressure (AP)	(a) systolic, and diastolic pressures	arterial catheter	250	Derived from pressure waveform by PRIMITIVE processor
	(b) mean pressure	analog averager module	1/10	
	(c) pressure data loss			
3. Cardiac output (CO)	cardiac output			Derived from ECG and pressure waveforms using systolic and model and pressure PRIMITIVE output
4. Mean venous pressure (VP)	mean venous pressure	venous pressure analog averager module	1/10	
5. PVC count (PV)	(a) count of premature ventricular contractions			Derived from ECG CYCLE output
6. Temperature (TP)	rectal temperature	analog module	1/10	
7. Ejection time (EJ)	ejection time			Derived from pressure waveform by PRIMITIVE processor
8. Peripheral vascular resistance (VR)	peripheral vascular resistance			Ratio of cardiac output mean arterial pressure

*From Glaeser, D. H., Trost, R. F., Brown, D. B., Kyle, A. C., Lenahan, M. S., Walker, C. K., Wilson, C. S., and DeBakey, M. E.: Comput. Biomed. Res., *8*: 336–361, 1975.

patient after cardiac surgery. Both Caceres'[10, 11] and Warner's[100] groups also have devoted a considerable effort to obtaining on-line electrocardiographic diagnoses of a more detailed nature, which might be applied to cardiograms transmitted from remote locations to the central computer for detailed analysis and diagnosis. These functions presumably will be useful in aiding less experienced physicians, surgeons, or paramedical personnel in the detection of myocardial infarction and in the discrimination between supraventricular and ventricular arrhythmias.

There have been several important attempts to integrate the computer into a postoperative monitoring system by organizing a number of these measurement techniques directed at the assessment of the cardiovascular system into an evaluation package.[57, 70, 74, 100] In the system developed by Glaeser and his colleagues,[25] an ingenious hierarchial system of minicomputers serves to preprocess signals acquired from the patient. These are then transmitted to a somewhat larger minicomputer which serves as a mass storage device for the data from several patients and generates trend displays, processes arrhythmias, and sends appropriate physiologic and data quality alarm messages to the physician and nursing personnel at the bedside. The advantage of this type of system is that it permits continuous monitoring rather than intermittent sampling and allows integration of data from several sources, such as fluid intake and blood gases, to be available for physician decision making. More impor-

tant, it is theoretically more efficient than a single large computer system as it uses separate specialized minicomputers for data preprocessing and analytic functions. The types of trend displays offered by this system and their source are shown in Table 1.

An interesting experiment in the use of an on-line computer facility to evaluate the automated treatment of critically ill patients has been carried out by Sheppard et al.[69, 70] This group has attempted to use a process-control computer capable of analog-to-digital conversion in a surgical intensive care unit for patients who have undergone cardiac surgery (Fig. 2). At the time of cardiac surgery, catheters are placed in the left atrium and in a peripheral artery. In the postoperative period a baseline cardiac output determination is made, using indicator dilution techniques, and an attempt is made to compute the K_1 constant in Warner's equation (see Fig. 1) so that future estimates of cardiac output can be made by the pressure pulse method. Since, as indicated earlier, there are frequent changes in this constant owing to changes in the patient's vascular tone, the indicator dilution technique has to be used several times in the course of the patient's evaluation to reset this constant to an approximate value. Kirklin's group also measures the patient's arterial pressure and heart rate as well as the right and left atrial pressure, and these are correlated with hourly determinations of the drainage from chest tubes and with urine output. A monitor program has been written that dictates and carries out a set of

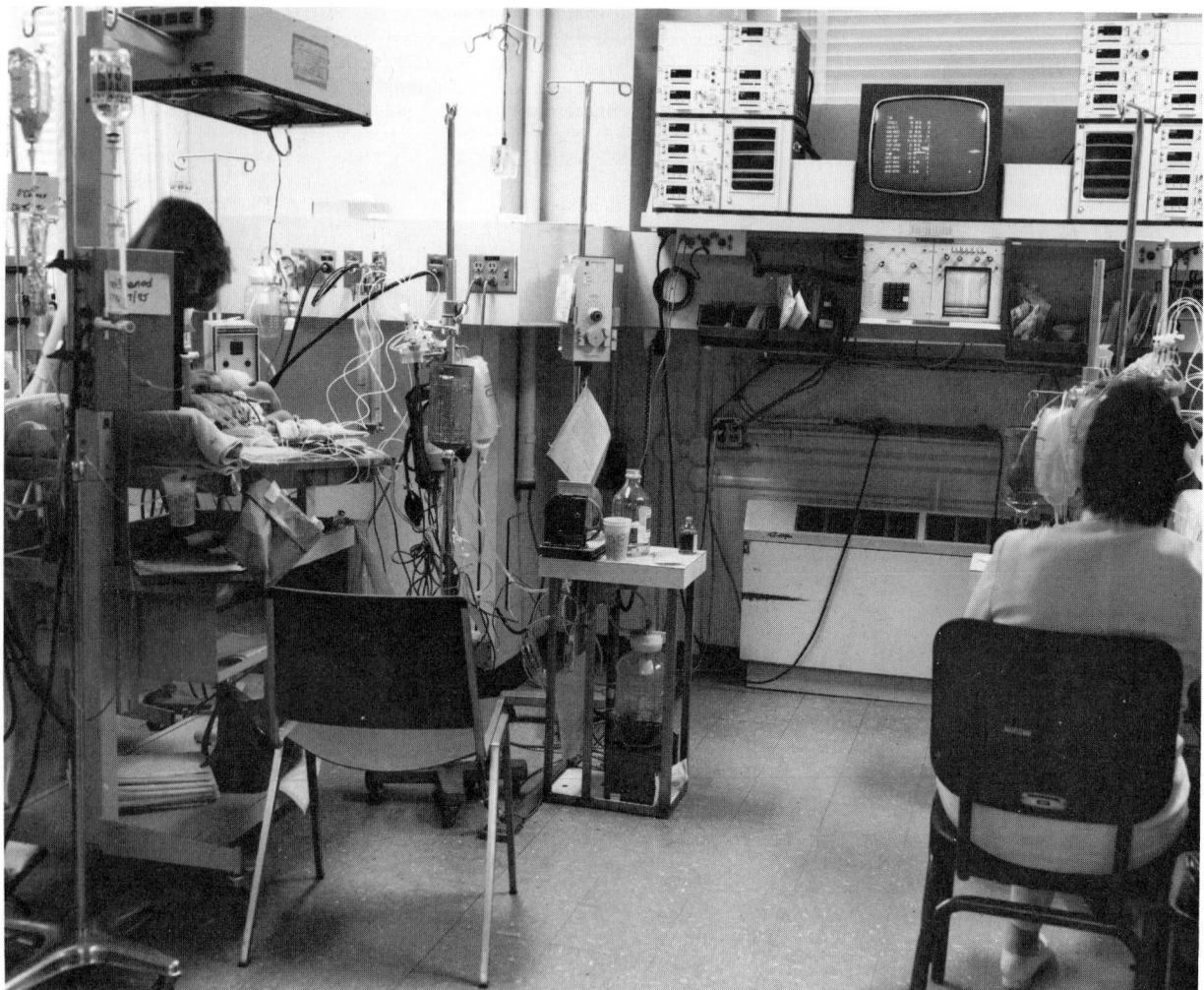

Figure 2. Computer-based monitoring system for automated volume replacement therapy in cardiac surgical patients. Note computer interface and display scope, and instrumented weighing device for measurement of chest tube drainage and urine output. Computer controlled fluid infusion pump is mounted on IV stand. (Photograph courtesy of L. C. Sheppard and J. W. Kirklin, University of Alabama. To be published in Anesthesiology.)

rules that have been established for the infusion of blood in patients after open intracardiac surgery. The assumptions on which these rules are based are related to the fact that left atrial pressure, under most circumstances, provides an adequate measure of the left ventricular end-diastolic pressure, and that end-diastolic pressure is in turn related to the intraventricular volume and distensibility.

As an integral part of their analytic program, they have developed computer-controlled servo devices for automated infusion of fluids based on the computer output.[69] By evaluating the mean left atrial pressure as a function of the cardiac output and work, a logical decision-making process is initiated which regulates the infusion of blood or crystalloid solution. The blood is administered in small increments which never exceed 20 ml., and the physician is capable of setting the level or limit beyond which he will not permit left atrial pressure to be increased by volume infusion. A similar program evaluates the measure of urine out-

put on an hourly basis. If this output is less than prescribed limits, the program automatically infuses a small amount of mannitol at a predetermined rate provided by the level of left atrial pressure. In addition, instructions are given to the surgical staff by the computer that will lead them to consider the use of cardiac inotropic agents. Warnings are also displayed if the augmentation of blood volume does not result in the maintenance of an adequate cardiac output in the face of increased left atrial pressure, and an attempt is made to lead the physician to distinguish between cardiac tamponade and decreased myocardial contractility.

A second major area in which on-line techniques have been effectively utilized to assess clinical function has been the measurement of respiratory parameters in the critically ill postoperative patient. The approaches in this area have been at two different levels. The first has been the use of noninvasive sensors to automate the routine postoperative monitoring of patients who have undergone major operative trauma, and the second has been the attempt to use more elaborate physiologic measurements of respiration to derive physiologically significant indices of respiratory dysfunction.

In the first area, Lewis and his colleagues[39, 41] have attempted to design a relatively simple system using entirely nondestructive techniques to measure respiratory rate and volume, and to correlate these measurements with those obtained from automated cuff blood pressure measurements using Korotkoff sounds, electrocardiographic determination of heart rate and rhythm, and tympanic membrane temperature. This system also permits information from blood gas determinations to be entered via a digital keyboard, so that they can be displayed together with the processed cardiorespiratory data for evaluation by the physician. Some data analysis is possible, because differential diagnosis of various acid-base disorders can be obtained on request from the system.

Emphasis on the second approach has motivated Osborn and his associates[55, 56, 57] and Peters and his group[34, 62, 63] to provide bedside monitoring and respiratory system analysis of patients undergoing thoracic and cardiac surgical procedures. In this application a pneumotachygraph is placed on the respiratory line, either at the endotracheal tube of patients who are intubated, or in the face mask of a patient who is breathing without intubation. Continuous sampling of the gas mixture is carried out, using mass spectrographic analysis of O_2 and CO_2, as well as dynamic measurements of the airway pressure and flow. In this way respiratory flows, pressures, and gas composition can be continuously monitored after analog-to-digital conversion by the computer. The computer program also permits the computation of respiratory mechanics and gas exchange, including oxygen consumption, carbon dioxide production, respiratory quotient, and the physiologic dead space. By combining digital entry of the venoarterial oxygen content difference, it is possible to obtain estimates of the cardiac output (using the Fick method) as well as the percentage of venoarterial admixture across the lung.[56] These data as well as pressure-volume plots can be displayed at frequent time intervals, and pulmonary work per minute, compliance, and resistance computed, along with the ratio of dead space to tidal volume. Osborn and his colleagues[55] have shown that such computer monitoring of the pressure-volume relationship during inspiration (Fig. 3) can be especially valuable in providing evidence of occult airway obstruction, and Peters' group[62, 63] showed that the dynamic aspects of this relationship also can be used to evaluate the effect of utilizing various respirators to produce an adequate ventilatory volume.

Such continuous airway monitoring based on the patterns of the airway pressure flow relationship can provide data on the immediate status of respiratory function which can be lifesaving at times, and can also contribute to the making of sound clinical decisions.[34, 55]

Using a similar set of on-line measurements, Peters[62, 63] has developed indices that may be used as a forewarning of deterioration of pulmonary function. He has attempted to apply his system to the analysis

of pulmonary parameters with these limits in mind, so as to suggest criteria by which the physician may determine the need for ventilatory assistance.

An example of the value of this type of application of computer-based data acquisition and analysis is shown in Figure 4, in which the histograms of measured compliance (Fig. 4A) and total work per liter of ventilation (Fig. 4B) are compared for patients on and off respiration therapy.[63, 67] It is clear that compliance is not a good discriminator of the need for mechanical ventilation, but that the computation of total work per liter ventilation separates patients requiring respiratory support from those who do not, with almost no overlap. Peters' present work has been directed to the design and construction of a portable computer interface which can acquire ventilatory data and transmit it to a remote special purpose computer for processing, with return of the derived data to the physician.[62, 63] An even more impressive demonstration of the potentialities of remote physiologic data transmission was provided by Osborn, who arranged for data transmission using his physiologic interface from the Mount Sinai Hospital in New York to the computer at the Institute for Medical Sciences in San Francisco with return of on-line information. For reasons related to the limitations of present day commercial phone communications and expense, this is not a cost-effective means of physiologic monitoring, but it proves the feasibility of a central computer facility serving many remote intensive care units, when technologic advances reduce transmission costs and increase communication reliability.

In an important application of Osborn's system for respiratory monitoring, Lamy and his colleagues[38] used this computer monitoring system to evaluate the pathologic mechanisms of hypoxemia and the response to changing inspired oxygen tension and positive end-expiratory pressure in patients with the adult respiratory distress syndrome. They showed that the computer-generated data can be used to distinguish those patients with fixed right to left shunts from those with ventilation inequalities as the primary cause of their

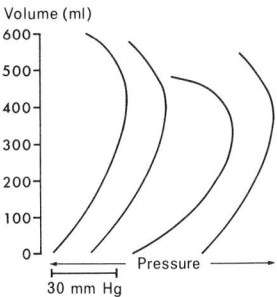

Figure 3. Selected pressure-volume curves of respiration from an on-line computer-based monitoring system, showing two normal curves followed by one of respiratory obstruction (increased nonelastic resistance). The final curve was taken after aspiration of secretions from the tracheobronchial tree. (From a system described by Osborne, J. J., et al. *In* Stacy, R. W., and Waxman, B. D. (Eds.): Computers in Biomedical Research, Vol 3. New York, Academic Press, 1969.)

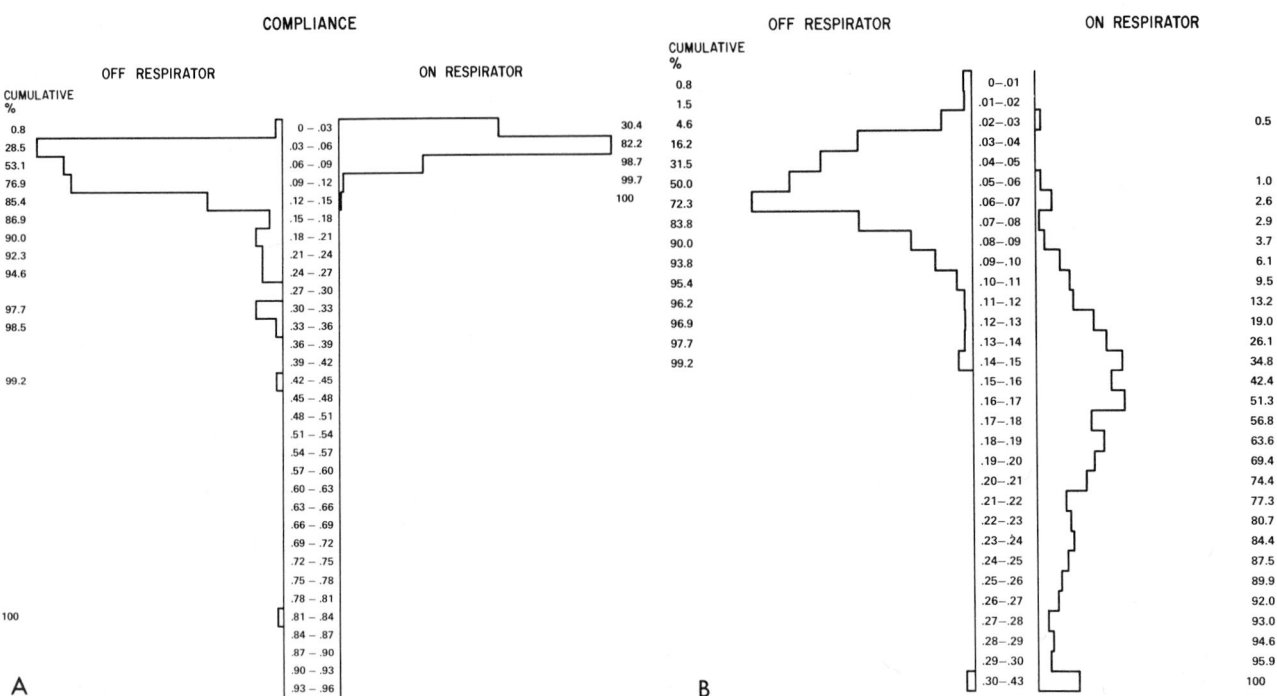

Figure 4. *A*, Computer-generated histogram of lung compliance of patients on and off respirator. *B*, Computer-generated histogram of total respiratory work per liter ventilation of patients on and off respirator. (Courtesy of R. M. Peters and A. R. Shapiro, University of California at San Diego.)

respiratory dysfunction. However, in a related study from the same institution, Eberhardt et al.[20] showed that while carefully selected data for research purposes can be generated from a computer-based respiratory monitoring system, in ordinary routine clinical monitoring single automated measurements of the mechanical parameters of ventilation and gas exchange appear to be insufficiently precise to detect clinically useful changes in the patient's respiratory status, and the prognostic capability was poor. These data indicate the continuing need for the development of error detection and on-line multivariable pattern recognition algorithms before this methodology can become an effective tool for the routine management of the critically ill patient. These studies of engineering efficiency are consistent with the earlier observations of Raison[65] and Weil[73] on alarm detection. They noted that most false alarms arose from external sources that originated from patient movements or nursing operations rather than from the sensing or data detection components of the monitoring system. These studies pointed out the need for the development of on-line techniques of continuous multivariable trajectory or time series analysis which can delineate significant trends while rejecting artifactual transients. It is also important to emphasize that the application of computer-based monitoring is not likely to reduce the need for physician or paramedical personnel but may allow them to make better and more efficient judgments concerning the patient's condition.

The elegant computer-based patient monitoring systems that have been described represent the highest level of sophistication reached thus far in the area of on-line computer-based monitoring. However, a simpler, less elegant, but considerably less expensive approach using a small digital computer has been developed by Siegel and his colleagues[82] for use in a wide variety of care situations related to the assessment of the critically ill general surgical patient. This system is based on the premise that judgmental decisions are generally made by the physician on the basis of his evaluation of the patient's physiologic status at certain nodal points in time, and that the data so obtained can contribute to the physician's ability to recognize clinical patterns, which in turn will then help him choose the frequency and the timing of subsequent evaluations. The additional premise behind this limited system is that in a general hospital setting, acutely ill patients may be found in a variety of physical locations, on the wards, in the intensive care unit, in the emergency room, or in the operating room. In order to make the initial assessment and continuing observation meaningful in the usual surgical setting, it is important to be able to evaluate the physiologic status of the patient wherever he is, rather than necessarily moving him to a special unit where such facilities are available. For this application a portable "shock cart" containing monitoring and recording devices has been designed (Fig. 5). It permits bedside cardiac catheterization with interval measurement of blood pressure, cardiac output, electrocardiogram, and arterial and venous blood gas determinations. The raw data from these physiologic measurements are manually entered into a small portable computer or into a terminal connecting with a time-shared, nationally available computer system.[80] These systems are preprogramed to compute the relevant physiologic variables, and to compare the patient's values with the means of previously studied groups.[77, 79, 80] The second assumption used by these workers in devising such an intermittent monitoring system is that not only does the surgeon wish to obtain information for the determination of parameters delineating the current physiologic status of his patient and their difference from previous measurements over time, but he also needs to be able to assess his patient's physiologic status relative to the patterns of abnormality found in the various forms of critical illness, in order to have sufficient diagnostic and prognostic information on which to base a clinical decision.

The Ultimate Purpose of Computer-Based Patient Monitoring

All of these approaches to computer-based patient monitoring have raised nearly as many questions as they have answered. The principal question, which has been addressed by Maloney[45] and Stacy,[91] is whether, considering the human effort involved in designing and implementing such systems, the share of the available financial resources for medical care required for these implementations, and the patient inconvenience and trauma caused by the use of the present generation of invasive sensors, these techniques really do materially increase our understanding of the patient's disease process, and whether they do in fact produce better patient care. Serious questions have also been raised as to whether the limited medical resources in this country would not be better spent in the recruiting and training of nurses or new types of paramedical personnel, who might actually provide a more intensive level of patient care.

From this collective consideration of the successes and failures of the current approaches has come a more or less general agreement: that the purpose of the application of computer techniques to patient monitoring activities must be to extract more information than is currently obtained by the ordinary measurement of cardiac, respiratory, and metabolic information. The computer should organize this information in a form that is easily understood by the physician, and should provide an analysis of various physiologic systems and their interrelationship in the critically ill. By presenting patterns of abnormalities present in individual patients and relating these to a data bank of similar patient information and patterns, the computer should increase the surgeon's understanding of the physiologic abnormalities so that he may prevent crisis situations from developing, and better handle those crises which in fact do develop.

The ultimate application of computer technology to the pressing problems of patient care should also permit the doctor to evaluate therapeutic measures in an individual patient in a situation where the usual type of clinical or experimental controls cannot be ethically applied. The need to apply the concept of system analysis to the study of critically ill patients in order to elucidate the adequacy of the performance of physiologic subsystems, as well as the reserve capacity of these systems, and to describe and predict system failures has been well stated by both Kirklin[36] and Stacy.[91] Their guideposts point out the directions for future research and development in computer-based patient monitoring.

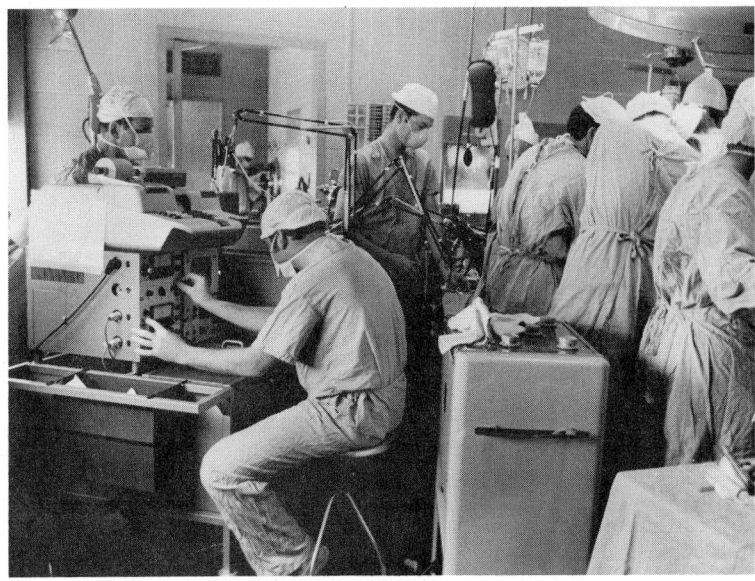

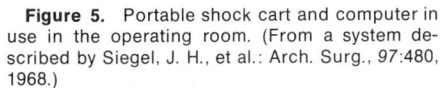

Figure 5. Portable shock cart and computer in use in the operating room. (From a system described by Siegel, J. H., et al.: Arch. Surg., 97:480, 1968.)

THE USE OF COMPUTER TECHNOLOGY IN THE DERIVATION OF STATISTICAL INDICES OF PATIENT STATUS

The investigation and care of critically ill patients often requires the physician to assimilate and interpret data obtained from a large number of variables, each of which represents a particular kind of measurement, such as blood pressure, heart rate, serum electrolyte concentrations, changing chest x-ray findings, and alterations in electrocardiograms. In order to interpret this enormous amount of information, the physician needs to be able to segregate the important aspects of a patient's clinical picture in such a way as to permit the division of the total patient population with a particular disease entity into subgroups that may have different prognoses or different responses to therapy. Much of this kind of clinical subgrouping is done intuitively on the basis of recognition of different patterns of symptoms or signs. Recently attempts have been made to utilize the computer to delineate physiologic patterns that may have diagnostic or prognostic significance.

One of the earliest attempts to apply computer techniques to the evaluation of a particular group of patients with regard to their risk category at surgery was carried out by Siegel and Williams,[86] who attempted to evaluate the interaction between normalized indices of cardiac and peripheral vascular function as a predictor of the operative risk of patients with cirrhosis and portal hypertension who required portal decompressive surgery. Using simple analytic geometric techniques applied to the use of a small stand-alone computer system, they attempted to deal with the functional interrelationships between oxygen consumption and vascular tone, and the relationship between stroke work and central venous pressure.[83, 86] They noted that one could define indices of cardiac ventricular function and relative peripheral shunting which between them could permit the preoperative selection for surgery of patients with cirrhotic portal hypertension with regard to their statistical chance of surviving operation.

Numerical Taxonomy

Using a somewhat more sophisticated approach, a number of workers have attempted to use mathematical techniques of measuring the similarity or dissimilarity among groups of patients with different disease entities on the basis of multivariable data of various types. These techniques, which are related to the measurement of distances between sets of patient data in a multidimensional space, are known generally as "numerical taxonomy." The application of these techniques to both the quantitative and qualitative data used in the preoperative assessment of patients undergoing pelvic surgery has been carried out by Neurath et al.[54] in an attempt to assist in the establishment of a correct differential diagnosis. A more elaborate attempt to represent multidimensional data of both a qualitative and quantitative nature obtained from patients with a presumptive diagnosis of acute myocardial infarction has been done by Thompson and Woodbury.[95] These workers attempted to generate so-called planar maps showing the interrelationship between symptom and sign complexes in patients with myocardial infarction. These techniques were also used to examine the improvement of patients as their clinical status changed. A similar approach has been used to relate symptom and sign complexes of patients with cirrhosis to the etiology of their liver disease.[107] These patient maps have been very useful in defining the relationship between some of the physiologic and clinical aspects of patients with myocardial infarction or cirrhosis, but have not been very easy to comprehend in terms of defining a physiologic state that would enable patient classification at a given moment in time.

Linear Discriminant Analysis and Sequential Order Techniques

In addition, a number of what can best be described as classification procedures have been applied to the critically ill in the attempt to develop a prognostic index which might discriminate between patients in various types of shock with good or poor chances of survival. Shoemaker et al.[71] have utilized a physiologic "cut-point" analysis and Afifi and his colleagues,[2, 3, 4] Chang et al.,[12] and Shubin and associates[72] have attempted to use techniques of multivariate linear discriminant function analysis to determine a discriminant score which might prognostically separate shock survivors from nonsurvivors.

In the latter type of analysis the various cardiovascular, respiratory, and metabolic variables obtained from a given patient, such as mean blood pressure (MBP), arterial carbon dioxide tension ($PaCO_2$), or lactic acid (LAC), are arranged as a linear combination of variables:

$$Z = a_0 + a_1 (MBP) + a_2 (PaCO_2) \ldots + a_k (LAC)$$

in which Z represents the discriminant score and the coefficients $a_1, a_2, \ldots a_k$ are determined from the data so that the difference between the mean values of Z for survivors and for nonsurvivors is maximized. The constant a_0 establishes a reference value at which the difference between survivors and nonsurvivors is zero.

From this type of discriminant scoring it is theoretically possible to compute an estimate of the probability of survival for a given patient by inserting his individual values in this equation, modified by the derived coefficients obtained from the difference between the mean values of the survivors and nonsurvivors.[72]

While some of the earlier studies by Afifi[3, 4] were flawed by the unsubstantiated assumption that the populations of surviving and nonsurviving shock patients each represented a multivariate normal distribution, i.e., a bell-shaped distribution curve in all physiologic dimensions, their present discriminant analysis is largely free of such errors. However, the assumption that the prognosis of a *new* individual patient can be predicted by this type of analysis remains to be statistically demonstrated, since their previous studies[3, 4, 72] and those of others[23, 79, 81] show that the choice of physiologic variables capable of providing survival discrimination differs in various types of shock. Therefore, the major decision as to the specific prospective variable selection in a new shock patient must be made on clinical and physiologic grounds and is not entirely dependent on the intrinsic data but on physician judgment.

In a related area Shapiro and Peters[67] have compared a standard linear discriminant analysis approach with two other statistical techniques of data classification to computer-generated data on pulmonary mechanics (Fig. 4A and B) in order to assist the physician in making the therapeutic decision as to whether a patient needs to be placed on a respirator. They evaluated the same human data by the linear discriminant analytic method and by a technique known as the Nearest Neighbor Rule, which estimates the odds that a given patient will require a respirator by asking what proportion of previously studied patients who were similar to the patient being evaluated required respirator therapy. In addition, they compared both of the above techniques with a procedure known as Kendall Sequential Order Statistics, in which a sequential analysis of each physiologic variable obtained (e.g., compliance, total work per liter, etc.) is made to determine the extent to which it will completely separate patients in the two groups. The variable which best separates the two groups is selected first, then the variable with the best ability to classify the remaining patients is selected next, and so on until all the variables are used or until no patients remain unclassified. Shapiro and Peter's study[67] showed a good degree of agreement among all three techniques on their original patient data. However, when new patient data were analyzed, the sequential order technique made fewer errors in classification but had a tendency to allocate a moderate number of patients to an unclassified group in which no prognostic information could be obtained.

The point of all of these techniques is that to a greater or lesser extent, they can quantify the physician's past experience and permit him to reference it in determining similarities or dissimilarities between his previous classifications of clinically significant entities and a new patient whom he is treating. The problem in their use is that they are not free from any original judgmental error in classifying the reference population of patients into arbitrary groups which may obscure the future definition of new patients. Also, they do not necessarily provide new data-dependent information concerning the physiologic significance of the reasons for the statistical classification, which may be useful to the physician in evaluating his therapy and altering it along rational lines.

Cluster Analysis

In an attempt to deal with the problem of arriving at data-dependent physiologic groupings, Siegel et al.[81] applied cluster analysis techniques[23] to studies of physiologic data from critically ill patients. Their objective was to quantify the pattern and severity of the state of physiologic decompensation and to develop a method of tracking the multivariable trajectory of recovery after the stress of major surgery, sepsis, or other critical illness. They utilized an interactive method to analyze a computer data bank of clinical, physiologic, and therapeutic variables to establish a physiologic frame of reference within which to evaluate the complex nature of the abnormalities present in patients with severe sepsis and septic shock. The data obtained by these workers originated from a large number of sources, including bedside cardiac catheterization studies, patient records, laboratory determinations, and physicians' and nurses' notes. Their patients were studied serially during the course of their treatment, and each set of measurements was centered in time around the determination of cardiac output. Since all of the information in a given set was related in time, the data were therefore cross-sectional with regard to the measurement sets of all patients studied and longitudinal with regard to many sets of an individual patient. A basic assumption behind their application of computer technology was that just as a physician's clinical status designation of a patient may be different from one time period to the next, so the multivariable data set obtained at each time period may reflect a different physiologic state. One of the advantages of the application of computer techniques to this type of analysis is that although most investigators have difficulty in evaluating relationships between data that are displayed in more than two dimensions, the computer has no difficulty in holding "in mind" data interrelationships in 3 or 1000 dimensions at the same time. It can therefore take a multivariable data set centered around a moment in time, and compare it with multivariable data sets from other time periods from the same patient, or from different patients (Fig. 6). By ordering all of these multivariable data sets in the high-dimensional space represented by the number of data directions, the computer can also permit the projection of these data-inferred interrelationships onto a hyperplane so that the relevant patterns can be evaluated by the physician or researcher. In addition, each of these multivariable data sets can be manipulated according to any desired mathematical or statistical technique and ordered in temporal sequence.

The basic statistical methodology behind the cluster technique of multivariable physiologic analysis has evolved around the definition of a physiologic frame of reference for the delineation of a state of normal compensation for the older high-risk patient, and a metric by which one may measure the magnitude and direction of a specific patient's departure from the reference state (R state).[81] As described in detail by Friedman and his colleagues,[23] in choosing the control population on whom to develop a concept of physiologic stability, Siegel et al.[77] delineated a group of 158 multivariable observation data sets from 56 older preoperative general surgical patients with a wide range of intercurrent diseases but without any major physiologic abnormality which would produce acute cardiovascular or cardiorespiratory decompensation. These data were compared to 437 multivariable data sets from 92 patients with severe sepsis, septic shock, hypovolemic shock, or cardiogenic shock.

After some preliminary screening they chose from these multivariable data a simultaneously obtained set of 11 physiologic variables which reflected aspects of cardiovascular and cardiopulmonary compensation.[77] These were cardiac index (CI), heart rate (HR),

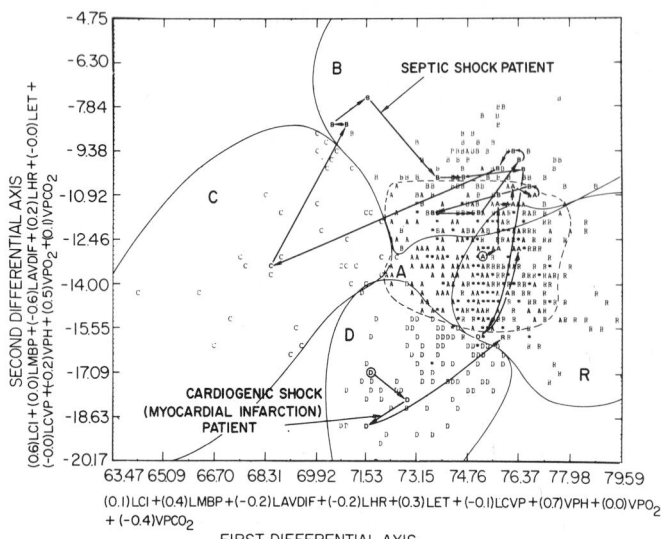

Figure 6. Patient sample groups (A, B, C, D, and R) projected from nine-dimensional hyperspace onto plane defined by linear discriminant axes. L before a variable indicates log transformation prior to a normalization with respect to R. (From Siegel, J. H., Farrell, E. J., Goldwyn, R. M., and Friedman, H. P.: The surgical implications of physiologic patterns in myocardial infarction shock. Surgery, 72:126–141, 1972.)

mean blood pressure (MBP), arteriovenous oxygen difference (A-V Diff), systolic ejection time (ET), right atrial mean pressure (CVP), mixed venous pH (VpH), PCO_2 (VpCO$_2$), and Po_2 (VpO$_2$) and two parameters derived from the analysis of the shape characteristics of the central indicator dilution curve, the cardiac mixing time (tm), which was shown to be directly related to the durational aspects of left ventricular contractility, and the dispersive time (td), which was shown under ordinary circumstances to reflect the mean transit time through the pulmonary vascular bed.[78]

They used the eleven variable physiologic data sets of the control population to establish the frame of reference and the metric by which to evaluate change from control in various forms of acute illness. Their technique was to normalize all of the 695 individual multivariable data sets from all 148 patients by the mean and standard deviation of that variable obtained from the 158 eleven-dimensional data sets of the control group. This statistical device enabled the scaling of all variables such as MBP, pH, CI, etc. in standard deviations from control, rather than in individual units such as mm Hg, pH units, or liters per minute per square meter. All of the individual normalized multivariable data sets were then subjected to a cluster analysis procedure,[23] in which data-inferred groupings of patient data sets were selected by a criterion which partitions the physiologic space of the eleven variables into regions. The patient samples grouped within a region were most like the eleven-dimensional mean of that group and most different from the multidimensional mean of other groups.

Their studies of this classification technique showed that, compared to the reference control group (R-state), the entire spectrum of clinical severity in patients with trauma, sepsis, or cardiogenic shock could be viewed in terms of four pathophysiologic states (A, B, C, and D) (Fig. 6).[77] The prototype patient of each of these abnormal states can be described by the physiologic pattern of the multivariable means of the group

(Fig. 7). In this figure each pathophysiologic pattern (dark line) is compared to the perfect circle (heavy circle) of the normalized control mean (R state). The specific individual variable abnormalities manifested by the prototype patient of each state can be evaluated by their difference from the R-state mean in standard deviations, increased or decreased (light circles).

Observing these prototype patterns, one can see that the A-state patient represents a compensated stress response characteristic of an adequate reaction to sepsis, surgery, or trauma. In this A-state pattern there is a statistically significant increase in cardiac index and heart rate, and a decrease in ejection time. Important also is the increase in myocardial contractility reflected by the decrease in cardiac mixing time (tm) and a more rapid pulmonary dispersive transit time (td). However, there is no significant change in any of the parameters of oxygen consumption (A-V Diff, VpO$_2$) or peripheral metabolism (VpCO$_2$ or VpH). Indeed, the net increase in cardiac flow adequately meets all of the body demands.[77, 79]

The B- and C-states are physiologic patterns of increasing severity characteristic of deteriorating stages in the septic process. In the B-state, a hyperdynamic cardiovascular pattern fails to supply peripheral needs adequately, and in spite of an increased cardiac output, the arteriovenous oxygen difference narrows, oxygen consumption often falls, and a metabolic acidosis with a fall in venous pH ensues. The C-state is seen when a respiratory decompensation is superimposed on the unbalanced septic process seen in the B-state. There is a profound septic shock with a fall in MBP in spite of a normal level of cardiac output, due to a fall in the vascular tone. A combined metabolic and respiratory acidosis occurs which is matched by a corresponding impairment in oxygen exchange.[79] In contrast, in the cardiogenic or D-state patient, a primary cardiac rather than a primary peripheral failure pattern occurs. There is a fall in cardiac contractility reflected by the lengthening of the cardiac mixing time (tm). The pulmonary dispersive mean transit time (tm) also increases as the cardiac index decreases. A marked rise in arteriovenous oxygen difference (A-V diff) occurs, which is generally proportionate to the fall in cardiac flow, and reflects the severity of the decrease in perfusion. Hypotension and acidosis may also occur, but are not characteristic statistical features of this pattern of physiologic abnormality.

It is unlikely that any individual patient will be exactly like the prototype patient whose values represent the multivariable patterns of means which define the characteristic physiologic states. However, the value of these prototype states is that they provide a grid which can be placed over the real physiologic continuum so that a given real patient can be classified, and his physiologic motion in this continuum can be quantified by study of his specific changing physiologic pattern.

Clearly these serial multivariable patterns are defining something about the time-course trajectory of these patients' response to injury or surgical stress.[76] They describe his movement through a multidimensional physiologic hyperspace, where the various regions, R, A, B, C, and D, represent different types of physiologic or pathophysiologic accommodations. As is shown in Figure 8, each region represents a specific set of patterns describing various kinds of compensated or decompensated responses to stress. The value of the prototype mean patterns shown in Figure 7 is not merely that they summarize the type of pathophysiologic response, but more important that they provide a scale by which change can be measured. Using this metric, it is possible to quantify precisely a patient's physiologic position at a given time by his "distance" from each of the "prototype" state means (R, A, B, C, and D) (Fig. 8). Since these distances are all normalized with respect to the reference of the control R-state, and since each state mean represents a different kind of response (A—compensated stress response, B—unbalanced septic response, C—decompensated septic shock, and D—cardiogenic decompensation), the nature and degree of a specific patient's pathophysiologic inadequacy can be inferred from the absolute distance from a given state or from the distance ratios between various states (Fig. 8).

By studying the sequential movements of different kinds of surgical patients as they moved in this physiologic hyperspace, Siegel and his colleagues[76] were able to define the statistical envelope of acceptable and nonacceptable time courses in a number of disease entities. In a study of patient recoveries after coronary artery bypass surgery, they showed that there were three types of recovery trajectories (Fig. 9A). There were two acceptable recovery trajectories, type I in which the patient's response to bypass surgery was movement into a normal stress response A-state with rapid recovery to the preoperative control R-state, and type II in which the patient had a transient myocardial depression into the cardiogenic D-state with a slower recovery trajectory through the A- and R-states. Both trajectories are associated with acceptable clinical courses, although a type II recovery should

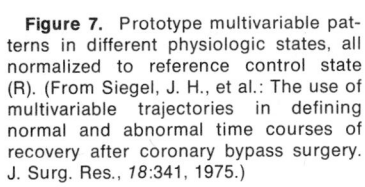

Figure 7. Prototype multivariable patterns in different physiologic states, all normalized to reference control state (R). (From Siegel, J. H., et al.: The use of multivariable trajectories in defining normal and abnormal time courses of recovery after coronary bypass surgery. J. Surg. Res., *18*:341, 1975.)

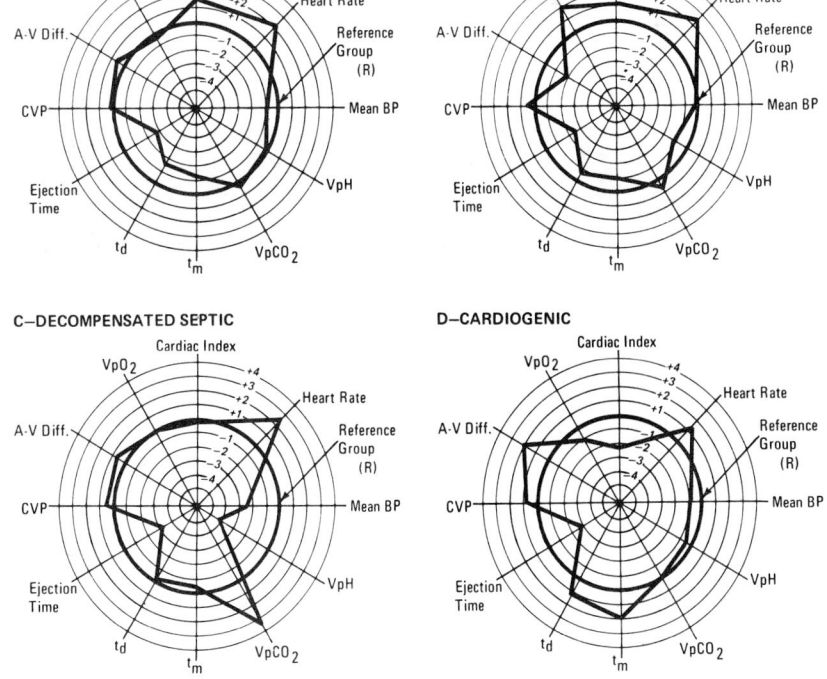

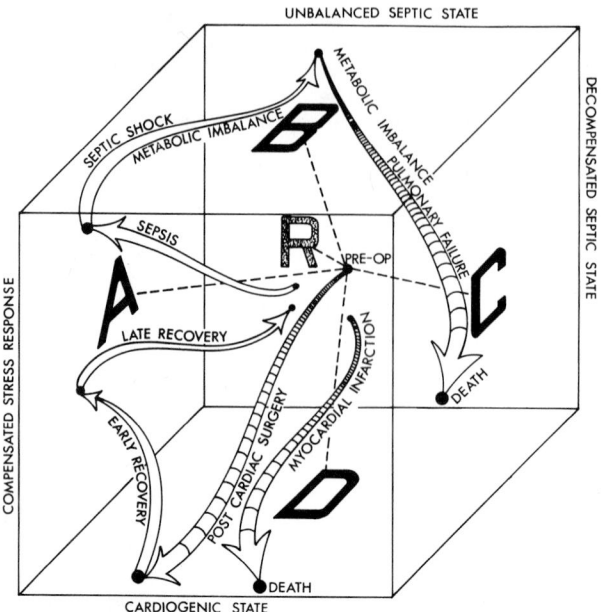

Figure 8. Diagram of patient time-course trajectories in physiologic state space. (From Siegel, J. H., et al.: The use of multivariable trajectories in defining normal and abnormal time courses of recovery after coronary bypass surgery. J. Surg. Res., *18*:341, 1975.)

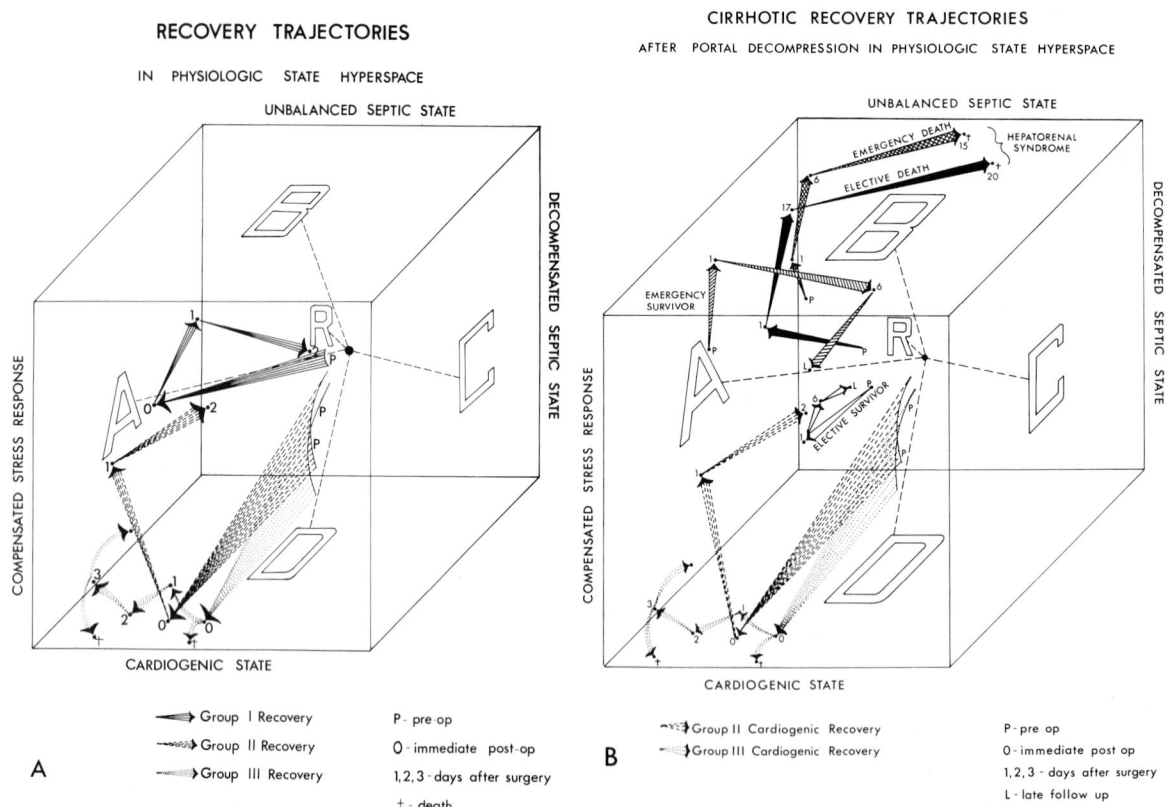

Figure 9. *A,* Three different types of recovery trajectories in patients undergoing coronary artery bypass surgery. *B,* Recovery trajectories of four cirrhotic patients after portal decompressive surgery. Compared with Group II and Group III cardiogenic recoveries from *A.* (From Siegel, J. H. *In* Siegel, J. H., and Chodoff, P. (Eds.): The Aged and High Risk Surgical Patient: Medical, Surgical, and Anesthetic Management. New York, Grune & Stratton, Inc., 1976.)

give the physician some concern. However, there is also an unacceptable type III recovery, in which the postcoronary bypass patient falls out of the statistical envelope of the least acceptable type II recovery. This type of trajectory is always associated with serious clinical complications or death.

The value of this type of serial analysis of recovery is that the physiologic evidence of transition from an acceptable recovery trajectory to a pathologic one usually occurs some time before a clear clinical pattern is evident. At worst, their study[76] showed that appearance of a type III trajectory can alert the surgeon to the significance of what may be an unclear clinical trend, and at best it demonstrated that the alteration in the recovery trajectory in response to a therapeutic maneuver can be used by the surgeon to gauge the effectiveness of his therapy. This is shown in Figure 10, in which the time trajectories of the ratio of the patient's physiologic distances between the prototype mean of the cardiogenic D-state and the normal stress response A-state (D/A ratio) are compared for three coronary bypass patients with a recovery pattern different than the statistical envelope of the least acceptable, type II recovery trajectory. Patient LD shows an excellent type I physiologic recovery which was associated with a normal clinical course. Patient BS had an immediate postoperative type III recovery which fell below the standard deviation envelope of the usual type II recovery and clinically required intra-aortic balloon counterpulsation (IAB) to be maintained. Furthermore each time the IAB was discontinued for a short period as a test, the D/A ratio fell (down arrows), until sometime on the second postoperative day, when a sustained trajectory rise occurred, associated with clinical stability. In contrast, patient HD, whose preoperative D/A ratio was below the lowest point in the statistical recovery trajectory envelope of type II

patients, could not be resuscitated after circulatory bypass and died in surgery.

In other types of pathologic conditions, the patient's response to surgical stress is associated with a totally different recovery trajectory. Figure 9B shows the trajectories of four patients with cirrhotic liver disease and portal hypertension who underwent portal decompression surgery. Lack of recovery in these patients and the development of a fatal hepatorenal syndrome was associated with a nonrecovery trajectory into a progressively worsening unbalanced hyperdynamic B-state.

Time Series Analysis

A relatively new type of statistical analytic technique which shows great promise of providing important physiologic information of potentially great value in studies of surgical physiology is time series analysis. These techniques[9, 59, 60, 89, 98] permit the analysis of the cross correlation and lag-time correlation between two or more physiologic variable time streams. By examination of the relevant cross products of the variables over time, time series techniques can permit the study of normal diurnal variations. Also, the precise definition of the temporal relationship of the interaction of one or more hormones in normal or abnormal rhythm can be detected by these techniques. As an example, Vagnucci et al.[96] have applied this evolving analytic technology to the study of the time pattern of hormonal interrelationships between aldosterone, cortisol, growth hormone, and plasma renin in normal patients and in a patient with an aldosterone-producing adenoma. These preliminary data suggest a different cross correlation pattern between aldosterone secretion and renin activity, and between aldosterone and cortisol secretion in the patient with a functioning aldosterone producing tumor compared to controls. However, the application and validation of these techniques in quantifying biologic phenomena are in their infancy and their great potential needs to be demonstrated by further investigative work.

These type of data suggest that the application of various multivariable statistical techniques may provide us with a means for quantitative characterization of the nature of the specific system failures and their interactions. In addition, as noted by Stacy,[91] this quantitative information should provide the input for appropriate statistical and other types of mathematic models by which the computer may assist the surgeon in evaluating the probability that a given individual will move into a crisis situation.

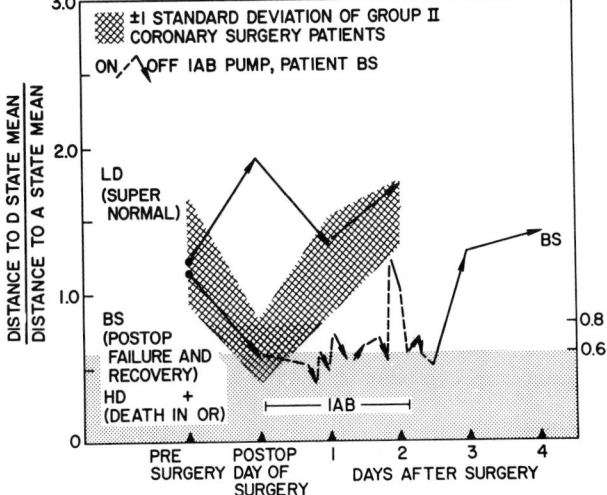

Figure 10. Time trajectories of D/A ratios of three patients with recovery patterns different from usual Group I or Group II patients. Shown against ± standard deviation of Group II time trajectories. (From Siegel, J. H., et al.: The use of multivariable trajectories in defining normal and abnormal time courses of recovery after coronary bypass surgery. J. Surg. Res., *18*:341, 1975.)

THE USE OF COMPUTER TECHNOLOGY IN THE DELINEATION OF PHYSIOLOGIC MODELS

The principle behind the application of mathematical modeling to physiologic systems is an attempt to extract more information from the observed data by fitting them with a set of equations that can be used to describe quantitatively particular aspects of the system. There are two general kinds of modeling techniques, *stochastic* models and *deterministic* models.

Stochastic models are statistical in nature and generally apply principles of probability to the analysis of data samples. This does not mean that the process being described by the model is necessarily random in nature; rather, it may be the result of a very complex set of deterministic reactions—so complex indeed that the process can only be characterized statistically. The best known examples of this approach are related to the use of Baye's theory to reproduce the process of a sequential differential diagnosis by computer techniques[29, 101, 102] and the "random walk" model of indicator dilution.[109] The time series analysis described earlier also lends itself well to the development of probability models of a stochastic nature.[9, 60]

Much greater use has been made of deterministic modeling, possibly because the statistical weighting factors required for the practical use of stochastic models in clinical situations are largely unknown. Although few of the deterministic models that have been used to solve biologic problems are pure, it is conceptually useful to classify them as being of one of three types—representational, functional, or physical.

Representational models are largely concerned with fitting an observed biologic signal with a mathematical function and then trying to relate changes in the model parameters to the biologic phenomena. Examples of this approach can be seen in curve fitting by use of Fourier series to derive transfer functions across various vascular beds,[18] using a lagged normal density function to model arterial dye dilution,[7] and the application of gamma variate functions to the central aortic indicator dilution curve.[31] This approach can often be useful in quantitatively characterizing a biologic signal for analytic purposes, but suffers from the disadvantage that it is often difficult to interpret the parameters of a representational model in physiologic terms. Another problem, which can arise with any model but is more frequently found in representa-tional models, is that because the model does not really describe the system it may not produce a good fit over the entire biologic range of variation. This is true of the gamma variate function that has been applied to predict operative mortality in the elderly from the indicator dilution curve.[31] It approximates the dye curve over the physiologic range of function, but provides a poor and inconsistent representation of the very low output pathophysiologic dye curves found in myocardial infarction shock and of the very high output curves found in patients with hyperdynamic septic shock or cirrhotic liver disease.[78]

Mathematical representations of biologic signals have often been developed into true functional models in an attempt to characterize various aspects of the system generating the signal. Such models can be considered as attempts to describe the general biochemical or physiologic functions of the system in circumstances where it is difficult to develop or test sufficiently detailed mathematical expressions of the mechanical or physiochemical properties, or control mechanisms, that are aspects of the system. Examples of this approach to solving certain surgical problems by using relatively simple functional models for the analysis of the volume of distribution of various radioisotopic materials in intracellular, extracellular, and intravascular body compartments have been presented by Moore.[51] These techniques define compartment models that rely on the interpretation of the exponential decay curve of an indicator substance. This approach has been used by Zollinger et al.[100] to measure the rate and volume of exchange between plasma and interstitial fluid in human hemorrhage.

A more sophisticated model of this functional type has been used by Spencer, Long, and Kinney[90] and Long et al.[43] to evaluate the metabolic utilization of glucose in critically ill patients (Fig. 11). Their model is an attempt to describe the kinetics of glucose metabolism in man in terms of a multipool system in which there are several body compartment sizes for

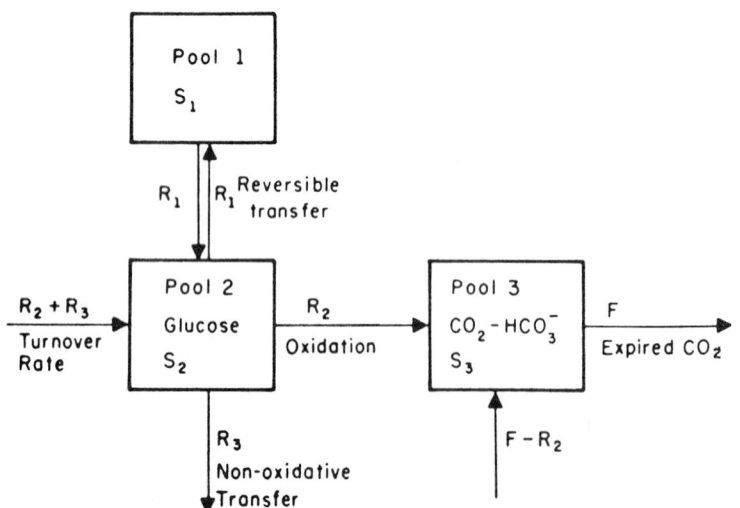

Figure 11. Three-pool functional model of ^{14}C glucose decay and $^{14}CO_2$ appearance for kinetics of glucose metabolism in man. (From Spencer, J. L., et al.: I&EC Fundamentals, *10*:2, 1971.)

metabolically exchangeable carbon, with different transfer rates between compartments. This model describes the system as being composed of two glucose pools, and one pool of carbon representing the labile carbon dioxide stores of the body (carbon dioxide and bicarbonate). One glucose pool is considered as being freely exchangeable with blood glucose (S_2), and the other represents a carbon source of potential glucose bound as glycogen, lactate, glycoproteins, and so forth, which is not well mixed with blood glucose (S_1). The two glucose pools have a reversible transfer (R_1) between them, but the CO_2-HCO_3^- pool (S_3) represents a one-way oxidation reaction (R_2) from the freely exchangeable glucose pool. By using ^{14}C-labeled glucose and measuring the decay in specific activity over time in blood glucose and expired carbon dioxide and fitting the observed curves with the model, the investigators were able to compute model parameters reflecting the size and rate of exchange of each of the pools. Their data suggested that major injury more than doubles the glucose pool sizes and the glucose turnover rate, as well as the size of the carbon dioxide pool. The utility of applying this functional model to a problem in human metabolism is that it not only provides great insight into the nature of alterations in carbohydrate metabolism in the critically ill, but also has considerable clinical significance, since it demonstrates that in spite of a tendency to hyperglycemia the injured patient is capable of markedly increasing the oxidation rate of glucose.

A functional model of a somewhat different type has been used by Siegel et al.[78] to explain the dynamic interrelationships between cardiac and pulmonary vascular function in various forms of human shock. By modifying and conceptually expanding the representational approach used by Bassingthwaighte et al.[7] to describe indicator dilution, these workers have attempted to analyze the indicator dilution curve obtained across the central circulation into four independent functions that can be parametrically represented (Fig. 12). In addition to the all-over flow that quantifies the cardiac output, three other elementary dilution functions with a physiologic interpretation are used to fit the observed dye curve: mixing, dispersion, and delay. The delay function is primarily related to the transit of dye particles through large vessels with laminar flow, the mixing function appears related to the dynamic aspects of the ventricles, and the dispersive function reflects the characteristics of the small vessel pulmonary vascular bed. This model was applied to the analysis of more than 1300 dye curves from nearly 300 patients with a variety of shock states and other forms of critical illness having a circulatory component. The authors were able to demonstrate both clinically and experimentally that the dynamic characteristics of the mixing parameter appeared related to the durational aspects of myocardial contractile function, thus providing an index of cardiac performance (Fig. 13). Compared to a group of preoperative high-risk patients, patients with myocardial infarctions showed prolonged mixing times (tm) and had reduced ejection fractions (EF), but septic and cirrhotic patients with hyperdynamic states showed reduced mixing times and increased ejection fractions.

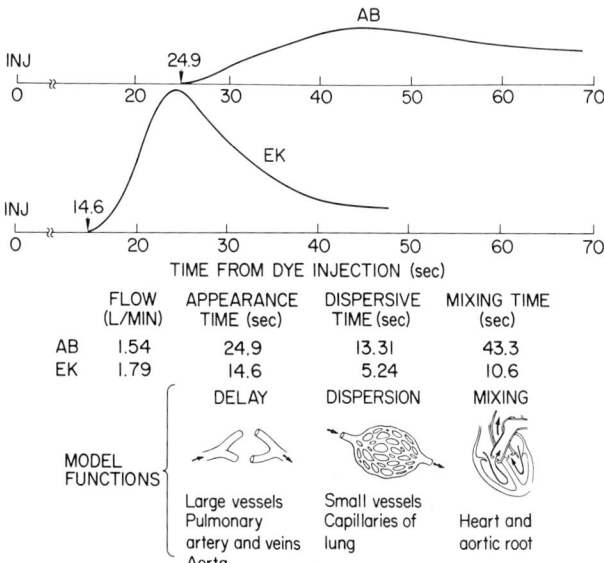

	FLOW (L/MIN)	APPEARANCE TIME (sec)	DISPERSIVE TIME (sec)	MIXING TIME (sec)
AB	1.54	24.9	13.31	43.3
EK	1.79	14.6	5.24	10.6

Figure 12. Dye curves and model parameters from two patients with acute myocardial infarction shock, prior to IAB. (From Siegel, J. H., Farrell, E. J., Goldwyn, R. M., and Friedman, H. P.: The surgical implications of physiologic patterns in myocardial infarction shock. Surgery, 72:126–141, 1972.)

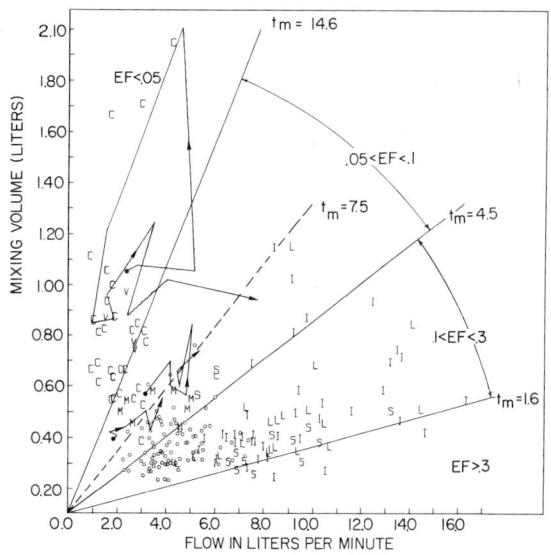

Figure 13. Ventricular mixing mean transit time (t_m) as model parameter reflecting myocardial contractile function in high-risk and critically ill patients. M = myocardial infarction; C = infarction shock; V = old myocardial infarction with left ventricular aneurysm; O = control preoperative; I = sepsis; S = septic shock; L = cirrhotic liver disease with portal hypertension. Trajectories show response to intra-aortic balloon counterpulsation of three patients with myocardial infarction shock who survived shock episodes. (From Siegel, J. H., et al.: Quantifying the need for cardiac support in human shock by a functional model of cardiopulmonary vascular dynamics: with special reference to MI. J. Surg. Res., 13:166, 1972.)

When myocardial depression or failure occurred, the tm lengthened and EF fell, even though cardiac output remained at normal or increased levels. Siegel and his colleagues[77, 78] also used this model to examine the relationship between cardiac mixing and nonmixing central volumes in patients with myocardial infarction shock. These investigators were able to show that those patients with prolonged duration of cardiac mixing, who also showed evidence for a cardiac nonmixing volume, producing a large increase in the dispersive mean transit time, were not capable of responding to conservative measures for the treatment of their infarct shock, but instead required assisted circulation if there were to be any possibility for resuscitation. Their work suggests that the application of such inferential techniques may make it possible to quantify the response to therapy in this difficult group of patients (see Fig. 13), and perhaps to indicate when emergency myocardial revascularization procedures may be necessary in addition to temporary circulatory support.

In some sense the most intellectually elegant mathematical approach to the description of biologic phenomena is provided by physical modeling. In modeling of this type, an attempt is made to model each significant element of the system by an appropriate mathematical term. The analysis of the arterial pressure pulse to obtain stroke volume by deriving a constant for the resistance and compliance factors of the proximal aorta described earlier is an example of such modeling in its simplest form. A lumped-parameter physical model of the human vascular system has been described by Goldwyn and Watt[27] for arterial pressure pulse analysis. More elaborate physical models of pulse wave transmission along the arterial tree that could be used in man have been derived by Streeter et al.,[93] by Patel,[61] by Noordergraaf,[105] and by Snyder and Rideout.[88] Gomez and his colleagues[28] have modeled the continuous distribution of tidal volume throughout the lung, and Moreno et al.[53] have developed a very sophisticated physical model that permits the description of venous return to the right heart and its modification by the hepatic fibrotic changes induced by cirrhotic liver disease.

Simulation Models

Simulation is an interesting and important extension of computer-based modeling which has been mainly confined to physical models because of their preciseness in describing biologic phenomena. A particularly valuable application of this approach with direct relevance to clinical surgical problems is the study of computer simulation of arterial dynamics in the human leg undertaken by Raines et al. (Fig. 14).[64] These workers evaluated the effects of alterations in arterial dimensions, compliance, flow distribution, blood viscosity, and resistance changes due to vasoconstriction or vasodilation on the characteristics of the distal arterial pressure pulse using one-dimensional nonlinear equations of fluid motion modeled on a digital computer. Their technique enabled them to simulate various geometric and physical properties of the arterial tree of the lower extremity in health and disease. It has had direct application in the interpretation of the significance of clinical pressure pulse

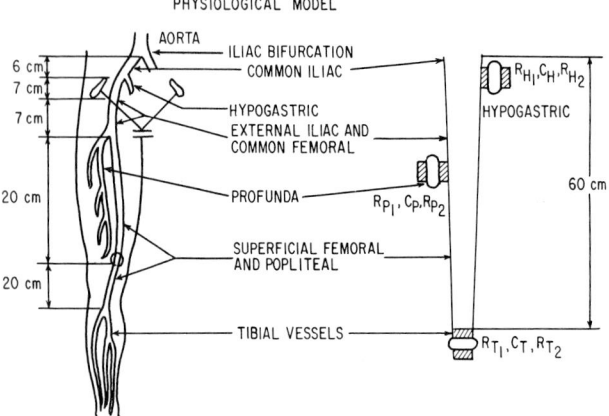

Figure 14. Structure of human arterial tree of lower extremity and computer simulation model. (From Raines, J. K., et al.: Structure of human arterial tree of lower extremity and computer simulation model. J. Biomech., 7:77, 1974.)

waves in patients with peripheral arteriosclerotic occlusive disease.

In another very useful area of simulation Maloney et al.[46] and Villamil et al.[99] have attempted to develop a computer-based model simulating the biochemical interactions involved in the maintenance of acid-base homeostasis in blood. More recently, Deland, Wolf, and Dell[19] have combined their model of body fluid homeostasis as input to what they describe as a "behavioral" model of the human kidney. This simulation functions like the kidney with regard to input and output, but does not mimic the detailed physical and chemical mechanisms by which the real kidney accomplishes its task (Fig. 15). Using this complex simulation they have developed a research and teaching tool which permits abnormal cases to be "treated" by medical students at a computer terminal (Fig. 16). The results of therapy can be evaluated in simulation and experiments designed to test clinical hypotheses.

A third major area of simulation applied to problems in human physiology with clinical potential has been concerned with gas transport in the lungs[24, 28, 58] and respiratory regulation.[21, 30, 42, 108] In this area Siegel and Farrell[75] have developed a complex model of cardiopulmonary function to study the respiratory regulation of blood gases in the critically ill patient (Fig. 17). This simulation permits the evaluation of the interaction of the nonlinear complex processes of respiration and pulmonary perfusion and their control in the setting of human pathophysiology in the various shock states described earlier in this chapter. It includes functions which describe the metabolic exchange rate and blood transport of oxygen, carbon dioxide, and acid; the respiratory capability of the lung with regard to resistance, compliance, ventilation, and perfusion; the pulmonary blood flow, blood volume, and veno-arterial shunt; the alveolar-capillary diffusion of gases across the pulmonary interstitial space; and the ventilatory control sensitivity

GENERALIZED SIGNAL FLOW DIAGRAM, BEHAVIORAL KIDNEY MODEL

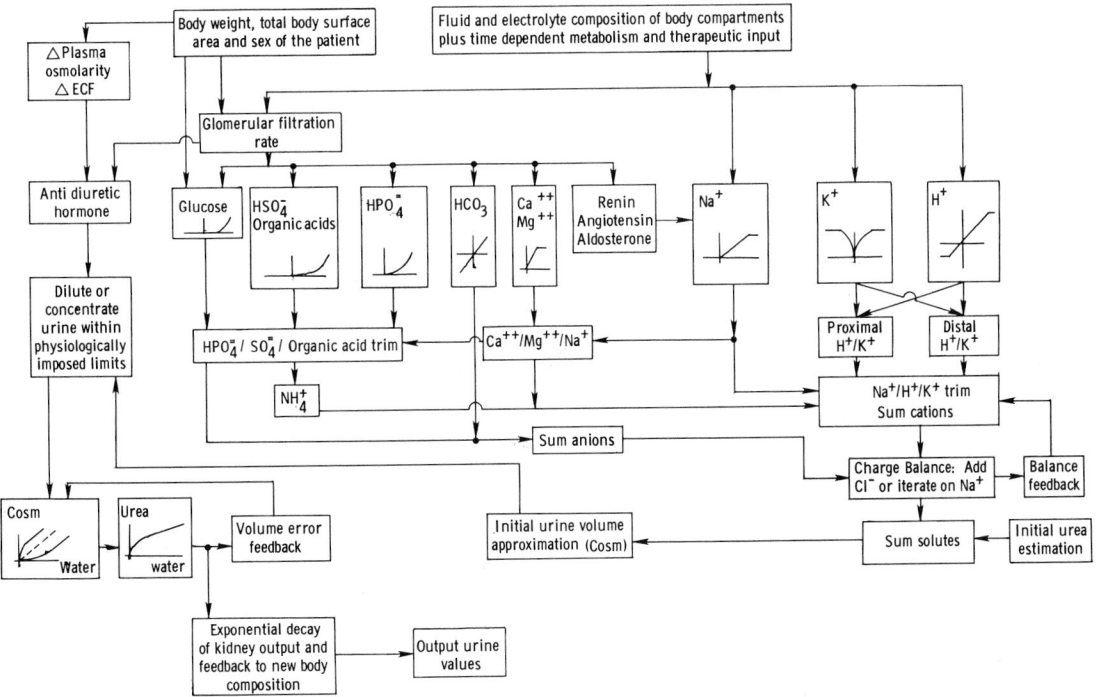

Figure 15. Behavioral model of functions of human kidney. (Courtesy of E. C. DeLand, University of California at Los Angeles.)

Figure 16. Application of behavioral model of kidney to study of response to ingestion of water or saline (above); and response to infusion of isotonic saline in severely dehydrated patient with acidosis (below). (Courtesy of E. C. DeLand, University of California at Los Angeles.)

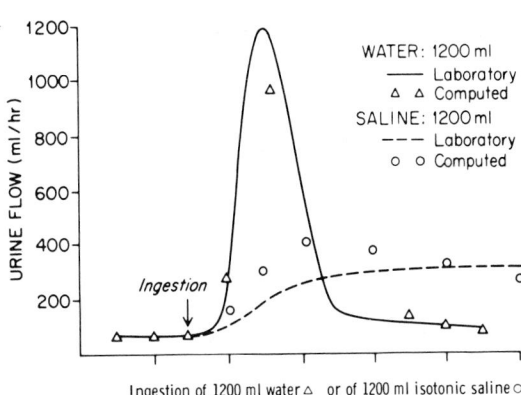

Ingestion of 1200 ml water △ or of 1200 ml isotonic saline ○ Data from Pitts, Physiology of the Kidney and Body Fluids, Yearbook Publishers, Chicago, 1963, 2nd Edition.

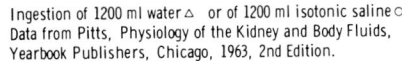

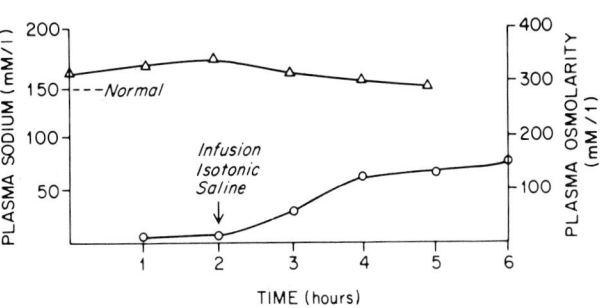

Severe dehydration with acidosis. Kidney remains essentially shutdown until expansion of extracellular fluid volume (Computed).

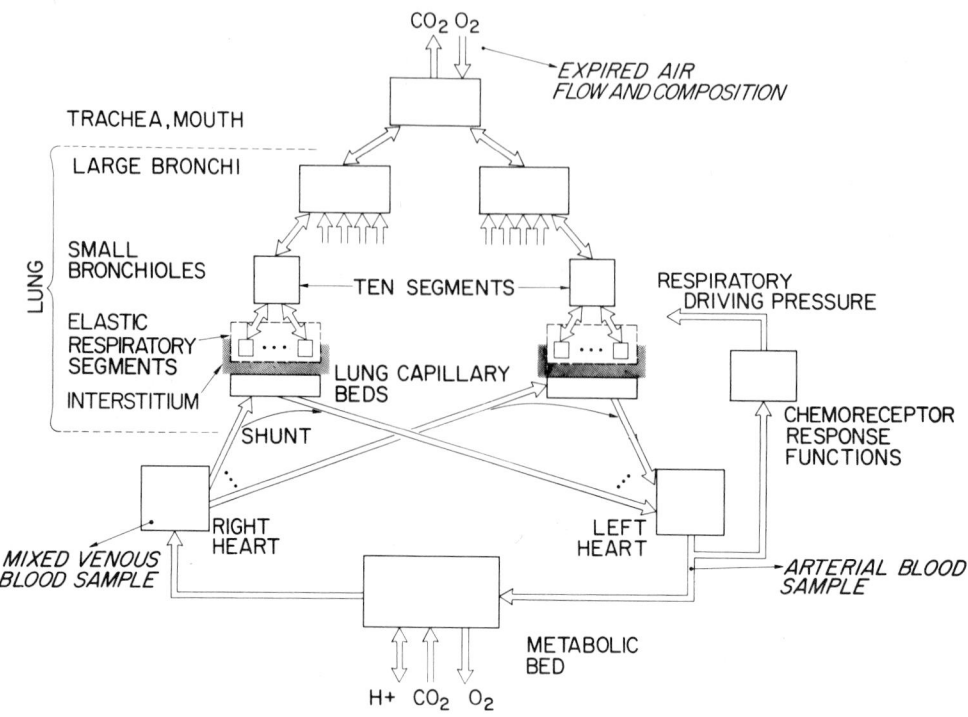

Figure 17. Model of cardiopulmonary interaction and respiratory control. (From Farrell, E. J., and Siegel, J. H.: Investigation of cardiorespiratory abnormalities through computer simulation. Comput. Biomed. Res., 5:161, 1973.)

to changes in arterial carbon dioxide and oxygen tensions, and pH. These investigators have used this simulation to explore systematically how alterations in cardiac output and alveolar ventilation, and their respective distributions, interact in the patient with the post-traumatic lung syndrome (Fig. 18), and thus to understand how the transitions between the prototype pathophysiologic states shown in Figure 7 can occur.[75, 79] Their present studies are directed at its use as a predictor of the patients' response to cardiorespiratory support measures in various forms of pulmonary insufficiency, under conditions where the real patients' physiologic data form the starting point for the simulation of various therapeutic measures. Although at present no computer simulation application has produced entirely reliable predictive models for anticipating patient responses to therapy, it seems likely that in the near future the evolution of this technique will permit the development of automated treatment diagnostics which can be utilized to guide the surgeon's approach to the physiologic care of the critically ill.

Another important area where computer technology may be of use in solving surgical problems related to modeling is image processing, in which scanning algorithms provide models to enable the recognition and retrieval of roentgenographic images. These techniques may serve to permit enhancement of difficult

vascular patterns preparatory to vascular surgery, and the utilization of computer techniques to compute the volumes and dynamic aspects of the ventricles of the heart[5, 14, 15, 32, 33] and the alterations in the distribution of coronary and pulmonary blood flow.[17] Studies along these lines suggest that areas of dyskinetic or nonfunctioning myocardium may be identified by these techniques[14, 32, 33] and this may perhaps assist in the evaluation of patients for whom coronary artery revascularization procedures or ventricular aneurysmectomy is considered.

COMPUTER-ASSISTED INSTRUCTION IN SURGICAL EDUCATION

A number of interesting attempts have been made to apply computer technology in the area of programed learning as related to undergraduate surgical education. Notable in this regard are the studies of Fonkalsrud et al.[22] in which fourth-year medical students at the University of California at Los Angeles were permitted to interact with the computer to obtain instruction as to how to proceed with a sequential evaluation of surgical patients. These programs were an effort to let students learn how to establish the correct diagnosis as efficiently as possible, and to teach them how to recommend the most logical course of treatment for a specific condition. Another computer-based instructional program along these general lines is that described by Williams et al.,[106] which has been used in the Ohio State University College of Medicine pilot medical school project. The Ohio State programs were designed to produce a computer-based tutorial evaluation system to permit students to engage in an independent study program which enables the integration of a multidisciplinary curriculum. The approach used also permits both the students and the faculty to evaluate student responses and the efficiency of programed learning, and to obtain a detailed cost effectiveness analysis for this method of teaching. Recently, Warner et al.[103] have implemented a program for computer-assisted instruction in clinical decision making which uses a model of history taking and diagnosis based on Baysean conditional probability. This program was used in an experimental project for teaching medical and surgical problems to first- and second-year medical students at the University of Utah and was enthusiastically received by the students. While in none of these studies has it been possible to show a statistically significant computer-derived advantage in terms of quantitative knowledge learned by the student, the qualitative data have suggested that computer-based education programs may facilitate closer student guidance, provide an earlier introduction to clinical problems, and present the student with an opportunity for continuing self-evaluation.

COMPUTER APPLICATIONS TO DELIVERY OF HEALTH CARE AND CONTINUING MEDICAL EDUCATION IN SURGERY

It is ideally only a short step from the development of computer-based systems designed for clinical research to their application in delivery of health care. Unfortunately, this step has been difficult to achieve in practice. Unquestionably, the patient monitoring systems described earlier are being used in patient care, as are the computer-based assessment systems used in the development of physiologic indices, but these applications have been limited to a few institutions with specially trained personnel, where they have been accepted primarily because of their research interest and only then secondarily applied as a service medium for patient care. The main barriers to the widespread use of computer-based care systems lie in three areas: (1) the need to delineate indices of patient status which provide the surgeon or intensive care specialist with essential information concerning patient status that he *cannot obtain* without the computer analysis of patient data; (2) the need to combine the technology with a program of continuing education and training for medical and paramedical personnel in the techniques of physiologic data collection and analysis, so that they can interpret the computer output; and (3) the cost of maintaining a large system and the need to justify this cost as a necessary expense of

Figure 18. Application of cardiorespiratory model to study of interrelationship of changing cardiac output and reduction in alveolar exchange volume in adult respiratory distress syndrome. (From Siegel, J. H., et al.: Chapter 25. *In* Siegel, J. H., and Chodoff, P. (Eds.): The Aged and High Risk Surgical Patient: Medical, Surgical, and Anesthetic Management. New York, Grune & Stratton, Inc., 1976.)

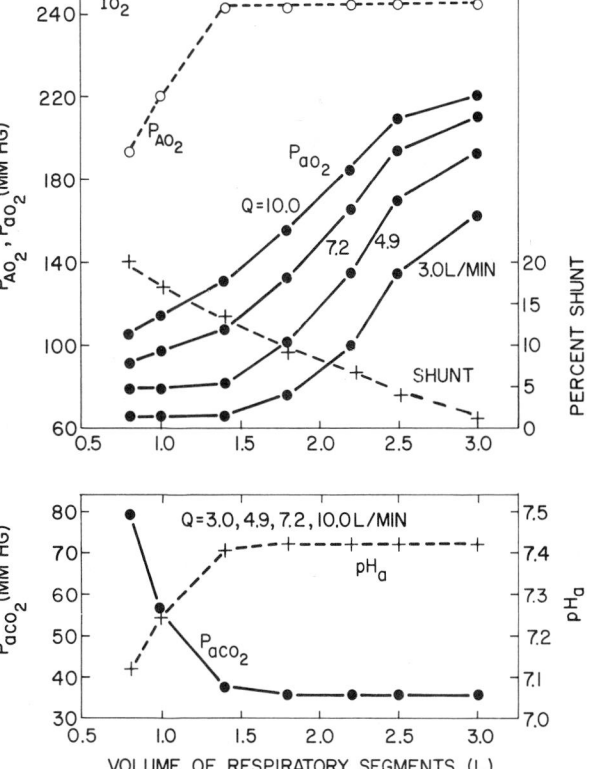

good patient care to federal, state, and private third-party hospital reimbursement sources who must pay the bill. A number of important attempts have been made to define the price tag involved in the allocation of computer time to patient care services.[44, 70] The real questions raised by such studies, however, are those related to medical cost and quality effectiveness rather than merely the cost of utilization. There are many examples of an anecdotal nature demonstrating the value of computer-based monitoring, and as shown earlier, there are also important investigations yielding computer-derived indices of prognostic or therapeutic significance. However, as yet it remains to be demonstrated statistically that computer utilization of this sort will effectively provide a better understanding of the patient's clinical problems and a greater patient salvage rate than can be obtained by careful bedside observation and judgment with present manual techniques.

The answers to these important questions will in the end determine the future of computer technology as applied to health care delivery. Nevertheless, there have been a number of important and interesting approaches to the task of utilizing computer techniques in the area of patient care and continuing education as it relates to patient care. A considerable amount of work has been devoted to computerization of the medical record so as to obtain a uniform medical history that can be used as a data base from which the physician or surgeon can begin his evaluation. Notable contributions in this area have been made by Weed,[104] Slack et al.,[87] Mayne et al.,[49] Warner et al.,[103] and Barnett.[6] A considerable effort has also been expended in addressing the problem of how best to use the computer in clinical decision making, and in defining the logical process of arriving at a differential diagnosis.[29, 102, 103] In a specific application to surgical problems, Mauney et al.[48] developed an automated interviewing technique that is suitable for use with patients in a surgical outpatient clinic, to assist the physician or paramedical personnel in arriving at a differential diagnosis and in selecting suitable diagnostic studies with which to confirm an initial impression. In a related approach Chodoff and Drews[13] have attempted to utilize automated techniques for preanesthetic interviewing of patients prior to elective surgery. Their approach is based on a series of decision modules in which the computer selects possibilities on the basis of weighted criteria in order to determine whether additional diagnostic and therapeutic procedures must be carried out.

In an extension of this type of approach, a number of workers have attempted to use the computer as a consultant in assisting the physician to understand complex metabolic problems. Most notable in this regard is the work of Bleich,[8] who developed a program to assist the physician in evaluating the significance of acid-base disorders. In this ingenious program, the physician is queried concerning the specific biochemical abnormalities and certain clinical features present in his patient. The program then computes the remaining acid-base data based on the Henderson-Hasselbalch equation, and suggests the possible cause of the specific disorder, as well as providing some recommendations regarding treatment, with appropriate references. The program is designed for remote operation from distant locations, and has undergone extensive testing in a number of institutions.

A somewhat more elaborate research endeavor more directly related to surgical problems is the CARE system designed by Siegel and colleagues,[80, 84, 85] which is now operational on a national time-sharing service. In this application the computer is used more as a "living textbook" applied to the problem of care organization, record keeping, and assessment of critically ill or injured patients. This program, which also is based on the manual entry of data, interrogates the surgeon concerning the specific aspects of the patient's major disease process and intercurrent diseases. It also demands certain relevant biochemical and hematologic data, and on the basis of this information produces a problem-oriented history (Fig. 19), as well as providing estimates of the magnitude of acute fluid deficits (Fig. 20) and the probable maintenance requirements of fluid, electrolytes, calories, and protein. In addition, it provides the surgeon with a series of therapeutic suggestions and cautions related to the specific disease entity as manifested in that patient, as well as to particular intercurrent disease problems that are present (Fig. 21). Once the initial assessment of a patient has been entered, the program also establishes a 15-day data bank for continuing patient management. This bank includes interrogative programs for entry of nurses' and physicians' notes, intake and output data, and laboratory studies. Using a set of regression equations derived from the metabolic studies of Moore,[52] and physiologic equations from Consolazio,[16] it computes daily estimates of fluid, electrolyte, and nitrogen balances derived from the primary input and output data. Modifying factors are introduced based on intercurrent diseases and changes in the patient's status, as well as on alterations in the cumulative balance of metabolic data. Attention is called to specific abnormalities in serum electrolytes, renal clearances, and metabolic and clinical data, and a continuing set of therapeutic suggestions and cautions is available for the physician's instruction as desired. Programs are also available under this system for the computation and evaluation of selected hemodynamic and respiratory data and for physiologic state classification and analysis of recovery trajectories.[76, 77]

None of these approaches to patient care is designed to provide all the mechanisms of consultation, but merely to apply information from the literature and clinical experience to guide the management of specific patient abnormalities. However, in the CARE system[80, 84, 85] the time-shared aspects were intended to provide a medium of consultation by which the responsible surgeon may present patient data to a remote, but more experienced consultant, in a form that enhances the latter's ability to provide a meaningful consultation. These systems were thought of as providing a framework around which a continuing teaching and training program for doctors in outlying hospitals and residents could be designed. At the present moment, however, while there are several large hospital and regional systems for medical record keeping,[1, 8, 49, 97] no system for patient management decisions has been ex-

```
            INITIAL ASSESSMENT OF THE CRITICALLY ILL
                         PROBLEM HISTORY
           PATIENT JAMES       SMITH         NUMBER 2222222
                    HOSPITAL BGH    RACE - WHITE
    AGE 36. YRS   SEX M   BODY WT  72.0 KG   BSA 1.97 SQ M   BLOOD TYPE O-
           DATE 08/13/74           TIME   9 HOURS  0 MINUTES

    BLOOD PRESSURE 124/ 70  HEART RT  70/MIN  RESP RT 12/MIN  TEMP 100.0 F

    PATIENT'S MAJOR ACUTE PROBLEM:
               MAJOR SOFT TISSUE INJURY W-W/O FRACTURES

    INJURY TO:
                   CHEST AND ABDOMEN
                   EXTREMITY
                   MULTIPLE TRAUMA
                   FACE OR JAW
    INJURY OCCURRED  5 HOURS 45 MINUTES PRIOR TO ADMISSION TO UNIT
    PERITONEAL TAP REVEALS NON-CLOTTING BLOOD
    FRACTURE OF:
                   JAW
                   RIGHT FLAIL CHEST
                   LEFT  FLAIL CHEST
                   RIGHT CLAVICLE
                   LEFT  CLAVICLE
    MAJOR HEMORRHAGE ASSOCIATED WITH INJURY
    THERE IS EVIDENCE OF PULMONARY TRAUMA

    GOOD URINE OUTPUT IS PRESENT
    PATIENT HAS ABDOMINAL DISTENTION
    BOWEL SOUNDS:    ABSENT
    NO FLATUS PASSING
    ASCITES ABSENT
    PATIENT HAS PAIN:
           PAIN CHARACTER   - STEADY
           MAIN LOCATION    - LEFT  UPPER QUADRANT
           MAIN RADIATION   - BACK

    PATIENT HAS NO DISEASE ASSOCIATED WITH MUSCLE WASTING IN ADDITION TO
           ACUTE PROCESS
    ATRIAL/VENTRICULAR RATE     70/ 70
    ELECTROCARDIOGRAM:
               NORMAL SINUS RHYTHM
    SEPSIS SITES:
               NONE
    WHITE CELL COUNT  16000.  CELLS/CUMM
    PATIENT LOSSES ARE ALL EXTRACORPOREAL.

    ESTIMATED VOLUME OF BLOOD LOSS          1000.00  ML
    BLOOD REPLACEMENT                        500.00  ML
    COLLOID REPLACEMENT                      500.00  ML
    ELECTROLYTE REPLACEMENT                  400.00  ML
```

Figure 19. Problem-oriented initial assessment history of patient sustaining major traumatic injury. (From Siegel, J. H., et al.: Chapter 28. *In* Siegel, J. H., and Chodoff, P. (Eds.): The Aged and High Risk Surgical Patient: Medical, Surgical, and Anesthetic Management. New York, Grune & Stratton, Inc., 1976.)

```
           PATIENT JAMES       SMITH         NUMBER 2222222
                    HOSPITAL BGH    RACE - WHITE
    AGE 36. YRS   SEX M   BODY WT  72.0 KG   BSA 1.97 SQ M   BLOOD TYPE O-
           DATE 08/13/74           TIME   9 HOURS  0 MINUTES

              INITIAL ESTIMATED BODY COMPARTMENT VOLUMES

    TOTAL BODY WATER (EXPECTED VALUE)          40.81 LITERS
    INTRACELLULAR WATER (EXPECTED VALUE)       21.54 LITERS
    EXTRACELLULAR WATER (EXPECTED VALUE)       19.27 LITERS
    BLOOD VOLUME (EXPECTED VALUE)               5.21 LITERS
    BLOOD VOLUME (PRESENT ESTIMATE)             5.21 LITERS
    PLASMA VOLUME (EXPECTED VALUE)              3.13 LITERS
    PLASMA VOLUME (PRESENT ESTIMATE)            3.37 LITERS
    RED CELL VOLUME (EXPECTED VALUE)            2.08 LITERS
    RED CELL VOLUME (PRESENT ESTIMATE)          1.84 LITERS

            SUMMARY OF ALTERATIONS IN BODY COMPOSITION
    PLASMA VOLUME            107.8% OF EXPECTED
    BLOOD VOLUME            100.0% OF EXPECTED
    RED CELL VOLUME          88.2% OF EXPECTED
    SERUM OSMOLALITY         98.0% OF NORMAL (SD 3%)      *

    THE FOLLOWING IS SUGGESTED INITIAL FLUID VOLUME REPLACEMENT FOR THIS
    PATIENT.  THIS SUGGESTED VOLUME AND ITS RATE OF ADMINISTRATION SHOULD
    BE ADJUSTED TO MAINTAIN 30 TO 50 ML/HR OF URINE UNLESS RENAL FAILURE
    OCCURS.
    THE ESTIMATED BLOOD LOSS, ASSUMING PLASMA REFILL, IS 1025. ML.
    IN ADDITION  410. ML OF BALANCED SALT SOLUTION (EG: RINGERS LACTATE)
    SHOULD BE GIVEN TO ACCOMMODATE FOR ASSOCIATED THIRD SPACE LOSSES.  THE
    DIFFERENCE BETWEEN THE SUM OF THE RESUSCITATIVE VOLUMES OF BLOOD AND
    COLLOIDS, 1000. ML, ALREADY GIVEN AND THE ESTIMATED BLOOD LOSS SHOULD
    BE ADMINISTERED TO REPLACE THE BLOOD VOLUME DEFICIT.  THE  400. ML OF
    CRYSTALLOID ALREADY GIVEN WILL CONTRIBUTE TO THE REPLACEMENT OF THE
    ESTIMATED THIRD SPACE LOSS.  NEVERTHELESS, A GREATER DEFICIT MAY STILL
    EXIST SINCE COMPLETE PLASMA REFILL MAY NOT HAVE OCCURRED.  THEREFORE,
    FURTHER REPLACEMENT SHOULD BE GUIDED BY CLINICAL CONSIDERATIONS AND
    VITAL SIGNS.
```

Figure 20. Estimates of expected body compartment volumes and estimated blood loss and replacement for patient shown in Figure 19 with volume replacement indicated based on a hematocrit fall from 40 to 35 per cent. (From Siegel, J. H., et al.: Chapter 28. *In* Siegel, J. H., and Chodoff, P. (Eds.): The Aged and High Risk Surgical Patient: Medical, Surgical, and Anesthetic Management. New York, Grune & Stratton, Inc., 1976.)

THERAPEUTIC SUGGESTIONS AND CAUTIONS

PART 3

CAREFUL EVALUATION OF THE PATIENT WITH POSSIBLE BLUNT TRAUMA INVOLVING THE ABDOMEN OR LOWER CHEST WALL SHOULD INCLUDE A DIAGNOSTIC PERITONEAL TAP. AN EASY WAY TO FOLLOW THE PATIENT FOR POSSIBLE INTRAPERITONEAL BLEEDING IS TO PLACE A #18 OR LARGER INTRACATH INTO THE PERITONEAL CAVITY CONNECTED TO A SYRINGE. THIS CAN BE LEFT IN PLACE FOR 24-36 HOURS IF NECESSARY AND ASPIRATED OR IRRIGATED PERIODICALLY. THIS IS ESPECIALLY IMPORTANT WITH A HEAD INJURY WHERE NORMAL ABDOMINAL REFLEXES MAY BE ABSENT. THE APPEARANCE OF NON-CLOTTING BLOOD ON PERITONEAL TAP OR IRRIGATION IS AN INDICATION FOR SURGICAL EXPLORATION.

CHECK FOR TRAUMATIC PNEUMOTHORAX OR HEMOTHORAX BY CAREFUL EXAM AND ERECT OR LATERAL DECUBITUS CHEST X-RAYS. IF PRESENT INSERT A THORACOSTOMY TUBE AND PLACE UNDER CONTINUOUS WATERSEAL SUCTION. IT IS IMPORTANT TO REEXPAND THE LUNG FULLY AS SOON AS POSSIBLE. IF MAJOR INTRATHORACIC BLEEDING IS PRESENT THE STERILELY COLLECTED THORACOSTOMY DRAINAGE CAN BE FILTERED AND RE-INFUSED FOR EMERGENCY VOLUME REPLACEMENT.

WITH INJURIES TO THE CENTRAL NERVOUS SYSTEM PRODUCING COMA, OR IN FACE AND JAW INJURIES, SPECIAL ATTENTION MUST BE PAID TO THE AIRWAY AND THE ADEQUACY OF VENTILATION. WHEN IN DOUBT INTUBATE, OR DO A TRACHEOSTOMY, AND ASSIST VENTILATION. IF YOU ELECT ANOTHER COURSE, IT IS ESSENTIAL TO FOLLOW ARTERIAL PO2 AND PCO2 CLOSELY. A PO2 OF UNDER 80 IS UNACCEPTABLE IN A PATIENT WITH CNS INJURY. A PCO2 GREATER THAN 49 INDICATES INEFFECTIVE VENTILATION REQUIRING ASSISTANCE. HOWEVER, WITH CNS INJURY IT IS ALSO ESSENTIAL THAT PCO2 BE MAINTAINED BETWEEN 25 AND 35 MM HG TO PRODUCE MAXIMUM CEREBROVASCULAR DILITATION, WITHOUT INDUCING FURTHER EDEMA. THE USE OF GAS MIXTURES CONTAINING 2% CO2 MAY BE USEFUL IN THIS REGARD.

THE DEVELOPMENT OF POST TRAUMATIC PULMONARY INSUFFICIENCY, EITHER ALONE OR IN COMBINATION WITH SEVERE SEPSIS, IS A SERIOUS COMPLICATION WITH A HIGH INCIDENCE OF MORTALITY. PROPHYLACTICALLY, USE COLLOID CONTAINING SOLUTIONS PREFERENTIALLY IN VOLUME REPLACEMENT, MONITORING CVP CAREFULLY. THE PRESENCE OF A LOW ARTERIAL PO2 ON ROOM AIR WITH A WIDE ALVEOLAR-ARTERIAL O2 GRADIENT AS THE INSPIRED OXYGEN CONCENTRATION IS INCREASED, AND THE PRESENCE OF A NORMAL OR EVEN LOW PCO2, ARE OBJECTIVE SIGNS OF SIGNIFICANT VENTILATION-PERFUSION ABNORMALITIES, WHICH ARE USUALLY DUE TO A REDUCTION IN THE FUNCTIONAL RESIDUAL CAPACITY OF THE LUNG. THE FALL IN FRC IS ASSOCIATED WITH A REDUCED LUNG COMPLIANCE AND AN INCREASE IN PULMONARY SHUNTING. THE MEASUREMENT OF VENTILATION ALONE MAY NOT BE SUFFICIENT TO DETECT THIS COMPLICATION, SINCE THESE PATIENTS TEND TO HYPERVENTILATE IN AN ATTEMPT TO COMPENSATE FOR THE LARGE PULMONARY VENO-ARTERIAL SHUNT. INCREASING THE INSPIRED O2 CONCENTRATION TO MORE THAN 60%, OR TO A LEVEL WHERE THE ARTERIAL PO2 IS GREATER THAN 150 IS ALSO NOT BENEFICIAL AND MAY NOT IN FACT LEAD TO FURTHER ENDOTHELIAL DAMAGE AND A PROGRESSIVE INCREASE IN THE A-AO2

Figure 21. Portion of therapeutic suggestions and cautions based on problem presented in initial assessment history in patient with traumatic injury shown in Figure 19. (From Siegel, J. H., et al.: Chapter 28. *In* Siegel, J. H., and Chodoff, P. (Eds.): The Aged and High Risk Surgical Patient: Medical, Surgical, and Anesthetic Management. New York, Grune & Stratton, Inc., 1976.)

tensively tested in a quantitative way that would provide statistical information concerning both its cost effectiveness and its quality effectiveness in improving patient care.

THE MODERN SURGEON AND THE COMPUTER: PERSPECTIVE ON THE FUTURE

The surgical applications of modern computer technology have increased considerably. In contrast to earlier uncritical efforts, most present approaches to surgical problems show considerable sophistication and understanding of the limitations of technology. While the contemporary investigations into areas related to patient care are far from definitive, in general they have been productive of important information which has in turn permitted a kind of bootstrap elevation of the level of surgical use of computers to define and solve diagnostic and postoperative surgical physiologic problems. The most successful aspect of the use of computer technology has been its demonstrated capability of assimilating and processing enormous amounts of physiologic data in a short period of time, and we can expect to see this use enhanced to permit the surgeon to relate the present patterns of patient response to past experience in a quantitative manner and in an on-line environment. This use can also be anticipated to provide the surgeon with new types of data correlations, which he can use to refine his diag-

nostic ability to recognize clinical patterns and their therapeutic implications.

An important area for rapid development is in the field of image processing. It seems highly probable that the next few years will see great enhancement of x-ray, ultrasonic, electrocardiographic, and radionucleotide imaging by computer techniques. These will provide the surgeon with critical information about regional and organ blood flows by nondestructive methods, which will permit functional assessments of the need for and effectiveness of vascular reconstructive surgery. Another critical area ready for exploration appears to be the use of computer-based models to analyze acute cardiorespiratory dysfunction and to control ventilatory therapy in an intensive care setting.

Other types of adaptive control models may be expected to assist in the management of the acutely ill diabetic patient with hyperglycemia, ketosis, and hyperosmolar coma; and in controlling transplant rejection. However, the most exciting prospect of computer application to surgical patient care appears to lie in the very real possibility of effective clinical computer simulation of various types of therapeutic interventions in the critically ill pre- or postoperative patient. These simulated therapeutic trials may help the surgeon to define his real therapeutic approach with greater sophistication and with an improved chance of success.

Obviously, to use the computer genie as a reliable

servant, the modern surgeon must master its command, and to do so he must impose an intellectual rigor on his own logical processes. He must learn to respect, analyze, and criticize data, and to understand the relevant physiologic interactions and stress responses which result in the observed data patterns. The computer is a powerful tool by which to extend the power of the intellect, and one which can permit us to visualize the likely implications of a given course or action. Since the surgeon is action oriented by nature and training, he has a moral obligation to attempt to project the logical consequences of his clinical decisions, and to remember or retrieve the lessons of the past, so that he will not repeat the mistakes of others. In this regard, the computer properly mastered and commanded may yet prove the surgeon's most faithful assistant in the long journey into the future.

SELECTED REFERENCES

Computer-Based Monitoring

Sheppard, L. C., and Kirklin, J. W.: Cardiac surgical intensive care computer system. Fed. Proc., 33:2326, 1974.
This excellent paper describes an elaborate computer-based monitoring system that has been used to implement an exciting experiment in automated therapy for patients who have undergone cardiac surgery. It provides the reader with an understanding of the logical decisions required in an approach to programed therapy.

Stacy, R. W.: The comprehensive patient-monitoring concept. *In* Stacy, R. W., and Waxman, B. D. (Eds.): Computers in Biomedical Research. Volume 3. New York, Academic Press, 1969, p. 253.
This thoughtful article explores the future of computer-based monitoring and provides insight into the real purpose of monitoring and how this goal can be achieved.

Multivariable Data Analysis

Friedman, H. P., Goldwyn, R. M., and Siegel, J. H.: The use and interpretation of multivariate methods in the classification of stages in serious infectious disease processes in the critically ill. *In* Elashoff, R. M. (Ed.): Perspectives in Biometrics I. New York, Academic Press, 1975, pp. 81–122.

Siegel, J. H., Farrell, E. J., Fichthorn, J., Lajos, T. Z., Lee, A. B., Schimert, G., and Eberhardt, R. C.: The use of multivariable trajectories in defining normal and abnormal time courses of recovery after coronary bypass surgery. J. Surg. Res., 18:341, 1975.

Siegel, J. H., Farrell, E. J., Goldwyn, R. M., and Friedman, H. P.: The surgical implications of physiologic patterns in myocardial infarction shock. Surgery, 72:126, 1972.
These papers describe the development of a data-dependent physiological classification of critically ill patients based on a multivariable cluster analysis. They derive pathophysiologic patterns in various shock states and demonstrate how these physiologic state classifications can be used as a means of quantifying patient recovery trajectories.

Modeling

Moore, F. D., Hartsuck, J. M., Zollinger, R. M., and Johnson, J. R.: Reference models for clinical studies by indicator dilution. Ann. Surg., 168:671, 1968.
The principles behind the use of compartment models for the study of the dilution of an isotopic tracer in various body pools are clearly and rationally presented. This excellent article provides a good introduction for the student interested in the application of modeling concepts to clinical problems.

Simulation

Raines, J. K., Jaffrin, M. Y., and Shapiro, A. H.: A computer simulation of arterial dynamics in the human leg. J. Biomech., 7:77, 1974.

This study develops a model based on sound anatomic and physiologic principles which is capable of explaining the alteration in the pulse wave form in human peripheral vascular disease. It has direct application in the diagnosis of arteriosclerotic occlusion disease of the lower extremities.

Siegel, J. H., and Farrell, E. J.: A computer simulation model to study the clinical observability of ventilation and perfusion abnormalities in human shock states. Surgery, 73:898, 1973.
This simulation provides a computer-based model which is capable of describing the interactions between ventilation and perfusion of the lungs, cardiac function, and peripheral metabolism in producing the observed patterns of physiologic dysfunction in critically ill patients. It has been used to simulate the response to ventilation therapy in patients suffering from the adult respiratory distress syndrome.

Patient Care

Barnett, G. O.: Computers in patient care. N. Engl. J. Med., 279:1321, 1968.
This article covers the essential features necessary in a patient care system. It serves as a general introduction to the mysteries and problems of hospital-wide computer systems primarily directed at organizing patient-oriented services.

Bleich, H. L.: The computer as a consultant. N. Engl. J. Med., 284:141, 1971.
This fine work describes a central computer system that permits physicians and surgeons at remote locations to obtain accurate and precise consultation about problems of acid-base balance. It discusses the problems of consultation by computer.

Siegel, J. H., and Fichthorn, J.: Computer based care of the aged or high risk patient: Automated assistance in fluid management, metabolic balance, and cardiopulmonary regulation. *In* Siegel, J. H., and Chodoff, P. (Eds.): The Aged and High Risk Surgical Patient: Medical, Surgical, and Anesthetic Management. New York, Grune and Stratton, Inc., 1976.
This paper describes a computer-based consultation system to assist in the care of the critically ill patient suffering from a variety of acute surgical diseases. It integrates the quantitative data concerning fluid and electrolyte replacement therapy from the literature with an ongoing metabolic balance obtained from the patient to provide a "living textbook" which the surgeon may consult in arriving at his present care decisions.

REFERENCES

1. Abrahamsson, S., Bergstrom, S., Larson, K., and Tillman, S.: Danderyd Hospital computer system. II. Total regional system for medical care. Comput. Biomed. Res., 3:30, 1970.
2. Afifi, A. A., and Azen, S. P.: Statistical Analysis: A computer Oriented Approach. New York, Academic Press, 1972, pp. 252–259.
3. Afifi, A. A., Chang, P. C., Liu, V. Y., Luz, V. Y., Weil, M. H., and Shubin, H.: Prognostic indexes in acute myocardial infarction complicated by shock. Am. J. Cardiol., 33:826, 1974.
4. Afifi, A. A., Sacks, S. T., Liu, V. Y., Weil, M. H., and Shubin, H.: Accumulative prognostic index for patients with barbiturate, glutethemide, and meprobamate intoxication. N. Engl. J. Med., 285:1497, 1971.
5. Baker, O., Khalaf, J., and Chapman, C. B.: A scanner-computer for determining the volumes of cardiac chambers from cinefluorographic films. Am. Heart J., 62:797, 1961.
6. Barnett, G. O.: Computers in patient care. N. Engl. J. Med., 279:1321, 1968.
7. Bassingthwaighte, J. B., Ackerman, F. H., and Wood, E. H.: Application of lagged normal density curve as a model for arterial dilution curves. Circ. Res., 18:398, 1966.
8. Bleich, H. L.: The computer as a consultant. N. Engl. J. Med., 284:141, 1971.
9. Box, G. E. P., and Jenkins, G. M.: Time Series Analysis, Forecasting and Control. San Francisco, Holden Day, 1970.
10. Caceres, C. A., and Hochberg, H. M.: Performance of the computer and physician in the analysis of the electrocardiogram. Am. Heart J., 79:439, 1970.
11. Caceres, C. A., Steinberg, C. A., Abraham, S., Carbery, W. J., McBride, J. M., Tolles, W. E., and Rikli, A. E.: Computer extraction of electrocardiographic parameters. Circulation, 25:356, 1962.

12. Chang, P., Afifi, A. A., Liu, V. Y., Nishijima, H., Weil, M. H., and Shubin, H.: Prognostic indices for the assessment of patients with gram-negative bacteremia and shock. *In* Urbascheck, B., Urbascheck, U., and Neter, E. (Eds.): Gram-negative Bacterial Infections and Mode of Endotoxin Actions—Pathological, Immunological, and Clinical Aspects. New York, Springer-Verlag, 1974, pp. 237–247.

13. Chodoff, P., and Drews, J. H.: Experiences with a new automated technique for interview and decision making in anesthesiology. J.A.M.A., *218*:85, 1971.

14. Chow, C. K., Kaneko, T., and Siegel, J. H.: Automated quantification of the contractile dynamics of myocardial wall segments by image processing or cardiac cineangiography. IBM Research, RC4271, 1973.

15. Clayton, P. D., Harris, L. D., Rumel, S. R., and Warner, H. R.: Left ventricular videometry. Comput. Biomed. Res., 7:369, 1974.

16. Consolazio, C. F., Johnson, R. E., and Pecora, L. J.: Physiological Measurements of Metabolic Functions in Man. New York, McGraw-Hill Book Company, 1963.

17. Coulam, C. M., Dunnette, W. H., and Wood, E. H.: A computer-controlled scintiscanning system and associated computer graphic technique for study of regional distribution of blood flow. Comput. Biomed. Res., *3*:201, 1970.

18. Coulam, C. M., Warner, H. R., Wood, E. H., and Bassingthwaighte, J. B.: A transfer function analysis of coronary and renal circulation calculated from upstream and downstream indicator-dilution curves. Circ. Res., *19*:879, 1966.

19. Deland, E. C., Wolf, M. B., and Dell, R. B.: A behavioral model of kidney function. Proceedings of the Society for Computer Simulation, Conference on Mathematics of a Large Scale Simulation, 1974.

20. Eberhardt, R. C., Lamy, M. L., Kamm, B., Fallat, R. J., and Osborn, J. J.: On the engineering accuracy and prognostic effectiveness of a computer-based patient monitoring system. Critical Care Med., in press, 1976.

21. Farrell, E. J., and Siegel, J. H.: Investigation of cardiorespiratory abnormalities through computer simulation. Comput. Biomed. Res., *5*:161, 1973.

22. Fonkalsrud, E. W., Hammidi, I. B., and Maloney, J. V., Jr.: Computer-assisted instruction in undergraduate surgical education. Surgery, *62*:141, 1967.

23. Friedman, H. P., Goldwyn, R. M., and Siegel, J. H.: The use and interpretation of multivariate methods in the classification of stages in serious infectious disease processes in the critically ill. *In* Elashoff, R. M. (Ed.): Perspectives in Biometrics I. New York, Academic Press, 1975, pp. 81–122.

24. Fry, D.: A preliminary lung model for simulating the aerodynamics in the bronchial tree. Comput. Biomed. Res., *2*:11, 1968.

25. Glaeser, D. H., Trost, R. F., Brown, D. B., Kyle, A. C., Lenahan, M. S., Walker, C. K., Wilson, C. S., and DeBakey, M. E.: A hierarchial minicomputer system for continuous post surgical monitoring. Comput. Biomed. Res., *8*:336, 1975.

26. Goldwyn, R. M., Friedman, H. P., and Siegel, J. H.: Iteration and interaction in computer data bank analysis: A case study in the physiologic classification and assessment of the critically ill. Comput. Biomed. Res., *4*:6, 1971.

27. Goldwyn, R. M., and Watt, T. B.: Arterial pressure pulse contour analysis via a mathematical model for the clinical quantification of human vascular properties. IEEE Trans. Biomed. Engin., *14*:11, 1967.

28. Gomez, D. M., Brisco, W., and Cumming, G.: Continuous distribution of specific tidal volume throughout the lung. J. Appl. Physiol., *19*:683, 1964.

29. Gorry, G. A., and Barnett, G. O.: Sequential diagnosis by computer. J.A.M.A., *205*:849, 1968.

30. Grodins, F. S., and James, G.: Mathematical models of respiratory regulation. Ann. N.Y. Acad. Sci., *100*:852, 1963.

31. Gudwin, A. L., Goldstein, C. R., Cohn, J. D., and Del Guercio, L. R. M.: Estimation of ventricular mixing volume for prediction of operative mortality in the elderly. Ann. Surg., *168*:183, 1968.

32. Harris, L. D., Clayton, P. D., Marshall, H. W., and Warner, H. R.: A technique for the detection of asynergistic motion in the left ventricle. Comput. Biomed. Res., 7:380, 1974.

33. Herman, M. V., Heinle, R. A., Klein, M. D., and Gorlin, R.: Localized disorders in myocardial contraction. N. Engl. J. Med., *277*:222, 1967.

34. Hilberman, M., Schill, J. P., and Peters, R. M.: On-line digital analysis of respiratory mechanics and the automation of respirator control. J. Thorac. Cardiovasc. Surg., *58*:821, 1969.

35. Jurado, R. A., Matucha, D., and Osborn, J. J.: Output estimation by pulse contour methods: Validity of their use for monitoring the critically ill patient. Surgery, *74*:358, 1973.

36. Kirklin, J. W.: Systems analysis in surgical patients with particular attention to the cardiac and pulmonary subsystems. Fifteenth Macewen Memorial Lecture, University of Glasgow. Glasgow University Publications 139, 1970.

37. Kouchoukos, N. T., Sheppard, L. C., McDonald, D. A., and Kirklin, J. W.: Estimation of stroke volume from the central arterial pressure contour in postoperative patients. Surg. Forum, *20*:180, 1969.

38. Lamy, M., Fallat, R. J., Koeniger, E., Dietrich, H. P., Ratliff, J. L., Eberhart, R. D., Tucker, H. J., and Hill, J. D.: Pathology and mechanism of hypoxemia in adult respiratory distress syndrome. N. Engl. J. Med., in press, 1976.

39. Lewis, F. J., Deller, S., Yokochi, H., Rosi, P. S., Quinn, M. L., Kite, M., and Rabin, S.: Automatic monitoring in the postoperative recovery room. Surg. Gynecol. Obstet., *130*:333, 1970.

40. Lewis, F. J., Shimizu, T., Scofield, A. L., and Rosi, P. S.: Analysis of respiration by an on-line digital computer system: Clinical data following thoracoabdominal surgery. Ann. Surg., *164*:547, 1966.

41. Lewis, F. J., and Welch, J. A.: Respiratory mechanics in postoperative patients. Surg. Gynecol. Obstet., *120*:305, 1965.

42. Lloyd, B. B., and Cunningham, D. J. C.: A quantitative approach to the regulation of human respiration. *In* Cunningham, D. J. C., and Lloyd, B. B. (Eds.): The Regulation of Human Respiration. Philadelphia, F. A. Davis Company, 1963.

43. Long, C. L., Spencer, J. L., Kinney, J. M., and Geiger, J. W.: Carbohydrate metabolism in man: Effect of elective operations and major injury. J. Appl. Physiol., *31*:102, 1971.

44. MacDonald, L. K., Gardner, R. M., Pryor, T. A., and Dag, W. C.: An exploratory study of the costs and cost implications in the operation of a MEDLAB time-sharing computer system. A physiological measurement facility. Comput. Biomed. Res., *3*:586, 1971.

45. Maloney, J. V., Jr.: The trouble with patient monitoring. Ann. Surg., *168*:605, 1968.

46. Maloney, J. V., Jr., DeHaven, J. C., Deland, E. C., and Bradham, G. B.: Examples of a large-model simulation of the blood biochemical system. J. Chronic Dis., *19*:411, 1966.

47. Maseri, A., Caldini, P., Permutt, S., and Zierler, K.: Frequency function of transit times through dog pulmonary circulation. Circ. Res., *26*:527, 1970.

48. Mauney, M., Fallon, H., Goertze, G., Marler, G. E., and Pulver, R. W.: Using: A primer for writing medical data base for the clinical decision support system. Progr. Brain Res., *33*:155, 1970.

49. Mayne, J. G., Weksel, W., and Sholtz, P. N.: Toward automating the medical history. Mayo Clin. Proc., *43*:1, 1968.

50. Milhorn, H. T., Jr., and Brown, D. R.: Steady-state simulation of the human respiratory system. Comput. Biomed. Res., *3*:604, 1971.

51. Moore, F. D., Hartsuck, J. M., Zollinger, R. M., and Johnson, J. E.: Reference models for clinical studies by isotopic dilution. Ann. Surg., *168*:671, 1968.

52. Moore, F. D., Oleson, K. H., McMurrey, J. D., Parker, H. V., Ball, M. R., and Boyden, C. M.: The Body Cell Mass and Its Supporting Environment. Philadelphia, W. B. Saunders Company, 1963.

53. Moreno, A. H., Katz, A. I., and Gold, L. D.: An integrated approach to the study of the venous system with steps toward a detailed model of dynamics of venous return to the right heart. IEEE Trans. Biomed. Engin., *16*:308, 1969.

54. Neurath, P. W., Enslein, K., and Mitchell, G. W., Jr.: Design of a computer system to assist in differential preoperative diagnosis for pelvic surgery. N. Engl. J. Med., *280*:745, 1969.

55. Osborn, J. J.: Monitoring respiratory function. Crit. Care Med., 2:217, 1975.

56. Osborn, J. J., Beaumont, J. O., Raison, J. C., and Abbott, R. P.: Computation for quantitative on-line measurements in an intensive care ward. *In* Stacy, R. W., and Waxman, E. D. (Eds.): Computers in Biomedical research. Volume 3. New York, Academic Press, 1969, p. 207.

57. Osborn, J. J., Beaumont, J. O., Raison, J. C. A., Russell, J., and

Gerbode, F.: Measurement and monitoring of acutely ill patients by digital computer. Surgery, 64:1057, 1968.

58. Paiva, M., and Demeester, M.: Gas transport in the air phase of the lung simulated by a digital computer. Comput. Biomed. Res., 3:675, 1971.

59. Parzen, E.: On empirical multiple time series analysis. Proc. Fifth Berkeley Symposium Math. Statist. Prob., 1:305, 1967.

60. Parzen, E.: Multiple time series modeling. In Krishnacah, P. R. (Ed.): Multivariate Analysis II. New York, Academic Press, 1969, pp. 389–410.

61. Patel, D. J., de Freitas, F. M., and Fry, D. L.: Hydraulic input impedance to aorta and pulmonary artery in dogs. J. Appl. Physiol., 18:134, 1963.

62. Peters, R. M., and Hilberman, M.: Respiratory insufficiency diagnosis and control of therapy. Surgery, 70:280, 1971.

63. Peters, R. M., Hilberman, M., Hogan, J. S., and Crawford, D. A.: Objective indications for respirator therapy in post-trauma and post-operative patients. Am. J. Surg., 124:262, 1972.

64. Raines, J. K., Jaffrin, M. Y., and Shapiro, A. H.: A computer simulation of arterial dynamics in the human leg. J. Biomech., 7:77, 1974.

65. Raison, J. C. A., Beaumont, J. O., Russell, A. G., Osborn, J. J., and Gerbode, F.: Alarms in an intensive care unit: An interim compromise. Comput. Biomed. Res., 1:556, 1968.

66. Sarnoff, S. J., and Mitchell, J. H.: The control of the function of the heart. In Handbook of Physiology. Section 2, Circulation. Volume 1. Baltimore, Williams & Wilkins Company, 1962.

67. Shapiro, A. R., and Peters, R. M.: Statistical approaches to determining the need for respirator therapy. Proc. San Diego Biomed. Symp., 13:325, 1974.

68. Sheppard, C. W., and Householder, A. S.: The mathematical basis of the interpretation of tracer experiments in closed steady-state systems. J. Appl. Physics., 22:510, 1951.

69. Sheppard, L. C., Kirklin, J. W., and Kouchoukos, N. T.: Computer controlled interventions for the acutely ill patient. In Stacy, R. W., and Waxman, B. D. (Ed.). Computers in Biomedical Research. Volume 4. New York, Academic Press, 1974, pp. 135–148.

70. Sheppard, L. C., Kouchoukos, N. T., Kurtts, M. A., and Kirklin, J. W.: Automated treatment of critically ill patients following operation. Ann. Surg., 168:596, 1968.

71. Shoemaker, W. C., Elwyn, D. H., Levin, H., and Rosen, A. C.: Early prediction of death and survival in postoperative patients with circulatory shock by nonparametric analysis of cardiorespiratory variables. Crit. Care Med., 2:317, 1974.

72. Shubin, H., Chang, P., Freund, V., Portugal, L., Schriver, J. A., and Weil, M. H.: Cumulative prognostic index: Patients with hypovolemic shock. In press.

73. Shubin, H., and Weil, M. H.: Efficient monitoring with a digital computer of cardiovascular function in seriously ill patients. Ann. Intern. Med., 65:453, 1966.

74. Shubin, H., Weil, M. H., Palley, N., and Afifi, A. A.: Monitoring the critically ill patient with the aid of a digital computer. Comput. Biomed. Res., 4:460, 1971.

75. Siegel, J. H., and Farrell, E. J.: A computer simulation model to study the clinical observability of ventilation and perfusion abnormalities in human shock states. Surgery, 73:898, 1973.

76. Siegel, J. H., Farrell, E. J., Fichthorn, J., Lajos, T. Z., Lee, A. B., Schimert, G., and Eberhardt, R. C.: The use of multivariable trajectories in defining normal and abnormal time courses of recovery after coronary bypass surgery. J. Surg. Res., 18:341, 1975.

77. Siegel, J. H., Farrell, E. J., Goldwyn, R. M., and Friedman, H. P.: The surgical implications of physiologic patterns in myocardial infarction shock. Surgery, 72:126, 1972.

78. Siegel, J. H., Farrell, E. J., and Lewin, I.: Quantifying the need for cardiac support in human shock by a functional model of cardiopulmonary vascular dynamics: With special reference to myocardial infarction. J. Surg. Res., 13:166, 1972.

79. Siegel, J. H., Farrell, E. J., Miller, M., Goldwyn, R. M., and Friedman, H. P.: Cardiorespiratory interactions as determinants of survival and the need for respiratory support in human shock states. J. Trauma, 13:602, 1973.

80. Siegel, J. H., and Fichthorn, J.: Computer based CARE of the aged or high risk patient: Automated assistance in fluid management, metabolic balance, and cardiopulmonary regulation. In Siegel, J. H., and Chodoff, P. (Eds.): The Aged and High Risk Surgical Patient: Medical, Surgical, and Anesthetic Management. New York, Grune and Stratton, Inc., 1976.

81. Siegel, J. H., Goldwyn, R. M., and Friedman, H. P.: Pattern and process in the evolution of human septic shock. Surgery, 70:232, 1971.

82. Siegel, J. H., Greenspan, M., Cohn, J. D., and Del Guercio, L. R. M.: A bedside computer and physiologic nomograms: Guides to the management of the patient in shock. Arch. Surg., 97:480, 1968.

83. Siegel, J. H., Greenspan, M., and Del Guercio, L. R. M.: Abnormal vascular tone, defective oxygen transport, and myocardial failure in human septic shock. Ann. Surg., 165:504, 1967.

84. Siegel, J. H., and Strom, B. L.: The computer as a "living textbook" applied to the care of the critically injured patient. J. Trauma, 12:739, 1972.

85. Siegel, J. H., and Strom, B. L.: An automated system to aid the physician in the care of the desperately sick patient. In Stacy, R. W., and Waxman, B. D. (Ed.): Computers in Biomedical Research. Volume 4. New York, Academic Press, 1974, pp. 115–134.

86. Siegel, J. H., and Williams, J. B.: A computer based index for the prediction of operative survival in patients with cirrhosis and portal hypertension. Ann. Surg., 169:191, 1969.

87. Slack, W. V., Hicks, G. P., Reed, C. E., and Van Cura, L. J.: A computer-based medical-history system. N. Engl. J. Med., 274:194, 1966.

88. Snyder, M., and Rideout, V.: Computer modeling of the human systematic arterial tree. J. Biomech., 1:341, 1968.

89. Sollberger, A.: Statistical aspects of diurnal biorhythms. Acta Anat., 23:97, 1955.

90. Spencer, J. L., Long, C. L., and Kinney, J. M.: A model for glucose metabolism in man. I & EC Fundamentals, 10:2, 1971.

91. Stacy, R. W.: The comprehensive patient-monitoring concept. In Stacy, R. W., and Waxman, B. D. (Eds.): Computers in Biomedical Research. Volume 3. New York, Academic Press, 1969, p. 253.

92. Starmer, C. F., McHale, P. A., Cobb, F. R., and Greenfield, J. C., Jr.: Evaluation of several methods of computing stroke volume from central aortic pressure. Circ. Res., 33:139, 1973.

93. Streeter, V. L., Keitzer, W. F., and Bohr, D. F.: Pulsatile pressure and flow through distensible vessels. Circ. Res., 13:3, 1963.

94. Thompson, H. K., Starmer, C. F., Whalen, R. E., and McIntosh. H. D.: Indicator transit times considered as a gamma variate. Circ. Res., 14:502, 1964.

95. Thompson, H. K., Jr., and Woodbury, M. A.: Clinical data representation in multidimensional space. Comput. Biomed. Res., 3:58, 1970.

96. Vagnucci, A. H., Wong, A. K. C., and Liu, T. S.: Time series analysis of hormonal patterns in human plasma. Comput. Biomed. Res., 7:513, 1974.

97. Van Brunt, E. E.: The Kaiser-Permanente medical information system. Comput. Biomed. Res., 3:477, 1970.

98. Van Cauter, E., and Huyberechts, S.: Problems in the statistical analysis of biologic time series: The cosinor test and the periodogram. J. Interdiscipl. Cycle Res., 4:41, 1973.

99. Villamil, M. F., Deland, E. C., Henney, R. P., and Maloney, J. V., Jr.: Anion effects on cation movements during correction of potassium depletion. Am. J. Physiol., 229:161, 1975.

100. Warner, H. R., Gardner, R. M., and Toronto, A. F.: Computer-based monitoring of cardiovascular functions in postoperative patients. Circulation, 37(Suppl. 2):68, 1968.

101. Warner, H. R., Rutherford, B. D., and Houtchens, B.: A sequential Bayesean approach to history taking and diagnosis. Comput. Biomed. Res., 5:256, 1972.

102. Warner, H. R., Toronto, A. F., and Veasy, L. G.: Experience with Baye's theorem for computer diagnosis of congenital heart disease. Ann. N.Y. Acad. Sci., 115:558, 1964.

103. Warner, H. R., Woolley, F. R., and Kane, R. L.: Computer assisted instruction for teaching clinical decision-making. Comput. Biomed. Res. 7:564, 1974.

104. Weed, L. L.: Medical Records, Medical Education, and Patient Care. Cleveland, Case Western Reserve University Press, 1970.

105. Westerhof, N., Bosman, F., DeVries, C. J., and Noordergraaf, A.: Analog studies of the human systemic arterial tree. J. Biomech., 2:121, 1969.

106. Williams, T. E., Folk, R. L., Prior, J. A., and Zollinger, R. M.: The O. S. U. pilot medical school. Surgery, 70:47, 1971.

107. Winkel, P., Paldam, M., and Tygstrup, N.: A numerical taxonomic analysis of symptoms and signs in 400 patients with cirrhosis of the liver. Comput. Biomed. Res., 3:657, 1971.

108. Yamamoto, W., and Hiri, T.: Phasic air movement model of respiratory regulation of carbon dioxide balance. Comput. Biomed. Res., 3:689, 1971.

109. Zierler, K. L.: Circulation times and the theory of indicator-dilution methods for determining blood flow and volume. In Handbook of Physiology. Section 2, Circulation, Volume 1. Baltimore, Williams and Wilkins Company, 1962, p. 585.

110. Zollinger, R. M., Jr., Skillman, J. J., and Moore, F. D.: Alterations in water, colloid, and electrolyte distribution after hemorrhage. In Fox, C. L., and Nahas, G. C. (Eds.): Body Fluid Replacement in the Surgical Patient. New York, Grune & Stratton, 1970.

13

RADIOISOTOPE TECHNIQUES FOR DIAGNOSIS OF SURGICAL DISORDERS

Robert H. Jones, M.D.

Use of radioisotopes for diagnosis of disease is a relatively new but rapidly developing area of modern medicine. These studies, which usually require only an intravenous injection, provide an innocuous approach to relating organ structure and function in patients. A large variety of radioisotope techniques have been devised for measurement of function and detection of disease in various organs. A number of radioisotope procedures provide reliable diagnostic information that otherwise could be obtained only by approaches imposing much greater risk and discomfort upon patients. Management of many surgical disorders can be facilitated by proper understanding and use of these radionuclide diagnostic procedures. This chapter emphasizes those techniques of greatest application in surgical patients.

GENERAL PRINCIPLES

Only a few of the large number of radionuclides available possess suitable physical and chemical properties for clinical studies. These agents may be used as simple compounds or attached to an organic substance as a radioactive label. Radiopharmaceuticals preferentially exclude or accumulate in regions of disease by mechanisms of active transport, phagocytosis, compartmental localization, simple diffusion, or capillary blockade. The accuracy of a radionuclide test depends primarily upon the magnitude of difference in radioactivity in diseased relative to normal organ tissues. The efficiency of present radioactivity detection instruments permits use of minute amounts of radiopharmaceuticals that do not alter organ function during measurement.

Radiation burdens, rather than pharmacologic properties, limit the dosage of radiopharmaceuticals. The potentially harmful effects of radioactive substances became apparent with use of Thorotrast, a colloidal suspension of thorium dioxide. The heavy thorium atom made this preparation a suitable radiographic contrast material that found widespread clinical use between 1928 and 1945. In addition to angiographic studies, Thorotrast permitted visualization of the liver and spleen, which selectively accumulated the colloid by phagocytosis. The usual amount of Thorotrast administered produced a weekly radiation burden of 1.5 rads to the liver and 2.5 rads to the spleen from thorium and its 11 radioactive daughter elements. After a 20-year latent period, tumors began to appear in patients subjected to this low but persistent irradiation. Kuisk and colleagues collected reports of 65 patients with *hepatic* malignant disease related to thorium administration. Unlike thorium, which remains permanently in the body and has a 14-trillion-year physical half-life, common radionuclides used for patient studies have biologic and physical half-lives measured in *hours or days*. The brief exposure to radioactivity produces a total-body irradiation ranging from 0.1 to 0.5 rads for common radionuclide studies. This amount of radiation approximates that of standard radiographic studies and remains within limits considered to be safe. Although radioactive substances should not be needlessly administered, the relatively small body radiation appears justified whenever a radioisotope study promises potential benefit to the patient.

The *Geiger counter* developed in 1928 for radioactivity detection has now largely been replaced by the more sensitive scintillation detector systems. In these detectors, gamma rays emitted by radionuclides within a patient are focused through apertures in a lead collimator onto a sodium iodide scintillation crystal that emits light in response to the radiation energy. A photomultiplier tube, which converts light from these crystals into an electrical impulse, is a vacuum tube coated on its inner surface with a substance with loosely bound electrons that dislodge in response to light. The weak electrical impulses generated by photomultiplier tubes are amplified and filtered electronically before storage. The *rectilinear scanner* developed by Cassen in 1953 is the standard detecting instrument for clinical scanning. This instrument moves a single scintillation counter over the region of interest and exposes film with an intensity pattern similar to the distribution of radioactivity detected. This technique creates a two-dimensional image of the intensity of radioactivity within the body. Scans usually include only the area about the organ of interest, but total-body scans with minification of the image can depict radioactivity in the entire body for bone, bone marrow, and soft tissue scans. Other scintillation detectors of more recent design, such as the System 77 and the Anger camera, simultaneously detect radioactivity from a number of crystals or from a single large crystal with electronic impulse positioning. These instruments permit dynamic imaging or measurement of changing radioactivity within regions of an organ.

Interpretation of scan data does not require recognition of patterns specific for various disorders. Rather, if the mechanism of radiopharmaceutical distribution within an organ is understood, diseases that might alter the normal distribution become apparent. As in all diagnostic procedures, radioisotope scanning must be related to other clinical data and particularly to information gained by careful history and physical examination. These studies are not short cuts to rapid diagnosis, but when properly used they can provide objective information useful in diagnosis and management of patients with many surgical disorders.

THYROID SCANNING

Active iodine uptake by the thyroid gland provides a method for imaging this organ, and assessment of thyroid function with radioactive iodine represents one of the first applications of isotopes in medicine. Of the several radioisotopes of iodine, ^{131}I possesses the most suitable properties for clinical use. The thyroid metabolism of radioactive iodine is identical to that of stable iodine, and scanning with this agent provides a method for assessing regional thyroid function.

One principal use of thyroid scanning is identification and localization of functioning thyroid tissue. Thyroid tissue may be present in masses located in the region from the base of the tongue to the superior mediastinum, and retrosternal extension of thyroid tissue is a particularly common cause of superior mediastinal masses (Fig. 1). Diagnosis by scanning aids selection of the operative approach best suited for excision of these masses. Not all aberrant thyroid tissue metabolizes iodine, and lack of function on scan does not exclude the possibility of thyroid tissue within a mass.

Thyroid scanning is useful for localization and evaluation of function of metastases after thyroidectomy in patients with thyroid carcinoma. The presence of functioning thyroid tissue limits uptake of iodine by metastases, and scanning rarely demonstrates metastases in the preoperative evaluation of patients suspected of thyroid carcinoma. However, after total thyroidectomy, metastases may demonstrate sufficient function to permit localization by scan, and administration of TSH several days prior to study enhances iodine uptake by functioning metastases. Total-body scanning permits localization of functioning thyroid metastases (Fig. 2). In evaluation of metastatic thyroid carcinoma, a thyroid scan is necessary in the immediate postoperative period for proper interpretation of subsequent scans. Even after total thyroidectomy, residual functioning thyroid tissue commonly remains in the neck, and postoperative determination of the size and location of this tissue permits later differentiation from local recurrence of carcinoma. In addition to localization, assessment of the degree of function in metastases of thyroid carcinoma permits a prediction of the benefit of radioactive iodine treatment. Radioactive iodine is indicated for treatment of

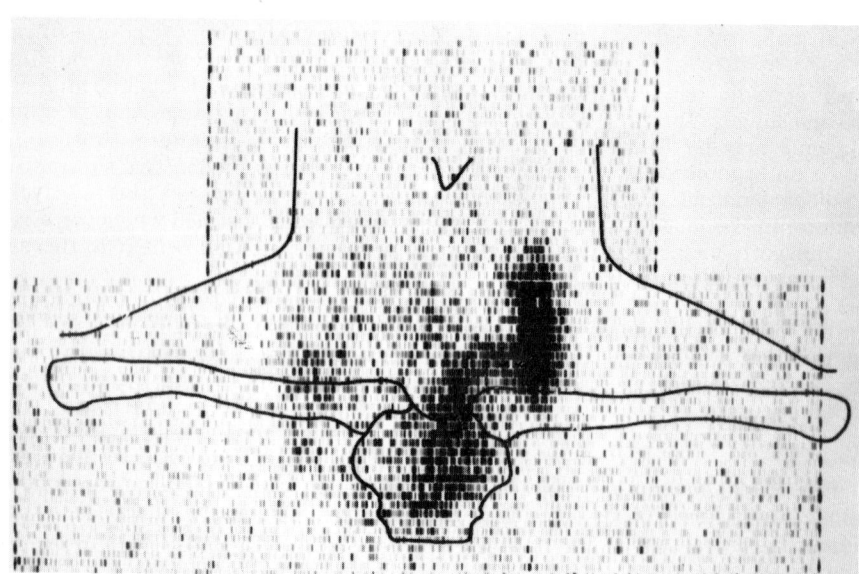

Figure 1. A diffusely enlarged right thyroid lobe was palpable in this patient with a superior mediastinal mass observed on chest radiograph. The thyroid scan shows diffuse enlargement and decreased uptake in the right thyroid lobe consistent with a nodular goiter. Thyroid tissue extends well below the sternal notch, suggesting that the superior mediastinal mass was composed of thyroid tissue. (Courtesy of Duke University Medical Center, Department of Radiology and Division of Nuclear Medicine.)

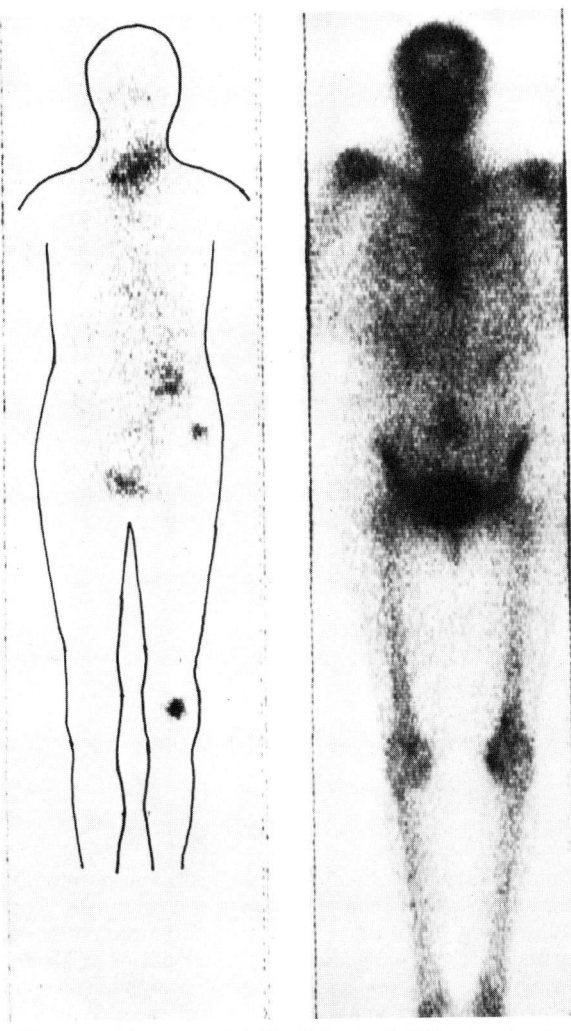

Figure 2. A bone scan (*right*) obtained with ⁹⁹ᵐTc stannous pyrophosphate demonstrated several areas of increased uptake in this patient following total thyroidectomy for follicular carcinoma of the thyroid. Following TSH stimulation, a ¹³¹I total body scan (*left*) demonstrated iodine uptake in the metastatic thyroid carcinoma in the left knee and iliac bone. Residual thyroid tumor was apparent in the neck. A therapeutic dose of radioactive iodine was administered for treatment of the metastases.

metastatic thyroid carcinoma only when iodine uptake by metastases can be demonstrated by scan.

Although evaluation of the function within palpable thyroid nodules is a common use of radioiodine scanning, the technique is not sufficiently specific to justify routine clinical use. Solitary hypofunctioning nodules are generally benign and may be cysts, adenomas, or regions of focal thyroiditis. However, carcinoma of the thyroid also most often presents as a nodule with decreased function, and 10 to 25 per cent of all hypofunctioning nodules contain malignant tissue. Nodules that demonstrate function are less likely to prove malignant, but some well-differentiated carcinomas may demonstrate normal or even increased iodine up-

take on scan. The management of most patients with palpable thyroid masses is not influenced by thyroid scan documentation of the location, size, and function of the nodules. However, demonstration of function in thyroid nodules by scan may justify nonoperative therapy in patients who have an unusually great risk for anesthesia.

LUNG SCANNING

Early isotope procedures used radioactive gases for measurement of pulmonary perfusion and ventilation but did not permit sufficient anatomic resolution to be of significant clinical value. In 1964, the use of radioactive particles for measurement of regional pulmonary perfusion was introduced, and this technique has become an important diagnostic study, particularly in patients with pulmonary embolism. Human serum albumin aggregated into 10 to 50 μ particles is labeled with radioactive iodine, technetium, or indium. After intravenous injection, these particles pass through the right heart and distribute in the lungs proportional to regional blood flow. These particles remain in the precapillary arterioles for a time sufficient to permit detection of the radioactivity, and then fragment and disappear from the lungs with a half-life of about 6 hours. The number of pulmonary vessels occluded during study has been estimated to be less than 0.1 per cent, and no detectable alteration in pulmonary function or histologic injury occurs after injection. Pulmonary scans may be safely performed even in patients with severe respiratory distress.

Lung scanning is particularly useful for the initial evaluation of symptoms suggestive of pulmonary embolism. Pulmonary embolism is incorrectly diagnosed more frequently than any other common disease, and less than one third of fatal cases diagnosed at postmortem examination are recognized prior to death. Clinical manifestations of this disorder are vague and frequently mimic symptoms of other diseases. The chest radiograph and electrocardiogram are often normal or may show only nonspecific changes in pulmonary embolism. Lung scanning sensitively depicts regional pulmonary perfusion, and a normal lung scan provides strong evidence for a diagnosis other than pulmonary embolism. The size and location of pulmonary emboli determine the lung scan appearance. Scattered small emboli produce crescent-shaped defects along a pleural surface (Fig. 3). Occluded segmental arteries cause perfusion defects in corresponding anatomic regions (Fig. 4). Embolism involving lobar arteries causes large, obvious perfusion deficits. In most patients with pulmonary embolism, lung scanning demonstrates bilateral involvement of vessels of various sizes. In addition to diagnosis, serial lung scans objectively document the response to treatment of pulmonary embolism and detect incomplete restoration of pulmonary perfusion and recurrent pulmonary embolism. Proper utilization of lung scanning can increase the diagnostic accuracy in pulmonary embolism and greatly aid management of this disorder.

All diseases altering pulmonary perfusion cause abnormal lung scans, and the distribution of radioac-

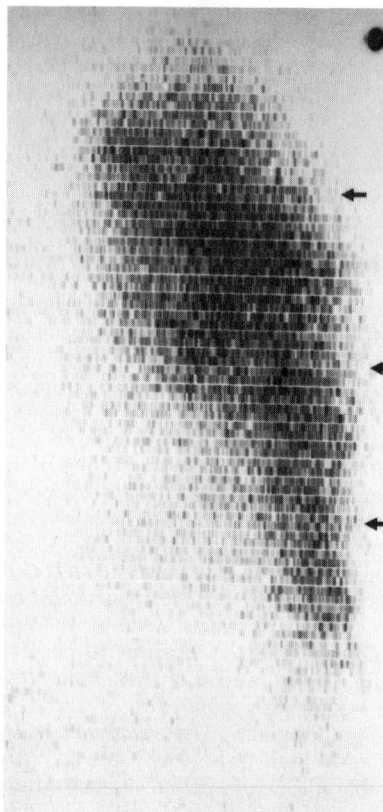
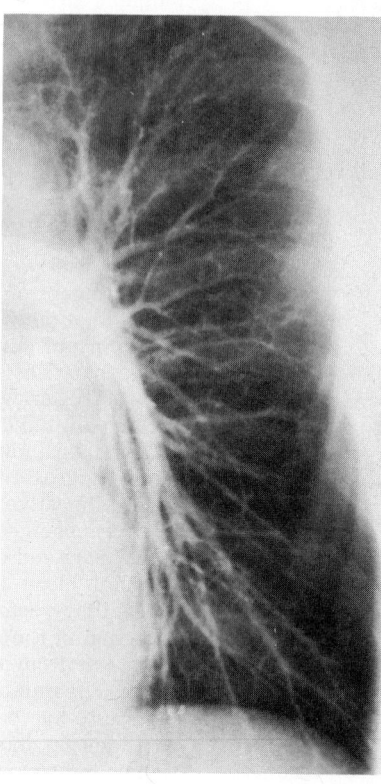

Figure 3. The lung scan in this patient with pulmonary embolism demonstrates *peripheral defects* suggestive of occlusion of multiple *small* pulmonary arteries. Pulmonary emboli located in small peripheral pulmonary arteries are *not* demonstrated by the selective left pulmonary angiogram in this patient.

tivity in the lungs quantitates regional blood flow. In patients with mitral stenosis, the degree of increased perfusion in apical lung regions indexes the severity of stenosis. Lung scans in patients with subclavian to pulmonary artery shunts for treatment of congenital heart disease demonstrate a shift of pulmonary arterial perfusion away from the side of the shunt. Thrombosis of the shunt can be recognized by a return of a normal distribution of blood flow to each lung on scan. Lung scans provide a more accurate assessment of regional function than the chest radiograph and are particularly useful for evaluating response to treatment in patients with bronchiectasis, cystic lung disease, congenital vascular abnormalities, and lobar emphysema.

Experimental and clinical studies indicate an excellent correlation of lung scan determinations of regional pulmonary perfusion with other methods of measurement. Recognition of the cause of perfusion defects observed on lung scan requires interpretation of the scan with a simultaneous chest radiograph. Pneumonitis that may appear minimal on a radiograph often causes a marked perfusion defect on scan similar to that in pulmonary embolism. Also, patients with asthma or obstructive lung disease frequently demonstrate uneven pulmonary perfusion secondary to bronchoconstriction and underventilation of lung regions. Ventilation scanning using an inert radioactive gas may aid in the differentiation of patients with regional perfusion abnormalities secondary to uneven ventilation (Fig. 5). If an infiltrate on chest radiograph or a history of asthma hinders lung scan interpretation, a pulmonary angiogram may be essential for diagnosis

of pulmonary embolism. The lung scan and pulmonary angiogram are complementary procedures that usually depict similar patterns of pulmonary arterial perfusion (Fig. 6). Because of greater patient risk and discomfort, pulmonary angiography should be performed only in patients in whom lung scan diagnosis is not conclusive.

LIVER SCANNING

Radiopharmaceuticals used for liver scanning depend upon referential uptake and secretion of compounds by the polygonal liver cells or phagocytosis of small particles by Kupffer cells. *Rose bengal* is a dye similar to Bromsulphalein (BSP) that is selectively secreted by liver cells. Rose bengal labeled with ^{131}I can be used to assess liver function in patients with jaundice, which prohibits the colorimetric determination of BSP. This agent has been particularly valuable in diagnosis of biliary atresia in infants with jaundice. Because ^{131}I rose bengal is concentrated in bile, scans with this dye demonstrate radioactivity in the functioning gallbladder and bile ducts and may aid the diagnosis of liver masses near the gallbladder (Fig. 7). A second isotope method for evaluation of liver function utilizes Kupffer cell sequestration of labeled particles of about 1 μ size. Reticuloendothelial cells of other organs also phagocytize these particles, and the spleen is also visualized on a normal liver scan made by this technique. A sulfur colloid labeled with technetium-99m is the agent commonly used for liver scanning by this approach. Most liver diseases decrease

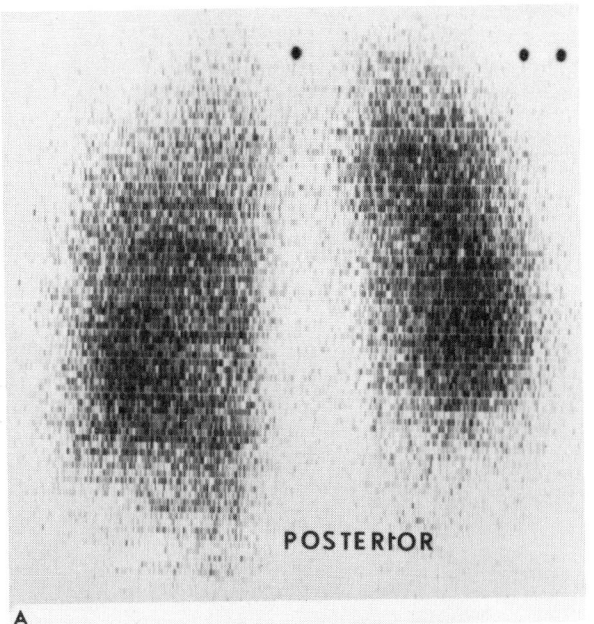

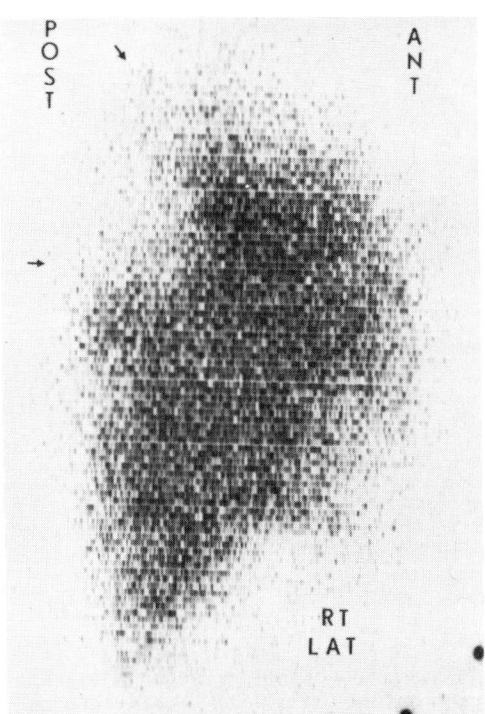

Figure 4. *A,* The lung scan in this patient with pulmonary embolism demonstrates decreased radioactivity in the right upper lung, which is in the area of perfusion of the apical and posterior segmental arteries. *B,* A pulmonary angiogram in this patient demonstrates the embolism as an intraluminal filling defect in the apical and posterior segmental arteries.

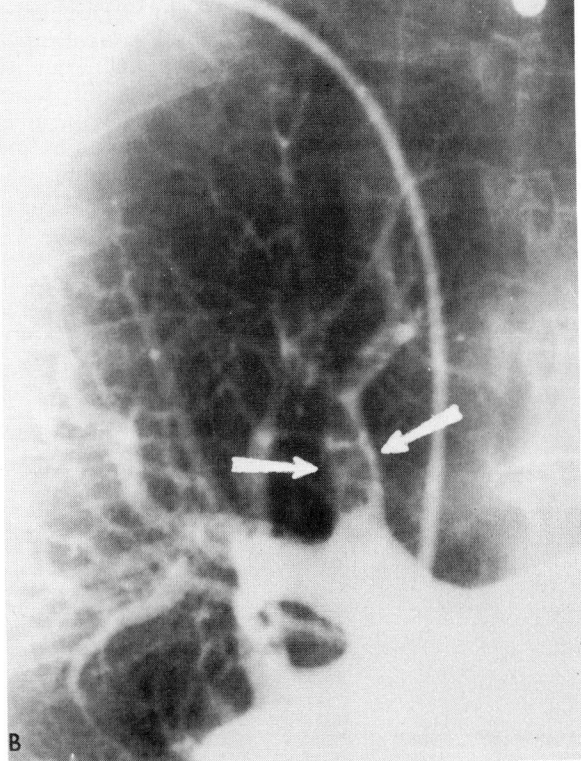

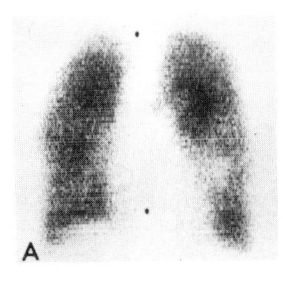

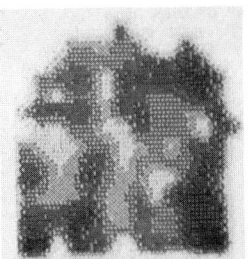

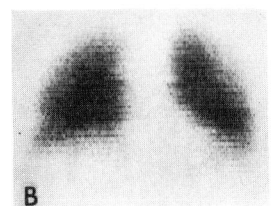

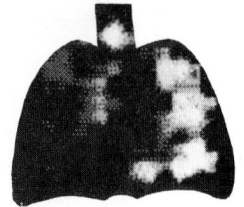

Figure 5. Ventilation-perfusion studies were performed in two patients with normal chest radiographs and peripheral perfusion defects on lung scan. An even distribution of ventilation and perfusion was observed in patient *A,* suggesting that perfusion defects were secondary to depressed ventilation in these regions. The ventilation-perfusion study in patient *B* demonstrated three areas of the left lung that had excessive ventilation compared to perfusion, compatible with pulmonary emboli at these locations.

PERF   VENT / PERF

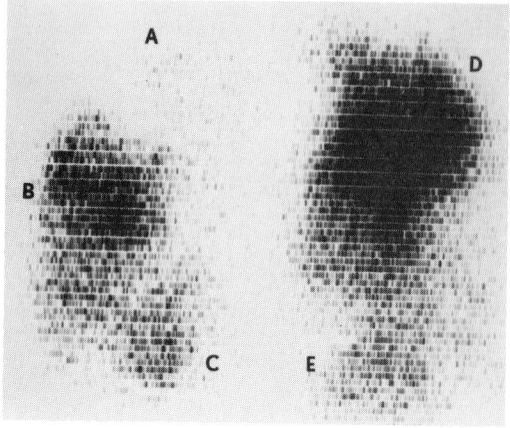
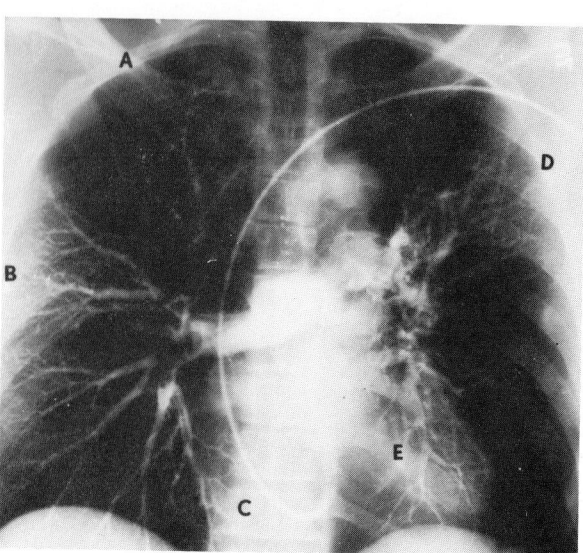

Figure 6. The lung scan and pulmonary angiogram in this patient with bilateral pulmonary embolism demonstrate the usual close correlation between the two studies of pulmonary perfusion. The letters on the two studies mark comparable lung regions.

the function of both Kupffer and polygonal liver cells, and liver scans by both approaches usually demonstrate similar abnormalities. Because of practical radiopharmaceutical features, the particle sequestration method is most commonly used.

The most important use of liver scanning in surgical patients is detection of hepatic metastases. Liver scanning has demonstrated an accuracy of approximately 80 per cent for the evaluation of hepatic metastases in a large number of studies reviewed by Lunia and co-workers. Jhingran and colleagues compared the efficacy of liver scanning with that of alkaline phosphatase and BSP determinations in the detection of metastatic carcinoma in 284 patients with a known

pathologic diagnosis. Abnormal alkaline phosphatase values were observed in 71 per cent of patients with hepatic metastases, but values were also abnormal in 41 per cent of patients with normal livers. BSP determinations revealed an 81 per cent accuracy in diagnosis of metastatic cancer but also produced a 61 per cent incidence of false positives. Liver scanning was 83 per cent accurate in detection of metastatic liver cancer, with a false-positive rate of only 9 per cent. These figures suggest that liver scanning is equally sensitive and more specific for detection of metastatic liver carcinoma than either alkaline phosphatase or BSP determinations. An additional value of liver scanning is the anatomic location of areas of decreased

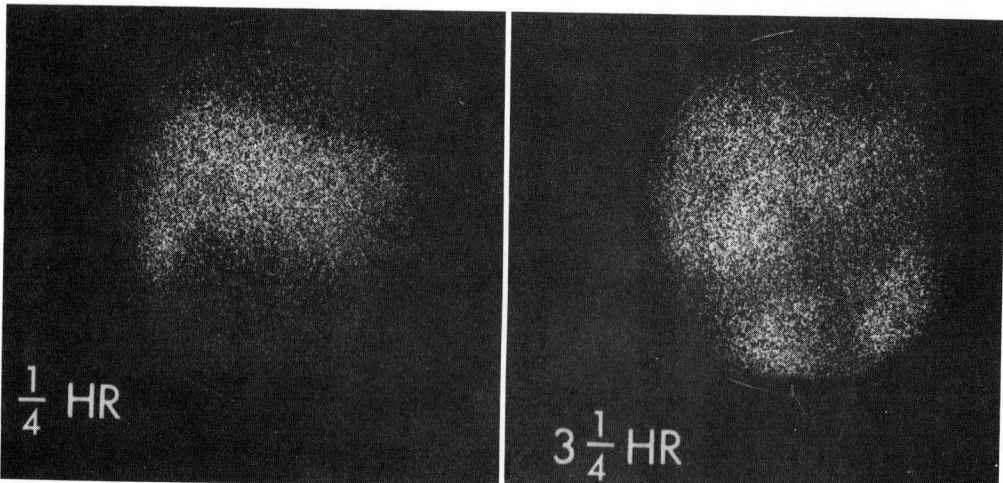

Figure 7. An ^{131}I-rose bengal study was performed in this child with a cystic mass palpable in the right upper quadrant of the abdomen. After 15 minutes, tracer outlines the liver, with upward displacement of the liver edge adjacent to the palpable mass. Three hours later, excretion of tracer into bile results in diffuse radioactivity in the gastrointestinal tract. In addition, a high concentration of tracer appears in the mass adjacent to the liver, indicating the structure to be bile-filled. Surgical exploration confirmed the diagnosis of choledochal cyst.

function, which aids selection of regions for needle liver biopsy. Liver biopsies guided by scan data should make it possible to diagnose more hepatic metastases than are found by random liver biopsy alone (65 to 75 per cent).

Approximately one third of all patients with malignant disease have hepatic metastasis, which may be present without clinical manifestations. Carcinomas of the gastrointestinal system, pancreas, lung, breast, uterus, ovary, and kidney are tumors that commonly metastasize to the liver. Preoperative liver scanning is not practical in each patient suspected of these tumors, but alkaline phosphatase determinations should be obtained. Liver scans should be performed in patients with elevated alkaline phosphatase values in whom presence of liver metastases might alter surgical therapy. In addition to metastatic carcinoma, liver scan defects may be caused by primary hepatic carcinoma, cysts, hamartomas, abscesses, granulomas, vascular malformations, and traumatic injury. Cirrhosis characteristically causes a diffuse decrease in tracer accumulation in the liver and increased phagocytosis by reticuloendothelial cells of other organs. However, generalized involvement of the liver with metastatic carcinoma can produce a similar picture

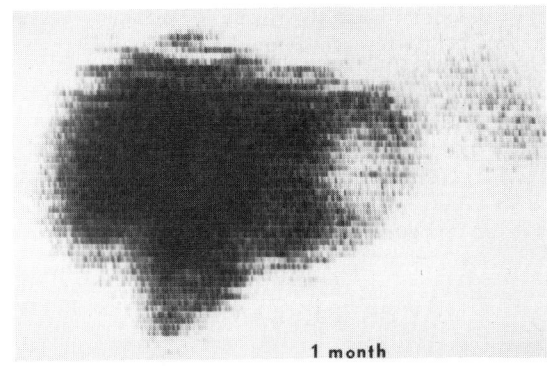

1 month

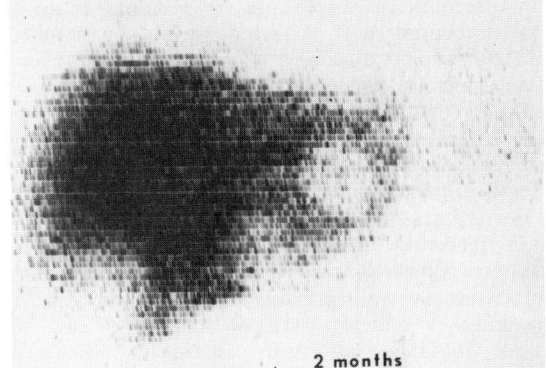

2 months

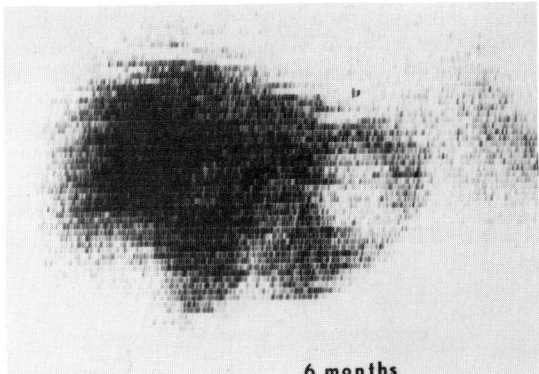

6 months

Figure 9. Serial liver scans in this patient with carcinoma of the rectum metastatic to the liver objectively document progression of the hepatic metastasis and aid in determination of prognosis.

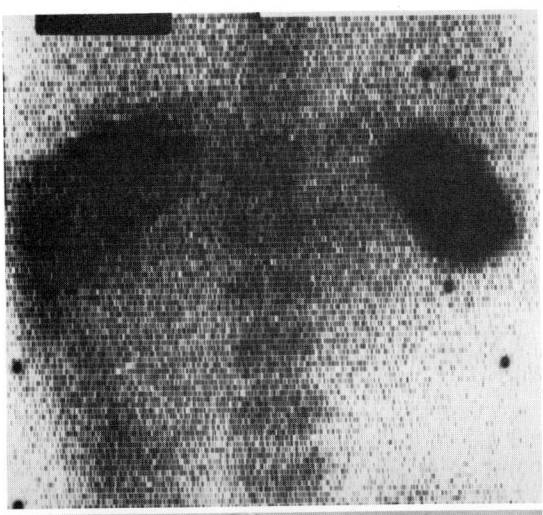

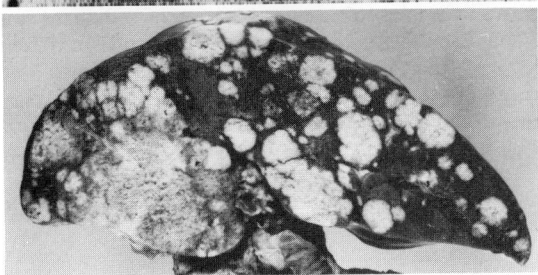

Figure 8. Destruction of Kupffer cells caused by replacement of a large portion of the liver by metastatic adenocarcinoma of the pancreas decreases liver phagocytosis in this patient. Posterior liver scan demonstrates decreased tracer accumulation in the liver and increased phagocytosis by the spleen and bone marrow of the vertebral bodies. This appearance on liver scan is present in any disease causing significant destruction of liver reticuloendothelial cells.

(Fig. 8). Definitive diagnosis of liver scan defects requires biopsy and histologic examination.

In addition to detection of metastases, changes in size of defects on liver scan provide objective documentation of response to chemotherapeutic agents to aid determination of prognosis (Fig. 9). An infrequent but important use of liver scanning is determination of organ position in patients with situs inversus or other congenital malformations of the abdominal organs. A liver scan in combination with a lung scan provides a method for diagnosis of subdiaphragmatic abscesses. The small space between the right lung base and liver dome cannot be separated on combination liver-lung scans in normal subjects. Abnormal subdiaphragmatic fluid collections separate the lung and liver and produce a zone of decreased radioactivity between the two organs on liver-lung scan (Fig. 10). Small collections of pus may occupy insufficient space to produce a positive liver-lung scan, and a normal study does not exclude the possibility of a subdiaphragmatic abscess. However, positive studies provide objective evidence of this disorder, which is often difficult to recognize by other approaches.

BRAIN SCANNING

Over the past 20 years, brain scanning has evolved from a complicated investigative technique to an integral component in the routine evaluation of patients with neurologic disorders. Lesions are identified by brain scanning as regions of high radioactivity compared to low activity in surrounding normal tissue. The preferential localization of radioactive tracers in abnormal regions depends upon disruption of the blood-brain barrier that limits penetration of tracers in normal tissue. The most common agent used for brain scanning is ^{99m}Tc pertechnetate, which may achieve a tumor-to-brain ratio of approximately 22 to 1. Unfortunately, radiopharmaceuticals do not localize in any manner characteristic of a specific pathologic process but detect alterations in the blood-brain barrier caused by tumor, intracerebral hemorrhage, infarction, abscess, granuloma, or arteriovenous malformations. Therefore, it is not possible to delineate the etiology of various abnormalities observed by brain scanning.

Although isotope localization is not specific for any disorder, predictions of the pathologic process may be made from the location, size, and shape of the abnormality observed. *Tumors* usually appear spherical or oval in shape, and margins of the lesions may be dis-

crete in neoplasms such as meningiomas or quite indistinct in highly invasive neoplasms such as gliomas (Fig. 11). Cerebral *infarcts* may be recognized as wedge-shaped defects extending into the periphery. A *subdural hematoma* often presents as a peripheral crescent pattern of increased radioactivity. Lesions that correspond to a specific arterial blood supply are more likely to be of a cerebral vascular etiology, whereas lesions that extend across the midline or beyond the zone of a single arterial supply are more likely to be neoplasms. A brain abscess may show increased uptake about the periphery with little accumulation in the center of the abscess, which lacks blood flow (Fig. 12).

Images of the dynamic flow of radioactive tracer through cerebral vessels display less anatomic resolution than cerebral angiography but are obtained with much less patient discomfort. These dynamic studies are useful in combination with static brain images in differentiation of cerebral vascular abnormalities from brain tumors. Although great variability may occur in dynamic studies, certain patterns are typical of abnormalities when observed. Cerebral infarcts may present an area of decreased activity in the region of the involved vessel during the arterial phase, which may be followed during the venous phase by increased activity in the ischemic area indicative of slow flow through collateral circulation. Subdural hematomas typically demonstrate a peripheral deficit of radioactivity throughout the entire study corresponding to the size and location of the lesion. Occasionally a rim of compressed normal brain tissue may display a zone of peripheral increased activity. *Arteriovenous malformations* demonstrate a zone of early increased activity that disappears at an increased rate (Fig. 13). *Abscesses* frequently are avascular and rarely show increased activity. The appearance of primary and metastatic neoplasms on flow study is variable and not usually helpful in differentiating these lesions.

The timing of the static brain scan relative to onset of cerebral vascular disease affects scan results. In patients with cerebral infarction or cerebral hemorrhage, brain scan may be normal soon after the episode (Fig. 14). The lesion typically demonstrates greatest radionuclide accumulation 2 to 3 weeks after the episode, and within several months the lesion may not appear on brain scan. Studies of subdural hematomas demonstrate only a 50 per cent rate of detection shortly after the episode of hemorrhage. However, approximately 10 days after bleeding, the accuracy of scan in subdural hematoma detection increases to 80 to 90 per cent.

BONE SCANNING

Complexes of ^{99m}Tc, tin, and a linear polyphosphate produce a highly specific bone-seeking radiopharmaceutical that accumulates in bone with kinetics similar to the inorganic phosphate ion. Any process increasing bone metabolism enhances tracer accumulation, and inflammatory as well as neoplastic pro-

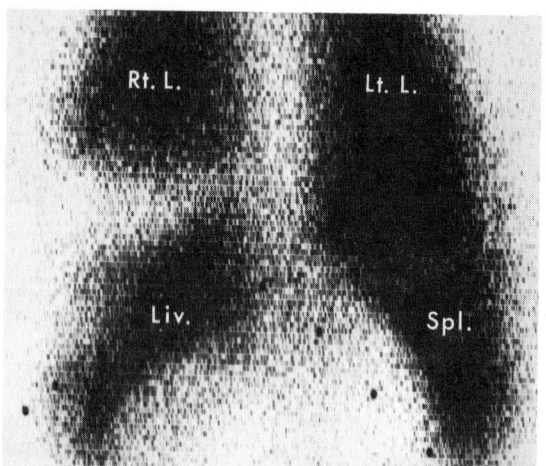

Figure 10. This liver-lung scan in a patient several weeks after a gunshot wound to the liver demonstrates abnormal separation of the liver and right lung and is diagnostic of a *subdiaphragmatic fluid collection* or abscess.

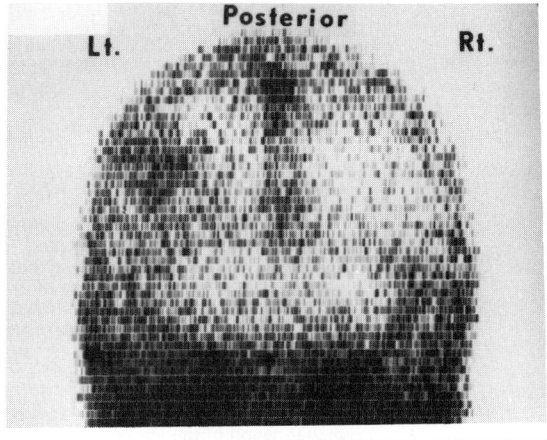

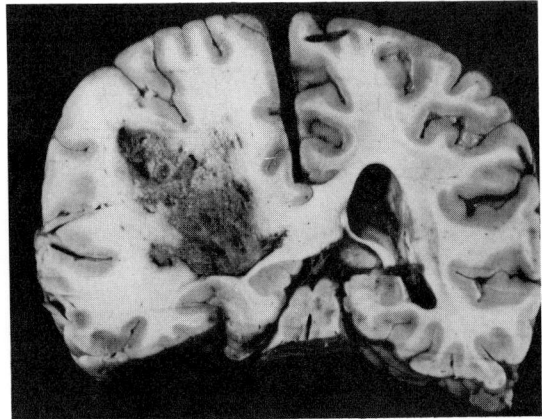

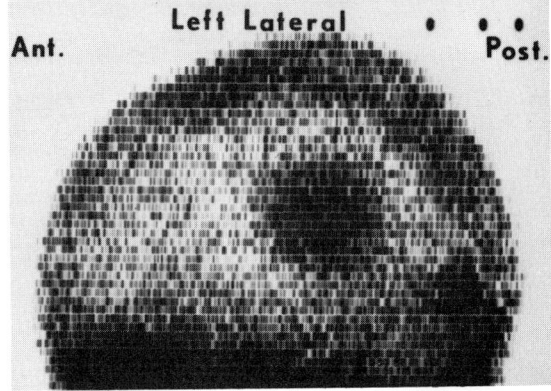

Figure 11. The irregular border of this brain scan lesion in the left hemisphere suggests a malignant neoplasm. Pathologic examination confirmed the presence of a large glioblastoma.

Figure 12. The rim of increased radioactivity surrounding the brain lesion in this patient represents the typical appearance of a brain abscess.

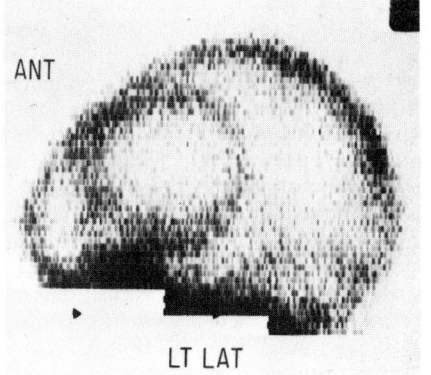

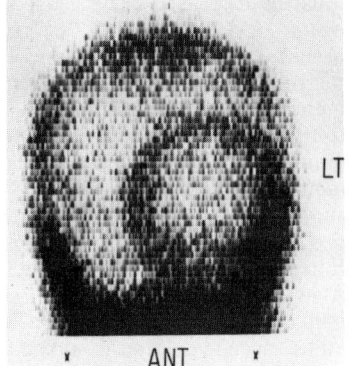

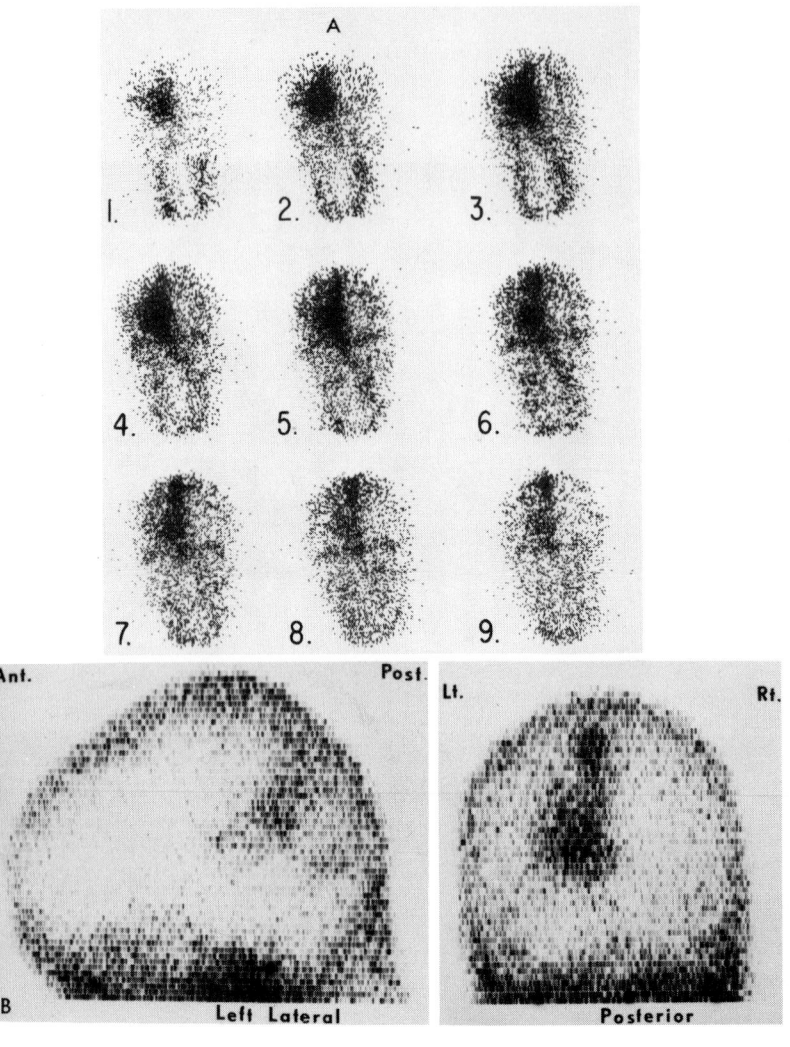

Figure 13. *A,* This dynamic brain study demonstrates radioactivity detected from the posterior view of the head and neck at 1-second intervals during passage of a bolus of technetium-99m pertechnetate through the carotid arteries and intracranial vessels. The early appearance of radioactivity in the left hemisphere is typical of the arteriovenous malformation present in this patient. *B,* The static brain scan in this patient with an arteriovenous malformation of the left occipital lobe demonstrates an increased amount of tracer localized in that region.

cesses result in increased tracer uptake. Conventional radiographs provide relatively insensitive detection of bone metastases, and the calcium content of bone must be increased or decreased about 50 per cent for a lesion to be apparent. Carcinomas of the prostate, breast, kidney, stomach, and lung commonly metastasize to bone, and metastatic disease can be documented by bone scanning in a large number of patients with these disorders at the time of initial diagnosis. The extent of metastatic disease documented by scan frequently exceeds involvement suggested by symptoms (Fig. 15). Documentation of the sites of systemic involvement of carcinoma aids selection of the proper treatment for these patients. Also, bone scanning permits selection of an optimal biopsy site when histologic confirmation of bone metastases is desired in patients with carcinoma. Elevated bone metabolism associated with trauma, osteomyelitis, or arthritis increases ^{99m}Tc stannous pyrophosphate accumulation, and this sensitivity for most inflammatory processes makes bone scanning a useful procedure in patients with undiagnosed musculoskeletal pain. Osteomyelitis may be apparent on bone scan several weeks before changes appear on a radiograph.

CARDIAC SCANNING

Technetium-99m stannous pyrophosphate, which is an agent commonly used for bone scanning, has been recently observed to accumulate in acutely infarcted myocardial tissue (Fig. 16). Greatest affinity for the radiopharmaceutical occurs from one to seven days after infarction and corresponds to the time of maximum calcium influx into the mitochondria of injured myocardial cells. Myocardial scanning appears to be particularly useful for documentation of myocardial infarction in patients following cardiac surgery. Dynamic cardiac studies, radionuclide angiocardiograms, may also be performed using a gamma-camera to record passage of a radioactive bolus through the heart. The resulting images of blood flow aid recognition of abnormal hemodynamics and are particularly useful in patients with congenital heart disorders. These studies provide indicator dilution curves from each cardiac chamber, from which useful hemodynamic information may be derived. The technique also provides a noninvasive approach for evaluation of cardiac function by measurement of the wall motion and ejection fraction of the left ventricle (Fig. 17).

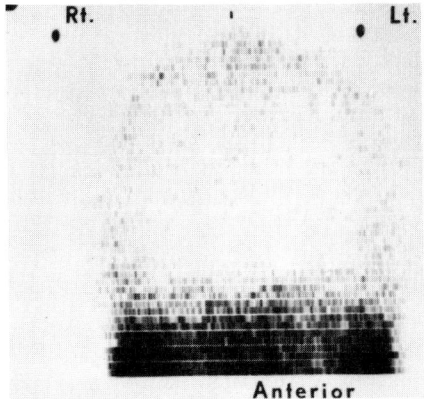

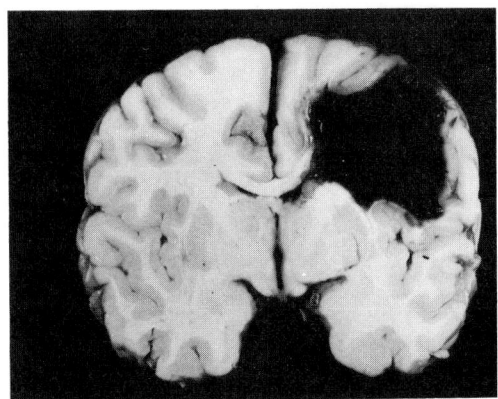

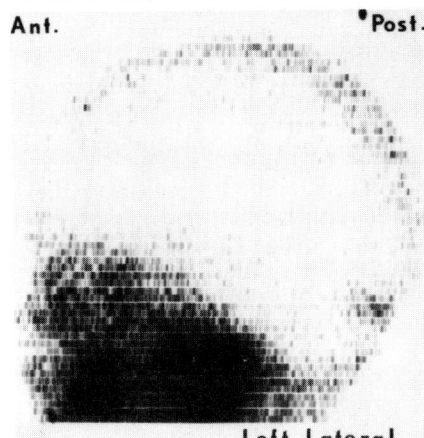

Figure 14. A brain scan in this 12-year-old boy obtained 12 hours after onset of neurologic symptoms appears normal. The patient died shortly after this study, and pathologic examination demonstrated a massive intracranial hemorrhage.

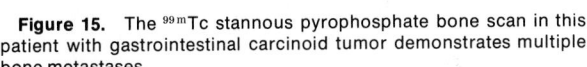

Figure 15. The ^{99m}Tc stannous pyrophosphate bone scan in this patient with gastrointestinal carcinoid tumor demonstrates multiple bone metastases.

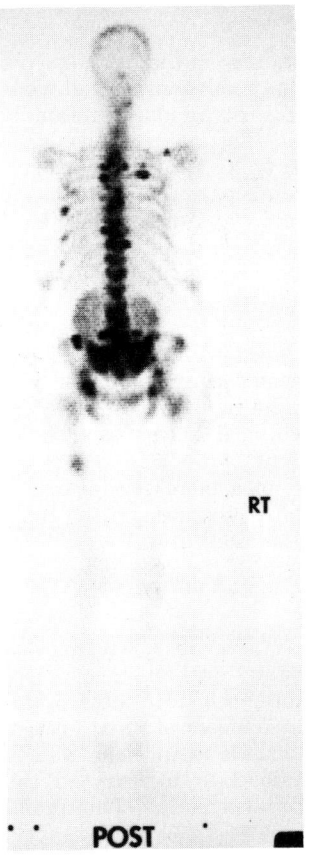

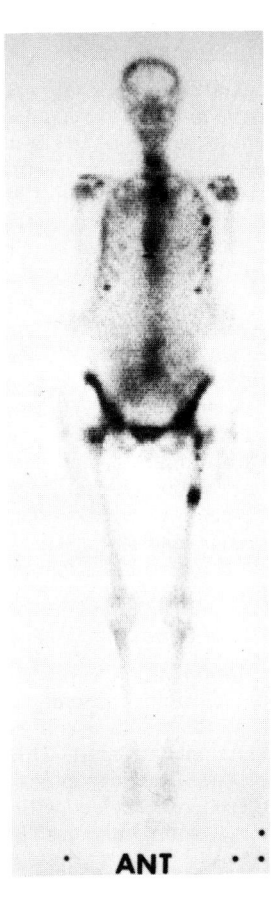

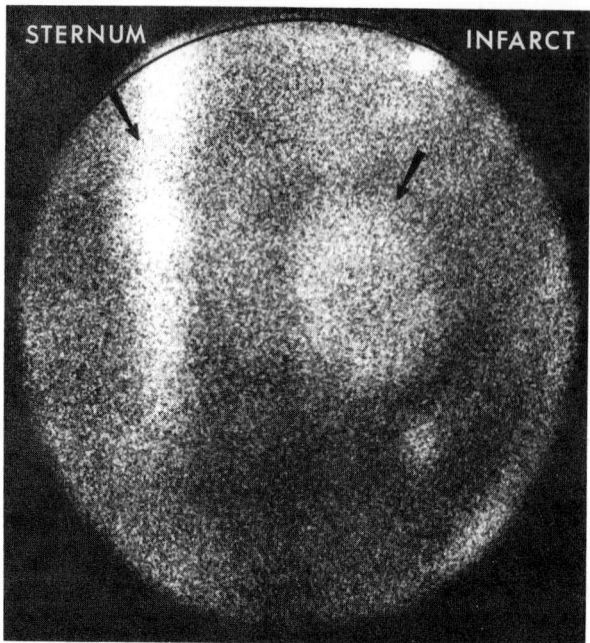

Figure 16. A myocardial scan performed with ^{99m}Tc stannous pyrophosphate shows normal bone accumulation in the sternum and ribs. Abnormal tracer accumulation in the apex of the heart localizes the area of acute myocardial infarction in this patient.

pharmaceutical selectively accumulates in functioning renal tubular cells, and most renal diseases cause scan defects. Renal scanning may be used for documenting congenital abnormalities in the size, shape, and position of the kidneys. Renal scanning also provides serial assessment of the amount of parenchymal injury in patients with renal trauma. It occasionally proves useful for detection of mass lesions of the kidney, but frequently the findings are of little diagnostic benefit, since both malignant tissue and benign masses such as cysts and adenomas commonly cause defects on scan.

The combination of dynamic assessment of renal blood flow using ^{99m}Tc pertechnetate and measurement of excretory function using ^{131}I Hippuran offers a useful approach for evaluation of transplanted kidneys. Regular use of this procedure in the postoperative period aids in the differential diagnosis of acute tubular necrosis, vascular compromise, and acute rejection.

Pancreatic and Parathyroid Scanning

The rapid protein metabolism that occurs in the pancreas and parathyroid glands provides a method for selective radionuclide accumulation within these organs. Selenomethionine, synthesized with selenium-

OTHER PROCEDURES

Gallium Scanning

Gallium-67 citrate accumulates in the liver, spleen, bone marrow, bone, and kidneys following intravenous administration. The tracer also accumulates in rapidly dividing cells and localizes selectively in neoplastic tissue. However, gallium scanning has not proved sufficiently accurate in the diagnosis of carcinoma to merit widespread clinical use. This tracer also selectively accumulates in areas of inflammation, probably by transport into the region as a haptoglobin or transferrin complex. Gallium-67 citrate has been used for localization of occult abscesses and has been suggested for evaluation of patients with intra-abdominal abscesses (Fig. 18). However, competing activity of ^{67}Ga in the liver, spleen, and kidneys often hinders accurate diagnosis, and the technique proves accurate in only about one half of patients with intra-abdominal abscess. Until development of a more specific radiopharmaceutical, ^{67}Ga remains the best tracer currently available for abscess localization despite its limitations.

Renal Scanning

Renal angiography and intravenous or retrograde pyelography provide adequate evaluation of most renal disorders. Renal scanning is of value only in unusual situations in which assessment of renal disease by these radiographic methods is insufficient. Chlormerodrin labeled with radioactive mercury is the agent commonly used for renal scanning. This radio-

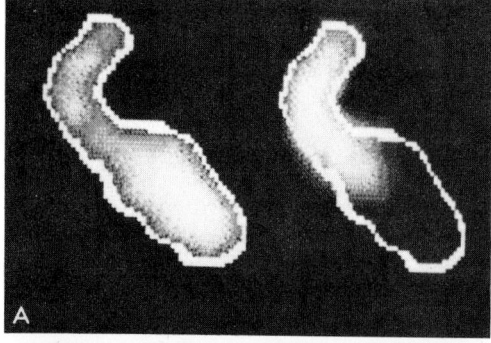
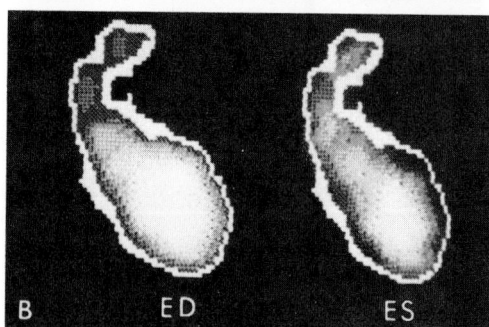

Figure 17. Images of end-diastole (ED) and end-systole (ES) were obtained during passage of a ^{99m}Tc-pertechnetate bolus through the left ventricle. Patient A with aortic stenosis and an increased left ventricular ejection fraction demonstrates a large amount of left ventricular wall motion from end-diastole to end-systole. Patient B with severe coronary artery disease and a low left ventricular ejection fraction demonstrates diffuse left ventricular hypokinesis during left ventricular contraction.

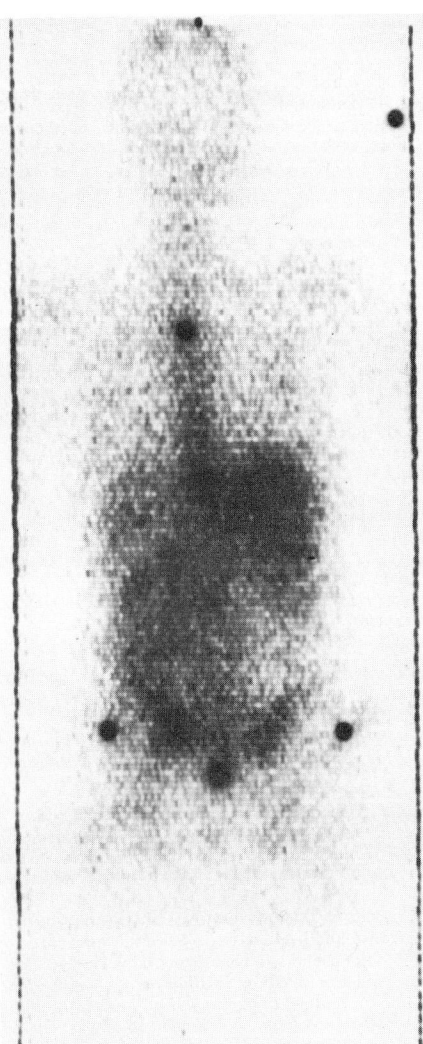

Figure 18. This anterior scan from the head to the knees was obtained two days after gallium-67 citrate administration in a patient with regional enteritis and chronic abdominal pain. Normal tracer accumulation outlines the bones, spleen, and liver. Abnormal tracer accumulation appears along the right side of the abdomen and extends into the pelvis. A large intra-abdominal abscess found at operation coincided with the region of increased gallium-67 citrate localization.

75 replacing the sulfur in methionine, enters the same metabolic pathways as the precursor amino acid. Within an hour after intravenous injection of seleno-methionine, the pancreas accumulates about 7 per cent of the injected dose and demonstrates a concentration nine times greater than that within the liver. The parathyroid concentration of this agent approaches seven times that of blood or thyroid tissue. However, the high total radioactivity that surrounds the pancreas and parathyroid glands makes imaging of these organs difficult.

In most reported studies, pancreas scanning proves about 90 per cent accurate in documentation of absence of pancreatic disease and only 50 per cent accu-

rate in recognition of patients with an abnormal pancreas. Only about 50 per cent of parathyroid glands demonstrated to be abnormal by excision can be recognized by preoperative scan. This low rate of accurate diagnosis does not justify use of parathyroid scanning in surgical patients. Routine clinical application of pancreas and parathyroid scanning awaits development of radiopharmaceuticals with a high selective uptake by these organs.

Meckel's Diverticulum Scan

Gastric mucosa selectively secretes $^{99m}TcO_4^-$, probably by the cellular mechanism responsible for Cl^- excretion. Ectopic gastric mucosa in the distal esophagus or in a Meckel's diverticulum may be imaged after ^{99m}Tc pertechnetate administration (Fig. 19). However, only about one fourth of patients with a Meckel's diverticulum have sufficient ectopic gastric mucosa to produce a positive scan. The technique, which is useful only when positive, may aid evaluation of patients with occult gastrointestinal bleeding.

Thrombus Detection

Iodine-125 fibrinogen has been the most widely used tracer for detection of venous thrombosis. Following intravenous administration, this agent disappears from the circulating fibrinogen pool with a half-life of about one week. For a period of about a week following the onset of venous thrombosis, sufficient fibrin deposition persists to permit incorporation of radioactive fibrinogen into the thrombus. Both legs may be

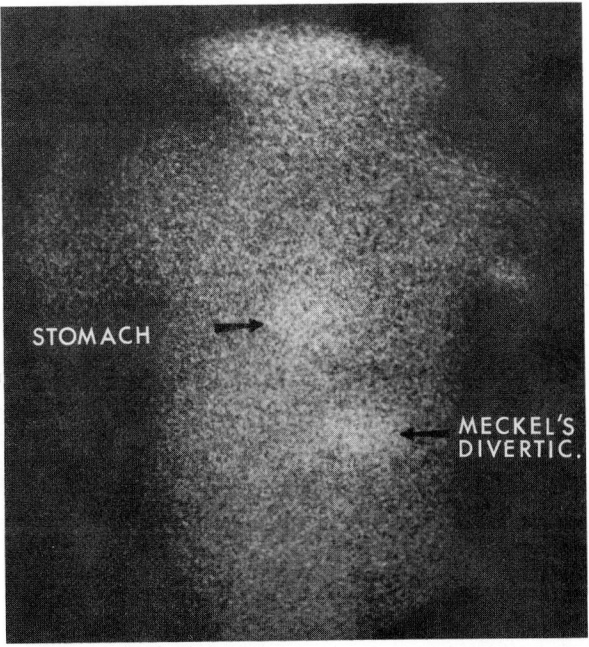

Figure 19. This anterior body image was obtained following ^{99m}Tc-pertechnetate administration in a child with occult gastrointestinal bleeding. Two areas of increased tracer accumulation are apparent in the abdomen. The upper area corresponds to the stomach and the lower area represents ectopic gastric mucosa in a Meckel's diverticulum. A Meckel's diverticulum was found at operation in this patient.

counted daily for one week after a single administration of tracer, and an increase in radioactivity provides an indication of the extent of thrombosis and the change of the process with time. The simplicity of the technique permits screening studies in groups of patients with disorders that predispose to venous thrombosis. Approximately 30 per cent of older patients undergoing major operative procedures develop evidence of venous thrombosis when studied by the ^{125}I fibrinogen technique.

SELECTED REFERENCES

Baum, S., and Bramlet, R.: Basic Nuclear Medicine. New York, Appleton-Century-Crofts, 1975.
This short text provides a cohesive summary of clinical radionuclide studies and is directed primarily to physicians with little previous training in nuclear medicine procedures.

Bonte, F. J., Parkey, R. W., Graham, K. D., and Moore, J. G.: Distributions of several agents useful in imaging myocardial infarcts. J. Nucl. Med., *16*:132, 1975.
These investigators first noted ^{99m}Tc stannous pyrophosphate accumulation in acutely infarcted myocardial tissue. This paper describes basic experimental observations with myocardial infarction imaging.

DeLand, F., and Wagner, H. N., Jr.: Atlas of Nuclear Medicine. Volume I: Brain. Philadelphia, W. B. Saunders Company, 1969.
This work collects instructive clinical examples that illustrate the use of brain scanning in evaluation of neurologic disorders.

DeLand, F., and Wagner, H. N., Jr.: Atlas of Nuclear Medicine. Volume II: Lung and Heart. Philadelphia, W. B. Saunders Company, 1970.
This companion volume well illustrates the clinical use of lung scanning.

Freeman, L. M., and Blaufox, M. D. (Eds.): Seminars in Nuclear Medicine. New York, Grune & Stratton, Inc., 1971–1976.
This excellent series of monographs contains original and review articles that provide thorough, current information on radionuclide techniques.

Freeman, L. M., and Johnson, P. M.: Clinical Scintillation Imaging. New York, Grune & Stratton, Inc., 1975.
This is an excellent current textbook and general reference source.

Harvey, W. C., Podoloff, D. A., and Kopp, D. T.: [67]Gallium in 68 consecutive infection searches. J. Nucl. Med., *16*:2, 1975.
This article reviews gallium-67 studies in 68 patients with infection and 37 patients with intra-abdominal infections. In the latter group, the false positive rate was only 4 per cent, but the false negative rate was 42 per cent.

James, A. E., Jr., Wagner, H. N., Jr., and Cooke, R. E.: Pediatric Nuclear Medicine. Philadelphia, W. B. Saunders Company, 1974.
This book emphasizes specific applications and limitations of nuclear medicine procedures in children.

Jhingran, S. G., Jordan, L., Monroe, F. J., and Haynie, T. P.: Liver scintigrams compared with alkaline phosphatase and BSP determinations in the detection of metastatic carcinoma. J. Nucl. Med., *12*:227, 1971.
This study of 284 patients compares techniques for detection of metastatic carcinoma in the liver.

Kakkar, V.: The diagnosis of deep vein thrombosis using the ^{125}I fibrinogen test. Arch. Surg., *104*:152, 1972.
This study summarizes use of ^{125}I fibrinogen in 784 patients. In 669 elective surgical patients, a 28 per cent incidence of positive studies was observed. The fibrinogen test was positive in 54 per cent of 50 patients with hip fractures, which was the group with greatest predisposition to venous thrombosis.

Kuisk, H., Sanchez, J. S., and Mizuno, N. S.: Colloidal thorium dioxide (Thorotrast) in radiology with emphasis on hepatic cancerogenesis. Am. J. Roentgenol., *99*:463, 1967.
This article reviews reports of malignancy associated with Thorotrast use.

Lunia, S., Parthasarathy, K. L., Bakshi, S., and Bender, M. A.: An evaluation of ^{99m}Tc-sulfur colloid liver scintiscans and their usefulness in metastatic workup: A review of 1,424 studies. J. Nucl. Med., *16*:62, 1975.
This study reviews liver scans on 1115 patients. Histopathologic evaluation of the liver was available in 581 patients and correlated with the liver scan in 77 per cent of this group.

Pierson, R. N., Jr., Kriss, J. P., Jones, R. H., and MacIntyre, W. J.: Quantitative Nuclear Cardiography. New York, John Wiley & Sons, Inc., 1975.
This text by a number of authors describes the large number of radionuclide studies applicable to patients with cardiovascular disease.

Subramanian, G., Rhodes, B. A., Cooper, J. F., and Sodd, V. J.: Radiopharmaceuticals. New York, Society of Nuclear Medicine, 1975.
This book summarizes current knowledge of the distribution kinetics of radiopharmaceuticals currently used for patient studies.

Tofe, A. J., Francis, M. D., and Harvey, W. J.: Correlation of neoplasms with incidence and localization of skeletal metastases: An analysis of 1,355 diphosphonate bone scans. J. Nucl. Med., *16*:986, 1975.
This study reviews findings in 1355 patients with diphosphonate bone scans. Patients with carcinoma of the breast, lung, and prostate demonstrated skeletal involvement in 67 per cent, 64 per cent, and 62 per cent, respectively, at the time of initial evaluation by bone scan. However, these percentages do not reflect accurately the extent of diffuse carcinoma at time of initial diagnosis, since many of these studies were performed late in the course of the disease.

Wagner, H. N., Jr.: Nuclear Medicine. New York, H. P. Publishing Co., Inc., 1975.
This well-illustrated book is directed primarily to the practicing physician.

14

WOUND HEALING: BIOLOGIC AND CLINICAL FEATURES

John W. Madden, M.D.

The response of living tissues to injury forms the foundation of all surgical practice. Indeed, from a biologic viewpoint, tissue injury and its sequelae participate in a majority of general medical problems. Although the cardiologist discusses complications of myocardial infarction in physiologic terms (congestive heart failure, chronic arrhythmia, embolism, and so forth), the ultimate outcome may depend entirely on the healing reactions of the heart. The gastrointestinal surgeon attacks abnormal physiology by removing or rerouting segments of gut; the vascular surgeon restores peripheral blood flow with clever reconstructions or replacements of peripheral blood vessels. Although directed toward correcting physiologic abnormalities, these therapeutic manipulations depend entirely on the body's ability to repair tissue damage. Unfortunately, because wound healing represents such a basic response of living organisms to life and, as a rule, produces successful restoration of tissue integrity, the biology of repair is taken for granted or ignored by some physicians.

Historical Aspects

The passive attitude toward the biology of repair has historical roots. The history of wound healing is, of course, the history of mankind. The earliest medical writings deal extensively with wound care. Seven of the 48 case reports included in the Smith Papyrus (1700 B.C.) describe wounds and their management. Empirically, the ancient physicians of Egypt, Greece, India, and Europe developed gentle methods of treating wounds. They appreciated the necessity of removing foreign bodies, suturing, covering wounds with clean materials, and protecting injured tissues from corrosive agents.

During the fourteenth century, with the widespread use of gunpowder and the increasing frequency of bullet wounds, a new era of wound treatment emerged. Instead of maintaining a caretaker's attitude in wound management and relying on natural processes for repair, surgeons assumed an aggressive posture. Active and dramatic action was taken to "help

wounds heal." Applications of boiling oil, burning oil, hot cautery, and scalding water replaced gentle washing with warm, boiled water and the application of mild salves. Cleanliness was forgotten. Needless to say, this "let's-do-something-about-it" attitude toward wound healing produced disastrous results.

In the mid-sixteenth century. Ambroise Paré, the great French army surgeon, rediscovered gentle methods. As in so many great biologic contributions, chance played a key role. During the Battle of Villaine, the supply of oil was exhausted, and Paré was forced to apply milder treatments to amputation wounds. To his surprise these wounds healed rapidly without the expected complications. From this beginning, the modern era of gentle wound care evolved. John Hunter, William Stewart Halsted, Alexis Carrel, and many other great clinical biologists demonstrated that minimizing tissue injury produces rapid and effective healing. The majority of technical advances in wound care over the past century have been based on a "minimal interference" concept: If the surgeon can remove all impediments, normal wound healing processes will produce the best possible result.

In the vast majority of clinical situations this elegant, simple concept is sound. The greatest portion of this chapter will be devoted to exploring the normal phenomenon of wound healing and demonstrating ways to allow the normal course of events to occur. Unfortunately, however, the normal response of tissues to injury does not always produce a perfectly functional result. The same processes that establish strength and integrity in incisions of bowel or abdominal wall also produce fibrous stricture of the esophagus, rheumatic valvular disease, cirrhosis of the liver, incarcerated tendons, keloids, intestinal adhesions, and a host of other abnormalities. If effective methods of controlling the shape, size, and physical properties of scars existed, a new phase of wound management could evolve. The pathophysiologic phenomena created by scar formation would no longer be considered inevitable. Effective control would replace minimal interference as a guiding principle. To some observers, the stage seems set for this new era in wound management. Experimentally, the wound healing process can be altered effectively, eliminating or reducing the pathophysiologic consequences of scar formation. Current methods of controlling scar formation will be discussed briefly at the close of this chapter.

BIOLOGIC CONSIDERATIONS

Wound healing represents a highly dynamic, integrated series of cellular, physiologic, and biochemical events which occur exclusively in whole organisms. Although individual components of the wound healing reaction (cell multiplication, cell migration, collagen synthesis, collagen crosslinking, and so forth) occur in tissue culture or even in cell-free systems, wounds do not heal in a bottle nor do single events occur in isolation. Examining all processes simultaneously, however, can be confusing. For the purposes of this discussion, wound healing will be separated into several natural components and later discussed as an integrated whole. Again, although all wounds heal by the same basic processes, clinical wounds are of two distinct types—simple closed wounds and open wounds with or without tissue loss. For organizational purposes, each of these clinical situations will be discussed separately.

CLOSED WOUNDS

Morphologic Events

Inflammation. Disruption of tissue integrity by accidental trauma or the surgeon's knife initiates a series of striking morphologic changes. After a transient vasoconstriction, all local small vessels dilate. As dilatation occurs, capillaries become abnormally permeable to proteins and plasma leaks into the site of injury. Coincident with vasomotor changes, alterations occur at the interface between white blood cells and endothelium. White cells begin sticking to endothelial surfaces, particularly small venules, and actively move through the vessel walls. Within hours after injury, the wound space fills with a highly cellular, inflammatory exudate composed of white cells, red cells, soluble plasma proteins, and fibrin strands. White cells, actively motile during this period, begin engulfing cell fragments and debris. The duration and intensity of this inflammatory response depend on the amount of local tissue damage. Obviously, extensive tissue injury or the presence of foreign materials or bacteria can prolong the inflammatory phase for months. In the usual clean incision, however, acute inflammation subsides within a few days.

Removing cellular debris and injured tissue fragments seems an essential part of wound healing and the white cells serve this function. At first, the polymorphonuclear leukocytes predominate. After several days, however, the proportion of monocytes increases significantly. During the initial migration of white cells, the ratio of granulocytes to monocytes in blood and extracellular exudate is identical. Granulocytes, however, are short-lived and the active movement of

white cells into the wound is transient. As the granulocytes die, lyse, and release acid hydrolases into the local environment, the proportion of monocytes increases. Monocytes, of course, can continue their scavenging activity for weeks. Differential survival rates, therefore, seem to account for the shift in cell population.[101]

The precise role each inflammatory cell type plays in the wound-healing process remains obscure, but studies using specific anticellular antisera suggest that wound healing proceeds normally in the absence of both polymorphonuclear granulocytes and lymphocytes. In contrast, monocytes must be present to create normal fibroblast production and invasion of the wound space.[33,49]

Epithelialization. While dead material is being removed from deeper areas, important events occur at the edges of epithelial wounds. In skin wounds, the epidermis immediately adjacent to the wound edge begins thickening within 24 hours after injury. Marginal basal cells lose their firm attachment to underlying dermis, enlarge, and begin to migrate down and across the defect. Fixed basal cells in a zone near the cut edge undergo a series of rapid mitotic divisions and daughter cells emigrate presumably directed in their migrations by contact guidance along fibrin strands and by contact inhibition.[71] Within 48 hours, the entire wound surface is re-epithelialized. Deeper recesses of the wound contain only fibrin strands and inflammatory cells at this point. After bridging the wound defect, migrating epithelial cells lose their flattened appearance, become more columnar in shape, and increase mitotic activity. Layering of epithelium is re-established and surface cells keratinize. The epithelial-mesenchymal interface, however, never regains a normal architecture.[40]

This remarkable response of epithelial cells to injury is not confined to surface areas. Injury to any epithelial element can initiate epithelial migration. For instance, if sutures remain in skin wounds for more than a few days, epithelial cells migrate down the suture tracts. Subsequent epithelial thickening and keratinization may produce marked foreign body reactions and sterile abscesses. Even subcuticular sutures that incise hair follicles or sweat glands can become surrounded by epithelial tracts and produce epithelial cysts.[72]

Cellular Phase. As the inflammatory reaction subsides and the epithelial surface thickens, a new cell type appears in the wound depths. Beginning the second or third day, spindle-shaped cells with oval nuclei become increasingly abundant and by 10 days dominate the cell population. Shortly after this cellular invasion, collagen fibers appear in the wound. Conclusive data indicate that this new cell type, the fibroblast, synthesizes and secretes collagen molecules. Although as a rule the active fibroblast is described as a stellate or spindle-shaped cell, direct observations of living material demonstrate that fibroblasts can assume almost any configuration. The electron microscopic appearance, however, is characteristic. In addition to a diffuse Golgi apparatus and large mitochondria with irregular cristae, fibroblasts contain an extensively developed and dilated

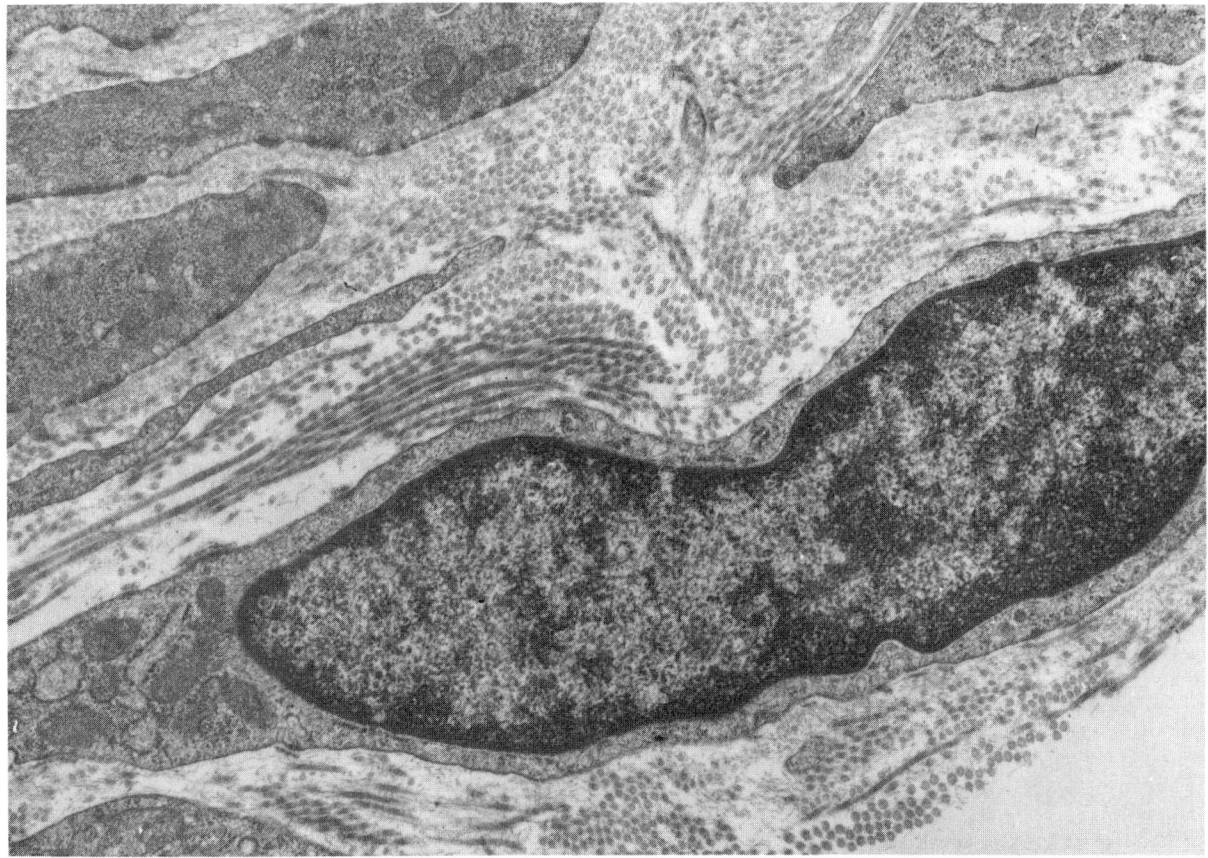

Figure 1. Normal resting fibroblast from human connective tissue. Note the large, smooth oval nucleus, normal mitochondria, and a small amount of rough endoplasmic reticulum. The cell is surrounded by collagen fibrils cut in longitudinal and cross-section. The cell fragments seen in the upper left are typical smooth muscle cells. Electron micrograph × 22,000. (Courtesy of Edward C.Carlson, Ph.D.)

rough endoplasmic reticulum. The long intercommunicating cisternae are bound by curved double rows of polysomes attached to ergastoplasmic membranes.

Although the origin of wound fibroblasts is controversial, recent data indicate that almost all fibroblasts seen in healing wounds are derived from local mesenchymal cells, particularly those associated with blood vessel adventitia. If circulating cells are capable of becoming fixed fibroblasts, as some authors suggest, they play a negligible role in wound healing. The most convincing evidence for the local origin of fibroblasts comes from Ross's recent experiments with parabiotic rats.[84]

At the time local fibroblasts begin moving into the wound, the wound space is filled with fibrin strands. Although migratory fibroblasts appear to use the fibrin network as a scaffolding, whether or not the fibrin strands provide orientation or contact guidance is still debated. Unlike ameboid cells, however, epithelial cells and fibroblasts require a solid or semisolid substrate for their gliding movements. Fibroblasts and epithelial cells move by forming adhesive contacts with the substratum, not by cytoplasmic flow. The leading edge of a moving fibroblast demonstrates the

largest number of attachments and consists of a thin, fanlike membrane, 5 to 10μ wide. This ruffled membrane undergoes continual folding movements that beat inward from the edge. Moving cells require a normal endoplasmic, microtubular architecture, and power is generated by contracting microfilaments within the cell.[9]

In isolated cells, ruffled membranes form intermittently on all areas of the cell surface and the cell moves randomly within a small area. When the ruffled membranes of two cells meet, each cell contracts slightly, the ruffled membranes disappear at the area of contact, and cell migration in that direction ceases. Cell edges free of cellular contact, however, continue to form ruffled membranes and cells move in the direction of ruffling. Although ruffled membrane formation and contact inhibition force populations of cells to migrate into cell-free spaces, neither phenomenon provides orientation or directional movement to single cells. In tissue culture, cell orientation and movement are influenced significantly by substrate orientation. Fibrin strands, glass fibers, and even grooves cut in glass or plastic surfaces orient cells. This peculiar behavior, termed contact guidance, may operate on many levels of substrate organization. Thus, the phenomena of contact inhibition and contact guidance may direct the fibroblast invasion of the wound space, by means of either the fibrin network or an undetected substrate orientation.

Because the first recognizable collagen fibers are associated with fibrin strands, some observers have suggested that fibrin is somehow converted to collagen. Quite the opposite is true. Fibroblasts do not contain fibrinolytic enzymes. Large amounts of fibrin, blood clot, or dead tissue actually produce a physical barrier preventing fibroblast penetration and delaying collagen fiber production. Fortunately, the fibroblast has help.

Rapid capillary proliferation is a prominent feature of all early wound healing. In closed or open wounds, new capillaries form by the budding of existing venules. Endothelial cells proximal to the injury undergo rapid mitosis. The distal cells lose their attachments to the basement membrane and move out into the injured area. Unlike fibroblasts, endothelium moves as a contiguous sheet. Only the leading cells develop ruffled membranes; cell membranes of the followers remain in intimate contact. Because endothelial cells proliferate from many points, a rich network of small vessels is established quickly. Endothelial cells contain a potent plasminogen activator. Thus, as fibroblasts advance into the injured area, followed closely by proliferating capillaries, fibrinolysis occurs, destroying the fibrin network.

Fibroplasia. The fixed cellular phase of wound healing lasts several weeks. By the fourth or fifth week, however, the absolute number of wound fibroblasts has decreased markedly. In addition, the rich capillary network has dwindled to a few well-defined capillary systems. Throughout the life of the scar, a modest number of cells remain associated with scar material, but these fibrocytes no longer possess the active endoplasmic reticulum characteristic of fibroblasts.

As the fibroblast population decreases, collagen fibers become the dominant anatomic feature of wounds. The first collagen fibers appear at 4 or 5 days. Quickly, the wound space fills with small, randomly oriented fiber bundles. Fiber bundles enlarge gradually and produce a massive, dense collagenous structure (the scar) binding the severed tissues together firmly.

In time past, our morphologic discussion of wound healing might have stopped here. For years, many biologists suggested that the important events in wound healing occurred quickly and stopped abruptly. Every careful observer with a personal wound knows this statement is false. All scars, deep or superficial, slowly and progressively change in bulk and form over many years. In certain unfortunate individuals, skin wounds enlarge producing massive keloids or hypertrophic scars; in others, color fades, bulk decreases, normal pigmentation returns, and the scar all but disappears. Scar tissue in most abdominal incisions remains firm and strong forever; occasionally however, abdominal scars thin, spread, lose strength, and incisional hernias develop.

The phenomenon of scar remodeling is basic to the function of injured tissues. The gross appearance of remodeling scars suggests that collagen fibers are, in some fashion, altered or rewoven into different architectural patterns with time. Unfortunately, classic light and electron microscopic techniques are not adequate to investigate remodeling except in unusual situations. Development of the scanning electron microscope, however, has provided a powerful tool suitable for investigating fiber architectural changes. Scanning electron micrographs demonstrate that scar fiber patterns do change slowly for many months.[26] Because remodeling represents such an important clinical property of scars, the phenomenon will be discussed in greater depth in connection with wound·chemistry.

Chemical Events

Inflammation. Although investigated extensively, the chemistry of local inflammation remains controversial. Since the early 1900s, a series of experimental studies have demonstrated conclusively that local substances released by injury produce vasodilatation and increased small vessel permeability. Initially, histamine was considered the primary mediator of inflammatory vascular responses. Histamine, liberated from mast cells, granulocytes, and platelets, produces local vasodilatation and increases small vessel permeability. Although present in early inflammatory exudates, histamine acts for short periods (less than 30 minutes) and local sources are depleted rapidly. In the rat, serotonin (5-hydroxytryptamine), also found in mast cells, has a local action similar to that of histamine. In man, however, the local effects of serotonin are negligible. Because of their short duration of action, it seems unlikely that these amines are responsible for prolonged inflammatory reactions.[101]

Recently, the kinins, a series of biologically active peptides, and the prostaglandins, principally PGE_1

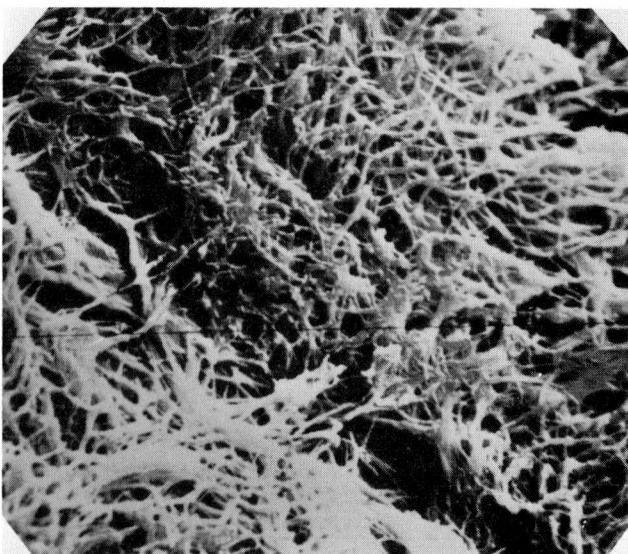

Figure 2. Collagen fibers in a 10-day-old sutured rat skin wound. Note the small size and random arrangement of fibers. Scanning electron micrograph × 4500. (From Forrester, J. C., Zederfeldt, B. H., Hayes, T. L., and Hunt, T. K.: J. Trauma, *10*:770, 1970.)

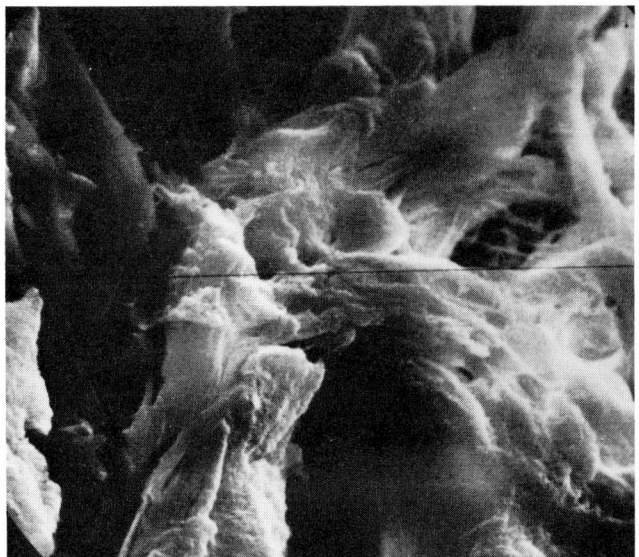

Figure 3. Collagen fibers in a 100-day-old sutured rat skin wound. Note the large, irregular masses of collagen, a significant morphologic change from the 10-day-old wound shown in Figure 2. Scanning electron micrograph × 4500. (From Forrester, J. C., Zederfeldt, B. H., Hayes, T. L., and Hunt, T. K.: J. Trauma, 10:770, 1970.)

and PGE_2, have been implicated in local inflammatory vascular responses. Kallikrein, an enzyme found in plasma and in granulocytes, releases bradykinin and kallidin from the α_2-globulin of plasma. In the presence of kinins and the complement system, local cells produce a variety of prostaglandins. The prostaglandins seem to be the final mediators of acute inflammation, including the reversible small vessel permeability, and may play a chemotactic role for fibroblasts and white cells as well.[99] Aspirin and indomethacin are potent inhibitors of prostaglandin biosynthesis, and the anti-inflammatory action of these drugs may result from their effects on prostaglandin metabolism.

The second phase of inflammatory response, local invasion of white blood cells, may also have chemical mediators. The evidence, however, is even more controversial. Leukotaxine, claimed to be a peptide formed in damaged tissue by the enzymatic destruc-

tion of albumin, was thought to be a chemotactic agent, attracting leukocytes into the damaged area. Although large concentrations of certain isolated peptides can cause leukocyte attraction in tissue culture and other experimental preparations, they do not show chemotactic activity in concentrations found in damaged tissue. Extracts of white blood cells and even certain forms of collagen cause leukocyte chemotaxis in experimental situations. Their role in wound healing, however, is unclear.

Ground Substance. Mature and developing scars contain the same basic extracellular components as all mesenchymal tissue: fibrous proteins, prinicipally collagen; and glycosaminoglycans – mucopolysaccharides, mucoproteins, and glycoproteins. Although the metabolism of both classes may be highly interrelated, their chemistry and kinetics will be discussed separately.

All connective tissues contain variable amounts of glycosaminoglycans. These huge macromolecules, composed chiefly of carbohydrate and a variable amount of protein, are of seven major types. Heparin may be included in this classification, but, is not a structural component of connective tissue. All glycosaminoglycans occur in the form of protein polysaccharide complexes with molecular weights between 7.5×10^5 and 10×10^5. The polysaccharide components are attached to a central protein core and the whole molecule has the configuration of a test tube or bottle brush. The highly charged, sulfated compounds influence local cellular environment significantly. For instance, the water of hydration shell around these molecules is huge and must produce significant effects on extracellular fluid composition.[47]

Early histochemical studies and hexosamine determinations suggested that during the first 3 or 4 days of healing, wounds synthesized large amounts of glycosaminoglycans. During the next few days, as collagen appeared in the wound, hexosamine content decreased sharply. Investigators concluded that the production and deposition of mucopolysaccharides prepared and directed the fibroblasts to produce collagen. Unfortunately, hexosamine values alone do not reflect accurately glycosaminoglycan content of wounds. Detailed analysis of the types of hexosamine-containing compounds present shows conclusively that the early increase reflects the appearance of serum glycoproteins carried into the wound with the initial inflammatory exudate, not locally synthesized compounds.[23]

TABLE 1.   Mucopolysaccharides of Connective Tissue

	Synonyms	Disaccharide Repeating Unit
Chondroitin	—	Glucuronic acid + Galactosamine
Chondroitin 4-sulfate	Chondroitin sulfate A	Glucuronic acid + 4 Sulfo galactosamine
Chondroitin 6-sulfate	Chondroitin sulfate C	Glucuronic acid + 6 Sulfo galactosamine
Dermatan sulfate	Chondroitin sulfate B Heparin	Iduoronic acid + 4 Sulfo galactosamine
Heparin sulfate	Heparitin sulfate Heparin monosulfate	Glucuronic acid + Glucosamine (Contains N and O sulfate groups)*
Hyaluronic acid	—	Glucuronic acid + Glucosamine
Keratin sulfate	Kerato sulfate	Galactose + 6 Sulfo glucosamine

*The structure of this compound is not completely clear.

TABLE 2. Collagenolytic Activity of Human Tissues*

Note the uniformly positive response of the wound margin and granulation tissue. No scar younger than 14 days was positive; however, scars were positive as long as 31 years after the initial injury.

Tissue	Collagenolysis	
	Positive	Negative
Normal skin	17	12
Wound margin	10	0
Granulation	8	0
Eschar	3	3
Healed scar (including 3 keloids which were positive)	23	9
	61	24

*From Riley, W. B., and Peacock, E. E., Jr.: Proc. Soc. Exp. Biol. Med., *124*:207, 1967.

Although human wounds have not been analyzed rigorously, careful studies of animal wounds provide an entirely different picture of glycosaminoglycan metabolism. Minor differences occur in various animal models, but, generally, the hyaluronic acid content of wound tissue remains relatively constant or decreases during the first 3 weeks of healing. In contrast, chondroitin-4-sulfate and dermatan sulfate concentration increases progressively from the fourth through the twenty-first day.[8] No sharp drop in concentration occurs with the appearance of collagen fibers. As yet, no clear-cut role has been established for glycosaminoglycans in wound healing. Several important possibilities exist, however, and will be discussed in a subsequent section.

Collagen Chemistry. Because of the importance of the fibrous proteins, particularly collagen, in scar formation, the study of wound healing requires a basic understanding of collagen chemistry. Until 1968, collagen was considered a single protein. Improved methods of protein separation and extensive sequencing of the peptide chains of collagen, however, have demonstrated at least four distinct types of collagen in mammalian tissues.[67] In spite of their differences in primary and secondary structure, all collagens have certain common and unique features. The collagen molecule (sometimes called tropocollagen) is a rigid rod 3000 Å long and 15 Å wide. This single functional unit is not a simple polypeptide. Instead, each molecule is composed of three polypeptide chains wound together in a characteristic helical relationship. Each of the chains has a glycine residue in every third position along the peptide backbone. Finally, all collagens contain two unique acids—hydroxyproline and hydroxylysine. Elastin contains minute amounts of hydroxyproline as does the C_{1q} component of complement, but for all practical purposes, this imino acid is the exclusive property of collagen and represents approximately 12 per cent of the molecule. The other imino acid, proline, comprises another 12 per cent of most collagens. Although the ratio of hydroxyproline to proline can vary tremendously between collagens from different species or even between collagens from different tissues within the same animal, proline and hydroxyproline taken together always represent about 25 per cent of the acid residues.[42] Thus, over half the molecule is composed of only three acids, glycine, hydroxyproline, and proline.

Collagen is a protein of unique character, and with a uniqueness comes confusion. Because of historial development and common usage, the language of collagen chemistry becomes complicated jargon to the uninitiated. Initially, structural studies were performed on the collagen derived from skin and tendon. Studies on the submolecular structure of this common collagen, now termed Type I, revealed that two of the three polypeptide chains composing the fundamental molecular structure are identical; the third contains a different sequence of amino acids. By convention, the identical chains are called α_1 and the dissimilar chain α_2. To confuse matters even more, native Type I collagen molecules often contain strong covalent bonds between individual polypeptide chains. As a result, two chains linked together covalently were separated and called β-chains. If, upon further separation, the individual components of the β-fraction are

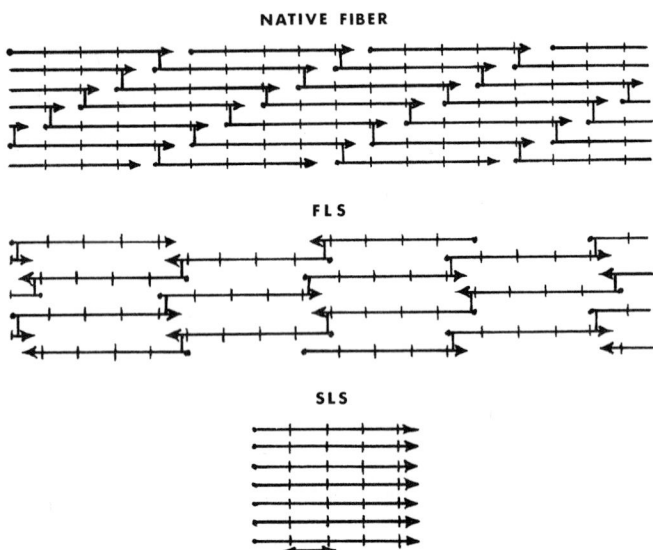

NATIVE FIBER

FLS

SLS

680

2990 Å

Figure 4. Schematic representation of the principal forms of tropocollagen aggregation. The upper figure shows the quarter-stagger, overlapping arrangement of the tropocollagen molecules in the native fiber. Overlapping produces the characteristic 680 Å banding seen in electron micrographs. The center figure represents the fibrous-long-spacing (FLS) form of collagen. Note that the same intermolecular crosslinks are present as in the native fiber. The lower figure represents the segment-long-spacing (SLS) variety of collagen. The tropocollagen molecules are aggregated side to side in parallel array. (From Peacock, E. E., Jr., and Van Winkle, W., Jr.: Surgery and Biology of Wound Repair, 2nd ed. Philadelphia, W. B. Saunders Company, 1976.)

identical to the α_1 chains, the two-chain fragment is called β_{11}; if one of the separate chains is an α_1 and the other an α_2, the chain designation becomes β_{12}; and so on. If all three individual chains are linked with covalent bonds, the isolated fragment is called a gamma chain.

In 1968, a second type of collagen was identified in hyaline cartilages. This collagen, called Type II, is composed of three identical polypeptide chains resembling the α_1 chain of Type I collagen but differing slightly in amino acid sequence.[97] Recently, studies on infant dermis have demonstrated a collagen (Type III) with an α_1 chain distinctly different from Type I and Type II.[14] Type III collagen has now been identified in aorta, lung, adult skin, and scar tissue in addition to infant dermis. Finally, collagen derived from basement membrane seems to be distinctly different from other collagens and has been designated Type IV.[44] Presumably, each of these different forms of the collagen molecule has distinct biological properties influencing the physical characteristics of connective tissues. As yet, however, the specific biological role of each collagen type has not been defined.

Because of the primary amino acid sequence, the α-chains of collagen assume a left-handed helical configuration. The three helices are then twisted into a right-handed "superhelix."[81, 82] Although most of the molecule is rigid, small portions at either end are nonhelical; these regions may be important in determining the biological properties of different collagens.[93]

The rigidity and strength of the triple helical structure and the molecular interactions discussed below are directly responsible for the physical properties of all mesenchymal tissues, including scars.

Collagen, one of the few animal proteins constructed specifically to become insoluble, represents the major structural protein of all vertebrates. Over 30 per cent of the total protein content of most animals is collagen. Specific differences in collagens from different species and from different tissues within the same animal exist, but the rigid rodlike molecular configuration is retained in all collagen types.

The tremendous adaptability of collagen to the structural requirements of animals resides in its aggregation properties. If a dilute solution of collagen molecules is allowed to stand under a variety of conditions, molecules aggregate quickly to form long fibers. Under the electron microscope, collagen fibers possess a striking band pattern with major repeating units at 680 Å. The elegant banding pattern originates in the precise lateral arrangement of collagen molecules. In native collagen fibers, molecules aggregate in a head-to-tail arrangement with adjacent molecules overlapping by approximately one quarter of their length. Recent data suggest that larger fibers are composed of microfibrils, in turn composed of groups of five molecules interrelated in a specific fashion.[91]

As normal collagen molecules aggregate to form fibers, another important event occurs. Initially, collagen molecules in fiber aggregates are held together with weak intermolecular forces, primarily hydrogen bonds. At this point, molecules can be disaggregated and solubilized in cold solutions of low ionic strength. The fibers themselves have very little tensile strength. Over a period of hours or days, however, the fibers increase their strength tremendously and alter their solubility characteristics significantly.

The analysis of the solubility properties of collagen molecules represents a brilliant chapter in collagen biology, and the information obtained is central to our understanding of how wounds heal. Unfortunately, language again becomes a problem. In the early 1950s Schmitt and his associates observed that a small fraction of collagen present in the skin of growing animals was soluble in cold solutions of low ionic strength. When rewarmed, the soluble collagen aggregated into normal collagen fibrils. When cooled again after a short time interval, most of the collagen redissolved. If molecules were allowed to remain in the aggregated state for a longer period, fibers no longer dissolved in cold salt solutions, but could be solubilized with dilute mineral acids. After long time intervals, only agents known to disrupt covalent bonds were capable of dissolving collagen fibers. With increased insolubility, the tensile strength of the fibers increased enormously.

The differential solubility of collagen molecules occurs not only in the test tube but also in normal tissues.[88, 89] In young growing animals synthesizing collagen rapidly, sequential extractions of skin yield up to 10 per cent neutral salt-soluble collagen and a larger percentage of acid-extractable collagen; the remainder is insoluble. In adult animals, the neutral salt-soluble fraction is almost nonexistent; acid-extractable collagen represents a few percentage points; and a majority of the material is insoluble. Unfortunately, the names given to these fractions (neutral salt-soluble, acid-soluble, and insoluble collagen) can be misleading. There is no evidence that any collagen in a warm-blooded animal at 37° C. is truly soluble. In order to demonstrate saline solubility, biologic materials must be cooled to 4° C., a condition not compatible with life. Soluble collagen, therefore, represents an artifact useful in identifying the bonded state of collagen molecules; it does not represent collagen molecules floating unattached in the intermolecular spaces. How collagen may be transported from the cell to the area of aggregation will be discussed below.

Through the work of many investigators, we now have a much clearer picture of how solubility and strength changes occur in collagen fibers. Newly synthesized collagen molecules present in the extracellular space aggregate with other single molecules or join larger established fibers. Initially, the only forces holding the three chains and the adjacent molecules together are weak hydrogen bonds. With time, strong covalent bonds form between individual chains and between adjacent molecules. Collagen molecules extracted with cold neutral salt solutions have no intermolecular covalent bonds. Molecules extractable with dilute acids have intermolecular bonds, but of a weak and unstable nature. Insoluble collagen, representing the majority of mature collagen in mesenchymal tissues, contains stronger intermolecular bonds. These strong intermolecular and intramolecular covalent bonds join the individual molecules together, creating a huge polymer, the mature collagen fiber. The ultimate strength of scars depends on this extracellular bonding process.

Although the nature of the intramolecular and intermolecular covalent bonds in collagen fibers remains the subject of intense investigation, at least some of the bonding reactions are established. Normal collagen contains several aldehyde groups located near the N-terminal end of the molecule. Aldehydes react with each other and with many other chemical groups. As an example, two aldehydes can join in an aldol condensation reaction, forming a covalent bond and regenerating an aldehyde group; data suggest that this reaction may produce intramolecular bonds.[11] In addition, aldehyde groups react with amino groups, forming Schiff bases and destroying the aldehyde; data suggest that this reaction may produce intermolecular bonds.[6] Although Schiff bases are relatively weak covalent bonds, reducing the base produces a stable, strong, carbon-to-nitrogen bond. Many other forces, including hydrogen bonding, electrostatic forces, bonding to noncollagenous components, and covalent bonds formed by as yet undetected mechanisms, may be involved in collagen maturation.[41] The aldehyde reactions, however, are responsible for a great deal of collagen's strength and, as we shall see, may be manipulated to the surgeon's advantage.

Mature collagen fibers contain more than just aggregated collagen molecules. Collagen molecules contain several carbohydrate residues, important in transporting the intracellular molecule to the extracellular space, which may serve as links to larger carbohydrates in glycosaminoglycan mole-

a1 H-Gly-Tyr-Asp-Glu-Lys-Ser-Ala-Gly-Val-Ser-Val-Pro-Gly-
a2 PCA-Tyr-Ser-Asp-Lys-Gly-Val-Ser-Ala-Gly-Pro-Gly-Pro-
a1 H-Gly-Tyr-Asp-Glu-Lys-Ser-Ala-Gly-Val-Ser-Val-Pro-Gly-
Lysyl
Amine Oxidase
Lysine
δ-Semialdehyde
α-Amino Adipic Acid
2 Mols Aldehyde
Aldol
Condensation
Cross-link

Figure 5. The postulated formation of intramolecular crosslinks. Note the crosslink between the lysines in the α_1 and α_2 chains at the amino-terminal end of the three polypeptide chains shown at the top. The postulated steps in the formation of this crosslink are shown in the lower portion of the figure. Note that after formation of the crosslink, an aldehyde group is available for further interaction. (From Peacock, E. E., Jr., and Van Winkle, W., Jr.: Surgery and Biology of Wound Repair, 2nd ed. Philadelphia, W. B. Saunders Company, 1976.)

cules. Because the size, strength, and orientation of collagen fibers determine the ultimate strength and physical characteristics of scar tissue, factors influencing fiber organization will be discussed in greater detail in subsequent sections.

Collagen Metabolism. During the period when fibroblasts are dividing and invading the wound space, little collagen is synthesized. Only after fibroblasts have reached a significant density (between the second and third day as a rule) can collagen synthesis be detected chemically. Collagen fibers are not seen histologically until the fourth or fifth day. Interestingly enough, fibroblasts in monolayer tissue culture behave the same way. During the log phase of growth, little, if any, collagen synthesis occurs; after confluence is attained and mitotic rate decreases, however, collagen is produced in large amounts.

Collagen is synthesized within the fibroblasts on large polyribosomes. Although as yet unproven, most investigators assume that the same DNA-messenger RNA control systems

Lysine-Derived Aldehyde
Hydroxylysine
reduction
Labile Schiff Base
Stable Cross-link

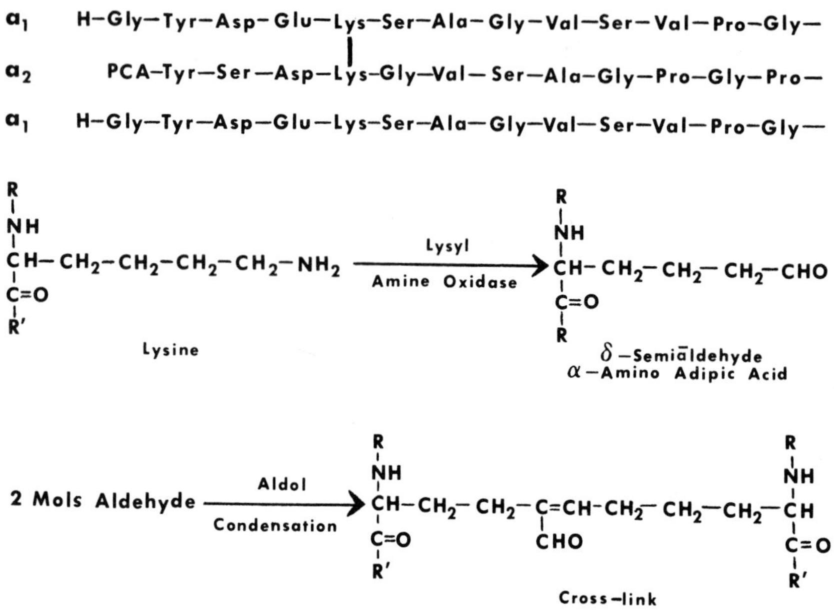

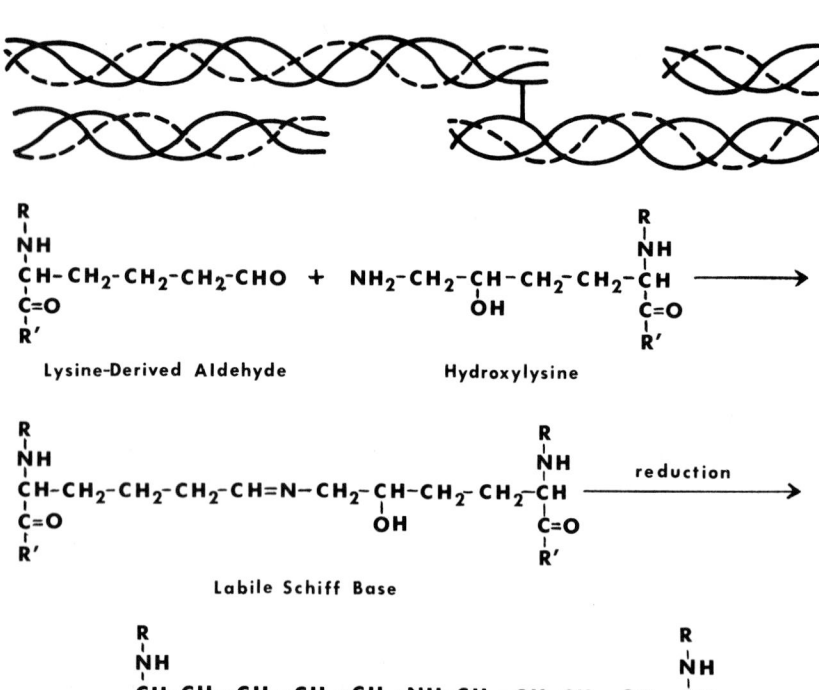

Figure 6. The postulated formation of intermolecular crosslinks. At the top, an intermolecular crosslink is shown between schematic representations of two tropocollagen molecules. In the lower part of the figure, the proposed reactions leading to labile and stable intermolecular crosslinks are shown. (From Peacock, E. E., Jr., and Van Winkle, W., Jr.: Surgery and Biology of Wound Repair, 2nd ed. Philadelphia, W. B. Saunders Company, 1976.)

work in collagen synthesis as in bacterial enzyme synthesis. We do know, however, that individual amino acids are assembled into the polypeptide chains of collagen by means of a soluble or transfer RNA. Synthesis begins at the amino-terminal end and proceeds sequentially toward the carboxy-terminal end. Whether the three polypeptide chains of collagen are synthesized and assembled simultaneously or whether chains are synthesized separately and assembled later is unknown.[83]

Recent evidence demonstrates that the peptides initially synthesized within the cell are much longer than the peptides recoverable from aggregated collagen molecules. Each collagen peptide is synthesized with a large nonhelical extension on either end of the rigid central section.[28] The nonhelical peptides, in contrast to the rigid central section of Type I collagen, contain cysteine.[68] The rapid association of the nonhelical ends and the formation of disulfide bonds facilitates "registration" and helical assembly of the rigid central section.[92]

Collagen synthesis contains some unique features not present in the synthesis of other proteins. Neither hydroxyproline nor hydroxylysine is incorporated directly into the collagen molecule. A precursor molecule, protocollagen, rich in proline but without hydroxyproline, is synthesized first. Later, an enzyme, peptidyl proline hydroxylase (PPH), hydroxylates specific proline residues in the assembled polypeptide.[43] This reaction is specific for collagen synthesis and, as we shall see, inhibiting enzyme activity has profound effects on scar tissue.

During hydroxylation, the oxygen atom in the hydroxyl group comes from molecular oxygen. In addition, PPH requires α-ketoglutarate as a co-substrate and ferrous iron as a co-factor. An electron donor is required and, under normal circumstances, ascorbic acid serves this purpose.[78] If PPH activity is inhibited by using ferrous iron chelators (α,α-dipyridyl, 1-10-phenanthroline) or by depriving the cells of oxygen, the cytoplasm fills with proline-rich peptides, and collagen synthesis and excretion are inhibited specifically.[37] If cells required to synthesize collagen rapidly are deprived of ascorbic acid, the same phenomenon occurs. The mechanism of lysine hydroxylation is less well known but is also enzymatically controlled.

A second unique metabolic reaction in collagen synthesis is of significant interest to the surgeon. In the discussion of collagen crosslinking, aldehyde reactions were prominent. Mesenchymal tissues contain an enyme, lysyl amine oxidase (LAO), that causes oxidative deamination of the ϵ-amino groups of lysine.[90] The resultant aldehydes produce intermolecular and intramolecular covalent bonds as described. LAO requires copper ions as co-factors. Copper depletion or chelation prevents aldehyde formation and subsequent crosslinking. In addition, a class of compounds called lathyrogens specifically inhibits covalent bonding by inhibiting LAO activity or by chelating the resultant aldehydes.[73] The biologic effects of these compounds will be discussed in a subsequent section.

After the collagen peptides have been synthesized, hydroxylated, and assembled, several small carbohydrates have been added, and aldehydes have been formed, the molecules make their way into the extracellular space. Precisely how this occurs is debated. The best data indicate that molecules are secreted directly into cisternal spaces and, either by direct communication of the ergastoplasmic membrane with the cell membrane or by vesicle formation and fusion with cell membranes, find their way outside the cell.[83]

Once the collagen molecules are outside the cell, the mechanisms responsible for their biologic behavior are less well understood. The assembled molecule with nonhelical extensions, called procollagen, is presumably excreted from the cell by the mechanisms described. Prior to molecular aggregation, the nonhelical extensions are cleaved from the

molecule by a specific enzymatic process. The specific proteolytic enzyme, procollagen peptidase, may exist in one or a variety of forms. A deficiency in procollagen peptidase is found in several recessive genetic disorders of animals and man. Dermatosparaxis is a genetic disorder of cattle characterized by extreme fragility of the skin and other organs.[50] Because dermatosparactic animals lack normal procollagen peptidase, procollagen molecules accumulate in the skin. The large nonhelical extensions prevent normal aggregation and maturation of collagen, leaving mature collagen fibers weak and disorganized.[28] A form of the Ehlers-Danlos syndrome is also associated with failure to cleave the nonhelical portions of collagen. Large amounts of procollagen are found in the tissues, resulting in weak mesenchymal structures.[53]

Because the orientation and weave of collagen fibers determines the mechanical properties of scars, factors influencing the architecture of collagen fibers determine scar physiology. From our previous discussion, collagen molecules obviously contain enough information within the primary, secondary, and tertiary molecular structure to undergo aggregation, fiber formation, and crossbonding without further help from the cell. And yet fiber architecture within different mesenchymal tissues and within scars is not the chance arrangement seen in test tubes. For instance, layering of collagen fibers in the cornea is a precise orthogonal arrangement, each successive laminar layer of small collagen fibrils oriented at right angles to ones above and below. In contrast, the huge collagen bundles of tendons are oriented with their long axes parallel to the lines of stress. Although the scar tissue between repaired tendon ends is at first randomly oriented, with time the collagen bundles align with the normal tendon fascicles.

Electron microscopic studies of fibroblast-fiber interactions demonstrate an intimate relationship between the cell processes and fiber bundles. In developing scars, small fibers are often seen in direct apposition to the cell membranes. This relationship is, at times, so intimate that some authors have suggested fibers actually form within the cell or as a part of the cell membrane. Although the best morphologic data indicate that fiber formation is entirely extracellular, cell processes may in some fashion help orient fiber bundles.

Another indirect way in which cells may influence fiber size and orientation is through their production of glycosaminoglycans.[13] As noted earlier, the specific role of mucopolysaccharides in wound healing is unknown. However, in vitro studies demonstrate that collagen fibers precipitated in the presence of dermatan sulfate have a greater average diameter than those formed in the presence of chondroitin-4-sulfate. In the cornea, where keratan sulfate is the principal glycosaminoglycan, collagen fibers are extremely fine. Heavier fibers of skin are associated with dermatan sulfate. Although the evidence to date is indirect, presence and orientation of ground substance molecules may play an important role in scar collagen architecture.

Finally, the demonstration of a precursor form of collagen and of a specific protease associated with the conversion to native molecules suggests that fiber formation may be controlled by biochemical as well as physical factors. As yet, the biological significance of procollagen and procollagen peptidase is unknown. This aspect of collagen metabolism is being investigated intensively. If the procollagen–procollagen peptidase system is a significant factor controlling fiber aggregation and size, surgeons may be able to control this aspect of scar formation pharmacologically.

So far we have discussed the synthesis of collagen molecules and the formation of fibers, both constructive events. For years, biologists knew that in some fashion collagen must also be destroyed or degraded in normal tissues. Until the early 1960s, the mechanism for collagen destruction went undetected. The experiments of Gross and his collaborators, however, provided a new dimension to our understanding of how morphogenic changes occur in growing organisms and, more important to our discussion, how wounds change in bulk and form.

Using a substrate of native collagen and tissue culture techniques, Lapiere and Gross demonstrated that the involuting tail of tadpoles produces a powerful and specific collagenase.[32] This enzyme splits the collagen molecule into two fragments, across all three chains, approximately one fourth of the distance from the carboxyl end. Even in tissues destroying collagen at a rapid rate, collagenase is produced in minute amounts. Since this initial observation, collagenase has been demonstrated in a variety of human and animal tissues, including involuting uterus, human rheumatoid synovial membrane, and human scars.[25] Additional data suggest that under certain conditions several other cellular proteases may also destroy collagen. In human tissues, collagenase activity has been demonstrated in epithelial tissues and in mesenchymal tissue associated with epithelial structures. Collagen destruction represents a major factor in normal scar remodeling and may be significant in several abnormal wound healing conditions. The relationship of collagen destruction and collagen turnover to wound remodeling will be discussed in a subsequent section.

Physical Events

From the surgeon's point of view, all of the morphologic and chemical events of wound healing lead to a single important conclusion: *Wounds become stronger with time.* The re-establishment of tissue integrity and strength produced by normal healing reactions allows the surgeon to perform modern manipulative therapy. Rate of strength gain and the ultimate strength of wounds determine what suture material should be used, when sutures should be removed, how patient activity should be resumed, and why certain incisions may be more appropriate than others.

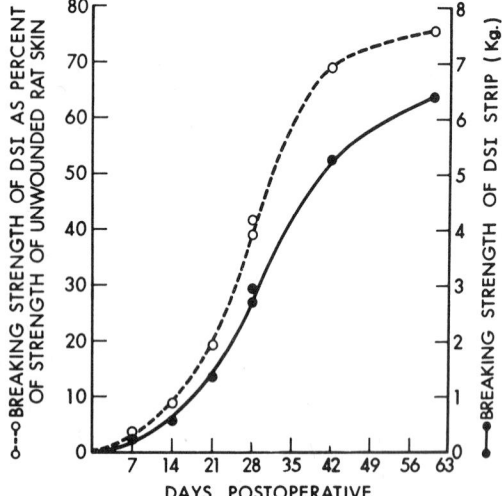

Figure 7. Increase in breaking strength of a healing rat skin wound shown in absolute terms and as a percentage of comparable unwounded skin. Note the prolonged gain in strength. The strength of the wound reached only 80 per cent of the strength of unwounded skin. DSI = dermal skin incision. (From Levenson, S. M., et al.: Ann. Surg., *161*:293, 1965.)

Like so much of the material presented here, most of the information on strength relationships in healing wounds comes from animal experimentation. Although major clinical differences exist between all species, most biologic events in healing seem comparable. The magnitude and timing of specific features, however, may differ significantly.

All measurable mechanical properties of physical objects depend on the direction and rate of application of force. Although many mechanical parameters, including stress-strain curves, elastic versus inelastic or plastic stretch, and energy absorption curves, have been utilized to measure physical properties of scars, the two commonly used parameters are burst strength and tensile strength. These measurements are not interchangeable. Tensile strength measures load per cross-sectioned area at rupture, burst strength measures load required to break the wound regardless of dimension. Failure to appreciate this simple difference produces erroneous interpretation of available data. For instance, because of thickness, the burst strength of back skin and eyelid skin differs significantly; the tensile strength, however, is comparable. Burst strength can provide valid comparisons between tissues and wounds only if the physical dimensions are comparable.

Strength gain in incised wounds begins immediately after suture. By 2 days, burst strength in incised rat skin wounds reaches 50 to 100 gm. per linear centimeter. Note that the wound space contains only fibrin strands, a few capillary loops, white cells, and a few fibroblasts at this point. The epithelial surface, however, does consist of a confluent sheet of cells. Experimental studies indicate that intercellular forces, adhesion of globular proteins, and fibrin polymerization can produce forces of this magnitude.[85]

With the appearance of collagen fibers on the third day, rate of gain in strength increases rapidly. By 21 days, burst strength has reached over 1 kg. per linear centimeter.[36] In spite of a generally held misconception, gain in strength does not stop here. Carefully performed studies even fail to reveal a plateau in strength at this point.[52] Instead, skin wounds continue to gain strength at a relatively rapid and constant rate for over 4 months and at a slower rate for over 1 year. In spite of its rediscovery every 10 or 15 years, this significant behavior, first measured experimentally by Howes and his co-workers in 1939, is still omitted from many discussions of wound healing.[35] Prolonged gain in strength is not limited to skin wounds. Muscle and fascial wounds gain strength slowly,[22] and rate of gain in strength for tendon injuries is even slower.[65] In spite of prolonged strength gain, wounds rarely, if ever, regain the strength of normal tissues. In addition, strength is not the only important physical parameter of scars. Normal elasticity, so important in tissue function, is lost in scars. The products of wound healing, although strong, often convert an elastic, pliable tissue to an inelastic, brittle mass.

Relationship of Chemical and Physical Events

The physical properties of scars depend on the collagen fibers they contain. Although other components of mature

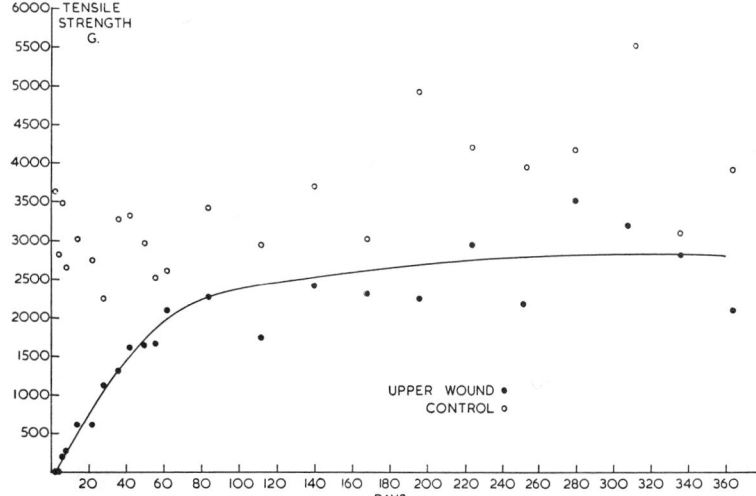

Figure 8. Breaking strength of a wound in the upper dorsal aponeurosis compared to the strength of unwounded fascia (open circles). Note that fascial wounds behave as skin wounds and gain strength steadily for months. (From Douglas, D. M.: Br. J. Surg., *40*:79, 1952.)

scars (cells, epithelium, blood vessels, and ground substance molecules) contribute to wound strength, the magnitude of collagen's contribution is overwhelming. The best evidence comes from two sources.

In scurvy, small amounts of collagen are produced in normal tissues. However, if tissues are stressed by injury, rate of collagen synthesis is inadequate to produce scars. As discussed, ascorbic acid is the normal electron donor required for peptidyl proline hydroxylase activity. Data also suggest that fibroblasts of animals deprived of ascorbic acid contain very little PPG.[69] Scurvy, then, represents a deficiency in scar collagen synthesis. After wounding in scorbutic animals, epithelialization occurs normally and the wound space fills with fibroblasts, capillaries, and large concentrations of glycosaminoglycans. All the normal products of wound healing except collagen are present, and yet the wound gains little strength.

The second source of evidence supporting the primary importance of collagen in strength gain comes from studies on the effects of lathyrogenic agents in healing wounds. Beta-aminopropionitrile (BAPN), the most powerful known osteolathyrogen, specifically inhibits the production of lysine-derived aldehydes during collagen synthesis. When BAPN is given to wounded animals, collagen molecules are synthesized and excreted at a normal rate. Extracellular collagen aggregates normally but intermolecular and intramolecular covalent bonds do not form with time.[73] Although lathyrogenic collagen fibers appear normal under the electron microscope, physical strength is greatly diminished.[51] The best data indicate that BAPN has no effect on the synthesis or function of other connective tissue components. If animals with incised wounds are treated with BAPN, the morphologic events of wound healing occur normally. In spite of the normal appearance, however, as long as the animals are treated with BAPN, wounds develop no increase in strength after the third or fourth day.[74] Thus, not only collagen fibers, but also normal intermolecular covalent bonding reactions are required for normal strength gain in healing wounds.

Although most investigators agree that collagen and its fibers are primarily responsible for scar strength, the precise way in which the molecule is utilized remains debatable. Scars could gain strength at least three ways: the density of collagen fibers could increase with time by adding more and more collagen to the wound; the fibers present could get stronger with time by increasing the density of intermolecular covalent bonding or by increasing bonding with noncollagenous components; or the architectural arrangement of the collagen fibers could change with time, producing a new, stronger configuration.

Experiments using radioactively labeled compounds demonstrate that scar collagen accumulates rapidly in rat skin wounds during the first three weeks of healing. After three weeks, however, further net accumulation does not occur.[62] Comparing net scar collagen accumulation with strength gain shows a positive correlation during the first three weeks, but no correlation thereafter. In muscle wounds, scar collagen accumulation can be correlated with strength gain only during the first six weeks.[3] Obviously, the total amount of scar collagen present is not per se responsible for changes in wound strength.

Although indirect, the evidence for the second alternative—increasing strength of individual fibers—is more convincing. Using thermal shrinkage temperatures, an indirect measurement of intermolecular bonding density, collagen

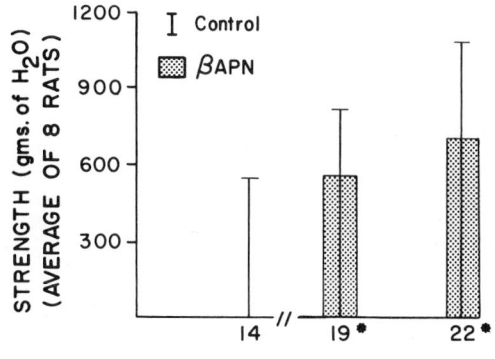

Figure 9. The effect of beta-aminopropionitrile (BAPN) on burst strength of rat skin wounds. From day 14 through 19, 100 mg. of BAPN was administered to experimental animals. BAPN prevents gain in strength completely; strength gain resumes when BAPN is discontinued. (From Peacock, E. E., Jr., and Madden, J. W.: Surgery, *60*:7, 1966.)

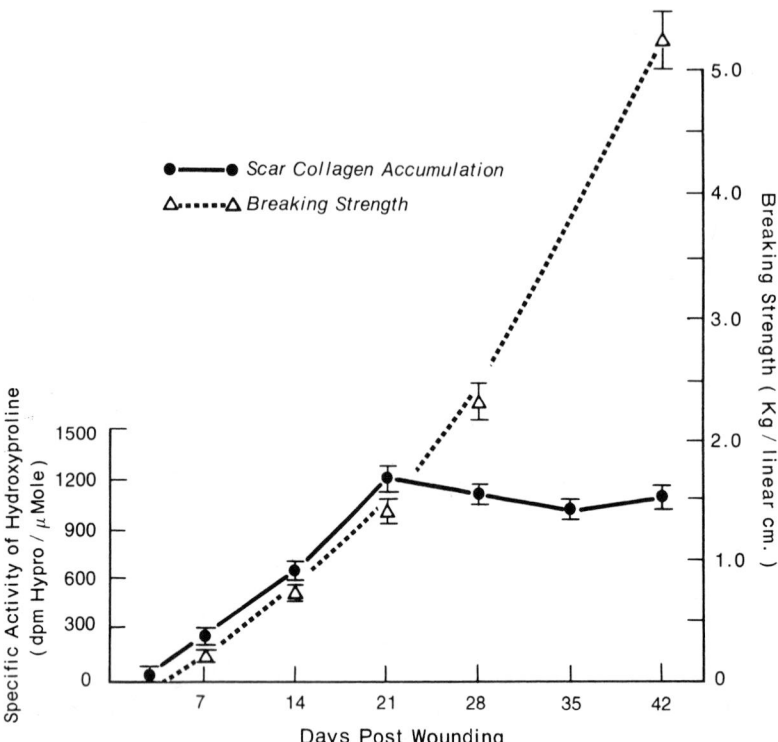

Figure 10. The breaking strength of rat skin wounds compared with net scar collagen accumulation. Note that over the first 3 weeks, strength and collagen content correlate. After 3 weeks, however, the wound continues to gain strength rapidly, but net scar collagen accumulation stops. There is no correlation between content and strength after 3 weeks. (From Madden, J. W., and Peacock, E. E., Jr.: Ann. Surg., *174*:511, 1971.)

fibers from older wounds show a denser crosslinking than fibers from younger wounds. Moreover, the addition of artificial intermolecular crosslinks with formaldehyde or other tanning agents increases the strength of younger much more than older wounds, suggesting that the crosslinking density of younger fibers has not reached saturation.[52] Although indirect, this evidence indicates that the gradual production of stronger fibers plays an important role in long-term strength gain.

The final possibility—gradual alteration in architectural pattern of scar collagen fibers—has much support. As previously discussed, scanning electron microscopic studies of healing skin wounds, as well as gross anatomic observations, show a gradual alteration in fiber anatomy with time. How could these architectural changes occur? Again, two possibilities exist; either the old scar collagen fibers are taken apart and the older molecules recombined into new fibers, or older fibers are destroyed and newly synthesized molecules woven into new fiber patterns.

Evidence for the first possibility is slight. Several investigators have demonstrated that a few collagen molecules synthesized some distance from wounds may be utilized in scar production. By this phenomenon, perhaps older molecules could be reutilized to produce new fibers. Currently, no direct evidence supporting this hypothesis exists.

The second hypothesis, simultaneous degradation and synthesis of scar collagen, requires demonstrating prolonged scar collagen turnover, even in scars with a stable histologic appearance. Utilizing the conversion of radioactively labeled proline to labeled hydroxyproline, the rate of scar collagen synthesis and deposition has been measured directly. Rate of new collagen deposition in rat skin wounds remains significantly elevated over control skin values for at least 3 months.[61] Simultaneous measurements of net scar collagen accumulation and net rate of new collagen deposition demonstrate that a prolonged, dynamic equilibrium exists between rapid scar collagen synthesis and degradation. Rapid turn-

over of scar collagen continues for months.[62] Although as yet the kinetics of collagen metabolism have not been measured directly in human wounds, indirect evidence suggests that rapid collagen turnover is a prominent feature of human scars. Thus, despite a stable histologic appearance and a constant collagen content, scar collagen metabolism remains dynamic for long periods. Interestingly enough, although the strength of skin wounds fails to correlate with total collagen content, strength gain correlates with the dynamic parameters of scar metabolism (rate of new collagen deposition and rate of turnover) through at least 3 months. The signifi-

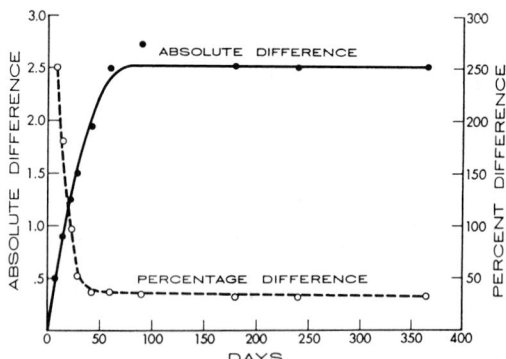

Figure 11. The difference between breaking strengths of fresh and formalin-fixed wounds as a function of time after injury. During the first 6 weeks, formalin tanning produces larger strength gains than during the later phases of healing. This represents indirect evidence that crosslinking density in collagen fibers increases with time. (From Levenson, S. M., et al.: Ann. Surg., *161*:293, 1965.)

cance of scar collagen turnover in remodeling wounds will be discussed in the next section.

In summary, the ultimate strength of scars depends on the physical properties of collagen fibers. Although many other tissue components including glycosaminoglycans may be influential in determining fiber size and orientation, and in providing interfiber support, the weave and crossbonding characteristics of collagen fibers seem paramount. Incised wounds gain strength slowly over prolonged periods. Although at first correlated with collagen content, ultimate scar strength seems to relate more to the intermolecular bonding characteristics of individual fibers and to the fiber weave. Finally, architectural changes in scar collagen fibers seem to correlate with rapid and prolonged scar collagen turnover.

Scar Remodeling

As discussed previously, all scars slowly and progressively change in bulk and form. As a rule, scar remodeling determines the physiologic function of injured tissues. During the early phases of wound healing, the wound space is filled completely with randomly oriented fibers. All injured tissues, regardless of the surgeon's carefully placed sutures, are bound together in a single unit by strong collagen fibers; in effect, all injured tissues form a single wound. Because the abdomen can function normally in the presence of a scar that welds peritoneum, muscle, fascia, subcutaneous tissue, and skin into one unit, both the patient and the surgeon are satisfied. Unfortunately, this result is not satisfactory in many other situations. For example, if a wound of the hand involves skin, palmar fascia, lumbrical muscle, tendon, periosteum, and bone, all injured components are united quickly by scar. Integrity and strength are re-established, but active motion of the finger is impossible. In order to function, cut tendon ends must be joined together with strong scar tissue, but the character of scar linking tendon with surrounding immobile structures must be altered to permit gliding. During the latter phases of wound healing, scars do change their anatomic arrangement. In the case of a lacerated flexor tendon, the random mat of collagen fibers becomes oriented in much more specific ways with time.[55] Scar collagen between tendon ends orients in parallel bundles resembling normal tendon. This physical weave establishes a strong union between the tendon ends capable of transmitting powerful longitudinal forces. In contrast, collagen fibers lying adjacent to gliding

surfaces enlarge, but retain their random orientation, creating a loose areolar configuration. Thus, over the course of many months, initial randomly oriented collagenous tissue is rewoven into structures resembling the preinjury condition (parallel collagen bundles between tendon ends, peritenon-like structures surrounding gliding surfaces).

In spite of intense investigation, the mechanisms responsible for long-term changes in scar architecture remain obscure. In all probability, the prolonged metabolic turnover of scar collagen demonstrated in animals exists in man and provides the biochemical mechanism for remodeling. Human scar tissue contains large amounts of collagenase, demonstrated in wounds as young as 14 days and as old as 31 years. Human wounds obviously have the capacity for collagen destruction. Additional indirect evidence for the equilibrium state of scar collagen in human wounds comes from clinical observations in scurvy. Classic descriptions of the disease describe wounds closed for years opening "as if they were freshly made." Ascorbic acid deficiency inhibits the rapid synthesis of collagen; it does not influence collagen destruction. A prolonged dynamic equilibrium between scar collagen synthesis and destruction could explain this phenomenon as well as several other abnormal wound healing reactions. For instance, slight alterations in the equilibrium could produce the abnormally large amounts of collagen seen in keloids and retroperitoneal fibrosis, in addition to the abnormally small amounts seen in scurvy.[76]

Given prolonged turnover, the mechanisms controlling remodeling are still poorly understood. Clinical observations in man suggest that physical forces play an important role. Incisions crossing lines of changing dimension produce large hypertrophic scars; incisions within normal skin creases where tension is minimal produce small, well-healed wounds. And yet, mild traction on healing wounds seems to increase the rate of gain in strength. Recently, the influence of tension on remodeling scar tissue has been demonstrated experimentally.[5] As yet, however, how the magnitude, rate of application, duration, frequency, and direction of stress application influences the ultimate size and physical properties of scar tissue remains unknown. In bone remodeling, local electrical fields produced by the deformation of bone crystals influence the orientation of bone matrix.[7] The influence of local fields in normal soft tissue healing, however, has not been documented. How physical forces and local environmental conditions direct scar remodeling remains an important area of inquiry.

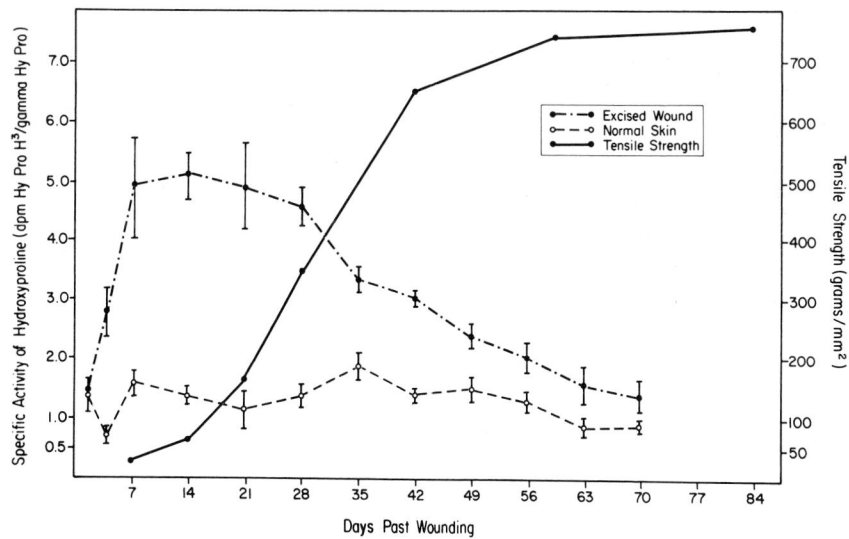

Figure 12. The relationship of rate of collagen synthesis to tensile strength of rat skin wounds. Note that the net rate of collagen synthesis and deposition remains elevated throughout the study period. In spite of a stable collagen content, incised wounds continue to synthesize and deposit collagen rapidly for prolonged intervals. Unlike net scar collagen content, net rate of new collagen deposition correlates with strength gain throughout the study interval. (From Madden, J. W., and Peacock, E. E., Jr.: Surgery, *64*:288, 1968; tensile strength curve taken from Levenson, S. M., et al.: Ann. Surg., *161*: 293, 1965.)

OPEN WOUNDS

Open wounds with or without tissue loss present entirely different clinical problems than incised and sutured wounds. Although the basic morphologic and chemical processes operating in the closed wound participate in healing open wounds, contraction becomes an important feature and epithelialization assumes a more prominent role. Interestingly enough, these two processes seem independent.[96]

Incised wounds allowed to remain open begin the healing process normally. An inflammatory exudate collects on the surface; marginal epithelial cells mobilize, divide, and migrate down the edges; injured venules bud, forming capillary networks; and fibroblasts invade the injured area. Early physicians, impressed with the finely granular nature of the new surface, named this material granulation tissue. After 3 or 4 days, the wound surfaces can be closed with sutures or other mechanical devices, and healing proceeds normally. Careful bacteriologic investigations demonstrate that heavily contaminated wounds left open can show a marked reduction in bacterial concentration during the first 3 to 6 days. In many instances, delayed closure of contaminated wounds can prevent clinical infection. This technique, developed during World War II, has become increasingly popular.

If delayed closure is not performed or if tissues have been lost, a remarkable change in the physical dimensions of the wound occurs with time. After a delay of 2 or 3 days, the wound margins move toward each other, making the surface defect smaller. The remarkable propensity of open wounds to contract has been recognized for centuries. Only recently, however, have the mechanisms responsible for wound contraction been investigated extensively.

Clinical observations in animals and man demonstrate that skin wounds contract by stretching the surrounding skin to close the defect, not by the production of new skin. In areas where skin is relatively loose, and mobile structures are not nearby, wound contraction produces minimal deformity. For instance, a 10 × 10 cm. defect high on one buttock contracting to 2 × 2 cm. causes little functional impairment. In contrast, where mobile skin is important, contraction produces serious functional abnormalities. A 4 × 4 cm. defect on the dorsum of the hand contracting to 2 × 2 cm. can cause a permanent extension deformity of the fingers. Because contraction seems limited by the tension developed in skin surrounding the defect, simply pulling the wound edges together with skin hooks reproduces the ultimate deformity. Thus, contraction of a defect in the upper eyelid can produce ectropion; of the antecubital space, a flexion contracture of the elbow; of the axillary skin, an adduction contracture of of the arm. Obviously, the contraction of open wounds produces serious deformity in man and controlling this relentless process becomes an important part of the surgeon's task.

Because skin is normally under mild tension, excision of full-thickness skin produces a defect slightly larger than the sample removed.[10] After a delay of 2 or 3 days, the dermal edges begin moving toward each other. Between day 5 and 10, wound edges move rapidly, but slow again by 2 weeks. In a rectangular or square defect, the midpoints of the sides move more rapidly than the corners, and the ultimate scar is stellate. Only three possible explanations for this event exist; either the dermal wound edges are pulled together by a force originating in the open bed, the edges are pushed toward the center by forces at the periphery, or contraction occurs by a combination of both. Although at first glance a rather simple problem, distinguishing between the possibilities is difficult.

Even though large amounts of collagen are produced by the granulating surface, neither normal collagen synthesis nor strong covalent bonding between collagen fibers is required for normal wound contraction.[39] Open skin wounds in scorbutic animals and man produce small amounts of collagen but contract normally.[1] In addition, inhibiting covalent bonding with lathyrogenic agents has no effect on contraction.[38] Collagen fibers themselves are not composed of contractile proteins. Where, then, does the force originate?

Wherever the application occurs, the force of wound contraction comes from living cells. Cytotoxic agents in nonlethal doses, particularly the cytochrome poisons, inhibit wound contraction significantly and the effect is reversible. Any treatment that inhibits cell motility has significant effects on wound contraction. Moreover, single cells and cell sheets moving on solid substrates can generate forces capable of closing open wounds. Where the cells responsible for wound contraction reside, however, is debated.

In the early 1950s, Grillo and his associates implicated a group of large cells immediately beneath the advancing dermal edge.[31] Excising the central granulating surface of open wounds in guinea pigs had no effect on contraction. Excising the dermal edge itself, however, re-established the initial size of the wound, leaving a smaller central area.[98] Repeated excisions of central mass had no effect; repeated excisions of the picture frame area always eliminated contraction. Irradiating the local area during the phase of active fibroblast division retarded contraction significantly. Although irradiation of wound margin and central granulation tissue separately was not possible, these studies do support the involvement and local origin of living cells.

Unfortunately, repeating the excision experiments in other species produces different results. In rabbits, excising the central granulating mass or separating the dermal edge from the wound base enlarges the contracting wound to the original dimensions.[2] In addition, inhibiting contraction with external splints and releasing the wound edges after a few days produces contraction at a rate far too fast to be explained by cell movements alone. Incising the wound base prior to releasing the splint eliminates the rapid marginal movement. Therefore, rapid contraction in the splinted wound seems to result from forces built up during splinting.

Recently, Gabbiani and co-workers have identified a specific cell type in granulation tissue which may rep-

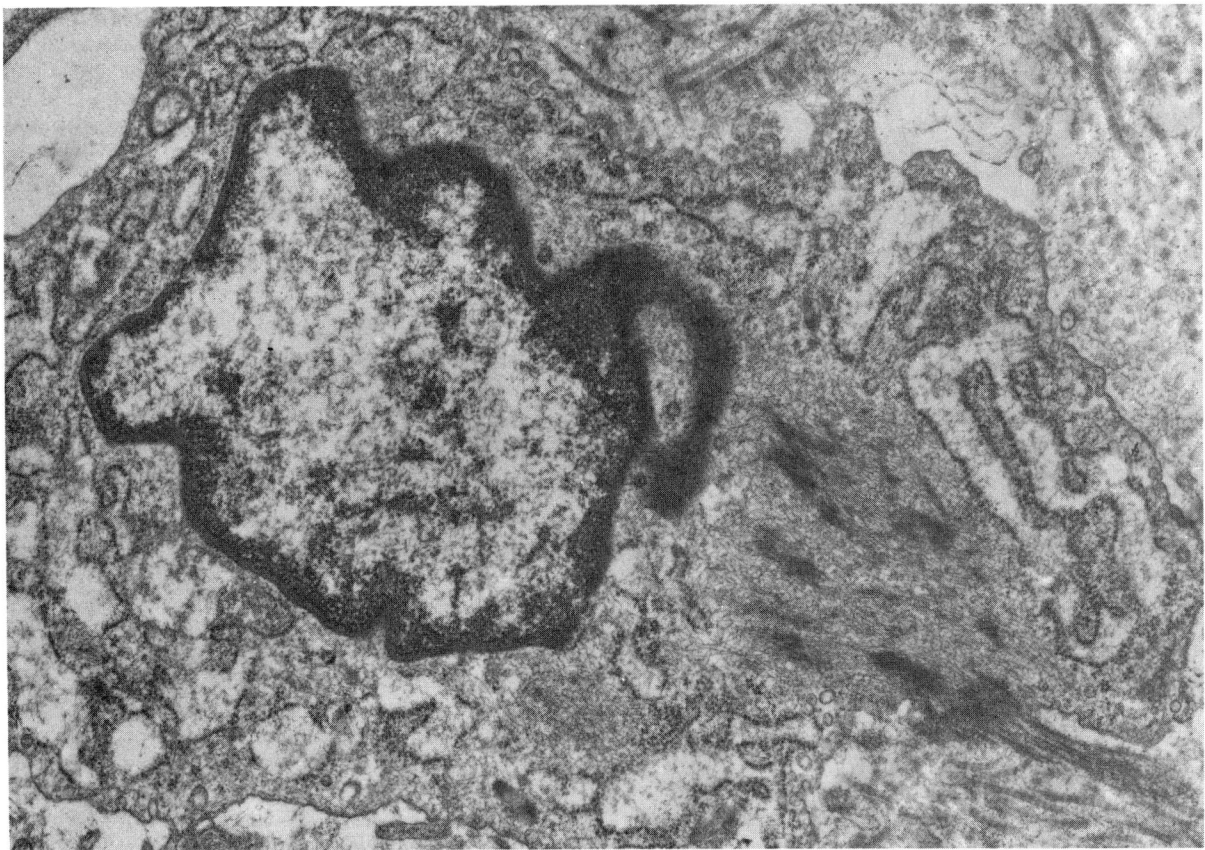

Figure 13. Atypical fibroblast (myofibroblast) from patient with plantar fasciitis. Compare this cell with the fibroblast illustrated in Figure 1. Note the highly irregular nucleus, the large amount of rough endoplasmic reticulum, and, most important, the dense collection of myofilaments. There are numerous dense bodies adjacent to and intermingled with the myofilaments. No basal lamina is seen and the cell is surrounded by numerous collagen fibrils. This cell has ultrastructural features intermittent between a fibroblast and smooth muscle cell. Electron micrograph × 25,000. (Courtesy of Edward C. Carlson, Ph.D.)

resent the contractile element responsible for wound contraction.[30] This unique cell combines the ultrastructural features of the fibroblast and smooth muscle cell. Modified fibroblasts (myofibroblasts) have been identified in contracting tissues from several animal species and in a variety of human fibrocontractive diseases.[54, 56, 57] Although impossible to prove using morphological criteria alone, a variety of data support the concept that atypical cells resembling smooth muscle supply the motive force for wound contraction. Biochemical measurements demonstrate that granulation tissue from contracting wounds contains as much actomyosin as does the uterus.[29] Human anti–smooth muscle sera label the cytoplasm of myofibroblasts.[34] Granulation tissue containing significant numbers of modified fibroblasts contracts actively *in vitro*, behaving as vascular smooth muscle tissue.[64] Finally, topically applied anti–smooth muscle agents inhibit wound contraction completely.[60] The mechanism of wound contraction remains an exciting area for investigation. Over the next few years, the nature of the cells involved in wound contraction and their relationship to pathophysiological conditions will be clarified.

Although the precise mechanism of wound contraction remains controversial, the factors responsible for initiating and inhibiting the contraction process are central to wound management. Forces of contraction act to close the wound until balanced by equal tension in the surrounding skin. Although tensions in surrounding tissue may lessen with time, for all practical purposes the wound contracts until fixed tissues prevent further contraction. Certain biological manipulations are known to influence the contraction process. Contrary to popular opinion, epithelialization per se does not inhibit wound contraction.[96] Contraction can be minimized by replacing missing skin immediately with thick skin grafts or pedical flaps. The ultimate area of the defect following coverage depends upon several important factors. Full thickness skin grafts inhibit the contraction mechanism most effectively.[87] Thin split-thickness grafts inhibit wound contraction, but only slightly. The thicker the graft, the larger the ultimate area. Once contraction has begun, replacing missing skin is much less effective in inhibiting the contraction process.[95] A combination of immediate skin coverage plus mechanical splinting, by skeletal structures in the area or by external devices, is the most effective method of minimizing wound contraction.[96] Obviously, the control of wound contraction resides in the interphase between the injured area and the moving dermal margin or grafted dermal tissue. The precise mechanism of this interaction, however, has not been defined.

In areas of fixed tissues and little excess skin (the skin over the skull or lower leg) maximal contraction cannot close a significant defect. Sufficient skin simply cannot be pulled into the wound. The wound surface either remains uncovered as a chronic open ulcer, or closes by epithelialization. In full-thickness defects, epithelialization occurs by the same mechanisms discussed under the closed wound. The magnitude of the process and its consequences, however, are entirely different. Even in partial-thickness injuries, where cells from the dermal appendages aid in epithelialization, the results are far from satisfactory.

Open wounds are covered by dried or denatured plasma proteins and dead cells, the scab. In thermal injuries, denatured dermal collagen may remain in place and constitute an eschar. In either case, epithelialization occurs beneath the surface covering. In thermal injuries with an intact eschar, migrating epithelial cells secrete collagenase, destroying the intact collagenous connections. Underneath a scab, the epithelial cells migrate on the collagenous tissue in the wound base.

Although epithelial sheets have remarkable migratory capacities, the extent of their migrations is not infinite. Cells can migrate 1, 2, and even 3 cm. from the wound edge under special circumstances, but they rarely cover larger defects. If the area is too large to be covered by epithelialization and contraction, the wound becomes a chronic open ulcer. Over long periods of time, open wounds of this type can develop a highly malignant form of squamous cell carcinoma. Adequate coverage can prevent this disastrous complication.

Like normal skin, epithelialized scar tissue represents a superficial epidermal layer and a deeper collagenous base. Epithelial cells on a base of scar tissue, however, have little resemblance to skin. Normally, epidermis is bound tightly to dermis through a strong undulating basement membrane. The rete pegs and epidermal appendages (hair follicles, sweat glands, sebaceous glands) provide a strong epidermal-dermal junction. Junction of epithelium with scar tissue, however, is a flimsy affair with little strength. Even minor shearing forces produce epithelial separation and loss. Unlike normal skin, epithelialized scar tissue responds to stress by deteriorating, not by a compensatory increase in strength. Although some animals can regenerate a few hair follicles and sebaceous glands with time, scar tissue in man lacks epidermal appendages. Epithelialized scar remains a poor substitute for skin.

Local and Systemic Factors

Secondary Wound Healing and Wound Hormones. A number of imaginative biologists have suggested through the years that injured tissues produce specific wound hormones. These substances, allegedly circulating freely in blood, increase the rate of healing at distant sites. To date, there are no critical experimental data to support this contention. In most instances, observed differences in healing rates result from other factors discussed in the following sections. These experiments, however, did produce a significant observation on the behavior of dehisced and resutured wounds.

In the early 1940s, Botsford noted that incised wounds allowed to heal for short periods undisturbed, then dehisced and immediately resutured, developed strength at a significantly faster rate than primary wounds.[12] The experiments of Dunphy, his associates, and others established that this secondary wound healing phenomenon was related entirely to local factors at the wound site and was not associated with circulating wound hormones.[86] Interestingly enough, excising the skin wound as a strip 14 mm. wide with the wound at the center and reapproximating the fresh edges abolishes rapid gain in strength. Excising a narrower skin strip with the wound reduces but does not completely inhibit increased rate of gain in strength. Small increases in rate have been noted in wounds dehisced months after the original incision. Collagen content of excised secondary wounds seems to be the same as or even lower than that of primary wounds of the same age. Time-related features of scar collagen metabolism, however, seem to explain secondary healing. As discussed previously, primary wounds require several days to prepare for collagen synthesis and continue to synthesize and deposit collagen at elevated rates for prolonged periods. Dehiscing and resuturing wounds seems to have no effect on rate of new collagen deposition.[63] Experiments in rats demonstrate that strength gain in wounds dehisced and resutured at different times correlates with the rate of collagen deposition at the time of dehiscence. Thus, in the dehisced and resutured wound, as well as the primary wound, gain in strength seems to depend less on collagen content than on rate of new collagen deposition.

General Nutrition Factors. Incised wounds in animals fed a protein-free diet for prolonged periods gain strength slowly. Although plasma restores normal wound kinetics, the plasma protein concentration fails to correlate with local wound abnormalities. Feeding DL-methionine or cystine alone prevents delayed healing.[100] This effect seems unrelated to collagen synthesis, and the mechanism of protein depletion effects on wound healing is obscure. Although discussed frequently, the magnitude of the effect of protein depletion on wound healing in man remains unknown.

Vitamin and Trace Element Deficiencies. The relationship of vitamin C to wound healing has been discussed frequently in this chapter. Although most species synthesize adequate amounts of ascorbic acid, primates and the guinea pig lack this ability. Experimental studies indicate that collagen synthesis can proceed at low rates in ascorbic acid-deficient animals. When circumstances require rapid synthesis, however, ascorbic acid depletion has profound effects on collagen production. Providing relatively small amounts of vitamin C

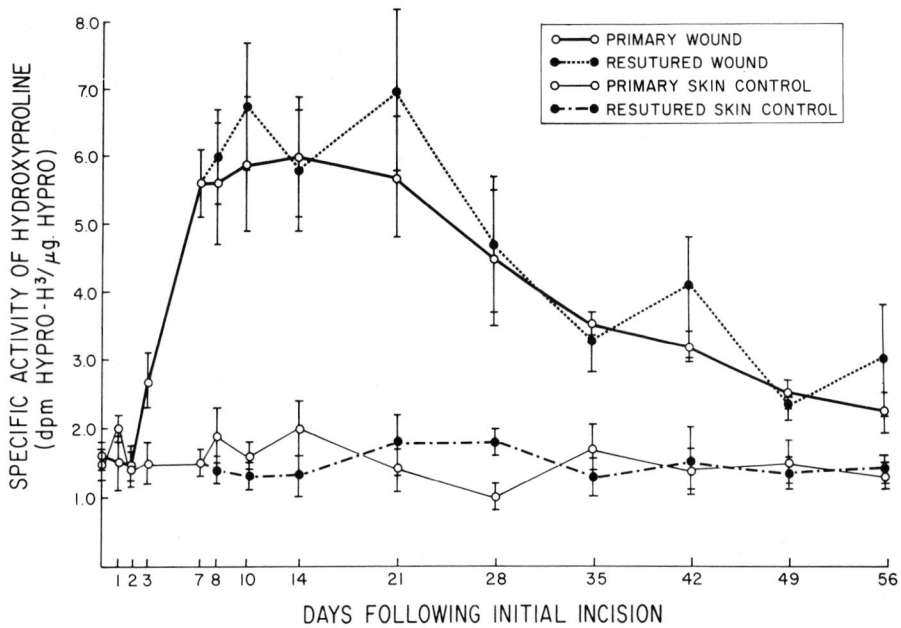

Figure 14.   Comparison of the net rate of new collagen deposition in primary and in dehisced-resutured rat skin wounds. Note that dehiscence has no effect on rate of new collagen deposition. During the first 3 days of primary healing, rate of synthesis is low and strength gain is minimal. During the first 3 days of secondary healing, however, rate of synthesis is maximal and strength gain is rapid. (From Madden, J. W., and Smith, H. C.: Surg. Gynecol. Obstet., *130*:487, 1970. By permission of Surgery, Gynecology & Obstetrics.)

restores normal healing; saturation is unnecessary. Although we have discussed the function of ascorbic acid in collagen synthesis, physiologic abnormalities in scurvy are not limited to collagen metabolism. Ascorbic acid, a strong reducing agent, seems to be involved in several other oxidation-reduction systems. Normal wound healing requires adequate amounts of ascorbic acid, but deficiency states are rare in the Western world except in alcoholics or severely malnourished individuals. Vitamin A and vitamin A deficiencies have been implicated in abnormal wound healing phenomena. Although the full implications of vitamin A deficiency have yet to be explored, vitamin A seems to be a specific antagonist to certain abnormalities created by cortisone and its derivatives.[24]

The role of metals in wound healing is being studied intensively. Copper and ferrous iron are required for normal collagen metabolism, but deficiency states are rarely, if ever, seen. Zinc and other divalent cations are co-factors in many metabolic reactions, and deficiency states in animals do retard epithelialization and strength gain. Relative zinc deficiency has been suggested as one cause of poor epithelialization in children with large burns. The data, however, are equivocal at present.[15, 77]

Anemia, Blood Loss, and Oxygen Tension. Many clinicians feel strongly that significant anemia delays healing. Unfortunately, this hypothesis is difficult to verify experimentally. The literature contains data to support both sides of a debate. The importance of tissue oxygen tension in healing, however, is established. Prolonged low tissue oxygen tension impairs healing significantly.[94] Perhaps the equivocal results with experimental anemias may be explained by differences in local oxygen tension. Adequate tissue perfusion seems to be more important than the oxygen-carrying capacity of the blood for normal healing. Hemorrhage or anemia alone may not alter tissue oxygen tension; hypovolemia, vasoconstriction, and elevated blood viscosity, however, can have profound effects on local oxygen tension. Environmental temperature also influences local oxygen tension in the skin and affects wound healing. Wounds gain strength significantly faster at higher than at lower room temperatures. Local blood flow seems critical because reducing local vasoconstriction by denervating the skin abolishes the effect of temperature on healing.

Stress, Steroids, and Anti-inflammatory Agents. Although wide variations exist between species and between individuals, ACTH, cortisone, and other glucocorticoids can have profound effects on healing rate.[4] Cortisone and its derivatives decrease the rate of protein synthesis, stabilize lysosomal membranes, and inhibit the normal inflammatory reaction. In most species studied, including man, high doses of corticoids limit capillary budding, inhibit fibroblast proliferation, and decrease the rate of epithelialization. Experimentally, steroids given prior to or immediately after wounding have the greatest effect.[66] As a rule, even with high doses of steroids, wound healing reactions go to completion; only the time scale is altered. All phases of healing proceed much more slowly, and most clinicians agree that patients receiving chronic steroid therapy who undergo surgical procedures have a greater risk of delayed healing. If careful adjustments are made for the altered time scale, however, wound complications can be minimized.

The other commonly used anti-inflammatory agents (salicylate derivatives, phenylbutazone) have minimal effects on healing. Experimentally, huge doses of aspirin delay strength gain significantly, but pharmacologic doses have no effect.[48]

Cytotoxic Drugs and Radiation. Chronic tissue changes induced by radiant energy of short wavelength have profound effects on healing and will be discussed elsewhere in this volume. Acute radiation effects and effects of other cytotoxic agents, however, also influence healing rate. Most cytotoxic agents show their greatest effect on dividing cells. From our previous discussion, it is clear that any agent that inhibits the division of local fibroblasts or epithelial cells should prevent or delay healing. Fortunately, the systemic administration of nitrogen mustard, thioTEPA, 5-fluorouracil, and other antimetabolites rarely causes high enough tissue concentrations to influence cell division in wounds. However, the chronic, local application of these agents (particularly 5-fluorouracil) can completely prevent healing. Similarly, high doses of radiation, especially during the first 3 days, delay strength gain significantly.

WOUND CARE

A major portion of this volume is devoted to the care of wounds in special tissues. Indeed, all technical considerations in surgery may be viewed as methods of minimizing the surgeon's interference with normal healing. Therefore, no attempt will be made in this section to review specific healing problems in each tissue. From our discussion of biologic behavior, however, certain general principles in the care of all wounds are evident. Although wound infections and surgical bacteriology will be discussed specifically in another chapter, factors delaying normal healing create conditions conducive to local sepsis.

Because almost all biologic phenomena associated with healing require the active participation of cells, local environmental conditions must be optimal for cellular metabolism. Any local diminution of blood supply will delay or prevent healing. Gross alterations in local tissue perfusion are easily recognized, but significant changes in tissue oxygen tension may be caused by subtle factors. Drying of exposed tissues not only kills surface cells, but also destroys normal blood flow in small vessels some distance from the surface. Because local inflammation alters vessel permeability, a suture initially encircling tissue under slight tension may become a garrote, choking off all local blood flow, as injured tissues swell. In addition, external pressure from carelessly applied dressings can decrease local tissue perfusion significantly. To allow healing to proceed normally, care must be taken to insure adequate tissue perfusion.

Preparing local tissues for surgery requires a thoughtful surgical biologist. The thick cornified layer of epidermis protects intact skin and underlying tissues from many noxious substances. When the epidermal layer is injured, deeper tissues are exposed to the surgeon's mistakes. Ethyl alcohol, iodine, ether, and other commonly used preparation solutions placed on the intact skin have minor effects; the same materials poured into an open wound kill cells on contact. Open wounds must be protected from all substances harmful to living cells. A good rule of thumb: never put anything in a wound that could not be placed in your own conjunctival sac with safety.

Rapid and complete invasion of the wound space by fibroblasts is a critical step in normal healing. As noted, dead tissue fragments, hematomas, foreign bodies, and fluid collections act as physical barriers, preventing normal fibroblast penetration. Space-occupying lesions prolong inflammation, encourage bacterial growth, and delay gain in strength significantly. Therefore, thorough removal of all dead materials and prevention of fluid collections are primary goals in good wound management. Tissue fragments and foreign objects loosely attached to the wound surface can be removed with careful saline irrigations. As a rule, however, dirty, traumatic wounds must be debrided carefully, using forceps, sharp tools, and, most important, time. Primarily healed abdominal wounds, functional extremities, and cosmetically acceptable facial scars are the surgeon's reward for the hours spent meticulously debriding traumatic wounds; infection, fibrosis, hypertrophic scars, and foreign body granulomas await the careless operator.

Although not discussed specifically, the rational choice of suture materials was implicit in our discussion of the biologic behavior of wounds. Only two questions need be asked: How much strength is needed? How long must the suture supply mechanical strength? Because wounds gain strength and remodel slowly, tissue unions requiring initial and prolonged strength should be made with suture material that retains strength for the desired period. In addition, the tissues coapted should be of sufficient mechanical strength to produce the desired result. Although several absorbable, synthetic materials have been introduced recently, the most commonly used absorbable suture is catgut, a collagenous preparation made from the submucosa of sheep intestines. Plain or untanned catgut retains strength for approximately one week. Preparations tanned with chromic acid retain most of their physical strength for approximately three weeks, depending upon local environment. As noted, most wounds develop less than 15 per cent of their ultimate tensile strength by three weeks. If this degree of physical integrity is sufficient, absorbable sutures are appropriate. If suture material must supply appreciable amounts of wound strength for longer periods, nonabsorbable materials are indicated.

Determining how much strength a suture must supply in each specific instance is difficult. Like most biological systems, the human body is over-engineered. Dense connective tissues are probably ten times stronger than needed to absorb the stresses of everyday living. Even when disease alters the physical properties of connective tissues significantly (i.e., Ehlers-Danlos syndrome, etc.), affected individuals do not have gaping wounds constantly. In many clinical situations, including the majority of abdominal incisions, 15 per cent of the ultimate tensile strength may be sufficient to resist normal stress.

One additional factor determines the magnitude of strength required. Significant pain inhibits the full activity of most voluntary muscles. Therefore, injured tissues are splinted internally, if normal pain mechanisms are functioning. If pain is totally eliminated, generated stresses can be much higher. As an example, many of us have had the unfortunate experience of having an entire inguinal hernia repair disrupted at the close of the procedure. Characteristically, the patient strains maximally during extubation and a frightening series of popping sounds is felt or heard! On immediate re-exploration, the sutures are either broken, or more commonly, have actually pulled out of the dense connective tissue in which they were placed. Because the patient is without pain during this interval, he can make stresses sufficient to disrupt the repair. Once the full pain mechanism is restored, however, the same mechanical repair is entirely sufficient to resist the stresses applied by the patient. Over-engineering and protective behavior following injury enable surgeons to close abdominal incisions and other stressed wounds successfully using a variety of materials.

Because a nonabsorbable suture, even monofilament steel or nylon, can act as a nidus for infection, absorbable materials have an advantage in contaminated or potentially contaminated wounds. Absorbable materials, however, cause a more intense tissue reaction. If minimal reaction is desired, use nonabsorbable materials.

A thorough understanding of wound healing biology provides a rational approach to suture removal. As noted, skin epithelial cells migrate down suture tracts, causing inflammation and sterile abscesses. In addition, skin sutures present for long periods tend to injure underlying skin, creating additional scarring. Therefore, when cosmesis is important, skin sutures should be removed early. Adequate strength to prevent wound spreading during remodeling can be obtained by placing permanent, buried subcuticular sutures in the lowest portion of the dermis. Where cosmesis is not a problem, skin sutures should remain in place until strength sufficient to resist local tissue tension and minor trauma has been attained. Timing varies widely in different areas of the body and in different individuals. The surgeon who always removes skin sutures on the same day in all areas and in all individuals will eventually have wound problems. For instance, the tensions on a simple horizontal laceration of the upper eyelid are minimal. Strength attained by fibrin strands and epithelialization are usually sufficient to prevent dehiscence, and sutures can be removed in 24 to 48 hours. In contrast, a vertical wound on the dorsal thorax may require 21 days to acquire sufficient strength to resist local tissue tension and strain produced by body movements. When doubt exists, removing several sutures and testing wound strength gently is helpful.

Epithelial cells will not spread on surfaces composed of dead material or tissue burdened with excessive number of bacteria. Granulating wounds awaiting epithelialization must be kept free of dead material. Careful débridement with forceps and sharp instruments can be invaluable. If small areas of dead tissue are too numerous or too small for gross mechanical removal, frequent wet-to-dry dressings can produce effective débridement. Dressings on epithelializing wounds must be applied carefully, however. As noted, the interface between epithelial cells and deeper scar is fragile and never regains normal epidermal-dermal strength. Migrating cells and recently epithelialized surfaces must be protected from mechanical trauma. Moreover, epithelialized scar tissue and fresh skin grafts are quite susceptible to bacterial invasion. As crusts develop and small suture abscesses occur, they must be removed mechanically. The care of skin grafts and consideration of dressings will be covered in greater depth in other chapters.

As discussed, wound contraction can produce serious functional impairment. The most effective method of preventing contraction is early coverage of open surfaces. The techniques used will be discussed in detail elsewhere. The timing, however, is equally important. Although fresh wounds covered with thick split-thickness or full thickness grafts do remodel and contract with time, the magnitude of contraction is small. Wounds allowed to remain open for long periods contract to a maximum. The only effective method of preventing contraction at present is early coverage. From our discussion of the mechanisms responsible, treating a fully contracted and epithelialized wound requires the excision of all the products of wound healing, re-creation of the original defect, and resurfacing of the newly created wound as soon as possible.

Finally, the prolonged metabolic activity of wounds can be used to the surgeon's advantage. As discussed, wounds reopened months after initial incision gain strength at a more rapid rate than primary wounds. Even though strength increases may be minimal, the secondary wound healing phenomenon can be used profitably. When rapid gain in strength is desirable, old incisions should not be excised. Rather, the new incision should remain within the old scar, In addition, because wounds change in color, bulk, and strength slowly, scar revision or reconstructive procedures should be delayed until scar reactivity is minimal. Bulky, prominent scars present 3 months after injury may become smooth, flat, and inconspicuous by 1 year. When reconstructive or cosmetic procedures are contemplated, patience is a virtue.

CONTROLLING THE HEALING PROCESS

In most cases, normal healing re-establishes tissue integrity quickly and effectively. Organ function is preserved, satisfying both the patient and the surgeon. There are situations, however, in which the surgeon wishes he had some control over the healing process. For instance, an effective method of increasing rate of gain in strength could prevent dehiscence and evisceration, disastrous complications of abdominal surgery. Increasing the rate of epithelialization in open wounds could reduce mortality in burned patients. Effective control of the remodeling process could insure normal function after tendon injury, prevent fibrous stricture of the esophagus following lye burns, and eliminate stenosis of hollow organs. More important, the same scarring process seen in healing wounds seems to be involved in a variety of human diseases. Cirrhosis of the liver, retroperitoneal fibrosis, Dupuytren's contracture, interstitial pulmonary fi-

brosis, post-traumatic epilepsy, rheumatic valvular disease, and a host of other pathologic conditions of man result from inappropriate fibrous tissue production. Effective methods of controlling scar formation would be extremely valuable.

Because of the obvious practical implications, many surgeons have searched for methods of accelerating healing through the years. In the early 1900s, Alexis Carrel noted that extracts of embryonic tissues increased mitotic activity of cultured fibroblasts. This simple observation stimulated surgeons to homogenize tissues of all varieties, both embryonic and adult, and to inject or apply extracts to wounds. After decades of experimentation, only one of these substances, cartilage powder, has been shown to affect healing unequivocally. Dried powdered cartilage from many species produces significant increases in breaking strength of animal and human wounds.[80] The effect, dose-related and demonstrable within 4 days, can be produced with local applications or by injecting saline extracts at a distance from the wound. Recent data suggest that polymers of N-acetyl glucosamine may be the effective agent.[79] By 7 days, cartilage-treated wounds are 20 per cent stronger than controls. Although the absolute strength gain remains constant for several weeks, the percentage change drops to a small value as the absolute strength of the wound increases. The mechanism of cartilage action is unknown. However, histologic studies suggest that fibroblast density and collagen formation are increased during the early phases of repair. Cartilage powder, implanted within polyvinyl sponges, stimulates rapid production of collagen. No direct measurements of rate of scar collagen synthesis or of scar collagen turnover have been performed, however.

Although supplying supernormal amounts of ascorbic acid, protein, or methionine fails to accelerate gain in strength, increasing local oxygen tension stimulates healing significantly. Animals in a 40 per cent oxygen environment have stronger wounds at 7 days than animals breathing air.[94] The oxygen effect seems unrelated to carbon dioxide concentration. Again, however, the magnitude of acceleration is slight, amounting to less than 15 per cent at 7 days.

Unfortunately, neither cartilage powder nor increased oxygen tension increases strength gain sufficiently to satisfy most clinicians. As discussed, incised wounds gain less than 5 per cent of their ultimate strength by 7 days and less than 15 per cent by 3 weeks. A 20 per cent increase or even a 100 per cent increase at 2 or 3 weeks may be of little clinical significance. Even with the increase, suture material would provide significant strength to the wounds. Gains of 300 per cent or 500 per cent by 3 weeks, however, could be of tremendous value.

Although of limited clinical usefulness, these experiments do demonstrate that wounds can be induced to gain strength more rapidly. Because the ultimate strength of scars depends on collagen molecules, crosslinking density, and fiber weave, agents influencing collagen metabolism should have significant effects on healing. Currently, agents known to affect crosslinking are much too nonspecific and toxic for clinical application. However, biologic agents may exist that influence crosslinking even under normal conditions. For instance, the rate of conversion of uncrosslinked collagen to insoluble collagen differs significantly between tissues, between individuals, and even in the same individual at different ages. Data suggest that these differences may result entirely from altered environmental conditions. However, if rate of crosslinking is determined, even in part, by enzymatic reactions, pharmacologic agents might be found that alter crosslinking rates and influence wound strength significantly. Influencing fiber weave in soft tissue healing remains an unexplored area. In bone remodeling, local electrical field changes seem to influence the architecture of bone matrix significantly.[7] Electrical fields, of course, can direct molecular orientation in vitro. Their influence on collagen fiber architecture in scars, however, is unknown. Tension and stress seem to produce significant alterations in scar metabolism, but as yet too little is known to use these modalities rationally.[5]

Although methods of effectively accelerating wound healing are desirable, techniques of inhibiting the fibrotic process might be more beneficial to man. Pathologic fibrosis produces significant pathophysiologic change by altering the form or physical properties of tissue. Normally pliant heart valves stiffened with scar become incompetent. Distensible gut replaced by firm, unyielding scar becomes an inefficient conduit. Therefore, methods of preventing collagen synthesis or altering the physical properties of collagen fibers might reverse or prevent pathophysiologic changes.

The techniques used must be specific in their effects on collagen and selective in their effects on scar tissue. All metabolic inhibitors of protein synthesis (puromycin, actinomycin D) decrease collagen synthesis. Unfortunately, they also inhibit the synthesis of other proteins; the effect is nonspecific and quite toxic to living cells. Selectivity can occur only if metabolic processes unique to collagen are interfered with. As discussed, the hydroxylation of proline is unique. Peptidyl proline hydroxylase activity requires molecular oxygen, α-ketoglutarate, ascorbic acid, and ferrous iron. No method of producing instant scurvy exists, but altering ferrous iron metabolism has profound effects on collagen synthesis. In tissue culture preparations, ferrous iron chelators specifically inhibit the synthesis of collagen without affecting noncollagenous protein metabolism.[18] More important, systemic administration of ferrous iron chelators in animals prevents silica-induced hepatic fibrosis, alters collagen content in implanted polyvinyl sponges, and reduces wound strength significantly.[16] Because most of the iron chelators tested so far have disturbing side effects, no human data are available; the effects of ferrous iron chelation on collagen metabolism in man are unknown.

Several other techniques can specifically inhibit collagen synthesis. Because the oxygen utilized in proline hydroxylation comes from molecular oxygen, cells grown in a nitrogen atmosphere fail to hydroxylate protocollagen and secretion of collagen stops. This technique has no future in clinical medicine. Recent observations, however, suggest another technique with wider application. Several analogs of proline (3,4-dehydroproline, cis-hydroxyproline) are incorporated into proteins but not hydroxylated.[16] In high enough concentrations, proline analogs prevent collagen formation and seem to have minimal effects on noncollagenous protein synthesis. Several authors have claimed that administering proline analogs to animals inhibits collagen synthesis and affects scar formation significantly.[20, 46] The effects of proline analogs in vivo, however, are controversial and the effects in human beings remain unknown.[17, 58]

The physical properties of scars can be altered without affecting rate of collagen synthesis. As noted, collagen fibers achieve their tremendous tensile strength by forming intermolecular covalent crosslinks. A class of compounds, the osteolathyrogens, specifically inhibit intermolecular covalent crosslinking in newly synthesized collagen. Beta-aminopropionitrile, a compound found in the stems and seeds of plants of the genus Lathyrus, prevents the formation of lysine-derived aldehydes by inhibiting lysyl amine oxidase activity. Under the influence of lathyrogens, collagen molecules are synthesized and excreted at normal rates, but the aggregated fibers fail to form crosslinks. Lathyrogenic collagen, therefore, has little tensile strength and is disrupted easily. Penicillamine, a powerful copper chelator liberated during the alkaline hydrolysis of penicillin, is lathyrogenic but produces its effects by a different mechanism.[70] Rather than inhibiting aldehyde formation, penicillamine chelates the resultant aldehydes, preventing aldol condensation reactions or Schiff base formation. In animals, systemic administration of BAPN or penicillamine inhibits gain in strength of incised wounds.[74] More important, BAPN prevents or reverses pathophysiologic changes in animal models of fibrotic diseases. Induced lathyrism prevents the stiff joint of immobility, improves gliding after tendon injury, prevents esophageal stenosis following lye burns, and restores esophageal diameter in fixed esophageal stenosis.[19, 21, 27, 59] Experience with BAPN in man is limited, but systemic administration does inhibit intermolecular crosslinking in scar collagen.[75] In one clinical series, BAPN produced significant allergic reactions; in another, no toxicity was demonstrated.[45] Whether or not lathyrogenic agents can alter pathophysiology in man remains untested.

Each of the anticollagenous agents discussed affects collagen metabolism specifically. To be clinically effective, however, specificity alone is insufficient; agents must selectively affect the scar. The dynamic metabolism of scar collagen, however, can provide selectivity and establish a useful therapeutic ratio. Because the techniques described affect only newly synthesized collagen, a differential turnover rate between scar collagen and normal tissue produces selectivity. Scar tissue turning over five times as rapidly as normal tissue responds selectively to short periods of anticollagenous therapy.[74] Theoretically, any fibrotic condition meeting the following criteria could be treated with effective anticollagenous agents: (1) Pathophysiology should be related directly to alterations in form or physical properties of fibrotic tissues. (2) Rate of new collagen deposition or turnover should be significantly higher in diseased than in normal tissues. (3) Formation of pathologic fibrous tissue should be limited to a short period of time. Interestingly enough, many common surgical problems meet these criteria.

To date effective control of the healing process in man has not been achieved. However, experimental data suggest that clinical control of the healing process is feasible. With time,

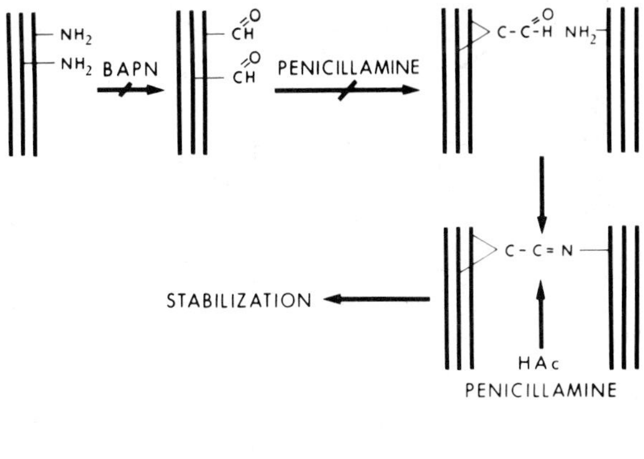

Figure 15. Schematic representation of the formation of intramolecular and intermolecular crosslinks in collagen and the effective points of lathyrogenic interference. Note that beta-aminopropionitrile blocks aldehyde formation while penicillamine interferes with aldehyde reactions. (From Peacock, E. E., Jr., and Van Winkle, W., Jr.: Surgery and Biology of Wound Repair, 2nd ed. Philadelphia, W. B. Saunders Company, 1976.)

clinically useful methods of controlling scar formation and wound contraction will be developed. Until these tools are in our possession, the skillful surgeon must utilize the biological information covered in this chapter to regain maximum function in injured parts. At the moment we have no pharmacologic crutch to support poor wound management.

SELECTED REFERENCES

International Review of Connective Tissue Research. New York, Academic Press. 1963 to current.

A continuing series of volumes is published under this title. Each volume contains monographs by several authors devoted to current connective tissue research problems. Most of the articles will interest serious students.

McMinn, R. M. H.: Tissue Repair, New York, Academic Press, 1969.

This scholarly monograph reviews the morphologic aspects of injury and repair in detail. Although the book is not oriented toward the surgeon, McMinn provides a rich source of anatomic information invaluable for the serious student.

Peacock, E. E., Jr., and Van Winkle, W., Jr.: Surgery and Biology of Wound Repair, 2nd ed. Philadelphia, W. B. Saunders Company, 1976.

This monograph is by far the most comprehensive work on wound healing available. Written by a surgeon and a biologist, this volume reviews current data on the biology of repair and extends basic biologic concepts to all phases of surgery. The practical consideration given to difficult wound healing problems should be vauable to any practicing clinician. This volume is recommended to all physicians with more than a passing interest in repair.

Trinkaus, J. P.: Cells into Organs. Englewood Cliffs, N.J., Prentice-Hall, Inc., 1969.

Although written for the student embryologist, this monograph contains a superb review of cell behavior. The author discusses mechanisms of cell locomotion, directional movements, chemotaxis, mechanisms of cell adhesion, and cell segregation in a clear, authoritative fashion. This small volume makes fascinating reading for any physician, but is particularly useful for the student of wound healing.

REFERENCES

1. Abercrombie, M., Flint, M. H., and James, D. W.: Wound contraction in relation to collagen formation in scorbutic guinea pigs. J. Embryol. Exp. Morphol., 4:167, 1956.
2. Abercrombie, M., James, D. W., and Newcombe, J. F.: Wound contraction in rabbit skin, studied by splinting the wound margins. J. Anat., 94:170, 1960.
3. Adamsons, R. J., Musco, F., and Enquist, I. F.: The relationship of collagen content to wound strength in normal and scorbutic animals. Surg. Gynecol. Obstet., 119:323, 1964.
4. Alrich, E. M., Carter, J. P., and Lehman, E. P.: The effect of ACTH and cortisone on wound healing. Ann. Surg., 133:783, 1951.
5. Arem, A., and Madden, J. W.: Effects of stress on healing wounds: I. Intermittent non-cyclical tension. Surg. Res., 20:93, 1976.
6. Bailey, A. J., Fowler, L. J., and Peach, C. M.: Identification of two interchain crosslinks of bone and dentine collagen. Biochem. Biophys. Res. Commun., 35:663, 1969.
7. Becker, R. O., and Bassett, C. A. L.: Generation of electric potential by bone in response to mechanical stress. Science, 137:1063, 1962.
8. Bentley, J. P.: Rate of chondroitin sulfate formation in wound healing. Ann. Surg., 165:186, 1967.
9. Bhisey, A. N., and Freed, J. J.: Ameboid movement induced in cultured macrophages by colchicine or vinblastine. Exp. Cell Res., 64:419, 1971.
10. Billingham, R. E., and Russel, P. S.: Studies on wound healing with special reference to the phenomenon of contracture in experimental wounds in rabbits' skin. Ann. Surg., 144:961, 1956.
11. Bornstein, P., Kang, A. H., and Piez, K. A.: The nature and loca-

tion of intramolecular cross-links in collagen. Proc. Nat. Acad. Sci., 55:417, 1966.
12. Botsford, T. W.: The tensile strength of sutured skin wounds during healing. Surg. Gynecol. Obstet., 72:690, 1941.
13. Bryant, W. M., Greenwell, J. E., and Weeks, P. M.: Alterations in collagen organization during dilatation of the cervix uteri. Surg. Gynecol. Obstet., 126:27, 1968.
14. Chung, E., Keels, E. M., and Miller, E. J.: Isolation and characterization of the cyanogen bromide peptides from the α (III) chain of human collagen. Biochemistry, 13:3459, 1974.
15. Chvapil, M.: Zinc and wound healing. In Zederfeldt, B. (Ed.): Symposium on zinc. Lunds, Sweden, A. B. Tika, 1974.
16. Chvapil, M.: Pharmacology of fibrosis: Definitions, limits, and perspectives. Life Sci. [I], 16:1345, 1975.
17. Chvapil, M., Madden, J. W., Carlson, E. C., and Peacock, E. E., Jr.: Effect of cis-hydroxyproline on collagen and other proteins in skin wounds, granuloma tissue, and liver of mice and rats. Exp. Molec. Pathol., 20:363, 1974.
18. Chvapil, M., Ryan, J. N., Madden, J. W., and Peacock, E. E., Jr.: Effect of chelating agents, proline analogs, and oxygen tension in in vivo and in vitro experiments on hydroxylation, transport, degradation, and accumulation of collagen. In Vogel, H. G. (Ed.): Connective Tissue and Ageing, 1:195, 1973. International Congress Series, No. 264. Amsterdam, Excerpta Medica.
19. Craver, J. M., Madden, J. W., and Peacock, E. E., Jr.: Biological control of physical properties of tendon adhesions: Effect of β-aminopropionitrile in chickens. Ann. Surg., 157:697, 1968.
20. Daly, J. M., Steigher, E., Prockop, D. J., and Dudrick, S. J.: Inhibition of collagen synthesis by the proline analogue cis-4-hydroxyproline. J. Surg. Res., 14:551, 1973.
21. Davis, W. M., Madden, J. W., and Peacock, E. E., Jr.: A new approach to the control of esophageal stenosis. Ann. Surg., 176:469, 1972.
22. Douglas, D. M.: The healing of aponeurotic incisions. Br. J. Surg., 40:79, 1952.
23. Dunphy, J. E., and Jackson, D. S.: Practical applications of experimental studies in the care of primarily closed wounds. Am. J. Surg., 104:273, 1962.
24. Ehrlich, H. P., and Hunt, T. K.: Effects of cortisone and vitamin A on wound healing. Ann. Surg., 167:324, 1968.
25. Eisen, A. Z., Bauer, E. A., and Jeffrey, J. J.: Animal and human collagenases. J. Invest. Dermatol., 55:359, 1970.
26. Forrester, J. C., Zederfeldt, B. T., Hayes, T. L., and Hunt, T. K.: Wolff's law in relation to the healing skin wound. J. Trauma, 10:770, 1970.
27. Furlow, L. T., Jr., and Peacock, E. E., Jr.: Effect of β-aminopropionitrile on joint stiffness in rats. Ann. Surg., 165:442, 1967.
28. Furthmayer, H., Timpl, R., Stark, M., Lapiere, C. M., and Kuhn, K.: Chemical properties of the peptide extension in the α-chain of dermatosparactic skin collagen. FEBS Letters, 28:247, 1972.
29. Gabbiani, G., Hirschel, B. J., Ryan, G. B., Statkov, P. R., and Majno, G.: Granulation tissue as a contractile organ: A study of structure and function. J. Exp. Med., 135:719, 1972.
30. Gabbiani, G., Ryan, G. B., and Majno, G.: Presence of modified fibroblasts in granulation tissue and their possible role in wound contraction. Experimentia, 27:549, 1971.
31. Grillo, H. C., Watts, G. T., and Gross, J.: Studies in wound healing: I. Contraction and wound contents. Ann. Surg., 148:145, 1958.
32. Gross, J., and Lapiere, C. M.: Collagenolytic activity in amphibian tissues: A tissue culture assay. Proc. Nat. Acad. Sci., 48:1014, 1962.
33. Heppelston, A. G., and Styles, J. A.: Activity of a macrophage factor in collagen formation by Silica. Nature, 214:521, 1967.
34. Hirschel, B. J., Gabbiani, G., Ryan, T. B., and Majno, G.: Fibroblasts of granulation tissue: Immunofluorescent staining with anti-smooth muscle serum. Proc. Soc. Exp. Biol. Med., 138:466, 1971.
35. Howes, E. L., Harvey, S. C., and Hewitt, W. J.: Rate of fibroplasia and differentiation in the healing of cutaneous wounds in different species of animals. Arch. Surg., 38:934, 1939.
36. Howes, E. L., Sooy, J. W., and Harvey, S. C.: The healing of wounds as determined by their tensile strength. J.A.M.A., 92:242, 1929.
37. Hurych, J., and Chvapil, M.: Influence of chelating agents on the biosynthesis of collagen. Biochim. Biophys. Acta, 97:361, 1965.

38. Jacques, J.: Wound contraction in experimental lathyrism. Br. J. Exp. Pathol., 50:486, 1969.

39. James, D. W., and Newcombe, J. F.: Granulation tissue resorption during free and limited contraction of skin wounds. J. Anat., 95:247, 1961.

40. Johnson, F. R., and McMinn, R. M. H.: The cytology of wound healing of body surfaces in mammals. Biol. Rev., 35:364, 1960.

41. Joseph, K. T., and Gowri, C.: Nature of the covalent cross-links in collagen. J. Sci. Indust. Res., 29:504, 1970.

42. Josse, J., and Harrington, W. F.: Role of pyrrolidine residues in the structure and stabilization of collagen. J. Molec. Biol., 9:269, 1964.

43. Juva, R.: Hydroxylation of proline in the biosynthesis of collagen. Acta Physiol. Scand. (Suppl.) 308:1, 1968.

44. Kefalides, N. A.: Isolation of a collagen from basement membrane containing three identical α-chains. Biochem. Biophys. Res. Comm., 45:226, 1971.

45. Keiser, H. R., and Sjoerdsma, A.: Studies on beta-aminopropionitrile in patients with scleroderma. Clin. Pharmacol. Ther., 8:593, 1968.

46. Lane, J. M., Bora, F. W., Prockop, D. J., Heppenstall, R. B., and Black, J.: Inhibition of scar formation by the proline analog cis-hydroxyproline. J. Surg. Res., 13:135, 1972.

47. Laurent, T. C.: The interaction between polysaccharides and other macromolecules. 9. The exclusion of molecules from hyaluronic acid gels and solutions. Biochem. J., 93:106, 1964.

48. Lee, K. H.: Studies on the mechanism of action of salicylate. II. Retardation of wound healing by aspirin. J. Pharm. Sci., 57:1042, 1968.

49. Leibovich, S. J., and Ross, R.: The role of the macrophage in wound repair. Am. J. Pathol., 78:71, 1975.

50. Lenaers, A., Ansay, M., Nusgens, B. V., and Lapiere, C. M.: Collagen made of extended α-chains, procollagen, in genetically-defective dermatosparactic calves. Eur. J. Biochem., 23:533, 1971.

51. Levene, C. I., and Gross, J.: Alterations in state of molecular aggregation of collagen induced in chick embryos by β-aminopropionitrile. J. Exp. Med., 110:771, 1959.

52. Levenson, S. M., Geever, E. F., Crowley, L. V., Oates, J. F., Berard, C. W., and Rosen, H.: The healing of rat skin wounds. Ann. Surg., 161:293, 1965.

53. Lichtenstein, J. R., Martin, G. R., Kohn, L. D., Byers, P. H., and McKusick, V. A.: Defect in conversion of procollagen to collagen in a form of Ehlers-Danlos syndrome. Science, 182:298, 1973.

54. Madden, J. W. On the contractile fibroblast. Plast. Reconstr. Surg., 52:291, 1973.

55. Madden, J. W., Wound healing: The biological basis of hand surgery. Clin. Plast. Surg., 3:3, 1976.

56. Madden, J. W., and Carlson, E. C.: Atypical fibroblasts, wound contraction and human fibrocontractive disease. Proceedings of the International Symposium on Wound Healing. Rotterdam, 1974.

57. Madden, J. W., Carlson, E. C., and Hines, J.: Presence of modified fibroblasts in ischemic contracture of intrinsic musculature of the hand. Surg. Gynecol. Obstet., 140:509, 1975.

58. Madden, J. W., Chvapil, M., Carlson, E. C., and Ryan, J. N.: Toxicity and metabolic effect of 3,4-dehydroproline in mice. J. Toxicol. Appl. Pharmacol. 26:426, 1973.

59. Madden, J. W., Davis, W. M., Butler, C., II, and Peacock, E. E., Jr.: Experimental esophageal lye burns. 2. Correcting established strictures with β-aminopropionitrile and bougienage. Ann. Surg., 178:277, 1973.

60. Madden, J. W., Morton, D., Jr., and Peacock, E. E., Jr.: Contraction of experimental wounds: I. Inhibiting wound contraction using a topical smooth muscle antagonist. Surgery, 76:8, 1974.

61. Madden, J. W., and Peacock, E. E., Jr.: Studies on the biology of collagen during wound healing. I. Rate of collagen synthesis and deposition in cutaneous wounds of the rat. Surgery, 64:288, 1968.

62. Madden, J. W., and Peacock, E. E., Jr.: Studies on the biology of collagen during wound healing: III. Dynamic metabolism of scar collagen and remodeling of dermal wounds. Ann. Surg., 174:511, 1971.

63. Madden, J. W., and Smith, H. C.: Rate of collagen synthesis and deposition in dehisced and resutured wounds. Surg. Gynecol. Obstet., 130:487, 1970.

64. Majno, G., Gabbiani, G., Hirschel, B. J., Ryan, G. B., and Statkov, P. R.: Contraction of granulation tissue in vitro: Similarity to smooth muscle. Science, 173:548, 1971.

65. Mason, M. L., and Allen, H. S.: The rate of healing of tendons. An experimental study of tensile strength. Ann. Surg., 113:424, 1941.

66. Meadows, E. C., and Prudden, J. F.: A study of the influence of adrenal steroids on the strength of healing wounds. Surgery, 33:841, 1953.

67. Miller, E. L.: A review of the biochemical studies on the genetically distinct collagens of the skeletal system. Clin. Orthop., 92:260, 1973.

68. Monson, J. M., and Bornstein, P.: Identification of a disulfide-linked procollagen as the biosynthetic precursor of chick-bone collagen. Proc. Nat. Acad. Sci., 70:3521, 1973.

69. Mussini, E., Hutton, J. J., Jr., and Udenfriend, S.: Collagen proline hydroxylase in wound healing, granuloma formation, scurvy and growth. Science, 157:927, 1967.

70. Nimni, M. E.: A defect in the intramolecular and intermolecular cross-linking of collagen caused by penicillamine. J. Biol. Chem., 743:1457, 1967.

71. Odland, G., and Ross, R.: Human wound repair: I. Epidermal regeneration. J. Cell. Biol., 39:135, 1968.

72. Ordman, L. J., and Gillman, T.: Studies on the healing of cutaneous wounds. I. The healing of incisions through the skin of pigs. Arch. Surg., 93:857, 1966.

73. Page, R. C., and Benditt, E. P.: A molecular defect in lathyritic collagen. Proc. Soc. Exp. Biol. Med., 124:459, 1967.

74. Peacock, E. E., Jr., and Madden, J. W.: Some studies on the effect of β-aminopropionitrile on collagen in healing wounds. Surgery, 60:7, 1966.

75. Peacock, E. E., Jr., and Madden, J. W.: Some studies on the effects of β-aminopropionitrile in patients with injured flexor tendons. Surgery, 66:215, 1969.

76. Peacock, E. E., Jr., Madden, J. W., and Trier, W. C.: Biological basis for the treatment of keloids and hypertrophic scars. South. Med. J., 63:755, 1970.

77. Pories, W. J., Henzel, J. H., Rob, C. G., and Strain, W. H.: Acceleration of healing with zinc sulfate. Ann. Surg., 165:432, 1967.

78. Prockop, D. J.: The intracellular biosynthesis of collagen. Arch. Intern. Med., 124:563, 1969.

79. Prudden, J. F., Migel, P., Hanson, P., Friedrich, L., and Balarsa, L.: The discovery of a potent pure chemical wound-healing accelerator. Am. J. Surg., 119:560, 1970.

80. Prudden, J. F., Wabarsky, E. P., and Balarsa, L.: The acceleration of healing. Surg. Gynecol. Obstet., 128:1321, 1969.

81. Ramachandran, G. N., and Sasisekharan, V.: Refinement of the structure of collagen. Biochem. Biophys. Acta, 109:314, 1965.

82. Rich, A., and Crick, F. H. C.: The molecular structures of collagen. J. Molec. Biol., 3:483, 1961.

83. Ross, R.: The fibroblast and wound repair. Biol. Rev., 43:51, 1968.

84. Ross, R., Everett, N. B., and Tyler, R.: Wound healing and collagen formation. VI. The origin of the wound fibroblast studied in parabiosis. J. Cell Biol., 44:645, 1970.

85. Rovee, D. T., and Miller, C. A.: Epidermal role in the breaking strength of wounds. Arch. Surg., 96:43, 1968.

86. Savlov, E. D., and Dunphy, J. E.: The healing of the disrupted and resutured wound. Surgery, 36:362, 1954.

87. Sawhney, C. P., and Monga, H. L.: Wound contraction in rabbits and the effectiveness of skin grafts in preventing it. Br. J. Plast. Surg., 23:318, 1970.

88. Schmitt, F. O., Gross, J., and Highberger, J. H.: State of aggregation of collagen. Soc. Exp. Biol. Symp., 9:148, 1955.

89. Schmitt, F. O., Gross, J., and Highberger, J. H.: Tropocollagen and the properties of fibrous collagen. Exp. Cell Res., 3(Suppl.):326, 1955.

90. Siegel, R. C., Pinnell, S. R., and Martin, G. R.: Crosslinking of collagen and elastin. Properties of lysyl oxidase. Biochemistry, 9:4486, 1970.

91. Smith, J. W.: Packing arrangement of tropocollagen molecules. Nature, 205:356, 1965.

92. Speakman, P. T.: Proposed mechanism for the biological assembly of collagen triple helix. Nature, 229:241, 1971.

93. Stark, M., Rauterberg, J., and Kuhn, K.: Evidence for a non-helical region at the carboxyl terminus of the collagen molecule. FEBS Letters, 13:101, 1971.

94. Stevens, F. O., and Hunt, T. K.: Effect of changes in inspired ox-

ygen and carbon dioxide tensions on wound tensile strength: An experimental study. Ann. Surg., *173*:515, 1971.

95. Stone, P. A., and Madden, J. W.: Effect of primary and delayed split skin grafting on wound contraction. Surg. Forum, *25*:41, 1974.

96. Stone, P. A., and Madden, J. W.: Biological factors affecting wound contraction. Surg. Forum, *26*:547, 1975.

97. Trelstad, R. L., Kang, A. H., Igarashi, S., and Gross, J.: Isolation of two distinct collagens from chick cartilage. Biochemistry, *9*:4993, 1970.

98. Watts, G. T., Grillo, H. C., and Gross, J.: Studies in wound healing: II. The role of granulation tissue in contraction. Ann. Surg., *148*:153, 1958.

99. Weeks, J. R.: Prostaglandins. Ann. Rev. Pharmacol., *12*:317, 1972.

100. Williamson, M. B., and Fromm, H. J.: Effect of cystine and methionine on healing experimental wounds. Proc. Soc. Exp. Biol. Med., *80*:523, 1957.

101. Willoughby, D. A.: Some views on the pathogenesis of inflammation. *In* Montagna, W., Bentley, J. P., and Dobson, R. (Eds.): The Dermis, Advances in Biology of Skin. New York, Appleton-Century-Crofts, 1970, Vol. X, pp. 221–230.

15

BURNS:
Including Cold, Chemical, And Electrical Injuries

Curtis P. Artz, M.D.,
and Dabney R. Yarbrough, III, M.D.

THERMAL INJURY

Injuries have always constituted one of man's chief medical problems; most of the earliest known medical writings contain references to the treatment of burns and other injuries. Burns may vary from minor first-degree wounds to the most severe form of injury to which man is liable. The magnitude of the injury determines the extent of the physiologic changes. Unlike other wounds that can usually be closed either immediately or in a few days, the deep burn requires time for removal of the eschar before closure. The persistence of this dead tissue furthers the injury, and additional systemic derangements occur. An extensive burn is a catastrophic illness—catastrophic in the overwhelming insult to the patient, catastrophic in its psychologic aspects, and catastrophic in cost and suffering to the family involved.

In general, there is no injury that is treated less expertly by the medical profession at large than a burn. The care of all phases of an extensive burn injury taxes the skill and knowledge of the surgeon to the utmost. Attention to the numerous details so necessary in ideal burn care is often not appreciated, nor does the surgeon have the time or team of assistants to execute them. Burns of more than 30 per cent of the body surface are best treated in special centers.

During the year 1974, according to data obtained from the National Safety Council, 2 million people suffered burn injury. This was approximately twice the rate reported for 1967. Three hundred thousand persons were disabled by their burn injuries, and over 30,000 people required prolonged hospitalization, with an average hospital stay of 64 days. From the foregoing statistics, it is obvious that burns are a major disease entity in the United States. Although the number of deaths is small in comparison to the number caused by the great killers—heart disease, cancer, and stroke—the number of working years lost is appreciable because of the younger age group in which burns take their toll.

HISTORY

Interest in injuries caused by fire reaches back to the early days of mankind. Hippocrates proposed the use of warm, vinegar-soaked dressings to relieve the pain, and later treated burns by tanning with solutions of oak bark. Fabricius Hildanus, in Switzerland, gave the first printed extensive description of burns, their classification, and their treatment in his book *De Combustionibus* in 1607.[3] Baraduc, in 1863, maintained that in burns the decrease of the circulating blood volume was the most probable cause of death and that the viscosity of the blood was increased. Underhill, in 1923, studied fluid requirements and tried to outline necessary replacement solutions according to the size of the burned surface and the age and general condition of the patient. One of the greatest disasters from fire was the Cocoanut Grove fire in Boston in 1942. This stimulated fundamental research on the systemic response to burning by Cope and Moore. They demonstrated that the fluid loss was inside the patient and not exclusively outside, which provided an explanation for the hidden fluid loss in burns.

For years, replacement therapy with dextrose in water, plasma, and blood was determined by changes in the hematocrit, and many patients died of so-called burn shock due to inadequate fluid therapy. In 1951, Evans proposed the use of a formula for estimating fluid requirements based on the size of the patient and the percentage of body surface burned. A refinement of this led to the development of the currently popular Brooke formula. Many types of local treatments have been used. Lisfrank, in 1835, recommended wet dressings containing sodium and calcium chloride. Syme, in 1833, proposed the use of dry cotton wool dressings applied with a firm degree of pressure, later known as the so-called pressure dressing. Tannic acid was used with the idea of coagulating the wound as early as 1858. Interest in the escharotics was renewed by Davidson in 1925, who made great claims for spraying tannic acid on the burn wound. It was believed that this technique decreased the fluid loss, relieved the pain, and produced a better eschar. This method was finally abandoned in 1942, when McClure pointed out that it was toxic to the liver and produced an eschar that enclosed infection.

The modern era of local burn care was initiated by Allen and Koch in 1942, who advocated and popularized the use of petrolatum gauze, bulky, occlusive dressings, and strict immobilization. This technique of local care was the one in vogue until Wallace, in 1949, reintroduced the exposure method in Great Britain. Pulaski and Artz and Blocker evaluated this method in the United States and outlined its indications and contraindications.

In 1954 septicemia was first emphasized as a common cause of death in burns by Liedberg, Reiss, and Artz.[11] Before this time it was believed that most patients died from burn shock or burn toxins. The classic work of Teplitz and Moncrief in 1964 characterized the pathogenesis of invasive burn wound infection. The clearer understanding of burn wound sepsis made possible by their work ushered in a new and successful era of topical control of burn wound sepsis. The introduction of these modes of therapy represented the first real clinical breakthrough in the problem of invasive burn wound infection. Reverdin introduced his method of pinch grafts for burn wound closure in 1870. Real advances in burn management were the introduction of the Brown electric dermatome in 1949 and the updated air-driven model by Hargest in 1964, which permits almost any physician to obtain skin easily for early wound closure.

CAUSES

In children under 3 years of age, most burns are due to scalds. In those from 3 to 14 years, flame burns, due to clothing catching fire, predominate; in persons from 15 to 60 years, industrial accidents account for a large number of burns; in those over 60 years of age, accidents associated with momentary blackouts, smoking in bed, or houses catching fire are the most common. About 80 per cent of burn accidents occur in the home. Home accidents are 15 times more common than burns in industry. Many burns in infants result from boiling water or hot coffee. A common burn seen in the southern part of the United States is in the little girl who, clothed only in a housecoat, backs up against an open fire. The housecoat ignites, the child runs, fans the flames, and becomes the victim of a severe burn.

At least half of all burning accidents could be prevented. One of the great needs in the United States is a more active program for the prevention of burns.

CLASSES OF BURN INJURY

Several classifications have been used to differentiate various depths of burns (Fig. 1). In recent years, it has been common practice to divide burns into three categories: first degree, second degree, and third degree. First- and second-degree burns are known collectively as partial-thickness burns, and third-degree burns as full-thickness burns.

Since the systemic and local changes are directly related to the amount of tissue destroyed, this classification is probably an oversimplification. Greater clarity might result if second-degree burns were further divided into superficial second-degree and deep dermal burns. Third-degree burns should be classified as full-thickness skin loss and as deep third-degree burns in which the injury involves the underlying subcutaneous tissue, muscle, or bone.

A *first-degree burn* involves only the epidermis. It is characterized by erythema that appears after a variable latent period. A first-degree burn may follow

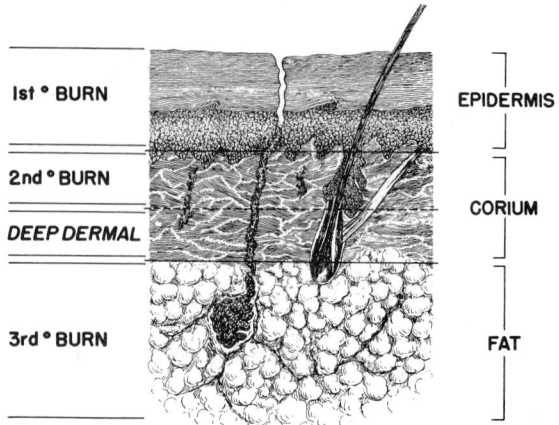

DIAGRAM OF SKIN: DEPTH OF BURN

Figure 1. Schematic outline of cross section of skin. First-degree burns involve only the epidermis and heal rapidly. Second-degree burns involve the upper portion of the corium and many islets remain that proliferate to cover the area in about 14 days. Deep dermal burns extend into the corium, and the only epithelium remaining is the lining of the sweat glands and hair follicles. Third-degree burns involve the full thickness of skin and extend down to subcutaneous fat. (From Artz, C. P., and Moncrief, J. A.: The Treatment of Burns, 2nd ed. Philadelphia, W. B. Saunders Company, 1969.)

prolonged exposure to bright sunlight or instantaneous exposure to more intense heat. Because tissue damage is so superficial, minimal systemic derangements occur. Pain and a slight amount of edema are the chief problems. The uncomfortable burning sensation and pain usually subside after 48 hours unless the first-degree burn is quite extensive, as in a severe sunburn. Since this is only a superficial injury, the capacity of the skin to prevent infection is retained. Healing usually takes place uneventfully. Within 5 to 10 days the epidermis peels off in small scales. There may be residual redness for a few days, but no scarring results.

A *second-degree burn* is a deeper injury than a first-degree burn. It involves all of the epidermis and much of the corium. Most second-degree burns are characterized by blisters, and are usually accompanied by considerable subcutaneous edema. The rate of healing is dependent upon the depth of skin destruction and on whether or not infection occurs. In superficial partial-thickness burns, healing usually occurs uneventfully within a period of 10 to 14 days unless infection supervenes. Deep dermal burns are injuries that extend deep into the corium. Epithelial regeneration takes place principally from the epithelial lining of the sweat glands and hair follicles. In the event of infection, deep dermal burns are readily converted to full-thickness injury. If the wound is properly protected, however, it will be covered with a thin layer of epithelium in 25 to 35 days. There may be thick scarring. Not infrequently, this thin epithelium is injured, giving rise to denuded areas and further scar formation. When the thin epithelial covering of a deep dermal burn is stretched by motion, blister formation may occur.

The deep dermal burn is of significant clinical importance. It is difficult to diagnose. It causes physiologic derangements that are more severe than those following superficial second-degree injury. It heals spontaneously if kept free from mechanical and bacterial trauma. If infection occurs, the burn is converted into full-thickness injury and grafting is necessary. Many burns commonly diagnosed as third-degree burns are really only deep dermal burns. By newer methods of local chemotherapy such as Sulfamylon and silver sulfadiazine, bacterial growth is controlled and epithelialization occurs.

A *third-degree burn* is a very severe form of injury. The entire dermis down to the subcutaneous fat is destroyed by coagulation necrosis. Thrombosis occurs in the small vessels of the underlying tissue. Increased capillary permeability and edema are greater than in the second-degree burn. In 2 or 3 weeks, the full-thickness dead skin liquefies, partially by autolysis and partially by leukocytic digestion. This process is accompanied by suppuration. Capillary tufts and fibroblasts organized into granulating tissue are found beneath the eschar. Deep third-degree burns are considerably different from the third-degree burns that involve only full-thickness skin loss. If the burn extends into the subcutaneous fat, liquefaction occurs in that area. Burns deep into the muscle cause increased destruction of red blood cells. The physiologic derangements that occur in deep third-degree burns may be severe even when the injury is of limited extent.

Full-thickness burns are treated by removal of the eschar and application of a skin graft to cover the wound. If grafting is not performed, a thick layer of granulating tissue will form, followed by severe contracture. The only method of epithelialization in this type of burn is slow proliferation from the wound edges, which occurs at the rate of about $\frac{1}{8}$ inch per week. The granulations become soft, overgrown, and infected, thus hindering epithelialization. After months and even years, the wound might heal, but not without considerable scarring and disfigurement.

DETERMINATION OF DEPTH OF BURN

Even in the most experienced hands, the diagnosis of the depth of burn is not entirely accurate because there are no definite clinical criteria for the depth of burn. This difficulty might be expected because there are various gradations of injury in the extensive burn. In addition, thickness of the skin varies with age and body location. The central area of the burned surface may be full-thickness, with a surrounding zone of deep dermal and superficial second-degree burn and first-degree burn at the periphery. One depth of injury seems to fade into the other in such a way that definite demarcation and gradation are almost impossible.

First-degree burns usually occur after gas explosions, brief contact with hot liquids, or quite prolonged exposure to sunlight. They appear as a simple erythematous flush. First-degree burns are dry and quite painful; blistering seldom occurs.

Second-degree burns are caused by short periods of exposure to intense flash heat or contact with hot liquids, or they may form the peripheral zone of a deeper flame burn. They are frequently characterized by the formation of blisters. The surface is mottled red or pink in appearance and it is usually moist because a plasma-like fluid exudes from the injured area. A second-degree burn is quite painful and sensitive to the air. In a deep dermal burn, the surface may be moist but the exudate that forms is not so profuse as in the superficial second-degree burn. The surface has a mottled appearance with a predominance of white rather than red or pink areas.

Third-degree burns are generally caused by flames or contact with hot objects. Because the outer layer of the skin is involved in the coagulation necrosis, the third-degree burn is usually dry and dead white or charred in appearance. The skin feels leathery in contrast to the moist, soft surface of a partial-thickness burn. Third-degree burns are not very painful; in fact, the area is almost insensible because the terminal nerve endings are inactivated by the deep injury. The impairment in sensation has been used clinically as a test for depth of skin loss. One of the best ways of differentiating between second- and third-degree areas is by pulling on a hair. If the hair pulls out easily and painlessly, it is a third-degree burn.

EXTENT OF BURN INJURY

The extent of a burn is usually expressed as a percentage of the total area of body surface. In 1924, Berkow presented data concerning percentage surface area of various parts of the body. Lund and Browder found that Berkow tables were not applicable to all ages; they determined the changes in percentage of body surface of various parts that occur during different stages of development from infancy through childhood and devised a special chart. The most accurate method for determining percentage of body surface burn is to map out the areas of injury on a Lund and Browder chart (Fig. 2). This is best done after the burn wound has been cleansed and all the loose, devitalized epithelium removed.

A rapid and popular method for estimating per cent of body surface burn is by use of the Rule of Nines (Fig. 3). This rule, first devised by Pulaski and Tennison, divides the body surface into areas representing 9 per cent or multiples of 9 per cent. The head and neck are graded as 9 per cent; the anterior trunk, twice 9, or 18 per cent; the posterior trunk, 18 per cent; each lower extremity, 18 per cent; each upper extremity, 9 per cent; and the perineum, 1 per cent. This is a good rapid method of estimating the percentage of a body surface burn, but is not nearly so accurate as the use of the Lund and Browder chart.

PROGNOSIS

It is extremely difficult to determine prognosis with any degree of accuracy in any specific burn. Mortality increases with the severity of burning and with advancing age. At one time, few patients survived burns involving more than one third of the body surface, but

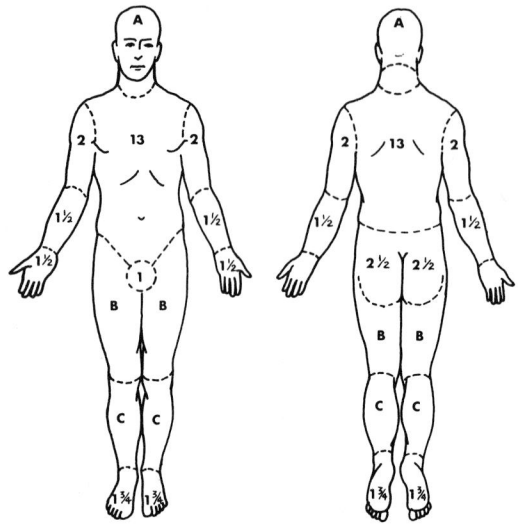

Relative Percentages of Areas Affected by Growth
(AGE IN YEARS)

	0	1	5	10	15	ADULT
A: ½ of head	9½	8½	6½	5½	4½	3½
B: ½ of thigh	2¾	3¼	4	4¼	4½	4¾
C: ½ of leg	2½	2½	2¾	3	3¼	3½

Total Per Cent Burned _____ 2° + _____ 3° = _____

Figure 2. Classic Lund and Browder chart. The best method for determining percentage of body surface burn is to mark the areas of injury on a chart, and then compute total percentage according to the patient's age. Every emergency room should have such a chart for the plotting of the burned area soon after the patient is admitted.

this is no longer true. With modern treatment, for many patients with burns of up to 50 or 60 per cent of the body surface, and for those more extensively burned, the outlook is not entirely hopeless. The prognosis of the burned patient should be guarded if the percentage of second- and third-degree burn is more than 40. It may be several days or weeks before the ultimate outcome can be predicted. Frequently, extensively burned patients survive the initial few weeks after the injury only to succumb later to complications. In severe injuries, prediction of survival should be withheld until about 30 days after the burn.

Pruitt and others published an excellent study of 1100 burned patients treated at the United States Army Surgical Research Unit at the Brooke Army Medical Center from 1950 to 1960. They constructed a mortality contour plot from the data in this series for ease in approximating expected mortality. This graphic illustration of mortality trends according to age in years and percentage of burns is reproduced in Figure 4.

PATHOPHYSIOLOGY

The Nature of Thermal Injury

Burns are the result of the transfer of heat to body tissues. The transfer may result from direct contact or

indirectly from radiant heat. The extent of tissue injury resulting from heat transfer is dependent upon several factors, including the temperature of the heat source, the duration of application of the heat, and the conductivity of the tissue involved. Tissue factors important in determining the degree of tissue conductivity are the water content of the tissue, the presence of local natural secretions and oils, the pigmentation of the tissue, the thickness of the skin, and the efficiency of protective heat transfer mechanisms such as blood flow through the tissue.

Because of the variability of these factors, the specific amount of heat necessary to cause significant skin injury varies widely. In general, thermal injury to skin at temperatures below 45° C. is minimal even with exposure times of as long as 20 minutes. Exposure of skin to temperatures above 60° C. for as brief a period as 1 minute ordinarily results in full-thickness injury. Experimental work utilizing a radiant heat source indicates that a 0.54-second exposure of human skin to 3.9 calories per square centimeter per second results in a partial-thickness burn, and increasing the heat to 4.8 calories per square centimeter per second produces full-thickness skin destruction.

Although the exact nature of the biochemical and physical changes in response to thermal injury that result in cellular death is not well delineated, presumably they are related to denaturation of protein and inactivation of critical enzyme systems. Experimentally, oxygen consumption of skin can be shown to decrease with stepwise exposure to increasing temperatures. Similarly, under the same conditions, it has been noted that glucose utilization decreases and lactate production increases. Certain enzyme systems,

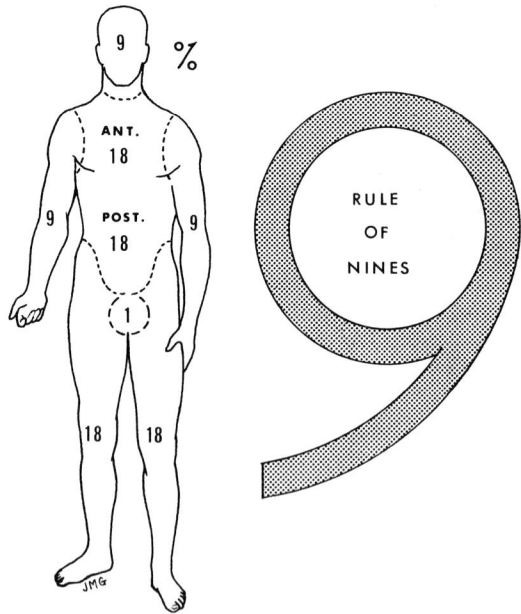

Figure 3. Schematic outline of the Rule of Nines. The use of this rule provides a rapid method for determining percentage of body surface burned, but it is of limited accuracy.

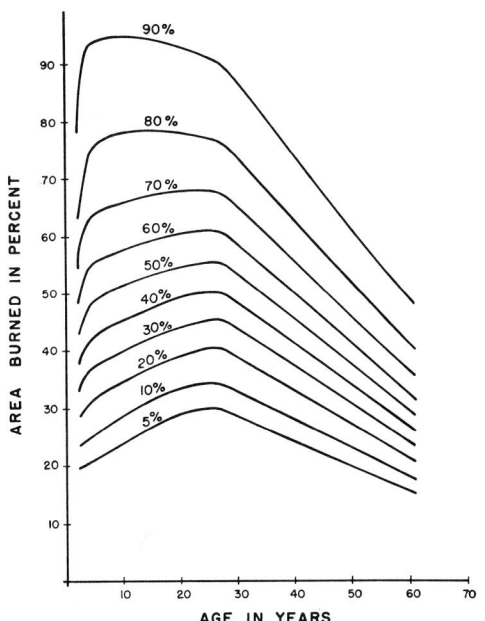

Figure 4. Mortality contours after Pruitt. The per cent mortality that can be expected at varying age with different areas of body surface burn is shown by these contours.

particularly those involved in the Krebs cycle, can be shown to be inactivated by exposure to critical amounts of heat. The activity of other enzymes appears relatively resistant to heat. For example, the enzyme aldolase shows no significant decrease of activity after heating, while fumarase shows a marked decrease in activity in response to heating at low temperatures for brief periods of time. Blockage of the Krebs cycle due to the above mechanisms would obviously result in a decrease in the efficiency of production of energy-rich substrates such as adenosine triphosphate and in turn might be postulated to have an effect on the energy-dependent metabolic processes of the cell.

Effects of Thermal Injury

The effects of burn injury can be grouped into three general categories: the effects on the skin, the effects on the vascular system and blood elements, and the general hemodynamic changes and metabolic response.

Effects on the Skin. In contrast to the usual view of the skin as a relatively inert protective envelope, the intact skin is a highly complex, metabolically active organ (the largest of the human body), critical to the maintenance of body homeostasis. The most important normal functions of the skin are as a protective barrier against heat and water loss from the body and in the prevention of invasive bacterial infection.

Intact human skin functions as a highly efficient barrier to the evaporative loss of water and heat. Normal intact skin is capable of limiting the evaporative loss of water from the body surface to approximately 5

per cent of the theoretical maximum that would occur without the protective skin. A hexane-soluble lipid complex in the skin has been identified as being of primary importance in this function.[8] The average transcutaneous water loss through intact skin is 700 to 1000 ml. daily, or approximately 15 ml. per square meter per hour, water losses through areas of full-thickness burn may reach values as high as 200 ml. per square meter per hour. Second-degree or partial-thickness burns similarly impair the effective function of the skin as a barrier to water vapor loss, although not to the same extent as full-thickness burns.[16, 23]

From these facts it readily can be seen that the evaporative loss of water from the body surface is markedly increased in the burned patient. The average evaporative water loss in an adult patient with a burn of 40 per cent of total body surface is approximately 100 ml. per square meter of body surface per hour.

The evaporative loss of water through areas of second- and third-degree burn is accompanied by a corresponding marked increase in heat loss by the body. Each gram of water evaporated from the body surface represents the loss of approximately 0.575 kcal. In major burn injuries, total energy expenditures occasioned by the increased evaporative loss of water from the body surface may reach 7000 kcal. per day. The marked increase in the rate of heat loss noted in patients with large burn injuries is accompanied by a significant rise in oxygen consumption, reflecting an increase in metabolic rate and energy expenditure in an attempt to maintain thermal homeostasis. These factors are critical in the consideration of caloric intake and fluid therapy of the severely injured patient. Since the evaporated water is essentially electrolyte-free, underestimation of the rate of vaporizational water loss in the burned patient may rapidly result in severe degrees of hypertonic dehydration. This circumstance is often initially manifested by increasing hypernatremia and azotemia.

A second major protective function of the skin is the prevention of invasive bacterial infection. Although the skin harbors a large population of both transient and resident bacteria, the occurrence of invasive infection through intact, unwounded skin is a rare development seen only in very unusual circumstances. This protection against invasive infection by environmental organisms is essentially abolished by full-thickness thermal wounding of the skin. Formerly, it was believed that intact, dry eschar provided effective protection against invasive infection. Present-day understanding of the pathogenesis of burn wound sepsis, however, has led to the realization that even dry, intact eschar serves as fertile soil for invasive infection.[22] The ability to prevent invasive burn wound sepsis is retained to a great extent in partial-thickness burn injury, but sometimes invasive sepsis does occur.

Effects on the Vascular System and Blood Elements. The most dramatic and clinically apparent physiologic alteration resulting from thermal injury is the loss of vascular integrity and the marked increase in capillary permeability occurring primarily in and around the area of burn injury (Fig. 5). Fluid and protein escape from the injured vessels at a rapid rate, resulting

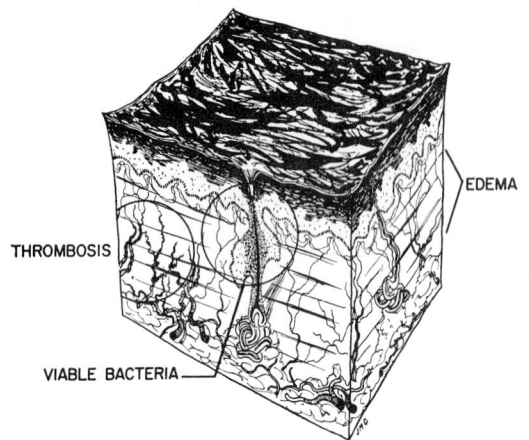

EDEMA

THROMBOSIS

VIABLE BACTERIA

Figure 5. Diagrammatic outline of changes occurring in the subcutaneous tissue beneath a full-thickness burn. Although the surface and all layers of the skin may be burned, viable bacteria remain in the crypts and hair follicles. Thrombosis occurs in the small vessels beneath the burned surface. An outpouring of fluid in and around burned areas produces a massive edema. Thrombosis and edema prevent the transport by way of the blood of host defense mechanisms to the area. With this limitation of the defense mechanisms and the excellent pabulum of the burned tissue, viable bacteria proliferate rapidly. The local pathologic changes in a third-degree burn provide an ideal environment for infection.

in a marked diminution of blood volume and a corresponding increase in interstitial fluid volume. Most of the volume loss is into the interstitial space, with resulting edema formation. Smaller amounts of protein and fluid are lost into the blebs and bullae of second- and third-degree burn areas and from the weeping surface of the second-degree burn. Although the increase in capillary permeability is most marked in the area of burn injury, the phenomenon appears to be a generalized one, with leakage of fluid from the capillaries occurring even in areas remote from the burn.[1]

The composition of the fluid lost through the capillaries is similar to that of plasma, although the protein content is somewhat lower. Generally, the amount of fluid lost is proportional to the extent and depth of the burn. The volume loss is greatest in extensive third-degree burns, usually in the range of 10 per cent of body weight.

Initially, the fluid that escapes into the burned area is carried away from the local site by the lymphatic drainage, but soon the rate of fluid loss exceeds the ability of the lymph channels to withdraw it. It accumulates in the interstitial spaces and produces edema, not only of the wound, but also of the area surrounding the wound. A large amount of fluid can be hidden when it is sequestered deep in the soft tissue and about the burned areas. A uniform 2-cm. increase in diameter of a lower extremity as a result of edema after burning may represent the sequestration of as much as 2400 ml. of fluid.[4]

The rate of fluid loss in the burned patient is greatest immediately after injury, and most of it occurs in the first 24 hours. Capillary permeability returns to near normal approximately 48 hours after injury, and resorption of edema fluid begins. This is frequently noted clinically as a period of diuresis.[2]

The loss of large volumes of this protein-rich fluid from the circulation, even though hidden to some extent, represents the same physiologic threat to life as acute external hemorrhage and calls forth many of the same physiologic responses. The major differences lie in the rate of volume reduction and the great preponderance of plasma volume loss in the burn as opposed to hemorrhage. The clinical picture produced by this volume depletion is essentially the same as that seen in hemorrhagic shock. With extensive volume losses, as seen in major burns, these events may progress to ischemia of the kidneys, oliguria, and, occasionally, acute renal tubular necrosis. The marked plasma loss secondarily results in hemoconcentration, usually of marked degree. Hemoconcentration in turn leads to the phenomenon of sludging. The physiologic results of sludging, although not well documented in humans, appear to lead to a further decrease in peripheral tissue perfusion and oxygenation as well as a diminution in functional red cell mass.

In addition to the losses of plasma there is a diminution of the red cell mass. This loss is associated primarily with deep burns. The diminution in red cell volume is usually gradual and is proportional to the depth and extent of burns. Red cell volume losses are about 10 per cent of total red cell mass in the first 24 hours after injury. Loss of red cell mass is a result of the following factors: (1) direct hemolysis of red cells by heat; (2) trapping of red cells by thrombosis of blood vessels within the area of burn, with later destruction; (3) alterations in red cell morphology caused by the effects of heat, with subsequent sequestration and destruction by the reticuloendothelial system; and (4) loss of effective red cell mass by sludging. Severe red blood cell destruction is often evidenced by the appearance of free hemoglobin in the plasma and urine. Later, decreases in red cell mass are caused primarily by failure in production and losses from the granulating surfaces. The cumulative losses in red cell mass over the entire course of illness of a burned patient may amount to as much as 185 per cent of the estimated normal. Even though significant amounts of red cells may be destroyed in a short time after injury, transfusion of whole blood is rarely necessary during the first 72 hours. The reason for this is that plasma is lost at a much greater rate than red cells, resulting in hemoconcentration. Transfusion of whole blood at this point may cause a further increase in the viscosity of blood, with consequent accentuation of the phenomenon of sludging. Transfusion may become necessary later as hemoconcentration is corrected and normal blood volume is restored. Multiple transfusions are usually required in the later open wound phase in most patients with severe burn injuries.

General Hemodynamic Changes and Metabolic Response. This response generally comprises three phases: (1) the early hypovolemic or shock phase (persisting approximately 48 hours); (2) an intensely catabolic phase prior to completion of closure of the burn wound; and (3) a final anabolic or restorative phase following closure of the burn wound. The pathophysiologic mechanisms underlying the hypovolemic or shock phase of burn injury have been described. The physiologic characteristics of this phase are relatively little different from those seen in hemorrhagic shock, the most notable difference being the relative prolongation of the plasma volume loss in the severe burn injury. The principal hemodynamic characteristics of this phase are tachycardia, hypotension, subnormal cardiac output, and vasoconstriction. Cardiac output in the shock phase may fall to 30 to 50 per cent of estimated normal values. Return to normal levels may not occur for several days despite seemingly adequate volume replacement. The decrease in cardiac output seen during the early phase after burn injury appears to be a result of both hypovolemia and the presence of a circulating myocardial depressant factor, which has been demonstrated by Baxter.

The early changes in renal function noted after burn injury are chiefly caused by hypovolemia, renal vascular constriction, and adrenocortical activity. They are manifested clinically as oliguria, decreased glomerular filtration rate, decreased free water clearance, sodium retention, and increased potassium excretion. These effects, however, are often obscured by therapy. Inadequate therapy during the shock phase may lead to acute renal failure, just as in hemorrhagic shock.

The endocrine effects of greatest importance to the shock phase are related to stimulation of adrenal activity. Studies of urinary excretion of hydroxycorticoids have shown an immediate increase after injury with a tendency to remain equal to or higher than the normal ranges throughout the burn course. The 17-ketosteroid excretion pattern, however, usually shows a sudden rapid rise after injury with a later fall to normal or below-normal values during the chronic open wound phase. In general, the adrenocortical response appears to parallel the severity of the burn. It appears that the increase in adrenocortical function is mediated by cerebral or hypothalamic activity and the anterior pituitary elaboration of ACTH. Instances of insufficient adrenal response in burns are documented but unusual; therefore, at present it would appear that the use of adrenal steroids in the management of the shock phase of burn injury has little physiologic justification. A prompt and sustained increase in urinary catecholamine and aldosterone excretion has also been noted.

Many of the events noted above persist to a lesser degree for prolonged periods of time as a result of the continued stressful stimuli of a large open burn wound and severe infection. Thus, the transition into the catabolic or open wound phase of burn injury is often not clearly demarcated.

The clinically most obvious metabolic defect in the open wound phase is a severe negative energy balance associated with negative nitrogen balance. The tremendous energy deficits incurred during the catabolic phase of burn injury would appear, at least in part, to relate to the markedly increased evaporative water loss and its attendant heat loss via the burned skin. This metabolic driving force may result in an increase in caloric requirements of up to 4000 and more calories per day and thus is of prime importance in the

hypermetabolism of the burn syndrome. Recent work indicates that although increased evaporative water loss is an important factor in the increased energy expenditure of the burned patient, other presently unidentified mechanisms are important in the causation of the hypermetabolic state commonly encountered in the burned patient. Patients with extensive burns frequently lose a pound or more a day for the first month.

Factors affecting the duration and magnitude of the negative nitrogen balance and energy deficits during this time are the extent and depth of the burn, the severity of accompanying wound infection, the nutritional regimen, and the duration of the open wound phase. Although the degree of negativity of the nitrogen balance can be diminished somewhat by various therapeutic measures, attainment of positive nitrogen balance prior to closure of the burn wound is rarely possible. The importance of newer methods of supplying calories and amino acids intravenously during this period of time has yet to be fully assessed. Close attention must be paid to the nutritional management of burned patients during the open wound phase of burn injury. After the wound has been closed, positive nitrogen balance soon follows and the restorative or anabolic phase of injury is entered.

FIRST AID

A person whose clothes are on fire should not run, as this only fans the flames. He should not remain standing, since this position may cause him to inhale flames or cause the hair to be ignited. A burned person should be placed in a horizontal position, and then rolled in a blanket or rug to smother the flames. Coats or other garments may be used for this purpose.

The initial step in the care of the burned patient is to cover the wound. This minimizes contamination and inhibits pain by preventing the air from coming in contact with the injured surface. The use of towels soaked in ice water will bring almost immediate relief from burn pain.[21] The cold may also have some value in arresting the effect of the heat on the tissue. Any burn involving more than 5 per cent of the body surface should be seen by a physician. Medicaments and home remedies should not be applied to the burn. A clean sheet or cloth may be used as an emergency dressing. The patient suffering from respiratory arrest due to smoke inhalation should receive artificial respiration by positive-pressure breathing with the mouth-to-mouth technique.

MINOR BURNS

Minor burns include those partial-thickness burns of less than 10 per cent of the body surface and full-thickness burns of less than 2 per cent of the body surface. Fluid replacement usually is not required except in infants, and the burns should be treated with local cleansing and the appropriate type of wound care. Usually, a grease gauze dressing is applied. In burns of 10 to 20 per cent of the body surface, intravenous fluids are occasionally required, particularly in children. During the first 24 hours, lactated Ringer's solution may be given intravenously in the amount of 2 ml. per kilogram of body weight for each per cent of burned surface.

The chief aim of the local care of minor burns is to make the patient as comfortable as possible. Although exposure is a good method of local care, most patients with minor burns treated on an outpatient basis should have a well-applied occlusive dressing that will permit them to continue their activities. They should return for redressing 3 to 5 days later. Antibiotics are rarely necessary.

EARLY SYSTEMIC MANAGEMENT

The emergency room care of a patient with a major burn should be the orderly execution of several established routine procedures. These include a quick history, estimation of the extent and depth of burn, drawing a sample of blood for crossmatching and baseline laboratory determinations, insertion of a cutdown cannula and an indwelling urinary catheter, determination of the need for tracheostomy, administration of antibiotics and tetanus immunization, and planning of fluid therapy.

History

A brief history should include when, where, and how the accident happened and information about the status of the patient's health before the injury. When the accident may have legal implications, a color photograph should be taken of the injured areas.

Immediate Procedures

As soon as the patient has been examined, a large-bore needle should be inserted into an accessible vein and a blood sample drawn for crossmatching, hematocrit, blood urea nitrogen, and other specific laboratory determinations. Lactated Ringer's solution should be administered through this needle until a cutdown cannula is in place. To make the patient more comfortable, eliminate apprehension, and alleviate pain associated with cleansing the burn wound, morphine may be given through the venipuncture needle. Narcotics should always be given intravenously; when given subcutaneously to a burned patient with circulatory deficiency, the narcotic is poorly absorbed and therefore ineffective.

Tracheostomy

A mechanically clear airway must be assured from the beginning. The need for a tracheostomy can usually be determined while the history is being obtained. A tracheotomy must be performed if there is severe respiratory obstruction. It is also indicated in the initial management when respiratory tract injury is suspected. The presence of established pulmonary damage may be manifested by hoarseness, coughing, rapid respirations, or cyanosis. A history of the patient being burned in a close space, or the appearance of redness in the posterior pharynx, may suggest respiratory damage. Singeing of the nasal hairs, stridor, or rales in the chest may give indication of pulmonary ir-

ritation. Although some deep burns of the face and neck may require a tracheostomy later, it is usually not indicated in the first 24 hours. Addition of a tracheostomy to the already complicated condition of the burned patient frequently gives rise to many other problems. Patients with burns about the head and neck may do very well without a tracheostomy, which is always associated with increases in water loss and infection, and requires additional nursing care.

Intravenous Administration

Since the life of a burned patient frequently depends upon the infusion of replacement solutions, it is wise to plan initially the utilization of various routes of administration. An intravenous cannula should be inserted in adult patients with greater than 20 per cent burn injury, and in children with greater than 10 per cent. Intravenous fluids may be required for as long as 12 days. During this time, thrombosis may occur in several veins and necessitate a change in infusion site from one vein to another. Good veins for intravenous infusion may be difficult to find; therefore, a plan for saving veins should be worked out before therapy is started.

When intravenous cannulas are inserted into the saphenous vein, superficial phlebitis is common after 4 or 5 days. If available, one of the best areas for the cannula is the cephalic vein in the shoulder area. Although it is more difficult to perform a cutdown in this area, it is the best site for prolonged administration of intravenous fluids because of the lesser incidence of phlebitis. Additionally, insertion of an intravenous cannula in this location provides easy access to the central venous system for monitoring central venous pressure during resuscitation.

When a cannula has to be inserted into a leg vein, it is wise to start as far distally as possible. If thrombosis of the vein occurs, the cannula may be moved proximally. The use of femoral vein catheters frequently precludes subsequent use of the saphenous vein. This route is not void of complications, such as edema of the lower extremity, septic thrombophlebitis, deep venous thrombosis, erosion of the vein wall, and tubing embolism. The use of a femoral catheter should be reserved for the time when no other veins are available. It should not be left in place longer than 7 days because complications are frequent after this period.[13]

In summary, important factors in the consideration of the location of phlebotomy sites in the burned patient include: (1) cutdowns in veins of the upper extremities are preferable to those in the lower extremities because of the lesser incidence of phlebitis; (2) cutdowns performed through burned tissue should be avoided if at all possible; and (3) advancement of the cannula to the superior vena cava is desirable so that central venous pressure can be monitored. Although central venous pressure can also be monitored in the inferior vena cava, readings obtained are much less reliable.

Indwelling Urinary Catheter

In all burns involving more than 25 per cent of the body surface, the most reliable method for determining the adequacy of fluid therapy is insertion of an indwelling catheter into the bladder and hourly measurement of the urinary output. As soon as the catheter is not absolutely necessary, it should be removed. In most instances, it can be discontinued after 72 hours. While it is in place, the patient should receive the appropriate antibacterial therapy to prevent urinary infections.

Fluid Therapy

Burns differ from most conditions characterized by losses of water and electrolytes in that the rate, volume, and composition of fluid losses can be anticipated. Clinical shock is a preventable syndrome if adequate therapy can be initiated soon after injury. Several factors influence the amount and type of fluid therapy. These include extent and depth of burn, weight, age, and general physical status of the patient, and degree of respiratory tract involvement.

No mathematical formula exists by which all burns can be treated. A given formula should be regarded only as a means of providing an order of magnitude of fluid requirements, and not as outlining a course of action that must be followed blindly. Without a predetermined estimate, gross errors are often made, usually in the direction of overtreatment. Because the volume and rate of fluid losses are predictable, several fluid formulas for estimating the types and amounts of therapy have been devised. These include the Evans formula, Moore's budget, the Massachusetts General Hospital formula, the Parkland Hospital regimen, and the Brooke formula. The Moore budget and the Massachusetts General Hospital formula favor larger quantities of colloids and less electrolyte solution. The Parkland regimen uses no colloids and accomplishes the entire replacement therapy with a balanced salt solution. The Brooke formula is a middle-of-the-road one, and at the present time is the most popular. In accordance with current knowledge of fluids in burns, however, this formula requires certain specific adjustments. It seems most adequate for a burn of up to 40 per cent in an adult. In more extensive burns, it is probably wise to increase the colloid estimate at the expense of the electrolyte requirement. Certainly in infants a larger proportion of the replacement solution should be given as colloids than is estimated in the Brooke formula. Each individual clinician should use the formula with which he is most familiar. There is an advantage to selecting one method of estimated fluid requirements in burns and gaining as much experience with it as possible. The Brooke formula estimates the following for the first 24 hours following injury:

Colloids (plasma, Plasmanate, or dextran):
    0.5 ml. per kilogram per percentage of body surface burn

Electrolyte solution (lactated Ringer's):
    1.5 ml. per kilogram per percentage of body surface burn

Water requirement (dextrose in water):
    2000 ml. for adults, for children correspondingly less

Water requirements in children vary. The following is a rough guide to daily water requirements in infants and children: during the first 2 years, 120 ml.

per kilogram; second to fifth year, 100 ml. per kilogram; fifth to eighth year, 80 ml. per kilogram; eighth to twelfth year, 50 ml. per kilogram.

It is important that burns of more than 50 per cent of the body surface be calculated as 50 per cent burns, or excess quantities of fluid will be given. In the second 24 hours after injury, about one half the colloid and electrolyte requirement of the first 24 hours is needed.

After the requirements are estimated, a number of factors must be considered before proceeding with therapy. Young children and elderly adults will not tolerate excessive fluids and therefore should receive minimal amounts. Patients with pre-existing cardiovascular or renal disease should be treated similarly. When there has been respiratory tract irritation, pulmonary edema is a threat.

Most of the calculated colloid requirement should be given early. Relatively more colloids should be given to burns of greater magnitude. Plasma, Plasmanate, albumin, and blood have been used as colloid therapy in burns. In recent years, it has become evident that less blood is required in the first 72 hours than was formerly believed. It is doubtful that any blood should be used in a patient with a second-degree burn. Occasionally, in those with deep burns of more than 50 per cent of the body surface and with burns associated with electrical injury, one unit of blood is advisable in the first 72 hours. Thereafter, the blood requirements should be determined by the hematocrit.

Because of its protein content, plasma is preferred as a colloid solution by most clinicians. When plasma is not available, Plasmanate or albumin may be used.

Because of the tendency of metabolic acidosis to develop in the early period after injury, lactated Ringer's solution, a balanced salt solution, is preferred to normal saline for fulfilling the electrolyte requirement.[19]

A profound paralytic ileus not infrequently accompanies severe burns; therefore, oral fluids should be withheld for 2 days in patients treated by intravenous infusion. Although most well-treated burned patients are thirsty during the first 48 hours, withholding oral fluids is indicated because of the fear of gastric distention and dilatation followed by vomiting and aspiration.

Clinical Appraisal of Therapy. After an approximation of fluid requirements has been made, some thought must be given to the order in which the various solutions should be administered. The first 8-hour period is the most important because the most rapid fluid losses occur soon after thermal injury. Generally, one half of the first 24-hour fluid requirement is given in the first 8 hours, one fourth in the second 8-hour period, and one fourth in the third 8-hour period. Fluid therapy so planned should be calculated for the period following injury rather than the period following admission to the hospital. If the patient's treatment has been delayed, initial fluid therapy should be given as colloid. Sometimes it is advisable to give the colloid solution in one vein and lactated Ringer's in another. The initial fluids should be given rather rapidly, at least 1 liter in the first hour. Thereafter, the rate of administration should be determined by the rate of urinary flow. Unfortunately, there are no laboratory determinations that serve as adequate guides to therapy. Sometimes in the first 48 hours, observations of the hematocrit are helpful. Severe thirst, collapsed veins, and hypotension obviously denote a fluid deficiency. The best guide to the rate of fluid infusion is the urinary output, which should be measured and recorded hourly. The ideal output in an adult is 30 ml. per hour. The rate of infusion should be increased if the urinary volume falls below 15 ml. per hour and decreased if it exceeds 50 ml. per hour. Excess water and electrolytes in amounts that will produce a urinary output of more than 50 ml. per hour may lead to overexpansion of the interstitial space. Too often, the clinician feels that the patient must be doing well if he is excreting 100 ml. of urine per hour. With such an output the intake must be more than is necessary, and additional troublesome edema may develop. Excessive fluid administration is a more common error than inadequate fluid therapy. A decreasing blood pressure and decreasing urinary output mean that colloids should be given. A decreasing urinary output with a normal blood pressure indicates that additional electrolyte solution or water is required. Gross hemoglobin in the urine is an indication that the burn is quite deep. In such instances, a high renal output should be forced to flush the kidney tubules. This may be accomplished with a high intake; sometimes mannitol is used.

Regular auscultation of the lungs and chest roentgenograms to detect the early signs of pulmonary edema should be routine.[10]

Central venous pressure monitoring has proved to be an extremely valuable technique in managing rapidly changing hypovolemic states. In general, the central venous pressure is indicative of the balance between volume input and cardiac output. The central venous pressure is probably best considered an indication of right ventricular function rather than blood volume per se. Central venous pressure depends upon the interaction of three factors: blood volume, cardiac function, and vascular resistance. Changes in any one of these three components can result in changes in the central venous pressure. To obtain satisfactory measurements, the proximal end of the cannula must be placed central to any venous valves. This ordinarily implies placement in the superior vena cava. Placement in the right atrium or ventricle should be avoided, as incidences of perforation of the heart by the catheter, resulting in cardiac tamponade, have been described. Generally, a central venous pressure in the range of 6 to 12 cm. of saline indicates good balance between volume input and cardiac output. Often more important is the trend of central venous pressure, whether rising or falling. An excessively high venous pressure indicates that the rate of volume input is exceeding the rate of loss or that the right side of the heart is being overloaded. An abnormally low or falling central venous pressure suggests that the rate of fluid loss from the vascular system exceeds the rate of fluid infusion.

Electrolyte determinations are of little value in guiding fluid therapy during the initial 48 hours. Hematocrit determinations during this period offer some guide to the clinical evaluation of fluid replacement, but should not be the sole determinant for the types and amounts of therapy. After 48 hours, the serum sodium concentration should be determined daily. In extensively burned patients, the serum sodium, potassium, chloride, and carbon dioxide-combining power should be followed each day or every other day. The nonprotein nitrogen frequently is a guide to prognosis; few patients survive with a persistent level above 100 mg. per 100 ml. In burns about the face or inhalation injury, blood gas determinations are of considerable value.

Therapy After 48 Hours. After 48 hours, most of the fluids given should be electrolyte-free water and blood. A hematocrit of less than 36 per cent is an indication for additional blood. Hyponatremia is usually present in spite of the large sodium load in the interstitial space. A normal serum sodium in burned patients is associated with a good clinical response and is desirable. The insensible water loss after the first 48 hours may be quite marked, as much as 5000 or 6000 ml. per day in an adult. After the acute stress of the burn injury, the body has a tendency to retain sodium, and very little is excreted by the kidneys. The loss of water by the insensible route and by the urine may be relatively greater than the loss of sodium. This means that the water load is diminishing more rapidly than the sodium load, and therefore a rise in serum sodium may occur. A serum sodium concentration of 135 mEq. per liter is usually ideal in the first few days after injury. When the serum sodium rises to 145 mEq. per liter or more, additional electrolyte-free water must be given. When insufficient water is infused, the serum sodium may rise rapidly and lead to severe hypernatremia.

After the first 48 hours, many burned patients will take oral fluids and regulate their own intake. When food cannot be taken orally, after 72 hours it may be necessary to give 40 or 80 mEq. of potassium each day.

Antibiotics and Tetanus Immunization

Although there are different opinions concerning the use of antibiotics initially in burns, it is doubtful that such therapy is indicated. Many believe that penicillin therapy for the first 5 days prevents infection by the beta hemolytic streptococcus. It is doubtful that prophylactic antibiotics are necessary in a clean hospital environment. If a streptococcal infection does develop, and this is rare, it is easily abated by the use of penicillin. Routine antibiotic therapy in burns only permits the growth of resistant organisms. Except in certain instances, antibiotics should be withheld until there is some evidence of infection. A concentrated effort should be made to determine the offending organism and the appropriate antibiotic administered. When patients have a concomitant disease or injury indicating antibiotics, they should be used.

Since tetanus may be a complication of burns, appropriate immunization against tetanus must be given to all patients with full-thickness burn injury.

WOUND MANAGEMENT

The chief problem in the management of large burn wounds is the control of infection. This emphasizes the importance of local care. The aim in the treatment of first- and second-degree burns is to provide an environment of cleanliness so that the areas will heal free from infection. The aim in the local management of third-degree burns is the early removal of dead tissue and closure of the wound with a skin graft as soon as possible. Every effort should be aimed at minimizing further contamination and achieving a surgically clean wound. All personnel who come in contact with the patient must be masked. The patient should be taken to a clean dressing room or operating room where aseptic technique can be followed in the initial management of the wound. In the extensively burned patient, fluid and electrolyte replacement should take precedence over local care. Intravenous morphine provides adequate analgesia for cleansing the wound; a general anesthetic is contraindicated. The burned area should be cleansed thoroughly. All debris and detached epidermis must be removed. Some type of bland soap and warm water may be used for initial cleansing.

There are many acceptable methods of local care. These may be classified primarily as occlusive dressings, exposure, initial excision, Sulfamylon cream, or silver nitrate soaks. Most surgeons use all methods. The type selected varies with each individual patient. In many instances, some areas will be treated by one method and other areas by another in the same patiet. At times, treatment of a burn may be started by one method of local care and then changed to another during the course of therapy. It is impossible to dictate any particular method. All are acceptable, and it is up to the physician to select the one most desirable for a particular patient at a particular time. The choice of method is determined by the location of the burn, size of the injury, depth of the burn, type of patient, facilities available, and patient's response. Only certain small full-thickness burns lend themselves to initial excision. Most patients treated on an outpatient basis do better when the wounds are dressed. Exposure, Sulfamylon cream, and silver nitrate soaks require more nursing care than other methods.

Occlusive Dressings

The aim of a good dressing is to cover the open wound to protect it from infection. It should not necessarily be a pressure dressing because pressure does not really inhibit the loss of fluid.

The material placed next to the wound must not macerate the tissue or damage the remaining viable epithelium. Several types of fabric are available; commercially prepared nylon fabric, Carbowax gauze, dry fine-mesh gauze, and lightly impregnated petrolatum gauze are satisfactory.

The dressing must be occlusive to prevent the invasion of bacteria. It should be absorptive to keep the wound surface dry and thereby inhibit the growth of bacteria. It should be bulky and applied with even, resilient compression so that it eliminates dead space, gives vascular support, and produces a splinting effect (Fig. 6). Many hospitals prepare thick, one-piece dressings of various sizes. Such burn pads are useful and practical, as they save a great deal of time during

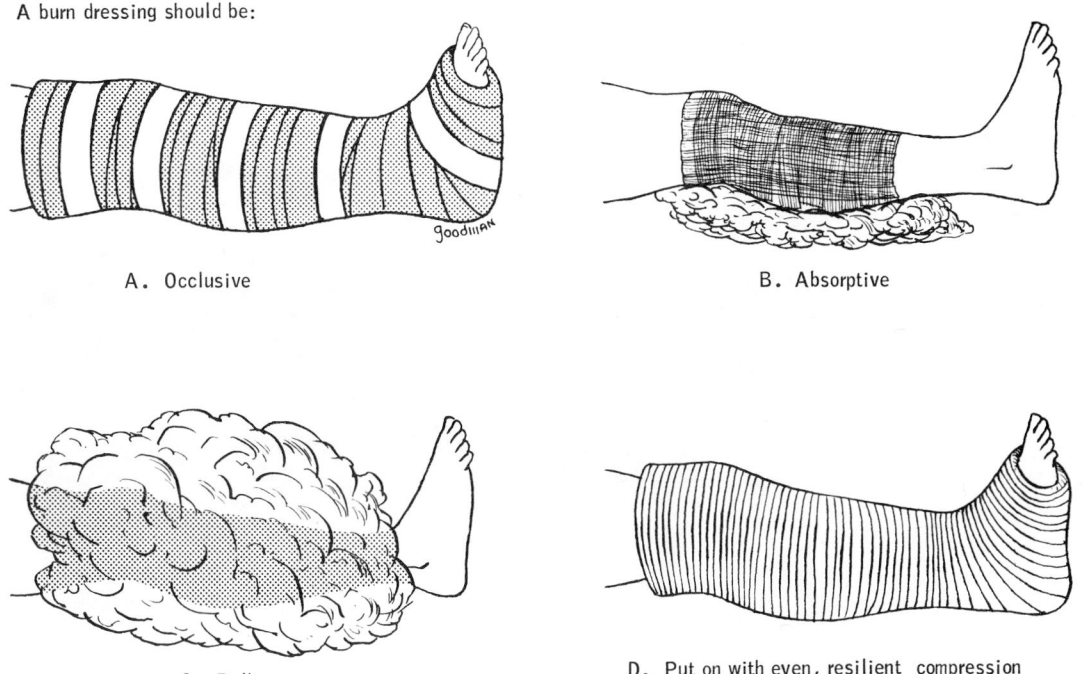

A burn dressing should be:

A. Occlusive

B. Absorptive

C. Bulky

D. Put on with even, resilient compression

Figure 6. Important aspects of a satisfactory burn dressing. *A,* It should be applied in such a way that it occludes the entire injury from outside invasion by bacteria. *B,* The dressing should be absorptive, so that the wound surface will be kept dry and thereby the growth of bacteria will be inhibited. *C,* It is important that the dressing be bulky, so that it provides a splint for the part and does not soak through within a short period. *D,* It should be put on with even, resilient compression to be comfortable and provide support to the vascular system.

dressing changes. The initial dressing frequently can be left in place for 5 days. In general, burn dressings should be changed every 4 or 5 days. The principal indications for the occlusive dressing method of burn wound management at the present time are the treatment of minor burns in outpatients, the protection of major burn wounds when the patient must be transported, as in the transfer of a patient from a small community hospital to a burn center, and the coverage of sloughing wounds prior to grafting.

Exposure

The accepted technique for the exposure method includes initial cleansing of the burn wound and placing the patient in bed on clean sheets in the position that best exposes the affected areas. Sterile sheets are unnecessary. The exudate of a partial-thickness burn dries in 48 to 72 hours and forms a hard crust. Epithelial regeneration proceeds beneath this crust unless impeded by infection. In 14 to 21 days, the crust separates spontaneously, leaving an unscarred, well-healed surface. The evolution of a full-thickness burn treated by exposure is different. Surface exudation is minimal and crust formation does not occur. The dead tissue of the full-thickness burn becomes dehydrated and is converted to a thick, tough eschar after about 72 hours of exposure.

The technique of exposure may be different in every patient because different configurations of the burned surface pose individual problems. Much of the success of exposure depends upon the ingenuity of the surgeon and nursing staff in achieving a good protective cover. This protective cover must be managed in such a way as to minimize softening, maceration, and cracking.

Burns of the face are easily exposed (Fig. 7). In full-thickness burns, removal of eschar may be hastened by application of saline soaks beginning on the eighth to the tenth day. Burns of the anterior aspect of the neck should be positioned with the neck in extension; this minimizes maceration. In almost every instance, cracks will occur in the region of the thyroid cartilage because of deglutition. Fortunately, these cracks are rarely troublesome because the excellent blood supply of the neck promotes rapid healing.

Burns that are circumferential are difficult to position. In a circumferential burn of the upper extremity, the part may be tied to an intravenous pole. This provides elevation and reasonably comfortable exposure. Skeletal traction is another frequently used technique that facilitates the exposure treatment of circumferential burns of extremities. Circumferential burns of other areas of the body must be exposed on one side and then turned and exposed on the other. This is usually accomplished by the use of a turning frame; probably the best is the circular electric bed. If the patient is turned every 4 hours, a fairly good protective covering will form.

One of the problems in the exposure of full-thickness circumferential burns is the tight or constricting eschar. As the burned skin dries, it contracts and the coagulated protein forms a stiff, inelastic eschar. A tight, constricting eschar on a circumferential burn of the chest will greatly limit respiratory exchange and can result in fatal hypoxia. Similarly, a circumferential full-thickness burn of an extremity unyielding to the pressure of edema fluid within it forces pressure occlusion of the arterial supply to distal tissues. Both problems can be solved by escharotomy of the burned skin down to the deep fascia.[9]

Exposure ends in partial-thickness burns when the

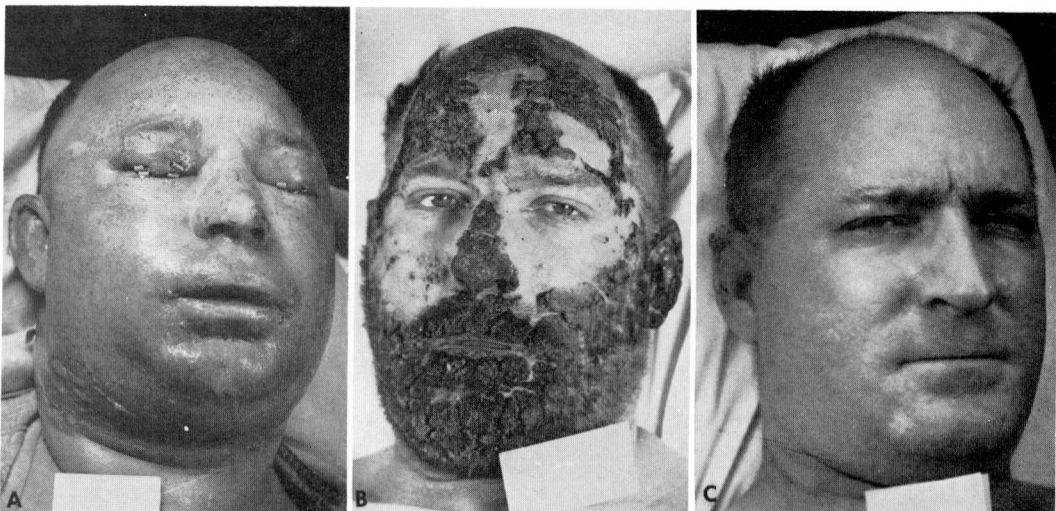

Figure 7. Second-degree burn of the face treated by exposure. *A,* The burned face has been cleansed and all detached epithelium removed. Massive edema was present when this photograph was taken at 48 hours. *B,* At 8 days post burn, the edema has disappeared and the entire burned surface is covered by a crust. Part of this crust has separated. *C,* Appearance of the face 19 days post burn. There is very little evidence of scarring. All the crust has desquamated except a little on the right ear. Second-degree burns of the face do extremely well when treated by exposure.

crust desquamates and falls off. Exposure ends in full-thickness burns when the eschar begins to soften and is ready for removal.

Initial Excision

Initial excision during the first day or two post burn is a desirable procedure because it permits removal of all dead tissue soon after injury and encourages early closure of the wound. It has two distinct disadvantages: in the first few hours or even days, it is difficult to determine accurately the extent of the full-thickness injury, and surgical excision of extensive areas may compound the initial injury. Although extensive initial excision has been tried, it is not recommended. In patients with burns not exceeding 15 per cent of the body surface, however, in whom there is definite evidence that the injury is full-thickness, initial excision followed by grafting 4 days later is an excellent method of local care.

An alternative technical method of initial excision that has been practiced with some degree of success in recent years is the method of tangential excision. In this technique, sequential excision of the upper layers of the burn wound is carried out until viable tissue is reached as manifested by the appearance of capillary bleeding. The excised area may then be autografted or heterografted immediately or treated with one of the topical antibacterial agents until the excised wound surface is judged to be ready for grafting. Although this technique is currently not widely practiced, preliminary results reported by Janzekovic and Monafo are quite encouraging. Further experience with this technique of burn wound excision is necessary to evaluate results fully.

Sulfamylon Cream

Abundant laboratory and clinical experience attests to the fact that Sulfamylon cream locally applied is an effective method of minimizing infection in burn wounds. This chemotherapeutic agent has the unique property of penetrating the thick heavy eschar and thereby diminishes the growth of bacteria beneath the burned skin. Sulfamylon cream is prepared as a 10 per cent concentration of Sulfamylon acetate (para-aminomethylbenzene sulfonamide acetate) in a water-soluble base. It is effective against a wide range of organisms, both gram-positive and gram-negative, and is particularly effective against anaerobes. Sulfamylon is soluble in water, actively diffuses into avascular tissue, is locally nontoxic, and is broken down to produce p-carboxybenzene sulfonamide, an acid salt. Application of Sulfamylon in a water-soluble base, which itself is 43 per cent water, has resulted in a significant decrease in the evaporative water loss from the burned surface.

Although the application of this material is simple, definite procedures and close observation of the patient are required. After the burn wound has been cleansed, the Sulfamylon cream is applied with a gloved hand to a thickness of 5 mm. over the entire wound. During the first 48 hours after injury, the exudate from the wound may cause the cream to slip off, and reapplication may be necessary two or three times a day. The cream should be washed from the wound surface at least once daily and the entire wound examined. This can be done most conveniently in a Hubbard tank. The cream is easily removed with water, movement is encouraged, and the patient has an increased sense of well-being. The usual procedure is to place the patient in a Hubbard tank each morning, wash off the cream, and reapply cream shortly thereafter. There is occasionally a local burning sensation for 15 to 20 minutes after the material has been applied, but this is usually not severe and does not require analgesia. The eschar remains on the burn wound longer than usual. It may be necessary after 30 days to excise the eschar in the operating room. The use of Sulfamylon has markedly decreased the conversion of deep partial-thickness burns to full-thickness wounds.[15]

Sulfamylon is a strong carbonic anhydrase inhibitor and thus impairs the effectiveness of the renal tubular buffering mechanism in maintaining normal body pH. In extensively burned patients, the continuous use of Sulfamylon acetate with its carbonic anhydrase inhibitory effect may lead to a metabolic acidosis due to the partial blockage of bicarbonate production. Frequently, the earliest clinical warning sign of a developing metabolic acidosis in patients being treated with Sulfamylon is tachypnea. Initially, the metabolic acidosis may be compensated for by hyperventilation with little resultant change in the arterial pH. When tachynpnea is noted in extensively burned patients, treatment should be discontinued and any residual cream on the burned surface should be removed whether or not laboratory analysis reveals acidemia. If severe uncompensated metabolic acidosis is noted, it easily can be reversed by administration of appropriate amounts of sodium bicarbonate intravenously. After control of the acidosis, treatment usually can be reinstituted safely within 24 to 48 hours. This complication of Sulfamylon therapy is, of course, more frequent and more severe in patients with renal or pulmonary disease whose compensatory mechanisms are impaired.[14]

Silver Sulfadiazine

Silver sulfadiazine is a relatively new topical antibacterial agent that has been investigated extensively in the management of the burn wound. Fox initially noted that combination of the silver ion with sulfadiazine appeared to increase the bacteriostatic activity of the sulfonamides significantly. Silver sulfadiazine has been proven to be effective against a wide variety of gram-negative organisms, including Pseudomonas aeruginosa. Overall bacterial control utilizing silver sulfadiazine appears to be at least as good as with either silver nitrate or Sulfamylon. Importantly, the side-effects and complications of silver sulfadiazine therapy appear to be significantly less than those encountered with either silver nitrate or Sulfamylon.

Silver sulfadiazine does not appear to be a significant carbonic anhydrase inhibitor and therefore the metabolic acidosis seen with Sulfamylon does not result. Pain upon application is minimal as compared with Sulfamylon. Renal complications theoretically may still occur as a result of absorption of the sulfanomide through the burn wound. The renal complications may result either from the precipitation of the sulfa crystals in the renal tubules with subsequent obstruction or as a hypersensitivity phenomenon. In any event, the rate of significant complications associated with the use of silver sulfadiazine appears to be extremely low. To summarize, present evidence indicates that silver sulfadiazine is an extremely safe and convenient drug to use in the topical therapy of the burn wound. Bacterial control appears to compare favorably with any of the other currently used topical antibacterial agents. The technique of its use is essentially the same as that used with Sulfamylon.

Silver Nitrate Soaks

Another effective topical antibacterial compound for use in burns is 0.5 per cent silver nitrate. Like Sulfamylon cream, this agent diminishes infection in and around the burn wound. Its indications for use are similar to those for Sulfamylon. It prevents the growth of bacteria and does not interfere with epidermal proliferation.

The application of silver nitrate soaks is more involved than the Sulfamylon treatment, and requires more nursing personnel. The wound is cleansed and then the aqueous solution is applied in a large dressing directly to the burn wound. Approximately 40 layers of four-ply, 9-inch dressing gauze are soaked with the solution of 0.5 per cent silver nitrate and closely applied to the wound surface with elastic wrappings of gauze or stockinette. This dressing complex is kept dripping wet by the addition of silver nitrate solution every 3 or 4 hours between daily changes of the dressing. A patient treated by wet dressings must be covered with a layer or two of dry cotton sheeting or a blanket to minimize evaporation and the loss of heat through the dressing. Each day as the dressing is changed any loose eschar is gently pulled away.

There are several disadvantages with this technique, although in burn centers with sufficient personnel and facilities these problems are well managed. Silver nitrate stains black when it is exposed to light; therefore, bed clothing, nurses' and physicians' clothing, and the materials in the ward must be segregated for the laundry. The sodium and chloride ions are rapidly diluted in the serum and they are also depleted with the use of these dressings. In children with large burns, this may occur within a matter of a few hours. Potassium deficiency is also seen, although it usually does not occur as rapidly. Calcium deficits have been noted. Electrolyte determinations must be done frequently in extensively burned patients treated in this manner. It is absolutely essential that supplementary sodium, chloride, potassium, and calcium be given. These supplements may be administered intravenously at first and later orally. Calcium lactate, 4 to 8 gm., should be given each day. If the serum calcium falls below 9 mg. per 100 ml., supplementary calcium gluconate should be given. After the fourth postburn day, 40 to 80 mEq. of potassium is necessary. Ten grams of sodium chloride and 30 to 50 ml. of molar sodium lactate are administered daily by mouth for burns covering 50 per cent of the body surface. This dosage is increased if the burns are of greater extent. These dosage schedules are for adults; correspondingly smaller doses are indicated for infants and children.[18]

Removal of Eschar

The ultimate aim in the treatment of full-thickness burns is to remove the eschar and apply a skin graft as soon as feasible. The technique for removal of eschar depends upon the extent of the burn and the type of local care employed. When occlusive dressings are used, the eschar softens and comes off earlier because of bacterial proliferation and autolysis beneath the eschar. When antibacterial agents such as Sulfamylon and silver nitrate are used, the eschar remains tightly adherent for a much longer period of time because bacterial growth is minimized.

If exposure or dressings are used, the eschar will usually begin to soften about the fourteenth day. Wet soaks may hasten its removal. If the patient is burned over more than 40 per cent of the body surface, the eschar should be allowed to remain intact until all the surrounding deep dermal burn has healed. It may be necessary then to take the patient to the operating room and as gently as possible, under anesthesia, remove the dead, leathery eschar. In burns of lesser extent, removal of the eschar under anesthesia should be accomplished between the twenty-fifth and thirtieth days.

Wound Coverage

A split-thickness skin graft should be applied to the third-degree burned areas as soon as the eschar is removed and the recipient site is prepared.

Preparation of Recipient Site. The aim in preparing a recipient site is to obtain a wound surface on which an excellent graft take may be expected. It is almost impossible, and certainly unnecessary, to sterilize a granulating surface for a good graft take. If the amount of purulent material and bacterial contamination is minimal, a graft will usually take unless the surface is colonized by group A beta hemolytic streptococci.

Several methods may be employed to prepare the recipient site for grafting. In some instances frequent changes of dry dressings will achieve the desired result. Soaking the patient in a Hubbard tank daily cleanses the wound and removes debris. Wet dressings changed every 4 hours provide a good technique for preparing the recipient site. If xenografts or allografts are available, their application every 3 or 4 days is an excellent method of treating the recipient site.

When grafting has been delayed, soft, pale, heaping granulations are often present. Skin grafts do not take well on such granulations. They must be shaved down to the base and a dressing applied for 2 days. In old burns with a considerable amount of fibrous tissue beneath old granulations, it is advisable to excise the entire area down to the subcutaneous tissue or underlying fascia, and graft 2 days later.

Grafting. Certain sites have priority for skin coverage. Areas around joints are covered before large flat surfaces, except in the extensively burned patient in whom rapid wound coverage must be obtained to save life. In most instances, skin should be placed first around the eyes, on the hands, and on other areas of motion such as the knees, elbows, and axillae. When only the lower extremity is burned, priority should be given to the area around the knee, then the lower part of the leg, with the larger surface on the thigh being grafted later.

In extensive burns, flat surfaces should be covered with thin skin, approximately 0.010 to 0.012 inch in thickness. Skin for areas over joints should be somewhat thicker, about 0.015 inch.

The donor site should be the most accessible area from which skin can be taken and the site then properly exposed. This exposure is both effective and desirable. In extensively burned patients, every available area of skin should be used as a donor site. As soon as the wound is ready for grafting, as much as possible of the area should be covered at the first grafting procedure. It may be necessary to take skin from the dorsum of the foot, the arms, the unburned areas between granulating surfaces. It is frequently possible to graft anterior wounds from donor sites on the anterior surface at the first grafting procedure; then 10 to 14 days later the patient can be turned on his abdomen, and skin removed from the posterior aspect of the body to cover recipient sites in that area.

DERMATOMES. A variety of instruments are available for obtaining a split-thickness skin graft. The use of the electric dermatome is one of the outstanding advances in the care of burns in the past several years. Recently, this instrument has been equipped with an air-driven motor in place of the electric one. This new air-driven dermatome is much easier to use and cuts more evenly. With this instrument, large sheets of split-thickness skin can be obtained rapidly. When skin must be taken from irregular areas, infiltration of the subcutaneous tissue with saline provides an even, firm surface for cutting the grafts.

The drum-type dermatomes are useful over certain areas of the body, particularly the chest and abdomen. The wide sheets of skin available with the drum dermatome are particularly useful around joints, in the popliteal areas, and especially on the dorsum of the hand. In many grafting procedures, both types of dermatomes may be advantageous.

Some surgeons like to use the mesh dermatome when skin is in short supply (Fig. 8). This dermatome permits a small piece of skin to be stretched to cover a larger surface. It has been of most value in treating children with extensive injuries.[12]

APPLICATION OF SKIN. There are many methods for the application of a skin graft. If the area is small, it is usually wise to apply a sheet of skin and suture it in place. When large flat surfaces are to be covered, the skin may be placed on the wound and then pushed into position so that there is little space between the sheets. In areas of motion, especially on the hands and around joints, it is usually wise to suture large sheets of skin in place.

The best graft take is achieved when a skin graft is exposed. The skin is merely placed over the recipient site and no dressing is applied (Fig. 9). It usually begins to adhere within a matter of a few hours. Once or twice each day any serum that collects beneath the graft is rolled out by the use of a cotton-tipped applicator. When the patient is cooperative and the surface is one that lends itself to exposure of graft, this technique should be used. Unfortunately, many areas are not suitable for exposure and a dressing must be applied. The application of the dressing is most important because it maintains the graft in place. A large, bulky dressing applied with even, resilient compression should be used. In some instances, it is wise to use a stent dressing, particularly on uneven surfaces or areas of motion. The dressing should be changed about 4 or 5 days after grafting.

DONOR SITES. For many years, the accepted method of treatment of donor sites was the application of a large, bulky dressing. Infection frequently occurred in the moist surfaces underneath this dressing. In more recent years, it has been found advantageous to treat donor sites in the burned patients by the exposure method. Immediately after the skin has been removed, the donor area is covered by fine-mesh gauze. A moist gauze pad is applied for hemostasis. At the end of the operation, the gauze pad is removed but the fine-mesh gauze is left over the wound. Sometimes it is wise to apply a light dressing over the gauze and remove it 24 hours later. Blood will clot in the interstices of the gauze and form a firm coagulum. This coagulum dries, hardens in 48 hours, and serves as a good protective covering. Epithelialization proceeds beneath the coagulum, and the area usually heals within 14 days.

Air Bed

One of the most gratifying advances in burns has been the development of the air fluidized bed. Burned patients suffer tremendously from discomfort. The air bed has made the course of many burned patients a less difficult one. Air is circulated through a large bed of ceramic spheres. By controlling the temperature and the flow rate, it is possible for the patient to be made more comfortable. He is kept warm and he rests better because he seems to float in the bed. The use of the bed is especially advantageous in the care of donor sites taken from the back, in burns of the posterior aspect of the body, and in the prevention of pressure ulcers (Fig. 10).

Allografts and Xenografts

In severely burned patients, providing temporary skin cover with allografts (homografts) may be lifesaving. Allografts persist for 15 to 30 days and serve as a biologic skin dressing, preventing infection and the loss of body fluids. In some patients, autografts may be available to cover a portion of the wound and allografts may be used for the remainder. The decision to use allografts is always determined by the size of the wound and the general condition of the patient. In seriously ill patients, it is wise to apply allografts to close the wound until the nutritional status improves and autografts may be obtained. If it seems impossible to obtain autografts to close the wound in a reasonable period, the use of allografts as biologic skin covering is indicated. Allografts may be taken from live donors or recently deceased bodies.

Recently, split-thickness porcine skin xenografts (heterografts) have been shown to be a satisfactory substitute for allograft skin as a biologic wound dressing (Fig. 11). Previously, the major disadvantage of allografts was the limited availability of skin donors and the consequent difficulty of procuring and main-

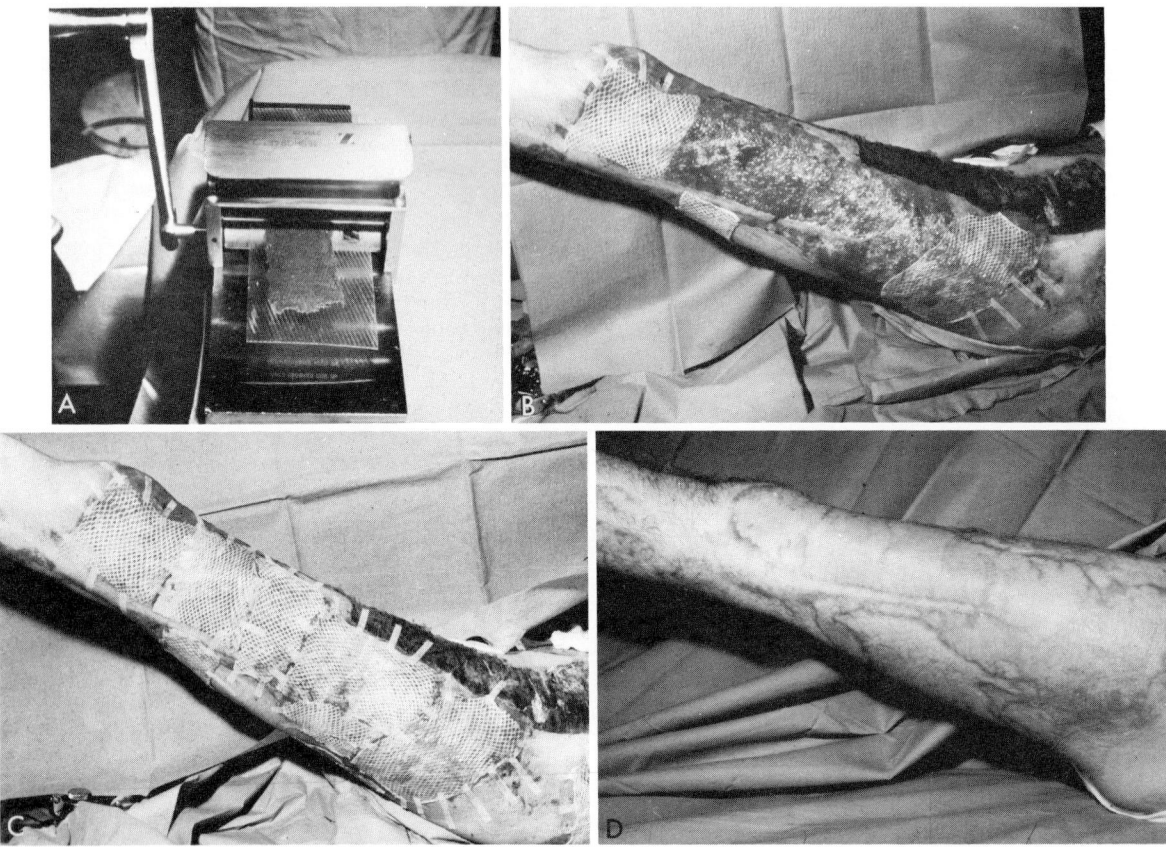

Figure 8. *A,* Mesh dermatome in action. The skin is perforated by the sharp knives on the roller. *B,* Area of skin placed over the lateral aspect of the knee after it has been put through the mesh dermatome at 1½ to 1. *C,* Complete area of grafting over the lateral aspect of the left leg with skin meshed 1½ to 1. The skin was about 1/15,000 of an inch in thickness. It was held in place by Steri-strips. *D,* Appearance of mesh grafted area after it was completely healed.

taining an adequate supply of split-thickness allografts. Biologic acceptance and rejection of xenografts is essentially similar to that of allografts from a clinical point of view. Areas in which porcine skin xenografts have proved most valuable include the primary treatment of second-degree burns and on granulating wounds as a biologic wound dressing. Wound care is frequently simplified and patient comfort markedly enhanced when xenografts are used. Additionally, xenograft application appears to control bacterial growth effectively on granulating surfaces in most instances and to promote epithelialization of wounds. Frequently, a dramatic improvement in the patient's metabolic status becomes apparent when open, infected granulating wounds are covered with xenografts.

NUTRITIONAL SUPPORT

The maintenance of blood volume of extensively burned patients during the grafting period is important. It is sometimes necessary to give transfusions as often as every other day. The hematocrit must be de-

termined twice weekly and sufficient blood given to maintain it at about 38 per cent.

A strongly negative nitrogen balance is characteristic of the severely burned patient because of the large nitrogen losses and low nitrogen intake. The duration and magnitude of negative nitrogen balance are influenced by the severity of the burn as well as by the nutritional regimen used (Fig. 12). Along with the negative nitrogen balance, there occurs a rapid pulse rate and elevated body temperature as a consequence of increased metabolic activity. Hypermetabolism occurs in burns, and the degree is directly related to the extent of injury. Years ago Cuthbertson demonstrated that the increased loss of nitrogen following long bone fractures really came from systemic sources rather than from damaged tissues at the site of injury. This concept has been confirmed in burns, in which the main source of catabolized protein is skeletal muscle. It is recognized that amino acids, primarily alanine, are released from muscle beds, transported to the liver, and converted to new glucose. This provides a constant flow of readily available fuel to maintain function in glucose-dependent tissues. Because glycogen stores are limited and fatty acids cannot be con-

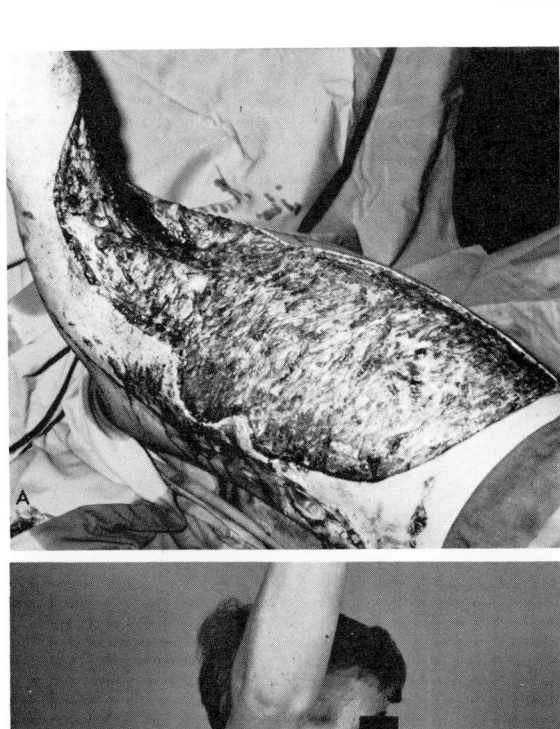

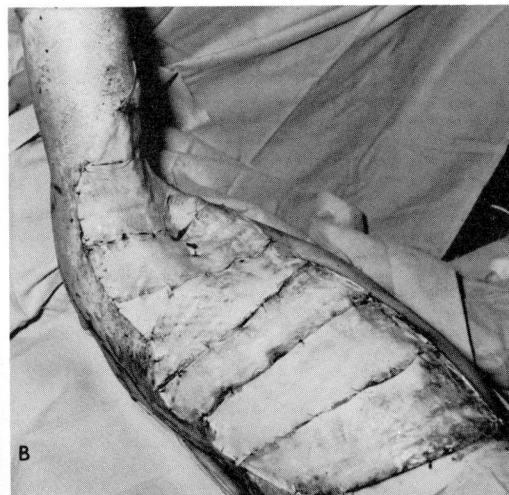

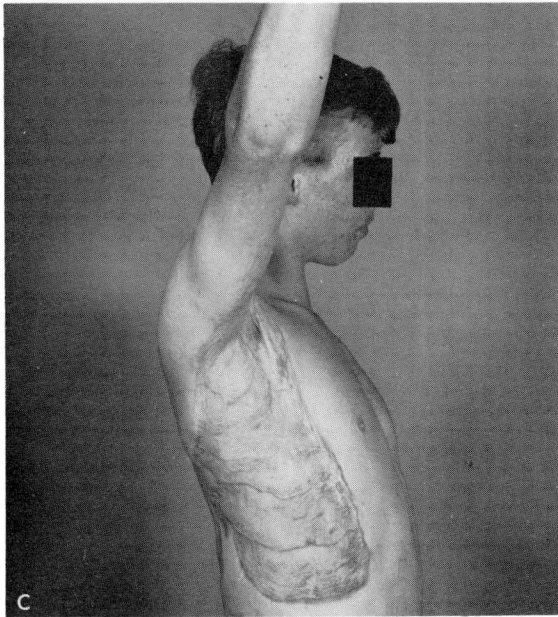

Figure 9. *A,* Area on arm, axilla, and right chest of electrical injury has been excised. This has left a large open wound. A dressing was applied for 3 days. *B,* On the large open wound sheets of split-thickness skin have been placed in lay-on fashion. A few sutures of 4–0 silk are used to hold the grafts in place. This grafted area was completely exposed; no dressing was applied; the right arm was suspended by tying it to an intravenous standard. *C,* Complete healing of area after grafted area was treated by exposure. There is no evidence of contracture in the axilla.

verted to new glucose, this alanine cycle provides an ongoing supply of glucose at the expense of body protein. Every effort should be made to provide the patient with protein and calories by the best means available.

Hypermetabolism essentially exhausts the patient. It appears that hypermetabolism is caused by catecholamines. Catecholamines are elevated following thermal injury, and adrenergic activity has been related to the extent of burn and to the oxygen consumption of the patient. It appears that increased catecholamines, that is, increased adrenergic activity, are in part the calorigenic mediators responsible for the post-traumatic, hypermetabolic response following thermal injury. Cold, pain, anxiety, and hypovolemia are potent afferent stimuli that augment the catecholamine response. The clinician hopes that he can minimize these by good burn care. He attempts to refuel the pa-

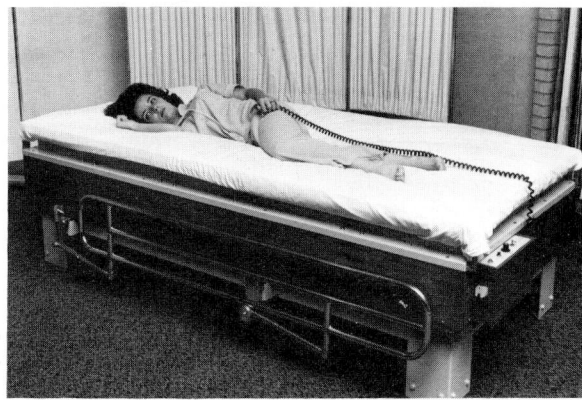

Figure 10. The air-fluidized bed. This bed allows the patient almost to float. The temperature of the air can be controlled.

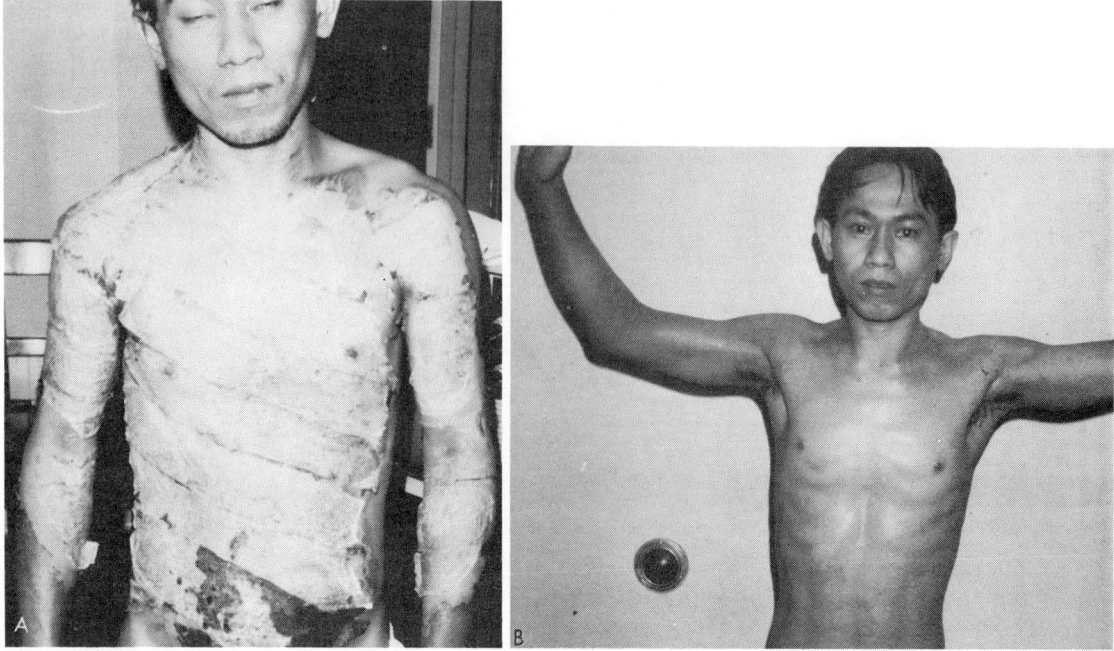

Figure 11. Use of porcine xenograft as dressing for second-degree burn. *A*, Xenograft in place. *B*, Completely healed burn in 21 days. The xenografts were removed and reapplied every 3 or 4 days.

tient by any and every method available (Fig. 13). If the patient is not too ill, this is usually done with a high protein, high caloric diet. In other instances, the use of predigested proteins and other formulae through a nasogastric tube may be very beneficial. If these fail, then careful consideration should be given to utilization of hyperalimentation fluid by means of central vein administration. It is recognized that one

of the complications of hyperalimentation is infection, and certainly this is quite true in the burned patient. On the other hand, however, to maintain an appropriate intake for survival the clinician may have to accept the chance of infection and utilize a hyperalimentation regimen. Sometimes the use of jejunostomy may be very beneficial.

Severely burned patients may lose as much as one

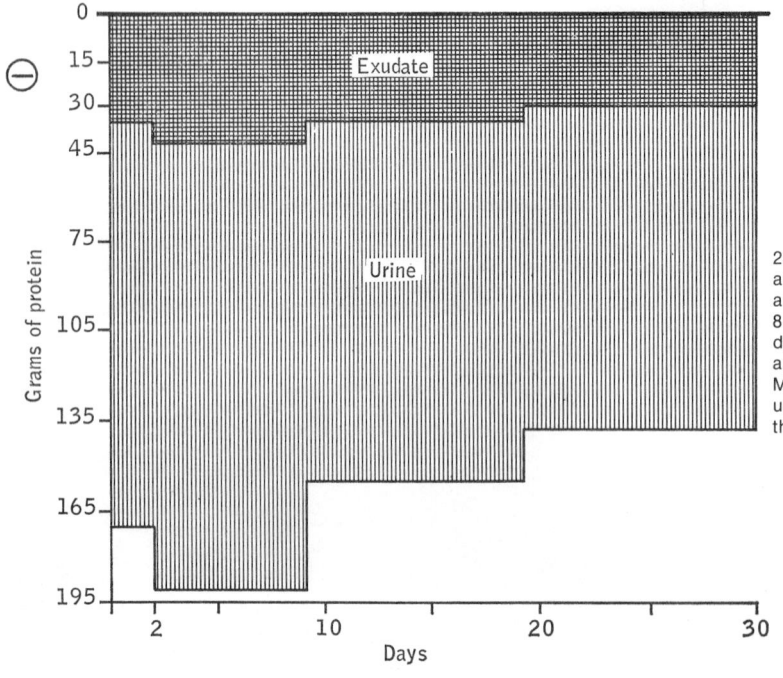

Figure 12. Composite protein losses typical of a 25 per cent second- and third-degree burn in an average adult male. The losses in grams of protein are plotted from the zero line down. During the first 8 days, the loss of protein approximates 190 gm. per day. Extensive losses continue for the first 30 days and then diminish as wound coverage is achieved. Most of the protein is lost in the urine, but the exudate is usually responsible for 15 to 20 per cent of the loss.

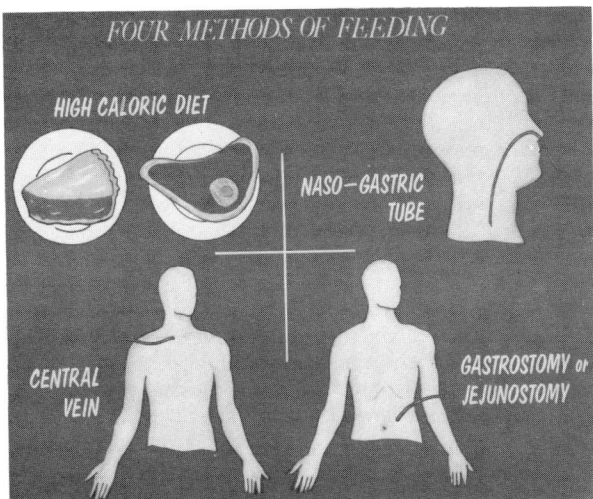

Figure 13. Various methods of feeding burned patients to maintain a positive nitrogen balance.

pound a day for the first 30 days post burn (Fig. 14). As soon as the wound is closed, positive nitrogen balance can be achieved and a weight gain program started. One of the most important factors in the re-covery of the extensively burned patient is his accep-tance of a large intake of protein and calories each day. The use of narcotics after the first two days should be discouraged because they have a tendency to interfere with the patient's nutritional intake.

COMPLICATIONS

An extensively burned patient has suffered a severe form of trauma and, therefore, is prone to a variety of complications.

Infection

Infection remains a cardinal problem in the treat-ment of burns. The infection of gravest import is burn wound sepsis. The concept of burn wound sepsis as defined by Moncrief and Teplitz in 1964 is essentially that there is proliferation and active invasion of the burn wound by microorganisms in the quantity of 100,000 or more per gram of tissue. Initially, the mi-croorganisms contaminating the surface of the wound and existing in the hair follicles and sweat glands begin to proliferate rapidly and by 48 hours post burn have often reached a sizable magnitude. This initial colonization and proliferation usually involve pri-marily staphylococci. Beginning about the fifth post-burn day, gram-negative bacilli are noted in increas-

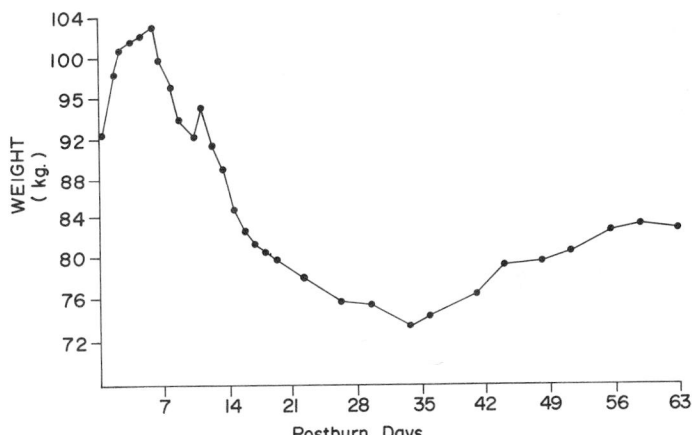

Figure 14. Weight curve and nitrogen loss data of a patient with a 70 per cent partial-thickness burn. (From Artz, C. P., and Moncrief, J. A.: The Treatment of Burns, 2nd ed. Philadelphia, W. B. Saunders Company, 1969.)

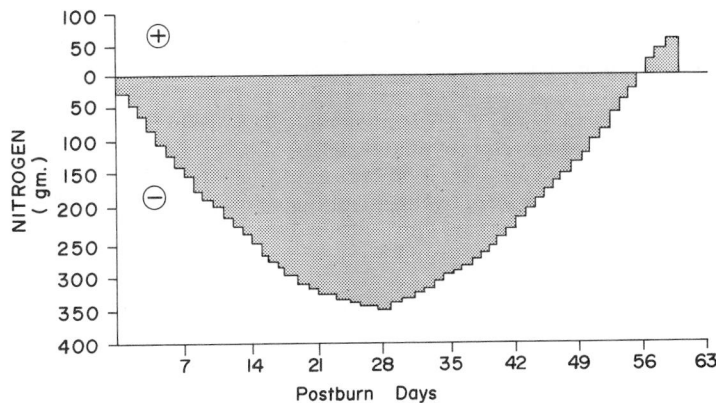

**TABLE 1.   Nitrogen Required for Equilibrium
at Various Phases after Burning***

Postburn Period	Approximate Amount of Nitrogen for Equilibrium in gm. per sq.m.
7–17 days	20–25
3–40 days	13–16
60–70 days	3–9
90–100 days	3–7

*From Soroff, H. S., Pearson, E., and Artz, C. P.:
Surg. Gynec. Obstet. *112*:159, 1961. By permission of
Surgery, Gynecology & Obstetrics.

ing numbers and are usually the predominant
organism by the end of the first week. Although the
bacterial spectrum of the burn wound appears to have
changed somewhat in recent years as a result of the
use of various topical antibacterial agents, *Pseudomonas aeruginosa* remains the most commonly implicated organism in burn wound sepsis.

In second-degree burns and donor sites, local infection can usually be controlled by appropriate systemic
antibiotic therapy and frequent changes of wet dressings.

The source of systemic infection in the burned patient is usually the wound itself, but it may involve
the bladder, the lungs, or aseptic thrombus. It is not
uncommon in extensively burned patients when an
indwelling catheter has been in place for a prolonged
period of time for a septic thrombus to develop. The
most common affecting organism in septic phlebitis is
Staphylococcus aureus. Such a thrombus usually responds to removal of the catheter, excision of the entire infected vein, and the administration of an appropriate antibiotic in large doses.

Another important facet of the host defense mechanism, namely the complement pathway, also undergoes alterations. In burns this so-called alternate
pathway, an important defense against pseudomonas
infection, appears to be blocked.

There now appear on the horizon several potential
immunotherapeutic tools for the specific bolstering of
defense mechanisms in burned patients. It is in this
area that advances are anticipated within the next
few years.

The first symptom of overwhelming sepsis is an
increase in the already febrile state, clouding of the
sensorium, and paralytic ileus. Intermittent disorientation rapidly becomes more profound, and persistent
abdominal distention is a prominent feature. Biopsies
of the full-thickness burn wound may be helpful in
diagnosing invasive burn wound sepsis. When the patient becomes septic, every effort should be made to
obtain a diagnosis as to the origin of the sepsis and the
primary offending organism. Sputum cultures, urine
cultures, blood cultures, and wound biopsy cultures
are most important.

Treatment consists of massive doses of systemic antibiotics chosen on the basis of the predominant causative organism. This may mean the simultaneous ad-

ministration of two or three antibiotics. If the eschar
is intact, the administration of the appropriate antibiotic in a subeschar fashion, as introduced by Baxter,
may be highly beneficial. The maximum daily dose of
the antibiotic selected according to the sensitivity of
the major offending organism is mixed with 500 ml. of
saline and allowed to flow into the subeschar area
through multiple portals by means of long spinal
needles (Fig. 15). Every effort should be made to
remove gently the devitalized tissue. If there is a large
open wound without eschar, it should be covered with
xenografts.

Clinicians involved in the treatment of burns have
long recognized the fact that burned patients appear
peculiarly susceptible to infection. During the past few
years there has been increasing scientific evidence to
support this thesis. One of the most productive areas
of current research in burns is in the field of the immune response and what can be done to enhance it.

The first protector against the entry of microorganisms is the integument, which is not only a mechanical and chemical barrier, but through the secretion of
surface immunoglobulin in body secretions, an immunologic barrier as well. Once the organisms have
entered the body, the inflammatory reaction is activated. It is well documented that burns impair many
facets of this reaction, particularly leukocyte chemotaxis and margination. In very large burns there is
hardly any inflammatory reaction in response to a
challenge applied to unburned skin. There is also evidence that, although the phagocytic capacity of neutrophils may remain normal, the complex intracellular killing mechanism of the neutrophil is impaired.
One of the key factors in host defenses is the thymic-
dependent lymphocyte or T-cell. There are many ways
of measuring T-cell function, one of the most common
ones being by skin tests of delayed hypersensitivity.
Skin tests remain essentially normal under 20 per
cent total body burn, but as the size of the injury
increases, the ability to respond to recall antigens in-

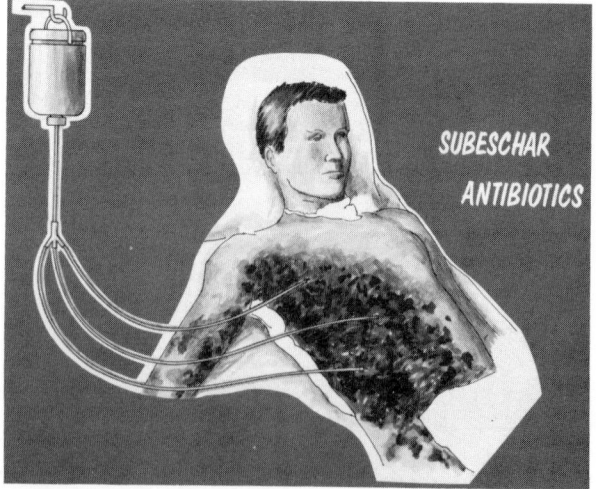

Figure 15.   Schematic diagram of a method of administering antibiotics in burned patients whose eschar is intact. The appropriate
antibiotic is given by clysis in the subeschar area.

volving prior exposure is abolished for about two weeks. If the injury is over 50 per cent of the body surface, the ability of the body to respond to a primary challenge is practically abolished. The other central lymphoid cell that reacts to infection is the bursa-dependent lymphocyte or B-cell. B-cells elaborate classic antibody immunoglobulin, which eliminates organisms by acting as opsonins, agglutinins, and precipitins. The serum IgG level of burned patients is severely depressed and returns to normal by about four weeks post burn. By contrast, the levels of serum IgM remains normal.

In the past several years, fungal infections have assumed increasing importance in burns. Prolonged survival of patients with severe burns increases the time at risk during a period when there is a progressive decrease in resistance to infection. Widespread use of topical and systemic antibiotics, while leading to a better control of bacterial infection, predisposes to the development of fungal infections. There has been a study in progressive increase in disseminated candidiasis. It is well known that there is an increase in incidence of Candida in stool cultures after patients have been treated with broad-spectrum antibiotics.

Therapeutic measures to control Candida have not been very satisfactory. Topical application of Mycostatin may be added to the usual topical antibacterial agents. Oral Mycostatin has been used in patients with urinary tract involvement. It is generally believed that this continuing systemic antibiotic therapy is desirable when candidemia is present. But it must be remembered that the incidence of bacterial sepsis in these patients is so high that this continuing antibiotic therapy is not always possible. Currently, the most popular therapy for systemic candidiasis is Amphotericin B. The results with this agent have not been very satisfactory.

Phycomycetes and *Aspergillus* species also invade burn wounds. An important characteristic of fungal invasion is the sudden appearance in a second-degree burn wound of violaceous or black spots. Frequently these are mistaken for focal areas of hemorrhage. Systemic sepsis may be the first indication of invasive fungal disease. Whenever a suspicious-appearing lesion is seen, a biopsy should be taken. Histologic examination is the most rapid method of making the diagnosis of invasive fungal infection. The primary treatment for this complication is radical excision. Invasion into unburned subcutaneous tissue requires a wide débridement of all the grossly abnormal tissue. If a muscle biopsy is positive for fungus, the mandatory treatment is wide débridement followed by daily observation and frequent wound biopsies.

In all serious infections every effort should be made to provide the best supportive therapy possible. This means an adequate amount of water and frequent blood transfusions. Since infection inhibits the regenerative power of the bone marrow, frequent transfusions are usually necessary to maintain the hematocrit at 38 per cent or above. A major decision at this time concerns the use of hyperalimentation. Although infection associated with hyperalimentation is a real threat to survival, diminution in body fuel may be an even greater threat. Certainly if the patient is septic

and unable to consume a reasonable intake, hyperalimentation should be instituted.

Acute Gastric Dilatation

This complication is more common than is usually recognized and may occur during the first week after injury. It is characterized by vomiting, upper abdominal distention, and dyspnea. It is important to recognize this complication immediately; burned patients frequently aspirate after regurgitation of fluids, and aspiration in a critically ill patient may lead to death.

Curling's Ulcer

An acute ulceration occurring in the stomach or duodenum associated with burns has come to be known as Curling's ulcer. It is almost invariably associated with extensive burns or moderate burns with significant sepsis. The understanding of this entity has been clarified in recent years by the study of McAlhaney[17] at the Institute of Surgical Research. He comments about his studies as follows:

Early and serial fiberoptic gastroduodenostomy in over 70 burned patients was used to determine the actual incidence and natural history of the acute gastroduodenal lesions after thermal injury. Diffuse erosive gastritis was discovered as early as five hours postburn in 83% of patients and acute duodenal mucosal disease or duodenitis was noted in 63% of patients. Mucosal lesions were not discovered in patients with burns of less than 30%. The fundus and body of the stomach were always involved, whereas the antrum was involved in approximately 1/3 of the patients. Gastric and duodenal ulcers were noted to evolve from early superficial mucosal disease after 72 hours postburn in approximately 25% of patients. Acute ulcerations were responsible for significant gastrointestinal bleeding, but bleeding from erosive gastritis was rarely life-threatening. The morphologic and histologic characteristics of these acute lesions and their early occurrence suggest an ischemic insult to the gastroduodenal mucosa. Histochemical evaluation of gastric muco-substances documented that acute gastric mucosal disease was encountered despite normal quantities of cellular muco-substance. Gastric acid output early postburn was not predictive of acute gastric disease, although gastric acid was present in all patients. Acute duodenal ulcers, however, were only discovered in patients with acid output greater than 3 ml/hr. In addition, life-threatening complications of hemorrhage and perforation developed only in patients with acid outputs of greater than 3 ml/hr. Because of this, the effectiveness of hydrogen on neutralization was assessed in a prospective randomized study. The conclusions of this warrant the recommendation that early administration of antacids and maintenace of intragastric pH at 7 by pH tape testing should be used in all burned patients with greater than 35% total body surface injury. After dietary intake is resumed, antacid should be given after meals and twice nightly.

Should hemorrhage occur, management should be similar to the treatment of bleeding from a chronic duodenal ulcer. The same indications for surgical intervention that apply to a chronic bleeding duodenal ulcer should apply to Curling's ulcer. In such instances, the best surgical procedures seems to be vagotomy and hemigastrectomy.

Pulmonary Complications

With the increasing success in controlling burn wound sepsis as a cause of death in the burned patient, the importance of various pulmonary complications has become strikingly accentuated. In general, pulmonary complications can be grouped in the following categories:

1. Acute upper respiratory obstruction
2. Inhalation injury
3. Postburn pulmonary insufficiency
4. Atelectasis and pneumonia

These complications frequently present a somewhat confusing and overlapping clinical picture in the burned patient.

Acute respiratory obstruction may occur within a few hours after injury as a result of edema of the upper airway. It is usually seen in burns around the face and neck. For years this type of injury was treated with tracheostomy. In the past few years there has been a marked change in attitude toward tracheostomy in burns. It has become evident that the tracheostomy is a ready avenue for invasive infection. More precise studies with blood gases, the use of an indwelling nasotracheal tube for a few days, and better techniques in maintaining pulmonary toilet, have led to the concept that whenever possible, a tracheostomy should be avoided. In edema of the upper airway, a nasotracheal tube, if it can be inserted, is the best method of management. If the edema or pulmonary difficulty has not subsided in four or five days, a tracheostomy may be necessary.

Inhalation injury to the lower airway is usually caused by the inhalation of large amounts of irritating noxious products of combustion. True burns of the lower respiratory mucosa are rarely seen. Diagnostic clues to the presence of this type of injury include physical evidence of respiratory difficulty and arterial hypoxemia. Whenever inhalation injury is suspected, the patient should receive special pulmonary care. Frequent arterial blood gases are necessary.

When there is a question about airway pathology, fiberoptic bronchoscopy may be of great help. It aids in the diagnosis of upper airway edema and of early inhalation injury. In addition, xenon lung scans may be helpful in the early diagnosis of inhalation injury.

Initially, support may be given by means of a nasotracheal tube. If the difficulty is prolonged, a tracheostomy will be necessary. Usually, the management of inhalation injury is ventilatory support, humidification of inspired air, broad-spectrum antibiotics, and pharmacologic doses of steroids (30 mg. per kg. of body weight of Solu-Medrol initially, followed by one fourth this dose every 6 hours for 48 hours).

The phenomenon of post-traumatic pulmonary insufficiency has assumed an increasingly important place in the list of major complications seen in patients after any major injury. Arterial hypoxemia is usually the earliest warning followed by clinically evident respiratory insufficiency and pulmonary changes on the chest roentgenograms. Treatment frequently requires the administration of an oxygen-enriched atmosphere by mask, endotracheal tube, or tracheostomy and sometimes assisted ventilation using a mechanical ventilator.

Miscellaneous Complications

Fecal impaction is particularly common in the burned patient. Prolonged immobilization and dehydration lead to the development of impaction. Cystitis and urethritis are complications of prolonged use of indwelling catheters. Urinary catheters should be removed as early as possible.

In deep circumferential injury of the extremities and of the chest, troublesome constriction may occur when the eschar dehydrates and contracts. Circumferential chest eschars must be incised to permit adequate expansion of the chest. Relaxing incisions should be made in constricting eschars in the extremities to prevent vascular insufficiency of the distal extremities.

Decubitus ulcers are likely to develop in the extensively burned patient. They may occur in the sacral region, over the anterior superior iliac spine, on the posterior aspect of the head, and on the back of the heel.

COLD INJURY
(FROSTBITE AND RELATED CONDITIONS)

Cold injury is trauma produced by exposure to cold and includes such entities as chilblain, frostbite, immersion foot, and trench foot. The type of injury produced is dependent upon the degree of cold to which the body is exposed, the duration of the exposure, and environmental factors that intensify the effect of the low temperatures.

Chilblain results from exposure to temperatures above freezing associated with high humidity. The term immersion foot implies a cold injury of the feet resulting from prolonged exposure, usually in excess of 12 hours, in water at temperatures below 50° F. Trench foot results from prolonged exposure to cold at temperatures from just above freezing to 50° F. and wetness of the feet. The term frostbite is applied when crystallization of the tissue fluids occurs in the skin or subcutaneous tissue. It is produced by exposure at temperatures of freezing or below. High-altitude frostbite results from exposure at high altitudes to temperatures usually varying from −20 to −80° F. The areas most commonly affected are the feet and toes, hands and fingers, and ears and nose.

Cold injury occurs sporadically in the civilian population, but is of primary concern in the military service. It has been recognized as a problem of military importance since the days of Alexander of Macedonia. Napoleon's famous surgeon, Bajon Larrey, classically described the role that cold injury played in the defeat of Napoleon's army in Poland in 1812. It was of considerable military significance in World War II, in aerial battles and in the Battle of Ardennes Forest during December, 1944, and at the Chosen Reservoir during the Korean conflict in 1951. Among United States troops, there were approximately 92,000 cases of cold injury during World War II and more than 9000 during the Korean War.

Pathogenesis

There are two main theories concerning the pathogenesis of frostbite. The first postulates that the tissue injury is secondary to vasoconstriction, vasodilatation, edema, sludging of erythrocytes in capillaries, and thrombosis with subsequent necrosis of tissue.

The second theory postulates that the tissue injury is due to the direct action of the cold on tissue cells, a true thermal injury. Most surgeons favor the vascular theory in the pathogenesis of cold injury in man.

Tissues do not show the same degree of susceptibility to cold injury. Nerves and striated muscle are highly sensitive; skin, fascia, and connective tissue are quite resistant, but not so resistant as compact bone or tendon. Blood vessels are highly susceptible to injury, which results in leakage of plasma into the surrounding tissue. This difference in resistance has resulted in the observation in humans and animals of muscle gangrene without necrosis of the overlying skin after exposure to cold.

Signs and Symptoms

The clinical manifestations and course subsequent to rewarming vary with the severity of the cold injury, which may be classified into four degrees; first degree, hyperemia and edema; second degree, hyperemia with blister formation; third degree, necrosis of skin and subcutaneous tissue; and fourth degree, complete necrosis and loss of tissue.

In *first-degree frostbite,* the skin becomes mottled blue or purple, then red. Swelling begins within 3 hours; the edema persists for 10 days or more. Desquamation of the superficial layers of the skin begins 5 to 10 days after injury, and may persist for many months.

Second-degree frostbite is characterized by hyperemia and edema with vesicle formation appearing 12 to 24 hours after rewarming (Fig. 16). The edema is usually not marked and disappears within 5 days. The blisters dry and form black eschars within 11 to 24 days. Throbbing and aching pain are noted 3 to 20 days after injury. The eschar gradually desquamates, revealing an intact skin which is thin, soft, and easily injured (Fig. 17).

Third-degree frostbite involves the full thickness of the skin and extends into the subcutaneous tissue, leading to ulceration. Vesicles may be present at the periphery of the area of damage. Edema of the entire part may occur. This usually disappears in about 6 days. Most patients have burning, aching, throbbing, or shooting pains, which may persist for 5 weeks. The skin overlying the area of third-degree frostbite forms a black, hard, dry eschar. This eschar finally desquamates and the remaining ulcer epithelializes. Healing occurs in about 2½ months.

Fourth-degree frostbite is characterized by destruction of the entire part including the bone. Edema may extend far beyond the area of frostbite. There may be severe paresthesia, which appears 3 to 13 days after rewarming. The injured tissues become black, dry, shriveled, and mummified. Usually, the area has the appearance of dry gangrene. The line of demarcation becomes apparent in about 1 month, and extends down to the bone in 2 months or more.

Production of Cold Injury

Cold is the specific agent in cold injury and is the immediate cause of tissue damage. A variety of environmental and host factors influence the incidence, types, and severity of the injury. Weather is a predominant influence in the causation of cold injury. Low temperatures and low relative humidity favor frostbite, whereas higher temperatures together with moisture are usually associated with trench foot.

Wind chill is considered to be one of the important factors in the production of cold injuries. Wind velocity greatly increases wind chill. For example, a temperature of 38° F., with a wind velocity of 10 miles an hour, has the same effect on exposed flesh as a temperature of 0° F. at a wind velocity of 1 mile an hour.

Conditions that decrease the internal heat supply include those that mechanically obstruct blood flow to the extremities, such as constrictive clothing or other pressure-producing objects. Tight or stiff clothing is especially harmful if individuals must remain in cramped quarters with arms and legs flexed. Wet clothing is especially dangerous. Environmental protection, including shelter and the quality and quantity of clothing, has a profound effect upon the development of cold injuries.

The majority of cold injuries are of the nonfreezing type and are generally associated with wetness, with the ambient temperatures several degrees above freezing.

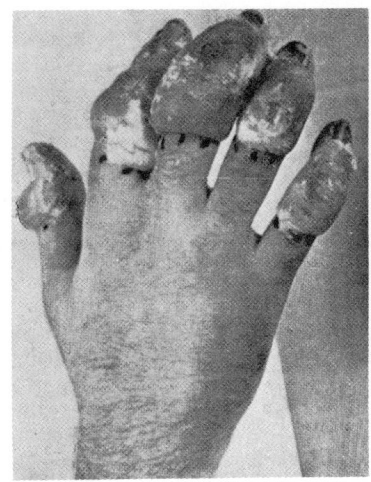
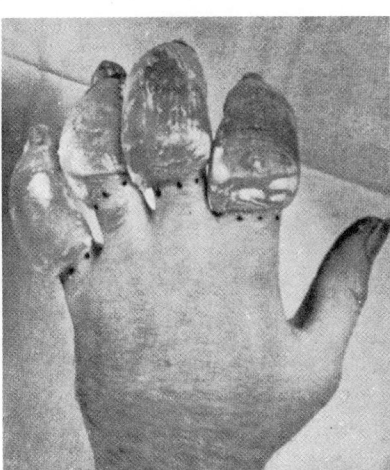

Figure 16. Severe blistering occurring with high-altitude frostbite 24 hours after injury.

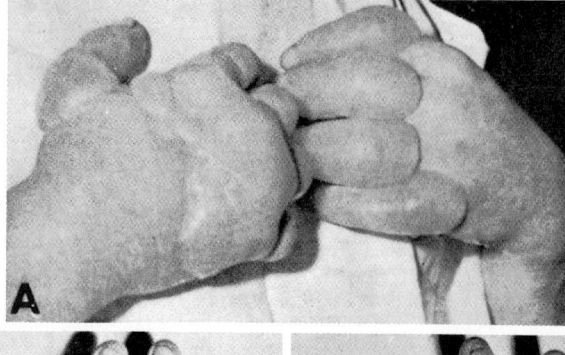

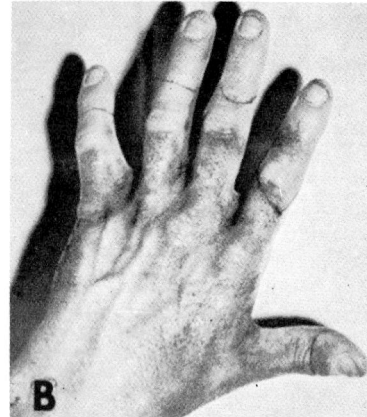

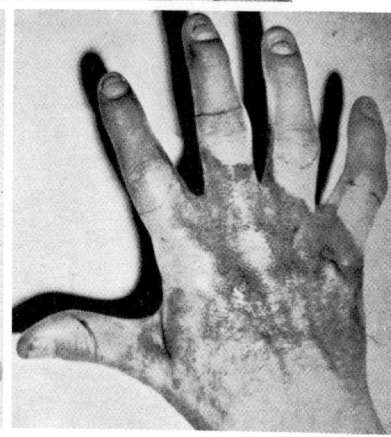

Figure 17. *A*, Severe blistering following high-altitude frostbite 24 hours after injury. *B*, Appearance of hands 2 months later. The lost nails show regeneration and the skin is beginning to recover its normal surface markings. Sensory disturbances and loss of sweating persisted for many months.

Treatment

The treatment of cold injury remains somewhat controversial. Anticoagulant therapy would appear to be the treatment of choice if the vascular theory of pathogenesis is correct. A few investiagors believe heparin is of value; the majority do not. Although the early use of heparin may be of value, its efficacy was not proved in the treatment of frostbite in Korea. Sympathetic nerve interruption, like other methods of increasing the blood supply to a frozen extremity, was for a long time condemned without trial. Several investigators believe that lumbar blocks, sympathectomy, or the use of vasodilators such as Priscoline are of value, but extensive use of vasodilators in the treatment of frostbite in Korea did not prove to be of significant value. Lumbar blocks and early sympathectomy were also of little or no value. The trial of unilateral sympathectomy in bilateral cold injury of the feet resulted in no significant difference in the amount of tissue loss and the residuals in the two feet.

Sympathectomy has been proved to be of value in the management of the late sequelae of frostbite, including chilblain and the complicating causalgia-like syndrome occasionally seen years after frostbite.

The treatment of cold injury may be divided into the emergency management and later hospital management. Initially, all constricting items of clothing such as boots, gloves, and socks should be removed. The injured parts, if still frozen, should be rapidly rewarmed by immersion in warm water at 90 to 104° F., and the general body warmth is maintained. Large vesicles or bullae are covered with a loose, dry dressing. Petrola-

tum dressings must not be applied. A booster dose of tetanus toxoid and penicillin should be administered.

Definitive treatment includes absolute bed rest for those with cold injury of the feet. The patient should be kept in bed until subsidence of edema or complete drying of vesicles has occurred. Patients with third-degree injury remain in bed longer, until areas of ulceration have been epithelialized; those with fourth-degree injury, until treated surgically.

All lesions are exposed to the air, and a ward temperature of 70 to 74° F. should be maintained. Smoking is discouraged. Active physical therapy is instituted at the bedside as soon as possible. Attention is directed toward the position of the feet and movement of the fingers, toes, and other major joints to prevent ankylosis. Second-, third, and fourth-degree lesions are cleansed daily with a mild antiseptic solution such as aqueous Zephiran solution. Superficial débridement of broken vesicles or necrotic tissue must be accomplished frequently. Suppurative eschars and partially detached toenails are removed. Lesions must first be cleansed with hydrogen peroxide solution, and then soaked in normal saline for 30 minutes before débridement is started. The necrotic eschar on digits is bivalved early to prevent contracture and further tissue damage. Patients with third- and fourth-degree injuries are given antibiotic therapy until their lesions have dried.

Buerger's exercises may be started as soon as the lesions show signs of healing. As soon as the eschar has desquamated, whirlpool therapy should be started and continued for 2 weeks. Emergency amputations are seldom indicated except in unusual cases with extensive wet gangrene and general sepsis. The part is not ready for amputation until the edge of the eschar has separated from the normal tissues by the ingrowth of epithelium. There is no specific therapy for cold injury; prevention is the only cure.

CHEMICAL INJURY

Most chemical injuries occur in laboratories and industrial plants. In time of war, chemical burns are caused by phosphorus, magnesium, and vesicant gases. Acute injury to the skin resulting from chemical agents is similar to that caused by heat. In fact, injurious effects of the chemical are sometimes due in part to the development of heat. The lesions produced by a chemical agent present a pathologic picture showing different degrees of destruction from a central zone of necrosis to a peripheral hyperemic zone.

Alkali burns are usually caused by sodium hydroxide, potassium hydroxide, or calcium oxide. Alkalis exert their pathologic effect in three ways: by saponifying the fat, by extracting considerable water from the cells because of their hygroscopic nature, and by dissolving and uniting with the proteins of the tissues to form alkaline proteinates. The initial treatment for burns caused by a strong alkaline solution is washing with large quantities of water. Pouring the water over the area permits the fluid to carry away excess alkaline agents as well as the heat of dissolution. In lime burns, the dry lime should be brushed away before washing so that the calcium oxide will not unite with water to form calcium hydroxide, a reaction that produces a tremendous amount of heat.

Concentrated acids withdraw water from cells and precipitate proteins to form acid proteinates. Sulfuric acid converts the corroded tissue into a greenish black or dark brown slough. Nitric acid causes a yellow color, which becomes a yellowish brown. Hydrochloric acid is a much more severe caustic than nitric or sulfuric acid and stains the skin yellowish brown. Trichloroacetic acid is the most corrosive of all organic acids. It forms, a white, soft slough. Phenol, a destructive and poisonous organic acid, causes an initial white slough that turns to a greenish black or copper color. Acid burns should be treated by diluting or removing the acid as rapidly as possible, usually by irrigation with large quantities of water. After removing the maximal amount of acid by washing, the remainder may be neutralized by a weak solution of baking soda.

Alkalinizing solutions should never be utilized prior to copious irrigation with large quantities of water because of the intense exothermic reaction that follows irrigation with neutralizing solutions in the presence of significant amounts of acid. The extent and depth of the burn wound might thus be unduly increased.

Phosphorus burns are extremely painful and a common injury of modern warfare. White phosphorus ignites spontaneously in air and is rapidly oxidized to phosphorus pentoxide. With the addition of water from the tissues, there is the formation of meta- and ortho-phosphoric acids. Burning phosphorus is easily extinguished by water, but reignites after drying. Phosphorus penetrates deep into the tissues. The particles of phosphorus continue to cause damage until washed or picked out of the wound. The wound can be seen to emit smoke if the phosphorus is exposed to air, and in the dark the wounds glow with a blue-green color. When the injury is extensive there may be hepatic and renal damage.

Emergency treatment of phosphorus burns is accomplished by rapid removal of the contaminated clothing, irrigation with warm water, and débridement of the visible imbedded particles. Burned areas should then be dressed with water-soaked gauze pads. At the hospital following removal of the dressings, the burns should be irrigated with warm water or with a dilute solution of sodium bicarbonate, then rinsed with 1 per cent copper sulfate solution. The copper phosphate coating formed by the irrigation with copper sulfate makes any retained particles easier to identify. When copper sulfate is used, great care must be taken to wash it from the wound and to maintain adequate urinary flow by the use of either an appropriate fluid load or mannitol.

Magnesium burns produce ulcers that are small at first but gradually enlarge to form an extensive lesion. Magnesium may be a rapid, or slow-burning ember, depending upon the size of the particles involved. If the slow-burning embers penetrate deeper than the outer layers of the skin, they must be excised completely and the resulting wound closed by skin grafting.

Mustard gas and lewisite are war gases that cause severe blister formation. Early care consists of washing with large amounts of water. Later definitive care is the same as that for other second-degree burns.

Hydrofluoric acid burns should be treated by the subcutaneous injection of a 10 per cent solution of calcium gluconate. The fluoride ion penetrates rapidly, causing liquifaction of cellular membranes and decalcification of bones. Local injections of calcium gluconate with formation of insoluble calcium fluoride decreases pain and may prevent deeper tissue destruction.

ELECTRICAL INJURY

Damage after electrical injury is frequently referred to as an electrical burn. Because there is usually damage to the deeper tissues by the electricity, an electrical injury more nearly simulates crush injury than does a thermal burn (Fig. 18).

The most important factors in determining the effect of the passage of an electric current through the human body are the type of circuit, the voltage and the amperage of the current, the resistance of the body, the path of the current through the body, and the duration of contact. The type of electrical circuit involved may be either direct current or alternating current. Whereas direct current produces muscular spasms only at the start and stop of the current flow, alternating current produces muscular contraction and relaxation with each cycle. The greater the volt-

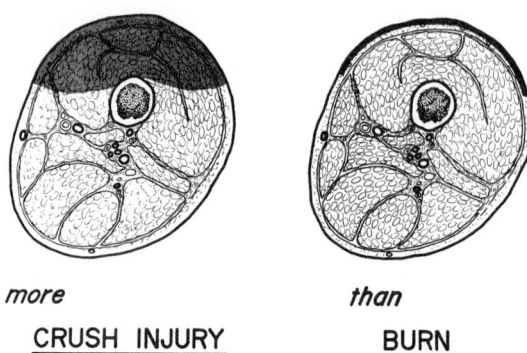

more   *than*

CRUSH INJURY   BURN

Figure 18. Schematic outlines emphasizing that electrical injury is a deep injury and is more like a crush injury than a thermal burn.

age, the greater its effect on the body. Deaths have been reported from contact with 60-volt circuits, while contact with circuits of less than 24 volts is generally safe except under unusual conditions.

Current amperage is the measure of current flow per unit time. This value ordinarily determines the severity of the injury, other factors being equal. A current of as little as 100 milliamperes may result in ventricular fibrillation under proper circumstances. Respiratory arrest due to central nervous system damage may occur at even lower amperage.

The resistance to current flow offered by the body varies with the tissue involved. The lowest resistances are offered by nerve tissue, blood, lymph, and cerebrospinal fluid, while bone offers the highest resistance. The resistance of dry intact skin is quite high but varies with the thickness, cleanliness, and degree of moisture. The resistance of dry skin is 20 times that of saline-moistened skin.

Damage associated with electricity may be divided into three categories.

Electric contact injury caused by an electric current passing through the skin produces damage to the skin's subcutaneous tissue, muscle, and other deeper structures. It is well known that the current follows blood vessels and that thrombosis even at some distance from the original injury is common.[24] This thrombosis is at least partly responsible for the fact that more tissue is always destroyed by an electrical

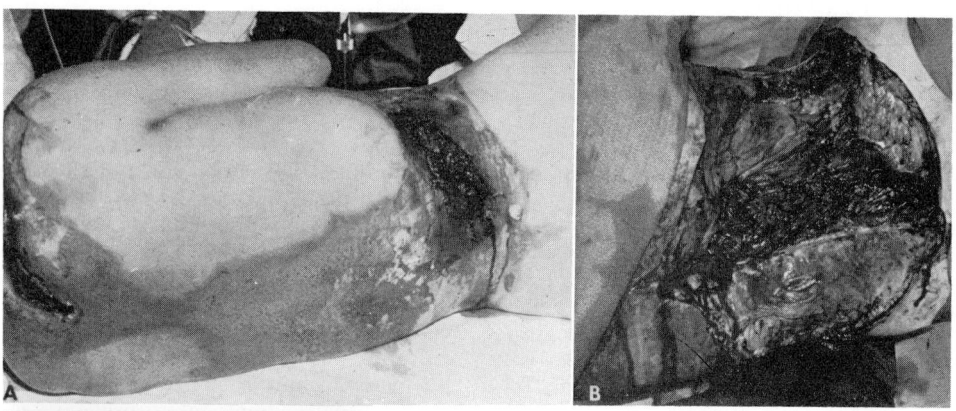

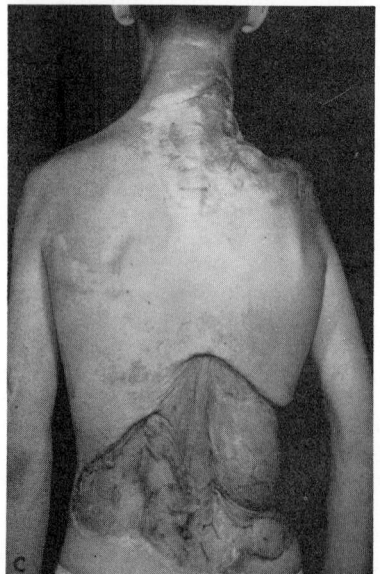

Figure 19. Severe electrical injury. *A,* Massive deep injury seen in the right flank and the right shoulder region. *B,* Within the first 24 hours the dead tissue of the flank was excised. It was necessary to remove skin, subcutaneous tissue, a large amount of muscle mass, and some bone. The fascia overlying the right kidney was exposed. *C,* Complete wound coverage achieved. The right kidney is supported only by fascia, subcutaneous tissue, and skin. Further reconstructive procedures will be necessary. This patient received 60,000 volts, was in the hospital 60 days, required 60 pints of blood, and lost 60 pounds in weight. Massive electrical injuries require early excision of dead tissue.

injury than is apparent at first inspection. Necrosis of blood vessel walls frequently leads to secondary hemorrhage. The histologic appearance of the dead muscle varies. Immediate heat coagulative changes give a pale appearance to the muscle. As time progresses, some muscle becomes soft. The death of muscle bundles is usually very uneven. It is not infrequent after the first 5 or 6 days to find nonviable muscle present where there is a good nutrient artery in normal conditions supplying the muscle bundle. One of the delayed effects of electrical injury, especially about the head, is the development of cataracts.[7]

Electrothermal burns that result from the electrical generation of heat outside the skin, such as flash or arc burns, occur by the leaping of an electric arc from the conductor to the skin. These are mainly associated with high-tension current. They are severe burns of the skin caused by high-intensity heat of short duration.

Flame burns resulting from the ignition of clothing by electrical sparks or arcing are associated with electrical injury, the lesion varying according to the type of accident. Many times all three types of injury may be evident in the same patient.

The treatment of electrothermal burns and flame burns associated with ignition of clothing is the same as for any similar thermal injury. The management of a true electrical injury is entirely different. Such an injury must be treated more like a crush injury. Renal damage is more common, and therefore massive replacement therapy is essential. In many instances, the use of an osmotic diuretic is indicated. Electrical injury frequently requires the use of whole blood in the first 24 hours. If there is a massive amount of dead tissue, an emergency operation to amputate the part or remove the dead tissue may be necessary.[5]

One of the most important factors in the management of the local wound is the incision of the overlying damaged skin to ascertin whether or not there is deeper injury such as dead muscle. If dead muscle is present, it must be excised. Failure to remove extensively damaged muscle may lead to clostridial myositis and death. After excision, a dressing should be applied and the wound reinspected with possible further débridement 4 days later (Fig. 19).

With small, low-intensity electrical injuries the areas should be kept clean and observed for several days. Many of these heal without much difficulty. Areas with moderate electrical injury may be observed until they are well demarcated at 7 or 8 days after injury and then excised.[25]

SELECTED REFERENCES

Artz, C. P., and Moncrief, J. A.: The Treatment of Burns, 2nd ed. Philadelphia, W. B. Saunders Company, 1969.
This is a rather concise treatise primarily on the treatment of burns. It is up-to-date and written in easily understandable language. It covers the entire field of burns from the practical aspect of management. Most of the data and treatment practices are derived from work at the Army Burn Center at Brooke Army Hospital, Fort Sam Houston, Texas. It is composed of 17 chapters and includes such topics as musculoskeletal changes in burns, anesthesia in the severely burned patient, and office treatment of burns, as well as the general problems of initial care, replacement therapy, metabolic responses, and grafting. It has a particularly good chapter on the pathology of burns.

Feller, I.: International Bibliography on Burns. Ann Arbor, American Burn Research Corporation, University of Michigan, 1969.
This is a very detailed bibliography on burns. It includes an excellent reference guide to anyone who is interested in looking up various facets of burn research or the methods of treatment of burns in different countries. It is kept up-to-date with supplements, the most recent of which appeared in 1971. The entire book with supplements is about 485 pages.

Lynch, J. B., and Lewis, S. R. (Eds.): Symposium on the Treatment of Burns. St. Louis, The C. V. Mosby Company, 1973.
This is a symposium on the treatment of burns presented and then put together under the sponsorship of the Educational Foundation of the American Society of Plastic and Reconstructive Surgeons. Drs. Lynch and Lewis are outstanding plastic surgeons who have spent an abundant part of their lives studying and treating burned patients. They have brought together some of the real leaders in burn care, and this volume is an overall dissertation on the most important facets of burns. It has sections on pathophysiology, anesthesia, electrical injury, burn unit patient team interaction, silver nitrate and Sulfamylon, silver sulfadiazine, gentamicin, isolation systems, and skeletal suspension. It contains some of the most up-to-date material currently available in book form.

Matter, P., Barclay, T. L., and Koníčková, Z. (Eds.): Research in Burns (Transactions of the Third International Congress on Research in Burns, Prague, September 1970). Berne, Hans Huber Medical Publisher, 1971.
This book provides some of the most up-to-date information on burns, since it is a compendium of all the papers presented at the most recent International Congress on Burns. It is a very well edited book with a limited number of illustrations. It contains approximately 150 articles, which include most of the data on metabolic response and burn wound management that one might expect from investigators from all over the world. There are particularly good sections on skin replacement and local treatment. It is of more value for the physician interested in a particular facet of investigative work in burns than for the clinician.

Moncrief, J. A.: Burns. N. Engl. J. Med., 288:444–454, 1973.
This is a two-part article, written as Medical Progress in the New England Journal of Medicine to bring the pathophysiologic concepts surrounding burns up to date. This superb article is a summary of our current knowledge on resuscitation, burn wound sepsis, topical therapy, evaporative water loss, pulmonary changes, toxic factors, and Curling's ulcer. Dr. Moncrief spent months covering 14,000 articles on burns published since 1964. It is a great compendium of our knowledge of the body's response to burn injury.

Monafo, W. W.: The Treatment of Burns. St. Louis, Warren H. Green, Inc., 1971.
This is a small book of 267 pages dealing primarily with the treatment of burns. It covers techniques that have evolved from individuals who were taught to treat burns by the late Carl Moyer. It has some excellent chapters in it on burn shock and wound care, and it is filled with practical techniques in the care of the burned patient.

Muir, I. F. K., and Barclay, T. L.: Burns and Their Treatment. Chicago, Year Book Medical Publishers, 1962.
This brief book on burns, of about 150 pages, is a very practical treatment manual and outlines in explicit fashion the way burns are treated in most of the burn centers in Great Britain. There is little concerning the pathophysiology of burns except that associated with fluid replacement in the early periods. It has an excellent section on burns of special areas.

Polk, H. C., Jr., and Stone, H. H.: Contemporary Burn Management. Boston, Little, Brown and Company, 1971.
This 444-page volume containing 30 chapters is written by a variety of scientists, many of whom present alternative viewpoints. The entire volume is on care and techniques of care, including some very special cares on various methods of topical wound care. The section on grafting is outstanding.

Wilmore, D. W., Long, J. M., Mason, A. D., Jr., Skreen, R. W., and Pruitt, B. A., Jr.: Catecholamines; mediator of the hypermetabolic response to trauma. Ann. Surg., 180:653–669, 1974.
This is an article concerning the effect of catecholamines. It presents a new discovery as to the mediator of the hypermetabolic response in surgical injury. Undoubtedly it will go down in history as a classic on burns. For a clear understanding of how the body's physiologic mechanisms handle burn injury, this offers the most up-to-date information available.

REFERENCES

1. Arturson, G.: Pathophysiologic aspects of the burn syndrome with special reference to liver injury and alterations of capillary permeability. Acta Chir. Scand. (Suppl.), *274*:1, 1961.
2. Artz, C. P.: A symposium on burns. J. Trauma, *5*:241, 1965.
3. Artz, C. P.: Historical aspects of burn management. Surg. Clin. North Am., *50*:1193, 1970.
4. Artz, C. P., and Moncrief, J. A.: The Treatment of Burns. Philadelphia, W. B. Saunders Company, 1969.
5. Baxter, C. R.: Present concepts in the management of major electrical injury. Surg. Clin. North Am., *50*:1401, 1970.
6. Fox, C. L., Jr.: Silver sulfadiazine—a new topical therapy for Pseudomonas in burns. Arch. Surg., *96*:184, 1968.
7. Jaffe, R. H.: Electropathology. Arch. Pathol., *5*:837, 1928.
8. Jelenko, C.: Studies in burns. I. Water loss from the body surface. Ann. Surg., *165*:83, 1967.
9. Kaplin, I., and White, W. L.: Incisional decompression of circumferential burns. Plast. Reconstr. Surg., *28*:609, 1961.
10. Lee, A. B., and Kinney, J. M.: Ventilatory management of the pulmonary burn. Ann. N. Y. Acad. Sci., *150*:738, 1968.
11. Leidberg, N. C.-F., Reiss, E., and Artz, C. P.: Infection in burns. III. Septicemia, a common cause of death. Surg. Gynecol. Obstet., *99*:151, 1954.
12. MacMillan, B. G.: The use of mesh grafting in treating burns. Surg. Clin. North Am., *501*:1347, 1970.
13. Moncrief, J. A.: Complications of burns. Ann. Surg., *147*:443, 1958.
14. Moncrief, J. A.: Topical therapy. Surg. Clin. North Am., *50*:1301, 1970.
15. Moncrief, J. A., Lindberg, R. B., Switzer, W. E., and Pruitt, B. A.: The use of a topical sulfonamide in the control of burn wound sepsis. J. Trauma, *6*:407, 1966.
16. Moncrief, J. A., and Mason, A. D., Jr.: Evaporative water loss in the burned patient. J. Trauma, *4*:180, 1964.
17. Czaja, A. J., McAlhany, J. C., Jr., Andes, W. A., and Pruitt, B. A., Jr.: Acute gastric disease after cutaneous thermal injury. A.M.A. Arch. Surg., *110*:600, 1975.
18. Moyer, C. A., Brentano, L., Gravens, D. L., Margraf, H. W., and Monafo, W. W.: Treatment of large human burns with 0.5 per cent silver nitrate solution. Arch. Surg., *90*:812, 1965.
19. Moyer, C. A., Margraf, H. W., and Monafo, W. W., Jr.: Burn shock and extravascular sodium deficiency—treatment with Ringer solution with lactate. Arch. Surg., *90*:799, 1965.
20. Munster, A. M.: Alterations of the host defense mechanism in burns. Surg. Clin. North Am., *50*:1217, 1970.
21. Ofeigsson, O. J.: Water cooling: First aid treatment for scalds and burns. Surgery, *57*:391, 1965.
22. Order, S. E., and Moncrief, J. A.: The Burn Wound. Springfield, Ill., Charles C Thomas, Publisher, 1965.
23. Roe, C. F.: Metabolic problems in burned patients. Evaporative water and heat loss. J. Trauma, *10*:180, 1964.
24. Skoog, T.: Electrical injuries. J. Trauma, *10*:816, 1970.
25. Sturim, H. S.: The treatment of electrical burns. Surg. Gynecol. Obstet., *128*:129, 1969.

16

PRINCIPLES OF OPERATIVE SURGERY: ANTISEPSIS, TECHNIQUE, SUTURES, AND DRAINS

Raymond W. Postlethwait, M.D.

ANTISEPSIS AND TECHNIQUE

Wound infection has been a major problem for surgeons since surgery began. An elaborate ritual has gradually evolved that surgeons and their associates observe in their efforts to prevent wound infections. Despite these efforts, infections still develop, and although our understanding of sepsis has improved, many infections in clean wounds are still unexplainable; our knowledge is obviously incomplete. In addition, the scope of surgery has broadened so greatly that operations are performed when resistance is known to be decreased. Indeed, in operations such as transplantation of organs, the immune mechanisms may have had to be deliberately suppressed. Finally, there is no general agreement on all the factors relative to the cause and prevention of infections.

Wound infections may be classified in many ways, such as by the causative organism, the type of operation, the tissue or organ involved, or the extent of the infection. The latter causes difficulty in the interpretation of the reported incidence of postoperative sepsis, as many authors consider only a purulent discharge to indicate infection. Others may include a stitch abscess or even erythema of the wound edges as infection.

Many papers have been written on various aspects of wound infections, so that only representative ones will be noted. Antisepsis and the prevention of infections will be discussed under the general headings of (1) the infecting organisms, (2) the patient and his disease, (3) environment, equipment, and personnel, (4) conduct of the operation, and (5) the role of antibiotics.

HISTORICAL ASPECTS

The situation regarding wound infection should be put in perspective up to the time of Lister, the logical starting point for any discussion of wound sepsis. Surgeons may be accustomed to the idea that wound suppuration had always been as rampant as indicated by the writings in the middle of the nineteenth century. Actually, for centuries wounds had been closed with sutures, adhesive straps, and bandages, with primary healing following more often than not. In the latter part of the eighteenth century and first half of the nineteenth century, hospitals were being built in increasing numbers and the sick and injured crowded into them before even the rudiments of isolation precautions were understood. In addition, the development of firearms and a growing humanitarian concern for the wounded conscripts brought to hospitals the injured who previously would have been slain or left to die on the battlefield. As a result, hospitalism or infections of all degrees of severity became of increasing concern as the morbidity and mortality became truly horrendous.

Surgeons still attempted primary closure, but less and less frequently. Finally the wounds were packed open in anticipation of laudable pus but with the hope of eventual recovery. In hospitals, only the most urgently required operations were performed. It was recognized that the same dangers were not associated with wounds treated away from the hospital.

Two men, separately and unknown to each other, anticipated the eventual outcome. In America, Oliver Wendell Holmes and, in Vienna, Ignaz Philipp Semmelweis were appalled by the high mortality caused by puerperal fever. Strangely enough, in each instance the death from infection of a physician, injured during participation in the autopsy on an infected subject, brought their attention to the fact that infection was being transmitted directly. Both excluded in detail other causes, such as the air and the food, in their classic papers. Both recognized that something was being transferred from the infected patient to the uninfected, usually by the attending physician's hands. Both urged washing of the hands, changes of clothing, and even remaining away from patients after attending one with puerperal sepsis. Finally, both were doubted by many of their colleagues and forced to defend their concept.

After Pasteur's discovery of bacteria, Lister was prompt to recognize the implications in wound infections, publishing his first description of the "antiseptic principle" in 1867. The system of dilute carbolic acid dressings, sprays, and soaks was not promptly accepted by other physicians and Lister had to defend his methods repeatedly. The Germans, however, were receptive, and this eventually led to the introduction by von Bergmann of steam sterilization in 1886 and of an elaborate aseptic ritual in 1891. By 1899, Kocher was able to report a 2.3 per cent infection rate in clean wounds.

The reception in America of these developments between 1867 and 1900 was slow, as the average American surgeon had insufficient basic biologic background to accept the germ theory, a necessary prerequisite to proper application of the new techniques. In the late 1860s, however, several American surgeons became strong proponents of Listerism: Andrews in Chicago, Yandell in Louisville, Weisse in New York, and Warren in Boston. Opponents as prominent as Gross of Philadelphia made acceptance slow, but publications, particularly by younger surgeons, gradually influenced opinion. The list includes Schuppert, Agnew, Keen, Grandle, Gerster, Homans, and Penn.

Halsted[21] was a champion of aseptic and meticulous surgical technique. In his paper in 1913, he describes his early use of silk, starting about 1882, which was prompted by the technique used by Kocher. The same article describes Halsted's role in development of the surgeon's glove.

Sutures have been used for centuries. The Edwin Smith Papyrus written nearly 4000 years ago describes the use of sutures. Suśruta around 600 B.C. described many materials for suturing, and the contributions since then have been many.

THE INFECTING ORGANISMS

Type

Early in the 1950s, many surgeons were alarmed by the apparent increase in postoperative wound infec-

tions, particularly those due to *Staphylococcus aureus*. This was attributed, at least in part, to emergence of antibiotic-resistant strains, especially in the hospital-acquired group. In some hospitals, as many as 80 per cent of postoperative infections were caused by *Staphylococcus aureus*. A careful analysis was made of four standard operations (herniorrhaphy, hysterectomy, gastrectomy, and appendectomy) performed over a 21-year period in a representative hospital.[4] Slight variation in the infection rate did occur from year to year, but in this institution there was actually no increase in the percentage of infections, nor was there an increase in those due to *Staphylococcus aureus*.

The organisms recovered from 100 consecutive wound infections have been reported and the distribution may be fairly typical for most hospitals.[14] Of the 100 infections, 48 were due to Staphylococcus, 3 were caused by Streptococcus, and the remaining were produced by a number of enteric bacteria. The number of times each was cultured was *Escherichia coli* 20, *Proteus vulgaris* 8, Pseudomonas 8, *Aerobacter aerogenes* 8, enterococci or anaerobic streptococci 33, *Bacteroides fusiformis* 4, *Clostridium welchii* 2, Corynebacterium 2, and *Bacillus subtilis* 1. Another representative study of 247 infections over a 5-year period recovered *Staphylococcus aureus* from 138, hemolytic streptococci from 6, and enteric organisms as follows: *Escherichia coli* 99, Proteus 25, and Pseudomonas 11.[32]

The incidence of various organisms will vary with a number of factors, one of these being the intensity of the efforts to prevent infection.[25] A study along these lines demonstrated in a 3-year period that the wound infections caused by *Staphylococcus aureus* decreased from 83 per cent in the first year to 52 per cent in the third, while infections due to the gram-negative organisms increased. At the same time, the overall infection rate decreased from 2.02 to 1.14 per cent.

It should be noted that recently organisms formerly considered as nonpathogenic have been recognized as the cause of infections. An example is the emergence of Serratia as the causative agent in infected arterial grafts and septicemia. In addition, reports are now ap-

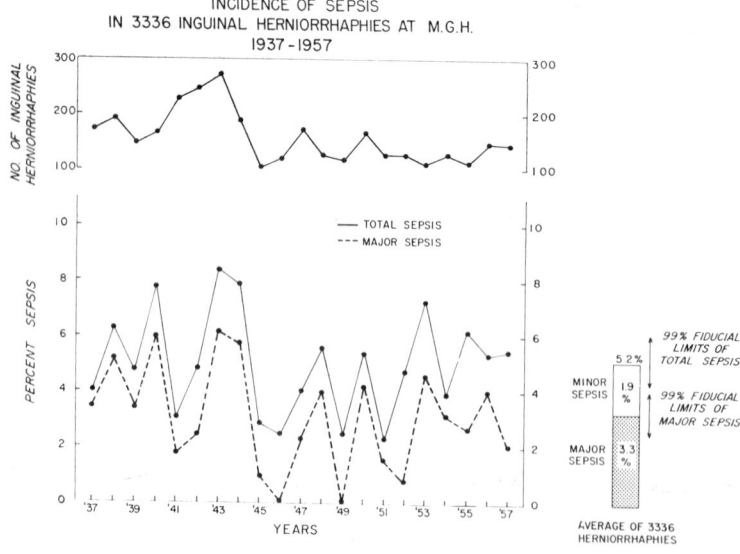

Figure 1. An analysis of the incidence of wound infections over a 20-year period in one hospital shows variation from year to year but no real increase. (From Barnes, B. A., et al.: Ann. Surg., 154:585, 1961.)

pearing indicating the important role of anaerobic organisms in many surgical infections.[39]

Number of Organisms

The type and virulence of the organism will influence the development of infection, as will the number of organisms present. The minimum pus-forming dose of *Staphylococcus pyogenes* by intradermal injection in human volunteers has been determined.[17] No pus formation was ever seen with *fewer than 1 million organisms,* and the minimum pus-forming dose was estimated to be between *2 and 8 million organisms to cause infection consistently.* Preformed toxin or excess plasma in the injection site did not alter the dose required, but a silk suture did (to as few as 100 organisms), and the virulence enhancement by a suture was therefore estimated to be of the order of at least 10,000 times. Exactly why the foreign body is so deleterious is not clear. It was noted that only 7 hours of logarithmic growth are required to convert a hundred to a million cocci. Perhaps in some way the foreign body reaction interferes with sterilization of a small inoculum.

In experimental animals, it has also been demonstrated that the viability in days of a small number of organisms in the tissues is a function of the inoculum size.[27] A single fine silk tie about a small vessel will cause inflammation well above the control level and fewer than 100 organisms on a suture will cause pus formation in over half the animals. Incisions in guinea pigs contaminated with staphylococci in increasing doses gives a sigmoid-shaped curve of the degree of infection related to the number of bacteria.

The body can, therefore, dispose of a huge number of virulent bacteria in normal circumstances, provided there is no interference with this process. Bacteria are a necessary but not a sufficient condition for the development of septic complications, and other factors must be present.[4] The wound surface may be visualized as presenting a gradient of resistance at different points ranging from excellent, where there is minimal cell destruction and good blood supply, to poor, where there is strangulation of tissue and poor blood supply.[27]

Frequency of Contamination

One classification of wounds according to the probability of contamination is as follows: (1) *clean,* operation under aseptic circumstances, no break in technique, no transection of gastroenteric, tracheobronchial, or genitourinary systems, and no apparent inflammatory reaction in the vicinity; (2) *clean-contaminated,* same as preceding but with opening or transection of viscera containing bacteria; (3) *contaminated,* as a result of violence, associated with gross spillage from a hollow viscus, or complicated by a major break in technique; (4) *dirty,* continual drainage of fecal, tracheobronchial, or genitourinary discharge or actual drainage of purulent material. Contamination is practically inevitable in the last two groups and is mainly a matter of degree. The first two groups theoretically might be sterile, but experience has shown that even in clean operations, careful bacteriologic studies will yield bacteria from most wounds. For example, in one extensive epidemiologic study, cultures of 350 wounds in clean operations resulted in bacterial growth in 68 per cent.[26] In another very careful study seeking the source of contaminating staphylococci, 50 wounds were cultured after the fascia was closed. All wounds contained bacteria and 46 had coagulase-positive staphylococci, with an average of 5.8 strains (phage types) per wound. The surgeon must therefore assume that all operative wounds will contain bacteria.

Sources of Bacteria

The sources of organisms that may contaminate the wound are numerous; a few will be noted here and others below. The patient himself is an obvious source, as well as the hospital ward personnel. Outside the hospital only 15 to 20 per cent of the people are nasal carriers of virulent staphylococci, whereas in the hospital environment, about 40 per cent will be carriers on any one examination and 80 per cent if repeated nasal cultures are made. In spite of good housekeeping, the organisms are found throughout the ward, on food tables, beds, and similar locations, and some investigators believe that sepsis due to *Staphylococcus aureus* is most frequently associated with ward cross infection.

A study of the staphylococcal epidemiology of a surgical ward showed a random fluctuation of staphylococcal strains, and the only consistent source of contamination was the open infection.[6] If the patient had an open infection, the area around him was heavily contaminated. The staphylococcus appeared to obey the rule of inverse square: the greater the distance from a septic focus, the less likely the infecting strain is to be found. It has been noted repeatedly that antibiotic therapy has little or no effect on the total incidence of carriers.

The patient may, therefore, carry with him to the operating room many organisms capable of causing

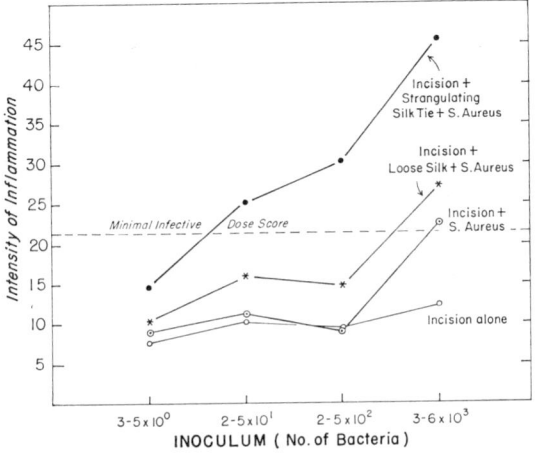

Figure 2. The degree of inflammation is related to the size of the inoculum; a foreign body in the form of a piece of loose silk increases the inflammatory reaction, and avascular tissue distal to a strangulating silk tie causes a marked increase in the inflammatory reaction. (From Howe, C. W.: Surg. Gynecol. Obstet., *123*:507, 1966.)

sepsis, and these may be in his nose and throat and on his skin, gown, bedclothes, and stretcher. Some of the contamination can be prevented by measures such as isolation and rigid housekeeping; some cannot be prevented. Meticulous measures designed to prevent infection may include, among other things, scrupulous preparation of the patient, a transition zone into the operating room with transfer to another stretcher, a clothing change, and further preparation in the operating room.

The possibility of infecting a closed wound from ward sources is more remote but does exist. Infections will seldom develop in clean wounds when dressings are removed after 48 hours and the wound left exposed. Years ago, it was shown experimentally that the surface of a carefully closed wound swabbed with bacteria within 6 hours nearly always became infected.[16] With increasing time, the percentage and severity of infections steadily decreased until about the fifth day, when it was no longer possible to cause infection.

A number of interesting epidemiologic studies have been reported, some a search for a single specific source of infection and others a general investigation of a hospital. For example, an increase in the infection rate leading to an intensive study may result in the eventual identification of one surgeon, nurse, or anesthetist as a nasal carrier of the pathogenic staphylococci. One important study attempted to identify the source of the staphylococci cultured from the patient's wound before closure.[6] Cultures of numerous possible sources and phage typing of the staphylococci recovered led to the following conclusions. The hands of the scrub team were the source in 6 per cent of the cases and the nose and throat of the scrub team in 14 per cent. The nose or skin of the patient was the source in 50 per cent and the air just over the wound in 68 per cent. As 5.8 strains were cultured from each wound, more than one source was possible. If the strain was found in the air and any other specific source, it was attributed to the latter.

The above discussion pertains mainly to clean wounds and to infection by staphylococci. In operations when a hollow viscus such as the colon is opened, the source of the bacteria is evident and the measures that may be used in an attempt to prevent infection are more obvious. In addition, factors such as a transient bacteremia from any of several sources may lead to wound infection.

Other Factors Influencing Infection

Certain specific and general factors that are determinants in the infection process should be noted here. One important study on nonspecific defense reactions in bacterial infections is of particular interest.[33] This was based on the fact that defense against infection entails either prevention of any lodgment of the pathogen whatsoever or its destruction in the primary lodgment before it can produce a manifest infection. The experimental model employed provided a fairly precise means of quantitating the degree of inflammatory reaction; i.e., the mean diameters of the mature lesions were roughly linear to the log dose of bacteria. This facilitated numerical comparison of infectivity

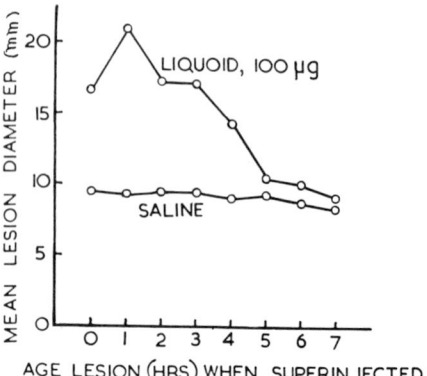

Figure 3. Superinjection experiment of Miles, showing the infection enhancement effect of Liquoid, an anticoagulant and anticomplement, which decreases with time. (From Miles, A. A.: Ann. N.Y. Acad. Sci., 66:356, 1956.)

under the influence of modifying agents. The studies included the effect of dehydration shock and of local injection of epinephrine or Liquoid (an anticoagulant and anticomplement; chemically, sodium polyanetholsulfonate). The degree of enhancement of the inflammatory reaction was from twofold to 100,000-fold. Accordingly, the body agents inhibited (blood supply or blood constituents) are responsible for killing from 50 to 99.99 per cent of the bacteria. The most important finding was that the decisive period was the first 2 or 3 hours after bacterial lodgment. This indicated that, although the discernible changes of infection in the wound may develop only after 24 hours or more, the ultimate presence or degree of infection is determined within the first few hours.

The same phenomenon was demonstrated in a study of the effect of antibiotics on experimental wounds with dermal injections of bacteria.[6] Penicillin, for example, given an hour before or at the time of bacterial lodgment afforded protection so that the lesion was no larger than the control. Penicillin injected an hour after lodgment gave a moderate effect; by 3 hours, the penicillin had little effect. The importance of this short period of effective antibiotic activity is obvious.

Some of the general factors in the etiology of sepsis either cannot be controlled or can be modified only to a limited extent. The duration of hospitalization preoperatively has a direct effect. The Cooperative Study Group[12] found an infection rate of 6.0 per cent in patients hospitalized 2 days or less, while the rate was 14.7 per cent in those hospitalized 3 weeks or more before operation. This must be related, at least in part, to the high carrier rate in hospital wards, as noted above. The duration of operation also is a direct factor; wound cultures show a gradual buildup in the number of bacteria recovered up to 3 hours, when there is a leveling off.[6] Some reports have related the place of the patient on the operating schedule to the infection rate, but this is largely a reflection of the activity in the operating room. Emergency operations are more likely to be followed by infection. The season of the year had no effect on the incidence of infection in the Cooperative Study,[12] but others found an increase during cold weather.

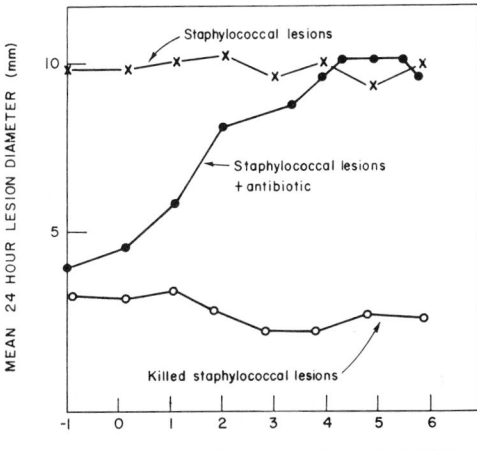

Figure 4. A demonstration of the principle that many determinants of wound infection act within the first 3 hours. Prophylactic antibiotics should be given before bacterial lodgment when possible. (From Burke, J. F.: Surgery, 50:161, 1961.)

THE PATIENT AND HIS DISEASE

Many of these factors are such that the surgeon cannot alter the probability of infection. Age, for example, appears to be directly related to the frequency of postoperative infection. Obesity has been found to be a contributing factor by some[12] but not by others. Certain diseases such as diabetes, cirrhosis, leukemia, and uremia have been associated with increased risk of infection.

The disease and the operation required may be such that opportunities to prevent infection are greatly modified. These are taken into account in the classification of operations noted above. Drainage of an abscess associated with perforated appendicitis gives no chance to keep the wound per se from becoming infected, although measures are taken to limit and prevent spread of the infection. Even with great care, resections of the colon will lead to more wound infections than the cleaner operations, since the colon is the locus of a large concentration of bacteria.

A discussion of resistance and immunity is beyond the scope of this summary, but advances in this area in preventing infection are suggested by several reviews.[6, 18] Some indications of the range of possible alterations can be obtained from one classification of the deficiencies or abnormalities in host resistance, which was as follows:[1]

  I. Abnormalities of deposition of phagocytic cells in contaminated foci
    A. Abnormality of mediators
      1. Complement deficiency
      2. Possible factor in old age or prematurity
    B. Abnormality of vascular response
      1. Drug-induced
      2. Radiation-induced
      3. Nutritional deficiencies
    C. Abnormality of blood flow to affected area
      1. Anatomic variation
      2. Foreign bodies, hematoma, necrotic tissue

      3. Low flow states
        a. Shock, injury
        b. Drug-induced
        c. Mechanical obstruction
  II. Abnormalities involving opsonic substances
    A. Antibody deficiencies
      1. Lack of prior experience
      2. Hereditary abnormalities
        a. Agammaglobulinemia
        b. Dysgammaglobulinemia
      3. Acquired abnormalities
        a. Decreased synthesis
        b. Consumptive states
    B. Complement deficiencies
      1. Hereditary
      2. Acquired, consumptive, or drug-induced, especially locally
  III. Abnormalities of phagocytic cells
    A. Insufficient production or release
    B. Abnormalities of phagocytosis
    C. Abnormalities of intracellular killing
      1. Hereditary
      2. Acquired
        a. Abnormal degranulation
        b. Abnormal lysosomal enzymes
      3. Cyclic variation in normal persons

An example of possible preventive or therapeutic application in the immunologic sphere is the recent development of a vaccine for Pseudomonas, containing purified antigens of seven immunotypes. A dramatic decrease in mortality due to Pseudomonas sepsis in burned patients has been reported when this vaccine has been employed. As has been pointed out, however, this approach offers difficulties because of the many different antigenic groups of organisms; for example, there are more than 150 different serologic types of *Escherichia coli.*[18] Another example is a recent report in which immunologic capacity was determined in preoperative patients considered to have a high risk of infection, the possibility being suggested that specific or nonspecific stimulation of cell-mediated immunity might alter their risks of infection.[30] Still another pertinent study showed the cyclic variation in neutrophil bacterial killing ability, although phagocytosis remained active. Periods of impaired killing correlated well with septic episodes. A defect in intracellular enzymes was suggested as the cause.[2]

THE ENVIRONMENT, EQUIPMENT, AND PERSONNEL

In spite of improvements in operating rooms, the possibility of complete sterilization remains remote. A number of factors have contributed to the reduction in the number of bacteria, such as isolation of the operating suite from all other hospital traffic. A most significant advance has been air conditioning that will deliver air under positive pressure to obtain a complete change of air every 5 to 10 minutes. The air is forced through filters which will remove particulate matter larger than 0.3 μ, so that the air is essentially sterile. The air does not remain sterile, however, as careful studies have shown.[10] With an Anderson sampler, an average of 3.8 viable bacteria per cubic foot of air was recovered, with an average of 0.015 coagulase-positive staphylococci per cubic foot.

Hart[23] since 1936 has advocated the use of *ultraviolet radiation* to reduce the number of airborne bacteria and thereby decrease the frequency of clean wound infections. The killing of airborne organisms has been amply demonstrated by Hart and confirmed by the Cooperative Study[12] designed to test the efficiency of ultraviolet radiation. The latter study showed a reduction in infections in refined clean wounds from 3.8 per cent in the controls to 2.9 per cent in the radiated group. The rates for all operations were 7.5 and 7.4 per cent, respectively. Hart has reported an infection rate of only 0.34 per cent in more than 23,000 clean operations.

The cleaning of the operating room, cleaning and sterilization of instruments, preparation and sterilization of packs, and the many other minutiae that are the duties of the operating room staff are too extensive to discuss here. Recent improvements include the ultrasonic instrument cleaner, effective gas sterilization, and better detergent germicidal solutions. Sources of difficulty existent in the past, such as unsterile sutures, are now rarely, if ever, encountered. Other factors and possible sources of infection should be noted, such as preparation of the skin, gowns, drapes, gloves, and masks.

It has been demonstrated convincingly that the patient's skin cannot be completely sterilized.[29] The transient bacteria on the skin surface can be killed with appropriate solutions, but the resident bacteria about the hair follicles and in the sebaceous glands cannot be destroyed. During the operation, the resident bacteria come to the surface and this plus the bacterial fallout from the air is a source of infection. The ideal antiseptic agent should therefore be effective against all micro-organisms, both resident and transient flora, and the effect should be sustained throughout the operation. It should be easily applied, nonirritating, and nonsensitizing, and should not be inactivated by common materials such as alcohol, soap, or organic matter.

The mercurial antiseptics have low bactericidal power and are not generally used. Ethyl alcohol, 70 per cent by weight, is an effective germicidal. Benzalkonium chloride, a quaternary ammonium compound, is active in fairly high dilutions, nonirritating, stable, a good wetting agent, and relatively inexpensive. It is incompatible with soap and is counteracted by organic matter, especially blood serum. Hexachlorophene is a phenol derivative that is highly bactericidal but acts slowly and is inactivated by alcohol.

Davies in 1839 first referred to the use of iodine in wounds.[28] In recent years, iodine complexed with polyvinylpyrrolidone has been used most extensively. The germicidal activity covers the gamut of bacterial strains and most pathogenic fungi. The iodine is released at a very slow rate, prolonging the germicidal action at least 4 hours after a single application. It is not inhibited by pus, but the activity may be shortened by blood or serum. Little irritation and no sensitivity occur. The effectiveness has been demonstrated by bacteriologic studies.[28]

The same principles of preparation of the patient's skin apply to the scrub of the surgical team's hands and arms. Studies have shown that the number of bacteria on the hands can be reduced by scrubbing with the iodine compound just discussed. The reduction may plateau at about 80 to 90 per cent of the original count, although one study showed 100 per cent effectiveness in the majority of the participants.[28] Restoration of the bacterial count on the hands, while gloved, is slow but does occur.

Although the hands may not be a frequent source of contamination, many studies, including our own, have shown that approximately a third of the gloves worn during an operation are punctured or torn. One interesting study showed that as many as 18,960 staphylococci could pass through a single needle hole from the gloved finger in 20 minutes.[11] This information indicates that the hands of the scrub team are a possible source of contamination that can be controlled, at least in part, by attention to scrub technique and to maintenance of intact gloves.

Drapes for the patient and gowns for the scrub team are important in prevention of sepsis. The time-

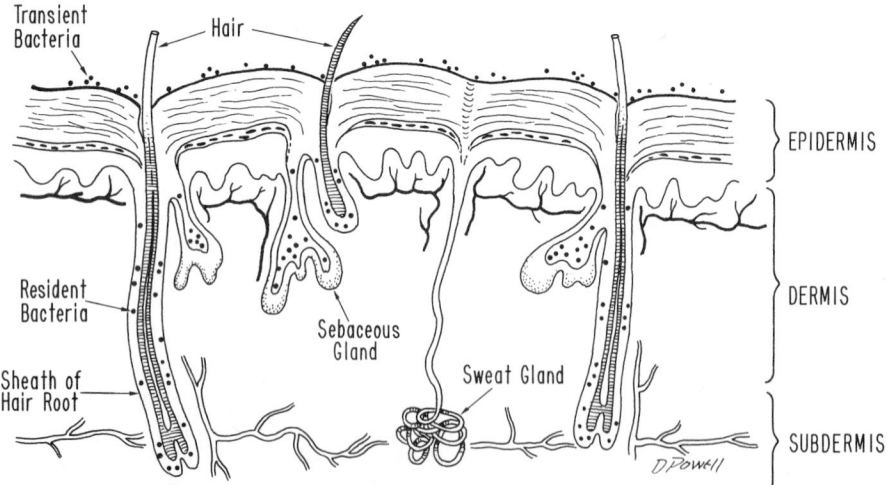

Figure 5. Lovell's concept of the transient bacteria on the surface, which are easily removed, and the deep resident bacteria, which cannot be destroyed by skin antiseptics.

honored cloth draps have the disadvantage of allowing penetration by bacteria when wet. Waterproof paper drapes are now available. Bacteriologic studies showed little or no penetration of paper drapes, compared to marked bacterial penetration of muslin.[15] For the patient, an additional safety measure is the application of an adherent plastic sheet over the operative area, through which the incision is made.

The possibility of isolating the operative area of the patient in the completely sterile atmosphere of a large plastic balloon has been explored, a maneuver used in germ-free animal research. Although this offers possibilities, the technique may be too expensive and cumbersome.

Bacteriologic studies of operating rooms have repeatedly shown that the number of bacteria in the air and indirectly in the wound is related to the activity and number of personnel in the room.[19] With careful cleaning, few bacteria come from the floor, tables, lights, and other equipment, and the source must be the persons in the room. Many bacteria are shed from the skin, particularly from the area below the waist. Impervious clothing has been suggested, but the comfort of the operating team limits the extent of application of this preventive measure.

Face masks are crucial barriers in the transmission of bacteria from the nose and mouth. A precise method of determining the filtering efficiency of masks has been developed.[19] One of the fiberglass masks available showed a filtering efficiency of 99.7 per cent. Other masks ranged in efficiency down to 15 per cent for one of the gauze masks. Other factors are, of course, involved, such as the fit of the mask to the face and the comfort of breathing through the mask.

CONDUCT OF THE OPERATION

An extensive discussion of surgical technique would be inappropriate here. Basically, however, from the standpoint of technique, any factor that may interfere with wound healing will enhance the possibility of wound infection. Some of these factors have been dramatically demonstrated, such as the experiment noted above in which a foreign body, a single silk suture, had an enhancement factor of at least 10,000 times. Other examples include the experiments demonstrating that wounds made with a knife heal better and are less susceptible to infection than those made by an electrosurgical knife.

Meticulous operative technique is largely a matter of respect for tissues and awareness of the healing process. Incisions and dissections are performed with the knife when feasible, as fewer cells are killed than with rough, blunt dissection. Bleeding vessels are clamped with as little adjacent tissue as possible and tied with the finest appropriate ligature to avoid necrosis of a large mass of tissue distal to the tie. Hemostasis is as complete as the particular situation will allow, as a blood clot is a foreign body and an excellent culture medium for bacteria. Sutures are foreign bodies but a necessary adjunct in surgery. The selection of the proper suture is important, but an even greater requirement is the proper use of sutures. Since their function is to appose tissues, the spacing of sutures, the depth of the bite taken, and the tension applied on tying should accomplish this without strangulation of the tissue or excessive foreign body implantation. Exposure of the operative field is important and the proper incision will do much to insure this, but retraction will be required and should be as gentle as possible.

During the course of the operation, if a hollow viscus is to be opened or other sources of contamination are to be exposed, protective gauze or plastic should be used to shield the adjacent normal tissues. In closure, dead space should be eliminated, as this is another fertile ground for bacterial growth. Needless to say, devitalized tissue is removed when possible.

A number of technical maneuvers apply to particular situations. For example, if an abdominal wound has been contaminated and infection is anticipated, the peritoneum and fascia may be closed and the subcutaneous tissues and skin left open to be closed secondarily.

PROPHYLACTIC ANTIBIOTICS

With the advent of bacteriostatic and bactericidal drugs, surgeons hoped that surgical infections, at least in clean wounds, could be completely prevented. This has not proved to be true, and currently most surgeons acknowledge that the complications caused by the antibiotic are greater than the likelihood of infection in clean operations such as herniorrhaphy. In "clean-contaminated" and contaminated operations, prophylactic antibiotics have a definite and beneficial place.

Two factors have bearing on the use of prophylactic antibiotics. First, the surgeon usually does not know the exact type of the potentially infecting bacteria, nor does he know the sensitivity of the organism to the antibiotic selected. Past clinical experience does give some indication of the flora to be expected in many situations, and broad-spectrum antibiotics provide an appropriate drug until sensitivities can be determined. Secondly, the experimental work already noted indicates the great importance of time; within 2 or 3 hours the determination has been made as to whether the bacterial lodgment will be successfully resisted by the tissues or whether infection will develop.[33] Experimentally, the importance of administering the antibiotic before, at the time of, or within 3 hours of the bacterial implantation if the infection is to be prevented or altered has been demonstrated.[6]

The clinical studies reported of prophylactic antibiotic use have frequently been so poorly controlled as to be worthless. Some recent reports are of value. In one study of potentially contaminated operations, three doses were administered, consisting of 600,000 U penicillin G, 1.0 gm. methicillin, and 200 mg. chloramphenicol.[5] One dose was given 1 to 2 hours before operation, one during operation, and one in the recovery room. The wound infection rate was 8 per cent in the treated group and 27 per cent in the placebo group, a result that is statistically significant. A definite beneficial effect has been demonstrated with other drug combinations and also with single antibiotics (penicillin and cephalothin), with essentially the same time schedule of administration. There appears to be little doubt that prophylactic antibiotics, properly chosen and administered, have a potentially important role in the prevention of infection in clean-contaminated wounds.

No controversy exists about the necessity for prompt antibiotic administration in infected patients, such as those with perforated appendicitis with abscess or peritonitis.

Another application of antibiotic prophylaxis is prior to colon surgery, in which a high rate of infection can be anticipated. Some controversy has existed as to the effectiveness, as opposed to the complications, of this antibiotic usage. Two recent randomized studies, however, indicate significant benefit in the prevention of infection. One group administered neomycin and tetracycline[40] and the other gave neomycin and erythromycin base.[35] The drugs should be given over a period of 24 to 36 hours preoperatively and for not more than 48 hours, as emergence of resistant strains may occur. Ulcerative and granulomatous colitis contraindicate these oral antibiotics because of enhanced absorption.

Wound irrigation in the prevention of infection has been practiced for many years. The use of topical antibiotic agents may be of value. In recent experimental studies, a mixture of neomycin sulfate, polymyxin B, and bacitracin was used.[20] Effective results against a variety of organisms were obtained with these poorly absorbed antibiotics. To my knowledge, no well-controlled clinical study has been reported, but the experimental evidence is sufficient to justify clinical application. An important basic principle remains: the most efficient antibiotic cannot compensate for inadequate and poor surgical technique.

SUTURES

The choice of material and size of sutures and ligatures is largely dependent upon the purpose to be achieved. In some situations, any of a variety of sutures may serve equally well, and the choice is then governed by the training, experience, and judgment of the surgeon. In other cases, the range is limited. To illustrate, essentially every type of suture material available has been used successfully for gastrointestinal anastomosis. If, however, the surgeon wishes a precise mucosal approximation in a gastroenterostomy, for example, very fine absorbable suture will serve well to hold the apposition until the rapidly regenerating mucosa is healed. For the seromuscular layer, where the strength of the anastomosis lies, a strong nonabsorbable suture is better, as it will hold

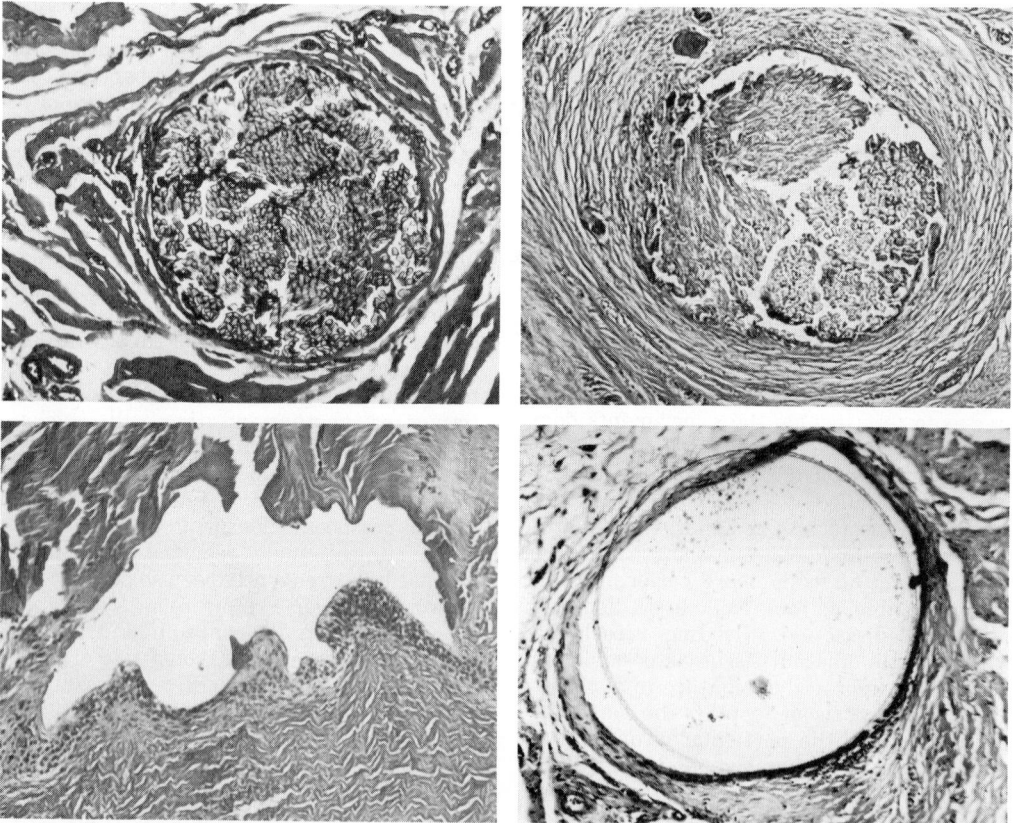

Figure 6. Sutures recovered from patients at second operation or autopsy. *Top left,* Silk from abdominal wall muscles 14 months after operation. *Top right,* Cotton in abdominal scar 2 years after cholecystectomy. *Bottom left,* Site of wire suture from recurrent hernia 6 years after first repair. *Bottom right,* Nylon in abdominal wall 6 months after operation.

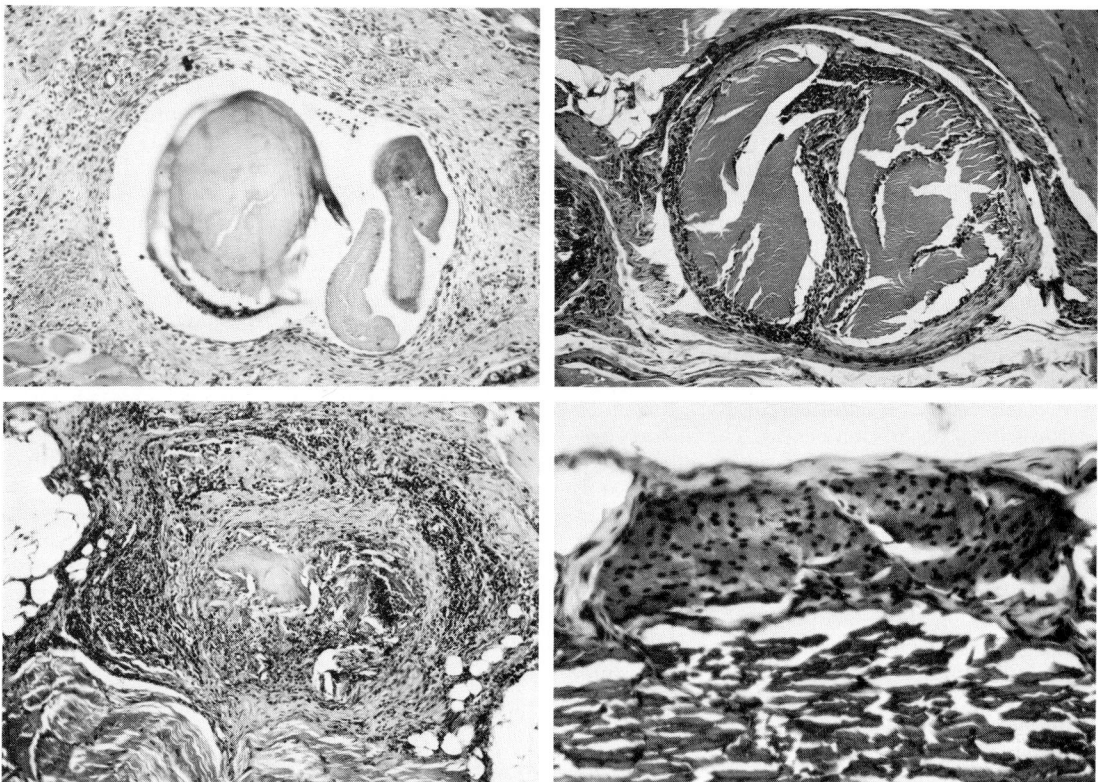

Figure 7. Catgut. *Top left,* Chromic 0000 after 14 days shows fragmentation although absorption has just started. *Top right,* Chromic 00 at 28 days with invasion in cracks in suture by mononuclear cells. *Bottom left,* Plain 00 after 28 days shows a mixed cellular response during absorption. *Bottom right,* The ghostlike cells marking the site of an absorbed chromic suture 4 months after implantation.

until adequate tensile strength returns. An extreme comparison would be cataract surgery, where the suture should be absorbed rapidly, as compared to the anastomosis of the aorta and graft, where the suture should remain and maintain tensile strength forever. It is obviously impossible to list the exact suture for each situation, if for no other reason than the disagreement among surgeons that could be anticipated. In addition, a basic principle is that the method of use of a suture is much more important than the suture itself. Some knowledge of available suture materials is of value, however.

Suture material should have and maintain adequate tensile strength until its purpose is served. The suture should stimulate minimal tissue reaction and should not create a situation favorable to bacterial growth. It should be nonelectrolytic, noncapillary, nonallergenic, and noncarcinogenic. The material should handle comfortably and naturally to the surgeon and a knot should hold securely without fraying or cutting. It should be inexpensive and easily sterilized without alteration. All sutures fulfill some of the criteria and some sutures meet nearly all of the requirements.

Sutures are generally classified as absorbable and nonabsorbable. The absorbable are some form of catgut or the newly developed synthetic polymers and, depending on several factors noted below, disappear from the tissues in a matter of months. Nonabsorbable materials such as silk, cotton, wire, and the other syn-

thetic sutures remain in the tissues indefinitely, although some alteration of the suture may occur.

Prior to a discussion that includes tissue reaction, it should be noted that the histologic reactions to all sutures are essentially the same for the first 5 to 7 days, as these changes are secondary to the trauma of passage of the needle and the suture.

Catgut and Collagen

Chemically, surgical gut or catgut consists essentially of collagen and is obtained from the small intestine, either the submucosal layer of sheep or the serosal layer of cattle. In order mainly to improve uniformity, extruded collagen sutures have been prepared from the deep flexor tendons of cattle. Catgut and collagen may be plain or chromic, the latter being exposed to chromate compounds that produce increased intermolecular bonding, resulting in a suture that is stronger and more slowly absorbed than the plain type. Iodine is also occasionally used in the treatment of these sutures for reasons noted below.

The extruded collagen sutures are smoother and more uniform and have less tendency to fray than catgut, but for practical purposes the two can be considered together. The sutures handle comfortably and hold a knot well. Both are strong, in the 00 size for example, having a straight-pull breaking strength of around 10 pounds and a knot breaking strength of about half this amount. In a recent study of ours, gut implanted in tissues lost about one third of its initial strength by the end of a week. At the end of 4 weeks, chromic gut size 0 had lost 60 per cent of its initial strength and size 000 had lost 66 per cent. With implantation in the same tissue (in this experiment, the abdominal wall muscles of rabbits), a wide range in the rate of loss of tensile strength is found, apparently a biologic variation dependent on the subject's reaction to the suture. The rates are different in other sites, slower in the subcutaneous tissues, for example, and extremely rapid if the suture is exposed to material such as gastric juice. The rate of loss of strength can be decreased to some extent by increasing the chromic acid treatment. Plain gut loses strength more rapidly.

The reaction to gut is similar to that caused by other sutures until absorption begins. The initial reaction consists of histiocytes, lymphocytes, fibroblasts, and a few polymorphonuclear leukocytes and capillaries; gradually these elements are replaced by maturing fibrous tissue. When absorption begins, the mononuclear cells usually become predominant, attached to the surface of the suture, at times invading cracks that develop. In some instances, particularly with plain gut, the reaction is more acute, with polymorphonuclear leukocytes predominating; apparently this reflects the rapidity of absorption. Foreign body giant cells are commonly seen and an occasional animal will show a predominantly eosinophilic reaction. After the gut can no longer be seen, for several weeks the site can be identified by a mass of mononuclear cells with faintly brownish granules in the cytoplasm.

Gut is usually employed in those situations in which a strong suture is needed only during the first week or two of healing, and in those procedures in which absorption of the suture is desirable. Typically, gut is used when a good possibility of infection exists, the rationale being that with infection the gut is absorbed rapidly, whereas a nonabsorbable suture might remain as a focus of infection.

Allergy to gut has been alleged but never convincingly demonstrated. A special form of gut, iodine-treated, has been shown to decrease the suture line implantation of transplantable tumors in experimental animals. Parenthetically, few studies have been directed toward the physiochemical aspects of catgut absorption, although one investigation showed, by histochemical staining techniques, both acid hydrolytic and collagenolytic activity about the suture.[36]

Silk

Silk is a continuous protein filament produced by various silkworms, particularly the species *Bombyx mori*. The silk is usually dyed and coated with a wax or resin. The small fibers are either twisted or braided to produce a suture of the desired size and strength.

Halsted adopted silk as a suture and established the principles for its use after Kocher began using silk because of the high infection rate with catgut. Whipple popularized the use of silk, and today silk remains the most commonly used nonabsorbable suture. Silk handles comfortably and holds a knot well. In like sizes, silk is not quite as strong as gut, and is also weaker than the synthetic sutures, but is a little stronger than cotton. In tissues, silk loses strength slowly; in our studies the loss was to a third of the initial strength in 6 months.

After the initial reaction subsides, the silk suture usually remains compact and is surrounded by a layer of mature connective tissue. Within this at the periphery of the suture almost invariably is a mononuclear reaction, which varies in depth and intensity. The reaction consists of fibroblasts, histiocytes, and lymphocytes with occasional giant cells and a few capillaries. The depth of the reaction from the periphery of the suture may be only a few layers of cells in thickness. This reaction persists for years. In infrequent samples, the fibers are separated by a granulomatous reaction and very uncommonly by mature fibrous tissue. Although classified as nonabsorbable, silk will slowly disappear from the tissues; the rate is variable, however, and the process may take many years.

Silk has a wide range of applications in surgery because it handles and knots well, maintains strength adequately, and causes a modest tissue reaction. If used as a continuous suture, the capillarity of the multifilament strand may allow an infectious process to travel along the entire suture. Should infection develop in a clean wound closed with interrupted silk, the sutures are extruded or have to be removed, as they act as a focus for infection.

Cotton

Cotton has been used clinically as suture, although it is less popular than silk. Cotton sutures are the plied and twisted yarns from the staple filament of the cotton plant. Cotton handles and knots well. While not as strong as gut or silk, it maintains its strength in tissues better than silk. The tissue reaction is similar to that for silk, with the exception that individual cotton fibers frequently detach from the main mass of sutures. As each separated fiber stimulates its own response, the overall reaction is thereby increased.

The major advantage of cotton is its low cost, but it has not replaced silk to any great extent. Cotton may handle a little less well and may have a slight tendency to cut through the tissues, but otherwise cotton could be substituted for silk in many operations.

Metals

The experimental and clinical details of wire suture usage have been reported.[3] Stainless steel is available and widely used as either multifilament or monofilament sutures. Stainless steel wire has become a popular suture and is used in a variety of operations. Some surgeons dislike wire because of the difficulties in handling it. Wire does hold a knot well. It is strong, and as long as it does not fragment, there is little loss of strength in tissues. As claimed by its proponents, wire causes very little tissue reaction, although our studies suggest some cutting action. The disadvantages are the handling, the fragmentation, and, if used for fascial closure in a thin patient, the presence of an easily palpable suture that occasionally pushes out through the skin.

Synthetic Materials

Since the first report on the use of nylon for sutures,[34] additional synthetic materials have been developed and a wide range of applications found for these

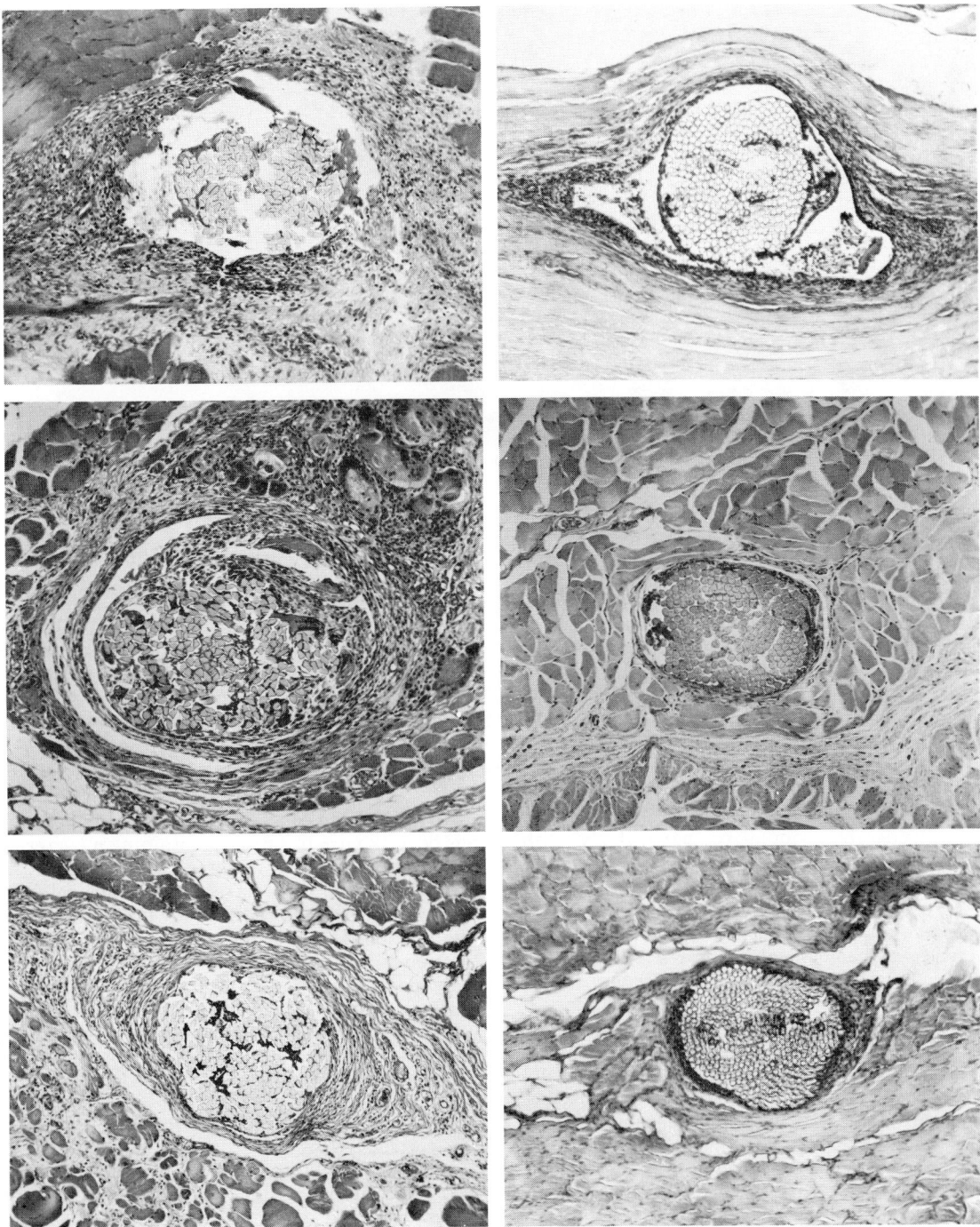

Figure 8. *Left* panel is silk, *right* is Dacron. *Top,* at 7 days; *middle,* at 14 days; *bottom,* at 42 days. The reaction to silk is more marked at each interval.

sutures. The most popular are nylon, Dacron, and polypropylene. These are long-chain polymers that can be extruded as filaments of the desired size. The nylon is available as both multifilament and monofilament but usually the latter is employed. Dacron is usually employed as a multifilament suture, and polypropylene as a monofilament. The monofilament, particularly the larger sizes, may be somewhat stiff to handle.

The major disadvantages of the synthetic sutures are that they are difficult to knot securely and that they tend to untie in the tissue. This does vary with the suture; monofilament nylon is the least satisfactory from this standpoint. If additional throws in the knot must be made, this results in a bulky mass, which may off-set some of the other advantages of these sutures. The synthetic sutures are stronger than gut, silk, or cotton

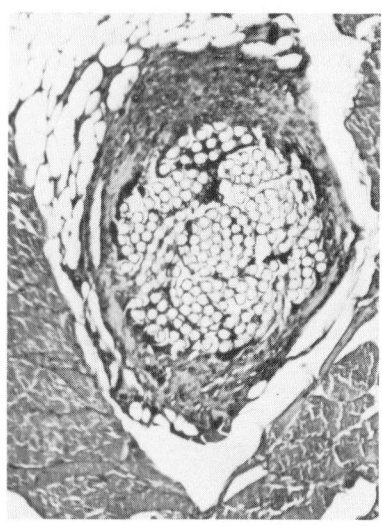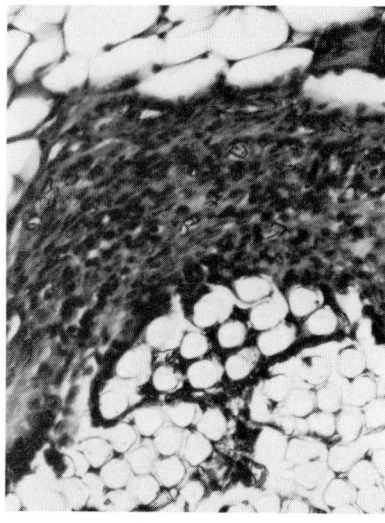

Figure 9. A Teflon-coated Dacron suture after 6 weeks. The irregular light granules of shed Teflon can be seen in the higher-power photomicrograph on the right, and the increased reaction over plain Dacron is obvious.

but weaker than wire in comparable sizes. In our implantation studies extending over a period of 2 years, the synthetic sutures lost little or no strength.

The tissue reaction is similar for the entire group, consisting essentially of a thin, firm connective tissue capsule. Occasional collections of mononuclear cells will be found near the suture, but the overall reaction is remarkably bland.

The advantages of synthetic sutures are their strength, which is retained, and the low tissue reaction. The one disadvantage is the difficulty with knots.

Teflon-coated, multifilament Dacron sutures have attained considerable popularity, particularly with cardiovascular surgeons. The coating was applied originally to decrease capillarity. These handle well, knot somewhat better than plain Dacron, and are quite strong. Teflon, however, is shed from the Dacron, and this increases the amount of tissue reaction. After a year or so, only a typical Dacron suture remains.

Polyglycolic and Polyglactic Acid. These materials are a decided advance in suture composition: synthetic filaments that are absorbed by body tissues. Polyglycolic acid is a polymer of glycolic acid (hydroacetic acid), which is extruded as filaments. Polyglactic acid is similar chemically, being a copolymer containing lactic acid. The handling properties, absorption characteristics, and rate of loss of strength are also similar, so that these sutures may be described together.

The suture handles much like silk, knots easily, and holds the knot well. The initial breaking strength is greater than catgut of the same size. In tissues, the breaking strength loss is almost a straight line to zero strength after 21 days. Absorption by the body tissues is well advanced by two months and nearly always complete within four months. The pattern, however, is completely different from that of catgut. After the initial reaction subsides, the suture is surrounded by a thin rim of fibrous tissue. Between the filaments are histiocytes, fibroblasts, and a few lymphocytes. Later, giant cells may be prominent. Without the reaction changing or expanding, the fibers simply decrease in number until finally only a few fragments of suture

can be seen with polarized light, with a tiny cluster of cells in the region.

The experimental evidence and now extensive clinical experience with these synthetic absorbable sutures suggest that they will probably replace catgut. The advantages of the synthetic sutures include uniformity, minor tissue reaction, and predictable decrease of strength and absorption as compared to the erratic behavior of catgut.

Other Sutures and Closures

An interesting concept of the prevention of infection has been the use of sutures containing a bacteriostatic or bactericidal agent. Sutures impregnated with benzalkonium compounds have been demonstrated to protect against staphylococci in our preliminary studies. The results suggest the necessity for continued investigation.

Cyanoacrylate compounds have been extensively investigated as physiologic tissue adhesives in recent years. Clinical application, however, has been quite limited.

DRAINS AND DRAINAGE

The provision of a mechanical means for the removal of the contents of body organs, cavities, or tissues has many applications. Catheterization of the urinary bladder and the insertion of a nasogastric tube are examples of well-established types of drainage. More complicated, but equally accepted, is the insertion of a tube or tubes into the pleural cavity after thoracotomy. The latter also illustrates clearly the basic reasons for drainage: obliteration of dead space and the removal of material foreign or harmful to a particular location.

The more specialized types of drainage such as those used for hydrocephalus, for an infected joint, or for an infected and obstructed kidney will be described in appropriate sections. This discussion will focus mainly on intraperitoneal drainage, for here opinions differ as

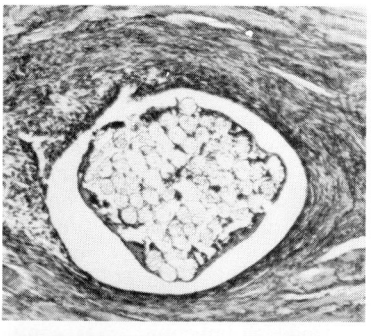
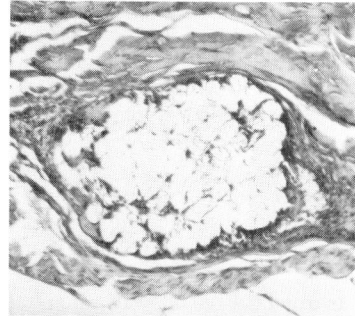
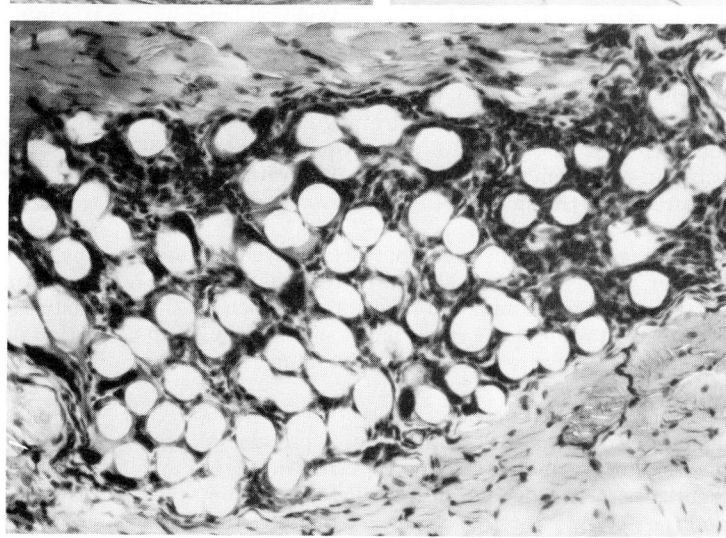

Figure 10. Polyglycolic acid suture. *Top left,* After 7 days. *Top right,* After 14 days. *Bottom,* After 28 days the reaction is almost completely confined to the cellular invasion of the interstices of the suture.

to the necessity for drainage, at least after some operations. In these situations, rigid guides are difficult to formulate and surgical judgment must play a dominant role.

General Indications for Drainage

To the basic reasons for drainage noted above, i.e., obliteration of dead space and the removal of material foreign or harmful to a particular location, should be added the operations or lesions in which such factors might be reasonably expected to develop. In other words, at times the purpose of drainage is to prevent complications. With these principles in mind, drainage should be considered in the following:

1. Abscess cavity with thick, shaggy walls that must collapse and heal from the deepest portion, such as a perforated appendix with localized abscess formation.

2. Insecure closure of a hollow viscus, as an anastomosis, because of size, tension, poor blood supply, infection, or general metabolic abnormalities in the patient.

3. Insecure closure in an anatomic location where the organ lacks a strong serosal covering, is extraperitoneal, or is fixed so that it is not readily covered by omentum, mesentery, or neighboring bowel.

4. Anticipated leakage, as from the gallbladder bed or pancreas where minute ducts may be cut and not identified at operation.

5. After trauma when débridement may necessarily be incomplete, foreign bodies missed, and massive contamination inevitable.

Generalized peritonitis per se is not an indication for drainage, if for no other reason than that "drainage of the general peritoneal cavity is physically and physiologically impossible." Yates[42] in 1905 reached this conclusion in one of the classic papers of surgical literature. He traced the history of drainage, beginning with the cannulas described by Hippocrates and Celsus. Chassaignac in 1859 introduced the use of soft rubber tubes. After gauze had been used for capillary drainage, Kehrer in 1882 placed the gauze within a rubber sheath to avoid adhesions, the first cigarette drain. Kellogg in 1895 described the forerunner of the present sump type of drain, and Heaton in 1898 applied constant suction to a siphon drain. Yates, after a detailed review of the reports on the principles, indications, methods, and results of drainage, described his experimental observations of drainage in dogs. These convincingly showed a drain to be promptly walled-off and isolated from the general peritoneal cavity. Localized drainage was possible, and Yates indicated that the purpose of the drain should be to "extraperitonealize" the affected area.

Specific Indications for Drainage

Spleen. Splenectomy is usually a reason for drainage to prevent subphrenic accumulation because hemostasis may be difficult to obtain, transudation from the raw area of the splenic fossa may be marked, and injury to the tail of the pancreas may occur. The advisability of drainage after splenectomy was questioned in a retrospective analysis of 130 splenectomies.[9] The total complication rate was 55 per cent in those drained and 5 per cent in those not drained. Subphrenic abscess developed in 10 of the 54 patients who were drained and in none of the 76 patients who were not. A similar study found 25 per cent complications in the drained versus 12 per cent in nondrained.[13] Five of 48 drained had a subphrenic abscess, compared to one patient of 58 not drained. Subphrenic abscess was most frequent after splenectomy for hematologic disease, when immunity might be reduced. Another study of 533 patients showed the incidence of infection to be increased by drainage after splenectomy.[7] It was also found in animal experiments that bacteria placed on the skin around the drain could be cultured from the splenic bed in 56 per cent of the subjects after 72 hours.

Drainage should, therefore, not be employed routinely after splenectomy but should be reserved for those patients who have injury to other organs such as the pancreas, in whom hemostasis is not satisfactory, or in whom other definite conditions exist that are conducive to infection.

Pancreas.   The majority of operations on the pancreas, other than internal drainage of a pseudocyst and possibly total pancreatectomy, require drainage. Pancreatic secretions even from tiny ducts can be marked, and the activated enzymes are extremely irritating to the neighboring tissues. Pancreatic abscess obviously requires drainage.

The digestive action of the exocrine enzymes in acute hemorrhagic pancreatitis has been emphasized, and the usual drains may be ineffective in preventing progressive extension of the necrotizing process.[41] A triple-lumen sump drain has been used with improved results. In addition, the effectiveness of the drain was demonstrated experimentally.

Biliary Tract.   Drainage is usually carried out after biliary tract surgery, although occasionally after simple cholecystectomy it may be omitted. Small accessory ducts may be present between the liver and gallbladder, and these are difficult to identify at the time of operation. The tie on the cystic duct may slip off and thus be a source of a bile accumulation. In my experience, it has been impossible to anticipate the amount of bile drainage. When a suction-type drain has been used, the drainage amounts to 200 ml. or less in most patients, but in others it may be considerably more, up to 4000 ml. While the peritoneum can absorb bile that is not infected, drainage is a safety valve that appears to be indicated. Other surgeons disagree and insert no drain after cholecystectomy.

After more extensive operations such as common duct exploration or reconstruction, drainage is certainly indicated because of the probability of bile leakage.

Duodenal Stump.   Of those complications directly related to the operation, leakage of the duodenal stump is responsible for as many as half of the deaths following gastric resection. One analysis of 369 Billroth II type gastrectomies showed duodenal stump perforation to be unpredictable and often fatal.[38] Prophylactic drainage did not increase the incidence of duodenal stump leakage, provided earlier diagnosis if perforation did occur, obviated the need of emergency operation, and lowered the mortality.

Prophylactic drainage has generally been advocated when closure of the stump has been difficult and when there is some reason, such as impaired blood supply, for concern about the probability of a breakdown of the closure. Certainly in this situation drainage or catheter duodenostomy is advisable. Parenthetically, it should be pointed out that in operations for duodenal ulcer, a difficult duodenal closure can usually be anticipated and an alternative operation selected.

Appendicitis.   Simple acute appendicitis does not require drainage. Perforated appendicitis with localized abscess formation, however, represents the typical lesion that always needs drainage, provided operative treatment is elected. Although it would be inappropriate here to discuss operative versus nonoperative therapy for periappendiceal abscess, prior to the antibiotic era many patients were successfully treated with nasogastric suction and intravenous fluids, with rapid resolution of the abscess. This form of treatment may still be advantageous in selected patients, excluding the very young and the very old.

The major problem concerns drainage with perforated appendicitis and generalized peritonitis. As noted above, the general peritoneal cavity cannot be drained, and no attempt should be made to do so. One survey of experiences with appendectomies in children led the authors to conclude that the use of intraperitoneal drainage in generalized peritonitis is to be condemned.[31] Some pediatric surgeons, however, insert a drain along the right colonic gutter and another into the pelvis in this situation.[24] Generally, we would agree with the latter procedure.

Intestinal Anastomosis.   With few exceptions, anastomoses in the gastrointestinal tract should be sufficiently secure that the question of drainage is not entertained. In unusual situations, such as caudal pancreaticojejunostomy, drainage should be used, since sealing of the suture line may not be prompt and secure.

Anterior resection of the lower part of the sigmoid and the proximal portion of the rectum with primary anastomosis requires drainage. The rectal wall is thin and has no serosal covering, the anastomotic line is extraperitoneal, where the tissues are less resistant to infection, and the hollow of the sacrum is an area in which blood and fluid tend to accumulate. The technique for an anatomic, dependent route of drainage has been described.[37] An incision is made posterolateral to the anus, dissection is carried bluntly but carefully to the hollow of the sacrum, and the drain is placed along the tract. Suction drains placed in the pelvis and brought out through the abdominal wall appear to be an equally satisfactory and less traumatic method of drainage.

Wound Drainage.   Not infrequently, intraperitoneal drainage may not be required, but contamination of the wound has occurred and the possibility of a wound infection is high. Here, the peritoneum and fascia may

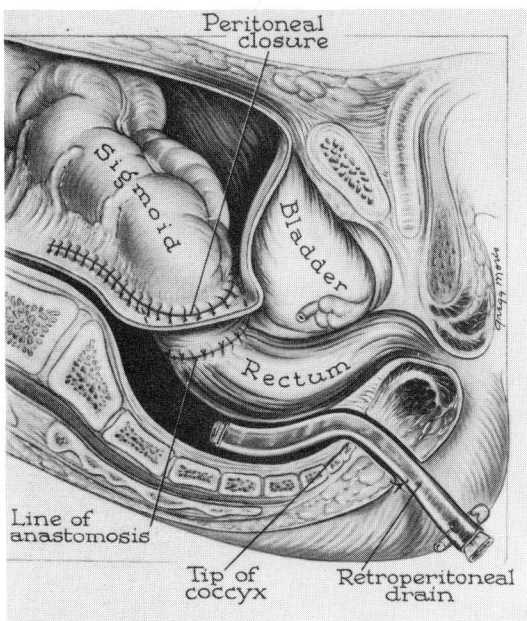

Figure 11. Method of drainage described by Schaupp for a specific operation: drainage of the presacral space after anterior resection and extraperitoneal anastomosis. (Modified from Mathewson and Richards in Schaupp, W. E.: Am. J. Surg., *118*:627, 1969.)

be closed and the subcutaneous tissues drained. Although it is not a form of drainage per se, at times the wound may be left open down to the fascia and closed secondarily.

Other Drainage.   The use of tubes with multiple perforations, attached to a low-pressure suction device, and placed in wounds or under skin flaps when oozing of blood or transudation of fluid is expected, is not unique to the abdomen. This technique is particularly useful after radical mastectomy or radical neck dissection.

Types of Drains

The most commonly used and probably most innocuous drain is a very thin rubber tube, usually 1/2 or 1 inch in diameter, called a Penrose drain. Because of capillary action and to provide greater bulk, gauze may be placed inside the Penrose drain to form a cigarette drain. Rubber or plastic catheters of various sizes and design are also used as drains.

The sump drain is utilized because adjacent tissues frequently seal off the openings in a single-bore drain and the sump drain allows air to enter the drained area with the object of displacing fluid into the drain. The sump drains are double-lumen, the ingress portion being smaller than the egress. Triple-lumen sump drains have been described, designed so that suction can be applied to one lumen, an irrigating solution introduced through a second, and air allowed to enter through the third opening. A somewhat similar triple-lumen tube is made by placing a double-lumen tube within a Penrose drain. This has recently been described as a sump-Penrose drain.[22] An interesting study of the efficiency of drains was reported in which solution was dripped in through a catheter in the left

upper quadrant of the abdomen in dogs. Drains were placed in Morison's pouch and recovery of the fluid was 40 per cent with a Penrose drain, 39 per cent with a tube drain, 58 per cent with a sump drain, and 72 per cent with the sump-Penrose drain.

Several types of tube and sump drains are commercially available, at least one with an ingenious device attached that provides constant low negative pressure.

The choice of the drain and its composition depend on the purpose and location of the drainage. Generally, however, the drain should be soft and pliable so that it will not encroach on important structures. It should not be irritating to the tissues and should not weaken or decompose on exposure to the drained fluid.

Insertion of Drains

Certain basic principles underlie the placement of drains. With few exceptions, intraperitoneal drains should not be brought out through the primary incision, as this favors the development of a wound infection, increases the incidence of dehiscence, and may lead to postoperative hernia. The stab wound or incision for the drains must be adequate: if it is too tight, drainage cannot take place; if it is too loose, bowel or omentum may herniate alongside the drain. Ideally, placement of the stab wound would provide dependent drainage by gravity, but this can seldom be accomplished. The wound is therefore placed to give the drain the most direct route of exit, not crossing vessels and preferably not crossing bowel.

The exit tract in the abdominal wall also should be direct. If the muscle and fascial layers are incised lateral to a rectus incision, for example, closure of the major wound will then restore the layers to normal position and the drain will be kinked. The peritoneum and fascia should therefore be pulled into approximately normal position while the stab wound is being made.

Most surgeons believe that a drain should not be in contact with a suture line, if for no other reason than that it might block off omentum that could seal a small leak. The deep end of a drain may be fixed in position, if necessary, with a very fine, plain catgut suture. The outside of the drain must be fixed to keep it from slipping back into the wound.

Drains should obviously be left in place until they have served their purpose. The length of time will

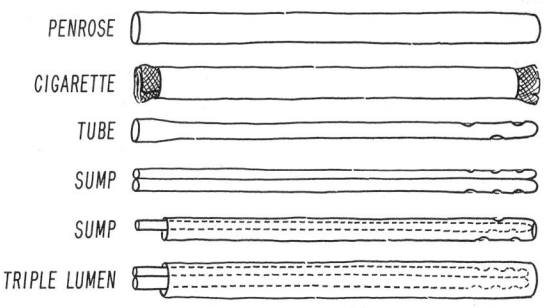

Figure 12. The most commonly used drains. Ties are placed on the triple-lumen drain to hold the outer Penrose drain in place.

vary considerably, but generally the drain should be removed when drainage has become small in amount. If used prophylactically, as for the duodenal stump, the drain should be left in place as long as the danger of perforation exists—at least 8 to 10 days.

Complications of Drains

If they are properly used, it is doubtful that drains cause an increased incidence of anastomotic leakage or duodenal stump perforation. A very firm drain may encroach on an adjacent structure, as already mentioned. The possibility does definitely exist that bacteria may be introduced along a drain to lodge and proliferate in the drained area.

A vessel may be cut when the stab wound is made; it may be temporarily compressed by the drain, and then later be the site of annoying or even dangerous hemorrhage. Bowel may herniate alongside a drain, with resulting obstruction.

The drain tract is always infected, and occasionally an abdominal wall abscess will form after removal of the drain, unless the superficial part of the site is kept open until the deeper portion heals.

An unfortunate complication is loss of a drain in the wound, particularly if it is unrecognized. For this reason, the number of drains used and the date of removal of each one must be carefully documented.

SELECTED REFERENCES

Burke, J. F.: Wound infection and early inflammation. Monogr. Surg. Sci., 1:301, 1964.
The author surveys his own work and that of others in a review of factors in wound infection, such as the source of the organisms and the determinants of the events after bacterial lodgment.

Cohen, L. S., Fekety, F. R., Jr., and Cluff, L. E.: Studies of the epidemiology of staphylococcal infection. VI. Infections in the surgical patient. Ann. Surg., 159:321, 1964.
This is an example of a well-conducted epidemiologic study of wound infections in one hospital over a period of 16 months.

Cooperative Study Group: Postoperative infections. Ann. Surg. (Suppl.), 160:1, 1964.
An extensive cooperative study in five hospitals involving 15,613 operations is reported. Although it was designed to evaluate the effects of ultraviolet radiation, many other important factors in wound infection are included.

Halsted, W. S.: The employment of fine silk in preference to catgut and the advantages of transfixing tissues and vessels in controlling haemorrhage. J.A.M.A., 60:1119, 1913.
This classic paper on the silk technique includes other measures utilized to promote healing of the wound.

Hermann, G.: Intraperitoneal drainage. Surg. Clin. North Am., 49:1279, 1969.
This carefully considered, objective survey of drainage brings up to date the work of Yates. In addition to the general use of drains, specific situations are described as well as technique and complications.

Miles, A. A.: Nonspecific defense reactions in bacterial infections. Ann. N.Y. Acad. Sci., 66:356, 1956.
This deservedly often quoted work is an example of a relatively simple experimental model yielding important clinically applicable information.

Yates, J. L.: An experimental study of the local effects of peritoneal drainage. Surg. Gynecol. Obstet., 1:473, 1905.
This classic paper on drainage is of value not only for its historic and informational content but as an interesting example of the medical literary style of the period.

REFERENCES

1. Alexander, J. W.: Surgical infections—pathogen versus host. J. Surg. Res., 8:225, 1968.
2. Alexander, J. W., and Meakins, J. L.: A physiological basis for the development of opportunistic infections in man. Ann. Surg., 176:273, 1972.
3. Babcock, W. W.: Metallic sutures and ligatures. Surg. Clin. North Am., 27:1435, 1947.
4. Barnes, B. A., Behringer, G. E., Wheelock, F. C., and Wilkins, E. W.: Postoperative sepsis: Trends and factors influencing sepsis over a 20-year period reviewed in 20,000 cases. Ann. Surg., 154:585, 1961.
5. Bernard, H. R., and Cole, W. R.: The prophylaxis of surgical infections: The effect of prophylactic antimicrobial drugs on the incidence of infection following potentially contaminated operations. Surgery, 56:151, 1964.
6. Burke, J. F.: Wound infection and early inflammation. Monogr. Surg. Sci., 1:301, 1964.
7. Cerise, E. J., Pierce, W. A., and Diamond, D. L.: Abdominal drains: Their role as a source of infection following splenectomy. Ann. Surg., 171:764, 1970.
8. Cohen, L. S., Fekety, F. R., Jr., and Cluff, L. E.: Studies of the epidemiology of staphylococcal infection. VI. Infections in the surgical patient. Ann. Surg., 159:321, 1964.
9. Cohn, L. H.: Local infections after splenectomy: Relationship of drainage. Arch. Surg., 90:230, 1965.
10. Cole, W. R., and Bernard, H. R.: Quantitative air sampling, a contrast with the settling-plate method for the study of bacterial air contamination in operation rooms. Surgery, 51:658, 1962.
11. Cole, W. R., and Bernard, H. R.: Inadequacies of present methods of surgical skin preparation. Arch. Surg., 89:215, 1964.
12. Cooperative Study Group: Postoperative infections. Ann. Surg. (Suppl.), 160:1, 1964.
13. Daoud, F. S., Fischer, D. C., and Hafner, C. D.: Complications following splenectomy with special emphasis on drainage. Arch. Surg., 92:32, 1966.
14. Dineen, P.: A critical study of 100 consecutive wound infections. Surg. Gynecol. Obstet., 113:91, 1961.
15. Dineen, P.: Penetration of surgical draping material by bacteria. Hospitals, 43:931, 1969.
16. DuMortier, J. J.: The resistance of healing wounds to infection. Surg. Gynecol. Obstet., 56:762, 1933.
17. Elek, S. D., and Conen, P. E.: The virulence of Staphylococcus pyogenes for man. A study of the problems of wound infection. Br. J. Exp. Pathol., 38:573, 1957.
18. Feingold, D. S.: Hospital-acquired infections. N. Engl. J. Med., 283:1384, 1970.
19. Ford, C. R., Peterson, D. E., and Mitchell, C. R.: An appraisal of the role of surgical face masks. Am. J. Surg., 113:787, 1967.
20. Glotzer, D. J., Goodman, W. S., and Geronimus, L. H.: Topical antibiotic prophylaxis in contaminated wounds. Experimental evaluation. Arch. Surg., 100:589, 1970.
21. Halsted, W. S.: The employment of fine silk in preference to catgut and the advantages of transfixing tissues and vessels in controlling haemorrhage. J.A.M.A., 60:1119, 1913.
22. Hanna, E. A.: Efficiency of peritoneal drainage. Surg. Gynecol. Obstet., 131:983, 1970.
23. Hart, D.: Bactericidal ultraviolet radiation in the operating room. Twenty-nine year study for control of infections. J.A.M.A., 172:1019, 1960.
24. Hermann, G.: Intraperitoneal drainage. Surg. Clin. North Am., 49:1279, 1969.
25. Hnatko, S. I., MacDonald, G. R., and Rodin, A. E.: A study of sepsis in surgical wounds. Can. Med. Assoc. J., 88:543, 1963.
26. Howe, C. W.: Bacterial flora of clean wounds and its relation to subsequent sepsis. Am. J. Surg., 107:696, 1964.
27. Howe, C. W.: Experimental studies on determinants of wound infection. Surg. Gynecol. Obstet., 123:507, 1966.
28. Joress, S. M.: A study of disinfection of the skin: A comparison of povidone-iodine with other agents used for surgical scrubs. Ann. Surg., 155:296, 1962.
29. Lovell, D. L.: Skin bacteria: Their location with reference to skin sterilization. Surg. Gynecol. Obstet., 80:174, 1945.
30. MacLean, L. D., Meakins, J. L., Taguchi, K., Duignan, J. P., Dhillon, K. S., and Gordon, J.: Host resistance in sepsis and trauma. Ann. Surg., 182:207, 1975.
31. Maddox, J. R. J., Johnson, T. M., and Grass, R. E.: Appendectomies in a children's hospital. Arch. Surg., 89:223, 1964.
32. Maitland, A. E.: Postoperative infection. Br. J. Surg., 52:931, 1965.

33. Miles, A. A.: Nonspecific defense reactions in bacterial infections. Ann. N.Y. Acad. Sci., *66*:356, 1956.

34. Nichols, H. M., and Diack, A. W.: An experimental study of nylon as a suture material. Western. J. Surg., *48*:42, 1940.

35. Nichols, R. L., Broido, P., Condon, R. E., Gorbach, S. L., and Nyhus, L. M.: Effect of preoperative neomycin-erythromycin intestinal preparation on the incidence of infectious complications following colon surgery. Ann. Surg., *178*:453, 1973.

36. Salthouse, T. N., Williams, J. A., and Willigan, D. A.: Relationship of cellular enzyme activity to catgut and collagen suture absorption. Surg. Gynecol. Obstet., *129*:691, 1969.

37. Schaupp, W. E.: Drainage of low anterior anastomoses. Am. J. Surg., *118*:627, 1969.

38. Stengel, B. F., Close, A. S., and Thomas, W. D.: The influence of prophylactic drainage on the results of duodenal stump perforation. Surg. Gynecol. Obstet., *117*:623, 1963.

39. Stone, H. H., Kalb, L. D., and Geheber, C. E.: Incidence and significance of intraperitoneal anaerobic bacteria. Ann. Surg., *181*:805, 1975.

40. Washington, J. A., II, Dearing, W. H., Judd, E. S., and Elveback, L. R.: Effect of preoperative antibiotic regimen on development of infection after intestinal surgery: Prospective, randomized, double-blind study. Ann. Surg., *180*:567, 1974.

41. Waterman, N. G., Walsky, R., Kasdan, M. L., and Abrams, B. L.: The treatment of acute hemorrhagic pancreatitis by sump drainage. Surg. Gynecol. Obstet., *126*:963, 1968.

42. Yates, J. L.: An experimental study of the local effects of peritoneal drainage. Surg. Gynecol. Obstet., *1*:473, 1905.

17

SURGICAL INFECTIONS AND CHOICE OF ANTIBIOTICS

W. A. Altemeier, M.D., and J. Wesley Alexander, M.D., Sc.D.

Despite the marked progress made in surgery and microbiology since Lord Lister's time, infections continue to present major challenges in the practice of surgery. Approximately one third of the surgical patients in a busy general hospital today are affected with infections of various types and degree of severity. Some of these infections develop spontaneously, requiring the patient's hospitalization for effective treatment. Others develop in or adjacent to wounds resulting from surgical operations, accidental trauma or violence, and many occur postoperatively in areas remote from the operative wound, for example, pneumonia or cystitis. Following burn injury or renal transplantation, infection is the leading cause of death, and it is a major cause of morbidity and mortality following trauma and most types of major operative procedures.

As serious as these current problems are, however, it is almost impossible for today's medical students to imagine the unbelievable conditions and confusion that existed in hospital practice 100 years ago or to appreciate the significance of the revolutionary contributions of Leeuwenhoek, Schwann, Pirogoff, Pasteur, Koch, Lister, Hunter, Kocher, Bergmann, Fleming, Domagk, Florey, and others. For exciting and interesting reading, the student of today is referred to historical sources for the developments of our knowledge by these great men.

Before the studies of Louis Pasteur and their application in surgical practice by Joseph Lister over 100 years ago, most if not all surgical wounds became infected. The most common complications of wounds were erysipelas, "hospital gangrene," septicemia, and tetanus. The extent and significance of infection at that time are exemplified by the 92 per cent mortality reported for amputations of the femur following trauma during the Crimean War as the result of "hospital gangrene." The results of injuries in the American Civil War were similar in their morbidity and mortality. The mortality was so high that elective surgery was avoided or was limited to minor or superficial operations. For example, few elective thyroidec-

tomies were done before 1890, largely because of the high morbidity and mortality resulting from infection and hemorrhage.

Lister has been generally recognized as the discoverer of antiseptic principle in surgery, and his paper, "On the Antiseptic Principle in the Practice of Surgery," published in 1867, revolutionized the practice of surgery. He was guided and stimulated by the work of Pasteur on the nature of fermentation and putrefaction, and of Schwann, who had shown that putrefaction could be prevented by heat and was therefore due to living organisms of some type. Lister's concepts and techniques, however, met with widespread disbelief during the latter part of the nineteenth century and were generally resisted.

The concept of Lister's *antisepsis* was extended by Bergmann to *asepsis* by his introduction of the principle of steam sterilization in 1886 and his elaborate aseptic ritual in 1891. His principle of aseptic surgery was based upon the exclusion of all bacteria from the wound made by the surgeon, permitting healing to take place without significant contamination and with a very low incidence of infection. His contributions were related to the observations and work of many men other than Lister, such as Oliver Wendell Holmes, Semmelweis, and Theodor Kocher. It is interesting to note that Kocher also emphasized the primary importance of contact contamination in the development of infections, and this led to the general use of rubber gloves in surgical operations as introduced by Halsted in the United States in 1890.

Microbiology has also contributed significantly to the control of infections in surgical practice through the development of modern chemotherapy by the clinical introduction and use of Prontosil by Domagk in 1935 and penicillin by Fleming in 1928 and Florey in 1941.

With the introduction of antibiotic therapy, it was hoped that serious infections complicating surgical practice would be eliminated. Unfortunately this has not occurred. Not only has the problem of postoperative wound and hospital-acquired infections continued, but widespread antibiotic therapy has increased the complexity of the difficulties related to the prevention and control of surgical infections. In this regard, increasing numbers of infections are being encountered in modern hospital practice as the result of iatrogenic factors. The past generation of surgeons has seen the emergence of increasing numbers of serious infections related to a complex combination of factors, including the performance of more complicated and longer operations, an increase in the number of geriatric patients with accompanying chronic or debilitating diseases, and increased utilization of diagnostic and treatment modalities that result in greater bacterial exposures or that suppress normal host resistance. Unfortunately, many infections have resulted from laxity in aseptic technique, disregard for established surgical principles, and unwarranted reliance upon prophylactic antibiotic therapy. Not only are these infections of medical significance, but they represent an important economic burden amounting to billions of dollars, both to the individual and to modern society.

For these and other reasons, the physician must keep in mind that the modern general hospital is a complex community in which are concentrated people who have been admitted with a variety of infections, as well as many others who are unusually susceptible to postoperative wound infections and hospital-acquired infections. In this environment, however, it is now possible to prevent infection routinely in the great majority of planned operative wounds, an achievement that was one of the great milestones of surgery. Thus, the modern surgeon cannot escape his responsibility to deal with infections and must realize that knowledge of many aspects of microbiology, immunology, and pharmacology is essential to complement his surgical skills. Because of their importance in today's complex practice, emphasis will be placed on the relationships between therapy and the pathophysiologic mechanisms in infections. A basic understanding of how the body defends itself against infection is essential to the rational application of surgical and other therapeutic principles to the control of infection.

HOST RESISTANCE TO MICROBIAL INFECTIONS

All higher animals live in a sea of potentially pathogenic bacteria, viruses, and fungi, which are normal inhabitants of their epithelial surfaces. The vast majority of microbes in contact with the host are denied entrance into the internal milieu, but epithelial function is by no means perfect, and viable microbes frequently gain entrance into sterile tissues. Such intrusion is usually of little consequence, but may result in clinical infection, sometimes with devastating consequences if the host's defenses are depressed or if an overwhelmingly large number of pathogenic organisms gain entrance. The host-pathogen interaction may vary considerably owing to differences between microbial species, but the defense mechanisms against each are generally similar (Fig. 1).

From the time that bacteria enter tissues, an inflammatory response contributes to their localization and containment. Usually, injury of the tissue is involved, and the early events are characterized by a biphasic vascular response. Mediators of the vascular response include endotoxin, histamine, the kinin system, slow-reacting substance, and other vasoactive substances derived from bacteria, cells, and serum proteins, especially those of the complement system. These chemical stimuli cause constriction of the vascular sphincters, venular and capillary dilatation, increased permeability to plasma proteins, and slowing of flow with resulting local acidosis and hypoxia. The endothelial surfaces become altered so that granulocytes and monocytes marginate on the endothelium, and the leukocytes emigrate through intercellular junctions by the process of diapedesis.

Among the exuded plasma proteins at new inflammatory foci are many that play an important role in the body's defense. Specific antibody directed toward a given microbe is frequently present because of past experience of the host with that organism. The so-called natural antibodies, exemplified by those directed against the enteric bacilli, probably represent no more than a result of past exposure to the specific or cross-reacting antigens.

Antibody against a microbe will combine with specific surface antigens, and this complex will activate complement which otherwise will not be activated by bacteria. Complement is an inclusive term for 11 chemically distinct serum proteins of the classical pathway and three or more additional proteins belonging to the alternative pathway which, acting together, serve as a biologic amplification system for the interaction between antigen and antibody (Fig. 2). When complement is activated by antigen-antibody complex, a series of enzymatic reactions are produced that in their fullest expression damage or lyse the cell wall of the bacterium, prepare it for phagocytosis, release chemotactic substances, and produce immune adherence. Complement and specific antibody, acting together, may kill several species of gram-negative bacteria and a few species of gram-positive bacteria in vitro. The effects of antibody and complement, however, are relatively insignificant in vivo in the absence of an adequate cellular response, and their major function in defense against microbial invasion is to prepare the microbes for phagocytosis and intracellular destruction, a process usually called opsonization. There is some evidence that a few species of bacteria activate the complement system in the absence of specific antibody. Other humoral factors have little direct effect on bacteria, although lysozyme occasionally has a synergistic action with antibody and complement.

The nature of the stimulus determines somewhat the characteristics of an inflammatory cellular exudate, but granulocytes are the predominant cells of the early lesion. The deposition of neutrophils at an inflammatory focus appears to be solely a function of the vascular response, and unless the stimulus for this response is continued, mononuclear phagocytes soon become relatively more numerous. The life span of these cells is considerably longer than that of neutrophils; the half-life of a neutrophil in tissues has been estimated to be only 24 hours.

Both mononuclear phagocytes and granulocytes are

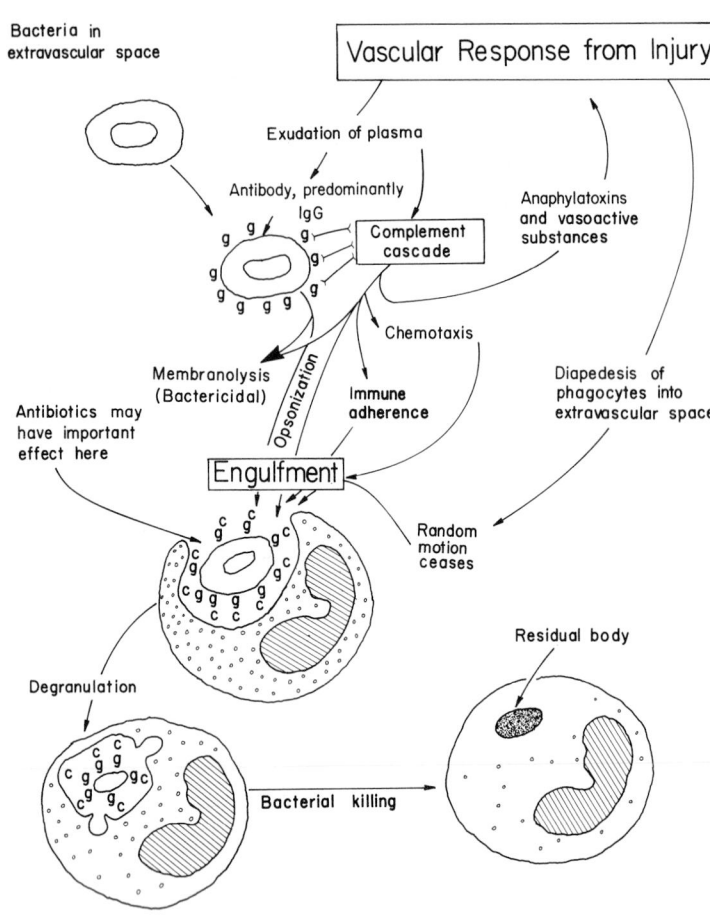

Figure 1. Schematic drawing of early physiologic events and response to bacterial contamination. Note the important interrelationships between specific antibody, complement, and the phagocytic cells in destruction of bacteria.

capable of phagocytosis and intracellular destruction of bacteria, but the neutrophil plays the dominant role in man, being the most essential phagocytic cell of the body that protects man from overwhelming microbial invasion. An estimated 20 to 50 billion neutrophils are circulating in the normal human adult at any given time, and an equal number are sequestered or margin-ated on vascular walls. These, however, represent only a fraction of the number held in the bone marrow reserve. Vast numbers of neutrophils are lost into the gastrointestinal, respiratory, and genitourinary tracts daily.

Once in the extravascular tissues, phagocytes move about randomly until they come within a relatively

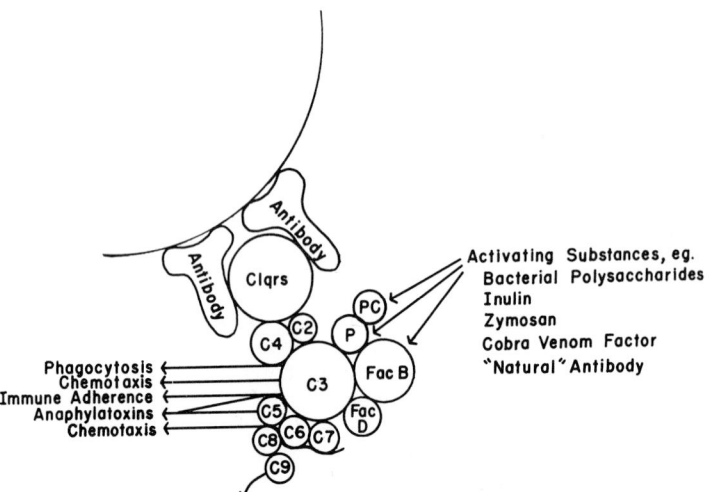

Figure 2. Schematic representation of the complement pathway. The classic pathway can be activated by antigen-antibody complex, whereas the alternative pathway is activated by a variety of substances such as those listed on the right. C1 to C9 are components of the classic pathway, PC = properdin convertase, P = properdin, Fac B = Factor B (C3 proactivator), and Fac D = Factor D (C3 proactivator convertase).

short distance of an attractive particle, when they become affected by chemotactic forces and abandon their random motion, a phenomenon involving a chemical concentration gradient that affects the gel-sol state of the cell membrane.

After a phagocyte has made contact with a microbe, phagocytosis will usually follow. Particle uptake by phagocytes is strikingly dependent upon the presence of antibody and complement for most bacteria. Specific antibody in the absence of complement can act as an opsonizing agent, but the bulk of evidence indicates that antibody serves primarily to activate the complement system, the latter having a far greater direct influence upon the opsonization of bacteria. Complement may also play an important role in intracellular killing.

Once phagocytosis has occurred, the opportunity for destruction of the bacterium is finally at hand. Although the process was described by Metchnikoff before 1900, precise mechanisms of bacterial killing by phagocytic cells remained poorly studied until recent years, and many questions are still unanswered. After ingestion of a bacterium, the membranes confining the lysosomal granules fuse with the phagosome, the portion of the plasma membrane surrounding the ingested bacterium. This causes emptying of hydrolytic enzymes into the vacuole, or phagolysosome, the process being called degranulation. A large number of hydrolytic enzymes and cationic proteins are present in lysosomes which may have an antibacterial effect. Among these are *peroxidases, cathepsins, lysozyme, lipases, proteases,* and *nucleases.* The low pH within the phagolysosome in itself tends to have a destructive effect on many bacteria as well as providing an optimal pH for activity of the lysosomal enzymes. An oxidation process involving the production of H_2O_2 and superoxide is also believed to be important in the destruction of many microbes. Certain bacteria such as Mycobacterium, Salmonella, and Brucella often successfully resist intracellular digestion by these enzymes and may remain viable intracellularly for long periods of time, especially in mononuclear phagocytes.

Resistance to infection caused by most viruses and fungi, *Pneumocystis carinii,* and certain bacteria characterized as intracellular pathogens is accomplished by participation of the lymphoid system, predominately the thymic dependent lymphocytes or T cells which are responsible for delayed hypersensitivity reactions. Effectiveness of this system is in part a result of the ability of activated T cells to activate macrophages. The role of this system in infections appears to be minor except in patients who are immunodepressed, e.g., in patients receiving steroid therapy or treatment with cytotoxic drugs.

Specific adaptive immunity follows an initial experience of the host with antigens of the offending organism, but details of this process are too extensive for presentation in this chapter. Several recent reviews of the subject are available. The various components of normal host resistance are strongly interrelated and interdependent. Like blood coagulation or complement activity, a defect or abnormality in any one of the steps may lead to malfunction of the entire system.

This summary is obviously a brief and greatly simplified introduction to a complex subject, but it provides a structure upon which the following discussion on surgical infections will be built.

CAUSES OF INFECTION

Infection resulting from surgical treatment is related either to intrinsic abnormalities in host defense, interference with the host defense process, or overloading the normal capabilities of the system. Each occurs frequently.

Bacterial Factors

The deposition and growth of bacteria within wounds are obvious prerequisites for the development of infection, and the kind and numbers of bacteria contribute significantly to the establishment of overt infection, or the lack of it. Several bacterial species have surface components that contribute to their pathogenicity by inhibiting phagocytosis (e.g., the capsules of Klebsiella and Pneumococcus). Other bacteria, notably the enterobacteria, have surface components that are toxic, and still others, such as certain strains of clostridia and streptococci, produce powerful exotoxins. The development of infection is thus somewhat dependent upon the toxins produced by the organism and its ability to resist phagocytosis and intracellular destruction. With highly virulent and pathogenic organisms, such as *Streptococcus pyogenes* group A or *Pasturella pestis*, relatively few may be required to establish an infection.

Careful studies of the bacterial flora of clean surgical wounds taken at the time of closure have shown that one or more types of organisms can be cultured from most wounds. Because devitalized tissues and foreign materials are invariably present, far fewer organisms are necessary to cause infection in wounds than in normal tissues. Even so, overt infection is unusual unless cardinal surgical principles have been violated or exceptionally large numbers of organisms have been introduced into the wound. Studies of traumatic wounds in healthy subjects have shown that bacterial contamination with greater than 10^5 organisms frequently results in infection, whereas contamination with less than 10^5 organisms usually does not. The normal defense mechanisms therefore are of great importance in the prevention of infection and at its inception.

Decreased Delivery of Phagocytes

Virtually any condition that contributes to a decreased delivery of phagocytic cells to an area of bacterial contamination will promote the development of infection. These conditions are of extreme importance to the surgeon and include: (1) a diminution in blood flow, as may be found in vascular occlusive states, in hypovolemic shock, or following the use of vasopressors; (2) the presence of devitalized tissue, foreign bodies, hematomas, and seromas; (3) a decreased vascular reactivity, as may be found in uremic conditions, old age, or patients receiving high doses of steroids; and (4) decreased delivery of phagocytes accompanying decreased production, as is found during nitrogen mustard therapy, irradiation, or granulocytopenic states. Recent studies have shown that abnormal chemotaxis may be a contributing factor in the development of some infections.

Abnormal Serum Factors (Opsonins)

At any site of injury, there is an exudation of plasma proteins into the area. The specific antibody and complement contained therein may act as strong opsonizing agents for phagocytosis of contaminating bacteria. If the host has had no prior experience with the offending organism, he will have little or no specific antibody, and the rate of phagocytosis by competent leukocytes will be minimal. Specific immunization might help in certain instances in which the species of contaminating organism could be anticipated far in advance, but one seldom has this opportunity. Patients who produce little or no gamma globulin (agammaglobulinemia) or respond abnormally to an antigenic stimulus (dysgammaglobulinemia) are occasionally encountered. In such cases, the early result is similar to those in which the host has had no prior experience with the offending organism, but infection is prolonged because the patient cannot respond by synthesizing specific antibody. Dysgammaglobulinemia or hypogammaglobulinemia can accompany nutritional deficiencies and many diseases associated with immunosuppressive therapy, competing antigenic stimuli, or multiple myeloma.

Several substances will promote the development of infection because of an anticomplement activity. Among these are heparin, mucin, hemoglobin, and sodium polyanethol sulfonate (Liquoid). Each of these, when administered locally with bacteria, will contribute to an increase in susceptibility to infection.

Disorders of the complement system which decrease levels or interfere with activation of C3 when the appropriate stimuli are applied also result in an increased susceptibility to infection. It has recently been shown that both specific antibody and components of the complement system can be reduced during acute severe infection, presumably by a consumptive process. When this occurs the lowered levels of opsonins may contribute both to progression of the existing infection and the development of superinfections. Complement levels and activity can be significantly reduced as a result of chronic malnutrition or acute starvation associated with stress.

Abnormal Ingestion by Phagocytes

Defects in the ingestive phase of leukocyte function have been implicated in uremia, ketosis, hyperglycemia, prematurity, certain malignancies (notably leukemias), and several immunologic deficiency diseases.

Abnormal Intracellular Killing

Even when the process of ingestion of bacteria is normal, intracellular killing may occur at a decreased rate. This type of abnormality was first discovered to occur in the congenital chronic granulomatous disease of childhood, but acquired defects of intracellular killing by the leukocytes of patients with severe thermal or traumatic injury, patients with malnutrition, and patients receiving immunosuppressive ther-

apy have also been demonstrated. In these conditions, phagocytosis by peripheral leukocytes has usually occurred at a normal or increased rate. In patients with large burns, the development of sepsis has usually occurred at times when neutrophil function was abnormal (Fig. 3). Of potential biologic importance is a cyclic variation in the function of neutrophils from normal persons, which is apparently accentuated by certain diseases, injuries, or drug therapies (Fig. 4). It has been suggested that this relative abnormality may be of etiologic importance in the genesis of spontaneous infection.

The acute starvation associated with traumatic injury or surgical therapy does not seem to adversely affect phagocytic function, nor is the production of specific antibody altered to any significant degree.

PREVENTION OF INFECTION

Prevention of septic complications is far more practical than treating them once they have become es-

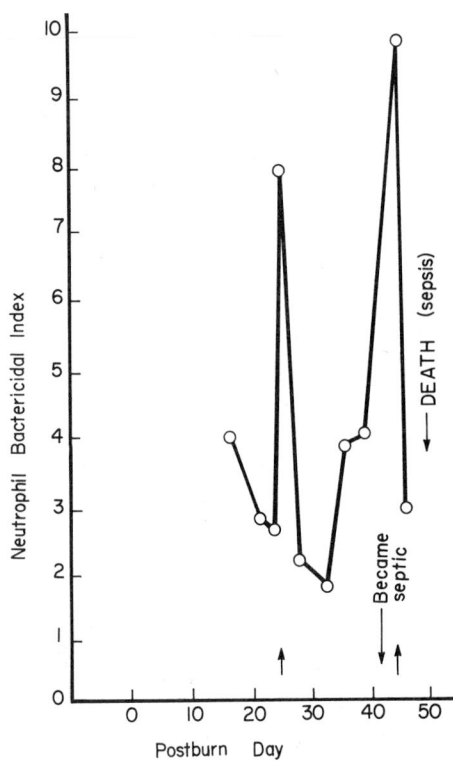

Figure 3. The development of invasive sepsis and septicemia in this 10-year-old girl with a 54 per cent burn was related to a relative inability of her neutrophils to kill ingested bacteria. The results of serial tests of neutrophilic function are expressed as a neutrophil-bactericidal index. The normal range for this value is 0.5 to 2, and increasing values for the index reflect worsening of the antibacterial function of neutrophils. Note that this patient had a cyclic variation in the antibacterial function of her neutrophils as well as an overall abnormality. (From Alexander, J. W., Dionigi, R., and Meakins, J. L.: Ann. Surg., *173*:206, 1971.)

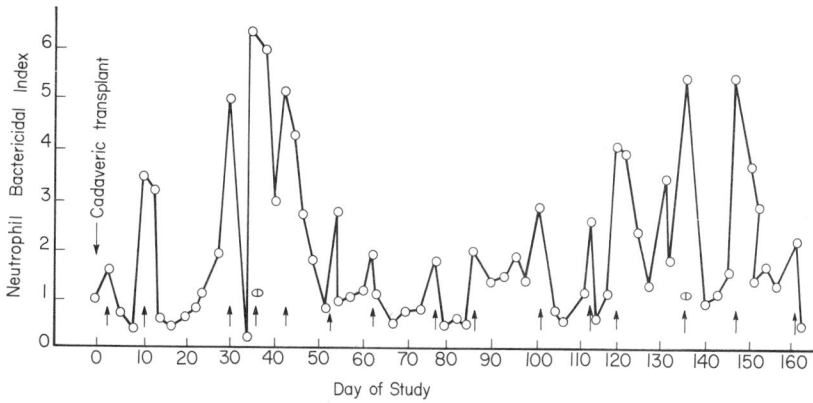

Figure 4. Serial tests of neutrophilic function from a patient who received a cadaveric renal transplant. Most of the determinations are in the abnormal range, suggesting that the immunosuppressive drugs depress neutrophilic antibacterial function. In addition, note that there are apparently two basic cycles of variation of neutrophilic function, one with a periodicity of approximately 2 weeks (arrows) and the other with a periodicity of approximately 100 days. These cycles are felt to be of clinical importance, since septic complications in these patients and burn patients appear to occur only at times when neutrophilic function is poor. (From Alexander, J. W., Dionigi, R., and Meakins, J. L.: Ann. Surg., 173:206, 1971.)

tablished. Fortunately, strict adherence to the principles of wound care and application of knowledge concerning the pathogenesis of wound infections can prevent the vast majority of infectious complications in surgical practice.

Avoidance of Predisposing Conditions

Bacterial Contamination. The most obvious means for controlling the bacterial population of any surgical incision is by minimizing contamination during operation through the use of strict aseptic techniques. Engineering and architectural advances have helped to limit airborne contamination to very low levels, but these have often not been followed by reductions in wound infection rates. At the present time, the two greatest sources of significant microbial contamination of operative wounds are exogenous contact from the hands of the operating team or errors in sterile operative technique, and endogenous contamination from the patient's skin and various tracts. Of the two, endogenous contamination is responsible for a greater number of infections in all types of wounds except those classified as "clean-electives."

As many as 90 per cent of the members of an operative team puncture or tear their gloves at some time during an operation. These gloves must be changed immediately to avoid bacterial contamination of the wound since the hands can never be sterilized by scrubbing. Even though the numbers of organisms present after a surgical scrub are low, they tend to increase with the length of the operation, and the numbers of organisms inside gloves at puncture sites increase remarkably when blood has gained entrance. These so-called minor infringements must not go unnoticed and should receive immediate attention, just like major breaks in technique.

Organisms reaching the wound from the patient's skin may be kept to a minimum by surgical prepara-

tion of the operative area for 10 minutes, with sterile gloves and a germicidal soap, and by painting the region with a bactericidal solution such as tincture of iodine and alcohol. Once the skin incision has been made, the wound edges should be covered immediately with towels held in position with towel clips or sutures. An alternative method currently in use is the application of sterile plastic film to the entire operative area, with the incision made through the plastic. This does not seem to offer any advantage over the wound towel method, and bacterial growth may occur at an accelerated rate beneath the impervious plastic cover, especially if the skin is contaminated with blood. Patients often harbor pathogenic bacteria on their skin at the time of admission, but more important, they tend to accumulate increasing numbers of pathogenic bacteria from the hospital environment with increasing length of hospitalization. It is not surprising, therefore, that patients who have been hospitalized for a relatively long period before operation tend to have a higher incidence of infection than those patients in whom the preoperative hospitalization has been relatively short.

Another very important but not always heeded source of bacterial contamination of the surgical wound is endogenous contamination at the time of transection of the gastrointestinal, respiratory, or genitourinary tract. Bacterial contamination occurs to varying degrees any time a hollow viscus is transected, but exceptional efforts to minimize the amount of contamination can result in a gratifyingly low occurrence of bacterial infection. Before a hollow viscus is entered, the operative area should be carefully isolated from the remainder of the operative field. A completely different set of instruments should be used for that portion of the operation until the hollow viscus is closed. At closure of the hollow viscus, all instruments, towels, and sponges that may have come into contact with the contaminating bacteria must be removed from the operative field. The gowns and gloves of the operative team should be changed. By strict observance of aseptic technique in clean-contaminated cases, the incidence of operative infections can be markedly reduced.

Laxity in isolation procedures and indifference in caring for patients with open infections, burns, tracheostomies, indwelling intravenous catheters, and urinary catheters are also frequent causes of nosocomial infection. Airborne infections of these sites occur less frequently in hospitals than those caused by person-to-person transfer, and the use of aseptic technique during such procedures as tracheostomy and wound care and continuous intravenous therapy is important for the prevention of hospital-acquired infections.

Wound Care. Infections in wounds associated with injury or planned operative procedures have a profound effect on the morbidity and mortality. Every patient deserves meticulous wound care, but this is particularly true in those instances in which there may be an impairment of host defense, since every wound transecting the gastrointestinal tract and a large percentage of so-called "clean surgical wounds" are contaminated by viable and potentially pathogenic bacteria.

All devitalized tissues and foreign bodies should be removed. When complete debridement is not possible, the wound should not be closed, since foreign bodies left in a wound may decrease the minimal infective dose of a bacterial inoculum 10,000-fold or more. Nearly a million viable staphylococci are necessary to produce a clinical infection when injected subcutaneously or intradermally into normal tissue, but when these same organisms are introduced on a piece of suture material, as few as 100 can produce a significant infection. Similar results have been shown with the enhancement of clostridial infections by devitalized muscle and sterile foreign bodies. It is easy to see that in grossly contaminated wounds, not only must all foreign bodies be removed, but careful consideration must be given to the introduction of new foreign bodies such as prostheses, grafts, and suture materials. In contaminated wounds, experimental studies have shown that monofilament suture materials are preferable to multifilament ones, all other things being equal. At the present time, the best nonabsorbable sutures for use in contaminated wounds are considered to be polypropylene and nylon. Of the absorbable materials, chromic catgut is probably superior.

The presence of hematomas, seromas, or dead spaces favors bacterial localization and prevents the delivery of phagocytic cells to such bacterial foci. One mistake frequently encountered in closing contaminated wounds is leaving a dead space between the layers rather than providing adequate drainage. Where a large potential dead space occurs in an operative wound which is not infected, the best method for preventing seromas is to provide a system of closed catheter suction drainage. Open drainage of wounds may increase rather than decrease the degree of contamination and the incidence of infection.

In heavily contaminated wounds or in wounds in which all of the foreign bodies or devitalized tissues cannot be satisfactorily removed, the use of delayed primary closure will, in most instances, minimize the development of serious infection. With this technique, the subcutaneous tissues and skin are left open and "packed" loosely with gauze after fascial closure. The number of phagocytic cells at the wound edges progressively increases to reach a peak about 5 days after the injury. Capillary budding is intense at this time, and closure may usually be successfully accomplished even in the face of heavy bacterial contamination, since phagocytic cells can be delivered to the site in large numbers. It has been shown experimentally that the number of organisms required to initiate an infection in a surgical incision progressively increases as the interval of healing increases, up to the fifth postoperative day.

Systemic Factors. Host resistance has been found to be abnormal in a variety of systemic conditions and diseases, including leukemia, diabetes mellitus, uremia, prematurity, burn injury, following trauma, advanced malignancy, old age, obesity, malnutrition, and several diseases of inherited immunodeficiency. When treating surgical patients with these or similar problems, extraordinary precautions should be taken to prevent the development of wound infections. These should include correction or control of the underlying defect whenever possible.

Recent studies have indicated that malnutrition, even when subclinical, can result in a significant impairment of host defense mechanisms. Since many surgical patients have some degree of malnutrition, one of the most important things a surgeon can do to prevent infection is to correct any evidence of malnutrition before surgical therapy or as soon thereafter as possible using either oral or intravenous hyperalimentation regimens. Alimentation by the oral route appears to be preferable, when possible.

The administration of many drugs, including steroids, antimetabolites, and anticancer agents, has been found to be associated with an increased incidence of septic complications. Unnecessary use of these drugs is to be avoided in the surgical patient. The role of antibiotics in opportunistic infections will be discussed later.

Immunotherapy

Active and passive immunization procedures for the prevention of surgical infections have merit in specific instances.

Tetanus is one condition in which the use of immunotherapy has had outstanding success in prevention of the disease. After a full course of active immunization, most persons are protected against the development of tetanus for years and many for a lifetime. In such persons, a booster injection of toxoid invariably elicits protective levels of antibody for as long as 20 years, and the administration of antitoxin for the prophylaxis of tetanus in these patients is not indicated except under unusual circumstances. For those persons who have not been actively immunized against tetanus before the time of their injury, it is important that they receive tetanus antitoxin. The use of antitoxin obtained from human donors has superseded the administration of antitoxin obtained from animals, and by comparison represents an extremely safe therapeutic measure. At the time of injury, 250 to 500 units of human tetanus antitoxin should be administered intramuscularly, the dose depending on the severity of the injury. If the patient is seen more than 24 hours after injury, the dose should be increased. Simultaneous administration of the initial injection of tetanus toxoid for active immunization is indicated in every case. A careful follow-up is necessary to insure completion of the course of active immunization. Tetanus antitoxin does not prevent infection with *Clostridium tetani*, but it does inactivate the toxin produced. Therefore, careful surgical débridement with removal of all devitalized tissue is clearly the most important means of prevention. The administration of systemic antibiotics has been recommended in the past for the prevention of tetanus, but this is of secondary importance and usually unnecessary.

A recently developed Pseudomonas vaccine has been evaluated clinically for the prevention of serious Pseudomonas infection in burned patients. While the material has not yet been approved as a commercial product for general distribution, its effectiveness has been impressive (Table 1). The use of a polyvalent hyperimmune pseudomonas globulin for the treatment of pseudomonas bacteremia also appears to be effective in these patients. The development of this vaccine may serve as a basis for the development of other vaccines against troublesome opportunistic infections. Its effectiveness has also been proved for the prevention of Pseudomonas infections in patients with leukemia, but it has not been helpful in cystic fibrosis.

Gas gangrene antitoxin is not recommended for prophylaxis for clostridial myositis and other infections, the main reliance in prevention being early and adequate surgical management of the wound and maintenance of a good blood supply. Other specific bacterial vaccines may be of benefit in selected cases in which other treatment modalities have failed. The use of pooled human gamma globulin for the prevention of bacterial infections should be limited to those patients who have agammaglobulinemia or a dysgammaglobulinemia.

Because opsonic proteins of the complement system may be reduced in patients with malnutrition and in patients with severe acute infections, it is sometimes indicated to administer these by passive therapy. This can best be accomplished by the transfusion of whole blood or plasma. In such patients, hemotherapy with red cell components and plasma protein derivatives may be less desirable.

Chemotherapy

The use of systemic prophylactic chemotherapeutic and antibiotic agents has continued to be a controversial subject among surgeons, mostly because of a lack of understanding of the basic principles involved. There is little doubt that the administration of therapeutic doses of antimicrobial agents is capable of preventing infection in experimental wounds contaminated by specific and highly sensitive bacteria, and there is evidence that it can attenuate or prevent infection developing in some clinical situations. The decision for the use of prophylactic antibiotic therapy, however, must be based upon the weight of evidence for possible benefit against the weight of evidence for possible adverse effects. Indiscriminate or blind use of antibiotics is discouraged because it may lead to secondary or superimposed infection with antibiotic-resistant strains of organisms, serious hypersensitivity reactions, and postponement of indicated surgical treatment. Their use may also mask the signs and symptoms of established infections, making diagnosis more difficult. An equal or even greater problem caused by the frequent use of antibiotics is the development of large numbers of antibiotic-resistant strains within the hospital environment.

Prophylactic antibiotics are clearly contraindicated in the management of patients undergoing clean surgical operations in which no obvious bacterial contamination has occurred. The incidence of wound infections in elective clean operations such as herniorrhaphy and thyroidectomy is less than 1 per cent when careful, gentle, meticulous, aseptic technique is practiced. When infections do occur, they can usually be traced to poor surgical technique or errors in aseptic technique. Prophylactic antibiotic therapy is no substitute for careful surgical technique using established surgical principles, and its indiscriminate or general use is not in the best interest of the patient. A more discriminating, limited, purposeful, and intelligent

TABLE 1. Effect of Immunotherapy on Colonization by and Infection with *Pseudomonas aeruginosa* in Patients with Burn Injuries Greater than 20 Per Cent Surviving an Initial Five Days of Hospitalization without Pseudomonas Sepsis*

Vaccine Category	Number of Patients	Colonization at Any Site (%)	Blood Cultures Positive for Pseudomonas (%)	Deaths from Pseudomonas Infection (%)
Antecedent control	75	72.2	18.7	14.7
Low dose, submaximal	40	72.5	15.0	12.5
Maximal dose	96	73.2	8.25	3.1
Maximal plus hyperimmune α-globulin given to patients with Pseudomonas bacteremia	186	66.1	5.9	0.0

*Adapted from Alexander, J. W., and Fisher, M. W.: J. Infect. Dis., *130* (Suppl.): S152, 1974.

use of antibiotic therapy should be adopted. Experience has emphasized the fact that antibiotic agents can be used effectively only as adjuvants to adequate surgery.

There are several clinical situations, however, in which the administration of prophylactic systemic antibiotic therapy will usually be of benefit. In principle, these situations almost always involve a brief period of contamination by organisms which can be predicted with reasonable accuracy. As examples, prophylactic systemic antibiotics are usually recommended in the following:

1. Accidental wounds with heavy contamination and tissue damage. The early administration of penicillin to burn patients has been considered by some authorities to be effective in preventing invasive infections of the wound by hemolytic streptococci and pneumococcus.

2. Accidental wounds requiring surgery in which treatment is unavoidably delayed.

3. Injuries in which adequate débridement cannot be accomplished, and contaminated or devitalized tissue must of necessity remain.

4. When known gross bacterial contamination has occurred in any wound.

5. Resection and anastomosis of the colon and small intestine.

6. Penetrating injuries of a hollow intra-abdominal viscus.

7. In operative procedures categorized as "clean-contaminated," when there is transection or resection of a hollow viscus of the gastrointestinal tract, biliary tract, respiratory tract, or genitourinary tract, with varying degrees of bacterial contamination, the decision for the use of antibiotic therapy must be based upon careful consideration of the evidence for and against its effectiveness. Evaluation should include an estimate of the degree of contamination, the status of nonspecific host resistance, the age of the patient, underlying disease conditions, associated drug therapy, and the length and severity of the operation. Each patient must be evaluated independently.

8. When emergency operation is indicated in patients with pre-existing or recently active infection.

9. When pre-existing valvular heart damage is present in a patient, in order to prevent the development of bacterial endocarditis.

10. Vaginal hysterectomy.

11. Common duct exploration in the presence of acute inflammation.

12 Cardiovascular surgery with placement of a prosthesis.

13. Amputation of an extremity with impaired blood supply, particularly in the presence of a current or recent ulcer.

14. Gastrectomy for carcinoma.

15. Operations entering the oral-pharyngeal cavity in continuity with neck dissections.

16. In injuries prone to clostridial infection because of extensive devitalization of muscle, heavy contamination, and impairment of blood supply.

17. In patients with open fractures, penetrating joint injuries, and joint protheses.

PROPHYLAXIS FOR OPERATIONS ON COLON

The administration of oral nonabsorbable antibiotics for the suppression of growth of intestinal bacteria has been successful in some hands and detrimental in others. At the Cincinnati General Hospital, one serious consequence of their administration has been shown to be the emergence and overgrowth of virulent antibiotic-resistant bacteria, particularly *Staphylococcus aureus* UC/18. Staphylococcal enterocolitis following antibiotic bowel preparation may develop as a serious nosocomial infection. Staphylococcal wound infection may also occur. Our own experience has led us to conclude that thorough mechanical cleansing of the intestinal tract is more important than prophylactic antibiotic bowel preparation, and is preferable, provided systemically administered antibiotic therapy is given immediately before, during, and after the operation. For this purpose, we have effectively employed a combination of aqueous penicillin and tetracycline given intravenously. Therapeutic doses should be given from the very beginning and continued for the first 3 or 4 days postoperatively, at which time they should be discontinued. For the average adult this means 3 to 4 million units of aqueous penicillin and 1.0 gm. of tetracycline daily given intravenously in three or four divided doses. Intermittent intravenous therapy is probably preferable to continuous intravenous therapy. If oral antibiotics are to be given as a preparation for colon surgery, neomycin plus erythromycin or neomycin plus tetracycline begun shortly before surgery seems to be the preferable combinations at the present time.

Prophylactic antibiotic therapy is clearly more effective when started preoperatively and continued through the intraoperative period. This procedure produces therapeutic levels of the antibiotic agents at the operative site throughout the procedure and in any seromas and hematomas that may develop subsequently. Antibiotics started as late as two to six hours after bacterial contamination are markedly less effective. Failure of the effectiveness of prophylactic antibiotic agents has resulted in part from a lack of appreciation of the importance of the timing and dosage of these agents, which are critical determinants.

Prophylactic antibiotic therapy is generally ineffective in those clinical situations where contamination is apt to continue to occur. Examples are as follows:

1. In patients with tracheostomies or tracheal intubation to prevent pulmonary infections.

2. In patients with indwelling urinary catheters.

3. In patients with indwelling central venous lines.

4. In most open wounds, including burn wounds. Some authorities feel that a brief 3- to 5-day course of penicillin therapy should be given to patients with severe burn injury to prevent infections with *Streptococcus pyogenes*, but others feel this is unnecessary and may lead to infections with more resistant organisms.

5. In immunologically deficient patients or those receiving immunosuppressive therapy unless there are other indications for systemic antibiotic therapy.

The use of topical antibiotics has proven to be effective in some instances in diminishing the incidence of infection in contaminated wounds. They should be considered as an alternative to the use of systemic prophylactic antibiotics, especially when it is desirable to avoid the latter, and as a complement to their use when heavy contamination has occurred. They may be particularly useful in those situations where the indications for systemic prophylactic antibiotics are marginal.

DIAGNOSIS OF SURGICAL INFECTIONS

The diagnosis of established surgical infections is often not difficult, but several types, such as abscesses of the retroperitoneal tissues, subphrenic space, liver, and pancreas, and deep-seated wound or abdominal infections, may tax the ingenuity of the most astute clinician. Accurate and prompt diagnosis with evaluation of the patient is a necessary prerequisite for adequate treatment, and in many instances, for survival.

By far the most important part of the evaluation of a patient suspected of having a surgical infection is a careful history and physical examination. Many times the lesion will be characterized by the cardinal signs of inflammation, but this is not always the case, especially when infection is deep-seated or has been attenuated by intensive immunosuppressive or antibiotic therapy. In the latter instances, massive pyogenic abscesses may occur in the absence of fever, tenderness, or leukocytosis. The most important physical finding in localizing an infection is the presence of a tender mass.

Urinalysis and complete blood count should be done on all patients suspected of having a surgical infection, since these measures may aid greatly in the diagnosis. Intra-abdominal infections are frequently mimicked by pyelonephritis, and the presence of diabetes mellitus will usually be detected by urinalysis. This is particularly important, since both infection and diabetes are difficult to control when they occur together. Occasionally, infections caused by hemolytic bacteria such as *Streptococcus pyogenes* and *Clostridium welchii* may become associated with a profound anemia. An elevation of the leukocyte count may or may not be helpful in the diagnosis of surgical infections. With most infections, it will be elevated, but in many conditions, such as typhoid fever, overwhelming infection, concomitant antibiotic therapy, and immunosuppressive drug treatment, the leukocyte count may be within the normal or subnormal range. In overwhelming infections and infections developing in the face of antibiotic therapy, there is often a shift to the left and toxic granulation of the cells even though the total leukocyte count is not elevated. Blood cultures may help to establish the etiologic agent in a surgical infection but do not help to pinpoint its location. In patients with chills, several blood cultures should be obtained at frequent intervals during the infection, since a single culture may often be negative. Roentgenographic examinations may aid in localizing deep-seated abscesses.

Whenever possible, pus or infectious exudate from the area of the infection should be examined to establish an etiologic diagnosis since this may be helpful in selecting the correct method of therapy. In deep-seated abscesses, pus can be obtained by needle aspiration or at the time of definitive drainage. Surface infections can be examined directly. In patients with life-threatening pulmonary infections complicating surgery, securing samples for examination by transtracheal aspiration is advisable. In this setting, sputum cultures as routinely done are of extremely limited value. Urine samples from females suspected of having urinary tract infection may be best obtained for definitive culture by suprapubic aspiration. To the experienced observer, gross examination of the pus with notation of its odor, color, and consistency will give important diagnostic suggestions. A foul odor to the pus, for example, is almost diagnostic for an anaerobic infection. Thick creamy pus suggests an infection caused by *Staphylococcus aureus,* whereas a greenish discharge from an open wound suggests infection with *Pseudomonas aeruginosa.* Infections with rapid onset after surgery associated with wound edema and discharge of a thin watery pus are often caused by Streptococcus or Clostridium species. Microscopic examination of a smear of the material after Gram staining, Ziehl-Neelsen staining, or other technique often yields immediate information regarding the etiologic agent and can aid substantially in the selection of the best antibiotic agent (Table 2).

In many types of infection, however, the etiologic agent may not be apparent on direct smear, and therefore immediate culture of the purulent material using aerobic and anaerobic technique should always be made. Whenever an abscess is drained, it should first be aspirated with a syringe and needle to obtain material for culture. The air should be excluded and the needle should be occluded, as for a blood gas measurement, and the syringe containing the pus transported to the laboratory as soon as possible. Satisfactory results can usually be obtained, since pus is an excellent transport medium, especially for anaerobic organisms. Cultures, particularly anaerobic cultures, must then be placed immediately into the appropriate media and incubated. Material kept in the refrigerator or at room temperature will frequently yield inconclusive or even false results, particularly when mixed infections are present. A direct smear of the pus onto a blood agar plate will often yield characteristic colonies within a few hours. If direct sensitivity tests are performed on the plated material, definitive antibiotic sensitivity results can be obtained within 12 to 24 hours in most instances when this information can be critical to the management of the patient.

Biopsy of the lesion in granulomatous infections may provide valuable information in establishing the definitive diagnosis. Utilization of the fluorescent antibody technique for identifying organisms in tissue sections has added significantly to the value of biopsied material. Other tests such as skin tests and examination of the patient's serum for specific antibodies may be of additional help when indicated.

TABLE 2.   Initial Choice of Antibiotics for Severe and Life-Threatening Infections Based Upon Results of Preliminary Gram Staining and Before Definitive Antibiotic Sensitivity Testing

Type of Bacteria Found on Gram Staining	Source	Initial Choice of Antibiotic
Gram-positive cocci in clumps (staphylococci)	Any source	Nafcillin and penicillin or a cephalosporin; give gentamicin or lincomycin if allergic to erythromycin
Gram-positive cocci in chains (streptococci)	Any source	Penicillin G
Gram-positive rods	Any source	Penicillin G, usually with tetracycline
Gram-negative rods	Lower respiratory tract	Gentamicin or kanamycin
	Urinary tract	Ampicillin with or without gentamicin or kanamycin
	Surgical wound (abdominal)	Penicillin and a tetracycline or ampicillin and gentamicin
	Surgical wound (chest)	Ampicillin and gentamicin
	Septicemia	Ampicillin or a cephalosporin and gentamicin or kanamycin
	Deep abscess	Same as septicemia. Treat with single agent if not severe and/or well drained
Mixed flora – gram-positive and gram-negative	Human bite	Penicillin and tetracycline
	Septicemia	Penicillin and gentamicin, or penicillin and chloramphenicol, or clindamycin and gentamicin
	Severe cellulitis or peritonitis following abdominal surgery	

TREATMENT OF SURGICAL INFECTION

Prevention is obviously the best form of therapy, but postoperative infections will occur occasionally even with the best means of preventive management. Other types of surgical infections arise spontaneously and require surgical management, as indicated earlier.

Surgical Intervention

The primary principle of the surgical treatment of infections is incision and drainage of localized collections of pus. The old adage "never let the sun set on an undrained abscess" is as true today as it ever was. In considering surgical intervention, one must take into account the location of the infection, the presence or absence of complicating cellulitis, the complication of disseminating sepsis, the duration of the lesion, and the presence or absence of complicating disease. Surgical drainage permits the removal of bacteria, dead leukocytes, and necrotic tissues, and the access of new phagocytes, antibiotic agents, and serum opsonins to the remaining infecting bacteria. When incision and drainage are employed as a method of treatment, it is essential that complete decompression be obtained. The incision must be large enough to accomplish free drainage, with the use of mechanical drains whenever these are indicated. Walls between loculations must be broken down or these areas drained separately. Dependent drainage is a cardinal principle to be practiced whenever possible. Needle aspiration of abscesses does not provide free drainage, and should not be done except for the purpose of establishing a diagnosis or localizing the site of an abscess. Like any

other operation, surgical drainage of an abscess should be accomplished under controlled and otherwise aseptic conditions to prevent the introduction of additional types of microbes into an already infected area. Synergistic infections or superinfections may occasionally develop under these conditions, becoming considerably more recalcitrant to treatment.

A thorough search should always be made for the underlying cause of the infection as well as for other systemic and local diseases that may be contributory. Surgeons should not neglect evaluation or consideration of local complications of systemic diseases such as malignant disease, diabetes mellitus, Cushing's disease, malnutrition, hypogammaglobulinemia or agammaglobulinemia, and chronic granulomatous disease of childhood.

Occasionally, surgical decompression of a rapidly progressing and fulminating infection by radical incision and drainage or amputation becomes necessary when other means of controlling a life-threatening infection fail. Examples of this include gas gangrene or clostridial myositis, anaerobic crepitant cellulitis, and acute hemolytic streptococcal gangrene. Total excision of specific chronic or indolent infections may also become necessary in rare instances.

Chemotherapy and Antibiotic Therapy

In the treatment of infections in which there is a localized collection of pus, antibiotic agents serve only as an adjunct to surgical drainage. Their widespread use in the treatment of abscesses has contributed little to any increase in survival, and their primary beneficial effect has been through the decreased incidence of complications and shortened convalescence.

In contrast, antibiotic therapy may have a primary role in the management of the patient when certain infections are manifested by diffuse cellulitis. In such instances, early and effective therapy usually results in resolution of the infection with minimal complications. Antibiotic therapy for diffuse cellulitis should be aggressive, but close observation of the patient must be made for signs and symptoms of any associated abscess that may develop. Failure of the systemic signs and symptoms of infection to recede within 48 to 72 hours after the beginning of specific antibiotic therapy often indicates the development of a collection of purulent material or metastatic infections.

Mechanisms of Action of Antibiotic Agents. The extreme clinical importance of the antimicrobial agents has stimulated studies in molecular biology to compound a substantial body of information concerning the biologic reactions of antibiotics and their degradation productions in both man and experimental animals. Perhaps even more attention has been given to the effect of these agents upon their intended targets, the microbes. Antimicrobial agents can conveniently be divided into those which affect the structure of the bacterial cell walls and those which affect protein synthesis, whether it is mediated by effects on the ribosome or on nucleic acid synthesis. While it is beyond the scope of this chapter to review this body of knowledge in depth, the principal mechanisms of action have been summarized in Table 3. In addition to the recognized role of antibiotics in the biochemical events of the organism, their effects on the host must be taken into consideration when they are administered. Weinstein and Dalton have presented an excellent review of this subject.

Selection of Antibiotic Agents. Because of the widely varying spectrum of sensitivity to the currently available antibiotic agents (Table 4), early identification of the offending organism and antibiotic sensitivity testing are essential for the most effective use of these agents. Sensitivity studies may be done by the serial dilution technique or the disc method with commercially prepared discs. The latter is considerably easier to perform but not as sensitive or as reliable. Its usefulness, however, can be increased when consideration is given to the size of the zone of inhibition, the completeness of the inhibition, and the controlled concentration of antibiotic in the disc. Under these circumstances the disc method provides valuable information, and experience has shown a strong correlation between the results obtained by in vitro sensitivity tests by the disc method and the clinical response obtained.

So-called "shotgun" therapy is to be discouraged except possibly in severe established infections when death of the patient appears probable before sensitivity tests would be available. Even in these instances, it is far more acceptable to use two antibiotics covering a broad spectrum of activity rather than many antibacterial agents in large dosage. A knowledge of bacterial sensitivity patterns associated with a presumptive diagnosis as to the offending organism will frequently lead to selection of the proper antibi-

otic (Table 5). Direct examination of stained smears of the pus obtained by incision and drainage or needle aspiration of the lesion will often reveal the nature of the infecting organism, as already noted (see Table 2). In critical situations when there is an immediate need for information concerning antibiotic sensitivity of the organism, direct sensitivity tests may be done, as mentioned before, by plating the purulent exudate directly on a blood agar plate and simultaneously testing with sensitivity discs. Definitive information can thus usually be obtained within 12 hours. Unfortunately, the results of culture and sensitivity tests in many laboratories are unnecessarily delayed, and a report may not be available to the attending physician for several days.

Administration of Antibiotic Agents. In minor infections, antibiotic therapy is often unnecessary and may even be contraindicated, but in patients with severe systemic infections, antibiotics should be administered as soon as possible after a definitive diagnosis has been made. In infections, the agents should be administered preferably by the intravenous or intramuscular route. When the intravenous route is used, injection of the antibiotic agent at intermittent intervals seems to be preferable to continuous infusions, since higher levels are usually obtained in the blood and extracellular fluids. It is important to recognize that antibiotic agents have their greatest effect upon actively growing bacteria but little or no effect on phagocytized organisms. Bacteria may remain viable intracellularly for prolonged periods of time even in the presence of very high concentrations of antibiotics in the extracellular fluid. Microbes damaged by antibiotics before phagocytosis, however, have been shown to be more readily killed by the phagocytic cells.

Complications of Antibiotic Therapy. Treatment with antibiotic agents is not without danger. In addition to a false sense of security and inappropriate reliance upon their effectiveness, complications may occur during or following their use (see Table 3). Untoward reactions may be toxic, associated with hypersensitivity reactions, or due to idiosyncrasies. All of the antibiotics commonly used have at one time or another produced one or more of these types of adverse reactions.

Toxic reactions are related to overdosage and can be easily managed by decreasing the dosage of the drug or discontinuing it. When sensitization occurs, severe allergic reactions may accompany administration of the drug. Penicillin sensitivity is the classic example of this type of reaction, and many patients still die in this country from this cause each year. Although often unreliable, the clinical history of past sensitivities is the only practical source of information available to the clinician treating acute infections. Recently developed in vitro tests and skin sensitivity tests may be of value in determining drug sensitivities after recovery, but the time requirement for their performance precludes their usefulness in patients with acute, severe infections. Persons who have had a hypersensitivity reaction to one drug are more prone to have hypersensitivity reactions to other therapeutic agents. Several antimicrobial agents such as chloramphenicol and the sulfonamides are capable of producing agranulocytosis or aplastic anemia. Regularly repeated blood counts

TABLE 3. Properties and Dosages of Selected Antimicrobial Agents

Drug and Usual Adult Dosage	Mode of Action	Complications of Use and Major Untoward Reactions
Sulfonamides 4 to 6 gm. per day in 4 to 6 divided doses for short-acting forms; less for longer-acting forms	Bacteriostatic. Competitive antagonism with PABA causing inhibition of one-carbon transferase activity which inhibits nucleotide synthesis and, therefore, DNA synthesis. Drug of choice for meningococcal, nocardial, and many urinary tract infections	Allergic reactions Urinary tract calculi Blood dyscrasias Nephrotoxicity Neuritis
Penicillins Penicillin G 2 to 30 million units per day parenterally in 4 to 6 divided doses	Bactericidal. All penicillins inhibit cell wall synthesis, causing protoplasts. Not acid-stable. Because of the high osmotic pressure in the bacteria, they absorb water from isotonic body fluids and burst. Requires growing cells for effect. Probably acts by interference with transpeptidase activity, causing prevention of crosslinkage in cell walls. Urinary excretion of all penicillins blocked by probenecid	Allergic reactions frequent CNS irritability and convulsions with high doses
Penicillin V 400,000 units q 4 to 6 hours orally	Acid-resistant and absorbed from GI tract	Allergic reactions frequent
Methicillin (parenteral only) 4 to 12 gm. per day in 4 to 6 divided doses. Dosage frequently higher than other semisynthetics	First penicillinase-resistant penicillin available for clinical use (1960). Not acid-stable. 18 to 30% bound to serum protein	Allergic reactions Bone marrow depression CNS effects
Oxacillin 2 to 12 gm. per day in 4 to 6 divided doses	Acid-stable	Allergic reactions CNS effects Cholestatic jaundice
Nafcillin 2 to 12 gm. per day in 4 to 6 divided doses	Acid-stable. Good tissue levels obtainable. High biliary excretion	Allergic reactions CNS effects
Cloxacillin 2 to 12 gm. per day in 4 to 6 divided doses	Differs from oxacillin only by a single Cl⁻ ion, but serum concentration twice as high after oral administration. 95% bound to serum proteins	Allergic reactions CNS effects
Dicloxacillin 1 to 4 gm. per day in 4 to 6 divided doses (oral only)	Best absorption of all the synthetic penicillins from the GI tract; therefore, good oral drug for penicillinase-producing staphylococci	Allergic reactions
Ampicillin 2 to 12 gm. per day in 4 to 6 divided doses	Acid-resistant and well absorbed. High biliary excretion. Mode of action against gram-negative bacteria similar to that of penicillin against susceptible gram-positive bacteria. Effectiveness may be from a better ability to penetrate the cell walls of gram-negative bacteria. Some binding to serum proteins (20 to 25%). Destroyed by penicillinase	Allergic reactions (rash in 9.5% given by oral route) CNS effects Diarrhea
Carbenicillin 4 to 30 gm. per day in 4 to 6 divided doses	Bactericidal. Same as penicillin but useful for Pseudomonas	Allergic reactions frequent Neutropenia rare
Cephalosporins Cephalothin, cephazolin, and cephaloridine 2 to 6 gm. per day in 4 to 6 divided doses parenterally Cephalexin May be given orally, 1 to 4 gm. per day.	Bactericidal. Inhibits cell wall mucopeptide synthesis by inhibiting final crosslinkage of peptidoglycan monomers. Resistant to penicillinase but can be degraded by cephalosporinase. Cephaloridine not bound to serum proteins. Best levels obtained with cephazolin	Resembles penicillin in structure. May cause allergic reactions in an occasional patient who is sensitive to penicillin (10%). Destroyed by cephaloridinease. Cephaloridine is nephrotoxic, cephalothin and cephazolin less so. Neutropenia rare

c_i should be used to monitor the bone marrow response when these agents are used. Other drugs such as kanamycin, gentamicin, polymyxin, and colistin can produce renal damage and uremia, particularly in persons with previously existing renal disease. Streptomycin, dihydrostreptomycin, kanamycin, and gentamicin may all produce ototoxicity when given in large doses or for a prolonged period. Tetracycline may cause severe yellow staining and deformity of the teeth when given to infants; this may also occur in infants born to mothers given tetracycline therapy in the prenatal period. Other antibiotics such as erythromycin, tetracycline, and ampicillin may produce diarrhea, and clindamycin therapy has occasionally been associated with severe colitis.

The administration of any antibacterial agent may produce a suppression of susceptible microbes with the emergence and overgrowth of those strains resistant to the antibiotic administered and the spontaneous development of secondary or superimposed infections by bacteria, fungi, or viruses. The development of diarrhea in most instances is related to a change in the bacterial flora of the intestine. An overgrowth with strains of *Staphylococcus aureus* may occur in the intestine during antibiotic therapy, but it is seen most frequently when nonabsorbable antibiotics have been

TABLE 3. Properties and Dosages of Selected Antimicrobial Agents (*Continued*)

Drug and Usual Adult Dosage	Mode of Action	Complications of Use and Major Untoward Reactions
Polymyxin B and Colistimethate 1.5 to 5 mg./kg./day in 2 divided doses IM	Bactericidal. Does not require cell growth for effect. Affects cell membrane permeability, acting as a cationic detergent. Also interferes with cellular oxidative phosphorylation	Nephrotoxic reactions frequent Neuritis and neurotoxicity Allergic reactions rare
Aminoglycosides Streptomycin IM only, 1 to 2 gm. per day in 2 to 4 divided doses	Bactericidal. Inhibits protein synthesis. Primary action on ribosomes. Causes misreading of m-RNA or interferes with association of 30S and 50S subunits	Vestibular-auditory nerve damage, deafness Bacterial resistance develops readily Peripheral neuropathy, blood dyscrasias rarely
Kanamycin IM only, 1 to 1.5 mg./kg./day in 2 to 3 divided doses	Same as streptomycin	Ototoxicity frequent; nephrotoxic occasionally, allergic reactions, peripheral neuropathy and blood dyscrasias rarely
Gentamicin 1.5 to 3 mg./kg./day IM in 4 divided doses	Same as streptomycin	May cause vestibular damage and deafness. May be nephrotoxic
Chloramphenicol 1 to 4 gm. per day in 2 to 6 divided doses PO, IM, or IV	Bacteriostatic. Inhibits protein synthesis. Interferes with assembly of amino acids in peptide synthesis, probably through an effect on RNA or on formation of the peptide bond	Occasionally aplastic anemia, thrombocytopenia, and neutropenia. May cause peripheral and optic neuropathy. May cause immunosuppression in clinical doses
Tetracyclines PO 1 to 2 gm. per day in 4 to 6 divided doses; IV 1 gm. per day in 4 to 6 divided doses	Bacteriostatic. Inhibit protein synthesis by blocking transfer of amino acids from the aminoacyl RNA to polypeptide. Inhibit bacterial enzyme synthesis. Efficient chelators of heavy metals; Mg^{++} may be important	Catabolic agent; may cause increased BUN. GI disturbances. Stains teeth in children and can affect bones. Degradation products nephrotoxic. Photosensitivity reactions. May cause hepatotoxicity in excess dosage. Allergic reactions, blood dyscrasias, visual disturbances, and interference with protein metabolism rarely seen
Erythromycin (Macrolide family) 1 to 4 gm. per day in 4 divided doses	Bacteriostatic. Selectively inhibits protein synthesis. Useful for treatment of L-forms and Mycoplasma	GI and hepatic disturbances. Resistance may develop during therapy
Clindamycin 1 to 2 gm. per day in 4 divided doses PO; 300–600 mg. IM TID or QID	Bacteriostatic. Inhibits protein synthesis by binding to 50S subunits of ribosomes and inhibits peptide bond formation. Action may be similar to that of erythromycin and chloramphenicol	GI disturbances, diarrhea, severe colitis, allergic hepatic dysfunction, skin rash.
Novobiocin 1 to 2 gm. per day in 4 divided doses	Bacteriostatic. Binds divalent ions, especially Mg^{++} resulting in markedly reduced RNA synthesis	Allergic reactions. Liver damage frequent. Blood dyscrasias occasionally. Bacterial resistance develops readily
Amphotericin B IV 250 μg./kg./day initially Raise dose gradually to maximum of 1.5 mgm./kg./day Total dose maximum of 3–4 gm.	Fungistatic or fungicidal by interacting within cell membranes	Highly nephrotoxic. Fever, anemia, GI symptoms common. Hypotension, liver damage, and blood dyscrasias occasionally seen

administered orally for intestinal antisepsis. Staphylococcal enterocolitis in its severest form is a dire emergency and must be treated by immediate fluid replacement and antistaphylococcal agents. The emergence of resistant organisms is particularly prone to occur when antibiotics are administered for the treatment of lesions subject to contamination from external sources, such as open wounds, leg ulcers, burns, and avulsion injuries. Superinfections with viruses and fungi have become increasingly more frequent and are especially difficult to treat. When systemic, they are usually associated with diminished host resistance and except in immunologically deficient patients they almost invariably occur during a course of antibiotic therapy.

Immunotherapy

Until recently, the usefulness of specific immunotherapy in the practice of surgery was limited primarily to administration of antitoxins against tetanus, rabies, and snake poisons. However, the successful use of a polyvalent Pseudomonas hyperimmune globulin in burn patients has led to a rekindling of interest in this approach to controlling opportunistic infections that occur in patients with diminished host resistance. Other specifically directed vaccines have occasionally

TABLE 4.   Choice of Antibacterial Agents for Treatment of Surgical Infections*

Infecting Microorganism	Agent of First Choice	Alternative Agents
Gram-Positive Cocci		
Diplococcus pneumoniae	Penicillin G	Erythromycin; a cephalosporin; gentamicin
Staphylococcus aureus		
Non-penicillinase-producing	Penicillin G	A cephalosporin; erythromycin; lincomycin
Penicillinase-producing	Dicloxacillin or nafcillin, or other peni-cillinase-resistant penicillins	A cephalosporin; gentamicin; erythromy-cin; clindamycin
Peptostreptococcus	Penicillin G	Erythromycin; clindamycin
Streptococcus faecalis (Enterococcus)	Penicillin G (with streptomycin for endo-carditis or septicemia)	Vancomycin or erythromycin with strepto-mycin
Streptococcus pyogenes Groups A, B, C, and D	Penicillin G	Erythromycin; a cephalosporin; clindamycin
Streptococcus viridans	Penicillin G with or without streptomycin	Erythromycin with or without streptomy-cin, vancomycin, or a cephalosporin
Gram-Positive Bacilli		
Bacillus anthracis (anthrax)	Penicillin G	Erythromycin; a tetracycline
Clostridium tetani	Penicillin G	A cephalosporin; a tetracycline; erythro-mycin
Clostridium welchii (Bacillus perfringens) (gas gangrene)	Penicillin G	Clindamycin; a tetracycline; a cephalo-sporin; erythromycin
Corynebacterium diphtheriae	Penicillin G	Erythromycin; a tetracycline
Listeria monocytogenes	Ampicillin	Penicillin; erythromycin; a tetracycline
Gram-Negative Bacilli		
Alcaligenes faecalis	Penicillin G or a tetracycline and streptomycin	Chloramphenicol; kanamycin
Bacteroides fragilis	Chloramphenicol or clindamycin	A tetracycline or erythromycin or carbenicillin or penicillin
Bacteroides melaninogenicus or *oralis*	Penicillin	Erythromycin; clindamycin
Bordetella (Haemophilus) pertussis (whooping cough)	Ampicillin	A tetracycline or chloramphenicol
Brucella species (brucellosis)	A tetracycline	Chloramphenicol
Calymmatobacterium granulomatis	A tetracycline	Streptomycin; chloramphenicol; ampicillin
Enterobacter (Aerobacter) species	Kanamycin	Gentamicin; a tetracycline with or without streptomycin; a polymyxin; carbenicillin
Escherichia coli		
Enteropathogenic	Kanamycin (oral)	A tetracycline
Sepsis	Ampicillin or gentamicin	Kanamycin; a polymyxin; a tetracycline; a cephalosporin
Haemophilus ducreyi (chancroid)	A tetracycline	A sulfonamide; streptomycin
Haemophilus influenzae	Ampicillin	Chloramphenicol with or without strepto-mycin; a tetracycline; a cephalosporin
Klebsiella pneumoniae	A cephalosporin	Kanamycin; a polymyxin; chloramphenicol
Mima, Herellea	Kanamycin; a tetracycline	A polymyxin; a tetracycline; kanamycin
Pasteurella pestis (bubonic plague)	A tetracycline	Streptomycin
Pasteurella tularensis (tularemia)	Streptomycin	A tetracycline; chloramphenicol
Proteus mirabilis	Ampicillin	Cephalosporin; kanamycin
Proteus (other species)	Kanamycin	Gentamicin; chloramphenicol; a tetracy-cline and streptomycin; cephalosporin
Providencia species	Carbenicillin	Gentamicin
Pseudomonas aeruginosa	Gentamicin or tobramycin	Polymyxin B; carbenicillin
Pseudomonas pseudomallei	A tetracycline with or without a sulfonamide	Chloramphenicol with or without a sul-fonamide; kanamycin
Salmonella species	Chloramphenicol	Ampicillin
Serratia species	Gentamicin	Kanamycin; chloramphenicol; carbeni-cillin
Shigella species	Ampicillin	A tetracycline; oral kanamycin
Vibrio cholerae (cholera)	A tetracycline	An erythromycin; chloramphenicol
Acid-Fast Bacilli		
Mycobacterium leprae	A sulfone	Amithiozone
Mycobacterium tuberculosis	Isoniazid combined with either amino-salicylic acid or ethambutol, with or without streptomycin	Pyrazinamide; cycloserine, ethionamide; viomycin; kanamycin; capreomycin; ery-thromycin
Mycoplasma	Erythromycin	A tetracycline; chloramphenicol
L-Forms of Bacteria	A tetracycline	Chloramphenicol; erythromycin
Actinomycetes		
Actinomyces israeli	Penicillin G and a sulfonamide	A tetracycline
Nocardia species	A sulfonamide	A tetracycline
Fungus		
Candida albicans	Amphotericin B	None
Cryptococcus neoformans	Amphotericin B	None
Coccidioides immitis	Amphotericin B	None
Histoplasma capsulatum	Amphotericin B	None
Mucor	Amphotericin B	None
Fusospirochetes	Penicillin G	Erythromycin; a tetracycline

*Modified from Med. Lett. Drugs Ther., *13*:37, 1971.

TABLE 5. Selection of Antibiotics Based Upon Most Likely Organism for
Selected Infections

Type of Infection	Most Likely Organism	Initial Choice of Antibiotic
Superficial Infections		
Erysipelas	Streptococcus	Penicillin
Acute necrotizing fasciitis	Polymicrobic, usually with anaerobes	Penicillin and tetracycline or gentamicin
Acute lymphangitis	Streptococcus	Penicillin
Meleney's synergistic gangrene	Streptococcus and Staphylococcus	Penicillin
Breast abscess	Staphylococcus, but often polymicrobic	A penicillin, tetracycline
Subcutaneous abscess (not hospital-acquired)	Staphylococcus	A penicillin or cephalosporin
Human bite (infected)	Polymicrobic, spirochetes important	Penicillin and tetracycline
Abscess of hand	Staphylococcus	Penicillin and nafcillin or dicloxacillin or a cephalosporin
Abdominal wound (GI and GU tract entered)	Polymicrobic; Bacteroides important	Penicillin and tetracycline
(GI and GU tracts not entered)	Staphylococcus	Nafcillin or other penicillinase-resistant penicillin
Deep Intra-abdominal Infections		
Peritonitis following appendicitis or injury to intestine	Polymicrobic; anaerobes important	Penicillin and tetracycline, or a cephalosporin
Perirectal, appendiceal, intra-abdominal, retroperitoneal, or subphrenic abscess	Polymicrobic; anaerobes important	Penicillin and tetracycline, or a cephalosporin
Cholecystic abscess and cholangitis	Polymicrobic; clostridia important	Penicillin and tetracycline, or a cephalosporin
Crepitant myositis	Clostridia	Penicillin and tetracycline or cephalosporin, erythromycin
Enterocolitis following antibiotic bowel preparation	Staphylococcus	Nafcillin or other penicillinase-resistant penicillins or cephalothin
Septicemia		
Septicemia following burn injury		
First 2 weeks	Staphylococcus	Gentamicin or penicillinase-resistant penicillin
After 2 weeks	Gram-negative rod, often Pseudomonas	Gentamicin
Septicemia following GU instrumentation	E. coli	Ampicillin and gentamicin or kanamycin
Septicemia from contaminated IV solutions or associated with indwelling intravenous catheters	Enteric bacteria, often Pseudomonas, Serratia, or Mimeae	Cephalothin and gentamicin or kanamycin
Septicemia from superinfections during antibiotic therapy	Gram-negative pathogens or Candida	Cephalothin and gentamicin. If Candida, stop antibiotic therapy, and if life-threatening, give amphotericin B
Pulmonary Infections		
Primary pneumonia	Pneumonococcus	Penicillin
Pneumonia complicating respirator treatment or intubation	Gram-negative pathogen, often Pseudomonas	Gentamicin

been of value in the management of infections resistant to all other forms of therapy. As emphasized earlier, patients suspected or proven to have reduced levels of opsonic proteins in their blood may benefit by replacement therapy with whole blood or plasma.

Supportive Therapy

Recent studies have emphasized the critical role of nutritional therapy in the management of surgical patients. Nutritional repletion in the malnourished individual can correct many abnormalities of host defense, including abnormal vascular responsiveness, diminished antibacterial activity of phagocytic cells, and low levels of opsonic proteins. Because of this, a vigorous approach to nutritional supplementation in the infected patient should be emphasized. In the sick, septic patient who is unable to eat, intravenous hyperalimentation administering a caloric, amino acid, vitamin, and mineral intake of 50 per cent or more above basal requirements should be instituted as soon as possible.

CLASSIFICATION OF SURGICAL INFECTIONS

The anatomic location of a lesion often provides valuable clues concerning the etiologic agent (see Table 5). For example, the majority of wound infections are caused by *Staphylococcus aureus* or a mixed bacterial flora. Intra-abdominal infections associated with perforation of the gastrointestinal tract are always polymicrobial and usually involve aerobic and anaerobic gram-negative enteric bacteria as well as gram-positive anaerobic bacteria. Infections arising in the genitourinary tract are predominantly from gram-negative organisms, and the most common of these is *Escherichia coli*. A spreading subcutaneous cellulitis most frequently results from infection with *Streptococcus pyogenes* but may be caused by *Staphylococcus aureus*.

The following discussion of etiologic agents includes those considered to be most important but is not intended to be a complete review.

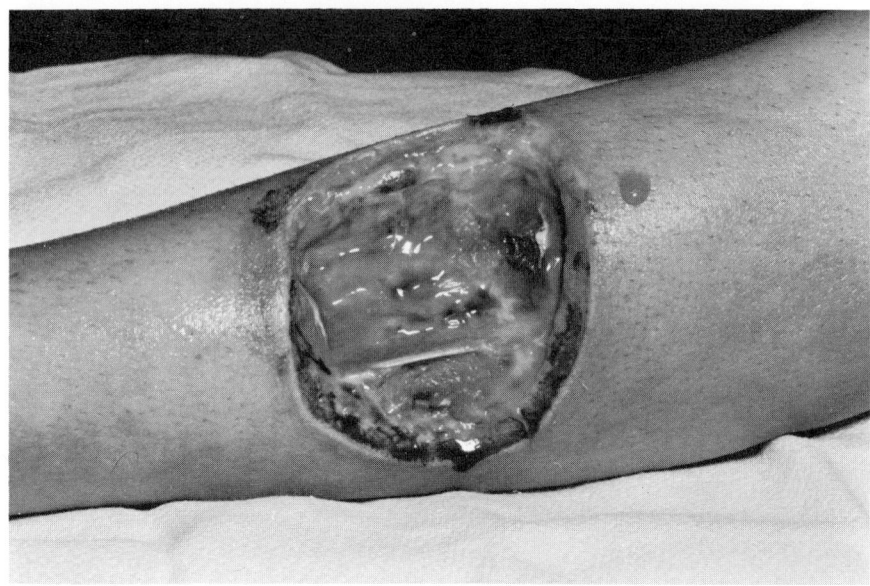

Figure 5. Acute postoperative localized wound infection caused by the hemolytic *Staphylococcus aureus*. Note thick, creamy pus.

Staphylococcal Infections

A large number of infections encountered in surgical practice are caused by *Staphylococcus aureus* (Fig. 5). It is an important pathogen in postoperative wound infection and in infections following penetrating wounds. The lesions produced by *S. aureus* are characteristically localized with an indurated area of cellulitis that undergoes central necrosis and abscess formation with a thick, creamy, odorless, and yellow or cream-colored pus. Bacteremia may occur, with the development of metastatic abscesses. Fever and leukocytosis are usually present. Those infections acquired during the course of hospitalization are often caused by antibiotic-resistant bacteria of increased virulence.

The treatment of established infections caused by *S. aureus* in those which have progressed to abscess formation includes adequate surgical drainage and active supportive therapy with heat, rest, and elevation of the affected part. A spreading cellulitis is occasionally seen with staphylococcal infections and should be treated vigorously with appropriate antibiotic therapy. When staphylococcal infections occur in postoperative incisions, the wound should be opened widely to facilitate free drainage of the purulent material. Drainage is promoted by loosely packing the abscess cavity with fine-mesh or iodoform gauze at the time of drainage. Antibiotic therapy in all cases should be started at or before the time of operation for the establishment of drainage. The preferred route of administration will depend upon the clinical circumstance.

Streptococcal Infections

A variety of streptococcal organisms produce infections seen in surgical practice. The most frequent of these is *Streptococcus pyogenes* (Group A, beta hemolytic) although others such as *S. viridans* (alpha hemolytic), Peptostreptococcus, aerophilic streptococcus, and *S. faecalis* (Group D enterococci) may be encountered.

The lesions caused by *S. pyogenes* are characteristically invasive with a rapid course. Full-blown infections are often seen within 12 to 24 hours after the time of contamination, but may occur as late as 1 or 2 weeks. The infections are characterized by diffuse cellulitis, lymphangitis, lymphadenitis, and extension of the inflammation along fascial planes. A thin, watery pus may develop, but frank abscess formation rarely occurs. Gangrenous processes may be caused by thrombosis of small vessels. Bacteremia occurs rather frequently, and is usually heralded by the development of chills, high fever, a rapid, thready pulse, and general signs of toxemia.

Several specific disease syndromes are related to streptococcal infection. Among these are erysipelas, which is most often produced by the hemolytic streptococci. It usually occurs in the epifascial tissues and skin, although it may develop at other sites of trauma or surgical incision. After an incubation period of 1 to 3 days, fever, chills, rapid pulse, and severe toxemia develop, associated with a spreading superficial cellulitis that has a characteristic appearance with an indurated, raised, and irregular margin. These infections are often self-limited, and improvement is seen within a period of 4 to 8 days.

Acute, recurrent lymphangitis may also result from infection with *S. pyogenes*, which usually has its portal of entry through small cracks in the skin. This syndrome is characterized by a sudden onset of high fever, chills, and painful swelling of the leg with regional adenopathy.

Surgical scarlet fever occurs with a typical scarlatiniform eruption 2 to 4 days after injury or operation and results from local wound infection by hemolytic streptococci that produce the erythrogenic toxin.

Streptococcal gangrene is a spreading, invasive,

epifascial and subcutaneous infection that usually occurs in the lower extremities and is associated with thrombosis of nutrient vessels and, slough of the overlying skin (Fig. 6). The development of clear, bullous lesions which later coalesce and become filled with hemorrhagic fluid is typical. Necrotizing fasciitis caused by streptococci is occasionally associated with cutaneous gangrene. Treatment of this condition is dependent upon wide surgical incision and drainage in association with adjuvant antibiotic therapy. A chronic type of infection may develop with multiple draining sinuses intercommunicating with areas of underlying necrotic fascia.

The microaerophilic streptococcus causes infections that develop and progress relatively slowly. Chronic burrowing ulcer and chronic progressive cutaneous gangrene are both results of infection by this type of organism. The former is characterized by surface ulcerations and communicating and burrowing sinus tracts. In both conditions, there is minimal sign of systemic toxicity, but marked pain at the site of infection is characteristic. Radical incision and drainage or excision is almost invariably necessary for eradication of the infection. Without surgical treatment, antibiotic therapy is inadequate.

Infections Caused by Gram-Negative Bacilli

A variety of gram-negative bacteria indigenous to the genitourinary and gastrointestinal tracts of humans may cause surgical infection. Wound infection by these organisms usually results from operative contamination of spilled gastrointestinal content and may be related to improper surgical technique. In other instances of wound infection or invasive systemic infection, these organisms act as opportunistic invaders and most frequently cause infection when there is impairment of the host defense mechanism, as previously discussed. They are frequent pathogens when there has been bacterial contamination from exogenous sources of incompletely removed devitalized tissue in burns and in infections associated with perforations of the gastrointestinal or genitourinary tract (Fig. 7). Gram-negative infections are often polymicrobic, with both anaerobic and aerobic organisms, but are often not recognized as such because anaerobic cultures are infrequently done on a routine basis in clinical practice. Postoperative wound infections caused by enteric bacilli usually have a longer incubation period than those caused by the Staphylococcus or Streptococcus. Surgical treatment of these infections, like those caused by gram-positive organisms, includes the establishment of free drainage with the administration of antibiotic agents as indicated.

Infections with a species of Bacteroides may be associated with thrombophlebitis developing in regional veins adjacent to areas of infection or in systemic veins such as the iliofemoral and may be related to the heparinase activity of the organism. Occasionally, there is no other local clinical or pathologic change to suggest infection by this organism, and it is discovered only by blood culture or culture of the thrombus. Treatment should include the administration of heparin and tetracycline and surgical removal of the thrombi. When only protoplastic or L-forms of the Bacteriodes are present, diagnosis is particularly difficult because of problems of cultivation and identification.

Clostridial Infections

Infections with anaerobic clostridia may cause three diseases of major consequence in surgical practice: gas gangrene or clostridial myositis, clostridial cellulitis, and tetanus.

Clostridial cellulitis is a serious septic process of

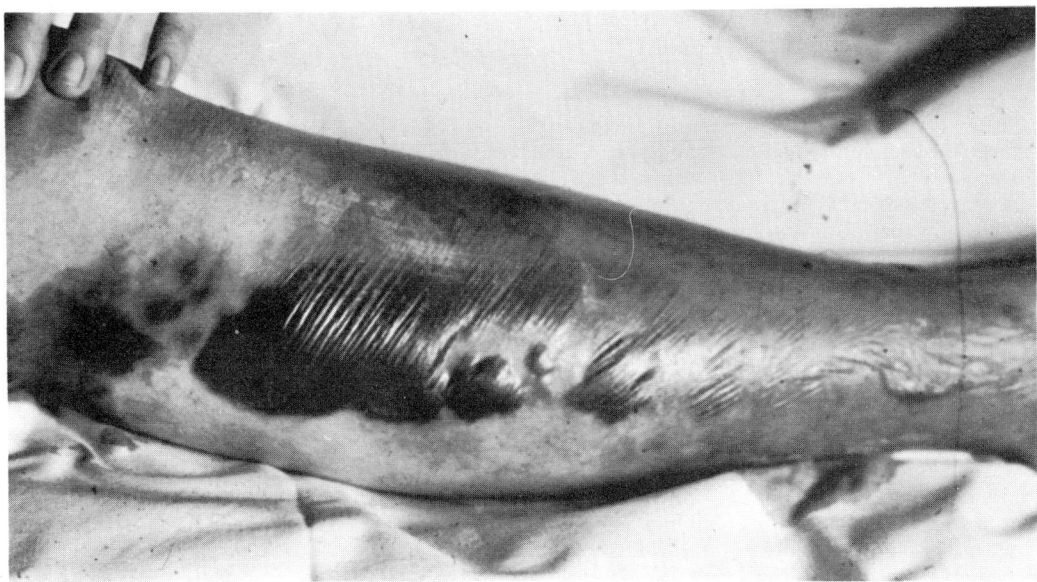

Figure 6. Acute, far-advanced hemolytic streptococcal cellulitis of the lower leg associated with high fever and prostration. Note patchy necrosis of skin and bullae.

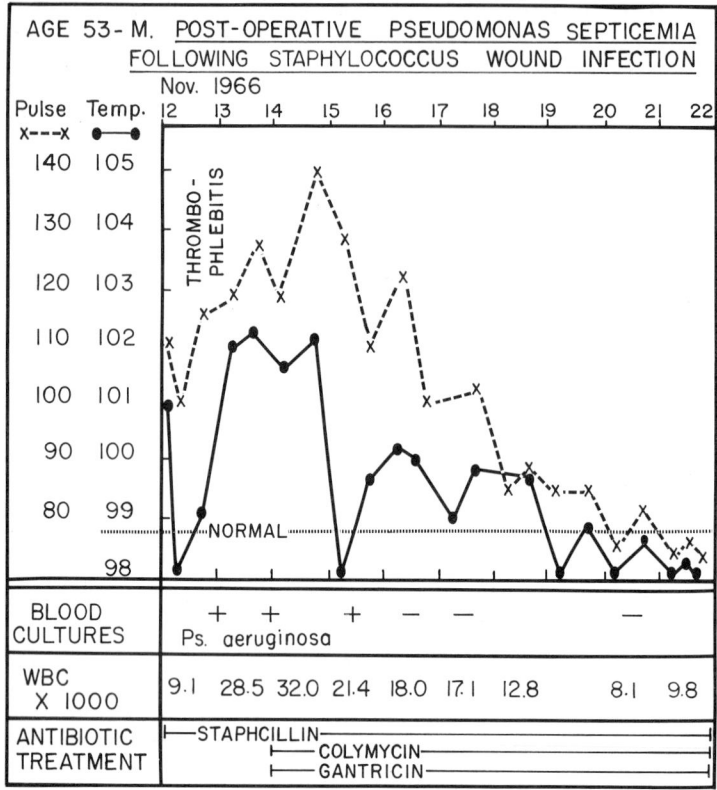

Figure 7. Chart showing course of 53-year-old diabetic male with *Pseudomonas aeruginosa* septicemia complicating acute thrombophlebitis of the arm related to continuous intravenous infusion. Recovery followed appropriate antibiotic therapy.

areolar tissues caused by one or more of the clostridia, most commonly *Clostridium welchii*. The infection is characterized by a crepitant cellulitis that spreads rapidly along fascial planes. Eventually, necrosis and sloughing of areolar tissues, fascia, and skin may occur as a result of thrombosis of neighboring blood vessels (Fig. 8). Pain about the wound is characteristic, as is a gray or reddish brown discharge. The symptoms associated with clostridial cellulitis are similar to those of clostridial myositis but occur to a lesser degree. Treatment should include extensive surgical decompression with elevation of skin flaps superficial to the fascia and the administration of systemic antibiotic agents in large doses, usually penicillin and one of the tetracyclines.

Clostridial myositis primarily involves muscle and is characterized by spreading gangrene and profound toxemia. A rapidly fatal course may develop in the absence of prompt therapy. This spectacular disease is usually associated with delayed or inadequate surgical care and impaired blood supply. The chief etiologic agents are *C. welchii*, *C. novyi*, *C. septicum*, and *C. sordellii*. Gas formation with crepitation within the muscles is characteristic, but may be absent. Swelling and pain occur early, usually within the first 24 hours after injury. The infected muscle becomes soft, swollen, and dark red. There is frequently a foul-smelling, brown, watery exudate containing bubbles of gas. Early diagnosis is facilitated by examination of the discharge, which usually contains many large gram-positive rods, usually without spores. Prostration is often far out of proportion to the degree of fever. The patient may become listless, sweat profusely, and have a grayish pallor. Stupor and delirium occur as the disease progresses, and marked anemia may develop. Surgical treatment should be prompt, with extensive

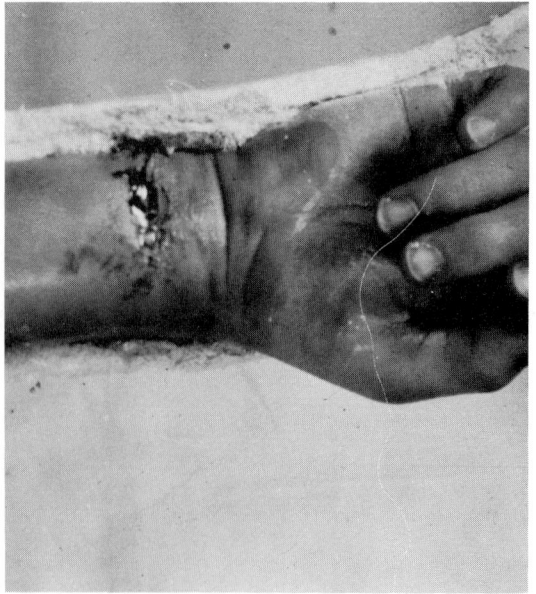

Figure 8. Gas gangrene of forearm and arm secondary to compound fracture-dislocation of the right wrist. Crepitation was evident.

decompression of all involved muscle compartments by incision and fasciotomy, or amputation of the part if irreversible gangrenous changes have developed in the extremity. The toxemia associated with gas gangrene is related primarily to the exotoxins produced by the clostridia, but antitoxin therapy directed toward neutralizing these toxins in clinical practice has been relatively ineffective. While antibiotic therapy cannot be depended upon to prevent gas gangrene or to cure an established infection, its use is recommended as an adjunctive measure to surgical operation. Hyperbaric oxygen therapy may be useful as an adjunct to surgical therapy in selected cases.

Tetanus, caused by *C. tetani*, is another serious anaerobic infection. It is unusual in that the entire clinical disease is caused by a powerful exotoxin released by the growing bacteria, the toxin being one of the most potent known to man. The incubation varies from 4 to 21 or more days. A prodromal period is often seen at the onset of the illness, being characterized by restlessness, yawning, headache, stiffness of the jaw muscles, and tetanic intermittent contractions in the region of the wound. Tonic spasm of the skeletal muscles with generalized tetanus usually follows within 12 to 24 hours and causes the classic facial distortion, opisthotonos, and rigidity. Clonic contractions may result from the slightest stimulation, and respiratory arrest may occur suddenly in association with these convulsive seizures. A rapid pulse, sweating, and salivation are accompanying symptoms. There is seldom depression of mental acuity, making it a particularly agonizing disease to the patient. Death usually results from respiratory arrest.

Treatment is best directed toward prevention, both by proper surgical therapy of wounds and by a program of active or passive immunization. Persons who have already received a full course of active toxoid immunization during their life are protected by a booster shot of tetanus toxoid at the time of injury. Wounded persons who have not been immunized previously should be given 500 units of tetanus immune globulin and started on a program of active toxoid immunizations immediately. The established disease is treated by local and intravenous administration of tetanus antitoxin and local excision or débridement of the wound as soon as possible. With the availability of human tetanus antitoxin, treatment as well as prophylaxis has been more effective. External stimuli must be kept to a minimum, and medical personnel must be in constant attendance so that respiratory arrest may be immediately treated when it develops. The convulsive seizures may be difficult to control, but a short-acting barbiturate used carefully as a continuous intravenous drip has proved to be most useful. Nasotracheal intubation and tracheostomy are to be done as indicated to preserve the airway and support artificial or assisted respiration. Curare-like drugs may be of benefit. Antibiotic therapy is of no value in the treatment of established tetanus per se, associated or complicating infections, including bacterial pneumonitis.

Other Anaerobic Infections

Anaerobic streptococcal (Peptostreptococcus) infections may occur as acute or chronic lesions, and they are usually characterized by the development of marked induration, foul-smelling and thick pus, progression along muscle bundles or along fascial planes, and extending necrosis. Streptococcal myositis is an infrequent type of this infection.

Various strains or species of Bacteroides produce a variety of surgical infections, including peritonitis, putrid abscesses, empyema, sepsis, parametritis, ovarian abscesses, etc. Infections of soft tissues caused by these gram-negative anaerobic bacilli have been associated with necrosis, spreading crepitation, and sometimes brownish or gray discoloration.

Mixed Bacterial Infections

Many surgical infections have a mixed bacterial etiology. The human bite is an example of a serious mixed infection. The introduction of human saliva into a deep puncture wound that contains crushed tissue, either as a result of a cut on the fist by the teeth of an intended victim or by deliberate biting, may be followed by the development of an unusually severe mixed infection involving the skin and underlying subcutaneous tissues, fascia, tendon, joint, and bone. These infections are almost always polymicrobic, and oral spirochetes usually participate with other aerobic and anaerobic mouth bacteria to produce a synergistic and locally destructive lesion. The infection is usually characterized by high fever, marked swelling and tenderness, and a thick, foul-smelling, purulent exudate associated with necrosis of the underlying areolar and fibrous tissues. Radical surgical decompression, systemic antibiotic therapy, and purposeful splinting of the parts are important for treatment.

Prevention is again the most effective treatment. The recent bite wound should be left open after its thorough debridement, the part immobilized with a dressing incorporating a splint, and appropriate antibiotic therapy instituted. Primary tenorrhaphy or neurorrhaphy should not be attempted under conditions of a fresh human bite.

Nonclostridial Crepitant Cellulitis

This is another type of mixed infection usually found as a complication of wounds that have been contaminated by gastrointestinal or genitourinary discharges. A wide variety of etiologic agents have been associated with this condition, including the anaerobic Bacteroides, the anaerobic Streptococcus, and many strains of the coliform group. The infection is characterized by necrosis of the areolar and fascial tissues with progressive gangrenous changes in the skin secondary to thrombosis of nutrient vessels. Crepitation of the wound results from the formation of gas by the bacteria. Surgical decompression with extensive surgical incisions, combined with intensive antibiotic therapy, is recommended for control of this condition (Fig. 9).

Synergistic Gangrene

The chronic progressive cutaneous gangrene first described by Meleney is an infrequent but important type of mixed infection caused by the synergistic action of the aerobic hemolytic *Staphylococcus aureus* and a microaerophilic nonhemolytic streptococcus. It

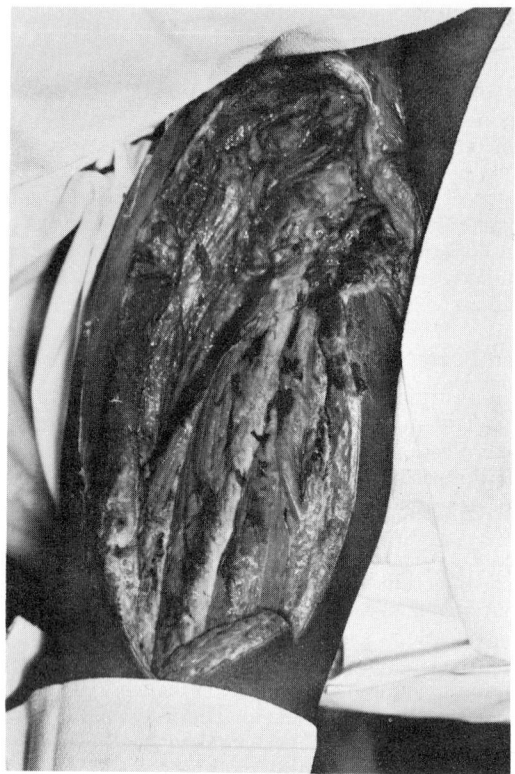

Figure 9. Mixed aerobic and anaerobic infection of medial posterior aspect of thigh complicating rectal injury. The bacterial flora included the anaerobic Streptococcus and *Bacteroides melanigenicum* which contributed to the grayish black discoloration of the infected tissue.

usually starts around stay sutures or wounds as a complication after an incubation period of 1 to 2 weeks. It is characterized by a wide area of pale red cellulitis with a purplish central area that finally becomes gangrenous and ulcerates. The ulceration gradually enlarges as its purplish black and very painful margin extends peripherally.

Treatment depends upon correct diagnosis and should include radical excision of the ulcerated lesion, systemic antibiotic therapy with penicillin or erythromycin, and delayed skin grafting. Local bacitracin therapy may be of some value before or after excision. Similar lesions may be caused occasionally by the synergistic action of a microaerophilic streptococcus with other strains of bacteria such as proteus.

Peritonitis and Abscess

Infections that follow perforation of the gastrointestinal or genitourinary tract or result from contamination by their contents are frequently polymicrobic, and many combinations of etiologic agents have been found. As many as four, five, or more different types of aerobic and anaerobic bacteria have been cultured simultaneously from the area of infection. The symbiotic and synergistic action between an anaerobic streptococcus and a Bacteroides species occurs with considerable frequency. This is usually not appreci-

ated, since the anaerobic streptococcus and the Bacteroides are anaerobic organisms that are difficult to culture and identify.

Mycotic Infections

Actinomycosis. Infections caused by *Actinomyces bovis* or *israelii* occur infrequently but may present particularly challenging diagnostic and therapeutic problems. The lesion is typically a granulomatous infection characterized by suppuration and discharge of pus through multiple sinus tracts (Fig. 10). Sulfur granules are characteristically found in the purulent discharge and their identification may be a valuable aid in diagnosis.

Recently, actinomycotic infections have not been considered as true mycotic lesions. Three principal forms of infection are recognized clinically: cervicofacial, thoracic, and abdominal. All may be associated with extensive burrowing sinuses and cutaneous fistulas. Treatment involves incision and drainage of abscesses and prolonged therapy with penicillin and sulfadiazine or another antibiotic regimen.

Blastomycosis. Blastomycosis, caused by yeastlike organisms of the genus Blastomyces, is usually a progressive, indolent, cutaneous infection with ulceration. It is characterized by a chronic ulceration with multiple small "daughter" abscesses along the advancing margin and a tendency for central healing of the lesions as the margins progress. Systemic spread with distant metastases may occur, giving a grave prognosis. Radical excision with skin grafting of the cutaneous lesion is recommended. In systemic lesions stilbamidine or large doses of sodium or potassium iodide may be of benefit.

Moniliasis. Primary infections by *Candida albicans* are encountered infrequently in normal individuals, but this pathogen is being seen in recent years with

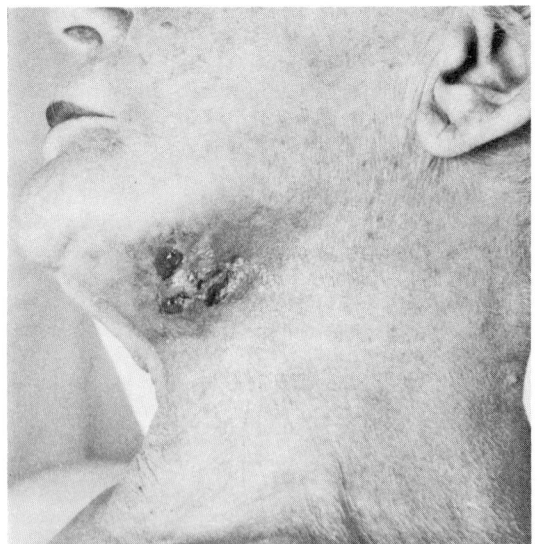

Figure 10. Cervicofacial actinomycosis with granuloma and multiple draining sinus tracts. Diagnosis established by demonstration of sulfur granules in hang-drop preparation and by anaerobic cultivation of *Actinomyces bovis*.

increasing frequency as an opportunistic invader. Secondary infections with this organism are particularly prone to occur in diabetic patients and others receiving intensive or prolonged broad-spectrum antibiotic therapy, especially in patients already debilitated by their underlying disease. Control of diabetes, if present, is essential. Amphotericin B is used in the treatment of systemic infections, and topical application of gentian violet or nystatin may be useful for local infections.

Other Fungi. Infections caused by other fungi are occasionally encountered in the practice of surgery, such as coccidioidomycosis and sporotrichosis. Coccidioidomycosis, caused by *Coccidioides immitis*, usually occurs as a pulmonary infection resembling pulmonary tuberculosis. Diagnosis is usually possible through recognition of the organisms in smears of sputum or local discharges and biopsied material. Skin sensitivity tests may be helpful. Sporotrichosis, caused by *Sporotrichum schenckii*, is a rare disease that follows contamination of a wound, usually on the extremities. It is characterized by a primary area of ulceration, regional nodular lymphangitis, and secondary ulcerations along the course of the involved lymphatic. Systemic invasion is very rare. Treatment with large doses of potassium iodide solution may be helpful.

Systemic infections with Aspergillus or Mucor as opportunistic invaders are also seen occasionally in debilitated patients.

Viral Infections

The most important viral infection of surgical significance is rabies. Rabies is a fatal encephalitis caused by a neurotropic virus that is inoculated by means of a bite from another rabid animal. It has been reported after bites from a variety of domestic as well as wild animals. The incubation period varies between 2 weeks and several months, and is related to the distance between the site of the injury and the brain. The established disease is characterized by maniacal excitement, progressive psychosis, and paralysis of the muscles of deglutition, followed by agitation and finally stupor. With a single possible exception, established rabies has been invariably fatal and the only means of treatment is through prophylaxis. Wounds caused by the bite of any suspected animal should be cleansed and debrided thoroughly. Whenever possible, the animal responsible for the bite should be impounded and observed for at least 14 days. If it has been killed, the brain should be examined for the presence of rabies virus particles. When the animal cannot be impounded or examined, a series of rabies vaccinations should be administered to the patient.

SELECTED REFERENCES

Alexander, J. W.: Antibiotic agents and the immune mechanisms of defense. Ann. N. Y. Acad. Med., *51*:1039–1045, 1975.
Current knowledge in this area is reviewed.

Alexander, J. W.: Emerging concepts in the control of surgical infections. Surgery 75:934–946, 1974.
Prevention and treatment of surgical infections must now include support of the immune system if further advances are to be made.

Alexander, J. W.: Nosocomial infections. *In* Current Problems in Surgery. Chicago, Yearbook Medical Publishers, 1973.
The prblem of nosocomial and hospital-acquired infections in surgical patients is reviewed in this monograph.

Alexander, J. W.: Nutrition and surgical infections. *In*, Ballinger, W. (Ed.): American College of Surgeons Manual of Surgical Nutrition. Philadelphia, W. B. Saunders Company, 1975, pp. 386–395.
Nutritional support is probably one of the most important aspects of therapy in the treatment of chronic or resistant infections. This chapter discusses the relationship between nutritional status and surgical infection and presents recommendations for nutritional therapy to provide or supplement treatment of infections in the surgical patient.

Alexander, J. W., and Fisher, M. W.: Immunization against pseudomonas infection after thermal injury. J. Infect. Dis., *130*(Suppl.): S152–S158, 1974.
A five-year experience with immunization to prevent serious Pseudomonas infection in burn patients shows good effectiveness of both a heptavalent vaccine and hyperimmune antipseudomonas gammaglobulin.

Alexander, J. W., and Good, R. A.: Immunobiology for Surgeons. Philadelphia, W. B. Saunders Company, 1970.
This monograph was written to provide a brief but comprehensive review of this important aspect of modern surgery. In it are included topics of cellular immunity, nonspecific immunity, and humoral immunity, with chapters on adaptive immunity, immunosuppression, immunologic aspects of cancer, transplantation, infections, and other subjects pertinent to surgery.

Alexander, J. W., McClellan, M. A., Ogle, C. K., and Ogle, J. D.: Consumptive opsonopathy: Possible pathogenesis in lethal and opportunistic infections. Ann. Surg., in press.
The findings of this study provide evidence that bacterial infection causes a consumption of opsonin proteins of the alternative pathways, which may result in a reduced ability of the patient's serum to opsonize bacteria and thereby further increases susceptibility to infection.

Alexander, J. W., and Meakins, J. L.: A physiological basis for the development of opportunistic infections. Ann. Surg., *176*:273–287, 1972.
Importance of defects in host resistance in the pathogenesis of surgical infection is emphasized in this article which focuses on neutrophil function.

Altemeier, W. A.: Bacteriology of surgical infections. Clinical and experimental considerations. Moscow, Vingt-quatrieme Congres de la Societe Internationale de Chirurgie, 1971, pp. 53–70.
An etiologic classification of the numerous and varied types of microorganisms capable of producing surgical infections is presented. Included are considerations of the changes in the patterns in bacterial etiology of wound infections associated with the widespread use of antibiotic therapy.

Altemeier, W. A.: Bodily response to infectious agents. J.A.M.A., *202*:1085, 1967.
A review of the subject of bodily responses to infectious agents which concludes that the dimension of surgical infection in the practice of surgery is real, significant, continuing, and demanding. It emphasizes the essentiality of the medical student's acquiring knowledge for proper hospital conduct and procedure.

Altemeier, W. A.: Control of wound infections. J. R. Coll. Surg. Edinb., *11*:271, 1966.
A report of the clinical experience and laboratory studies in the epidemiology of postoperative wound infections during a 15-year period, which will be valuable to students, residents, and clinical surgeons.

Altemeier, W. A.: The significance of infection in trauma. Bull. Am. Coll. Surg., *57*, 1972.
The 1971 Scudder Oration in Trauma of the American College of Surgeons, which emphasizes the complexity of surgical infection and the significance and importance of both bacterial and nonbacterial factors as causes of wound infections.

Altemeier, W. A., and Berkich, E. J.: Wound sepsis and dehiscence. *In* Hardy, J. (Ed.): Critical Surgical Illness. Philadelphia, W. B. Saunders Company, 1971.
A review of the causes of wound sepsis and dehiscence with a discussion of their prophylaxis and therapy.

Altemeier, W. A., Burke, J. F., Pruitt, B. A., Jr., and Sandusky, W.: Manual on control of infections in surgical patients. Committee on Control of Surgical Infections of the Committee on Pre- and

Postoperative Care, American College of Surgeons. Philadelphia, J. B. Lippincott Company, 1976.
A manual written by the Committee on Control of Infections of the Pre- and Postoperative Care Committee of the American College of Surgeons. The volume is a summary of the reports and discussions of world-wide authorities in the field of surgical infections. The aim of the manual is to provide clinical surgeons, surgical housestaff, students, nurses, anesthesiologists, infection committees, and epidemiologists with an up-to-date and readily available source of information useful in the prevention and control of surgical infections in hospital practice.

Altemeier, W. A., and Fullen, W. D.: Prevention and treatment of gas gangrene. J.A.M.A., *217*:806, 1971.
An analysis of a series of 54 cases of gas gangrene which discussed the clinical picture, etiology, incidence, methods and pitfalls in diagnosis, differential diagnosis, and treatment of this spectacular and dreaded complication of wounds.

Altemeier, W. A., and Furste, W. L.: Gas gangrene. Int. Abstr. Surg. Gynecol. Obstet., *84*:507, 1947.
This extensive review continues to be a standard for the subject of clostridial infections.

Altemeier, W. A., Hummel, R. P., Hill, E. O., and Lewis, S.: Changing patterns in surgical infections. Ann. Surg., *178*:436–445, 1973.
This is a recommended article which describes a series of interesting changes that have occurred during the past 28 years. Included have been a marked increase in the incidence of gram-negative infections superimposed on or secondary to antibiotic therapy, and an increasing incidence of infections by bacteria formerly considered to have little or no virulence.

Altemeier, W. A., McDonough, J. J., and Fullen, W. D.: Third day surgical fever. Arch. Surg., *103*:158, 1971.
The importance of the continuous intravenous infusion of fluids as a source of serious and life-threatening infection in surgical patients is demonstrated with the frequent and striking temporal relationship of the onset of the sepsis to the third day after the patient's operative procedure.

Altemeier, W. A., Todd, J. C., and Inge, W. W.: Gram-negative septicemia: A growing threat. Ann. Surg., *166*:228, 1967.
Review of gram-negative sepsis during a 12-year period shows that there has been a progressive increase in its incidence. The cause, clinical picture, treatment, and results are emphasized.

Armstrong, D. (Ed.): Infectious diseases: Diagnosis and treatment. New York, Medcom Press, 1975.
This short multi-authored textbook on infectious disease presents a good general description of antimicrobial agents and their use in selected infections. An up-to-date review is also available on the pharmacology of antimicrobial agents.

Beard, N. S., Jr., Armentrout, S. A., and Weisberger, A. S.: Inhibition of mammalian protein synthesis by antibiotics. Pharmacol. Rev., *21*:213, 1969.
An extensive review of the biochemical mechanisms of action of antibiotics that inhibit protein synthesis. Included in this group are most clinically useful antibiotics.

Bennett, J.V., and Brachman, P. (Eds.): Nosocomial Infections. Boston, Little, Brown and Company, 1976.
This multiauthored text provides a cross-section and computation of data related to hospital-acquired infections. It is highly recommended.

Burke, J. F.: The effective period of preventive antibiotic action in experimental incisions and dermal lesions. Surgery, *50*:161, 1961.
An important study which demonstrates the importance of definite short periods when developing staphylococcal dermal or incisional wound infection may be suppressed by antibiotics. It emphasizes the fact that antibiotics give maximum suppression if given before bacteria gains access to the tissues.

Dubos, R. J., and Hirsch, J. G.: Bacterial and Mycotic Infections of Man, 4th ed. Philadelphia, J. B. Lippincott Company, 1965.
This expanded edition contains a wealth of information pertaining to clinical infections of all types. It is a good text for in-depth review.

Edsall, G.: Current status of tetanus immunization. Arch. Environ. Health, *8*:731, 1964.
The author emphasizes that while active immunization for tetanus is extremely effective for prevention of the disease, frequent immunizations not only are unnecessary, but can cause complications. His recommendations for infrequent booster shots in adequately immunized persons have now been generally accepted.

Finegold, S. M., Davis, Z., Ziment, I., and Jacobs, I.: An outline to chemotherapy. Hosp. Phys., *6*:75, 1970.
For the student who wishes a brief guide for antibiotic therapy in renal disease, this article is an excellent one. The table on antibiotic dosages in renal failure includes most of the antibiotics that might be considered in clinical practice.

Finland, M.: Changing ecology of bacterial infections as related to antibacterial therapy. J. Infect. Dis., *120*:419, 1970.
Opportunistic infections not only have become more frequent, but their seriousness is often related to previous antimicrobial therapy. The experience of the Boston City Hospital is presented to emphasize the shifting patterns of nosocomial infections.

Fullen, W. D., Hunt, J., and Altemeier, W. A.: Prophylactic antibiotics in penetrating wounds of the abdomen. J. Trauma, *12*:282, 1972.
A study which emphasizes the effectiveness of antibiotic therapy in the management of penetrating abdominal wounds, with the greatest effect obtained when the administration of the antibiotics is started prior to the operative exploration.

Hart, P. D., Russel, E., and Remington, J. S.: The compromised host in infection. II. Deep fungal infection. J. Infect. Dis., *120*:169, 1969.
This study emphasizes the important marked increase in recent years in the numbers of fungal infections in the compromised host. Both the presentation of the authors' own material and their review of the literature are of value.

Jawetz, E.: The use of combinations of antimicrobial drugs. Ann. Rev. Pharmacol., *8*:151, 1968.
Antagonism and synergism between antibiotics are reviewed, with a plea for the use of combinations of antibiotics only in exceptional situations.

Klainer, A. S., and Beisel, W. R.: Opportunistic infections: A review. Am. J. Med. Sci., *258*:431, 1969.
Opportunistic infections are considered in their typical circumstances to demonstrate the possibility of anticipating their development, to establish a precise diagnosis, and to formulate a rational plan of therapy. Deficiencies of host resistance and their contribution to the wide variety of clinical pictures which may be presented with opportunistic infections are emphasized. This is an excellent review for those interested in the subject.

Roe, E., Jones, R. J., and Lowbury, E. J. L.: Transfer of antibiotic resistance between *Pseudomonas aeruginosa, Escherichia coli,* and other gram-negative bacilli in burns. Lancet, *1*:149, 1971.
The conclusive evidence for the transfer of antibiotic resistance between various genera of bacteria in burn wounds in vivo is an extremely important observation that provides a strong argument against the indiscriminate use of antibiotics or the use of prophylactic antibiotics for marginal indications. The authors' observations are particularly pertinent to clinical situations in which infections occur in open wounds or in sites subject to contamination from external sources, such as tracheostomies and indwelling urinary catheters.

Seelig, M. S.: Mechanisms by which antibiotics increase the incidence and severity of candidiasis and alter the immunological defenses. Bact. Rev., *30*:442, 1966.
Mechanisms by which the pathogenicity of an organism is increased in the clinical situation are explored.

Swenson, R. M., and Sanford, J. P.: Clinical implications of the mechanism of action of antimicrobial agents. Intern. Med., *16*:373, 1970.
This review will be particularly helpful for those students who are interested in molecular biology related to the anti-infective drugs. It is a well-referenced and sound scientific discussion.

Weinstein, L., and Dalton, A. C.: Host determinants of response to antimicrobial agents. N. Engl. J. Med., *279*:467, 524, 580, 1968.
This group of papers should be a must for anyone using antimicrobial drugs, since it helps to put into perspective the important interrelationship of differences in the host and its response to the agent. It is a well-referenced and excellent review.

18

BITES AND STINGS

Kenneth P. Ramming, M.D.

SNAKEBITE

The subject of snakebites and their treatment extends far back into history. It has been only in recent decades that a systematic study of the problem has evolved and a scientific rationale of treatment has been formulated. Snakebite constitutes a medical emergency, and familiarization with basic principles of diagnosis and treatment is essential.

Incidence

The World Health Organization estimates that as many as 300,000 snakebites occur throughout the world each year, causing perhaps 30,000 to 40,000 deaths. The largest number of fatal snakebites occur in Southeast Asia (about 25,000). The mortality in South America is 3000 to 4000 annually.[9] In the United States, approximately 45,000 snakebites are reported each year, of which about 7000 are treated as venomous, with only 14 to 15 deaths resulting.[27, 38]

At least one venomous snake species is indigenous to every state in the United States except Maine, Alaska, and Hawaii. The largest number of snakebites occur in Texas. States having the highest incidence per 100,000 population are, in order: North Carolina, Arkansas, Texas, Georgia, West Virginia, Mississippi, Louisiana, and Oklahoma. Few occurrences are reported in New England. More than 90 per cent of all snakebites occur from April through October.[9, 27, 38] Males between the ages of 5 and 19 are most often afflicted.

About 10 per cent of snakes relative to the United States are poisonous. Pit vipers, including rattlesnakes, copperheads, and cottonmouths, account for 99 per cent of all venomous bites. The diagnosis and management of bites from this group are essentially the same. Coral snakes and snakes from other areas of the world in captivity in the United States are responsible for the remainder of venomous bites.[9]

Identification of venomous snakes in the United States is relatively simple. As shown in Figure 1, pit vipers have a characteristic pit located between the eye and the nostril on each side of the head. They are also identified by elliptical pupils, two well-developed fangs which protrude from the maxilla, and single subcaudal plates. Harmless snakes have round pupils, no pits, no fangs, and double subcaudal plates. The one exception to this rule is the coral snake, an indigenous poisonous snake with round eyes and no fangs. It has brightly colored bands of red, yellow, and black, and is the only snake to have adjacent red and yellow bands ("red touching yellow means a dangerous fellow").[27-29] Information on venomous snakes in the United States is summarized briefly in Table 1.

Biology

The fangs of pit vipers are long, hollow tubes set forward in the maxilla, ideal for deep delivery of venom. Pit vipers can control the position of the fangs and the amount of venom injected, and this may account for some variability in the toxic effects of different bites. The fangs of the coral snake are fixed. Large snakes produce more venom than small ones.[8, 28, 36]

Snake venoms are complex mixtures of polypeptides with diverse pharmacologic effects. Enzymes such as phospholipase A, hyaluronidase, ATPase, 5-nucleotidase, and DPN are found in venom. Phospholipase A is the most potent contributor to toxicity, converting lecithin to lysolecithin, a substance very destructive to tissues. Local damage, neurotoxicity, hemolysis, histamine release, and possibly anaphylaxis have been attributed to this enzyme. Hyaluronidase aids in spreading venom by lysis of ground substance. ATPase and 5-nucleotidase depress metabolism and contribute to shock. Other enzymes isolated from some venoms are cholinesterase, L-amino acid, oxidase, protease, phosphomonoesterase, RNAase, and DNAase. Also present in venoms are polypeptide elements that have a direct toxic effect on cells. Crotoxin, for instance, has been implicated in causing hemolysis, paralysis, bradykinin release, and direct toxicity to cardiac muscle. Collectively, snake venoms have effects on every organ system. In most cases, however, the deleterious effects are directed toward the blood and the cardiovascular, nervous, and respiratory systems.[8, 9, 37]

Clinical Manifestations

In Crotalus (pit viper) bites there is an almost immediate, intense destruction of local tissue. Edema and erythema result, provoking a subjective sensation of intense pain. Permeability of blood vessels is altered and extravasation of plasma and blood into tissues results in ecchymosis and bulla formation.

CHARACTERISTICS OF SNAKES

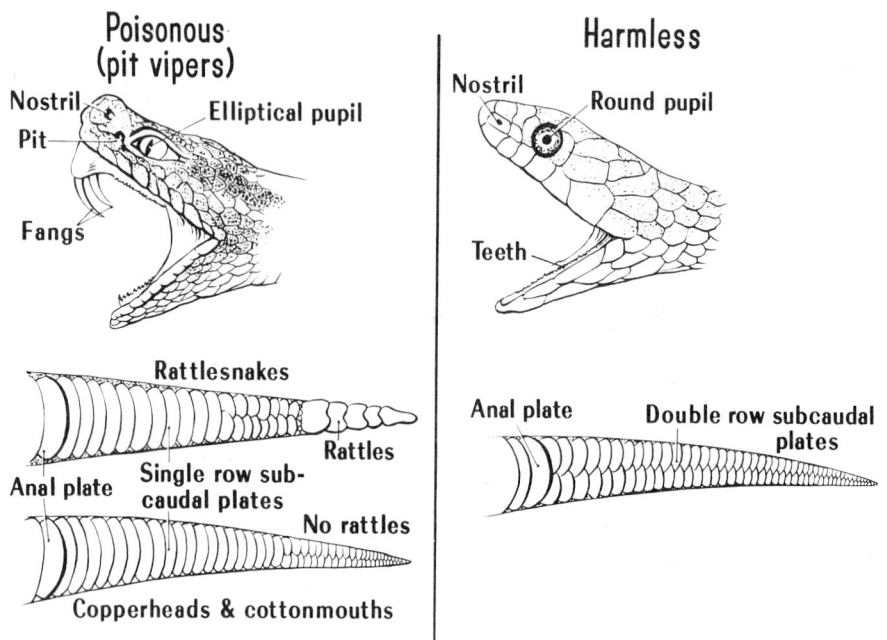

Figure 1. Characteristics that differentiate poisonous pit vipers from nonpoisonous snakes. (From Parrish, H. M.: Public Health Rep., *81*:269, 1966.)

Slough occurs at the wound site. When large amounts of venom are injected, severe systemic effects ensue. Often massive tissue necrosis and edema of an entire extremity result. Red blood cells respond by swelling and becoming spherical, and some are lysed. The hematocrit falls, and platelets may be markedly reduced. Bleeding, coagulation, and prothrombin times are increased. Hematuria, melena, hematemesis, epistaxis, and hemoptysis may result. Blood vessel walls are altered, and there is increased resistance in postcapillary veins, resulting in pooling of blood in the lungs and chest. Pulmonary edema may result, and bleeding may occur in the peritoneum or pericardium. All these, together with direct toxic effects on the heart, contribute to the clinical picture of peripheral vascular collapse. The renal lesion of crotalid envenomation is a glomerulonephritis, often accompanied by progressive, proliferative endarteritis and cortical ne-

TABLE 1. Classification of Poisonous Snakes Indigenous to the United States

Family	Genus	Common Name	Identification	Characteristics
Crotalidae	Crotalus	Large rattlesnake (diamondback, mojave, timber, sidewinder, pacific, prairie)	Broad head, many coloration patterns, light belly; often has diamond markings. Rattles; up to 6 feet in length.	Can strike long distance. Potent cytotoxic venom. Accounts for most severe bites and fatalities.
	Sistrurus	Small rattlesnake (pigmy, massasauga)	Less than 3 feet in length.	Rattler often small and audible only at close range. Bites cause severe pain, swelling, few fatalities.
	Ancistrodon	Copperhead	Pink, russet, or orange-brown with dark brown or reddish crossbands. Head is triangular, yellow to copper with pale sides. Two to 3 feet in length.	Accounts for most bites in eastern United States. Fatalities almost unknown.
		Cottonmouth	Olive or brown with wide black crossbands. Yellow belly marked with gray. White interior of mouth. Around 4 feet in length.	Semiaquatic. Belligerent, aggressive behavior. Rare fatalities, but severe tissue destruction by venom.
Elapidae	Micrurus	Coral snake	Complete rings of yellow, black, red, and sometimes white with red and yellow adjacent. Less than 4 feet in length.	Frequently bites are not envenomated. Little local reaction at bite site, but neurotoxin-induced respiratory paralysis in several hours is usually fatal.

crosis. Necrosis of the tubular epithelium appears to be a direct local effect of the toxin.[10] This, along with profound circulatory collapse and intravascular hemolysis, accounts for the occurrence of acute renal failure frequently seen in rattlesnake bite. A systemic anaphylaxis has also been described.[9, 36]

Elapidae (coral snake) venoms cause less tissue damage and far greater neuromuscular changes. Reaction about the bite is frequently absent, pain is minimal, and symptoms are systemic, such as numbness, nausea, vomiting, euphoria, salivation, paresthesia, ptosis, weakness, abnormal reflexes, depression, dyspnea, and respiratory arrest. In most experimental preparations, the first changes in electrical conduction induced by crude venom occur at the neuromuscular junction, but with low doses, changes of varying degree occur. The ultimate clinical catastrophe, which can come on with acute suddenness, is total respiratory paralysis.[29, 36]

Some 200 strains of bacteria have been isolated from snake venom. Ledbetter found clostridia in 48 of 100 venoms cultured, and in 43 of 50 fangs, but coagulase-positive Staphylococcus was not found. The most prevalent gram-negative organisms were Aerobacter, Proteus, and Pseudomonas.[26]

Management

Therapy for snakebite must be initiated early. Correct diagnosis is essential. Pit vipers usually leave characteristic paired puncture wounds made by fangs, whereas bites of nonpoisonous snakes often leave teeth marks in the shape of a "U." Bites by poisonous snakes usually cause immediate and intense pain. A convenient classification for bites by pit vipers is that of Wood and associates as modified by Parrish.[27, 41]

Grade 0 — no venation: fang or tooth marks; minimal pain; edema and erythema of less than 1 inch in 12 hours; usually no systemic involvement.

Grade 1 — minimal venation: fang or tooth marks; severe pain; 1 to 5 inches of surrounding edema in first 12 hours; usually no systemic involvement.

Grade 2 — moderate venation: fang or tooth marks; severe pain; 6 to 12 inches of surrounding edema and erythema in first 12 hours; systemic involvement sometimes present, as neurotoxic symptoms, nausea, giddiness, shock, palpable regional lymph nodes.

Grade 3 — severe venation: fang or tooth marks; severe pain; more than 12 inches of surrounding edema and erythema; systemic symptoms as hypotension, generalized petechiae and ecchymosis, shock.

Grade 4 — very severe venation: fang or tooth marks, multiple; local edema may be present beyond involved extremity to ipsilateral trunk; systemic symptoms always present, may include renal failure, coma, blood-tinged secretions.

In Parrish's nationwide survey, 27 per cent of venomous snakebites were classified Grade 0; 37 per cent were Grade 1; 22 per cent were Grade 2; and 14 per cent were Grades 3 and 4.[27]

The management of snakebite should follow a rational sequence. The following are suggested as guidelines.

1. Retard Absorption of the Venom. A tourniquet should be applied several inches above the bite. It must be emphasized that the tourniquet should occlude venous and lymphatic return *but not arterial flow.* Snyder has shown that a tourniquet reduces the uptake of ^{131}I-labelled venom in animals by two thirds. Loosening the tourniquet every 15 minutes actually increases the spread of venom, and it should be left in place for up to 2 hours without release. Immobilization of the bitten extremity aids in slowing the spread of venom.[38, 39] The use of alcohol, a vasodilator, should be avoided. Immersion of the bitten extremity in ice would theoretically seem to be beneficial by inducing vasoconstriction. However, the mortality and morbidity in experimental animals have been increased by prolonged exposure to ice. In addition, the application of ice has led to numerous tragic excesses of therapy, including many cases of limb loss where the bite was not even envenomated. *Therefore, the use of cryotherapy is absolutely contraindicated.*[18, 28-31, 41]

2. Remove as Much Venom as Possible from the Wound. Small incisions $1/4$ inch long and $1/8$ to $1/4$ inch deep are made over the bite and mechanical suction is employed. Cruciate incisions heal poorly and are not required. Suction by mouth may be used if necessary. Venom is not absorbed through intact oral mucosa, but will be absorbed through any mucosal laceration. Digestive juices neutralize any swallowed venom. Over 50 per cent of venom can be removed in 15 minutes by this measure.

Huang et al. noted that much of the injected venom remains in the subcutaneous tissue compartment following envenomation. In a series of 54 patients seen in the hospital within 2 hours of the snakebite, wide excision of the bitten area was performed. Skin flaps were elevated and the ecchymotic subcutaneous tissue removed. This greatly reduced systemic toxicity (no antivenin was necessary in this series), and the clinical judgment as to whether fasciotomy would be necessary was facilitated.[24] Snyder, Glass, and others have also advocated excision of the bite.[21, 39]

3. Neutralize the Venom. Polyvalent antivenin (Wyeth) should be given intravenously,[28, 30, 41] or intraarterially,[38] not intramuscularly or locally at the wound site. A useful guide for administration is no antevenin for Grade 0; 10 ml. (one ampule) for Grade 1; 30 to 40 ml. for Grade 2; and 50 ml. or more for Grades 3 and 4.[28] A form of antivenin was developed in horses by Calmette in 1848, and the material used today is still an equine serum. In sensitive patients skin tests should be done first, but in severe cases withholding the antivenin may be more dangerous than administering it. The incidence of serum sickness in recipients of more than two ampules of antivenin is significant.

4. Prevent or Reduce the Effects of the Venom. Appropriate infusions of saline, plasma, blood, and vasopressor drugs should be instituted to prevent shock. Blood coagulation studies should be obtained and fibrinogen replacement may be required. Fasciotomy may become necessary to prevent ischemic necrosis in a grossly edematous limb.

Previous studies have shown that small to moderate doses of corticosteroids may prolong life but do not affect mortality. However, Glass has recommended massive doses of hydrocortisone (1 gm. intravenously every 4 hours) at the first sign of systemic toxicity. With this regimen, coupled with early wide wound incision and fasciotomy, he has achieved good functional limb salvage, particularly in patients with known sensitivity to antivenin.[20, 21]

5. Prevent Complications. Broad-spectrum antibiotics are given to combat infection, and tetanus toxoid or tetanus immune globulin is administered. Vomiting, excessive salivation, and convulsions are treated symptomatically. Assisted ventilation may be necessary and renal function must be monitored.

Patients bitten by coral snakes should be admitted to the hospital for careful observation for at least 48 hours, as the effects of this venom are characteristically slow to develop. The wound should be carefully washed, for small amounts of the highly toxic venom may remain on the skin. The only commercially available coral snake antivenin is Soro Anticlapidico manufactured by Instituto Butantan, São Paulo, Brazil, and is available from most zoos and reptile houses in this country. Twenty milliliters should be given at once, and 120 ml. or more administered if signs of venenation develop. If respiratory paralysis occurs, intubation and assisted respiration will be required. Intravenous fluid maintenance, urinary catheter, Levin tube, antibiotics, and tetanus prophylaxis will be required. It is encouraging that some patients suffering respiratory paralysis from coral snake venom have recovered completely.[29]

RABIES

Rabies has been considered an invariably fatal, terrifying disease for centuries. As early as the first century A.D., Celsus recognized the infectivity of the bite of a mad dog and recommended cauterization of such wounds. Since the classic work of Pasteur in the 1880s and the development of the first rabies vaccine, the incidence of this disease has declined appreciably. Yet the increasing incidence of rabies virus in wildlife reservoirs and the dread complications of the clinical syndrome in humans continue to keep rabies an ever-present menace to mankind.

Incidence

Approximately 2 million people are bitten by animals annually, 500,000 by dogs.[25] The incidence of rabies in humans has declined markedly in recent years (nine cases being reported in the United States from 1963 through 1968 in contrast to 230 cases between 1946 and 1963).[32] This is the result of an intensive vaccination program for pets, primarily dogs and cats.

In the United States today, wild carnivorous animals are the most frequent source of rabies infection for man. Seventy-nine per cent of all confirmed animal rabies cases in 1973 occurred in wildlife, particularly skunks, bobcats, foxes, and bats. Though dogs and cats account for only 20 per cent of animal rabies, bites by these animals are responsible for most of the approximately 30,000 postexposure rabies prophylactic treatments administered annually.[11] The cost of animal bites to society, in terms of funds expended and man hours lost, is substantial.[5]

Biology

The rabies virus is a large, nonfilterable particle that measures 75×180 mμ. Infected nervous tissue or salivary gland tissue is the best source of the virus. At refrigerator temperature, the virus may remain active for several weeks and at subfreezing temperatures for one or more years. Rabies virus is inactivated by exposure to a temperature of 56° C. for an hour or less. It is rapidly destroyed by sunlight or ultraviolet radiation, and is readily inactivated by formalin, bichloride of mercury, strong acids, and quaternary ammonium compounds. It is not affected by any antibiotics or common bacteriostatic agents.[42]

The virus is usually transmitted through a break in the skin or by direct contact with the mucous membrane. Airborne infection is possible, has been reported clinically in humans in areas inhabited by rabid bats, and has accounted for the death of one laboratory technician handling infected tissue.[43] The virus may persist in the inoculation site for several days. Progression of the virus occurs passively through the nerve-associated spaces. In the central nervous system, the virus is found in the gray matter and appears to multiply in the neurons. The incubation period is usually 3 to 6 weeks but has been reported to range from 6 days to 23 months. Since the virus travels in association with nervous structures, those areas rich in nerve endings (the fingers and face) provide rapid access for the rabies virus, and multiple facial or finger bites have the shortest incubation periods.[42]

The human disease is characterized by three phases: a prodromal phase, an acute excitement phase, and a paralytic phase. The prodromal phase is nonspecific and may be manifested by fever, headache, malaise, anorexia, and sore throat. The most notable clinical symptom of rabies is related to swallowing, with violent and painful contractions of the muscles of deglutition. The excitement phase is marked by increasing nervousness, insomnia, anxiety, and apprehension. Convulsive seizures are common, and unusual behavior patterns may appear. If the patient survives, the paralytic phase (due to neuronal death) follows. Depressive or paralytic symptoms may predominate at any time during the course of the disease. Hypoxia, cardiac arrhythmias, hemiparesis, and coma are usually present. Although the almost invariable outcome is death, the actual cause of death has never been clearly established. Patients usually die within 4 to 10 days, but delayed clinical courses of up to 133 days have been observed,[6] and one complete recovery has been reported.[22]

At autopsy dark inclusion bodies (Negri bodies) are found in the brain in the area of the thalamus and lentiform nucleus.[42] False-negative results of tests to demonstrate these bodies in animals have occurred, and a human death has been ascribed to this error. The fluorescent antibody test as described by Goldwasser and associates is currently used, and a diagnosis may be obtained in a few hours.[35] Inoculation of mice and demonstration of the virus or Negri bodies in their nervous tissue is still a valuable diagnostic test.

Therapy

The management of dog and animal bites embodies the application of the usual surgical principles in the care of soft tissue injury (cleansing, antisepsis and, if necessary in severe bites, débridement of necrotic tissue). The most pressing medical decision will be whether or not to treat the bitten patient for rabies. In cases in which the biting animal is known and confined, this problem is resolved, as therapy can be deferred during an observation period in which the animal will or will not exhibit death from rabies. Rabies virus might be demonstrated in saliva or glands during this time. However, when the biting animal is not captured, this decision must be made on the basis of the incidence of rabies in that species in the locale, and especially on the behavior of the biting animal.

Animal rabies can be classified as *furious* or *dumb*. In furious rabies, animals show a prolonged excitation phase, becoming increasingly apprehensive and nervous. This is the most dangerous phase, as a dog may show no recognition of its master and exhibit only an insane desire to bite. In wild animals, the daytime appearance of abnormal behavior (loss of fear of humans and attacks on livestock or man) should induce a high order of suspicion. In dumb rabies there is a very short excitation phase, after which the animal becomes apathetic, appears to seek solitude, and eventually succumbs to progressive paralysis, coma, and death.[42]

Rabies is not endemic in rodents. Bites by rats, mice, chipmunks, squirrels, rabbits, or other rodents have never been proved to produce human rabies, and postexposure prophylaxis is currently not indicated. However, rabies is endemic in bats in every state except Hawaii, and all persons bitten by a bat that escapes should receive postexposure prophylaxis.[11, 19] The rationale for treatment is based on the severity and location of the attack, the immune status of the attacking animal, the clinical status of the attacking animal, and occasionally on the immune status of the victim. Once the decision to treat the patient is made, therapy should be instituted promptly according to the guidelines for postexposure prophylaxis set forth in Table 2.

Local Treatment. Repeated swabbing and flushing with soap and water followed by 1 per cent benzalkonium chloride will reduce rabies in the wound site. This gives significant protection up to 12 hours after the bite. Fuming nitric acid cauterization should be avoided. The infiltration of antirabies serum under the wound itself has been effective in animals, and should be administered in severe bites. A minimum of 5 ml. of serum should be injected.

Systemic Treatment. Rabies virus is poorly antigenic. In clinical infections, it appears that the virus must reach the brain before high antirabies antibody levels are achieved. Although the virus may be eliminated ("autosterilization") by this immune response, the course of the disease is unfortunately not altered. The rationale for postexposure prophylaxis is therefore to give vaccine to induce an immune response against rabies, and to administer antiserum (passive transfer) to effect immediately elevated antibody levels while the body mounts its own immune response to the vaccine.[6, 11]

Duck embryo vaccine, which is the only licensed vaccine currently available in the United States, causes fewer side effects than the older spinal cord preparations derived from those of Pasteur, which induced a high incidence of allergic reaction to nervous tissues retained in the vaccine.[9] However, 100 per cent of patients treated will experience local symptoms of pain and erythema, and 33 per cent have experienced systemic symptoms of fever and malaise (based on a review of 424,000 treatments). Less than 0.5 per cent have anaphylaxis, and the incidence of fatal complications is very small. Antihistamines will ameliorate most reactions. Corticosteroids interfere with the development of active immunity and should not be used. Twenty-one doses of vaccine, given subcutaneously in the abdomen or lateral thigh, followed by two booster injections, is the recommended treatment.[11, 14, 33]

For years the only available hyperimmune serum (ARS) was of equine origin, which produced serum sickness in approximately 15 per cent of children and up to 40 per cent of adults. The recommended dose is 40 international units (IU) per kg of body weight. Up to 50 per cent of the antiserum should be used to infiltrate the wound and the rest is given intramuscularly. Recently a hyperimmune rabies immune globulin obtained from human volunteers, HRIG, has been licensed. Since allergic reactions to this are minimal, it is the treatment of choice when available. The recommended dose of HRIG is 20 IU per kg.[11, 23, 34]

A well-documented complete recovery from clinical rabies in an 8-year-old boy bitten by an infected bat has been accomplished. The success of this treatment resulted from the anticipation of complications in the natural course of the disease, such as hypoxia, convulsions, elevated intracranial pressure, arrhythmias, and aspiration, followed by aggressive treatment of each as they occurred.[22] This landmark case dispels the absolute finality of this dreaded disease, and at long last lends hope to both the victim of rabies and the physicians treating him.

HUMAN BITES

Human bites are relatively rare, but can constitute serious clinical problems. The three types are: (1) a genuine bite in which the assailant sinks his teeth into the victim, producing puncture wounds, lacerations, or avulsion of tissue (particularly of the tip of the nose, the earlobe, or the tongue); (2) abrasion and laceration of the knuckles and hand which occurs from the clenched fist striking the victim's mouth and teeth; and (3) a self-inflicted bite, usually of the tongue or lip, occurring often after falls or seizures.

Bacteriology

Infection is the most severe complication of human bites. The human mouth contains many more pathogenic organisms than those of most animals, and can be a reservoir for Staphylococcus, Streptococcus, an-

TABLE 2.   Specific Systemic Treatment of Rabies*

| Nature of Exposure | Status of Biting Animal (Irrespective of Whether Vaccinated or Not) | | Recommended Treatment |
	At Time of Exposure	During Observation Period of 10 Days	
No lesions; indirect contact	Rabid	—	None
Licks:			
Unabraded skin	Rabid	—	None
Abraded skin, scratches, and unabraded or abraded mucosa	Healthy	Clinical signs of rabies or proved rabid (laboratory)	Start vaccine† at first signs of rabies in the biting animal
	Signs suggestive of rabies	Healthy	Start vaccine† immediately; stop treatment if animal is normal on fifth day after exposure
	Rabid, escaped, killed, or unknown		Start vaccine† immediately
Bites:			
Mild exposure	Healthy	Clinical signs of rabies or proved rabid (laboratory)	Start vaccine†‡ at first signs of rabies in the biting animal
	Signs suggestive of rabies	Healthy	Start vaccine† immediately; stop treatment if animal is normal on fifth day after exposure
	Rabid, escaped, killed, or unknown	—	Start vaccine†‡ immediately
	Wild (wolf, jackal, fox, bat, etc.)	—	Serum‡ immediately, followed by a course of vaccine†
Severe exposure (multiple, or face, head, finger, or neck bites)	Healthy	Clinical signs of rabies or proved rabid (laboratory)	Serum‡ immediately; start vaccine† at first sign of rabies in the biting animal
	Signs suggestive of rabies	Healthy	Serum‡ immediately, followed by vaccine; vaccine may be stopped if animal is normal on fifth day after exposure
	Rabid, escaped, killed, or unknown	—	
	Wild (wolf, jackal, pariah dog, fox, bat, etc.)	—	Serum‡ immediately, followed by vaccine†

*From Habel, K.: Med. Clin. North Am., *51*:693, 1967.

†Practice varies concerning the volume of vaccine per dose and the number of doses recommended in a given situation. In general, the equivalent of at least 2 ml. of a 5 per cent tissue emulsion should be given subcutaneously daily for 14 consecutive days. Many laboratories use 20 to 30 doses in severe exposures. To ensure the production and maintenance of high levels of serum-neutralizing antibodies, booster doses should be given at 10 days and at 20 or more days following the last daily dose of vaccine in *all* cases. This is especially important if antirabies serum has been used, in order to overcome the interference effect.

‡In all severe exposures and in all cases of unprovoked wild animal bites, antirabies serum or its globulin fractions together with vaccine should be employed. This is considered by the Expert Committee on Rabies as the *best* specific treatment available for the postexposure prophylaxis of rabies in man. As with vaccine alone, it is important to start combined serum and vaccine treatment as early as possible after exposure, but serum still should be used no matter what the time interval. Serum should be given in a single dose (40 I.U. per kilogram of body weight) and the first dose of vaccine given at the same time. Sensitivity to the serum must be determined before its administration.

aerobic Streptococcus, gonococcus, Vincent's bacillus, fusiform bacillus, spirochetes, tetanus bacillus, gas gangrene bacillus, *Treponema pallidum,* and others. Heavy contamination of the wound should be assumed and treatment directed toward its eradication.

Therapy

All wounds should be cultured, thoroughly scrubbed with bacteriostatic soap, and liberally irrigated with sterile saline. Examination of damage to deep structures should be made, and tendon injury noted. Damaged tissues should be debrided. Severed tendons and nerves should not be sutured primarily.

Despite the potential for infection, with the advent of antibiotic therapy, soft tissue wounds of the head and face area, properly cleansed and debrided, can usually be sutured primarily when seen within 6 hours of injury. This applies even when cartilage of the nose or ear is exposed. Good cosmetic effects usually result. All other wounds should be left open. Attempts to reattach totally avulsed segments of ear or nose rarely are successful. Broad-spectrum antibiotics in therapeutic dosage are routinely given systemically and are modified subsequently on the basis of the organism cultured. Tetanus toxoid is administered.

All patients should be observed carefully for signs of cellulitis or gangrene, especially in bites of the fingers. Wounds seen late with cellulitis and secondary infections require hospitalization for massive antibiotic therapy, immobilization, and débridement.

Avulsed wound defects will require plastic surgery repair after infection subsides.[7, 13, 31]

SPIDER BITES

Black Widow Spider Bite

The black widow spider *(Latrodectus mactans)* is found everywhere in the United States except Alaska. The female is distinguished by a shiny black globular body with a red hourglass mark on the abdomen (Fig. 2). These spiders prefer dry, dimly lighted places, and are most commonly found around houses and buildings, under stones and lumber piles, between cracks and crevices, and in debris. Sixty-three deaths occurred between 1950 and 1960 from the bite of this spider.

Frequently a definite history of bite cannot be obtained. The venom is primarily neurotoxic and centers in the spinal cord. A victim may recall a pinprick sensation followed by dull and somewhat numbing pain. Slight local swelling and tiny red fang marks may be found. In a severe bite, pain in the chest soon results from upper extremity bites, and abdominal rigidity follows lower extremity bites. Spasms soon appear in all major muscle groups, and abdominal rigidity, suggesting an acute abdominal emergency, though it is usually nontender, occurs. Intense pain and spasms continue, usually resolving in 24 to 48 hours. Ptosis, dizziness, conjunctivitis, respiratory distress, nausea, and skin rash may occur. A burning sensation in the soles of the feet may be present during convalescence. Mortality is 4 per cent, usually resulting from shock or respiratory arrest.

Therapy. Therapy in adults consists of narcotics for relief of the agonizing pain and muscle relaxants to relieve muscle spasms. Infusion of 10 per cent calcium gluconate will give temporary relief of spasm but methocarbamol (Robaxin) is the drug of choice, 10 ml. being administered intravenously over a 5-minute period with another ampule started in saline drip.[16, 17, 37] In children under 6, in debilitated or aged adults, or in cases of severe invenomation, antivenin (Lyovac) is given. One ampule in 50 ml. of saline is usually sufficient.

Brown Recluse Spider Bite

The brown recluse spider *(Loxosceles reclusa)* is widely disseminated through the southern and central United States, and its range is increasing. Rocks, barks, and woodpiles are the common habitats in the southern states, while in cooler climates they have moved indoors and are found in closets, cellars, and used clothing. They are 10 to 15 mm. long, light tan to dark brown in color, and have flat bodies with a species-specific, dark, violin-shaped band over the dorsal cephalothorax (Fig. 3).[15, 16]

Biology. The venom is necrotizing and hemolytic and contains a spread factor (probably hyaluronidase). Shortly after inoculation of venom into guinea pigs, capillary dilation and pooling of blood occur, followed by the presence of hyalinized thrombi at 24 hours and coagulation necrosis and subcutaneous abscesses by 72 hours. In humans, edema and thickening of vascular endothelium is seen at 18 hours, followed by progressive endothelial thickening and occlusion. Sludging with perivascular infiltrate occurs at the periphery of the lesion. Hemolysis, hemoglobinuria, hemolytic anemia, and renal failure can develop.[15, 16, 37]

The patient may or may not have severe pain at the time of the bite, which frequently occurs in bed. After several hours a painful red area appears with a pale, mottled, cyanotic center which may blister. A zone of hemorrhage with induration and a surrounding halo of erythema which may be very extensive develop. Pain is severe. A central black eschar forms by 6 or 7 days, and soon there is a slough, leaving an open ulcer which may continue to enlarge. Deep and wide necrosis of fat undermining the skin about the eschar is a characteristic finding in this lesion, as shown in Figure 4.[1, 15, 17]

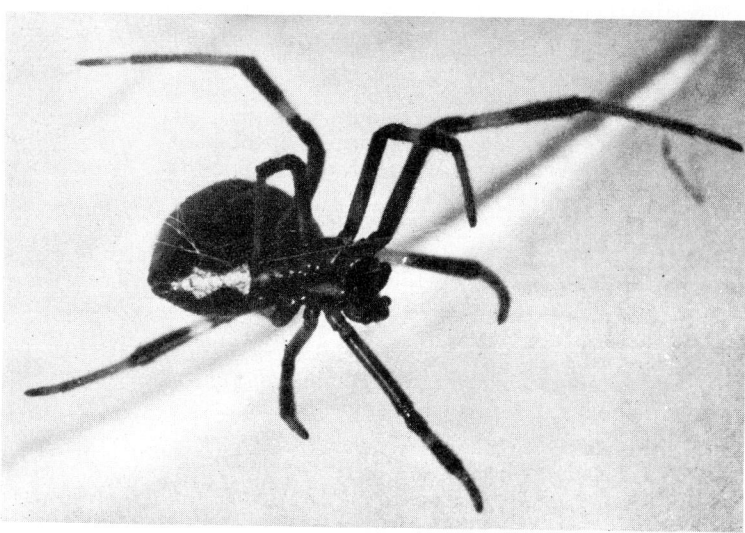

Figure 2. The female black widow spider has a shiny, black, globular body with a red hourglass mark on the abdomen. (From Paton, B. C.: Surg. Clin. North Am., *43*:537, 1963.)

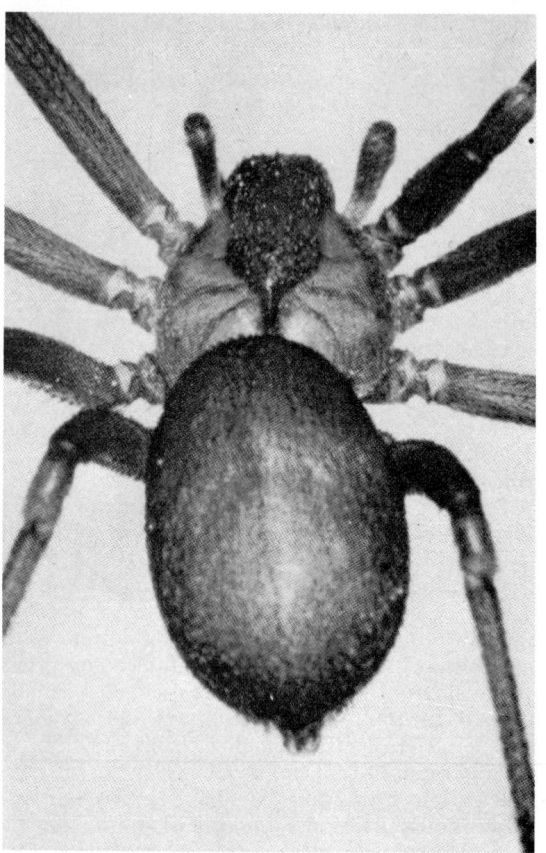

Figure 3. The brown recluse spider is 10 to 15 mm. long, is light tan to dark brown in color, and has a species-specific dorsal, dark, violin-shaped band. (From Dillaha, C. J., Jansen, G. T., Honeycutt, W. M., and Hayden, C. R.: J.A.M.A., *188*:33, 1964.)

BITES OF BEES, WASPS, HORNETS, AND OTHER INSECTS

Incidence

Arthropods of the order Hymenoptera include the honeybee, bumble bee, wasp, yellow jacket, yellow and black hornet, ant, and sawfly. Probably more than 100,000 species of this order exist, and more bites are inflicted upon man by these creatures than by any other venomous group. Their venom is just as toxic as that of the rattlesnake, and more deaths result from insect bites in the United States yearly than from all snakebites. Less venom is injected in insect bites, and severe allergic reactions rather than direct toxic effects of the venom account for most fatalities. Bees, wasps, hornets, and ants account for 65 per cent of deaths, spiders 31 per cent, and scorpions 4 per cent.

Biology

All insects of Hymenoptera, except the bee, retain their sting and can sting repeatedly, injecting a portion of the venom sac contents each time. The barbed stinging apparatus of the honeybee cannot be withdrawn, and as the bee attempts to escape it is disemboweled. The remaining anchored sting is driven farther into the skin by rhythmically contracting muscles attached to it, and venom from the sac can be injected for as long as 20 minutes.

Insect venoms, like those of snakes, contain a mixture of protein-like substances of varying antigenicity, kinins, histamine, and serotonin. Humans vary greatly in their reaction to insect bites, and these characteristics govern therapy. In general, the more rapid the onset of symptoms, the more severe the reaction is likely to be. Stings of the head, face, and neck tend to cause more serious effects. A transient,

Severe systemic symptoms may occur, especially in small children, with fever, malaise, weakness, nausea, vomiting, and petechiae developing early. Fatalities have been reported.

Therapy. Severe systemic symptoms must receive supportive therapy as given for the black widow spider bite. Antibiotics are always administered. No specific antivenin exists.

The administration of steroids has not stopped the progression of necrotic lesions in animal studies, and they should not be used for this purpose in humans. Steroids have been given to ameliorate systemic toxicity, though absolute guidelines for their use do not exist. Antihistamines, low molecular dextran, heparin, EDTA, and epsilon-aminocaproic acid are *not* agents of proved benefit, and their use at this time is *not* recommended.[1, 3, 4]

In most patients the primary problem will be care of the progressive, painful, necrotizing ulcer. Early excision of the bite is the best way of eliminating this, as the toxin diffuses slowly. Excision must be complete in order to avoid recurrence of the lesion. Large ulcers seen late are treated with wide débridement, which must include the necrotic fat. Skin grafting is often necessary.[1, 3, 15, 16, 31]

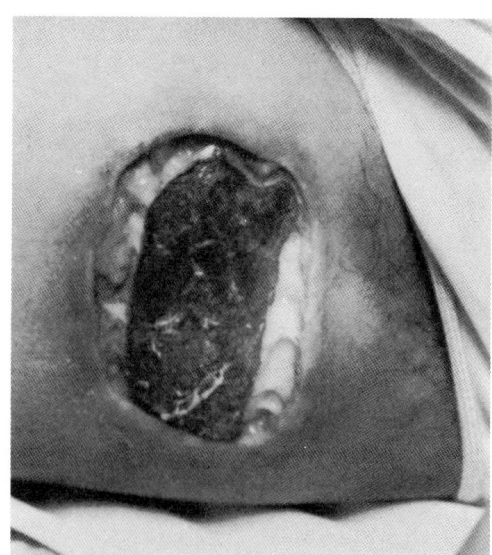

Figure 4. A central black eschar surrounded by deep necrosis of fat which undermines the skin is seen about 7 days after a brown recluse spider bite. (From Hershey, H. R., and Aulenbacker, C. E.: Ann. Surg., *170*:300, 1969.)

painless papule may result, or violent, diffuse burning pain can occur together with itching, paresthesias, areas of anesthesia, and headache. Urticaria, edema, erythema, and intense angioneurotic edema may appear as histamine is liberated by the toxin. The site of the sting can swell and may become septic or gangrenous. Muscular weakness, spasm, twitching, and paralysis may be seen. Respiratory distress, cyanosis, dysphagia, ocular palsies, apprehension, fever, nausea, bradycardia or tachycardia, and shock will occur in severe cases. A delayed hypersensitivity reaction resembling serum sickness may occur 10 to 14 days after injury.

Therapy

In 50 cases of fatal anaphylaxis resulting from insect bites over a 10-year period, 62 per cent of the patients were dead in the first hour. Inadequate or no treatment was the rule. In a similar survey of 100 nonfatal cases of severe anaphylaxis, 87 per cent of the patients received treatment in the first hour after the bite. The most frequent types of systemic reactions in these survivors were general urticaria (74 per cent), syncope (65 per cent), and respiratory tract obstruction (38 per cent).

Local Care. The retained sting shaft, if present, should be scraped off with a blade. The wound is washed with soap and water. Cellulitis or gangrene may require débridement. Local injection of lidocaine (Xylocaine) in uncomplicated cases has relieved persistent pain.

Toxic Reactions. In multiple bites, the total amount of injected toxin may be sufficient to cause severe systemic symptoms, principally diarrhea, vomiting, faintness, edema, muscle spasms, or convulsions. Supportive therapy as sedation, intravenous fluids, antibiotics, and antihistamines may be necessary. The toxic effects of the venom can be counteracted by calcium gluconate infusion.

Allergic Reactions. Immediate treatment is the key to success. Epinephrine 1:1000, 0.3 to 0.5 ml. for adults, is given subcutaneously. This is short-acting, and the dose may have to be repeated at 15- to 20-minute intervals. An antihistamine is also injected immediately. In severe cases, intravenous fluids, pressor agents, plasma expanders, and respiratory assistance may be required.

Prevention. All patients with a history of severe reaction to insect bites should be desensitized according to the directives of the Insect Allergy Committee of the American Academy of Allergy. This should be instituted 14 days after a severe bite. Sensitive patients should wear long-sleeved clothing, avoid obvious hazards, and carry a kit containing 10-mg. isoproterenol tablets for sublingual use, epinephrine aerosol for inhalation, and tweezers to remove the sting.[2, 9, 16, 37, 40]

SELECTED REFERENCES

Christy, N. P. (Ed.): Poisoning by venomous animals. Am. J. Med., *42*:107, 1967.
  This monograph presents a lucid review of the biochemical composition and physiologic effects in humans of animal venoms. Current aspects of therapy are clearly presented. The historical development of clinical treatment is of particular interest.

Corey, L., and Hattwick, M. A. W.: Treatment of persons exposed to rabies. J.A.M.A., *232*:272, 1975.
  This is a short, informative guide to therapy which presents the most recent concepts of treatment in a concise fashion. It is the most up-to-date such reference available.

Frazier, C. A.: Insect Allergy. St. Louis, Warren H. Green, Inc., 1969.
  This thorough and factual book contains detailed information about the toxicology, physiology, and therapy associated with insect allergy in humans. Complete and containing many references, this well-illustrated volume is probably the definitive work on insect allergy for clinicians.

Russell, F. E.: Venomous animal injuries. Curr. Probl. Pediatr., *3*:1, 1972.
  This is a very complete, detailed, yet practical overview of the pharmacology and therapy of bites from all classes of venomous animals. The section on marine animals, often not included in similar presentations, is particularly useful.

U. S. Department of the Navy, Bureau of Medicine and Surgery: Poisonous Snakes of the World. Washington, D.C., U.S. Government Printing Office, 1968.
  Concise and practical, this monograph presents in outline form information about the identification, habits, and habitats of poisonous snakes throughout the world. The plates, many in color, are excellent. Treatment from first aid to surgery is thoroughly covered.

White, D. L.: Rabies 1970. N. Y. J. Med., *70*:2456, 1970.
  A complete review of the current epidemiologic and microbiologic status of rabies today is presented. The immunology of rabies, rabies prophylaxis, and therapy are covered in detail.

REFERENCES

1. Auer, A. I., and Hershey, F. B.: Surgery for necrotic bites of the brown spider. Arch. Surg., *108*:612, 1974.
2. Barnard, J. H.: Studies of 400 Hymenoptera sting deaths in the United States. J. Allergy Clin. Immunol., *52*:259, 1973.
3. Berger, R. S.: A critical look at therapy for brown recluse spider bite. Arch. Dermatol., *107*:298, 1973.
4. Berger, R. S., Millikan, L. E., and Conway, F.: An *in vitro* test for Loxosceles reclusa spider bites. Toxicon, *11*:467, 1973.
5. Berzon, D. R., and DeHoff, J. B.: Medical costs and other aspects of dog bites in Baltimore. Public Health Rep., *89*:377, 1974.
6. Bhatt, D. R., Hattwick, M., Gerdsen, R., Emmons, R. W., and Johnson, H. N.: Human rabies. Am. J. Dis. Child., *127*:862, 1974.
7. Brandt, F. W.: Human bites of the ear. Plast. Reconstr. Surg., *43*:130, 1969.
8. Buckerl, W., Buckley, E., and Deulofeu, V. (Eds.): Venomous Animals and Their Venoms. New York, Academic Press, 1968.
9. Christy, N. P. (Ed.): Poisoning by venomous animals. Am. J. Med., *42*:107, 1967.
10. Chugh, K. S., Aikat, B. K., Sharma, B. K., Dash, S. C., Matthew, M. T., and Das, K. C.: Acute renal failure following snakebite. Am. J. Trop. Dis. Hyg., *24*:692, 1975.
11. Corey, L., and Hattwick, M. A.: Treatment of persons exposed to rabies. J.A.M.A., *232*:272, 1975.
12. Crick, J., and Brown, F.: Efficacy of rabies vaccine prepared from virus grown in duck embryo. Lancet, *1*:1106, 1970.
13. Curtin, J. W., and Greely, P. W.: Human bites of the face. Plast. Reconstr. Surg., *28*:394, 1961.
14. Ellenbogen, C., and Slugg, P.: Rabies neutralizing antibody: Inadequate response to equine antiserum and duck-embryo vaccine. J. Infect. Dis., *127*:433, 1973.
15. Fordon, D. W., Wingo, C. W., Robinson, D. W., and Masten, F. W.: The treatment of brown spider bite. Plast. Reconstr. Surg., *40*:482, 1967.
16. Frazier, C. A.: Diagnosis and treatment of insect bites. Clin. Sympos., *20*:75, 1968.
17. Frazier, C. A.: Insect Allergy. St. Louis, Warren H. Green, Inc., 1969.
18. Gill, K. A.: The evaluation of cryotherapy in the treatment of snake envenomization. South. Med. J., *63*:552, 1970.
19. Girard, K. F.: Rabies in Massachusetts—eleven years in retrospect. N. Engl. J. Med., *288*:319, 1973.
20. Glass, T. G.: Snakebite. Hosp. Med., 1971, pp. 31–51.
21. Glass, T. G.: Early debridement in pit viper bite. Surg. Gynecol. Obstet., *136*:774, 1973.

22. Hattwick, M. A. W., Weis, T. T., Stechschulte, C. J., Baer, G. M., and Gregg, M. B.: Recovery from rabies. Ann. Intern. Med., 76:931, 1972.

23. Hattwick, M. A. W., Rubin, R. H., Music, S., Sikes, R. K., Smith, J. S., and Gregg, M. B.: Postexposure rabies prophylaxis with human rabies immune globulin. J.A.M.A., 227:409, 1974.

24. Huang, T. T., Lynch, J. B., Larson, D. L., and Lewis, S. R.: The use of excisional therapy in the management of snakebite. Ann. Surg., 179:598, 1974.

25. Jones, R. C.: Rabies: Present attitudes. Postgrad. Med., 43:141, 1968.

26. Ledbetter, E. O., and Kutscher, A. E.: Aerobic and anaerobic flora of rattlesnake fangs and venom. Arch. Environ. Health, 19:770, 1969.

27. Parrish, H. M.: Incidence of treated snakebites in the United States. Public Health Rep., 81:269, 1966.

28. Parrish, H. M., and Carr, C. A.: Bites of copperheads (Ancistrodon contortrix) in the United States. J.A.M.A., 201:927, 1967.

29. Parrish, H. M., and Kahn, M. S.: Bites by coral snakes: Report of 11 representative cases. Am. J. Med. Sci., 253:561, 1967.

30. Parrish, H. M., and Dannell, H. D., Jr.: Bites by cottonmouths (Ancistrodon piscivorus) in the United States. South. Med. J., 60:429, 1967.

31. Paton, B. C.: Bites—human, dog, spider, and snake. Surg. Clin. North Am., 43:537, 1963.

32. Rubin, R. H., Gregg, M. B., and Sikes, R. K.: Rabies in citizens of the United States 1963–1968. Epidemiology, treatment and complications of treatment. J. Infect. Dis., 120:268, 1969.

33. Rubin, R. H., Hattwick, M. A. W., Jones, S., Gregg, M. B., and Schwartz, V. D.: Adverse reactions to duck embryo rabies vaccine. Ann. Intern. Med., 78:643, 1973.

34. Rubin, R. H., Sikes, R. K., and Gregg, M. B.: Human rabies immune globulin. J.A.M.A., 224:871, 1973.

35. Russell, F. E.: Pharmacology of animal venoms. Clin. Pharmacol. Ther., 8:849, 1967.

36. Russell, F. E.: Clinical aspects of snake venom poisoning in North America. Toxicon, 7:33, 1969.

37. Russell, F. E.: Venomous animal injuries. Curr. Probl. Pediatr., 3:1, 1973.

38. Snyder, C. C., Pickins, J. E., Knowels, R. P., Emerson, J. L., and Hines, W. A.: A definitive study of snakebite. J. Florida Med. Assoc., 55:330, 1968.

39. Snyder, C. C., Straight, R., and Glenn, J.: The snakebitten hand. Plast. Reconstr. Surg., 49:275, 1972.

40. Sobotka, A. K., Valentine, M. D., Benton, A. W., and Lichtenstein, L. M.: Allergy to insect stings. J. Allergy Clin. Immunol., 53:170, 1974.

41. U.S. Department of the Navy, Bureau of Medicine and Surgery: Poisonous Snakes of the World. Washington, D.C., U.S. Government Printing Office, 1968.

42. White, D. L.: Rabies 1970. N. Y. J. Med., 70:2456, 1970.

43. Winkler, W. C., Fashinell, T. R., Feffingwell, L., Howard, P., and Conomy, J. P.: Airborne rabies transmission in a laboratory worker. J.A.M.A., 226:1219, 1973.

19

TRAUMA: MANAGEMENT OF THE ACUTELY INJURED PATIENT

Martin S. Litwin, M.D., and Theodore Drapanas, M.D.

The care of the acutely injured has traditionally been considered the province of the military. Methods developed principally during wartime have led to progressive reductions in war wound mortality (Fig.1). Recently, however, trauma has become a major civilian problem. As a result of the widespread use of the automobile and the general availability of firearms, a trauma epidemic is sweeping the United States (Fig. 2). In 1970 more than 100,000 persons died as a result of external violence. For every person killed by some type of trauma, 10 to 15 more required hospitalization for periods ranging from a day to many months. These patients occupy at least 12 per cent of the total general hospital space. From 1899, when the first person was killed by an automobile, through 1965, the death toll from motor vehicles was 1.56 million. In World War II, total battle deaths amounted to 292,000. From the beginning of action in Vietnam in 1962 through December, 1965, there were 1550 combat deaths, while during the same period, accidents alone resulted in 10,000 deaths in all branches of the United States Armed Forces, a ratio of 6:1.

Because of the common occurrence of severe injury and the fact that with proper treatment many injured patients can be saved, care of the acutely injured patient is one of the most important areas in which a young surgeon should have early experience.

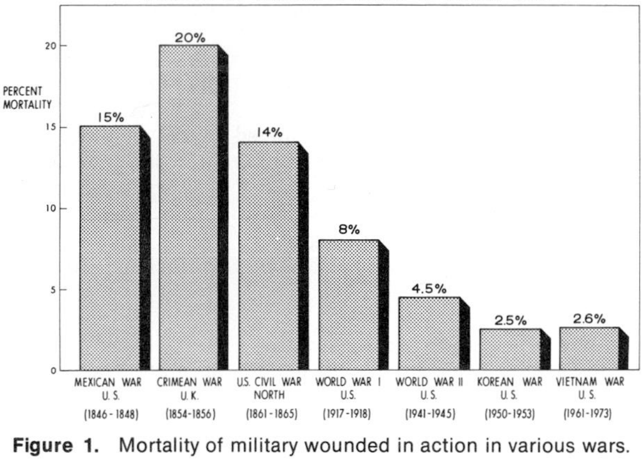

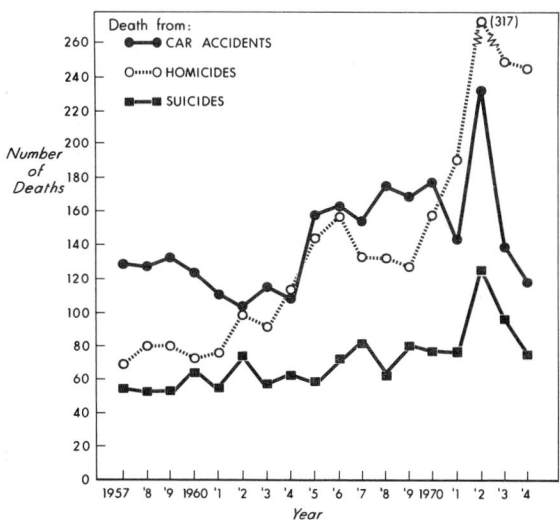

Figure 2. Number of violent deaths seen by Orleans Parish Coroner, 1957–1974. Dramatic decrease since 1972 in the number of deaths from car accidents began after enactment of a 55 m.p.h. speed limit. (Courtesy Orleans Parish Coroner's Office, New Orleans, La.)

MORTALITY OF WOUNDED IN ACTION IN VARIOUS WARS

Figure 1. Mortality of military wounded in action in various wars.

HISTORICAL ASPECTS

The development of standards of treatment for the acutely injured has been closely related to several significant medical discoveries (Table 1). Despite these advances, organized care of the acutely injured is a comparatively recent innovation. The Continental Congress established a medical service for the Continental Army on 27 July 1775. However, the physicians of the newly created Medical Department were not given military rank, and Dr. Benjamin Church of Massachusetts was appointed its first Director General and Chief Physician. He hastily established large general hospitals for more efficient treatment of larger numbers of individuals than had been possible in the regimental hospitals of the state militia. Because of questionable associations with the British, he was shortly relieved of his responsibilities and Dr. John Morgan was appointed. In 1781, authority was granted to hire nurses, orderlies, and other paramedical personnel necessary for the orderly functioning of a large hospital.

Surgeons in the eighteenth century were completely unaware of the causes and effects of infection. By the late eighteenth century, it was realized that miniballs were not poisonous, and they were often allowed to remain in place when they could not be easily located. When battle injuries involved fractures, especially when open fractures occurred, amputation was frequently done. The mortality for such procedures was often as high as 65 per cent when the leg was removed at mid-thigh. Additionally, there were severe difficulties in keeping up with the demand for supplies, and there was little experience with the maintenance of the health of large numbers of gravely ill and injured men in crowded hospitals.

During the War of 1812, the U.S. Army Medical Department was formally established by Act of Congress, but it was not until 1847 that military rank was given to medical officers. As late as 1854, when the Crimean War began, care of military and civilian casualties in the British Army was an even more random and haphazard process than in the United States. Medical officers were still attached to specific regiments, and there were no medical corps, military nurses, or trained orderlies. All hospitals were civil organizations. As a result, fully 20 per cent of the British who fell wounded in the Crimea died as a result of their wounds. It was then that Florence Nightingale (1820–1910), on her own initiative, introduced women nurses into the hospitals at Scutari.

Conditions were slightly better during the American Civil War, when 14.1 per cent of the Northern troops who were wounded died as a result of their injuries. In 1873 the first British Army Medical Corps was organized, and in 1884 medical officers rather than nonmedical personnel assumed command of the Corps.

In 1867 Lister published convincing evidence that the use of antiseptic techniques led to an amazing improvement in wound healing, and in 1889 Crile published work indicating that intravenous infusions could rapidly restore blood pressure after massive hemorrhage.

Treatment of acute injuries changed little, however, until World War I. During the early years of the war, conservative treatment of wounds was universal. Tetanus, gas gangrene, and the hemolytic streptococcus took their toll without hindrance, and mortality for compound fractures of the femur approached 80 per cent. It became obvious that something must be done. Gradually, the process of excision of the tissue lining the tract of a wound became an established principle. The years of World War I further represented a period during which an attempt was made to apply fundamental physiologic principles to shock treatment. New emphasis was given to the use of intravenous plasma replacement. However, the average time required for evacuation of a patient from the battlefield to a site

TABLE 1. Outstanding Medical Discoveries of Importance in Care of The Acutely Injured

Priests of Asklepieia	1000 B.C.	Cleansed and bandaged sword wounds
Hippocrates	500 B.C.	Distinguished between primary and secondary wound healing
Alexandria School (Greek)	300 B.C.	First used ligature to control bleeding
Claudius Galenus	130–201	Irrigated and used sutures to reapproximate clean wounds
Ambroise Paré	1510–1590	Cleansed traumatic wounds and discontinued cauterization; repopularized ligature for bleeding blood vessels
John Collins Warren	1846	First used general anesthetic to perform surgical procedure
Ignaz Semmelweis	1847	Proved that puerperal fever did not occur with proper antisepsis
Louis Pasteur	1864	Proved existence of atmospheric germs
Joseph Lister	1867	Discovered that antisepsis markedly improved wound healing
Robert Koch	1877	Discovered that different bacteria caused different types of infection
Karl Landsteiner	1900	Discovered blood grouping
Richard Lewisohn	1915	Discovered sodium citrate as an anticoagulant
World War I	1917–1918	Débridement of gunshot wounds, use of blood transfusions and intravenous fluids
Alexander Fleming	1929	Discovered penicillin
World War II	1941–1945	Management of thoracic and vascular injuries
Korean conflict	1950–1953	Improved management of vascular injuries, liberal use of whole blood
Vietnam War	1961–1973	Rapid resuscitation and evacuation

where definitive therapy could be started was 10 hours.

As far as the treatment of the acutely injured patient is concerned, the years 1923 to 1941 were noteworthy chiefly for a newly awakened interest in the possible role of capillary contractility and permeability in the etiology of shock.

Compared to that in previous wars, the mortality in World War II for patients with battle wounds who reached a medical facility dropped markedly, to 4.5 per cent. This was due to prompt evacuation, the use of whole blood, and, during the later years of the war, the use of antibiotics. Stress was placed on the maintenance of primary treatment facilities near the battle zone with sufficient bed capacity and staff to provide care long enough for the patient to achieve a well-stabilized state prior to evacuation. Mortality and morbidity were both shown to rise if patients with serious wounds were evacuated within 10 days after wounding.

During the Korean conflict, the fatality rate for those wounded in action who reached medical treatment facilities was only 2.4 per cent, and the ratio of patients hospitalized with wounds to those killed in action was 2.8:1. The lower mortality rate in the Korean conflict as compared to that of previous wars has been ascribed to a number of factors: shorter evacuation time, the administration of large quantities of resuscitative fluids preoperatively and during surgery, and the routine use of antibiotics. Because of the availability of helicopters, the average evacuation time from injury to admission was only 3.6 hours, and from admission to surgery, 3.0 hours. However, the single greatest difference in the management of casualties in Korea from that in previous wars appeared to be the administration of large quantities of blood throughout the resuscitative period.

In the Viet Nam conflict the principles originally defined during World War II and in Korea were considerably refined. The mortality among wounded reaching medical facilities remained at 2.6 per cent but the ratio of hospitalized patients with wounds to the number of individuals killed in action rose markedly to 4.15:1. This dramatic achievement was brought about largely by the more prompt and more efficient treatment of hemorrhagic and traumatic shock. Through the combined efforts of the Army, Navy, and Air Force, the Armed Services Whole Blood Procurement Laboratory supplied from the United States an almost unlimited amount of fresh whole blood on a daily basis. Additionally, there were continued efforts at even earlier evacuation from field of battle to the proper facility where an adequate initial definitive procedure could be accomplished. The availability of highly qualified surgeons, modern equipment, and advanced surgical techniques also contributed significantly to these dramatic changes. With the availability of swift, reliable helicopter evacuation, the time between wounding and effective treatment was reduced to 35 minutes. In World War II and in Korea, most wounded men who died did so within 4 to 6 hours after wounding, before treatment. In Viet Nam, such patients arrived at medical facilities alive. The helicopter made evacuation from *first echelon* (emergency care) to *second echelon* (continued resuscitation) or *third echelon* (full resuscitation and initial definitive surgery) stations optional. Helicopters are now being used extensively in civilian practice throughout the United States for the early transportation of severely injured patients. Yesterday's battlefield lessons are once again serving as blueprints for today's trauma surgeon.

MULTIPLE INJURIES

The magnitude of the problem of trauma in the United States is not generally appreciated. *Trauma is the leading cause of death in the first three decades of life and ranks fourth among causes of death overall.* Automobile accidents alone kill more Americans each year than were lost during the entire Korean War.

In a recent study it was found that among a group of 1678 injured occupants in 1000 automobile crashes, 65 per cent sustained multiple injuries. Until 1973, the number and mortality rate of patients in this multiple trauma category constantly increased.

Many of the lessons that have already been learned about the management of patients with multiple injuries are not commonly appreciated outside military practice and large trauma centers. This is unfortunate, because there is no field of medicine in which the rewards of intelligent, immediate, purposeful treatment are greater than in the early care of the severely injured. The patient with multiple injuries is in desperate physiologic straits, and his survival is directly dependent upon a coordinated, carefully planned team approach to diagnosis and treatment. As with all team approaches, the patient is best managed when the overall responsibility for his care rests with one physician. Division of responsibility or attention only to the particular area in which the physician has special knowledge may decrease awareness of complications and will hinder the evaluation of the patient's overall problems. Meticulous and detailed attention to total patient care during the early phases of the patient's injury is of paramount importance, and the physician who is called upon to treat a patient with multiple injuries should be capable of initially dealing with all the acute derangements that are present.

Priorities

In many instances, the margin between survival and death is narrow enough to require that a priority list be established for every patient who is admitted to the emergency room with multiple injuries. The physician who understands these priorities and can initiate steps in diagnosis and therapy with priorities in mind will usually perform creditably in the initial management of the patient.

1. The most dramatic and urgent symptom in the acutely injured patient is *asphyxia*. It is quickly fatal if not relieved, and death can ensue in minutes.

2. *Hemorrhage* is next in importance and should be rapidly controlled by whatever means are necessary.

3. Perhaps of equal importance with the control of hemorrhage is the *sealing of open or sucking chest wounds* because these can produce death almost as rapidly as asphyxia.

4. Next in order of importance is the treatment of *shock*. Although replacement of circulating blood volume is usually indicated in the patient with multiple injuries, not all patients presenting with hypotension and shock have had blood loss.

5. The *splinting of fractures* is an important factor in the control of shock and in preventing further injuries during movement of the patient.

6. Rapid *evaluation of the patient for further injuries* should be performed, and adequate treatment instituted.

7. Last in the order of priority but not least in importance is the *continuous observation* of the patient, preferably by the same physician who treated him initially, and evaluation for latent injuries that may appear more obvious with the passage of time.

Airway Maintenance. Maintenance of an adequate airway should hold the highest priority in the management of the patient with multiple injuries (Fig. 3). This is particularly true in patients who have multiple injuries about the head and neck, and in patients who have suffered thoracic trauma. A simple unstable fracture of the mandible may lead to death if an airway is not promptly provided. Many patients, particularly those involved in automobile accidents, have consumed alcohol or have a full stomach; in such persons aspiration poses a serious danger.

The simplest method of obtaining an adequate airway is by insertion of an oropharyngeal tube. Patients with intact gag reflexes, even though they are unconscious, may gag and vomit during insertion of the tube, and aspiration may occur. Under these conditions, particularly when question exists concerning the status of the stomach, it is safer to insert a cuffed endotracheal tube and thereby prevent aspiration. Endotracheal tube insertion in the unconscious patient is easily performed if the appropriate laryngoscope, endotracheal tubes, and suction apparatus are available, as they should be in every emergency room. Tracheostomy may also be of great benefit in some patients and

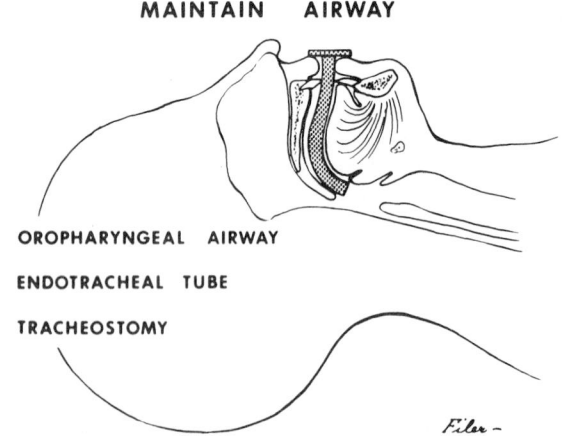

MAINTAIN AIRWAY

OROPHARYNGEAL AIRWAY

ENDOTRACHEAL TUBE

TRACHEOSTOMY

Figure 3. Techniques of maintaining adequate airway in the emergency room. Oropharyngeal airway is preferred in unconscious patients. This may be replaced by endotracheal tube with inflated cuff to prevent aspiration. Tracheostomy rarely, if ever, should be performed in such patients without preliminary insertion of endotracheal tube.

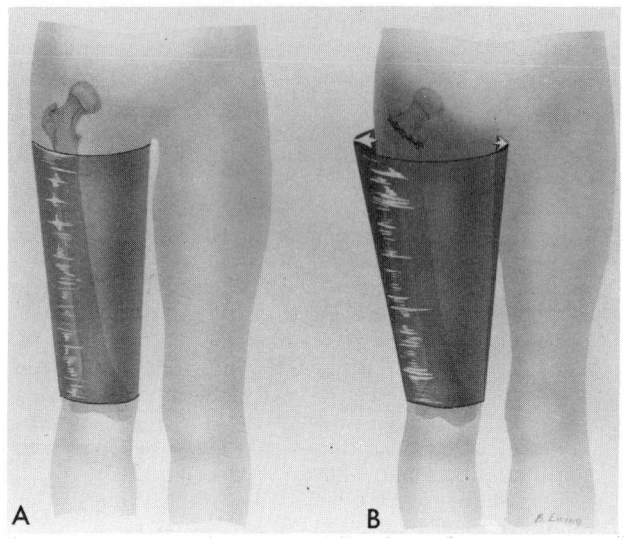

Figure 4. Large amounts of blood may be lost into the soft tissues surrounding a fracture. Using the geometric formula for the volume in a truncated cone, it has been calculated that when a normal adult *(A)* suffers an intertrochanteric fracture of the femur and when the amount of blood lost into the surrounding soft tissues is sufficient to increase the radius of the upper thigh by only 1 cm. *(B)*, then approximately 1.5 liters of blood will have been lost from the vascular system.

will further facilitate care of the airway and lungs; however, tracheostomy is a hazardous procedure in a patient who is thrashing about because of asphyxia, pain, or head injury. Except under the most extreme emergency conditions, a tracheostomy is best performed after endotracheal intubation has been successfully accomplished and the airway reestablished.

Control of Hemorrhage. The second item on the priority list is to control hemorrhage. Hemorrhage may be overt or occult. In controlling overt hemorrhage, the most efficient emergency maneuver is to apply pressure over the bleeding point and to elevate the part. This will usually suffice to control the bleeding and a tourniquet is rarely needed. However, when a major vessel has been lacerated, a tourniquet may be necessary.

Concealed or occult hemorrhage is more difficult to diagnose. It is not generally realized that patients with fractures may lose a considerable amount of blood into the soft tissues (Fig. 4). For example, it has been estimated that approximately one to two units of blood are lost into the soft tissues of the thigh following a shaft fracture of the femur. A patient with such an injury, particularly if he is young, may not manifest signs of shock until he is taken to the operating room for open reduction of the fracture. A catastrophic and precipitous fall in blood pressure may then occur as anesthesia is induced. An axiom in patients with multiple fractures is that they have lost at least two units of blood into the soft tissues surrounding the fracture. Patients with major pelvic trauma may also lose considerable quantities of blood into the pelvic space and the retroperitoneal area.

Sucking Chest Wounds. The immediate care of a patient who has a sucking chest wound usually makes the difference between death and survival. The hole in the chest wall should be closed by any available maneuver without particular consideration of bacterial contamination. In a sucking chest wound, particularly if the hole is large, not only does collapse of the lung on the involved side occur, but on inspiration there is a shift of the mediastinum to the opposite side (Fig. 5), which results in a marked decrease in ventilation of the normal lung. There is a marked loss in vital capacity, which in turn leads to rapid arterial desaturation, anoxia, and death. A sucking chest wound is usually an indication for immediate thoracotomy after the wound has been sealed. Closure of large defects may be challenging but can usually be accomplished by the use of adjacent muscle flaps.

Shock. Shock is present, whether obvious or not, in every patient with multiple injuries. It is, therefore, mandatory to withdraw samples of blood for typing and cross matching and then to start an intravenous infusion through a large-bore needle. The signs and symptoms of shock, when they are well established, are usually easy to recognize. Most are the result of low peripheral blood flow and excess adrenal sympathetic activity. For this reason, a rapid infusion of either normal saline or lactated Ringer's solution should be started in every patient with impending or actual shock. The solution should be administered rapidly so that within a period of 15 minutes between 1 and 2 liters will have been given. Shires and others have shown that the use of balanced salt solutions, e.g., Ringer's lactate, may significantly reduce the requirement for whole blood in the patient with hemorrhagic hypotension. In a patient who has lost whole blood, a marked reduction in the extracellular fluid space may occur. Balanced salt solution appears to correct this functional reduction in extracellular fluid. However, crystalloids have a dilutional effect on plasma protein concentration and lead to a decrease in intravascular oncotic pressure. Thus, large quantities may induce interstitial pulmonary edema. For this reason, amounts of Ringer's lactate larger than those recommended should be given only with great care.

After adequate crystalloid has been given, the administration of plasma expanders should be considered when shock is suspected. Plasma solution or 1.25 per cent albumin in a balanced salt solution may be used. Because of its ability to improve tissue blood flow and oxygen delivery, to expand plasma volume, and to prevent deep venous thrombosis, dextran-40 (Rheomacrodex) in amounts up to 1 liter may also be of benefit in treatment of severely injured patients.

The best primary therapy for hemorrhagic shock continues to be adequate replacement of properly cross-matched, type-specific whole blood. When properly typed and cross-matched whole blood is not immediately available, low-titer, Rh-negative, type O blood can be administered until type-specific blood can be obtained. When large quantities of blood must be administered, the blood given should be as fresh as possible. Induction of clotting abnormalities may thereby be at least partially prevented. If hemothorax is present, the aspirated blood may be citrated, filtered, and transfused. Autotransfusion devices have recently been developed for intraoperative reinfusion of such blood.

In the past, the use of vasopressors in treatment of

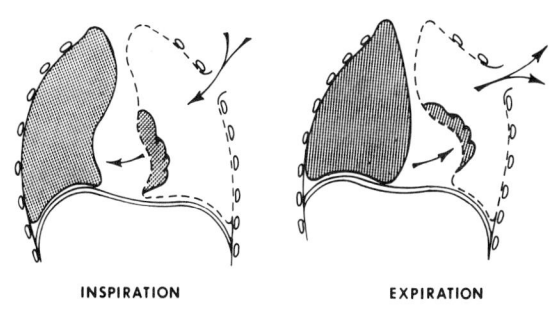

OPEN CHEST WOUNDS

INSPIRATION   EXPIRATION

Figure 5. Physiologic derangements in open chest wounds. With inspiration there is shift of the mediastinum to the normal side as air enters the involved pleural cavity and pleural pressure equilibrates with atmospheric. This limits alveolar ventilation on the normal side. With expiration, the mediastinum shifts to the involved side.

hemorrhagic shock was widespread. It now appears that their use is rarely, if ever, warranted in the emergency treatment of hypovolemic shock. The use of vasodilators in treatment of shock is still highly experimental and at this time has no place in the clinical treatment of shock.

In monitoring an acutely injured patient, pulse rate, arterial blood pressure, central venous pressure, and hourly urinary output should be followed closely (Table 2). Even though pulse rate in a healthy adult may increase as a result of the anxiety associated with a traumatic episode, it is unusual for arterial blood pressure to drop for more than a brief, transient period. For this reason, the physician must first determine whether under normal circumstances the patient has hypertension. It is distinctly possible for such a patient to have a "normal" blood pressure but to have a severe blood volume deficit. In an adult patient who is usually normotensive, a prolonged drop in blood pressure usually indicates the loss of at least 1200 to 1500 ml. of blood from the intravascular compartment.

Urinary output will cease once arterial blood pressure has dropped to approximately 60 mm. Hg systolic, but when arterial pressure is above this level, hourly urinary output serves as a reliable indicator of renal perfusion and renal function. Optimal hourly urinary output ranges from 30 to 50 ml. per hour.

Measurement of central venous pressure is an extremely helpful adjunct in monitoring a severely injured patient. Even though arterial blood pressure after trauma may be normal, it is quite possible that intravascular volume replacement has not been ade-

TABLE 2. Useful Parameters for Monitoring Adequacy of Blood and Fluid Replacement

1. Pulse rate
2. Arterial blood pressure
3. Central venous pressure
4. Hourly urinary output

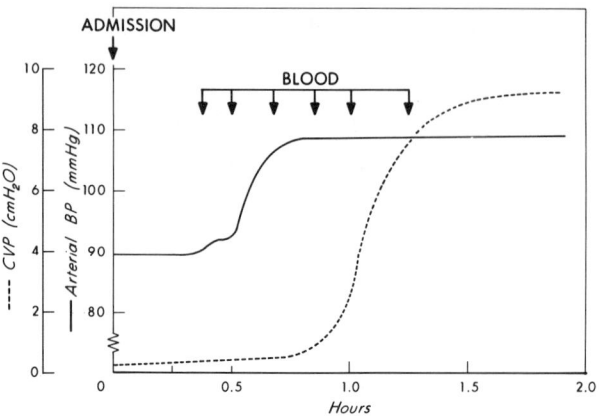

Figure 6. Value of the central venous pressure measurement. Recorded data from a patient with a large pelvic hematoma, the result of multiple pelvic fractures, are shown. Although arterial blood pressure promptly returned to normal after three units of blood were given (arrows), the central venous pressure remained at extremely low levels (<1 cm. H_2O) until five units of blood had been administered and blood volume had been restored. Frequently the central venous pressure is a better index of the adequacy of volume replacement than the arterial blood pressure.

quate (Fig. 6). This is indicated by an unusually low central venous pressure. Normal central venous pressure in the right atrium of a healthy adult is approximately 2 cm. H_2O but may range as high as 5 cm. H_2O. When intravascular volume is below normal, it is not unusual for central venous pressure to be 0 or even negative during inspiration. When such is the case, administration of appropriate fluids is indicated until the central venous pressure begins to rise and may be safely continued until it reaches 10 cm. H_2O.

Fractures. All fractures should be splinted to avoid further trauma to the soft tissues and also to relieve pain. Splinting usually can be easily performed in the emergency room. If the patient has other more serious injuries, the splinted fracture may be then ignored until his condition has stabilized. In open fractures (compound fractures) a sterile dressing should be applied to avoid further contamination of the wound, but exploration will eventually be necessary for adequate débridement and removal of foreign material at the site of fracture. Several different types of splints should be available in any emergency ward (Fig. 7).

Further Evaluation. Once the patient's airway patency is assured, hemorrhage and shock have been adequately controlled and treated, and fractures have been splinted, the physician may then carefully examine and evaluate him for possible occult injuries. Such an examination should be performed in a systematic fashion by investigating and evaluating the thorax, abdomen, genitourinary tract, central nervous system, and finally the musculoskeletal system. While many injuries will become apparent as the patient is evaluated, some may not appear obvious for a considerable period of time. For this reason, the patient should be continuously observed and his vital signs monitored, preferably by the same physician who saw him initially. In this fashion, any change in the patient's physical findings may be more accurately evaluated.

To review briefly the priorities in initial management of a patient with multiple injuries: first, the airway should be maintained; second, hemorrhage should be controlled; third, open or sucking chest wounds should be sealed; fourth, adequate treatment for shock should be instituted; fifth, fractures should be splinted; sixth, a more complete examination of all the body viscera should be performed; and finally, sev-

enth, the patient should be under continuous observation for as long as is necessary to be absolutely certain that he has no other injuries.

The various diagnostic and therapeutic maneuvers in the emergency area for a typical patient with multiple injuries are shown in Figure 8.

MECHANISMS OF INJURY

Penetrating Chest Injury

Sharp penetrating injury may be due to any of a variety of weapons—swords, spears, knives, bullets, and so forth. Penetration of the abdomen is, of course, serious; however, unless major blood vessels are injured and severe hemorrhage ensues, such injuries are not immediately life-threatening. Penetration injury into the thorax constitutes a much more immediate threat to life. When the thoracic cavity is entered and the lung penetrated, an air leak with pneumothorax results. This in turn leads to lung collapse, ineffective oxygen exchange, and severe respiratory distress. If

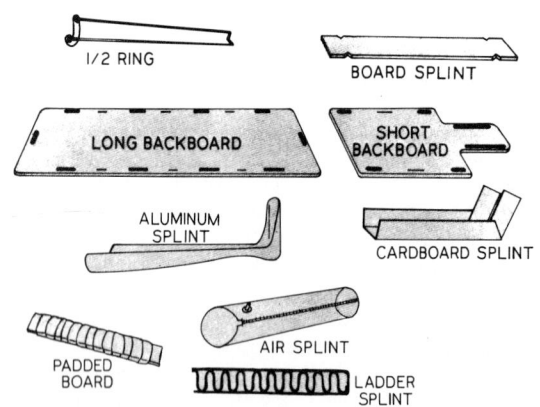

Figure 7. Types of splints that should be available in ambulances and in emergency rooms. (From Committee on Injuries of American Academy of Orthopedic Surgeons: Emergency Care and Transportation of the Sick and Injured. Chicago, American Academy of Orthopedic Surgeons, 1971.)

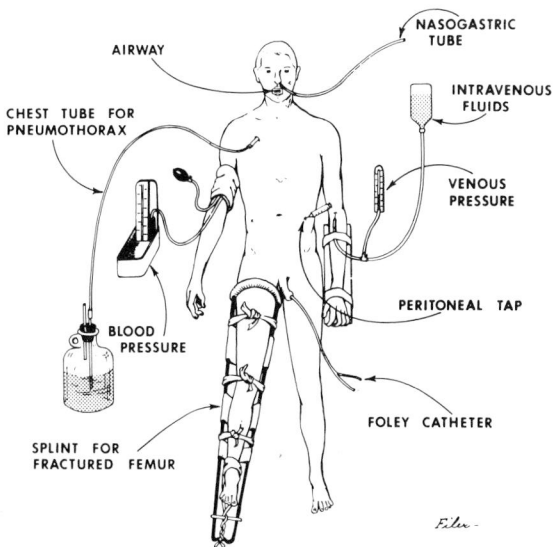

Figure 8. Emergent diagnostic and therapeutic maneuvers in a patient with multiple injuries. Shown in this patient are an oropharyngeal tube for the maintenance of an airway, a nasogastric tube for gastric decompression, a closed thoracostomy tube for treatment of tension pneumothorax on the right side, a Thomas splint for immobilization of a fractured femur, a Foley catheter for monitoring urinary output, peritoneal tap for occult abdominal injury, monitoring of central venous pressure, and administration of intravenous crystalloid solutions. Such diagnostic and treatment modalities should be rapidly instituted in patients with multiple injuries, depending on the extent and areas involved.

the heart is penetrated, blood leaking into the pericardial sac may cause pericardial tamponade. (See also Thoracic Trauma in Chapter 55.)

Blunt Chest Injury

In our modern society, automobile injuries constitute the most common cause for blunt chest injury. Flail chest, also known as "steering wheel injury," results when the driver of an automobile is suddenly thrown forward into the steering column, or when the side of an automobile is crushed into the driver or a passenger. Numerous ribs are fractured, usually lateral to the sternum on both sides, and an isolated floating or "flail" segment, consisting of the anterior severed rib segments and costal cartilages and the sternum, is produced. The flail segment in lateral injuries is usually confined to one hemithorax and consists of several ribs that have been fractured in at least two spots. When the patient creates a negative intrathoracic pressure by inspiring, this flail segment moves inward rather than forward and upward as in normal respiration. Such paradoxical motion prevents the formation of a negative intrathoracic pressure; hence the lungs cannot expand, the patient cannot inspire, and adequate oxygen exchange cannot take place.

The severity of the respiratory insult in a patient with flail chest depends on the condition of his respiratory system prior to injury as well as on the size of the flailing segment. A middle-aged male with a long history of smoking and moderate emphysema will be less able to endure a respiratory insult than a young man who has never smoked and who has run 2 miles daily before injury.

Blunt injury to the chest may also result in myocardial contusion; this is not immediately life-threatening unless the myocardium has ruptured. Post-traumatic myocarditis usually occurs several days after injury and can be diagnosed by its typical electrocardiographic pattern.

Of more pressing importance in the acutely injured patient who has suffered blunt injury to the chest is the possibility of aortic rupture. When deceleration occurs very suddenly, the heart and proximal attached aorta are thrown forward violently. Shearing injury to the aorta may occur posteriorly at the point where the aorta passes from its mediastinal to a retropleural position. Such injury should always be suspected when the chest film reveals widening of the mediastinal shadow. When this is noted, aortography should be carried out immediately, and if the injury is present, surgical intervention with pump-oxygenator standby should not be delayed.

Sudden deceleration may also result in shearing injury to the intima of the aorta and the rapid progression of a traumatic dissecting aneurysm. Diagnosis of this condition is made in the same way as diagnosis of an arteriosclerotic dissecting aneurysm. Pulses and blood pressures in the upper extremities may be unequal, and there may be excruciating chest pain. When the coronary ostia are involved in the dissection, death usually occurs quickly.

Like the heart, the lungs also may be thrown forward in deceleration injuries, and a bronchial tear or complete laceration of any of the bronchi may result. Air is forced into the mediastinum and a classic crunch may be heard on auscultation of the chest. Subcutaneous emphysema also occurs at the back of the neck. When laceration of the lung has occurred and tension pneumothorax is present, immediate insertion of a large-bore needle into the appropriate pleural space to allow escape of accumulated air is lifesaving.

Direct trauma to the chest may result in the occurrence of a "sucking chest wound," in which a portion of the chest wall has been either blown or torn away, and lung tissue is exposed. When this happens, the natural elasticity of the lung leads to sudden and complete collapse of the lung on the involved side. The intermittent negative pressure created in the opposite pleural space as a result of respiratory movement leads in turn to marked intermittent shifts in the mediastinum. Such mediastinal shifts are associated with ineffective respiratory exchange and with marked cardiac arrhythmias. A sucking chest wound constitutes a serious emergency, and the chest wall defect must be sealed airtight as soon as possible. (See also Thoracic Trauma in Chapter 55.)

Penetrating Abdominal Injury

Penetrating wounds of the abdomen may be due to penetration by any sort of foreign object. Until recently, the punji stick, a sharpened bamboo spike, was a frequent cause of penetrating injury in the military. All penetrating injuries of the abdomen are, of course, potentially lethal, but the danger is not immediate unless there is associated major vascular injury. A gunshot wound that simultaneously penetrates both a major artery or vein and the colon is particularly lethal because of the contamination produced at the vascular repair site. When a major blood vessel is involved in a penetrating abdominal wound, immediate surgical exploration is indicated to control hemorrhage. Rapid bleeding causes all of the classic signs and symptoms of hypovolemic shock.

Blunt Abdominal Injury

As the use of the automobile has become more widespread, blunt trauma to the abdomen has become increasingly common. Either sudden deceleration or sudden compression of the abdomen may result in injury to abdominal viscera. When the body is traveling forward at a high rate of speed and stops suddenly as a result of impact with a stationary object, organs that are loosely fixed continue to travel forward. Such stress frequently results in severe injury, most often at the renal pedicle, the root of the mesentery, or sites where the duodenum and colon pass from free-hanging intraperitoneal positions to fixed retroperitoneal positions. Occasionally a branch of the superior mesentery artery may also be sheared off by this mechanism. When an artery, such as the renal artery, is acutely stretched during deceleration, the adventitia and muscular coats may remain intact and only the intima may be lacerated. Arterial thrombosis quickly occurs and acute renal failure, possibly with complete renal necrosis, results. The base of the vascular pedicle at the spleen may also be partially avulsed during sudden deceleration. When this occurs intraperitoneal hemorrhage ensues.

Because of its position, the duodenum is apt to undergo an unusual type of injury. During sudden deceleration, the first portion of the duodenum is thrown forward simultaneously with the jejunum, which has the ligament of Treitz as its flexion point. At the same time, intra-abdominal pressure usually increases markedly. This pressure is transmitted to the duodenum, which is now closed either by the pylorus or by the peritoneal flexion point at one end and the ligament of Treitz at the other. Posterior retroperitoneal rupture of the duodenum may then result. When duodenal disruption is incomplete and only the mucosa and submucosa are torn, bleeding beneath the mucosa and through the submucosa may result in the accumulation of a large submucosal hematoma. The hematoma may be large enough to obstruct the duodenal lumen and cause intestinal obstruction. The classic "coiled-spring" pattern seen in the duodenum on an upper gastrointestinal series is diagnostic.

Other areas in the abdominal cavity that are liable to injury during sudden deceleration include the ileum at the ileocolic junction; the right colon and the descending colon where this organ passes from relatively free-hanging intraperitoneal positions to fixed retroperitoneal positions; and the portion of the pancreas where the head and the body meet and also where the pancreas makes contact with the superior mesenteric artery. Occasionally, unusually acute deceleration may lead to disruption of the common bile duct from the duodenum, avulsion of the cystic duct from the common bile duct, or rupture of the gallbladder.

When blunt force is applied to the abdomen, a tremendous amount of energy may be transmitted directly to the abdominal viscera, which are in turn acutely and suddenly compressed. In this situation, capsular disruption and organ laceration of the liver and spleen commonly occur. Splenic laceration may be associated with acute, sudden, exsanguinating intra-abdominal hemorrhage for which the only treatment is immediate laparotomy and splenectomy. Compression lacerations of the liver may also be acutely life-threatening, particularly when they have extended posteriorly into the hepatic veins and vena cava or into the hilum through the hepatic artery or its major branches.

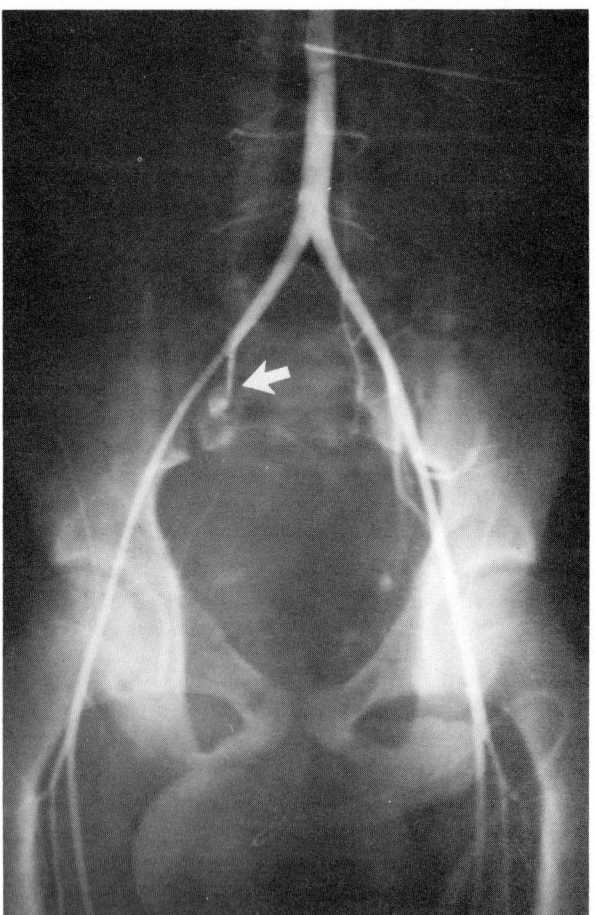

Figure 9. Aortogram in a man who was struck by an automobile. Hypotension recurred in spite of massive blood replacement. At the time of operation, a large retroperitoneal hematoma was found and the lacerated right hypogastric artery (arrow) was ligated. The patient fully recovered.

Acute compression injury to the abdomen is frequently associated with the fractures of the pelvis. Large amounts of blood may be lost into the retroperitoneum when the hypogastric arteries are involved in such injury (Fig. 9). Shock developing after pelvis fracture should lead one to suspect this diagnosis. When hemorrhage continues, and the bleeding point has been demonstrated by arteriography, autologous blood clots may be injected retrograde through an arterial catheter directly into the lacerated vessel. Alternatively, hypogastric artery ligation may be required.

Gunshot Wounds

Gunshot wounds constitute one of the most serious forms of penetrating injury seen in man. The severity of the injury suffered is related not only to the tissues penetrated and to those in the vicinity of the injury but also to the weapon used.

The severity of the injury resulting from a bullet is directly proportional to the amount of energy it delivers to the tissues. The amount of kinetic energy possessed by a traveling bullet may be calculated by using the formula $KE = \dfrac{mv^2}{2g}$, where m is mass of the missile, v is the velocity of the missile, and g is the gravitational acceleration. Thus, the kinetic energy is directly proportional to the mass of the bullet multiplied by the square of the velocity. Beyer has classified bullet velocities of less than 1200 feet per second (f.p.s.) as *low*, those from 1200 to 2500 f.p.s. as *medium*, and velocities in excess of 2500 f.p.s. as *high*. Bullet velocity is the most important factor determining the extent of tissue destruction. When the mass is greatly increased, however, as in a .45 caliber bullet, it too becomes an important factor in determining the severity of the injury produced. The most extensive tissue damage is produced when both velocity is high and mass is great.

Since the severity of injury resulting from gunshot wounds is directly proportional to the kinetic energy imparted to the tissues, the severity of the injury will be directly related to the muzzle velocity of the firearm and the weight of the bullet expelled (Table 3). Thus, an M16 rifle with a muzzle velocity of 3250 f.p.s. will produce a much more severe injury than a .22 caliber rifle with a muzzle velocity of 1000 f.p.s. even though both utilize the bullets of approximately the same size, shape, and weight. On the other hand, a .45 caliber automatic pistol with a muzzle velocity of 860 f.p.s. will produce a much more severe injury than a .22 caliber rifle with a muzzle velocity of 1000 f.p.s. Even though the muzzle velocity of the latter is greater than the muzzle velocity of the former, the more severe injury results from the markedly larger, heavier slug expelled from the .45 caliber pistol.

Nondisintegrating bullets that pass completely through the tissues do not deliver all of their energy. Such bullets cause less tissue destruction than those of similar weight and velocity that do not pass completely through.

A soft bullet that disintegrates on contact with the tissue imparts all of its energy to the tissue and produces a much more serious local injury. Since fragments of shattered bone serve as secondary missiles that trasmit all their energy to the surrounding tissues, the bullet that strikes bone will produce a more serious injury. A bullet that tumbles and strikes the tissues broadside at a velocity comparable to that of a bullet that spins and rolls from a rifled gun barrel will also cause greater tissue injury because more of its energy is imparted to the tissues at the larger area of exposed surface. In close-range shotgun blasts, a large mass of pellets is expelled with a great amount of energy over a relatively wide area. Usually such injuries are exceedingly severe (Fig. 10).

When a bullet strikes soft tissue, *shock waves* are immediately transmitted to the tissues involved (Fig. 11). These shock waves spread out from the missile tract through tissue at the speed of sound and cause extensive local tissue damage. Tissue damage far from the primary tract may also result (Fig. 12). In addition, a temporary tract much wider than the primary missile tract is formed by sudden expansion. The vacuum thus formed sucks foreign debris into the primary tract and may also cause local blood vessel and nerve damage. Since most rifles expel bullets of great mass at a medium or high velocity, gunshot wounds produced by rifles are considerably more severe and usually require much more extensive débridement along and around the missile tract than do gunshot wounds produced by .32, .38, and .45 caliber hand guns (Fig. 13). The latter are those most commonly available to civilians. Exceptions to this generalization are the .357 magnum and the .44 magnum pistols.

TABLE 3. Masses and Muzzle Velocities of Frequently Used Bullets

Cartridge (caliber)	Mass of Bullet (grains)	Muzzle Velocity (ft./sec.)
.22 short and long	29	1000
.22 long rifle	40	1150
5.56 mm. (M16 – Southeast Asia)*	55	3250
.25	50	820
.270 Winchester*	130	3140
.30 Mauser*	86	1420
.30-30 Winchester*	170	2200
.30-06*	150	2300
.30-40 Krag*	180	3030
.30 (World War II)		
Garand M1*	120	2800
M1-A1 carbine*	110	1975
7.62 mm. (M14 – Korea and NATO)*	150	2500
.32	90	800
8 mm. Mauser*	170	2530
9 mm. Luger	125	1150
.357 magnum	158	1430
.38 revolver	150	750
.38 special	158	870
.38 automatic	95	970
.44 magnum	240	1470
.45	250	860

*Rifle.

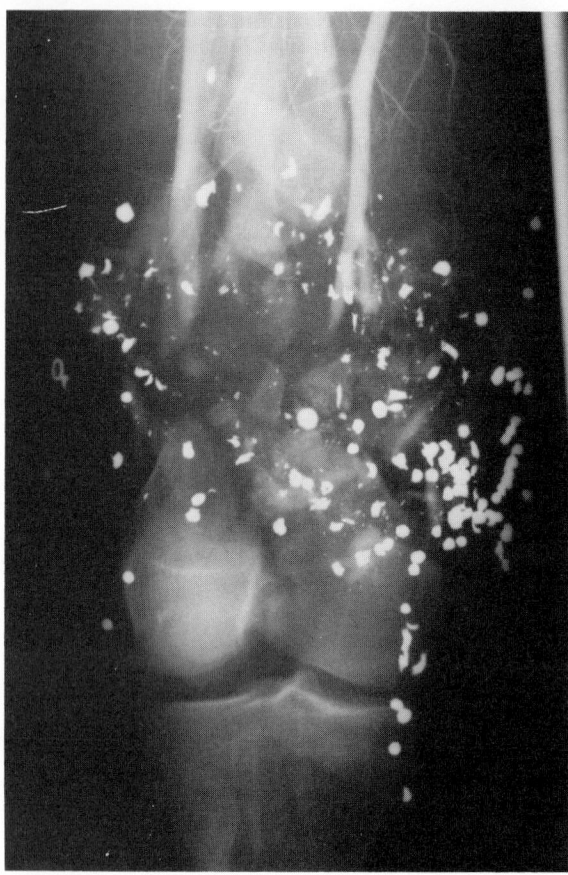

Figure 10. Close-range shotgun blast injury of the leg. Soft tissue damage was extensive and particles of bone were blasted through the anterior surface of the thigh. It was not possible to accomplish adequate repair. Mid-thigh amputation was necessary. The patient is now walking satisfactorily on an artificial limb.

Figure 11. Mechanism of tissue injury in gunshot wounds. *A*, Primary passage of a bullet results in distraction of the skin surrounding the point of entry and development of a conical primary missile tract. *B*, Transmission of kinetic energy by the bullet causes this primary missile tract to undergo sudden expansion; at the same time the skin contracts back over the primary port of entry. *C* and *D*, Shock waves are transmitted from the cavity of injury over a wide area and the vacuum formed sucks foreign debris into the injury tract.

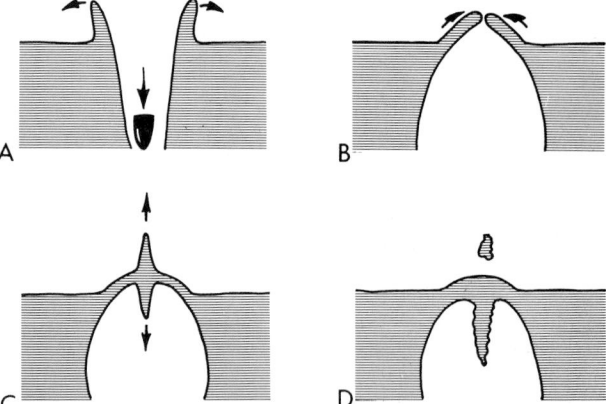

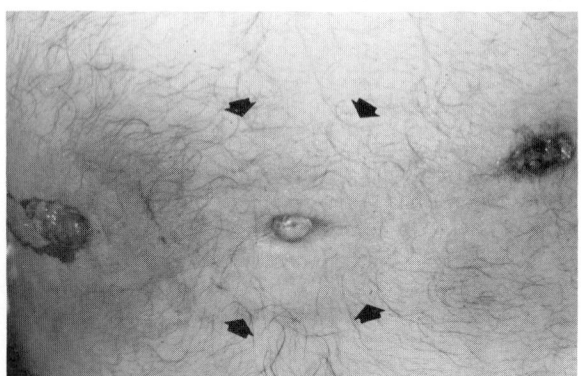

Figure 12. Typical appearance of gunshot wound of the abdomen requiring débridement. The wound of entrance (right) and the larger wound of exit (left) produced by a .44 magnum bullet (mass, 244 grains) fired from a rifle (muzzle velocity 1800 f.p.s.) at approximately 20 feet is shown. An exceedingly large area of tissue was destroyed (arrows). After extensive débridement and packing, the wound was closed secondarily. Concussive injury to the colon required no treatment, and the patient recovered.

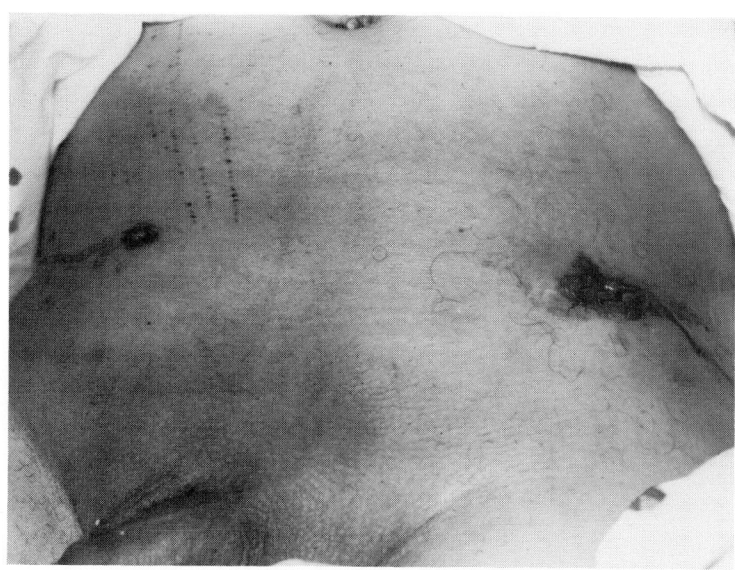

Figure 13. Typical appearance of gunshot wound of abdomen requiring no débridement. The wound of entrance (left) and the larger wound of exit (right) produced by a .45 caliber bullet (mass, 250 grains) fired from a pistol (muzzle velocity 860 f.p.s.) at close range (8 ft.) is shown. The abdominal cavity was traversed, and injuries of multiple loops of small bowel, the colon, the urinary bladder, and the lower pole of left kidney required emergency surgery. This patient survived.

DIAGNOSTIC PROCEDURES

The problem of accurate diagnosis in severely injured patients with obscure lesions continues to plague the surgeon. Aspiration of various accessible body cavities may be of great assistance in both diagnosis and treatment.

Thoracentesis

Appropriate anterior and lateral x-ray views of the chest are first taken to determine the site of the fluid. Thoracentesis is then performed with the patient sitting erect in bed or on a stretcher, but not on a chair, since an occasional patient may faint during the procedure. The skin is carefully prepared with an appropriate antiseptic and a small wheal is raised with a local anesthetic at the desired puncture site. A large-bore (16- to 18-gauge) needle attached to a large syringe through a three-way stopcock is then inserted through the intercostal space. Care should be taken to insert the needle over the lower rib bordering the space rather than under the upper rib in order to avoid laceration of the intercostal artery. To prevent laceration of the underlying lung and possible pneumothorax, care should also be taken not to insert the needle too deeply.

With this technique, the presence of blood in the chest cavity can easily be verified. When air is present in the thorax, particularly when it is under positive pressure (tension pneumothorax), insertion of a needle into the pleural space will result in immediate equalization of the pleural and atmospheric pressures. Partial re-expansion of the involved lung and improved respiration will occur almost immediately. Continued aspiration will aid in further expansion of the lung.

Abdominal Paracentesis

Intra-abdominal injury is frequently present in patients who are so critically ill that complete diagnostic studies are not advisable. Potentially lethal abdominal conditions may exist with only a few early clues indicating their presence. All too frequently, serious abdominal injury may be masked by a concurrent head injury and unconsciousness. In other patients, obvious injuries to the extremities and thorax may be so striking that serious delays in treatment of blunt abdominal injuries may occur. Indeed, Williams and Zollinger, in a review of 200 patients with abdominal trauma, stated that "88% of deaths from nonpenetrating abdominal wounds were due to hemorrhage.... of perhaps the most significance was the delay in diagnosis and treatment in half the patients who died."

Probably the most valuable adjuncts in the diagnosis of acute abdominal disease or injury are diagnostic peritoneal tap and peritoneal lavage.

The patient, shortly after voiding, or after catheterization if he is unable to void, is placed in a supine position. The abdomen is carefully examined, and scars or other possible points of fixation of the bowel to the abdominal wall are carefully avoided in order to prevent penetration with the needle during paracentesis. Simple skin preparation is performed bilaterally over the flanks with any of the common antiseptics. Intracutaneous skin wheals are raised by injection of a local anesthetic through a 25-gauge needle at each puncture site. A long, 18-gauge, short-beveled spinal needle attached to a 10-ml. syringe is inserted through the abdominal wall (Fig. 14). When the peritoneum is entered, a slight "give" of the needle can be felt. Gentle suction is intermittently applied to the syringe, and the needle is slowly advanced and its position carefully changed in the search for the desired fluid. If a positive tap is obtained, the needle is withdrawn and the procedure terminated. One tenth of 1 ml. of fluid is considered a positive tap, especially if additional fluid can be obtained in other puncture sites. A positive tap can be obtained with as little as 100 ml. of blood in the peritoneal cavity.

Puncture anteriorly through the rectus sheath should be avoided for a number of reasons: (1) a rectus sheath hematoma may result, owing to puncture through the inferior epigastric vessels; (2) because

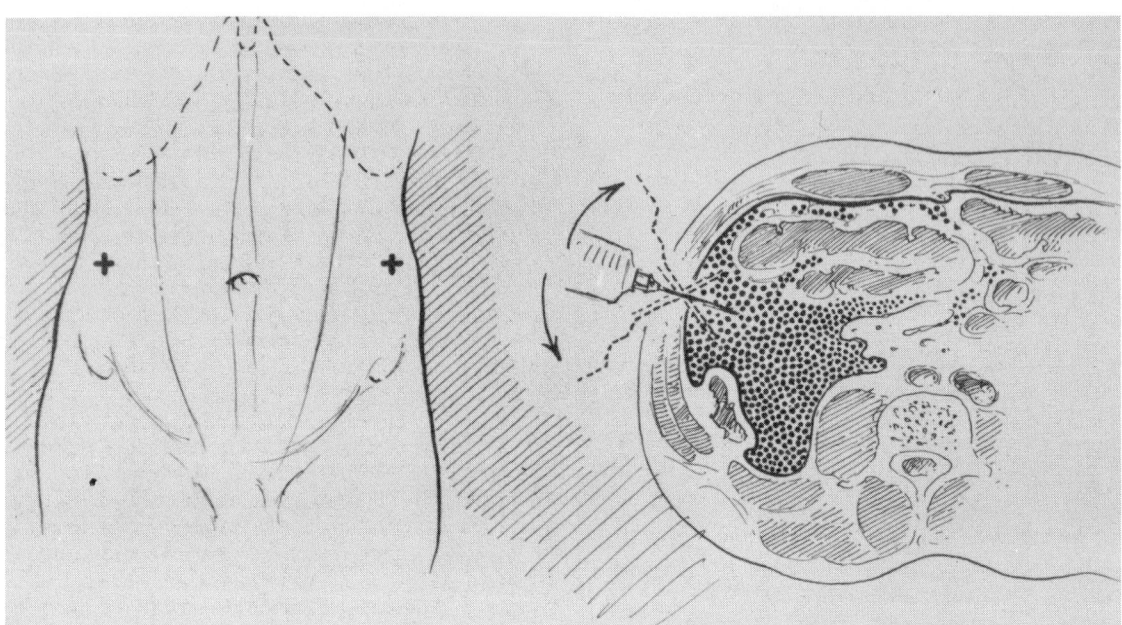

Figure 14. Techniques of bilateral flank taps. The preferred areas of insertion of the peritoneal tap needle are shown. (From Drapanas, T., and McDonald, J.: Surgery, 50:742, 1961.)

gas-filled loops of bowel will tend to float anteriorly in an abdomen containing fluid or blood, the chance of needle penetration of the bowel is higher; and (3) aspiration laterally along the peritoneal gutters will increase the chances of success of the tap if only small amounts of fluid are present.

A refinement in the technique of the peritoneal tap is the use of the Potter needle, a short-beveled needle inserted with a stylet. As the peritoneal cavity is entered, the stylet is withdrawn. A syringe is then attached and aspiration performed. Unlike a classic hypodermic needle, the Potter needle has a side hole just above the end hole. This increases the possibility of obtaining a positive tap, if fluid is present.

Complications attendant to peritoneal tap are rare. They include rectus sheath hematoma, aspiration of bowel content, mesenteric hematoma, and continued leakage from penetrated bowel, particularly if the bowel is obstructed or if the abdomen is punctured at a point of fixation of the bowel wall to the anterior peritoneum. On theoretical grounds, peritoneal taps should probably be avoided in the presence of obstructed and distended bowel, when the elevated intraluminal intestinal pressure may tend to cause continued leakage. Puncture of the urinary bladder may be avoided by insuring that the bladder is empty.

For peritoneal tap an accuracy rate of approximately 80 to 90 per cent may be anticipated. Almost all failures with this technique are false-negative ones, e.g., failure to aspirate fluid when it is present. *It should be emphasized that a peritoneal tap is valuable only if positive.* A negative tap does not exclude the presence of intra-abdominal visceral injury, bleeding, or fluid, and it is very dangerous to attach any significance to a negative tap.

To increase the possibility of obtaining a positive tap, Root and others have devised a technique of *peritoneal lavage.* A small lavage catheter (plastic or rubber) is inserted through a small incision in the linea alba, and 20 to 30 ml. per kilogram of sterile saline or Ringer's solution is slowly infused through this catheter. The catheter is then attached to a drainage bottle in a dependent position and the fluid is permitted to drain back into the bottle. Aliquots of fluid obtained are centrifuged and the sediment is observed for abnormal cells. This technique can be anticipated to improve the yield of positive taps, but it is more time-consuming than simple needle aspiration and there is greater potential hazard attendant to its use. The technique is particularly useful in patients whose abdominal findings are minimal and who are not in acute distress from extensive blood loss but in whom retroperitoneal injury is suspected. Root and his associates have also found it useful in the early diagnosis of pancreatic injury.

Lumbar Puncture

Lumbar puncture is best performed on a firm bed or table. The patient should be curled up on his side, and his back should be at a 90-degree angle to the surface on which he is lying. The knees are drawn up and the head lowered so that the knees and forehead are almost touching. A wide area over the lower back is prepared in sterile fashion and the spine is located by palpation. At the spot where an imaginary line drawn between the iliac crests crosses the spinal column, a small skin wheal is raised with a local anesthetic (Fig. 15). A long spinal needle can then easily be passed gently through the dura mater into the subarachnoid space. Since the spinal cord ends at approximately the level of the first lumbar vertebra (L1), there is little danger of damaging the cord during this procedure.

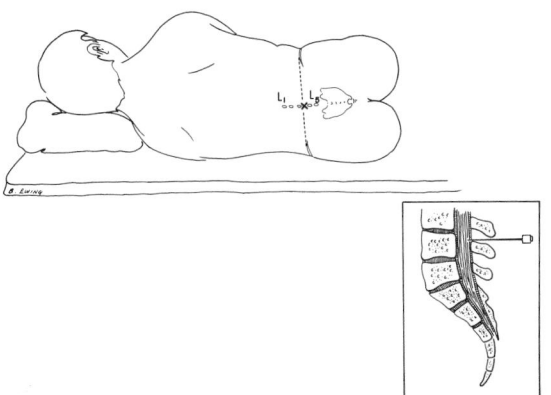

Figure 15. Technique of lumbar puncture. A long spinal needle is inserted at a point midway between the posterior superior iliac spines. Generally this line is at the level of the second or third lumbar interspace and is well below the level of the spinal cord.

Spinal taps at higher levels should be performed very carefully and only by those especially trained in the procedure. Because the dura seals rather slowly and a continued spinal fluid leak usually results in severe headache when the patient assumes the erect position, spinal tap should be performed with a needle of as small caliber as possible, preferably 22-gauge.

Pericardicentesis

When the venous pressure is elevated, the pulse pressure is narrow, and a pulsus paradoxicus is noted, acute cardiac tamponade should immediately be suspected. The patient may be fully conscious, but his anxious facies and shocklike state should further indicate this diagnosis. Acute cardiac tamponade is most likely to be present when penetrating injury of the chest has occurred. In such a situation, removal of as little as 20 to 30 ml. of blood may be lifesaving. Pericardicentesis should be undertaken immediately, and valuable time should not be wasted in obtaining chest x-rays, which will be of little use.

The patient should be in a supine position. The upper abdomen and lower chest are quickly prepared in sterile fashion, and a small wheal is raised with a local anesthetic just to the left of the xiphoid process where the lowest costal cartilage joins the sternum. With a medium 18- or 19-gauge needle on a large syringe, the pericardial sac can be entered with ease by passing the needle cephalad at an angle to the skin of approximately 45 degrees and aiming high for the tip of the patient's left scapula (Fig. 16). If blood is present under pressure in the pericardium, the plunger of the syringe will be pushed out very quickly for a short distance. The peritoneal sac should then be gently aspirated and all free blood removed. If blood continues to accumulate, the needle or a small plastic catheter may be left in place for a short period to allow continued decompression. Prolonged accumulation of blood may necessitate operative closure of the myocardial laceration.

Occasionally, during pericardicentesis, the needle may pass into one of the chambers of the heart. This possibility can be minimized by monitoring passage of the aspirating needle with a sterile electrocardiogram lead attached to the base of the needle. Additionally, intracardiac blood can easily be differentiated from blood that has collected in the pericardial sac by its tendency to clot. Since the fibrin has been removed from blood in the pericardial sac by its contact with the beating heart, it will not clot.

Central Venous Catheter Insertion

In the acutely injured patient, a catheter placed directly into the superior vena cava is an important route for determination of central venous pressure and for rapid administration of blood or fluids. This catheter may be passed through the cephalic, subclavian, or external jugular vein. A long premeasured plastic catheter may also be passed through any of the antecubital veins of the arm, but this is often difficult because of obstruction by valves or sharp angles at venous junctions.

The cephalic vein may be exposed directly through a small incision about one fingerbreadth lateral to the deltopectoral groove, and approximately two fingerbreadths below the clavicle. The vein should be tied off distally in the subcutaneous tissues just before it enters the axillary vein, and an appropriate plastic catheter is passed directly into the superior vena cava or into the right atrium.

The subclavian and external jugular veins can be entered by direct puncture. The patient is placed in slight Trendelenburg position and the head rotated sharply to the side. This position, accompanied by either straining or performance of the Valsalva maneuver, will cause marked dilation of the external jugular vein. The external jugular vein can be entered with a large needle, and a plastic catheter may be passed through this needle directly into the superior vena cava.

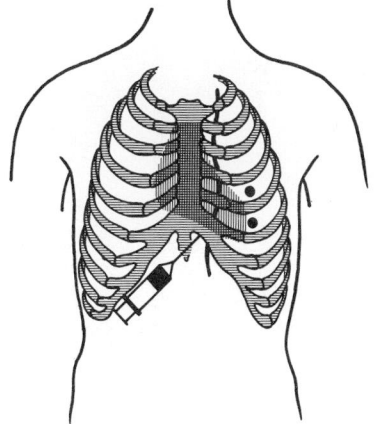

Figure 16. Technique of pericardicentesis. The subxiphoid approach is preferred (shown). Alternative sites for aspiration in the fourth and fifth intercostal spaces are also shown (circles). There is increased hazard of producing a pneumothorax with the latter approaches. (From Hewitt, R. L., Smith, A. D., Jr., Weichert, R. F., III, and Drapanas, T.: Arch. Surg., *101*:683, 1970.)

Percutaneous catheterization of the subclavian vein may be the preferred technique. It is only slightly more difficult than external jugular vein catheterization but subsequently is more comfortable for the patient. With the patient in the same position as for catheterization of the external jugular, and the shoulders thrown back maximally, a small local anesthetic wheal is raised in the skin at the inferior margin of the midpoint of the clavicle. A large-bore needle attached to a small syringe is advanced parallel to the skin and medially toward a finger pressed firmly into the suprasternal notch (Fig. 17). Slight negative pressure is exerted on the syringe, so that blood will appear when the vein has been entered. Once entry is adequate, a plastic catheter is inserted into the superior vena cava or the right atrium. The needle is then withdrawn and the catheter firmly anchored to the skin.

Certain precautions must be observed when inserting and while using a central venous catheter. Because of the negative pressure exerted during inspiration, air may be sucked into the chest, causing air embolism. Therefore, great care must be exercised to insure that all connections are secure. Since the needle through which the plastic catheter is inserted is sharp, the catheter may be cut off and embolize to the heart. No attempt should ever be made to pass a sharp needle over a catheter, and catheters must not be withdrawn through the needle. Because of the increasing incidence of bacterial and fungal growth on the catheter tips, especially when they must remain in place for long periods, all central venous catheters should be handled with absolutely sterile technique. In addition, an antibiotic ointment should be applied to the puncture wound, and a sterile gauze dressing should be affixed firmly over the site.

Sinogram

It is often difficult to determine whether a stab wound of the abdomen has violated the peritoneal cavity. Because of the shutter-like action of superimposed muscle layers, probing of such an injury tract is not a satisfactory method of determining whether the peritoneum has been penetrated. When the probe can be passed into the peritoneal cavity, it may be assumed that peritoneal penetration has occurred, but inability to pass a probe through an injury tract is insufficient reason to assume that peritoneal penetration has not occurred. While immediate exploration may not necessarily be indicated, such patients must be observed closely for signs of increasing peritoneal irritation. When it occurs, abdominal exploration should be performed forthwith.

In another method that may be of use in determining whether an injury of the abdominal wall has entered into the peritoneal cavity, a Foley catheter is inserted into the external injury tract, and the balloon is distended or a purse-string stitch is tied tightly at the base of the catheter so as to occlude tightly the external entry site. A radiopaque dye is then injected through the catheter under a mild degree of pressure and an x-ray is taken simultaneously. If the peritoneum has been penetrated, the dye can be seen to enter into the peritoneal space. There are several disadvantages to this method of diagnosis, however. It is somewhat painful, and the dye used is relatively irritating to the normal tissues. This often leads to the development of local muscle spasm and makes future evaluation of the patient's abdominal signs more difficult. This latter problem can be obviated by irrigation of the wound with copious amounts of saline following dye injection. Many surgeons are not familiar with this technique.

Pyelography

Visualization of the upper urinary tract is dependent on the selective renal excretion of certain inorganic iodine preparations. Of equal importance is the functional ability of the kidneys to excrete the dye

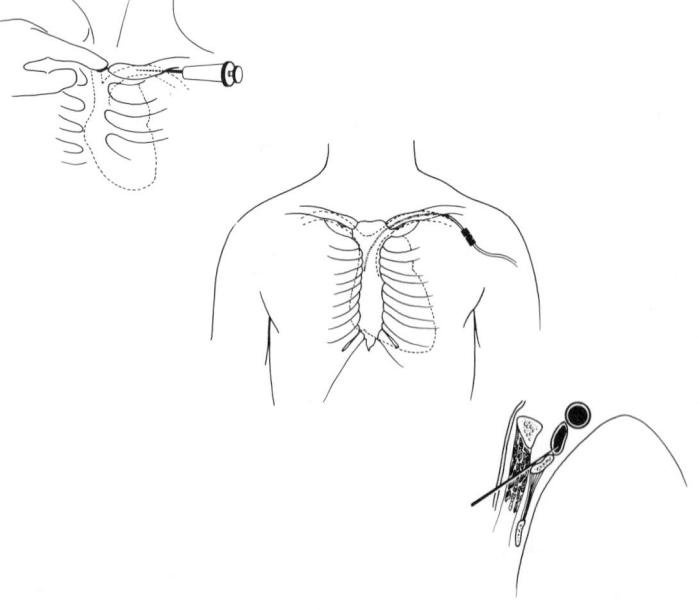

Figure 17. Technique of rapid administration of central venous pressure catheter through the infraclavicular approach. A large, 14-gauge, 3-inch, short-bevel needle is inserted beneath the midpoint of the clavicle and passed over the first rib, aimed toward the finger placed in the suprasternal notch. As the subclavian vein is entered, the syringe is aspirated to confirm the free flow of blood, and a plastic catheter is then inserted through the needle for a distance of approximately 6 to 8 inches into the superior vena cava. This technique also permits simultaneous administration of large volumes of fluids and blood. Catheter placement should always be confirmed by x-ray.

in a concentration sufficient to be visualized on x-ray examination. Severe toxic reactions may occur in patients with hypersensitivity to the dye or in those who have marked degrees of renal damage; therefore, the history of allergic phenomena should be determined prior to dye administration. When allergic history is negative, an intravenous sensitivity test may be done by injecting 1 ml. of the dye intravenously and observing the patient for allergic manifestations. In an acutely injured patient, it may be necessary to forego sensitivity tests in order to obtain much needed information as soon as possible.

An appropriate dye is administered intravenously, and serial x-rays of the abdomen are taken at 15 minutes, 30 minutes, 45 minutes, and 1 hour after injection. Dyes used include Diodrast and Hypaque, the dosages of which are calculated on the basis of body weight. Damage to various portions of the upper urinary tree will cause loss of dye into the soft tissue surrounding the area of damage.

When patients are allergic to the intravenous dye, consideration should be given to retrograde pyelograms; however, materials to which the patients are sensitive intravenously should not be used for retrograde pyelography. Various other opaque media may be used for this maneuver.

In diagnostic pyelography, extensive x-ray examinations for prolonged periods are often done in association with prolonged dehydration of the patient to allow better concentration of the dye in the lower urinary passages. In an acutely injured patient, however, this is not possible, and a 15 minute postinjection film to determine secretory status of both kidneys, the presence of both kidneys, and damage to the upper excretory system is usually all that is needed prior to surgical intervention.

Cystography

Following intravenous pyelography the radiopaque dye will concentrate in the urinary bladder. Occasionally this will demonstrate large bladder lacerations. However, the dye contained within the bladder must be under a slight amount of pressure to cause extravasation into perivesical tissues.

In the normal bladder, pressure is elevated only during micturition. For this reason, radiopaque dye should be instilled into the urinary bladder through a Foley catheter. After intravenous pyelography has been done, approximately 50 ml. of 50 per cent Hypaque is diluted in 200 ml. of normal saline. The balloon of the Foley catheter is inflated and pulled snugly down against the bladder neck. The diluted dye solution is then instilled through the catheter into the bladder under slight pressure. A bladder laceration will appear on x-ray as an extravasation of dye from the bladder into the adjacent perivesical tissues.

Arteriography

When an extremity has been injured and peripheral signs indicate that arterial blood supply has been compromised, arteriography should be performed. In addition, penetrating injury in the immediate vicinity of a major blood vessel is often associated with localized damage to the arterial wall or an acute arterio-venous fistula even though peripheral pulses are normal. For this reason, the arterial blood supply to such areas should always be clearly visualized.

A site should be selected proximal to the injury where pulsations in a major artery can be felt with ease. After adequate skin preparation using sterile technique, a small intradermal skin wheal is raised with an appropriate local anesthetic. A medium-bore (17- or 18-gauge) needle is passed directly into the artery. After an initial sensitivity test with the contrast material, 20 ml. of an appropriate radiopaque dye is injected as rapidly as possible. X-rays are taken under the extremity immediately after termination of the injection and at 5-second intervals thereafter.

In general, arteries of the leg can best be visualized by injection into the common femoral artery just distal to the inguinal ligament and those in the arm by injection into the axillary or subclavian artery. Because of the small tissue mass that must be penetrated by the x-rays, 35 per cent Diodrast or 50 per cent Hypaque is usually adequate dye concentration for visualization of arterial blood vessels in the extremities.

Aortography

When it is necessary to visualize the entire arterial tree or portions of the arterial system that lie above the inguinal ligament but below the diaphragm, dye may be injected directly into the lumbar aorta (lumbar aortogram). With the patient lying prone, a large cutaneous area over the back, centered at about the last thoracic vertebra, is prepared and draped in sterile fashion. After an initial intravenous test with the contrast material, an intracutaneous wheal is raised with a local anesthetic at a point 2 cm. below the left twelfth rib and 5 cm. to the left of the midline. A long, large-bore (16-gauge) needle is inserted at an angle of approximately 45 degrees from a midline sagittal plane. If the needle is pointed slightly cephalad, it should enter the aorta just above the renal arteries.

Initially, a small amount of dye is injected and a test film taken to determine that the tip of the needle is in the aorta. If such is shown, 30 ml. of the contrast material is then injected as rapidly as possible under pressure, and films are taken at intervals to determine the status of the arterial tree.

For visualization of the aortic arch or its branches, or any of the areas of the lumbar or thoracic aorta, a catheter may be passed retrograde through a cutdown in the brachial or superficial femoral artery (retrograde aortogram) and dye injected through this catheter. A similar, generally preferable procedure is the percutaneous technique of Seldinger. A large-bore (14-gauge) needle is used to enter the artery and a semirigid cardiac catheter is inserted over a Seldinger guide. Both are advanced under fluoroscopic vision to the appropriate arterial site. After the guide is withdrawn, rapid dye injections may be done and appropriate x-rays taken.

Blood Volume Measurement

Blood volume determination is extremely useful and is relatively accurate in healthy patients. Regrettably, this measurement is notably unreliable when performed on patients in shock. The procedure is performed by injection of Evans blue dye, human serum albumin labeled with radioiodine ^{131}I, or red cells labeled with isotopes of chromium, phosphorus, or iron. It must be emphasized that in shock there are continuous fluxes of both red cells and plasma into and out of the intravascular compartment. For this reason, blood volume determination is of little use in the acutely injured patient who continues to bleed, is simultaneously receiving blood transfusions, and remains in shock.

CENTRAL NERVOUS SYSTEM INJURY

Central nervous system injury may be to the brain or to the spinal cord. Because of concussive shock to the brain or actual destruction of brain tissue, craniocerebral injuries are more immediately life-threatening than those of the spine. However, end results from spinal cord injury usually involve much greater incapacity. Once transection of the spinal cord has occurred, peripheral reinnervation by the nervous system does not occur. Decompression or resolution of traumatic intracranial lesions usually results in complete recovery. (See also Chapter 43, Neurosurgery.)

Spinal Cord Injury

Penetrating injuries that completely sever the spinal cord will result in total muscular paralysis and loss of sensation below the level of injury. Little can be done for this type of damage other than to secure local hemostasis and to prevent infection by appropriate débridement, closure, and administration of antibiotics.

Blunt injury to the spine, however, when cared for properly, will often heal with complete recovery (Fig. 18). Accurate and early diagnosis is therefore of great importance. While some controversy may exist over the safety and necessity of lumbar puncture in the presence of head injury, such is not the case when attempts are being made to diagnose spinal cord compression. To determine whether the spinal cord is compressed, a spinal tap should be done in the lumbar area. After a manometer has been attached to the lumbar puncture needle, the external jugular veins are compressed for a few seconds (Queckenstedt test). Normally, this jugular compression leads to an increase in the intracranial cerebrospinal fluid pressure, which is in turn transmitted to the lumbar area. Pressure on the spinal cord and blockage of the sub-

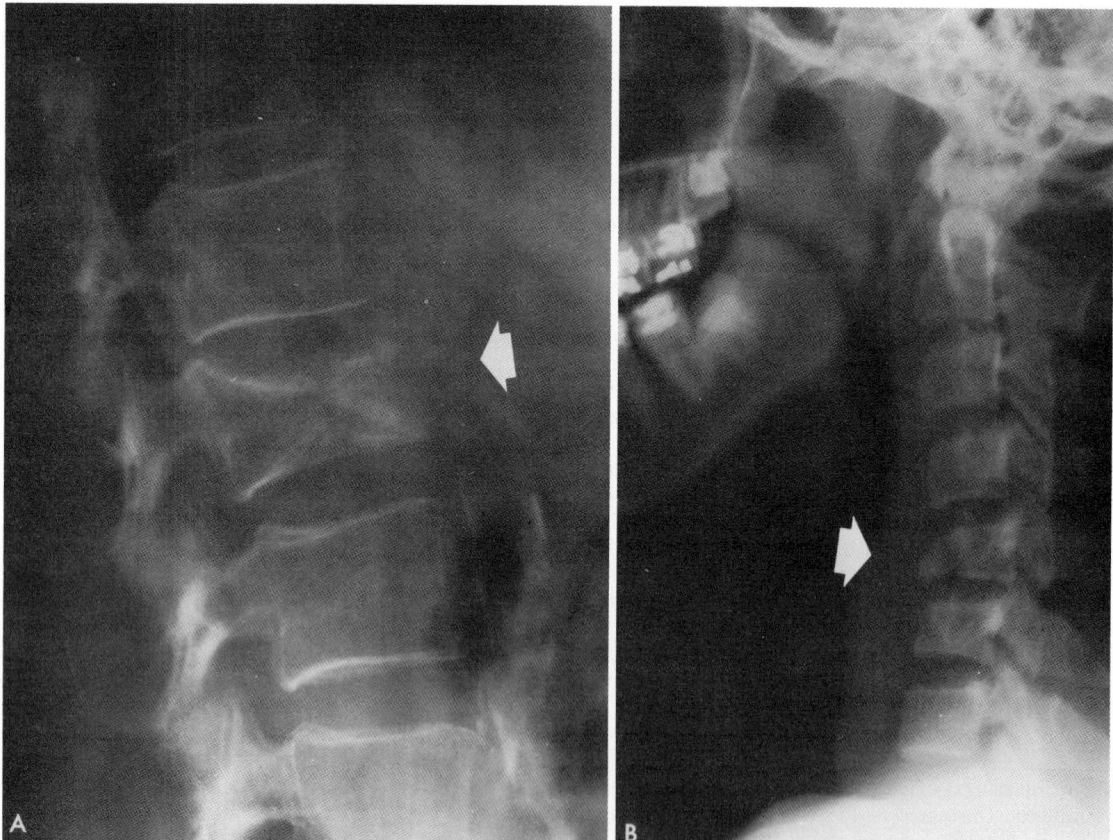

Figure 18. A, Typical compression fracture of the twelfth thoracic vertebra. Such injuries heal promptly with bed rest and immobilization, and no spinal cord injury is anticipated. B, Compression fracture of fifth cervical vertebra, which is unstable. Flexion of the neck should be avoided in such patients in order to avoid cervical cord injury. Treatment consisted of cervical traction with the neck in moderate extension. Complete healing without neurologic residual occurred.

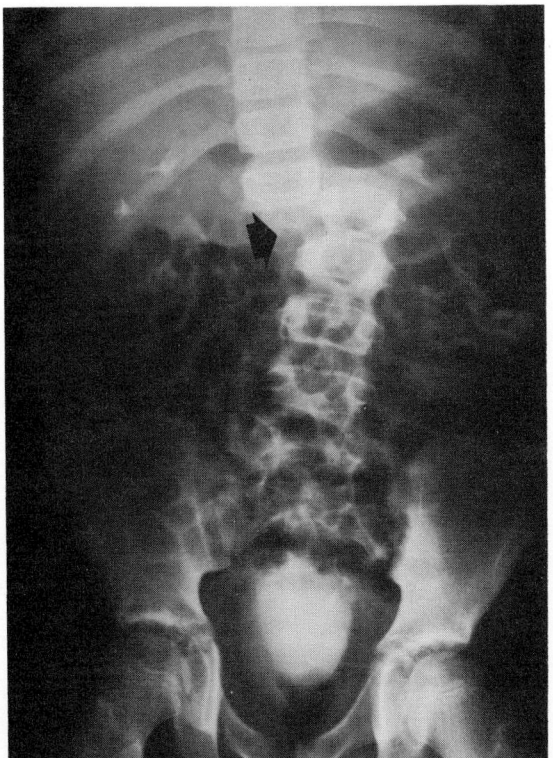

Figure 19. Fracture dislocation of spine between the twelfth thoracic and first lumbar vertebrae. Complete transection of the lower portion of spinal cord and cauda equina occurred in this patient, with permanent lower limb paralysis and neurogenic bladder and rectum. Such fractures are markedly unstable and care is necessary in transporting such patients to avoid further injury.

dural space about the spinal cord will prevent a rise in the cerebrospinal fluid pressure. When there has been damage to the spinal column, this test is diagnostic of a mechanical block. This may be further confirmed by having the patient perform a Valsalva maneuver or cough. This increased intra-abdominal pressure is transmitted directly through the epidural veins to the lumbar cerebrospinal fluid, and the cerebrospinal fluid pressure rises if there is pressure on the spinal cord.

Compression of the spinal cord by impingement from fractured or dislocated vertebral bodies results in sensory and motor impairment below the level of the cord involvement. In any type of injury in which bilateral sensory and motor changes are noted, spinal column injury must be suspected (Fig. 19). In the absence of external signs of penetrating injury, spinal cord compression is likely. In such patients, blood pressure may also drop as a result of loss of vascular sympathetic tone in the involved area. Placement of the patient in the Trendelenburg position will aid in overcoming this hypotension ("spinal shock").

Patients with spinal cord injury must be moved with extreme care to prevent flexion, extension, or rotation of the spinal column. Any such movement may cause further damage to the cord and extension of an otherwise reversible lesion to an irreversible one. Place-

ment of Crutchfield tongs into the calvarium or application of halter traction and suspension of appropriate weights should be employed as an initial maneuver (Fig. 20). When this is done, care should be taken to assure that the head and vertebral column are in a neutral position. Weights should be added gradually in 5-pound increments and reduction is achieved. When weights totaling 50 pounds have been added and reduction is still unsatisfactory, operative reduction should be considered.

X-rays are of use in the diagnosis of spinal fracture or dislocation, but positioning in the x-ray department may result in further cord damage unless a physician is in attendance at all times. If marked sensory and motor changes are noted, the patient should be placed on a Stryker frame even before x-rays are taken. Acute surgical decompression of the spinal cord is indicated under the following circumstances: (1) x-ray evidence of impingement of a bony fragment on the spinal cord; (2) progressive development or failure of rapid improvement of a severe neurologic deficit; (3) presence of a neurologic lesion with a positive Queckenstedt test; (4) foreign bodies remaining after a penetrating wound; (5) injuries of the conus medullaris or cauda equina; and (6) inability to reduce vertebral dislocations with cervical traction.

If treatment of spinal cord injuries has been proper and suspension has been initiated early, sensory and motor regeneration occurs rapidly. Early and judicious treatment is often followed by complete recovery.

Head Injury

Head injury constitutes a more serious and immediate threat to life than does injury to the peripheral nervous system. Penetrating injuries of the head associated with stabs involve only local injury and are frequently not fatal (Fig. 21). However, gunshot wounds of the head usually lead to death of the patient. Penetration by a bullet not only causes exten-

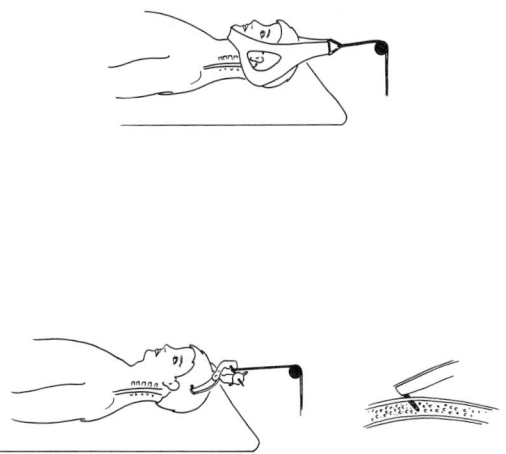

Figure 20. Techniques of cervical traction for cervical spinal fracture. Shown are the use of a head halter for temporary traction and the application of Crutchfield tongs for prolonged traction. Inset shows penetration of the outer table of the skull by the Crutchfield tongs, which permits strong traction in order to effect reduction.

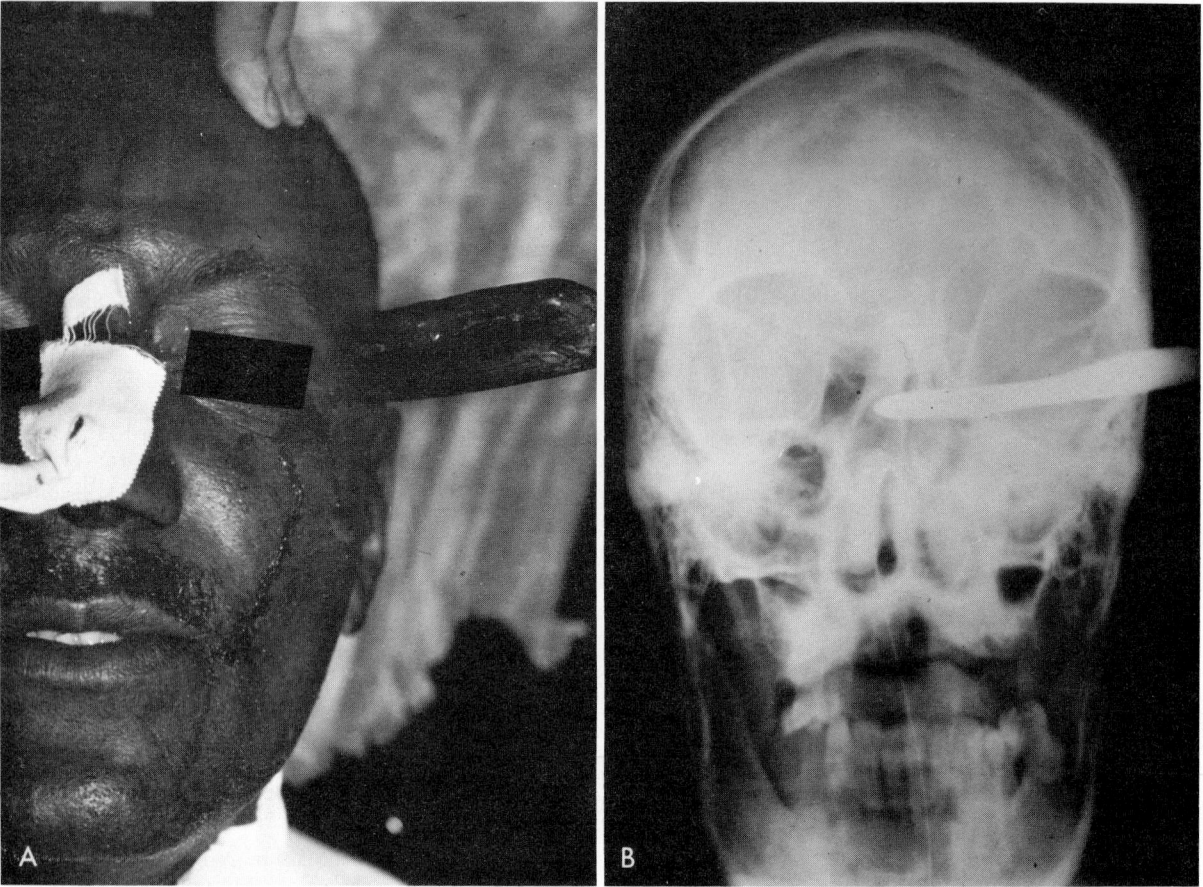

Figure 21. Stab wound of head *(A)* and x-ray appearance *(B)*. Patient was completely asymptomatic except for a complaint of headache. After exploratory craniotomy to insure hemostasis, he recovered completely.

sive direct damage to the brain, but also the shock wave developed may cause severe destruction distant from the point of entry of the bullet.

Blunt injury to the skull may be of varying severity (Fig. 22) and often constitutes a much more vexing clinical problem than do gunshot wounds. Typically, the patient suffers an injury to the skull that results in a short period of unconsciousness. He may then regain consciousness for a short "lucid" interval, after which time his level of consciousness may rapidly decrease. When damage to the brain has been severe, this "lucid" interval may not intervene. While the patient is unconscious, his respiratory rate, pulse rate, and blood pressure must be closely observed. A rapidly developing subarachnoid hemorrhage or subdural hematoma causes a sudden and marked rise in cerebrospinal fluid pressure. The increased pressure compresses the brain tissue and further depresses the level of consciousness. Pressure on the vital centers in the medulla also leads quickly to an elevation in blood pressure, a decrease in pulse rate, and a decrease in respiratory rate. Temperature increase is usually a preterminal event.

Because of the possibility of the development of such catastrophic pathologic lesions, patients who have been rendered unconscious must be kept under close observation for at least 24 hours. Even then, one cannot be absolutely certain that a chronic subdural hematoma will not develop. In addition to vital signs, eye signs are of considerable aid in determining the severity of head injury. All of the eye muscles except the superior oblique and the external rectus are innervated by the oculomotor (III) nerve. For this reason, oculomotor paralysis leads to external deviation and a slight downward rotation of the ipsilateral eye. When the nerve is completely paralyzed, the ipsilateral pupil will be dilated and fixed and the contralateral pupil will be constricted. When only the abducens (VI) nerve is involved, however, pupillary reaction is not involved; muscles innervated by the oculomotor and trochlear (IV) nerves remain intact, and the eye deviates inward. If a constricted pupil begins to dilate progressively, the presence of a progressively expanding lesion is obvious, and it should be treated immediately by appropriate surgical evacuation. Under such circumstances the level of consciousness of the patient

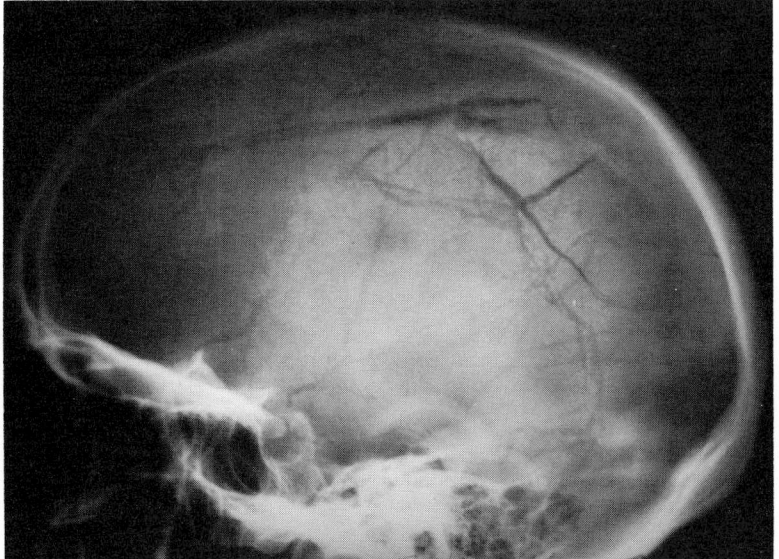

Figure 22. Multiple fractures of the skull. Lateral skull film shows extensive linear fractures resulting from closed head injury. This patient was observed closely, and complete healing resulted with no neurologic disability.

will be markedly depressed. If his level of consciousness remains good, changes observed are likely to be due to involvement of the peripheral portions of the nerve or of the orbit.

Because of the possibility of cerebellar herniation through the foramen magnum, lumbar puncture is contraindicated in the presence of cerebral tumor. This hazard also exists after craniocerebral injury but is much less likely to occur. However, little information can be gleaned from a spinal tap performed after head injury. In the patient who has suffered a severe head injury, the spinal fluid will almost always be bloody, and differentiation of subarachnoid hemor-

rhage, cerebral hemorrhage, cerebral contusion, and cerebral concussion is not possible on this basis. When continued bleeding or a rapidly expanding intracranial hematoma is suspected, cerebral arteriography with appropriate x-ray views is the most certain way to verify the diagnosis (Fig. 23). Occasionally a radioactive brain scan may also be of some assistance. In the acutely injured patient, such specialized tests as echoencephalography, pneumoencephalography, and electroencephalography are of little use.

If a rapidly expanding intracranial hematoma is strongly suspected, early trephination is the safest and most certain diagnostic measure. It is also the

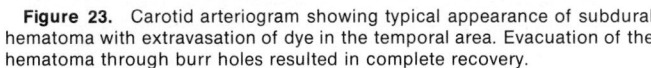

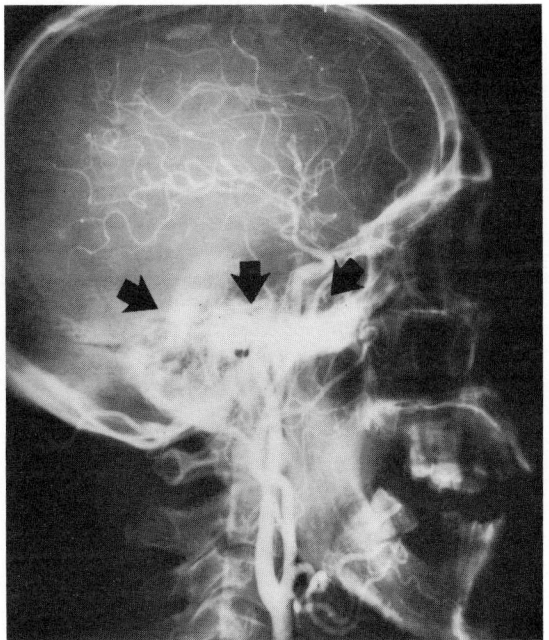

Figure 23. Carotid arteriogram showing typical appearance of subdural hematoma with extravasation of dye in the temporal area. Evacuation of the hematoma through burr holes resulted in complete recovery.

TABLE 4. Types of Common Brain Injuries

Lesion	Clinical Findings	X-rays	Treatment	Recovery
Concussion	Retrograde amnesia, no localization	Usually negative	Observation	Usually complete
Contusion	Prolonged unconsciousness, cerebral edema	May have fractures	Observation, measures to treat cerebral edema, may require decompression	Prolonged disability, permanent neurologic sequelae or death
Intracerebral hematoma	Unconsciousness, rapid increase in intracranial pressure	May have multiple fractures of skull	Decompression of hematoma	Variable prolonged disability, mortality 75%, occasional complete recovery
Subdural hematoma	Slow or rapid progression of localized neurologic findings. May be bilateral (contre coup)	Fracture usually not present	Emergency burr holes or craniotomy	Mortality about 25%, recovery variable, may recur, requiring craniotomy
Epidural hematoma	Brief unconsciousness, lucid interval followed by rapid progression of neurologic localizing signs, pupillary changes	Temporal fracture	Emergency burr holes, ligation of bleeding meningeal artery	Mortality 10–20%, prompt surgery lifesaving, full recovery anticipated

best method for relieving rapidly increasing intracranial pressure due to hemorrhage or intracerebral hematoma.

The more common types of brain injuries encountered and the usual findings are outlined in Table 4.

NECK INJURIES

Penetration by either knives or bullets causes the majority of injuries to the neck. Because so many vital structures lie within this relatively small anatomic area, routine exploration of any significant penetrating injury is advisable. Time need not be wasted in attempts to diagnose the extent of an obviously severe injury, and exploration of all such lesions should be performed under general anesthesia. An expanding hematoma, a neurologic deficit, and the presence of subcutaneous emphysema are all obvious indications for exploration. Large hematomas in the neck usually result when major blood vessels are lacerated (Fig. 24). These may compress the trachea and even cause airway obstruction unless surgical intervention is prompt.

When injury is obviously less severe, the demand for immediate action is less pressing. Thorough physical examination should then be performed to define the extent of injury more precisely. Vagus and recurrent laryngeal nerve injuries can be detected by vocal cord examination, and phrenic nerve damage by fluoroscopic visualization of diaphragmatic motion. Other major nerves in the neck that are likely to be injured are the hypoglossal and spinal accessory nerves as well as the brachial and cervical plexuses. Generally, an attempt should be made to repair primarily all severed and lacerated nerves in the neck. An end-to-end anastomosis should be performed with fine stitches inserted into the perineurium.

Any neck injury may be more extensive than is

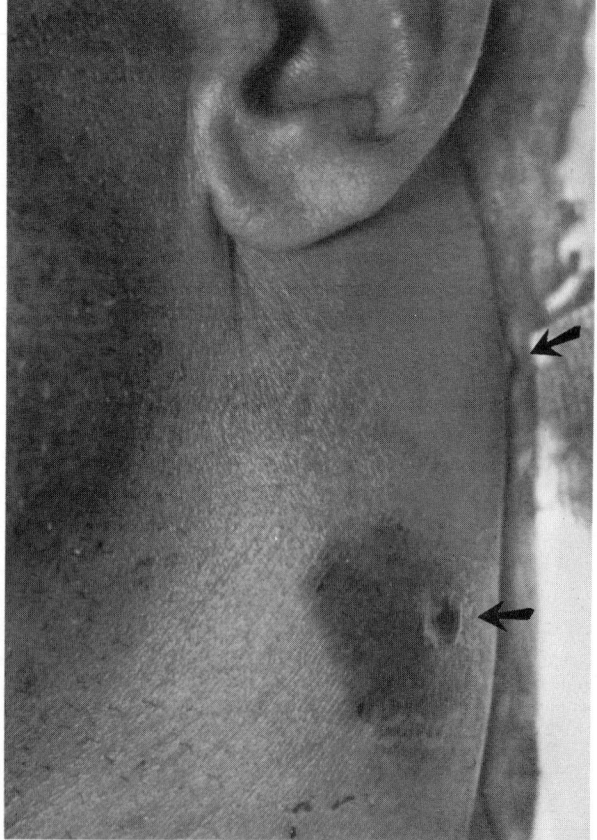

Figure 24. Gunshot wound of the neck from a .25 caliber pistol. Beneath the point of entry (lower arrow), the internal jugular vein was partially severed, and the bullet exited posteriorly (upper arrow). A moderate-sized hematoma was evacuated, and the lacerated vein repaired. Recovery was prompt and uncomplicated. In patients with penetrating neck injuries, care must be taken to prevent intraoperative air embolism.

readily apparent on examination, and often major damage in a neck wound is on the side contralateral to the point of entry of the foreign object. For this reason, all injury tracts in the neck must be widely opened and thoroughly explored under adequate general endotracheal anesthesia. False aneurysms commonly develop between major blood vessels after penetrating stab injuries or after a bullet has passed nearby. Injury tracts in the vicinity of major vessels of the neck should all be carefully examined, and proper care should be taken to verify that blood vessels are intact and tissue is viable. Hematomas lying on major vessels should never be disturbed until both proximal and distal control has been gained. Severed major lymphatic channels may be ligated without consequence.

When immediate exploration is not necessary, an esophagram should be done to verify that the esophagus has not been penetrated. Injuries to either the trachea or the esophagus should be closed primarily. An esophageal suture line may be protected, if need be, by passing a small feeding tube, and a tracheal closure may be protected by performing a tracheostomy. To insure adequate drainage, drains should be left in place for a short time after completion of all procedures in the neck.

Most patients admitted to a hospital after blunt cervical trauma have associated severe head or chest injuries that divert the physician's attention from the neck. However, severe injuries, other than cervical spine fractures, may also exist in the neck. Sharp blows may result in fractures of any of the cartilages of the larynx or of the trachea. Such injuries cause upper respiratory obstruction, and endotracheal intubation or tracheostomy should be done when indicated. A more severe neck injury that can be associated with blunt trauma is closed injury to the carotid artery. When the artery is forcibly stretched or compressed against a vertebra, the intima may be fractured and disrupted. Five unique clinical features have been recognized that characterize this injury: (1) hematoma in one of the upper triangles of the neck; (2) Horner's syndrome on the side of the injury; (3) transient ischemic attacks identical to those seen in patients with carotid artery occlusive disease; (4) lucid interval; and (5) monoplegia or hemiplegia in an alert patient. Successful treatment of this injury depends on early diagnosis and prompt surgical exploration.

THORACIC INJURIES

When thoracic injuries are present, their management should occupy a high priority. Thoracic injuries may involve the *thoracic wall,* the *lungs,* and the *mediastinum* (Table 5). Often a combination of injuries is present, such as multiple fractured ribs with flail chest, pneumothorax, hemothorax, and cardiac contusion. The average patient possesses considerable physiologic reserve, and often injuries such as pulmonary contusion may be masked until an additional insult, such as atelectasis resulting from painful shallow breathing, produces a catastrophic change in the patient's condition. The presence of multiple fractured

TABLE 5. Unexpected Complications in Thoracic Trauma

Cardiac tamponade
Ruptured bronchus and trachea
Ruptured esophagus
Thoracic duct injury
Great vessel injury
Ruptured diaphragm
Respiratory distress syndrome
Extrathoracic injury

ribs should always alert the physician to the presence of a flail chest, even though such may not be immediately apparent. Similarly, crepitus beneath the skin (subcutaneous emphysema) is almost always associated with pneumothorax. Bleeding from a pulmonary parenchymal injury is often slow because of the lower pressure in the pulmonary circuit and may not be manifest until some time after the initial evaluation of the patient has been accomplished. After blunt trauma, complete transection of the aorta may occur without obvious shock and with minimal findings in the chest x-ray. In such instances, the hematoma surrounding the aortic rupture may be contained by the pleura, only to rupture hours or even days after the injury with further expansion of the hematoma due to the arterial pressure. Too often, the statement that "the patient appeared to be doing well when he had a cardiac arrest" is made. Such is the nature of injury involving the thoracic viscera.

Diagnosis

The diagnosis of thoracic injuries is relatively easy when compared to the diagnostic problems involved in the patient with blunt abdominal trauma. This is largely due to the ease of roentgenographic evaluation of the thorax, the ability to detect myocardial contusion by electrocardiography, the ability to measure arterial blood gases and pH, the ease of auscultation of the lungs, and the ready accessibility of the pleural cavity to needle aspiration and drainage, if needed.

With the advent of improved techniques for the instantaneous determination of arterial pH and gas tensions, primarily pO_2 and pCO_2, combined with an understanding of the physiologic principles involved, the physician is often in a much better position to follow the patient's course and make appropriate adjustments in therapy. In the management of extremely ill patients, multiple arterial punctures can be avoided by inserting a small intra-arterial catheter via the percutaneous route, preferably into the femoral artery through the groin, for serial monitoring of blood gases. The catheter can be left in place for days as long as frequent irrigations with heparinized saline solution are done as a precaution against clotting.

Hemothorax

The diagnosis of hemothorax can be made readily. In addition to dullness in the bases on percussion, and diminished or absent breath sounds, the chest roentgenogram will reveal not only the presence of blood or fluid, but also the quantity (Fig. 25). Howev-

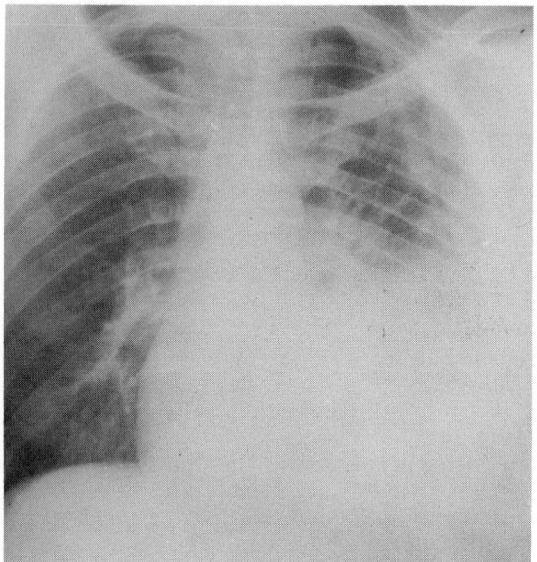

Figure 25. Hemothorax on the left side in patient with closed-chest trauma and fractured ribs. Closed thoracotomy tube drainage in the eighth intercostal space in the posterior axillary line resulted in the evacuation of 2000 ml. of blood with prompt expansion of the lung and no further bleeding.

28 French) and in a dependent position, preferably in the eighth intercostal space in the midaxillary line (Fig. 26). Such tubes should always be attached to an underwater seal in order to avoid the introduction of air into the pleural cavity and a resultant pneumothorax.

The procedure is performed with the patient sitting erect in bed or lying supine with the side slightly elevated. The skin over a wide area is prepared with an antiseptic, and a small wheal is raised with a local anesthetic over the eighth intercostal space at the midaxillary line, where a small skin incision is made. A chest tube is grasped with a curved hemostat at the tip to be inserted and is bluntly pushed through the skin incision into the pleural space. The tube is advanced posteriorly and upwards until at least 6 to 8 inches lies within the chest. The tube should be kept clamped during the procedure, and after insertion may be connected to a suction pump or underwater seal drainage. It should be firmly affixed at its base with skin sutures tied about the tube; this will prevent inadvertent removal. Posterior tubes should not be in-

er, such a diagnosis may be difficult when chest x-rays are taken in the supine position. When the patient is supine, blood will be spread thinly through the pleural cavity, and large quantities may be present before significant changes occur in the x-ray. It has been estimated that in the erect position a minimum of 500 ml. of blood must be present in the pleural space before it can be detected radiographically. When question arises as to the presence of intrapleural blood, particularly if the patient is unable to sit for an erect film, lateral decubitus x-rays of the chest will more readily reveal the presence of fluid. Should question still exist, simple needle aspiration of the pleural cavity in its most dependent position may be diagnostic.

Except for small accumulations of blood, most patients with hemothorax require the insertion of a chest tube for rapid evacuation of the blood and expansion of the lung. This also permits the physician to monitor carefully the extent of the bleeding by measuring directly, minute by minute, the volume of blood drained through the chest tube into the chest bottle.

The blood that enters the pleural cavity usually remains liquid for considerable periods of time. However, in the presence of air (hemopneumothorax), clotting may occur, and the blood cannot be aspirated with a needle or a chest tube. If the volume of clotted blood is large, the lung will remain collapsed. As organization of the thrombus progresses, a fibrothorax will result, producing marked restriction of the ability of the lung to expand with respiration and diminishing the pulmonary reserve. For this reason, all significant quantities of blood in the pleural space should be evacuated as soon as possible.

Technique of Chest Tube Insertion. When a chest tube is to be placed, it should be as large as possible (20 to

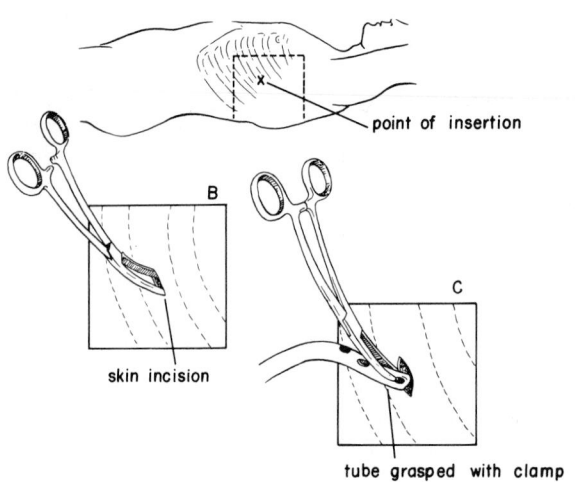

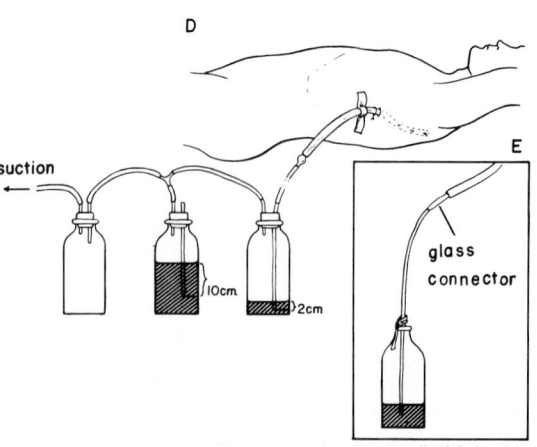

Figure 26. Technique of rapid insertion of large intercostal catheter for drainage of hemothorax. The tube is inserted in the eighth intercostal space in the midaxillary line and attached to underwater seal.

serted posterior to the posterior axillary line, since those so inserted cause a great deal of discomfort when the patient lies flat.

In most patients with hemothorax resulting from injuries to the lung, bleeding will cease promptly. It is rare that more than 1 to 2 liters of blood is evacuated unless a major pulmonary blood vessel has been injured. Continued brisk bleeding from the chest tube should alert the physician to the possibility of injury to an intercostal artery or to the great vessels in the mediastinum. In these instances, the bleeding is usually more profuse because of the systemic arterial pressure in such vessels.

There is little excuse at present for "observing" a patient with hemothorax or avoiding prompt drainage of such a complication. A misconception commonly held is that blood in the pleural cavity provides tamponade and protects against further bleeding. Introduction of an amount of air into the pleural cavity equivalent to the volume of blood removed, as has been advocated in the past, should not be done.

Pneumothorax

The presence of subcutaneous emphysema should always alert the physician to the possible presence of pneumothorax. In most cases, pneumothorax is readily visible radiographically (Fig. 27), but the presence of only a small amount of air in the pleural cavity should not lull the physician into believing that nothing further need be done. After trauma, continuous leakage

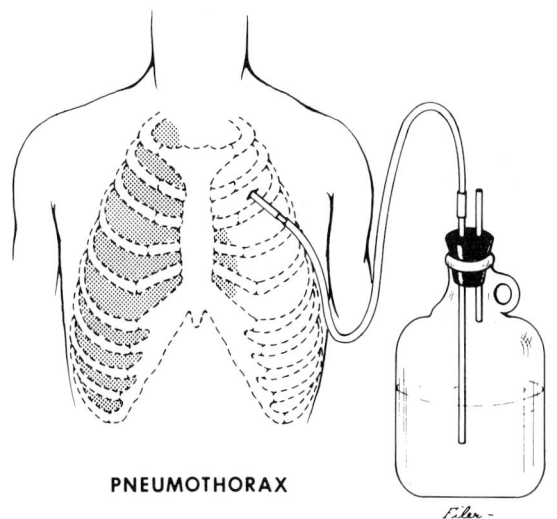

PNEUMOTHORAX

Figure 28. Preferred site for insertion of the intercostal catheter in the midclavicular line anteriorly at the level of the second intercostal space. The catheter is attached to underwater seal. In extensive leaks, suction should also be applied to the bottle by means of a thoracic pump.

of air may result in conversion of a small pneumothorax into a large one, or even into a tension pneumothorax. Pneumothorax resulting from trauma should always be drained with a chest tube when the patient is initially seen in the emergency department.

Technique of Anterior Chest Tube Insertion. The technique for insertion of a chest tube for drainage of pneumothorax is similar to that for drainage of hemothorax, except that the tube is placed in the first or second intercostal space anteriorly in the midclavicular line (Fig. 28). When hemothorax and pneumothorax coexist, two chest tubes should be inserted, one in the eighth interspace in the midaxillary line for drainage of the blood, and the other in the second interspace anteriorly for the evacuation of air.

To insert the anterior chest tube, a small skin wheal is raised with a local anesthetic after sterile preparation, and the skin is incised over the third intercostal space. The skin is pulled up with the sterile-gloved left hand so that the incision overlies the second intercostal space, and a large trocar is inserted in a cephalad direction over the top of the third rib into the pleural space. An 18F catheter that has been previously clamped is then quickly inserted through the trocar, and the trocar is rapidly removed, with the catheter left in place. The catheter is attached to underwater seal drainage or to an appropriate suction device, and the clamp on the catheter is removed. The tube should be firmly fixed with stitches to the skin at its base to prevent its removal.

In more than 90 per cent of patients with uncomplicated pneumothorax after trauma, rapid lung expansion will follow placement of the chest tube and underwater seal drainage. Serial chest x-rays should be obtained to insure that the lung has promptly expanded. The tubes should be left in place for at least 24 to 48 hours to insure that air does not reaccumulate. If any question of continued air leakage exists,

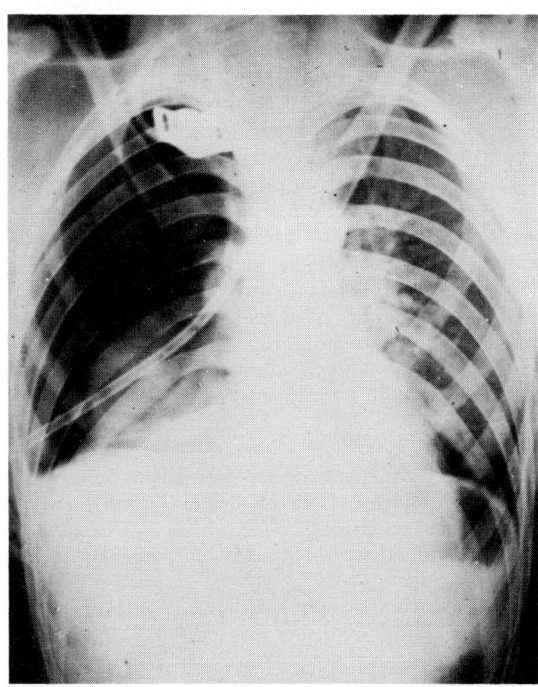

Figure 27. Extensive pneumothorax (right) in a patient with closed thoracic trauma and fractured ribs. This x-ray shows an intercostal catheter that had been inserted a few minutes previously for drainage of blood, but the lung remains collapsed. Another catheter was inserted in the second interspace anteriorly and the lung promptly expanded.

preliminary clamping of the tube for 4 to 8 hours, followed by chest x-ray, is advisable before the tube is removed.

In a small percentage of patients, the air leak may be of such magnitude that simple underwater seal does not suffice. Under these circumstances, the use of a high-volume, low-pressure thoracic drainage pump attached to the air outlet of the chest bottle will permit more rapid withdrawal of air and prevent the development of tension pneumothorax. Continued air leakage of large magnitude should alert one to the possibility of a major rupture of the trachea or a bronchus. Such injuries are best treated by immediate thoracotomy and suture.

Flail Chest

Any patient who has sustained multiple fractures of the ribs should be considered to have a flail chest, even though the flail may not be immediately apparent (Fig. 29). Too often in the past such patients were managed by adhesive strapping to "stabilize" the thoracic wall. This usually led to diminished alveolar ventilation, atelectasis, hypoxemia, and serious physiologic derangements (Fig. 30). A flail can be best observed by careful inspection of the thorax anteriorly and from oblique and lateral angles with the patient completely disrobed. Under such conditions, even a small flail may be readily detected. Often, however, there is associated contusion of the soft tissues of the chest wall, which may hide the portion involved in the "paradoxical motion" or flail.

Patients sustaining a flail chest of even moderate proportions who are unable to maintain an arterial

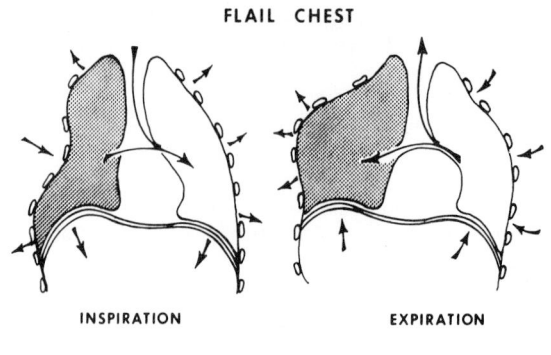

FLAIL CHEST

INSPIRATION   EXPIRATION

PENDULUM AIR

Figure 30. Physiologic derangements in flail chest. On inspiration there is a collapse of the flail segment, preventing expansion of the lung and resulting in ineffective alveolar exchange. There is also a shift of the mediastinum toward the opposite side. On expiration the flail segment "paradoxically" moves out, with shift of the mediastinum toward the involved side.

pO_2 of 60 mm. Hg are best treated by endotracheal intubation or tracheostomy and the use of volume-controlled ventilations with a respirator ("internal splinting"). If the flail is minimal, setting the respirator to "assist" the patient may be sufficient. The patient should be carefully observed and blood gases sequentially monitored. Should there be little improvement, it is probably best to reset the respirator to controlled ventilation so that it takes over all respiratory effort. Control of respirations is almost always needed when there is any significant flail or when the patient has associated head injury and difficulty in breathing.

With intermittent positive-pressure respiration the lungs can be promptly expanded and adequate alveolar ventilation obtained. The use of stabilizing apparatus such as towel clips applied to the ribs or sternum, wires, sandbags, or adhesive strapping is rarely, if ever, indicated at present, except possibly when there are markedly unstable, severe, and bilateral injuries involving both rib and sternum.

The management of a patient on the ventilator requires knowledge not only of the fundamentals of pulmonary physiology but also of the numerous complications attendant to the use of the ventilator.

Pulmonary Contusion

Pulmonary contusion is usually the result of blunt trauma to the chest. Contusion may be quite localized or it may be disseminated, with bilateral involvement (Fig. 31). The full evolution of the contusion may not be readily apparent on x-ray for at least 2 to 3 days after injury, during which time the patient may appear to be doing well. As the full pattern emerges, there is progressive deterioration of respiratory function and hypoxia with a dropping arterial pO_2. Radiologic criteria that are useful in the diagnosis of pulmonary contusion include the presence of soft "fluffy" densities with peribronchial and perivascular infiltration. With extensive injury there may be com-

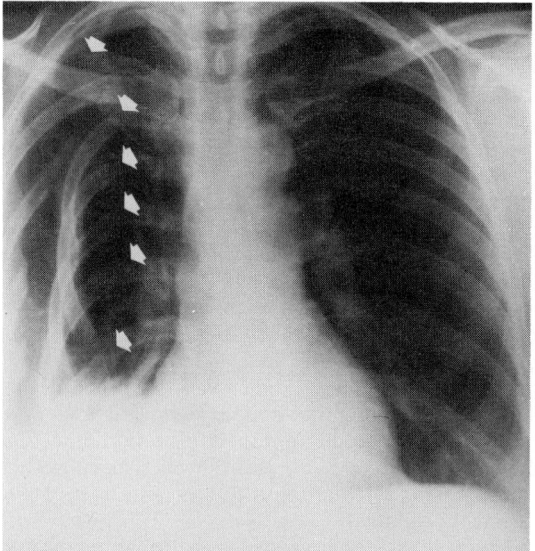

Figure 29. Flail chest (right). Multiple fractured ribs are shown with a free-floating "flail" segment. Arrows point to the multiple posterior fractures, and the marked displacement of the entire lateral rib cage can be seen. In order to produce a flail of such magnitude, ribs are usually fractured in at least two places. Treatment consisted of respirator support for a 3-week period, resulting in complete recovery with no deformity of the thorax.

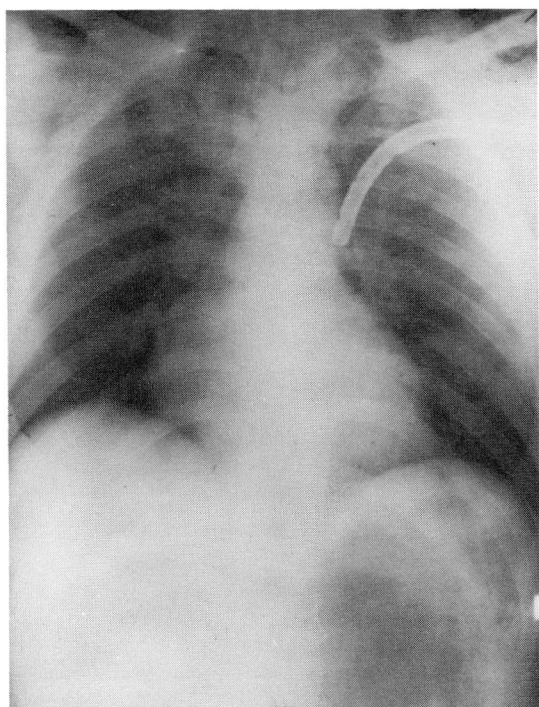

Figure 31. Typical x-ray appearance of bilateral pulmonary contusion. A chest tube is also shown inserted on the left for treatment of a partial pneumothorax. Bilateral fluffy infiltrates are present, particularly in the upper portions of the lung.

plete opacification of entire segments or lobes, or even the entire lung; this results from intra-alveolar hemorrhage, congestion, and edema. Pulmonary effusion may also be associated with severe contusion and is usually sanguineous in nature. The resolution of the entire pathologic process may take up to 7 to 10 days. The appearance of the pulmonary infiltration on x-ray for longer periods may indicate the presence of pneumonitis superimposed on the pulmonary infiltration.

In mild pulmonary contusion, no treatment may be required except for good pulmonary hygiene, periodic use of intermittent positive-pressure breathing (IPPB), and administration of supplemental oxygen. In rib fracture, intercostal rib block with a local anesthetic may be helpful in relieving the pain of breathing and may result in improved respiratory excursion and alveolar ventilation. In severe pulmonary contusion, inadequate alveolar perfusion may cause severe respiratory distress. Cyanosis may rapidly supervene, with a marked drop in oxygen saturation and arterial pO_2. In such instances, intubation or a tracheostomy may be required, and the institution of controlled positive-pressure ventilation may be lifesaving.

Adult Respiratory Distress Syndrome

During the past few years, extensive studies in young soldiers injured in the Vietnam conflict have provided a description of a syndrome that has been variously labeled as *adult respiratory distress syndrome, congestive atelectasis, "shock" lung, posttraumatic pulmonary insufficiency, and hypoxic hyperventilation* (Fig. 32). It is not yet clear why severe injury that is unrelated to the thorax may produce progressive impairment of ventilation, but this does occur, and its causes are probably multiple, including microemboli from multiple blood transfusions, fat embolism, shock, the effects of resuscitative fluids in the lung, neurogenic factors, vasoactive agents released into the circulation that affect the lung, oxygen toxicity, intravascular coagulation, and sepsis.

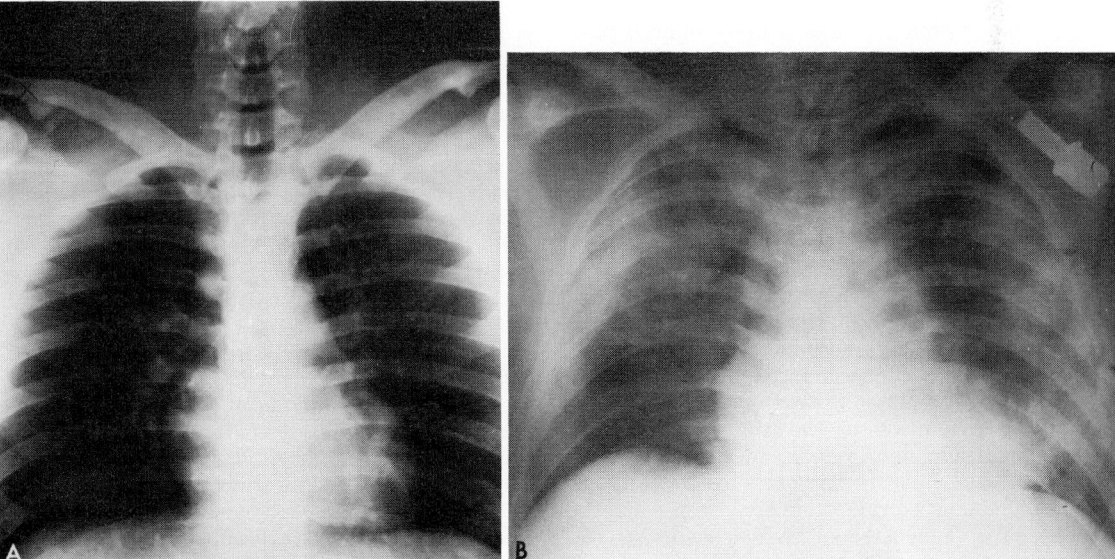

Figure 32. Adult acute respiratory distress syndrome. This patient had multiple abdominal and extremity injuries without direct thoracic injury. *A,* Normal chest film on admission. *B,* Bilateral pulmonary infiltrates with marked pulmonary insufficiency 4 days after admission. The patient required ventilator support for a 10-day period for treatment of this syndrome, along with administration of colloids and diuretics and restriction of fluids and antibiotics.

The clinical picture and course have been well defined by Moore and others. The clinical course of such patients can be divided into four phases:

1. *Injury, resuscitation, and alkalosis.* In this phase there is a mild metabolic acidosis, the result of injury. Compensatory hyperventilation occurs and dissolved carbon dioxide is excreted at an increased rate. This produces respiratory alkalosis, which is further aggravated by the alkalinizing effects of bicarbonate infusion given during resuscitation and the metabolism of citrate in banked blood to form more bicarbonate.

2. *Stabilization and respiratory distress.* Hyperventilation continues and there may be an increase in cardiac output. Because of the development of arteriovenous shunting within the lungs and hypoperfusion of groups of pulmonary alveoli, arterial pO_2 drops markedly.

3. *Pulmonary insufficiency.* Within 48 to 72 hours after injury, there may be overt pulmonary insufficiency. As the pattern progresses further, infiltrates are seen within the lungs and increasing arteriovenous shunting continues. The pO_2 also continues to drop and may be unresponsive to administered oxygen.

4. *Bradycardia and asystole.* With further anoxia, there is generalized tissue hypoperfusion. This results in failure of cellular metabolism, cardiac arrhythmias, and death.

Along with increased arteriovenous shunting, there are decreased pulmonary compliance, increased rate of breathing with high oxygen requirements, and decreasing arterial oxygenation despite decreasing arterial carbon dioxide. This syndrome, because of the excess work of breathing it causes, may eventually exhaust patients who have multiple associated injuries. In such instances, the extreme energy costs may be partially avoided by the early use of controlled ventilation with a respirator.

Recently, the problem of *microembolism* as a result of multiple transfusions in these acutely injured patients has received considerable attention (Fig. 33). Swank has developed a method of estimating the number of aggregates of platelets and leukocytes in banked blood, the so-called "screen filtration pressure." These small emboli can often be demonstrated in the pulmonary capillaries after intravenous infusion of large amounts of banked blood. In Vietnam, Berman showed a close correlation between elevated arterial screen filtration pressures and arterial hypoxia in seriously injured casualties. In similar studies, McNamara also found considerable debris in banked blood that was filtered primarily by the pulmonary capillary bed and secondarily by the peripheral capillary bed. He related the postoperative hypoxemia in these casualties to the volume of blood received. In addition, he was able to show a rapid increase in the screen filtration pressure in banked blood with increasing storage time (Fig. 34). Barrett and others have demonstrated that transfusion of microaggregate-rich blood causes a striking increase in pulmonary arteriovenous shunting and a decrease in pulmonary diffusing capacity. It may well be that the administration of large quantities of blood with

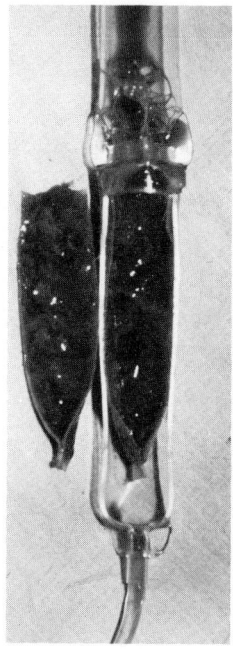

Figure 33. Cross-section of standard blood transfusion filter following passage of one unit of 12-day-old human whole blood. A considerable amount of amorphous debris was removed by this filter, but great quantities of microaggregates passed through the nylon screen mesh.

these particles plays a major role in development of post-traumatic pulmonary insufficiency.

Blaisdell has attempted to determine the mechanisms by which microembolism could affect pulmonary function, and has described (1) the release of vasoactive and bronchial constrictive substances from platelet aggregates; (2) mechanical vascular obstruction by these aggregates within the pulmonary capillaries, producing ischemia, interstitial edema, hemorrhage, and decreases in pulmonary surfactant; and (3) the initiation of intravascular coagulation. He has suggested that the common intermediary pathway in these situations is initiated by intravascular coagulation, activated by the cellular debris from transfused blood. The appearance of intravascular coagulation, however, has been difficult to document.

Pathologic examination in patients who have died of post-traumatic pulmonary insufficiency has consistently shown increased lung weight, marked interstitial edema, intra-alveolar hemorrhage, and pulmonary congestion. When combined with the enthusiasm, particularly in Vietnam casualties, for the use of large quantities of crystalloid solutions such as Ringer's lactate or saline, these findings have suggested that *excess fluid administration* may also play a role in producing this syndrome. Gump and his associates have further shown that, in patients with shock and sepsis, extravascular lung water is abnormally increased along with an acute increase in total body water. Not only does the interstitial edema reduce pulmonary compliance, but fluid overload may also alter the colloid osmotic pressure of the blood, further aggravating the transcapillary leakage into the tissues, particularly in the interstitial spaces of the lung. Undoubtedly, excess utilization of resuscitative electrolyte solutions plays a significant role in the development of this syndrome.

Finally, the role of *fat embolism* as a possible participant in the development of this syndrome has been again emphasized by Collins and his associates, who found that the arterial hypoxemia occurring after serious injuries was directly related to the number and location of the wounds. This was particularly true for those wounds located in areas where fat stores were present, such as the bone marrow in multiple fractures. Fat embolism is a well-documented entity and closely resembles post-traumatic pulmonary insufficiency; furthermore, its existence is difficult to prove in many patients with this syndrome. Fat embolism should be suspected when fat droplets are noted on sputum smear or in the urine sediment.

A special Dacron wool filter, interposed in the infusion line, for patients who are receiving large quantities of banked blood has proven effective in preventing post-transfusion respiratory failure (Fig. 35). These filters are highly efficient in the removal of microaggregates of platelets and other debris down to 15 μ in size. It is not surprising, therefore, that, in patients who have received five or more units of banked blood for resuscitation, this particulate matter may be trapped in lungs, initiating many of the findings characteristic of the acute respiratory distress syndrome. This phenomenon has been well recognized for a number of years in patients who have been on cardiopulmonary bypass for correction of cardiac defects,

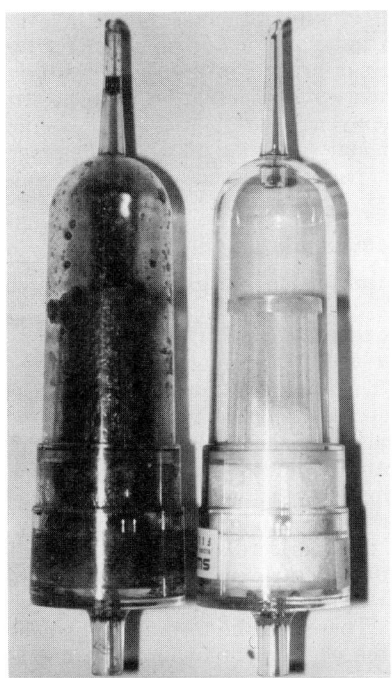

Figure 35. Dacron wool (Swank) blood transfusion filter (right). Spike at upper end is inserted into blood transfusion container and standard intravenous set is inserted into the lower part of filter. Particles passing this filter are 15 μ in diameter or smaller. Up to 2000 ml. of 21-day-old human blood may be completely filtered, even under pressure. Such filters are useful when transfusion of large quantities of blood is anticipated, particularly in the emergency room. Appearance of a Dacron (Swank) filter (left) after filtration of approximately 1500 ml. of whole blood. Numerous microaggregates are evident. (From Dawidson, I., Barrett, J. A., Miller, E., and Litwin, M. S.: Ann. Surg., *181*:51, 1975.)

and the term "perfusion lung" is well accepted. Many institutions that handle large numbers of patients with multiple injuries have found the use of these filters highly effective in preventing post-traumatic pulmonary insufficiency.

The treatment of the acute post-traumatic pulmonary distress syndrome (Table 6) includes (1) use of continuous positive-pressure ventilations; (2) administration of diuretics to reduce excess body water; (3) restriction of intravenous fluids containing large amounts of crystalloids; (4) administration of colloids such as albumin to restore the colloid osmotic pressure

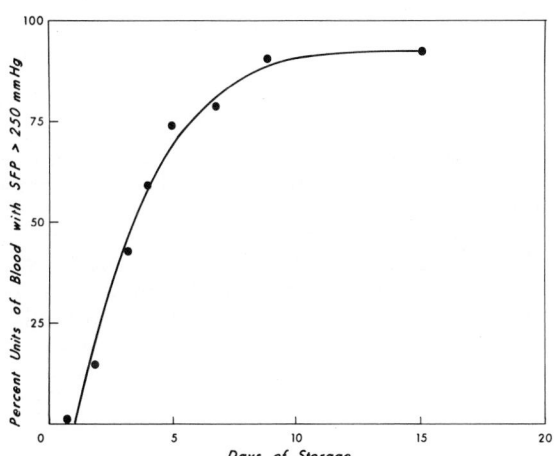

Figure 34. Screen filtration pressure of stored, banked blood. On successive dates following withdrawal of fresh blood, which was stored in citrate, aliquots were obtained and studied by the screen filtration technique. The marked rise in screen filtration pressure occurred within 48 hours and reached a peak after 8 to 10 days of storage. This is due to large amounts of particulate matter and aggregated platelets in stored blood. (Modified from McNamara, J. J., Boatright, D., Burran, E. L., Molot, M. D., Summers, E., and Stremple, J. F.: Ann. Surg., *174*:58, 1971.)

TABLE 6. Acute Respiratory Distress Syndrome: Treatment

1. Continuous positive-pressure ventilation
2. Diuretics
3. Fluid restriction
4. Colloids (albumin)
5. Steroids
6. Heparin (in disseminated intravascular coagulation)
7. Antibiotics

of blood; (5) administration of steroids in large doses to reduce the inflammatory intrapulmonary process; (6) judicious use of heparin in instances in which disseminated intravascular coagulation is suspected; and (7) use of prophylactic antibiotics to prevent superimposed pulmonary infection, to which these patients are susceptible, particularly those on prolonged respirator management.

Cardiac Tamponade

Cardiac tamponade is usually associated with penetrating thoracic injury but occasionally also occurs after blunt thoracic trauma. Tamponade may develop hours after the acute injury and may often be unsuspected. The usual clinical signs of increased venous pressure, decreased intensity of heart sounds, hypotension, and diminished pulse pressure are often seen in patients with multiple injuries, and the unwary physician may ascribe these findings to massive blood loss rather than to tamponade. Since only a small quantity of intrapericardial blood is required to reduce venous return (as little as 50 to 100 ml.), enlargement of the heart shadow on x-ray *rarely* occurs in acute tamponade. Therefore, reliance upon the heart size as shown in the chest roentgenogram is not helpful in making the diagnosis.

In all patients with blunt or penetrating thoracic trauma, the presence of shock should alert the physician to the possibility of cardiac tamponade, particularly in the face of normal or increased central venous pressure. Should any question exist concerning the presence of tamponade, pericardiocentesis can readily be performed. Aspiration of a small quantity of nonclotting blood from the pericardial sac confirms the diagnosis, and it may also markedly improve the patient's condition. In some patients, a single aspiration may suffice as definitive therapy; however, should tamponade recur or bleeding into the pericardial sac continue, emergency thoracotomy should be performed to suture the cardiac laceration. All penetrating cardiac injuries produced by gunshot wounds that result in cardiac tamponade require immediate exploration because of the severity of the injury. In a study of 57 patients treated for cardiac tamponade at the Charity Hospital of Louisiana in New Orleans, it was concluded that prompt treatment is the most important factor in the survival of patients with penetrating cardiac injuries. Pericardiocentesis was preferable to operation in certain patients with small puncture wounds, and in most of these it represented definitive treatment. Thoracotomy was reserved for (1) continued bleeding, (2) failure to respond to aspiration, (3) recurrent tamponade after aspiration, (4) cardiac arrest, and (5) all gunshot wounds.

Cardiac Contusion

Cardiac contusion should be suspected in *all* patients with blunt thoracic trauma. Among 210 patients suffering nonpenetrating chest injuries, Jones et al. found that 21 per cent had cardiac contusions. Life-endangering cardiac complications occurred in 29 per cent of these patients and four patients died as a result of the contusion. The injury usually results from a sudden blow to the sternum or anterior rib cage

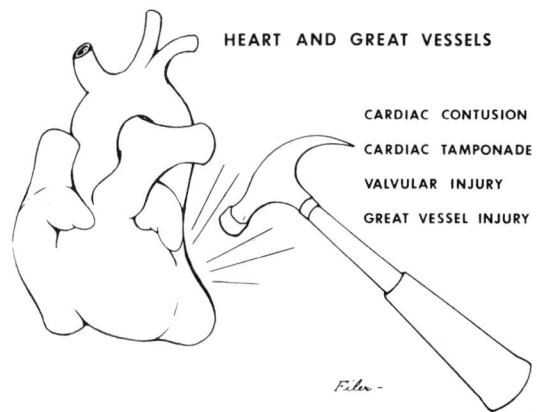

Figure 36. Types of injuries to the heart and great vessels. Penetrating or blunt thoracic trauma may cause major injury to the heart and mediastinal structures. Cardiac contusion often is not diagnosed. In cases of severe thoracic trauma, an electrocardiogram is mandatory.

and transmission of this energy to the anterior surface of the heart (Fig. 36). Acute compression of the heart between the sternum and the spine in crushing chest injuries may also lead to cardiac contusion. Pathologic findings in such patients include ecchymotic areas over the left or right ventricle, intramural hemorrhage, and even traumatic coronary artery thrombosis or laceration. If the injury is severe, the myocardium may be ruptured. The contused myocardium may be unable to respond with an appropriate cardiac output under stress conditions and is more vulnerable to the development of arrhythmias during periods of shock and hypoxia. Irreversible arrhythmia may develop. When there is associated thoracic wall injury or intrapulmonary injury or both, chest pain and alterations in cardiac output may be erroneously ascribed to the associated injuries. Even though the clinical and diagnostic features of cardiac contusion are similar to those of myocardial infarction, its diagnosis is frequently missed. Prompt recognition and treatment of specific conditions, particularly cardiac arrhythmia, is of utmost importance.

The most common arrhythmia is atrial flutter or fibrillation. In addition, there is a high incidence of supraventricular and ventricular arrhythmia. Electrocardiography is the most accurate method of establishing the diagnosis of cardiac contusion in severely injured patients. Since the diagnosis is made by electrocardiography, this should be done immediately in all patients who sustain blunt thoracic injury. Serial electrocardiographic changes revealing evolution of ST-T segment changes over the precordial leads are also helpful in confirming this diagnosis and in predicting prognosis after injury.

Primary objectives in the management of cardiac contusions include prompt correction of hypovolemia and hypoxia, control of injuries that contribute to hypovolemia, and appropriate control of arrhythmias. Treatment is similar to the treatment of myocardial infarction, and includes bed rest, limitation of physical activity until electrocardiographic findings have stabilized, and the administration of oxygen and morphine. Because of the increased risk of bleeding into the myocardium, anticoagulants are absolutely contraindicated in myocardial contusion.

Patients with a diagnosis of cardiac contusion should be followed carefully for long periods of time, since delayed complications may appear months or years later. Those who recover can be expected to have normal cardiac functions unless there has also been an associated coronary thrombosis. In the latter instance, permanent fibrosis of a portion of ventricle may occur.

Great Vessel Injury

In patients with massive penetrating or blunt thoracic injuries, the existence of shock should lead to the suspicion of a major vascular injury within the mediastinum. Initial x-rays are helpful, particularly if there is marked widening of the mediastinum. Unfortunately, the latter is not an accurate guide, since many conditions can produce widening of the mediastinum in patients with thoracic trauma. Mediastinal widening is most commonly seen when an inadequate portable x-ray falsely shows enlargement of the mediastinal area or when a mediastinal hematoma is present. The presence of massive hemothorax in association with a mediastinal hematoma is almost diagnostic of injury to the great vessels, especially when bleeding continues after the insertion of a chest tube.

A common location for injury to the thoracic aorta is just distal to the ligamentum arteriosum, which is a point of fixation of the aorta. With sudden deceleration injuries, a shearing force may be applied to this region, resulting in intramural rupture, rupture of the muscular coat, or even complete transection of the aorta at this point. Ruptures can also occur in other areas along the aortic arch but with less frequency. The sudden development of unequal pulses in the upper extremities or inequality of pulses in the arms compared to those in the legs should immediately alert one to the possibility of severe thoracic aortic injury.

Should any suspicion exist concerning the possibility of great vessel injury, particularly if there is widening of the mediastinal shadow, there is little reason for continued "observation" of the patient. The use of arteriography in the diagnosis of these injuries has permitted the salvage of many patients with major aortic injury. A retrograde aortogram in a patient with a complete transection of the thoracic aorta has a fairly typical appearance (Fig. 37). In addition to the widened mediastinum, disruption in the continuity of the aorta can be clearly seen. The patient should be taken immediately to the operating room, and reanastomosis of the transected aorta should be performed. To avoid ischemic damage to the brain and spinal cord, left heart bypass should be used during the period of aortic occlusion required for repair of the defect.

All major penetrating injuries involving the mediastinum should be explored. Examples of such injuries include gunshot and knife wounds directed toward the mediastinum either from the root of the neck or from the parasternal area. Various surgical approaches may be utilized in the operative management of such injuries (Fig. 38).

Rupture of Trachea and Bronchi

Rupture of the trachea or one of the major bronchi is a relatively uncommon complication of severe closed thoracic trauma. The manifestations of this type of injury are well recognized and include uncontrolled pneumothorax, with or without hemothorax, and progressive mediastinal and subcutaneous emphysema. However, there remains a significant group of injuries in which fracture of the bronchial cartilages occurs without extensive leakage of air because the mucosa and membranous wall of the bronchus remain intact or because such tears become sealed by adjacent structures. It is possible that such occurs in some patients with crushing chest wounds who recover completely with no residual ill effects. It appears more likely, however, that the injured bronchus, now lacking its normal cartilaginous support, becomes progressively involved with scarring. This results in stenosis, stricture, or even eventually complete occlusion.

This diagnosis should be strongly suspected in any patient with a severe thoracic injury in whom there is

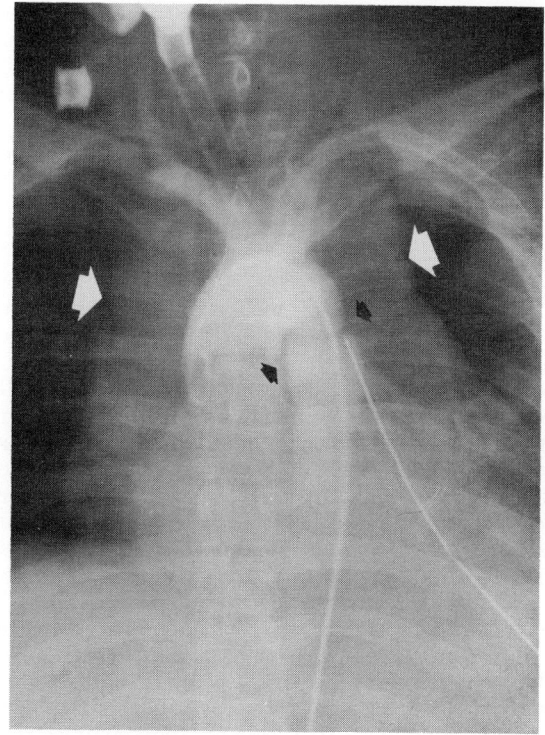

Figure 37. Rupture of the aortic arch was suspected because of widening of the mediastinum on routine chest film (large arrows). A retrograde arteriogram obtained by transfemoral passage of a Seldinger catheter confirms complete transection of the aortic arch (small arrows) just beyond the ligamentum arteriosum. In this instance the patient had a huge mediastinal hematoma. Thoracotomy was performed with the aid of left heart bypass; the aortic injury was repaired, and the patient recovered. (From Drapanas, T., Hewitt, R. L., Weichert, R. F., III, and Smith, A. D.: Ann. Surg., 172:351, 1970.)

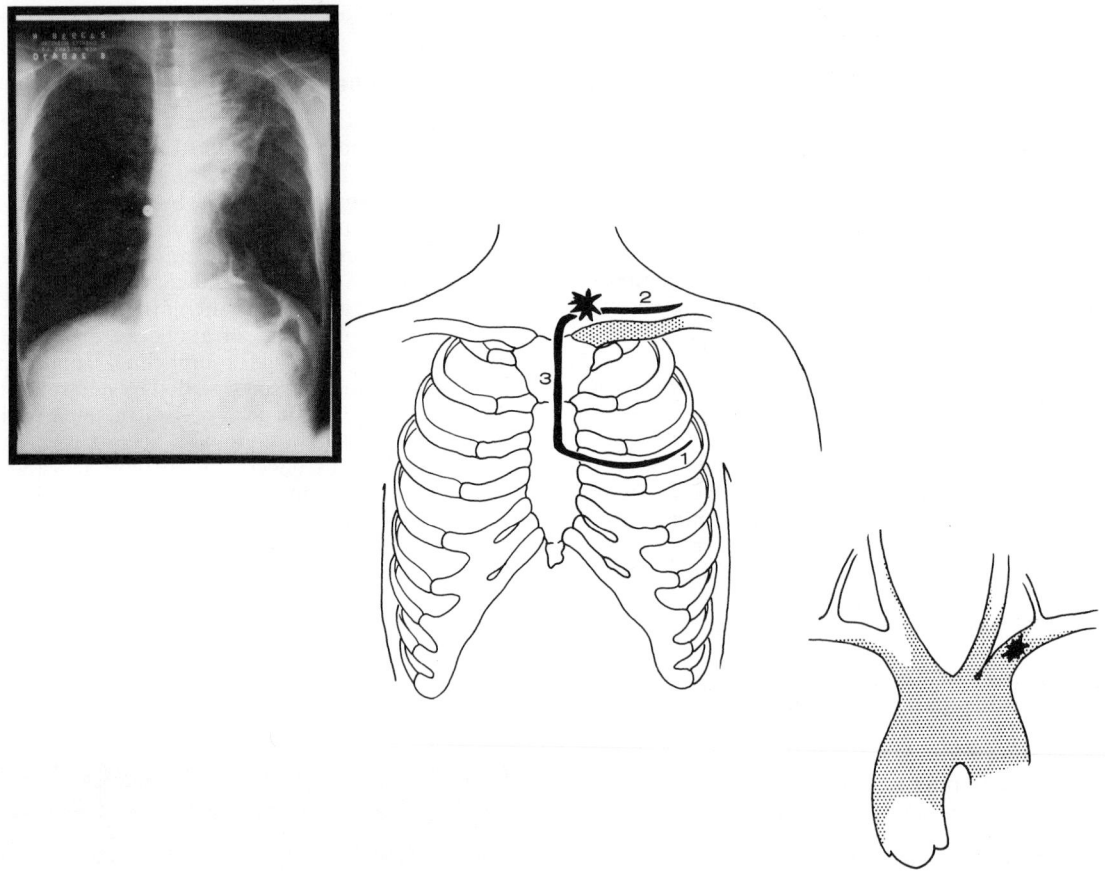

Figure 38. Gunshot wound of the root of the neck, with mediastinal hematoma. The incision used for exploration is shown in this patient. The through-and-through injury of the left subclavian artery was repaired and the hematoma evacuated. Adequate exposure is necessary in this type of injury in order to obtain proximal and distal control of the injured vessels prior to exploration of the hematoma. (Courtesy of R. L. Hewitt.)

evidence of mediastinal emphysema or a massive pneumothorax that cannot be easily controlled by the insertion of an underwater-sealed intercostal chest tube. In such patients, emergency bronchoscopy will often reveal the site of injury, usually in the lower thoracic trachea, the tracheal bifurcation, or the major bronchi within 2 to 3 cm. of the trachea. Major rupture of the trachea and central bronchi can also occur without pneumothorax, particularly if the mediastinal pleura has not ruptured at the time of the injury. Massive mediastinal emphysema that spreads to the neck and along the subcutaneous tissue planes, eventually to include the entire thorax, abdomen, and scrotum, is a well-recognized complication of mediastinal rupture of the tracheobronchial tree.

Once the diagnosis has been established, proper therapy is emergency thoracotomy and repair of the major bronchial or tracheal laceration. In instances of complete transection of the bronchus, all efforts should be made to restore continuity by bronchial anastomosis or replantation.

As has been emphasized, the diagnosis of major bronchial injury may not be readily apparent. A patient who suffered a severe crushing injury to the chest is shown in Figure 39. After abdominal explora-

tion, a chest film in the recovery room showed evidence of pulmonary contusion on the right and an apparently normal lung on the left (Fig. 39A). However, in retrospect, there was evidence of hyperaeration and trapping of air in the left lung, which produced complete and massive atelectasis of that lung a few days after the injury (Fig. 39B). Complete disruption of the bronchial cartilage had occurred, but the mucosa had remained intact, so that a major air leak was prevented (Fig. 39C). Complete bronchial collapse with obstruction led to the rapid onset of bronchiectasis. Such acute changes within the bronchi are reversible, if prompt surgical correction can be performed (Fig. 39D).

Esophageal Injuries

Penetrating injuries are the most common injuries to the esophagus. The cervical, thoracic, or intra-abdominal portion of the esophagus may be involved.

Cervical Esophagus. Penetrating cervical esophageal injuries may produce devastating results if the diagnosis is missed. Because of the location of the esophagus in the neck, just anterior to the prevertebral fascia, extravasation from the wound will rapidly produce mediastinitis unless repair and drainage are performed. For this reason, a carefully performed esophagram with a water-soluble radiopaque dye (Gastrografin) and esophagoscopy followed by exploration should be done in all penetrating injuries near the esophagus. Blunt injuries of the cervical esophagus are extremely rare because of the protected location of the esophagus between the trachea and spine high in the neck and between the great vessels and spine lower down.

Thoracic Esophagus. Penetrating injuries of the thoracic esophagus may also be easily missed, particularly when there are other injuries within the thoracic cavity. Diagnostic clues include the presence of mediastinal emphysema and fever and the finding of widening of the mediastinum and bilateral or unilateral pleural effusion on chest x-ray. Diagnosis can often be made from x-rays taken after the patient has swallowed a water-soluble, radiopaque dye (Gastrografin). Such x-rays will demonstrate leakage of the contrast material from the esophageal defect (Fig. 40).

Esophagoscopy should also be performed, but caution should be taken to avoid further tearing of the esophagus.

Intra-abdominal Esophagus. Injuries to the intra-abdominal portion of the esophagus may simulate an acute abdomen. X-ray examination after barium swallow may demonstrate barium under the diaphragm, or an abnormal air-fluid level above the gastric air bubble.

Another diagnosis to be considered in the acutely injured patient is spontaneous or postemetic rupture of the esophagus occurring as a result of violent retching or vomiting (Boerhaave syndrome). The mechanism for this syndrome has not been clearly established, but it is presumed that sudden retching may subject the supradiaphragmatic portion of the esophagus to transient peaks of high, bursting pressure. This results in rupture of the mucosa and the muscularis, usually on the posterolateral wall of the lower thoracic esophagus within 2 to 3 inches of the diaphragm. The presence of

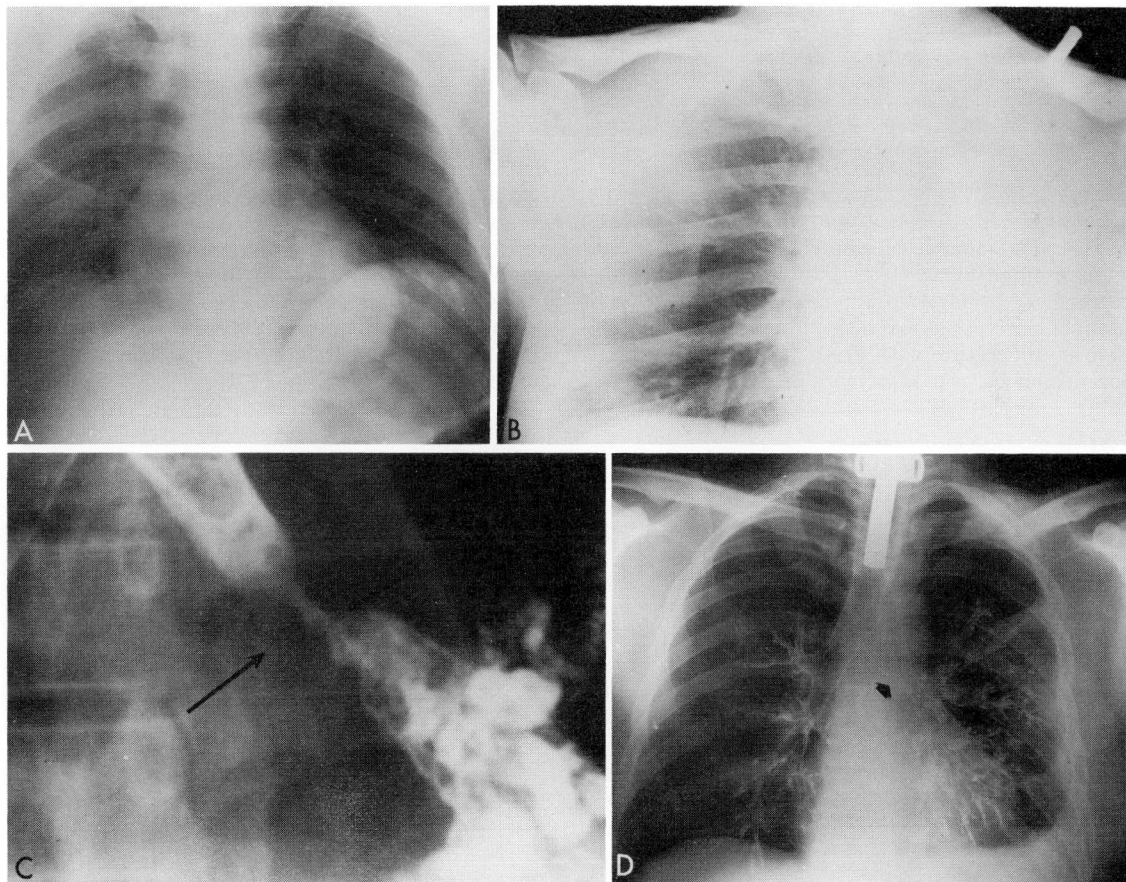

Figure 39. The evolution of a bronchial injury after thoracic trauma. *A,* Hyperaeration over the left lung was misinterpreted on the admission chest film as "normal." *B,* Film obtained 3 days later shows complete atelectasis in the left lung. Complete bronchial collapse has occurred, with absorption of the trapped alveolar air. *C,* Bronchogram obtained 3 weeks after admission confirms complete collapse of the left main bronchus, with marked bronchiectasis distal to this point. Complete repair of the transected bronchus was performed by left thoracotomy. *D,* Complete expansion of the lung with a normal bronchogram 1 year after admission. The site of the bronchial anastomosis is shown by the arrow; there is only a minimal narrowing of the suture line. The patient is asymptomatic. (From Drapanas, T., Siewers, R., and Feist, J. H.: N. Engl. J. Med., *975:*917, 1966.)

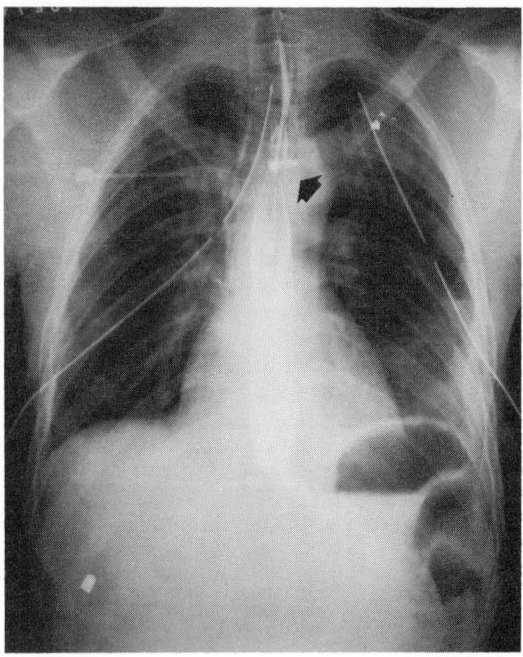

Figure 40. Gunshot injury to the thoracic esophagus. Barium swallow shows leakage of contrast material (arrow) at the level of the aortic arch. The injury was caused by a .32 caliber pistol bullet, which is seen on the lower portion of the film lying in the lumen of the duodenum after having passed down the esophagus, through the stomach, and into the duodenum by normal peristalsis.

a "mediastinal crunch" on auscultation of the lower thorax is pathognomonic of esophageal rupture, as is mediastinal emphysema.

Treatment of esophageal injuries, if the diagnosis can be made early, is immediate exploration of the involved area and suture with drainage. In late or misdiagnosed injuries, repair is more difficult because of

the local inflammatory response and associated friability of the esophageal wall. In this circumstance, wide drainage is mandatory. Danger of development of an esophageal fistula persists for some time, and supportive nutrition by intravenous hyperalimentation or by gastrostomy may be indicated.

Traumatic Rupture of the Diaphragm

In severe crushing thoracic or abdominal injuries, traumatic rupture of the diaphragm may occur, usually through the central tendinous portion. The diagnosis may often be obscured by associated injuries. Herniation of the abdominal viscera into the thorax, particularly in injuries involving the left hemidiaphragm, may be misinterpreted as hemopneumothorax (Fig. 41A). The unwary physician may institute chest tube drainage to evacuate blood and fluid, only to be greeted by drainage of gastric or intestinal contents if the tube penetrates the herniated hollow abdominal viscera. Such injuries should be suspected when the diaphragm cannot be clearly delineated, particularly on a lateral chest film.

Since the liver usually provides tamponade of rents in the right diaphragm, injuries on this side of the diaphragm are less obvious than those on the left. Complete herniation of the liver into the thorax may occur, however.

Additional clues to the diagnosis include the presence of abnormal bowel sounds on auscultation of the chest, a friction rub over the lower thorax, and abnormal position of the abdominal viscera as determined by gastrointestinal series or barium enema (Fig. 41B). Should doubt still exist, pneumoperitoneum should be created by instillation of 300 to 500 cc. of air. Prompt appearance of partial pneumothorax on an upright chest x-ray will confirm the diagnosis.

Treatment consists of emergency operation and repair of the rent. The transthoracic approach gives the best exposure and offers the best opportunity for a surgeon to repair the defect. However, when there are

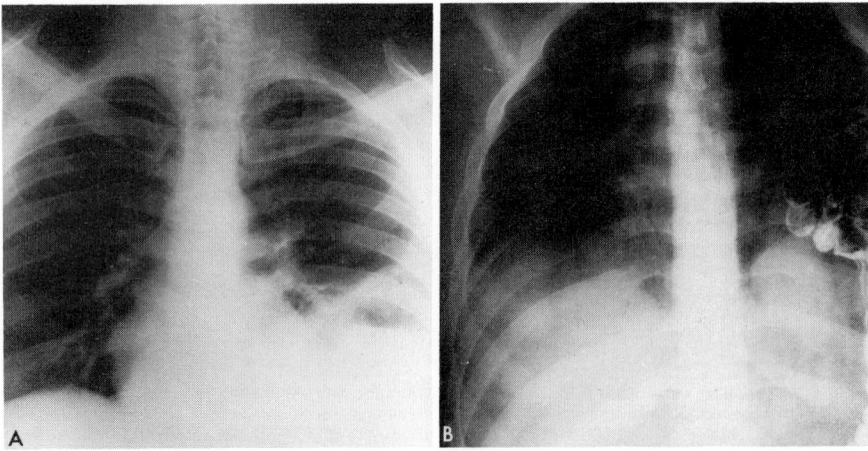

Figure 41. Traumatic rupture of the left diaphragm is seen in this patient following closed compression injury to the lower left thorax. The presence of an air-fluid level immediately after injury is pathognomonic of diaphragmatic rupture *(A)*. *B,* Barium enema confirms the presence of colon in the left chest. Transthoracic repair was performed, with complete recovery.

associated intra-abdominal injuries, the surgical approach should be transabdominal so that the abdominal viscera may be examined. Repair through the transabdominal approach is more difficult but can usually be performed satisfactorily.

ABDOMINAL INJURIES

Patients with abdominal injuries may usually be managed on a more elective basis than those with chest injuries. However, abdominal injuries involving major hemorrhage from solid viscera constitute surgical emergencies almost as grave as severe thoracic injuries. When rupture or thrombosis of the arterial supply to these organs has occurred, blood flow must be re-established within a very short time if major ischemic damage is to be prevented. As elsewhere, total disruption or lacerations of major blood vessels require immediate operation.

Penetrating Injuries

Penetrating injuries of the abdomen due to knives or other sharp objects are usually easier to deal with than similar penetrations in the chest, and simple suture of such wounds will usually suffice. Gunshot wounds are much more difficult injuries to treat. Multiple viscera are usually involved, and when the bullet is of high velocity or great mass, surrounding damage will necessitate extensive débridement of tissue that has been destroyed by the concussive forces. Wounds caused by small-caliber, low-velocity bullets can be handled in much the same way as simple knife stab wounds. When a major blood vessel has been lacerated at the same time that intestinal perforations have occurred, great care must be taken to irrigate the area thoroughly to remove contaminating material and prevent infection of the vascular suture line (Fig. 42).

Blunt Injury

Because great shearing forces are generated, deceleration is most likely to produce shearing injury to the renal pedicle, the splenic pedicle, or the intestines at points where they pass to fixed retroperitoneal positions. Acute abdominal compression, on the other hand, leads to transmission of massive pressures to the intra-abdominal viscera and will cause explosive injuries of the liver and spleen or blowout injuries and intraperitoneal contamination from the intestines (Fig. 43).

Liver and Biliary Tree

Small lacerations of the liver may be simply drained to prevent the development of bile peritonitis; if the laceration is large, the hepatic capsule may first be sutured. Injuries to the extrahepatic biliary tree may also be simply sutured and drained. If there has been partial or complete transection of a major biliary duct, a T tube should be inserted for drainage and to serve as a stent. The duct should be repaired over this drainage tube, which is left in place for at least 10 days and until the ducts have healed and the cholangiogram is normal.

Gunshot wounds of the liver may be treated as lacerations. However, when the bullet is of large caliber or the velocity is exceedingly great, the explosive impact will result in severe shattering of the liver substance and multiple severe lacerations of the hepatic capsule. Occasionally, such injuries are so extensive that hepatic resection is necessary.

Compression injury to the abdomen usually causes solitary lacerations into the liver substance. Deceleration, however, may be associated with avulsions of the extrahepatic biliary tree. Solitary deep lacerations are particularly dangerous when they extend deep into the liver substance across major hepatic arterial branches or into the hepatic veins and vena cava.

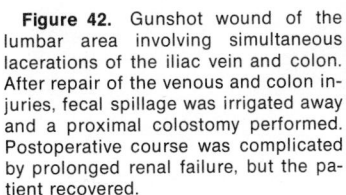

Figure 42. Gunshot wound of the lumbar area involving simultaneous lacerations of the iliac vein and colon. After repair of the venous and colon injuries, fecal spillage was irrigated away and a proximal colostomy performed. Postoperative course was complicated by prolonged renal failure, but the patient recovered.

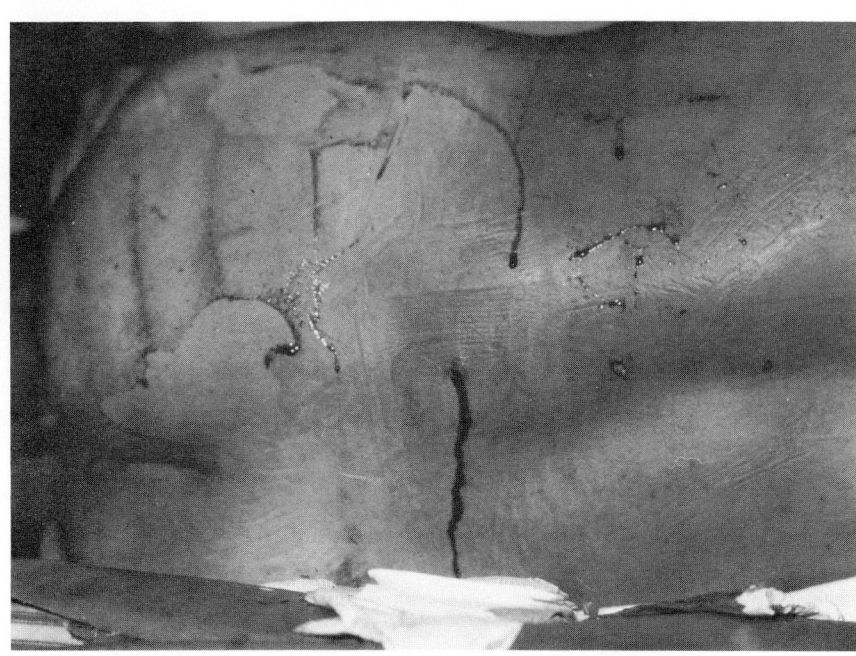

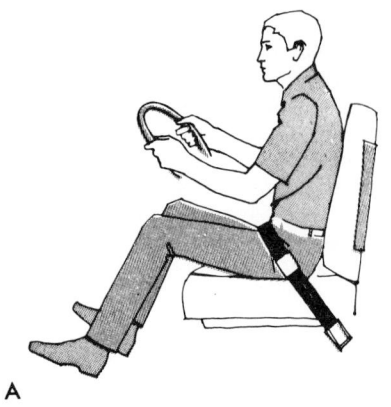

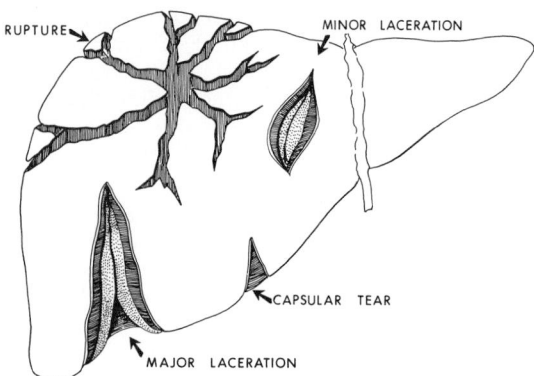

Figure 44. Types of hepatic injuries commonly encountered. The most serious type of injury is the stellate fracture of the dome of the liver, which if extensive enough usually requires hepatic lobectomy.

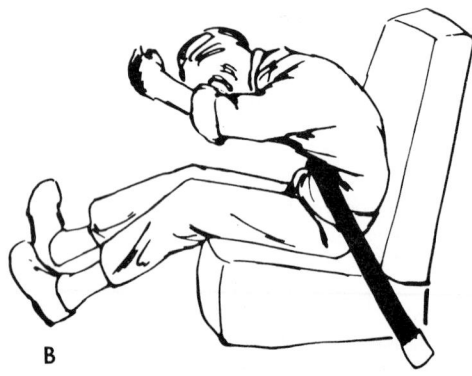

Figure 43. Mechanism of seat belt injury. A sudden deceleration force across the seat belt produces compression injury to hollow and solid intra-abdominal viscera. Common injuries encountered include rupture of the small bowel, hematoma of the mesentery, avulsion of the renal arteries, thrombosis of the aorta, and transection of the neck of the pancreas. Although these serious injuries can occur when seat belts are used, the injury would have been far more serious had the seat belt not been used, and it is doubtful whether the patient would have survived. (From Committee on Injuries of American Academy of Orthopedic Surgeons: Emergency Care and Transportation of the Sick and Injured. Chicago, American Academy of Orthopedic Surgeons, 1971.)

Treatment of this condition is immediate abdominal exploration and splenectomy.

Occasionally after blunt trauma the splenic pulp may be injured without laceration of the capsule. A subcapsular hematoma may then form over a period of days, weeks, or even months (Fig. 45). Ultimately, spontaneous rupture will occur and exsanguinating hemorrhage ensue unless there is appropriate surgical intervention. It is possible to diagnose this condition before splenic rupture by arteriography of the splenic vessels (Fig. 46). A splenic hematoma may also displace the gastric air bubble medially on abdominal scout films and this further suggests the diagnosis (Fig. 47). Elective splenectomy should be performed once the diagnosis has been made.

Such injuries constitute surgical emergencies and must be managed immediately in the operating room to prevent exsanguination. Various types of liver injuries are depicted in Figure 44.

Spleen

Because of its relatively free-hanging position, the spleen is the organ most commonly injured in blunt abdominal trauma. Acute abdominal compression most often results in laceration of the splenic capsule, whereas deceleration commonly results in partial or complete avulsion of the splenic pedicle. In patients who have suffered blunt trauma to the abdomen, a high level of suspicion of splenic injury should be maintained. Diagnosis can best be made from the history of abdominal trauma and by finding blood in the peritoneal cavity during abdominal paracentesis.

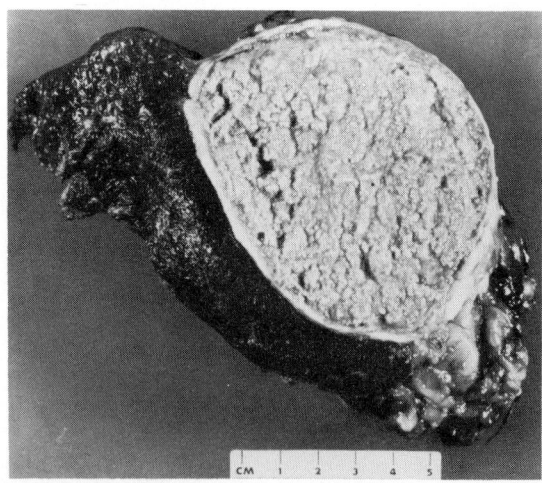

Figure 45. "Occult" rupture of the spleen, 1 month after injury. The mechanism of injury is usually blunt trauma resulting in parenchymal rupture without intraperitoneal hemorrhage because of an intact splenic capsule. The organizing hematoma is shown. (From Drapanas, T., Yates, A. J., Breckman, R., and Wholey, M.: Arch. Surg., 99:298, 1969.)

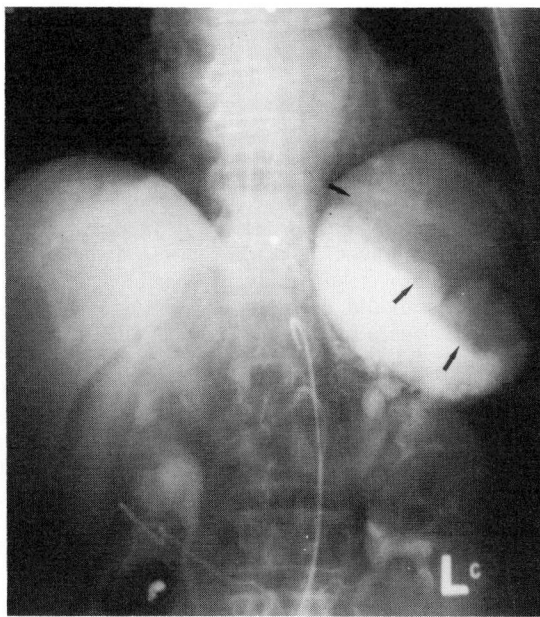

Figure 46. The use of arteriography for the diagnosis of splenic hematoma. There is medial displacement of the spleen during the venous phase of the retrograde celiac angiogram. The large hematoma is shown in the left upper quadrant. (From Drapanas, T., Yates, A. J., Breckman, R., and Wholey, M.: Arch. Surg., 99:298, 1969.)

Pancreas and Duodenum

Simple lacerations of the pancreas made by a knife or a similar object may be closed primarily with a few silk stitches in the pancreatic capsule. Bullet injuries of the pancreas, however, are much more liable to

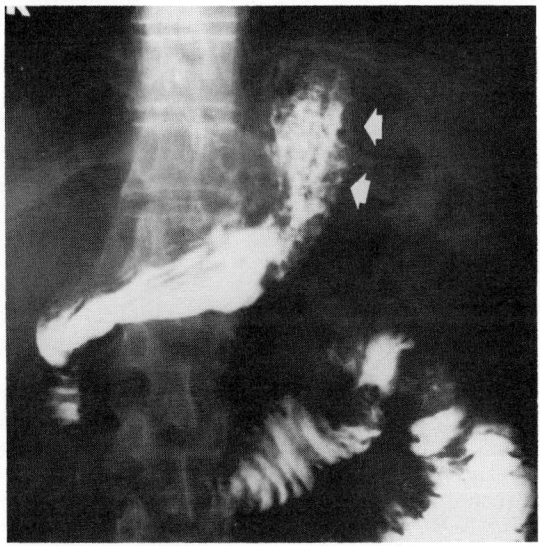

Figure 47. Medial displacement of the stomach (arrows) following blunt abdominal trauma in this patient led to the diagnosis of large splenic hematoma and delayed rupture of the spleen. Splenectomy was successfully performed. (From Drapanas, T., Yates, A. J., Breckman, R., and Wholey, M.: Arch. Surg., 99:298, 1969.)

necrosis and fistula formation. Bullet wounds of the pancreas should be closed in a manner similar to knife wounds, and a drain or large continuous sump catheter should be inserted as far as the area of the pancreatic damage. In such injuries, necrosis of the pancreatic capsule is usually a late occurrence after the operation; therefore, pancreatic drains and sumps should not be removed for at least 10 days after insertion.

Gunshot wounds in the vicinity of the pancreas frequently involve the duodenum; simple closure should be performed after the edges have been debrided to normal tissues. When extensive devitalizing injury to both the duodenum and pancreas has occurred, it is occasionally necessary to perform a pancreatico-duodenectomy (Whipple procedure). Damage to the tail of the pancreas can be treated by local resection of the tail, with care being taken to ligate the main pancreatic duct adequately. After resection of the pancreatic tail, a drain should always be left in the bed of the pancreas to allow external drainage of any leak that may occur.

Blunt injury to the pancreas usually occurs at the junction of the body and head in immediate juxtaposition to the superior mesenteric artery. Lacerations may extend partially through the pancreas, but when trauma is more severe, complete transection may result. Depending on the severity of the injury, several procedures may be used to obtain satisfactory closure (Fig. 48). For severe injuries, the most satisfactory procedure appears to be distal pancreatic resection and anastomosis of a Roux-en-Y loop of small intestine ("living sucker") to the area of trauma. This permits the pancreas to drain through the ampulla of Vater, or, if the pancreatic repair has not been satisfactory, the Roux-en-Y loop provides effective retrograde drainage of the pancreatic duct.

If duodenal injury is suspected, careful exploration of the retroperitoneal portion should also be performed. The second portion of the duodenum is best visualized after the Kocher maneuver and the third and fourth portions may be inspected by exposure of the duodenum through the root of the mesentery or by mobilization of the hepatic flexure of the colon. Perforation of the duodenum should always be suspected when air appears to be present in the retroperitoneal area. Lacerations of the duodenum may be repaired directly. An intramural hematoma of the duodenum, as evidenced by the external bluish and thickened appearance of the duodenal wall, may be removed by incising the serosa and alternately scooping and sucking the blood clot with the fingers and the suction tip. The serosa may then be reapproximated. A submucosal hematoma has a classic "coiled spring" pattern when seen on upper gastrointestinal series and usually partially obstructs the duodenum (Fig. 49).

Stomach, Small Intestine, and Colon

Perforations of the stomach, small intestine, and right colon may be sutured in two layers. Perforations of the left colon may in certain instances also be sutured in two layers, provided significant peritoneal infection or fecal contamination has not occurred and multiple associated injuries are not present. Experience gained in civilian practice has proved that simple

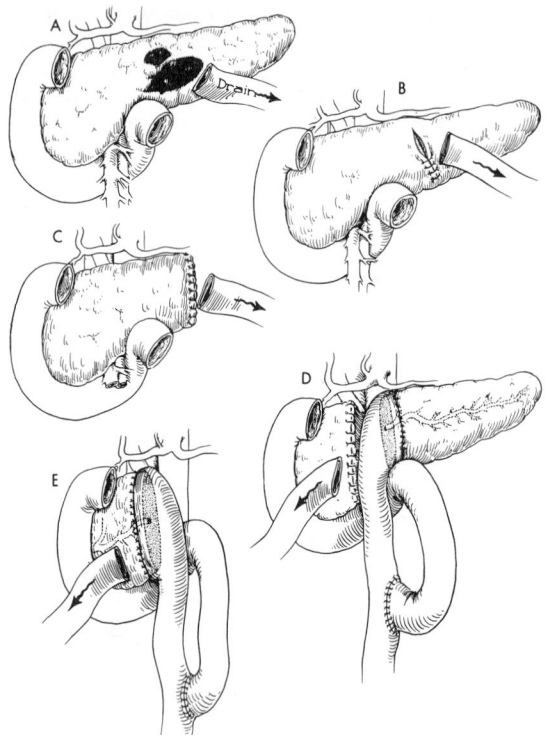

Figure 48. Techniques of treatment of pancreatic injuries. *A,* Simple drainage of pancreatic contusion. *B,* Suture of a pancreatic laceration, along with adequate drainage. *C,* Complete transection of the wide portion of the body of the pancreas, treated by distal pancreatic resection and drainage. *D,* In transection of the pancreas at the neck, a Roux-en-Y loop of jejunum is used to drain the distal end of the pancreas, the proximal end being oversewn and drained. *E,* Resection of the distal three fourths of the pancreas following injury to the level of the neck, with Roux-en-Y drainage of the proximal end. In our experience, pancreaticoduodenectomy for such injuries is rarely, if ever, indicated and is useful only in patients who have devitalizing injuries to *both* duodenum and pancreas. (From Diagnosis and Management of Abdominal Trauma, by Jordan, G. L., and Beall, A. C., Jr., in Current Problems in Surgery, edited by Ravitch, M. M., et al. Copyright © 1971, Year Book Medical Publishers. Used by permission.)

perforations of any viscus may safely be sutured with a minimum of danger to the patient.

When the stomach, small intestine, or right colon is injured by a bullet, débridement of the edges of each penetration in the intestine should extend to clean, viable intestine. The hole should then be closed transversely to insure maximal size of the intestinal lumen. Penetration by small-caliber, low-velocity bullets of the transverse, descending, and sigmoid colon may be closed by a similar technique, provided fecal contamination of the peritoneum has not occurred. A temporary proximal diverting colostomy may be performed to allow the injured areas to heal completely and to protect the closure site from breakdown. Proximal diverting colostomy should always be performed when left colon injuries are due to large-caliber or high-velocity bullets or when the surgeon has any doubt

concerning the wisdom of primary closure. Such injuries are associated with greater fecal contamination of the peritoneum, and the risk of breakdown of the suture line is markedly increased because of the increased destruction of surrounding bowel wall by the missile.

Recent experience indicates that when there is no fecal spillage, when there is negligible destruction of surrounding tissue, and when vital vascular structures are not involved, colostomy may not be necessary and primary closure may be possible. However, such decisions should be made only by one who has had *wide experience* in the treatment of such injuries. Many surgeons continue *routinely* to perform proximal diverting colostomies for all gunshot wounds of the left colon.

Injuries involving simultaneously multiple loops of intestine and major vascular structures are the most difficult of all abdominal injuries to manage. When the stomach, small intestine, or right colon is involved, both vascular and intestinal injuries may be repaired primarily. The peritoneal cavity must be copiously irrigated to remove all contaminating material and to prevent infection of the vascular suture line. Because of the increased incidence of infection and breakdown of the vascular suture line, bullet wounds involving major vascular structures and the left colon are exceedingly difficult problems. Great care must be taken to insure that the intestinal perforations are properly closed, that the vacular closure is adequate, and that a proximal diverting colostomy is done (see Fig. 42).

Deceleration or compression injuries of the intestines usually result in greater intraperitoneal contamination than do those due to penetrating trauma. This undoubtedly results from the fact that intraluminal contents under pressure are frequently expelled into the peritoneal space. Following blunt injuries to the abdomen, ruptured hollow viscera may be reapproximated in simple fashion by means of routine intestinal anastomotic procedures. Compression of the large intestine is usually associated with massive peritoneal contamination. Such injuries should be repaired, peritoneal contaminants should be removed by copious saline irrigation, and a temporary proximal diverting colostomy should be performed to protect the suture line, or the area of injury may be exteriorized (Fig. 50). Lesions of the right colon are often amenable to primary resection (Fig. 51*A*).

Rectum

The rectum is rarely injured in blunt abdominal trauma, even in severe pelvic fractures. However, penetrating injury from bullets or various sharp objects inserted per rectum is a relatively common occurrence. Because of the solid nature of the rectal contents and the heavy bacterial contamination, suture of penetrating rectal injuries should always be followed by proximal diverting colostomy and presacral drainage (Fig. 51*B*).

Mesentery and Vascular Structures

Acute deceleration may result in a shearing type of injury to the renal vascular pedicle, the splenic pedi-

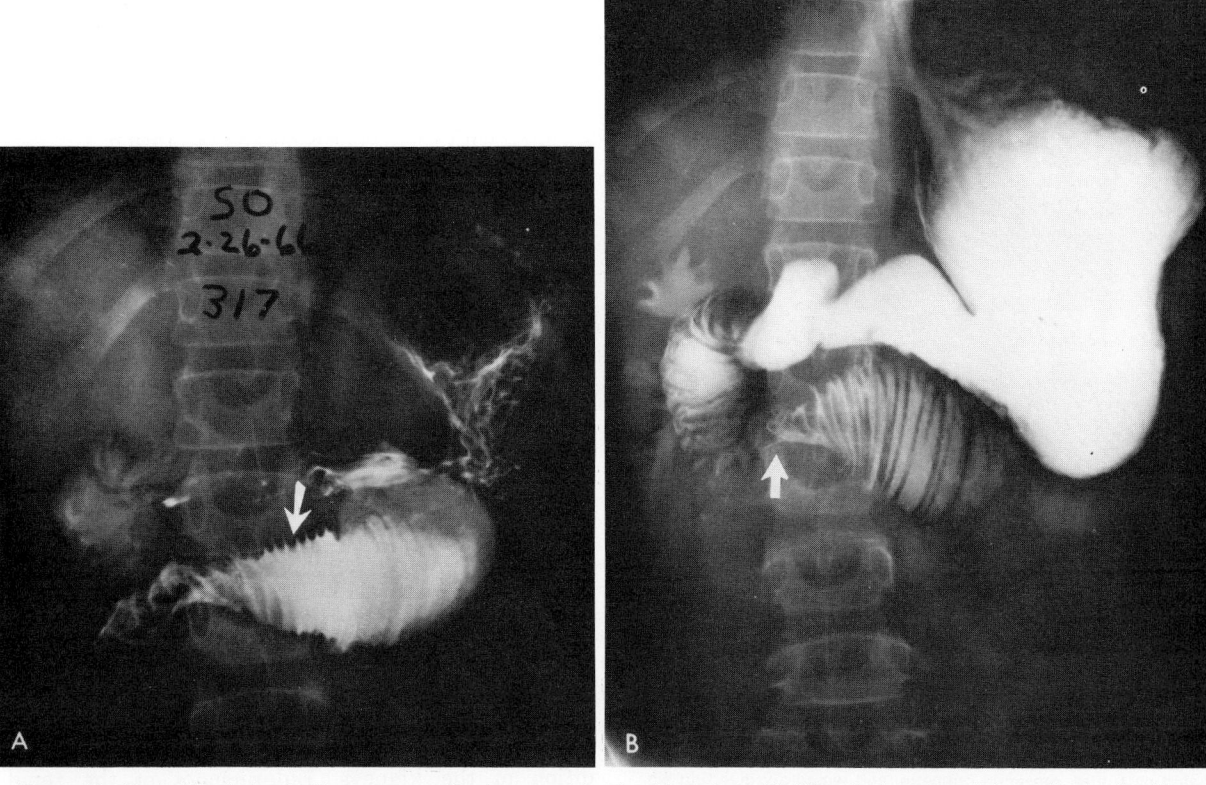

Figure 49.   Typical "coiled spring" appearance of an intramural duodenal hematoma *(A)*. When the hematoma is large, the duodenal lumen may be partially or completely obstructed *(B)*. (Courtesy of Dr. Charles Nice, Professor and Chairman, Department of Radiology, Tulane University School of Medicine.)

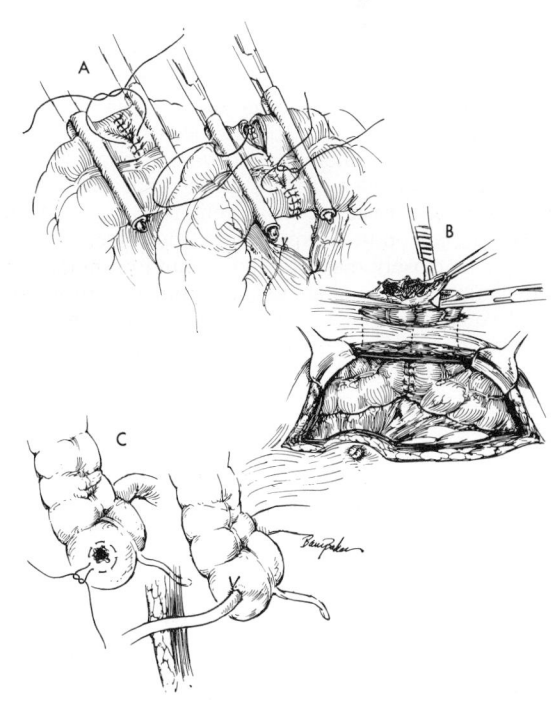

Figure 50.   Treatment of injuries to the colon. *A,* Resection and an anastomosis of an injured area. *B,* Exteriorization of the damaged colon with subsequent resection of devitalized tissue. The colostomy can be closed once the patient's condition has stabilized, usually after 2 to 3 weeks. *C,* Perforating injury of the cecum treated by tube cecostomy. (From Diagnosis and Management of Abdominal Trauma, by Jordan, G. L., and Beall, A. C., Jr., in Current Problems in Surgery, edited by Ravitch, M. M., et al. Copyright © 1971, Year Book Medical Publishers. Used by permission.)

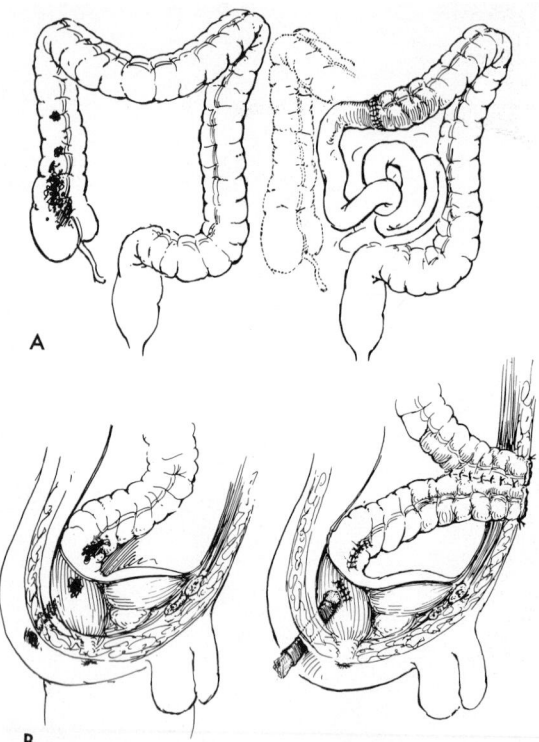

Figure 51. Additional methods for management of colon injuries. *A,* Resection of the right colon for gunshot wounds, with a primary end-to-end anastomosis. *B,* A penetrating wound of the rectum treated by suture, presacral drainage, and temporary diverting sigmoid colostomy. (From Diagnosis and Management of Abdominal Trauma, by Jordan, G. L., and Beall, A. C., Jr., in Current Problems in Surgery, edited by Ravitch, M. M., et al. Copyright © 1971, Year Book Medical Publishers. Used by permission.)

cle, or the superior mesenteric artery or any of its branches. Thrombosis associated with intimal injury should be repaired as soon as possible to prevent ischemic damage distal to the occlusion. Mesenteric blood vessels or splenic blood vessels may be safely ligated, but injuries of the superior mesenteric artery or the renal arteries must be repaired.

During abdominal exploration, the retroperitoneum should be closely inspected for expanding hematomas. Stationary hematomas usually indicate retroperitoneal contusion, but expanding hematomas may indicate severe vascular or renal injury. Expanding hematomas should always be thoroughly explored to insure the integrity of major vascular structures in the area and also to determine whether the hematoma is dissecting down from the chest. Frequently, intrathoracic aortic lacerations will dissect posteriorly behind the parietal pleura and present in a subdiaphragmatic position.

URINARY TRACT INJURY

Even though the kidneys are relatively well protected in the renal fossae, sharp blows to the flanks

are frequently associated with renal contusion or fracture. Such is not the situation with acute frontal compression of the abdomen. Since the kidneys float relatively freely, they may be thrown forward in acute deceleration. Resulting stretching of the renal artery may lead to renal arterial thrombosis. Gunshot wounds in the vicinity of the kidney may also be associated with renal contusion and laceration.

The first overt manifestation of urinary tract injury is hematuria. When the patient is severely injured, an initial urine sample should be obtained by passage of a Foley catheter into the bladder. If the urine specimen is bloody or if no urine flow is detected, damage to the urinary tract must be suspected. On the basis of urinalysis alone, it is not possible to gauge the location or the severity of such damage. In general, traumatic lesions of the urinary tract are relatively easy to diagnose, once their presence is suspected (Fig. 52).

Kidneys

Penetrating injuries near the flanks may be associated with renal contusion or lacerations. When renal injury is suspected, intravenous pyelography should be performed immediately to determine the functional capacity of both kidneys, and also to determine whether the patient has two kidneys. *It is a catastrophe to remove inadvertently a solitary kidney after traumatic injury.* Since chronically diseased kidneys are more apt to be damaged than normal kidneys, important information can also be obtained from the pyelogram about the anatomic and functional condition of the kidneys. Enlargement of the renal shadow on a routine abdominal film, extravasation of dye into the perirenal area on intravenous pyelogram (Fig. 53), and appearance of blood in the urine all indicate damage to the kidney or the upper urinary tract. Injury to the renal pelvis is often seen in association with renal injury, but ureteral injury is relatively uncommon. Interruption of the renal arteries bilaterally will lead to acute cessation of urinary output. This latter condition is best diagnosed by renal arteriography.

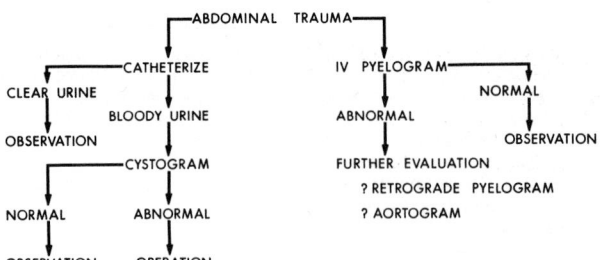

Figure 52. Flow diagram for the diagnosis of injury to the genitourinary tract. In general, patients suffering *blunt* abdominal trauma should have an intravenous pyelogram. If the patient is unable to void, he should be catheterized. In the presence of clear urine and bilateral function on an intravenous pyelogram, observation may be safely carried out. When *penetrating* injury is present, and the urine is bloody, cystography and intravenous pyelography should be performed for further evaluation of possible bladder, ureteral, and renal injuries.

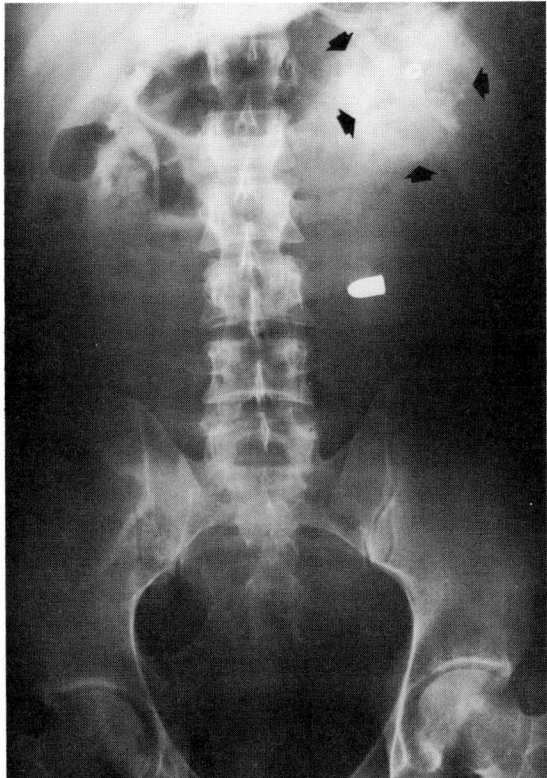

Figure 53. Typical appearance of extravasation of dye following intravenous pyelography for a gunshot injury to the left kidney. Nephrectomy was required. The bullet was in the left psoas muscle.

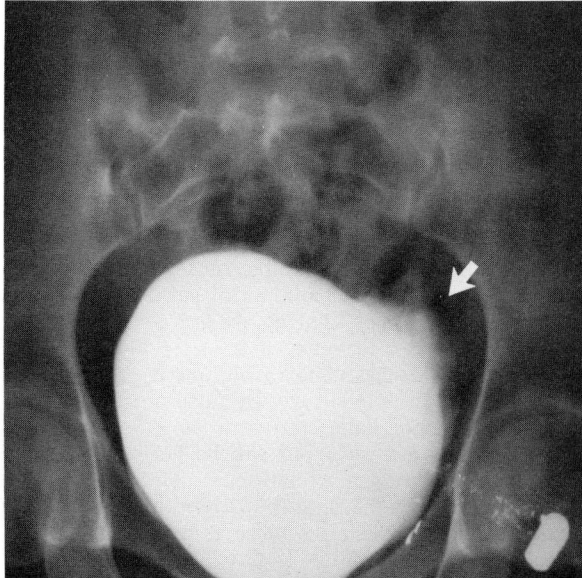

Figure 54. Laceration of urinary bladder following abdominal gunshot wound. The bullet did not penetrate the peritoneum, and the radiopaque dye appeared only in the perivesical tissues (arrow), not in the free peritoneal space.

Ureters

Ureteral injuries usually result from penetrating injury and hardly ever follow blunt abdominal trauma. Diagnosis is made when dye extravasation is noted during pyelography. Surgical repair should be done.

Bladder

Injury to the urinary bladder occurs quite commonly after compression injury of the abdomen, particularly when the compression has occurred acutely in the presence of a full bladder. Penetrating injuries in the lower abdomen may also be associated with bladder laceration (Fig. 54). To diagnose the condition, a radiopaque dye should be instilled under slight pressure into the urinary bladder through a Foley catheter. A bladder laceration will appear on x-ray as an extravasation from the bladder into the adjacent perivesical tissues (Fig. 55). Surgical repair is indicated once the diagnosis has been made.

Urethra and Seminal Vesicles

Urethral lacerations are common when the bony pelvis has been fractured, particularly when the fracture involves the pubic rami. If one experiences difficulty in passing a catheter through the urethra in an acutely injured patient and a pelvic fracture is noted

on x-ray, it may be assumed that the urethra has been torn. A suprapubic cystostomy must then be done. Frequently, difficulty in inserting a urethral catheter may be the result of urethral stricture or prostatic gland enlargement. In such cases, it may be necessary to resort to the passage of filiform catheters. Injury to the seminal vesicles as a result of blunt trauma is uncommon, but may occur. No specific therapy is indicated.

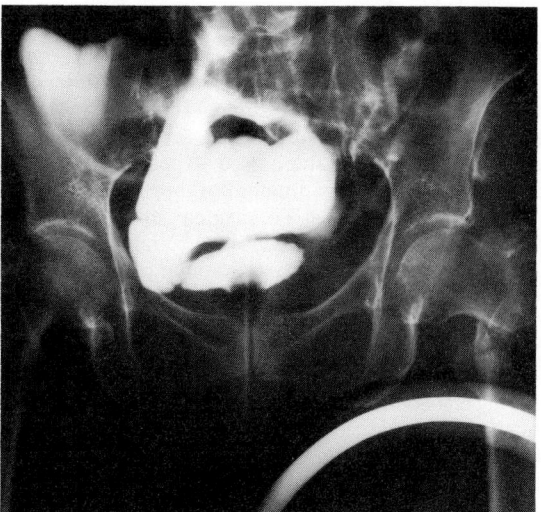

Figure 55. Rupture of bladder following blunt trauma. Appearance on cystography. Marked extravasation of the contrast medium within the peritoneal cavity is shown.

INJURIES TO THE AORTA AND VENA CAVA

Penetrating wounds of the abdominal aorta or vena cava are usually not diagnosed until operation, since the posterior peritoneum provides some degree of tamponade of the vascular wound. A retroperitoneal hematoma is usually the sign that alerts one to the possibility of a severe penetrating injury of the major vessels. Therefore, prior to dissection of a retroperitoneal hematoma, certain conditions must be met. Necessary blood and dependable routes for its administration, vascular clamps, arterial sutures, adequate assistance, and proper lighting are prerequisites to exposing the aorta and vena cava. After bleeding has been controlled, most penetrating aortic injuries can be repaired by simple suture. Because of the rapidity with which hemorrhage can occur, however, controlling bleeding until suturing can be performed often taxes all of the surgeon's faculties.

Despite the lower pressure within the vena cava, caval injuries are usually more difficult to manage than aortic injuries. This is due largely to the difficulty in obtaining proximal and distal control, the tendency of venous lacerations to extend, and the presence of great numbers of large collateral branches, i.e., lumbar veins, splenic veins, and renal veins.

Often, control of bleeding from a caval injury can be gained by finger pressure or by pressure with sponge sticks above and below the injured area. Alternatively, a tangential occlusion clamp can be applied and the injured area excluded from the remaining cava. If the bleeding point can be readily controlled, simple interrupted stitches with fine vascular sutures on an atraumatic needle may control the hemorrhage. If there is extensive injury to the vena cava below the renal veins, ligation and interruption of the vena cava may be safely done. An occasional postoperative sequela of this procedure is lower extremity edema due to venous thrombosis.

Perhaps the most difficult to treat of the injuries of the aorta and vena cava are those occurring between the diaphragm and the renal vessels. In this location, these blood vessels are relatively inaccessible because of the costal margin and the overlying viscera, including stomach, pancreas, and mesentery. Standard abdominal incisions do not suffice to approach these areas, and a thoracoabdominal incision may be needed. On the right side, good exposure can be obtained by reflecting the duodenum and right colon anteriorly (Fig. 56). A better surgical approach to the proximal aorta and vena cava is through a left thoracoabdominal incision, with the spleen, pancreas, and stomach reflected anteriorly (Fig. 57). Another approach for control of hemorrhage from injuries to the proximal vena cava, particularly in that portion adjacent to the liver and involving the hepatic veins, has been described by Blaisdell and his associates. This consists of the addition of a thoracotomy, cannulation of the right atrium, and insertion of a long tube with a balloon attached, which is advanced retrograde into the area of injury. Inflation of the balloon will provide tamponade at the site of the tear of the vena cava but will still permit flow from the lower extremities and kidneys and to the heart. After repair of the caval in-

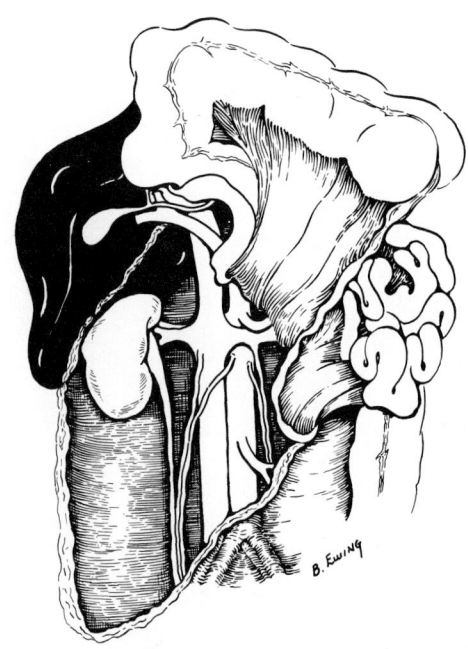

Figure 56. Approach to the upper abdominal aorta and inferior vena cava by reflection of the duodenum and colon. (From Weichert, R. F., III, and Hewitt, R. L.: J. Trauma, *10*:649, 1970.)

jury, the tube can be removed and the atriotomy closed. During repair of any vena caval laceration, care must be exercised to prevent *air embolism*.

Air Embolism

When the head is elevated and penetrating injuries are present in the neck or upper thorax, passage of air into the venous system and air embolism is an ever-present danger. Tracheal, bronchial, or pulmonary injuries and tension pneumothorax may also lead to air embolism. Intraoperative air embolism may occur when the patient is either prone or in the Trendelenburg position, and there are injuries about the liver, hepatic veins, and upper abdominal vena cava. Air embolism occurring under these circumstances results from the negative intrathoracic pressure created on inspiration. Such negative pressure sucks air through the injury site into the veins. The air then passes into the right atrium and the pulmonary circulation. Cardiac output is thereby compromised, and small vessel circulation is blocked. Air embolism may also occur in injured patients when air is inadvertently pumped into the vascular system from a transfusion bottle or an autotransfusion apparatus. Entry of a large amount of air into the venous system leads to sudden vascular collapse. Passage of air bubbles into the coronary circulation usually causes ventricular fibrillation and sudden death. In addition to vascular collapse, classic physical signs of venous air embolism include a peculiar hissing sound over the precordium followed almost immediately by a churning noise in the heart.

Transcutaneous ultrasonic cardiac auscultation with a Doppler flowmeter is the most sensitive technique for detecting air embolism. When an air bubble passes through an ultrasonic beam directed through the right atrium or ventricle, amounts of air as small as 0.25 ml. will lead to a shift in the audible frequency.

Obviously, air embolism should be prevented. Penetrating neck injuries should be tightly sealed, and if possible, patients with such injuries should be put into slight Trendelenburg position. Venous pressure in the upper part of the body will then be greater than negative intrathoracic pressure on inspiration. Surgical procedures about the liver, hepatic veins, or inferior vena cava should be performed with the upper part of the body slightly elevated or only after the proximal vena cava has been occluded. When there are injuries of the thorax with damage to the respiratory system, care should be taken to insure that air under pressure does not accumulate in closed spaces. If it is necessary for blood transfusions to be pumped in under positive pressure, they should be watched closely to insure that air is not inadvertently pumped into the venous system from the blood administration set. Though not applicable during massive autotransfusion, the use of plastic transfusion packs will partially obviate this problem.

Once the diagnosis of air embolism is made, a central venous catheter should be passed quickly into the right atrium. Air at the site may then be mechanically aspirated. When air is distal to the right atrium or bubbles have passed into the arterial circulation, hy-

perbaric oxygenation is an effective means for resolving all intracirculatory air.

EXTREMITY INJURIES

Traumatic penetration of an extremity, with hemorrhage due to massive disruption of major blood vessels, constitutes the only situation in which extremity injuries may be immediately life-threatening. Sharp transection or complete avulsion of an extremity may also involve major blood loss, but if treatment is prompt, there is not immediate threat to life.

All *penetrating injuries* of the extremities, and especially those caused by high-velocity bullets, should be cleansed and meticulously debrided. Soft tissue injuries should be cleansed of foreign material and debrided extensively to the point where normal muscle that bleeds on being cut is encountered. However, *low velocity missile injuries produced by most civilian handguns rarely require such extensive débridement.* No maneuver contributes as much to the prevention of tetanus or gas gangrene infection as complete débridement of all devitalized muscle tissue. Because of the possibility of hidden lacerations or development of arteriovenous fistulas, injuries near all major blood vessels should be thoroughly explored. If blood vessels have been lacerated, these should be adequately debrided and then closed primarily if enough length can be obtained. When primary closure is not possible, a strip of autogenous saphenous vein will serve as an adequate arterial replacement.

Bullet wounds, particularly those resulting from missiles that deliver large quantities of energy to the tissues, are frequently associated with long bone fractures that result when the long bones are struck by the bullet. These fractures should always be treated as open (compound) fractures. Débridement must be adequate to insure that minimal contamination persists.

Blunt injury to the extremities almost always results in induction of long bone fractures. Initially, simple (single fracture line) or comminuted (several fracture lines and several bony fragments) fractures should be stabilized as simply as possible. Bony fractures may be reduced at almost any time during the initial 24 hours after injury, and other more serious injuries take priority over treatment of fractures. Temporary splints may be applied until other more pressing procedures have been performed, and proper reduction done at a later time. Open reduction of fractures should always be performed under sterile conditions in the operating room. When possible, general anesthesia rather than local anesthesia should be used for simple reductions, with the anesthetic introduced directly into the fracture site. The risk of infecting the fracture hematoma by this latter technique is very high, and when such infection occurs, osteomyelitis and nonunion result. Compound or "open" fractures (bone exposed to air), whether simple or comminuted, should be adequately cleansed and debrided and then reduced. Introduction of metallic foreign bodies into the area of an open fracture to aid in stabilization is contraindicated because of the possibility of infection.

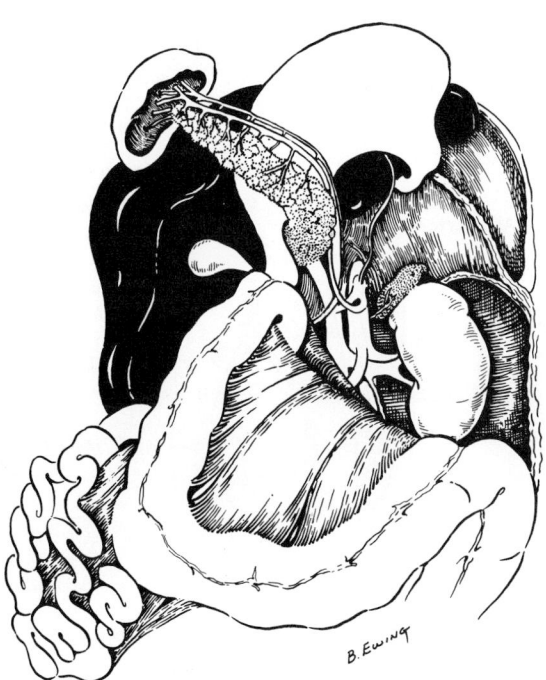

Figure 57. Alternative approach to more proximal areas of the aorta and vena cava through a left thoracoabdominal incision. The spleen, pancreas, and stomach are elevated anteriorly. The splenic flexure is deflected inferiorly. Adequate exposure of the upper abdominal viscera and vascular structures can be obtained in this fashion. (From Hewitt, R. L. *In* Ballinger, W. F., and Drapanas, T.: Practice of Surgery—Current Review. St. Louis, The C. V. Mosby Co., 1972.)

Peripheral Nerve Injury

Peripheral nerves are most often injured by direct laceration. Clean, fresh lacerations may be reapproximated immediately. When the wound is heavily contaminated and macerated, limited débridement to preserve severed nerve ends and delayed reapproximation may be the best management.

Peripheral nerve injury often occurs in association with certain fractures. Direct injury by the bony fragments to both the median and radial nerves frequently accompanies supracondylar fractures of the humerus. In these cases, the nerves are usually bruised rather than severed, and proper reapproximation of the humerus usually leads to disappearance of neurologic signs. Supracondylar fractures of the femur may lead to similar injury of the tibial nerve, but more often damage to the popliteal artery is the more severe injury and the one that necessitates surgical exploration. Fractures of the lateral tibial plateau may be associated with contusion of the common peroneal nerve. Proper reduction of these fractures usually leads to complete recovery of nerve function, but more severe damage may result in a permanent foot drop.

Stabs or gunshot wounds to the base of the neck or pelvis that penetrate the brachial or pelvic plexus, respectively, usually lead to permanent neurologic damage. When the bullet is of large caliber or high velocity, concussion damage may also occur to any nerve plexus or peripheral nerve near the bullet's path. It is unusual for such concussion to lead to complete devascularization, and complete recovery of nerve function may be expected.

Limb Reimplantation

Recently developed techniques now make it possible to reimplant severed extremities. When such a patient is seen in the emergency room, the ambulance driver or other attendants must immediately be sent back to the scene of the accident to retrieve the amputated part. The severed limb should be adequately cleansed and the wound edge debrided. At the same time, arterial perfusion of the limb with a solution of dextran 40 (Rheomacrodex), heparin, and normal saline should be started so as to remove formed blood elements and prevent intravascular clotting. The limb should be immersed in a container of ice water to reduce muscle metabolism. Reimplantation is accomplished in the operating room under strictly sterile conditions as soon as possible (see also Chapter 45).

PERIPHERAL VASCULAR INJURIES

The increased salvage of life and limb after acute vascular injuries during the past three decades is largely attributable to the principles of diagnosis and therapy evolved from military experience. In civilian practice, diagnostic problems continue to exist largely because of differences in patient populations and in mechanisms of injury and because few physicians treat a large enough number of injuries to gain adequate experience. Of 226 arterial injuries encountered during a 30-year period at the Charity Hospital of Louisiana in New Orleans, penetrating arterial injuries occurred in 90 per cent of the patients, while blunt trauma produced injury in 10 per cent (Fig. 58). Penetration, perforation, transection, and lateral lacerations are the usual forms of injury among patients with penetrating wounds, whereas fracture of the intima with obstruction and thrombosis is the usual type of arterial injury following blunt trauma.

Four types of arterial injuries may be produced by penetrating or blunt trauma (Figs. 59 to 62). Injuries to major arteries should always be repaired, if possible. Results of suture repair of the injury appear to be superior to results after ligation. Other important factors that influence the end result in arterial injury include: (1) time lag, (2) practical difficulty, such as the experience of the surgeon in the management of vascular injuries; (3) associated injuries; (4) site of the wound; (5) type of injury of lesion; and (6) infection. The phenomenon of edema following obstruction of arterial flow has been well documented. Following prolonged ischemia, incision of the fascia (fasciotomy) to decompress muscle will often prevent muscle necrosis. Care should be taken to insure that *all* fascial compartments have been incised. During the Korean War, notable progress was made in the repair of large defects in injured arteries when vein autografts were

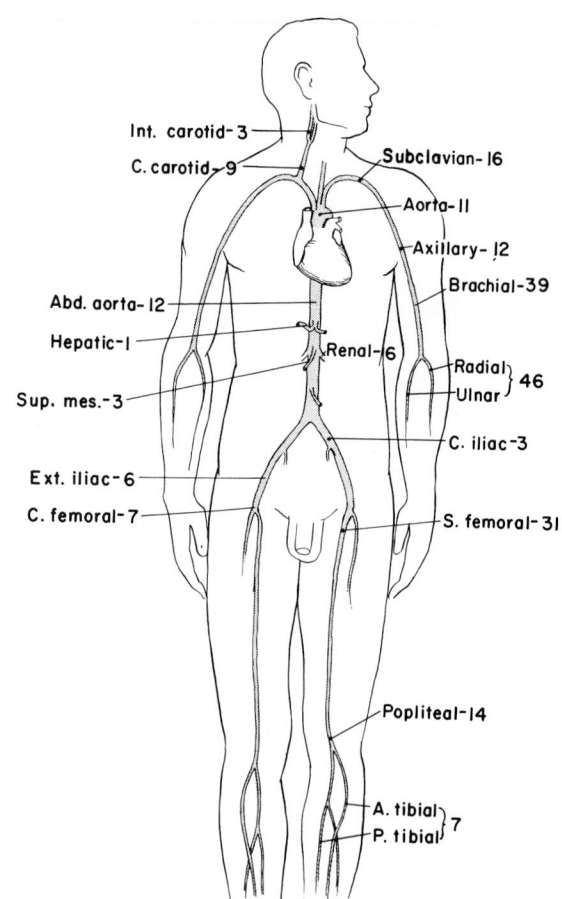

Figure 58. Distribution of 226 arterial injuries encountered at Charity Hospital. (From Drapanas, T., Hewitt, R. L., Weichert, R. F., III, and Smith, A. D.: Ann. Surg., *172*:351, 1970.)

LATERAL TEAR

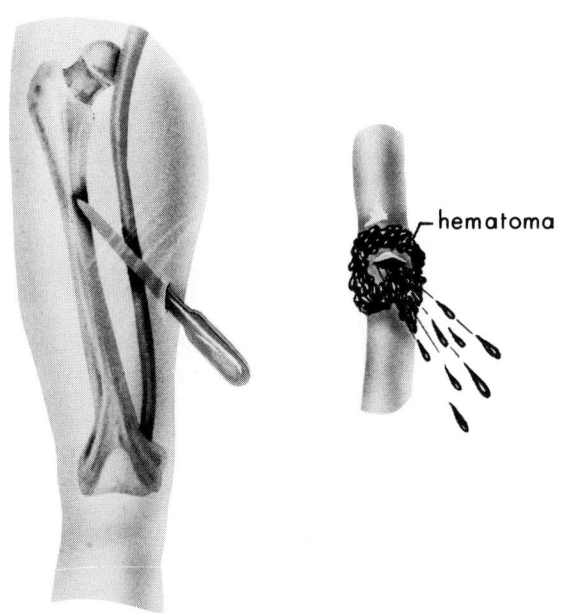

Figure 59. Illustration of major arterial injury with large pulsating hematoma.

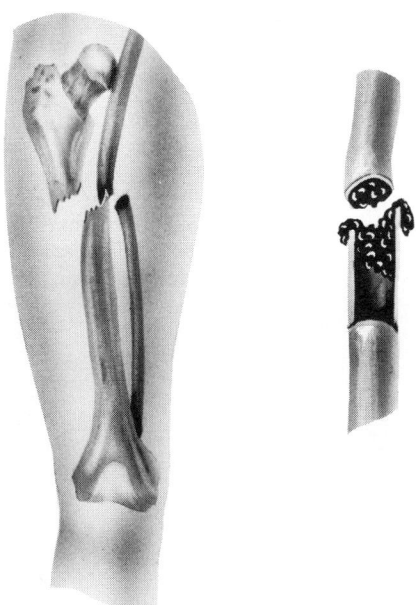

Figure 60. Avulsion and transection of major artery due to displaced bone fragment. Often in such patients there is no large hematoma because of retraction of the cut ends and cessation of bleeding.

used for patients with acute injury. Reduction of time lag also led to further improvement in surgical results.

In Vietnam, improved results have been attributable to two main factors: a further reduction in time lag by efficient helicopter evacuation and the availability of surgeons experienced in vascular surgery. While arterial injuries in Vietnam have been more serious than in the past because of the use of very high-velocity bullets, early recognition and prompt repair appear to

most influence successful management of patients with acute arterial injuries once they reach the hospital. If immediate repairs of all acute arterial injuries are performed, the development of serious complications, including arteriovenous fistulas and false aneurysms, can largely be prevented.

Careful examination may often result in the diagnosis of unsuspected arterial injury. Ischemia distal to an arterial injury may be observed in only one quarter

Figure 61. Contusion of major artery by bullet. Shock waves from high-velocity missile in close proximity to the artery produce an area of contusion with intimal damage. Treatment consists of resection of at least 1 to 2 cm. on both sides of the contused area with either anastomosis or interposition of a vein graft.

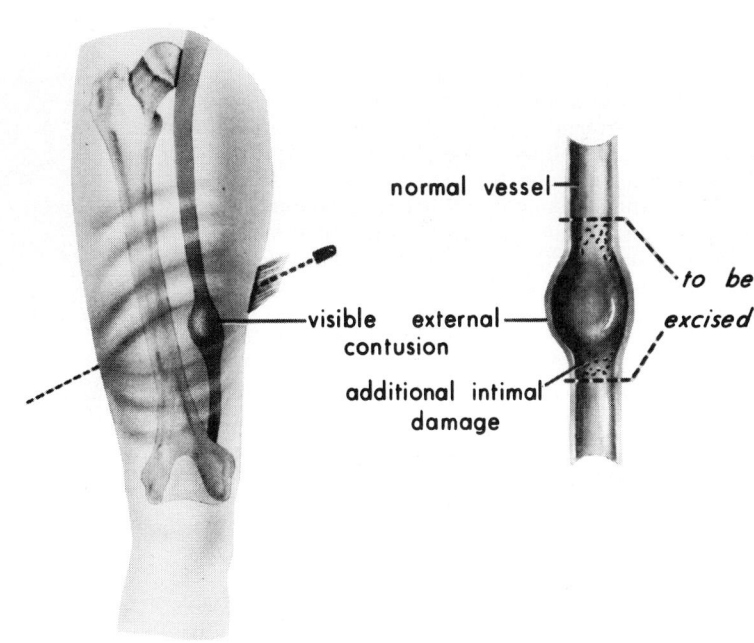

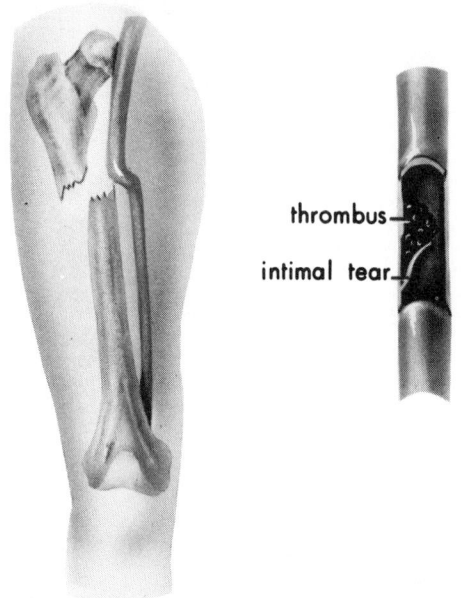

Figure 62. Intimal tear due to stretching of a major artery. The muscular coat and adventitia remain intact. The intimal tear presents as a flap, with resultant thrombosis. Treatment consists of arteriotomy, suture of the intimal tear, and evacuation of the clot.

tween injury and successful repair and may also be related to venous injury or thrombosis or both. When a major vessel injury has been present for more than 6 hours and a successful arterial repair has been performed, a concomitant fasciotomy should always be done. Fasciotomies should be extensive enough to include all fascial compartments within the extremity. In the lower extremity, where this complication is most apt to occur, fasciotomies should be done into all four compartments (Fig. 67).

When one suspects that a major vascular injury exists, operative exploration should be performed even though the arteriogram may be normal and distal pulses are present.

Disruption of the intima of the aorta just distal to the mesenteric artery, with intimal dissection, thrombosis, and occlusion of the distal aorta, is a relatively uncommon aortic injury and is usually due to blunt trauma. Treatment consists of repair or insertion of an aortofemoral bypass graft (Fig. 68).

Renal artery thrombosis is also apt to occur after blunt abdominal trauma (Fig. 69). If the diagnosis can be made early, blood flow to the kidneys may be successfully restored. When there is extensive renal injury and repair has been delayed, nephrectomy with later renal transplantation may be necessary.

to one third of patients with aortic wounds, while the remainder of patients with such injuries will have palpable pulses beyond the injury. Inferior vena caval or aortic injuries are usually accompanied by the presence of distal pulses and apparently adequate distal blood flow.

Arteriography is helpful in the diagnosis and determination of the site of most arterial injuries and may also provide information of use in choosing the surgical approach (Figs. 63 to 65). It should be done without delay when the patient's condition and the presence of active bleeding do not contraindicate its performance. Arteriography may also be of help in the evaluation of an arterial repair after operation.

The severity of an arterial injury often determines the type of arterial repair to be performed and to an extent may also influence the ultimate result (Fig. 66). Most injuries can be repaired by simple suture or resection and anastomosis. When an anastomosis cannot be made without tension, an autogenous vein graft should be used. Recognition of the importance of preventing tension on the arterial suture line has resulted in increasing use of vein grafts among civilian as well as military casualities. Synthetic grafts such as Dacron and Teflon should be avoided in traumatic vascular injuries of the extremities because of the high thrombosis rate and the increased incidence of infection.

A distressing complication frequently encountered after successful vascular reconstruction is the development of marked edema of the extremity. This most often occurs in the lower extremities and may progress to produce necrosis of entire muscle groups. It is caused by ischemic damage to capillaries and muscles during the period of interruption of the blood flow be-

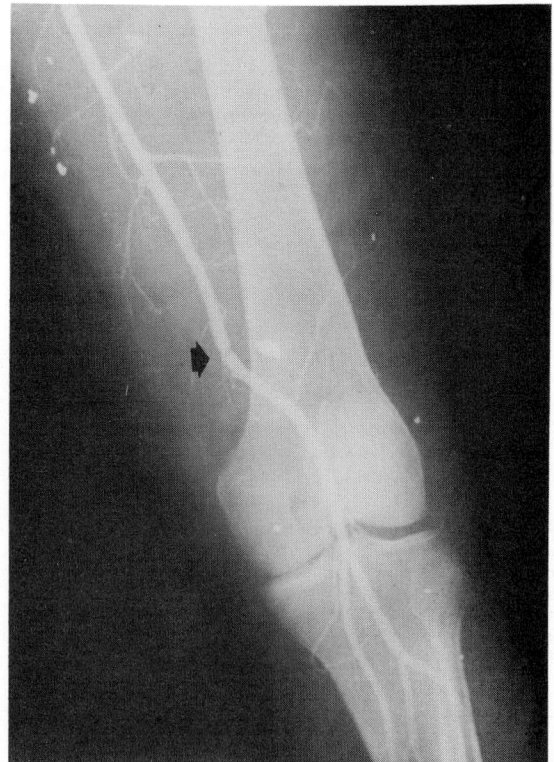

Figure 63. Injury by .22 caliber bullet of the lower femoral artery at the region of adductor canal. Arteriography showed the *distal* pulses to be normal, but the area of arterial injury is shown (arrow) adjacent to the bullet. The ankle pulses disappeared shortly after this. Exploration of the artery revealed marked contusion and intimal fracture, which required resection and anastomosis.

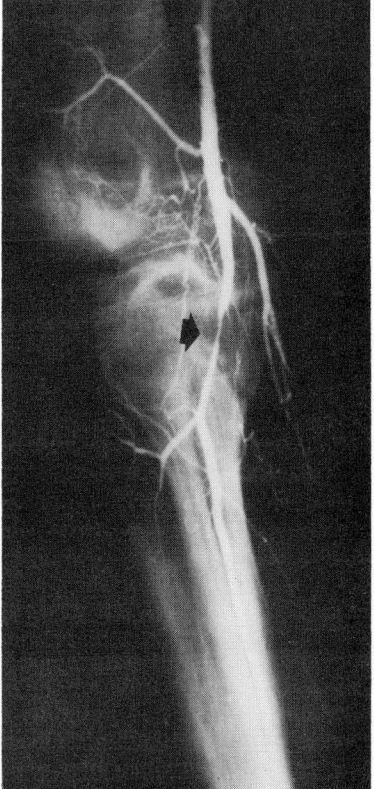

Figure 64. Rupture of the tibial plateau with arterial injury. This was misinterpreted initially as spasm of the popliteal artery (arrow). Within a few hours, however, ischemic changes noted in the lower extremity forced the decision for exploration. An intimal tear was present that required resuture of the intima and evacuation of the hematoma. We now feel that all such injuries should be promptly explored.

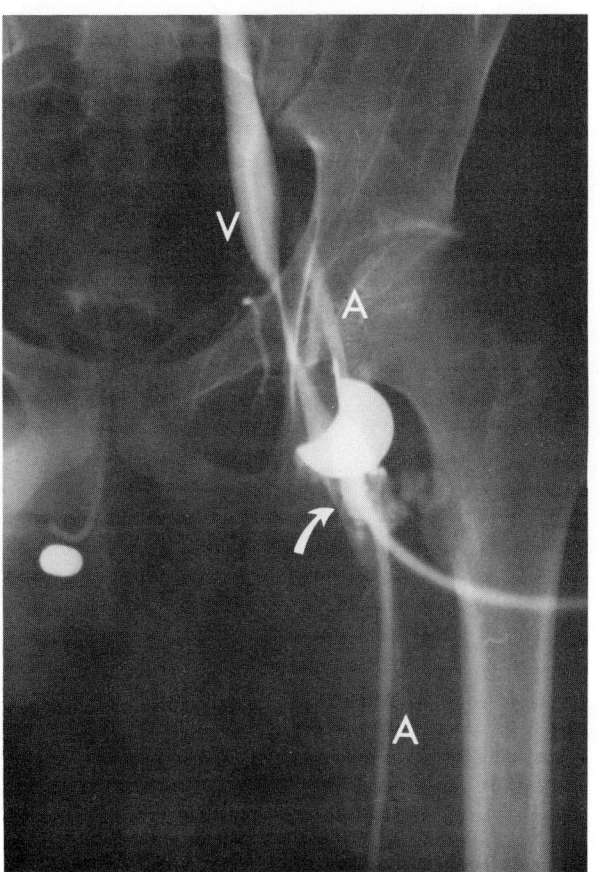

Figure 65. Acute arteriovenous fistula between the femoral artery and vein following a gunshot wound. The needle through which the radiopaque dye is injected is present in the femoral artery (A). The common femoral vein and the external iliac vein (V) opacify almost immediately, owing to passage of the dye through an acute arteriovenous fistula (arrow). A small hematoma is present in the area of the arterial injury and the .32 caliber bullet can be seen lodged in the right buttock. Treatment consisted of emergency repair of the arterial and venous injuries. Recovery was complete.

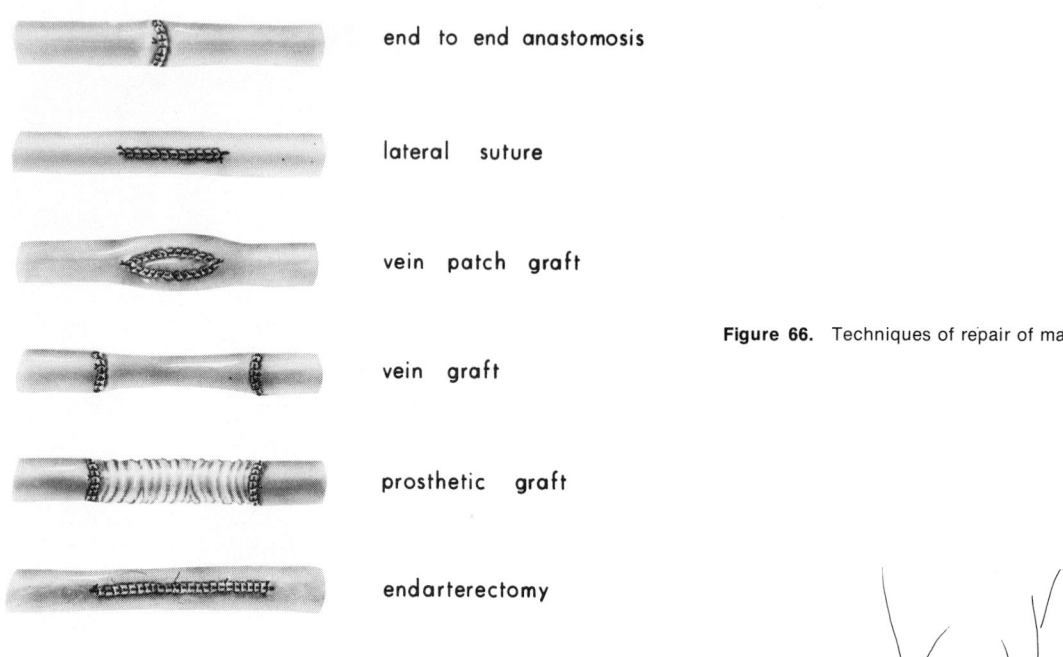

end to end anastomosis

lateral suture

vein patch graft

vein graft

prosthetic graft

endarterectomy

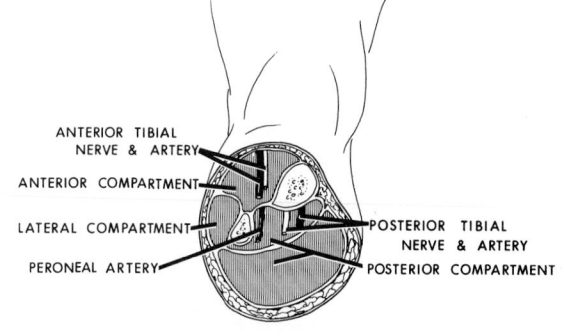

Figure 66. Techniques of repair of major arterial injuries.

Figure 67. Fascial compartments of the lower limb. The four compartments are clearly shown. Fasciotomy is required in major vascular injuries to the lower extremity, particularly if reconstruction is delayed beyond 6 hours after injury. (From Hewitt, R. L.: Milt. Med., *134*:617, 1969.)

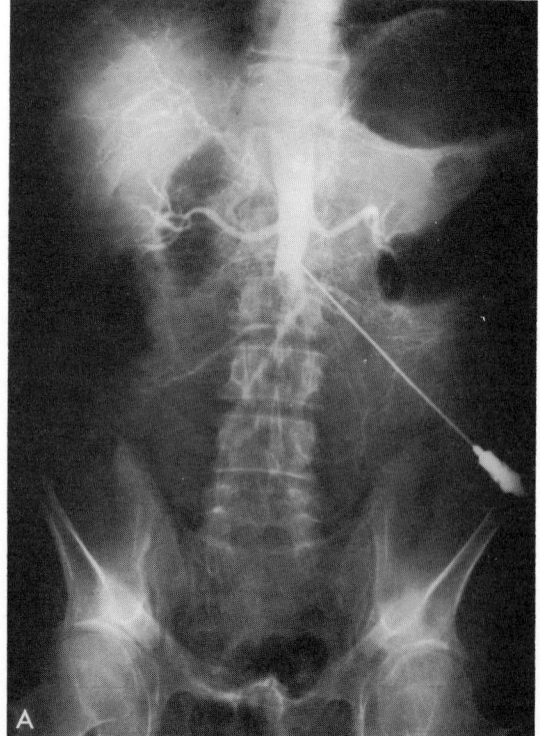

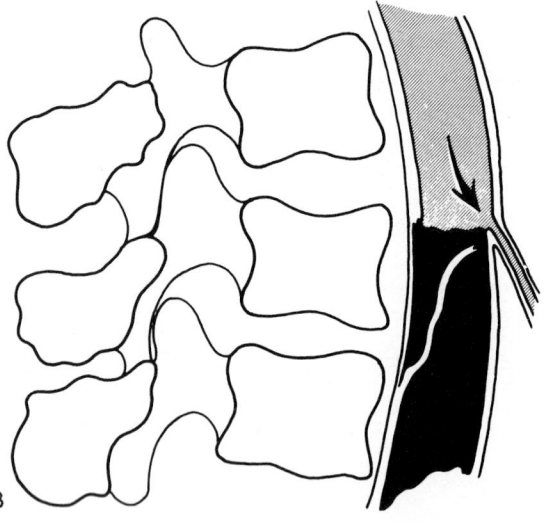

Figure 68. An acute flexion injury following a motorcycle accident resulted in thrombosis of the abdominal aorta distal to the renal arteries, shown by translumbar arteriography *(A)*. *B,* Diagram of the mechanism of injury, with elevation of an intimal flap and thrombosis. Treatment in this patient consisted of aortofemoral bypass necessitated by extensive atherosclerosis in the remaining aorta. (From Drapanas, T., Hewitt, R. L., Weichert, R. F., III, and Smith, A. D.: Ann. Surg., *172*:351, 1970.)

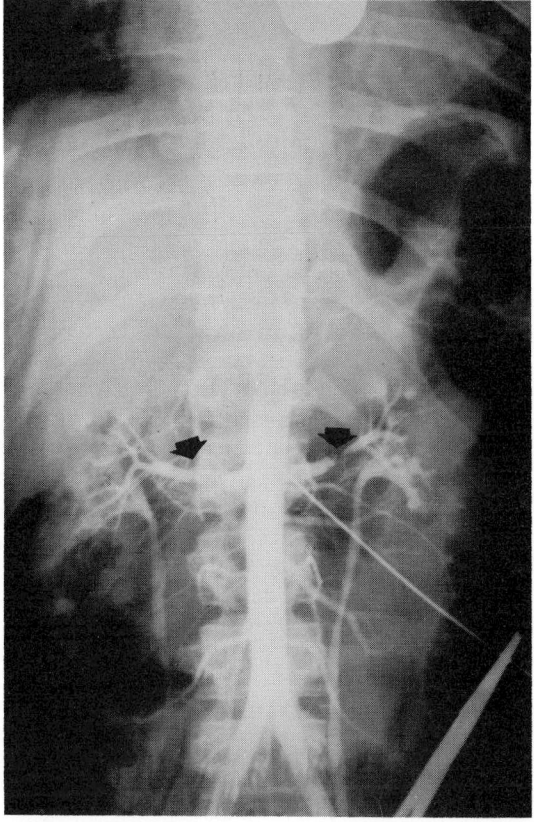

Figure 69. Avulsion of both renal arteries (arrows) following deceleration injury. This patient presented with hematuria. Emergency surgery with reconstruction of renal arteries was required. (From Drapanas, T., Hewitt, R. L., Weichert, R. F., III, and Smith, A. D.: Ann. Surg., *172*:351, 1970.)

TETANUS PROPHYLAXIS

Tetanus occurs only rarely in acutely injured patients admitted to hospitals today. The great decrease in the incidence of tetanus in the past 50 years is the result of a massive educational drive and immunization courses initiated by local and national medical societies and by the United States Armed Forces.

The Subcommittee on Prophylaxis Against Tetanus of the Committee on Trauma of the American College of Surgeons has published specific recommendations for tetanus immunization that should be strictly followed (Figs. 70 and 71). Regardless of the active immunization status of the patient, however, immediate meticulous surgical care of all wounds, including removal of all devitalized tissue and foreign bodies, is absolutely essential. It is then the responsibility of the attending physician to determine whether the patient requires prophylaxis for tetanus. Every patient should receive tetanus toxoid intramuscularly at the time of injury, as an initial immunizing dose or as a booster for a previously immunized patient, unless he has received a booster or has completed his initial immunization within the past 12 months. Since antigen concentration varies in different products, close attention should be paid to information available on each vial of toxoid.

For passive immunization, the prophylactic dose of human tetanus immune globulin now regularly used in adults is 250 units intramuscularly. For wounds in children, the dosage should be calculated in terms of body weight (4.0 units per kilogram). When wounds in adults are severe, neglected, or old, a dose of 500 units of human tetanus immune globulin is advisable. In all cases in which the injury is severe and the risk of potential tetanus infection is higher, a dose in excess of that recommended may be indicated, and antibiotic prophylaxis may also be advisable. Should infection continue, a repeat of the initial dose after 3 weeks may be indicated. *It cannot be stressed too strongly that tetanus is the result of a local infection; therefore, proper initial wound care is of paramount importance in avoiding the development of this disease.* Human tetanus immune globulin is only adjunctive to this procedure.

Prior to the availability of human tetanus immune globulin, equine antitoxin was used as the sole measure for passive human tetanus immunization. In spite of skin testing, marked sensitivity reactions with anaphylaxis and death often resulted. To overcome this problem, bovine antitoxin was often substituted for the equine antitoxin; however, it was found that severe cross-sensitivity existed in about 50 per cent of patients who received the bovine material. Both of these antitoxins were foreign proteins that were rapidly destroyed, and some question existed as to their effectiveness and duration of activity. Desensitization of some patients was attempted, but this probably resulted in rapid inactivation of the antitoxin, and little or no effect was produced.

Since human tetanus immune globulin is now widely available (Homo-Tet, Savage Laboratories;

Specific measures for patients with wounds

I. Previously immunized individuals

A. When the patient has been actively immunized within the past ten[2] years:
1. To the great majority, give 0.5 cc of adsorbed tetanus toxoid[1] as a booster unless it is certain that the patient has received a booster within the previous five years.
2. To those with severe, neglected, or old (more than 24 hours) tetanus-prone wounds, give 0.5 cc of adsorbed tetanus toxoid[1] unless it is certain that the patient has received a booster within the previous year.

B. When the patient has been actively immunized more than ten[2] years previously:
1. To the great majority, give 0.5 cc of adsorbed tetanus toxoid[1].
2. To those with severe, neglected, or old (more than 24 hours) tetanus-prone wounds:
   a) Give 0.5 cc of adsorbed tetanus toxoid[1] [3],
   b) Give 250 units[4] of tetanus immune globulin (human)[3],
   c) Consider providing oxytetracycline or penicillin.

II. Individuals NOT previously immunized

A. With clean minor wounds in which tetanus is most unlikely, give 0.5 cc of adsorbed tetanus toxoid[1] (initial immunizing dose).

B. With all other wounds:
1. Give 0.5 cc of adsorbed tetanus toxoid[1] (initial immunizing dose)[3],
2. Give 250 units[4] of tetanus immune globulin (human)[3],
3. Consider providing oxytetracycline or penicillin.

NOTE: With different preparations of toxoid, the volume of a single booster dose should be modified as stated on the package label.

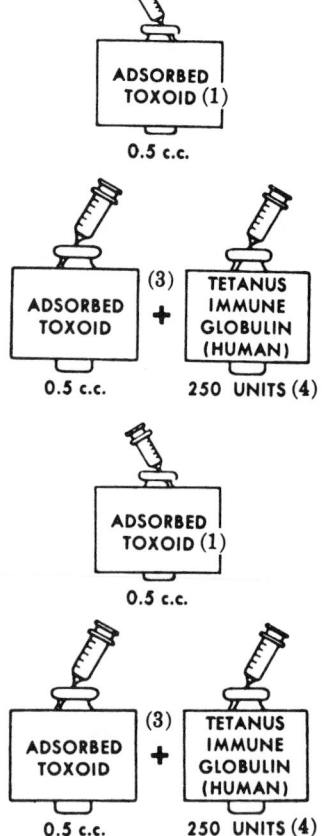

(1) The Public Health Service Advisory Committee on Immunization Practices in 1972 recommended DTP (diphtheria and tetanus toxoids combined with pertussis vaccine) for basic immunization in infants and children from two months through the sixth year of age, and Td (combined tetanus and diphtheria toxoids: adult type) for basic immunization of those over six years of age. For the latter group, Td toxoid was recommended for routine or wound boosters; but, if there is any reason to suspect hypersensitivity to the diphtheria component, tetanus toxoid (T) should be substituted for Td.
(*Morbidity and Mortality Weekly Report, Vol. 21, No. 25, National Communicable Disease Center*)

(2) Some authorities advise six rather than 10 years, particularly for patients with severe, neglected, or old (more than 24 hours) tetanus-prone wounds.

(3) Use different syringes, needles, and sites of injection.

(4) In severe, neglected, or old (more than 24 hours) tetanus-prone wounds, 500 units of tetanus immune globulin (human) are advisable.

PRECAUTIONS regarding passive immunization with tetanus antitoxin (equine):

If the patient is not sensitive to tetanus antitoxin (equine), and if the decision is made to administer it for passive immunization, give at least 3000 units.

Do not administer tetanus antitoxin (equine) except when tetanus immune globulin (human) is not available within 24 hours, and only if the possibility of tetanus outweighs the danger of reaction to heterologous tetanus antitoxin.

Before using tetanus antitoxin (equine), question the patient for a history of allergy and test for sensitivity. If the patient is sensitive to tetanus antitoxin (equine), do not use it, as the danger of anaphylaxis probably outweighs the danger of tetanus; rely on penicillin or oxytetracycline. Do not attempt desensitization, as it is not worthwhile.

Figure 70. Recommendations of Committee on Trauma, American College of Surgeons, for tetanus prophylaxis. (From "A guide to prophylaxis against tetanus in wound management." Bull. Am. Coll. Surg., 57:33, 1972.)

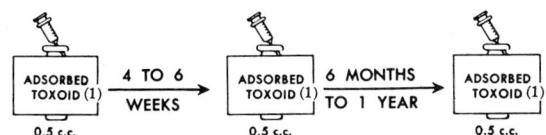

Figure 71. Technique for active immunization of patients with tetanus. (From "A guide to prophylaxis against tetanus in wound management." Bull. Am. Coll. Surg., 57:32, 1972.)

Hyper-Tet, Cutter Laboratories; IMMU-tetanus, Parke, Davis; Pro-Tet, Lederle Laboratories; Tetanus Immune Globulin, Wyeth Laboratories and Armour Pharmaceutical), and because of the critical danger of anaphylaxis, administration of antitoxin of animal origin is currently contraindicated unless human tetanus immune globulin is unavailable.

SELECTED REFERENCES

Ballinger, W. F., II, Rutherford, R. B., and Zuidema, G. D.: The Management of Trauma, 2nd ed. Philadelphia, W. B. Saunders Company, 1973, p. 795.
This book is a revision of an earlier edition, and the same high standards are maintained. There is excellent basic and detailed information on the pathophysiology of changes in traumatic injury. Not only is the type large and clear and the sentence structure easy to understand, but also the illustrations are profuse and highly illustrative of the points that are made. The chapter on the pathophysiology of shock remains outstanding, with a detailed discussion of the modern concepts of shock and shock therapy. The chapters dealing with injury to specialized sensory organ systems are unique to this book and contain numerous photographs and diagrams.

Beyer, J. C. (Ed.): Wound Ballistics. Washington, D.C., Department of the Army (Office of the Surgeon General), 1963.
During the interim between World Wars I and II, active research on a probable mechanism of wound production by high-velocity missiles was conducted. The need for more data on battle wounds was recognized by the Conference on Missile Casualties at the Division of Medical Sciences of the National Research Council in the fall of 1943, and a recommendation was made to the Surgeon General that a battle casualty survey team be organized. This book represents a detailed presentation of the team's findings. Indeed, the editor was the Chief of the Battle Casualty Survey Team in Korea. Excellent detailed descriptions are given of ballistic characteristics of wounding agents, mechanisms of wounding, and pathologic findings in many soldiers killed during World War II and in Korea. There are numerous illustrations of various types of firearms, missiles, and effects of various missiles on tissues, both in the experimental laboratory and on the battlefield.

Blaisdell, F. W., and Schlobohm, R. M.: The respiratory distress syndrome: A review. Surgery, 74:251–262, 1973.
This excellent review by an outstanding authority was the keynote address at the 34th Annual Meeting of the Society of University Surgeons on February 8-10, 1973. Pathologic and physiological changes of the adult respiratory distress syndrome are described, and recommended treatment is presented. The principal feature in treatment consists of positive-pressure ventilation. If progressive pulmonary deterioration occurs on intermittent positive-pressure ventilation, positive end-expiratory pressure (PEEP) may be indicated. The exact etiology of this syndrome is still controversial, but positive-pressure ventilation represents a major advance in treatment. This paper is necessary reading for all surgeons and medical students.

Committee on Trauma, American College of Surgeons: Early care of the Injured Patient. Philadelphia, W. B. Saunders, Company, 1972, p. 441.
This monograph is a ready reference for physicians on the care of severely injured patients and for use in the emergency department and in the hospital. It contains sections on injury assessment, resuscitation, and mass casualty management. Excellent individual chapters encompass emergency therapy of all types of injuries to specific anatomic areas. The section on fractures and dislocations is particularly recommended. This easy-to-read, concise monograph should be in the library of all medical students and all physicians who deal with severely injured patients.

Finck, P. A.: Ballistic and forensic pathologic aspects of missile wounds. Conversion between Anglo-American and metric-system units. Milit. Med., 130:545, 1965.
This excellent paper provides a means of interpreting and converting some of the various factors involved in the kinetic energy of projectiles, and includes useful conversion tables. Such data are of great value in the interpretation of gunshot wounds. Representative cases are presented that illustrate that tissue damage produced by a projectile is related to the character of the tissue struck; the shape, components, weight, and velocity of the missile; and the interface presentation of the bullet and the surface struck.

LoCicero, J., Tajima, T., and Drapanas, T.: A half century of experience in the management of colon injuries: Changing concepts. J. Trauma, 15:575, 1975.
A total of 773 patients who sustained colon injuries during the period between 1927 and 1974 were reviewed. Mortality from colon injuries declined steadily from 68 per cent during the initial 15-year period of the study to 9 per cent during the last 15-year period of the study. Three methods of therapy were used: (1) primary repair, (2) repair with proximal colostomy, and (3) exteriorization. During the last 15 years primary repair was used in 44 per cent of the patients; repair with proximal decompressive procedure was utilized in 22 per cent; and exteriorization was performed in 33 per cent of the patients. The selective use of primary repair was associated with lower mortality, fewer complications, and a shorter hospital stay. A plea is made for the selective use of primary repair of colon injuries in patients in good general condition when the local injury to the colon appears to warrant such an approach. Colon injuries associated with extensive involvement of the colon and mesentery, including devascularization, are still best treated by exteriorization or resection and colostomy.

Moore, F. D., Lyons, J. H., Jr., Pierce, E. C., Jr., Morgan, A. P., Jr., Drinker, P. A., MacArthur, J. D., and Dammin, G. J.: Posttraumatic Pulmonary Insufficiency. Philadelphia, W. B. Saunders Company, 1969.
The cause of death in previously young healthy patients who have been acutely injured is often a peculiar, progressive, and highly lethal form of respiratory failure. The purpose of this excellent monograph was "to assemble the clinical syndrome as it is seen in patients after resuscitation from tissue injury." The syndrome has been divided into four relatively distinct phases: (1) injury, resuscitation, and alkalosis; (2) circulatory stabilization and beginning respiratory difficulty; (3) progressive pulmonary insufficiency; and (4) terminal hypoxia with hypercarbia and asystole. Pathophysiology, pathogenesis, and prevention are discussed in great detail. Much practical information is given, including details of the use and operation of various types of ventilators.

Shires, G. T.: Care of the Trauma Patient. New York, McGraw-Hill Book Company, 1966.
This excellent monograph, written by members of the Department of Surgery at the University of Texas Southwestern Medical School, represents the first authoritative text specifically devoted to recommendations for the care of the severely injured patient. The literature is surveyed, and in addition, detailed descriptions of every conceivable type of injury and its management are presented. Numerous original diagrammatic illustrations and others taken from the literature clearly illustrate many of the points made. This detailed, easily read book should have a place on every surgeon's book shelf.

Shires, G. T., Carrico, C. J., and Canizaro, P. C.: Shock. Philadelphia, W. B. Saunders Company, 1973, p. 166.
This fine monograph represents a summary of the most current literature on clinical and physiological manifestations of shock. The discussion on pathophysiological responses to shock, especially the pulmonary responses, is particularly outstanding. The section on volume replacement in shock therapy is heavily weighted toward Dr. Shires' previous work and views on Ringer's lactate therapy; however the remainder of this section contains an outstanding discussion on adjunctive therapeutic methods. This small volume is strongly recommended for those interested in the etiology and therapy of shock in severely injured patients.

Smith, L. L., and Moore, F. D.: Refractory hypotension in man–is this reversible shock? N. Engl. J. Med., 267:733, 1962.

Patients in severe refractory hypotension were studied by hemodynamic and biochemical techniques. Four groups were discernible on the basis of the etiologic factor in their refractory hypotension: those with unrecognized volume deficit, those with severe sepsis, those with myocardial failure, and those with local vascular complications of extensive operations. Monitoring of central venous pressure and the hourly urinary output, together with observations of skin color and capillary blood flow, was more important than blood volume measurements in assessing tissue perfusion and blood volume adequacy. Postmortem examination of all patients who died disclosed an adequate anatomic explanation for death in all. None presented evidence of "irreversible shock" as seen in the dog. These observations emphasize that refractory hypotension in man should not be considered a primary diagnosis or ascribed to a single cause.

Williams, R. W., Burns, G. T., Andersen, M. N., Reading, G. P., Border, J. R., Mindell, E. R., and Schenk, W. G.: Mass casualties in a maximum security institution. Ann. Surg., 179:592, 1974.

This paper is a general discussion of the surgical experience encountered during the 1971 Attica uprising. The organizational experience is well described. It is unusual for the student to have direct access to the information contained in this excellent description. The paper is recommended reading for all general surgeons, particularly those who may face a mass-casualty situation resulting from multiple high velocity gunshot wounds.

REFERENCES

1. Allen, T. W., Reul, G. J., Morton, J. R., and Beall, A. C.: Surgical management of aortic trauma. J. Trauma, 12:862, 1972.
2. Anderson, C. B., Connors, J. P., Mejia, D. C., and Wise, L.: Drainage methods in the treatment of pancreatic injuries. Surg. Gynecol. Obstet., 138:587, 1974.
3. Ashbaugh, D. G., Petty, T. L., Bigelow, D. B., and Harris, T. M.: Continuous positive pressure breathing (CPPB) in adult respiratory distress syndrome. J. Thorac. Cardiovasc. Surg., 57:31, 1969.
4. Barrett, J., Dawidson, I., Dhurandhar, H. N., Miller, E., and Litwin, M. S.: Pulmonary microembolism associated with massive transfusion: II. The basic pathophysiology of its pulmonary effects. Ann. Surg. 182:56, 1975.
5. Beall, A. C., Jr., Diethrich, E. B., Crawford, H. W., Cooley, D. A., and DeBakey, M. E.: Surgical management of penetrating cardiac injuries. Am. J. Surg., 112:686, 1956.
6. Beebe, G. W., and DeBakey, M. E.: Battle casualties: Incidence, mortality, and logistic considerations. Springfield, Ill., Charles C Thomas, Publisher, 1952, p. 77.
7. Berman, I. R., Gutierrez, V. S., Burran, E. L., and Boatright, R. D.: Intravascular microaggregation in young men with combat injuries. Surg. Forum, 20:14, 1969.
8. Blair, E., Topuzlu, C., and Davic, J. H.: Delayed or missed diagnosis in blunt chest trauma. J. Trauma, 11:129, 1971.
9. Cass, A. A., and Ireland, G. W.: Management of renal injuries in the severely injured patient. J. Trauma, 12:516, 1972.
10. Cornell, W. P., and Ebert, P. A.: Penetrating wounds of the abdominal wall: A new diagnostic technic. Am. J. Roentgenol. 96:414, 1966.
11. Dawidson, I., Barrett, J. A., Miller, E., and Litwin, M. S.: Pulmonary microembolism associated with massive transfusion. I. Physiologic effects and comparison in vivo of standard and Dacron wool (Swank) blood transfusion filters in its prevention. Ann. Surg., 181:51, 1975.
12. Dawidson, I., Barrett, J. A., Miller, E., and Litwin, M. S.: Effects of intravascular cellular aggregate dissolution in postoperative patients. Ann. Surg., 182:776, 1975.
13. DeMuth, W. E.: Mechanism of shotgun wounds. J. Trauma, 11:219, 1971.
14. Doty, D. B., Anderson, A. E., Rose, E. F., Go, R. T., Chiu, C. L., and Ehrenhaft, J. L.: Cardiac trauma: Clinical and experimental correlations of myocardial contusion. Ann. Surg., 180:452, 1974.
15. Drapanas, T., and McDonald, J.: Peritoneal tap in abdominal trauma. Surgery, 50:742, 1961.
16. Duncan, S. E., Klebanoff, G., and Rogers, W.: A clinical experience with intraoperative autotransfusion. Ann. Surg., 180:296, 1974.
17. Dziemian, A. J., and Herget, C. M.: Physical aspects of primary contamination of bullet wounds. Milit. Surg., 106:294, 1950.
18. Ebert, P. A., Gaertner, R. A., and Zuidema, G. D.: Traumatic diaphragmatic hernias. Surg. Gynecol. Obstet., 125:59, 1967.
19. Engleman, R. C., and Joy, R. T.: Two Hundred Years of Military Medicine. Fort Detrick, Maryland: The Historical Unit, U.S. Army Medical Department, 1975, p. 56.
20. Finck, P. A.: Ballistic and forensic pathologic aspects of missile wounds. Conversion between Anglo-American and metric-system units. Milit. Med., 130:545, 1965.
21. Fullen, W. D., Selle, J. G., Whitely, D. H., Martin, L. W., and Altemeier, W. A.: Intramural duodenal hematoma. Ann. Surg., 179:549, 1974.
22. Gillett, M. C.: History of the Army Medical Department, 1775–1818. Fort Detrick, Maryland: The Historical Unit, U. S. Army Medical Department (unpublished manuscript).
23. Gould, R. J., and Thorwarth, W. T.: Retroperitoneal rupture of the duodenum due to non-penetrating abdominal trauma. Radiology, 80:743, 1963.
24. Gourin, A. F., and Garzon, A. A.: Diagnostic problems in traumatic diaphragmatic hernia. J. Trauma, 14:19, 1974.
25. Gump, F. F., Mashima, Y., and Kinney, J. M.: Water balance and extra vascular lung water measurements in surgical patients. Am. J. Surg., 119:515, 1970.
26. Hardy, J. D., and Bane, J. W.: Arterial injury and massive blood loss. A case report of management of pelvic gunshot injury with femoro-subscrotal-femoral bypass and 116 units of blood. Ann. Surg. 181:245, 1975.
27. Heaton, L. D., Hughes, C. W., Rosegay, H., Fisher, G. W., and Feighny, R. E.: Military surgical practices of the United States Army in Viet Nam. Curr. Probl. Surg., Nov., 1966.
28. Hewitt, R. L., Smith, A. D., and Drapanas, T.: Acute traumatic arteriovenous fistulas. J. Trauma, 13:901, 1973.
29. Hewitt, R. L., Smith, A. D., Jr., Weichert, R. F., III, and Drapanas, T.: Penetrating cardiac injuries: Current trends in management. Arch. Surg., 101:683, 1970.
30. Jernigan, W. R., and Gardner, W. C.: Carotid artery injuries due to closed cervical trauma. J. Trauma, 11:429, 1971.
31. Jones, J. W., Hewitt, R. L., and Drapanas, T.: Cardiac contusion: A capricious syndrome. Ann. Surg., 181:567, 1975.
32. Jordan, G. L., Jr., and Beall, A. C., Jr.: Diagnosis and management of abdominal trauma. Curr. Probl. Surg., Nov., 1971.
33. Lim, R. C., Trunkey, D. D., and Blaisdell, F. W.: Acute abdominal aortic injury. Arch. Surg., 109:706, 1974.
34. Lucas, C. E.: Prospective clinical evaluation of biliary drainage in hepatic trauma. Ann. Surg., 174:830, 1971.
35. Margolies, M. N., Ring, E. J., Waltman, A. C., Kerr, W. S., and Baum, S.: Arteriography in the management of hemorrhage from pelvic fractures. N. Engl. J. Med., 287:317, 1972.
36. McNamara, J. J., Boatright, D., Burran, E. L., Molot, M. D., Summers, E., and Stremple, J. F.: Changes in some physical properties of stored blood. Ann. Surg., 174:58, 1971.
37. Mendelson, J. A.: Use of whole blood and blood volume expanders in U.S. military facilities in Viet Nam, 1966–1971. J. Trauma, 15:1, 1975.
38. Nance, F. C., Wennar, M. H., Johnson, L. W., Ingram, J. C., and Cohn, I.: Surgical judgment in management of penetrating wounds of the abdomen: experience with 2212 patients. Ann. Surg., 179:639, 1974.
39. Naylor, R., Coln, D., and Shires, G. T.: Morbidity and mortality from injuries to the spleen. J. Trauma, 14:773, 1974.
40. Olsen, W. R., and Hildreth, D. H.: Abdominal paracentesis and peritoneal lavage in blunt abdominal trauma. J. Trauma, 11:824, 1971.
41. Parvin, S., Smith, D. E., Asher, W. M., and Virgilio, R. W.: Effectiveness of peritoneal lavage in blunt abdominal trauma. Ann. Surg., 181:255, 1974.
42. Persky, L., and Hoch, W. H.: Genitourinary tract trauma. Curr. Probl. Surg., Sept., 1972.
43. Ravitch, M. M., and Blalock, A.: Aspiration of blood from the pericardium in the treatment of acute cardiac tamponade after injury. Arch. Surg., 58:463, 1949.
44. Relihan, M., and Litwin, M. S.: Morbidity and mortality associated with flail chest injury: A review of 85 cases. J. Trauma, 13:663, 1973.
45. Reul, G. J., Greenberg, S. D., Lefrak, E. A., McCollim, W. B., Beall, A. C., and Jordan, G. L.: Prevention of post-traumatic pulmonary insufficiency. Arch. Surg., 106:386, 1973.
46. Ring, E. J., Waltman, A. C., Athanasoulis, C., Smith, J. C., and

Baum, S.: Angiography in pelvic trauma. Surg. Gynecol. Obstet., *139*:375, 1974.

47. Roman, E., Silva, Y. J., and Lucas, C.: Management of blunt abdominal injury. Surg. Gynecol. Obstet., *132*:7, 1971.

48. Root, H. D., Hauser, C. W., McKinley, C. R., LaFave, J. W., and Mendiole, R. P., Jr.: Diagnostic peritoneal lavage. Surgery, *57*:633, 1965.

49. Sheely, C. H., Mattox, K. L., Reul, G. J., Beall, A. C., and DeBakey, M. E.: Current concepts in the management of penetrating neck trauma. J. Trauma, *15*:895, 1975.

50. Sheldon, G. F., Lim, R. C., and Blaisdell, F. W.: Use of fresh blood in treatment of critically injured patients. J. Trauma, *15*:670, 1975.

51. Skinner, D. C.: Traumatic renal artery thrombosis. Ann. Surg., *177*:264, 1973.

52. Smith, A. D., Woolverton, W. C., Weichert, R. F., and Drapanas, T.: Operative management of pancreatic and duodenal injuries. J. Trauma, *11*:570, 1971.

53. Swank, R. L.: Alterations of blood on storage: Measurement of adhesiveness of "ageing" platelets and leukocytes and their removal by filtration. N. Engl. J. Med., *265*:728, 1961.

54. Thomas, A. N., and Stephens, B. G.: Air embolism: A cause of morbidity and death after penetrating chest trauma. J. Trauma, *14*:633, 1974.

55. Traylor, F. A., Morgan, W. W., Lucero, J. I., and Owens, J. C.: Abdominal trauma from seat belts. Am. Surg., *35*:313, 1969.

56. Trunkey, D. D., Shires, G. T., and McClelland, R.: Management of liver trauma in 811 consecutive patients. Ann. Surg., *179*:722, 1974.

57. Weaver, A. W., Sankarian, S., Fromm, S. H., Lucas, C. E., and Walt, A. J.: Management of penetrating wounds of the neck. Surg. Gynecol. Obstet., *133*:49, 1971.

58. Weichert, R. F., III, and Hewitt, R. L.: Injuries to the inferior vena cava: Report of 35 cases. J. Trauma, *10*:649, 1970.

59. Williams, J. W., and Sherman, R. T.: Penetrating wounds of the neck: Surgical Management. J. Trauma, *13*:435, 1973.

60. Williams, R. D., and Zollinger, R. E.: Diagnostic and prognostic factors in abdominal trauma. Am. J. Surg., *97*:575, 1959.

20

SURGICAL COMPLICATIONS

James D. Hardy, M.D.

Most operations are successful and the patient progresses smoothly to complete convalescence and rehabilitation. In a certain number of instances, however, complications develop. These may be minor and easily treated, so that recovery is not delayed, or they may be major, hospitalization may be prolonged, and death may ensue. Virtually any operation may be associated with both preventable and nonpreventable complications. This is not to say that the deeply experienced surgeon, operating upon a good-risk patient, will not in general have fewer and less severe postoperative problems than will the surgeon of lesser experience, operating upon the poor-risk patient. Thus, the incidence and severity of problems that arise after operations are influenced by many factors. Certain complications, such as pulmonary embolism, may follow any major operation, but in addition each specific type of operation has its own special problems. The purpose of this discussion is to survey both the postoperative problems common to virtually all major operations and those special problems that are peculiar to specific operations.

PROBLEMS COMMON TO ALL MAJOR OPERATIONS

The complications that may be associated with almost all major surgical operations include hypovolemic shock, respiratory insufficiency, cardiac failure and cardiac arrest, electrolyte imbalance and oliguria, postoperative jaundice including liver failure, infection, defective wound healing, disorders of consciousness, alimentary tract dysfunction, vascular complications, and miscellaneous other problems (Fig. 1).

POSTOPERATIVE SHOCK

There are numerous causes of significant systemic arterial hypotension during the postoperative period. These include acute respiratory insufficiency, cardiac failure, electrolyte imbalance, invasive infection, and vascular complications such as pulmonary embolism. Acute respiratory insufficiency is excluded on the basis of the chest x-ray and arterial blood gas values and pH. Cardiac failure is excluded on the basis of the central venous pressure, by measurement of the pul-

monary wedge pressure with a Swan-Ganz catheter, and by actual measurement of the cardiac output when feasible. Heart failure is treated by digitalis, diuretics, positive pressure assisted ventilation, often with a degree of positive end-expiratory pressure (PEEP), and fluid restriction. Electrolyte imbalance is

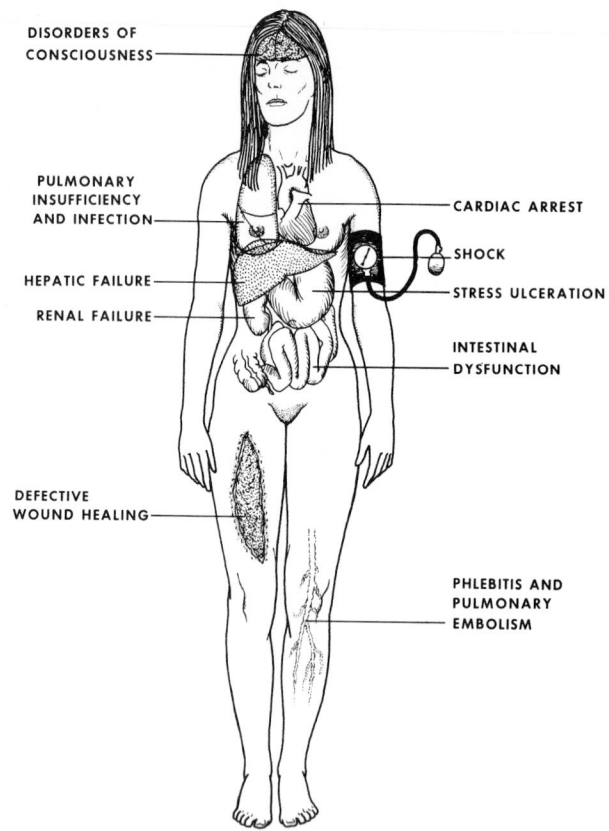

COMPLICATIONS WHICH MAY FOLLOW ANY MAJOR OPERATION

DISORDERS OF CONSCIOUSNESS

PULMONARY INSUFFICIENCY AND INFECTION

HEPATIC FAILURE

RENAL FAILURE

DEFECTIVE WOUND HEALING

CARDIAC ARREST

SHOCK

STRESS ULCERATION

INTESTINAL DYSFUNCTION

PHLEBITIS AND PULMONARY EMBOLISM

Figure 1. The importance of a good technical performance at operation cannot be overemphasized, for many postoperative complications owe their genesis to an imperfect operation itself. Certain operations are more likely to be followed by specific complications than are other operations; however, the complications shown in the illustration may upon occasion follow almost any major operation.

424

excluded by plasma chemistry measurements, and invasive infection is detected on clinical grounds and, in due course, by the blood cultures. However, the commonest cause of shock in the early postoperative period is hypovolemia. This inadequate circulating blood volume may reflect a blood volume deficit prior to operation, unreplaced loss during operation, or continuing hemorrhage in the postoperative period whether apparent to the observer or not. Therefore, when the patient who has had a major operation exhibits serious hypotension, and the effects of anesthesia or of excessive sedation have been excluded by brief assessment, it is wise to assume that the most likely cause of such hypotension is a blood volume deficit, to be corrected by the transfusion of matched blood. Among the numerous other signs of hypovolemia, in addition to the reduced arterial blood pressure, are a weak or thready pulse, a rapid heart rate, diminished capillary filling, a reduced or absent urine output, pallor of skin and mucous membranes, and anxiety. When hypovolemia is suspected, a central venous pressure catheter should be introduced for monitoring the central venous pressure, a urethral catheter should be inserted for the measurement of urine output every hour or every half hour, and at times it is useful to insert a catheter into a brachial, radial, or femoral artery for the continuous measurement of intra-arterial pressure.

Three important considerations arise when there is definite evidence of hypovolemia, as reflected in a reduced systemic arterial blood pressure and a low central venous pressure, plus the collateral evidence just mentioned. First, it must be reasonably well established that there is hypovolemia; second, the source of the hemorrhage must be identified; and third, the cause of the bleeding must be considered. The probability that hypovolemia exists is usually not difficult to determine, but the site and cause of hemorrhage may be hard to find. If the operation involved the thoracic cavity, the chest x-ray will usually suggest the presence of any significant amount of blood, but an operation within the abdomen may be followed by fairly massive hemorrhage without convincing overt external evidence. Even if drains were placed and there is substantial bleeding from the abdomen, it is sometimes hard to be certain whether the bleeding is due to a hemorrhagic diathesis with abnormal coagulation, or to an unligated artery or, less often, a vein. While the surgeon will wish to avail himself of all facilities available for the assessment of the efficiency of blood clotting in such a patient, he can gain a fairly accurate evaluation by two simple measurements: if the smear of the peripheral blood shows an adequate number of platelets and if the blood clots promptly on standing in a test tube, the odds are strongly in favor of an unligated blood vessel, and reoperation will often be necessary.

Management of Postoperative Shock

The management of the postoperative shock due to hypovolemia depends upon whether there was a preoperative deficit that has simply been accentuated by the vasodilatation caused by the anesthetic agent, or whether there was unreplaced loss during operation,

or whether there is continuing hemorrhage in addition, perhaps, to unreplaced loss during operation.

The surgeon often knows whether or not there is a distinct possibility that hemorrhage is continuing. If the operative field was completely dry at the time of closure and if no significant blood vessels were thought to have been inadequately managed, shock associated with an abdominal operation often reflects a relatively modest deficit and will usually respond adequately to one or two units of blood. It should be remembered that the adult has a blood volume of approximately 5 to 7 liters and that if serious shock is present the patient has usually lost approximately one fourth to one third of his total blood volume. Adequate blood replacement will produce a rise in the systemic arterial blood pressure, a slowing of the pulse, an increase in the central venous pressure, and an increase in urine output. It is not uncommon for these various indices to respond favorably to the transfusion, only to drift downward again over the course of the next hour or so. This usually reflects a continuing blood loss, and it often indicates the need for exploration of the wound. Again, bleeding from the chest can usually be identified with chest roentgenograms, in addition to the fact that most intrathoracic operations are drained with one or two large-bore plastic catheters to make certain that all blood and fluids are removed from the chest, to maintain full expansion of the lung on the involved side. Open-heart operations, with the use of prolonged cardiopulmonary bypass, are frequently attended by abnormal blood coagulation, and reoperation for hemorrhage is not uncommon. If the rate of postoperative hemorrhage through the drainage tubes into the underwater collection bottle exceeds 100 to 200 ml. per hour over a period of several hours, the chest should be re-explored. While it often happens that at re-exploration only minor bleeding points are found, there may be many of these and the extensive use of electrocautery may reduce the blood loss to a level that is readily tolerated and all hemorrhage eventually ceases.

For operations in the abdomen, however, the available guides may not be dependable. One may have to decide the issue concerning re-exploration on the basis of the fact that the patient is not responding satisfactorily to the transfusions that have been given. In general, it is much better to explore promptly, before prolonged hypovolemia has resulted in serious metabolic deficits, even if occasionally exploration turns out to have been unnecessary. Actually, the experienced observer will rarely be wrong in his diagnosis of continuing blood loss.

The precise amount of blood to be given is, simply, "enough." Since it is impossible to determine the exact volume of blood that is being lost from drain sites or into the abdomen, chest, or alimentary tract, physiologic measurements must be depended upon to indicate the volume replacement that is required. Blood is transfused until the arterial blood pressure has risen to a normal level, until the central venous pressure has risen to a moderate level (from 100 to 200 mm. of saline), until the urine output is consistently at least 25 ml. and preferably 40 to 50 ml. per hour, until the pulse rate has slowed, and until the general overall appearance of the patient is becoming satisfactory. If the blood pressure remains low after the central venous pressure has risen to 20 cm. of saline, digitalization should be considered and other causes of hypotension excluded. Prompt and effective treatment will usually prevent the development of cardiac arrest.

ACUTE RESPIRATORY INSUFFICIENCY

The patient undergoing a major operation is exposed to numerous respiratory hazards. Inadequate respiration often poses a much more immediate hazard than does a moderate rate of blood loss, since it takes longer for such blood loss to precipitate a potentially catastrophic set of circumstances. Failure to achieve effective respiration for only a few minutes may cause severe hypotension and even cardiac arrest. For this reason the experienced surgeon is most attentive to the quality of respiration in his patient during and immediately after operation, and for the first several days thereafter. Of course, the anesthesiologist will be following the patient for at least a brief period after operation, but it is a surgeon's obligation to see that the entire hospital course is satisfactory from every standpoint.

Acute respiratory insufficiency in the postoperative patient may be caused by defective ventilation, diffusion, or perfusion (Table 1). Perhaps the commonest cause of inadequate respiration in the recovery period is the prolonged effect of preanesthetic medication and of the anesthetic that was used at the operation, or excessive pain medication in the postoperative period. The patient exhibits hypoventilation, which results in a characteristic fall in arterial Po_2 and a rise in Pco_2. The problem is readily corrected by increasing the minute volume of respiration, whether by urging the patient to breathe deeply or by reintubation with a nasotracheal tube.

Pre-existing lung disease predisposes to postoperative respiratory insufficiency, a fact that is especially important in the chronic heavy smoker. Furthermore, since prolonged anesthesia induced by almost any agent will result in a temporary reduction in lung function, the operation must be planned so as to preserve a safe margin of respiratory reserve. The pulmonary secretions stimulated by an irritating anesthetic agent will further impair ventilation, and it is not infrequent that some pulmonary aspiration of gastric contents occurs, even when the stomach was considered empty.

The transfusion of large amounts of homologous blood has been shown to result in the passage of minute blood emboli and detritus through the usual commercial transfusion set filters. This material passes into the lungs and may occlude a substantial number of small pulmonary vessels. The administration of excessive fluid to the patient can result in pulmonary edema which of itself might not be significant but, when added to the various other possible causes of pulmonary dysfunction, may represent a serious additional impairment of lung function. Finally, the presence of an inevitable degree of atelectasis, perhaps associated with accompanying pneumonitis, and possibly aggravated by a mild degree of cardiac failure, may produce respiratory distress in the early and intermediate postoperative period. These and still other causes of postoperative respiratory embarrassment are often loosely diagnosed as "bronchospasm," though of course an element of bronchospasm per se may also exist.

Management of Postoperative Respiratory Insufficiency

The proper management of this condition will depend upon the cause or causes involved in the given case. Fortunately, the most common cause is inadequate pulmonary ventilation, and measures to increase ventilation will rectify the problem. However, when underlying lung disease exists, difficulties may arise, especially in older patients who may have chronic pulmonary emphysema or fibrosis or other pre-existing pulmonary disease. The aged patient has less strength to clear the often thick and tenacious postoperative bronchial secretions, and a degree of cardiac failure may exist.

Perhaps the first consideration is to appreciate preoperatively that a postoperative respiratory problem may develop. This will permit preoperative treatment designed to improve lung function to the maximal degree possible, as monitored by arterial blood gas values. Measures that can be most helpful are cessation of smoking for at least several days and preferably one month prior to an elective operation, daily exercises with the inhalation therapist employing bronchial dilators and antibiotics, and the use of diuretics and digitalization in patients with a degree of heart failure and fluid retention. The operation should then be performed expeditiously and with an appropriate type of anesthesia that causes minimal impairment of lung function. Postoperatively, the blood gas values should again be employed to detect early any significant degree of respiratory insufficiency. Actually, it is often wise to leave the endotracheal tube in place until the patient is fully awake, or for 24 hours or more, if there is any tendency to respiratory insufficiency. This has substantially reduced the incidence of cardiac arrest in the postanesthetic recovery room. The maximal benefit of leaving the endotracheal tube used at operation in place for a prolonged period of time is usually achieved by the end of

---

TABLE 1.   Causes of Postoperative Respiratory Insufficiency

1. Inadequate pulmonary ventilation due to prolonged effects of anesthesia, tracheal or bronchial obstruction, sedation, pain, age, or general debility
2. Pre-existing lung disease plus smoking
3. Retained pulmonary secretions with atelectasis
4. Pneumonitis
5. Excessive fluid administration and pleural effusion
6. Pulmonary edema due to left heart failure
7. Pulmonary embolism
8. Bronchospasm
9. Homologous blood syndrome

perhaps 48 hours, and of course the tube is always removed at the earliest safe interval after operation. After this time, retention of secretions in the lungs becomes a serious factor, since it is rarely possible to aspirate the pulmonary secretions as effectively as the patient himself can cough them out of the smaller bronchi, where the respiratory obstruction usually occurs. If the endotracheal tube must be left longer than 5 to 7 days, a tracheostomy may be elected, but with the objective of removing the tracheostomy tube at the earliest feasible moment. Extensive use is made of positive-pressure ventilation, using humidified air and the ultrasonic nebulizer, employing bronchodilators and antibiotics. If pulmonary aspiration of gastric fluid is known to have occurred, steroid therapy may be useful to reduce the inflammatory reaction in the lungs. If there is evidence of excessive fluid retention, diuretics and digitalis may be employed. Although the simple positive-pressure ventilator will prove adequate in most cases, in some instances it is valuable to use a volume respirator that will produce a sufficient pressure to give a set volume of ventilation. In the patient whose lungs are relatively rigid and stiff, with a reduced pulmonary compliance, a much higher pressure is required to achieve a given desired minute volume of ventilation. Positive end-expiratory pressure (PEEP) can be useful in improving oxygenation of the blood and in reducing pulmonary edema, but PEEP is also associated with a significant risk of pneumothorax. Lastly, it will often be useful to enlist the assistance of the members of the anesthesia department and the division of pulmonary medicine and inhalation therapy. Frequent chest x-rays are useful to exclude significant collections of fluid in the thorax and to indicate the general trend of the pulmonary disorder.

When patients are severely hypoxic, cardiac function may be impaired to the extent that significant arterial hypotension develops. Under such circumstances the heart frequently exhibits ventricular arrhythmia, which can be extremely serious and even lead to *cardiac arrest* in ventricular fibrillation or complete standstill. To avoid profound hypotension, while respiration is being improved, a vasopressor drug may be required. An isoproterenol drip is useful for this purpose but, in the presence of serious ventricular arrhythmia, this drug can prove hazardous also. One cannot state which drug or combination of drugs may be required in a given case, but isoproterenol (Isuprel) represents a good initial choice. If this drug produces unacceptable arrhythmia, even in the presence of a lidocaine drip, it may be advisable to shift to a very dilute drip of norepinephrine for a period of time, using lidocaine drip or procainamide (Pronestyl) to control arrhythmia. If severe hypotension is not relieved by isoproterenol, a dopamine drip or a dilute norepinephrine drip should be used, but with care to avoid subcutaneous infiltration which can produce skin necrosis. As soon as respiration has improved, permitting the Po_2 to rise from perhaps 40 to 50 mm. Hg to 70 to 80 mm. Hg, the heart action will improve and the patient can be gradually weaned off the vasopressor drug support. The improvement in lung compliance will be reflected in the reduced amount of positive pressure necessary to achieve a given tidal volume of respiration.

Effective short-term, artificial extracorporeal respiratory support will be available in a few years, and then it should be possible to give the patient in acute respiratory distress a sufficient degree of respiratory assistance to permit recovery of his own lungs over a period of several days.

ELECTROLYTE IMBALANCE AND OLIGURIA

The general problems of electrolyte and acid-base imbalance are discussed at length elsewhere in this volume, as is acute renal insufficiency. Nevertheless, these complications are so common and important in postoperative patients that some consideration must be accorded them in any survey of postoperative problems.

Electrolyte Imbalance

Electrolyte imbalance in the early postoperative period often reflects a preoperative deficit or excess of water or electrolytes that was not completely corrected and has persisted into the postoperative period. For example, the patient who enters the hospital with severe and prolonged vomiting, secondary to alimentary tract obstruction, may receive only partial replacement of the water and salts that have been lost, before operation is prudently performed to abolish further risk of prolonged intestinal distention with the attendant danger of gangrene of the bowel. The patient may progress through the operation without a serious fall in blood pressure, but thereafter the dissipation of the effects of anesthesia and other general measures of support may permit postoperative hypotension due to volume or salt deficits. In other cases, the prolonged use of cardiopulmonary bypass may cause a serious lowering of the serum potassium level, especially in patients who have been given diuretics preoperatively or who have been on a restricted diet. Thus adequate sodium, calcium, and potassium levels should be established in the postoperative period to achieve a satisfactory circulatory rate and heart action. The common types of postoperative fluid imbalance are presented in Table 2. The recognition that a given abnormality exists will usually suggest the proper treatment. The decision for water and electrolyte replacement is based on the need for additional volume, as determined from clinical evidence of the state of hydration as well as urine output, plus repeated measurements of the plasma electrolytes. Measurements of central venous pressure changes are useful, but a considerable excess of noncolloid solution can be given without producing a substantial rise in venous pressure. In fact, one of the most frequent states of postoperative fluid and electrolyte imbalance is that caused by the administration of excessive amounts of fluids, such as Ringer's lactate. It is not uncommon to observe a weight gain of several pounds and at times as much as 15 to 20 pounds, without abnormal increase in the central venous pressure.

TABLE 2. **Classification of States of Water and Electrolyte Imbalance**

Water and Salt Depletion	Acid-Base Imbalance
Pure water depletion	1. Acidosis
Pure sodium chloride depletion	Respiratory (retention of CO_2)
Mixed water and sodium chloride depletion	Metabolic (all causes other than respiratory, such as in diabetic acidosis, diarrhea, or uremia)
Deficits of other ions	2. Alkalosis
Potassium	Respiratory (hyperventilation)
Calcium	Metabolic (all causes other than respiratory)
Magnesium	
Water and Salt Excess	
Water excess	
Sodium chloride excess	
Water and sodium chloride excess	

Acid-Base Imbalance

The major states of acid-base imbalance are also shown in Table 2. We have already mentioned respiratory acidosis, which usually results from inadequate minute respiratory volume but may also attend diffusion and perfusion deficits. It is not rare to encounter a serious respiratory alkalosis, especially in patients in whom hyperventilation is produced by positive-pressure ventilation, or in those who have spontaneous respiratory alkalosis due to hyperventilation. A more sinister form of alkalosis is occasionally met in patients with "traumatic lung" and respiratory insufficiency. States of metabolic alkalosis and acidosis are also common. Metabolic alkalosis is most often encountered in the presence of prolonged pyloric obstruction with vomiting of hydrochloric acid and potassium from the stomach, commonly associated with some loss of sodium as well. The alkalosis is usually corrected preoperatively but may remain inadequately corrected and persist into the postoperative period. In fact, it may be further aggravated by prolonged postoperative nasogastric tube suction with inadequate or improper salt replacement. Metabolic alkalosis is also frequently found associated with states of potassium depletion, perhaps unrecognized and uncorrected preoperatively. The metabolic alkalosis is corrected by the infusion of adequate amounts of chloride ion as sodium chloride solution, and by the administration of adequate amounts of potassium chloride. Marked metabolic acidosis may result from inadequate tissue perfusion owing to a low cardiac output, from diabetic acidosis, or from renal failure with the accumulation of fixed acids normally eliminated by adequate renal function.

The diagnosis of these various states of acid-base imbalance is made on a clinical basis and by measurement of the arterial blood gases and pH, as well as plasma electrolytes and carbon dioxide-combining power. Actually, the specific clinical situation will usually suggest the state of acid-base imbalance that is most likely to develop.

Third Space Losses. Large volumes of fluid may be lost into the peritoneal cavity, into the distended gut in mechanical obstruction and ileus, or into sites of injury, such as around soft tissue and bone in trauma of the extremities or beneath burn wounds. These losses must be replaced, since these transudates are temporarily not available to maintain plasma volume.

Oliguria

The hourly urine output is a cornerstone of the objective assessment of the general state of the blood volume and of cardiopulmonary and renal function in the critically ill surgical patient. A urine output in the range of 30 to 50 ml. per hour, with a satisfactory specific gravity, constitutes substantial evidence that circulatory and renal function are reasonably good. Hypovolemia, inadequate cardiac output, severe hypoxia with the development of metabolic acidosis, and renal failure per se may all result in a reduced urine output.

When the patient exhibits marked oliguria, the surgeon must investigate the cause promptly and institute appropriate corrective measures. The urine output may have ceased abruptly, it may have gradually diminished in volume and then continued at a low and inadequate rate suggestive of hypovolemia, or it may have become bloody and then ceased altogether, suggesting serious renal damage.

When the urine output ceases abruptly, having previously been adequate, one must consider first the possibility that the catheter is obstructed and the urine from the bladder is simply not being transmitted to the outside. The catheter should be irrigated or replaced. If bladder drainage is found satisfactory, the possibility of unilateral or bilateral ureteral injury during operation must be considered and ruled out by appropriate roentgenographic studies of the urinary tract. Having excluded mechanical possibilities such as obstruction of the catheter or ureters or bladder injury ("postrenal"), one must consider whether the oliguria is "prerenal" (hypovolemia, cardiac failure) or "renal" (renal injury).

If the urine remains clear but the volume simply begins to decline over a period of several hours, additional blood or fluid replacement is usually indicated, especially if the central venous pressure has declined or has remained low. If the patient is losing a significant amount of blood by any route, blood transfusion is almost certainly needed, especially if the arterial blood pressure has also declined. Obviously, if the patient is in shock, the urine output will be scant indeed in most instances. However, if the central venous pressure is adequate and the arterial blood pressure is good, and the patient is still excreting an inadequate amount of urine, a single dose or even two doses of furosemide (40 to 100 mg.) may be given intravenously to determine whether or not the kidneys are capable of excreting urine. If little effect is realized from the infusion of blood or other fluid, with or without a potent diuretic, the possibility of significant renal damage must be seriously considered and renal sodium excretion should be measured. Normally, the kidney is very efficient in conserving sodium if no sodium is being given. Therefore, the loss of more than 30 mEq. of sodium per liter of urine excreted is highly suggestive of renal damage in the form of acute tubular necrosis. Such tubular necrosis is usually caused by hypoxia, whether inflicted by inadequate respiration or by inadequate kidney perfusion as a result of hypovolemia or reduced cardiac output from other causes. Blood incompatibilities can also result in tubular damage and severe oliguria. Massive cortical necrosis can result in permanent anuria. Kidney perfusion can be estimated by renal scan, or by selective renal arteriograms when indicated.

If optimal blood and fluid replacement has been achieved and severe oliguria persists, with a high sodium loss, acute tubular necrosis must be suspected and proper steps taken. Thus, fluid intake thereafter must be restricted to approximately 800 ml. per day. A highly concentrated carbohydrate and fat diet, providing perhaps 1000 calories in a small volume of fluid, will reduce protein catabolism and diminish the liberation of cellular potassium and the hazard of hyperkalemia. By rule of thumb, the patient in acute renal insufficiency should be allowed to lose approximately 1 pound per day.

If the urine output does not increase and the blood urea nitrogen level approaches 150 mg. per 100 ml., the serum potassium level approaches 6.5 mEq. per liter, or the serum creatinine level reaches 15 mg. per 100 ml., either peritoneal dialysis or hemodialysis should be initiated before clinical signs of uremia develop. If the patient has not had an abdominal condition that precludes the use of peritoneal dialysis, this procedure may prove adequate to gain time for renal function to return. Often the kidneys have not suffered severe damage, and adequate urine output may be restored in 3 to 5 days. However, if severe tubular necrosis has occurred, a period of 10 to 21 days may be required for adequate renal function to return. During this time the patient should be kept in the best possible condition, and this will usually require some form of dialysis, whether peritoneal dialysis or hemodialysis with the artificial kidney. Patients who have just undergone an operation or sustained major trauma, perhaps with sepsis, may exhibit marked catabolism, and the potassium and BUN levels may rise far more rapidly than they would in the nontraumatized and nonseptic patient in chronic renal failure. Here dialysis must be performed early and often to achieve a successful outcome and, even so, the mortality of renal failure in the traumatized patient remains in the range of 50 per cent. When diuresis does begin it may be temporarily excessive, and fluid balance must be carefully maintained. Incidentally, the body fluid shifts which occur during hemodialysis can pose a considerable hazard for the critically ill patient whose circulatory equilibrium is precariously balanced.

POSTOPERATIVE JAUNDICE

Postoperative jaundice of varying degrees is common in the postoperative period (Table 3). In a prospective study, Evans et al.[8] found an overall incidence of 20 per cent (3.7 per cent severe and 16.5 per cent mild jaundice). An excellent review with a full bibliography was published by Van Thiel and Lester,[22] and by Morgenstern.[18] The serum bilirubin level may

TABLE 3. Some Causes of Postoperative Jaundice

1. Hemolysis
2. Operative stress superimposed upon pre-existing liver disease
3. Liver hypoxia during operation — hypoxemia or underperfusion
4. Leakage of bile into peritoneal cavity
5. Viral hepatitis
6. Drug or anesthetic toxicity
7. Extrahepatic biliary tract disorder
8. Hepatic infection with abscesses
9. Septicemia
10. Pulmonary embolism

rise moderately for several days, level off, and then decline. Even mild jaundice should be viewed with definite interest but without serious concern in most patients, especially those who have received several blood transfusions. The rise in the serum bilirubin level usually represents hemolysis. If intra-abdominal disease was the indication for the operation, other possibilities must be considered. Significant quantities of blood in the peritoneal cavity or in the retroperitoneal space, as with ruptured abdominal aortic aneurysm, can produce hemolytic jaundice. However, other and more serious causes, exclusive of liver failure, which will be considered in the next paragraph, may exist. Leakage of bile into the peritoneal cavity, from liver trauma, cholecystectomy, or a leaking gastroenteric anastomosis, will permit transperitoneal absorption of bile, often with evidence of associated sepsis. Mechanical stenosis or obstruction of the common bile duct, by dissection or perhaps pancreatitis, may also produce jaundice, as can inadvertent ligation of the major hepatic arterial blood supply. Even thoracic operations may precipitate acute cholecystitis or pancreatitis. In some poorly understood manner, severe sepsis may also cause jaundice, even in the absence of gross liver infection per se. Pulmonary embolism may cause a rise in the serum bilirubin level, and the obscure intraductal cholestasis may develop. Fortunately, most of these causes of jaundice will recede if appropriate nonoperative management is elected. Mechanical obstruction may require operation for repair of common bile duct stricture or for gallstones.

Jaundice Due to Hepatic Disease

In addition to the causes just presented, plus still others, the jaundice may be due to liver disease per se and this can be serious or even fatal. The etiology may be drug toxicity (e.g., chlorpromazine), operative stress superimposed upon pre-existing liver disease, homologous serum hepatitis from a previous blood transfusion, or liver hypoxia during the operative experience. Thus, significant postoperative jaundice, in the absence of probable hemolysis, must be viewed with serious concern. Subclinical, preoperative hepatic insufficiency, secondary to cirrhosis or perhaps heart disease, is not uncommon, and severe hypoxemia or prolonged hypotension can produce a state of severe hepatic insufficiency. Even the normal liver can be critically damaged by prolonged shock, and the condition is often aggravated by the use of a norepinephrine drip.

The anesthetic agent itself may have caused liver damage, and it is now generally accepted that halothane may rarely be hepatotoxic when used a second or third time. In the very occasional patient, the first anesthetization with halothane appears to produce a sensitivity phenomenon, and later use of the agent triggers the allergic reaction and produces liver damage that can prove fatal.

However, significant postoperative jaundice due to anesthetic or other drug toxicity is uncommon. Much more often, the rise in serum bilirubin level secondary to liver disease per se is caused by prolonged shock or other hypoxia, and it is not truly rare following open-heart surgery and heart valve replacement in patients with long-standing heart disease. Liver injury is reflected not only in jaundice but also in the serum transaminase level and other indices of liver function. An artificial heart valve can produce hemolysis on occasion.

Management of Postoperative Jaundice

Mild jaundice is common and usually subsides without event. However, if jaundice persists or increases, all efforts must be made to make an accurate diagnosis, to permit appropriate management. If the bilirubin level continues to rise to a level of, say, 10 mg. per 100 ml., the possibility of significant impairment of liver function must be considered. Blood volume and cardiopulmonary function should be rendered optimal, and nutritional support should be provided with dextrose infusions. The progress of the hepatic injury should be followed with frequent measurements of the serum transaminase and bilirubin levels. If the jaundice progresses to serum bilirubin levels of 25 mg. per 100 ml. or greater, the patient will frequently exhibit clinical signs of hepatic failure if the jaundice is due to liver damage per se. Renal failure may also develop, the so-called hepatorenal syndrome. In recent years there has been some use of exchange transfusion for acute hepatic failure with coma, since the previously used extracorporeal perfusion of pig or human livers proved cumbersome, did not significantly increase the number of survivors, and has not recently enjoyed wide application. The condition of a patient in hepatic coma may indeed be improved by exchange transfusion, though the relief is only temporary and death will ensue unless liver function improves. Unfortunately, an artificial liver is not yet available, largely because of the complexities involved in normal liver function. Thus, at present the prognosis for a patient in severe liver failure is guarded, at best.

INFECTION

Infection is a major cause of postoperative morbidity and mortality. Moreover, surveys have indicated that the development of a serious postoperative infection results in an average cost of approximately $7000 to the national economy, a figure derived from medical costs plus work days missed. At one time it was believed that the advent of effective antibiotics would in large part abolish serious infection in surgical patients. Unfortunately, although appropriate antibiotic therapy does provide assistance of considerable magnitude, infection still constitutes a major cause of death on most surgical services. It is standard surgical procedure to clear up infections to the extent possible preoperatively, to minimize contamination during the course of the operation, and to take every precaution against the introduction or spread of infection postoperatively. Yet, irrespective of preventive measures taken in all these directions, in a certain number of patients mild, moderate, or life-threatening infections will develop. Of course, in some the contamination and infection will have existed preoperatively.

Diagnosis of Postoperative Infections

The hallmark of developing infection is fever, usually associated with leukocytosis exhibiting a shift to the left. An increase in the pulse rate usually occurs. The patient who had no infection preoperatively and acquires no infection postoperatively may show a mild rise in the body temperature to perhaps 99 to 100° F., but the temperature curve will rarely rise above this level. Therefore, careful daily examination of the clinical chart for changes in body temperature, pulse rate, and perhaps respiratory rate will identify the probable presence of infection before localizing signs have appeared. The fever of suppurative infection may be low in the morning, but rises in the afternoon and evening.

The timing of the development of evidence of infection in the postoperative period often affords an important clue to the probable source and location of the infection. For example, the patient in whom significant fever develops within 24 to 48 hours of operation often has pulmonary atelectasis and associated pneumonitis, which can be abolished by effective coughing and other measures designed to clear the small bronchial passages and achieve full expansion of the lungs. Antibiotic therapy is usually employed to assist in this general therapeutic endeavor. When the fever appears several days after operation, time having been allowed for the development of sepsis within the operative area itself, one must suspect the possibility of infection within the coelomic cavity where the dissection was performed, or in the body wall itself (the wound). The site of infection within the chest can usually be determined or at least suspected from roentgenograms. However, infection within the abdomen can exist in multiple locations and may even require surgical exploration for identification. The most common sites of major pus collections are the subdiaphragmatic spaces, the pelvis, and the liver. The lateral gutters and pockets among adherent loops of bowel represent other sites. Fever due to urinary tract infection may occur at any time, even the day of operation in certain urinary tract procedures. Exploration of the common bile duct in the presence of stones may often cause entry of bacterial organisms into the bloodstream and produce gram-negative shock the very day of operation. Again, fever that develops several days after operation is usually caused by wound infection, phlebitis, infection around intravenous catheters, or, rarely, parotitis.

Stress Ulceration. Stress ulceration is discussed elsewhere in this volume. It may follow a variety of severe metabolic stresses, including severe burns (Curling's ulcer), intracranial trauma (Cushing's ulcer), respiratory insufficiency with hypoxia, prolonged shock, and still other conditions. However, *infection* appears to be a major contributing factor in approximately two-thirds of patients, many of whom are first met in the intensive care unit. Routine gastroscopy among patient populations at high risk has shown that the incidence of ulceration is considerably higher than had been suspected when hemorrhage was the only diagnostic criterion.

Treatment of stress ulcer hemorrhage remains unsettled, but several modalities are commonly used and with some success—this despite the fact that the onset of massive stress ulcer bleeding heralds a set of circumstances which often terminate fatally. Prophylactic treatment with oral antacids is probably useful. With the onset of hemorrhage, lavage of the stomach with iced isotonic saline solution reduces the temperature below the optimum level for pepsin digestion and cleanses the stomach. The selective intra-arterial infusion of Pitressin has stopped the bleeding in some patients. Operative intervention most often consists of oversewing or undersewing of the ulcer, truncal vagotomy, and distal gastrectomy.

Subphrenic Abscess. The commonest site of intra-abdominal abscess formation is *beneath the diaphragm,* on one side or the other. It is not always appreciated that the subphrenic space is dependent in position and of large potential size (Fig. 2). Unfortunately, a large collection of pus may exist in either the right or the left subphrenic space with few localizing symptoms. However, when intraperitoneal soiling is followed by a septic course, and especially if lung infection or pelvic abscess has been virtually excluded, the subphrenic space should always be suspected.

The importance of subdiaphragmatic abscess is emphasized by two studies. DeCosse et al.[7] analyzed subphrenic abscess in 60 patients. Of the 52 patients in whom the abscess had followed an operation, 22 had followed gastric surgery and 11 biliary tract surgery. Many abscesses actually represented infected hematomas. Twenty-one patients died after surgical drainage of the abscess (43 per cent). The mortality rate in patients whose suppuration was adequately drained was 25 per cent, but it was 55 per cent in patients whose abscess was not adequately drained. Mackenzie et al.[16] studied subphrenic abscess in children: 4 of 19 consecutive patients died, and appendicitis caused 11 of the 19 infections.

The diagnosis of subphrenic abscess is made on the basis of history and appropriate investigations. Shoulder pain or hiccups may reflect diaphragmatic irritation. Fist percussion may elicit tenderness on the involved side, but on the right a liver abscess should be excluded by liver scan. Chest x-ray may reveal a (sterile) pleural effusion on the involved side, and fluoroscopic examination may disclose fixation of this hemidiaphragm. A liver scan may reveal a space between this organ and the diaphragm, and at times needle aspiration produces pus. Ultrasound may be

DRAINAGE OF SUBPHRENIC ABSCESS

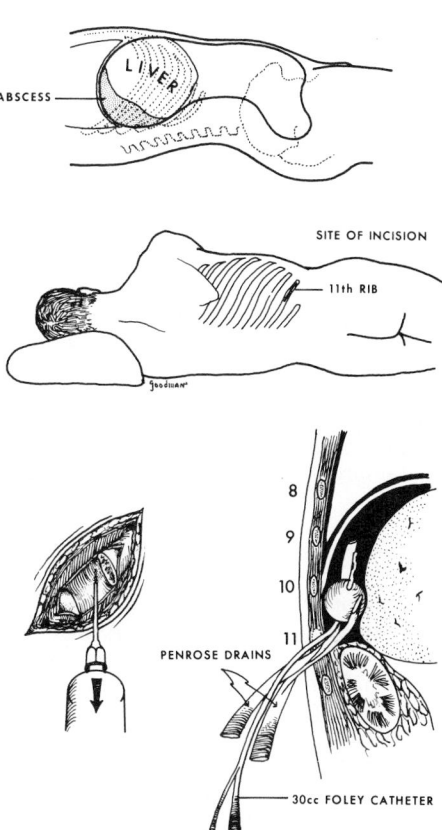

Figure 2. Intra-abdominal abscesses can be difficult to identify and to localize. If the abscess cannot be detected in the pelvis by rectal or vaginal examination, and if the liver scintiscans are normal, a subphrenic location should always be suspected. The posterior approach for drainage is preferred. The pleural cavity and the free peritoneal cavity are avoided. Note that the precise location of the pus is identified by needle aspiration before an incision is made. A Foley catheter should be left in place until the size of the cavity has diminished to the size of the 30 cc. bag, as demonstrated by roentgenograms after injection of a radiopaque medium.

helpful. If all other diagnostic measures fail, surgical exploration should be performed on clinical grounds alone.

The abscess may be approached anteriorly on either side, but usually it is preferable to drain through the bed of the partially excised eleventh rib (Fig. 2).

Pseudomembranous Enterocolitis. This is a condition characterized by severe diarrhea that may be bloody, abdominal pain and distention, and usually fever. A cast of the colon mucosa may be passed, and circulatory collapse and death may ensue. In some respects, the toxicity may resemble that of a patient with the "toxic megacolon" of idiopathic ulcerative colitis.

Pseudomembranous enterocolitis was described prior to the antibiotic era,[10] often following shock, and the writer has seen bloody diarrhea followed by mucosal loss in instances of severe colonic ischemia. However, most often this relatively rare colon disorder seems to appear in patients who have been on broad-spectrum antibiotics which have suppressed the normal colonic bacterial flora and permitted massive overgrowth of *Staphylococcus aureus*.[6] Actually, the entire gastrointestinal tract may be involved, but the lesions are best seen in the visually accessible colon at proctoscopy. The pseudomembrane need not include major elements of the mucosa, but it often does.

Treatment consists of prompt presumptive diagnosis, including gram stain of the stool for staphylococci. All previous antibiotics are stopped, since there is some evidence that a toxic effect of the agents themselves may be an etiologic factor. Antibiotics effective against resistant strains of staphylococci are initiated in large doses. The circulation is supported by intravenous fluids. Retention enemas of a saline suspension of normal stool have been used to restore normal bacterial flora to the colon. If Pseudomonas species are found, appropriate antibiotic therapy should be given. If prompt improvement is not forthcoming, the prognosis is poor.

Management of Postoperative Infection

Local signs of *wound infection* consist of pain and tenderness, swelling, warmth, and erythema. Early in the course, the characteristic swelling may not be visible, especially if the infection lies deep in the wound. However, swelling of the wound at the involved site is usually apparent, and at times the actual drainage of small amounts of fluid from the site of the infection in the wound can be noted. In contrast to an infected wound, the healthy wound that is several days old usually is neither spontaneously painful nor excessively tender.

The entire wound may not be infected initially. Therefore to permit precise drainage of the pus, the point of maximal tenderness should be identified by palpation. If no more than a week or 10 days has elapsed since operation, the healing incision can simply be spread open with a hemostat without the need for anesthesia. Effective drainage to the extent necessary will abolish the local and systemic evidence of infection and accelerate wound healing. The insertion of a drain for 48 to 72 hours is frequently desirable, but the common practice of packing the wound open with some form of gauze can be abused to the extent that wound healing is unnecessarily delayed and a poor cosmetic result ensues. If systemic evidence of infection persists after drainage, either the local drainage was inadequate or other sources of infection exist and must be detected. While some purulent collections do slowly resolve spontaneously, convalescence and wound healing are usually facilitated by surgical drainage when possible. Furthermore, undrained pus may at any time produce a serious bloodstream invasion. Sputum, pus, urine, and blood specimens should be cultured and bacterial sensitivities to antibiotics determined as soon as possible. Meanwhile, a broad-spectrum antibiotic in effective dosage should be started.

The appearance of excessive febrile states, especially with shaking chills, suggests bloodstream invasion, and repeated blood cultures should be obtained to identify the offending organisms in order to obtain antibiotic sensitivities. The blood should be drawn as quickly after the chill has occurred as possible, since it has been found that it is at the time of the chill that cultures are most likely to be positive. If there are no chills, the blood culture should be taken at the time of maximal temperature rise. Again, fever due to infection usually is maximal in the afternoon and evening, with an almost normal temperature in the morning. Significant fever throughout the entire 24 hours suggests a truly serious infection.

After the specific organism has been identified and appropriate antibiotics initiated, vigilance should not be lessened. Whereas the appropriate antibiotic may subdue the initial organism that was cultured, either the flora causing the infection or its antibiotic sensitivities may be shifting continuously, and the physician must persevere until all evidence of infection has been absent for a period of several days. Above all, the therapy should not be stopped too soon and the patient discharged, since stopping of the antibiotics too soon may permit resurgence of the infection after the patient is no longer under close observation.

The use of "prophylactic antibiotics" has been a subject of controversy for years. In general, prophylactic antibiotics are not recommended in otherwise clean cases in which a postoperative infection would entail relatively little risk of life. On the other hand, prophylactic antibiotics are often used in most major vascular cases and whenever a hollow viscus has been opened with possible bacterial contamination of the wound to some degree. A combination of penicillin and streptomycin is preferred, but cephalothin (Keflin) is used if the patient is sensitive to penicillin. Whether or not these antibiotics reduce the incidence of infection is not certain, but we have had a gratifyingly low rate of infection in clean wounds and, most important, those associated with an artificial prosthesis in the heart or a fabric arterial graft. The antibiotic therapy is augmented by instillation of the appropriate agent directly into the wound at operation.

To conclude, there are a number of measures that can be employed to minimize the possibility of significant postoperative infection. Preoperative and postoperative pulmonary exercises are important in preventing lung infection. Adequate hydration and mouth care should reduce the incidence of the admittedly rare parotitis, and early mobilization of the patient should diminish the incidence of phlebitis. However, the most productive means of reducing postoperative infections is to avoid infection in the area of the dissection and in the body wall itself. This implies the clearing up of various infections preoperatively and the meticulous avoidance of contamination of the wound by hand or by leakage of bronchial or alimentary tract material at the time of operation. Careful attention to hemostasis and the avoidance of mass ligatures that devitalize large amounts of tissue enhance convalescence. While any single one of these measures may appear relatively insignificant, it is by employing all possible precautions that the experienced surgeon minimizes infection and attendant complications and achieves superior morbidity and mortality rates.

DEFECTIVE WOUND HEALING

Wound complications have always represented a prominent cause of postoperative morbidity, but they are less frequently a cause of mortality than they once were. Infection has already been considered; here attention will be directed to complications of clean wounds.

Thoracotomy incisions made between the ribs usually heal promptly, though occasionally there is clear evidence that the deeper layers of muscle and even the ribs have separated. However, the skin usually remains intact, despite drainage of serosanguineous fluid from the pleural cavity, and healing slowly occurs. There is no bowel to eviscerate or become obstructed, and the lung does not herniate, as a rule. Paradoxical motion may be visible with respiration, but the resulting physiologic defect is usually not sufficient to embarrass respiration. The favorable healing of the posterolateral thoracotomy wound derives from its several muscle layers, the relatively thin layer of subcutaneous fat, and the usual absence of infection. Of course, these wounds do occasionally separate and then must be reclosed at a second operation.

In contrast to the intercostal approach, the median sternotomy or sternum-splitting incision frequently exhibits poor healing, and infection is not rare. First, secure healing involves bony union, which occurs slowly and thus requires wire sutures. Secondly, there is little available musculature to suture anterior to the sternum. Reclosure may be required if complete separation occurs, but usually prolonged observation and administration of appropriate antibiotics achieves an adequate result. The skin sutures should be left until healing has clearly occurred.

The abdominal wound is subject to a considerable variety of complications, some minor and some very serious. In addition to inadequate technical closure or hematoma formation or infection, all of which may result in partial or major separation of the wound margins, increased intra-abdominal pressure due to excessive coughing, vomiting, gaseous distention, or intraperitoneal accumulation of fluid may cause partial or complete wound separation. Inadequate technical closure may represent excessive tension on the sutures, poor placement of the sutures, or sutures of excessive or inadequate size. Other causes of poor healing include previous irradiation and metabolic derangements such as Cushing's disease, diabetes mellitus, malignant disease with starvation, and uremia. To be sure, an occasional wound will separate when none of these conditions exists and the cause is attributed simply to "poor tissues for closure." When a wound separates, the sutures usually have pulled through on one side or the other; they rarely break except in husky young men when suture material of inadequate strength was used.

A common-sense approach will do much to achieve good and prompt wound healing without complications. The incision should be no longer than needed. Infection and hematoma and excessive tension should be avoided. Drains should exit through a separate incision or "stab wound." A suction tube should be placed beneath large skin flaps to prevent fluid collections so that the skin can become adherent to the underlying tissues.

The management of abdominal wound *separation* will depend upon multiple factors. When the deeper layers have separated, as indicated by the escape of serosanguineous fluid between the skin sutures, the surgeon has the choice of nonoperative management, with acceptance of a late incisional hernia, or of reoperation with formal closure of all layers. If the patient is young and in good general condition, the wound usually should be reclosed. However, often the patient has serious other problems and is old, in which case it may be elected to accept a probable late hernia. If the bowel appears between the skin sutures, however, or on the abdominal wall after the skin sutures have been removed, formal repair under major anesthesia is obligatory. Also, if small bowel obstruction develops as a result of partial wound separation, reoperation is mandatory. While it is always hard to tell the patient that he must have another operation so soon after the first, the decision must be made on the basis of sound surgical principles and all other considerations are secondary. Since the layers of the wound are often friable or even unidentifiable in the disrupted wound, a single-layer, through-and-through closure, with strong suture material such as wire, is often employed. Reclosure of wounds is usually successful and little increase in the mortality rate is caused by reoperation per se, though death may result from the underlying problems that precipitated evisceration.

TABLE 4. Causes of Abdominal Wound Dehiscence

1. Imperfect technical closure
2. Increased intra-abdominal pressure from gut distention, ascites, coughing, vomiting, or straining
3. Hematoma with or without infection
4. Infection
5. Metabolic diseases such as diabetes mellitus, uremia, Cushing's disease, and malignant disease with starvation
6. Tissues inadequate for strong closure

DISORDERS OF CONSCIOUSNESS

The patient subjected to general anesthesia undergoes an induced loss of consciousness. This loss of consciousness is usually profound, as required to provide sufficient anesthesia to permit an operation that will not be painful or remembered. Thereafter a normal mental state should be achieved promptly, but this recovery can be arrested at any point along the line. Although the surgeon is usually not concerned if the patient does not wake up immediately following cessation of the anesthetic agent, since respiration can be adequately supported by leaving the endotracheal tube in place and using whatever assisting mechanical ventilation is required, the attending staff will feel increasing anxiety as several hours pass without progressive recovery from anesthesia. If all reflexes are present and the pupils are round and equal and react promptly to light, and especially if the patient reacts to painful stimuli, it can usually be assumed with some confidence that complete recovery will soon occur. Nevertheless, there are those patients who do not recover promptly or even at all, and it is the purpose here to examine some of the reasons why the patient may fail to regain promptly the mental status he enjoyed preoperatively.

The most common cause of delayed recovery is excessive or prolonged effects of the anesthetic agent itself. The length of action of various anesthetic agents varies considerably, and the length of action of a given anesthetic agent in patients of the same general habitus likewise varies considerably. Furthermore, the obese patient who has absorbed large amounts of a fat-soluble anesthetic agent into the fat depots will metabolize or excrete the agent more slowly than will the lean person who has relatively small fat deposits. Therefore, the first consideration in slow awakening is to reappraise the possible effects of the anesthetic agent that was used and of any other drugs such as opiates or tranquilizers that might have been administered during the immediate postoperative period.

Unfortunately, many states of disturbed consciousness are due not to the anesthetic agent, but to more serious considerations. Perhaps the most common and serious complication is inadequate oxygenation of the brain during the period of anesthesia or the immediate postoperative period. This cerebral hypoxia may have resulted from a restricted oxygen supply in the gas mixture during operation, various types of pulmonary insufficiency, or a reduced oxygen-carrying capacity of the blood. It may have been caused by a diminished cerebral perfusion itself, owing to a reduced cardiac output, whether secondary to intrinsic myocardial disease or to arrhythmia or hypotension from other causes such as hypovolemia. Elderly patients frequently have cerebral atherosclerosis and, if the blood pressure is allowed to decline in a patient whose brain blood flow was already critically low because of atherosclerotic narrowing of important cerebral blood vessels, oxygenation may be inadequate to maintain normal cerebral function and integrity. Still other causes of altered brain activity found postoperatively are various types of embolism such as atherosclerotic plaques, blood clots, fat embolism, and even air embolism in open-heart surgery or other situations in which significant amounts of air enter the bloodstream. For example, it has been shown that a certain amount of air can traverse the pulmonary circuit and enter the systemic circulation. Finally, intracranial hemorrhage or thrombosis may have occurred during the course of the operation without its being detected.

In addition, alterations in cerebral metabolism must also be considered. Profound hypoglycemia, abnormalities in acid-base and electrolyte balance, dysfunction of adrenal or other endocrine glands, and the enzymatic alterations caused by hepatic failure, drugs, or thermal extremes should be excluded. Invasive infection may have been initiated during intraoperative manipulations in an infected field, and the obtunded mental state may reflect septicemia.

The occasional patient will exhibit a type of psychiatric or hysterical withdrawal that is difficult to differentiate from organic brain disorder due to various of the causes just described. Usually, however, an experienced neurologist can by careful examination determine whether the patient is in a trance or whether actual organic brain disorder exists.

It frequently happens that the patient has responded satisfactorily after the anesthesia experience, but then several days later exhibits aberrations in affect and personality structure. These changes are usually not due to brain damage sustained under anesthesia. In the elderly patient they may be due to senile atherosclerosis, and recovery may be anticipated in a few days or perhaps when he is back at home in familiar surroundings. The occasional patient will develop a frank postoperative psychosis that will require psychiatric attention. Even so, late development of mental changes may also be due to serious tissue hypoxia or other metabolic changes. Abnormal behavior in the postoperative period should never be ignored but should prompt careful observation and continuous pursuit of diagnostic possibilities that may disclose some serious underlying metabolic states that must be treated promptly. *As a minimum, arterial blood gas values should be determined to exclude hypoxia.*

Management of Postoperative Disorders of Consciousness

If it is concluded that the failure of the patient to awaken promptly is due to the prolonged effect of anesthesia, and if the blood pressure and other vital signs are stable, all that is required is watchful waiting with careful maintenance of adequate pulmonary ventilation. If specific antidotes to the anesthetic agent that was used are available, these may be given cautiously, but in general the effects are simply allowed to dissipate spontaneously. If it is judged that definite brain damage has occurred during the course of the operative experience, an entirely different situation exists. At this point it is essential to make certain that everything possible is done to avoid subjecting the brain to further damage in the form of inadequate cardiac output or inadequate respiration. Furthermore, if there is reason to believe that a plaque may have been dislodged into the cerebral arterial supply, perhaps in an operation upon the aortic valve, carotid arteriography should be used to explore the possibility of removing the plaque or embolus or any carotid thrombi that may have formed. However, the first step will generally be to request neurologic consultation. While the effective therapeutic modalities available for the treatment of brain damage are limited, it is important to establish a baseline neurologic evaluation, so that changes may be noted and all treatment possibilities explored. The patient in whom relatively minor brain damage has occurred, owing to underperfusion or hypoxia from a variety of causes, will usually be obtunded for perhaps 24 to 72 hours or so, and then rapidly regain a normal state of consciousness without apparent sequelae. Although few reports of psychologic testing are available to indicate what the state of cerebration is in such patients years later, grossly they appear to be normal after recovery.

In marked contrast, the patient in whom severe brain injury has occurred will commonly show abnormalities of limb reflexes and posture, pupil size and reflexes, and facial expressions, and may even exhibit convulsions, coma, and decerebrate rigidity. But even these relatively severe manifestations of cerebral hypoxic damage may be reversible, and an aggressive and hopeful outlook is essential for the management of such patients. The writer has, over the years, followed many patients who made a complete clinical recovery when all observers would have expected permanent evidence of substantial brain injury. The most important consideration that arises in the patient with serious and prolonged brain dysfunction is the maintenance of adequate respiration, the prevention of pulmonary sepsis and hypoxia, and the maintenance of nutrition and function of the alimentary tract and kidneys. Unfortunately, significant brain damage is always a serious complication and many patients do not recover.

ALIMENTARY TRACT DYSFUNCTION

Most patients exhibit some change in alimentary tract function and in alimentation after major operations, regardless of what region of the body was operated upon. This relative loss of appetite and the development of distention with gas pains are in part due to the anesthetic agent, but the total metabolic assault of the operation has a cumulative effect. Fortunately, it is not necessary that food be ingested every day, and most patients promptly recover normal alimentary tract function, divest themselves of excessive gas, and are ready for food intake on the second, third, or fourth postoperative day. However, if such patients are fed before return of their desire for food, or the readiness of their gastrointestinal tract to accept it, gastric stasis may result in nausea and vomiting. There is also the definite hazard of pulmonary aspiration of some of the vomited material, especially in weak, elderly, or obtunded patients.

If the alimentary tract dysfunction is prolonged, however, as may occur after extensive intra-abdominal operations and especially when intraperitoneal sepsis develops, several problems arise. First, the stomach and upper reaches of the small bowel must be kept decompressed by gastrointestinal suction to prevent pooling of the several liters of bile, gastric juice, pancreatic juice, and succus entericus that enter the upper reaches of the alimentary tract each day. If the stomach becomes overdistended with this material, the serious syndrome of acute gastric dilatation and even shock may develop, and at the least the patient may vomit repeatedly with the risk of pulmonary aspiration. Furthermore, paralytic ileus of the intestine, not necessarily a primary problem but often secondary to other intra-abdominal or neurologic disorders, can produce much discomfort from gas pains. In the immediate postoperative period, the gut distention is almost certainly due to paralytic ileus alone, but as the days and perhaps even weeks pass, this ileus may give way

to mechanical obstruction caused by fibrous adhesions secondary to the operation. At this point, it often becomes difficult to decide whether to continue nonoperative management of "paralytic ileus" or to operate to correct mechanical small bowel obstruction and prevent gut strangulation with possible perforation. This decision often requires considerable clinical experience and judgment.

For many years most abdominal surgeons have almost routinely passed a nasogastric tube for continuous suction during the first 48 to 72 hours postoperatively. However, recently there has been a trend away from this practice, with the use of the nasogastric tube confined to those patients who vomit or who are otherwise uncomfortable and in whom there is evidence of gastric distention. Since approximately 70 per cent of the gas that distends the small bowel represents swallowed air, the use of a nasogastric tube with continuous suction does much to reduce the degree of small bowel distention and to lessen gas pains. We continue to insert a nasogastric tube in most patients who have undergone a major operation, to reduce the risk of pulmonary aspiration if for no other reason. When a tube is used, it is usually left in place for about 48 to 72 hours, or until the patient has active bowel sounds and is passing flatus. Once the tube has been removed, the patient is permitted a liquid intake, followed by an increasingly liberal diet, to full normal intake. Although the appetite center is in the hypothalamus, the alimentary tract and the appetite are closely related, and appetite does not usually return until normal alimentary tract function has returned. During the period when the patient is not taking an adequate oral intake, the daily fluid requirements are supplied by the intravenous route.

Fecal impaction is a relatively common complication, even in vigorous patients if they have lain in bed for a period of days. It is especially common in old people who are bedridden. The patient has the sensation of never completely emptying the rectum at stool, even though diarrhea may occur around the impaction and often with fecal incontinence. When these symptoms are complained of, the possibility of bacterial overgrowth due to broad-spectrum antibiotics should at least be considered but, more important, a rectal examination should be performed to exclude fecal impaction. If it is found, multiple oil enemas followed by soapy water should be given. Oral saline cathartics may also be useful. However, it is often necessary to break up the impaction digitally before it can be removed. This can be very painful and an opiate should be given prior to the manipulation. Rarely is major anesthesia required.

Inadequate nutritional intake is often a result of alimentary tract dysfunction. No serious attention need be given to nutrition when prompt recovery is anticipated, though perhaps 1000 calories will be given incidentally in the intravenous fluids. In contrast, if the patient has a condition that may well deplete his metabolic reserves over a period of several weeks or months, such as a high-output small bowel fistula, prompt and unceasing attention must be given to the introduction of calories and protein by every route available. This represents a subject of considerable dimensions and is mentioned here only as an admonition that in many clinical circumstances the outcome is ultimately decided on the basis of the nutrition achieved and the assiduous conservation of the patient's general metabolic reserves. If one reflects that he himself prefers not to miss three meals in one day, he will view with concern the fact that patients in the hospital may go for days or weeks without significant alimentation. Patients with increased metabolic requirements, such as those in febrile states, are less able to withstand long periods of starvation than are those who merely fail to take nourishment.

Miscellaneous Postoperative Problems

A wide variety of other postoperative problems may develop upon occasion. These include vascular problems, neurologic deficits from strokes or improper pressure upon nerves as a result of the patient's position during the operation, the leaving of foreign bodies in wounds, the dislodgement and embolization of catheters placed in veins, needle breakage with retention of a metal foreign body in the patient, skin burns due to the use of electrocautery with improper grounding during operation, skin necrosis due to subcutaneous infiltration of a norepinephrine drip in the postoperative period, various complications associated with the use of the nasotracheal tube, nasogastric tubes, or urinary catheters, and still other uncommon problems. We have not mentioned the most common problem, namely, the pain produced by the operation itself. When the patient complains of excruciating pain, it is wise to believe him and to search carefully for a possible abnormal cause of this pain. For example, an offending cast should be removed sufficiently to determine whether or not excessive pressure is being exerted on the tissues beneath. The usual wound is not spontaneously painful after the first 48 to 72 hours.

Hiccups (singultus) can be very annoying in the postoperative period. This symptom may be due to gastric distention, to irritation of the diaphragm, or to metabolic disorders affecting the brain, among other causes. Fortunately, modern tranquilizing drugs, such as chlorpromazine (Thorazine) will control hiccups in most cases. Where this drug fails, carbamazepine[17] or diazepam (Valium)[9] may prove efficacious. Nonetheless, it is wise to pass a nasogastric tube and provide continuous suction for 24 hours if the symptoms are associated with gastric distention. If the patient is febrile, subdiaphragmatic infection should be considered.

Decubitus ulcers ("bed sores," "pressure sores") can present a vexing problem in the debilitated patient, who is often malnourished. Not infrequently the development of severe decubitus ulcers reflects insufficient nursing attention to keep the patient turned and to prevent prolonged pressure on body prominences, usually the sacrum, greater trochanters of the femur, the lateral malleoli of the fibulae, and the heels. However, despite the best of nursing care, pressure sores will develop in some patients, especially paraplegics. Fortunately, good nursing care, foam rubber protectors, sheep's wool, air mattresses, water mattresses, and nutritional adjuvants have reduced the incidence and severity of these indolent lesions.

PROBLEMS RELATED TO SPECIFIC OPERATIONS

The foregoing discussion has involved consideration of problems that may develop after almost any major operation. Brief consideration will now be accorded specific problems that may follow specific operations, owing to the nature and location of the dissection involved.

Operations upon the Neck

Operations performed upon the neck are associated with special complications. Since the operation is frequently performed for some type of malignant neoplasm, the thin skin flaps fashioned in the course of the dissection at times permit complications that can be disastrous.

The most important complication that may follow an operation upon the face, jaw, or neck is that of postoperative respiratory distress due to hemorrhage in the depths of the wound. This is especially true following thyroidectomy, since once the deep cervical fascia has been reapproximated with sutures there is a little opportunity for hematoma of increasing size to expand outward, unless drains achieve a ready egress of the liquid blood. Unfortunately, the blood often clots in the drainage tract and thereafter a large unsuspected hematoma may compress the pharynx and trachea to produce severe respiratory embarrassment and even asphyxia. Moreover, the large blood collection may be almost invisible externally. Therefore, it is important to achieve meticulous hemostasis in operations involving the neck—above all in the hypertensive patient who has a somewhat greater chance of postoperative oozing than does the patient with a normal blood pressure level. If in the postoperative period the patient complains of difficulty in swallowing or is continually clearing his throat, or says that he has the sensation of choking, the closest possible attention must be paid to the wound and, if there is any doubt, the sutures should be removed and the depths of the wound explored with the sterile-gloved finger to make certain that hematoma has not formed. If it becomes necessary to open the wound and to evacuate a clot, and if the situation is not completely satisfactory, an endotracheal tube should be reinserted for 24 to 48 hours, until the situation has stabilized. With the airway thus secured, tracheostomy should rarely be necessary.

A second serious complication, especially after jaw resection with associated radical neck dissection, is infection, often with sloughing of the skin flaps and exposure of the carotid vessels. A pharyngeal fistula may develop and preoperative radiation may further impair healing. Carotid erosion may produce massive hemorrhage that can be controlled only at the risk of producing contralateral hemiplegia. The management of this problem has been well discussed by Callison and Edgerton.[3]

Further complications involve injury to important nerves, such as the recurrent laryngeal, hypoglossal, and superior laryngeal. Damage to the recurrent nerve on only one side produces dysphonia but usually not respiratory distress. Fortunately, the dysphonia of unilateral recurrent nerve injury can now be largely or completely abolished by Teflon paste injections (Arnold). Hypoglossal nerve injury causes disturbance in both swallowing and, to an extent, phonation, but the patient gradually compensates to a degree. Injury to the superior laryngeal nerve impairs sensation in the pharynx, especially the epiglottis and uvula, and strangling may accompany attempts to swallow food. Again, compensation occurs here also in a matter of months, but this injury can be much more disabling than is generally realized. Hypoparathyroidism follows excision of excessive amounts of parathyroid tissue at thyroidectomy. This deficit is temporary in many or most cases, and only temporary administration of 12 gm. of calcium lactate in divided doses, at times with 50,000 units of vitamin D per day, is required. In some patients, however, the hypocalcemia is permanent, but becomes better tolerated in time. In still others a relative or subclinical parathyroid deficiency may persist, which may become overt in the presence of excessive demands for calcium, as in pregnancy.

Still another complication of neck dissection, especially on the left side, is a thoracic duct fistula. The fistula will usually close in a matter of days and reoperation is not often necessary. Local compression may expedite closure of the fistula, since there are numerous alternate sites for thoracic duct lymph to reenter the venous circulation.

PULMONARY RESECTION

Pulmonary resection represents a common type of operation within the thorax, and its complications are representative of those of many other thoracic procedures. The most frequent postoperative complications of pulmonary resection are hemorrhage into the thorax, atelectasis and pneumonitis, pneumothorax that causes pulmonary compression, respiratory insufficiency, empyema, and bronchopleural fistula.

The *hemorrhage* into the thorax may not be great in volume, but it poses several problems. First, the bleeding can cause hypovolemia and hypotension, which have been discussed previously. Second, if the blood is allowed to clot in the thorax, compressing the lung and reducing lung volume and vital capacity, the benefits of the operation may be less than might otherwise have been expected, for if the blood clots, it will not emerge through the drainage tubes inserted at operation, and another operation will often be required to evacuate this blood. Therefore, postoperative hemorrhage should be prevented to the extent possible by careful hemostasis throughout the operation and particularly at the time of closure.

Pneumothorax is usually managed effectively by insertion of a tube above and anteriorly, so that air will be permitted to escape from the uppermost portion of the thorax when the patient is lying supine. If both air and fluid are present, a second tube is inserted below for dependent drainage. Any operation that involves lung tissue can result in some degree of air leak, but this will usually close in 24 to 48 hours. However, if a *bronchopleural fistula* develops, especially if associated with tuberculosis or malignant neoplasm, the bronchopleural fistula may remain open for a long while and may even require a second operation with additional bronchus resection for closure.

Infection in the pleural space that causes pus to accumulate is called empyema, and this is usually drained with a tube using an underwater seal. If such closed drainage is not successful, thoracotomy may be required.

In addition to these complications that come from the lung itself, total removal of a lung may be associated with some degree of postoperative dyspnea and *respiratory insufficiency*. A reduced oxygen tension in the arterial blood, with associated hypercarbia, can produce serious cardiac arrhythmias. These complications are best avoided by careful preoperative assessment of pulmonary function.

OPEN-HEART OPERATIONS

Open-heart operations involve a wide variety of technical procedures, but the general postoperative complications of all of them are remarkably similar. Among the complications is *bleeding* from the operative field, which is more serious in this particular operation than in most others because of coagulation problems attendant upon use of the heart-lung machine, the transfusion of homologous blood, and certain congenital coagulation defects. The hemorrhage can result in hypovolemia and low cardiac output, assuming that the low output does not also result from failure to correct the cardiac disorder for which operation was performed. The blood may also produce cardiac tamponade, which can be hard to distinguish from heart failure per se, since both are associated with a high central venous pressure and a low arterial blood pressure. Optimal cardiopulmonary bypass, meticulous attention to hemostasis, adequate tube drainage, and appropriate blood replacement usually are successful in controlling hemorrhage. The use of plastic drainage tubes is preferred because their patency is readily visualized and occlusion by clots occurs less readily than in rubber tubes.

Disorders of consciousness and related neuropsychiatric deficits have become less common as the precision and safety of cardiopulmonary bypass and blood filtration have improved. In 166 open-heart cases (1973–1974), Bethune et al.[1] had three deaths and eight patients who exhibited neurologic or psychiatric abnormalities, none of which was permanent.

Respiratory distress is also a common postoperative problem after open-heart surgery. This can be caused by blood loss but it also is frequently due to cardiac or pulmonary insufficiency, or both. Chronic heart disease may have produced extensive lung disorder, which is further aggravated by cardiopulmonary bypass and the usual postoperative atelectasis. Thus, even if the heart lesions have been fully corrected, a low Po₂ may persist for days. For this reason, it is often desirable to leave the endotracheal tube in place for 24 to 72 hours, with assisted positive-pressure mechanical ventilation.

Arrhythmias represent still another serious postoperative problem in some patients.[5] These may result from technical factors at operation, cardiac ischemia, hypoxia, or abnormal electrolyte concentrations, especially potassium. Rose et al.[21] found that 37 of 50 patients studied (74 per cent) had at least one postoperative arrhythmia. In 28 (56 per cent) an arrhythmia was present postoperatively that had not been present preoperatively. The most common arrhythmias were atrial fibrillation and multiple premature ventricular contractions. A total of 79 different arrhythmias were met in these 37 patients. Once the patient had left the operating room, an electrolyte imbalance was rarely incriminated as an etiologic factor; rather, digitalis effects and a nonspecific effect of the operative trauma appeared to play the more important roles. Management consists of providing the best possible respiration and optimal blood volume, judicious use of cardiac drugs, careful maintenance of a normal serum potassium level, and the use of a lidocaine drip to suppress excessive ventricular irritability. Third-degree heart block is treated with a pacemaker.

Low cardiac output syndromes are fairly common after major open-heart surgery. These are usually due to inadequate blood volume, heart failure that is perhaps due to incomplete correction of the cardiac defects, or to tamponade, arrhythmia, or defective respiration. The use of central venous pressure and left atrial pressure measurements, to ensure that blood volume is adequate, assists in avoiding hypovolemia, which is the most common cause of a low cardiac output.

BILIARY TRACT OPERATION, PANCREATIC RESECTION, AND SPLENECTOMY

Biliary Tract

Operations upon the biliary tract are followed by a variety of complications that are peculiar to this particular area of dissection. Postoperative hemorrhage, excessive bile drainage, ascending cholangitis due to manipulation within an infected common bile duct, pancreatitis, and even postoperative hepatic insufficiency may result. Common bile duct injury is not frequent, but it is a serious long-term complication of cholecystectomy and of other operations in the region of the common bile duct. Postoperative fever is frequently due to subhepatic or subphrenic collections of infected bile or to hepatic sepsis including liver abscesses. When a T tube is used, there are occasional minor problems in extracting the tube. Common duct stones are frequently overlooked and may require a second operation if one of the ingenious new techniques for removing such stones through the inlying catheter or T tube is not successful.

However, efforts to dissolve residual bile stones by a continuous drip of cholic acid through the T tube were reported by Way[23] to have been successful in almost two thirds of cases. If the chemical lysis was effective, the cholesterol stones disappeared after 10 to 14 days of infusion. Some stones diminished in size and then abruptly disappeared, as if they had passed into the duodenum. As to be expected, patients with multiple residual common duct stones or those with stones larger than 1.5 cm. were less likely to have a successful result. Other surgeons have reported some success with a heparin drip.

Finally, there is the so-called postcholecystectomy syndrome, which represents, in effect, a continuation of the symptoms for which the patient underwent cholecystectomy in the first place. This set of symptoms may be due to an erroneous original diagnosis, with the symptoms actually having been due to some other condition such as peptic ulcer, diaphragmatic hernia, or angina pectoris. However, the most common cause of the postcholecystectomy syndrome is a stone or stones in the common bile duct, in the remaining portion of the cystic duct, or the lower portion of the gallbladder that was left behind, infections in the general neighborhood of the common duct, common bile duct injury with stricture, or even the very rare cystic duct neuroma. When the patient was operated upon for jaundice and no definite stones were found, it is always possible that a malignant tumor in the head of the pancreas or intrahepatic disease was overlooked.

The close association between pancreatitis and biliary tract stones has been known for many years, and frequently the patient with gallbladder or common duct stones is first admitted with an attack of acute pancreatitis. In general, the attack of pancreatitis should be allowed to subside completely before operation is performed to remove the gallbladder and to explore the common bile duct. The operation can be more safely carried out during a quiescent period, and the actual dissection and common duct exploration can be more effectively executed at that time.

Pancreatic Resection

The most serious complication of pancreatic resection is a pancreatic duct fistula. Since the operation involves anastomosis of the upper jejunum to the common bile duct, to the stomach, and to the remaining portion of the pancreas, any of these suture lines can leak. The digestive enzymes, plus associated sepsis, may produce hemorrhage in the depths of the wound with serious or fatal results.

Some pancreatic fistulas close spontaneously without major sequelae. Fortunately, in recent years the operative techniques have become so standardized in some surgical centers as to permit a low mortality rate from pancreatic resection, a development that has encouraged a more liberal use of the operation. Even so, the 5-year survivals after resection of pancreatic carcinoma involving only the ampullary region or the tissues immediately adjacent to it are few, and in most hands pancreatic resection involves a mortality rate of 10 to 20 per cent.

Splenectomy

Splenectomy is basically a simple operation and its complications are not particularly severe. Hemorrhage can occur, as can pancreatitis due to trauma to the tail of the pancreas. If care is not exercised, the greater curvature of the stomach can be injured in the course of ligating the vasa brevia between the stomach and the spleen. However, the most important complication of splenectomy is infection in the splenic bed. It has seemed that this complication occurs more frequently after splenectomy than after other clean operations within the abdomen, and it is well to place antibiotics in the left subphrenic space. Nonetheless, postsplenectomy infection is less common in our hospital now than it was a decade ago. If hemostasis is complete at the time of closure, drainage is not routinely employed.

ALIMENTARY TRACT OPERATIONS

Esophagus

The most serious early complication of esophageal operations is leakage at the suture line, and a major leak often proves fatal. The thoracic esophagus gets its blood supply primarily from arteries that enter perpendicularly, and excessive mobilization of the remaining esophagus, to which the stomach or jejunum or colon is to be anastomosed, can result in ischemic necrosis at the anastomosis. Thus, while it is wise to transect the esophagus well above the apparent extent of the tumor, the remaining esophagus should be denuded only to the extent necessary for precise suture placement. If the esophagogastric anastomosis has a good blood supply and undue tension is avoided at the time of anastomosis and prevented in the postoperative period by fixing the stomach in the thorax, satisfactory healing will occur in most instances.

Assuming that the anastomosis has healed satisfactorily, the later complications of esophageal resection are stenosis or stricture of the anastomosis and esophagitis with mucosal erosion due to reflux of the material from the stomach. It is advisable to perform a pyloroplasty at the time of the original operation, since the routine division of the vagus nerves might otherwise result in gastric stasis.

Stomach

The commonest early complication of operations upon the stomach is hemorrhage, either anastomotic, from a residual ulcer, into the free peritoneal cavity from the spleen, or from unligated vessels. Bleeding from the anastomosis can usually be expected to cease in a few hours, but this is not always the case. Unfortunately, continued or recurrent bleeding from the ulcer for which the operation was performed may require reoperation. If vagotomy and pyloroplasty and oversewing of the bleeding ulcer were employed at the first operation, a distal subtotal gastric resection with excision of the ulcer or its exclusion with a Billroth II anastomosis is preferred. Whatever the procedure elected, the bleeding must be abolished.

The next most important complication of gastric surgery is leakage at a suture line, including dehiscence of the duodenal stump if a Billroth II anastomosis was employed. This and other causes of infection produce much of the major morbidity following

TABLE 5. Postoperative Complications Following Gastric Surgery* (604 Cases)

Deaths	37
Hemorrhage	29
Continuing (11)	
Anastomotic (9)	
Intermediate (2-20 POD) (9)	
Gastric retention	14
Proximal loop syndrome	21
Duodenal stump dehiscence (15)	
Subacute and chronic (6)	
Anastomotic leakage	7
Marked dumping and/or diarrhea	29
Severe malnutrition	28
Intraperitoneal infection (including abscess)	14
Wound complications	76
Infection and abscess (55)	
Evisceration (21)	
Jaundice	18
Hemolytic and absorptive (14)	
Obstructive (4)	
Common bile duct injury	2
Marginal ulceration	15
Fistulas (other than duodenal)	10
Jejunal (1)	
Pancreatic (2)	
Gastrocutaneous (5)	
Gastrocolic (2)	
Internal hernia	1
Intussusception	1
Pancreatitis	6
Pulmonary complications	54
Total	362

*Elective operations comprised 82 per cent of the total cases, while 18 per cent were emergency procedures. (From Hardy, J. D.: Problems associated with gastric surgery. A review of 604 consecutive patients with annotation. Am. J. Surg., *108*:699, 1964.)

gastric surgery. Adequate surgical drainage, antibiotics, and nutritional support will be successful in the majority of patients.

Failure of the stomach to empty represents a prominent problem of the later postoperative period. There are numerous causes of gastric retention, even when only vagotomy-pyloroplasty was performed. First, the vagotomy effect may result in marked loss of gastric tone and contractions, and many days may elapse before the stomach resumes its propulsive capacity, assuming that the pyloroplasty or gastrojejunostomy was technically satisfactory. If distal subtotal gastrectomy was performed, especially of a Billroth II type, poor emptying may be due to marked distention of the proximal loop with distortion of the gastrojejunal anastomosis, stenosis of the anastomosis itself, adhesions involving the loops of jejunum near the anastomosis, infection or pancreatitis surrounding the anastomosis, or any of a variety of other mechanical defects that may involve the gastrojejunal region. Special complications of gastric resection for peptic ulceration include the dumping syndrome, diarrhea and malnutrition, and especially recurrent ulceration due to inadequate control of the ulcer diathesis. Bezoars may form secondary to cellulose accumulation, orange ingestion being a cause.[12, 20]

It may be noted that even a gastrostomy presents hazards, consisting mainly of intraperitoneal leakage, and there has been a trend away from gastrostomy for postoperative decompression of the stomach. The inflated balloon of a Foley type gastrostomy catheter may obstruct the duodenum. Nasogastric tube suction is safer and is effective.

Small Bowel

Operations upon the small bowel are most often performed for obstruction, whether due to the adhesions or to hernias, which together account for a majority of the cases of small bowel obstruction. However, small bowel resection may also be required for inflammatory disease or tumors. Occasionally a very large part of the small bowel must be resected for gangrene due to inadequate blood supply, occasioned either by obstruction of the arterial or venous blood supply or by volvulus associated with congenital malrotation or adhesions.

Enteric anastomoses may disrupt and produce a fistula and peritonitis, though this is rare unless ischemia, infection, or distention existed. Major small bowel fistulas are associated with a mortality rate of approximately 20 to 30 per cent. In brief, management consists of adequate external drainage, control of infection, nutritional support in all its forms, and protection of the skin from erosion by the digestive enzymes. Operative intervention for attack upon the fistula itself is undertaken only after careful analysis, and only when nonoperative measures have proved inadequate. However, judicious operation can be most helpful in an appropriate situation. Intestinal *insufficiency* will result if excessive amounts of small bowel are resected. When total colectomy is performed, with a permanent ileostomy, numerous minor and even major problems may attend the ileostomy before it is finally stabilized. A special problem consists of high-volume and even explosive and salt-depleting output from the ileostomy, upon occasion. The most common causes of this ileostomy "diarrhea" are recurrent inflammation of the residual bowel, partial small bowel obstruction, and intraperitoneal sepsis. When these possible causes have been excluded, Hill et al.[13] believe the next most important consideration to be the amount of ileum that was resected. They recommend the use of codeine phosphate, Lomotil, and the oral administration of sodium chloride tablets. When possible, an end-to-end anastomosis of the small bowel should be performed to avoid a blind loop, which may gradually enlarge and produce stasis with bacterial growth and the destruction of vitamin B_{12} with resulting anemia and other problems.

The resection of a massive amount of the small bowel frequently results in gastric hypersecretion.[19, 24] This hypersecretion, involving both volume and hydrochloric acid, may be intermittent,[15] and it would appear to be related to a loss of inhibitory effects of intestinal hormones upon gastric secretion.[14] A succinct review of this problem with an excellent bibliography has recently appeared.[2] One of the complications of this gastric hypersecretion is peptic ulceration with

hemorrhage. The use of antacids does not always prevent this complication, and gastric surgery may be required.

Large Bowel

The most sinister complication of resection of the large bowel is leakage at the suture line. Whereas leakage at the suture line of the small bowel may produce a small bowel fistula, which will cause some sepsis and will usually produce water and electrolyte losses if the fistula is fairly high, the breakdown of a colon anastomosis may introduce into the peritoneal cavity such a sinister and massive bacterial flora that death may result even if proximal colostomy is performed and good external drainage established. Massive antibiotic coverage is indicated. If the colon heals satisfactorily initially, because of a good blood supply at the suture line and the absence of surrounding infection or infiltrating tumor, the anastomosis may continue to scar down and may eventually become so stenotic that obstruction occurs and reoperation is required. This is rare, however. Hemorrhage is not usually a problem after colon operations, with the exception of abdominoperineal resection. Other complications include injury to the bladder, ureter, or duodenum.

A colostomy may be associated with various local complications. These involve necrosis of the colostomy itself, or its retraction beneath the skin, or obstruction just beneath the skin due to an improper technique. Late complications of the colostomy include inadequate evacuation of the fecal material, stricture at the skin level, herniation around the colostomy, prolapse of the colostomy through the stoma, and prolapse of the small bowel behind the colostomy within the abdomen to produce intestinal obstruction. Whereas an ileostomy may result in excoriation of the surrounding skin, due to the digestive enzymes contained in small bowel contents, feces from the colostomy rarely produce serious erosion of the surrounding skin.

RADICAL MASTECTOMY

The radical operation for the removal of the breast and the underlying musculature is representative of operations performed upon the surface of the body in which tension upon the suture line exists. Skin sloughs are common, fluid tends to accumulate beneath the flaps, and if the sutures are removed too early the skin margins may separate over a considerable distance. Thus, careful attention and judgment are required to achieve optimal healing of the wound. Excessive tension must be avoided, even if a skin graft must be used. Since the collection of considerable amounts of fluid beneath the skin flaps will prevent their becoming adherent to the underlying tissue, in addition to placing tension on the suture line, this fluid should be aspirated continuously with appropriately placed tubes or catheters. Incidentally, we have not been impressed that creation of excessively thin skin flaps at operation has materially contributed to the long-term results of radical mastectomy for carcinoma of the breast, and ischemic flaps are apt to slough.

Infection does not often constitute a serious threat to life after radical mastectomy, but it does contribute to postoperative morbidity. For example, if the operative field becomes infected and there is poor healing of the skin, delayed skin union results. Axillary contractures may develop. If late skin grafting becomes necessary, a considerable period of wound preparation may be required, causing excessive hospital expense to the patient that would have been avoided by primary healing. Furthermore, there is reason to believe that the development of infection in the axilla may result in an increased incidence of late swelling of the arm.

Injury to various nerves may not be immediately apparent after operation, but these complications do become obvious and troublesome as the patient increases the activity of the involved arm. The nerves most often injured are the long thoracic nerve of Bell to the serratus anticus muscle and the thoracodorsal nerve to the latissimus dorsi. Rarely, elements of the brachial plexus itself are injured in dissecting the axilla free of tissue containing lymph nodes, and the axillary vein and the axillary artery can also be injured. These problems are avoided by careful dissection and a sure knowledge of the anatomy of the area. Actually, injury to the long thoracic nerve or to the thoracodorsal nerve does not occasion major morbidity, but these deficits should be avoided when possible.

The late complications include skin contractures in the axilla, lymphedema, and years later lymphangiosarcoma in a markedly swollen arm. The swelling of the arm may range from a mild swelling to a truly massive edema. This edema usually involves the arm more than it does the hand itself, and it is due either to the great reduction of lymph drainage channels or to axillary vein thrombosis or to both. Usually axillary vein thrombosis is absent, and the lymphedema is perhaps due in part to subclinical infection. Nevertheless, this condition may develop in patients who have had perfect and immediate healing of the radical mastectomy wound, and the etiology in many patients is obscure.

Treatment of the lymphedema is essentially nonoperative. One helpful procedure is to wrap the arm from the fingers to the shoulder with an elastic bandage at bedtime, to reduce the degree of swelling during the night. The bandage may be removed during the day, because of its obvious detraction from the patient's appearance, and reapplied at night. This will tend to reduce the swelling to some extent. The patient should avoid exposure of the involved extremity to excessive sunlight, since sunlight appears to cause the development of cellulitis in some patients. Various operations have been recommended to reduce the swelling, including radical excision of much of the edematous subcutaneous tissue and fat that produce most of the swelling. However, we have never employed these procedures and consider them ill advised in most instances. In general, the swelling can be fairly well controlled with the use of elastic bandages, and the patient will become more tolerant of the condition as time passes after the original operation and the malignant tumor does not recur.

SELECTED REFERENCES

Artz, C. P., and Hardy, J. D.: Management of Surgical Complications, 3rd ed. Philadelphia, W. B. Saunders Company, 1975.
Forty-two authorities contributed to this volume, which covers a wide spectrum of surgical complications and their management.

Berk, J. L. (Ed.): Symposium on a physiologic approach to critical care. Surg. Clin. North Am., 55:1–753, 1975.
This monograph contains a wealth of information on the care of the critically ill patient. Emphasis is upon the derangements in respiratory, cardiovascular, and renal dynamics in these patients. Contributions include an explanation of the use of the Swan-Ganz catheter (Drs. Swan and Ganz) and an especially fine discussion of cardiovascular physiology (Dr. Levy). Also of much interest are the three articles on the low cardiac output state.

Cammerer, R. C., Anderson, D. L., Boyce, H. W., Jr., and Burdick, G. E.: Clinical spectrum of pseudomembranous colitis. J.A.M.A., 235:2502, 1976.
Five cases of pseudomembranous colitis are reported, together with observations on clinical, endoscopic, and histologic features. The authors conclude that individualized therapy is imperative. They believe that antibiotics themselves, rather than specific organisms and especially staphylococci, are often the causal agents.

Danielson, R.: Differential diagnosis and treatment of oliguria in posttraumatic and postoperative patients. Surg. Clin. North Am., 55:697, 1975.
This article describes the physiologic aspects of postrenal, prerenal, and renal failure, as well as the laboratory and clinical observations in surgical causes of oliguria. Diagnosis and treatment of acute renal failure are emphasized.

Fleming, W. H., Plummer, A. L., and Hatcher, C. R., Jr.: Current management of postoperative pulmonary insufficiency. Am. Surg., 40:200, 1974.
This timely report correlates the treatment of postoperative pulmonary insufficiency in a university setting with that in combat casualties. Standards for routine monitoring of surgical patients are outlined, as well as the authors' criteria for use of the respirator. Application of these principles resulted in a decrease in postoperative morbidity, elimination of wet lung syndrome as a cause of death, and a dramatic decrease in deaths caused by postoperative pulmonary insufficiency in both a university hospital and a hospital in which combat casualties were treated.

Rose, M. R., Glassman, E., and Spencer, F. C.: Arrhythmias following cardiac surgery: Relation to serum digoxin levels. Am. Heart J., 89:288, 1975.
In this clinical study of 50 patients, 37 (74 per cent) had at least one arrhythmia following cardiac surgery. In 28 patients (56 per cent) an arrhythmia was present postoperatively which was not present preoperatively. The authors concluded that serum digoxin levels may have been a factor, but they were often normal.

Shires, G. T., Carrico, C. J., and Canizaro, P. C.: Shock. Major Problems in Clinical Surgery. Volume 13. Philadelphia, W. B. Saunders Company, 1973.
This comprehensive monograph is based upon clinical and animal studies in the area of shock. Treatment of the shock state receives particular emphasis.

REFERENCES

1. Bethune, D. W., English, T. A. H., and Milstein, B. B.: Letter: Delirium after surgery. Br. Med. J., 4:408, 1974.
2. Buxton, B.: Small bowel resection and gastric acid hypersecretion. Gut, 15:229, 1974.
3. Callison, J. R., and Edgerton, M. T.: Radical neck dissection with sloughing, infected flaps, exposed vessels, and pharyngeal and thoracic duct fistulae. In Hardy, J. D. (Ed.): Critical Surgical Illness. Philadelphia, W. B. Saunders Company, 1971.
4. Cammerer, R. C., Anderson, D. L., Boyce, H. W., Jr., and Burdick, G. E.: Clincal spectrum of pseudomembranous colitis. J.A.M.A., 235:2502, 1976.
5. Danielson, G., and Ellis, F. H.: Low cardiac output and cardiac arrhythmias after open-heart surgery. In Hardy, J. D. (Ed.): Critical Surgical Illness. Philadelphia, W. B. Saunders Company, 1971.
6. Dearing, W. H., Baggenstoss, A. H., and Weed, L. A.: Studies on the relationship of *Staphylococcus aureus* to pseudomem-

branous enteritis and to postantibiotic enteritis. Gastroen-terology, *38*:441, 1960.

7. DeCosse, J. J., Poulin, T. L., Fox, P. S., and Condon, R. E.: Sub-phrenic abscess. Surg. Gynecol. Obstet., *138*:841, 1974.

8. Evans, C., Evans, M., and Pollock, A. V.: The incidence and causes of postoperative jaundice. A prospective study. Br. J. Anaesth., *46*:520, 1974.

9. Fariello, R. G., and Mutani, R.: Treatment of hiccup. Lancet, *2*:1201, 1974.

10. Finney, J. M. R.: Gastroenterostomy for cicatrizing ulcer of the pylorus. Bull. Johns Hopkins Hosp., *4*:53, 1893.

11. Hardy, J. D.: Problems associated with gastric surgery. A review of 604 consecutive patients with annotation. Am. J. Surg., *108*:699, 1964.

12. Henderson, R. P.: Recurrent gastric bezoar in a postgastrectomy patient. J. Miss. State Med. Assoc., *16*:42, 1975.

13. Hill, G. L., Mair, W. S. J., and Goligher, J. C.: Cause and manage-ment of high volume output salt-depleting ileostomy. Br. J. Surg., *62*:720, 1975.

14. Johnson, L. R., and Grossman, M. L.: Intestinal hormones as inhibitors of gastric secretion. Gastroenterology, *60*:120, 1971.

15. Klein, M. S., and Winawer, S. J.: Intermittent basal gastric hypersecretion following small bowel resection. Am. J. Gas-troenterol., *61*:470, 1974.

16. Mackenzie, M., Fordyce, J., and Young, D. G.: Subphrenic abscess in children. Br. J. Surg., *62*:305, 1975.

17. McFarling, D. A., and Susac, J. O.: Carbamazepine for hiccoughs. J.A.M.A., *230*:962, 1974.

18. Morgenstern, L.: Postoperative jaundice. An approach to a diag-nostic dilemma. Am. J. Surg., *128*:255, 1974.

19. Osborne, P., Frederick, P. L., Sizer, J. S., et al.: Mechanism of gas-tric hypersecretion following massive intestinal resection. Clinical and experimental observations. Ann. Surg., *164*:622, 1966.

20. Rigler, R. G., and Grininger, D. R.: Phytobezoars following partial gastrectomy. Surg. Clin. North Am., *50*:381, 1970.

21. Rose, M. R., Glassman, E., and Spencer, F. C.: Arrhythmias fol-lowing cardiac surgery: Relation to serum digoxin levels. Am. Heart J., *89*:288, 1975.

22. Van thiel, D. H., and Lester, R.: Postoperative jaundice. Mecha-nism, diagnosis and treatment. Surg. Clin. North Am., *55*:409, 1975.

23. Way, L. W.: Retained common duct stones. Surg. Clin. North Am., *53*:1139, 1973.

24. Winawer, S. J., Broitman, S. A., Molochow, D. A., et al.: Success-ful management of massive small bowel resection based on absorption defects and nutritional needs. N. Engl. J. Med., *274*:72, 1966.

21

ACUTE POSTOPERATIVE RENAL FAILURE: PROPHYLAXIS AND MANAGEMENT

Samuel R. Powers, Jr., M.D.

Acute postoperative renal failure is a serious, frequently lethal complication of both elective surgery and accidental injury. The continuing mortality of approximately 60 per cent for established postoperative acute renal failure is all the more surprising when viewed within the context of recent advances in dialytic therapy and renal transplantation. Early recognition and prompt correction of the physiologic derangements which constitute the clinical setting for the development of acute renal failure provide the only opportunity for reducing the large number of deaths due to this disorder. The problem is to distinguish the many vagaries of renal function which constitute normal responses to surgical stress from those which will lead to renal failure. These functional alterations may be superficially similar in both situations and can be differentiated only by the severity and duration of the physiologic disturbance. Fortunately, the modern clinical laboratory can provide the surgeon with the necessary quantitative measurements of renal function which a few years ago were available only in sophisticated research laboratories. Liberal application of these methods, combined with a thorough understanding of their interpretation, is the modern foundation for successful prevention of acute renal failure. Once renal failure becomes established, the course of the disease cannot be significantly modified by therapeutic interventions and the mere supportive nature of dialytic therapy is insufficient to reverse the high mortality.

HISTORICAL PERSPECTIVE

Clinical recognition of post-traumatic and postoperative acute renal failure as a separate entity associated with injury of peripheral tissues has occurred in only the very recent past. The third edition of this textbook, published in 1943, included a new chapter entitled "War Injuries." The chapter begins with the statement: "War, which is now raging, has immensely stimulated interest in war wounds and at the same time, it is revealing new types of injuries and developing new types of treatment." Under the heading "Types of War Injuries" is listed: "6: Crushing injuries caused by burial beneath fallen masonry and buildings. In addition to the direct damage which may result from such injuries (e.g., fractures), there now is recognized a new syndrome, the crush syndrome, in which death follows severe crushing injury of the soft tissue of an extremity by reason of renal failure, anuria and uremia." This syndrome, also known as the "crush kidney," was further defined in an article by Lucke.[13]

Improvements in the understanding of the prevention of acute renal failure are characteristic of many major advances in surgery that occurred as a result of experience gained in the treatment of war injuries. The first recognition of the true nature of this disorder appeared in a classic paper by Oliver,[16] who demonstrated that the disruption of tubular architecture was associated with renal ischemia. These studies provided an essential background for the clinical investigation of acute renal failure so that during the next military conflict in Korea, a surgical research team was assigned to study the response of the kidney to massive injury. These encyclopedic research efforts were published in a monumental document under the subheading "Post Traumatic Renal Insufficiency."[12] These studies demonstrated that the commonest cause of delayed death in those patients who had been successfully resuscitated from severe injury was the development of acute renal failure. At that time, 1 in every 200 seriously injured soldiers developed acute renal failure, with mortality approaching 90 per cent. The clinical frequency of postoperative acute renal failure following various surgical procedures in civilian practice was reported by Kiley soon after the publications from the Korean War.[10] Subsequent intense clinical and laboratory investigations led to improvement in our ability to prevent this disorder, as indicated by an occurrence of only 1 in 600 in the Viet Nam conflict. The mortality of established renal failure improved little, if at all.

DEFINITIONS OF ACUTE RENAL FAILURE

The generic name, *acute renal failure*, implies any acute disorder that results in inability of the kidneys to maintain the integrity of the internal environment. This general designation must be distinguished from the syndrome of *acute postoperative renal failure*, which is a specific clinical entity. Nevertheless, all of the conditions that may result in failure of renal function in the postoperative period must be considered in the differential diagnosis. The multiplicity of disorders which may produce the varieties of acute renal failure may be conveniently divided into three major groups: (a) prerenal; (b) renal, and (c) postrenal. Each of these may present with either oliguria or polyuria, but all have in common a rising blood urea nitrogen and serum creatinine. The fundamental problem in surgical patients is to distinguish a normal kidney trying to correct an abnormal internal environment (prerenal) from a kidney that has lost the ability to maintain homeostasis (renal) from an obstructive uropathy (post-

renal). The first condition is corrected by adjusting the internal environment to a more normal state, whereas the second demands the use of a mechanical extracorporeal kidney to maintain the internal environment while the patient's kidneys recover in their own time, uninfluenced by the therapeutic interventions of the surgeon. The third, or postrenal, acute renal failure responds to relief of the obstruction. Our current understanding of the mechanism involved in the various forms of acute renal failure is a triumph of the sciences of microscopic anatomy and physiology. Familiarity with these recent advances provides the basis for the successful management of postoperative patients with disturbances of renal function.

ANATOMIC AND PHYSIOLOGIC DETERMINANTS OF RENAL FUNCTION

The anatomic configuration of the individual nephrons within the kidney is the basis for current concepts of renal function (Fig. 1). The glomerular capillary tuft surrounded by the relatively impermeable Bowman's capsule permits the escape of variable quantities of an ultrafiltrate of the plasma which passes through the kidney (renal plasma flow, RPF). The total quantity of fluid which passes across the cap-

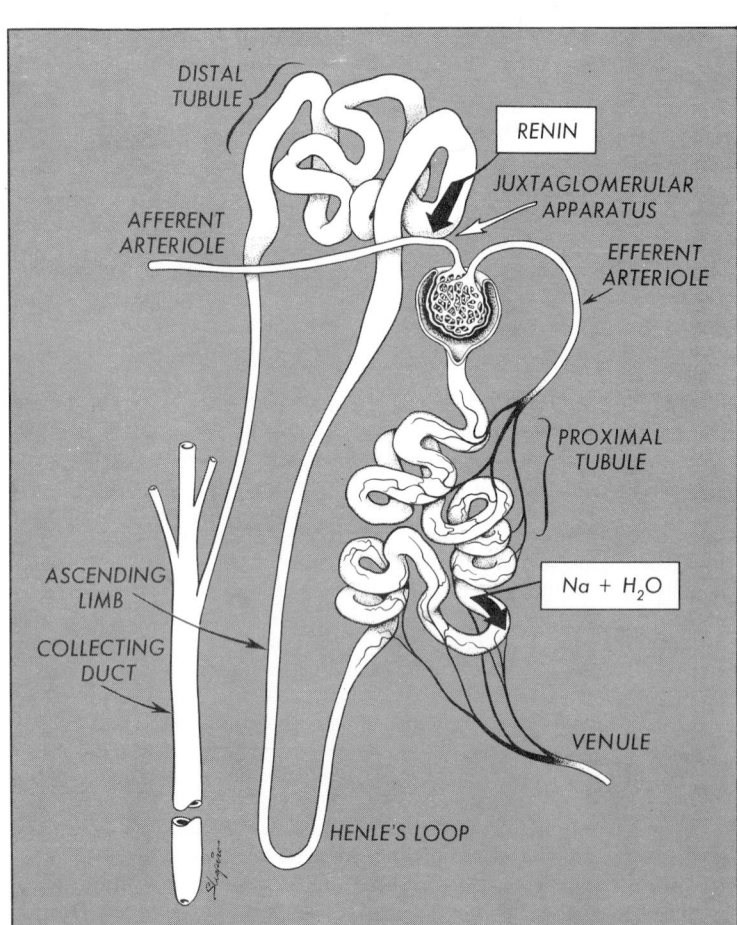

Figure 1. Principal functional and anatomic features of a typical nephron. The intimate relation between afferent arteriole, distal tubule, and juxtaglomerular apparatus is an essential feature of the tubular glomerular feedback loop. The proximal tubule accounts for the greatest fraction of sodium and water resorption.

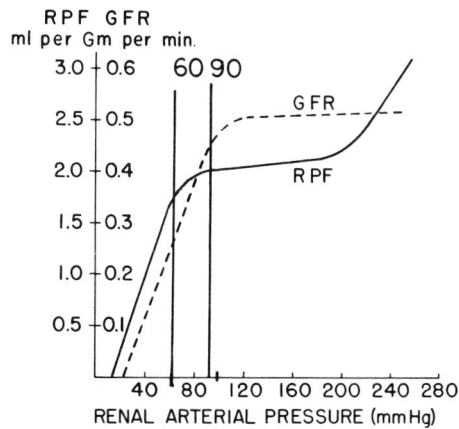

Figure 2. Autoregulation of GFR with varying arterial mean pressure. GFR begins decline when mean arterial pressure falls below 90 mm. Hg and is reduced to approximately one-half when mean pressure reaches 60 mm. Hg. (Adapted from Ochwadt, B.: Prog. Cardiovasc. Dis., *3*:501, 1961.)

illary tuft (glomerular filtration rate, GFR) depends upon a balance between the net hydrostatic forces between the capillary and the surrounding Bowman's capsule and the opposing osmotic forces due to the presence of plasma protein within the capillary and its absence in capsular fluid. If the sum of these forces is equal to zero, then all filtration ceases, even though adequate quantities of plasma continue to perfuse the kidney. The hydrostatic pressure in Bowman's capsule is normally vented through the renal tubule, and the osmotic forces are fixed by the level of plasma proteins. Therefore, the variable which is normally responsible for the quantity of glomerular filtrate is the hydrostatic pressure within the glomerular capillary. This pressure depends upon the difference in vascular tone of the afferent and efferent arterioles. Adjustments in these two resistances can maintain glomerular capillary pressure at a constant level in spite of wide fluctuations in systemic arterial pressure (Fig. 2). When, for example, systemic blood pressure falls, glomerular capillary pressure is maintained by a decreased resistance in the afferent arteriole and an increased resistance in the efferent arteriole. The result of these changes is to force a greater fraction of the total renal plasma flow through the capillary wall as a filtrate so that although total renal blood flow decreases, the glomerular filtration rate remains relatively constant. When mean arterial pressure falls below approximately 40 mm. Hg, even this compensatory mechanism is inadequate to maintain glomerular filtration. The relation between mean arterial pressure and glomerular filtration rate is shown in Figure 2. As pressures fall below the critical level, the quantity of filtrate decreases below that necessary to clear the body of metabolic nitrogenous waste products, and renal failure supervenes. There is strong evidence to support the concept that adjustments in the vascular tone of the afferent and efferent arterioles, which maintains glomerular filtration of each nephron at a constant level, resides in part in a tubular-glomerular feedback system, which adjusts the filtration rate to

the volume resorptive rate of the nephron.[14] The success of this control mechanism depends upon the anatomic coupling of the macula densa cells of the distal convoluted tubula with specialized structures in the adventitia of the afferent arteriole which, taken together, make up the juxtaglomerular apparatus. This structure is the site for renin production which, when locally converted to angiotensin II, becomes a powerful constrictor of the afferent arteriole. The signal which activates this mechanism appears to be related to a high sodium flux in the distal convoluted tubule. This feedback mechanism normally functions to preserve body sodium chloride by sensing excessive sodium loads in the distal convoluted tubule and causing a constriction of the afferent arteriole. This constriction results in a reduction in the glomerular filtration rate and a consequent curtailment of sodium loss. The tubuloglomerular feedback mechanism may, in extreme circumstances, produce a reduction of glomerular filtration rate below the level necessary to remove nitrogenous wastes and may be responsible for the oliguria and azotemia characteristic of certain forms of acute renal failure.

Conservation of body sodium is normally accomplished by the proximal tubule, which resorbs approximately 85 per cent of the glomerular filtrate. Further sodium is removed by active transport in the loop of Henle, with final adjustment of the sodium concentration in the distal convoluted tubule being determined by the level of aldosterone and other factors. Failure of the tubular epithelium to resorb sodium constitutes one of the characteristics of acute renal failure and accounts for the failure of the concentrating mechanism of the kidney. The anatomic configuration responsible for this function of the nephron is the path of the collecting tubule from the cortex to the depth of the medulla. The collecting duct traverses a region of interstitial fluid made hypertonic as a result of sodium that has been pumped out of the tubule lumen. The osmotic force of this hypertonic interstitial fluid acting across the tubular epithelium, modulated by antidiuretic hormone, results in the passive transfer of water out of the collecting duct into the interstitium. The final quantity and composition of urine is, therefore, a result of microscopic, anatomic inter-relations between glomerular blood supply, distal tubule juxtaglomerular apparatus, and the long course of the collecting duct from cortex through medulla. Acute renal failure occurs when the quantity of fluid filtered at the glomerulus is inadequate to remove nitrogenous wastes. The glomerular filtration rate is, in turn, determined by the systemic blood pressure and, to some extent, by the tubuloglomerular feedback mechanism controlled by the renin angiotensin system. Recognition of developing acute renal failure depends upon a measurement of the glomerular filtration rate, sodium resorption, and urine solute concentration.

THE GLOMERULAR FILTRATION RATE

The kidney can be considered to have three principal functions: filtration, sodium absorption, and water resorption (Fig. 3). Any one or more of these

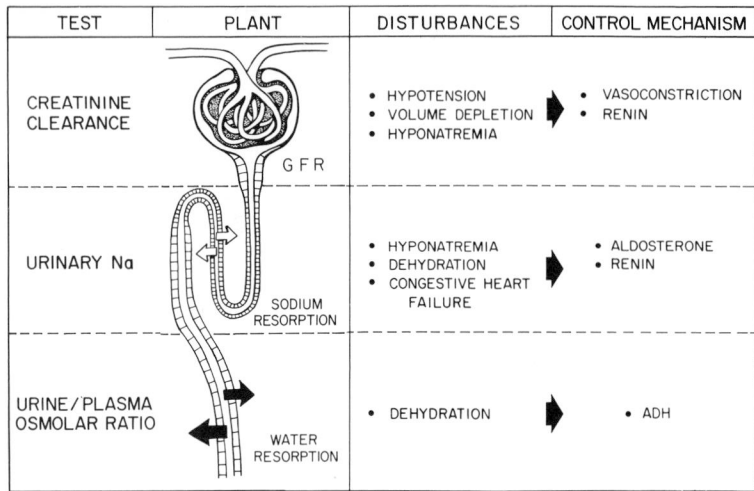

TEST	PLANT	DISTURBANCES	CONTROL MECHANISM
CREATININE CLEARANCE	GFR	• HYPOTENSION • VOLUME DEPLETION • HYPONATREMIA	• VASOCONSTRICTION • RENIN
URINARY Na	SODIUM RESORPTION	• HYPONATREMIA • DEHYDRATION • CONGESTIVE HEART FAILURE	• ALDOSTERONE • RENIN
URINE/PLASMA OSMOLAR RATIO	WATER RESORPTION	• DEHYDRATION	• ADH

Figure 3. The three principal functions of the nephron and the corresponding tests of each. The control mechanisms serve to maintain the constancy of the internal environment following disturbances of the volume and composition of the extracellular space. The complete control systems are much more complex than indicated involving prostaglandins and other vasoactive substances.

functions can be disturbed in the various forms of acute renal failure and each can be assessed by standard, clinical laboratory methods. The glomerular filtration rate (GFR) is conveniently determined from a one-hour timed creatinine clearance. Creatinine is removed from the body by filtration alone and, therefore, all creatinine which appears in the urine must have passed through the glomerular filtration mechanism at the concentration that exists in plasma. The calculation of GFR is straightforward. If the one-hour urine collection contains 60 mg. of creatinine, then the kidney must have excreted 1 mg. of creatinine per minute. If the concentration of creatinine in plasma is 1 mg. per 100 ml., then 100 ml. of plasma must have been filtered each minute to produce the 1 mg. of urinary creatinine each minute. The GFR under this circumstance would be 100 ml. per minute. The general formula for calculating GFR is GFR (ml. per min.) = UV/P, where U equals the urine creatinine concentration (mg./100 ml.), V equals the urine volume per minute (ml./min.), and P equals the plasma creatinine concentration (mg./100 ml.). This measurement is the cornerstone for evaluation of renal function in the postoperative patient and should be carried out routinely on all patients suspected of either incipient or developing acute renal failure.

The glomerular filtration rate for normal, healthy young adults is generally above 100 ml. per minute but may fall to values as low as 40 ml. per minute during periods of hypotension and still be sufficient to remove the products of nitrogen metabolism. Values of the GFR below 30 ml. per minute are generally associated with acute renal failure.

EVALUATION OF TUBULAR FUNCTION

Determination of the GFR includes a measure of the concentration of creatinine in both urine and plasma. The ratio of these two numbers, the urine/plasma creatinine ratio, is one of the reliable measurements of tubular function. The normal kidney working at max-

imum concentrating effort will produce a urine/plasma creatinine ratio of around 100. The presence of established acute renal failure generally results in urine/plasma ratios of 10 or less.

A more direct measurement of the adequacy of tubular function is obtained from the urine/plasma sodium ratio. A prime function of the tubules is to regain sodium lost from the body in the glomerular filtrate. The magnitude of this task and its importance for the maintenance of body homeostasis is appreciated by estimating the total amount of sodium which is filtered through the glomeruli in each 24-hour period. The total glomerular filtrate is approximately 200 liters, each liter containing roughly 150 mEq./L. of sodium. The total quantity of sodium passed through the glomeruli is, therefore, 30,000 mEq. per 24 hours. Under normal circumstances, all but approximately 50 mEq. are resorbed into the body by means of both passive diffusion in the proximal tubules and active sodium pumping. This is accomplished by the normal kidney to produce a resultant urine/plasma sodium ratio of around 0.1. Failure of the tubular sodium exchange mechanism yields a urinary concentration of sodium which is close to, if not identical with, that found in plasma. The urine/plasma sodium ratio is a particularly useful test of tubular function, since the sodium concentration in the serum is quite constant and is not affected by changes in catabolic rate and by breakdown of body tissues. Estimates of tubular function based on concentration of urea and creatinine in the urine are more difficult to interpret, since they are influenced by nitrogen metabolism and the amount of these substances appearing in the urine is determined by factors other than the adequacy of tubular function.

EVALUATION OF CONCENTRATING ABILITY

The final function of the kidney, in addition to filtration and tubular resorption, is the ability to concentrate the urine. The measure of concentration is the urine/plasma osmolar ratio. Resorption of water takes place in the collecting tubules which pass throughout the whole depth of the kidney from cortex to medulla. During this passage, the tubule is exposed to the hypertonic environment of the medulla, and it is the elevated osmolarity of the peritubular fluid which allows water to be passively absorbed back into the body. The interstitial fluid in the medulla of the kidney is hypertonic owing to its elevated sodium concentration, a consequence of active sodium transport from inside the tubule to the interstitial fluid.

A further requirement for urine concentration is that the collecting tubule be permeable to water, a factor controlled by ADH. In the presence of this hormone, water passes freely out of the collecting tubule into the renal interstitium until the osmolarity is equal on the two sides on the tubular cells. The ability to concentrate the urine, therefore, depends first upon adequate tubular function to pump sodium from the tubular lumen to the interstitium and also upon normal collecting tubules and the presence of ADH. The normal kidney acting under maximal stress can produce a urine/plasma osmolar ratio of greater than 1.3. On the other hand, failure of the tubular mechanism or the absence of an effective action of ADH results in a urine which is isosmotic with plasma. The functional assessment of the kidneys is, therefore, carried out by a single, one-hour timed urine collection and a single serum sample. From these, the urine/plasma ratios of sodium, creatinine, and total osmolarity are obtained and, in addition, a one-hour creatinine clearance can be calculated. A summary of the normal values obtained from such studies as well as the values obtained in a typical patient with acute postoperative renal failure is shown in Table 1. Taken together, these measurements can be referred to as the "one-hour renal function test."

Measurement of the hourly urine volume is not by itself a reliable test of renal function. On the other hand, an inappropriate urine volume is frequently the first clinical evidence that renal failure may be developing. The operational word in this measurement is "inappropriate." Patients suffering from volume depletion will uniformly demonstrate an appropriate oliguria, whereas patients who have received an excess of electrolyte replacement solution during the intraoperative period will usually present an appropriate polyuria. Either finding is evidence for a normal functional renal mechanism. The presence of severe oliguria in a patient who is normovolemic and the presence of polyuria in a patient who is volume depleted are examples of inappropriate urine volume and signify a probable acute renal failure. Proper postoperative fluid management and normal kidneys will result in a urine volume between 30 and 60 ml. per hour. Gross deviation either below or above these values should alert the clinician to the possibility of impending renal dysfunction. The one-hour renal function provides a definitive answer to the clinical suspicion of impending renal failure.[7] This decision must be made promptly. Severe derangement of renal function, allowed to persist for more than two hours, constitutes a true medical emergency and if not immediately corrected, may lead to irreversible damage.

On the other hand, prompt correction of all disorders of the internal environment, along with the addition of specific prophylactic measures, will frequently reverse impending renal failure during its functional phase and permit resumption of normal renal function. Indications for performing the "one-hour renal function test" should be liberal and the necessary chemical determinations should be available on a 24-hour-a-day basis. Indirect methods of assessment such as the use of a fluid load may delay the proper biochemical evaluation and should not supplant a function test. Further, a transient increase in urine volume does not necessarily exclude the presence of developing acute postoperative renal failure, nor does a failure to respond to a small fluid challenge result in a firm diagnosis. Attempts to manipulate the urinary volume may lead to the pernicious administration of one of the loop diuretics in an attempt to maintain renal function. Therapeutic intervention in this situation, as in all of clinical medicine, should await accurate diagnosis.

TABLE 1. Typical Results from the "One-Hour Renal Function Test"

A. Common Values Obtained from Oliguric Patients with Normal Kidneys

	Urine	Plasma	U/P	GFR (ml./min.)
Creatinine (mg./100 ml.)	100	1	100	
if urine volume = 30 ml./hr. (0.5 ml./min.)				50
Osmols (mOsm./L.)	400	300	>1.3	
Sodium (mEq./L.)	20	140	0.14	

B. Common Values Obtained from Patients with Acute Renal Failure

	Urine	Plasma	U/P	GFR (ml./min.)
Creatinine (mg./100 ml.)	20	2	10	
if urine volume = 10 ml./hr. (0.16 ml./min.)				1.6*
Osmols (mOsm./L.)	300	290	1.03	
Sodium (mEq./L.)	110	130	0.9	

*If urine volume = 100 ml./hr. (1.6 ml./min.), GFR = 16.

THE CLINICAL SETTING FOR ACUTE POSTOPERATIVE RENAL FAILURE

Effective prophylaxis for the development of acute postoperative renal failure begins with a prompt recognition of the high-risk clinical settings for the development of this disorder. Acute post-traumatic renal failure was first described by Bywaters[4] in association with severe shock and crushing injuries of skeletal muscle. Repeated clinical assessment of patients developing "traumatic anuria" revealed that hemorrhagic hypotension alone was rarely, if ever, associated with renal failure, whereas the combination of hypotension and crushing injuries resulted in a high incidence of this disorder. This conclusion is easily confirmed in civilian hospital practice by reviewing the incidence of acute renal failure in patients who suffered hypotension as a result of gastrointestinal hemorrhage from a duodenal ulcer. The incidence in this group of patients is almost zero. In the period following World War II, the syndrome of acute postoperative renal failure was observed in various clinical settings, in addition to massive muscle necrosis. The relative frequency of acute renal failure in a wide variety of clinical disorders was described by Kiley,[10] who noted that the single most common operative procedure in civilian practice which was associated with acute postoperative renal failure was a complicated operation on the biliary tract.

A remarkably high incidence of renal failure was seen in patients subjected to both elective and emergency resection of abdominal aortic aneurysms.[10] These patients were of great theoretical interest, since the common denominator appeared to be the placement of a clamp across the aorta just distal to the renal arteries. The probability that renal failure would develop as a postoperative complication increased with the length of time that the aortic clamp was in place. An early study of patients subjected to aortic aneurysmectomy[18] revealed an incidence of acute renal failure approaching 30 per cent when the aortic clamp remained in place for over 100 minutes. Experimental studies suggested that the aortic clamp induced stimulation of the rich plexus of autonomic nerves surrounding the origin of the renal arteries and that blockade of these nerves by pharmacologic means resulted in significant protection of the kidney.

The presence of circulating, abnormal globin pigment has been frequently associated with the development of acute renal failure. These pigments may arise from hemoglobin following a transfusion reaction or from myoglobin following crush injury. This clinical observation provides the basis for one of the experimental methods for producing acute renal failure.[15]

The appearance of visible globin pigments in the urine in association with a period of hypotension or traumatic injury suggests that the patient is at a greatly increased risk for the development of renal shutdown.

These varying clinical settings can be generalized into several initiating factors and predisposing events which are associated with a markedly increased incidence of acute postoperative renal failure. These factors are shown in Table 2.

TABLE 2. Factors Associated with the Development of Acute Renal Failure

1. Hypotension
2. Abnormal globin pigments
3. Increased sympathetic tone

Especially IF
A. Patient is dehydrated
B. Patient is hyponatremic
C. Items 1, 2, and 3 are allowed to persist for several hours

HYPOTENSION

A fall in mean arterial pressure sufficient to exceed the autoregulatory mechanism of the kidney will result in a fall in GFR (Fig. 2). Hypotension to this level will not in itself lead to acute renal failure but sustained hypotension may cause the kidney to become vulnerable to other factors which will result in renal damage. Moderate degrees of hypotension can be tolerated as long as the GFR, as measured by a one-hour creatinine clearance, remains above 30 ml. per minute. A mean arterial pressure below the 60 mm. Hg level necessary to sustain an adequate GFR should be immediately corrected.

ABNORMAL GLOBIN PIGMENT

Visible discoloration of the urine from abnormal globin pigments is apparently innocuous as long as the rate of tubular urine flow is sufficient to dilute and wash out this material. Maintenance of a urine volume in an excess of 60 ml. per hour should be assured by a combination of fluid loading, osmotic diuresis, and, under certain circumstances, the use of a loop diuretic. The simultaneous occurrence of hypotension, oliguria, and myoglobinuria describes an extremely high-risk clinical setting.

INCREASED RENAL VASCULAR RESISTANCE

Peripheral crushing injuries as well as operative procedures which stimulate the renal and splanchnic nerves will result in a disproportionate increase in renal vascular resistance at a time when cardiac output and total peripheral resistance may still be within the normal range. Increased renal vascular resistance may continue for several days after apparently adequate resuscitation as judged by normal blood pressure and cardiac output, which places the kidney at increased risk for the development of acute renal failure.[19]

Awareness of the clinical settings which place the kidney at increased risk for the development of acute renal failure is the primary requirement for successful prophylaxis. All patients in this clinical setting require a "one-hour renal function test" for the determination of GFR and urine/plasma, creatinine sodium, and osmolar ratios. Prompt, accurate correction of these specific underlying disorders will result in the virtual elimination of postoperative renal failure as a surgical complication.

CURRENT CONCEPTS FOR THE PATHOGENESIS OF ACUTE RENAL FAILURE

Evaluation of renal hemodynamics in both experimental animals and man following hemorrhage and trauma has shown a preferential ischemia of the superficial layers of the renal cortex.[9] This response of the outer cortical vessels was first demonstrated by Barger[2] by means of the radioactive gas technique and subsequently confirmed by Silastic injection of the renal vasculature and digestion of the renal tissue to form a corrosion cast. Following severe hypotension, there was a failure of the small subcortical vessels to fill with the injected material. The blood supply to the nephrons in the superficial cortex differs from that in the deeper portions of the kidney in several important respects (Fig. 4). Blood leaving the glomerular capillaries by way of the efferent arterioles passes directly to the subcapsular region, where it enters the peritubular capillaries, which surround the tubule, and then goes directly into the renal vein. In addition, the juxtaglomerular apparatus of these subcortical nephrons is rich in renin, with the concentration of this material decreasing as the deeper regions of the cortex are approached. Finally, approximately 85 per cent of the renal blood flow passes through this superficial area with the remainder of the kidney, particularly the medulla, being relatively ischemic. The effect of prolonged, severe hypotension on these nephrons has been studied in experimental animals using the micropuncture technique. In addition to a severe reduction in GFR, the resorptive capacity of the proximal tubule was markedly reduced. Persistence of impaired tubular resorption leads to an increased sodium load at the cells of macula densa, which triggers afferent arterial constriction and a further reduction in GFR. A normally functioning tubuloglomerular feedback system acting in the presence of hypotension initiates a vicious cycle where ischemia of the proximal tubule cell interferes with sodium resorption, resulting in an increased sodium delivery to the distal tubule which, in turn, is associated with renin release, formation of angiotension, and further reduction of subcapsular blood flow. Decreased flow through the efferent arterioles further aggravates proximal tubular ischemia, compromising the ability of these cells to resorb sodium. A positive feedback loop is established, with ever-increasing quantities of renin being released at the afferent arteriole. Indirect evidence to support this concept is obtained from the work of Oken, who demonstrated that experimental animals subjected to long-term saline loading with consequent near-total renal renin depletion were protected from the development of acute renal failure.

Vander[23] noted that renal artery hypotension following partial cross-clamping of the aorta above the renal arteries resulted in renin release from the kidneys. The release of renin could be blocked by the simultaneous administration of the osmotic diuretic mannitol. In a later study of experimental acute renal failure,[22] the administration of mannitol reduced renin production. There is, therefore, considerable circumstantial evidence that acute renal failure is associated with renin release from the kidney and, further, that substances which interfere with renin release are associated with protection of the kidney.

The role of renin in the development of acute renal failure may be of secondary importance rather than the prime etiologic factor. Thiel[21] investigated glycerol-induced acute renal failure in rats depleted of renin by chronic saline loading. During the initial four hours after glycerol injection, these animals showed the same apparent renal ischemia, cessation of filtration, and tubular collapse seen in rats that were not renin depleted. Despite this initial ischemia, renal function returned rapidly with individual nephron GFR reaching 75 per cent of normal within the succeeding 12 hours. He concluded that renin depletion prevented the protracted afferent arteriolar constriction that was responsible for the final pathophysiologic state in this model of acute renal failure. These studies are consistent with previously mentioned tubular glomerular feedback loop. The initial insult caused failure of the proximal tubule with an elevated sodium load to the distal tubule, causing renin release. The renin-induced afferent arteriolar spasm resulted in severe protracted reduction in GFR. This hypothesis of a two-step development of acute renal failure provides an intriguing explanation for the occurrence of the clinically puzzling syndrome of high-output renal failure. In this disorder, a normal or excessively high urine volume is associated with progressive azotemia and all of the metabolic derangements associated with acute renal failure. Slight variations in the effectiveness of the tubular glomerular feedback loop might result in a high urine volume even though only a small fraction of nephron population remained open. A GFR of 5 ml. per minute, clearly within the range of severe acute renal failure, will nevertheless produce a total filtrate of 300 ml. per hour. If the tubular mechanism resorbs two thirds of this filtrate, the urine volume would still be 100 ml.

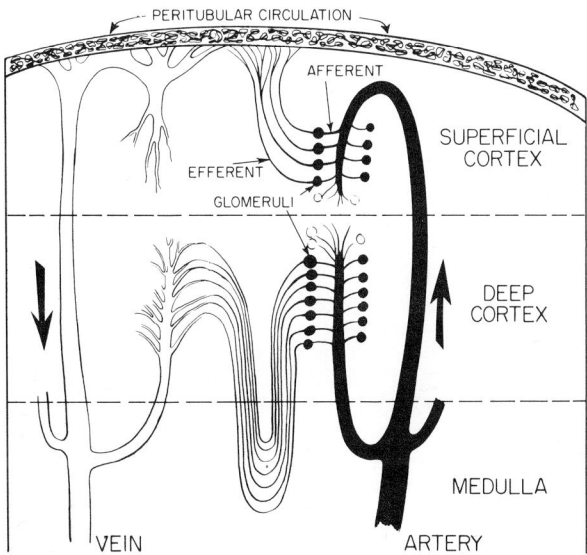

Figure 4. Schematic representation of the different blood supplies to nephrons in different portions of the renal cortex. Eighty-five per cent of the total renal blood flow perfuses the superficial cortical nephrons and passes directly from the efferent arterioles to the peritubular capillaries without coming into contact with the loop of Henle. The juxtaglomerular apparatus of the nephrons in this region of the cortex is rich in renin. The more deeply placed nephrons contain little renin and have large efferent arterioles which pass deeply into the medulla along with the loops of Henle. These nephrons make up the countercurrent multiplier system responsible for the renal concentrating mechanism.

per hour or 2400 ml. per day. The syndrome of high-output renal failure is, therefore, only a minor variant of oliguric renal failure. These considerations may also explain the apparent temporary reversal of acute renal failure occasionally noted following the administration of a loop diuretic. A transient increase in urine volume to apparently normal levels may occur because these drugs block tubular resorption of sodium. There is no improvement in GFR and little change in the course of the renal lesion. This error can be avoided if renal function is evaluated by a one-hour timed urine collection before the loop diuretic. This somewhat simplistic explanation is not entirely consistent with other studies which demonstrate complex interrelations between angiotension production, prostaglandins, and neurotransmission. Nevertheless, from a practical standpoint, pharmacologic intervention that blocks renin release from the kidney appears to be effective in the prevention of acute renal failure in man.

THE PREVENTION OF ACUTE RENAL FAILURE

Acute renal failure will generally be prevented when the GFR is maintained above 60 ml. per minute and when the renin angiotensin system is not activated. Both of these situations will usually prevail when the mean arterial blood pressure has been restored to normal levels, vasoconstriction has been reversed, and a high rate of urine flow obtained. In most clinical situations, all of these will be assured if the blood volume is restored to normal, and sufficient balanced electrolyte solution is administered to maintain the volume and composition of the extracellular space. On the other hand, hypotension, oliguria, and renal vasoconstriction that persist for more than a few hours place the kidney at an increased risk which is progressively less responsive to volume replacement. The kidney may then pass through a stage of functional renal failure where the administration of mannitol may facilitate the partial return of renal function in association with adequate volume replacement.[8, 16]

RESTORATION OF MEAN ARTERIAL PRESSURE

The relation between GFR and arterial pressure shown in Figure 2 relates to the mean pressure. Measurements of blood pressure in which the systolic pressure is the sole criterion of adequate resuscitation can be misleading. Figure 5 shows an arterial pulse

tracing from a patient recovering from traumatic shock. The systolic blood pressure is recorded at 60 mm. Hg, whereas the mean arterial pressure is only 25 mm. Hg. GFR at this pressure will be zero. Patients who fall into this high-risk category for the development of acute renal failure should have their blood pressure monitored by means of an intra-arterial cannula and strain gauge transducer. Blood pressure must be restored to a mean pressure of at least 80 mm. Hg and maintained at that level by adequate volume replacement.

MAINTENANCE OF EXTRACELLULAR FLUID

Replacement of shed blood may not be sufficient to maintain the extracellular space at a normal level. Extracellular fluid deficit may result in a decrease in GFR with a consequent contraction of the urine volume. Although ECF depletion is not a primary cause of acute renal failure, the administration of large volumes of electrolyte solution has been shown to minimize the severity of experimental acute renal failure.[6] Maintenance of an adequate extracellular fluid volume following hemorrhagic hypotension may require the administration of a balanced electrolyte solution in quantities in considerable excess of measured losses.[5] Surgical patients who are about to undergo operative procedures that have a high risk for the development of acute renal failure can generally be protected from this disorder by the prior administration of adequate volume of a balanced electrolyte solution. An adequate extracellular volume is indicated by a urine volume in excess of 40 ml. per hour and a normal central venous pressure. Hyponatremia must be corrected, since decreased serum concentrations of sodium are generally associated with a contraction of the extracellular space.

PREVENTION OF RENIN RELEASE

Normal renal perfusion with an adequate GFR is generally sufficient to prevent renin release unless direct stimulation of the renal nerve takes place, as in operations for an abdominal aortic aneurysm. In these high-risk situations or in the presence of massive soft tissue crushing injury, the administration of mannitol appears to be effective. The drug will exert its maximum prophylaxis if administered prior to the insult. A good practice is to include 50 gm. mannitol in the initial intravenous infusion of all patients admitted in

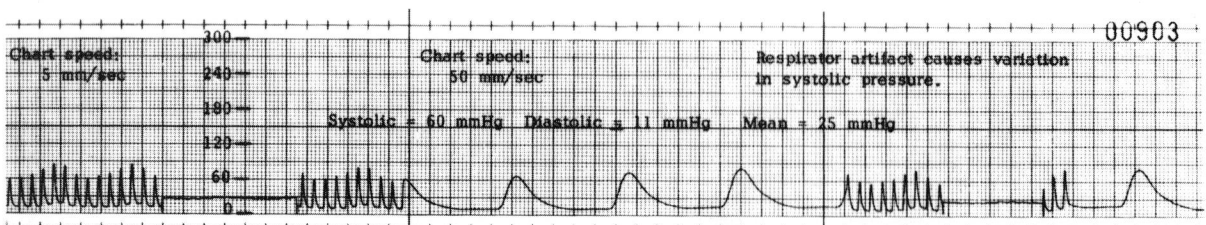

Figure 5. Arterial pulse wave tracing from a patient in shock. The mean arterial pressure is well below the value required for any glomerular filtration to occur.

traumatic shock associated with crushing injuries and in all patients subjected to aortic surgery.

A Physiologic Guide for the Prevention of Acute Renal Failure

Effective prevention of acute renal failure depends upon the liberal use of physiologic tests of renal function in all high-risk situations. In the usual clinical setting, a high-risk situation is defined as one in which a patient presents with an inappropriate urine volume. The order of procedure begins with optimizing the internal environment, for, if this is successful, a normal kidney will produce a normal quantity of urine of normal composition. Failure of the kidney to provide a normal quantity and composition of urine when the internal environment is normal suggests the preliminary diagnosis of impending acute renal failure. Prompt, energetic measures to reverse the physiologic abnormality before renal failure becomes established may still be accomplished. The sequential steps in this process are best provided by a table of decisions where specific physiologic tests are followed by corrective measures and the response to these measures then serves to indicate further tests or to establish a diagnosis. These steps should be pursued in an orderly fashion without jumping immediately to the inappropriate use of a loop diuretic for every patient who becomes oliguric. The loop diuretics, ethacrynic acid, and furosemide are effective agents for increasing urine flow in postoperative and post-trauma patients. These drugs are so effective that they may induce a large urine loss at a time when the patient's condition is in a critical balance and the additional loss of fluid and electrolytes will deplete the extracellular space to a dangerous degree. Precisely because these agents are effective and usually produce a gratifying increase in urine volume, there is a tendency to omit the step-by-step evaluation of renal function which would lead to a correct diagnosis for the cause of oliguria, and to proper corrective measures. With very few exceptions, oliguria in the immediate postoperative period is due to extracellular fluid volume depletion. If a diuretic is indicated in the orderly course of resuscitation, the use of mannitol will produce a moderate increase in urine volume which will not risk a further reduction in glomerular filtration rate. Under special circumstances where there is a concern about a pre-existing overexpansion of the extracellular fluid volume and a risk of congestive heart failure from fluid overload, the use of loop diuretics may be considered. Evidence for such overexpansion should be obtained from either a central venous pressure measurement or preferably a measurement of pulmonary capillary wedge pressure with a balloon-tipped, flow-directed pulmonary artery catheter. A safe rule to guard against the indiscriminate and dangerous use of loop diuretics is that these agents should not be administered to an oliguric patient until a direct measure of central venous or left atrial pressure has been carried out. Loop diuretics administered to a volume-depleted patient may eventuate in acute renal failure by causing the patient literally to urinate himself into shock.

ACUTE RENAL FAILURE DUE TO MECHANICAL OBSTRUCTIONS TO THE OUTFLOW OF URINE

Postoperative and post-trauma patients with a sudden onset of anuria must be considered to have mechanical obstruction of the ureters. Accidental direct injury to the ureters is an uncommon but ever-present cause of the syndrome of postrenal acute renal failure. The operating surgeon will invariably be certain that no damage to the ureters could possibly have occurred, since recognized damage would, of course, have been corrected. Nevertheless, this condition must be suspected whenever operative or traumatic injury of the retroperitoneal or pelvic area has taken place. Absolute anuria is rarely seen in the renal form of acute renal failure and never in the prerenal form. This diagnosis can only be established with certainty by cystoscopy and retrograde catheterization of the ureters. Prompt recognition of this condition followed by a return of the patient to the operating room and surgical correction of the obstructed ureters will generally result in complete salvage of renal function. Other causes of postrenal failure include traumatic rupture of the bladder with extravasation into the perivesicle space and the placement of a urethral catheter through a false passage into the periurethral tissues. In each case, the diagnosis can be suspected by irrigating a small amount of saline into the urethral catheter and the diagnosis confirmed by the injection of a small quantity of radiopaque dye. When mechanical obstruction has been ruled out as a possible cause of the anuric state, an orderly investigation of renal function should be performed, as indicated in Table 1.

Therapy of Established Postoperative Acute Renal Failure

The diagnosis of acute renal failure is established when the glomerular filtration rate remains less than 30 ml. per minute after the mean arterial blood pressure has been restored to greater than 80 mm. Hg. Elevations in the blood urea nitrogen and serum creatinine concentrations are the consequences of established acute renal failure, not the criteria for diagnosis. Reliance on these measurements of biochemical abnormalities will result in an unnecessary delay in arriving at the correct definition of impaired renal function. As soon as this diagnosis can be made with certainty, a program of therapy should be immediately undertaken. The therapy can be divided into three general categories: (1) therapy directed at the maintenance of a normal internal environment; (2) therapy directed at preventing late systemic complications; and (3) adjustment of the dosage of administered drugs to compensate for their impaired excretions.

TABLE 3. A Physiologic Guide for the Prevention and Recognition of Acute Renal Failure

A. Indication if urine volume < 30 ml./hr.

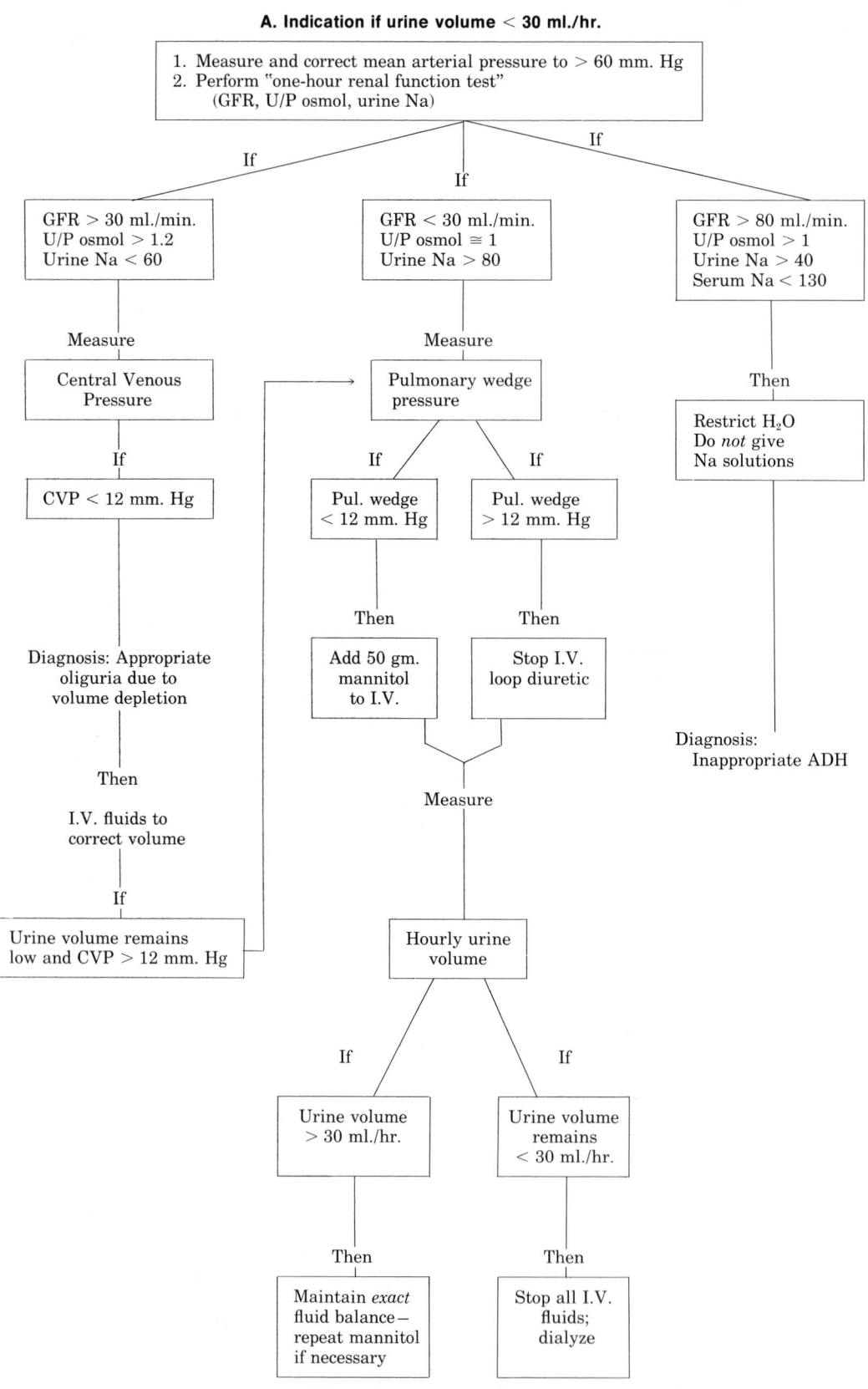

Table continued on opposite page

TABLE 3. A Physiologic Guide for the Prevention and Recognition of Acute Renal Failure—*Continued*

B. Indication if urine volume > 60 ml./hr.

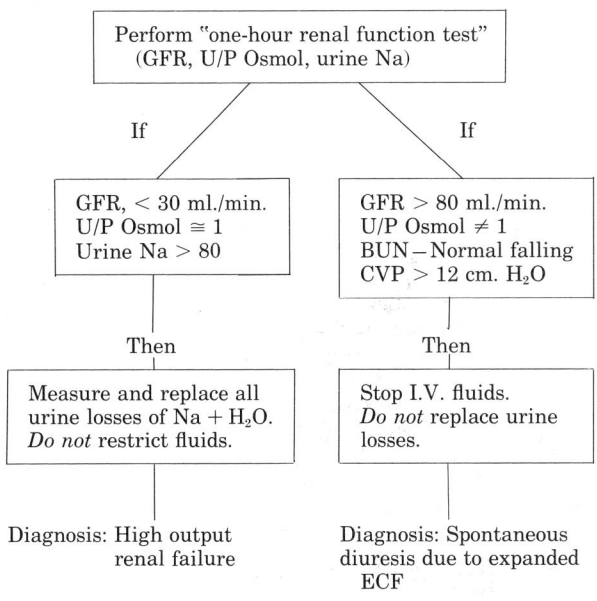

Perform "one-hour renal function test" (GFR, U/P Osmol, urine Na)

If / If

GFR, < 30 ml./min.
U/P Osmol ≅ 1
Urine Na > 80

GFR > 80 ml./min.
U/P Osmol ≠ 1
BUN—Normal falling
CVP > 12 cm. H_2O

Then / Then

Measure and replace all urine losses of Na + H_2O. *Do not* restrict fluids.

Stop I.V. fluids. *Do not* replace urine losses.

Diagnosis: High output renal failure

Diagnosis: Spontaneous diuresis due to expanded ECF

THERAPY DIRECTED AT MAINTENANCE OF A NORMAL INTERNAL ENVIRONMENT

Cessation of renal function in the postoperative patient has more rapid and more serious consequences than cessation of renal function associated with nephrotoxic drugs or with renal transplantation. In one reported series, 95 per cent of patients who developed acute renal failure following renal transplantation survived, compared to only 31 per cent of patients who developed acute renal failure as a postsurgical complication.[11] The difference in mortality is most likely due to the different clinical states of the patients at the time acute renal failure occurred. The patient receiving a renal transplant begins with a normal internal environment, whereas the postoperative patient has often suffered tissue damage, hypotension, fluid and electrolyte imbalance, and sepsis. Successful management of the postoperative patient with acute renal failure begins with meticulous and precise restoration of a normal internal environment. Certain abnormalities of the internal environment pose immediate threats to survival, whereas treatment of others may be delayed for several days.

Potassium

The most immediate threat to survival of the patient with postoperative acute renal failure is a rapidly rising concentration of serum potassium. Potassium is liberated from tissue cells at an accelerated rate in the postoperative period owing to an accelerated catabolic state, and directly as a result of tissue injury. Death from cardiac standstill may occur within a matter of hours after the onset of acute renal failure. Myocardial dysfunction associated with abnormalities of the electrocardiogram may develop more rapidly than the clinical laboratory can provide the chemical evidence for hyperkalemia. For this reason, continuous electrocardiographic monitoring assumes prime importance in the detection of this disorder. Nursing personnel in the intensive care unit must be trained to recognize the early electrical changes in time to institute corrective therapy. Management of potassium intoxication begins with cessation of all administered postassium ions, including the cancellation of balanced electrolyte solutions which often contain potassium ions, and of all drugs such as aqueous penicillin which contain a potassium salt. Patients able to take oral medications can usually be managed by the administration of the exchange resin Kayexalate, 20 gm. given 3 or 4 times a day, along with 20 ml. of 70 per cent sorbitol solution. When oral ingestion is not possible, the resin can be administered as an enema. If the potassium concentration rises so rapidly that pronounced ECG changes occur, emergency measures are required. The most effective treatment is the intravenous administration of a 10 per cent solution of calcium chloride injected very slowly to a total dose of 10 ml. This agent may be especially hazardous if the patient has been receiving digitalis. Reduction in the serum level of potassium can also be accomplished by administering glucose and insulin. Five hundred ml. of a 10 per cent solution along with 10 units of regular insulin will result in a temporary reduction in potassium levels. These emergency measures should be used during preparation for hemodialysis, which provides the only effective method of removing potassium from the body.

Water

The next most serious threat to the patient with oliguric renal failure is water. Most patients enter the phase of oliguric acute renal failure with conspicuous overhydration due to repeated fluid challenges delivered in the vain hope of restoring renal function. Frequent performance of the "one-hour renal function test" will help to establish an early diagnosis and reduce the likelihood of this complication, although its occurrence must still be presumed in a majority of instances. The actual daily water requirement of the totally anuric patient is less than is generally appreciated. Basal insensible water loss from skin and lungs amounts to approximately 12 ml. per kg. per day. This loss is partially offset by the production of metabolic water resulting from the metabolism of glucose. This "metabolic water" may approach 400 ml. per day so that the patient's net deficit is as little as 500 ml. A useful guide to the adequacy of water replacement is the constancy of the serum sodium. If there are no extrarenal losses from the gastrointestinal tract, the concentration of sodium in the serum is determined entirely from the patient's water balance. If extrarenal losses occur from tube drainage or fistulae, these should be carefully collected, their volume and sodium concentration measured, and the losses exactly replaced. Reliance on body weight may be hazardous. Maintenance of a constant weight is an indication of continuing overhydration, since the starving patient should lose approximately 0.5 to 1.0 kilogram per day.

Nitrogen Catabolism

A major advance in the management of established postoperative renal failure is the concept of prophylactic dialysis described by Teschan.[20] Early effective dialysis will usually prevent death from hyperkalemia, edema, and rapidly developing uremia. Dialysis is best performed by the technique of hemodialysis, utilizing a surgically placed arterial venous shunt consisting of Silastic catheters placed in a peripheral artery and an adjacent peripheral vein. These catheters can be connected directly to the hemodialysis unit or can be connected together to form a small arteriovenous fistula in the periods between dialytic therapy. The aim of dialytic therapy is to maintain a normal blood urea nitrogen, rather than to allow it to rise to crisis levels before instituting dialysis. An alternative method of dialytic therapy makes use of the large peritoneal surface area. Unfortunately, the peritoneal cavity of many postoperative patients is partially obliterated as a result of adhesions or infection, and the surface area is too small to provide effective dialysis. Nevertheless, peritoneal dialysis may be life-saving in those patients whose cardiovascular status will not support the added burden of hemodialysis.

A second major advance in the management of the metabolic consequences of acute renal failure was reported by Abel. He demonstrated that intravenous hyperalimentation with a solution containing essential amino acids and adequate calories would stabilize the serum levels of potassium, magnesium, and phosphate, and also decrease the rate of blood urea nitrogen elevation.[1]

Present experience indicates that early, aggressive, repeated dialysis can generally prevent the metabolic derangements associated with acute renal failure.

THERAPY DIRECTED AT LATE SYSTEMIC COMPLICATIONS

Dialysis has been effective in minimizing deaths due to the metabolic consequences of acute renal failure but have had less effect on the late complications of this disorder. The most serious late complications are associated with bleeding, sepsis, and drug intoxication.

Bleeding

Massive gastrointestinal hemorrhage accounts for the majority of deaths in patients with acute postoperative renal failure, although it is somewhat less frequent in patients who have been managed by early aggressive prophylactic dialysis. This complication results from a multiplicity of factors, including coagulation defects associated with acute renal failure and stress ulceration of the gastric mucosa. Repeated measurements of coagulation factors with replacement by appropriate blood fractions may be helpful in reversing this defect, and the administration of prophylactic antacids will result in a substantial decrease in the incidence of stress ulceration. Frequent aspiration of gastric contents for determination of pH, followed by administration of sufficient antacid solution to maintain the gastric pH above 6, is the most effective prophylactic measure. The presence of gastrointestinal bleeding at a time when further dialysis is necessary to maintain the internal environment poses a special problem. Regional heparinization, which maintains adequate anticoagulant levels for the blood within the dialysis equipment and then neutralizes the anticoagulants as the blood returns to the patient, will assist in controlling this dangerous situation. In spite of all efforts, recurrent bleeding during hemodialysis remains a significant problem.

Sepsis

A major cause of late death in patients with acute renal failure is systemic sepsis. Infections may arise from necrotic tissue in the operative site or from undetected abscess cavities. Careful inspection of all wounds and the liberal use of scanning techniques will detect foci of sepsis and permit their early correction. Careful aseptic technique in the use of intravenous and urethral catheters will minimize the chance for introduction of pathogenic organisms. The low mortality associated with the treatment of acute renal failure following transplantation may be largely due to the careful isolation techniques routinely employed in the management of these patients.

THERAPY DIRECTED AT PROPER DRUG DOSAGE

Patients suffering from acute renal failure frequently receive medications that are normally excreted by the kidney. Digitalis and many of the antibiotics are common examples. Continuation of the usual dosage schedule of these drugs will result in toxic concentrations, which may be a cause of late death. The most effective prevention of these complications is obtained by frequent determinations of blood levels of each administered drug. Techniques for determination of antibiotic blood levels are now available in most institutions and should be freely utilized. If these tests are not available, a useful approximation of proper dosage can be obtained from the tables provided by Bennett.[3]

RECOVERY FROM ACUTE RENAL FAILURE

Recovery of renal function in the patient with acute postoperative renal failure will be indicated by the onset of an increased urine flow. Management of the patient at this time becomes more difficult rather than less. A urine volume of 1000 ml. per day does not necessarily mean that the GFR has returned to normal. Continued dialysis may still be necessary to maintain the blood urea nitrogen at a normal level. Accurate maintenance of water and salt balance may be difficult. Large volumes of urine containing substantial quantities of sodium can result in volume depletion, hypotension, and the return to a further period of acute renal failure. Accurate daily measurements of urine volume and electrolyte concentration with meticulous replacement will prevent this disastrous complication. Restoration of normal renal function as determined by the "one-hour renal function test" is the best indication that recovery has taken place and that the patient's kidneys are again capable of maintaining the integrity of the internal environment.

SELECTED REFERENCES

Hollenberg, N. K., Epstein, J., Rosen, S. M., Basch, R. I., Oken, D. E., and Merrill, J. P.: Acute oliguric renal failure in man: Evidence for preferential renal cortical ischemia. Medicine, 47:455, 1968.
This study demonstrated that regional changes in renal blood flow will result in cortical ischemia. The technique of xenon washout can be applied to both experimental animals and man and has provided much of the data for the modern hypothesis of the development of acute renal failure.

Abel, R. M., Abbott, W. N., and Fischer, J. E.: Intravenous essential L-amino acids and hypertonic dextrose in patients with acute renal failure. Am. J. Surg., 123:632, 1972.
A major advance in the management of established acute renal failure has been the stabilization of the blood levels of potassium, magnesium, and phosophate and a slowing of the rate of increase of blood urea nitrogen by administration of essential amino acids and glucose. These biochemical changes were associated with a decrease in mortality and improvement in wound healing. The details of this new therapeutic tool are carefully outlined.

Eliahou, H. E., and Bata, A.: The diagnosis of acute renal failure. Nephron, 2:287, 1965.
A classic description of the biochemical basis for the diagnosis of acute renal failure. The most useful tests of renal function in the clinical setting of an intensive care unit are provided.

REFERENCES

1. Abel, R. M., Abbott, W. N., and Fischer, J. E.: Intravenous essential L-amino acids and hypertonic dextrose in patients with acute renal failure. Am. J. Surg., 123:632, 1972.
2. Barger, A. C.: Renal hemodynamic factors in congestive heart failure. Ann. N.Y. Acad. Sci., 139:276, 1966.
3. Bennett, W. N., Singer, I., and Coggins, C. H.: Guide to drug usage in adult patients with impaired renal function. J.A.M.A., 223:991, 1973.
4. Bywaters, E. G. L., and Beall, D.: Crush injuries with impairment of renal function. Br. Med. J., 1:427, 1941.
5. Carrico, C. J., Colin, C. D., Lightfoot, A., Allsman, A., and Shires, G. T.: Extracellular volume fluid replacement in hemorrhagic shock. Surg. Forum, 14:10, 1963.
6. Chedru, M. F., Baetheke, R., and Oken, D. E.: Renal cortical blood flow and glomerular filtration rate in myohemoglobinuric acute renal failure. Kidney Int., 1:232, 1972.
7. Eliahou, H. E., and Bata, A.: The diagnosis of acute renal failure. Nephron, 2:287, 1965.
8. Flores, J., DiBona, D. R., and Beck, C. H.: The role of cell swelling in ischemic renal damage and the protective effect of hypertonic solute. J. Clin. Invest., 51:118, 1972.
9. Hollenberg, N. K., Epstein, J., Rosen, S. M., Basch, R. I., Oken, D. E., and Merrill, J. P.: Acute oliguric renal failure in man: Evidence for preferential renal cortical ischemia. Medicine, 47:455, 1968.
10. Kiley, J. E., Powers, S. R., and Beebe, R. T.: Acute renal failure. Eighty cases of renal tubular necrosis. N. Engl. J. Med., 262:481–486, 1960.
11. Kjellstrand, C. M., Simmons, R. L., Shideman, J. R., Bufelneier, T. J., Von Hartitizsch, B., and Najarian, J. S.: Acute tubular necrosis after renal transplantation. DHEW Pub. No. (NIH) 74–608, 1973.
12. Ladd, M.: Battle Casualties in Korea: Studies of the Surgical Research Team. Post traumatic renal insufficiency. Vol. 4. U.S. Army Medical Service Graduate School, Walter Reed Medical Hospital, 1956, pp. 193–233.
13. Lucke, B.: Lower Nephron Nephrosis. Milit. Surg., 99:371–396, 1946.
14. Mason, J., and Thurau, K.: Physiological mechanisms responsible for the adjustment of renal function during acute renal failure. VIth International Congress of Nephrology, pp. 104–105, 1975.
15. Muller, D. C.: The mechanism of acute renal failure after injury and transfusion reaction and its prevention by solute diuresis. Surg. Clin. North Am., 45:499, 1965.
16. Oliver, J., MacDowell, M., and Tracey, A.: The pathogenesis of acute renal failure associated with traumatic and toxic injury, renal ischemia, nephro-toxic damage and the ischemuric episode. J. Clin. Invest., 30:1305–1438, 1951.
17. Powers, S. R.: Bull. N.Y. Acad. Med., 1959.
18. Powers, S. R., Boba, A., and Stein, A.: The mechanism and prevention of distal tubular necrosis following aneurysmectomy. Surgery, 42:156–162, 1957.
19. Rosenberg, I. K., et al.: Renal insufficiency after trauma and sepsis. A prospective and functional ultra-structural analysis. Arch. Surg., 103:175, 1971.
20. Teschan, P. E., Baxter, C. R., O'Brien, T. F., Freyhof, J. N., and Hall, W. H.: Prophylactic hemodialysis in the treatment of acute renal failure. Am. Intern. Med., 53:992, 1960.
21. Thiel, G., McDonald, F. D., and Oken, D. E.: Micro-puncture studies of the basis for protection of renin depleted rats from glycerol induced acute renal failure. Nephron, 7:67, 1970.
22. Vander, A. J.: Effect of catecholoamines and the renal nerves on renin secretion in anesthetized dogs. Am. J. Physiol., 209:659, 1965.
23. Vander, A. J., and Miller, R.: Control of renin secretion in the anesthetized dog. Am. J. Physiol., 207:537, 1964.

22

TRANSPLANTATION

I

HISTORICAL ASPECTS

Delford L. Stickel, M.D., and H. F. Seigler, M.D.

DEFINITIONS AND CLASSIFICATIONS

A number of terms are used in various classifications of transplants.[3, 10, 16] The terms transplant and transplantation are used broadly in reference to any removal or partial detachment of a part of the body and its implantation into or onto the body of the same or a different individual. As used here, *graft* is synonymous with transplant, *host* and recipient are synonymous, and transplantation does not include the use of prostheses, synthetic materials, or artificial devices that may be fixed within or attached to the body but that do not comprise human or animal cells or tissues. The following classifications are applicable to therapeutic transplantation in man and to experimental transplantation generally within the animal kingdom.

According to the genetic relationship between donor and recipient there are four classes of transplants: (1) *autograft*—donor and recipient the same individual; (2) *isograft* or *syngeneic* graft—donor and recipient genetically identical individuals of the same species (a graft between monozygotic twins or between animals of a highly inbred strain); (3) *allograft* or *homograft*—donor and recipient genetically dissimilar individuals of the same species; and (4) *xenograft* or *heterograft*—donor and recipient individuals of different species. The terms homograft and heterograft are older than their respective modern synonyms, allograft and xenograft, but all four of these terms are acceptable and widely used clinically and experimentally. Grafts between human monozygotic twins are usually described as such; stating the twin relationship is more specific than using the term isograft or syngeneic graft. In discussions of genetic and immunologic aspects of transplantation, the prefixes *auto-, syn-, allo-,* and *xeno-* are used in forming adjectives (-geneic and -immune) and nouns (-antigen, -antibody, -immunity, -graft, and less frequently -transplant). The prefix *iso-* is ambiguous because it is used with two distinctly different meanings, as discussed by Gorer.[7] The term isograft as defined earlier derives from geneticists' use of the term isogenic in referring to genetically *identical* individuals, whereas for over 70 years immunologists have used iso- to refer to immunity to antigens of blood and tissues of genetically *dissimilar* individuals of the same species (isoimmune, isoantigen, isoantibody, and so forth).

According to the site of implantation, transplants are *orthotopic* if surrounded by the same kind of tissues or located in the same part of the body after transplantation as before; otherwise, they are *heterotopic*. The following are examples of orthotopic transplants: corneal transplants; skin grafts that cover a surface defect; and intrathoracic transplants of heart and lung and subdiaphragmatic transplants of liver with normal anatomic vascular connections. Some examples of heterotopic transplants are subcutaneous or intramuscular grafts of endocrine tissue, and grafts of the liver or a kidney to the lower abdomen or the pelvic region. Replanted extremities, the subject of a separate chapter, are an example of orthotopic autografts.

According to technique of implantation, transplants are classified as follows: *anastomosed* grafts—the circulation of the host established in the graft at the time of transplantation by vascular anastomosis; *pedicled* grafts—the graft connected to the donor site at least temporarily by a pedicle containing blood vessels; *free* grafts—isolated pieces of tissue devoid of vascular, nervous, and lymphatic connections at the conclusion of the transplant procedure; and *infused* grafts—the graft established by means of an infusion of a cell suspension into the bloodstream, a body cavity, or tissues of the host. Infusion is a commonly employed experimental technique of grafting hematopoietic and lymphoid cells. Bone marrow is transplanted by intravenous infusion, and the infused cells populate the bone marrow spaces. Blood transfusion is, of course, the most frequent example of use of this method.

Pedicled grafts are usually autografts, but in parabiosis of experimental animals the pedicles may be allografts or syngeneic grafts.

Grafts may be *viable* or *nonviable* when implanted. Nonviable grafts of bone, cartilage, and blood vessels are therapeutically functional although rendered nonviable by freezing, drying, chemical, or other preservative processes.

Transplants may also be classified in a number of other ways: with reference to the anatomy, histology, and cytology of the graft; as to whether the graft was from an embryonic or a mature donor; as to whether the recipient was immunologically immature (early fetal) or mature (postnatal and adult); as to whether or not the implantation site was privileged, i.e., a site that protects the graft from rejection (e.g, anterior chamber of the eye, within the brain or testis, in a micropore diffusion chamber); as to whether the graft was neoplastic or non-neoplastic tissue; according to technique and duration of preservation and storage of the graft; as to whether the purpose was therapeutic or experimental; and so forth.

HISTORICAL ASPECTS

The idea of grafting parts of the body from one person to another has inspired a number of legends. The following quotation is from a translation of a Chinese document written about 300 B.C.:

One day two men, Lu and Chao, called on the surgeon Pien Ch'iao. He gave them a toxic drink and they were unconscious for three days. Pien Ch'iao operated and opened their stomachs and explored the heart; after removing and interchanging their organs he gave a wonderful drug and the two men went home recovered.[17]

The fifteenth century Italian poet, Calenzio, referred to slaves donating noses to their masters.[3, 17] The transplantation of a whole leg by Saints Cosmas and Damian was the inspiration of several Renaissance paintings.[3, 17] According to this legend, the leg of a dead black man was successfully used to replace the cancerous leg of a white man. The distinction between the real and the imaginary was not always clear. Tragically, in 1492 two boys were bled to death in a vain attempt to save the life of Pope Innocent VIII by means of transfusion of young blood.[17]

The oldest evidence of grafting that could have been of some therapeutic benefit is seen in the remains of trephined prehistoric skulls. The trephine holes were usually small, but in the Bronze Age skull shown in Figure 1, a rather large defect evidently was filled by implanting the removed fragment as an orthotopic autograft.[8] In this specimen, the cut margin showed no sign of healing, so the operation may have been fatal. Recovery from primitive skull trephination is well documented, however, both archeologically and in studies of primitive peoples in modern times, and it is conceivable that such trephination was sometimes therapeutically effective.

There is archeologic evidence that teeth were transplanted in man in ancient Egypt, Greece, pre-Columbian North and South America, Rome, and perhaps China.[12] Transplantation of teeth was described by Arabian writers around A.D. 1000,[12] by Ambroise Paré in Paris in the sixteenth century,[12] and by John Hunter in the eighteenth century (see later). Transplanted teeth did not live; the results were poor and the practice waxed and waned.

Ancient Hindu surgeons described methods for repairing defects of the nose and ears using techniques of grafting simi-

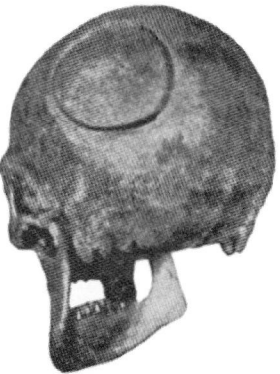

Figure 1. Orthotopic autograft of bone in Bronze Age skull. (From Guthrie, D.: A History of Medicine. Philadelphia, J. B. Lippincott Company, 1946.)

lar to those used in modern times. The following technique for nasal reconstruction is quoted from a translation of the Suśruta Sanhita, a document written about 700 B.C.[12, 16, 17]

When a man's nose has been cut off or destroyed, the physician takes the leaf of a plant which is the size of the destroyed parts. He places it on the patient's cheek and cuts out of this cheek a piece of skin the same size (but in such a manner that the skin at one end remains attached to the cheek). Then he freshens with his scalpel the edges of the stump of nose and wraps the piece of skin from the cheek carefully all around it, and sews it at the edges. Then he places two thin pipes in the nose where the nostrils should go, to facilitate breathing and to prevent the sewn skin from collapsing. Thereafter he strews powder of sapan wood, licorice-root and barberry on it and covers it with cotton. As soon as the skin has grown together with the nose, he cuts through the connection with the cheek.[2]

The use of Indian methods appears to have spread to Greece and Rome. The use of adjacent flaps to repair various facial defects is described in Greco-Roman writings of the first century A.D.[16] In 1794 English surgeons stationed in India described nasal reconstruction as they had seen it performed by an Indian surgeon, the technique quite similar to that described more than 1000 years earlier.[16]

During the sixteenth century the Italian surgeon Tagliacozzi reconstructed the nose using a flap from the arm.[3, 5, 12, 16, 17] This extremely painful procedure was used to replace noses cut off in combat or for punishment, or destroyed by syphilis. The technique is still in use, known as the Tagliacotian flap or the Italian method.[5] In considering but discarding the idea of grafting tissue donated by another person, Tagliacozzi made the following remarkable statement:

The singular character of the individual entirely dissuades us from attempting this work on another person. For such is the force and the power of individuality, that if anyone should believe that he could accelerate and increase the beauty of union, nay more, achieve even the least part of the operation, we consider him plainly superstitious and badly grounded in physical sciences.[15]

During the eighteenth century, the Scottish surgeon John Hunter revived the practice of transplantation of teeth,[3, 12, 16] and about this operation he wrote: "Success of this operation is founded on the disposition of all living substances to unite when brought in contact with one another, although they are of different structure and even though the circulation is carried in one of them."[3] He reported success with autografts and allografts of chicken testes and other tissue transplantation experiments, but he failed to observe a difference between autografts and allografts. In other animal experiments, he observed that the ends of severed Achilles tendons grew together after suturing.

In 1770 Missa reported successful transplantation of the extensor tendon of the middle finger to the extensor tendon of the index finger.[12, 16] According to Woodruff's[16] comprehensive review, reports of the following kinds of grafts were first published during the nineteenth century: free grafts of skin, tendon, nerve, cartilage, cornea, adrenal, thyroid, parathyroid, ovary, and adipose tissue; and pedicled grafts of muscle, tendon, nerve, and portions of the gastrointestinal and urinary tracts. Some of these grafts were performed only in experimental animals, but most were attempted with various degrees of success in man. Many of the developments in human transplantation were made possible by two developments during the last half of the century: the use of ether and other general anesthetics, and acceptance of Lister's principles of antiseptic surgery. Some of the accomplishments and limitations of transplantation in the nineteenth century are illustrated in reports of skin and corneal transplantation.

Skin Grafts

The first well documented report of successful free autografts of skin was in 1804 by Baronio, who experimented with sheep, although free autografts of human skin may have been used successfully centuries before.[3, 5, 12, 16] In 1822 Bunger reported successful use of a free full-thickness human skin autograft to repair a nasal defect.[5, 12, 16] In 1870 Reverdin reported the observation that small grafts of epidermis on a granulating surface increased in size and grew out to coalesce with adjacent grafts.[5, 12, 16] In 1886 Thiersch in Germany described the resurfacing of wounds with large sheets of split-thickness skin.[5, 12, 16] Such grafts are still sometimes called Thiersch's grafts, although essentially the same procedure was reported 14 years earlier by Ollier in France.[12, 16]

In 1863 Paul Bert, a student of Claude Bernard, reported that autografts, allografts, and xenografts behaved differently.[5, 16] The significance of these observations received little attention, however; nineteenth century authors (including Baronio and Reverdin) generally failed to observe that the results of allografts and autografts of skin were different. Skin allografts were used to some extent clinically, as illustrated in a story by Winston Churchill of his donating a small piece of skin to a wounded fellow officer in 1898.[5] There appear to have been three reasons for the mistaken belief that skin allografts grew permanently, a belief still widely held as late as the third decade of the twentieth century: (1) for a week or more skin allografts are indistinguishable from autografts; (2) it is difficult to distinguish between permanent survival of a small skin graft and ingrowth of adjacent host skin to cover the area of a sloughed graft; and (3) corneal allografts do survive permanently.

Corneal Transplants

Corneal xenografts attempted early in the nineteenth century were unsuccessful. A successful corneal allograft between two gazelles was subsequently reported by Bigger in 1835,[12, 16] but the essentiality of using a cornea from the same species was not recognized until the period 1872 to 1880 when successful corneal allografts were reported in animals and in man. Refinements of operative techniques, methods of preservation of grafts, and systems of graft procurement were subsequently developed. During the period of 1925 to 1945 corneal transplantation emerged as a widespread and generally accepted therapeutic practice.[5, 12, 16]

Advances in the twentieth century include the first reports

of the following kinds of transplants in man or animals: vascular anastomosed grafts of blood vessels, kidney, spleen, pituitary, heart, lung, liver, portions of the gastrointestinal tract, and pancreas; free grafts of fascia, heterotopic dermis, and pituitary; and infused grafts of hematopoietic and lymphoid cells.[12, 16] The development of transplantation during the twentieth century has depended on advances in surgical techniques, in our understanding of the problem of rejection, and in means of graft preservation and storage and artificial life support.

SURGICAL TECHNIQUES

Among the many surgical techniques that have contributed to the development of transplantation during this century, the technique of vascular anastomosis by suturing stands out as especially significant. Prior to 1900 there had been occasional reports of successful repair of vascular injuries and of successful reunion of the ends of completely severed vessels by means of suturing and by other techniques.[12, 16] The first reports of consistently reliable vascular anastomosis by suturing were those of Carrel (a French surgeon working in Chicago and New York) and Guthrie between 1902 and 1912. In a large number of animal experiments, these authors immediately used this technique successfully in the transplantation of blood vessels and whole organs including heart, spleen, ovaries, various endocrine glands, extremities, and the head and neck.[3, 5, 10, 12, 16, 17] Technical success was proved, for instance, with autografts of kidneys that functioned and supported normal health indefinitely. These authors also made observations contrasting autografts with allografts. Carrel thus clearly recognized the problem of rejection as he wrote in 1910:

Should an organ, extirpated from an animal and replanted into its owner by a certain technique, continue to functionate normally, and should it cease to functionate when transplanted into another animal by the same technique, the physiological disturbance could not be considered as brought about by the surgical factors. The changes undergone by the organ would be due to the influence of the host, that is, the biological factors.[4]

After 1910 Carrel contributed further to the development of transplantation by work in the fields of tissue culture and organ perfusion. Guthrie[17] suspected that rejection was an immune process, and Carrel,[5] in observing the work of Murphy, was encouraged that the problem would be overcome. The work of Carrel and Guthrie received the greatest attention, but successful organ transplantation by vascular anastomosis was reported by other authors about the same time.[3, 5, 10, 12, 16, 17]

PROBLEM OF REJECTION

The immunity theory of graft rejection was postulated by several authors during the first decade of this century. The reader should keep in mind, however, that a number of other theories were considered as this subject was debated for over 40 years. Loeb in particular, as late as 1945, favored a different theory of allograft rejection.[5, 16] The immunity theory was questioned largely because there was no direct evidence that circulating antibody—the traditional hallmark of immunity — was involved in the rejection process. Antibodies had been demonstrated in response to allografts of tumor but not allografts of normal tissues, and attempts to confer allograft immunity passively with serum were unsuccessful. The rather extensive history of studies relating to the nature and prevention of graft rejection will be briefly summarized under six subtopics.

Genetics of Transplantation Antigens, Tissue Typing, and Crossmatching

The antigens responsible for graft rejection and the genetic control of these antigens have been most extensively studied in the mouse. In studies of transplanted tumors during the first two decades of this century, Jensen,[3, 5, 16] Tyzzer,[12, 16] and Little[12, 16] reported the influence of genetic factors. Numerous authors studied grafts of tumors and of normal tissues in highly inbred strains of mice, and Gorer in England was a major contributor to this work from 1937 to 1961. In 1948 Gorer, Lyman, and Snell described H-2 as a genetic locus controlling strong histocompatibility antigens in the mouse;[16] subsequently this locus and numerous minor histocompatibility loci were characterized in great detail. In a subsequent section of this chapter, Amos gives an account of this work in the mouse, similar but less extensive studies of the genetics of transplantation antigens of other animal species, and rather extensive recent work pertaining to the HLA locus of man.

The work of Landsteiner during the first four decades of this century with erythrocyte ABO and Rh antigens was a necessary basis for blood banking and blood transfusing, which came into extensive use during and after World War II. The development of blood transfusion contributed to progress with the problem of graft rejection in three respects. (1) The A and B erythrocyte antigens are widely distributed in tissues and are transplantation antigens that must be considered in the selection of tissue and organ donors. (2) By analogy with typing and crossmatching for blood donor selection, one of the major approaches to the problem of graft rejection has been tissue compatibility testing. (3) The serum of patients who have received multiple blood transfusions frequently contains antibodies to human leukocytes. It is now known that these are HLA antibodies, and serum from such patients was the principal source of antibodies in early studies of the HLA system.

The Second-Set Phenomenon

In 1903 Jensen observed that a second graft did not survive as long as the first when a mouse received two grafts of a tumor separated by an interval of several days, and he suggested that immunity accounted for the difference.[3, 5, 16] This effect of a prior graft was not always observed with transplants of tumor, however; under certain conditions survival of the second graft was prolonged, as will be discussed later. Holman used skin allografts to treat a burned patient and reported in 1923 that a second group of pinch grafts from the same donor was rejected more rapidly than the first.[5, 10, 16] Referring to immunologic memory, he postulated that "each group of grafts develops its own antibody." In 1943 Gibson and Medawar in England reported similar observations with burn patients, and use of the term "second set" dates to this report.[3, 5, 10, 16] In subsequent controlled experiments with rabbits, Medawar demonstrated the immunologic specificity of the phenomenon, which was observed uniformly only when the same donor was used for both the first and second sets of grafts. The specificity of the second-set phenomenon had been described by Shinoi[14] in Japan in 1932. Medawar also contrasted the histologic characteristics of first- and second-set rejections—differences that later were attributed to the predominance of cellular (first-set) vs. humoral (second-set) mechanisms of rejection. Numerous authors working with inbred mice and various other biologic systems subsequently established firmly that acceleration of rejection of the second graft depends upon antigenic identity or similarity between the first and second grafts.

Cellular Immunity

In 1914 Murphy reported lymphocytic infiltrates in host tissues surrounding rejecting transplanted tumors.[5, 16] He postulated that the small lymphocyte was responsible for the rejection and he used radiation and treatment with benzol to modify the process. The concept of cellular immunity effected by "killer" lymphocytes—as a process distinguishable from humoral immunity effected by circulating antibody—was not firmly established, however, until experiments were performed in which certain forms of immunity were observed to be transferable to an unimmunized subject by lymphoid cells and not by serum. In 1939 Potter et al. and in 1954 Mitchinson reported such transfer of immunity to tumor allografts in mice.[16] In 1942, 1945, and 1953, Landsteiner and Chase reported transfer of cellular immunity in man.[16] Their studies were with tuberculin hypersensitivity and cutaneous hypersensitivity to simple compounds. In 1954 Billingham, Brent, and Medawar reported the use of lymphoid cells to transfer immunity to skin and other tissue grafts in mice.[16] Immunity was not conferred if the transferred cells were killed by heat, ultrasonication, irradiation, or other means. Although passive in a sense, such transfer of immunity required the activity of viable cells and this phenomenon was designated "adoptively acquired immunity" to distinguish it from passive immunity produced by injections of antibody. Subsequent studies of numerous authors have firmly established that normal immunologic responsiveness comprises two distinguishable mechanisms. (1) The cellular mechanism is dependent upon the thymus, and the products of this mechanism are "sensitized" or "killer" lymphocytes that are reactive with antigen. (2) The humoral mechanism is dependent upon the bursa of Fabricius of chickens and upon anatomically undefined sites in other species, and the products of this mechanism are the immunoglobulins—antibodies that may be circulating or cell-bound. Studies regarding these two mechanisms have recently been reviewed by Good,[6] who himself has made a number of original experimental and clinical contributions, particularly in regard to defining the nature of various immunologic deficiency states. The transplantation of bone marrow and lymphoid tissue in the treatment of hematologic and immunologic deficiency states is emerging from these developments.

Humoral Immunity

Although the cellular immune mechanism was emphasized in establishing the immunity theory of graft rejection, the importance of the humoral mechanism has become increasingly evident as refined methods for the detection and characterization of immunoglobulins have been developed. During the last two decades the humoral mechanism has been shown to be important to the problem of graft rejection in three major aspects:

1. Circulating antibody is unquestionably the principal effector of xenograft rejection and second-set allograft rejection, particularly hyperacute, immediate rejection due to a high degree of presensitization. Less conspicuously, the humoral mechanism is also operative along with the cellular mechanism in first-set allograft rejection. (See also the subsequent section of this chapter by Amos and the section on renal allografts.)

2. Alloantibodies have been used as the basic reagents in the development of serologic tests for histocompatibility. (See earlier under Genetics of Transplantation Antigens.)

3. "Enhancing" or "blocking" antibodies are potentially useful as a means of preventing rejection. A number of authors have observed that the growth of transplanted tumors is enhanced by a previous graft of the same tumor or by prior exposure of the recipient to substances derived from tumor tissue. Casey in 1932 called the phenomenon "enhancement," and Kaliss in 1953 reported that the effect is transferable to normal animals by injections of serum.[16] The effect was subsequently shown to be due to an immunoglobulin, and enhancing or blocking antibodies have been used experimentally to prolong the survival of grafts of normal (non-neoplastic) tissues. The potential for using such antibodies clinically to prevent graft rejection is discussed by Amos in a subsequent section of this chapter.

Chimerism and Tolerance, Natural and Acquired

A chimera is an organism carrying within it healthy living tissues of two or more genetically different individuals.[10] The term and the concept date from Greek mythology, but the actual existence of such a state was reported first by Owen in 1945.[10, 16] He reported that dizygotic cattle twins sometimes each carry two different types of erythrocytes, and he postulated that the marrow of each individual had become populated by cells of both in utero when the circulation of the two placentas was mixed. (Such circulatory union had been demonstrated by Lillie in 1916.[10]) Owen successfully exchanged skin grafts and in 1955 Simonsen reported that kidneys as well as skin could be successfully transplanted between such cattle twins.[3] In 1953 Dunsford discovered a human twin carrying both A

and O erythrocytes but the other member of the pair had died in infancy.[10, 16] In 1959 Woodruff and Lennox reported successful exchange of skin grafts between dizygotic human twins showing blood chimerism with types A and O.[10, 16] Allografts on a chimera from donors other than the chimeric mate were rejected in the normal manner. Thus, immediately upon discovery of naturally occurring chimerism—a naturally occurring allograft as it were—the essential experiments were performed to demonstrate that a natural chimera is specifically nonreactive to the tissue antigens of its chimeric mate. Such nonreactivity, specifically limited to particular antigens, is referred to as specific immunologic tolerance or simply tolerance. In contrast, immunosuppression is nonspecific suppression of immune responses to antigens generally.

The most common example of naturally occurring tolerance is the normal state of nonreactivity to self antigens, i.e., to the antigens of one's own body. Autoimmune diseases are the consequence of abnormal reactivity to self antigens. Burnet conceived recognition of self antigens as one of the aspects of embryologic maturation of the immunologic system.[10, 16]

The creation of states of *acquired tolerance*, i.e., induced specific immunologic tolerance, has been achieved largely by exposure of embryonic, fetal, or early postnatal hosts to grafts that the normal adult animal would immunologically reject. Before tolerance was defined immunologically, Murphy in 1912 observed that rat sarcomas grew on chick embryos but not in the mature organism, and he observed that the chick acquired the adult capacity to reject the tumor about 5 days before completion of shell life.[5, 16] In 1929 Danforth and Foster reported successful skin grafts between newborn Rhode Island Red and Plymouth Rock chicks.[10] In 1950 Cannon and Longmire reported similar observations, but they noted additionally that the percentage of take was only 1 per cent if the grafts were peformed on chicks 3 days old and was nil at the age of 14 days.[10, 16] Billingham, Brent, and Medawar systematically studied the phenomena of actively acquired tolerance between inbred strains of mice of various ages before and after birth and concluded in 1953 that in mice the transition occurs at about the time of birth.[10] Grafts established on the fetus survived permanently and the host was tolerant to other grafts from the donor strain; grafts performed more than a day or two after birth were rejected and the rejection of subsequent grafts from the donor strain was accelerated.

In subsequent studies, these authors reported "breaking" tolerance, i.e., reversing tolerance and terminating the chimeric state, by injecting lymphoid cells of normal adult host-strain mice into tolerant animals. The reversal of the tolerant state in these experiments was marked by the sloughing of long-established grafts of skin and other tissues from the donor strain.

Because animals rendered tolerant prenatally or neonatally were normal except for being chimeras and for being specifically nonreactive to antigens of the donor, many studies have been directed toward the objective of inducing tolerance in the adult by methods that would be applicable to therapeutic transplantation in man. Lasting tolerance has been produced in adult mice that were temporarily immunosuppressed at the time of initial exposure to donor antigens, but tolerance is readily produced by this means only if the donor-recipient incompatibility is weak. Immunity, not tolerance, usually results if the incompatibility is strong. Also studied have been phenomena similar and probably related to tolerance, namely, *immunologic paralysis* and antigen overload — specific nonreactivity to antigens that have been administered in massive dosage compared with the ordinary immunizing dose. The potential for using tolerance and related phenomena clinically to prevent graft rejection is discussed further by Amos in a subsequent section of this chapter.

Immunosuppression

The therapeutic benefits of renal and other allografts in man are largely dependent upon methods of nonspecific suppression of immune responses that have been developed during the last three decades. Total-body irradiation had been used extensively to prevent rejection of grafts in experimental animals when in 1959 this method was used successfully in the first human renal allografts from living, related donors in Paris and in Boston[10] (see the section on renal allografts). Shortly thereafter, the purine analog azathioprine came into almost universal use for clinical immunosuppression, on the basis of studies that followed the report by Schwartz and Dameshek in 1959 that 6-mercaptopurine blocked the capacity of rabbits to form antibody.[3] Around midcentury numerous authors reported the efficiency of adrenal cortical steroids in reversing the manifestations of various immunopathologic disease states. Hume used ACTH or steroids in eight of the nine cadaver renal allografts he reported prior to 1960.[16] In 1964 Marchioro et al. reported the successful use of prednisone to reverse established manifestations of renal allograft rejection,[3] and this drug continues to be one of the most potent immunosuppressants available. Antilymphocyte serum (ALS) has been the most recently introduced major immunosuppressant. ALS had been studied by a number of authors previously when Woodruff and Anderson in 1963 reported its efficacy in prolonging skin allograft survival in rats.[3] In 1967 Starzl reported the first clinical use of ALS. Numerous other methods of immunosuppression have been introduced, as discussed by Simmons, Foker, and Najarian in a separate section of this chapter.

GRAFT PRESERVATION AND STORAGE AND ARTIFICIAL LIFE-SUPPORT SYSTEMS

The structural integrity and for most transplants the viability of the graft must be maintained during the interval from removal to implantation. For vital organ transplantation, the life of the organism must also be maintained during periods of temporary graft failure and periods of awaiting the availability of a suitable graft. Methods of sustaining life for these purposes are basically similar to methods used during operations for surgical repair or revascularization of vital organs. Whether the life to be sustained in these circumstances is that of a graft, a part of the body being surgically repaired, or the whole organism, basically two approaches are available: (1) methods that reduce or bring to a reversible standstill the need for oxygen and other metabolic requirements and (2) systems that support active metabolism and that are all or in part artificial or in vitro. The first three methods to be discussed are in the first category, and the last four are in the second. For a particular situation, the two approaches may be combined; hypothermic perfusion is a common example of such a combination.

Simple Cooling: Hypothermia

At temperatures in the range of 0 to 4° C., tissues remain viable in the absence of circulation 10 or more times longer than at normal body temperature. Use of this simple method has accompanied the development of techniques of grafting, and clinically this method has been particularly useful in preserving skin, cornea, kidney, and blood. The physiology of hypothermia of the whole body and of particular organ systems was studied extensively by many authors during the period 1950 to 1960 following the introduction of hypothermia as a means of extending the time limits of safely interrupting the circulation of the heart, brain, liver, kidney, and other parts of body. Perfusing an organ with a cold perfusate (usually a balanced electrolyte solution) is used widely as a means of rapid cooling, within seconds, to temperatures that by surface cooling could be achieved only after a number of minutes and at the expense of loss of viability. Such perfusion is mentioned here to distinguish it from perfusion designed to support metabolism (see later).

Freezing

Mammalian cells are ordinarily killed by freezing and thawing. Although Luyet and Hartung had reported in 1941 that ethylene glycol and glycerol protected cells from freeze-thaw damage,[9, 16] studies of preserving cell viability by freezing were not undertaken widely until after 1949 when Polge et al. in England reported observing accidentally that glycerol protected spermatozoa of fowl from injury by freezing.[16] During the ensuing decade this property of glycerol was studied by numerous investigators, and suspensions of various kinds of cells were successfully frozen and thawed with protection by glycerol, dimethyl-sulfoxide, or other cryoprotective substances. Useful applications of this method include the following three: (1) Blood erythrocytes can be frozen for many months, thawed, washed, and used for transfusion purposes. The method is too expensive for routine use but is in use for special purposes. (2) Suspensions of tissue culture cells can be preserved indefinitely by freezing; this obviates the expense and risk of loss and change of character associated with prolonged active culture. (3) Commercial cattle breeding has been facilitated with the use of frozen sperm.

Split-thickness skin, cornea, other thin tissue slices, and organs of small animals have been successfully established as viable grafts after freezing, prolonged storage, and thawing with the aid of cryoprotective substances, or after ultrarapid freezing and thawing without the use of such substances.[9, 11, 12, 16] For reasons of convenience and graft quality, however, fresh skin and cornea preserved by simple cooling are still preferred for therapeutic use.

Formidable obstacles stand in the way of successful freeze preservation of organs even as large as canine kidneys. Systems have not yet been successfully devised for simulating for all cells within such organs the conditions that are readily obtained with thin tissue slices and with cell suspensions. Attempts to preserve organ viability by freezing have been thwarted by difficulties in controlling the rate of movement of cryoprotective substances into and out of cells and the rate of freezing and thawing. Luyet has recently written a historical review of the biophysics of freeze preservation of tissues.[9]

Chemical Inhibition of Metabolism

Phenothiazine derivatives, magnesium compounds, and other chemical substances have been used adjunctively for tissue and organ preservation because of their reversible inhibition of certain metabolic processes.[11, 16] This approach to preservation has been of quite limited usefulness, however.

Tissue Culture

The work of Carrel for three decades beginning in 1910 was a major contribution to the technology of tissue culture,[11, 12] which during the nineteenth century had had only elementary beginnings. By emphasizing meticulous aseptic technique he successfully overcame the problem of bacterial contamination that had limited the development of tissue culture previously. He maintained a line of chick embryo fibroblasts in active culture for over 30 years. There have been scattered attempts to maintain parathyroid and other tissues in culture for subsequent grafting, but such methods are not in general use. Tissue culture has been useful principally in providing an understanding of the basic requirements of living mammalian cells being maintained for prolonged periods of time in an artificial environment.

Organ Perfusion

In 1938 Carrel and Lindbergh reported the use of perfusion in maintaining viability of organs of small animals for various periods of time up to 3 days.[11, 16, 17] They used cell-free perfusates and called the method "organ culture," a logical extension of Carrel's work with tissue culture. The discovery of heparin and the development of blood transfusion provided a basis for perfusing organs with blood under conditions designed to simulate fully the natural internal environment of the organ with normothermic metabolism. Numerous investigators have succeeded in maintaining normal viability and function for a few hours; but when organ perfusion with whole blood is attempted for longer periods the quality of the circulation deteriorates, largely because of the embolization of vessels with cellular and amorphous deposits and because of swelling, which may be unexplained.

In 1968 Belzer et al. reported preservation of kidneys for 72 hours by hypothermic pulsatile perfusion with plasma from which lipoproteins had been removed by freezing, thawing, and filtration. This and other methods of renal preservation are described by Belzer in a subsequent section of this chapter, and organ preservation is the subject of a recent book.[11]

Artificial Vital Organs

The history of the development and use of the pump-oxygenator is given in the chapter on the heart, and of the artificial kidney in the section on renal allografts in this chapter. Both were first used successfully clinically at about the middle of the present century. The need for such artificial organs in conjunction with transplantation is obvious. The use of a pulsatile pump-membrane oxygenator for renal allograft preservation, as noted earlier, is an example of the relatedness of these technologies.

Other Methods

A number of other methods of temporary life support have been attempted.[11] Some of these other methods have been rather ingenious, but none as yet have reached general clinical application. Crossed circulation between two individuals has been frequently used experimentally and occasionally clinically. Crossed circulation incidentally accomplishes a rather massive cross grafting of immunologically competent lymphocytes. Lavender maintained cadaver kidneys temporarily inside a plastic chamber attached to the arm of the prospective recipient at the site of the arteriovenous cannulation tubes that had been used for dialysis. One purpose of this method was to avoid transplantation if the kidney failed to function for reasons of either inadequate preservation or immunologic incompatibility. Other semiartificial perfusion systems have been used. Notable examples include the use of a real lung or liver from the same or a different species in an extracorporated perfusion circuit for the temporary support of a patient or an experimental animal. Such semiartificial systems incidentally expose the recipient to antigens by way of the bloodstream and thus have some of the characteristics of an allograft or xenograft. Grafts have been temporarily "stored" by transplanting them into massively immunosuppressed individuals of a related species prior to the definitive transplantation procedure. Hyperbaric oxygenation has been used adjunctively in various methods of preservation.

OTHER DEVELOPMENTS

There have been numerous other contributions to the development of transplantation; this review is selective, not exhaustive. Part of this development has been that of "spin-off," applications to other fields of knowledge. Examples include the use of immunosuppressive agents for purposes not related to transplantation, improved understanding of functions of the thymus, and new methods of treating immunologic deficiency diseases and other immunopathologic states. Finally, the development of transplantation has stimulated the interest of the general public[10, 17] and has raised a number of questions in fields other than medicine and biology, particularly in law, sociology, economics, and theology. An example of response to such questions was the development of the Uniform Anatomical Gift Act to facilitate postmortem donation of tissues and organs for medical and other scientific uses.[13] Enactment into law in all of the 50 states was accomplished in the remarkably short period of less than 3 years. Therapeutic transplantation is still in a very active state of development. A broad range of interests will undoubtedly continue to be stimulated by further development of this form of treatment.

SELECTED REFERENCES

Calne, R. Y.: Renal Transplantation. London, Edward Arnold, Ltd., 1967.
  The first portion of this book is devoted to historical and basic biologic aspects of tissue transplantation and the remaining sections to a review of renal transplantation. The author has had extensive personal experience with both clinical and experimental aspects of transplantation.

Converse, J. M., and Casson, P. R.: The historical background of transplantation. *In* Rapaport, F. T., and Dausset, J. (Eds.): Human Transplantation. New York, Grune & Stratton, Inc., 1968.
  The authors present a history of the principal developments in transplantation from ancient to modern times, and they include some details not included in the other histories cited.

Moore, F. D.: Give and Take. Philadelphia, W. B. Saunders Company, 1964.
  In this volume is presented a concise review of developments in basic biology and in medicine and surgery that apply to therapeutic renal transplantation. Interesting aspects of historic renal transplants in Boston are described by the author, who was there at the time and has communicated personally with scientists there and elsewhere who have made notable contributions. For the student, this book is an informative introduction to the subject of transplantation, and for the lay reader, a readily understood account of some interesting developments in biology and medicine.

Norman, J. C. (Ed.): Organ Perfusion and Preservation. New York, Appleton-Century-Crofts, 1968.
  This volume consists of the 67 papers presented during a conference on the subject in Boston in 1968. Collectively these papers amount to a comprehensive historical review and description of current developments in the technology of tissue and organ preservation.

Peer, L. A.: Transplantation of Tissues. Baltimore, Williams & Wilkins Company, 1955.
  This is a comprehensive two-volume review of the subject. The most exhaustive reviews are those pertaining to transplantation of skin, teeth, cornea, fascia, bone, cartilage, and other connective tissues.

Woodruff, M. F. A.: The Transplantation of Tissues and Organs. Springfield, Ill., Charles C Thomas, Publisher, 1960.
  This monograph is a comprehensive and exhaustive review of both experimental and clinical transplantation. Over 4000 references are conveniently listed at the end with cross referencing from text to reference and from author's name to pages in the text. A truly monumental work, this text reflects the experience of the author as a clinical surgeon and as a basic scientist.

Worshofsky, F.: The Rebuilt Man. New York, Thomas Y. Crowell Company, 1965.
  This book is a brief historical review of the development of transplantation from ancient to modern times. Written by a science writer for lay readers, the discussion is well documented by references to and quotations from the scientific literature.

REFERENCES

1. Bettmann, O. L.: A Pictorial History of Medicine. Springfield, Ill., Charles C Thomas, Publisher, 1956, p. 211.
2. Bhisragratna, K. K.: The Sushruta Sanhita, An English Translation Based on the Original Sanscrit Text. Calcutta, Bose, 1916.
3. Calne, R. Y.: Renal Transplantation. London, Edward Arnold, Ltd., 1967.
4. Carrel, A.: Remote results of replantation of the kidney and the spleen. J. Exp. Med., *12*:146, 1910.
5. Converse, J. M., and Casson, P. R.: The historical background of transplantation. *In* Rapaport, F. T., and Dausset, J. (Eds.): Human Transplantation. New York, Grune & Stratton, Inc., 1968.
6. Good, R. A., and Gabrielsen, A. E.: The thymus and other lymphoid organs in the development of the immune system. *In* Rapaport, F. T., and Dausset, J. (Eds.): Human Transplantation. New York, Grune & Stratton, Inc., 1968.
7. Gorer, P. A.: Transplantese. Ann. N.Y. Acad. Sci., *87*:604, 1960.
8. Guthrie, D.: A History of Medicine. Philadelphia, J. B. Lippincott Company, 1946, p. 12.
9. Luyet, B.: Preservation and storage of living cells at low temperatures. *In* Rapaport, F. T., and Dausset, J. (Eds.): Human Transplantation. New York, Grune & Stratton, Inc., 1968.
10. Moore, F. D.: Give and Take. Philadelphia, W. B. Saunders Company, 1964.
11. Norman, J. C. (Ed.): Organ Perfusion and Preservation. New York, Appleton-Century-Crofts, 1968.
12. Peer, L. A.: Transplantation of Tissues. Baltimore, Williams & Wilkins Company, 1955.
13. Sadler, A. M., Jr., Sadler, B. L., Stason, E. B., Jr., and Stickel, D. L.: Transplantation—a case for consent. N. Engl. J. Med., *280*:862, 1969.
14. Shinoi: Specificity of second set phenomenon. Tokyo J. Med. Sci., *46*:11, 1932.
15. Tagliacozzi, G.: De curtorum chirurgia per insitionem. Venice, 1597, p. 61.
16. Woodruff, M. F. A.: The Transplantation of Tissues and Organs. Springfield, Ill., Charles C Thomas, Publisher, 1960.
17. Worshofsky, F.: The Rebuilt Man. New York, Thomas Y. Crowell Company, 1965.

II

TRANSPLANTATION ANTIGENS

D. Bernard Amos, M.D.

Enthusiasm for transplantation, like enthusiasm for different forms of cancer therapy, especially immunotherapy, has waxed and waned depending upon the energies and optimisms of its proponents, since long-term results often fall short of expectations. An outstanding example from the past of an apparently successful procedure soon abandoned was the transplantation of teeth as practiced by John Hunter. This procedure enjoyed immediate popularity, but was gradually discredited as a practice when it became apparent that the transplanted teeth had died.

Steady gains have been made, especially during the last decade. The transplantation of cornea and of bone is taken as much for granted now as is blood transfusion, the most widely practiced form of transplant. The transplantation of kidney is being increasingly accepted throughout the world as a practical means of treating end-stage renal disease, while occasional long-surviving grafts of liver, heart, and bone marrow give an indication of the potential widespread applicability of organ and tissue transplantation.

However, *rejection* spoils the record of corneal grafts, kills bone and skin homografts, and has prevented any wide-scale attempt to transplant heart, lung, and liver. The threat of rejection and knowledge of the miseries suffered by patients experiencing chronic, uncontrollable rejection dissuade some nephrologists from recommending transplantation as a preferable alternative to dialysis for the treatment of kidney disease. This section will be concerned almost exclusively with the recognition of foreign tissue, factors provoking recognition and the initiation of rejection, and the nature of the antigens thought to be responsible. A subsequent section will discuss the immune response and how it may be circumvented. When the problems of rejection are solved, and undoubtedly they will be, transplantation will be the treatment of choice of countless thousands of patients, as it potentially offers a relatively inexpensive and immediate relief from many diseases for which the only alternative is palliation.

ANTIGENICITY AND THE RECOGNITION OF FOREIGNNESS

Autotransplants and grafts between monozygotic twins succeed, while grafts between all other individuals or between members of different species fail except under special circumstances. The special cases include transplants to a few especially favored sites and transplants to recipients who have a natural or an acquired immunologic unresponsiveness. The reason for the distinction between grafts between twins and grafts between other close relatives is that blood and tissue cells carry certain identification markers or antigens that are recognized as foreign unless they exactly match those already present in the recipient. A donor and recipient may be identical with respect to all detectable antigenic markers and graft rejection will still occur, since other antigens for which no test can be made at present will be different.

Some antigens, or combinations of antigens, are much more potent than others. The variation between the response to different antigens has given rise to the concepts of antigenic strength and of "minor" and "major" antigens. It is possible, although not easy, to obtain a measure of antigenic strength in certain situations. Antigenic strength or immunogenicity is well documented for some of the red cell antigens. Blood group A is a "strong" or major antigen and the trans-

fusion of A blood into an O or B recipient leads to an acute transfusion reaction; in contrast, the M and N antigens on the red cell are so feeble they rarely give rise to severe immune reactions. Even within a single antigenic system there are wide variations in antigenic strength, the A_1 antigen, for example, being stronger than A_2 is even further modified when it occurs in the combination A_2B. Variants A_3 and A_4 are progressively weaker than A_2 in terms of the transfusion reactions produced and in their ease of detection.

Many blood group antigens outside the ABO system are very potent but are of little relevance to transfusion practice; these are the so-called private or public blood groups. Although some of these have been associated with disease, e.g., hemolytic disease of the newborn, and can cause severe transfusion reactions, the public blood group antigens may be present on over 99 per cent of individuals and the private in less than 0.1 per cent.

Thus, as far as the red cell is concerned, antigens may be classified into three groups: strong antigens of clinical importance, strong antigens of little clinical relevance because of their peculiar distribution, and weak antigens.

Documentation of the strength and distribution of tissue antigens is more sketchy, especially in the human where studies of these antigens have only recently been started. It is helpful to be able to refer to animal systems where tissue antigens or tissue and red cell systems are known from serologic or transplantation studies extending over many years.[56] The most intensively studied mammal is the mouse; therefore, reference will be made to studies on mouse antigens before returning to a consideration of man.

The mouse has the tremendous advantage of extensive inbreeding, and more than 75 inbred lines or distinctive sublines are available. Many of the lines or strains are well characterized with respect to transplantation antigens and to many other factors, such as complement levels, immunologic responsiveness to defined antigens, tumor susceptibility, and resistance to infection or to x-irradiation. Because they have been inbred for many generations, members of an inbred strain are almost as alike as monozygotic twins; therefore, animals from the same strain behave alike in transplantation studies. Grafts exchanged between members of different inbred strains are usually rejected, and the time taken for rejection to occur gives a measure of the strength of the antigenic diversity between them. Generally speaking, the greater the number of antigens differentiating donor from recipient, the faster and more severe the rejection. The most potent single system of antigens is called H-2.[27] Other antigens such as H-1, H-3, and H-4 are less potent, are serologically difficult to identify, and are best detected by graft rejection in selected combinations of especially bred mice, called congenic lines. A congenic pair differs only by one small segment of chromosome determining the particular antigen to be studied. A special codified designation is given to these lines; A. SW and A. CA are congenic with respect to each other and with respect to the A strain. More than 99 per cent of the genome is A; the remainder carries the histocompatibility-2 locus of the remote ancestral SW or CA mouse, respectively.

From studies with hybrids between inbred lines, certain laws of transplantation have been laid down. These laws were established over a long period of time by numerous investigators and have been summarized by Snell[55] as follows:

1. Grafts within inbred strains are successful.

2. Grafts between different inbred strains fail.

3. Grafts from either parental line to the first generation hybrid (F_1 hybrid) between them are successful.

4. Grafts from animals produced by crossing two similar F_1 animals (F_2 hybrids) onto the F_1 hybrid are also successful.

5. Grafts from a parental line are accepted by some members of the F_2 hybrid population and rejected by others.

6. Grafts from a parent to the resistant back-cross formed by crossing the F_1 hybrid to the other parent may also be successful, but the proportion of successful takes is somewhat lower.

These various crosses are summarized in Table 1, which diagrams the inheritance of an antigen A and its alternative or allelic form a. The first parent (P_1), being from an inbred stock, is uniform (homozygous) with respect to A; therefore all its gametes carry the information for A. The other parent (P_2), being from a different strain, is homozygous for the allele a and its gametes are also uniform. The F_1 hybrid resulting from a mating between P_1 and P_2 inherits both A and a. All F_2 hybrids carry both antigens and are said to be heterozygous. Since F_1 are heterozygous with respect to A and a, they cannot recognize tissues carrying either of these antigens and so cannot reject a graft. When F_1 hybrids are crossed with each other, half the gametes carry the gene for A and the remainder the gene for a. The gametes can fuse in any of four possible combinations, AA, Aa, aA, or aa. Of these four gametic combinations, Aa and aA are indistinguishable and are called phenotypically identical. There are thus four genotypes but only three phenotypes. A graft from an AA (or an Aa) donor will be recognized as foreign by a recipient carrying only aa; one fourth of all F_2 recipients will be of this genotype, and thus 25 per cent of grafts will fail because A is foreign. Frequently, two strains differ by more than one antigen. If the genes for the different antigens are on different chromosomes (unlinked), there will be a random assortment of characters. The proportion of successful grafts will be $(3/4)^n$ where n is the number of unlinked transplantation or histocompatibility (H) genes. For the back-cross, only two phenotypes can exist, Aa or aa. Fifty per cent of the back-cross mice will reject a graft carrying antigen A and the general formula is $(1/2)^n$. When n is large, as it usually is when skin grafts are transplanted, the proportion of successful grafts is usually very small.

In practice, the number of antigens differentiating two strains is usually measured by transplanting tumor, for the very practical reason that tumor grafts are very easily performed, and recently induced tumors share many of the antigens of the donor. Thus, results obtained with newly derived tumors can be extrapolated to other tissues. After repeated passage, the tumor grows faster and seems to be able to overcome the host's resistance to some of the weaker factors. This is variously called tumor progression, antigenic simplification, or antigen loss. "Antigen loss" is a partial misnomer, since the continued presence of otherwise undetectable antigens can be shown by preimmunization; a weak or abortive reaction can be turned into an effective one.

Note that the "laws" on transplantation, as listed here, apply only to inbred populations and their hybrids. They cannot be directly applied to outbred populations, such as man, because the gametes are not identical and the offspring do not receive a complete set of genetic information from each parent. Hence, grafts from human parent to child are rejected, often violently. The animal studies do, however, provide a logical genetic basis on which to build information about more complex outbred populations, and most of the information we have about strong histocompatibility antigens in man derives from the animal studies.

METHODS OF DETECTION OF ANTIGENS

The presence of transplantation antigens can be detected in several different ways. Transplantation of organs or tissues is the most direct test of antigenicity but gives only a crude definition of the antigens involved. Since some of the H-2 and many of the non-H-2 antigens, notably H-5, H-6, H-14, and the so-called beta, iota, and kappa antigens, are readily detected on red cells, hemagglutination has been widely used for detecting these antigens, especially in the past.[3] Some-

TABLE 1. Inheritance of Antigen A

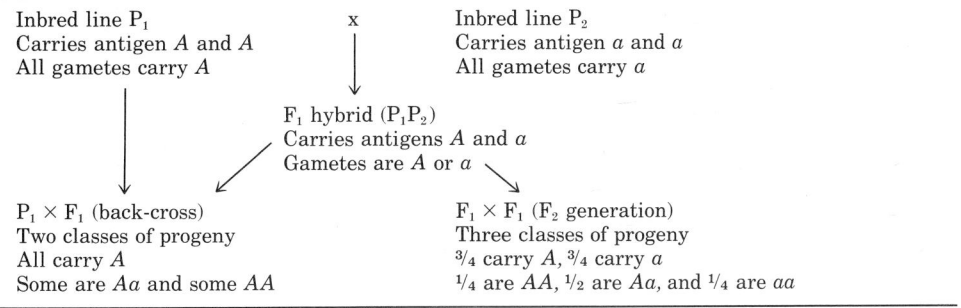

times the agglutination reaction is complete in saline. Other antigens can be detected only in media that reduce the negative surface charge or zeta potential. If the combination of antigen and antibody is weak, a high surface charge on the cell will prevent agglutination, especially by the 7S gamma globulins with their relatively short spanning reach. The macroglobulins because of their pentagonal form can span greater distances; hence, they can react even when the cells are in strong repulsion. Suspension of cells in low ionic strength media, or the addition of high molecular weight compounds, such as fluid from pseudomucinous ovarian cysts, various dextrans, and polyvinylpyrrolidone, has been used to facilitate red cell agglutination by reducing the zeta potential.[33] Centrifugation provides an additional mechanism for bringing the cells closer together and thus facilitating agglutination by antibody.[73] However, some antigens are either absent from red cells or present in only trace concentrations in some mouse strains, and nucleated cells are now frequently used in tests for the presence of antigen, since their antigenic representation appears to be more complete. Leukoagglutination has been employed to demonstrate H-2 antigens[2] but is technically difficult, and leukocyte cytotoxicity is now the method of choice. The two-stage method is the most sensitive.[36] In the first stage, suitable target cells, usually from lymph nodes, are incubated with antibody and then washed. In the second stage, complement is added to the washed, sensitized cells. After incubation, the target is tested for its ability to exclude a vital dye, such as trypan blue, eosin, nigrosin, or ethidium bromide. An alternative indicator is provided by the ability of the cell to retain fluorescein added to the suspension in the form of fluorescein diacetate.[14] Complement fixation with platelet antigen is rarely used in the mouse, but is becoming popular in testing human HLA antigens. In this test, antibody is allowed to react with the platelets in the presence of a known amount of complement.[18] Sensitized red cells are then added. If complement has been fixed, the red cells remain intact; if the complement is still present, the red cells lyse.

Very different in principle are tests for lymphocyte *reactivity*. Most widely used is the mixed lymphocyte culture reaction (MLR) in which lymphocytes from two donors are mixed together and incubated.[11] Changes in morphology or in the ability of responding cells to take up radioactive precursors of nucleic acid or protein are determined. In general, the greater the antigenic diversity between the lymphocyte donors, the greater the response. Of considerable interest is the finding that stimulation is usually an attribute of the K zone of H-2.[61]

Also widely used in animal studies of the aggressiveness associated with incompatibility is the spleen or lymph node weight gain assay.[69] Foreign (allogeneic) lymphocytes are injected intravenously or intraperitoneally and the spleen is removed and weighed after a predetermined interval. In a more sensitive variant of this procedure, lymphoid cells are injected into the footpad; an increase in weight of the popliteal node is determined. Less used are the kidney capsule test and the irradiated hamster test. In the first of these tests, the lymphocytes are injected into the sub-capsular space of the kidney; the lesion is examined histologically.[30] In the second test, a mixture of lymphocytes from two allogeneic donors is injected intradermally into a lethally irradiated hamster.[59] The interaction results in palpable induration. The hamster test is of particular interest, since the lymphoid cells used can come from man, mouse, or any other species. One other interesting test has been used in guinea pigs or humans to test for reactivity of these species. This is the normal lymphocyte transfer (NLT) test in which blood lymphocytes are injected intradermally.[16] This test can be made unidirectional by pretreating the lymphocytes with mitomycin C.

The MLR, which is the most widely used measure of lymphocyte reactivity, is imperfectly understood. If conducted with unmodified lymphocytes from two different individuals, it is bidirectional; that is to say, clones from both cell populations respond. As usually performed, one population is treated by x-irradiation or by exposure to mitomycin C and so can no longer incorporate thymidine into DNA. Cells prevented from dividing in this manner can still stimulate. Cells killed by freezing and thawing, by heat, or by other means do not stimulate; most nonlymphoid cells and at least some lymphoid tumors also fail to stimulate. From these observations, it is clear that the MLR is not a simple test for the presence of antigen. Many materials, highly antigenic in the sense of being able to absorb antibody or to initiate an immune response in vivo, fail to stimulate at all or stimulate very feebly. Further, the MLR seems to be triggered only by certain classes of antigen. This is especially true in man, in whom only HLA seems to stimulate, and even then, strong stimulation is given only by lymphocytes, macrophages, and vascular endothelium.

The irradiated hamster test also appears to produce lymphokines and thus to result in an accumulation of PMN. Injection of a single nonimmune lymphoid population into the skin of a guinea pig or human produces inflammatory changes, but those changes too appear to depend on the participation of two different lymphocyte populations: donor and host. In man, NLT reactions become visible by 8 hours and usually reach a peak within 48 hours. Inflammation appears to be in part a consequence of a reaction of the injected cells against the host, since some response (although diminished) is seen in anergic recipients.[7] It must also be in part a reaction of the host against the injected cells, since the reactions to mitomycin-treated cells are also diminished. Mixtures of allogeneic lymphocytes provide a strong and rapid response in anergic subjects, so this test can be made to parallel the irradiated hamster test.

Reactivity against a target monolayer, usually of tumor or of fibroblasts, also provides a test for lymphocyte activity.[18] Reactivity is most effective when the lymphocytes are from specifically immunized donors. The target cells can be labeled with isotope. This test determines the cytotoxic activity of immune lymphocytes, whereas the other procedures measure proliferation or reactivity of normal cells and are more nearly reflective of some function of genetic disparity than of the state of immunity. Of potential clinical interest is the finding that cytotoxic lymphocytes are generated in vitro during the course of an MLR. In addition, the cells that have reacted in MLR are now educated and respond rapidly when exposed to cells from the original stimulating donor or to cells from a donor having similar antigens. This is the basis of the primed lymphocyte test (PLT) now being evaluated for use in the selection of transplant donors.

Each of these tests has been used for certain specific situations. All of the procedures, serologic or involving cellular reactivity, have inherent technical problems, and reliable results come only with experience and due attention to adequate experimental design and control. All the tests measure some feature of genetically controlled diversity, but it is far from certain that all measure similar attributes.

SPECIFIC ANTIGENS IN MICE
(THE H-2 SYSTEM)

Mouse histocompatibility antigen systems are denoted by the symbol H followed by a number, thus H-1, H-2, and so forth. The alleles or alternative forms are designated by a superscript letter (H-2[a], H-2[b]), and the specific antigens by an upper-case letter in the older literature (H-2B, H-2D) or, more recently, by an arabic numeral (H-2.2, H-2.4).[44]

The most potent murine transplantation antigens belong to the H-2 system. This system was first described by Gorer, Lyman, and Snell, who, in a very elegant study, gave a positive identification to the gene controlling a strong antigen.[32] They showed that the antigen was present on red cells as well as on the tumor and that the determinant gene was on the same chromosome as the gene for a tail abnormality. Since the antigen on the red cell had previously been recognized by Gorer as antigen II, the transplantation or *histocompatibility* antigen was named H-2. At first it was believed to be a simple factor existing in several allelic forms and not much more complex than the human A and B antigens. By transplantation, Snell soon found that there were many different variants or alleles of the H-2 gene,[70] and Gorer and his colleagues showed that each H-2 allele controlled at least two, and probably more, specific antigens.[6] The serologic and transplantation tests almost always, but not invariably, agreed.

The H-2 system was soon compared to the human Rh system because of its complexity, and, like Rh, its exact genetic constitution is still controversial. The genetic control of H-2 was soon distinguished from that of Rh. Whereas Fisher and Race postulated the existence of three genes controlling Rh and Wiener argued there was only one, Gorer and his colleagues were soon able to prove that H-2 was complex by identifying recombinants within H-2.[34] Animals resulting from recombination had some of the characteristics of each parent on the same chromosome. At least two of the determinants, those for antigens D and K, have been separated from each other repeatedly by crossing over, and recombinants having D but not K or K but not D were among the first to be recovered. Although the respective antigens are now designated 4 and 11, the determinants on the chromosome are still identified as the D region and the K region. "Gene,"

"locus," and "region" are operational descriptions, and H-2 includes a whole series of genetic determinants, so the designation H-2 "region" is appropriate. It is probable, because of the high frequency of recombination between D and K and from differences between the chemical properties of molecules carrying D and K antigenic activity, that at least two H-2 genes, or cistrons, each coding for a different polypeptide responsible for serologic specificity, are represented.

The present concept of H-2 is that it includes at least five major regions called K, I, S, G, and D, but this number may shortly be expanded to eight.[44] The conservative view of H-2 would restrict it to the five regions listed; of these five regions, K and D include genetic loci controlling the production of glycoproteins and the H-2 antigens, which are present on the majority of tissues and cells. The amount of antigen present on the cell surface varies greatly, being highest on peripheral lymphoid cells and in low concentration on tissues such as kidney and muscle. The H-2 antigens are present on all peripheral B and T lymphocytes. This distinguishes them from antigens controlled by genes in the I region (Ia antigens) which are primarily expressed on B cells and can be demonstrated on T lymphocytes only indirectly, e.g., by absorption.

The I region has been divided into three subregions, IA, IB, and IC. IA includes loci regulating the immune response to a number of antigens, most intensively studied being a series of branched chain, synthetic polypeptides.[49] All animals appear to recognize the antigen being studied by producing IgM antibodies. However, only animals with the appropriate Ir allele can develop a mature response by switching to IgG production. The deficiency can be overcome by transferring bone marrow or fetal liver cells from an immunocompetent donor or by presenting the antigen on an appropriate carrier molecule. Most of the Ia antigens are controlled by genetic loci in the IA subregion but at least three Ia antigens are also controlled by genes in IC. The IB region was recognized by differences in the ability of various mice to respond to a myeloma protein. Since the evidence for the existence of the IB region rests solely upon the reactions of one recombinant (h4), very little information is available about the region and no Ia antigens have been firmly localized to it. The S region controls the production of a serum protein, Ss, which is related to the C4 component of complement.[66] The Ss protein is also under the control of a gene, Slp, which has not been separated from Ss by recombination, and which further regulates the amount in serum through hormonal mechanisms. The G region is at present distinguished only by loci controlling red cell antigens, but is also believed to code for other specificities involved in skin graft rejection and possibly for MLR stimulation.

Besides the important Ir genes, which have obvious immunologic functions, other genes within the H-2 complex are also biologically active. Among the known activities are the induction of strong homograft reactions following transplantation, the ability to stimulate lymphocyte proliferation in the mixed lymphocyte reaction (MLR) with allogeneic lymphocytes, and also one or more genes regulating the level of the response in MLR, genes responsible for graft versus host reactions, and for the generation of cytotoxic effector (T) cells, loci conferring susceptibility to viral leukemia and possibly for viral attachment. It has also been proposed that the histocompatibility antigens are responsible for self-recognition in the generation of diversity of immunologic responsiveness. Interestingly, modification of self can occur following exposure to virus or to any of several simple haptens.[87] The modified self antigens can be strongly immunogenic.[66] Although this type of reaction has been studied only in model systems, it may indicate one of the mechanisms for self recognition in autoimmune or autoaggressive reactivity.

To add complexity to an already complicated situation, at least three genetic loci coding for histocompatibility antigens are known to lie immediately adjacent to the H-2 region and may come to be recognized as components of H-2. These are the loci identified as H-31 and H-32, which have been mapped between the D region of H-2 and the locus for thymic leukemia (T1) antigens lying about 0-5 crossover units from it, and H-33, which maps on the other side of the K region, between K and the gene (tf) for tufted hair.

The precise regulation of these varied functions is somewhat uncertain. Klein has summarized the uncertainty, saying, "The distinction between region and subregion in the H-2 complex is not very great . . . subregions of the same region . . . are both topographically and functionally related." It is clear that the MHC, as typified by H-2, must be treated in different ways by different investigators. The geneticist is interested in the fine detail. He wants to know, for example, which of the genes are structural and which are regulatory and how they relate functionally to each other. The transplant surgeon needs to know the overall immunogenicity of the haplotype bearing the complex and how to overcome it.

The precise details of H-2 itself are likely to remain the center of controversy until the products of H-2 are adequately defined. A start has been made by isolating soluble materials with antigenic properties, but, because of the minute amounts of purified material available for study, chemical sequence analysis is only available for the products of the D and K region genes.

The soluble products studied for antigenic activity are best made by extraction of isolated cell membranes with proteolytic enzymes such as papain,[25, 53] detergents such as deoxycholate,[50] or with high concentrations of salts such as potassium chloride[60] which seem to facilitate autolytic release.[46] EDTA has also been used sucessfully to release antigen.[29] At least 90 per cent of the complete antigen appears to be associated with the cell membrane; hence the use of isolated plasma membrane as a starting material gives an initial purification step with little loss of antigenicity.[37, 81] The washed membrane is then treated by various solubilizing procedures to give an extract.[47, 52] The solubilized material is usually purified by chromatographic separation as, for example, with DEAE-cellulose. Separate peaks of activity have been described by a number of investigators.[15, 82] The antigenic material has a molecular weight between 30,000 and 50,000 and contains approximately 10 per cent carbohydrate with little or no lipid.[47, 52] Since the molecule contains carbohydrate, affinity columns, notably Concanavalin A, also offer a convenient means

of initial purification. Two separate proteins are noncovalently bound. One is a small (11,000) dalton β_2 microglobulin molecule, the other is the 35,000 dalton H-2 or HLA molecule proper. Sequence analysis of D-end and K-end specificities of H-2 and also of the HLA-A and HLA-B loci on man has been partially completed at the time of writing. There is considerable sequence homology between β_2 microglobulin and part of the Fc portion of IgG. This led to speculation that the histocompatibility antigens might be similar to immunoglobulins, but sequence comparisons of H-2 or HLA with mouse or human globulin show only about 20 per cent homology, indicating the relationship is not close. On the other hand, there is considerable homology between the D and K region products of H-2, between the A and B locus products of HLA, and also between HLA and H-2. This confirms the homology between H-2 and HLA and indicates that the histocompatibility genes evolved independently from the immunoglobulin genes. Variability has been established in several sequences and the serologic reactivity of the histocompatibility antigens may therefore be a function of the tertiary structure of the molecule.

Only six carbohydrate residues have been detected, and two of these, fucose and mannose, are present in only trace amounts.[52] It has been shown that one of the carbohydrates, sialic acid, is not part of the antigenic site, since its removal by neuraminidase does not abolish the absorptive capacity of the product for antibody.[65] Sialic acid does seem to play a part in the antigenic property of the whole cell, however, since treatment of live cells with neuraminidase increases complement fixation and renders the cell more vulnerable to attack by antibody.[35] The increased reactivity of neuraminidase-treated cells seems to be related more to development of reactivity to minor antigens than to profound changes in H-2 or HLA and may be a function of the reduction of the surface charge or zeta potential, since many weak reactions are potentiated by low ionic strength. Carbohydrates, including sialic acid, and glycolipids may be more directly involved in the composition of some non-H-2 and non-HLA antigens; certainly the human antigen 5b, described by van Rood and chemically characterized by Bruning, appears to have properties and chemical compositions very different from those of HLA.[17a] The identity of many, if not most, of the non-H-2 and non-HLA antigens has not been well established. In the absence of good markers for these antigens, it is impossible to know how free from contamination the purified products of any antigen are. These considerations, together with the low concentration of antigen in the starting material, the retention of unsolubilized antigen on the membrane, and the loss of antigen product at each stage in purification, add to the problems of recovery of the antigens.

Scientists are not yet agreed that the soluble antigens are direct products. Since the "purified" antigen is usually a glycopeptide, the possibility exists that the antigenic portion is carbohydrate, although as far as H-2 is concerned, this appears to be less and less likely. However, it is still possible that the primary product of the H-2 or HLA "genes" is transferase enzymes that attach polysaccharides or short-chain glycopeptides that determine antigenic specificity to a carrier polypeptide.[4] Conversely, the serologic activity may be due to attributes of the carrier molecule, and some of the biologic attributes, such as the elicitation of delayed-type responses, would be properties of the side chains.

Isolation, identification, and sequence analysis of the primary product itself is essential before we can say how many such products are made by a given cell and thus how many codons (3-nucleotide message units of DNA) are involved. Until then, all interpretation is speculative and the nonspecialist should remember only that *H-2 is a complex system located on a segment of a known (the IXth) linkage group, is intimately associated with many important attributes such as resistance or susceptibility to disease, and, because H-2 and the human HLA systems apparently have so much in common, information relating to H-2 may have very direct relevance to man.* It is because of the possibility that knowledge of H-2 may have great practical application that so much attention is being paid to this system.

HUMAN HISTOCOMPATIBILITY ANTIGENS AND THE HLA SYSTEM

Knowledge of human transplantation begins—and almost finishes—with HLA.[8] The little direct knowledge of antigens other than HLA will be summarized separately later. Suffice it to say at present that many such antigens exist, that some can be detected serologically, and that the existence of others can be inferred from observations on graft rejection between HLA-identical siblings. Immunity to non-HLA antigens (excluding, of course, A and B blood antigens) seems to be considerably weaker and easier to suppress than is immunity to HLA.

In 1958, Dausset described an antigen on human leukocytes detectable by agglutinins present in serum obtained from several donors immunized by blood transfusions. The antigen he detected, now known to be present in about 50 per cent of Caucasians, was then called Mac.[21] This designation was later changed to HLA-2 or HLA-Mac. Early detection methods were crude, sera were scarce and impure, and knowledge developed slowly until Payne and Rolfs and van Rood and van Leeuwen found leukoagglutinins in the serum of multiparous women.[55, 79] Van Rood and his associates rapidly accumulated information about several interrelated series of antigens which were named 4a and 4b, 6a and 6b, 7a, b, c, and d, and 8a.[80] All these factors are now known to be components of the HLA system. Payne and her colleagues developed a system independently, designating their antigens HLA-A1, -2, -3, and -4.[13] Dausset and his colleagues, using some common sera and some collected locally, described a large and complex series of specificities, and other investigators, including Ceppellini, Terasaki, Walford, Batchelor, and Amos, were also active in developing new techniques, defining new specificities, and redefining the old. Several attempts at genetic studies were made but, because of the complexities of the system and the relatively poor reliability of the tests, little was done to resolve the problems of genetic control of the antigens. At first it appeared as if a large number of loci were involved, but most investigators noticed interrelationships between different systems of different specificities. Dausset and the Ivanyis, without the benefit of family studies to guide them, made the sweeping assertion that all the antigens studied by them were components of a single genetic system.[24] This system was called Hu-1 by them. Bach and Amos immediately confirmed the validity of this assumption.[10] They studied serologic reactions in a number of large families and compared mixed lymphocyte culture reactions, skin graft survival times, and segregation patterns of the antigens. Serologically, about 25 per cent of the children appeared to have inherited the same two alleles from their parents. Lymphocytes from these genotypically identical pairs failed to stimulate in mixed culture, and skin grafts between them survived for many days longer than grafts between nonidentical pairs. The data all fitted the concept that there was only one locus and that this was a powerful transplantation locus. An international terminology was agreed upon with the help of the World Health Organization. The name of the locus was changed to HLA and seven of the specificities were designated. These were HLA-1, -2, -3, -5, -7, -8, and -9. Designations 4 and 6 were reserved for the antigens 4a and 4b which had not been adequately defined. Later, HLA-10, -11, -12, and -13 were added to the series. The development of information about HLA has followed a unique course necessitating a degree of collaboration unusual in biomedical science. Collaboration focuses around international workshops which are held at approximately two-year intervals. The number of participating groups and the scope of the workshops have progressively increased. The Fourth Workshop, held in 1970, greatly increased the number of known specificities. This information was used in studies of the HLA antigens of indigenous populations during the 1972 Fifth Workshop. The Sixth Workshop, held in 1975, studied reactions of antisera to a third allelic series of HLA antigens and also categorized a number of alleles contributing to stimulation in MLR. Following this workshop, the WHO Terminology Committee revised the nomenclature. The WHO committee now recognizes four genetic loci within the HLA system. These are HLA-A, HLA-B, HLA-C, and HLA-D. HLA-A and HLA-B are the former first or LA locus and the former second or Four locus, respectively. The former numbers used for these series are retained. The HLA-C locus was previously known as the third or AJ locus, while HLA-D was variously known as MLR-S, MLC, or LD1 locus. HLA-C appears to define a series of antigens detected serologically, whereas HLA-D is defined in terms of the ability of lymphocytes to stimulate and has no exact serologic equivalent. It is recognized that human B lymphocytes carry serologically detectable antigens and that the distribution of some of these closely follows the distribution of the HLA-D alleles. Indeed, it is believed that the HLA region includes at least three loci whose products are primarily expressed on B lymphocytes.[20, 48] One of these loci is in proximity to HLA-A, one segregates in recombination with HLA-B, and one with HLA-D. This information is still preliminary and no official designations are expected before the Seventh Workshop, to be held in 1977. Two gene products have, however, been identified by immunochemical procedures. These are membrane-associated proteins of MW of approximately 30,000 daltons; they do not carry a β_2-microglobulin component and appear to be similar to the Ia antigens of the H-2 region.

The most widely recognized specificities are given official HLA designations (HLA-A1, HLA-B7, etc.). Less well defined specificities carry the prefix w (HLA-Aw30, HLA-Bw35, etc.), while other specificities are provisional and carry the prefix w. A list of currently recognized HLA specificities is given in Table 2. Note that the HLA designation is not an abbreviation for human leukocyte antigen or histocompatibility locus A but is merely a convenience designation.

As a result of extensive family studies conducted during the Fourth Histocompatibility Testing Workshop, it was agreed that the specificities could be arranged in the form of two segregant series. In many respects, the HLA determinants behave as if they consist of two closely linked loci or subloci—comparable to the D series and the K series antigens of the mouse. Each series appears to exist in various allelic forms. In this convention, the maximal number of antigens present on a diploid cell is four. Each HLA-determining chromosome is said to control the production of two specificities, one being a product of the first series and the other of the second, the combined product being designated a haplotype (Table 3). Proponents of this hypothesis believe that crossing over (recombination) between the two segregant series occurs with a frequency approaching 1 per cent. In many populations, reasonably good equilibrium has been attained between the series; however, there are some notable exceptions, especially with respect to HLA-1 and 8, 3 and 7, 2 and 5, and 2 and 12.[1] There is also a tendency for HLA-2 to be frequently associated with some of the less frequent and less well defined specificities. The cause and significance of this disequilibrium is still obscure. A blood group system that seems to be analogous is that of the MN and Ss factors.

M and N can be regarded as two alleles controlled by one locus and S and s as alleles at a closely linked locus.[58] Like HLA, M and N show considerable quantitative and qualitative variability when examined carefully, and an undeterminant series of alleles have been described. The variant M_2 of M is present in about one fourth of American Negros, M^c is an infrequent form easily confused with M_1, and many other variants are known. This is a fascinating system notable for the effect that some of the variants have on the expression of the homologous allele. M_1N cells react less strongly with anti-N than do MN cells. Cross-reacting antibodies have also been described; anti-M^v reacts strongly with M^vN cells, reacts less strongly with MN cells, M^vM, or NN, and does not react at all with MM cells. Similar effects may be operating in HLA. For example, cells from a subject typed as negative for HLA-2 stimulated the formation of an anti-2-like antibody when injected into a 2-minus recipient. On retesting, her cells failed to react

TABLE 2. Complete Listing of Recognized HLA Specificities*

New	Previous†	New	Previous	New	Previous	New	Previous
HLA-A1	HL-A1	HLA-B5	HL-A5	HLA-Cw1	T1	HLA-Dw1	LD 101
HLA-A2	HL-A2	HLA-B7	HL-A7	HLA-Cw2	T2	HLA-Dw2	LD 102
HLA-A3	HL-A3	HLA-B8	HL-A8	HLA-Cw3	T3	HLA-Dw3	LD 103
HLA-A9	HL-A9	HLA-B12	HL-A12	HLA-Cw4	T4	HLA-Dw4	LD 104
HLA-A10	HL-A10	HLA-B13	HL-A13	HLA-Cw5	T5	HLA-Dw5	LD 105
HLA-A11	HL-A11	HLA-B14	W14			HLA-Dw6	LD 106
HLA-A28	W28	HLA-B18	W18				
HLA-A29	W29	HLA-B27	W27				
HLA-Aw19	Li‡	HLA-Bw15	W15				
HLA-Aw23	W23	HLA-Bw16	W16				
HLA-Aw24	W24	HLA-Bw17	W17				
HLA-Aw25	W25	HLA-Bw21	W21				
HLA-Aw26	W26	HLA-Bw22	W22				
HLA-Aw30	W30	HLA-Bw35	W5				
HLA-Aw31	W31	HLA-Bw37	TY				
HLA-Aw32	W32	HLA-Bw38	W16.1				
HLA-Aw33	W19.6	HLA-Bw39	W16.2				
HLA-Aw34	Malay 2	HLA-Bw40	W10				
HLA-Aw36	Mo	HLA-Bw41	Sabell				
HLA-Aw43	BK	HLA-Bw42	MWA				

*The previously reserved specificities W4 (4a) and W6 (4b) remain w4 and w6. These specificities are closely associated with the B locus.

†For a more comprehensive listing of equivalents see "Table of Equivalent Nomenclature" *In* Dausset, J., and Colombani, J. (Eds.): Histocompatibility Testing. Copenhagen, Munksgaard, 1972, p. 7.

‡HLA-Aw19 includes at least HLA-A29, Aw30, Aw31, Aw32, Aw33, and Aw34 (?).

TABLE 3. Inheritance of HLA Haplotypes

	Father		Mother	
	A	B	C	D
Haplotype				
Antigens HLA	1–8	3–7	2–12	9–13
	1	2	3	4
Children	A + C	A + D	B + C	or B + D
Antigens	1, 8, 2, 12	1, 8, 9, 13	3, 7, 2, 12	3, 7, 9, 13

Any other child must also be AC, AD, BC, or BD

with a variety of anti-2 sera but could absorb anti-2 activity from many of these sera. This is but one of many known examples of anomalous and, at present, unpredictable reactivity encountered in the HLA system.

There are interrelationships within each of the series, usually referred to as cross reactions. These interrelationships were shown most clearly by absorption and elution studies of certain widely reactive but apparently monospecific sera.[9] New cross reactivities are constantly being found, and it is quite possible that the whole description of HLA may have to be revised as more information is obtained. It appears as if most of the antigens can be arranged in a relatively few cross-reactive sets. One such series or set would include HLA-A1, -3, -10, and -11 and another would include HLA-A2, the subgroups of HLA-Aw23,24 and HLA-A28. Cohesive series of this type would be expected if a single amino acid substitution in the ligand distinguished one specificity from another member of the same series.

The effects of cross reactivity between different HLA specificities are still being evaluated in terms of their effects on the induction of immunity and on transplantation rejection. Cross reactivity would occur if two antigens, say HLA-A3 and HLA-A11, resembled each other very closely. A recipient of genotype HLA-A-1-8, 3-7 might accordingly react less vigorously to a graft from a donor who was 1-8, 11-7 than he would to a graft having the antigens 1-8, 9-7, since antigens 3 and 9 are not known to be cross-reactive. This appears a likely possibility but is still unproved. The converse is also possible. Certain grafts, known to be incompatible, survive and function surprisingly well. Failure of the recipient to react vigorously against the transplant may be due in part to other cross reactivities not well recognized at present. Recognition is a highly individual characteristic determined by factors not fully understood. Thus, one individual may be unable to distinguish between two specificities that another clearly regards as distinct. Our serum RA reacts with all HLA-B7 and all HLA-B8-containing cells; in this serum, anti-7 cannot be separated from anti-8 by absorption so that even HLA-B7 and HLA-B8 can be cross-reactive under certain conditions. Many other sera, previously regarded as containing mixtures of different specific antibodies, are now known to contain cross-reactive antibodies, indicating shared sequences or other similarities between apparently unrelated antigens.

At the same time that these cross-reactive series are beginning to emerge, some of the original antigens are being split into subcomponents. The recent history of HLA is confounded by the discovery that what appeared at first to be a single specificity is made up of two or more distinct entities. This happens when the reactions of a cross-reactive antibody are described first. The original HLA-9-containing sera, such as Hunt, Tuckerman, HM, reacted with many members of the cell donor panel. As more specific sera became available, the specificity now known as HLA-9 was defined. As new sera were produced, some reacting with only a proportion of HLA-9 positive cells were found and the older sera were found to be cross-reactive. It now seems clear that HLA-9 comprises two separate but cross-reactive specificities, HLA-Aw23 and HLA-Aw24, and more recently HLA-10 has also been split, probably into at least three subspecificities.[22] Even HLA-2, once regarded as the best defined of the HLA series, appears to be a composite of two or even three antigens. Antigen splitting is being regarded as a possible cause of rejection of an apparently compatible graft. Two people, previously regarded as being HLA-9-positive, may later be shown to have different components of 9.

Because of the cross reactivities, it has been suggested that HLA may have much in common with Rh. The widely cross-reactive specificities as typified by 4a and 4b, or our serum BH and HLA-2, or Walford's sera Thompson and HLA-7, have points of resemblance to C and c and E and e of the Fisher-Race terminology of Rh, with some of the infrequently reacting sera corresponding to anti-f or anti-ce of this system. In both systems, deciding which is the "correct" answer is not simple. In Rh practice, the question is almost completely academic, but in HLA, it is of extreme relevance to transplantation to find a solution to these complexities.

Typing for Transplantation

There are sharply divided viewpoints among biologists and clinicians regarding the relevance of tissue typing to transplantation; members of both groups have alternated in their feelings.[56] The evidence can be divided into three parts: that derived from grafts between HLA-identical siblings, that from grafts between family members who differ by one (called haploidentical) or two (haplodistinct) HLA alleles, and that from grafts exchanged between unrelated individuals.[63] The most informative grafts have been those of kidney or of skin.[84] With rare exceptions, kidney grafts from HLA-identical siblings (where HLA identity has been determined from the inheritance patterns of the alleles, i.e., genotypically HLA-identical) are marked by smooth convalescence, early rehabilitation, good function, and freedom from severe rejection episodes.[72] Grafts between family members differing at one (or two) alleles generally succeed, but a certain proportion provoke violent rejection.[57] Some grafts run a smooth course, some a violent and abruptly terminated one. Thus, even where donor and recipient are close family relations, there is a considerable degree of uncertainty as to the outcome of a transplant; the uncertainty is considerably greater when both haplotypes are mismatched, but a proportion of such transplants are highly successful.

IR genes on tissue transplantation in rodents and polygenic control with at least some loci being unlinked to HLA seems likely. Studies on Ir genes in man are much more difficult to carry out. First, the choice of antigens is restricted to those that are clearly noninjurious. The majority of ethical antigens have multiple antigenic sites. Then, whereas an inbred mouse strain is homozygous, a human is generally heterozygous and has two HLA haplotypes, each of which can contribute to an immune response; within a family there are four haplotypes. Finally, although many HLA recombinants are known, few have progeny and so fine mapping is much more laborious. It is not surprising that attempts to show association between HLA and immune responses on a population level have been unsuccessful. However, within the family, especially in three-generation families in which some individuals are atopic, HLA-associated responses to a variety of antigens have been demonstrated and HLA is clearly linked to IR genes.[12a, 17a, 75] From the same data, it is possible to infer that the level of immune response to a variety of other antigens is not associated with HLA.

Such studies do not relate directly to human transplant rejection. They do indicate the existence of human response genes and illustrate the manner in which information about the response to tissue may be developed. There is evidence that the level of MLR is under control of regulation genes. Obviously, if genes regulating responsiveness to HLA haplotype products could be identified, a new approach to transplantation would be to select a recipient whose response genes would not permit them to recognize donor antigens. This appears to be one potential use for HLA typing.

Another feature of HLA which may prove very relevant to transplantation is called linkage disequilibrium. It has earlier been pointed out that the number of possible permutations of HLA-A, B, and C alleles on a haplotype is large; a minimum estimate would be 4000 different possible haplotypes. In practice, some haplotypes are very frequent and some are rare or absent. In Caucasians, HLA-A1 is most frequently associated with HLA-B8, HLA-A2 with B12 or B5, HLA-A3 with B7, and so on. These associations are much more frequent than could be expected by chance. The association coefficient between two linked loci is called delta. High delta values exist not only between the A and B loci, but are also present between the B and D loci. HLA-B8 and Dw3, and HLA-B7 and Dw2 are notable examples. Delta between B locus and C locus alleles is even higher, extreme examples being between HLA-Bw35 and Cw4 or between HLA-B12 and Cw4. Finally, the high delta between HLA-D and B cell determinants has already been commented on, antisera correlating with HLA-Dw2 and HLA-Dw3 being among the best documented.

The cause of high delta values is still being sought. The simplest explanation is that they represent founder effects. In a somewhat inbreeding population, such as that of rural England or in The Netherlands of the eighteenth century, the number of different haplotypes would be quite small. When such a population increases, as in the settlement of the Americas, the earliest settlers would make the largest contribution to the gene pool. Since the overall recombinational frequency in the HLA haplotype is less than 1 per cent, it would take many generations for the loci to reach a random assortment, or equilibrium. However, there are other explanations; one is from a parallel with the mouse where the 17th chromosome which carries the H-2 haplotype may be positively selected. The possible implication of histocompatibility antigens in the response of a mother to her fetus or to semen has been discussed.[26, 28] Some HLA haplotypes appear to be associated with specific diseases, for example with juvenile diabetes, which would introduce negative selection pressures unless compensated for.

The implication of high delta values is that by improved characterization, truly identical haplotypes may in the future be identified by typing. Assume that the HLA region carries more loci than we are currently aware of and that some of these are important for transplantation, either because they determine structural membrane proteins or by virtue of their interrelationship with other loci on the haplotype. Now, linkage disequilibrium is by no means absolute. Two haplotypes that carry the antigens -A2 and -B12 may type alike serologically, yet differ in many other respects and be quite incompatible for transplantation. Let us further assume that the number of possible 2-12 haplotypes is finite, say, less than 10. With the ability to recognize more points on the haplotype, we could identify the different subclasses of 2-12 haplotype and obtain a far greater compatibility than by matching just for the antigens 2 and 12. This could most easily be accomplished by typing B cells, since these lymphocytes appear to carry several additional markers. Thus, even though we might still fail to identify as yet unknown immunogenic loci, the chance of compatibility would be improved.

This has been a highly speculative section and the issues discussed are obviously for pursuit by a limited number of sophisticated laboratories, but the possibilities discussed must obviously be explored. Another line of investigation to be pursued is the attempt to locate those loci within the haplotype that contributes most to the immunogenicity of a transplant. We know, from family studies, the overwhelming importance of the HLA system in organ, bone marrow, and tissue transplantation. We still do not know which components of the haplotype are the most immunogenic. It may prove to be the HLA antigens themselves, or, as Yunis and Amos have suggested, another locus, HDR, may be responsible for eliciting strong cellular responses to transplants.[83] The HDR determinant is thought to control a product that is not detected serologically or in the MLR, but that is responsible for provoking first-set graft rejection. To give a clearer concept, it is helpful to introduce three new terms. Serologically detectable (SD) specificities are the antigens recognized as belonging to the HLA, H-2 (or other) systems. Lymphocyte specificities (LAD) are recognized by MLR, graft versus host, cell-mediated cytotoxicity, inhibition of macrophage migration, and similar reactions. The major histocompatibility complex (MHC) is then defined as a segment of chromosome that determines the individual SD and LAD components belonging to the complex. This concept does not imply that SD antigens are never involved in cellular recognition or that LAD factors are never detectable serologically but does suggest that SD is usually detected by antibody and LAD are not so readily detected by conventional serologic tests. The response of a patient immunized by transfusion or pregnancy and who is producing antibody will be predominantly against the SD component (i.e., HLA) of the human MHC. Antibodies formed against the HLA antigens as a result of blood transfusion or a prior transplant are involved in hyperacute rejection. Since graft rejection commonly has some elements of both first- and second-set reactions, compatibility for both HLA and HDR is desirable. If this concept is correct, most of the anomalies between serotyping, MLR, and graft survival can be explained. HLA typing within families would have predictive value, since HLA and HDR are closely linked. Outside the family, HLA would have less predictive value, since HLA and HDR would be in a state of equilibrium.

The hypothesis relates the major role of HLA incompatibility to second-set or antibody-mediated hyperacute rejection, MLR to lymphocyte proliferation in the MLC and in graft versus host assays, and HDR to cell-mediated immunity. For easy acceptance of a graft of kidney, heart, or nonreticular tissue, compatibility for HLA, to avoid antibody-mediated reactions, and for HDR, to avoid cell-mediated rejection, appears to be necessary. With bone marrow, compatibility for MLR may also be important since a recombinant incompatible for a first-series antigen but nonstimulatory in MLR was involved in a successful bone marrow transplant.[31] It is obvious that if this hypothesis is correct, serotyping alone has only limited predictive value.

There are various ways in which LAD can be assayed. For example, one of the oldest measures of genetic distance between individuals is the MLR. HLA identical subjects do not stimulate; HLA-D homozygotes do not stimulate individuals who share an HLA-D allele; subjects differing at one allele do not stimulate and subjects who differ at two alleles stimulate more strongly.[39] The MLR should thus be a useful test for measuring immunogenicity, but this has not proved to be the case, and the HLA-D locus appears to contribute little to transplant rejection; neither is the MLR capable of fine discrimination between individuals. An offshoot of the MLR is the primed lymphocyte test (PLT). This is based on the observation of Ginsberg,[31a] Häyry,[38] and others that lymphocytes responding to an allogeneic stimulation respond more rapidly to a second stimulation, and that specific cytotoxic cells are stimulated by the first response and are much more numerous during the second. Two uses can be made of this information: (1) A series of donors can be used to provide stimulating cells for the secondary MLR. Subjects who most resemble the original stimulating donor will give the strongest secondary response. (2) The reactivity of the cytotoxic cells can be assessed to determine specificity of stimulation.

HLA typing for compatibility continues to be important, however, because correlation between phenotypic identity of donor and recipient and prolonged survival is very strong. It is also essential to avoid giving grafts to recipients possessing antibodies directed against the HLA determinants of the graft. Because of the complexity of HLA and the probably high polymorphism of HDR, the skill of the clinician in controlling immunosuppression will continue to be the most important factor in obtaining good graft survival. The real breakthrough in transplantation that will allow grafting of lungs and other highly antigenic organs may come from the establishment of tolerance, enhancement, or some other highly selective procedure, rather than from tissue typing as it is currently performed. An adequate definition of HDR could also be of great prognostic value.

Complicating donor selection in the absence of compatibility are the effects of previous exposure to cross-reactive antigens. Cross reactivity to HLA follows blood transfusion and probably exposure to antigens in the environment. Cross-reactive antibodies can be identified by testing serum from the recipient with cells from the intended donor. The serum from the recipient should be freshly drawn, since antibodies can develop within five days of exposure in a previously sensitized subject. The test system must also be as sensitive as possible, since even weak reactions that appeared to be inconsequential have given a warning of hyperacute rejection on at least two occasions. Hypersensitivity to products of the hypothetical HDR antigen cannot be detected serologically, but a proportion of transplants fail acutely in the absence of detectable preformed antibody and occasional HLA-identical grafts undergo very severe rejection crises.

This section gives an account of current lines of research in HLA. Until some of the uncertainties mentioned are cleared up, there is likely to be little obvious advance in matching. Despite considerable advances in resolution of the HLA specificities, there has been little advance in the overall survival of cadaveric kidneys. The contrasting findings, in two reported series, of increased survival with four-antigen matching, is extremely encouraging. Further progress along this line could rapidly follow advances in long-term storage that would permit a wider choice of donor-recipient pairs.

Antigens of Other Systems and of Other Species

Most other species appear to have a system that is comparable to the HLA–MLR–HDR complex. This has been found true for sheep, cattle, pigs, dogs, chickens, and rats. In the rat, the major complex is called AgB.[54] Responses to immunosuppressive drugs and the ability of lymphocytes to stimulate in mixed culture are attributes of AgB incompatibility. The dog has a comparable system called DLA, and a similar system, PLA, has been reported for pigs. The general pattern in mammals thus seems to be of a single complex system controlling a series of attributes. Some species appear to be exceptional. No major locus has been identified in the Syrian hamster, probably because of serologic difficulties in this species. It was at one time felt that the available strains all shared the same major H locus, but rapid skin graft rejection and strong cellular reactions are being found between certain inbred hamster strains. No serologic definition has been made of the major locus in the guinea pig, but a strong transplantation antigen system is known to be closely linked to an immune-responsiveness gene.[12] It appears that the analog of HDR is expressed in this system, whereas the analog of HL-A is not; however, this could be due to a deficiency in the serologic detection system. The rabbit remains relatively complex and inadequately explored; MLR appears to be lost rapidly upon inbreeding. The mouse appears to be paradoxical in its MLR, but this may be fallacious. Mouse strains of the same H-2 type may or may not stimulate, and responsiveness between two strains of the same H-2 type cannot be predicted a priori. This is explicable if MLR-S is different in different mouse strains of the same H-2 type. At least some of the stimulation appears to come from a locus (M) that is not linked to H-2. Four alleles of the M locus have been postulated. M locus incompatibility is not correlated with any known effect on transplantation.

The simplest overall concept of major histocompatibility loci is that mammalian and avian species have all inherited, and modified within rather narrow limits, an information system that includes a polymorphic series of serologically detectable antigens comparable to HLA. However, there is a strong possibility that a polymorphic MLR system and a polymorphic HDR system have also evolved in close relationship to the serologically detectable factors.

In addition to the major gene complexes, all species appear to possess an almost infinite variety of minor antigens. In the mouse, the list is extremely long. Antigens 1 to 33 have been given formal designations in the H system, but antigens unique to plasma cells, to lymphocytes, to thymus, and to lymphoma cells have also been described.[76] Similarly, antibodies specific to neutrophils and to platelets in man have been documented.[43, 78] Some of these antigens are associated with graft rejection; others are of questionable significance. Many other antigens common to particular

tumors and tissues, to embryonic cells, and to red cells have been partially defined. Those antigens that are system-restricted will obviously play a part only in the rejection of grafts of the organ or tissue involved and will be detectable only in that tissue. These antigens are unlikely to present a serious problem. The majority of antigens described to date are quite widely distributed and may still have wide variations in their relative content in different tissues. The amount of antigen present on a given tissue appears to be a direct attribute of the particular genetic system. It may be necessary to consider specific minor locus antigens (which would include the human red cell antigens) in the transplantation of various organs, especially in the presence of preformed antibodies. A red cell crossmatch as well as a white cell crossmatch should be a prerequisite for any transplant. It has, for example, recently been found that an antigen, G55, not related to HLA, can be detected in the cytotoxic system, and that this antigen is, or is closely related to, the red cell antigen Le[a].[27] So far, such antigens appear to play a very secondary role in transplantation and major emphasis is likely to remain on the HLA complex.

CONCLUSION

In the early stage of white cell and tissue typing, the abundance of antibodies and lack of precise genetic information made it appear that many antigenic systems could be detected on human tissues. Improved techniques and reagents showed that most of the antigens detected belonged to a single system—HLA. This system behaves as if it is controlled by two closely linked genes. It thus appeared that matching for four antigens, two homologous antigens of the first segregant series and two of the second, would suffice to ensure major locus compatibility. However, phenotypic identity for four antigens in an unrelated donor does not give compatibility approaching that between HLA-identical siblings when skin is exchanged; data with respect to kidney are only just beginning to accumulate for evaluation. A reappraisal of the available data suggests that the major gene complex in man consists of three elements: HLA, which determines the serologic specificities, MLR-S, which controls lymphocyte stimulation, and HDR, which determines cell-mediated reactions of the delayed type. The evolution of information regarding the specificities of man and other species is summarized, with some suggestions as to what more is needed.

REFERENCES

1. Allen, F., Amos, D. B., Batchelor, R., Bodmer, W., Ceppellini, R., Dausset, J., Engelfriet, C., Jeannet, M., Kissmeyer-Nielsen, F., Morris, P., Payne, R., Terasaki, P., van Rood, J. J., Walford, R., Zmijewski, C., Albert, E., Mattiuz, P., Mickey, M. R., and Piazza, A.: Joint Report of Fourth International Histocompatibility Workshop. *In* Histocompatibility Testing 1970. Copenhagen, Munksgaard; 1970, pp. 2–47.
2. Amos, D. B.: The agglutination of mouse leukocytes by isoimmune sera. Br. J. Exp. Path., 34:464, 1953.
3. Amos, D. B.: Some iso-antigenic systems of the mouse. *In* Proceedings of the 3rd Canadian Cancer Conference. New York, Academic Press, 1959, p. 241.

4. Amos, D. B.: Genetic aspects of human HL-A transplantation antigens. Fed. Proc., 29:2018, 1970.

5. Amos, D. B.: Anderson, E. E., Glenn, J. F., Gunnells, J. C., Lancaster, S. L., MacQueen, J. M., Robinson, R. R., Seigler, H. F., Stickel, D. L., and Ward, F. E.: Selection of donors for kidney transplantation. Transplant. Proc., 3:993, 1971.

6. Amos, D. B., Gorer, P. A., and Mikulska, Z. B.: An analysis of an antigenic system in the mouse (the H-2 system). Proc. R. Soc. London (Biol.), 144:369, 1955.

7. Amos, D. B., Nicks, P. J., Peacocke, N., and Sieker, H. O.: An evaluation of the normal lymphocyte transfer test in man. J. Clin. Invest., 44:219, 1965.

8. Amos, D. B., and Ward, F. E.: Immunogenetics of the HL-A system. Physiol. Rev., 55:206, 1975.

9. Amos, B., and Yunis, E.: Human leukocyte antigenic specificity HL-A3: Frequency of occurrence. Science, 165:300, 1969.

10. Bach, F. H., and Amos, D. B.: Hu-1: Major histocompatibility locus in man. Science, 156:1506, 1967.

11. Bach, F. H., and Voynow, N. K.: One-way stimulation in mixed leukocyte cultures. Science, 153:545, 1966.

12. Benacerraf, B., Bluestein, H. G., Green, I., and Ellman, L.: Specific immune response genes of guinea pigs. In Progress in Immunology. New York, Academic Press, 1971, pp. 485–494.

12a. Blumenthal, M. N., Amos, D. B., Noreen, H., Mendell, N. R., and Yunis, E. J.: Genetic mapping of Ir locus in man: Linkage to second locus of HLA. Science, 184:1301, 1974.

13. Bodmer, J., Coukell, A., Bodmer, W., Payne, R., and Shanbrom, E.: A new allele for the LA series of HL-A antigens. In Histocompatibility Testing 1970. Copenhagen, Munksgaard, 1970, pp. 175–185.

14. Bodmer, W., Tripp, M., and Bodmer, J.: Application of a fluorochromatic cytotoxicity assay to human leukocyte typing. In Histocompatibility Testing 1967. Copenhagen, Munksgaard, 1967, pp. 341–350.

15. Boyle, W.: Soluble HL-A iso-antigen preparations. Transplant. Proc., 1:491, 1969.

16. Brent, L., and Medawar, P. B.: Tissue transplantation: A new approach to the "typing" problem. Br. Med. J., 2:269, 1963.

17. Brunning, J. W., Masurel, M., Brent, V. D., and van Rood, J. J.: Leukocyte antigenic fractions from placental tissue. In Histocompatibility Testing 1967. Copenhagen, Munksgaard, 1967, pp. 303–306.

17a. Buckley, C. E., III, Dorsey, F. C., Corley, R. B., Ralph, W. B., Woodbury, M. E., and Amos, D. B.: HL-A linked human immune response genes. Proc. Natl. Acad. Sci., 70:2157, 1973.

18. Canty, T. G., and Wunderlich, J. R.: Quantitative in vitro assay of cytotoxic cellular immunity. J. Natl. Cancer Inst., 45:761, 1970.

19. Colombani, M., Colombani, J., Dehay, C., and Dausset, J.: A microtechnique of platelet complement-fixation. Results obtained with sera and eluates as the source of antibody. In Histocompatibility Testing 1970. Copenhagen, Munksgaard, 1970, pp. 553–559.

20. Cresswell, P., and Ayres, J. L.: HLA antigen: Rabbit antisera reacting against all A series or all B series specificities. Eur. J. Immunol., 6:82, 1976.

21. Dausset, J.: Iso-leuco-anticorps. Acta Haematol. (Basel), 20:156, 1958.

22. Dausset, J., and Colombani, J. (Eds.): Histocompatibility Testing 1972. Copenhagen, Munksgaard, 1973.

23. Dausset, J., and Hors, J.: Analysis of 221 renal transplants: Influence of cross-reactions between donor and recipient HL-A antigens. Transplant. Proc., 3:1004, 1971.

24. Dausset, J., Ivanyi, P., Colombani, J., Feingold, N., and Legrand, L.: The Hu-1 system. In Histocompatibility Testing 1967. Copenhagen, Munksgaard, 1967, pp. 189–202.

25. Davies, D. A. L.: The molecular individuality of different mouse H-2 histocompatibility specificities determined by single genotypes. Transplantation, 8:51, 1969.

26. Diczfalusy, E. (Ed.): Immunological Approaches to Fertility Control. Stockholm, Karolinska Institute, 1974.

27. Dorf, M. E., Eguro, S., Cabrera, G., Yunis, E., Swanson, J., and Amos, D. B.: Detection of cytotoxic non-HL-A antisera. I. Relationship to anti-Le[a]. Vox Sang., 22:447–456, 1972.

28. Doughty, R. W., and Gelsthorp, K.: An initial investigation of lymphocyte antibody activity through pregnancy and in eluates prepared from placental material. Tissue Antig., 4:291, 1974.

29. Edidin, M.: The release of soluble H-2 alloantigens during disag-

gregation of mouse embryo tissue by a chelating agent. J. Embryol. Exp. Morphol., 16:519, 1966.

30. Elkins, W. L.: Specific and nonspecific lymphoid cell proliferation in the pathogenesis of graft-versus-host reactions. Transplant. Proc., 2:273, 1970.

31. Gatti, R. A., Meuwissen, H. J., Terasaki, P. I., and Good, R. A.: Recombination within the HL-A locus. Tissue Antig., 1:239, 1971.

31a. Ginsberg, H., and Lagunoff, D.: Aggregation and transformation of rat lymphocyte on rat embryo monolayers. J. Cell. Biol., 39:392, 1968.

32. Gorer, P. A., Lyman, S. A., and Snell, G. D.: Studies on the genetic and antigenic basis of tumour transplantation. Linkage between a histocompatibility gene and "fused" in mice. Proc. R. Soc. London (Biol.), 135:499, 1948.

33. Gorer, P. A., and Mikulska, Z. B.: The antibody response to tumor inoculation: Improved methods of antibody detection. Cancer Res., 14:651, 1954.

34. Gorer, P. A., and Mikulska, Z. B.: Some further data on the H-2 system of antigens. Proc. R. Soc., 151:57, 1959.

35. Grothaus, E. A., Flye, M. W., Yunis, E., and Amos, D. B.: Human lymphocyte antigen reactivity modified by neuraminidase. Science, 173:542, 1971.

36. Grothaus, E. A., Rauckman, E. J., and Amos, D. B.: Conditions affecting the performance of the lymphocyte cytotoxicity test. Transplantation, 2:145, 1971.

37. Haughton, G.: Transplantation antigen of mice: Cellular localization of antigen determined by the H-2 locus. Transplantation, 4:238, 1966.

38. Häyry, P., and Defendi, V.: Mixed lymphocyte cultures produce effector cells: Model in vitro for allograft rejection. Science, 168:133, 1970.

39. Jørgensen, F., Lamm, L. U., and Kissmeyer-Nielsen, F.: Mixed lymphocyte cultures with inbred individuals: An approach to MLC typing. Tissue Antig., 3:323, 1973.

40. Klein, J.: Biology of the Mouse Histocompatibility-2 Complex. New York, Springer-Verlag, 1975.

41. Koch, C. T., Frederiks, E., Eijsvoogel, V. P., and van Rood, J. J.: Mixed-lymphocyte-culture and skin-graft data in unrelated HL-A identical individuals. Lancet, 2:1334, 1971.

42. Lalezari, P., and Bernard, G. E.: A new neutrophil-specific antigen. Its role in the pathogenesis of neonatal neutropenia. J. Clin. Invest., 45:1741, 1966.

43. Lalezari, P., Thalenfeld, B., and Weinstein, W. J.: The third neutrophil antigen. In Histocompatibility Testing 1970. Copenhagen, Munksgaard, 1970, pp. 319–322.

44. Lengerová, A., and Vojtisková, M. (Eds.): Immunogenetics of the H-2 System. Basel, Karger, 1971.

45. Lilly, F.: The influence of H-2 type on Gross virus leukemogenesis in mice. Transplant. Proc., 3:1239, 1971.

46. Mann, D. L.: Panel on histocompatibility antigens. In Conference on Cellular Antigens. Heidelberg, Springer-Verlag, 1971.

47. Mann, D. L. and Fahey, J. L.: Histocompatibility antigens. Ann. Rev. Microbiol., 25:679, 1971.

48. Mann, D. L., Ableson, L., Harris, S., and Amos, D. B.: Detection of antigens specific for B lymphoid cultured cell lines with human alloantisera. J. Exp. Med., 142:84, 1975.

49. McDevitt, H. O., Bechtol, K. B., Grumet, F. C., Mitchell, G. F., and Wegmann, T. G.: Genetic control of the immune response to branched synthetic polypeptide antigens in inbred mice. In Progress in Immunology. New York, Academic Press, 1971, pp. 495–508.

50. Metzgar, R. S., Flanagan, J. F., and Mendes, N. F.: Serological studies of extracted human tissue isoantigens. In Histocompatibility Testing 1967. Copenhagen, Munksgaard, 1967, pp. 307–313.

51. Najarian, J., and Symonds, R.: Transplantation. Philadelphia, Lea and Febiger, 1972.

52. Nathenson, S. G.: Biochemical properties of histocompatibility antigens. Ann. Rev. Genetics, 4:69, 1970.

53. Nathenson, S. G., Shimada, A., Yamane, K., Muramatsu, T., Cullen, S., Mann, D. L., Fahey, J. F., and Graff, R.: Biochemical properties of papain-solubilized murine and human histocompatibility alloantigens. Fed. Proc., 29:2026, 1970.

54. Palm, J.: Classification of rat strains for AgB histocompatibility antigens. Transplant. Proc., 3:169, 1971.

55. Payne, R., and Rolfs, M. R.: Fetomaternal leukocyte incompatibility. J. Clin. Invest., 37:1756, 1958.

56. Pederson, N. C., and Morris, B.: The role of the lymphatic system

in the rejection of homografts. A study of lymph from renal transplants. J. Exp. Med., *131*:936, 1970.

57. Porter, K. A., Andres, G. A., Calder, M. W., et al.: Human renal transplantation. II. Immunofluorescent and immunoferritin studies. Lab. Invest., *18*:159, 1968.

58. Race, R. R., and Sanger, R.: Blood Groups in Man, 5th ed. Philadelphia, F. A. Davis, 1968.

59. Ramseier, H., and Streilein, J. W.: Homograft sensitivity reactions in irradiated hamsters. Lancet, *1*:622, 1965.

60. Reisfeld, R. A., Pellegrino, M. A., and Kahan, B. D.: Salt extraction of soluble HL-A antigens. Science, *172*:1134, 1971.

61. Rychlikova, M., Demant, P., and Ivanyi, P.: Further studies on mixed lymphocyte reaction in H-2 incompatibility. *In* Proceedings of the Symposium on Immunogenetics of the H-2 System. Basel, S. Karger, 1971, pp. 178–181.

62. Seigler, H. F., Amos, D. B., Ward, F. E., Andrus, C. H., Southworth, J. G., Hattler, B. G., and Stickel, D. L.: Immunogenetics of consanguineous allografts in man: I. Histocompatibility testing and skin allografts. Ann. Surg., *172*:2, 1970.

63. Seigler, H. F., Gunnells, J. C., Jr., Robinson, R. R., et al.: Renal transplantation between HL-A identical donor-recipient pairs: Functional and morphological evaluation. J. Clin. Invest., *51*:3200, 1972.

64. Shearer, G. M., Rehm, T. G., and Garbarino, C. A. Cell mediated lympholysis of triphenyl-modified autologous lymphocytes. J. Exp. Med., *141*:1348, 1975.

65. Shimada, A., and Nathenson, S. G.: Removal of neuraminic acid from H-2 alloantigens without effect on antigenic reactivity. J. Immunol., *107*:1197, 1971.

66. Shreffler, D. C.: Studies on genetic fine structure of the H-2 region. *In* Proceedings of the Symposium on Immunogenetics of the H-2 System. Basel, S. Karger, 1971, pp. 138–147.

67. Shreffler, D. C., and Klein, J.: Genetic organization and gene action of mouse H-2 region. Transplant. Proc., *2*:5, 1970.

68. Shreffler, D. C., and Passmore, H. C.: Genetics of the H-2 associated Ss-Slp trait. *In* Proceedings of the Symposium on Immunogenetics of the H-2 System. Basel, S. Karger, 1971, pp. 58–68.

69. Simonsen, M.: Graft versus host reactions. Their natural history, and applicability as tools of research. Progr. Allerg., *6*:349, 1962.

70. Snell, G. D.: A fifth allele at the histocompatibility-2 locus of mouse as determined by transplantation. J. Natl. Cancer Inst., *11*:1299, 1951.

71. Snell, G. D.,and Stimpfling, J. H.: Genetics of tissue transplantation. *In* Jackson Laboratory: Biology of the Laboratory

Mouse. New York, McGraw-Hill Book Company,1966, p. 457.

72. Stickel, D. L., Seigler, H. F., Amos, D. B., Ward, F. E., Price, A. R., and Anderson, E. E.: Immunogenetics of consanguineous allografts in man: II. Correlation of renal allografting with HL-A genotypes. Ann. Surg., *172*:160, 1970.

73. Stimpfling, J. H.: The use of PVP as a developing agent in mouse hemagglutination tests. Transplant. Bull., *27*:109, 1961.

74. Stimpfling, J. H., Reichert, A. E., and Hudson, P.: The serological properties of some H-2 recombinant alleles. *In* Proceedings of the Symposium on Immunogenetics of the H-2 System. Basel, S. Karger, 1971, pp. 10–17.

75. Svejgaard, A., Platz, P., Ryder, L. S., and Themsen, M.: HLA and disease associations—a survey. Transplant. Rev., *22*:3, 1975.

76. Takahashi, T. Old, L. J., and Boyse, M. D.: Surface alloantigens of plasma cells. J. Exp. Med., *131*:1325, 1970

77. Terasaki, P. I., Mickey, M. R., and McClelland, J. D.: Serotyping for homotransplantation. XIV. Provisionary evaluation of various antisera in predicting clinical outcome of kidney transplantation. *In* Histocompatibility Testing 1967. Copenhagen, Munksgaard, 1967, pp. 231–235.

78. van der Weerdt, Ch. M.: The platelet agglutination test in platelet grouping. *In* Histocompatibility Testing 1965. Copenhagen, Munksgaard, 1965, pp. 161–166.

79. van Rood, J. J., van Leeuwen, A., and Eernisse, J. G.: Leukocyte antibodies in the serum of pregnant women. Vox Sang., *4*:427, 1959.

80. van Rood, J. J., van Leeuwen, A., Schippers, A. M. J., Pearce, R., Blankenstein, M. V., and Volkers, W.: Immunogenetics of the group four, five and nine systems. *In* Histocompatibility Testing 1967. Copenhagen, Munksgaard, 1967, pp. 203–219.

81. Wilson, L. A., Amos, D. B., and Boyle, W.: Subcellular location of antigens. *In* Conference on Cellular Antigens. Heidelberg, Springer-Verlag, 1972.

82. Yamane, K., and Nathenson, S. G.: Biochemical similarity of papain-solubilized H-2^d alloantigens from tumor cells and from normal cells. Biochemistry, *9*:4743, 1970.

83. Yunis, E. J., and Amos, D. B.: Three closely linked genetic systems relevant to transplantation. Proc. Natl. Acad. Sci., *68*:3031, 1971.

84. Yunis, E. J., Gatti, R. A., and Amos, D. B. (Eds.): Tissue Typing and Organ Transplantation. New York, Academic Press, 1973.

85. Zinkernagel, R. M., and Doherty, P. C.: H-2 compatibility requirement for T-cell-mediated lysis of target cells infected with lymphocytic choriomeningitis virus. J. Exp. Med., *141*:1427, 1975.

III

RENAL ALLOGRAFTS

Delford L. Stickel, M.D., and H. F. Seigler, M.D.

HISTORICAL ASPECTS

The therapeutic use of renal allografts* is in an active state of development that is closely related to basic advances reviewed at the beginning of this chapter and in the sections on transplantation antigens, immunosuppression, and graft rejection. Woodruff[23] reviewed reports of 23 renal allografts in man that were published prior to 1959. All but one of these were reported after 1949. The first was by a Russian surgeon, Voronoy, who in 1936 unsuccessfully grafted a cadaver kidney into a patient with mercury poisoning. Hume in 1955 reported the results of nine cases. Included in this series was a cadaver donor graft that functioned 5½ months in the thigh of a recipient who received no immunosuppression. In 1954 Murray et al. performed the first transplant of a kidney between monozygotic twins.[9] The long-term success of this and subsequent renal transplants between monozygotic twins was followed by a great increase in clinical studies with renal allografts.

In 1959 Murray in Boston and Hamburger in Paris each performed a renal allograft using a nonidentical twin as the donor and a recipient immunosuppressed with total-body irradiation.[9] As immediate and long-term success was observed in these two cases, there were numerous further reports of the use of living related donors and immunosuppressed recipients. Total-body irradiation was used little after the first clinical use of azathioprine in 1961.[9] In 1964 Marchioro et al. reported the efficacy of prednisone in reversing established manifestations of threatened rejection,[3] and in 1967 the first clinical use of antilymphocyte globulin was reported by Starzl.[14]

Successful use of hemodialysis to substitute for renal function temporarily during a period of *acute* renal failure was developed by Kolff in the Netherlands during World War II.[9] In 1960 Quinton and Scribner[14] reported the successful use of permanently indwelling Silastic-Teflon arteriovenous shunts for *chronic* hemodialysis. A patient thus could be maintained as long as necessary—weeks, months, years—until a *cadaver* kidney suitable for grafting became available.

The shortcomings of immunosuppression stimulated the development of tissue compatibility testing. Prior to 1965 very unfavorable experiences had been reported with renal allografts that were incompatible for the ABO blood group antigens, and compatibility with

respect to these antigens was accepted as an absolute requirement in renal donor selection.[6] Subsequently the major human genetic locus, HLA, was identified as the principal other determinant of histocompatibility; and matching donor and recipient for HLA antigens and crossmatching for HLA antibodies in recipient serum were introduced as selection procedures for both living related and cadaver donors.

The *incidence of end-stage renal disease* in the United States was the subject of the 1967 Gottschalk Report (discussed by Bluemel[20]). The shortages of dialysis facilities that prompted this report have largely been overcome, but the report is still useful. In it the estimated incidence of death due to renal failure in the United States was 500 per million per year, composed mostly of patients who could not be benefitted by transplantation or dialysis because of conditions other than renal failure. It was estimated that, with 1967 selection criteria, 35 per million per year would be candidates for dialysis and transplantation. Since then progressively less strict selection criteria have been observed in actual practice,[17, 32] and the incidence of need for entry into dialysis-transplant programs now is estimated in the range of 50 to 75 per million per year. A continuing upward trend is evident as experience with these forms of treatment increases.

THERAPEUTIC APPROACHES TO END-STAGE RENAL DISEASE

Specific disease entities causing end-stage renal disease are listed in Table 1 and discussed under Re-

TABLE 1.   Original Renal Diseases of 15,921 Renal Allograft Recipients, as Reported to the Registry*

Original Renal Disease	Per Cent of Total
Glomerulonephritis	56.0
Pyelonephritis	13.1
Renal disease, unspecified	5.9
Polycystic disease	5.4
Nephrosclerosis	4.9
Two or more diseases reported	3.2
Congenital kidney disease, nonobstructive	1.4
Nephritis, secondary to drugs	1.3
Diabetic glomerulosclerosis	1.2
Familial nephropathy	1.2
All others	6.4
Total	100.0

*From Bergan, J. J., et al. J.A.M.A., *233*:787, 1975.

---

*The term "allograft" and the older but still acceptable term "homograft" are synonymous; a graft between genetically dissimilar individuals of the same species. In man allografts include all grafts from one person to another except those between monozygotic twins.

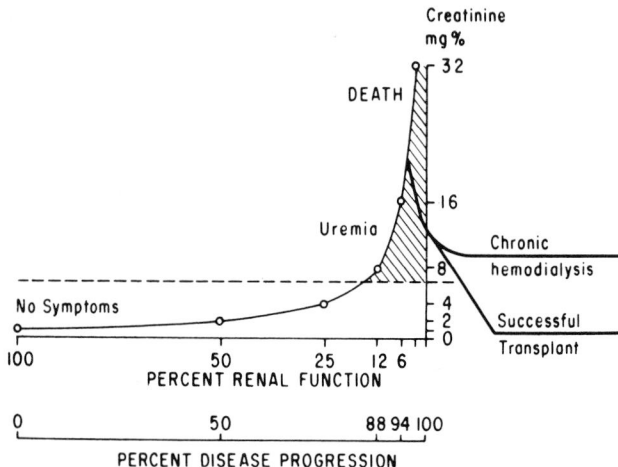

Figure 1. Natural course of renal failure. The time scale of the abscissa may be months, years, or decades. Not shown in this diagram is the course of the symptomatic recipient of a partially successful transplant. (From Maddock, R.: Low Protein Diets in Renal Failure. Salt Lake City, University of Utah Press, 1968.)

cipient Selection. As shown in Figure 1, whether renal insufficiency progresses over a period of months, years, or decades, dialysis and transplantation are the two basic means whereby life can be sustained when renal function is chronically below a level of about 5 per cent of normal. In practice, however, some combination of both dialysis and transplantation is usually included in planning treatment for an individual patient. The possible therapeutic approaches and some of their comparative advantages and disadvantages are as follows.

Sibling or Parental Donor Renal Allografts and Short-term Dialysis

Determination of whether or not a suitable sibling or parental donor will be available generally requires at most several weeks, and all or part of the selection process can transpire prior to the patient's first need for dialysis. Accordingly, living donor renal allografting usually entails only a short period of dialysis. This approach is considered first because it is the most effective means of treating terminal renal insufficiency—considerably more effective than either cadaver donor renal allografting or chronic dialysis without transplantation.

The prinicipal *disadvantage* of this approach is the undesirability of subjecting a healthy person to nephrectomy. In a multihospital survey of 1565 living donor nephrectomies, one death was reported (an incidence of 0.06 per cent), due to pulmonary embolus on the tenth postoperative day.[26] The mortality rate of the procedure has not been firmly established, but this is about the expected immediate risk associated with the procedure. The long-term risk of not having two kidneys (needing a spare and not having it) is slight but not negligible. Opinions vary regarding the weight of these risks, one view being to categorically exclude consideration of living donors. As is evident from the fact that approximately 30 per cent of transplanted kidneys being reported to the Registry are from living related donors,[2] the more generally held view is that the use of a suitable sibling or parental donor is the treatment of choice if such a donor is available.

Cadaver Donor Renal Allograft and Chronic Hemodialysis

Approximately 70 per cent of renal allografts being reported to the Registry are from cadaver donors, and this percentage has not greatly changed in recent years.[2] Despite its shortcomings, this means of treatment is restoring health to many patients. At the present time this approach envisions approximately a 50 per cent probability of failure of the graft during the first year, its removal, and return of the patient to chronic hemodialysis for a period of waiting for a second graft. The cycle may be repeated for a third graft, and so forth. Approximately 10 per cent of renal allografts are the second graft for the same patient and approximately one per cent are third grafts.[2]

Infrequently Utilized Donor Sources

Other donor sources deserve mention, but for a variety of reasons these comprise less than 3 per cent of renal allografts.[2] An *identical twin* donor is genetically highly desirable but is rarely available. The *patient's children* are genetically as suitable as the patient's parents, but for reasons of age the patient's children are seldom used as donors. *Other relatives* have little genetic advantage over unrelated donors. Very little use has been made of *living unrelated healthy donors*, partly because they have no genetic advantage over cadaver donors, and partly because of questions that arise about the motivation of persons who respond to an appeal for such donors. Rarely a *therapeutic nephrectomy* (for instance, nephrectomy for the treatment of ureteral fistula) will result in the removal of a normal kidney that can be used as a graft.

Chronic Dialysis without Transplantation

Chronic hemodialysis is best utilized as a means of maintaining patients waiting to receive renal allografts. Hemodialysis only partially eliminates the symptomatic and physiologic manifestations of chronic uremia, and the physical and psychologic adjustments to this form of treatment are difficult. Although gainful employment has been reported in up to 90 per cent of dialysis patients,[14] the health of even the best adjusted patients is less than robust, and incapacitating complications are frequent. The mortality is 5 to 15 per cent per year.[20] Nevertheless, chronic dialysis is selected for some patients with end-stage renal disease. A few have specific contraindications to transplantation, and in others various considerations affect the choice. Some patients elect indefinite dialysis because they perceive the side effects of immunosuppression and other morbidity and mortality of transplantation to be more disadvantageous than the shortcomings of dialysis. Age is a consideration. Patients over 60 generally tolerate chronic dialysis better than cadaver renal allografting, and age may reasonably be raised as a consideration for patients in their 50's or late 40's.[17]

RECIPIENT SELECTION

The reported renal diseases of allograft recipients are listed in Table 1. The predominant diagnostic category, glomerulonephritis, includes a number of different specific glomerulopathies, and glomerulonephritis was probably the true original disease in a significant number of those reported to the Registry as pyelonephritis.[2]

Inasmuch as dialysis and transplantation are in essence replacement therapy, the ideal recipient is a patient with primary renal disease, no uncorrectable complications of renal disease, and no other serious disease. At the other extreme of the spectrum of patients who might be considered for renal allografting are those whose death due to renal insufficiency appears certain but who have other serious incurable disease. Irreversible complications of uremia take the patient out of the ideal category but may or may not amount to a contraindication to renal allografting. Similar considerations apply to patients with cerebral or coronary[17] manifestations of atherosclerosis. Renal allografting in patients with the following diagnoses is the subject of a recent report from the Registry:[27] diabetes mellitus, gout, systemic lupus erythematosus, cystinosis, amyloidosis, oxylosis, Fabry's disease, familial nephritis, medullary cystic disease, and Alport's syndrome. Renal transplantation for oxylosis appears to be unwise on the basis of the results in the 10 patients in this report. The other diagnoses are not contraindications to renal allografting. Renal transplantation for insulin-dependent diabetics is the subject of a recent report.[32]

Contraindications to renal allografting occasionally develop in patients on dialysis awaiting a cadaver kidney. These include temporary problems such as infections and permanent contraindications such as disseminated cancer.

Conversely, progression of one or more of the complications of uremia while the patient is maintained on chronic dialysis may constitute a pressing indication to proceed with transplantation as soon as possible. Other conditions that may give a recipient priority consideration for an available and suitable cadaver kidney include problems of maintaining a functioning arteriovenous fistula or shunt, or the development of widely reactive HLA antibody in the patient, which makes it nearly impossible to identify an acceptable donor.

The age distribution of patients currently receiving renal allografts is similar to that reported in the ninth report of the Registry,[2] which was as follows among 5796 patients: to age 5 years, 1 per cent; 6 to 15 years, 8 per cent; 16 to 40 years, 68 per cent (with a peak in the range of 20 to 25 years); 41 to 50 years, 18 per cent; 51 to 60 years, 4 per cent; and over 60 years, 1 per cent. Age beyond 50 years is discussed in the preceding paragraph on dialysis and transplantation.

Excellent results can be achieved with renal allografting in preadolescent children.[2, 6, 17] There are, however, some special considerations that apply to such children. Access to vessels is difficult and dialysis is technically more difficult in children in other respects. Growth is impaired in children on chronic dialysis, and impaired growth is part of the steroid-induced Cushing syndrome which may occur after transplantation. The overall effect of the illness and the treatment effort upon both patient and members of the family is obviously different in children than in adults. These considerations of age are especially significant if use of a cadaver donor and chronic dialysis are planned, and prior to age five years the results of cadaver renal allografting are especially poor.[2]

Sex has no bearing on recipient selection. More than half of recipients under age 16 years are female, whereas approximately two thirds of those over 16 are male.[2]

PREOPERATIVE AND POSTOPERATIVE CARE OF UREMIC PATIENTS

A number of special considerations affect the care of the chronically uremic patient prior to the transplant operation, and before and after the other operations they need prior to transplantation. The topics in this section are discussed in more detail in recent reviews by Merrill[20] and by Seldin et al.[20]

Diet, Hydration, Electrolytes, and Acid-Base Balance

Moderate restriction of protein (40 gm. per day) is usually prescribed for the patient who is stabilized on maintenance hemodialysis. To prepare for a major operation upon a patient who has become severely debilitated, as for instance after a bout of severe infection, it may be desirable to induce weight gain. At the expense of increasing the frequency of dialysis, weight gain can be speeded by increasing dietary protein. Nitrogen balance can be maintained in adult patients with chronic uremia on an intake of as little as 20 gm. of protein per day provided the quality of the protein is good and total caloric intake is adequate. Such protein restriction minimizes the requirement for dialysis, and satisfactory experiences with this degree of protein restriction have been reported.

The severely diseased kidney characteristically excretes sodium and water at a fixed rate which varies little with variations of intake. During a diuretic salt-losing phase this fixed rate of excretion may be above the normal range of salt and water intake, but more commonly in uremia the problem is salt and water retention due to excessive intake. Salt and water retention aggravate hypertension and cardiac failure. Sodium restriction to 2 gm. per day or less is usually prescribed, and fluids are restricted to 600 to 800 ml. per day plus urine output. *Optimal hydration* is especially important immediately before transplant. Retention of excess salt and water is associated with massive, potentially dangerous diuresis from the transplanted kidney and predisposes to cardiopulmonary and thromboembolic complications. On the other hand, preoperative dehydration (resulting from excessive withdrawal of salt and water during dialysis or undue dietary restriction) results in oliguria of the transplanted kidney and obscures critically important post-transplant observations of urine output and renal function.

Restriction of dietary *potassium* to about 60 mEq. per day is prescibed to prevent hyperkalemia. More rigid restriction of intake is difficult to achieve. Orally administered resins that exchange sodium for potassium will effectively lower the serum potassium but at the expense of sodium input. The serum potassium frequently rises with dangerous rapidity postoperatively in the presence of renal insufficiency, especially after extensive procedures requiring blood transfusions. Under these circumstances measuring serum potassium more than once daily and frequent or continuous monitoring of the electrocardiogram are necessary precautions; otherwise, the first manifestation of hyperkalemia may be cardiac arrest. The cardiac effects of hyperkalemia can be reduced by intravenous administration of sodium bicarbonate, and such treatment is especially appropriate if acidosis is also present. The serum potassium can be lowered rapidly by the administration of enemas containing the resin noted earlier, but peritoneal dialysis or hemodialysis may be required. Intravenous glucose and insulin may be helpful, though quantitatively less effective than the other measures.

The metabolic *acidosis* that is characteristic of acute or chronic renal insufficiency is a consequence of impaired renal production of ammonia and bicarbonate. Acidosis is controlled acutely by intravenous sodium bicarbonate and chronically by dialysis and by such oral preparations as Shohl's solution (a mixture of sodium citrate and citric acid).

Hypertension

If salt and water retention is prevented, hypertension associated with end-stage renal disease and maintenance dialysis is seldom severe. Appropriate dietary restriction of sodium and effective dialysis are the principal means of preventing severe elevations of blood pressure and the complications of encephalopathy and retinopathy. Antihypertensive drugs are necessary in some patients. Reserpine derivatives should be avoided because the catecholamine-depleting effect of these drugs predisposes to troublesome hypotension under anesthesia, and this effect of the drug persists several weeks after it is discontinued. Hypertension that is not controlled by these measures and hypertension associated with elevations of plasma renin are definite indications for removal of the patient's own kidneys at the time of or prior to transplantation.

Cardiac Failure

If salt and water retention is prevented and if hypertension is controlled, dialysis patients usually have little difficulty with cardiac failure. Digitalis derivatives may be discontinued after the manifestations of heart failure have cleared. Persisting cardiac failure in the absence of salt and water retention or severe hypertension is indicative of coexisting primary cardiac disease. Functionally anephric patients maintained by dialysis require only about one fourth of the normal dose of digitalis derivatives, and toxicity from overdosage is a hazard.

Anemia and Blood Transfusions

The anemia of chronic uremia is due to a number of abnormalities, the most uniform one being impaired erythropoiesis associated with low serum levels of erythropoietin, which is produced by the kidneys and is essential to normal erythropoiesis. Toxic suppression of erythropoiesis in uremia has long been suspected but not conclusively proved. Another factor is blood loss from occult or demonstrable uremic ulcerations of the gastrointestinal tract. Some blood is also lost during hemodialysis. Shortened red cell life span also contributes to the anemia of uremia to a variable degree.

Antibodies reactive with HLA antigens are formed by the recipients of multiple blood transfusions, and such antibodies are associated with hyperacute rejection of renal allografts. The administration of blood transfusions to potential renal allograft recipients therefore should be minimized. The hematocrit of chronically dialyzed patients will frequently stabilize between 20 and 30 per cent without any maintenance blood transfusions. Furthermore, the effect of transfusing a uremic patient is transient; the hematocrit subsequently rapidly returns to the previous level. Accordingly, blood transfusions administered in preparation of the patient for a general anesthetic and a major surgical procedure should be given within a day or so of the scheduled operation. The hematocrit is ordinarily raised to approximately 30 per cent preoperatively except for emergency procedures when time is insufficient for such preparation. All blood transfused into potential allograft recipients should be in the form of washed, leukocyte-free erythrocytes and leukocyte-free plasma. Erslev and Shapiro[20] recently reviewed the anemia and the coagulopathy of chronic uremia.

Abnormal Blood Coagulation

The coagulation defect of chronic uremia is characterized by abnormal platelet adhesiveness, decreased platelet aggregation, abnormal prothrombin consumption, and prolonged bleeding time. These abnormalities are corrected by peritoneal dialysis or hemodialysis, and uremic bleeding associated with these abnormalities may be stopped by dialysis. Certain dialyzable substances inhibit platelet function. Other clotting factor deficiencies have been reported in uremia, but their occurrence and importance in uremic bleeding is variable.

Dialysis

The last hemodialysis is usually performed 1 or 2 days before a scheduled operation, but a patient on dialysis may undergo an emergency operation at any time on short notice. If hemodialysis happens to be in progress, the patient is disconnected from the machine and systemic heparinization is reversed with protamine.

Hemodialysis, if needed, is usually tolerated quite well postoperatively, but there are two circumstances wherein peritoneal dialysis is preferable: (1) Patients who are hemodynamically unstable tolerate peritoneal dialysis better than hemodialysis. This is especially true when a major objective of the dialysis procedure is the extraction of retained salt and water. (2) Peritoneal dialysis is preferred for patients who are vulnerable to hemorrhage from active gastrointestinal ulceration or from a fresh operative wound in which hemostasis is tenuous. The heparin used during hemodialysis, even when the effect is "regionalized" to the extracorporeal circuit by the administration of protamine in the venous line, unavoidably has some systemic effect on blood coagulation. This effect may be manifested most as "heparin rebound" two to four hours after hemodialysis when the effects of heparin persist and the effects of protamine have cleared. A review of dialysis was recently written by Bluemle.[20]

Drug Dosage

Renal insufficiency and dialysis affect the clearance of some drugs considerably, some moderately, and some not at all. Helpful summaries have been prepared to facilitate appropriate adjustment of drug dosage for chronically uremic patients.[20, 25]

RECIPIENT OPERATIONS OTHER THAN TRANSPLANTATION

Arteriovenous Fistulas and Shunts

Although hemodialysis may be performed several times through percutaneously inserted cannulas into a peripheral artery and vein, a surgically constructed fistula or shunt is necessary for chronic hemodialysis; and sometimes a shunt is desirable to facilitate acute hemodialysis.

In 1966 Brescia and Cimino (cited by Bluemle[20]) introduced the use of a surgically constructed internal *radiocephalic arteriovenous fistula*, and this is now the vascular access procedure of choice for chronic dialysis in patients with a normal radial artery and a large cephalic vein. The anastomosis and the appearance of the forearm during and between dialyses are illustrated in Figure 2. Other sites in the forearm, foot, or leg may be used. Use of a freshly created fistula for dialysis is best deferred one to four weeks for the development of increased flow and prominence of the affected vein. A delivery of 150 to 250 ml. per minute is needed during dialysis.

The most frequent complication of a radiocephalic fistula is thrombosis on the day of operation, the incidence of which should be less than 10 per cent if the

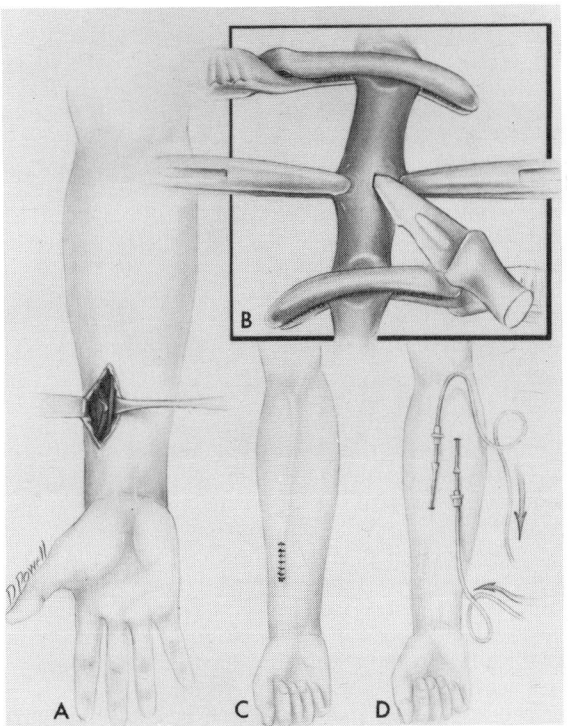
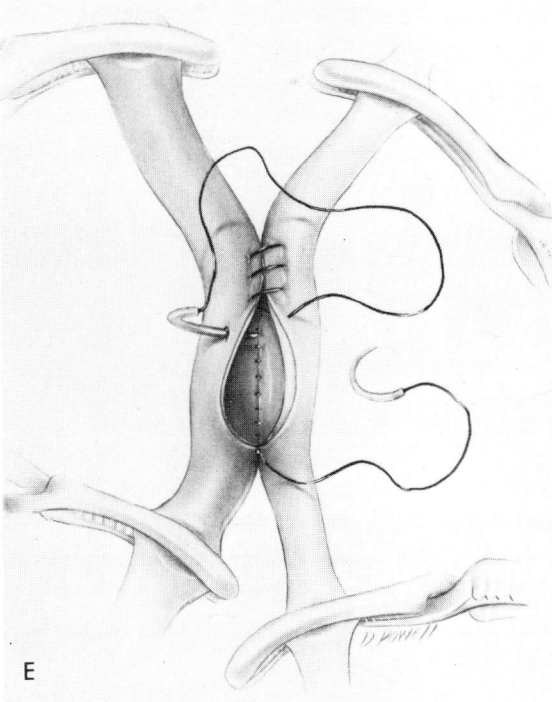

Figure 2. Arteriovenous fistula. *A,* Exposure of radial artery and nearby large subcutaneous vein. *B,* Incision of vessel. Preliminary dilation by an intraluminal injection of local anesthetic between clamps or tapes facilitates this step. *C,* Arm between dialyses. *D,* Arm during dialysis. *E,* The anastomosis. The opening in the vessels is 7 or 8 mm. long, and the suture is 6–0 or 7–0.

procedure is limited to vessels of adequate size. Other early complications include bleeding and wound infection. Late complications include thrombosis, inflow or outflow stenosis, and pseudoaneurysm. Cardiac failure caused or aggravated by excessive flow has been observed rarely and is an indication for surgical revision. Bloodstream infection originating at the fistula occurs rarely and is an indication for surgical closure. Endocarditis associated with such infections has been reported. Arterial insufficiency or venous stasis of the hand is observed occasionally, especially in diabetics.[32] Such complications are usually managed easily by surgical revision of the fistula.

If a satisfactory radiocephalic fistula cannot be created and maintained, a *bovine graft arteriovenous fistula* is the preferred vascular access procedure.[33] One of several acceptable techniques is illustrated in Figure 3. This procedure is indicated if the cephalic vein is initially thrombosed or congenitally small, or if a surgically uncorrectable problem develops with an established fistula. The graft material is nonviable, composed mostly of collagen remaining after enzymatic (ficin) processing of bovine carotid artery. The complications of bovine grafts and their management are similar to those of radiocephalic fistulas.

An external *arteriovenous shunt* may be used immediately and thus is particularly indicated for dialysis for acute (reversible) renal failure. A shunt may also be used temporarily during the period of maturation of a fistula. Shunts were originally used chronically but seldom are now. Since 1960 when Quinton and Scribner[14] reported successful chronic use of Teflon-tipped Silastic arteriovenous shunts, a number of variations have been reported in regard to the cannula tips, connecting tubing, and technique of insertion. The authors' technique is depicted in Figure 4. Other

sites on the forearm, ankle, leg, and thigh can be used. Most patients do not require anticoagulation to prevent clotting of the shunt.

Some occurrences of clotting and infection can be managed successfully without sacrifice of the shunt. Failures of shunts result mostly from thrombosis, infection, pseudoaneurysm, bleeding, and shunt extrusion as a foreign body. Shunts occasionally function satisfactorily without surgical revision for several years, but average shunt life is 6 to 12 months.[14] In contrast, fistulas typically function well for years. The problem of running out of usable vessels for shunt insertion is the principal reason for preferring fistulas for access for chronic dialysis. Moreover, most patients prefer fistulas because shunts require a ritual cleanliness, dressing changes, and keeping them dry during bathing and swimming.

Nephrectomy

The principal indications for removing the patient's own kidneys pertain to: (1) hypertension, (2) infection, (3) the prevention of glomerulonephritis in the renal allograft, and (4) symptoms of polycystic kidneys. Hypertension has already been discussed. Demonstrably infected kidneys should be removed prior to renal allografting. Polycystic kidneys may need to be removed because of great size or intermittent pain, infection, or hemorrhage.

Antibody reactive with glomerular basement membrane (GBM) is one cause of nephritis, and some patients with glomerulonephritis have demonstrable titers of such antibody, especially after removal of glomerulonephritic kidneys. It is thus reasonable, especially in patients whose glomerulonephritis has been recently active, to remove the patient's own kidneys, to look for the subsequent appearance of anti-GBM antibody, and to defer renal allografting until some arbitrary time (four to six months) after the antibody is no longer detectable. The effectiveness and appropriate timing of nephrectomy for the purpose of preventing glomerulonephritis in the renal allograft have not yet been fully elucidated, however. The pathogenesis of glomerulonephritis is the subject of a recent review by Fish et al.[20]

Nephrectomy may be performed transperitoneally, but in the presence of infection the retroperitoneal route is preferable. Practices vary in regard to removing the recipient's own kidneys prior to renal allografting, at the same time, subsequently, or not at all. If there is vesicoureteral reflux or other significant ureteral disease, the ureters should be removed; otherwise, the ureters should be retained. The patient's own ureters are useful in the management of urologic complications of renal allografting.

A comparison of the results of renal allografting with and without bilateral nephrectomy was reported from the Registry.[2] Living and cadaver donor graft survival data are shown in Figure 14. Patient and graft survival data were included in this report with respect to each of the following primary renal diseases of the recipients: glomerulonephritis, pyelonephritis, nephrosclerosis, polycystic disease, and lupus. Data favoring bilateral nephrectomy were statistically significant for pyelonephritis and polycystic disease, and

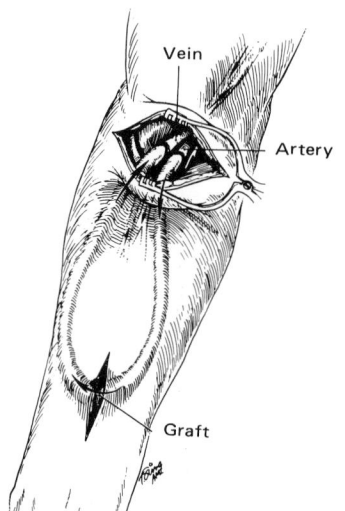

Figure 3. Bovine graft arteriovenous fistula. The looped graft lies in a subdermal tunnel in the right forearm after end-to-side anastomoses of its ends to brachial artery and basilic vein in the antecubital fossa. (From Lefrak, E. A., and Noon, G. P.: Ann. Surg., *182*: 782, 1975.)

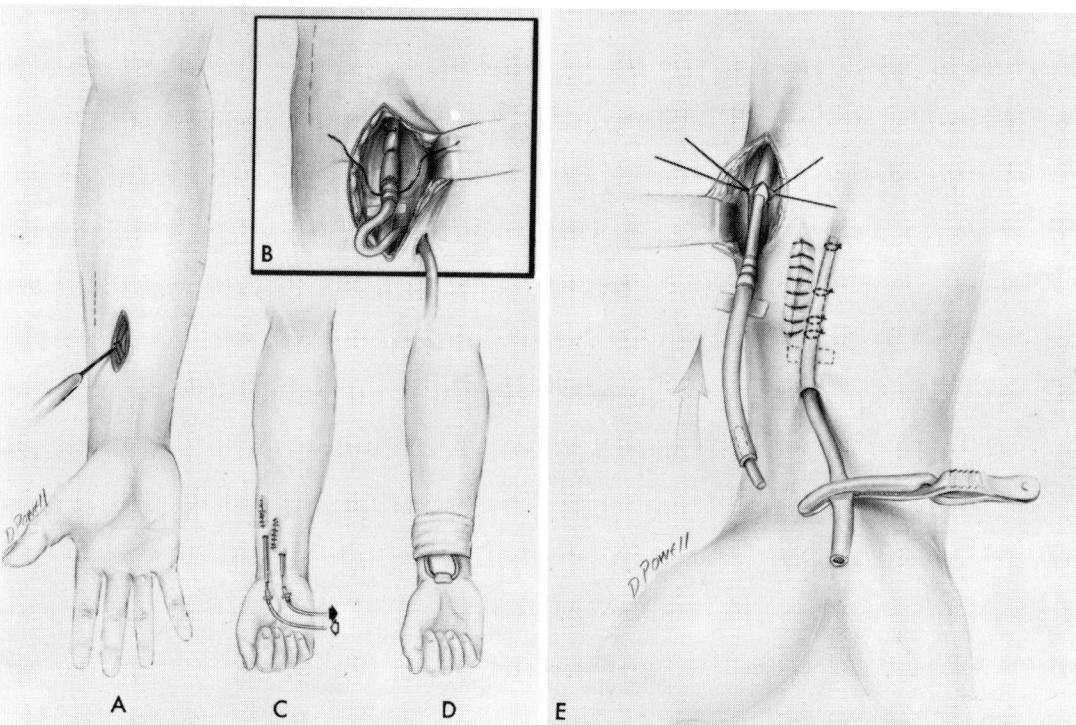

Figure 4. Arteriovenous shunt. *A*, Exposure of artery and vein. *B*, Cannulation of radial artery. *C*, Shunt in use during dialysis. *D*, Shunt incorporated in dressing between dialyses. If the shunt clots the patient will see clot retraction in the exposed tubing and seek immediate attention. *E*, Cannulation of vein. Note that incisions do not lie directly over the vessels. The cannulas are one-piece and all-Silastic (Extracorporeal Medical Specialties, Inc.).

in no category were the results better without bilateral nephrectomy. Nevertheless, there is at present no conclusive answer to the question of routinely vs. selectively performing bilateral nephrectomy before renal allografting.[32]

Lower Urinary Tract Operations

Any obstruction or other abnormality of the lower urinary tract should be corrected prior to transplantation. Significant uncorrectable abnormalities of the bladder and urethra constitute relative contraindications to renal allografting; however, there has been limited experience with connecting a renal allograft to an ileal loop.[14, 17, 21, 24] If such a loop is to be used it should be well established prior to the transplant operation.

Parathyroidectomy

Parathyroidectomy for hyperparathyroidism secondary to chronic renal insufficiency is necessary in about 5 per cent of renal allograft patients and is performed sometimes before and in others after renal allografting.

Renal osteodystrophy—bone disease associated with chronic uremia—is the result of two disorders of calcium physiology which may to varying degrees coexist: (1) impaired metabolism of vitamin D; and (2) hyperparathyroidism. Chief cell hyperplasia is the characteristic microscopic abnormality in the parathyroid glands, and the weight of the glands varies from slightly above normal to a hundredfold enlargement.

Both the hyperplasia and the gross enlargement frequently are distributed unevenly among the four glands. Following renal allografting the parathyroid glands may remain hyperactive, and restoration of normal renal function is sometimes followed by a rise in the serum calcium to levels greatly exceeding pretransplant values, as illustrated in Figure 5. Such persistence of hyperfunction has been called "autonomous" or "tertiary" hyperparathyroidism. Mild hyperparathyroidism after renal allografting may remain stable for a number of months or years, or may very slowly regress without surgical intervention.

The symptoms of hyperparathyroidism in the patient with chronic uremia are musculoskeletal pain, weakness, cramps, twitching, and pruritus. Bone tenderness may be present. The serum calcium and the product of the calcium and phosphorus may be either normal or elevated. The alkaline phosphatase is characteristically elevated unless the process is early. Radiographic decrease in bone density alone is consistent with osteomalacia (vitamin D deficiency); hyperparathyroidism is characterized by the changes of osteofibrosis cystica, resorption of the lamina dura of the teeth, subperiosteal resorption and erosion of the terminal tufts of the phalanges, degeneration of the acromial end of the clavicle, and pathologic fractures.

The effects of impaired gastrointestinal absorption of vitamin D can be largely overcome by an oral regimen of dihydrotachysterol and calcium gluconate; and an oral phosphate-binding agent such as aluminum hydroxide will, by lowering the plasma phosphate,

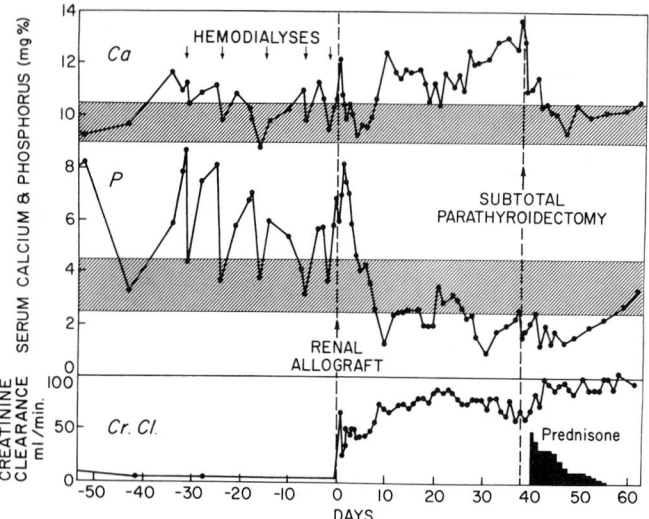

Figure 5. "Tertiary" hyperparathyroidism. Excessive parathyroid activity secondary to renal insufficiency did not regress following restoration of normal renal function. Mild residual hyperparathyroidism subsided during the 18 months following subtotal parathyroidectomy without further treatment. The subsequent course of this patient (L. D. No. 1[41]) is shown in Figure 11.

decrease the stimulus to parathyroid hyperactivity. Effective medical management is difficult or impossible, however, in the presence of hyperparathyroidism that is producing grossly evident bone disease or metastatic calcification. The originally established surgical procedure was to remove all of three parathyroid glands and one-half or more of the fourth, leaving in not more than about the equivalent of one normal gland. Even this much parathyroid tissue sometimes results in troublesome residual hyperparathyroidism, so total parathyroidectomy may be preferable. Successful autografting of fresh or cryopreserved (frozen) parathyroid to forearm muscle has been recently reported.[44] Total parathyroidectomy will therefore likely be increasingly preferred, with autografting to the forearm either immediately or after normal renal function is restored by a successful allograft. Calcium and phosphorus metabolism in uremia is discussed fully in a recent review by Stanbury.[20]

Other Operations

Pericardectomy is necessary occasionally in chronic hemodialysis patients in whom pericarditis develops despite optimal nonsurgical treatment. A fatal complication of uremic pericarditis is pericardial tamponade due to hemorrhage, occurring during heparinization for a dialysis procedure. *Cannulation of the thoracic duct* is sometimes performed to drain lymph as an immunosuppressive measure. *Thymectomy* and *splenectomy* have been nearly abandoned as measures to modify the immune response, but the spleen is sometimes removed because of thrombocytopenia or when it is accidentally injured. Finally, surgical intervention is frequently indicated in the care of the various *postoperative complications* of renal allografting.

LIVING RELATED DONORS

Immunologic Selection

Two genetic systems are of major importance in human organ transplantation: ABO on Chromosome 9

(C9), and HLA on Chromosome 6 (C6). C6 and C9 are *autosomes*, so neither ABO nor HLA is sex-linked.

Donor-recipient *ABO compatibility* is an absolute requirement.[6] ABO antigens are on cells other than erythrocytes, and a graft must not contain either A or B antigens that are absent in the recipient. Although isolated cases of successful ABO incompatible renal allografting have been reported, ABO incompatible kidneys characteristically undergo early irreversible rejection. The exact role of other red cell antigens in graft rejection is unclear; however, incompatibility for these antigens, if significant at all, seems to be adequately controlled by immunosuppressive therapy.

HLA is a complex genetic region composed of at least four* closely linked loci on the C6 autosome, and

---

*The four defined HLA loci are called HLA-A, -B, -C, and -D in recently established international nomenclature.[29] These designations, -A, -B, -C, and -D, must be distinguished from the designations A, B, C, and D that are customarily applied to the four parental haplotypes within a family, as in Figure 6. Where A to D refer to parental HLA haplotypes, each parental haplotype, A, B, C, *and* D, carries one gene of each of the HLA loci, -A, -B, -C, *and* -D *and* any additional HLA loci that have not yet been defined, *and* C6 genes outside the HLA region.

All four HLA loci are remarkably polymorphic. Approximately 20 alleles have been defined for HLA-A, 20 for -B, 5 for -C, and 6 for -D. Each individual, of course, expresses at most two alleles for each locus, and only one in the event of homozygosity. The map order (on C6) is: centromere-D-B-C-A.[29, 43]

The products of HLA-A, -B are serologically detectable cell membrane surface antigens. They are widely distributed on leukocytes and cells of most tissues, but not on erythrocytes. They are complex antigens with multiple reactive sites capable of provoking strong immune responses. They are inherited as mendelian dominant factors. Genetic studies of these two loci and most clinical HLA matching and crossmatching have utilized various serologic tests for these antigens.

Recently *HLA-C* was defined, and it too controls serologically detectable antigens.[29, 43] *HLA-D* is detectable by blastogenesis in cultures of mixtures of lymphocytes from different individuals.

probably additional loci not yet defined.[29, 43] HLA is the major histocompatibility system in man, comparable to H-2 in the mouse. The HLA system is involved in both the humoral and the cellular immune mechanisms of allograft rejection, as discussed by Amos in sections of this chapter on transplantation antigens and allograft rejection. For the selection of renal allograft donors, the principal immunologic tests are those of HLA matching and crossmatching.

A negative *HLA crossmatch* is an absolute requirement.[8] For this test donor lymphocytes or other donor tissue cells are reacted in vitro with recipient serum. In a positive crossmatch HLA antibodies in the recipient's serum react with antigens on donor cells. Reactive donor cells include those of vascular endothelium, and intraoperative hyperacute rejection of a renal allograft nearly always occurs if the HLA crossmatch is positive (see under Rejection). The circulating antibody causing a positive HLA crossmatch is an *acquired* characteristic, due to the recipient's prior exposure to HLA antigens through such experiences as blood transfusions, previous allografts, and pregnancies.

The term *HLA match* refers to the degree of similarity between two individuals with respect to their serologically detectable HLA antigens and other *inherited* HLA characteristics. For renal allografting the closest possible HLA match is desirable, but no minimum or absolute HLA match requirement has been established for either living or cadaver donors. With the important exception of grafts from HLA identical siblings (see below), all renal allografts are to some extent HLA incompatible.

HLA matching for the selection of a living related renal donor is most reliably based on genotyping all of the family members for HLA. A diagram of a hypothetical family is shown in Figure 6. The term *haplotype* refers to all of the genetic determinants on one chromosome. The letters A and B are customarily assigned to the father's two haplotypes and C and D to the mother's. The four possible genotypes of the offspring are then AC, AD, BC, and BD. In the family in Figure 6 there are two HLA-identical sibling pairs: a brother and sister who both inherited A and D, and two sisters who both inherited B and D. The seventh sibling illustrates the infrequent genetic event, *recombination*, in which the inheritance from one parent is composed of pieces of both haplotypes of that parent.

Potential donor-recipient pairs within a family therefore fall into three categories (in the absence of recombination): (1) *HLA identical*, with the same HLA haplotypes (e.g., AC-AC); (2) *HLA haploidentical*, a one-haplotype difference between them (e.g., AC-AD and AB-AD); and (3) *HLA non-haploidentical*, with a two haplotype difference (e.g., AC-BD). One fourth of sib-sib pairs are HLA identical, one half haploidentical, and one fourth non-haploidentical. All parent-child pairs are HLA haploidentical.

Renal allografts from ABO compatible, *HLA identical donors* are highly compatible and, with few exceptions, rejection of such grafts is easily prevented with safe, low-dosage immunosuppression. The exceptions comprise about 5 per cent of HLA identical renal allografts whose uncontrollable rejection evidently

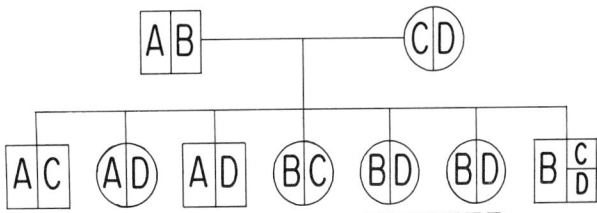

Figure 6. Inheritance of a complex genetic region. This diagram is applicable to *any* non-sex-linked genetic region of such complexity that no two of the four parental haplotypes (see text) are likely to be the same. It is thus applicable to HLA. Whatever the known or unknown specific characteristics of the different haplotypes, A,B,C, and D, each child inherits one entire haplotype en bloc from the father and one from the mother. Thus, whatever the complexity of the genetic region and its products, only four genotypes occur among the siblings—AC, AD, BC, and BD—and one fourth of sib-sib pairs will be identical with respect to the given genetic region. In this diagram there are two such sibling pairs, one sister-brother (AD-AD) and one sister-sister (BD-BD). The seventh sibling in this large hypothetical family illustrates the infrequent genetic event, *recombination*, which occasionally results in an exception to the rule that, for a given genetic region, there will be only four genotypes among the children within a family.

results from one or more non-HLA, non-ABO incompatibilities.[39] *HLA haploidentical donors* are generally much more likely to be compatible than HLA non-haploidentical donors, but some HLA haploidentical grafts are rejected despite intensive immunosuppression.[38, 41] If the choice of donor is to be from a number of HLA haploidentical family members, the selection is usually based on nonimmunologic criteria. (Immunologic testing for such a selection would resemble that described later for cadaver donor-recipient selection.) Data in Table 2 on renal allografts from *HLA non-haploidentical sibling donors*,[2] and data on larger numbers of test skin grafts from such donors[37] indicate that such siblings are no more compatible than unrelated donors, and increasingly such siblings are being excluded from consideration as renal donors.[22, 31, 41]

Other Aspects of Selection

The prospective donor must wish to donate after being fully informed at the beginning of the selection process as to the risks and the expected morbidity. The

TABLE 2. Survival of Renal Allografts from Sibling Donors*

Category of Sibling Donor	Sample Size	Grafts Functioning At One Year (Per Cent ± SE†)
HLA identical	561	78.6 ± 1.8
HLA haploidentical	189	70.5 ± 3.3
HLA non-haploidentical	28	50.6 ± 9.9

*From Bergan, J. J., et al.: J.A.M.A., *233*:787, 1975. The data in this table, omitted from the published twelfth report, were included in a reprint to all Registry participants.

†SE = standard error of the mean.

medical evaluation must include unequivocal documentation that the prospective donor is in good general health and in possession of two normal kidneys. Psychiatric evaluation may be considered optional but is desirable. The selected donor who fulfills the medical criteria and who is immunologically acceptable undergoes renal angiography. Utilization of the kidney with a single renal artery is technically the most desirable, but this is not an absolute requirement. Legally valid informed consent is secured.

Technique of Living Donor Nephrectomy

Najarian (cited by Stickel[41]) emphasized the importance of hydrating the donor prior to and during the procedure sufficiently to maintain a brisk diuresis until the moment when the donor kidney is removed. Intravenous fluids and mannitol are administered as necessary to achieve such a diuresis. The kidney is approached through the flank with resection of either the eleventh or twelfth rib. Local anesthetic is infiltrated around the renal artery to prevent vasospasm. The artery and vein are dissected free at their origins; dissection near the renal pelvis is avoided in order not to injure the blood supply of the ureter. Both vessels are ligated before they are divided in order to reduce the risk of hemorrhage. Upon removal, the kidney is immediately submerged in an ice-cold isotonic bath and is perfused with 200 to 500 ml. of a perfusate at 4° C. The perfusate consists of a balanced electrolyte solution with additives which vary from center to center.[6, 16]

CADAVER DONORS

Procurement of Kidneys

Cadaver kidneys are suitable for transplantation only if renal function is normal at the time of death and the donor is free of disease that can be transmitted to the recipient. These conditions are satisfied in only a small fraction of deaths in the general population. Nevertheless, if all kidneys at such deaths were actually removed for transplantation, they would greatly exceed the need. Shortages and delays are thus attributable to a lack of needed arrangements to make transplantable kidneys actually available. The enactment of the Uniform Anatomical Gift Act in all 50 states in the late 1960's overcame a number of legal barriers. Significant current developments include increasing acceptance of the concept that the person is dead if the brain is dead, and the organization of surgical teams to procure usable kidneys at nontransplanting community hospitals.

Donors over 80 years of age have been used successfully, but the success rate decreases somewhat with age of donor beyond 50 years (9th Registry report[2]). Kidneys from children at least 5 years old can be used in adults with little technical modification and with ultimate function about as good as that with kidneys from adult donors. Satisfactory results have been achieved with the use of one or both kidneys of donors 0 to 4 years of age with considerable modification of technique.

A variety of carcinomas[6] and infections[6, 16] — viral, bacterial, and fungal — have been transmitted by cadaver kidneys and have been reported as the cause of death of a number of renal allograft recipients. Transmission of thrombocytopenic purpura has also been reported.[6] Except for primary malignant tumors of the central nervous system and for basal cell carcinomas of the skin, malignancy in the donor contraindicates transplantation of the kidneys. Chronically indwelling catheters in the lower urinary tract also contraindicate kidney donation unless the urine is proved sterile. Hypertension, diabetes mellitus, renal stones, and other conditions in the potential donor that are associated with renal abnormalities are disqualifying considerations.

Multihospital *regional kidney-sharing organizations* provide a number of services that are provided poorly or not at all in the absence of such an organization. These services include (1) procuring kidneys in areas where the supply exceeds the need and transporting them to deficient areas, and in other ways reducing wastage of transplantable kidneys and shortening the time patients wait for their transplants; (2) early procurement of a kidney for the dialysis patient who has an urgent medical indication to be transplanted; (3) finding a kidney for the patient whose widely reactive HLA antibody reduces to virtually zero the probability of identifying a suitable donor locally; and (4) increasing the incidence of 3- and 4-antigen HLA matches between donor and recipient (see below). Population density and other considerations affect whether the geographical area encompassed by a regional organization is metropolitan, multistate, or international. Cooperation among a number of regional organizations is facilitated by computerized linkages of their lists of dialysis patients awaiting kidneys, and such cooperation is serving to increase the benefits stated above. There are practical limits to such cooperative arrangements, however. The quality of tissue typing and kidney preservation performed at the donor hospital must be known and acceptable to the staff at the recipient hospital. The current state of development of these two technologies is such that much of the necessary communication between donor and recipient hospitals is individualized — not transmissible by computer.

Technique of Cadaver Donor Nephrectomy

Although the two kidneys can be removed separately through a wide bilateral subcostal incision, the preferred technique is to remove them together en bloc with a segment of aorta and vena cava through a midline incision from xiphoid to pubis.[30] With the en bloc technique the ureteral blood supply is less subject to injury, and the renal blood vessels are made available with their entire length and any attached aorta and vena cava that might be needed for fashioning one or more Carrel patches, each containing the orifices of one or multiple small renal vessels. (The incidence of multiple renal arteries is 20 per cent on the left and 15 per cent on the right.[30]) With the transverse colon retracted superiorly, the renal structures are exposed through an incision in the posterior peritoneum over the infrarenal aorta. Exposure of the renal vasculature is facilitated by dividing the superior mesenteric artery, gonadal veins, and infrarenal vena cava. If on the left a single large artery and vein are found, the left kidney may be removed separately before the right one. Lymph nodes and a slice of spleen may need to be removed for tissue typing. Throughout the procedure vital systems are intensively supported as described below under Renal Preservation.

Renal Preservation

Renal preservation is discussed by Belzer in a separate section of this chapter. Some points concerning *three critical periods* are summarized here.

The *first* critical period is prior to nephrectomy, when the kidneys are still being perfused by the donor's circulation. During this period, which might be several hours or a day or more, the vital systems of the donor are increasingly subject to deterioration. Especially during the final hours, perfectly normal kidneys can deteriorate to useless ones in an hour or less. Blood pressure, hydration, urine output, and other parameters need to be monitored closely. During the interval from death of the donor to kidney removal, the circulation and respiration need to be vigorously supported to maintain normal renal perfusion. Terminal diabetes insipidus when present necessitates intensive fluid and electrolyte replacement.

The *second* critical period is the "warm ischemia time." For a given kidney this is the time from cessation of its circulation in the donor until the kidney is cooled upon removal. The warm ischemia time is essentially zero if the donor's circulation is maintained throughout the removal procedure. Warm ischemia times of 0 to 10 minutes are associated with diuresis during the transplant operation if the kidney was normal when removed from the donor and if the recipient's intraoperative blood pressure, blood volume, and hydration are normal. Warm ischemia times of 30 to 60 minutes are associated with postoperative acute tubular necrosis and need for dialysis temporarily — usually 10 to 20 days. If the warm ischemia time exceeds 60 minutes, the injury is virtually always acute cortical necrosis, which is irreversible. The maximum acceptable warm ischemia time at most centers is in the range of 10 to 40 minutes.

The *third* critical period is the "cold time," which begins when the kidney is removed from the donor, immediately immersed in an ice bath, and flushed for a few minutes with a refrigerated perfusate. Cold time ends when the graft is first perfused by the recipient's circulation. After the flush and before the implant procedure is commenced, there are two methods of renal preservation that may be used: (1) simple cold storage — the kidney in a sterile container under ice at 0° C; and (2) continuous pulsatile perfusion with oxygenated plasma at 6 to 8° C. Preservation of a kidney may be solely by one of these methods, or partly by one and partly the other. With simple cold storage alone the maximum acceptable cold time is approximately 24 hours, and immediate diuresis is frequently seen after cold storage of this duration. With pulsatile hypothermic perfusion the maximum acceptable cold time is extended to 48 to 72 hours. In metropolitan areas where both kidneys from a donor are ordinarily transplanted within 24 hours, simple cold storage may be used exclusively or predominantly. The advantages of perfusion are evident where more than 24 hours are likely to be needed for transportation of kidneys and recipients, HLA crossmatches, and all other necessary preoperative procedures.

Immunologic Selection of Recipients

As with living related donors, *ABO compatibility* and a *negative HLA crossmatch* between cadaver donor and recipient are absolute requirements. Some dialysis patients periodically require blood transfusions, and some have received previous renal allografts. These immunologic experiences result in a much greater incidence of positive HLA crossmatch than is encountered between potential living related donors and recipients. In a cadaver kidney procurement network, therefore, the immunology laboratories of all donor hospitals are periodically provided with updated serum samples from all potential recipients who have circulating HLA antibodies. HLA crossmatching is initially performed at the donor hospital prior to recipient selection and transportation of the kidney, and a confirmatory crossmatch is usually performed at the recipient hospital.

In a patient with circulating HLA antibody, the reactivity of the serum is expressed as the percentage of the general population with which the serum gives a positive HLA crossmatch. Reactivities throughout the range of 1 to 99 per cent are frequently observed. The reactivity of any given patient can vary from time to time, and monthly updates are advisable. The patient should not receive the kidney if the crossmatch is positive with either current serum or the patient's most widely and strongly reactive old serum. HLA crossmatch techniques are currently of such sensitivity that intraoperative hyperacute rejection is rarely seen after a negative crossmatch. Postoperatively, however, patients with preformed HLA antibodies at present or in the past may experience a higher incidence of accelerated humoral rejection than those whose sera have always been negative. As reported to the Registry,[2] in three groups of patients the percentages of one-year graft survival ±SE were as follows: (1) 55.3 per cent ± 1.2 in 1743 recipients with no preformed antibody; (2) 55.7 per cent ± 3.0 in 308 recipients with a 1 to 5 per cent reactive antibody; and (3) 44.3 per cent ± 2.2 in 524 recipients with a greater than 5 per cent reactive antibody. For the third group the difference was statistically significant with $p < 0.01$. From these data and other reports it appears that a widely reactive HLA antibody adversely affects the prognosis for renal allografting. Nevertheless, transplantation is permissible if the HLA crossmatch with the specific donor is negative.

The clinical significance of *HLA matching* is less with cadaver donors than with familial donors. Nevertheless, all cadaver donors and recipients are tissue typed for HLA-A, -B antigens, and the donor-recipient match for these antigens receives some consideration in recipient selection at most centers. (Techniques for matching for the other two HLA loci are not at present applicable to cadaver donors. See footnote on p. 484.)

An individual may have up to two antigens of the HLA-A locus (one of maternal and one of paternal origin) and up to two antigens of the HLA-B locus. Thus, up to four antigens will define an individual's HLA-A, -B phenotype. Fewer than four antigens will be detected if the individual is homozygous at either allele, or if any of the individual's antigens are not detectable by currently available tissue typing sera. Donor-recipient pairs will therefore be matched for 4,3,2,1, or 0 HLA-A, -B antigens. In random pairing, 0- and 1-antigen matches occur most frequently, and 4-antigen matches rarely. In a local group of 50 dialysis patients on the transplant waiting list, the frequencies of 4-, 3-, 2-, 1-, and 0-antigen matches were, respectively, 0.03, 1.1, 12, 45, and 42 per cent of random matches. It is thus evident that cadaver renal allografts with 3- or 4-antigen matches will be possible rarely unless the waiting lists of several institutions are cooperatively combined to yield potential recipient pools numbering in the hundreds or thousands.[35]

A correlation of HLA matching with cadaver renal allograft survival was recently reported by the Registry,[2] and the results are summarized in Table 3. The difference between 3- and 1-antigen matches was statistically significant at all time intervals after three months, with $p < 0.001$ at three years. The difference between 3- and 4-antigen matches was not significant. A similar correlation of HLA matching with graft survival was reported earlier from European centers.[2] Thus, the effect of HLA matching on clinical results at present appears to be limited but significant, and further development of methods appears to be worthwhile.

A number of *other immunologic tests* for selecting cadaver kidney recipients have been recently reported to be of some predictive value for prolonged graft survival, but these tests are not widely established. Some of them apply to specific donor-recipient pairs who are under consideration for renal allografting, and others purport to measure the general immune responsiveness of the potential recipient.

THE TRANSPLANT OPERATION

If the recipient is called to the hospital from home to receive a cadaver kidney, an interim history and physical examination and recheck of blood counts, blood chemistry determinations, electrocardiogram, chest x-ray, and the HLA crossmatch are obtained even if time is limited. Hydration of the recipient and the donor (living or cadaver), the procedure upon the donor, preoperative blood transfusions and dialysis, and recipient nephrectomies are discussed in preceding sections. The choice of anesthetic is a less important consideration than meeting the special physiologic requirements of patients with chronic renal failure and a newly implanted graft that is highly susceptible to acute renal failure; however, the potentially nephrotoxic agents methoxyflurane and enflurane should not be used.[28] Muscle relaxants are not contraindicated, but usually the required dose is considerably less than normal, whatever relaxant is selected, and prolonged postoperative apnea is frequently observed if normal doses are used.[28] Maintaining blood pressure, blood volume, and cardiac output is especially important in order not to add further ischemic insult to that which the graft necessarily sustains during the procedure prior to revascularization. Monitoring the central venous pressure is useful in determining amounts of blood, plasma, and intravenous fluids to administer during and after operation. If the recipient's own kidneys are to be removed, this part of the operation is performed first, usually through a separate transabdominal incision but sometimes through the transplant incision.

Meticulously careful surgical technique is particularly important considering the immunosuppressed state of the patient and the coagulation defects of chronic uremia. The iliac fossa is exposed retroperitoneally through an incision just above the inguinal ligament (Fig. 7). A left kidney is usually implanted on the right side and vice versa, but either kidney may be readily implanted on either side if the iliac vein is mobilized by dividing the hypogastric vein. Lymphatics that are divided should be ligated to prevent the development of a lymphocele. The kidney is first positioned, and then the vascular anastomoses are constructed without angulation or tension. The renal artery is anastomosed end-to-end to the hypogastric artery and the renal vein end-to-side to the external iliac vein. Within one minute after restoration of blood flow to the kidney, a normal color and tissue turgor return, and the flow of urine begins within five minutes in the absence of complications. Momentary compression of the renal vein produces immediate distention of the vein and the kidney, and this is a useful diagnostic maneuver. The recognition of complications that may be seen intraoperatively after restoration of renal circulation will be discussed in the section on differential diagnosis of hyperacute rejection. Ureteroneocystostomy is the most frequently used anastomosis to restore the urinary tract. There must be neither tension nor redundant length of ureter.[16, 18] Unnecessary length predisposes to kinking and to inadequate blood supply at the anastomosis.[21] To prevent obstruction at the ureteroneocystostomy, the tunnel through the bladder wall must be wide enough to allow a very free passage of the ureter.[1, 18, 21] Most surgeons drain the bladder with a ureteral catheter for several days and do not use a ureteral catheter.[1, 6, 18, 21] Practices vary in regard to draining the wound.[6, 16, 18, 21, 24] Metallic clip markers may be attached to the renal capsule for postoperative roentgen-

TABLE 3.   Cadaver Renal Allograft Survival and HLA Matching in 1301 Recipients with Four Antigens Identified*

No. of HLA Antigens Matched	n	Per Cent Graft Survival		
		1 yr.	2 yr.	3 yr.
4	77	56	48	43
3	375	48	40	48
2	532	49	42	37
1	317	47	38	27
	1301			

*From Bergan, J. J., et al.: J.A.M.A., *233*:787, 1975.

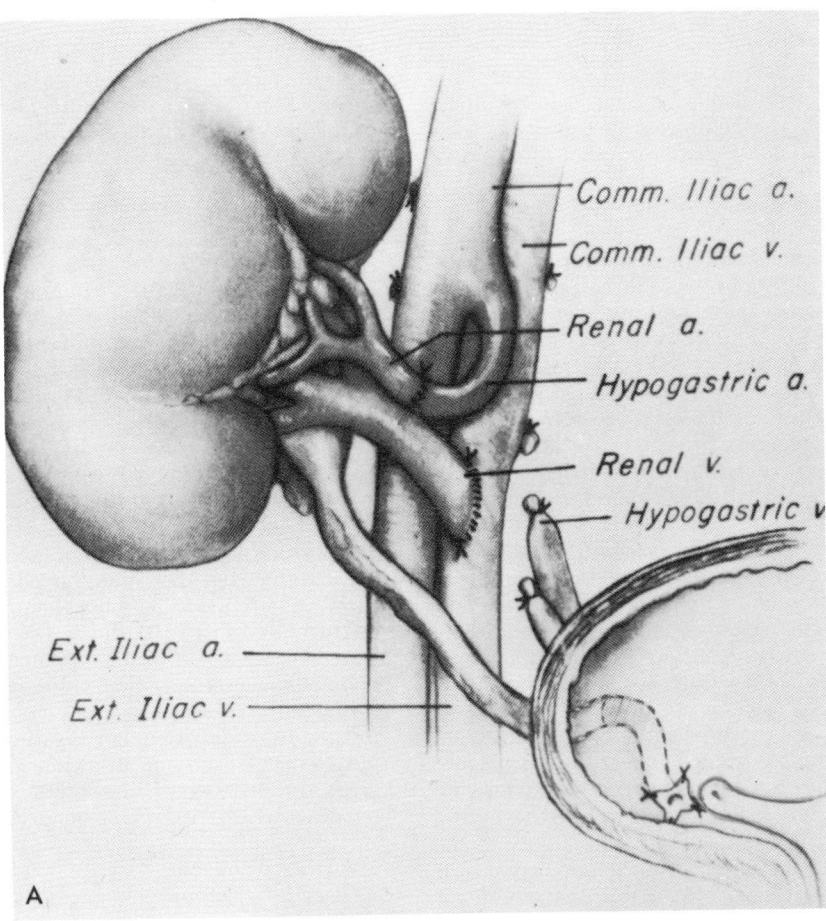

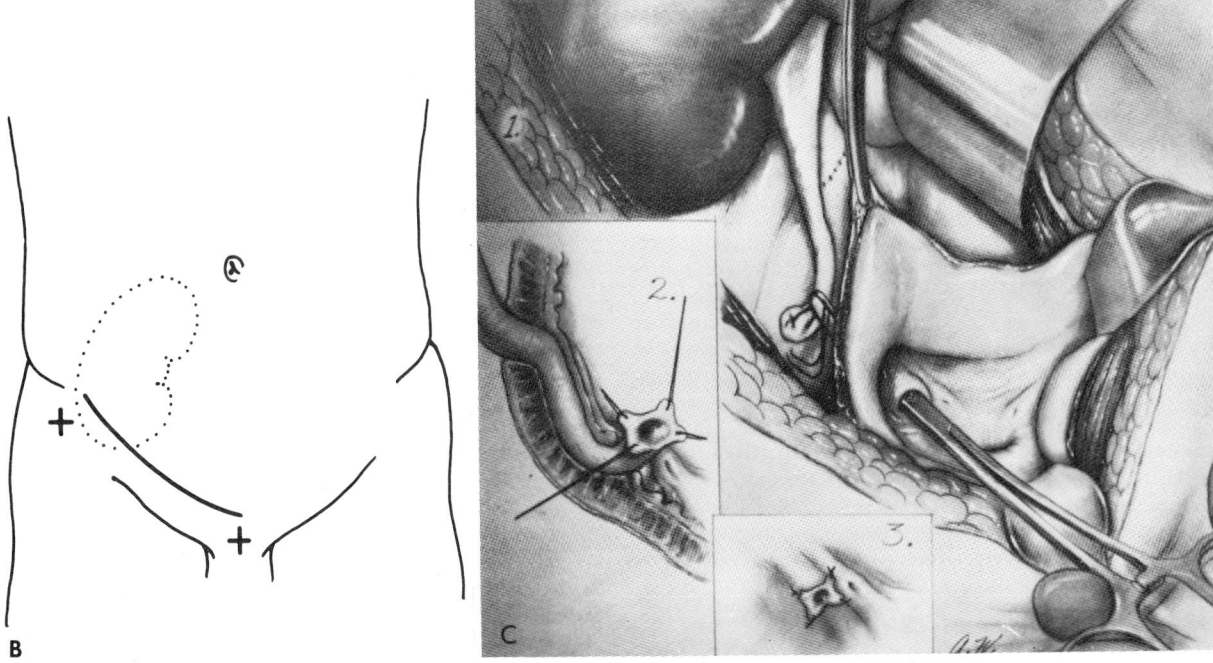

Figure 7. The transplant operation. The usual procedure is shown in this figure. Modifications are described in the text. *A*, The completed anastomoses of artery, vein, and ureter. *B*, The incision for implanting a left kidney into the right iliac fossa. *C*, Donor ureter passing through bladder wall and a submucosal tunnel for ureteroneocystostomy near orifice of patient's right ureter. (From Hume, D. M. *In* Rapaport, F. T., and Dausset, J. (Eds.): Human Transplantation. New York Grune and Stratton, 1968.)

ographic detection of changes in size of the graft (see Fig. 12).

Modifications of the transplant operation are frequently necessary for various reasons. Adult kidneys are implanted into most children by the usual technique, but for *small children* the implantation is performed by end-to-side vascular anastomoses either to the common iliac vessels or to aorta and vena cava—through a retroperitoneal approach. *Accessory renal arteries* should not be ligated because renal arteries are "end-arteries," and a life-threatening urinary fistula can result from the sloughing of a segment of the kidney supplied by a ligated accessory artery (with the possible exception of tiny polar arteries supplying less than 5 per cent of the renal parenchyma). Two renal arteries of equal or unequal size can be reconstructed for anastomosis as a single renal artery by the following technique: Longitudinal incisions in the walls of the two arteries at their cut ends are closed by a V-shaped suture line that forms one combined lumen proximal to the bifurcation resulting from the reconstruction. *Accessory veins* are ligated; it is safe to assume that collaterals to the principal vein are adequate. The infrequent anomaly *double ureter* is regularly associated with two renal pelves and two renal arteries and veins. The two ureters are in a common sheath that can obscure the fact that there are two. The sheath containing both is tunneled through bladder wall as for a single ureter, but within the bladder each ureteral orifice must be sutured to bladder mucosa. The *recipient's ureter* should be used to perform a ureteropyelostomy if adequacy of blood supply of the donor ureter is questionable, if the donor ureter was otherwise injured during nephrectomy, or if the donor ureteropelvic junction is congenitally abnormal.[18, 21]

REJECTION: IMMUNOPATHOLOGY

Manifestations of threatened rejection may appear at any time during the life of a graft. For a full description of the pathogenesis and pathology of renal allograft rejection the reader is referred to articles by Dammin,[14] Hume,[6] Najarian,[12] Porter,[13] and Rowlands.[15] Renal allograft rejection may be classified as *hyperacute* (early, beginning within minutes or hours of the time of implantation), *acute* (intermediate, beginning after the graft has functioned for a number of days or weeks), or *chronic* (late, manifested a number of months or years after transplantation). The distinctions between these patterns of rejection are not sharp, but there is good clinical, pathologic, and immunologic basis for this classification. Techniques used in a complete study of renal allograft tissue will include light, electron, and immunofluorescence microscopy. The immunofluorescence techniques used include those for the detection of immunoglobulins, complement, and fibrin.

Hyperacute Rejection

The cut surface of the hyperacutely rejected kidney is diffusely hemorrhagic, especially in the cortical region. The microscopic findings are intravascular fibrin, platelets, and polymorphonuclear cells in glomerular and peritubular vessels; interstitial hemorrhage and polymorphonuclear infiltrates; and necrosis, especially in the cortex (Fig. 8). Fibrin is conspicuous in immunofluorescence studies; immunoglobulins and complement may or may not be demonstrable.

Hyperacute rejection characteristically occurs in the presence of antibodies that are circulating in the recipient at the time of grafting and that react immediately with antigens of the graft. Such conditions exist (1) with experimental xenografts; (2) with experimental allografts in a recipient previously sensitized to antigens of the donor; (3) with clinical allografts across a major ABO blood group incompatibility; and (4) with clinical allografts bearing HLA antigens that are reactive with antibodies preformed in the recipient as a consequence of previous pregnancy, blood transfusion, or a previous renal allograft. The initiating event in most, if not all, cases of hyperacute rejection is the reaction of circulating antibody with antigens of the cell membrane of vascular endothelium throughout the kidney. Complement joins the antigen-antibody complexes. By immune adherence and chemotaxis, platelets and polymorphonuclear leukocytes are agglutinated intravascularly. Clotting probably is initiated by release of proteolytic enzymes from polymorphonuclear leukocyte and platelet breakdown. As postulated by Najarian,[12] hyperacute rejection could be initiated by endotoxin or by antigen-antibody complexes formed outside the kidney and trapped in the graft. In any event the main effector pathway in hyperacute rejection is blood coagulation, triggered very probably by an antigen-antibody reaction with involvement of complement.

Rejection that morphologically is hyperacute may be somewhat delayed in onset, beginning a day or more after grafting. Such a delay may be related to the kinetics of the particular reaction, or may be due to antibody produced subsequent to grafting. Such rejection is called *accelerated humoral rejection*, to distinguish it from intraoperative hyperacute rejection. To a variable degree and somewhat as a function of time, the lesions of hyperacute rejection are seen in association with the lesions of acute rejection.

Acute Rejection

Acute renal allograft rejection is classically observed experimentally in unmodified recipients (Fig. 9). The immunity is more conspicuously cellular than humoral, but antibody is involved in the process. Graft destruction is complete usually within two weeks. Acute rejection is modified by the effects of chronic uremia and immunosuppression, but the characteristic lesions are observed in clinical renal allografts. Acute rejection usually appears during the early weeks but may appear later. After the first year, episodes of acute (steroid-reversible) rejection are usually due to a reduction in dosage of maintenance steroids, but they may be triggered by other events.

Acute rejection sufficient to cause markedly impaired renal function is usually associated with gross enlargement of the graft, commonly to as much as two or three times the normal size. When subjected to open biopsy, the cortex bleeds less than normally. The most prominent gross abnormality of the cut surface is focal hemorrhage.

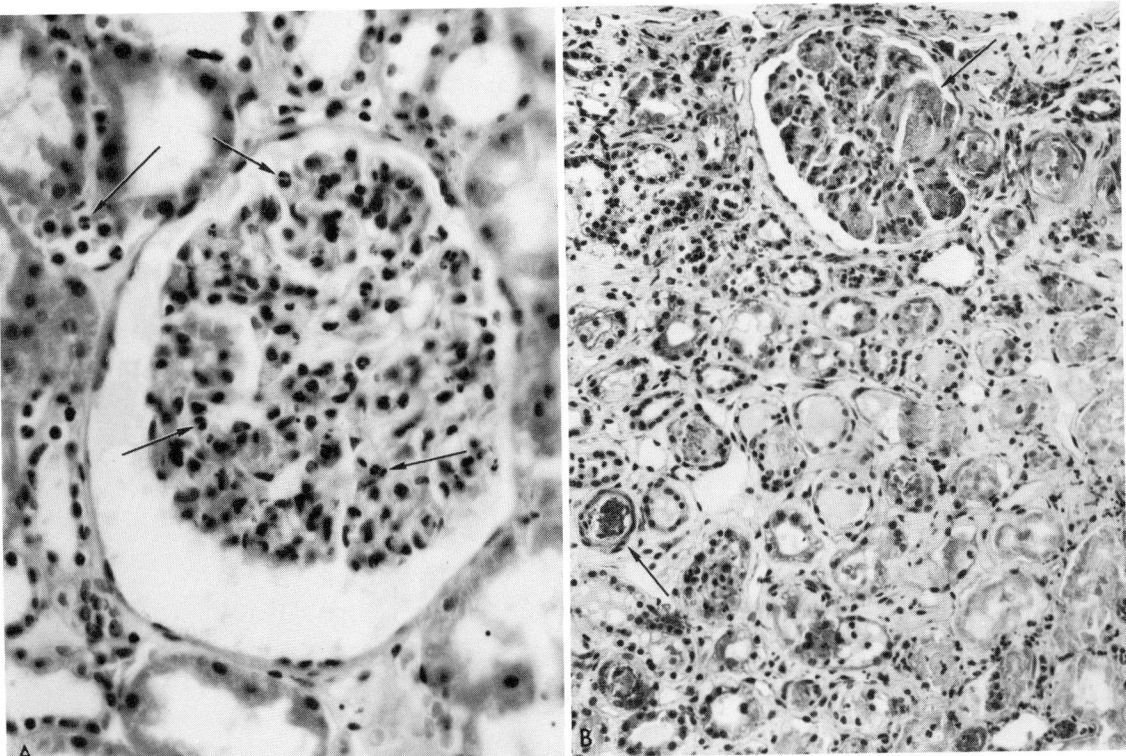

Figure 8. Hyperacute rejection. *A*, This glomerulus of a renal allograft (L. D. No. 56), biopsied approximately 15 minutes after blood flow was established, shows marked infiltration by neutrophils. There are approximately 30 in this section. Neutrophils are also present in the peritubular capillaries (H & E, ×400). *B*, This section from the same kidney 24 hours later when it was removed shows eosinophilic fibrin thrombi in arterioles and in glomerular tufts (see arrows). Tubular necrosis is also seen (H & E, ×180). (The materials for Figures 8, 9, and 10 were prepared in collaboration with Drs. R. C. McCoy and D. T. Rowlands.)

The earliest microscopic evidence of acute rejection is the adherence of small lymphocytes to the endothelium of peritubular capillaries and venules. Cytoplasmic continuity of these small lymphocytes and endothelial cells is seen by electron microscopy (Fig. 9*A*). Cell death occurs, and disruption of these vessels leads to tubular necrosis and interstitial infiltrates. In the early stages the cellular exudate is predominantly small lymphocytes. Later, the infiltrate becomes quite diverse with the appearance of large lymphocytes, plasma cells, macrophages, and polymorphonuclear leukocytes. The infiltrate is often associated with disruption of the tubular basement membrane. Interstitial edema is prominent. In arterioles and small arteries there are swelling of the intima and focal fibrinoid necrosis of the media. Immunoglobulins and complement can sometimes be demonstrated in the walls of arterioles. Proliferation of endothelial cells of interlobular arteries and plugging of the lumen by fibrin, platelets, and pyroninophilic lymphoid cells are seen. There is no sharp distinction between these arterial lesions and those of chronic rejection.

Chronic Rejection

The lesions of chronic rejection (Fig. 10) characteristically are seen in allografts that survive a number of months or years as a consequence of relative compatibility between donor and recipient, and immunosuppression which has prevented, arrested, or reversed acute rejection. The lesions of acute and chronic rejection are frequently seen in the same graft, especially during the latter part of the first year and during the second year. Grossly the chronically rejecting kidney may be enlarged, normal, or reduced in size. Endothelial proliferation of small arteries and arterioles is the most characteristic lesion, and some of these vessels may be completely occluded. Tubular atrophy is a frequent associated finding. Fluorescent staining reveals immunoglobulin and complement in the walls of many of the affected vessels.

Glomerular lesions are also commonly seen in association with late rejection and may appear earlier. These lesions include endothelial hypertrophy and proliferation, mesangial cell proliferation, irregularly thickened basement membranes, and fused epithelial foot processes. Glomerular fibrin deposition and clusters of plasma cells and lymphocytes surrounding glomerular vessels have also been described. Subendothelial deposits of immunoglobulins and complement are found on the basement membranes, and perivascular deposits of immunoglobulins have also been described. Whether this immunologic damage to

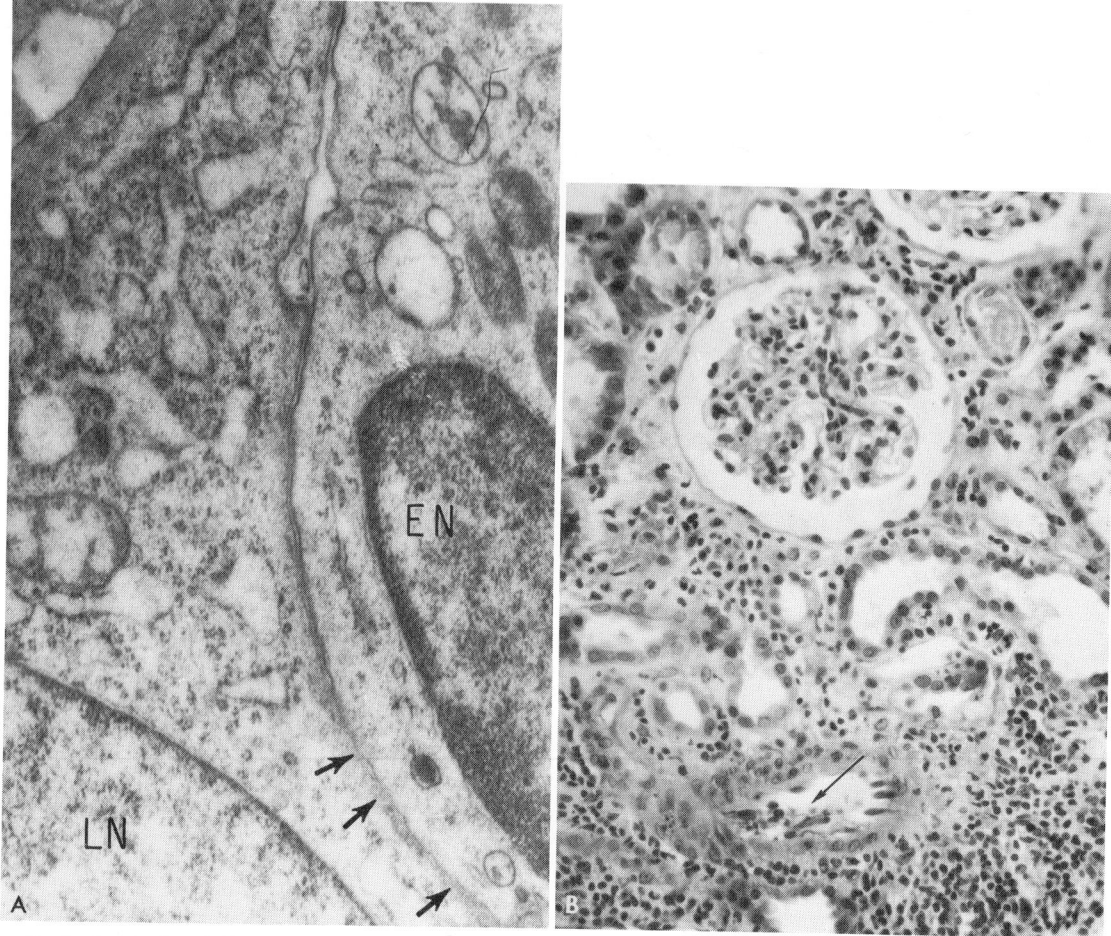

Figure 9.   Acute rejection. *A,* Electron micrograph of a biopsy of a functioning canine renal allograft 72 hours after grafting. Lymphocyte and endothelial cell nuclei are designated LN and EN. The two cells are in close apposition, and the arrows mark points of breakdown of both cell membranes, if not actual continuity of cytoplasm. (From Williams, P. L., Williams, M. A., Kountz, S. L., and Dempster, W. J.: J. Anat., *98:*545, 1964, Cambridge University Press, reprinted by permission. Note: Kountz et al. had earlier documented definite cytoplasmic continuity between such cells, in Nature, *199:*257, 1963.) *B,* Section from rejected renal allograft (L. D. No. 69) removed at 19 days, showing margination of round cells along the endothelium of a small artery (see arrow), and focal intense interstitial infiltrate of lymphocytes and plasma cells extending into the tubular epithelium (H & E, ×200).

glomeruli is a consequence of rejection or of the appearance of the patient's original glomerulonephritis is debatable.[19] Attempts to demonstrate IgG on the glomerular basement membrane by fluorescent antibody techniques have not always been successful in patients experiencing the nephrotic syndrome with chronically surviving renal allografts. A rise in titer of lymphocytotoxic antibody following removal of the renal allograft and the elution of HLA antibodies from the removed kidney suggest that the nephrotic syndrome can be a consequence of immunologic rejection without specific damage to the glomerular basement membrane.

REJECTION: DIFFERENTIAL DIAGNOSIS

Hyperacute Rejection

The manifestations of hyperacute rejection can appear during the transplant operation. For a number of

minutes after revascularization the cortical blood flow is grossly normal as judged by color and turgor of the kidney and by rapid swelling of the kidney upon momentary compression of the vein. Urine may be produced normally for a time. The graft then rather rapidly becomes blue, soft, and anuric, and it no longer swells when the vein is compressed. The characteristic polymorphonuclear infiltrates can be readily demonstrated by frozen section within 60 minutes of revascularization.[6] Hyperacute rejection must be distinguished from other conditions that cause early acute oliguria or anuria, particularly (1) obstruction of renal artery, vein, or ureter; (2) ischemic injury (acute tubular or cortical necrosis) due to suboptimal condition of the donor prior to removal of the graft, or to imperfect preservation during the interval prior to implantation; (3) ischemic injury due to an episode of shock in the recipient after implantation of the graft; and (4) oliguria due to suboptimal maintenance of hydration and blood volume of the recipient. Acute

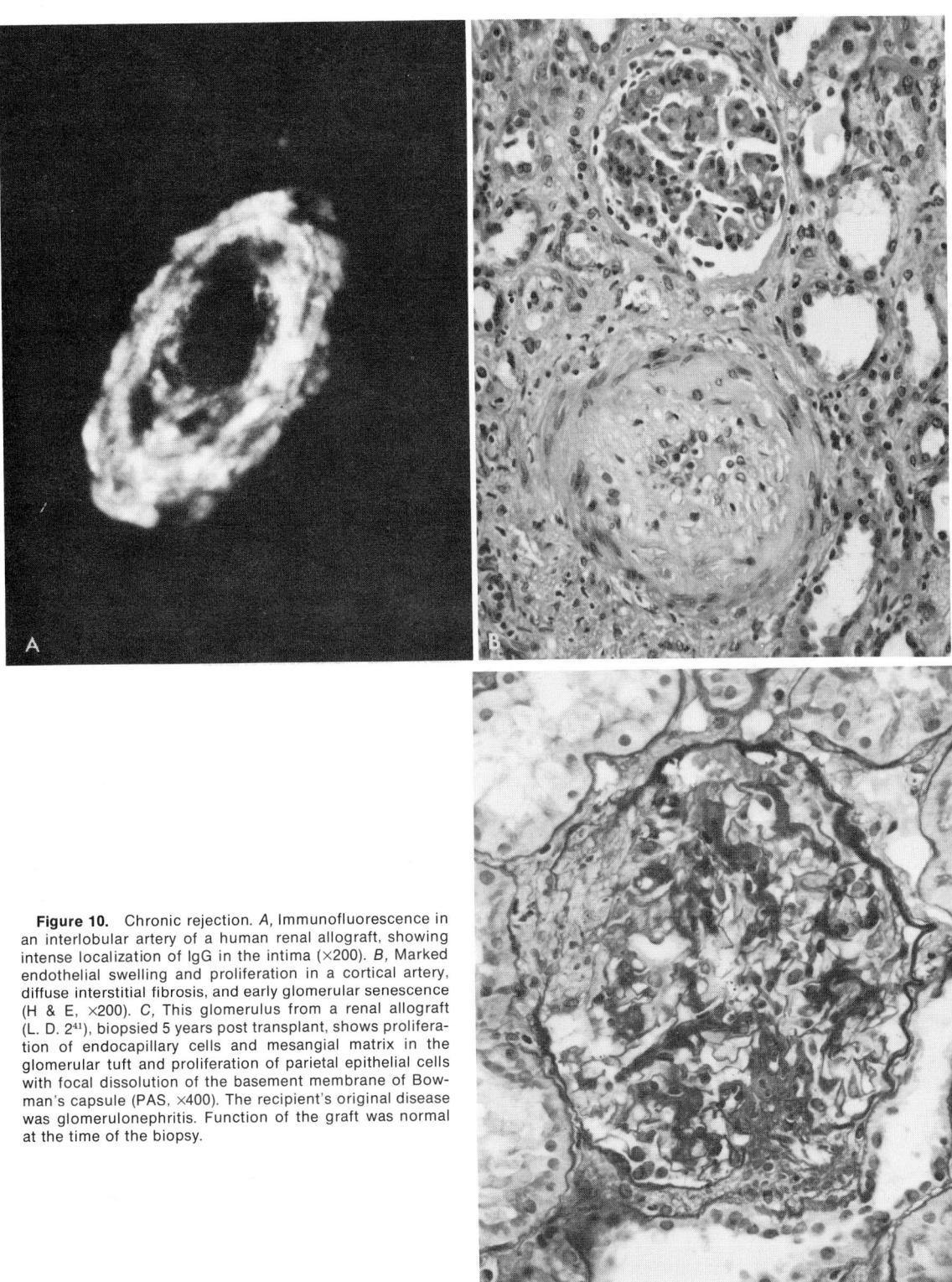

Figure 10. Chronic rejection. *A*, Immunofluorescence in an interlobular artery of a human renal allograft, showing intense localization of IgG in the intima (×200). *B*, Marked endothelial swelling and proliferation in a cortical artery, diffuse interstitial fibrosis, and early glomerular senescence (H & E, ×200). *C*, This glomerulus from a renal allograft (L. D. 2[41]), biopsied 5 years post transplant, shows proliferation of endocapillary cells and mesangial matrix in the glomerular tuft and proliferation of parietal epithelial cells with focal dissolution of the basement membrane of Bowman's capsule (PAS, ×400). The recipient's original disease was glomerulonephritis. Function of the graft was normal at the time of the biopsy.

cortical necrosis is characterized by reduced cortical blood flow and anuria but not an initial interval of relative normalcy typical of hyperacute rejection. Arterial obstruction is diagnosed by palpation of the extrarenal arterial tree. Venous obstruction is characterized by cyanosis, swelling, and great tenseness of the kidney. Mild acute tubular necrosis is characterized by relatively normal gross appearance and blood flow, and the onset of urine flow may be normal or delayed. Severe acute tubular necrosis is characterized by anuria or severe oliguria and grossly normal or somewhat impaired blood flow, but cortical color if abnormal is more grayish pink than blue. Intraoperative and early postoperative diagnosis of these complications is facilitated by constantly monitoring rate of urine flow beginning at the moment when the incision in the bladder is closed.

The clinical manifestations of postoperative accelerated humoral rejection are similar to those of early acute rejection. The distinction between the two is histologic.

Acute Rejection

The diagnosis of acute rejection is usually based upon the observation of a significant reduction in function of the graft in the absence of problems other than rejection. Urine flow and renal function should be monitored closely so that threatened rejection will usually be diagnosed and treated (Fig. 11) before the appearance of symptoms and physical signs. Early symptoms include pain at the graft, malaise with or without chills, and reduced urine output. Gross hematuria is rare. The blood pressure frequently is elevated. Fever,[5, 6] which is usually sustained and nonspiking, may be present. The allograft may be palpably enlarged, and overlying direct tenderness and peritoneal rebound tenderness may be pronounced. Weight gain due to salt and water retention is usually demonstrable, and pitting edema is frequent.

The plasma creatinine is the most important laboratory parameter to follow closely—daily as long as the patient is hospitalized and frequently on an outpatient basis thereafter. The creatinine clearance (which is a close approximation of the glomerular filtration rate) is conveniently computed daily from plasma and urine creatinine concentrations and the volume of 24-hour urine collections. Reduced renal blood flow, particularly cortical blood flow, may be an earlier indication of rejection, but renal blood flow is not monitored as easily as creatinine clearance and thus is not measured regularly. Sudden changes in function are more sharply evident in the creatinine clearance than in the plasma creatinine. The blood urea nitrogen is useful but is affected by a number of influences that do not affect the plasma creatinine, e.g., variation in dietary protein and fluid intake and dosage of steroids.

Certain manifestations of cortical ischemia due to rejection may appear as early as the reduction in the glomerular filtration rate. These include reduced hourly excretion rate of sodium, fluid and water retention, weight gain, and elevation of plasma renin.[6] The urinary sodium may drop to less than 10 mEq. per liter when dietary sodium is normal. If the lesion is

acute tubular necrosis, the urinary sodium will be much higher.

Other laboratory manifestations[6] of acute rejection include leukocytosis and proteinuria. During rejection the urinary sediment contains leukocytes, particularly lymphocytes, and cellular and other debris from damaged tubules. Examination of the urinary sediment is useful but not sufficiently specific or early in the rejection process to form by itself the basis of a diagnosis of acute rejection.

There have been numerous attempts to associate acute renal allograft rejection with changing titers of the recipient's HLA antibodies, with circulating levels of various components of complement, with the results of mixed lymphocyte cultures, and with inhibition of leukocyte migration. These tests, however, are not sufficiently predictive of functionally significant acute rejection to be helpful for purposes of diagnosis and treatment.[14]

The differential diagnosis of acute rejection includes arterial, venous, and ureteral obstruction or leak, and conditions affecting the parenchyma of the kidney such as acute cortical or tubular necrosis, infection, and recurrence of the recipient's original disease. Prerenal conditions such as dehydration, hypovolemia, and hypotension also can cause temporary renal functional impairment. Artifactual causes of apparent reduction in urine output and reports of impaired renal function must be kept in mind, e.g., an obstructed or leaking urinary catheter, an incomplete 24-hour collection of urine, or a laboratory error.

Anuria is characteristic of arterial, venous, or ureteral obstruction or cortical necrosis, whereas oliguria is more characteristic of rejection or tubular necrosis. These generalizations are of limited use diagnostically, however, because severe rejection or tubular necrosis will result in anuria, and the other conditions, if partial, can be seen with oliguria. Delayed drainage of bladder irrigation fluid can be mistaken for urine when the kidney is actually anuric.

Changes in size of the graft can be seen on roentgenograms taken with standard tube-to-kidney and kidney-to-film distances if metallic clip markers were placed on the kidney at the time of transplantation (Fig. 12). Significant enlargement is frequently but not always seen in association with acute rejection. Venous obstruction, which is rare, is the only other condition that typically causes sudden increase in size of the graft. Normal compensatory hypertrophy is observed as gradual enlargement during the first three to six months.

Significant partial ureteral obstructions may occur without early effect on function.[6, 18] Accordingly, an intravenous urogram (Fig. 12) is obtained routinely during the first week or as soon as function permits and at regular intervals thereafter. With a drip infusion of the contrast medium a satisfactory study is usually obtained if the creatinine clearance is at least 20 ml. per minute. A retrograde pyelogram may not be feasible because it is sometimes impossible to insert a catheter into a transplanted ureter at cystoscopy; and if an indwelling ureteral catheter is used at all (most surgeons do not), it is usually removed a few days post

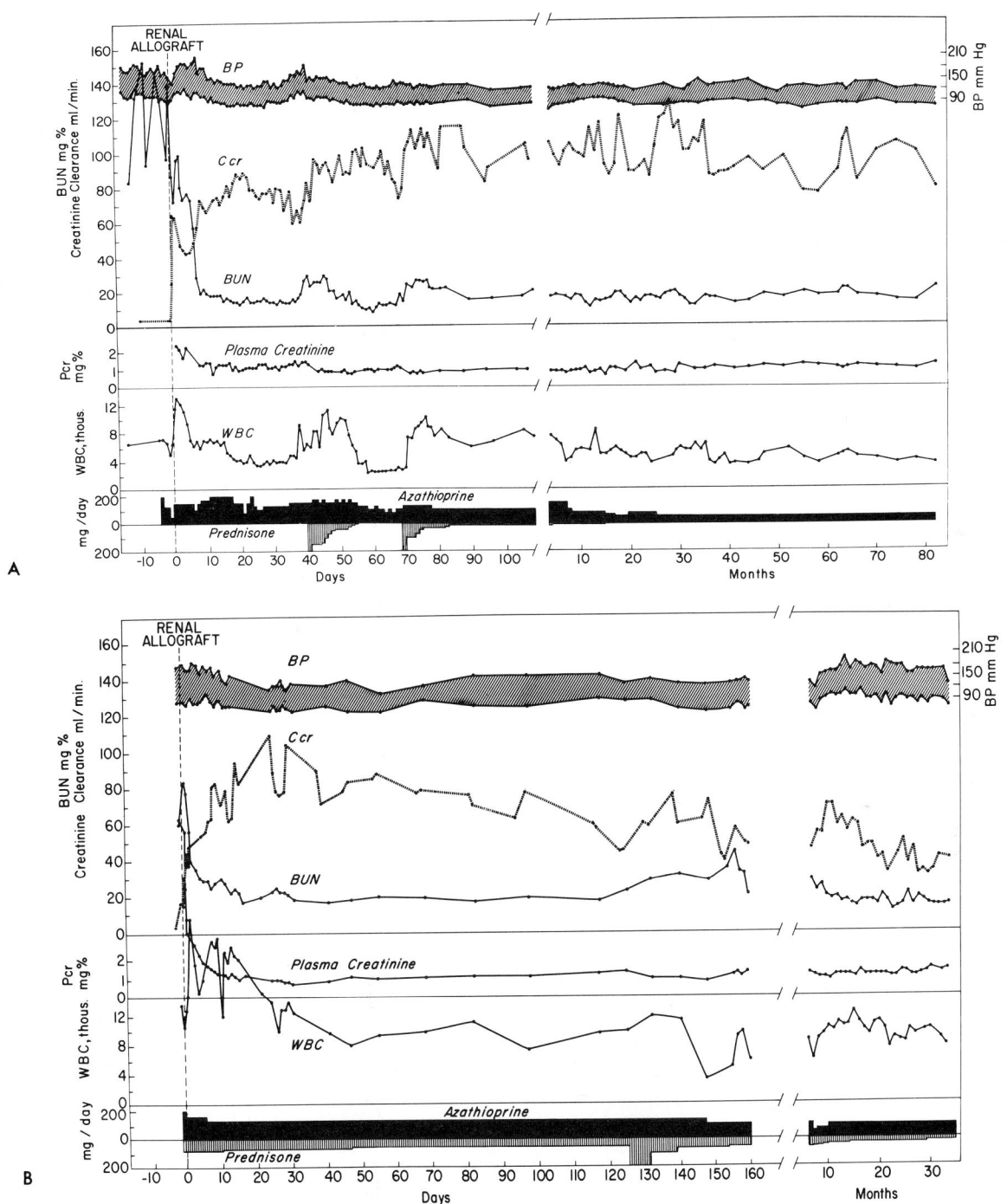

Figure 11. Clinical course. *A*, This patient (L. D. No. 1[41]) received an HLA Class 2 kidney from his brother. The two rejection episodes were mild, late in onset, and readily reversed without sustained high dosage steroids. Rehabilitation was early and complete. This patient is well 12 years post transplant. (See also Fig. 5.) *B*, This patient (C.D. No. 18), age 41 years when he received a cadaver kidney, experienced one episode of acute rejection at 4 months. At 5 years the Pcr was 2.0, and the daily prednisone, 20 mg. He died suddenly of unknown cause (no autopsy) 6½ years post transplant.

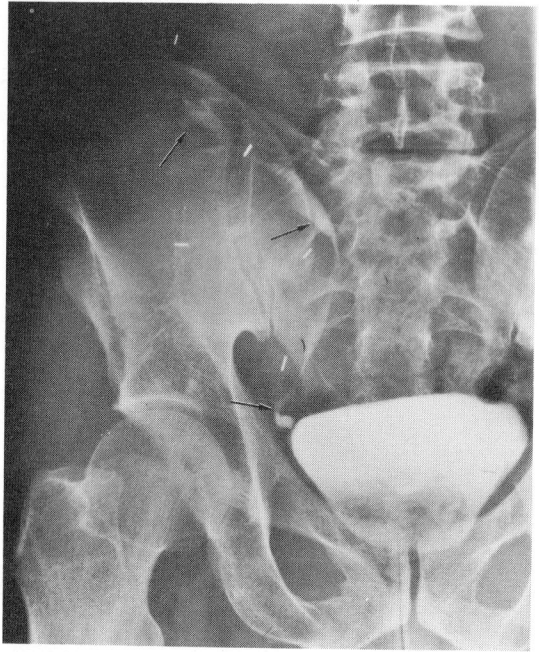

Figure 12. Intravenous urogram. The collecting system, ureter, and bladder are normal (see arrows). See also metallic clips placed on the renal capsule for following changes in size of the graft. This study was performed 4 years post transplant (L. D. No. 3[41]).

transplant. Surgical exploration is sometimes necessary to diagnose ureteral complications.

When there is little if any measurable renal function, it is useful to follow the condition of the graft by serial observations of blood flow. The methods that can be used include xenon washout, rapid-sequence scintillation photo-scanning (Fig. 13), and arteriography. The radioactive Hippuran renogram may show the initial vascular spike and some renal function in the absence of measurable excretion. During recovery from tubular necrosis the circulation is stable or improving, whereas the circulation progressively deteriorates as rejection develops. Rejection can appear and progress to complete destruction of the graft before there is time for recovery from tubular necrosis. Such rejection can sometimes be reversed by appropriate intensification of immunosuppression; however, when circulation deteriorates to the point of complete infarction of the graft, it should be promptly removed and the immunosuppression discontinued.

Chronic Rejection

The diagnosis is suspected after the first few months when slowly progressive deterioration of function is observed in the absence of other demonstrable cause and without response to steroids or other immunosuppression. In patients whose disease in their own kidneys was glomerulonephritis, recurrence of original disease must be considered. Renal biopsy is frequently helpful, but not always conclusive.

Renal Allograft Biopsy

Biopsy is useful when doubt exists clinically regarding diagnosis. Open biopsy of a renal allograft is readily accomplished under local anesthesia. Compared with needle biopsy, the open method has the advantages of allowing gross inspection of a portion of the graft and securing more tissue than can be obtained by needle. Because of the rather focal nature of rejection, even open biopsy may miss some of the lesions

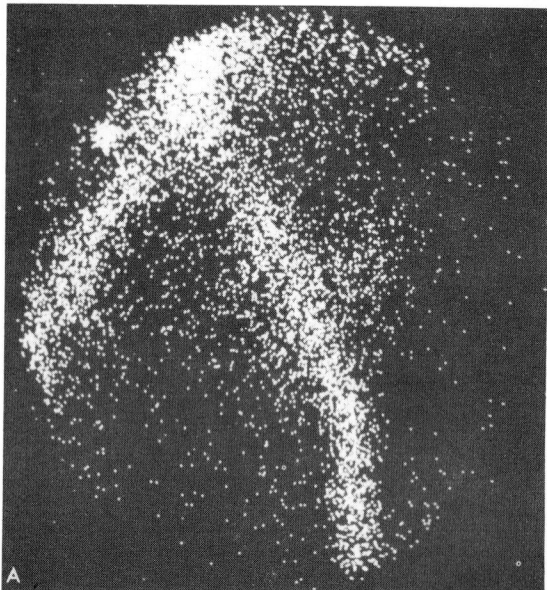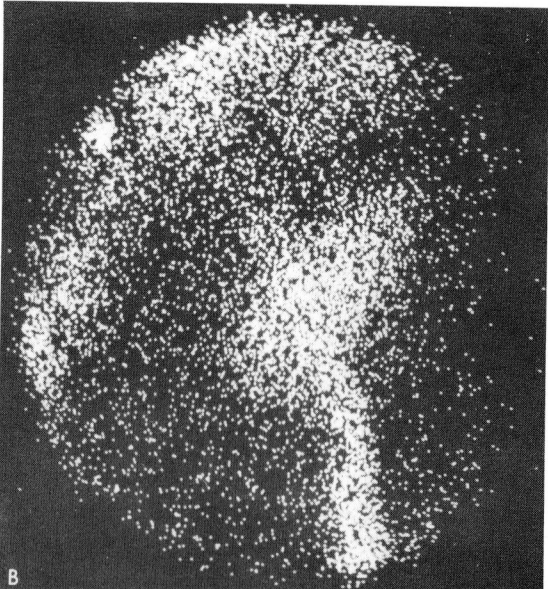

Figure 13. Rapid-sequence photoscan. This study was performed two days post transplant when the allograft (C. D. No. 68) had no measurable excretory function. *A,* At 12 seconds after intravenous injection of $Na^{99m}TcO_4$ the aorta and iliac arteries are seen clearly and the allograft faintly. *B,* Three seconds later the allograft and external iliac artery are clearly demonstrated. This study is done in conjunction with the standard radioactive Hippuran renogram.

that may be present. Needle biopsies can be performed with or without fluoroscopic placement of the needle in the cortex. The graft may be visualized by infusing contrast media as during an intravenous urogram. Alternatively, the cortex of the graft may be outlined with multiple metallic clips placed at the time of transplantation. The principal risk is the same as that of needle biopsy of native kidneys: perinephric or urinary tract hemorrhage. Rarely does such bleeding result in loss of a renal allograft.[3, 16]

Recurrence of Glomerulonephritis

With both acute and chronic allograft rejection, recurrence of glomerulonephritis is among the diagnoses to be considered. Clinical observations such as proteinuria greater than 2 gm. per day, microscopic hematuria, and failure to respond to steroid therapy are more characteristic of glomerulitis than acute rejection; but as with the original disease, renal biopsy is necessary for definitive diagnosis. Although some glomerular lesions of rejection may not be distinguishable from glomerulonephritis (see Chronic Rejection above), a distinction is usually possible, especially where sections from the patient's own kidneys are available for histologic comparison. The lesions of *crescentic membranoproliferative glomerulitis* characteristically occur most acutely and can progress to destruction of the graft during the first four months. *Lobular membranoproliferative glomerulonephritis* characteristically appears during the first year and may progress to graft destruction within a year or two. Electron *dense deposit membranoproliferative lesions* usually progress more slowly. The lesions of recurrent *IGA nephropathy* can be quite benign, associated with proteinuria and microscopic hematuria for years with renal function remaining normal or near normal. The incidence of recurrent glomerulonephritis appears to vary inversely with donor-recipient compatibility. An incidence of approximately 30 per cent was reported with early experiences with monozygotic twins (9th Registry report[2]). In a series of 46 HLA identical renal allografts followed by the authors for 1 to 11 years the incidence has been approximately 15 per cent,[39] whereas it has been approximately 5 per cent with HLA haploidentical grafts,[38] and less with cadaver grafts.

REJECTION: PREVENTION AND TREATMENT

Prevention

The prevention of rejection begins with pretransplant immunologic testing for donor-recipient selection, but some immunosuppression will be needed even with use of an HLA identical donor because certain unidentified non-HLA, non-ABO antigens contribute weakly but significantly to allograft rejection.

The purine analog, *azathioprine* (Imuran), is used at nearly all centers as the principal drug to prevent rejection. The initial "loading dose" of 4 to 8 mg. per kilogram should be administered at about the time of transplantation (within two days before and after) for full effect during the critical period when the recipient's immunologic system is first exposed to antigens of the graft. The maximum dose tolerated for maintenance varies considerably and is usually in the range from 0.5 to 2 mg. per kilogram per day. Azathioprine therapy is usually continued throughout the life of the graft unless liver dysfunction prompts its cessation. A 50 per cent reduction in the dose is advisable during periods of anuria because the excretion route is partially renal. This drug should be temporarily discontinued during periods of leukopenia. Leukocyte counts of less than 6000 per cu. mm. are unsafe if the patient is receiving as much as 40 mg. of prednisone daily. In patients stabilized on a maintenance dose of azathioprine, leukopenia sometimes develops paradoxically in response to acute infection. Leukocytosis due to infection or to the effects of steroids does *not* justify a higher dose than would otherwise be given.

At most centers at least one other major immunosuppressent, usually *prednisone*, is administered beginning at or prior to the time of transplantation. Because of the complications of steroids there is a current trend of decreasing dosage, with considerable variation among centers. Most regimens of maintenance steroids are in the following range for a 70-kilogram adult: 40 to 100 mg. per day of prednisone (or prednisone-equivalent) initially, with some reduction at the end of the first week and subsequent tapering to 30 to 80 mg. per day at one month; 20 to 60 mg. per day at three months; 15 to 30 mg. per day at six months; 10 to 30 mg. per day at twelve months; 10 to 20 mg. per day during the second year; and 5 to 15 mg. per day thereafter. The daily dose may be divided or given all at once. There are advocates of alternate day steroids for renal allograft immunosuppression, but a net advantage to this modification of the regimen has not been firmly established.

The third major immunosuppressant is *antilymphocyte globulin*.[6, 11, 17, 24, 32] Its well-established strong immunosuppressive effects in various experimental models and its mechanisms of action, which are different from the other two, are discussed in the section of this chapter on immunosuppression. It may be used in addition to full doses of the other two agents, or with a substantial reduction of steroids, particularly during the first month. Like the other two it has serious side effects, e.g., thrombocytopenia, that must be carefully weighed against the benefits. Aspects currently being clinically studied include methods of manufacture, refinement and standardization of the product, and clinical regimens of administration and monitoring.

Local irradiation of the graft has a definite though not intensive immunosuppressive effect.[6, 11, 24, 32, 41] It may be administered prophylactically during the first week after transplantation, or it may be used adjunctively with steroids to treat episodes of acute rejection.

The alkylating agent *cyclophosphamide* may be used as an alternative to azathioprine either from the beginning or when liver dysfunction necessitates discontinuance of azathioprine. Another regimen is to combine these two drugs, administering half of the usual dose of each.[40, 42]

Other methods of immunosuppression have been used clinically, but their use is not widely established because benefits have not been proved or because they have been difficult to manage clinically. These methods include splenectomy,[5, 6, 11, 32] total-body irradiation, thoracic duct drainage,[6, 11] extracorporeal irradiation of the blood,[6] and thymectomy.[5, 6, 19]

When immunosuppression is withdrawn from long-surviving canine renal allografts, some of the grafts are rejected and some are unaffected. Clinically *immunosuppression should be continued indefinitely unless the graft is to be sacrificed deliberately.* One patient was reported to have had a serious threatened rejection less than three weeks after elective withdrawal of azathioprine.[24] This attempt to withdraw was undertaken five years post transplant when the patient was well and being treated with low doses of this drug and no other immunosuppression. The authors have had similar experiences with patients who discontinued azathioprine or prednisone or both (some for medical reasons and others against medical advice). For recipients of HLA identical sibling grafts, total withdrawal of prednisone may be carefully attempted after the first year, but azathioprine or cyclophosphamide should be continued indefinitely. For all other recipients, any such attempt to withdraw steroids totally would be questionable because of the probability of precipitating an irreversible episode of acute rejection. Various immunologic tests to monitor chronic maintenance immunosuppression are under development, but their reliability for adjusting dosage has not been established.

Treatment of Hyperacute Rejection

If the diagnosis of hyperacute rejection is confirmed intraoperatively by frozen section, and the graft is anuric, it should be removed.

Because of the prominence of intravascular thrombosis in the pathogenesis of accelerated humoral rejection (postoperative hyperacute rejection), anticoagulation with heparin has been suggested as a therapeutic agent. The efficacy of such treatment remains to be established, however, and anticoagulation may cause bleeding in the fresh operative wound or interstitially in the renal allograft.

Treatment of Acute Rejection

Steroids are the most effective means of reversing established manifestations of acute rejection (see Fig. 11), and either the intravenous or the oral route may be used. By the intravenous route methyl prednisolone, 20 to 30 mg. per kg., is infused over a two- to four-hour period daily or on alternate days. By the oral route prednisone is increased to 2 to 3 mg. per kg. per day in divided doses. By either method the total dose should not be more than sufficient to restore renal function to the prerejection level. Regardless of the response, however, dosage is reduced after 3 to 10 days at these levels. The return to the prerejection level of maintenance oral steroids—or to a judiciously increased level—may be abrupt or by tapering during one to four weeks. Azathioprine is *not* increased during or after a rejection episode, and should be decreased if the rejection has severely impaired renal function. Local irradiation of the graft to a total dose of not more than 1500 rad, administered in doses of 150 rad on alternate days, may be used adjunctively with

steroids, as well as some of the other immunosuppressive measures mentioned earlier under Prevention of Rejection.

In the absence of other major complications a *second rejection episode* is usually managed with treatment similar to that for the first, though with greater consideration for the early and late morbidity and mortality attributable to steroids. Treating a third rejection episode during the first six months is accordingly more questionable, and thus is frequently though not always judged inadvisable.

The most frequent cause of *late acute rejection* is a reduction in the level of oral steroids. After six months it is therefore advisable to reduce oral prednisone in decrements of not more than 5 mg. per day, to wait at least one month before considering further reduction, and to follow every reduction with measurement of renal function at least weekly for at least one month. Two syndromes of late, steroid-reversible rejection are frequently seen: (1) an episode of rapid and severe reduction in renal function, triggered evidently by a small reduction in oral steroids; and (2) a small but measurable reduction in renal function following a reduction in oral steroids. The management of the first syndrome is by early diagnosis and treatment as for other acute rejection episodes. For the second syndrome oral steroids are increased to the earlier level unless it is decided that this would be excessive.

The host-graft interactions of an established renal allograft present a delicate balance of incompletely understood forces. Steroid-reversible episodes are occasionally seen without any apparent triggering event, or in association with an event that is not a provable cause, e.g., an acute infection, or an intercurrent major or minor surgical operation.

Treatment of Chronic Rejection

There is no known treatment for chronic rejection. Chronic rejection is thus one of the causes of end-stage renal disease, and its clinical course as diagrammed in Figure 1 may transpire over a period of weeks, months, or years. It is advisable to reduce immunosuppression as symptoms of renal failure increase. Doses of steroids and other drugs that were maintaining good renal function will be progressively less justifiable as renal function deteriorates.

Complications of Immunosuppression

The principal cause of death in renal allograft recipients is *infection*,[2, 6] and the incidence and seriousness of the infections correlate directly with intensity of immunosuppressive therapy. Infections occur both early and late in the post transplant course and are caused by a large variety of organisms. Diagnosis is frequently delayed because steroids mask many of the clinical manifestations. Treatment generally is similar to that which is appropriate in other patients. Immunosuppression should be reduced or terminated if necessary to improve host resistance to life-threatening infection. The use of "sterile rooms" for totally isolating the patient has been largely abandoned. Such measures do not protect the patient from endogenous microorganisms, and it has not been established that renal allograft patients really benefit from such an environment. Simple protective isolation is appropriate, however, in the early postoperative period and during periods of recovery from overdosage of immunosuppression.

Infections due to pyogenic bacteria occur most frequently in the urinary tract, the surgical wounds, and the lungs, but involvement of numerous other parts of the body has been reported. Tuberculosis has been reported. Oral and genital monilial infections are common, and systemic infections have been reported.[6] Other fungus infections reported include aspergillosis, blastomycosis, cryptococcosis, histoplasmosis, mucormycosis, and nocardiosis.[6, 24] Viral infections that have been reported include hepatitis,[6, 42] herpes simplex, and herpes zoster.[6] Hepatitis-associated antigen, acquired before or after transplant, was detected in the serum of one fifth of a series of allograft recipients. With few exceptions this infectious carrier state persisted indefinitely for periods of observation up to four years.[42] The cytomegalic virus is readily isolated from the urine and lungs of many transplant patients but pathogenicity is uncertain.[6] Pneumocystis carinii has been reported.[6] Pulmonary infestation with the parasite Strongyloides has been reported,[34] and the authors have seen this problem in a renal allograft recipient.

Frequent *side effects of steroid therapy* include diabetes mellitus, aseptic necrosis of the head of the femur[6, 11, 22] and other musculoskeletal abnormalities,[6, 24] cataract, serious mental disturbances, peptic ulcer, hypertension, and profound changes in facial appearance which greatly disturb some patients. The ill effects on bone of prednisone and of hyperparathyroidism are probably additive in causing musculoskeletal complications. Cushing's syndrome contributes very substantially to the mortality, morbidity, and delayed rehabilitation of renal allograft patients.

Despite careful monitoring of the white count, azathioprine sometimes produces serious *bone marrow depression* with leukopenia and thrombocytopenia which may be associated with purpura and serious cerebral, gastrointestinal, or other hemorrhage. This drug can also produce serious *hepatic dysfunction* which, unless quite mild, should prompt the substitution of another drug, e.g., cyclophosphamide.[40] The use of antilymphocyte globulin not infrequently must be discontinued because of *thrombocytopenia* or delayed or anaphylactoid *hypersensitivity reactions*. A significantly increased incidence of *neoplasia* has been reported in renal allograft recipients.[2, 11, 19, 24] The greatest increase, several hundred-fold that of the general population, is seen with reticulum cell sarcoma and bone marrow malignancy; however, the total incidence of malignancy in renal allograft recipients is less than 5 per cent, and a third of those reported are cutaneous carcinomas or carcinoma in situ of the cervix that is easily detected and effectively treated.[2]

OTHER ASPECTS OF POST-TRANSPLANT MANAGEMENT

The topics in this section are those not previously discussed in the paragraphs on rejection and the complications of immunosuppression, and under the heading Recipient Operations Other Than Transplantation. If the graft fails to function for a significant period of time, the paragraphs under the head Preoperative and Postoperative Care of Uremic Patients will be applicable. If treatment fails, the plan is usually to remove the graft, reinstitute dialysis, and plan another transplant.

Hydration, Blood Volume, and Diuretics

Mild deficits in hydration or blood volume that might be of no great consequence in other settings should be studiously avoided for the first week or two following renal transplantation. Such deficits cause oliguria and temporary impairment of renal function and thus may delay or obscure the diagnosis of more serious problems such as rejection for which prompt diagnosis and treatment are of critical importance. The central venous pressure (CVP) should be monitored until the patient's hydration and hemodynamics are stable. Volume deficits are frequently reflected in the CVP and renal function more than in systemic blood pressure and pulse rate. During the first day or two the need for plasma and extracellular fluid and electrolytes may considerably exceed measurable plus normal insensible losses. Evidently there is an occult difference of one to three liters between the ideal total body fluid volume that is optimal for chronic dialysis and that which is required intraoperatively and immediately following renal transplantation. Excessive volume must also be avoided; the capacity of the transplanted kidney to compensate is likely to be temporarily impaired.

Mild polyuria is desirable for the first week or so: 100 to 200 ml. per hour for the first 24 to 48 hours, and 75 to 150 ml. per hour thereafter. Initially there may be a rather massive diuresis,[6] and when this occurs the output should be replaced on at least an hourly basis until it becomes clear whether the diuresis is (1) an appropriate response of good renal function to excessive extracellular fluid or (2) an inappropriate diuresis resulting from impaired renal function. Serious, even fatal, dehydration can be the consequence of incomplete replacement of losses during a massive diuresis, and this is a hazard especially in children. If renal function is good the diuresis should be gradually reduced; replacement of two thirds of the urine volume of the previous hour until the output is in the desirable range is usually well tolerated.[6] Half-normal saline in 2.5 per cent glucose is usually a satisfactory intravenous fluid for replacing urine over a wide range of rates of urine flow. During massive diuresis sodium bicarbonate, about 25 mEq. per liter, is added to prevent acidosis. Use of 5 per cent glucose is avoided because glucosuria resulting from its rapid administration can perpetuate an osmotic diuresis. Measurement of serum electrolytes after the administration of each 2 to 5 liters of intravenous fluids is advisable. There is no need for potassium in the parenteral fluids except during sustained massive diuresis, and potassium is strictly contraindicated if there is any question of renal functional impairment. Fluid intake of course should be restricted in the presence of anuria or oliguria due to impaired renal function.

The most frequent uses of *diuretics* are the same in patients with renal allografts as in others: (1) to increase the rate of excretion of excessive salt and water; and (2) to stimulate urine flow and to decrease renal injury during the transplant operation and in other circumstances during or after temporary reduction or total interruption of renal blood flow. Mannitol, furosemide, and ethacrynic acid are the diuretics most frequently used intravenously. As in other clinical settings, the complications of the use of diuretics include acute and chronic water and electrolyte depletion states that can be minimized by adjustments in dosage and appropriate electrolyte and water replacement.

Hypertension

Mild to severe systemic hypertension[6, 19] can appear at any time during the life of the graft and is usually associated with moderate to severe manifestations of rejection. Other causes include recurrence of original nephritis or essential hypertension, side effects of prednisone, salt and water retention, or some combination of these. Occasionally the cause is a surgically correctable stenosis of the renal artery at the anastomosis, or proximal or distal to this point.[6] The renin mechanism may be operative in association with rejection and other parenchymal abnormalities when the renal artery and its principal branches are normal. The dietary and pharmacologic treatment of hypertension is essentially the same in renal allograft patients as in others.

Other Complications

The incidence of the *urologic complications* of urinary fistula and ureteral obstruction is quite variable, ranging from less than 5 per cent in some series to over 20 per cent in others.[1, 6, 18, 21, 32] Mortality is high, 30 to 70 per cent, except in the case of fistulas that close spontaneously in a few days. Mortality is especially high when fistula or obstruction is associated with moderate to severe rejection and high-dosage immunosuppression.[18] Under these circumstances prompt removal of the graft is less hazardous than attempting surgically to correct ureteral complications. If, however, renal function is good and the patient is receiving little immunosuppression, successful treatment of such complications is possible with acceptable risk. The recipient's own ureter may be used if the first procedure was ureteroneocystostomy.

The incidence of intraoperative and postoperative *vascular anastomotic* complications of hemorrhage and thrombosis is generally less than 3 per cent. Total infarction results unless the problem is recognized and corrected immediately. The arterial anastomosis may leak as a result of infection of the transplant wound, and in this situation reanastomosis is futile and risks further life-threatening hemorrhage. If an end-to-side iliac arterial anastomosis was used, this complication is a serious threat to the lower extremity, which may not survive ligation of the iliac artery if this is necessary to control hemorrhage from an infected suture line. Thrombosis due to defective anastomosis should be distinguished from an extension of thrombosis due primarily to rejection, cortical necrosis, or other renal parenchymal complication.

Early and late *thromboembolic* complications are principally intracranial and coronary arterial thrombosis, and peripheral venous thrombosis with or without pulmonary embolism. In renal allografts reported to the Registry[2] the mortality due to cerebrovascular accident was 3.3 per cent, and mortality due to myocardial infarction was 4.2 per cent. Considering the average age of the patients with these complications, approximately 40 years, the incidence greatly exceeds that in the general population. Deep venous thrombosis is usually on the side of the renal allograft, and it may propagate into the graft and cause loss of the graft. Because of the anatomic location of a renal allograft, the incidence of such thrombosis is probably influenced by technique of implantation,[6] and postoperatively the sitting position should be avoided for at least two or three weeks. Early ambulation and other measures to reduce venous stasis are important. Neither heparin nor Coumadin is administered prophylactically, but anticoagulation is indicated if deep venous thrombosis is diagnosed.

The term *transplant lung*[6] is applied to the syndrome of alveolar capillary block associated with few if any abnormalities on physical examination of the chest and with a chest x-ray that is normal or shows miliary or splotchy infiltrates. The P_{O_2} is low, and peripheral cyanosis may be observed. The P_{CO_2} is normal. The syndrome often is associated with an episode of rejection, and an autoimmune mechanism has been postulated. Cytomegalic viral and other undiagnosed pulmonary infections are also among the postulated etiologies. In any event it is a life-threatening complication, and transplant nephrectomy probably carries less risk than intensive immunosuppression.

A number of *other complications* occur occasionally but with an incidence that collectively is significant. A major hemorrhage can result from rupture[11, 16] of a swollen renal allograft in the early post-transplant period due to acute tubular necrosis or rejection. Diagnosis is made at exploration or at autopsy. Unless the rent is severe it is not necessary to sacrifice the graft. The mortality of pancreatitis in renal allograft patients is high.[6, 19] Cholecystitis has been observed, and under the effects of steroid a perforation of the gallbladder may not immediately be clinically evident. A lymphocele of the transplant wound is treated by simple drainage.[18] Migratory polyarthritis is observed occasionally, especially during steroid withdrawal.[6] Suicide[19] has been reported.

Late Follow-up

Rehabilitation is effectively promoted by early release of the patient from the hospital, but some of the aforementioned complications appear many weeks or months post transplant, and successful treatment depends upon prompt diagnosis. Late management therefore includes education of the patient and his family regarding (1) the purpose of all treatment and diagnostic tests in the follow-up plan; (2) the symptoms of complications and the importance of seeking early medical attention; and (3) the restorative effects of returning to pre-illness work and activity following temporary disability due to complications if these do occur.

Medical Records

A considerable volume of data is generated in the course of caring for even the uncomplicated renal allograft patient, and the traditional medical record by itself is not adequate. To facilitate long-term outpatient care as well as intensive inpatient care, frequently used data should be tabulated chronologically on large flow sheets.

RESULTS AND PROGNOSIS

Quality and Duration of Function of Renal Allografts

In the absence of complications, the glomerular filtration rate (GFR) of a renal allograft is normal for one kidney within 24 hours of the transplant operation, and within one week the GFR is well above normal. During the ensuing weeks compensatory anatomic hypertrophy develops both in the graft and in the remaining kidney of a healthy living donor. Within three to six months the combined GFR of the two kidneys reaches 130 to 190 per cent of the normal GFR of the donor prior to transplantation. A series of 10 renal allografts from HLA identical donors was studied by comparing the function of the allograft with the function of the kidney remaining in the donor a year or more posttransplant.[36] By all of the ordinary tests and a number of special renal function tests, the function of the allograft and that of the kidney remaining in the donor were equal in most comparisons. Some of the grafts were slightly impaired in ability to concentrate, but this abnormality was of no practical significance. Mild cellular infiltrates were not unusual, however, in biopsies of renal allografts in the presence of normal function.

If function of the renal allograft is normal, the acute manifestations of uremia clear rapidly and anemia and debilitation clear gradually over a period of several weeks. Severely disabling retinopathy and neuropathy will either clear completely or very markedly improve. Vitamin D metabolism returns to normal. A rapid spurt of growth is usually observed in children. Although renal allograft recipients are not encouraged to have children because of their own uncertain long-term prognosis and the uncertain genetic effects of immunosuppression, a number of males have fathered normal children, and a number of females have given birth uneventfully by cesarean section or vaginally to normal children.[2, 6]

A complete spectrum of quality and duration of function of renal allografts is observed between long-term normal function and early acute failure. For a full description of the results of this form of treatment it is necessary to read reports from a number of individual institutions, among which methods, results, and conclusions differ considerably.[4-8, 10, 11, 16, 17, 19, 22, 24]

For a brief overview of the collective experiences of many institutions, it is useful to refer to reports of the worldwide Human Renal Transplant Registry. The twelfth report[2] was on 16,444 renal allografts performed between 1951 and 1974 at 288 institutions including 164 in the United States. The functional survival of renal allografts is shown in Figure 14 and in Table 4. The results were reported by standard actuarial methods of computing life tables. If dialysis was resumed before the graft was removed, the end point of function was defined as the time when dialysis was resumed (excluding dialysis during a period of temporary functional failure of the graft). The shape of the curves is noteworthy. The incidence of both graft failure and other complications is highest during the first few months post transplant. Thereafter the incidence of problems diminishes progressively but remains appreciable for all categories of renal allografts for as long as they are followed. Rejection, suboptimal preservation of cadaver kidneys, technical complications, and infections are the most frequently

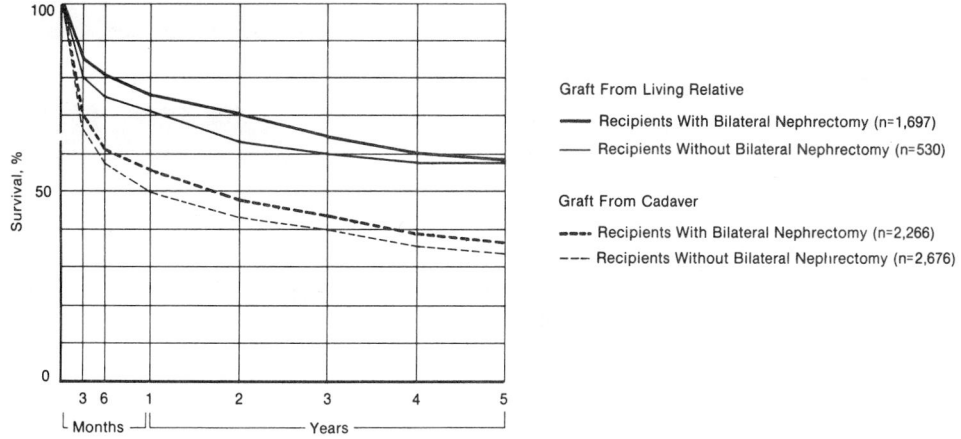

Figure 14. Results of renal allografts as reported from the Registry.[2] Functional survival of grafts from living relatives and cadavers with and without prior bilateral nephrectomy. See text here and under Recipient Operations Other Than Transplantation.

TABLE 4. Registry Data: Results of Renal Allografts*

Donor Source	Year Transplant Performed	Sample Size	One Year		Five Years	
			Graft Functioning (Per Cent ± SE)	Patient Living (Per Cent ± SE)	Graft Functioning (Per Cent ± SE)	Patient Living (Per Cent ± SE)
Sibling	1969	217	76.5 ± 2.9	82.6 ± 2.6	60.8 ± 3.7	71.1 ± 3.5
Sibling	1972	447	79.9 ± 1.9	90.9 ± 1.4	– –	– –
Parent	1969	234	69.2 ± 3.0	78.7 ± 2.8	42.0 ± 3.8	61.8 ± 3.8
Parent	1972	359	71.7 ± 2.4	86.6 ± 1.9	– –	– –
Cadaver	1969	847	54.2 ± 1.7	65.5 ± 1.7	35.2 ± 1.9	50.6 ± 2.0
Cadaver	1972	1707	50.6 ± 1.2	71.8 ± 1.2	– –	– –

*From Bergan, J. J., et al.: J.A.M.A., *233*:787, 1975. One-year and five-year follow-up for graft survival and patient survival. SE = standard error of the mean. Not shown are data from preceding and intervening years which confirm a substantial and continuing trend of improving patient survival for transplants performed from 1967 to 1972, but no such trend for graft survival. The better results with sibling donors than with parental donors are due to the preferential use of HLA-identical siblings.

reported causes of graft failure.[2] Specific factors affecting graft survival are discussed in more detail throughout this section. Immunogenetic factors are discussed under living and cadaver donor selection.

Life Expectancy of Renal Allograft Recipients

Patient survival exceeds graft survival.[2, 6, 7] Among 14,479 recipients of one or more renal allografts whose follow-ups were reported to the Registry, 6,781 (46.8 per cent) were alive with a functioning graft, and 2,979 (20.6 per cent) were surviving without graft function.[2] The differences between graft survival and patient survival are shown in more detail in Table 4. The trend of improving patient survival is a notable development with this form of treatment, attributable largely to increasing experience with avoidance of high-dosage immunosuppression where ill effects exceed benefits. The trend of improving patient survival is doubly remarkable because of the concomitant trend of increasing acceptance of various high-risk patients who previously would not have been accepted for dialysis and transplantation.[17, 32]

Rehabilitation of Renal Allograft Recipients

In the absence of complications the patient may leave the hospital and resume sedentary work less than two weeks post transplant, and after six weeks the patient will be physically unrestricted except for avoidance of trauma to the graft (which is protected only by the soft anterior abdominal wall). At the other extreme is the patient who struggles for weeks or months critically ill with a number of serious complications and who ultimately succumbs. Between these two extremes there is a complete spectrum of various degrees of rehabilitation.

The rate of rehabilitation in one series of recipients of kidneys from living related donors is shown in Figure 15. In this study the quality of rehabilitation was scored on a scale of "1," the patient in hospital or

totally incapacitated at home, to "5," the patient physically unrestricted and working full time in the pre-illness occupation or at an equal or higher level. The 10 patients in *Group I* had HLA identical donors. (The drop in the score of this group near the end of the second year was due to recurrence of original disease in one patient, nodular glomerulonephritis.) The donors for the five patients in *Group II* differed from the recipient at one HLA haplotype, and this haplotype was by test skin grafting shown to be antigenically weak. The 11 patients in *Group III* had parental or sibling donors who did not fulfill the criteria for inclusion in Groups I or II.[31] Similar results have been reported by others.[22, 31]

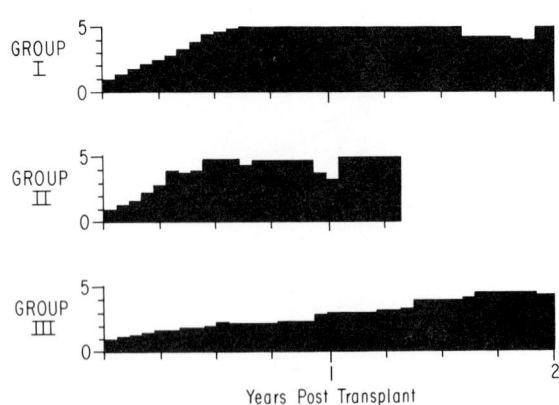

Figure 15. Rehabilitation of renal allograft recipients. Group I: HLA identical donors. Group II: HLA haploidentical donors selected prospectively by test skin grafts which demonstrated a *weak*, one-haplotype difference between donor and recipient. Group III: All other sibling and parental donors who did not meet the criteria for inclusion in Group I or II. See text. (From Stickel, D. L., et al.: Ann. Surg., *172*:160, 1970.)

Some recipients of cadaver kidneys are as well rehabilitated as the best of those whose donors were living and related. Overall, however, there is a considerable difference. Recipients of cadaver kidneys are about twice as likely to be poorly rehabilitated and half as likely to be completely normal as those whose donors were living and related (see ninth report from the Registry, cited in the twelfth report[2]).

SELECTED REFERENCES

Each of these references is an authoritative review, or a report on a rather large series of patients, or both. Numerous publications cited by author's name in the text are omitted from these references and the bibliography. At such points in the text the reader is referred to a publication in which the reference can be readily located. References marked with an asterisk (*) are described at the end of part I of Chapter 22.

1. Belzer, F. O., Kountz, S. L., Najarian, J S., Tanagho, E. A., and Hinman, F., Jr.: Prevention of urological complications after renal allotransplantation. Arch. Surg., 101:449, 1970.
2. Bergan, J. J., and other members of the Registry Advisory Committee: The 12th report of the human renal transplant registry. J.A.M.A., 233:787, 1975. (See also the 9th, 10th, and 11th reports cited in the 12th.)
*3. Calne, R. Y.: Renal Transplantation, 2nd ed. London, Edward Arnold, 1967.
4. Daussett, J., and Hors, J.: Analysis of 221 renal transplants: Influence of cross-reactions between donor and recipient HL-A antigens. Transplant. Proc., 3:1004, 1971.
5. Flanigan, W. J., Caldwell, F. T., Williams, G. D., Brewer, T. E., Glenn, W. E., Headstream, J. W., and Campbell, G. S.: Clinical patterns of renal allograft rejection. Ann. Surg., 173:733, 1971.
6. Hume, D. M.: Kidney transplantation. In Rapaport, F. T., and Dausset, J. (Eds.): Human Transplantation. New York, Grune and Stratton, 1968.
   This is both an exhaustive review of the subject and the report on extensive personal experience of the author who in Boston and in Richmond was for more than 20 years a leader in the development of transplantation both clinically and in the laboratory—prior to his untimely death in 1973.
7. Kountz, S. L., and Belzer, F. L.: The fate of patients after renal transplantation, graft rejection, and re-transplantation. Ann. Surg., 176:509, 1972.
8. Lucas, Z. J., Coplon, N., Kempson, R., and Cohn, R.: Early renal transplant failure associated with subliminal sensitization. Transplantation, 10:522, 1970.
*9. Moore, F. D.: Give and Take: The Development of Tissue Transplantation. Philadelphia, W. B. Saunders Company, 1964.
10. Morris, P. J.: Analysis of histocompatibility in cadaver renal transplantation. Transplant. Proc., 3:1030, 1971.
11. Murray, J. E., Wilson, R. E., Tilney, N. L., Merrill, J. P., Cooper, W. C., Birtch, A. G., Carpenter, C. B., Hager, E. B., Dammin, G. J., and Harrison, J. H.: Five years' experience in renal transplantation with immunosuppressive drugs: Survival, function, complications, and the role of lymphocyte depletion by thoracic duct fistula. Ann. Surg., 168:416, 1968.
12. Najarian, J. S., and Foker, J. E.: Mechanisms of kidney allograft rejection. Transplant. Proc., 1:184, 1969.
13. Porter, K. A.: Morphological aspects of renal homograft rejection. Br. Med. J., 21:171, 1965.
14. Rapaport, F. T., and Dausset, J. (Eds.): Human Transplantation. New York, Grune and Stratton, 1968.
15. Rowlands, D. T., Jr., and Bossen, E. H.: Immunological mechanisms of allograft rejection. Arch. Intern. Med., 123:491, 1969.
16. Salaman, J. R., Caine, R. Y., Pena, J., Sells, R. A., White, J. O., and Yoffa, D.: Surgical aspects of clinical renal transplantation. Br. J. Surg., 56:413, 1969.
17. Simmons, R. L., Kjellstrand, C. M., Buselmeier, T. J. and Najarian, J. S.: Renal transplantation in high-risk patients. Arch. Surg., 103:290, 1971.
18. Starzl, T. E., Groth, C. G., Putnam, C. W., Penn, I., Halgrimson, C. G., Flatmark, A., Gecelter, L., Brettschneider, L., and

Stonington, O. G.: Urological complications in 216 human recipients of renal transplants. Ann. Surg., 172:1, 1970.
19. Starzl, T. E., Porter, K. A., Andres, G., Halgrimson, C. G., Hurwitz, R., Giles, G., Terasaki, P. I., Penn, I., Schroter, G. T., Lilly, J., Starkie, S. J., and Putnam, C. W.: Long-term survival after renal transplantation in humans (with special reference to histocompatibility matching thymectomy, homograft glomerulonephritis, heterologous ALG, and recipient malignancy). Ann. Surg., 172:437, 1970.
20. Strauss, M. B., and Welt, L. G. (Eds.): Diseases of the Kidney, 2nd ed. 2 vol. Boston, Little, Brown and Co., 1971.
21. Weil, R., III, Simmons, R. L., Tallent, M. B., Lillehei, R. C., Kjellstrand, C. M., and Najarian, J. S.: Prevention of urological complications after kidney transplantation. Ann. Surg., 174:154, 1971.
22. Wonham, V. A., Winn, H. J., and Russell, P. S.: Serotyping and genetic analysis in the selection of related renal-allograft donors. N. Eng. J. Med., 284:509, 1971.
*23. Woodruff, M. F. A.: The Transplantation of Tissues and Organs, Springfield, Ill., Charles C Thomas, Publisher, 1960.
24. Woodruff, M. F. A., Nolan, B., Robson, J. S., and MacDonald, M. K.: Renal transplantation in man. Experience in 35 cases. Lancet, 1:6, 1969.

REFERENCES

25. Bennett, W. M., Singer, I., and Coggins, C. H.: A practical guide to drug usage in adult patients with impaired renal function. J.A.M.A., 214:1468, 1970.
26. Bergan, J. J.: Current risks to the kidney transplant donor. Transplant. Proc., 5:1131, 1973.
27. Bergan, J. J., and other members of the Registry Advisory Committee: Renal transplantation in congenital and metabolic diseases. J.A.M.A., 232:148, 1975.
28. Brown, J. H. J.: Anesthesia for renal transplantation, a review. Anesthesiol. Rev., 3:22, 1976.
29. Editorial: New nomenclature for the HLA system. J. Immunol., 116:573, 1976.
30. Freed, S. Z., Veith, F. J., Tellis, V., Whittaker, J., and Gliedman, M. L.: Improved cadaveric nephrectomy for kidney transplantation. Surg. Gynecol. Obstet., 137:101, 1973.
31. Jonasson, O., Lichter, E. A., Hamby, W. M., Smith, R. D., Gantt, C. L., and Nyhus, L. M.: Donor selection for renal transplantation based on genotypic analysis of HLA in a family. Arch. Surg., 101:219, 1970.
32. Kjellstrand, C. M., Shideman, J. R., Simmons, R. L., Buselmeier, T. J., vonHartitzsch, B., Goetz, F. C., and Najarian, J. S.: Renal transplantation in insulin-dependent diabetic patients. Kidney Int., 6:S15, 1974.
33. Lefrak, E. A., and Noon, G. P.: Surgical technique for creation of an arteriovenous fistula using a looped bovine graft. Ann. Surg., 182:782, 1975.
34. Liepman, M.: Disseminated Strongyloides stercoralis, a complication of immunosuppression. J.A.M.A., 231:387, 1975.
35. Pliskin, J. S.: On the probability of finding an HLA- and ABO-compatible cadaver organ for transplantation. Transplantation, 20:181, 1975.
36. Robinson, R. R.: Personal communication.
37. Seigler, H. F., Amos, D. B., Ward, F. E., Andrus, C. H., Southworth, J. G., Hattler, B. G., and Stickel, D. L.: Immunogenetics of consanguineous allografts in man: I. Histocompatibility testing and skin allografts. Ann. Surg., 172:151, 1970.
38. Seigler, H. F., Ward, F. E., McCoy, R. C., Gunnells, J. C., Gutman, R. A., Tisher, C. C., Weinerth, J. L., and Stickel, D. L.: Renal transplantation between HLA haploidentical donor-recipient pairs: Functional and morphological evaluation. Surgery, 79:241, 1976.
39. Seigler, H. F., Ward, F. E., Weinerth, J. L., McCoy, R. E., and Stickel, D. L.: Long term results with 45 living related renal allograft recipients genotypically identical for HLA. Surgery, 1977, in press.
40. Starzl, T. E., Putnam, C. W., Halgrimson, C. G., Groth, C. G., Booth, A. S., and Penn, I. Renal transplantation under cyclophosphamide. Transplant. Proc., 4:461, 1972.
41. Stickel, D. L., Seigler, H. F., Amos, D. B. Ward, F. E., Gunnells, J. C., Jr., Price, A. R., and Anderson, E. E.: Immunogenetics of consanguineous allografts in man: II. Correlation of renal allografting with HL-A genotyping. Ann. Surg., 172:160, 1970.

42. Torisu, M., Yokoyama, T., Amemiya, H., Kohler, P. F., Schroter, G., Martineau, G., Penn, I., Palmer, W., Halgrimson, C. G., Putnam, C. W., and Starzl, T. E.: Immunosuppression, liver injury, and hepatitis in renal, hepatic, and cardiac homograft recipients: With particular reference to the Australia antigen. Ann. Surg., *174*:620, 1971.

43. van Rood, J. J., van Leeuwen, A., Termijtelin, A., and Keuning, J. J.: The genetics of the major histocompatibility complex in man, HLA. *In* Katz, D. H., and Benacerof, B. (Eds.): The Role

and Products of the Histocompatibility Gene Complex in Immune Responses. New York, Academic Press, 1976.

44. Wells, S. A., Gunnells, J. C., Shelburne, J. D., Schneider, A. B., and Sherwood, L. M.: Transplantation of the parathyroid glands in man: Clinical indications and results. Surgery, *78*:34, 1975.

45. Williams, P. L., Williams, M. A., Kountz, S. L., and Dempster, W. J.: Ultrastructural and Haemodynamic studies in canine renal transplants. J. Anat., *98*:549, 1964.

IV

PRINCIPLES OF IMMUNOSUPPRESSION

John E. Foker, M.D., Ph.D., Richard L. Simmons, M.D., and John S. Najarian, M.D.

Clinical transplantation is becoming more beneficial to a wider range of patients. Kidney transplantation, for example, is now superior to chronic hemodialysis therapy for most patients with end-stage renal failure. More limited gains have also been made in heart, bone marrow, liver, and pancreatic islet cell transplantation. The technical ability to transplant these organs exists, so success depends on the ability to inhibit the normal rejection of foreign tissue. Although clinical immunosuppression cannot yet produce complete tolerance to a graft, many transplanted kidneys have functioned for as long as 10 years. Furthermore, immunosuppressive drugs are also used to treat certain diseases that involve immune reactions against the patient's own tissues. The principles of treatment for both graft survival and suppression of autoimmune diseases are similar, and they will be better understood by considering the mechanisms of the immune response.

THE SMALL LYMPHOCYTE

The small lymphocyte is the heart of the immune system. This cell can recognize foreign antigens and effectively decides whether a molecule or another cell belongs or is alien. By virtue of the great specificity in such recognition, self and non-self are judged accurately. The recognition of a foreign antigen stimulates the resting small lymphocyte to transform into a large active cell. This begins the many cellular and subcellular events that make up the immune response. Individual lymphocytes probably can recognize only one or a few closely related antigens. Consequently, early in the immune development of the individual, groups or clones of lymphocytes are formed that have rather discrete target specificities. The range of possible antigenic configurations is, therefore, matched by a panoply of lymphocyte clones arrayed against them.

It is not known how immune specificity is acquired during development, but small lymphocytes are fully competent cells that are resting and waiting to respond to an antigen (Fig. 1).

For the immunologically competent patient, the encounter between lymphocyte and antigen is most critical and marks the apparent beginning of an active immune response to an antigen. There are several functional subgroups of lymphocytes, so the circumstances and the consequences of the encounter between cell and antigen will vary. Nevertheless, lymphocyte activation is necessary to initiate the immune response and is the phase most susceptible to inhibition.

For the transplant patient, the lymphocyte-antigen encounter is the first point of possible immunosuppressive attack. The earlier developmental steps leading to the small lymphocyte have taken place and are no longer vulnerable. By birth the individual has full immunologic competence and has clearly defined self. The peripheral lymphoid tissues are established, and maturation can no longer be successfully impeded. This is an oversimplification, because cellular renewal takes place and opens the possibility of blocking an earlier maturational step. What step this might be, however, remains unknown and awaits a better understanding of lymphocyte development and replenishment.

Immunosuppression is less effective after the lymphocyte has responded to the antigen. The immune response is far more difficult to control after it has been fully activated. Specific agents such as preformed antibodies, activated killer lymphocytes, and antibody-armed macrophages, as well as nonspecific effectors like platelets, neutrophils, complement, and coagulation factors, are difficult to suppress. More importantly, many cells and molecules are involved, and the suppression of only one or two is ineffective. Consequently, clinical immunosuppression at present

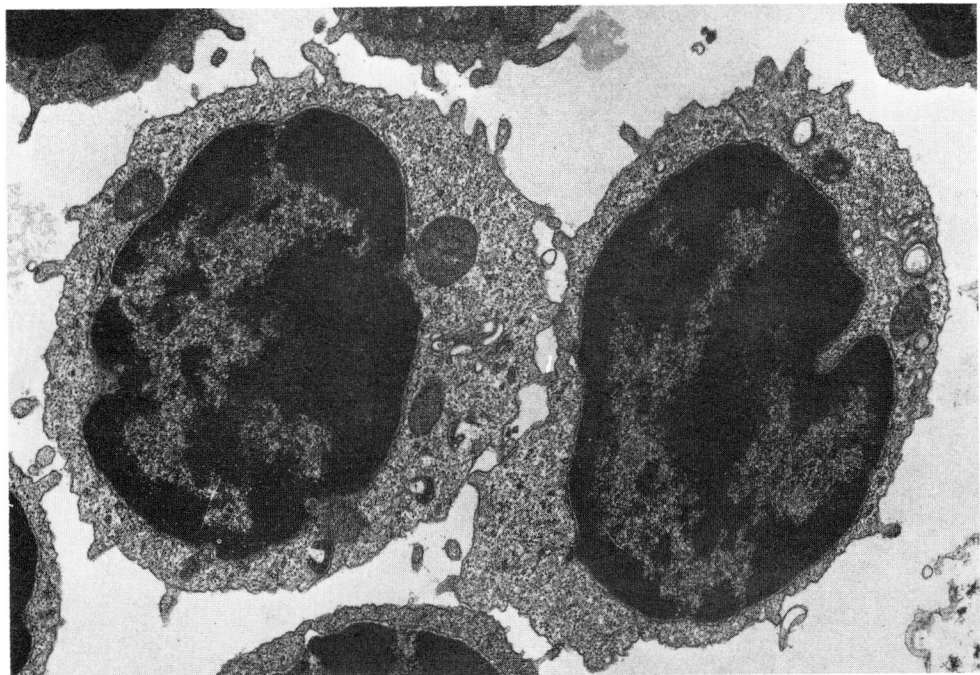

Figure 1. The morphology of these mouse small lymphocytes is typical of mammalian peripheral small lymphocytes from the blood, thoracic duct, lymph nodes, or spleen. The dense, inactive nucleus occupies much of the intracellular volume. The rim of cytoplasm contains ribosomes, a few inclusion bodies, and occasional mitochondria. The small lymphocytes are resting cells, awaiting immunological stimulation that will transform them into large active cells (×12,000).

relies on two general modes of action. The first is simply to reduce the peripheral lymphocyte population by nonspecific methods, and the second is to interfere with the subcellular response of the small lymphocyte to an antigen. The success of organ transplantation is mainly a result of the ability to inhibit the response of the small lymphocyte to the graft. In spite of the present benefit to patients, the full promise of transplantation will not be fulfilled until graft rejection can be specifically prevented while maintaining the integrity of the remaining immune system. Recipient tolerance of the transplanted organ without general immunosuppression is the ultimate goal. This too will probably be accomplished at the level of antigen-lymphocyte interaction.

THE ORIGINS OF THE SMALL LYMPHOCYTE

As a fuller understanding of the immune response is gained, it is easier to appreciate the difficulty of achieving effective immunosuppression. A review of the mechanisms involved will illustrate this difficulty and provide more understanding of the principles of immunosuppression. It will also reveal the considerable potential that exists for the development of other modes of inhibition, such as the induction of specific tolerance.

The origin of the immune system can be traced to a single hematopoietic stem cell in the extraembryonic yolk sac (Fig. 2). The stem cells multiply and migrate to various centers, including the fetal liver and bone marrow, for further differentiation. Within these centers, progenitor cells for erythrocytes, eosinophils, basophils, neutrophils, and lymphoid cells arise. The local microchemical environment determines which lines of cells will develop. Further proliferation of these progenitor stem cells probably depends on the action of hormones, which expand the population of specialized cells much like erythropoietin expands the erythrocyte line.

Following proliferation of the early stem cells, the lymphoid cell line next appears within two primary (or central) lymphoid organs. The epithelial cells of these organs further expand the cell populations and govern the eventual development of the peripheral small lymphocytes. The thymus is the primary organ where a lymphocyte subpopulation, called T lymphocytes, is matured and released to stock the peripheral lymphoid tissues. The second subpopulation that descends from the stem cells is the B cell line. The primary lymphoid organ that produces B cells in mammals is unknown, but in birds it is the bursa of Fabricius. Recent evidence suggests that the fetal liver may be the bursal equivalent in mammals. The bone marrow also serves as a source of predifferentiated B cells, although it is probably not the central origin of the B cell line.

The functional difference between T and B cells is considerable; most simply, T cells produce direct cell-to-cell immune damage, whereas B cells synthesize antibody. In actuality the differences are more com-

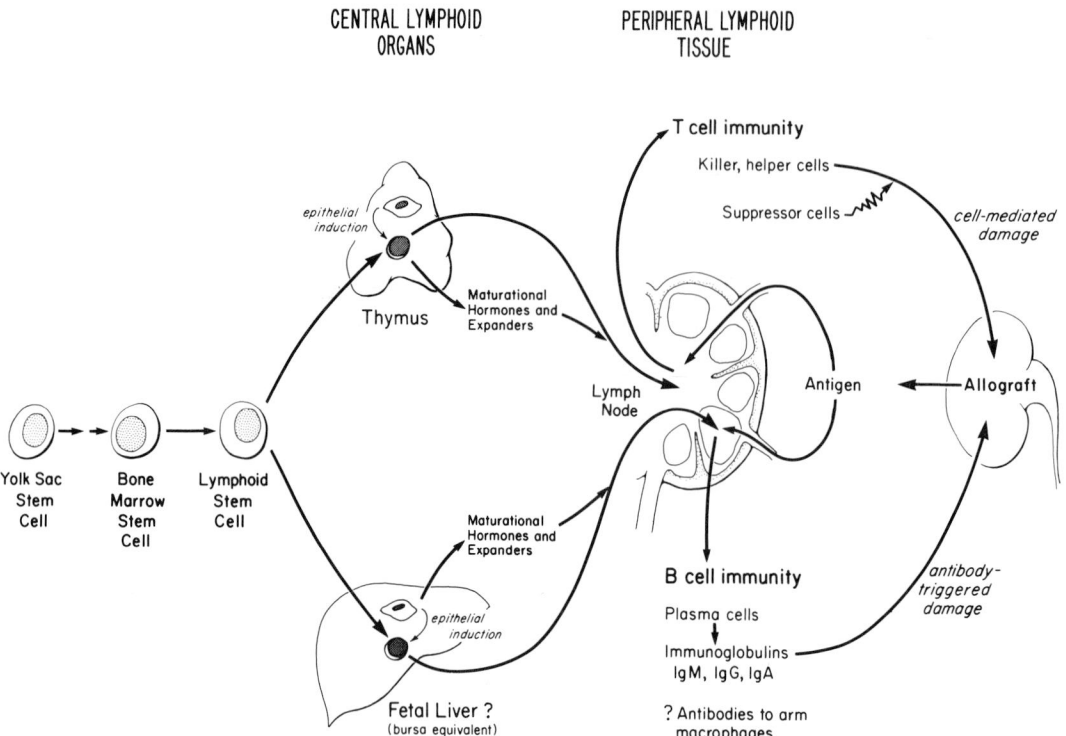

Figure 2. The extraordinarily complex developmental sequences of the immune system are encapsulated in this diagram. Certain of the known inducers, expanders, growth factors, and sites of maturation needed to establish the T and B cell lines are presented. Much of this takes place before birth, so transplant recipients are fully competent with established peripheral lymphoid populations in the lymph nodes, Peyer's patches, and spleen. Therefore, clinical immunosuppression consists principally of lymphocyte depletion and inhibition of the activation of antigen-stimulated lymphocytes.

plex. Both T and B cells have subpopulations with different immunologic activities and varying degrees of cooperation with other lymphocyte subgroups. The complexity of their behavior often blurs the distinction between T and B cells. Evidence for the existence of the T and B cells in human beings is based in part on the functional states that characterize congenital immunodeficiency diseases. The sex-linked agammaglobulinemia of the Bruton type, for example, is characterized by low levels of immunoglobulins, an absence of B cells in lymphoid tissues, and normal direct lymphocyte reactivity, all of which suggests that the bursal equivalent has failed to develop. Patients with Swiss type immunodeficiency, in contrast, have an absence of T cells and cell-mediated sensitivity; immunoglobulins are present, although depressed. Similar diseases can be produced experimentally. Neonatal bursectomy in chickens leads to agammaglobulinemia. Thymectomy in the newborn period, before the T cell populations are established in the outlying tissues, will produce a selective T cell deficiency state in a variety of animals.

The central lymphoid tissues are responsible for the development of peripheral lymphoid tissues, e.g., spleen, lymph nodes, Peyer's patches. Early in development, the thymus is the site of vigorous cell proliferation, and many of these cells migrate to the paracortical and medullary areas of lymph nodes. Other lymphocytes pass through the thymus and acquire T

cell characteristics during their temporary residence. How many T cells arise in the thymus and how many are simply matured there is unknown, but after T cells have migrated from the thymus they seldom return. There is evidence that the thymus produces a hormone-like substance (thymosin) that is necessary for the maintenance of the full functional capacity of the peripheral T cell system. These migrations and maturational events occur *in utero,* and humans are fully immunocompetent for T cell function before birth. The thymus begins to atrophy before puberty, but T cell function is by then well established in the periphery and will maintain itself. Only slight deterioration comes with age.

There are definite locations for T and B cells within the peripheral lymphoid tissues. The antibody-producing B cells reside in the germinal centers and medullary cords of the peripheral lymphoid tissues while the T cells populate mainly the deep cortical areas. The ontogeny of B cell immunocompetence in mammals is poorly understood, but their central lymphoid organ is probably the fetal liver. A humoral factor, similar to that secreted by the thymus, may be at work maturing and maintaining the population of immunocompetent B cells.

There is a behavioral difference between B and T cells that reflects their functional abilities. B cells are relatively sessile within the lymph nodes and the spleen, but the antibodies they secrete are mobile and able to interact with foreign antigens at distant sites. The T cells responsible for cell-mediated immunity are of necessity more peripatetic and must migrate to the periphery to neutralize foreign antigens. From the peripheral blood, T cells enter the lymph nodes or spleen via highly specialized regions in the postcapillary venules. The T cells then percolate through the lymphoid organs, enter the lymph, pass into the thoracic duct, and return to the bloodstream to begin circulating again in quest of an antigen. When an organ is transplanted into a patient, activation of both T and B cells occurs in the lymph nodes, which filter out graft antigens. Some transformation may also occur within the graft by circulating T lymphocytes enticed to remain there. The result is an assault on the graft by a variety of sensitized cells and antibodies.

Cell-to-Cell Interactions

The previous discussion barely hints at the intricacy of the ontogeny of the immune system. Once confronted with an antigen the response of the lymphocytes is equally complex. One facet of this complexity involves the cell-to-cell interactions that are required to produce the immune response. The number and dimensions of these cellular relationships remain unknown, but the evidence indicates that several exist. We have already mentioned the lymphocyte-epithelial cooperation that is important for the induction of lymphoid tissue differentiation and development in the thymus and bursa. How many more interactions are required to produce the many clones of small lymphocytes is completely unknown. Even after the immune system has completely developed and is fully competent, additional interactions are apparently necessary for the full expression of specific immunity.

Cellular cooperation of more than one kind may be required in the activation of the small lymphocytes by antigens. The reticular cells in the cortical area of the lymph node seem to bind antigens on their surface and retain them in an exposed position, which facilitates recognition by lymphocytes. Certain complex antigens, however, may first need to be partially digested by phagocytic cells before the antigenic information can be transferred to the lymphocyte. The nature of the transferred material is unclear, but most simply it would be the antigen itself. Some evidence indicates that the macrophage may produce an RNA molecule, with or without a portion of the antigen attached to it, which activates the lymphocyte. How much these mechanisms contribute to the development of transplantation immunity is unknown, but antigen processing is only one of the points in the initiation of the immune response where cell-to-cell interactions take place.

Even the recognition of foreign cells is a complex process. One group of antigens on the surface of the graft cells stimulates certain T cells to divide. There is evidence, however, that the proliferating cells do not destroy the graft. Rather, they may induce immunity in another group of T cells, which damage the foreign cells. The T cell immunity that develops, moreover, is expressed against another group of genetically linked cellular antigens. The first group of T cells has been called "helper" cells because their proliferative re-

sponse is necessary for the development of "killer" activity in a less frequently dividing T cell population. The details of the antigens involved are beyond the scope of this discussion, but it would seem that T-to-T cell interactions are among the kinds of cellular cooperation required to develop transplantation immunity (Fig. 3).

Not only do certain T cells augment the response of other T cells, but another type seems able to suppress the development of immunity. This third type of T cell, the suppressor cell, probably helps regulate the immune response and prevent an overreaction to a given immunologic stimulus. Suppressor cells are currently the subject of much investigation. Lymphocytes that apparently suppress antibody production have been generated experimentally, both in vitro and in vivo. If suppressor cells are able to inhibit the development of allograft immunity, it may open an avenue of promise for transplantation. The ability to stimulate an abundance of suppressor lymphocytes may be a way to produce effective immunosuppression without toxicity.

Although we have presented the T and B cell systems as independent of each other, they cooperate to enhance immunity against a specific antigen. Most transplantation antigens seem to be recognized by T cells, which can, of course, develop cellular immunity against them. In addition, helper T cells seem to enlist B cells to produce specific antibody against the graft antigens. It is unknown whether this is carried out by a specific subcategory of T cells or by those that help develop cellular immunity. Finally, as mentioned, T cells also act as suppressors for antibody formation. But this does not end the interactions—after immunity has been acquired, additional cellular cooperation

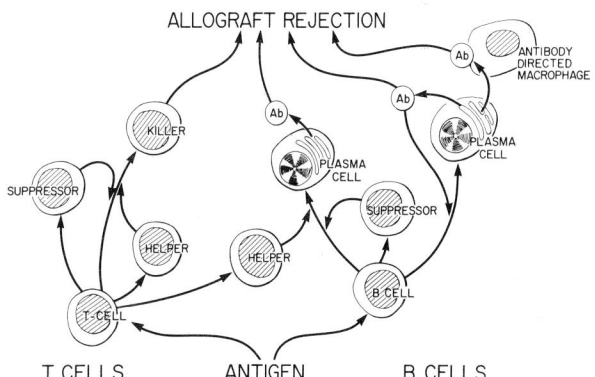

Figure 3. A diagrammatic portrayal of some of the many cellular interactions that take place during the development of allograft immunity. Antigen initiates the response in both T and B cells. Certain allograft antigens appear to be recognized mainly by T cells, which then act as helper cells to aid the response of both B and T cells. The immunologically specific agents of allograft damage include killer T cells, antibody molecules, and activated macrophages and lymphocytes given specificity by absorbed antibodies. Suppressor cells and antibody molecules modulate these pathways and provide a feedback inhibition of the immune response. The origins of the suppressor cells have not been clearly defined, but most seem to be from the T cell line.

contributes to the destruction of the graft. These interactions will take place during rejection.

Most of the various T and B cell interactions discussed so far have been uncovered relatively recently, and the significance for graft rejection has not been determined. As yet no method has been found that will specifically and effectively interfere with them and the development of transplantation immunity. Clinical immunosuppression at this time, therefore, depends on daily interference with the subcellular events in lymphocyte metabolism.

Subcellular Events

Mature small lymphocytes, whether T or B cells, appear to be in a resting, but immunologically ready, state. Antigenic stimulation of a clone of cells triggers a remarkable cellular transformation. Gene activation is followed by a prompt increase in RNA and protein synthesis. A host of membrane, cytoplasmic, and nuclear changes are included in the many subcellular events that occur within the first two hours. Over the suceeding hours the small lymphocyte transforms into a large, active cell, bulging with polysomes and organelles (Fig. 4). Included in the activation are the complex cellular changes of further differentiation and eventually division. Not only do these cells become activated and increasingly immunocompetent, but they also enter a proliferative cycle. It is during cell proliferation that the lymphocyte becomes most vulnerable to several of the commonly used immunosuppressive agents.

As lymphocytes transform from resting to dividing cells, they pass through distinct phases common to all cells (Fig. 5). Although the present subdivisions of the cell cycle are oversimplified, it has been found that susceptibility to the commonly used immunosuppressive agents varies over the different phases. The small lymphocyte is in a resting or G_0 phase. Antigenic stimulation activates the cell and moves it into the first gap or phase (G_1) of the proliferative cycle. The complex G_1 phase contains the commitment to cell division, but whether this occurs early or late in G_1 is unknown. After the cell becomes committed to divide, DNA synthesis (S phase) will occur. The gap (G_2) between the S phase and the final mitosis (M phase) is relatively short. After mitosis has occurred, the cells enter into the G_1 phase again and the cell cycle is complete.

Differentiation appears to progress with cell division and, with each successive cycle, the cells become more and more capable of eliminating the activating antigen. After successive divisions, B cells become plasma cells, which are the most efficient producers of specific antibody. A similar progression probably

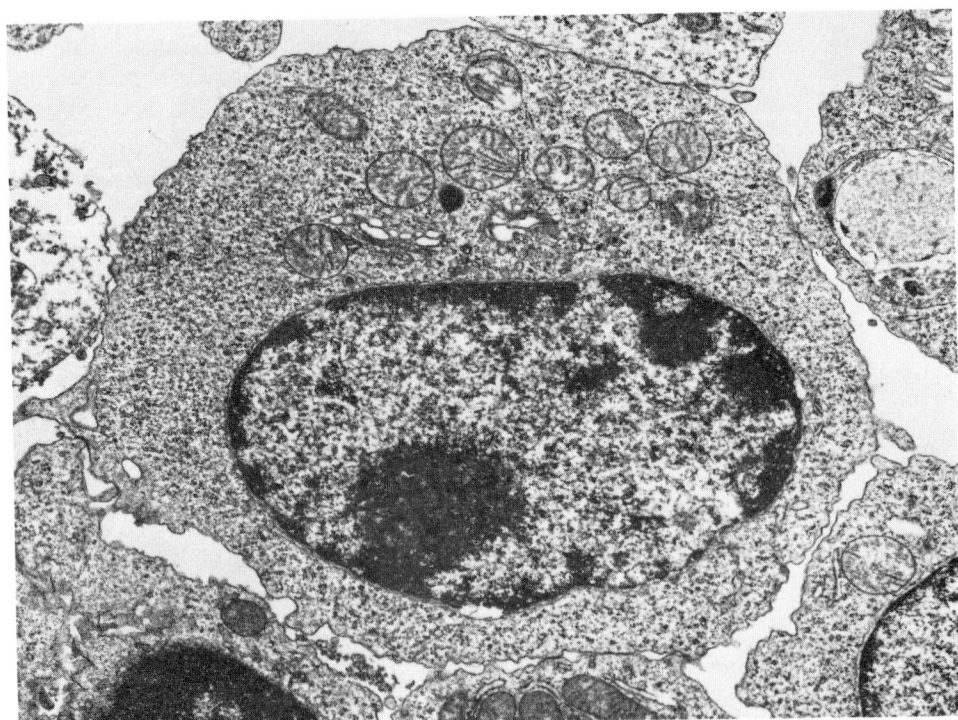

Figure 4. The transformed lymphocyte, 24 hours after stimulation, is a much larger, more active cell. The open nucleus is the site of increased RNA synthesis, and the enlarged cytoplasm contains abundant polysomes and mitochondria. Many subcellular changes take place in the conversion from resting to active lymphocytes. These biosynthetic events are vulnerable to the antimetabolites used to prevent allograft rejection. In addition, these cells begin to synthesize DNA at this time, increasing their susceptibility to antimetabolites, alkylating agents, and radiation (×12,000).

Lymphocyte Cell Cycle

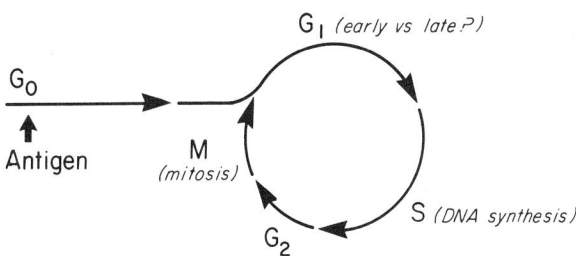

Figure 5. The phases of the cell cycle are depicted in this diagram. Following stimulation by an antigen, or other type of mitogen, small lymphocytes are activated. They are converted from the resting G_0 phase to the active G_1 phase. The G_1 phase lasts 10 hours or longer before DNA synthesis (S phase) begins. The S phase lasts about 10 hours and is followed by a short (2 to 4 hours) G_2 phase before mitosis (M phase). M phase is relatively brief, usually less than 2 to 3 hours, after which the cells are returned to the G_1 phase. The susceptibility of the cell to the immunosuppressive agents used in transplantation varies with the phase of the cycle. Periods of most intense nucleic acid synthesis, particularly S phase, are most vulnerable to the antimetabolites. As discussed in the text, the resting, G_0, lymphocyte is also susceptible to several of the clinically used immunosuppressive agents.

occurs among T cells, although the relationship between proliferation and differentiation in these cells is unclear at this time.

Much of the susceptibility of lymphocytes to immunosuppression results from the vast cellular changes that follow immune stimulation. The many biosynthetic events that take place make the lymphocytes vulnerable to the mistakes and inhibitions caused by the structural analogues, antimetabolites. Alkylating agents and radiation, although they do not depend on deception, produce cross-linkages and breaks in DNA strands, which interfere with cell differentiation and division. The subcellular actions of steroids are also complex. The actions of the individual immunosuppressive agents will be discussed in more detail in subsequent sections. The inhibitory effects of these agents, with the principal exception of antilymphocyte serum, are not specific for lymphocytes, and similar consequences can be expected for other differentiating and dividing cells.

GRAFT REJECTION

Graft rejection results from the participation of various combinations of immunologically specific and nonspecific cells. Immune T cells are a significant, or even major, cause of graft rejection, and they accomplish it in several ways. T cells can (a) be directly cytotoxic to graft cells, (b) help B cells produce antigraft antibody, and (c) enlist destructive activated macrophages. For their part, B cells produce antigraft antibodies that attach to the graft cells. Damage results from the activation of the complement, coagulation, and kinin pathways triggered by the antigen-antibody

combination. Vasoactive peptides, chemotactic factors, and thrombus formation then directly produce the damage. Neutrophils, platelets, and macrophages are called to the scene and release their many proteolytic enzymes. Furthermore, it has recently been found that certain antibodies will attach to other lymphocytes and macrophages, converting them to cells specifically active against the graft. Direct cell-to-cell toxicity results, but the importance of these armed cells to allograft destruction is not yet known.

The preceding abbreviated description of the development of allograft immunity, nevertheless, reveals many potentially vulnerable sites. Theoretically, the immune response can be suppressed in many ways, by (a) destroying the immunocompetent cells prior to transplantation, (b) making the antigen unrecognizable or even toxic to the reactive lymphocyte clones, (c) interfering with antigen processing by the recipient cells, (d) inhibiting lymphocyte transformation and proliferation, (e) limiting lymphocyte differentiation to killer or antibody synthesizing cells, (f) activating sufficient numbers of suppressor lymphocytes, (g) inhibiting destruction of graft cells by killer lymphocytes, (h) interfering with the combination of immunoglobulins with target antigens, or (i) preventing tissue damage by the nonspecific cells and molecules that are activated by sensitized cells or antigen-antibody complexes.

In fact, clinically useful immunosuppression largely depends on the destruction or elimination of the immunocompetent cells and on inhibiting the differentiation and proliferation of these cells. Methods of inducing specific immune tolerance by various antigen preparations prior to grafting, or by inhibiting sensitized cells and antibodies once they have been produced, have not been clinically successful. Furthermore, it is more difficult to inhibit the immune response after it is underway, and less clinical effect can be gained after sensitization has occurred. To be most effective, immunosuppression must be present at the time of transplantation, or even before. Nevertheless, some success can be achieved in reversing the exacerbations of the rejection reaction seen in clinical transplantation. Lesser but still significant benefits have even resulted from inhibiting such immunologically nonspecific cells as platelets.

METHODS OF IMMUNOSUPPRESSION

The true complexity of immune rejection is only beginning to be revealed, but many potential points for inhibition have already been exposed. At this time, however, a similar complexity does not exist in clinical immunosuppression. Virtually all clinical transplantation immunosuppression regimens include azathioprine, steroids, radiation, and antilymphocyte antibodies. Agents that are occasionally used or are purely experimental will be presented more briefly.

Clinical Immunosuppression

Antiproliferative Agents. Most of the commonly used immunosuppressive agents, including antimetabolites, alkylating agents, toxic antibiotics, and x-rays, have been borrowed from cancer chemotherapy for their antiproliferative activity. They inhibit the full expression of the immune response by preventing the differentiation and division of the immunocompetent lymphocyte after it encounters the antigen. The plethora of investigational immunosuppressive drugs has been reduced to a few for clinical use. All of them, however, fall into one of two broad mechanistic categories. Either they structurally resemble needed metabolites or they combine with certain cellular components, such as DNA, and thereby interfere with function. The former group, the antimetabolites, have a structural similarity to cell metabolites and either inhibit enzymes of that metabolic pathway or are incorporated during synthesis to produce faulty molecules.

The antimetabolites include purine, pyrimidine, and folic acid analogues that are most effective against proliferating and differentiating cells. They are given at the time of transplantation when the immunocompetent cells are first stimulated, and then for the life of the graft to interfere with the continuing stimulus to the immune system.

Alkylating agents and certain antibiotics include those compounds that combine with DNA and other cellular components. Although these agents would be useful in the pretransplant period to reduce the number of effective immunocompetent cells in the recipients, and thereafter to prevent proliferation, they are so toxic that their use has been limited to bone marrow transplantation and as occasional substitutes for azathioprine.

Purine Analogues. The purine analogue azathioprine (AZ) (Imuran) is the most widely used immunosuppressive drug in clinical organ transplantation. Azathioprine is 6-mercaptopurine (6-MP) plus a side chain to protect the labile sulfhydryl group. In the liver, the side chain is split off to form the active compound, 6-MP. The mechanism of action would seem to be similar for these two compounds; however, azathioprine seems to enjoy the advantage of slightly lower toxicity.

Full metabolic activity comes in the cell with the addition of ribose-5 phosphate from phosphoribosyl pyrophosphate to form 6-MP ribonucleotide. The structural resemblance of this molecule to inosine monophosphate is obvious, and 6-MP ribonucleotide inhibits the enzymes that begin to convert inosine nucleotide to adenosine and guanosine monophosphate (Fig. 6). In addition, the presence of 6-MP ribonucleotides slows the entire purine biosynthetic pathway by fraudulent feedback inhibition of an early step. The steric similarity to either adenosine or guanine nucleotides is not great enough to allow significant incorporation into DNA or RNA and synthesis of faulty molecules. The result of inhibiting these several enzymes, however, is to block the synthesis of cellular RNA, DNA, certain co-factors, and other active nucleotides.

The biologic activity of azathioprine and 6-MP is greatest when nucleic acid synthesis is most required. They will inhibit the development of both humoral and cellular primary immunity by interfering with the differentiation and proliferation of the responding lymphocytes. The inhibition of nucleic acid synthesis by azathioprine is most effective in these rapidly replicating cells. Once expansion of fully immunocompetent cells has been completed, nucleic acid synthesis is less important and the drug is less effective. The benefit of azathioprine may also result from a reduction of neutrophil production and macrophage activation. These effects would reduce the nonspecific inflammatory aspect of the immune reaction.

The toxicity of azathioprine results from the same mechanisms. The primary toxic effect of azathioprine is bone marrow suppression, leading to leukopenia. Again, it is the antiproliferative effect of inhibiting nucleic acid synthesis that affects this rapidly dividing cell population. Liver toxicity can also result, possibly because of the high rate of RNA synthesis by these cells, but because hepatic dysfunction does not seem to be dose related, the mechanism is unclear. Pancreatitis also occasionally occurs for unknown reasons.

Pyrimidine Analogues. Although pyrimidine analogues have been studied extensively as immunosuppressants in the laboratory, they have had only limited clinical use. The structure of 5-bromodeoxyuridine resembles thymidine, and it is incorporated into DNA (Fig. 7). Once incorporated, however, it does not have the precision in base pairing that thymidine has, and subsequent synthesis of DNA and RNA is defective. Although 5-bromodeoxyuridine will

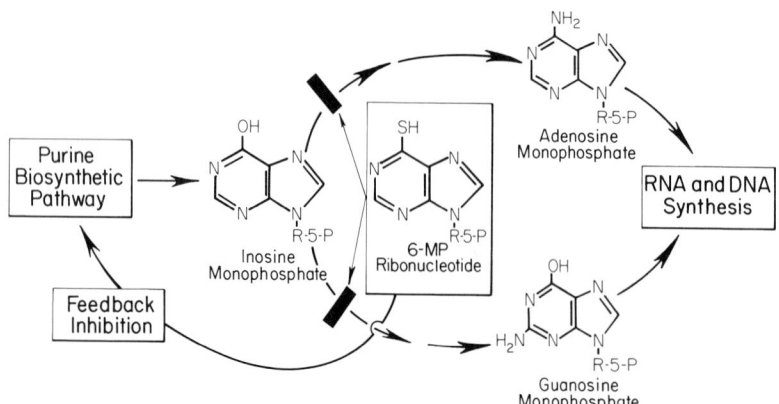

Figure 6. The mechanisms of action of the antimetabolites 6-mercaptopurine (6-MP) and azathioprine are similar. These molecules are converted in the cell to 6-MP ribonucleotide, which resembles inosine ribonucleotide in its steric configuration. Consequently, there is competition between these molecules in the pathways to adenosine monophosphate and guanosine monophosphate. Although 6-MP ribonucleotide is not extensively incorporated, it effectively inhibits the enzymes of these pathways, which reduces the precursors available for incorporation into RNA and DNA. In addition, 6-MP slows the purine biosynthetic pathway by feedback inhibition. The net effect of 6-MP and azathioprine is to greately reduce DNA and RNA synthesis by their competitive activity.

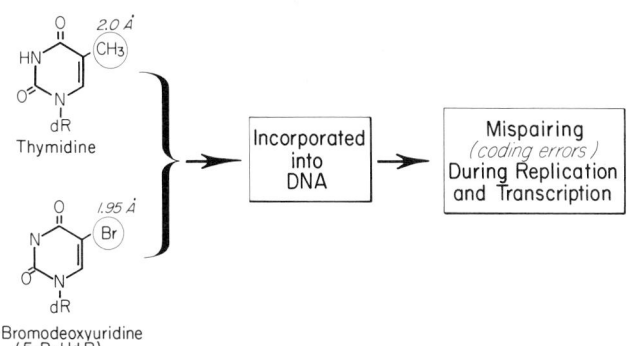

Figure 7. The mechanism of action of the antimetabolite 5-bromodeoxyuridine (5-BrUdR) results from its steric resemblance to thymidine. The bromine atom is similar in size to the methyl group and 5-BrUdR, therefore, competes with thymidine for incorporation into DNA. The incorporated 5-BrUdR does not have the same precision in subsequent base pairing, however, and DNA and RNA synthesis is faulty.

prolong animal skin grafts and act in synergy with antilymphocyte globulin, its use is experimental.

Another pyrimidine analogue, cytosine arabinoside, also inhibits DNA synthesis and, therefore, the proliferative phase of the immune response. This molecule has an altered sugar moiety and is confused with cytosine riboside. Experimentally, the immunosuppressive effect of cytosine arabinoside has been more easily demonstrated in primary humoral antibody responses than in cell-mediated reactions. Clinically it is used to prepare leukemic recipients for eventual bone marrow transplantation. With more experience this agent may become more widely employed.

Folic Acid Antagonist. The immunosuppressive effect of a diet deficient in pteroylglutamic acid was orginally noted by Little and set the stage for the use of the folic acid antagonists, aminopterin and methotrexate. Both drugs inhibit the enzyme dihydrofolate reductase and prevent the conversion of folic acid to tetrahydrofolic acid. This step is necessary for the synthesis of DNA, RNA, and certain coenzymes. Again, proliferating cell systems are most affected.

Some of the toxicity of aminopterin and methotrexate can be abrogated by the administration of folinic acid some hours or even days after the use of the antagonist. Nevertheless, the ratio of immunosuppression to toxicity has not justified their use in clinical kidney transplantation. The immune reactions that accompany bone marrow transplantation are more difficult to control, and methotrexate is used to both prevent and reverse the severe graft-versus-host reactions that occur. Methotrexate is usually used with one or more other drugs, so the toxic effects of methotrexate can be difficult to identify. Megaloblastic hematopoeisis, mucosal breakdown with severe gastrointestinal bleeding, and liver damage seem to be related to methotrexate therapy. These effects, even with high dosages of methotrexate, can usually be prevented by folinic acid (citrovorum rescue). Obviously, depression of the transplanted marrow may also result from the activity of methotrexate, although assigning the cause may be difficult in the complex clinical situation.

Alkylating Agents. The alkylating agents have highly reactive rings as part of the molecular structure. These unstable rings have electron-seeking points that combine with electron-rich nucleophilic groups such as the tertiary nitrogens in purines and pyrimidines, or with $-NH_2$, $-COOH$, $-SH$, and $-PO_3H_2$ groups on a variety of molecules. The high-energy rings of alkylating agents break and combine with these constituents to form stable covalent bonds. Obviously, many cell components have such groups, including DNA, RNA, and the enzymatic and structural proteins. Alkylation of DNA is probably the most detrimental. If the DNA strands are not repaired, chromosomal replication will be faulty in proliferating cells. Both DNA and RNA can be alkylated at several points, but a common site appears to be N-7 of the quanine ring (Fig. 8). Mispairing of DNA during replication may result from the presence of the alkylating agent itself, the clipping out of the alkylated quanine residue, or the cleavage of an alkylated quanine ring. Also, chain breaks and cross-linkages frequently interfere with chain replication.

The damage to DNA can be repaired, so these effects are apparently time-dependent. Consequently, the administration of alkylating agents just before and during stimulation by the antigen would most interfere with the ability of the immunocompetent cells to respond to that antigen. Continued use of the alkylating agents would also muffle the proliferative response of these cells in the face of a persistent stimulus. There are differences, however, in the response of T and B cells. The B cell seems to be more susceptible to cyclophosphamide than the T cell. This drug is a potent inhibitor of antibody formation, but its effect on skin or kidney rejection is much less spectacular. The reason for this apparent difference is unknown.

The usefulness of alkylating agents, which include nitrogen mustard, phenylalanine mustard, busulphan, and cyclophosphamide is limited by their toxicity. Even so, cyclophosphamide has been used with good results in renal transplantation when liver toxicity prohibited the use of azathioprine. Cyclophosphamide is frequently used in clinical bone marrow transplantation, where it potentiates the effects of radiation and enhances the disruption of DNA. When cyclophosphamide is used, lower doses of radiation are required to deplete the recipient bone marrow population and provide space for donor cells. When leukemia is the indication for bone marrow transplantation, cyclophosphamide will aid in the destruction of these cells.

Toxicity is high, however, and predictable reactions

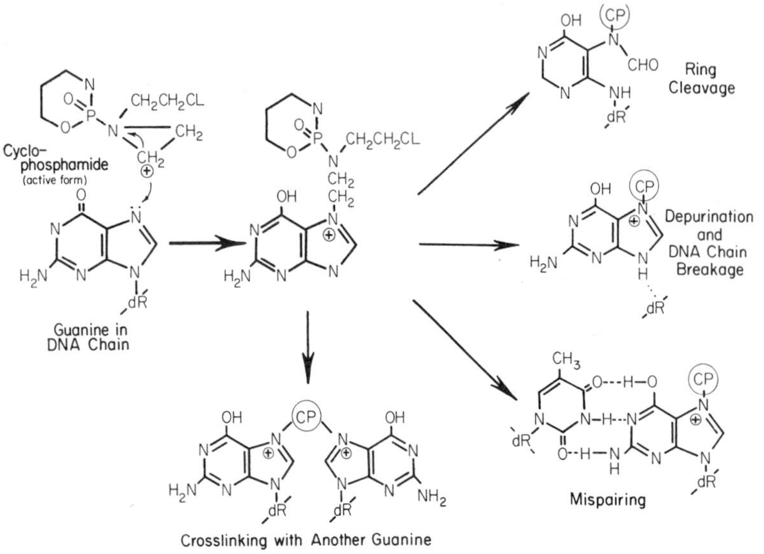

Figure 8. The alkylating agents have reactive rings that can combine with electron-rich points of a variety of molecules. The effect of the alkylating agents seems to be related to its DNA binding. Cyclophosphamide (CP), as an example, binds extensively to guanine molecules within the DNA chain. The guanine-CP complex has several possible consequences for the DNA strand. The ultimate effect of the four examples shown is to interfere with accurate base pairing and DNA replication.

occur, principally to rapidly replicating cell populations. Stomatitis, nausea, vomiting, diarrhea, skin rash, anemia, and alopecia are all common reactions. The more specific effects of cyclophosphamide administration are prompt fluid retention, occasionally severe hemorrhagic cystitis, and cardiac toxicity. The cardiac and edema problems suggest that even nonreplicating cell populations are adversely affected by this drug.

Antibiotics. The immunosuppressive antibiotics include the inhibitors of nucleic acid synthesis, and chloramphenicol and puromycin, which interfere with cellular protein synthesis. Actinomycin D binds to the guanine residue of DNA, thereby sterically interfering with RNA polymerase and, consequently, DNA-directed RNA synthesis. This potentially effective means of suppressing the development of immunity led to its use in reversing acute rejection of kidney grafts. The toxicity of actinomycin D has limited the overall clinical benefit, however, and it has been used less and less frequently.

Mitomycin C combines with cellular DNA and hinders replication. This compound would also be useful in inhibiting allograft immunity, but its toxicity has precluded clinical use. Mitomycin C, nevertheless, does contribute to clinical transplantation through the mixed lymphocyte reaction. In this laboratory test, the reactivity of recipient lymphocytes toward the cells of potential donors is measured. This determination will probably become increasingly important to the assessment of tissue matches prior to transplantation. The test is easiest to interpret when only the recipient lymphocytes can react. Pretreatment of the donor cells with mitomycin C blocks their replication, and only the recipient lymphocytes can respond. The reactivity of the recipient lymphocytes is usually measured by the incorporation of tritiated thymidine into DNA synthesis.

Both puromycin and chloramphenicol inhibit protein synthesis, and both can be immunosuppressive.

Puromycin structurally resembles an amino acid–charged transfer RNA molecule and is accepted into the ribosome. There is no amino acid to be donated, however, and the peptide chain is prematurely terminated. Although protein synthesis is obviously central to immunologic expression, it is so general a requirement for other cells that inhibition, and hence toxicity, will be widespread. Chloramphenicol has also been investigated experimentally. It is most potent in prokaryotic (bacterial) cell systems, and its effects on mammalian cells may be due to inhibiting mitochrondrial synthesis. Unfortunately, it is only weakly immunosuppressive and its potentially severe bone marrow toxicity precludes its use.

In general, only the antibiotic agents that are S phase specific and primarily affect DNA synthesis can be expected to be clinically successful. Inhibition would be concentrated on dividing cell populations, and generalized toxicity would be less likely. This would potentially allow a favorable benefit/toxicity ratio.

Adrenal Corticosteroids. Adrenal corticosteroids are the immunosuppressive agents most commonly used in clinical practice. They are effective in a variety of situations, from transplantation to the treatment of lupus erythematosus, childhood nephrotic syndrome, and asthma. Why steroids are beneficial for patients is not clear in most clinical situations. Experimentally, many effects have been described in a variety of cells from numerous species. Consequently, much of the uncertainty of mechanism of action stems from the difficulty in relating the many isolated in vitro effects to the patient. This is compounded by the variation in species susceptibility to steroids, which makes extrapolation difficult. In fact, direct evidence for immunosuppression by corticosteroids in human beings is lacking, and their benefit may be due primarily to inhibition of the inflammatory response. Despite this uncertainty about the mechanism of action, steroids are necessary for successful human transplantation and are commonly used to produce immunosuppression in other types of patients.

Many effects of steroids are known (Fig. 9). The problem is deciding which are primary and which are secondary actions. Steroids cross the cell membrane and bind to specific receptors in the cytoplasm of most cells, lymphocytes included. Many experiments have shown a correlation between binding affinity and steroid potency, specifically between binding and lymphocyte resistance or susceptibility. The steroid-receptor complex then enters the nucleus and interacts with DNA in an unknown way. Subsequently in lymphocytes, DNA, RNA, and protein synthesis are inhibited, as are glucose and amino acid transport. At a sufficient dosage, lymphocyte degeneration and lysis occur. Cytolysis can readily be produced in vivo, and T cells appear to be most susceptible. In some experiments the disintegration of nuclear membranes takes place within hours of exposure to steroids. Depletion of small T lymphocytes occurs in both the peripheral and the central lymphoid tissues. Although it is unclear why the resting small lymphocyte should be so susceptible, it would seem that the primary antilymphocyte action of steroids may be to deplete small lymphocytes before they are activated by antigen.

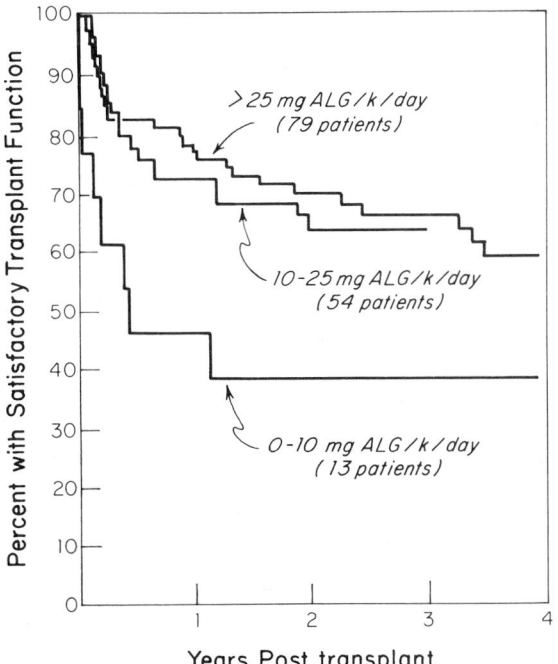

Figure 9. The effect of ALG on kidney allograft function in transplant patients at the University of Minnesota is shown in this graph. All kidneys were from cadavers and graft losses due to technical difficulties and hyperacute rejection were excluded. Although this is not a randomized study, improved function seems to occur in patients treated with ALG. The results with high doses (> 25 mg./kg./day) and medium doses (10 to 25 mg./kg./day) of ALG given for 14 days after transplantation do not seem to be significantly different. An accurate dose response analysis is not possible, however, because of the lack of a satisfactory assay for the potency of individual batches of ALG.

The functional effects of steroids are predictable, and all T cell responses are depressed. Paradoxically, the steroid-resistant thymocytes that remain after an injection of steroids have increased activity, but the net immunologic capability of the treated animal is reduced.

Although B cell activity and antibody production are relatively unaffected by steroids, many other cell types that participate in graft rejection are damaged. Neutrophil chemotaxis is inhibited, but whether or not suppression of phagocytosis occurs remains controversial. Similar results and controversies surround the effects on macrophages. It seems certain, however, that the accumulation of neutrophils, macrophages, and monocytes at sites of immune and inflammatory activity is reduced when steroids are given. Steroids also increase the membrane stability of digestive lysosomal particles in these cells, which reduces their inflammatory activity. These observations provide a basis for understanding the antiinflammatory action activity of steroids. Inflammation is so intertwined with any substantial immune reaction that the various effects are inseparable. The variety of immunologic activities that steroids will suppress means that their effectiveness against the rejection reaction is probably the sum of many influences. When these effects are understood at the molecular level, however, there may prove to be a common discrete point of inhibition.

The effectiveness of cortisone in suppressing the allograft reaction was first recognized by its prolongation of skin graft survival in rabbits. Increased skin graft survival was subsequently shown in mice and guinea pigs, but the results were not as conclusive in pigs, dogs, monkeys, and human beings when cortisone was used alone. In experimental kidney allografts, steroids have not been convincingly effective by themselves but are valuable in combination with such agents as azathioprine, nitrogen mustard, and antilymphocyte globulin. Similarly, steroids alone cannot prevent clinical allograft rejection but, together with other compounds, are potent in both preventing and reversing rejection reactions.

Steroid toxicity of some degree is frequent and commonly includes a cushingoid appearance. Other characteristic problems from steroid therapy are hypertension, weight gain, peptic ulcers and gastrointestinal bleeding, euphoric personality changes, cataract formation, hyperglycemia that may progress to steroid diabetes, and osteoporosis with avascular necrosis of bone. The appearance and severity of these complications vary considerably, but all too frequently they are life-threatening. Clinical transplantation will be improved tremendously when more specific means of immunosuppression are developed and present steroid dosages can be reduced.

Antilymphocyte Globulin. The use of antilymphocyte antibodies to suppress the immune response is an interesting aspect of the transplantation story. In experimental studies, antilymphocyte globulin is a potent immunosuppressive agent, yet evidence for its value in clinical transplantation is meager. This apparent contradiction results more from the difficulties that surround analysis of a complex clinical situation than from the ineffectiveness of antilymphocyte globulin. Evidence for the benefit of antilymphocyte globulin exists, but better designed studies will be needed to measure the effects accurately.

The ability of an antiserum to destroy white cells was noted as early as 1899 by Metchnikoff. After guinea pigs were stimulated with lymph node or spleen cells from either rats or rabbits, their serum would agglutinate and kill polymorphonuclear leukocytes of the donor species. In the same era, Flexner found that lymphoid depletion occurred in animals treated with anti–lymph node serum. It was only during the last decade, however, that the functional consequences of heterologous sera made against lymphoid tissue was investigated. Certain immunologic reactions, e.g., tuberculin sensitivity and allograft rejection, were found to be depressed. Monaco and Russell induced potent antisera that were very effective in prolonging skin grafts with strong histocompatibility differences, even including xenografts. Starzl was the first to use antilymphocyte serum in clinical kidney transplantation and, subsequently, these preparations have been widely used.

Antilymphocyte globulins (ALG) are produced when thoracic duct, peripheral blood, lymph nodes, thymus, or spleen lymphocytes are injected into animals of a different species. Cell membranes or cultured lymphocytes serve equally well to provide the antigenic stimulation. The addition of adjuvants, usually Freund's complete adjuvant, enhances the immunogenicity of the foreign lymphocytes and produces sera that are consistently more immunosuppressive. The rabbit, goat, and horse are commonly used to produce antisera for clinical transplantation.

Most of the relatively specific antibody against human lymphocytes resides in the IgG fraction. Further purification of the sera by separating the globulin fraction can be achieved by Cohn fractionation, column chromatography, or forced flow electrophoresis. The purified material can be administered intravenously, intramuscularly, or subcutaneously. Unlike the immunosuppressive drugs used clinically, the course of ALG is short, usually the first 10 to 14 days after transplantation.

The action of ALG seems to be directed mainly against the T cell. The suppression produced by ALG can be at least partially reversed by T cells, but not by bone marrow cells. Thymectomy will enhance the effect of ALG, and ALG decreases the number of circulating T cells. Even in vitro, ALG will reduce the number of T cells. As would be expected, ALG administration interferes most with the cell-mediated reactions – skin or renal allograft rejection, tuberculin sensitivity, and the graft-versus-host reaction. ALG can abolish pre-existing delayed hypersensitivity reactions, and larger doses will prolong the survival of some xenografts. ALG has a definite, but lesser, effect on humoral reactivity, and this, too, is concentrated on T cell–dependent antibody production.

The net effect of the relatively selective antilymphocyte activity of ALG is to enhance the activity of steroids, alkylating agents, and azathioprine against graft rejection. Most simply, the background of lymphocyte depression provided by ALG potentiates the

effect of these agents without adding to the toxicity against other rapidly dividing cell systems. The fact that ALG and the other immunosuppressive drugs reinforce each other means that large doses of ALG can be used as a priming agent, followed by small doses of the more toxic immunosuppressants for a more effective and safer clinical regimen.

Many theories have been used to explain why ALG is a powerful (at present the most potent) inhibitor of cell-mediated immunity but only weakly affects antibody formation. Most of the explanations can be discarded because the anti-T cell activity is more a function of the structure of the immune system than of the specificity of ALG itself. The spectrum of in vitro ALG activity can be easily shifted from anti-T to anti-B cell by changing the cells used to stimulate antibody production. Antithymus sera are richer in anti-T antibodies, anti–bone marrow sera have more anti-B cell activity, while antispleen and lymph node sera contain large amounts of both types of antibodies. When ALG is given to the transplant patient, however, there is poor penetration of the antilymphocyte antibodies in the lymphoid regions where most of the relatively sessile B cells reside. The circulating long-lived lymphocytes, which are overwhelmingly T cell in origin, therefore absorb the bulk of the antibody. Lymphocytes coated with ALG share the fate of erythrocytes coated with antibody. They are either lysed or cleared from the blood by reticuloendothelial cells in the liver and spleen. More prolonged administration of ALG will deplete the paracortical regions of the lymph nodes where T cells reside, but high doses will also reduce the B cells in the medullary regions and follicles of the nodes.

Antilymphocyte globulin is widely used in clinical transplantation with apparently beneficial results. Absolute proof of the effect of ALG is lacking, but the weight of the evidence suggests that it is of value. What the many studies show is that it is difficult to analyze one factor, here ALG, in a complex clinical situation. Several studies have shown an increased percentage, and length of survival and renal function were increased among cadaver allografts when high doses of ALG were given (Fig. 10). The studies were not randomized, however, and the treatment groups not strictly comparable. There are many considerations that must be balanced in such a study, including (a) the length of time on dialysis, (b) the presence of presensitization, (c) the number of patients with depressed immune response, (d) the condition of the recipient, and (e) the condition of the graft, if it is from a cadaver donor.

The factors influencing the results are so numerous that a broad randomized study may not be able to equalize them all. Such an attempt has been made, however, by the Medical Research Council of Canada with interesting results. There was no apparent effect of horse antithymocyte globulin on the one-year survival of either living related or cadaver kidney allografts. But these patients did show a decrease in the average number of acute rejection episodes, an improvement in renal function, and a decrease in the amount of steroids given. These results could be interpreted to mean that the effect of ALG is greatest on

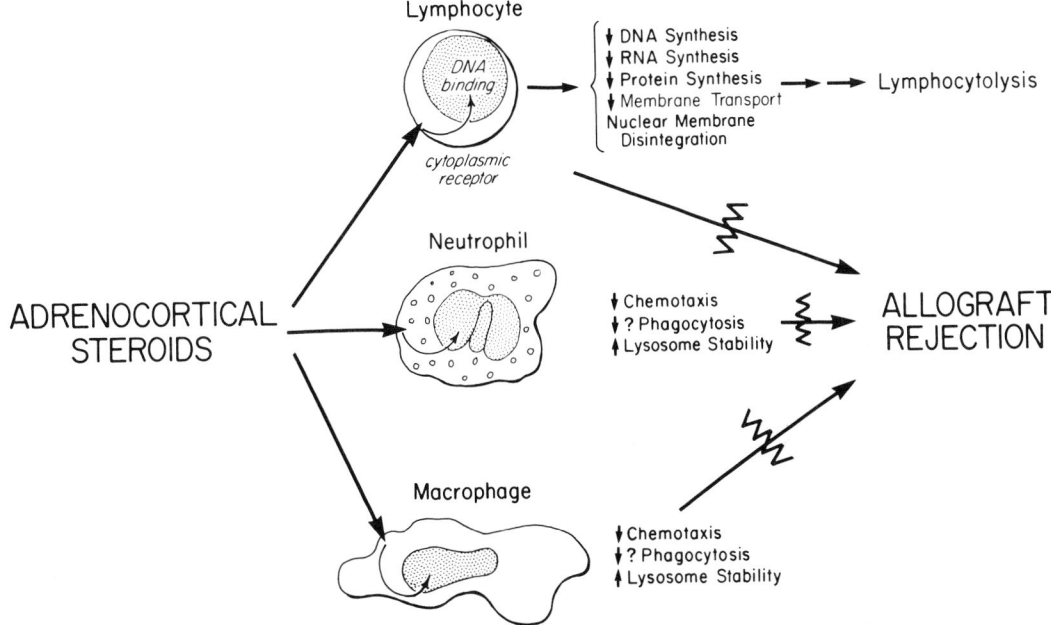

Figure 10. Adrenocortical steroids play an important role in clinical allograft immunosuppression. Many apparent sites of action have been located experimentally. These compounds bind to cytoplasmic receptors and this complex combines with DNA. How this relates to the many functional consequences of steroids presented in this diagram is unclear. In the complex clinical transplantation setting it is not possible to determine if the primary suppression of lymphocytes is more important than the anti-inflammatory effects on neutrophils and macrophages in the suppression of allograft rejection reactions. Nevertheless, they produce a significant portion of the immunosuppressive effect of current clinical therapy.

the early, cell-mediated rejection reactions and less on later, antibody-produced graft damage. Unanswerable at this time is how much ALG adds to the risk of infection in the immunosuppressed patient. The benefit of ALG may be offset by an increased susceptibility to infection, and this may account for the lack of improved patient survival in the clinical studies.

The use of ALG is not confined clinically to kidney transplantation, and beneficial results have also been reported in bone marrow transplantation. These studies have suggested that ALG pretreatment of the recipient is of value in suppressing the response to the donor cells and for enlarging the marrow space. Also in this situation, a potentiating effect with certain drugs, such as procarbazine, has been described. Furthermore, it seems that ALG may be useful in the treatment of the graft-versus-host reactions that arise in these patients.

The toxicity of any heterologous serum preparation prepared against human tissue depends on two factors: (1) its cross-reactivity with other tissue antigens, and (2) the ability of the patient to make antibodies against the protein itself. When administered intramuscularly, ALG produces an area of erythematous induration accompanied by high fever. This probably results from the combination of antibodies with cellular antigens at the injection site. Anemia and thrombocytopenia can also occur and presumably result from a reaction between ALG and host erythrocytes and platelets. Although prior absorption with human platelets and red cell stroma reduces the severity,

some cross-reactivity to these cells persists in most ALG preparations. Cross-reactivity to renal glomerular basement membranes has occasionally been found, but no evidence for functionally significant nephrotoxic serum nephritis has been presented. These cross-reactions can be reduced by using a purer lymphocyte suspension to stimulate ALG production. Either cultured lymphoblasts or thoracic duct lymphocytes will produce a more specific ALG than will the heterogenous cell populations found in the spleen or bone marrow.

Allergic reactions to the antiserum itself are the most common clinical problem associated with the use of ALG. Urticaria, anaphylactoid reactions, and serum sickness, including joint pain, fever, and malaise, all result from the patient's developing immunity to the heterologous globulin. To reduce the occurrence of these reactions, one can attempt to induce immunologic unresponsiveness to the foreign proteins in ALG by intravenous administration of a highly purified, deaggregated IgG fraction. This method has been used experimentally to produce tolerance to foreign proteins, and it is especially effective in the presence of the other immunosuppressive drugs used in renal transplantation. An additional, but so far rare, complication has been the development of a reticulum cell sarcoma at the site of ALG injection. This has occurred at least twice.

The major problem in the production of a standardized antihuman ALG is the inability to develop a method of assaying its in vitro immunosuppressive potency. Other immunosuppressive drugs are available in measurable quantities; therefore the response is more predictable. Unfortunately, individual laboratories make their own ALG preparations, and a standard method of assay has not been developed. Cytotoxic assays, the formation of cellular rosettes by antibody-coated cells, and animal assays for immunosuppressive activity have all been attempted, but their correlation with graft prolongation has been inconsistent. Standardization is important because two batches of ALG prepared by the same method will have varying degrees of immunosuppressive potency. A suitable assay is necessary to identify the better ALG preparations and make their use increasingly beneficial.

Radiation. Radiation was probably the first agent used to produce immunosuppression. Ionizing radiation (x-rays, alpha rays, beta rays) affects both cellular proteins and nucleic acids. Despite the fact that relatively small doses of irradiation may disrupt the secondary protein structure formed by hydrogen bonding and the tertiary conformation that results, biologically significant alterations of protein function seem to require very high dosages. Consequently, most of the immunosuppressive effects of x-radiation are caused by changes produced in nucleic acids. DNA is particularly vulnerable and, therefore, so is cellular replication. The most important of the several modes of damage is the production of scattered breaks in the deoxyribose-phosphate backbone of DNA (Fig. 11). Disruption of either the carbon-carbon bonds of the deoxyribotides or the bonds involving the phosphate groups produces breaks in one of the DNA strands. Occasionally both strands are broken at the same point. Other sites of damage, such as the bases themselves, are even less frequent.

Repair mechanisms exist to mend the breaks, but insufficient time may be available in the dividing cell. Therefore, the effectiveness of radiation is dependent upon the phase of the cell cycle in which the cell is found. Cells in the M or G_2 phase are most sensitive to irradiation. Presumably, DNA breaks that occur during these phases cannot be repaired quickly enough, and the synthetic events and precise apportionment of cellular components that occur during mitosis may become scrambled. Conversely, the early G_1 phase and the latter part of the S phase are the most resistant portions of the cell cycle. Although irradiation is, in general, most effective just prior to or during mitosis, lymphocytes are a special case. For reasons that are not known, these cells are also sensitive in their resting or G_0 phase and lysis of lymphocytes follows radiation of sufficent doses.

Despite the complexity of the subcellular mechanisms, the effect of irradiation on the immune response is predictable and depends greatly on its timing with relation to antigen exposure. The possibilities are best seen when a relatively simple response, antibody production against a defined antigen, is measured. When the antigen is given soon after irradiation, the immune response will be inhibited because there is insufficient time for the immunocompetent cell population to recover before the antigen is encountered. If radiation is given during the time of maximal

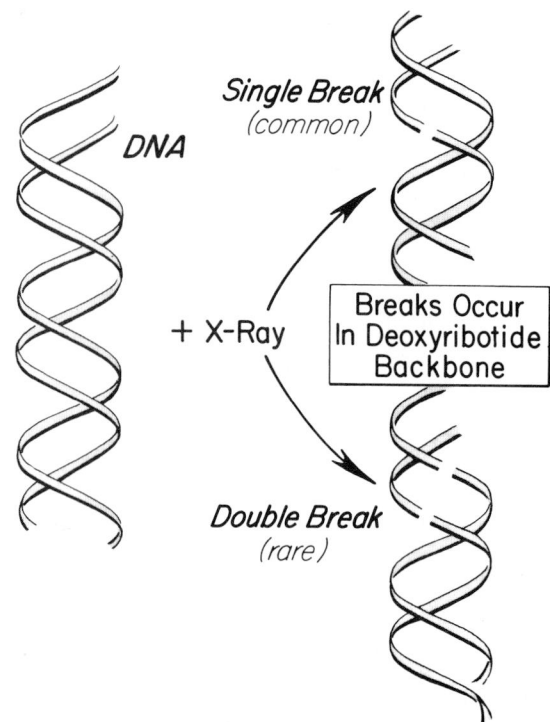

Figure 11. X-ray–induced damage of DNA molecules frequently induces single breaks in the deoxyribotide backbone of the DNA double helix. More rarely, irradiation induces double breaks within the backbone. These breaks can be repaired if sufficient time exists before mitosis.

proliferation of the immunocompetent population to an antigen (soon after antigen administration), the response will be strongly inhibited. On the other hand, if antigenic stimulation is delayed long enough for the precursor cells to recover from the radiation, there will even be a slight augmentation of the response. Radiation is also ineffective if given long after the antigen, when a mature population of antibody-synthesizing cells has been formed. Fully differentiated plasma cells, and presumably cytotoxic lymphocytes, are radioresistant. Although radiation is relatively ineffective in blocking the secondary response of an immunized animal, paradoxically an augmented antibody response may occur under certain circumstances. The timing of radiation must be carefully planned for the greatest immunosuppressive effect.

X-radiation has limited use in clinical transplantation. Effective suppression of the recipient's lymphoid tissues can be achieved, but the toxicity associated with the total body radiation is too great. Local irradiation of the graft, however, may provide some immunosuppressive effects. When given prior to transplantation, x-ray of the kidney may destroy the passenger leukocytes in the graft. These cells seem to be a potent source of antigen to the host and, thus, the stimulus is somewhat diminished. After transplantation, radiation of the graft may damage invading cells, as well as produce nonspecific anti-inflammatory effects. Although proof of the benefit is lacking, some centers irradiate the kidney graft at the onset of a rejection reaction.

Other methods of using radiation have been tried. Selective irradiation of circulating lymphocytes has been done experimentally by diverting blood via a shunt through an extracorporeal radiation source. The circulating lymphocytes are depleted and immunocompetence reduced. Selective irradiation has the advantages that the neutrophils remain active in clearing infection, and protein loss is avoided. The inefficiencies of the system, however, and the need for nearly continuous irradiation make this technique impractical for clinical use.

Total body radiation does have one application at present in clinical transplantation. It is used to eliminate the immune reactivity of patients in preparation for bone marrow transplantation. The toxicity is predictable. The rapidly replicating skin and gastrointestinal tract are universally affected, and nausea, vomiting, diarrhea, and skin changes occur. Late problems are also probably attributable to damage to the cellular genetic apparatus: growth retardation, vertebral deformities, sterility, cataracts, and a likely increased incidence of cancer.

Thymectomy. There is some evidence that the adult mammalian thymus continues to play a role, albeit a diminished one, in maintaining the immunologic responsiveness of the animal. Its extirpation, therefore, may enhance the effects of immunosuppressive agents or irradiation. Unfortunately, although thymectomy can be performed rather simply through a cervical incision, as well as by the classic trans-sternal route, it has not proved to be of use in clinical transplantation. In the early days of renal transplantation, Starzl tried thymectomy in a number of patients but had little improvement in results. It may be that a relatively small increment of benefit may be more apparent now when better results are regularly achieved. Perhaps thymectomy deserves another try. It must be conceded, however, that the thymus in an adult has largely completed its inductive functions and removal may have no measurable consequence. Furthermore, even if thymectomy could augment immunosuppression, it may not be desirable to produce greater general immunologic incompetence in transplant recipients. In summary, it seems unlikely that the admittedly small potential gain will stimulate another clinical trial of thymectomy unless it is shown to be important to the production of tolerance.

Lymphoid Extirpation. Immunity rapidly becomes systemic. It is not confined for long to the regional lymph nodes or to a single major lymphoid organ like the spleen. Experimentally, the acquisition of immunity can be delayed for only brief periods by interrupting the lymphatic channels, by placing grafts in sites with poor lymphatic drainage, or by excising local lymphoid tissue. In one of the earliest clinical experiments, transplanted kidneys were placed in plastic bags after completion of the vascular anastomoses. This approach failed, because vascularized organ grafts do not require lymphatic drainage to disseminate the antigen to awaiting lymphocytes. Excision of locally draining lymph nodes or the spleen is also ineffective as an immunosuppressive technique.

Thoracic Duct Drainage. Cannulation and drainage of the thoracic duct will successfully deplete the body of a large proportion of its circulating T lymphocytes. Such depletion will lead to prolongation of allograft survival, and to lesser, but real, decreases in the capacity for antibody synthesis. Thoracic duct cannulation and drainage have been used for clinical immunosuppression and, although it seems to produce prolongation of allografts, it is cumbersome, the indwelling cannula can become plugged or infected, and protein depletion may result. It is not used at the present time.

CLINICAL KIDNEY TRANSPLANTATION

From among the many possible methods of immunodepression, most clinical kidney transplant teams use azathioprine and prednisone almost exclusively. In addition, antilymphocyte globulin (ALG) is used at many centers, but other modes of therapy are seldom added. The treatment given at the University of Minnesota is representative of most antirejection regimens. Kidney recipients are given 2.5 mg. per kg. of azathioprine and 2 mg. per kg. of prednisone before transplantation. Azathioprine is begun at 5 mg. per kg. per day postoperatively and tapered to 3.0 mg. per kg. per day within a week and thereafter adjusted according to peripheral white blood count, platelet levels, and renal function. Recipients of identical antigen matches begin their prednisone dose at 1 mg. per kg. per day. Tapering continues over one year, and the maintenance dosage is about 0.3 mg. per kg. per day. ALG is given intravenously at 20 mg. per kg. per day for ideal matches and 30 mg. per kg. per day for others. The dosage is reduced if the platelet level is less than 200,000 per cu. mm. Treatment is continued for two weeks or until sensitivity to ALG appears. The kidney is given 250 R of local x-radiation on three alternate days following transplantation. When a rejection episode occurs, the prednisone dosage is increased to 2 mg. per kg. per day for three days. The kidney is given x-radiation again, unless the patient has already had 1500 R total dose. With improvement in renal function, the prednisone dosage is again tapered.

An important but unanswered question is how long immunosuppression therapy should be continued when the kidney functions well with no signs of rejection. Several successful instances of stopping medication have been reported, suggesting that some host-graft accommodation may take place. Rarely, this coexistence may even approach tolerance. This is unusual, however, and cessation of treatment has most frequently been followed by gradual or rapid rejection. At the present time immunosuppressive therapy should be considered a lifelong necessity.

CONSEQUENCES OF IMMUNOSUPPRESSION

Apart from the many specific immunologic and toxic effects of immunosuppressive drugs, there are several interesting and clinically important consequences of immunosuppression that must be considered.

Parameters of Immunosuppression. Obviously, the process of graft rejection can be prolonged, but are other parameters of immunocompetence concurrently depressed in the transplant patient? Can immunosuppression be measured in any other way than by the life of the graft? Our results have been both interesting and puzzling. During the first two weeks after kidney transplantation, an immunosuppressive effect can be detected. The response of the patient's circulating lymphocytes to either the mitogen phytohemagglutinin (PHA) or to foreign leukocytes is depressed. The loss of reactivity seems to be roughly proportional to the decrease in T cells among the peripheral lymphocytes and to the rise in null cells that occurs. The latter are lymphocytes, coated with ALG and consequently inhibited.

Overall, the depressed lymphocyte reactivity probably results from a combination of acute destruction of T cells by ALG and steroids, inactivation of other lymphocytes by masking with ALG, and inhibition of the lymphocyte proliferative response by azathioprine. Among these agents, ALG would seem to be the most responsible because lymphocyte reactivity begins to return shortly after the ALG course is ended. Surprisingly, peripheral lymphocytes from kidney graft recipients show a normal response to PHA and foreign lymphocytes shortly thereafter. Because the kidney grafts continue to survive, an immunosuppressive effect that is not measured by these assays must persist. At the present time, there is no way to monitor the level of immunosuppression achieved after the effect of ALG has disappeared. Nor is it possible accurately to predict incipient rejection, although some success has been claimed for the detection of a rise in lymphocyte-dependent antibodies immediately prior to rejection. Because the degree of immunosuppression cannot yet be measured, the dosages of immunosuppressive agents are regulated instead by the toxicity produced.

Infection. Immunosuppression understandably increases the risk of infection, but the consequences may offer some surprises. The routine post-transplant immunosuppression regimen does not necessarily result in a higher bacterial infection rate. In our series, the postoperative wound infection incidence is only 0.7 per cent. These patients seem to cope satisfactorily with the inevitable contamination during the operation despite the increased immunosuppressive therapy used at the time. When there are no severe rejection reactions and the graft maintains good function, the day-to-day bacterial challenge to the recipient is handled. Although urinary tract infections are frequent, they are usually mild and easily controlled by antibiotics. Occasionally, unexplained septic arthritis will crop up in these patients. And overwhelming pneumococcal sepsis has occurred in transplant patients without spleens.

We do not mean to imply that bacterial infection is an insignificant problem for transplantation patients. On the contrary, infection is still the most common complication of immunosuppression, and overall it is the most common cause of death in transplant recipients. Even so, increasing experience has both lowered the incidence of serious infection and lengthened the time before it occurs.

The recent report of the American College of Surgeons/National Institute of Health Organ Transplant Registry stated that sepsis was the primary cause of death in 47 per cent of all renal allograft recipients who died. Graft rejection not associated with sepsis accounted for less than 10 per cent of patient deaths. Rejection of a kidney graft should not be fatal, because the patient can be maintained on hemodialysis. The difficulties seem to arise with the treatment of rejection. Rejection causes decreased kidney function, which further potentiates the increased immunosuppression used to combat the rejection episode. The consequence is usually a severely immunodepressed patient, often with very few circulating polymorphonuclear leukocytes, who is highly susceptible to infection. In this setting, particularly if it is prolonged, severe bacterial infections and generalized sepsis can still occur.

Most of the deaths early in the history of kidney transplantation occurred in the first few post-transplant months as a result of highly pathogenic bacterial infections. For example, pneumococcal pneumonia has been reported to be the most common type of pneumonia in kidney recipients. Since then, improved antibiotics and greater skill in immunosuppression therapy have shifted the spectrum of organisms. There has been a relative increase in lethal infection caused by organisms that are normally weakly pathogenic. Antibiotics will eradicate the more aggressive bacteria, but they leave opportunistic organisms free to colonize the susceptible transplant patient.

The opportunistic organisms, which are normally eliminated by cellular mechanisms, can now blossom in the face of the relative T cell depression. Fungi are prominent opportunists, and they can cause urinary tract and pulmonary infections, skin lesions, and central nervous system involvement, as well as generalized sepsis. *Candida albicans* infections are probably the most common. The inevitable mucosal candidiasis can be satisfactorally prevented by oral mycostatin. Candida can become more deep-seated and the pneumonia, usually part of a mixed infection, can be lethal. Characteristically, it produces soft, bulky infiltrates, although invasion of pulmonary arteries can lead to infarction and wedge-shaped peripheral infiltrates. Candida sepsis is most often associated with indwelling catheters, but it can take a more entrenched systemic form.

Aspergillus species are probably the second most common cause of fungal infection and typically produce upper lobe pulmonary cavities. *Rhizopus oryzae*, *Histoplasma capsulatum*, and *Cryptococcus neoformans* also invade the lung and the latter occasionally causes meningitis. The indolent bacterium *Nocardia asteroides* occasionally infects, producing nodular pulmonary lesions. The protozoan *Pneumocystis carinii*, more commonly seen in patients undergoing cancer chemotherapy, usually causes an alveolar infiltrate with disproportionate dyspnea and cyanosis.

Standard patient isolation precautions are useless against these organisms, and prophylactic antibiotics are not available for most of them. Prevention is dependent upon avoiding excessive doses of immunosuppressive agents in a futile attempt to prolong the function of a rejected graft.

Viral Infections. Viral infections seem to be almost ubiquitous with kidney transplant recipients. The herpes group of DNA viruses are most commonly present. Infection or antibody response to cytomegalovirus (CMV) is found in up to 90 per cent of patients after renal transplantation. Herpes simplex infection occurs in about 25 per cent and herpes zoster in 10 per cent of graft recipients. Reports from England have shown that the Ebstein-Barr virus commonly infects transplant patients, but the clinical significance of this is unclear. Antigenic evidence for hepatitis B virus infection can be detected in 15 per cent of transplant patients. It seems almost certain that as detection methods improve, evidence will appear for other kinds of viral infections in these transplantation patients.

Several questions are raised by the recent appreciation of viral infections in kidney recipients. Are these infections of any consequence or are they merely laboratory curiosities? The case of the hepatitis B virus is particularly interesting. Transplantation and hemodialysis patients who have circulating HB antigen, paradoxically, usually have no symptoms of hepatitis. The reason that the disease is apparently much milder in these patients is unknown, but intriguing. It seems likely that liver damage is mediated by an immune reaction against viral antigens on the cell surface, and this may be reduced in these immunodepressed patients.

The situation with cytomegalovirus infection appears to be slightly clearer but no less intriguing. Most evidence suggests that cytomegalovirus infection usually produces a clinical illness characterized by fever, neutropenia, and frequently a decrease in kidney function and apparent rejection. The virus may be newly acquired from blood transfusions or from the foreign graft itself. It is far more likely that the apparently new infection is a reactivation of latent intracellular viruses. The finding that most normal adults have antibodies to CMV supports the latent virus hypothesis.

In transplant patients does the infection cause the rejection or does the rejection encourage viral activation? Rejection reactions are accomplished by bursts of lymphocyte proliferation. Cell division is known to activate latent viruses experimentally, and most immunosuppressive agents are mutagenic. Viral infections, on the other hand, can be associated with either an augmented or a depressed immune response. If the patient is able to produce antibody against virus, graft rejection is also enhanced. In preimmunized individuals, viruses seem to act as immunologic adjuvants and enhance the response to both virus and graft. When no antibody response accompanies the viral infection, a generalized immunodepression is usually present. At the present time it can only be said that viral infections and rejection reactions are clearly linked; which initiates and which follows is usually unknown.

A special case of CMV infection is worthy of note. The typical CMV infection is a mild febrile illness, followed by an antibody response and regression of viral symptoms. A rejection episode usually accompanies the viral infection and raises the controversy discussed in the previous paragraph. These patients remain asymptomatic but may continue to excrete CMV in urine or saliva despite the presence of antibodies to CMV. In certain patients, however, there is no antibody response or apparent rejection, and the infection can be lethal. The virus proliferates in many kinds of cells. Viral inclusion bodies have been found, for example, in the cells that rim the diffuse gastrointestinal ulcerations that can develop in these patients. The stomach and cecum are particularly vulnerable, but the ulcerations can be widespread. Viral infestation of the lungs and liver can cause a fulminant interstitial pneumonitis and hepatitis. Bone marrow involvement is manifested by leukopenia and thrombocytopenia. This group of severely immunodepressed patients is at the mercy of this usually trivial parasite, which would suggest that rejection is not essential for viral activation. Certainly the ability of the patient to respond to the virus is very important to his or her survival.

The other herpesviruses seem to behave in a similar manner. Transplant patients also have infections typical of herpes simplex and zoster. The infections may be more severe than in normal patients and, although the lesions may be localized, the viruses are systemic and can be recovered in the urine. Fever, neutropenia, and allograft rejection may accompany the infection, and antibody responses to the virus seem to be important for the patient.

We are not sure when the viral infections occur in relation to the clinical symptoms. With the exception of the hepatitis infection, these may represent activation of a normal intracellular viral flora rather than recent infection. In transplant patients, studies suggest that cytomegalovirus "infection" takes place about the time of transplantation, when the mutagenic antirejection drugs are begun at high levels. This obviously may result merely from activation of latent intracellular viruses.

Malignancy. Cancer has been an unexpectedly frequent companion of clinical transplantation. The incidence of cancer is not high enough, however, to contraindicate the transplant procedure. Tumors in kidney recipients have come from two general sources. Some have been unfortunately transplanted from cadaver donors in whom the cancer was unsuspected. These tumors usually can be treated simply by halting immunosuppression therapy and allowing rejection of the tumor tissue, as well as the kidney, to occur. The more common cancers are the primary tumors that appear in the immunosuppressed recipient. The data are still accumulating on these primary tumors, and precise frequencies are not yet available. It would seem, however, that the rate of development of malignancy in patients surviving renal transplantation may be as high as 30 times that of a similar, normal population.

Only certain tumors grow more readily in immunodepressed patients. Seventy-five per cent of the spontaneous cancers are either lymphoid or epithelial in origin. Carcinoma-in-situ of the cervix, carcinoma of the lip, and squamous or basal cell carcinomas account for about half of this group, while lymphomas, predominantly reticulum cell sarcomas, make up the remainder. It has been estimated that the risks to the transplant recipient of developing skin cancer, lymphoma, or reticulum cell sarcoma are increased by 4, 40, and 350 times, respectively. The lymphomas are unusual in both their frequency and their behavior. Almost 50 per cent of the immunosuppressed patients with lymphomas have brain involvement, which occurs in only 1 per cent of non–transplant-related cases of lymphoma. These lymphomas, moreover, are difficult to treat and have led to death in almost all cases. The superficial malignant lesions of the lip, skin, and cervix are usually successfully treated by standard operative techniques. There is no need to jeopardize the allografts by reducing the immunosuppressive therapy.

We do not know the reasons why transplant patients have an increased risk for cancer in general, and epithelial and lymphoid cancers in particular. It has been postulated that the surveillance and elimination by lymphocytes of tumor cells as they arise are important natural defenses of man against cancer. Certainly, this function would be depressed in transplantation patients who are immunodepressed by antirejection therapy. Despite this, two observations argue that this explanation is incomplete. First, only a few kinds of cancer are increased in these patients. Second, and perhaps more telling, is the finding that patients receiving hemodialysis have an increased risk of cancer, but the tumors arise with the usual spectrum and frequency distribution. Dialysis patients have decreased immunologic competence. Perhaps the inhibition of a surveillance mechanism contributes to their increased risk.

Transplant patients, however, must have additional factors operating that contribute to the development of cancer. They are immunosuppressed, which may be important, but the presence of the mutagen azathioprine is a more certain factor. Azathioprine, theoretically, either could act as a primary mutagen on dividing lymphocytes and epithelial cells or could contribute to the activation of viruses and their transformation of normal cells into tumors.

It is unclear what consequences steroids and ALG have, but at least two reticulum cell sarcomas have sprung up at the site of ALG injections. It would seem possible that the most important effect the immunosuppressive agents have on tumor development is to encourage viral transformation of normal into cancer cells. Cancers of the epithelium, for example, may be a consequence of herpesvirus transformation. This group of viruses is carcinogenic in animals, and circumstantial evidence exists for a role in human cervical cancer. Herpesviruses are usually dormant, but the stress of transplantation or the action of antimetabolite may activate them. The viruses might then either proliferate and cause a clinical viral illness or produce cellular transformation into cancer cells. Similar possibilities exist for the lymphomas. Several animal lymphomas are produced by RNA viruses, and transformation by related viruses could be occurring in these patients. Perhaps a simpler explanation would do. Active lymphoid proliferation occurs after transplantation, and cell division in the presence of the mutagenic immunosuppressants may carry an increased risk of transformation of normal cells into cancer.

Growth. The antiproliferative effects of immunosuppressive drugs would seem to make satisfactory growth in children unlikely after transplantation. Chronic renal failure itself is inhibitory to development, so these children are usually far behind their peers in size. After successful transplantation their growth response is highly variable and may depend on age, previous growth rate, renal function, and immunosuppressive drug regimen. Although many children return to a normal growth rate, unfortunately the growth that was lost during their original illness is not made up, so these children will always be smaller than their peers.

Wound healing is a specific case in this category, and is to all outward appearances normal. It is apparent clinically, however, that wound healing is severely affected when debilitation, chronic renal failure, and high steroid levels are present.

Pregnancy. Many arguments can be raised against the likelihood of a successful pregnancy and a normal child being born when one parent has received a kidney graft. Excessive steroid levels, the antigrowth and mutagenic effects of the immunosuppressive agents, and viral activation and infection all should be detrimental to the fetus. As usual, however, the story is complicated.

The Human Renal Transplant Registry by 1975 had reported on 132 graft recipients who had become parents. The experience at the University of Minnesota has been examined in detail and seems to be representative. Seventeen of our patients became pregnant after transplantation, and 12 children were born. Only one spontaneous abortion occurred. The children had a normal size distribution, and no congenital defects were found. There is no doubt, however, that azathioprine, and probably steroids, are mutagenic and that the risk of congenital abnormalities is real. Multiple defects have been reported in the child of a male transplant recipient. From the overall experience, the risk is not high, but the incidence is still unknown. Steroids also cause their own peculiar problems, and a few cases of severe neonatal adrenocortical insufficiency, as well as lymphopenia, have been reported.

Transplant recipients who are pregnant are often beset with medical problems. Toxemia has occurred in over half of the pregnancies, and bacterial and viral infections, particularly of the urinary tract, are common. Both of these factors may contribute to the higher incidence of premature labor that has been reported in these patients. Another important medical concern is the effect of the pregnancy on renal function. Although the data are insufficient to judge whether or not pregnancy is deleterious to kidney function, each series has apparent examples that show it may be true. An indication for the termination of pregnancy is the compromise of graft function. The increased risk of cancer, in particular of the cervix, in transplant patients has already been discussed. The effect of pregnancy on this tendency is unknown. Another important problem that must be faced is the decreased life expectancy of transplant recipients. Parenthood is a long-term obligation, and counseling of transplant patients should include a discussion of these considerations.

Tolerance. Many kidneys survive for years in their new host. That this represents an acquired tolerance, a specific nonreactivity to the graft antigens, has been suggested in the literature and is hoped for in immunosuppressive therapy. The question of tolerance has been raised earlier in this chapter, and the possible means of achieving it will be discussed in the following section on experimental immunosuppression. At this time acquired tolerance seems rarely, if ever, to occur. Reduction of immunosuppression, even after long accommodation of graft and host, almost invariably leads to rejection. Some adaptation must occur, however, and long-term graft survival can be achieved at immunosuppressive dosages that do not immunologically cripple the recipient or produce other severe toxic consequences.

EXPERIMENTAL IMMUNOSUPPRESSION

The complexity of the immune response gives rise to the hope that many potential points of vulnerability exist. New approaches are constantly being tried and old ones refined to produce better immunosuppressive therapy.

Antigen Recognition and Processing. An obvious, if difficult, approach to immunosuppression would be to alter or mask graft antigens. Evidence exists that by perfusing the organ, before transplantation, with concanavalin A (Con A) the host response to it may be reduced. Although the mechanism is not known, presumably Con A aggregates on graft cell surfaces and interferes in some way with host recognition. Subsequently, the cell membrane is cleared by normal repair processes but may no longer be as antigenic as before.

Many agents have been tried to blockade the reticuloendothelial system generally. Talc and gold, for example, can depress particle uptake and presumably antigen processing by these cells. The effect of talc and gold on graft survival, however, has been negligible.

Immunosuppression by Specific Antigens. The complications of immunosuppression constantly reinforce the importance of developing modes of immunosuppression that will be specific for the incompatible graft antigens. The immunosuppressive drugs and antilymphocyte globulin all act by suppressing the capacity of the immunocompetent cell to respond to any antigen. Thus, even ALG, with it predilection for cellular immunity, cannot select between T cells destined to reject an allograft and T cells necessary for immunity against viruses and tumors. The ability to produce a state of tolerance would obviously be of enormous benefit to the field of transplantation. Experimentally, a functional state of tolerance has been produced in two general ways; either manipulation of the stimulating antigens or infusion of specific antibodies has been successful.

A variety of conditions have been shown to predispose to the introduction of tolerance, rather than immunity, on exposure to antigen. The best example of antigen-directed immunologic unresponsiveness is the tolerance enjoyed by animals to their own body constituents. This apparently develops early, before or during maturation of the immune mechanism, and is usually maintained throughout life. Burnet, as part of his clonal selection hypothesis, considered this unresponsive state to result from direct contact between "self" antigens and the individual's own lymphocytes. The clones of lymphocytes reactive to "self" are eliminated, and tolerance ensues. He further predicted that specific unresponsiveness could be induced to foreign antigens if they were given very early in life. Experimental proof by Billingham, Brent, and Medawar followed and demonstrated tolerance to histocompatibility antigens after neonatal injection of replicating allogenic cells.

Obviously this opportunity has passed for transplant patients, but under certain carefully controlled conditions, tolerance has been produced experimentally in adult animals. Thus, hope exists for future progress in this area, and several techniques have yielded limited but encouraging results. Repeated injection of small, subimmunogenic doses of antigen or the use of very large amounts of antigen preparations has produced unresponsiveness. When these preparations are cleared of aggregated material, the tendency to induced tolerance is greater. Certain antigens (like serum proteins) are endowed with properties that are particularly favorable for the induction of immunologic unresponsiveness. These seem to be the ability to persist in the circulation and equilibrate within the extravascular spaces, thereby coming in contact with antigen-reactive cells in effective concentration. Whether or not this results in deletion of the antigen-reactive lymphocytes, however, is unknown.

Unfortunately, viral and bacterial antigens and transplantation antigens do not have these properties and, in addition, may possess multiple antigenic specificities. A diminished response to transplantation antigens can be induced in adult animals, but the antigen dose, physical state of the antigen, and route of injection all must be carefully chosen to avoid immunization. Tolerance is more easily produced to weak antigens; therefore, close histocompatibility matching is desirable. Irradiation, chemical immunosuppression, and antilymphocyte globulins have been used to inhibit the immune response and potentiate the emergence of a relatively unresponsive state. Although only modest successes have been achieved so far by these approaches, careful control of the conditions of antigen presentation may yet be important in the production of tolerance.

Recently, attempts to produce tolerance have utilized antigens tagged with radioactive compounds or alkylating agents. The purpose is to form a lethal combination with the specifically reactive lymphocyte clones and eliminate them. So far, only a hyporesponse state of short duration has been induced, but this approach may yet be fruitful.

In summary, the induction of tolerance by manipulating the presentation of the incompatible antigens is an attractive idea. So far, success for allografts has not been achieved, but it remains a promising pathway.

Immunosuppression by Specific Antibodies. Tolerance

can be easily defined. A conceptual understanding of tolerance is readily available by considering the lack of reactivity toward self. Understanding the subcellular mechanisms involved is far more difficult, and they are unknown at this time. Tolerance may result from the absence of the reactive clone of lymphocytes. An alternative to this is that tolerance is due to an antibody that interferes with the development of immunity. Certainly the immune system is regulated and subject to feedback control; the presence of an adequate level of antibody may block further activity. Experimentally, the immune response can be eliminated by the passive transfer of specific antibody prior to, or shortly after, giving the antigen.

Two general mechanisms for this phenomenon have been proposed. The first states that the antibodies formed are inactive and do not trigger the effector mechanisms, such as complement. These blocking antibodies have been best demonstrated in tumor immunology, where they have been shown to enhance the growth of transplanted tumors and prevent rejection. The second explanation is that these antibodies produce a negative feedback effect. The most striking example of this is the prevention of erythroblastosis fetalis in newborns by the administration of an Rh factor antiserum to the pregnant mother. The anti-Rh antibodies suppress the synthesis of antibodies in response to the foreign Rh antigens. Both of these mechanisms for production of tolerance require the presence of antibody to the antigen. While the appropriate antibodies cannot always be detected in animals following the induction of "tolerance," they are often present. Furthermore, antibodies are frequently detected in patients with well-functioning, long-term kidney allografts. Graft function is thought to be prolonged by the presence of a specific antibody that inhibits the development of truly effective antigraft immunity. If immunosuppression is reduced, however, the balance is tipped and the common result of graft rejection is observed. Consequently, the apparently paradoxical hypothesis that tolerance to an antigen requires the presence of antibodies to that antigen may yet be valid.

When applied to transplantation, the application of this theory has yielded some success. The best results, however, for experimental kidney graft prolongation has been following the administration of both graft-specific antigens and antibodies against them. Therefore, the distinction between antigen- and antibody-induced tolerance is blurred, and they may meet at virtually the same point in the subcellular response.

Immunosuppression by Cellular Mechanisms. Even more theoretical than the preceding are two recent proposals for inducing immunologic unresponsiveness. As previously mentioned, the ability to induce a sufficient number of suppressor T cells could effectively block graft rejection. A further requirement, of course, would be that the suppressor cells are antigen-specific, or general immunosuppression would result.

Additional leverage on the immune response may be gained by manipulating the genes that govern the response to histocompatibility antigens. Not all individuals respond in the same way to different histocompatibility antigens, and part of this difference may be ascribable to a specific genetic locus. Matching the immune response governing loci in a similar way to aligning histocompatiblity antigens may yield improved results.

Interference with Nonspecific Effectors. The combination of sensitized cells or antibodies with the foreign antigens marks the beginning of the active effort to dispose of the graft. The complex of sensitized cells, or antibodies, with the antigens triggers the recruitment of a multitude of effector systems. We have mentioned the cascading enzyme systems, the complement, clotting, and kinin pathways, as well as the cellular mediators, lymphocytes, macrophages, platelets, and polymorphonuclear leukocytes. These are enlisted both by the specific immunologic reaction itself and as a result of subsequent events. All play an active role in disposing of the allograft.

It is conceivable that one could reduce the effect of an immune response by (a) interfering with the complement, clotting, and kinin cascades that are activated by antigen-antibody complexes, (b) destroying factors secreted by activated cells (migration-inhibiting factor, chemotactic factor, cytophilic antibody, transfer factor, mitogenic factor), or (c) neutralizing the vascular permeability factors, lysosomal enzymes, lymphotoxins.

A number of agents or combination of agents that interfere with the expression of immunity have been tested. For example, anticomplementary drugs (vitamin A, cobra venom factor) are either ineffective or, if potent, are short-acting and are not clinically useful. Antimacrophage globulin, carrageen, and silica all destroy macrophages but are weak transplant immunosuppressants. Antibodies to lymphotoxins or migration-inhibitory factors and other effector molecules are still in very early experimental states of evaluation. Antihistamines and antiserotonin agents are also relatively weak immunosuppressant drugs. Anticoagulants (heparin) and agents that interfere with platelet aggregation (dipyridamole, aspirin), and fibrinolytic agents have been employed to interfere with the thrombosis of graft vessels. The antiplatelet agents have been found to improve long-term clinical function in both kidney and cardiac grafts and will undoubtedly be more widely used in the future. More information is needed on the role platelets play in the production of arterial narrowing, which seems often to limit graft survival.

The limited success with these agents reinforces the difficulty in attempting to interfere with the immune response after antibody has been synthesized, and large numbers of immunologically commited effector cells have been mobilized. In fact, it is difficult to inhibit the secondary or anamnestic response of any immune reaction. Successful interference with the effector mechanism of graft rejection is prohibited by both the complexity and the interdependence of the reaction. Many pathways and cellular participants need to be blocked. In addition, there are points of cross-activation between these pathways that make it difficult effectively to inhibit any or all of them. If true immunosuppression is to be achieved, with respect to a certain antigen, interference must take place during the early phases of the primary immune response.

SELECTED REFERENCES

Bach, J.-F.: The Mode of Action of Immunosuppressive Agents. Series of Frontiers of Biology, Vol. 41. New York, American Elsevier Publishing Company, Inc., 1975.
The most frequently used immunosuppressive agents are presented in detail from both experimental and clinical viewpoints in this monograph.

Dutton, R. W.: Suppressor T cells. Transplant. Rev., 26:39–55, 1975.
Suppressor cells are of potentially great importance to the field of transplantation, and they are introduced in more depth in this paper.

Feldmann, M.: Cell-to-cell interactions in the immune response. Ser. Haematol., 7:593–609, 1974.
Many cellular interactions are required for the immune response, and this article provides considerable information about them.

Foker, J. E., Simmons, R. L., and Najarian, J. S.: Allograft rejection. In Najarian, J. S., and Simmons, R. L. (Eds.): Transplantation, Philadelphia, Lea & Febiger, 1972, pp. 63–145.
This book section provides a more complete discussion of the development and expression of transplantation immunity and the pathologic consequences.

Monaco, A. P., and Codish, S. D.: Survey of the current status of the clinical use of antilymphocyte serum. Surg. Gynecol. Obstet., 142:417–426, 1976.
This lucid review is a summary of the current knowledge and questions about antilymphocyte serum.

Simmons, R. L., Balfour, H. H., Lopez, C., Mauer, S. M., Kjellstrand, C. M., Buselmeier, T. J., and Najarian, J. S.: Infection in immunosuppressed transplant recipients. Surg. Clin. North Am., 55:1419–1430, 1975.
Infection remains a major problem for transplantation patients, and this paper describes the many forms it can take.

Weigle, W. O.: Immunological unresponsiveness. Adv. Immunol., 16:61–122, 1973.
This paper summarizes many of the important experiments and concepts about tolerance.

V

PRESERVATION OF THE KIDNEY

Folkert O. Belzer, M.D.

With the increasing reliance upon renal transplantation as the treatment of choice for most patients with end-stage renal disease, *improved methods of organ procurement and organ preservation* have become necessary. If renal transplantation is to be offered as treatment for end-stage renal disease, large numbers of viable organs must be made available. The role of clinical renal preservation today is simple; namely, to preserve the kidney for the required time with the best possible function on reimplantation. Variables such as the number of transplants performed in a center and donor selection may determine the choice of preservation. Renal preservation can be divided into four different types: (1) simple hypothermic storage for up to 24 hours, (2) short-term preservation for up to 3 days, (3) intermediate preservation for 2 to 3 weeks, and (4) long-term preservation for months or years. Each will be discussed briefly.

Simple Hypothermic Storage

Simple hypothermic storage of cadaver kidneys has been used extensively and is an excellent method for clinical renal transplantation. Its advantages are its simplicity and low cost. After the kidney is removed from the cadaver donor, it is usually flushed with a chilled solution to develop rapid core cooling and is then stored at a temperature between 2 and 4° C until transplantation. If the kidney is obtained under the most ideal conditions with no or only minimal warm ischemia, the kidney can be stored for up to 24 hours. If warm ischemia has occurred, the safe time for storage is probably no more than 10 hours. Most published series report an average preservation time

of about 5 hours. Thus, if tissue typing is to be performed, the donor must be tissue typed prior to death and transplantation performed on an emergency basis. The ideal constitution of the washout solution to be used in the initial cooling of the kidney has been extensively studied. Collins and associates[5] have advocated using a flushout solution that is high in potassium and low in sodium. They based this on the hypothesis that tissues of nonhibernating animals passively leaked potassium and gained sodium when perfused with a cold electrolyte solution resembling extracellular fluids because of the cold sensitivity of the cells' sodium pump. Utilizing this intracellular type of solution, they showed that dog kidneys removed under optimum conditions and flushed out with this intracellular solution functioned immediately after transplantation after being stored for up to 30 hours. Other investigators[6] have shown, however, that the probable beneficial effects of the intracellular washout solutions are not due to the high potassium concentration but are actually due to the presence of high concentrations of nonionic (glucose) and ionic (magnesium sulfate) substances that are poorly permeable and osmotically active and, therefore, prevent cellular swelling. Thus, dogs' kidneys flushed out and stored in an extracellular type solution with equal amounts of glucose and magnesium sulfate tolerated cold storage equally well. The detrimental effect of the brief periods of warm ischemia in this type of renal preservation should be re-emphasized, even if the most optimum washout solution is used. In short, simple hypothermic storage is a clinically applicable method for renal preservation. Ideally, the kidney should be obtained from the so-called heart-beating cadaver to avoid warm ischemia. Immediately after nephrectomy, the kidney should be flushed out with a cooling solution containing adequate concentrations of poorly permeable substances such as glucose or mannitol. If warm ischemia has occurred, the kidney should probably be transplanted within 10 hours. Careful selection and adequate pretreatment of the donor (hydration, correction of hypotension, etc.) prior to death avoids the need for viability testing after the nephrectomy.

Short-Term Preservation

Short-term preservation, the second method of clinical renal preservation which has undergone extensive laboratory as well as clinical testing, is continuous pulsatile perfusion. Since its introduction in clinical renal transplant in 1967,[2] it has been used extensively in many renal transplant centers in the United States and abroad. The basic principles of continuous perfusion are: (1) pulsatile flow, (2) hypothermia, (3) oxygenation, and (4) a perfusate containing albumin as well as lipids[1] (Fig. 1). With minor modifications, all current units or methods make use of these basic principles. The composition of the ideal perfusate is still unknown. In the United States, the best results have been obtained with homologous specially prepared plasma,[3, 10] but in Europe albumin solutions have been found to be equally effective. In general, the perfusate must contain albumin to produce oncotic pressure during perfusion and should also contain fats, since, under the conditions of hypothermia, the kidney can use only fat or its derivatives as exogenous fuel.[7]

The advantages of continuous perfusion for transplantation are two-fold. First, short-term preservation provides enough time to make transplantation of the cadaver kidneys a semielective procedure except for donor nephrectomy. The average storage time in centers using pulsatile perfusion is around 30 hours, and kidneys have been successfully transplanted after

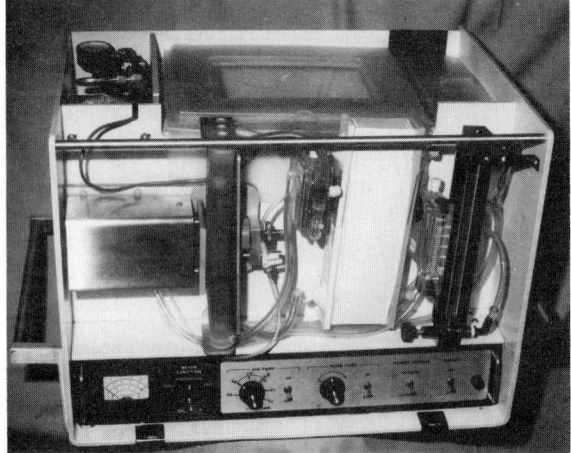

Figure 1. One of the newer portable battery-operated kidney preservation units. The perfusion circuit including a membrane oxygenator, pulsatile pump, cooling unit, and flow meter is supplied sterile and is disposable.

storage periods of up to 3 days. Thus, transplantation can be performed at a time most advantageous to the patient and to the surgical team, and no kidneys must be discarded because of time limitation. Since the actual transplant can be performed semielectively, a sudden influx of cadaver organs to a transplant center can be adequately managed, even by a small team.

The second advantage of continuous perfusion is that it allows viability testing to be performed prior to transplantation. Viability testing is not necessary if only ideal donors are used but becomes important if donors are accepted who have been in prolonged shock, who have been anuric for hours or even days, or who may already have had abnormal renal function prior to death. It has been shown that viability can be adequately insured if the following criteria are observed: (1) warm ischemia time of less than 1 hour, (2) adequate perfusion characteristics during preservation, including an acceptable flow rate and a low mean perfusion, (3) acceptable, although perhaps not normal, renal function of the donor at time of death, and (4) if a combination of cold storage and perfusion storage is used, an acceptable perfusate lactate level.[4, 8] All four of these criteria must be observed to insure viability. Satisfactory perfusion characteristics show only the absence of vasospasm and will not detect pre-existing degrees of anoxic damage, so that warm ischemia time must also be considered. Perfusion will not detect pre-existing damage in the donor and, for this reason, the donor's serum creatinine must be measured at the time of death. The serum lactate level after the kidney is placed on perfusion will determine the amount of damage that has occurred during the period of cold storage, as under anerobic conditions lactate is produced by the kidney. If any of these four criteria are not met, the kidney should not be used. This decision can be difficult at times, but the principle that no kidney is better than a bad kidney cannot be overemphasized.

Short-term preservation is probably the method of choice for large transplant centers where the higher cost and the specially trained personnel needed for this method of storage are compensated by the logistical advantages. Unfortunately, the extra time made available by this method of preservation has not improved donor-recipient matching utilizing currently available methods of tissue typing. The graft survival at one year will be no better than that of kidneys stored by simple hypothermia.

Intermediate Storage

The third method, intermediate-term storage allowing preservation for several weeks, is still in its infancy. The underlying problems appear to be simple but difficult to solve. In intermediate-term preservation, tissues of nonhibernators are subjected to conditions which only true hibernators have been able to tolerate by their adaptation through the process of evolution. For instance, the cellular and subcellular membranes of organs of homeotherms, in contrast to those of poikilotherms and hibernators, respond to hypothermia by transition from a liquid crystalline state to a solid gel state in a lipid portion of the membrane.[9] These changes disrupt the activity of en-

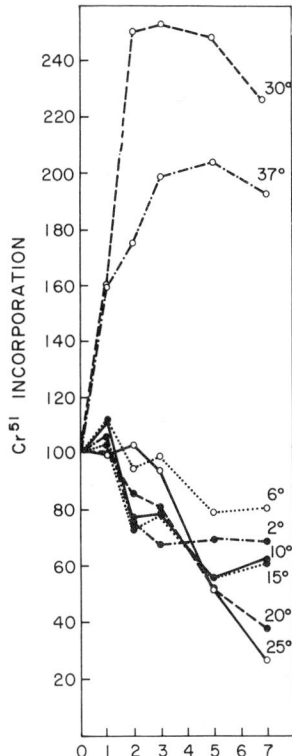

Figure 2. Viability of dog kidney cells as measured by ^{51}Cr incorporation after 7-day storage at different temperatures. It is obvious that in temperatures below 30° C. progressive cell death occurs.

preservation has been successfully accomplished, as only then will the more time-consuming methods of donor-recipient matching such as mixed lymphocyte culture be practical. In addition, it would be an enormous advantage if kidneys could be stored for the same period of time that blood is stored now.

Long-Term Preservation

Long-term preservation awaits a break-through in freezing of whole organs at temperatures below −79° C. The problems involved in freezing large organs, such as the human or dog kidney, are enormous. So far, there have been no published reports that such organs have been actually frozen for any length of time, thawed, and successfully implanted. Although this may become the procedure of choice in the distant future, this method probably depends upon the development of a nontoxic cryoprotective agent that will remain in liquid form at much lower temperatures than are currently possible. If such a cryoprotective agent can be found, the problems of uneven freezing and thawing of large organs could be solved.

SELECTED REFERENCES

Karow, A. M., Abouna, G. J. M., and Humphries, A. L.: Organ Preservation for Transplantation. Boston, Little, Brown and Company, 1974.
A good recent and detailed review in the field of organ preservation not only for the kidney but also of other organs such as the heart, liver, bone marrow, and pancreas.

zymes which are bound to membranes, thereby resulting in a metabolic imbalance that eventually results in irreversible injury. Other problems to be solved include the cold sensitivity of certain necessary enzyme systems and specific substrate utilization under conditions of hypothermia. At the present time, it is impossible not only to store a whole kidney for 7 or more days but even to maintain a kidney cell from a nonhibernator, such as the dog, in simple culture for a week or more. Figure 2 shows the effect of hypothermia on dog kidney cells. Excellent viability and growth are shown if the temperature is 30° C or higher, but if the temperature is dropped below 30° C, progressive cell death occurs. The graph shows some protective effect of hypothermia, but progressive cell death occurs with time.

If the cold injury can be identified and corrected, substrates and oxygen must be delivered to the organ and metabolic waste products must be removed. Thus, perfusion will be necessary for intermediate preservation. The next breakthrough in clinical renal transplantation will probably occur after intermediate-term

REFERENCES

1. Belzer, F. O., Ashby, B. S., and Dunphy, J. E.: 24-hour and 72-hour preservation of canine kidneys. Lancet, 2:536–539, 1967.
2. Belzer, F. O., Ashby, B. S., Gulyassy, P. F., and Powell, M.: Successful 17-hour preservation and transplantation of human-cadaver kidney. N. Engl. J. Med., 278:608–610, 1968.
3. Belzer, F. O., Ashby, B. S., Huang, J. S., and Dunphy, J. E.: Etiology of rising perfusion pressure in isolated organ perfusion. Ann. Surg., 168:382–391, 1968.
4. Belzer, F. O., Reed, T. W., Pryor, J. P., Kountz, S. L., and Dunphy, J. E.: Cause of renal injury in kidneys obtained from cadaver donors. Surg. Gynecol. Obstet., 130:467–477, 1970.
5. Collins, G. M., Bravo-Shugarman, M., and Terasaki, P. I.: Kidney preservation for transportation. Initial perfusion and 30 hours ice storage. Lancet, 1:219, 1969.
6. Downes, G. L., Hoffman, R., Huang, J. S., and Belzer, F. O.: Mechanism of action of washout solutions for kidney preservation. Transplantation, 16:46–53, 1973.
7. Huang, J. S., Downes, G. L., Childress, G., Felts, J., and Belzer, F. O.: Oxidization of C[14]-labeled substrates by dog kidney cortex at 10°and 38° C. Cryobiology, 11:387–394, 1974.
8. Johnson, R. W. G., Taylor, R. M. R., Swinney, J., Salvatierra, O., and Belzer, F. O.: Perfusate lactic acidosis, an essential parameter for evaluating human cadaver kidneys. Surg. Forum, 25:266–267, 1974.
9. Kountz, S. L., Cochrum, K. C., and Belzer, F. O.: Control of renal blood flow and sodium excretion in renal allografts by intrarenal infusion of acetylocholine. Surg. Forum, 19:210–212, 1968.
10. Toledo-Pereyra, L. H., Condie, R. M., Malmberg, R., Simmons, R. L., and Najarian, J. S.: A fibrinogen-free plasma perfusate for preservation of kidneys for one hundred and twenty hours. Surg. Gynecol. Obstet., 138:901–905, 1974.

VI

LIVER HOMOTRANSPLANTATION

Thomas E. Starzl, M.D., Ph.D., and Charles W. Putnam, M.D.

Treatment of terminal liver disease by transplantation was founded on the encouragement and knowledge provided by the steadily improving experience in renal transplantation.[17, 27] However, the liver is a far more complicated organ, and its malfunction leads to vastly more complex physiologic derangements. Liver patients are further handicapped, as are heart patients, by the lack of a satisfactory means of artificial support comparable to renal dialysis that could take over the organ's compromised functions during the wait for a suitable donor, or over the critical immediate postoperative period. The transplanted liver must function efficiently practically from the moment of anastomosis or the patient is lost.

Despite these and other difficulties, there has been enough progress in the laboratory and clinic to state that liver transplantation is now a feasible and legitimate, although imperfect, form of therapy, and one that may in certain cases be considered the treatment of choice. Human survivals up to 6 years have been achieved. A great deal has been and is being learned at a pace that suggests that liver transplants will soon have at least as much chance to succeed as kidney grafts now have.

KINDS OF LIVER TRANSPLANTATION

There are two general approaches to transplantation of the liver. With the first method, the host liver is removed and replaced with a homograft (orthotopic homotransplantation). The alternative technique is the insertion of an extra liver (auxiliary homotransplantation) at an ectopic site. Both procedures were developed in dogs and later studied in other species including rats, pigs, monkeys, and humans. The most encouraging results have been with orthotopic transplantation, for which reason most of this chapter will be concerned primarily with this replacement operation. However, in a special section near the end of the chapter, auxiliary hepatic transplantation also will be briefly considered.

IMMUNOLOGIC CONSIDERATIONS

Is the Liver a Privileged Graft?

When research in liver transplantation was in its early stages, it was suggested by Cannon[5] that if the liver played a significant role in graft rejection, hepatic homografts might enjoy a better fate than other transplants because presumably the grafted liver would not participate in its own repudiation. The case for this rather mystical view even seemed strengthened by certain experiences with laboratory animals. When immunosuppression in canine recipients was stopped after 4 months, a surprising number of animals continued to thrive either with no signs of rejection or with rejection episodes that waxed and waned remittently.[20, 27] One such dog lived in our laboratory with stable liver function for 11 years and 8 months after transplant. This phenomenon of "graft acceptance" had been noted in dogs with renal transplants,[17, 27] but less frequently.

If the liver thus seemed to be an immunologically favored organ for transplantation in dogs, its status in pigs as observed by Garnier,[9] Terblanche,[29] Calne[4] and in our own laboratory[27] was even more noteworthy. In some experiments with pigs not treated with immunosuppressive agents, identifiable homograft rejection did not occur. In other experiments, rejection was indolent and spontaneously reversed. These surprising results occurred in only a minority of animals. Nevertheless, they had to be attributed to some special privilege of the liver, since porcine skin[11] and kidney grafts[4] were regularly rejected in the usual way.

These observations in both dogs and pigs (and now in other animals) invited certain hypotheses in addition to the one stated above that the new liver helped create an internal milieu favorable to itself. Other possibilities[27] were that the liver was inherently less antigenic than other organs, that its relatively great antigenic mass was a beneficial factor, that its enormous regenerative capacity made it less susceptible than other tissues to the effects of chronic rejection, or, in the view of Calne,[3] that it possessed or released some special factor promoting the induction of specific immunologic tolerance.

Whatever the explanation, overstatement of the case for the liver's privileged status could lead to erroneous conclusions about the practical requirements for immunosuppressive therapy following hepatic transplantation in man. At a research level, another danger could stem from the notion that hepatic transplantation, especially in the pig, is somehow qualitatively unique. The fallacy of such a contention is obvious from the fact that even in the "easy" pig model, the majority of untreated liver recipients died from acute rejection.[27] In dogs and humans, control of hepatic rejection may be difficult or impossible in spite of very heavy immunosuppressive therapy.[20, 27]

Rejection Reversal

Instead of being unique, it is probable that liver homografts vary from other organs only by degree in the host immunologic response they evoke in all species including the pig. In this context, two key observations initially made with kidneys[17, 22] have been extended to the liver,[20, 27] and there is little doubt that they apply to other tissues as well. The first is the reversibility of rejection. In patients, reversal usually requires intensification of treatment, but it has sometimes been noted without any change in the pre-existing therapy, suggesting that such recoveries had an element of spontaneity. As mentioned earlier, "spontaneous remission" of rejection in the absence of all therapy has been seen both in dogs and in pigs, particularly the latter. The events with the liver in all three species are undoubtedly expressions of the same phenomenon, differing only quantitatively.

Graft Acceptance

The second observation of overriding practical and theoretical interest concerns what has already been referred to as "graft acceptance." In many of the human kidney recipients treated almost a decade ago,[17, 22, 27] it was shown that a melting away of host resistance to the homograft occurred surprisingly early after transplantation, often following an acute rejection crisis. This was manifested by eventual declines in the doses of immunosuppressive agents necessary to retain stable graft function. In many patients, the level of chronic immunosuppression has proved to be less than that which at the outset failed to prevent the onset of a severe rejection.

All treatment has been stopped without subsequent rejection by some of these human renal recipients whom we have now followed for many years, but such a drastic final step is known to be exceptionally dangerous. However, as described earlier, therapy has been successfully discontinued in dogs after kidney transplantation and even more consistently after liver replacement, indicating that graft acceptance may become very complete. In pigs, the barrier of natural host resistance is apparently low enough that the cycle of hepatic graft acceptance can be completed without any immunosuppression at all. Viewed in this way, the curious pig liver experiments become only a special example of, rather than an exception to, a general principle of transplantation. Perper and his associates[13] and subsequently other authors have provided evidence to support both this concept and the original idea that there is a slight but limited biologic advantage in transplanting the liver versus the kidney. Perper showed that a 3-day course of heterologous antilymphocyte globulin (ALG) treatment or other short-term therapeutic maneuvers in pigs permitted long-term acceptance of kidneys in precisely the same way as occurs with the liver in the absence of all iatrogenic intervention.

Explanations for Graft Acceptance

It is indisputable that some element of acceptance of various kinds of grafts occurs often in humans under the appropriate conditions of immunosuppression and that the degree to which this develops is a prime determinant of the long-term prognosis. Unfortunately, the reason for the change in the host-graft relationship is not known. More than one immunologic pathway may be involved.

Immunologic Tolerance. Schwartz and Dameshek[16] first suggested the possibility that the continuous presence of a transplanted organ in a host being treated with immunosuppressive therapy could lead to a selective loss of responsiveness to antigens. The suggestion is that specific lymphocyte clones, induced to replicate by the graft antigens, are thereby rendered more vulnerable to the killing effect of immunosuppressive agents than the rest of the lymphocyte population (Fig. 1). Inasmuch as the maintenance of such activated cell lines appears to be thymus-dependent even in adult life, at least in some experimental animals, it is reasonable to be curious about the effect of thymectomy as an adjuvant immunosuppressive measure. The results of thymectomy in a series of our

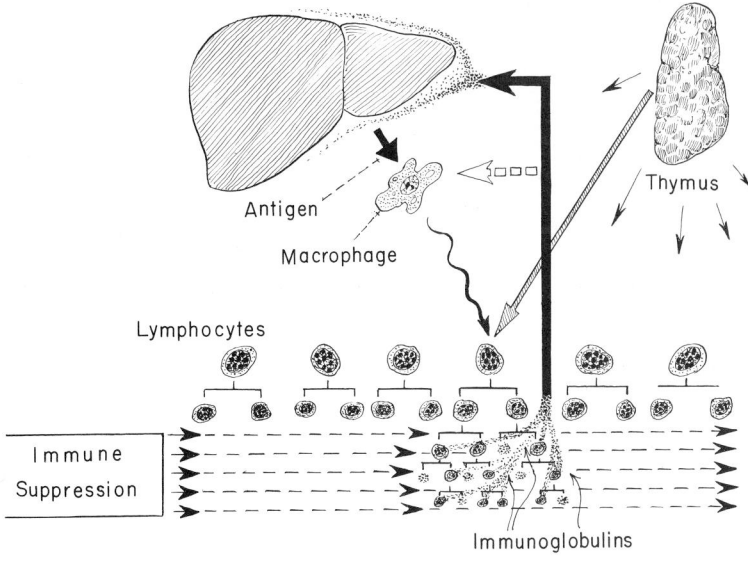

Figure 1. Hypothetical mechanims by which nonspecific immunosuppression may lead to selective abrogation of the host immune response. Special susceptibility to these agents of a fraction of the lymphoid population could lead to exhaustion of a clone, and hence, tolerance. Since maintenance of such cell lines even in adult life is apparently thymic-dependent in experimental animals, thymectomy would be expected to aid the process; this appears to be true in rodents, but such an effect of thymus removal has not been proved in dogs or humans (see discussion in text). A possible protective role of immunoglobulins elaborated by the replicating cells is also shown.

Antigen

Macrophage

Thymus

Lymphocytes

Immune Suppression

Immunoglobulins

human renal transplants were inconclusive.[23] While the patients with thymic excision did not have better survival or superior renal function, there were fewer and less severe histopathologic abnormalities when their grafts were examined long after transplantation.

The concept of specific, differential tolerance through "clone stripping" can partly explain the characteristic cycle of rejection and reversal occurring after whole-organ transplantation both in treated animals and man and in the weak and self-resolving crises in the untreated pig. Moreover, it is consistent with the fact that a wide variety of agents that are capable of general immunologic crippling can also provide specificity of action under the stipulated conditions of immunosuppressive treatment during presence of the antigen.

To date, few investigations have been performed in human recipients of chronically functioning renal homografts to establish the presence or absence of classic immunologic tolerance to their donor tissue. It would be interesting to know if skin from these donors would be accepted. One of the reasons why such a test has not been carried out in patients is the potential risk of precipitating an immune reaction that could damage the graft.[12] Of course, viable donor tissue is not available for such an experiment in liver recipients even if this were a desirable undertaking.

Amos and Bach[2] have provided evidence that at least some kidney recipients develop true tolerance to their donors. They performed mixed lymphocyte cultures with peripheral blood from a number of our renal recipients and their donors 2 to 4 years after transplantation. In some cases, the recipient lymphocytes no longer developed blast transformation when exposed to killed donor white cells, although they reacted vigorously to third-party cells. However, in other cases recipient lymphocytes retained their reactivity to donor cells. In experiments, dogs with tolerated kidneys may promptly reject skin or kidney grafts from the original donor.

Enhancement. These ambivalent findings do not disprove tolerance through "clone stripping" so much as they suggest that at least another mechanism of graft acceptance may be involved. One such mechanism, termed "enhancement," has been envisioned as a process in which immunoglobulins synthesized by the activated lymphoid tissues circulate to the target tissue and coat it or protect it in some way that is not yet understood (see Fig. 1). Antigraft antibodies, selectively capable of being absorbed by the nucleated cells of the original donor, have been detected in patients carrying well-tolerated renal transplants. Extensive immunoglobulin deposition has been demonstrated by immunofluorescence techniques in long-functioning kidney homografts,[15] but this latter finding usually has an adverse connotation rather than a favorable one.

The two foregoing mechanisms of graft acceptance by tolerance induction and enhancement are not mutually exclusive. The Seattle transplantation group headed by Marchioro, using the techniques developed by the Hellströms, has demonstrated changing host-graft relationships in kidney recipients that are consistent with a multifactorial graft-acceptance hypothesis.[14]

TISSUE TYPING

Another way by which clinical results might be improved would be effective donor-recipient matching of histocompatibility (HLA) antigens as discussed elsewhere in this chapter. Unfortunately, the state of our knowledge about human histocompatibility systems is still primitive. While a good match between siblings appears to provide a more favorable prognosis after renal transplantation than a poor match, our experience with unrelated subjects provides no such correlation[23] and has led us for the moment to ignore the question of HLA matching altogether in cadaveric cases. In liver transplantation, in which nonrelated cadaveric sources must be utilized exclusively, we have had some excellent results with poor histocompatibility matches and some discouraging results despite close matches.[26, 27] Not only has a correlation with tissue typing been absent with regard to clinical outcome, but no connection at all has been found between the quality of the match and the appearance of the hepatic homograft at subsequent histologic examination.[27] Until the discrimination of the matching methods in nonrelated cases is improved, it is difficult to justify denying a patient an available organ solely on the basis of poor serologic histocompatibility. Nor do we even use most favorable matching as an instrument of selection among candidates for transplantation. At the present time, a more valid criterion may be who has the most pressing need.

There is even reason to believe that screening procedures for preformed antigraft antibodies are not as critical in liver cases as with the kidney.[19] Preformed anti-red cell isoagglutinins that react against donor tissues and cytotoxins that can be detected by their lysis of donor lymphocytes immediately destroy many renal homografts that are transplanted in violation of such positive crossmatches.[17] The liver is very resistant to this so-called hyperacute rejection.[26] In our series, 3 liver transplantations were carried out in spite of red blood group incompatibility and 3 more were performed in confrontation of cytotoxic antibodies. There were no unequivocal hyperacute rejections.

THE PROCUREMENT OF ORGANS

In contrast to typing, the procurement of a fresh, functioning, nonischemic liver is of paramount advantage and provides the strongest correlation with success or failure.

The Source of Donors

In discussing homograft quality, the technical details of organ preservation become interwoven with, or even distinctly secondary to, ethical considerations about the conditions for the pronouncement of donor death and problems of cooperation by the medical and lay community. Unquestionably, one of the most important advances that have been made in transplantation has been social in nature, consisting of acceptance by the public of the concept of cadaveric organ removal. In turn, this was made possible by a willingness of many members of the medical profession to identify potential donors, to approach family members at a time of their bereavement, or to indicate in other ways their belief in the propriety of these efforts. By avoiding the glare of lay publicity, this can be and has been done impersonally and with restraint in many areas without exaggeration and without infringing on the personal right to privacy of the individuals involved.

Pronouncement of Death

After the donor has been identified and made available, an effort is made to maintain good liver perfusion up to the last possible moment in order to minimize the ischemic damage that even a short unperfused period may wreak under normothermic conditions. The extraordinary resuscitative efforts required in the donor to prevent circulatory depression in the face of a hopeless prognosis usually require explanation to relatives.

Ultimately, a final decision to discontinue supportive measures may be made after all is in readiness to proceed with the recipient. During the first years of liver transplantation at the University of Colorado, a considerable physiologic penalty was accepted because of criteria that required both brain death and cessation of heartbeat before commencing with organ removal. The price of this insistence was the loss of critical time, and variable ischemic damage both during the agonal stages of circulatory failure and in the minutes after cardiac arrest.[27]

The reason for accepting these conditions was the fear that the quality of terminal care for the donor might be compromised by the pronouncement of death in the presence of a heartbeat. In 1968 our criteria were liberalized in accordance with the concept of irreversible brain injury as it was first outlined and applied at the University of Louvain, Belgium, by Alexandre,[1] and later defended by the Harvard ad hoc committee.[7] Experience since then has convinced us that anxieties about terminal care were unfounded. Acceptance of the brain death concept alleviated one of the most serious problems in liver transplantation, for it virtually eliminated the interval of normothermic ischemic injury and often permitted the organ to be taken in the presence of an intact and effective circulation.

Preservation Techniques

The subsequent preservation of the liver is also of vital importance and has been accomplished by one or more preservation modalities, depending on circumstances, and always including organ hypothermia.[27] With the advantages conferred by the acceptance of brain death, it is often possible to maintain a naturally perfused liver in situ practically up to the moment of its excision. After removal, quick cooling may be accomplished by running a chilled electrolyte solution through the portal vein, thus lowering the donor organ temperature to about 10 or 15° C., which is sufficient for adequate preservation during the hour or so required for the vascular anastomoses in the recipient. In the event of a heart standstill before the recipient is ready, it is possible to employ the procedure used before 1968, when cardiac arrest was required before proceeding; by means of a heart-lung machine, circulation in the cadaver is reinstituted in combination with cooling (Fig. 2). Complicated preservation devices are no longer used.

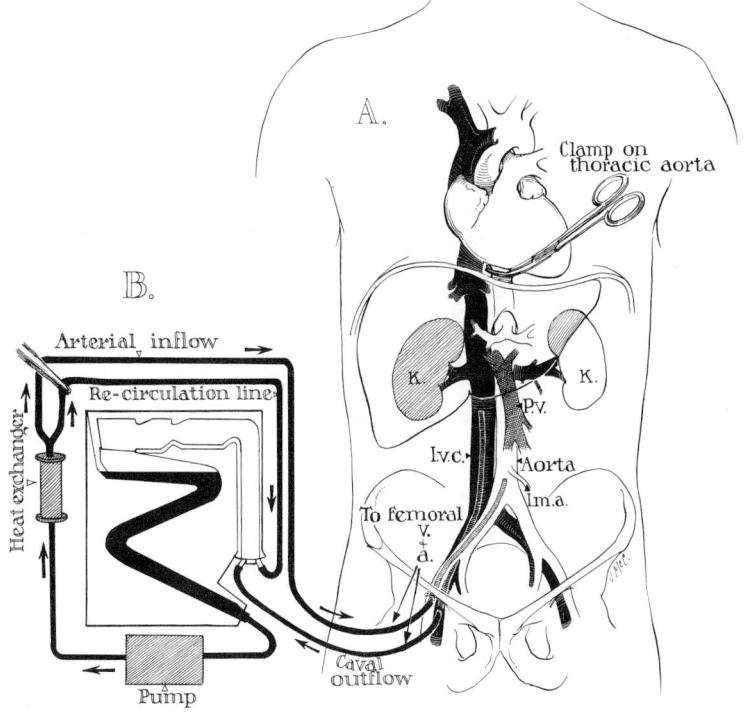

Figure 2. Technique of extracorporeal perfusion with a heart-lung machine. Catheters are inserted via the femoral vessels into the aorta and vena cava as soon as possible after death. The extracorporeal circuit is primed with a glucose or electrolyte solution to which procaine and heparin are added. The cadaver is thus anticoagulated with the first surge of the pump. Temperature control is provided by the heat exchanger. Cross-clamping the thoracic aorta limits perfusion to the lower part of the body.

SURGICAL TECHNIQUES OF ORTHOTOPIC TRANSPLANTATION

Species Differences

The procedure of liver replacement was first accomplished in dogs. The transition from animal experimentation to clinical application required some major technical adjustments and in at least one important and unexpected way demonstrated the need to be alert to the special requirements of human physiology. With removal of the host liver it is necessary to cross-clamp temporarily the great veins draining the intestines (portal vein) and the lower half of the body (inferior vena cava). If provision is not made for decompression of the distal venous pools during the anhepatic phase, dogs either die of shock on the operating table or expire at a later time because of irreparable damage to the mesenteric capillary bed. It was assumed that the same precaution would be necessary in humans and this was accomplished in the first five human recipients by plastic bypasses from the splenic or femoral vein or both to the external jugular veins. There was a dismaying incidence of pulmonary emboli, which caused or contributed to the death of three of the first five recipients. It was suspected either that the clots originated within the bypasses and were actually carried to the lungs during the operation or that they formed a short time later at or near the site where the femoral catheter had been inserted.

The omission of the venous decompression procedure in later patients did not produce any serious or long-lasting circulatory effects, including hypotension. Although a slight duskiness of the intestine developed in some recipients, it immediately disappeared when blood flow was restored through the reconstructed venous channels. One can explain the ease with which portal and vena caval cross-clamping was tolerated by man's inherently richer network of potential collateral channels for the return of blood to the right heart, and by the presumed additional increase in their size and ramifications in consequence of the underlying liver disease.[27] Venous decompression with bypasses has not been used in any recent case.

Vascular Anomalies

In planning a liver transplantation, the surgeon must be prepared for a high incidence of anatomic variations in either the graft or host structures.[27] These have been encountered in almost 40 per cent of our cases. Multiple arteries have been the most frequent anomalies. When these have been in the recipient, most commonly the graft celiac axis has been connected to the host aorta. When the multiplicity has been of the transplant vessels, multiple arterial anastomoses or other variant procedures have been used. There is no question that the need to improvise in these situations imposes an extra risk, particularly in very young recipients whose arteries are quite small and thin-walled even under the best technical circumstances.

Bile Duct Problems

The problems of obtaining adequate bile drainage and avoiding technical errors that may lead to leakage or obstruction may also be complicated by the presence of biliary tract anomalies, and the surgeon must be prepared to tailor his procedure to the individual case.

Choice of Biliary Drainage. In several of our first recipients who did not have biliary atresia, bile duct reconstruction was with choledochocholedochostomy over a T-tube stent (Fig. 3D). The method lost favor because of a high incidence of biliary fistula, and cholecystoduodenostomy after ligation of the common duct (Fig. 3A) became our first choice for a number of years. However, since November, 1973, the preferred technique has been cholecystojejunostomy with a Roux-en-Y loop (Fig. 3B), thus removing the homograft from the mainstream of the gastrointestinal tract and draining it through a defunctionalized jejunal limb. Alternatively, Roux-en-Y choledochojejunostomy (Fig. 3C) has been used for recently treated patients. In a number of cases it has been necessary to convert from cholecystojejunostomy to choledochojejunostomy (Fig. 3B and C) because of delayed obstruction at the cystic duct.[19, 26]

Bile Duct Anomalies. Ligation of the transplant common duct in conjunction with cholecystoduodenostomy may be dangerous if anomalies are not recognized. Communication between the cystic and common ducts may not always be at the point of their juncture (Fig. 4). In one patient the ducts were externally fused but separated by an internal septum; in 2 others the homograft cystic duct passed behind the common duct and descended for almost 2 inches as one compartment of a double-barreled lumen. In all 3 cases, biliary drainage was inadvertently obstructed when the common duct ligature closed both parallel passages, a technical error that subsequent surgery failed to correct and that proved fatal.

Some of the vascular and ductal anomalies could have been diagnosed preoperatively, resulting either in better planning for surgery or a decision not to operate at all. These earlier cases did not, however, have the benefits of the extensive arteriography and cholangiography that are now used routinely in the donor and sometimes in the recipient as well.

Hemorrhage

Other problems during and after operation may be caused by derangements in the coagulation mechanism that may result in either hemorrhage or thrombosis.[27] As one would expect, acute bleeding can be particularly troublesome during the actual liver transplantation. The very nature of the underlying hepatic pathologic process produces portal hypertension in nearly every patient, and the nature of the operation tends to exaggerate it. The usual consequence is mechanical bleeding that can rapidly assume nightmare proportions during the procedure. Many of the normal coagulation factors that might help control hemorrhage are dependent on the liver and are therefore defective in the diseased recipient. These coagulation factors may be even more deficient during the anhepatic phase, or subsequently they may be of dubious quality, depending on the state of preservation of the homograft, on how much ischemia it has suffered, and

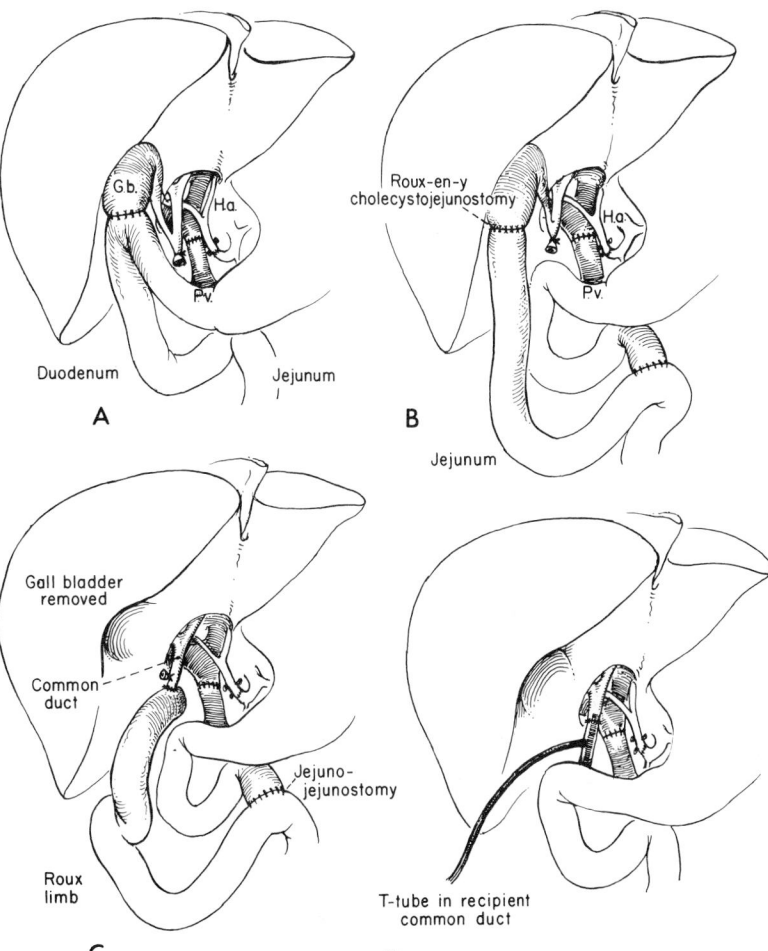

Figure 3. Techniques of biliary duct reconstruction used for most liver transplant recipients. *A,* Cholecystoduodenostomy. *B,* Cholecystojejunostomy. *C,* Choledochojejunostomy after removal of gallbladder. *D,* Choledochodochostomy. Note that T-tube is placed if possible in recipient common duct. (From Starzl, T. E., et al.: Surg. Gynecol. Obstet., *142*:487, 1976.)

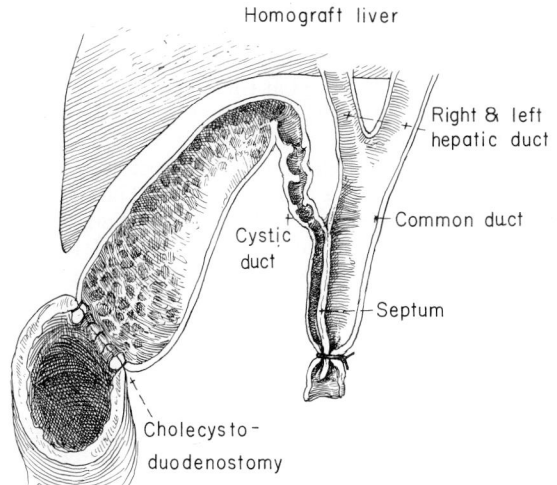

Figure 4. The anatomic basis for a technical error which cost the life of a patient. Distal ligation of the double-barreled extrahepatic duct system resulted in total biliary obstruction.

on how much immediate functional capability it has retained.

When hemorrhage occurs, the surgeon's challenge is to use any and all available hemostatic tactics—ligating, suturing, cauterizing—until the revascularized homograft can participate in what is hoped will be appropriate coagulation function. With our earlier patients, whose homografts were generally of less than optimal quality for the reasons stated earlier, an attempt was made to treat bleeding problems by administering thrombogenic agents. However, hypercoagulability was caused in some instances. The unacceptable incidence of pulmonary embolism in these patients led us to abandon this approach.

In retrospect, it is possible that the coagulability induced by exogenous thrombogenic agents might be prohibitively additive to the clotting brought about by the homograft which, when it begins to function, may overreact. Indeed, the better the condition of the transplant, the greater the risk of unwanted coagulation. Almost every series of liver transplants, including our own, has at least one example of thrombosis of the hepatic arterial circulation to which a rebound phenomenon may have contributed. The use of anticoagulants to forestall this emergency is dangerous. Documented intravascular clotting during the operation would be an indication for heparin, but such proof is hard to obtain. Moreover, heparinization is a double-edged maneuver; depressed clotting can have devastating effects on patients submitted to such major trauma and with so many potential bleeding sites.

In general, it is now considered best to avoid iatrogenic manipulation of the clotting process with either thrombogenic or anticoagulant agents. Instead, our current approach is to leave correction of coagulation abnormalities to natural processes, intervening only under special circumstances and for very specific indications.

Anesthesia

During operation, there are other metabolic abnormalities than those concerned with coagulation. These contribute to the complexity of anesthetic management. Not only is the procedure long and difficult, but even more important, it is an operation on the primary organ involved in the metabolism and detoxification of most common anesthetics. At any point during the operation, the liver is either inherently impaired, absent, or untried in its new setting. Hence, the task of the anesthesiologist is to administer correctly drugs that, first, are not hepatotoxic and, second, do not depend primarily on the liver for their degradation. In our cases, reliance has been placed mainly on combinations of volatile agents in nonexplosive concentrations. Such management permits use of the electrocautery, gives flexibility in lightening or deepening anesthesia, and allows anesthesia to be abruptly stopped if required by changing physiologic circumstances.[27]

Other Operative Problems

The foregoing are some selected difficulties associated with liver transplantation. There is a long list of other technical pitfalls: adrenal venous infarction, air embolism, and crushing of the right phrenic nerve by too high a clamp on the upper vena caval cuff, to mention but a few. The reader interested in a more detailed discussion of these and other surgical problems is referred to more detailed publications.[19, 26, 27] These technical matters have played a major role in the mortality encountered in our first cases. Even though deaths from such causes are theoretically avoidable, technical misadventures still constitute the leading cause of failure, as has been very well documented in our exhaustive study of the first 93 consecutive cases.[26]

IMMUNOSUPPRESSION

The immunosuppressive therapy in liver transplantation has borrowed heavily from the experience gained with human renal transplants. Two general treatment programs were evolved with the simpler kidney model and then applied to the liver recipients.

Double Drug Therapy

The first protocol, which was used from 1962 to 1966 for all organ recipients at the University of Colorado, consisted of "double drug" treatment with azathioprine and the synthetic adrenal cortical steroid, prednisone.[17] Evolution of the use of these two agents together, appreciation of their marked synergism, and demonstration that rejection could be readily reversed by increasing the steroid doses were among the advances that made clinical transplantation practical and that introduced what is known as the modern era of this field. But in spite of fair results with renal transplantation, the double drug therapy either did not prevent rejection of hepatic homografts or else it proved too toxic to permit host survival. Six patients treated with liver transplantation from 1963 to 1965 died in a month or less.

Triple Drug Therapy Including ALG

In 1966, heterologous antilymphocyte serum (ALG) was introduced clinically at our center as a third immunosuppressive agent, added to the drugs mentioned above.[24, 27] Since then, this triple drug therapy has been given to all our renal, hepatic, and cardiac recipients, even though not all transplant surgeons concede the need for ALG.

Almost all of our human liver recipients who achieved chronic survival were treated with the combination of azathioprine, prednisone, and intramuscular ALG. In the event of a rejection episode, it is the steroid component that has proved to be the agent most amenable to quick adjustment of dosage according to need. In the event that hepatotoxicity of azathioprine is suspected, we have been free to substitute the alkylating agent, cyclophosphamide, which has immunosuppressive qualities equivalent to azathioprine.[28]

Penalties of Immunosuppression

Some of the hypotheses of the actions of these immunosuppressive drugs have been discussed elsewhere[27] and reviewed earlier in this chapter. Suffice it to say, as was emphasized at the outset of this chapter, the method by which these agents are used in conjunction with the actual transplantation may conspire to permit selective abrogation of the host rejection response. If this were not true, there would be little hope of rehabilitating patients and returning them to life in an unrestricted environment, since each of the individual agents can cause general immunologic crippling more or less in proportion to the dose used.

Risks with All Organs. The most obvious penalty of a depressed immune system is heightened susceptibility to infection.[17, 27] However, it has also become obvious that chronically immunosuppressed patients have an increased vulnerability to de novo malignancies.[17, 27] In our own series of chronic survivors after renal transplantation, more than 5 per cent have developed either mesenchymal or epithelial malignant tumors. Almost all other major transplantation centers have recorded this complication, which is presumably due to failure of the depressed immunologic surveillance mechanism to identify the tumor tissues as alien and to eliminate them or restrict their growth.

Extra Risks for Liver Recipients. In addition to the foregoing general liabilities of immunosuppression, there are some special risks for the liver candidate. One is the fact that hepatic injury in all kinds of organ recipients has commonly been produced by the agents, individually or in combination, of the therapeutic regimen.[27] In some instances, virus hepatitis, apparently made chronic by the partial immunologic invalidism of the host, has been a plausible explanation. In others, hepatotoxicity of the drugs was probably responsible. With liver malfunction, dose control of some of the agents may become difficult, since the liver participates in their pathways of action or degradation. These hepatic factors are obviously important in any situation requiring immunosuppression, but they have heightened significance for a traumatized liver transplanted to a new and hostile environment.

It was mentioned in the preceding section that infection was a major risk to any immunosuppressed patient. In the liver recipient, postoperative sepsis of the graft itself has proved to be a special problem, without doubt partly because of the anatomic location of the orthotopically placed organ, interposed between the intestinal tract and the heart. Bacteria from the bowel, particularly of the gram-negative variety, can be brought into contact with the transplanted liver via the intestinal veins draining into the portal vein or, far more importantly, by retrograde spread up the duct system after passage through the biliary anastomosis (Fig. 5). In either event, the presence of nonviable hepatic tissue provides a perfect medium for bacterial growth. Eventually, partial gangrene of the transplant can result, with characteristic nonvisualizing areas on the liver scans (Fig. 6), gram-negative bacteremia, and all the findings of generalized sepsis.

Avoidance of Homograft Sepsis. Early in our clinical series, the above findings of graft and systemic infection led us to consider the essential problem to be one of bacterial invasion and thus prompted reductions of immunosuppression. Such decisions were tragically incorrect and were followed by necrosis and infection of large parenchymal areas. Experience soon taught that ischemia of portions of the liver was the initiat-

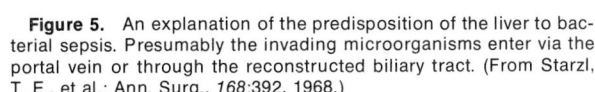

Figure 5. An explanation of the predisposition of the liver to bacterial sepsis. Presumably the invading microorganisms enter via the portal vein or through the reconstructed biliary tract. (From Starzl, T. E., et al.: Ann. Surg., *168*:392, 1968.)

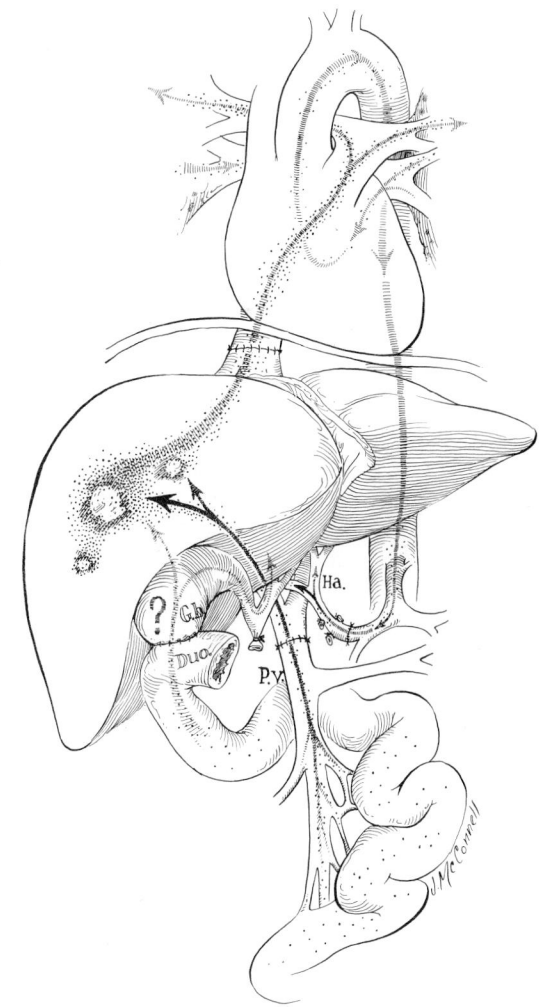

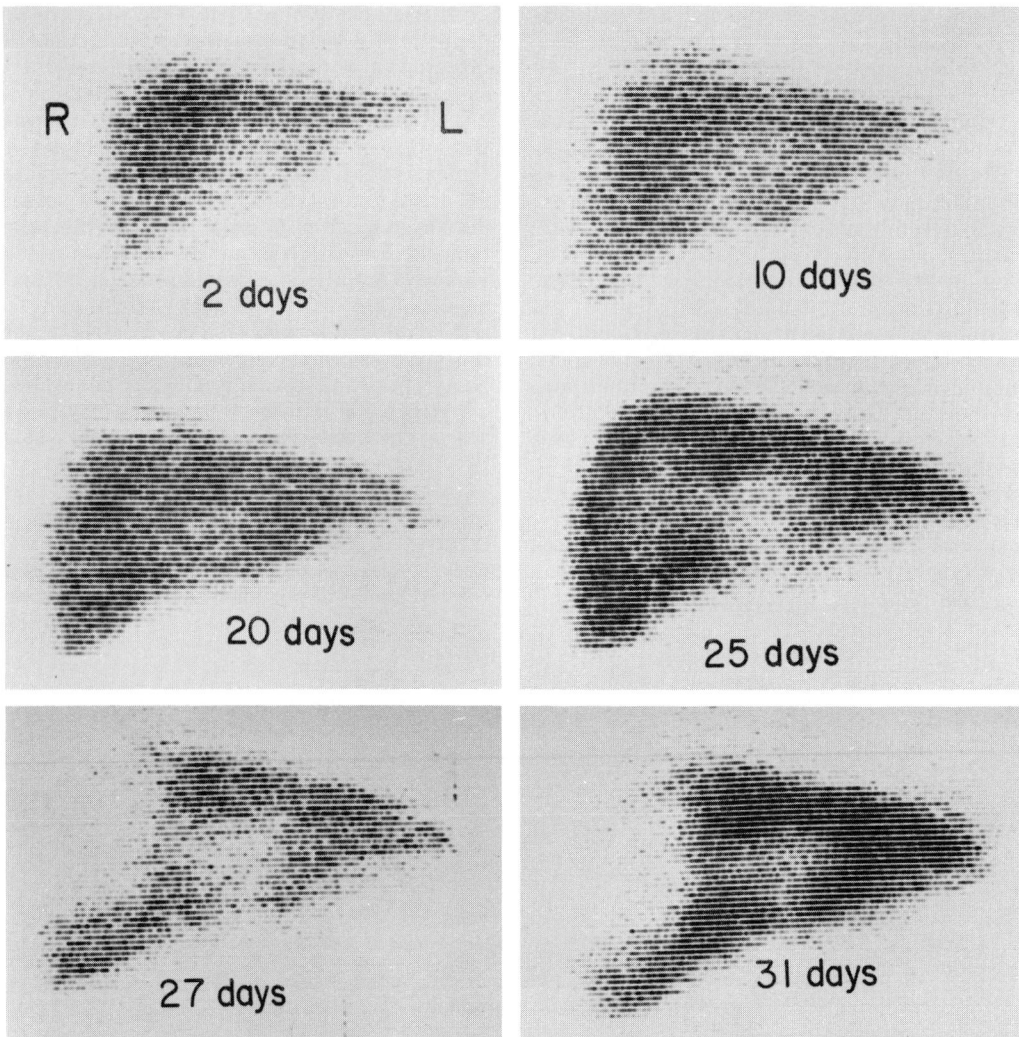

Figure 6. Postoperative technetium scans of the liver in a 13-month-old infant whose indication for orthotopic transplantation was biliary atresia. *2 days:* The small homograft is normal. *10 days:* An increase in size is evident although the general configuration of the organ is still normal. *20 days:* No further change is noted. *25 days:* The examination was conducted as an emergency when gram-negative septicemia developed and very high increases in the transaminases appeared. Areas of decreased isotope uptake are obvious in the right lobe and the central part of the liver. *27 days:* A striking extension of the process can be seen less than 48 hours later. A débridement procedure was carried out the same evening. *31 days:* Four days after débridement the radiographic appearance was improved.

ing event, and that the basis for the ischemia was rejection.[27] Consequently, immunosuppression should ordinarily be increased rather than reduced if this complication is thought to be impending. When this was done by giving substantially higher doses of prednisone (as noted, the only highly dose-maneuverable component of the immunosuppressive triad), the incidence of regional hepatic gangrene fell to nearly zero. It should be added that our prophylactic treatment protocol includes heavy antibiotic treatment for the first postoperative week, including agents effective against gram-negative bacteria, after which this therapy is stopped.

The other vitally important step in reducing homograft sepsis has been to use biliary reconstructive techniques that prevent systematic contamination by gastrointestinal contents (see Fig. 3B, C, and D).

INDICATIONS FOR LIVER REPLACEMENT

The understanding of regional hepatic gangrene that evolved illustrates well the learning process of caring for patients receiving a new kind of treatment. With the acquisition of experience, other important issues have also been clarified, including that of the indications for liver replacement. A brief summary of our first 93 consecutive recipients, treated from March, 1963, to November, 1974, can be used to illustrate these indications in the light of the results after a minimal potential follow-up of 14 months.[26] The 93 patients were aged 3 months to 68 years.

Hepatic Malignancy

The indication for 15 of these transplants was hepatoma, cholangiocarcinoma, intrahepatic duct cell carcinoma, or hemangioendothelial sarcoma. Seven of these patients died within 39 days from technical problems of one kind or other.

Six patients had more prolonged survival, but died after 76, 87, 143, 339, 400, and 432 days. In all 6, metastases were present and in 5, the recurrences were directly responsible for death. Two other more recently treated patients who had intrahepatic duct cell carcinomas are still alive after 22 and 16 months, but the recipient with the longer follow-up has extensive metastatic disease.

An additional unsuspected hepatoma was found in a 4-year-old child treated for extrahepatic biliary atresia. This child is still alive, now 6 years after the operation; she has no evidence of recurrence of neoplasia.

Because of the high rate of recurrent malignancy, it has become our policy to consider liver replacement for primary liver tumors only under the most exceptional circumstances, even though our experience and that of Daloze of Montreal and Calne of Cambridge have demonstrated the possibility of an occasional tumor cure.

Biliary Atresia

Far more desirable candidates are those without neoplasms, in spite of the fact that the technical difficulties in benign hepatic disease are more severe because the patients tend to be sicker and to have more advanced portal hypertension. Moreover, if the diagnosis is biliary atresia, an increased incidence of vascular anomalies can be expected to compound the difficulties, together with the small size of the structures to be anastomosed in these young patients.[27] Nevertheless, the longest survivors of liver transplantation in the world are those who had this disorder (Fig. 7). Of our own series of 40 patients with biliary atresia, treated 14 months or longer ago, including the child with the incidental hepatoma already mentioned, 11 lived for longer than 1 year and 7 are still surviving with completely normal liver function 16 months to 6 years after operation. Three of the late deaths after 13, 13½, and 30 months were from recurrent hepatic insufficiency caused in two instances by chronic rejection, but probably in the third by indolent viral hepatitis. The fourth late death after 41 months occurred a few weeks after a bout of Hemophilus septicemia, which had resulted in multiple organ damage.

The potential of liver transplantation for the treatment of biliary atresia will not be realized until the heavy early mortality is reduced. A recent analysis of the deaths within the first postoperative year has

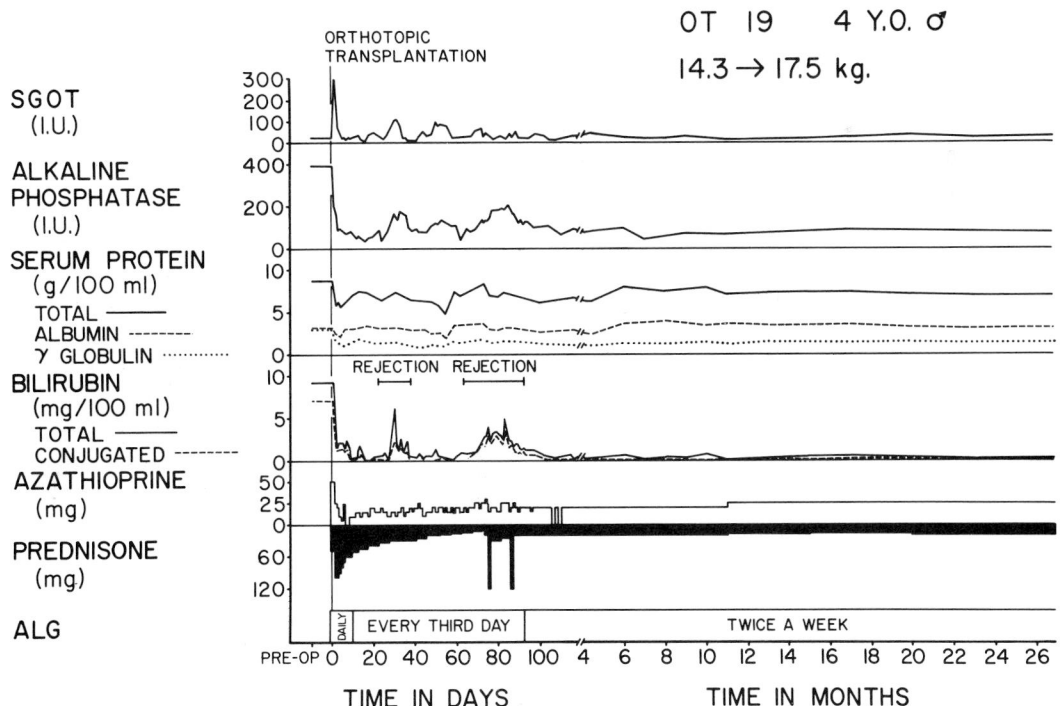

Figure 7. The course of a 4-year-old child after orthotopic liver transplantation for the indication of biliary atresia. Note the rejection episodes at 1 month and 2½ months, which were easily controlled. The patient, who died after 3½ years, was for a long time the longest-surviving liver recipient in the world. This distinction now belongs to another child whose original disease was biliary atresia and who has been followed for 6 years after transplantation.

shown the overwhelming contribution of technical and mechanical problems to the acute loss rate.[26] Inability to control rejection played a surprisingly minor role. With the use of microsurgical techniques and an increased alertness to biliary tract complications, there is no reason why these children should not be the best of all potential candidates for liver replacement.

Cirrhosis

Among the 93 consecutive patients treated with liver replacement, there were 18 with cirrhosis due to chronic aggressive hepatitis (9 children and 9 adults) and 9 with end-stage alcoholic cirrhosis. Six of the 18 patients with chronic aggressive hepatitis lived for at least 1 year. Only 1 of the 9 with alcoholic cirrhosis lived into the second postoperative year.

Undoubtedly, one reason for the bad experience with cirrhotic patients has been a reluctance to recommend such therapy except in the agonal stages of the disease. Now that the feasibility of long-term survival and rehabilitation has been demonstrated, transplantation at an earlier time probably should be considered, particularly in cases of postnecrotic cirrhosis in which the maximal value of medical management and of abstinence from alcohol has already been realized.

Other Indications

Periodic reassessment of the influence of the original host disease upon the outcome will also be necessary insofar as this factor influences future case selection. None of the diseases for which liver transplantation has been used so far can be categorically precluded as an indication for further trials, especially in children. The brightest chapter in liver transplantation has been in the treatment of inborn errors of metabolism in children, including our two cases of Wilson's disease (one patient is alive after 5 years, the other died after 6 years [Fig. 8]), our patient with alpha-1-antitrypsin deficiency (alive after 2¼ years), and Daloze's child with Niemann-Pick disease,[6] who is alive after 1½ years. It has become clear that the hepatic-based inborn errors of metabolism are all potentially curable with liver transplantation.

Other conditions for which transplantation has been performed include congenital biliary cirrhosis, primary biliary cirrhosis, secondary biliary cirrhosis, sclerosing cholangitis, the Budd-Chiari syndrome, and acute and chronic serum hepatitis due to the HB_sAg virus.

Even continued efforts to treat recipients with chronic HB_sAg antigenemia are probably warranted, especially if hyperimmune specific gamma globulin therapy can be offered. Without such treatment, it seems highly probable that the new liver will eventually be afflicted with the same disease that destroyed the native organ (Fig. 9).

Future Prospects

In a positive sense, the most important conclusion that has emerged from the experience with our first 93

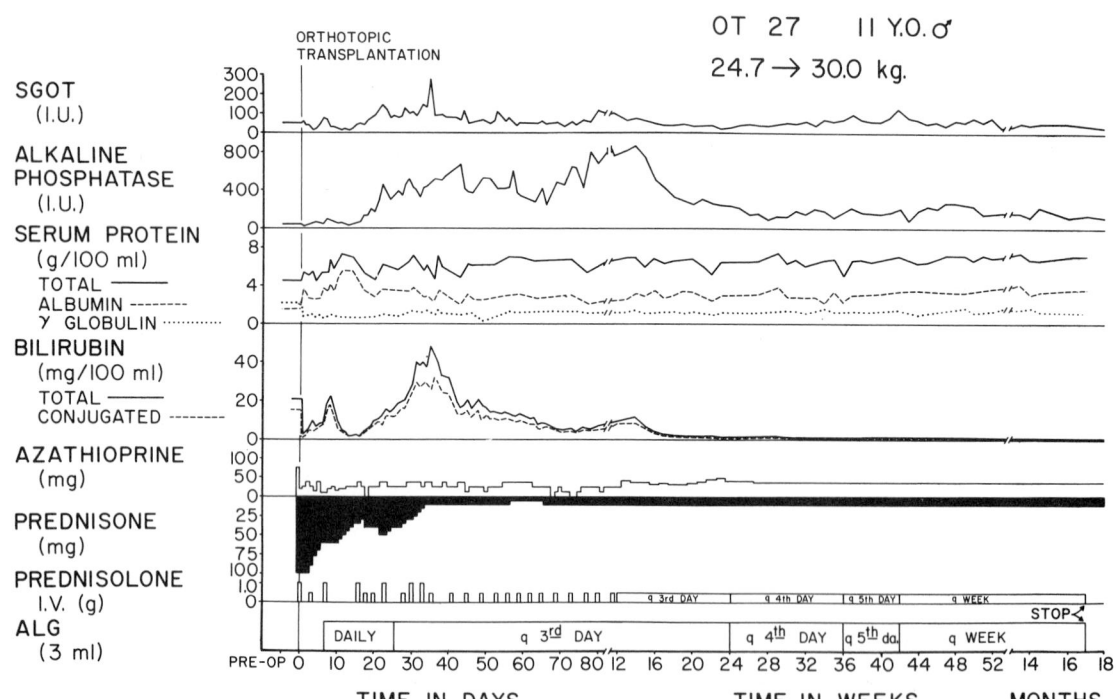

Figure 8. Course of a child with Wilson's disease and hepatic cirrhosis who was treated with liver replacement in July, 1969. He lived for six years without stigmata of recurrent Wilson's disease. Eventually his death was caused by chronic partial biliary duct obstruction of the homograft, which led to widespread intrahepatic sludge formation. (From DuBois, R. S., et al.: Lancet, 1:505, 1971.)

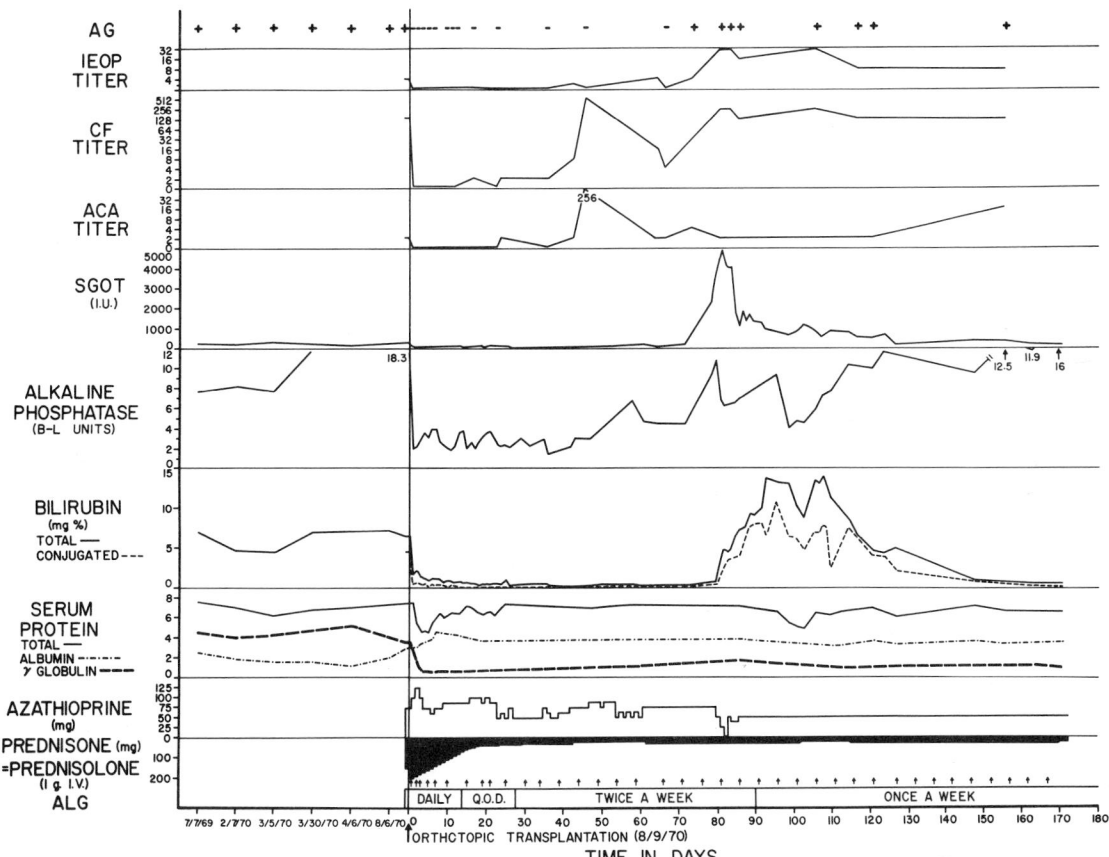

Figure 9. The course of a patient who was terminally ill with chronic aggressive hepatitis, Australia (Au) antigen-positive. She was treated by liver replacement. Note that all serologic evidence of serum hepatitis disappeared immediately after operation only to return some weeks later. AG, agarose gel micro-Ouchterlony test for Au antigen. IEOP, quantitative immunoelectro-osmophoresis test for Au antigen. CF, complement fixation test for Au antigen. ACA, anticomplementary activity, which is thought to reflect the presence of circulating antigen-antibody complexes; the test is not immunologically specific for Au antigen. Normal Bessey-Lowry (B-L) units for alkaline phosphatase are less than 3. This patient eventually developed a modified serum hepatitis in her homograft and died 20 months after transplantation. (From Torisu, M., et al.: Ann. Surg., 174:620, 1971.)

consecutive liver replacements was that prolonged survival repeatedly was possible. A total of 27 patients lived for at least a year following operation, and 16 of this group are still alive after more than 1 to almost 6 years. The outlook has slowly improved, although not to a satisfactory state. The first 25 recipients who formed the basis of a monograph on liver transplantation[27] included only 5 one-year survivors. The next group of 25 contained 6, and the group from 51 to 75 had 8 one-year survivors. There have already been 8 one-year survivors among the 18 patients beginning with number 76.

The chronic survivors, particularly those in recent times, have had remarkably stable liver function, and usually they have achieved complete social rehabilitation. Survival of more than a year after orthotopic liver transplantation has been recorded from other centers by Williams and Calne and their associates in England,[30] by Daloze and his colleagues in Canada,[6] and by Hume and his associates in the United States.[10]

In our own case material of 93 consecutive cases,[26] rejection of the liver as judged by classical histopathologic criteria played a surprisingly small role in the heavy overall mortality, accounting for less than 10 per cent of the deaths. Technical or mechanical problems, especially those of biliary duct reconstruction, were a far greater cause of failure, as were systemic infections. When abnormalities of liver function developed in the postoperative period, the nearly automatic diagnosis of homograft rejection proved in retrospect to have been wrong in most instances.

Further development of liver transplantation depends upon three kinds of progress. First, earlier decisions for transplantation will be necessary, especially in adult recipients. Second, there must be reduction of operative and early postoperative accidents and complications by more discriminating case selection, purely technical improvement, and better standardization of biliary duct reconstruction. The third area will be sharpening the criteria for the differential diagnosis of postoperative hepatic malfunction, including the liberal use of transhepatic cholangiography and needle biopsy. Only then can better decisions be made about changes in medication or about the need for secondary corrective surgical procedures.

The frequency with which liver transplantation is being used is steadily increasing. Within the next five years, it is virtually certain that this approach to the treatment of liver disease will become far more widely accepted.

AUXILIARY LIVER TRANSPLANTATION

Both in experimental animals and in patients, survival after auxiliary transplantation has been inferior to that with the orthotopic procedure. The reasons for these disappointing results have not been entirely clear, but plausible explanations have been advanced indicting both metabolic and mechanical factors.

Metabolic Considerations

When auxiliary liver transplantation was first attempted in immunosuppressed canine recipients, a curious and disquieting observation was soon made.[21] The extra organs underwent rapid shrinkage, which was usually evident within 2 weeks and which was

very advanced at all times after one month. Subsequent research has shown that the atrophy can be prevented if the homograft's portal inflow is provided with blood returning from the pancreas. The most important constituent of portal venous blood in maintaining liver health has been demonstrated unequivocally to be insulin.[18, 25]

Clinical Experience

In most of the early attempts at auxiliary liver transplantation, the homograft was not given an acceptable blood supply by the criteria just described. The results were uniformly poor.[27]

More recently, Fortner[8] has reported survival of more than one year in a child with biliary atresia whose auxiliary liver was furnished with both an arterial and an adequate splanchnic venous inflow similar to that shown in Figure 10.

This single success has demonstrated the feasibility of auxiliary liver transplantation. However, the technical difficulties of achieving optimal revascularization, the abdominal over-crowding by the addition of an extra large organ, and the consequent pulmonary complications that have plagued auxiliary transplant recipients have all suggested that the auxiliary procedure will play no more than a minor role in the exploitation of clinical liver transplantation.

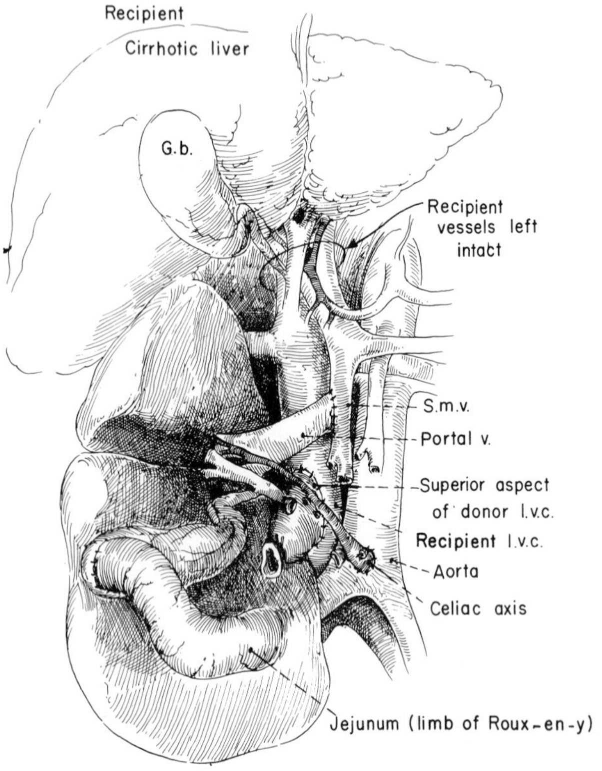

Figure 10. Auxiliary liver transplantation with a technique that provides an adequate blood supply for the homograft. Note that the transplant is given a double blood supply and that the venous component is from the nonhepatic splanchnic bed. Biliary drainage can be with a Roux-en-Y cholecystojejunostomy.

SELECTED REFERENCES

Starzl, T. E., Porter, K. A., Putnam, C. W., Schroter, G. P. J., Halgrimson, C. G., Weil, R., III, Hoelscher, M., and Reid, H. A. S.: Orthotopic liver transplantation in 93 patients. Surg. Gynecol. Obstet., *142*:487, 1976.
   The article contains a clinical-pathologic analysis of the first 93 consecutive cases of orthotopic liver transplantation carried out at the University of Colorado, with a minimum potential follow-up of 14 months. Emphasis was on the causes of failure and upon means of improving future results.

Starzl, T. E., and Putnam, C. W.: Experience in Hepatic Transplantation. Philadelphia, W. B. Saunders Company, 1969.
   The book summarizes the first clinical attempts at liver transplantation and contains a complete survey of the literature on liver transplantation up to the spring of 1969.

Williams, R., Smith, M., Shilkin, K. B., Herbertson, B., Joysey, V., and Calne, R. Y.: Liver transplantation in man: The frequency of rejection, biliary tract complications, and recurrence of malignancy based on an analysis of 26 cases. Gastroenterology, *64*:1026, 1973.
   The article is an exhaustive and well-written summary of the first 26 patients treated with liver replacement by the King's College-Cambridge English team.

REFERENCES

1. Alexandre, G. P. J.: Discussion of Murray, J. E.: Organ transplantation, the practical possibilities. *In* Wolstenholme, G. E. W., and O'Connor, M. (Eds.): Ethics in Medical Progress: With Special Reference to Transplantation. Boston, Little, Brown and Company, 1966, pp. 54–77.
2. Amos, D. B., and Bach, F. H.: Phenotypic expressions of the major histocompatibility locus in man (HL-A): Leukocyte antigens and mixed leukocyte culture reactivity. J. Exp. Med., *128*:623, 1968.
3. Calne, R. Y., White, H. J. O., Binns, R. M., Herbertson, R. M., Millard, P. R., Pena, J. R., Samuel, J. R., and Davis, D. R.: Immunosuppressive effects of the orthotopically transplanted porcine liver. Transplant. Proc., *1*:321, 1969.

4. Calne, R. Y., White, H. J. O., Yoffa, D. E., Binns, R. M., Maginn, R. R., Herbertson, R. M., Millard, P. R., Molina, V. P., and Davis, D. R.: Prolonged survival of liver transplants in the pig. Br. Med. J., *4*:645, 1967.
5. Cannon, J. A.: Transplantation Bull., *3*:7, 1956.
6. Daloze, P., Corman, J., Block, P., Delvin, E. E., and Glorieux, F. W.: Enzyme replacement in Niemann-Pick disease by liver transplantation. Transplant. Proc., 7:607, 1975.
7. Definition of irreversible coma: Report of the *ad hoc* committee of the Harvard Medical School to examine the definition of brain death. J.A.M.A., *205*:337, 1968.
8. Fortner, J. G., Beattie, J., Jr., Shin, M. H., Kawano, N., and Howland, W. S.: Orthotopic and heterotopic liver homografts in man. Ann. Surg., *172*:23, 1970.
9. Garnier, H., Clot, J. P., Bertrand, M., Camplez, P., Kunlin, A., Gorin, J. P., Goaziou, F. L., Levy, R., and Cordier, G.: Greffe de foie chez le proc: Approache chirurgicale (Liver transplantation in the pig: Surgical approach.) C. R. Acad. Sci. (Paris), *260*:5621, 1965.
10. Hume, D. M., Wolf, J. S., Lee, H. M., and Abouna, G.: Liver transplantation. Transplant. Proc., *4*:781, 1972.
11. Jaffe, W. P., Symes, M. D., and Terblanche, J.: Observations on the immunological reactions of pigs. In Read, A. E. (Ed.): The Liver. London, Butterworth & Co., Ltd., 1967, pp. 331–357.
12. Murray, J. E., Sheil, A. G. R., Moseley, R., Knight, P. R., McGavic, J. D., and Dammin, G. J.: Analysis of mechanism of immunosuppressive drugs in renal homotransplantation. Ann. Surg., *160*:449, 1964.
13. Perper, R. J., Bowersox, B. E., and VanGorder, T. J.: Prevention of rejection of porcine renal allografts. Transplant. Proc., *3*:488, 1971.
14. Pierce, G. E., Quadracci, L. J., Tremann, J. A., Hoe, R. E., Striker, G. E., Hellström, I., Hellström, K. E., and Marchioro, T. L.: Studies on cellular and humoral immune factors in human renal transplantation. Ann. Surg., *174*:609, 1971.
15. Porter, K. A., Andres, G. A., Calder, M. W., Dosseter, J. B., Hsu, K. C., Rendall, J. M., Seegal, B. C., and Starzl, T. E.: Human renal transplants. II. Immunofluorescent and immunoferritin studies. Lab. Invest., *18*:159, 1968.
16. Schwartz, R., and Dameshek, W.: Drug-induced immunological tolerance. Nature, *183*:1682, 1959.
17. Starzl, T. E.: Experience in Renal Transplantation. Philadelphia, W. B. Saunders Company, 1964.
18. Starzl, T. E., Francavilla, A., Halgrimson, C. G., Francavilla, F. R., Porter, K. A., Brown, T., and Putnam, C. W.: The origin, hormonal nature and action of portal venous hepatotrophic substances. Surg. Gynecol. Obstet., *137*:179, 1973.
19. Starzl, T. E., Ishikawa, M., Putnam, C. W., Porter, K. A., Picache, R., Husberg, B. S., Halgrimson, C. G., and Schroter, G.: Progress in and deterrents to orthotopic liver transplantation; with special reference to survival, resistance to hyperacute rejection, and biliary duct reconstruction. Transplant. Proc., 6:129, 1974.
20. Starzl, T. E., Marchioro, T. L., Porter, K. A., Taylor, P. D., Faris, T. D., Hermann, T. J., Hlad, C. J., and Waddell, W. R.: Factors determining short- and long-term survival after orthotopic liver homotransplantation in the dog. Surgery, *58*:131, 1965.
21. Starzl, T. E., Marchioro, T. L., Rowlands, D. T., Jr., Kirkpatrick, C. H., Wilson, W. E. C., Rifkind, D., and Waddell, W. R.: Immunosuppression after experimental and clinical homotransplantation of the liver. Ann. Surg., 160:411, 1964.
22. Starzl, T. E., Marchioro, T. L., and Waddell, W. R.: The reversal of rejection in human renal homografts with subsequent development of homograft tolerance. Surg. Gynecol. Obstet., *117*:385, 1963.
23. Starzl, T. E., Porter, K. A., Halgrimson, C. G., Andres, G., Hurwitz, R., Giles, G., Terasaki, P. I., Penn, I., Lilly, J., Starkie, S. J., Schroter, G. P. J., and Putnam, C. W.: Long term survival after renal transplant in humans: With special reference to histocompatibility matching, thymectomy, homograft glomerulonephritis, heterologous ALG, and recipient malignancy. Ann. Surg., *172*:437, 1970.
24. Starzl, T. E., Porter, K. A., Iwasaki, Y., Marchioro, T. L., and Kashiwagi, N.: The use of antilymphocyte globulin in human renal homotransplantation. *In* Wolstenholme, G. E. W., and O'Connor, M. (Eds.): Antilymphocytic Serum. London, J. & A. Churchill, Ltd., 1967, pp. 4–34.
25. Starzl, T. E., Porter, K. A., Kashiwagi, N., Lee, I-Y., Russell, W. J. I., and Putnam, C. W.: The effect of diabetes mellitus on portal blood hepatotrophic factors in dogs. Surg. Gynecol. Obstet., *140*:549, 1975.
26. Starzl, T. E., Porter, K. A., Putnam, C. W., Schroter, G. P. J., Halgrimson, C. G., Weil, R., III, Hoelscher, M., and Reid, H. A. S.: Orthotopic liver transplantation in 93 patients. Surg. Gynecol. Obstet., *142*:487, 1976.
27. Starzl, T. E., and Putnam, C. W.: Experience in Hepatic Transplantation. Philadelphia, W. B. Saunders Company, 1969.
28. Starzl, T. E., Putnam, C. W., Halgrimson, C. G., Schroter, G. P., Martineau, G., Launois, B., Corman, J. L., Penn, I., Booth, A. S., Jr., Porter, K. A., and Groth, C. G.: Cyclophosphamide and whole organ transplantation in humans. Surg. Gynecol. Obstet., *133*:981, 1971.
29. Terblanche, J., Peacock, J. H., Bowes, J., Davies, R., Tierris, E. J., Palmer, D. B., and Hunt, A. C.: The use of pigs as an experimental animal for orthotopic liver homotransplantation. Br. J. Surg., *54*:231, 1967.
30. Williams, R., Smith, M., Shilkin, K. B., Herbertson, B., Joysey, V., and Calne, R. Y.: Liver transplantation in man: The frequency of rejection, biliary tract complications, and recurrence of malignancy based on an analysis of 26 cases. Gastroenterology, *64*:1026, 1973.

VII

LUNG TRANSPLANTATION

Keith Reemtsma, M.D., and Henry M. Spotnitz, M.D.

HISTORICAL ASPECTS

Among the various organs, the lung was one of the last to be used in experimental transplantation. Demikhov[17] first investigated experimental pulmonary transplantation extensively. He developed techniques for transplantation of lobes and the intact lung in dogs. Metras[40] was the first to utilize the atrial cuff technique for the venous anastomosis. Juvenelle in 1951 performed the first successful orthotopic autograft, and function of this lung was demonstrable 35 months later.[48] In 1963 Hardy reported the first human pulmonary allograft.[34]

EXPERIMENTAL PULMONARY TRANSPLANTATION

Initial attempts at autogenous reimplantation of a single lung in dogs resulted in a 35 to 80 per cent mortality.[20] By contrast, dogs consistently survive unilateral pneumonectomy. Analysis of the anatomic and physiologic difficulties in reimplantation of the lung have resulted in important technical improvements, with reported long-term survival in excess of 80 per cent.[43] Pertinent results of studies in autogenous reimplantation of the canine lung will therefore be summarized prior to separate discussion of canine allografts and experiments in other animals.

TECHNICAL ASPECTS OF AUTOGENOUS REIMPLANTATION

The high early mortality has been due primarily to technical failures. Venous obstruction and the resultant pulmonary edema have been the most common cause of failure and decreased function.[2] A high incidence of thrombosis occurs with anastomosis of individual pulmonary veins. For this reason, individual lobes are less frequently reimplanted, and the atrial cuff technique is utilized in most lung reimplantations. This method does not prevent venous obstruction entirely, however. Decreased function and pulmonary hypertension were found in lungs in which excision and reanastomosis of a cuff of atrium containing the pulmonary veins were the only procedures.[7] Acute thrombosis, chronic fibrotic narrowing of the suture line, and fibrous plugs originating proximal to the anastomosis have been described.[55]

Thrombosis at the pulmonary artery anastomosis has not been observed frequently except in the presence of vascular stasis in the lung secondary to narrowing of the venous anastomosis. A pressure gradient across the arterial anastomosis is often demonstrable and is more severe when the contralateral pulmonary artery is occluded.[53] Veith has shown that this is due to the inability of the anastomosis to dilate, and he has advocated the creation of a distensible anastomosis by spatulating the ends of the pulmonary artery or by use of a vein patch in the anastomosis.[66, 69]

Bronchial complications have been observed in as many as 50 per cent of animals undergoing reimplantation.[19] Ischemia of the bronchial anastomosis is the major cause. Stone,[58] after division and reanastomosis of only the bronchus, found necrotic changes at most of the anastomoses. By 6 weeks, however, the majority of these changes had regressed and healing was occurring. Subsequent scar tissue formation may narrow the bronchus, but this must be severe to be functionally significant. Most investigators have found that if the bronchus is divided as close to the hilum as possible, the incidence of bronchial complications is markedly reduced.[2, 33] Ellis[24] has demonstrated that collateral blood flow via the pulmonary artery to the bronchus is present at the hilum but not more centrally. This would explain the lack of necrosis of the short bronchial stump. Others feel that reconstruction of the bronchial arterial supply is indispensable if bronchial complications are to be avoided.[41] A telescoped, overlapping bronchial anastomosis has also proved beneficial.[69]

Regeneration of the bronchial arterial supply occurs in three to four weeks.[47] Division of hilar lymphatics has been found to have no effect, and regeneration of lymphatics is demonstrable within two to three weeks.[25, 33]

FUNCTIONAL EVALUATION AND PATHOPHYSIOLOGY OF THE REIMPLANTED LUNG

Several methods have been employed to evaluate function of the reimplanted lung. Differential bronchospirometry with measurement of ventilation and oxygen uptake has been used most frequently.[30] Reliable separation of function of the reimplanted lung from that of the normal lung is difficult. Angiography has been used to evaluate circulation in the graft but gives little quantitative information. Right heart catheterization is employed to measure cardiac output and pulmonary vascular resistance. Balloon tamponade of the contralateral normal pulmonary artery and measurement of its effect on pulmonary resistance and cardiac dynamics also may be accomplished by this method. Arterial blood gas determinations are used routinely to evaluate the status of the graft. The xenon-133 scintiscan is one of the most promising methods of evaluation of lung transplants. It is noninvasive, and sedation of the animal may not be required. Both ventilation and perfusion are evaluated in a quantitative fashion.[35] Oxygen uptake and intrapulmonary shunts are not measured by this technique. The most stringent test of function has been simultaneous or delayed contralateral pneumonectomy or pulmonary artery ligation.[28, 69]

Function of the lung decreases immediately after reimplantation. Within 2 to 3 weeks the ventilation and oxygen uptake increase but do not return to normal in most instances.[19, 28, 30, 50] Perfusion of the graft is decreased also, especially to the upper lobe. However, in many instances abnormal vascular anastomoses are found in conjunction with the decreased perfusion.[35] In those lungs without structural abnormalities, perfusion also will return toward normal.

Pulmonary arterial hypertension is present to a variable degree in all reimplanted lungs and is a major cause of death.[3, 21, 28, 30, 45] Although hypertension decreases with time, the recovery phase is more prolonged, and pressure does not return to normal. Elevated pulmonary artery pressures may be secondary to arterial or venous stenosis, or vasoconstriction of the pulmonary vascular bed. Depending on whether pressures are measured proximal or distal to the anastomosis, the true source of the pulmonary hypertension may be difficult to determine. Nigro[45] demonstrated increased pulmonary artery pressures in the absence of angiographically demonstrable defects in the arterial or venous anastomoses. Ketonen has shown by xenon flow distribution studies that pulmonary blood flow may be substantially obstructed even though pressure gradients cannot be demonstrated at the pulmonary artery anastomosis. This obstruction could be eliminated with a Dacron patch.[38] Although reimplantation appears to increase pulmonary resistance,[42] Veith has demonstrated that the vascular bed will dilate in response to oxygen following the vasoconstriction produced by hypoxia.[65] Autografting without ligation of the contralateral pulmonary artery results in focal interstitial edema, producing patchy infiltrates on chest x-ray. This pattern is maximized by the third postoperative day, and usually disappears by day 7 to 21.[49, 64] This syndrome is identified as the "reimplantation response." Reimplantation of the left lung with simultaneous ligation of the right pulmonary artery provides an interesting model in which survival is totally dependent on the autotransplanted lung. Mortality in initial studies was high; the mechanism of death was right ventricular failure and acute pulmonary edema.[16, 42] Pulmonary resistance in this model was higher with autografts than with allografts, suggesting compromise of the pulmonary artery anastomosis.[16] Ebert, in unanesthetized dogs, showed in control animals that pulmonary artery systolic pressure increased only 10 per cent when cardiac output doubled during exercise. On the other hand, pulmonary artery pressure more than doubled in the autotransplanted group.[21] Veith demonstrated survival of 9 of 16 dogs when a distensible pulmonary artery anastomosis was constructed, incorporating a jugular vein patch.[70] Allgood examined the causes of death in this model. Small groups of animals were subjected to (a) clamping of the left hilum for 75 minutes, (b) reimplantation after flushing with heparin saline, (c) skeletonization of hilar structures, (d) division and reanastomosis of the left main bronchus, or (e) division and reanastomosis of the pulmonary artery and veins. All animals retained the capacity for pulmonary vasodilatation with increasing blood flow except the total reimplantation group.[3] Scrutiny of these results re-emphasizes the contention of some authors that the combination of atelectasis and ischemia is most damaging during transplantation.[57] Others emphasize that flushing the pulmonary artery also tends to produce pulmonary edema.[13] While denervation and division of bronchial arteries and lymphatics do not appear to be primary causes of pulmonary edema in this model, they may be contributory.

The denervation of the lung that occurs as a consequence of reimplantation has been of serious concern to many investigators, as it was feared that respiratory paralysis would occur. It is generally recognized that the Hering-Breuer reflex is absent in reimplanted lungs, and regression of the intrinsic pulmonary nerves and afferent autonomic stretch receptors has been demonstrated. Denervation also has been postulated as an explanation for the increased vascular resistance.

The fact that animals survive after bilateral reimplantation or unilateral reimplantation with simultaneous contralateral pneumonectomy lessens the functional significance of denervation.[26, 44] The rate and rhythm of respiration in the resting state after these procedures usually are altered. More important, however, is the fact that these animals will respond normally to hypoxia and hypercarbia.[54] The reinnervation of the reimplanted lung is a controversial subject. Recent observations suggest parasympathetic bronchoconstrictor nerves, with some ganglion cells distal to the bronchial suture line, regain function within 3 to 6 months of reimplantation. Sympathetic efferent function and afferent nerve function were not detected, even 28 months after reimplantation.[22] Other investigators have been unable to detect vagal function 22 months after reimplantation.[53] Presence of cough reflexes following bilateral reimplantation has been attributed to residual tracheal innervation.[44]

Lung compliance either decreases or remains unchanged. Mucous transport has been studied by means of tantalum particles and found to be subnormal up to 120 days following reimplantation, but subsequently it became normal. This was ascribed to the effects of denervation.[23] Ischemia of the lung while reimplantation is being accomplished is an important factor. Most investigators feel that 2 hours is the maximum allowable time in which to re-establish circulation. However, a correlation between increased pulmonary artery pressures, decreased surfactant activity, and an ischemia time greater than 60 minutes has been demonstrated.[27] At the other extreme, no functional differences were noted between lungs with ischemic times of 1 hour and those with 5 hours ischemic times.[65] Ardekarni found that after 4 hours of ischemia survival was 75 per cent. At 5 hours it had decreased to 50 per cent and was 33 per cent at 6 hours. Death in all cases was due to pulmonary edema.[5]

Histologically, the reimplanted lung assumes a normal appearance several weeks to months after operation. In the immediate postoperative period, varying degrees of atelectasis, intra-alveolar and interstitial edema, and necrosis of the bronchial mucosa are present.

EXPERIMENTAL PULMONARY ALLOGRAFTS

Without immunosuppression, pulmonary allografts are rejected in 5 to 8 days. Furthermore, the animal usually dies as a result of rejection even though the contralateral normal lung is not manipulated in any fashion. Function of the allograft is similar to that of the autografts until the fifth post-transplant day, when allograft function begins to decrease precipitously.[35, 36] Technically, allografts present a less formidable problem in dogs than do autografts. Veith has reported 100 per cent five-day survival of 37 dogs with left lung allografting by an optimized technique.[69] Veith has distinguished several distinct processes that may contribute to the clinical picture following allografting. The reimplantation response, which may produce diffuse infiltrates on chest x-ray, tends to peak within three days and subside spontaneously.[60]

Progressive appearance of pulmonary infiltrates after three days may represent either rejection or pneumonia. Sputum cytology and cultures are useful in distinguishing these processes. In true rejection, Veith distinguishes vascular and alveolar components. The vascular component results in perivascular cuffs of mononuclear cells and intimal hyperplasia with reduced blood flow. The alveolar component consists of an exudative process with reduced alveolar ventilation. Immunosuppression may be more effective against the vascular component than the alveolar component of allograft rejection.[64]

Histologically, untreated allografts show perivascular and peribronchial infiltrates of plasma cells and lymphocytes by the third day.[32] Intra-alveolar edema then appears, and by the tenth day necrosis of the alveolar wall and intra-alveolar hemorrhage are prominent, and progressive destruction of the pulmonary architecture then occurs. With immunosuppressive therapy the sequence of events is variable, and some lungs may appear the same as those in untreated animals. In others a mild perivascular infiltrate may appear transiently. In long-term survivors progressive thickening of the alveolar septum may occur.[62, 64] The rapid appearance of histological evidence of rejection is unique to lung allografts and raises the question of some sort of presensitization.[32]

Various drugs and methods have been investigated as means of increasing survival of pulmonary allografts. Cortisone and ACTH prolong survival slightly. Large, intermittent doses of methylprednisolone appear effective in control of infiltrates revealed by x-ray and attributed to rejection on clinical grounds.[62, 64] Total-body irradiation causes severe bone marrow depression when used in high enough doses to affect a rejection. Blumenstock has been successful in prolonging survival with methotrexate. Whole-body cobalt irradiation and marrow transplantation when combined with methotrexate appear to be somewhat more effective than methotrexate alone.[10] Drug toxicity with methotrexate has been a significant problem, and most investigators have used azathioprine. In animals that survive the first few days after transplantation, average survivals of 30 to 50 days have been obtained when either methotrexate or azathioprine was used.[27] Anderson demonstrated that infusion of immunosuppressive drugs into the pulmonary artery in addition to oral azathioprine increased survival over that obtained with oral therapy alone.[4]

Contralateral pulmonary artery ligation has demonstrated the ability of the allograft to function immediately. In animals that thus survived operation, the average survival when azathioprine was used was 60 days.[68] Pulmonary artery pressure consistently increases after transplantation, the smallest increase being reported by Veith using the anastomotic method discussed earlier.

Blumenstock[11] has performed serial function studies on animals surviving up to 64 months after allotransplantation, with methotrexate or azathioprine used as immunosuppressive agents. Function gradually declines. For example, oxygen uptake by the allograft was 32 per cent of the total at 2 months but by the eighth month had decreased to 8 per cent. In another case, the values were 36 per cent at 7 months but 0 at 18 months. These results suggest that chronic rejection also occurs in pulmonary allografts. The animal surviving 64 months died when contralateral pneumonectomy was attempted. Surfactant activity and compliance were both decreased 48 hours post transplant in one series.[72] The possible significance of alterations in surfactant production during lung transplantation has recently been reviewed.[8] Heterotopic allografting into the retroperitoneal space has proved of some interest as an auxiliary oxygenator.[9] Allograft function can be assessed by specialized tests such as pulmonary angiography for evaluation of arterial patency,[56] serial bronchoscopy for detection of stenosis of the bronchial anastomosis and analysis of exudates,[52] and alveolar lavage cytology that may anticipate rejection by detection of abnormal alveolar macrophages and increased extracellular fibrin.[1] The rosette inhibition test may prove valuable in distinguishing infection and rejection.[15]

LUNG PRESERVATION

Little work has been done in the field of lung preservation. After preservation for 24 hours in a hyperbaric chamber under hypothermia, three of five lungs were found to have normal breathing capacity as measured by spirometry when reimplanted.[29] Using similar techniques, Blumenstock found normal lungs at biopsy in 6 of 15 animals following preservation for 24 hours and subsequent allotransplantation.[12] Methotrexate was used for immunosuppression. The canine lung apparently is easily damaged by current perfusion techniques. Castagna et al. concluded that vascular flushing and perfusion of lung allografts is detrimental to survival and should be avoided.[13] Additional studies suggest that prevention of lung collapse during transplantation is more important to preservation of function than is ischemia.[57] Utilization of a perfusate resembling intracellular electrolyte composition apparently permits storage of canine allografts for 5 hours at 4° C. or 3 hours in situ in a cadaver.[39] Techniques for analysis of lung metabolism are being proposed as an index of success of lung preservation methods.[51]

PULMONARY TRANSPLANTATION IN OTHER ANIMALS

Haglin has criticized the use of the dog in experimental lung transplantation because of its increased blood coagulability, propensity to pulmonary hypertension, and lack of bronchial artery–to–pulmonary artery anastomoses. He has used baboons and has found no evidence of venous or bronchial anastomotic complications. Pulmonary artery thrombosis has been an infrequent finding.[31] Staged contralateral pneumonectomy has been successful in a high percentage of cases, in contrast to the experience in dogs. Right heart catheterization was normal in five of six animals studied 8 to 20 months after reimplantation and contralateral pneumonectomy. Simultaneous contralateral pulmonary artery ligation in the baboon has also produced results superior to those obtained in canine experiments. Baboons appear to be inferior to dogs in ability to clear interstitial edema in the first two weeks after lung allografts.[6, 37] Use of the membrane oxygenator for temporary support following pulmonary allografting has also been studied in the baboon.[14] Results in sheep and calves have not been significantly different from those in the dog.

CLINICAL PULMONARY TRANSPLANTATION

Hardy performed the first human lung transplant, and the recipient survived 18 days before succumbing to renal failure, demonstrating the technical feasibility of the operation.[34] In 1968 Derom's patient survived 10 months following transplantation. Furthermore, the patient's symptoms from his basic disease were definitely ameliorated.[18, 71] Thirty-seven lung transplants have now been performed in twenty-two transplant centers (December, 1975).

Twenty-two transplants have been done for chronic obstructive pulmonary disease, eight for restrictive disease, and two for pulmonary hypertension. Four lobar transplants have been performed, with living donors used in all cases. In three of these the lobe was subsequently removed, with survival of the recipient. Donors in the remaining cases have most often died of cerebrovascular causes. Three cardiopulmonary transplants have been done, one in an infant with congenital heart disease and two in adults with obstructive lung disease. In only one case was an attempt made to reconstruct the bronchial arteries. Degenerative changes have been noted at the bronchus and there have been three reported instances of dehiscence. The atrial cuff technique has been used for the venous anastomosis in all cases of lung transplantation. Excluding Derom's survivor of 10 months, Veith's survivor of six months,[61] and the three survivors of lobar transplantation, there have been 24 survivors beyond 2 days, the longest survival time being 57 days. Seventeen patients died of respiratory insufficiency. Seven of these deaths were due to problems related to the recipient's remaining lung. Compression of the transplant by the contralateral lung occurred three times, and in two cases high airway resistance in the transplant resulted in marked right-to-left shunting. High vascular resistance in the recipient lung, with consequent diversion of most of the cardiac output to the transplant, resulted in acute pulmonary edema of the graft and death in two cases. In the other six cases various factors such as ischemia, rejection, and pulmonary edema were present. Pneumonia was the cause of death or a significant factor in eleven cases.

Blood or tissue typing was not consistently performed. Azathioprine and corticosteroids were the main immunosuppressive agents used. Other drugs, in addition to antilymphocyte serum and radiation, also were employed. Considerable difficulty has been encountered in distinguishing rejection and infection, both clinically and morphologically.[59, 62, 63] In 16 patients who survived longer than 5 days, rejection was clinically recognized in four. The transplant was re-

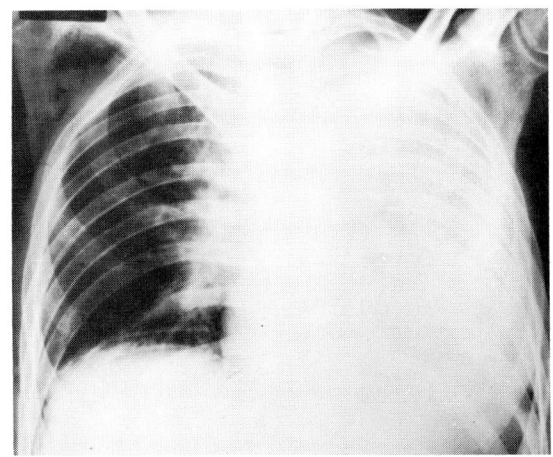

Figure 1. Well-expanded transplanted lung. The patient's left lung is completely opacified. (From Derom, F. R., et al.: J. Thorac. Cardiovasc. Surg., *61*:835, 1971.)

moved in three of these and the fourth was effectively treated during three separate rejection crises.

Several factors may have contributed to the long-term survival of Derom's patient. The recipient was young, aged 23, and had restrictive lung disease (silicosis). The donor was 40 years old, died of cerebrovascular causes, and was heparinized prior to removal of the lung. The lung was not flushed with any solution, and the ischemia time was only 55 minutes. Although chronic infection was present in the recipient's remaining lung, it was successfully controlled with antibiotics and did not interfere with function of the transplant (Figs. 1 and 2). The patient finally died of chronic rejection (Fig. 3).

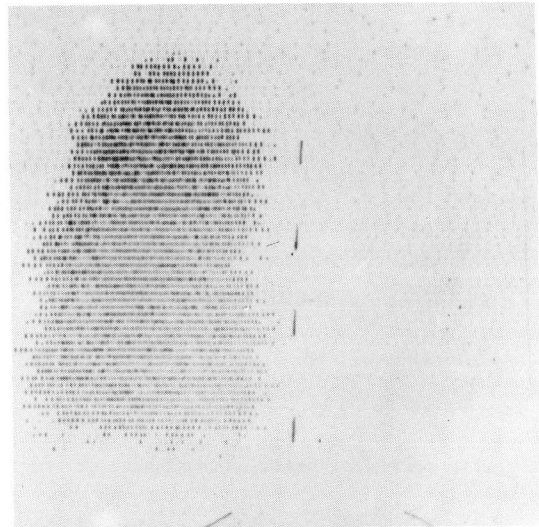

Figure 2. Pulmonary scan. There is near-normal blood flow to the transplanted lung but none to the patient's own left lung. (From Derom, F. R., et al.: J. Thorac. Cardiovasc. Surg., *61*:835, 1971.)

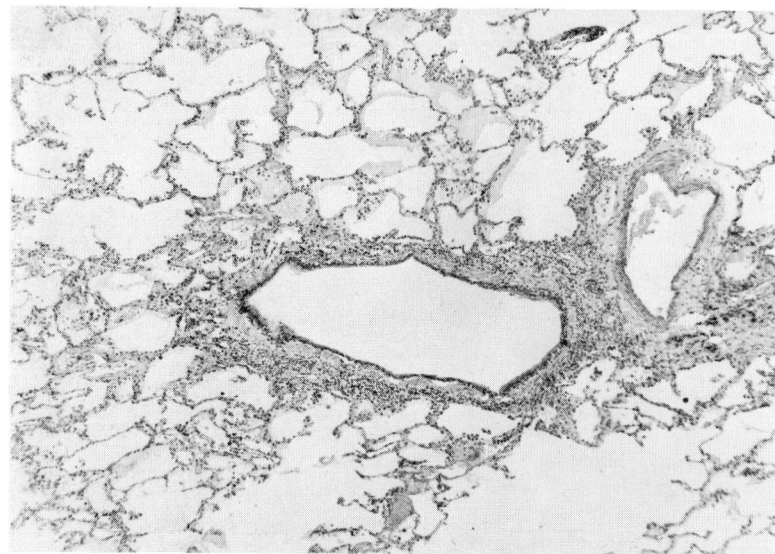

Figure 3. Histologic section of the transplanted lung 10 months after operation. There is moderate peribronchial lymphocytic infiltration. (From Derom, F. R., et al.: J. Thorac. Cardiovasc. Surg., 61:835, 1971.)

In summary, two primary obstacles have arisen in clinical lung transplantation. Early progressive respiratory insufficiency has been the most frequent and is due to abnormalities of the remaining diseased lung or to inadequacies of the transplanted lung. The second leading cause of death and complications has been pulmonary sepsis. As yet the precise nature of rejection and its role in graft failure has not been well defined.

ACKNOWLEDGMENT

We are grateful to Professor Dr. F. Derom of the University of Ghent, Belgium, for providing the illustrations of his case.

SELECTED REFERENCES

Trummer, M. R., and Berg, P.: Lung Transplantation. Springfield, Ill., Charles C Thomas, Publisher, 1968.
This excellent monograph discusses all aspects of pulmonary transplantation, with the greatest emphasis being placed on experimental data. Thorough discussions of technical details, functional evaluation, and efforts to enhance allograft survival are presented.

Veith, F. J., and Koerner, S. K.: The present status of lung transplantation. Arch. Surg., 109:734, 1974.
This is a comprehensive but concise review of both experimental and clinical lung transplantation as of July, 1974. Experience with 36 human transplants is reviewed in tabular form.

REFERENCES

1. Achterrath, U., Blümcke, S., Koerner, S. K., Yipintsoi, T., Siegelman, S. S., Chandler, P., Hagstrom, J. W. C., Torres, M., Cobbah, J. E., Fujii, P., and Veith, F. J.: Alveolar lavage cytology in transplanted lungs. I. Staining methods and findings in dogs with autografts and allografts without immunosuppression. J. Thorac. Cardiovasc. Surg., 69:510, 1975.
2. Alican, F., and Hardy, G. D.: Lung reimplantation. Effect on respiratory pattern and function. J.A.M.A., 183:849, 1963.
3. Allgood, R. J., Ebert, P. A., and Sabiston, D. C., Jr.: Immediate changes in pulmonary hemodynamics following lung autotransplantation. Ann. Surg., 167:352, 1968.
4. Anderson, J. M., Hannah, G., Neely, M. G., and Hutchinson, J.: Localized immunosuppression for pulmonary transplants. Br. J. Surg., 56:597, 1969.
5. Ardekarni, R. G., Faber, L. P., and Beattie, E. J.: Pulmonary function after various periods of ischemia in the canine lung. J. Thorac. Cardiovasc. Surg., 59:607, 1970.
6. Baker, R. R., Sabanayagam, P., Zarins, C. K., James, A. E., Hutchins, G. M., Byers, J. M., III, Katarajan, T. K., and Lee, J. M.: Functional and morphologic changes after lung allografting in baboons. Surg. Gynecol. Obstet., 137:650, 1973.
7. Benfield, J. R., and Coon, R.: The role of the left atrial anastomosis in pulmonary reimplantation. J. Thorac. Cardiovasc. Surg., 53:676, 1967.
8. Benfield, J. R., Drews, J. A., and Shors, E.: Transplantation of the lung: A symposium. Lung grafting and surfactant. Vasc. Surg., 8:298, 1974.
9. Blank, R. H., Rodewald, H., and Linberg, E.: Heterotopic transplanted lung allograft as an auxiliary oxygenator. Surgery, 71:902, 1972.
10. Blumenstock, D. A., and Ferrebee, J. W.: Transplantation of the lung — retrospect and prospect. Vasc. Surg., 8:266, 1974.
11. Blumenstock, D. A., Grosjean, D. V., Otte, H. P., and Mulde, M. A.: Experimental allotransplantation of the lung. J. Thorac. Cardiovasc. Surg., 54:807, 1967.
12. Blumenstock, D. A., Lempert, N., and Morgodo, F.: Preservation of the canine lung in vitro for 24 hours with the use of hypothermia and hyperbaric oxygen. J. Thorac. Cardiovasc. Surg., 50:769, 1965.
13. Castagna, J. T., Shors, E., and Benfield, J. R.: The role of perfusion in lung preservation. J. Thorac. Cardiovasc. Surg., 63:521, 1972.
14. Corso, P. J., Geelhoed, G. W., and Joseph, W. L.: Membrane lung oxygenation for temporary support of the failing transplanted lung. Trans. Am. Soc. Artif. Int. Organs, 19:525, 1973.
15. Cullum, P. A., Bewick, M., Shilkin, K., Tee, D. E., Ayliffee, P., Hutchison, D. C., Laws, J. W., Mason, S. A., Reid, L., Hugh-Jones, P., and MacArthur, A. M.: Distinction between infection and rejection in lung transplantation. Br. Med. J., 2:71, 1972.
16. Daicoff, G. R., Allen P. D., and Streck, C. J.: Pulmonary vascular resistance following lung reimplantation and transplantation. Ann. Thorac. Surg., 9:569, 1970.
17. Demikhov, V. P.: Experimental Transplantation of Vital Organs. New York, Consultants Bureau Enterprise, 1962, pp. 130–135.
18. Derom, F. R., Barbier, F., Ringoir, S., Versieck, J., Roux, G., Berzsenyi, G., Vermeire, P., and Vrints, L.: Ten month survival after lung homotransplantation in man. J. Thorac. Cardiovasc. Surg., 61:835, 1971.
19. Duvoisin, G. E., Fowler, W. S., Ellis, F. H., and Payne, W. S.: Causes of depressed pulmonary function following reimplantation of the canine lung. Chest, 58:102, 1970.
20. Duvoisin, G. E., Payne, W. S., and Ellis, F. H.: Influence of

surgical technique on results of pulmonary reimplantation. Chest, *58*:96, 1970.

21. Ebert, P. A., and Hudson, B. H.: Pulmonary hemodynamics following lung autotransplantation. J. Thorac. Cardiovasc. Surg., *62*:188, 1971.

22. Edmunds, L. H., Jr., Graf, P. D., and Nadel, J. A.: Reinnervation of the reimplanted canine lung. J. Appl. Physiol., *31*:722, 1971.

23. Edmunds, L. H., Jr., Stallone, R. J., Graft, P. R., et al.: Mucous transport in transplanted lungs of dogs. Surgery, *60*:15, 1969.

24. Ellis, F. H., Grindley, J. H., and Edwards, J. E.: The bronchial arteries. I. Experimental occlusion. Surgery, *30*:810, 1951.

25. Eraslan, S., Turner, M. D., and Hardy, J. D.: Lymphatic regeneration following lung reimplantation in dogs. Surgery, *56*:970, 1964.

26. Faber, L. P., Scaffa Pedreira, A. L., Pevsner, P. H., and Beattie, E. J.: The immediate and long-term physiologic function of bilateral reimplanted lungs. J. Thorac. Cardiovasc. Surg., *50*:761, 1965.

27. Fonkalsrud, E. W., Stevens, G. H., Rangel, D. M., Joseph, W. C., Yakeishi, T., and Torcornal, J.: Physiologic evaluation of allogenic canine lung transplants from living donors. J. Thorac. Cardiovasc. Surg., *57*:607, 1969.

28. Fujimura, S., Parmley, W. W., Tomoda, H., Norman, J. R., and Matloff, J. M.: Hemodynamic alterations after staged and simultaneous bilateral lung autotransplantation in dogs. Follow-up studies. J. Thorac. Cardiovasc. Surg., *63*:937, 1972.

29. Garzon, A. A., Cheng, L., Lichtenstein, S., and Karlson, K. E.: Functional evaluation of the lung preserved for 24 hours. Surg. Forum, *17*:208, 1966.

30. Garzon, A. A., Goldstein, S., Okadigwe, C., Paley, N., Minkowitz, S., and Karlson, K. E.: Lung autografts—long term functions. Ann. Surg., *179*:136, 1974.

31. Haglin, J. J., and Arnar, O.: Lung transplantation in the baboon. Ann. N. Y. Acad. Sci., *162*:404, 1969.

32. Halasz, N. A., Catanzaro, A., Trummer, M. J., Tisi, G. M., Saltzstein, S. L., Moser, K. M., and Hutchin, P.: Transplantation of the lung. Correlation of physiologic, immunologic, and histologic findings. J. Thorac. Cardiovasc. Surg., *66*:581, 1973.

33. Hardy, J. D., Eraslan, S., and Dalton, M. L.: Autotransplantation and homotransplantation of the lung: Further studies. J. Thorac. Cardiovasc. Surg., *46*:606, 1963.

34. Hardy, J. D., Webb, W. R., Dalton, M. L., and Walker, G. R.: Lung homotransplantation in man. J.A.M.A., *186*:1065, 1963.

35. Hutchin, P., Freezor, M. P., Walker, E. L., and Peters, R. M.: Ventilation and perfusion after transplantation of the lung—studies with intravenous xenon-133. J. Thorac. Cardiovasc. Surg., *61*:476, 1971.

36. Hutchin, P., and Walker, E. L.: Ventilatory and circulatory adjustments after transplantation of the lung. Ann. Surg., *175*:349, 1972.

37. James, A. E., Hutchins, G. M., Natarajan, T. K., Sabanayagam, P., Byers, J. M., III, Wagner, H. N., and Baker, R. R.: Evaluation of primate allografts following treatment with immunosuppression and ameroid constrictors. Am. J. Roentgenol., *120*:782, 1974.

38. Ketonen, P.: Immediate changes in the pulmonary blood flow after various vascular anastomoses in lung autotransplantation. Scand. J. Thorac. Cardiovasc. Surg., *6*:311, 1972.

39. Kondo, Y., Turner, M. D., Cockrell, J. V., and Hardy, J. D.: Ischemic tolerance of the canine autotransplanted lung. Surgery, *76*:447, 1974.

40. Metras, H.: Cited by Trummer, M. J., and Berg, P.: Lung transplantation. Springfield, Ill., Charles C Thomas, Publisher, 1968, p. 3.

41. Mills, N. L., Coyd, A. D., and Gheranpong, L.: The significance of the bronchial circulation in lung transplantation. J. Thorac. Cardiovasc. Surg., *60*:866, 1970.

42. Momma, K., Lindle, L. M., Fonkalsrud, E. W., Stevens, G. H., Rangel, D., and Yakeishi, Y.: Hemodynamics and blood gas exchange in allografted canine lungs. I. Immediate effects. Surgery, *67*:799, 1970.

43. Moss, G.: Simplified experimental unilateral pulmonary autotransplantation. J. Thorac. Cardiovasc. Surg., *65*:899, 1973.

44. Nasseri, M., Eisele, R., Stadtler, K., Keilbach, H., Blumcke, S., and Bucherl, E. S.: Neural supply of the autotransplanted lung with special reference to respiratory control after bilateral pulmonary reimplantation. Eur. Surg. Res., *2*:287, 1970.

45. Nigro, S. L., Reiman, A., Fry, W. A., Trockil, F., and Adams, W. E.: Alterations in cardiopulmonary physiology following autotransplantation of the lung. Surg. Forum, *12*:56, 1971.

46. Pain, M. C. F., DeBono, A. H., Glazier, J. B., Maloney, J. E., and West, J. B.: Measurement of function of the transplanted lung in the dog with the use of xenon-133. J. Thorac. Cardiovasc. Surg., *53*:707, 1967.

47. Pearson, F. G., Goldberg, M., Stone, R. M., and Colapinto, R. F.: Bronchial arterial circulation restored after reimplantation of canine lung. Can. J. Surg., *12*:243, 1970.

48. Portin, B. A., Rasmussen, G. L., Stewart, J. D., and Andersen, M. N.: Physiologic and anatomic studies 35 months after successful reimplantation of the lung. J. Thorac. Cardiovasc. Surg., *39*:380, 1960.

49. Rabinovich, J. J.: Bronchographic and angiologic observations in experimental autotransplantation of a lung or lung lobe. J. Thorac. Cardiovasc. Surg., *69*:806, 1975.

50. Reemtsma, K., Rogers, R. E., Lucas, J. E., Schmidt, F. E., and David, F. H., Jr.: Studies of pulmonary function in transplantation of the canine lung. J. Thorac. Cardiovasc. Surg., *46*:589, 1963.

51. Shimada, K., Davidson, W. D., and Benfield, J. R.: Metabolic changes in ischemic lungs for evaluation of graft viability. J. Thorac. Cardiovasc. Surg., *66*:137, 1973.

52. Shimada, K., Gondos, B., and Benfield, J. R.: Photofiberoptic bronchoscopic findings during lung transplant rejection. Arch. Surg., *106*:774, 1973.

53. Slim, M. S., Yacoubian, H. A., Simonian, S. J., and Sahyoun, P.: Bilateral reimplantation of canine lungs. Ann. Thorac. Surg., *1*:755, 1965.

54. Slim, M. S., Yacoubian, H. D., Wilson, J. C., Rubeiz, G. A., and Ghardin-Manymneh, L.: Successful bilateral reimplantation of canine lungs. Surgery, *55*:676, 1964.

55. Stevens, G. H., Rangel, D. M., Yakeishi, Y., and Fonkalsrud, E.: Technical problems in lung allotransplantation. Causes of pulmonary venous outflow obstruction. Arch. Surg., *99*:506, 1969.

56. Siegelman, S. S., and Veith, F. J.: Angiography of the transplanted lung. Am. J. Roentgenol., *120*:795, 1974.

57. Stevens, G. H., Sanchez, M. M., and Chappell, G. L.: Enhancement of lung preservation by prevention of lung collapse. J. Surg. Res., *14*:400, 1973.

58. Stone, R. M., Ginsberg, R. J., Colapinto, R. F., and Pearson, F. G.: Bronchial artery regeneration after radical hilar stripping. Surg. Forum, *17*:109, 1966.

59. Veith, F. J., and Hagstrom, J. W.: Alveolar manifestations of rejection—an important cause of the poor results with human lung transplantation. Ann. Surg., *175*:336, 1972.

60. Veith, F. J., and Koerner, S. K.: The present status of lung transplantation. Arch. Surg., *109*:734, 1974.

61. Veith, F. J., Koerner, S. K., Hagstrom, J. W., Attai, L., Bloomberg, A., Jacobson, E., Nagashima, H., Boley, S. J., and Gliedman, M. L.: Experience in clinical lung transplantation. J.A.M.A., *222*:779, 1972.

62. Veith, F. J., Koerner, S. K., Siegelman, S. S., Kawakami, M., Kaufman, S., Attai, L. A., Hagstrom, J. W., and Gliedman, M. L.: Diagnosis and reversal of rejection in experimental and clinical lung allografts. Ann. Thorac. Surg., *16*:172, 1973.

63. Veith, F. J., Koerner, S. K., Sprayregan, S., Siegelman, S. S., Blumcke, S., Crane, R., Hagstrom, J. W., and Gliedman, M. L.: Corticosteroids in clinical and experimental lung transplantation. Transplant. Proc., *7*:99, 1975.

64. Veith, F. J., Sinha, S. B., Blumcke, S., Dougherty, J. C., Becker, N. H., Siegelman, S. S., and Hagstrom, J. W.: Nature and evolution of lung allograft rejection with and without immunosuppression. J. Thorac. Cardiovasc. Surg., *63*:509, 1972.

65. Veith, F. J., Panossian, A., Bogartz, L., and Koerner, S.: Immediate and early functional adequacy of transplanted lungs. Surg. Gynecol. Obstet., *129*:493, 1969.

66. Veith, F. J., and Richards, K.: Mechanism and prevention of fixed high vascular resistance in autografted and allografted lungs. Science, *163*:699, 1969.

67. Veith, F. J., and Richards, K.: Lung transplantation with simultaneous contralateral pulmonary artery ligation. Surg. Gynecol. Obstet., *129*:708, 1969.

68. Veith, F. J., Richards, K., and Lalezari, P.: Protracted survival after homotransplantation of the lung and simultaneous contralateral pulmonary artery ligation. J. Thorac. Cardiovasc. Surg., *58*:829, 1969.

69. Veith, F. J., and Richards, K.: Improved technic for canine lung transplantation. Ann. Surg., *171*:553, 1970.

70. Veith, F. J., Siegelman, S. S., and Dougherty, J. C.: Long term survival after lung autotransplantation and immediate contralateral pulmonary artery ligation. Surg. Gynecol. Obstet., 133:425, 1971.

71. Vermeire, P., Tasson, J., Lamont, H., Barbier, F., Versieck, J., and Derom, F.: Respiratory function after lung homotransplantation with a ten-month survival in man. Am. Rev. Resp. Dis., 106:515, 1972.

72. Waldhausen, J. A., Giammona, S. T., Kilman, J. W., and Daly, L. J.: Effect of transplantation of canine lung on pulmonary compliance and surfactant. J.A.M.A., 195:1002, 1965.

VIII

PANCREAS AND PANCREATIC ISLET TRANSPLANTATION

Keith Reemtsma, M.D., and Collin Weber, M.D.

HISTORICAL ASPECTS

Transplantation of the pancreas has been considered potentially useful in the treatment of diabetes mellitus since the demonstration by von Mering and Minkowski[109] in 1889 that removal of the canine pancreas resulted in hyperglycemia. In 1892, Hedon[30, 31] reported successful vascularized autografts of segments of pancreas transplanted into subcutaneous tissue in dogs that then were subjected to removal of the remainder of the organ. At a second procedure, the vascular pedicle was divided, but the grafts survived, having become neovascularized, and recipient animals remained normoglycemic. Subsequent excision of grafts resulted in hyperglycemia. Historic studies by Ssobolew[100] in 1902, Ivy and Farrell[38] in 1926, Delezzenne[19] and Gayet[21] in 1927, and Houssay[33] in 1929 documented short-term endocrine function and histological survival of canine pancreatic allografts. However, in 1922, Banting and Best[5] reported successful reversal of hyperglycemia in a patient with diabetes mellitus given injections of a refined pancreatic extract, thus initiating the era of exogenous insulin therapy in the treatment of diabetes mellitus.

Interest in pancreas transplantation was revived in the 1930s when it became clear that exogenous insulin therapy did not prevent progression of blood vessel abnormalities in diabetics, primarily those found in the kidney, retina, and cardiovascular system.[15, 29, 46, 58, 67] In 1935, Murray and Bradley[74] published studies of subcutaneous axillary implants of fragments of human islet adenoma cells transplanted into a diabetic patient. Neither beneficial nor ill effects were observed. In the same year, Selle[97] described similar studies using subcutaneous implants of canine pancreatic fragments. In 1936, Bottin[10] reported functional survival of revascularized canine pancreatic allografts for one week. Browning and Resnick,[13] in 1951, observed short-term function of embryonic murine pancreatic allografts. In 1959, Brooks and Gifford[11] grafted minced pancreatic tissue from a stillborn infant into the quadriceps muscle of the diabetic mother. A transient reduction in insulin requirement was noted. The authors also reported extensive experimental studies of canine whole-organ allografts,[11] and they identified several technical difficulties of pancreas transplantation. Necrosis of grafts and surrounding structures, with autolysis and hemorrhagic pancreatitis, resulted in peritonitis and death in the majority of animals. Studies reported by Reemtsma and associates between 1962 and 1964[66, 91, 92] demonstrated that prior duct ligation with acinar atrophy reduced the incidence and severity of these technical complications but did not prolong allograft survival.

Familiarity with pancreatic and vascular surgery, coupled with success in renal transplantation, led to detailed experimental studies of canine whole-pancreas grafts in many laboratories,* testing a variety of organ preservation and implantation techniques and the relative efficacy of different immunosuppressive regimens in prolonging allograft survival. Various gastrointestinal and vascular reconstructions were developed; most employed intra-abdominal heterotransplantation, with vascular anastomosis to the iliac vessels. An area of continued concern and investigation related to development of methods for dealing with exocrine pancreatic secretions.

One technique, simple duct ligation, produced atrophy and fibrosis in the transplant, and some degree of impairment of endocrine function. Lillehei and associates[63, 64, 108] described gradual and persistent impairment of glucose tolerance in animals given duct-ligated pancreas transplants. Reemtsma[66, 90, 92] and DeGruyl[17] reported early impairment of glucose tolerance, with gradual improvement over one year to 75 per cent of baseline values.

Transplantation of the pancreas with duodenum, employing Roux-en-Y duodenojejunostomy or cutan-

---

*See references 3, 9, 17, 18, 36, 37, 39, 53, 62, 64, 65, 72, 82, 86, 95, 96, 106, and 108.

eous duodenostomy, as developed by Lillehei and associates,[36, 37, 57, 63, 65] was complicated by early and uncontrollable rejection of the duodenal segment. Subsequent attempts to transplant the pancreas without duodenum, utilizing pancreatic duct–jejunostomy or pancreatic duct–ureterostomy,[3, 22, 76] yielded encouraging results in terms of decreased indices of pancreatitis, fistula formation, and hemorrhage.[22, 108]

DeGruyl[17] demonstrated that histocompatibility was directly related to the duration of function of pancreas allografts. The work of Reemtsma[90-92] and Merkel[72] showed prolongation of graft survival by immunosuppression and graft irradiation. Idezuki[36, 37] and Tersigni[106] achieved successful 24-hour preservation of whole-pancreas grafts.

The first human cadaveric pancreatic allograft was transplanted in 1966 by Kelly et al.[41] The recipient was a patient with long-term juvenile-onset diabetes in terminal renal failure. Renal and pancreatic grafts were taken from a single cadaver donor. The allograft of body and tail of pancreas had demonstrable endocrine function for six days. Brazil[56] performed a similar pancreas allograft shortly thereafter, which functioned for five days. Lillehei and associates[63-65] subsequently reported a series of cases of pancreaticoduodenal allografts, with periods of endocrine function ranging from one to twelve months. Studies by Connolly[16] and Gliedman[22] demonstrated similar periods of graft function. To date, 45 pancreas allografts have been transplanted in human subjects.[8]

In spite of the encouraging results obtained in experimental and clinical studies, whole-organ pancreatic transplantation was not adopted widely and applied to the treatment of large numbers of human diabetics. Organ procural and storage were major obstacles. However, complications of pancreatitis, hemorrhage, and fistula formation in association with graft rejection remained serious problems and accounted for significant morbidity and mortality in all reported human studies. Because these problems were directly related to the presence of exocrine tissue in pancreatic grafts, extensive studies were undertaken in several laboratories to test the feasibility and efficacy of grafts of isolated pancreatic islets.

Moskalewski,[73] Hellerstrom,[35] and Lacy and Kostianovsky,[49] adapted and developed collagenase digestion techniques that permitted dispersion of minced pancreatic tissue into fragments from which islets could be separated. Successful tissue culture[2, 14, 32, 50, 55, 75, 113] and transplantation* of isolated rodent islets demonstrated long-term functional and morphological survival of islet isografts, with reversal of diabetic parameters comparable to that achieved with whole pancreas transplants. Islets were shown to be at least as vulnerable to rejection as intact pancreas grafts[6, 64, 79, 87]; immunosuppressive regimens and synthetic envelopment of islets in porous membrane chambers were associated with modest prolongation of graft survival.[64, 79, 87, 89, 102, 103, 112, 114] Associated studies of porcine and primate islet transplants were reported,[94,

---

*See references 1, 4, 7, 12, 25, 26, 42–44, 47, 55, 59–61, 80, 83, 86–88, 93, 101, 110, 111, 113, and 120.

[104] and recently published data[23, 34, 40, 55, 69] have suggested that human pancreatic islets can be isolated and preserved in vitro with evidence of insulin production and morphologic viability.

ANATOMIC AND HISTOLOGICAL ASPECTS

In the fetus, the pancreas arises as a ventral and dorsal bud of the foregut and fuses in a retroperitoneal position following rotation of the gut. In this position the adult pancreas is intimately related to the stomach, duodenum, jejunum, common bile duct, and spleen. The pancreas derives its arterial supply from branches of the celiac axis, and venous blood drains into tributaries of the portal vein. The exocrine product of the pancreas is drained via the ducts of Wirsung and Santorini into the second part of the duodenum through the ampulla of Vater.

Histologically the pancreas is a mixed endocrine-exocrine organ, composed of approximately one million islets of Langerhans,[51] 40 to 200 μ in diameter, dispersed within the substance of the acinar parenchyma. Islets contain beta cells that produce insulin, alpha cells (glucagon producing), delta cells (somatostatin producing),[85] and "c" cells (function unknown), which are in close apposition to one another as well as to surrounding acinar cells. Conventional and scanning electron microscopic studies[48, 77] have documented intimate "bridges" connecting all cell types within islets, implying the existence of physiologic interactions among them in the regulation of carbohydrate metabolism in the normal as well as the diabetic state.

Early reports[24] suggested that the pancreas, and particularly pancreatic islets, were less antigenic than other organs. However, recent studies have demonstrated that pancreatic allografts are rejected as rapidly as those of the skin and heart.[87] Rejection of whole pancreatic allografts results in autolysis, hemorrhagic pancreatitis, vascular thrombosis, or hemorrhage and fistula formation.[17, 64, 92] Microscopically, edema and interstitial round cell infiltrates are seen first in perivascular areas and spreading throughout the parenchyma, with apparent relative sparing of islets. Rejection of isolated islet allografts is more precipitous than that of whole pancreas allografts.[88, 114] The reasons for this finding are unknown; it has been suggested that highly dispersed tissues such as islets and bone marrow may be more vulnerable to host immunocytes than are intact organs.[119] Rejection of islet allografts and xenografts does not differ markedly; both are characterized by dense round cell infiltration and target cell autolysis.[114]

BIOLOGIC BASIS AND SURGICAL PRINCIPLES

The justification and stimulus for experimental and clinical studies of whole pancreas and pancreatic islet transplantation are twofold. First, in many patients with "brittle," juvenile-onset diabetes, adequate control of glucose homeostasis is exceedingly difficult to maintain, even with multiple insulin injections each day; and in this group, mortality and morbidity remain unacceptably high.[20, 81] Second, optimal dietary and insulin regimens do not prevent the occurrence of renal, retinal, and atherosclerotic disease in human diabetics.[15, 29, 46, 58, 67] Recent experimental studies[27, 28, 99, 118] are in accord with clinical observations[15, 29, 54, 67, 81, 84, 105] that the development of blood vessel disease can be slowed but not prevented in very carefully controlled insulin-dependent diabetics.

Forty years after the description of human diabetic glomerular intercapillary lesions by Kimmelstiel and Wilson,[46] the exact mechanism responsible for the development of these lesions remains unknown. The suggestion has been made[45, 99] that the occurrence of accelerated vascular disease in diabetic patients may reflect the fact that replacement therapy with exogenous insulin does not approach simulating the fine regulation of carbohydrate metabolism achieved by physiologically released insulin from a normal pancreas. It has been the hope that a transplanted pancreas or pancreatic islets might supply insulin to the body more homeostatically than do exogenous insulin injections, and that such fine modulation of insulin requirements and carbohydrate metabolism might result in adequate control of "brittle" diabetics and in the prevention and/or reversal of associated diabetic blood vessel abnormalities.

As Karl[40] and Barker[6] have pointed out, the long-term consequences of whole-pancreas or pancreatic islet transplantation are largely unknown. It is clear from experimental studies* that heterotopic whole-organ or pancreatic islet grafts will reconstitute basal normoglycemia and normal glucose tolerance. In the absence of rejection (isogeneic models), insulin production is maintained for long periods, with concomitant normalization of survival, growth, and fat and mineral metabolism.[60, 78, 79, 83, 90, 98, 101, 107, 110, 111, 113, 114] Relative hyperinsulinemia and persistent hyperglucagonemia have been observed in graft recipients[78, 83, 93, 111]; however, serious and uncontrollable endocrine aberrations have not been noted following pancreas transplantation. The most significant complicating factors have been and remain the management of exocrine pancreatic secretions following whole-pancreas grafting, the prevention of graft rejection, and the preservation of pancreatic tissue after organ harvesting and prior to implantation. Successful resolution of these problems may be achieved by the development of improved techniques for isolation, in vitro manipulation, tissue culture storage, and immunological modification of pancreatic islets. These studies have been stimulated by the recent observation that isolated islet as well as whole-organ pancreatic grafts appear to arrest the progression of renal structural and functional abnormalities in diabetic animals.[70, 71, 115-117]

An important consequence of studies of pancreas transplantation will be a clearer understanding of the pathophysiology of diabetes mellitus. Alexander Marble's definition of the disease must be regarded as an hypothesis to be verified:

Diabetes mellitus is a chronic, hereditary disease characterized by an abnormally high level of glucose in the blood and the excretion of that sugar in the urine. The basic defect is an absolute or relative lack of insulin which leads to abnormalities of metabolism, not only of carbohydrate but also of protein and fat.[68]

In addition to providing a unique opportunity to test the validity of this hypothesis under physiological, in vivo conditions, pancreas and pancreatic islet transplants may prove useful in the clinical management of severely diabetic patients, and possibly also in the prevention and/or reversal of associated blood vessel abnormalities in human diabetics.

SELECTED REFERENCES

DeGruyl, J.: Transplantation of the Entire Pancreas with Ligation of the Exocrine Ducts. Rotterdam, Kooyker Sci. Publ., 1975.
This very recent reference is a well-organized monograph summarizing extensive experimental studies of endocrine function and survival of duct-ligated canine whole pancreas auto- and allografts. The author clearly demonstrates that tissue typing is predictive of pancreas allograft survival, and that relatively normal long-term insulin responses can be achieved with duct-ligated pancreas transplants.

Lazarow, A., Wells, L. J., Carpenter, A. M., Hegre, O. D., Leonard, R. J., and McEvoy, R. C.: Islet differentiation, organ culture and transplantation. Diabetes, 22:877, 1973.
This excellent summary paper, the Banting Memorial Lecture of 1973, details results of in vitro and in vivo studies of animal and human pancreatic islets, spanning fully fifteen years. It has numerous relevant illustrations and references. Of special interest are the authors' observations that islets will survive (1) in tissue culture, as evidenced by insulin production and morphologic viability, and (2) following intraperitoneal isografting.

Lillehei, R. C., and Ruiz, J. O.: Pancreas. In Najarian, J. S., and Simmons, R. L.: Transplantation. Philadelphia, Lea and Febiger, 1972, p. 627.
This chapter is a complete and detailed summary of previous studies of whole-pancreas transplantation, with particular attention given to results of pancreatic allotransplantation in man. It describes various techniques for pancreas grafting; in addition, numerous charts and graphs outline the clinical course of patients following transplantation.

Marble, A., White, P., Bradley, R. F., and Krall, L. P. (Eds.): Joslin's Diabetes Mellitus. Philadelphia, Lea and Febiger, 1971.
This comprehensive text contains literally thousands of pertinent references covering every aspect of the pathophysiology of diabetes mellitus, as well as extensive documentation of the course and results of treatment of large numbers of diabetic patients. It summarizes the extent of our knowledge of diabetes mellitus, which is a prerequisite to progress and understanding in the field of pancreas and pancreatic islet transplantation.

REFERENCES

1. Amamoo, D. G., Woods, J. E., and Donovan, J. L.: Preliminary experience with pancreatic islet-cell implantation. Mayo Clin. Proc., 49:289, 1974.
2. Andersson, A.: Monolayer culture of pancreatic islets. In Falkmer, S., Hellman, B., and Taljedal, I. B. (Eds.): The Structure and Metabolism of the Pancreatic Islets. Oxford, Pergamon Press, 1970, p. 73.
3. Aquino, C., Ruiz, J. O., Schultz, L., and Lillehei, R. C.: Pancreatic transplantation without the duodenum in the dog. Am. J. Surg., 125:240, 1973.
4. Ballinger, W. F., and Lacy, P. E.: Transplantation of intact pancreatic islets in rats. Surgery, 72:175, 1972.
5. Banting, F. G., Best, C. H., Gollip, J. B., Campbell, W. R., and Fletcher, A. A.: Pancreatic extracts in the treatment of diabetes mellitus. Can. Med. Assoc. J., 12:141, 1922.
6. Barker, C. F.: Transplantation of the islets of Langerhans and

---

*See references 4, 9, 17, 43, 52, 55, 64, 76, 78, 88, 90, 92, 113, 114, and 120.

the histocompatibility of endocrine tissue. Diabetes, *24*:766, 1975.

7. Barker, C. F., Reckard, C. R., Ziegler, M. M., and Naji, A.: The liver as an immunologically privileged site for rat pancreatic islet allografts. Diabetes, *24* (Suppl. 2): 418, 1975.

8. Bergan, J. J.: A review of human solid organ transplantation. Bull. Am. Coll. Surg., *60*:24, 1975.

9. Bergan, J. J., Hoehn, J. G., Porter, N., and Dry, L.: Total pancreatic allografts in pancreatectomized dogs. Arch. Surg., *90*:521, 1965.

10. Bottin, J.: Transplantation du pancreas sur la circulation carotid-jugulaire chez le chien. Souroie et l'animal. Causes de la mort. C. R. Soc. Biol. (Paris), *121*:872, 1936.

11. Brooks, J. R., and Gifford, G. H.: Pancreatic homotransplantation. Transplant. Bull., *6*:100, 1959.

12. Brown, J., Molnar, I. G., Clark, W., and Mullen, Y.: Control of experimental diabetes mellitus in rats by transplantation of fetal pancreases. Science, *184*:1377, 1974.

13. Browning, H., and Resnick, P.: Homologous and heterologous transplantation of pancreatic tissue in normal and diabetic mice. Yale J. Biol. Med., *24*:141, 1951.

14. Chick, W. L.: Beta-cell replication in rat pancreatic monolayer cultures: Effects of glucose, tolbutamide, glucocorticoid, growth hormone and glucagon. Diabetes, *22*:687, 1972.

15. Colwell, A. R.: Relation of small blood vessel complications to treatment of diabetes: A review. *In* Siperstein, M. D., Colwell, A. R., and Meyer, K. (Eds.): Small Blood Vessel Involvement in Diabetes Mellitus. Washington, American Institute of Biological Science, 1964, p. 253.

16. Connolly, J. E., Martin, D. C. Steinberg, T., Gwinup, G., Gazzanigo, A. D., and Bartlett, R. H.: Clinical experience with pancreatico-duodenal transplantation. Arch. Surg., *106*:489, 1973.

17. DeGruyl, J.: Transplantation of the Entire Pancreas with Ligation of the Exocrine Ducts. Rotterdam, Kooyker Sci. Publ., 1975.

18. DeJode, L. R., and Howard J. M.: The function of the homotransplanted canine pancreas. Brit. J. Surg., *53*:364, 1966.

19. Delezzenne, C., Hallion, L., and Gayet, R.: Sur le mechanisme de la secretion pancreatique par un processus humoral, demontree par des transplantations du pancreas; experiences sur des animaux normaux. Ann. Physiol., *3*:508, 1927.

20. Drash, A.: Diabetes mellitus in childhood: A review. J. Pediatr., *78*:919, 1971.

21. Gayet, R., and Guillaumie, M.: La regulation de la secretion interne pancreatique par un processus humoral, demontree par des transplantations du pancreas. Experiences sur des animaux depancreates. C. R. Soc. Biol., *97*:1615, 1927.

22. Gliedman, M. L., Gold, M., Whittaker, J., Rifkin, H., Soberman, R., Freed, S., Tellis, V., and Veith, F. J.: Clinical segmental pancreatic transplantation with ureter-pancreatic duct anastomosis for exocrine drainage. Surgery, *74*:171, 1973.

23. Goldman, H., Colle, E., and Brazeau, P.: The investigation of the human pancreatic endocrine cell in long-term culture. Diabetes, *24* (Suppl. 2):421, 1975.

24. Gonet, A. E., and Renold, A. E.: Homografting of fetal rat pancreas. Diabetologia, *1*:91, 1965.

25. Gray, B. N.: Transplantation of isolated pancreatic islet tissue in experimental diabetes. Lahey Clin. Bull., *22*:146, 1973.

26. Griffith, R. C., Scharp, D. W., Ballinger, W. F., and Lacy, P. E.: A morphologic study of intrahepatic portal vein islet isografts. Diabetes, *24* (Suppl. 2):419, 1975.

27. Hagg, E.: Influence of insulin treatment on glomerular changes in rats with long-term alloxan diabetes. Acta Pathol. Microbiol. Scand., *82*:228, 1974.

28. Hansen, R. O., Lundbaek, K., Olsen, T. S., and Orskov, H.: Kidney lesions in rats with severe long-term alloxan diabetes. Lab. Invest., *17*:675, 1967.

29. Hardin, R. C., Jackson, R. L., Johnston, T. L., and Kelly, H. G.: The development of diabetic retinopathy: Effects of duration and control of diabetes. Diabetes, *5*:397, 1956.

30. Hedon, E.: Greffe sous-cutane du pancreas; son importance dans l'etude du diabete pancreatique. Arch. Physiol. Norm. Pathol., *5*:617, 1892.

31. Hedon, E.: Sur la pathogenie du diabete consecutif a l'extirpation du pancreas. Arch. Physiol. Norm. Pathol., *5*:245, 1892.

32. Hegre, O. D., Wells, L. J., and Lazarow, A.: Insulin content of fetal rat pancreases grown in organ culture and subsequently transplanted into maternal hosts. Diabetes, *21*:193, 1972.

33. Houssay, B. A.: Technique de la greffe pancreaticoduodenale au cou. C. R. Soc. Biol., *100*:138, 1929.

34. Hellerstrom, C., Andersson, A., Groth, C. G., Gunnarsson, R., Lundgren, G., Westman, J., and Ostman, J.: Structure and metabolism of human pancreatic islets maintained in tissue culture. Diabetologia, *11*:348, 1975.

35. Hellerstrom, C.: A method for the microdissection of intact pancreatic islets in mammals. Acta Endocrinol., *45*:122, 1964.

36. Idezuki, Y., Feemster, J. A., Dietzman, R. H., and Lillehei, R. C.: Experimental pancreaticoduodenal preservation and transplantation. Surg. Gynecol. Obstet., *126*:1002, 1968.

37. Idezuki, Y., Goetz, F. C., and Lillehei, R. C.: Experimental allotransplantation of the preserved pancreas and duodenum. Surgery, *65*:485, 1969.

38. Ivy, A. C., and Farrell, J. I.: Contribution to the physiology of the pancreas. I. Method for the subcutaneous autotransplantation of the tail of the pancreas. Am. J. Physiol., *77*:474, 1926.

39. Joison, J.: Pancreatic allotransplantation without cessation of blood flow. Surg. Gynecol. Obstet., *124*:1295, 1967.

40. Karl, R. C.: Transplantation of islets of Langerhans. Arch. Pathol., *99*:401, 1975.

41. Kelly, W. D., Lillehei, R. C., Merkel, F. K., Idezuki, Y., and Goetz, R. C.: Allotransplantation of the pancreas and duodenum along with the kidney in diabetic nephropathy. Surgery, *61*:827, 1967.

42. Kemp, C. B., Knight, M. J., Scharp, D. W., Ballinger, W. F., and Lacy, P. E.: Effect of transplantation site on the results of pancreatic islet isografts in diabetic rats. Diabetologia, *9*:486, 1973.

43. Kemp, C. B., Knight, M. J., Scharp, D. W., Lacy, P. E., and Ballinger, W. F.: Transplantation of isolated pancreatic islets into the portal vein of diabetic rats. Nature, *244*:447, 1973.

44. Kemp, C. B., Scharp, D. W., Knight, M. J., Ballinger, W. F., and Lacy, P. E.: Importance of implantation site of pancreatic islet isografts in treatment of experimental diabetes. Surg. Forum, *24*:297, 1973.

45. Kilo, C., Vogler, H., et al.: Muscle capillary basement membrane change related to aging and to diabetes mellitus. Diabetes, *21*:881, 1972.

46. Kimmelstiel, P., and Wilson, C.: Intercapillary lesions in the glomeruli of the kidney. Am. J. Pathol., *12*:83, 1936.

47. Kramp R. C., Congdon C. C., and Smith, L. H.: Recovery from experimental diabetes mellitus in mice after pancreas transplantation. Diabetes, *23*:183, 1974.

48. Lacy, P. E., and Greider, M. H.: Ultrastructural organization of mammalian pancreatic islets. Handbook Physiol. Sect., *71*:77, 1972.

49. Lacy, P. E., and Kostianovsky, M.: Method for the isolation of intact islets of Langerhans from the rat pancreas. Diabetes, *16*:35, 1967.

50. Lambert, A. E., Blondel, B., Kanazawa, Y., Orci, L., and Renold, A. E.: Monolayer cell culture of neonatal rat pancreas: Light microscopy and evidences for immunoreactive insulin synthesis and release. Endocrinology, *90*:239, 1972.

51. Langerhans, P.: Beitrage zur mikroskopischen Anatomie der Bauchspeicheldruse. Inaug. Disert. Berlin Lange., 1869.

52. Largiader, F.: Carbohydrate metabolism after pancreatic transplantation. Surg. Clin. North Am., *47*:1363, 1967.

53. Largiader, F., and Wegmann, W.: Experimental orthotopic transplantation of the pancreas. Transplant. Proc., *3*:497, 1971.

54. Lauvaux, J. P., Pirart, J., and Eisendrath, C.: The course of diabetic retinopathy: A statistical study on its development, progression and regression in 4,400 diabetics. Diabetologia, *11*:358, 1975.

55. Lazarow, A., Wells, L. J., Carpenter, A. M., Hegre, O. D., Leonard, R. J., and McEvoy, R. C.: Islet differentiation, organ culture and transplantation. Diabetes, *22*:877, 1973.

56. Leading article: Pancreas transplantation. Br. Med. J., *2*:262, 1969.

57. Lee, S., Tung, K. S. K., Koopmans, H., et al.: Pancreaticoduodenal transplantation in the rat. Transplantation, *13*:421, 1972.

58. Le Compte, P. M.: Vascular lesions in diabetes mellitus. J. Chron. Dis., *2*:178, 1955.

59. Leonard, R. J., Hegre, O., and Lazarow, A.: Intraperitoneal isotransplantation of dissociated fetal and neonatal pancreas:

Effect of age and quantity of donor islet on the reversal of alloxan-induced diabetes in the rat. Diabetes, 24 (Suppl. 2):419, 1975.

60. Leonard, R. J., Lazarow, A., and Hegre, O. D.: Pancreatic islet transplantation in the rat. Diabetes, 22:413, 1973.

61. Leonard, R. J., Lazarow, A., McEvoy, R. C., and Hegre, O. D.: Islet cell transplantation. Kidney Intern., 6:s-169, 1974.

62. Lichtenstein, I. L., and Barschak, R. M.: Experimental transplantation of the pancreas in dogs. J. Int. Coll. Surg., 28:1, 1957.

63. Lillehei, R. C., and Ruiz, J. O.: Pancreas. In Najarian, J. S., and Simmons, R. L.: Transplantation. Philadelphia, Lea and Febiger, 1972, p. 627.

64. Lillehei, R. C., Simmons, R. L., Najarian, J. S., Weil, R., Uchida, H., Ruiz, J. O., Kjellstrand, C. M., and Goetz, F. C.: Pancreatico-duodenal allotransplantation: Experimental and clinical experience. Acta Diabetol. Lat., 7:909, 1970.

65. Lillehei, R. C., Simmons R. L., Najarian, J. S., Weil, R., Uchida, H., Ruiz, J. O., Kjellstrand, C. M., and Goetz, F. C.: Pancreatico-duodenal allotransplantation: Experimental and clinical experience. Ann. Surg., 172:405, 1970.

66. Lucas, J. F., Rogers, R. E., and Reemtsma, K.: Homologous pancreatic transplantation in dogs: Report of new technique and studies of endocrine function. Surg. Forum, 13:314, 1962.

67. Marble, A: Relation of control of diabetes to vascular sequelae. Med. Clin. North Am., 49:1137, 1965.

68. Marble, A., White, P., Bradley, R. F., and Krall, L. P. (Eds.): Joslin's Diabetes Mellitus. Philadelphia, Lea and Febiger, 1971, p. 2.

69. Matas, A. J., Sutherland, D. E. R., Najarian, J. S., and Steffes, M. W.: Human neonatal pancreas: Suitability for transplantation. Diabetes, 24 (Suppl. 2):421, 1975.

70. Mauer, S. M., Steffes, M. W., Sutherland, D. E. R. Najarian, J. S., Michael, A. F., and Brown, D. M.: Studies of the rate of regression of the glomerular lesions in diabetic rats treated with pancreatic islet transplantation. Diabetes, 24:280, 1975.

71. Mauer, S. M., Sutherland, D. E. R., Steffes, M. W., Leonard, R. J., Najarian, J. S., Michael, A. F., and Brown, D. M.: Pancreatic islet transplantation: Effects on the glomerular lesions of experimental diabetes in the rat. Diabetes, 23:748, 1974.

72. Merkel, K. K., Kelly, W. D., Goetz, F. C., and Maney, J.: Irradiated heterotopic segmental canine pancreatic allografts. Surgery, 63:291, 1968.

73. Moskalewski, S: Isolation and culture of islets of Langerhans of the guinea pig. Gen. Comp. Endocrinol., 5:342, 1965.

74. Murray, M. R., and Bradley, C. F.: Two-island-cell adenomas of the human pancreas cultivated in vitro. Am. J. Cancer, 25:98, 1935.

75. Murrell, L. R.: Mammalian pancreatic islet tissue in organ culture. Cell Res., 41:350, 1966.

76. Nozawa, M., Weil, R., McIntosh, R. M., and Reemtsma, K: Vascularized transplantation of the rat pancreas without duodenum. Transplantation, 17:137, 1974.

77. Orci, L., Malaisse-Lagae, F., Ravazzola, M., Pouiller, D., Renold, A. E., Perrelet, A., and Unger, R.: A morphological basis for intercellular communication between alpha and beta cells in the endocrine pancreas. J. Clin. Invest., 56:1066, 1975.

78. Orloff, M. J., Lee, S., Charters, A. C., Grambort, D. E., Storck, L. G., and Knox, D.: Long-term studies of pancreas transplantation in experimental diabetes mellitus. Ann. Surg., 182:198, 1975.

79. Panijayanond, P., and Monaco, A. P.: Enhancement of pancreatic islet allograft survival with ALS and donor bone marrow. Surg. Forum, 25:379, 1974.

80. Panijayanond, P., Soroff, H. S., and Monaco, A. P.: Pancreatic islet isografts in mice. Surg. Forum, 24:329, 1973.

81. Paz-Guevara, A. T., Hsu, T. H., and White, P.: Juvenile diabetes mellitus after forty years. Diabetes, 24:559, 1975.

82. Pennell, R. C., Miller, E. C., and Milford, T.: Blood flow measurements in canine pancreatic allografts. Am. Surg., 35:871, 1969.

83. Pipeleers, D., Pipeleers-Marichal, M., and Kipnis, D.: Metabolic and morphologic studies of long-term islet transplanted rats. Diabetes, 24 (Suppl. 2):420, 1975.

84. Pirart, J., Lauvaux, J. P., and Eisendrath, C.: Diabetic retinopathy, nephropathy, neuropathy. Relation to duration and control: A statistical study of 4,400 diabetics. Diabetologia, 11:370, 1975.

85. Polak, J. M., Pearse, A. G. E., Grimelius, L., Bloom, S. R., and Arimura, A.: Growth hormone release-inhibiting hormone in gastrointestinal and pancreatic D-cells. Lancet, 1:1220, 1975.

86. Raussis, C., Choudhury, A., and Ogata, Y.: Influence of pancreatic duct anastomosis on function of autotransplanted canine pancreatic segments. J. Surg. Res., 10:551, 1970.

87. Reckard, C. R., and Barker, C. F.: Transplantation of isolated pancreatic islets across strong and weak histocompatibility barriers. Transplant. Proc., 5:761, 1973.

88. Reckard, C. R., Ziegler, M. M., and Barker, C. F.: Physiological and immunological consequences of transplanting isolated pancreatic islets. Surgery, 74:91, 1973.

89. Reemtsma, K.: Experimental islet cell grafting: A transplantation model. Transplant. Proc., 4:513, 1970.

90. Reemtsma, K., Giraldo, N., Depp, D. A., and Eichwald, E. J.: Islet cell transplantation. Ann. Surg., 168:436, 1968.

91. Reemtsma, K., Hewitt, R. L., Smith, P. E., and Weichert, R. F.: Studies of endocrine function following transplantation of the canine pancreas. Ann. N.Y. Acad. Sci., 120:656, 1964.

92. Reemtsma, K., Lucas, J. F., Rogers, R. E., Schmidt, F. E., and Davis, F. H.: Islet cell function of the transplanted canine pancreas. Ann. Surg., 158:645, 1963.

93. Ruiz, O. J., and Lillehei, R. C.: Pancreas transplantation. In Carey, L. C. (Ed.): The Pancreas. St. Louis, The C. V. Mosby Company, 1973, p. 351.

94. Scharp, D. W., Murphy, J. J., Newton, W. T., Ballinger, W. F., and Lacy, P. E.: Transplantation of islets of Langerhans in diabetic rhesus monkeys. Surgery, 77:100, 1975.

95. Seddon, J. A., and Howard, J. M.: The exocrine behavior of the homotransplanted pancreas. Surgery, 59:226, 1966.

96. Seddon, J. A., and Howard, J. M.: The endocrine function of the homotransplanted pancreas. Surgery, 59:235, 1966.

97. Selle, W. A.: Studies on pancreatic grafts made with a new technique. Am. J. Physiol., 113:118, 1935.

98. Sells, R. A., Calne, R. Y., Hadjiyanakis, V., and Marshall, V. C.: Glucose and insulin metabolism after pancreatic transplantation. Br. Med. J., 3:678, 1972.

99. Spiro, R. G.: Biochemistry of the renal glomerular basement membrane and its alternations in diabetes mellitus. N. Engl. J. Med., 288:1337, 1973.

100. Ssobolew, L. W.: Zur normalen und pathologischen Morphologie der inneren Secretion der Bauchspeicheldruse. Arch. Pathol. Anat. Klin. Med., 168:91, 1902.

101. Steffes, M. W., Sutherland, D. E. R., Mauer, S. M., Leonard, R. J., Najarian, J. S., and Brown, D. M.: Plasma insulin and glucose levels in diabetic rats prior to and following islet transplantation. J. Lab. Clin. Med., 85:75, 1975.

102. Steffes, M. W., Sutherland, D. E. R., Mauer, S. M., Najarian, J. S., and Brown, D. M.: Islet transplantation in diabetic rats receiving corticosteroids. Transplantation, 19:449, 1975.

103. Strautz, R. L.: Studies of hereditary-obese mice (ObOb), after implantation of pancreatic islets in millipore filter capsules. Diabetologia, 6:306, 1970.

104. Sutherland, D. E. R., Steffes, M. W., Bauer, G. E., McManus, D., Noe, B. D., and Najarian, J. S.: Isolation of human and porcine islets of Langerhans and islet transplantation in pigs. J. Surg. Res., 16:102, 1974.

105. Takazakura, E., Nakamoto, Y., Hayakawa, H., Kawai, K., Muramoto, S., Yoshida, K., Shimizu, M., Shinoda, A., and Takeuchi, J.: Onset and progression of diabetic glomerulosclerosis: A prospective study based on serial renal biopsies. Diabetes, 24:1, 1975.

106. Tersigni, R., Toledo-Pereyra, L. H., Merino, G. E., and Najarian, J. S.: Endocrine and exocrine functional viability of preserved and transplanted pancreaticoduodenal allografts. Surg. Forum, 26:456, 1975.

107. Teixeira, E., Sharkey, E., Colwell, J., and Bergan, J. J.: Insulin and glucose levels following pancreas allografting. Surg. Forum, 17:205, 1966.

108. Toledo-Pereyra, L. H., Costellanos, J., Lampe, E. W., Lillehei, R. C., and Najarian, J. S.: Comparative evaluation of pancreas transplantation techniques. Ann. Surg., 182:567, 1975.

109. von Mering, J., and Minkowski, O.: Diabetes mellitus nach pankreasextirpation. Arch. Exp. Pathol. Pharmacol., 26:371, 1889.

110. Weber, C., Greenwood, M. R. C., Zatrici, A., Hardy, M., Lerner, R., and Reemtsma, K.: Effects of islet transplantation on growth and glucose homeostasis in diabetic rats. Diabetes, 24 (Suppl. 2):419, 1975.

111. Weber, C. J., Lerner, R. L., Felig, P., Hardy, M. A., and Reemtsma, K.: The effect of pancreatic islet transplantation on insulin and glucagon levels in diabetic rats. Surg. Forum, 26:192, 1975.

112. Weber, C., Weil, R., McIntosh, R., Hogle, H., Warden, G., and Reemtsma, K.: Xenotransplantation of piscine islets into hyperglycemic rats. Surgery, 77:208, 1975.

113. Weber, C., Weil, R., McIntosh, R., and Reemtsma, K.: Transplantation of pancreatic islets from neonatal to adult rats. Transplantation, 19:442, 1975.

114. Weber, C., Zatriqi, A., Weil, R., McIntosh, R., Hardy, M. A., and Reemtsma, K.: Pancreatic islet isografts, allografts and xenografts: Comparison of morphology and function. Surgery, 79:144, 1976.

115. Weil, R., Nozawa, M., Koss, M., Weber, C., Reemtsma, K., and McIntosh, R.: Effect of pancreas transplantation on diabetic nephropathy in rats. Surg. Forum, 25:386, 1974.

116. Weil, R., Nozawa, M., Koss, M., Weber, C., Reemtsma, K., and McIntosh, R.: Pancreatic transplantation in diabetic rats. Renal function, morphology, ultrastructure and immunohistology. Surgery, 78:142, 1975.

117. Weil, R., Nozawa, M., Koss, M., Weber, C., Reemtsma, K., and McIntosh, R.: The kidney in streptozotocin diabetic rats. Arch. Pathol. Lab. Med., 100:37, 1976.

118. Wehner, H., Huber, H., and Kronenberg, K. H.: The glomerular basement membrane of the rabbit kidney in long-term treatment with heterologous insulin preparations of different purity. Diabetologia, 9:255, 1973.

119. Winn, H.: Humoral antibody in the allograft reaction. Transplant. Proc., 2:83, 1970.

120. Ziegler, M. M., Reckard, C. R., and Barker, C. F.: Long-term metabolic and immunological considerations in transplantation of pancreatic islets. J. Surg. Res., 16:575, 1974.

IX

CARDIAC HOMOTRANSPLANTS

Randall B. Griepp, M.D., and Norman E. Shumway, M.D., Ph.D.

Cardiac transplantation was first attempted in 1905 when Carrel and Guthrie performed a heterotopic transplant in a dog. The heart removed from a small dog was interposed in the carotid-jugular circulation of a large dog. The heart spontaneously defibrillated one hour after completion of the anastomoses and beat for an additional two hours, until intracavitary thromboses terminated the experiment. Following this isolated attempt, no further studies with cardiac transplantation were reported until 1933, when Mann conducted a systematic investigation of the technical aspects of heterotopic cardiac transplantation.[24] In a series of experiments in dogs, the donor heart was sutured into the neck vessels of the recipient (Fig. 1). The major technical problem encountered was distention of the heart prior to defibrillation. The hearts beat for one to eight days. When removed they were found to be friable and ecchymotic, and histopathologic examination revealed marked edema and lymphocyte, monocyte, and polymorphonuclear infiltration. The investigators concluded that it was a biologic rather than a technical factor that prevented the long-term survival of cardiac homotransplants.

Minor variations in technique were developed by Marcus in 1951,[25] Wesolowski in 1953,[30] and Downie, also in 1953,[11] but no real improvement in survival was achieved. In 1957 Sayegh and Creech utilized prenatal and neonatal puppy hearts as donor organs in an unsuccessful attempt to extend survival of the heterotopic heart homotransplant.[26] In the past decade a number of investigators have utilized the model of heterotopic cardiac transplantation to study the metabolism, physiology, pathology, and immunology of the transplanted heart. The technique is simple, and cardiopulmonary bypass is unnecessary. Conclusions reached with the heterotopic model, however, are not necessarily valid when applied to orthotopic cardiac

transplantation in which the graft provides its own blood supply as well as supporting the host circulation.

A second experimental approach to cardiac trans-

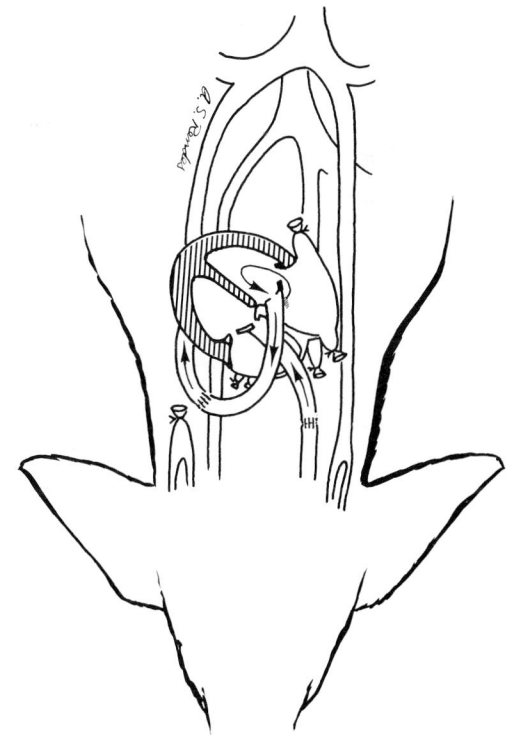

Figure 1. Technique developed by Mann for heterotopic cardiac transplantation in the neck. (From Najarian, J. S., Foker, J. E., and Simmons, R. L. (Eds.): Transplantation. Philadelphia, Lea & Febiger, 1972.)

plantation involved the placement of a second heart within the thorax in such a manner that part of the circulatory load was assumed by the second heart. This approach was most thoroughly investigated by Demikhov.[10] In one series of 22 experiments between 1951 and 1955 he performed end-to-side anastomoses between the donor and recipient venae cavae, pulmonary arteries, and aortas. The left atrial appendages were also connected. After satisfactory donor heart action was present, the recipient heart was excluded from the circulation by ligation of the recipient great vessels proximal to the anastomoses and tightening of a purse-string suture around the mitral valve. Two of Demikhov's dogs lived 11 and 15 hours, providing the first instances of total assumption of the circulation of a dog by a transplanted heart.

With the advent of cardiopulmonary bypass in the late 1950's, orthotopic cardiac transplantation became a possibility. In 1958 Golberg et al. attempted transplantation in three dogs.[13] Their longest survival was 21 minutes following discontinuation of bypass. In 1959 Webb et al. reported 12 technically successful canine transplants, but all the dogs succumbed within 7½ hours.[29] Arrhythmias and air embolism caused problems, but hemorrhage from suture lines was the limiting factor for survival. In 1959 Cass and Brock reported a single attempt at orthotopic homotransplantation in the dog.[6] Hemorrhage limited survival to a few minutes following discontinuation of cardiopulmonary bypass. In 1960 Lower and Shumway reported the first successful canine orthotopic cardiac transplant.[23] In a series of eight consecutive animals, five lived from 6 to 21 days following operation. At autopsy severe myocarditis characterized by round cell infiltration, necrosis, hemorrhage, and edema was present in all hearts. The essentials of the Lower and Shumway operative technique were preservation of the donor heart by immersion in a cold saline solution for several minutes following excision, and performance of the systemic and pulmonary venous anastomoses at the midatrial level, eliminating the tedious suture of both venae cavae and four pulmonary veins (Fig. 2).

Over the last decade the canine model for orthotopic transplantation has been utilized for physiologic and immunologic studies. These have shown that the transplanted heart functions adequately at rest and can meet the demands of moderate exercise until rejection supervenes.[8] Routine immunosuppressive treatment of recipients will prolong survival from an average of 7 days in untreated animals to 17 days in treated ones.[22] Intermittent use of immunosuppressive therapy for acute rejection episodes diagnosed on the basis of diminished electrocardiographic voltage will increase average survival to 75 days following transplantation.[21] Survival beyond one year has been achieved, and several animals have whelped normal litters of puppies following cardiac transplantation.

CLINICAL EXPERIENCES

Cardiac transplantation was first performed in man in 1964 by Hardy, who attempted transfer of a heart from a chimpanzee to a 68-year-old man in the terminal stages of cardiogenic shock.[20] Following grafting, the venous return overwhelmed the small primate heart, which was used because of the lack of a suitable human donor, and attempts at resuscitation were abandoned one hour following discontinuation of cardiopulmonary bypass. In December, 1967, Barnard performed the first successful human cardiac transplant.[2] The recipient was a 54-year-old man with end-stage arteriosclerotic heart disease. The heart was protected during the operation by antegrade coronary perfusion rather than retrograde coronary sinus perfusion as used in the chimpanzee transplant. The operation and immediate postoperative period proceeded satisfactorily, but pneumonia resulted in the patient's

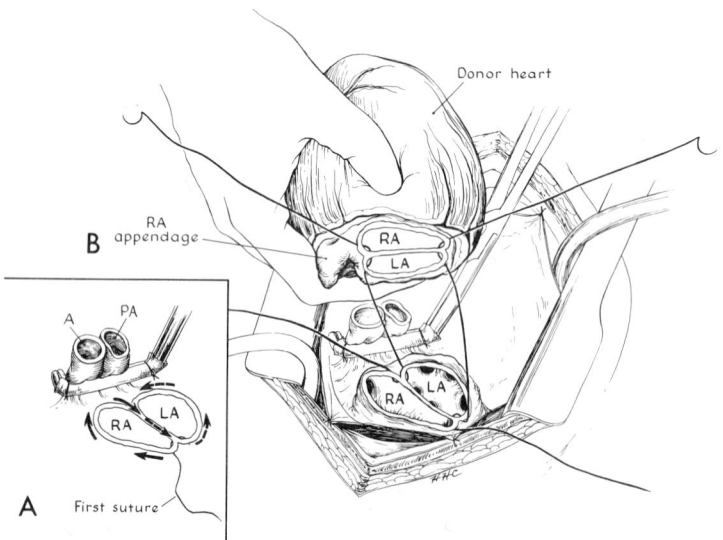

Figure 2. Technique developed by Lower and Shumway for canine orthotopic cardiac transplantation. Cannulation for cardiopulmonary bypass is via the external jugular vein and the femoral artery and vein. The venous anastomoses are combined into atrial anastomoses.

death 17 days following operation. By August, 1976, 314 cardiac transplants had been performed in man throughout the world. The wide variations in recipient selection, operative technique, and postoperative management render a complete analysis of this entire experience problematical. Since the authors' series represents approximately one third of the world experience, attention will be focused in the following pages on this relatively homogeneous group.

Recipient Selection and Operative Risk

Consideration of a patient for heart transplantation implies that he is in the final stages of myocardial decompensation. Cardiologic evaluation includes a history, focusing upon the duration and progression of disease; a physical examination; routine laboratory studies; an electrocardiogram; chest roentgenograms; complete right and left heart catheterization; selective coronary arteriography; and left ventriculography. A thorough etiologic, anatomic, and physiologic understanding of the patient's heart disease is required to decide whether the patient has had an adequate trial of appropriate medical therapy and whether a less radical surgical procedure might be of benefit. If no alternative therapy is available, further evaluation is undertaken to rule out operative contraindications.[16]

Absolute contraindications to heart transplantation include the presence of severe pulmonary hypertension, ongoing infection, or unrelated life-limiting conditions such as malignant neoplasm. Severe pulmonary hypertension characterized by a mean pulmonary artery pressure of greater than 60 mm. Hg or a pulmonary vascular resistance of greater than 10 Wood units is associated with a high incidence of acute right heart failure immediately following transplantation. The normal unhypertrophied right ventricle of the donor heart fails acutely when placed in series with a markedly elevated pulmonary vascular resistance, and death from intractable right heart failure follows within 72 hours. Similarly, a fulminant course is usually pursued by patients with an established infectious process at the time of operation, resulting in death from infection within days to weeks following transplantation.

Among the relative contraindications to heart transplantation is an age greater than 50 years or a history of significant cardiac disease of more than five years' duration. It became apparent quite early in our experience that the older patient, especially when chronically debilitated, tolerated the operative procedure and the rigors of postoperative immunosuppression poorly. Although rejection occurred no more frequently in this older and sicker group, infectious complications resulted in a substantial mortality during the first three postoperative months. A history of recurrent pulmonary infarction, particularly when coupled with roentgenographic evidence of pulmonary scar, appears to be an important predisposing factor to infection in the immunosuppressed patient, and is therefore another relative contraindication to heart transplantation. Patients with relatively recent pulmonary infarcts at the time of transplantation have frequently developed life-threatening infection within the ischemic segment. Patients with insulin-requiring diabetes mellitus are poor candidates for heart transplantation both because of the difficulty of controlling their diabetes while they are receiving corticosteroid therapy and because of the severity of concomitant peripheral vascular disease.

One hundred forty-eight patients have been accepted as transplant recipients in our series, and 109 of these have received one or more heart transplants. Ninety-nine of the recipients were male, and 10 were female. Coronary artery disease was the preoperative diagnosis in 72 recipients, idiopathic cardiomyopathy in 33 patients, post-traumatic aneurysm in 1 patient, and rheumatic heart disease in 3 patients. Preoperative hemodynamic studies in the graft recipients revealed an average cardiac index of 1.7 liters per min. per meter^2, an average left atrial pressure of 27 mm. Hg, an average pulmonary artery pressure of 38 mm. Hg, and an average pulmonary vascular resistance of 4.1 units. Thirty-seven patients died before a suitable donor became available. That the patients selected for transplantation are indeed terminal is verified by survival in this nontransplanted group: 85 per cent were dead within three months following selection, and only one patient lived for more than nine months.

The Cardiac Donor

The cardiac donor must be a relatively young individual who has suffered irreversible brain injury, but in whom the heart continues to beat. In our experience the average age of donors has been 30. Each has been in one of four diagnostic categories: blunt head trauma, gunshot wound of the head, intracranial hemorrhage, or primary intracranial tumor. The average period from hospital admission to certification of cerebral death has been 61 hours, following which an average of six hours has elapsed until cardiectomy has been performed. Certification of brain death is done by a group of physicians independent of the transplantation team. Neurologic evaluation is based on a history, physical examination, cerebral angiography, operative findings, and electroencephalogram. Although the criteria of the Harvard *ad hoc* Committee serve as guides for determination of cerebral death, these criteria are not considered restrictive.[1] All consulting neurosurgeons or neurologists must agree that there is irreversible loss of cortical and brainstem function. It is of note that one of the major contributions of cardiac transplantation to the field of medicine has been in increasing public acceptance of the concept of cerebral death, which has now received judicial recognition throughout the United States. In several states, legislation has been enacted which formally recognizes the concept of cerebral death.

Evaluation of the heart in a prospective donor is relatively straightforward. A careful history obtained from the family members and the personal physician, a physical examination of the heart, an electrocardiogram, and a chest film are all that is necessary in most cases. If any suggestion of cardiac disease is raised, cardiac catheterization and/or angiography are performed. In addition, in all males over the age of 30, and in all females over the age of 35, selective coronary arteriography is done routinely to rule out the presence of occult coronary atherosclerosis. In the first

20 donors used for cardiac transplantation in this series, the only preoperative factors with any deleterious effect on immediate postoperative graft function were increasing age of the donor and occurrence of a cardiac arrest at any time in the preoperative history.[15] The duration of hospitalization and of respiratory and vasopressor support, the donor weight, the highest systolic blood pressure, and the presence of ST-T wave abnormalities in electrocardiograms did not adversely prejudice postoperative graft function.

The primary consideration in management of the prospective organ donor is the maintenance of circulatory integrity in the absence of brainstem function. When loss of brainstem activity occurs suddenly, profound vasodilation and venous dilation occur, followed by cardiac arrest if appropriate steps are not taken. Infusion of large volumes (2 to 10 liters) of crystalloid or colloid solution coupled with the use of small doses of an alpha-adrenergic agent will restore normal circulatory dynamics. Hypothermia, with its potential influence on cardiac rhythm, must be avoided. Diabetes insipidus in these patients is managed readily with intramuscular administration of antidiuretic hormone. The clinical course of a cardiac donor is shown in Figure 3.

Tissue Typing

The discovery of the HLA system of human tissue antigens has made available to workers in transplantation a system of assessing the degree of tissue incompatibility between donors and recipients. In related-donor renal transplantation, HLA typing has been extremely valuable in selecting the relative

whose tissues most closely match those of the prospective recipient, and good correlation between graft survival and function and tissue compatibility has been demonstrated conclusively. In cadaver renal transplantation this relationship is much less firm. Although other investigators have reported a correlation between tissue compatiblity and survival in cardiac transplants,[12] no such relationship is evident in our experience.[28]

Operative Technique

In the first clinical cases of cardiac transplantation, the operative technique was identical to that developed in the animal laboratory (Fig. 4). With the accumulation of experience, although several features of the laboratory procedure were retained, some modifications have been found useful. The performance of the venous anastomoses at the midatrial level shortens and simplifies the operation in the human as in the dog, and stenoses of the venae cavae of pulmonary veins are avoided.

Several techniques to prevent ischemic damage to the myocardium during transplantation have been used, including antegrade coronary perfusion via the ascending aorta and retrograde perfusion via the coronary sinus; we find profound topical hypothermia both effective and simple. The excised donor heart is passed through a series of basins containing cold saline solution, and then while the anastomoses are performed, a slow infusion of ice-cold saline into the pericardial well maintains myocardial cooling. Anoxic intervals range between 35 and 75 minutes, a period well within the safe limits for profound hypothermic arrest.

In the dog, peripheral cannulation of the great vessels has been useful in providing an unobstructed operative field, whereas in the human central cannulation is preferable. The disparity in size between the recipient pericardium and the donor heart provides adequate operating room, and problems with wound healing in the groin of the immunosuppressed patient are avoided.

If the right atrium is opened by a posterior incision connecting the superior and inferior venae cavae, a nodal or coronary sinus rhythm may occur postoperatively, and Barnard therefore recommends a lateral incision in the right atrium.[3] By this maneuver the sinus node is isolated from the suture line by several centimeters, and injury to the internodal tracts of James is avoided. Sinus rhythm immediately postoperatively has been the rule since the adoption of this modification.

All patients in our series have had some degree of elevated pulmonary vascular resistance secondary to long-standing left ventricular failure. The increased load placed upon the transplanted right ventricle by an elevated pulmonary vascular resistance gives rise to several operative considerations. First, a patent foramen ovale must always be searched for in the donor heart, and if any opening is demonstrated, closure is required to prevent right-to-left shunting. Following restoration of coronary flow in the recipient, a considerable period of support by the heart-lung machine may be necessary to resuscitate the right ventricle completely and prepare it for the increased demands

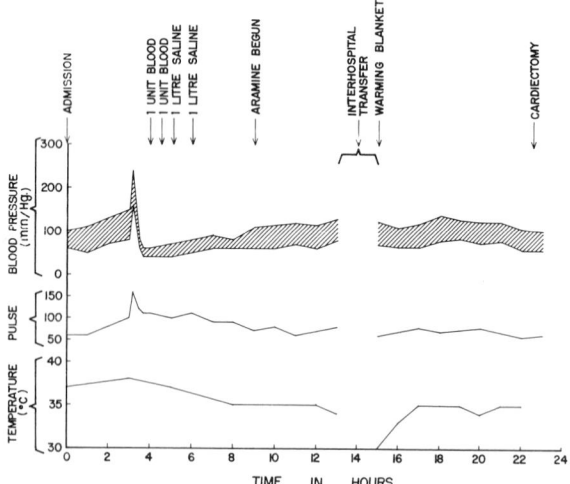

Figure 3. Vital signs in an 18-year-old male heart donor who sustained blunt trauma to the head in an automobile accident. Note acutely developing hypertension at three hours followed by severe hypotension, which presumably occurred at the time of infarction of the intracranial nervous tissue. Partial reversal of hypotension was achieved with intravenously administered fluid, but the restoration of a normal blood pressure required the addition of metaraminol (Aramine). (From Griepp, R. B., et al.: Surg. Gynecol. Obstet., *133*:792, 1971. By permission of Surgery, Gynecology & Obstetrics.)

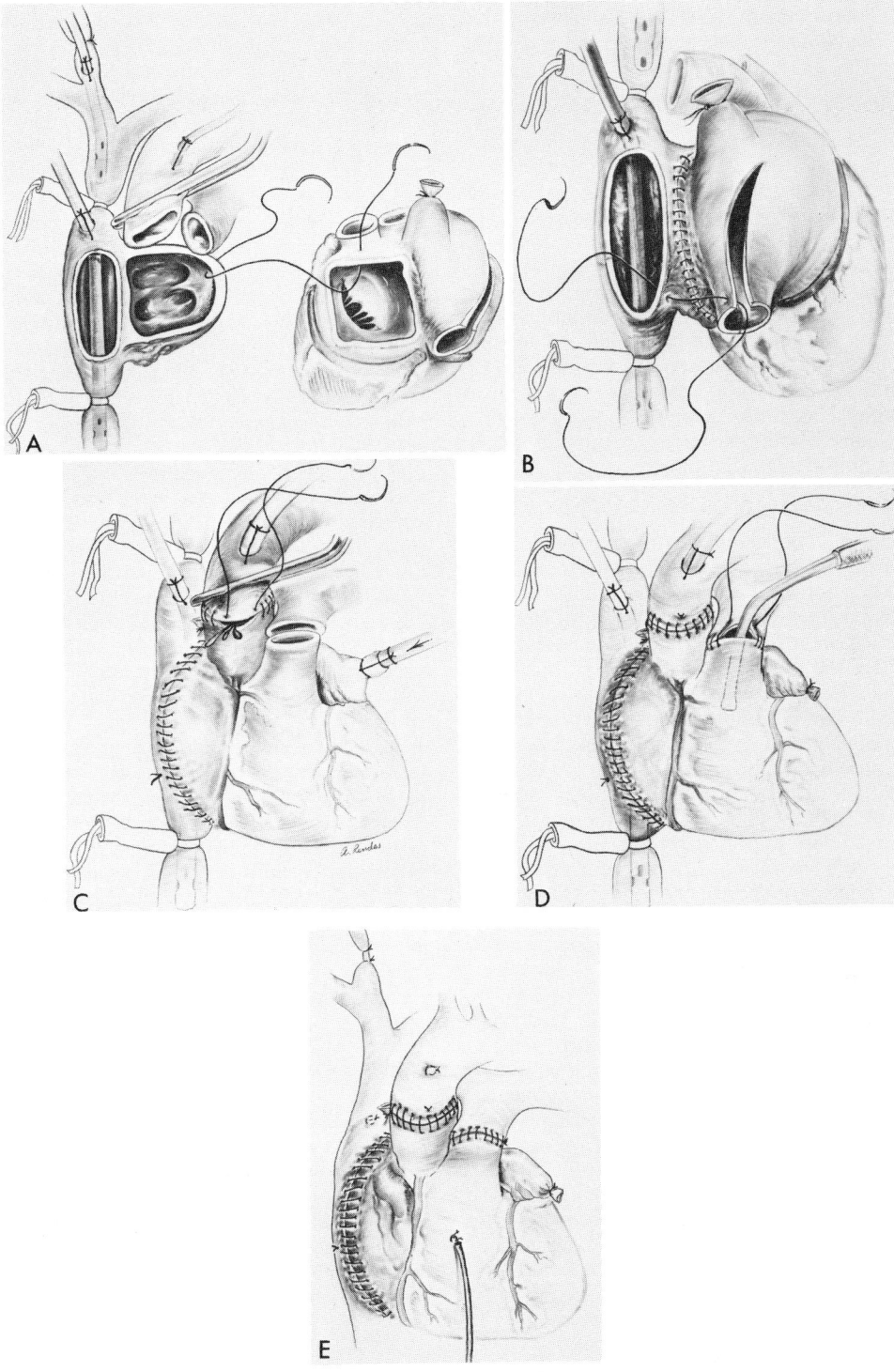

Figure 4. Operative technique utilized for human heart transplantation. *A,* Cannulation of the great vessels is performed, and the heart is isolated from the circulation with caval tapes and an aortic crossclamp. Since inception of the endomyocardial biopsy technique the superior caval cannula has been passed through the right atrium rather than through the superior vena cava as shown, thus preserving the superior vena cava for postoperative endomyocardial biopsies. The recipient heart is removed by severing the atria just posterior to the appendages and cutting the great vessels just above the semilunar valves. The donor atria are opened by connecting the pulmonary vein orifices and incising the right atrium laterally. The superior vena cava is ligated in the donor heart. *B,* The left atrial anastomosis is complete. Suturing of the right atrium follows. *C,* Following completion of the atrial anastomoses, the aortas are joined. A conduit for cold saline is tied into the left atrial appendage to cool the left heart and flush if free of air. *D,* The aortic crossclamp is removed and the pulmonary arteries are joined. A coronary sucker in the right ventricle returns coronary sinus drainage to the heart-lung machine. *E,* The operation is complete and the bypass cannulas are removed. A temporary pacing wire is sewn to the right ventricle.

to be placed upon it. Also, scrupulous attention must be given to removal of air from the left side of the heart prior to removal of the aortic crossclamp. Air remaining in the left heart will usually embolize to the right coronary artery, adding an additional insult to the already overburdened right ventricle.

The precarious state of the circulation in the recipient prior to transplantation is of prime consideration during the anesthetic induction and opening of the chest. Pharmacologic support with isoproterenol is useful during this critical period. It is preferable to avoid internal cardiac massage because of the high incidence of intracardiac thrombus in patients who are in the terminal stages of heart failure. In our series, intracardiac clot has been found in the left side of the heart in 60 per cent of the cases. In one patient in whom internal massage was necessary to maintain the circulation during cannulation for bypass, embolization to the femoral artery occurred, requiring operation six hours following transplantation.

Maintenance Immunosuppressive Therapy

The pattern of maintenance immunosuppressive therapy was initially derived from the experience with renal transplantation as well as with management of rejection in experimental animals with cardiac allografts. Inasmuch as myocardial function is frequently compromised in the early postoperative period as a result of periods of hypotension and myocardial ischemia in the organ donor, followed by the reversible but inevitable myocardial injury occurring during cardiac surgery, it is particularly important that additional immunologically mediated myocardial injury not be incurred during the first few days following operation. Accordingly, high-dose immunosuppression is used for two days following operation. Thereafter the aim of maintenance immunosuppressive therapy is not to prevent all occurrences of acute rejection, since in experimental animals intermittent use of immunosuppressive therapy during periods of maximal immunologic reactivity constitutes the most effective technique for inducing graft acceptance.[21] With the present regimen practically every patient will exhibit at least one episode of acute rejection, which suggests that this treatment is slightly less immunosuppressive than the least reactive patient required, consequently making certain that no patient will receive more immunosuppressive therapy than is necessary.

Corticosteroids and either azathioprine or cyclophosphamide are the primary immunosuppressive agents. Steroids are administered during operation and for the first two postoperative days as intravenous methylprednisolone. Thereafter oral prednisone is begun at a dose of 1.5 mg. per kg., tapering to approximately 1 mg. per kg. by two months following operation. Over the subsequent six months, oral prednisone is further tapered to approximately 0.7 mg. per kg. and the average long-term maintenance dose is 0.4 mg. per kg. The prolonged administration of prednisone is associated with a disturbing array of side effects, including diminished resistance to infection, vertebral osteoporosis, peptic ulcer, salt retention, and cutaneous friability. Consequently, every attempt is made to decrease the prednisone dosage to the lowest level

compatible with adequate myocardial function. In no patient have we been able to discontinue prednisone altogether.

Azathioprine is begun immediately preoperatively, and resumed postoperatively as soon as the patient takes oral medications. An optimal dose is 2 to 3 mg. per kg. per day, but occasional reduction in dosage is necessary owing to leukopenia, and in several patients azathioprine has been associated with significant hepatic toxicity requiring its discontinuation. The average long-term dose of azathioprine is 1.7 mg. per kg. We have observed repeatedly that the larger the dose of azathioprine the patient is able to tolerate, the less corticosteroids he will require. In those patients in whom azathioprine is poorly tolerated, and who consequently need high-dose corticosteroid maintenance therapy, the incidence of immunosuppressive side effects, particularly infection, is substantially increased.[19]

Cyclophosphamide was initially used in recipients of cardiac transplants as a substitute for azathioprine in patients who manifested hepatic toxicity from the latter agent. In a series of 17 patients in whom cyclophosphamide was utilized as the primary agent, the incidence of leukopenia was greater than that occurring in azathioprine-treated patients. As a consequence, we no longer use cyclophosphamide as a primary agent except in patients that have substantial evidence of hepatic dysfunction prior to transplantation.

In recent years it has become apparent that heterologous antisera directed against host lymphocytes are potent immunosuppressive agents. Initially we utilized antisera raised in horses against either splenocytes or thoracic duct lymphocytes. Subsequently we switched to equine antisera raised against human thymocytes and finally to antisera raised in rabbits against fresh human thymocytes. Our experience indicates that the latter preparation is the most potent immunosuppressive agent of the three in recipients of cardiac allografts.

Acute Rejection

With minimal maintenance immunosuppression, as described, acute episodes of cardiac rejection occur in practically every case. Most episodes occur within the first three months following transplantation. The incidence is one episode per 33 patient days during this period, decreasing thereafter to an average of one episode per 190 patient days during the remainder of the first postoperative year, and thereafter to an average of one per 465 patient days. In our early experience the diagnosis of acute rejection was based solely on indirect indices of myocardial function.[17] With the introduction of the endomyocardial biopsy, however, it has been possible to obtain histologic confirmation of allograft rejection as well as to monitor the effect of antirejection therapy.[7]

A simplified protocol for surveillance for rejection injury is currently employed. During the early postoperative period a standard 12 lead electrocardiogram is obtained, and the summation of QRS voltage in leads 1, 2, 3, VI, and V6 is calculated twice daily. Careful cardiac auscultation is also carried out on a routine basis. A fall in the electrocardiographic voltage of 10 to 20 per cent with the appearance of arrhythmias or of a new diastolic filling sound (usually an S3 gallop) is considered presumptive evidence of early rejection injury, and an endomyocardial biopsy is obtained forthwith. Microscopic examination of the specimen is performed within 18 hours. If clinical criteria are strongly suggestive of acute rejection injury, therapy is initiated immediately following the biopsy; in cases in which the evidence is less conclusive, treatment is deferred until the results of the biopsy have been obtained. Following initiation of antirejection therapy, biopsies are obtained every 5 to 7 days until satisfactory resolution of the process is apparent.

Inasmuch as the technique of endomyocardial biopsy has simplified immeasurably the management of cardiac allograft recipients, a brief outline of the technique seems warranted (Fig. 5). The patient is positioned supinely, and utilizing local anesthesia, a needle is introduced percutaneously into the right internal jugular vein. A guide wire is advanced through the needle, a sheath is advanced over the guide wire, and the bioptome is introduced into the jugular vein via the catheter sheath. Under fluoroscopic control the tip of the bioptome is advanced until it impacts on the intraventricular septum. Several small snippets of tissue are removed, and the specimens are submitted for routine histologic staining as well as staining with methylpyronin green. Histologic evidence of ongoing rejection injury consists of perivascular, interstitial, and subendocardial round cell infiltration and· edema. Small vessels may show evidence of endothelial cell injury, and in advanced cases, myocytolysis and myocyte necrosis may be apparent. Figure 6 demonstrates the characteristic findings in a biopsy specimen taken in the initial stages of an acute rejection episode, and

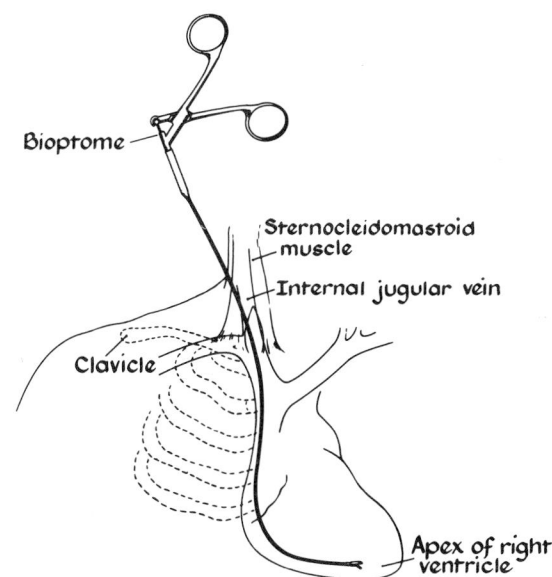

Figure 5. Technique for percutaneous endomyocardial biopsy. See text.

another taken following resolution of the episode with immunosuppressive therapy.

Treatment of an acute rejection episode consists of the intravenous administration of 500 to 1000 mg. of methylprednisolone and 200 to 500 mcg. of actinomycin D once or twice daily until evidence of rejection diminishes. In the treatment of severe acute rejection episodes, reinstitution or increase in the dose of antithymocyte globulin has proved a valuable adjunct. Because of the histologic findings of platelet and fibrin thrombi within the graft vasculature during severe

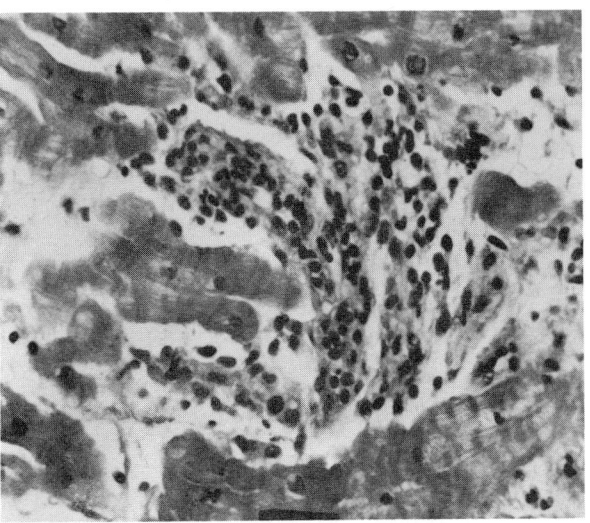

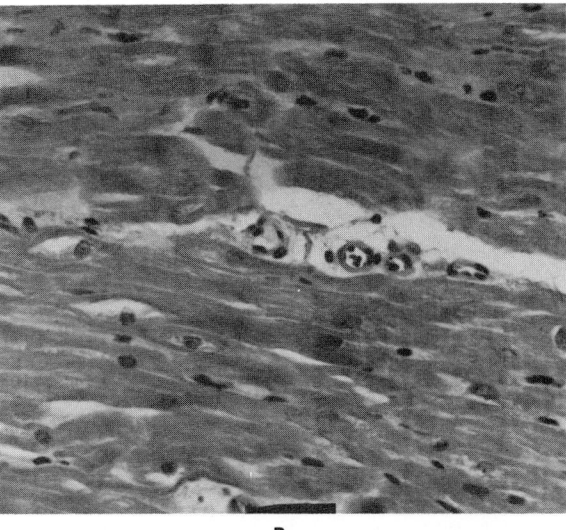

A   B

Figure 6. Tissue obtained by endomyocardial biopsy during acute allograft rejection and following its resolution. A, A dense infiltrate of mononuclear cells is evident within the interstitium, and some myocytolysis is evidenced by nonuniform staining of the myocardial elements. B, Resolution of acute rejection injury with no evidence of mononuclear cell infiltration and restoration of normal myocardial architecture.

acute rejection, systemic heparinization is also utilized.

In instances of severe rejection or delayed diagnosis, marked impairment of myocardial function may occur. Inasmuch as there are no routinely available interim support devices comparable to dialysis in renal transplantation, early and effective reversal of rejection episodes is mandatory. During periods of depressed myocardial function, administration of inotropic agents, such as isoproterenol and digoxin, and maintenance of adequate ventricular filling pressures with intravenous infusion constitute the primary support modalities. Demands on myocardial reserve must be diminished by bed rest and pharmacologic control of fever, if present.

Early diagnosis with institution of effective therapy is now possible in nearly all instances of acute cardiac rejection. In our series 95 per cent of all acute rejection episodes diagnosed have been satisfactorily reversed. It should be emphasized, however, that if diagnosis is delayed until low cardiac output or congestive failure becomes obvious, the treatment may be ineffective and death from myocardial insufficiency may result. The course and management of acute rejection episodes in a representative patient are shown in Figure 7.

Chronic Rejection

We have chosen to designate the progressive coronary arterial narrowing that occurs in the allografted human heart as chronic rejection or graft arteriosclerosis. Histologically, the lesions consist of intimal proliferation complicated in some patients by lipid deposition and formation of atheromatous plaques. The myocardial ischemia that occurs as a result of this process eventuates in death either acutely as a consequence of myocardial infarction or arrhythmia, or in some cases by a pathway involving congestive heart failure. In our early long-term survivors lesions of chronic rejection were ubiquitous findings at postmortem examination.[4] Figure 8 is a section of the left anterior descending coronary artery in a patient who died of an acute myocardial infarction 21 months following cardiac transplantation.

With the hypothesis that the process of chronic rejection involves intravascular microthrombosis and that hyperlipidemia contributes to the atheromatous form of the lesions, a vigorous prophylactic regimen was begun in 1970 for subsequently operated patients. This protocol consists of attempts to combat thrombosis by chronic administration of warfarin and dipyridamole, and control of serum lipid levels by restriction of dietary lipid and maintenance of normal body weight. The incidence of graft arteriosclerosis (determined either at autopsy or by annual coronary arteriography) in our first nine long-term survivors, who were not on the therapeutic regimen is compared in Figure 9 to that in the next 44 long-term survivors, all of whom were on the regimen.[19] The difference in the incidence of detectable arterial lesions between the two groups is highly significant. In patients on the therapeutic regimen for the prophylaxis of chronic rejection, only two patients have developed life-threatening forms of this lesion. One patient died as a consequence of coronary artery narrowing, and one patient required retransplantation.

Hemodynamics and Cardiac Allograft Physiology

In an attempt to confirm the clinical impression that cardiac allograft function is compromised in the early postoperative period, serial hemodynamic studies were performed in 10 cardiac recipients and are summarized in Figure 10.[27] In the first 24 hours after operation, cardiac index was moderately depressed to 1.8 liters per min. per meter.[2] By four days this value had increased to 2.4, and by seven days cardiac index was 3.0 liters per min. per meter[2], a value well within normal limits. The effectiveness of routine maneuvers designated to increase cardiac output was also evaluated during the first 24 hours following operation. Ventricular pacing was found to have virtually no effect on cardiac index unless the resting cardiac rate was less than 60 beats per minute. Atrial pacing, however, had a modest beneficial effect, increasing rate from an average of 81 beats per minute to 123 beats per minute and augmenting cardiac index from 1.9 to 2.3. In contrast, the infusion of a small dose of isoproterenol (2.2 mcg. per min.) resulted in a much more dramatic increase of cardiac index, from an average resting value of 2.0 to 5.6 liters per min. per meter[2]. Isoproterenol is extremely well tolerated in the early postoperative period, and its routine use for one to five days following operation makes a smooth postoperative course, free of the many complications of low cardiac output, more likely.

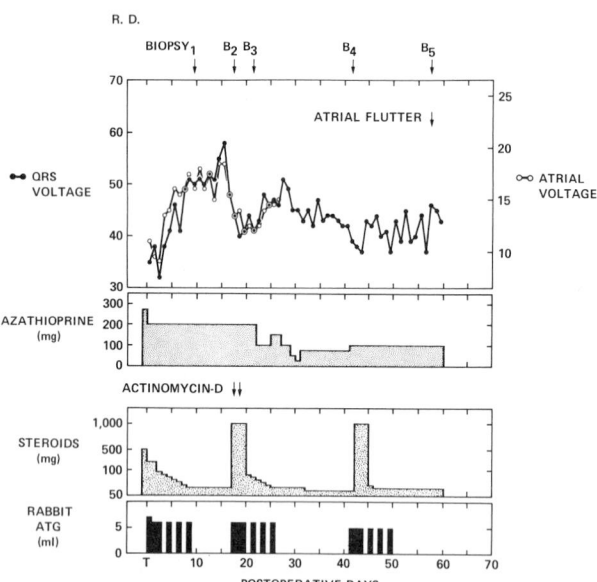

Figure 7. Summarized clinical course of a cardiac allograft recipient. Acute rejection episodes were diagnosed by biopsies 2 and 4 on postoperative days 18 and 42. Both episodes responded satisfactorily to increased immunosuppressive therapy. QRS voltages are the summation of the QRS voltage in leads I, II, III, V₁, and V₆. Atrial flutter occurred on postoperative day 58, but biopsy 5 showed no evidence of acute rejection injury and the arrhythmias resolved spontaneously 24 hours later.

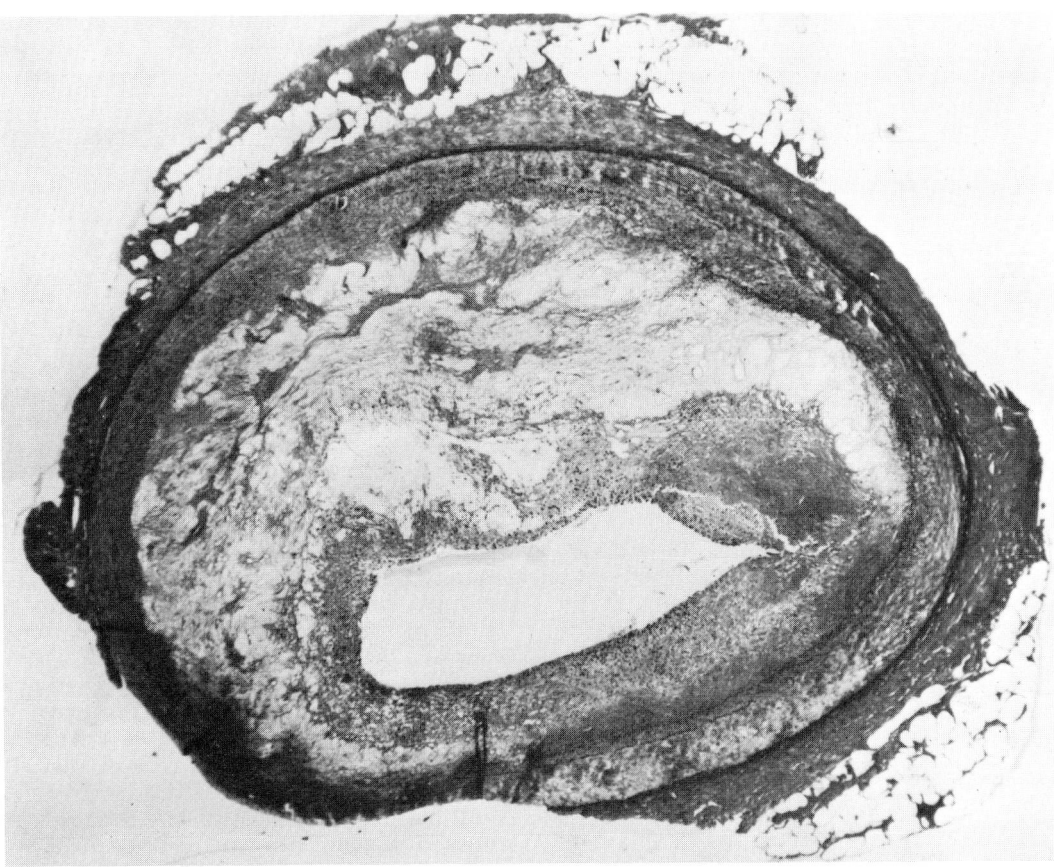

Figure 8. Cross-section of the left anterior descending coronary artery in a patient who died of an acute myocardial infarction 21 months following cardiac transplantation. Marked intimal thickening consisting of both cellular proliferation and atheromatous deposits is evident.

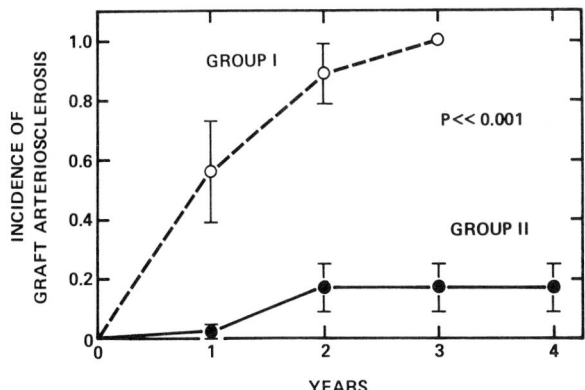

Figure 9. Incidence of graft arteriosclerosis determined either at autopsy or by annual coronary arteriography in two groups of cardiac allograft recipients. Group 1 consists of 9 three-month survivors who were not placed on the hypolipidemic antithrombotic prophylactic regimen. Group 2 consists of 44 three-month survivors who were placed on the prophylactic regimen. The vertical bars indicate the standard error of the determination at each time point. The probability that this difference in incidence in graft arteriosclerosis between the two groups is due to chance is < 10⁻⁶.

An assessment of late hemodynamic function has been carried out in a series of 10 patients one and two years following operation.[18] Intracardiac pressures were within normal limits at rest in all patients. Average cardiac index at rest was 2.5 liters per min. meter^2, increasing to 4.8 liters per min. per meter^2 with moderate supine exercise.

At the time of postoperative hemodynamic study, an attempt has been made to detect cardiac allograft reinnervation by positioning an electrode in the right atrium to allow monitoring of P waves arising from the recipient atrial remnant as well as from the grafted heart. Carotid massage, Valsalva maneuver, amyl nitrate inhalation, and intravenous administration of atropine are used to elicit autonomic discharge. In all patients studied up to five years postoperatively, appropriate responses to these maneuvers were noted in the rate of the recipient atrial remnant whilst the donor heart rate remained constant. Thus, reinnervation of the human cardiac allograft has yet to be demonstrated.

The means by which the denervated cardiac allo-

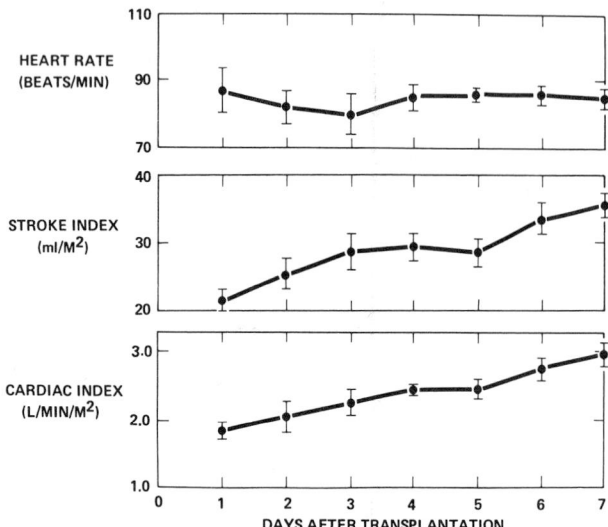

Figure 10. Serial hemodynamic measurements in 10 cardiac allograft recipients during the first postoperative week. See text.

TABLE 1. Primary Cause of Death in Sixty-five Patients Following Heart Transplantation

Pulmonary hypertension	3
Rejection, acute and/or chronic	22
Infection	32
Graft arteriosclerosis	4
Lymphoma	2
Cerebrovascular accident	2

Results

In August, 1976, 44 recipients of cardiac allografts in this series were alive, having survived for one week to 6½ years following transplantation. The causes of death in the remaining 65 patients are shown in Table 1. Acute right ventricular failure secondary to markedly elevated pulmonary vascular resistance resulted in the death of three patients early in the series prior to the recognition that severe pulmonary hypertension constitutes an operative contraindication. The deaths occurring from acute rejection and infection are closely inter-related, the first resulting from undertreatment and the other from overtreatment. The increased precision in the diagnosis and management of acute rejection made possible largely by endomyocardial biopsy, coupled with increased experience with immunosuppressive drugs, has reduced mortality from these causes.

All but one of the deaths from chronic rejection occurred in patients operated on prior to 1970, so it appears that our antithrombotic hypolipidemic prophylactic regimen has substantially decreased mortality secondary to coronary artery narrowing. Two patients died of lymphoma, a recognized complication of prolonged immunosuppressive therapy. Two long-term survivors died of cerebrovascular accidents.

Figure 11 depicts the survival of all patients in this series, contrasted with all patients who were accepted for transplantation but who died before an ABO compatible donor became available. One-year survival in the nontransplanted group was less than 3 per cent, whereas of the patients who received grafts, 49 per cent were alive at one year and 23 per cent at five years. Although overall one-year survival is 49 per

graft meets the demand for increased output during exercise involves two sequential although overlapping mechanisms. During the first three minutes of exercise, the heart rate increases modestly, but most of the increase in cardiac output is secondary to an increase in stroke volume associated with an elevation of left ventricular end-diastolic pressure. Several minutes later heart rate increases further while stroke volume remains stable. Left ventricular end-diastolic pressure peaks and then decreases slightly as left ventricular contractility (LV dp/dt) increases. Thus, in the denervated heart, increased stroke volume secondary to the Starling mechanism precedes increased heart rate and contractility secondary to catecholamine effect, whereas in the normal heart they appear simultaneously. It is probable that this difference is the consequence of a delay in an adrenergic response by the denervated heart until catecholamines are released into the circulation from extracardiac sites.

Retransplantation

Six patients have received a second cardiac allograft in our series.[9] In one patient, retransplantation was necessary within 24 hours of operation owing to an extremely unstable donor heart rhythm. Retransplantation was accomplished during the first two postoperative months in three patients who had drug-resistant, intractable acute rejection. In one patient, the second allograft was rejected within 14 days, whereas in the other two patients the second allograft was accepted. Cardiac retransplantation was performed in two patients two to five years postoperatively because of coronary artery insufficiency occurring as a consequence of graft arteriosclerosis. Following operation, one patient succumbed to a fungal infection that had been present preoperatively. In the second patient, retransplantation was successful.

STANFORD CARDIAC TRANSPLANTATION

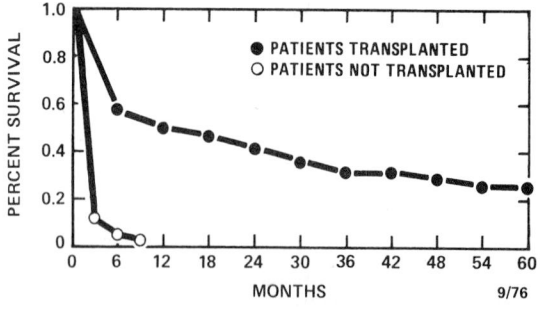

Figure 11. Survival of all patients who received cardiac allografts in this series. Also shown for comparison is the survival of 34 patients who were selected for cardiac transplantation but who died before a suitable donor became available.

STANFORD CARDIAC TRANSPLANTATION

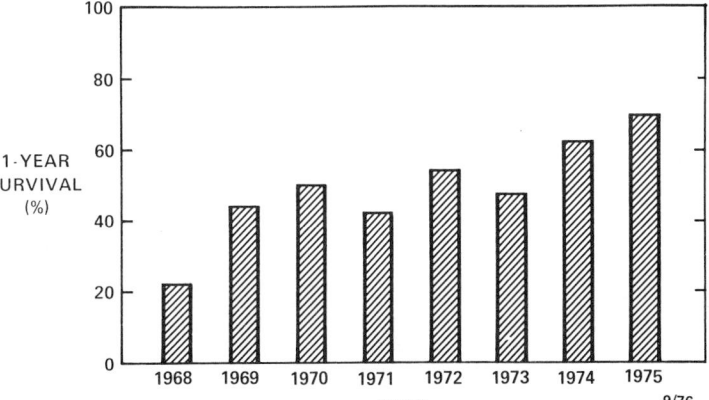

Figure 12. One-year survival by year in which the patients received their cardiac allografts. A clear trend for increasing survival from 22 per cent in 1968 to 65 per cent in 1975 is apparent.

cent, a steady improvement has been achieved, with a one-year survival of 22 per cent in patients operated on in 1968, compared with a 65 per cent one-year survival for patients operated on in 1975 (Fig. 12). Rehabilitation of the long-term survivors has been very encouraging, with 84 per cent restored to a New York Heart Association Functional Class I, and 72 per cent returned to full-time employment.

SUMMARY

Cardiac transplantation has undergone considerable maturation as a therapeutic procedure since its introduction in 1967. Operative contraindications are now recognized, and recipient selection is made on a more rational basis. Operative technique has been improved. The management of the cardiac donor has become routine, and public, judicial, and legislative recognition of the concept of cerebral death is a reality. The use of currently available immunosuppressive therapy has been refined, and, coupled with the increased sensitivity in the diagnosis of cardiac rejection made possible by endomyocardial biopsy, has resulted in successful diagnosis and treatment of the majority of acute rejection episodes. Coronary arterial narrowing secondary to chronic rejection appears to be held in check by restriction of dietary lipids and administration of antithrombotic agents. Late hemodynamic function of the grafted heart has been found adequate for normal activities and moderate exercise despite the functional disadvantages of denervation. Cardiac retransplantation is an option for cardiac recipients in whom acute or chronic rejection cannot be controlled. Patient survival is continuing to improve and is now equivalent to results of cadaver renal transplantation. Functional and vocational rehabilitation has been achieved in the majority of long-term survivors.

SELECTED REFERENCES

Cooper, D. K. C.: Experimental development of cardiac transplantation. Br. Med. J., *4*:174, 1968.
A concise article that thoroughly covers the experimental work in this field, with 132 bibliographic entries.

Najarian, J. S., Foker, J. E., and Simmons, R. L. (Eds.): Transplantation. Philadelphia, Lea & Febiger, 1972.
A comprehensive text on the general field of transplantation. The first section involves general considerations of the immune response, allograft rejection, and immunosuppression. The second section is devoted to clinical transplantation.

REFERENCES

1. A Definition of Irreversible Coma. Report of the Ad Hoc Committee of the Harvard Medical School to Examine the Definition of Brain Death. J.A.M.A., *205*:337, 1968.
2. Barnard, C. N.: The operation. A human cardiac transplant. S. Afr. Med. J., *41*:1271, 1967.
3. Barnard, C. N.: What we have learned about heart transplants. J. Thorac. Cardiovasc. Surg., *56*:457, 1968.
4. Bieber, C. P., Stinson, E. B., Shumway, N. E., Payne, R., and Kosek, J. C.: Cardiac transplantation in man. VII. Cardiac allograft pathology. Circulation, *41*:753, 1970.
5. Carrel, A., and Guthrie, C. C.: The transplantation of veins and organs. Am. Med., *10*:1101, 1905.
6. Cass, M. H., and Brock, R.: Heart excision and replacement. Guys Hosp. Rep., *108*:285, 1959.
7. Caves, P. K., Stinson, E. B., Billingham, M. E., Rider, A. K., and Shumway, N. E.: The diagnosis of human cardiac allograft rejection by serial cardiac biopsy. J. Thorac. Cardiovasc. Surg., *66*:461, 1973.
8. Chartrand, C., Dong, E., Jr., and Shumway, N. E.: Hemodynamics of the orthotopic homotransplanted heart. Surg. Forum, *19*:238, 1968.
9. Copeland, J. G., Griepp, R. B., Bieber, C. P., Billingham, M., Schroeder, J. S., Hunt, S., Mason, J., Stinson, E. B., and Shumway, N. E.: Successful retransplantation of the human heart. J. Thorac. Cardiovasc. Surg., in press.
10. Demikhov, V. P.: Experimental Transplantation of Vital Organs. Trans. Basil Haigh. New York, Consultants' Bureau, 1962, p. 126.
11. Downie, H. G.: Homotransplantation of the dog heart. Arch. Surg., *66*:624, 1953.
12. Fernbach, D. J., Nora, J. J., and Cooley, D. A.: Prospective tissue typing for heart transplants. Lancet, *1*:425, 1969.
13. Golberg, M., Berman, E. F., and Akman, O. C.: Homologous transplantation of the canine heart. J. Int. Coll. Surg., *30*:575, 1958.
14. Griepp, R. B., Stinson, E. B., Bieber, C. P., Reitz, B. A., Copeland, J. G., Oyer, P. E., and Shumway, N. E.: Control of graft arteriosclerosis in human heart transplant recipients. Surgery, in press.
15. Griepp, R. B., Stinson, E. B., Clark, D. A., Dong, E., Jr., and Shumway, N. E.: The cardiac donor. Surg. Gynecol. Obstet., *133*:792, 1971.
16. Griepp, R. B., Stinson, E. B., Dong, E., Jr., Clark, D. A., and Shumway, N. E.: Determinants of operative risk in human heart transplantation. Am. J. Surg., *122*:192, 1971.
17. Griepp, R. B., Stinson, E. B., Dong, E., Jr., Clark, D. A., and

Shumway, N. E.: Acute rejection of the allografted human heart: Diagnosis and treatment. Ann. Thorac. Surg., *12*:113, 1971.

18. Griepp, R. B., Stinson, E. B., Dong, E., Jr., Clark, D. A., and Shumway, N. E.: Hemodynamic performance of the transplanted human heart. Surgery, *70*:88, 1971.

19. Griepp, R. B., Stinson, E. B., Oyer, P. E., Bieber, C. P., Dong, E., Jr., and Shumway, N. E.: Management of long-term survivors of heart transplantation. Transplant. Proc. 7 (Suppl. I):595, 1975.

20. Hardy, J. D., Chavez, C. M., Kurrus, F. D., Neely, W. A., Eraslan, S., Turner, M. D., Fabian, L. W., Labecki, T. D.: Heart transplantation in man: Developmental studies in report of a case. J.A.M.A., *18*:114, 1964.

21. Lower, R. R., Dong, E., Jr., and Glazener, F. S.: Electrocardiograms of dogs with heart homografts. Circulation, *33*:455, 1966.

22. Lower, R. R., Dong, E., Jr., and Shumway, N. E.: Long-term survival of cardiac homografts. Surgery, *58*:110, 1965.

23. Lower, R. R., and Shumway, N. E.: Studies on the orthotopic homotransplantation of the canine heart. Surg. Forum, *11*:18, 1960.

24. Mann, F. C., Priestley, J. T., Markowitz, J., and Yater, W. M.: Transplantation of the intact mammalian heart. Arch. Surg., *26*:219, 1933.

25. Marcus, E., Wong, S. N. T., and Luisada, A. A.: Homologous heart grafts: Transplantation of the heart in dogs. Surg. Forum, *2*:212, 1951.

26. Sayegh, S. F., and Creech, O., Jr.: Transplantation of the homologous canine heart. J. Thorac. Surg., *34*:692, 1957.

27. Stinson, E. B., Caves, P. K., Griepp, R. B., Rider, A. K., Grahm, A. F., Dong, E., Jr., and Shumway, N. E.: The transplanted human heart in the early postoperative period. Surg. Forum, *24*:189, 1973.

28. Stinson, E. B., Payne, R., Griepp, R. B., Dong, E., Jr., and Shumway, N. E.: Correlation of histocompatibility matching with graft rejection and survival after cardiac transplantation in man. Lancet, *2*:459, 1971.

29. Webb, W. R., Howard, H. S., and Neely, W. A.: Practical method of homologous cardiac transplantation. J. Thorac. Surg., *37*:361, 1959.

30. Wesolowski, S. A., and Fennessey, J. F.: Pattern of failure of the homografted canine heart. Circulation, *8*:750, 1953.

X

AUTOTRANSPLANTATION

Samuel L. Kountz, M.D.

Autotransplantation is defined as the transfer of an organ or part of an organ from one location to another in the same organism. Autotransplantation is an ancient technique compared to other forms of transplantation, primarily because there is no problem of an immunologic rejection phenomenon. In general, autotransplantation is limited by dependence on the nutritional needs of the graft and the available blood supply in its new location. Some control of this phenomenon has been possible only in the last several years.

There is no specific discipline of autotransplantation in medicine, but rather it is a technique used by virtually all surgical specialties.

SKIN

Historically, the first documentation of an autotransplanted organ was the transfer of skin and subcutaneous tissue from the forearm to the face to form a new nose. This technique prompted the writing of the first textbook on plastic surgery, De Cutorum Chirurgia per Insitionem, in 1587 by Gasparo Tagliacozzi (Fig. 1).

Skin grafts may be of two types: free grafts, in which the skin is completely severed from its blood supply during transfer; and pedicle grafts, in which a new blood supply is provided at the recipient site before the graft is divided from its original blood supply. Free grafts may be of full or partial (split)

thickness, depending on the needs of the recipient site, the size of the site to be covered, and the availability of donor sites.

Split-thickness grafting is most commonly used today to cover areas of skin loss in third- and fourth-degree burns. The primary reason for using split-thickness skin grafts is that the donor site from which the graft is taken has the potential to heal completely on its own. In fact the same donor site can be used several times. Regrowth or healing of the donor site occurs from epithelium remaining in hair follicles and sweat glands, since the basal layer of skin is transferred in the graft; the epithelial islands left behind spread until the donor area is again covered.[27]

A variety of instruments have been devised to aid in obtaining split-thickness grafts of consistent thickness. Freehand grafts are obtained with a Blair knife, a large dermatome-like blade with a handle, but this instrument requires significant skill and experience if any but small, irregular grafts are required. The Reese dermatome is a drum to which a dermatome blade is attached. The drum and skin are painted with adhesive; then, when they are pressed together and elevated, the calibrated knife can cut a very consistent graft. The Brown dermatome is an electrically operated knife similar to barber clippers; the rapidly vibrating knife is protected by micrometer-like adjustments. Though delicate, when used properly it can take a consistently thick graft of unlimited length.

Choice and preparation of the donor site are important. In general, split-thickness skin grafts are taken

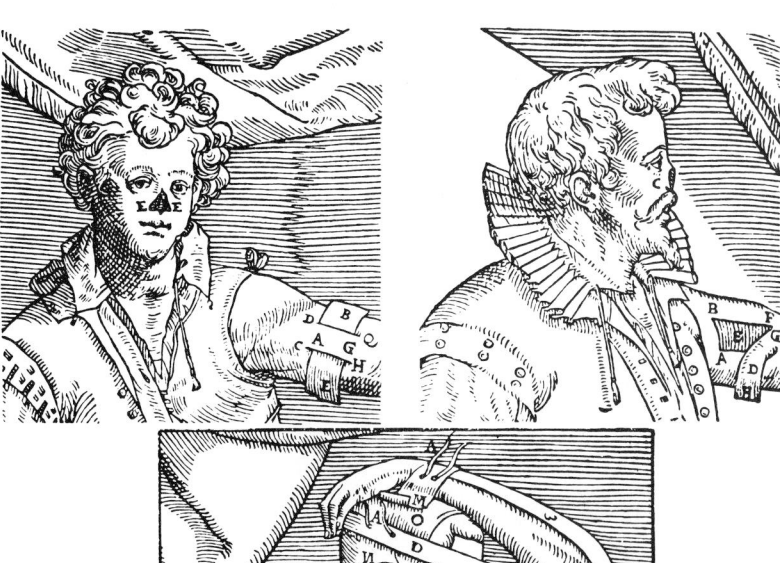

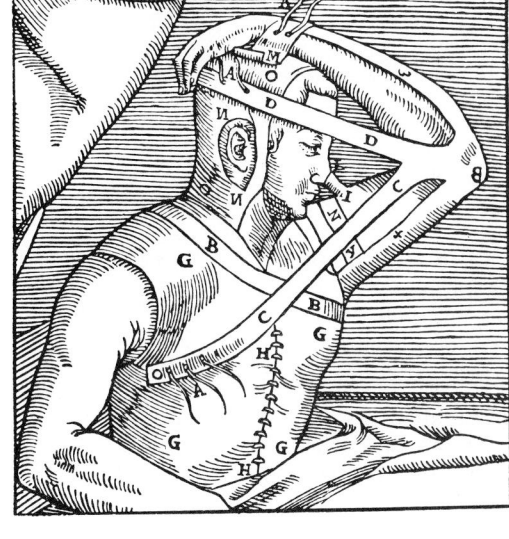

Figure 1. Reconstruction of the nose with a staged tubular pedicle graft. (From Tagliacozzi, G.: De Cutorum Chirurgia per Insitionem, 1587.)

from easily accessible, broad, flat areas such as abdomen, thigh, buttocks, medial arm, and chest. In desperate cases such as in a severely burned patient, virtually any bodily site may be used. The area must be free of hair (shaved) and sterile. A lubricating substance, usually liquid petrolatum, is spread over the surface to allow the cutting instrument to glide freely. After the skin is removed, it is placed on a saline-moistened board and cut to the desired size and shape. When a split-thickness graft is taken, the donor site is covered with antibiotic-impregnated gauze, bandaged, and left to re-epithelialize.

The recipient site must be able to provide immediate nourishment to the graft. The area to be covered must be a well vascularized soft tissue part, such as muscle, or it must be well covered with a layer of granulation tissue. Bleeding in the recipient site must be completely controlled. A blood clot separating the graft from its nutrient bed will prevent healing. The graft will not survive or take if placed directly on to bone, tendon, fat, or fascia. If these avascular areas need be covered by a skin graft, either time or special techniques must be used to allow growth of granulation tissue. For example, if an area of skull is to be covered, the outer table of bone must be chiseled away, exposing the vascular marrow cavity, or multiple holes must be drilled through the outer table. Granulations will then grow that will accept a graft. The other alternative is the pedicle graft, yet to be discussed.

Two requisites to healing determine the ultimate success of the graft and largely the manner in which the recipient site is dressed. The recipient site must be free of debris and there must be no bleeding. Furthermore, there must be no motion between the graft and recipient site during the early stages of healing until they have firmly adhered to one another. Healing in the split-thickness graft depends first on close approximation of the graft to the new recipient site so that the oxygen-laden serous exudate can reach the graft. Adhesion begins with accumulation of fibrin beneath the graft; the fibrin clot is then invaded by fibroblasts and capillary tufts, which ultimately invade the graft. Interruption of the plane between graft and recipient site will delay or prevent healing. Therefore, extreme care must be taken to avoid movement of the graft. In most cases, a stable, firm, well anchored pressure dressing suffices. For some body parts, immobilization, even in plaster, is often necessary. Excess serum will often accumulate beneath a loosely applied graft, and it must be removed by "rolling" the graft to expel the serum at the sides of the graft or by perforating the graft carefully to allow the serum to escape. Meshed grafts or "postage stamp" size pinch grafts obviate much of this problem.

If excess split-thickness skin is removed for which a future need may be anticipated, the skin can be stored for up to 4 weeks at 4° C. The skin is stored on rolls and immersed in normal saline to which an antibiotic has been added. If it is stored at temperatures above 4° C., deterioration of the cells will be accelerated. If the temperature is below 4° C., water crystallizes within the cells and destroys them. When needed, the skin can be removed from refrigeration and applied as a fresh free split-thickness graft.

Full-thickness free skin grafts are used when covering an area of cosmetic importance in which contraction must not occur, such as around the eyelid or an area subject to increased trauma, for example, the palmar surface of the hand or plantar surface of the foot. Several factors should be considered in the decision whether to use full- or partial-thickness grafts. Because it is thicker, a full-thickness graft requires more nutrition so that the likelihood of the graft's taking is less than with a partial-thickness graft. Since a full-thickness graft contains all the adnexal structures of the skin, the donor site cannot re-epithelialize on its own except from the periphery of a very small donor site. Most full-thickness donor sites must be closed by primary suture, or covered with a split-thickness graft. Size of the area to be covered is thus another consideration. Donor sites should generally conform in texture and color to the recipient area. Donor sites for full-thickness grafts are generally chosen from areas where the skin is loose or redundant or may easily be recovered. The posterior auricular fold, the loose skin of the lower neck, and flexor surfaces of joints such as the elbow, buttock, or groin are frequently used. When transferred to the recipient site, the graft must be completely free of subcutaneous fat to insure take. After the graft is placed, its care is the same as for the partial-thickness graft.

Pedicle grafts actually contain more than skin. They include blood vessels and subcutaneous tissue as well. Their constitution defines the primary reasons for their usefulness. Pedicle grafts are used when important structures need to be covered, especially those of poor vascularity such as bone or tendon, or in areas in which repeated trauma is expected, as in reconstructive surgery or nonunion of a bone fracture site. The grafts can be advanced, or moved, to the desired recipient site in the form of a tube or flap. Tubes may even be "walked" some distance in a series of procedures involving repeated division and reattachment nearer and nearer the desired recipient site.

For a more detailed discussion on pedicle flaps, the reader is referred to textbooks on plastic surgery. Basically, however, the technique of pedicle grafting involves a three-sided incision into skin and subcutaneous tissue, the unincised side being that closest to the vascular inflow and outflow. After the flap is undermined in the subcutaneous plane, it is rotated or transferred to the adjacent area needing the graft and is sutured into position. If the recipient area is near enough to the base of the flap, the base need not be divided, and the procedure is completed in a single step. However, if the area to be grafted is some distance from the preferred donor site, then the graft must be advanced as a tube in multistaged procedures in which the tube of skin is eventually severed completely from its original blood supply, but only after new vascularity at the recipient site is established. The donor site must be covered by a split-thickness graft or closed by primary suture, since full-thickness skin has been removed.

MUSCULOSKELETAL AUTOGRAFTS

Bone has been used as autogenously grafted material since Merrem replaced a portion of a dog's skull in 1809. Today it is quite frequently used in man for replantation of lost facial structures such as mandible, nose, brow, zygoma, and the floor of the orbit, and orthopedically to stimulate healing in fracture nonunion and in arthrodeses such as in spinal fusions.

Though initially it was believed that bone required its periosteal blood supply for survival in a new area, it is now known that all bone cells die except those nearest the surface and the bone is replaced by new bone after resorption in a fashion called "creeping substitution."[27] Cancellous bone is preferred and has a higher rate of survival than the harder, more compact cortical bone. The cancellous bone is more readily replaced by ingrowth of osteoclasts and osteoblasts and consequent new bone formation.[4]

Donor sites for bone grafts are determined primarily by the function required of the graft. The iliac crest is a preferred site because it is rich in cancellous bone, and its gentle curving shape makes it ideal for replacement of many facial structures. Ribs are used to replace mandible or to form stents when resection of vertebral bodies is necessary. Tibia is also occasionally used for orthopedic bone grafting procedures.

Recipient areas generally include any place where bone naturally occurs. When segments of mandible are removed for radical surgery for oral malignant disease, rib or iliac crest serves as very satisfactory replacement. Chips of bone placed between other bone ends, as in a joint fusion or in nonunion of a fracture, will stimulate new bone fusion and solidification of previously separated bone.

Cartilage finds its main uses in autotransplantation in plastic surgery. The donor sites are primarily the costochondral junctions of the anterior rib cage. Occasionally, nasal septum, external ear, and meniscus of the knee are used.

Recipient areas are those of cosmetic importance; for example, grafts may be used to create a new pinna for a deformed external ear, nasal support, orbital rim, maxilla, and mandible. When transplanted, cartilage grafts are not replaced in their host position but are nourished by adjacent blood supply since they have none of their own, and heal by fibrous union to adjacent structures.

Tendon grafts are often necessary to restore function to damaged hands and feet. When transplanted as a free graft, the tendon heals by vascularization from adjacent tissues as well as through the sutured tendon ends. Frequently used donor tendons are the palmaris longus of the forearm, the plantaris, and occasionally the triceps tendon. Recipient areas are determined by lost function, as in tendon laceration with delayed repair and shortening or severe scarring. Meticulous technique is required to prevent adhesions of the tendon to skin or deep structures.

Fascia lata from the thigh has been used as a tendon replacement to bolster an abdominal hernia repair and for leaflets to replace damaged cardiac valves. Its main value over synthetic or exogenous materials lies in the decreased susceptibility of natural tissue to infection.

Transfer of muscle groups is occasionally done in patients with paralysis due to nerve damage, e.g., transfer of muscle and tendon supplied by the radial nerve to an area supplied by a damaged ulnar nerve. Free muscle transplants will not survive as such but are replaced by fibrous tissue. Free muscle grafts are occasionally used, however, to control hemorrhage during neurosurgery and to aid in closure of atrial septal defects.

NERVE

Peripheral nerves are occasionally transplanted to supply an area of lost function, usually after trauma. The area of neuron distal to the injury degenerates after trauma, but the sheath cells remain viable. Regeneration from the point of injury through the remaining sheath can occur. Nerve regeneration progresses at approximately 1 mm. per day. Placement of the graft demands careful approximation of the ends of the nerve sheath. The grafted and recipient nerves must be of similar diameter. Sural nerve and greater auricular nerve have been used, the latter primarily to replace facial nerve in facial paralysis. Unfortunately, excellent results are rare.

ARTERIAL AND VENOUS GRAFTS

Carrel successfully transplanted autogenous veins in the arterial system in 1905, 2 years after the first unsuccessful attempts by Exner, which resulted in thrombosis.[11] After a long period of quiescence, use of autogenous grafting techniques gained momentum and enjoys a primary position in vascular surgery today.

Since the venous system has such a remarkable capacity for adaptation to changes in blood flow, obstruction of veins rarely becomes a surgical problem. When arteries are obstructed, the therapeutic objective is to restore blood flow to the area distal to the block. This can be accomplished, for example, by removal of the obstructing atherosclerotic plaque, resection of the obstructed segment of vessel, and replacement with autogenous or synthetic material, or by bypassing the obstruction with a graft connecting patent proximal and distal vessels. Choice of procedure involves many considerations, such as the diameter of the involved vessel, the length of segment involved, the condition of surrounding tissues (presence or absence of infection), and anticipated activity, as in an area of active joint motion. This section will be concerned with the indications for and uses of autogenous materials.

Venous grafts are the most commonly used substitutes for peripheral arteries.[6] Among the venous grafting procedures, those utilizing greater saphenous veins have several advantages. Saphenous vein is usually of sufficient diameter, the limit having been suggested as a minimum of 4 mm.,[30] to insure flow adequate to avoid thrombosis. Saphenous vein is consistently found to withstand arterial pressures without aneurysmal change or dilatation. When aneurysms occur in patients who have had saphenous vein grafts, technical failure is suggested. The vein grafts are normally flexible and are quickly incorporated into the host tissue. Nourishment of the graft comes from intraluminal blood flow. Femoral, popliteal, and upper extremity veins have been used but are generally inferior to saphenous veins, being more prone to dilatation.

Obtaining saphenous vein for use in grafting is a relatively simple procedure. An incision is made in the groin over the saphenofemoral junction, where the four main proximal saphenous tributaries are ligated and divided. Several small longitudinal incisions are then made over the course of the vein through which other connecting venous channels are ligated. After the desired length of vein is obtained and divided distally, the vein can be removed intact as one long tube. Great care is necessary to avoid damage to vessel wall and intima. When placed into the arterial tree, the vein graft must be reversed so that the blood flow does not close the venous valves, which have been left intact. The graft may then be sutured end to end to a divided artery or end to side to bypass an obstruction in an intact artery.

An example of a saphenous vein bypass in a subcutaneous tunnel providing flow between a patent right femoral artery and an obstructed left femoral artery is shown in Figure 2. In this elderly patient with concurrent coronary and pulmonary disease, a subcutaneous crossover graft was chosen instead of a procedure providing flow directly from the aorta to the femoral artery, which would have required a laparotomy. Crossover grafts utilizing saphenous vein have been used in patients with cerebral ischemia to bypass obstruction of cerebral vessels at the thoracic aortic arch, as well as in patients with peripheral ischemia.[5]

Though initially these grafts were used to bypass obstruction in the superficial femoral artery by grafting from the proximal femoral artery to the popliteal artery, improved vascular techniques in recent years have permitted successful grafting of long segments of saphenous vein to smaller arteries such as the anterior and posterior tibial arteries in the lower leg.[12] Maintenance of patency in the graft and surgical relief of ischemic ulceration of the foot or severe claudication depend on adequate patency of the vessel to which the graft is attached so that the peripheral vessel can receive the increased blood flow provided by the prosthesis. Without adequate "run-off," one can expect no improvement in symptoms, and thrombosis will almost certainly occur in the graft.

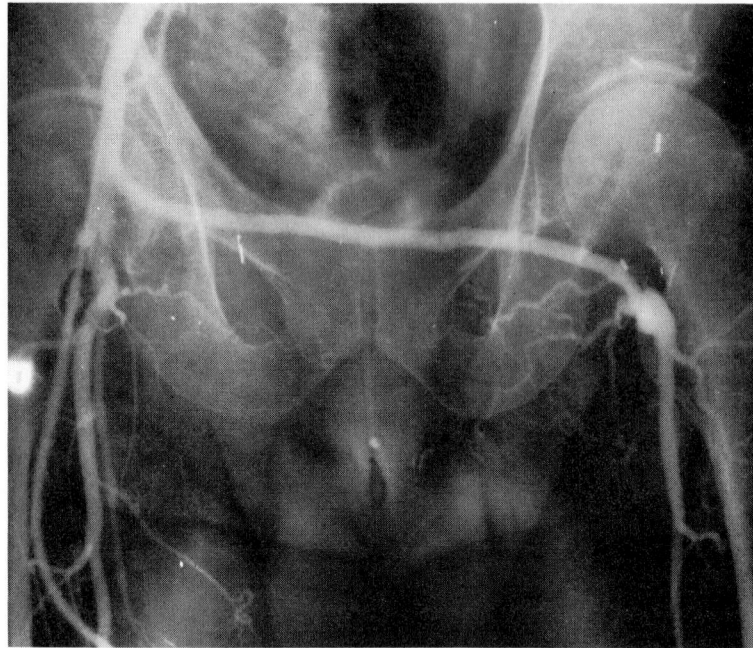

Figure 2. Operative arteriogram showing a subcutaneous saphenous vein bypass from the right femoral to the left femoral artery. (From Ehrenfeld, W. K., et al.: Ann. Surg., *167*:287, 1968.)

The techniques of saphenous vein bypass grafting have more recently been extended to cardiac surgery. Tubular segments of reversed saphenous veins are interposed between the aorta and a coronary artery to bypass a proximal obstruction (Fig. 3).[24] This technique, initiated by Favaloro in 1967, has recently achieved great popularity and has provided a new therapeutic possibility for many patients with atherosclerotic coronary artery disease.

In addition to tubular venous grafts, free patches of vein are also employed in the repair of arterial lesions.

When narrowing of the artery is an inherent part of the surgical problem, a patch of vein can be employed after the artery has been opened and the internal cause of the obstruction removed, to maximize the resulting diameter of the closed arteriotomy.[35] The technique is analogous to inserting a piece of material to increase the size of the waistband in a pair of pants. A diamond-shaped piece of vein is sutured into the diamond-shaped orifice of a longitudinal arteriotomy (Fig. 4). This technique minimizes any chance of stricture at the site of the arteriotomy.[34]

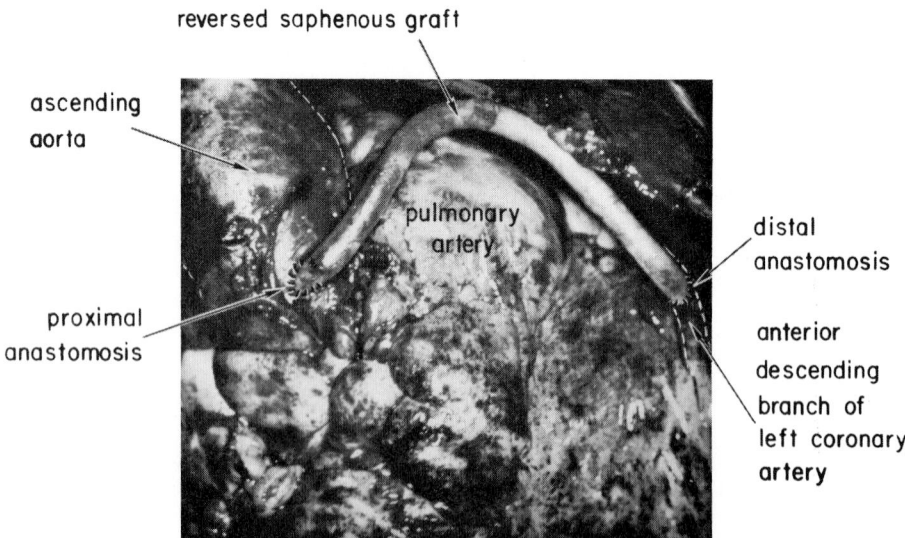

Figure 3. Saphenous vein bypass graft in a 51-year-old male with obstruction of the proximal left coronary artery. The saphenous vein graft carries blood from the aorta to the left anterior descending coronary artery, bypassing the arterial obstruction. (From Sanderson, R. G.: The Cardiac Patient: A Comprehensive Approach. Philadelphia, W. B. Saunders Company, 1972.)

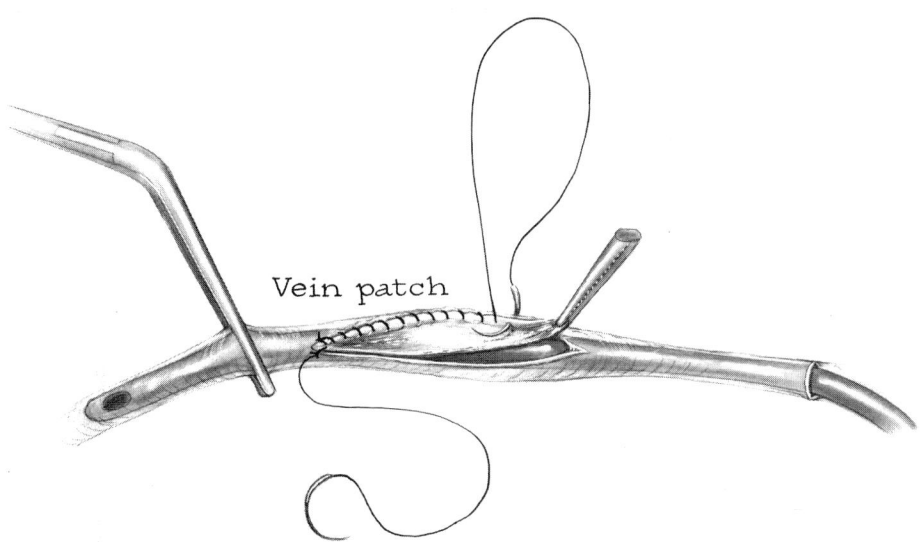

Figure 4. Application of a vein patch in closing an arteriotomy to avoid narrowing at the suture line. (From Wylie, E. J., Binkley, F. M., and Albo, R. J.: Am. J. Surg., *108*:215, 1964.

Though vein grafts are usually satisfactory, the ideal replacement material for a diseased artery is naturally another artery. Unfortunately, in patients needing these procedures arterial segments of sufficient length and diameter are rarely free from severe atherosclerosis. The hypogastric (internal iliac) artery is occasionally used. In 1967, Stoney et al.[28] reported a technique for obtaining artery suitable for grafting. External iliac artery is sectioned and replaced with a Dacron prosthesis, which works very satisfactorily in this location. The common iliac and hypogastric arteries are advanced to extend beyond the flexion crease of groin (Fig. 5). These arterial grafts are specifically useful in areas of extreme activity or in infected areas where no soft tissue support for the prosthesis is available, and when a vein of suitable size is unavailable or its removal would cause undesirable side-effects from venous stasis. The arterial graft has more strength and flexibility than synthetic grafts.[29, 33] Recently, Belzer and associates,[3] using a machine technique of hypothermic pulsatile kidney perfusion, have been able to reconstruct diseased segments of the renal artery ex vivo using microvascular techniques, then autotransplanting the kidney. This type of "work bench

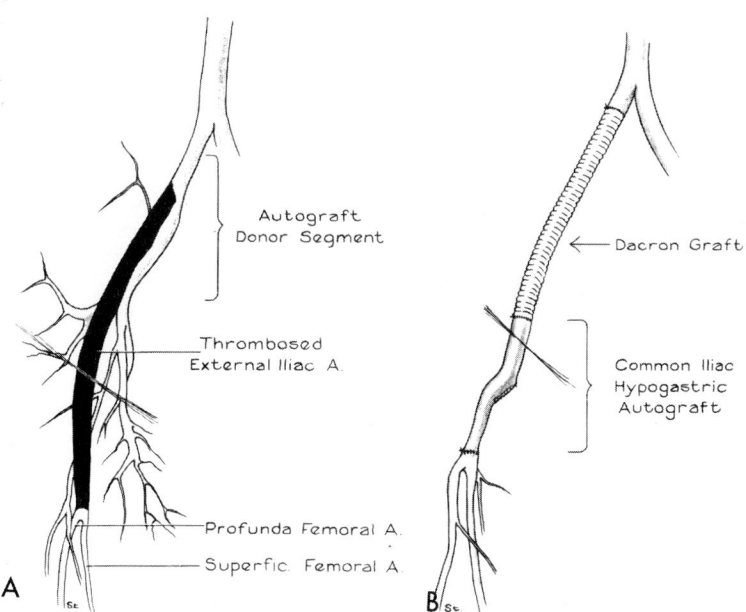

Figure 5. *A,* The normal iliac-hypogastric segment used for autograft replacement of the occluded segment. *B,* Artist's drawing showing reconstruction. (From Stoney, R. J., Ehrenfeld, W. K., and Wylie, E. J.: Surgery, *61*:377, 1967.)

surgery" has been performed for renal tumors and renal stones.

There are two reasons for use of autogenous material instead of synthetic grafts. First, clotting is far less likely to occur spontaneously in an endothelialized natural tube than in the rough inner surface of a knitted or woven Dacron prosthesis. This is especially true in areas of activity such as joints. Second, grafts of natural materials are far more resistant to infection. When organisms become established in the interstices of a prosthesis of synthetic fibers, the usual defenses against the infection are severely encumbered. Antibiotics are often of no avail. Grafts of artery or vein, however, allow for normal invasion of white blood cells. The phenomenon of healing of an arterial graft placed into an infected bed of a previous synthetic graft is well recognized.

Although autologous and synthetic materials have been used successfully in the arterial system, venous replacements still leave much to be desired.[15] Composite vein grafts made up of several small veins have been used to replace the venae cavae, but with modest results at best. The low pressures in the venous system apparently predispose the grafts to thrombosis. Long segments of saphenous vein have been used as crossover grafts to bypass deep femoral vein obstruc-

tion. No venous grafting techniques have met with universal success as yet, however.

ENDOCRINE GLANDS

The history of transplantation of endocrine glands began in 1771, when John Hunter observed vascularization of a testis transplanted to the peritoneal cavity.[17] Later, Berthold in 1849 demonstrated the endocrine function of the testis by castrating cocks and autotransplanting the testes to the peritoneal cavity in some animals while leaving others without testes. Those with autotransplanted testes developed normal secondary sexual characteristics of roosters, while the others, left without testes, did not. Though historically interesting, and scientifically important in defining the physiologic roles of the gonads, autotransplantation of ovaries or testes has little clinical importance today. Prior to the development of synthetic estrogens, multiple attempts at autotransplantation of ovaries were documented as being successful in preventing the undesirable effects of premature menopause following bilateral oophorectomy. Today, the widespread use of estrogen and progesterone compounds for purposes of birth control or relief of symptoms of meno-

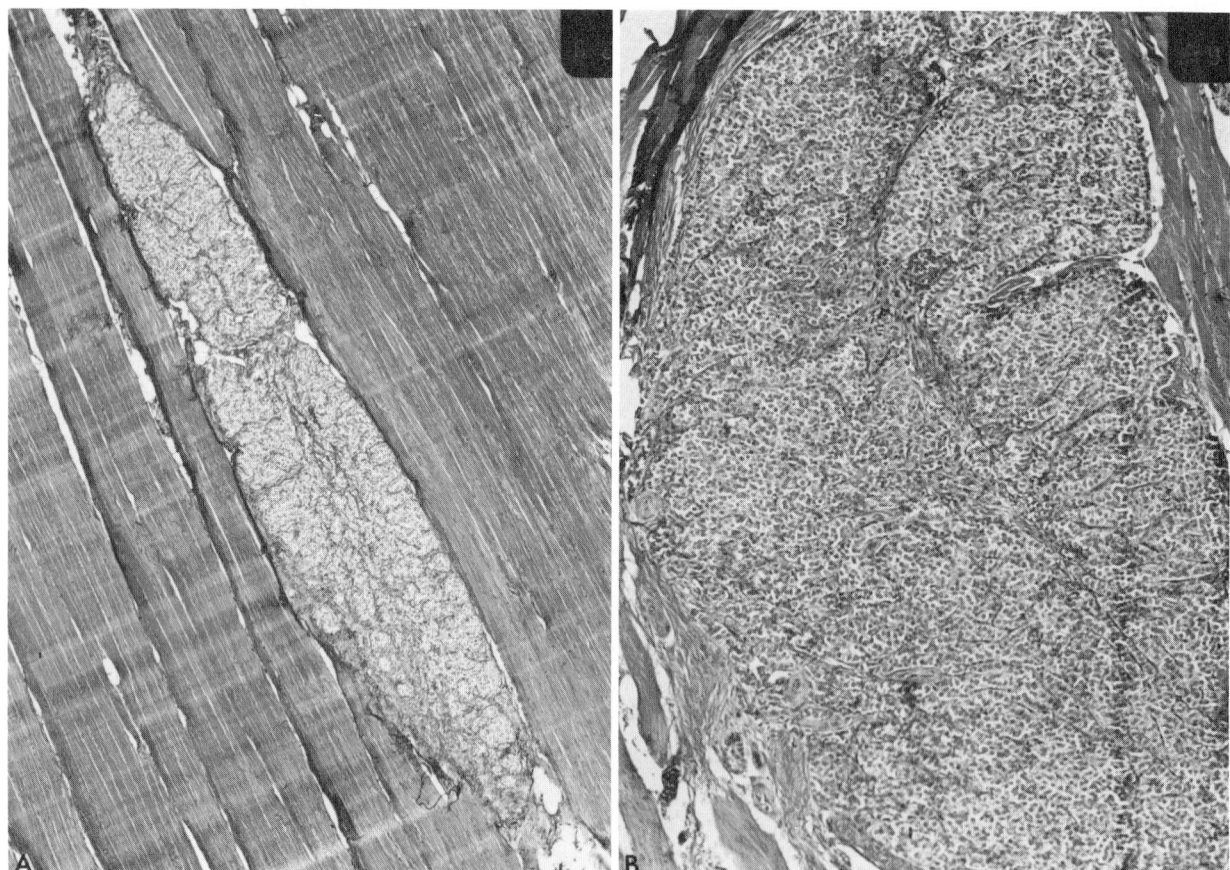

Figure 6. Histological section of a parathyroid graft within a muscle bed at magnification of 41× (A) and 100× (B). (Courtesy of Samuel A. Wells, Jr., M.D.)

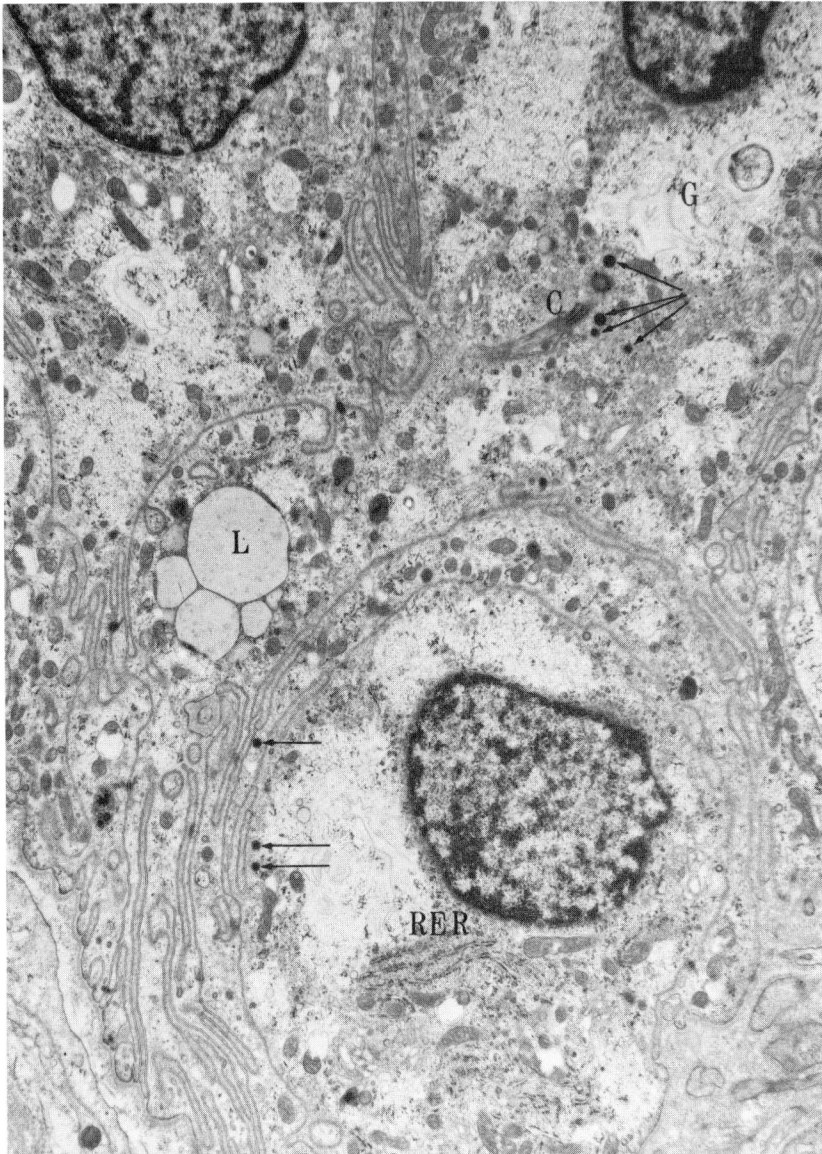

Figure 7. Low-power electron micrograph of three chief cells. Several secretory vacuoles are indicated by arrows, the rough endoplasmic reticulum by *RER*, glycogen by *G*, and lipid by *L*. Original magnification, ×10,680. (From Surgery, *78*:38, 1975.)

pause makes these medications among the most commonly used in medicine.

Experimentally, as well as clinically, attempts have been made to use virtually every endocrine gland for autotransplantation, including adrenal cortex and medulla, thyroid, parathyroid, pancreas, pituitary, and, as previously mentioned, ovary and testis.[17] Of these, only the testis and parathyroid glands are used clinically in any but the rare instance since excellent synthetic substitutes exist for the other organs. In 1975, Wells and associates[31] demonstrated histologically survival of parathyroid autotransplants in man (Figs. 6 and 7) and showed that such grafts produced parathyroid hormone (Table 1).

TABLE 1. PTH Levels (ng./ml.) in Antecubital Veins of Autografted Patients*

H.W.	L†	R	Arterial
1 min.	3.2	0.0	
3 min.	3.5	0.1	
5 min.	7.2	0.3	0.2
M.E.	L†	R	Arterial
1 min.	4.5	0.6	
3 min.	2.8	0.0	
5 min.	2.6	0.0	0.1

*Courtesy of Samuel A. Wells, Jr., M.D.
†Autografted arm.

Autotransplantation of the testis, in fact, is not done for reasons of endocrine function, but rather to insure successful spermatogenesis in an undescended testis. During intrauterine development, the testis is an intra-abdominal organ; it ordinarily descends through the inguinal canal into the scrotum at or near the time of gestational completion. Occasionally the normal descent of the testis is interrupted, with the testis left in an aberrant position. The position may vary widely, from inside the peritoneal cavity to the inguinal canal; the testis is termed cryptorchid when it is arrested in its normal descent and in other positions is called ectopic.[26] Operative intervention is necessary since spermatogenesis will not occur at normal body temperature of 98.6° F., but requires the slightly lower temperature in the scrotal sac. Operative interception, which consists of placing the testis with its blood supply intact into the scrotum, should be done when the patient is about 1 year old. After the age of 6, definite changes in the spermatogenic tubules can be demonstrated. The operation of choice consists of placing the testis through the scrotal septum, anchoring it to the opposite side. Inguinal hernia is commonly found coincident with undescended testis and can be corrected at the same time as the orchidopexy. An increased incidence of testicular carcinoma has been reported in undescended testes, but this is open to argument.

Parathyroid autotransplantation is a therapeutic measure taken as a result of inadvertent removal of the parathyroid, usually during thyroidectomy. After initiation of experimental parathyroid transplantation by Christiani in 1905,[17] Halsted made a series of unsuccessful attempts to autotransplant parathyroids in dogs; his experience prompted him to formulate what later became known as Halsted's law:[16] "Transplants of endocrine organs are normally unsuccessful unless a deficiency of greater than one-half is created." More specifically, unless an endocrine deficiency exists, transplantation of the organ will fail. Though this guided the thinking of surgeons for some time, gradually they began to advocate a thorough search of excised tissue at the time of thyroidectomy, to identify any tissue suspected of being parathyroid by frozen section, and prompt autotransplantation of the specimen into the body of the sternocleidomastoid muscle.[19] The viability of such a transplant was histologically proved in an autopsy reported in 1936.[25]

The symptoms of hypoparathyroidism precipitated by hypocalcemia and hypomagnesemia extend from tetany and psychologic disturbances to convulsions, coma, and death. Medical therapy for hypoparathyroidism is varied and complicated and includes vitamin D, calcium, aluminum hydroxide, probenecid, and a diet low in phosphorus.[10] Synthetic parathyroid hormone is not yet available.

Transplantation of the parathyroids is difficult because of their small size, and blood staining at surgery makes their brown color even less distinguishable. Toluidine blue dye, injected intravenously at the time of operation, is advocated as an aid to their recognition because it stains the parathyroid tissue selectively.[7] Knowledge of the normal parathyroid anatomy is essential: the superior parathyroid glands are at the midlateral portion of the thyroid lobe and the inferior glands are at the lower thyroid poles. The bifurcation of the inferior thyroid artery is a useful landmark, the glands usually being within 2 cm. of it. Important, too, is that the parathyroids are often located behind the sternum in the superior mediastinum.

HEMATOPOIETIC BONE MARROW

Earlier we discussed the use of cancellous bone grafts in orthopedic surgery. Another use for cancellous marrow has been growing in importance in recent years: transplantation of the immature hematopoietic cells in patients with secondary anemia.

Within 8 years of the discovery of x-rays by Röntgen in 1895, investigators began describing atrophy of lymphoid and bone marrow tissues following x-irradiation.[22] It was soon noted that x-rays had their effect on cells undergoing mitosis rather than on mature cells. Later, with the advent of radiomimetic chemotherapy and its increasingly frequent use in clinical medicine, clinical bone marrow depression of hematopoiesis became a more common and serious problem. These antimetabolites are generally used in the treatment of a wide variety of malignant diseases.

Though homograft bone marrow transplants have been performed clinically, their use is limited by the usual problems of homograft rejection. A second, often more potent, problem exists: the graft versus host reaction. The graft versus host reaction is, in a sense, the rejection of the recipient by the donor graft. This occurs by virtue of the fact that immunologically competent, antibody-producing cells are transplanted in the marrow, which will recognize the host as foreign and precipitate a rejection, usually resulting in death of the host. At autopsy in such cases, the marrow is seen to be thriving.

Both rejection of the graft and the graft versus host phenomenon are obviated by marrow exchange between identical twins. As of 1966, this rare operation had been performed only 13 times. Modest success was achieved in patients with aplastic anemia, and only little success in patients with leukemia.

Autotransplantation of hematopoietic marrow consists of aspiration of marrow into syringes that are stored at 4° C. while the patient receives chemotherapy or radiation therapy. When the therapy is completed the marrow is returned to the patient, either by intravenous infusion or directly to the marrow cavity. Only 50 ml. is required for this procedure. A complicating factor is that occasionally there are malignant cells in the bone marrow aspirate. Efforts then are taken to destroy them selectively prior to reinfusion of the specimen; this technique is still under investigation.

GASTROINTESTINAL TRACT

No other organ system is as well adapted for autotransplantation as the gastrointestinal tract, by virtue of the freely mobile intestines tethered on long vascular pedicles. Many surgical procedures are concerned with rearrangement of ducts and conduits, creating new passages where old ones were obstructed with scar or tumor, reversing the direction of peristalsis to retard passage of gastrointestinal contents, or substituting one organ for another, as when a loop of ileum serves to replace a urinary bladder. This section will be concerned primarily with the substitution of one organ for another, in particular, esophageal replacement by autogenous grafting.

Early attempts at esophageal replacement utilized tubes fashioned from skin from the anterior thorax. These required multiple-stage procedures and rarely resulted in any better than a poor swallowing mechanism.[13] Roux first used another segment of gastrointestinal tract to replace the esophagus in 1907 in an 11-year-old boy suffering from a caustic esophageal stricture.[23] After several other attempts at esophageal replacement, this field of surgery became quiescent until 1938, when stomach was shown to provide an adequate esophageal replacement.[1] Today stomach remains the most popular organ substitute in cases of esophageal cancer and is frequently used in benign disorders as well.[20]

The technique of gastroesophagostomy involves ligation and division of the left gastric, short gastric, and gastroepiploic arteries, leaving the right gastric artery to maintain blood supply. After division of the gastrohepatic and gastrolienal ligaments, vagus nerves, and the left gastric vein, the stomach is freely mobile. It may then be advanced through the esophageal hiatus to points well into the superior thorax. A pyloroplasty must accompany the procedure to facilitate emptying.[13]

Regurgitation of contents of the gastric pouch into the remaining esophagus is a common problem. This complication of esophagitis can be relieved by making the entire stomach an intrathoracic organ, leaving no part of the stomach in the abdomen. The stomach is then not subjected to the increased pressures of the abdomen, and reflux is less of a problem. Other complications of intrathoracic gastroesophagostomy include distress from distention of the intrathoracic gastric pouch and the dumping syndrome.

Stomach is preferred as an esophageal replacement for carcinoma because the procedure is simpler than other procedures. The operation takes less time, and it can always be completed at one stage in these patients, who almost always are debilitated. The procedure is usually palliative and the best statistics for lower esophageal carcinoma show a survival rate of only 17 to 34 per cent.[32] These survival statistics grow worse with tumors more proximally situated in the midesophagus and proximal esophagus, for which treatment relies almost entirely on radiation therapy.

For benign disorders of the esophagus, such as peptic or caustic stricture, the procedure of choice, which relieves the underlying cause and resulting illness, is esophageal resection and replacement or bypass with a segment of intestine.[32] Grimes has laid down the following criteria for satisfactory esophageal substitute: (1) its blood supply must be plentiful and easily preserved by careful handling; (2) it should possess an adequate luminal caliber; (3) its length after mobilization should allow spanning of the entire thorax, if

necessary; and (4) it should be able to resist the relentless effects of acid-peptic digestion.[14] Though stomach may at times satisfy these criteria, the use of jejunum, ileocolon, and right, transverse, and left colon has progressively gained in popularity in recent years.

When jejunum is used as the door organ, the usual procedure is to leave the proximal end exposed in the neck because the blood supply frequently is inadequate. After several days of observation, the proximal anastomosis to cervical esophagus is completed if the jejunum continues to appear viable at that time. A segment of jejunum immediately distal to the ligament of Treitz is chosen; the pattern of the vascular arcades from the superior mesenteric arterial supply is used to guide in the selection of the appropriate artery on which the graft's blood supply will be based (Fig. 8). Attention to venous drainage is just as important as consideration of the arterial supply. The graft is then brought behind the transverse colon through the esophageal hiatus, and proximal and distal anastomoses are completed. Since the vagus nerves are sectioned during the preparatory esophagectomy, a pyloroplasty should accompany the procedure (Fig. 8B).

Though all segments of the colon have been used to replace esophagus, the left colon is currently preferred by most surgeons for replacement of esophagus in benign disease as well as for bypass of the esophagus in cases of malignant disease.[9]

Colon grafting avoids the disadvantages of esophageal replacement by stomach, which are reflux esophagitis at the site of anastomosis, postural regurgitation of gastric secretions and bile, reduced gastric capacity, and nutritional disorders. In infants and children, jejunal grafts have received criticism because of inadequate blood supply, making their viability precarious, and because an alkaline esophagitis exists proximal to the anastomosis.[2]

Left colon is of ideal diameter, as well as being of adequate length to replace the entire thoracic esophagus.[14] Pressure symptoms from dilatation of left colon are rare and the blood supply to left colon, based on the middle colic or left colic arteries, is usually excellent, with good collateral circulation provided through the marginal artery (Fig. 9A). If the blood supply is based on the middle colic artery, the colon graft will be antiperistaltic; if it is based on the left colic artery, it will be isoperistaltic.

After the colon is freed from all its intra-abdominal connections except the blood supply, it may be carried to the cervical esophageal hiatus, as described with jejunum, or it may be carried in a subcutaneous presternal tunnel or in an anterior mediastinal substernal tunnel (Fig. 9B). The most favorable results have been obtained with placement in the normal posterior mediastinal position, but when bypassing an inoperable carcinoma in a debilitated patient, a substernal or subcutaneous route may be preferred.

Late evaluations of colon transplants have shown that the transplanted colon acts only as a conduit without peristalsis. Peptic ulceration has occurred in the distal colon grafts but has been attributed to anterior cologastrostomies, to lack of vagotomy or pyloroplasty or both, or to herniation of the stomach into the thorax.[18]

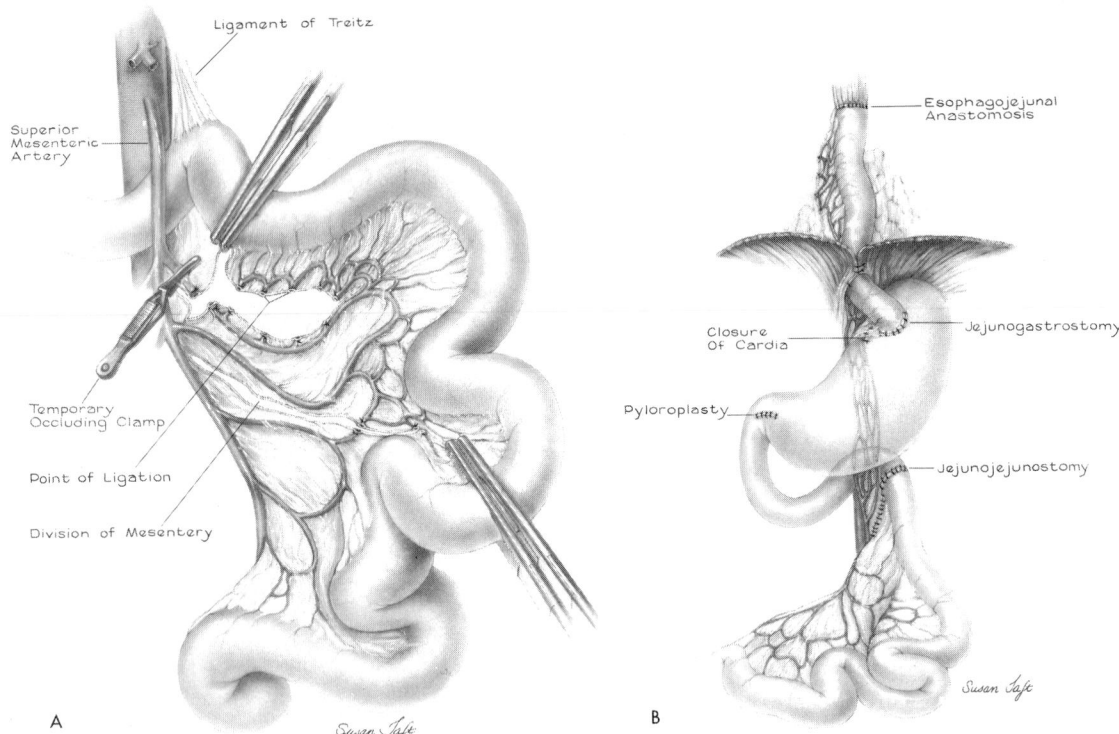

Figure 8. *A,* Preparation of the jejunal segment for interposition. The second artery in the jejunal mesentery has been divided after its temporary occlusion to insure that the one remaining artery in the pedicle can adequately nourish the segment. *B,* The position of the jejunal transplant at completion of the procedure. During reconstruction of the esophageal hiatus care is taken to avoid pressure on the vascular pedicle of the jejunal graft. (From Grimes, O. F.: Surgery, *61*:325, 1966.)

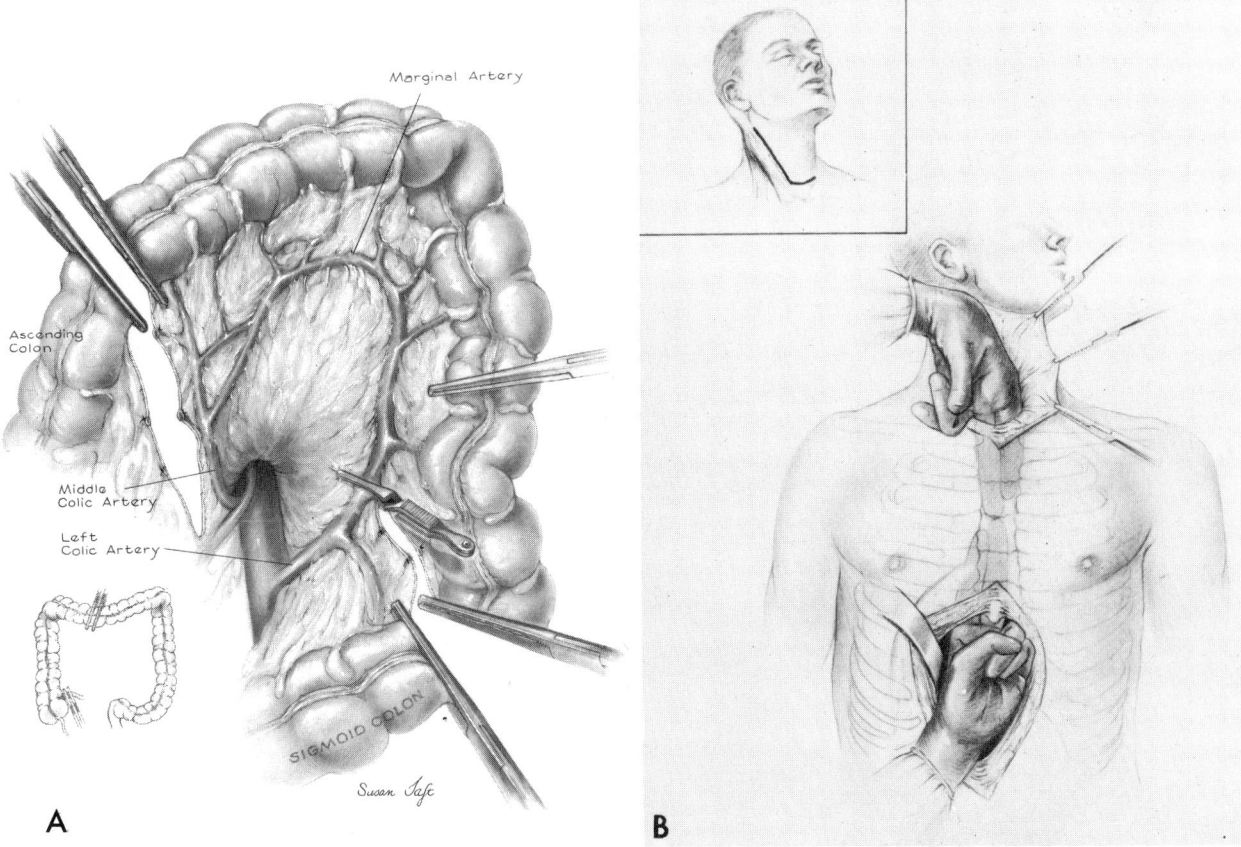

Figure 9. *A*, The middle colic or left colic artery used for blood supply to a left colon transplant. Note the rich collateral circulation via the marginal artery. *B*, A substernal tunnel is created by blunt dissection through which the colon transplant can be passed to the neck. (From Grimes, O. F.: Surgery, *61*:487, 1967.)

Free autografts using stomach and colon have been used to replace cervical esophagus. Their use is limited, however, and a careful search of the subclavian artery for satisfactory arterial blood supply to the free graft is necessary.[21]

SELECTED REFERENCES

Darling, R. C.: Peripheral arterial surgery. N. Engl. J. Med., *280*:26, 84, 141, 1969.
This three-part work constitutes a 6-year review of current literature dealing with all aspects of peripheral arterial disease and surgery. It includes 127 references.

Grimes, O. F.: Replacement of the esophagus. Am. J. Surg., *100*:278, 1960.

Grimes, O. F.: Surgical reconstruction of the diseased esophagus. I. Interposition of the jejunum. II. Interposition of the ileocolon and colon. Surgery, *61*:325, 487, 1967.
These articles present a comprehensive view of the surgical problems of esophageal replacement. They discuss historical and current considerations in the use of stomach and small and large bowel for esophageal substitution.

Wells, S. A., Jr., Gunnells, J. C., Shelburne, J. D., Schneider, A. B., and Sherwood, L. M.: Transplantation of the parathyroid glands in man: Clinical indications and results. Surgery, *78*:34, 1975.
This is an analysis of the results of parathyroid autotransplantation, describing techniques and documenting both histological and functional evidence of survival.

Wilkins, E. W., Jr., and Skinner, D. B.: Surgery of the esophagus. N. Engl. J. Med., *278*:824, 887, 1968.

This is a comprehensive review of esophageal surgery for the past 5 years. It includes 102 references and discusses all surgical problems involving the esophagus.

REFERENCES

1. Adams, W. E., and Phemister, D. B.: Carcinoma of the lower thoracic esophagus; report of a successful resection and esophagogastrostomy. J. Thorac. Surg., 7:621, 1938.
2. Belsey, R.: Reconstruction of the esophagus with left colon. J. Thorac. Cardiovasc. Surg., *49*:33, 1965.
3. Belzer, F. O., Salvatierra, O., Palubinskas, A., and Stoney, R. J.: Ex vivo renal artery reconstruction. Ann. Surg., *182*:456, 1975.
4. Boyne, P. J.: Autogenous cancellous bone and marrow transplants. Clin. Orthop., *73*:199, 1970.
5. Darling, R. C.: Peripheral arterial surgery. N. Engl. J. Med., *280*:26, 84, 141, 1969.
6. Darling, R. C., Linton, R. R., and Razzuk, M. A.: Saphenous vein bypass grafts for femoropopliteal occlusive disease: A reappraisal. Surgery, *61*:31, 1967.
7. Egdahl, R. H.: Surgery of the parathyroid glands. Surg. Gynecol. Obstet., *130*:901, 1970.
8. Ehrenfeld, W. K., Levin, S. M., and Wylie, E. J.: Venous crossover bypass grafts for arterial insufficiency. Ann. Surg., *167*:287, 1968.
9. El-Domeiri, A., Martin, N., and Beattie, E. J.: Esophageal reconstruction by colon interposition. Arch. Surg., *100*:358, 1970.
10. Escamilla, R. F., Kempe, C. H., Crane, J., Goldman, L., and Gordan, G. S.: Preliminary experiences with transplants of cultured parathyroid tissue in hypoparathyroidism. Ann. Intern. Med., *46*:649, 1957.
11. Exner, A.: Einige Tierversuche über Vereinigung und Transplan-

tation von Blutgefässen. Wien. Klin. Wochenschr., 16:273, 1903.

12. Garrett, H. E., and DeBakey, M. E.: Distal posterior tibial artery bypass with autogenous vein graft: A report of three cases. Surgery, 60:283, 1966.

13. Grimes, O. F.: Replacements of the esophagus. Am. J. Surg., 100:278, 1960.

14. Grimes, O. F.: Surgical reconstruction of the diseased esophagus. I. Interposition of the jejunum. II. Interposition of the ileocolon and colon. Surgery, 61:325, 487, 1967.

15. Haimovici, H., Hoffert, P. W., Zinicola, N., and Steinman, C.: An experimental and clinical evaluation of grafts in the venous system. Surg. Gynecol. Obstet., 131:1173, 1970.

16. Halsted, W. S.: Auto- and isotransplantation, in dogs, of the parathyroid glandules. J. Exp. Med., 11:175, 1909.

17. Krohn, P. L.: Transplantation of endocrine glands. In Peer, L. A. (Ed.): Transplantation of Tissues. Baltimore, Williams & Wilkins Company, 1959, Volume II, p. 401.

18. Malcolm, J. A.: Occurrence of peptic ulcer in colon used for esophageal replacement. J. Thorac. Cardiovasc. Surg., 55:763, 1968.

19. Matsuura, H., Sako, K., and Marchetta, F. C.: Successful reimplantation of autogenous parathyroid tissue. Am. J. Surg., 118:779, 1969.

20. Mullen, D. C., Young, W. G., Jr., and Sealy, W. C.: Results of twenty years' experience with esophageal replacement for benign disorders. Ann. Thorac. Surg., 5:481, 1968.

21. Nakayama, K., et al.: Experience with free autografts of bowel with new venous anastomosis apparatus. Surgery, 55:796, 1964.

22. Pegg, D. E.: Bone Marrow Transplantaion. Chicago, Year Book Medical Publishers, 1966.

23. Roux, C. K.: L'oesophago-jéjuno-gastromose; nouvelle opération pour rétrécissement infranchissable de l'oesophage. Sem. Méd., 27:37, 1907.

24. Sanderson, R. G.: The Cardiac Patient: A Comprehensive Approach. Phiadelphia, W. B. Saunders Company, 1972.

25. Shambaugh, P., and Cutler, E. C.: Survival of an autoplastic parathyroid transplant in a patient without parathyroid deficiency. Arch. Surg., 32:842, 1936.

26. Smith, D. R.: General Urology. Los Altos, Calif., Lange Medical Publications, 1969.

27. Stark, R. B.: Plastic Surgery. New York, Harper & Row, 1962.

28. Stoney, R. J., Ehrenfeld, W. K., and Wylie, E. J.: Autogenous replacement of the external iliac and common femoral arteries by common iliac-hypogastric advancement. Surgery, 61:377, 1967.

29. Stoney, R. J., and Wylie, E. J.: Arterial autografts. Surgery, 67:18, 1970.

30. Turcotte, J. G., Dent, T. L., and Fry, W. J.: Preparation for femoral popliteal bypass. Arch. Surg., 100:627, 1970.

31. Wells, S. A., Jr., Gunnells, J. C., Shelburne, J. D., Schneider, A. B., and Sherwood, L. M.: Transplantation of the parathyroid glands in man: Clinical indications and results. Surgery, 78:34, 1975.

32. Wilkins, E. W., Jr., and Skinner, D. B.: Surgery of the esophagus, I and II. N. Engl. J. Med., 278:824, 887, 1968.

33. Wylie, E. J.: Vascular replacement with arterial autografts. Surgery, 57:14, 1965.

34. Wylie, E. J., Binkley, F. M., and Albo, R. J.: Femoropopliteal endarterectomy. Am. J. Surg., 108:215, 1964.

35. Wylie, E. J., Perloff, D. L., and Stoney, R. J.: Autogenous tissue revascularization technics in surgery for renovascular hypertension. Ann. Surg., 170:416, 1969.

XI

IMMUNE MECHANISMS AND ALLOGRAFT DESTRUCTION

D. Bernard Amos, M.D.

Tissue cells carry cell-surface markers. If the markers on a grafted cell differ from those present in the host, they are rapidly recognized as foreign and a complex series of changes is initiated.[17] These processes lead, in most instances, to the formation of antibodies and to the appearance of activated or killer lymphocytes. Antibody production is the function of certain specialized cells called B cells, and of plasma cells derived from them; other reactive lymphocytes that are not producers of antibody are called T cells.[18] The origin of both cell types appears to be in the yolk sac and, later, in the bone marrow. Both are present in the spleen.[15]

Stem cells leave the marrow and enter the thymus. There they continue in a rapid state of cell division. In the mouse, where they have been most carefully studied, thymic lymphocytes can also be subdivided. The majority carry antigenic markers called theta and TL; thymic cells are also distinguishable by their extreme sensitivity to lysis by species-specific antibodies present in normal or immune guinea pig and rabbit serum (xenoantibodies).[10] Cells harvested directly from the thymus have a very feeble immunologic potential. When TL-positive lymphocytes leave the thymus, they lose their TL markers completely. They also become much less sensitive to xenoantibodies, although most if not all of them appear to retain their theta antigen. The loss of TL appears to be absolute, while the loss of xenoantigen is only apparent. It seems likely that additional sialic acid is added to the plasma membrane as the cells leave the thymus, since reactivity for guinea pig serum reappears if the cell is treated with neuraminidase. The second population of thymic lymphocytes do not have TL, are resistant to xenoantibodies, and have a higher H-2 content. These cells are immunologically competent and will produce splenomegaly in the graft versus host assay. Both classes of thymic lymphocytes undergo rapid cell division. Thymocytes leaving the thymus migrate to lymph nodes and spleen and may then recycle through the bloodstream and tissues.[12]

Whether B cells pass through the thymus or pass directly to the lymph nodes has not yet been clarified. They do not have a characteristic marker corresponding to TL, but in later development another antigen, PC, does appear.[47]

T cells, also known as thymus-dependent or thymus-derived cells, are responsible for delayed-type responses.[28, 32] In a typical delayed-type reaction, such as the tuberculin reaction, numbers of mononuclear cells appear in the vicinity of the antigen, where they set up an inflammatory response characterized by induration. Macrophages and other types are also found at the reaction site. The lesion usually takes 24 hours or longer to develop. In its most severe form, central necrosis and caseation of the center of the lesion occur, followed by fibrosis.[7]

Most immunologists would like to believe that T cells carry immunoglobin on their surfaces. This would be logical, since T cells do have specificity and the only known molecule that has specificity for antigen is the immunoglobulin (Ig) molecule. Attempts to demonstrate Ig on T cells have been disappointing. An apparent exception has been reported by Binns and Wigzell, who produced antibody to T rat lymphocytes in F_1 hybrid animals.[9] The antibody produced had specificity for a subpopulation of Lewis rat cells and appeared to be an anti-immunoglobulin. The Binns-Wigzell antibody differs from most antiglobulins in being an anti-idiotype. Anti-idiotype antibodies react against the variable portion of the Ig molecule. Conventional anti-immunoglobulins react against constant portions of the molecule and hence with all Ig molecules of a particular class. These findings represent a major advance in our knowledge of T lymphocytes and, if fully substantiated, will contribute greatly to our knowledge of delayed-type reactions and cellular immunity in general.

In contrast, B cells carry easily identified immunoglobulin heavy and light chains on their surface.[33] This attribute is used to separate the two populations and to distinguish between different subclasses of B cells, i.e., between those producing IgG and those producing IgM or IgA. If lymphocytes are passed through a column of beads coated with anti-immunoglobulin, the B cells are trapped and the T cells pass through. To remove B cells reactive against a specific antigen, the beads are coated with that particular antigen. The immunologic capacity of the passed cells is then assayed. While the majority of B lymphocytes bear Ig molecules on their surface and secrete the same Ig into the medium, there are exceptions. Some cells carry two surface Ig markers but secrete only one class of Ig, while in certain pathologic states, abundant B cells may be present but fail to secrete significant amounts of Ig, giving rise to hypogammaglobulinemia.[42] A few cells, null cells, carry neither B cell nor T cell markers; many of these cells, like many B cells, do have Fc receptors that allow binding to immunoglobulin complexed to antigen.

In the chicken, B cells develop in the bursa of Fabricius. Bursectomy at the time of hatching depletes most of the B cell population and the chick is unable to make antibody in the normal way. The earlier the bursectomy is carried out, the more severe the depression. T cell reactivity remains relatively normal. These chicks will reject skin grafts. There is no known analog of the bursa in mammals; the term B cell, however, can be equated with "bursal cell equivalent." Thymectomy in newborn rodents or newly hatched chicks depletes the host of T cells and results in delayed skin graft rejection. Antibody responses are usually still present though they may also be depressed. Tolerance is readily induced in thymectomized animals, especially if antilymphocyte serum is also given.[23] Adult thymectomy has a much less pronounced effect since many of the T cells already released from the thymus are very long-lived.

For induction of immunity to the great majority of antigens, the participation of T cells is required. This is true both for the induction of delayed responsiveness and for antibody production. Very few substances, such as pneumococcal polysaccharide and coli lipopolysaccharide, can induce an antibody response in the T-cell-depleted animal. The majority of antigens need the intervention of what is called a helper cell.[39] Whether this is a specific form of T cell and what the specificity of helper cells may be have not yet been discovered. The helper T cell appears to have undergone a stage in differentiation which distinguishes it from the more immature thymocyte.[43] It bears certain surface markers called, in the mouse, Ly antigens. The other major class of T cell known at present is the effector T cell, which carries other Ly markers. The T-cell-deficient animal corresponds approximately to the human with DiGeorge syndrome, and B cell deficiency is roughly analogous to Bruton-type agammaglobulinemia.

For a complete immunologic response both T cells and B cells are required.[15] The two systems act in part synergistically and in part antagonistically. The antagonism is of great importance for the control of the level of immunologic responsiveness. If there were no control, the clones of cells responding to an antigen would keep on replicating. An uncontrolled B cell response would in time produce an effect similar to that seen in myeloma.

The synergism and manner in which the immune response matures with time after sensitization have been shown in experiments with a mouse sarcoma, BP8. Lymph node cells harvested three days after immunization and mixed with the tumor did not affect its growth when reimplanted. When harvested five days after immunization, the lymph node cells began to kill the tumor. Their effectiveness reached a peak at about seven days. By 10 days, the effect was beginning to fade and by 14 days the tumoricidal effect was observed only when the lymphoid cell number was greatly increased. When hyperimmune antibody was added to the mixture, the effectiveness of the seven-day node cells was completely abolished; however, when antiserum was added to the 14-day node cells there was a potentiating of the cytotoxic effect. The antibody alone had a slight growth-promoting or -enhancing effect; curiously enough, so did low numbers of the 14-day cells when injected without added antibody.[19]

An example of a slightly different type of cooperation should be mentioned. Under certain circumstances antibody can potentiate the cytotoxic activity of cells from nonimmune hosts. This reactivity has the specificity of the antibody, while the host cell, whether it be polymorphonuclear leukocyte, macrophage, or lymphocyte, appears to exert its effect through the release of enzymes.[2]

That passively administered antibody can curtail further antibody production and control T cell reactivity has been known for many years. Transferred hyperimmune antibody has been found to have great practical application in the prevention of sensitization of Rh-negative mothers of Rh-positive children and in the prevention of graft versus host reactions from transplanted bone marrow.[4, 5] More recently, it has also been found that transferred T cells also have the property of curtailing antibody production.[22] There seems, therefore, good evidence that there is not one immunologic system but two. Each system is largely independent of the other; at times their effects combine and at others they exert a mutual control on each other.

The response to certain stimuli can be clearly regarded as a response of just one of these systems. The response to contact allergens such as dinitrofluorobenzene appears to involve only a T cell response while the response to pneumococcal polysaccharide can be a pure B cell reaction. The response to transplanted organs is compound; cytotoxic antibodies are formed and at the same time antigen-reactive cells infiltrate the graft to produce cytotoxic damage.

The sequence of changes that occurs after transplantation varies greatly, depending upon the site of implantation, the nature of the vascular connections, and the size, lymphoid content, and nature of the graft.

The greatest intensity of immunity is achieved where there is good lymphatic drainage of the graft area. The sequence of changes at the regional nodes has been identified in animals with a variety of antigens but the conclusions reached appear to be generally valid for tissue transplants in man. Antigen travels through lymphatic channels, in solution or trapped inside macrophages. If inside macrophages, it undergoes processing which may involve complexing to a low molecular weight RNA molecule to form what has been called a "super antigen." The antigen-laden macrophages form a cap around the germinal centers in the draining lymph node.[34] Within 24 hours, the node begins to undergo a complete metamorphosis. The orderly columns of small lymphocytes are replaced by masses of primitive-looking blastoid cells. These cells divide to form mature plasma cells and small lymphocytes. Similar changes but without plasma cell formation may also occur in the medullary and paracortical areas. By cannulation of the efferent lymphatic, increased traffic in macrophages, neutrophils, and red cells can be observed within a few hours after exposure to antigen. The afferent lymph is free from macrophages and for some hours after stimulation may be almost devoid of cells entirely. Later, small lymphocytes are found in considerable numbers with few or no macrophages passing through. The antigen-labeled macrophages disappear quite rapidly, probably passing directly into the bloodstream and thence to the liver. Most of the antigen injected appears to pass to the liver where it may sometimes be recovered years later. Nossal and Ada have shown that minute quantities of antigen remain deep within the germinal center apparently attached to the surface of dendritic follicular reticular cells.[34]

The interpretation is that those lymphocytes capable of responding to the specific antigen are stimulated to dedifferentiate into lymphoblasts and to divide in the presence of a suitable form of that antigen. Their progeny may be plasma cells and lymphocytes in a 1:1 ratio in the case of B cells; T cells may also give unlike daughter cells, but the separation is not morphologically apparent. T lymphocytes, as they differentiate, exhibit new cell surface (Ly) markers. Specialized T cells, such as T helper, T suppressor, and T effector cells, carry different Ly antigens.[18, 38] The T cells tend to migrate out from the node while the B cells remain and the plasma cells gradually die off. More than 90 per cent of the cells in the thoracic duct appear to be T cells. However, enough B cells migrate so that the other lymph nodes are seeded with immunocytes (T and B) of the stimulated clones. A secondary immune response tends to involve not only the draining node but nodes from other areas as well.

The importance of lymphatic drainage and events occurring in the node has been proved in many experimental situations in vitro and in vivo. In vitro, it is impossible to induce an immune response with dissociated lymphoid cells from a cesarean-derived piglet and even in conventionalized animals the induction is easier to accomplish in organ culture than with isolated cells. Intimate contact is absolutely necessary. In vivo, the most critical experiments showing the involvement of the lymphatic system are those of Barker and Billingham.[6] Skin pedicles were raised above the surface of the surrounding skin, connected to the circulation only by a single leash of vessels. The vessels always included an artery and a vein; they sometimes included a lymphatic vessel and sometimes did not. When the pedicle was secure, a graft of allogeneic skin was placed on it. If a lymphatic vessel had been left intact, the graft was destroyed normally. If the lymphatic vessel had been ablated, the graft persisted for the life of the pedicle. Most significantly, those grafts surviving where there was no lymphatic were promptly rejected if the animal was given a normal orthotopic, allogeneic graft. Thus the efferent arc of the immune response remained intact. Immune lymphocytes could pass from the artery and destroy the graft but the afferent arc had been interrupted and antigen leaving the graft was not entering the lymphoid system in sufficient concentration to trigger a response. Many other less elegant experiments lead to the same conclusion, including human experiments in which all the lymphatics supplying an extremity were severed whereafter allogeneic grafts survived for longer than anticipated, experiments in which skin grafts were placed on hamster cheek pouch epithelium and were not rejected unless the recipient had been sensitized, and experiments in which the removal of a graft after

24 hours did not in itself prevent sensitization but removal of the graft together with the regional node did stop the induction of immunity. However, in studies of renal allograft rejection in sheep, Pedersen and Morris showed sensitization of lymphocytes within the organ during the first 24 hours after transplantation.[36]

Immunization by the intraperitoneal route is almost as effective as immunization via the skin. This has been shown by injecting allogeneic spleen or tumor cells and measuring antibody levels. This route is probably highly effective because of the high content of macrophages in peritoneal exudate. These cells can pass freely into the lymphatics of the diaphragm. Intravenous injection is also effective, since a considerable proportion of the antigen reaches the spleen. The spleen itself appears to condition lymphocytes, since it has been found that congenitally spleenless mice have a deficient response to certain types of antigen.

The morphologic changes that occur in a transplant have also been well documented. The specificity of rejection was shown in England by Medawar[29] and in Japan, some years earlier, by Shinoi.[44] Rabbits received simultaneously several autografts and several allografts. All the allografts were rejected at the same time, but the autografts were left intact. If a few syngeneic tumor cells are mixed with a large number of allogeneic tumor cells and injected, the allogeneic cells are rejected while the few syngeneic cells escape harm and may even grow more vigorously. The specificity is, however, not absolute and there is wide cross reactivity. If a subject is sensitized by a prior skin graft or the injection of lymphocytes, and then skin grafts from several unrelated donors are placed, they may all undergo accelerated rejection (the so-called second-set response) and some may be even more violently thrown off by what is called the white graft reaction in which the immunity is so strong that the graft never heals.[41]

In first-set skin grafts, healing is complete within a few days and the allograft is indistinguishable from an autograft. By about the sixth day, lymphoid cells begin to appear around the small vessels, which themselves become tortuous and dilated. Large accumulations of mononuclear cells also appear deep in the dermis outside the graft itself. Sludging of blood in the capillaries becomes extreme and thrombosis occurs. Meanwhile, the lymphocytes have spread throughout the graft proper. Rejection is more rapid in a preimmunized recipient. The second graft barely establishes vascular connection before thrombosis and cellular infiltration set in. In the white graft there is no vascular connection and no cellular infiltration but a band of cells, including numerous neutrophils, may form deeper in the dermis. Another histologic picture is given when the rejection is very indolent. Called the blue graft because of its gross appearance when stained with hematoxylin, the graft is seen to be stuffed with lymphocytes with very little evidence of vascular damage. Often the epidermal layer and its appendages may remain intact despite the very heavy infiltration.[16]

Somewhat similar changes occur in other organs. Cuffing of small vessels, breaks in the media of arterioles or small arteries, and narrowing of the lumen with lymphocytic infiltration of the interstitium are common findings in chronically rejecting kidneys. Accumulations of platelets to form thrombi, and the presence of large numbers of neutrophils, are typical of acute or hyperacute rejection.[14]

There is general agreement on most of the statements made so far. The observations themselves appear to be valid, as far as they go. There is, however, controversy over the interpretation of the findings. The majority of investigators believe that rejection of grafts in the previously unsensitized host is almost exclusively a T cell function. This concept can be traced back to Medawar and his colleagues who stressed the similarity between the changes occurring in skin graft rejection and those observed in the tubular reaction. The relevant arguments were summarized by Brent.[11] The principal points were: (1) Antibodies could not be detected in the serum of reactive animals. (2) The cellular infiltration in the tuberculin reaction is roughly comparable to the cellular infiltration at a graft site. (3) Immunity to skin grafts can be readily transferred with cells from draining lymph nodes. (4) Immunity to skin grafts cannot be transferred even with high doses of serum from animals rejecting grafts.

More recent information has caused most of these concepts to be revised.

1. Cytotoxic, agglutinating, and often blocking antibodies can, by the use of more sensitive techniques now available, be demonstrated in the serum of men, dogs, rats, and mice receiving allografts of kidney or skin.[40, 49] These antibodies are often present at relatively low concentrations while the graft is intact. Antibody levels may rise after removal of the graft, and large quantities of antibody can usually be recovered from the graft tissue by acid elution. If care is taken to avoid anticomplementary effects, these antibodies can be shown to lyse fibroblasts, epithelial cells, and sarcoma cells, i.e., cell types formerly thought to be very resistant to lysis by antibody. The role of such lytic antibodies in organ rejection cannot be overlooked.[56]

2. The direct involvement of lymphoid cells in graft rejection is still by no means completely clear. It often appears as if a graft dies from ischemic necrosis following thrombosis of small vessels rather than by a piecemeal attack on the cells of the graft. In chronic rejection, vast numbers of lymphocytes can accumulate but sometimes appear to cause relatively little damage. Undoubtedly, T cells can cause tissue damage. How they do this is unknown, but they are known to release many factors into the surrounding fluid when they are stimulated. Resting lymphocytes are relatively deficient in mitochondria, microsomes, and lysosomes and their Golgi apparatus is not prominent. Upon activation, as for example after exposure to phytohemagglutinin (PHA) or to specific antigen, a sequence of changes occurs. This begins with an increased activity (and probably permeability) of the lymphocyte membrane, and the histones show increased activity of the cell. Lysosomal enzymes show a marked increase within 17 hours and the activated cell secretes products including blastogenic factor (BF), cytotoxic factor (CF), and macrophage migration-inhibiting factor (MIF), which all influence the behavior of other cells.[24] Blastogenic factor can recruit other lymphoid cells into the active state; cytotoxic

factor is, as its name implies, lytic for other cells; macrophage-inhibiting factor exerts its effect to reduce the mobility of macrophages. None of these factors has any specificity, nor do the T cells have any appreciable quantities of conventional antibody on their surface. That they do have specificity, however, is indicated by experiments in which specific tolerance was initiated in T cells as well as by many experiments in which T lymphocytes immunized against tumor cells from one mouse strain could kill other tumor cells from the immunizing strain but had little or no cytotoxic effect on tumor cells from a third party. Graft rejection in vivo is a dynamic process; by histologic studies it is possible to study only those cells present at the moment of fixation. Lymphocyte activation followed by dissolution of the active cell would not be detected by this means and there are some grounds for supposing that activated lymphocytes are destroyed on contact with their target in the so-called "allergic death" phenomenon. Alternatively, the proportion of actual killer cells may be quite small. In many experiments, 20 to 100 lymphoid cells were needed to destroy one target cell. However, if there is a selective retention of specific killer cells in a graft such that one killer cell could successively damage a series of targets, there would be little histologic evidence of infiltration. There is evidence to support this view.[8]

3. Adoptive transfer of immunity with lymphoid cells has been accomplished by many investigators. However, most of the studies have been with the transfer of both T and B cells under conditions in which the B cells could immediately initiate antibody production. The most efficient transfer occurs when cells from a draining lymph node are intimately mixed with the target cell, usually a tumor suspension.[55] Ten times as many cells are required if injected at a site remote from the target. Interesting observations on the effectiveness of lymphoid cells have also been made by the use of diffusion chambers. A diffusion chamber is a small plastic cylinder closed at each end by a membrane with a pore size large enough to allow the free passage of proteins but small enough to prevent the passage of cells. Target tissues, tumor, or fragments of embryonic tissue placed in such chambers are rapidly destroyed if immune lymphocytes are included inside the chamber.[52] So are the immune lymphocytes. Experiments to show that antibody could produce the same effect were at first unsuccessful. Later studies using tumor cells as a target showed that antibody could be lytic under the same conditions provided that the concentration reached was sufficiently high, and that complement was available.[3]

4. Passive transfer of immunity has not been very successful in destroying a graft. However, if the vascular permeability of the graft is artificially increased, antibody is effective.

Many of the experiments to show the actual cause of graft rejection are then inconclusive or counterbalanced by other experiments to show an opposite effect. To further illustrate this dilemma, consider the simplest in vivo system that can be devised, namely the rejection of ascites tumor cells by allogeneic mice. The free-cell suspension is injected into the peritoneal cavity and samples can be aspirated every day. With some tumors, massive phagocytosis by macrophages

can account for their removal. Other tumors cannot be phagocytosed. These macrophage-resistant tumors grow exponentially for a number of days and then suddenly regress. They do not appear to be sensitized by antibody, since they are not lysed when excess complement is added, but there is also no cytotoxic activity of the supernatant for other cells and there is no sudden influx of host cells before rejection occurs. One possible explanation was given by Prioleau and his colleagues, who recorded marked changes in lysosomal activity in tumor cells in contact with macrophages.[37] These experiments opened up the possibility that one of the attributes of the host defense system was to overactivate certain metabolic pathways of the target cell, thus leading to autolysis.

Critical examination of the lymphoid cells present in the ascites reveals that these cells are extremely active in tumor destruction. The cell involved is not adherent to nylon or plastic and has a very great specific reactivity for tumor cells.[8] The cytotoxic effector cells were found to be small to medium-sized lymphocytes which were not actively dividing. These cells, which carry T cell markers but also react with antibody to B cells,[46a] first bind to the target via receptors which are not immunoglobulin in nature. This process requires the participation of divalent Mg and Ca ions and lasts for about six minutes.[8] Within this time certain irreversible changes occur in the target, which then proceeds to die. The lymphocyte is released and can proceed to kill again. A variety of agents, including drugs which affect microtubular and microfilamentous structures, metabolic inhibitors, and antibodies to cell surface antigens, can inhibit binding of the cytolytic reaction. Thus, while we do not know exactly how the activated lymphocyte kills its target, the processes are becoming very sharply defined, and this knowledge is proving very useful in developing new agents for suppressing effector cell activity. It is interesting that all cells are not equally susceptible to lysis by cytotoxic cells. Some tumor cells are highly sensitive; others are very resistant. Fibroblasts are intermediate. The part played in vivo in the control of tumors is not known, but because similar cells can be recovered from rejected transplants, it appears that cytotoxic effector cells are strongly implicated in transplant rejection.

Thrombosis, cytolysis by antibody and complement, and autolysis by exogenous enzymes released from activated lymphocytes and macrophages or by sabotage from within all are possible mechanisms whereby target tissues are destroyed. At present, it appears that the process of organ graft destruction involves the cooperation of T cells, B cells, and probably other wandering cells including macrophages, neutrophils, and mast cells. The extent to which each component is utilized will depend upon the particular circumstance. Early in the response, T cell function would seem to predominate. In the first few days, antibody titers are very low. The affinity of early antibody is also low but this may be an advantage, as the antibody molecules can then dissociate from the target quite easily and attach to another cell. T cells leave the node after the fifth day and can produce their various factors in the vicinity of the target. One side effect of this is to increase vascular permeability and to allow more white cells and considerably more antibody and complement to enter the reaction area. In secondary responses, there is general agreement that circulating antibody plays a much more dominant role.[2]

A possible sequence of events in a first-set reaction is: Following the arrival of antigen at the lymph node, antibody production is initiated. Some of the antibody is released into the circulation. The levels in the serum and in the tissue spaces gradually build up but usually do not reach a high level. Absorption onto the graft and to a lesser extent adsorption to host cells also tend to keep the level of free antibody low. Immunization is not achieved if antigen is unable to reach the lymph nodes in an effective form and in adequate concentration.

Lymphoid cells—possibly elaborating, possibly transporting antibody—appear in the graft area together with polymorphonuclear cells and macrophages. The proportion of each depends upon the nature of the tissue grafted. Cells other than lymphocytes, even red cells, passively transport small amounts of antibody from the circulation. Much of this antibody diffuses off into the tissue fluid, but the "immune" cells have an affinity for antigen, probably from residual surface antibody. This cell-bound antibody acts as an attractive force holding host and target cell together. Other lymphocytes can attack the target in the absence of antibody. When any of the cells involved in the homograft reaction lyse, intracellular enzymes and (in the case of host cells) any antibody contained within the cell will be released. Many of the known lysosomal enzymes are cathepsins or soluble trypsin-like proteases. These enzymes are especially proteolytic for even mildly denatured proteins. The cells effectively attacked are therefore those on which an antibody-antigen reaction has occurred in the presence of complement. The surfaces of graft cells that have been sensitized by antibody are accordingly further damaged and disintegrate. During disintegration, their quota of intracellular enzymes is released. They also release small particles of antigen and soluble factors. This leads to the activation of macrophages and the stimulation of additional effector lymphocytes.

The reaction will be accelerated by the concentration of host cells. In this connection, the immobilization of macrophages and possibly of lymphocytes by MIF may be very important. The reaction may be accelerated or hindered by the presence of humoral antibody. Excess antibody will neutralize antigenic particles released from lysed graft cells and so prevent their reacting on the surface of remote host cells. The reaction will be damped down by antienzymes, by lack of complement, and by the presence of blocking antibodies.

The attraction of such a general theory is that it is independent of the nature of the host cell involved; it applies to macrophages as well as to plasma cells or lymphocytes. The graft cell will be attacked even though it is relatively insensitive to the lytic action of antibody. High concentrations of antibody are not needed. The reaction needs the presence of immune cells, antibody, and complement and so will be hampered in states or sites where any of these are lacking. The reaction does not depend upon vascular changes, although such changes may result from the reaction,

and indeed graft destruction can proceed perfectly well in the diffusion chamber where there is no question of vascular intervention.

Conceding, then, that the reaction of a host against a graft is a very complex one in which many factors are involved, each participating to an extent determined by the particular circumstances of the graft-host relationship, what steps can be taken to prevent rejection? These may be divided into three main categories: (1) nonspecific depressants of the immune response; (2) the induction of specific tolerance; and (3) intervention by blocking or enhancing antibodies.[1]

The nonspecific agents are well known. They include the various immunosuppressive or antibiotic drugs of which azathioprine, cyclophosphamide, and actinomycin D have been used most successfully. Although highly effective at preventing graft rejection, because these agents are nonselective they also depress immunity against microbial invaders. The transplant recipient is then very susceptible to infection and may also suffer from toxic side effects of the agents. Most of these drugs hinder cell replication and, although cell division is not absolutely essential for an immune reaction to occur, augmentation of immunity follows an increase in the number of reactive cells, thus magnifying their effect. The mode of action of the steroids in immunity is not thoroughly known. To some extent they may cause a reduction in the absolute number of lymphocytes, but their more important function seems to be to stabilize lysosomal membranes. It is now well established that lymphocytes secrete a variety of active compounds into the surrounding fluid; it is also presumed that many of the factors are proteolytic enzymes, so that stabilization of lysosomal membranes would tend to impair the release of such enzymes. If the concept that autolysis of graft cells can also be induced by substances released by host cells is correct, then cortisone should help to protect the graft from autolytic damage.

The other nonselective or partially selective agent widely used is antilymphocyte serum (ALS) and again its mode of action is not clear. ALS is usually produced in rabbits or horses against lymph node cells, thoracic duct cells, or lymphoid cell lines grown in culture.[48] Antithymus serum, ATS, is also widely used and may be somewhat more effective than ALS. There is evidence that ATS contains a small proportion of thymus-specific antibodies. These antibodies are presumed to have their greatest effect on the T cells, possibly by combining with specific receptor sites. ATS and ALS are cytotoxic for lymphocytes, but do not depend upon lympholysis for their effect. IgM antibodies, although highly cytotoxic in vitro, have little immunosuppressive effect, and many IgG antibodies with cytotoxic titers are also ineffective. ALS will induce blast transformation and inhibit macrophage or lymphocyte migration. It will also block the capacity of lymphocytes to form rosettes with red cells, presumably by interfering with the effectiveness of immunoglobulins on the cell membrane. The theory that it coated and thus blindfolded the surface of the lymphocytes has been discarded and it is generally thought that ALS produces a central inhibition. It is a most intriguing agent, exerting its greatest effect in the thymectomized host. Thymectomized, ALS treated mice can accept a rat or even a human skin graft for considerable periods. Mice treated in this way can also be rendered tolerant easily.[23]

Tolerance was originally used with reference to mice that had received an injection of live spleen cells from an allogeneic donor at birth. When these animals grew up, they would accept a skin graft from a mouse of the same strain as the spleen donor but not from one of an indifferent strain. They were later found to carry lymphoid cells from the donor strain and were thus also called chimeras. Elegant studies in rats have recapitulated in brief many years of studies in mice.[46] A phenomenon related to tolerance, antigen overload, has been known for many years. Mice treated with large doses of pneumococcus polysaccharide retain the polysaccharide in their circulation and fail to make antibodies against it. A third term, immunologic unresponsiveness, has been applied to the nonreactive state that follows the injection of a variety of soluble antigens, including serum albumin and disaggregated gamma globulin.[53] The three terms, tolerance, antigen overload, and unresponsiveness, are roughly synonymous.

Tolerance to soluble proteins can be achieved by injecting rather large or very small amounts of antigen.[54] In the intermediate range, immunity rather than tolerance may result. Tolerance is very difficult to induce with aggregates and so far it has been found difficult to induce it with soluble preparations of histocompatibility antigens. One of the problems is that the complete histocompatibility antigen molecule has a hydrophilic region which is inserted into the membrane and which makes it impossible to retain in soluble form in aqueous solution.[45] This may be one reason why the results have been disappointing. Another reason is that a skin graft is usually used for testing for tolerance. Skin of the mouse carries at least one potent antigen that is apparently tissue-specific, and for this reason it may prove easier to induce tolerance to solid organ grafts, which may lack such an antigen, than to skin. However, it remains a sad fact that the induction of tolerance to soluble preparations of transplantation antigen has not yet been found a practicable means of preventing graft rejection.

In contrast, enhancement, the Cinderella sister of tolerance, has already found successful clinical application. In the earlier part of this chapter, the concept that one part of the immunologic system helped in the control of the other was repeatedly emphasized. One further attribute of this regulatory system was not mentioned and is of especial relevance to enhancement. This is that high-avidity antibodies selectively suppress the formation of lower-avidity antibodies. The potential of enhancing antibody was first discovered by Kaliss and his colleagues, who were able to facilitate the growth of an incompatible tumor by pretreating the host with immune serum. It was later found that the enhancing effect developed only some weeks after immunization and also that minute quantities of antibody were effective.[21]

Just as there are low- and high-dose zones in tolerance, so there appear to be low- and high-dose zones in enhancement. High-dose tolerance (HDT) and high-dose enhancement (HDE) can be easily distinguished. There is no detectable antibody in HDT, and even

when it is possible to induce an antibody response by the injection of a cross-reactive antigen, the antibody is of very low affinity. The affinity of HDE antibody, by contrast, is high. The distinction between low-dose tolerance (LDT) and low-dose enhancement (LDE) may be very difficult. Small quantities of antibodies are now being detected in the form of complexes in a number of conditions once thought of as typical of tolerance. These include antinuclear antibodies and antithyroid antibodies in man, and antibodies to lymphocytic choriomeningitis or mammary tumor virus in the mouse. All of these were thought to be examples of natural tolerance, or of acquired tolerance to viruses passed on by the mother in uterine or neonatal life. Blocking or enhancing antibodies are now being found in chimeras, in animals and humans with cancer, and in dogs receiving kidney or bone marrow grafts, and a new phenomenon, that of autoenhancement, appears to be relatively commonplace. The deliberate induction of enhancement is practiced in the prevention of Rh sensitization, and has been used in kidney transplantation in rats and also in man by several investigators, and in human bone marrow transplants by Buckley et al.[13] Lucas has shown autoenhancement in rat kidney transplantation.[26] One of the recipient's kidneys was left in place at the time of transplantation. The transplanted kidney showed evidence of rejection after a few days but then recovered. The remaining autologous kidney was then removed and the transplant could support life in the absence of any immunosuppressive treatment of any kind.

Not enough is yet known about the specificity of enhancement to make it of immediately practicable clinical value. All hyperimmune sera appear to have enhancing capability and it is fairly clear that the blocking antibodies are not the same as the cytotoxic antibodies found in anti-HLA antisera. Some noncytotoxic sera can block lymphocyte reactivity when introduced into a mixed lymphocyte culture (MLC). Preliminary studies on the blocking of MLC responses between unrelated individuals suggest that the specificity is different from that of HLA, although it is known that the major locus is involved. This is one of the reasons for the suggestion made in a previous section that HLA, MLR-S, and HDR are three distinct loci, closely linked but subserving different functions. Selective immunosuppressive regimens to encourage the development of enhancing antibodies to the various components of the major histocompatibility complex and the deliberate production of high-titered immune sera for use in kidney and heart transplants are two real possibilities that would revolutionize the practice of clinical transplantation. Absorption of hyperimmune antisera by platelets removes antibody against HLA or H-2 antigens but leaves blocking activity intact. This suggests that blocking is against the components of the complex, such as Ia or B cell antigens.

In conclusion, it must be stressed that the immune response is the result of complex interactions between balanced systems typified by the T and the B cell systems.[30, 31] Disturbances of one or loss of equilibrium of one is likely to affect the balance of the other. The clinician, through an instinctive appreciation of his patient, can exert a very fine control over the immune system by his selective use of immunosuppressive drugs. The immunologist has the responsibility of learning how to selectively control the immune response so that only reactivity against the transplant is lost, and the pharmacologist could contribute information about the control of segments of immune response by drugs having specific activity against cells in the different phases of the immune response. These projected developments would provide two-edged information—that needed for the control of immunity to transplants, and the mirror image, that necessary for the induction of immunity to cancer.

SELECTED REFERENCES

Dausset, J. (Ed.): Histocompatibility Testing 1972. Copenhagen, Munksgaard, 1973.

Very different in scope from all previous Histocompatibility Testing volumes, this monograph is devoted to an analysis of the leukocyte antigens of more than 30 populations, many of them aboriginal. Besides giving a fascinating new aspect of anthropology, the data give interesting insights into the nature of leukocyte antigens in contrasting populations.

Lengerova, A., and Vojtiskova, M. (Eds.): Immunogenetics of the H-2 System. Basel, S. Karger, 1971.

This work presents data on the H-2 antigens of different strains and of other properties controlled by the same linkage group, and includes chapters on genetics of H-2 and cell interactions, on the chemistry of antigens on different cell types including spermatozoa, and on comparisons between different antigens.

Nathenson, S.: Biochemical properties of histocompatibility antigens. Ann. Rev. Genet., 4:69, 1970.

This comprehensive review deals with the general properties of cell-surface antigens with special reference to H-2 in the mouse. Included are descriptions of the location and subcellular distribution, biochemical properties, methods of solublization, and the characterization of subunits.

Terasaki, P. I. (Ed.): Histocompatibility Testing 1970. Copenhagen, Munksgaard, 1970.

Original papers on leukocyte genetics, serology of leukocyte antigens, chemical characterization of antigens, histocompatibility, maternal-fetal incompatibility, and mixed leukocyte culture and methodology, together with a joint report on the results of the Fourth International Histocompatibility Workshop. An extremely valuable reference book. This is the third in a series; earlier volumes with similar titles appeared in 1965 and 1967.

Journals largely devoted to studies of tissue and leukocyte antigens: Transplantation Proceedings, Tissue Antigens, Transplantation Reviews, and Cellular Immunology.

REFERENCES

1. Amos, D. B. (Ed.): Progress in Immunology. New York, Academic Press, 1971.
2. Amos, D. B.: The use of simplified systems as an aid to the interpretation of mechanisms of graft rejection. Progr. Allerg., 6:468, 1962.
3. Amos, D. B., and Wakefield, J. D.: Growth of mouse ascites tumor cells in diffusion chambers. II. Lysis and growth inhibition by diffusible isoantibody. J. Natl. Cancer Inst., 22:1077, 1959.
4. Bach, F. H., and Good, R. A. (Eds.): Clinical Immunobiology. Vol. I. New York, Academic Press, 1972.
5. Bach, F. H., and Good, R. A. (Eds.): Clinical Immunobiology. Vol. II. New York, Academic Press, 1974.
6. Barker, C. F., and Billingham, R. E.: The role of regional lymphatics in the skin homograft response. Transplantation, 5:962, 1967.
7. Bellanti, J. A., and Dayton, D. H. (Eds.): The Phagocytic Cell in Host Resistance. New York, Raven Press, 1975.
8. Berke, G., and Amos, D. B.: Mechanism of lymphocyte-mediated cytolysis. The LMC cycle and its role in transplantation immunity. Transplant. Rev., 17:71, 1973.
9. Binz, H., and Wigzell, H.: Shared idiotype determinants on B and T lymphocytes reactive against the same antigenic determinant. J. Exp. Med., 142:197, 1975.
10. Boyse, E. A., In Smith, R. T., and Landy, M.: Immune Surveillance. New York, Academic Press, 1970. p. 5.
11. Brent, L.: Tissue transplantation immunity. Progr. Allerg., 5:271, 1955.
12. Brent, L., and Holborow, J. (Eds): Progress in Immunology II. Vols. 2-5. New York, American Elsevier, 1974.
13. Buckley, R. H., Amos, D. B., Kremer, W. B., and Stickel, D. L.: Incompatible bone-marrow transplantation in lymphopenic immunologic deficiency. N. Engl. J. Med., 285:1035, 1971.
14. Busch, G. J., Braun, W. E., Carpenter, C. B., Corson, J. M., Galvanek, E. R., Reynolds, E. S., Merrill, J. P., and Dammin, G. J.: Intravascular coagulation (IVC) in human renal allograft rejection. Transplant. Proc., 1:267, 1970.
15. Cerottini, J. C., Nordin, A. A., and Brunner, K. T.: Cellular and humoral response to transplantation antigens. J. Exp. Med., 134:553, 1971.
16. Eichwald, E. J., Wetzel, B., and Lustgraff, E. C.: Genetic aspects of second set skin grafts in mice. Transplantation, 4:260, 1966.
17. Good, R. A., and Fisher, D. W.: Immunobiology. Stamford, Conn. Sinauer Associates, 1971.
18. Greaves, M. F., Owen, J. J. T., and Raff, M. C.: T and B Lymphocytes: Origins, Properties, and Roles in Immune Responses. New York, Academic Press, 1973.
19. Hutchin, P., Amos, D. B., and Prioleau, W. H.: Interactions of humoral antibodies and immune lymphocytes. Transplantation, 5:68, 1967.
20. Jerne, N.: The somatic generation of immune recognition. Eur. J. Immunol., 1:1, 1971.
21. Kaliss, N.: Dynamics of immunologic enhancement. Transplant. Proc., 2:59, 1970.
22. Katz, D. R., and Benacerraf, B.: The regulatory influence of activated T cell or B cell responses to antigen. Adv. Immunol., 15:2, 1972.
23. Lance, E. M., and Medawar, P. B.: Antilymphocyte serum: Its properties and potential. In Immunobiology. Stamford, Conn., Sinauer Associates, 1948, p. 248.
24. Lawrence, H. S., and Landy, M. (Eds.): Mediators of Cellular Immunity. New York, Academic Press, 1969.
25. Lindahl-Kiessling, K., and Osoka, D.: Lymphocyte Recognition and Effector Mechanisms. Proceedings of the Eighth Leukocyte Culture Conference. New York, Academic Press, 1974.
26. Lucas, Z. J., Markley, J., and Travis, M.: Immunologic enhancement of renal allografts in the rat. Fed. Proc., 29:2041, 1970.
27. Marshall, W. H., Valentine, F. T., and Lawrence, H. S.: Cellular immunity in vitro. J. Exp. Med., 130:327, 1969.
28. McClusky, R. T., and Cohen, S. (Eds.): Mechanism of Cell-Mediated Immunity. New York, John Wiley & Sons, Inc., 1974.
29. Medawar, P. B.: The behavior and fate of skin autografts and skin homografts in rabbits. J. Anat., 78:176, 1944.
30. Möller, G. (Ed.): Interaction between humoral antibodies and cell-mediated immunity. Transplant. Rev., 13:1-141, 1972.
31. Möller, G. (Ed.): T and B lymphocytes in humans. Transplant. Rev., 16:1-217, 1974.
32. Möller, G. (Ed.): Components of immune recognition: Detection and analysis. Transplant. Rev., 18:1-191, 1974.
33. Möller, G. (Ed.): Concepts of B lymphocyte activation. Transplant. Rev., 23:1-268, 1975.
34. Nossal, G. J. V., and Ada, G. L.: Antigens, Lymphoid Cells and the Immune Response. New York, Academic Press, 1971.
35. Nossal, G. J. V., and Ada, G. L.: Antigens, Lymphoid Cells and the Immune Response. New York, Academic Press, 1971.
36. Pederson, N. C., and Morris, B.: The role of the lymphatic system in the rejection of homografts. J. Exp. Med., 131:936, 1970.
37. Prioleau, W. H., Hutchin, P., and Amos, D. B.: Histochemical changes during rejection of C3H ascites tumor BP8 in C57BL mice. Cancer Res., 28:228, 1968.
38. Raff, M. C.: Cell surface immunology. Sci. Am., 5:30, 1976.
39. Rajewsky, K., and Pohlit, H.: Specificity of helper function. Progr. Immunol., 1:337, 1971.
40. Ramseier, H., and Lindermann, J.: Cellular receptors. Effect of alloantibodies on the recognition of transplantation antigens. J. Exp. Med., 134:1083, 1972.
41. Rapaport, F. T., Thomas, L., Converse, J. M., and Lawrence, H. S.: The specificity of skin homograft rejection in man. Ann. N. Y. Acad. Sci., 87:217, 1960.

42. Samter, M. (Ed.): Immunological Diseases, 3rd ed. Vols. I & II. Boston, Little, Brown and Company, 1976.

43. Sercarz, E. E., Williamson, A. R., and Fox, C. (Eds.): The Immune System: Genes, Receptors, Signals. New York, Academic Press, 1974.

44. Shinoi, K.: Study of skin homotransplantation. Tokyo J. Med. Sci., 46:39, 1932.

45. Shreffler, D. C., and David, C. S.: The H-2 major histocompatibility complex and the I immune response region: Genetic variation, function and organization. Adv. Immunol., 20:125, 1975.

46. Silvers, W. K., and Billingham, E. E.: Contributions of the rat to the immunobiology of tissue transplantation. Transplant. Proc., 2:152, 1970.

46a. Sullivan, K. A.: A bone marrow surface antigen shared by immune peritoneal exudate cells. Fed. Proc., 35:754, 1976.

47. Takahaski, T., Old, L. J., and Boyse, E. A.: Surface alloantigens of plasma cells. J. Exp. Med., 131:1325, 1970.

48. Taub, R. N.: Biological effects of heterologous antilymphocyte serum. Progr. Allerg., 14:208, 1970.

49. Tom, B. H., Huang, L. O., Jakstys, M. M., and Kahan, B. D.: Characteristics of the leukocyte-aggregation assay for cell-mediated immunity. Clin. Exp. Immunol., 20:131, 1975.

50. Triplett, E. L.: On the mechanism of immunologic self-recognition. J. Immunol., 89:505, 1962.

51. Unanue, E. R.: The regulatory role of macrophages in antigenic stimulation. Adv. Immunol., 15:95, 1972.

52. Weaver, J. M., Algire, G. H., and Prehn, R. T.: The growth of cells in vivo in diffusion chambers. II. The role of cells in the destruction of homografts in mice. J. Natl. Cancer Inst., 15:1737, 1955.

53. Weigle, W. O.: Immunobiological unresponsiveness. Adv. Immunol., 16:61, 1973.

54. Weigle, W. O., Chiller, J. M., and Habicht, G. S.: Immunological unresponsiveness, cellular kinetics and interactions. Progr. Immunol., 1:311, 1971.

55. Winn, H. J.: Immune mechanisms in homotransplantation. J. Immunol., 68:228, 1961.

56. Winn, H. J.: Humoral antibody in allograft rejections. Transplant. Proc., 2:83, 1970.

23

IMMUNOBIOLOGY OF NEOPLASTIC DISEASE; MELANOMA; SOFT TISSUE SARCOMAS

I

IMMUNOBIOLOGY AND IMMUNOTHERAPY OF NEOPLASTIC DISEASE*

Donald L. Morton, M.D., and Samuel A. Wells, Jr., M.D.

Cancer is a disease caused by the insidious progressive growth of abnormal cells. It spares no organ system, age group, or socioeconomic class, although these factors determine to some degree the way in which it is expressed. It will attack an estimated 50 million of the 200 million Americans currently alive, and with present methods of treatment 34 million of its victims will die of their disease. Thus, only one of every three cancer patients can be cured by single modality therapy, usually through surgical treatment or, less commonly, by radiotherapy or chemotherapy. Fortunately, recent developments in multimodality therapy for cancer appear to be significantly increasing the tumor-free survival of cancer patients, and are providing hope for the eventual control of this disease.[62] The most exciting improvements in cancer therapy have come from the use of combinations of surgery and adjuvant pre- and postoperative chemotherapy or immunotherapy for the solid neoplasms that had formerly been treated by operation alone, such as malignant melanoma, skeletal and soft tissue sarcomas, and breast cancer. These advances in therapy associated with recent developments in the basic biology of the neoplastic process have stimulated research

in the basic problems posed by cancer. The Conquest of Cancer program established by the United States Government in 1971 has furnished the impetus and guidelines for these studies. As a result, we can expect more progress in cancer therapy during the next decade than at any time in medical history.

Tumor immunology and immunotherapy are but one of the exciting new areas in cancer research. An example of the rapid progress in this field is perhaps best illustrated in Figure 1, which shows the increasing number of publications in tumor immunology from 1965 to 1975. Progress in this field is so rapid that reviews such as this are often outdated by the time they appear in print. This section is designed to introduce the student to the general principles of tumor immunology and immunotherapy and to provide a background for understanding future developments in this expanding field.

The concept that a neoplasm creates in its host an immune response similar to that of infectious diseases is not new. This was first suggested during the early 1900's by workers using random-bred laboratory animals. Strong immunity could be induced against transplantable rodent neoplasms. There followed a period of intense laboratory and clinical investigation in tumor immunology in the anticipation that these observations would subsequently lead to the control of malignant disease. However, it soon became evident that this immunity against tumors was not directed

*This investigation was supported by grants from the National Cancer Institute (DHEW) CA12582, CA12285, CA05262, and Medical Research Services, Veterans Administration.

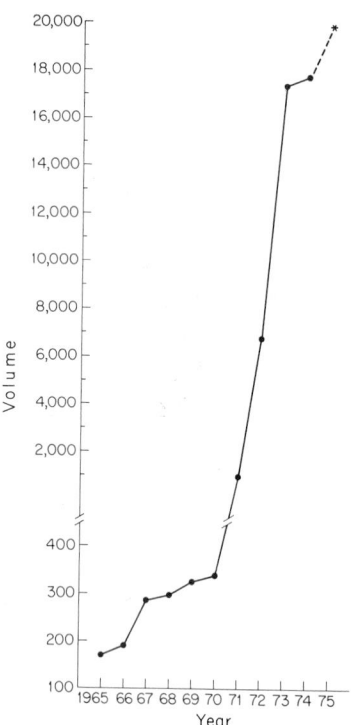

Figure 1. Increased incidence of literature about tumor immunology and immunotherapy by year (MEDLARS, Natl. Libr. Med.). (Broken line indicates hypothetical increase because actual figures were not available at time of printing.)

against tumor-specific antigens, but against normal histocompatibility antigens carried in the tumor cells. This fact was established by inducing similar immunity by immunization with normal tissues from the tumor donor. Thus, this tumor immunity was, in reality, homograft immunity directed against normal tissue antigens in the tumor due to genetic differences between the tumor donor and recipients.

Thereafter, interest in cancer immunology rapidly declined. During the long "dark ages" that followed, most immunologists and experimental oncologists even doubted the existence of the tumor-specific antigens that were to form the very foundation of this discipline of cancer research. However, interest was finally reawakened by the work of Foley in 1953[20] and of Prehn and Main in 1957.[87]

These investigators conclusively demonstrated tumor-specific antigens in methylcholanthrene-induced sarcomas of mice. Their work was aided by the development of inbred strains of laboratory rodents which, through many years of inbreeding, had reached the genetic homogeneity of monozygotic twins. In these animals, grafts of normal tissues were permanently accepted when transplanted between members of the same inbred strain. The search for tumor-specific immunity could now be carried out in an environment free of histoincompatibility due to genetic differences between the animals used in the tumor transplantation studies. It was this important advance in

immunogenetics, coupled with the use of techniques derived from transplantation biology, that paved the way for the first successful demonstration of *tumor-specific transplantation antigens* (TSTA).

Using inbred animals, researchers found that tumor-specific transplantation resistance could be induced by presensitization with a transplant of tumor tissue that was allowed to grow for a time and then excised (Fig. 2). The resultant tumor immunity developed by the animals was relative, not absolute. A challenge inoculation of 100,000 to 1 million tumor cells met with rejection, while 10 million or 100 million cells overwhelmed the immunologic defense and progressed to tumor formation. This set of circumstances was significantly different from the immunity developed against the histocompatibility antigens in which the immune recipient usually rejected any number of histoincompatible tumor cells. In this regard, histocompatibility antigens were considered to be strong antigens and tumor-specific transplantation antigens much weaker.

The next major discovery in tumor immunology was the finding that certain oncogenic DNA viruses (polyoma, SV-40, and adenovirus) produced tumor-containing common transplantation antigens. This common component rendered the viral-induced tumors susceptible to rejection in immunized animals.[76]

During the past decade, tremendous progress has been made in cancer immunology. Cancer-specific antigens have been demonstrated in almost every adequately studied viral- or chemical carcinogen-induced neoplasm, as well as in certain spontaneous tumors of laboratory rodents. These tumor-specific antigens, initially established by tumor transplantation experiments, have now been demonstrated by a variety of classic immunologic techniques, including complement fixation, gel diffusion, immune cytolysis, and immunofluorescence reactions. Thus has cancer immunology emerged as a new discipline, the conception of which resulted from the union of immunogenetics and tissue transplantation immunity. Its development

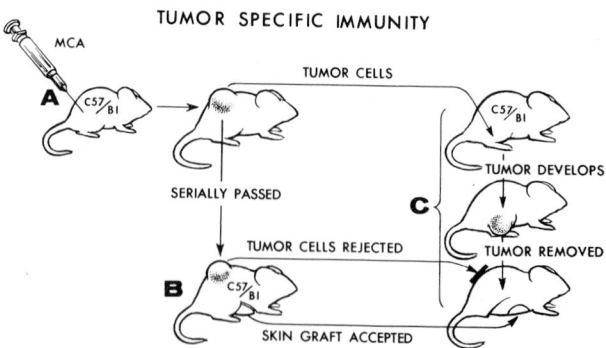

Figure 2. Tumor induced in mouse *A* with methylcholanthrene is serially passed in inbred mice of the same strain (*B*). Mouse *C* develops tumor-specific immunity following resection of a progressively growing neoplasm as demonstrated by the rejection of tumor cell challenge but acceptance of a normal skin graft from the tumor donor.

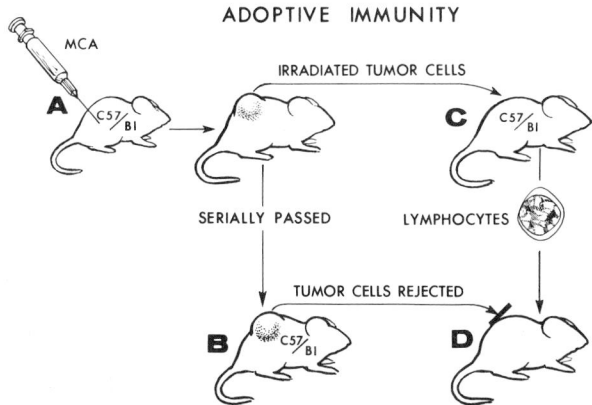

Figure 3. Tumor induced in a mouse A with methylcholanthrene is serially passed in inbred mice of the same strain (B). Mouse C is immunized with injections of nonproliferating x-irradiated tumor cells. Immune lymphocytes transferred from mouse C to mouse D confer specific immunity to subsequent tumor challenge.

has been nurtured by knowledge and techniques borrowed from the fields of classic immunology and viral oncology.

TUMOR-SPECIFIC IMMUNE MECHANISMS

The mediation of the rejection response against tumor cells is comparable to rejection of normal tissues transplanted to a histoincompatible recipient. Important in this regard is the well-established fact that sensitized lymphoid cells seem to exert a more efficient inhibitory effect on tumor cells than do humoral antibodies. This is shown by the phenomenon of adoptive immunity (Fig. 3), in which a normal animal receiving lymphocytes from a tumor-immune donor acquires resistance to tumor cell challenge.[77]

Although the exact mechanism by which immune lymphocytes destroy target cells is unknown, it is essential that close contact occur. The lymphocytes may act by secreting humoral antibody or by producing a special class of antibody which is bound to their surface. After attachment to the antigenic site on the cell surface, the lymphocytes may secrete a toxic factor (lymphotoxin) that causes a nonspecific lytic effect on the cell membrane, resulting in cell death. Contact must be established between the lymphocyte and tumor cell either by a special antibody that is bound to the lymphocyte surface or via a lymphocyte surface antigen-specific receptor. It has been shown that not only sensitized lymphoid cells, but immune peritoneal macrophages as well, are fully competent to destroy target cells in tissue culture or in vivo.

Recently, Pilch and Ramming[84] were able to transfer specific antitumor immunoreactivity to previously nonimmune mouse lymphoid cells by incubating them with RNA extracted from the lymphoid organs of guinea pigs immunized with a mouse tumor. Such procedures have great potential for increasing the effectiveness of the immune response to weakly antigenic tumors.

The ability of humoral antibodies to inhibit tumor growth varies with different cell types. Leukemias and lymphomas are most sensitive to cytotoxic antibodies, but inhibition of solid neoplasms by special classes of antibody also has been observed. There is a correlation between the sensitivity of a tumor to cytotoxic antibodies in vitro and its response to antibodies in vivo. It is clear that antigen density on the tumor cell surface influences the cytotoxic sensitivity. Cells with a higher concentration of surface antigen receptors are more sensitive to antibody lysis than cells with low concentrations of surface antigens. When there are few antigen receptor sites on the cell surface and, consequently, a greater distance between them, it becomes increasingly difficult for antibody and complement to become fixed and to disrupt the cell membrane to produce cell lysis.

Immunity is conferred with difficulty by the passive transfer of humoral antibody. Usually, it must be given prior to or immediately after tumor transplantation and is ineffective or weakly potent if injected several days later. The passive transfer of serum antibody sometimes can result in enhanced tumor growth, rather than the desired rejection, owing to afferent inhibition of the immune response by antibody complexing with antigens on the tumor cell surface, or other unknown mechanisms.[36, 48]

Although thymus-derived lymphocytes are assumed to be the main effector cells for tumor immunity, a recent demonstration in several systems showed that a thymus-independent cell was also involved in cytotoxic reactions. DeVries[10] found that most in vitro cytotoxicity in melanoma was due to non-T cells, and O'Toole[81] demonstrated that thymus-independent cells are necessary for cell-mediated immunity in human bladder cancer cytotoxicity assays. Some evidence for the participation of thymus-derived lymphocytes in tumor cytotoxicity has been reported in human leukemias and in animal tumor systems. Although it is likely that B-lymphocytes play a role in some systems, there is at present no evidence that this effector cell was a B-lymphocyte in the human systems.

The nature of the thymus-independent cell involved in tumor cytotoxicity reactions is unknown, but many believe it may be a K or killer cell, a special population of lymphoid cells that can mediate a cytotoxic event once armed by specific antibody against the target cells. This antibody-dependent cellular cytotoxicity (ADCC) also has been described as lymphocyte-dependent antibody (LDA),[31] arming,[103] and potentiation,[36] as well as K-cell cytotoxicity. Briefly summarized, this phenomenon consists of a cytotoxic event mediated by a nonimmune effector cell in the presence of antibodies specific for the target cells. The cell able to mediate ADCC (the K or killer cell) is not a thymus-derived lymphocyte and must have a receptor for the FC portion of immunoglobulin. The cytotoxic event is not complement-dependent and not phagocytic, although monocytes can mediate ADCC. Antibody able to induce ADCC is usually of the IgG class, but IgM antibody may also be effective. A few examples of ADCC have been described in human tumor systems by Hellstrom[36] and in transitional cell carcinomas of the urinary tract by Hakala.[31]

In addition to lymphoid cells, macrophages have been shown to be a key element in tumor immunity in animals. There appear to be at least two classes of tumoricidal macrophages, the nonspecifically activated macrophage, and the specifically armed macrophage. The activated macrophage was described by Hibbs et al.[38] in 1972 as a nonspecifically cytotoxic cell from animals infected with parasitic organisms, such as BCG. A number of microbes and microbial products have been shown to activate macrophages. These activated macrophages are specifically cytotoxic for tumor target cells and have little activity against normal cells in tissue culture. Whereas the nonspecifically activated macrophage is toxic for any cancer cell, the armed macrophage possesses specificity for the antigens of a specific tumor cell. These immune macrophages are cytotoxic only to the specific target cells to which they have been sensitized. The effect of the armed macrophage may be either to inhibit growth of tumor cells (cytostasis) or to cause lysis of the target cells. Normal macrophages can be armed by contact with specifically sensitized lymphocytes or by a serum that renders them specifically cytotoxic to tumor cells.

Thus, tumor immunity appears to be mediated by a variety of immune mechanisms, including humoral antibody, T- and B-lymphocytes, as well as K-cells and macrophages. The optimum interaction of this multifactoral system can result in tumor cell destruction. However, it has been demonstrated that a weak immune reaction against tumor mediated by either lymphoid cells[88] or antibody[96] can enhance tumor growth, both in vivo and in vitro. Much remains to be learned about the interaction of these various factors for causing tumor rejection.

METHODOLOGY FOR STUDY OF TUMOR-SPECIFIC IMMUNE REACTIONS

Concerning the methodology currently available, immunologic tests are usually divided into those done in vivo and those done in vitro. The detection of TSTA by the immune animal's ability to reject specific tumor challenge is by far the most commonly used in vivo test. Tumor-specific transplantation immunity has been produced in experimental animals by several methods, e.g., strangulation of a growing tumor by ligation at its base, complete tumor excision, immunization with large doses of irradiated tumor cells, or injection of small numbers of viable tumor cells that are insufficient to cause a progressively growing tumor. Recently, it was shown that soluble preparations of TSTA also can immunize animals effectively against tumor cell challenge.[40] The concomitant injection of immunologic stimulants, such as Freund's adjuvant or BCG (attenuated tubercle bacillus), often creates a stronger immunity than the injection of tumor cell antigens alone.

The most frequently used in vivo test for the study of human tumor immunology has been the use of cutaneous hypersensitivity reactions to extracts of human tumor cells. In this test, tumor cell extracts of membrane fractions of tumor cells, or solubilized preparations prepared with agents such as 3 molar potassium chloride extracts, are injected intradermally. The extent of reaction is read as any other delayed hypersensitivity test at 24 to 48 hours. Reactions have been demonstrated to a wide variety of human neoplasms using this technique, pioneered by Herberman, his associates, and Wells.[80, 111]

A second in vivo test, referred to as neutralization, is performed by mixing the target tumor cells with immune lymphoid cells from specifically sensitized donors.[92] Inhibition of tumor growth is influenced by several factors. Among these are the number of immune lymphoid cells, the target cell type, and the specificity of the immune lymphocytes for the cellular antigen.

In vitro tests can be further divided into those detecting immunity mediated either by humoral antibody or by lymphoid cells.[4] Of the humoral antibody tests, the indirect immunofluorescence test employing fluorescence-tagged antiglobulin to detect specific antibody binding has been used extensively. However, interpretation of the test requires experience, because nonspecific immunofluorescence occurs and quantitative differences must be appreciated. The test specificity can be enhanced by tagging a specific antibody directly with fluorescein and using this reagent to study the blocking reaction. Prior to exposure to fluorescent-labeled antibody, the tumor cells are incubated with test sera. Should the test sera contain specific antibody, then these unlabeled antibodies would attach themselves to the cellular antigen sites, thereby effectively blocking labeled-antibody attachment to the tumor cell. Therefore, lack of immunofluorescence on the tumor cell indicates specific antibody in the test serum.[68]

The immune cytotoxicity test is singularly useful for detection of cytotoxic antibody against cell surface antigens. Incubation of tumor cells plus test sera and complement results in cell death as quantitated by direct counting or other methods. Generally, murine leukemia and lymphoma cells are more sensitive to cytotoxic antibody than are solid tumor cells.[78]

Other classic serologic techniques for studying humoral antibodies, such as complement fixation and gel diffusion, are particularly useful in studying the antigens of viral-induced neoplasms.[76] A test used with increasing frequency is the iodine-125 antiglobulin assay devised by McKhann.[33] In principle, this test resembles the immunofluorescence test except that radioiodinated antiglobulin is used to detect specific antibody binding. The test is quantitated by radioactive counting of bound antiglobulin, thereby removing the subjective component inherent in the immunofluorescence test.

Other in vitro tests have been used to detect cellular immunity. Specific destruction of cultured normal or neoplastic target cells by immune lymphoid cells has been demonstrated.[34, 92] This reaction does not require humoral antibody or complement. Large ratios of lymphocytes to target cells are required, i.e., 200:1, perhaps because of the relatively small number of sensitized lymphocytes in a random lymphoid population.

Several techniques measuring isotope release from target cells destroyed by immune lymphocytes are being used to quantitate the cytotoxicity. Tritiated thymidine, chromium-51, and, lately, iodine-125 iododeoxyuridine have all been used to label target cells.

The phenomenon of lymphocyte transformation, whereby sensitized lymphocytes are exposed in vitro to the sensitizing antigens, develop into lymphoblasts, synthesize DNA, and ultimately divide, has been applied to tumor biology. The test mainly detects strong antigenic differences, although antigenic specificity has been detected in some human tumor systems with this test.[109]

ONCOGENIC AGENTS

Some of the known chemical, physical, and viral agents capable of inducing tumors in experimental animals are summarized in Table 1. Each of these oncogens will be briefly discussed.

Antigens of Chemically and Physically Induced Neoplasms

The study of chemical carcinogenesis began in 1775 with Percival Pott, who attributed the frequency of scrotal cancer in chimney sweeps to soot exposure. Passey was to confirm this hypothesis in 1922, when he induced skin cancer in mice with soot extracts. Four years previously, Yamagiwa had produced cancer experimentally by painting rabbit ears with a derivative of coal tar. Subsequently, there were several successful attempts at tumor induction by hydrocarbons, which led to the hope that a single compound

TABLE 1. Systems with Demonstrated Occurrence of Tumor-Specific Antigens Capable of Inducing Rejection Responses in Syngeneic Hosts

Chemical carcinogens
  3-Methylcholanthrene
  1,2,5,6-Dibenzanthracene
  9,10-Dimethylbenzanthracene
  3,4,9,10-Dibenzpyrene
  3,4-Benzpyrene
  p-Dimethylaminoazobenzene } no cross reactivity
Physical agents
  Films: Millipore filter
          Cellophane film
  Radiation: Ultraviolet
                  ^{90}Sr

Virus

DNA { Polyoma
      SV-40
      Adenovirus 12, 18   } cross reaction within
      Shope papilloma   each group

RNA { Mammary tumor agent
      Leukemia
        Gross
        Moloney
        Rauscher } cross reaction } cross reaction within each group
        Friend   between groups
        Graffi
        Rich
        Rous (Schmidt-Ruppin)

in the complex mixtures used might be responsible for the carcinogenesis. However, several polycyclic hydrocarbons since have been found to be carcinogenic. Attempts were made to correlate hydrocarbon structure and cancer-inducing potential, but no relationship has been found.

The greater frequency of skin cancer in those occupationally exposed to sunlight has been attributed to ultraviolet irradiation. Ionizing radiation was found to be carcinogenic in the 1920's, when subcutaneous sarcomas were induced by radium implantation in experimental animals. It soon became evident that radiation was also carcinogenic in man, when bone cancers developed in radium dial painters who licked brushes containing radioactive material. An apparent dose-response relationship in the carcinogenic effects of radiation in man was also found after the Nagasaki bombing, as evidenced by an increased rate of leukemia in survivors.

Foley in 1953[20] first clearly demonstrated specific antigenicity in this class of experimental tumors. He showed that ligation of the base of a growing tumor induced by the chemical carcinogen, methylcholanthrene, was followed by resistance to subsequent challenge with the same tumor. This work was confirmed by Prehn and Main,[87] who further showed that immune animals, while rejecting tumor transplants, would tolerate grafts of normal skin from the same inbred animal who donated the tumor (see Fig. 2). Here was strong evidence that the observed immunity was specific for the tumor and not attributable to genetic disparity among the inbred animals used. Klein[5] proved specific immunity conclusively by demonstrating that an animal with a tumor excised and transplanted serially in other inbred hosts would reject its own neoplasm, if first immunized repeatedly with irradiated cells from its own tumor.

It is well established that tumors induced by any of the chemical or physical carcinogens contain unique TSTA that do not cross-react with tumors induced in other inbred animals by the same agent. For example, in two inbred rats, A and B, injected with methylcholanthrene, tumors will develop with unique TSTA. A third animal, C, immunized against tumor A will, on challenge, reject line A tumor cells but tumor cells from rat B will grow unimpeded (Fig. 4). Even if a single animal is injected in two sites with the same carcinogen, the tumors arising will have different TSTA, and neither will immunize effectively against the other in secondary hosts. Several factors bear on the strength of the specific transplantation antigens induced by these agents. Tumors appearing soon after carcinogen injection have stronger antigens than those which appear after a longer latency period. Tumors induced by chemical carcinogens are more strongly antigenic than those induced by physical agents, such as cellophane films or Millipore filters. There also seems to be a species difference in that methylcholanthrene tumors induced in guinea pigs are more strongly antigenic than those induced in mice.

It is not known why chemical carcinogens are oncogenic. One hypothesis suggests that a local effect might stimulate single-cell malignant transformation.

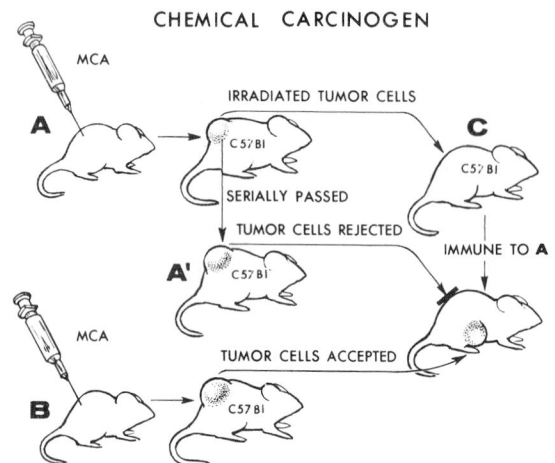

CHEMICAL CARCINOGEN

Figure 4. Mouse *C* immunized to methylcholanthrene tumor *A* is able to reject subsequent challenge of *A* tumor cells. Cells from tumor *B* induced by methylcholanthrene in another animal of the same inbred strain grow unimpeded in host *C*.

Such a mechanism seems to be operational, at least partially, since in vitro malignant transformation can be induced by these agents. A second hypothesis is based upon the finding that all chemical carcinogens so far tested proved to be immunosuppressive, not only to humoral antibody, but to cell-mediated immunity as well. This is readily shown by the prolongation of allogeneic skin grafts in animals receiving standard doses of methylcholanthrene compared to nontreated controls. That immunosuppression favors tumor growth is well established, but to what degree it is important in chemical carcinogenesis is unknown.

A third hypothesis implies that methylcholanthrene activates latent tumor viruses. One would have to assume that enough different viruses existed within each cell to account for the unique antigenicity expressed by carcinogen-induced tumors or that a single virus can induce different antigens, such as reported for adenocarcinomas induced by the mammary tumor virus.[64] As yet, there is little evidence to support this hypothesis, and even though viruses have been isolated from chemical carcinogen-induced tumors, it is possible that they are passenger viruses of little etiologic significance. Thus, there is some evidence to implicate all three mechanisms in the oncogenicity of chemical carcinogens, and it is likely that all play an active role.

Viral Carcinogenesis

Ellerman and Bang of Copenhagen successfully transmitted the erythromyeloblastic form of chicken leukemia by cell-free filtrates in 1908. Rous in 1911 succeeded in transmitting a solid chicken sarcoma with cell-free filtrates. Subsequently, several oncogenic viruses have been isolated from numerous species. There has been increasing evidence that both DNA and RNA viruses produce cancer in many animal species including primates.[89] DNA viruses of the herpes group have been shown to cause renal adenocarcinoma in frogs, infectious lymphomas in chickens, and highly malignant leukemias and lymphomas in monkeys. Type C RNA tumor viruses (oncornoviruses)

have been identified as the causative agent of leukemias and sarcomas in chickens, mice, rats, cats, and gibbon apes. A morphologically distinct B-type RNA virus induces mammary carcinomas in mice, and a related viral agent has been isolated from a Rhesus monkey breast tumor.

The search for similar tumor viruses in humans has become an area of intense investigation. The Epstein-Barr virus (EBV), a member of the herpesvirus group, has been shown to cause infectious mononucleosis in Western countries and is clearly associated with Burkitt's lymphoma in Africa and nasopharyngeal carcinoma in southern China.[50] Although viral particles are not found in the tumors, patients invariably have high antibody levels to EBV, and the viral genome has been demonstrated by molecular hybridization in both Burkitt's lymphoma and nasopharyngeal carcinomas. EBV nuclear antigens are expressed in all tumor cells, and cultured cells derived from the tumors often begin to produce viral particles. Despite the overwhelming evidence for a connection between EBV and Burkitt's lymphoma, its geographical restriction to central Africa suggests that additional factors, possibly host immunologic impairment induced by malaria, are necessary for its inception. Other DNA viruses suspected of playing a role in human cancer include herpes simplex virus, cytomegalovirus, and several recently isolated human papovaviruses.[28] The results of these studies, although encouraging, are preliminary and require additional confirmation.

A number of investigators have obtained evidence linking RNA tumor viruses to human cancer. Soluble antigens related to the mouse mammary tumor virus (MMTV) are detectable in sera of 25 per cent of human breast cancer patients but are not found in normal sera. MMTV also inhibits migration of leukocytes in tests of women with mammary tumors.[61] In addition, breast tumor tissues contain RNA related to MMTV gene sequences and have been reported to contain antigens related to Mason-Pfizer monkey virus (MPMV), the virus isolated from the Rhesus breast tumor.

A great amount of effort has been focused on the possibility of Type C RNA viruses in human leukemias.[21] Recently, an RNA tumor virus was isolated from cultured cells derived from a patient with myelogenous leukemia. This virus is related to several known primate RNA tumor viruses. Virus-like particles with antigenic and molecular similarities to primate RNA tumor viruses have been reported by several investigators in preleukemia bone marrow, lymphosarcomas, leukemias, and cultured embryonic cells of human origin. Antigens in human leukemia cells also have been shown to cross-react with viral structural proteins from Friend leukemia virus, simian sarcoma virus (SSV-1), and the endogenous baboon placenta virus. Recently proviral DNA sequences complementary to RNA from baboon virus have been detected in human leukemic cells.

Several reports suggest that human sarcomas contain antigens and RNA sequences related to mouse leukemia viruses. Human renal carcinomas, especially transitional cell tumors, also have been shown to contain neoantigens and virus-like particles similar to Type C RNA tumor viruses.[32] Current studies in many laboratories appear likely to substantiate and extend the preliminary evidence for both RNA and DNA viruses in human cancer. If tumor viruses in man can be definitely established as etiologic agents of human cancer, it may be possible to prevent certain tumors with viral vaccines. Similar vaccines have been shown to be extremely effective in immunizing primates, cats, and chickens against leukemia induced by several DNA and RNA tumor viruses.

Table 2 lists possible viruses associated with human cancer.

It has been found that experimental host animals must be injected early in life with most oncogenic viruses if a tumor is to occur later in life. There is immunologic immaturity of the host during this time, which allows viral transformation and tumor induction to proceed uninhibited by the host immune response. Adult animals injected with oncogenic viruses are almost always resistant unless they have been immunosuppressed. Two modes of oncogenic viral transmission, vertical and horizontal, have been described. *Vertical transmission* refers to passage from parent to

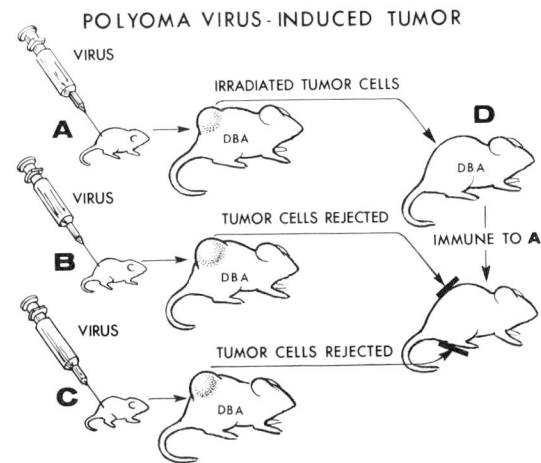

Figure 5. Mouse *D* immunized to polyoma virus-induced tumor *A* also rejects challenge of tumor cells from polyoma virus-induced tumors *B* and *C*.

TABLE 2. Evidence for Oncogenic Virus in Various Human Tumors

Tumor Type	Associated Virus	Nature of Evidence
Lymphomas	EBV	Viral antigens, viral gene sequences
	DNA herpesvirus	Serum antibody, virus in cultured cells
Leukemias	Type C RNA virus	Antigens related to murine and primate viruses, viral gene sequences, reverse transcriptase, virus in cultured tumor cells
Sarcomas	Type C RNA virus	Antigens related to murine and primate viruses, viral gene sequences, virus observed in liposarcoma culture, common tumor antigens
Breast carcinoma	Type B RNA virus	Antigens related to murine and primate mammary tumor viruses, viral gene sequences, serum antibody
Renal carcinoma	Type C RNA virus	Tumor antigens, virus-like particles, reverse transcriptase
Melanoma	Type C RNA virus	Common tumor antigens, gene sequences related to mouse melanoma virus

offspring, as occurs with the mouse mammary tumor virus which is transmitted through the milk, or to the Gross virus leukemia in AKR mice, which is transmitted by the gametes of either parent to the offspring. *Horizontal transmission* refers to passage to cohort cage members by way of excreta, touch, or air-borne particles, as occurs with polyoma virus of mice, feline leukemia virus of cats, and Marek's disease virus of chickens.

Antigens of Viral-Induced Neoplasms

Sjogren[100] showed in 1961 that TSTA were present on the cells of tumors induced in mice by the polyoma virus. In contrast to the noncross-reacting TSTA of chemical carcinogen-induced tumors, those present on tumor cells induced by an oncogenic virus cross-react with any other tumor cell induced by the same virus. For example, if three mice are injected with polyoma virus, in each mouse a tumor will develop that can effectively immunize a fourth normal mouse against challenge with the tumors of either of the other two mice (Fig. 5). It has been shown that this immunity exists even across species lines; i.e., a mouse immunized to a rat polyoma tumor will resist challenge of mouse polyoma tumor cells of the same mouse strain. Tumors induced by polyoma virus, however, do not contain antigens that cross-react with tumors induced by SV-40 virus or adenovirus 12, but some cross-reactivity does exist within the Friend, Moloney, and Rauscher groups of RNA viruses.[76]

The tumor antigens associated with neoplasms produced by the oncogenic DNA viruses (polyoma, SV-40, and adenoviruses) will be discussed together, since the immunologic findings with the different viruses within this group have been similar.[76] When a cell infected by a DNA virus undergoes malignant transformation, the virus itself has an aborted cycle and does not continue to replicate. Despite continued growth of the malignant cells, there is no subsequent evidence of virus production.

Although the neoplasms induced by the virus do not

produce infectious virus, new antigens appear in cells transformed by DNA viruses which persist in the transformed malignant cell. Two classes of antigens are found in the transformed cells—the tumor-specific transplantation antigens and the T or *neo-antigens.* The T antigens were first detected within the nucleus of the transformed cell by classic serologic techniques of complement fixation and immunofluorescence and are not related to any antigens of the intact viral particle or to those found in the normal cell prior to transformation; thus, they were named neo-antigens.

The other class of antigens found associated with these tumors is referred to as the transplantation antigen. It is recognized by the development of transplantation resistance following prior infection with the homologous virus or tumor cells induced by this virus. These transplantation antigens are considered to be different from the T antigens and viral antigens, since certain polyoma tumors, free of infectious virus, still elicit tumor-specific transplantation resistance without the production of detectable viral antibodies.

The mechanism of TSTA induction in cells transformed by oncogenic viruses is unknown. It appears likely, however, that the new transplantation antigens appearing on the surface of virus-induced tumor cells are determined by the viral and not the cellular genome, because of the wide cross-reactivity between the different tumors, as well as that across species lines. Since viral and TSTA are immunologically distinct, it is difficult to explain how virus infection stimulates tumor-specific transplantation resistance. One possible explanation for this could be that during the course of the previous viral infection, cells were transformed, inducing TSTA, but were rejected by the immune response thus stimulated.

The RNA tumor viruses differ considerably from the DNA viruses, both in structure and in manner of replication.[76] This type of oncogenic virus is best exemplified by the avian and murine leukemia and sarcoma virus and by the mouse mammary tumor virus. Most RNA viruses do undergo replication after transforming a cell, and there is continuous shedding of viral particles from the tumor cell surface. For this reason, it has been extremely difficult to distinguish tumor-specific antigens from viral antigens of the RNA tumor viruses. Some RNA viruses, however, have a complex relationship with the cell, whereby they induce transformation but cannot themselves replicate. This is particularly evident in certain strains of avian or murine sarcoma viruses that are able to induce tumors in foreign species, such as the hamster. Such tumors differ from the sarcoma virus-induced neoplasms in their natural host in that they contain little or no demonstrable infective virus. However, it is possible to recover the infectious virus by inoculating the hamster tumors induced by these sarcoma viruses back into the chicken or mouse that is the natural host for these viruses. Also, under certain circumstances both the avian and murine sarcoma viruses can transform cells of their natural host in such a way that they induce transformation but do not themselves replicate. However, formation of complete infective virus particles can be induced by the addition of specific leukemia virus, which aids in the intracellular manufacture of components necessary for complete maturation of the defective sarcoma virus particles. In this case, the rescued sarcoma viruses carry the antigenic specificity of the helper leukemia virus.

Despite the differences between the DNA and RNA tumor viruses, the tumor-specific antigens of neoplasms induced by each of these oncogenic virus groups are commonly cross-reactive. Thus, the antigens of tumors induced by any one oncogenic virus cross-react with other tumors induced by that same virus, but not with tumors induced by other oncogenic viruses.

Fetal Antigens

A third mechanism for induction of tumor-specific antigens not yet discussed has been suggested by finding that experimental tumors frequently show cross-reactivity with embryonic but not with adult tissue antigens. This led to the hypothesis that specific antigens are present in early embryonic life but become repressed with maturation. Upon malignant transformation, these antigens are derepressed and present as tumor-specific antigens. There has been some evidence in animals that SV-40, polyoma, and methylcholanthrene-induced tumor-specific antigens originate through such a mechanism. Also, a carcinoembryonic antigen has been described in human colon carcinomas.

THE CONCEPT OF IMMUNOLOGIC SURVEILLANCE

Considering the relative infrequency with which clinically apparent cancer occurs, one might assume that malignant cell mutants rarely develop. Such is unlikely. Malignant deviants are probably commonplace among the innumerable cell divisions occurring daily, but, for several reasons, few ever establish themselves successfully.

Burnet[8] hypothesized that an immunologic surveillance system exists in man that is capable of discerning foreignness on the surfaces of deviant cells and thereby eliminating them from the host. This policing mechanism was viewed as being mediated especially, but not exclusively, by the lymphoid system and ideally would be needed only to eliminate relatively small numbers of cells. It certainly seems logical that an immunologic response would be initiated against the sudden appearance of a "foreign" cancer cell much as it is against a bacterial, parasitic, or viral pathogen. Although there have been recent data that question the classic theory of immune surveillance presented by Schwartz,[94] we currently believe that the balance of evidence favors the existence of such a system.

Hereditary factors are important in determining the effectiveness of surveillance mechanisms against neoplasia. Genetic influences can determine the effectiveness of the immune response against foreign tumor antigens, i.e., C57Bl mice rarely have spontaneous malignant tumors, are not susceptible to polyoma tumor oncogenesis, and are highly resistant to noncogenic pathogens such as vaccinia. Guinea pigs and rabbits are also inherently resistant to polyoma tumor induction. It is perhaps presumptive to assume that this resistance is all immunologically mediated. In the case of viral oncogenesis, genetic factors at the cellular level, such as lack of viral receptors on the cell surface, have been demonstrated to be of importance for viral transformation in vitro.

EVASION OF IMMUNE SURVEILLANCE

One might well argue that if surveillance mechanisms exist immunologically or otherwise, why then do tumors ever develop? Actually, several mechanisms have been described whereby tumor cells might evade the host's defenses and grow progressively.

Old and Boyse[78] found that small numbers of tumor cells having foreign tumor-specific transplantation antigens were often capable of forming tumors in situations where large cell numbers would be rejected. It was hypothesized that a small number of cells would not be sufficiently immunogenic and would "sneak through" the host immune response as it arose. Such a mechanism might also be functional in newborn animals injected with oncogenic viruses. The immunologic immaturity known to exist in such hosts might allow the malignant induction process a head start.

A second mechanism known to exist in certain mouse strains is the reduction or loss of antigen at the cell surface known as *antigenic modulation*. Old and Boyse[77] described an antigen (TL) on certain murine thymus leukemia cells that disappears in an immune environment, but returns when the cells are grown in a nonimmune host. In the usual sense, such an antigen would not be described as a TSTA, because its presence does not lead to tumor rejection. Whether TSTA use this method to escape immunologic destruction is unknown. Workers in Klein's laboratory have described a similar process, in which there is a permanent quantitative reduction of antigenic expression in some Moloney leukemias, probably due to immunoselection. Such cells are more immunoresistant than other Moloney leukemia cells that have a greater antigen density on the cell surface.

Immunologic tolerance is another possible mechanism for the evasion of immune surveillance. Exposure of neonatal rodents to a specific antigen prior to the maturation of their immune systems can induce a state of specific immunologic nonresponsiveness to that antigen referred to as *tolerance*. Tolerance can be induced during formation of the germ layers. Such a mechanism is believed to be operational in AKR mice carrying the Gross virus, where either parent may transmit the agent. Tolerance also may be induced in the neonate through the passage of the mammary tumor virus (MTV) from mother to offspring. The former type of tolerance is referred to as *natural*, the latter type as *acquired*. Bittner discovered in 1936 that C3H female mice transmitted MTV through milk to their nursing young, which later induced mammary tumors in a high percentage of their adult female progeny. Several investigators attempted unsuccessfully to demonstrate the presence of TSTA in this tumor system before Morton[65] showed that the mammary carcinomas in these mice did contain common TSTA. He demonstrated that mice infected as neonates subsequently were tolerant to the MTV and therefore were unable to be immunized to it as adults. Newborn mice foster-nursed on non-MTV-carrying mothers from another strain were not tolerant to the virus, and as adults could be effectively immunized against it as well as against the MTV-induced mammary tumors. Also, the incidence of mammary tumors in these foster-nursed mice was much less than in those nursed by MTV-carrying mothers.

Immunosuppression, which accompanies old age, neonatal thymectomy, or the administration of x-rays, drugs, or antilymphocyte serum, is a fourth mechanism that increases the animal's susceptibility to the growth of malignant cells. Thus, certain strains of mice naturally resistant to adenovirus oncogenesis are no longer so after neonatal thymectomy or the administration of antilymphocyte serum during the viral induction period. Neoplasms also develop more frequently in immunosuppressed humans than in their normal counterparts.

Immunologic enhancement, as defined by Kaliss,[48] refers specifically to the establishment of a tumor homograft and its progressive growth as a consequence of the tumor's contact with specific antibodies in the host. These antibodies could be elicited by active immunization with lyophilized tumor tissues, but passive immunization with antibodies produced in another host of the same strain or even a foreign species also was effective. This phenomenon is not unique to tumor homografts, since by giving immune antibody to allogeneic graft recipients, prolongation of skin grafts can be achieved. These findings have been well confirmed, but the exact site at which antibody exerts its protective effect is unknown.

At least three possibilities have been proposed. In what has been termed *afferent enhancement,* there would be neutralization of the immunizing capacity of tumor cells due to coating of their antigens by enhancing antibody, which prevented interaction with the lymphoid system. Evidence supporting this hypothesis comes from the observation that splenectomy in the mouse interferes with active enhancement, presumably by decreasing the number of antibody-forming cells. *Central enhancement* would involve direct inhibition of the maturation and proliferation of immunocompetent cells, thereby decreasing their reactivity. *Efferent enhancement* would occur if humoral antibody alone or antibody complexed with antigen coated the antigenic sites of the target cells, preventing their recognition or destruction by sensitized lymphocytes. Much experimental evidence seems to support the fact that enhancing antibody acts on the efferent limb of the immune response.

Work incriminating immunologic enhancement as a prime factor aiding tumor growth has come from the Hellstroms'[36] laboratory, where the colony inhibition test is used. In this test, tumor cells are plated in Petri dishes with either specific humoral antibody and complement or immune lymphocytes added. Inhibition of tumor cell colony formation serves to index the specific activity of the antibody or the lymphoid cells. One study involved tumors induced in inbred Balb/c mice by the Moloney sarcoma virus (MSV). In animals injected with the virus prior to 10 days of age, progressively growing tumors developed, whereas those animals injected after 30 days of age showed tumor formation with subsequent regression.

The Hellstroms used the terms *progressors* and *regressors* to differentiate the two groups of mice. The tested lymphoid cells from both progressors and regressors inhibited colony formation equally well. However, the discovery that serum from progressors added to cultured tumor cells was able to block the inhibiting effect of the immune lymphocytes added subsequently was of great importance. Sera from animals of the same strain carrying tumors induced by other agents were unable to block the effects of the immune lymphocytes. This rules out a possible nonspecific factor that might occur in tumor sera generally.

To determine whether the blocking effect was on the tumor cells or the lymphoid cells, each, in turn, was incubated with progressor sera before the test. It was found that tumor cell growth was inhibited only when target cells were coated with antiserum. Incubation of lymphocytes with blocking serum did not prevent their cytotoxic effect. Further in vitro immunologic studies seem to indicate that the blocking factor is an antigen-antibody complex.[35] Regressor animals had this serum-blocking factor initially, but with tumor regression, cytotoxic antibodies developed that had no blocking effect over a wide range of concentrations.

In fact, the serum from regressor animals would neutralize the blocking effect of the progressor sera on immune lymphocytes in vitro and could induce tumor regression in vivo.[36]

CLINICAL EVIDENCE FOR TUMOR IMMUNITY IN MAN

It is logical to assume that human neoplasms contain cancer-specific antigens similar to those found in animal tumors, but until recently, there was little evidence for the existence of such antigens. The tumor transplantation techniques used to demonstrate the tumor-specific antigens of animal neoplasms have not been applicable to the study of human tumors because of the obvious lack of syngeneic recipients and the ethical limitations implicit in such human experiments. Nevertheless, for many years, clinicians have known that the growth of human cancer is greatly influence by host-tumor interactions.

There are a wide variety of well-documented clinical observations that suggest the existence of host defenses against cancer in man. Although there has been little direct evidence to support an immunologic basis for these clinical observations, they are most consistent with the hypothesis that immune defenses play a major role in controlling the growth of cancer in man.

The following clinical observations suggest the existence of host immunity against cancer:

1. The *spontaneous regression* of established tumors is a rare but well-documented phenomenon in which prolonged, apparently spontaneous regressions occur without treatment or are associated with minor viral or bacterial infections.[17] Spontaneous remissions are particularly frequent in neuroblastomas of children, malignant melanomas, choriocarcinoma, adenocarcinomas of the kidney, and soft tissue sarcomas, but have been observed in other tumors as well. Instances of spontaneous regression of metastatic lesions in the lung or elsewhere following removal of the primary tumor are also well documented and probably occur most frequently in hypernephromas. Prolonged remission or cure of patients following incomplete removal of their cancers is not uncommon.[101] Although other physiologic or endocrinologic changes could be responsible for these spontaneous regressions, they are most easily explained on an immunologic basis.

2. Delayed recurrence, 10 or 20 years after successful treatment of the primary tumor, with the development of rapidly progressive disease, strongly suggests the existence of host defenses that inhibited tumor growth during the tumor-free interval.

3. Cellular infiltration by histiocytes, plasma cells, lymphocytes, and eosinophils implies that certain tumors evoke cellular defense mechanisms. These striking cellular reactions are suggestive of specific immunologic reactions to some component of the tumor. There is a morphologic similarity between these reactions and those associated with rejection of transplanted tumors in man.[26] In most neoplasms, such cellular infiltration of tumors is associated with an improved prognosis. The highest survival rate from gastric cancers is associated with lymphoid infiltration around the tumor and sinus histiocytosis of the regional lymph nodes. In fact, clinical evidence indicates that these considerations have a higher correlation with survival from gastric cancer than adequacy of surgical removal of the tumor.[5]

4. Furthermore, cancer cells are frequently found in the washings of operative wounds or in postoperative wound drainage in patients undergoing definitive cancer surgery. The existence of host immune defenses is suggested by the observation that in many of these patients, recurrent cancer never develops.[90]

5. Apparently viable tumor cells frequently found in the blood or lymphatics of cancer patients seldom lead to metastatic lesions, and their presence cannot be correlated with prognosis. Since in many of these patients subsequent metastatic lesions never develop, these tumor cells are presumably destroyed by host defenses.

6. On the basis of the evidence gained in animal experimentation, the most direct method for establishing tumor-specific antigenicity would be to show that tumor cell explants are rejected in the tumor's own host. This has been attempted in man by several investigators. Surprisingly, most attempts to implant human neoplasms from the primary site to intracutaneous or subcutaneous areas of the same patient fail to take. The incidence of successful tumor growth varies between 10 and 25 per cent even in patients with advanced malignant disease. Southam's studies suggest that this resistance is relative rather than absolute, since challenges of greater than 100 million tumor cells will usually result in tumor growth.[102] However, the most direct evidence that humoral and cellular immune factors are responsible for the growth inhibition of tumor autotransplants is provided by Southam's studies, wherein the mixture of tumor cells with autologous leukocyte or plasma inhibited cancer growth in almost half of the patients studied.[102]

IMMUNODEFICIENCY IN THE DEVELOPMENT AND PROGRESSIVE GROWTH OF HUMAN CANCER

The observations just summarized suggest the existence of host immune defenses in human cancer. If the immune response is important in controlling the development and progression of this disease, then there should be some correlation between the general immune competence of human beings and resistance to cancer. Clinical data derived from several sources are consistent with this concept.

Human Tumor Allografts

The pioneering work of Southam and associates clearly demonstrated that allotransplants of tumor cells from tissue culture into normal human volunteers were promptly rejected, but delayed rejection was sometimes observed in cancer patients.

The importance of an intact immune response causing the rejection of human tumor allografts is illustrated by observations of patients with renal allografts. Patients receiving immunosuppressive drugs for kidney transplantation have shown increased susceptibility to the outgrowth of tumor allografts transplanted from the kidney donor. In these cases, the kidney graft derived from a patient who died of malignant disease was transplanted to a recipient who then received standard continuous immunosuppressive therapy. Metastatic cancer from the transplanted kidney developed in the recipient several months later. In one particularly interesting case, cessation of immunosuppressive therapy resulted in rejection of the kidney but not of the tumor tissue. When the rejected kidney, which contained a large mass of tumor tissue, was removed, however, the residual metastases gradually disappeared. Furthermore, there was no evidence of tumor reappearance when a second successful kidney transplant was performed nine months later, even though the patient was placed on a full program of immunosuppressive therapy. Thus, complete destruction of the allografted cancer tissue seems to have been accomplished by the host immune system during a relatively brief period of normal function, but only after the bulk of tumor tissue had been reduced.[112]

A comparable situation to that which exists in the case of accidental tumor transplantation occurs with choriocarcinoma. Choriocarcinoma is a malignant growth arising from trophoblastic elements of the placenta. The tumor proliferates, invades the uterine wall, and disseminates to remote organs. Since choriocarcinoma is of fetal genotype, it contains histocompatibility genes of both maternal and paternal origin. Thus, the presence of paternal transplantation antigens on the choriocarcinoma tumor cells makes this tumor an allograft. Nevertheless, untreated choriocarcinoma is associated with a high mortality, illustrating an allografted human tumor that contains transplantation antigens foreign to the host but is not necessarily rejected. However, a number of regressions of metastatic choriocarcinomas have been reported following hysterectomy and removal of a large tumor mass.[23] Moreover, choriocarcinomas are very sensitive to chemotherapeutic agents, and appropriate chemotherapy has resulted in a five-year survival of greater than 75 per cent. These two observations may be related in that both primary tumor removal and chemotherapy temporarily alter the tumor-host relationship in such a fashion as to favor the host. When this occurs, an effective immune response may promote rejection of the tumor allograft. An immunologic basis is further suggested by a report of metastatic choriocarcinoma that failed to regress following chemotherapy. It did regress when the patient was immunized with her husband's leukocytes and was given antiserum prepared in rabbits against her husband's seminal fluid.[23]

Congenital and Acquired Immunologic Deficiency States

Additional evidence for the importance of the host immune response in human cancer comes from observations of an increased incidence of spontaneous malignancy developing in patients with immune deficiency.

Human beings with congenital immunologic deficiency disorders, such as ataxia telangiectasia and Wiscott-Aldrich syndrome, have a high incidence of spontaneous neoplasms, usually involving the lymphoreticular system and estimated to occur at a frequency roughly 10,000 times that in a normal age-matched population.[83] Such tumors constitute a major cause of death in these patients. Evidence of immunologic deficiency almost always precedes the appearance of tumors, but the question of cause and effect remains.

Reports of a greatly increased incidence of malignant neoplasms developing in patients on immunosuppressive treatment for renal homografts provides further evidence for the importance of immunologic factors in malignancy. Immunosuppressed organ homograft recipients have a 5 to 6 per cent risk of developing de novo cancers. Although initially it was thought that these malignancies were lymphomas or reticulum cell sarcomas, more recent data indicate that 67 per cent are of epithelial origin and only 33 per cent of mesenchymal origin. However, the mesenchymal malignancies have a latency period of approximately 20 months, compared to 32 months for epithelial lesions. This predominance of epithelial malignancies somewhat weakens the hypothesis proposed by Schwartz[94] that the increased frequency of malignancy in organ homograft recipients was due to activation of a latent virus caused by the host's immunologic reaction against the organ transplant. This alternative view was quite consistent with the earlier reported predominance of lymphoma and reticulum cell sarcoma malignancies in these patients, but less compatible with the present data. In addition, it has been observed that cancers can develop in nontransplant patients treated with immunosuppressive therapy for other illnesses, such as psoriasis[83] and Hodgkin's disease.[2] Although a cause-effect relationship has not been definitely demonstrated, the frequent association of lymphomas with psoriatic patients chronically treated with methotrexate must be regarded with considerable suspicion.[83]

CORRELATIONS BETWEEN PROGNOSIS AND IMMUNOCOMPETENCE IN CANCER PATIENTS

Evidence thus far presented suggests that the patient's immune response or lack of response is important in controlling the development and progression of malignant disease. Why does cancer develop? Obviously, where clinical cancer is observed, the immunoprotective mechanisms have either failed or been overwhelmed. It is, therefore, relevant to inquire into the general functional status of the cancer patient's immunologic system. Such studies can be grouped into two categories — those concerned with humoral antibody production and those dealing with cell-mediated immune reactions.

Humoral antibody formation to known antigenic substances has been studied by many investigators who have concluded that, in most patients with either solid or lymphoreticular neoplasms, the ability to form humoral antibodies to a variety of antigenic substances, even in the presence of advanced disease, is not impaired. Thus, there is no evidence to implicate a defect in humoral antibody production in most cancer patients.

Cell-mediated immune reactions of cancer patients have been measured by the ability of these patients to manifest delayed cutaneous hypersensitivity to a variety of common skin test antigens to which most normal persons are reactive by virtue of previous exposure, such as mumps, tuberculin, streptokinase, or streptodornase. In addition, the ability of these patients to manifest a primary immune response following exposure to a new antigen for the first time has been evaluated. An important method tests the ability of these patients to develop delayed cutaneous hypersensitivity to the contact sensitizer dinitrochlorobenzene (DNCB). Such studies show that the cell-mediated immune reaction was significantly impaired in patients with advanced lymphoreticular neoplasia. These results were not surprising, since lymphoreticular malignant diseases usually diffusely involve the immune effector system. However, a similar impairment in cell-mediated immune reactions was also found in patients with localized and far-advanced solid neoplasms that did not involve the immune system. These observations clearly indicate a defect in cell-mediated immune reaction in patients with neoplasia.

More recent studies demonstrated a significant correlation between cell-mediated immunologic reactivity as measured by the ability to manifest delayed cutaneous hypersensitivity following sensitization to DNCB and the postoperative course of cancer patients.[43, 66] It was found that more than 95 per cent of normal control volunteers, patients with benign neoplasms, and those free of disease five years or more following cancer surgery could all be sensitized to this chemical. However, only 72 per cent of all cancer patients who presented themselves as candidates for definitive cancer surgery were able to be sensitized to DNCB; the remaining 28 per cent exhibited cutaneous anergy to this chemical. The anergic patients had a uniformly poor prognosis following surgical therapy. More than 95 per cent of these patients either were found to have inoperable disease because of local or metastatic spread, or had recurrent disease within six months of surgery.

Most patients who were immunologically competent, as evidenced by their ability to be sensitized to DNCB, had a much improved prognosis. Eighty-four per cent of these patients were found to have localized tumors that could be resected and were free of disease for at least six months following surgery. There appeared to be considerable differences, however, in the pattern of DNCB reactivity in patients with different histologic types of solid tumors. Patients with epidermoid carcinomas of either the cervix, mouth, pharynx, or larynx showed a very strong correlation between a positive DNCB reponse and a good prognosis following cancer surgery. Most patients who could be sensitized to this chemical had operable disease and were free of disease for at least six months after surgery, whereas those who were anergic had a uniformly poor prognosis. In contrast, there appeared to be little correlation between positive DNCB tests and recurrence after surgery for skeletal and soft tissue sarcomas. Most sarcoma patients were immunologically competent regardless of whether they were free of disease at six months or had early recurrence.

Thus, it is evident that patients with severe impairment of the cell-mediated immune reaction, as exhibited by cutaneous anergy to 100 micrograms of DNCB, have a poor prognosis after surgical therapy regardless of the histologic type of their neoplasm. However, the prognostic significance of an intact cellular immune response is very much related to the histologic type of neoplasm being studied. The explanation for these differences in cutaneous reactivity with various tumor types is unknown, although it is possible that these patterns of cutaneous reactivity are indicative of some important differences in the etiology of different types of neoplasms.

Recent studies have done much to clarify the immunosuppression produced by malignant disease. Sequential evaluation of general immune competence in cancer patients revealed that variations in immune reactivity correlated with body burden of cancer. Patients who, on sequential testing with DNCB, converted from a reactive to an anergic status were usually found to have progressive malignant disease. Conversely, patients with conversion from an anergic to a reactive status were observed to have control of tumor as frequently as those patients who were reactive initially and maintained their reactivity during the postsurgical observation period.[13] Thus, it was evident that the defect in systemic immunity was a result of the neoplastic process and that the immunosuppression could be reversed by successful therapy. Additional studies of lymphocyte function in patients with malignant disease revealed that lymphocytes from cancer patients were depressed when compared to normal individuals and that the degree of depression correlated to the extent of the malignancy.[28, 41] Most recently, serum factors have been found in cancer patients that have the ability to inhibit the function of lymphocytes from normal individuals in tissue culture and undoubtedly contribute to the immunosuppression observed in cancer patients.[9, 24] Thus, at this time it appears that the immunosuppression caused by malignancy is the result of a humoral factor released by the cancer cell itself, or a response by the body to the cancer cell that is capable of depressing normal host cellular immunity as measured by delayed cutaneous hypersentivity and lymphocyte function.

EVIDENCE FOR TUMOR-SPECIFIC ANTIGENS IN HUMAN NEOPLASMS

Since the tumor transplantation techniques used to demonstrate tumor-specific antigens in animal neoplasms have not been applicable to man, it was necessary to study human tumor antigens by other methods. Early attempts to detect tumor-specific antigens in human neoplasms depended primarily upon serologic analysis of antisera against human tumor tissue produced in foreign species, such as the rabbit. Because of the antigenic disparity between man and rabbit, antibodies were formed against normal tissue antigens that contaminated the immunizing material. Thus, it was difficult or impossible to sort out the tumor-specific antibodies and to distinguish between qualitative and quantitative differences in the antigenic composition of normal versus neoplastic tissues. For this reason, most of the earlier reports suggesting the presence of tumor-specific antigens by these methods were not widely accepted. However, recent reports indicate that this method can be used successfully to demonstrate fetal antigens in human neoplasms.

Fetal Antigens and Human Neoplasms

The concept of neoplastic transformation accompanied by dedifferentiation and reversion to an embryonic state is not new. This concept has been expressed by many investigators during the past century, but it is only during the past decade that antigens specific for fetal tissues have been described in various human neoplasms. Embryonic or fetal antigens are normal embryonic constituents produced during fetal development. Their production appears to be repressed shortly after birth, and in the adult they are either barely detectable or not found at all. However, when adult tissues undergo malignant transformation, the production of these primitive embryonic constituents is resumed. The participation of these fetal antigens in terms of the tumor-host relationship from an immunologic standpoint is unclear at the present time, although they may have great importance in possible diagnostic tests for malignancy.

Alpha₁-Fetoprotein (AFP)

In 1964, Tatarinov[105] reported the detection of a protein with the electrophoretic mobility of an alpha₁-globulin circulating in sera from patients with primary hepatoma, but not in normal sera. Since this protein was antigenically identical to a constituent of normal fetal serum, it was termed alpha₁-fetoprotein (AFP). Many reports subsequently confirmed the association of AFP with hepatomas, and less frequently with totipotential tumors of the testis and ovary. However, it was not until a highly sensitive radioimmunoassay was developed that AFP became detectable in a large proportion of hepatoma patients.[98] Using radioimmunoassay detection, AFP elevations can be expected in approximately 80 per cent of hepatoma patients, with some variation depending on race and geographic area. High circulating AFP concentrations are found in association with hepatoma, totipotential germinal cell tumors, and occasionally with carcinoma of the stomach. However, the highly sensitive tests also have detected relatively low levels of AFP in a few patients with a variety of neoplasms, or occasionally with nonmalignant hepatic disorders, but always in association with normal pregnancy. Thus, while AFP determinations are valuable in diagnostic tests, they must be interpreted in the light of other clinical information, especially when relatively low levels are found. Perhaps the greatest potential value of AFP determinations will be as a determinant of response to surgery or chemotherapy in hepatoma patients, since a drop in AFP serum concentrations may provide an index of therapeutic response. A fall in AFP levels, followed by a rise to that approaching preoperative levels, would be expected with recurrence of hepatoma.[97]

It is of interest to note that many of the nonmalignant diseases in which relatively low AFP elevations have been found are associated with an increased risk of subsequent development of hepatoma. Perhaps this is analogous to the finding that in dimethylaminoazobenzine (DAB) induction of rat hepatomas, there is an initial peak of AFP synthesis without concurrent liver cell malignancy, followed by a second peak of AFP production, at which time the hepatic tumor becomes manifest. It is tempting to speculate that human AFP production in nonmalignant hepatic disorders is in some way similar to the initial AFP peak in DAB-induced rat hepatomas. However, it has yet to be shown that patients who produce AFP elevations during a period of hepatic insult are at a greater risk of subsequently developing primary liver cell cancers.[99]

Carcinoembryonic Antigen (CEA)

Gold and Freedman[22] reported the discovery of a new tumor-associated antigen in adenocarcinoma of the human colon in 1965. These studies were well controlled because colon cancer usually does not extend intramurally for more than 6 to 7 cm. Therefore, normal colon taken from surgical specimens beyond these points was available as control tissue from the same donors who supplied the cancer material. In this manner, the problem of alloantigenic differences between donors of normal and tumor tissues was overcome. Antitumor antisera were prepared in rabbits and rendered tumor-specific either by absorption with an excess of corresponding normal tissue extract, or by the phenomenon of acquired immunologic tolerance. These heterologous antisera were then used to detect CEA by a variety of serologic procedures. As a result, CEA was found in human adenocarcinoma arising from entodermally derived digestive system epithelium and embryonic and fetal gut, pancreas, and liver throughout the first two trimesters of gestation. The predominant cellular localization of CEA in digestive system tumors and fetal gut, as demonstrated by immunofluorescence, was closely associated with the glycocalyx of the cell membrane. CEA, initially purified by Krupey et al.,[54] was characterized as a perchloric acid–soluble glycoprotein that contained approximately 55 per cent carbohydrate with beta-globulin mobility on electrophoresis and a molecular weight of approximately 2000 daltons.

In 1969, Thomson[107] described a sensitive radioimmunoassay for detection of CEA. Using this technique, he reported that while 35 of 36 patients with known colorectal cancer had serum CEA elevations, CEA was not detected in the sera of patients with nonentodermally derived cancers or patients with a variety of other nonmalignant disease. Subsequently, several investigators[114] using a variety of detection techniques reported that CEA elevations were not seen as frequently in association with colorectal cancer as initially reported, and that CEA could be detected in association with a variety of other malignant and nonmalignant disorders. This discrepancy in apparent incidence of CEA elevations in colorectal cancer patients was probably related to the fact that the earlier studies included a patient population with advanced disease. It is now known, as reported by Dhar et al.,[11] that as few as 20 per cent of patients with tumors localized to the bowel wall have a demonstrable CEA elevation, whereas close to 100 per cent of patients with widespread metastases have elevated levels. The fact that CEA elevations have been reported in association with a much greater variety of pathologic conditions than initially envisioned is the central issue underlying an ongoing controversy concerning the specificity of the CEA test. The problem is at least partly explained by the fact that a variety of reagents and assays have been used by different investigators. This is important because many "nonspecific cross-reacting," or "CEA-like" molecules have been found which vary slightly in composition, electrostatic charge, and molecular weight. There are at least seven such substances, some of which are present in relatively large concentrations in perfectly normal tissue. The problem is further compounded by the fact that there are probably several antigenic sites on a given CEA molecule, some of which may have either A, B, Lewis-a, or Lewis-b blood group activity. Ongoing intensive investigations in this area will be of great interest. Meanwhile, commercially available CEA assays are of great potential value in two situations:

1. As a diagnostic tool, CEA by itself cannot be used as a diagnostic test, since elevations may be found in association with a variety of malignancies, especially adenocarcinomas of any site as well as some nonmalignant illnesses such as cirrhosis, ulcerative colitis, emphysema, and even in normal smokers. However, it is important that while relatively high CEA elevations tend to be seen with entodermally derived adenocarcinomas that are often advanced, much lower levels are the rule in association with localized disease, other neoplasms, or nonmalignant conditions. Thus, as with any clinical test, CEA determinations are only of diagnostic value when the actual plasma concentration is known and interpreted in the light of other clinical information.

2. As a prognostic tool, CEA level is usually a reflection of tumor burden in any given individual with a neoplasm. Thus, the disappearance of this antigen from the circulation would be expected to follow successful cancer surgery. The reappearance of this antigen during the postoperative period is strong evidence for recurrence, and may precede any other clinical evidence of recurrence by months.[58] Whether or not reappearance of circulating CEA following surgery can be used as a basis for a second look operation or further therapy is at present under investigation.

Other Fetal Antigens

AFP and CEA are detectable in relatively high concentrations in fetal gastrointestinal organs, tend to disappear or are barely detectable after the perinatal period, and recur in association with malignancy. It probably is not accidental that these markers are invariably found in the fetus. Fetal and cancer tissues are similar in two major respects; both involve rapidly proliferating cells and both, to varying degrees, are composed of undifferentiated cells.

Of these two factors, the latter seems to bear the most consistent relationship to the appearance of fetal type proteins or glycoproteins. After partial hepatectomy, massive regeneration and cell proliferation occur, with no or minimal production of AFP. However, a relatively small neoplasm may be associated with a several hundred thousand–fold AFP elevation. Morphologic or functional cellular dedifferentiation, or a return to the primitive state, may be an essential hallmark of malignancy. Thus, there may be a wide variety of fetal antigens, some of which might be specific for malignancy of a specific organ, such as AFP, and others that are shared by neoplasms arising in an organ.

Preliminary evidence to support this concept comes from reports by Edynak and his colleagues[12] describing a common fetal antigen in a wide variety of human neoplasms, as well as in normal tissue adjacent to breast carcinomas, in fetal tissues, in human umbilical cord serum, and in fetal calf serum. This antigen was widely distributed in 75 to 95 per cent of human cancers, including carcinomas of the breast, head and neck, ovary, kidney, and genitourinary tract, in all categories of sarcomas tested, and in the cells and sera of patients with leukemia. Although the antigen was found in the extracts of 15 of 20 benign tumors, it could not be demonstrated in extracts from 172 normal or diseased tissues, even though it was detectable in the unconcentrated sera of 10 per cent of cancer patients. Its potential usefulness as a universal diagnostic test for malignancy is obvious.

Another fetal antigen, the oncofetal antigen (OFA), was described by Irie et al.[46] using the immune adherence (IA) technique. OFA was first demonstrated on melanoma cells and later on a variety of malignant cells in vivo. The antigen is not present on normal biopsy tissues but may appear on normal tissues during their adaptation to the tissue culture process. OFA differs from CEA and alpha$_1$-fetoprotein in that it is barely perceived in the fetal digestive tract, but is very apparent in fetal brain tissue and, in contrast to

AFP, is not found in fetal liver or in umbilical cord serum. None of the previously described cancer-associated antigens has been shown to be cross-reactive with fetal brain tissues.[46] OFA could be demonstrated in fibroblasts from cancer patients and noncancer patients, whereas a similar fetal antigen recently described by The et al.[106] could not.

EVIDENCE FOR TUMOR-SPECIFIC IMMUNE RESPONSES IN HUMAN CANCER

Since most of the fetal antigen systems have been defined by means of antisera produced in a foreign species such as the rabbit, their possible role in influencing tumor growth in the human host is unknown. Many of them may not be immunogenic in man, but may be important as possible diagnostic tests for the presence of malignancy. Until recently, there was little direct evidence that human tumors contained tumor-specific antigens capable of eliciting a specific immune response in the cancer patient. The transplantation techniques used to demonstrate tumor-specific antigens in animal tumors have not been applicable to man because of the lack of syngeneic recipients, as well as ethical and moral limitations. Therefore, the demonstration of tumor-specific antigens in human neoplasms has depended primarily upon a variety of sensitive in vitro immunologic techniques previously used to establish the existence of tumor-specific antigens in animal neoplasms. Tumor-associated antigens have been shown in a variety of human neoplasms by use of these sensitive immunologic techniques to detect antibodies or lymphocytes in the blood of cancer patients specifically reactive with the antigens of autologous tumor tissue. Such studies revealed that most, if not all, human neoplasms contain tumor-associated antigens that are capable of inducing an immune response in the tumor-bearing host.

Past studies by Graham and Graham[27] and Finney[19] suggested that the sera of cancer patients did contain antibodies reactive with autologous tumor tissue. However, in many cases, suitable controls were not employed to exclude the role of bacterial, fungal, viral, or mycoplasma contaminants in these reactions. More recent studies clearly indicate the existence of cellular and humoral immune responses in patients to their cancers.

A wide variety of human neoplasms have been shown to elicit humoral antibodies or cell-mediated immune responses in cancer patients by many different immunologic techniques. Detailed review of the wide variety of neoplasms in which tumor-associated antigens have been detected is beyond the scope of this chapter, but Table 3 illustrates the large number of different types of human neoplasms to which patients have shown evidence of humoral or cell-mediated immunity. Some specific types of human neoplasms that are of particular interest from an historical standpoint will be discussed in greater detail.

At the present time, the antigenic specificity of the different types of tumor-associated antigens on human neoplasms remains largely undetermined. However,

TABLE 3. Human Neoplasms Associated with Host Immune Reactions Demonstrated by Various Immunologic Techniques

Bladder carcinoma
Breast carcinoma
Burkitt's lymphoma
Colon carcinoma
Leukemia
Lung carcinoma
Malignant melanoma
Neuroblastoma
Renal carcinoma
Skeletal and soft tissue sarcomas

the demonstration of antibody and complement fixed to the surface of the human cancer cell in vivo[28, 44, 45] clearly indicates that these immune responses to human cancer do have in vivo significance and are not in vitro artifacts.

Burkitt's Lymphoma

Burkitt's lymphoma was one of the first human tumors that was clearly shown to be immunogenic in the autologous host.[37, 51, 52] This malignant disease occurs primarily in African children but also is observed sporadically in other parts of the world. It has a peculiar predilection for growth in the jaw and facial bones. The epidemiology of this tumor in a relatively limited geographic area led Burkitt to suspect it was an arthropod-borne infectious disease. This hypothesis was strengthened by the finding of virus particles morphologically similar to the herpes group in cell lines derived from Burkitt's lymphoma. The virus has been designated as the Epstein-Barr virus (EBV) after the EB-1 line of Burkitt cells in which it was first observed. Whether EBV is the etiologic agent in Burkitt's tumor or merely a passenger virus is uncertain, because similar particles also have been observed in tissue cultured cells from patients with nonmalignant diseases, such as infectious mononucleosis, and in peripheral leukocytes from healthy donors. While the etiologic role of EBV in malignancy remains in question, it does appear to cause infectious mononucleosis.

The participation of immune factors in the course of Burkitt's lymphoma was suggested by the observation of spontaneous regressions and the high incidence of long-term remissions in patients receiving short-term therapy with small doses of chemotherapeutic agents. Experimental evidence supporting the role of host immune responses was provided by the demonstration of antibodies in the sera of patients with Burkitt's lymphoma. These serum antibodies were reactive with antigens on autologous lymphoma cells, as well as antigens on tissue culture cells derived from these tumors. A variety of different immunologic techniques, including immunofluorescence, immunodiffusion, and complement fixation, have been used to study the immune response to this tumor. Each patient's serum was found to react with his own tumor and with the tumors of other patients. Thus, common antigens have been demonstrated in tumors from different patients with Burkitt's lymphoma. Subsequent studies revealed that the antigens involved in these reactions were quite different, although all were induced by EBV. High incidences and titers of antibody also were detected in the sera of patients with carcinoma of the postnasal space, or infectious mononucleosis, but were seen less frequently in normal sera and sera from patients with other diseases.

The various types of antigens associated with the Burkitt's lymphoma system include the following:[37, 51, 82]

1. Antibodies to EBV-induced capsid antigens are detected by cytoplasmic fluorescence staining of acetone-fixed smears of lymphoblastoid cells. Antibodies to this antigen have no correlation with the clinical course and are found in normal sera as well as in the sera of patients with a wide variety of other diseases.

2. Antibodies to membrane antigens located on the cell surface or viable lymphoblastoid cells are demonstrated by immunofluorescence. These antigens are detected on cells of lymphoma biopsies, as well as on continuous cultures from them. They are not found on cells from bone marrow aspirates of patients with Burkitt's lymphoma, or on allogeneic lymph node cells or allogeneic leukemia cells of various kinds. The clinical course of patients with Burkitt's lymphoma appears to correlate with the antibody to membrane antigens, in that high titers are found with regression of Burkitt's lymphoma but tend to decrease with recurrence of disease.

3. Antibodies to EBV-induced early antigens are demonstrated by immunofluorescence in acetone-fixed lymphoblastoid cells shortly after infection with concentrates of EBV. Antibodies to these antigens are found primarily in the sera of patients with Burkitt's lymphoma, nasopharyngeal carcinoma, and infectious mononucleosis who have active disease.

4. Antibodies to the precipitating antigen are detected by immunodiffusion reactions with an antigen prepared by concentrates of lymphoblastoid cells derived from Burkitt's lymphoma. These antibodies also are found in sera from patients with active disease and may disappear from the serum following regression of Burkitt's lymphoma but reappear with recurrence of the disease.

5. Antibodies to a nuclear antigen are found in some sera. This antigen is present in all cells carrying the EBV genome.

Thus, there are a wide variety of serologic responses to EBV-induced antigens in patients with Burkitt's lymphoma, infectious mononucleosis, and carcinoma of the postnasal space.

In addition to antitumor antibodies, cell-associated immune responses to Burkitt's lymphoma have been demonstrated by delayed hypersensitivity reactions to autologous tumor extracts.

Malignant Melanoma

Malignant melanoma is a disease whose clinical behavior might lead one to expect that it is influenced by immunologic factors.[30, 63] Clinical observations possibly indicative of the importance of host immunity in malignant melanoma include the following: unexpec-

tedly high rate of spontaneous regressions; observations that transfusions of blood from patients with spontaneous regression sometimes induce regressions of malignant melanoma in recipients of the transfusions; and reports that therapeutic cross-transplantation of tumors and sensitized leukocytes is sometimes successful.

Direct experimental evidence of immunologic factors in malignant melanoma was provided by Morton and Malmgren,[63] who demonstrated a common tumor antigen in malignant melanoma that was immunogenic in patients with this disease. These initial immunofluorescence studies were soon confirmed and extended by a variety of immunologic techniques, including colony inhibition, immune cytotoxicity, and complement fixation. The sera of patients with malignant melanoma contained antibodies that were reactive with their own autologous melanoma cells but that would also frequently cross-react with melanomas from other patients. These cross-reactions suggested the presence of a common melanoma antigen shared by most or all malignant melanomas. Immunofluorescence studies revealed this antigen to be intracytoplasmic, but cross-reactions observed by the membrane-immunofluorescence test[66] and by immune cytolysis indicated that a common antigen also was found at the cell surface. Lewis and his associates[56] presented evidence of a second group of cell-surface antigens in human melanomas that are individually distinct for each melanoma, in addition to the common melanoma antigen just described.

There appears to be a correlation between the clinical status of the melanoma patient and the incidence of antimelanoma antibodies in his serum. Patients with a localized melanoma were more likely to have antibody in their sera than those patients with disseminated disease.[56, 66] Furthermore, in some patients who were observed frequently throughout their clinical course, the antibody disappeared from the serum as the disease progressed.

Antimelanoma antibodies also were found in lower incidence and titer in the sera of normal blood bank donors. These findings cannot be adequately explained at the present time. However, all animal neoplasms induced by the same virus are known to contain the same tumor-specific antigens; therefore, it is possible that the observed sharing of antigens among melanomas may similarly indicate a common viral etiology. The reactivity of normal sera then would be explainable by antibodies produced in response to an asymptomatic infection with this hypothetical melanoma virus or a closely related agent.

Additional evidence for a common melanoma-specific antigen was provided by studies of cellular immunity using the lymphocyte microcytotoxicity tests[34, 103] and delayed hypersensitivity reactions in skin tests of melanoma patients with their own autologous tumor extracts.[18, 42] Cellular immunity was demonstrable by microcytotoxicity tests regardless of the clinical status of the patient,[34] whereas the skin test reactivity appeared to be correlated with the stage of disease. The cross-reactivity observed between one patient's melanoma and another patient's lymphocytes by the microcytotoxicity technique supports the presence of common cell-surface antigens among human malignant melanomas.

Neuroblastoma

An immune response to neuroblastomas in children has been suspected from clinical observations because of the unusually high incidence of spontaneous regressions of these neoplasms and the observations that even inadequate tumor therapy frequently results in tumor regression. Hellstrom[36] used the colony inhibition technique exclusively in immunologic studies with this neoplasm. Lymphocytes from patients with neuroblastomas were found to inhibit in vitro colony formation of the malignant cells regardless of whether the tumor cells were tested against autologous lymphocytes or the lymphocytes from other patients so afflicted. Furthermore, the lymphocytes from mothers of children with neuroblastoma produced inhibition of the neoplastic cells in tissue culture regardless of whether the explanted tumor cells were obtained from their own offspring or from other children. These results suggest either that neuroblastomas are induced by a virus that infects both mothers and children or that mothers may be immunized during pregnancy by antigens from the fetal tumors. Subsequent studies revealed that the blood lymphocytes from these patients were found to inhibit neuroblastoma cells independently, whether the lymphocytes were derived from patients with active disease or from those who were symptom-free following therapy. However, sera from patients with active disease could specifically nullify the inhibitory effect of the lymphocytes upon the neuroblastoma cells, while such inhibition was absent from sera of patients free of disease. In addition, sera from patients who were tumor-free were sometimes directly cytotoxic to neuroblastoma cells, although these cytotoxic sera were never capable of blocking the cytotoxic effect of the lymphocytes upon the tumor cells. Furthermore, when cytotoxic sera were mixed with known blocking sera, they would inhibit the blocking effect of such sera on cytotoxic lymphocytes; thus, they were called "blocking sera."[36]

Human Sarcomas: Soft Tissue and Skeletal Sarcomas

Immunofluorescence studies of human osteosarcomas by Morton and Malmgren[68] initially demonstrated the presence of specific antibody in the sera of these patients that was reactive not only with each patient's own osteosarcoma, but also with the osteosarcomas of other patients. Shortly thereafter, these studies were extended to other types of human skeletal and soft tissue sarcomas, and an antigen was found that was common to all types of sarcomas regardless of histologic type. Subsequent investigations by complement fixation, immune cytotoxicity, colony inhibition, and lymphocyte transformation confirmed the presence of a common antigen shared by all histologic types of human sarcomas.[14, 34, 66, 109]

A possible relationship between the sarcoma antigen and an infectious agent was suggested by the observation of a high incidence of antibody to this an-

tigen in the sera of immediate family members and close friends of sarcoma patients.[6, 14, 68] The presence of a common antigen in human sarcomas, by analogy with animal virus-induced tumors, as well as the presence of antibodies in close associates of sarcoma patients, suggested that the antigen might be viral-induced. Tissue culture cell lines were established from several different histologic types of skeletal and soft tissue sarcomas in order to further investigate this hypothesis.

The viral hypothesis was strengthened by finding that one of the cell lines, derived from a liposarcoma, contained Type C viral particles morphologically similar to the avian and murine sarcoma viruses.[68] Furthermore, cell-free filtered extracts of the original sarcomas, or tissue cultures derived from human sarcomas, consistently induced the formation of the new sarcoma antigen on normal human embryonic fibroblasts in tissue culture.[15] Moreover, some extracts induced morphologic alterations in these fibroblastic cultures.[68] Collectively, these observations strongly suggest the association of the virus with human sarcomas, but the role of this agent in the etiology of these neoplasms remains to be proved.[14]

Additional immunologic studies using complement fixation techniques were undertaken to determine whether there was any relationship between the antisarcoma antibody titer and the clinical status of the malignant disease.[66] Serial serum samples were obtained from tumor-bearing patients and assayed for antisarcoma antibodies. Analysis of sera from patients who enjoyed long-term survival after treatment for sarcoma showed a persistently elevated antisarcoma antibody titer (Fig. 6). Little variation was noted, and persistence of antibody was evident three to four years after removal of the primary tumor.

Analysis of sera obtained from patients before and after surgery showed that in those who had treatment and remained free of recurrence, antisarcoma antibody titers rose after surgery and remained elevated

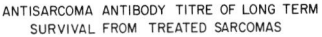

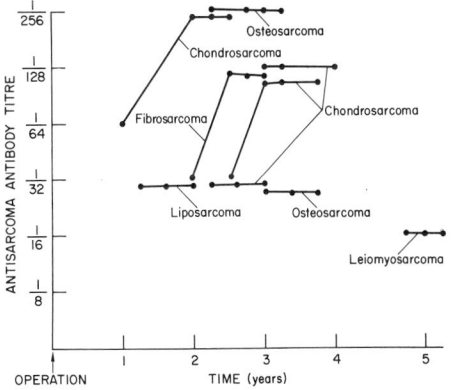

Figure 6. Antisarcoma antibody titers determined by complement fixation against the HuSA-1 liposarcoma antigen. Serial serum samples obtained following resection of the primary sarcoma in patients who remained free of disease. (From Morton, D. L., et al.: Ann. Surg., 172:740, 1970.)

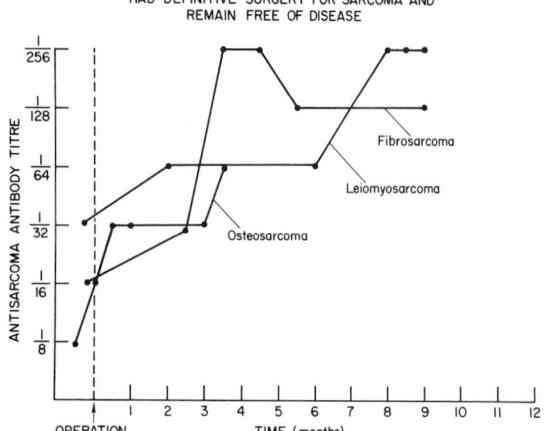

Figure 7. Antisarcoma antibody titers determined by complement fixation against the HuSA-1 liposarcoma antigen. Serial serum samples obtained following resection of the primary sarcoma in patients who remained free of disease. (From Morton, D. L., et al.: Ann. Surg., 172:740, 1970.)

(Fig. 7). In contrast, studies of a group of treated patients in whom metastatic disease subsequently developed revealed that although in some cases the titers rose after surgery, the titer of antisarcoma antibody declined in all cases as the disease became widespread (Fig. 8). Furthermore, antisarcoma antibody titers increased and remained elevated in patients who had pulmonary resections for metastatic sarcomas and subsequently remained free of disease. However, in those patients in whom resections were done and additional pulmonary metastases subsequently developed, the titers declined to nondetectable levels.

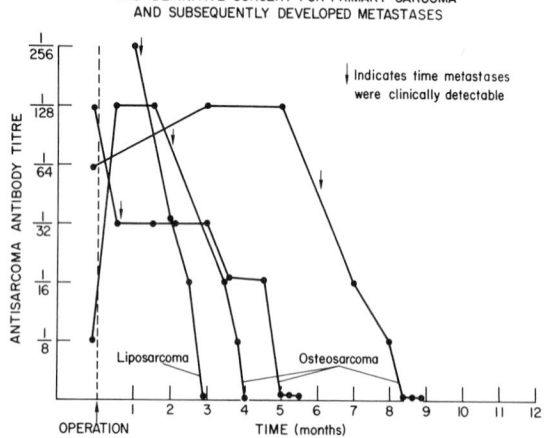

Figure 8. Antisarcoma antibody titers determined by complement fixation against the HuSA-1 liposarcoma antigen. Serial serum samples obtained following resection of the primary sarcoma in patients in whom recurrent disease with pulmonary metastases developed. The time at which pulmonary metastases were detected on the chest x-ray is indicated by arrows. (From Morton, D. L., et al.: Ann. Surg., 172:740, 1970.)

Although it is unclear from available data whether the antisarcoma antibody titer fell before or after the development of radiologically detectable metastasis, patients with progressive metastatic disease have always shown a progressive decline in their antisarcoma antibody titers. Thus, a remarkable correlation has been observed between the antibody titer and the clinical course of patients with human skeletal and soft tissue sarcomas.

Other Types of Human Neoplasms

Immunologic studies with a wide variety of other types of human neoplasms, including leukemias and carcinomas of the colon,[22, 34] breast, lung, endometrium, ovary, testis, bladder, and kidney, indicated the presence of an active humoral and cellular immune response to these neoplasms.[7, 34] These studies consistently demonstrated the presence of immune reactions directed against each patient's own neoplasm. Cross-reactions were seen with antigens found in other neoplasms of the same histologic type, but not with tumors of different histologic types. Immunologic reactions were not seen, however, against control cultures of normal tissues derived from patients whose tumors were reactive.

The possibility that isoantigens to normal HLA histocompatibility antigens or blood group antigens could be the explanation for these findings was excluded by the observation that a reaction could be demonstrated against each patient's own autologous tumor cells, as well as the tumor cells of other patients. Furthermore, reactions were observed with tumor cells, but not with normal control tissues derived from the same patient, when one patient's serum or lymphocytes were tested against the tumor and normal control tissues of other patients.

ORIGIN AND SIGNIFICANCE OF HUMAN TUMOR ANTIGENS

Thus, it appears that most, if not all, human cancers contain tumor-associated antigens capable of inducing a host immune response. Each patient's serum antibodies or lymphocytes react not only with his own tumor but also with other tumors of the same histologic type from different patients. There are several possible explanations for the observation that tumors of the same histologic types have cross-reacting antigens, while tumors of different histologic types do not.

Tissue or Organ-Specific Antigens

The existence of organ-specific antigens that are capable of being autoantigenic are well known for organs such as thyroid and brain, where they are associated with thyroiditis and encephalomyelitis. Other tissue-specific antigens also probably exist in other organs and may be found in tumor cells derived from these organs. In most cases, it is not possible to exclude tissue-specific immune responses from tumor-specific activity in human neoplasms.

Fetal Antigens

Fetal antigens could be the explanation for many of the cross-reactions observed between tumors of the same histologic type, since these antigens may be tissue- or organ-specific, detectable on malignant or embryonic cells, but not expressed on normal adult cells. In fact, this explanation appears to be correct for some of the common antigens found in colonic carcinomas and for the oncofetal antigen present in a large number of different types of human cancer.[46] The carcinoembryonic antigens may result either from derepression of gene products normally found only in the embryonic state or from the failure of the cancer cell to form certain normal cellular components that normally mask these fetal antigens. It is important to note that such antigens may be viral-induced, since a virus could be responsible for turning on production of the fetal antigen or for turning off the synthesis of some hypothetically masking, normal cell-surface constituents.

Viral-Induced Antigens

All animal neoplasms, regardless of histologic type, induced by a given virus, share a common tumor antigen. This antigen is different from the tumor antigens associated with neoplasms induced by other viruses. By analogy with animal virus-induced neoplasms, it is possible that the common antigens found in human neoplasms of the same histologic type are due to a common viral etiology. Although there are no data at this time that adequately prove or disprove this hypothesis, the common antigens in Burkitt's lymphoma are induced by the Epstein-Barr virus. Also, the findings with human sarcomas strongly suggest a viral-associated antigen. This explanation would explain both the high incidence of antibodies in the relatives and close associates of sarcoma patients, and the lower frequency and titer of antibodies in normal blood bank donor sera. The observations of cytotoxic lymphocytes in the blood of mothers of patients with neuroblastoma would also be compatible with the hypothesis. The concept of a fetal antigen being responsible for these immunologic reactions in mothers of patients with neuroblastoma cannot explain this finding in associates of sarcoma patients, however.

IMMUNOPREVENTION OF CANCER

Tumor transplantation experiments in laboratory animals have clearly demonstrated that immunization prior to tumor challenge is much more effective in inhibiting tumor growth than immunotherapy initiated after a neoplasm is established and growing. Thus, immunoprophylaxis should be more successful than immunotherapy.

The prevention of a viral-induced cancer by immunologic means could be based upon immunization against either the oncogenic virus itself or against the tumor-specific antigens of the viral-induced neoplasm. Nonspecific enhancement of the immune response by immune adjuvants or specific immunization with tumor-specific antigens might also be effective against neoplasms induced by physical or chemical carcinogens.

Theoretically, it should be possible to develop a vaccine prepared from purified tumor-specific antigens to prevent certain types of human neoplasms, since all neoplasms of the same histologic type share common tumor antigens.[69] Similarly, a viral vaccine could be developed *if* human neoplasms are caused by an oncogenic virus and *if* this virus could be isolated. However, the practical application of this approach is hampered by two basic problems. First, each different histologic type of neoplasm appears to have a different tumor-specific antigen, and it would be necessary to develop a vaccine for each neoplasm arising from every organ site such as breast, colon, or lung. Secondly, it is unlikely that all human neoplasms are caused by the same virus. Therefore, it would probably be necessary to develop a separate vaccine for each type of viral-induced human neoplasm.

Unfortunately, preventive immunization with a vaccine prepared from either tumor-viral antigens or tumor-specific antigens would take many decades to develop and to test because of the intrinsic characteristics of human cancer. The incidence of each individual tumor type is quite low, and the latency period for most human neoplasms is probably quite long, based upon measurable growth rates. For example, carcinoma of the breast typically occurs between the ages of 30 and 70. Thus, if one wanted to test a vaccine against breast cancer, its effectiveness could not be reasonably assessed in less than two decades. For these reasons, a preventive vaccine based upon specific immunization against cancer is an unrealistic short-term goal.[69]

In contrast, a tumor vaccine based upon nonspecific immunization might be feasible much sooner. Well-documented animal studies have shown that nonspecific stimulation of the immune response by agents such as BCG significantly decreases the development of many different types of spontaneous neoplasms in several strains of mice. These agents also increase immune reactivity against a wide variety of antigens in viral and chemical carcinogen-induced neoplasms.[3, 79] Furthermore, animal studies suggest that BCG may actually prevent the outgrowth of neoplastic cell clones even when immunization is carried out after infection with oncogenic viruses. Therefore, nonspecific stimulation of the immune response would have a great advantage over a specific vaccine, since theoretically it could be effective against all types of human neoplasia.[69] It would seem, then, that nonspecific immunization eventually may become useful for immunoprophylaxis against cancer in man. Preliminary evidence suggesting the validity of this approach comes from the studies of Rosenthal and associates,[93] who report a significant lowering of acute leukemia incidence in children receiving BCG vaccine when compared to control groups.

IMMUNOTHERAPY FOR HUMAN CANCER

Numerous attempts at immunotherapy for human cancer have been undertaken since the turn of the century. Although an occasional striking regression was obtained, in most cases the results were not impressive or consistent, and confidence in this treatment modality declined until recently. However, studies of the past decade generated increasing evidence for the participation of immune responses in human cancer and have stimulated new interest in immunotherapy.

Surgery as Immunotherapy

Cancer surgery is perhaps the most frequently used form of immunotherapy. Present evidence suggests that the effectiveness of the host's immune defenses is limited because the growing neoplasm seems to be able to evade an immune attack by producing specific and nonspecific immunosuppression in the cancer patient to enhance its growth. The growing neoplasm constantly sheds soluble tumor-associated antigens into the blood and these antigens circulate alone or as antigen-antibody complexes. These serum antigens can inhibit the lymphocyte-mediated destruction of tumor cells in vitro and may play a similar role in vivo.[36] In addition to this tumor antigen-specific blocking, a growing neoplasm often causes a nonspecific and generalized suppression of the cancer patient's immune competence. Humoral factors produced by or in response to the neoplasm can be found in the sera of cancer patients and are thought to be the cause of the general immune depression. These concepts are illustrated in Figure 9. The extent of the immunosuppression correlates with the stage of disease and level of tumor burden; it is reversible by removal of the growing neoplasm. Therefore, any therapeutic maneuver that lowers tumor burden may reverse both specific and nonspecific immunosuppression and alter the immune balance in favor of the patient. In this respect, cancer surgery is immunotherapy because it effectively removes the cancer cell mass that produces the immunodepression and allows the patient's immune responses to recover.

Once the tumor mass has been removed, the immune mechanisms may deal with the clinically silent micrometastases present in many patients with presumably localized solid tumors. These host defenses are quite capable of destroying small numbers of tumor cells on the order of 1 to 10 million, but not masses of 100 million or more. Unfortunately, the metastatic foci present in most patients are too great for the host's natural immune defenses and progressive growth will occur. Therefore, many attempts have been made to further stimulate the patient's immune response against his cancer by a variety of methods. These methods will be discussed under the following general classifications: (1) *Nonspecific immunotherapy:* Nonspecific stimulation of the immune system in an attempt to increase the patient's response to his tumor. (2) *Active immunotherapy:* Active immunization with tumor cell vaccines in an attempt induce specific autoimmunity against cancer. (3) *Passive immunotherapy:* Administration of lymphoid cells or antiserum from another host that has been specifically immunized against the patient's cancer tissues in an attempt to increase the cancer patient's level of immunity.

Nonspecific Stimulation of the Immune Response

The rationale for this method of immunotherapy is based upon the observation that certain substances, such as mixed bacterial toxins and fractions of the tubercle bacillus, have the ability to nonspecifically stimulate host resistance to most viral, fungal, and bacterial agents. The exact mechanism of action is unknown, but it does appear to increase the immune responses to a wide variety of antigens, including tumor-specific antigens.

One of the earliest and most impressive examples of this type of therapy was Coley's series of experiments at the turn of the century.[74] Coley became interested in the possible therapeutic value of nonspecific immune therapy when a patient with a recurrent inoperable sarcoma of the neck enjoyed a seven-year regression after two attacks of erysipelas. Coley next attempted to produce erysipelas in patients with recurrent cancer. This led him to develop Coley's toxins. The toxins were combinations of living or heat-killed streptococcus and *Bacillus prodigiosus* that were mixed in varying proportions and then injected directly into a tumor or, in some cases, were given intravenously. Impressive regressions and long-term cures were attributed to these agents, even though more recent experiments with similar preparations were never as impressive.

BCG. In the past few years, attenuated tubercle bacillus or BCG has been used in the treatment of patients with acute leukemia and malignant melanoma. Mathé reported a significant improvement in survival in patients with acute leukemia who were treated with BCG vaccine after complete remissions had been induced by standard chemotherapeutic agents.[59]

Morton and his colleagues treated patients by direct injection of BCG vaccine into metastatic nodules of malignant melanoma.[67] Regressions of the tumor nodule occurred only in patients who were immunologically competent. The criterion for cellular immune competence was based upon the patient's ability to display a hypersensitivity response to DNCB and/or a positive tuberculin test reaction after initiation of treatment. Approximately 90 per cent of the melanoma nodules directly injected with BCG were observed to regress. Moreover, the nodules at sites distant from the BCG inoculation also regressed in approximately 20 per cent of patients who were immunologically

CANCER   SURGERY   AS   IMMUNOTHERAPY

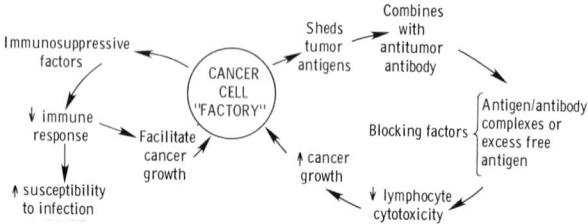

Figure 9. Schematic depiction of a method by which the cancer cell "factory" could enhance its own growth by producing immunosuppression of the host. Since cancer surgery removes the cancer cell "factory," the site of production of specific antigen and nonspecific immunosuppressants, the host immune response is allowed to return to normal function.

competent. Patients showing regression of uninjected nodules had disease remission of one to seven years.[70] Response to immunotherapy in these patients also was associated with a rising titer of antimelanoma antibodies. Sequential biopsies of tumor nodules following BCG inoculation revealed regression of these nodules to be associated with a granulomatous infiltration of lymphocytes, monocytes, and fibroblasts surrounding and infiltrating the melanoma cells (Fig. 10).

Additional studies indicated that the response to immunotherapy in melanoma patients occurred primarily in those whose disease was limited to the skin, subcutaneous tissue, and regional lymph nodes.[70] Patients who had large amounts of tumor metastatic to the parenchymal organs, such as the lung, liver, and brain, generally had little response to BCG immunotherapy. However, from the natural history of malignant melanoma in man, we know that many of these patients who seemed to have disease limited to the skin and subcutaneous tissues when initially seen also

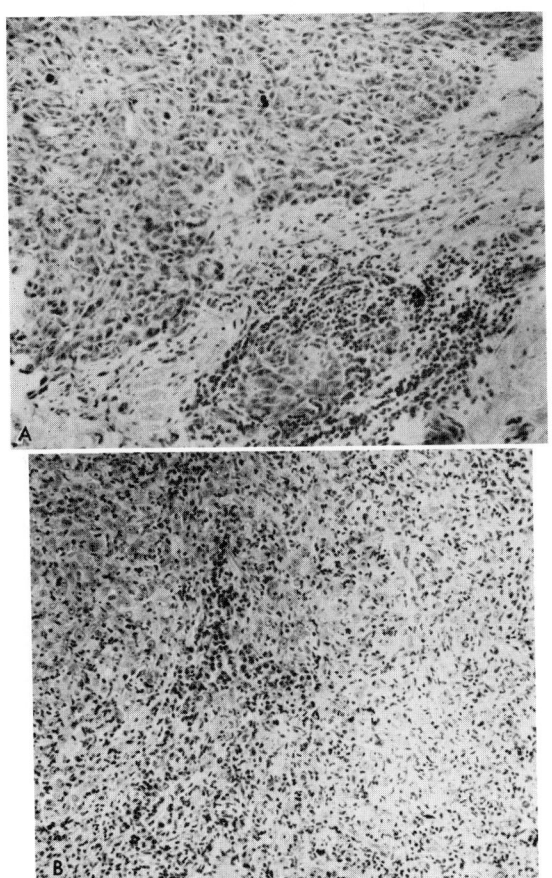

Figure 10. *A*, Subcutaneous metastases of malignant melanoma prior to immunotherapy with BCG. Note the absence of lymphocytic and monocytic infiltration among the tumor cells. *B*, Subcutaneous metastases which had decreased in size from 10 mm. to 5 mm. during the six-week period following immunotherapy with BCG injections into other melanoma nodules. This nodule was *not* injected with BCG. Note the marked lymphocytic and monocytic infiltration among the melanoma cells. (From Morton, D. L., et al.: Ann. Surg., *172*:740, 1970.)

had subclinical disease at metastatic sites in other organs. Since 15 to 20 per cent of these patients remained free of disease for long periods of time following BCG immunotherapy, we must conclude that the immunotherapy was successful in eliminating the smaller metastatic sites of melanoma in the parenchymal organs. Thus, BCG immunotherapy appears to have both a systemic and local effect. Of major significance, of course, is the fact that BCG immunotherapy of malignant melanoma demonstrates that a human cancer, even when disseminated, can be made to regress for long periods of time. This fact alone indicates the feasibility of cancer immunotherapy for subclinical microscopic disease in man.

Having demonstrated the effectiveness of BCG immunotherapy in patients with Stage III malignant melanoma, studies were undertaken to determine the usefulness of BCG immunotherapy as an adjunct to primary surgical resection of regional lymph node metastases in malignant melanoma. Patients who have metastases to the regional nodes in this disease have a high incidence of distant clinically silent micrometastases that will result in an 80 per cent recurrence rate within five years. However, postoperative immunotherapy with BCG appears to significantly lower the recurrence rate in these patients, as shown in Figure 11.[16]

There is currently great interest in the use of BCG as an adjuvant to surgical resection and chemotherapy of malignant disease.[73] Intralesional BCG has been effective in the treatment of intradermal local recurrences of breast carcinoma following mastectomy. Recent reports by McKneally and associates[60] described the use of intrapleural BCG administered as a surgical adjunct following pulmonary resection for lung cancer. Preliminary analysis of recurrence and survival data indicate that intrapleural BCG has a definite beneficial effect. Extensive data from M. D. Anderson Hospital and Tumor Institute by Gutterman, Hersh, and their associates[30] suggest that BCG effectively prolongs the remission rate following surgery or chemotherapy for a variety of solid tumors, including colon cancer, breast carcinoma, and malignant melanoma. MER, a methanol extractable residue of BCG, is a nonliving extract that appears to have some of the antitumor activity of the living organism.[110]

The mechanism of tumor regression following immunotherapy with BCG in melanoma is unclear. BCG does not have direct antitumor activity, because it does not cause tumor regression in tuberculin-negative patients. Both specific and nonspecific immune reactions are probably involved. BCG is known to be a potent immunologic adjuvant capable of increasing host immune response to a wide variety of tumor-specific antigens. Nevertheless, the fact that the observed regressions of melanoma only occurred after direct injection of nodules in tuberculin-positive patients suggests that a large part of the antitumor effect is nonspecific and results from the delayed hypersensitivity reaction occurring within the melanoma nodule. In addition, a specific immune response to the melanoma antigens also occurs in some patients, since the appearance of lymphocyte infiltrates and regression of uninjected melanoma nodules observed in these

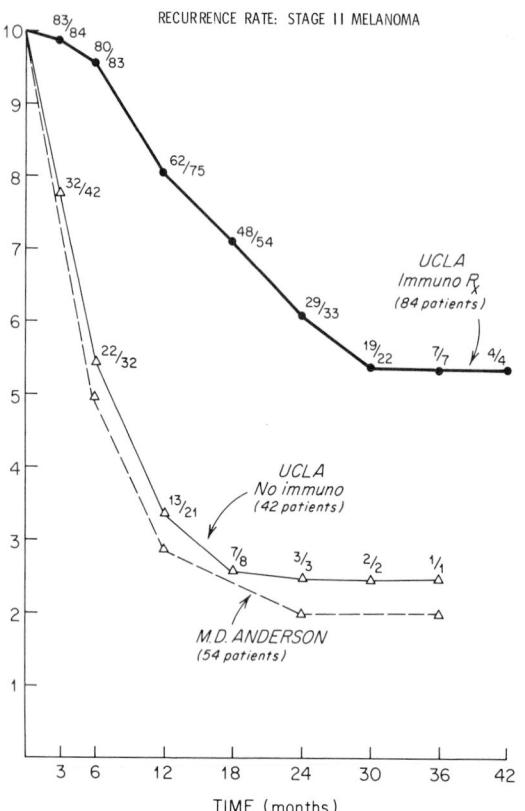

Figure 11. Recurrence rate, Stage II melanoma of Life Table Analyses comparing patients treated by immunotherapy with patients treated by operation alone. Numbers separated by slash (/) indicate number of patients free of disease/over number of patients at risk of recurrence during that time interval. (Reprinted, by permission, from Eilber, F. R., Morton, D. L., Holmes, E. C., Sparks, F. C., and Ramming, K. P.: Adjuvant immunotherapy with BCG in treatment of regional lymph node metastases from malignant melanoma. N. Engl. J. Med., 294:237, 1974.)

patients accompanied the rising titer of antimelanoma antibodies.

DNCB and Other Local Immunotherapeutic Agents. Other evidence that the induction of delayed hypersensitivity reactions by any agent (DNCB, BCG, or PPD) results in tumor regression in tumor nodules or tumor tissue comes from the studies of Klein in patients with basal and squamous cell carcinomas of the skin.[49] The induction of delayed hypersensitivity reactions to DNCB in these neoplasms resulted in the resolution of more than 90 per cent of multiple superficial basal cell or squamous cell carcinomas. The deeper squamous cell lesions responded similarly, though some required a second course of immunotherapy or surgical excision to effect complete cure. Interestingly, the intensity of the inflammatory reaction to DNCB correlated directly with the degree of malignancy of the lesions. Malignant lesions responded more intensely than premalignant lesions, which in turn reacted more vigorously than normal skin.

Corynebacterium parvum. Corynebacterium parvum is a gram-positive anaerobic organism. In contrast to

BCG, C. parvum is not used as a viable organism, but is formalin- or heat-killed.[47, 75, 95] Also in contrast to BCG, it can be administered intravenously. C. parvum is a potent macrophage stimulator but a strong T-cell suppressor when given intravenously. Conversely, when injected intradermally or intralesionally, it is a T-cell stimulator. Therefore, the mechanism of action is determined, once more, by the route of administration in another of the immunostimulating agents. C. parvum, like BCG, is very effective when given intralesionally, and has been shown to be effective when combined with tumor cells and injected into a region that is drained by the same lymph nodes that drain the tumor. It has been used effectively as a surgical adjuvant in animals, but there is less clinical experience available for its use in man. C. parvum has been evaluated extensively as an adjunct to chemotherapy by Israel and his associates,[47] who have reported that this agent increased both the incidence of remissions and the duration of remissions in patients. Patients receiving C. parvum maintained their immunologic competence better than those who received chemotherapy alone and had a prolonged survival. Additional clinical trials with this interesting agent are currently underway.[75]

Levamisole. Levamisole is a recently discovered immunotherapeutic agent that seems to have an entirely different mechanism of action from C. parvum and BCG. Levamisole is a chemical compound that was originally developed as an antihelmintic and has been used extensively in Western Europe and other parts of the world to treat intestinal infestations in man. Its effect on the immune system was discovered by accident. There has been some reluctance to prescribe it as a nonspecific immunostimulating agent, since it appears to have little effect on the intact normal immune system. The most dramatic effects have been seen in certain patients who have a depressed immune function. In these instances, Levamisole has been shown to enhance macrophage chemotaxis and return T-cell levels to normal. It appears to augment depressed delayed cutaneous hypersensitivity reactions in man and seems to improve symptomatology of systemic lupus, rheumatoid arthritis, and herpes simplex.

Two of many extensive clinical trials are of sufficient duration to merit mention. Rojas reported an impressive increase in the disease-free interval and survival in patients with locally unresectable breast cancer treated by radiation therapy and levamisole.[91] Another study used levamisole as a surgical adjuvant following pulmonary resection for lung cancer.[1] There appeared to be an impressive difference between the control group and the patients treated with levamisole, particularly in those patients who had large primaries, vascular invasion, or regional lymph node metastasis. Clinical trials are currently being undertaken with levamisole, BCG, and C. parvum to determine their use as nonspecific immunotherapeutic agents in man.[75]

Active Immunotherapy Using Tumor Cell Vaccines

Numerous attempts have been made to immunize patients against their own tumors or tumors of similar histologic types. The rational basis for this approach is the assumption that a growing neoplasm does not induce a maximal immune response to the tumor-specific antigens it contains. Efforts have been made to increase the patient's immunity by altering the tumor antigens in such a way that they become more antigenic, or by stimulating the patient's lymphoreticular system with adjuvants that improve his immune system capabilities.

In model experiments with animal neoplasms, immunologic adjuvants, such as BCG vaccine or Freund's adjuvant, act as potent stimulants of the immune system and can enhance resistance to neoplastic growth (Fig. 12). Similar autoimmunization procedures to autologous tumor cells have been used to stimulate immune responses against human cancer (Fig. 13). However, the results obtained from clinical application of active immunotherapy have not been impressive for patients with advanced disease. Studies of patients with earlier disease may improve these results considerably.[71]

Efforts to increase the antigenicity of tumor vaccines have included alteration of the antigen by treatment with neuraminidase[39] by freeze-thaw techniques, by heating, and by the addition of a highly antigenic carrier protein. The theoretical basis for the latter approach was dependent upon experiments with other weakly antigenic substances. It was found that an immune response could be elicited from a normally nonantigenic substance if this substance was coupled with a highly antigenic protein carrier. The antibodies formed against this complex were specifically directed against the previously nonantigenic substance, as well as the foreign protein portion of the complex. Preliminary reports, using rabbit gamma globulin as a carrier protein attached to autologous tumor cells, suggested some therapeutic benefit, but more recent studies with a large number of patients have failed to confirm the effectiveness of the therapy.

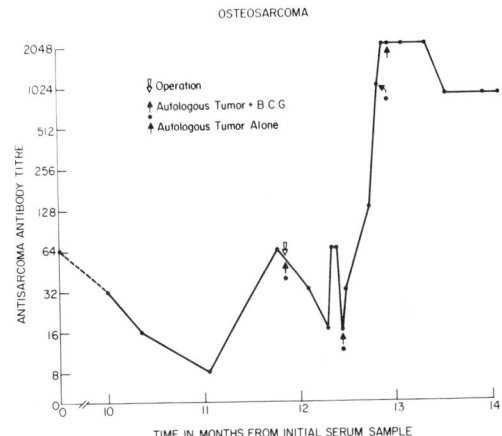

Figure 13. Antisarcoma antibody titers determined by complement fixation against the HuSA-1 liposarcoma antigen on serial serum samples from a 14-year-old boy with a primary osteosarcoma of the right femur in whom pulmonary metastases developed 10 months after resection of the primary, for which a left pneumonectomy was performed and immunotherapy initiated. (From Morton, D. L., et al.: Ann. Surg., 172:740, 1970.)

Studies with animal neoplasms have shown that living tumor cells administered intradermally in numbers insufficient for progressive growth are generally the most effective immunogens. Until recently, the possibility of growth at the inoculation site has inhibited the use of live tumor cell vaccines in man. However, it would seem that in certain tumors that share common tumor antigens, such as skeletal and soft tissue sarcomas, one patient could be immunized with an allogeneic vaccine of living tumor cells from another patient. An immune response would then be induced against the foreign HLA transplantation antigens on the tumor cells causing their rejection. In addition, this immunization should induce a strong immune reponse against a common cross-reacting tumor-specific antigen. Our experience with such live allogeneic tumor cell vaccines has confirmed their safety and effectiveness in skeletal and soft tissue sarcomas (Fig. 14).[108] A vaccine composed of irradiated allogeneic leukemia cells combined with BCG has been shown to prolong the remission rate in acute leukemia by Mathé and associates[59] and in acute myeloblastic leukemia by Powles[86] and by Holland and Bekesi.[39]

Passive or Adoptive Immunotherapy

Since patients with cancer develop two types of immune responses to their neoplasms, humoral antibodies and cell-mediated immune responses, passive immunotherapy is logically based upon the administration of either antitumor serum or lymphoid cells.

Current dogma in tumor immunology suggests that cell-mediated immune responses are primarily responsible for tumor cell destruction and that humoral antibodies play a secondary role. In some cases the humoral antibodies are thought to enhance tumor

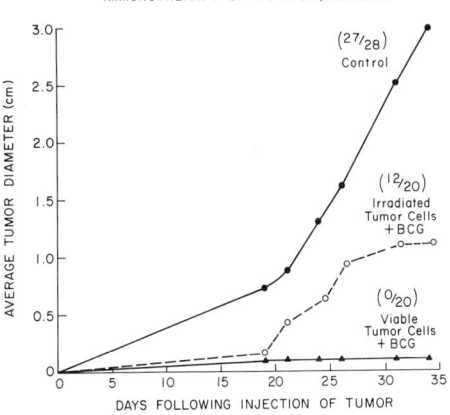

Figure 12. Immunotherapy experiments with a transplantable liposarcoma in syngeneic strain 2 guinea pigs: 1×10^5 liposarcoma tumor cells were inoculated intramuscularly into the leg and immunotherapy was initiated intradermally in four sites on the back with 1×10^6 living of 1×10^7 irradiated tumor cells mixed with BCG. (From Morton, D. L., et al.: Ann. Surg., 172:740, 1970.)

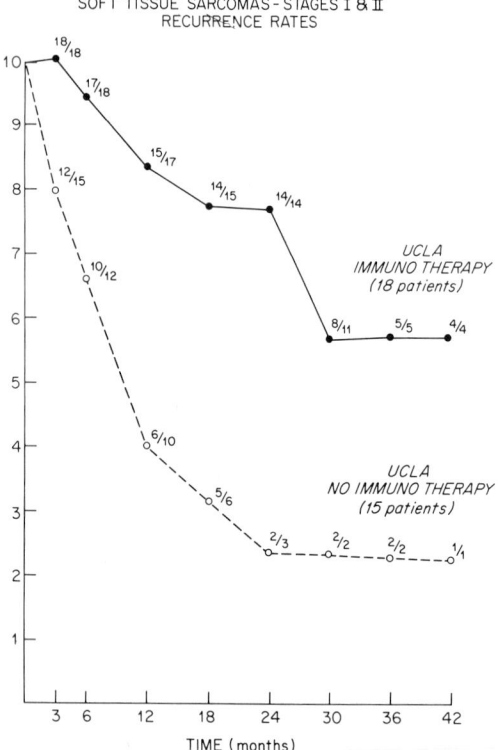

SOFT TISSUE SARCOMAS – STAGES I & II
RECURRENCE RATES

Figure 14. Time to recurrence in soft tissue sarcomas, Stages I and II by Life Table Analyses. Numbers separated by slash (/) indicate number of patients free of disease/over number of patients at risk of recurrence during that time interval. (From Townsend, C. M., Jr., Eilber, F. R., and Morton, D. L.: Skeletal and soft tissue sarcomas: Results of treatment with adjuvant immunotherapy. J.A.M.A., 1976, in press.)

growth because of their ability to inhibit cellular immunity. Therefore, most recent attempts at passive or adoptive immunotherapy have employed lymphoid cells.

Passive immunotherapy of human cancer with antiserum produced in a foreign species has been tried over the years, but the results have been discouraging. Such antiserum was usually very toxic because it contained antibodies against normal tissue antigens of the host. However, this problem may be resolved with the successful isolation and purification of tumor-specific transplantation antigens from human cancers so that the antisera produced will have specificity directed against the tumor-specific transplantation antigens of the tumor cells. Another potential source of antiserum may be from those patients cured of the malignant condition who demonstrate high titers of cytotoxic antibodies, or antibodies that are capable of conferring the antibody-dependent cell-mediated cytotoxicity reactions on normal lymphocytes. In some animal tumor systems, such antiserum has been shown to be effective for inducing regression of established tumors. Although not currently effective for

human cancer, this method of immunotherapy should receive more serious consideration in the future.[113]

The possibility for adoptive immunotherapy using lymphoid cells or fractions of lymphoid cells has stimulated a great deal of interest. In animal studies with highly inbred mice, experiments have indicated that transferred lymphocytes which persist in the host have a significant immunotherapeutic effect. However, this practice is difficult to apply in man, because of rejection due to HLA differences between the donor and the recipient. Several clinical studies have been performed in an effort to induce remissions in cancer patients with lymphocytes from patients who have undergone a complete remission. Sumner and Foraker reported one of the only successes by this means when they transfused a melanoma patient with whole blood from a second patient who had undergone a complete remission.[104]

Another method of immunotherapy with specifically sensitized lymphocytes has been undertaken in the following manner. Patients with incurable cancer were paired according to blood type and tumor type. Tumors from patients in Group A were transplanted subcutaneously to patients in Group B, and vice versa. Following sensitization to each other's tumor, transfusions of peripheral lymphocytes from patients in Group B to patient in Group A, or vice versa, were begun and continued daily for variable periods of time. The response rate following this type of immunotherapy from three groups of investigators was approximately 15 to 20 per cent.[43, 53, 72] The logistic difficulties of this type of immunotherapy and the relatively low response rate make it unlikely that it will be used much in the future.

One particularly appealing method for adoptive immunotherapy concerns the transfer of information molecules that arouse a specific immune response in the recipient's own immune system. The two reported substances that apparently have this remarkable ability are Lawrence's transfer factor[55] and the immune RNA described by Pilch. Recent reviews of the use of these substances in immunotherapy have been published.[57, 85] Use of such extracts from lymphoid cells is particularly attractive, because they do not contain HLA specificities and, therefore, are not rejected by the recipient.

Immune RNA is an informational molecule that is extracted from the lymphoid organs of specifically sensitized donors. It is capable of transferring immunologic capabilities to unsensitized lymphocytes. A heterologous species, such as the sheep, is immunized with human tumor cells and the resultant RNA that is formed is extracted from the sheep lymph nodes. This extract is used for immunotherapy. Immune RNA generated in this manner is capable of transferring the ability to kill tumor cells to normal lymphocytes in vitro. In essence, the immune RNA instructs the lymphocytes to destroy the tumor cells. A number of trials are now ongoing to evaluate the effects of immune RNA on a variety of human neoplasms. At the present time, it is known that immune RNA is well tolerated in humans, although it is too early to draw any definite conclusions.[85]

Transfer factor is also capable of transferring immunity from one human to another.[55] Extracted from human leukocytes, it can transfer immunity against skin grafts, tuberculosis, and a variety of antigens. Transfer factor is effective for treating certain immune deficiency diseases, chronic fungal infections, and certain viral illnesses. It has been used in a variety of clinical trials for human cancer, including malignant melanoma, breast cancer, renal cell carcinoma, and sarcoma.[57] However, the results to date are mostly anecdotal, although sufficiently encouraging to result in a design for prospective clinical trails. Since the activity of transfer factor cannot be evaluated except in man, there is considerable difficulty in standardizing this agent; however, it is theoretically very appealing for cancer therapy.

Thus, a large amount of data has accumulated during the past few years implicating the immune response as an important component of the host-tumor interaction. Results from several clinical trials indicate that immunotherapy may be a useful adjunct to other forms of cancer therapy, such as operation and chemotherapy. It has become clear that immunotherapy as it is currently used has limited effectiveness as a single therapeutic modality. Obviously, its rational application to human cancer must depend upon a better knowledge of the nature of tumor-specific antigens in human neoplasms and of the host's response to these antigens. Our knowledge of the clinical application of immunotherapy is still quite limited, and there are many unknown factors to be defined, such as optimum dose of the immunotherapeutic agents, the optimum duration of treatment, and even its basic mechanisms of action. Nevertheless, the future of immunotherapy for human cancer is bright, and results should improve as more is learned about the immune response to cancer.

At the present, nonspecific immunotherapy with BCG vaccine and with *C. parvum* is clinically useful in certain specific situations in the treatment of malignant melanoma, skin cancer, lung cancer, and leukemia.

CANCER IMMUNITY: PRESENT STATUS AND FUTURE SIGNIFICANCE

During the past decade, it has become increasingly apparent that cancer cells have acquired new antigens during neoplastic transformation that are not found in their normal counterparts. These antigens may be of many different types.

Fetal antigens are those substances produced as a result of dedifferentiation and reversion of the cell to a primitive embryonic state. These embryonic antigens are constituents of the normal fetus during embryonic development, but their production is repressed in the normal adult organ. The participation of the fetal antigens in terms of the tumor-host relationship is unclear. However, they probably have their greatest importance as a diagnostic tool to detect malignancy at its earlier stage before other diagnostic findings occur, or to detect recurrence of a neoplasm following surgical treatment and thereby provide the basis for further therapy.

Other types of tumor-associated antigens that play a major role in tumor-specific immunity include those antigens located on the cell surface. In the case of viral-induced neoplasms, these antigens are common to all neoplasms induced by the same virus. Another class of tumor-specific antigens that frequently appear in chemical carcinogen-induced neoplasms are individually distinct for each neoplasm. Many neoplasms appear to possess both common and individually specific tumor antigens.

Human cancers, like animal neoplasms, appear to contain tumor-associated antigens that are capable of eliciting a specific immune response in the cancer patient. There is considerable clinical evidence that the cancer patient's immune response to these tumor-specific antigens is important in controlling the growth of his neoplasm. Some of these clinical observations that are readily explainable on an immune basis are: (1) There are well-documented instances of spontaneous regression or prolonged remissions of human neoplasms. (2) Immunodeficiency, either congenital or acquired, is associated with an increased incidence of cancer. (3) Cancer patients in whom immunodeficiency develops have more rapidly growing neoplasms and poor prognosis.

Laboratory studies indicate the importance of the patient's specific immune response to these tumor-specific antigens. Serologic studies reveal a remarkable correlation between the titers of antitumor antibody and clinical course in patients with melanomas and sarcomas.

Lymphocytes specifically sensitized to tumor-specific antigens appear to be present at all stages of malignant disease. However, it is likely that their effectiveness in mediating inhibition of tumor cell growth is dependent upon circulating serum factors, which are probably antigen-antibody complexes or free antigens that inhibit the activity of sensitized lymphocytes. These blocking factors, found in the sera of patients with growing tumors, can be neutralized by specific antibodies frequently found in the sera of patients who are free of malignant disease. Thus, both cellular and humoral immune responses are probably important in controlling the growth of human cancer.

Quantitative factors are very important in the tumor-host relationship, since immunity against cancer is relative rather than absolute. An immune response is quite effective for destroying small numbers, 1 to 10 million, of tumor cells, whereas 100 million cells almost uniformly result in progressive tumor growth. Since a neoplasm only 1 cm. in diameter contains approximately a billion tumor cells, by the time most tumors are clinically detectable they have already outgrown the patient's immune defenses. Surgical therapy, radiation therapy, and chemotherapy may owe their effectiveness to the role they play in reducing tumor mass to a level that can be controlled by host immunity. Evidence for this hypothesis comes from observations that cancer cells are often found in the washings of operative wounds, in the regional lymphatics, or circulating in the blood of patients who are cured of their neoplasms by local removal of the tumor mass or local radiation therapy. Thus, it appears likely that much of the success of cancer therapy is dependent upon the effectiveness of the patient's immune response. It is not surprising, therefore, that patients who are defective in their cell-mediated immune responses are likely to have a poor prognosis after cancer operations.

Many empiric attempts at immunotherapy of human cancer have been made in the past, employing active and passive immunization. Although an occasional impressive regression may have resulted from these attempts, the therapeutic potential of immunotherapy is in its earliest stages of development at the present time. Obviously, the rational application of immunotherapy to human cancer will depend, to a large extent, upon a better knowledge of the nature of tumor-specific antigens in human neoplasms and methods for increasing the immune response against these antigens. Since it has been difficult or impossible to cause regression of large established tumors in animals by immunologic means, it is unlikely that immunotherapy alone will ever play the major role in the treatment of cancer. Furthermore, by the time most tumors are clinically detectable, they have already outgrown the patient's immune defenses, and it is unlikely that immunotherapy alone will ever bolster host defenses sufficiently to reverse this process in the patient with advanced disease. However, immunotherapy is a logical adjunct to definitive surgery for several reasons:

1. Patients who have only a small focus of cancer cells remaining after surgical removal of the bulk of tumor are those most likely to benefit from immunotherapy, because the tumor mass that must be destroyed by host responses is smallest at that time.

2. The specificity of the immune response for cancer cells provides a possible therapeutic tool that will have selectivity for small foci of cancer cells not possible with other currently available treatment modalities, such as chemotherapy or irradiation.

3. Surgical patients are most likely to respond to any immunotherapeutic maneuvers, since the cancer patient's general immunologic competence is greatest when the disease is localized.

4. Immunotherapy would be expected to complement rather than interfere with other currently available methods for managing cancer recurrences following operation, such as irradiation and chemotherapy.

5. Since both irradiation and chemotherapy are immunosuppressive agents, immunotherapy should logically precede these treatment modalities. However, both of these modalities have been shown to induce an intensified immune response when immunization is carried out under special conditions. Therefore, with increasing knowledge of the influence of these agents upon the immune mechanisms and their more rational application, the results of cancer therapy may correspondingly improve.

Evaluation of the cell-mediated immunologic reactivity in cancer patients may provide a more rational basis for future control of malignant disease. Presumably, such information would be helpful in planning immunotherapy, since active immunization in an immunologically competent patient and passive immunotherapy in an anergic patient would appear to have the greatest potential for success.

SELECTED REFERENCES

Burnet, F. M.: The concept of immunologic surveillance. Prog. Exper. Tumor Res., *13*:1, 1970.
Dr. Burnet, a Nobel laureate, discusses the concept of immunologic surveillance. According to this concept, the immune system functions as a policing mechanism for detecting and eliminating neoplastic cells that develop as a result of spontaneous mutation or under the influence of carcinogens. Since these cells develop tumor-specific antigens on their surfaces, they elicit an immune response that leads to their rejection.

Everson, T. C., and Cole W. H.: Spontaneous Regression of Cancer. Philadelphia, W. B. Saunders Company, 1966.
This monograph discusses in considerable detail the well-documented cases of spontaneous regression of human cancer.

Hellstrom, K. E., and Hellstrom, I.: Lymphocyte-mediated cytotoxicity and blocking serum activity to tumor antigens. Adv. Immunol., *18*:209, 1974.
Lymphocytes specifically cytotoxic to their own tumor cells in tissue culture can be demonstrated in the blood of most cancer patients. The presence of these cytotoxic lymphocytes cannot be correlated with the stage of disease. However, patients with growing neoplasms were found to have factors in their serum that specifically inhibit the cytotoxic effect of lymphocytes on tumor cells. This paper discusses these factors, which may be circulating antigen-antibody complexes.

Morton, D. L.: Cancer immunotherapy: An overview. Sem. Oncol., *1*:297, 1974.
Since the early 1900's, the concept that immunity to cancer might be acquired in the same manner as immunity to infectious diseases has formed an important concept of the biology of neoplastic disease. This paper reviews the basic rationale for immunity against cancer in man and the possible usefulness of this knowledge in the therapy of cancer. The use of BCG as immunotherapy for malignant melanoma is discussed.

Schwartz, R. S.: Another look at immunologic surveillance. N. Engl. J. Med., *293*:181, 1975.
Dr. Schwartz's interesting paper expresses concern that the "modern" theory of immune surveillance is in danger of being accepted as "fact" rather than theory. He suggests that a theory must be challenged by experiments designed to refute its validity until no challenge remains.

Shuster, J., Liverstone, A., Banjo, C., Silver, H. K. B., Freedman, S. O., and Gold, P.: Immunologic diagnosis of human cancers. Am. J. Clin. Pathol., *62*:243, 1974.
The authors review the concept of fetal antigens and their possible usefulness in diagnoses of cancer. Fetal antigens are substances produced as a result of the dedifferentiation and reversion of the cell to a primitive embryonic state. The embryonic or fetal antigens are constituents of the normal fetus during embryonic development, but their production is repressed shortly after birth, and they are not found in the normal adult. However, during neoplastic transformation, there is reversion of the cell to an embryonic state with renewed production of these fetal antigens. Therefore, these antigens have great importance as a possible diagnostic tool to detect malignancy at its earlier stage before other diagnostic findings occur, or to detect recurrence of a neoplasm following surgical treatment and thereby provide a basis for further therapy.

Reviews of cancer immunology may be consulted for a more detailed discussion of the immunobiology of neoplastic disease:

Golub, S. H.: Host immune response to human tumor antigens. *In* Becker, F. F. (Ed.): Cancer—A Comprehensive Treatise. Vol. 4. New York, Plenum Press, 1975, pp. 259–300.

Malmgren, R. A., and Morton, D. L.: Viral and immunologic studies of human neoplasms. Pathobiol. Ann., *63*:81, 1971.

Old, L. J., and Boyse, E. A.: Antigens of tumors and leukemias induced by virus. Fed. Proc., *24*:1009, 1965.

Pilch, Y. H., Meyers, G. H., Jr., Sparks, F. C., and Golub, S. H.: Prospects for the Immunotherapy of Cancer. Part I: Basic Concepts of Tumor Immunology. Current Problems in Surgery. Chicago, Year Book Medical Publishers, Inc., 1975.

Pilch, Y. H., Myers, G. H., Jr., Sparks, F. C., and Golub, S. H.: Prospects for the Immunotherapy of Cancer. Part II: Current Status of Immunotherapy. Current Problems in Surgery. Chicago, Year Book Medical Publishers, 1975.

Southam, C. M.: Areas of relationship between immunology and clinical oncology. Am. J. Clin. Pathol., *62*:224, 1974.

REFERENCES

1. Amery, W.: Immunopotentiation with Levamisole in resectable bronchogenic carcinoma: A double-blind controlled trial. Br. Med. J., 3:461, 1975.
2. Arseneau, J. C., Sponzo, R. W., Schnipper, L. E., Bonner, H., Young, R. C., Canellos, G. R., Johnson, R. E., and DiVita, V. T.: Nonlymphomatous malignant tumors complicating Hodgkins disease. N. Engl. J. Med., 287:1119, 1974.
3. Bast, R. C., Zbar, B., Borsos, T., and Rapp, H. J.: BCG and cancer. N. Engl. J. Med., 290:1413, 1974.
4. Berkelhammer, J.: In vitro testing in tumor immunotherapy. Sem. Oncol., 1:397, 1974.
5. Black, M. M. Opler, S. R., and Speer, F. D.: Structural representations of tumor-host relationships in gastric carcinoma. Surg. Gynecol. Obstet., 102:599, 1956.
6. Boddie, A. W., Jr., Urist, M. M., Townsend, C. M., Jr., Holmes, E. C., and Morton, D. L.: Cellular immunity to tumor-associated antigens in sarcoma patients and their relatives. Surg. Forum, 36:154, 1975.
7. Bubenik, J., Perlmann, P., Helmstein, K., and Moberger, G.: Cellular and humoral immune responses to human urinary bladder carcinomas. Int. J. Cancer, 5:310, 1970.
8. Burnet, F. M.: Immunological Surveillance. New York, Pergamon Press, 1970.
9. Chretian, P. B., Catalona, W. G., Twomey, P. L., and Sample, W. F.: Correlation of immune reactivity and clinical status in cancer. Ann. Clin. Lab. Sci., 4:331, 1974.
10. DeVries, J. E., Cornain, S., and Rumke, P.: Cytotoxicity of non-T versus T-lymphocytes from melanoma patients and healthy donors on short- and long-term cultured melanoma cells. Int. J. Cancer, 14:427, 1974.
11. Dhar, P., Moore, T. L., Zamcheck, N., and Kupchik, H.: Carcinoembryonic antigen (CEA) in colonic cancer.: Use in pre- and postoperative diagnosis and prognosis. J.A.M.A., 221:31, 1972.
12. Edynak, E. M., Old, L. J., Vrana, M., and Lardis, M. P.: A fetal antigen associated with human neoplasia. N. Engl. J. Med., 286:1178, 1972.
13. Eilber, F. R., Nizze, A., and Morton, D. L.: Sequential evaluation of general immune competence in cancer patients: Correlation with clinical course. Cancer, 35:660, 1975.
14. Eilber, F. R., and Morton, D. L.: Etiology of human skeletal and soft tissue sarcomas: A summary of immunologic and virologic studies. In Bones and Joints. Baltimore, Williams & Wilkins, 1976.
15. Eilber, F. R., and Morton, D. L.: Immunologic studies of human sarcomas: Additional evidence suggesting an associated sarcoma virus. Cancer, 26:588, 1970.
16. Eilber, F. R., Morton, D. L., Holmes, E. C., Sparks, F. C., and Ramming, K. P.: Adjuvant immunotherapy with BCG in treatment of regional lymph node metastases from malignant melanoma. N. Engl. J. Med., 294:237, 1976.
17. Everson, T. C., and Cole, W. H.: Spontaneous Regression of Cancer. Philadelphia, W. B. Saunders Company, 1966.
18. Fass, L., Herberman, R. B., Ziegler, J. L., et al.: Cutaneous hypersensitivity reactions to autologous extracts of malignant melanoma cells. Lancet, 1:116, 1970.
19. Finney, J. W., Byers, E. H., and Wilson, R. H.: Studies in tumor autoimmunity. Cancer Res., 20:351, 1960.
20. Foley, E. J.: Antigenic properties of methylcholanthrene-induced tumors in mice of the strain of origin. Cancer Res., 13:835, 1953.
21. Gallo, R. C., and Todaro, G. J.: Oncogenic RNA viruses. Sem. Oncol., 3:81, 1976.
22. Gold, P., and Freedman, S. O.: Specific carcinoembryonic antigens of the human digestive system. J. Exp. Med., 122:467, 1965.
23. Gold, P.: The role of immunology in human cancer research. Can. Med. Assoc. J., 103:1043, 1970.
24. Golub, S. H.: Host Immune Response to Human Tumor Antigens. New York, Plenum Press, 1975.
25. Golub, S. H., O'Connell, T. X., and Morton, D. L.: Correlation of in vivo and in vitro assays of immune competence. Cancer. Res., 34:1833, 1974.
26. Grace, J. T., Jr., and Kondo, T.: Investigations of host resistance in cancer patients. Ann. Surg., 148:633, 1958.
27. Graham, J. B., and Graham, R. M.: Antibodies elicited by cancer in patients. Cancer, 8:409, 1955.
28. Green, M., and Wold, W. S. M.: Oncogenic DNA viruses: Replica-

29. tion, tumor gene expression, and role in human cancer. Sem. Oncol., 3:65, 1976.
29. Gupta, R. K., and Morton, D. L.: Suggestive evidence for in vivo binding of specific antitumor antibodies of human melanomas. Cancer Res., 35:58–62, 1975.
30. Gutterman, J. U., Mavligit, G. M., and Hersh, E. M.: Chemoimmunotherapy of human solid tumors. Med. Clin. North Am., 60:441, 1976.
31. Hakala, T. R., and Lange, P. H.: Serum induced lymphoid cell-mediated cytotoxicity against human transitional cell carcinomas of the urinary tract. Science, 184:795, 1974.
32. Hakala, T. R., Lange, P. H., Castro, A., Elliott, A., Fraley, E. E.: Cell-mediated cytotoxicity against human transitional cell carcinomas of the genitourinary tract. Cancer, 34:1929, 1974.
33. Harder, F. H., and McKhann, C. F.: Demonstration of cellular antigens on sarcoma cells by an indirect ^{125}I-labeled antibody technique. J. Natl. Cancer Inst., 40:231, 1968.
34. Hellstrom, I., Hellstrom, K. E., Sjogren, H. O., and Warner, G. A.: Demonstration of cell-mediated immunity to human neoplasms of various histological types. Int. J. Cancer, 7:1, 1971.
35. Hellstrom, I., Sjogren, H. O., Warner, G. A., and Hellstrom, K. E.: Blocking of cell-mediated tumor immunity by sera from patients with growing neoplasms. Int. J. Cancer, 7:226, 1971.
36. Hellstrom, K. E., and Hellstrom, I.: Lymphocyte mediated cytotoxicity and blocking serum activity to tumor antigens. Adv. Immunol., 18:209, 1974.
37. Henle, G., and Henle, W.: Immunofluorescence in cells from biopsy specimens and tissue cultures. J. Natl. Cancer Inst., 39:1027, 1967.
38. Hibbs, J. B., Lambert, L. J., and Remington, J. S.: Possible role of macrophage mediated nonspecific cytotoxicity in tumor resistance. Nature (New Biol.), 235:48, 1972.
39. Holland, J. F., and Bekesi, J. G.: Immunotherapy of human leukemia with neuraminidase-modified cells. Med. Clin. North Am., 60:539, 1976.
40. Holmes, E. C., Kahan, B. D., and Morton, D. L.: Soluble tumor-specific transplantation antigens from methylcholanthrene-induced guinea pig sarcomas. Cancer, 25:373, 1970.
41. Holmes, E. C., and Golub, S. H.: Immunologic defects in lung cancer patients. J. Thorac. Cardiovasc. Surg., 71:161, 1976.
42. Holmes, E. C., Roth, J. A., and Morton, D. L.: Delayed cutaneous hypersensitivity reactions to melanoma antigen. Surgery, 78:160, 1975.
43. Humphrey, L. J., Lincoln, P. M., and Griffen, W. O., Jr.: Immunologic response in patients with disseminated cancer. Ann. Surg., 168:374, 1968.
44. Irie, K., Irie, R. F., and Morton, D. L.: Evidence for in vivo reaction of antibody and complement to surface antigens of human cancer cells. Science, 186:454, 1974.
45. Irie, K., Irie, R. F., and Morton, D. L.: Detection of antibody and complement complexed in vivo on membranes of human cancer cells by mixed hemadsorption. Cancer Res., 35:1244, 1975.
46. Irie, R. F., Irie, K., and Morton, D. L.: A membrane antigen common to human cancer and fetal brain tissues. Cancer Res., 36:3510, 1976.
47. Israel, L., and Edelstein, R. L.: Nonspecific Immunostimulation with Corynebacterium parvum in Human Cancer. Baltimore, Williams and Wilkins, 1974.
48. Kaliss, N.: Immunological enhancement of tumor homografts in mice. A review. Cancer Res., 18:992, 1958.
49. Klein, E., Holtermann, O., Milgrom, H., Case, R. W., Klein, D., Rosner, D., and Djerassi, I.: Immunotherapy for accessible tumors utilizing delayed hypersensitivity reactions and separated components of the immune system. Med. Clin. North Am., 60:389, 1976.
50. Klein, G.: The Epstein-Barr virus and neoplasia. N. Engl. J. Med., 293:1353, 1975.
51. Klein, G., Clifford, P., Klein, E., Smith, R. T., Minowada, J., Kourilsky, F. M., and Burchenal, J. H.: Membrane immunofluorescence reactions of Burkitt's lymphoma cells from biopsy specimens and tissue cultures. J. Natl. Cancer Inst., 39:1027, 1967.
52. Klein, G., Sjogren, H. O., Klein, E., and Hellstrom, K. E.: Demonstration of resistance against methylcholanthrene-induced sarcomas in the primary autochthonous host. Cancer Res., 20:1561, 1960.

53. Krementz, E. T., and Samuels, M. T.: Tumor cross-transplantation and cross-transfusion in the treatment of advanced malignant disease. Bull. Tulane Univ. Med. Fac., 26:263, 1967.

54. Krupey, J., Gold, P., and Freedman, S. O.: Purification and characterization of carcinoembryonic antigens of the human digestive system. Nature, 215:67, 1967.

55. Lawrence, H. S.: Transfer factor. Adv. Immunol., 11:195, 1969.

56. Lewis, M. G., Ikonopisov, R. L., Nairn, R. C., Phillips, T. M., Fairley, H. G., and Bodenham, D. C.: Tumour-specific antibodies in human malignant melanoma and their relationship to the extent of the disease. Br. Med. J., 1:547, 1969.

57. LoBuglio, A. F., and Neidhart, J. A.: Transfer factor: A potential agent for cancer therapy. Med. Clin. North Am., 60:585, 1976.

58. Mach, J. P., Jaeger, P., Bertholet, M. M., Ruegsigger, C. H., Loosli, R. M., and Pettavel, J.: Detection of recurrence of large-bowel carcinoma by radioimmunoassay of circulating carcinoembryonic antigen (CEA). Lancet, 2:535, 1974.

59. Mathé, G., Amiel, J. L., Schwarzenberg, L., Schneider, M., Cattan, A., Schliemberger, J. R., Hayat, M., and deVassal, F.: Active immunotherapy for acute lymphoblastic leukemia. Lancet, 1:697, 1969.

60. McKneally, M. F., Maver, C., and Kausel, H.: Regional immunotherapy of lung cancer with intrapleural BCG. Lancet, 1:377, 1976.

61. Moore, D. H.: Mammary Tumor Virus. New York, Plenum Press, 1975.

62. Morton, D. L.: What's new in cancer therapy? Bull. Am. Coll. Surg., 62:1977, in press.

63. Morton, D. L., Malmgren, R. A., Holmes, E. C., and Ketcham, A. S.: Demonstration of antibodies against human malignant melanoma by immunofluoresence. Surgery, 64:233, 1968.

64. Morton, D. L., Miller, G. F., and Wood, D. A.: Demonstration of tumor-specific immunity against antigens unrelated to the mammary tumor virus in spontaneous mammary adenocarcinomas. J. Natl. Cancer Inst., 42:289, 1969.

65. Morton, D. L.: Acquired immunological tolerance and carcinogenesis by the mammary tumor virus. I. Influence of neonatal infection with the mammary tumor virus on the growth of spontaneous mammary adenocarcinomas. J. Natl. Cancer Inst., 42:311, 1969.

66. Morton, D. L., Holmes, E. C., Eilber, F. R., and Wood, W. C.: Immunological aspects of neoplasia: A rational basis for immunotherapy. Ann. Intern. Med., 74:587, 1971.

67. Morton, D. L., Eilber, F. R., Malmgren, R. A., and Wood, W. C.: Immunological factors which influence response to immunotherapy in malignant melanoma. Surgery, 68:158, 1970.

68. Morton, D. L., Malmgren, R. A., Hall, W. T., and Schidlovsky, G.: Immunologic and viral studies in human sarcomas. Surgery, 66:152, 1969.

69. Morton, D. L.: Horizons in tumor immunology. Surgery, 74:69, 1973.

70. Morton, D. L., Eilber, F. R., Holmes, E. C., Hunt, J. S., Ketcham, A. S., Silverstein, M. J., and Sparks, F. C.: BCG immunotherapy of malignant melanoma: Summary of a seven-year experience. Ann. Surg., 108:635, 1974.

71. Morton, D. L., Eilber, F. R., Joseph, W. L., Wood, W. C., Trahan, E., and Ketcham, A. S.: Immunological factors in human sarcomas and melanomas: A rational basis for immunotherapy. Ann. Surg., 172:740, 1970.

72. Nadler, S. H., and Moore, G. E.: Clinical immunologic study of malignant disease; response to tumor transplants and transfer of lymphocytes. Ann. Surg., 164:482, 1966.

73. Nathanson, L.: Use of BCG in the treatment of human neoplasms: A review. Sem. Oncol., 1:337, 1974.

74. Nauts, H. C., Fowler, G. A., and Bogatko, F. H.: A review of the influence of bacterial infection and of bacterial products (Coley's toxins) on malignant tumours in man. Acta Med. Scand., S276:5, 1953.

75. Oettgen, H. F., Pinsky, C. M., and Delmonte, L.: Treatment of cancer with immunomodulators: Corynebacterium parvum and Levamisole. Med. Clin. North Am., 60:511, 1976.

76. Old, L. J., and Boyse, E. A.: Antigens of tumors and leukemias induced by virus. Fed. Proc., 24:1009, 1965.

77. Old, L. J., Boyse, E. A., Clark, D. A., and Carswell, E. A.: Antigenic properties of chemically-induced tumors. Ann. N.Y. Acad. Sci., 101:80, 1962.

78. Old, L. J., Boyse, E. A., and Stockert, E.: Antigenic properties of experimental leukemias. I. Serological studies in vitro with spontaneous and radiation-induced leukemias. J. Natl. Cancer Inst., 31:977, 1963.

79. Old, L. J., Benacerraf, B., Clark, D. A., Carswell, E. A., and Stockert, E.: The role of the reticuloendothelial system in the host reaction to neoplasia. Cancer Res., 21:1281, 1961.

80. Oren, R. K., and Herberman, R. B.: Delayed cutaneous hypersensitivity reactions to membrane extracts of human tumor cells. Clin. Exp. Immunol., 9:45, 1971.

81. O'Toole, C., Stejskal, V., Perlmann, P., and Karlsson, M.: Lymphoid cells mediating tumor-specific cytotoxicity to carcinoma of the urinary bladder. Separation of the effector population using a surface marker. J. Exp. Med., 139:437, 1974.

82. Pearson, G., Dewey, F., Klein, G., Henle, G., and Henle, W.: Relation between neutralization of Epstein-Barr virus and antibodies to cell membrane antigens induced by the virus. J. Natl. Cancer Inst., 45:989, 1970.

83. Penn, I.: Chemical immunosuppression and human cancer. Cancer, 34:1474, 1974.

84. Pilch, Y. H., and Ramming, K. P.: Transfer of tumor immunity with ribonucleic acid. Cancer, 26:630, 1970.

85. Pilch, Y. H., Fritze, D., and Kern, D. H.: Immune RNA in the immunotherapy of cancer. Med. Clin. North Am., 60:567, 1976.

86. Powles, R.: Immunologic maneuvers in management of acute leukemia. Med. Clin. North Am., 60:463, 1976.

87. Prehn, R. T., and Main, J. M.: Immunity to methylcholanthrene-induced sarcomas. J. Natl. Cancer Inst., 18:769, 1957.

88. Prehn, R. T.: The immune reaction as a stimulator of tumor growth. Science, 176:170, 1972.

89. Rapp, R.: Viruses as etiologic factors in cancer. Sem. Oncol., 3:49, 1976.

90. Roberts, S. S., Hengesh, J. W., McGrath, R. G., Valaitis, J., McGrew, E. A., and Cole, W. H.: Prognostic significance of cancer cells in circulating blood: A ten-year evaluation. Am. J. Surg., 113:757, 1967.

91. Rojas, A. F., Feierstein, J. M., Mickiewicz, E., et al.: Levamisole in advanced human breast cancer. Lancet, 1:211, 1976.

92. Rosenau, W., and Morton, D. L.: Tumor-specific inhibition of growth of methylcholanthrene-induced sarcomas in vivo and in vitro by sensitized isologous lymphoid cells. J. Natl. Cancer Inst., 36:825, 1966.

93. Rosenthal, S. R., Crispin, R. G., Thorne, M., et al.: BCG vaccination and leukemia mortality. J.A.M.A., 222:1543, 1972.

94. Schwartz, R. S.: Another immunologic surveillance. N. Engl. J. Med., 293:181, 1975.

95. Scott, M. T.: Corynebacterium parvum as an immunotherapeutic anticancer agent. Sem. Oncol., 4:367, 1974.

96. Shearer, W. T., and Parker, C. W.: Humoral immunostimulation. V. Selection of variant cell lines. J. Exp. Med., 142:1133, 1975.

97. Shuster, J., Livingstone, A., Banjo C., Silver, H. K. B., Freedman, S. O., and Gold, P.: Immunologic diagnosis of human cancers. Am. J. Clin. Pathol., 62:243, 1974.

98. Silver, H. K. B., Gold, P., Feder, S., Freedman, S. O., and Shuster, J.: Radioimmunoassay for human alpha₁-fetoprotein. Proc. Natl. Acad. Sci. U.S.A., 70:526, 1973.

99. Silver, H. K. B., Gold, P., Javitt, N. B., Freedman, S. O., and Finlayson, N. C.: Alpha₁-fetoprotein in chronic liver disease. N. Engl. J. Med., 291:506, 1974.

100. Sjogren, H. O., Hellstrom, I., and Klein, G.: Transplantation of polyoma virus-induced tumors in mice. Cancer Res., 21:329, 1961.

101. Solomon, H. A., and Kreps, S. I.: Twenty-six years of survival following cancer of sigmoid with prolonged liver metastases. J.A.M.A., 144:221, 1950.

102. Southam, C. M., Brunschwig, W., Levin, A. G., and Dixon, Q. S.: The effect of leukocytes on transplantability of human cancer. Cancer, 19:1743, 1966.

103. Sulit, H. L., Golub, S. H., Irie, R. F., Grooms, G. A., and Morton, D. L.: Human tumor cells grown in fetal calf serum: Influences on the tests for lymphocyte cytotoxicity, serum blocking and serum arming effects. Int. J. Cancer, 17:461, 1976.

104. Sumner, W. C., and Foraker, A. C.: Spontaneous regression of human melanoma, clinical and experimental study. Cancer, 13:79, 1960.

105. Tatarinov, Y. S.: Content of embryo-specific alpha-globulin in the blood serum of human fetus, newborn, and adult man in primary cancer of the liver. Vopr. Med. Khim., 11:20, 1965.

106. The, T. H., Huiges, H. A., Schraffordt-Koops, H., Lamberts, H.

B., and Nieweg, H. O.: Surface antigens on cultured malignant melanoma cells as detected by a membrane immunofluorescence method with human sera. Lack of tumor-specific reactions on melanoma cells. Ann. N.Y. Acad. Sci., *257*:1296, 1975.

107. Thomson, D. M. P., Krupey, J., Freedman, S. O., and Gold, P.: The radioimmunoassay of circulating carcinoembryonic antigen of the human digestive system. Proc. Natl. Acad. Sci. U.S.A., *64*:161, 1969.

108. Townsend, C. M., Jr., Eilber, F. R., and Morton, D. L.: Skeletal and soft tissue sarcomas: Results of treatment with adjuvant immunotherapy. J.A.M.A., 1976, in press.

109. Vanky, F., Stjernsward, J., and Nilsonne, U.: Cellular immunity against human sarcoma. J. Natl. Cancer Inst., *47*:1145, 1971.

110. Weiss, D. W.: MER and other mycobacterial fractions in the immunotherapy of cancer. Med. Clin. North Am., *60*:473, 1976.

111. Wells, S. A., Melewicz, F. C., Christiansen, C., and Ketcham, A. S.: Delayed cutaneous hypersensitivity reactions to extracts of carcinomatous cells of the cervix uteri. Surg. Gynecol. Obstet., *136*:717, 1973.

112. Wilson, R. E., Hager, E. B., Hampers, C. L., Corson, J. M., Merrill, J. P., and Murray, J. E.: Immunologic rejection of human cancer transplanted with renal allograft. N. Engl. J. Med., *278*:479, 1968.

113. Wright, P. W., Hellstrom, K. E., Hellstrom, I., and Bernstein, I. D.: Serotherapy of malignant disease. Med. Clin. North Am., *60*:607, 1976.

114. Zamcheck, N., and Kupchik, H.: The interdependence of clinical investigations and methodological development in the early evolution of assays for carcinoembryonic antigen. Cancer Res., *34*:2131, 1974.

II

MALIGNANT MELANOMA

Loren J. Humphrey, M.D.

While skin cancer is the most common malignant tumor, it ranks relatively low in mortality. In general, this is due to the fact that basal cell and squamous cell carcinoma of the skin seldom contribute to death of the patient. Contrariwise, approximately 9000 cases of melanoma were diagnosed in 1975 and 5000 patients succumbed in its disseminated phase. Malignant melanoma is rare in individuals under 20 and occurs most commonly between the ages of 30 and 60. Statistics show an equal occurrence in men and women, although the survival is better for females. Caucasians are afflicted more frequently than blacks. For the lay person and indeed for the physician, other types of pigmented lesions create problems in early recognition.

PIGMENTED LESIONS

A fundamental problem for the patient, as well as the physician, is the existence of pigmented lesions of variable size, shade, and location normally found on the human body. Owing to the extreme variation in shades of color, the patient may present with concern over a brownish pigmented spot that is no more than a "freckle" of melanin accumulated as a result of the stimulating effect of sunlight. Obviously, this normal response to sunlight must not be confused with Hutchinson's melanotic freckle or true nevi. The decision by the clinician as to which pigmented lesion deserves biopsy for definitive histopathologic diagnosis requires a recognition at least of the types of nevi difficult to distinguish from malignant melanoma.

In general, *blue nevi* are small without distinctive pigmented color, whereas cellular blue nevi are noted for being more darkly pigmented. The competent pathologist has no problem in determining the benignancy of these lesions. Similarly, the so-called juvenile melanomas now referred to as *spindle* and *epithelioid cell nevi* are benign lesions that may present as pinkish to tan nodules. The most common form of nevus in the adult is the *intradermal nevus.* Pigment in the lesion varies so that the color of different nevi and within various areas of a single nevus may vary from dark tan to brown to gray and black. While these nevi are generally hairy, they may present as flat, raised, or rarely papillary in appearance. In contrast, the *junctional nevus* is slightly raised, if at all, and a tan-brown color without hair. Of all the nevi, this lesion is the most worrisome, in that, while benign as such, it is thought to give rise to malignant melanoma. Junctional nevi are more common in children and decrease with age.

In addition to nevi mentioned above, one must remember that seborrheic keratosis (Fig. 1) may present as a pigmented lesion; in addition, an occasional basal cell carcinoma may be pigmented. Finally, malignant melanoma, which is described as a flat, darkly pigmented lesion without hair, may present at times as a slightly raised lesion, a brown lesion, and even a lesion with hair (Fig. 2).

The average person has approximately 13 nevi; the clinician must recognize indications for excision or biopsy, since clearly all nevi need not be excised. Therefore, nevi that grow, change color, ulcerate, itch, or bleed, as well as those in an area of continual irritation such as bra line, belt line, and those on palms, feet, and genitals should be considered malignant melanoma until proved otherwise by histologic examination.

Appreciation of the various locations of primary

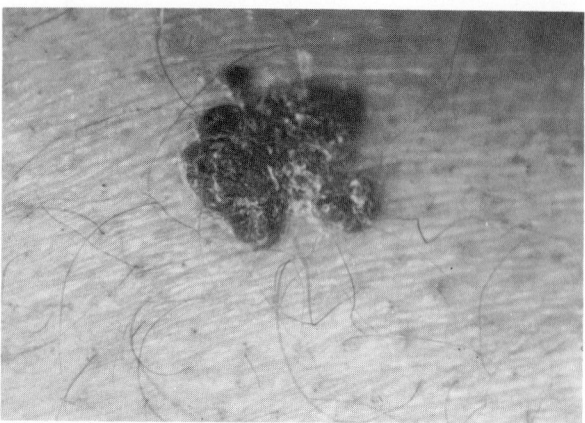

Figure 1. Seborrheic keratosis of the arm. Note slightly scaly effect over otherwise suspicious appearing melanoma.

TABLE 1. Life Table for All Patients with Melanoma by Site of Primary Lesion*

Location	Age Adjusted Survival	
	5 Years	10 Years
Head and Neck	32.9%	24.7%
Upper Extremity	37.5%	32.1%
Trunk	17.3%	6.8%
Lower Extremity	51.5%	43.3%

*From C. O. Knutson et al.; "Melanoma," in M. M. Ravitch, Current Problems in Surgery. Copyright © 1971 by Year Book Medical Publishers, Inc., Chicago. Adapted by permission.

malignant melanoma does not aid in diagnosis except as pointed out above, but survival rates definitely relate to location. Of the 95 per cent of patients presenting with an identifiable primary lesion, about 30 per cent present with melanoma on the lower extremity, 15 per cent on the upper extremity, and 35 per cent on the head and neck area and extracutaneous locations. The prognosis for the patient with malignant melanoma as it relates to location is shown in Table 1.

DIAGNOSIS

Microscopic examination of biopsy material is required to establish the diagnosis of malignant melanoma. Owing to difficulty with certain lesions, a pathologist with competence in this field is essential, and consequently the conscientious pathologist frequently obtains consultative opinions. The suspected

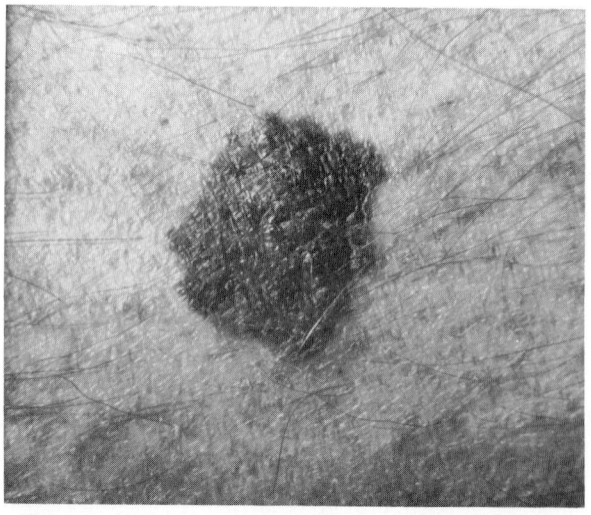

Figure 2. Malignant melanoma of the arm. Note variegated color in slightly raised lesion with a few hairs.

lesion is generally removed by excisional biopsy, including a margin of normal skin. In certain cosmetic areas such as the face, a punch biopsy may be obtained.

Consonant with a complete diagnosis is a thorough description of the lesion as to the level and depth of invasion. This microstaging of melanoma is essential in guiding the surgeon in a definitive surgical approach. The description of melanomas by level of extension in relation to histological landmarks as described by Clark et al.[2] has been related to survival. In their description, Level I involves the epidermis, Level II the upper papillary dermis, and Level III the entire papillary dermis, with even a few cells spreading into the reticular dermis. Level IV penetrates the reticular dermis, while Level V extends into the subcutaneous tissue. The current trend is to utilize this description in place of the previous categorization according to type, i.e., superficial spreading melanoma, nodular melanoma, and lentigo-maligna-melanoma. Recent data suggest that this latter categorization is of little value compared to description by levels, and at the same time, one must be aware of the limitations of determining depth of invasion by level. For example, a "Level I melanoma" is not truly malignant melanoma.

Furthermore, levels lose their significance somewhat when dermal papillae are quite elongated; in particular, skin from the sole of the foot, the knee, and the elbow frequently has indistinctly recognizable levels. Owing to these constraints, direct measurement of depth of invasion as described by Breslow[1] adds to the value of histologic microstaging. For comparison of Clark's levels versus depth of invasion, see Table 2.

With the diagnosis of malignant melanoma and information relative to depth of invasion of the primary, the physician must complete clinical staging preoperatively in order to finalize treatment plans. Stage I melanoma is confined to the primary site; in Stage II, in addition to the primary site, the melanoma has metastasized to regional lymph nodes. Melanoma that has spread to sites beyond the regional lymph nodes is classified as Stage III. Appropriate classification by stage requires the physician to re-examine with great care the lymph node area to which the primary is likely to drain. Obviously, those on the trunk may spread to one or more lymph node areas. Further, the precision in clinical staging is wanting, in that any but hard and enlarged nodes require excision to deter-

TABLE 2. Composite Measurements of the Mean Depth, Width and Cross-sectional Area (Product of Width Times Depth)*

Level		Free of Disease 5 Yrs.	Recurred or Metastasized
II	<0.76	45 (7)†	0
	0.76–1.50	7 (3)	2 (1)
III	<0.76	9 (3)	0
	0.76–1.50	7	5 (3) (1)‡
	1.51–2.25	4 (3)	1
	2.26–3.00	3 (2)	4 (1)
	>3.00	1 (1)	2 (1) (1)‡
IV	<0.76	0	0
	0.76–1.50	4 (2)	2
	1.51–2.25	9 (3)	5 (3) (1)‡
	2.26–3.00	0	6 (1)
	>3.00	2 (2)	11 (6) (4)‡
V	2.26–3.00	1	0
	>3.00	1	7

*From Breslow, A.: Ann. Surg., *182*:572, 1975.

†Number treated with prophylactic node dissection.

‡Number with positive nodes in prophylactic dissection. There is great heterogeneity with each group, especially in Levels III and IV.

mine accurately whether to classify the patient's disease as Stage I or Stage II. The physical examination should also concentrate on "in-transit melanoma" (skin and subcutaneous lesions between primary site and regional node area) as well as a search for distant subcutaneous nodules, lymphadenopathy in the other areas, and organomegaly.

Liver enzymes and chest x-ray complete the workup and should be performed in every patient with the diagnosis of malignant melanoma. Further search for disseminated disease is completed by brain, bone, and liver/spleen scans. On the other hand, owing to the expense and lack of precision of isotopic scans, one must exert judgment in the decision to order complete. survey of the body in search of metastases. Certainly in the patient with identifiable distant metastatic disease, a complete survey by isotopic scans is indicated. In addition, locally or regionally recurrent disease should prompt a complete survey, since aggressive surgery to control once again the disease would be modified in the presence of distant metastases. For

Stage I and II melanoma, the judgment to order a complete survey must be individualized, since Felix et al.[3] have shown that considerable error exists in the accuracy of isotopic scans in the patient free of symptoms.

TREATMENT

Appropriate therapy is determined by the preoperative workup as described above. Hence the surgeon has obtained a histologic diagnosis including the level and depth of invasion. Clinical staging by physical examination and scans when indicated determines if the patient's disease is "curable." Re-excision of the primary site with a 5-cm. margin to include the deep fascia is ideal treatment. Many authors point out that carrying the dissection below the deep fascia is not necessary. On the other hand, since in removing the primary lesion initially, the subcutaneous tissue was violated, generally to an uncertain depth, the deep fascia serves as a boundary below which previous dissection has not occurred. In addition, 5-cm. margins are impossible in the face, although one must still take very adequate margins of normal skin. For primary sites near regional lymph nodes, re-excision should be performed in continuity with the regional lymph node dissection. Since it is impossible to determine accurately if the patient is Stage I or II without submitting the lymph nodes to histologic examination, level and depth of invasion of the primary lesion should be used as determinants of possible spread. Hence, lymph node dissection is definitely indicated for Level II and III lesions with a depth of invasion of 1.0 mm. or greater. A careful scrutiny of the data reported by Wanebo et al.[10] emphasizes the problem facing the surgeon whose patient has a primary lesion with a depth of invasion of 0.6 to 1.0 mm.

Note particularly that of patients whose primary lesion had a measured depth of invasion from 0.6 to 1.0 mm., 9 per cent (2 of 22 patients) had regional lymph node metastases. Further note that the 5-year survival free of disease was 100 per cent. However, one must keep in mind that this survival rate was achieved by performing lymph node dissection. For this reason, we feel that good risk patients with potential spread to only one lymph node–bearing area and depth of invasion of at least 0.6 mm., should have

TABLE 3. Correlation Between the Measured Depth of Invasion and Incidence of Regional Node Metastases with Overall 5-Year Cure*

Clark's Level	1955–1964		January, 1972–March, 1974		Total	Per Cent Positive Nodes
	Positive Nodes	Number of Dissections	Positive Nodes	Number of Dissections		
I			0	0		
II	1 (5.3%)	19	0 (0%)	9	28	4%
III	2 (4%)	46	2 (13%)	16	62	7%
IV	8 (25%)	44	9 (36%)	25	69	25%
V	3 (75%)	4	4 (67%)	6	10	70%

*Wanebo et al.: Cancer, *35*:666, 1975.

lymph node dissection at the time of re-excision of the primary site. With the likelihood of spread to more than one area and depth of invasion from 0.6 to 1.0 mm., benefit versus morbidity and mortality risk factors must be weighed on an individual basis. Obviously, all Level IV and V lesions require lymph node dissection. Such an approach eliminates the spurious arguments of prophylactic versus therapeutic lymph node dissection, since one does not know the status of the lymph nodes until several days postoperatively in these patients with a significant statistical chance of having metastases to regional lymph nodes.

With the successful utilization of multimodal therapy at the time of treatment of the primary therapy for sarcomas,[8] several clinical trials are underway using adjuvant immunotherapy for melanoma patients with a significant risk of recurrence. In these studies, patients with Stage I disease have not been included. On the other hand, utilization of immunotherapy at the time of curative surgery for Stage II melanoma is being carried out at several centers. Although early data came from phase one, nonrandomized studies, trials of a prospective randomized type are underway; for example, Morton et al.[7] reported that 13 of 14 patients with Stage II melanoma treated by lymphadenectomy and BCG immunotherapy were free of disease at two years.

Historical controls from the M. D. Anderson Hospital's experience showed only a 30 per cent survival at two years. Interestingly, Jewell et al.[4] reported similar results using an allogeneic vaccine rather than BCG as immunotherapy. Should the prospective randomized studies now being done support the phase one results, adjuvant immunotherapy at the time of lymphadenectomy for Stage II melanoma will become accepted treatment.

Finally, proper treatment of the patient with malignant melanoma must include the patient with disseminated melanoma (Stage III). For regional recurrences, individualization of treatment must be employed. Frequently wide re-excision or multiple excisions are beneficial, although any recurrence of melanoma should be considered as a local sign of other as yet occult metastases, and hence systemic therapy should be considered (see below for Stage III). Those 17 per cent of patients who experience recurrence limited to the extremity (apparently) should be considered for regional perfusion with chemotherapy.[6]

The patient with Stage III melanoma should be considered for immunotherapy, although not every patient is a candidate for such treatment. However, those without brain metastases and those with small metastatic lesions appearing at least one year after treatment of the primary lesions are more likely to benefit. When large, readily excisable lesions are found, removal should be performed prior to immunotherapy. The effect of such a "debulking" maneuver can be appreciated by scrutinizing Figure 1 of the paper by Jewell et al.[4] One can note that the 6- to 24-month survival of Stage III melanoma patients treated by Morton[7] was greater than that of those treated with allogeneic vaccine by Jewell,[4] although survival at 30 months was comparable.

In addition to using different immunotherapy in

their study, Morton and co-workers made a point of removing as much tumor as feasible, whereas Jewell and colleagues did not "debulk" the patient of tumor. Note further, however, that Jewell's Figure 1 shows that both studies achieved a 40 per cent 2-year survival of Stage III melanoma patients, compared to a 20 per cent 2-year survival of Stage III melanoma patients at Ellis Fischel Hospital (historic controls). Further support for the use of immunotherapy for Stage III melanoma can be seen in the data presented by Seigler et al.[9]

Following failure of or relapse from immunotherapy and for patients not considered candidates for immunotherapy, one should evaluate the feasibility of chemotherapy for each patient. Owing to the frequent appearance of new drugs, such patients should be referred to a chemotherapist. In general, one can expect some benefit in 20 to 30 per cent of the patients for 3 to 9 months.

From the above data, it can be appreciated that the proper treatment of the patient with malignant melanoma not only requires proper staging but must be individualized with a sophisticated understanding of the biology of malignant melanoma.

SELECTED REFERENCES

Jewell, W. R., Thomas, J. H., Sterchi, M., and Humphrey, L. J.: Critical analysis of treatment of stage II and stage III melanoma patients with immunotherapy. Ann. Surg., in press.

The authors have presented data from several centers with respect to stage II and stage III malignant melanoma. Hence, the student can gain an understanding of the prognosis of the patient who has lymph node metastasis as well as of the patient who has recurrent and disseminated malignant melanoma. While immunotherapy rightfully should be considered as experimental, this is a modality that should be offered to the patient with stage III melanoma. In this report, immunotherapy used by several experts is presented.

Knutson, C. O., Hori, J. M., and Spratt, J. S., Jr.: Melanoma. *In* Ravitch, M. M. (Ed.): Current Problems in Surgery. Chicago, Year Book Medical Publishers, 1971.

This is a very comprehensive review of virtually all aspects of malignant melanoma. The student who wishes to have an in-depth understanding of the biology of malignant melanoma should very carefully review the numerous tables in this report. From this, one will have a greater understanding of the effect of location, age, sex, etc. on the spread of disease and survival of patients with this disease. Only recent information such as level and depth of invasion and treatment of recurrent and stage III malignant melanoma is not covered comprehensively, and the student should expect to look further for this information.

Wanebo, H. J., Woodruff, J., and Fortner, J. G.: Malignant melanoma of the extremities: A clinicopathologic study using levels of invasion (microstage). Cancer, 35:666, 1975.

Undoubtedly, the precise significance of level and depth of invasion is yet to be resolved; nevertheless, the current status and importance of microstaging are presented very nicely in this reference. In correlating both level and depth of invasion, the author has clearly pointed out the contributions made by the experts who brought to the surgical literature the importance of levels and depth of invasion.

REFERENCES

1. Breslow, A.: Tumor thickness, level of invasion and node dissection in stage I cutaneous melanoma. Ann. Surg., *182*:572, 1975.
2. Clark, W. H., Jr., From, L., Bernardino, E. A., and Mihm, M. C.: The histogenesis and biologic behavior of primary human malignant melanoma of the skin. Cancer Res., *29*:705, 1969.
3. Felix, E. L., Sindelar, W. F., Bagley, D. H., Johnston, G. S., and

Ketcham, A. S.: The use of bone and brain scans as screening procedures in patients with malignant lesions. Surg. Gynecol. Obstet., *141*:867, 1975.

4. Jewell, W. R., Thomas, J. H., Sterchi, M., and Humphrey, L. J.: Critical analysis of treatment of stage II and stage III melanoma patients with immunotherapy. Ann. Surg., in press.

5. Knutson, C. O., Hori, J. M., and Spratt, J. S., Jr.: Melanoma. *In* Ravitch, M. M. (Ed.): Current Problems in Surgery. Chicago, Year Book Medical Publishers, 1971.

6. Krementz, E. T., Sutherland, C. M., Carter, R. D., and Ryan, R. F.: Malignant melanoma in the American negro. Ann. Surg., in press.

7. Morton, D. L., Eilber, F. R., Holmes, E. C., Hunt, J. S., Ketcham,

A. S., Silverstein, M. J., and Sparks, F. C.: BCG immunotherapy of malignant melanoma: Summary of a seven year experience. Ann. Surg., *180*:635, 1974.

8. Pratt, C. B., Huster, H. O., Fleming, I. D., and Pinkel, D.: Coordinated treatment of childhood rhabdomyosarcoma with surgery, radiotherapy and combination chemotherapy. Cancer Res., *32*:606, 1972.

9. Seigler, H. F., Shingleton, W. W., Metzgar, R. S., Buckley, C. E., III, and Bergoc, P. M.: Immunotherapy in patients with melanoma. Ann. Surg., *170*:352, 1973.

10. Wanebo, H. J., Woodruff, J., and Fortner, J. G.: Malignant melanoma of the extremities: A clinicopathologic study using levels of invasion (microstage). Cancer, *35*:666, 1975.

III

SOFT TISSUE SARCOMAS

LaSalle D. Leffall, Jr., M.D.

The *soft tissues* constitute nearly half of the body weight, and thus represent the single greatest amount of tissue in the human body. Present in every organ of the body and primarily concerned with support and locomotion, they include the mass situated between the epidermis and the parenchymal organs. These consist of connective tissues and lymphatic vessels, smooth and striated muscle, fat, fascia, synovial structures, and reticuloendothelium. Soft tissue sarcomas are relatively uncommon neoplasms constituting only about 1 per cent of malignant tumors. These sarcomas differ widely in incidence and site and can be classified into many categories with different histopathological characteristics. There are more than 20 types of soft tissue sarcomas, each with distinguishing histologic and biologic behavior with varying tendencies for local infiltration and distant metastases.[30] A classification of these neoplasms is shown in Table 1. These tumors are derived from tissues arising from primitive mesenchyme. Although technically not soft part sarcomas since they arise from ectoderm (peripheral nerves), malignant neurilemomas are included because they present as soft tissue tumors. Liposarcomas, fibrosarcomas and rhabdomyosarcomas occur most commonly, with other types presenting less frequently (Table 2).[19, 30] Soft part sarcomas may develop at any site in the body. They are not encapsulated but possess a pseudocapsule of compressed malignant and normal cells. These tumors extend along fascial planes, muscle bundles, and nerve sheaths beyond the gross tumor. If local excision or simple enucleation is performed, local recurrence is high, up to 70 to 80 per cent. Distant metastases occur most frequently to the lungs by the hematogenous route. Some of these tumors, especially synovial sarcoma and rhabdomyosarcoma, may metastasize to regional lymph nodes in 10 to 20 per cent of patients.

Major Types

Liposarcomas can become the largest of all soft tissue sarcomas and are the most common neoplasms noted in most series (Fig. 1). The well-differentiated liposarcoma may have 5-year survival rates of 70 to 80 per cent, whereas the survival rate for poorly differentiated lesions is about 20 per cent. Liposarcomas are quite radioresponsive and are usually best treated by surgery and irradiation.[17, 24]

Fibrosarcomas are the second most common soft tissue sarcomas noted, although they appear to be the most common histologic type found in blacks (Fig. 2).[3, 27] The histologic differentiation of fibrosarcomas from other lesions of fibrous tissue origin may be difficult, but it is important in order to determine proper treatment. Fibromatoses are connective tissue hyperplasias that infiltrate locally, do not metastasize, and tend to recur if not adequately excised. They may be seen at any age and are circumscribed but not encapsulated and usually arise from fascia.[29] The term "aggressive fibromatosis" is often used to better define the marked cellularity and aggressive local behavior of the lesion.[34] Adequate surgical excision is the treatment of choice. Some examples of fibromatoses are (1) desmoids, (2) nodular or pseudosarcomatous fasciitis, and (3) plantar fibromatosis. These lesions are locally invasive but do not metastasize.

Desmoids are usually located on the anterior abdominal wall arising from the musculoaponeurosis of the rectus abdominis muscle and its sheath. It is more frequent in women in the child-bearing years and may have its onset near the time of pregnancy. It may also arise in surgical scars. Extra-abdominal desmoids occur most often in the region of the shoulder and thighs and are more aggressive than those in the abdominal area (Fig. 3). Both abdominal and extra-abdominal desmoids are benign, do not metastasize to

TABLE 1.   Classification of Soft Tissue Sarcomas*

Cell of Origin	Type of Tumor	Subtypes
Fat cell	Liposarcoma	Well-differentiated Myxoid Round cell Pleomorphic
Fibroblast	Fibrosarcoma	Well-differentiated Poorly differentiated Dermatofibrosarcoma Protuberans
Histiocyte	Fibroxanthosarcoma (malignant fibrous histiocytoma)	
Smooth muscle	Leiomyosarcoma	Leiomyoblastoma
Striated muscle	Rhabdomyosarcoma	Embryonal Botryoid Alveolar Pleomorphic
Osteoblast	Osteosarcoma	"Classic" Parosteal (juxtacortical)
Chondroblast	Chondrosarcoma	
Endothelium of blood vessels	(Hem)Angiosarcoma	Hemangio- endothelioma (malignant) Hemangiopericytoma (malignant)
Endothelium of lymph vessels	Lymphangiosarcoma	
Synovial cells	Synovial sarcoma	
Pluripotential mesenchyme	Malignant mesenchymoma	
Ectoderm (peripheral nerve)	Malignant neurilemoma	
Uncertain	Alveolar soft part sarcoma	
	Malignant granular cell tumor	
	Kaposi's sarcoma	
	Clear-cell sarcoma of tendon sheath and aponeuroses	
	Epithelioid sarcoma (acidophilic fascial sarcoma)	

*Modified from Ackerman, L. V., and Rosai, J.: The pathology of tumors, part four; grading, staging, and classification of neoplasms. Ca., 21:373, 1971.

TABLE 2.   Relative Incidence of Soft Tissue Sarcomas

Type	Percentage
Liposarcoma	25
Fibrosarcoma	20
Rhabdomyosarcoma	15
Synovial sarcoma	10
Leiomyosarcoma	5
Mesenchymoma	5
Malignant neurilemoma	5
Angiosarcoma	2
Kaposi's sarcoma	2
Extraskeletal osteogenic sarcoma and chondrosarcoma	2
Other	9
	100

and treated as sarcoma. The clinical course is fairly typical. The lesion is usually solitary and subcutaneous in location on the trunk or arms with a very short duration between appearance and excision of the tumor. The lesion rapidly enlarges and is generally excised within two weeks. Recurrences are rare after local excision.

Plantar fibromatosis is a benign lesion of fibrous tis-

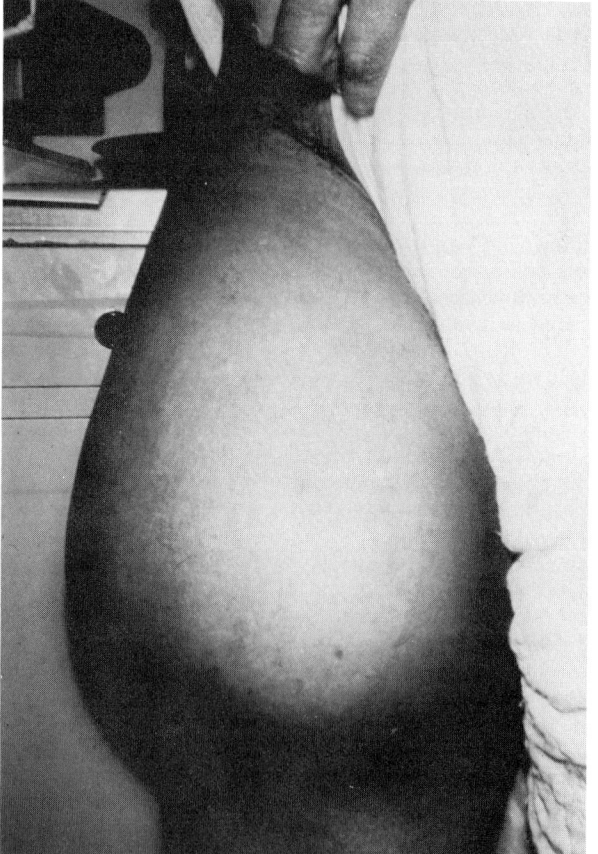

Figure 1.   This huge mass in the right anterior thigh proved to be a liposarcoma.

distant organs, and have a great tendency for local recurrence. Wide excision is the treatment of choice. Large nonresectable tumors may be controlled by irradiation.

Nodular (pseudosarcomatous) fasciitis originates from the fascia, affects middle-aged adults, and is most commonly located on the forearm.[4, 26] It is a benign lesion of fibroblasts that may be incorrectly diagnosed

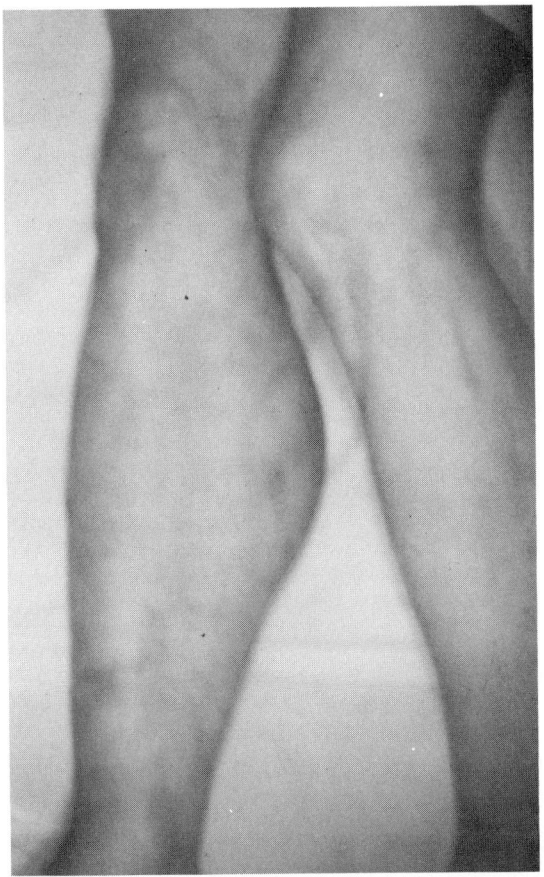

Figure 2. This tumor of the calf of the right leg represents a fibro-sarcoma.

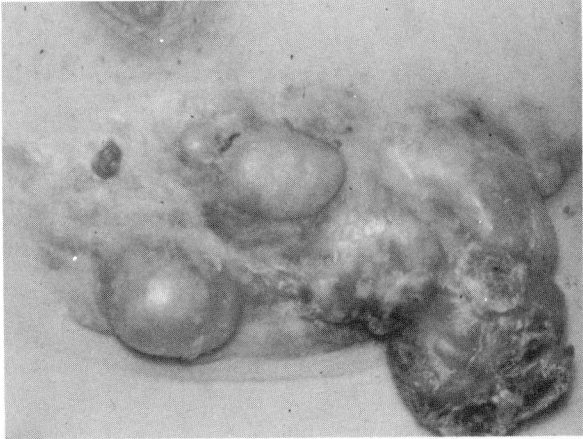

Figure 4. Dermatofibrosarcoma protuberans of the right breast.

sue proliferation that characteristically replaces varying portions of the plantar aponeurosis, with eventual invasions of the overlying skin. Wide excision is essential to prevent recurrence.

Dermatofibrosarcoma protuberans (storiform fibrous histiocytoma) is considered to be a very low-grade fibrosarcoma.[22] It tends to recur locally but rarely metastasizes. The tumor develops as a protuberant lesion, most often arising from the skin of the trunk (Figs. 4 and 5). The tumor involves the dermis, although it may invade the subcutaneous tissue. Histologically the cartwheel or storiform arrangement of fibroblasts is quite characteristic of the lesion. Wide local excision is the treatment of choice.

Rhabdomyosarcomas are divided into four subtypes: (1) pleomorphic, (2) embryonal, (3) botryoidal, and (4) alveolar. It may spread to lymph nodes in 10 per cent of cases (Fig. 6). The pleomorphic type occurs most frequently and is usually found in patients over 35 years of age. Embryonal rhabdomyosarcoma is the most common soft tissue sarcoma in infants and children.[29] It is far more prevalent under the age of 6 years, and about 50 per cent occur in the head and neck region. Sarcoma botryoides occurs in young children in the genitourinary tract and presents as a grapelike or polypoid edematous mass. Alveolar rhabdomyosar-

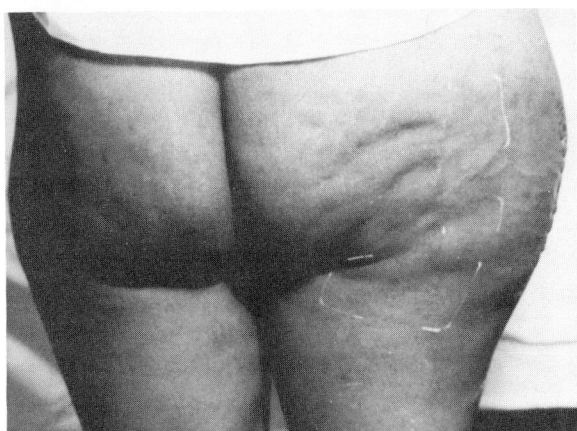

Figure 3. An extra-abdominal desmoid is responsible for the enlargement of the right lateral thigh.

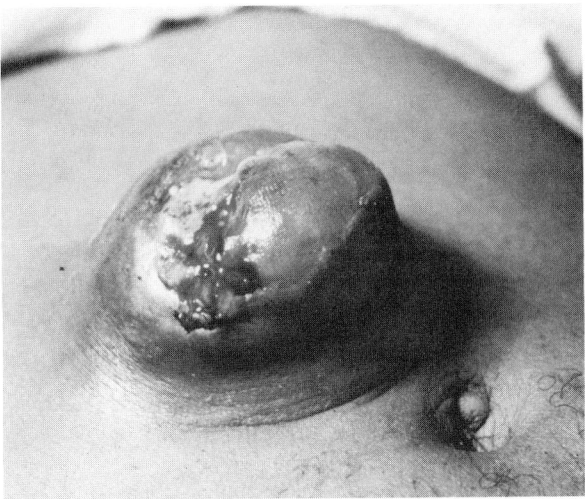

Figure 5. Dermatofibrosarcoma protuberans of the anterior abdominal wall.

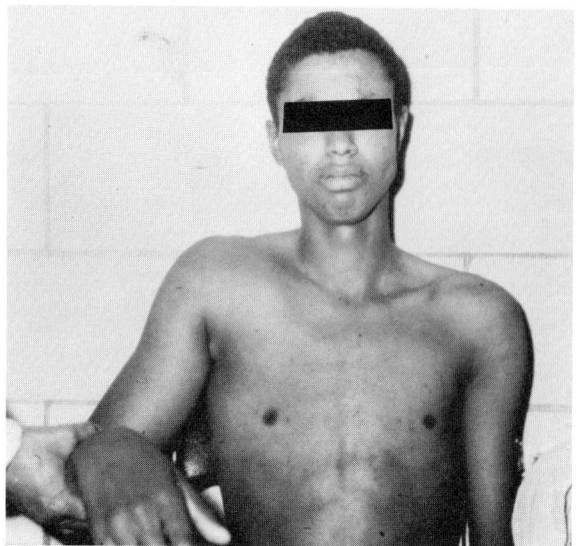

Figure 6. The swelling of the right anterior axillary region is produced by bulky metastatic embryonal rhabdomyosarcoma from a malignant neoplasm of the upper arm.

coma is a highly malignant tumor occurring in young adults.

Other Types

Synovial sarcomas are the most common soft tissue sarcomas of the hands and feet and affect chiefly young adults. They occur in the vicinity of joints but seldom involve the synovial lining of the joint itself (Fig. 7). Lymph node matastases occur in 20 per cent of cases.[19]

Malignant neurilemoma is uncommon, and metastases are slow but widespread.[11] About 50 per cent arise in patients with multiple neurofibromatosis (von Recklinghausen's disease). These tumors produce pain, tenderness, and paresthesias. Wide resection of the involved nerve is indicated. Lymphangiosarcoma occurs rarely and may be secondary to postmastectomy lymphedema or to chronic congenital and idiopathic lymphedema. Leiomyosarcomas rarely occur in the soft tissue and are most common in other locations. They may arise in the smooth muscle of blood vessels (Fig. 8).[15] Although not common, fibroxanthosarcoma is being encountered with increasing frequency (Fig. 9).[16]

Kaposi's sarcoma is a malignant blood vessel tumor and is thought to be multicentric in origin.[6] It occurs predominantly in adult males. In 75 to 85 per cent of cases the primary tumor arises in the skin. The disease usually begins with bluish red macules in the skin of the extremities, which progress to plaques and then nodules and tumors associated with nonpitting edema and eventual extension to the viscera. Two unusual features of this disease are the high frequency of a second primary cancer and the presence of diabetes mellitus. Irradiation is the treatment of choice, al-

though surgery and chemotherapy may be used in selected cases.

Clinical Manifestations

The most common presenting symptom is a painless mass that gradually enlarges until it becomes painful or interferes with function. However, the growth rate of these tumors varies. Trauma may call attention to an unsuspected sarcoma but has not been proved to be an etiological factor. Although uncommon, hypoglycemia has been described with some soft tissue sarcomas.[20, 23] Physical examination usually reveals a firm, non-tender tumor mass that may appear fairly well circumscribed because of its pseudocapsule. These neoplasms occur most often in the lower extremity, especially in the medial upper thigh, but may occur in other locations such as the upper extremities, trunk, retroperitoneum, head, and neck. There is a predilection for some types to originate in certain areas: (1) rhabdomyosarcomas—upper thigh or arm; (2) liposarcomas—thigh, shoulder, and retroperitoneum; (3) synovial sarcomas—feet, hands, and knees; and (4) dermatofibrosarcoma protuberans—trunk.[19]

Diagnosis

Biopsy is essential to establish the diagnosis and institute proper therapy. Adequate tissue must be obtained for histopathologic study. Excisional biopsy is used for lesions up to 3 cm. in size. Incisional or wedge

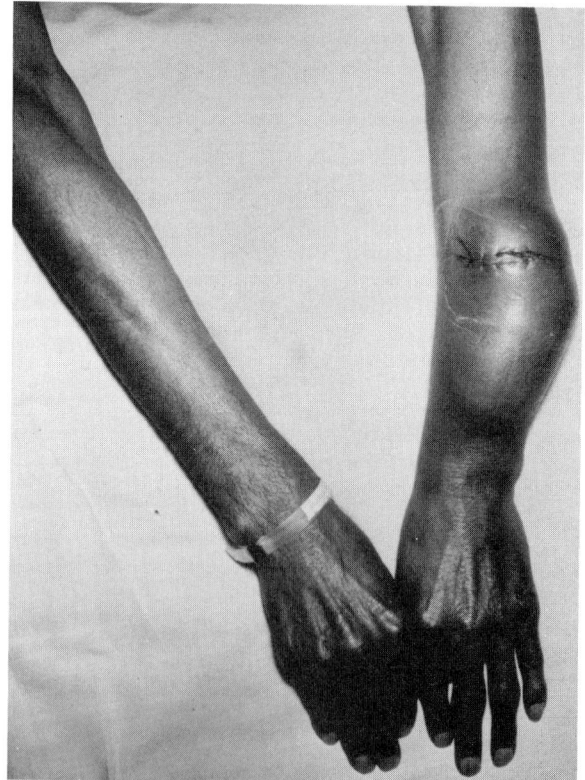

Figure 7. The tumor on the dorsal aspect of the left forearm represents a synovial sarcoma. The sutured wound is the side of incisional biopsy.

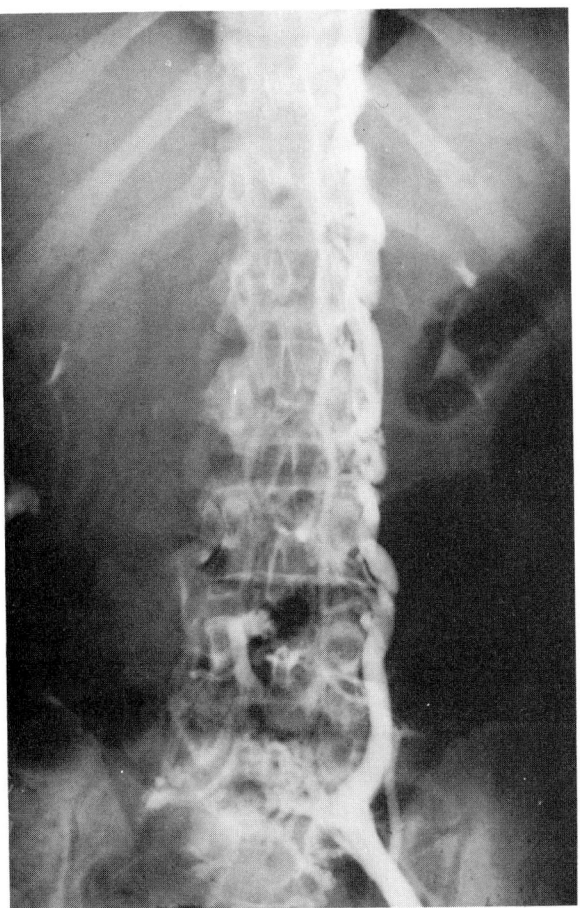

Figure 8. This inferior vena cavagram reveals nonfilling of the inferior vena cava and a dilated left ascending lumbar vein secondary to a retroperitoneal leiomyosarcoma probably arising from the inferior vena cava.

portant in helping to determine the type of treatment (1) histologic type, (2) histologic grade, (3) anatomic location, (4) status of tumor bed (primary or recurrent), (5) mode of spread, (6) size, and (7) mobility. Simple enucleation must be avoided because this increases the chance for spread and decreases the chance for cure. Wide excision is essential because these sarcomas spread by infiltration along muscle and fascial planes. Recurrent tumors behave in a more virulent manner than primary ones, and inadequate removal increases the likelihood of local recurrence. The surgical modalities are wide local excision, muscle group excision, and amputation. The wide excision must be three-dimensional in scope to obtain adequate margins in all directions around the tumor, if possible. Ideally, the surgeon should be cutting through normal tissue at all times and should remove the sarcoma encompassed by normal tissue. In order to obtain good margins, major blood vessels may have to be sacrificed, with replacement by prosthetic or autologous grafts. Muscle group excision may be used for some sarcomas requiring the removal of all involved muscles from their origin to insertion. The decision to treat a patient by amputation is often very difficult. Generally the amputation site is above the joint of in-

biopsy is used for larger lesions. Needle biopsy may be used, but often insufficient tissue is obtained to make a definitive diagnosis and incisional biopsy must be utilized. It is usually better not to rely on frozen section diagnosis but to await the results of permanent sections to afford the pathologist the best chance to make the correct diagnosis.[5] Accurate histologic diagnosis is mandatory before proper therapy can be given. Chest x-rays and tomograms are necessary to exclude pulmonary metastases. Soft tissue x-rays of the tumor can help differentiate a primary bone tumor from a soft tissue sarcoma invading bone. Angiography may demonstrate tumor vessels characteristic of malignant tumors and can help to determine relationships of the sarcomas to bone, nerves, and blood vessels that are helpful in planning surgical excision (Figs. 8 and 10).

Management

The treatment of choice for soft part sarcomas is adequate surgical resection in order to eradicate the disease and decrease the incidence of distant spread and local recurrence.[5, 28] The following factors are im-

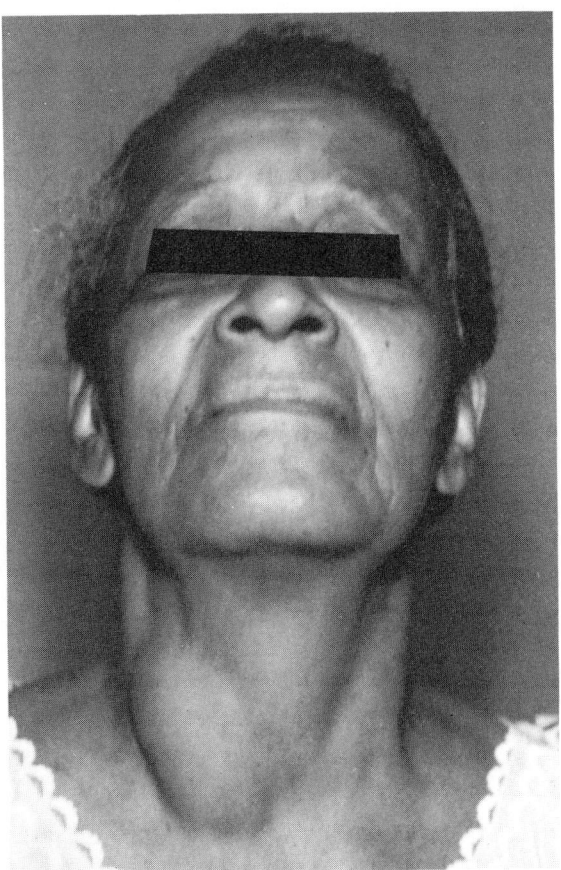

Figure 9. This slowly enlarging mass in the right lower neck proved on biopsy to be a malignant fibrous histiocytoma (fibroxanthosarcoma).

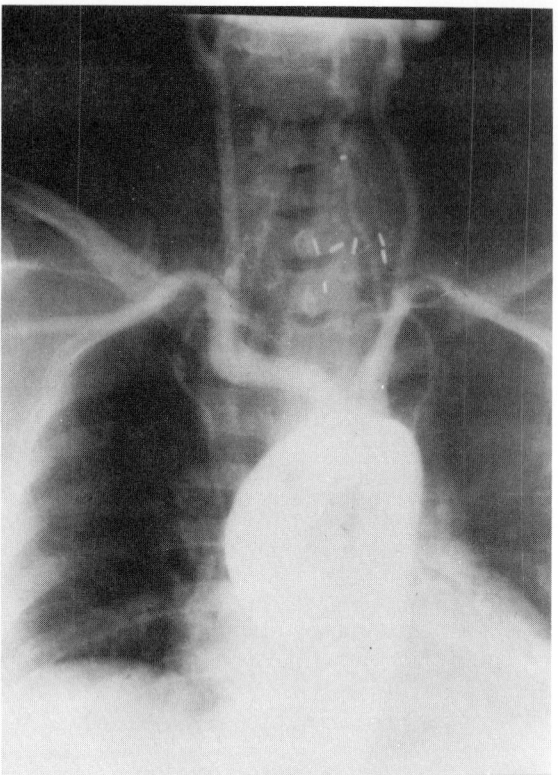

Figure 10. Retrograde aortogram reveals tortuosity and lateral displacement of the left common carotid artery secondary to a recurrent desmoid tumor that also displaces the trachea to the right and invades the superior mediastinum.

volved muscle groups. For sarcomas near the pelvic or shoulder girdle, hemipelvectomy or interscapulothoracic amputation may be indicated, whereas midhumeral or midthigh amputations are used for lesions below the elbow or knee. Adequate surgical resection of soft tissue sarcomas is often not technically feasible in lesions below the elbow or knee when the lesion is close to major neurovascular structures. Attempted wide surgical excision is often unsuccessful because the margin of normal tissue is very thin at one or more points, even though for most of the specimen the margin appears generous. Further adequacy of margin is difficult to assess for those that are diffusely infiltrating. These factors account for a local recurrence rate of 25 to 30 per cent following wide surgical excision.[2] In such cases, amputation has often been the recommended treatment of choice. In recent years an alternative to amputation has become available.

Radical, high-dose precision radiation therapy (6000 to 7000 rads in 6 to 7 weeks) with or without limited surgical excision has been effective in treating early to moderately advanced soft part sarcomas.[18, 23, 32] For those tumors like synovial sarcoma and rhabdomyosarcoma with increased likelihood of lymph node metastases, irradiation is also given to regional lymph node depots (5000 rads in 5 weeks). Of 100 patients with soft tissue sarcomas treated by local excision and irradiation, 58 per cent of those observed for 5 years were free of disease. All recurrences appeared within 3 years. The local recurrence rate following this type of treatment was 20 to 25 per cent, which compares favorably with that reported following radical surgical excision, 25 to 30 per cent. In all of the patients with extremity lesions, amputation had been recommended. In addition, about 75 per cent of these patients retained a functional extremity free of pain and edema. Irradiation cannot be given to the full width of the extremity if a functional limb is to be expected. Low-grade nonmetastasizing tumors such as desmoids, if not amenable to surgical resection, which is the treatment of choice, can often be treated successfully by radical dose irradiation.[10] It has been shown that most soft tissue sarcomas, including well-differentiated tumors, are radioresponsive. The most important factor affecting disease-free survival rates is the histopathologic grade of the tumor. If limited surgery and radical dose radiation are used, amputation may be reserved for irradiation failures.

The combination of selected surgery, irradiation, and chemotherapy has produced marked improvements in the treatment of embryonal rhabdomyosarcoma in children.[7, 9, 12, 25, 35] With this regimen, amputations are rarely indicated for tumors of the extremities. When surgical treatment is not applicable, intensive irradiation and chemotherapy may produce local tumor control. The most effective chemotherapeutic combination is VAC (vincristine, actinomycin D, and cyclophosphamide) for a 1- to 2-year period. Current results indicate that over 50 per cent of children with inoperable or metastatic embryonal rhabdomyosarcoma can be successfully treated and achieve eradication of their disease. The addition of adriamycin and imidazole carboxymide to the combination therapy program for adults with soft tissue sarcomas has resulted in significant improvement in their response as well. Hyperthermic perfusion with chemotherapeutic agents combined with radiation therapy and surgical excision may also be of value in the treatment of soft part sarcomas.[31] Al-

TABLE 3.   Prognosis in Soft Tissue Sarcomas Treated by Surgery at Memorial Hospital (1968)*

Histologic Type	Survivals			
	5 Years		10 Years	
Spindle cell sarcomas	68/112	62%	37/83	45%
Liposarcoma	44/73	60%	24/43	56%
Rhabdomyosarcoma	41/69	59%	24/52	46%
Fibrosarcoma	64/83	77%	33/46	71%
Synovial sarcoma	26/56	46%	8/33	24%
Neurosarcoma	10/17	59%	7/14	50%
Embryonal rhabdomyosarcoma	6/17	35%	4/12	33%

*Modified from McNeer, G. P., Cantin, J., Chu, F., and Nickerson, J. J.: Effectiveness of radiation therapy in the management of sarcoma of the soft somatic tissues. Cancer, 22:391, 1968.

though irradiation and chemotherapy have added significantly to our therapeutic armamentarium, adequate surgical excision remains the treatment of choice and the most effective method of eradicating localized tumor. When total surgical excision of the sarcoma is not feasible, limited resections (tumor debulking procedures) may be performed, to be followed by irradiation and possibly chemotherapy. Curative surgical resection should be considered in patients who have pulmonary metastases. Patients with metastatic pulmonary lesions that have a tumor-doubling time greater than 40 days should be considered for surgical resection even though lesions are multiple and bilateral.[13, 14] In such patients, the primary lesion must be under control and the lungs represent the only site of distant spread. The presence of a new primary cancer of the lung must also be kept in mind.

The survival rates for soft tissue sarcomas vary. Five- and ten- year survivals after surgical therapy are presented in Table 3. In most series, survival rates are somewhat lower than those listed here, with overall 5-year survival rates of 30 to 50 per cent, depending on the type of sarcoma.[21] However, further improvement in survival can be expected with appropriate combination therapy using surgery, irradiation, and chemotherapy. This has already been observed in the increased survival of patients with embryonal rhabdomyosarcoma. The role of immunotherapy has not yet been determined.

SELECTED REFERENCES

Enzinger, F. M.: Recent Trends in Soft Tissue Pathology. *In* Tumors of Bone and Soft Tissue. Chicago, Year Book Medical Publishers, 1965, pp. 315–332.
This chapter discusses the different pathological lesions that present as soft part sarcomas. It is of value in obtaining additional information about the less commonly encountered lesions as well as the subtypes of those sarcomas that occur most commonly.

Pack, G. T., and Ariel, I. M.: Tumors of the Soft Somatic Tissues, Treatment of Cancer and Allied Diseases. New York, Paul B. Hoeber, 1958.
In this classic book, Pack and Ariel discuss possible etiological factors, diagnosis, and treatment of tumors of the soft somatic tissues. Relying on their vast experience in the management of all types of soft tissue sarcomas, these authors present data that should be of value to both medical students and practitioners. Although this book was published almost 20 years ago, it remains one of the most important sources of information about soft part sarcomas.

Stout, A. P.: Sarcomas of soft tissues. Ca, *11*:210–231, 1961.
In this monograph, Stout, an international authority on tumors of the soft somatic tissues, discusses incidence, types, and behavior of these neoplasms. As a surgical pathologist with years of experience studying soft tissue sarcomas, he presents important factors about these neoplasms in a concise and interesting manner.

Suit, H. D., and Russell, W. O.: Radiation therapy of soft tissue sarcomas. Cancer, *36*:759–764, 1975.
This article emphasizes the role of radiation therapy in the clinical management of patients with soft tissue sarcomas. Irradiation, when combined with limited surgery or used alone, has proved to be quite effective in the treatment of early to moderately advanced soft part sarcomas.

Wilbur, J. R., Sutow, W. W., Sullivan, M. P., and Gottleb, J. A.: Chemotherapy of sarcomas. Cancer, *36*:765–769, 1975.
This article details the development of intensive treatment techniques with combination chemotherapy, irradiation, and selected surgery, which have produced dramatic improvements in the treatment of soft tissue sarcomas. This has been best demonstrated in children with embryonal rhabdomyosarcoma and to a lesser degree in adults with other soft tissue sarcomas.

REFERENCES

1. Ackerman, L. V., and Rosai, J.: The pathology of tumors, part four; grading, staging and classification of neoplasms. Ca., *21*:373, 1971.
2. Cantin, J., McNeer, G. P., Chu, F., and Booher, R. J.: The problem of local recurrence after treatment of soft tissue sarcomas. Ann. Surg., *168*:47–53, 1967.
3. Crawford, M., Chung, E. B., Leffall, L. D., Jr., and White, J. E.: Soft part sarcomas in negroes. Cancer, *26*:503–512, 1970.
4. Culbertson, J. D., and Enterline, H. T.: Pseudosarcomatous fasciitis: A distinctive clinicopathologic entity. Ann. Surg., *151*:235, 1960.
5. Das Gupta, T. K., and Brasfield, R. D.: Soft tissue tumors: Classification and principles of management. Ca., *18*:259, 1968.
6. Davis, J.: Kaposi's sarcoma. Present concept of clinical course and treatment. N.Y. State J. Med., *68*:2067–2073, 1968.
7. Donaldson, S. S., Castro, J. R., Wilbur, J. R., and Jesse, R. H.: Rhabdomyosarcoma of head and neck in children. Cancer, *31*:26–35, 1973.
8. Enterline, A. T., Culbertson, J. D., Rochlin, D. B., and Brady, L. W.: Liposarcoma. A clinical and pathological study of 53 cases. Cancer, *13*:932–950, 1960.
9. Grosfeld, J. L., Clatworthy, H. W., Jr., and Newton, W. A.: Combined therapy in childhood rhabdomyosarcoma: An analysis of 42 cases. J. Pediatr. Surg., *4*:637–645, 1969.
10. Hill, D. R., Newman, H., and Phillips, T. L.: Radiation therapy of desmoid tumors. Am. J. Roentgenol., *117*:84–89, 1973.
11. Jacobs, R. L., and Barmada, R.: Neurilemoma: A review of the literature with six case reports. Arch. Surg., *102*:181–186, 1971.
12. Johnson, D. G.: Trends in surgery for childhood rhabdomyosarcoma. Cancer, *35*(Suppl.):916–920, 1975.
13. Joseph, W. L.: Criteria for resection of sarcoma metastatic to the lung. Cancer Chemother. Rep., *58*:185–296, 1974.
14. Joseph, W. L., Morton, D. L., and Adkins, P. C.: Prognostic significance of tumor doubling time in evaluating operability in pulmonary metastatic disease. J. Thor. Cardiovasc. Surg., *61*:23–32, 1971.
15. Jurayj, M. N., Midell, A. I., Bederman, S., Gruen, J., and O'Brien, P. H.: Primary leiomyosarcomas of the inferior vena cava. Report of a case and review of the literature. Cancer, *26*:1349–1353, 1970.
16. Kempson, R. L., and Kyriakos, M.: Fibroxanthosarcoma of the soft tissues. A type of malignant fibrous histiocytoma. Cancer, *29*:961–975, 1972.
17. Kinne, D. W., Chu, F. D., Huvos, A. G., Yagoda, A., and Fortner, J. G.: Treatment of primary and recurrent retroperitoneal liposarcoma. Twenty-five year experience at Memorial Hospital. Cancer, *31*:53–64, 1973.
18. Lindberg, R. D., Martin, R. G., and Romsdahl, M. M.: Surgery and postoperative radiotherapy in the treatment of soft tissue sarcomas in adults. Am. J. Roentgenol., *123*:123, 1975.
19. Morton, D. L.: Soft tissue sarcomas. *In* Holland, J. F., and Frei, E., III, Cancer Medicine. Philadelphia, Lea & Febiger, 1973, pp. 1845–1861.
20. Mars, H., Schumacher, P. O., and McCormack, L. J.: Intra-abdominal extrapancreatic neoplasm (leiomyosarcoma) associated with severe recurrent hypoglycemia. Cancer, *20*:1155–1160, 1967.
21. McNeer, G. P., Cantin, J., Chu, F., and Nickerson, J. J.: Effectiveness of radiation therapy in the management of sarcoma of the soft somatic tissues. Cancer, *22*:391, 1968.
22. McPeak, C. J., Cruz, T., and Nicastri, A. D.: Dermatofibrosarcoma protuberans: An analysis of 86 cases, five with metastasis. Ann. Surg., *166*:803–816, 1967.
23. McPeak, C. J., and Papaioannou, A. N.: Nonpancreatic tumors associated with hypoglycemia. Arch. Surg., *93*:1019–1024, 1966.
24. Perry, H., and Chu, F.: Radiation therapy in the palliative management of soft tissues sarcomas. Cancer, *15*:179–183, 1962.
25. Pratt, C. B., Hustu, H. O., Fleming, I. D., and Pinkel, C.: Coordinated treatment of childhood rhabdomyosarcoma with surgery, radiotherapy and chemotherapy. Cancer Res., *32*:606–610, 1972.
26. Price, E. B., Silliphant, W. M., and Shuman, R.: Nodular fasciitis—a clinicopathologic analysis of 65 cases. Am. J. Clin. Pathol., *35*:122, 1961.
27. Pritchard, R. J., Soule, E. H., Tayler, W. F., and Ivins, J. C.: Fibrosarcoma—a clinicopathologic and statistical study of 199 tumors of the soft tissues of the extremities and trunk. Cancer, *33*:888–897, 1974.

28. Shiu, M. H., Castro, E. B., Hajdu, S. I., and Fortner, J. G.: Surgical treatment of 297 soft tissue sarcomas of the lower extremity. Ann. Surg., *182*:597–602, 1975.

29. Soule, E. H., Mahour, G. H., Mills, S. D., and Lynn H. B.: Soft tissue sarcomas of infants and children: A clinicopathologic study of 135 cases. Mayo Clin. Proc., *43*:313, 1968.

30. Stout, A. P., and Lattes, R.: Tumors of the soft tissue: Atlas of tumor pathology, Series 2, Fasc. I. Washington, D. C., Armed Forces Institute of Pathology, 1967.

31. Stehlin, J. S., de Ipolyi, P. D., Giovanella, B. C., Gutierrez, A. E., and Anderson, R. F.: Soft tissue sarcomas of the extremity—multidisciplinary therapy employing hyperthermic perfusion. Am. J. Surg., *130*:643–646, 1975.

32. Suit, H. D., and Lindberg, R.: Management of patients with sarcoma of soft tissue. Tex. Med., *67*:60–63, 1971.

33. Suit, H. D., Russell, W. O., and Martin, R. G.: Sarcoma of soft tissue—clinical and histopathologic parameters and response to treatment. Cancer, *35*:1478–1483, 1975.

34. Wilkins, S. A., Jr., Waldron, C. A., Mathews, W. H., and Droulias, C. A.: Aggressive fibromatosis of the head and neck. Am. J. Surg., *130*:412–415, 1975.

35. Wilbur, J. R., Sutow, W. W., Sullivan, M. P., and Gottlieb, J. A.: Chemotherapy of sarcomas. Cancer, *36*:765–769, 1975.

24

THE BREAST

Richard E. Wilson, M.D.

HISTORICAL NOTES

The breast has always been a symbol of womanhood and ultimate fertility. As a result, both disease and surgery of the breast evoke a fear of mutilation and loss of femininity. Cosmetic considerations, false vanity, and fear of infertility have hindered early diagnosis and prompt treatment of breast cancer from times of earliest recorded history until today.

Herodotus, a Greek historian who just preceded Hippocrates, tells of Atossa, daughter of Cyrus and wife of Darius, who had a small breast tumor which she concealed until it reached a point of ulceration and widespread disease. The skilled physician Democedes (525 B.C.) was sent for and he was successful in curing her, although his technique was never revealed. This often-repeated presenting history of the patient with untreated breast cancer is common in our "modern" civilization, but the outcome is rarely as successful as that attributed to Democedes.

In the Edwin Smith Surgical Papyrus,[12] the earliest known medical record (3000–2500 B.C.), description is made of bulging tumors of the breasts that were differentiated from abscess and mastitis. While drainage of breast abscesses was practiced, there is no evidence that operative procedures were utilized for treating breast cancer in Egypt. Hippocrates, likewise, considered cancer of the breast incurable, and a classic description of a woman succumbing to late breast cancer appears in his volume, *Diseases of Women.* Celsus, a Roman scholar in the first century A.D., emphasized the danger of operating on the breast if cancer was present rather than leaving the tumor in place, a point stressed 1800 years later by Haagensen. Celsus also argued against removal of the pectoral muscles when breast amputation was to be attempted. Galen wrote, "Cancerous tumors are found . . . in the breasts of women, after cessation of menstruation, which, so long as it is regular, preserves good health." He conceived of melancholia as the cause of cancer. He did recommend surgical excision of readily removable breast tumors and gave a remarkable description of the spreading of breast cancer: "We have often seen in the breast a tumor exactly resembling the animal called the crab. . . . We have often cured this disease in its early states, but after it has reached a large size, no one has cured it without operation." Leonides of Alexandria was the first to stress that nipple retraction was an important clinical sign of breast cancer, and he described the technique for surgical and cautery excision of the breast that probably was most used through the Dark Ages.

It was not until the sixteenth century that further understanding and progress was made in the surgical management of breast cancer. Vesalius placed the anatomy of the breast and axilla in proper perspective and advocated wide surgical excision with ligature control of bleeding vessels rather than cautery. Fabricius was critical of any partial excision of breast cancer, advocating radical surgery or none at all. Severinus was one of the first surgeons to remove enlarged axillary lymph glands at the time of breast amputation.

It remained for Le Dran in the eighteenth century to point out that at its earliest stage, breast cancer was a local lesion; that it spread to regional nodes via lymphatics; that early operation provided the best chance for cure; and that axillary nodal involvement was associated with a poorer prognosis. Petit stressed block dissection and the need for wide excision with careful axillary nodal removal. He was skilled enough to be successful in this technique and recognized the poor prognosis associated with supraclavicular nodal involvement. Velpeau, in 1856, raised the issue that is still pertinent: "To destroy a cancerous tumor by surgical means is usually an easy matter, and but little danger in itself; but the question arises, whether such a proceeding affords a chance of radically curing the patient?"

Thereafter, a parade of eminent surgeons urged more extensive excision of breast tumors, when operable, leading up to the present concepts of radical mastectomy. Syme, in 1842, recommended wide excision of cancers even when they were small. Moore, in 1867, had the advantage of the dawning of microscopic pathology when he stressed that local recurrence after breast amputation was due to disseminated tumor fragments not removed at the time of the initial operation. He advocated that "It is not sufficient to remove the tumor . . . mammary cancer requires careful extirpation of the entire organ." He outlined the essential principles of radical mastectomy except for pectoral muscle removal. Lister described division of these muscles for adequate removal of the axillary glands, and Gross, in 1880, supported Moore's radical operation and extended it to include pectoral fascia excision. Gross was one of the first prominent American surgeons to be convinced that early, thorough operative procedures could cure women with breast cancer, and he was able to apply careful histologic study to his thesis. Volkmann, in 1875, described wide excision of breast skin and pectoral fascia, extending the procedure to include the muscles themselves in far advanced cases. The absence of local or distant recurrence in some of these patients encouraged other prominent German surgeons such as Billroth and Heidenhain to espouse the concept of pectoral muscle excision with total mastectomy.

Halsted first described his technique for excision of the pectoralis major muscle along with axillary nodal removal and mastectomy in 1890–91 in an obscure report of wound healing.[53] He pointed out the error of trying to determine muscle involvement by gross examination, yet for many years he felt that the pectoralis minor muscle could be left in place. It was Meyer[82] who added the removal of both muscles to his operative procedure in 1894. Halsted and his associates extended the radical mastectomy to include cervical, supraclavicular, and anterior mediastinal dissection with excision of part of the chest wall in some cases, but his enthusiasm for these more extensive features of the operative procedure waned as results did not support them. As Lewison[72] so aptly pointed out, "The fertile mind of Halsted was, so to speak, made up of all the minds of the preceding ages."

Radical mastectomy achieved wide usage for the treatment of breast cancer in the twentieth century, but Haagensen[45] pointed out that patient selection was essential if proper therapy was to be provided for women presenting with a wide variety of primary disease. He showed that certain cases were "categorically unoperable." His writings and teachings were the perfect complement to the enthusiasm of Halsted for radical mastectomy. He identified those "grave" signs of widespread local disease and subtle evidences of incurability of breast cancer by local excision that have fostered more rational selection of therapy on an individual basis and have encouraged investigation of many other approaches to the primary treatment of breast cancer. Today's clinicians are no more certain of their stand on the treatment of breast cancer than were their earlier counterparts. The surgeon now has modern statistical methods, histopathologic studies, and the choice of a variety of agents, not just surgery, to help him select the most successful therapy for a given patient.

ANATOMY AND PHYSIOLOGY

The breast, in most simplistic terms, is a modified sweat gland lying on the pectoral fascia and the musculature of the chest wall over the upper anterior rib cage, surrounded by a layer of fat and encased in a skin envelope (Fig. 1). Breast tissue extends toward the axilla, forming the so-called axillary tail of Spence. Each mammary gland consists of 12 to 20 glandular lobes or acini, much like a bunch of grapes, with the stems representing the ramifying ductal system. The ducts are surrounded by specialized connective tissue, the periductal tissue, which is under hormonal control and is different from the general stroma of the breast.

Each lactiferous duct enlarges as it picks up more ductules and runs towards the nipple. Each duct has an ampullary dilatation beyond which it branches before opening onto the surface of the nipple. The nipple is surrounded by pigmented circular skin called the areola, which contains contractile smooth muscle fibers to facilitate nipple contraction. Although it appears that each duct is lined by a single layer of epithelial cells, there is actually a second, flat layer of cells that acts as a basement layer of epidermis. This "reserve layer" reproduces the lining cells, and can proliferate in various pathologic conditions, such as cystic hyperplasia and ductal carcinoma. Fibrous septa run from the fascia around the breast lobules, through the overlying fat to the superficial fascia and dermal layer of the skin. These suspensory ligaments (Cooper's ligaments) of the breast permit considerable mobility of the breast itself. The deep fascia is contiguous with the superficial pectoral fascia, completely enveloping the breast within the skin and subcutaneous fat and also with the superficial cervical and abdominal fascia (Camper's).

The male breast consists of rudimentary, short ducts without any well-developed acini. The nipple and areola are proportionately smaller than in the female and much less fat is present between the ductules and the surface of the pectoral fascia.

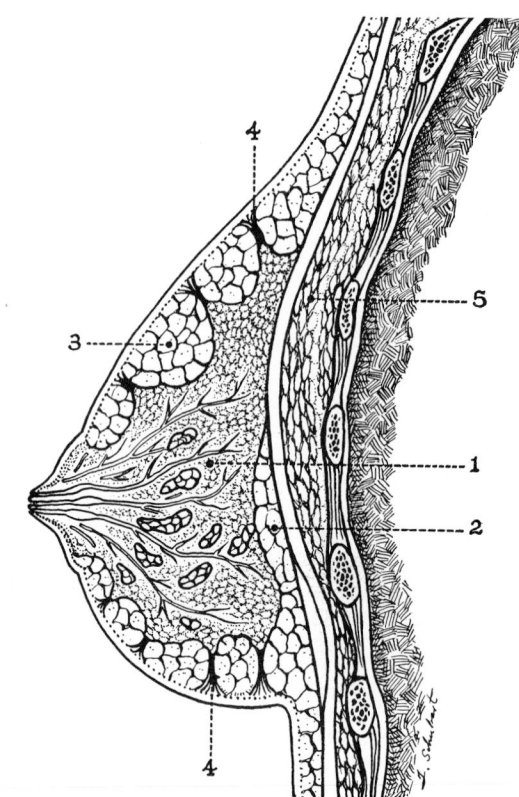

Figure 1. Sagittal section of the normal breast, showing its relation to the chest wall and the rib cage. *1*, The mammary gland tissue. *2*, Retromammary fat separating the breast from the pectoral fascia. *3*, The investing envelope of subcutaneous fat separating the breast from the overlying skin. *4*, The fibrous septa that fix the breast tissue to the overlying skin (Cooper's ligaments). *5*, Fat and pectoral muscle layer beneath the deep fascia. The ductal system begins in the periphery of the breast and ducts enlarge as they approach the nipple. There is an ampullary dilatation before the duct enters the nipple proper. (From Ackerman, L. V., and del Regato, J. A.: Cancer Diagnosis, Treatment and Prognosis, 4th ed. St. Louis, The C. V. Mosby Company, 1970.)

Breast Lymphatics

The lymphatic network of the breast is exceedingly rich and drainage is extensive in many directions from the breast itself. Lymphatic channels of the skin overlying the breast are valveless and communicate, although sluggishly, with the subepithelial plexus, which flows toward the subareolar plexus of lymphatics. Fine lymphatic ducts flow from the subareolar plexus, along the lactiferous ducts in the periductal connective tissue. The flow in these lymphatics is unidirectional, toward the perilobular or interlobular network and then along the major venous channels to the draining lymph nodes. The valvular periductal lymphatics carry lymph rapidly to the lymph nodes as a result of wavelike contractions. Reverse flow out to the skin or along the chest wall occurs only in the presence of obstruction in deeper channels.

There are three main pathways for the lymphatic channels arriving in the breast to enter lymph nodes (Fig. 2): the axillary, interpectoral, and internal mam-

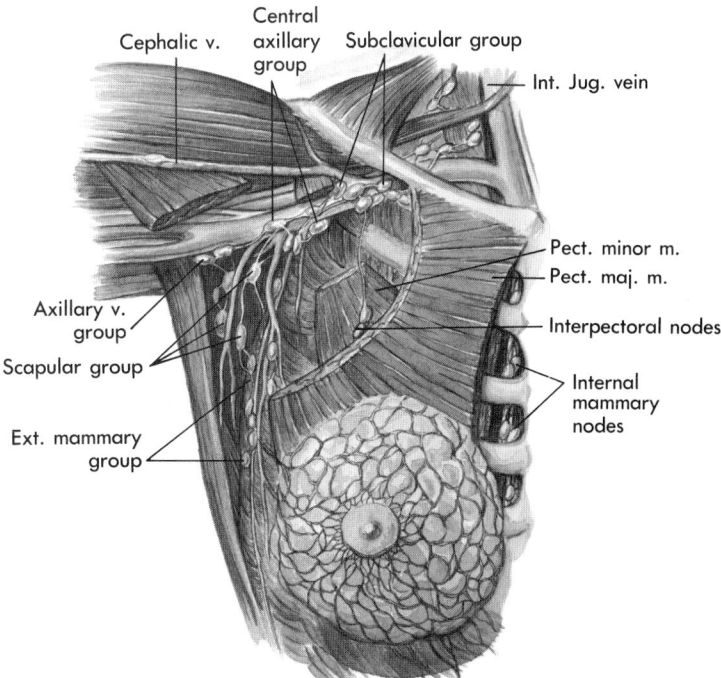

Figure 2. The distribution of lymph node drainage from the breast. The subareolar lymphatics progress radially to the draining lymph nodes. The major drainage is laterally through the external mammary group and then upward to the central axillary group of nodes before reaching the apex of the axilla. Direct drainage through the pectoral musculature to the subclavicular nodes can occur. The central and medial portions of the breast communicate directly with the internal mammary nodes. (From Spratt, J. S., Jr., and Donegan, W. L.: Cancer of the Breast. Philadelphia, W. B. Saunders Company, 1967.)

mary pathways. The major and primary route of drainage is the axillary pathway.[95] Lymphatics from the lobules and ducts pass through the axillary fascia along with the lateral thoracic blood vessels to the lateral or external mammary group of nodes, which are closest to the breast. Scapular and lower axillary vein nodes are the next stop in the progression of flow toward the apex of the axilla. The central nodes are along the main portion of the axillary vein, and highest axillary nodes include the subclavicular lymph glands, which lie beneath the clavicle on top of the first rib and medial to the pectoralis minor muscle.

Lymphatics draining the posterior breast accompany the acromiothoracic vessels and pass through the interpectoral group of nodes between the pectoralis major and the pectoralis minor, ending in the highest axillary nodes. These channels may drain the subareolar plexus directly and frequently connect with supraclavicular and higher internal mammary lymph nodes. The internal mammary lymph nodes lie along the internal mammary vessels in the intercostal spaces and behind the costal cartilages. They are primarily in the first to third interspaces, but are variable in their number, size, and distribution. They drain lymphatic channels that pass through the intercostal muscles from the medial half of the breast and the subareolar plexus.

The internal mammary lymph nodes and the highest axillary nodes drain toward the medial end of the clavicle near the junction of the subclavian and internal jugular veins. Tumor involvement in this important sentinel node produces retrograde spread to the supraclavicular glands as well as extension to the mediastinal nodes. Internal mammary nodes also drain directly into the anterior mediastinum by multiple interlocking channels.

Less frequent pathways of lymphatic drainage are via the lymphatic plexus on the rectus sheath from the lower and medial portions of the breast and in an anterolateral pathway to the opposite axilla.

Breast Development and Physiology

The healthy breast shows remarkable variation in gland structure. During a woman's menstrual life it is affected and altered daily as a result of the multiple pituitary and ovarian hormones. It appears that interaction of the various endocrine secretions rather than any single hormone is responsible for the structural alterations in the breast.

The breast at birth is a rudimentary organ consisting only of ducts. At the time of puberty, under the influence of estrogen and progesterone in the ovary as well as trophic pituitary hormones, active budding of the ducts with acinar formation begins (Fig. 3). Cyclic changes in the breast occur during each menstrual cycle, but usually not all the lobules undergo these changes. The ducts shrink at the menses, with desquamation of some epithelial cells, and then a few days after completion of the menstrual period the ductal system begins to proliferate again. The periductal connective tissue becomes rich in pale mucus with lymphocyte infiltration, and the ductal epithelial cells increase in size and number. Variations of this cyclic balance are often observed, with resultant dilatation and hypertrophy of ducts, hyperplasia of the periductal connective tissue, and increased lymphoid infiltrates. These abnormal responses form the basis for many benign pathologic conditions.

During pregnancy, glandular tissue of the breast replaces the fat as the lobules proliferate maximally and alveoli form. The placental hormones are the main stimuli for this hyperplasia, and their sudden

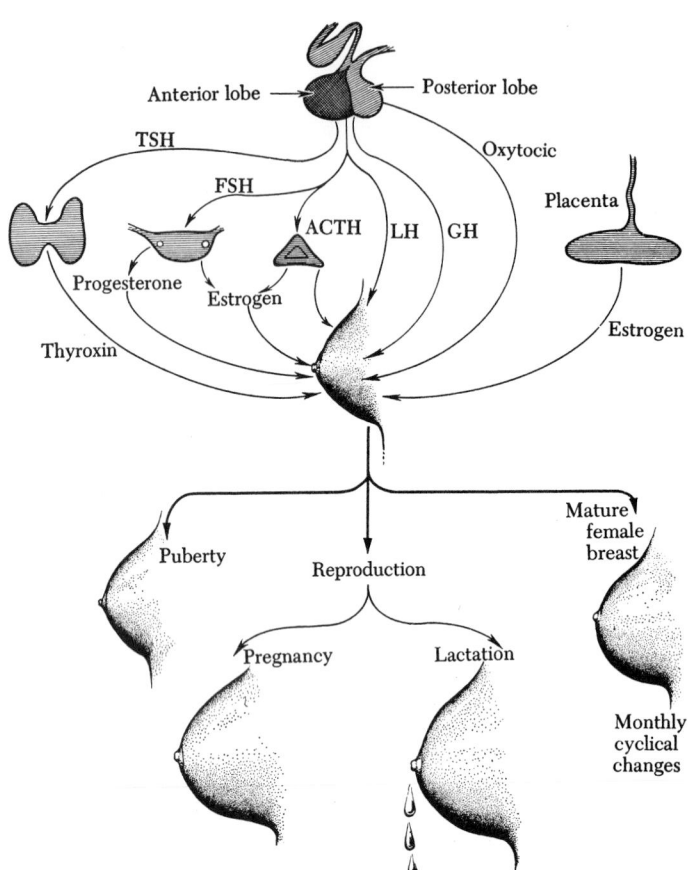

Figure 3. The breast is subject to a multiplicity of hormonal factors that affect its development and normal function. The most profound changes occur during pregnancy and lactation, when there is maximal hormonal activity. (From Jessiman, A. G. *In* Warren, R.: Surgery. Philadelphia, W. B. Saunders Company, 1963.)

withdrawal at the time of delivery, along with prolactin secretion from the anterior pituitary, is responsible for the onset of lactation. Milk is produced by shedding of the surface of the alveolar cells and there is lymphocytic invasion of the lobules. Although involution follows lactation, it is never complete and some of the glandular hypertrophy remains until the menopause, when glandular tissue is replaced by connective tissue.

In the involuting breast, there is loss of parenchyma and an increase in fibrous tissue. The periductal fibrous tissue becomes thickened in the senile breast and lobular outline disappears. Ductal dilatation is common and small cysts often develop as the enlarged acini, emptied of their hyperplastic epithelium, fail to return to their normal size. Involutional abnormalities in the breast thus take the form of lobular irregularities, epithelial proliferation, cystic dilatation of the ducts, and epithelial metaplasia in the duct wall lining. The disordered hormonal balance resulting in the menopause greatly affects the delicate structure of the breast, which is so responsive to these hormones.

BREAST EXAMINATION

Patient History

Public education and fear of cancer are responsible for more frequent self-examination of the breast on the part of the female population. It is now more common to have a patient discover an abnormality in her breast than in years past. It is wise to obtain certain data from the patient before examining the breast itself.

The patient's age, parity, nursing history, menopausal status, and family history are important. Questions about previous breast or pelvic surgery, particularly oophorectomy or hysterectomy, are essential, as is information about the observed pathologic change and any adjunctive therapy that might have been used. The age of onset of menses and present menstrual status are significant, since many breast lesions will show great alteration during the menstrual cycle.

Specific questions about the patient's complaint should elicit whether or not there is a lump or mass in the breast, and whether or not it is painful. The time course of the complaint, the presence of breast swelling or heaviness, a history of trauma, waxing and waning of the complaint with menstrual periods, and a previous history of similar problems are all important facts to be obtained. If there is a lump in the breast, then its rate of growth, whether or not the breast or axilla has become enlarged, and whether the overlying skin has become inflamed or discolored are of interest. Whether or not there is nipple discharge, and its character, frequency, and timing, should be questioned with any breast complaint, and the patient should be asked about constitutional symptoms, such as weight loss, anorexia, bone pain, fever, cough, and chest pain. A careful drug history, particularly of any hormonal therapy, must be obtained. If contraceptive medication has been used, the length of time it has been taken, the exact name of the drug and its dosage, the schedule of its use, and the time of the most recent breast examination are of value.

Inspection

In order to perform a proper physical examination there must be adequate privacy so that the patient can be relaxed, the examining area must be well lighted so that subtle changes in the skin can be identified, and the patient should be able to lie down or sit up as the examiner wishes. Careful inspection of both breasts should be the initial procedure. Variation in symmetry, size, shape, skin color, and venous patterns should be observed. The examiner must pay special attention to the nipple, looking for excoriation, inversion, discharge, edema, or redness. The skin of the breast may show diffuse edema, as seen with cellulitis; peau d'orange or "pigskin" edema (Fig. 4), as seen with underlying lymphatic obstruction; or dimpling, tethering, or retraction due to contraction of Cooper's ligaments by tumor growth in the deeper portions of the breast. Retraction of the skin is best seen when the patient sits up, with hands either on the iliac crests or crossed behind the neck, and with hyperextension of the back to tighten the pectoralis fascia. On occasion, retraction of the skin can be accentuated

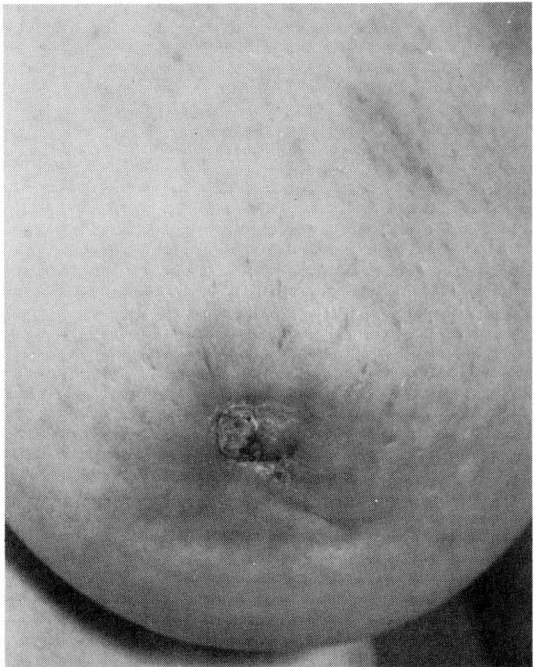

Figure 4. The breast of a patient with untreated Paget's disease of the nipple and associated peau d'orange. There is some lymphatic involvement of the skin superior to the nipple, demonstrated by the darker area at the periphery of the breast. Despite this extensive involvement, no palpable mass was present in the breast. Mammograms of this patient's breasts are seen in Figure 6B.

when the patient leans forward. At other times, gentle traction on the breast by the examiner may demonstrate it (Fig. 5D). It is an important observation because it is very unusual with benign lesions except fat necrosis, and it may identify a carcinoma too small to be clearly palpable.

Palpation

Palpation of the breast is most efficient when the patient lies down, preferably with a small pillow or towel under the shoulder and with her arm raised while the medial half of the breast is examined and with her arm down at her side during examination of the lateral half of the breast (Fig. 5A and B). Gentle palpation with fingertips is essential and a systematic examination, quadrant by quadrant, must be carried out. Changes in skin temperature, turgor, and thickness should be noted. The object of breast palpation is to search for a mass lesion that is discrete from the surrounding breast stroma. A mass that is smooth, moveable, firm, and totally separable from the adjacent lobular tissue is easily identified and probably benign. It is much more difficult to decide whether firm, irregular areas, within a breast containing cystic hyperplasia, truly represent separate lesions or are a part of the diffuse process. Such cystic changes are most common in the upper outer quadrants and in the axillary tail of the breast and are often symmetric. They are least active just after the menstrual period and re-examination at that time can be very useful. Examination by an experienced physician and often re-examination may be required to decide whether an area in the breast represents a dominant or discrete mass. Many newer techniques have been developed to aid in this decision and they will be discussed. Like cystic hyperplasia, carcinomas also are most common in the upper outer quadrant of the breasts; the most experienced physician can diagnose accurately only about 70 per cent of carcinomas by examination. Even the most questionable lesion must be re-examined and if uncertainty remains as to its presence, biopsy should be performed, as with all more definite lesions.

Regional lymph node drainage sites should always be routinely evaluated at the time of breast examination. It is advantageous to examine both the supraclavicular and axillary areas bilaterally with the patient in both the sitting and supine positions. In the neck, the area directly behind the sternoclavicular junction and the medial half of the clavicle usually contains involved lymph nodes. The neck should be examined with the examiner standing both behind the patient and in the front. When the axilla is examined, it is essential to support the patient's arm so that the musculature of the shoulder girdle is relaxed. The palpating fingers should be slid up to the very apex of the axilla with the arm abducted. Then the arm is brought down to the patient's side and the examiner's fingertips slide down over the normal axillary fat pad and on to the surface of the rib cage to the lower axilla (Fig. 5C). Thus all abnormal lymph glands within the axillary contents can be compressed against the rib cage and easily palpated. This examination may have to be repeated several times and comparison with the opposite side may be necessary for accuracy. When ex-

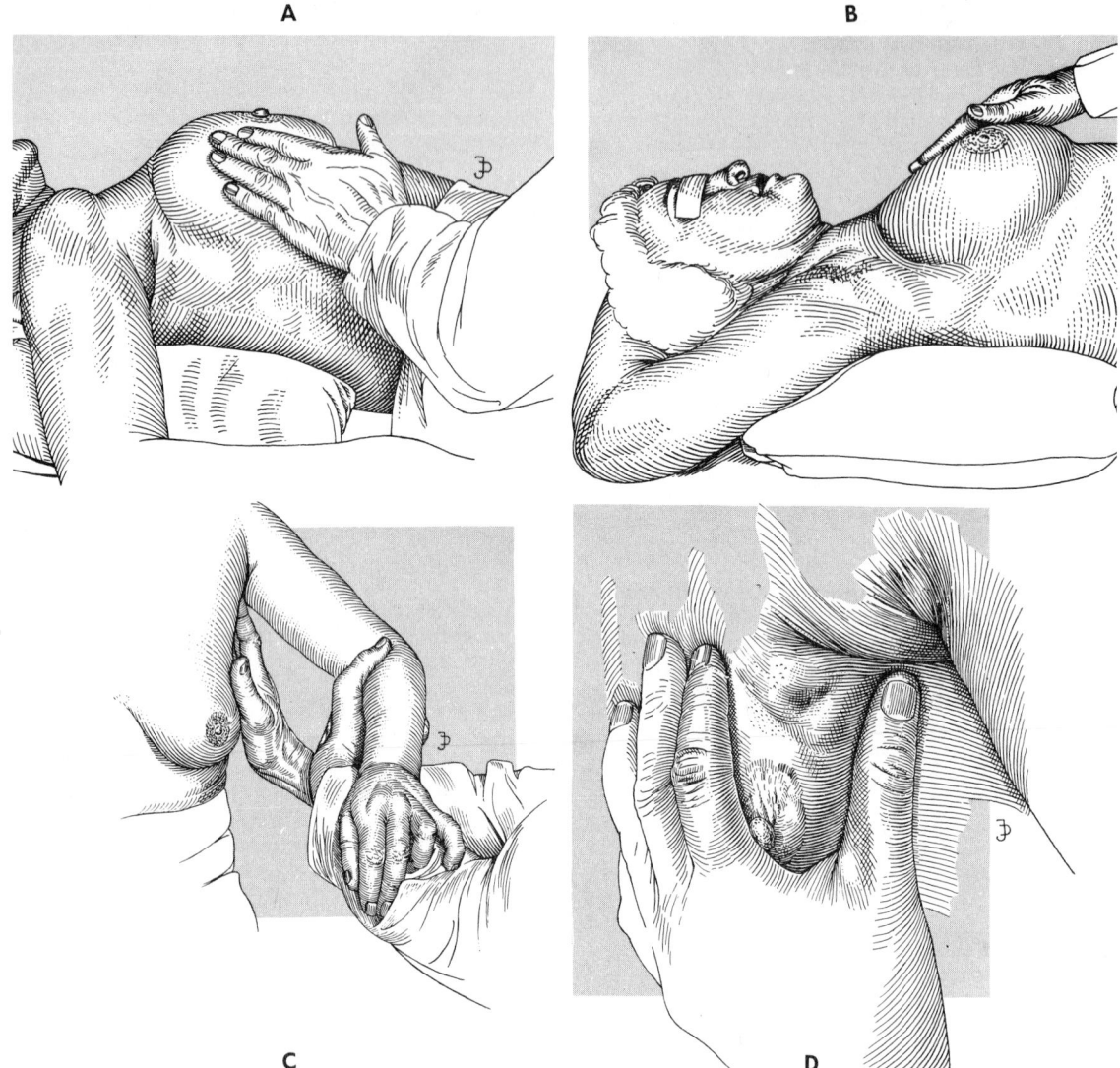

Figure 5. Palpation of the breast and demonstration of skin dimpling. *A,* When the lateral portion of the breast is palpated, the patient lies with her arm at her side and the shoulder slightly elevated on a firm pad. Palpation should be performed with the gentle pressure of the fingertips rather than with the flat of the hand. *B,* Palpation of the medial half of the breast is best accomplished with the arm above the head and the shoulder slightly elevated on a firm pillow. *C,* Examination of the axilla is best performed with the patient sitting and the arm supported by the examiner. The patient's arm should be elevated as the examiner inserts his fingertips into the highest portion of the axilla, and then as the arm is brought downward the axillary contents are palpated against the chest wall. *D,* Dimpling of the skin demonstrated by gently compressing the skin on each side of the lesion. (From Dunphy, J. E., and Botsford, T. W.: Physical Examination of the Surgical Patient, 4th ed. Philadelphia, W. B. Saunders Company, 1975.)

amining the right axilla, the left hand should be used for palpation; the right hand should be used to palpate the left axilla. As with any other examination by palpation, the examiner must be in a completely comfortable position so that his sense of touch is not distracted by extraneous discomfort. Size, consistency, and number of lymph nodes in each axilla should be noted, and also their mobility. Internal mammary lymph nodes are not palpable until they become so involved with metastatic tumor that they protrude into the intercostal spaces. When the breast is being exam-

ined for the presence of tumor, it is wise to palpate the liver edge at the same time, since its evaluation should be a routine feature of breast examination.

Nipple Examination

Since all lobules of the breast communicate with it, the nipple may provide important information about each area in the breast. The skin of the nipple should be critically examined, since papillomas, eczema, and infection can occur in the nipple. These must be differentiated from Paget's disease[90] of the nipple, which always is associated with an underlying carcinoma, often undetected by palpation. In Paget's disease, the nipple has either a dry, scaling surface that bleeds on contact or a red, weeping eczematoid appearance (see Fig. 3). Haagensen[45] has supported the concept that lesions involving the nipple, with or without the areola, are usually Paget's disease, while those involving areola or skin only are usually benign. Microscopic study is necessary for the definitive diagnosis of Paget's disease.

Nipple inversion is quite common in normal breasts, but recent appearance of unilateral retraction or inversion of the nipple is most worrisome. In a normal breast, an inverted nipple can always be everted to the normal position. If this is not possible, or if a mass can be palpated beneath the inverted nipple, biopsy is indicated.

Nipple discharges always are abnormal except during lactation, but they do not always indicate malignancy. Serous, colorless discharge can occur during normal menstrual cycles, result from intraductal papilloma, or accompany early pregnancy. A blood discharge is usually associated with either intraductal papilloma or ductal carcinoma. Milky discharge may persist after lactation has finished and is of no consequence in the diagnosis of breast cancer. Other systemic hormonal abnormalities such as acromegaly can produce this kind of discharge. Yellow discharge may indicate a galactocele or cystic hyperplasia and is rarely associated wtih carcinoma.

Bloody discharge is the most common type, present 50 to 75 per cent of the time in most studies. It is the only type of drainage from the nipple in which cancer must be seriously suspected; yet it is unusual for a bloody discharge, in the absence of a mass, to be associated with malignancy in patients under 50 years of age. When a discharge is present, the quadrant from which it comes should be sought by gentle palpation. This may reveal a mass or dilated duct that would not otherwise be palpable. In over half the cases of chronic discharge, the site of discharge in the breast can be found even if no mass is palpable. Papanicolaou smear is helpful in nipple discharge only if it is positive. A negative Papanicolaou smear should not be considered adequate reassurance that a given lesion is benign. Transillumination may be useful in identifying a cyst along the course of a dilated duct. Fourteen per cent of patients with discharge had malignant disease of the breast in Funderburk's[39] series, and 9 per cent in Spratt's[106] experience. Funderburk[39] has recommended the use of a ductogram with contrast radiography, rather than more extensive procedures, to localize sources of discharge or permit local excision of a lesion. Surgical exploration of the subareolar area is indicated if the source of the discharge cannot be found and if no mass is present in the subjacent breast. Probing of the duct combined with palpation usually identifies the responsible lesion, permitting proper therapy.

Self-Examination

Women should be instructed to examine their own breasts in a systematic manner after the age of about 25. Examination is best performed at the same time in each menstrual cycle, preferably just after the completion of the menses when the breast is least engorged. The patient should lie down, with a pillow or towel behind the shoulder, just as for examination by the physician. The ipsilateral arm should be placed up and behind the head and the opposite hand should gently palpate the breast circumferentially with the fingertips. The breasts should be inspected in the mirror as well, to identify any dimpling or asymmetry. Women must be encouraged to report abnormalities to their physician, since early diagnosis and prompt treatment offer the best chance for successful control of malignant disease of the breast.

Mammography, Xeroradiography, and Thermography

Although diagnostic radiography of the breast is not a new concept, it has achieved widespread acceptance in the past decade. Special and careful techniques are necessary with fine-grain x-ray film; views are taken of each breast from the superior and medial aspects, with the inferior and lateral surfaces of the breast against the cassette, respectively. Mammography offers an opportunity on a screening basis to identify breast cancer prior to the appearance of clinical signs and symptoms. As the accuracy is increased and cost is reduced, it will become more practical for mass screening. Where it has been used as a community enterprise with an interdisciplinary approach, 80 per cent of the patients in whom breast cancer was found had an early stage of the lesion; Egan and his colleagues[29] found clinically undetected cancer by mammography in 10 per cent of these patients and 92 per cent had no tumor in axillary nodes. Mammography is particularly useful in the older woman with large, fatty breasts, where bulky soft tissue makes palpation difficult but where the high fat content makes x-ray identification of a malignant lesion easier. Younger women have dense, active breast stroma that obscures lesions from radiographic examination. Mammography is also very important in examining the opposite breast in women who have already had a breast cancer. Egan reports identification of twice as many bilateral cancers in a 5-year period when mammography was available as compared to an earlier series.[29] Women with previous breast cancer and relatives (mothers, sisters, children, and nieces) of patients who have had breast cancer are in a high-risk group and should represent the first target of a screening program with mammography to identify occult carcinoma. Stevens and Weigen[107] reported a 4.5 per thousand cancer recognition rate over a 5-year period from combined physical and x-ray examination of previously mastectomized women, which is twice the yield in patients without previous breast cancer in the same interval. Interpretation of mammograms requires special experience, as emphasized by Gershon-Cohen and colleagues.[42] Benign lesions are usually well circumscribed, homogeneous, and often surrounded by a zone of fatty tissue (Fig. 6). Calcification, if present, is usually coarse and confined to the periphery of the lesion. The more definite radiologic signs of breast cancer are mass lesions with poorly defined margins, particularly when the edges are ei-

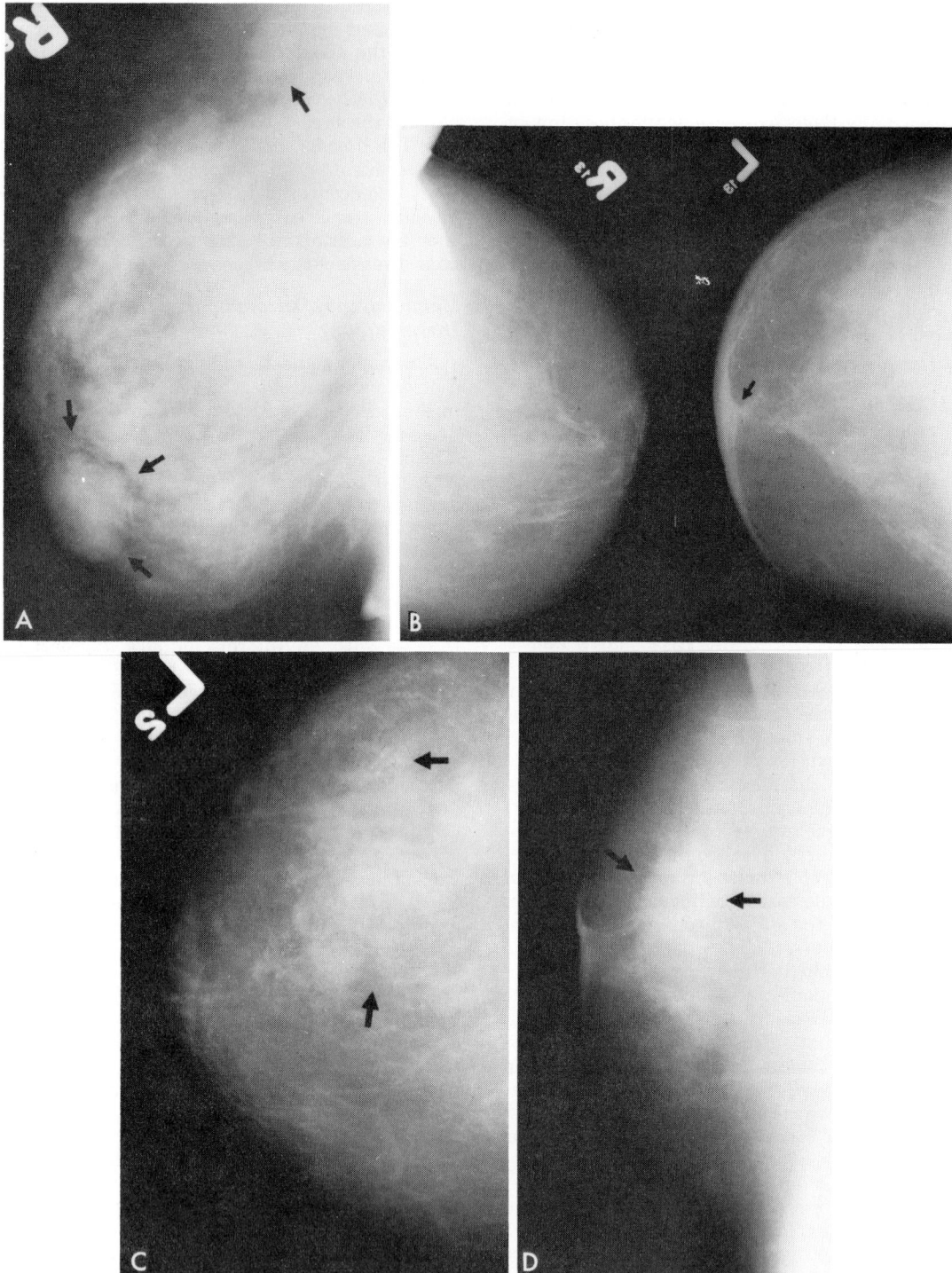

Figure 6. Mammograms of benign and malignant lesions. *A,* This benign fibroadenoma has relatively uniform density and well-defined margins and shows no increase in vascularity. The skin overlying this lesion is very thin. The upper arrow points to a second fibroadenoma in the breast. *B,* The right and left mammogram of the patient whose left breast is seen in Figure 4. The left breast shows heavily thickened skin that takes on the clinical appearance of peau d'orange. The opposite breast shows the normal thickness of skin for this patient. Despite the extensive disease in the nipple (arrow) and surrounding lymphatics, there is no clear mass in the underlying breast tissue. Diffuse thickening is present in each breast. *C,* This mammogram demonstrates diffuse, stippled calcification in a large malignant lesion. This fine calcification is typical of malignant disease, whereas coarse vascular calcification is not. *D,* This mammogram reveals a malignant lesion deep within the breast that produces nipple retraction by extension along the ducts to the areola. The borders of the tumor are poorly defined and extend into the surrounding atrophic breast tissue. (Courtesy of Dr. A. Lewicki, Department of Radiology, Peter Bent Brigham Hospital.)

ther spiculated or irregular. Fine, stippled soft tissue and periductal calcification, not vascular calcification, are also important findings. Thickening and retraction of the overlying skin can be seen by mammography in some cases of breast cancer. Less certain findings are increased ductal and stromal activity and ductal dilatation secondary to obstruction. Serial mammograms may be particularly useful in certain cases, so that progression of a possible abnormality may be identified.

Xeroradiography[124] consists of making x-ray images on a selenium plate instead of a photographic plate, producing a positive impression with accentuation of density differences. Xeroradiography and mammography should be considered equivalent diagnostic procedures. Wolfe[124] reports a false negative rate of only 4.7 per cent; 30 per cent of the carcinomas in his large series were occult, and 37 per cent of these were identified by the presence of calcifications alone.

Thermography and ultrasonography are physical techniques employed in early detection of breast cancer. In general, these techniques are less accurate than mammography and currently serve as preliminary screening devices for mammograms in a large population.[73] Thermography is based on the observation that the breast with a malignant lesion has increased skin temperature and radiation of heat. Infrared camera equipment identifies the increased surface temperature and records the variations by scanning the breast. A temperature-controlled ambient atmosphere is required, which is time-consuming for contemplated large-scale screening. Better spatial resolution will reduce the scan time and increase the accuracy of the interpretation.[26]

Bone Studies

In patients with primary breast cancer, despite normal chest x-rays and the absence of skeletal symptoms, about 10 per cent will have occult bone metastases. Charkes et al.[19] identified such metastases by ^{87m}Sr scanning in 9 per cent of their patients, despite normal bone x-rays. They reported a significant correlation between positive bone scans and the presence of greater than 6 involved axillary nodes. Bone scans are superior to standard metastatic skeletal x-rays, but as Galasko and Doyle[40] pointed out, x-rays must be taken in patients with positive scans to avoid "false" positive interpretation due to benign disease. Available isotopes and imaging techniques are constantly improving; Barrett and Smith[7] have recently shown that ^{99m}Tc polyphosphate could detect 99 per cent of bone lesions, compared to 56 per cent with ^{18}F and 29 per cent with bone x-rays. They found the gamma camera superior to the scanner.

BENIGN BREAST DISEASE

Congenital and Developmental Abnormalities

Although the normal location of the breast is the anterior thorax, breast tissue with or without a nipple or just a nipple and areola alone can occur anywhere along the milk line, which is an ectodermal thickening appearing at 6 weeks' gestation running from the midclavicle to the midportion of the inguinal ligament. Total lack of breast tissue (amastia) or of a nipple (athelia) is unusual. Supernumerary nipples (polythelia) and breasts (polymastia) are quite common and are most frequent on the anterior chest wall, below and medial to the normal breasts. Either the supernumerary breast or nipple can occur alone and they may be present in both men and women. When polymastia is present in women, the additional breast tissue can respond normally in the postpartum period and even secrete milk when a nipple is present.

Since the breast is a secondary sex organ, it is responsive to ovarian and pituitary secretion during development. Breast tissue is sufficiently responsive at birth that persistence of placental estrogen in the newborn may produce an infantile mastitis that is self-limiting, but may develop into cellulitis in rare cases. Precocious puberty and breast hypertrophy accompany adrenal cortical and ovarian tumors in childhood and may be among the earliest manifestations of the underlying endocrinopathy. Unless mammary underdevelopment results from ovarian agenesis or some other defect of estrogen production, little can be gained by estrogen administration. Massive virginal hypertrophy occurs when pubertal growth persists, resulting in breasts weighing as much as 35 to 40 pounds. Surgical therapy for either underdeveloped breasts or hypertrophied, pendulous breasts should not be attempted until full growth has been achieved.

Gynecomastia is development of a female-type breast in a male. It is usually unilateral and occurs in young men; there is no relationship to hormonal dysfunction in unilateral gynecomastia. When bilateral gynecomastia is seen, a systemic etiology must be searched for. It is common in hepatic cirrhosis associated with high levels of circulating estrogen and, of course, after estrogen administration for prostatic malignancy. It is rarely necessary to be concerned about malignancy in the usual case of gynecomastia. The mass of breast tissue is rubbery, nontender, and moveable from the underlying muscle. It often presents a serious psychological problem in an otherwise healthy young man and is best removed if it fails to resolve in a few months. Removal can easily be performed under local anesthesia through a circumareolar incision, with virtually no residual scar. These breasts show proliferation of fibrous stroma and ducts without acinar growth. In older men, the breast mass is often more irregular and biopsy is always required to rule out a carcinoma. In this situation, simple excision of the breast mass as a biopsy is the treatment of choice.

Inflammatory Disease: Acute Mastitis and Breast Abscess

Acute mastitis due to bacterial infection most commonly occurs within the first few weeks of lactation. Infection usually results from staphylococci or streptococci entering the breast through abraded or lacerated nipple surfaces or by way of the lactiferous ducts as they enter the nipple. Lymphatic involvement results in either cellulitis or frank abscess formation. Streptococcal infections tend to produce a diffuse cellulitis, even to the point of an erysipelas of the breast with systemic toxic manifestations. Cessation of nursing, local heat, and appropriate antibiotics may control this type of cellulitic infection without the development of an abscess. *Staphylococcus aureus* infections usually suppurate as they invade deeply, and abscess formation is more common with this organism. Multiple abscesses may occur as the infection dissects between fibrous septae, and serious destruction of breast tissue can result. Early and adequate drainage is essential if fluctuation occurs, with care being taken to drain each abscess cavity that has formed. Either several septae can be opened through a single circumareolar incision or multiple incisions may be required. The red, hot, tender mass beneath the skin in early acute mastitis becomes softer and less painful as suppuration occurs and that is the indication for wide drainage. The most important consideration in the management of acute mastitis is its prevention. Strict adherence to nipple hygiene is essential during breast feeding and any cracks or inflamed areas should be promptly treated. If some redness develops, an ice pack to the area and either the use of a breast pump or continued suckling is recommended to prevent stasis and intraductal growth of bacteria.

Chronic abscesses are rare and can easily simulate carcinoma. The usual cause of chronic mastitis with abscess formation is tuberculosis, which is secondary to pulmonary or chest wall disease. The lesion is "cold" and is not tender; multiple sinus tracts to the skin surface develop and cystic cavitation of the breast results. The diagnosis can be made only by biopsy. Adequate drainage and antitubercular therapy can avoid the need for mastectomy.

Occasionally a chronic, well circumscribed breast abscess can result from inadequately drained postpartum mastitis. This lesion may be present intermittently, especially if there are repeated episodes of inadequate drainage. The edema, induration, and severe local scarring can easily simulate a malignant process. Wide local drainage with excision of the most extensively involved portions of the wall and careful histologic proof that this is a benign lesion are necessary, as well as appropriate antibiotics, in order to achieve complete healing of these chronic abscesses.

Fat Necrosis

The development in the breast of a firm, hard lump that is often tender and rarely enlarges after it is first noticed may represent fat necrosis. It is usually impossible to differentiate this lesion from carcinoma either by physical examination or mammography. Skin retraction, irregularity of the edges, and fine, stippled calcification may all be present. About half the time, a history of trauma can be obtained, and often hemorrhage into the fat is observed at the time of biopsy. It usually occurs in fat, pendulous breasts and may be related to prolonged pressure in a given site. Occasionally, the fat may liquefy in the early stages, giving a cystlike structure, but the longer-standing lesions of fat necrosis are scarred and contracted. Excisional biopsy is the treatment of choice and is usually required for the diagnosis to be certain. Histologically, the early lesion shows saponification of the fat with clouding of the fat cells, rather than true necrosis. More extensive fat necrosis is associated with a chronic inflammatory reaction; foreign body giant cells and lymphocytes infiltrate the center of the lesion and many foamy macrophages and new connective tissue growth surround the central core.

Mammary Duct Ectasia

This condition has several stages of involvement, and has a variety of names, including plasma cell mastitis, comedomastitis, and chronic abscess simulating carcinoma. It is a benign lesion that may be virtually impossible to differentiate from carcinoma by its gross appearances. Nipple retraction, skin adherence and edema, and axillary adenopathy may accompany a hard, diffuse mass within the breast. The primary pathologic finding is subacute inflammation of the ductal system, usually beginning in the subareolar area with ductal obstruction. The ducts become distended and filled with debris and fatty material and the epithelium is atrophic rather than hypercellular. Sheets of plasma cells in the periductal fat can be present during some stages of the disease. The periductal inflammation, due to irritating lipid eroding through the ducts, produces the initial inflammatory reaction, which may never be seen by the physician, since the patients present at a later time with the gross appearance of a breast carcinoma.

This disease usually appears around or after the menopause and there is often a history of difficult nursing. Multiple biopsies may be required to rule out carcinoma, and Ackerman and del Regato[2] described a case in which an underlying carcinoma was masked by this lesion.

Galactocele

This problem usually occurs after cessation of lactation and represents obstruction of a duct distended with milk and desquamated epithelial cells. The galactocele usually lies beneath the areola, and the ampullary portions of the duct are the sites of the obstruction. On palpation the duct is found to be enlarged, it is often tender, and it sometimes can be emptied by properly placed pressure. It cannot be adequately drained in this manner, however, and will fill up once again. It is best excised, since it may be the site of future sepsis and if left in place can calcify and become confused with a malignant lesion. Galactoceles drained early after their formation show a milky, clear material with a well-formed capsule. Later on, the material is greenish yellow and thick and it looks purulent but is usually sterile.

Cystic Hyperplasia

This is the most common lesion in the female breast and its nomenclature has been fraught with controversy in the past. Cystic lobular hyperplasia and fibrocystic disease of the breast are two descriptions that are acceptable, but unquestionably the term cystic mastitis should be discarded since inflammation is not present. Cystic hyperplasia represents a variant of the normal cyclic changes in the breast that occur with menstruation. Hormonal imbalance to some degree, probably excessive estrogen production and deficient corpus lutein activity, produces exaggerated responses in the breast. This hyperplasia usually presents bilaterally in the upper outer quadrants of the breasts and is most painful in the premenstrual period. Nonovulatory cycles may provoke the most pain and discomfort and the condition is commoner in the later years of reproductive life.

Patients with cystic hyperplasia usually complain of pain or a lump in the breast. The breasts are frequently tender in many locations, axillary adenopathy is rare, and multiple lumps or nodules are frequently scattered about both breasts but inseparable from the rest of the granular induration. Bilateral involvement is common but not necessarily equal. The palpable lumps usually represent larger cysts that are tense and consequently not fluctuant. Cysts may appear rapidly and then maintain their size or shrink after the next menstrual flow. Although the natural course of the disease varies, there is usually a cessation of active disease at the time of the menopause. About 15 per cent of patients with chronic cystic disease present with nipple discharge; usually the discharge is clear, but occasionally a bloody discharge occurs. With transillumination one can identify large cysts but not rule out a concomitant carcinoma. That, indeed, is the essence of the clinician's problem with fibrocystic disease. Cystic hyperplasia is exceedingly common and it can coexist with carcinoma of the breast, which is also a very common lesion. Whether or not cystic hyperplasia is a precancerous lesion is unsettled and probably purely an academic question. No one will deny the possibility that some lesions of cystic lobular hyperplasia may develop into carcinoma, but there are no clear data as to how often this may occur. The practical difficulty lies not with whether a given lesion will become malignant, but rather with whether a lesion in the present represents a benign disease of cystic hyperplasia or an already present carcinoma. Although clinical experience, Papanicolaou smear of discharge, and mammography all contribute to this decision, the ultimate answer must be obtained after biopsy and histologic examination of any persistent discrete lump in the breast.

It is not unusual, after a single large cyst has been excised, for no further cyst formation to occur. If additional cysts do develop, however, after an initial biopsy with a proven diagnosis of cystic hyperplasia, it is permissible to carry out needle aspiration and evacuation of the dirty, gray-green fluid filling the cyst. Many of these large cysts no longer have any functional wall and there may be no recurrence after aspiration. If either blood or no fluid at all is obtained from an apparent cystic mass, or if the cyst recurs over the subsequent month or two, then open biopsy is indicated. Smears of cyst fluids should be obtained, but they are often unsatisfactory because of the paucity of cells. A positive Papanicolaou smear is, of course, most significant, and should be immediately followed by biopsy.

Breast tissue involved with cystic hyperplasia is rubbery in consistency, yellowish white in color, and not encapsulated. It is not gritty to cut, as is carcinoma, and there are often many small cysts scattered through the tissue. The classic diffuse cystic disease is called Schimmelbusch's disease, while a single, tense, large, blue dome cyst is known as a Bloodgood cyst.[43] Some ducts are distended with grayish green desquamated cells that extrude from their cut surface like toothpaste.

The major microscopic appearances of cystic hyperplasia are: (1) Glandular hyperplasia, primarily involving ducts. (2) Cyst formation, usually small, related to ductal dilatation and failure of hyperplastic ducts to fully involute (Fig. 7). Hemorrhage into a cyst or obstruction of a dilated duct with continued secretion causes larger cysts to form. (3) Papillary formation in cysts due to hyperplasia of the epithelium, which may reach such a degree of proliferation that the ductal lumen is full of cells. (4) Apocrine epithelium, appearing as large eosinophilic cells, lining the ductal lumen, representing a form of dedifferentiation to more primitive sweat gland epithelial cells. (5) Con-

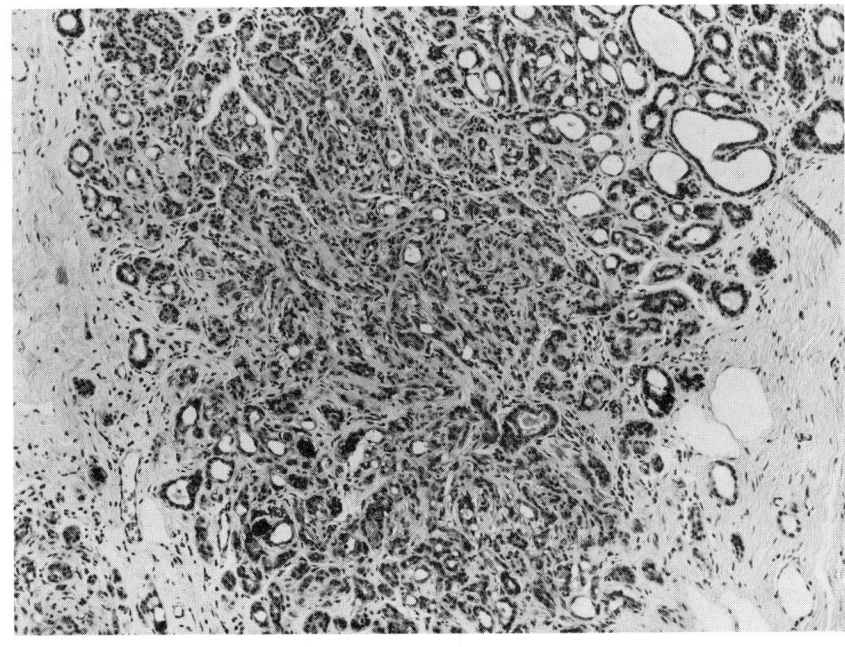

Figure 7. Cystic disease of the breast. ×180, H and E. The primary lesion in this breast is sclerosing adenosis, but there are enlarged cystic structures with ductal dilatation on the periphery of this section. The extensive scar tissue and apparent distortion of the ductal system might appear confusing on initial glance, but the uniformity of the cells and the evidences of ductal dilatation, even though compressed, differentiate this lesion from that of carcinoma. (Courtesy of Dr. J. M. Corson, Department of Pathology, Peter Bent Brigham Hospital.)

nective tissue hyperplasia of both the periductal tissue and the fibrous stroma, which may distort acinar patterns. (6) Lymphocytic infiltration, which is common but not always present. (7) Sclerosing adenosis. This is a form of the disease more common in younger women and most likely to be confused with carcinoma on histologic study (Fig. 7). It is more solid and fibrous than most cystic hyperplasia and when the fibrosis is so intense that lobules and epithelial cells lose their orientation, the appearance on frozen section is most like that of scirrhous carcinoma. However, there are no mitoses, the nuclei are very regular, and there are actually small compressed cystic spaces between cells.

Management of cystic lobular hyperplasia is best accomplished by frequent examination of the patient by the physician, as well as self-examination by the patient. Hormonal therapy should be discouraged, in order to reduce the amount of estrogen stimulation. Yearly mammograms will serve to aid in the identification of any new lesions and provide an excellent adjunct to the physical examination of these women. Any new or changing lesion must be treated as a potential carcinoma regardless of the underlying cystic hyperplasia.

Intraductal Papilloma

These benign lesions of the lactiferous duct walls occur centrally beneath the areola in 75 per cent of the cases. They most commonly produce a bloody nipple discharge, sometimes associated with pain, and are solitary proliferations of ductal epithelium, in contrast to the papillomatous changes associated with cystic disease of the breast, which can occur in many sites simultaneously. These papillomas may be soft, small, and difficult to palpate beneath the areola or the nipple, and often must be located by compression or milking of the specific duct in which it lies so as to express some blood from the nipple. Ductograms, as discussed earlier,[38] can also be very useful in identifying such papillomas. If a patient presents with a small, palpable mass and bloody nipple discharge, there is a 95 per cent chance that she has an intraductal papilloma. When no mass can be felt, then Paget's disease of the nipple, adenoma of the nipple, or a deeper lying carcinoma with ductal invasion must be sought. Intraductal papillomas can become secondarily infected; then the mass becomes fixed to adjacent tissue and the differential diagnosis becomes more difficult.

Intraductal papillomas should be treated by excision of the duct as a wedge resection. If the mass can be palpated, location of the wedge to be excised is simple. If no mass can be felt, the duct from which blood is expressed should be gently probed and excision carried out along the probe until the papilloma is identified. If no papilloma can be found in a suspected duct that has been dissected along a probe, then a blind wedge resection should be performed of that portion of the breast from which the secretion appeared. Simple mastectomy is not justified for this lesion. Intraductal papillomas are always benign but other papillomas may arise in a breast after one has been excised. Intraductal papillary carcinoma is rare and probably arises de novo in the duct; invasion through the duct wall must be identified to confirm this diagnosis. Although most intraductal papillomas are in the range of 0.4 to 1 cm. in size, large papillomas have been identified, up to 10 cm. in size.

Fibroadenoma

Fibroadenoma is a common, well-circumscribed lesion of the breast that tends to occur in younger women or girls. The peak age incidence is 21 to 25 years, and multiple fibroadenomas occur 15 per cent of the time. The fact that they can be produced by estrogen in animals would indicate some relationship between excessive hormone levels and fibroadenomas. They are characterized as being freely moveable, smooth, lobulated, and independent from the surrounding breast tissue, without any fixation to the overlying skin no matter what size they attain within the breast. These lesions are usually painless but can be tender to palpation and do not regress after a menstrual cycle. The nipple is always normal and there is no associated discharge. In adolescence, exceedingly large tumors have been reported that can be confused with virginal hypertrophy. Rapid growth of fibroadenoma has been seen at the time of pregnancy and lactation, or just prior to the menopause, when estrogen stimulation is highest.

Fibroadenomas are best treated by excisional biopsy because of their continued growth and the need to be certain of the diagnosis. They are well-encapsulated, fleshy, and homogeneous with fibrous whorls, and they bulge from the capsule on being cut. They are described as either pericanalicular or intracanalicular in origin and are primarily fibromas. Since both cystic hyperplasia and fibroadenoma are related to estrogen stimulation, it is common to have them occur simultaneously. The pericanalicular type is firmer and smaller, with an increase in ducts and fibrous stroma over normal breast tissue. The intracanalicular type of adenoma tends to grow larger and has extensive invagination into the duct system, producing great distortion of the ducts with polypoid masses of connective tissue. Because the connective tissue may be so profuse and loosely adherent, the tumor has been referred to as an intraductal myxoma.

Cystosarcoma Phyllodes

This is a rare variant of fibroadenoma often referred to as a giant fibroadenoma. When it was first described in 1838 by Müller[86] it received its name because the tumor contained large cysts and was fleshy, a connotation for the term sarcoma at that time. Large surface clefts were thought to resemble leaves in a book; this accounts for the choice of the term "phyllon" (leaf). Most of these tumors are benign, but a few develop true sarcomatous potential. The treatment of these tumors will be discussed under the section on sarcomas of the breast.

Cystosarcomas occur most commonly in women in an age group between that of the peak incidence of fibroadenoma and that of the peak incidence of breast carcinoma. They are usually large, bulky tumors with the breast having the typical "tear-drop" appearance as the skin is stretched over the lesion. Despite the size of the tumor, skin involvement does not occur, but the skin is usually red, shiny, and warm, and large

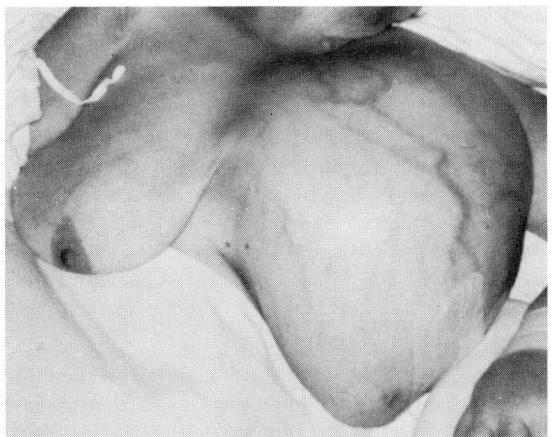

Figure 8. A patient with massive involvement of the left breast with cystosarcoma phyllodes. Notice the large distended veins and the stretching of the skin over the very large mass in the breast. On the lateral undersurface of the breast, an ulceration of the skin has occurred as a result of necrosis of the tumor with secondary infection, a common problem with this lesion when it grows exceedingly large. This lesion was invasive of the chest wall and was a malignant type of cystosarcoma.

dilated veins are easily visible overlying the tumor (Fig. 8). Axillary gland metastases are also rare, a fact that serves to distinguish this tumor from carcinoma on physical examination. It would be very unusual to see a carcinoma 10 to 15 cm. in diameter, totally replacing the breast tissue, that invaded neither the overlying skin, the pectoral fascia, nor the axilla. Occasionally, the thinning and distention of the skin over the tumor produces necrosis of the skin. Likewise, the tumor itself may outgrow its blood supply because of its rapid growth, and areas of necrosis with overlying inflammatory reaction occur. Even when malignant sarcomatous degeneration is present, distant metastases from this tumor are unusual.

CARCINOMA OF THE BREAST

EPIDEMIOLOGY

Breast carcinoma is the most common form of cancer in women in the United States. It is the leading cause of death among women 40 to 44 years old, and is one of the leading causes of death in women from age 30 onward. About 89,000 women were first diagnosed as having breast cancer in the year 1974 in this country, and approximately 32,500 women died of breast cancer in the United States in the same year. Whereas the death rates from cancer of the uterus and stomach and, to a much lesser degree, colon and rectum have declined in the past two decades, deaths from breast cancer occur at approximately the same rate (Fig. 9). Relative survival rates of women with breast cancer have begun to improve (Fig. 10); with a rising incidence of breast cancer, there is a stable mortality in white females but not in blacks (Fig. 11). The incidence of breast cancer is of such proportion that in

New York State 6 per cent of newly born girls, or one of 17, might be expected to develop breast cancer at some time during their lives.[104]

The mortality rate from breast cancer varies in different locations in the world (Fig. 12). In the United States, the relative 10-year survival rate for all women treated for breast cancer between 1955 and 1964 was 50 per cent; it was 73 per cent for localized disease and 37 per cent for regional disease (Fig. 13). Among women in the United States, breast cancer death rates are higher among nonwhites than whites through age group 45 to 49, but lower thereafter (Fig. 14). In the male, the nonwhite individual has a higher mortality from breast cancer throughout life.

Breast cancer mortality is much higher in developed countries (with the exception of Japan) than in undeveloped countries (see Fig. 12). Even within New York City, women in the high-income socioeconomic class have a higher mortality from breast cancer than do those in a lower income group. In a comparison of the same groups, a smaller proportion of the women of

TRENDS IN AGE-STANDARDIZED*FEMALE CANCER DEATH RATES BY SITE-UNITED STATES
1930-1973

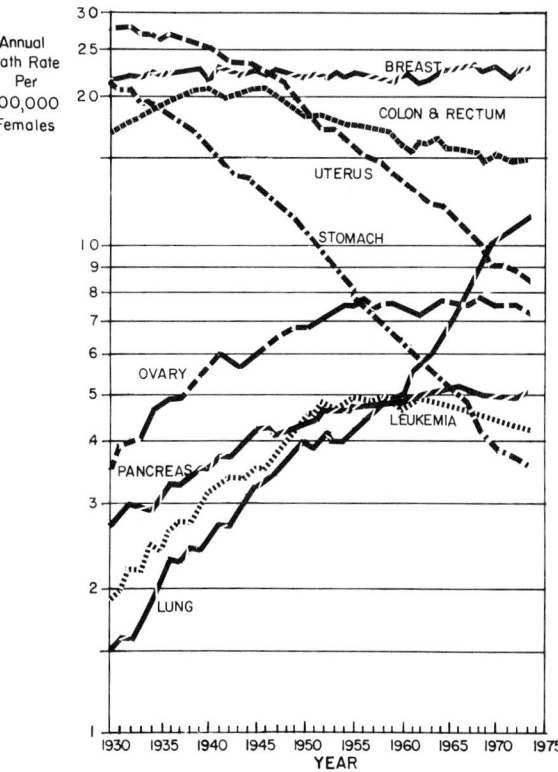

*Standardized on age distribution of population of United States, 1940

Figure 9. This chart demonstrates stability of the mortality rate for breast cancer in American women as compared with the falling rate for gastric and uterine carcinoma and the rising rate from ovarian cancer, leukemia, and lung cancer. Breast cancer has for the past twenty-five years been the most common cause of death from malignancy in women in the United States. (Chart provided by the American Cancer Society.)

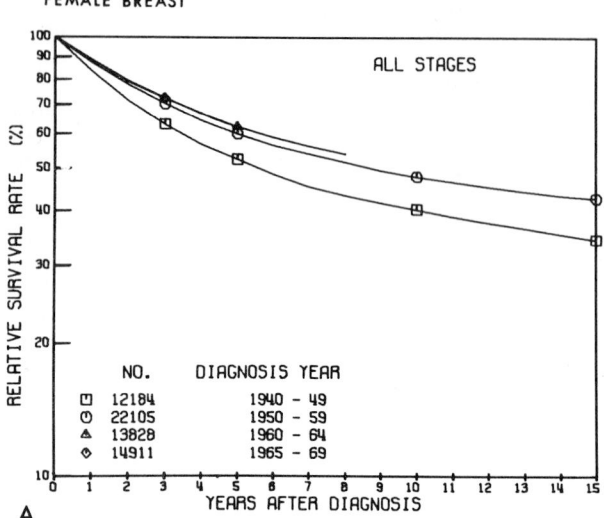

FEMALE BREAST

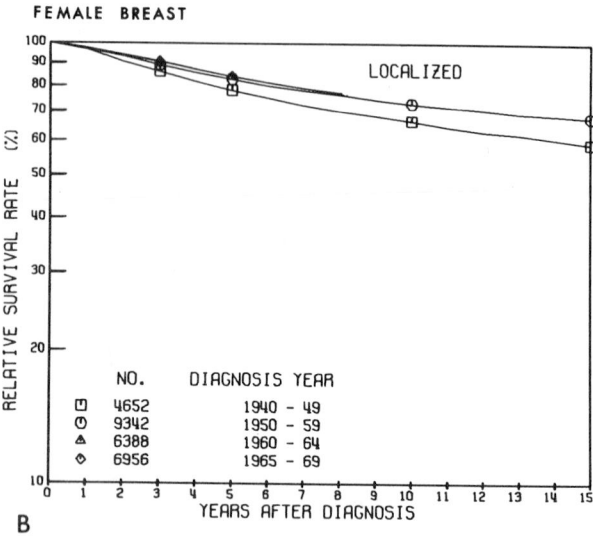

FEMALE BREAST

Figure 10. Relative survival data for patients with breast cancer diagnosed from 1940 through 1969. *A,* Data for the entire group of patients. After the definite improvement in results from the first to the second decade of the study, there has been no change since 1960. The five-year survival rate for 1960–64 was 63 per cent as compared with 53 per cent in the first decade. *B,* Data from patients with localized disease (no lymph node involvement) also showed improvement in survival since the 1940–49 decade. Differences are less for this subset. Five-year survival was 84 per cent in 1965–69 as compared with 78 per cent in 1940–49. (From Axtell, L. M., Cutler, S. J., and Myers, M. H. (Eds.): End Results in Cancer, Report #4. DHEW Publication No. (NIH) 73–272. Washington, D. C., 1972.)

the higher socioeconomic class had had pregnancies before age 20, and fewer had three or more children.

Because breast cancer mortality rates are much lower for Japanese women, intense interest has been centered upon that population group. Even though Japanese women migrate to Hawaii or to the continental United States, they and their United States-born daughters have maintained a far lower incidence than the remainder of the American population, although the incidence has risen. The best explanation

to date for this difference between Japanese and American women is that dietary factors and obesity may affect the tissue concentrations of fat-soluble estrogenic hormones. Wynder[125] has demonstrated excellent correlation between fat intake and breast cancer mortality; Japanese women have the lowest dietary fat levels of any major population group. The greatest variation between Japanese and American women in breast cancer mortality was in those beyond 50 years of age[30] (Fig. 15). This may reflect the more modern type of dietary regimen of the younger generation of Japanese women. Continued observation will be necessary to determine whether these findings persist as these younger women pass through the menopause.

Numerous investigations to identify epidemiologic features of high-risk populations have demonstrated that two major factors influence the development of breast cancer: (1) a woman who has had a previous breast cancer is at a higher risk of developing cancer in the opposite breast, and (2) a history of breast cancer in the immediate family places a woman at a greater risk.[125] A woman with a previous breast cancer under the age of 50 has a 0.7 per cent chance per year of developing a second breast cancer. The occurrence rate for breast cancer is 15 times greater in sisters of breast cancer patients whose mothers also had breast

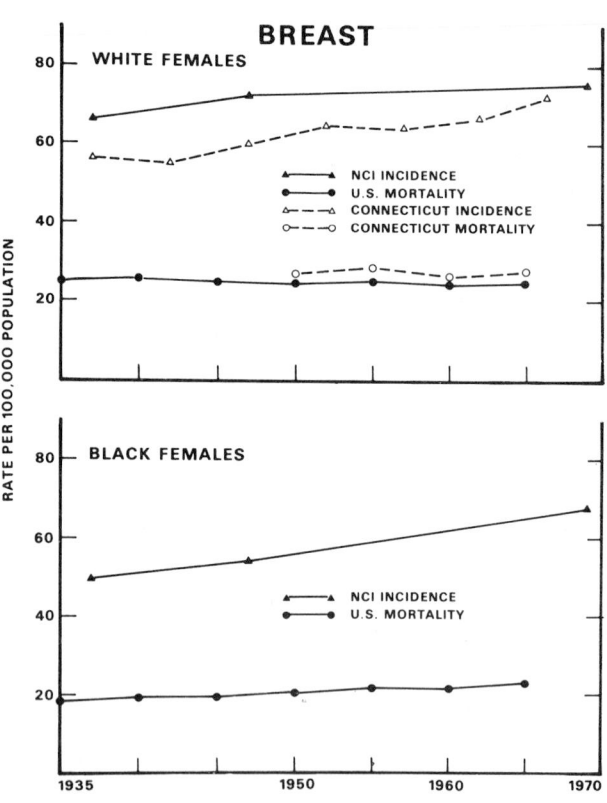

Figure 11. Trend of breast cancer incidence and mortality, 1935 to 1969. Although the incidence for both black and white females in the United States continues to rise, the mortality for white females has been stable for the past 35 years. There is a slight increase in the mortality rate for black females, but its proportion to the incidence rate is the same as for white females. (From Cutler, S. J., and DeVesa, S. S. *In* IARC Scientific Publication #7, FIC Proceedings No. 18, Lyon, France, 1973, pp. 15–33.)

FEMALE BREAST CANCER DEATH RATES FOR VARIOUS COUNTRIES, 1970-1971

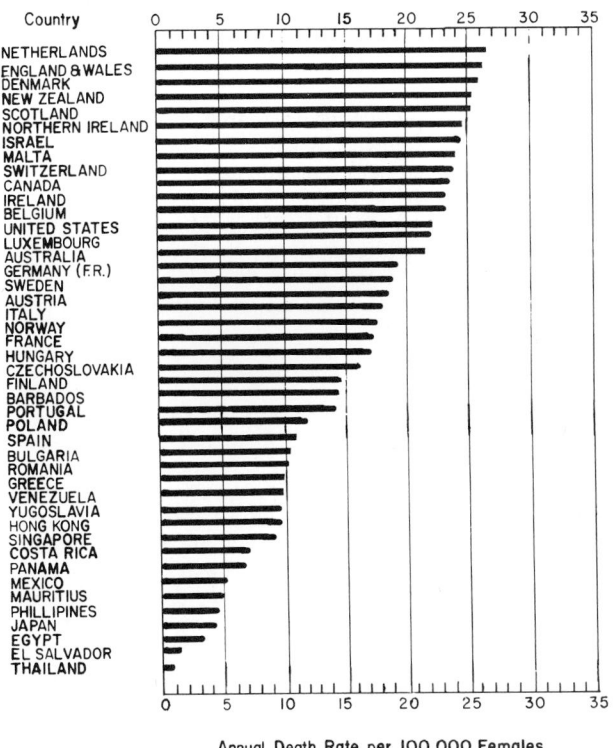

Figure 12. The death rate from cancer of the breast is highest in the Western industrialized countries, as demonstrated in this chart. The exceedingly low incidence in Japan is apparent. (Chart provided by the American Cancer Society.)

nursing by no means clearly reduce the incidence of breast cancer. Patients in whom breast cancer develops do not appear to differ from other women with respect to lactation if it is realized that breast cancer patients tend to be of low parity. In those parts of the world where lactation is responsible for interruption of the menstrual cycle for as long a time as the gestation period, pregnancy is protective, but lactation is not. A

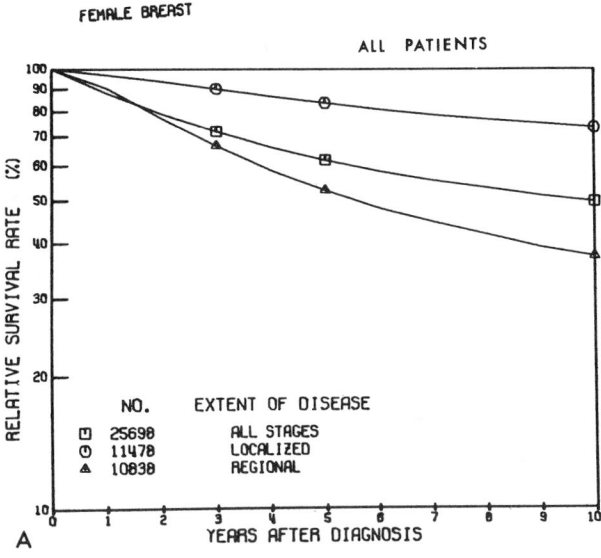

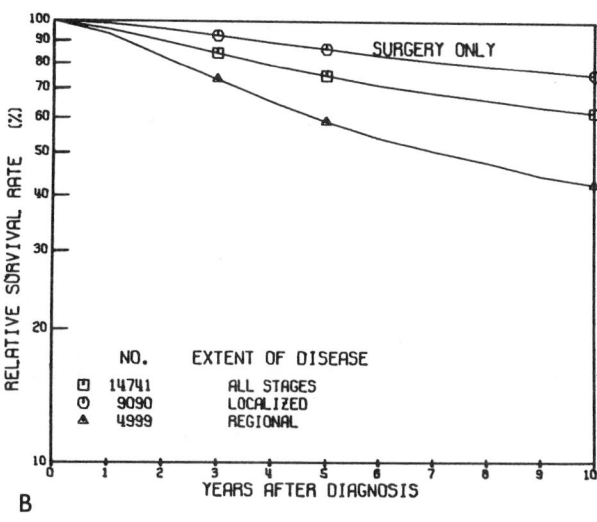

Figure 13. Relative survival data for patients operated upon between 1955 and 1964. A, Results for all patients treated in that decade showed a 10-year survival of 37 per cent. Women with localized disease (no lymph node involvement) had a 55 per cent 10-year survival and those with regional disease (lymph nodes involved) had a 29 per cent 10-year survival. B, When treatment was by surgery only, the overall 10-year survival was 47 per cent. Women with localized disease had a 57 per cent 10-year survival and those with regional disease had a 33 per cent 10-year survival. (From Axtell, L. M., Cutler, S. J., and Myers, M. H. (Eds.): End Results in Cancer, Report #4, DHEW Publication No. (NIH) 73–272. Washington, D. C., 1972.)

cancer than in the normal population.[25] These findings of familial relationship have been observed in all demographic studies. Breast cancer develops at an earlier age in descendants of breast cancer patients; daughters of breast cancer patients have elevated serum levels of prolactin and estrogen (estrodiol + estriol).[59] Malignancy of the thyroid, endometrium, and ovary has a higher incidence in women with breast cancer.

Infertile women have a somewhat higher risk of developing breast cancer, as do women who do not have their first pregnancy until the age of 30. Likewise, long-term nursing (for more than a total of 36 months in a lifetime) has been considered by some investigators to reduce the risk of breast cancer to a slight degree. This factor of long-term nursing, with its suppression of ovulation, relates to the major known factor associated with a lower risk of breast cancer: that a lower rate of breast cancer exists for women who have been castrated before the age of 47, as reported by Wynder.[125] Feinleib[30] showed that in women castrated before age 40 the risk of developing breast cancer was one-quarter that of the normal population. MacMahon[78] has further stated that the ovary is clearly the prime target for etiologic investigation in breast cancer. He pointed out that lactation and

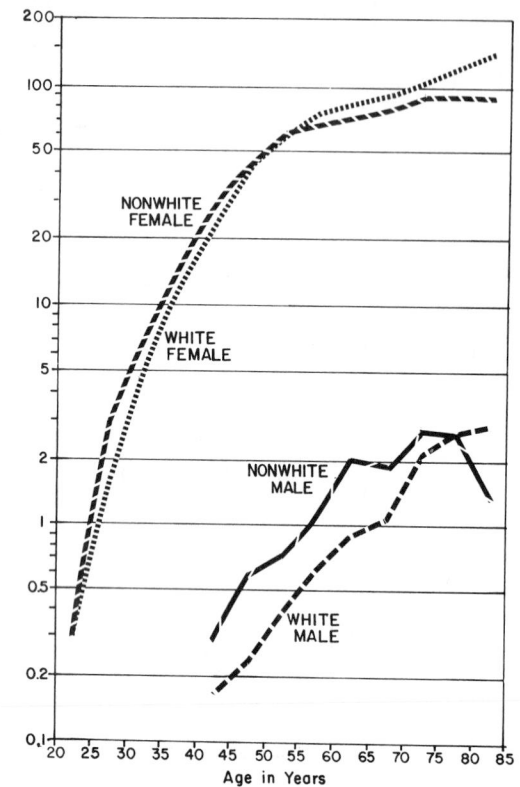

BREAST CANCER DEATH RATES
BY AGE, RACE, AND SEX, U.S. 1971-73

Figure 14. Comparison of death rates for both females and males from breast cancer indicates that there is a reduction in mortality for females after age 55. For white males, however, there is no change in mortality with age, while the rate is reduced over age 60 for nonwhite males. Ninety-two per cent of non-white patients in the United States are Negro. (Chart provided by the American Cancer Society.)

the greatest number of cases occurs in women between the ages of 45 and 59. There is clearly a break in the rising slope of the incidence rate at the menopausal age and then a slower rise in incidence until age 80. This provides further evidence of the importance of hormonal factors in the incidence and development of breast cancer.

The natural history of untreated breast cancer has been recently reviewed by Bloom.[10] The mean survival from all reported series of untreated breast cancer is 39.9 months, with a range of 30.2 to 46.2 months. In Bloom's series from the Royal Marsden Hospital, which closely parallels others, the importance of the histologic grade of the tumor in determining the ultimate survival of the patient was demonstrated (Fig. 17).

PATHOLOGIC CLASSIFICATION

The role of a pathologic classification of breast carcinoma is to provide standardization for therapy of operable breast cancer and to offer a method of determining prognosis. Simple histopathologic classification of breast cancer cannot be expected to achieve this in itself, but when clinical staging and histologic grading are added to the morphologic typing of the tumor, then a more accurate method of prognostication can be expected.

present concept is that the setting for breast cancer development may be in the decade after puberty. The early timing of the first pregnancy may serve to virtually terminate the high risk for tumor induction. Estriol is noncarcinogenic, whereas estrone and estradiol have been shown to be carcinogenic. During pregnancy, estriol production increases proportionately over production of carcinogenic estrogen. The overall effect might be a relative fall in carcinogenic estrogens triggered by pregnancy occurring before age 18, the time of greatest susceptibility of the breasts to carcinogenesis. The reduction in the incidence of breast cancer is equivalent, whether the first pregnancy occurs before the age of 18 or oophorectomy is performed by age 35. Later pregnancies have much less effect than does the timing of the first pregnancy. Epidemiologic studies continue to unravel the complexities of the biologic setting for malignant disease of the breast.

The incidence of breast cancer has shown a progression with rising age (Fig. 16). There are fewer women at risk in each decade, so that the incidence continues to rise although the number of actual cases is progressively fewer after the age of 60. In the United States

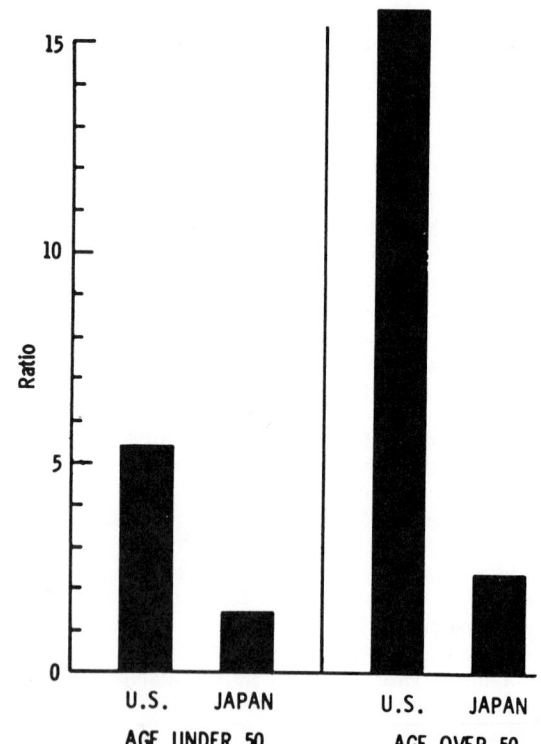

Figure 15. The death rate from breast cancer in women under 50 years of age is much more similar for the United States and Japanese populations than that for women over 50 years of age. These data were taken for the year 1963. (From Wynder, E. L.: Cancer, *24*:1235, 1969.)

FEMALE BREAST CANCER INCIDENCE RATES AND DISTRIBUTION OF CASES BY AGE

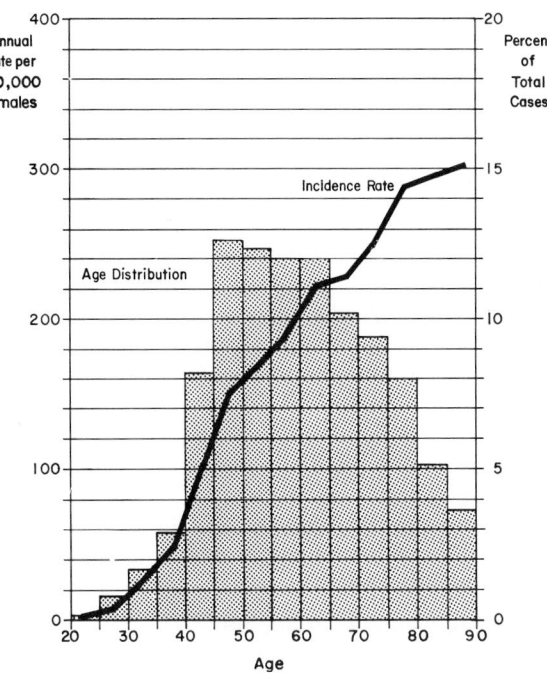

Figure 16. The incidence of breast cancer among women in the United States shows a continued rise from age 30 through the eighth decade. The previously identified reduction in incidence at the time of the menopause is no longer seen in these most recent data. As indicated in Figure 14, the mortality rate is reduced after the menopause. (Chart provided by the American Cancer Society.)

3. Adenocarcinoma with fibrosis (scirrhous carcinoma)
4. Medullary carcinoma with lymphoid infiltration

III. Carcinoma of lobules
  A. Noninfiltrating
  B. Infiltrating

A few additional rarer varieties such as mucoid or colloid carcinoma, sweat gland carcinoma, epidermoid carcinoma, and adenoid cystic carcinoma of the breast can be added, and further subgroups could be made of those already listed. Before discussing the various types of cancer in this list, a few points should be clarified. Comedocarcinoma consists of intraductal, non-papillary collections of cancer cells, often with central necrosis, so that extrusion of sebaceous-like material occurs on cut section of the fresh tumor. This is the origin of the term "comedo." Noninfiltrating carcinoma is synonymous with the standard term carcinoma-in-situ, and it applies to both lobular and ductal cancer. There can be no rigidity to morphologic classification because tremendous variation has always been observed within each breast tumor; the final classification is based on the experience of the pathologist and the findings in the majority of the areas sampled.

Paget's Disease

This unique form of breast cancer begins as a weeping eczematoid lesion of the nipple, which is usually red and thickened.[90] The surface can be either scaly and crusted or moist and oozing. The areola and surrounding skin can be involved as well. A subareolar mass may not be palpable when the nipple lesion first

Many attempts have been made to establish a practical classification of breast cancer on morphologic criteria.[43, 45] The classification presented by Foote and Stewart in 1946,[36, 108] and recently adopted with slight modification by the World Health Organization, has the attributes of simplicity, diagnostic accuracy, and general acceptability, and provides the clinician with an appreciation of the biologic activity of the carcinoma. Foote and Stewart have stressed the fact that cancer of the breast can arise from either the lobule, the ducts, or the nipple, with the tumor arising from ductal epithelium in the majority of cases. They also identified two major biologic properties of breast cancer: either the carcinoma has the ability to infiltrate diffusely or it tends to remain localized. Their list is:

I. Carcinoma of the nipple
  Paget's disease
II. Carcinoma of the ducts
  A. Noninfiltrating
    1. Papillary
    2. Comedo
  B. Infiltrating
    1. Papillary
    2. Comedo

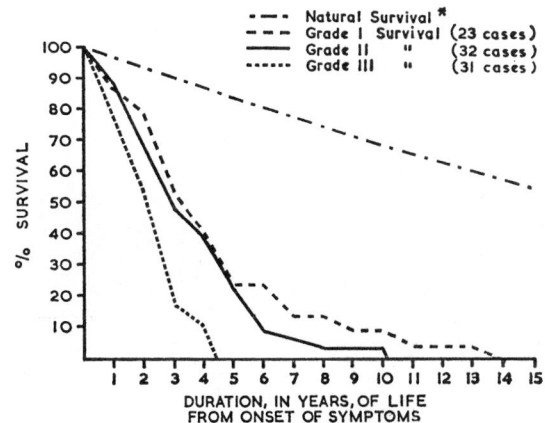

Figure 17. The natural history of untreated breast cancer at the Middlesex Hospital, London, according to histologic grade of the tumor. These 86 patients were cared for between 1902 and 1933. The clear difference in survival from the apparent onset of disease depending upon the histologic grade of the tumor is an important consideration in evaluating various modes of therapy. At 3 years, 52 per cent of patients with Grade I, 37 per cent of patients with Grade II, and 16 per cent of patients with Grade III disease were alive. At 5 years, 22 per cent of women with tumors of low- or intermediate-grade malignancy were alive, whereas none with Grade III tumors were alive. (From Bloom, H. J. G., et al.: Br. Med. J., 2:213, 1962.)

presents, but eventually a tumor will develop beneath the nipple in most cases. Whereas other breast carcinomas that involve the skin carry a particularly poor prognosis, this is not the case with Paget's disease. This tumor is most likely an intraductal carcinoma, developing in the minute ducts of the nipple, which then grows upward into the skin to produce the typical gross lesion and downward into the subjacent breast tissue to produce the mass. The better prognosis may result from the fact that the diagnosis is made relatively early in the course of the disease because of the local symptoms.

There are three special microscopic features of this lesion:[3] (1) Paget's cells; (2) epidermoid hypertrophy; and (3) round cell infiltration in the subepidermis (Fig. 18). The Paget cells are distinctly large, clear, and vacuolated, with small dark nuclei. They are seen alone or in clusters in the deeper layers of the epidermis, but arise from duct cell epithelium and proceed to spread outward within the duct and thence into the epidermis. Mucin stains can confirm the identity of the ductal cells in both locations. The epidermis may be two to three times its normal thickness and the hypertrophy occurs before any ulceration takes place. Round cells and plasma cells infiltrate the superficial portion of the epidermis in the vicinity of the Paget cells.

Noninfiltrating Papillary Duct Cell Carcinoma

This is a rare type of carcinoma-in-situ that can arise from a duct of any size in the breast, often from many sites in the same breast. It is difficult for the pathologist to differentiate this lesion from a benign intraductal papilloma or the papillomatosis of cystic hyperplasia of the breast. The loss of cell polarity and the relationship of the various cells to each other are the keys to the diagnosis.

Noninfiltrating Comedocarcinoma

This tumor constitutes less than 1 per cent of cases of ductal carcinoma of the breast and is also a type of carcinoma-in-situ. It has comedos or small casts of desquamated tumor cells that extrude from the cut surface of the ducts. The cells are more anaplastic than those of the noninvasive papillary type and usually arise in the smaller ducts. This tumor is also called intraductal carcinoma; cells completely pack ductal lumina, distending them and producing focal calcification of the walls (Fig. 19). The walls of these distended ducts tend to become thickened and hypertrophied, particularly with elastic tissue.

Infiltrating Papillary Carcinoma

This tumor tends to be bulky, slowly growing, and circumscribed, presenting as a soft, cystic mass or several such masses within the breasts. It is a progression of the noninfiltrating type and does not arise from a pre-existing intraductal papilloma. Axillary nodal involvement is a late finding, as is invasion of the skin or pectoral fascia, despite the large size these tumors may attain. Microscopically, the papillary growth is more vascular and anaplastic than in the noninfiltrating type, and the tumor can be seen extending through the thickened duct wall and growing into the surrounding connective tissue.

Infiltrating Comedocarcinoma

This is a more common type of duct cell carcinoma, since it is rare for the comedocarcinoma to remain in situ. In order to separate this variety of tumor histologically from simple adenocarcinoma of the breast, the intraductal component must be seen. Calcification in this tumor is common at focal sites, and well-differentiated tumor cells are often seen in the ducts, just as in the in situ lesions. The tumors are

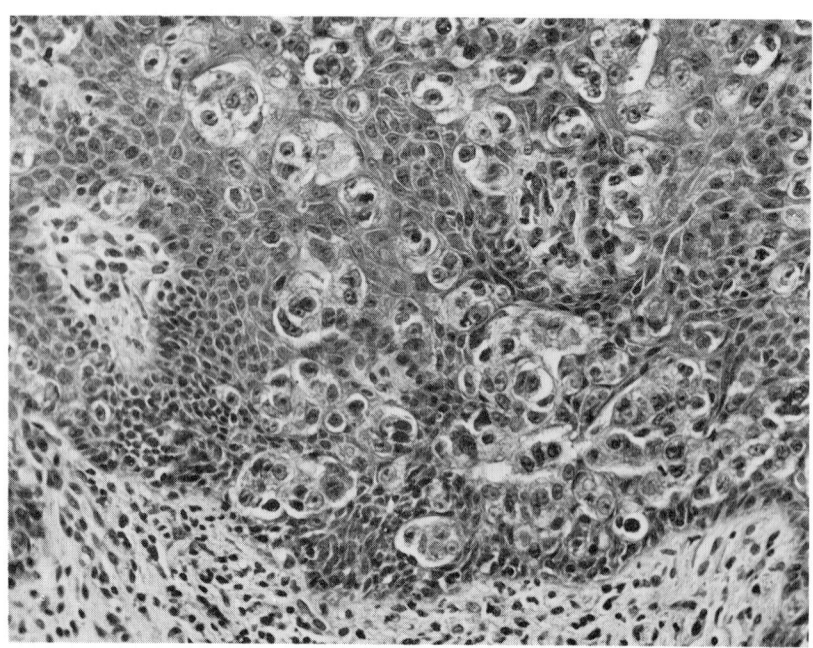

Figure 18. The microscopic appearance of Paget's disease of the nipple. ×400, H and E. The large typical Paget cells invade the dermis and are accompanied by a lymphocytic infiltration. The tumor cells have dark nucleoli and clear cytoplasm. (Courtesy of Dr. J. M. Corson, Department of Pathology, Peter Bent Brigham Hospital.)

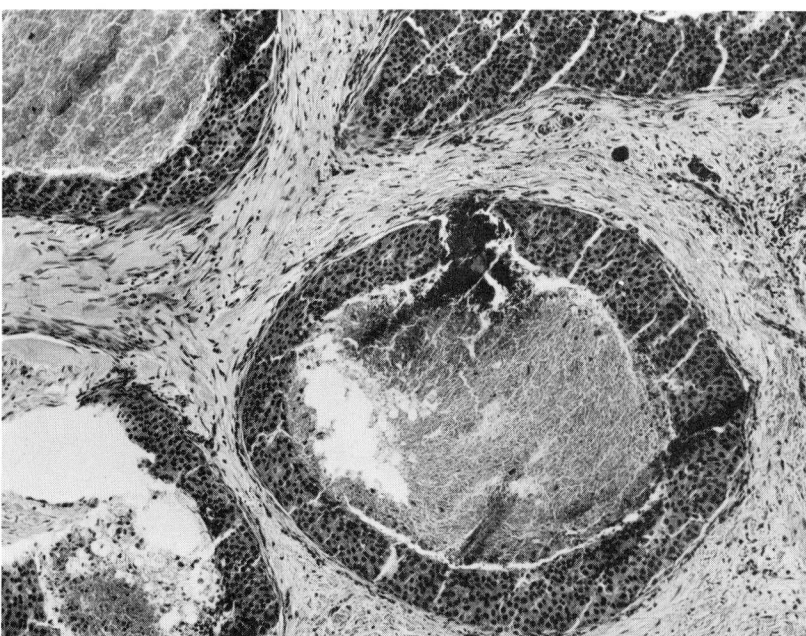

Figure 19. Microscopic appearance of intraductal carcinoma-in-situ. ×180, H and E. The ducts are packed with malignant cells and debris, and calcification is present in the duct walls. There is no evidence in these ducts of invasion through the duct wall into the surrounding tissue. (Courtesy of Dr. J. M. Corson, Department of Pathology, Peter Bent Brigham Hospital.)

usually large but do not ulcerate through the skin; infection of the ducts may be evident, with some inflammatory changes in the breast on physical examination.

Infiltrating Adenocarcinoma with Fibrosis

This is the most common type of breast carcinoma, accounting for about 75 per cent of the total number of cases. It is generally referred to as scirrhous adenocarcinoma and is hard to the touch because of the marked desmoplastic response with fibrosis. The tumor is very infiltrative and adheres to overlying skin and fat as well as to the deep fascia. The cut surface is exceedingly gritty and does not bulge at all after incision. Yellow, chalky streaking is common on the gray tumor background. When the surgeon touches the tip of the scalpel blade to a biopsy specimen of this tumor, the fixation to fat is evident because the entire piece of tissue moves as one. This is an important gross distinction from fibroadenoma or cystic disease, which does not transmit the motion of the scalpel tip. Rapid lymphatic spread occurs through the breast and it is very difficult to identify the boundaries of the scirrhous carcinoma since multiple satellite masses within the breast are common.

On microscopic study, great variability exists in the pathologic picture. All degrees of differentiation, from anaplasia to well-differentiated tumor with attempts at adenoid formation, can occur in different areas of the same breast. The tumor cells are often spherical in clumps within the dense fibrous stroma (Fig. 20). Areas of hemorrhage and necrosis with calcification are common. Attempts at grading depend on the predominant differentiation and whether or not blood vessels are involved.

Medullary Carcinoma with Lymphoid Infiltration

This is a bulky tumor with well-defined edges, usually measuring at least 4 cm. in diameter. It is soft and generally centrally located deep in the breast. Hemorrhages and cyst formation are common and apparent encapsulation is a frequent finding. These tumors tend to be less invasive than the scirrhous ones and they are usually not adherent to the skin despite their size. Since axillary involvement and distant spread is late, the prognosis is more favorable for medullary carcinoma. Because these tumors can be so slow-growing, the patient, when first seen by the physician, may have a fungating, ulcerated breast tumor of this type that has been disregarded for years and yet may still be free of apparent metastases. These women are the most favorable group referred to by Bloom in his studies of untreated carcinoma of the breast (see Fig. 17). Stewart showed that only 11.5 per cent of women with medullary carcinoma were dead of cancer in 5 years, compared with 56 per cent for scirrhous carcinoma.[108]

A characteristic microscopic feature of this carcinoma is the intensive infiltration of the scanty stroma with small lymphocytes (Fig. 21). The tumor cells have large vesicular nuclei and delicate cytoplasm, and there are numerous mitoses. The tumor cells are arranged in anastomosing nests or masses of cells and in some cases the lymphocytic infiltrate makes up the bulk of the tumor. Sharp borders are usually seen in the tumor, but no true capsule is present.

Lobular Carcinoma

This rare type of breast cancer arises from the lobular tissue rather than the ductal epithelium. The noninfiltrating type is a carcinoma-in-situ. It has been shown by Gallagher and Martin to often accompany duct cell carcinoma on whole-organ section and is frequently multicentric in origin.[41] These in situ carcinomas may be concentrated in the upper quadrant of the breast and may present just as enlarged lobules. Microscopically, in a lobule or group of lobules there may be acinar cells heaped up in a disordered fashion,

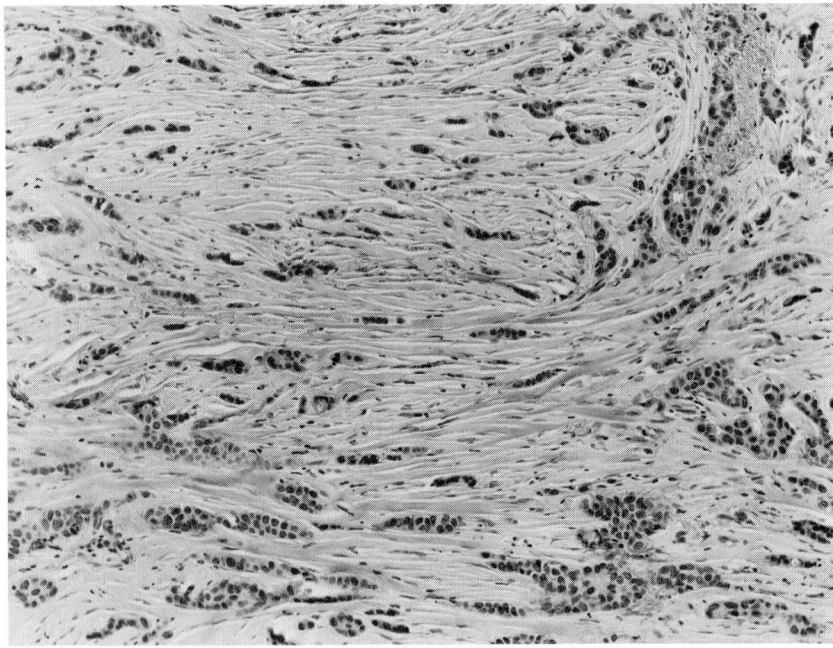

Figure 20. Histologic appearance of scirrhous carcinoma. ×180, H and E. Small cords of tumor cells are surrounded by the extensive desmoplastic reaction of the tumor as it invades widely throughout the breasts. (Courtesy of Dr. J. M. Corson, Department of Pathology, Peter Bent Brigham Hospital.)

usually with a few mitoses. As the lesion becomes enlarged, typical solid masses appear in the lobules as the disordered clumps of cells coalesce. Small areas of necrosis may be present. As the process continues, invasion of the parenchyma and lobules occurs. The infiltrating form of lobular carcinoma may be grossly and microscopically indistinguishable from scirrhous carcinoma, and only when a preinvasive lobular nodule of tumor can be identified histologically can the diagnosis be certain.

Mucinous Carcinoma

This tumor has gelatinous material within it and has sharply delineated margins. It feels like a well-circumscribed, jelly-filled cystic mass on palpation. Mucinous carcinomas are usually large, bulky tumors and are either reddish brown or purplish in color with slimy material present on the cut surface. The mucin is produced by the tumor cells and is variable in amount. Some tumors appear in microscopic section as

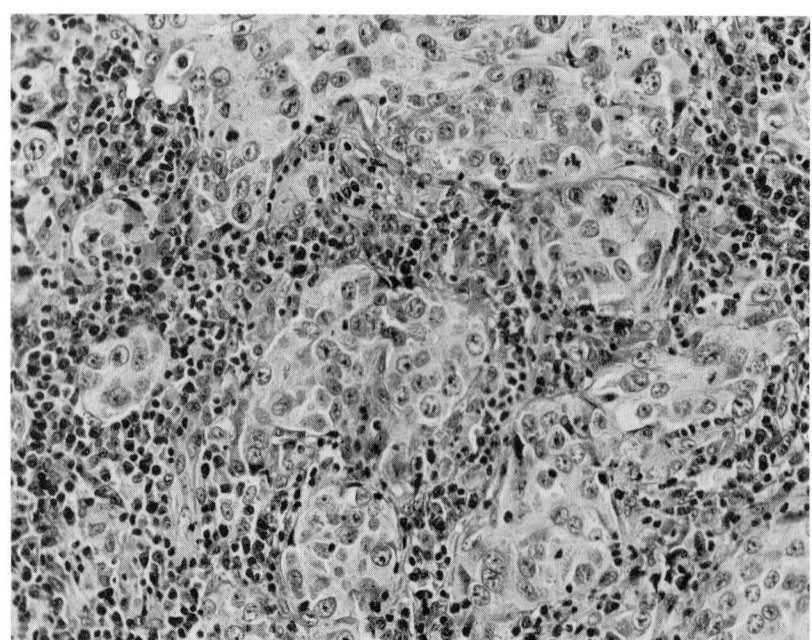

Figure 21. Medullary carcinoma of the breast. ×400, H and E. Numerous clusters of lymphocytes are distributed throughout the tumor field. These are typical small lymphocytes, whereas the tumor cells have large nuclei with light-staining cytoplasm and are arranged in anastomosing nests between the extensive lymphocyte infiltration. (Courtesy of Dr. J. M. Corson, Department of Pathology, Peter Bent Brigham Hospital.)

small clumps of tumor cells in a sea of mucoid material. The cells are often well differentiated and may even have a signet ring appearance. Signet cell types tend to grow more rapidly. The incidence of lymph node metastasis and distal spread is similar to that seen in medullary carcinoma, but the prognosis is not as good.

Sweat Gland Carcinoma

A primitive tubular type of cell of epidermal origin is probably the common basic cell for sweat and mammary glands. Sweat gland tubules can occur in normal breast tissue, anastomosing with small lactiferous ducts. The tubules have cells with eosinophilic cytoplasm and are lined by an inner layer of columnar cells. Intracystic papillary processes are commonly found in these sweat glands and small peripheral carcinomas of the breast have these characteristics. Their clinical behavior is similar to that of breast cancer.

Epidermoid Carcinoma of the Breast

This tumor is rare and appears to arise from metaplasia of ductal epithelium. It is usually far advanced when identified, and within the breast can frequently be traced back to metaplastic, well-differentiated, squamous epithelium. These tumors form typical intracellular bridges and epithelial pearls of squamous carcinoma as in other parts of the body.

Adenoid Cystic Carcinoma of the Breast

This is an extremely rare tumor of the breast and is related to the cylindroma of salivary glands and the respiratory tract.[122] It is of low-grade malignancy and rarely metastasizes, but local recurrence is frequent if therapy is inadequate. Microscopically, there is usually a trabecular pattern with hyaline material between the acinar clusters of cells.

Inflammatory Carcinoma

This is a clinical description of a very lethal and aggressive form of breast cancer that is not specifically related to any histologic type. The tumor cells are usually very undifferentiated and the subdermal lymphatics are widely involved with carcinoma. As a result, there is an acute onset of redness, pain, and swelling of the breast due to lymphatic blockade and lymphangitis. The breast is hot and grossly appears to be involved with cellulitis. Not only are skin lymphatics full of tumor cells but so are the surface veins and the axillary nodes on many occasions. It most commonly occurs post partum in younger women with the full breasts of lactation and the associated engorgement and widely patent lymphatic and venous channels. The prognosis is very grave and treatment is usually inadequate to control the disease.

Ackerman[2] has stressed a more formalized classification of breast cancer, which is a modification of Tornberg's system. The tumor types in this classification are dependent on the same criteria as those stressed by Foote and Stewart,[36] that is, the ability to metastasize and the cell type. The classification is:

Type I. Nonmetastasizing (noninvasive)
  1. Intraductal (comedo) carcinoma without stromal invasion

Type II. Rarely metastasizing (always invasive)
  1. Pure extracellular mucinous or colloid carcinomas
  2. Medullary carcinomas with lymphocytic infiltration
  3. Well-differentiated adenocarcinomas

Type III. Moderately metastasizing (always invasive)
  1. Adenocarcinoma
  2. Intraductal carcinoma with stromal invasion
  3. Any other carcinomas not specifically classified in the other groups

Type IV. Highly metastasizing (always invasive)
  1. Undifferentiated carcinomas
  2. Any tumor that definitely invades blood vessels

This type of staging is dependent on a term known as "grading" of the malignancy process, whereas the Foote and Stewart classification is dependent upon the tumor type per se. Grading is performed on the basis of histologic changes in the periphery of the tumor. Three factors are most critical: (1) structural differentiation, such as tubular formation; (2) regularity and size, shape, and staining of the nuclei; and (3) frequency of hyperchromasia and mitosis. From these three major factors, three important grades can be derived: Grade I—a mature and well-differentiated tumor; Grade II—moderately mature and partially differentiated tumor; and Grade III—immature and undifferentiated. It is important to recognize that in addition to the grade of the tumor itself there are other important aspects in predicting the prognosis that are related to the size and location of the tumor, margination of tumor growth, and the status of the regional lymph nodes. As already mentioned, vascular invasion and inflammatory malignancies are of particularly grave prognosis but would not necessarily appear in the grading or the clinical staging.

CLINICAL STAGING

Clinical staging can be defined as an attempt by the surgeon to identify the extent of the malignant lesion, based on the physical examination and laboratory studies prior to any operative procedure. Since decisions for patient management must be made from the best available data for any given individual, clinical staging of cancer serves as the primary method for comparing techniques of therapy. Whereas histologic typing and grading are important in understanding what happens to a patient with breast cancer, the clinical stage is the guide to treatment.

There are three methods of clinical staging in use at the present time, the Manchester System, the Columbia Clinical Classification, and the TNM (tumor, nodes, metastases) System. The TNM System is achieving more widespread acceptance, since it is applicable to many different malignant diseases and serves to define most clearly the status of the disease in a given patient. It is also most applicable to computer storage of data. By their very nature, the clinical staging systems amplify the various features of the primary tumor that are important in prognosticating results of therapy. None of the systems take into account the quadrant of the breast that the lesion is located in, the age of the patient, the length of time that the tumor has been present, or the characteristics of the palpable tumor margin in the breast, all of which features may play a role in the ultimate result.

The Manchester System was developed in 1940 at the Christie Hospital and Holt Radium Institute in Manchester, England. It is a four-stage system:

Stage I: The growth is confined to the breast.
Stage II: The growth is confined to the breast, but palpable, mobile lymph nodes are present in the axilla.
Stage III: The growth extends beyond the mammary parenchyma as shown by:
   a. Skin invasion or fixation over an area large in relation to the size of the breast or skin ulceration.
   b. Tumor fixation to the underlying muscle or fascia; axillary nodes, if present, are mobile.
Stage IV: The growth extends beyond the breast area as shown by fixation or matting of the axillary nodes, complete fixation of tumor to chest wall, deposits in supraclavicular nodes or in the opposite breast, satellite nodules, or distant metastasis.

The Columbia Clinical Classification is based on extensive experience of Haagensen and Stout[45, 48] at Columbia-Presbyterian Medical Center in New York City. These authors established certain criteria for operability in patients with breast cancer and defined those features of the primary disease that influenced the probability of surgical cure. The Classification is as follows:

Stage A: No skin edema, ulceration, or solid fixation of tumor to the chest wall; axillary nodes not clinically involved.
Stage B: No skin edema, ulceration, or solid fixation of tumor to the chest wall; clinically involved axillary nodes, but less than 2.5 cm. in transverse diameter and not fixed to overlying skin or deeper structure of axilla.
Stage C: Any one of five grave signs of comparatively advanced carcinoma:
   1. Edema of skin of limited extent (less than one third of the skin over the breast).
   2. Skin ulceration.
   3. Solid fixation of tumor to chest wall.
   4. Massive involvement of axillary lymph nodes (2.5 cm. or more in transverse diameter).
   5. Fixation of the axillary nodes to overlying skin or deeper structures of the axilla.
Stage D: All other patients with more advanced breast carcinoma, including:
   1. A combination of any two or more of the five grave signs listed in Stage C.
   2. Extensive edema of skin (involving more than one third of the skin over the breast).
   3. Satellite skin nodules.
   4. The inflammatory type of carcinoma.
   5. Supraclavicular metastasis, clinically.
   6. Parasternal metastasis, clinically.
   7. Edema of the ipsilateral arm.
   8. Distant metastasis.

The TNM System, first presented by the International Union against Cancer, has been adopted by the Joint Committee on Cancer Staging and End Results Reporting, organized in 1959 by the American College of Surgeons. It is based on the clinical observations related to tumor (T), regional lymph nodes (N), and distant metastasis (M). The TNM System is described as follows:

T (Primary Tumor)
   T1: Tumor of 2 cm. or less; skin not involved or involved locally in Paget's Disease.
   T2: Tumor 2 to 5 cm. in size.
   T3: Tumor greater than 5 cm. in size.
   T4: Tumor of any size with any of the following: skin infiltration, ulceration, peau d'orange, skin edema, pectoral muscle or chest wall attachment.

N (Regional Lymph Nodes)
   N0: No clinically palpable axillary lymph nodes.
   N1: Clinically palpable but movable axillary nodes (N1a—metastasis not suspected, N1b—metastasis suspected).
   N2: Clinically palpable, fixed, axillary nodes (metastasis suspected).
   N3: Homolateral supra- or infraclavicular nodes considered to contain metastasis; edema of the arm.

M (Distant Metastasis)
   M0: No distant metastasis.
   M1: Clinical and radiographic evidence of metastasis except those to homolateral axillary or infraclavicular lymph nodes.

Staging
   Stage I: T1, N0 or N1a, M0
   Stage II: T1, N1b, M0; or T2, N0, M0
            T2, N1a, M0; or T2, N1b, M0
   Stage III: Any T3 with any N, M0
            Any T4 with any N, M0
            Any T with N2 or N3, M0
   Stage IV: Any T, any N with M1

At the Peter Bent Brigham Hospital, a TNM Staging Sheet as well as a diagram for locating the mass within the breast is completed for each patient with primary breast cancer and remains as a part of the hospital record (Fig. 22). It provides an accurate description of the primary tumor for anyone examining the patient on follow-up examination as well as eliminating the need for retrospective staging.

DIAGNOSIS OF BREAST CARCINOMA

The most common initial evidence of breast cancer is a lump in the breast, usually painless and frequently discovered by accident. Most breast lumps are discovered by the patient herself, but a fair number are identified by the physician during the routine examination. Spratt and Donegan[106] reported that in 774 patients with mammary carcinoma, a painless lump was the initial symptom in 66 per cent of the cases, a painful breast mass in 11 per cent, nipple discharge in 9 per cent, nipple crusting or retraction in 5 per cent, and local edema in 4 per cent. Ackerman and del Regato[2] noted the presence of a lump to be the first sign in 78 per cent of 100 consecutive patients with breast cancer, while local pain was the initial finding

NAME _____ **NO.** _____

AGE _____ **DATE** _____

T _____ **N** _____ **M** _____

STAGE _____

For Addressograph Plate

Mid-line

1
3cm.
2
3
4
5
1cm.
6

1
3cm.
2
3
4
5
1cm.
6

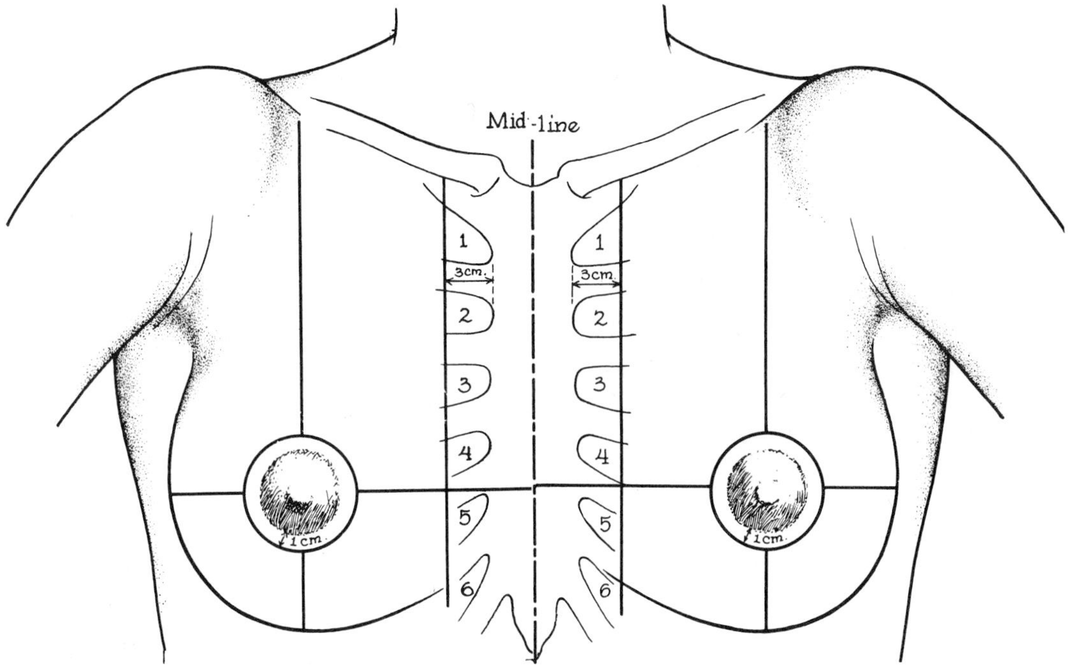

T
(Local Tumor)

T₁ Tumor of 2 cm. or less in its greatest dimension: Skin not involved or involved locally with Paget's disease.

T₂ Tumor over 2 cm.; or with skin attachment; or nipple retraction. No pectoral muscle or chest wall attachment.

T₃ Tumor of any size with any of the following: skin infiltration, ulceration, peau d'orange, skin edema, pectoral muscle or chest wall attachment.

N
(Regional Lymph Nodes)

N₀ No clinically palpable axillary lymph node(s).

N₁ Clinically palpable axillary lymph nodes that are not fixed.

N₂ Clinically palpable homolateral axillary or infraclavicular lymph node(s) that are fixed to one another or to other structures.

M
(Distant Metastasis)

M₀ No distant metastasis

M₁ Clinical and radiographic evidence of metastasis except those to homolateral axillary or infraclavicular lymph nodes.

Figure 22. This staging chart is utilized in the record of the patient with a breast mass at the Peter Bent Brigham Hospital. In addition to diagraming the mass in the proper position, the specific T, N, and M classifications are noted and then the stage is determined. On the back of this sheet, a detailed description of the various stages with a summation of the TNM system for breast cancer has been reproduced so that this information will be available to the student or house officer.

in 12 per cent, nipple soreness, discharge, or retraction in 11 per cent, and an axillary mass in 4 per cent. Other less common accompanying complaints included breast enlargement, ulceration of the breast, local erythema of the breast, diffuse breast soreness, arm edema, breast abscess, or skin puckering.

Although the initial complaints of a patient with breast cancer are usually related to the breast itself, occasionally systemic metastatic disease to the skeleton, axilla, supraclavicular area, or lungs causes the initial symptoms or signs of disease. Carcinoma of the breast presents a variety of biologic aspects in relation to host-tumor relationships. Some breast cancers metastasize before the primary tumor can even be identified; others remain locally invasive for years without ever manifesting distant spread, despite the absence of treatment. Most patients with breast cancer fall between these two extremes; generally, breast cancer can be considered to be a tumor that tends to spread early in the course of its primary growth by both lymphatic and hematogenous routes and with widely spread metastases. Multicentricity of origin within one or both breasts is frequent.

Clinicians have recognized that one of the key indices of the biologic relationship between the tumor and the host is the interval between primary therapy and the appearance of metastatic lesions. In some women, metastatic disease appears only a scant few months after the primary tumor is first diagnosed, while in others it may take 10 to 20 years for a metastatic focus to come to light. This interval between primary treatment of the breast cancer and the appearance of metastatic disease is referred to as the Free Interval and is a valuable prognosticator of response to treatment of metastatic breast cancer.

Breast cancer is most commonly found in the upper outer quadrant of the breast (47 to 50 per cent); the upper inner quadrant is the site for about 12 to 15 per cent of cases. Cancer is less common in the lower quadrants, being present in the lower inner quadrant in only 2 to 5 per cent and in the lower outer quadrant in 6 to 12 per cent. Centrally located breast cancer is beneath the nipple and areola, or presents as Paget's disease, and accounts for 15 to 22 per cent of cases in various series. Some slight increase in incidence of left-sided cancer has been repeatedly noted. Primary breast cancer presents as bilateral simultaneous disease in 1 to 2 per cent of cases, and very rarely the tumor may arise in a previously undetected axillary supernumerary breast. In these cases, the tumor is often considered to be in an axillary node with an unknown primary site.

The accuracy of diagnosis of breast cancer on physical examination is only 70 per cent in the most experienced hands; thus any discrete lump or mass in the breast must be considered as possibly representing a carcinoma. Tumors do not generally become palpable until they are greater than 1 cm. in diameter; it has been estimated by calculations of tumor doubling time that it takes approximately 5 years for a tumor to reach this size from the single cell stage. Any fixation of the locally invasive tumor to fibrous strands produces tethering, dimpling, or skin retraction, all very positive findings in breast cancer. Subdermal lym-

phatics, when involved, produce a characteristic peau d'orange appearance of the skin over a breast cancer, with edema and breast elevation or shortening. Asymmetry of the involved breast is common, with deviation of the nipple or flattening due to retraction or swelling as common causes. The dramatic skin changes of inflammatory carcinoma have already been described. The nipple may be affected early in the disease with a bloody discharge, changes already mentioned as characteristic of Paget's disease, or nipple retraction due to tumor fixation beneath the surface. Axillary adenopathy to varying degrees may accompany the breast mass and the finding tends to increase the likelihood of the correct diagnosis. Nonetheless, the accuracy rate of correctly determining whether axillary lymph nodes contain malignant lesions is far lower than that for diagnosing the primary lesion of the breast. Ackerman[2] found the examiner to be correct only 54 per cent of the time when no tumor was present in lymph nodes, while the correct diagnosis was made 85 per cent of the time when the axillary tissue was histologically positive for carcinoma. Fixation to the chest wall, diffuse peau d'orange, edema, and ulceration are all very late signs of breast cancer. Ackerman and del Regato[2] have compiled a summary of clinicopathologic correlates for prognosis in carcinoma of the breast (Table 1).

Mammography can be particularly important in two aspects of the diagnosis of breast cancer. Screening procedures have been mentioned, and they are particularly valuable in high-risk populations (patients with previous breast cancer or with relatives having breast cancer) and when a mass is palpable in the breast but the diagnosis is uncertain. The fine calcifications, irregular borders, and variable density of the mass lesion and the increased vascularity of adjacent tissue with overlying skin edema are suggestive findings indicating a malignant lesion of the breast. All methods of diagnosis have just one goal, to stress the need for definitive diagnosis by biopsy at the earliest time in the course of the patient's disease.

TREATMENT OF PRIMARY BREAST CANCER

GENERAL PRINCIPLES

The basic task in treating patients with primary breast cancer is to select a procedure that has the best chance of curing the greatest number of patients with the least disability and fewest untoward side effects. Fortunately, long-term survival is common after prompt treatment of breast cancer, and many surgical techniques have been devised. On the other hand, approximately half of all patients presenting with untreated breast carcinoma have occult metastases and are no longer curable by local treatment to the breast, but their identification is not possible at the present time. The mode of treatment chosen should ideally: (1) prevent the development of distant metastatic disease in those patients whose tumors have not yet seeded the lymphatics or the bloodstream; (2) prevent local recurrence of disease; and (3) eliminate extensive local surgery for those patients who will not benefit from it.

This discussion of the various approaches for treat-

TABLE 1. Clinicopathologic Correlations in Carcinoma of Breast*

Clinical Findings	Pathologic Findings
Lump: small, painless, hard	Smaller the cancer, less chance of axillary metastasis; hardness directly related to amount of connective tissue or inflammation present
Attachment to skin	Tumor growing just beneath skin
Discharge from nipple	If bloody, cancer has grown into a major duct, is Paget's disease or intraductal cancer
Prominent veins in region of tumor	Tumor blocking venous return
Edema, orange-skin appearance to skin	Tumor growing in subdermal and dermal lymphatics
Fixation to chest wall	Invasion of pectoral fascia and rarely of muscle
Satellite nodules	Extensive dermal and subdermal lymphatic involvement
Hard supraclavicular node	Usually metastasis; rule out benign lesions by biopsy
Contralateral axillary lymph nodes	Usually metastasis; rule out benign lesions by aspiration or formal biopsy
Fixed masses in axilla	Tumor growing in nodes, breaking through capsule, and growing in loose fat
Edema of arm	Tumor blocking lymphatics and venous return
Horner's syndrome (miosis, enophthalmos, and narrowing of palpebral fissure)	Metastatic tumor pressing on or invading cervical sympathetic chain
Diffuse chest pain, dyspnea	Tumor involving pleura and probably lung
Girdle chest pains (lumbar or sciatic pains)	Questionable metastasis to vertebrae or sacroiliac region
Marked, extreme weight loss	May mean distant metastasis, possible to liver

*From Ackerman, L. V., and del Regato, J. A.: Cancer—Diagnosis, Treatment, and Prognosis. 4th ed. St. Louis, C. V. Mosby Company, 1970.

ing primary breast cancer will review the aspects of points 1 and 2. Although the importance of the third point is recognized by all who treat breast cancer, techniques for identifying patients whose disease is already disseminated are crude. Haagensen has stressed repeatedly the grave signs of breast cancer, the crux of his staging system. He has educated and warned surgeons of the dangers of unwise operations. His triple biopsy technique[49] is the ultimate step in safely exploring the tissues of the patient before advancing to definitive surgery. Hormonal, biochemical, radiologic, and isotopic evaluations may also be helpful in identifying some women in this group. Bulbrook and co-workers[16, 57] have pioneered in efforts to define the hormonal patterns in patients with breast cancer and to delineate those women who will fare less well with their disease. These studies revealed that women with low resting levels of the 17-ketosteroid metabolite etiocholanolone, in relation to the urinary excretion products of 17-hydroxycorticosteroids, tended to have a poorer prognosis. Jensen et al.[65] have documented the presence of estrogen receptors in human and experimental breast cancers, and Rosen et al.[102] have shown that invasive lobular carcinomas have the highest frequency of estrogen receptor protein.

Unfortunately, no serum factor has been identified that can detect already disseminated breast cancer. The serum alkaline phosphatase may be very helpful in identifying hepatic metastasis. Not all patients with liver involvement have elevated alkaline phosphatase, lactic dehydrogenase, and serum glutamic oxalacetic transaminase levels, but when they are elevated they are important indicators. Paget's disease of bone will produce elevated alkaline phosphatase levels, but metastatic bone lesions are much less likely to cause elevation of the level of this enzyme in the serum. Serum calcium levels are rarely elevated until the patient has widespread bone disease detectable by history and radiologic examination.

Radiologic studies of patients presenting with breast masses may reveal occult metastatic lesions. The chest x-ray is most valuable, but any site of skeletal pain must be evaluated. In the absence of symptoms, it is rare for a metastatic bone survey to identify metastatic disease in patients presenting with primary breast cancer who have a normal chest x-ray. The advantages of bone scanning over skeletal x-ray examination have already been presented. As bone scan capabilities are made more widely available and the accuracy of their interpretation increases, isotopic bone scans will probably become a standard component of the preoperative evaluation of suspicious breast masses. Bone scans are capable of detecting occult bone metastases about 6 to 8 weeks before standard bone x-rays.[103] Liver scanning is of particular value when the liver is palpably enlarged and liver function tests are abnormal, but it is not capable of detecting metastatic foci less than 1 cm. in diameter. In all instances of preoperative evaluation, the validity, cost, and utilization of hospital beds must be balanced against the specific value of the findings for a given patient.

BIOPSY OF BREAST LESIONS

Examination of abnormal breast tissue under the microscope is the only certain way to determine proper management. A discrete, palpable mass in the breast, regardless of its mobility, the length of time it has been present, or the benign nature of any previous biopsy, must be considered the prime indication for biopsy. Persistently encrusted, inflamed, or eczematoid lesions of the nipple and bloody nipple discharge are also important biopsy indications. Occasionally, suspicious areas will be identified by mammography without any palpable disease; biopsy of these sites can identify early malignant disease. Smooth, chronically cystic lesions, in a patient with previous proven cystic hyperplasia of the breast, may be aspirated with reasonable safety, provided that the mass disppears after aspiration, and that the cyst does not reappear within the next 1 to 2 months. If these criteria are not met, it is wiser to biopsy the breast once again. It is rare for a woman to question the wisdom of breast biopsy; the great majority of breast lumps are found by the patient and she does not want false reassurance from the surgeon.

The most satisfactory biopsy is obtained by surgical technique under general anesthesia. The lesion is always deeper within the breast than it appears to be by palpation. Comfort, hemostasis, and reconstruction of the breast contour are best accomplished with proper anesthesia, but the major reason is that the most satisfactory tissue sample is obtained in this manner.

As the roles of hospital facilities and medical care delivery undergo change, breast biopsies are being performed more frequently on an ambulatory basis. Only those women with a proven malignancy would then be thoroughly evaluated for metastatic disease and the number of hospital admissions for breast masses could be reduced to about 20 per cent of the present level. There are obvious psychological advantages for the patient with this approach, and there may be less patient delay when she knows that a simple biopsy under local anesthesia is the first step in the diagnosis and management of a breast lump. There is adequate evidence that a delay of up to four days from outpatient biopsy to mastectomy in no way increases the complication rate or alters long-term survival statistics.[1] Tissue should be submitted for estrogen receptor protein determination, as well as histological diagnosis, on all biopsy specimens, whether they are obtained under local or general anesthesia.

Excisional biopsy can be performed for smaller lesions, under 2 cm. or less, and those that appear to be benign. Unless the plan for primary therapy of breast cancer is to be local excision of the mass combined with radiotherapy, total excision of a specific malignant lesion for biopsy provides no advantage to the patient. If the diagnosis is uncertain after examination of the initial frozen section, then total removal of the palpable lump may be indicated. Incisional biopsy is usually adequate for diagnosis of breast cancer, and it limits both the size of the incision and the lymphatic massage that occurs with more extensive biopsy.

The incision for breast biopsy should be placed in the circumareolar position when possible, since it is more cosmetic and less scarring of the breast tissue results if a benign lesion is found. If carcinoma is proved by biopsy and a simple or radical mastectomy is to be performed, it permits skin flaps to be made more easily because it is centrally placed. If the circumareolar incision is not used, incisions should be made in Langer's lines that concentrically encircle the areola. Dissection can be carried out at the junction

between subcutaneous fat and breast tissue until the mass is identified. The breast, because of its rubbery, fibrous consistency, is best incised with a scalpel; the recognition of the texture and the consistency of the breast tissue is of value to the experienced surgeon. The gritty, invasive character of carcinoma is very easily recognized. If carcinoma is detected, the incision should be closed more snugly than usual to facilitate repreparation of the skin. If the lesion is benign, careful approximation of the cut edges of breast tissue, utilizing absorbable suture material and a cutting-edge needle, can minimize the scarring and make future examinations more accurate. Drainage of breast biopsy sites for 24 hours usually speeds the healing process by reducing hematoma formation.

Needle biopsy of the breast under local anesthesia should be reserved for those malignant lesions which are far advanced and are not suitable for primary surgical management. It is difficult to obtain an accurate tissue diagnosis from soft, small, mobile lesions by needle biopsy and the proper diagnosis may be delayed because of falsely negative information. There is a small group of patients with other systemic disease for whom general anesthesia constitutes too great a risk. Percutaneous needle biopsy or sometimes an open biopsy by needle or scalpel with local anesthesia is indicated in these patients to identify the specific breast disease and then permit planning of the patient's complex management. Needle biopsy can be performed in the ward or outpatient department to facilitate rapid histologic diagnosis. The Vim-Silverman needle or one of its modifications is most commonly used; the technique consists of passing the trochar with its obturator into the surface of the tumor mass, substituting the cutting blade for the obturator, advancing the blade into the mass, and then shearing off a tumor core as the shaft is rotated and advanced on the blade.

When aspiration of a cyst is to be accomplished under the circumstances already described, local anesthesia is used and an 18-gauge needle on a 20-ml. syringe is advanced through a small wheal raised in the overlying skin. The usual benign cyst fluid is dirty gray in color and does not contain grossly visible blood. The cyst should collapse immediately upon aspiration, and a small dressing may be applied.

The most expeditious timing of breast biopsy is as a prelude to further operative procedures, particularly when general anesthesia is desired for the biopsy. There are specific situations, however, when biopsy may precede definitive therapy by a matter of 2 to 4 days; this should not be construed as deleterious to the patient. In addition to those patients for whom general anesthesia is not justified unless the diagnosis is certain, no more than a biopsy should be performed in those patients for whom a clear and accurate statement of malignancy cannot be made by the pathologist on the basis of a frozen section. Permanent tissue sections from paraffin blocks can be cut more thinly and stained more efficiently to allow a more certain diagnosis. No mastectomy, radical or simple, should be performed for malignant disease unless the pathologist's decision is unqualified. Very rarely, simple mastectomy may be performed as a biopsy if the patient has had multiple previous breast biopsies and malignancy is strongly suspected or if she has had prior mastectomy of the opposite breast and new, poorly defined disease is present in the second breast.

The triple biopsy has been devised by Haagensen and Obeid[49] as a way of identifying that patient with apparently operable local disease in whom in fact sufficient nodal spread has occurred that her condition is considered not "curable" by radical mastectomy. The biopsies are performed under local anesthesia several days prior to the contemplated mastectomy. In addition to the breast lump itself, the nodes sampled and histologically studied are the highest axillary nodes and the ipsilateral internal mammary chain of nodes at the level of the first three intercostal spaces. Although this triple biopsy has not gained general acceptance, its principles have been provocative.

SURGICAL AND COMBINED APPROACHES FOR TREATMENT

The fact that several options are available for the treatment of primary, potentially curable breast cancer indicates that there is no unanimity of opinion as to the best one and that all have their inadequacies. The choice of surgical procedure ranges from simple excision of the mass to superradical mastectomy; the problem confronting the surgeon is to select a treatment that offers, in prospect, the greatest chance for cure of the disease with the least disability. Any compromise with adequacy of treatment to achieve what may be construed as less disability is unjustified, but there is a lack of clear-cut evidence to indicate that the extent of mammary gland and lymphatic ex-

tirpation or irradiation correlates with long-term cure or survival.

Radical Mastectomy

At the start of the twentieth century, Halsted[53] and Meyer[82] independently developed the technique of radical mastectomy. They stressed certain aspects of the operation: (1) en bloc dissection of all tissues; (2) removal of pectoral muscles; (3) axillary node dissection; and (4) wide excision of skin around the breast tumors. Over the ensuing years, these principles have formed the basis for the surgical approach to primary breast cancer (Figs. 23 to 25). Haagensen[47] has stressed the need for careful patient selection to rule out those who are already incurable, if the best results are to be achieved. He also has urged that the operation be performed in a meticulous fashion with four essential features: (1) meticulous dissection of thin skin flaps with sacrifice of virtually all skin over the breast; (2) dissection off the chest wall of subcutaneous tissue, skin, and both pectoral muscles, allowing them to fall laterally; (3) dissection of the axilla as the last step, with sacrifice of the thoracodorsal neurovascular bundle; and (4) skin grafting of the chest wall defect in essentially all patients. There is little doubt that most surgeons do not adhere to these strict technical facets in performing a radical mastectomy. The major point of contention is whether or not one believes that the precise manner in which the operation is performed is responsible for better survival in this disease. Those patients who, in retrospect, are found to have microscopic involvement of only one or two nodes close to the breast, in the external mammary group, may derive further specific benefit from this operation,

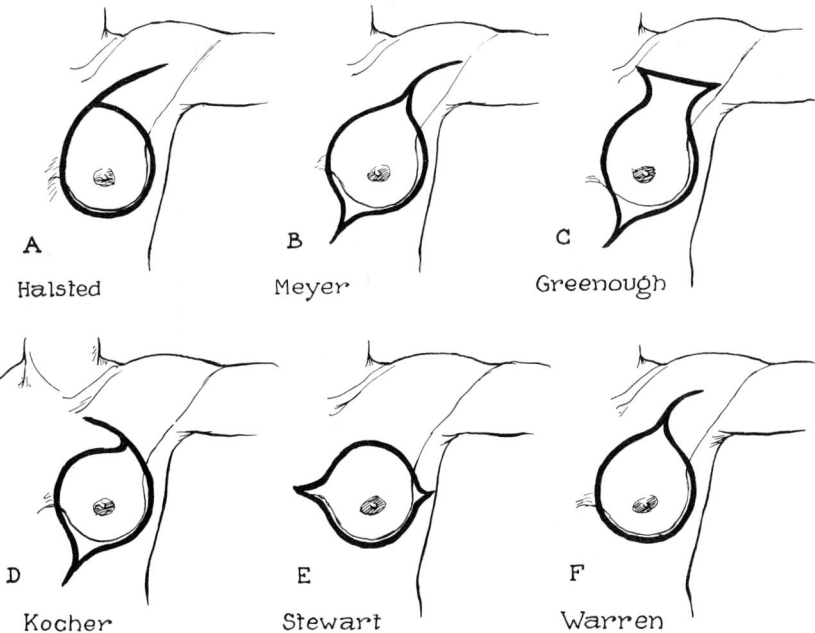

Figure 23. Various standard incisions for radical mastectomy. The type of incision chosen by the surgeon may depend on the location of the lesion within the breast and the preference of the surgeon. Each of these is designed to remove the total breast, a wide margin of skin around the tumor mass, the pectoral musculature, and the axillary nodal tissue. (From Geschickter, C. F.: Diseases of the Breast. Philadelphia, J. B. Lippincott Company, 1943.)

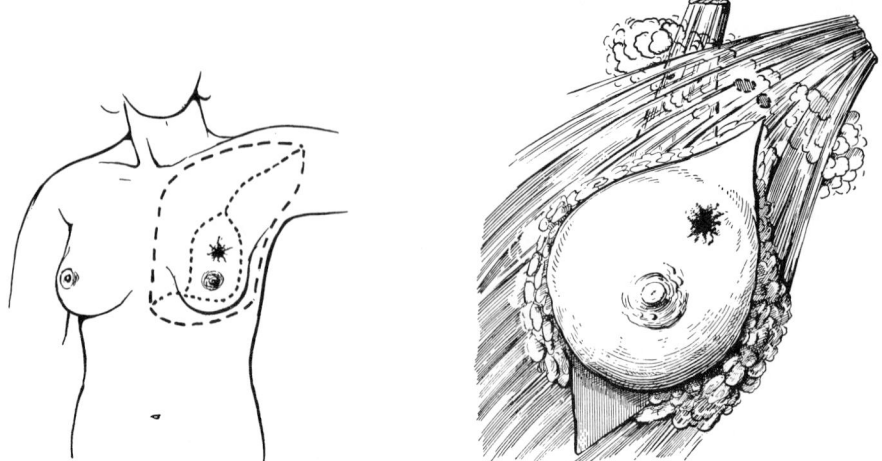

Figure 24.   Radical mastectomy. *A,* The small dotted lines indicate the incision in the skin and the tumor excision performed. The heavier dotted lines indicate the extent of the skin flaps in the area of dissection. *B,* The surgical specimen comprises both pectoral muscles, the fatty axillary contents containing lymph nodes, and the breast including the tumor mass and surrounding skin. (From Jessiman, A. G. *In* Warren, R.: Surgery. Philadelphia, W. B. Saunders Company, 1963.)

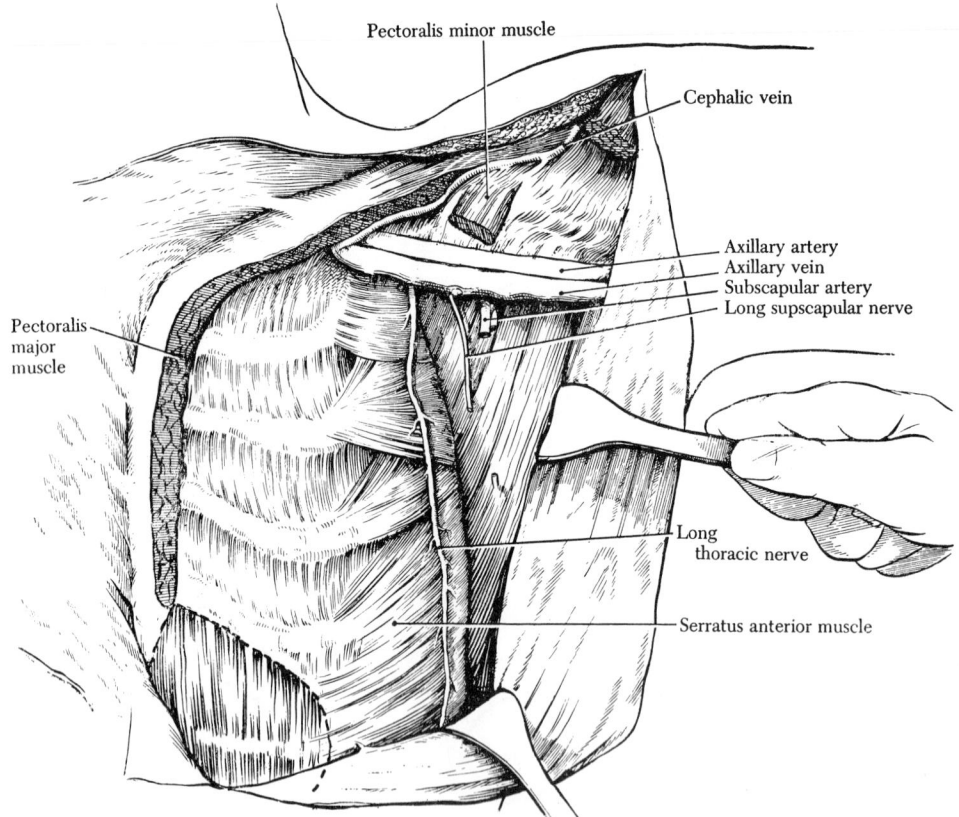

Figure 25.   The appearance of the chest wall following standard radical mastectomy. The axillary vessels have been dissected free of their nodal and fatty tissue and the long thoracic nerve supplying the serratus anterior muscle is preserved. The thoracodorsal nerve supplying the latissimus muscle is generally preserved, but this depends upon the degree of axillary involvement. Some of the anterior rectus sheath has been removed with the specimen as well. Following modified radical mastectomy, the axillary dissection appears identical, but pectoral muscles remain intact. (From Jessiman, A. G. *In* Warren, R.: Surgery. Philadelphia, W. B. Saunders Company, 1963.)

since they are known to have as favorable a prognosis as those without any nodal involvement.[64] The skin margin around the primary tumor should be at least 8 cm., without consideration as to whether or not a skin graft will be required. The pectoral muscles should be divided from their insertions before the axillary vein is dissected. The nodal dissection should start at the axillary apex, the medial aspect of the vein, and move laterally until the vein leaves the axilla at the border of the latissimus dorsi muscle. The axilla should be considered as being in two segments: the apical portion being medial to the subscapular muscle and the lateral portion being between the latissimus dorsi and subscapular muscles. The long thoracic and thoracodorsal nerves are usually spared. Skin grafting should be performed to cover the chest wall defect in preference to closing the skin flaps with undue tension and risking necrosis and secondary sepsis. Edema and limitation of motion of the arm as well as longer hospitalization often are the end results of wound infection and graft necrosis. Early active arm motion, beginning on the first postoperative day, is essential to avoid eventual limitation of activity.

Modified Radical Mastectomy or Simple Mastectomy with Axillary Dissection

This procedure is often referred to as the Patey operation,[92] and it differs from the classic radical mastectomy only in that the pectoralis major muscle is left functionally intact. In addition to Patey, Auchincloss,[5] Handley,[54] and Madden[79] have all been advocates of this procedure. Patey removed the pectoralis minor with the axillary and interpectoral nodes, whereas Auchincloss left the pectoralis minor as well as the major muscles intact, removing nodes between them as well as dissecting the axillary vein. The breast excision, including excision of overlying skin, skin flap dissection, and the need for skin grafting, is essentially the same as with the standard radical mastectomy. Although the en bloc type of removal of axillary lymph nodes is not achieved by this modified operation, full sampling of the lymph nodes is accomplished, with a somewhat better functional and cosmetic result. At the Peter Bent Brigham Hospital, our present philosophy is that modified radical mastectomy serves effectively to remove the primary lesion. This prevents further dissemination and lessens the chance for local recurrence, while removal of axillary lymph nodes and their histological examination identifies those patients who are candidates for adjuvant therapy by virtue of their poorer prognosis.[84] This operative procedure also facilitates later breast reconstruction if that is desired. We have not identified any significant difference in survival or recurrence rates compared with our patients treated by standard radical mastectomy. A recent report by Papatestas and Lesnick[91] showed identical results for these two procedures.

Extended Radical Mastectomy

Dissatisfaction with the results of the standard radical mastectomy, coupled with Handley's findings that in 21 per cent of outer quadrant tumors and 43 per cent of central or inner quadrant tumors there was internal mammary node involvement,[54] led to attempts to include the internal mammary chain of nodes with the specimen. Wangensteen[114] first performed en bloc excision of internal mammary, mediastinal, and supraclavicular nodes with the classic radical mastectomy, but the increased mortality and morbidity made this procedure unacceptable. Urban[112] has advocated the removal of the ipsilateral half of the sternum and a portion of ribs two through five with the underlying pleura and the internal mammary nodes (Fig. 26). The mortality and complication rate after this procedure has been no greater than for the classic mastectomy.[24] Urban utilizes it primarily in patients with central and inner quadrant tumors.

Simple Mastectomy, with or without Radiotherapy

Simple mastectomy is designed to remove only the breast tissue and nipple, and less overlying skin than is excised in the radical mastectomy. Skin grafting is not usually required, nor is axillary node sampling a standard aspect of this procedure. Crile[22] has been a provocative spokesman for this procedure without the concomitant use of radiotherapy to the lymph node drainage areas.

The combination of radiotherapy and simple mastectomy as primary treatment for operable breast cancer has been championed by McWhirter.[81] His concept was to avoid dissemination of malignancy by not operating in an involved axilla and to include internal mammary nodes in the initial treatment of the cancer. His first report of this work was in 1948, at which time he utilized orthovoltage (250 kV) therapy delivering 3500 R to the axillary, supraclavicular, and internal mammary lymph nodes. Kaae and Johansen[68, 69] utilized McWhirter's technique of combined simple mastectomy and postoperative irradiation in a randomized trial comparing this approach with extended radical mastectomy without radiotherapy. The axillary and supraclavicular lymph nodes were treated with 400 kV while the internal mammary chain received 250 kV therapy. The midaxillary dose was usually 3800 to 4000 R, slightly more radiation than McWhirter's patients received.

Excision of Tumor Mass and Radiotherapy

A more extreme reversal of the principles of radical extirpation of the breast is exemplified by recent reports of simple excision of the tumor mass from the breast, followed by supervoltage radiotherapy to the breast and draining lymph nodes. The advent of supervoltage radiotherapy has made this approach more practical with its greater efficiency and skin-sparing effects. Guttmann's[44] fine results with Haagensen's patients whose disease was otherwise operable except for positive supraclavicular or axillary apex nodes on triple biopsy have also stimulated the investigation of radiotherapy as a primary treatment of operable breast cancer. In addition to external beam radiation, implants of iridium or other radioactive materials into the mass, particularly when the tumor is not totally removed, can increase the tumor dose to the range of 8000 R.[115] The most recent reports of local tumor resection and radical radiotherapy have been by Peters,[93] Rissanen,[100] and Wise et al.,[123] each of these series

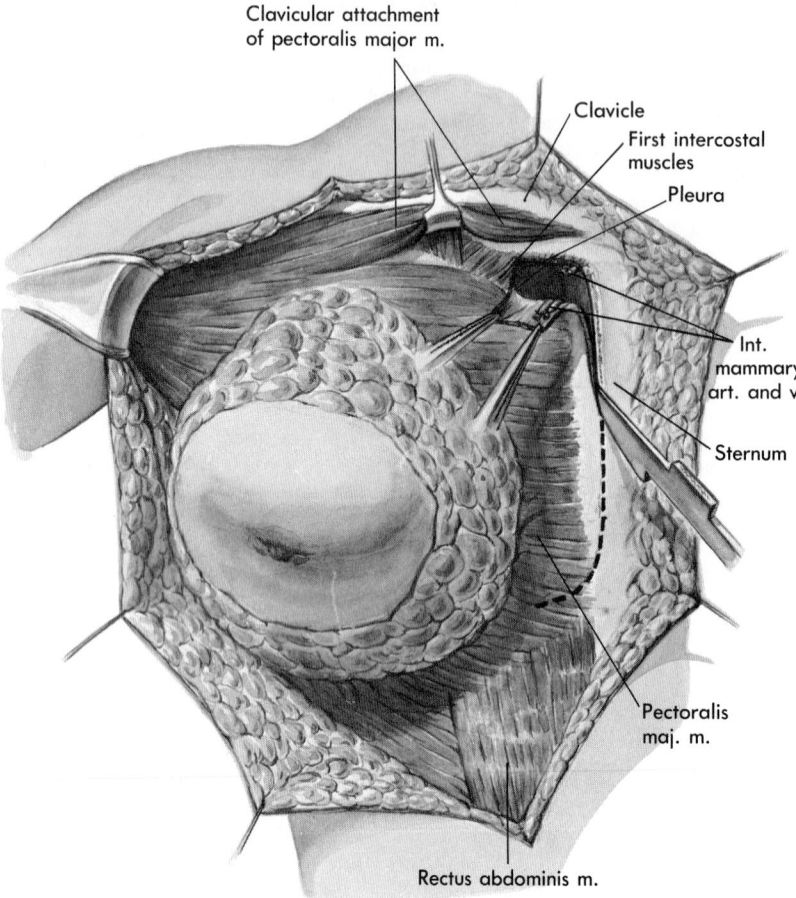

Clavicular attachment
of pectoralis major m.

Clavicle

First intercostal
muscles

Pleura

Int.
mammary
art. and v.

Sternum

Pectoralis
maj. m.

Rectus abdominis m.

Figure 26. Operative procedure for extended radical mastectomy. In addition to the excision of the pectoralis musculature and the breast, the sternum is split on the side of the lesion and the internal mammary vessels are ligated at the level of the first rib. The second, third, fourth, and fifth ribs are removed in their chondral portions and the intercostal vessels are ligated at the edge of this dissection. The internal mammary node chain is removed with this specimen, the parietal pleura being removed as well. The pleura is sutured to the intercostal muscles to close the mediastinum. The defect in the chest wall can be closed with the skin flaps or with a prosthesis. The remainder of the mastectomy is carried out as for a standard radical mastectomy with the axillary dissection. (From Spratt, J. S., and Donegan, W. L.: Cancer of the Breast. Philadelphia, W. B. Saunders Company, 1967.)

compares this conservative surgical and radiotherapeutic approach with classic radical mastectomy.

Adjunctive Therapy in the Treatment of Primary Breast Carcinoma

Experience over the past 75 years with radical mastectomy and more recently with various modifications of surgical excision has consistently shown that less than 50 per cent of women treated for apparently curable lesions will be alive 10 years later. This propensity for early dissemination has encouraged the search for adjuncts to the treatment of the primary tumor in hopes of altering potential metastatic disease. Three types of adjunctive therapy have been utilized: (1) radiotherapy; (2) chemotherapy; and (3) oophorectomy or castration.

Radiotherapy

PREOPERATIVE RADIOTHERAPY. The concept of this treatment is that radiotherapy prior to surgical excision of the breast might sterilize peripheral portions of the tumor, reducing local recurrence rate and dissemination at the time of mastectomy. This may be considered of greatest value in larger tumors of borderline operability. A tumor dose of 4000 R to draining nodes and 3500 to 4000 R to the breast with supervoltage therapy was administered by White et al.[116] to 50 cancer patients. In all but eight surgical specimens,

marked damage to or complete absence of tumor cells was noted. There was no difference in survival rates between patients with positive nodes treated preoperatively and those treated postoperatively, but the local recurrence rate was 8.8 per cent for the former and 20.5 per cent for the latter group. Lindgren et al.,[74] investigating the role of preoperative radiotherapy in alternate patients among 503 women with operable breast cancer, used 170 kV therapy and a skin dose of 1500 R to each of two opposing ports covering the chest wall and the axilla. Postoperative x-ray therapy was also given to all women. Preoperative irradiation did not affect 5- and 10-year survival rates, nor did it significantly alter local recurrence rates.

POSTOPERATIVE RADIATION THERAPY. The goal of postmastectomy radiotherapy to the unresected draining lymph nodes and the chest wall is primarily to reduce local recurrences.[118] There is no evidence that survival rates have been altered by these techniques, even though lymph node metastasis can be eradicated. One of the most thorough investigations of this question was performed at the Christie Hospital and Holt Radium Institute in Manchester; the 10-year follow-up results have recently been reported by Easson.[27] After standard radical mastectomy for curable lesions, 1461 patients were divided into two groups, those who would receive radiotherapy shortly after mastectomy (treated) and those whose radiotherapy was withheld until local recurrence required it (watched). Two different techniques of radiation were used: from 1948 to 1952 the quadrate technique, which concentrated on the chest wall and axillary apex; and from 1953 to 1955 the peripheral technique, which irradiated the three lymph node areas but not the skin flaps. The 10-year survival rate in all groups, watched or treated, quadrate or peripheral therapy, was 45 per cent. When the groups were further subdivided into those with positive or negative axillary lymph nodes, no differences existed between treated and watched subgroups, either. There are, however, two equally important considerations in these data: (1) 35 per cent of the watched patients died of metastatic disease without ever manifesting local recurrence; and (2) therapy of local recurrence that did appear in the watched group was effective, since at the time of death, the incidence of uncontrolled local recurrence in the treated and watched groups was the same. Fletcher et al.[35] have stressed the advantages of preoperative or postoperative radiotherapy in reducing local recurrence rate after mastectomy. More recently, Fisher et al.[32] reported the results of the National Surgical Adjuvant Breast Project's cooperative trial on postoperative radiotherapy. Like Easson's, their conclusions were that survival of treated and untreated groups was unaltered, but there was a significant reduction in the rate of local and regional tumor recurrence in 5 years in treated patients as compared to untreated control patients.

Chemotherapy

The use of chemotherapy as an adjunct to primary treatment of breast cancer represents one of the most exciting new aspects of cancer care. The 10-year follow-up results[34] for a prospective randomized trial of patients receiving thioTEPA only on the day of radical mastectomy and for the subsequent two days showed a significant increase in survival at 5 years for premenopausal women with four or more positive axillary nodes. Survival differences persisted for the full 10 years, but it was not significant at that time. Two important randomized trials are now in progress to evaluate the role of other agents, various times of therapy, and the effectiveness of drug combinations. The National Surgical Adjuvant Breast Project trial under the direction of Dr. Bernard Fisher presented preliminary data in 1975.[33] l-Phenylalanine mustard is being used in this trial for two years, with no postoperative radiation, after radical mastectomy in women with positive axillary nodes. This drug was well tolerated and had mild myelosuppressive effects. Life-table methods were used to evaluate data: treated patients had a failure rate of 9.7 per cent, compared with 22 per cent for controls (p = 0.01). The differences were most apparent for premenopausal women with four or more positive nodes, where the recurrence rate in treated patients was 8 per cent, compared to 42 per cent in controls (p = 0.008). Dr. Gianni Bonadonna in Milan has reported on an adjuvant program with a combination of Cytoxan, methotrexate, and 5-fluorouracil after radical or extended radical mastectomy.[11] This treatment plan was extended for one year after mastectomy and although it represents more aggressive therapy, the results appear even more definite than those with l-phenylalanine mustard. All groups of patients treated, both premenopausal and postmenopausal women, showed significant reduction in recurrence followed to 28 months at present. The relapse rate in the treated patients was 5.3 per cent (11/207), compared with 24 per cent in controls (43/179) (p = 0.000001). Equally effective results were obtained for large lesions treated with extended radical mastectomy or smaller lesions treated with standard radical mastectomy. Only patients with positive axillary nodes were treated and, likewise, no postoperative radiotherapy was given. Continued clinical trials with adjuvant chemotherapy in higher risk patients will serve to define the effect of such drugs on survival after mastectomy.

Oophorectomy

In 1939 Taylor[109] concluded that prophylactic oophorectomy was not advantageous, but his study, like many others, was a retrospective analysis. A randomized prospective trial was carried out by the National Surgical Adjuvant Breast Project in premenopausal women (under 50 years of age) with operable carcinoma of the breast.[97] Patients with surgical oophorectomy (154) were compared with 121 who received thioTEPA and 82 given a placebo. At no time up to 5 years, regardless of classification by nodal status, could any increase in survival rate or lengthening of time to first recurrence be demonstrated for the women who had had an oophorectomy. These same conclusions were reported from the cooperative study in the Greater Boston hospitals and reported in 1969.[88]

RESULTS OF TREATMENT

Proper evaluation of treatment of breast cancer requires careful identification of the clinical staging of the disease prior to operation, and preferably a randomized, prospective comparison of one modality with another in the same institution by the same surgeon. These rather idealistic criteria have only rarely been fulfilled, but now that the orthodox technique of radical mastectomy has been successfully challenged, several such trials are in progress. The study of Kaae and Johansen[68, 69] fails to demonstrate any superiority of survival with extended radical mastectomy as compared with simple mastectomy and irradiation (McWhirter technique). This was a prospective randomized trial carried out in Copenhagen. A large clinical trial in progress in Edinburgh,[14] comparing radical mastectomy and simple mastectomy plus irradiation (all women are castrated in this study), has shown a 76 per cent survival rate for patients treated with radical mastectomy and a 66 per cent survival rate for those treated with simple mastectomy plus radiotherapy. These figures involve only the first 100 patients in each group, and at the present time the differences are not statistically significant. When the mortality percentages within each treatment group are plotted, it is noted that for each year a slight increase in mortality occurred among women treated with simple mastectomy and radiotherapy, but again, these differences were not statistically significant as compared with the mortality (yearly) in women treated with radical mastectomy. Continued follow-up and statistical evaluation are in progress for this important clinical trial.

Brinkley and Haybittle,[13] in a randomized, prospective clinical trial, compared modified radical mastectomy plus radiation with radical mastectomy plus radiation in the treatment of Stage II disease. The modified radical mastectomy in this series is so designated because the simple mastectomy included removal of an adequate sampling of axillary lymph nodes by the surgeon. No significant differences existed between the groups in either survival or recurrence-free rates after 5 years. Rissanen[100] in 1969 reported the results of a nonrandomized, retrospective comparison of patients with TNM Stage I disease treated with either radical mastectomy and radiotherapy or local tumor excision and radiotherapy. All radiotherapy was with orthovoltage, and the 5- and 10-year survival rates were not statistically different for these two highly selective and curable groups. Wise et al.[123] have recently reported a nonrandomized comparison between local tumor excision plus irradiation and radical mastectomy with or without postoperative radiotherapy. Stage I and II cases were treated in 96 patients by local excision and 207 patients by radical mastectomy. The 5- and 10-year survival rates, using the Berkson-Gage type of calculation, were: Stage I—5 years: local excision, 95 per cent, radical mastectomy, 80 per cent; 10 years: local excision, 62 per cent, radical mastectomy, 73 per cent; Stage II—5 years: local excision, 71 per cent, radical mastectomy, 71 per cent; 10 years: local excision, 53 per cent, radical mastectomy, 55 per cent. No significant differences existed in survival at either 5 or 10 years for the two groups.

A 10-year international cooperative study of the treatment of operable breast cancer by various modalities has recently been reported.[17, 24, 47, 48, 55, 69, 83, 118] Although statistical comparison between the seven different case series would hardly be conclusive, there was no striking difference between them, particularly in the Stage B lesions (Table 2). The recurrence rates for five of the seven series are included in Table 3. In Haagensen's series,[47] 39 patients were excluded from treatment by radical mastectomy because regional lymph nodes were found to be positive by triple biopsy.

This further selection may have helped to reduce the local recurrence rate in his series. There is no difference in recurrence rates for the other patients. Guttmann[44] has treated 148 women, proved inoperable by Haagensen's triple biopsy technique, with supervoltage radiotherapy alone. At 5 years, 60 per cent were alive. Despite these good results from radiotherapy, Haagensen[46] has abandoned the triple biopsy technique after 17 years and now prefers to perform radical mastectomy in all Stage A and B cases, following the operation with internal mammary node radiation in patients with either Stage B lesions, a tumor in the inner half of the breast, or a tumor greater than 3 cm. in diameter. Radiation is given to the axillary apex and the supraclavicular area if the axillary nodes are positive, and to the chest wall as well if more than eight axillary nodes are involved.

At the present time, survival and recurrence rates appear to be similar for a variety of methods of treatment of primary, operable breast cancer. Until proper scientific assessment of these different modalities is accomplished, there is no evidence to suggest that any one technique is superior to another. Inadequate local treatment of the primary lesion may produce a higher incidence of local recurrence and reduced survival, as was demonstrated by the clinical trial from Guy's Hospital, in which wide tumor excision and radiotherapy were compared with radical mastectomy.[58] Controversy about radical mastectomy has stimulated important investigations into biologic and epidemiologic features of breast cancer that will ultimately improve its treatment. The ultimate survival of patients with breast cancer is clearly related to the clinical stage of the disease at the time of its first treatment, as shown so well in Table 4, taken from Haagensen's most recent publication.[50] As seen in Figure 27, the patient with primary breast cancer is at greater risk for mortality than the normal population for about 7 years after primary treatment, after which time the survival curve parallels that of the normal population. The more advanced the stage of the disease, the greater the reduction in survival. A summation of the various options available in the management of primary breast cancer according to its clinical stage at the time of presentation is provided in Figure 28.

TABLE 2. Results of Treatment in Mammary Carcinoma — 10-Year Survival Columbia Clinical Classification*

Columbia Clinical Classification	Miller Simple Mastectomy		Handley and Thackray Conservative Radical Mastectomy		Butcher Radical Mastectomy		Haagensen and Cooley Radical Mastectomy		Dahl-Iversen and Tobiassen Extended Mastectomy		Williams and Stone—Total Mastectomy +Axillary Dissec.+ Irrad.		Kaae and Johansen McWhirter Method	
	No. of Patients	% 10-Year Survival	No. of Patients	% 10-Year Survival	No. of Patients	% 10-Year Survival	No. of Patients	% 10-Year Survival	No. of Patients	% 10-Year Survival	No. of Patients	% 10-Year Survival	No. of Patients	% 10-Year Survival
A	105	40	77	61	216	56	344	69	352	57	68	59	159	50
B	34	26	58	25	135	30	138	37	75	24	57	46	28	32
Totals	212		143		425		556		476		142		199	

*From Kaae, S., and Johansen, H.: Ann. Surg., *170*:895, 1969.

TABLE 3. Carcinoma of the Breast Local Recurrence within 10 Years*

Columbia Clinical Classification	Method of Treatment	Parasternal Recurrence % 10 Years	Chest Wall Recurrence % 10 Years	Axillary Recurrence % 10 Years	% Patients with Local Recurrence 10 Years
Stage A	Total mastectomy +ax. dissection +irradiation Williams and Stone	0	12	10	22
	Conservative radical mastectomy Handley and Thackray	5	12	2	16
	McWhirter method Kaae and Johansen	1	10	8	19
	Extended radical mastectomy Dahl-Iversen and Tobiassen	2	10	8	20
	Radical mastectomy Haagensen and Cooley	4	3	0	7
Stage B	Total mastectomy +ax. dissection +irradiation Williams and Stone	0	12	14	26
	Conservative radical mastectomy Handley and Thackray	6	22	0	26
	McWhirter method Kaae and Johansen	0	11	18	29
	Extended radical mastectomy Dahl-Iversen and Tobiassen	0	16	16	32
	Radical mastectomy Haagensen and Cooley	5	13	1	18

*From Kaae, S., and Johansen, H.: Ann. Surg., *170*:895, 1969.

TABLE 4. Radical Mastectomy for Breast Carcinoma: Correlation of Extent of Axillary Metastases with 10-Year Survival*

Columbia Clinical Classification	Number of Axillary Nodes with Metastases	Number of Patients	10-Year Survival	
			Number	Per Cent
Stage A	None	418	320	76.5
	1 to 3	131	89	68
	4 to 7	30	10	33
	8 or more	29	6	20
	Total	608	425	70
Stage B	None	48	34	70
	1 to 3	61	27	44
	4 to 7	37	14	38
	8 or more	40	5	12
	Total	186	80	43
Stage C	None	17	8	47
	1 to 3	21	6	29
	4 to 7	9	4	44
	8 or more	29	3	10
	Total	76	21	30
Stage D	None	1	0	
	1 to 3	2	1	
	4 to 7	1	0	
	8 or more	8	1	
	Total	12	2	17
Total		882		

*From Haagensen, C. D.: Surgery, *76*:685, 1974. Summary of Haagensen's Personal Series, 1935 – July, 1963.

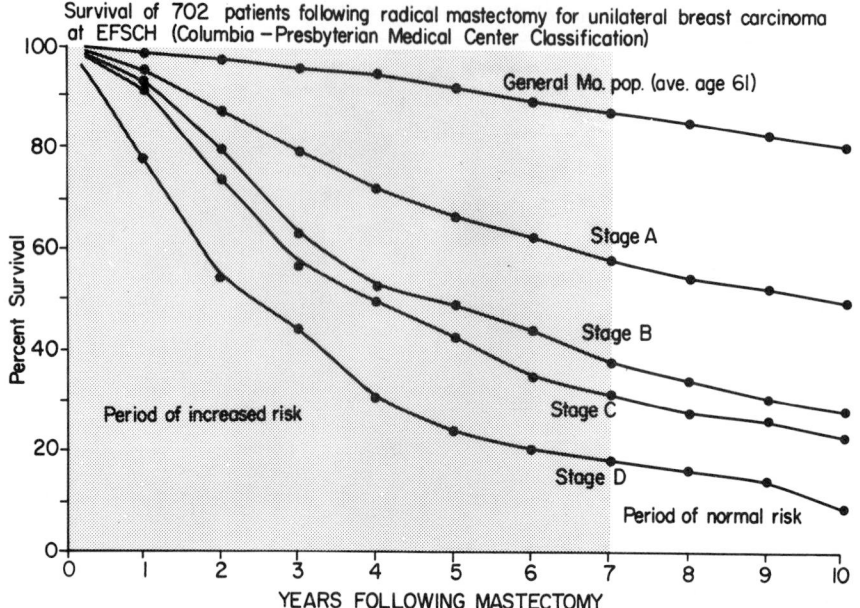

Figure 27. Survival according to the Columbia Clinical Classification for 704 patients after radical mastectomy at the Ellis Fischel State Cancer Hospital. The survival rate for a comparable age group in the general population is indicated for Missouri. After 7 years, the survival curves are parallel to the general population for women having breast cancer. The period of increased risk and greatest mortality is in the first 5 years; between 5 and 7 years it begins to approach the normal risk. (From Spratt, J. S., and Donegan, W. L.: Cancer of the Breast. Philadelphia, W. B. Saunders Company, 1967.)

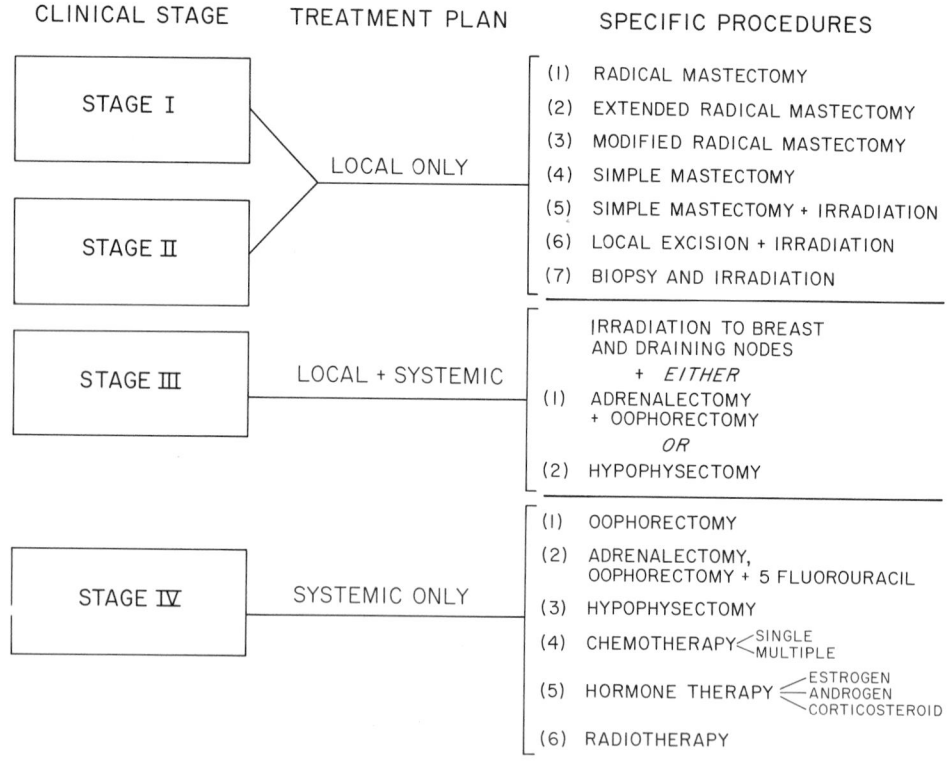

Figure 28. This diagram provides a general outline of the various methods of management for primary carcinoma of the breast according to the stage at the time of presentation. Many options are available for treatment of Stage I and II disease, therapy being directed toward local cure. The addition of radiation to the chest wall or draining lymph nodes or both can be considered as feasible for any of the surgical procedures listed. Stage III disease would appear to be best treated by both local and systemic approaches with local therapy being radiation, systemic therapy comprising either adrenalectomy with oophorectomy or hypophysectomy. Breast cancer presenting as Stage IV involvement without prior treatment of the primary tumor has generally been treated in a systemic manner at the outset, again with a large variety of approaches.

Special Problems in Primary Breast Cancer

Cancer in Pregnancy and Lactation

The prognosis of carcinoma of the breast appearing during pregnancy and lactation is considered to be poor. One reason for this may be the relatively younger age group in which these cancers occur and another is the higher incidence of nodal involvement in these patients. Rissanen reported that 75 per cent of 33 patients with breast cancer during pregnancy and lactation had axillary metastasis; 43 per cent survived 5 years.[99] In White and White's study[117] only two of 25 such women with axillary metastasis survived 5 years. Peters[94] studied 271 patients with breast cancer associated with pregnancy, a group that constituted 3.8 per cent of the total breast cancer population of the Ontario Cancer Institute. When women were matched for age and stage of breast disease, pregnant women had only a slightly less favorable yearly survival rate up to 10 years, as seen in Figure 29A. The author found, however, that those women treated for breast cancer during the second half of pregnancy did significantly less well than those treated in the first half of pregnancy or in the first 6 months postpartum, regardless of the time of onset of the disease. In patients treated for breast cancer, those who had subsequent pregnancies had significantly better 10-year survival (55 per cent vs. 27 per cent) than women in a matched series who did not become pregnant after mastectomy (Fig. 29B). Peters' plan of management for patients presenting with carcinoma of the breast during pregnancy and lactation is:

1. Proven carcinoma during the first half of pregnancy should be treated with radical mastectomy, without radiation or interruption of pregnancy.

2. Patients with carcinoma of the breast identified during the second half of pregnancy require more individual consideration. Small lesions are not treated until after delivery; if rapid growth occurs or the lesion is already Stage III when seen, pregnancy is terminated, lactation is suppressed by administration of androgens, and then the breast lesion is treated.

3. Cancers arising during lactation are treated in a conventional manner after suppression of lactation.

4. Breast cancer patients under 35 are encouraged to plan pregnancies after a one-year interval following mastectomy.

Bilateral Breast Cancer

Bilateral, simultaneous breast cancer has a prognosis based essentially on the evidence of spread of disease in either breast. The prognosis for clinically detectable simultaneous disease is worse than for unilateral disease. Urban[113] advocates the identification of the occult second primary at its earliest stages by biopsy of a generous area of the opposite breast at the time of the first mastectomy for proven carcinoma of the breast. He performed biopsies of the opposite breast in 73 per cent of patients undergoing radical mastectomy. If no lesion was palpable in the opposite breast he removed a wedge of the upper outer quadrant as well as the mirror image of the site where the proven cancer was. Simultaneous breast cancer was proved in 10 per cent of the group, and 14.3 per cent of

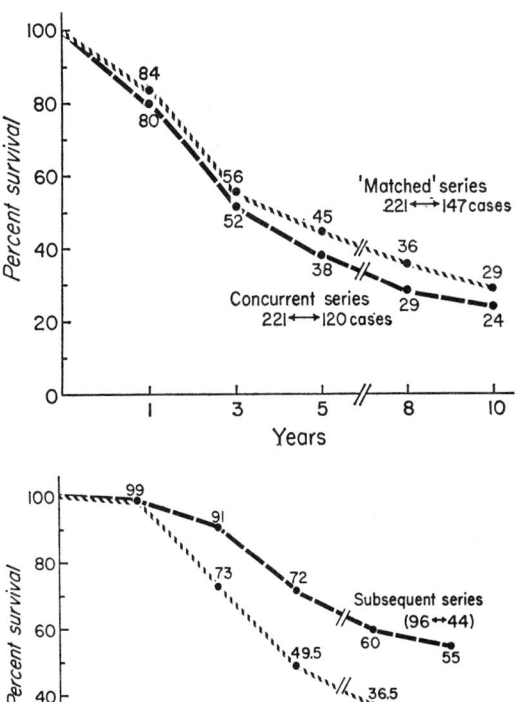

Figure 29. *A,* Two hundred twenty-one patients in whom breast cancer developed during pregnancy or lactation (from the years 1933–1961) were compared with a matched series of nonpregnant patients at the same stage and age. The survival rate parallels the control series and runs about 5 per cent lower for the entire 10-year period. The numbers given for "current" and "matched" series indicate the patients at risk for the entire 10-year time. *B,* The survival curves of 96 patients who became pregnant subsequent to the primary treatment of breast cancer (from the years 1933–1961), as compared with a matched group of 96 patients of similar age and clinical stage of disease who did not become pregnant after mastectomy. There is a highly significant difference in the survival of these patients at 10 years. (From Peters, M. V. *In* Forrest, A. P. M., and Kunkler, P. B. (Eds.): Prognostic Factors in Breast Cancer. Baltimore, Williams & Wilkins Company, 1968.)

the whole series had bilateral breast cancer. Fifty of 57 patients with simultaneous breast cancer detected in this manner were living and well at the time of the report, although only 12 were more than 5 years from operation.

Robbins and Berg[101] stated that approximately 1 per cent of patients treated for primary breast cancer developed a detectable breast cancer in the opposite breast each year. They demonstrated that primary breast cancer was five times more likely in patients who had undergone a previous mastectomy than in the normal female population. Urban[113] observed that 9 per cent of patients with extended radical mastectomy developed a second primary within 10 years.

Identification of a second primary in the opposite breast is the single most important function of follow-up care after mastectomy. Yearly mammography, frequent physical examinations, monthly self-examination by the patient, and early biopsy of any suspicious lesions are essential. In selected situations, when multiple biopsies have already been performed and evaluation of the breast is difficult, simple mastectomy of the opposite breast, with or without insertion of any inlying Silastic prosthesis, may be justified.

Cancer of the Male Breast

Cancer occurring in the male breast, because of early and diffuse lymphatic and nodal involvement, tends to have a poorer prognosis than that in the female. About 1 to 2 per cent of cases of breast cancer occur in males, and breast cancer accounts for 0.7 per cent of all cases of cancer in men. Gynecomastia is not a concomitant of breast cancer in the male, but biopsy of the lump in the breast must not be delayed because of uncertainty of the diagnosis. Nipple retraction, discharge, and ulceration may all occur in cancer of the male breast. This disease tends to be relatively slow-growing in the man and excellent survival data have been achieved with radical mastectomy. When regional nodes are negative, good results have been reported by Cortese and Cornell[21] in a small series, and even 6 of 10 patients with positive axillary nodes survived 5 years or longer. In Holleb's review,[60] men with infiltrating ductal carcinoma confined to the breast alone had a survival of 80 per cent at 5 years. Since these lesions are centrally located beneath the nipple, all males at the Peter Bent Brigham Hospital with breast cancer have received radiotherapy after mastectomy. When the patient has locally inoperable or recurrent disease, orchiectomy is very effective, producing a 45 per cent objective remission rate in Holleb's series.

MANAGEMENT OF METASTATIC CARCINOMA OF THE BREAST

The chance for excellent palliation and long-term survival is greater with metastatic breast carcinoma than with any other late malignant disease, with the possible exception of choriocarcinoma of placental origin in females. Careful follow-up of patients after therapy for their primary disease should be directed toward identification of metastasis as well as observation of the opposite breast for a possible secondary primary cancer. Recurrent disease can occur locally in the axilla, neck, chest wall, or internal mammary chain, or at distant sites. Bruce[15] has shown that the majority of patients who develop recurrence tend to do so in the first 5 years (86 per cent), and that by 10 years 97 per cent of patients have manifested their recurrence. Some women, however, have developed metastasis more than 20 years after mastectomy. Although local recurrence may be solitary, particularly when there are small subcutaneous nodules in the area of the incision, it usually is not. Multiple sites of metastatic disease often become clinically apparent si-multaneously, as though a total reversal in host-tumor relationship had occurred.

There are three general patterns of metastatic disease: (1) soft tissue—including lymph nodes, opposite breast, or chest wall; (2) bone; and (3) viscera—including pleura, lungs, liver, retroperitoneum, and brain. Although combinations of these three major groupings frequently occur, in the majority of patients the disease seems to be dominant and produce the most symptoms in one area. Occasionally, a woman will have widespread bone involvement without any lesions in other tissues, or both lungs will have innumerable metastatic foci and lymphangitic involvement, yet no skeletal lesions are present. Brain metastases are less common, but meningeal involvement is not; many women with metastatic breast cancer who arrive at the hospital in semicoma in reality have hypercalcemia secondary to extensive osteolytic bone disease.

In general, once metastatic disease is found, it is usually much more widespread than is initially apparent. This observation has led most clinicians to look to systemic therapy for the palliative management of metastatic breast cancer. There are many therapeutic alternatives and the choice is often dependent upon the experience and capabilities of the physician involved in the care of such patients. The prime objective, as with any palliative therapy, must be improvement in the quality of survival, with length of survival being a secondary consideration. The major types of modalities in current use are: (1) hormonal therapy, (2) endocrine organ ablation, (3) chemotherapy, and (4) radiotherapy. These may be used alone or in various combinations. There are two general concepts of management: the first is to use sequential therapy in hopes of obtaining several remission periods, and the other is to utilize two or more of these approaches simultaneously in a more aggressive manner in order to obtain remission in a larger number of patients. These are by no means mutually exclusive; decisions must be based on the general status of the patient, the sites of involvement, the specific symptoms of the patient, and the previous therapy she has received.

Hormonal Therapy

Androgen, estrogen, corticosteroids, progestational agents, and thyroid hormone have been used to alter the growth rate and produce remissions of metastatic breast cancer. Loeser[75] in 1939 first described the therapeutic effects of androgen in metastatic breast cancer and many other reports soon appeared. Haddow[51] in 1944 reported significant response to estrogen therapy in 75 patients. Nathanson and Kelley[87] in 1952 confirmed the value of estrogen administration for palliation of disseminated disease. A large cooperative investigation, instituted by the American Medical Association,[110] demonstrated that estrogen produced 36 per cent regressions in postmenopausal women, while androgen therapy was responsible for objective remissions in 20 per cent of premenopausal women and 21 per cent of postmenopausal women. Estrogen has been most effective for soft tissue and visceral disease in older women, whereas androgen is most helpful for younger women with skeletal involvement. Androgen therapy has many undesirable side-effects, the most dangerous of which is its interconversion to estrogen at about 1 per cent of the administered dose.[89] This may result in physiologic administration of estrogen to young women and is a frequent cause of hypercalcemia after androgen treatment. Some physicians utilize these two sex hormones alternatively, and they have also been combined.[71] Kennedy[70] considers estrogen therapy as a primary approach to treatment of metastatic breast cancer in postmenopausal women and oophorectomy in premenopausal women. Sequential treatment is planned from that point, depending upon the initial responses.

Corticosteroids have fewer side-effects than androgen and estrogen and have not been demonstrated to stimulate growth of the metastatic cancer, a potential problem whenever androgen or estrogen is used. They are particularly useful in the management of hypercalcemia, along with vigorous fluid therapy and phosphate administration, if necessary. The usual remission with corticosteroid therapy is for about 6 months, and at one time this served as the primary hormonal therapy for patients with metastatic breast cancer at the Peter Bent Brigham Hospital. In 79 patients receiving this therapy for more than 60 days, a 57 per cent response rate was achieved, and 47 per cent of 190 patients given a major course of corticosteroids had an objective remission.[84] Although most patients at this clinic now are treated with adrenalectomy, corticosteroids in the form of prednisone constitute an important alternative.[119]

Neither progestational agents nor thyroid hormone has produced sufficiently clear remissions to justify continued use, and severe hypercalcemia has been noted after progesterone therapy. The combinations of progestins and estrogen have been more encouraging, particularly in estrogen responders who have become resistant to further therapy. Crowley and MacDonald[23] reported a 27 per cent further objective response in such patients when 1000 mg. of Delalutin was added to the continued estrogen dosage.

Endocrine Organ Ablation

Oophorectomy, hypophysectomy, and adrenalectomy, with or without oophorectomy, are various procedures that have been utilized. Therapeutic oophorectomy, because of its simplicity, was for many years the only ablative therapy available. It was first described in 1896 by Beatson[8] and in most institutions is considered the initial procedure of choice in premenopausal women with recurrent breast cancer.[70] There seems to be little choice between surgical oophorectomy and radiotherapeutic castration, except that the effect is immediate with oophorectomy, whereas it takes about 2 months for ovarian suppression to be completed after radiation. Little can be gained by oophorectomy as a solitary procedure in the postmenopausal period, since essentially no estrogen secretion occurs in most postmenopausal ovaries.[6] About 40 to 50 per cent of patients who are within 10 years of the menopause will have a salutary response to therapeutic oophorectomy. Because cortical stromal hyperplasia can persist until the eighth decade of life, it has been the practice at the Peter Bent Brigham Hospital to perform oophorectomy in all patients undergoing adrenalectomy, regardless of their age.[84, 85, 119]

Adrenalectomy and Hypophysectomy. In 1945, Huggins and Scott[63] reported the control of metastatic carcinoma of the prostate with bilateral adrenalectomy, and in 1952 they reported its use as a means of obtaining regression of metastatic breast cancer.[62] Also in 1952, Luft, Olivecrona, and Sjögren[76] described successful treatment of metastatic cancer of the breast with surgical hypophysectomy. The Joint Committee on Endocrine Ablative Procedures in Disseminated Mammary Carcinoma compared the relative values of adrenalectomy and hypophysectomy.[77] No statistical differences were noted in either response rates or length of remission between the two modalities. The Free Interval and the response to previous oophorectomy were observed to be important clinical predictors of remission.

One of the advantages of hypophysectomy is that oophorectomy is not necessary, but diabetes insipidus occurs in about 20 per cent of the cases. In Ray's series[98] of 630 patients treated by hypophysectomy, one of the largest series reported, the mortality was 7.3 per cent in the first 218 patients, but it later fell to 2 per cent. The palliative success rate in his series was 42 per cent. Jessiman et al.,[66] reporting a series of 77 patients from the Peter Bent Brigham Hospital, had a 40 per cent objective response rate. Many of these early patients were in a preterminal state and the mortality was 9.1 per cent.

Several modifications of surgical hypophysectomy have been utilized to reduce the complexity of the procedure in women with extensive metastatic disease; however, total destruction of the pituitary appears necessary for effective remission. Edelstyn[28] inserted yttrium-90 into the pituitary fossa at the completion of surgical hypophysectomy with an increase in the response rate from 24 to 54 per cent. Forrest[37] utilized a ^{90}Y transnasal screw-type implant, but could not show any real advantage to this technique over simpler forms of therapy. Stereotactic cryohypophysectomy has been reported by Rand,[96] and radiofrequency stereotactic hypophysectomy by Zervas,[126] who obtained a 29 per cent response rate in 66 patients.

Adrenalectomy has gained more widespread popularity than has hypophysectomy; its inherent risk is less, its side-effects are fewer, and it is a more familiar procedure to most surgeons dealing with breast cancer. Atkins,[4] comparing the two procedures in a recent clinical trial, found that they produced equal response rates in women with metastatic disease after previous mastectomy. In patients with metastatic disease with an untreated primary lesion (Stage IV with "0" Free Interval), the response rate to adrenalectomy was negligible, but hypophysectomy was capable of producing its usual remission rate in these women. At the Peter Bent Brigham Hospital, women in this category were observed to have similarly poor responses, until 5-FU was administered at the time of adrenalectomy.[52, 85, 121] It was in the group of Stage IV women with "0" Free Interval that chemotherapy was first combined with adrenalectomy, and the objective response rate was risen until it now stands at 63 per cent (22 of 35 cases). Over the past 15 years adrenalec-

TABLE 5.   The Effect of Chemotherapy (5-Fluorouracil) on Objective Response Rates to Adrenalectomy for Metastatic Carcinoma of the Breast in Various Patient Categories*

Category	With Chemotherapy		Without Chemotherapy		Comparison Significance (P)
	No.	Objective Response (%)	No.	Objective Response (%)	
Adrenalectomy	158	58	80	40	<0.02
Zero free interval	35	63	12	0	<0.001
Free interval less than 1 year	73	52	31	16	<0.002
Free interval less than 2 years	101	52	43	23	<0.003
Age under 40	18	44	6	0	NS
Age over 40	140	59	74	43	<0.05
Less than 1 year after menopause	32	47	10	10	NS
Bone metastases predominate	60	67	35	34	<0.005
Skin and soft tissue metastases	12	58	12	50	NS
Pleura and lung metastases	36	53	11	55	NS
Visceral metastases	50	50	22	36	NS

*From Moore, F. D., et al.: Surgery, 76:376, 1974.

tomy has been performed in more than 400 patients with active and symptomatic metastatic breast cancer at the Peter Bent Brigham Hospital, with an operative mortality of 1.5 per cent and an overall objective response rate, for a minimum of 6 months, of 52 per cent. As shown in Table 5, about two thirds of the patients had had 5-FU with adrenalectomy. Since 1967 this has been the standard practice and the results have improved most noticeably in those patients with shorter Free Intervals and skeletal metastases.

Women with liver metastases showed a 39 per cent response rate and those with lung metastases had a 28 per cent response rate. Some representative examples of the bony, liver, and lung responses are seen in Figures 30 to 32. These adrenalectomies were all performed through a routine posterior, bilateral approach. Fraccia[38] reported a 5.8 per cent mortality rate, Harris and Spratt[56] a 9 per cent mortality rate, and Silverstein et al.[105] a 5.6 per cent mortality rate; these are somewhat higher than the 1.5 per cent rate

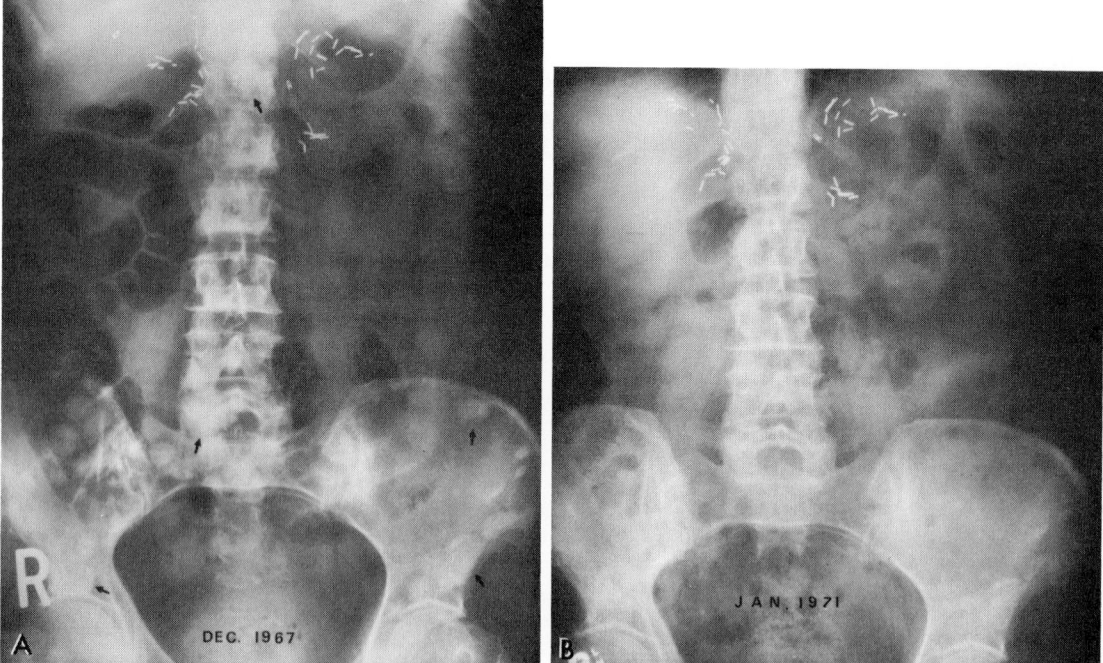

Figure 30.   The effect of adrenalectomy on bone metastases in a patient with advanced breast cancer. *A,* At the time of adrenalectomy this patient had widespread osteoblastic and osteolytic metastases as indicated by the arrows. *B,* Four years later the bones remain well healed without any residual evidence of metastatic disease. She has continued on chemotherapy throughout this entire time. (Courtesy of Dr. A. Lewicki, Department of Radiology, Peter Bent Brigham Hospital.)

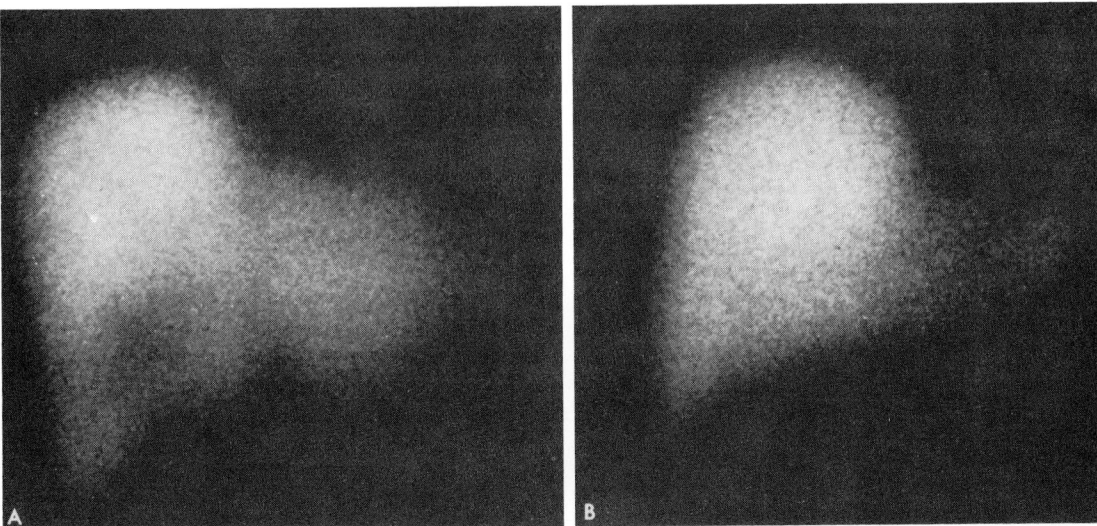

Figure 31. The effect of adrenalectomy on liver metastases. *A,* This patient had a large mass of metastatic disease in the right lobe of the liver (December, 1969). *B,* Six months later the liver scan had assumed a normal configuration. This scan was performed with technetium-99m. A liver scan made in May, 1971, 1½ years from the time of adrenalectomy, was normal. (Courtesy of Dr. S. J. Adelstein, Department of Nuclear Medicine, Peter Bent Brigham Hospital.)

observed at the Peter Bent Brigham Hospital. In all of these series, adrenalectomy was accomplished by the transabdominal route, a technique possibly associated with a higher complication and mortality rate.

All patients treated with adrenalectomy should have an oophorectomy if it has not been previously performed. The value of therapeutic oophorectomy as a predictor of adrenalectomy or hypophysectomy response is by no means as certain as it once was considered to be.[105] Younger women with more aggressive metastatic disease may fail to respond to oophorec-

tomy and then lose the opportunity to be treated with the more potent ablative procedures. Consequently, the policy at the Peter Bent Brigham Hospital has been to perform simultaneous oophorectomy and adrenalectomy in all nonoophorectomized patients rather than staging these two operations.

Biochemical discriminants have been extensively evaluated as a means of selecting those patients who might respond to either hypophysectomy or adrenalectomy. Bulbrook et al.[16] first utilized a discriminant based on the analysis of resting urinary hormone

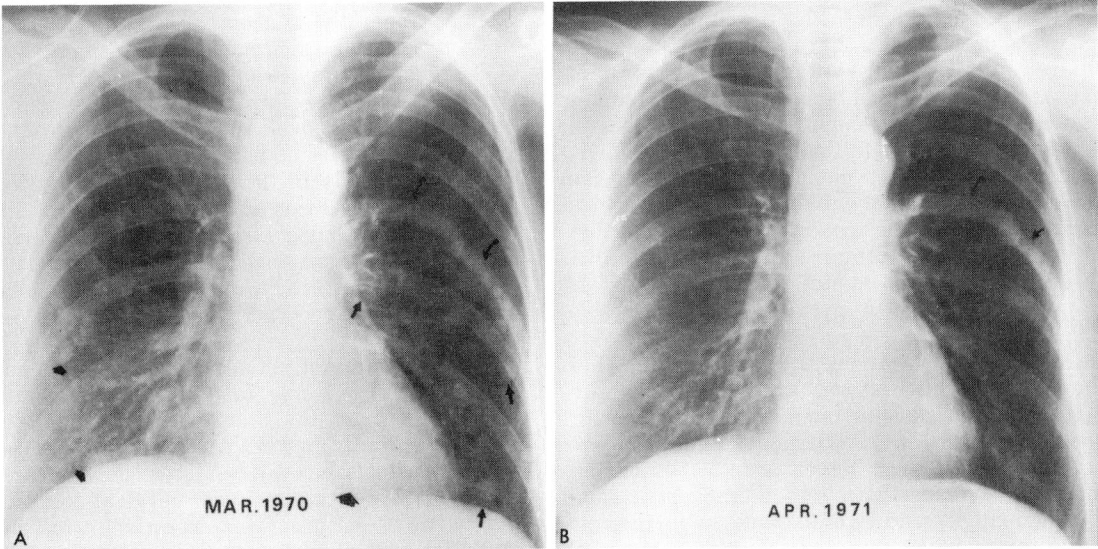

MAR. 1970   APR. 1971

Figure 32. The response of pulmonary metastases to adrenalectomy. *A,* Diffuse nodular densities are present in the lung field of this patient, as demonstrated by the straight arrows. In addition, a pathologic fracture of the left sixth rib is present. *B,* Chest x-ray more than a year after adrenalectomy indicates complete disappearance of all pulmonary nodules and healing of the pathologic fracture. (Courtesy of Dr. A. Lewicki, Department of Radiology, Peter Bent Brigham Hospital.)

excretion values, in which the etiocholanolone level was the outstanding feature. A strongly positive discriminant correlated with palliative responses. A similar type of linear discriminant was derived from the urinary steroid excretion values in response to an ACTH stimulation test by Wilson et al.,[119] and the Free Interval affected this calculation. A specificity of 80 per cent and a selectivity of 75 per cent were possible with this function. More recently, Dao and Libby[25] studied the ability of metastatic tumor tissue to enzymatically sulfurylate dehydroepiandrosterone and estradiol-17β. Of 44 patients, 13 women whose tumors did not have sufficient sulfokinase activity to conjugate dehydroepiandrosterone more efficiently than estradiol-17β failed to respond; in the rest of the patients, whose tumors did not conjugate dehydroepiandrosterone more efficiently, adrenalectomy produced remission.

Jensen's demonstration of estrogen receptor protein (estrophilin) in hormone-responsive breast cancers[65] holds exciting promise for better selection of therapy in patients with metastases. It appears that tumors lacking estrophilin cannot respond to hormonal manipulation. The objective response rate to endocrine therapy or ablation among estrophilin-positive tumors is in the range of 50 per cent.[9] A preliminary report by Horwitz et al.[61] showed that the presence of both estrogen and progesterone receptors correlated more accurately with a response.

Chemotherapy

Combination chemotherapy has been more effective than single agents in the treatment of metastatic breast cancer. Responses with single agents have generally achieved partial remissions of 10 to 30 per cent. Canellos et al.[18] have shown that cyclical combination therapy using methotrexate, 5-fluorouracil, cyclophosphamide, and prednisone resulted in a significant antitumor response in 68 per cent of the patients, with a complete remission in 28 per cent. The median duration of antitumor response was 9 months. Metastases in soft tissue, lymph nodes, and the lung were most responsive. Jones et al.[67] have reported the use of Adriamycin and Cytoxan with a response rate (minimum time of one month) of 80 per cent and a complete remission rate of 12 per cent. The survival data for these patients are shown in Figure 33. The median duration of response was 10 months. Actuarial survival for the entire group of 12 patients was 70 per cent at 12 months. In both of these series of combination therapy, the toxicity was acceptable and the drugs proved to be safe for outpatient administration.

Radiotherapy

The well-known effectiveness of orthovoltage therapy in treating local chest wall and nodal recurrence, as well as painful skeletal metastases, has been further augmented by the widespread availability of supervoltage equipment. Solitary, locally recurrent tumor is best treated with radiotherapy of a small field. In a small percentage of patients, no further metastatic disease will occur and this single approach suffices. Recurrence in multiple intracutaneous areas of chest wall, referred to as cancer-en-cuirasse, can be treated either by irradiation of large tangential fields

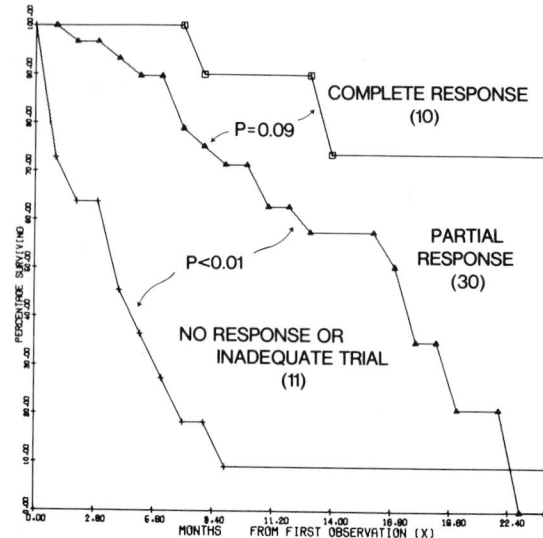

Figure 33. Actuarial survival curves for patients with metastatic breast cancer treated by combination chemotherapy (Adriamycin and cyclophosphamide). A total of 51 patients were treated who had received no prior chemotherapy; the numbers in parentheses represent the number of patients in each group. A complete or partial response significantly affected the survival time of patients. In this study, there was an 80 per cent objective response rate (complete, 12 per cent; partial, 68 per cent) with a mean response duration of 10 months. (From Jones, S. E., et al.: Cancer, 36:90, 1975.)

or superficial beam treatment, particularly by electrons. This is one of the most difficult types of metastatic disease to treat because it is so widespread in the skin lymphatics. Radiotherapy is the only effective means of palliation for brain metastasis from breast cancer. High doses of corticosteroids are given during the initial phases of therapy to the brain to reduce edema. Generally, the entire brain is treated when any intracranial lesion has been identified.

Osseous metastasis can be particularly well treated with a short course of radiotherapy. Often, only a dose of 1800 to 2000 R over 3 to 5 days is required, resulting in rapid relief of pain, stabilization of damaged bone, particularly in the spine, pelvis, ribs, and long bones, and prevention of subsequent pathologic fractures. When pathologic fractures do occur, particularly in the femur, aggressive therapy with internal fixation, local radiotherapy, and systemic hormonal therapy can achieve good palliative results with return of function.[20]

A special area of potential advantageous combination of therapy exists in the management of Stage III carcinoma of the breast (see Fig. 28). These lesions are locally inoperable, but the presence of distant metastasis has not yet been demonstrated. The prognosis is dismal for 5-year survival, but local control of the breast lesion is imperative. A full course of radiation to the breast and the lymph nodes, combined with early adrenalectomy and oophorectomy and postoperative chemotherapy, is the plan of management for these patients at the Peter Bent Brigham Hospital.

SARCOMA OF THE BREAST

Cystosarcomas account for the majority of sarcomas of the breast, although fibrosarcomas, liposarcomas, rhabdomyosarcomas, and hemangiosarcomas have been observed rarely. Lymphosarcoma has been known to arise primarily in the breast in both sexes, and Hodgkin's disease can involve the breast tissue without any contiguous spread from axillary nodes.

The majority of cystosarcomas are not malignant. In the report of McDivitt et al.,[80] only 14 of 73 cases (19 per cent) were malignant; Treves and Sunderland[111] found 23 per cent of their cases to be malignant. Cystosarcomas are usually slow-growing and frequently present as a large lobular mass in the breast without skin fixation, peau d'orange, ulcerations, or axillary adenopathy (see Fig. 8). The majority of metastases from malignant forms of cystosarcoma and other sarcomas result from blood vessel invasion, although local recurrence in the chest wall is common with inadequate excision. The treatment of cystosarcoma is surgical. Since the tumor's malignant propensity is often difficult to identify by biopsy or even after mastectomy, excision should tend to be conservative. Simple mastectomy is adequate for benign lesions, but radical mastectomy should be performed if malignancy is demonstrated by biopsy. Simple mastectomy is much more effective for borderline cases than local excision alone; it reduces the incidence of local recurrence if a tumor is eventually found to be malignant. If local recurrence occurs after local excision or simple mastectomy, surgical re-excision is still the best therapy. In the series reported by Treves and Sunderland,[111] 41 patients with benign tumors had no further treatment; of 18 patients with borderline disease, four had local recurrences; 8 of 18 patients with obvious malignant disease died with metastasis. The prognosis for patients with other types of sarcomas generally is less favorable because of early blood-borne pulmonary metastases.

SELECTED REFERENCES

Ackerman, L. V., and del Regato, J. A.: Cancer—Diagnosis, Treatment, and Prognosis. 4th ed. St. Louis, The C. V. Mosby Company, 1970.
The chapter on breast cancer in this book provides an excellent up-to-date review of present concepts in epidemiology, treatment, and prognosis. The broad clinical experiences of the authors are added to the various viewpoints expressed in the literature. This chapter is well illustrated and contains an excellent bibliography.

Anderson, W.: Boyd's Pathology for the Surgeon. 8th ed. Philadelphia, W. B. Saunders Company, 1967.
The chapter on the breast offers a fine review of pathologic correlations of the breast and its diseases and places them in perspective for the surgeon. The differential diagnosis of malignant breast disease and the discussion of cystic hyperplasia of the breast are particularly noteworthy.

Geschickter, C. F.: Diseases of the Breast. Philadelphia, J. B. Lippincott Company, 1943.
This book was an earlier attempt at compiling a general review of all problems of breast disease and providing a basis for their management. Its clinical-pathologic correlations are particularly outstanding and the section on benign cystic disease is classic.

Haagensen, C. D.: Diseases of the Breast. Philadelphia, W. B. Saunders Company, 1956; 2nd ed., 1971.
This book stands as the classic volume on diseases of the breast. The meticulous concern of the author for surgical technique and his clear understanding of the limits of surgical management in breast cancer are key features in the development of his surgical philosophy. The extensive experience of a single surgeon with breast cancer provides excellent data to support his contentions.

Haagensen, C. D., Cooley, E., Miller, E., Handley, R. S., Thackray, A. C., Butcher, H. R., Jr., Dahl-Iverson, E., Tobiassen, T., Williams, I. G., Stone, J. R., Kaae, S., and Johansen, H.: The treatment of early mammary carcinoma: A cooperative international study. Ann. Surg., 170:875, 1969.
This series of articles represents a cooperative international 10-year review of the management of operable breast cancer. Simple mastectomy alone, simple mastectomy with radiotherapy, modified radical mastectomy, radical mastectomy with and without radiotherapy, and extended radical mastectomy are all evaluated in their current settings. This series of articles provides 10-year survival statistics, but these various surgical approaches were independently studied without statistical comparisons.

Lewison, E. F.: The surgical treatment of breast cancer, an historical and collective review. Surgery, 34:904, 1953.
This is by far the most thorough and enlightening historical review of the surgical approach to breast cancer. Abundant quotations and descriptions from ancient manuscripts provide fascinating reading. The surgical events in progress in the nineteenth century leading up to Halsted's development of the classic radical mastectomy are clearly documented. A superb historical bibliography is supplied, as well as original drawings of the Halsted radical mastectomy by Max Brödel.

MacMahon, B., Cole, P., and Brown, J.: Etiology of human breast cancer. J.N.C.I., 50:21, 1973.
This is an authoritative and current review of the epidemiological features associated with breast cancer. Proven risk factors and theoretical etiologic mechanisms are objectively presented.

Moore, F. D., Woodrow, S. I., Aliapoulios, M. A., and Wilson, R. E.: Carcinoma of the Breast, A Decade of New Results with Old Concepts. Boston, Little, Brown and Company, 1967.
This monograph was first published as a Progress Report in the New England Journal of Medicine in 1967. Its primary purpose was to review the experience with primary and metastatic cancer of the breast at the Peter Bent Brigham Hospital from January, 1954, to December, 1963, and to relate this experience to the current literature. The objective of the authors was to formulate a rational program for the management of breast cancer in its various stages based upon such a retrospective review. Approximately equal numbers of patients with primary and metastatic disease were considered in this review and the follow-up was excellent.

Spratt, J. S., Jr., and Donegan, W. L.: Cancer of the Breast. Philadelphia, W. B. Saunders Company, 1967.
This more recent book compiles the extensive personal experience of the authors with breast cancer primarily in the state-operated cancer hospital. The statistical considerations, the illustrations, the chapter-by-chapter bibliographies, and the breadth of the clinical information are the major advantages of this volume.

Stewart, F. W.: Tumors of the Breast. Subcommittee of Oncology of the Committee of Pathology of the National Research Council, Section IX, Fascicle 34. Washington, D.C., Armed Forces Institute of Pathology, 1950.
This detailed description of the surgical pathology of breast disease is the recognized classic review of the subject. The extensive personal experience of the author is reflected in the monograph and the basis for his classification of breast disease is revealed.

REFERENCES

1. Abramson, D. J.: 857 breast biopsies as an outpatient procedure: Delayed mastectomy in 41 malignant cases. Ann. Surg., 163:478, 1966.
2. Ackerman, L. V., and del Regato, J. A.: Cancer—Diagnosis, Treatment, and Prognosis. 4th ed. St. Louis, The C. V. Mosby Company, 1970.
3. Anderson, W.: Boyd's Pathology for the Surgeon. 8th ed. Philadelphia, W. B. Saunders Company, 1967.
4. Atkins, H., Bulbrook, R. D., Falconer, M. A., Hayward, J. L., MacLain, K. S., and Schurr, P. H.: Ten years' experience of steroid assays in the management of breast cancer. Lancet, 2:1255, 1968.

5. Auchincloss, H.: Significance of location and number of axillary metastases in carcinoma of the breast; a justification for a conservative operation. Ann. Surg., *158*:37, 1963.

6. Barlow, J. J., Emerson, K., Jr., and Saxena, B. N.: Estradiol production after ovariectomy for carcinoma of the breast; relevance to the treatment of menopausal women. N. Engl. J. Med., *280*:633, 1969.

7. Barrett, J. J., and Smith, P. H. S.: Bone imaging with 99mTc polyphosphate: A comparison with 18F and skeletal radiography. Br. J. Radiol., *47*:387, 1974.

8. Beatson, G. T.: On the treatment of inoperable cases of carcinoma of the mamma: Suggestions for a new method of treatment, with illustrative cases. Lancet, *2*:104, 1896.

9. Block, G. E., Jensen, E. V., and Polley, T. Z.: The prediction of hormonal dependency of mammary cancer. Ann. Surg., *182*:342, 1975.

10. Bloom, H. J. G.: Survival of women with untreated breast cancer—past and present. *In* Forrest, A. P. M., and Kunkler, P. B. (Eds.): Prognostic Factors in Breast Cancer. Edinburgh, E. & S. Livingstone, Ltd., 1968, pp. 3–19.

11. Bonadonna, G., Brusamolino, E., Valagussa, P., Rossi, A., Brugnatelli, L., Brambilla, C., DeLena, M., Tancini, G., Bajetta, E., Musumeci, R., and Veronesi, U.: Combination chemotherapy as adjuvant treatment in operable breast cancer. N. Engl. J. Med., *294*:405, 1976.

12. Breasted, J. H.: The Edwin Smith Surgical Papyrus. Volume I. Chicago, University of Chicago Press, 1930.

13. Brinkley, D., and Haybittle, J. L.: The treatment of stage II carcinoma of the female breast. Lancet, *2*:291, 1966.

14. Bruce, J.: Operable cancer of the breast, a controlled clinical trial. Cancer, *28*:1443, 1971.

15. Bruce, J., Carter, D. C., and Fraser, J.: Patterns of recurrent disease in breast cancer. Lancet, *1*:433, 1970.

16. Bulbrook, R. D., Greenwood, F. C., and Hayward, J. L.: Selection of breast cancer patients for adrenalectomy or hypophysectomy by determination of urinary 17-hydroxycorticosteroids and aetiocholanolone. Lancet, *1*:1154, 1960.

17. Butcher, H. R., Jr.: Radical mastectomy for mammary carcinoma. Ann. Surg., *170*:883, 1969.

18. Canellos, G. P., Devita, V. T., Gold, G. L., Chabner, B. A., Schein, P. S., and Young, R. C.: Cyclical combination chemotherapy for advanced breast carcinoma. Br. Med. J., *9*:218, 1974.

19. Charkes, N. D., Malmud, L. S., Caswell, T., Goldman, L., Hall, J., Lauby, V., Lightfoot, W., Maier, W., and Rosemond, G.: Preoperative bone scans; use in women with early breast cancer. J.A.M.A., *233*:516, 1975.

20. Coran, A. G., Banks, H. H., Aliapoulios, M. A., and Wilson, R. E.: The management of pathologic fractures in patients with metastatic carcinoma of the breast. Surg. Gynecol. Obstet., *127*:1255, 1968.

21. Cortese, A. F., and Cornell, G. N.: Carcinoma of the male breast. Ann. Surg., *173*:275, 1971.

22. Crile, G., Jr.: Results of simple mastectomy without irradiation in the treatment of operative stage I cancer of the breast. Ann. Surg., *168*:330, 1968.

23. Crowley, L. G., and MacDonald, I.: Delalutin and estrogens for the treatment of advanced mammary carcinoma in the postmenopausal woman. Cancer, *18*:436, 1965.

24. Dahl-Iverson, E., and Tobiassen, T.: Radical mastectomy with parasternal and supraclavicular dissection for mammary carcinoma. Ann. Surg., *170*:889, 1969.

25. Dao, T. L., and Libby, T. R.: Conjugation of steroid hormones by breast cancer tissue and selection of patients for adrenalectomy. Surgery, *66*:162, 1969.

26. Dodd, G. D., Zermeno, A., Marsh, L., Boyd, D., and Wallace, J. D.: New developments in breast thermography. High spatial resolution. Cancer, *24*:1212, 1969.

27. Easson, E. C.: Post-operative radiotherapy in breast cancer. *In* Forrest, A. P. M., and Kunkler, P. B. (Eds.): Prognostic Factors in Breast Cancer. Edinburgh, E. & S. Livingstone, Ltd., 1968, pp. 118–127.

28. Edelstyn, G., Gleadhill, C., and Lyons, A.: A rational approach to hypophysectomy. Br. J. Surg., *52*:953, 1965.

29. Egan, R. L.: Roles of mammography in the early detection of breast cancer. Cancer, *24*:1197, 1969.

30. Feinleib, M., and Garrison, R. J.: Interpretation of the vital statistics of breast cancer. Cancer, *24*:1109, 1969.

31. Fisher, B., Ravdin, R. G., Ausman, R. K., Slack, N. H., Moore, G. E., and Noer, R. J.: Surgical adjuvant chemotherapy in cancer of the breast: Results of a decade of cooperative investigation. Ann. Surg., *168*:337, 1968.

32. Fisher, B., Slack, N. H., Cavanaugh, P. J., Gardner, B., and Ravdin, R. G.: Postoperative radiotherapy in the treatment of breast cancer: Results of the NSABP clinical trial. Ann. Surg., *172*:711, 1970.

33. Fisher, B., Carbone, P., Economou, S. G., Frelick, R., Glass, A., Lerner, H., Redmond, C., Zelen, M., Band, P., Katrych, D., Wolmark, N., and Fisher, E. R.: l-phenylalanine mustard (LPAM) in the management of primary breast cancer. N. Engl. J. Med., *292*:117, 1975.

34. Fisher, B., Slack, N., Katrych, D., and Wolmark, N.: Ten year follow up results of patients with carcinoma of the breast in a co-operative clinical trial evaluating surgical adjuvant chemotherapy. Surg. Gynecol. Obstet., *140*:528, 1975.

35. Fletcher, G. M., Montague, E. B., and White, E. C.: Evaluation of irradiation of the peripheral lymphatics in conjunction with radical mastectomy for cancer of the breast. Cancer, *21*:791, 1968.

36. Foote, F. W., and Stewart, F. W.: A histologic classification of carcinoma of the breast. Surgery, *19*:74, 1946.

37. Forrest, A. P. M., Stewart, H. J., Benson, E. A., Ker, H., Jones, V., Kunkler, P. B., and Campbell, H.: Controlled studies in advanced breast cancer. *In* Forrest, A. P. M., and Kunkler, P. B. (Eds.): Prognostic Factors in Breast Cancer. Edinburgh, E. & S. Livingstone, Ltd., 1968, pp. 186–196.

38. Fraccia, A. A., Randall, H. T., and Farrow, J. H.: The results of adrenalectomy in advanced breast cancer in 500 consecutive patients. Surg. Gynecol. Obstet., *125*:747, 1967.

39. Funderburk, W. W., and Syphax, B.: Evaluation of nipple discharge in benign and malignant diseases. Cancer, *24*:1290, 1969.

40. Galasko, C. S. B., and Doyle, F. H.: The detection of skeletal metastases from mammary cancer. A regional comparison between radiology and scintigraphy. Clin. Radiol., *23*:295, 1972.

41. Gallager, H. S., and Martin, J. E.: Early phases in the development of breast cancer. Cancer, *24*:1170, 1969.

42. Gershon-Cohen, J., Berger, S. M., and Hermel, M. B.: Roentgenography and the management of breast cancer. Am. J. Roentgenol., *89*:51, 1963.

43. Geschickter, C. F.: Diseases of the Breast. Philadelphia, J. B. Lippincott Company, 1943.

44. Guttmann, R. J.: Survival and results after two-million volt irradiation in the treatment of primary operable carcinoma of the breast with proved positive internal mammary and/or highest axillary nodes. Cancer, *15*:383, 1962.

45. Haagensen, C. D.: Diseases of the Breast. Philadelphia, W. B. Saunders Company, 1956; 2nd ed., 1971.

46. Haagensen, C. D., Bohnslay, S. B., Guttmann, R. J., Habif, D. V., Kister, S. J., Markowitz, A. M., Sanger, G., Tretter, P., Wiedel, P. D., and Cooley, E.: Metastasis of carcinoma of the breast to the periphery of the regional lymph node filter. Ann. Surg., *169*:174, 1969.

47. Haagensen, C. D., and Cooley, E.: Radical mastectomy for mammary carcinoma. Ann. Surg., *170*:884, 1969.

48. Haagensen, C. D., Cooley, E., Miller, E., Handley, R. S., Thackray, A. C., Butcher, H. R., Jr., Dahl-Iverson, E., Tobiassen, T., Williams, I. G., Stone, J. R., Kaae, S., and Johansen, H.: The treatment of early mammary carcinoma: A cooperative international study. Ann. Surg., *170*:875, 1969.

49. Haagensen, C. D., and Obeid, S. J.: Biopsy of the apex of the axilla in carcinoma of the breast. Ann. Surg., *149*:149, 1959.

50. Haagensen, C. D.: The choice of treatment for operable carcinoma of the breast. Surgery, *76*:685, 1974.

51. Haddow, A., Watkinson, J. M., and Paterson, E.: Influence of synthetic oestrogens upon advanced malignant disease. Br. Med. J., *2*:393, 1944.

52. Hall, T. C., and Wilson, R. E.: A safe and effective method of administering 5-fluorouracil to adrenalectomized patients. Surg. Gynecol. Obstet., *123*:978, 1966.

53. Halsted, W. S.: The treatment of wounds with especial reference to the value of the blood clot in the management of dead spaces. Johns Hopkins Hosp. Rep., *2*:255, 1890–91.

54. Handley, R. S.: The early spread of breast carcinoma and its bearing on operative treatment. Br. J. Surg., *51*:206, 1964.

55. Handley, R. S., and Thackray, A. C.: Conservative radical mastectomy (Patey's operation). Ann. Surg., *170*:880, 1969.

56. Harris, H. S., Jr., and Spratt, J. S.: Bilateral adrenalectomy in

metastatic mammary cancer. An analysis of sixty-four cases. Cancer, 23:145, 1969.

57. Hayward, J. L.: Steroid excretion in early breast cancer. Br. J. Surg., 51:224, 1964.

58. Hayward, J.: Conservative surgery in the treatment of early breast cancer. Br. J. Surg., 61:770, 1974.

59. Henderson, B. E., Gerkins, V., Rosario, I., Casagrande, J., and Pike, M. C.: Elevated serum levels of estrogen and prolactin in daughters of patients with breast cancer. N. Engl. J. Med., 293:790, 1975.

60. Holleb, A. I., Freeman, H. P., and Farrow, J. H.: Cancer of the male breast. Parts I and II. New York J. Med., 68:544, 656, 1968.

61. Horwitz, K. B., McGuire, W. L., Pearson, O. H., and Segaloff, A.: Predicting response to endocrine therapy in human breast cancer: A hypothesis. Science, 189:726, 1975.

62. Huggins, C., and Bergenstal, D. M.: Inhibition of human mammary and prostatic cancers by adrenalectomy. Cancer Res., 12:134, 1952.

63. Huggins, C., and Scott, W. W.: Bilateral adrenalectomy in prostatic cancer. Ann. Surg., 122:1031, 1945.

64. Huvos, A. G., Hutter, R. V. T., and Berg, J. W.: Significance of axillary macrometastases and micrometastases in mammary cancer. Ann. Surg., 173:44, 1971.

65. Jensen, E. V., Block, G. E., Smith, S., Kyser, K., and DeSombre, E. R.: Estrogen receptors and breast cancer response to adrenalectomy. Prediction of Response in Cancer Therapy. NCI Monograph 34, 1971.

66. Jessiman, A. G., Matson, D. D., and Moore, F. D.: Hypophysectomy in the treatment of breast cancer. N. Engl. J. Med., 261:1199, 1959.

67. Jones, S. E., Durie, B. G. M., and Salmon, S. E.: Combination chemotherapy with adriamycin and cyclophosphamide for advanced breast cancer. Cancer, 36:90, 1975.

68. Kaae, S., and Johansen, H.: Simple versus radical mastectomy in primary breast cancer. In Forrest, A. P. M., and Kunkler, P. B. (Eds.): Prognostic Factors in Breast Cancer. Edinburgh, E. & S. Livingstone, Ltd., 1968, pp. 93–102.

69. Kaae, S., and Johansen, H.: Simple mastectomy plus postoperative irradiation by the method of McWhirter for mammary carcinoma. Ann. Surg., 170:895, 1969.

70. Kennedy, B. J.: Endocrine therapy of breast cancer. J.A.M.A., 200:971, 1967.

71. Kennedy, B. J., and Brown, J. H.: Combined estrogenic and androgenic hormone therapy in advanced breast cancer. Cancer, 18:431, 1965.

72. Lewison, E. F.: The surgical treatment of breast cancer, an historical collective review. Surgery, 34:904, 1953.

73. Lilienfeld, A. M., Barnes, J. M., Barnes, R. D., Brasfield, R., Connell, J. F., Diamond, E., Gershon-Cohen, J., Haberman, J., Isard, H. J., Lane, W. Z., Lattes, R., Miller, J., Seaman, W., and Sherman, R.: An evaluation of thermography in the detection of breast cancer: A cooperative pilot study. Cancer, 24:1206, 1969.

74. Lindgren, M., Borgström, S., and Landberg, T.: Preoperative radiotherapy in operable breast cancer. In Forrest, A. P. M., and Kunkler, P. B. (Eds.): Prognostic Factors in Breast Cancer. Edinburgh, E. & S. Livingstone, Ltd., 1968, pp. 103–117.

75. Loeser, A.: Male hormone in the treatment of cancer of the breast. Act. Union Int. Cancer, 4:375, 1939.

76. Luft, R., Olivecrona, H., and Sjögren, B.: Hypophysectomy in man. Nord. Med., 47:351, 1952.

77. MacDonald, I.: Endocrine ablation in disseminated mammary carcinoma. Surg. Gynecol. Obstet., 115:215, 1962.

78. MacMahon, B., Cole, P., and Brown, J.: Etiology of human breast cancer: A review. J. Natl. Cancer Inst., 50:21, 1973.

79. Madden, J. L.: Modified radical mastectomy. Surg. Gynecol. Obstet., 121:1221, 1965.

80. McDivitt, R. W., Urban, J. A., and Farrow, J. H.: Cystosarcoma phyllodes. Johns Hopkins Med. J., 120:33, 1967.

81. McWhirter, R.: The value of simple mastectomy and radiotherapy in the treatment of cancer of the breast. Br. J. Radiol., 21:599, 1948.

82. Meyer, W.: An improved method of the radical operation for carcinoma of the breast. Med. Rec., 46:746, 1894.

83. Miller, E.: Simple mastectomy for mammary carcinoma. Ann. Surg., 170:879, 1969.

84. Moore, F. D., Woodrow, S. I., Aliapoulios, M. A., and Wilson, R. E.: Carcinoma of the Breast, A Decade of New Results with Old Concepts. Boston, Little, Brown and Company, 1967.

85. Moore, F. D., VanDevanter, S. B., Boyden, C. M., Lokich, J., and Wilson, R. E.: Adrenalectomy with chemotherapy in the treatment of advanced breast cancer: Objective and subjective response rates; duration and quality of life. Surgery, 76:376, 1974.

86. Müller, J.: Ueber Den feinein Bau und die Sormen der krankhaften Geschwulste, 1938.

87. Nathanson, I. T., and Kelley, R. M.: Hormonal treatment of cancer. N. Engl. J. Med., 246:135, 1952.

88. Nevinny, H. B., Nevinny, D., Rosoff, C. B., Hall, T. C., and Muench, H.: Prophylactic oophorectomy in breast cancer therapy. Am. J. Surg., 117:531, 1969.

89. Nissen-Meyer, R., and Sanner, F.: Excretion of oestrone, pregnanediol and pregnanetriol in breast cancer patients. I. Excretion after spontaneous menopause. Acta Endocr., 44:325, 1963.

90. Paget, J.: On disease of the mammary areola preceding cancer of the mammary gland. St. Bartholomew Hosp. Rep., 10:87, 1874.

91. Papatestas, A. E., and Lesnick, G. J.: Treatment of carcinoma of the breast by modified radical mastectomy. Surg. Gynecol. Obstet., 140:22, 1975.

92. Patey, D. H.: A review of 146 cases of carcinoma of the breast operated on between 1930 and 1943. Br. J. Cancer, 21:260, 1967.

93. Peters, M. V.: Wedge resection and irradiation: An effective treatment in early breast cancer. J.A.M.A., 200:134, 1967.

94. Peters, M. V.: The effect of pregnancy in breast cancer. In Forrest, A. P. M., and Kunkler, P. B. (Eds.): Prognostic Factors in Breast Cancer. Edinburgh, E. & S. Livingstone, Ltd., 1968, pp. 65–80.

95. Pickren, J. W., Rube, J., and Auchincloss, H.: Modification of conventional radical mastectomy; a detailed study of lymph node involvement and follow-up information to show its practicality. Cancer, 18:942, 1965.

96. Rand, R. W., Dashe, A. M., Paglia, D. E., Conway, L. W., and Solomon, D. H.: Stereotactic cryohypophysectomy. J.A.M.A., 189:255, 1964.

97. Ravdin, R. G., Lewison, E. F., Slack, N. H., Dao, T. L., Gardner, B., State, D., and Fisher, B.: Results of a clinical trial concerning the worth of prophylactic oophorectomy for breast carcinoma. Surg. Gynecol. Obstet., 131:1055, 1970.

98. Ray, B.: Hypophysectomy as palliative treatment for disseminated carcinoma. J.A.M.A., 200:974, 1967.

99. Rissanen, P. M.: Carcinoma of the breast during pregnancy and lactation. Br. J. Cancer, 22:663, 1968.

100. Rissanen, P. M.: A comparison of conservative and radical surgery combined with radiotherapy in the treatment of stage I carcinoma of the breast. Br. J. Radiol., 42:423, 1969.

101. Robbins, G. F., and Berg, J. W.: Bilateral primary breast cancer. Cancer, 17:1501, 1964.

102. Rosen, P. P., Menendez-Botet, C. J., Nisselbaum, J. S., Urban, J. A., Mike, V., Fracchia, A., and Schwartz, M. K.: Pathological review of breast lesions analyzed for estrogen receptor protein. Cancer Res., 35:3187, 1975.

103. Rubin, P.: Status of bone scanning for bone metastases in breast cancer. Cancer, 24:1338, 1969.

104. Seidman, H.: Cancer of the breast, statistical and epidemiological data. Cancer, 24:1355, 1969.

105. Silverstein, M. J., Byron, R. L., Jr., Yonemoto, R. H., Riihimaki, D. U., and Schuster, G.: Bilateral adrenalectomy for advanced breast cancer: A 21 year experience. Surgery, 77:825, 1975.

106. Spratt, J. S., Jr., and Donegan, W. L.: Cancer of the Breast. Philadelphia, W. B. Saunders Company, 1967.

107. Stevens, G. M., and Weigen, J. F.: Survey mammography as a case finding method for routine and post-mastectomized patients. A five-year study. Cancer, 24:1201, 1969.

108. Stewart, F. W.: Tumors of the Breast. Subcommittee of Oncology of the Committee of Pathology of the National Research Council, Section IX, Fascicle 34. Washington, D.C., Armed Forces Institute of Pathology, 1950.

109. Taylor, G. W.: Evaluation of ovarian sterilization for breast cancer. Surg. Gynecol. Obstet., 68:452, 1939.

110. Therapeutic Trials Committee, American Medical Association. Androgens and estrogens in the treatment of disseminated mammary carcinoma. J.A.M.A., 172:1271, 1960.

111. Treves, M., and Sunderland, D. A.: Cystosarcoma phyllodes of the breast; a malignant and a benign tumor. Cancer, 4:1286, 1951.

112. Urban, J. A.: Clinical experience and results of excision of the internal mammary lymph node chain in primary operable breast cancer. Cancer, *12*:14, 1959.

113. Urban, J. A.: Bilateral breast cancer. Cancer, *24*:1310, 1969.

114. Wangensteen, O. H., Lewis, F. J., and Arhelger, S. W.: The extended or super-radical mastectomy for carcinoma of the breast. Surg. Clin. North Am., *36*:1051, 1956.

115. Weber, E., and Hellman, S.: Radiation as primary treatment for local control of breast carcinoma. J.A.M.A., *234*:608, 1975.

116. White, E. C., Fletcher, G. H., and Clark, R. L.: Surgical experience with preoperative irradiation for carcinoma of the breast. Ann. Surg., *155*:948, 1962.

117. White, T. T., and White, W. C.: Breast cancer in pregnancy; report of 49 cases followed five years. Ann. Surg., *144*:384, 1956.

118. Williams, I. G., and Stone, J.: Total mastectomy with axillary dissection and irradiation for mammary carcinoma. Ann. Surg., *170*:892, 1969.

119. Wilson, R. E., Crocker, D. W., Fairgrieve, J., Bartholomey, A. F., Emerson, K., and Moore, F. D.: Adrenal structure and function in advanced carcinoma of the breast. II. The relation of steroid excretion to adrenal morphology and the outcome of adrenalectomy, with description of a new discriminant function. J.A.M.A., *199*:134, 1967.

120. Wilson, R. E., Piro, A. J., Aliapoulios, M. A., and Moore, F. D.: Evaluation of adrenalectomy and hypophysectomy in the treatment of metastatic cancer of the breast. Cancer, *24*:1322, 1969.

121. Wilson, R. E., Piro, A. J., Aliapoulios, M. A., and Moore, F. D.: Treatment of metastatic breast cancer with a combination of adrenalectomy and 5-fluorouracil. Cancer, *28*:962, 1971.

122. Wilson, W. B., and Spell, J. P.: Adenoid cystic carcinoma of the breast: A case with recurrence and regional metastasis. Ann. Surg., *166*:861, 1967.

123. Wise, L., Mason, A. Y., and Ackerman, L. V.: Local excision and irradiation—an alternative method for the treatment of early breast cancer. Ann. Surg., *174*:392, 1971.

124. Wolfe, J. N.: Analysis of 462 breast carcinomas. Am. J. Roentgenol., *121*:846, 1974.

125. Wynder, E. L.: Identification of women at high risk for breast cancer. Cancer, *24*:1235, 1969.

126. Zervas, N. T.: Stereotaxic radiofrequency surgery of the normal and the abnormal pituitary gland. N. Engl. J. Med., *280*:429, 1969.

RECONSTRUCTIVE SURGERY OF THE BREAST

Nicholas G. Georgiade, M.D.

In recent years there has occurred a tremendous reactivation of the concept of the breast as an object of sensuous pleasure. The psychological stress placed on this aspect of the female form has produced an increased awareness of the surgical possibilities that exist for the improvement of the breast form. The hypoplastic breast can be readily augmented with the newer softer silastic implants. In the last decade refined surgical techniques have made possible the correction of hypermastia, ptosis, and asymmetry of the breast. In the last few years the problem of fibrocystic disease of the breast has been adequately treated by a subcutaneous mastectomy, retaining the nipple-areola with immediate reconstruction of the breast utilizing a silastic prosthesis. The newest development has been the reconstruction of the breast following modified and radical mastectomy

HISTORICAL ASPECTS

Augmentation Mammaplasty

Although augmentation mammaplasty is a relatively recent operative procedure, as early as 1895 Czerny unsuccessfully attempted to augment the breast. In the 1940s and 1950s use of free grafts of autogenous fat, dermis-fat grafts, and dermis-fat pedicle flaps was advocated by Berson,[7] Maliniac,[41] Barnes,[6] and Longacre,[37] but due to the problems experienced these techniques have been abandoned. Paraffin, as used by Gersuny in 1900,[20] resulted in severe complications, as has the use of silicone in recent times. Both the polyvinyl alcohol sponge (Ivalon) as introduced by Pangman[49] and the polyvinyl ether (Etheron) prostheses at first exhibited a satisfactory aesthetic appearance; however, infection, contracture, and hardening of the implants resulted in distorted small firm breasts. In 1963 Cronin and Gerow[11] reported on the first Silastic gel prostheses backed with Dacron mesh. For the last decade this type of prosthesis has been the one of choice and has undergone numerous modifications in design with regard to sizes and shapes, inflatable and self-contained, with and without backing. The newest prostheses, which are constructed of a very thin Silastic skin and filled with a thinner gel, give the best aesthetic results and produce the fewest complications.

Hypermastia and Ptosis

As early as the sixth century Paulus Aegineta[2] has been credited with amputation of part of the breast as a method of reduction mammaplasty. In 1912 Lexer[36] described the bilateral amputation of the breasts with free areolar grafts. Thorek[66] popularized the use of this method followed by Dartigues,[13] Adams,[1] and Clarkson.[10]

The removal of skin and subcutaneous tissue was first performed by Pousson[53] in 1897. Dehner,[14] Girard,[23] Gobell,[24] Maliniac,[40] and Lewis[35] advocated removal of portions of skin and subcutaneous tissue, with attachment of the breast tissue to either the pectoralis fascia or the ribs or both. Although these methods resulted in reduction of breast tissue with elevation of the ptotic nipple, the aesthetic results were poor because of the resultant scarring and inadequate support of the breasts.

Aubert[4] in 1923 reported successful cases of transposition of the nipple, which concept provided the basis of the modern reduction mammaplasty. Because of the problem of nipple necrosis, Joseph[31] and Schreiber[60] suggested two-stage procedures.

Axhausen[5] and Biesenberger[8] dissected skin flaps from the underlying breast tissue, partially removed the glandular tissue, transposed the nipple, and molded a new breast form. The Bisenberger method was modified by Gillies and McIndoe,[21] Maliniac,[38] and Ragnell,[54] who recommended a two-stage glandular resection.

Since these skin flap methods resulted in frequent sloughing of nipples and necrosis of skin, newer methods were sought. Strömbeck[65] introduced the use of a horizontal dermal bipedicle flap for transposition of the nipple. Similar procedures were described by Skoog,[63] Pitanguy,[50, 51] and Gerow.[19] McKissock[45] utilized a vertical dermal bipedicle flap for transposing the nipple. A superiorly based flap has been used by Weiner[67] and Georgiade[18] to transpose the nipple superiorly. In the correction of ptosis Regnault[55] and Goulian[25] recommended the use of the dermal pedicle technique with augmentation of the breast with a Silastic gel prothesis.

Reconstruction after Subcutaneous Mastectomy

Freeman[16] was the first to recommend subcutaneous mastectomy for fibrocystic disease of the breast utilizing a submammary incision followed by augmentation with a polyurethane prosthesis. Zybliski[70] and Marino[43] used the dermal pedicle technique to reposition the nipple, which method was further modified by Georgiade,[18] Goulian,[26] and Weiner.[67]

Reconstruction after Radical Mastectomy

Early reconstruction of the breast following mastectomy was attempted by the use of local flaps and the tubed pedicle flaps by Kleinschmidt,[32] Gillies,[22] and Alexander.[3] Reinhard,[57] Holdsworth,[28] and Pontes[52] utilized the remaining breast to reconstruct the missing breast. A flap transferred from the buttocks was used by Orticochea.[48] Snyderman[64] was the first to augment the missing breast with a Silastic gel prosthesis. Bohmert[9] has been successful in reconstructing the breast using a lateral abdominal flap.

Blood Supply to the Nipple

The surgeon must be aware of the blood supply to the nipple. The dermal pedicle flap was recommended by Schwarzman,[61] who stressed the importance of the dermal blood supply to prevent necrosis of the nipple. The three major types of periareolar plexuses have been described by Marcus[42] and Maliniac.[39] Montagna[46] demonstrated that the patterns of cutaneous blood supply were extremely irregular and that the thickness of the dermal layer, the type of skin perfused, and the association with underlying structures affected these vascular fields. Although skin is supplied by some subcutaneous vessels, actually the blood vessels in these plexuses are interconnected at the various levels of dermis and connections exist as A-V shunts. Thus, to prevent necrosis of the nipple and the glandular tissue, the surgeon must preserve the dermal and subdermal blood supply of the nipple-areola complex and maintain continuity of the cutaneous blood supply with the glandular tissue and dermal pedicle.

SURGICAL TECHNIQUES

HYPOMASTIA AND INTERRELATED DEFORMITIES

The correction of hypomastia should produce a breast contour that appears normal in all dimensions, proportionate in size, and of a softness simulating that of the natural breast.

Prostheses

The prostheses most generally used for breast augmentation consist of a thin-walled, smooth, seamless Silastic envelope containing a low viscosity silicone fluid. The inflatable prostheses, which can be filled to the desired size with either Dextran* or saline, is of necessity constructed of a thicker Silastic envelope to minimize the possibility of leakage of fluid. The prefilled prostheses are available in a variety of shapes and sizes, including round, oval, and elongated to simulate the axillary tail of the breast, and may have a flat, low, or teardrop profile. The prostheses may have a tab on the back for attachment to the chest wall or may have Dacron backing to allow attachment to the chest wall by fibrous proliferation, although some authors feel this is undesirable.[68]

Surgical Methods

The surgical method of insertion varies and usually is performed utilizing one of the following techniques. The inframammary approach is used most extensively. An incision, 5 cm. in length, is placed approximately 5½ cm. below the nipple just superior to the inframammary crease (Fig. 2A). The breast tissue is dissected posteriorly to the pectoralis muscle and fascia, and retraction and elevation of the breast tissue permit extension of the dissection along the pectoralis fascia extending superiorly to the axillary tail. The medial dissection is completed short of the perforating vessels and the bleeding points are controlled meticulously with electrocautery. An appropriate-sized prosthesis is inserted and properly oriented, and the operative area is closed carefully in layers. A tight occlusive dressing is applied and maintained for one week, at which time the skin sutures are removed and a snug brassiere (without any wires) is placed over the breasts to be worn night and day for one month (can be removed for bathing). The patient is instructed regarding restriction of abduction of arms during this period of time (Fig. 2B to E).

The axillary approach described by Hoehler[27] has the advantage of breast augmentation without any visible scars on the breast, since a 6-cm. incision is made in the anterior line in the shadow of the pectoralis muscle. Scissors are used to dissect to the pectoralis fascial plane, and the dissection proceeds to the inframammary area utilizing a urethral sound. A round prosthesis is inserted, as orientation is not necessary. It is felt by some surgeons that the round

---

*Cutter Laboratories, Berkeley, California.

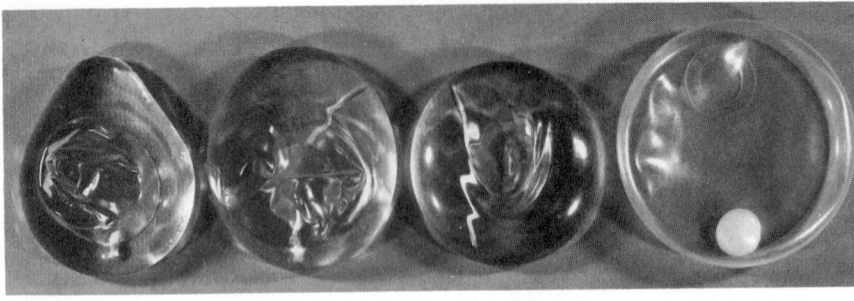
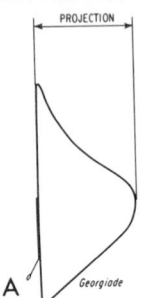
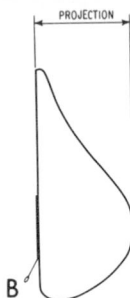
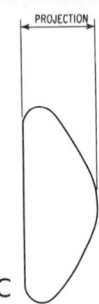
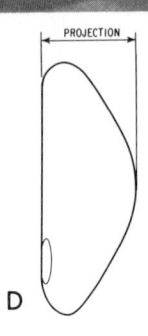

Figure 1. *A*, 225 ml. Georgiade natural-contour mammary implant which has an extra soft Silastic shell filled with a soft silicone gel. These produce both a natural appearing and naturally soft feeling breast. *B*, 255 ml. oval mammary implant of a Silastic shell filled with silicone gel. This implant has a wider base. *C*, 190 ml. round mammary implant of a Silastic shell filled with silicone gel. In the author's opinion the round implants do not provide the natural appearing contour of the breast. *D*, 400 ml. inflatable round mammary prosthesis which consists of a thicker Silastic outer shell and is filled with sterile saline solution to the desired volume. Although these prostheses have been improved in recent years, there still exists the possibility of leakage. These prostheses are coated a number of times to minimize the possibility of leakage and as a result they do not have as soft a feel to palpation. (Prostheses supplied by Surgitek, Medical Engineering Corporation, Racine, Wisconsin.)

prosthesis does not produce a natural looking breast. The proper horizontal alignment of the prosthesis is difficult with this technique and it is more difficult to establish adequate hemostasis because the majority of the perforating vessels are at nipple level or in the inferior portion of the breast tissue.

A periareolar or transareolar approach is used by some surgeons.[30] However, the advisability of this approach is questioned by many surgeons, because the dissection is carried directly through the breast tissue, thus interfering with the normal ductal system of the nipple.

In all of the methods the prosthesis usually is placed superior to the pectoralis muscle and fascial plane. If the patient has a limited amount of breast tissue, the prosthesis may be placed subpectorally; however, postoperatively the prosthesis will not have the same appearance and abduction of the arms will often cause shifting of the prosthesis superiorly, producing an unusual appearing mammary area.

Local anesthesia is used routinely for the augmentation mammaplasty procedure. Initially, the patient is given 15 mg. of morphine or 100 mg. of Demerol intramuscularly one half hour before surgery. An intravenous line is inserted and the patient is given 5 mg. of Valium intravenously prior to local infiltration with 0.5 per cent Xylocaine containing 1:200,000 epinephrine. The operative area is prepared with three layers of Betadine* surgical scrub followed by three layers of Betadine solution. An additional 5 mg. of Valium is given intravenously prior to the incision and dissection. As the dissection continues, additional Valium may be administered depending on the patient's response.

---

*Purdue Frederick Co., Norwalk, Conn.

Complications

Hematoma is the most common of the infrequent complications and usually develops during the first 48 hours but may develop as late as the fifth postoperative day. The procedure of choice is removal of the prosthesis, evacuation of the hematoma, irrigation of the operative area, coagulation of bleeding points, reinsertion of the prosthesis followed by closure of the operative area, application of Elastoplast support, and placement in a suitably-sized brassiere. The patient will usually recover satisfactorily without further difficulty.

Infection has not been a problem postoperatively, since every patient is started immediately postoperatively on a broad-spectrum antibiotic, usually 250 mg. Keflex every six hours until she returns on the seventh postoperative day, at which time the antibiotics are discontinued.

Extrusion of the prosthesis has been reported; however, in the author's opinion this probably occurs because of the insertion of too large a prosthesis, causing overstretching of the skin with too much tension in the area of closure and resultant wound separation.

Firmness of the breast may occur, usually unilaterally, and may be a result of a breast hematoma that was unnoticed or not evacuated, resulting in a thicker capsule formation than desirable around the prostheses. In many instances no direct cause for the firmness can be established. Massage of the postoperative breasts initiated two to three weeks postoperatively appears to limit the capsular constriction. Insertion of 40 mg. of triamcinolone prior to insertion of the prostheses is used routinely to minimize the initiation of the fibrous response around the prostheses. The use of prostheses without a Dacron backing allows greater motion of the prostheses with less capsular contraction.[68]

Figure 2. *A,* The types of incisions used to perform an augmentation mammaplasty: (1) inframammary; (2) axillary; (3) periareolar; (4) transareolar. *B* and *C,* Preoperative front and lateral views of a 35-year-old patient with hypoplastic breasts. *D* and *E,* Five-month postoperative view of same patient who had an augmentation mammaplasty with insertion of a prosthesis through an inframammary incision.

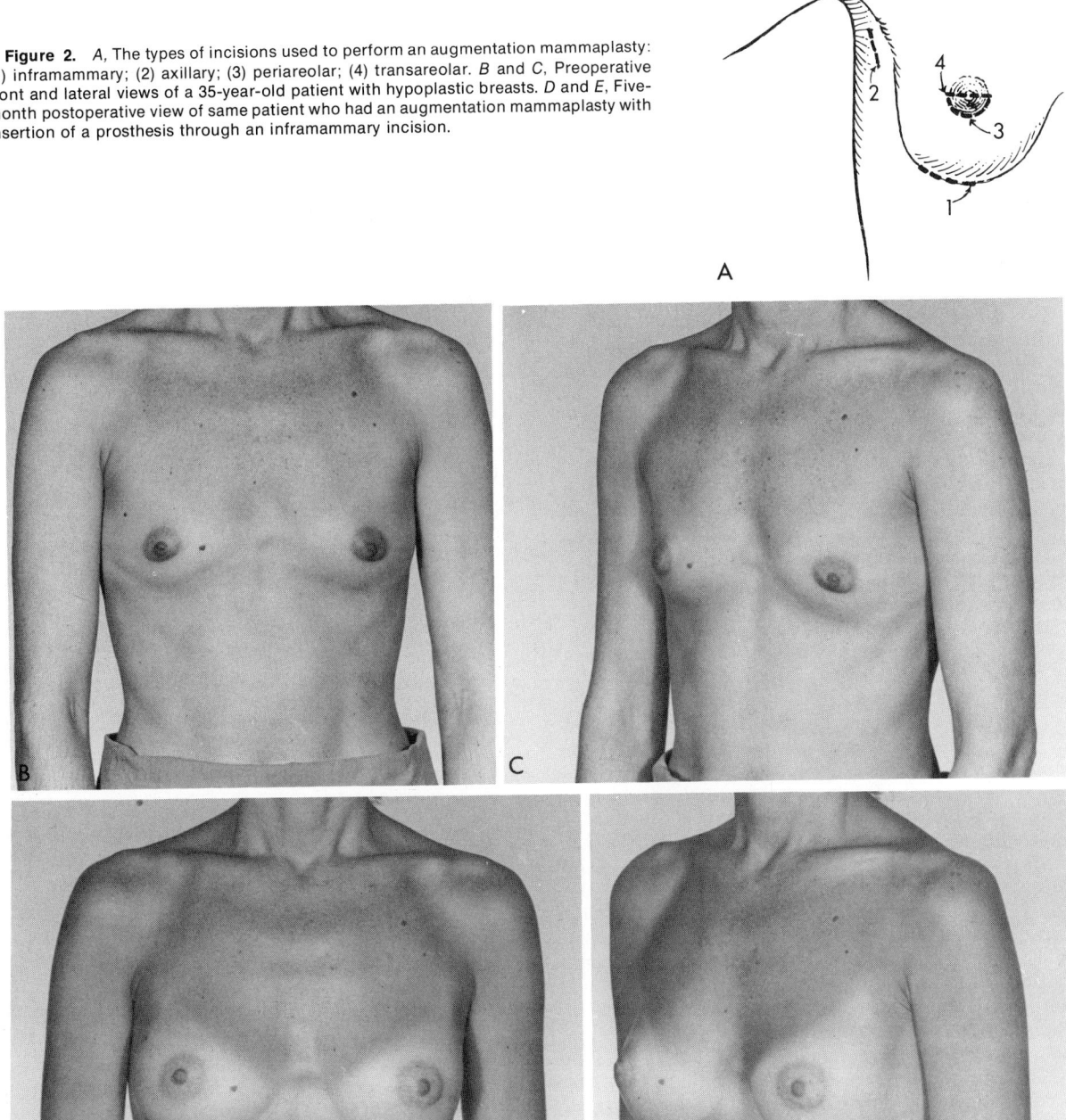

MAMMARY HYPERPLASIA WITH ASSOCIATED PTOSIS

The main goal of all techniques for reduction of the hyperplastic ptotic breast is removal of sufficient breast tissue to construct a normal appearing breast with simultaneous positioning of the nipple-areola complex in a suitable position on the chest. In order to maintain a viable nipple-areola complex, an adequate blood supply to that area is maintained by the use of either the underlying breast tissue or a dermal pedicle flap to transpose the nipple-areola complex.

Surgical Techniques

The early technique of Biesenberger,[8] a one-stage method for reduction of the breast, consisted of dissection of thick skin flaps, excision of an S-shaped portion of the lateral half of the breast, with transposition of the nipple on the remaining medial pedicle. The breast tissue is repositioned with draping and tailoring of the skin to cover the new breast cone. In this method Biesenberger relied on the blood supply from the intercostal perforating arteries for nipple viability. However, since the lateral thoracic artery is frequently involved in the blood supply to the nipple and the stroma, there is significant incidence of both nipple and breast tissue necrosis.

At present, dermal pedicle flaps are used for the transposition of the nipple and areola because viability of the nipple can be maintained by the dermal circulation. The horizontal dermal flap was developed first by Strömbeck[65] and Skoog;[63] the vertical dermal flap was introduced by McKissock,[45] and subsequently the superiorly based dermal flap was used.[18, 67]

Strömbeck established the new position of the nipple at a distance of approximately 19 to 22 cm. from the upper sternal notch just lateral to the midclavicular line. With the patient in the standing position, the skin flaps and the dermal areolar flap are outlined on the breast with brilliant green, using a pattern fashioned after the method of Wise.[69] A split thickness skin layer is excised, leaving a bipedicle horizontal dermal areolar flap. The predetermined amount of skin and breast tissue is excised, including only a sufficient quantity of underlying breast tissue to allow the dermal flap with the nipple-areola portion of the pedicle to be transposed into the newly created site (Figs. 3 and 4). The Strömbeck technique is best suited for the breast with moderate hypertrophy, with transposition of the nipple 6 to 10 cm. superiorly. The advantages of the Strömbeck method are: the shape of the breast is excellent; the nipple transfer on the lateral and medial pedicle ensures adequate blood supply and sensation. Necrosis of the skin flaps does not occur because of the absence of skin undermining. A complication that may result is inversion of the nipple due to excessive removal of breast substance from the new nipple site or undue traction of the horizontal dermal pedicle.

Vertical dermal flaps (McKissock[45] type) carrying the nipple-areola can be used in moderately hypertrophied breasts. The areola is aligned in its new position using the same technique previously described. Premarking of the breast is again performed with the

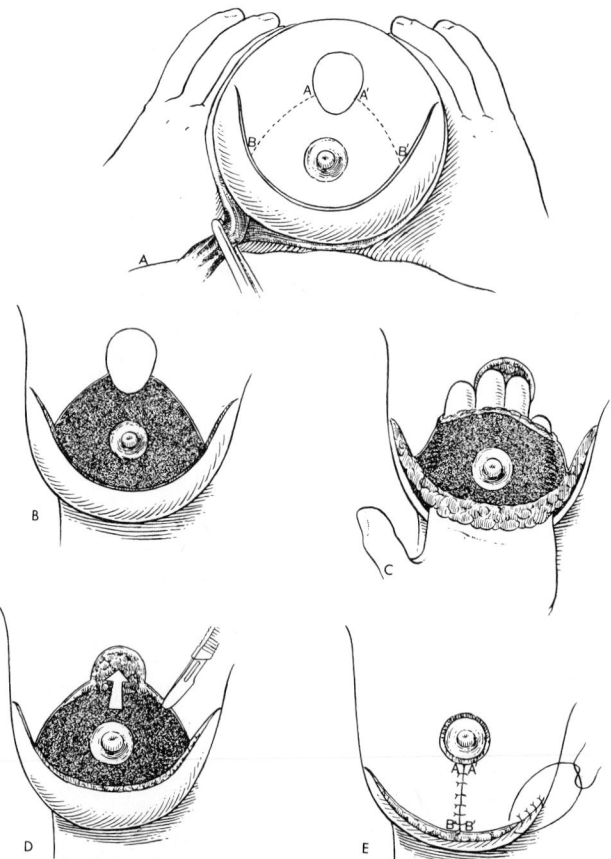

Figure 3. *A*, Diagram of Strombeck technique. The breast is tensed utilizing a sponge clamped at the base of the breast and tensed by the hands. Points A and B will be approximated to points A′ and B′ in the final stage. *B*, A split thickness skin graft has been removed within this area and the new area of the nipple-areola is excised. *C*, The bipedicle areola-nipple flap is shown. *D*, The dermal pedicle flap is advanced superiorly. A lateral dermal-epidermal incision may be necessary to allow advancement of the areola-nipple. The skin and breast inferior to this flap are excised down to the pectoralis muscle. *E*, Points A, A′ and B, B′ are shown approximated. A breast flap of 5 to 6 cm. is considered to be satisfactory. (From Georgiade, N. G.: Correction of the pendulous hypertrophied breast. *In* Georgiade, N. G. (Ed.): Reconstructive Breast Surgery. St. Louis, The C. V. Mosby Co., 1976.)

patient standing, utilizing a "keyhole" type pattern of the author's design. The vertical flaps are outlined extending inferiorly to the inframammary crease. The flaps are designed so that the lateral flap diverges more than the medial flap; in approximating the flaps the line of closure and resultant scar will be less conspicuous. The split thickness skin graft is removed from the vertical dermal flap and the previously determined amount of skin and underlying breast tissue is excised, and in order to assure symmetry the tissue removed bilaterally is weighed. A suction drain is inserted following adequate hemostasis with electrocautery. The advantage of the vertical dermal flaps is that they are more easily and suitably constructed to position the nipple-areola in its new position.

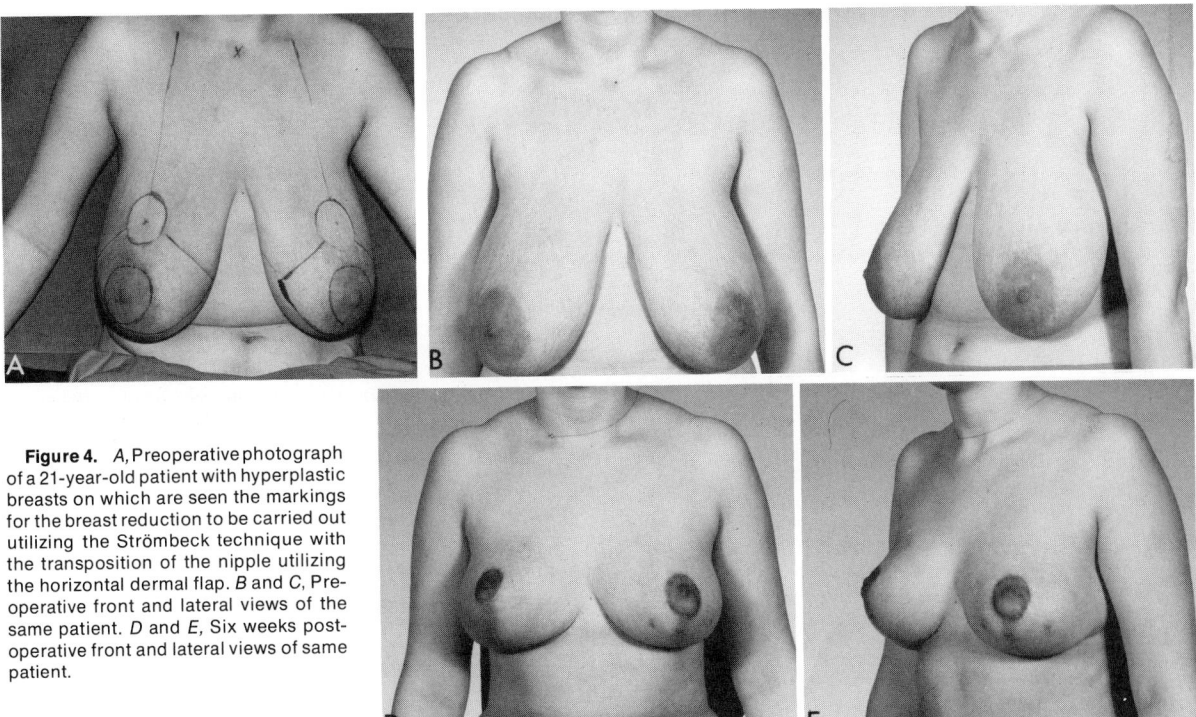

Figure 4. *A*, Preoperative photograph of a 21-year-old patient with hyperplastic breasts on which are seen the markings for the breast reduction to be carried out utilizing the Strömbeck technique with the transposition of the nipple utilizing the horizontal dermal flap. *B* and *C*, Preoperative front and lateral views of the same patient. *D* and *E*, Six weeks postoperative front and lateral views of same patient.

The superiorly based vertical dermal nipple-areola flap is used quite often when there is a slight to moderate ptosis and hypertrophy. The author has restricted the use of this flap to procedures in which the maximum superior movement of the nipple is 5 cm. in order not to jeopardize adequate blood supply to the nipple. This technique is performed in a similar manner to the bipedicle dermal flap with the exception that in the markings only a superiorly based flap is utilized, with a 3-cm. extension of the dermis inferior to the areola. The vascular supply to the nipple is via the dermal and subdermal plexus of vessels.

The small to moderate ptotic hypertrophied breast can be corrected by the technique described by Mouly and Dufourmentel,[47] Schatten,[59] and Regnault.[56] This technique, which utilizes an oblique lateral resection of skin and breast tissue, appears to yield a more central prominence and coning of the breast. Breast tissue is removed from all quadrants of the breast and a thicker portion of breast tissue is left inferior to the nipple in order to increase its forward projection and minimize the chance of postoperative inversion of the nipple. If this technique is performed on too large a breast, the laterally displaced scar is objectionable to many patients because of its extension inferior to the mammary crease and laterally toward the axilla. The eventual positioning of the nipple is also not as easily determined and only finally determined at the time of closure following the breast resection.

In women who have massive, hypertrophied, pendulous breasts, the treatment of choice is amputation of the breasts with the immediate application of free nipple grafts.[44, 58] The age of this group of women will vary from the adolescent female to the middle-aged. In all cases, the tremendous size of the breasts limits physical activity and causes back and shoulder pain and frequently skin excoriations in the inframammary area. Associated severe psychological problems are also quite common. The use of horizontal bipedicle flaps or long vertical flaps as previously described does not yield a satisfactory breast contour and one cannot be assured of adequate blood supply to the nipple-areola.

Subcutaneous Mastectomy with Immediate Reconstruction

Freeman[16] in 1962 recommended treating fibrocystic disease of the breast by subcutaneous mastectomy followed by augmentation with a polyurethane prosthesis. A number of procedures employing the dermal pedicle technique to reposition the nipple in conjunction with the subcutaneous mastectomy have been described by Georgiade,[18] Goulian,[25] and Letterman and Schurter.[34] The development of a new-shaped, thin-shelled Silastic prosthesis for use in this procedure has resulted in an aesthetically pleasing, natural-shaped breast reconstruction. The preoperative markings for positioning of the nipple on the breast have been simplified by the use of the author's pattern.[18] In all breast surgery involving upward movement of the nipple, the surgeon must be aware that there is always a tendency for the nipple to be displaced upward as the breast tissue repositions itself downward postoperatively. A sufficient dermo-fat flap must be retained beneath the nipple-areola to assure the required circulation. Subcutaneous mastectomy

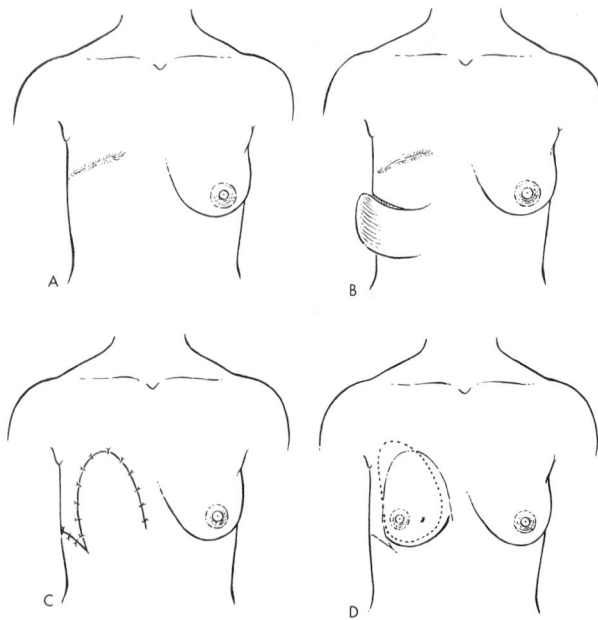

Figure 5. *A,* Appearance of a typical scar following a modified radical mastectomy. *B,* A large lateral flap extending posteriorly and vertically based and delayed once is used to bring "new" tissue into the tight scarred area in order to allow a larger prosthesis to be inserted at the next stage. *C,* The previously delayed lateral flap is shown transferred into its final position on the chest. *D,* The dotted lines show the position of the preferred type of prosthesis inserted under the previously transferred flap. (Drawings after the method of H. Bohmert.)

with immediate reconstruction of the breast should be the procedure of choice in the treatment of fibrocystic disease of the breast.

Breast Reconstruction Following Mastectomy

Freeman[15] and Hueston[29] have reported immediate reconstruction following mastectomy for malignant disease of the breast. This procedure has not attained widespread acceptance as yet, but in the future the plastic surgeon will likely work in conjunction with the general surgeon in planning the mastectomy in order to achieve the best aesthetic reconstructive results. The areola-nipple complex can be banked in the groin for future use as a full thickness graft. When this is done, histologic serial sections of the underlying dermis of the areola-nipple complex should be obtained.

Bohmert[9] has successfully reconstructed the breast utilizing a lateral abdominal flap which, after delay of the flap, is transferred into the area of the chest to be reconstructed (Fig. 5). These flaps are subsequently followed by an augmentation with a Silastic prosthesis and areola reconstruction using full thickness skin grafts from the labia minora (Fig. 6).

If there is sufficient skin and underlying tissue, the author has been reconstructing the breast by the in-

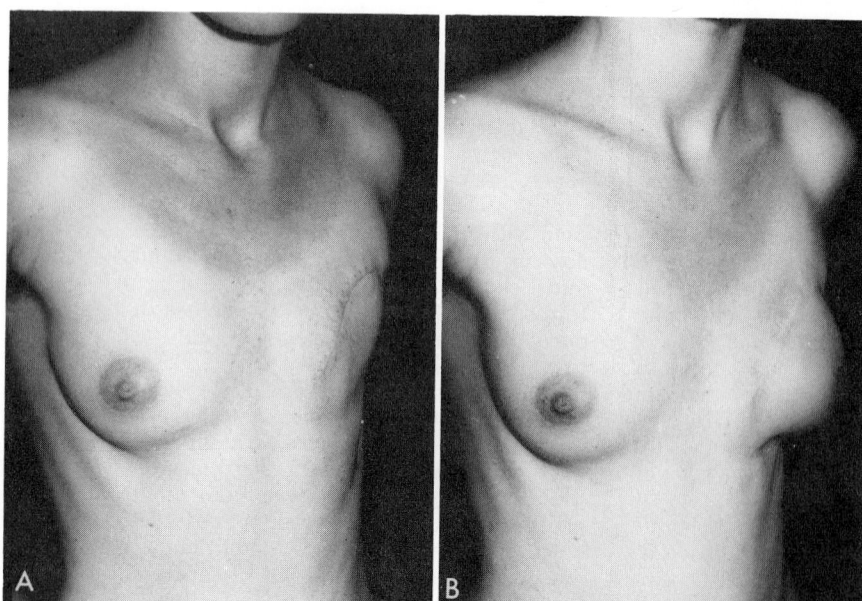

Figure 6. *A,* Preoperative view of patient following mastectomy. *B,* Postoperative view of patient with breast reconstruction utilizing lateral flap method of Bohmert. (Photographs courtesy of H. Bohmert.)

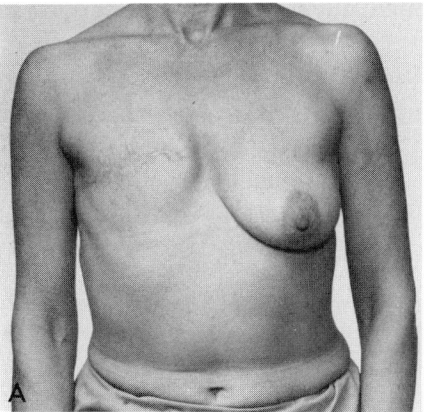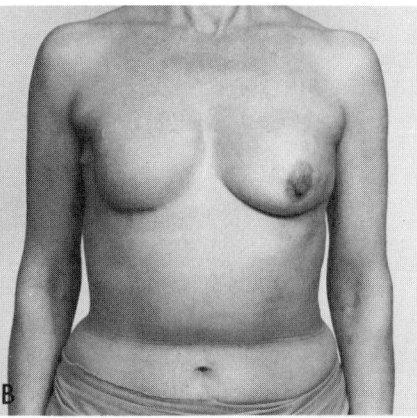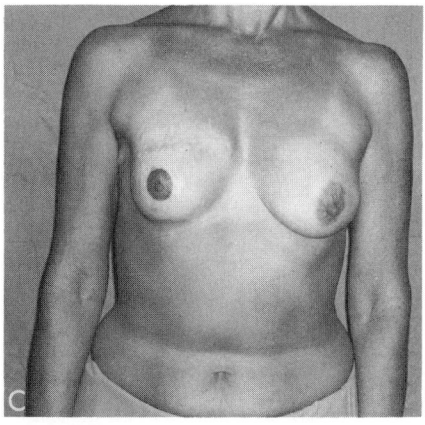

Figure 7. *A*, Preoperative view of a 47-year-old patient who had a right mastectomy performed on October 29, 1973, for lobular carcinoma. On July 16, 1974, a 125 ml. Georgiade Surgitek prosthesis was inserted in the right breast. At the same time a subcutaneous mastectomy was performed on the left breast and a 150 ml. Georgiade Surgitek prosthesis was inserted. *B*, On January 9, 1975, the above prostheses were replaced— on the right side a 200 ml. Georgiade Surgitek soft-shell "tear drop" prosthesis was inserted and on the left side a 185 ml. Georgiade Surgitek prosthesis was inserted. This view on February 6, 1975, shows the results. *C*, A front view showing the areola-nipple complex which was tatooed on the right breast on August 18, 1975. (From Georgiade, N. G.: Reconstruction of the breasts following mastectomy. *In* Georgiade, N. G. (Ed.): Reconstructive Breast Surgery. St. Louis, The C. V. Mosby Co., 1976.)

sertion of Silastic implants.[17] This method entails several operative procedures. A moulage is obtained of the entire chest and a prosthesis is specially designed to fill in all of the chest defect including the subclavicular and axillary defect. A preliminary, suitably-sized prosthesis is inserted to stretch the skin. The nipple-areola complex can be reconstructed in several ways. If the remaining breast tissue is too large and should be recontoured, quite often a portion of the areola can be excised and utilized to construct a new nipple on the opposite side undergoing reconstruction. A labial mucosa graft can also be used or the nipple-areola can be tattooed on the breast surface (Fig. 7).

SELECTED REFERENCES

Georgiade, N. G. (Ed.): Reconstructive Breast Surgery. St. Louis, Mo., The C. V. Mosby Company, 1976.
This most recent well-illustrated book includes chapters by a number of plastic surgeons who are well known for their expertise in reconstructive surgery of the breast. The newest techniques of augmentation and reduction mammaplasty, correction of ptosis, subcutaneous mastectomy with immediate reconstruction, and reconstruction of the breast after mastectomy are presented.

Lalardrie, J. P., and Jouglard, J. P.: Chirurgie Plastique du Sein. Paris, Masson et Cie, 1974.
This well-illustrated French book presents various methods of reconstructive breast surgery compiled from the world literature. It supplies an extensive bibliography.

Maliniac, J. W.: Breast Deformities and Their Repair. New York, Grune and Stratton, 1950.
This reference was the first comprehensive book on reconstructive surgery of the breast written by a plastic surgeon. The history, anatomy, and updated studies of the arterial blood supply of the breast were presented.

Thorek, M.: Plastic Surgery of the Breast and Abdominal Wall. Springfield, Ill., Charles C Thomas, Publisher, 1942.
This book provides the early history of breast reconstruction and

the surgical methods of breast reconstruction at the time it was written.

REFERENCES

1. Adams, W. M.: Free composite grafts of the nipples in mammaplasty. South. Surg., *13*:715, 1947.
2. Aegineta, P.: The Seven Books of Paulus Aegineta, Vol. 2, Book 6. Section 46, p. 334. Translated from the Greek by Francis Adams. London, Syndenham Society, 1847.
3. Alexander, J. E., and Block L. I.: Breast reconstruction following radical mastectomy. Plast. Reconstr. Surg., *40*:175, 1967.
4. Aubert, V.: Hypertrophie mammaire de la puberté, résection partielle restauratrice. Arch. Franco-Belges Chir., *3*:284, 1923.
5. Axhausen, G.: Über Mammaplastik. Med. Klin., *22*:976, 1926.
6. Bames, H. O.: Augmentation mammaplasty by lipo-transplant. Plast. Reconstr. Surg., *11*:404, 1953.
7. Berson, M. I.: Derma-fat-fascia transplants used in building up the breasts. Surgery, *15*:451, 1944.
8. Biesenberger, H.: Eine Neue Methode der Mammaplastik. Zentralbl. Chir., *55*:2382, 1928.
9. Bohmert, H.: Personal communication.
10. Clarkson, P., and Jeffs, J.: Modern mammaplasty. Br. J. Plast. Surg., *20*:297, 1967.
11. Cronin, T. D., and Gerow, F. J.: Augmentation mammaplasty: A new "natural feel" prosthesis. Transactions of the Third International Congress of Plastic Surgery. Amsterdam, Excerpta Medica, 1967, pp. 41–49.
12. Czerny, V.: Plastischer Ersatz der Brustdrüse durch ein Lipom. Zentralbl. Chir., *27*:72, 1895.
13. Dartigues, L.: État actuel de la chirurgie. Esthétique mammaire. Monde Med., *38*:75, 1928.
14. Dehner, J.: Mastopexie zur Beseitigung der Hängebrust. München Med. Wochenschr., *55*:1878, 1908.
15. Freeman, B. S.: Personal communication.
16. Freeman, B. S.: Subcutaneous mastectomy for benign breast lesions with immediate or delayed prosthetic replacement. Plast. Reconstr. Surg., *30*:676, 1962.
17. Georgiade, N. G.: Reconstruction of the breasts following mastectomy. *In* Georgiade, N. G. (Ed.): Reconstructive Breast Surgery. St. Louis, Mo., The C. V. Mosby Company, 1976.
18. Georgiade, N. G., and Hyland, W.: Simultaneous correction of

ptosis of the breast, subcutaneous mastectomy and augmentation mammaplasty. Plast. Reconstr. Surg., 56:121, 1975.

19. Gerow, F. J., Spira, M., and Hardy, S. B.: A simplified design for reduction mammaplasty. Plast. Reconstr. Surg., 53:271, 1974.

20. Gersuny: quoted by Thorek, M.: Plastic Surgery of the Breast and Abdominal Wall. Springfield, Ill., Charles C Thomas, 1942.

21. Gillies, H., and McIndoe, A. H.: The technique of mammaplasty in conditions of hypertrophy of the breast. Surg. Gynecol. Obstet., 68:658, 1939.

22. Gillies, H., and Millard, D. R.: Principles and Art of Plastic Surgery. Vol. 1, Boston, Little, Brown and Company, 1957, p. 413.

23. Girard, C.: Über Mastoptose und Mastopexie. Langenbecks Arch. Klin. Chir., 92:829, 1910.

24. Göbbell, R.: Mamma pendula and Mastodynie. Med. Gesellsch. Kiel, June 18, 1914.

25. Goulian, D.: Dermal mastopexy. Plast. Reconstr. Surg., 47:105, 1971.

26. Goulian, D., and McDivitt, R.: Subcutaneous mastectomy with immediate reconstruction of the breasts. Plast. Reconstr. Surg., 50:211, 1972.

27. Hoehler, H.: Breast augmentation: The axillary approach. Br. J. Plast. Surg., 26:373, 1973.

28. Holdsworth, W. G.: A method of reconstructing the breast. Br. J. Plast. Surg., 9:161, 1956.

29. Hueston, J., and McKenzie, G.: Breast reconstruction after radical mastectomy. Austr. N. Z. J. Surg., 39:367, 1970.

30. Jones, F. R., and Tauras, A. A.: A periareolar incision for augmentation mammaplasty. Plast. Reconstr. Surg., 51:641, 1973.

31. Joseph, J.: Zur Operation der Hypertrophischen Hängebrust. Dtsch. Med. Wochenschr., 51:1103, 1925.

32. Kleinschmidt, O. In Joseph, J.: Nasenplastik und Sonstige Gesichtsplastik nebst einem Anhang uber Mammaplastik. Leipzig, Kabitzsh, 1931.

33. Letterman, G., and Schurter, M.: Will Durston's "Mammaplasty." Plast. Reconstr. Surg., 53:48, 1974.

34. Letterman, G., and Schurter, M.: Inframammary-based dermofat flaps in mammary reconstruction following a subcutaneous mastectomy. Plast. Reconstr. Surg., 55:156, 1975.

35. Lewis, G. K.: A method of mastopexy with fascia lata transplants. J. Int. Coll. Surg., 26:346, 1956.

36. Lexer, E.: Die Freien Transplantation. Stuttgart, Ferdinand Enke, 1919.

37. Longacre, J. J., DeStefano, G. A., and Holmstrand, K.: Breast reconstruction with local derma and fat pedicle flaps. Plast. Reconstr. Surg., 24:563, 1959.

38. Maliniac, J. W.: Asymmetrical breast deformities. Ann. Surg., 99:743, 1934.

39. Maliniac, J. W.: Arterial blood supply of the breast. Arch. Surg., 47:329, 1943.

40. Maliniac, J. W.: A mammaplastic substitute for amputation in hypertrophies. Surgery, 26:573, 1949.

41. Maliniac, J. W.: Use of pedicle dermofat flap in mammaplasty. Plast. Reconstr. Surg., 12:110, 1953.

42. Marcus, G. H.: Untersuchungen uber die Arterielle Blutversorgung der Mamilla. Arch. Klin. Chir., 179:361, 1934.

43. Marino, H.: Glandular mastectomy: Immediate reconstruction. Plast. Reconstr. Surg., 10:204, 1952.

44. McCormack, R. M., and Bales, H. W.: A natural contour reduction mammaplasty for huge breasts. In Georgiade N. G. (Ed.): Reconstructive Breast Surgery. St. Louis, Mo., The C. V. Mosby Co., 1976.

45. McKissock, P. K.: Reduction mammaplasty with a vertical dermal flap. Plast. Reconstr. Surg., 49:245, 1972.

46. Montagna, W., and Parakkal, P. F.: The structure and function of skin. New York, Academic Press, 1974, pp. 142–155.

47. Mouly, R., and Dufourmentel, C.: Mammaplasty by the lateral method. Trans. Int. Congr. Plast. Reconstr. Surg., Melbourne, Butterworths, 1971, p. 1173.

48. Orticochea, M.: Use of the buttock to reconstruct the breast. Br. J. Plast. Surg., 26:304, 1973.

49. Pangman, W. J., and Wallace, R. M.: Use of plastic prosthesis in breast plastic and other soft tissue surgery. West. J. Surg. Obstet. Gynecol., 63:503, 1955.

50. Pitanguy, I.: Breast Hypertrophy. Trans. 5th Int. Congr. Plast. Reconstr. Surg. Melbourne, Butterworths, 1971, pp. 1180–1187.

51. Pitanguy, I.: Surgical treatment of breast hypertrophy. Br. J. Plast. Surg., 20:78, 1967.

52. Pontes, R.: Single stage reconstruction of the missing breast. Br. J. Plast. Surg., 26:377, 1973.

53. Pousson, M.: "De la Mastopexie." Bull. Soc. Chir. Paris, 13:507, 1897.

54. Ragnell, A.: Operative correction of hypertrophy and ptosis of the female breast. Acta Chir. Scand., Suppl. 113, 1946.

55. Regnault, P.: The hypoplastic and ptotic breast: A combined operation with prosthetic augmentation. Plast. Reconstr. Surg., 37:31, 1966.

56. Regnault, P.: Reduction mammaplasty by the "B" technique. Plast. Reconstr. Surg., 53:19, 1974.

57. Reinhard, W. In Thorek, M. (Ed.): Plastic Surgery of the Breast and Abdominal Wall. Springfield, Ill., Charles C Thomas, 1942.

58. Rubin, L. R.: The surgical treatment of the massive hypertrophic breast. In Georgiade, N. G. (Ed.): Reconstructive Breast Surgery. St. Louis, Mo., The C. V. Mosby Co., 1976.

59. Schatten, W. E., and Hartley, J. H., Jr.: Reduction mammaplasty by the Dufourmentel-Mouly method. Plast. Reconstr. Surg., 48:306, 1971.

60. Schreiber, F.: Operation der Hängebrust. Beitr. Z. Klin. Chir., 147:56, 1929.

61. Schwarzmann, E.: Die Technik der Mammaplastik. Chirurg, 2:932, 1930.

62. Serafin, D.: Anatomy of the breast. In Georgiade, N. G. (Ed.): Reconstructive Breast Surgery. St. Louis, Mo., The C. V. Mosby Co., 1976.

63. Skoog, T.: A technique of breast reduction, transposition of the nipple on a cutaneous vascular pedicle. Acta Chir. Scand., 126:453, 1963.

64. Snyderman, R. K.: Reconstruction of the female breast following radical mastectomy. Plast. Reconstr. Surg., 47:565, 1971.

65. Strömbeck, J. O.: Mammaplasty: Report of a new technique based on the two pedicle procedure. Br. J. Plast. Surg., 13:79, 1960.

66. Thorek, M.: Possibilities in the reconstruction of the human form. N. Y. Med. J., 116:572, 1922.

67. Weiner, D. L., Aiache, A. E., Silver, L., Tittiranonda, T.: A single dermal pedicle for nipple transposition in subcutaneous mastectomy, reduction mammaplasty or mastopexy. Plast. Reconstr. Surg., 51:115, 1973.

68. Williams, J. E.: Experiences with a large series of Silastic breast implants. Plast. Reconstr. Surg., 49:253, 1972.

69. Wise, R. J.: A preliminary report on a method of planning the mammaplasty. Plast. Reconstr. Surg., 17:367, 1957.

70. Zbylski, J. R., and Parsons, R. W.: A method of adenectomy and breast reconstruction for benign disease. Plast. Reconstr. Surg., 37:38, 1966.

25

THE THYROID GLAND

I

HISTORICAL ASPECTS AND ANATOMY

Timothy S. Harrison, M.D.

The extirpation of the thyroid gland for goitre typifies, perhaps better than any operation, the supreme
triumph of the surgeons' art.

—Halsted

The thyroid has inevitably attracted the attention of
surgeons because of its predisposition to development
of goiter. As a consequence, few surgical developments
equal that of thyroid surgery as a sensitive and accurate reflection of the maturation of surgical thinking
and technique.

The first operations on the thyroid were primarily
for simple goiter, and much experience was gained
that later proved of importance in the surgical management of hyperthyroidism. Until the introduction of
antithyroid drugs in the 1940s, partial thyroidectomy
for toxic goiter was practiced widely but not always
with gratifying results. Although special indications
remain for surgical treatment of hyperthyroidism,
most thyroid surgery today is for neoplastic disease
and multinodular goiter.

HISTORICAL ASPECTS

The first successful thyroidectomy on record appears to
have been performed about A.D. 952 in Zahra, an Arab city of
Spain, by a Moorish physician, Albucasis, who was well
known throughout the Moslem world of his time, including
Baghdad, one of the leading intellectual centers of the day.
He was a remarkable man, both prolific and courageous. He
recorded many of his medical ideas in his subsequently
famous book, *al-Tasrif*, which was translated into Latin,
French, and Hebrew and is today regarded as one of the
treasures of medical history emanating from the Arab world.
Albucasis is thought to have been the first to introduce many
surgical innovations, among them the use of catgut and cotton sutures. He also accomplished successful small intestinal
anastomoses by amputating the bodies of horned ants from
their locked pincers, which were left applied to the seromuscular layers of the bowel. Halsted's quotation of Mandt is
responsible for bringing Albucasis' successful thyroidectomy

to modern attention, and it is of some interest that the
translation of *al-Tasrif* available to Mandt's sources records
Albucasis as a "bold and, one may say, venturesome operator."[8]

For hundreds of years no basic progress in thyroidectomy
was made, and the surgical literature of the late nineteenth
century is replete with descriptions of fatalities from thyroid
surgery, generally resulting from massive and uncontrollable
hemorrhage. From Leipzig in 1848 comes the statement: "If
we review all we know concerning operations upon hard
goitres we can only regard with tremendous aversion these
foolhardy performances." Samuel D. Gross, the famed nineteenth century Philadelphia surgeon, wrote in 1866, "Can
the thyroid in the state of enlargement be removed? Emphatically experience answers *no*. Should a surgeon be so foolhardy to undertake it...every stroke of the knife will be
followed by a torrent of blood and lucky it would be for him if
his victim lived long enough for him to finish his horrid
butchery. No honest and sensible surgeon would ever engage
in it."[8]

In this technical and professional void, the dedicated genius of Theodor Kocher, Professor of Surgery in Berne, was
the primary force that moved thyroid surgery forward. Io-
dine-deficiency goiter was a common disease in mountainous
Switzerland, and more than 5000 patients were operated
upon in Kocher's clinic, of which approximately 4000 were
his own. Kocher advocated gentle, meticulous surgery, with
sparing of the parathyroid glands and anatomic appreciation
of the recurrent laryngeal nerve. With application of these
principles, the surgical mortality decreased from more than
50 per cent to approximately the current figure of 0.2 per
cent, representing a remarkable achievement. Even more important than these technical perfections was the discovery by
Kocher that *total* thyroidectomy was followed by the development of myxedema, and he demonstrated that this distressing complication could be prevented by subtotal thyroidectomy. For his monumental contributions to the advancement
of medical understanding and care in diseases of the thyroid
gland, Kocher was awarded the Nobel Prize in 1909.

As scientific medicine began to emerge in the United
States at the turn of the century, it was largely to the German and Swiss university clinics that interested Americans
were attracted. The Johns Hopkins University School of Medicine was intentionally patterned after the German schools,
and it is not surprising that its first professor of surgery,

William S. Halsted, was a frequent and discerning visitor in the university clinics of Germany and Switzerland. Halsted was outspoken in his admiration of Kocher's surgical technique, and it was largely the exquisite surgery of the thyroid gland practiced by Kocher that so thoroughly captivated Halsted's interest in the thyroid. Stimulated by Kocher's example, he undertook considerable historical research on thyroid surgery and evolved his own method of thyroidectomy. He described this work in a historical paper of superb dimensions, "The Operative Story of Goitre,"[8] which to this day remains a model of surgical thinking based on scholarship of the highest quality. It is clearly the definitive account of the evolution of thyroidectomy in English. Moreover, it is an example of surgical insight that even casual students of thyroid surgery will find uniquely compelling.

With the technique of thyroidectomy largely established, knowledge of the physiologic function of the thyroid provided the basis for further effective treatment of its disorders. In 1891, Murray, an English physician, administered a glycerin extract of sheep thyroid to a myxedematous patient, with resulting improvement. In 1896, Baumann established the presence of a high iodine content in an acid hydrolysate of thyroid tissue, and Oswald's preparation of iodothyroglobulin 8 years later suggested that the iodine was bound in large part to a releasable protein substance. Thyroxin itself was isolated by Kendall in 1915, and its synthesis was accomplished by Harington and Barger in 1927. In 1953, the important discovery of 3,5,3′triiodothyronine was made by Gross and Pitt-Rivers and by Roche, Lissitsky, and Michel almost simultaneously. This compound proved to be more potent in a variety of its effects than thyroxin itself.

Of particular importance to safe thyroid surgery was the advent of effective antithyroid drugs. Thiouracil was introduced in 1943 by the MacKenzies and Astwood et al. while several other groups of investigators were contributing information in the same field. The discovery of additional and improved antithyroid drugs made possible preoperative control of hyperthyroidism. With these drugs, safe surgical control of thyrotoxicosis became a reality, and this advance removed the remaining acute threat inherent in the surgery of the thyroid gland.

ANATOMY

Embryologically, the thyroid appears about the third week, when the embryo is only 3.5 to 4.0 mm. in

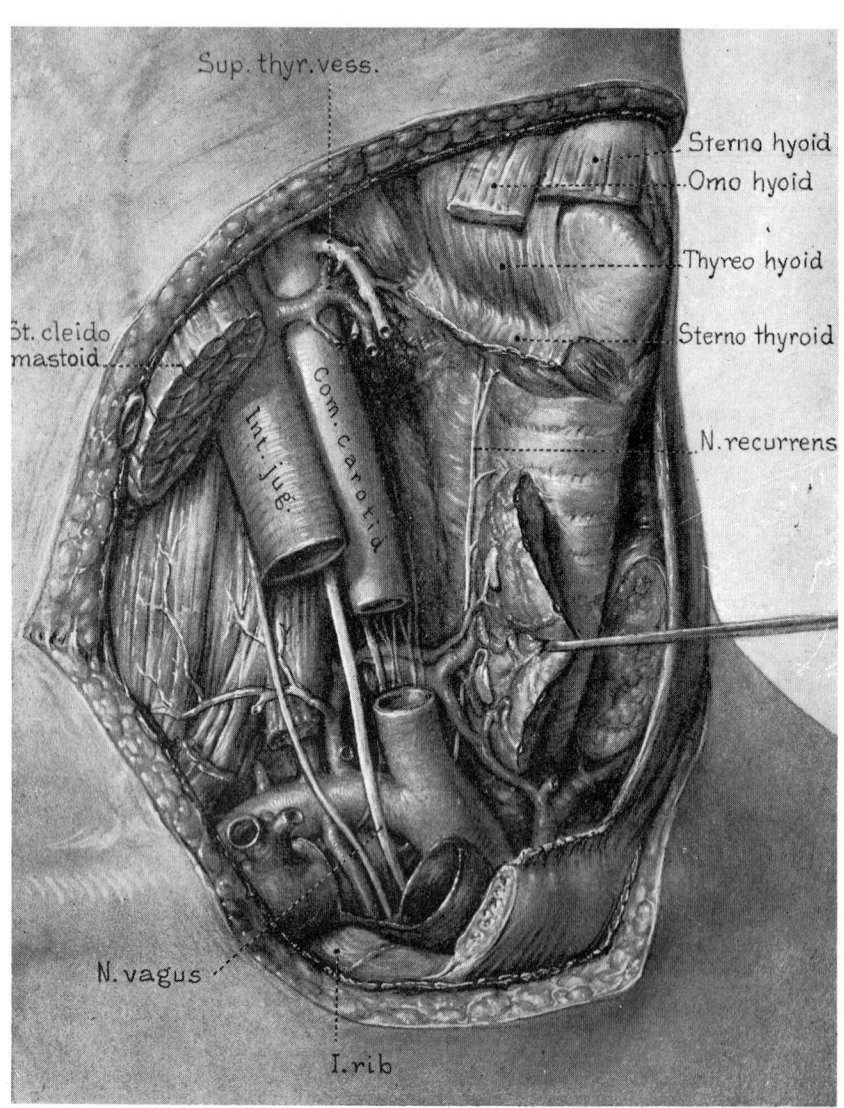

Figure 1. Dissection showing anatomic structures of the neck, especially those in the region of the thyroid gland. The nerve to the left of the vagus is the phrenic. Note location of parathyroid glands and recurrent laryngeal nerve. The amount of thyroid gland on the right side of the trachea is about twice the amount that is left after subtotal thyroidectomy. (Drawings from dissections made by Mr. Max Brödel for Dr. W. S. Halsted; from Rienhoff, W. F., Jr.: Diseases of the Thyroid Gland and Parathyroid Glands. Monographs from Volume VI, Lewis' Practice of Surgery. Hagerstown, Md., W. F. Prior Company, 1953.)

length. It begins as a proliferation of epithelial cells in the floor of the developing pharynx at a point indicated by the foramen cecum, a dimple-like depression at the base of the tongue. As the thyroid primordium descends, it acquires mesodermal contributions such as the parafollicular C cells, which will ultimately secrete calcitonin. The thyroid then emerges as a bilobed diverticulum connected to the pharynx by the thyroglossal duct, which eventually becomes obliterated in most cases. With further descent, the thyroid eventually reaches its definitive location in front of the hyoid bone and the laryngeal cartilages and assumes its fully developed configuration of two lateral lobes usually joined by a median isthmus. At the end of the third month of fetal development, follicles containing colloid become visible, and it is probable that the gland begins to release thyroid hormone at this time.

The normal thyroid weighs about 20 gm. and is attached to the anterior and lateral aspects of the trachea by loose connective tissue. The isthmus joins the two lobes, and its upper margin lies just below the cricoid cartilage. The two thyroid lobes are found along the lower half of the lateral margins of the thyroid cartilage. The thyroid is surrounded by a thin, fibrous capsule that penetrates the gland, forming pseudolobules.

The *blood supply* of the thyroid is primarily through the *inferior thyroid artery,* a branch of the subclavian, and the *superior thyroid artery,* arising from the external carotid (Fig. 1). The *thyroidea ima* artery may also be present, varying in size from a minute vessel to one the size of the inferior thyroid and arising from either the innominate artery or the aortic arch and coursing upward anterior to the trachea to the inferior border of the thyroid. The excellent blood flow of the thyroid, presumably related to its endocrine function, is in the

range of 4 to 6 ml. per gram per minute, or approximately 50 times as much blood per gram as in the body as a whole.

The *microscopic* appearance of the thyroid shows numerous follicles (acini) filled with proteinaceous colloid. The wall of the acinus is composed of a single layer of cuboidal cells resting on a basement membrane that is richly supplied with capillaries. The acini are arranged in subunits of 20 to 40, which are demarcated by connective tissue to form lobules, each supplied by an individual artery. The height of the epithelial cells lining the follicles varies with the state of functional activity but normally is about 15 μ. The size of the follicles also varies but approximates 200 μ. in diameter. In any microscopic slide, the follicles vary widely in size since they are cut at different planes in the section.

Migration of thyroid tissue into the anterior *mediastinum* is frequent. Substernal goiter may develop in this location and often is continuous with the cervical thyroid. Rarely, posterior mediastinal thyroid tissue is found, and from it may arise large goiters of the posterior mediastinum that are usually not continuous with the cervical thyroid gland.

Occasionally, fully developed children or adults may have a *sublingual thyroid* that represents the only thyroid tissue and can be confirmed by iodine-131 scan. Thus, a knowledge of the developmental anatomy of the thyroid is helpful in alerting the surgeon to hazards otherwise inherent in this condition. Total removal of such a sublingual thyroid would be disastrous if the surgeon were not aware that it represented all of the thyroid tissue present. Such a patient would require permanent thyroid hormone replacement.

For references, see page 692.

II _____

PHYSIOLOGY

Timothy S. Harrison, M.D.

The primary function of the thyroid is the production of sufficient thyroid hormone for appropriate regulation of cellular metabolism throughout the body. The formation of normal amounts of these substances and the synthesis of the specific protein—thyroglobulin—that serves as a matrix in which thyroid hormones are formed and stored are dependent upon the availability of adequate quantities of exogenous iodine. In the normal American diet, about 200 μg. of iodine is ingested daily, and in the steady state approximately 150 μg. is excreted in the urine each 24

hours. The normal pathways of iodine metabolism are shown in Figure 1.

Thyroid-Stimulating Hormone. Thyroid-stimulating hormone (TSH, thyrotropin) is the major regulator of both the anatomic and physiologic status of the thyroid. It is a protein secreted by the adenohypophysis and has a molecular weight of approximately 25,000. The production of TSH seems to be clearly related to a thyrotropin-releasing factor (TRF), which has been obtained from the brain, except the cerebellum, and particularly from the hypothalamus of a

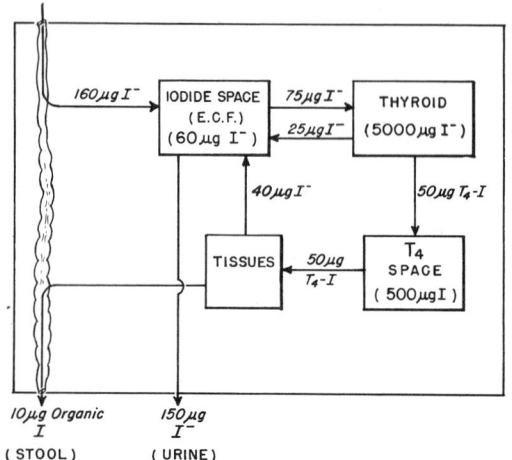

Figure 1. Schema depicting normal pathways of iodine metabolism in a state of iodine balance. Note that the major proportion (approximately 90 per cent) of body iodine stores is present in the thyroid (predominantly in the organic form). Approximately 10 per cent is present as iodide. Arrows indicate daily flux of iodine from one compartment to another. In this example, one third of the iodide entering the iodide space (75/225) is accumulated by the thyroid. Peak thyroidal uptake of ^{131}I should be 33 per cent. The rate of turnover of T_4-iodine peripherally would be 10 per cent per day. (From Ingbar, S. H., and Woeber, K. A. *In* Williams, R. H. (Ed.): Textbook of Endocrinology, 5th ed. Philadelphia, W. B. Saunders Company, 1974.)

Both T_3 and T_4 are bound to plasma proteins in the blood. The body metabolism correlates most closely with the concentration of free hormone, since the total concentration represents the large fraction that is also attached to plasma proteins. It is interesting that the amount of triiodothyronine (T_3) that is unbound is normally about 10 times that of T_4, and T_3 is removed from the blood more rapidly. Peripheral (extrathyroidal) conversion of T_4 to T_3 also takes place physiologically, suggesting that T_3 is a specific stimulus for certain thyroid hormone effects. Circulating thyroxine exists in free and bound (to thyroid-binding globulin, TBG) forms, whereas circulating T_3 is less bound and thus more labile. The major steps in the biosynthesis of thyroid hormone are depicted in Figure 3.

Thyroglobulin. Thyroglobulin is an iodized glycoprotein with a molecular weight of about 660,000. It represents the storage form of thyroxin. Present in the follicles, it does not normally appear in the circulation but is hydrolyzed as necessary by a mixture of cathepsins, yielding iodinated amino acids, especially 3,5,3'-triiodothyronine (T_3) and 3,5,3',5'-tetraiodothyronine (thyroxin, T_4), the active thyroid hormones. The structure of the more important thyroid components is shown in Figure 4.

Thyroid Hormone Release

Given the unique capacity of the thyroid gland to concentrate iodine selectively from the blood and to utilize it in the biosynthesis of thyroxin and triiodothyronine, it is the circumstances controlling the release of thyroid hormone that are particularly fascinating to students of thyroid disease. Receptor cells in the an-

number of species, including man. TRF causes an increased production of thyroid hormone, but only if the pituitary is intact; therefore, the increase in thyroxin production is assumed to be the result of TSH stimulation. The normal secretion rate of TSH is estimated to be about 125 mμg. per day, with about half of euthyroid persons showing measurable amounts in the blood. Evidence suggests that the hormone is degraded in the kidney, with little excretion in the urine. Removal of TSH produces hypovascularity and atrophy of the thyroid, with diminished production of thyroxin. When secreted in normal amounts, TSH causes thyroxin to be produced in appropriate quantities for normal body metabolism. The pathways of TSH production and its effects are shown diagrammatically in Figure 2.

Thyroxin and Triiodothyronine. Within the thyroid gland, iodide is oxidized to a higher-valence form that is highly reactive and exists only temporarily to combine immediately with tyrosyl groups of intrathyroid proteins to form monoiodotyrosine (MIT) and diiodotyrosine (DIT). These compounds then yield a variety of iodothyronines, including 3,5,3'-triiodothyronine (T_3) and thyroxin (T_4). T_4 and T_3 are the primary hormonally active compounds secreted by the thyroid gland and in combination with thyroglobulin are stored in the thyroid acini. Thyroglobulin does not normally enter the circulation, and its products are hydrolyzed by proteases and peptidases. Neither MIT nor DIT enters the blood, since the action of an iodotyrosine deiodinase removes their iodide.

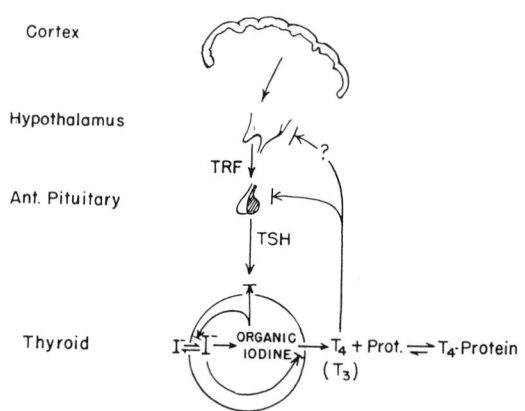

Figure 2. Schema of the homeostatic regulation of thyroid function. Secretion of TSH is regulated by a negative feedback mechanism acting directly on the pituitary and is normally inversely related to the concentration of unbound hormone in the blood. Release of TSH is induced by the thyrotropin-releasing factor (TRF), secretion of which appears to set the level of pituitary feedback mechanism. Factors regulating secretion of TRF are uncertain, but may include the free hormone in the blood and stimuli from higher centers. Autoregulatory control of thyroid function is also shown. High concentrations of intrathyroidal iodide decrease the rate of release of thyroidal iodine. In addition, the magnitude of the organic iodine pool inversely influences the iodide transport mechanism and the response to TSH. (From Ingbar, S. H., and Woeber, K. A. *In* Williams, R. H. (Ed.): Textbook of Endocrinology, 5th ed. Philadelphia, W. B. Saunders Company, 1974.)

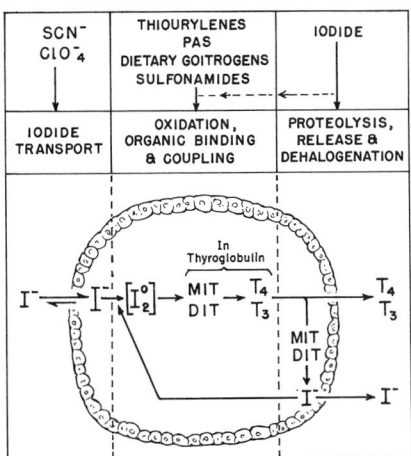

Figure 3. Schema of the major steps in thyroid hormone biosynthesis. In this schema, the follicular outline is intended merely to differentiate the intrathyroidal from the interstitial compartment and should not be construed as indicating that the reactions shown necessarily occur in the follicular lumen. Note that the concentration of intrathyroidal iodide maintained by the iodide transport mechanism is greater than that in the extracellular fluid. The processes of iodide oxidation, organic binding, and coupling of iodotyrosines are grouped together, since they appear to be closely related oxidative reactions. The precise proportions of the iodide liberated from iodotyrosines by dehalogenation that are reutilized or released into the extracellular fluid are unknown. Shown above are the major inhibitors of the several steps in hormonal biosynthesis. As indicated by the dashed line, large quantities of iodide inhibit organic binding and coupling, but this effect is usually transient. (From Ingbar, S. H., and Woebar, K. A. In Williams, R. H. (Ed.): Textbook of Endocrinology, 5th ed. Philadelphia, W. B. Saunders Company, 1974.)

hypothalamic nuclei. Very likely these receptors are involved in a feedback control of the release of a hypothalamic releasing factor, which when transported to the anterior pituitary by the hypophyseal portal system influences the "setting" of the pituitary feedback system for the release of thyrotropic hormone and consequently of thyroid hormone. A variety of central nervous system stimuli of thyroid hormone secretion are thought to act by effecting release of thyrotropin-releasing factor. There is cogent experimental evidence that psychic factors[15] and electrical stimulation of discrete hypothalamic locations[10] stimulate thyroid hormone secretion, and no doubt other stimuli will be described as more sophisticated insight into basic neurophysiologic possibilities is attained. When such central nervous system stimuli coexist with the pituitary feedback control, the central nervous system stimuli to thyroid secretion will supervene. This knowledge is of fundamental importance in understanding the distorted hypersecretion in thyrotoxicosis, to which subsequent reference will be made. It is most logical to believe that, in general, central nervous system effects on thyroid function are mediated through the hypothalamic thyrotropin-releasing factor. This probably occurs by increasing the "set point," beneath which low thyroid hormone levels stimulate the release of pituitary thyrotropin.

An important realization is that thyroid hormone is released much more quickly in response to thyroid-

terior lobe of the pituitary and hypothalamus are exquisitely sensitive to changes in the concentration of thyroid hormone in the circulating blood. When thyroid hormone levels fall, the pituitary releases into the circulation increased quantities of thyroid-stimulating hormone (TSH), which stimulates the release of sufficient thyroid hormone to restore normal levels of plasma thyroid hormone. The converse of this situation is also true; that is, if excessive circulating thyroid hormone reaches the pituitary gland, the release of thyrotropin and consequently of thyroid hormone is markedly decreased, with gradual restoration of normal plasma levels of thyroid hormone. This is the essence of the pituitary feedback control of thyroid hormone secretion. One of the many experimental methods that have been used to elucidate these features has been inhibition of radioiodine release from the neck after microinjections of thyroxin directly into the anterior lobe of the pituitary gland. The same minute quantities of thyroxin have no effect when injected peripherally.

From a succession of brilliant investigative discoveries in Sweden, the United States, and Britain, it is now clear that receptor cells sensitive to changes in circulating thyroid hormone concentration exist not only in the pituitary but also in some of the anterior

THYROID HORMONES AND RELATED COMPOUNDS

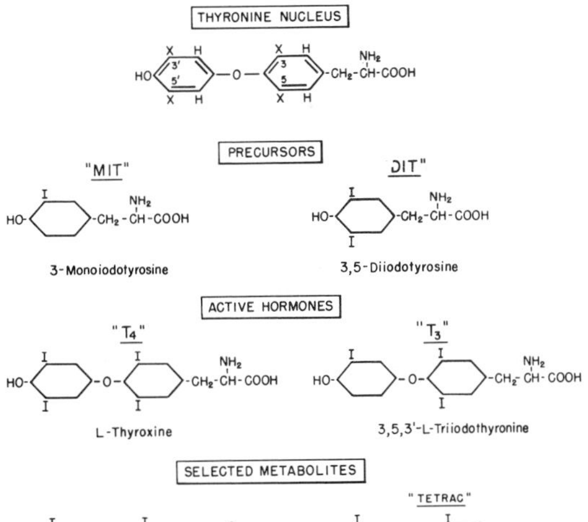

Figure 4. Structural formulas of thyroid hormones and related compounds. The structure of the thyronine nucleus of the hormonally active iodinated amino acids, T3 and T4, is shown above. Iodinated thyronines are formed through the oxidative coupling of the precursor iodotyrosines, MIT and DIT, in varying combination. 3,5,3'-Triiodothyropyruvic acid is derived by oxidative deamination from T₃. "Tetrac" is derived from T₄ by oxidative deamination followed by decarboxylation. (From Ingbar, S. H., and Woeber, K. A. In Williams, R. H. (Ed.): Textbook of Endocrinology, 5th ed. Philadelphia, W. B. Saunders Company, 1974.)

stimulating hormone than was originally thought.[23] These so-called "short-term" reactions of the thyroid were demonstrated as technical refinements permitting their measurement were developed. Formerly, a conventional method of measuring thyroid secretion experimentally was the determination of release rates of radioactivity from the necks of animals of a variety of species whose thyroids had trapped administered radioiodine. These semilogarithmic release curves have been invaluable in unfolding much of what is known about thyroid physiology, and they rest on extremely sound experimental evidence evolved principally by the late Geoffrey Harris and his colleagues at Oxford. Nevertheless, such release curves suffer from a time resolution of at least 30 minutes under the best circumstances, and generally of 1 hour. Thus, it was not that the thyroid gland was sluggish in its response, but that the only techniques available for defining the events of thyroid secretion were slow to respond. When methods were devised that counted radioactivity in every consecutive drop of the total thyroid venous effluent, it soon became apparent that thyroid response can occur in a matter of a few seconds. Whenever such delicate measurements can be applied, other endocrine glands are being found to be capable of similar speed of response.

One controversial physiologic point clarified by the study of short-term thyroid reactions is the effect of epinephrine on thyroid secretion. For many years it was held, on the basis of inadequate evidence, that epinephrine stimulated secretion of thyroid hormone. Indeed, currently published authoritative texts on the thyroid continue to make this assertion. With the information now available, it is clear that although the thyroid vasculature is uniquely sensitive to epinephrine, the actual release of radioiodine from the thyroid proceeds quite *independently* of the epinephrine effect except for an evanescent on and off burst when epinephrine administration is commenced and finished. This burst is a statistically and functionally inconsequential fragment of the total radioactivity released from the thyroid in these conditions.

TESTS OF THYROID FUNCTION

The variety of tests that provide objective evidence of the status of thyroid function is increasing constantly. It is generally agreed that no single procedure consistently yields a reliable basis for a diagnosis, and therefore a combination of the various tests is generally indicated. Most frequently, the tests combine to provide a correct overall assessment of thyroid function.

Basal Metabolic Rate (BMR)

It has long been recognized that hyperfunction of the thyroid gland is associated with an increase in oxygen consumption. With this increase in basal metabolism, a corresponding increase in energy expenditure occurs, with resultant heat production. Clinically, this is reflected by weight loss and is associated with an increased intake of calories to provide the additional energy. Since the direct measurement of heat loss

from the body is difficult, it is usually assessed indirectly by measuring the oxygen consumption. Under truly *basal* conditions, the amount of oxygen utilized is relatively constant. The energy equivalent of a liter of oxygen is 4.83 Calories, or equal to a respiratory quotient of 0.82. Basal oxygen consumption is slightly higher in males than in females; it declines rapidly from infancy to the third decade, with a slower decline thereafter; and the BMR is related to body surface area. Each of these factors must be considered in determination of the final value. The results are expressed as a percentage difference from predicted normal values, and the BMR is generally between −10 per cent and +10 per cent in healthy subjects. Emphasis should be placed upon the fact that a series of disorders can alter the BMR, including fever, neoplastic disease, hypertension, diabetes, heart failure, and pulmonary insufficiency, as can the presence of drugs. Body heating of large amounts of ingested or intravenously administered fluid, as in diabetes insipidus, will also raise the BMR.

Thyroid Uptake of Iodine-131

This test is very commonly employed in assessment of thyroid function. Following oral ingestion of ^{131}I, the maximal uptake is near its peak at 24 hours. A dose of 2 to 15 µg. of ^{131}I is usually given orally, and the thyroidal content of ^{131}I is determined with a suitable detector. The normal value was approximately 30 per cent (range, 15 to 45 per cent) in 24 hours but in recent years has been a little lower.

Circulating Thyroxine and Triiodothyronine

The most useful index of thyroid function now available is the direct measurement of circulating thyroid hormones (thyroxine [T_4] — normal range, 4.6 to 11.5 µg per 100 ml. and triiodothyronine [T_3] — normal

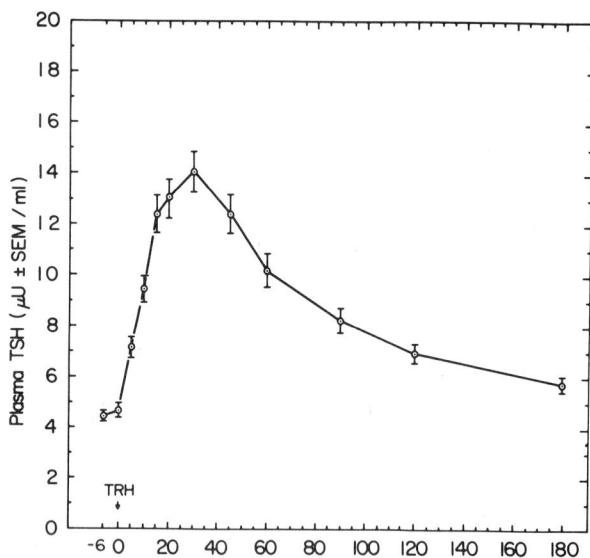

Figure 5. The plasma TSH response in man following the administration of synthetic TRF (thyrotropin releasing factor). This is a convenient test for pituitary TSH responsiveness. (From Anderson, M. S., and Bowers, C. Y.: N. Engl. J. Med., *285*:1279, 1971.)

range, 80 to 220 μg. per 100 ml.). Both can be measured most specifically and easily by radioimmunoassay, but in many centers the use of a T_3 resin binding test is still employed as an indirect measurement of circulating thyroid hormone.

Resin Triiodothyronine Uptake (Resin-T₃)

This test measures the competitive binding for radioactive T_3 between serum thyroxin-binding globulin (TBG) and a resin. The radioactive T_3 added to the system will be bound preferentially by the resin if the thyroid hormone binding sites on TBG are saturated with endogenous T_3 and T_4, and the T_3 "uptake" by the resin will be high. The resin uptake of T_3 is directly proportional to the fraction of free T_4 in the serum and inversely related to the TBG binding sites. The uptake is high in thyrotoxicosis and low in hypothyroid states. The test serves as an indirect measurement of the unbound fraction of T_4 and is valuable since it is simpler to perform than other measurements of T_4.

Thyroid Releasing Factor (TRF) Stimulation Test

Administration of TRF will, in man and other species, cause a release of thyrotropin (TSH) from the pituitary with an associated increase in circulating TSH levels.[2] This is an excellent test of pituitary thyrotropin reserve and is especially valuable in defining pituitary failure as a cause of hypothyroidism.

Thyroid Suppression Test

This test evaluates the integrity of the pituitary-thyroid axis. It is based upon the principle that the administration of thyroid hormone will not suppress the patient's thyroid function when normal homeostatic mechanisms are disrupted. After an initial radioactive iodine uptake test, triiodothyronine is administered in a dose of 100 μg. daily for 7 days. The radioactive iodine uptake test is then repeated, and if the radioactive iodine uptake is less than 20 per cent, this provides good evidence that thyrotropin suppression is present. Values above 20 per cent in 24 hours indicate a disturbance of homeostatic control, which might be present in hyperthyroidism or occur in the presence of thyroid neoplasms. Care should be taken not to administer this test to persons in whom excessive metabolic activity induced by the test would lead to complications, including patients with cardiac conditions or vascular disease.

Thyrotropin Stimulation Test

This test is employed to differentiate primary thyroidal failure from thyroid hypofunction as a result of inadequate TSH stimulation. If an increase in radioactive iodine uptake of 10 per cent or more, or a rise in thyroxine of at least 2 μg. per 100 ml., can be demonstrated, then it is likely that the thyroid can respond to exogenous TSH stimulation. Thyrotropin is given in a dose of 5 to 10 units intramuscularly to assess primary thyroid insufficiency or diminished

TABLE 1. Classification of Hypothyroidism by Level of Lesion

	Hypothalamus	Pituitary (primary)	Thyroid
Serum TSH	low	low	high
Serum TSH after TRH:	increase	no response	exaggerated increase
Thyroid response* to exog. TSH:	increase	increase	no response

*In thyroid radioiodine uptake and serum thyroxine.

thyroid reserve. Increased amounts of TSH may be necessary in the presence of pituitary failure.

Using TSH determinations at rest and after TRH (thyrotropin-releasing factor) stimulation, coupled with a dependable index of thyroid hormone release following TSH administration, it is possible to define the site of the lesion in hypothyroidism. Table 1 shows findings to be expected in each form of hypothyroidism.

Serum Cholesterol Determination

Although the serum cholesterol level is known to vary widely in both normal and diseased states, the value is usually elevated in patients with hypothyroidism and certainly in those with frank myxedema. In most patients with primary myxedema, the serum cholesterol is definitely increased. Moreover, serial measurements of serum cholesterol values are of help in following the progress of patients treated for hypothyroidism.

Thyroid Biopsy

Not infrequently, biopsy of the thyroid gland is indicated in order to establish a firm pathologic diagnosis. Both needle and open biopsy techniques may be employed. Open biopsy is the superior biopsy and needle biopsy is the simpler. Needle biopsy has been criticized as a technique when neoplastic disease is suspected. Some have found needle biopsy useful in the diagnosis of Hashimoto's disease. Biopsy can establish a diagnosis of benign and malignant tumors, chronic thyroiditis, nodular goiter, and hyperthyroidism.

Other Tests

In addition to the tests mentioned here, there are a variety of other tests that evaluate thyroid function, including measurements of thyroid iodide clearance rates, absolute iodine uptake, and the urinary excretion of radioiodine[131] for the use of which there are special indications. Determination of thyroid antibodies is of particular interest in thyroiditis and in Graves' disease.

For references, see page 692.

III

HYPERTHYROIDISM

Timothy S. Harrison, M.D.

In the strictest possible sense, hyperthyroidism develops when thyroid hormone secretion rates are stimulated to exceed normal, and the thyroid-pituitary feedback system is already maximally suppressed. Increasing the pituitary threshold for thyroid hormone suppression is the probable basic mechanism underlying many forms of hyperthyroidism, although this can be a difficult point to substantiate. Only the sustained varieties of hyperthyroidism require surgical treatment.

THYROTOXICOSIS (GRAVES' DISEASE, EXOPHTHALMIC GOITER)

Thyrotoxicosis has been known since its original description by Parry in 1786, with later additions by Graves in 1835 and von Basedow in 1840. It is usually not difficult to make the diagnosis of thyrotoxicosis. The classic history of irritability, weight loss, heat intolerance, and emotional instability is usually striking, especially when coupled with the presence of a goiter, exophthalmos, and other eye signs. A host of laboratory examinations are now available to confirm the diagnosis. Basal metabolic rate, serum protein-bound iodine, thyroidal radioiodine uptake, triiodothyronine red cell binding capacity, serum thyroxin (T_4), serum triiodothyronine (T_3), and plasma levels of thyrotropin can be helpful. No single laboratory test is consistently superior to all the others. Furthermore, occasionally a test may yield results in the diagnostic range in one thyrotoxic patient, and at the upper limit of normal in another. Thus, if a patient's T_3 is clearly elevated, this test may be the cheapest and most straightforward laboratory substantiation of the diagnosis. However, as not infrequently happens, if the T_3 and T_4 are at the upper limit of normal, and a 24- and 48-hour uptake of a trace amount of radioiodine is in the diagnostic range for hyperthyroidism, then clearly radioiodine uptake is the better test for both diagnosis and evaluation of the patient's response to treatment. If for some reason a patient has been taking appreciable amounts of stable iodine, either in the diet or by medication, PBI levels will not reflect thyroid hormone secretion rates accurately. The PBI may, in these circumstances, be capriciously high and the radioiodine uptake low. In this instance, triiodothyronine binding capacity or serum thyroxin and triiodothyronine determination would be more apt than either protein-bound iodine or radioiodine uptake. Thus, of the available tests, one or two of these especially suited to the individual patient's situation should be selected as the most direct laboratory confirmation of the disease.

Graves' classic article, describing six patients, all of whom were recently pregnant women, can easily be found in most medical libraries. In it he mentions that in one patient "the emotional disturbance preceded the onset of the tachycardia by several weeks." This observation is of great interest because the emotional disturbance stimulating the occurrence of thyrotoxicosis is quite different from that resulting from the excessive thyroid hormone of established hyperthyroidism. Students of the thyrotoxicosis, beginning with Parry, who originally described the disease, have consistently been impressed by the emotional background of thyrotoxicosis. Many excellent descriptions of the emotional patterns surrounding hyperthyroidism exist.[15] It is well known that during times of stress, such as the World War II air attacks on London, the incidence of thyrotoxicosis rises sharply. Physicians in European countries hard pressed by the war, Yugoslavia for example, noted the same phenomenon.

For several reasons, the precise cause-and-effect relationship between what is broadly characterized as emotional disturbance and thyrotoxicosis is not always easy to establish. Susceptibility to the development of thyrotoxicosis in response to emotional upheaval appears to vary rather widely. It has not been possible to predict such susceptibility, but there is little doubt that thyrotoxicosis does not develop in the majority of persons who experience emotional upheavals pronounced enough to produce thyrotoxicosis in susceptible persons. It has been emphasized previously that one should not confuse the anxiety, irritability, tremulousness, and lability of temperament secondary to the presence of excessive thyroid hormone with the emotional background preceding the development of thyrotoxicosis. The more subtle emotional reactions to sudden fright, acute grief, or other psychically disturbing events preceding thyrotoxicosis are apt to be "bottled up" by the patient and less obvious than the behavioral results of excessive thyroid hormone.

Several important considerations arise in the management of hyperthyroidism and in acquainting patients with their disease. A logical question is, for example, Why not control the hyperthyroidism with antithyroid drugs and allow the central nervous system stimulation of pathologically high thyroid secretion rates to subside? Another question is, Why not keep a patient on antithyroid drugs forever? The most limiting feature of extended use of the antithyroid drugs is the occasional development (in about 1 in 200 patients) of irreversible agranulocytosis. The smooth control of thyrotoxicosis by antithyroid drugs is admirable, and short-term trials with the antithyroid drugs should be used. However, these agents succeed in inducing a *permanent remission* of Graves' disease in only a small minority of adults and in about 20 per cent of children. Thus, it appears to be a difficult matter to stop the augmented secretion of thyroid hormone in hyperthyroidism once the mechanism has been stimulated by the central nervous system.

Insights into the pathophysiology of thyrotoxicosis

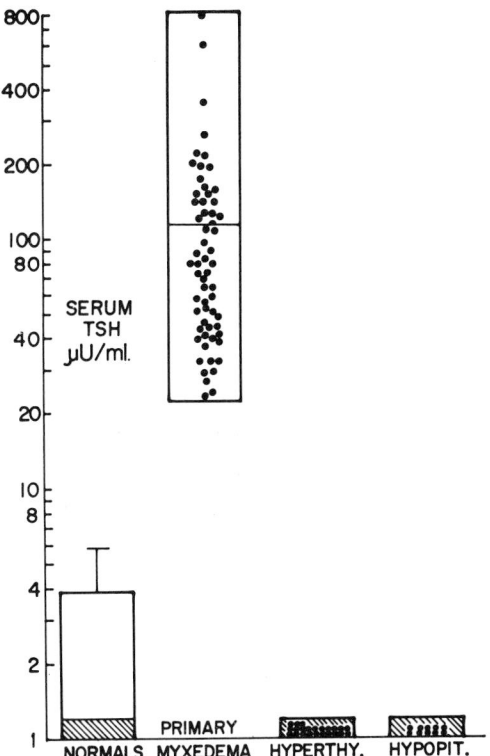

Figure 1. Serum thyrotropin (TSH) levels are shown in various types of thyroid disorder. Note that in myxedema the levels are high, indicating an attempt by the pituitary to stimulate thyroids incapable of responding. Of added interest are the suppressed levels seen in hyperthyroidism. These indicate a resetting upwards of the thyroid hormone level effective in stimulating pituitary TSH release or some independent stimulus to the thyroid in hyperthyroidism. (From Heashman, J. M., and Pittman, J. A., Jr.: Ann. Intern. Med., 74:481, 1971.)

are now accumulating at a rapid rate. In part, this is due to the availability of radioimmunoassay analytical techniques for measuring circulating pituitary thyrotropic hormone. This technique has permitted the identification of thyrotropin-secreting pituitary chromophobe adenomas.[9]

Of great pathophysiologic interest has been the discovery of a long-acting thyroid-stimulating substance (LATS) in the serum of about 60 per cent of patients with thyrotoxicosis. This substance now appears to be a globulin, immune in origin, and possibly a modified form of the parent thyrotropin molecule. It does not appear to be an abnormal thyroid-stimulating hormone of pituitary or central nervous system origin.[19] Recently a number of other immune globulins that stimulate thyroid secretion have been found in the serum of thyrotoxic patients. This increases the suspicion that these immune globulins are implicated in the pathogenesis of thyrotoxicosis.

MANAGEMENT

The *management* of hyperthyroidism can be approached in several different ways. The thyroid hyper-

secretion of thyrotoxicosis can be controlled by antithyroid drugs, by destruction of most of the thyroid gland with radioiodine, or by surgical removal of a large part of the gland. Each method causes a reduction of the net secretion rate of thyroid hormone to euthyroid levels. It is curious that each of these treatments is reasonably effective, and it is interesting that recurrences of hyperthyroidism are not more frequent than they actually are. Selective *block* of central nervous stimulation of excessive thyroid secretion, allowing the thyroid-pituitary feedback system to monitor a consistently euthyroid condition, would be the definitive treatment, and it may be possible in the future. Until that time, it behooves all physicians to recognize the potential benefits and hazards inherent in drug therapy as well as in radioiodine and surgical treatment of hyperthyroidism. With appropriate data, the physician is in the best possible position to achieve agreement with the patient on which treatment is the best choice.

Antithyroid Drugs

Some patients with hyperthyroidism can be managed with antithyroid drugs. The majority of these agents produce their effect by interference with the organic binding of iodine by the thyroid and by prevention of coupling of iodotyrosines in the thyroid gland. The primary agents employed are propylthiouracil, methimazole (Tapazole), methylthiouracil, and carbimazole (Neo-mercazole). Of these, propylthiouracil and Tapazole are the most commonly used. They are thought to be degraded relatively rapidly, primarily in the thyroid gland, and then excreted, thereby requiring administration at relatively frequent intervals to maintain an effective concentration. It is of interest that these compounds are excreted in breast milk; they are also capable of crossing the placenta and can thereby inhibit fetal thyroid function. A standard dose of propylthiouracil is 100 mg. orally three times daily, although smaller or larger doses may be required, depending upon the clinical situation. Generally, clinical improvement begins within 2 weeks after administration of the drug, and restoration of a normal metabolic rate is often accomplished within 6 weeks. When the metabolism returns to normal, the dosage can frequently be reduced.

In the long-term use of antithyroid drugs, the question of the time necessary to control the syndrome arises. It is to be remembered that there is no evidence that antithyroid drugs affect the *basic* pathogenesis of thyrotoxicosis. Moreover, the natural history of diffuse toxic goiter is usually one of remission and exacerbation. Therefore, withdrawal of therapy may be followed by quiescence if the patient is already in a remission. Contrariwise, the hyperthyroidism may return if the basic mechanisms producing the disease are still active when the drug is withdrawn. A decrease in the size of the thyroid gland is suggestive of quiescence, and in addition, the thyroid suppression test is of assistance in determining resumption of physiologic control. Some recommend the performance of suppression tests at 6-month intervals, with cessation of drug treatment when the tests revert to normal.[13]

Recurrence of hyperthyroidism following drug withdrawal is variable, and reports in the literature indicate an incidence of up to 72 per cent.[13] Another objection to the use of antithyroid agents is the drug sensitivity that occurs. Rash and drug fever both are seen, but the most dangerous reaction is agranulocytosis (with an incidence of less than 1 per cent). Other reactions include peripheral neuritis, hepatitis, arthralgia, myalgia, lymphadenopathy, and psychoses.

Radioiodine

In the early days of the use of radioactive iodine, well-advised caution prevailed because of the recognized susceptibility of the thyroid gland to development of malignant tumors, as, for example, after cervical x-irradiation for hypertrophic lymphoid tissues such as tonsils and adenoids in adolescents. It is gratifying that thus far this has not proved to be a detraction with radioiodine treatment of the thyroid, and it now seems clear that thyroid carcinoma is no more likely to develop in radioiodine-treated patients than in patients from any randomly selected population. Reports of limited trials of radioiodine treatment for thyrotoxicosis in *children* are now beginning to appear.[12]

The problem that has caused the greatest difficulty with universal use of radioactive iodine treatment for thyrotoxicosis is the unpredictable and conspicuous development of permanent hypothyroidism. The precise incidence of this complication varies in different series, but a number of patients treated with radioactive iodine for thyrotoxicosis will be made permanently hypothyroid. One of the particularly difficult aspects of this hypothyroidism is that it may not develop until several years after treatment, at a time when the patient is no longer being followed. The symptoms of hypothyroidism in these circumstances may appear gradually, and the clinical manifestations may be so insidious that the danger that the patient will not seek medical attention has proved to be real. Nevertheless, radioactive iodine treatment of thyrotoxicosis is a simple, effective, and highly useful method for the control of this disease. Certainly in those patients too ill for surgery, radioiodine can be recommended confidently as the treatment of choice, since it consists only of swallowing the appropriate amount of iodine-131 (usually 140 to 160 μg. per gram of estimated glandular weight).[13] Because of the great ease of administering this treatment, it is hoped that the efforts to diminish post-treatment hypothyroidism will be successful. At present, the incidence of post-radioiodine hypothyroidism at 10 years is at least 40 per cent (Fig. 2), and reported figures range up to 70 per cent.[18] More accurate means of calculating the radiation delivered to the epithelial cells of the thyroid are needed so that more effective dosage regimens can be devised.

Subtotal Thyroidectomy

The fact that surgery is effective in controlling hyperthyroidism is unquestioned, and in most series the incidence of postoperative hypothyroidism in adults is under 10 per cent,[13] although it may be higher.[18] However, as with radioactive iodine treatment,

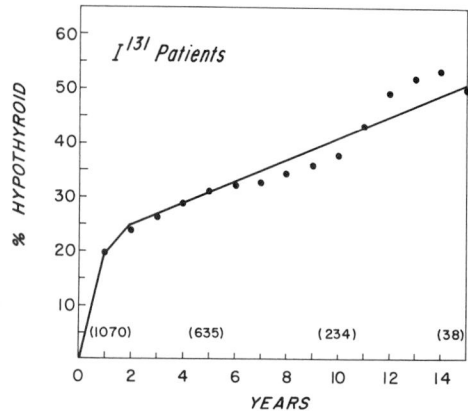

Figure 2. Onset of hypothyroidism after ^{131}I therapy in 86 patients followed for more than 10 years (only hypothyroid patients are included). The number of years between ^{131}I treatment and the diagnosis of hypothyroidism is plotted against the cumulative fraction of the 86 patients who were hypothyroid at the end of each year. (From Dunn, J. T., and Chapman, E. M.: N. Engl. J. Med., *271*:1037, 1964.)

subtotal thyroidectomy treatment of hyperthyroidism is not free of imperfections. Permanent hypoparathyroidism and damage to the laryngeal innervation rarely follow subtotal thyroidectomy. Hypothyroidism may follow surgery, but the best evidence seems to indicate that it is not as apt to occur *late* as that after radioiodine treatment. Both subtotal thyroidectomy and radioactive iodine treatment are attended by a modest risk of recurrence of hyperthyroidism. This complication is seen slightly more frequently, in about 10 per cent of cases, after subtotal thyroidectomy. In either instance, it can best be treated effectively with a therapeutic dose of radioactive iodine, since repeated surgery on the thyroid increases the risk of nerve damage.[1] Occasionally, a patient with hyperthyroidism suffers from a uniquely virulent thyrotoxicosis, and if any glandular remnant is left, may experience multiple recurrences. In this situation, total ablation of the thyroid with radioactive iodine is the safest method of control. In recurrent hyperthyroidism, serum TSH should always be measured to exclude the presence of TSH-secreting pituitary adenomas.

The *preoperative preparation* for control of hyperthyroidism is essential in the conduct of safe thyroid surgery. Treatment with propylthiouracil, or one of its derivatives, is effective, and there need be no haste in operating. The usual dosage of propylthiouracil is in the range of 100 mg. three times daily, although larger doses may be necessary, especially if *rapid* control is desired. Surgery performed too soon after control of thyrotoxicosis is associated with a risk of thyroid crisis, and it is preferable to schedule operation about 2 months after a euthyroid status has been achieved. Rarely, patients are resistant to the usual antithyroid drugs, and perchlorate or other less ideal agents may be necessary. If iodine alone is used to control the thyrotoxicosis, surgery must be scheduled before the well-known escape from iodine control occurs.

It is customary to treat controlled thyrotoxic patients with small amounts of iodide and iodine, 15 drops of Lugol's solution (a combination of potassium iodide, 10 gm. per 100 gm., and iodine, 5 gm. per 100 gm.), two or three times daily for 10 days prior to surgery to decrease the "vascularity" of the gland. Many prefer to use thyroid hormone rather than iodine. Adequate doses of thyroid hormone will suppress the TSH increase seen with propylthiouracil and will decrease the thyroid vascularity stimulated by that mechanism.

Beta Adrenergic Receptor Blockade with Propranolol. For over 70 years it has been known that several forms of sympathetic nervous system blockade will ameliorate some of the major cardiac effects of hyperthyroidism.

This awareness has led to the use of beta-adrenergic receptor blockade in thyrotoxicosis. When used alone, beta-receptor blockade will decrease the pulse rate and allay the tremor of hyperthyroidism, but oxygen consumption of these same patients is not affected. One should therefore avoid the use of propranolol for extended control of hyperthyroidism, since hypermetabolism and weight loss will continue with beta-receptor blockade.

The most important role emerging for beta blockade in hyperthyroidism is the further resolution of tachycardias that have incompletely resolved with antithyroid drugs in conventional doses. On a cost-effective basis, combined beta-receptor blockade and antithyroid drugs, or beta blockade alone, will decrease the number of preoperative visits and the length of hospital stay for patients undergoing surgery for control of hyperthyroidism. Beta-receptor blockade should not be used in patients with significant myocardial disease because it may precipitate myocardial failure.[14, 17, 20, 25]

Technique of Operation. Precise knowledge of the surgical anatomy of the thyroid is crucial to the surgeon performing thyroid surgery. The *recurrent laryngeal nerve,* the *superior laryngeal nerve,* and the *parathyroid glands* exist in such intimate proximity to the usual thyroidectomy dissection that a fastidious awareness of the fine points of the surgical anatomy is necessary if they are to be spared needless injury. The technique of subtotal thyroidectomy is depicted in Figures 3 to 5.

The *recurrent laryngeal nerve* lies adjacent to the postero-

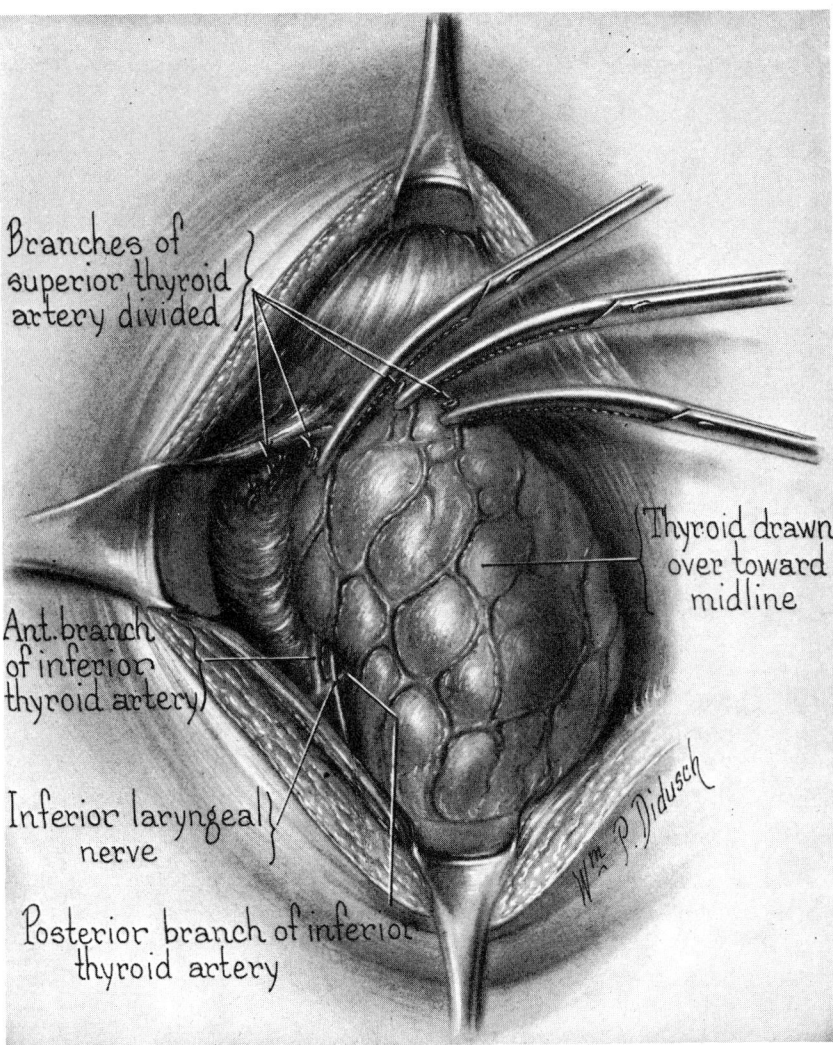

Figure 3. Dislocation of upper right pole caudalward and rotation anteriorly with ligated branch of superior thyroid artery are shown, as is relation of inferior thyroid artery to recurrent laryngeal nerve. Sentinel clamp should be placed on parenchyma of gland just above recurrent laryngeal nerve. (From Rienhoff, W. J., Jr.: Diseases of the Thyroid Gland and Parathyroid Glands. Monographs from Volume VI, Lewis' Practice of Surgery. Hagerstown, Md., W. F. Prior Company, 1953.)

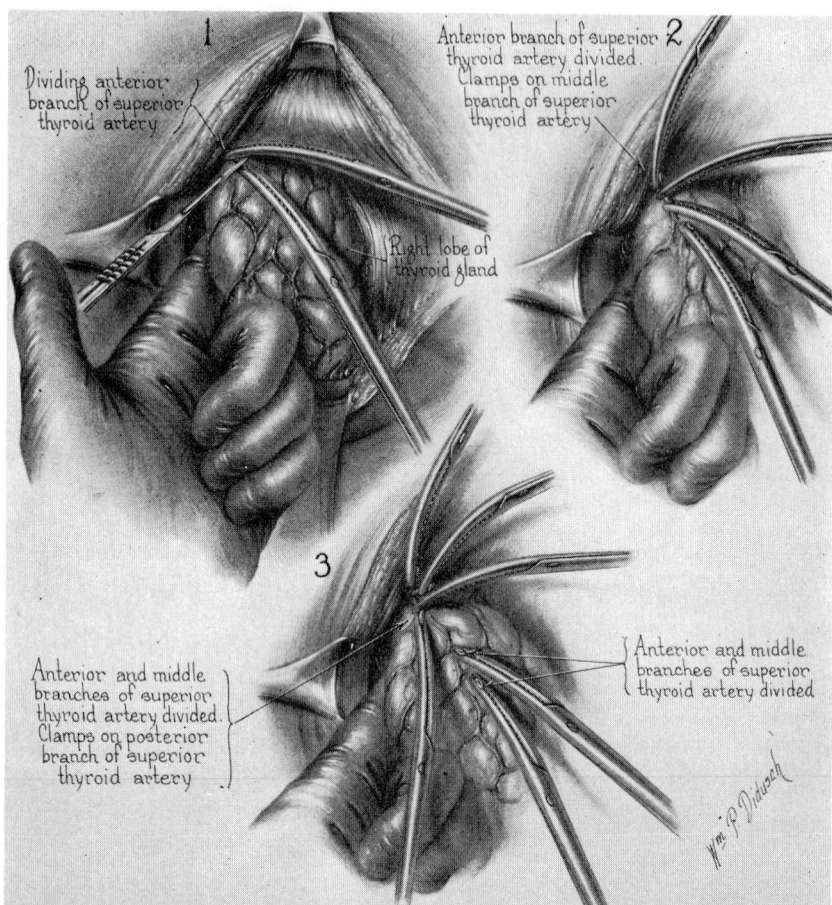

Figure 4. Evolution of superior artery from bed with ligation of branch of superior thyroid artery. The entire upper pole may thus be displaced from under the umbrella-like blood vessels without cutting across the gland parenchyma. (From Rienhoff, W. F., Jr.: Diseases of the Thyroid Gland and Parathyroid Glands. Monographs from Volume VI, Lewis' Practice of Surgery. Hagerstown, Md., W. F. Prior Company, 1953.)

Figure 5. Completely mobilized gland held in fingers of left hand of operator is resected from the midline lateralward. The amount of thyroid tissue remaining can thus be exactly determined, the actual size here shown being approximately $2 \times 2 \times 4$ cm. (From Rienhoff, W. F., Jr.: Diseases of the Thyroid Gland and Parathyroid Glands. Monographs from Volume VI, Lewis' Practice of Surgery Hagerstown, Md., W. F. Prior Company, 1953.)

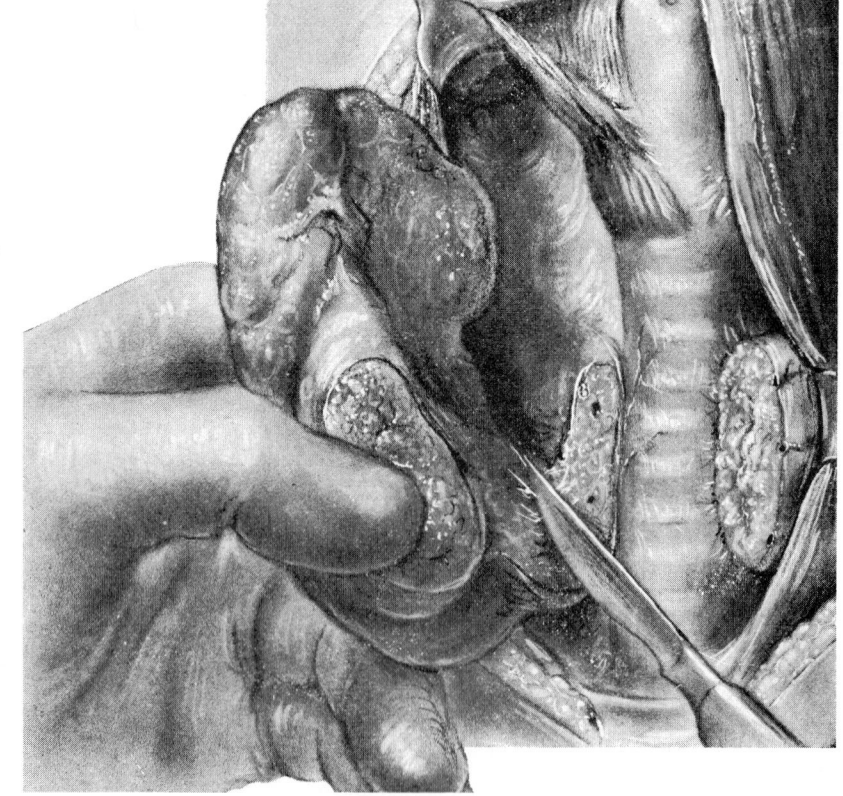

medial aspect of the thyroid near the small groove between the lateral aspects of the trachea and esophagus. This nerve contains the motor fibers innervating the abductor muscles of the true vocal cords. If conduction through the nerve is blocked by operative division or trauma, immediate hoarseness is apparent, and the voice never recovers its customary timbre and focus even though effective phonation can be achieved eventually. One of the most overlooked features of importance of the anatomy of the recurrent laryngeal nerve is that in 50 per cent of meticulous cadaver dissections the nerve is found to consist of more than a single trunk, sometimes as many as four or five, at the level of the usual thyroidectomy dissection.[22] Thus, it behooves the surgeon to avoid damaging not just one vertically oriented nerve in this anatomic location but *any* vertically oriented nerve in the region. Some authors have stressed the importance of the unexpectedly close proximity of a common bifurcation of the recurrent laryngeal nerve to the superior pole of the thyroid. The two branches are thought to innervate adductor and abductor musculature of the nerve and are far from its customary anatomic location. As noted, the hoarseness following unilateral vocal cord palsy does tend to improve with time. *Bilateral* recurrent nerve injury, with acute paralysis of both vocal cords, is a far more serious situation since the unrelieved adduction of the true vocal cords may obstruct the airway and require emergency tracheostomy. Bilateral vocal cord paralysis, fortunately extremely rare, results in permanent hoarseness of debilitating degree.

Considerable controversy has long existed concerning the advisability of *deliberate* exposure of the recurrent laryngeal nerve. Many hold the view that specific exposure of the nerve will diminish the likelihood of its injury. It is interesting that Kocher commented on this problem, and after describing the technical details of his operation said: "By following this method the recurrent laryngeal nerve can often be beautifully dissected out; but injury to it can with certainty be avoided without this direct exposure. Since we have adhered strictly to this procedure [his operation for thyroidectomy], the hoarseness, formerly so frequently observed after operation, has now become exceptional."[78] It is significant that in the current reports in the surgical literature on the best means to avoid recurrent laryngeal nerve injury Kocher's sound surgical advice has been virtually forgotten, and reference to it is rarely made. Elaborate electroneurographic devices for use at the operating table to aid the attempt to spare the nerve have been described. Others hold a strong conviction, also on the basis of extensive clinical experience, that deliberate exposure of the recurrent nerve increases the likelihood of trauma to it. Williams[48] studied 100 consecutive thyroidectomies in which the continuity of the nerve was confirmed by direct vision during surgery and normal vocal cord function confirmed by direct laryngoscopy postoperatively. He later found that in seven patients unilateral palsy of one recurrent nerve developed; in two it was irreversible. Edema following traumatic thrombosis of vasa nervorum on the surface of the nerve, followed by nerve infarction or fibrosis, is believed to be the cause of this delayed complication, and this is an argument against deliberate exposure of the nerve. Unquestionably, the recurrent laryngeal nerve will often be seen without a deliberate search for it, and just as certain is the fact that surgeons performing total thyroidectomies, regardless of the technique employed, are apt to injure the recurrent laryngeal nerve in 1 to 3 per cent of the instances in which the nerve is exposed to risk. It remains a situation in which each surgeon will find the approach that suits him best.

As important as sparing the recurrent laryngeal nerve from operative injury is the preservation of the *parathyroid glands.* Clearly, technical precision greatly decreases the incidence of permanent hypoparathyroidism. Normal parathyroid glands and their blood supply are usually recognizable in the operative field. Their brownish yellow coloration is dis-

tinctively different from that of fat which may lie adjacent to them and from that of the thyroid gland itself, and the glands are quite different in color and shape from lymph node tissue, with which they are sometimes confused. Extracapsular thyroidectomy exposes adjacent parathyroids to surgical trauma, and it is well to remember that the parathyroids are notoriously fragile and easily injured.

With these considerations in mind, it behooves the surgeon to be alert for parathyroid glands, particularly when dissecting the posterior surface of the thyroid. The inferior parathyroids are usually the more easily seen and often can be found by following the origin of their arterial supply from the inferior thyroid artery. There is less variability in the location of the superior parathyroids, which may be found posteromedial to the inferior portion of the superior pole of the thyroid gland. Usually there are four parathyroid glands, but there may be as many as seven. The inferior parathyroids originate from the third pharyngeal pouch, from which the thymus also arises, and therefore it is logical that the inferior parathyroids may migrate large distances into the anterior mediastinum, within the substance of the thymus gland or adjacent to it. While it is essential for the surgeon searching for hyperfunctioning parathyroids to realize that such glands may be far removed from the thyroid, it is little comfort to a careless surgeon to realize that such was not the case in a patient with permanent hypoparathyroidism following total thyroidectomy.

Although some embryologic purists hold that it is not possible for a parathyroid to occur in the thyroid gland itself, if one concedes that the fourth pharyngeal pouch contributes to the development of the thyroid, the possibility of an intrathyroid parathyroid must be recognized. There is no question that a straightforward, accurate total thyroid lobectomy will on rare occasion yield a thyroid lobe containing within its capsule a parathyroid gland with no discernible independent blood supply. Such parathyroids may be surrounded microscopically by thyroid tissue. This realization obviously has important implications in the surgical management of hyperparathyroidism.

The external branch of the *superior laryngeal nerve* is another structure vulnerable to surgical injury during thyroidectomy. In fact, this nerve was found in intimate proximity to the superior thyroid artery and vein in 85 per cent of cadaver dissections in which its course was followed carefully.[4] This relationship is depicted in Figure 6, where it can be seen that there is a layer of deep cervical fascia, an extension of which forms the thyroid capsule, interposed between the superior thyroid vessels and the nerve. This fascia is not dense in this portion of the neck and is not adequate protection against mass ligation of all of the structures at the superior pole of the thyroid. During this part of the thyroidectomy, individual ligation of the superior thyroid artery and vein often makes visible the superior laryngeal nerve, as the superior aspect of the thyroid is rotated from its bed. As with the recurrent laryngeal nerve, it is not essential to see the nerve in order to spare it from injury. Nevertheless, the nerve is observed in a high proportion of routine thyroid lobectomies.

The consequences of superior laryngeal nerve injury, while more subtle than those following recurrent laryngeal nerve injury, are deserving of attention. Coursing in the external branch of the superior laryngeal nerve are motor fibers to the cricothyroid muscle. It is the function of the cricothyroid muscle to maintain the tone of the true vocal cord. Thus, when the cricothyroid is paralyzed, the mobility of the vocal cord is unimpaired, unlike the situation following recurrent laryngeal nerve injury. However, with heavy or protracted use of the voice, such as operatic singing or 60 minutes of speaking, it loses its timbre and focus and becomes "tired" and less resonant. While many can compensate for such a tendency by spacing the conversational use of their voice, in some crucial situations this is not possible. In the past, many

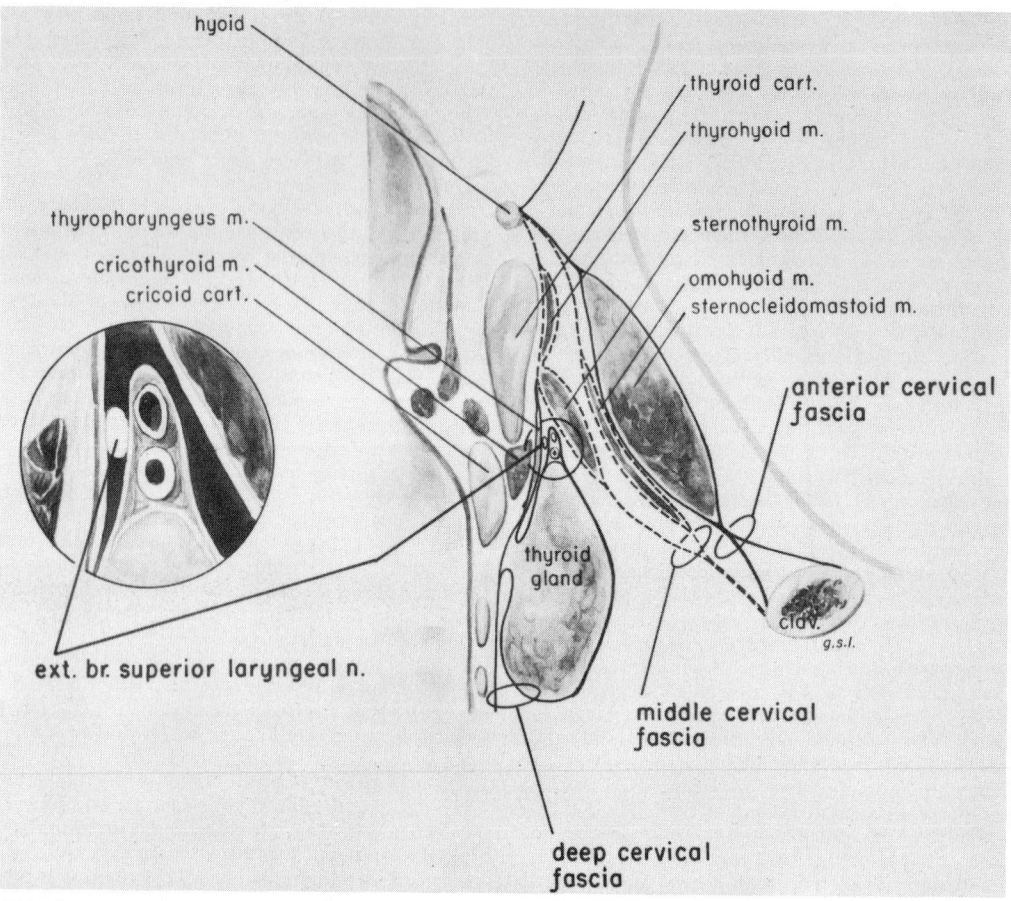

Figure 6.   This diagram represents a frontal plane of the lateral neck in the region of the thyroid gland. Depicted are the fascial relationships of the structures of the neck, and in particular the proximity of the superior thyroid artery and vein to the deep cervical fascia and to the external branch of the superior laryngeal nerve is shown. (From Durham, C. F., and Harrison, T. S.: Surg. Gynecol. Obstet., *118*:38, 1964.)

injuries to the superior laryngeal nerve have been overlooked because surgeons and patients alike have been willing to ascribe such voice fatigue and loss of timbre to tracheitis and chronic laryngitis following thyroidectomy. Instances of these latter conditions are probably quite rare, and scrupulous examination and careful history will probably reveal more cases of superior laryngeal nerve injury.

The most famous case illustrating this point is that of Amelita Galli-Curci, one of the world's great lyric sopranos of the 1920s. Airway obstruction from a large goiter threatened to ruin her operatic career, and so she underwent operation under local anesthesia for removal of the goiter. Four days after operation, in an interview in the Chicago *Tribune*, she said, "I cannot tell you how happy I am. My voice is free again, unbridled after years of struggle with the 'potato.' The result of my operation is just short of marvelous. Even now when I am not fully recovered I need hardly to open my mouth to obtain the pure tones difficult when the 'potato' was in my throat." Plans were made for Galli-Curci's return to the stage as Mimi in Puccini's *La Boheme.* Of the available accounts of the performance, that of *Time* is the most graphic: "No audience ever wanted to applaud a singer's voice more than did the 3400 who bought out the Chicago Civic Opera House last week to hear Galli-Curci sing Mimi in *La Boheme.* When the garret door opened upon Puccini's heroine, frail and pathetic in a grey ruffled gown, they shouted and clapped for a full minute. But the applause they gave her later was

less shattering and was more for her nerve than for her singing. Veterans grieved that her upper voice had crumbled, found her middle register competent but a little breathless. The passages when she caught her old fluency and full tones were too rare to give much hope . . . critics returned to their desks to write the obituaries of a great voice."

THYROID STORM

A sometimes important feature of thyrotoxicosis treated by any modality is thyroid crisis or thyroid storm. In the era before preoperative control of thyrotoxicosis was possible, thyroid storm was frequent, severe, and life-endangering and thwarted many measures directed to it. It is now a much milder phenomenon but continues to occur not only after operations for hyperthyroidism but also in patients with undiscovered hyperthyroidism and in thyrotoxic patients with active infections.

The manifestations of thyroid storm include hyperthermia, tachycardia, intense irritability, profuse sweating, hypertension, extreme anxiety, and eventual prostration, hypotension, and death, all of which are impressively adrenergic phenomena, and each of which has been produced experimentally by either epinephrine or norepinephrine administration. It is pertinent that clinical hyperthyroidism and experimentally administered thyroid hormone excess both greatly augment many actions of catecholamines.

It is thought that thyroid storm represents an acute adrenergic outburst in an organism tremendously sensitized to the effects of adrenergic amines. This is supported by the fact that through the years sympatholytic treatment has been the most effective. Reserpine and guanethidine have been used to dissipate the thyroid crisis gently and effectively.[3] Beta-adrenergic receptor blockade with propranolol will decrease the tachycardia and tremor. Oxygen should be administered, as well as liberal amounts of intravenous glucose. Intravenous use of sodium or potassium iodide (1 to 2.5 gm.) is also recommended. Large doses of adrenal steroids (cortisol or one of its analogs) have been advised and used but may be unnecessary. Rosenberg's suggestion that steroids be given when refractory hypotension develops seems apt because such hypotension may be a reflection of adrenal cortical insufficiency.[21] In this connection, it is important to remember that cortisol breakdown is accentuated by excess of thyroid hormone. In addition, there are adrenergic varieties of peripheral vasodilatation, both neurogenic and humorally mediated by peripheral beta-adrenergic receptors. Hence, hypotension resulting from circulating epinephrine may be greatly exaggerated in the circumstances of thyrotoxicosis. Hypotension in thyroid storm, therefore, is a development of concern, for which either of these mechanisms may be responsible. As such, it may be improved with sympatholytic treatment, but if not, therapeutic trial with intravenous cortisol is indicated. Vigorous antithyroid treatment to diminish thyroid hormone secretion should be used when appropriate. Fortunately, thyroid storm is much less common now than previously, and the results of treatment are improved.

HYPERTHYROIDISM IN PREGNANCY

Thyroid function tests are altered in pregnancy because of an increase in thyroid-binding globulin. For this reason, serum T_4 levels tend to be high in pregnancy. Awareness of this and measurement of both serum T_3 and basal metabolic rate are therefore most helpful in establishing the diagnosis of hyperthyroidism in the pregnant female.

Management of the pregnant hyperthyroid patient has evoked controversy. Radioiodine treatment is absolutely contraindicated because destruction of the fetal thyroid would result from its use. Antithyroid drugs in conventional doses carry a risk of fetal goiter developing, which may obstruct the airway of the newborn infant. Low-dose treatment with antithyroid drugs minimizes this risk.[7, 16] The cause-and-effect relationship of mental retardation in the newborn with antithyroid medication has been suggested but is difficult to substantiate.

In the mid trimester of pregnancy, subtotal thyroidectomy after a short course of antithyroid drugs and propranolol has been effective. So far as can be determined, the risks to mother and fetus from surgery are comparable to those of nonoperative treatment.[24]

MALIGNANT EXOPHTHALMOS

Although exophthalmos frequently occurs in hyperthyroidism, fortunately malignant exophthalmos is rare. It is a serious problem and difficult to manage. The infiltrative edema that occurs in the orbital tissues may also involve those in the periorbital region, and occasionally pretibial myxedema is an accompanying finding. Recommended forms of treatment include massive administration of prednisone, external irradiation to the orbit or pituitary gland, and surgical decompression of the orbit. Rarely, cryosurgical destruction of the pituitary may be indicated.

HYPERTHYROIDISM IN MULTINODULAR GOITER

Patients with long-standing multinodular goiter may become hyperthyroid. This form of hyperthyroidism is generally not as striking or as marked as that seen with classic Graves' disease. Exophthalmos is quite unusual. The hyperthyroidism may develop insidiously and appears to be unrelated to psychic disturbance. In such patients, treatment with radioactive iodine is highly unreliable, probably because blood flow through such goiters is not as homogeneous or symmetric as it is in the diffuse thyroid hyperplasia of thyrotoxicosis. As a consequence, the uptake of radioactive iodine by the goiter is irregular. Hence, many hyperfunctioning thyroid epithelial cells escape effective radiation and the hyperthyroidism continues. For this reason, subtotal thyroidectomy has emerged as the treatment of choice for the hyperthyroidism due to multinodular goiter. This approach has the added feature of removing a goiter that is cosmetically unappealing. The same principles guiding the preoperative preparation of the patient with diffuse toxic goiter should apply to those with multinodular goiter.

HYPERFUNCTIONING THYROID ADENOMA

Hyperfunctioning adenomas often are first appreciated on a thyroid scan, where they appear as "hot" nodules. Such nodules may be noticed by the patient in a very casual way. Often the patient is still euthyroid because, even though the adenoma is hypersecreting independently of the pituitary feedback system, the suppression of thyroid secretion from the normal gland serves to maintain a physiologic net secretion rate of thyroid hormone. Only when the normal gland can no longer be suppressed and the adenoma continues to increase its secretion rate of thyroid hormone will laboratory or clinical evidence of hyperthyroidism appear.

Thyroid nodules of various forms require a clear understanding for treatment, and these features are discussed in detail later in this chapter. For purposes of control of hyperthyroidism, eventual or achieved, surgical excision of the hyperfunctioning adenoma is simple, safe, and effective. If the patient is clinically hyperthyroid, preoperative control with antithyroid drugs, using the same principles mentioned previously, is wise. Hot nodules have been treated effectively with therapeutic doses of radioactive iodine, and from the functional standpoint the results are good. A disadvantage of this approach is that a precise pathologic diagnosis of the lesion is not provided.

APATHETIC HYPERTHYROIDISM

Attention should be drawn to some forms of hyperthyroidism most often seen in elderly patients, in whom the diagnosis is not suspected because of the insidious onset of the disease, which can be quite atypical. Diffuse myopathy, myocardial failure, and cachexia without adequate explanation all may be found to have occult hyperthyroidism as their basis, especially in older patients. In such situations, the various thyroid function tests may be invaluable in establishing the diagnosis. The principles of treatment are the same as in Graves' disease, and it is to be expected that with a larger proportion of elderly patients more of them will be found suitable for radioactive iodine treatment.

For references, see page 692.

IV

THYROIDITIS

Timothy S. Harrison, M.D.

Inflammatory conditions affecting the thyroid gland are not uncommon. For reasons that will become apparent, classification of the subacute and some of the chronic forms of thyroiditis is difficult. In some situations, it is not possible to assign to certain forms of subacute and chronic thyroiditis a name that will be equally acceptable to all authorities. Part of the problem is semantic, and part of it reflects an incomplete understanding of the pathogenesis of the several conditions involved. If one bears in mind the clinical potential inherent in the several diagnostic possibilities, inappropriate treatment of the patient involved will be avoided, even though precise terminologic agreement may be absent.

Acute Thyroiditis (Specific Thyroiditis, Bacterial Thyroiditis)

The thyroid gland is rarely involved by bacterial infection. Such a condition may occur after infections of the mouth, pharynx, or neighboring lymph nodes. Generally, these infections respond to specific antibacterial treatment, but if not, thyroid abscesses should be drained. Also rare are infections such as tuberculosis, actinomycosis, and syphilis. The primary treatment in each of these conditions is chemotherapeutic.

Subacute Thyroiditis (De Quervain's Disease)

This is a disease of moderately abrupt onset, often following an upper respiratory infection. The thyroid becomes acutely congested, swollen, and mildly tender. Clinically, the patient experiences repeated remissions and exacerbations over a period of up to a few months. Seldom are the patients hypothyroid, and the radioactive iodine uptake is usually normal but occasionally may be slightly depressed. The leukocyte count is normal or depressed, and the erythrocyte sedimentation rate is elevated. Most often this condition is attributed to a viral infection, and ordinarily thyroid antibodies are not present. On microscopic examination of biopsy sections, giant cells may be present. Spontaneous recovery is frequent, and if the patient is acutely uncomfortable, a short course of hydrocortisone may bring symptomatic relief. Residual nodules seldom occur. Because of the possibility of recovery of normal thyroid function, this condition should not be treated by subtotal thyroidectomy.

Hashimoto's Disease (Lymphocytic Thyroiditis, Struma Lymphomatosa)

This disorder, first described by Hashimoto in 1912, most commonly occurs in middle-aged women. Its incidence appears to be definitely increasing.[5] The thyroid is firm and rubbery with many lobular projections. The clinical manifestations should arouse suspicion of the diagnosis. In the early stages of the evolution of the disease, mild hyperthyroidism may be present. This hyperthyroidism represents release of stored hormone and the radioiodine uptake will be normal or low. The hyperthyroidism will pass and should not be definitively treated.[6] In the later and chronic stage, hypothyroidism, which may be marked, is the most common presenting problem.

Of considerable interest has been the demonstration of circulating antibodies in some patients with Hashimoto's thyroiditis. These antibodies are reactive either to thyroglobulin itself or to antigens from the thyroid epithelial cell. The disorder is generally considered an "autoimmune" disease, and the possibility is a very strong one. However, the point has been made that these antibodies might be a reflection of the response of thyroid epithelium to certain types of viral infection or other as yet unrecognized pathogenic factors.

In the early stages of the disease, the laboratory tests of thyroid function may give the illusion of hyperthyroidism. The uptake of radioiodine by the thyroid may be slightly elevated, as may be the serum protein-bound iodine. However, if serum thyroxin and triiodothyronine are normal, the rise in protein-bound iodine may be a result of release from the diseased thyroid of relatively noncalorigenic iodinated compounds. A radioactive scan of the thyroid usually shows irregular uptake, with some areas devoid of iodine-131.

Some of the nodules occurring in thyroiditis are hard and closely simulate those of malignant disease. Thus, the surgeon's opinion concerning such nodules is often sought. It is well to recognize that the incidence of papillary adenocarcinoma is increased in chronic thyroiditis. With this consideration, one is well advised to insist upon adequate biopsy of the thyroid, best obtained by open biopsy. Open biopsy has two advantages: (1) it permits complete removal of the nodule; and (2) other suspicious areas of the thyroid (which may be missed on physical examination) can be evaluated. During the course of the biopsy, the muscles and fascia overlying the thyroid gland are often noted to be adherent to the thyroid parenchyma. If the scarred thyroid is beginning or threatening to constrict the trachea, it is a simple matter to divide the thyroid isthmus and relieve actual or potential tracheal constriction.

Percutaneous needle biopsy has often been recommended and used for the diagnosis and for following the course of thyroiditis. The major objection is that the technique is a blind one, and the tissue obtained is often inadequate. Thus, the most crucial area in a gland with thyroiditis may be overlooked or ignored completely.

The microscopic pathologic appearance is characterized by diffuse lymphocytic infiltration of the thyroid with minimal to extensive obliteration of the acini. Typical lymphoid follicles are present throughout the gland. In the later stages, fibrosis is a characteristic feature (Fig. 1).

The opinion is frequently expressed that subtotal thyroidectomy should be performed in chronic thyroiditis in order to remove as much of the disease as possible. This practice is mentioned only for condemnation. In some of the lymphoid varieties of thyroiditis, the thyroid will recover its function with time, and needless subtotal thyroidectomy will only decrease or completely destroy this possibility. Frozen section diagnosis of thyroid nodules in general has been unreliable, but with newer rapid fixation and staining techniques it is somewhat improved. Frozen sections in thyroiditis are, however, notoriously misleading, and close cooperation between pathologist and surgeon is necessary to avoid inappropriate thyroidectomy.

The *treatment* of Hashimoto's disease is dependent upon its severity. In some patients, no therapy is indicated; in others, thyroid hormone administration is appropriate to combat hypothyroidism. In still others, pressure symptoms may require surgical relief, and surgery is also indicated for large glands that present a cosmetic problem.

Riedel's Struma (Chronic Thyroiditis)

This type of thyroiditis is rare. The presenting symptoms are usually those of profound hypothyroidism, and it is usually irreversible. The gland tends to be so hard that differentiation from malignant thyroid tumors by open biopsy is often wise. Morphologically, there is dense fibrosis throughout the gland with a minimum of other cells. There is speculation as to whether or not this disease is an end stage of Hashimoto's disease, but currently the weight of evidence appears to favor the belief that it is a separate pathophysiologic entity. The treatment is administration of thyroid hormone, which relieves the hypothyroidism but does not affect the lesion.

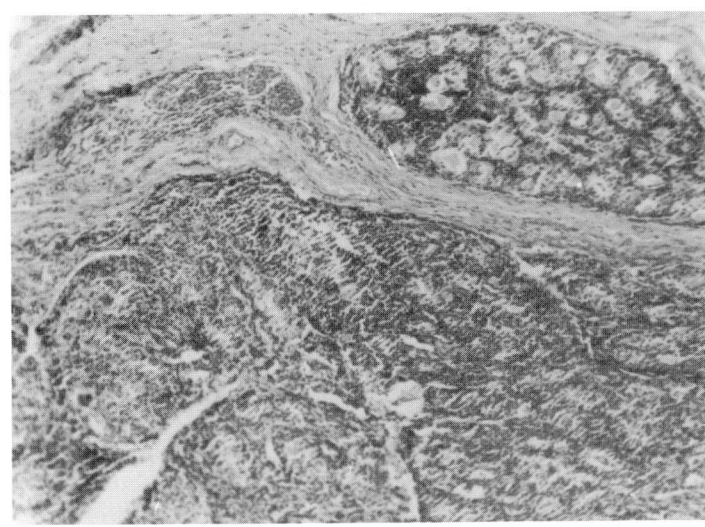

Figure 1. Photomicrograph of a section from the thyroid of a patient with the fibrous variant of Hashimoto's thyroiditis. × 80.

SELECTED REFERENCES

Halsted, W. S.: The operative story of goiter. Johns Hopkins Hosp. Rep., *19*:71, 1929. Reprinted in Halsted, W. S.: Surgical Papers. Baltimore, The Johns Hopkins Press, 1924, Volume II, p. 257.
This is the definitive history of thyroid surgery in the English language. The article also describes, with superb plates, the steps in Professor Halsted's operations on the thyroid gland.

Hayek, A., Chapman, E. M., and Crawford, J. D.: Long term results of I-131 treatment of thyrotoxicosis in children. N. Engl. J. Med., *283*:949, 1970.
An effort to treat childhood thyrotoxicosis with radioactive iodine is evaluated. The considerations involved are briefly but cogently reviewed. It is by no means certain that radioiodine treatment of childhood thyrotoxicosis will become widespread, but the author's attempt to evaluate its potential in this group is commendable.

Ingbar, S. H., and Woeber, K. A.: The thyroid gland. *In* Williams, R.H. (Ed.): Textbook of Endocrinology, 5th ed. Philadelphia, W. B. Saunders Company, 1974.
This chapter in an excellent text of endocrinology presents an outstanding review of the anatomy, physiology, biochemistry, and clinical derangements of the thyroid gland. It provides a superb description of the tests of thyroid function and their interpretation. It is a valuable resource for all aspects of the thyroid gland.

Lidz, T., and Whitehorn, J. L.: Psychiatric problems in the thyroid clinic. J.A.M.A., *139*:698, 1949.
Of the many descriptions of the emotional background of thyrotoxicosis, this one is the most vivid and apt. The history of thyrotoxicosis is treated briefly but effectively.

Michie, W., Pegg, C. A. S., Hamer-Hodges, D. W., et al.: Beta blockade and partial thyroidectomy for thyrotoxicosis. Lancet, *1*:1009, 1974.
This recent study from Aberdeen, Scotland, documents carefully the safety and ease of the preoperative use of beta-adrenergic receptor blockade in hyperthyroidism. Three groups of hyperthyroid patients were studied. In one antithyroid drugs and iodine were used. In the second group, propranolol and iodine were used, and in the third group, propranolol was the sole agent used. Duration of treatment was significantly shorter for the propranolol groups. Control of pulse rate was adequate in all three groups. No complications or deaths were encountered in any group. Recurrence of hyperthyroidism at one year was comparable in all three groups. This study provides an excellent contemporary view of the usefulness and role of beta-receptor blockade in the preoperative control of hyperthyroidism.

Nofal, M. M., Beierwaltes, W. H., and Patno, M. E.: Treatment of hyperthyroidism with sodium iodide I-131. J.A.M.A., *197*:605, 1966.
The incidence of hypothyroidism in 848 patients treated for hyperthyroidism with I-131 was compared with that in 121 patients treated surgically. With follow-up periods up to 16 years, at least 51 per cent of those treated with I-131 and 28 per cent of those managed surgically became hypothyroid. Estimates in this series suggest that at 10-year follow-up the incidence of hypothyroidism will be 70 per cent in those treated with I-131, as contrasted with 43 per cent of those treated with subtotal thyroidectomy. This series is a large and carefully evaluated one.

Rustad, W. H.: The Recurrent Laryngeal Nerves in Thyroid Surgery. Springfield, Ill., Charles C Thomas, Publishers, 1956.
This monograph describes in detail the surgical anatomy of the recurrent laryngeal nerves. The information is based on meticulous cadaver dissection, and the potential for variation in the course and number of recurrent laryngeal nerves is described.

Soderberg, U.: Temporal characteristics of thyroid activity. Physiol. Rev., *39*:777, 1959.
This review presents the evidence and significance of short-term reactions of the thyroid gland. The literature pertinent to this subject is reviewed critically.

Williams, A. F.: Recurrent nerve lesions. Surgery, *43*:435, 1958.
This study of recurrent nerve lesions resulting from thyroidectomy is objective and well done. One of the important points is that delayed paralysis of an injured nerve may occur several days following thyroidectomy.

REFERENCES

1. Abraham, E., and Harrison, T.: Complications of thyroid surgery. Lebanese Med. J., *23*:553, 1970.
2. Anderson, M. S., and Bowers, C. Y.: Synthetic thyrotropin releasing hormone. A potent stimulator of thyrotropin secretion in man. N. Engl. J. Med., *285*:1279, 1971.
3. Dillon, P. T., Babe, J., Meloni, C. R., and Canary, J. J.: Reserpine in thyrotoxic crisis. N. Engl. J. Med., *283*:1020, 1970.
4. Durham, C. F., and Harrison, T. S.: The surgical anatomy of the superior laryngeal nerve. Surg. Gynecol. Obstet., *118*:38, 1964.
5. Furszyfer, J., Kurland, L. T., and Woolner, L. B., et al.: Hashimoto;s thyroiditis in Olmstead County, Minnesota, 1935–1967. Mayo Clin. Proc., *45*:586, 1970.
6. Gluck, F. B., Nusynowitz, M. L., and Plymate, S.: Chronic lymphocytic thyroiditis, thyrotoxicosis, and low radioactive iodine uptake. N. Engl. J. Med., *293*:624, 1975.
7. Goluboff, L. G., Sisson, J. L., and Hamburger, J. I.: Hyperthyroidism associated with pregnancy. Obstet. Gynecol., *44*:107, 1974.
8. Halsted, W. S.: The operative story of goiter. Johns Hopkins Hosp. Rep., *19*:71, 1929. Reprinted in Halsted, W. S.: Surgical Papers. Baltimore. The Johns Hopkins Press, 1924, Volume II, p. 257.
9. Hamilton, C. R., Adams, L. C., and Maloof, F.: Hyperthyroidism due to thyrotropin-producing pituitary chromophobe adenoma. N. Engl. J. Med., *283*:1077, 1970.
10. Harris, G. W., and Woods, J. W.: Electrical stimulation of the hypothalamus and thyroid activity. Nature, *178*:80, 1956.
11. Harrison, T. S., Silver, D. M., and Zuidema, G. D.: Thyroid and adrenal medullary function in chronic "executive" monkeys. Endocrinology, *78*:685, 1966.
12. Hayek, A., Chapman, E. M., and Crawford, J. D.: Long term results of I-131 treatment of thyrotoxicosis in children. N. Engl. J. Med., *283*:949, 1970.
13. Ingbar, S. H., and Woeber, K. A.: The thyroid gland. *In* Williams, R. H. (Ed.): Textbook of Endocrinology. 5th ed. Philadelphia, W. B. Saunders Company, 1974.
14. Lee, T. L., Coffey, R. J., Mackin, J., et al.: The use of propranolol in surgical treatment of thyrotoxic patients. Ann. Surg., *177*:643, 1975.
15. Lidz, T., and Whitehorn, J. L.: Psychiatric problems in the thyroid clinic. J.A.M.A., *139*:698, 1949.
16. Mestman, J. H., Manning, P. R., and Hodgman, J.: Hyperthyroidism and pregnancy. Arch. Intern. Med., *134*:434, 1974.
17. Michie, W., Pegg, C. A. S., Hamer-Hodges, D. W., et al.: Beta blockade and partial thyroidectomy for thyrotoxicosis. Lancet, *1*:1009, 1974.
18. Nofal, M. M., Beierwaltes, W. H., and Patno, M. E.: Treatment of hyperthyroidism with sodium iodide I-131. J.A.M.A., *197*:605, 1966.
19. Ochi, Y., and De Groot, L. J.: Long acting thyroid stimulator of Graves' disease. N. Engl. J. Med., *278*:718, 1968.
20. Pegg, C. A. S., Stewart, D. J., Bewster, P. D., et al.: The surgical management of thyrotoxicosis. Br. J. Surg., *60*:765, 1973.
21. Rosenberg, I. N.: Thyroid storm (Editorial). N. Engl. J. Med., *283*:1052, 1970.
22. Rustad, W. H.: The Recurrent Laryngeal Nerves in Thyroid Surgery. Springfield, Ill., Charles C Thomas, Publisher, 1956.
23. Soderberg, U.: Temporal characteristics of thyroid activity. Physiol. Rev., *39*:777, 1959.
24. Talbert, L. M., Thomas, C. G., Jr., and Rankin, P.: Hyperthyroidism during pregnancy. Obstet. Gynecol., *36*:779, 1970.
25. Turner, P., Granville-Grossman, F. L., and Smart, J. V.: Effect of adrenergic receptor blockade on the tachycardia of thyrotoxicosis and anxiety state. Lancet, *2*:1316, 1965.
26. Williams, A. F.: Recurrent nerve lesions. Surgery, *43*:435, 1958.

V

NODULAR GOITER AND BENIGN AND MALIGNANT NEOPLASMS OF THE THYROID

Colin G. Thomas, Jr., M.D.

HISTORICAL ASPECTS

Until the early part of the twentieth century, management of toxic goiter remained the primary therapeutic problem in thyroid disease. There was little effort to distinguish between nodular goiter and thyroid cancer. Although thyroid cancer was first described in the English language by Burns in 1811, it was regarded as a medical curiosity and received little emphasis until the middle of the twentieth century. Increased interest in the disease was associated with the ability to better evaluate thyroid function with radioactive iodide and the finding of Cole and associates in the early 1940s of a high incidence of thyroid cancer in surgically removed nodular goiter, i.e., 17 per cent in nodular goiter and 24 per cent in solitary nodules. This awakened interest led to further studies of the genesis, incidence, and natural history of thyroid cancer and the realization that thyroid carcinoma comprises a spectrum of diseases rather than a single entity.

CLASSIFICATION

The objective of classifying any disease is to provide clarification of its biologic characteristics as related to etiology, natural history, and therapy. Classification of thyroid disease is compromised by disagreement as to the relationship between diffuse goiter and adenomatous goiter, and whether an "adenoma" is truly a benign neoplasm or whether all these lesions result from the physiologic consequences of continual stimulation of the thyroid by thyrotropic hormone. Terms in the older literature such as "lateral aberrant thyroid," "benign metastasizing goiter," and "malignant adenoma" are descriptive but not enlightening. With better appreciation of thyroid physiology and the mechanisms of carcinogenesis, a classification is proposed that is based upon correlation of earlier studies of Marine and subsequent experimental and clinical observations.[8, 18] This classification presents a unified concept of the known biologic characteristics of goiter and has implications for diagnosis, therapy, and prognosis (Table 1). Adenomatous goiter and thyroid neoplasms are not singular entities arising de novo, but represent a spectrum of disease. The biologic behavior of a particular entity will vary with its etiology, morphology, functional status, and autonomy of growth. These factors are in turn influenced by the ge-

netic composition, sex, and age of the host. Cognizance of this spectrum is essential in order that therapeutic measures be concordant with the natural history of the disease.

INCIDENCE OF ADENOMATOUS GOITER AND THYROID CANCER

Adenomatous (nodular) goiter is a worldwide disease, its incidence varying from high—in Switzerland, the Andes, India, and the Congo basin—to low, depending on the genetic composition of the population and the intensity and duration of the goitrogenic stimuli to which the population is subjected. Adenomatous goiter remains a very common disorder in the United States despite widespread use of iodine prophylaxis and the virtual disappearance of iodine deficiency. Approximately 4 per cent of the adult population have clinically palpable nodules, and the prevalence increases in the later decades of life. Autopsy findings in adults disclose an even higher incidence of thyroid disease, with some type of nodular enlargement in more than 50 per cent (Table 2).[25]

In the United States, carcinoma of the thyroid has been estimated to be responsible for 0.5 to 1 per cent of

---

TABLE 1. Classification of Benign and Malignant Thyroid Disease

I. Diffuse Enlargement of the Thyroid
II. Benign Lesions of the Thyroid
  A. Adenomatous goiter
  B. Follicular adenoma
  C. Hyperfunctioning adenoma
III. Malignant Lesions of the Thyroid
  A. Well differentiated (from follicular epithelium)
    1. Papillary or papillary-follicular
      a. Encapsulated or occult sclerosing
      b. Invasive
    2. Follicular
      a. Encapsulated
      b. Invasive
  B. Medullary with amyloid (from parafollicular cells)
  C. Undifferentiated (anaplastic, small cell, spindle, giant cell)
  D. Others (epidermoid, sarcoma, lymphoma, metastatic)

TABLE 2. **Histologic Nature of Nodules Found at Autopsy in Patients with Clinically Normal Thyroid Glands**

Nodule	Number	Per Cent
Adenomatous goiter	263	32
Thyroiditis	42	5.1
Adenoma	272	33
Carcinoma	17	2.1
Metastatic carcinoma	15	1.8
No nodules	211	26
Total	820	100.0

*Data from Mortensen, J. D., Bennett, W. A., and Wooner, L. B.: J. Clin. Endocrinol., 15:1270, 1955.

all cases of clinical cancer, to have an incidence of 25 cases per 1 million population per year, and to account for approximately 1100 deaths annually.[11] There appears to be an increase in the frequency of the clinical diagnosis of thyroid cancer,[5] but because of the long natural history of the disease, this has not yet been reflected by change in the death rate. In routine autopsies, the mean overall incidence of thyroid cancer is 0.08 per cent.[31] However, when special attention is given to the thyroid the incidence rises to 5.7 per cent.[29] Most of these cancers have little clinical significance, and few are responsible for the death of the patient. Similarly, until recently the coincidence of Graves' disease and thyroid cancer was considered to be extremely rare. Careful examination of glands removed surgically reveals papillary carcinoma in approximately 1 per cent. In patients undergoing surgical excision of nodular goiter, the incidence of carcinoma varies between 4 and 17 per cent.[7, 35]

ETIOLOGY AND PATHOGENESIS OF THYROID NEOPLASMS

The concept of initiating and promoting factors facilitates the understanding of neoplastic growth in the endocrine system and is particularly applicable to the thyroid.[14] This concept postulates that an initial stimulus (initiating factor) may be followed by a permanent change in cell DNA characteristics. This alteration in cell potential may follow contact with a carcinogen or radiation injury, or perhaps may have a genetic basis. A subsequent growth stimulus (thyrotropic hormone in normal or excessive amounts) may serve as a promoting factor, with the ultimate development of an invasive neoplasm. At times, excess trophic stimuli, by increasing the likelihood of mutants, seem to satisfy all requirements for both the initiation and promotion of neoplastic growth.

An equally important concept in the understanding of neoplastic growth is that of progression.[6, 34, 35] A neoplasm is not the consequence of an abrupt transition from normal controlled to unrestrained cellular growth, but is frequently more evolutionary in character. Initially, only hyperplastic changes are seen. With

continual stimulus, probably change in DNA characteristics aided by the processes of mutation and selection, cells may evolve that, although initially dependent, ultimately become autonomous in their growth characteristics. Although usually such autonomy is accompanied by loss of cellular differentiation, acceleration of growth, loss of adhesiveness, and ability to invade, an autonomous tumor may remain localized and well differentiated. Furthermore, a neoplasm consists of a heterogeneous cell population in which promotion and progression occur as a continuum. Early in the biologic evolution of such a lesion, withdrawal of trophic hormones or promoting factors may be followed by regression or inhibition of growth. Later in its development only temporary regression follows withdrawal of promoting agents, either because of continued progression and evolution of tumor development or because of ascendancy of those cells that are autonomous. Ultimately, a highly autonomous and anaplastic neoplasm with unrestrained growth develops.

These concepts of the biology of thyroid neoplasms may be illustrated by an analysis of tumor development in the experimental animal. Neoplasms of the thyroid occur spontaneously in a number of species. Through the common denominator of thyrotropin stimulation, an increased frequency and a spectrum of tumors have been produced. Depending upon genetic factors, presence of a carcinogen or initiating factor, and type of goitrogen, neoplasms will vary in their time of genesis, functional status, and growth potential. Iodine deficiency, thiourea, and radioiodine alone or in combination have all produced thyroid neoplasms. Initially, such tumors are dependent upon thyrotropin for growth. With continued stimulation and as aided by retransplantation into hosts with decreasing levels of thyrotropin, they ultimately become autonomous.[18] In some animals carcinogenesis is apparently accelerated by the coincidental administration of chemical carcinogens or ionizing irradiation. All of the circumstances leading to the development of thyroid neoplasms in the experimental animal have in common a persistent stimulus by thyrotropin.[18]

An analysis of conditions under which thyroid neoplasms are known to occur in man discloses instances of an initiating factor, a goitrogenic stimulus, and progression from a well-differentiated to an undifferentiated tumor.

Radiation as an Initiating Factor in Man. The association between irradiation to the neck region and the subsequent development of thyroid neoplasia is well established. Infants and children are more susceptible than adults. The risk of thyroid neoplasia increases linearly over a dose range of 20 to 1100 r to the thyroid.[10] The incidence of thyroid cancer has been estimated to be as high as 1 to 7 per cent of patients exposed.[10, 26] In 1950 Hempleman et al. reported that children with thyroid cancer had an increased incidence of exposure to radiation.[18] Winship collected 878 cases of thyroid cancer occurring before the age of 15 and noted a history of irradiation, usually directed to the thymus or cervical lymph nodes, in 70 per cent. The average interval between irradiation and the diagnosis of cancer was 8.5 years.[40] Radiation exposure later in life associated with the treatment of acne and cervical arthritis has also been implicated, with an average interval of 12.3 years between radiation injury and the development of well-differentiated cancer. Data from a study of Hiroshima survivors indicate thyroid carcinoma to be more prevalent among those who were exposed to ionizing radiation, and an increased incidence of thyroid nodules and cancer has been observed among the Marshall Islanders exposed to radiation fallout. There does not appear to be an increased risk in patients receiving therapeutic ^{131}I for Graves' disease. This is apparently related to the relatively high dose, which appears sufficient to destroy the proliferative ability of thyroid epithelia.

Iodine Deficiency.   The most convincing evidence for the relationship of iodine deficiency to the development of thyroid cancer in man is seen in certain areas of endemic goiter and iodine deficiency where the incidence of thyroid cancer has been many times its incidence in other parts of the world. Following several decades of iodine administration with reduction of goiter incidence, there has been decrease in age-specific mortality rates.[18] However, iodine prophylaxis of goiter in endemic regions has not eliminated malignant neoplasms of the thyroid gland. This is in keeping with the observation that in several areas of the world iodine deficiency has not been associated with an increased incidence of thyroid cancer.

Goitrogenic Stimuli.   Drugs that block the production of thyroxin in the animal give rise initially to a hyperplastic gland which may ultimately become neoplastic. Although carcinoma has not developed in man following administration of goitrogenic drugs, there are people in whom an inherent metabolic block in the biosynthesis of thyroid hormone has resulted in goitrous cretinism or varying degrees of hypothyroidism. Histologically, the thyroid glands of these persons show an intense degree of nodular hyperplasia and in some patients frank cancer has occurred. These cancers are usually of the well-differentiated papillary-follicular variety.

Progression.   The exact mechanism of progression from well differentiated to undifferentiated in thyroid cancer is unknown. However, radiation injury in conjunction with increased stimulation by thyrotropin appears to provide optimal conditions for such transformations.[6] After moderate doses of radiation to the thyroid, bizarre nuclear forms containing unusually large quantities of DNA have been found.[38] These changes have also been observed after small doses of radiation followed by the administration of thiouracil. Small doses of radiation that do not impair physiologic function produce latent changes that become evident only with an added stimulus for cell division. The transition from well-differentiated to poorly differentiated thyroid cancer characterized by increasing degrees of autonomous and aggressive behavior of the cells occurs in the natural evolution of thyroid cancer in approximately 5 per cent of patients.[28] Progression appears to be enhanced by a combination of irradiation and hypothyroidism.[6, 34, 35] The available data do not establish whether or not the incidence of progression can be decreased in many by the administration of thyroid hormone.

BIOLOGIC CHARACTERISTICS OF ADENOMATOUS GOITER AND THYROID CANCER

ADENOMATOUS GOITER, ADENOMA, HYPERFUNCTIONING ADENOMA

The term nodular goiter is purely descriptive, referring to a number of pathologic processes that cause asymmetric enlargement of the thyroid. By common usage the term includes adenomatous and colloid nodular goiter, which are further categorized as solitary or multiple, and nontoxic or toxic. The etiologic relationships between diffuse goiter, adenomatous (nodular) goiter, adenoma, and hyperfunctioning adenoma are unclear. Studies done in the experimental animal and correlated with pathologic findings in man indicate that these entities may have a common genesis and represent a response to continual or intermittent thyrotropin stimulation.[8, 32] In most areas of the world, iodine lack remains the commonest cause of deficient thyroid hormone synthesis. This is no longer true in the United States. The etiologic factors are multiple and complex and may be complementary, including dietary goitrogens (food and drugs), water pollution, sex, and calcium, fluoride, and chloride intake. Also important is a genetic predisposition to goiter characterized by inborn metabolic errors resulting in defective biosynthesis of thyroid hormone. Metabolic deficiencies include iodide transport defect, iodide organification defect (Pendred syndrome—goiter and deafness), deficiency of the enzyme dehalogenase, iodotyrosyl coupling defect, and abnormal plasma iodopeptide level.

The natural history of adenomatous goiter is that of a diffuse, soft goiter of childhood or adolescence—more common in females—that persists into adult life. The goiter may have become larger with pregnancy. Thyrotropic hormone stimulation results initially in diffuse hyperplasia, later in focal areas of hyperplasia and regression, and ultimately in the development of a solitary or multinodular goiter. These nodules present a spectrum of pathologic findings, e.g., cellular nonfunctioning adenomas, localized colloid nodules (microfollicular and macrofollicular), nodules with degenerative changes, and relatively acellular hyperfunctioning nodules. Focal (lobular) areas of hyperplasia may enlarge and with progressive growth persist as an adenoma. Such an adenoma, although initially dependent upon TSH, ultimately achieves a stage of autonomy—a benign "adenoma" with follicles of varying size and histologic appearance, e.g., fetal adenoma, papillary adenoma, Hürthle cell adenoma, follicular adenoma, or macrofollicular adenoma. These lesions are multivariates of adenomatous goiter rather than specific disease entities.

The initial phase of diffuse hyperplasia is difficult to reconcile with the subsequent development of nodules with adjacent normal parenchyma. The nodular enlargement of the thyroid as a consequence of continual or intermittent stimulation may be related to the lobular anatomic peculiarities of the thyroid, with 20 to 40 follicles being bound together by connective tissue and supplied by a single artery and vein. This type of blood supply with arteriovenous anastomoses permits a highly dynamic blood flow, influenced by vasohumoral mechanisms, and may account for the altered sensitivity of follicular epithelium to thyrotropic stimuli. The location of adenomatous changes in general corresponds to the blood supply to the lobules.[21]

The multinodular goiter is the end result of years of thyroid stimulation. In its early stages, the thyroid may be diffusely involved and lobular or bosselated in configuration, representing varying degrees of hyperplasia and involution. At this stage of development, the goiter is still dependent upon thyrotropin. Function, as measured by uptake of radioiodide or the endogenous production of thyroxin, may be completely suppressed by the administration of thyroid hormone, e.g., 75 to 100 μg. of triiodothyronine daily. In later stages some degree of autonomy may develop, as evidenced by a persistent 24-hour uptake of radioiodide of at least 10 per cent or the maintenance of a normal level of circulating thyroxin despite the administration of triiodothyronine.[23] With further increase in the mass of autonomously functioning thyroid tissue, and if the progression is not mitigated by degenerative changes, hyperthyroidism (Plummer's disease) ensues. Plummer observed in 1913 that diffuse, multinodular goiter antedated the development of hyperthyroidism by an average of 15 years.

Why some individuals develop a solitary nodule (follicular adenoma), others a hyperfunctioning nodule, and still others a multinodular goiter consisting of a spectrum of nodules needs further clarification. Although the solitary nodule occurs most often in the third and fourth decades and the multinodular goiter in later years, solitary nodules may become manifest only late in life and occasionally multinodular goiter is observed during early adulthood.

Unless there is a severe deficit in the biosynthesis of thyroid hormone (goitrous hypothyroidism), the patient will remain euthyroid both clinically and by the usual function tests. Symptoms are related to the presence of the mass, which if sufficiently large may provoke local discomfort, dyspnea, dysphagia, and occasionally chest discomfort when it is located substernally. Because of the slowly progressive nature of their development over many years, goiters may achieve a relatively large size and remain essentially asymptomatic.

Although functioning and nonfunctioning adenomas have been considered to be common findings in the genesis of nodular goiter,[32] a phase of dependency upon TSH cannot always be demonstrated. Small foci of hyperplastic and hyperfunctioning nodules have been observed to be present at the outset and have been proposed as representing a form of benign endocrine neoplasia[24] or an embryonic rest.[8]

Hyperfunctioning adenomatous goiter (hot nodules, toxic nodules, autonomous nodules) characteristically occurs as a solitary nodule in the third or fourth decade of life.[15] The lesion predominates in women. Although these nodules meet many of the criteria of a neoplasm, namely, autonomy of growth and function, invasive features are almost unknown. Histologically, these nodules exhibit a rather loose papillary pattern with columnar epithelium. Their hyperfunctional status is not suggested by their morphologic appearance except by the atrophy of any remaining normal parenchyma. The nodule may continue to function autonomously until it attains sufficient size to produce hyperthyroidism, or it may undergo necrosis with partial or temporary regression. Hyperfunctioning nodules are readily identified by thyroid scanning techniques because of the localization and intense uptake of the radioisotope (Fig. 1). Hormonal output (secretory activity) appears to be related to the size of the nodule, and if the mass is large enough hyperthyroidism results. A mass 3 to 4 cm. in diameter is required,

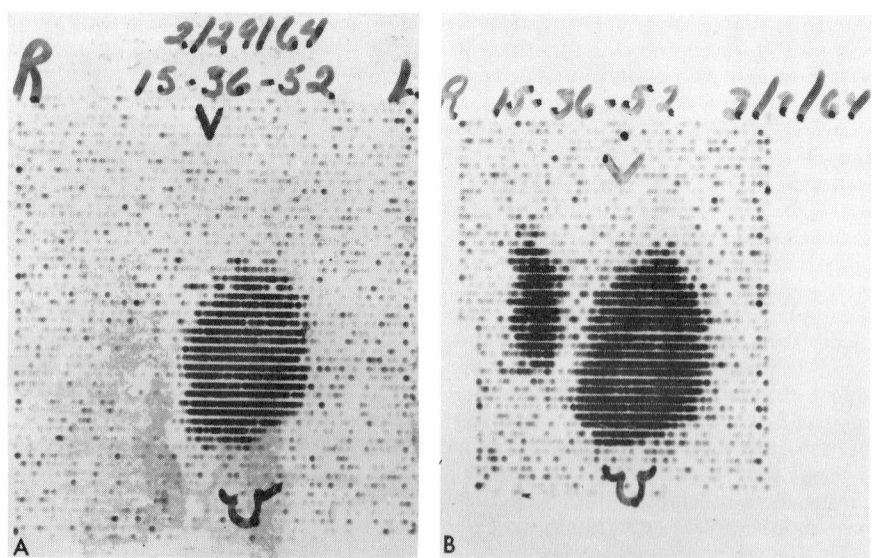

Figure 1. *A*, Radioiodide scan of hyperfunctioning adenoma with complete suppression of function in the remainder of the gland. *B*, The functional capacity of the suppressed normal parenchyma is indicated by the uptake of the radioisotope following stimulation with thyrotropin.

although occasionally multiple nodules may produce the same result. Hyperfunctioning nodules have also been reported to be capable of secreting only triiodothyronine and consequently producing hyperthyroidism with a normal serum thyroxin level and ^{131}I-labeled T_3 resin uptake.

The implication of these concepts is that the ideal treatment for nodular goiter is one of prophylaxis. This should be instituted at that phase of development when deficient hormone biosynthesis is manifested by a diffuse goiter. TSH may be elevated at this and subsequent stages of development. Removal of a portion or all of a nodular goiter merely aggravates the underlying disease. Treatment with replacement doses of thyroid hormone needs to be initiated not only to maintain a euthyroid state, but also to prevent the further development of adenomatous changes in the remaining "normal" parenchyma.

THYROID CANCER

Cognizance of the biology of thyroid cancer is important to its diagnosis as well as to its management. Cancer of the thyroid is not a single entity but a spectrum of lesions with highly variable biologic potentials. In general, the course of the disease will be related to (1) tumor morphology; (2) age of onset; (3) sex; (4) extent of disease; (5) presence of initiating and promoting factors; and (6) modes of therapy.[4, 35] As an example, encapsulated follicular adenocarcinoma of the thyroid behaves essentially as a benign disease and is accompanied by a near-normal life expectancy.[1] Similarly, well-differentiated papillary-follicular adenocarcinoma with cervical lymph node metastases arising in a 30-year-old woman may pursue a remarkabley indolent course. In contrast, a tumor of identical morphology but arising later in life or in the male usually is much more aggressive and is associated with a shorter survivorship. Undifferentiated cancers are usually associated with a rapid progression and early demise.[34] All thyroid carcinomas, however, are capable of causing death, and unfortunately only generalizations can be made with reference to the biologic potential of any specific type. It is obvious that all therapeutic measures must be not only concordant but also evaluated with reference to the natural history of the disease.

From a therapeutic as well as prognostic standpoint, it is useful to classify thyroid cancer as (1) well-differentiated, namely papillary or follicular, arising from follicular epithelium; (2) solid carcinoma with medullary stroma arising from parafollicular cells; (3) undifferentiated cancer (anaplastic, spindle cell, small cell, giant cell); and (4) others such as squamous cancer, lymphoma, and metastatic carcinoma (see Table 1). The variation in the biology of well-differentiated tumors warrants further division into papillary carcinomas that are (a) occult sclerosing or encapsulated and (b) frankly invasive. Follicular carcinoma similarly should be recognized as being (a) encapsulated and (b) invasive. Such classification of well-differentiated carcinomas is indicated because of the implications for therapy and prognosis.

Well-Differentiated Thyroid Cancer

Papillary and papillary-follicular carcinomas account for 60 per cent of all cases of thyroid cancer. Pathologically, few papillary or follicular tumors are homogeneous; usually they consist of a mixture of both elements. Gross as well as microscopic examination (predominant cell pattern) provides criteria for classification. Well-differentiated lesions, whether papillary or follicular, may be circumscribed or encapsulated, indicating their indolent rate of growth, and are difficult to differentiate from noninvasive adenomas. These neoplasms are characterized by well-differentiated thyroid epithelial cells growing in a papillary pattern as a frond with its contained blood supply. There may be considerable infolding of the epithelial cells, with some being surrounded by colloid-like material. This papillary pattern may be mixed with well-formed acini, again containing colloid (Fig. 2E). Frankly invasive papillary and follicular carcinomas are more likely to be grossly infiltrative and firm and gritty on cut surface because of the associated desmoplastic reaction. A characteristic feature of papillary carcinoma is psammoma bodies—crescentic basophilic calcific bodies—which probably represent necrotic or hyalinized epithelial cells. Multiple small tumor foci may be present throughout both lobes.[28] Cervical lymph node, lung, and bone metastases may resemble the primary tumor or have quite a different papillary or follicular pattern.

Follicular carcinoma, constituting about 20 per cent of all cases of thyroid cancer, resembles normal follicular epithelium with acini of varying sizes. The acini may or may not contain colloid. Papillary elements may be present. Differentiation of encapsulated follicular adenocarcinoma from follicular adenoma can be made only by careful study and demonstration of capsular or blood vessel invasion (Fig. 3D). Other follicular carcinomas may be frankly invasive.

Ultrastructural studies of well-differentiated carcinomas have demonstrated chiefly nuclear abnormalities, increased numbers of mitochondria, and reduced endoplasmic reticulum. Follicular carcinoma is characterized by a number of intraluminal microvilli and their secretory potential is suggested by the presence of apical intracellular granules. Papillary carcinoma does not possess the same evidence of secretory activity.

Although papillary and follicular carcinomas can be separated on a morphologic basis, it is more difficult to do so on a biologic basis. Considerable emphasis has at times been placed upon the distinguishing characteristics of follicular and papillary carcinoma, viz., that papillary carcinoma is prone to spread to cervical lymph nodes and follicular carcinoma is more likely to metastasize to lungs or bones. They possess many more features in common than those that identify them as separate entities. Both tumors arise early in life with a distinct predilection for the female. Papillary carcinoma is prominent from the second through the seventh decades, with a slight peak in the third decade; follicular carcinoma has a similar age distribution but with a higher incidence somewhat later in life (Fig. 4). Important criteria of biologic activity are tumor size and evidence of encapsulation. Occult

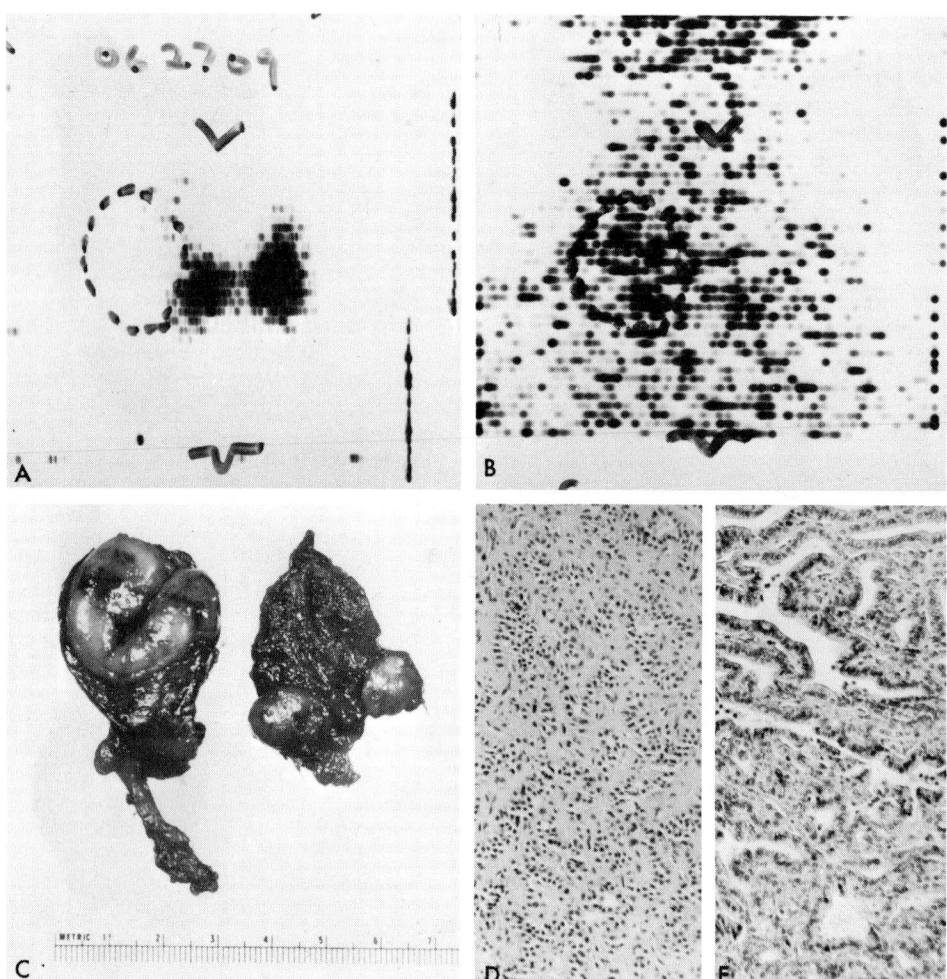

Figure 2. Scanning (*A*, iodide-125; *B*, selenium-75 selenomethionine); *C*, gross; and *D* and *E*, microscopic (×130) characteristics of a pleo-morphic papillary-follicular carcinoma in a 47-year-old woman who had received radiation therapy for acne 20 years previously. In addition to the gross neoplasm involving both the right and left lobes, there were multiple small tumor foci throughout the entire gland in keeping with multi-focal sites of origin or intraglandular metastasis.

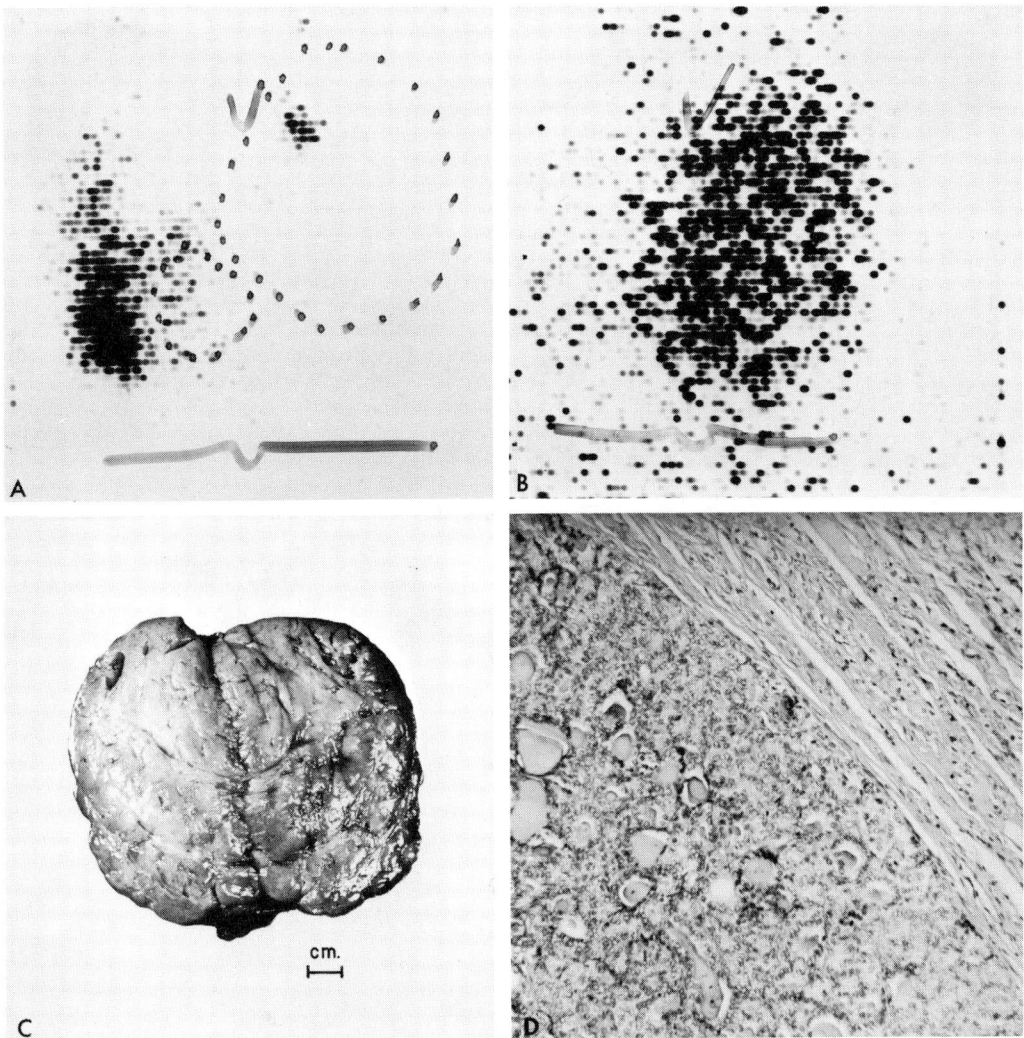

Figure 3.   Scanning characteristics (*A*, ¹²⁵I; *B*, ⁷⁵Se-selenomethionine); *C*, gross; and *D*, microscopic (× 130) findings in a 67-year-old woman with an encapsulated follicular adenocarcinoma of the thyroid.

sclerosing papillary adenocarcinomas, although occasionally productive of lymph node metastasis, are usually indolent in their growth, with a good prognosis. Similarly, in encapsulated follicular adenocarcinoma the survival rate is essentially that of the normal population. Histologic characteristics alone may not indicate the relative indolence or aggressiveness of a particular tumor. These findings must be correlated with the age and sex of the patient as well as the original size and circumscription of the neoplasm.

Well-differentiated adenocarcinomas of the thyroid arising in childhood or in the female before the fifth decade are characterized by slow growth of the primary tumor and of metastases.[3, 4, 40] There is little tendency for the tumor to spread through the capsule of the thyroid until late in the course of the disease. Early extension to regional lymph nodes is not uncommon. The primary tumor may be inconspicuous, with cervical node metastases being the presenting complaint. Survival curves depict little difference between

papillary and follicular neoplasms in women in this age group.[4] In contrast, well-differentiated tumors arising later in life, particularly in the male sex, are much more aggressive and associated with a poorer prognosis.[4]

Differences exist between thyroid cancer in children and in adults.[3] In association with exposure of children to ionizing radiation secondary to treatment of hyperplastic tonsils and enlargement of the thymus—a prevailing practice from 1920 to 1955, there was an increased incidence of thyroid cancer in this age group. Younger patients have predominantly well-differentiated cancers which tend to be more advanced at the time of diagnosis, i.e., extension to regional lymph nodes. Pulmonary metastases may occur; however, bone metastases are exceedingly uncommon. The disease is twice as common in the female. The most striking biologic characteristic of childhood thyroid cancer is the excellent survivorship. In association with surgical treatment the life expectancy of an indi-

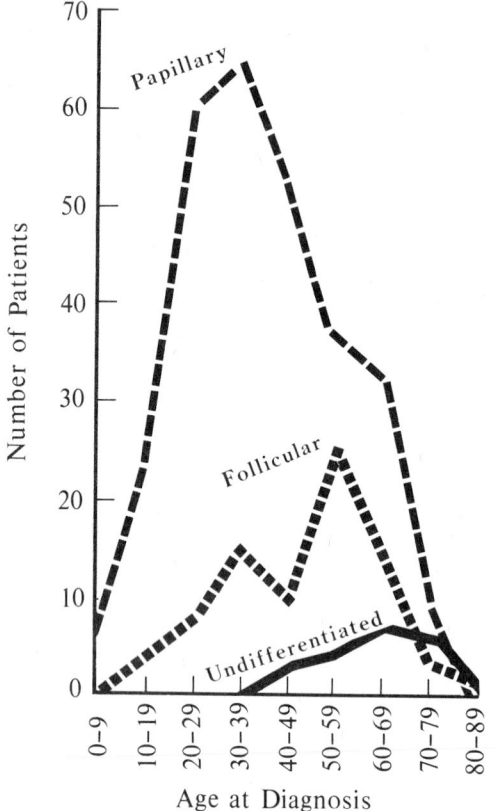

Figure 4. Age incidence and relative frequency of various types of thyroid cancer. (Modified from Hirabayashi, R. N., and Lindsay. S.: J. Clin. Endocrinol., *21*:1596, 1961.)

small cell, and spindle cell.[35] Histologically, these tumors present as solid sheets of epithelial cells with no resemblance to the cell of origin and with little evidence of follicle formation or papillary pattern (Fig. 6). Pleomorphism and frequent mitoses are common. The small cell tumors may be difficult to differentiate from lymphosarcoma. Their striking response to radiotherapy suggests that the lesion is a lymphoid rather than an epithelial neoplasm. As already discussed, these undifferentiated tumors may represent progression from well-differentiated adenocarcinomas. Clinical manifestations appear most frequently during the sixth and seventh decades (Table 3), with these tumors representing approximately 15 per cent of all cases of thyroid cancer. The predilection for females is not so striking as in the well-differentiated cancers. These neoplasms may develop after a long-standing history of antecedent goiter. At the time of diagnosis many of them will already have extended to regional lymph nodes or into the soft tissues of the neck, or metastasized to lung, bone, or other tissues. The tumors are usually independent of thyrotropin, as shown by their failure to collect iodide and to be influenced by the hormonal status of the patient. More than 75 per cent of patients with undifferentiated thyroid cancer will be dead within 3 years after the diagnosis (see Fig. 18). Although the prognosis is poor, an aggressive surgical attack for those lesions confined to the thyroid and cervical lymph nodes is occasionally rewarding and is warranted. External irradiation provides worthwhile palliation in some undifferentiated thyroid cancers.

vidual younger than 20 years of age at time of diagnosis of well-differentiated cancer is the same as that of the normal population (Fig. 5). The reasons for the differences in the behavior of well-differentiated thyroid cancer in the adult and child are not apparent. There are no differences in the histopathology. Progression to an undifferentiated tumor rarely occurs and may account for this greatly improved survivorship. In view of the age of onset, TSH may play a more active role as a promoting factor in the disease and these neoplasms may be more dependent upon TSH than those in the adult. Thus, TSH suppression may contribute to the better survivorship in this age group. It is of interest that the original observations on TSH dependency were made in children.

From the viewpoint of the surgeon, encapsulated or circumscribed well-differentiated cancer and invasive papillary or follicular tumors behave in a sufficiently similar way that the principles of surgical treatment are the same for both neoplasms.

Medullary Carcinoma

See Chapter on Medullary Carcinoma and Multiple Endocrine Neoplasia.

Undifferentiated Thyroid Cancer

In sharp contrast to the biologic characteristics of well-differentiated thyroid cancer are those of the poorly differentiated tumors—anaplastic, giant cell,

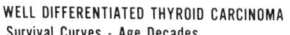
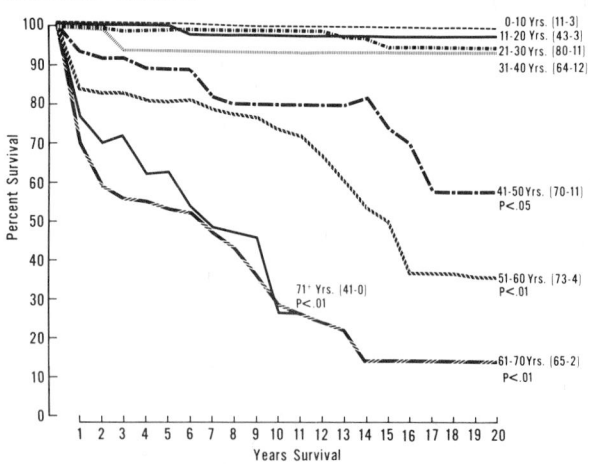

Figure 5. The survival curves for patients with well-differentiated thyroid carcinoma show the differences from the expected survival of normal individuals with the same sex distribution for each decade. The survival of the normal population is expressed as 100 per cent for 20 years. For example, for patients who were 51 to 60 years old at diagnosis, there was a difference of 62 per cent from the normal (expected) survival at 20 years, P < 0.01. The numbers in the parentheses indicate how many patients there were of each decade and the number alive 20 years from the time of diagnosis. (From Buckwalter, J. A., and Thomas, C. G., Jr.: Ann. Surg., *176*:573, 1972.)

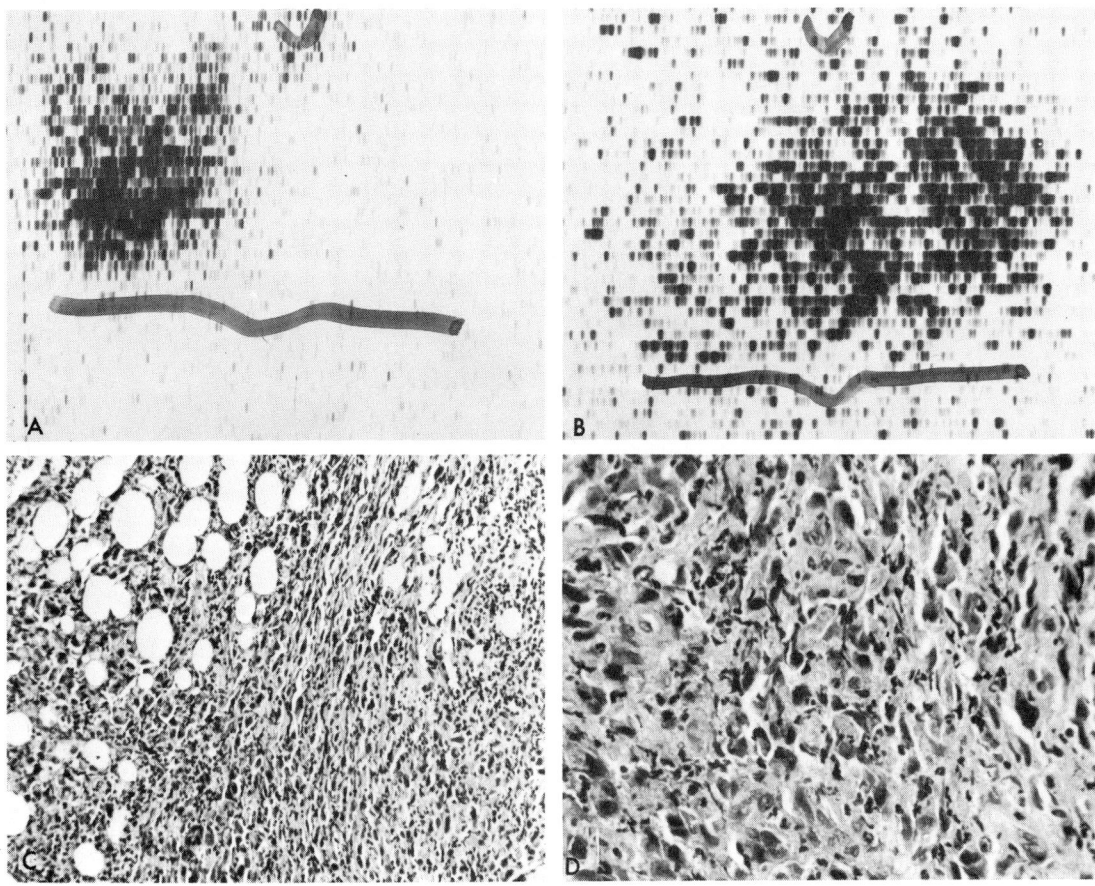

Figure 6. Scanning characteristics (*A*, ^{125}I; *B* ^{75}Se-selenomethionine) and microscopic findings (*C*, × 50; *D*, × 130) in a 77-year-old woman with undifferentiated carcinoma arising in the left lobe of the thyroid.

Lymphoma

Lymphoma is an uncommon form of malignant disease that may arise within the thyroid gland. It may remain localized, extend to involve regional lymph nodes, or be a manifestation of systemic disease. It usually presents as a large goiter of recent onset with obstructive symptoms, having its greatest incidence in

TABLE 3.   Clinical Symptoms in Patients with Thyroid Cancer*

Clinical Symptoms	Percentage of Patients with Symptoms			
	Papillary	Follic-ular	Medul-lary	Undiffer-entiated
None	73	63	50	28
Neck pain	10	5	0	72
Tightness, fullness, increased size of neck	8	11	25	15
Hoarseness	6	0	25	43
Dysphagia	6	16	50	25
Dyspnea	2	0	0	43

*From Beahrs, O. H., and Kubista, T. B. *In* Cancer Management: A Special Graduate Course on Cancer. Philadelphia, J. B. Lippincott Company, 1968, pp. 573–579.

women in their seventh decade. Lymphoma appears to be superimposed upon Hashimoto's thyroiditis in some patients, and may be difficult to differentiate therefrom on a morphologic basis. The lesion may be confined to one lobe of the thyroid, and differentiation from carcinoma is not possible without histologic examination. In the majority of cases, however, both lobes are involved. When lymphoma is confined to the thyroid, thyroidectomy is indicated and should be followed by postoperative irradiation. In those circumstances in which the disease extends beyond the thyroid, involving strap muscles as well as regional lymph nodes, biopsy will establish the nature of the disease. In lesions extending beyond the thyroid, radiation is the most effective therapy.

The prognosis of lymphoma is generally considered poor although unpredictable, dependent upon cell type and whether the lesion is localized to the thyroid, invasive beyond the thyroid, or a manifestation of systemic disease. Small cell lymphosarcoma is associated with long-term survival, whereas reticulum cell sarcoma has a poorer prognosis. Involvement of the thyroid by reticulum cell sarcoma is frequently a manifestation of systemic disease. There is very limited experience in the treatment of lymphoma of the thyroid by current radiotherapeutic techniques, i.e., therapy to the primary site and staging the extent of the disease by appropriate biopsy. With such staging and carefully directed radiotherapy, survival may be better than is indicated by previous experience.

CLINICAL ASPECTS AND DIAGNOSIS OF THYROID CANCER

Symptoms and Findings

The symptoms of thyroid cancer correlate well with the biologic characteristics of a particular tumor (see Table 3). Differentiation from nodular goiter is facilitated by a history of previous irradiation to the head or neck. The well-differentiated tumors are less frequently associated with a previous history of long-standing goiter than are the undifferentiated carcinomas. Well-differentiated cancers characteristically grow slowly and commonly present as an asymptomatic mass confined to one lobe or the isthmus of the thyroid gland. At times enlargement of cervical lymph node(s) may be the presenting complaint. The thyroid mass has usually been identified by the patient, or during a routine physical examination. Occasionally, the mass is of sufficient size to produce tracheal compression, dysphagia, or local pressure symptoms. More rapidly growing tumors that are highly invasive, e.g., undifferentiated thyroid cancer, are more frequently associated with local symptoms, e.g., cervical discomfort or fullness, tightness, pain referred to the ear or angle of the jaw because of involvement of the superficial cervical plexus, dysphagia, dyspnea, rarely stridor, and hoarseness. Hoarseness is usually secondary to invasion of the recurrent laryngeal nerve. Indirect laryngoscopy confirms loss of vocal cord function in patients with hoarseness and in some who are asymptomatic. One half of patients with medullary cancer and over 70 per cent of those with undifferentiated cancer will be symptomatic (see Table 3).

When examining the thyroid gland, it is important to procure a three-dimensional concept of its size and overall consistency. The examiner stands behind the patient and by digital pressure dislocates the trachea and thyroid gland to the side of the lesion. The mass within the thyroid is then palpated between the thumb, placed behind the sternocleidomastoid muscle, and the index and long fingers, in front of and overlying the thyroid (Fig. 7). The findings on physical examination are related to the type of neoplasm. Well-circumscribed, encapsulated, follicular-papillary or follicular adenocarcinoma is soft to firm in consistency and from one to several centimeters in diameter. Invasive and infiltrating papillary or follicular carcinoma, in contrast, is frequently quite hard and more likely to be poorly defined or irregular. The latter lesions are frequently associated with enlarged cervical lymph nodes, solitary or multiple, along the course of the internal jugular vein. The primary tumor within the thyroid may be too small to be palpable and manifested only by an increased consistency of one lobe. The cervical lymph node metastases from well-differentiated papillary-follicular lesions may be their chief manifestations. Because of their histologic similarity to normal thyroid tissue, such metastases at one time were classified as "lateral aberrant thyroid." However, careful examination discloses this well-differentiated tissue to be within a lymph node, a metastasis from a small or occult primary carcinoma of the thyroid. Advanced disease is characterized by more extensive metastases involving lymph nodes of the superior deep jugular chain, posterior cervical triangle, and contralateral side of the neck. Poorly differentiated neoplasms frequently extend through the thyroid capsule, producing a woody infiltration of strap muscles or surrounding vessels and skin. A bruit is uncommon over the primary tumor. However, metastatic follicular carcinoma involving bone or soft tissue is sometimes associated with a palpable thrill and audible bruit. Only metastatic renal carcinoma produces similar physical findings.

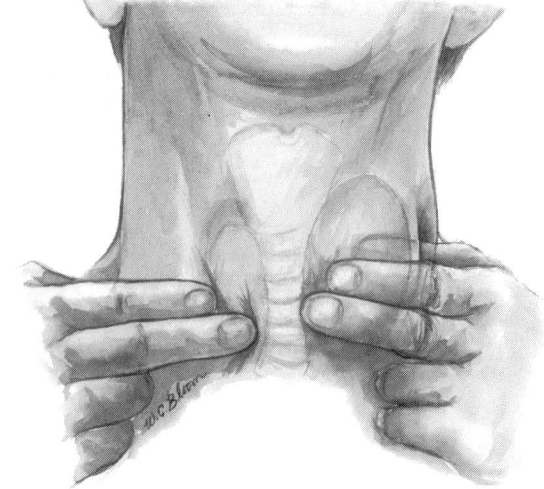

Figure 7. Technique of examination of the thyroid. The trachea and thyroid are displaced to the left by pressure on the contralateral lobe. Palpation of the left lobe between thumb, index, and long fingers provides a three-dimensional concept of its size, consistency, and topography.

Radiographs of the neck may show tracheal compression or displacement, depending upon the size of the mass (Fig. 8). Focal calcification, which is more common in long-standing nodular goiter, may also be seen with thyroid cancer. Thyroid cancer tends to remain localized to the neck, and distant metastases are uncommon. Pulmonary metastases present as a diffuse infiltrate or well-localized nodules. Bone metastases, which frequently are asymptomatic, may cause pain or neurologic deficit secondary to a compression fracture of the spine. In patients dying from thyroid cancer, extensive local disease with invasion of the trachea is common.[30] Distant metastases in these patients are also more frequent, regardless of the histologic appearance of the tumor. Lung and bone are the most common metastatic sites; other viscera are involved less often. In such advanced disease, the histologic appearance may be a poor criterion of the aggressiveness of the tumor. There may be evidence of progression from a well-differentiated to an undifferentiated neoplasm.

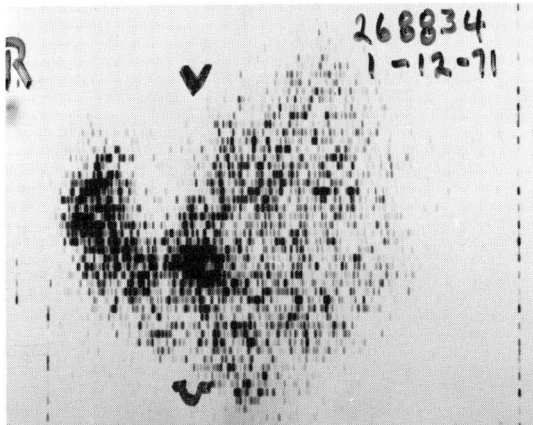

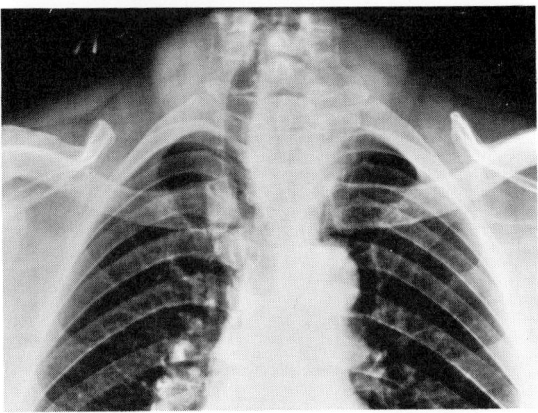

Figure 8. Characteristics of radioiodide scan in 59-year-old male with multinodular goiter. Note heterogeneity of radionuclide uptake in left lobe with area of hyperfunction near medial portion of lobe. The roentgenogram discloses extension to the superior mediastinum with displacement and compression of the trachea.

Hormonal and Biochemical Characteristics of Thyroid Cancer

Because of the functional reserve of normal thyroid parenchyma, the laboratory values for serum thyroxin, protein-bound iodine, ^{131}I T_3 resin uptake, and free thyroxin index reflect the euthyroid status of the patient and are usually within normal limits. Rarely is enough of the normal parenchyma destroyed to produce hypothyroidism. Hyperthyroidism, if it does occur, is usually coincidental and is most likely to be associated with an occult carcinoma. Most thyroid cancers are characterized by a lack of iodide uptake, and may be distinguished by this characteristic from adenomatous goiter.[9] Abnormal soluble iodoproteins have occasionally been observed in patients with both well-differentiated and undifferentiated thyroid cancer. These proteins, for the most part, have been iodoalbumins. At times, the abnormal iodoproteins may give rise to a spuriously elevated P.B.I., suggesting the diagnosis of subacute thyroiditis. Antithyroglobulin antibodies are no more elevated in thyroid cancer than in other diseases of the thyroid, excluding thyroiditis.

Medullary carcinoma is unique in that, because of the output of thyrocalcitonin, serotonin, or prostaglandins, presenting symptoms may be manifestations of the action of these hormones. Of the hormones elaborated by medullary carcinoma, the most common is thyrocalcitonin, which may be associated with parathyroid adenoma and hyperparathyroidism.

Thyroid Scanning in the Diagnosis of Cancer

The affinity of the thyroid gland for iodide permits the functional activity of the gland to be mapped after administration of a radioactive isotope. Cancer of the thyroid, in contrast to normally functioning thyroid parenchyma, is characterized by a lack of affinity for radioiodide. Consequently, scanning of the gland following administration of radioiodide or technetium-99m provides an index of the functional status of the "nodule" and helps differentiate between benign and malignant lesions (see Figs. 2, 3, and 6). There are, however, distinct limitations to this technique. The intimate relationship of the nodule to the surrounding normal parenchyma usually precludes detection of a lesion smaller than 1 cm. Because of contiguous overlying normal parenchyma, the scan may not accurately reflect iodide uptake within the nodule. Photoscanning techniques permitting oblique views may provide a more accurate index of the radionuclide content of a nodule (Fig. 9). Colloid nodules, cysts, and follicular adenomas may also exhibit lack of iodide uptake and cannot be differentiated from malignant tumors by scanning alone. The positive correlation between the lack of iodide uptake within a nodule and thyroid cancer is in the range of 10 to 20 per cent.

Thyroid cancer, as compared to normal parenchyma, is characterized by an increase in cell density as well as an increased rate of cell replication. These features can be appraised by scanning the thyroid following the intravenous administration of selenium-75 selenomethionine (see Figs. 2, 3, and 6).[36] A localized uptake and positive scan have been found primarily in thyroid cancer, highly cellular follicular adenomas, and localized granulomatous or chronic thyroiditis. However, a homogenous uptake of ^{75}Se-selenomethionine corresponding to the configuration of the thyroid is most characteristic of chronic thyroiditis (Fig. 10). Thyroid scans with ^{75}Se-selenomethionine are most valuable in evaluating lesions that have a high probability of being carcinoma. The incidence of cancer in lesions that are cold on iodide scanning and demonstrate selective concentration of ^{75}Se-selenomethionine approximates 50 per cent.[36] Lesions that fail to selectively concentrate ^{75}Se-selenomethionine and that exhibit some uptake of radioiodide are most likely to be a manifestation of adenomatous goiter, and either observation or a trial of suppressive therapy with thyroid hormone is justified.

Regional or whole-body scans may be utilized to identify functioning bone or pulmonary metastases (Figs. 11 and 12). A positive scan is more likely to be procured after removal of the normal thyroid gland or stimulation of metastases by thyrotropic hormone or both. In the patient who has undergone surgical treatment of well-differentiated thyroid cancer and who has no clinical evidence of residual disease, there is no in-

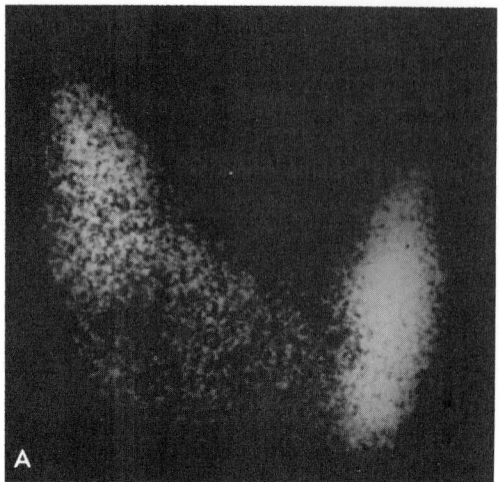
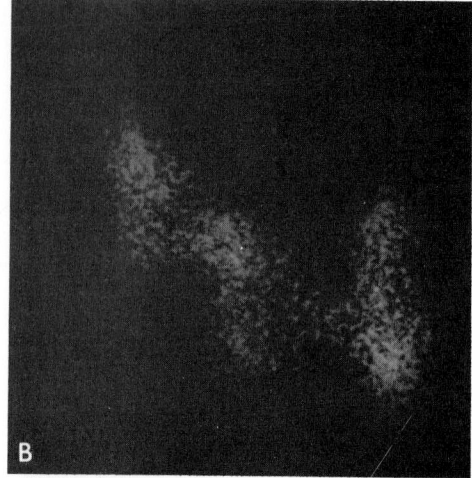

Figure 9. Anteroposterior and oblique photoscans of the thyroid using ^{99m}Tc. A 1 cm. palpable hypofunctioning nodule in the right lobe (*A*) is demonstrated to be nonfunctioning in an oblique view (*B*). This technique has advantages over rectilinear scanning, permitting better appraisal of the intrinsic radioactivity of a nodule.

dication for performing whole-body scanning as a screening procedure.

Ultrasonography. B-mode ultrasonography identifies interfaces between tissues of different densities by measuring the amplitude and timing of echoes reflected from them.[2] A homogeneous liquid within a cystic structure can be distinguished from the surrounding tissue, permitting distinction between thyroid nodules that are solid or cystic in composition (Table 4).[27] Cysts that are "pure" can usually be differentiated from those that have a solid component (mixed). They may present as a painful mass in the thyroid secondary to hemorrhage into an existing nodule or as a "solitary" asymptomatic nodule. Accurate interpretation of echograms requires careful correlation with the patient's history, physical examination, and the radionuclide scan (Fig. 13). The accuracy of diagnosis by echography is estimated to be between 80

and 90 per cent, with areas as small as 1 to 2 mm. being detected.

The incidence of cysts in patients with a solitary thyroid nodule has been reported to be from 7 to 25 per cent.[2, 27] There are insufficient data to give precise figures as to the incidence of cancer in cystic lesions. Since most cysts represent degenerative changes in adenomatous goiter, the incidence of cancer is probably quite low. However, some well-differentiated carcinomas may have a cystic component and may present as a "mixed" cyst.

Needle Biopsy and Identification of Thyroid Disease

Needle biopsy has been advocated as a means of distinguishing between malignant and benign lesions of the thyroid.[16] The limitations of needle biopsy are related primarily to the adequacy of the sample and

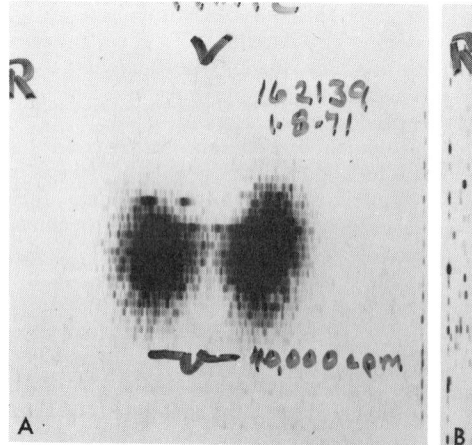
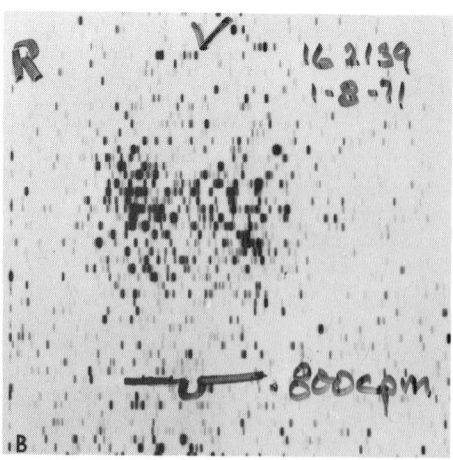

Figure 10. Characteristic scans (*A*, technetium-99m; *B*, ^{75}Se-selenomethionine) in chronic thyroiditis.

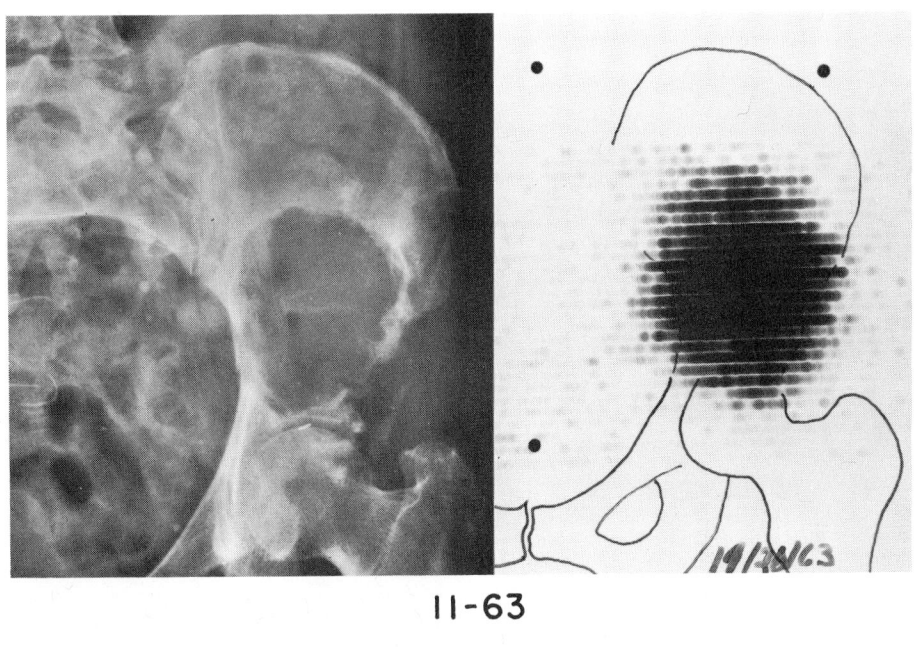

11-63

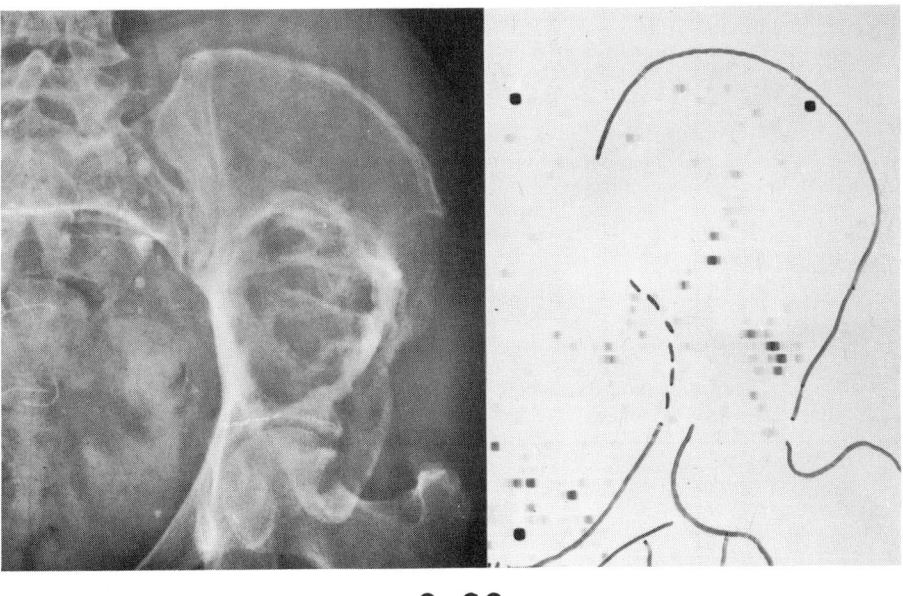

6-66

Figure 11. Follicular adenocarcinoma of the thyroid metastatic to the left ilium with functional autonomy demonstrated by the radioiodide scan. Following therapy with 200 mc. [131]I, there is partial reossification of the osteolytic lesion as well as negligible uptake of radioiodide.

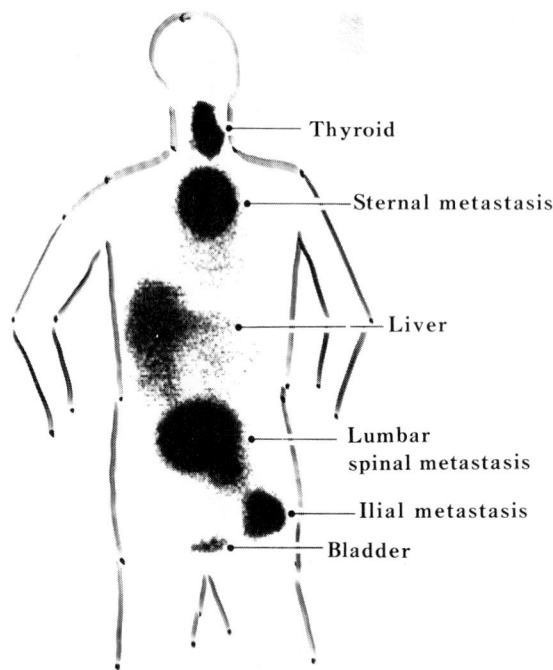

Figure 12. Total-body scan in woman with follicular adenocarcinoma metastatic to sternum, lumbar spine, and left ilium. Scan procured 120 hours after 10 units of TSH and 48 hours after oral administration of 101 mc. ¹³¹I.

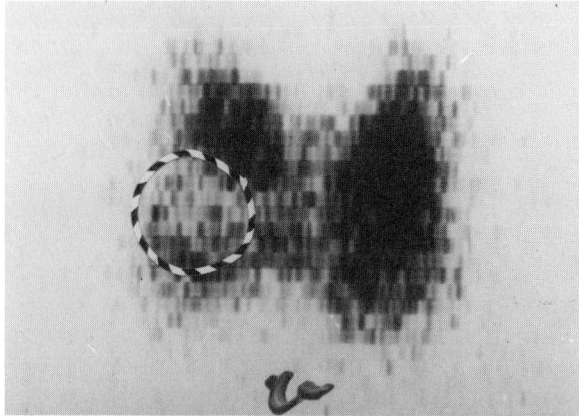

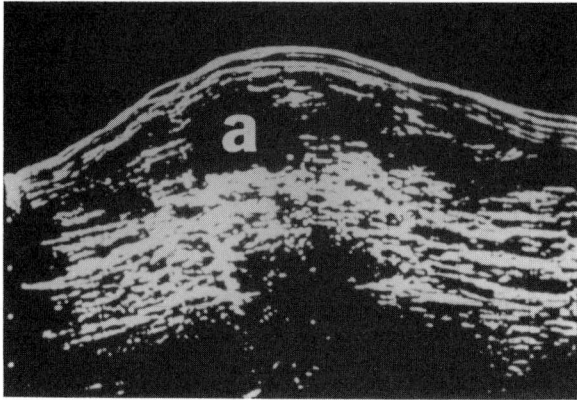

Figure 13. Scanning characteristics and B-mode ultrasonographic findings in a patient with a 3 cm. solitary thyroid nodule. The nodule was nonfunctioning and sonolucent (a) indicating a cystic lesion.

the accuracy of the pathologic diagnosis. The thyroid does not have a homogeneous distribution of disease, and needle biopsy may not be representative. Pathologists may have difficulty in distinguishing between a benign nodule and well-differentiated thyroid carcinoma. Although there has been concern about implanting cancer in the needle tract, this has been an infrequent complication. Needle biopsy is most valuable in confirming the diagnosis of chronic thyroiditis where it has a high degree of sensitivity and specificity. It has a more limited role in older, poor-risk surgical patients with a solitary nodule. A diagnosis of

cancer by needle biopsy is a more conclusive finding than that of an adenoma or adenomatous goiter.

Differential Diagnosis

With asymmetric thyroid enlargement, cancer is suggested by: (1) a history of radiation therapy to head or neck; (2) a history of rapid thyroid enlargement; (3) a hard, fixed mass in the region of the thyroid; (4) evidence of invasion or infiltration of adjacent structures; (5) an immobile vocal cord; (6) discretely enlarged and firm cervical lymph nodes; and (7) an elevated serum thyrocalcitonin level. With such strong evidence of thyroid cancer, only the histologic type and extent of the disease must be determined in order to select the appropriate therapy.

More frequently the patient presents with an asymptomatic unilateral thyroid mass that is considered to be of recent origin. The differential diagnosis includes (1) adenomatous goiter which may be nonfunctioning, hypofunctioning, or normally functioning; (2) adenoma; (3) hyperfunctioning adenoma (autonomously functioning thyroid lesion); (4) cyst; (5) Hashimoto's thyroiditis; (6) granulomatous (subacute) thyroiditis; and (7) thyroid cancers. Knowledge of the natural history of each of these entities, a careful ex-

TABLE 4. Correlation of Echographic and Pathologic Findings in 155 Patients with Thyromegaly*

	Ultrasound			Pathologic Findings		
	Cyst	Solid	Mixed	Cyst	Solid	Mixed
Carcinoma	1	20	2	...	20	4
Adenoma	...	57	1	...	57	1
Cystadenoma	3	2	8	...	...	13
Colloid nodule	1	16	...	...	16	1
Cyst	22	3	...	25	...	...
Thyroiditis	...	7	...	...	7	...
Goiter	...	10	...	...	10	...
Goiter and cyst	2	...	...	2	...	...

*From Rosen, I. E., and Walfish, P. G.: The application of ultrasound to the study of thyroid enlargement. Arch. Surg., 110:940, 1975. Copyright 1975, American Medical Association.

TABLE 5.   Causes of Unilateral Thyroid Enlargement, Selected Laboratory and Clinical Findings

	T_4	^{99}Tc or ^{125}I Scan	Echogram	^{75}Selenomethionine Scan	Consistency	Topography
Adenomatous goiter	N	Hypo-nonfunctioning	Solid	+, −	Soft to firm	Nodule(s)
Cyst	N	Nonfunctioning	Cyst	−	Firm to hard	Nodule
Adenoma	N	Nonfunctioning	Solid	++	Soft to firm	Nodule
Hyperfunctioning adenoma	N–↑	Hyperfunctioning	Solid	−	Firm	Nodule
Well-differentiated carcinoma	N	Nonfunctioning	Solid	++	Firm to hard	Nodule
Undifferentiated carcinoma	N	Nonfunctioning	Solid	+++	Hard	Diffuse involvement
Hashimoto's thyroiditis*	N–↓	Heterogeneous uptake	Solid	+++	Firm (bosselated)	Thyroid lobe
Subacute thyroiditis	N–↑	Hypo-nonfunctioning	Solid	+++	Firm-hard (tender)	Thyroid lobe

*TSH elevated, + thyroglobulin antibodies, P.B.I.-T_4 discrepancy.

amination of the thyroid gland, and appropriate laboratory studies will usually result in a clinical diagnosis more precise than "solitary thyroid nodule" (Table 5).[37] Since adenomatous goiter, the most common cause of thyroid enlargement, has its greatest incidence in women and increases in frequency with age, the younger the patient, particularly if a male, the greater the likelihood of a mass being cancer. A thyroid nodule in a euthyroid child has approximately a 50 per cent chance of being malignant in contrast to approximately a 5 per cent chance in persons in the seventh decade of life.

The natural history of adenomatous goiter and thyroid cancer is of limited value in differentiating between these entities in any one patient. Thyroid scanning with radioiodide (or ^{99m}Tc) and ^{75}Se-selenomethionine helps to differentiate these lesions. Hyperfunctioning nodules may occur in essentially any age group, although they are more frequently found during the third and fourth decades. They are characteristically "hot" on scintiscan, with suppression of radioiodide uptake in the remaining thyroid tissue (see Fig. 1). They may be multiple. The question of treatment is related not so much to the possibility of malignancy as to the natural history of the lesion and its potential for producing hyperthyroidism.

Subacute and Hashimoto's thyroiditis can ordinarily be differentiated by their characteristic clinical picture and laboratory findings (see Fig. 10). Rarely, the clinical course and alteration in thyroid function seen in subacute thyroiditis have been simulated by thyroid cancer.

Thyroid cysts are differentiated from solid nodules by ultrasound studies (Fig. 13). A cyst may be managed by aspiration, with histologic studies of fluid content to determine the presence of an underlying papillary adenocarcinoma. The presence of a mass after aspiration is evidence of a solid cellular component and subsequent treatment should be that of a "cold" solid nodule. Recurrence following aspiration constitutes an indication for excision because of comesis and/or the possibility of an associated neoplasm.

The greatest problem is to differentiate carcinoma of the thyroid from a nonfunctioning adenomatous nodule or an adenoma. Since thyroid enlargement, either diffuse or nodular, that is not due to a primary neoplasm or inflammatory disease probably represents a response of the thyroid to increased TSH, regression of such a goiter may follow the administration of exogenous thyroid hormone. The older the nodule, the less likely it is to respond to TSH withdrawal, because of autonomy or the development of degenerative changes. Regression is unusual in individuals over 40 years. Thus, in a young woman with a solid solitary mass that exhibits some iodide uptake and has no clinical characteristics of malignancy, a trial of suppressive therapy is justified, viz., 75 to 100 μg. of triiodothyronine or 0.2 to 0.3 mg. of thyroxin daily. The administration of triiodothyronine is of some advantage, since adequacy of TSH suppression may be appraised by measuring the fall in serum thyroxin to a hypothyroid range. About 10 to 15 per cent of goiters of this type will respond with complete resolution. Unless regression is complete within 6 months, cancer must be excluded by surgical excision.[37]

Patients in the older age group with a multinodular goiter may be difficult to evaluate, since calcification, fibrosis, and nonfunction are common. There is rarely change in size of the thyroid following suppressive therapy except that the nodules become more apparent (Fig. 14). A history of rapid growth of the gland, with changes in physical characteristics and topography, as well as the absence of function, is suggestive of a malignant neoplasm and the need for surgical removal.

Patients with a history of exposure to thyroid irradiation should have a careful examination of the thyroid gland, a thyroid scan, serum thyroid hormone and TSH levels, and thyroglobulin determinations. The scan serves primarily as a basis for subsequent evaluation. A palpable mass warrants a surgical approach similar to that in other patients with a solitary thyroid nodule. An abnormal scan in the absence of a palpable mass is not an indication for thyroidectomy. Patients without positive physical findings are observed. Although TSH suppression is logical, there are no data indicating that this will reduce the incidence of thyroid carcinoma. Suppressive therapy seems most appropriate in those patients with an elevated TSH level. The peak incidence of radiation-associated thyroid cancer is from 10 to 20 years. Carcinoma occurring as late as 30 years after exposure has been reported.

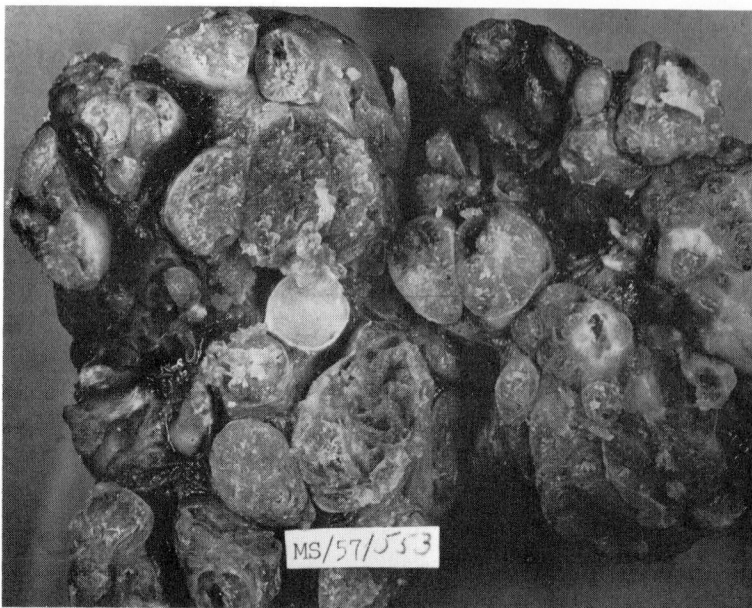

Figure 14. Gross findings in a patient with a multinodular goiter who had been given suppressive therapy for three years. There was regression of normal thyroid parenchyma and persistence of the adenomatous goiter (follicular adenoma, cyst formation, and degenerative changes are evident).

Metastatic carcinoma occasionally involves the thyroid, masquerading as a primary cancer or nodular goiter. Involvement of the thyroid is usually indicative of widespread metastatic disease. Rarely is the thyroid the sole site of metastasis. When particular attention has been paid to the thyroid in patients dying of metastatic malignant disease, the incidence of thyroid metastases has varied from 3.9 to 24 per cent.[31] The most common primary neoplasm having metastases to the thyroid is carcinoma of the kidney, followed in frequency by neoplasms of the gastrointestinal tract, lung, and breast.

MANAGEMENT

ADENOMATOUS GOITER, ADENOMA, AND HYPERFUNCTIONING ADENOMA

The management of adenomatous goiter based on an understanding of its pathogenesis should be one of prophylaxis. During that phase of the disorder when the gland becomes diffusely enlarged and when the adenomatous changes are still dependent on TSH stimulation, regression of the goiter follows suppressive treatment with full replacement doses of thyroid hormone, e.g., thyroxin, 0.2 to 0.3 mg. daily, or triiodothyronine, 75 to 100 μg. daily. Failure of regression of a uninodular mass is an indication for surgical excision to distinguish the lesion from invasive cancer. Differentiation of highly cellular follicular adenomas from follicular adenocarcinoma, which may have similar clinical as well as scanning characteristics, can be made only histologically. When the adenomatous goiter is removed, the underlying pathogenic mechanisms remain. With a life expectancy of more than 10 to 15 years, the patient who is untreated has a 10 to 15 per cent chance of developing a recurrent adenoma-

tous goiter.[20] To prevent this, permanent thyroid hormone replacement is necessary.

Surgical removal of a nontoxic multinodular goiter is performed primarily for the relief of pressure symptoms, respiratory tract obstruction, or dysphagia, or for cosmetic reasons. Less frequently multinodular goiter is removed because it is producing hyperthyroidism or because of the possibility of carcinoma. Because of the slowly progressing enlargement of the goiter with the gradual encroachment upon the airway, symptoms may develop insidiously and considerable tracheal compression may exist by the time the patient seeks medical consultation. Narrowing of the trachea may interfere with pulmonary drainage, predisposing to the retention of bronchial secretions and intercurrent respiratory tract infections. Most of these patients with goiters of many years' duration have pathologic changes that are no longer dependent upon continued thyrotropic stimulus, representing the end result of such stimulation. Therefore, withdrawal of thyrotropic stimulation by the administration of thyroid hormone is unsuccessful in causing regression of these goiters of long duration, which are present most often in the older age group (see Fig. 14).

There is little justification for the prophylactic removal of nodular goiter to preclude the development of thyroid cancer. The mortality rate of thyroidectomy is from 0.1 to 0.5 per cent, or 1 to 5 deaths per thousand. The risk of cancer and cancer deaths in patients with multinodular goiter is similar. The available data do not indicate that prophylactic thyroidectomy should be done for all multinodular goiters for either theoretical or practical reasons.[39]

There have been relatively few long-term observations on the natural history of hyperfunctioning nodules (autonomously functioning thyroid lesions).[39] Hyperfunctioning nodules sometimes regress spontaneously, probably representing hemorrhage into the acellular stroma. The chief indication for treatment is related to the propensity of the patient to develop hyperthyroidism. Consideration must be given to size of the lesion (lesions less than 3 cm. are rarely associated with hyperthyroidism), the life expectancy of the patient, and the practicability of periodic observation of the patient to detect evidence of hyperthyroidism. In general, the larger the mass and the younger the patient, the more warranted is surgical excision. Euthyroid patients in the older age group with small nodules (less than 2 cm.) may be observed, remembering the possibility that these patients may eventually develop hyperthyroidism. Radioiodide has been used as therapy, but in patients with a life expectancy of more than 20 years it is not recommended because of (a) the unpredictability of the dosage, (b) the mass remaining in the thyroid, and (c) the effect of irradiation on the remaining thyroid parenchyma. Rarely, a hyperfunctioning nodule is functioning cancer.

THYROID CANCER

The objective of surgical treatment in a patient in whom a clinical diagnosis of thyroid cancer has been made is to establish the diagnosis and to completely excise the neoplasm, with preservation of parathyroid function and without injuring the recurrent laryngeal nerves. Consideration needs to be given to the biologic behavior that characterizes the different types of thyroid cancer, i.e., the indolent growth of occult sclerosing papillary cancer; the more aggressive behavior of medullary carcinoma, with its multiple sites of involvement and predilection for dissemination to cervical lymph node; and the rapid extension and poor prognosis of the undifferentiated cancers. The operation performed should be selected with these characteristics in mind and on the basis of the extent of the disease. In patients succumbing to this disease, one third die because of persistent or recurrent disease in the neck. Every effort should be made to remove the tumor from about the trachea at the initial operation. Recurrent disease in cervical lymph nodes more readily lends itself to excision at a second operation.

In the removal of a solitary mass confined to one lobe of the thyroid, incisional biopsy or enucleation of the nodule is to be condemned because of the danger of tumor dissemination as well as the possibility of providing the pathologist with an inadequate specimen. Complete lobectomy with removal of pericapsular lymph nodes and preservation of the recurrent laryngeal nerve is the procedure of choice. The lesion should be examined for gross (invasion) and microscopic (frozen section) evidence of cancer. Differentiation of benign from malignant lesions may also be facilitated by determining the ratio between radioiodide content of the thyroid "tumor" and that of normal paranodular parenchyma.[9] In the event of a benign lesion, i.e., adenomatous goiter, adenoma, or thyroiditis, no further surgery is indicated. The desirability of supplemental thyroid hormone to reduce the incidence of the disease in the opposite lobe should be considered.

A pathologic diagnosis of "cancer" of the thyroid should be regarded as unacceptable. The surgeon and pathologist should make every effort to further categorize the lesion in order to plan the most appropriate treatment.

Occult sclerosing papillary adenocarcinoma as well as encapsulated follicular adenocarcinoma is treated by lobectomy with removal of a margin of normal thyroid parenchyma at the isthmus or medial portion of the contralateral lobe. Frequently, follicular adenocarcinoma cannot be readily differentiated at the time of operation from its benign counterpart, "follicular adenoma." However, if the lesion is found to be encapsulated on gross and microscopic examination and there is no evidence of involvement of regional lymph nodes as determined by careful appraisal at the time of surgery, a subsequent diagnosis of follicular adenocarcinoma based upon evidence of vascular and capsular invasion is not an indication for additional surgery. The prognosis of these patients following lobectomy is excellent.

Invasive papillary-follicular carcinomas of the thyroid more often exhibit gross evidence of infiltration at the site of origin and involve the opposite lobe, as manifested by multifocal sites of carcinoma.[28] In addition, there is a higher incidence of cervical lymph node metastases. Because of these characteristics, which can usually be determined in the operating theater, a lobectomy on the side of the primary lesion and a near-total thyroidectomy on the contralateral side is recommended. The parathyroid glands on the contralateral side should be identified and an adequate blood supply maintained by preserving the posterior capsule of the lobe. Attention to this point in technique will usually prevent the development of postoperative hypoparathyroidism.

The indication for removal of cervical lymph nodes is the presence of metastatic cancer. Knowledge of common routes of lymphatic flow facilitates inspection at operation of the appropriate lymph nodes (Fig. 15). Carcinoma of the thyroid is unique in that routes of lymphatic drainage are singularly available for examination at the time of removal of the primary tumor. The extent of the neck dissection will depend upon the magnitude of node involvement as well as the location of the primary lesion. In those neoplasms arising from the inferior pole without capsular invasion, and with two or three lymph node metastases along the recurrent laryngeal nerve and no evidence of enlarged lymph nodes along the course of the midjugular or inferior jugular chain, excision of pretracheal areolar tissue as well as of the lymphatic tissue along the recurrent nerve is indicated. More extensive involvement of lymph nodes along the internal jugular vein requires a modified type of neck dissection, with removal of lymphatic drainage peculiar to the thyroid (Fig. 15). Excision of extensively involved nodes along the internal jugular vein can be done more completely by removal of the vein. Unless the sternocleidomastoid muscle is involved by direct extension, it can be preserved along with the eleventh nerve. The deformity-producing type of radical neck dissection so necessary for cancer of the larynx, tongue, or floor of the mouth is not required for the removal of cancerous lymph nodes involved in well-differentiated carcinoma of the thyroid.

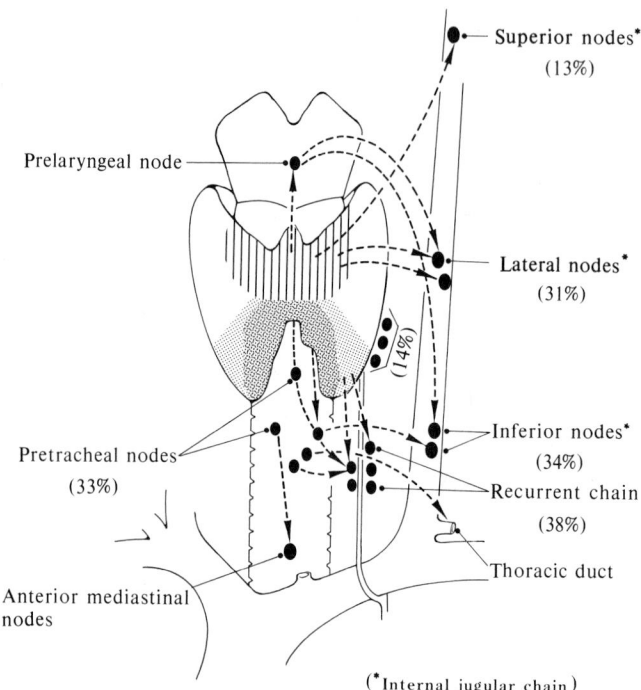

Superior nodes*
(13%)

Prelaryngeal node

Lateral nodes*
(31%)

(14%)

Inferior nodes*
(34%)

Pretracheal nodes
(33%)

Recurrent chain
(38%)

Thoracic duct

Anterior mediastinal
nodes

(*Internal jugular chain)

Figure 15. Routes of lymphatic flow and sites of metastasis in 52 patients with metastases from well-differentiated adenocarcinoma of the thyroid.

Massive involvement of cervical lymph nodes is occasionally associated with extension to mediastinal lymph nodes. The question arises as to the advisability of extending the node dissection to include the mediastinum. Superior mediastinal node dissection is indicated only in patients with well-differentiated tumors when all the cancer can be removed from the neck, there are no distant metastases, and the patient is a good surgical risk with a life expectancy of at least 10 years. At present there is insufficient clinical experience to evaluate the effect of this procedure on survival. Mediastinal metastases from well-differentiated thyroid cancer are infrequent. In the author's experience, mediastinotomy has been carried out in less than 1 per cent of patients operated upon for thyroid cancer. Mediastinal node dissection for treatment of poorly differentiated thyroid cancer is not indicated.

Papillary adenocarcinomas of the thyroid have been reported in thyroglossal duct cysts. These rare lesions have a sex and age distribution similar to that of well-differentiated papillary-follicular carcinoma arising in the thyroid gland. The diagnosis is usually made on pathologic examination of the surgical specimen. The principles of treatment are the same as for a comparable neoplasm arising in the thyroid, viz., complete excision of the thyroglossal duct mass and of the regional lymph nodes when involved.[22]

Medullary (solid) carcinoma of the thyroid with amyloid occupies an intermediate position, between well-differentiated and undifferentiated thyroid cancer, with regard to prognosis. Because of the propensity for multicentric involvement and metastases to cervical lymph nodes, the same general principles apply in its management as for invasive papillary or follicular adenocarcinoma.

Undifferentiated carcinoma of the thyroid is frequently so extensive at the time of diagnosis that only biopsy is indicated. However, when the lesion is grossly confined to the primary site, with or without extension to regional nodes, the results of an aggressive surgical attack, though poor, warrant thyroidectomy and a radical neck dissection.[34] The objective is to remove as much gross neoplasm as possible without injuring the recurrent nerves or producing hypoparathyroidism. The effectiveness of postoperative irradiation and/or chemotherapy is enhanced by following this recommendation.[12] Because of the propensity for undifferentiated carcinomas to invade the trachea,[30] every effort should be made to remove all of the neoplasm from about the trachea at the initial operation.

Technical Considerations in Surgical Management of Thyroid Cancer

Operations upon the thyroid gland are best performed with general endotracheal anesthesia. If the goiter is large and causes tracheal deviation or compression, manipulation of the gland at operation may further compromise the tracheal lumen and an endotracheal tube will insure an adequate airway. Special attention should be given the patient with a large cervical, substernal, or retrotracheal goiter whose airway may be compromised. In order to avoid further tracheal compression or laryngospasm during induction, sedatives should not be administered to the patient until he is under the direct observation of the anesthesiologist, and intubation should be done with topical anesthesia while the patient is awake. In the poor-risk patient, thyroidectomy may be performed very satisfactorily with bilateral deep cervical block. Here again, however, insertion of an endotracheal tube under topical anesthesia may be necessary.

A low collar incision with reflection of platysma superiorly to the hyoid and inferiorly to the manubrium permits separation of the strap muscles in the midline to expose the underlying thyroid gland. Appropriate retraction of the strap and the sternocleidomastoid muscles will disclose the middle thyroid vein(s), which is ligated and divided. The inferior thyroid artery is identified inferior to this vein. The recurrent nerve is visualized in the neck at the tracheal-esophageal groove well below the lower pole of the thyroid.* The recurrent nerve(s) is visualized throughout its course. It can almost always be dissected free from an overlying tumor within the thyroid. Direct invasion, however, does constitute an indication for its excision with the primary tumor.

Following division of the inferior thyroid veins, the lobe can be rotated medially to expose the recurrent laryngeal nerve, which is freed from the overlying thyroid gland by sharp dissection. Parathyroid gland(s) that can be identified and is extracapsular should be gently dissected from the thyroid, with preservation of its blood supply. Juxtacapsular lymph nodes should be removed in conjunction with the lobe. Identification of the superior pole vessels is facilitated by dividing the suspensory ligament of Berry, separating the superior thyroid artery and vein from the adjacent cricothyroid muscle so as to avoid injury to the external branch of the superior laryngeal nerve. Dissection of the superior pole of the thyroid at a level above the cricothyroid articulation avoids injury to the recurrent nerve, which enters the larynx posterior to this point.

Following identification of the recurrent nerve and ligation of the superior thyroid artery and vein and penetrating branches of the inferior thyroid artery, the lobe is removed from its fascial attachment to the trachea by sharp dissection so as to bare the underlying trachea and its investing fascia. The dissection is carried medially to include the pyramidal lobe and the isthmus of the thyroid.

Hemostasis is achieved with fine silk and the wound is closed with the same. Suction catheters or Penrose drains may be employed if there is considerable "dead space" or if the wound is not completely dry.

Near-total to total thyroidectomy is accomplished by carrying out a comparable procedure on the contralateral side. Unless there is gross involvement of the posterior aspect of the opposite lobe, a near-total thyroidectomy with preservation of the posterior capsule of the thyroid in the region of the parathyroids is advocated in order to lower the incidence of postoperative hypoparathyroidism.[4, 13] If parathyroid glands are excised they should be cut into 1 mm. pieces and individually implanted into pectoral or forearm muscles.

---

*On the right side, because of the anomalous origin of the right subclavian artery from a persistent sixth aortic arch, in approximately 1 per cent of patients it will arise directly from the vagus at the level of the cricothyroid articulation.

Complications of Surgical Management of Thyroid Cancer

The complications of radical thyroid surgery are related to those of operations about the head and neck, e.g., obstruction of the airway, postoperative bleeding, pneumomediastinum and pneumothorax, injury to phrenic nerve or cervical sympathetics, thoracic duct fistula, and those peculiar to the thyroid, viz., injury to the recurrent laryngeal nerve and parathyroid insufficiency. In general, these complications are infrequent and radical surgery is quite safe.[13]

Postoperative Hemorrhage. Arterial hemorrhage into the operative wound, though rare, constitutes a serious complication, since the resulting tracheal compression may produce asphyxia. It is manifested by obvious swelling of the wound or the complaint of dyspnea. The skin and fascial layers of the wound should be opened and the hematoma immediately evacuated, sometimes at the bedside. Hemostasis is secured under appropriate operative conditions. Rarely is a tracheostomy indicated if the hematoma has been properly evacuated. Venous bleeding is more gradual in onset and less likely to compromise the airway.

Recurrent Nerve Paralysis. Near-total or total thyroidectomy requires identification of both recurrent laryngeal nerves from well below the thyroid to the point at which they pass beneath the cricothyroid articulation to enter the larynx. There may be direct invasion by cancer, or temporary postoperative paresis may follow overzealous dissection, exposure, and manipulation of the nerve(s) by the surgeon. With injury to the laryngeal nerves, the vocal cords are ordinarily found in one of two positions, midline or cadaveric. The latter implies a position midway between the midline and the position of extreme abduction. If only one recurrent nerve is paralyzed, the cord occupies the midline position in most instances. Unilateral recurrent nerve injury, although it may result in permanent hoarseness, is usually well tolerated. Unless there are other factors compromising the airway, it does not ordinarily require tracheostomy. Damage to both recurrent laryngeal nerves produces airway obstruction and is an indication for tracheostomy.

Additional difficulty in the immediate postoperative period may be anticipated if the superior laryngeal nerve has also been damaged. Besides being responsible for adduction of the cords by innervating the arytenoid and cricothyroid muscles, the superior laryngeal nerve supplies sensation to the larynx and pyriform sinus. This loss of sensation increases the chance of aspiration.

Hypoparathyroidism. Implicit in the performance of total thyroidectomy for thyroid cancer is the preservation of one or more parathyroid glands with an intact blood supply provided by the inferior thyroid artery. Deliberate sacrifice of all parathyroid tissue is unwarranted. The incidence of hypoparathyroidism is variable, ranging from a negligible incidence after near-total thyroidectomy to 12.5 per cent after total thyroidectomy.[13] Acute hypoparathyroidism is not difficult to recognize and manage; however, chronic hypoparathyroidism, if uncontrolled or unrecognized, may be associated with serious sequelae such as cataracts, convulsions, mental deterioration, or psychosis.

Parathyroid insufficiency may be either transient or permanent. It is usually manifested 24 to 72 hours after surgery, but occasionally 5 to 7 days may elapse before symptoms present themselves. The time of onset of symptoms may not necessarily be related to the severity or permanency of the hypoparathyroidism. A positive Chvostek sign (provided it was absent preoperatively) commonly precedes other symptoms and findings. This may be the only manifestation of minor and usually transient degrees of parathyroid insufficiency. Hypocalcemia should also be suspected when paresthesias involve fingers, toes, or the circumoral region. A positive Trousseau sign usually indicates a more serious degree of hypocalcemia and the need for therapy.

For immediate treatment of tetany or severe symptoms or findings, intravenous calcium gluconate (10 to 20 ml. of a 10 per cent solution) is given. For more continuous therapy, 20 to 40 ml. of this solution in a liter of 0.9 per cent saline or 5 per cent dextrose may be given until symptoms and signs have abated. As soon as the patient can take oral medication, vitamin D_2 should be started at 50,000 to 150,000 units per day in conjunction with calcium by mouth (calcium lactate powder, 12 to 25 gm. per day or calcium carbonate—Titralac—9 tablets per day). Chronic hypocalcemia may be followed by opacity of the lens in as short a period as 2 to 3 weeks. Consequently, it is mandatory that adequate treatment not merely render the patient asymptomatic, but restore serum calcium levels to normal.

Postoperative Management of Thyroid Cancer

Any patient operated upon for thyroid carcinoma should be given thyroid hormone in dosage sufficient to maintain him in a euthyroid state. This prevents the development of hypothyroidism and also may play a role in minimizing or controlling recurrent disease in patients with well-differentiated lesions. TSH suppression may also reduce the chance that a well-differentiated cancer will progress to one that is poorly differentiated. Evaluation with radioiodide scintiscan in the immediate postoperative period will identify any remaining remnant of thyroid, whether in the region of the posterior capsule, pyramidal lobe, or superior pole, and provides an important baseline for future evaluation of recurrent disease.

The use of ^{131}I has been recommended following surgical removal of thyroid cancer.[17] However, there is no justification for its prophylactic use because of the good results from surgical treatment and the potential hazards related to radioiodide. Iodine-131 should be reserved for recurrent tumors that are autonomous and unresectable, and cannot be controlled by hormonal suppression.[34] After surgical excision of thyroid carcinoma, reevaluation for evidence of recurrent disease should be performed at periodic intervals, viz., 6 to 12 months. Particular attention is directed to the most likely sites of recurrence—neck, cervical lymph nodes, and lungs. Because a thyroid carcinoma may change its biologic characteristics, the functional status of recurrent cancer should be determined by radioiodide scintiscan.

Recurrence of undifferentiated carcinoma of the neck is most often extranodal and can rarely be excised. Such patients are candidates for external irradiation and/or chemotherapy.[12]

Since patients treated for thyroid carcinoma are frequently in the childbearing age, the question arises as to whether pregnancy is deleterious. There is no evidence at present that pregnancy changes the course of the disease.

Recurrent Disease. Carcinoma of the thyroid possesses biologic characteristics that merit special emphasis when considering palliative treatment or management of recurrent disease. The well-known propensity of certain types of tumor to invade locally, and for others to metastasize to regional lymph nodes, bone, or lung, influences the type of treatment that is indicated. Palliative therapy should be considered only when the primary tumor and regional lymph nodes cannot be surgically removed from the neck and upper mediastinum or when there are metastatic deposits elsewhere in the body. However, thyroid cancer is unique in that there are patients who, despite fairly widespread incurable disease, may with appropriate therapy have a life expectancy approaching that of the normal population.[4, 34] Consequently, the presence of pulmonary or bony metastases or both does not necessarily signify short survival or even contradict a surgical attack on the primary tumor. In fact, removal of the primary tumor and involved cervical lymph nodes may not only prevent death from local invasion and tracheal compression but also facilitate the management of distant metastatic disease.

One or more of the following measures may be employed in the management of patients with recurrent or persistent disease that is not amenable to complete excision: (1) thyrotropin suppression; (2) radioiodide therapy; (3) tracheostomy; (4) external irradiation; and (5) chemotherapy. The first two measures are based upon the unique biologic characteristics of thyroid cancer, viz., the retention of sufficient function by the tumor to trap and organify iodides, and the dependency of certain thyroid tumors upon trophic hormones for genesis, growth, and progression. Both of these characteristics may be utilized in the management of well-differentiated thyroid cancer.[33] Irradiation and chemotherapy may be indicated in selected patients. Undifferentiated thyroid cancer is best palliated by irradiation and chemotherapy.[12] Finally, because of the propensity of thyroid cancer to obstruct the trachea by invasion or compression, tracheostomy has a definite role in palliative care.

Thyrotropin Suppression and Radioiodide Therapy. Because of the demonstrated role that thyrotropin plays in the genesis of some thyroid neoplasms, it has seemed logical to attempt control of inoperable thyroid cancer by suppressing the output of thyrotropin.[6, 33, 34] By exploiting the feedback mechanism that regulates the output of thyrotropin and thyroxin, the output of thyrotropin can be effectively suppressed by the administration of exogenous thyroid hormone. L-Triiodothyronine or its equivalent is administered by mouth to tolerance, i.e., approximately 100 to 150 μg. daily. Most patients tolerate 100 μg. of triiodothyronine without symptoms of hyperthyroidism and many can be maintained at levels of 150 μg. daily. In patients who are being treated by thyrotropin suppression, periodic evaluation of the extent of the disease should be done by measuring serum thyroxin and TSH and performing a radioiodide uptake and scintiscan.

The most important complication of such treatment is factitious hyperthyroidism. The adequacy of thyrotropin suppression is established by measuring ^{131}I uptake, TSH, and the fall in endogenous secretion of thyroxin.

Therapy of inoperable metastatic thyroid cancer by means of thyrotropin suppression is particularly applicable to (1) patients in the younger age groups in whom tumor growth is likely to be indolent and in whom the genetic and functional hazards of intensive radioiodide therapy are considerably greater than in older patients; (2) patients harboring neoplasms with considerable mass or with extensive pulmonary involvement in whom large amounts of radioiodide would be required or in whom radioiodide therapy might be followed by pulmonary fibrosis; and (3) patients with well-differentiated neoplasms in whom there is insufficient uptake of radioiodide. The responsiveness of the neoplasm may be measured by a decrease in size of a palpable mass and radiologic regression or disappearance of pulmonary or bony metastases (Fig. 16). Symptomatic relief from pain and recovery of neurologic deficits may also be useful

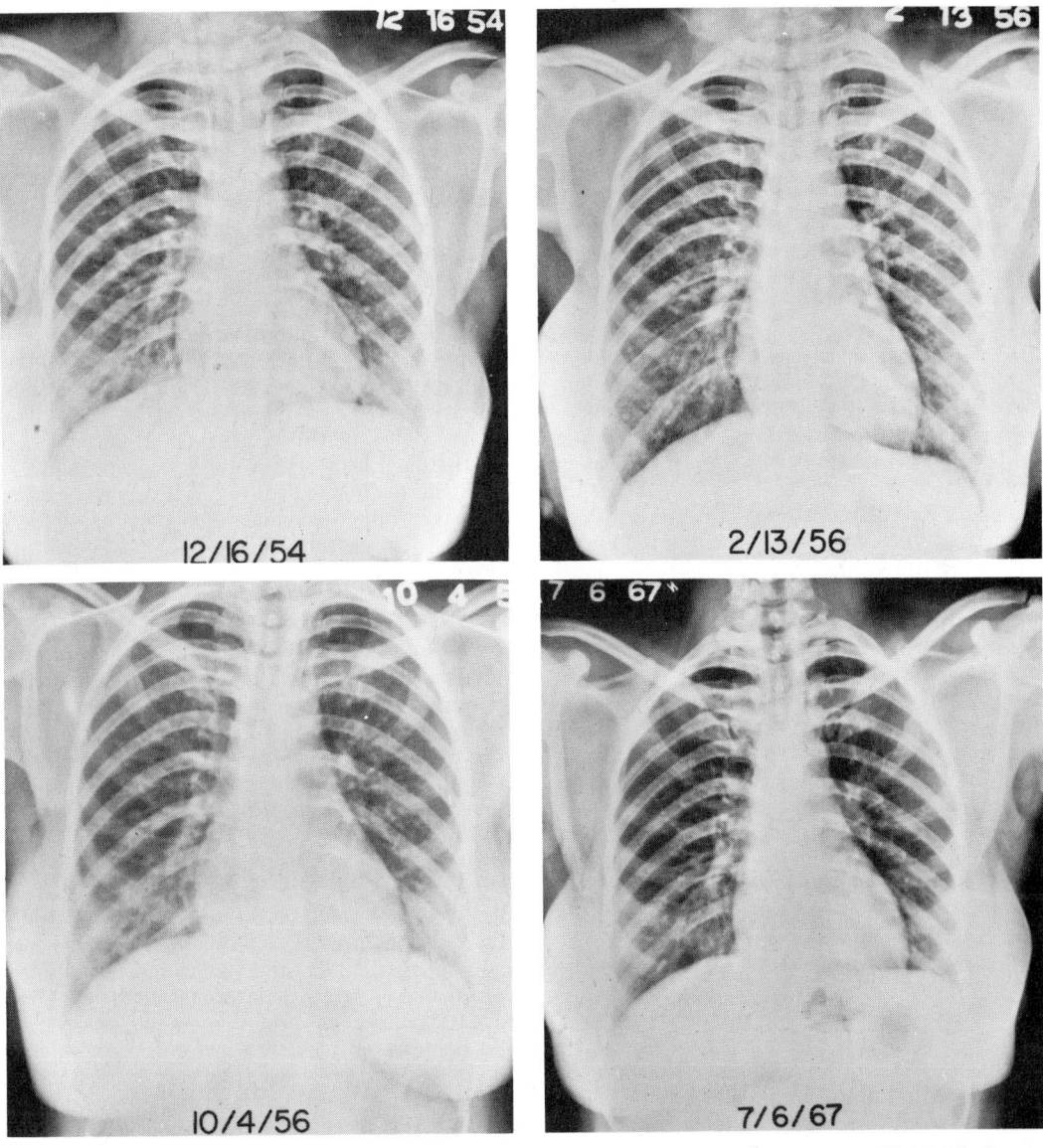

Figure 16.   Chest roentgenograms demonstrating bilateral diffuse lower lobe metastases which concentrated [131]I (12/54). These metastases regressed following suppressive therapy with desiccated thyroid (2/56), and then recurred in association with a period of hypothyroidism (10/56). The metastases again regressed following therapy with triiodothyronine. The patient has remained asymptomatic with essentially a normal chest x-ray on 125 μg. of triiodothyronine daily (7/67).

guides. Assuming that adequate doses of thyroid hormone are given, the dependent status of thyroid cancer can usually be determined within 3 to 6 months. This is a relatively brief period in the life of most well-differentiated thyroid cancers. In addition to the author's own experience,[33] Crile has noted that most of the papillary carcinomas and some encapsulated angioinvasive carcinomas and follicular adenocarcinomas have responded to administration of desiccated thyroid by cessation of growth or regression. Others, however, have observed recurrent disease in a number of patients despite the prophylactic administration of thyroid hormone.

A lack of response to thyrotropin suppression does not contraindicate subsequent attempts at treatment with radioiodide, since lesions may exhibit considerable dichotomy between growth and function. Function may be inhibited without comparable regression in growth, and tumors may have autonomy of both function and growth. Autonomously functioning metastases may grow during the administration of more than adequate replacement doses of thyroid hormone, and collect sufficient ^{131}I to make treatment with the same feasible (see Fig. 11).

Radioactive iodine has been extensively used during the past two decades in the treatment of thyroid cancer. Although occasionally dramatic effects have been obtained, in general the results have been disappointing. Because of the radiation hazards, particularly in childhood and in the reproductive period, radioiodide therapy should be used only when less noxious methods are ineffective. In general, radioiodide treatment should be reserved for (1) patients with functioning tumors in whom thyrotropin suppression has failed to cause cessation or regression of growth; (2) patients in whom there is autonomy of function, which may be manifested by associated hyperthyroidism or inability of thyrotropin inhibition to suppress function; (3) older patients with functioning tumors in whom the lesions are likely to be more aggressive and in whom some of the radiation hazards are less important; and (4) patients with rapidly progressive lesions in whom greater risks are warranted in an effort to control the disease.

As already indicated, patients who are candidates for therapy with radioiodide harbor neoplasms that may be controlled by thyrotropin suppression. These two forms of therapy may sometimes be used simultaneously with a complementary effect.

Tracheostomy.   Tracheal obstruction is a relatively common cause of demise from thyroid cancer. Tracheostomy may be beneficial not merely to prolong life, but also to enable the patient to live more comfortably during his remaining months or years. The caliber of the normal trachea provides a large reserve airway. Symptoms are not usually present unless there is a reduction of at least 75 per cent. Tracheostomy is indicated when there is sufficient compromise of the tracheal lumen to result in labored breathing or stridor. In patients without symptoms, laminograms of the trachea or a laryngogram may be helpful in delineating the relative constriction of the larynx or trachea. Prophylactic tracheostomy may be indicated if a patient with a narrowed tracheal lumen is to un-

dergo radiation therapy, since the lumen may be further compromised by local edema and slough of neoplastic cells that have invaded the trachea.

Hypophysectomy and Pituitary Stalk Section.   The biologic characteristics of thyroid cancer suggest that surgical ablation of pituitary function might be effective treatment. However, since thyrotropin suppression can be readily accomplished by the administration of exogenous thyroid hormone, hypophysectomy and pituitary stalk section are unnecessarily hazardous. Furthermore, in those few patients in whom it has been performed, the benefits have not been striking.

External Irradiation in the Management of Thyroid Cancer.   As has been indicated, surgery is the primary treatment for cancer of the thyroid. Well-differentiated thyroid cancer (papillary or follicular or both) is somewhat similar to normal thyroid tissue in its insensitivity to external irradiation. When all gross neoplasm has been removed from the neck, radiotherapy as an adjunct to the surgical treatment of this type of thyroid cancer to eliminate remaining microscopic neoplasm is of no benefit. However, external irradiation may have a palliative role in those well-differentiated lesions, primary or recurrent, not amenable to management by surgical excision, thyrotropin suppression, or radioiodide. In view of the aforementioned relative radioresistance of this type of neoplasm, a small amount of tissue enabling the administration of a higher radiation dose is preferable. External irradiation plays a primary role in the management of patients with poorly differentiated cancers. These lesions are frequently so extensive that they cannot be removed by surgery. Control of the massive infiltrating tumors of this type is difficult. With the use of orthovoltage therapy, skin tolerance was formerly a limiting factor, as was previous surgery, which enhanced the propensity for postirradiation induration, necrosis, and subcutaneous fibrosis. Tracheal and laryngeal reactions also constituted limitations. The availability of newer methods of irradiation (linear accelerator, cobalt) has changed the outlook considerably and enabled the interstitial radiation dose to be much greater without causing the reactions cited above. Poorly differentiated thyroid cancers (small cell, giant cell) vary considerably in their radiosensitivity. Small cell carcinoma has responded so favorably in some series as to raise the question whether the lesion was a lymphoma rather than carcinoma.

Lymphoma of the thyroid, when confined to the thyroid gland, is ordinarily treated by total thyroidectomy. Any lymphoma of the thyroid should be carefully and completely evaluated for other sites of involvement, and the surgical bed and adjacent uninvolved lymph node areas should be prophylactically irradiated.

Chemotherapy.   There is limited experience in the management of thyroid cancer by chemotherapeutic agents. Since papillary and follicular tumors in general have a metabolism comparable to that of normal thyroid tissue, they are not particularly sensitive to the currently available carcinolytic drugs. Furthermore, these tumors are best handled by the means already described. Treatment of the more aggressive solid and anaplastic tumors is in keeping with cancer chemotherapy in general.[12]

PROGNOSIS IN THYROID CANCER

Prognosis in carcinoma of the thyroid is a function of the biologic characteristics of the neoplasm, with several factors playing important roles: (1) histology; (2) sex; (3) age of patient; (4) size of tumor; (5) encapsulation; (6) extent of disease; i.e., parenchymal and extracapsular invasion, lymph node and systemic metastases; and (7) treatment (Figs. 17 and 18).[1, 34]

The microscopic anatomy of a well-differentiated thyroid cancer (papillary-follicular carcinoma) does not in itself indicate whether it will behave as an indolent or highly invasive and rapidly growing lesion. Age, sex, tumor size, and extent of disease are other important prognostic factors. However, an anaplastic histologic pattern, whether present in all or in a portion of the neoplasm, is almost always associated with a poor prognosis.

The influence of sex and age, perhaps reflecting the endocrine and immune status of a patient, is clearly seen in well-differentiated adenocarcinomas. Such cancers arising in the female below the age of 40 are associated with a near-normal life expectancy (Figs. 5 and 17). It is therefore difficult to evaluate the role of surgical treatment in these patients. In contrast, well-differentiated tumors arising in the male or female over the age of 40 are more aggressive and associated with a shorter life expectancy. Buckwalter observed a survival rate of 60 per cent at 20 years for women (mean age 44.4), as compared with 20 per cent for men (mean age 46.8). Similarly, a survival rate of 55 per cent was noted at 20 years for patients below 40 and 22 per cent for those over 40 years of age.[4] Age and sex did not seem to influence the course of patients with undifferentiated cancer.[34]

Occult papillary carcinoma, even with lymph node metastases, is associated with an excellent survival.

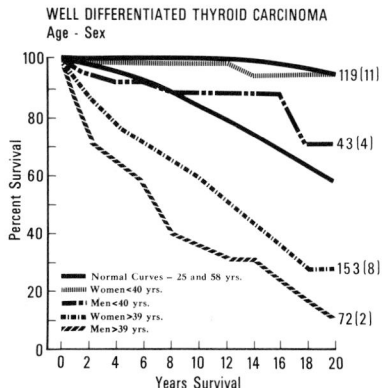

Figure 17. Effect of age and sex on survivorship in thyroid cancer.

Most of these tumors also arise in the female in the younger age group. Similarly, the smaller the primary tumor, the better the prognosis.[18]

The extent of disease, as indicated by "encapsulation" in contrast to invasion of thyroid parenchyma by the primary tumor with lymph node and systemic metastases, also relates to survival. Malignant lesions that are grossly well circumscribed with an apparent capsule may differ little on gross examination from their benign counterpart, follicular adenoma. The differential diagnosis is made by the histologic findings of capsular and vascular invasion. Such tumors, although pathologically possessing the criteria of malignancy, are more likely to behave clinically as benign lesions and are associated with a normal life expectancy.[1] However, those follicular carcinomas that clearly exhibit gross parenchymatous invasion, those with extensive vascular invasion, and most papillary carcinomas that have extended beyond the thyroid all have a poorer prognosis.[4]

The impact of various forms of surgical treatment on survival is difficult to evaluate. This is particularly true with regard to radical thyroidectomy and prophy-

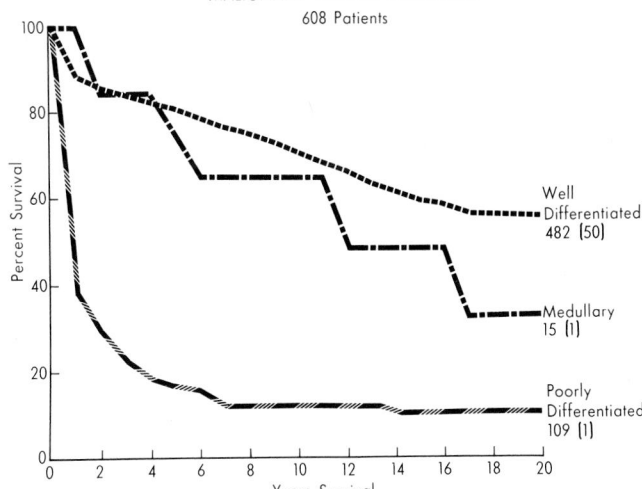

Figure 18. Survival curves of patients with well and poorly differentiated and medullary thyroid malignancies.

lactic node dissection. In well-differentiated tumors that are confined to the site of origin in the thyroid without extension to regional lymph nodes, there are no differences in survival in patients treated by partial thyroidectomy, lobectomy, and total thyroidectomy. Neck dissection seems an effective method of controlling well-differentiated thyroid cancer that has spread to regional lymph nodes.[4] The prognosis does not seem to be improved by more radical surgery.

There are no prospective randomized clinical studies of the effectiveness of various modes of surgical treatment—that is, lobectomy versus total thyroidectomy. It is apparent that with the variation in the biologic features of the disease, unless this aspect is carefully considered, the limited experience of any one observer may bias his conclusion, depending upon that spectrum of neoplasms that he evaluates.

The therapeutic impact of thyroid hormone administration has not been appraised in a prospective controlled study. However, there are a number of reports of well-documented regression of well-differentiated thyroid cancer. It is difficult to evaluate the effect of thyroid hormone administered on a prophylactic basis. Several observers have been impressed with the effectiveness of this approach. Recurrence of well-differentiated thyroid cancer despite the prophylactic administration of the thyroid hormone has, however, been documented. The prophylactic administration of ^{131}I following the surgical treatment of well-differentiated carcinoma has also been reported to be effective. Again, the studies are uncontrolled and, in view of the known hazards of such therapy and the good results from surgery alone, this type of prophylaxis is difficult to justify.

SELECTED REFERENCES

Beahrs, O. H., and Pasternak, B. M.: Cancer of the thyroid gland. Curr. Probl. Surg., Dec., 1969.
The vast experience of the surgeons at the Mayo Clinic in the management of thyroid cancer is nicely recounted in this article. The authors' approach, which is representative of that of most surgeons, appears to be well supported by their results.

Buckwalter, J. A., Thomas, C. G., and Freeman, J. B.: Is childhood thyroid cancer a lethal disease? Ann. Surg., 181:632, 1975.
The biologic characteristics of thyroid cancer in childhood are reviewed, emphasizing differences between neoplasms arising in the child and those occurring in older age groups. Implications regarding therapy and factors associated with the excellent survivorship in this age group are presented.

Dobyns, B. M.: Goiter. Curr. Probl. Surg., Jan., 1969.
This small monograph provides an excellent review of the underlying mechanisms of goiter formation, with an emphasis on its pathophysiology. It is well illustrated and written by a man who has had a lifelong interest in diseases of the thyroid.

Hedinger, C. E.: Thyroid Cancer. U.I.C.C. Monograph Series, Volume 12. New York, Springer-Verlag, 1969.
This monograph is composed of papers on thyroid cancer presented at the International Conference on Thyroid Cancer held in Switzerland in 1968. It is a comprehensive report covering controversial issues, pathologic characteristics, epidemiology, and experimental observations. A clinical classification of thyroid cancer is given and the results of treatment are reviewed with respect to factors influencing survivorship.

Miller, J. M., and Block, M. A.: Functional autonomy in multinodular goiter. J.A.M.A., 214:3, 1970.
This brief paper on multinodular goiter presents a new understanding of the disease based upon the studies with radioactive iodine. It provides a physiologic basis for observations made by Plummer in 1910.

Taylor, S.: The evolution of nodular goiter. J. Clin. Endocr., 13:1232, 1953.
This paper presents a scholarly discussion of the anatomy, etiology, and evolution of simple and nodular goiter. The author's conclusions are based on observations from surgical specimens examined histologically and complemented by radioautography.

Thomas, C. G., Jr., and Buckwalter, J. A.: Thyroid cancer. In Longmire, W., Jr. (Ed.): Advances in Surgery. Chicago Year Book Medical Publishers, Inc., 1976.
A comprehensive review of thyroid cancer with discussions of biology, diagnosis, available therapy, and prognosis.

REFERENCES

1. Beahrs, H. H., and Pasternak, B. M.: Cancer of the thyroid gland. Curr. Probl. Surg., Dec., 1969.
2. Blum, N., Goldman, A. B., Herskovic, A., and Hernberg, J.: Clinical applications of thyroid echography. N. Engl. J. Med., 287:1164, 1972.
3. Buckwalter, J. A., Thomas, C. G. Jr., and Freeman, J. B.: Is childhood thyroid cancer a lethal disease? Ann. Surg., 181:632, 1975.
4. Buckwalter, J. A., and Thomas, C. G. Jr.: Selection of surgical treatment of well differentiated thyroid carcinomas. Ann. Surg., 176:565, 1972.
5. Carroll, R. E., Haddon, W., Jr., Handy, J. H., and Wieben, E. E.: Thyroid cancer: Cohort analysis of increasing incidence in New York state, 1941–1962. J. Natl. Cancer Inst., 33:277, 1964.
6. Crile, G., Jr.: The endocrine dependency of certain thyroid cancers and the danger that hypothyroidism may stimulate their growth. Cancer, 10:1119, 1957.
7. DeGroot, L. J., Greer, M. A., and Utiger, R. D.: Thyroid nodules. In Inglefinger, F. J., Ebert, R. V., Finland, M., et al. (Eds.): Controversies in Internal Medicine II. Philadelphia, W. B. Saunders Company, 1974.
8. Dobyns, B. M.: Goiter. Curr. Probl. Surg., Jan., 1969.
9. Dobyns, B. M., and Bertozzi, G.: Identification of cold thyroid lesions at operation and its place in the surgical management of carcinoma of the thyroid. Ann. Surg., 172:703, 1970.
10. Foster, R. S.: Thyroid irradiation and carcinogenesis. Am. J. Surg., 130:608, 1975.
11. Gordon, T., Crittenden, M., and Haenszel, W.: End results and mortality trends in cancer. Part II. Washington, D.C., U.S. Dept. of Health, Education and Welfare, 1962.
12. Gottlieb, J. A., and Hill, C. S., Jr.: Chemotherapy of thyroid cancer with adriamycin. N. Engl. J. Med., 290:193, 1974.
13. Gould, E. A., Hirsch, E., and Brecher, I.: Complications arising in the course of thyroidectomy. Arch. Surg., 90:81, 1965.
14. Hall, I. V.: Role of initiating and promoting factors in pathogenesis in tumors of the thyroid. Br. J. Cancer, 2:273, 1948.
15. Hamburger, J. I.: Solitary autonomously functioning thyroid lesions. Am. J. Med., 58:740, 1975.
16. Hansen, J. B.: Fine needle biopsy. N. Engl. J. Med., 291:851, 1974.
17. Harness, J. K., Thompson, N. W., Session, J. C., and Beierwaltes, W. H.: Differentiated thyroid cancer—treatment of distant metastases. Arch. Surg., 108:410, 1973.
18. Hedinger, C. E.: Thyroid cancer, U.I.C.C. Monograph Series, Vol. 12. New York, Springer-Verlag, 1969.
19. Hirabayashi, R. N., and Lindsay, S.: Carcinoma of the thyroid gland: A statistical study of 390 patients. J. Clin. Endocrinol., 21:1596, 1961.
20. Jenny, H., Block, M. A., Horn, R. E., and Miller, J. M.: Recurrence following surgery for benign thyroid nodules. Arch. Surg., 92:525, 1966.
21. Johnson, N.: The blood supply of the thyroid gland. II. The nodular gland. Aust. N. Z. J. Surg., 23:4, 1954.
22. LiViola, V. A., Perzin, K. H., and Savetsky, L.: Carcinoma arising in median ectopic thyroid (including thyroglossal duct tissue). Cancer, 34:1303, 1941.
23. Miller, J. M., and Block, M. A.: Functional anatomy in multinodular goiter. J.A.M.A., 214:3, 1970.
24. Miller, J. M., Horn, R. C., and Block, M. A.: The evolution of toxic nodular goiter. Arch. Intern. Med., 113:122, 1964.
25. Mortensen, J. D., Bennett, W. A., and Woolner, L. B.: Gross and microscopic findings in clinically normal thyroid glands. J. Clin. Endocrinol., 15:1270, 1955.

26. Refetoff, S., Harrison, J. H., Karanfilski, B. T., Kaplan, E. L., DeGroot, L. J., and Bekerman, S.: Continuing occurrence of thyroid carcinoma after irradiation to the neck in infancy and childhood. N. Engl. J. Med., 292:171, 1975.
27. Rosen, I. E., and Walfish, P. G.: The application of ultrasound to the study of thyroid enlargement. Arch. Surg., 110:940, 1975.
28. Russell, W. O., Ibanez, M. L., Clark, R. L., and White, E. C.: Thyroid carcinoma, classification, intraglandular dissemination and clinicopathological study based upon whole organ sections of 80 glands. Cancer, 16:1425, 1963.
29. Sampson, R. J., Woolner, L. B., et al.: Occult thyroid carcinoma in Olmstead County, Minn., prevalence at autopsy compared with that at Hiroshima and Nagasaki, Japan. Cancer, 34:2072, 1974.
30. Silverberg, S. G., Hutter, R. V. P., and Foote, F. W., Jr.: Fatal carcinoma of the thyroid: Histology, metastases and causes of death. Cancer, 25:4, 1970.
31. Silverberg, S. G., and Vidone, R. A.: Carcinoma of the thyroid in surgical and postmortem material—analysis of 300 cases at autopsy and literature review. Ann. Surg., 164:291, 1966.
32. Taylor, S.: The evolution of nodular goiter. J. Clin. Endocrinol., 13:1232, 1953.
33. Thomas, C. G., Jr.: The dependency of thyroid cancer: A review. Ann. Surg., 146:879, 1957.
34. Thomas, C. G., Jr., and Buckwalter, J. A.: Poorly differentiated neoplasms of the thyroid. Ann. Surg., 177:632, 1973.
35. Thomas, C. G., Jr., and Buckwalter, J. A.: Thyroid cancer. In Longmire, W., Jr. (Ed.): Advances in Surgery. Chicago, Year Book Medical Publishers, Inc., 1976.
36. Thomas, C. G., Jr., Pepper, F. D., and Owen, J.: Differentiation of malignant from benign lesions of the thyroid gland using complementary scanning with [75]Selenomethionine and radioiodide. Ann. Surg., 170:396, 1969.
37. Thomas, C. G., Jr., Buckwalter, J. A., Staab, E. V., and Kerr, C. Y.: Evaluation of the dominant thyroid masses. Ann. Surg., 183:463, 1976.
38. Vickery, A. L.: Thyroid alterations due to irradiation. In Hazard, J. B., and Smith, D. E. (Eds.): The Thyroid. Baltimore, Williams & Wilkins Co., 1964.
39. Welch, C. E.: Therapy for multinodular goiter. J.A.M.A., 195:95, 1966.
40. Winship, T., and Roxvall, R. V.: Thyroid carcinoma in childhood: Final report on a twenty year study. Clin. Proc. Child. Hosp., 26:11, 1970.

VI

THE MULTIPLE ENDOCRINE NEOPLASIAS*

Samuel A. Wells, Jr., M.D. and Stephen B. Baylin, M.D.

Tumors of the endocrine system most often develop within a single gland. There are clinical disorders, however, which are characterized by the concurrence of multiple neoplasms involving several endocrine tissues. These diseases almost always occur familially in a Mendelian autosomal dominant pattern.

MULTIPLE ENDOCRINE ADENOMATOSIS TYPE I

The first description of associated endocrinopathies was Jacob Erdheim's report in 1903 of an acromegalic patient who at necropsy was found to have a pituitary eosinophilic adenoma and four enlarged parathyroid glands. In 1927, Cushing and Davidoff reported a patient with simultaneous neoplasms of the pituitary (esosinophilic adenoma), parathyroids (two adenomas), and pancreas (islet cell adenoma). Rossier, in 1939, described two sisters afflicted with multiple endocrine tumors; the male members of this sibship seemed to have peptic ulcer disease without apparent endocrine involvement. In 1954, Wermer[19] described the familial

occurrence of tumors involving the pituitary gland, parathyroids, and pancreatic islets. The disease has been subsequently termed multiple endocrine adenomatosis type I (MEA-I). In the family studied by Wermer, the father and four of nine children were affected. Four of the five patients had pituitary tumors, three were hypercalcemic, four had peptic ulcer disease, and three had pancreatic adenomas. He proposed that the syndrome in this family was caused by a dominant autosomal gene with a high degree of penetrance.

The peptic ulcer diathesis frequently associated with MEA-I almost always seems to be associated with the pancreatic endocrinopathy. In 1955, Zollinger and Ellison[20] reported two cases of severe recurrent peptic ulcer disease associated with pancreatic islet cell tumors. The ulcer disease was markedly resistant to standard operative treatment and was characterized by the secretion of hydrochloric acid in large volumes. It was proposed by these investigators that the islet cell tumors of the pancreas were ulcerogenic. In 1960, Gregory and associates demonstrated that an extract from a non-beta cell adenoma of the head of the pancreas excised from a patient afflicted with this disease stimulated acid secretion from a denervated gastric pouch. The extracted substance was like neither histamine nor insulin in its action, and these investigators concluded that the material resembled an-

*Supported in part by a grant (RR-30) from the General Clinical Resources Center Program of the Division of Research Resources, National Institute of Health and NIH Contract CB-63994-39.

tral gastrin in its chemical and physiologic properties. McGuigan in 1968 demonstrated by radioimmunoassay that gastrin was indeed the hormone produced by these pancreatic tumors. It was also subsequently shown that a marked elevation in the serum gastrin concentration was associated with this disease.

PATHOGENESIS

The disease has been described in all age groups subsequent to the first decade. The majority of women develop the disease in the third decade, whereas the peak incidence for males is in the fourth. It is unknown whether the parathyroid, the pancreas, and the pituitary gland derangements are all governed by the same gene, or whether a single endocrine gland anomaly is genetically determined, which then induces pathologic changes in other endocrine tissues. Most likely the former situation is the case, but there has been some evidence that the excess production of either insulin, gastrin, or glucagon by the pancreatic islets could lead either directly or indirectly to stimulation and perhaps neoplastic development in the parathyroid and pituitary glands.

CLINICAL PRESENTATION

The clinical manifestations of MEA-I are protean and depend partly on which endocrine glands are involved. Of 85 patients reviewed in Ballard's series,[1] the most frequent mode of clinical presentation was peptic ulcer disease or its complications. Manifestations of hypoglycemia represented the second most common presenting feature, while symptoms due to altered parathyroid function and complaints referable to pituitary dysfunction (headaches, visual field defects, and secondary amenorrhea) least often led to the diagnosis. It is important to note, however, that the mode of clinical presentation did not actually portray the incidence of involvement of the various endocrine organs.

Parathyroids

Evidence of hyperparathyroidism occurs in approximately 90 per cent of cases and is the most common endocrine abnormality. Although the majority of reported patients (50 to 60 per cent) with parathyroid disease have multiple gland involvement, complete dissection of the neck has often not been undertaken, and the incidence of generalized parathyroid disease is probably much higher. A large percentage of patients with hyperparathyroidism have kidney disease, usually consisting of renal or ureteral lithiasis and/or nephrocalcinosis. Surprisingly, there is little evidence of skeletal involvement. Parathyroid chief-cell hyperplasia is the characteristic pathologic lesion in this syndrome.

Pancreas

Pancreatic tumors are present in approximately 80 per cent of patients and commonly are multicentric in origin. Of reported series, approximately 40 per cent of patients with pancreatic involvement have had beta cell lesions and symptoms of hypoglycemia. Because few patients in initial reports were evaluated by simultaneously measuring immunoreactive insulin and fasting blood glucose levels, it is difficult to determine the true incidence of beta cell tumors. In Ballard's series, non-beta cell tumors were more frequent, with only 25 per cent of pancreatic neoplasms being of the beta cell type.

Approximately 10 per cent of beta cell tumors are malignant, whereas 60 per cent of non-beta cell tumors are. It has been reported and subsequently confirmed that metastatic non-beta cell neoplasms occasionally regress following total gastrectomy for the Zollinger-Ellison syndrome.[4] This is unusual, however, as metastatic disease is usually associated with tumor progression and death.

It was noted by Ballard that there was a high incidence of associated watery diarrhea in patients with non-beta cell tumors of the pancreas and MEA-I. At one time this was thought to be the result solely of a large volume of gastric juice released into the gut. It has become apparent, however, that this symptom can occur in the absence of gastric hypersecretion and in all likelihood is due to some hormonal substance secreted by the pancreatic tumor. High concentrations of vasoactive intestinal polypeptide (VIP) have been immunochemically identified in the plasma of non-MEA-I patients with the watery diarrhea syndrome.

Pituitary

Pituitary tumors, usually chromophobe adenomas, occur in 60 to 70 per cent of cases. Secondary amenorrhea in women and hypogonadism in men are the most common manifestations of altered pituitary function, while less often headache and visual disturbances are presenting features. Acromegaly occurs in approximately 30 per cent of patients.

Adrenal

Forty per cent of patients have adrenal cortical involvement, including adenomas, miliary adenomas, hyperplasia, multiple adenomas, and multinodular hyperplasia. Adrenal cortical hyperfunction rarely occurs clinically, however.

Thyroid

Thyroid disorders are relatively infrequent, occurring in 10 to 15 per cent of patients. While thyroid carcinomas and thyrotoxicosis have been reported, the most common lesions are functioning thyroid adenomas and colloid goiters.

DIAGNOSIS

The parathyroid and the pituitary hyperfunction can be diagnosed by standard clinical evaluation combined with laboratory and radiologic tests. The diagnosis of the Zollinger-Ellison syndrome depends on the demonstration by radioimmunoassay of an inappropriately elevated basal serum gastrin level or a brisk increase following secretin or calcium ion infusion. The diagnosis of insulin-secreting tumors of the pancreas depends on establishing that inappropriate levels of immunoreactive insulin are present when the patient is in a hypoglycemic state during a prolonged fast.

TREATMENT

Parathyroids

The most commonly accepted surgical procedure for the treatment of generalized parathyroid hyperplasia has been the subtotal (3½ gland) resection of parathyroid tissue. An alternative procedure which might prove to have greater utility has been the performance of total parathyroidectomy with associated parathyroid autografting into the forearm musculature[18] (see also Chapter 26).

Pancreas

The standard accepted surgical procedure for patients with the Zollinger-Ellison syndrome associated with non-beta cell pancreatic tumors is total gastrectomy. Patients with hyperinsulinism associated with solitary tumors are best treated by resection of the neoplastic tissue. Multiple insulinomas or more rarely beta cell hyperplasia can also cause hyperinsulinism in MEA-I patients, and preoperative arteriography is useful in localizing the neoplastic pancreatic tissue and defining its extent. The operative procedure of choice can then be determined. Pituitary tumors, either functioning or nonfunctioning, may require ablation surgically or by x-ray therapy.

MULTIPLE ENDOCRINE NEOPLASIA TYPE II

The term multiple endocrine neoplasia type II (MEN-II)[15] is used to describe patients with a triad of inherited neoplasms, including medullary carcinoma of the thyroid gland (MCT), pheochromocytoma(s), and parathyroid hyperplasia. This syndrome, although rare, is being increasingly recognized in the families of patients with medullary thyroid carcinoma. Some 10 kindreds have now been reported, and the syndrome becomes a diagnostic consideration in all patients initially diagnosed as having either pheochromocytoma(s) or MCT.

Medullary carcinoma of the thyroid gland was first described as a distinct clinical entity by Hazard and associates in 1959.[5] Its characteristic histologic appearance, including the presence of an amyloid-like material and its rather specific production of the polypeptide hormone thyrocalcitonin (TCT), is now well recognized. In the early 1960s Sipple[14] reported the unusually high incidence of pheochromocytomas, often bilateral, in patients with thyroid malignancy. The association of hyperparathyroidism with the syndrome was subsequently demonstrated, and it was clarified that the thyroid tumors were of medullary histology. Schimke and his co-workers documented the familial nature of the disorder and established that the trait was inherited in a mendelian autosomal dominant pattern with an extraordinarily high gene penetrance. In the late 1960s several investigators established that medullary thyroid carcinoma produced large concentrations of the peptide hormone thyrocalcitonin (TCT). This finding supported the suggestion that MCT was a tumor of the parafollicular cells of the thyroid gland, since these cells were known to be the source of the hormone in species other than human. The secretion of TCT by the tumor with resultant elevated levels of plasma TCT is now recognized as the single best diagnostic test for the presence of MCT.

A variant of MEN-II (MEN-II-B or MEN-III) is composed of medullary carcinoma of the thyroid gland and pheochromocytomas without hyperparathyroidism. Additionally these patients have a marfanoid habitus, characteristics facies, and multiple mucosal neuromas involving the eyelids, lips, and tongue. The disease most often occurs sporadically with no familial pattern.[9]

PATHOGENESIS

The two multiple endocrine neoplasia syndromes and particularly MEN-II have provided exciting information as to the embryologic tissue of origin of many endocrine cells and endocrine tumors. Elegant studies by Pearse[13] have demonstrated that the parafollicular cells of various species embryologically derive from neural crest tissue. Parafollicular cells and MCT cells have the biochemical features of a cell line designated by Pearse as the "APUD" cell system (A = amines, for the presence of amines such as serotonin and dopamine; PU = precursor uptake for the fact that these cells can actively take up precursors to serotonin and dopamine in vitro; and D = decarboxylase for the presence of the amine synthesizing enzyme L-aromatic decarboxylase). The medullary portion of the adrenal gland which gives rise to pheochromocytomas in patients with MEN-II also comes from the neural crest and has APUD cell characteristics. The inheritance of simultaneous MCT and pheochromocytomas may result from a single defect or a combination of defects in neural crest tissue. The nature of this defect has yet to be more precisely defined.

The presence of the parathyroid abnormality in MEN-II is less well understood. Parathyroid cells do not appear to be derived from neural crest tissue and do not have the biochemical features of "APUD" cells. It is possible that chronic stimulation of the parathyroid by the hypocalcemic effects of excess TCT from MCT accounts for the eventual hyperplasia. On the other hand, some workers have reported elevated levels of circulating PTH early in the course of MEN-II patients and in family members who have no other signs of the syndrome. Additionally, patients with spontaneous (nonfamilial) MCT and MEN-II-B rarely have hyperparathyroidism, thereby raising the possibility that the parathyroid lesions could be a primary rather than a secondary feature in MEN-II.

CLINICAL FEATURES

Frequency of Associated Tumors

Although any of the neoplasms that make up the syndrome may account for the initial symptoms that bring the patient to the physician's attention (i.e., MCT-producing thyroid nodules, pheochromocytomas producing headaches and/or hypertension, or parathyroid hyperplasia producing hypercalcemia), the thyroid tumor is the constant feature of MEN-II, being present in virtually 100 per cent of affected individuals. The presence of the other two lesions is more variable and definitive figures are lacking; however, approximately 40 per cent of patients have pheochromocytoma(s) and 60 per cent have parathyroid hyperplasia.[8]

Pathologic and Histologic Features

Histologically, MCT in patients with MEN-II is no different from the tumor which arises spontaneously without associated endocrinopathies. However, in virtually all patients with MEN-II or MEN-II-B the thyroid tumors are bilateral, whereas medullary tumors occurring otherwise seldom are. Medullary carcinoma constitutes 5 to 10 per cent of all types of thyroid malignancies, and approximately 80 per cent of MCT patients have no family history of the disease. The tumor typically appears as a circumscribed whitish tan nodule on the surface of the thyroid gland. Histologically, the tumor consists of sheets or cords of round or spindle shaped cells separated by a variable amount of amorphous stromal material.

When MCT lesions are stained with Congo red and examined for amyloid-like material, the typical apple green birefringence is often found scattered throughout the amorphous stromal portions. While this finding is frequent, it is not needed to diagnose MCT histologically. The amyloid-like material is thought to be composed of aggregates of a prohormone of thyrocalcitonin synthesized by the tumor cells. From a clinical standpoint, MCT can be diagnosed on a biochemical basis alone, as discussed in detail below. Very early stages of the tumor have been detected by such means and a "premalignant" or hyperplastic stage (C-cell hyperplasia) has now been defined.

The pheochromocytoma (s) of MEN-II are characterized by their tendency to manifest in the second and third decades of life and by the high incidence of bilaterality (70 per cent). The lesion is almost always limited to the adrenal medulla and is almost always benign. The histology of the pheochromocytomas in MEN-II is typical of that found in the spontaneous or nonfamilial setting.

The parathyroid lesions in MEN-II consist primarily of generalized hyperplasia, and single parathyroid gland involvement is rare. Also, it is important to note that enlarged parathyroid glands can be found in patients with MEN-II who do not have biochemical evidence of hyperparathyroidism.

Clinical Findings and Natural History

It must be emphasized that the optimal management of patients with the MEN-II syndrome entails diagnosis of the disease by biochemical parameters before clinical signs are apparent. Obviously, however, for initial detection of a family with MEN-II, one or more patients with clinical features of the disease must be recognized and suggest the need for intense screening of other and usually younger family members.

While any of the lesions in MEN-II can produce symptoms in a given patient and lead to the diagnosis, the MCT is the lesion which most often is detected first. Most commonly the patient presents with a multinodular thyroid gland, although occasionally only a single nodule is felt. By palpation, there is little to distinguish these lesions from other thyroid neoplasms. Firm and enlarged lymph nodes in the cervical region suggest a metastatic tumor.

The MCT cells are capable of great biosynthetic activity and have been reported to secrete ACTH, MSH, serotonin, and prostaglandins. Accordingly, certain syndromes may exist with MCT and suggest the presence of this tumor. It is important to recognize that the syndromes are rare, and, since they unfortunately occur with advanced disease, they are not usually useful for diagnosing early lesions. Approximately 30 per cent of patients with MCT have clinically significant diarrhea. Occasionally bouts of diarrhea can be associated with flushing, abdominal cramping, and carcinoid-like symptoms. Any investigation of a patient suspected of having endocrine or hormonally induced diarrhea should include a consideration of MCT. Likewise, the syndrome of ectopic ACTH production must include MCT in the differential diagnosis. Although rare, patients with this tumor and all of the features of excess ACTH production have been well described in the literature.[12]

Two radiologic features of MCT may suggest the presence of the tumor. First, both primary and metastatic lesions of this malignancy have a propensity to calcify, with a characteristic dense, irregular distribution of calcium throughout the neoplasm. This finding contrasts with the faint homogeneous calcification seen in other types of thyroid tumors. Cervical films may demonstrate calcification in a primary thyroid lesion or a metastatic lesion in a cervical lymph node. Again, it must be stressed that the existence of tumor masses large enough to calcify in this manner is a parameter of advanced and long-standing disease and is not useful for making an early diagnosis. Secondly, MCT may metastasize to the mediastinum, appearing as a retrosternal mass or mediastinal widening on chest x-ray.

The pheochromocytomas in MEN-II may be either clinically silent or product dramatic clinical symptoms. As discussed later, it is important to diagnose these tumors by biochemical means and to remove them first, thereby avoiding unexpected hypertensive crises that can accompany the discharge of catecholamines during anesthesia induction for thyroid surgery. Symptoms produced by the adrenal lesions can include vague feelings of anxiety and nervousness, episodic whole body diaphoresis, palpitations, and severe pounding frontal headaches.

Hyperfunction of the parathyroid glands in patients with MEN-II is the most variable component of the syndrome. It is not uncommon to find one or more enlarged glands at the time of neck surgery for MCT in a patient who has never had documented hypercalcemia. Clinical recognition of the parathyroid lesions often stems from the finding of asymptomatic hypercalcemia during routine blood studies. The most common symptom of the altered calcium homeostasis in patients with MEN-II is the presence of asymptomatic or symptomatic renal stones. More advanced signs of hyperparathyroidism, such as osteitis fibrosa cystica and nephrocalcinosis, are unusual.

The course of patients with MEN-II is essentially that of the thyroid lesion. MCT is an aggressive malignancy in terms of its metastatic potential. This is vividly illustrated by the studies of Melvin et al.[10] Members of an MEN-II kindred operated upon for tumors as small as 1 to 10 mm. and detected only through abnormalities of the blood TCT had a 50 per cent incidence of metastatic lesions in the cervical lymph nodes.

Although the mortality rate for MCT is lower than for undifferentiated thyroid tumors, it is higher than for papillary or follicular neoplasms. The 10-year survival is approximately 50 per cent. The behavior of MCT is extremely variable between individuals and even within MEN-II kindreds.

Hill and his colleagues[7] have categorized the postoperative courses of MCT patients into three clinical groups. Group 1 patients underwent surgery for disease localized to the neck and had no further problems with tumor. The average survival time was 111 months. Group 2 patients had surgery at the same clinical stage, but exhibited progressive spread of disease postoperatively with early signs of recurrent and residual disease. Patients in the subgroup 2-a had a more deliberate course, with periods of quiescence of demonstrable disease spread and an average survival time of 75 months. Group 2-b patients had a much more explosive downhill course after surgery, with relatively early death from disseminated disease and an average survival time of 22 months. Group 3 patients had a latent period, often as long as 10 years or more, between the time of initial surgery and the appearance of metastatic disease. The average survival time was 107 months for such patients. At present, there is no known method for detecting which patients will do well and which will do poorly.

DIAGNOSIS

When the proper clinical setting for suspicion of MCT or of MEN-II exists, precise diagnosis depends upon familiarity with the biochemical activity of the potential lesions. For MCT the production of TCT by the cells holds the key for diagnosis. With the advent of radioimmunoassay techniques for this hormone, Tashjian et al.[16] documented that virtually all patients with clinically detectable medullary carcinoma have elevated circulating TCT levels. In the laboratories of most investigators, TCT levels in normal individuals are difficult to detect and probably are less than 0.2 ng. per ml. of plasma. Patients with palpable MCT lesions or with clinically apparent metastatic disease all have levels above normal and generally greater than 1.0 ng. per ml. With extensive disease basal values can be over 1000 ng. per ml.

Thus, in patients suspected of having MCT on clinical grounds, a single determination of plasma TCT can establish the diagnosis. Although elevated blood levels of this hormone have been reported in patients with other tumors (small cell lung carcinoma, carcinoid tumors, and breast carcinoma), for practical purposes in the proper clinical setting, elevated TCT levels are specific for MCT. When a kindred has been proven to have MEN-II, screening family members in an effort to identify early states of MCT requires more than obtaining a basal level of blood TCT. Melvin et al.[11] identified the fact that minimal elevations of plasma TCT can be indicative of MCT that is clinically undetectable by palpation or by thyroid scan. Indeed, tumors no larger than 1.0 mm. in size can be so diagnosed. These workers also found that some patients with normal basal levels had an abnormally brisk rise in blood TCT levels following a calcium ion infusion (15 mg. per kg. over four hours). These patients also proved to have small medullary tumors in the thyroid. Small but progressive elevations of TCT detected in patients followed serially with the calcium infusion test were useful in the diagnosis of the premalignant phase termed C-cell hyperplasia.

Most recently the peptide pentagastrin (Ayerst) has proved to be more potent than the standard four-hour calcium ion infusion in stimulating TCT secretion from medullary carcinoma cells.[6] Following a bolus intravenous injection of pentagastrin (0.5 μg. per kg.), peak TCT levels are detectable in 1 to 3 minutes, compared to 30 minutes following the beginning of calcium ion (15 mg. per kg. over four hours) infusion. Furthermore, peak TCT levels following pentagastrin are two- to threefold higher than peak levels following calcium infusion (Fig. 1). Pentagastrin stimulation has been successful in detecting MCT in MEN-II patients who have had no clinical or radiologic evidence of MCT and no elevations of TCT following calcium ion infusion (Fig. 2).[6, 17]

Another biochemical feature of MCT is the presence of high levels of the enzyme histaminase in MCT tissue.[2] Approximately 50 per cent of all patients with MCT also have abnormal circulating levels of this enzyme. Although the factors governing which patients have abnormal blood histaminase levels are not completely known, there is a positive correlation with the presence of metastatic disease (Fig. 3). Patients who have abnormal levels prior to surgery, and especially those whose levels do not return to normal postoperatively, have a high incidence of persistent disease or of subsequent recurrent disease.[3]

The diagnosis of pheochromocytoma in MEN-II depends on careful analysis of the levels of urinary catecholamines and catecholamine metabolites. This is especially important, since this lesion can be unsuspected clinically. As a rule, one of three determinations has a high probability of diagnosing the lesion; these include the measurement of (a) 24-hour urine total catecholamines, (b) metanephrines, or (c) vanillylmandelic acid (VMA). Because of their constant location in the adrenal medulla, pheochromocytomas in MEN-II can have a number of patterns of catecholamine secretion that makes simultaneous measurement of all of the above products most useful. These tumors in MEN-II often produce a preponderance of epinephrine to norepinephrine, as opposed to

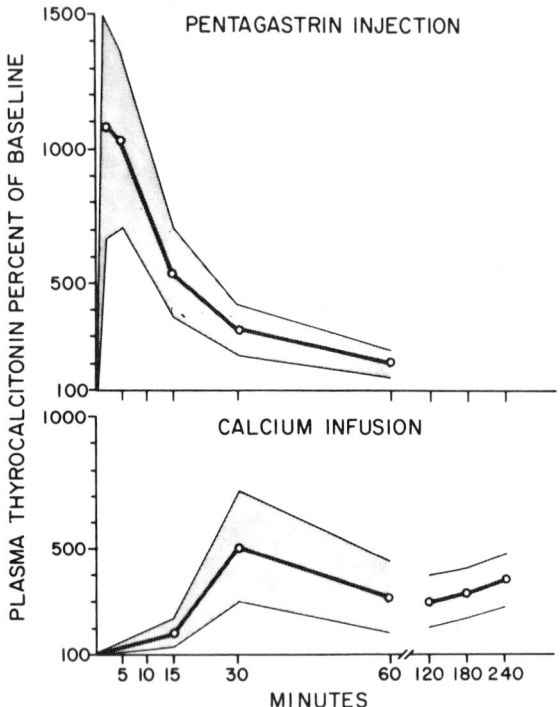

Figure 1. Combined responses of seven patients with elevated base line levels of plasma TCT to pentagastrin injection and calcium infusion. Each patient received both tests on separate days with pentagastrin injection being the initial test in four of the patients and calcium infusion being the initial test in three of the patients. Details of the test procedures are given in the text. Responses are expressed as the per cent increase in immunoreactive TCT above initial base line levels. Open circles and solid lines represent the mean responses, and the shaded areas indicate the range of the standard errors. (From Hennessy, J. C., et al.: J. Clin. Endocrinol. Metabol., *39*:487, 1974).

pheochromocytomas outside the adrenal. When available, quantitation of the ratio of epinephrine to norepinephrine can be useful, as in some cases the epinephrine levels alone may be increased. Secondly, with large pheochromocytomas in the adrenal, the catecholamines may be largely metabolized in the tumor. This leads to a situation in which total urinary catecholamines may be normal while metanephrines and VMA determinations are frankly elevated.

Several test agents (histamine, tyramine, and glucagon) have been used to provoke catecholamine discharge from silent pheochromocytomas. In MEN-II patients, these tests have not proved particularly helpful, since many false negative responses occur. Cases have occurred in which provocative testing was negative, yet a hypertensive crisis with arrhythmias occurred during anesthesia prior to a neck exploration for thyroid carcinoma. Thus, careful analysis of urinary catecholamines and all of the catecholamine metabolites remains the best diagnostic maneuver to rule out the adrenal tumor.

Invasive procedures to localize pheochromocytomas in MEN-II also may have limited use. Since the tumors are usually intraadrenal and often bilateral, the surgical approach should always allow for careful

exploration of both adrenals. This somewhat negates the need for arteriography or venography to localize the lesions. Noninvasive techniques such as intravenous pyelography with tomography or sonography of both kidneys can be helpful if the tumors are relatively large.

The diagnosis of hyperparathyroidism in MEN-II depends largely on serial measurements of blood calcium levels. Determination of peripheral PTH levels can be misleading, since increased values have been reported in members of involved kindreds who have neither hypercalcemia nor MCT. Any history of recurrent renal stones should, of course, make the search for hyperparathyroidism even more vigorous.

SURGICAL MANAGEMENT

It is unusual that one is able to diagnose and treat cancer in an early preclinical stage. From previous experience with large kindreds, it is known that the detection of an elevated blood TCT level (>1.0 ng. per ml.) following pentagastrin stimulation in an asymptomatic, clinically "normal" patient is virtually diagnostic of medullary carcinoma of the thyroid gland. This has been demonstrated repeatedly in patients with no mass palpable in the thyroid gland, normal thyroid scans, and undetectable levels of TCT in the peripheral blood even following calcium infusion. The-

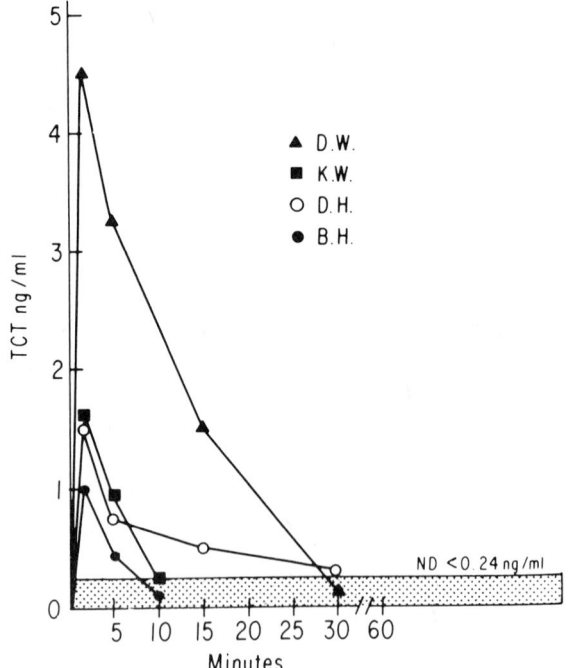

Figure 2. Thyrocalcitonin response to pentagastrin stimulation in four children (D. W., K. W., D. H., and B. H.) with a family history of multiple endocrine neoplasia type II. In none of the four children was a thyroid mass present and all had normal ^{131}I thyroid scans and no increase of TCT following calcium infusion. At surgery, however, all were found to have foci of medullary thyroid carcinoma bilaterally. (From Wells, S. A., Jr., et al.: Ann. Surg., *182*:362, 1975).

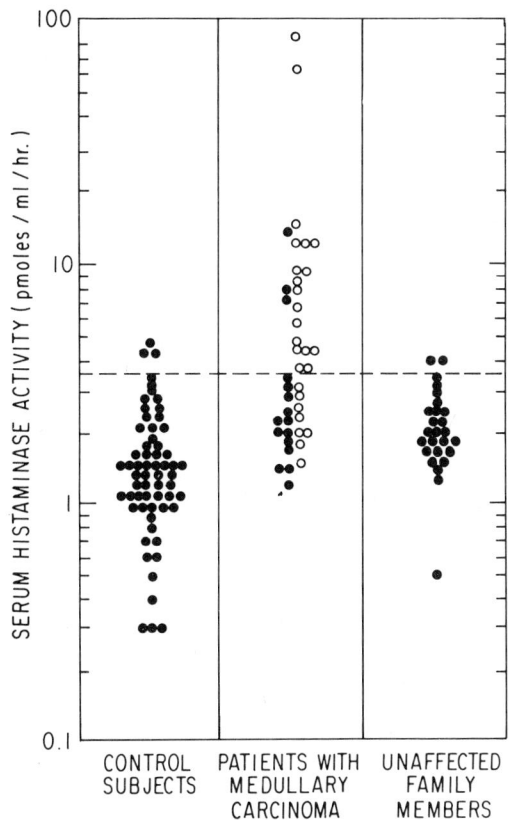

Figure 3. Serum-histaminase activity in 62 controls, 42 patients with medullary thyroid carcinoma, and 26 relatives of patients who were clinically normal. (From Lancet, 1:455, 1972.)

oretically, the MCT in most affected members of an MEN-II kindred should be diagnosed in the "preclinical state." Such patients at surgery have usually had MCT confined to the thyroid gland with no evidence of metastases to regional lymph nodes. When members of a kindred are screened beginning at a young age, it is the MCT that will almost always be diagnosed first. The necessity of ruling out an associated pheochromocytoma(s) prior to surgery has been emphasized previously.

Should the presence of a pheochromocytoma(s) be diagnosed, then bilateral adrenal exploration is mandatory. Patients should be explored through the abdomen, utilizing a bilateral subcostal incision. Both adrenal glands must be completely evaluated to be sure that bilateral lesions do not exist. Although extra-adrenal lesions are very rare in MEN-II, the sympathetic chain and organ of Zuckerkandl must be examined to be sure that no pheochromocytomas are present in these locations. The state of adrenal medullary hyperplasia has been described in MEN-II, and some investigators have advocated bilateral total adrenalectomy on the basis of this histologic picture. It has not been our policy to routinely biopsy the contralateral, normal-sized adrenal gland after resecting a unilateral pheochromocytoma. If patients are followed carefully at six-month or yearly intervals, these lesions can be diagnosed before they are clinically threatening.

Prior to surgery for pheochromocytomas, preoperative preparation has usually been that of adrenergic blockade with the alpha blocker phenoxybenzamine (40 to 200 mg. a day). Rarely, beta-adrenergic blockade with propranolol (40 mg. a day) has been necessary when tachycardia develops with phenoxybenzamine. Intraoperative control is most effectively achieved with sodium nitroprusside or phentolamine. Bilateral adrenalectomy obviously requires long-term glucocorticoid and mineralocorticoid replacement.

The surgical treatment of medullary carcinoma of the thyroid gland is total thyroidectomy. It is unwise to leave any thyroid tissue, because recurrent disease can be expected. In early disease, even that diagnosed by biochemical means (calcium infusion or pentagastrin injection), it is always wise to resect the lymph nodes in the central zone of the neck from the thyroid cartilage to the sternal notch as far laterally as the jugular veins. Should obvious lymphatic disease exist lateral to the jugular veins, then total thyroidectomy should be combined with a neck dissection. Generally the larger the lesion and the longer it has been clinically apparent, the greater the incidence of lymph node metastases. The efficacy of an adequate surgical resection can be ascertained postoperatively by repeating the pentagastrin stimulation test and determining levels of blood TCT peripherally.

Hyperparathyroidism

Whereas at one time it was thought that patients with familial MCT and hyperparathyroidism had parathyroid adenomas as the associated lesion, it is now appreciated that almost invariably the parathyroid glands are hyperplastic and there is generalized involvement. If patients are found to be hypercalcemic preoperatively, then one can expect to find enlargement of parathyroid glands at the time of thyroid surgery; however, enlarged parathyroid glands are often seen in the absence of an elevated serum calcium concentration. Although the operative procedure of choice has been a subtotal (3½ gland) parathroidectomy, it has been our policy recently to perform total parathyroidectomy with an autograft of parathyroid tissue into the forearm musculature[17] (see also Chapter 26).

Postoperative Follow-up

In MEN-II, the medullary carcinoma is the disease that is most frequently lethal for the host. As mentioned previously, the behavior of this disease is variable, being more virulent in some patients than others. With the radioimmunoassay for TCT, a specific tumor marker can be followed, and invariably the detection of an elevated level of this hormone in the peripheral blood following surgery is indicative of recurrent or persistent MCT. It is the policy of most physicians following a sizable number of MCT patients to perform pentagastrin stimulation tests or calcium infusion tests once a year after surgery. If an elevated TCT level is detected in the plasma of a patient when it was previously undetectable, then it is useful to perform a selective venous catheterization with pentagastrin stimulation to detect the site(s) of tumor recurrence. This is done by simultaneously placing catheters into both innominate veins, the hepatic vein, and a peripheral vein and then injecting pentagastrin intravenously. Blood samples are simultaneously drawn at 1, 2, 3, 5, and 10 minutes, and plasma TCT levels are determined by radioimmunoassay. An elevated level in any of the sampled sites indicates the presence of MCT. If one detects an elevated TCT level in the hepatic vein, then this is diagnostic of metastatic MCT involvement. If the disease is confined to the neck in patients following initial thyroid surgery, then a second exploration and neck dissection may be indicated.

The ideal treatment of nonresectable metastatic MCT is unclear. This tumor is known to be radioresistant, and there has been very little data assessing its responsiveness to chemotherapeutic agents. Some investigators have indicated that these neoplasms are responsive to doxorubicin hydrochloride. Responsiveness of these neoplasms to chemotherapeutic agents can be readily assessed by measuring TCT serially during treatment.

SELECTED REFERENCES

Ballard, H. S., Frame, B., and Hartsock, R. J.: Familial multiple endocrine adenoma-peptic ulcer complex. Medicine, 43:481, 1964.
This paper represents an extensive evaluation of patients with MEA-I. It covers all aspects of the disease, including a historical review, clinical manifestations, pathology, genetic aspects, diagnosis, and management.

Harrison, T. S., and Thompson, N. W.: Multiple endocrine adenomatosis-I and II. Curr. Prob. Surg., August, 1975.
This monograph gives an up-to-date discussion of clinical presentation and management of both MEA-I and MEN-II.

Khairi, M. R. A., Dexter, R. N., Burzynski, N. J., et al.: Mucosal neuroma, pheochromocytoma and medullary thyroid carcinoma: Multiple endocrine neoplasia type 3. Medicine, 54:89, 1975.
This monograph discusses the most recently described variant of MEN-II. The authors have a large number of personal cases and have collected others from the literature. These cases are grouped together to give an excellent discussion of the clinical manifestations of this specific syndrome.

Melvin, K. E. W., Tashjian, A. H., Jr., and Miller, H. H.: Studies in familial (medullary) thyroid carcinoma. Recent Prog. Horm. Res., 28:399, 1972.
This paper is devoted to the genetic aspects, pathophysiology, early diagnosis utilizing the thyrocalcitonin radioimmunoassay, and surgical management of MEN-II.

REFERENCES

1. Ballard, H. S., Frame, B., and Hartsock, R. J.: Familial multiple endocrine adenoma-peptic ulcer complex. Medicine, 43:481, 1964.
2. Baylin, S. B., Beaven, N. A., Engelman, K., et al.: Elevated histaminase activity in medullary carcinoma of the thyroid gland. N. Engl. J. Med., 283:1239, 1970.
3. Baylin, S. B.: Medullary carcinoma of the thyroid gland: Use of biochemical parameters in detection and surgical managment of the tumor. Surg. Clin. North Am., 54:309, 1974.
4. Friesen, S. R.: A gastric factor in the pathogenesis of the Zollinger-Ellison syndrome. Ann. Surg., 168:483, 1968.
5. Hazard, J. B., Hawk, W. H., and Crile, G., Jr.: Medullary (solid) carcinoma of the thyroid: A clinico-pathologic entity. J. Clin. Endocrinol. Metab., 19:152, 1959.
6. Hennessy, J. F., Wells, S. A., Jr., Ontjes, D. A., et al.: A comparison of pentagastrin injection and calcium infusion as provocative agents for the detection of medullary carcinoma of the thyroid. J. Clin. Endocrinol. Metab., 39:47, 1974.
7. Hill, C. S., Jr., Ibanez, M. L., Samaan, N. A., et al.: Medullary (solid) carcinoma of the thyroid gland—an analysis of the M.D. Anderson Hospital experience with patients with the tumor, its special features and its histogenesis. Medicine, 52:141, 1973.
8. Keiser, H. R., Beaven, M. A., Doppman, J., et al.: Sipple's syndrome: Medullary thyroid carcinoma, pheochromocytoma, and parathyroid disease. Ann. Intern. Med., 78:561, 1973.
9. Khairi, M. R. A., Dexter, R. N., Burzynski, N. J., et al.: Mucosal neuroma, pheochromocytoma and medullary thyroid carcinoma: Multiple endocrine neoplasia type 3. Medicine, 54:89, 1975.
10. Melvin, K. E. W., Miller, H. H., and Tashjian, A. H., Jr.: Early diagnosis of medullary carcinoma of the thyroid by means of calcitonin assay. N. Engl. J. Med., 285:1115, 1971.
11. Melvin, K. E. W., Tashjian, A. H., Jr., and Miller, H. H.: Studies in familial (medullary) thyroid carcinoma. Recent Prog. Horm. Res., 28:399, 1972.
12. Melvin, K. E. W., Tashjian, A. H., Jr., Cassidy, C. E., et al.: Cushing's syndrome caused by ACTH and calcitonin-secreting medullary carcinoma of the thyroid. Metabolism, 19:831, 1970.
13. Pearse, A. G. E.: Common cytochemical and ultrastructural characteristics of cells producing polypeptide hormones (of the APUD series) and their relevance to thyroid and ultimobranchial C-cells and calcitonin. Proc. R. Soc. (Biol.), 170:71, 1968.
14. Sipple, J. H.: The association of pheochromocytoma with carcinoma of the thyroid gland. Am. J. Med., 31:163, 1961.
15. Steiner, A. L., Goodman, A. D., and Powers, S. R.: Study of a kindred with pheochromocytoma, medullary thyroid carcinoma, hyperparathyroidism and Cushing's disease. Multiple endocrine neoplasia type 2. Medicine, 47:371, 1968.
16. Tashjian, A. H., Jr., Howland, B. G., Melvin, K. E. W., et al.: Immunoassay of human calcitonin. Clinical management, relation to serum calcium in studies in patients with medullary carcinoma. N. Engl. J. Med., 283:890, 1970.
17. Wells, S. A., Gunnells, J. C., Shelburne, J. D., et al.: Transplantation of the parathyroid glands in man. Clinical indications and results. Surgery, 78:34, 1975.
18. Wells, S. A., Ontjes, D. A., Cooper, C. W., et al.: The early diagnosis of medullary carcinoma of the thyroid gland in patients with multiple endocrine neoplasia type II. Ann. Surg., 182:128, 1975.
19. Wermer, P.: Endocrine adenomatosis: Peptic ulcer in a large kindred. Am. J. Med., 35:205, 1963.
20. Zollinger, R. M., and Ellison, E. H.: Primary peptic ulceration of the jejunum associated with islet cell tumors of the pancreas. Ann. Surg., 142:709, 1955.

26

THE PARATHYROID GLANDS

Samuel A. Wells, Jr., M.D.

HISTORICAL ASPECTS

In 1880 a Swedish medical student, Ivar Sandström, first described the parathyroid glands in several animals including man. His discovery went unnoticed until 1891, when the glands were rediscovered by Gley, who also demonstrated that their removal led to tetany. Years later MacCallum and Voegtlin noted a decrease in blood calcium levels of thyroparathyroidectomized animals and found that the tetany that frequently ensued could be corrected by the infusion of calcium salts. In the same year as Gley's discovery, von Recklinghausen described a characteristic disease of bone that later was found to be caused by hyperparathyroidism. The first to describe the association of bone disease and parathyroid neoplasia was Askanazy who in 1904 studied a woman with pains in the extremities and spontaneous fractures. At autopsy, she was found to have both the generalized osteitis fibrosa cystica described earlier by von Recklinghausen and an "incidental" tumor lateral to the thyroid gland. In 1907 Erdheim studied several patients who had died of osteomalacia and correctly concluded that the marked parathyroid hyperplasia observed was secondary to the bone disease. Thereafter, the theory evolved that all parathyroid tumors, single as well as multiple, arose to compensate for various osseous abnormalities. Schlagenhaufer in 1915 argued that it was unlikely for compensatory hypertrophy to involve only a single gland and suggested that some parathyroid tumors were primary and caused secondary changes in the skeleton. Mandl confirmed this hypothesis 10 years later when he excised a parathyroid adenoma from a Viennese streetcar conductor who was admitted to the hospital clinic with hypercalcemia, hypercalciuria, roentgenographic changes of von Recklinghausen's bone disease, and a broken leg. After surgery the calcium in the blood and urine decreased, the bones became more dense and pain-free, and the patient became ambulatory. Within six years, however, his disease recurred and became progressively worse, ultimately resulting in his death. At the time of the recurrence he underwent a second neck exploration but no abnormal parathyroid tissue was found then or at necropsy three years later. The first case treated successfully in the United States was reported in 1929 by Barr, who proposed the term "hyperparathyroidism" for this disease.

Biologically active parathyroid extracts were first prepared independently by Hanson in 1924 and Collip in 1925. Albright's studies on calcium homeostasis and bone metabolism are classic, and he was the first to fully appreciate the frequency of renal complications in hyperparathyroidism. Parathyroid hormone was isolated and purified by Rasmussen and Craig and Aurbach in 1959. Copp in 1962 described calcitonin (thyrocalcitonin), a potent hypocalcemic agent, which was subsequently found to originate from the parafollicular cells of the thyroid gland. In 1963 Berson and Yalow developed a radioimmunoassay for parathyroid hormone.

EMBRYOLOGY

Phylogenetically, the parathyroids appear relatively late, being first seen in the Amphibia. In man the superior parathyroids arise from the fourth pharyngeal pouch and the inferior parathyroids from the third.[18] During the branchial complex stage, the glands are intimately associated with the derivatives of their respective pouches—the inferior parathyroids with the thymus and the superior parathyroids with the lateral thyroid complex. As the embryo grows, the inferior parathyroids migrate caudally owing to the descent of the thymus cord. Typically, the separation of these glands from the thymus becomes complete when they lie posterior to the lower pole of the thyroid lobe. This migration is extremely variable, however, and results at one extreme in the parathyroids being found embedded in the pharyngeal mucosa or at the more common extreme in their residing in the thoracic cavity, usually adherent to the thymus gland. Rarely, the parathyroids become completely enclosed within the thyroid parenchyma during migration of the lateral thyroid complex (Fig. 1E).

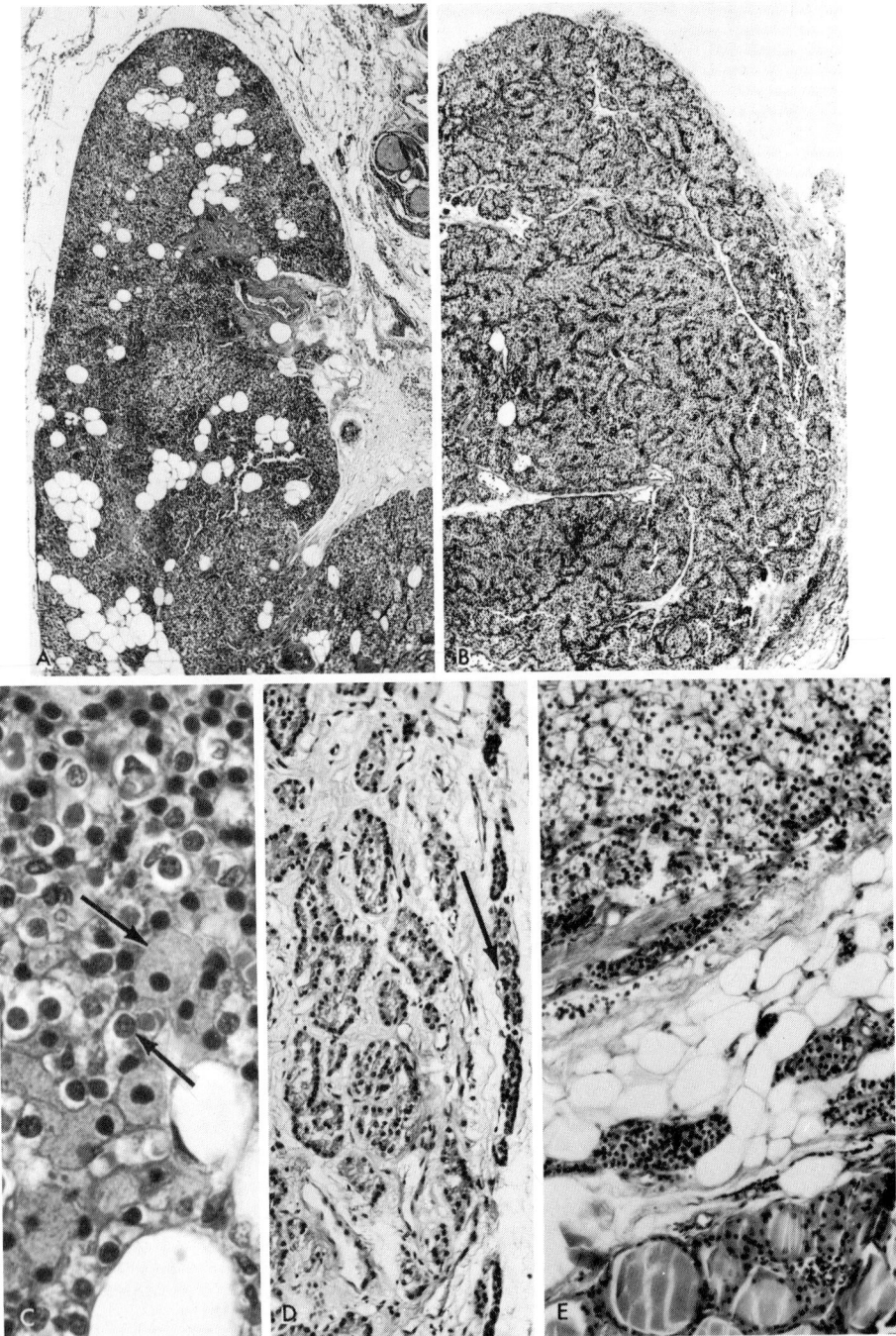

Figure 1. *A,* Normal parathyroid. A moderate amount of fat is visible throughout the gland. × 35. *B,* Primary chief cell hyperplasia. The gland is slightly enlarged, and virtually all the fat has been replaced by parathyroid cells. × 35. *C,* Normal parathyroid. The chief cells predominate and have cytoplasm that varies from dark-staining to clear. A chief cell with light cytoplasm is marked by the lower arrow. A few large oxyphilic cells are present (upper arrow). ×530. *D,* Parathyroid adenoma. The tumor has an acinar pattern suggestive of a thyroid adenoma. To the right is a thin remnant of the normal parathyroid tissue (arrow). × 115. *E,* Parathyroid adenoma (intrathyroidal). Visible are the thyroid (lower), the remnant of normal parathyroid (center), and the adenoma (upper). × 120. (Courtesy of D. J. E. Oertel, Armed Forces Institute of Pathology, Washington, D.C.)

ANATOMY

Typically, there are four parathyroid glands. In Alveryd's series of 354 adults studied at autopsy, 90.6 per cent had four glands, 3.7 per cent had five, 5.1 per cent had three, and 0.6 per cent had two glands.[2] Similar findings have been reported by others. In only one of Alveryd's 18 patients with three identified parathyroid glands was the combined weight of the glands sufficiently high to suggest that none had been overlooked. Alveryd therefore concluded that nearly all persons have four or more parathyroid glands. In the 109 cases of Norris and the 35 cases of Boyd, in which parathyroids were identified by studying serial sections of embryos, at least four parathyroid glands were found in every specimen. Norris considered supernumerary glands the result of the separation of parathyroid remnants when the glands pulled away from the pouch structures during the branchial complex phase.

The vascular supply to the parathyroid glands is usually from the inferior thyroid artery but it can arise from the superior thyroid artery, the thyroid ima artery, and arteries in the larynx, trachea, esophagus, or mediastinum or from anastomoses between these vessels. The inferior, middle, and superior thyroid veins drain the parathyroid glands.

About 50 per cent of all parathyroids will be found adjacent to the area where the inferior thyroid artery enters the thyroid parenchyma. The superior parathyroids are usually located on the posterior surface of the upper two thirds of the thyroid lobe, while the inferior glands are anterolateral to the thyroid lobe and closer to the lower pole. Approximately 10 per cent of parathyroid glands are located in the mediastinum, usually at the thoracic inlet. In about 80 per cent of patients the position of both the superior and inferior parathyroid glands on one side does not deviate more than 2 cm. from the position of the glands on the opposite side. The normal glands tend to be flat and ovoid but on enlargement they become globular. Normally, they measure 5 to 7 mm. by 3 to 4 mm. by 0.5 to 2 mm. The combined weight of the parathyroids is 90 to 130 mg. and the upper glands generally are smaller than the lower. In adults the parathyroids are usually reddish brown to yellow, whereas in the newborn they are gray and semitransparent.

HISTOLOGY

The main cell of primate parathyroid glands and the only cell of many species of lower animals is the chief cell, two types of which have been described. The light chief cell is supposedly hormonally inactive, while the dark chief cell is considered to be the main source of parathyroid hormone. This functional separation is controversial, however, and many feel that both cell types contribute to hormone production. Through infancy and early childhood, the parathyroid glands are composed almost entirely of chief cells (Fig. 1C). The acidophilic oxyphil cells (Fig. 1C) appear in the parathyroids near puberty and increase in number with age. Normally present but few in number are the polygonal water-clear cells which have little visible cytoplasm. The oxyphil cells and the water-clear cells are derived from chief cells, and both are apparently capable of secreting parathyroid hormone. Also, an abundant number of fat cells are present within the parenchyma of the adult parathyroid gland (Fig. 1A).

CALCIUM AND PHOSPHATE METABOLISM

Calcium is a constituent of all animal fluids and it is involved in a variety of physiologic processes, ranging from blood coagulation and bone formation to milk production. It constitutes about 2 per cent of the adult body weight and almost all of the total quantity is contained in the skeleton. Plasma calcium measures 9.0 to 10.5 mg. per 100 ml. (4.5 to 5.2 mEq. per liter) and is about equally divided between an ionized and a protein-bound phase. Five per cent is bound to organic anions. Of greatest importance is ionized calcium, which is most immediately related to the activity of the parathyroid glands. Calcium is absorbed in the upper small intestine in the inorganic form; the daily requirement is approximately 1 gm.

The adult body contains about 700 gm. of phosphate, most being located in the bones and teeth. Plasma phosphate measures 2.5 to 4.3 mg. per 100 ml. The plasma levels of calcium and phosphate vary inversely one with the other. Normally, the relationship is such that the product of plasma calcium and phosphate (measured in milligrams per 100 ml.) is constant and ranges between 30 and 40. The daily requirement of phosphate is 1 gm.

PHYSIOLOGY

Two polypeptides, *parathyroid hormone* (molecular weight 9500) and *calcitonin* (molecular weight 3600), are the principal hormones regulating calcium metabolism. The rate of secretion of parathyroid hormone is not under the control of any known trophic hormone. It is, however, inversely related to plasma calcium concentration but is uninfluenced by the levels of plasma phosphate. The hormone mainly affects the skeleton and kidney. In the former, it causes a shift of calcium from bone to the extracellular fluids. This is a direct effect and although the exact mechanism of bone resorption is unknown, it appears to be mediated by the osteoclast. In the kidney, parathyroid hormone directly increases the tubular excretion of phosphate and enhances calcium reabsorption from the glomerular filtrate. There is suggestive evidence that parathyroid hormone increases the absorption of calcium from the gastrointestinal tract but if so, this action is significantly less than its effect on the bone and kidney. The hormone activity is mediated by cyclic 3'5'-adenosine monophosphate (3'5'-AMP) produced through specific hormonal activation of the enzyme adenyl cyclase in the bone and kidney.

The secretion of calcitonin is a direct function of plasma calcium concentration. The primary action of this hormone is to inhibit bone resorption, but the biochemical mechanism by which this is accomplished is unknown.

The D vitamins are biologically active sterols that promote the absorption of calcium and phosphate from the gastrointestinal tract. They also enhance bone resorption and exert a growth-promoting effect that is not explained by mineral retention. The physiologic effect of vitamin D on the kidney is at present unclear.

DISORDERS OF THE PARATHYROID GLANDS

HYPERPARATHYROIDISM

The cause of spontaneous hyperfunction of the parathyroid glands is unknown and, as with many endocrine neoplasms, overactivity is recognized not because of anatomic enlargement but because of the peripheral effects of excess hormone. Primary hyperparathyroidism occurs when the normal feedback control by serum calcium is lost and there is autonomous production of parathyroid hormone. Secondary hyperparathyroidism occurs most commonly in patients with renal disease but also compensates for the true hypocalcemia associated with some diseases of the gastrointestinal tract, bone, or other endocrine organs. There is a defect in mineral homeostasis leading to a compensatory increase in parathyroid gland function and size. Occasionally with prolonged compensatory stimulation, a hyperplastic gland develops autonomous function. This state is referred to as tertiary hyperparathyroidism.

Primary Hyperparathyroidism

Parathyroid Adenoma. Primary hyperparathyroidism develops most frequently in persons between the ages of 35 and 65. It occurs three times more commonly in females than in males and is especially common in postmenopausal women. It is extremely rare in childhood. In the majority of cases a single adenoma composed predominantly of chief cells is the offending lesion (Table 1). Water-clear cell adenomas are much less frequent, and oxyphil cell adenomas are rare and frequently nonfunctional. Some pathologists do not classify adenomas histologically because on careful search all cell types can be found. At frozen section examination there is little fatty stroma and the adenoma is surrounded by a rim of normal parathyroid tissue (Fig. 1D). Numerically, the tumors appear more commonly in the inferior than in the superior glands. Recently, Lloyd[15] has shown that patients with bone disease alone have a higher serum calcium, a greater tumor weight, and a shorter duration of symptoms than patients with only renal disease. On the basis of these observations he proposed that there were two different types of parathyroid tumors: one growing rapidly, being highly active, and causing overt bone disease; and the other growing slowly, being of low activity, and causing kidney stones. There was no characteristic tumor histology associated with either type of disease.

Primary Hyperplasia. This phenomenon occurs in two forms: primary water-clear cell hyperplasia and primary chief cell hyperplasia. Albright[1] described water-clear cell hyperplasia in 1934. Clinically it is indistinguishable from the hyperparathyroidism associated with adenomas, but the gross appearance at operation is characteristic. All four glands are diffusely enlarged and dark brown with uneven surfaces and numerous pseudopods. The cut surface appears cystic. Microscopically the glands are composed almost entirely of water-clear cells.

Primary chief cell hyperplasia was first described by Cope in 1958.[6] Some pathologists consider the disease to be characterized by generalized hyperplasia while others feel that all four glands are adenomatous. There may be a great difference between the sizes of the glands and frequently the superior are larger than the inferior. The glands are often nodular and reddish brown, and grossly they are characterized by the presence of fibrous septa within the gland substance. Histologically, chief cells predominate (Fig. 1B), but there also are nests of water-clear or oxyphil cells. In Cope's original series several patients had associated endocrine disturbances including insulin- and noninsulin-producing islet cell adenomas, pituitary tumors, adrenal hyperplasia, and thyroid adenomas. Pancreatitis and peptic ulcer disease occur much more commonly in persons with this pathologic entity than in the general population.

Parathyroid Carcinoma. Carcinoma of the parathyroid glands is rare, with only 50 unequivocal cases described in Holmes' 1969 review.[12] In more than 90 per cent of the cases the disease is functional and presents as primary hyperparathyroidism, usually with a markedly elevated serum calcium. About 50 per cent of the patients have palpable neck masses. At operation the tumor is characteristically hard and surrounded by a dense, white fibrous tissue. The presence of mitoses on histologic examination greatly strengthens the diagnosis. Frequently at the initial operation, it is not appreciated that malignant disease exists and inadequate resection is done. Adequate surgical treatment entails removal of the thyroid isthmus and the ipsilateral lobe, skeletonization of the trachea, and excision of involved muscle and nerve. Ipsilateral radical neck dissection is also indicated because of the high incidence of regional lymph node

TABLE 1.   The Pathologic Classification of Primary Hyperparathyroidism*

	Per Cent
Neoplasia	
Benign	
Single adenoma	83.0
Multiple adenoma	4.3
Carcinoma	1.7
Hyperplasia	
Wasserhelle or water-clear cell	7.6
Chief-cell†	3.6

*Based upon 751 cases. From Rasmussen, H. *In* Williams, R. H. (Ed.): Textbook of Endocrinology, 5th ed. Philadelphia, W. B. Saunders Company, 1974.

†Associated with polyendocrine disorders. The reported incidence may be too low because some authors classify this disorder as multiple adenoma.

metastases. Fifty per cent of the patients in Holmes' review survived 5 years but only 13 per cent lived for 10 years.

Hypercalcemia and Malignancy. When hypercalcemia occurs in association with nonparathyroid malignant disease, it is usually due to osseous metastases. Albright first suggested that localized nonparathyroid malignant tumors might produce parathyroid hormone, and subsequently there have been reports confirming his supposition.[22] In most cases, however, it has not been possible to measure parathyroid hormone, in either the patient's plasma or tumor, thereby suggesting that there were other causes of the hypercalcemia. In addition to parathyroid hormone, vitamin D (or its metabolites), nonvitamin D sterols, prostaglandins, and osteoclast-activating factors from leukocytes have been proposed as inducing an elevated serum calcium. The extent to which any of these substances might be operational in causing hypercalcemia clinically is at present unclear, but it certainly seems likely that there are several factors which account for this syndrome in cancer patients.

Familial Hyperparathyroidism. The familial occurrence of hyperparathyroidism is well established. In its simplest form it occurs as a single disease with no associated abnormalities,[7] while in its more complex form, it presents as a part of one of the multiple endocrinopathy syndromes. Multiple endocrine adenomatosis type I (MEA-I) is characterized by the association of parathyroid hyperplasia, pituitary adenomas, pancreatic neoplasms, and occasionally tumors of the thyroid or adrenal cortex. Many patients with MEA-I also have the Zollinger-Ellison syndrome. Multiple endocrine neoplasia type II (MEN-II) is a concurrence of parathyroid hyperplasia, medullary carcinoma of the thyroid gland, and pheochromocytoma(s). Each of the multiple endocrinopathy syndromes is characterized by an autosomal dominant pattern of inheritance. They are discussed at greater length in Chapter 6.

Secondary Hyperparathyroidism

Since the initiation of maintenance dialysis and renal transplantation the course of patients with chronic renal disease has been altered. One of the frequent complications found in such patients has been the development of secondary hyperparathyroidism, which is commonly associated with metastatic calcification and a variety of bone lesions collectively referred to as renal osteodystrophy. Occasionally the medical management is unsatisfactory or the disease is incapacitating and surgical removal of the hyperfunctioning parathyroid tissue may be necessary. Almost invariably the histopathology of the offending lesion is generalized hyperplasia.

Clinical Presentation (Signs and Symptoms)

Hyperparathyroidism presents in a variety of ways. It is diagnosed more frequently today than a decade ago because it is being sought more aggressively. Most hospitals now include calcium and phosphorus determinations as part of their admission screening laboratory evaluation and as a consequence many asymptomatic patients with the disease are discovered each year. The incidence of the disease in a clinical population has recently been reported to be 1 in 1000.

TABLE 2. Presenting Symptoms in Patients with Hyperparathyroidism*

	Percentage
Skeletal symptoms	8.0
Fracture	1.0
Local bone tumor	0.5
Urinary symptoms	60.0
Hypertension	1.0
Gastrointestinal symptoms	10.0
Muscular weakness or generalized fatigue	6.0
Psychiatric complaints	4.0
Discovered on routine chemical screening	3.0–8.0

*From Rasmussen, H. *In* Williams, R. H. (Ed.: Textbook of Endocrinology, 5th ed. Philadelphia, W. B. Saunders Company, 1974.

The usual symptomatic case of hyperparathyroidism seen by the physician is in the chronic phase with signs and symptoms from secondary changes in the genitourinary system and skeleton. The most common presenting symptoms are those shown in Table 2. The earliest complaints, such as muscle weakness, anorexia, nausea, constipation, polyuria, and polydipsia, occasionally cause the patient to seek medical advice, but it is unusual for these vague symptoms to lead to the correct diagnosis.

Renal Complications. Renal complications are generally the most severe clinical manifestations of hyperparathyroidism. Usually the presenting symptoms are related to nephrolithiasis, which occurs in about 65 per cent of cases; conversely, about 5 to 10 per cent of patients presenting with nephrolithiasis have hyperparathyroidism. Patients complain of back pain, hematuria, and the passing of renal calculi, most of which are composed of calcium phosphate or calcium oxalate. Nephrocalcinosis represents calcification within the parenchyma of one or both kidneys and is much less common than nephrolithiasis, occurring in only 5 to 10 per cent of patients. It is very unusual for nephrolithiasis and nephrocalcinosis to occur together. Although renal stones can be removed surgically, there is nothing that can be done for nephrocalcinosis, and after definitive treatment of hyperparathyroidism, there is rarely improvement of this condition. Renal damage is much more common in patients with evidence of nephrolithiasis, and especially nephrocalcinosis, but it can occur in the absence of renal calcification. If renal impairment is severe preoperatively, it tends to remain unchanged or become progressively worse postoperatively; mild degrees of renal damage are usually functional and reversible. Careful evaluation of renal function in patients with hyperparathyroidism reveals an incidence of some degree of renal damage in 80 to 90 per cent.

The incidence of hypertension in patients with hyperparathyroidism was about 70 per cent in Hellstrom's series of 139 patients, and the persistence of high blood pressure postoperatively correlated closely with the degree of preoperative renal impairment.

Hypertension with its associated clinical complications (heart failure, cerebral hemorrhage, and renal insufficiency) was responsible for death in 30 per cent of the patients having persistent hypertension after parathyroid surgery. Hellstrom's investigation demonstrates in a striking fashion the importance of this complication in hyperparathyroidism and the urgency of early diagnosis and treatment if the late cardiovascular and renal sequelae are to be minimized.

Musculoskeletal Complications. Musculoskeletal symptoms usually are mild and rather vague and include weakness, hypotonia, and bone or joint pain, but in severe cases of bone involvement actual fractures may occur or shortening of stature may be evident. The earliest roentgenographic skeletal change is subperiosteal resorption, which occurs most commonly in the phalanges of the hand (Fig. 2), the distal third of the clavicle, and the distal ulna. Generalized demineralization also occurs. X-rays of the skull may show a washed-out granular appearance with diffuse miliary osteolytic areas (Fig. 3). Bone cysts (Fig. 4) and os-

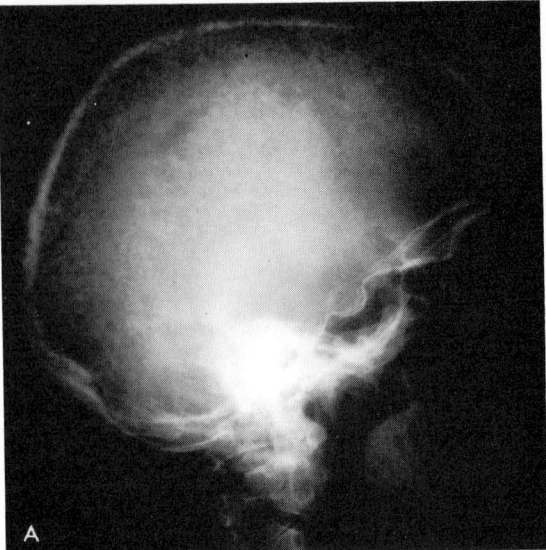

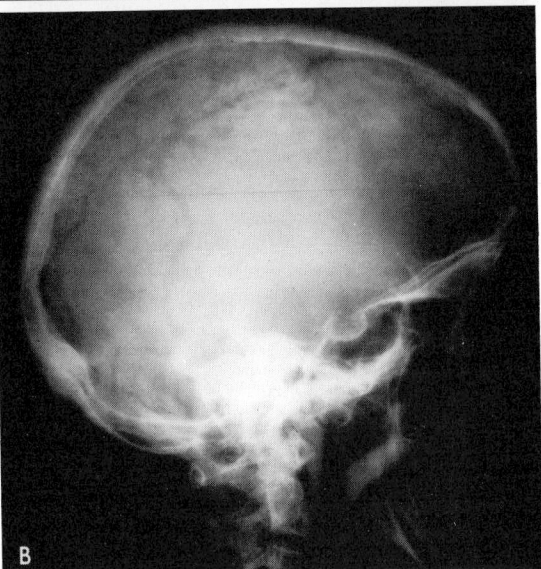

Figure 3. *A*, Skull x-ray from a patient with hyperparathyroidism. There is demineralization imparting a salt-and-pepper texture to the calvarium with obliteration of the normal vascular grooves of the inner table. The cortex of the ascending ramus and alveolar ridge of the mandible are severely demineralized. *B*, Two years after removal of parathyroid adenoma there is restoration of normal bone mineralization. (Courtesy of Dr. Peter Shimkin, National Institutes of Health, Bethesda, Md.)

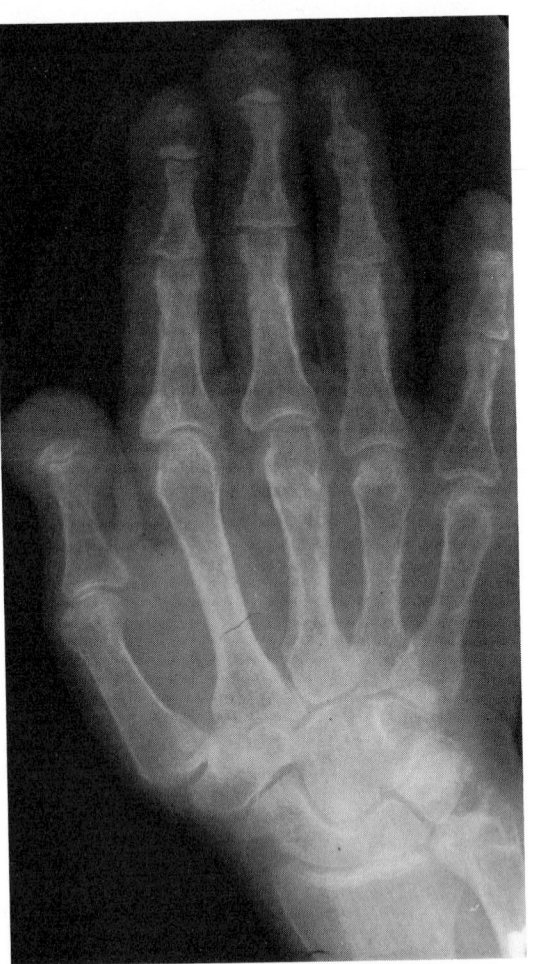

Figure 2. Hand x-ray. Note uniform demineralization with concomitant soft tissue clubbing, severe erosion of distal phalanges, and cyst at base of middle phalanx, index finger. Subperiosteal cortical resorption is best shown along the metacarpal shaft of the fifth digit. (Courtesy of Dr. Peter Shimkin, National Institutes of Health, Bethesda, Md.)

teoclastomas are a distinctive finding. These commonly occur in the central medullary part of the shaft of the long bones, the metacarpals, and the ribs.

Gastrointestinal Manifestations. The gastrointestinal effects of hyperparathyroidism include anorexia, constipation, nausea and vomiting, peptic ulcer, and pancreatitis. Chronic duodenal ulcer associated with hyperparathyroidism was first reported by Rogers[21] in 1946. Subsequently there have been several cases reported, in most of which there have been duodenal

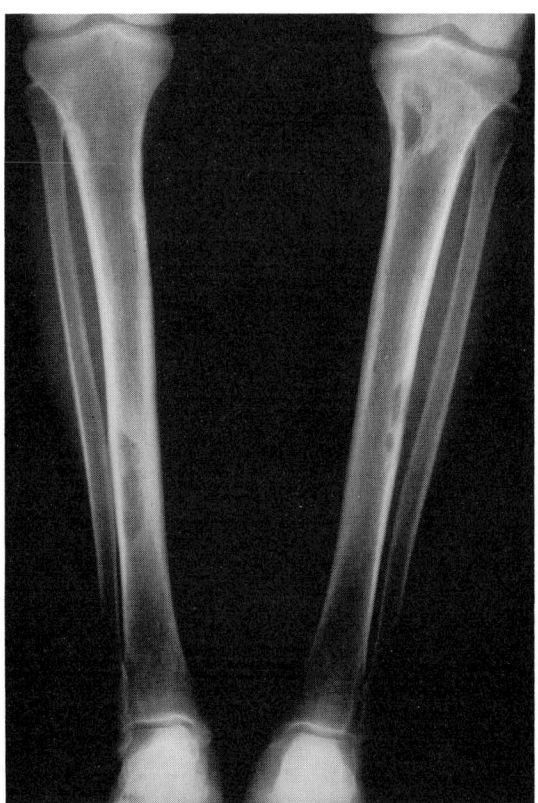

Figure 4. Lower leg x-ray. Multiple bone cysts (brown tumors) are present. The cortical location and sharp margins are characteristic. (Courtesy of Dr. Peter Shimkin, National Institutes of Health, Bethesda, Md.)

rather than gastric ulcers and hyperplasia of the parathyroid glands rather than adenomas. The reported incidence of peptic ulcers complicating hyperparathyroidism is about 10 per cent. Many feel that this approaches the incidence of peptic ulcer in the general population and that there is no increased frequency of ulcer disease in patients with hyperparathyroidism. Furthermore, most published series have failed to separate the cases of peptic ulcer occurring familially, as with the multiple endocrine adenomatosis syndrome, in which there is a definitely increased incidence, from nonfamilial cases of hyperparathyroidism. There have been, however, several cases reported in which intractable ulcers have healed or become manageable following the removal of hyperfunctioning parathyroid tissue. Thus, the true relationship between hyperparathyroidism and peptic ulcer is not fully settled, but most reviewers feel that a special relationship exists between the two.

The incidence of pancreatitis in patients with hyperparathyroidism is about 7 per cent; this is greater than could be accounted for by mere coincidence. Pancreatitis seems to be especially common in cases of acute hyperparathyroidism and in cases of parathyroid carcinoma. The etiology of the pancreatitis is unknown.

Acute Hyperparathyroidism. Most patients presenting with hyperparathyroidism are chronically ill with complaints referable to the kidneys or skeleton.

Rarely, however, patients may become acutely ill with urgent symptoms which sometimes prove fatal.[14] The terms "acute hyperparathyroidism" and "acute hyperparathyroid crisis" have been used to describe this clinical dilemma. The onset is usually characterized by rapidly developing muscular weakness, nausea and vomiting, weight loss, fatigue, drowsiness, and confusion. Males and females are equally affected. The serum calcium is almost always elevated, in the range of 16 to 20 mg. per 100 ml., and azotemia is usually present. This clinical picture not only is associated with hyperparathyroidism but also is seen in patients with acute hypercalcemia accompanying other diseases. The offending lesion is most often a single parathyroid adenoma, but hyperplasia, carcinoma, and multiple adenomas have all been causative. The lesions are usually large and in about one third of the patients a tumor is palpable in the neck preoperatively, which is not surprising since larger adenomas are usually associated with higher calcium values than are smaller ones. The etiology of this sudden increase in parathyroid activity is unknown; there have been cases reported in which sudden hemorrhage into an adenoma was associated with the crisis but this is uncommon. The treatment of choice is immediate surgical removal, which is curative in about 90 per cent of the patients. If the diagnosis is missed or if treatment is unduly delayed, the mortality approaches 40 per cent. Rarely, surgical therapy is not immediately possible because the patient is too ill with accompanying disease, and medical therapy must be instituted. This measure is a temporizing one, however.

Physical Findings

Few physical findings aid in the diagnosis. Patients rarely have palpable lesions in the neck. With longstanding hypercalcemia, there may be band keratopathy and extraosseous calcification.

Laboratory Findings

Hypercalcemia is almost always present, and calcium determination is the single biochemical test that most frequently leads to the diagnosis. There have been patients reported who were not hypercalcemic, "normocalcemic hyperparathyroidism," but this entity is controversial. Plasma phosphate is reduced in about 50 per cent of patients and hypercalciuria is usually present, especially late in the disease. An elevated serum alkaline phosphatase is found in 30 per cent of hyperparathyroid patients, being most commonly associated with osteitis. Hyperchloremia is a little-known but helpful diagnostic clue. Values below 102 mEq. per liter are seldom found in patients with hyperparathyroidism. All of these biochemical findings may be altered if significant renal damage develops.

Special Diagnostic Tests

Determination of Tubular Reabsorption of Phosphate. Parathyroid hormone increases the renal clearance of phosphate by decreasing its tubular reabsorption. It would be expected that a test demonstrating this alteration should be of value in identifying patients with hyperparathyroidism, but of the many such tests based on this phenomenon, none is sufficiently specific to distinguish uniformly between normal and hyperparathyroid subjects. Intravenous calcium infusion usually decreases the phosphate clearance less markedly in hyperparathyroid patients than in normal persons, and this modification has been used diagnostically by several investigators with some success. It is not completely satisfactory, however, since normal responses have been observed in some patients with hyperactive glands while changes typical of hyperparathyroidism have been found in normal subjects.

Glucocorticoid Suppression Test. Most cases of hypercalcemia due to hyperparathyroidism are resistant to the oral administration of glucocorticoids. Hypercalcemia due to other causes such as hypervitaminosis D, sarcoidosis, the milk-alkali syndrome, or metastatic cancer usually is suppressed by glucocorticoid administration but this is variable. The test is helpful in the differential diagnosis of hypercalcemia but considered alone is of little diagnostic value.

Determinations of Parathyroid Hormone Levels in the Blood. Berson and Yalow[4] first described a radioimmunoassay for parathyroid hormone in 1963. The method is based on the ability of unlabeled hormone in human plasma to inhibit competitively the binding of bovine parathyroid hormone labeled with iodine-131 to antibodies against bovine parathyroid hormone. The authors detected elevated levels of hormone in the peripheral blood of almost all patients with chronic renal disease and about half of the patients with parathyroid adenomas. Egdahl[9] found elevated peripheral levels of parathyroid hormone in each of 12 patients with parathyroid adenomas or hyperplasia. The hormone levels rose during operative manipulation of the hyperfunctional glands but fell sharply postoperatively. As a diagnostic parameter, an elevated peripheral plasma parathyroid hormone level is present in 70 to 80 per cent of hyperparathyroid patients. In practically all patients, however, concentrations of parathyroid hormone are inappropriately high relative to serum calcium.

Of greatest help in localizing parathyroid neoplasms has been the radioimmunoassay measurement of parathyroid hormone in plasma obtained by selective venous catheterization. Parathyroid adenomas have been localized in the neck and mediastinum by detecting increased hormone levels in the superior vena cava, jugular and innominate veins. Selective catheterization of the inferior thyroid veins has offered the greatest sensitivity in correctly localizing hyperfunctioning tissue (Fig. 5). This technique has been especially helpful in patients with persistent or recurrent hyperparathyroidism following previous parathyroid exploration when the anatomy is distorted and localization is helpful in preventing injury to important structures during a second exploration.[23] The one disadvantage of radioimmunoassay is that it takes several days to determine hormone levels in the submitted samples.

Renal Cyclic Adenosine Monophosphate (R-CAMP). Parathyroid hormone exerts its effect on target organs, bone, and kidney by activating adenylate cyclase and elevating tissue concentrations of cyclic 3'5'-AMP (CAMP). This parathyroid hormone action

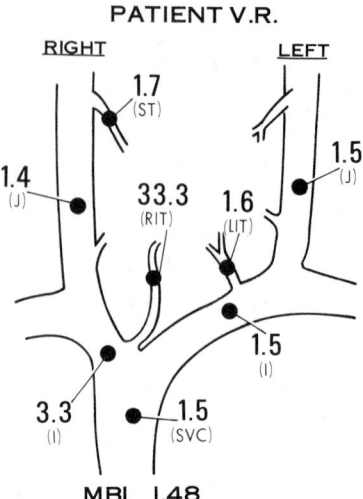

Figure 5. Patient V.R. Parathyroid hormone radioimmunoassay values of plasma samples obtained at selective venous catheterization. A right inferior parathyroid adenoma was found at operation. J = jugular; I = innominate; SVC = superior vena cava; ST = superior thyroid vein; LIT = left inferior thyroid vein; RIT = right inferior thyroid vein; MBL = mean background level of parathyroid hormone in the peripheral circulation.

on the kidney leads also to an increase in urinary excretion of CAMP. In primary hyperparathyroidism, the mean urinary excretion of the nucleotide is elevated, and conversely in hypoparathyroidism, the rate of excretion is decreased. The sensitivity of CAMP measurement can be increased by determining the fraction of the nucleotide actually contributed by the action of parathyroid hormone on the proximal nephron as differentiated from the total urinary cyclic AMP, including that derived from the plasma. Although there are few clinical reports evaluating the utility of this test, it promises to be most helpful in differentiating hyperparathyroid patients from normals and from other hypercalcemic patients without hyperparathyroidism.

Arteriographic Localization. Parathyroid adenomas were first demonstrated arteriographically by Seldinger in 1954. This technique has been utilized by several investigators to localize abnormal parathyroid glands (Fig. 6), but the results are usually negative with small adenomas and the test has not achieved general use diagnostically.

Isotopic Labeling. Cobalt-57 cyanocobalamin and selenium-75 selenomethionine localize selectively in the parathyroid glands of humans. The specificity of [57]Co B[12] has been insufficient to permit localization by photoscanning. Selenium-75 selenomethionine has been used successfully to detect large parathyroid tumors but, like the arteriogram, the test is not sufficiently sensitive to detect the more commonly occurring small adenomas.

Differential Diagnosis

Several other diseases cause hypercalcemia and must be differentiated from primary hyperparathyroid-

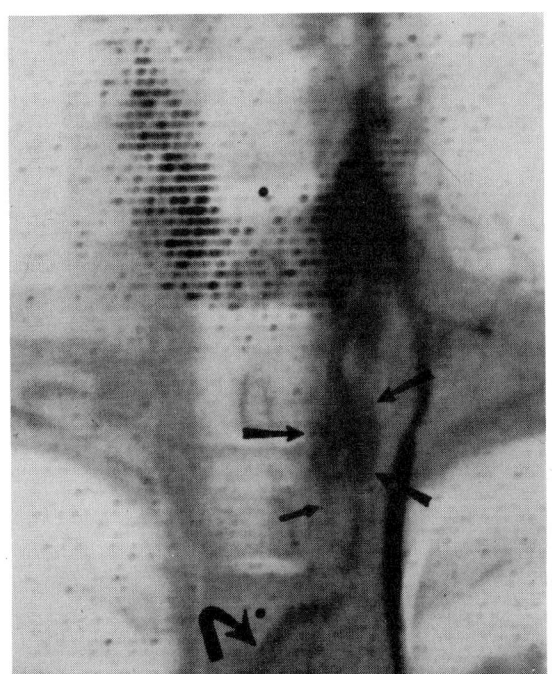

Figure 6. Late phase of an inferior thyroid arteriogram. The left lower parathyroid adenoma stain is indicated by the four small arrows. The normal thyroid gland blush is superior and is identified as such by superimposition of the thyroid scan. The curved arrow denotes the draining inferior thyroid vein. (Courtesy of Dr. Peter Shimkin, National Institutes of Health, Bethesda, Md.)

ism if unnecessary neck exploration is to be avoided. The milk-alkali syndrome, vitamin D intoxication, and hypercalcemia secondary to immobilization can usually be diagnosed by the history. Hyperthyroidism can usually be diagnosed clinically and confirmed by thyroid function tests. In sarcoidosis and multiple myeloma, globulin levels are usually elevated, and each of these diseases usually has characteristic roentgenographic features, as does Paget's disease of bone. Malignant tumors without osseous metastases when associated with hypercalcemia, are the most difficult to differentiate from primary parathyroid adenomas or hyperplasia, especially if the offending carcinoma has not been diagnosed. Table 3 lists several diseases commonly accompanied by abnormalities of calcium homeostasis.

Treatment

The only curative treatment of primary hyperparathyroidism is surgery. In the usual patient, the diagnosis is not difficult and no special preoperative management is necessary. Before subjecting a patient to an operation, the surgeon obviously should be confident of the diagnosis and should have adequate experience to systematically explore the neck, recognizing in the process all normal and abnormal parathyroid tissue. The patient should be made fully aware of the possible postoperative complications, especially if bone disease and an elevated serum alkaline phosphatase level are present, because the hypocalcemia that frequently follows resection in these patients is most dis-

TABLE 3. Chemical Findings in Diseases of Calcium and Skeletal Homeostasis*

	Findings												
	Plasma							Urine					
Disease	Ca	Mg	P	Ptase	TP	BUN	Cl	Ca	TRP†	HOP‡	AA§	CA¶	AcA**
Hyperparathyroidism	↑	N↓	↓N	N↑	N	N↓	↑	↑N	↓N	↑N	↑N	↓	↓
Hypoparathyroidism	↓	N	↑	N	N	N	N	↓	↑	↓	N	N	N
Vitamin D intoxication	↑	↑	N↑↓	N↑	N	N↑	N↑	↑	↓N	–	N	N↓	N↓
Sarcoidosis	↑	–	↓N	N	↑	N	N	↑	↓N	–	–	↓	–
Milk alkali syndrome	↑	N	N	N	N	↑	↓	N	N↓	N	–	↓	–
Multiple myeloma	N↑	N	N↑	N↑	↑	↑	N↓	↑	↓	N	–	–	–
Acute bone atrophy	↑	N	↑N	N	N	N	N	↑	N	–	–	N	N
Paget's disease	N↑	N	N	↑↑	N	N	N	↑	N	↑	–	N	N
Osteoporosis	N	N	N	N	N	N	N	N↑	N	N↑	N	N	N
Osteomalacia	↓	↑N↓	↓	↑	N	N	N↑	↓	↓N	↓	↑	N	↓N
Malignant neoplasm with osseous metastasis	↑	N	N	N	N	N	N	↑	N	↑	N	N	N
Malignant neoplasm without osseous metastasis	↑	N	↓N	N↑	N	N	↑	N↑	↓N	↑	–	↓	↓
Hyperthyroidism	↑N	N	N↓	N↑	N	N	N	↑	N	↑	N	↓	N
Osteopetrosis	N	N	N	N	N	N	N	↓	N	↓	N	N	N
Idiopathic hypercalciuria	N	N	↓	N	N	N	N	↑	↓N	N	N	N	N

*From Rasmussen, H. *In* Williams, R. H. (Ed.): Textbook of Endocrinology, 5th ed. Philadelphia, W. B. Saunders Company, 1974.

　†TRP, tubular reabsorption of phosphate.

　‡HOP, hydroxyproline excretion.

　§AA, amino acid excretion.

　¶CA, renal concentrating ability.

　**AcA, renal acidifying ability.

turbing. A second exploration of the neck because of failure to find the lesion at the initial procedure is very difficult and should be avoided by an assiduous primary operation. If reoperation is required, not only is parathyroid tissue more difficult to identify but damage to the recurrent laryngeal nerve is more likely.

General anesthesia is employed and the neck is opened through a transverse cervical incision. After the strap muscles are separated in the midline, a chosen lobe of the thyroid gland is elevated and rotated medially. The tissues inferior to the thyroid lobe are cleaned down to the trachea to expose the recurrent laryngeal nerve and the inferior thyroid artery. In the majority of patients the nerve lies in the tracheoesophageal groove, less commonly lateral to the trachea, and rarely anterolateral to the trachea, where it is especially vulnerable to injury. A direct laryngeal nerve may be given off in the neck without looping around the right subclavian artery. The external branch of the superior laryngeal nerve is the most important tensor of the vocal cords and it usually lies immediately adjacent and medial to the vascular pedicle of the superior thyroid lobe. With mobilization of the lobe, care must be taken not to injure this nerve. Four or more parathyroid glands may be present and abnormal, and the reconnaissance of the neck area requires great patience. One also needs the help of an experienced pathologist because frozen section identification of the parathyroid glands is helpful. The upper parathyroid glands are more easily found and are usually located far dorsally on the surface of the thyroid lobe at the level of the upper two thirds of the gland. The lower glands are larger than the upper and less constant in location, being normally distributed from well above the upper half of the thyroid to well within the mediastinum. The lower glands are usually more anterior than the upper glands. If the upper glands are identified and normal but both of the lower glands cannot be found, then the thymus pedicle in the lower neck should be carefully examined and removed. The majority of parathyroid adenomas located in the mediastinum can be removed through the cervical incision, as they are usually adherent to this thymic tissue at the thoracic inlet. If no parathyroid tissue is found after the thymus pedicle is removed, the surgeon should mobilize, examine, and palpate both lobes of the thyroid gland, for occasionally a parathyroid is completely encapsulated within the thyroid parenchyma. Removal of a thyroid lobe on the side where a parathyroid gland is not found is occasionally indicated as a last resort but should by no means be a substitute for the meticulous search for parathyroid tissue. It is also helpful to follow the branches of the inferior thyroid artery, especially if one is enlarged, as these often lead to an abnormal parathyroid gland or adenoma. Because of the possibility of multiple gland involvement, every effort must be made to identify all four parathyroids. To be sure that one has actually identified parathyroid tissue small biopsies of the suspected glands should be taken. The organs must be handled with extreme care, however, as they are delicate structures and their blood supply is easily damaged.

Hurvitz[13] reported the use of toluidine blue dye as a selective vital stain for the parathyroid glands at the time of surgery. Others have reported varying degrees of success with this agent. Unfortunately, myocardial toxicity occurs with the drug and there has been one reported incident of possible neurotoxicity.

If after diligent search in the neck, including exploration of the upper mediastinum, retroesophageal area, carotid sheaths, and thyroid gland, no parathyroid adenoma has been found, a decision must be made regarding mediastinotomy. Most surgeons favor delay of this procedure, reasoning that the blood supply to the hyperfunctional gland might have been damaged during manipulation or that the pathologist will find the abnormal gland on further sectioning of the submitted tissues. Others have favored attack of the mediastinum at the time of the negative cervical exploration. Mediastinotomy is indicated in only about 1 to 2 per cent of patients.[17] If this procedure is decided upon it should probably not be done earlier than two to four weeks after the neck operation, assuming that serum calcium levels remain elevated. Dent has suggested that when serum calcium transiently drops following surgery, a parathyroid adenoma has been left near the operative field, its blood supply being temporarily compromised. In Hellstrom's series of parathyroid adenomas, 15 patients required subsequent mediastinal exploration following negative exploration of the neck. Six of the 15 patients were found to have parathyroid adenomas still confined to the neck. This emphasizes the importance of finding the offending parathyroid tissue at the first exploration.

In mediastinal exploration the centralmost part of the surgical scar is opened and a midline vertical incision is made from the jugular fossa to the level of the third intercostal space. After the sternum is split longitudinally in the midline, the two sternal halves are separated. The remaining thymus tissue is first isolated and examined because an adenoma will most likely be found associated with this structure located in front of the great vessels. In parathyroid adenomas that are true mediastinal organs, the blood supply is often from the mediastinal vessels and not the inferior thyroid artery. If the anterior mediastinal exploration is negative, the posterior mediastinum is next examined, especially posterior and lateral to the trachea. The location of 20 mediastinal parathyroid tumors in Nathaniels' series is depicted in Figure 7.

Upon removal of a parathyroid adenoma or hyperplastic glands, the serum calcium drops to normal within 24 to 48 hours. If bone disease is present, then the drop might be marked with the onset of circumoral tingling, carpopedal spasm, and even seizures. The alkaline phosphatase may remain elevated for a longer period of time if significant bone disease exists. The overall mortality of the operation is about 0.1 per cent, death most commonly occurring in patients with severe renal disease. Long-term administration of calcium and vitamin D supplements is required in 0.5 per cent of patients, and 0.5 per cent have permanent unilateral vocal cord paralysis.

Differentiation of "Adenomatous" from "Hyperplastic" Disease. Although the true incidence of primary

POSITION OF INDIVIDUAL MEDIASTINAL GLANDS

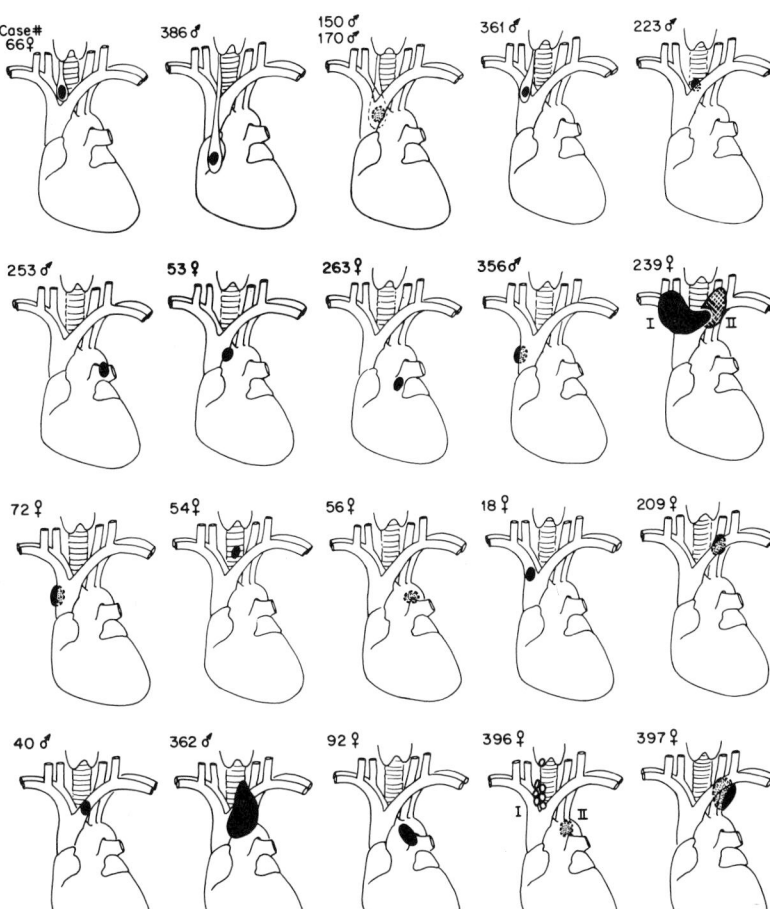

Figure 7. Schematic representation of the position of 20 mediastinal parathyroid tumors uncovered by mediastinotomy. (From Nathaniels, E. K., Nathaniels, A. M., and Wang, C. A.: Ann. Surg., *171*:169, 1970.)

parathyroid hyperplasia is unknown, there are those[10, 19] who feel that most patients with hyperparathyroidism have generalized involvement and they recommend subtotal (3 1/2 gland) parathyroidectomy in all cases of hyperparathyroidism. Most, however, think that primary parathyroid hyperplasia is uncommon and that the subjection of all hyperparathyroid patients to subtotal parathyroidectomy is unwarranted.

After locating all four parathyroid glands, the surgeon must decide which are grossly normal and which abnormal. Usually one finds a single large parathyroid gland associated with three normal-sized or smaller parathyroid glands. In this situation, one should remove the single large parathyroid gland, and a portion of the ipsilateral normal parathyroid gland for submission to frozen section. If the large parathyroid gland is interpreted as being hypercellular or an "adenoma," and the smaller gland as being normal, then the sites of the remaining parathyroid glands should be marked with a nonabsorbable suture and the neck closed. Almost invariably these patients will do well and will not develop recurrent hypercalcemia.

A difficult situation arises when more than one parathyroid gland is found to be grossly enlarged. In those cases where patients have primary parathyroid hyperplasia and all four parathyroid glands are found to be enlarged, the procedure of choice formerly had been to perform a three and one-half gland parathyroidectomy. There are few reported long-term evaluations of patients receiving this treatment, but in the series of Castleman and Cope[5] where such patients were followed postoperatively from two to ten years, half developed recurrent hypercalcemia and almost all had hypercalciuria with or without bacilliuria. It is also possible that the half gland remaining in the neck will not function and the patient will be permanently hypoparathyroid. Because of these possibilities, we have recently elected to perform a total parathyroidectomy and concomitant parathyroid autograft in this group of patients.

In the uncommon situation where two or three parathyroid glands are enlarged, and yet the other parathyroid gland(s) is small, we have elected to resect three parathyroid glands, carefully marking the location of the remaining normal sized parathyroid.

This is a most unusual and difficult situation and probably represents a state of parathyroid "hyperplasia" rather than "double adenomas." These patients occasionally require repeat neck explorations for recurrent hypercalcemia.

It should be mentioned here that while the pathologist can readily identify parathyroid tissue from other tissue by frozen section, it is often difficult for him to discriminate between parathyroid "adenomas" and hyperplasia. Even upon carefully reviewing the permanent sections, one cannot be sure histologically whether a given parathyroid gland is hyperfunctional or not. The most reliable index of abnormality is the surgeon's determination of gland size by visual observation.

Management of Secondary Hyperparathyroidism. Wilson[25] recently reported the experience at the Peter Bent Brigham Hospital, where 800 patients with chronic renal disease have been treated over the last seven years. Twenty-eight patients required the removal of hyperfunctioning parathyroid tissue. There were four major indications: (1) persistent and symptomatic hypercalcemia in prospective renal transplant patients; (2) pathologic fractures secondary to osteodystrophy; (3) symptomatic hyperparathyroidism including bone pain, ectopic calcification, and intractable itching; and (4) less commonly, progressive and symptomatic hypercalcemia in patients with well functioning renal transplants. In Wilson's series five patients died as a result of progression of their renal disease or its complications and three other patients died of septic complications of their subsequent renal transplant. In the remainder of the patients, surgery afforded complete relief of the hyperparathyroidism and associated complaints. Although most surgeons perform subtotal parathyroidectomy, some prefer total parathyroidectomy.

Parathyroid Transplantation. There are certain clinical situations in patients with hyperparathyroidism where one would like to reduce the total parathyroid mass and yet still have a portion of parathyroid tissue to maintain the patient in normal calcium homeostasis. As mentioned above, parathyroid hyperplasia, either primary or secondary, has been a malady most frequently treated by subtotal parathyroidectomy. Should patients develop hypercalcemia after this treatment, then a second neck exploration with all of its attendant risks is usually required. It had previously been demonstrated in animals that parathyroid glands could be transplanted as autografts or as allografts if the hosts were immunosuppressed.[24] The success of the transplantation depended on the freshly removed parathyroid tissue being sliced into very small pieces for subsequent implantation into a muscle bed. This technique has been applied in patients with both primary and secondary parathyroid hyperplasia.[25] A total parathyroidectomy is performed and approximately 20 to 25 parathyroid pieces are autografted to the forearm musculature. Should the patient subsequently develop hypercalcemia from the grafted parathyroid tissue, a few of the pieces can be removed under local anesthesia. That the transplanted parathyroid tissue functions is documented by the patient's maintaining normocalcemia with the grafted tissue as the only source of parathyroid hormone. Furthermore, large concentrations of parathyroid hormone are detectable in the antecubital vein draining the graft bed compared to normal parathyroid hormone levels in the contralateral antecubital vein (Fig. 8). This technique has also been used for transplanting a parathyroid allograft from father to son (Fig. 9).

It has also been demonstrated that parathyroid glands can be viably frozen in dimethyl sulfoxide and autologous serum for as long as nine months.[26] This ability offers the surgeon great versatility, for in those cases where he is uncertain about the amount of parathyroid tissue remaining in the neck following resection of hyperparathyroid tissue in a patient undergoing reoperation, a portion can be frozen viably to await the postoperative course. Should the patient become hypocalcemic, then parts of the frozen autologous parathyroid tissue can be reimplanted under local anesthesia. The histologic appearance of a frozen and grafted autologous parathyroid gland biopsied 18 months after implantation is shown in Figure 10.

Medical Management of Hypercalcemia. In patients with acute parathyroid intoxication who are too ill to undergo immediate surgery or in patients with hypercalcemia occurring with nonresectable malignant disease, medical management is indicated. These patients usually present with weakness, disorientation, progressive uremia, and coma. Dehydration is often a contributory factor in the development of hypercalcemia and uremia, and therefore extracellular fluid restoration should be instituted immediately. Several agents have been used to decrease serum calcium, among them EDTA, phosphate salts, sodium sulfate, mithramycin and calcitonin. Of these, phosphate salts are the most widely used today. They can be given either intravenously or orally, the latter route being preferred, since intravenous administration, especially in azotemic patients, has resulted in profound hypocalcemia and death. The exact mode of action of the calcium-lowering ability of phosphates is unknown, but it has been proposed that increased phosphate leads to increased deposition of bone mineral.

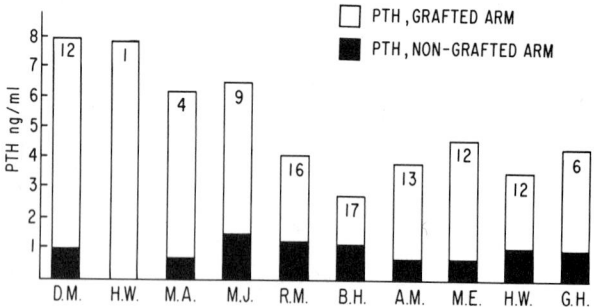

Figure 8. Parathyroid hormone (PTH) values in 10 patients with either primary or secondary parathyroid hyperplasia who have undergone total parathyroidectomy and parathyroid autotransplantation to the forearm musculature. The numbers at the top of each bar denote the time in months following total parathyroidectomy and transplantation. (From Wells, S. A., Jr., Gunnells, C., Shelburne, J. D., Schneider, A. B., and Sherwood, L. M.: Transplantation of the parathyroid glands in man: Clinical indications and results. Surgery, 78:34–44, 1975.)

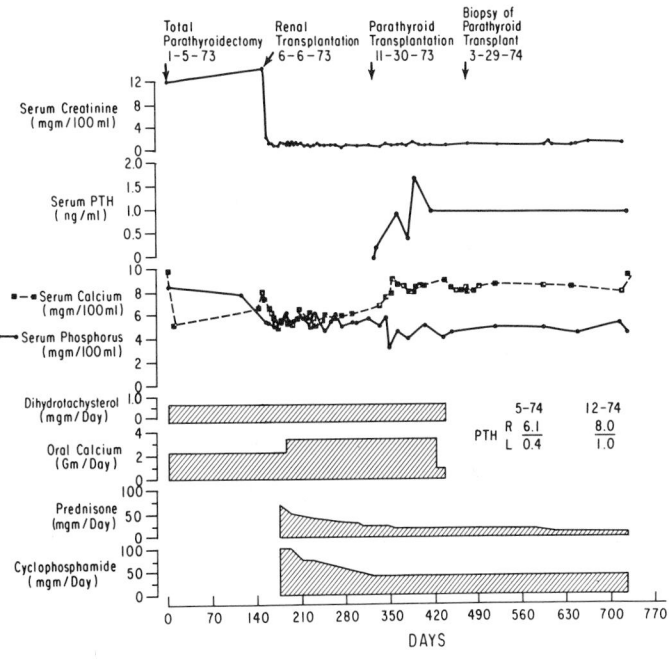

Figure 9. The clinical course of patient D. M., who received a kidney transplant from his father five months after undergoing a total parathyroidectomy for renal osteodystrophy. Because the serum calcium concentration could not be elevated despite large doses of oral calcium and dihydrotachysterol replacement therapy, he received a two-gland parathyroid allograft from his father. This was associated with an increase in the serum calcium concentration to normal, an elevation of the serum parathyroid hormone level to normal, and the detection in May and December, 1974, of large concentrations of parathyroid hormone in the vein draining the parathyroid graft bed. Also, the patient was asymptomatic without calcium and Vitamin-D replacement therapy.

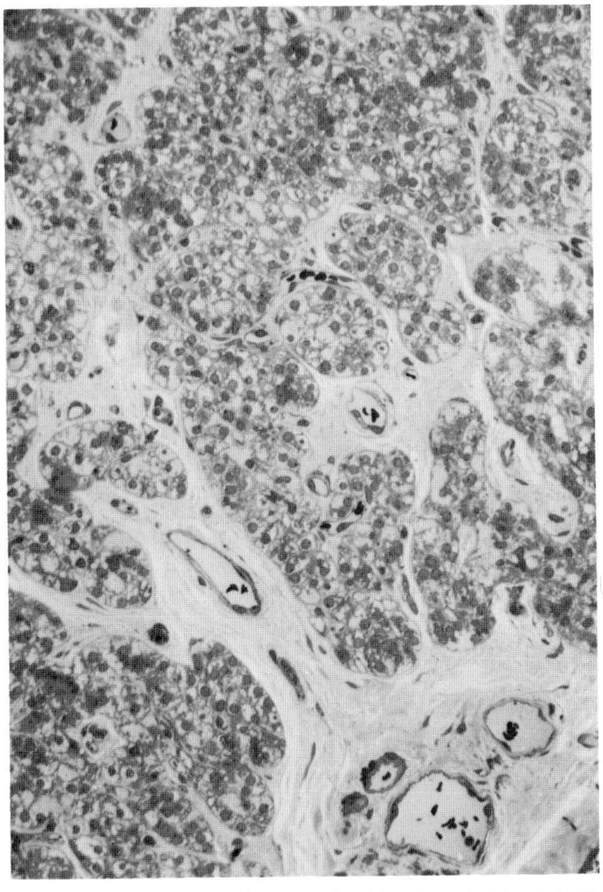

Figure 10. Histology of a parathyroid autograft biopsied 18 months after implantation. The parathyroid tissue had been frozen for six weeks prior to grafting. Hematoxylin and eosin stain, × 200.

HYPOPARATHYROIDISM

The most common cause of hypoparathyroidism is damage to the parathyroid glands during thyroid surgery and it occurs more commonly with total thyroidectomy. It is not at all unusual for patients undergoing operative procedures on the thyroid gland to experience a drop in serum calcium after surgery. This probably represents bruising or compromise of the blood supply of the parathyroids, and the hypocalcemia is transient. Serum calcium reaches its lowest level in about 48 to 72 hours and returns to normal two to three days thereafter. The sooner after surgery the drop in serum calcium occurs and the longer it persists, the greater is the likelihood that all parathyroid glands have been damaged and the poorer the prognosis for recovery. The major signs and symptoms of hypocalcemia are directly attributable to the reduction of plasma ionized calcium, which leads to increased neuromuscular excitability. Clinically, the earliest manifestations are numbness and tingling in the circumoral area, fingers, and toes. Mental symptoms are common and patients are anxious, depressed, or occasionally confused. Tetany may develop and it is characterized by carpopedal spasms, tonic clonic convulsions, and laryngeal stridor which may prove fatal. On physical examination contraction of the facial muscles is elicited by tapping on the facial nerve anterior to the ear (Chvostek's sign). This sign is present in a small number of normal persons. Trousseau's sign is elicited by occluding blood flow to the forearm for 3 minutes. The development of carpal spasm indicates hypocalcemia.

A far less common cause of hypoparathyroidism is idiopathic lack of function. There have been about 150 cases reported, most of which occurred in childhood and some of which appeared to be familial. Hypoparathyroidism in newborns frequently results from prenatal suppression of fetal parathyroid glands by the hyperparathyroid mother. In DiGeorge's syndrome[8] there is congenital absence of the parathyroid glands and the thymus. In addition to hypocalcemia, these children suffer from absence of the thymus-dependent lymphoid system.

The treatment of acute hypocalcemia is intravenous administration of calcium gluconate or calcium chloride. Vitamin D and oral calcium are utilized for long-term management.

SELECTED REFERENCES

Alveryd, A.: Parathyroid glands in thyroid surgery. Acta Chir. Scand. (Suppl.), *389*:1–120, 1968.
This is a thorough monograph discussing the anatomically important relationships of the normal and abnormal parathyroid glands, i.e., location, weight, blood supply, number, and so forth. There is also an informative section on the technique of locating the parathyroid glands at surgery.

Mallette, L. E., Bilezikian, J. P., Heath, D. A., and Aurbach, G. D.: Primary hyperparathyroidism: Clinical and biochemical features. Medicine, *53*:127, 1974.
This is an excellent recent article that covers the general area of hyperparathyroidism. It is especially strong in discussing in depth the laboratory diagnosis of hyperparathyroidism. It also covers the most recent diagnostic tests and localization procedures utilized in hyperparathyroidism.

Pyrah, L. N., Hodgkinson, A., and Anderson, C. K.: Primary hyperparathyroidism. Br. J. Surg., *53*:245, 1966.
This excellent article is clinically oriented and covers all aspects of primary hyperparathyroidism. The secondary complications, diagnostic tests, operative technique, and problem of reoperation for recurrent disease are all thoroughly discussed.

REFERENCES

1. Albright, F., Bloomberg, E., Castleman, B., and Churchill, E. D.: Hyperparathyroidism due to diffuse hyperplasia of all parathyroid glands rather than adenoma of one. Clinical studies on three such cases. Arch. Intern. Med., *54*:315, 1934.
2. Alveryd, A.: Parathyroid glands in thyroid surgery. Acta Chir. Scand. (Suppl.), *389*:1–120, 1968.
3. Ballard, H. S., Frame, B., and Hartsock, R. J.: Familial multiple endocrine adenoma–peptic ulcer complex. Medicine, *43*:481, 1964.
4. Berson, S. A., Yalow, R. S., Aurbach, G. D., and Potts, J. T.: Immunoassay of bovine and human parathyroid hormone. Proc. Natl. Acad. Sci., *49*:613, 1963.
5. Castleman, B., and Cope, O.: Primary parathyroid hyperplasia. Bull. Hosp. Joint Dis., *12*:368, 1951.
6. Cope, O., Keynes, W. M., Roth, S. I., and Castleman, B.: Primary chief cell hyperplasia of the parathyroid glands. A new entity in the surgery of hyperparathyroidism. Ann. Surg., *148*:375, 1958.
7. Cutler, R. E., Reiss, E., and Ackerman, L. V.: Familial hyperparathyroidism. N. Engl. J. Med., *270*:859, 1964.
8. DiGeorge, A. M.: Congenital absence of the thymus and its immunologic consequences: Concurrence with congenital hypoparathyroidism. Birth Defects Orig. Art. Series, *4*:116, 1968.
9. Egdahl, R. H., Canterbury, J. M., and Reiss, E.: Measurement of circulating parathyroid hormone concentration before and after parathyroid surgery for adenoma or hyperplasia. Ann. Surg., *168*:714, 1968.
10. Haff, R. C., and Ballinger, W. F.: Causes of recurrent hypercalcemia after parathyroidectomy for primary hyperparathyroidism. Ann. Surg., *173*:884, 1971.
11. Hellstrom, J., and Ivemark, B. I.: Primary hyperparathyroidism. Acta Chir. Scand. (Suppl.), *294*:1–111, 1962.
12. Holmes, E. C., Morton, D. L., and Ketcham, A. S.: Parathyroid carcinoma. A collective review. Ann. Surg., *169*:631, 1969.
13. Hurvitz, R. J., Perzik, S. L., and Morgenstern, L.: In vivo staining of the parathyroid glands. Arch. Surg., *97*:722, 1968.
14. Lemann, J., and Donatelli, A. A.: Calcium intoxication due to primary hyperparathyroidism. Ann. Intern. Med., *60*:447, 1964.
15. Lloyd, H. M.: Primary hyperparathyroidism: An analysis of the role of the parathyroid tumor. Medicine, *47*:53, 1968.
16. Mallette, L. E., Bilezikian, J. P., Heath, D. A., and Aurbach, G. D.: Primary hyperparathyroidism: Clinical and biochemical features. Medicine, *53*:127, 1974.
17. Nathaniels, E. K., Nathaniels, A. M., and Wang, C.: Mediastinal parathyroid tumors. A clinical and pathological study of 84 cases. Ann. Surg., *171*:165, 1970.
18. Norris, E. H.: The parathyroid glands and the lateral thyroid in man: Their morphogenesis, histogenesis, topographic anatomy and prenatal growth. Contrib. Embryol., *26*:247, 1937.
19. Paloyan, E., Lawrence, A. M., Baker, W. H., and Straus, F. H.: Near-total parathyroidectomy. Surg. Clin. North Am., *49*:43, 1969.
20. Pyrah, L. N., Hodgkinson, A., and Anderson, C. K.: Primary hyperparathyroidism. Br. J. Surg., *53*:245, 1966.
21. Rogers, H. M.: Parathyroid adenoma and hypertrophy of the parathyroid glands. J.A.M.A., *130*:22, 1946.
22. Potts, J. T.: Production of parathyroid hormone by non-parathyroid tumors. J. Clin. Endocrinol., *27*:140, 1967.
23. Wells, S. A., Doppman, J. L., Bilezikian, J. P., Shimkin, P. M., Powell, D., Ketcham, A. S., and Aurbach, G. D.: Repeated neck exploration in primary hyperparathyroidism: Localization of abnormal glands by selective thyroid arteriography, selective venous sampling, and radioimmunoassay. Surgery, *74*:678, 1973.
24. Wells, S. A., Burdick, J. F., Hattler, B. G., Christiansen, C., Pettigrew, H. M., Abe, M., and Sherwood, L. M.: The allografted parathyroid gland: Evaluation of function in the immunosuppressed host. Ann. Surg., *180*:805, 1974.
25. Wells, S. A., Gunnells, J. C., Shelburne, J. D., Schneider, A. B., and Sherwood, L. M.: Transplantation of the parathyroid glands in man: Clinical indications and results. Surgery, *78*:34, 1975.
26. Wells, S. A., and Christiansen, C.: The transplanted parathyroid gland: Evaluation and cryopreservation and other environmental factors which affect its function. Surgery, *75*:49, 1974.
27. Wilson, R. E., Hampers, C. L., Bernstein, D. S., Johnson, J. W., and Merrill, J. P.: Subtotal parathyroidectomy in chronic renal failure. A seven year experience in a dialysis and transplant program. Ann. Surg., *174*:640, 1971.

27

THE PITUITARY AND ADRENALS

H. William Scott, Jr., M.D.

PITUITARY

The pituitary (or hypophysis) has been of interest to surgeons since the recognition by Marie[99] in the 1880s that acromegaly was caused by a pituitary tumor. It was soon learned that pituitary tumors may produce blindness, disorders of growth and metabolism, and obstruction to the ventricular system. Problems in the management of pituitary tumors were a great stimulus to the development of neurosurgery as a specialized surgical field.

Although Schloffer[126] in 1907 did the first successful operation on the pituitary, the pioneering work of the great neurosurgeon Harvey Cushing[29-32, 34] forms the basis for much that has been learned about the physiology of the gland and surgical treatment of its disorders. Schloffer, Cushing, Hirsch, and other surgeons in the early part of this century devised transnasal approaches to the pituitary. Both transorbital and supraorbital extradural approaches to the gland were devised by Krause, Frazier, and others[147] in the period before World War I and later modified by Cushing. The intradural approach to the pituitary was introduced in 1920 by Heuer and subsequently modified by Dandy.[37]

Because of the environmental relationships of the pituitary and its tumors and cysts, the difficulties they present in treatment were felt by Cushing to "offer the most baffling problem which confronts the neurosurgeon." His early technical difficulties with hypophysectomy led him to develop new techniques for hemostasis. Among these are the familiar Cushing clip[33] which he applied to bleeding points or to vessels before their transection, and in 1926, in collaboration with W. T. Bovie,[16] he introduced electrocoagulation as a hemostatic method. His contributions to knowledge of the pituitary endocrinopathies were of fundamental importance to endocrinology.

Modern neurosurgeons have a choice of several surgical approaches for hypophysectomy, which may be either intradural or extradural, intracranial or transsphenoidal. Destruction of pituitary tumors by ionizing radiation was used by radiologists early in the century, but has become much more effective since the availability of supervoltage sources, cobalt-60, and the Bragg peak proton beam. Fraser et al.[51] in the early 1950s began to use a method of yttrium (^{90}Y) implantation to destroy the pituitary. This method has been greatly improved by Harper and his associates[66] by the use of stereotactic-vision fluoroscopy with an image intensifier to permit accurate injection of strontium-90–yttrium-90 into the pituitary via the transsphenoidal route. Rand et al.[116] have applied the technique of cryosurgery for pituitary ablation with stereotactic control. In the last several years the techniques of microsurgery using the operating microscope have been applied to transsphenoidal hypophysectomy by Hardy[64] and appear to have extended the accuracy and safety of the operation (Fig. 1).

ANATOMY AND EMBRYOLOGY

The normal pituitary gland is a small structure that weighs about a half gram, is roughly spherical in shape, and has dimensions of about $10 \times 13 \times 6$ mm. It lies within the sella turcica, a cavity in the sphenoid bone at the base of the brain. The sella is covered by a tough fibrous reflection of the dura mater, the diaphragma sellae, through which the pituitary stalk and its accompanying vessels reach the gland. In addition to the stalk, the pituitary consists grossly of the anterior lobe or adenohypophysis and the posterior lobe or neurohypophysis. The pars intermedia that is present in the pituitary of lower animals is virtually absent in the human gland. The terminology recommended by the International Commission on Anatomical Nomenclature for the divisions of the pituitary gland is given in Table 1.

Immediately beneath the sella turcica in which the pituitary gland lies is the sphenoid sinus. Immediately anterior to the pituitary stalk is the optic chiasm. Immediately lateral to the gland and its stalk lie the cavernous sinuses with the intracranial portion of the internal carotid arteries. Superiorly the pituitary stalk joins the hypothalamus.

The pituitary gland receives its blood supply from two sources. Arterial blood reaches it from branches of the superior hypophyseal artery, which is a branch of the internal carotid artery. Venous blood enters the pituitary by a physiologically important portal system that originates in specialized vascular structures of the median eminence and other components of the hypothalamus. Venous tributaries of this hypothalamic system course down the pituitary stalk to the sinusoidal capillaries of the anterior lobe of the pituitary.

The blood supply of the posterior lobe arises from the inferior hypophyseal arteries. Venous blood from both pituitary lobes drains into the cavernous sinus by multiple small veins.

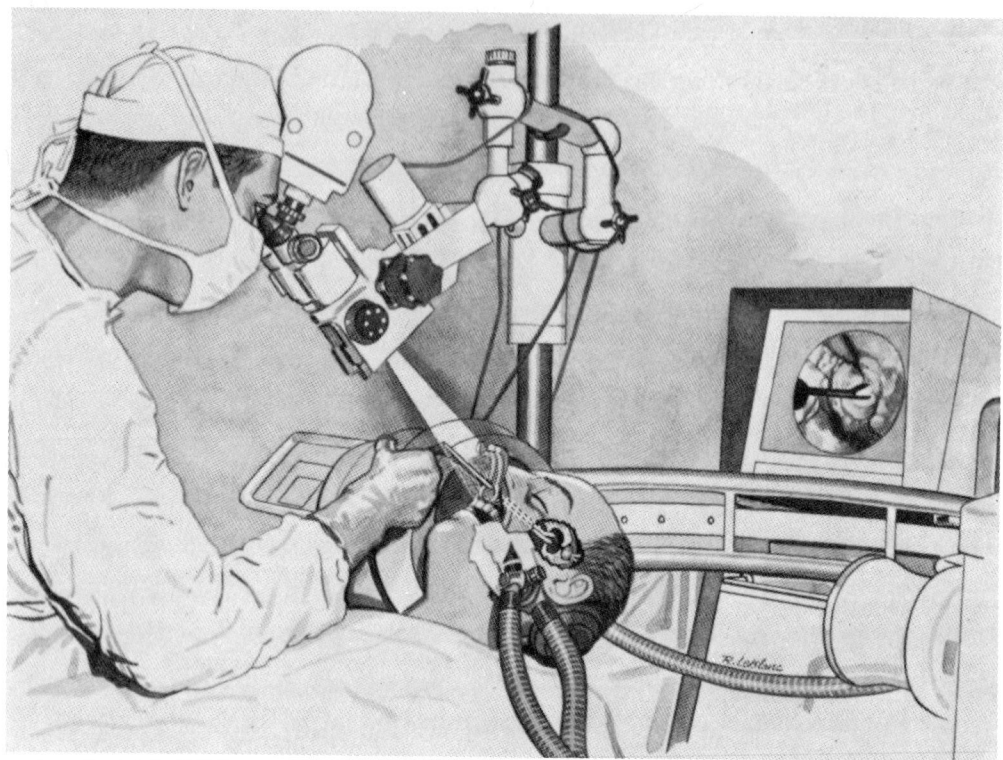

Figure 1. Operative setup for transsphenoidal hypophysectomy with combined use of televised radiofluoroscopic control and the binocular operating microscope. (From Hardy, J.: J. Neurosurg., *34*:582, 1971.)

Embryologically, the pituitary is formed in early fetal life from the fusion of a primitive evagination of the roof of the primitive stomodeum, Rathke's pouch, and an outpouching of the floor of the third ventricle, which is destined to become the neurohypophysis. The portion of the primitive stomodeum known as Rathke's pouch undergoes much more extensive proliferation and forms the anterior lobe of the pituitary. A pair of lateral buds that arise from Rathke's pouch extend upward to invest the neural stalk with cells that later become the pars tuberalis. The connection of Rathke's pouch with the oral cavity, or stomodeum, is separated by the development of the sphenoid bone. The lumen of Rathke's pouch is nearly completely obliterated by proliferation of the cells of the anterior and posterior lobes of the hypophysis. The lumen may persist as small clefts or colloid-filled cysts at the junc-

tion between the neurohypophysis and the pars distalis of the anterior lobe.

The human anterior pituitary contains several distinct cell types, which are responsible for the secretion of at least seven independent hormones: prolactin (LTH); corticotropin (ACTH); growth hormone (GH) or somatotropin (STH); thyrotropin (TSH); melanocyte-stimulating hormone (MSH); and the two gonadotropins (GTH), follicle-stimulating hormone (FSH) and luteinizing hormone (LH), or in the male, interstitial cell-stimulating hormone (ICSH). The posterior lobe of the pituitary secretes two hormones: antidiuretic hormone or vasopressin (ADH) and oxytocin.

There is currently considerable controversy concerning the various cell types of the anterior hypophysis and the specific hormone secreted. The three primary cell types of classic

TABLE 1. Divisions of Pituitary Gland*

Adenohypophysis Lobus glandularis		Pars distalis	Anterior lobe
		Pars tuberalis	
		Pars intermedia	
Neurohypophysis	Lobus nervosus (neural lobe)	Processus infundibuli	Posterior lobe
	Infundibulum (neural stalk)	Pediculus infundibularis (stem) Bulbus infundibularis (bulb) Labrum infundibularis (rim) or Median eminence of the tuber cinereum	

*Terminology recommended by the International Commission on Anatomical Nomenclature. (From Daughaday, W. H. *In* Williams, R. H. (Ed.): Textbook of Endocrinology, 5th ed. Philadelphia, W. B. Saunders Company, 1974.)

histology, acidophils (or eosinophils), basophils, and chromophobes, were based on eosin-methylene blue staining characteristics. These have been divided into multiple subgroups by special staining techniques and electron microscopy. Investigation of the function of the cells by use of specialized staining methods and cytochemical and immunologic techniques, as well as experimental animal and clinical data, suggests that at least seven specific cell types exist. One of the seven known anterior lobe hormones is thought to be secreted specifically by each cell type and the evidence for specificity is quite strong. Current data suggest that the acidophilic cells and their subgroups are associated with the production of growth hormone (GH), while the basophilic cells and their subgroups are associated with secretion of thyrotropin (TSH), follicle-stimulating hormone (FSH), luteinizing hormone (LH) or its male analog (ICSH), and corticotropin (ACTH). Melanocyte-stimulating hormone (MSH) may also be a product of the basophil series. Some evidence suggests that the subgroups of the acidophil series secrete prolactin (LTH). Corticotropin (ACTH) is also thought to be secreted by certain subgroups of the chromophobe cellular series. Clinical evidence in support of this hypothesis is based on the fact that the pituitary adenomas that develop after bilateral adrenalectomy for Cushing's disease are invariably chromophobe in type.

Current evidence indicates that the hormones identified with the posterior lobe of the pituitary are produced in the supraoptic nuclei (ADH) and paraventricular nuclei (oxytocin) of the hypothalamus and are transported to the neurohypophysis for storage and secretion.[104, 151]

PHYSIOLOGY

The anterior pituitary has been often called the "master gland" of the endocrine system. It regulates the activity of multiple subsidiary endocrine organs by secreting tropic hormones. These specific tropic hormones may induce hypertrophy and hyperplasia in the target gland and their absence may result in atrophy of the cells of the target gland. The hormones secreted by the target gland commonly serve to promote homeostasis by negative feedback control of the secretion of the pituitary tropic hormones.

With at least five of the pituitary hormones, secretion is controlled by polypeptide-releasing factors produced in the hypothalamus and transmitted to the anterior pituitary via the hypophyseal portal system. For example, corticotropin-releasing factor (CRF) is currently thought to stimulate the production of ACTH and MSH by the pituitary. Other known hypothalamic releasing factors include those which release thyrotropin (TSF), somatotropin (GH), prolactin (LTH), and the gonadotropins (GTH). The gonadotropins, ACTH, and TSH stimulate endocrine organs that produce hormones, and these hormones in turn operate by the negative feedback mechanism to suppress the secretion of their respective pituitary hormones (Fig. 2).

One of the major functions of the endocrine system is to maintain the constancy of the *milieu intérieur*. Endocrine control systems vary from simple to extremely complex biologic mechanisms (the interested student is referred to the discussion of this subject by Rasmussen[117]). An important general concept is that of feedback control and particularly negative feedback. According to Rasmussen,[117] one of the simplest types of endocrine control systems is one in which a hormone acts on specific cells and promotes the release of a substance into extracellular fluid which in turn regulates the secretion of the hormone. An important feature of feedback in the biochemical sense is that input to the system is usually a concentration and output usually a rate of change of concentration. In the simpler endocrine control systems, there is usually absence of direct hypothalamic or pituitary control. In the highest order of complexity, the activity of the endocrine target organ is controlled by the anterior pituitary, the activity of which is regulated in turn by the hypothalamus. The regulation of adrenocortical function by ACTH is an example of this type. The final endocrine product is the feedback effector rather than some substance produced as a result of its action on target cells. Further, the site of feedback control is primarily at the hypothalamic level, although there is evidence that some feedback control is exerted at the level of the anterior pituitary. Adrenocortical, thyroid, and gonadal functions are regulated by this type of organization.

Mammalian hormones fall into three main chemical classes: steroid, polypeptide, and amine. Many have been isolated in pure form and have been actively characterized. Both the hypothalamic releasing factors and the pituitary hormones are polypeptides.

ANTERIOR LOBE HORMONES

Corticotropin (ACTH) and Melanocyte-Stimulating Hormone (MSH)

The isolation and purification of ACTH and MSH have occupied biochemists for many years. In 1956 Shepard and co-workers[137] established the primary structure of ACTH and determined the amino acid sequence of porcine corticotropin. In all species that have been examined, the hormone consists of a single unbranched sequence of 39 amino acids. The ACTH molecule was synthesized by Schwyzer and Sieber.[128] Melanocyte-stimulating hormone is found to exist in the pituitaries of nearly all species as two peptides: alpha-MSH contains 13 amino acids; beta-MSH exhibits species variations in the size of amino acid sequence. The first three amino acids of ACTH are identical to the structures of alpha-MSH. According to Lerner,[86] beta-MSH contains 22 amino acids in man and is biologically less active than alpha-MSH.

ACTH must be synthesized promptly to meet the body's needs under conditions of stress, as it is not stored in the adenohypophysis in any great concentration. According to Daughaday,[39] the entire human pituitary has been found to contain only about 50 units of ACTH, which is equivalent to 0.25 mg. of the active peptide. ACTH may be detected in plasma by bioassay in hypophysectomized rats. More recently, methods of radioimmunoassay for plasma corticotropin have been developed. ACTH leaves the plasma rapidly; the biologic half-life is only about 25 minutes. Under basal conditions ACTH is secreted in greater concentrations in the morning than in the afternoon and evening. Its secretion is increased by stress and by adrenalectomy and is greatly elevated in Cushing's disease. It is

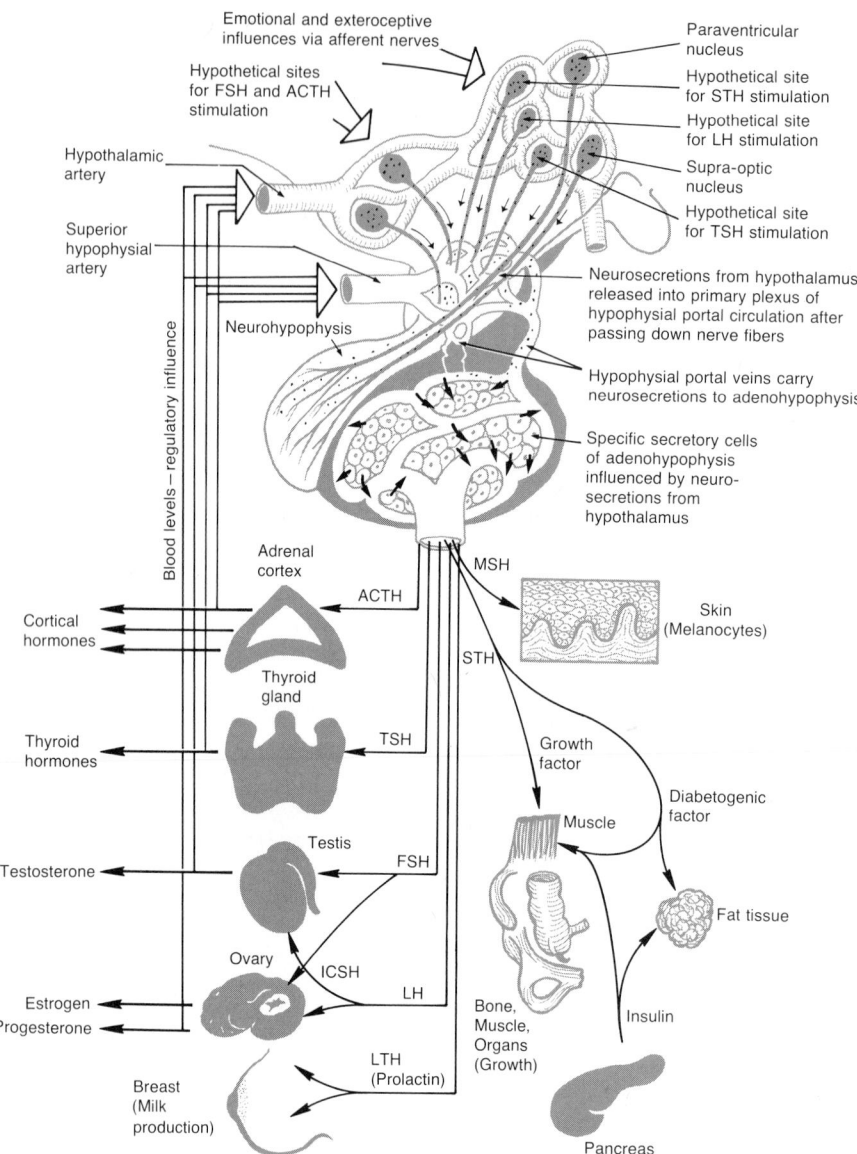

Figure 2. Anterior pituitary hormones.

suppressed by administration of exogenous corticosteroids. The concentration of plasma ACTH in normal subjects and in patients with various endocrine conditions is shown in Figure 3.

Although the biologic actions of ACTH are not limited to the adrenal, its primary effect is on the adrenal cortex. It produces changes in adrenal cortical structure, chemical composition, and enzymatic activity, as well as stimulation of the release of cortical steroid hormones. In the adrenal cortex, ACTH causes increased protein synthesis, increased formation of steroid hormones from acetate and cholesterol, and increased synthesis of active phosphorylase, and by multiple other mechanisms enhances steroid synthesis and hydroxylation. To produce these effects corticotropin binds with specific receptors on the surface of the

adrenal cortical cell and is one of the many hormones now known to act through the intracellular mediation of cyclic AMP (adenosine-3',5'-phosphate) as shown by Sutherland and his associates.[123] Cyclic AMP, according to Liddle[91] serves as a cofactor in activating key enzymes of the adrenal cortex called protein kinases. The most thoroughly studied protein kinases are composed of two subunits that are metabolically inactive when combined. One subunit serves as a receptor for cyclic AMP and the other is potentially catalytic. The attachment of cyclic AMP to the receptor results in dissociation of the receptor subunit from the catalytic subunit, which then acts to catalyze the transfer of phosphate groups from ATP to certain proteins. Presumably, these phosphorylated proteins stimulate the rate-limiting step in steroidogenesis and, in addition,

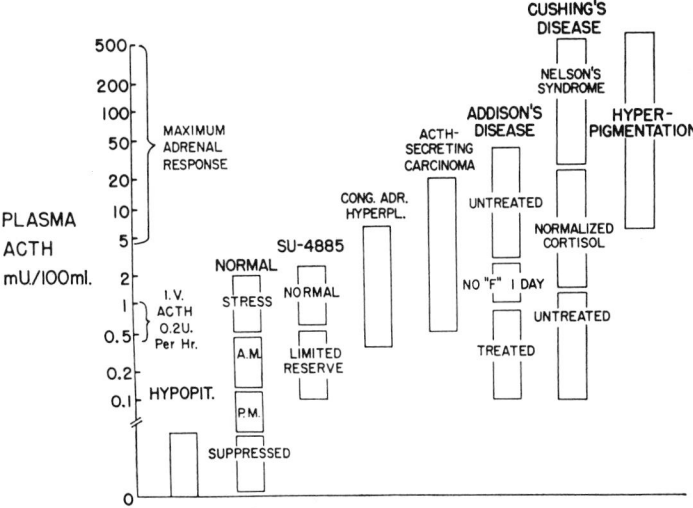

Figure 3. A diagram illustrating the concentration of plasma ACTH in normal human beings and in a number of endocrine conditions. Nelson's syndrome refers to patients with pituitary tumors after adrenalectomy. Results from postoperative patients without hyperpigmentation or tumor who were receiving replacement cortisol are labeled "normalized cortisol." (From Liddle, G. W., Island, D., and Meador, C. E.: Rec. Progr. Hormone Res., 18:125, 1962. Used by permission of Academic Press, Inc.)

induce adrenocortical growth. The extra-adrenal effects of ACTH include mobilization of free fatty acids from fat depots, an increased rate of fat oxidation and enhancement of ketogenesis, production of hypoglycemia, increase in muscle glycogen, and reduction in plasma amino acid levels. Further, ACTH inhibits the degradation of corticosteroids and prolongs the biologic half-life of plasma cortisol. Under conditions of stress, corticotropin has a dual role: it stimulates corticosteroid production and also inhibits degradation of active adrenal hormones.

It is well known that MSH can lead to an intense darkening of the human skin. The evolutionary importance of MSH in this regard in fish, amphibians, and other lower animals is probably more important than the hormone's role in man. In human beings MSH has no rapid effects on the dispersal of melanin granules, but increases pigmentation by promoting melanin synthesis. While α-MSH has not been detected in normal human plasma, β-MSH is present in extracts of normal plasma in a concentration of about 0.1 ng. per ml. Greatly increased concentrations of MSH are present in plasma under pathologic conditions. According to Daughaday,[39] patients with untreated Addison's disease have from 0.5 to 1.1 ng. per ml. of β-MSH, and in Cushing's syndrome β-MSH concentration can rise as high as 6 ng. per ml. Although the predominant hypothalamic control is thought to be exerted by MSH inhibiting factor and an MSH releasing factor is postulated by some, in man MSH shares the same feedback inhibition by cortisol with ACTH, and the secretion of the two hormones is closely interlocked. MSH may have actions unrelated to pigmentation that have not yet been established.

Gonadotropins (GTH)

Two pituitary hormones have primary action on the gonads. Follicle-stimulating hormone (FSH) promotes follicular development in the ovaries and spermatogenesis in the testes. Luteinizing hormone (LH) in the female is called the interstitial cell–stimulating hormone (ICSH) in the male. This substance promotes

luteinization in the ovaries and supports the function of the Leydig cells of the testes. Each of these hormones is a glycoprotein with a molecular size of 30,000. The gonadotropins are virtually absent from the pituitaries of children.

The cellular actions of LH and FSH on the ovaries, corpora lutea, and granulosal cells have been extensively studied. In corpora lutea, steroidogenesis is promoted by LH by conversion of cholesterol to pregnenolone. According to Daughaday,[39] LH binds with specific receptors in the cell membrane, activating the adenyl-cyclase-cyclic AMP intracellular messenger system. The initial actions of ICSH (LH) in the male on the Leydig cells of the testes are comparable, but the end product is testosterone rather than progesterone. The cellular actions of FSH are less well defined.

The secretion of FSH and LH is regulated by the hypophysiotropic hormone (or hormones) of the hypothalamus and by the negative feedback of the sex steroids. Daughaday states that a single hypothalamic hormone, LH releasing hormone (LRH), also stimulates release of FSH. The possibility of another hypothalamic hormone acting solely on FSH release has not been entirely eliminated.

The hypothalamus is directly concerned with the initiation of the secretion of gonadotropins that occurs at puberty. Many clinical examples of disturbances of this mechanism are recognized; precocious puberty may be a complication of midbrain lesions, and delayed puberty occurs in various types of hypothalamic diseases.

At puberty the concentration of the pituitary gonadotropins rises, and similar high levels are maintained in men and women during the reproductive period. In women, FSH stimulates the development of the follicle, but the simultaneous action of LH apparently increases the maturation of the follicle and its secretory activity and is responsible for subsequent ovulation. In males, FSH is primarily concerned with the integrity of testicular tubular structure and spermatogenesis, while LH (ICSH) is required for interstitial cells and the secretion of testosterone. There are no known clinical syndromes related to excess production of FSH or LH.[39]

Prolactin (LTH)

The primary function of this hormone is to stimulate and maintain lactation. Prolactin has been isolated in very pure form from the pituitaries of a variety of animals, and its physical properties in various species are remarkably similar. The molecule consists of a single chain of 205 amino acids with one free amino acid group. Prolactin resembles growth hormone in that it affects many tissues. While it is capable of initiating and sustaining lactation, by itself it has little effect on the mammary gland. Full lactation requires the interplay of many other hormones. Estrogens and progesterone are necessary for proliferation of the mammary ducts and alveoli. Growth hormone, ACTH, and cortisol must be present for the ovarian steroids to exert their full effects. When the mammary gland has been thus prepared, prolactin brings about milk secretion. Finally, in some species oxytocin seems to be necessary to force the milk into the terminal collecting ducts and to make it available for the suckling infant. In human females, growth hormone does not seem to be required for lactation.

In lower animals, prolactin induces changes in maternal behavior that are important for the helpless young. In some birds, it promotes the nesting behavior. The pathways by which prolactin induces these changes have not been established. Various growth-hormone-like effects of prolactin have been observed in experimental animals and in man. These include nitrogen retention, impairment of carbohydrate tolerance, hypocalciuria, and even skeletal growth. As yet there is no known role of this hormone in males.[39]

Growth Hormone (GH)

The isolation of growth hormone from the pituitary glands of various species in the last 25 years has resulted in sufficient purity for current characterization. Human growth hormone is the smallest of the growth hormone molecules that have been examined. It is composed of a single chain of 188 amino acids without carbohydrate substituents. The human pituitary is particularly rich in growth hormone. Present extraction methods show that between 4 and 10 mg. of growth hormone are present per gland. It is interesting that there is no significant change in growth hormone content of the pituitary with age. Human GH can be measured readily in plasma by immunoassay.

With radioimmunoassay, the level of circulating growth hormone in an adult at basal conditions has been found to be less than 3 ng. per milliliter. The turnover of growth hormone in plasma is rapid. It has a plasma half-life of only about 25 minutes. Stimuli to secretion of growth hormone include a rapid fall in blood sugar, as may be induced by insulin, prolonged fasting, or the experimental drug 2-deoxyglucose, a glucose inhibitor that stimulates the secretion of growth hormone. Other stimuli include exercise, trauma, major surgical operation, acute febrile illness, and the administration of certain amino acids, especially arginine. This observation has given rise to the

reasonable concept that secretion of growth hormone induced by amino acids is the mechanism for stimulating protein synthesis when precursor is available. Many facets of protein metabolism have been examined after administration of somatotropin, but the primary action of the hormone has not yet been localized. A tremendous investigational effort has gone into the study of the biologic actions of growth hormone. The growth of tumors, progress of wound healing, growth of hair and teeth, and regeneration of liver can occur in the absence of growth hormone. The preparation and testing of human growth hormone in normal subjects and in patients with pituitary dwarfism indicates that the hormone clearly causes major metabolic changes: nitrogen balance becomes strongly positive; sodium, chloride, potassium, magnesium, and phosphorus are retained concomitant with the positive nitrogen balance. Further, GH produces an increase in protein synthesis and deposition, proliferation of epiphyseal cartilage with an increase in synthesis of chondroitin sulfate, and an increase in breakdown of fatty depots with a rise in nonesterified fatty acids in plasma.

Extensive studies strongly suggest that growth hormone exerts its effect on cartilage through a component of plasma, somatomedin (sulfation factor), which stimulates cartilage directly. This is a simple peptide with a molecular weight of 4000. In normal plasma it circulates with the large molecular-size plasma protein. Somatomedin is thought to be responsible for the increased synthesis of collagen and other proteins in cartilage. It also promotes cell replication (DNA synthesis) and synthesis of ribonucleic acids.

When growth hormone is administered to fasting normal and hypophysectomized subjects, little change occurs in plasma glucose and insulin concentrations. However, when glucose is administered a few hours after GH, impairment in glucose removal from plasma can be demonstrated. Thus, GH has diabetogenic properties and can block the ability of insulin to increase glucose removal from plasma by muscle. The diabetogenic action of human growth hormone tends to be masked by the presence of normal pancreatic reserve.[39]

Thyroid-Stimulating Hormone (TSH)

Thyrotropin increases the size of the thyroid, enhances its vascularity and its metabolic activity, and leads to the secretion of the thyroid hormone. Deficiency of TSH can produce all the characteristic features of primary thyroid deficiency or myxedema. Chemically, TSH is a glycoprotein with a molecular weight of about 25,000. It is currently thought to be composed of a single polypeptide chain with a number of intrachain disulfide linkages. A variety of methods of bioassay of TSH are used. These are based on the effects of TSH on the thyroid and include increase in thyroid weight, increase in follicle cell size, reduction in iodine content, promotion of iodine-131 uptake or release, increase in weight of incubated thyroid slices, promotion of tadpole metamorphosis, and various other effects. More recently, sensitive radioimmunoassay techniques have been applied to the measurement of TSH. Normal human plasma contains less than 1 to

5 μg. of TSH per milliliter. Studies with ¹³¹I-labeled human TSH show a half-life of 54 minutes, and the pituitary secretory rate of TSH has been estimated to be about 110 μg. per day. The secretion of TSH by the anterior pituitary is partially determined by the level of circulating thyroid hormone and partially by influences transmitted from the hypothalamus by thyrotropin-releasing factor. There is evidence that the negative feedback control of thyrotropin secretion exercised by the thyroid hormone takes place in both the hypothalamus and pituitary.

In addition to the effects mentioned, thyrotropin has profound effects on thyroid hormonogenesis; TSH increases iodide clearance from plasma and enhances the formation of iodotyrosine and iodothyronine, thyroglobulin proteolysis, and the release of thyroxin and triiodothyronine (T_3) from the thyroid gland. The extrathyroidal effects of TSH include promotion of lipolysis in adipose tissue; thyrotropin preparations in various animal species have induced exophthalmos due to deposition of edema fluid in the retro-orbital tissues. It is questionable, however, whether exophthalmos is entirely due to the action of TSH. In patients with hyperthyroidism and exophthalmos, the plasma frequently contains a long-acting thyroid-stimulating substance (LATS) that is not found in the pituitary and an exophthalmos-producing substance (EPS) that has been separated from TSH by chromatography of pituitary extracts from animals. The precise hormonal cause of exophthalmos remains controversial.[39]

POSTERIOR LOBE HORMONES

Vasopressin or Antidiuretic Hormone (ADH)

The major physiologic role of this hormone relates to its potent antidiuretic activity. The structure of ADH and that of oxytocin were discovered by du Vigneaud and his associates in 1954.[41] Both hormones contain eight amino acid residues arranged with a five-member S—S bonded ring and a tail composed of three amino acids. Both stress and dehydration provide the stimulus for release of ADH. The graphic studies of Verney[144] established the role of the hormone in the conservation of body water. Verney demonstrated that an increase of only 1 to 2 per cent in effective osmotic pressure in plasma in the distribution of the internal carotid artery results in the release of ADH and the formation of a concentrated urine. Osmoreceptors localized in the anterior hypothalamus are believed to stimulate ADH release by nerve impulses transmitted along the axons of the pituitary stalk to the posterior pituitary. Suppression of the release of ADH occurs with a water load that dilutes plasma and extracellular fluid. In the absence of ADH, a profuse water diuresis occurs, with excretion of a urine hypotonic to the body fluids. This serves to restore osmolality of body fluids to normal levels. The direct renal effect of ADH is to increase tubular reabsorption of water. ADH secretion is controlled by a negative feedback system which includes the kidney and central nervous system and which preserves within narrow limits the total solute concentration of the body fluids. When infused in quantities considerably larger than those required for maximal antidiuresis, ADH causes contraction of smooth muscle. In pharmacologic amounts, its vascular effects are widespread and result in generalized increase in vascular resistance. The resultant rise in blood pressure is responsible for the name "vasopressin," which was given to the antidiuretic hormone by early investigators. Recently vasopressin has been used in the control of bleeding from the gastrointestinal tract, especially in patients with gastric or esophageal varices.[85]

Oxytocin

This second neurohypophyseal hormone has been long known to have its predominant effect in contraction of the uterine musculature in late pregnancy. Oxytocin shares some of the physiologic actions of vasopressin. Oxytocin is weakly antidiuretic but is potent in its milk-ejection activity in the lactating human breast. In spite of many investigations of the physiologic actions of oxytocin, the precise functions of this hormone have not been established in human subjects. Exactly how oxytocin affects the uterine musculature and the musculature of the mammary ducts is not known. The nonpregnant human uterus is much less responsive to oxytocin than the uterus of late pregnancy. The pharmacologic uses of oxytocin include the induction of labor at term and the control of postpartum hemorrhage and postpartum uterine atony. Oxytocin may also be used to relieve painful engorgement of the breasts during lactation. When it is given in large pharmacologic doses, it has a transient vasodilating effect on vascular smooth muscle, causing a drop in peripheral vascular resistance and in blood pressure. This effect is quickly blocked by small doses of vasopressin. Oxytocin is not known to have any function in the male.[85]

CLINICAL CONDITIONS

Pituitary Anterior Lobe Deficiency

In children, severe anterior pituitary deficiency, whether caused by congenital abnormalities, pituitary granulomas, tumors, or suprasellar cysts (craniopharyngiomas), can result in a complex of clinical endocrine deficiency states, including dwarfism, gonadal and genital underdevelopment, hypothyroidism, and adrenocortical insufficiency, with or without diabetes insipidus. The term panhypopituitarism should be reserved for cases in which the functions of both the anterior and posterior lobes are affected. Tumors and cysts that encroach on the optic chiasm in such cases can produce optic atrophy with associated visual loss.

In less severe anterior pituitary deficiency, failure of gonadotropic production is usually the principal problem. In children, this can result in normal or increased stature with eunuchoid habitus. In males, absence of pituitary stimulus to testicular maturation causes failure of pubertal development and of appearance of secondary sex characteristics. The penis remains small, the scrotum fails to develop mature rugae, and the prostate and seminal vesicles remain infantile. The larynx fails to enlarge and the voice retains high pitch. Epiphyseal closure is delayed and, if growth hormone is adequate, arms and legs become disproportionately long. Eventually, the epiphyseal lines do close, but often not until the third decade of life. Axillary and pubic hair does not appear or is sparse; the beard does not grow; frontal baldness does not develop. There is failure of normal libido and potency. Osteoporosis may be observed in these eunuchoid patients and is probably due to lack of the protein anabolic effect of testosterone.

Hypogonadotropic hypogonadism is much less common in girls. When it does occur, eunuchoid proportions, failure of female pubertal changes, and amenorrhea are characteristic. In young girls hypogonadotropic hypogonadism is most commonly the result of craniopharyngioma.

In adults, severe symptoms of anterior pituitary deficiency occur only when destruction of the anterior lobe is nearly complete. Lesions that destroy the adenohypophysis without any extrasellar effect usually cause only hypogonadism until about 75 per cent of the lobe is destroyed. Progression of the destructive process produces increasing severity of hypogonadism, with loss of potency and libido, accompanied by manifestations of thyroid and adrenal insufficiency, such as weakness, fatigue, anorexia, cold intolerance, and hypoglycemia. In addition to gonadal atrophy, regression of secondary sexual characteristics occurs in adults with severe anterior lobe deficiency. The external genitalia shrink; vaginal epithelium becomes atrophic; the uterus regresses to infantile size and breasts atrophy. In males the penis decreases in size, the testes become soft and the scrotum loses its normal rugae, and the prostate becomes atrophic. There is loss of facial, extremity, and body hair, especially from the chest and axillary and pubic areas. In women the pubic and axillary hair appears to be largely under the control of adrenal androgens, and noticeable loss of hair in these areas may not occur except in very severe anterior pituitary deficiency.

In both sexes there may be varying degrees of muscular wasting with premature senility and the development of wrinkled, dry skin involving especially the face and forehead. Normal skin pigment often fades, and a peculiar pallor or fawnlike color is common.

In addition to pituitary tumors and cysts, postpartum or posthemorrhagic necrosis of the gland can cause severe anterior pituitary insufficiency. Simmonds[138] described fatal cases of pituitary infarction as early as 1914, and 35 years later Sheehan[136] emphasized the importance of pregnancy as a cause for pituitary hyperplasia and enhanced vulnerability to a sudden decrease in blood supply by spasm or thrombosis.

"Sheehan's syndrome" is the clinical term for postpartum acute hypopituitarism, most commonly due to necrosis of the anterior lobe secondary to shock that accompanies severe postpartum bleeding. Usually the neurohypophysis survives this form of pituitary necrosis, but in severe cases it may be affected, with diabetes insipidus as one of the prominent clinical manifestations.

One of the endocrine tests for anterior pituitary insufficiency that has wide clinical usage is based on the effect of the drug metyrapone (Metopirone) on the pituitary-adrenocortical axis. Metyrapone in appropriate dosage (750 mg. orally every 4 hours) blocks the activity of the enzyme 11-β-hydroxylase in the adrenal cortex and selectively inhibits the conversion of 11-desoxycortisol (compound S) to cortisol.[90] The drop in plasma cortisol concentration normally stimulates a rise in pituitary ACTH secretion, which causes a rise in adrenocortical secretion of compound S. The latter has little or no inhibitory effect on ACTH secretion, and its excess production is readily detected in urine by the Porter-Silber method as an increase in 17-hydroxycorticosteroids or 17-ketogenic steroids. In severe pituitary insufficiency no significant rise in plasma or urinary 17-hydroxycorticoids occurs. This test has further value in differentiating adrenal cortical hyperplasia and tumor (as discussed in the section on the adrenals) in patients with Cushing's syndrome.

Management of the various types of anterior hypopituitarism involves both treatment of the specific cause, such as excision of pituitary tumor or suprasellar cyst, and appropriate hormonal substitution therapy. Hypophysectomy for pituitary tumor frequently enhances the severity of pituitary insufficiency. Currently, hormonal substitution therapy is quite efficient in relieving the various anterior pituitary deficiency states. Human growth hormone, which has recently become available, should be enormously valuable in treatment of pituitary dwarfism. The human gonadotropins (isolated from female urine) may be used in management of hypogonadotropic hypogonadism. The more severe forms of anterior lobe deficiency require maintenance with testosterone or estrogens, accompanied by thyroid and adrenocortical substitution.

Posterior Lobe Deficiency: Diabetes Insipidus

Injury by neoplastic compression or trauma to the hypothalamic supraoptic nuclei or the pituitary stalk, or destruction of the pituitary's posterior lobe, either singly or in combination, can impair secretion of antidiuretic hormone (ADH), and diabetes insipidus may result. This may be transitory, as is usual after hypophysectomy, unless the hypothalamic structures are damaged, in which case a chronic problem develops. The clinical syndrome consists of uncontrolled water diuresis, polyuria, and polydipsia. A dilute, hypotonic urine is excreted in large volume. In older children and adults urinary volumes of 5 to 15 liters per day are common. The large water loss is due to the absence of ADH effect on reabsorption of water in the distal renal tubules. Severe thirst demands a large volume of water intake without which severe dehydration may rapidly ensue. Severe salt loss is usually prevented by unimpaired aldosterone activity.

Nephrogenic diabetes insipidus, a rare hereditary defect in renal tubular function, as well as other forms of renal disease causing polyuria, can be differentiated from diabetes insipidus by the prompt relief of the latter condition by ADH administration.

Treatment of severe chronic diabetes insipidus may require the use of long-acting ADH preparations such as vasopressin tannate in oil given intramuscularly or other posterior pituitary preparations by nasal spray. The thiazide diuretics have an *antidiuretic* effect in diabetes insipidus, which has been of benefit in managing some patients.[85]

Syndrome of Excessive Antidiuretic Hormone (ADH)

Prolonged excessive exposure to vasopressin by human subjects results in water retention with concomitant weight gain and dilution of body fluids. A sodium diuresis results from increase in glomerular filtration rate and suppression of aldosterone secretion as a consequence of expanded volume of body fluid. Schwartz and associates[127] first described a clinical syndrome which had these features in two patients with bronchogenic carcinomas and postulated that an inappropriate and excessive secretion of ADH was responsible.

Since this description the syndrome has been reported in a variety of pathologic states usually involving lung or brain. According to Leaf and Coggins,[85] patients with tuberculous meningitis, brain tumors, head injuries, pneumonia, and intrathoracic tumors may all show this type of asymptomatic hyponatremia. The exact nature of the antidiuretic substance and whether it derives from the neurohypophysis or other sources are not usually known in these cases. In two reports, however, assays of tumors showed potent antidiuretic activity.

Gigantism and Acromegaly

Hyperfunction of the acidophilic cells of the anterior pituitary, with excessive production of somatotropin or growth hormone (GH), causes gigantism if the disorder begins before puberty and acromegaly if the onset is later in life. Usually an acidophil adenoma is the underlying pathophysiologic factor in both patterns of abnormal growth. Less commonly chromophobe or mixed chromophobe-acidophil tumors are to blame.

Before the epiphyseal plates are fused, hypersecretion of GH causes proportionate growth of the long bones, and gigantism results. The growing period in pituitary giants is longer than in normal children since epiphyseal closure is apt to be delayed by accompanying hypogonadism. According to Daughaday,[39] giants who survive into adult life have the long extremities of eunuchoidism combined with mildly acromegalic features. Almost all of the recorded giants with extreme height have died in early adult life of infection or secondary pituitary insufficiency (Fig. 4).

Acromegaly develops when a GH-producing pituitary tumor begins to function after the epiphyseal plates have closed. The onset most commonly is between the third and fifth decades. The disease is two to three times more common in women. In most acromegalics there is little increase in height. The syndrome usually develops slowly and insidiously over a period of years. The frequency of some of the manifestations and associations of acromegaly is given in Table 2.

The changes in facial appearance and in the acral parts usually develop so gradually that they are often

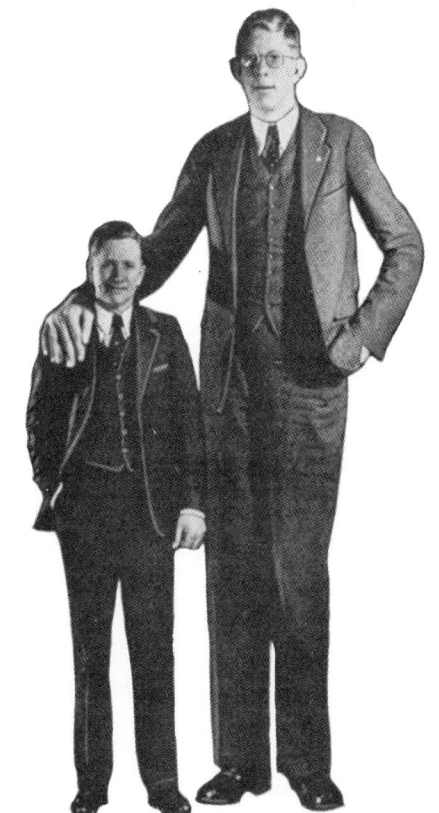

Figure 4. Gigantism. The "Alton Giant," Robert Wadlow, age 22, height 8 feet, 11 inches, weight 475 pounds. (From Cole, W. H., and Zollinger, R. M.: Textbook of Surgery, 8th ed. New York, Appleton-Century-Crofts, 1963; courtesy of Peters Shoe Company.)

unrecognized by the patient and his family and friends until the syndrome is far advanced. The earliest manifestations noted by the patient may be that larger shoes, hats, and gloves are required to fit him. Headaches are a complaint of most patients and may result from stretching of the diaphragma sellae by the growth of the pituitary tumor. Loss of vision occurs in two thirds of acromegalics. It is caused by compression of the inferior and medial portions of the optic nerves and chiasm by the expanding tumor and is at first bitemporal hemianopsia but may progress to total blindness.

The striking physical changes of acromegaly are most obvious in the face, skin, and skeleton, especially the skull and the hands and feet (Fig. 5).

The facial features coarsen, with enlargement of nose and lips. The skull enlarges, the orbital ridges and malar eminences become very prominent, and the lower jaw elongates to produce the characteristic prognathous appearance. The skin of the whole body thickens and becomes leathery. Skin appendages, hair follicles, and sebaceous and sweat glands increase in size, and body hair increases in amount. Although skeletal overgrowth is generalized, with thickening of the calvarium and the cortices of both long and flat

TABLE 2. Acromegaly: Frequency of
Manifestations*

	Per Cent
Parasellar manifestations	
Enlarged sella	93
Headache	87
Visual impairment	62
Uncinate fits	7
Rhinorrhea	15
Pituitary apoplexy	
Papilledema	3
Growth hormone excess	
Weight gain	39
Hypermetabolism	70
Hyperhidrosis	60
Impaired glucose tolerance	25
Clinical diabetes mellitus	12
Acral growth	100
Prognathism	Common
Arthritic complaints	
Osteoporosis	Common
Soft tissue growth	100
Hypertrichosis	53
Pigmentation	40
Fibroma molluscum	27
Visceromegaly	Common
Goiter	25
Disturbances of other hormones	
Lactorrhea (?prolactin excess)	4
Hyperadrenocorticism	Rare
Hyperthyroidism	Rare
Increased libido	38
Decreased libido, male	23

*From Daughaday, W. H. In Williams, R. H. (Ed.):
Textbook of Endocrinology, 5th ed. Philadelphia, W. B.
Saunders Company, 1974.

bones, it is most noticeable in the enlargement, thickening, and bony "tufting" of the phalanges. Osteophytic changes occur in the joints as well as periarticular soft tissue thickening, causing arthralgia and limiting articular function. Peripheral neuropathies may occur as a result of entrapment of nerves at sites of bony overgrowth or by proliferation of endoneural and perineural fibrous tissue.

Visceral enlargement also occurs in acromegalics. The cardiac enlargement commonly observed is often associated with hypertension, myocardial hypertrophy, and progressive congestive heart failure, especially in older patients. Hepatomegaly may be detected on clinical examination. Enlargement of the kidneys, spleen, pancreas, thyroid, parathyroids, and other viscera is usually observed at autopsy. Microscopic examination shows increased size of structures such as the islets of Langerhans, the glomeruli, and the renal tubules.

Diabetes mellitus develops in about 25 per cent of acromegalics, and about one third exhibit a decrease in glucose tolerance. There is evidence that GH is an insulin antagonist. Serum insulin levels are usually elevated in acromegaly. According to Daughaday,[39] it is possible that diabetes develops only in those acromegalic patients who have a hereditary disposition to the disease, and in the remaining group of acromegalics insulin secretory reserve is adequate to compensate for the diabetogenic effects of excess secretion of growth hormone.

As the acidophil tumor enlarges, compression of the remaining elements of the normal gland may cause certain secondary features of hypopituitarism. Diminished thyrotropin and gonadotropin secretion may result. Despite reduced TSH secretion, certain clinical features suggest hyperthyroidism in acromegalics. Increased basal metabolic rate and increased sweating occur, but since specific measurements of thyroid function such as protein-bound iodine and radioiodine thyroidal uptake are normal, it is likely that the hypersecretion of growth hormone causes these symptoms.

Decreased gonadotropin secretion is the usual consequence of acidophilic pituitary tumors. As previously mentioned, sexual immaturity is common in pituitary giants. According to Daughaday,[39] about a third of men with acromegaly become impotent and in most women with the syndrome amenorrhea develops. Occasionally, inappropriate lactation occurs in young women with acromegaly, which suggests excess production of prolactin. Adrenocortical function is usually normal.

In some patients with pituitary tumors that produce gigantism or acromegaly, there is an increased incidence of adenomas of the parathyroids, pancreatic islets, and adrenal cortex, and an association with the genetic syndrome of multiple endocrine adenomatosis.[8]

X-rays of the skull in acromegalic patients usually show enlargement of the sella turcica and erosion and atrophy of the clinoid processes. The cranial bones show great thickening, the mandible is elongated, and the paranasal sinuses are greatly enlarged (Fig. 6.) X-rays of the large hands show widening of the bones with cortical thickening and tufting of the terminal phalanges. The spine shows osteoarthritic changes, and hyperostosis is especially prominent on the anterior aspect of vertebral bodies.

The most precise diagnostic test is the measurement of elevated concentrations of growth hormone in the peripheral blood by radioimmunoassay after administration of glucose. In normal persons, hyperglycemia causes suppression of GH secretion, and the hormone virtually disappears in peripheral blood. In acromegaly and gigantism, elevated serum GH levels (> 5 mμg. per milliliter) can be measured and are not suppressed by glucose infusion. In two thirds of these patients an elevated serum phosphorus is found (> 4.5 mg. per 100 ml.).

Treatment of a GH-producing tumor by hypophysectomy is most clearly indicated when expansion of the tumor causes shrinkage of the fields of vision; prompt operative removal of the pituitary tumor can prevent blindness. Progressive disfiguring growth without visual impairment, with or without headache, suggests a trial of radiation therapy directed at the pituitary tumor. This can currently be accomplished by external sources such as conventional x-ray therapy, ^{60}Co, or the proton beam. Transsphenoidal implantation of ra-

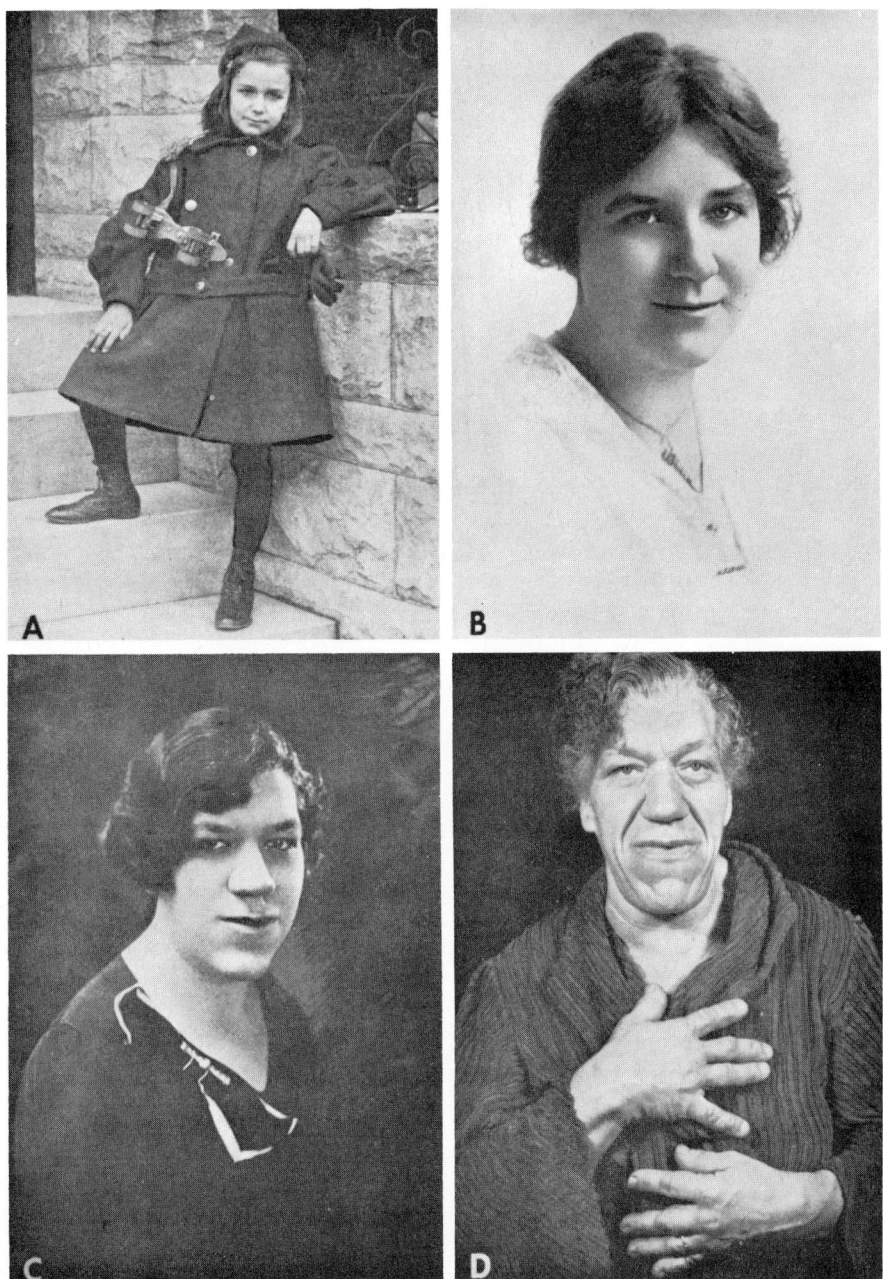

Figure 5. The progression of acromegaly is illustrated in these photographs. *A,* Normal, age 9 years; *B,* age 16 years, with possible early coarsening of features; *C,* age 33 years, well established acromegaly; *D,* age 52 years, end-stage acromegaly with gross disfigurement. (From Clinical Pathological Conference. Am. J. Med., *20:*133, 1956.)

dioactive yttrium (^{90}Y) has been advocated by Harper et al.[66] and by Fraser and Wright.[52] In 44 patients with acromegaly treated by ^{90}Y implants, Fraser and Wright recorded 16 satisfactory results, 24 partial remissions, and satisfactory responses in 4 patients. Regression of the acromegalic facies and reduction in GH secretion to normal levels were observed in the patients who obtained good responses.

Hypophysectomy has been advocated in treatment

of acromegaly and used extensively by Hamberger et al.[63] in Sweden and by Ray and his associates[119] in this country. In a group of 24 patients reported by Ray et al., results were good or satisfactory in 19, while 5 had partial responses or inadequate follow-up. Transitory diabetes insipidus occurred in 19 patients after operation, and in 4 patients prolonged treatment of diabetes insipidus was necessary. Postoperative cerebrospinal fluid rhinorrhea developed in 4 patients. All patients

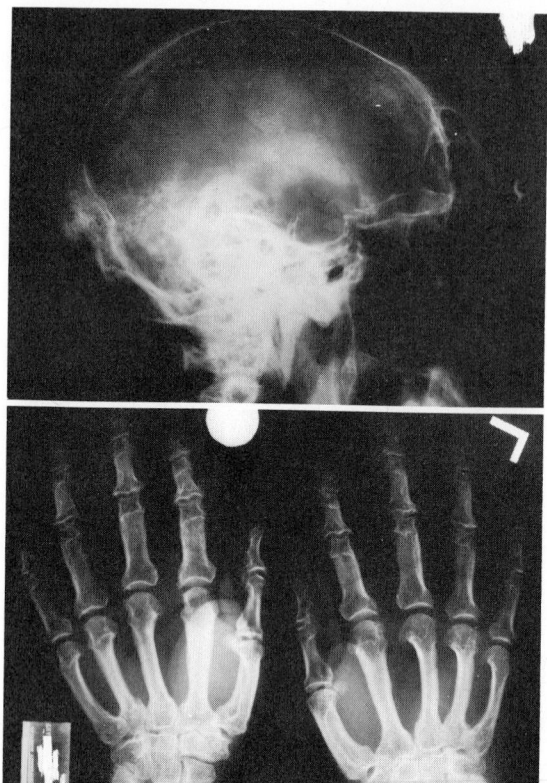

Figure 6. X-rays of skull and hands in acromegaly, far advanced.

required full hormonal replacement therapy including cortisone and thryoid and sex steroids or gonadotropins.

Surgical hypophysectomy in treatment of acromegaly is most clearly indicated when the tumor is large, extends upward above the sella turcica, and threatens vision. In the last several years the introduction of the techniques of microsurgery using the operating microscope have increased the accuracy and safety of transsphenoidal excision of the pituitary.[64] Hardy has reported that 40 acromegalic patients with varying sizes of pituitary tumor were treated by transsphenoidal surgical exploration and excision; favorable results were obtained in 35 cases (87.5 per cent).[65] This new approach may increase the indications for and usefulness of surgical hypophysectomy.

Cushing's Disease

Cushing's syndrome is discussed in detail later in this chapter. The term "Cushing's disease" is reserved for endogenous hypercortisolism caused by excessive ACTH production by the pituitary which stimulates adrenocortical hyperplasia.

Infrequently, a pituitary tumor (basophil or chromophobe) that secretes excess ACTH autonomously is the cause of Cushing's disease. In the majority of cases it currently appears that a true neoplasm of the pitu-

itary is absent and that the corticotropin-releasing factor (CRF) of the hypothalamus stimulates excessive ACTH secretion by the pituitary despite the usually efficient, negative feedback, self-regulating effect of cortisol on the hypothalamic center and on the pituitary. The exact cause of Cushing's disease is unknown.

Hardy has questioned these concepts because of his experience with 10 cases of Cushing's disease in which transsphenoidal surgical exploration of the pituitary has yielded 10 tumors.[65] Eight of these patients were cured and one improved by excision of the tumor; in five of these selective excision of 3- to 10-mm. "microadenomas" was done without inducing hypopituitarism. The remaining patient had a malignant tumor which invaded the base of the brain.

Differential diagnosis of Cushing's syndrome, including precise endocrinologic methods, and other aspects of treatment are discussed in the next section of this chapter.

Persistent Lactation

Inappropriate lactation may occur as a result of pituitary tumors and suggests the excessive secretion of prolactin (LTH) by the tumor cells. It may accompany acromegaly or may develop in combination with amenorrhea following pregnancy (Chiari-Frommel syndrome). Persistent lactation may also occur in nonacromegalic women with pituitary tumors (Forbes-Albright syndrome). The lactorrhea is accompanied by amenorrhea, which is a constant feature of the syndrome and is thought to be due to gonadotropin deficiency.[39, 104]

Inappropriate lactation with gynecomastia has also been observed recently in several men with pituitary tumors.[104]

The clinical association of inappropriate lactation with pituitary tumors seems to be well established, but the exact mechanism of the hormonal etiology remains to be clarified. Although hypersecretion of prolactin (LTH) is widely suspected as the cause, accurate objective data are needed to establish this suspicion.

Nonfunctioning Pituitary Tumors and Craniopharyngiomas (Suprasellar Cysts)

The most common variety of pituitary tumor is the chromophobe adenoma, and most of these are nonfunctioning adenomas. While rarely they may produce ACTH and be the primary cause of Cushing's disease, clinical experience indicates that a chromophobe tumor is more apt to occur *after* bilateral adrenalectomy used in treatment of Cushing's disease (Nelson's syndrome).[103]

In most instances chromophobe tumors cause compression of the normal elements of the anterior pituitary lobe and give rise to progressive manifestations of anterior pituitary deficiency, which have been described previously. Occasionally, chromophobe tumors occur as part of the genetic syndrome of multiple endocrine adenomatosis.[8]

Craniopharyngiomas or suprasellar cysts[76] are neoplasms of developmental origin that originate from the embryonically primitive Rathke's pouch. Histologically, they are usually composed of masses of squamous cells that form a tough lining around cystic cavities, or they may include solid elements that are indistinguishable from the ameloblastomas or adamantinomas of the jaw. The much more common cystic tumors contain an oily secretion resembling motor oil which consists of squamous epithelial detritus. The cysts may originate in the pituitary or above it and commonly cause compressive damage to the optic chiasm, the anterior pituitary lobe, the pituitary stalk, and the infundibular structures of the hypothalamus. The larger cysts may obstruct the ventricular system and can extend backward into the middle cranial fossa. Calcification occurs frequently in craniopharyngiomas and helps in radiologic diagnosis. Treatment of both chromophobe tumors and craniopharyngiomas consists of surgical excision.

HYPOPHYSECTOMY IN TREATMENT OF DIABETIC RETINOPATHY AND METASTATIC CANCER OF BREAST AND PROSTATE

The therapeutic possibilities of hypophysectomy or induced pituitary insufficiency as a means of arresting the progression of diabetic retinopathy were raised in 1953 by Poulsen,[113, 114] who observed regression of retinopathy in a patient with postpartum hypopituitarism (Sheehan's syndrome). In 1955 Luft and Olivecrona[95] in Sweden reported that hypophysectomy was effective in treatment of diabetic retinopathy. Since diabetic retinopathy is a leading cause of blindness and conventional therapy has not been very effective in its management, the reports by Poulsen and by Luft and Olivecrona led to an extensive trial of hypophyseal ablation in patients with the diabetic ocular disorder.[54] A variety of methods of interference with pituitary function have been used, including surgical excision of the gland, ^{90}Y implantation, cryohypophysectomy, hypophyseal stalk section, and pituitary ablation by Bragg peak proton beam irradiation. In Field's[47] collective review in 1968 of more than 600 patients with diabetic retinopathy treated by the various methods of pituitary ablation, satisfactory ocular re-

sults were observed in 48 to 75 per cent of patients treated.

Results of pituitary ablative procedures in patients with *diabetic retinopathy* are very difficult to assess. The variations in the status of ocular disease at the time of institution of treatment and the difficulty of conducting rigidly controlled clinical trials of therapy are major problems. Two fairly well controlled studies have been carried out: Lundbaek et al.[97] in Denmark used transsphenoidal hypophysectomy, while Oakley and his associates[105] at Hammersmith Hospital in London used transsphenoidal ^{90}Y implantation for pituitary ablation. Results were compared with those in carefully matched patients who did not have pituitary ablation. Each study supported the value of treatment by induced pituitary insufficiency.

The excellent summary of the role of hypophyseal ablation and the difficulty of evaluation of results in diabetic retinopathy by Sweet and Field[141] is recommended to interested students.

Hypophysectomy in palliation of *metastatic carcinoma of breast and prostate* was initially tried by Luft et al.[96] in Sweden and Ray[120] in this country after the demonstration by Huggins and his associates[73, 74] that bilateral adrenalectomy could provide palliation in certain advanced cases of these "endocrine-dependent" tumors.

The same techniques available for pituitary ablation in patients with diabetic retinopathy have been used extensively in patients with recurrent and metastatic carcinomas of breast and prostate.

In selected patients, hypophysectomy and adrenalectomy both are useful procedures in palliative treatment of advanced carcinoma of the breast and the prostate. In a large number of patients with advanced breast cancer studied by Fracchia et al.[49] the responses to various palliative treatments of recurrences were assessed and compared with the effects of hypophysectomy. The comparative responses to treatment in these patients with advanced metastic breast cancer are summarized in Table 3.

In the study by Fracchia et al.,[49] 38 per cent of patients with advanced breast cancer had an objective

TABLE 3. Response to Previous Treatment and to Hypophysectomy
(Patients with Advanced Carcinoma of the Breast)*

	No. of Patients	Response to Previous Treatment	Response to Hypophysectomy No.	Response to Hypophysectomy Per Cent	Failure to Previous Treatment	Response to Hypophysectomy No.	Response to Hypophysectomy Per Cent
Oophorectomy	35	18	3	17	17	2	12
Radiation castration	13	6	2	33	7	3	43
Oophorectomy and adrenalectomy	20	11	1	9	9	0	
Testosterone	69	13	4	31	56	14	25
Estrogen	23	4	2	50	19	6	32
Corticosteroid	44	8	3	38	36	9	25
Chemotherapy	31	5	1	20	26	4	15

*From Fracchia, A. A., et al.: Surg. Gynecol. Obstet., *133*:241, 1971. By permission of Surgery, Gynecology & Obstetrics.

period of palliation after hypophysectomy, while 35.4 per cent of a similar group treated by bilateral adrenalectomy had a similar objective response. There was no significant difference between the ablative procedures in the mean duration of response. It would appear that neither adrenalectomy nor hypophysectomy has a distinct advantage as to frequency or duration of response. According to Fracchia and his associates, the most important prognostic indicators for the selection of patients are the length of the clinically free interval (from mastectomy to recurrence) and the anatomic site of metastases. If an estrogen receptor can be identified in metastatic tissue, the likelihood of a beneficial response to adrenalectomy or hypophysectomy is about 50 per cent. Hypophysectomy is preferred by this group when the patient has diminished cardiopulmonary reserve, nodular pulmonary or pleural metastases, or cutaneous metastases in the line of incision for adrenalectomy.

Scott and his associates[134, 135] have made extensive studies of the management of disseminated prostatic cancer by total adrenalectomy and by hypophysectomy. Their studies, along with those of Ray,[118] Luft and Olivecrona,[95, 96] Smith,[139] Murphy,[102] and many others, have shown that objective and subjective evidence of benefit may be expected after hypophysectomy in approximately 40 per cent of patients with metastatic prostatic cancer. Remissions after bilateral adrenalectomy in patients with advanced prostatic cancer seem to be less frequent and of shorter duration.

In a study by Murphy et al.[102] at Roswell Park of 34 patients with disseminated prostatic cancer treated by surgical or cryosurgical hypophysectomy, those patients who had objective evidence of suppression of human growth hormone (HGH) had a 42 per cent rate of satisfactory remission. In contrast, those patients who had no evidence of HGH suppression had no significant remission of the malignant disease. In 12 patients with disseminated prostatic cancer treated by bilateral adrenalectomy, Murphy and his associates found significantly less response than after hypophysectomy.

THE ADRENALS

More than a century has passed since Thomas Addison[1] described the syndrome of adrenal insufficiency that bears his name. He described the clinical manifestations with such clarity in the 11 cases he reported, and elaborated the etiologic conditions so pointedly, that little can be added even today. Efforts to provide substitutive therapy in adrenal cortical insufficiency were made as early as 1856.[17] However, it remained for Kendall[80] and Reichstein[121] in the late 1930s to elaborate the biochemical studies that led to the many important discoveries concerning the synthesis and pathophysiology of the adrenal cortical steroids. Although epinephrine has been recognized as an important hormonal product of the adrenal medulla since the nineteenth century, the isolation of norepinephrine in tissues by von Euler and his associates[145] in 1946, and in the adrenal gland by Holtz

et al.[72] in 1947, and the subsequent elucidation of its role and that of the other catecholamines in physiologic and pathophysiologic states form an equally important contribution to knowledge of adrenal function. As a consequence, the clinician of today can approach the diagnosis of adrenal disease with much more accuracy and sophistication than he could even a few short years ago. This, coupled with the ability to provide adequate replacement for total absence of the adrenal glands, has extended the field of adrenal surgery remarkably.

SURGICAL ANATOMY AND EMBRYOLOGY

The two adrenal glands in man sit as caps over the upper poles of the kidneys. The convex surface of the kidney produces a concave impression on the inferior surface of each gland. The right suprarenal gland is roughly triangular in outline, and its anterior surface touches the inferior vena cava posteriorly and medially, the liver laterally, and the upper pole of the right kidney inferiorly. The left adrenal is crescentic in its outline and lies between the anteromedial border of the left kidney and the left lateral edge of the aorta. The glands are a darker yellow color and firmer than the perirenal fat in which they lie. They are situated in the upper extension of a compartment enclosed by Gerota's fascia and are held in position by numerous fibrous bands as well as vascular attachments. Their relationship to the kidney has been overemphasized. When the kidney is depressed inferiorly, the suprarenal glands remain in a relatively fixed position.

The weight of the normal adrenal gland may vary considerably but usually is in the range of 3 to 5 gm. In the male the adrenal gland is usually 30 per cent heavier than its female counterpart. The glands vary from 40 to 60 mm. in length, 20 to 30 mm. in width, and 2 to 8 mm. in thickness except at the bases where they are considerably thicker. The sectioned gland is seen grossly to consist of an outer cortical layer and an inner medullary portion which constitutes approximately 10 per cent of its weight. The outer cortex is yellowish in color and has a firmer consistency than the reddish brown medullary portion.

The adrenal glands have an abundant arterial supply via branches of the inferior phrenic artery superiorly, the aorta medially, and the renal artery inferiorly. In addition, branches from the ovarian or internal spermatic artery on the left side and from the intercostals bilaterally are found in many patients. As many as 50 or 60 small adrenal vessels have been observed in some subjects. These vessels break up into large sinusoids, and blood flows of 6 to 7 ml. per gram of tissue per minute have been measured.[48] After traversing the gland, the blood drains into large venous lacunae in the medulla from which it is collected into a large venous trunk as well as a number of smaller veins. On the right, the short adrenal veins drain directly into the inferior vena cava, while the left adrenal vein drains either into the left renal vein or into the vena cava. A small vein on each side courses along with the inferior phrenic vessels, and on the left small venous channels leave the cortex to join the vena cava and the splenic and pancreatic veins, and in this way a small part of the venous return reaches the portal system.

The lymphatic channels of the adrenals form two plexuses, one directly under the capsule and another one in the medulla. The lymphatics of the right adrenal drain into lymph nodes near the aorta and near the crus of the diaphragm. On the left side, they connect with lymph nodes at the origin of the left renal artery and with the lymph nodes along the aorta. The nerve supply is derived primarily from the splanchnic nerves. These nerves then form the suprarenal plexuses and connect with the renal and celiac plexuses and celiac ganglia. Stimulation of the adrenal nerves brings about a prompt release of medullary hormones without influencing cortical activity.[48]

Histologic examination of the cortex reveals three distinct areas as viewed from the periphery medially. The zona glomerulosa, a thin outer layer of short loops of glomeruloid clusters of irregularly arranged cells lying just beneath the capsule of the adrenal, apparently secretes materials having to do with electrolyte exchange. Next, the zona fasciculata, which is the widest cortical zone, consists of radially oriented strands of cells that elaborate hormones having to do with organic metabolism. Most centrally located is the zona reticularis, with its netlike cords of cells, which borders on the edge of the medulla and which elaborates hormones with androgenic and estrogenic effects. In contrast to the cortex, the medulla is structurally uniform, consisting of networks of anastomosing cords of polyhedral cells that secrete the hormonally active catecholamines, epinephrine, norepinephrine, and dopamine, and other precursors which currently seem to be biologically inert. Epinephrine makes up approximately 75 to 80 per cent of the medullary secretion, and its inotropic effect on the myocardium causes an increase in cardiac output, whereas norepinephrine exerts a pressor effect by increasing peripheral resistance by vasoconstriction.

Embryologically, development of the adrenal gland represents the union of certain cells from the neural crest which form the adrenal medulla and cells from the splanchnic mesoderm which compose the cortex. These two elements in lower vertebrates such as the fish are permanently separated. In embryos at the 5 to 6 mm. stage, the mesothelium at the upper level of the mesonephros proliferates and sends cords of cells laterally into the mesenchyme of the dorsal mesentery. Crowder[28] states that there are three different types of cells composing the adrenal cortex, two of which derive from the coelomic epithelium and one which arises from the Bowman's capsule cells of the mesonephron. The fetal cortex is composed of the same cell types as the adult cortex, but proportions and arrangements differ. Crowder maintains that both in the fetus and in the adult all three types of cells of the cortex are renewed from the glomerulosa and migrate inwardly. Somewhat later (about the 18 mm. stage) than is the case with the adrenal cortex, the chromophil cells of the medulla begin to develop. The medullary cells are ectodermal in origin and derive from sympathetic ganglia. The cells are of two types, sympathoblasts, which eventually give rise to mature sympathetic ganglion cells, and pheochromoblasts, which subsequently develop into the characteristic chromaffin cells of the adrenal medulla. By the 20 mm. stage in the human embryo, these chromaffin cells migrate along the lateral dorsal mesentery and penetrate the cortical anlage. At the 100 mm. stage, the chromaffin cells have reached the central vein and have formed a true medulla.

During the third and fourth months of fetal life the adrenals are enormous in size and actually exceed the kidneys in total mass. Most of this enlargement is due to the growth of the fetal cortex. Subsequently, the adrenals grow less rapidly than the developing adjacent structures and at the sixth month of fetal life are only half as large as the kidneys. At birth, the adrenals are approximately one third as large as the kidneys.

The cells of the fetal cortex are most closely related to the zona reticularis. The normal human fetal adrenal cortex accounts for approximately 80 per cent of the total adrenal mass throughout most of fetal life. At birth and occasionally immediately preceding birth, the fetal zone undergoes rather marked changes. These changes are characterized by necrosis, hemorrhage, vascular engorgement, loss of cellular detail, and fragmentation of cells. This degeneration is compen-

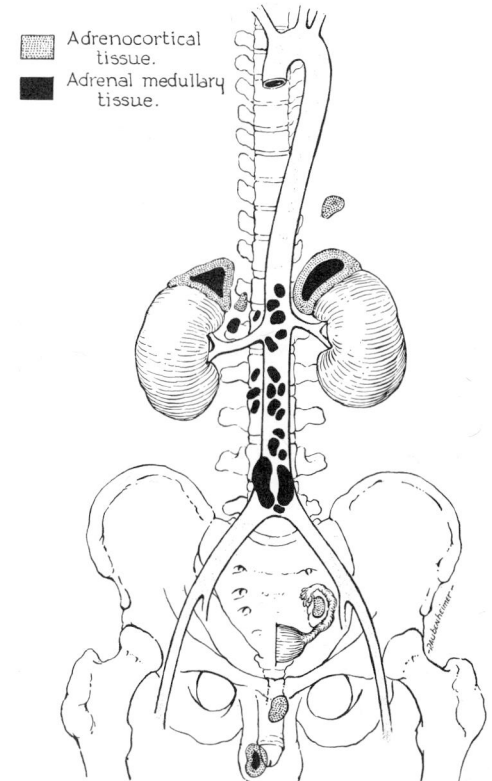

Figure 7. Extra-adrenal sites of adrenal cortical and medullary tissue. (From Forsham, P. H. *In* Williams, R. H. (Ed.): Textbook of Endocrinology, 5th ed. Philadelphia, W. B. Saunders Company, 1974.)

sated for in part by proliferation of the zona fasciculata, and by the fifth to sixth postnatal week the adrenal cortex has obtained a more adult type of appearance. By the end of the first year of life there is total disappearance of the fetal adrenal cortex. The rate of disappearance is the same for premature and full-term infants and, therefore, seems to be related to the changes induced by birth and not by the actual age of the adrenal cortex. In hemicephalia, hydrocephalus, and cephalomeningocele, the adrenals are usually smaller than normal, while in congenital syphilis, kwashiorkor, pancreatic fibrosis, hypertrophic pyloric stenosis, and congenital heart disease, there tends to be a prolonged persistence of the fetal adrenal cortex. Evidence at present indicates that the biosynthetic capabilities of the human fetal adrenals in both the definitive and fetal zones are essentially similar to those of adult man (Fig. 7).

PHYSIOLOGY

The adrenal cortex can both synthesize cholesterol and take it up from the circulation. Cholesterol is found in abundance in adrenocortical cells, chiefly in cytoplasmic lipid droplets, and is the substrate from which the cortical steroid hormones are synthesized. There is little utilization of available cholesterol in steroidogenesis unless the adrenocortical cell is stimulated by an extra-adrenal regulator (Fig. 8).

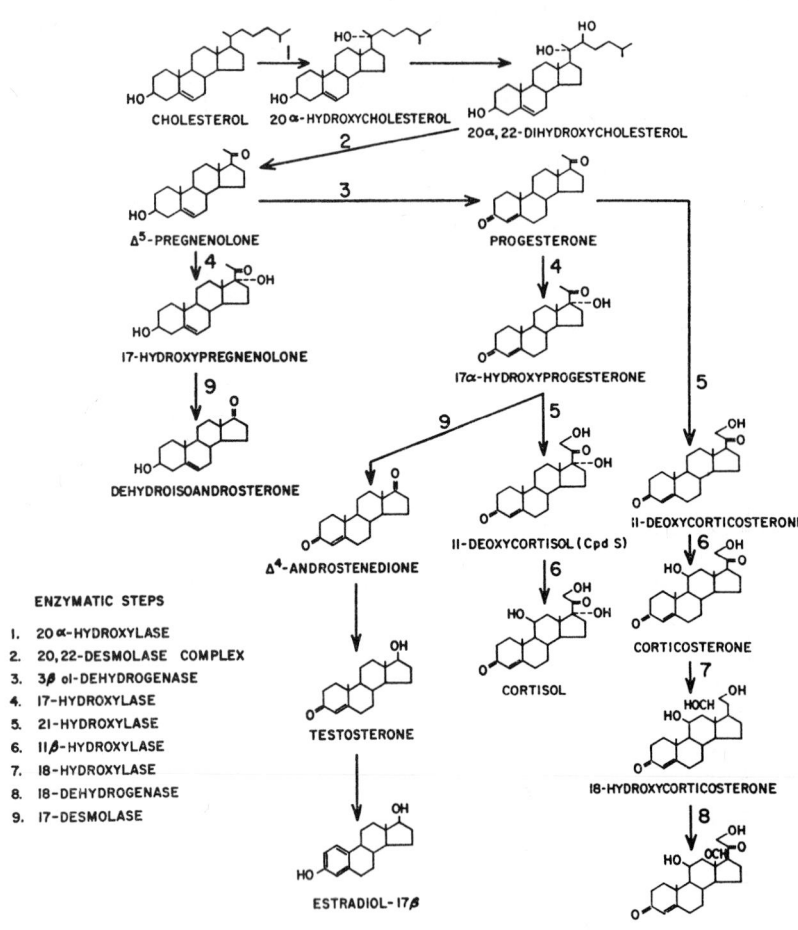

Figure 8. Major biosynthetic pathways for adrenal steroids. (From Temple, T. E., and Liddle, G. W.: *Ann. Rev. Pharmacol., 10*:199, 1970.)

The rate-limiting step and the best known pathway in biosynthesis of steroids in the adrenal cortex are represented by the conversion of cholesterol to *pregnenolone*. The latter is efficiently transformed by a stable group of enzymes into the major biologically active corticosteroids. The major steps in the subsequent hormonal syntheses are indicated in the diagram (Fig. 8).

A side reaction results in conversion of some pregnenolone to 17-hydroxy pregnenolone and then to the relatively weak androgen dehydroepiandrosterone (DHEA).

The conversion of pregnenolone to *cortisol* by the zona fasciculata first entails dehydrogenation of the 3 beta-hydroxyl group of pregnenolone and subsequent isomerization to form *progesterone*. As indicated in Figure 8 progesterone is enzymatically converted to 17 alpha-hydroxyprogesterone which subsequently is converted by the 21-hydroxylase system to 11-deoxycortisol ("substance S" of Reichstein). Substance S is converted by the action of 11 beta-hydroxylase to cortisol (compound F). Progesterone is also converted by the zona fasciculata to small amounts of *corticosterone* as a by product of cortisol synthesis.

The conversion of pregnenolone to *aldosterone* by the zona glomerulosa involves intermediate enzymatic synthesis of corticosterone. Some of this steroid is acted on by 18-hydroxylase to form 18-hydroxycorticosterone and then by 18-hydroxysteroid dehydrogenase to form aldosterone. The zona glomerulosa lacks the capacity to form 17 alpha-hydroxyprogesterone and therefore cannot synthesize cortisol. Only the zona glomerulosa contains the enzyme 18-hydroxysteroid dehydrogenase and only cells of the glomerulosa can synthesize aldosterone.

Only cortisol and aldosterone among the adrenocortical steroids appear to be essential for good health. The adrenal produces in addition to dehydroepiandrosterone small amounts of the classical androgens, *androstenedione* and *testosterone,* and minute amounts of *estrogen* (estradiol-17β). In normal subjects the conversion of pregnenolone to cortisol, corticosterone, aldosterone, and dehydroepiandrosterone occurs so rapidly that only these hormones constitute physiologically important secretions.

No secretory nerves to the adrenal cortex have been demonstrated in man, in contrast to the rich supply to the medulla. Growth of the adrenal cortex, as well as secretory activity of all its hormones except aldosterone, is regulated by the pituitary hormone adreno-corticotropin (ACTH). The basophilic cells of the pituitary increase in number after adrenalectomy and thus are presumably a source of corticotropin. The anterior pituitary may show sheaths of basophils in patients who have died of Addison's disease, and their excess has been associated with elevated blood levels of corticotropin. The classic concept of the mechanism of secretion of ACTH in response to stress is diagramatically shown in Figure 9. Among the stresses which have been found to induce increased pituitary-adrenal activity are severe trauma, pyrogens, acute hypoglycemia, injections of histamine, electric shock, and acute anxiety.

The corticotropin releasing factor (CRF) of the hypothalamus stimulates the release of ACTH by the pituitary. Experimental evidence suggests that hypothalamic secretion of CRF is stimulated by cholinergic neurons and inhibited by adrenergic neurons. In normal subjects who are not under stress and who have normal sleeping habits there is a diurnal or circadian rhythm in the secretion of ACTH by the pituitary and the responsive secretion of cortisol by the adrenal cortex. The normal individual has higher blood ACTH and cortisol concentrations in the morning than in the evening. The "long loop," negative feedback action of cortisol is to suppress ACTH secretion and, conversely, if cortisol levels fall below normal the corticotropin-producing cells of the anterior pituitary are released from this suppressive effect, ACTH secretion occurs and continues until normal cortisol levels are restored. This has been described as a classic example of a "servo mechanism" which is important in maintaining homeostasis.

For practical purposes Liddle proposes that ACTH secretion by the pituitary with the hormonal response of the adrenal cortex is regulated by three factors: cortisol and cortisol-like steroids, a "biologic clock," and stress.[91]

Among the various adrenal steroids, apparently only hydrocortisone (cortisol) has a physiologically significant role in regulating the rate of ACTH secretion. The reciprocal relationship between these two hormones maintains the constancy of plasma cortisol within rather narrow limits in the absence of stress.

Both organic and inorganic metabolism are affected by the adrenal cortical steroid hormones. The organic functions are controlled by the glucocorticoids, especially the catabolic cortisol and corticosterone; the 17-ketosteroids, such as dehydroepiandrosterone, which are anabolic and androgenic; estrogens in small amounts; and various precursors of active corticoids. The inorganic functions include sodium retention and potassium excretion and are principally influenced by the mineralocorticoids aldosterone and desoxycorticosterone. The adrenal corticoids have both specific actions and permissive functions in affecting metabolic processes.

According to Williams,[151] there is considerable functional overlap between glucocorticoids and mineralo-corticoids. For instance, aldosterone has 500 times the activity of cortisol in sodium retention, yet only one third its gluconeogenetic potency. Cortisol, however, has a significant effect on electrolyte metabolism, since it is secreted in a quantity of about 20 mg. per day, as contrasted to 150 μg. per day of aldosterone.

Cortisol is the most important glucocorticoid. It enhances gluconeogenesis and in excess produces protein depletion and diabetes. It also induces a centripetal distribution of fat, hyperlipemia, and hypercholesterolemia. It enhances water diuresis and assists in maintenance of the homeostasis of extracellular fluid volume by preventing the shift of water into the cell. Its hematologic effects are to increase the number of circulating erythrocytes, platelets, and neutrophils while reducing the number of eosinophils, basophils, and lymphocytes.

Physiologically, cortisol maintains the homeostasis of muscle protein and function. In its absence, striated muscles become weak, and with excess cortisol muscle protein is depleted. In the central nervous system cortisol lowers the threshold for electrical excitation. Psychiatric disturbances are common both with lack of cortisol and with its excess. In the gastrointestinal tract, gastric acidity is increased by cortisol, and peptic ulcer formation is enhanced, possibly also by gastric mucus suppression, in the presence of excess cortisol. Cortisol blocks new bone formation at the level of the protein matrix, antagonizes the action of vitamin D, impedes the absorption of calcium from the gut, and increases the urinary clearance of calcium; thus, in excess it enhances every phase of osteoporosis.

A most important physiologic effect of cortisol on the cardiovascular system is its "permissive" effect in sensitizing the arterioles to the pressor effects of norepinephrine and related compounds. Prolonged excess of cortisol enhances atherosclerosis. The glucocorticoids reduce the inflammatory process and the cellular

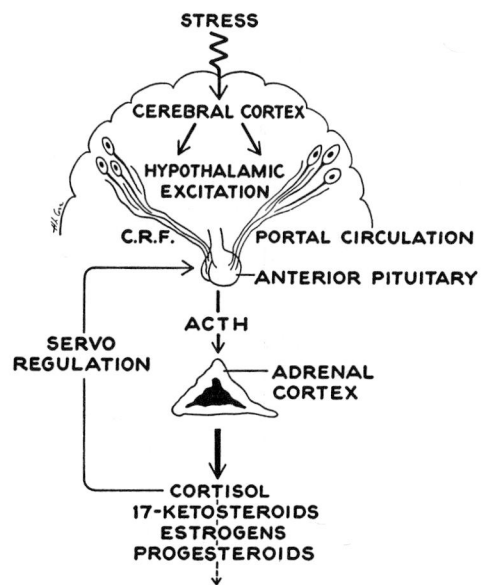

STRESS

CEREBRAL CORTEX

HYPOTHALAMIC EXCITATION

C.R.F.   PORTAL CIRCULATION

ANTERIOR PITUITARY

ACTH

SERVO REGULATION

ADRENAL CORTEX

CORTISOL
17-KETOSTEROIDS
ESTROGENS
PROGESTEROIDS

ALDOSTERONE

Figure 9. Schematic representation of mechanisms involved in the release of corticotropin from the anterior pituitary gland. (From Forsham, P. H. *In* Williams, R. H. (Ed.): Textbook of Endocrinology, 5th ed. Philadelphia, W. B. Saunders Company, 1974.)

response to injury, and cortisol inhibits hypersensitivity responses to antigen-antibody complexes. In excess, it reduces the production of antibodies, lyses plasma cells and lymphocytes, and depresses immunologic responses.

The half-life of free cortisol in plasma is normally about 90 minutes. Its principal site of metabolic degradation is the liver, where it undergoes enzymatic reduction and conjugation. The Porter-Silber chromogens or 17-hydroxycorticosteroids (17-OHCS) are easily measured urinary metabolites of cortisol and related glucocorticoids.

The anabolic, androgenic 17-ketosteroids enhance the synthesis of proteins from amino acids and antagonize the catabolic effects of the glucocorticoids. When they are present in excess, increases in muscle mass, virilization, hirsutism, acne, deepening of the voice, and other masculinizing features result. The 17-ketosteroids are metabolized in the liver and are excreted in the urine chiefly as sulfate conjugates.

The mineralocorticoids, aldosterone and desoxycorticosterone, effect sodium retention and potassium loss. Sodium is exchanged for potassium and hydrogen ion in the renal tubule, and similar exchanges that take place in sweat glands, salivary glands, and intestinal mucosa and in general between intracellular and extracellular fluid are controlled by these corticoids. Aldosterone, which has 30 times the sodium-retaining potency of desoxycorticosterone, is secreted by the zona glomerulosa of the adrenal cortex. This part of the cortex maintains its integrity after hypophysectomy and is apparently not controlled by ACTH. Rather, aldosterone secretion is closely related to the renin-angiotensin system (see Fig. 21) of the renal juxtaglomerular apparatus and responds to and delicately controls intravascular and extravascular fluid volumes. The effects of aldosterone on the sodium pump of the renal countercurrent multiplier system are demonstrated in Figure 10.

The adrenal medullary secretory activity is dependent on stimulation or excitation of its sympathetic nerves. In contrast to cortical secretion, there is no known direct hormonal control over the medullary secretion. Epinephrine, norepinephrine, and dopamine are secreted by at least two types of chromaffin cells in the medulla. These catecholamines are synthesized from tyrosine by pathways indicated in Figure 11.

The physiologically more significant compounds are norepinephrine and epinephrine. Apparently the cells that store norepinephrine are incapable of methylating this catecholamine. Most of the extra-adrenal chromaffin tissues, including sympathetic ganglia and nerve endings, also largely lack the methylating mechanism. Accordingly, these extra-adrenal tissues produce chiefly norepinephrine and dopamine.

The catecholamines differ in their pharmacophysiologic effects, although a good deal of overlap exists. Their effects and differences are summarized in Table 4. Epinephrine has greater excitatory, hyperglycemic, and metabolic effects and induces fright. Both compounds enhance the liberation of free fatty acids from fat depots and raise the circulating plasma levels. The catecholamines are normally metabolized rapidly by ortho-methylation and oxidative deamination. About

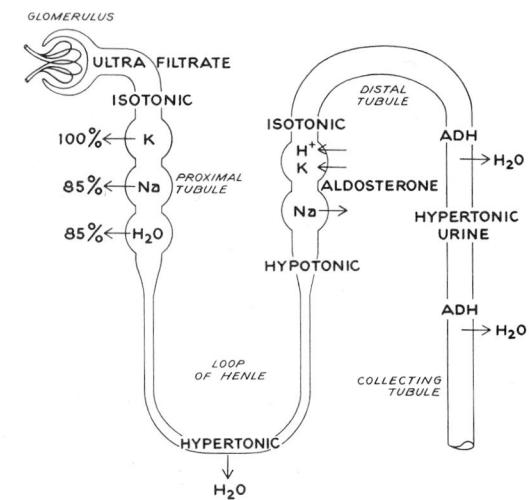

Figure 10. Diagrammatic representation of the renal tubular action of aldosterone and antidiuretic hormone (ADH). Glucocorticoid action enhances glomerular filtration. (From Forsham, P. H. *In* Williams, R. H., (Ed.): Textbook of Endocrinology, 5th ed. Philadelphia, W. B. Saunders Company, 1974.)

40 per cent of the catecholamine secretion appears in the urine as conjugated 3-methoxy,4-hydroxymandelic acid (VMA).

RADIOGRAPHIC DIAGNOSIS

Except in unusually large tumors of the adrenal gland, adrenal tissue is not well seen on plain roentgenograms of the abdomen. Although the kidney and suprarenal gland are surrounded by a relatively radiolucent fat pad, the radiodensity of the suprarenal gland in relationship to the upper pole of the kidney and to the medial structures does not make its outline immediately and easily apparent. With enlargement of the adrenal gland the most usual roentgenographic sign seen on the plain abdominal or KUB film is displacement of the renal mass inferiorly and laterally, with the kidney on the same side as the tumor shifting its upper pole to a more lateral position. Sometimes even in bilateral adrenal hyperplasia in which no tumor is present, the upper pole of the kidney may be subtly changed in its position and can be visualized in the plain roentgenogram.

As previously mentioned, the normal adrenal glands are small, yellowish, flattened, roughly triangular-shaped structures lying at the upper extension of the perinephric fascia and capping the upper pole of each kidney. Each gland lies superior and medial to the upper pole of the kidney and presents as a slightly curved triangular mass surrounded by adipose tissue. The gland tends to adhere to the upper condensation of Gerota's fascia, and the mass of the perirenal fat tends to become more evident when the patient is placed in the upright position, thus allowing the kidney to drop inferiorly and delineating the margins of the adrenal to a better advantage.

The upright film with the presence of contrast me-

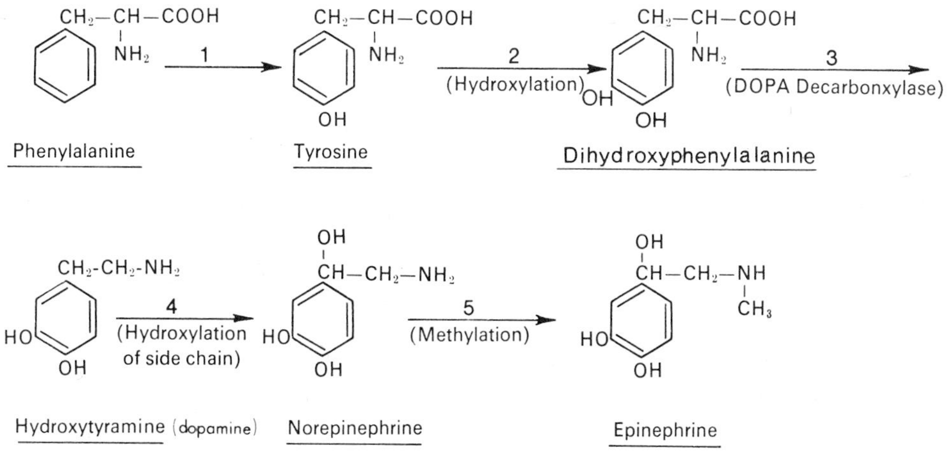

Figure 11. Biosynthesis of norepinephrine and epinephrine.

dium in the kidney will in most instances delineate the separation of the kidney and the adrenal if the adrenal is enlarged. Laminagraphy will greatly improve the delineation of the contours of the adrenals, particularly when combined with the presence of contrast medium in the kidney. However, additional procedures are often required to demonstrate adrenal enlargement.

Retroperitoneal pneumography has long been a valuable procedure for delineation of the outlines of the adrenal gland. Gas directly injected around the kidney was first introduced by Carelli in 1921.[19] Refinements in technique and the utilization of more highly soluble gases have eliminated many of the previous complications of this type of study. The use of

carbon dioxide or nitrous oxide has reduced the hazards of gas embolism. The availability of image intensification has also greatly increased the diagnostic accuracy of this technique. The authors prefer a direct needle injection of nitrous oxide or carbon dioxide into the perirenal or presacral fat, with control of the volume of gas by image intensification to delineate the adrenals (Fig. 12). With this technique, not only adrenal tumors but also adrenal hyperplasia can be recognized.

In the last several years there has been a tendency to use arteriography extensively in diagnosis of adrenal tumors. Flush aortograms and selective renal arteriograms can be precisely diagnostic in the larger tumors. Occasionally catheterization of the inferior phrenic artery is possible, and small tumors may be visualized by selective anteriography. Retrograde adrenal phlebography has been advocated recently, but in the authors' opinion the technique presents a risk of adrenal infarction and extravasation of contrast material that is unattractive.

SURGICAL APPROACHES TO THE ADRENAL GLAND

Four different surgical approaches to the adrenals have been advocated. The choice of approach must be individualized on the basis of the diagnostic findings and the physical characteristics of the patient. Cahill,[18] one of the pioneers in adrenal surgery, has advocated the transabdominal approach because of the advantage of simultaneous bilateral exploration through a single incision. However, this approach is more time-consuming, more difficult, and associated with greater morbidity in the obese patient than some of the other

TABLE 4. Comparison of Pharmacologic Effects of Norepinephrine and Epinephrine*

Norepinephrine		Epinephrine
++++	Pressor effect	+
+++	Lipolysis	++
±	Increased cardiac output	++
+	Hyperglycemia	++++
++	Increased basal metabolic rate	++++
+	Eosinopenia	++++
0	Central nervous system excitation	++++

*From Forsham, P. H. *In* Williams, R. H. (Ed.): Textbook of Endocrinology, 5th ed. Philadelphia, W. B. Saunders Company, 1974.

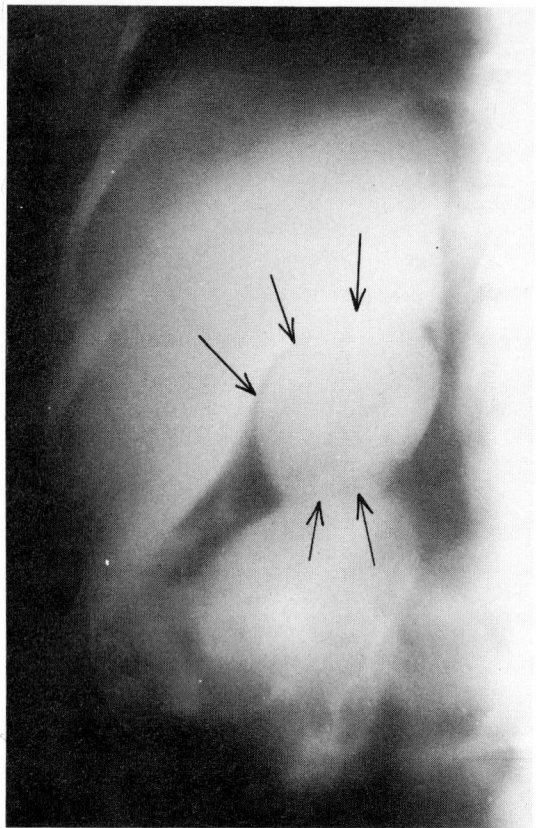

Figure 12. Radiographic visualization of adrenal tumor using retroperitoneal carbon dioxide insufflation. (From Scott, H. W., Jr., et al.: Ann. Surg., *162*:505, 1965.)

tumor who have intercurrent abdominal disease that needs correction (Fig. 13).

The thoracoabdominal approach affords the most optimal exposure of a single adrenal and the contents of the ipsilateral renal fossa. It is indicated when large tumors are encountered, especially pheochromocytomas and adrenal carcinomas. This approach, however, does have the drawback of providing less than optimal exposure of the contralateral adrenal (Fig. 14).

The most commonly used approach is that originally described by Young,[153] a bilateral posterior approach. In Young's approach to the adrenal gland the patient is placed on the operating table in the prone position and the trunk is flexed. Usually a subperiosteal resection of the eleventh or twelfth rib or both is done. This approach has the advantage of being extraperitoneal, extrapleural, and subdiaphragmatic (Fig. 15). It is particularly advantageous when bilateral adrenalectomy is to be carried out and when there may be an adrenal cortical adenoma or aldosteroma in which exposure of both adrenal glands is a necessity. The main disadvantage is the limited operative exposure afforded. The postoperative morbidity is usually impressively reduced as compared to that with other approaches.

The posterolateral approach affords a wide field of operation with direct access to the suprarenal region on one side at a time, and is extremely useful when adrenal tumor has been accurately localized prior to operation or when the patient is too large or obese for an approach by either the anterior or the posterior route.

approaches. It is most useful in thin patients, especially those with pheochromocytoma in whom exploration of sites of aberrant adrenal tissue is contemplated, and in patients of normal habitus with adrenal

CLINICAL CONDITIONS

Adrenal cortical insufficiency may be primary, as in Addison's disease, or secondary, as a result of pituitary corticotropic insufficiency. It may be overt or latent, organic or functional. Whether primary or secondary, the clinical syndromes manifest deficiences in

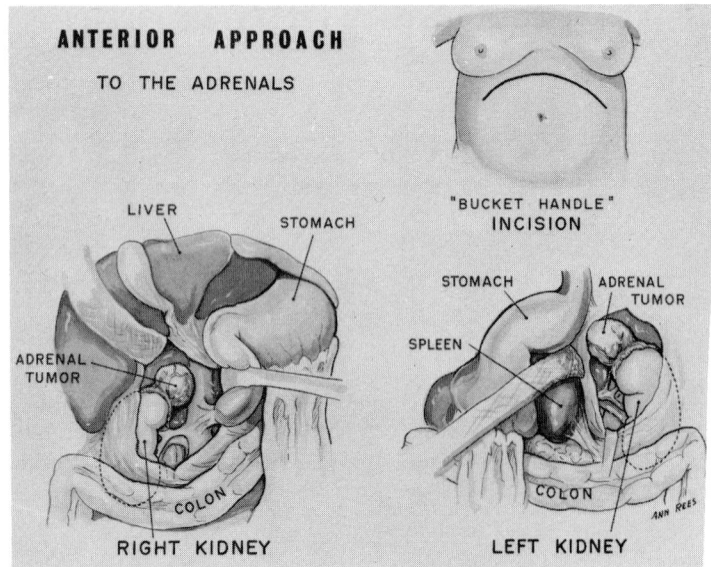

Figure 13. Anterior approach to the adrenals. (From Surgical considerations in hypertension, by Scott, H. W., Jr., and Foster, J. H. in Current Problems in Surgery, edited by Ravitch, M. M., et al. Copyright © 1964, Year Book Medical Publishers. Used by permission.)

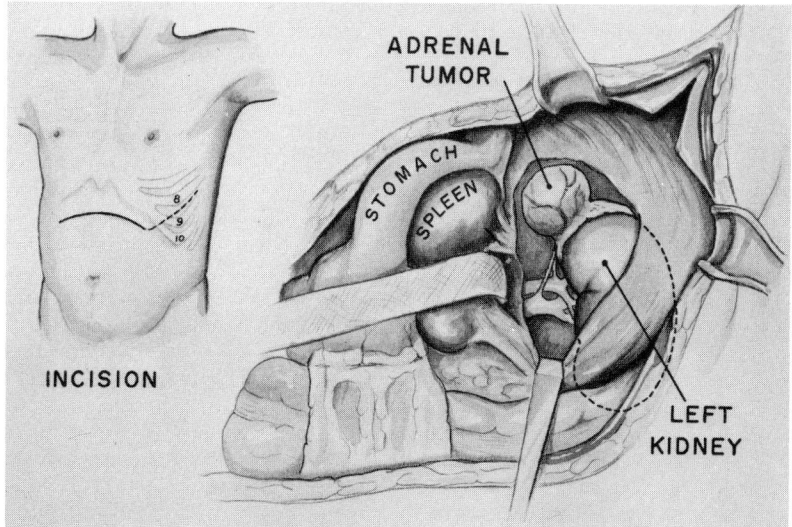

Figure 14. Thoracoabdominal approach to adrenal tumor. (From Scott, H. W., Jr., Foster, J. H., Liddle, G. W., and Davidson, E. T.: Ann. Surg., *162*:505, 1965.)

adrenal steroids. In 1855 Thomas Addison[1] wrote: "The leading and characteristic features of the morbid state to which I would direct attention are anaemia, general languor, and debility, remarkable feebleness of the heart's action, irritability of the stomach and a peculiar change of color in the skin occurring in connection with a diseased condition of the 'suprarenal capsules.'" His brilliant descriptions of the clinical manifestations of this disease require essentially no alterations even today. However, our understanding of the metabolic aspects and the effects of this syndrome are considerably more complete. A classification of the etiologic agents is presented in Table 5.

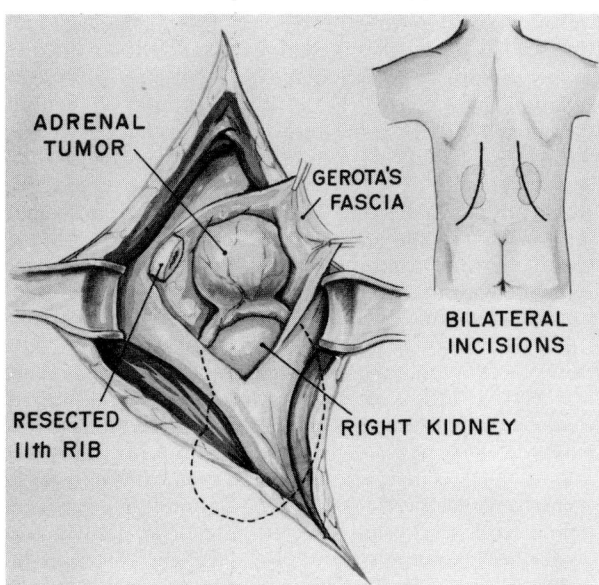

Figure 15. Posterior approach to the adrenals with bilateral incisions. (From Scott, H. W., Jr., Foster, J. H., Liddle, G. W., and Davidson, E. T.: Ann. Surg., *162*:505, 1965.)

ACUTE ADRENAL INSUFFICIENCY (ADDISONIAN CRISIS)

Acute loss of adrenal function is attended by profound changes in blood pressure, electrolytes, and carbohydrate metabolism. This dramatic condition often demands emergency and heroic methods of treatment. The syndrome is classically manifested by anorexia, nausea, vomiting, headache, diarrhea, abdominal pain, dehydration, hypotension, hypoglycemia, marked weakness, and extreme lethargy. Hyperpyrexia normally is present, with coma and vascular collapse rapidly following. Acute adrenal cortical failure may follow hemorrhage into the adrenals as a result of trauma, infection, tumor, or adrenal vascular thrombosis. Hemorrhage into the adrenal glands of the newborn is responsible for about 1 per cent of neonatal deaths, occurring most commonly after a difficult labor and fetal anoxia. The Waterhouse-Friderichsen syndrome may be seen in meningococcal septicemia and in other severe infections with organisms such as pneumococcus, staphylococcus, and hemolytic streptococcus, and with other bacteremic and viremic states including smallpox and diphtheria. Laboratory study in these patients usually shows hyponatremia, hyperkalemia, hypoglycemia, and azotemia.

The fever in meningococcal septicemia rises rapidly, with cyanosis, petechial rash, stiffness of the neck, convulsions, and coma soon developing. The Waterhouse-Friderichsen syndrome rarely affects adults and almost never results in permanent adrenocortical insufficiency.

The treatment of the adrenal crisis is aimed at: (1) provision of adequate cortical hormone, (2) control of infection, and (3) support of the cardiovascular system. In babies and young children an immediate intravenous injection of 50 mg. of hydrocortisone is followed by a maintenance infusion of 100 to 200 mg. of hydrocortisone (adults may require more) dissolved in 5 per cent dextrose and normal saline of appropriate

**TABLE 5.   Adrenal Insufficiency Syndromes
— Classication of Adrenal Cortical Hypofunction****

I. Primary—deficiency of corticosteroids, aldosterone, and adrenal androgen
   A. *Acute*—Addisonian crisis
      1. Impaired adrenal secretory capacity—the demand for hormone exceeds the amount that can be produced
      2. Adrenal "apoplexy"—trauma, overwhelming infection, hemorrhage
      3. Adrenalectomy
      4. Atrophy due to prolonged steroid therapy
   B. *Chronic*—Addison's disease
      1. Complete
         a. Primary atrophy of the adrenal
         b. Destruction or replacement of cortical tissue by various diseases, e.g., tuberculosis, amyloidosis, etc.
         c. Adrenalectomy
      2. Incomplete
         a. Partial replacement of the gland, e.g., tumor, infection, hemorrhage
         b. Reduced adrenal cortical function—inanition (?), cachexia
II. Secondary—reduced cortisol secretion as a result of ACTH deficiency
   A. Hypopituitarism—Complete, fractional, or unitropic deficiency of ACTH production
   B. Inhibition of ACTH synthesis and/or release due to glucocorticoid administration or hypothalamic-portal system defect
III. Altered adrenal cortisol metabolism
   A. Spontaneous and induced defects of cortisol synthesis—reduced or absent capacity to secrete cortisol as seen in the adrenogenital syndrome or after specific drugs
   B. Accelerated cortisol catabolism—thyroid storm; insulin-induced hypoglycemia

*From Frawley, T. F. *In* Eisenstein, A. B. (Ed.): The Adrenal Cortex. Boston, Little, Brown and Company, 1967.

volume and administered by intravenous drip over a period of 24 to 48 hours. Infection, which so commonly accompanies this syndrome, should be treated with appropriate antibiotics. If hypotension persists after the initiation of the hydrocortisone, a phenylephrine (Neo-Synephrine) drip, 5 to 10 mg. per liter, may be added to maintain blood pressure. Because these patients are usually hypovolemic, blood transfusions may be necessary if the shock persists. After the emergency period of treatment, hydrocortisone dosage is reduced by daily decrements, as described by Liddle,[88] until oral therapy with hydrocortisone in the range of 0.3 mg. per kilogram can be initiated. The addition of 0.05 to 0.1 mg. of *fluoro*hydrocortisone daily is adjusted to maintain normal blood pressure. The need for maintenance dosage on a long-term basis must be determined by careful endocrine studies.

CHRONIC ADRENAL INSUFFICIENCY (ADDISON'S DISEASE)

Addison's disease is relatively rare. The death rate from this disorder in the United States is approxi-

mately 0.3 per 100,000. It is predominantly a disease of adult life. The majority of cases occur between the second and the fifth decades and males and females are affected with equal frequency. Basic to the physiopathology of the disease is a loss of adrenal cortical substance. Prior to 1950, 70 to 88 per cent of cases of Addison's disease were ascribed to adrenal tuberculosis while the remaining cases were felt to be due to primary atrophy of the gland.

Currently, tuberculosis probably accounts for about 50 per cent of cases of Addison's disease. In the remainder, various other lesions may be encountered, including bilateral tumor metastasis, leukemic infiltration, amyloidosis, hemochromatosis, histoplasmosis, coccidioidomycosis, cryptococcosis, blastomycosis, reticuloendotheliosis, giant cell granuloma, diphtheria, measles, scarlet fever, smallpox, typhoid fever, influenza, syphilis, malaria, amebiasis, and pyogenic infections. In addition, in rare instances familial Addison's disease has been described.

In Addison's disease due to tuberculosis of the adrenals, the lesions are always found bilaterally, since the disease does not become symptomatic until 90 per cent or more of the glandular tissue has been destroyed. Although fibrosis is usually present, calcification of the caseous material occurs on rare occasions and may be demonstrated on x-ray examination. Tuberculosis of the adrenal glands is always secondary to an extra-adrenal focus and, therefore, pulmonary or renal tuberculosis or both should be looked for.

Addison's disease is usually insidious in its onset. Mild to severe weight loss is invariably present. Easy fatigability and muscular weakness occur in almost every case. The muscular weakness, which is commonly improved by sleep and rest, also improves markedly when glucocorticoid administration restores carbohydrate metabolism to normal. Hyperpigmentations has been commonly observed in this disease. It is present in approximately 90 per cent of patients with Addison's disease. It is most marked in exposed areas of the skin, particularly in scars and on mucosal surfaces. The hyperpigmentation in patients with primary adrenal cortical insufficiency results from increased release in the pituitary gland of peptide hormones (MSH) that cause the melanocytes to darken. Hyperpigmentation improves with treatment. Vitiligo is said to occur in 10 to 20 per cent of patients with Addison's disease. Hypotension, which is seen in approximately 90 per cent of patients with the disease, results from a combination of dehydration, decreased plasma volume, and diminished peripheral vascular tone. Symptomatically, it is reflected by syncope, vertigo, weakness, and postural hypotension. The symptoms most commonly presented by the patient are those associated with the gastrointestinal tract: anorexia, nausea, and vomiting are present in the majority of cases. Abdominal pain may be seen in a few instances along with constipation or diarrhea. Hypoglycemic symptoms are described in approximately 60 per cent of patients with Addison's disease. The mental and "nervous" symptoms in Addison's disease are undoubtedly due in large measure to hypoglycemic episodes. Loss of libido, impotence, and reduced virility reflect

TABLE 6. Laboratory Data Commonly Found in Addison's Disease

1. Increased urinary sodium and chloride excretion
2. Increased serum sodium concentration
3. Increased serum potassium concentration
4. Decreased plasma 17-hydroxycorticosteroids
5. Decreased urinary 17-ketosteroid and 17-hydroxycorticosteroid excretion
6. Hypoglycemia
7. Abnormal electroencephalogram
8. Low-voltage electrocardiogram with prolonged PR and QT intervals, with nonspecific T wave changes
9. Basal metabolism decreased
10. Anemia

the decreased androgenic function. Amenorrhea is noticed frequently in the female. The common laboratory findings in Addison's disease are depicted in Table 6.

Radiographically, skull films may aid in the differential diagnosis between primary and secondary adrenal cortical insufficiency. Enlargement of the sella turcica or erosion of the clinoids or both often occur with pituitary tumors, and adrenal insufficiency may be secondary to destruction or failure of the anterior pituitary. Calcification of the pinna of the ear has been described in Addison's disease but also is seen in other conditions. Calcification of costal cartilages has been reported by Jarvis in 93 of 104 patients with Addison's disease.[78] The chest film may reveal the source of the tuberculous infection, while the cardiac silhouette is ordinarily decreased in size in this condition. Abdominal films will reveal calcification of the adrenal in about 12 per cent of patients.

The definitive diagnosis of adrenal insufficiency is largely, if not entirely, dependent upon the results of laboratory tests that measure adrenal function. The test procedures generally used can be divided into two categories, as shown in Table 7. The diagnosis of Addison's disease can be best confirmed by the poor response to adrenal stimulation using an intravenous infusion of ACTH over a period of 8 hours, with simultaneous measurement of urinary corticosteroid excretion.

The treatment of chronic adrenal insufficiency is dependent upon the relative deficiencies of the various corticosteroid compounds. The addisonian patient normally does not require special dietary measures; however, with extreme physical activity, compensation in total caloric requirement should be made. During periods of stress or infection, foods that are high in carbohydrates and contain considerable sodium are to be preferred. If the addisonian patient works in a hot environment or travels to a region of high ambient temperatures, the need for salt and fluids must be recognized and the losses compensated. In adults, the usual maintenance dose of steroid necessary in complete adrenal insufficiency is approximately 20 to 40 mg. of hydrocortisone daily. Usually two thirds of the dosage is given in the morning and the remainder in the late afternoon or evening. If weakness, hypoglycemia, or other symptoms of adrenal insufficiency appear, the steroid dosage must be increased. The predominance of gastrointestinal symptoms in adrenal insufficiency makes these an excellent clinical indicator of insufficient maintenance dosage. Therefore, when nausea and vomiting occur, the patient should take additional steroid medication. As far as other corticosteroids are concerned, symptoms as listed in Table 8 give an adequate guideline for replacement therapy.[53]

TABLE 7. Tests of Adrenal Function

Indirect
1. Impaired water diuresis
2. Salt deprivation
3. Serum Na:K ratio; salivary Na:K ratio
4. Absolute level of circulating eosinophils
5. Insulin-glucose tolerance test
6. Fast, 12 to 18 hour

Direct
1. Basal levels of urinary steroid excretion
2. Plasma level of cortisol
3. Response to ACTH stimulation

TABLE 8. Selection Basis for Specific Steroid Therapy*

1. Glucocorticoids
   Weakness
   Hypoglycemia
   Anorexia and gastrointestinal disturbances
   Central nervous system disturbances
   Hyperpigmentation
   Impaired water tolerance
   Drugs
   a. Hydrocortisone 10–40 mg. by mouth daily in divided doses
   b. Cortisone 25–50 mg. by mouth daily in divided doses
2. Mineralocorticoids
   Dehydration and weight loss
   Hypotension and small heart size
   Weakness
   Low serum sodium, high serum potassium
   Elevated urinary, salivary, sweat sodium
   Drugs
   a. Deoxycorticosterone acetate in oil 3–5 mg. intramuscularly daily
   b. Deoxycorticosterone trimethylacetate 50–100 mg. intramuscularly every 4–6 weeks
   c. Fluorohydrocortisone acetate 0.1–0.2 mg. by mouth daily
   d. Sodium chloride 3–6 gm. daily
3. Androgenic-Anabolic Hormones
   Anemia
   Impotence
   Diminished axillary and pubic hair
   Weakness and decreased muscle mass
   Drugs
   a. Fluoxymestrone 2 mg. by mouth daily 5 days per week
   b. Testosterone cyclopentylproprionate 50 mg. intramuscularly every 4–6 weeks

*From Frawley, T. F. *In* Eisenstein, A. B. (Ed.): The Adrenal Cortex. Boston, Little, Brown and Company, 1967.

TABLE 9.　Clinical Patterns of Hyperadrenocorticism*

Adrenal Secretion	Principal Hormone	Results of Excessive Secretion
Glucocorticoid	Hydrocortisone	Cushing's syndrome
Mineralocorticoid	Aldosterone	Hyperaldosteronism (Conn's syndrome)
Androgen	Androstenedione	Virilism in females
	Dehydroepiandro-sterone	Precocious puberty in males
Estrogen	Estradiol-17B	Feminization in males

*From Harrison, J. H., and Desautels, R. E.: *In* Davis, L., (Ed.): Christopher's Textbook of Surgery, 8th ed. Philadelphia, W. B. Saunders Company, 1964.

HYPERADRENOCORTICISM

Clinical syndromes of hyperadrenocorticism are much more common than adrenal cortical insufficiency. Since the adrenal gland is capable of secreting glucocorticoids, mineralocorticoids, androgens, and estrogens, the spectrum of manifestations of disease in hyperadrenocorticism is wide. The clinical patterns of hyperadrenocorticism are listed in Table 9.

Cushing's Syndrome

The syndrome described by Harvey Cushing[35] in 1932 was based on a series of patients he had studied with manifestations of adiposity, amenorrhea, hypertrichosis, purplish striae, hypertension, polyphagia, polydipsia, polycythemia, and susceptibility to infections. In four of the eight patients in his series, basophil adenomas of the pituitary were found at autopsy, and Cushing ascribed the syndrome to pituitary basophilism.

Anderson and her co-workers[6] in 1938 were among the first to present evidence that the probable common denominator in all cases of Cushing's syndrome was hyperactivity of the adrenal cortex. Subsequently, owing largely to the work of Anderson, Albright,[4] Thorn,[142] and other endocrinologists, it has become well established that the fundamental hormonal basis of the syndrome described by Cushing is *hypercortisolism.*

Aside from cases due to the use of steroid hormones in medical therapy, hypercortisolism occurs spontaneously from three causes: (1) bilateral adrenal cortical hyperplasia under the stimulatory effect of increased secretion of adrenocorticotropin (ACTH) by the pituitary, which may or may not contain an adenoma; (2) bilateral adrenal cortical hyperplasia under the stimulus of ectopic ACTH secreted by a nonendocrine tumor, such as certain carcinomas of the lung; (3) adrenocortical tumor.

In recent years it has been the impression of some physicians that the incidence of Cushing's syndrome is on the increase. However, it appears more likely that this represents better implementation of diagnostic methods that promote wider recognition of the disease rather than an absolute increase. In spite of the increased number of reported cases, Cushing's syndrome still remains comparatively rare. The incidence of spontaneous Cushing's syndrome is probably about six per million population. It occurs more frequently in young adults and is three to five times more common in females than in males.

During the period 1952 through 1976 at Vanderbilt University Medical Center, more than 200 patients with Cushing's syndrome unrelated to the medicinal use of steroids were studied and treated. The age range was 9 months to 71 years, and two thirds of the patients were females. Sixty-three per cent of this group of patients proved to have pituitary-dependent hypercortisolism (Cushing's disease), 24 per cent had hypercortisolism caused by adrenocortical tumors, and 13 per cent had hypercortisolism due to nonendocrine tumors that produced ACTH (ectopic ACTH syndrome). In the group of patients with adrenocortical tumors causing Cushing's syndrome, one third of the tumors proved to be carcinomas.

In a study of Cushing's syndrome reported by Heeg,[69] the incidence of the pituitary-dependent syndrome and the syndrome caused by adrenocortical tumor was similar to that in the Vanderbilt experience, but almost two thirds of Heeg's patients with adrenocortical tumor had malignant lesions.

The manifestations of Cushing's syndrome caused by adrenocortical tumor in a series of 28 patients are summarized in Table 10.

As can be readily discerned from the table, several patients had only a few of the classic manifestations of the syndrome as originally described by Cushing; even obesity and hypertension were occasionally absent.

There is little essential difference in the frequency or pattern of distribution of the various clinical manifestations of Cushing's syndrome whether it be due to adrenocortical tumor, pituitary-dependent adrenocortical hyperplasia, or the ectopic ACTH syndrome. Rapidly growing malignant tumors of the adrenal cortex that produce cortisol and malignant tumors of extraendocrine origin that produce ACTH may induce the clinical syndrome in florid fashion in a very short period of weeks or months. A much more gradual evolution of the syndrome, commonly developing over a period of many months or even a few years, is more apt to occur in patients with benign adrenocortical tumors or pituitary-dependent adrenal hyperplasia.

TABLE 10.　Incidence of Clinical Manifestations in 28 Patients with Cushing's Syndrome due to Adrenocortical Tumor

	No. Patients	Per Cent
Central obesity	26/28	93
Hypertension	26/28	93
Weakness	23/28	82
Hirsutism	22/28	79
Impaired glucose tolerance	22/28	79
Mental aberrations	16/28	57
Osteoporosis	15/28	54
Ecchymoses	16/28	57
Edema	13/28	46
Striae	10/28	36
Menstrual abnormalities	9/12	75

Excessive production of corticoids in Cushing's syndrome results in a catabolic effect which leads to protein depletion and diminution in the mass of connective tissue and muscle of the patient. The thinness and delicateness of the skin and increased capillary fragility that are manifested by easy bruisability and abdominal striae are characteristic of the severe protein depletion. Children usually show growth retardation, muscular weakness, and osteoporosis with loss of strength of bones, and pathologic fractures are common. Cutaneous striae result where the protein-depleted corium of the skin is stretched and split by underlying accumulations of adipose tissue. (Patients with Cushing's must be separated from normal parturient women in whom the enlarging uterus causes splitting of the corium.) The accelerated protein breakdown results in increased gluconeogenesis and diminished carbohydrate tolerance. Overt diabetes may result from these processes. Another common result of altered protein and carbohydrate metabolism is impairment of wound healing. The integument is sometimes so friable it may be denuded merely by removal of adhesive tape.

The serum gamma globulin tends to be decreased, and this coupled with altered metabolism of protein and carbohydrate makes these patients particularly subject to infections. Accompanying the excessive protein breakdown is abnormal accumulation of fat with deposition especially in the face, neck, back, and trunk. The cervicodorsal fat pad has been characterized as a "buffalo hump."

Accumulation of fat in the face often produces the characteristic "moon facies." Fat accumulation in the trunk is often strikingly severe in contrast to the muscular wasting and thinning of the arms and legs which usually occur simultaneously.

Weakness and easy fatigability are directly related to protein catabolism and the severe depletion of muscle mass. Hypertension, often with associated headache, develops most likely because of salt and water retention with expansion of extracellular volume. There is a distinct tendency in many of these patients to development of metabolic alkalosis with attendant hypokalemia.

Amenorrhea is a common symptom in adolescent girls and premenopausal women. Hirsutism, acne, and other aspects of virilization occur in women, and precocious sexual development can occur in boys (Fig. 16).

Emotional instability is frequently observed in patients with Cushing's syndrome and more severe mental disorders which extend to the psychoses are not uncommon.

Endocrinologic Diagnosis of Cushing's Syndrome. Although the clinical symptoms alone may be sufficiently clear to suggest the diagnosis of Cushing's syndrome, it is often necessary and certainly always desirable to confirm the clinical impression by precise studies of adrenocortical function and pituitary-adrenal relationships. These studies are of fundamental importance in differentiating Cushing's syndrome due to pituitary-dependent adrenocortical hyperplasia, extraendocrine tumor, and adrenocortical tumor. Furthermore, some degree of help may be offered in preoperative differentiation of Cushing's syndrome due

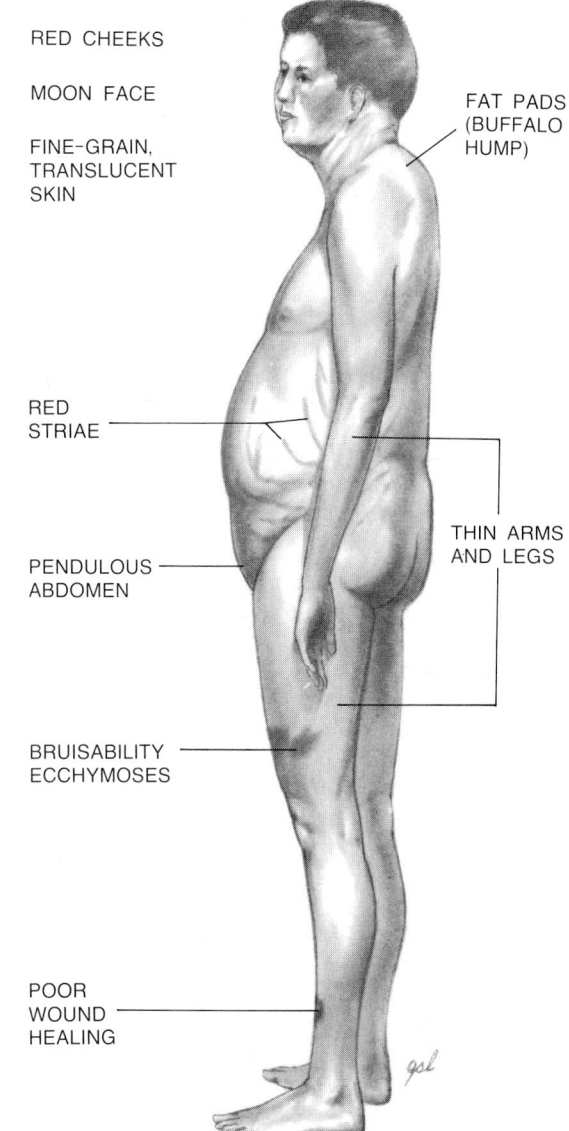

RED CHEEKS

MOON FACE

FINE-GRAIN, TRANSLUCENT SKIN

FAT PADS (BUFFALO HUMP)

RED STRIAE

THIN ARMS AND LEGS

PENDULOUS ABDOMEN

BRUISABILITY ECCHYMOSES

POOR WOUND HEALING

Figure 16. Cushing's syndrome.

to adrenal adenoma and that caused by adrenal carcinoma.

The cortisol secretion rate is considered by Cope,[26] O'Neal,[106] and others to be the best index of hypercortisolism. It is determined by the isotopic dilution method, measuring a cortisol metabolite in the urine after a known amount of cortisol with a radioactive label is injected. However, the technical validity of the method is questionable and clinical use is limited.

A more widely available laboratory estimation of the activity of the adrenal cortex in producing cortisol is the measurement of the daily urinary excretion of 17-hydroxycorticosteroids (17-OHCS). Normal adults excrete 3 to 12 mg. of 17-OHCS in 24 hours and patients with Cushing's syndrome usually excrete in excess of 12 mg. per day. The accuracy of the urine collection and at the same time an adjustment for body weight can be obtained by relating the quantity of 17-OHCS to the quantity of creatinine in the urine. Normal persons excrete 3 to 7 mg. and patients with Cushing's syndrome almost always excrete more than 10 mg. of 17-OHCS per gram of creatinine.[84, 88]

Plasma cortisol levels in normal subjects show characteristic diurnal variations. Cortisol levels measured in the early morning are approximately twice as high as those measured in the late evening. These diurnal variations in plasma cortisol levels correlate with plasma ACTH concentrations in normal subjects. Characteristically, normal subjects have evening values of plasma cortisol concentrations less than 7 μg. per 100 ml. On the contrary, patients with Cushing's syndrome do not have the normal diurnal variation in plasma cortisol levels. Although the early morning plasma cortisol levels in patients with Cushing's syndrome may fall within the normal range, late evening values are distinctly elevated (usually well above 12 μg. per 100 ml.).[13, 110]

The most reliable test in establishing the diagnosis of Cushing's syndrome in our opinion is the dexamethasone suppression test devised by Liddle.[87, 88] This is based on the urinary 17-OHCS response to small doses of the potent synthetic steroid dexamethasone, which has 30 times the potency of cortisol and which, like cortisol, can suppress ACTH secretion by the pituitary. In normal subjects, 0.5 mg. of dexamethasone orally every 6 hours causes a drop in urinary secretion of 17-OHCS to less than 2.5 mg. per day in 48 hours. Patients with Cushing's syndrome show resistance to suppression at this small dosage of dexamethasone. In the experience at Vanderbilt this abnormal resistance to the suppressive effect of dexamethasone in low dosage is characteristic of patients with Cushing's syndrome.

When the diagnosis of Cushing's syndrome has been established, it is then necesary to determine the etiology of the adrenocortical hyperfunction. Cushing's syndrome due to excess pituitary ACTH secretion can

be differentiated by the patient's response to dexamethasone in large dosage. In such patients when dexamethasone is given in oral doses of 2 mg. every 6 hours for 2 days, pituitary ACTH secretion is inhibited and urinary 17-OHCS secretion is completely or almost completely suppressed.

On the contrary, the patient who has adrenocortical tumor that produces cortisol autonomously characteristically shows no evidence of urinary or plasma 17-OHCS suppression with high-dose dexamethasone administration.[87, 88]

Since patients with the ectopic ACTH syndrome produced by nonendocrine tumors also show resistance to high-dose dexamethasone suppression, they must be differentiated from patients with Cushing's syndrome due to autonomous adrenocortical tumors. This can be done by measuring the plasma ACTH concentration. In this situation if the patient has a high plasma ACTH, he has Cushing's syndrome due to autonomous secretion of ACTH by an extraendocrine nonpituitary tumor. If the plasma ACTH concentration is low (less than 1.0 mU. per 100 ml.), the test indicates the presence of an adrenocortical tumor. In such a situation the cortisol produced autonomously by the adrenal tumor causes chronic suppression of pituitary ACTH secretion. Furthermore, this usually leads to atrophy of the contralateral adrenal cortex (Fig. 17).[88, 101]

Other endocrine studies that are helpful in the diagnosis of Cushing's syndrome and the endocrinologic differentiation between ACTH-dependent adrenocortical hyperplasia and adrenocortical tumor include the metyrapone (SU-4885) test, the ACTH stimulation test, and measurement of urinary 17-ketosteroid levels. The drug metyrapone (Metopirone) blocks 11 β-hydroxylation in the adrenal cortex and thus impairs the conversion of compound S (17-hydroxy-11-desoxycorticosterone) to cortisol. When patients with Cushing's syndrome are tested with this drug, those with pituitary-dependent adrenocortical hyperplasia show an increased output of urinary 17-OHCS, while pa-

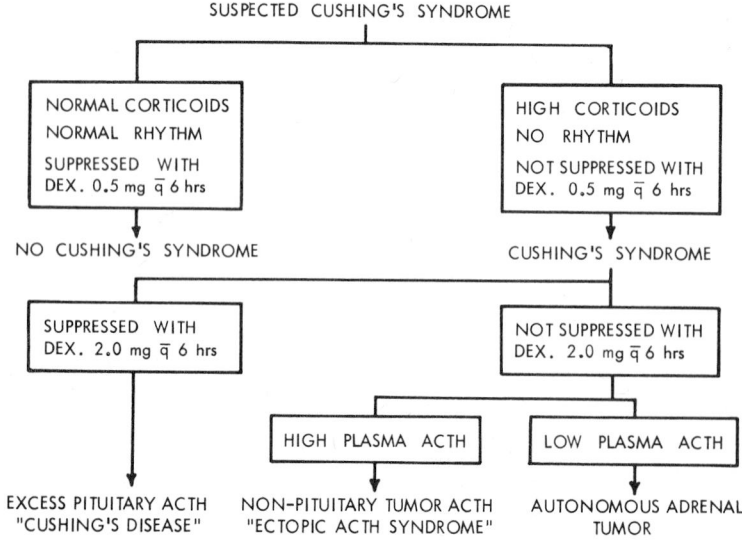

Figure 17. Protocol for evaluation of patients with suspected Cushing's syndrome. (From Scott, H. W., Jr., et al.: Ann. Surg., *173*:892, 1971.)

tients with the ectopic ACTH syndrome have a variable response, and those with adrenocortical tumor characteristically fail to respond.[88, 90]

The standard ACTH stimulation test offers further diagnostic information. In response to an 8 hour infusion of 50 units of ACTH, normal subjects excrete 20 to 40 mg. of 17-OHCS in urine in the subsequent 24 hours, while patients with Cushing's syndrome due to adrenocortical hyperplasia respond by excreting more than 50 mg. of 17-OHCS per 24 hours.[88, 122]

On the other hand, only about half of the patients who prove to have benign adrenal adenoma have shown an increase in urinary 17-OHCS secretion after intravenous infusion of 50 units of ACTH. Furthermore, patients with adrenal carcinoma that causes Cushing's syndrome are characteristically unresponsive to ACTH stimulation, although rare exceptions have been recorded.[129]

Additional help in the endocrinologic recognition of adrenal cortical carcinoma as a cause of Cushing's syndrome can be obtained from measurements of urinary 17-ketosteroids. Normal 24 hour 17-ketosteroid excretion averages 10 ± 5 mg. for females and 15 ± 5 mg. for males. While slight increases in these levels of 17-ketosteroid excretion occur in many patients with Cushing's syndrome due to a benign adrenal adenoma, extremely high levels of urinary 17-ketosteroid excretion (in the range of 40 to 100 mg. per 24 hours) are commonly associated with adrenal cortical carcinoma.[106, 130]

Treatment and Results

PITUITARY-DEPENDENT HYPERCORTISOLISM WITH BILATERAL ADRENOCORTICAL HYPERPLASIA (CUSHING'S DISEASE). In those patients whose endocrinologic evaluation indicates the diagnosis of Cushing's syndrome due to excess pituitary ACTH secretion, the anterior pituitary may show cytologic abnormalities characterized by basophilic cytoplasmic hyalinization, vacuolization, and degranulation. Cushing[35] described these changes originally as "pituitary basophilism." True basophilic adenomas have rarely been found, but mixed basophilic and chromophobe tumors and pure chromophobe tumors are not rarities in Cushing's disease. Their precise incidence is unknown. As mentioned above, Hardy has used microsurgical techniques in pituitary exploration in 10 patients with Cushing's disease and found a pituitary tumor in each patient.[65]

Among 119 patients with Cushing's *disease* studied by Liddle and his associates at Vanderbilt from 1952 through 1976, none had clinical or unequivocal radiologic evidence of pituitary tumor when initially seen. Other authors have found an incidence of pituitary tumors in Cushing's *disease* ranging from 5 to 17 per cent, but the criteria for diagnosis of pituitary tumors in such cases are quite variable.[103]

Histologically, bilateral hyperplasia of the zona fasciculata of the adrenal cortex is present in almost all patients with Cushing's disease. Unilateral adrenocortical hyperplasia has been reported on rare occasions. A small percentage of patients with Cushing's disease exhibit no structural abnormality of the adrenal glands, grossly or microscopically.

Earlier in our experience at Vanderbilt, bilateral total adrenalectomy was used in treatment of most cases of pituitary-dependent hypercortisolism. Elimination of the pituitary's target organ, the adrenal cortex, is the most dependably accurate means of effecting prompt regression of Cushing's syndrome in these patients. The addisonian state that is produced as a substitute for Cushing's syndrome can be managed currently with considerable ease and accuracy. More recently, however, with the use of radioactive cobalt (^{60}Co), the linear accelerator with its photon beam, and Bragg peak proton beam therapy, pituitary irradiation has been found by Liddle and his group to be increasingly satisfactory in controlling Cushing's disease, and bilateral adrenalectomy has been reserved for the most severe cases and for those which fail to respond satisfactorily to pituitary irradiation.

In the entire Vanderbilt University Hospital series of patients with Cushing's disease, 81 have been treated by pituitary irradiation either here or in other hospitals. Their courses of treatment at Vanderbilt have averaged 4500 rads to the pituitary. Prior to 1968 these patients were treated by cobalt. Since that date they have been treated by the 6 mev accelerator. Approximately a third of the patients treated by pituitary irradiation have sustained endocrinologic cure of hypercortisolism. Another third have been improved to the extent that adrenalectomy has been deferred, and the remainder have failed to respond satisfactorily. The recent more beneficial results of pituitary irradiation achieved by the photon beam of the 6 mev linear accelerator have encouraged us to continue the policy in management of patients with Cushing's disease which is outlined above.

Thirty-eight patients with Cushing's disease have been submitted to adrenalectomy at Vanderbilt. Twenty-four of these had had a trial of pituitary irradiation without relief of hyperadrenocorticism. In eight of these patients, chiefly from our earlier experience, operations involving less than total adrenalectomy were done with resulting incomplete relief of hypercortisolism. Bilateral total adrenalectomy was reserved for the most severe cases and for failures of pituitary irradiation. In 29 patients with total bilateral adrenalectomy there was one postoperative death. Two of 28 survivors had incomplete relief of hypercortisolism and required additional therapy for its control. One patient with recent operation is improved and another with early improvement died suddenly at home three months after operation. The 24 other adrenalectomized patients, followed six months to 20 years, were considered endocrinologic cures of Cushing's disease. One patient in the group who had not received pituitary irradiation developed signs of expanding pituitary tumor after adrenalectomy (Nelson's syndrome) with satisfactory response to radiation therapy.

This experience, coupled with the poor results described by Egdahl et al.[42] and by others in patients with Cushing's disease treated by subtotal adrenalectomy, has convinced us that the only absolutely dependably curative surgical procedure in this form of Cushing's syndrome is total bilateral adrenalectomy.

Those who are cured of Cushing's disease by total adrenalectomy require life-long substitution therapy with both glucocorticoid and mineralocorticoid.

In the early part of this series, bilateral adrenalectomy was carried out transperitoneally through a long transverse upper abdominal incision, using techniques of exposure of the glands similar to those described by Ian Aird.[3] As noted above, one postoperative death occurred, in a 55-year-old woman with florid Cushing's syndrome, hypertension, and severe purpuric manifestations who had persistent bleeding from the adrenal fossae following adrenalectomy. In two other patients, cardiac arrest occurred during operation, but resuscitation in each instance was successful, and complete recovery ensued.

In the last 15 years we have used the bilateral posterior retroperitoneal approach for removal of the adrenals in all patients with Cushing's syndrome associated with bilateral adrenal cortical hyperplasia. There has been no mortality and less postoperative morbidity with this operative approach.[131]

As a medical alternative to bilateral adrenalectomy, Liddle and his group[107] have used the adrenocorticolytic drug o,p'DDD in treatment of eight patients with Cushing's disease. Three to six grams of the drug were given daily for four to six months and followed by smaller maintenance doses for as long as five years. Each patient so treated was considered to be cured of hyperadrenocorticism. The chief side effect of the drug was recurrent nausea, which was a problem for four of the eight patients.

Ideal objectives in treatment of Cushing's syndrome have been previously outlined by Orth and Liddle.[107] In brief they include (1) removal of any functional tumor which threatens health; (2) reduction of excessive cortisol secretion to normal; (3) preservation of normal pituitary and adrenal function; (4) avoidance of permanent dependence on hormonal substitution therapy.

All of these objectives may be achieved when Cushing's syndrome is cured by successful surgical removal of a localized, noninvasive, unilateral tumor of the adrenal cortex, or in the very rare instances when the hypercortisolism can be cured by removal of an extraendocrine ACTH-producing tumor which has similar favorable characteristics.

In the pituitary-dependent hypercortisolism of Cushing's disease Hardy has recently demonstrated in several cases that these ideal objectives can also be achieved by successful identification and removal of ACTH-secreting microadenomas of the hypophysis.[65] Hardy's observations and accomplishments represent an exciting new validation of Harvey Cushing's original ideas about the pituitary's role in the disease that he described. Obviously many questions remain to be answered concerning the frequency and localization of microadenomas in pituitary-dependent hypercortisolism as well as the frequency with which it is feasible to remove them.

ADRENOCORTICAL TUMOR. In a 24-year period at Vanderbilt Medical Center, 39 patients with Cushing's syndrome due to adrenocortical tumor were studied and treated. There were 32 females and 7 males in this group. Ages ranged from 9 months to 71 years with an average of 35 years; seven of the patients were children under 15 years of age.[130]

In this series, the endocrinologic diagnosis of an adrenal tumor as the cause of Cushing's syndrome was accurately made before operation in each instance. Excepting several of the early patients for whom data are incomplete, the laboratory findings consistently observed in the patients with Cushing's syndrome due to adrenocortical tumor in this series included basal elevation of urinary 17-OHCS levels, resistance to high-dose dexamethasone suppression, loss of diurnal rhythm in plasma cortisol concentrations, and subnormal levels of plasma ACTH activity.

While efforts to differentiate between benign and malignant adrenocortical tumors before operation were not made on endocrinologic grounds alone, some help was provided in this regard by the characteristic unresponsiveness of adrenocortical carcinomas to ACTH stimulation, combined with extremely high basal urinary 17-ketosteroid levels. In 24 of the 25 patients who proved to have benign adrenal adenomas, the basal urinary 17-ketosteroid levels were in the normal range or were only slightly elevated. Only one patient with histologically benign adrenal adenoma in this group had high basal urinary 17-ketosteroid levels. Fifteen of the 25 patients showed marked elevations in 17-OHCS excretion in response to ACTH infusion.

In contrast, among 14 patients with adrenocortical carcinoma, 12 showed extremely high basal urinary 17-ketosteroid levels (ranging from 40 to 100 mg. per 24 hr.). Only one patient with adrenal carcinoma had basal urinary 17-ketosteroids in the range below 40 mg. per 24 hr. Furthermore, there was no response to ACTH infusion in twelve patients with adrenal carcinoma in whom the test was done prior to operation. The test was omitted in two patients.

In addition to these endocrinologic features which may identify adrenocortical carcinoma before operation, clinical data may also contain helpful information. Patients with adrenocortical carcinomas tend to have rapid onset of the florid manifestations of Cushing's syndrome, with the alarming development of virilizing changes, particularly hirsutism in the female. Virilizing changes may develop rapidly and be readily apparent also in young boys with adrenal carcinoma, but are not apt to be detected in normal adult males. Finally, it is clear that carcinoma is more prevalent in the very young and very old patients who have Cushing's syndrome due to adrenal tumor. In the seven children 15 years of age and under in this series, four had adrenal carcinoma. Among the four adults in the series whose ages were 60 years or above, there were two patients with adrenal carcinoma.

Before operation, the side of the adrenal tumor was accurately determined in 35 of 39 patients. In six instances (five carcinomas and one large adenoma) a large tumor was readily palpated on clinical examination. In each of the 39 patients in this series intravenous pyelography was done, and it served to localize the tumor in 20 instances. However, confirmation of the pyelographic study, with added information concerning the size and shape of the tumor, has been ob-

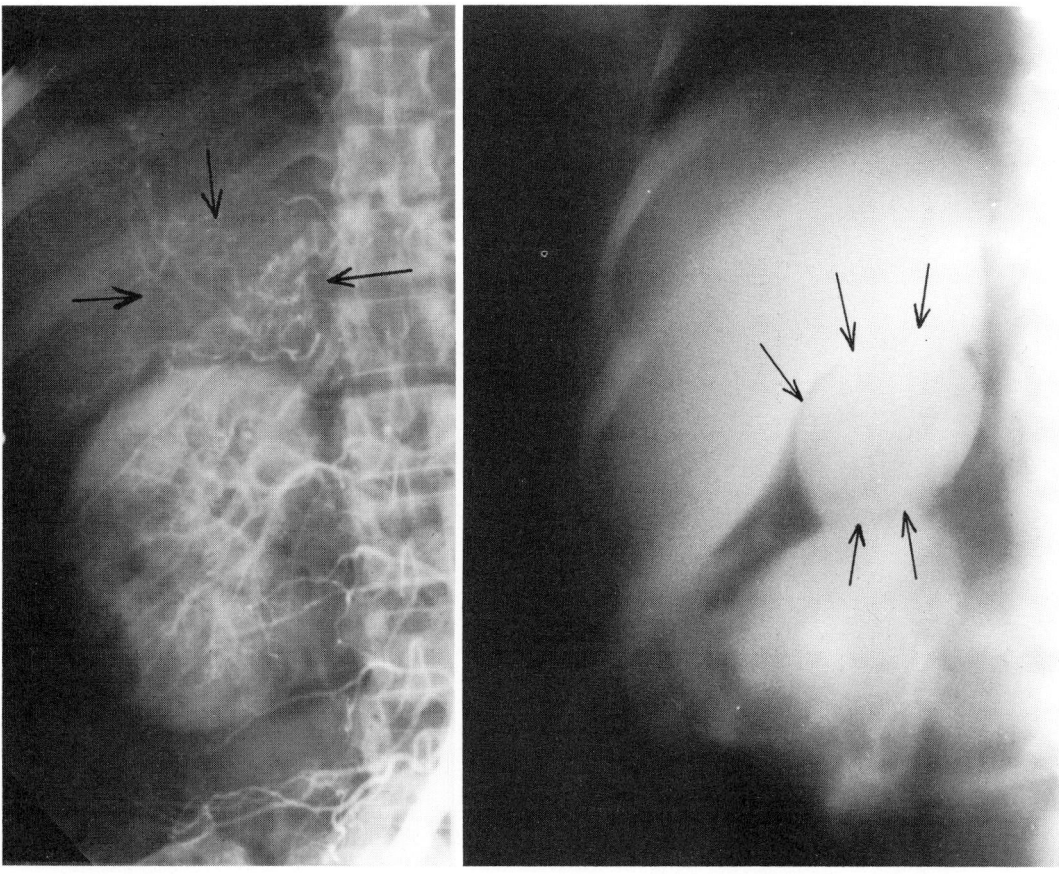

Figure 18. *Left,* Tumor vessels above right kidney shown on flush aortogram. *Right,* Confirmation of adrenal adenoma in same patient by retroperitoneal pneumography.

tained in the last 20 years by use of retroperitoneal pneumography and arteriography (Fig. 18). The retroperitoneal pneumogram using nitrous oxide or carbon dioxide has silhouetted and localized the smaller adrenal tumors that do not displace the kidney downward or rotate its axis laterally. Tomography has supplied added help alone and when combined with retroperitoneal pneumography. In the last 10 to 12 years flush aortography and selective adrenal arteriography have replaced retroperitoneal pneumography in diagnosis of adrenal tumors in our radiology department, and the lesions have been accurately localized in each of the last 35 patients in this series (Fig. 19). In the earlier part of the series, prior to the introduction of currently accurate radiologic methods, the site of small adrenal adenomas in three patients and a large (70 gm.) bilateral adrenal adenoma in a fourth could not be determined before operation.

In the first seven patients of the series, a transabdominal approach was used to remove the adrenal tumors. In most patients a long transverse or "buckethandle" incision was used, which was extended across the costal margin into a lower intercostal space in 3 patients with large tumors.[129, 130]

In the last 15 years, with increased accuracy in dif-

ferentiating between benign and malignant adrenal tumors and more accurate visualization of the lesions by better radiologic methods prior to operation, we have preferred to use the posterior retroperitoneal approach in patients with benign tumors. We have reserved the anterior abdominal approach with thoracoabdominal extension for the removal of adrenal carcinomas. In our experience the posterior retroperitoneal approach to the adrenal area provides excellent exposure and is associated with less postoperative morbidity than is a transabdominal or abdominothoracic procedure. In the last 32 patients of this series, our surgical approach to the adrenal area in patients with Cushing's syndrome due to adrenal tumor has been guided by these considerations.

When a benign adenoma appears likely after clinical, endocrinologic, and radiologic evaluation, it has been our practice to use the posterior retroperitoneal approach. After induction of anesthesia and intubation, the patient is placed in the prone decubitus position with the operating table broken at the hips and a firm pillow placed under the pelvis. Bilateral posterolateral incisions of the Hugh Young type are made and each adrenal fossa is explored simultaneously, usually through the bed of the resected eleventh rib.

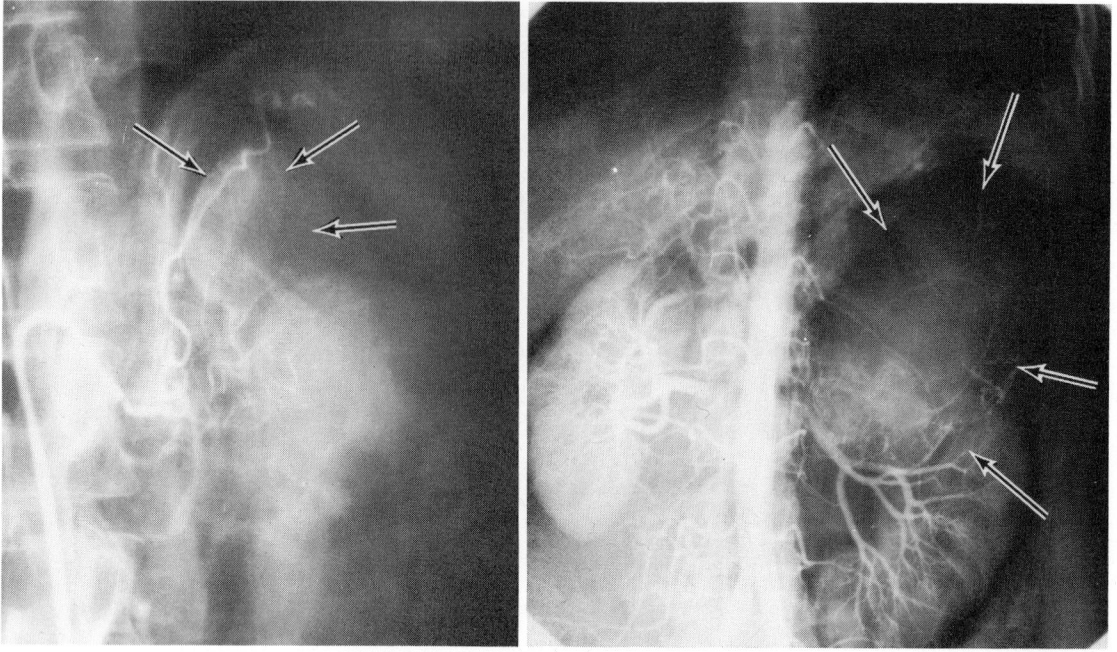

Figure 19.   *Left,* Selective arteriogram outlining small adrenal adenoma. *Right,* Flush aortogram showing large adrenal carcinoma.

The possibility of bilateral adenoma, as emphasized by Mark Hayes,[68] can be accurately confirmed or excluded.

We believe it is a sound principle to appraise the gross status of each adrenal gland before proceeding to remove a tumor involving one or both glands. Biopsy of the normal or atrophic adrenal, contralateral to a single cortical tumor, can provide corroborative histologic information and a more accurate appraisal of the anatomic status of the gland. This appraisal, however, may have limited value in predicting the functional status of adrenocortical tissue.

When a carcinoma of the adrenal causing Cushing's syndrome appears likely on preoperative study, we have employed the abdominothoracic approach to the adrenals and to the tumor. Usually the abdominal component of the incision is made first. After confirmation of the location of the tumor, search for intra-abdominal metastases, and appraisal of resectability have been made, the incision is extended across the costal margin into the eighth or ninth intercostal space. The incision divides the diaphragm, providing wide exposure of the adrenal fossa on the side of the tumor. While simple excision suffices in the cure of benign adrenocortical adenoma, radical nonmanipulative en bloc resection, rather than enucleation, is indicated in the management of adrenal carcinomas, which are usually highly malignant (Fig. 20).

In 39 patients with adrenocortical tumors the lesions were removed successfully in all but two. A child with a massive right adrenal carcinoma, which involved the kidney, liver, inferior vena cava, aorta, and retroperitoneal lymph nodes, died in the early postoperative period after radical resection of the growth.

In another patient, the massive invasive extent of adrenal carcinoma with metastases precluded resection and only a biopsy was done. This patient and all other patients in the series, excepting the child, survived operation and the immediate postoperative period. The operative mortality rate in the series was 2.5 per cent.

Operative and postoperative complications in the 38 survivors included a wound infection in four patients, transient pleural effusion in another, and lower lobe atelectasis and fever in another; hepatitis developed 6 weeks after operation in another patient, who recovered after steroid therapy. Ureteral injury occurred at operation in one patient and was repaired successfully with no residual uropathy.

Following removal of the adrenocortical tumors in this series of patients, a careful regimen of adrenal substitution therapy was instituted. Since the patient's normal adrenal tissue becomes relatively atrophic and nonfunctional when a cortisol-producing tumor of the adrenal cortex is present, therapy must be continued until the remaining normal cortical tissue resumes adequate functional activity. All patients are followed carefully and are gradually weaned from adrenal substitutes over periods of several weeks to several months as determined by follow-up studies of clinical recovery and adrenocortical function.

The follow-up period in the 38 patients who survived operation extends from 6 months to 23 years. Among the 25 patients with benign adrenocortical adenomas, one patient died at home, suddenly, of an unexplained cause 2½ months after apparently successful surgical treatment. Another patient died of intestinal obstruction 17 months after excision of an

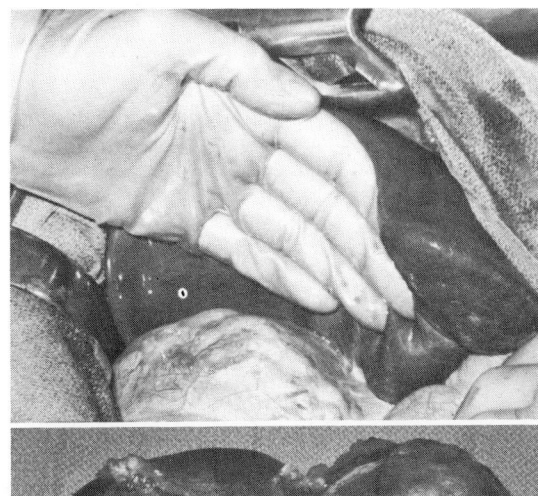

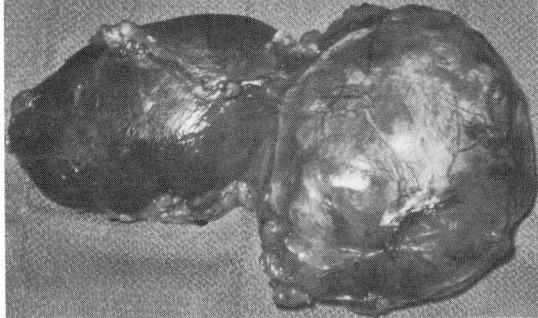

Figure 20. *Above,* Abdominothoracic exposure of right adrenal carcinoma. *Below,* The carcinoma and right kidney were resected en bloc. (From Scott, H. W., Jr., et al.: Ann. Surg., *173*:892, 1971.)

adenoma; he had been completely relieved of Cushing's syndrome in the interval. A third patient was well for 10 years after removal of adrenal adenoma and died of myocardial infarction at the age of 67. The remaining 22 patients who underwent removal of histologically proven benign adrenal adenoma causing Cushing's syndrome have survived for 6 months to 23 years. In general, the prominent stigmata of Cushing's syndrome have disappeared in this group of patients. The more florid manifestations regressed promptly; however, a complete return to "normal" status has often required several months.

Among the 13 patients with adrenal carcinoma who survived operation, removal of a massively invasive tumor was not attempted in two, and only palliative resections were done in two other patients in whom widespread metastases were present at the time of operation. Each of these patients died within 8 to 10 months after operation with progressive malignant disease and persistent Cushing's syndrome. Very little palliation was obtained in these patients by operation or use of the adrenocorticolytic chemotherapeutic agent o,p'DDD. In the nine other patients with adrenal carcinoma, resection abated the symptoms of Cushing's syndrome for periods of 10 months to 16 years. In four of these patients Cushing's syndrome and carcinoma recurred, after 3 years in three and after 12

years in the fourth. One of these patients died after radical resection of the recurrent tumor. Another patient underwent successful resection of the recurrent growth 12 years after initial removal of the carcinoma, with remission of Cushing's syndrome for 18 months. The syndrome and the tumor, which subsequently recurred, were controlled for her last 18 months by o,p'DDD. In the third patient, the drug provided two additional years of fairly good control of both Cushing's syndrome and metastatic tumor following the initial recurrence three years after resection. A fourth patient who had a resectable massive recurrence a year after primary resection in another hospital has survived four years with intermittent o,p'DDD therapy and repeated operative removal of tumor recurrences. The five remaining patients are currently alive and well with no stigmata of Cushing's syndrome and no evidence of recurrent tumor from 18 months to 16 years after operation.[130]

ECTOPIC ACTH SYNDROME. The management of patients with Cushing's syndrome due to an extraendocrine tumor that produces ACTH is apt to be most unsatisfactory. In the majority of such cases, the source of the ectopic ACTH is a highly malignant tumor, which has most often reached an incurable stage by the time the manifestations of Cushing's syndrome are recognized. The ectopic ACTH that stimulates the adrenal cortex to produce hypercortisolism is not responsive to dexamethasone suppression. The incidence of extremely high corticosteroid levels is greater in this syndrome than with the other varieties of Cushing's syndrome.[101]

Liddle[88] has pointed out that many patients with this syndrome lack the characteristic Cushingesque central obesity. The only explanation that has been offered for this is that these patients eat poorly and fail to gain weight as a result of the advanced primary malignant tumor.

The logical treatment of the ectopic ACTH syndrome is removal of the primary tumor that produces the ACTH. Unfortunately, this is rarely possible because of the invasive and metastatic state of the tumor.

In the period 1961 through 1970 at Vanderbilt, the diagnosis of Cushing's syndrome due to ectopic ACTH production by an extraendocrine tumor was made in 17 patients.[107] While most patients had advanced forms of lung cancer, especially the oat cell variety, there were a few cases of other cancers such as prostate and pancreas. One patient had a non-beta cell islet carcinoma of pancreas that produced ACTH, melanocyte-stimulating hormone, and gastrin; she had both the Zollinger-Ellison and Cushing syndromes. None of these patients were cured of the malignant tumor and survival was limited to a few months.

Palliation of the syndrome can be achieved by bilateral total adrenalectomy or by the adrenocorticolytic drug o,p'DDD. In a cooperative study among a group of endocrinologists representing multiple clinics, 11 of 105 patients with this form of Cushing's syndrome appear to have been cured by surgical removal of their ACTH-secreting tumor. The prognosis in most cases is very poor.[92, 107]

Aldosteronism

In 1952, Grundy, Simpson, and Tait[61] detected biologically and isolated chromatographically an amorphous fraction of the adrenal cortical extract that had shown mineralocorticoid activity. Because of its extremely potent effect upon electrolyte metabolism, this material was tentatively given the name "electrocortin." Later isolation of the compound in pure crystalline form, with the identification of its chemical structure as the 18-aldehyde of corticosterone, brought about a change of the name to aldosterone.

In 1955, Conn[23] described a clinical syndrome, which he designated "primary aldosteronism," of mineralocorticoid excess induced by adrenocortical elaboration of excessive amounts of aldosterone and characterized by abnormally large amounts of urinary aldosterone and normal amounts of 17-hydroxycorticoids and 17-ketosteroids. The symptomatology of Conn's syndrome in its full-blown state includes intermittent or recurrent bouts of muscular weakness, occasionally progressing to flaccid paralysis of the lower extremities; headache, usually severe; polydipsia and polyuria with nocturia; and paresthesias consisting of prickling and tingling of hands and feet and bouts of carpopedal spasm. The most prominent physical finding in the syndrome is hypertension, which may vary from a mild, benign form to malignant hypertension with papilledema and hemorrhagic retinopathy. Chvostek's and Trousseau's signs may be present (17 per cent). Zimmermann[155] has described a dramatic clinical sign that should alert the physician to the possibility of the presence of aldosteronism. This is the production of carpal spasm at the time the blood pressure cuff is inflated, coupled with the recording of hypertension (Table 11).

Women are afflicted more commonly than men in a ratio of 2.5:1. Although children and young adults occasionally have primary aldosteronism, the majority of patients are within the age range of 30 to 50 years.

The clinical syndrome of primary aldosteronism is most commonly produced by functioning benign adrenal cortical adenoma, usually single but occasionally multiple, and bilateral in 10 per cent of instances. These adenomas are usually small, 1 to 3 gm., and well

TABLE 11. Presenting Complaints in Primary Aldosteronism*

Complaint	%
Muscle weakness	73
Polyuria or nocturia	72
Headache	51
Polydipsia	46
Paresthesia	24
Visual disturbances	21
Intermittent paralysis	21
Tetany	21
Fatigue	19
Muscle discomfort	16
No symptoms	6

*From Conn, J. W., Knopf, R. F., and Nesbit, R. M.: Am. J. Surg., 107:159, 1964.

encapsulated, although large lesions up to 90 gm. in weight have been reported. More recently, bilateral adrenal hyperfunction, with or without gross or microscopic evidence of hyperplasia, has been described as the cause of elevated aldosterone secretion and hypertension. This has been more common in young adults and in children. The least common cause of primary aldosteronism has been an adrenal cortical carcinoma.

The small cortical adenomas that commonly are found to be the cause of the syndrome are usually soft, orange to yellow, spherical lesions. On microscopic examination, the adenomas are composed of uniform clear cells of the type seen in the zona glomerulosa of the adrenal cortex, from which they are believed to arise. In contrast to other endocrine tumors, there appears to be very little correlation between the size of the adenoma and the rate of aldosterone production.

The characteristic laboratory findings in primary aldosteronism are hypokalemia, hypernatremia, and alkalosis, accompanied by large urine volumes with low specific gravity (80 per cent) and a neutral or alkaline reaction. Proteinuria is commonly observed (85 per cent). The typical changes of hypokalemia are usually present in the electrocardiogram. With a normal salt intake, urinary potassium levels are usually elevated to 30 mEq. per liter or more. Urinary aldosterone excretion (of the free hormone) is increased in most instances from the normal 2 to 12 μg. per 24 hours to the range of 12 to 40 μg. per 24 hours.

Measurement of the rate of aldosterone secretion by radioisotopic techniques has become accepted as the most accurate laboratory method for establishing the diagnosis of hyperaldosteronism. Coppage and his associates[27] found the rate of secretion of aldosterone in 15 normal subjects on unrestricted diets with liberal sodium intakes to range from 95 to 249 μg. per day. Normal persons on low-sodium diets and patients with either primary or secondary hyperaldosteronism are found to have secretory rates greatly in excess, up to 2000+ μg. per day, of this normal range.

In making a diagnosis of primary aldosteronism, the syndrome must be differentiated from the various secondary states of excess aldosterone secretion which may occur in decompensated cirrhosis of the liver, the nephrotic syndrome, congestive heart failure, and various hypertensive diseases. The common use of the chlorothiazide diuretics in the management of hypertension results in symptoms that may obscure or be confused with Conn's syndrome (Table 12).

The recognition of the significant combination of hypertension and hypokalemia associated with metabolic alkalosis in the absence of the stigmata of Cushing's syndrome, or the states that produce secondary aldosteronism, becomes the initial basis for the diagnosis of the primary disorder. It has been repeatedly stressed that the diagnosis of this disease largely depends on precise laboratory studies. Hypokalemic alkalosis is usually present and is accompanied by excessive urinary potassium losses. In the presence of normal salt intake, hypernatremia is commonly observed. Conn[24] has demonstrated that secondary hyperaldosteronism may occur in patients with advanced essential hypertension, renovascular hypertension, and unilateral renal disease with malignant hyperten-

TABLE 12. Causes of Secondary Aldosteronism*

I. Angiotensin excess
  A. Decreased pressure at baroreceptor of juxta-glomerular apparatus
    1. Shrunken effective arterial blood volume
      a. Volume depletion
        1) Low sodium intake
        2) Diuretic therapy
        3) Hemorrhage
        4) Vomiting, diarrhea
        5) Salt wasting, e.g., adrenal insufficiency
      b. Edematous states
        1) Cirrhosis with ascites
        2) Nephrotic syndrome
        3) Congestive heart failure (rarely)
        4) Idiopathic edema
      c. Pregnancy (?mechanism)
    2. Obstruction to renal blood flow
      a. Renovascular hypertension (occasionally)
      b. Accelerated—malignant hypertension
    3. Insensitivity to angiotensin (Bartter's syndrome)
  B. Decreased sodium at macula densa, e.g., hyponatremia
  C. Increased renin substrate, e.g., estrogen administration
  D. Renin-producing renal tumor
II. ACTH excess
  A. Exogenous administration (transient)
  B. Non-salt-losing congenital adrenal hyperplasia
    1. Partial 17-hydroxylase deficiency
    2. Partial 21-hydroxylase deficiency
III. "Pseudo" aldosteronism
  A. Licorice ingestion
  B. Other mineralocorticoid excess
    1. Cushing's syndrome
    2. Adrenal tumors
    3. Complete 17-hydroxylase deficiency
  C. Excess renal sodium conservation (Liddle's syndrome)

*From Kaplan, N. M.: Am. J. Clin. Pathol., 54:316, 1970.

sion. In secondary aldosteronism, potassuric hypokalemic alkalosis may be present, but hypernatremia is absent and hyponatremia is common.

The double isotope derivative assay for aldosterone secretion described by Kliman and Peterson[81] makes the investigation of aldosterone secretion rate more reliable, and therefore, in evaluation of patients, fewer aldosterone secretion rate determinations are necessary. Although making the spadework of evaluation easier and more uniform, this new method does not add to the differentiation between primary and secondary aldosteronism.

The role of angiotensin in circulatory homeostasis has recently been clarified.[40] In addition to its role in constriction of the arterioles, angiotensin stimulates the adrenal glands and causes the production of aldosterone. Renin produced by the renal juxtaglomerular cells acts on a liver substrate α_2 globulin to form angiotensin I, which is then converted by a plasma enzyme into the active peptide, angiotensin II. The relationships of renin, angiotensin, and aldosterone in primary and secondary aldosteronism are shown in Figure 21.

With the development of a bioassay for the measurement of human plasma renin activity levels, the diagnostic criteria for primary aldosteronism have been sharpened. Only those hypertensive patients with an elevated aldosterone secretion rate on high sodium intake and a low plasma renin activity on a low-sodium diet can be considered to fulfill the present criteria for the diagnosis of primary aldosteronism. The relationships between aldosterone secretion rate and plasma renin activity in primary and secondary aldosteronism under different conditions of salt balance are shown in Figure 22. The major differentiating finding is a low plasma renin activity on a low-sodium diet in patients with primary aldosteronism. The value of plasma renin activity in differentiating primary from secondary aldosteronism has led to a practical approach to the diagnosis of primary aldosteronism. Definitive diagnosis can be made only by demonstrating inappropriately and autonomously elevated aldosterone secretion rate, but this determination in every hypertensive patient is not practical at present. Priority for evaluation should be given to patients who manifest hypokalemia and the classic clinical findings. In patients in whom the diagnosis is suspected, plasma renin activity response to low-sodium diet should be tested first. This determination yields diagnostically crucial information and is less expensive and more efficient as a screening procedure than determination of

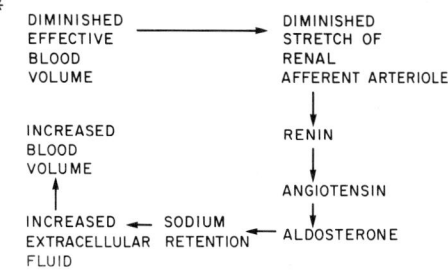
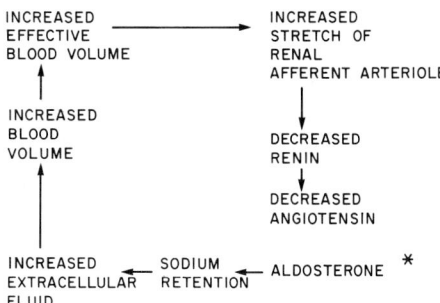

Figure 21. Pathogenesis of hyperaldosteronism—primary and secondary types.

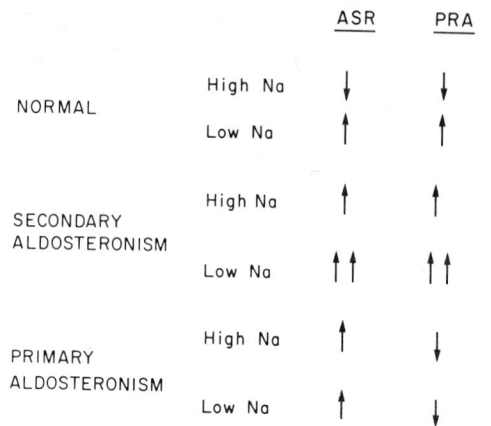

Figure 22. Effects of variation in sodium intake on aldosterone secretion rate (ASR) and plasma renin activity (PRA) in the normal subject and in states of hyperaldosteronism.

the aldosterone secretion rate. In patients unable to increase plasma renin activity in response to a low-sodium diet and upright posture, the aldosterone secretion rate while on a high-sodium diet should be determined.

Considerable interest in normokalemic primary hyperaldosteronism has been demonstrated recently; these patients demonstrate elevated aldosterone production with elevated aldosterone excretion rate consistently, but usually not to the high degree seen in those patients with hypokalemic changes. The hypertension in these patients and the entire gamut of the symptomatology seem to be less pronounced than in those with adenomas. At operation these patients appear to have either normal or hyperplastic glands, but do not demonstrate the presence of adenoma. The renin levels tend to be higher than in the adenomatous group, although still decreased as compared to normal. This group represents about 25 per cent of all patients with primary aldosteronism. The consistency of laboratory findings is such that one cannot accurately differentiate patients in this group from those in the adenoma group before operation.

Conn[24] attributes the renal defect in tubular reabsorption of water in hyperaldosteronism, as well as the kidney's ability to acidify the urine normally, to the effect of chronic depletion of body potassium on renal function and structure. The histopathologic lesions have been designated "kaliopenic nephropathy." These are concentrated in the proximal tubules and consist mainly of vascular degeneration progressing in severe cases to tubular necrosis and calcification. Much of the tubular lesion is thought to be reversible with potassium repletion.

Because of the small size of the adenomas that cause primary aldosteronism, preoperative efforts to determine the site or the side of the tumor are not likely to be successful, although the less common larger tumors may be identified by the use of retroperitoneal pneu-

mography, aortography, or pyelography, alone or in combination. Adrenal phlebography has been associated with adrenal damage and subsequent hypocorticism in a significant number of cases. Thus, enthusiasm for this procedure has waned. Isotopic techniques employing the gamma camera with ^{131}I-labeled cholesterol appear promising in the identification of adenomas. After the diagnosis is established, efforts to eliminate severe hypokalemic alkalosis are in order and usually require large amounts of supplemental potassium, up to 300 mEq. per day, for many days. Failure to correct the severe electrolyte imbalance prior to operation may increase the likelihood of arrhythmias, respiratory paralysis, and irreversible shock with the stress of anesthesia and operation. Zimmermann[155] attributes these complications to inadequate repletion of severe potassium deficits. He also warns against the use of the curare-like compounds during anesthesia in these patients because of the synergistic effects of such drugs and potassium deficiency.

In the surgical treatment of primary aldosteronism, careful bilateral exploration of the adrenal glands seems to be clearly indicated. This can be accomplished by the posterior eleventh rib approach with the greatest ease and lowest postoperative morbidity. A grossly detectable adenoma in either gland is excised. If no adenoma can be found and the clinical and laboratory diagnosis of primary aldosteronism is unequivocal, the right adrenal gland should be removed and carefully sectioned. If an adenoma still cannot be found, the surgeon should remove half of the left adrenal and carefully section it. It is very important, however, that the surgeon leave the patient a viable half adrenal gland. It is not justifiable to substitute addisonian disease, with its well known hazards, for primary aldosteronism. If primary aldosteronism cannot be cured surgically, it can be managed medically with good results.

Correction of hypertension has been complete in about 70 per cent of patients. An additional 25 per cent of patients have had significant reductions in blood pressure, although not to normal levels. Only 5 per cent of the patients who have had adenomas removed have been unimproved. Correction of the hypokalemia, however, is the rule.

In a 13-year period at Vanderbilt, 16 patients with primary aldosteronism were identified and submitted to operation. The average age of the patients was 41 years, with a range from 21 to 56 years; three fourths were females. Preoperative blood pressures ranged from 160 to 240 systolic and 90 to 140 diastolic. Serum potassium concentrations averaged 2.7 mEq. per liter, with a range of 1.8 to 3.9 mEq. per liter. Ninety-six per cent of the patients were hypokalemic, and 90 per cent showed changes in the electrocardiogram indicative of electrolyte imbalance.

Aldosterone excretion was measured in two patients in this group, whereas in the remaining patients, aldosterone secretion rates were determined by a double isotope derivative method. The normal aldosterone secretion rate in our laboratory is less than 150 μg.

per day in a patient equilibrated on a 100 mEq. sodium diet. The range in these 14 patients was 169 to 10,000 μg. per day, with an average of 397 μg. per day, excluding the 10,000 μg. per day value. This latter value was measured in a young woman in the sixth month of pregnancy.[57]

Plasma renin activity was also measured in eight patients by modification of the bioassay of Boucher.[15] After 4 days of a 10 mEq. sodium diet and after having been upright for at least 4 hours, normal subjects have a plasma renin activity greater than 600 ng. per 100 ml. The range of values in these patients with primary aldosteronism was 0 to 401 ng. per 100 ml., with an average of 127 ng. per 100 ml.

Adrenal adenomas were present in 14 of these 16 patients. Two patients had no demonstrable abnormality of the adrenal gland, and no ectopic adrenal tissue with adenoma could be found at operation. In two thirds of the patients, the adenoma was in the right adrenal, and one patient had bilateral tumors. This is in contrast to Conn's series,[22] which demonstrated a 2 to 1 ratio of left over right. In each instance bilateral adrenal exploration was carried out, and in the last 12 patients the bilateral posterior retroperitoneal approach was used. In the 14 patients in whom adrenal adenomas were found and removed, hypertension and other manifestations of hyperaldosteronism regressed rapidly, although in a few patients mild hypertension persisted for 6 to 12 months.

Medical management of aldosteronism has recently been greatly enhanced. Liddle and his associates[89] have successfully treated several patients with the experimental adrenal inhibitor aminoglutethimide. In vitro studies in Liddle's laboratory and in that of Kahnt and Neher[79] have shown that this drug inhibits a very primitive step in the steroid biosynthetic pathway, the step at which cholesterol is converted to 20α-hydroxycholesterol. Since this step occurs in the pathway for all hormonal steroids, aminoglutethimide is an inhibitor of all adrenal steroids, including both aldosterone and cortisol. Cortisol inhibition leads to a compensatory increase in ACTH, so that cortisol deficiency is not a problem. The renin-angiotensin system, however, is inactive in patients with primary aldosteronism, and so there is no compensatory response of the aldosterone-regulating mechanism. As a result, aminoglutethimide brings about a net reduction in aldosterone secretion in patients with primary aldosteronism. Another aldosterone antagonist, spironolactone, has been used widely in recent years in medical therapy of aldosteronism. While the standard treatment of primary aldosteronism is surgical excision of the adrenocortical adenoma, Liddle has found that chronic treatment with spironolactone can control this disorder when operative risk is great or when an adenoma is not found.[91]

Conn[25] has recently suggested that 10 to 20 per cent of patients with so-called essential hypertension probably harbor a small aldosterone-secreting cortical tumor. Evaluation of a large series of relatively unselected hypertensive patients has led us to believe that probably no more than 3 per cent of such patients actually fulfill the present criteria for the diagnosis of primary aldosteronism. However, until the currently accurate diagnostic methods are applied on a wide scale, the true incidence of aldosteronism in essential hypertension must remain unknown.

Congenital Adrenal Hyperplasia (Adrenogenital Syndrome)

This syndrome is an inherited inborn error of metabolism and is related to specific enzymatic defects in biosynthesis of steroids by the adrenal cortex. The enzymatic steps in biosynthesis of cortisol, aldosterone, and adrenal androgens and estrogen are outlined in Figure 8. Individual enzymatic deficits can cause both deficiency of synthesis of specific corticosteroids and compensatory overproduction of others in response to extra-adrenal regulators (ACTH). The full details of the currently known alterations in steroidogenesis in all types of these congenital syndromes have been succinctly summarized by Liddle.[91] Congenital adrenal hyperplasia occurs frequently in siblings, but the parents show no evidence of endocrine dysfunction, and consanguinity is rare. Childs[20] has deduced that this syndrome is due to a non-sex-linked recessive mutant gene, which can express itself clinically only in homozygous offspring. The detection of the disease in twins, first cousins, and half-sisters is in accordance with this mode of inheritance. The greater frequency of the disease in females is an artifact caused by the difficulty in diagnosis in males. Childs has found there is at least one affected child per 62,500 persons in the state of Maryland. Discovery of the efficiency of cortisone therapy by Wilkins et al.[149] and the more recent elucidation of the enzymatic defects concerned with this syndrome have greatly improved our understanding of the diagnosis, pathophysiology, and treatment of the disease.

Congenital bilateral adrenal cortical hyperplasia produces pseudohermaphroditism in females and macrogenitosomia praecox in males. This may manifest itself in the prenatal period or in the postnatal years:

1. *Prenatal:* Pseudohermaphroditism in females; macrogenitosomia praecox in males.

2. *Postnatal:* Virilism in females; virilism (hypermasculinization) in males; feminization in males; feminization in females (isosexual precocity).

The exact set of symptoms arising in each individual depends upon the enzymatic block present in the biosynthesis of cortisol and aldosterone. The four major types of congenital adrenal hyperplasia are (1) the simple virilizing form, (2) the sodium-losing form, (3) the hypertensive form, and (4) the 3β-hydroxysteroid dehydrogenase defect. The relative frequency of these four forms is demonstrated in Table 13.

The "simple virilizing" type is ascribed to 21-hydroxylase deficiency and is the most common variety. In some families the metabolic deficits are quite mild. Because of the impaired cortisol synthesis there is hypersecretion of ACTH by the pituitary gland, which in turn leads to adrenal hyperplasia. The excess secretion of the adrenal androgens and the virilism that is characteristic of this syndrome are responses to hypersecretion of ACTH. In the male infant the internal and external genitalia are quite normal, though the penis may be slightly enlarged. Female infants present as pseudohermaphrodites in that they have a small phallus but otherwise normal external and in-

TABLE 13. Relative Incidence of the Different Types of Congenital Adrenal Hyperplasia*

Authors	Simple Virilizing			Salt Losing			Hypertensive			Total		
	M	F	Total	M	F	Total	M	F	Total	M	F	Total
Wilkins	14	64	78	10	35	45	2	5	7	26	104	130
Prader et al.	19	35	54	18	19	37	–	–	–	37	54	91
Raiti, Newns	13	16	29	11	17	28	1	0	1	25	33	58
Total	46	115	161	39	71	110	3	5	8	88	191	279

Note: One must also add 1 male with partial 3β-ol-dehydrogenase defect in Wilkins' series and 3 cases with "lipoid hyperplasia" in Prader's series.

*From Baulieu, E. E., Peillou, F., and Migeon, C. J. *In* Eisenstein, A. B. (Ed.): The Adrenal Cortex. Boston, Little, Brown and Company, 1967.

ternal genitalia. The phallus may be represented by any extreme from a simple hypertrophied clitoris to a penile-appearing organ, with scrotum-like labia without testes and a urogenital sinus opening at the end of the phallus. The genital abnormality may be so extreme as to present the appearance of a cryptorchid male, but the chromosome structure is that of the female with congenital adrenal hyperplasia. In such cases the müllerian tubercle fails to descend normally and the vagina and the urogenital sinus can be at a considerable distance from each other. Sometimes the müllerian tubercle fails to canalize, and so no communication with the vagina can be demonstrated. The degree of masculinization depends both upon the time in fetal life in which the androgens begin to exert their influence and upon the degree of androgen secretion. The postnatal development of children with this disorder is one of progressive virilization. In boys the penis continues to grow rapidly and its large size is certainly obvious by the second year. The scrotum expands also, but the testes remain infantile. In girls the gonads remain infantile and the external genitalia become virilized. The clitoris enlarges and may reach a length of 2 to 3 inches and may have erections. The labia majora grow and project forward and appear like a split scrotum. Pubic hair usually appears in patients of both sexes at about 3 years of age and acquires a more masculine distribution. Axillary hair usually appears a few years later, and a mustache may appear between 9 and 12 years of age (Fig. 23).

Other characteristics including the skin changes of acne, light brown coloration generally, and deep pigmentation in the anogenital regions are also noted. The skeletal changes include premature epiphyseal closure, with complete absence of the female contour. Patients usually have a short, stocky build with wide thorax and shoulders and narrow pelvis. The limbs are short in relation to the trunk, which is usually of normal length. Muscular development is extremely good, and these patients are usually stronger than children of their own age; most have a rather athletic build when they get older. In adult life the clinical picture remains essentially a progression of the childhood traits; the physique remains masculine, and the female is, of course, bothered by considerable increase in facial and body hair. The infertility in these persons is attributed to hypogonadism, and the males have obviously hypoplastic testes. Primary amenorrhea is always a feature in the females, although, infrequently, scanty menses have been reported. In the simple virilizing form, the usual clinical picture is that of a female child with ambiguous external genitalia. The establishment of the correct sex assignment for this group is essential early in life.

The salt-losing form of congenital adrenal hyperplasia is also more frequent in females than in males. In addition to the virilization seen in the simple type, these children also have symptoms of acute adrenal insufficiency. Because of equilibrium with the maternal circulation, the symptoms usually do not appear until the infant is approximately 5 to 10 days of age. A lack of appetite, apathy, vomiting, diarrhea, hypoglycemia, dusky color of the skin, convulsions, and sudden circulatory collapse are common features. Many of the deaths have been due to a combination of hypovolemia and hyperkalemia. Laboratory studies in these children show low serum sodium and bicarbonate and high serum potassium; excretion of 17-ketosteroids and pregnenetriol is increased. The salt-losing type is also associated with a defect of 21-hydroxylase.

In the hypertensive form, there is a defect of the enzyme 11β-hydroxylase. This leads to a deficient cortisol synthesis and to hypersecretion of ACTH. The patients exhibit virilization as well as a mildly elevated blood pressure, although in a few cases the blood pressure has been quite high. It has been suggested that the hypertension is due to excessive secretion of desoxycorticosterone.[10]

A rare type of adrenogenital syndrome is associated with 3β-hydroxysteroid dehydrogenase defect. This causes a block in the synthesis of cortisol at a much earlier stage and is manifested by virilization, but to a smaller degree in females than in the other types of perineal hypospadias in males. The presence of perineal hypospadias in males suggests a role of this enzyme in androgen synthesis by the testes as well as by the adrenals. Of the six patients reported, three were hypospadic males and three were females with hypertrophy of the clitoris and labial fusion but no development of a urogenital sinus. In five of these patients there was a marked urinary salt loss, and four died in early infancy. Diagnosis of this condition can be expedited by the following measures: (1) determination of nuclear sex chromatin is extremely helpful when combined with endocrine studies to establish the sex in this type of ambiguous external genitalia and to differentiate this from other forms of pseudohermaphroditism; (2) radiologic and cystoscopic examination of the lower genitourinary tract should be done; (3) increased excretion of 17-ketosteroids and pregnene-

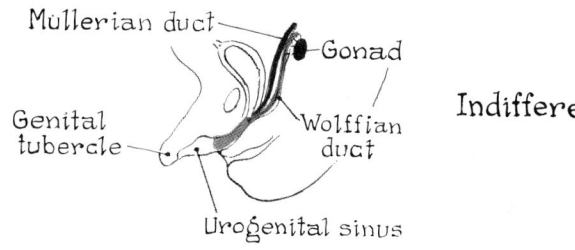

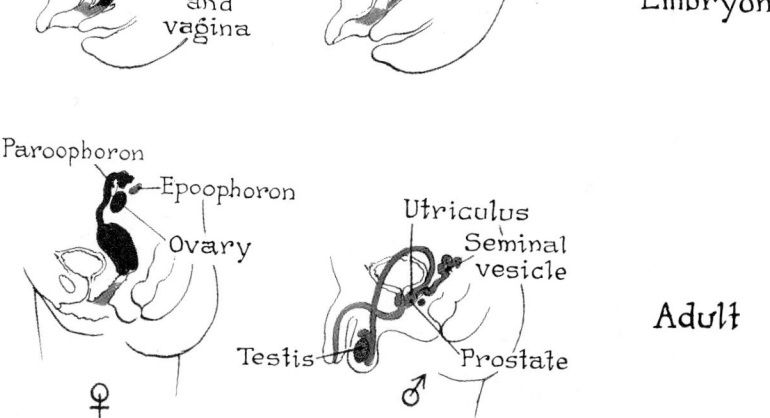

Figure 23. Differentiation of gonads and genital ducts from the indifferent stage to the male and female adult stage. (From Wilkins, L.: The Diagnosis and Treatment of Endocrine Disorders in Childhood and Adolescence, 3rd ed., 1966. Courtesy of Charles C Thomas, Publisher, Springfield, Ill.)

triol, along with normal or diminished excretion of corticosteroids, should be demonstrated; (4) suppression of abnormal urinary excretion of steroids with cortisol or dexamethasone stimulation is pathognomonic of the syndrome. When uncertainty still exists, exploratory operation must be undertaken in order to determine the true nature of the gonads. Wilkins has demonstrated in recent years the efficacy of cortisone or hydrocortisone in treatment of patients with bilateral adrenal hyperplasia.[148] With this therapy there is a striking reduction in the secretion of adrenal androgens, presumably on the basis of inhibition of ACTH production by the anterior pituitary.

Using the level of urinary 17-ketosteroid excretion as a guide, dosage has to be individualized throughout the period of treatment. The dosage level employed should be the least amount of cortisone necessary to suppress the 17-ketosteroid excretion to a normal level for the age and sex of the patient (Table 14). This usually is in the neighborhood of 50 mg. per day in older children and 25 mg. in infants and younger children. Maximal suppression of 17-ketosteroid excretion should occur within approximately 5 to 10 days after initiation of treatment, and maintenance doses are usually half the initial dosage. Oral cortisol is usually less effective in maintenance therapy than that given intramuscularly, and the dosage needed, accordingly, is two to three times greater. The length of therapy is presumably for lifetime. It is essential in this syndrome that diagnosis and accurate therapy be initiated as soon as possible so that the child can be raised in its genetic sex orientation.

Feminizing Tumors of the Adrenal Cortex

In rare instances, tumors of the adrenal cortex may produce feminizing effects. Most of these tumors are highly malignant. Of the 52 cases of feminizing tumors reported in males, the tumor was a carcinoma in 41 and an adenoma in 7; in 4 it could not be deter-

TABLE 14. Urinary Excretion of 17-Ketosteroids in Patients with Untreated Congenital Adrenal Hyperplasia*

| Age | Urinary 17-Ketosteroids | |
	Untreated Patients	Normal Subjects
0–1 month	1–5	0.5–2.5
2–6 months	1–10	<0.5
7–12 months	3–10	<0.5
1–5 years	4–30	0.5–2.0
6–9 years	11–40	1–3
10–15 years	16–50	3–8
Over 15 years		
♂	23–80	6–18
♀	21–75	4–15

*From Wilkins, L.: Arch. Dis. Child., 37:231, 1962.

TABLE 15. Incidence of Signs and Symptoms of Feminizing Tumors in the Male (52 Patients)*

Sign or Symptom	Per Cent
Gynecomastia	98
Palpable tumor	58
Atrophy of testis	52
Diminished libido and/or potency	48
Pain at site of tumor	44
Tenderness of breast	42
Pigmentation of areolae	27
Obesity	27
Feminizing hair change	23
Atrophy of the penis	20
Elevation of the blood pressure	16
Increasing skin pigmentation	12
Varicocele	11
Acne	8

*From Gabrilove, J. L., Sharma, D. C., Wotiz, H. H., and Dorfman, R. I.: Medicine, *44*:37, 1965.

mined whether the tumor was malignant or benign. These tumors almost always occur in males; only two cases have been reported in young females. Most feminizing tumors occur in patients between 25 and 45 years of age, although several patients as old as 50 to 66 years of age have been reported. Gynecomastia is the most common symptom. The incidence of this and other symptoms is listed in Table 15. The gynecomastia is usually rather prominent, with tender fullness of both breasts, although on occasion it may be unilateral. In addition to this, the patients exhibit impotence and loss of libido but very few other hypoandrogenic features. A palpable tumor is present in many patients, and local pain due to neoplastic growth is frequent. Calcification in the tumor has occurred in four patients. Urinary estrogen levels are usually markedly elevated and are higher in patients with carcinoma than in those with adenoma. In several patients, estrogen excretion was increased 100-fold. Although these are feminizing tumors, the levels of urinary 17-ketosteroid excretion are also elevated in most cases. Urinary gonadotropin excretion has shown no significant variation from the normal in the cases in which it has been measured. In the malignant tumors there are two cell types. The predominant type closely resembles the cells of the zona reticularis. The cells are variable in size and shape; sometimes fusiform or spindle shapes are most common, but usually the cells are eosinophilic, rounded, and polygonal. They contain an abundance of finely granular cytoplasm and small hyperchromatic nuclei, located generally in a central position. Upon differential staining the tumor cells show characteristics of the cells of the zona recticularis. The second cell type is much larger, and more polygonal in shape, containing large amounts of homogeneous, clear or slightly foamy cytoplasm. The nuclei are large, bizarre, and hyperchromatic. These elements closely resemble the cells of the zona fasciculata although they are lacking in the characteristic cord or columnar arrangement. The diagnosis of malignancy is based upon capsular invasion,

venous invasion, and distant metastasis. The testes show profound changes, with total absence of spermatogenesis and no recognizable spermatogonia. Sertoli cells are not significantly altered and Leydig cells are not found. The hypophysis appears normal but slightly enlarged.

The feminizing tumor should obviously be removed as soon as the diagnosis is established, and postsurgical radiotherapy is usually advisable. Because some of these tumors also produce increased amounts of cortisol, substitution therapy postoperatively is usually indicated. After operation gynecomastia regresses and libido usually returns to normal, as does spermatogenesis. Unfortunately, in most cases metastases appear in a short time, with or without return of urinary steroids to the preoperative levels. Recurrence and spread of tumor often occur within one year of primary operation. In rare instances in which the tumor was an adenoma, cures have been obtained.

Pheochromocytoma

Considerable progress has been made in the last 15 years in the recognition and management of pheochromocytoma, undoubtedly the most dramatic and treacherous of the various surgically correctable causes of hypertension. Although the tumor was described as early as 1886 by Frankel,[50] and given its name, pheochromocytoma or "black celled tumor," by Pick[111] in 1912, it was not until 1922 that the clear demonstration of the association of the tumor with hypertension of a paroxysmal nature was made by Labbe and his associates.[83] While Roux[125] in France and Charles Mayo[100] in this country are credited with early successful surgical removal of pheochromocytomas during the 1920s, the first correct preoperative diagnosis of the tumor was apparently made in 1929 by Pincoffs[112] in Baltimore, with subsequent successful removal of the lesion by A. M. Shipley. In 1929 Rabin[115] demonstrated an epinephrine-like substance in a pheochromocytoma, and for a time the syndrome of paroxysmal hypertension was thought to be the only manifestation of the "epinephrine-producing" tumor of the adrenal medulla. However, in 1938 Binger and Craig[12] and Palmer and Castleman[108] described instances of pheochromocytoma with sustained hypertension. In 1946 the studies of U. S. von Euler and his associates[145] demonstrated the presence of norepinephrine at the terminals of adrenergic nerve fibers and in the adrenal medulla, and in 1949 Holton[71] and in 1950 Goldenberg[55] demonstrated the presence of norepinephrine in pheochromocytomas. It thus became apparent that the clinical manifestations of these neoplasms were related at times to their secretion of norepinephrine as well as epinephrine.

The tumor originates in a majority of cases in the adrenal medulla and less frequently in the cells of the extra-adrenal paraganglion system which are disseminated along the paravertebral axis from the pelvis to the base of the skull. The cell of origin is regarded by Pearse[109] as part of the neuroendocrine group of cells which he calls the APUD system. The cells of this system are able to secrete polypeptide hormones and are, whether by origin or functional similarity, very much alike in character. Multiple endocrine neoplasia, type

II, is a genetic disorder involving multifocal tumor formation in this system of polypeptide secreting cells. Its expressions include pheochromocytoma, medullary carcinoma of thyroid, parathyroid hyperplasia or tumors, and multiple mucosal neuromas, which may occur in combination or singly in several members of a kindred. Familial pheochromocytoma also occurs in association with neuroectodermal dysplasias which include von Recklinghausen's disease, tuberous sclerosis, Sturge-Weber's syndrome, and Lindau-von Hippel disease. In these various familial syndromes, bilateral adrenal pheochromocytomas are prone to occur. However, in its most frequent form the tumor occurs as a single lesion of adrenal medullary origin without familial associations (Table 16).

From the work of von Euler and others[146] it has become clear that the clinical manifestations of pheochromocytoma are related to the secretory output of catecholamines by the tumor. In normal man there are three naturally occurring catecholamines: dopamine, norepinephrine, and epinephrine. Each of these can be identified in adrenal medullary tissue, but at postganglionic sympathetic nerve endings apparently only dopamine and norepinephrine can be identified in other than the most minute concentrations. It has been suggested that efficient methylation of norepinephrine to form epinephrine occurs only in the well-organized tissue of the adrenal medulla. In normal man at rest, the adrenal medulla is said to secrete 0.07 μg. per kilogram per minute of epinephrine and 0.02 μg. per kilogram per minute of norepinephrine.[62] In tumors, amounts of these catecholamines greatly in excess of normal levels occur and ratios vary widely. For a time it was thought that pheochromocytomas that occur in the periphery could produce only norepinephrine, while tumors of the adrenal medulla could produce both epinephrine and norepinephrine. Goodall reported two epinephrine-producing pheochromocytomas of the organ of Zuckerkandl at the aortic bifurcation which were studied by von Euler.[56] In general, it would appear that, despite these rare exceptions, the majority of extra-adrenal pheochromocytomas are pure norepinephrine producers, while the tumors that arise in the adrenal medulla for the most part produce both epinephrine and norepinephrine; very rarely, pure epinephrine-producing tumors of the adrenal medulla and the periphery are encountered.

Pheochromocytomas are relatively uncommon tumors but are by no means rarities. The incidence has been variously determined as 0.4 to 2 per cent of all hypertensive persons, but some investigators believe the actual incidence to be higher. Kvale[82] identified pheochromocytomas as a cause for hypertension in 2 per cent of 900 hypertensive patients in a study reported in 1954. Barbeau[9] collected 626 cases of pheochromocytoma for a review of the literature in 1957. Graham[58] calculated that 600 to 800 people die yearly as a result of untreated pheochromocytoma.

The majority of pheochromocytomas occur in adults, but about one fifth of reported cases have occurred in children. In the latter, according to Zimmermann,[155] 39 per cent of the tumors are either bilateral or multiple. The tumor occurs in women with greater frequency than in men, and many cases are first recognized during pregnancy. The reported age incidence is from 5 months to 82 years. Chong et al.[21] recently reported 138 patients with pheochromocytoma who were operated on at the Mayo Clinic between 1926 and 1970. There were 63 males and 75 females. The tumor was extra-adrenal in 10 per cent, bilateral in 4.4 per cent, multiple in 7 per cent, and malignant (proven by metastases) in 18 patients (13.4 per cent).

Grossly, most pheochromocytomas are well encapsulated tumors of yellow-brown or reddish brown color. Often an attenuated adrenal gland can be seen overlying a portion or all of the tumor. Microscopically, the structure is somewhat variable. The cells are usually large and polyhedral or irregularly shaped, with granular, slightly acidophilic cytoplasm and a large eccentric vesicular nucleus. For the most part, the cells are arranged in an alveolar pattern, but this is by no means constant. Pleomorphism and lymphatic, blood vessel, and capsular invasion frequently occur and

TABLE 16.   Pheochromocytoma: Location of Tumors

Location	Adult* No.	Adult* Per Cent	Child No.	Child Per Cent
Total cases	207		76	
Right adrenal		44.5		33
Left adrenal		33.8		14.5
Bilateral		8.7		19.7
Bilateral plus extra-adrenal				4.0
Right side, extra-adrenal		3.4		1.3
Left side, extra-adrenal		2.4		7.9
Adrenal and extra-adrenal		0.5		9.2
Multiple		1.5		5.3
Aorta (organs of Zuckerkandl)		3.8		3.8
Intrathoracic		0.9		1.3
Celiac ganglion		0.5		

	Adult, Per Cent	Child, Per Cent	Familial, Per Cent
Bilateral	9 } 10.5	24 } 39	50
Multiple	1.5	15	9
Extra-adrenal	11.5	15	14
Total, per cent	22	54	73

Bilateral, Familial, Neurofibromatosis†

	Adult No.	Adult Per Cent	Child No.	Child Per Cent
Total cases	543		83	
Bilateral		7		24
Familial		2.6		10
Familial bilateral		1.7		2.4
Bilateral, not familial		5.3		21
Neurofibromatosis		4.8		1.4

*From Graham, J. B.: Surg. Gynecol. Obstet., *92*:105, 1951. By permission of Surgery, Gynecology & Obstetrics.
†See Hume, D. M.: Am. J. Surg., *99*:458, 1960.

cannot be considered signs of malignancy. The majority of these tumors are benign, and only the finding of direct invasion of surrounding structures and distant metastases provides the justification for the diagnosis of malignancy.

The tumors vary greatly in size and weight. The largest on record weighed 2000 gm. with its contained cystic fluid. Usual weight range is from 1 to 75 gm. For reasons that are unknown, right-sided tumors are more common than those on the left, and the incidence of bilaterality or of multiplicity of pheochromocytoma ranges from 7 to 11 per cent of reported cases.

The symptoms and signs of pheochromocytoma are those which result from the release of excessive amounts of the catecholamines (epinephrine or norepinephrine or both). While epinephrine and norepinephrine are similar in metabolic action, epinephrine is 30 to 100 times more potent than norepinephrine is in this regard (Table 17).

Ahlquist's division of adrenergic responses into those of alpha and beta receptors has clarified the understanding of the action of epinephrine and norepinephrine.[2] His work was verified by the discovery that adrenergic blocking agents are specific for either alpha or beta receptors. Alpha receptors are generally excitatory and beta receptors inhibitory in the periphery. Pure alpha stimulation causes peripheral arteriolar constriction with attendant rise in blood pressure. Cardiac effects of alpha stimulation are produced by

reflex changes, most notably a vagal-mediated bradycardia. Beta stimulation causes peripheral vasodilation with lowering of diastolic pressure. Cardiac receptors are purely of the beta variety and produce tachycardia and inotropism.

Norepinephrine is a relatively pure alpha stimulator, although it has some cardiac beta stimulatory properties that are usually seen only after alpha blockade. Epinephrine has a mixed effect. It is a more potent alpha stimulator than norepinephrine, but it also has a strong beta stimulant effect. Dopamine has an anomalous effect: cardiac beta stimulation with a specific renal vasodilation that is neither alpha nor beta.

The catecholamines produce a general hypermetabolic effect which seems to account for the feeling of "nervousness" common in patients with pheochromocytoma. The two more specific effects are glycogenolysis, primarily in the liver, and elevation of serum free fatty acids from increased activity of a triglyceride lipase enzyme found in adipose tissue. Both of these effects have been shown by Robison and coworkers[123] to be mediated by stimulation of adenyl cyclase, causing an increase in cyclic $3',5'$ adenosine monophosphate (cyclic AMP) which acts as a secondary messenger to stimulate activity of the target enzyme.

Paroxysms of hypertension occur in 30 to 50 per cent of patients with pheochromocytoma. These represent episodes of massive release of hormone, either epinephrine or norepinephrine or both, and are precipitated by a variety of stimuli, including various forms of stress such as trauma, exercise, massage of tumor, sexual intercourse, and emptying of bladder. Paroxysms are characterized by extreme levels of hypertension, blanching, occasionally flushing, tachycardia, syncope, sweating, angina, and headache.

Three clinical patterns of hypertension occur with pheochromocytomas: First, there is the "classic" situation in which blood pressure is normal between hypertensive paroxysms. This was long thought to be the only manifestation of the tumor. Second, blood pressure may be elevated in a sustained fashion without paroxysms and resemble essential hypertension. Third, blood pressure may be elevated constantly and in addition extreme paroxysmal hypertensive crises are superimposed.[133]

The signs and symptoms of hypermetabolism are evident in many patients with pheochromocytomas and reflect the intensive metabolic activity of the catecholamines secreted by the tumor. Symptoms simulating hyperthyroidism, with tremor, tachycardia, and elevated basal metabolic rate, may be present. The manifestations of diabetes, including glycosuria and a diabetic type of glucose tolerance curve, may occur. Weight loss is quite common in these persons and the majority of patients with pheochromocytoma are thin. Fever, vasomotor phenomena, headache, angina, nausea, and anxiety attacks are quite common. Death is apt to occur during a paroxysmal episode. The causes of death from pheochromocytoma include cerebrovascular accident, congestive heart failure with pulmonary edema, and ventricular fibrillation. Rarely, a malignant pheochromocytoma has recurred after its

TABLE 17. Comparison of the Effects of Epinephrine and Norepinephrine*

Effector	Norepinephrine	Epinephrine
Heart	Positive inotropic	Positive inotropic
Isolated	Positive chronotropic	Positive chronotropic
In vivo	Positive inotropic	Positive inotropic
	Negative chronotropic	Positive chronotropic
Blood pressure		
Systolic	Increase	Increase
Diastolic	Increase	Slight increase
Peripheral resistance	Increase	Slight increase or decrease
Cardiac output	Slight increase or unchanged	Increase
Liver	Vasoconstriction	Vasodilation
Skeletal muscle	Vasoconstriction	Vasodilation
Skin	Vasoconstriction	Vasoconstriction
Kidneys	Vasoconstriction	Vasoconstriction
Intestinal smooth muscle	Relaxation	Relaxation
Sweat glands	Slight activation	Activation
Pupils	Slight dilation	Dilation
Central nervous system, nervousness and apprehension	No effect	Marked effect
Basal metabolic rate	Slight increase	Increase
Blood sugar	Slight increase	Increase
Plasma nonesterified fatty acid level	Increase	Increase

*From Scott, H. W., Jr., et al.: Surg. Gynecol. Obstet., *120*:707, 1965. By permission of Surgery, Gynecology & Obstetrics.

TABLE 18. Symptoms and Signs of Pheochromocytoma[*]

	Approximate Per Cent	
	Adult	Child
Symptoms:		
Persistent hypertension	65	92
Paroxysmal hypertension	30	8
Headache	80	81
Sweating	70	68
Palpitation, nervousness	60	34
Pallor of face	40	27
Tremor	40	
Nausea	30	56
Weakness, fatigue	25	27
Weight loss	15	44
Abdominal or chest pain	15	35
Dyspnea	15	16
Visual changes	10	44
Constipation	5	8
Raynaud's phenomenon	5	
Convulsions	3	23
Polydipsia, polyuria		25
Puffy, red, cyanotic hands		11
Signs:		
BMR over +20 per cent	50	83
Fasting blood sugar over 120 mg./100 ml.	40	40
Glycosuria	10	3
Eye ground changes	30	70

[*]From Hume, D. M. *In* Astwood, E. B., and Cassidy, C. E. (Eds.): Clinical Endocrinology. Volume II. New York, Grune and Stratton, 1968.

operative removal, and widely distributed metastases have caused the patient's death (Table 18).

Since the introduction of the histamine provocative test by Roth and Kvale[124] in 1945, a variety of pharmacologic tests have been devised as aids in diagnosis of pheochromocytoma. The histamine test is based on the direct stimulating effect of the drug on chromaffin cells, with release of catecholamines; a prompt rise in blood pressure usually occurs in a patient who has a pheochromocytoma. Phentolamine (Regitine), introduced in 1949 by Longino, Grimson, et al.,[94] causes a fall in blood pressure in patients with pheochromocytoma by blocking the effector cell for catecholamines. Other pharmacologic tests based on the patient's blood pressure responses to such drugs as methacholine (Mecholyl), benzodioxane, Dibenamine, and tetra-ethylammonium bromide have been developed but have not proved to be of much additional value in diagnosis of these tumors. In the last decade the indirect pharmacologic tests have been used less and less and have been supplanted to a great extent by direct chemical methods of estimating the levels of the catecholamines and metabolites in plasma and urine.

The metabolic pathways for the catecholamines, as they pass from synthesis to degradation, are outlined in Figure 24. Primary interest in pheochromocytoma revolves around the metabolites of norepinephrine and epinephrine, specifically normetanephrine, meta-nephrine, and VMA. The two enzymes involved are monamine oxidase, a mitochondrial enzyme, and catechol O-methyl transferase, a cytoplasmic enzyme. Monamine oxidase is found specifically in the sympathetic nerve endings and the adrenal medullary cell. However, circulating catecholamines are broken down by both enzymes and 40 per cent excreted as VMA and 40 per cent as metanephrines.

Laboratory confirmation of the diagnosis of pheochromocytoma can usually be made quite easily by measurement of free catecholamines, vanillyl mandelic acids (VMA), and metanephrines in 24-hour collections of the patient's urine (Table 19). Urinary free catecholamines were elevated above 100 μg. per 24 hours in 28 patients in the clinical series of 35 patients with pheochromocytoma studied at Vanderbilt University.[132] In all but two of these, the elevations were repeatedly in excess of 200 μg. per 24 hours, most commonly in the range of 300 to over 1000 μg. per 24 hours. Urinary VMA was elevated above 12 mg. per 24 hours in 15 patients and was below 10 mg. per 24 hours in three others in the series. Urinary metanephrines, elevated above 1.3 mg. per 24 hours, are considered to be the most accurate indicator of pheochromocytoma at the Mayo Clinic,[21] while the endocrine laboratory at Vanderbilt favors free catecholamines. Harrison has emphasized the reliability and accuracy of measurement of urinary free catecholamines and metanephrines in the differential diagnosis of pheochromocytoma and the inaccuracy and unreliability of the commonly used colorimetric reaction for VMA.[67]

Once the diagnosis of pheochromocytoma has been established, the next clinical problem is that of localization of the tumor. By far the great majority develop in the adrenal medulla, and even those which originate in extra-adrenal chromaffin tissue have a predilection for the renal fossae. Cervical, mediastinal, and pelvic sites of origin occur with rarity, but there are several reports of pheochromocytoma originating in such bizarre sites as the jugular foramen and the wall of the urinary bladder.

In attempting to localize a pheochromocytoma, intravenous pyelography should always be used but cannot be counted on to locate the tumor unless it is quite large. Abdominal laminagrams occasionally indicate the tumor's density or identify flecks of calcification in the lesion. Retroperitoneal pneumography with carbon dioxide as used in the past can contribute valuable localizing information, either alone or combined with aortography. Aortography represents both a diagnostic localizing procedure and a provocative procedure. Although deaths have been reported with its use, at present a selective catheterization technique combined with the availability of blocking agents has made this an extremely valuable procedure in the demonstration of pheochromocytomas, particularly those which are extra-adrenal. This procedure in experienced hands is a safe and valuable diagnostic asset. Mahoney[98] and his associates have described an ingenious localizing technique based on vena caval catheterization with plasma catecholamine determinations on blood samples drawn at intervals as the catheter is passed along the cava.

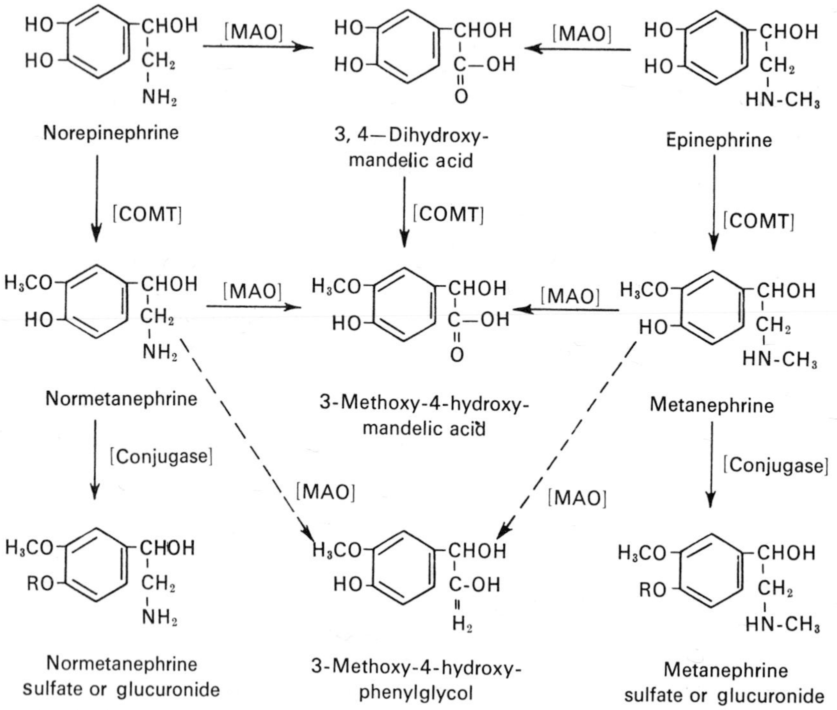

Figure 24. Steps in metabolic degradation of epinephrine and norepinephrine. MAO = monoamine oxidase. COMT = catechol-O-methyl-transferase.

TABLE 19. Normal Values for Excretion of Catecholamines and Metabolites

Catecholamines	10–100 μg./24 hrs.
Norepinephrine	10–70 μg./24 hrs.
Epinephrine	0–20 μg./24 hrs.
Vanillylmandelic acid (VMA)	1.8–7.0 mg./24 hrs.
Normetanephrine and	
metanephrine	Less than 1.3 mg./24 hrs.

Retrograde adrenal phlebography has been found useful by many radiologists in demonstrating a variety of adrenal lesions, including pheochromocytoma. Concern about the hazard of extravasation of contrast media has limited its use in some clinics including our own. However, Harrison points out that extravasation is rarely now seen as technical sophistication has developed and it is uncommon to have a severe hypertensive reaction result from the study.[67] During the past decade at Vanderbilt, we have come to rely preferentially on contrast arteriography in most patients with suspected pheochromocytoma.[132] While rapid injection of hypertonic iodinated contrast medium is a powerful pharmacologic stimulus for catecholamine release from the pheochromocytoma, if the procedure is carried out with appropriate precautions, including monitoring of vital signs and electrocardiogram with full preparation for carrying out whatever resuscitation may be required, excellent results can be safely obtained.

An effective radioscanning technique for pheochromocytoma would be a great diagnostic asset. Anderson et al. have worked on the problem for many years.[5] Recently they demonstrated that ^{14}C tagged dopamine given intravenously is concentrated in pheochromocytoma and a scanning method with a gamma-ray-emitting isotope for the tumor may soon be available. They have adapted the ^{131}Iodocholesterol adrenal cortical scanning procedure to demonstrate adrenal pheochromocytoma by a definite negative impression of the lesion.[93] Unfortunately, the technique is not applicable to extra-adrenal tumors.

Localization of pheochromocytoma before operation can currently be accomplished by one or more of these diagnostic procedures in a majority of patients. However, it must be emphasized that careful surgical exploration remains the most dependable localizing method of all.

Preoperative preparation of patients with pheochromocytoma during the last decade has usually included the use of adrenergic blocking agents. Of the various drugs which produce alpha-adrenergic blockade, the most widely used are phenoxybenzamine (Dibenzyline) and phentolamine. Beta-adrenergic blockade is produced by only a few known drugs, all derivatives of the beta stimulator, isoproterenol; propranolol is in general use for this purpose.

Phenoxybenzamine produces alpha-adrenergic blockade with relatively minor side effects. Its action is slow. It appears to inactivate the alpha-adrenergic receptor by forming a stable bond with it. Peak effect occurs one to two hours after oral administration. The drug is generally given orally in daily doses of 20 to 200 mg. The effects of daily administration are cumulative for five to seven days. Phentolamine is a 2-substituted imidazoline which causes rapid and transient alpha-adrenergic blockade. Onset of action after intravenous administration is within 30 seconds, peak effect is within 5 minutes, and duration of action is 30 to 60 minutes. Absorption after oral administration is erratic. Accordingly, it is usually given by intravenous infusion. The initial dose is 1 to 5 mg., but the rate of administration may vary from 2 to 50 mg. per hour and must be titrated against blood pressure. Phentolamine is useful in the acute control of hypertension in pheochromocytoma, but is inferior to phenoxybenzamine for long-term use.

Propranolol induces a competitive beta-adrenergic blockade with a half life of several hours. It is usually given orally in doses of 10 to 40 mg. every 6 to 8 hours. The intravenous preparation is used primarily for intraoperative administration; the dose is 1 to 3 mg. over several minutes with electrocardiographic monitoring.

The clinical indications for the use of alpha and beta blockade vary from one clinic to another. In the last 10 years we have tended to use alpha blockade with phenoxybenzamine for 4 to 10 days in most patients with pheochromocytoma. Beta blockade with propranolol has rarely been needed. The most clear indication for beta blockade is the patient in whom tachycardia or tachyarrhythmia occurs after alpha blockade. In a pure epinephrine-producing tumor beta blockade is also indicated. However, propranolol should be given only after alpha blockade is established. Spontaneous restoration of normal plasma volume can occur during several days of alpha blockade and thus reduce operative risk. However, the extent to which operative intervention should be delayed by maintenance of alpha or beta blockade remains controversial.

Anesthetic management in most clinics in recent years has begun with adrenergic blockade. It should be emphasized that complete blockade is not obtainable, and the patient must still be protected from excessive catecholamine release at operation. Thiopental and nitrous oxide are generally used for induction, with deep halothane anesthesia for maintenance in most patients. A lidocaine drip is used to control arrhythmias with phentolamine supplementation if needed. Aggressive blood and fluid replacement is used during operation in anticipation of hypotension after removal of the tumor. Usually 50 to 75 gm. of albumin and two to three liters of Ringer's lactate are given during operation. At Vanderbilt an effort is made to avoid the use of norepinephrine infusions during or after operation.[132, 143]

Operative procedure has been based on the need for wide exposure and nonmanipulative dissection in removal of pheochromocytomas. An anterior transperitoneal approach that permits examination of both adrenal glands and a search of the paraspinal axis is desirable. With large (> 6 cm. diameter) tumors, extension of the incision across the costal margin into the eighth or ninth intercostal space greatly improves exposure. At Vanderbilt we have used either a midline or transverse thoracoabdominal incision in the majority of patients with adrenal pheochromocytomas. There have been no deaths during operation. We believe the safety and excellence of the exposure justify the slight increase in morbidity.

At operation, even though the site of the tumor has been well localized preoperatively, careful examination of the contralateral adrenal and the renal fossa, the paraspinal axis, and the pelvis in search of additional tumors should be made. A left adrenal tumor may be approached by reflecting the mobilized spleen and the pancreatic tail medially and the splenic flexure inferiorly, or by dividing the gastrocolic omentum and retracting the tail of the pancreas, spleen, and stomach upward. The right adrenal is approached by mobilizing the hepatic flexure of the colon, displacing it inferiorly, and dividing the lateral peritoneal attachments of the duodenum to permit the latter and inferior vena cava to be retracted medially. Careful, gentle dissection with early control of the tumor's blood supply is highly desirable. A technique which "dissects the patient away from the tumor" and minimizes manipulation of the lesion will reduce the release of catecholamines and the risk of operation. When a large adrenal tumor (> 6 cm. in diameter) presents, the possibility of carcinoma must be considered and wide exposure using a thoracoabdominal incision is mandatory to permit radical en bloc, non-manipulative resection of the tumor with the ipsilateral kidney and, if necessary, in the case of left adrenal tumors the tail of the pancreas and spleen. An upper abdominal incision is first made, the abdomen and contralateral adrenal explored, and the incision then carried across the costal margin into the eighth or ninth intercostal space with division of the diaphragm on the side of the tumor. This permits truly excellent exposure of a large pheochromocytoma (Fig. 25).

Postoperative complications are rather frequent. In general the hazards of operation combine those peculiar to pheochromocytoma with those of any large upper abdominal or thoracoabdominal procedure.

In the 138 patients with pheochromocytoma treated surgically at the Mayo Clinic from 1926 through 1970, the mortality rate of the primary operation was 2.9 per cent.[21] Two of the deaths were due to massive uncontrollable bleeding from inferior vena cava or common iliac veins. In the other two deaths, cardiac arrest occurred during operation. These four deaths occurred prior to 1965.

In a 26-year period (1950–1976) at Vanderbilt University Affiliated Hospitals, 46 patients with pheochromocytoma were observed. Ages ranged from 9 to 78 years. There were 31 females and 15 males. Familial occurrence of tumors presented as multiple endocrine neoplasia, type II, in three patients and two others had the associated findings of von Recklinghausen's cutaneous neurofibromatosis and Lindau-von Hippel disease respectively. The remainder had no familial or neuroectodermal dysplastic associations. In 11 patients seen in the earlier years of this period, clinical diagnosis of pheochromocytoma was not made and the tumor was discovered at autopsy by the pathologist. Among the 35 patients in whom the clinical diagnosis was made, 33 had removal of primary pheochromocytomas with a single postoperative fatality. In two patients with metastatic malignant tumors, only biopsy of metastases was done to establish pathologic diagnosis prior to chemotherapy.[132]

Pathologic classification of pheochromocytomas as benign or malignant is based on the presence or absence of proven metastases. This practice is followed because histologic pattern does not accurately predict biologic behavior.

The results for patients who survived operative removal of pheochromocytoma have varied with age, familial relationships, and the benign or malignant characteristics of the tumor. Patients with familial pheochromocytoma and those in the childhood age group have an increased tendency to have bilateral tumors as well as synchronous and metachronous multiple extra-adrenal tumors.

Follow-up has been completed through 1976 in all but two patients of the Vanderbilt series. In these exceptions, a single benign adrenal pheochromocytoma was removed in 1957 and 1963 and each patient remained normotensive and asymptomatic for a period of 11 years and 18 months respectively before they were lost to follow-up. Each of the four patients with malignant pheochromocytoma who were clinically managed received x-ray therapy and various chemotherapeutic agents and died with disseminated metastases 9 months, 2, 3, and 11 years after the diagnosis was made. In two of these patients histologically benign pheochromocytoma had initially been removed 11 and almost 6 years, respectively, prior to death from metastatic disease. In the 27 remaining patients with benign pheochromocytoma, up-to-date follow-up extends from 1 to 20 years. In this group are three adults with MEN, type 2, and the only child in the series, a 9-year-old boy with no identifiable familial associations. Each had bilateral adrenal pheochromocytomas removed with satisfactory courses on maintenance

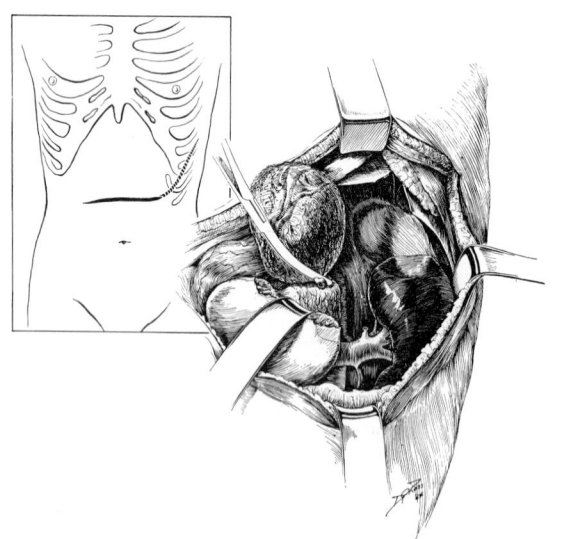

Figure 25. Left thoracoabdominal approach for pheochromocytoma. (From Scott, H. W., Jr., et al. Surg. Gynecol. Obstet., *120*:707, 1965. By permission of Surgery, Gynecology & Obstetrics.)

steroids in the last one to four years. One of the two patients with MEN, type 2, is known to have widely distributed metastases of medullary thyroid carcinoma. Each of these four patients is normotensive.

Among the 23 other patients who had a single benign pheochromocytoma removed, 14 who have been followed from 12 months to 20 years have remained normotensive and asymptomatic with no evidence of recurrence of pheochromocytoma. However, in the nine other patients, hypertension has persisted or developed in the period of follow-up after excision of the tumor. One of these patients had malignant hypertension with diffusely severe renal arteriolosclerosis and nitrogen retention at the time her small para-aortic pheochromocytoma was excised. She sustained no improvement from removal of the tumor and died in uremia three months later. Catecholamines were normal after operation in this patient and have been in the normal range in each of the other eight patients who have developed hypertension during the follow-up period. In each instance hypertension has been controlled satisfactorily with antihypertensive drugs. Three of these patients are on digitalis preparations and one also has an enlarged heart which has been attributed to catecholamine myocardiopathy. Diabetic glucose tolerance tests which existed before operation in nine patients have reverted to normal in seven after removal of the pheochromocytoma.[132]

Pheochromocytoma can simulate any hypertensive syndrome. Although it is an uncommon cause of high blood pressure, all hypertensives should be screened for the tumor. Follow-up for life is mandatory in all patients with surgically treated pheochromocytoma.

Neuroblastoma

Excepting leukemia and tumors of the central nervous system collectively, neuroblastoma is the most common malignant tumor that occurs in infancy and early childhood. Although it most commonly arises in the adrenal medulla, neuroblastoma can develop from sympathetic tissue anywhere in the body. While it may occur in the brain, it is much more common in structures outside the central nervous sytem. In a group of 217 cases of neuroblastoma, excluding those of the central nervous system, studied by Gross, Farber, and Martin,[60] 40 per cent of the tumors were found to originate in the adrenal, 11 per cent in the thorax, 6 per cent in the pelvis, 5 per cent in retroperitoneal sympathetics, and 2 per cent in the neck. Although neuroblastomas are highly malignant, metastasize early, and have an exceedingly serious prognosis, they are not uniformly fatal. Spontaneous regression of the tumor may rarely occur, and therapeutic efforts have resulted in a number of cures.

Pathology. In the development of the sympathetic nervous system and the adrenal medulla, the precursor cell known as the sympathogon forms the ganglionic anlage. The sympathoblast derives from the ganglion crest and migrates into the visceral areas to form the anlage of the sympathetic nervous system and adrenal medulla, finally differentiating into unipolar and multipolar neuroblasts. Further differentiation produces mature ganglion cells. Neoplasia in this cellular system may produce an extremely primitive tumor which can be designated a sympathogonioma or a sympathoblastoma. Collectively, these malignant tumors are called neuroblastomas. Neoplastic changes in the ganglion cell may produce a benign tumor, the ganglioneuroma, and rarely an intermediate type of tumor that contains both immature and mature ganglion cells and has been called ganglioneuroblastoma. The highly malignant neuroblastoma is much more common than the benign ganglioneuroma.

Grossly, neuroblastoma, whether originating in the adrenal medulla or in the areas of the sympathetic nervous system, usually has a nodular or lobulated surface with a rubbery, firm consistency. The tumors are often grayish-red in color, with a fine vascular network over the surface. Areas of hemorrhagic necrosis are frequent. The neuroblastoma of the adrenal medulla may arise on either side of the vertebral column but has a strong tendency to invade across the midline. The tumor may extend upward and downward in the retroperitoneal plane and up through the diaphragmatic hiatuses in the retropleural plane. It usually grows rapidly to large size. Often the growth will infiltrate adjacent viscera such as the kidney, body of the pancreas, or root of the mesentery. At times the tumor may remain relatively well localized and seemingly encapsulated, but in most instances extensive retroperitoneal invasion occurs early.

Metastasis takes place by lymphatic and blood stream invasion. In addition to regional nodes, there is a predilection for metastasis to the skeletal system, and often extensive replacement of bone marrow occurs. Metastases to the skull and orbits from this tumor were described by Hutchinson in 1907 and came to be known as the Hutchinson syndrome, whereas diffuse invasion of the liver by the tumor was described by Pepper a few years earlier and has in the past been referred to as the Pepper syndrome. These eponymous terms have no longer any real value except for historic interest. Gross points out that the tumor had metastasized by the time the patient was hospitalized in 60 per cent of cases of neuroblastoma observed at Boston Children's Medical Center. Pulmonary metastases tend to occur later in the course of the disease than do those to bone marrow, liver, orbit, and skin.

Microscopically, neuroblastomas are highly cellular tumors consisting of broad sheets of small cells with dark, round nuclei between wide areas of pale fibrillar stroma. Rosette formation is characteristic of many neuroblastomas, with clusters of cells in ringlike formation in the center of which neurofibrils may be demonstrated with phosphotungstic acid-hematoxylin stain. In the less differentiated and more malignant forms of neuroblastoma, the cells are usually a little smaller and often no rosettes or fibrils can be identified. Conversely, in the less malignant and more favorable varieties of the tumor there may be areas in which ganglion cells are present, suggesting that the tumor is a neuroblastoma that is differentiating into a ganglioneuroma. This remarkable although rare tendency of neuroblastoma was first recognized by Cushing and Wolbach.[36]

Clinical Aspects. While neuroblastomas may occur at any age in children, they are most commonly found in infants and very young children. Eighty per cent of reported cases have been observed in the first five years of life. The tumor occurs with equal frequency in boys and girls. Children with adrenal neuroblastomas usually present with a complaint of painless abdominal swelling accompanied by pallor, fatigue, loss of appetite, and often weight loss of several months' duration. All too often the presenting complaints represent manifestations of distant metastases, with the development of headache and vomiting from cerebral metastases, the pain and deformity of a pathologic fracture, or the proptosis of an orbital site of spread.

The principal finding on abdominal examination with adrenal neuroblastoma is the presence of a firm nodular mass occupying one side of the abdomen. Unlike Wilms' tumor, from which adrenal neuroblastoma must always be differentiated, the neuroblastoma is not reniform in shape or smooth in outline. Rather, the neuroblastoma usually presents as a nondescript, nodular, vaguely rounded mass which often does not permit clear delineation of contour on physical examination. Often the tumors are fixed in the flank and do not move with inspiration. There may be a palpable extension of the mass across the midline. Other significant physical findings are apt to be those associated with the metastases of the tumor.

Laboratory studies often show a mild degree of anemia. It is very rare for urinalysis to show any abnormalities. In a very small percentage of cases with invasion of the renal pelvis, hematuria may present. If a profound anemia is present, bone marrow invasion should be suspected, and marrow aspiration may reveal metastatic neuroblastoma. Chemical analysis of 24-hour collections of urine for the metabolites of norepinephrine and its precursors, dopamine and dopa, may show abnormally high levels of homovanillic acid (HVA) and 3-methoxy-4-hydroxymandelic acid (VMA). According to Williams and Greer,[150] most neuroblastomas produce excessive quantities of these compounds.

Roentgenologic Examination. Plain films of the abdomen may show a nonspecific radiopaque mass above a kidney. Calcification can be detected as fine, stippled or flocculent densities in about half of these tumors, being more common in older children than in infants. Intravenous or retrograde pyelography commonly shows displacement of the kidney and deformity of the pelvis, but Gross states that such studies may fail to differentiate with certainty between neuroblastoma, Wilms' tumor, and retroperitoneal teratoma. Hiller of the Royal Children's Hospital in Melbourne has shown that angiography may be helpful in this differentiation.[70]

A skeletal survey and films of the chest are mandatory parts of the evaluation of the patient with suspected neuroblastoma. According to Snyder,[140] skeletal metastases are found at the time of initial examination in about 35 per cent of cases. The preferential sites of bony metastases are the skull, femur, humerus, vertebrae, pelvis, and ribs, in descending order of frequency. The moth-eaten spotty rarefactions of neuroblastoma's bony metastases have a characteristic roentgenographic appearance (Fig. 26). The more extensive lesions tend to be symmetrically distributed.

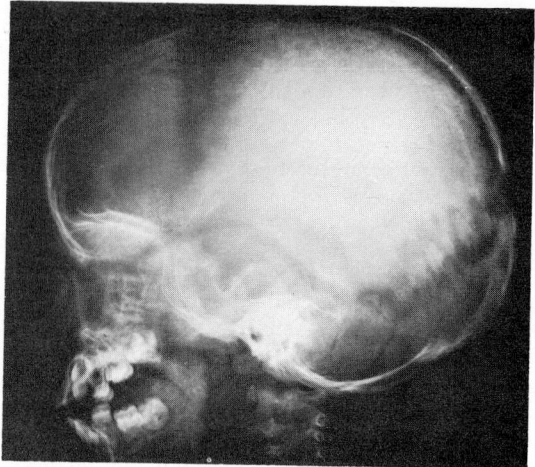

Figure 26. Roentgenogram of child's skull with changes characteristic of neuroblastoma metastatic to brain, skull, and facial bones.

Proliferative bone lesions may occur and at times may produce sclerosing changes in the skull, spine, or pelvis that resemble Paget's disease.

Treatment. Unless contraindicated by extensive metastases, primary treatment of adrenal neuroblastoma in infants and children is always surgical resection of the tumor. During the last three decades, the experience of Ladd and Gross and their associates at Boston Children's Medical Center has demonstrated the value of very radical resection of the lesion and the surrounding tissues invaded by it when it is technically feasible. If total removal of the tumor cannot be safely done, Gross[59, 60] advises that as much of the bulk of the tumor as possible be resected. In either case, whether total or subtotal resection has been possible, postoperative radiation therapy should be used.

The surgical approach most commonly used is a long, transverse, supraumbilical abdominal incision which is extended into the loin on the side of the lesion; occasionally, an extension of the incision across the costal margins into a lower interspace is needed to provide optimal exposure. In assessing the resectability of the tumor, the surgeon should look for metastases in liver and other abdominal viscera and should inspect and palpate the posterior and medial attachments of the lesion. Because of the close proximity and early invasion of the renal capsule and kidney, the resection usually involves removal of the kidney with the tumor. Accordingly, assurance of the functional integrity of the contralateral kidney is always in order. As with the operation for Wilms' tumor of the kidney, early ligation of the hilar vessels is desirable before extensive operative manipulation of the tumor. Unless the lesion has metastasized or invaded diffusely, radical surgical removal of the contents of the renal fossa is indicated. On the left side, large tumors may compromise the splenic vessels and the tail of the pancreas, often necessitating resection of the tail of the pancreas and spleen with the kidney and tumor (Fig. 27). On the right side, invasion in and around the vena

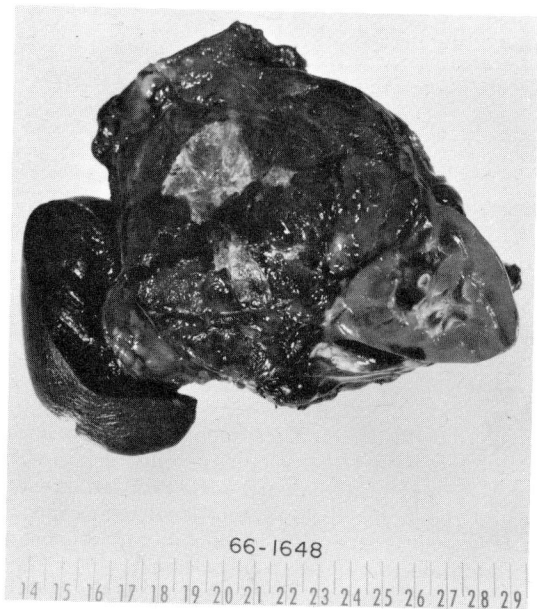

66-1648

14 15 16 17 18 19 20 21 22 23 24 25 26 27 28 29

Figure 27. Photograph of gross specimen removed at operation from two-year-old child with left adrenal neuroblastoma involving kidney, spleen, and tail of pancreas.

cava may prevent complete removal of the lesion. Unless the tumor is so friable, necrotic, and vascular that it cannot be resected with safety, subtotal removal of a diffusely invasive tumor can be accomplished by dividing the tumor tissue lateral to the great vessels between clamps. The residual tumor should be outlined by clips to aid the roentgenologist in postoperative radiotherapy.

Most neuroblastomas are radiosensitive, and to date the best results have occurred when the combination of surgical resection and radiotherapy has been used. At Boston Children's Medical Center, Gross, Neuhauser, and Wittenborg[152] for years began radiotherapy on the day of operative removal of the neuroblastoma. In Gross' large series there were no significant wound complications from early postoperative irradiation with air doses to the skin of 1400 to 1800 R in 7 to 10 days. Many radiologists advise a second comparable series in 3 months.

Radiotherapy of individual metastatic sites in skin or bone may provide transitory palliative relief of pain and parental anxiety, but unfortunately, in most instances not much more. Widespread metastases to skin or skeleton cannot be safely treated with "spray" x-ray therapy because of the depressant effect of extensive radiation on the hematopoietic system. Complications of radiation therapy in these tumors must be equated with the theoretically curative potential of such postoperative therapy. In general, with widespread skeletal metastases, radiotherapy has very little to offer, and the prognosis after radiation in widespread osseous lesions is uniformly bad.

Chemotherapy has proved to be increasingly valuable in treatment of disseminated neuroblastoma and as an adjunct to surgical resection. Farber and his as-

sociates[45] initiated the use of treatment with nitrogen mustard and folic acid antagonists as early as 1951 and have subsequently observed remission or objective regression of extensive tumor in sporadic cases with a variety of other chemotherapeutic agents. Bodian[14] has had enthusiasm for vitamin B_{12} in large doses. However, none of the many agents that have been used has proved to be consistently effective.

Two of the more promising newer drugs that have been tried in treatment of neuroblastoma are the alkylating agent cyclophosphamide and the alkaloid vincristine sulfate. Transitory objective tumor regression has been reported in fewer than half of children with neuroblastoma who have received one or the other of these drugs. However, the combination of the two drugs was reported by James and his associates[77] to provide objective tumor regression in each of nine children with unresectable neuroblastomas, and "complete remission" for periods as long as 12 to 26 months in seven of the group. In two of these youngsters with this treatment, subsequent complete surgical excision of the primary tumor was accomplished.

Results and Prognosis. Despite the lethal potential and continued high fatality rate of neuroblastoma, patients with this malignant neoplasm have shown an increased number of favorable responses to treatment in the last two decades. As pointed out by Gross, Farber, and Martin,[60] prior to 1930 neuroblastoma was considered a hopeless condition; with no effort to treat it, there were no cures. As surgeons and radiologists mounted a combined attack on the problem in the period of 1930 to 1950, a few cures began to appear. In the period since 1950, with an aggressive approach to the tumor, combining surgery, radiotherapy, and chemotherapy, the cure rate has definitely increased. At Memorial Hospital for Cancer and Allied Disease in New York, Dargeon[38] found 28 long-range survivors in 236 cases of neuroblastoma (12 per cent). During a similar period of time at Vanderbilt, there are 7 long-term survivors in a series of 44 patients (15 per cent). By 1959 Gross and his associates were able to report a cure rate of 36.7 per cent for all patients with the tumor who entered the Boston Children's Medical Center during the period 1950 to 1957. Judgment of response to therapy, however, must take cognizance of spontaneous regression of the tumor. In 1964 Everson[44] collected a total of 28 well-documented cases of complete spontaneous regression of neuroblastoma with prolonged survival.

Other factors that apparently influence response to treatment include age of patient and location of tumor and its metastases, as well as type of treatment used. Gross reports that in those cases in which there are no demonstrable metastases and the treatment has consisted of total excision of the tumor followed by local x-ray therapy, a cure rate of 88 per cent has been obtained. Babies under a year of age have had the best response to treatment. In those cases in which total removal of the tumor has not been possible, partial surgical removal followed by radiation and tumor chemotherapy has provided a cure rate as high as 64 per cent. Unfortunately, if skeletal metastases are present, few cures have been observed, even with the most aggressive therapy. However, recent reports of

TABLE 20.   Comparison of Duration of Response*
(Patients with Advanced Carcinoma of the Breast)

	6 Mos.		12 Mos.		18 Mos.		24 Mos.	
	No.	Per Cent	No.	Per Cent	No.	Per Cent	No.	Per Cent
Hypophysectomy, 203 patients	68	33.4	50	24.6	32	15.7	25	12.3
Adrenalectomy or combined oophorectomy and adrenalectomy, 500 patients	177	35.4	92	18.4	59	11.8	30	6

*From Fracchia, A. A., et al.: Surg. Gynecol. Obstet., *133*:241, 1971. By permission of Surgery, Gynecology & Obstetrics.

James and his associates on the remarkable responses to the combination of cyclophosphamide and vincristine, both with and without surgery and radiation, bring a further note of optimism.

ADRENALECTOMY IN TREATMENT OF METASTATIC CANCER OF PROSTATE AND BREAST

Bilateral total adrenalectomy for advanced disseminated carcinoma was first employed by Huggins and Scott[74] for prostatic cancer in 1945. The surgical risk was high, and the postoperative maintenance of their early patients was very difficult, since the patients were operated on before the advent of cortisone and its facilitation of substitution therapy after total adrenalectomy. In 1951 Huggins and Bergenstal[73] described bilateral total adrenalectomy for metastatic carcinoma of the breast. The theoretical basis for the operation in patients with these "endocrine-dependent" cancers was the fact of the common embryonic origin of the gonads and the adrenal cortex and the belief that these were the only endocrine organs that have the capacity to synthesize androgenous steroid hormonal substances.

No very large series of patients with disseminated prostatic cancer treated by adrenalectomy has been reported, but the current feelings of urologists are well summarized by Fergusson,[46] who believes that a previous response to orchiectomy and antiandrogen therapy increases the potential for response to bilateral total adrenalectomy; however, the low rate of response and the short duration of remission in those who do respond make the value of adrenalectomy in advanced prostatic cancer extremely limited. The greater value of hypophysectomy in this disease has been previously discussed.

Several large series of patients with advanced breast cancer treated by bilateral total adrenalectomy attest to the value of adrenalectomy in selected patients. A comparison of the responses of women with advanced breast cancer to adrenalectomy (alone or combined with oophorectomy) and to hypophysectomy in the study reported by Fracchia et al.[49] is shown in Table 20. Both hypophysectomy and adrenalectomy are useful palliative procedures in selected patients. As seen in the table, at the 6 month level, adrenalectomy appears to have a slightly better response rate,

whereas the 12, 18, and 24 month remissions are slightly higher in the hypophysectomy series. The longer the free interval between the initial mastectomy and the first appearance of local recurrence or metastasis, the greater the likelihood of a response to either adrenalectomy or hypophysectomy.

Criteria for adrenalectomy in metastatic breast cancer include a free interval of two years or more, a previous response to therapeutic oophorectomy or irradiation castration in premenopausal women or an abnormally high vaginal smear index in postmenopausal women, and presence of estrogen receptors in metastatic tissue. If an estrogen receptor can be identified, the likelihood of a beneficial response to adrenalectomy or hypophysectomy is reported to be about 50 per cent. In Fracchia's study, the poorest responses were in patients with metastases to the central nervous system, nodular pulmonary and pleural lesions, jaundice, myelophthisic anemia, and hypercalcemia. The highest remission rate was noted in patients in whom the disease did not affect vital areas, but was limited to soft tissue and bone without evidence of hypercalcemia.

SELECTED REFERENCES

Addision, T.: Disease of suprarenal capsules. London Med. Gaz., *43*:517, 1849.
  This is the original classic description of the syndrome of adrenal insufficiency subsequently named after its illustrious author. The superb clinical description has never been excelled.

Conn, J. W.: Primary aldosteronism: A new clinical syndrome. J. Lab. Clin. Med., *45*:6, 1955.
  In a presidential address this leading endocrinologist describes the physiology, physiopathology, and clinical manifestations of mineralocorticoid excess due to adenoma or hyperplasia of the glomerulosa cells of the adrenal cortex. The syndrome now bears his name.

Cushing, H.: The basophil adenomas of the pituitary body and their clinical manifestations (pituitary basophilism). Bull. Johns Hopkins Hosp., *50*:137, 1932.
  This is the classic description by the late great neurosurgeon and surgical physiologist, Harvey Cushing, of the disease that has come to bear his name. This article stimulated great interest in the endocrine disturbance and promoted intensive investigation by endocrinologists and biologists of its etiology and pathogenesis.

Eisenstein, A. B. (Ed.): The Adrenal Cortex. Boston, Little, Brown and Company, 1967.
  This book has 26 contributing authors who are expert in their

areas of discussion. It is an in-depth treatment of the subject and an excellent reference work.

Liddle, G. W.: Tests of pituitary-adrenal suppressibility in the diagnosis of Cushing's syndrome. J. Clin. Endocrinol., *20*:1539, 1960.
This important report by an endocrinologic expert demonstrates how knowledge of adrenocorticotropin and cortisol relationships can lead to specific clinical diagnosis in patients suspected of having Cushing's syndrome; further, it establishes the basis for differentiating the several causes of the syndrome.

Netter, F. H.: The Ciba Collection of Medical Illustrations. Volume 4, Endocrine System and Selected Metabolic Diseases. Summit, N. J., Ciba Pharmaceutical Company, 1965.
This volume contains 222 full color plates painted by a superb medical artist. Dr. Netter depicts in his graphic and vivid anatomic style the anatomy, physiology, and pathophysiology of the endocrine system and a selection of metabolic diseases. The text accompanying Dr. Netter's sketches has been contributed by a group of authorities. It summarizes the fundamental physiology and physiopathology with an emphasis on clinical manifestations of the endocrinopathies and metabolic derangements.

Robison, G. A., Butcher, R. W., and Sutherland, E. W.: Cyclic AMP, New York, Academic Press, 1971.
In this book, Dr. Sutherland, distinguished Nobel laureate, tells how cyclic AMP was discovered. He and his collaborators present a profound discussion of the current knowledge of hormones and their cellular action with a critical review of present knowledge of the many roles of cyclic AMP in biologic processes. The book contains over 1500 references, more than half the papers published since 1968.

Wilkins, L.: The Diagnosis and Treatment of Endocrine Disorders in Childhood and Adolescence, 3rd ed. Springfield, Ill, Charles C Thomas, Publisher, 1966.
This is one of the classics of endocrinology and provides a rich source of reference and clinical experience with endocrinopathies in the pediatric age group.

Wilkins, L., Lewis, R. A., Cline, R., and Rosenberg, E.: The suppression of androgen excretion by cortisone in a case of congenital adrenal hyperplasia. Bull. Johns Hopkins Hosp., *86*:249, 1950.
This is a landmark report by this great pediatric endocrinologist and his colleagues of the clinical use of cortisone as a means of suppressing pituitary function and adrenocortical hyperplasia. This concept of therapy opened a new area of investigation and treatment of endocrinopathies.

Williams, R. H. (Ed.): Textbook of Endocrinology, 5th ed. Philadelphia, W. B. Saunders Company, 1974.
This superb textbook, edited by a leading endocrinologist, contains chapters on each organ system by experts in the field. It is a rich source of fundamental physiology, biochemistry, and pathology as applied to the normal and abnormal functions of the endocrine system correlated with clinical manifestations.

REFERENCES

1. Addison, T.: Disease of suprarenal capsules. London Med. Gaz., *43*:517, 1849.
2. Ahlquist, R. P.: A study of adrenotropic receptors. Am. J. Physiol., *153*:586, 1948.
3. Aird, I.: Bilateral anterior transabdominal adrenalectomy. Br. Med. J., *2*:708, 1955.
4. Albright, F., Parson, W., and Bloomberg, E.: Therapy in Cushing's syndrome. J. Clin. Endocrinol., *1*:375, 1941.
5. Anderson, B. G., Beierwaltes, W. H., Harrison, T. S., Ansari, A. N., and Buswick, A. A.: Labelled dopamine concentration in pheochromocytoma. J. Nucl. Med., *14*:781, 1973.
6. Anderson, E., Haymaker, W., and Joseph, M.: Hormonal and electrolyte studies of patients with hyperadrenocortical syndrome (Cushing's syndrome). Endocrinology, *23*:398, 1938.
7. Apgar, V., and Papper, E. M.: Pheochromocytoma—anesthetic management during surgical treatment. Arch. Surg., *62*:634, 1951.
8. Ballard, H. S., Frame, B., and Hartsock, R. J.: Familial multiple endocrine adenoma-peptic ulcer complex. Medicine, *43*:481, 1964.
9. Barbeau, A., et al.: Le phéochromocytome bilateral: présentation du'un cas et revue de la littérature. Un. Med. Can., *87*:165, 1958.
10. Baulieu, E. E., Peillon, F., and Migeon, C. J.: Adrenogenital syndrome. *In* Eisenstein, A. B. (Ed.): The Adrenal Cortex. Boston, Little, Brown and Company, 1967, p. 601.
11. Bergenstal, D. M., Hertz, R., Lipsett, M. B., and Moy, R. H.: Chemotherapy of adrenocortical cancer with o,p' DDD. Ann. Intern. Med., *53*:672, 1960.
12. Binger, M. W., and Craig, W. M.: Atypical case of hypertension with tumor of adrenal gland. Proc. Mayo Clin., *13*:17, 1938.
13. Bliss, E. L., Sandberg, A. A., Nelson, D. H., and Eik-Nes, K.: The normal level of 17-hydroxycorticosteroids in the peripheral blood of man. J. Clin. Invest., *32*:818, 1953.
14. Bodian, M.: Neuroblastoma. Pediatr. Clin. North Am., *6*:449, 1959.
15. Boucher, R., et al.: New procedures for measurment of human plasma angiotensin and renin activity levels. Can. Med. Assoc. J., *90*:194, 1964.
16. Bovie, W. T.: Electro-surgery as an aid to the removal of intracranial tumors: With a preliminary note on a new surgical-current generator. Surg. Gynecol. Obstet., *47*:751, 1928.
17. Brown-Sequard, C. E.: Arch. Gen. Med., *8*:385, 1856. Cited by Olmstead, J. M. D.: Charles-Edouard Brown-Sequard. Baltimore, Johns Hopkins Press, 1946. p. 91.
18. Cahill, G. F.: Hormonal tumors of the adrenal. Surgery, *16*:233, 1944.
19. Carelli, M. D.: Sur le pneumopéritoine et sur une méthode personelle pour voir le rein sans pneumopéritoine. Bull. Soc. Med. Hop. Paris, *45*:1409, 1921.
20. Childs, B., Grumbach, M. M., and Van Wyk, J. J.: Virilizing adrenal hyperplasia: A genetic and hormonal study. J. Clin. Invest., *35*:213, 1956.
21. Chong, G. C., ReMine, W. H., Van Heerden, J. A., Sheps, S. G., and Harrison, E.: Current management of pheochromocytoma. Ann. Surg., *179*:740, 1974.
22. Conn, J. W.: Aldosteronism in hypertensive disease. Med. Times, *98*:116, 1970.
23. Conn, J. W.: Primary aldosteronism: A new clinical syndrome. J. Lab. Clin. Med., *45*:6, 1955.
24. Conn, J. W.: Evolution of primary aldosteronism as a highly specific clinical entity. J.A.M.A., *172*:1650, 1960.
25. Conn, J. W., Cohen, E. L. Rovner, D. R., and Nesbit, R. M.: Normokalemic primary aldosteronism. J.A.M.A., *193*:101, 1965.
26. Cope, C. L., and Pearson, J.: Clinical value of the cortisol secretion rate. J. Clin. Pathol., *18*:82, 1965.
27. Coppage, W. S., Island, D. P., Conner, A. E., and Liddle, G. W.: The metabolism of aldosterone in normal subjects and in patients with hepatic cirrhosis. J. Clin. Invest., *41*:1672, 1962.
28. Crowder, R. E.: Development of the adrenal gland in man with special reference to origin and all of the locations, cell types, and evidence in favor of cell migration (theory). Contrib. Embryol., *36*:193, 1957.
29. Cushing, H.: Sexual infantilism with optic atrophy in cases of tumor affecting the hypophysis cerebri. J. Nerv. Ment. Dis., *33*:704, 1906.
30. Cushing, H.: The hypophysis cerebri—clinical aspects of hyperpituitarism and of hypopituitarism. J.A.M.A., *53*:249, 1909.
31. Cushing, H.: Partial hypophysectomy for acromegaly with remarks on the function of the hypophysis. Ann. Surg., *50*:1002, 1909.
32. Cushing, H.: The function of the pituitary body. Am. J. Med. Sci., *139*:473, 1910.
33. Cushing, H.: The control of bleeding in operations for brain tumors, with the description of silver clips for the occlusion of vessels inaccessible to the ligature. Ann. Surg., *54*:1, 1911.
34. Cushing, H.: The Pituitary Body and Its Disorders. Philadelphia, J. B. Lippincott Company, 1912.
35. Cushing, H.: The basophil adenomas of the pituitary body and their clinical manifestations. Bull. Johns Hopkins Hosp., *50*:137, 1932.
36. Cushing, H., and Wolbach, S. B.: The transformation of a malignant paravertebral sympathicoblastoma into a benign ganglioneuroma. Am. J. Pathol., *3*:203, 1927.
37. Dandy, W. E.: Selected Writings of Walter E. Dandy. Springfield, Ill., Charles C Thomas, Publisher, 1957.
38. Dargeon, H. W.: Neuroblastoma. J. Pediatr., *61*:456, 1962.
39. Daughaday, W. H.: The adenohypophysis. *In* Williams, R. H. (Ed.): Textbook of Endocrinology, 5th ed. Philadelphia, W. B. Saunders Company, 1974.

40. Davis, J. O.: The regulation of aldosterone secretion. In Eisenstein, A. B. (Ed.): The Adrenal Cortex. Boston. Little, Brown and Company, 1967, p. 203.
41. Du Vigneaud, V.: Hormones of the posterior pituitary gland: Oxytocin and vasopressin. Harvey Lect., 50:1, 1954–1955.
42. Egdahl, R. H., and Melby, J. C.: Recurrent Cushing's disease and intermittent functional adrenal cortical insufficiency following subtotal adrenalectomy. Ann. Surg., 166:586, 1967.
43. Elkington, S. G.: Pituitary adenoma: Preoperative symptomatology in a series of 260 patients. Br. J. Ophthalmol., 52:322, 1968.
44. Everson, T. C.: Spontaneous regression of cancer. Ann. N. Y. Acad. Sci., 114:721, 1964.
45. Farber, S., and Toch, R.: Chemotherapy of disseminated neuroblastoma in children. Am. J. Dis. Child., 82:239, 1951.
46. Fergusson, J. D.: Endocrine-control therapy in prostatic cancer. Br. J. Urol., 30:397, 1958.
47. Field, R. A.: Hypophysectomy in diabetic retinopathy. In Astwood, E. B., and Cassidy, C. E. (Eds.): Clinical Endocrinology II. New York. Grune and Stratton, 1968.
48. Forsham, P. H.: The adrenals. In Williams, R. H. (Ed.): Textbook of Endocrinology, 4th ed. Philadelphia, W. B. Saunders Company, 1974.
49. Fracchia, A. A., Farrow, J. H., Miller, T. R., Tollefson, R. H., Greenberg, E. J., and Knapper, W. H.: Hypophysectomy as compared with adrenalectomy in the treatment of advanced carcinoma of the breast. Surg. Gynecol. Obstet., 133:241, 1971.
50. Frankel, F.: Ein Fall von doppelseitigen, vollig latent verlaufenen Nebennierentumor und gleichzeitiger Nephritis mit Veranderungen am Circulations-apparat und Retinitis. Arch. Pathol. Anat., 103:244, 1886.
51. Fraser, R., Joplin, G. F., and Steiner, R. E.: Pituitary ablation with Y90 implants for diabetic retinopathy. Diabetes, 11:482, 1962.
52. Fraser, T. R., and Wright, A. D.: Treatment of acromegaly and Cushing's disease by Y90 implant for partial ablation of the pituitary. In Astwood, E. B., and Cassidy, C. E. (Eds.): Clinical Endocrinology II. New York, Grune and Stratton, 1968, p. 78.
53. Frawley, T. F.: Adrenal cortical insufficiency. In Eisenstein, A. B. (Ed.): The Adrenal Cortex. Boston, Little, Brown and Company, 1967, p. 439.
54. Goldberg, M. F., and Fine, S. I. (Eds.): Symposium on the Treatment of Diabetic Retinopathy. U. S. Department of Health, Education and Welfare. Public Health Service Publication No. 1890. Washington, U. S. Government Printing Office, 1968.
55. Goldenberg, M., et al.: Pheochromocytoma and essential hypertensive vascular disease. Arch. Intern. Med., 86:823, 1950.
56. Goodall, M. C., and Stone, C.: Adrenaline and noradrenaline producing tumors of the adrenal medulla and sympathic nerves. Ann. Surg., 151:244, 1960.
57. Gordon, R. D., Fishman, L. M., and Liddle, G. W.: Plasma renin activity and aldosterone secretion in a pregnant woman with primary aldosteronism. J. Clin. Endocrinol., 27:385, 1967.
58. Graham, J. B.: Pheochromocytoma and hypertension. Surg. Gynecol. Obstet., 92:105, 1951.
59. Gross, R. E.: The Surgery of Infancy and Childhood. Philadelphia, W. B. Saunders Company, 1953, p. 616.
60. Gross, R. E., Farber, S., and Martin, L. W.: Neuroblastoma sympatheticum. Pediatrics, 23:1179, 1959.
61. Grundy, H. M., Simpson, S. A., and Tait, J. F.: Isolation of highly active mineralocorticoid from beef adrenal extract. Nature, 169:795, 1952.
62. Guyton, A. C.: Textbook of Medical Physiology, 5th ed. Philadelphia, W. B. Saunders Company, 1976.
63. Hamberger, C. A., Hammer, G., Norlen, G., and Sjögren, B.: Hypophysectomy in acromegaly. J. Clin. Endocrinol., 19:1500, 1959.
64. Hardy, J.: Transsphenoidal hypophysectomy. J. Neurosurg., 34:582, 1971.
65. Hardy, J.: Transsphenoidal surgery of hypersecreting pituitary tumors. Int. Congress Series No. 303. Diagnosis and treatment of pituitary tumors. Proceedings of a conference held in Bethesda, Md., USA, January, 15–17, 1973. Amsterdam, Excerpta Medica.
66. Harper, P. V., Strandjord, N., and Paloyan, E., et al.: Destruction

of the hypophysis with a Sr90-Y90 needle. Ann. Surg., 160:743, 1964.
67. Harrison, T. S., Gann, D. S., Edis, A. J., and Egdahl, R. H.: Surgical disorders of the adrenal gland: Physiologic background and treatment. New York, Grune and Stratton, 1975.
68. Hayes, M., and Goldenberg, I. S.: Operative treatment of adrenal cortical hyperfunctionary diseases. Ann. Surg., 154:33, 1961.
69. Heeg, M. M.: Urological spectrum of adrenal surgery. J. Urol., 96:427, 1966.
70. Hiller, H.: Personal communication.
71. Holton, P.: Noradrenaline in adrenal medullary tumors. Nature, 163:217, 1949.
72. Holtz, P., Credner, K., and Kroneberg, G.: Ueber das sympathicomimetische pressorische Prinzip des Harns ("Urosympathin"). Arch. Exp. Pathol. Pharmakol., 204:224, 1947.
73. Huggins, C. B., and Bergenstal, D. M.: Surgery of the adrenals. J.A.M.A., 147:101, 1951.
74. Huggins, C. B., and Scott, W. W.: Bilateral adrenalectomy in prostatic cancer. Ann. Surg., 122:1031, 1945.
75. Hume, D. M.: Pheochromocytoma in the adult and in the child. Am. J. Surg., 99:458, 1960.
76. Ingraham, F. D., and Scott, H. W., Jr.: Craniopharyngiomas in children. J. Pediatr., 29:95, 1946.
77. James, D. H., Hustu, O., Wrenn, E. L., Jr., and Pinkel, D.: Combination chemotherapy of childhood neuroblastoma. J.A.M.A., 194:123, 1965.
78. Jarvis, L., Jenkins, D., Sosman, M., and Thorn, G.: Roentgenologic observations in Addison's disease. Radiology, 62:16, 1954.
79. Kahnt, F. W., and Neher, R.: Adrenal steroid biosynthesis in vitro. Helv. Chim. Acta., 49:725, 1966.
80. Kendall, E. C.: The chemistry and partial synthesis of adrenal steroids. Ann. N. Y. Acad. Sci., 50:540, 1949.
81. Kliman, B., and Peterson, R. E.: Double isotope derivative assay of aldosterone in biological extracts. J. Biol. Chem., 235:1639, 1960.
82. Kvale, W. F., et al.: Present-day diagnosis and treatment of pheochromocytoma. J.A.M.A., 164:854, 1957.
83. Labbe, M., Tinel, J., and Doumer, A.: Crises solaires et hypertension paroxystique en rapport avec une tumeur surrénale. Bull. Soc. Med. Hop. Paris, 46:982, 1922.
84. Laidlaw, J. C., Reddy, W. J., Jenkins, D., Haydar, N. Abu, Renold, A. E., and Thorn, G. W.: Advances in the diagnosis of altered states of adrenocortical function. N. Engl. J. Med., 253:747, 1955.
85. Leaf, A., and Coggins, C. H.: The neurohypophysis. In Williams, R. H. (Ed.): Textbook of Endocrinology. 5th ed. Philadelphia, W. B. Saunders Company, 1974.
86. Lerner, A. B., and McQuire, J. S.: Melanocyte stimulating hormone and adrenocorticotrophic hormone. N. Engl. J. Med., 270:539, 1964.
87. Liddle, G. W.: Tests of pituitary-adrenal suppressibility in the diagnosis of Cushing's syndrome. J. Clin. Endocrinol., 20:1539, 1960.
88. Liddle, G. W.: Cushing's syndrome. In Eisenstein, A. B. (Ed.): The Adrenal Cortex. Boston, Little, Brown and Company, 1967, p. 543.
89. Liddle, G. W.: Management of aldosteronism. Am. J. Clin. Pathol., 54:331, 1970.
90. Liddle, G. W., Estep, H. L., Kendall, J. W., Jr., Williams, W. C., Jr., and Townes, A. W.: Clinical application of a new test of pituitary reserve. J. Clin. Endocrinol., 29:875, 1959.
91. Liddle, G. W., and Melmon, K. L.: The adrenals. In Williams, R. H. (Ed.): Textbook of Endocrinology, 5th ed. Philadelphia, W. B. Saunders Company, 1974.
92. Liddle, G. W., Nicholson, W. E., Island, D. P., et al.: Clinical and laboratory studies of ectopic humoral syndromes. Recent Progr. Hormone Res., 25:283, 1969.
93. Lieberman, L. M., Beierwaltes, W. H., Conn, J. W., et al.: Diagnosis of adrenal diseases by visualization of human adrenal glands with 131I-19-iodocholesterol. N. Engl. J. Med., 185:1387, 1971.
94. Longino, F. H., et al.: Effects of a new quaternary amine and a new imidazole derivative on the autonomic nervous system. Surgery, 26:421, 1949.
95. Luft, R., and Olivecrona, H.: Hypophysectomy in man: Experience in severe diabetes mellitus. J. Clin. Endocrinol., 15:391, 1955.

96. Luft, R., Olivecrona, H., and Sjögren, B.: Hypopfysektomi pa manniska. Nord. Med., 47:351, 1952.

97. Lundbaek, K., Malmros, R., Andersen, H. C., Rasmussen, J. H., Bruntse, E., Poul, H. M., and Jensen, V. A.: Hypophysectomy for diabetic angiopathy: A controlled clinical trial. In Goldberg, M. F., and Fine, S. L. (Eds.): Symposium on Treatment of Diabetic Retinopathy. U. S. Department of Health, Education and Welfare. Public Health Service Publication No. 1890. Washington, D.C., U. S. Government Printing Office, 1968.

98. Mahoney, E. M.: Localization of (adrenal and extra-adrenal) pheochromocytomas by vena caval blood sampling. Surg. Forum, 14:405, 1963.

99. Marie, P.: Sur deux cas d'acroméglie. Rev. Med., 6:297, 1886.

100. Mayo, C. H.: Paroxysmal hypertension with tumor of retroperitoneal nerve. J.A.M.A., 89:1047, 1927.

101. Meador, C. K., Liddle, G. W., Island, D. P., Nicholson, W. E., Lucas, C. P., Nuckton, J. G., and Luetscher, J. A.: Cause of Cushing's syndrome in patients with tumors arising from "nonendocrine" tissue. J. Clin. Endocrinol., 22:693, 1962.

102. Murphy, G. P., Reynoso, G., Schoonees, R., Gailani, S., Bourke, R., Kenny, G. M., Mirand, E. A., and Schalch, D. S.: Hypophysectomy and adrenalectomy for disseminated prostatic carcinoma. J. Urol., 105:817, 1971.

103. Nelson, D. H., and Sprunt, J. G.: Pituitary tumors postadrenalectomy for Cushing's syndrome. Proceedings of the International Congress of Endocrinology, 2nd. London. 1964. International Congress Series, No. 3, 1965.

104. Netter, F. H.: The Ciba Collection of Medical Illustrations. Volume 4. Endocrine Systems. Summit, N. J., Ciba Pharmaceutical Company, 1965.

105. Oakley, N. W., Jopkin, G. F., Kohner, E. M., and Fraser, T. R.: The treatment of diabetic retinopathy by pituitary implantation of radioactive yttrium. In Goldberg, M. F., and Fine, S. L. (Eds.): Symposium on Treatment of Diabetic Retinopathy. U. S. Department of Health, Education and Welfare, Public Health Service Publication No. 1890. Washington, D.C. U. S. Government Printing Office, 1968.

106. O'Neal, L. W.: Surgery of the Adrenal Glands. St. Louis, The C. V. Mosby Company, 1968.

107. Orth, D. N., and Liddle, G. W.: Results of treatment in 108 patients with Cushing's syndrome. N. Engl. J. Med., 285:243, 1974.

108. Palmer, R. S., and Castleman, B.: Paraganglioma of adrenal gland stimulating malignant hypertension. Report of a case. N. Engl. J. Med., 219:793, 1938.

109. Pearse, A. G. E.: The cytochemistry and ultrastructure of polypeptide hormone producing cells of the APUD series and their embryologic physiologic and pathologic implications of the concept. J. Histochem. Cytochem., 17:303, 1969.

110. Perkoff, G. I., Eik-nes, K., Nugent, C. A., Fred, H. L., Nimer, R. A., Rush, L., Samuels, L. T., and Tyler, F. H.: Studies of the diurnal variation of plasma 17-hydroxycorticosteroids. J. Clin. Endocrinol., 19:432, 1959.

111. Pick, L.: Das Ganglioma embryonale sympathicium. Klin. Wochenschr., 19:16, 1912.

112. Pincoffs, M. C.: A case of paroxysmal hypertension associated with suprarenal tumor. Trans. Assoc. Am. Physicians, 44:295, 1929.

113. Poulsen, J. E.: The Houssay phenomenon in man: Recovery from retinopathy in a case of diabetes with Simmonds' disease. Diabetes, 2:7, 1953.

114. Poulsen, J. E.: Diabetes and anterior pituitary insufficiency. Final course and postmortem study of a diabetic patient with Sheehan's syndrome. Diabetics, 15:73, 1966.

115. Rabin, C. B.: Chromaffin cell tumor of suprarenal medulla. Arch. Pathol., 7:228, 1929.

116. Rand, R. W., Dashe, A. M., Paglia, D. E., Conway, L. W., and Solomon, D. H.: Stereotactic cryohypophysectomy. J.A.M.A., 189:255, 1964.

117. Rasmussen, H.: Organization and control of endocrine systems. In Williams, R. H. (Ed.): Textbook of Endocrinology, 5th ed. Philadelphia, W. B. Saunders Company, 1974.

118. Ray, B. S.: Some inferences from hypophysectomy on four hundred and fifty human patients. Arch. Neurol., 3:121, 1960.

119. Ray, B. S., Horwith, M., and Mantalen, C.: Surgical hypophysectomy as a treatment for acromegaly. In Astwood, E. B., and Cassidy, C. E. (Ed.): Clinical Endocrinology II. New York, Grune and Stratton, 1968.

120. Ray, B. S., and Pearson, O. H.: Hypophysectomy in treatment of disseminated breast cancer. Surg. Clin. North Am., 42:419, 1962.

121. Reichstein, T., and Shopper, C. W.: The hormones of the adrenal cortex. Vitamins Hormones, 1:345, 1943.

122. Renold, A. E., Jenkins, D., Forsham, P. H., and Thorn, G. W.: The use of intravenous ACTH: A study of quantitative adrenocortical stimulation. J. Clin. Endocrinol., 12:763, 1952.

123. Robison, G. A., Butcher, R. W., and Sutherland, E. W.: Cyclic AMP, New York, Academic Press, 1971.

124. Roth, G. M., and Kvale, W. F.: Tentative test for pheochromocytoma. Am. J. Med. Sci., 210:653, 1945.

125. Roux, C.: Cited by Barbeau, A., et al.[9]

126. Schloffer, H.: Erfolgreiche Operation eines Hypophysentumors auf nasalem Wege. Wein. Klin. Wochenschr., 20:621, 1907.

127. Schwartz, W. B., Bennett, W., Curelop, S., and Bartter, F. C.: A syndrome of renal sodium loss and hyponatremia, probably resulting from inappropriate secretion of antidiuretic hormone. Am. J. Med., 23:529, 1957.

128. Schwyzer and Sieber. Quoted by Daughaday, W. H.: The adenohypophysis. In Williams, R. H. (Ed.): Textbook of Endocrinology, 5th ed. Philadelphia, W. B. Saunders Company, 1974.

129. Scott, H. W., Jr., Foster, J, H., Liddle, G. W., and Davidson, E. T.: Cushing's syndrome due to adrenocortical tumor. Ann. Surg., 162:505, 1965.

130. Scott, H. W., Jr., Foster, J. H., Rhamy, R. K., Klatte, F., and Liddle, G. W.: Surgical management of adrenocortical tumors with Cushing's syndrome. Ann. Surg., 173:892, 1971.

131. Scott, H. W., Jr., Liddle, G. W., Mulherin, J. L., McKenna, T. J., Stroup, S. L., and Rhamy, R. K.: Surgical experience with Cushing's disease. Ann. Surg., in press.

132. Scott, H. W., Jr., Oates, J. A., Nies, A. S., Burko, H., Page, D. L., and Rhamy, R. K.: Pheochromocytoma: Present diagnosis and management. Ann Surg., 183:587, 1976.

133. Scott, H. W., Jr., Riddell, D. H., and Brockman, S. K.: Surgical management of pheochromocytoma. Surg. Gynecol. Obstet., 120:707, 1965.

134. Scott, W. W.: Endocrine management of disseminated prostatic cancer including bilateral adrenalectomy and hypophysectomy. Trans. Am. Assoc. Genitourin. Surg., 44:101, 1952.

135. Scott, W. W., and Schirmer, H. K. A.: Hypophysectomy for disseminated prostatic cancer. In Boyland, E., et al.: On Cancer and Hormones. Chicago, University of Chicago Press, 1962.

136. Sheehan, H. L., and Summers, V. K.: The syndrome of hypopituitarism. Q. J. Med., 18:319, 1949.

137. Sheppard: Quoted by Daughaday, W. H.: The adenohypophysis. In Williams, R. H. (Ed.): Textbook of Endocrinology, 5th ed. Philadelphia, W. B. Saunders Company, 1974.

138. Simmonds, M.: Ueber Hypophysisschwund mit todlichen Ausgang. Dtsch. Med. Wochenschr., 40:322, 1914.

139. Smith, E. J. R., Gurling, K. J., and Baron, D. N.: The effect of hypophysectomy in advanced carcinoma of the prostate. Br. J. Urol., 31:181, 1959.

140. Snyder, W. H., Jr., et al.: Retroperitoneal tumors in infants and children: Report of 88 cases. A.M.A. Arch. Surg., 63:26, 1951.

141. Sweet, W. H., and Field, R. A.: Production of hypopituitarism in the treatment of diabetes. In Goldberg, M. F., and Fine, S. L. (Eds.): Symposium on Treatment of Diabetic Retinopathy. U. S. Department of Health, Education and Welfare, Public Health Service Publication No. 1890. Washington, D.C. U. S. Government Printing Office, 1968, p. 722.

142. Thorn, G. W., Renold, A. E., and Winegrad, A. I.: Some effects of adrenal cortical steroids on intermediary metabolism. Br. Med. J., 2:1009, 1957.

143. Van Way, C. W., III, Scott, H. W., Jr., Page, D. L., and Rhamy, R. K.: Pheochromocytoma. Current Problems in Surgery, June, 1974. Chicago, Year Book Medical Publishers, Inc., 1974.

144. Verney, E. B.: The absorption and excretion of water: The antidiuretic hormone. Lancet, 2:739, 781, 1946.

145. von Euler, U. S.: Specific sympathomimetic ergone in adrenergic nerve fibres (sympathin) and its relations to adrenaline and nor-adrenaline. Acta Physiol. Scand., 12:73, 1946.

146. von Euler, U. S.: Increased urinary excretion of noradrenaline in cases of pheochromocytoma. Ann. Surg., 134:929, 1951.

147. Walker, A. E.: A History of Neurological Surgery. Baltimore, Williams & Wilkins Company, 1951.

148. Wilkins, L.: The Diagnosis and Treatment of Endocrine Dis-

orders in Childhood and Adolescence, 3rd ed. Springfield, Ill., Charles C Thomas, Publisher, 1966.

149. Wilkins, L., Lewis, R. A., Klein, R., and Rosenberg, E.: The suppression of androgen excretion by cortisone in a case of congenital adrenal hyperplasia. Bull. Johns Hopkins Hosp., 86:249, 1950.

150. Williams, C. M., and Greer, M.: Homovanillic acid and vanilmandelic acid in diagnosis of neuroblastoma. J.A.M.A., 183:836, 1963.

151. Williams, R. H. (Ed.): Textbook of Endocrinology, 5th ed. Philadelphia, W. B. Saunders Company, 1974.

152. Wittenborg, M. H.: Roentgen therapy in neuroblastoma. Radiology, 54:679, 1950.

153. Young, H. H.: Genital Abnormalities. Hermaphroditism and Related Adrenal Diseases. Baltimore, Williams & Wilkins Company, 1937.

154. Zimmermann, B.: The endocrine glands. In Cole, W. H., and Zollinger, R. M. (Eds.): Textbook of Surgery, 8th ed. New York, Appleton-Century-Crofts, 1963, p. 1092.

155. Zimmermann, B., and Moran, W. H.: Aldosterone. Am. J. Surg., 99:503, 1960.

28

THE ESOPHAGUS

I

HISTORICAL ASPECTS AND ANATOMY

F. Henry Ellis, Jr., M.D., Ph.D.

Esophageal surgery has been influenced profoundly by two major twentieth century developments. The introduction of techniques permitting operations on the intrathoracic portion of the esophagus clearly paved the way for all subsequent advances, while the perfection and clinical application of sophisticated techniques of measuring normal and abnormal esophageal function have provided a scientific basis for the specialty.

HISTORICAL ASPECTS

Before transthoracic operations were possible, only the cervical esophagus could be treated surgically, and insofar as is known, the earliest operations on this organ were limited to cervical esophagotomy for removal of foreign bodies. By the latter part of the nineteenth century, malignant lesions of the cervical esophagus became amenable to surgical ablation largely through the efforts of Billroth[3] and Czerny.[11] A pharyngoesophageal diverticulum was first resected in 1886,[70] and transabdominal procedures for the relief of esophageal achalasia were performed in the early 1900s,[28, 50] as were staged reconstructive operations for corrosive stricture and malignant lesions.[68] A successful one-stage, transpleural esophageal resection and esophagogastrostomy for carcinoma remained an unattainable goal until Ohsawa's report in 1933.[54] In the United States, the first successful esophagogastrectomy for cancer was performed by Marshall of the Lahey Clinic in 1937.[49] Thereafter, all aspects of thoracic surgery progressed rapidly. Advances in anesthesia, blood replacement, and surgical technique lowered the mortality and morbidity rates of esophageal surgery to acceptable levels.

Despite these major advances, it was not until after World War II that esophageal surgeons became aware of the many complexities of esophageal function which are so often disturbed by disease and by surgical intervention. Through the efforts of Code and associates[7] and of Ingelfinger,[34] the heretofore poorly understood physiology of this important organ was carefully detailed, and the information disseminated. As a result, the surgeon can now emphasize function as well as technique. Proper patient selection has been facilitated, and the surgeon can base his operative efforts on sound physiologic grounds. A prerequisite for safe and effective esophageal surgery is a clear understanding of normal and abnormal esophageal physiology.

ANATOMY

The esophagus is a long muscular tube extending from the pharynx at the level of the sixth cervical vertebra to the stomach within the abdomen (Fig. 1). In the neck, the esophagus begins at the level of the cricopharyngeus muscle, which is bordered superiorly by the oblique fibers of the inferior pharyngeal constrictor muscle. This muscle passes upward and backward from its origin on the thyroid cartilage to insert into a median raphe (Fig. 2). The cricopharyngeus muscle runs transversely across the posterior wall of the esophagus, connecting the two lateral borders of the cricoid cartilage, and inferiorly blends into the circular and longitudinal muscle fibers of the upper esophagus. The esophagus occupies a midline position in the neck immediately behind the trachea. After entering the thorax, the esophagus inclines posteriorly with the trachea behind the great vessels and curves slightly to the left to pass behind the left main bronchus. From there it inclines slightly to the right as it continues in the posterior mediastinum. It again deviates to the left behind the pericardial sac to run anterior to the thoracic aorta, crossing it to the left of the midline. It reaches the abdomen through the esophageal hiatus, a noose of diaphragmatic muscle most often made up chiefly of the right diaphragmatic crus. Less frequently both right and left crura give equal contributions to the hiatal muscular noose.

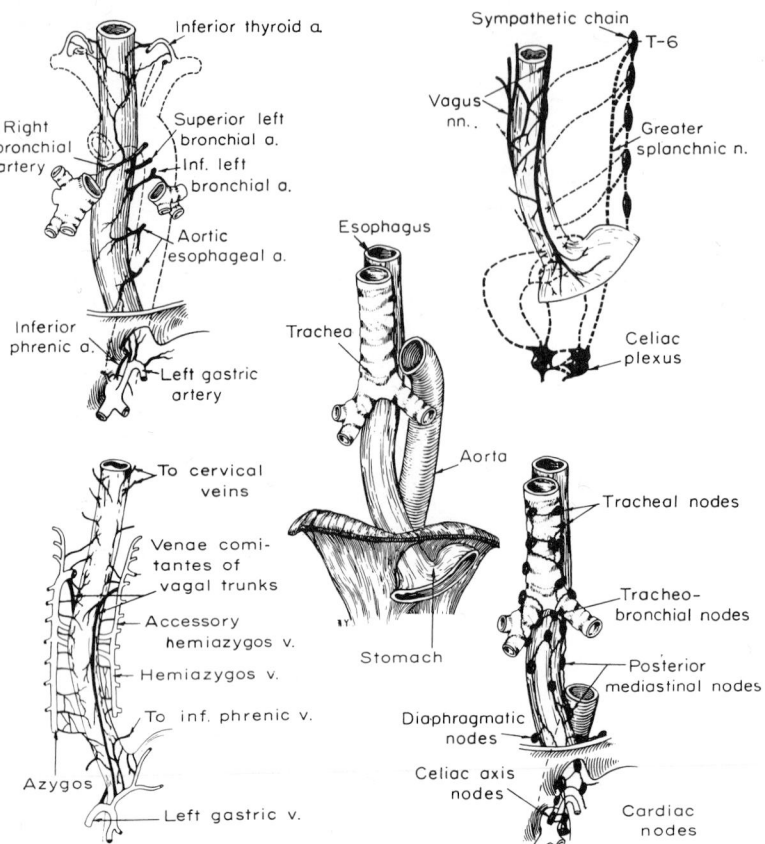

Figure 1. Anatomy of human esophagus. Arterial supply (*upper left*), venous drainage (*lower left*), innervation (*upper right*), and lymphatic system (*lower right*).

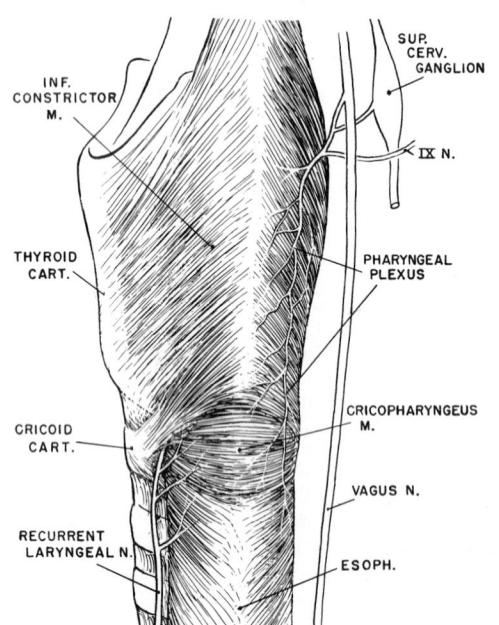

Figure 2. Anatomy of pharynx and upper esophagus. Posterolateral view. (From Ellis, F. H., Jr.: Surg. Clin. North Am., *51*:553, 1971.)

An esophageal segment of variable length lies within the abdomen where it joins the stomach at the esophagogastric junction, a point often referred to as the "cardia" (Fig. 3). This term is vague and lacks precise meaning, including such anatomic areas as the lower esophagus, esophagogastric junction, and upper portion of the stomach. The true esophagogastric junction is best described as that point at which the esophageal tube meets the gastric pouch and is best identified by the oblique sling fibers of the stomach sometimes called the loop of Willis or the collar of Helvetius. The junction of squamous with columnar epithelium is an inaccurate identification of the esophagogastric junction, for the distal 1 to 2 cm. of esophagus is lined by columnar epithelium (Fig. 4).[32]

Another important anatomic structure related to the esophagogastric junctional zone is the diaphragmaticoesophageal or phrenoesophageal membrane or ligament. This structure, described by Laimer[38] in 1883, is composed largely of mature collagenous fibers and is a continuation of the transversalis fascia of the abdominal parietes. A contribution to this structure is provided by fascia arising from the upper surface of the diaphragm, while additional support is provided by the pleura above and the peritoneal reflection below. The fibers themselves fan out and insert into the circumference of the lower 2 to 3 cm. of the esophagus and the uppermost portion of the stomach at the esophagogastric junction.

The muscular wall of the esophagus is composed of an inner circular layer and an outer longitudinal layer without a surrounding serosal covering. Striated muscle fibers make

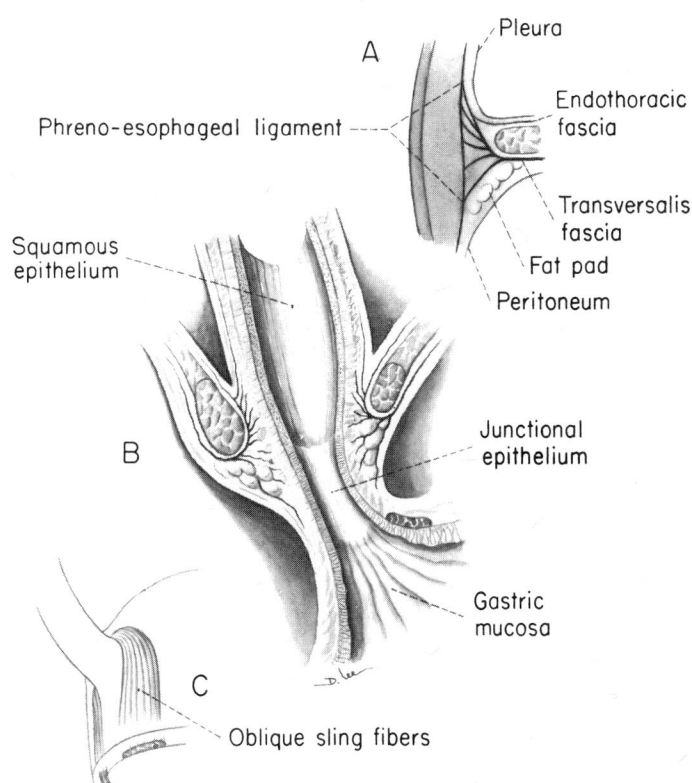

Figure 3. Gross anatomy of region of the esophagogastric junction. *A*, Details of origin and insertion of phrenoesophageal membrane. *B*, Cross section of distal esophagus and proximal stomach. *C*, Oblique gastric sling fibers. (From Payne, W. S., and Ellis, F. H., Jr. *In* Schwartz, S. I. (Ed.): Principles of Surgery. New York, McGraw-Hill Book Company, 1969.)

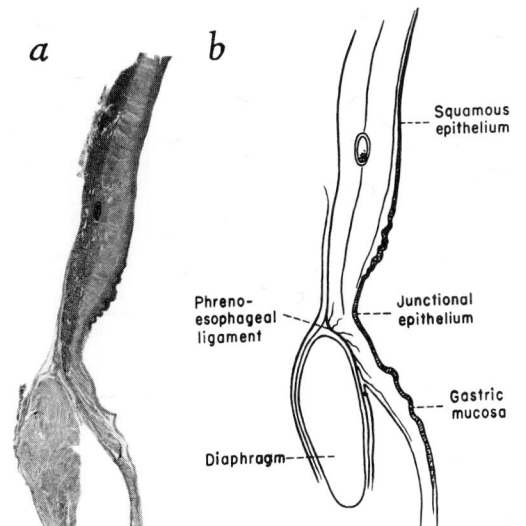

Figure 4. Microscopic anatomy of the esophagogastric junction region. *a*, Photomicrograph. Hematoxylin and eosin. × 1. *b*, Schematic representation, showing origin and insertion of the phrenoesophageal ligament, diaphragm, and mucosal lining.

a considerable contribution to the outer longitudinal coat in the upper portion of the esophagus, whereas smooth muscle predominates in the lower third. With few exceptions,[58] it has not been possible to identify any increase in the thickness of the muscle layers of the distal esophageal wall in the segment that corresponds to the physiologic lower esophageal sphincter. A prominent submucosa containing mucous glands, blood vessels, Meissner's plexus of nerves, and a rich network of lymphatic vessels is present. The mucosal lining is characteristically made up of squamous epithelium, although ectopic islands of gastric mucosa have been identified, particularly in the proximal portions of the esophagus. The distal 1 or 2 cm. of the esophageal lumen is lined by columnar epithelium.

The cervical esophagus is supplied by the inferior thyroid arteries,[67] while the thoracic portion is supplied by branches from the aorta itself and by esophageal branches of the bronchial arteries. These esophageal vessels are supplemented by others descending from vessels at the base of the neck, by ascending branches from arteries on the abdominal side of the diaphragm, and sometimes also branches from the intercostal arteries.

Subepithelial and submucous venous channels course longitudinally to empty above and below into hypopharyngeal and gastric veins.[5] They also penetrate the esophageal muscle, from which they receive branches and leave the esophagus to form a periesophageal plexus, the longest trunks of which accompany the vagus nerves. The drainage from the cervical esophagus empties ultimately into the inferior thyroid and vertebral veins, that from the thoracic portion into the azygos and hemiazygos veins, and that from the abdominal portion mostly into the left gastric vein.

The lymphatic vessels, in a pattern completely independent from that of the blood vessels, tend to run longitudinally in the wall of the esophagus before penetrating the muscle layers to reach regional nodes. Hence, malignant lesions of the mid or upper esophagus may metastasize first to cervical nodes, and lesions of the lower esophagus to gastric and celiac nodes. Once the lymphatic channels leave the esophagus, however, they go to the nearest group of nodes, which within the thorax are usually identified by their location as tracheal, tracheobronchial, posterior mediastinal, and diaphragmatic.

The nerve supply of the esophagus is from both the vagi and the sympathetic chains. The recurrent nerves supply the upper portion of the esophagus, which also receives branches from the ninth, tenth, cranial root of the eleventh, and sympathetic nerves. The vagal trunks send branches to the remaining voluntary muscle and parasympathetic preganglionic fibers to the smooth muscle. Along most of the esophagus, the vagus nerves lie on either side, forming a plexus about it. As the hiatus is approached, the two major trunks emerge, the left one coming to lie anteriorly and the right one posteriorly. The vagal plexuses are joined by mediastinal branches from the thoracic sympathetic chain and the splanchnic nerves. The lower end of the esophagus and the esophagogastric junctional region also receive branches from the periarterial plexuses along the left gastric, hepatic, and left inferior phrenic arteries.

For references, see page 808.

II

PHYSIOLOGY

F. Henry Ellis, Jr., M.D., Ph.D.

The esophagus functions as a channel through which ingested material is conveyed from the pharynx to the stomach. At either end of the tube are regulatory mechanisms that assist in this function, primarily by permitting one-way passage only, except under unusual circumstances. Current knowledge of the physiology of the esophagus has been gained by the special use of recording techniques to detect and record intraesophageal pressures. In routine tests, three or four pressure-detecting units (fine, water-filled, polyethylene tubes with openings spaced at 5-cm. intervals attached to strain-gauge manometers) are positioned at various points in the esophagus. Accuracy of pressure recording is enhanced by the infusion of fluid into the recording catheter unit by a constant infusion pump.[60] Measurements are made when the esophagus is at rest and after swallowing, the resting pressures being measured while the units are being withdrawn in a stepwise fashion from the stomach into the esophagus before the recording of deglutitory measures.

At the upper end of the esophagus is a 3-cm. zone of increased pressure which relaxes promptly with swallowing and contracts thereafter as a wave of high pressure passes through it (Fig. 1). This is the upper esophageal sphincter, which is composed of the cricopharyngeus muscle and a few centimeters of the upper cervical esophagus. Contractions of the sphincter are in peristaltic sequence with those of the pharynx above and the esophagus below, and the peristaltic pressure sweeps in an orderly fashion down the entire body of the esophagus. Pressures reach an intensity of 50 to 100 cm. of water and are slightly more forceful in the lower esophagus (Fig. 2). Resting pressures in the body of the esophagus are normally less than atmospheric pressure, reflecting negative intrathoracic pressure. There is a zone of increased pressure at the lower end of the esophagus, measuring 3 to 5 cm. (Fig. 3). It is located in the region of the hiatus, and in response to a swallowing effort relaxation of this zone of increased pressure can be identified, followed by sphincteric contraction. This constitutes the lower esophageal sphincter.

There is considerable controversy concerning the exact mechanism by which gastroesophageal competence is maintained. Factors that have been suggested as important include the diaphragm, the valve flap mechanism, the gastric sling fibers, the oblique angle of entry, and the mucosal rosette. Most important of all, however, is the physiologic sphincter at the lower

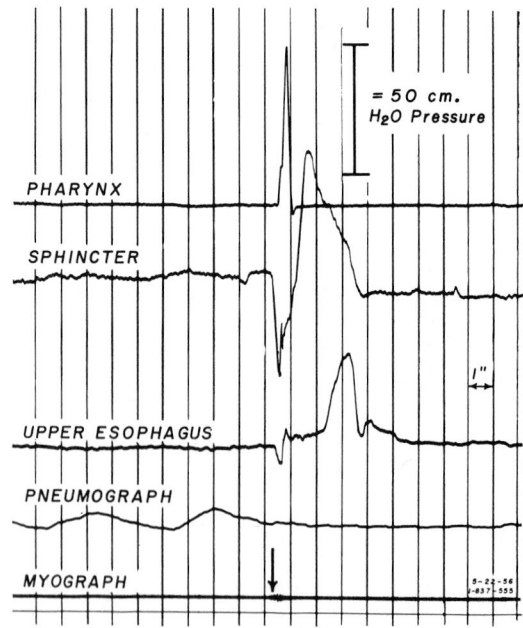

Figure 1. Swallowing pressures at pharyngoesophageal junction. Note relaxation of pressure in sphincter as pressure in pharynx increases. Pressure passes as wave through sphincter into upper part of esophagus. (From Code, C. F., et al.: An Atlas of Esophageal Motility in Health and Disease, 1958. Courtesy of Charles C Thomas, Publisher, Springfield, Ill.)

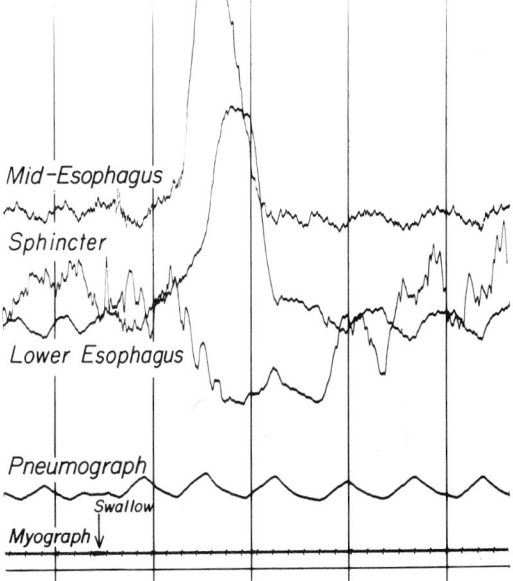

Figure 2. Esophageal and lower sphincteric response to swallowing. Note peristaltic sequence of pressure elevations in mid and lower esophagus accompanied by relaxation of sphincter.

end of the esophagus, for, in its absence, none of the other suggested mechanisms individually or together can prevent gastroesophageal reflux. It is likely that in most humans the musculature of the intrinsic sphincter in combination with prominent folds of gastric mucosa at the esophagogastric junction contributes to the reflux barrier.

The details of esophageal innervation are still uncertain. Whereas the cervical esophagus may be innervated in part by the recurrent nerves, cricopharyngeal function is probably dependent on a nerve derived from the pharyngeal branch of the vagus through the pharyngeal plexus.[46] Peristalsis in the body of the esophagus is under vagal control because division of these nerves produces low simultaneous pressures after deglutition. The lower esophageal sphincter, however, may continue to relax on swallowing even after lower thoracic vagotomy and sympathetic denervation, so it must possess a high degree of autonomy.[48]

The adaptive response of the lower sphincter to graded increases in intragastric pressure has been shown to be under vagal control.[40] Normally the ratio of increment of sphincter pressure to the increment of

intragastric pressure in response to abdominal compression in greater than one. In addition, the lower sphincter is under hormonal control, as evidenced by its enhancement in response to gastrin administration[24] and its reduction in response to secretin, cholecystokinin, and glucagon.[14]

While esophageal manometry is the key to an understanding of esophageal function and to the diagnosis of abnormal function, other techniques are useful in studying esophageal function. Esophagoscopy (to be discussed in detail in another section) is an integral part of the diagnosis of a patient with suspected esophageal disease. Cinefluorography is particularly useful in studies of the pharynx and upper esophagus where events occur extremely rapidly. Radiographic studies, however, are not the best way to identify the presence or absence of pathologic reflux. The pH reflux test is probably the most sensitive measure of esophageal reflux.[2] Less useful is the acid perfusion test, which not uncommonly gives false positive and false negative results.

For references, see page 808.

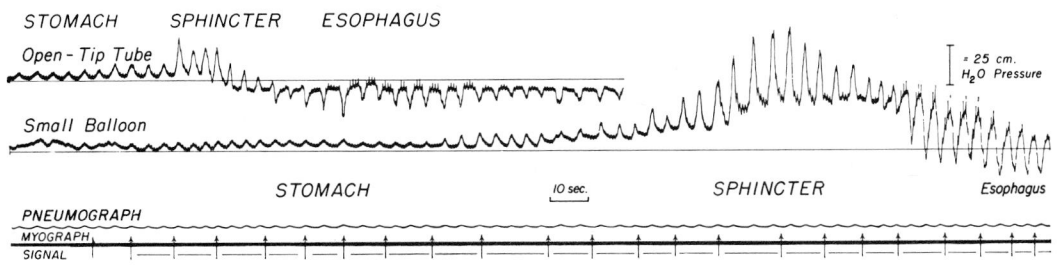

Figure 3. Pressure profile of normal gastroesophageal sphincter detected by withdrawal of open-tip tube and small balloon.

III _____

DISORDERS OF ESOPHAGEAL MOTILITY

F. Henry Ellis, Jr., M.D., Ph.D.

The widespread use of esophageal function tests has clarified the nature of a variety of esophageal diseases. As a result, most benign conditions of the esophagus can now be classified according to their specific abnormal motility patterns. This has significant therapeutic implications, for not only can heretofore undiagnosable esophageal symptoms be explained by distinct disease entities but also surgical therapy can be directed along proper physiologic lines. The implications are therefore quite clear. No work-up of a patient complaining of esophageal symptoms as a result of benign disease can be considered complete without a study of esophageal motility.

UPPER SPHINCTER

A number of diseases involving the central nervous system give rise to esophageal symptoms due to abnormalities of pharyngoesophageal function. Patients with bulbar poliomyelitis[35] or those who suffer a cerebrovascular accident[1] may complain of dysphagia, as do some patients with multiple sclerosis.[12] Abnormalities of sphincteric relaxation are said to characterize such lesions. Diseases that directly affect muscular activity also may result in swallowing difficulties. Most common among these diseases are muscular dystrophy, myasthenia gravis, dermatomyositis, and the myopathy of thyrotoxicosis.[39, 59] In such patients, failure to develop effective pharyngeal peristalsis seems to be the most common cause of swallowing difficulties. Preoperative study of esophageal function may help to identify those patients who might be aided by cricopharyngeal myotomy by identifying those with abnormal cricopharyngeal function.[51, 52]

Difficulty in swallowing has been reported after extensive operations on the oropharyngeal region. Spasm of the cricopharyngeus muscle has been considered contributory to the swallowing difficulty, and cricopharyngeal myotomy is currently advisable when extensive resections of this sort are performed.[53]

Although the term cricopharyngeal achalasia has been suggested as applicable to swallowing difficulties, particularly when there are pharyngoesophageal diverticula, motility studies have failed to provide confirmation. Rather, a type of incoordination has been observed in patients with upper esophageal pouches, characterized by an abnormal temporal relationship between pharyngeal contraction and pharyngoesophageal sphincteric relaxation and contraction.[20] In these patients, sphincteric contraction occurs before completion of the contraction of the pharynx, suggesting a possible etiologic role. A detailed discussion of pharyngoesophageal diverticulum and its surgical management is presented later.

BODY OF ESOPHAGUS AND LOWER SPHINCTER

Achalasia

Esophageal achalasia is a disease of unknown etiology characterized by absence of peristalsis in the body of the esophagus and failure of the lower esophageal sphincter to relax in response to swallowing. It was first described in 1674 by Thomas Willis, who prescribed forceful dilation as the treatment of choice.[72]

Although the cause of the disease is unknown, there is general agreement that it has a neurogenic basis. Pathologic evidence in support of this theory is provided by demonstration of disintegration or absence of ganglion cells of Auerbach's plexus in the esophagus in many patients with this disease,[6] an abnormality demonstrable at all levels of the thoracic esophagus although more prominent in the body of this organ in the majority of patients. Not only is the cause of the ganglion cell abnormalities obscure but it is not known whether they represent a primary or secondary manifestation of the disease. That the primary site of the disorder may be in the extraesophageal nerve supply—the vagus nerve itself or its central nuclei—has been suggested by pathologic studies of biopsy and autopsy material and by experiments involving selective destruction of the motor nuclei of the vagus nerve in the cat and dog.[6, 31, 42]

In Brazil and other South American countries where the leishmaniacal forms of *Trypanosoma cruzi* exist, changes in Auerbach's plexus have been demonstrated in patients with Chagas' disease who appear to have an esophageal condition indistinguishable from achalasia.[37]

Achalasia of the esophagus occurs at an annual incidence rate of 0.6 per 100,000,[15] with equal frequency in the two sexes. It may occur at any age but is seen most often between the ages of 30 and 50 years. The natural history of the disease has been well documented.[16] The earliest and most constant symptom is obstruction to swallowing or dysphagia, which at first may be intermittent but becomes more constant as the disease progresses. As a rule, the patient experiences more difficulty with cold than with warm food, and often solid foods are said to pass more easily at first than do liquids. Pain is a relatively infrequent symptom, occurring in a little more than one fourth of the patients. It is more likely to occur in the early stage of the disease and becomes less noticeable as the esophagus dilates. Regurgitation is a common symptom, particularly noticeable at night when the patient is reclining. Pulmonary complications in the form of aspiration pneumonitis may develop as a direct result of regurgitation. An increased susceptibility to the development of carcinoma of the esophagus has been described in patients with this disease, particularly those who have had it for long periods without proper treatment.[16, 75]

The earliest evidence of esophageal achalasia is that of obstruction at the cardia with slight esophageal dilatation proximally. As the disease progresses, the classic roentgenologic signs develop (Fig. 1). The esophagus is dilated, and the lower portion of the lumen appears conical and narrowed for a short distance, with a beaklike extension directed into the narrowed segment. Although esophageal achalasia in its more advanced forms has roentgenographic characteristics that distinguish it from carcinoma, it may not be differentiated thus in its early stages. Esophagoscopy is essential to distinguish early achalasia from carcinoma or from benign esophageal stricture.

Confirmation of the clinical diagnosis of esophageal achalasia can be provided by studies of esophageal motility.[4] These studies show slight elevation of pressures in the esophagus, a reflection of esophageal dilatation, and lack of peristalsis in the body of the esophagus after deglutition. The swallowing effort is accompanied by feeble elevations in pressure that are simultaneous throughout the body of the esophagus. In contrast to its normal behavior, the lower esophageal sphincter fails to relax in response to swallowing efforts (Fig. 2). The lower sphincter exhibits higher than normal resting pressures and responds excessively to the administration of gastrin.[9] In some patients the motility pattern exhibits some of the features of diffuse spasm of the esophagus, as evidenced by powerful, repetitive, nonperistaltic esophageal contractions in response to swallowing. The term vigorous achalasia has been applied to this manifestation of the disease.[63]

The disordered esophageal motility characteristic of esophageal achalasia cannot be restored to normal, and so effective therapy must be directed to relief of the distal esophageal obstruction. Since diet and drugs are ineffective, it must be accomplished either by forceful dilation or by surgical means. Forceful dilation of the esophagogastric junction may be performed by hydrostatic (Fig. 3), pneumatic, or mechanical dilation. At the Mayo Clinic, hydrostatic dilation has been successful in relieving the symptoms of patients with esophageal achalasia in 81 per cent of cases.[62] This method, however, is not without risk. Complications occurred in 4.6 per cent of cases, usually as a result of esophageal perforation.

Limitations of medical therapy, including the use of forceful dilation, have led to surgical efforts to relieve the symptoms of patients with this disease. Such techniques have included excisional or bypassing procedures and denervation operations. The latter were ineffective, and the uniform development of severe esophagitis after any procedure that destroys or bypasses the inferior esophageal sphincter has rightly led to their abandonment.

Current surgical therapy stems historically from the double cardiomyotomy first carried out by Heller in 1913.[28] The simplest and most effective modification of the Heller operation involves a longitudinal incision through the muscle layers of the distal esophagus using a thoracic approach (Fig. 4). The incision is carried onto the stomach only far enough to ensure

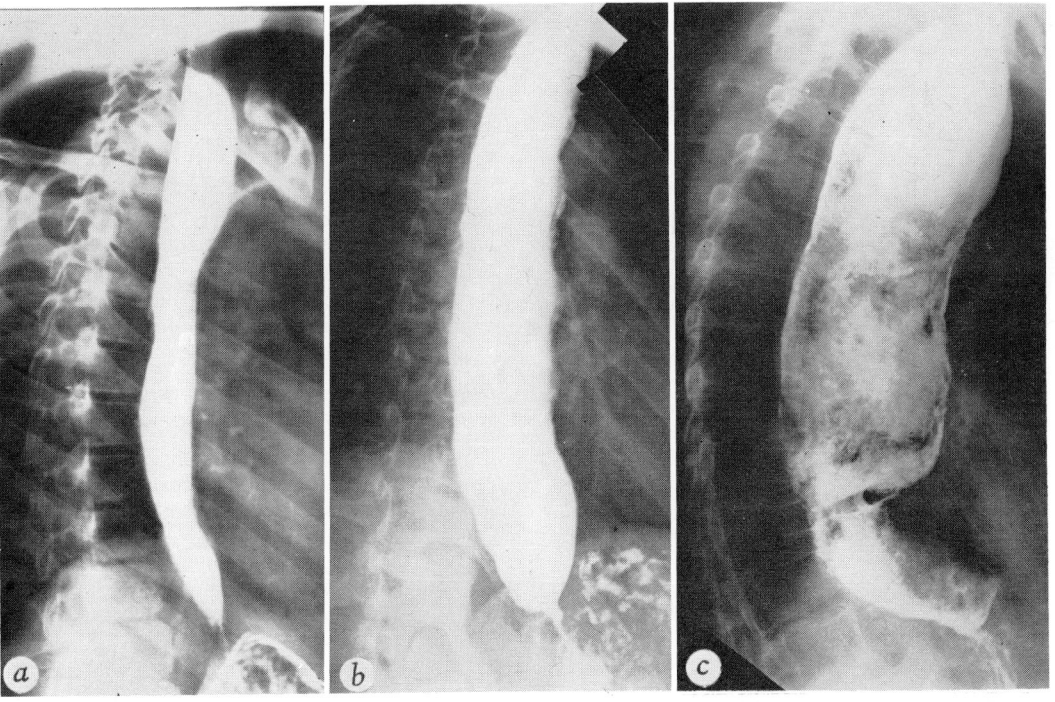

Figure 1. Roentgenographic appearance of (a) mild, (b) moderate, and (c) severe achalasia of the esophagus. (From Olsen, A. M., et al.: J. Thorac. Surg., 22:164, 1951.)

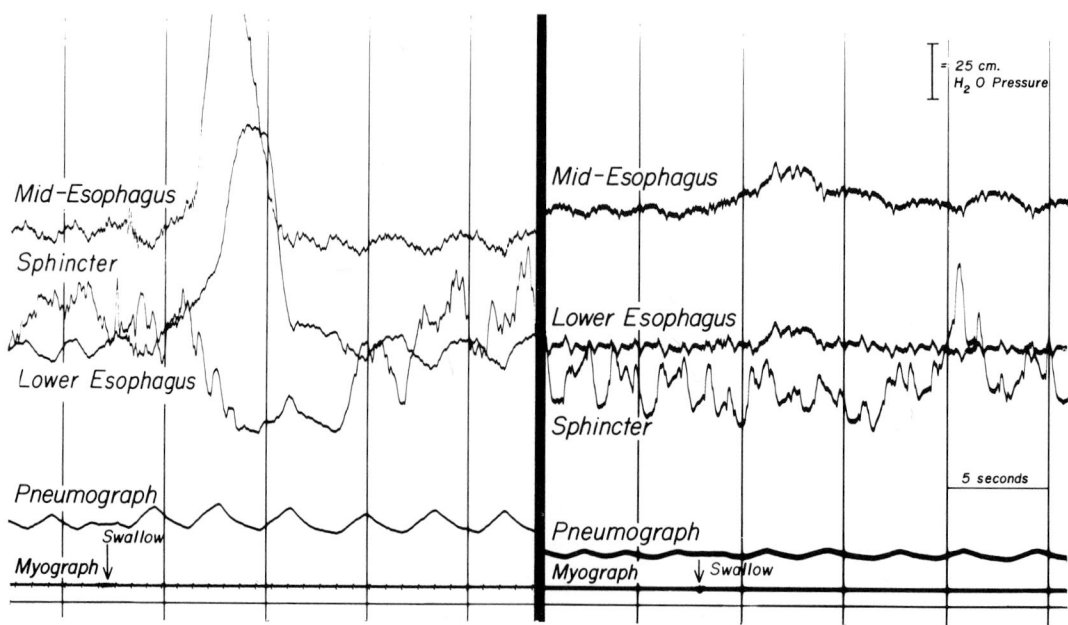

Figure 2. Deglutitive responses in body and lower sphincter of esophagus in health (*left*) and in achalasia (*right*). Note normal peristalsis and sphincteric relaxation in health, and absence of both peristalsis and sphincter relaxation in achalasia.

complete division of the distal esophageal musculature (Fig. 4*A*). The mucosa is freed in such a fashion as to allow it to pout through the incision (Fig. 4*B*). To avoid a postoperative diaphragmatic hernia, damage to the esophageal hiatus and its supporting structures should be avoided. The addition of such ancillary procedures as vagotomy, pyloroplasty, or fundoplica-

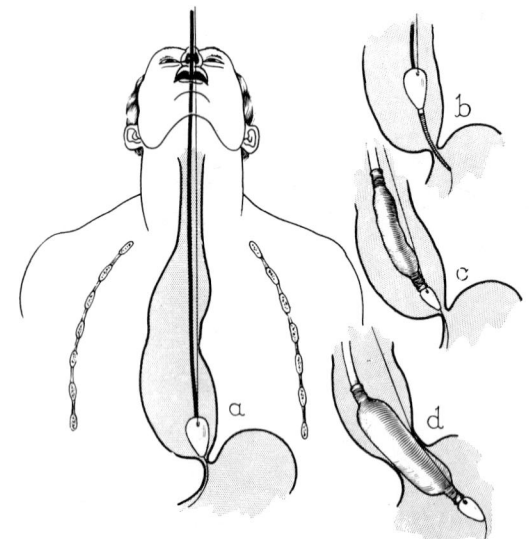

Figure 3. Method of performing hydrostatic dilation. *a*, Passage of 41 F olive-tipped bougie into stomach. *b*, Passage of 50 or 60 F sound into stomach, guided by flexible wire spiral. *c*, Passage of hydrostatic dilator into cardia. *d*, Distention of hydrostatic dilator across cardia. (From Olsen, A. M., et al.: J. Thorac. Surg., 22:164, 1951.)

tion are not only unnecessary but inadvisable. In fact, care is taken to preserve the vagus nerves. Over 90 per cent of patients operated on by this technique have been helped by the operation, and the incidence of reflux esophagitis is minimal.[17, 18]

Because of its uniformly good results, esophagomyotomy has become the primary treatment of choice in the hands of many in the management of this disease. Others still prefer treatment by dilation as preliminary therapy, reserving operation for patients who have failed to improve after dilation or when a recurrence of symptoms develops. Treatment by dilation has proved unsatisfactory in the management of achalasia in children and has proved to be a dangerous procedure in patients with a huge, dilated tortuous esophagus and in those with vigorous achalasia. An operative approach is clearly indicated in those patients who have associated conditions requiring operation, such as an esophageal hiatal hernia or an esophageal diverticulum.

Diffuse Spasm of the Esophagus and Hypertensive Gastroesophageal Sphincter

While esophageal achalasia is a manifestation of esophageal hypomotility, diffuse spasm of the esophagus and hypertensive gastroesophageal sphincter are conditions characterized by hypermotility of the esophagus. Very little if any evidence exists to suggest that the conditions are in any way related, and diffuse esophageal spasm is not an early stage of esophageal achalasia but rather a totally different type of motility disturbance.

Differentiation from esophageal achalasia can usually be made clinically, for pain is far more pronounced in diffuse spasm, dysphagia occurring inter-

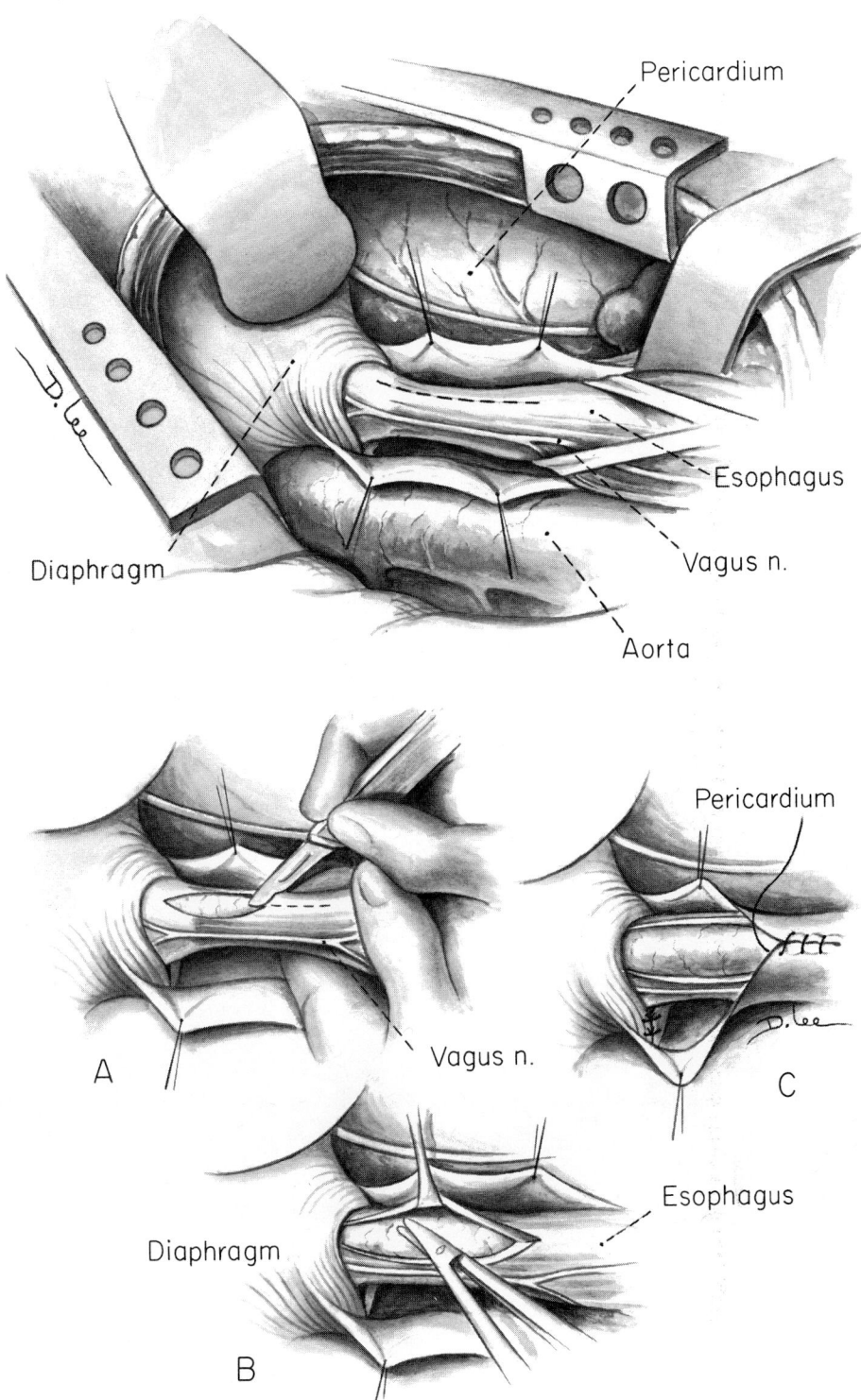

Figure 4. Technique of esophagomyotomy. *Upper panel:* Operative exposure. Dotted line indicates intended line of incision. *Lower panel:* A, Beginning the incision. B, Dissection of mucosa from muscularis. C, Restoration of esophagogastric junction to intra-abdominal position with suture narrowing of esophageal hiatus if necessary. (From Ellis, F. H., Jr., et al.: Ann. Surg., *166*:640, 1967.)

TABLE 1. Differential Diagnosis of Achalasia, Diffuse Spasm, and Vigorous Achalasia*

Symptom or Sign	Incidence, According to Diagnosis		
	Achalasia	Diffuse Spasm	Vigorous Achalasia
Pain	Uncommon	Almost always	Frequent
Obstruction	Always	Sometimes	Nearly always
Regurgitation	Common	Rare	Frequent
Retention	Frequent	Never	Frequent
Nervousness	Uncommon	Almost always	Occasional
Radiologic findings			
Diffuse dilatation	Common	Never	Occasional
Segmental spasm	Uncommon	Frequent	Common

*From Sanderson, D. R., Ellis, F. H., Jr., Schlegel, J. F., and Olsen, A. M.: Dis. Chest, *52*:514, 1967.

mittently or not at all (Table 1). The pain varies from a sensation of discomfort beneath the lower half of the sternum to severe, colicky substernal pain extending through the back or into the neck, shoulders, or arms, mimicking cardiac pain. The pain may be provoked by eating, or it may come on spontaneously, even awakening the patient at night. Patients so afflicted tend to be high-strung and nervous, and the diagnosis of psychoneurosis is often entertained. Symptoms are more likely to be troublesome than truly incapacitating. Even during an attack the patient seldom seems seriously ill.

Unfortunately, abnormalities of the esophageal roentgenogram occur in less than half the cases. When they are present, however, they are quite striking and explain why in the past a variety of descriptive terms, including curling, corkscrew esophagus, pseudodiverticulosis, and idiopathic muscular hypertrophy of the esophagus, were used (Fig. 5). A small diaphragmatic hernia is frequently present, and an epiphrenic diverticulum commonly co-exists. Diffuse spasm may occur independently or may coexist with hypertensive gastroesophageal sphincter. Because esophageal roentgenograms may appear normal in patients with these disorders, the diagnosis usually rests on the results of esophageal motility studies. In patients with diffuse spasm, the abnormality is usually localized in the lower half or third of the body of the esophagus,

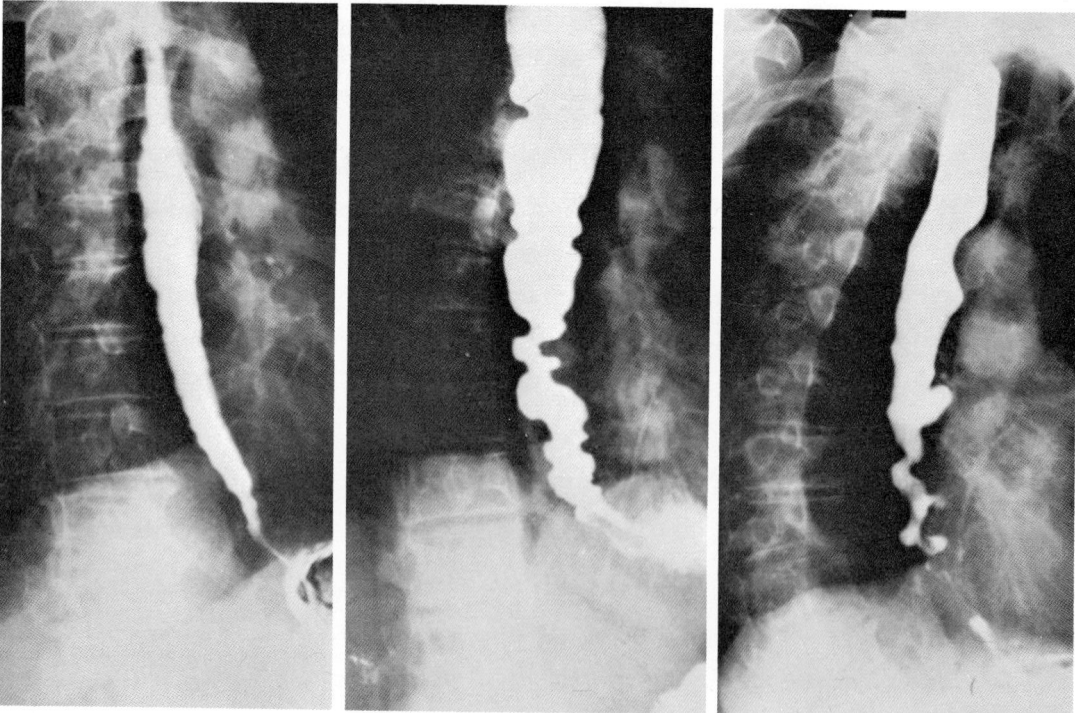

Figure 5. Esophageal roentgenograms from three patients with diffuse spasm of esophagus. (From Olsen, A. M., et al.: J. Thorac. Surg., 22:164, 1951.)

where peristaltic waves are replaced by simultaneous, repetitive, and occasionally prolonged increases in pressure in response to deglutition[8] (Fig. 6). Most patients show no abnormality of the sphincters unless there is a hypertensive gastroesophageal sphincter in which case resting pressures are excessive, and sphincteric relaxation may be poor, or premature contraction may occur.[57]

The hyperactive character of these motility disturbances led to the use of an extended modified Heller myotomy in patients with severe symptoms, since other forms of treatment are unsuccessful.[19] A similar approach had been used earlier by Lortat-Jacob[44] in patients with "diffuse nodular myomatosis of the esophagus." The technique resembles in most respects that employed for achalasia of the esophagus (Fig. 7). The myotomy is more extensive, however, its limits being defined before operation by the extent of the disease as determined by esophageal motility studies. Occasionally, the incision may reach the aortic arch. If the lower sphincter is normotensive, it should not be included in the myotomy in order to prevent postoperative reflux. Surgical repair of an associated diaphragmatic hernia is essential when one is present. Concomitant excision of epiphrenic diverticula is recommended, although in all likelihood the symptoms are due more to the underlying motility disturbance than to the diverticulum in such instances. Although the majority of patients are benefited by the operation and usually maintain an initially good result over the years, the results are not as good as those after esophagomyotomy for achalasia of the esophagus, only 70 to 80 per cent of the patients so treated being benefited.[19,55] For this reason, patients should be selected carefully for the operation, the ideal candidate being an emotionally stable individual with serious disability from the disease but without evidence of associated gastrointestinal problems. There should be demonstrable evidence of the severity of the disease in the form of a markedly abnormal esophageal motility pattern, ideally, associated with roentgenographic evidence of esophageal spasm.

Hypotensive Inferior Esophageal Sphincter

When the resting pressure at the lower esophageal sphincter is low (less than a mean of 12 cm. of water using an infused system), gastroesophageal reflux is facilitated. The sphincter may exhibit normal pressures at rest, yet reflux occurs if its adaptive response to increases in intra-abdominal pressure is abnormal. The close relationship between the level of pressure at the lower sphincter and the presence or absence of reflux is now generally recognized.[10] While the most common accompaniment of gastroesophageal reflux is a sliding esophageal hiatal hernia, other conditions characterized by low sphincteric pressures and reflux exist. Operations on the sphincter or specific diseases such as scleroderma (vide infra) will lower sphincteric pressures and result in gastroesophageal incompe-

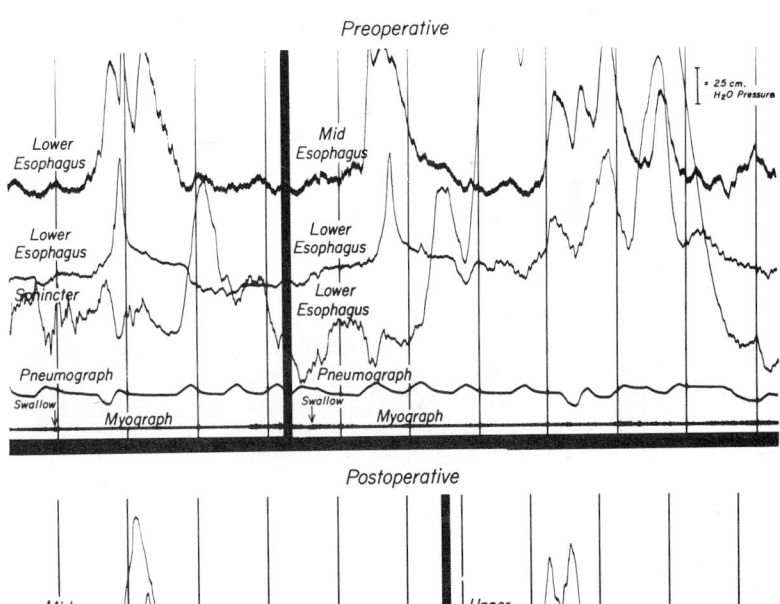

Figure 6. Deglutitive responses in body and sphincter of esophagus before (*upper panels*) and after (*lower panels*) esophagomyotomy. Amplitude, duration, and repetitiveness of contractions have been reduced by operation. (From Ellis, F. H., Jr., et al.: Surgery, *48*:155, 1960.)

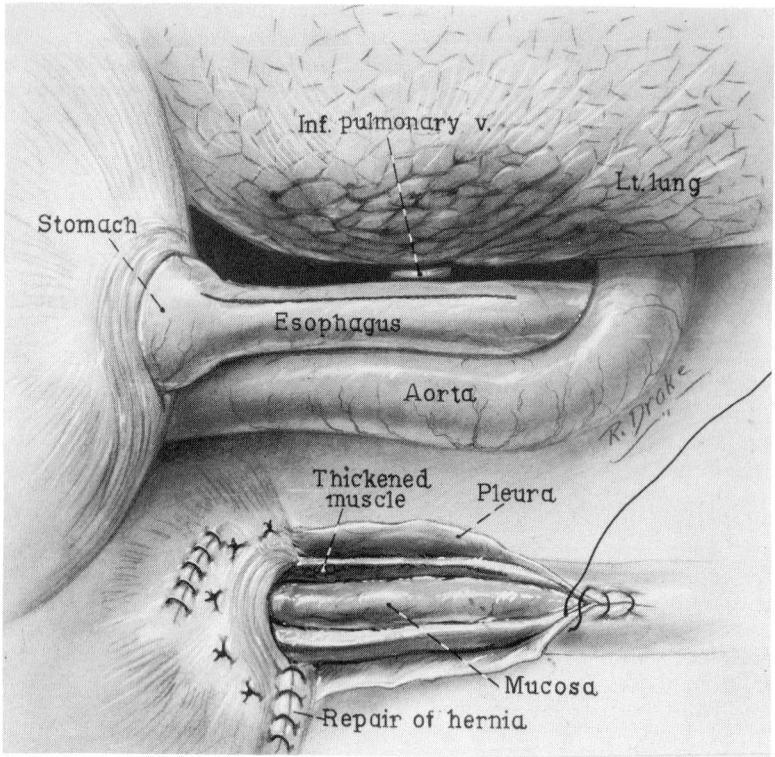

Figure 7. Technique of esophagomyotomy and hiatal hernia repair of diffuse spasm of the esophagus and a small hiatal hernia. (From Ellis, F. H., Jr., et al.: Surgery, *48*:162, 1960.)

tence. Primary sphincteric incompetence in the absence of hiatal hernia or other obvious causes is being recognized with increasing frequency.[30] It has been suggested, though not confirmed, that hypotension of the lower sphincter may be the result of gastrin deficiency.[41] Because of the hazards of reflux esophagitis and its deleterious consequences, surgical therapy may be required to restore competence if medical therapy fails. These techniques will be discussed in a subsequent section.

Miscellaneous Disturbances

Sometimes systemic diseases involve the esophagus, and scleroderma is probably the most common one to give rise to significant abnormalities of this organ.[23] It usually affects the connective tissues of the body, and when the esophagus becomes involved, the characteristic changes are fragmentation and homogenization of the submucosal connective tissue elements coupled with atrophy of the smooth muscle. Motor failure of the esophagus is the characteristic finding on esophageal motility studies. These findings may often precede the development of significant symptoms. Symptoms, when they develop, are the result of involvement of the lower esophageal sphincter with loss of gastroesophageal competence and consist of regurgitation, heartburn, and ultimately dysphagia when esophageal stricture develops. As the disease progresses, fibrosis and shortening of the esophagus ensue with the development of a hiatal hernia of the short esophagus type, a condition that is quite clearly secondary to gastroesophageal reflux and esophagitis.

Medical treatment consists of efforts to minimize the

deleterious effects of gastroesophageal reflux. When medical therapy is ineffective and an esophageal stricture is present, forceful dilation may be required for the relief of symptoms. Only when dilation fails should surgery be undertaken. The details of the surgical management of esophageal stricture are discussed later in this chapter.

While dysphagia may occur in most of the so-called collagen diseases, it is encountered most frequently in dermatomyositis, an incidence of 60 per cent having been reported in one series.[13] A generalized muscular defect may be demonstrated by esophageal motility studies in patients with this disease. In contrast to scleroderma, skeletal as well as smooth muscle is involved. Motility abnormalities occur in the body of the esophagus that resemble those seen in scleroderma. Usually, however, the integrity of the lower sphincter is maintained. Remission of the disease may occur after administration of corticosteroids.

Swallowing dysfunction is common in patients with neuromuscular disorders. Reference has already been made to the effect of certain of these conditions on the upper esophageal sphincter. The most striking abnormalities can be seen in patients with disorders that are primarily myotonic in origin, such as myasthenia gravis and myotonia dystrophica.[21] Rarely do esophageal motility studies give normal results in such patients. The amplitude of the peristaltic waves is decreased in myasthenia gravis, and they disappear in the lower esophagus during repetitive swallowing. Motor failure of the esophagus also occurs in myotonia dystrophica, a condition in which both smooth and striated muscles are affected.

A variety of nonspecific abnormalities may be seen in patients with central and peripheral neurologic disorders, usually involving changes in peristalsis. An increase in the number of simultaneous waves may occur, or esophageal spasm may be demonstrated. Some of these changes are seen in patients with hemiplegia or Parkinson's disease. In amyotrophic lateral sclerosis, the most common finding is occurrences of feeble peristaltic contractions in place of the vigorous contractions seen normally.[66] Contractions are simultaneous and may be repetitive. Sphincteric changes are relatively less common. In multiple sclerosis, a variety of abnormalities may be noted, including poor relaxation of the lower esophageal sphincter, simultaneous deglutition waves, incoordination of swallowing complexes, and diffuse spasm of the esophagus.[12] Some patients with diabetic neuropathy of long standing have been found to have a decreased amplitude of peristaltic contraction throughout the esophagus and lowered sphincteric pressures.[65] Neuropathy associated with alcoholism also has been implicated in esophageal dysfunction, a lack of primary peristalsis in the distal one third of the esophagus being the most common abnormality.[73]

For references, see page 808.

IV

DIVERTICULA AND MISCELLANEOUS CONDITIONS OF THE ESOPHAGUS

F. Henry Ellis, Jr., M.D., Ph.D.

DIVERTICULA

Esophageal diverticula can be classified by location, mode of development, and status as true or false diverticula. They commonly occur at three separate sites and are appropriately classified as pharyngoesophageal, midthoracic, and epiphrenic diverticula. Those at the upper and lower ends of the esophagus are often referred to as pulsion diverticula, and they are usually the consequence of an underlying esophageal motility disturbance. Such pouches consist primarily of esophageal mucosa and submucosa, and hence the classification of false diverticula. Midthoracic diverticula have been called traction diverticula and usually occur at the level of the tracheal carina. In contrast to the other two groups, they are more likely to include all layers of the esophageal wall and are known as true diverticula.

Pharyngoesophageal Diverticulum

The most common diverticulum of the esophagus arises at its upper end between the oblique fibers of the inferior constrictor muscle of the pharynx and the transverse fibers of the cricopharyngeus muscle. First described by Ludlow in 1767,[45] the condition has been well recognized for many years. After Ludlow's description, Zenker's name became associated with it, and in 1875, he and von Ziemssen collected 22 cases from the literature and added five of their own.[77] Diverticula arising in this location usually occur in elderly persons. They clearly represent an acquired abnormality, although a congenital weakness or deficiency in the supporting musculature of the area has been postulated as a possible cause. Studies of esophageal motility in patients with pharyngoesophageal diverticulum, however, have demonstrated an incoordination in the swallowing mechanism whereby pharyngeal contraction occurs after closure of the cricopharyngeus sphincter (vide supra). This may well prove to be the cause of the pharyngeal pouch.[20]

The chief symptoms are dysphagia, regurgitation, and noisy deglutition. Pulmonary manifestations may result from aspiration of the diverticular contents during nocturnal regurgitation. The diverticulum inevitably enlarges, and ultimately, if it is untreated, total esophageal obstruction occurs. The diagnosis is made roentgenographically (Fig. 1). One stage resection (Fig. 2) has for many years been the preferred method of treatment.[69] The procedure is readily accomplished through a left vertical or transverse cervical incision. The diverticulum is exposed by retracting the thyroid gland medially and the carotid sheath laterally. After the sac is dissected up to its neck, it is divided and removed, the pharyngeal mucosa is closed with sutures or an automatic stapler, and the edges of the muscle layer are approximated carefully. The operation carries minimal risk even in debilitated and elderly patients. Recurrence is rare. A simpler and equally effective approach, particularly for the small pharyngeal pouch, is that of cricopharyngeal myotomy (Fig. 3). The exposure is the same as for diverticulectomy and involves a longitudinal incision through the cricopharyngeus muscle extending caudally onto the esophagus itself, the total length of the incision

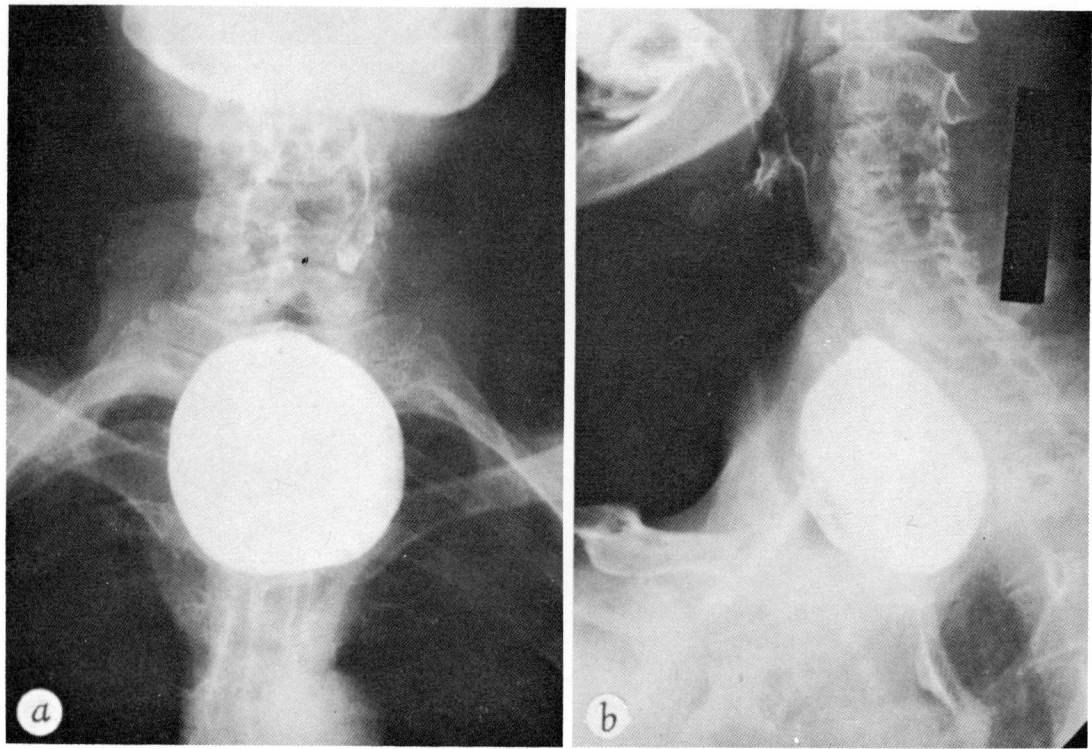

Figure 1. Classic (*a*) posteroanterior and (*b*) lateral roentgenologic appearance of pharyngoesophageal diverticulum in same patient.

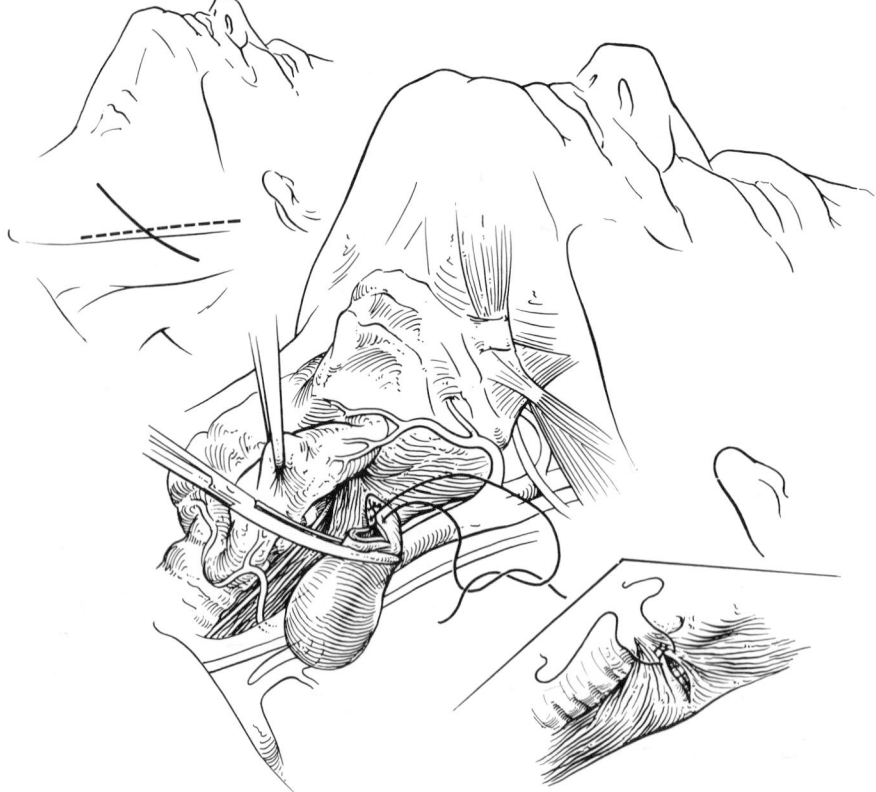

Figure 2. Procedure for removal of pharyngoesophageal diverticulum.

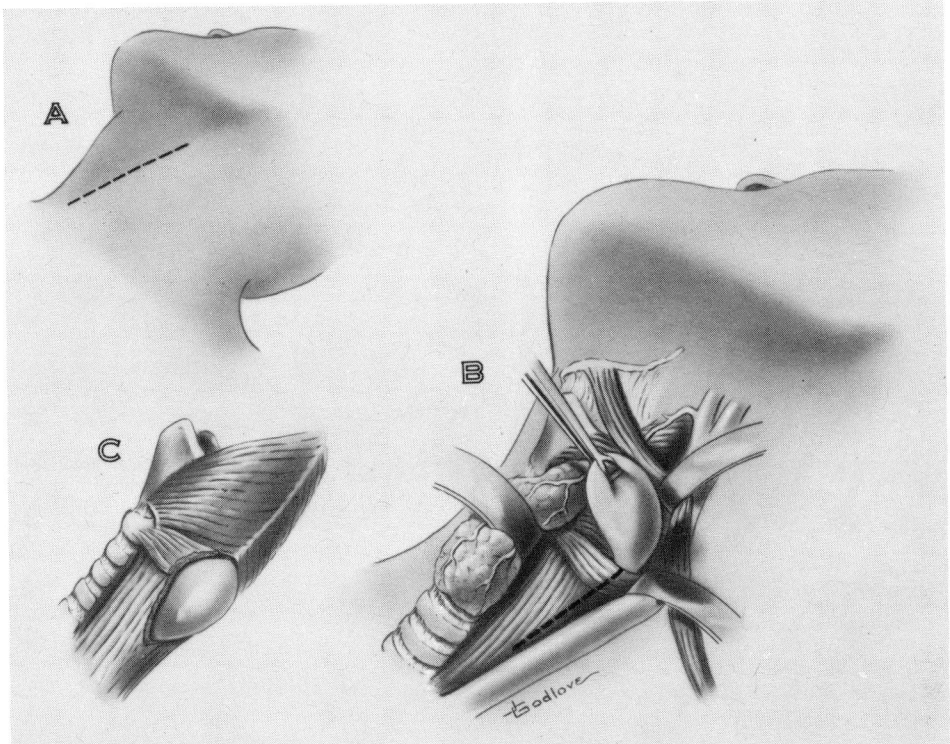

Figure 3. Technique of cricopharyngeal myotomy. *A*, Site of skin incision. *B*, Exposure of diverticulum. Dotted line indicates proposed myotomy. *C*, Completed operation. (From Ellis, F. H., Jr., et al.: Ann. Surg., *170*:343, 1969.)

being about 3 or 4 cm. The success of this operative approach lends credence to the theory that such diverticula are the result of incoordination of the pharyngoesophageal sphincter mechanism.[20]

Midthoracic Diverticula

Diverticula seldom develop in the midthoracic part of the esophagus and rarely produce symptoms. When they do, they are usually caused by granulomatous infections of the mediastinal lymph nodes, particularly those in the subcarinal and parabronchial regions. Only rarely will such a diverticulum give rise to significant complications, the most serious of which is a tracheobronchial esophageal fistula. When fistulas develop between the esophagus and the lower respiratory tract, excision and closure of the communication with interposition of normal tissues are usually successful in preventing recurrence.[74]

Epiphrenic Diverticulum

Located just above the diaphragm are epiphrenic diverticula, sometimes called supradiaphragmatic diverticula. They not only are less common than the upper pharyngeal pouches but are less likely to produce symptoms. The pathologic anatomy is very similar to that of upper pharyngeal pouches, and they also are frequently associated with underlying motility disturbances of the esophagus, usually esophageal acha-lasia or diffuse spasm.[22] Dysphagia and regurgitation are common symptoms, as is true for upper esophageal pouches, but many patients have no symptoms at all. Roentgenographic examination of the esophagus is usually quite characteristic, but complete evaluation of the patient should include studies of esophageal motility. Operation is usually indicated when symptoms are progressive and severe, and involves resection of the diverticulum accompanied by a long extramucosal esophagomyotomy (Fig. 4). Recurrence is rare after such a combined procedure, and the clinical results are usually excellent.

Diverticulosis

More uncommon even than midesophageal traction diverticula are examples of a condition termed "intramural diverticulosis of the esophagus."[27] Radiographs of the esophagus demonstrate multiple tiny outpouchings along the course of the esophagus, and the commonest symptom described by patients with such findings is dysphagia. The condition is often secondary to other esophageal diseases, such as esophageal web, reflux esophagitis, and disturbances in esophageal motility, and therapy should be directed toward relieving the underlying cause. Roentgenographically, the appearance is usually confused with inflammatory lesions of the esophagus, particularly monilial esophagitis.

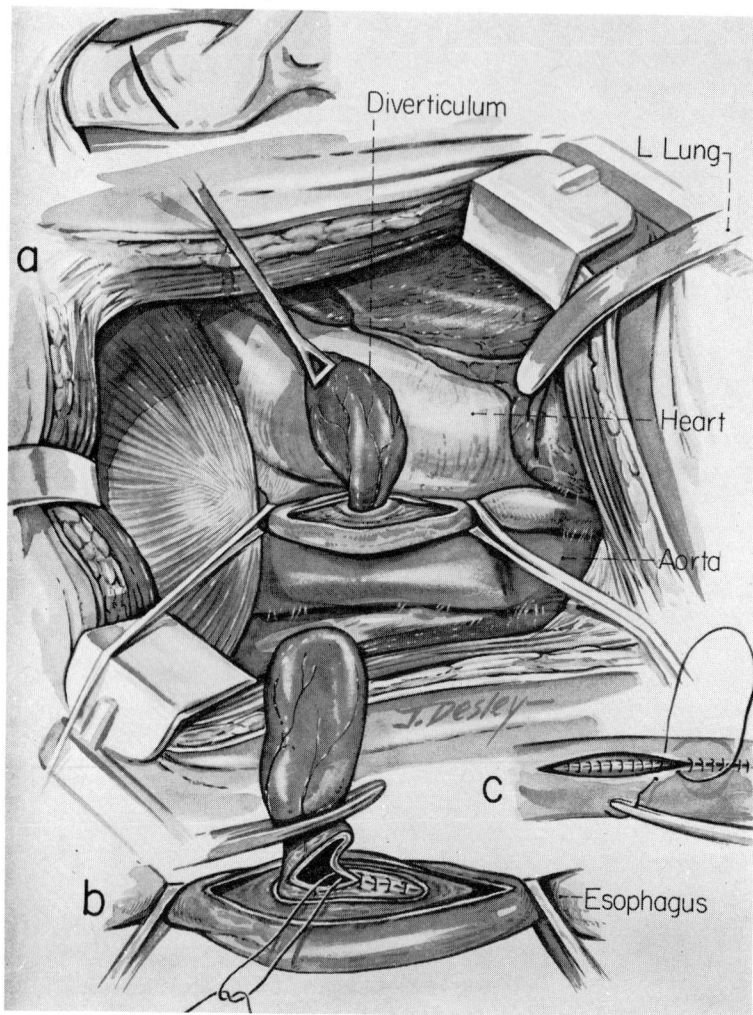

Figure 4. Surgical treatment of epiphrenic diverticulum. *A,* Exposure through bed of non-resected left eighth rib. *B,* Removal of diverticulum and closure of mucosa. *C,* Closure of esophageal musculature over mucosal suture line.

Illustration continued on opposite page

MISCELLANEOUS CONDITIONS OF THE ESOPHAGUS

Paterson-Kelly Syndrome

In 1919 Paterson[56] and Kelly[36] independently described a clinical state with which the names of Plummer and Vinson later became associated in the United States. The typical patient is a middle-aged, edentulous woman with atrophic oral mucosa, spoon-shaped fingers with brittle nails, and a long-standing history of anemia and dysphagia. The cause of the dysphagia is usually a fibrous web partially obstructing the esophageal lumen a few millimeters below the introitus. A high incidence has been reported in the Scandinavian countries, and because of the iron-deficiency anemia the term "sideropenic dysphagia" was used. A dietary deficiency has been established as the cause, and the condition responds well to iron therapy and forceful dilation of the stricture. In approximately 10 per cent of affected persons, a malignant lesion of the oral cavity, hypopharynx, or esophagus develops.[76] The syndrome is relatively imprecise and covers a broad range of clinical entities. Not all patients are anemic or malnourished, nor are they all found to have an esophageal web. Some upper esophageal webs must certainly be congenital in origin even though a more common location for esophageal rings and webs is the lower portion of the esophagus.

Lower Esophageal Rings and Webs

While congenital webs of the distal esophagus are extremely rare, the association of a ringlike constriction of the lower esophagus with a sliding esophageal hiatal hernia is being recognized more and more frequently (Fig. 5). The roentgenographic characteristics of the lesion have been described by Schatzki and Gary,[64] who pointed out that while the majority of patients in whom this abnormality is demonstrated are symptomatic, dysphagia may occur if the degree of narrowing produced by the ring is 20 mm. and is almost always present if the lumen is 13 mm. or less in diameter. While many etiologic theories have been proposed, the cause of the condition is unknown. The lesion may either be muscular or mucosal in nature, the latter occurring characteristically at the squamocolumnar junction.[26] Because of the intact mucosa overlying the ring, endoscopy may fail to disclose it. Obstruction resulting from the esophageal ring can

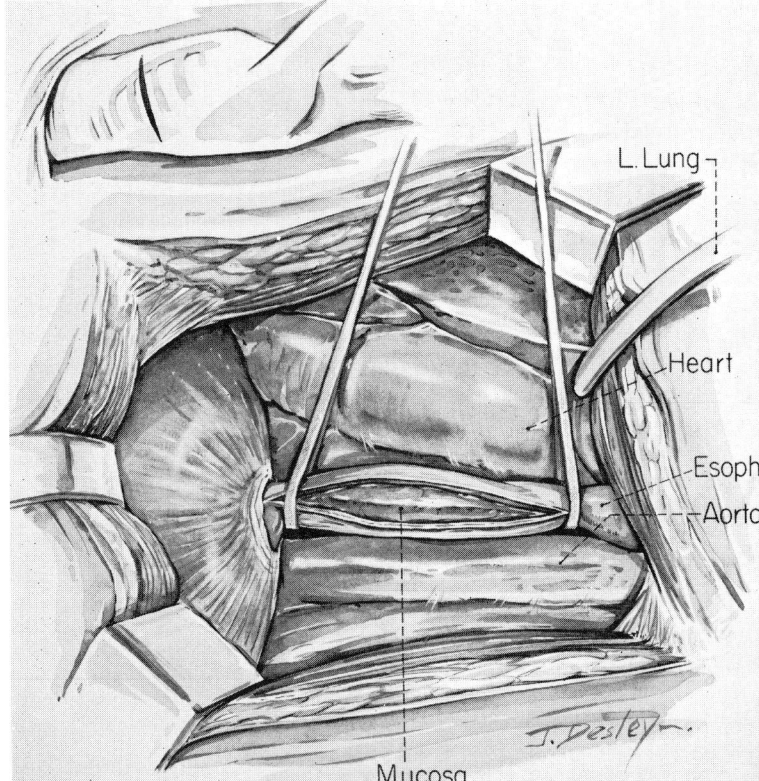

Figure 4. *Continued.* Long myotomy done concomitantly after site of diverticular excision was rotated out of the field. The incision extends almost to the aortic arch. If a diaphragmatic hernia is present, it should be repaired at the same time. (From Payne, W. S., and Clagett, O. T.: Curr. Probl. Surg., April, 1965. Copyright © 1965, Year Book Medical Publishers. Used by permission.)

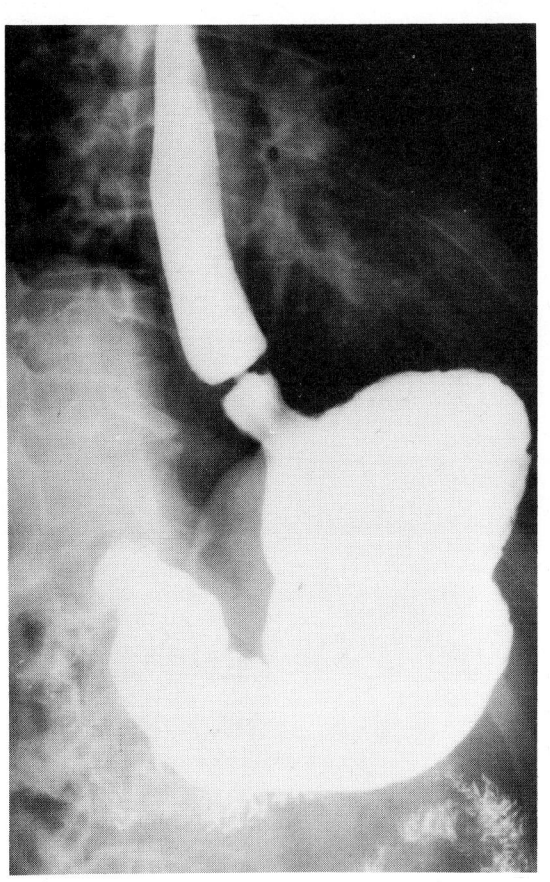

Figure 5. Esophageal roentgenogram of a patient with a small diaphragmatic hernia and a typical "Schatzki ring."

usually be relieved by peroral bougienage.[61] If symptoms of reflux are also present because of the sliding esophageal hiatal hernia, this should be repaired surgically. At the time of hiatal hernia repair, the ring can be excised or radially incised or ruptured digitally through a small gastrotomy,[71] and recurrence is rare.

Emetogenic Injury

A common cause is believed to be responsible for both esophagogastric mucosal lacerations (Mallory-Weiss syndrome[47]) and spontaneous rupture of the esophagus (Boerhaave syndrome). The latter condition will be discussed in a later section. This consists of a sudden increase in intra-abdominal pressure, the result of an explosive vomiting effort against a closed glottis. A history of prolonged retching or vomiting often but not always associated with alcoholism is characteristic.

When such a mechanism leads to gastroesophageal mucosal lacerations, painless gastrointestinal bleeding may ensue. Early diagnosis can be facilitated by roentgenographic studies to exclude the possibility of other lesions and by endoscopy to identify the site of bleeding. Although the bleeding may be self-limited, surgical exploration may be required if it persists. The upper end of the stomach should be exposed through a long gastrotomy, and after manual evacuation of clots and the insertion of proper retractors for exposure, the lacerated areas should be repaired with sutures.[33] Prompt arrest of bleeding can be expected with this technique.

INFLAMMATORY LESIONS

Increasing numbers of cases of esophageal moniliasis are now being reported, undoubtedly as a result of the increasingly widespread use of immunosuppressive therapy, steroids, and antibiotics. The symptoms are those of painful dysphagia, and the radiographic features include an irregular, ragged mucosal pattern with numerous small indentations and protrusions sometimes referred to as a "cobblestone" esophagus.[25] Treatment should be devoted to supportive measures and to correction of the underlying predisposing factors, with discontinuation of immunosuppressive drugs, steroids, or antibiotics. If the infection does not subside spontaneously, oral use of nystatin is indicated.

Other infections which, in the past, were occasionally reported as involving the esophagus include tuberculosis and syphilis. While bona fide cases of Crohn's disease of the esophagus have been difficult to document, some probable examples of this condition are reported in the literature.[43] Since the esophagus, like the skin, is covered with squamous epithelium, it is not surprising that certain dermatologic disorders are associated with esophageal manifestations, particularly pemphigoid vulgaris, bullous pemphigoid, or benign mucous membrane pemphigoid.

SELECTED REFERENCES

Code, C. F., and Schlegel, J. F.: Motor action of the esophagus and its sphincters. In Handbook of Physiology. Section 6, Alimentary Canal. Baltimore, Williams & Wilkins Company, 1967, Chapter 90, pp. 1821–1839.

This superb summary by two of the pioneers in the field of esophageal manometry provides the reader with all the information necessary for a basic understanding of the normal function of the esophagus and its sphincters.

Earlam, R.: Clinical Tests of Oesophageal Function. London, Crosby Lockwood Staples, 1976.
A new text incorporating all that is new and useful in analyzing the patient with esophageal disease.

Ellis, F. H., Jr., and Olsen, A. M.: Achalasia of the Esophagus. Philadelphia, W. B. Saunders Company, 1969.
This monograph represents a modern summary of all aspects of this interesting disease. Emphasis is on the surgical management of esophageal achalasia which the authors prefer to forceful dilation as primary therapy.

Payne, W. S., and Olsen, A. M.: The Esophagus. Philadelphia, Lea and Febiger, 1974.
Those interested in the esophagus have long awaited a modern summary of diagnosis and treatment of diseases of this organ. This monograph, based on the extensive experience of the Mayo Clinic, more than fulfills this need. It is currently the best of the available texts on the subject and is already a classic.

Zaino, C., Jacobsen, H. G., Lepou, H., and Ozturk, C. H.: Pharyngoesophageal Sphincter. Springfield, Ill., Charles C Thomas, Publisher, 1970.
Anatomic texts on the esophagus are rare and unusually dull. This is an exception and concerns a long-neglected anatomical region of this important organ.

REFERENCES

1. Akl, B. F., and Blakeley, W. R.: Late assessment of results of cricopharyngeal myotomy for cervical dysphagia. Am. J. Surg., 128:818, 1974.
2. Benz, L. J., Hootkin, L. A., Margulies, S., Donner, M. W., Cauthorne, R. T., and Hendrix, T. R.: A comparison of clinical measurements of gastroesophageal reflux. Gastroenterology, 62:1, 1972.
3. Billroth, T.: Ueber die Resection des Oesophagus. Arch. Klin. Chir., 13:65, 1871.
4. Butin, J. W., Olsen, A. M., Moersch, H. J., and Code, C. F.: Study of esophageal pressures in normal persons and patients with cardiospasm. Gastroenterology, 23:278, 1953.
5. Butler, H.: Veins of oesophagus. Thorax, 6:276, 1951.
6. Cassella, R. R., Brown, A. L., Jr., Sayre, G. P., et al.: Achalasia of the esophagus: Pathologic and etiologic considerations. Ann. Surg., 160:474, 1964.
7. Code, C. F., Creamer, B., Schlegel, J. F., et al.: An Atlas of Esophageal Motility in Health and Disease. Springfield, Ill., Charles C Thomas, Publisher, 1958.
8. Creamer, B., Donoghue, F. E., and Code, C. F.: Pattern of esophageal motility in diffuse spasm. Gastroenterology, 34:782, 1958.
9. Cohen, B. R., and Guelrud, M.: "Cardiospasm" in achalasia: Demonstration of supersensitivity of the lower esophageal sphincter. Abstract. Gastroenterology, 60:769, 1971.
10. Cohen, S., and Harris, L. D.: Does hiatus hernia affect competence of the gastroesophageal sphincter? N. Engl. J. Med., 284:1053, 1971.
11. Czerny: Neue Operationen: Vorläufige Mittheilung. Zbl. Chir., 4:433, 1877.
12. Daly, D. D., Code, C. F., and Andersen, H. A.: Disturbances of swallowing and esophageal motility in patients with multiple sclerosis. Neurology, 12:250, 1962.
13. Donoghue, F. E., Winkelmann, R. K., and Moersch, H. J.: Esophageal defects in dermatomyositis. Ann. Otol., 69:1139, 1960.
14. Earlam, R. J.: Clinical Tests of Oesophageal Function. London, Crosby Lockwood Staples, 1976, pp. 93–126.
15. Earlam, R. J., Ellis, F. H., Jr., and Nobrega, F. T.: Achalasia of the esophagus in a small urban community. Mayo Clin. Proc., 44:478, 1969.
16. Ellis, F. G.: The natural history of achalasia of the cardia. Proc. R. Soc. Med., 53:663, 1960.
17. Ellis, F. H., Jr.: Management of oesophageal achalasia. Clin. Gastroenterol., 5:89, 1976.
18. Ellis, F. H., Jr., and Olsen, A. M.: Achalasia of the Esophagus. Philadelphia, W. B. Saunders Company, 1969.
19. Ellis, F. H., Jr., Schlegel, J. F., Code, C. F., et al.: Surgical treatment of esophageal hypermotility disturbances. J.A.M.A., 188:862, 1964.
20. Ellis, F. H., Jr., Schlegel, J. F., Lynch, V. P., et al.: Crico-

pharyngeal myotomy for pharyngo-esophageal diverticulum. Ann. Surg., *170*:340, 1969.

21. Fischer, R. A., Ellison, G. W., Thayer, W. R., et al.: Esophageal motility in neuromuscular disorders. Ann. Intern. Med., *63*:229, 1965.

22. Garcia, J. B., Bengochea, J. B., and Wooler, G. H.: Epiphrenic diverticula of the esophagus. Certain considerations about its surgical treatment. J. Thorac. Cardiovasc. Surg., *63*:114, 1972.

23. Garrett, J. M., Winkelmann, R. K., Schlegel, J. F., and Code, C. F.: Esophageal deterioration in scleroderma. Mayo Clin. Proc., *46*:92, 1971.

24. Giles, G. R., Mason, M. C., Humphries, C., and Clark, C. G.: Action of gastrin on the lower esophageal sphincter in man. Gut, *10*:730, 1969.

25. Gonzales, G.: Esophageal moniliasis. Am. J. Roentgenol., *113*:233, 1971.

26. Goyal, R. K., Bauer, J. L., and Spiro, H. M.: Nature and location of lower esophageal ring. N. Engl. J. Med., *284*:1175, 1971.

27. Hammon, J. W., Jr., Rice, R. P., Postlethwait, R. W., and Young, W. G., Jr.: Esophageal intramural diverticulosis. A clinical and pathological survey. Ann. Thorac. Surg., *17*:260, 1974.

28. Heller, E.: Extramuköse Cardioplastik beim chronischen Cardiospasmus mit Dilatation des Oesophagus. Mitt. Grenzgeb. Med. Chir., *27*:141, 1913.

29. Helsper, J. T., Lance, J. S., Baldridge, E. T., and Vap, J. G.: Cricopharyngeal achalasia. Am. J. Surg., *128*:521, 1974.

30. Hiebert, C. A.: Primary incompetence of the gastric cardia. Am. J. Surg., *119*:365, 1970.

31. Higgs, B., Kerr, F. W., and Ellis, F. H., Jr.: The experimental production of esophageal achalasia by electrolytic lesions in the medulla. J. Thorac. Cardiovasc. Surg., *50*:613, 1965.

32. Higgs, B., Shorter, R. G., and Ellis, F. H., Jr.: A study of the anatomy of the human esophagus with special reference to the gastroesophageal sphincter. J. Surg. Res., *5*:503, 1965.

33. Hinchey, E. J., and Hreno, A.: Postemetic gastroesophageal laceration with hemorrhage. Surg. Gynecol. Obstet., *126*:324, 1968.

34. Ingelfinger, F. J.: Esophageal motility. Physiol. Rev., *38*:533, 1958.

35. Kaplan, S.: Paralysis of deglutition, post-poliomyelitis complication treated by section of cricopharyngeus muscle. Ann. Surg., *133*:572, 1951.

36. Kelly, A. B.: Spasm at entrance to oesophagus. J. Laryngol., *34*:285, 1919.

37. Köberle, F.: Enteromegaly and cardiomegaly in Chagas disease. Gut, *4*:399, 1963.

38. Laimer, E.: Beitrag zur Anatomie des Oesophagus. Med. Jahr. Wein., 1883, pp. 333–388.

39. Leach, W.: Generalized muscular diseases presenting as pharyngeal dysphagia. J. Laryngol., *76*:237, 1962.

40. Lind, J. F., Warrian, W. G., and Wankling, W. J.: Responses of the gastroesophageal junctional zone to increases in abdominal pressure. Can. J. Surg., *9*:32, 1966.

41. Lipshutz, W. H., Gaskins, R. D., Lukash, W. M. and Sode, J.: Pathogenesis of lower-esophageal-sphincter incompetence. N. Engl. J. Med., *289*:182, 1973.

42. Lise, M., Perrino, G., Cordioli, G. P., and Cagol, P. P.: The autonomic nervous system in esophageal achalasia. Chir. Gastroenterol., *6*:103, 1972.

43. LiVolsi, V. A., and Jaretzki, A., III: Granulomatous esophagitis. A case of Crohn's disease limited to the esophagus. Gastroenterology, *64*:313, 1973.

44. Lortat-Jacob, J. L.: La myomatose nodulaire diffuse de l'oesophage. Acquis. Méd. Récent., 1950, pp. 103–111.

45. Ludlow, A.: Obstructed deglutition, from a preternatural dilatation of, and bag formed in, the pharynx. Med. Soc. Phys., *3*:85, 1762–1767.

46. Lund, W. S.: A study of the cricopharyngeal sphincter in man and in the dog. Ann. R. Coll. Surg. Engl., *37*:225, 1965.

47. Mallory, G. K., and Weiss, S.: Hemorrhages from lacerations of the cardiac orifice of the stomach due to vomiting. Am. J. Med. Sci., *178*:506, 1929.

48. Mann, C. V., Code, C. F., Schlegel, J. F., et al.: Intrinsic mechanisms controlling the mammalian gastro-oesophageal sphincter deprived of extrinsic nerve supply. Thorax, *23*:634, 1968.

49. Marshall, S. F.: Carcinoma of the esophagus: Successful resection of lower end of esophagus with reestablishment of esophageal gastric continuity. Surg. Clin. North Am., *18*:643, 1938.

50. von Mikulicz, J.: Zur Pathologie und Therapie des Cardiospasmus. Dtsch. Med. Wochenschr., *30*:17, 50, 1904.

51. Mills, C. P.: Dysphagia in pharyngeal paralysis treated by cricopharyngeal sphincterotomy. Lancet, *1*:455, 1973.

52. Mitchell, R. L., and Armanini, G. B.: Cricopharyngeal. myotomy: Treatment of dysphagia. Ann. Surg., *181*:262, 1975.

53. Mladick, R. A., Horton, C. E., and Adamson, J. E.: Cricopharyngeal myotomy: Application and technique in major oral-pharyngeal resections. Arch. Surg., *102*:1, 1971.

54. Ohsawa, T.: The surgery of the oesophagus. Arch. Jap. Chir., *10*:605, 1933.

55. Paris, F., Benages, A., Berenguer, J., Blasco, E., Garrido, G., Parrilla, P., Ridocci, M. T., and Carbonell, C.: Pre- and postoperative manometric studies in diffuse esophageal spasm. J. Thorac. Cardiovasc. Surg., *70*:126, 1975.

56. Paterson, D. R.: A clinical type of dysphagia. J. Laryngol., *34*:289, 1919.

57. Pedersen, S. A., and Alstrup, P.: The hypertensive gastroesophageal sphincter. A manometric and clinical study. Scand. J. Gastroenterol., *7*:531, 1972.

58. Pera, C., Suner, M., and Capdevila, J.: Anatomical demonstration of the lower esophageal sphincter: A biometrical analysis of 300 specimens. Bull. Soc. Int. Chir., *34*:285, 1975.

59. Pierce, J. W., Creamer, B., and MacDermot, V.: Pharynx and oesophagus in dystrophia myotonica. Gut, *6*:392, 1965.

60. Pope, C. E., II: Effect of infusion on force of closure measurements in the human esophagus. Gastroenterology, *58*:616, 1970.

61. Postlethwait, R. W., and Sealy, W. C.: Experiences with the treatment of 59 patients with lower esophageal web. Ann. Surg., *165*:786, 1967.

62. Sanderson, D. R., Ellis, F. H., Jr., and Olsen, A. M.: Achalasia of the esophagus: Results of therapy by dilation, 1950–1967. Chest, *58*:116, 1970.

63. Sanderson, D. R., Ellis, F. H., Jr., Schlegel, J. F., et al.: Syndrome of vigorous achalasia: Clinical and physiologic observations. Dis. Chest, *52*:508, 1967.

64. Schatzki, R., and Gary, J. E.: Dysphagia due to diaphragm-like localized narrowing in the lower esophagus ("lower esophageal ring"). Am. J. Roentgenol., *70*:911, 1953.

65. Silber, W.: Diabetes and oesophageal dysfunction. Br. Med. J., *3*:688, 1969.

66. Smith, A. W., Mulder, D. W., and Code, C. F.: Esophageal motility in amyotrophic lateral sclerosis. Mayo Clin. Proc., *32*:438, 1957.

67. Swigart, L. L., Siekert, R. G., Hambley, W. C., and Anson, B. J.: The esophageal arteries: An anatomic study of 150 specimens. Surg. Gynecol. Obstet., *90*:234, 1950.

68. Torek, F.: The first successful resection of the thoracic portion of the esophagus for carcinoma: preliminary report. J.A.M.A., *60*:1533, 1913.

69. Welsh, G. F., and Payne, W. S.: The present status of one-stage pharyngo-esophageal diverticulectomy. Surg. Clin. North Am., *53*:953, 1973.

70. Wheeler, W. I.: Pharyngocele and dilatation of pharynx with existing diverticulum at lower portion of pharynx lying posterior to the oesophagus, cured by pharyngotomy, being the first case of the kind recorded. Dublin J. Med. Sci., *82*:349, 1886.

71. Wilkins, E. W., Jr., and Bartlett, M. K.: Surgical treatment of the lower esophageal ring. N. Engl. J. Med., *268*:461, 1963.

72. Willis, T.: Pharmaceuticae rationalis: Sive diatraba de medicamentorum, operationibus in humano corpore. London, Hagae-Comitis, 1674.

73. Winship, D. H., Caflisch, C. R., Zboralske, F. F., et al.: Deterioration of esophageal peristalsis in patients with alcoholic neuropathy. Gastroenterology, *55*:173, 1968.

74. Wychulis, A. R., Ellis, F. H., Jr., and Andersen, H. A.: Acquired nonmalignant esophagotracheobronchial fistula: Report of 36 cases. J.A.M.A., *196*:117, 1966.

75. Wychulis, A. R., Woolam, G. L., Andersen, H. A., and Ellis, F. H., Jr.: Achalasia and carcinoma of the esophagus. J.A.M.A *215*:1638, 1971.

76. Wynder, E. L., Hultberg, S., Jacobsson, F., and Bross, I. J.: Environmental factors in cancer of the upper alimentary tract; a Swedish study with special reference to Plummer-Vinson (Paterson-Kelly) syndrome. Cancer, *10*:470, 1957.

77. Zenker, F. A., and von Ziemssen, H.: Krankheiten des Oesophagus. *In* von Ziemssen, H.: Handbuch der Speciellen Pathologie und Therapie. Volume 1. Leipzig, F.C.W. Vogel, 1875, pp. 1–208.

V

ESOPHAGOSCOPY

Bradley M. Rodgers, M.D.

Used in conjunction with the radiologic examination of the esophagus, esophagoscopy is an invaluable diagnostic technique for the gastroenterologist and surgeon and has provided a method of direct evaluation and treatment of many esophageal disorders.

Chevalier Jackson stated that it is an "unquestionable fact, that whereas any medical graduate can be taught to introduce the bronchoscope safely, teaching the beginner to introduce the esophagoscope is fraught with graver responsibilities than the teaching of anything else in the whole realm of surgery." Because it is a difficult and potentially dangerous procedure, esophagoscopy should be attempted only by a physician familiar with the anatomy of the esophagus and skilled in the specialized techniques of endoscopy. The more recent addition of flexible fiberoptic esophagoscopes has added further to the value and safety of this examination.

HISTORICAL ASPECTS

The earliest recorded attempts to directly examine the esophagus in a living subject were the efforts of Semeleder and Stoerk in 1866. Semeleder designed a forceps with spoon-shaped blades for viewing the upper esophagus. His confidence in this instrument was so great that he offered himself to Stoerk as an experimental subject. In 1868 Waldenberg reported the use of a gum elastic esophagoscope for viewing the cervical esophagus. In the same year, using an elongated urethroscope, Kussmaul became the first to visualize the esophagus directly. This report demonstrated the feasibility of introducing a rigid tube throughout the length of the esophagus. In 1881 Mikulicz, working with the Viennese electro-optician Joseph Leiter, introduced an instrument employing a distal electric light source for illumination. This was the forerunner of the modern esophagoscope. Killian reported the first case of removal of a foreign body through an esophagoscope in 1902. Subsequent technical modifications have included the Hopkins' rod lens optical system. Hirschowitz introduced flexible fiberoptic endoscopy in 1958.

All students of the art of esophagoscopy owe a lasting debt to the efforts of Dr. Chevalier Jackson for defining the exacting technique of esophagoscopy and developing its high degree of efficiency and safety. One would be remiss in attempting to perform esophagoscopic examinations without first consulting one of Jackson's invaluable textbooks on this subject.

ANATOMY AND PHYSIOLOGY

Embryologically, the esophagus develops as a portion of the foregut, from which the trachea arises ventrally as a diverticulum. Initially it is lined with ciliated columnar epithelium, but prior to birth this is converted to a stratified squamous epithelium. The average length of the esophagus in the adult is 40 cm. Excepting the pylorus, the esophagus is the narrowest and most muscular segment of the alimentary tract. The musculature of the upper third of the esophagus is striated and under voluntary control. This gradually progresses to the involuntary smooth muscle of the distal third. Lacking a serosa, the esophagus is invested in loose areolar tissue and is freely mobile except where fixed at the level of the cricopharyngeal sphincter and of the diaphragm. The lumen of the esophagus opens and closes rhythmically with changes in intrathoracic pressure caused by respiratory excursions of the diaphragm.

The esophagus has its origin at the level of the sixth cervical vertebra at the cricopharyngeal sphincter. In traversing the thoracic cavity, the esophagus lies in close approximation to several vital organs (Fig. 1). On entering the thorax, the esophagus lies posterior to and slightly to the left of the trachea. It crosses to the right as it passes posterior to the arch of the aorta and the tracheal bifurcation. At the level of the tenth thoracic vertebra, it curves to the left and anteriorly to pass in front of the aorta and through the esophageal hiatus in the diaphragm.

There are three areas of physiologic narrowing of the esophagus that are of importance to the esophagoscopist. The most important of these is the cricopharyngeal sphincter. The tonic contraction of the cricopharyngeus muscle pulls the cricoid cartilage posteriorly against the cervical spine. This is the principal anatomic factor contributing to the perforation of the esophagus during esophagoscopy. The second area of physiologic narrowing occurs at the point at which the esophagus passes behind the arch of the aorta and left main stem bronchus. This area is rarely noticed as a constriction by the esophagoscopist unless the aorta is markedly dilated. By "feeling" with the tip of the esophagoscope, however, the operator may easily locate the aortic pulsations transmitted through the wall of the esophagus. The third area of constriction is referred to as the diaphragmatic "pinchcock," where the esophagus passes through the diaphragmatic hiatus. This area is viewed as a tight narrowing by the esophagoscopist and must be carefully traversed.

The act of swallowing is a complex, integrated series of voluntary and involuntary muscular contractions propelling a bolus of food through the cricopharyngeal constrictor, along the length of the esophagus, and through the diaphragmatic sphincter into the stomach. These movements are ordinarily not observed by the esophagoscopist, but evidence of their failure in the form of dilation of the esophagus is readily appreciated.

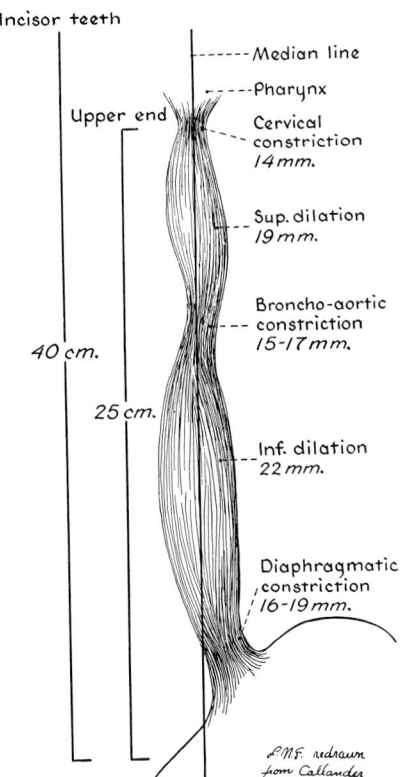

Incisor teeth

Median line

Pharynx

Upper end

Cervical constriction 14mm.

Sup. dilation 19mm.

Broncho-aortic constriction 15-17mm.

40 cm.

25 cm.

Inf. dilation 22mm.

Diaphragmatic constriction 16-19mm.

Figure 1. Normal anatomic landmarks of the esophagus. (From Boies, L. R. Hilger, J. A., and Priest, R. E.: Fundamentals of Otolaryngology, 4th ed. Philadelphia, W. B. Saunders Company, 1964.)

INDICATIONS AND CONTRAINDICATIONS

When used in conjunction with barium x-ray studies, esophagoscopy is indicated in the evaluation of all patients with symptoms of esophageal disease. Such symptoms might include dysphagia, substernal discomfort, regurgitation, nausea, vomiting, hematemesis, weight loss, or gagging. Esophagoscopy is particularly useful whenever symptoms persist despite a negative x-ray study or whenever there is question of a

lesion on x-ray. In the former situation, the esophagoscopist may be able to identify an esophageal web or esophagitis. Often esophagoscopy is helpful in differentiating between benign and malignant strictures of the esophagus and should provide a tissue diagnosis. Conceived as a method of removing foreign bodies from the esophagus, this remains today a primary indication for immediate esophagoscopy. The ease, safety, and rapidity with which esophagoscopic examinations can be performed with the flexible fiberoptic esophagoscope have allowed a more aggressive approach to the direct diagnosis of upper gastrointestinal bleeding from esophageal varices.

Contraindications to esophagoscopy are few. For many years the presence of thoracic aortic aneurysms or severe hypertension was thought to preclude esophagoscopy. However, with newer techniques and a greater awareness of these problems, even these conditions should not cause a patient to be denied esophagoscopy in the most urgent situations, such as esophageal foreign body. One contraindication to esophagoscopy is the presence of acute corrosive or necrotizing esophagitis from ingestion of caustic substances. In such patients, the edema and inflammation of the esophagus greatly increase the likelihood of perforation from a complete esophagoscopy examination.

INSTRUMENTATION

The standard Jackson rigid esophagoscope is constructed of a hollow metal tube with a beveled blunt tip (Fig. 2). It differs from the rigid bronchoscope by incorporating an integral drainage canal into the wall for intermittent aspiration. The standard size esophagoscopes used for adults are 9 mm. by 45 cm. or 9 mm. by 53 cm. For infants, the 4 mm. by 30 cm. esophagoscope is more appropriate. For older children, the 6 mm. by 35 cm. or the 7 mm. by 45 cm. esophagoscope may be used. For removal of foreign bodies from the upper esophagus, the shorter esophageal speculum is useful. Ancillary equipment should include aspirating tubes, sponge carriers, brushes, silk-woven and mercury-filled bougies, and various forward and side-grasping forceps for biopsy and foreign body removal.

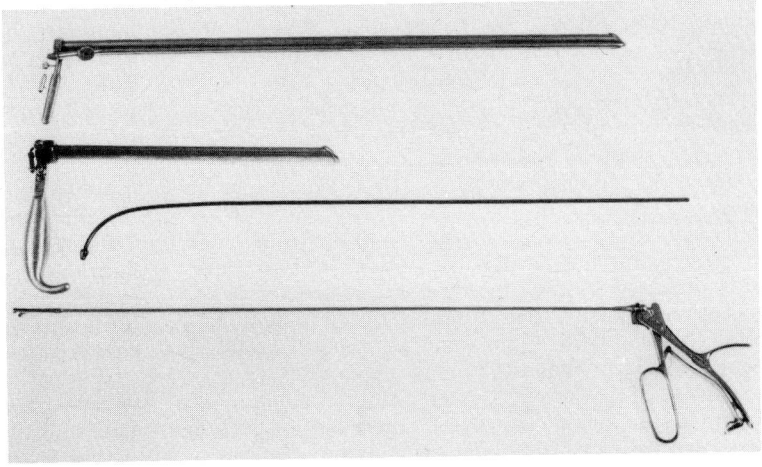

Figure 2. Basic esophagoscopic instrumentation. Top to bottom: standard Jackson esophagoscope, esophageal speculum, aspiration cannula, biopsy forceps.

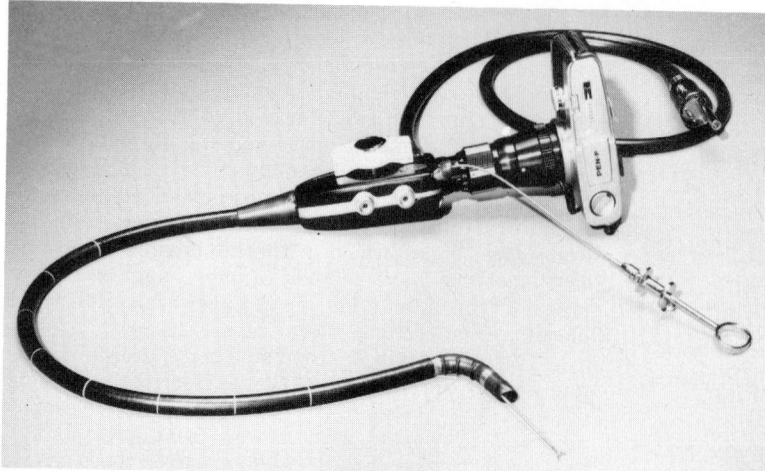

Figure 3. Flexible esophagofiberscope. (Courtesy of Olympus Corporation of America.)

Care must be taken to assure that all of these instruments are of suitable length for the esophagoscope chosen.

Recent technical advances have allowed the development of the flexible fiberoptic esophagoscope (Fig. 3). Less suited for removing most foreign bodies, or esophagal dilatation, the flexible esophagoscope nonetheless has introduced a new realm of convenience and safety to the field of esophagoscopy. Once considered a surgical procedure, esophogoscopy may be performed safely at the bedside with these instruments. Flexible esophagoscopes allow irrigation, insufflation, biopsy, and brushing for cytology to be performed in addition to magnified observation of the esophagus.

TECHNIQUE

Most esophagoscopic procedures can be performed quite satisfactorily under topical anesthesia of the hypopharynx. Topical anesthesia with tetracaine (Pontocaine) or lidocaine (Xylocaine) may be preferred to general anesthesia because of the possibility of aspiration of gastric contents, but the choice of anesthesia should be made on an individual basis. Situations that may require prolonged manipulation or observation, such as difficult foreign body extractions, should be done under general anesthesia. General anesthesia administered through an endotrocheal tube is preferred for infants and small children, because of the compressibility of the adjacent trachea.

Thorough preoperative preparation of the patient is of importance for the safe performance of esophagoscopy. The stomach and esophagus must be completely emptied of retained secretions. Occasionally, as in cases of achalasia, this may require esophageal lavage and drainage for several days prior to the anticipated procedure. Psychologically, the patient must be carefully prepared for the procedure and instructed in cooperation and relaxation. Administration of pentobarbital (Nembutal), 0.1 gm., and atropine, 0.5 mg., 1 hour prior to esophagoscopy may aid in alleviation of anxiety. Unless there are extenuating circumstances, esophagoscopy should always be preceded by barium x-ray studies of the esophagus, including a lateral x-ray of the cervical esophagus, to help outline this difficult area for the esophagoscopist.

The actual performance of esophagoscopy with the Jackson esophagoscope requires skill and gentleness derived only from experience under careful guidance. Jackson divided the technique into four steps for convenience, and the beginner is well advised to consult his complete description of each step.

Step one begins with the insertion of the esophagoscope down the posterior pharyngeal wall into the right pyriform sinus. The patient's head is held by an assistant, with the occiput well above the level of the table and slightly extended. *Step two* is the most difficult and critical moment of the procedure. The cricopharyngeal sphincter is located and with steady, gentle pressure the esophagoscope is carefully insinuated through this area. An open lumen must always be visualized. Insertion of a silk-woven bougie through the sphincter may help to locate and relax it and guide the esophagoscope through this narrow area. *Step three* involves passage of the esophagoscope through the thoracic esophagus. The patient's head should be lowered and turned as required for constant visualization of the lumen. Careful attention should be paid to the color of the mucosa and the mobility of the esophageal wall. The mucosa, which is pink in the upper esophagus, assumes a paler hue as the esophagogastric junction is approached. Suspicious areas may be biopsied or brushed for pathologic examination and secretions may be collected for cytologic examination. The *fourth step,* during which the esophagoscope is passed through the diaphragmatic hiatus into the stomach, requires the patient's head to be lowered and moved to the right. As with the cricopharyngeal area, a lumen finder will often aid in identifying and relaxing this sphincter.

As with the rigid esophagoscope, most procedures with the flexible fiberoptic esophagoscope may be performed under topical anesthesia, except in small infants and children. The flexible esophagoscope is most easily passed with the patient in the sitting or semi-sitting position. The scope is guided into the posterior pharynx with the index finger of the operator's hand. The tip is then flexed slightly anteriorly and the scope advanced into the upper esophagus. This maneuver

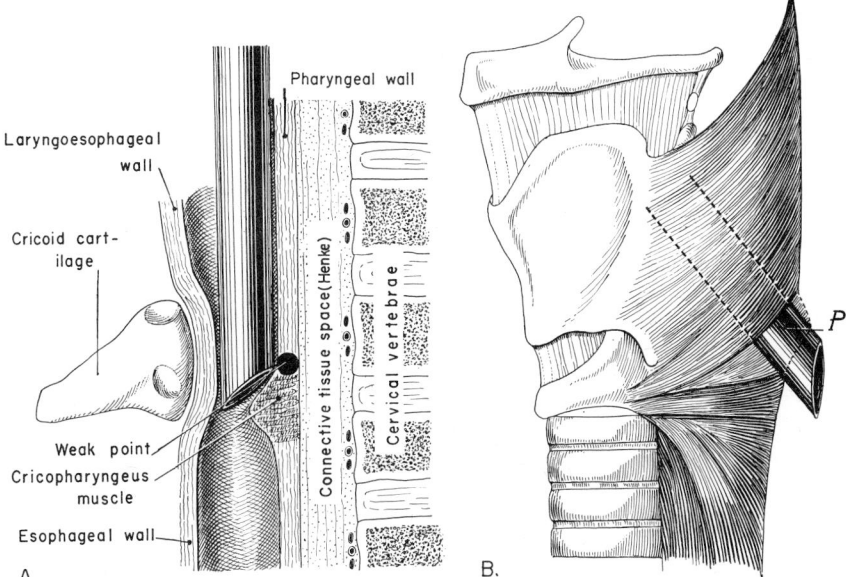

Figure 4. Schematic illustration of the anatomic basis for high esophageal perforation with the esophagoscope. (From Terracol, J., and Sweet, R. H.: Diseases of the Esophagus. Philadelphia, W. B. Saunders Company, 1958.)

may be facilitated by asking the patient to swallow as the esophagoscope approaches the cricopharyngeal sphincter. In order to avoid damage to the flexible esophagoscope, a small plastic "bite block" is placed around the esophagoscope prior to starting the procedure. With gentle insufflation of air, the esophagus is distended and the esophagoscope can be guided under direct vision through the length of the esophagus. Directed biopsy or brush cytology may be obtained through the operating side channel of the esophagoscope. The development of special forceps has allowed retrieval of small foreign bodies from within the esophagus utilizing this esophagoscope. Because the flexible esophagoscope is passed blindly through the cricopharyngeal region, this region should be carefully inspected on retrieval of the esophagoscope.

COMPLICATIONS

Complications incident to esophagoscopy are largely to be avoided with careful technique. During esophagoscopy in infants, dyspnea may result from the use of too large a tube, which may encroach upon the more compressible trachea of these patients. The most frequent serious complication following esophagoscopy is perforation of the esophageal wall, usually *at the level of the cricopharyngeal sphincter* (Fig. 4). This injury manifests itself by pain in the neck and substernal area, fever, and crepitation in the neck and supraclavicular area. While antibiotic management without drainage has been advocated,[5] most observers recommend immediate drainage combined with antibiotic therapy.[3] Less commonly, the *thoracic* esophagus may be perforated, with resulting pneumothorax and mediastinitis. Treatment of this complication generally requires drainage of the pleural cavity and administration of antibiotics. When perforation of the esophagus is associated with *obstruction* distal to the perforation or is through a diverticulum, the leak is not apt to

close unless definitive therapeutic measures are taken. For this reason, Groves and others advise immediate appropriate surgical therapy for the distal pathology.[3]

SELECTED REFERENCES

Berry, L. H.: Gastrointestinal Pan-endoscopy. Springfield, Ill., Charles C Thomas, Publisher, 1974.
   This comprehensive volume, with many expert contributers, completely covers the past and present developments in gastrointestinal endoscopy. A thorough section on the indications and contraindications to esophagoscopy is included in addition to an excellent review of the historical developments in this field. Dr. Berry gives an excellent description of the techniques involved in the use of the flexible as well as rigid esophagoscopy equipment.

Jackson, C.: Difficulties and pitfalls in the insinuation of the esophagoscope. Ann. Otol., 45:1109, 1936.
   This delightful paper was presented by Dr. Jackson before the Nineteenth Annual Meeting of the American Bronchoscopic Society. In it, he describes all of the common pitfalls of the esophagoscopist and important ways of avoiding them. It is excellent reading for any student of modern esophagoscopy.

Jackson, C., and Jackson, C. L.: Bronchoesophagology. Philadelphia, W. B. Saunders Company, 1950.
   This volume is the classic text on the subject of esophagoscopy. It is extraordinarily complete in every detail of the technique and its uses and should be considered required reading for the physician performing these procedures.

REFERENCES

1. Bautista, A., and DuLuca, V. J.: Endoscopic photography, biopsy and cytology of the esophagus and stomach with the Olympus fiberesophagoscope. Gastroenterology, 60:294, 1970.
2. Brick, J. B.: Esophagoscopy by and for the internist: A review of results of a thousand cases. Am. J. Med. Sci., 241:288, 1961.
3. Groves, L.: Instrumental perforation of the esophagus. What is conservative management? J. Thorac. Cardiovasc. Surg., 52:1, 1966.
4. Killian, G.: On direct endoscopy of the upper air passages and oesophagus. Br. Med. J., 2:269, 1902.
5. Mengoli, L. R., and Klassen, K. P.: Conservative management of esophageal perforation. A.M.A. Arch. Surg., 91:238, 1965.
6. Patterson, E. J.: History of bronchoscopy and esophagoscopy for foreign body. Laryngoscope, 36:157, 1926.
7. Waye, J. D.: The current status of esophagoscopy, gastroscopy and duodenoscopy. Mt. Sinai J. Med., 42:57, 1975.

VI

PERFORATION OF THE ESOPHAGUS: SPONTANEOUS (BOERHAAVE'S SYNDROME), TRAUMATIC, AND FOLLOWING ESOPHAGOSCOPY

David B. Skinner, M.D.

Rupture of the esophagus, an uncommon condition, is a difficult clinical problem. It can be an unexpected cause of rapid death in otherwise healthy people, is often difficult to diagnose, and continues to be a challenging surgical problem. Spontaneous rupture of a normal esophagus was first reported under dramatic circumstances by Boerhaave in 1704 in the Netherlands. In Meade's *A History of Thoracic Surgery,*[7] Van Swieten is cited as providing the first English language description of Boerhaave's observation: ". . . the illustrious Baron Wassenaer, Lord High Admiral to the Republick, after intense straining in vomiting, broke asunder the tube of the esophagus, near the diaphragm, so that after the most excruciating pains, the aliments which he swallowed passed, together with the air, into the cavity of the thorax, and he expired in 24 hours."

Pathophysiology

Compared to the incidence of esophageal rupture, spontaneous or instrumental perforation of other portions of the normal alimentary tract is unusual. Consideration of the causes for this difference provides guidance to understanding and management. The esophagus differs from the remainder of the alimentary tract in having no serosal layer. Both serosal and submucosal layers containing collagen and elastic fibers provide strength to the gut wall. The absence of serosa in the esophagus makes it more likely to rupture at lower pressures than the rest of the gut. The distal esophagus lies immediately beneath the left thoracic pleura, and the middle esophagus lies beneath the right pleura. As pressures in the thoracic cavities are less than atmospheric, the gradient across the esophageal wall is greater than intraluminal esophageal pressure. Ruptures of the lower esophagus nearly always perforate into the left thoracic cavity, and ruptures of the mid-esophagus perforate into the right thoracic cavity. There are no surrounding soft tissues to buttress the esophagus in these locations. The esophagus must periodically adjust to rapid forced increases in diameter. During vomiting, the lower esophagus almost momentarily increases in diameter by five times or more.[4] Swallowing of a large bolus requires rapid increase in the esophageal lumen. This combination of factors—the absence of serosa, a pressure gradient across the esophageal wall caused by negative intrathoracic pressures, and the need for rapid dilatation during vomiting and ingestion—pro-vides the setting in which rupture of the esophagus is prone to occur.

Classification and Incidence

Perforations of the esophagus are classified according to etiology and location. The incidence of perforation resulting from a particular cause varies depending upon the patient population treated by the reporting hospital or physician. Several recent reports suggest that the frequency of esophageal perforation is increasing. For example, Sawyers and colleagues report that esophageal perforations have increased from 1 in 20,000 admissions to 1 in 8,000 admissions at the Vanderbilt University Hospitals.[10]

The etiologic classification is listed in Table 1. Commonly recognized categories include spontaneous rupture, instrumental perforation, traumatic perforation, and perforation of intrinsic esophageal disease. Spontaneous or strain-induced rupture is rare and occurs less commonly than traumatic or instrumental perforations in several large series. Ruptures in 8 of 64 patients reported by Sawyers et al. were caused spontaneously in a normal esophagus, and 16 of 68 esophageal perforations described by Rosoff and White were attributed to this cause.[9] In these reports, the incidence of spontaneous esophageal rupture was approximately one in each 75,000 hospital admissions. A large experience with 47 cases of strain-induced perforation has been presented by Abbott and co-workers.[1]

TABLE 1.   Causes of Esophageal Perforation

I. Spontaneous or strain-induced
II. Instrumental
   A. Esophagoscopy
   B. Dilatations
   C. Intubation
III. Traumatic
   A. Penetrating missile
   B. Foreign body swallowed
   C. Blunt chest or abdominal injury
   D. Surgical dissection
   E. Ingested caustic agents
IV. Intrinsic esophageal disease
   A. Carcinoma
   B. Acid-peptic ulceration
   C. Other

All ruptures occurred in the lower third of the esophagus, the common location for spontaneous perforation.

Instrumental perforations of the esophagus may occur during esophagoscopy, esophageal dilatation, or the passage of upper alimentary tract tubes. It is estimated that the risk of perforation during esophagoscopy is approximately 1 in 150 procedures.[2] The incidence may be less when the flexible fiberoptic esophagoscope is used routinely, but this does not eliminate the problem of instrumental perforation. Factors that contribute to the frequency of endoscopic perforation include the type and effectiveness of anesthesia, and failure to deflate an endotracheal tube cuff if present. The risk is greater in elderly patients suffering from cervical arthritis. Instrumental perforation may occur at any level, but is most common just above the cardia and in the cervical esophagus. Spasm or hypertrophy of the cricopharyngeal sphincter in addition to arthritic vertebral osteophytes explains the frequency of cervical perforations, and the forward and left lateral bend of the distal esophagus contributes to perforation at the lower end. Perforation is also likely to occur at the level of intrinsic esophageal disease. Once inflammation or neoplasm has penetrated the submucosa, the strength of the esophageal wall is markedly decreased. Accordingly, patients undergoing esophagoscopy or dilatation are routinely warned of this potential danger, and they must be evaluated shortly following the procedure so that perforation may be detected promptly when it occurs.

Traumatic disruption of the esophagus may be subdivided into five additional categories. Perforations resulting from penetrating wounds of the neck, chest, or abdomen are reported with increasing frequency in recent years, particularly in urban hospitals. In several reports the incidence of these injuries is now the highest for all causes.[8, 9] The level of the injury depends upon the location of the penetrating wound. Rupture of the esophagus from nonpenetrating external trauma is uncommon, but must be considered following blunt trauma to the chest or upper abdomen. Ingestion of foreign bodies accounts for a small number of esophageal perforations. These perforations are at the levels at which foreign bodies commonly lodge – the cervical region just below the cricopharyngeal sphincter, the level of the aortic arch, and the distal esophagus just above the cardia. Ingestion of corrosive agents, especially lye, may cause perforation of the esophagus in severe cases. The fifth category of traumatic esophageal perforation results from surgical dissection around the esophagus in the course of other operations. The incidence of esophageal perforation during the performance of abdominal vagotomy is estimated at approximately 0.5 per cent in several series.[10, 13] Esophageal perforation may occur in the course of hiatal hernia repair or other procedures involving esophageal dissection. Perforation of the cervical esophagus during anterior spinal fusion is reported.

Rupture of the esophagus may occur as a complication of primary esophageal disease. Carcinoma of the esophagus may penetrate full thickness through the esophageal wall and cause a mediastinal or pleural cavity perforation. Benign esophageal ulcerations, particularly penetrating gastric ulcers in distal esophagus lined with columnar epithelium, may perforate completely through the esophageal wall. The location of such perforations depends on the level of the intrinsic disease.

Symptoms

Symptoms of esophageal rupture are usually dramatic and signal a catastrophic event. Death may occur within 24 hours in untreated cases. Early collapse of the patient is common. Pain related to the level of perforation is almost a universal complaint. As in the case of Admiral Wassenaer, this is generally severe and of such intensity and distribution that it may mimic the abdominal pain of a perforated gastroduodenal ulcer or severe pancreatitis, and the chest pain of dissection of the aorta or myocardial infarction. Nausea is a common complaint. Vomiting may precede the onset of pain in cases of spontaneous rupture, but disruption of the normal esophagus can occur without prior vomiting. Emesis following the onset of pain often contains blood. Hematemesis and pain also occur following forceful vomiting in the Mallory-Weiss syndrome in which the mucosal laceration is on the stomach side of the cardia where complete disruption is rare.[6] Evidence of perforation is not part of this syndrome. When a strain-induced tear occurs below the cardia, bleeding rather than perforation is the dominant feature. The reverse is true for tears above the cardia. If perforation occurs into the pleural cavity with resulting pneumohydrothorax, the respiratory symptoms predominate – dypsnea, cyanosis, air hunger, and other symptoms related to a collapsed lung and possible tension pneumothorax.

Physical Findings

Usually fever develops shortly after the onset of pain, and the patient rapidly becomes acutely ill. An early change in vital signs, tachycardia, tachypnea, and hypotension, and clinical evidence of shock are common. When the perforation is limited to the mediastinal tissues, rales in the lung bases are frequently heard. The sound of air in the mediastinum crackling with each heartbeat while the patient holds his breath is occasionally present. This is called the mediastinal crunch sound of Hamman. More extensive mediastinal emphysema is palpable as crepitus at the base of the neck. In time this may extend to cause subcutaneous emphysema over the chest wall and neck. If the perforation has penetrated the pleural cavity, findings include those of pneumothorax and pleural effusion. Absence of breath sounds is observed on the affected side with dullness to percussion over the lower thoracic cavity and a normal or increased percussion note in the upper chest. Evidence of tension pneumothorax with tracheal shift and limited excursion of the hemithorax occurs in severe cases. In addition to the chest findings, patients with thoracic perforations may have spasm, guarding, and tenderness of the upper abdomen and complain of abdominal pain. An ileus may develop rapidly along with gastric distention. Perforations limited to the neck cause much less severe abnormalities, often limited to fever, local tenderness and spasm, and crepitus. Abdominal perforations present the findings of an acute abdominal emergency but are frequently accompanied by mediastinal emphysema and lower chest abnormalities as well.

Diagnosis

Unfortunate delays in diagnosis occur when rupture of the esophagus is not suspected, and the patient is treated promptly for another incorrect diagnosis such as myocardial infarction, dissecting aortic aneurysm, or perforated abdominal viscus, which may cause similar catastrophic symptoms. When the diagnosis of ruptured esophagus is suspected by analysis of symptoms and physical findings, the confirmation is generally easy. Chest radiograph alone may be diagnostic when a hydropneumothorax is seen combined with air dissecting in the mediastinum. When emphysema is limited to the mediastinum, the chest x-ray findings are more subtle. Mediastinal widening may be prominent (Fig. 1). Air in the mediastinum outlined against the left pleural surface and collapsed lung produces a characteristic shadow behind the heart. This may be accentuated by pneumonitis in the partially collapsed basal segments of the left lower lobe.

Esophageal radiographic contrast studies should be performed promptly. Iodized oil (Lipiodol) or a water-soluble medium such as Gastrografin is used initially to prevent contamination of the mediastinum and pleura with barium if a perforation is demonstrated. Occasionally these substances fail to show the perforation. If nothing is seen during Lipiodol or Gastrografin swallow but the diagnosis is highly suspected, the examination should be repeated with barium (Fig. 2). Even when perforation is obvious by chest radiographs, the esophageal contrast study is essential to document the level and extent of perforation. Generally an upright abdominal radiograph is taken to exclude perforation into the abdomen.

Usual laboratory findings include an elevation in the white blood cell count, and hemoconcentration due to fluid loss. Aspirated pleural fluid may contain a high amylase level due to swallowed saliva. When the perforation is near the cardia, pleural fluid may be acidic, although neither of these findings is consistent. Serum electrolyte abnormalities and hypoalbuminemia, when present, reflect the duration of the perforation or pre-existing malnutrition, a common problem in alcoholic patients susceptible to esophageal rupture during vomiting. An electrocardiogram is performed to exclude a concomitant myocardial infarction causing a portion of the pain and symptoms. Arterial blood-gas determinations provide a useful guide to the

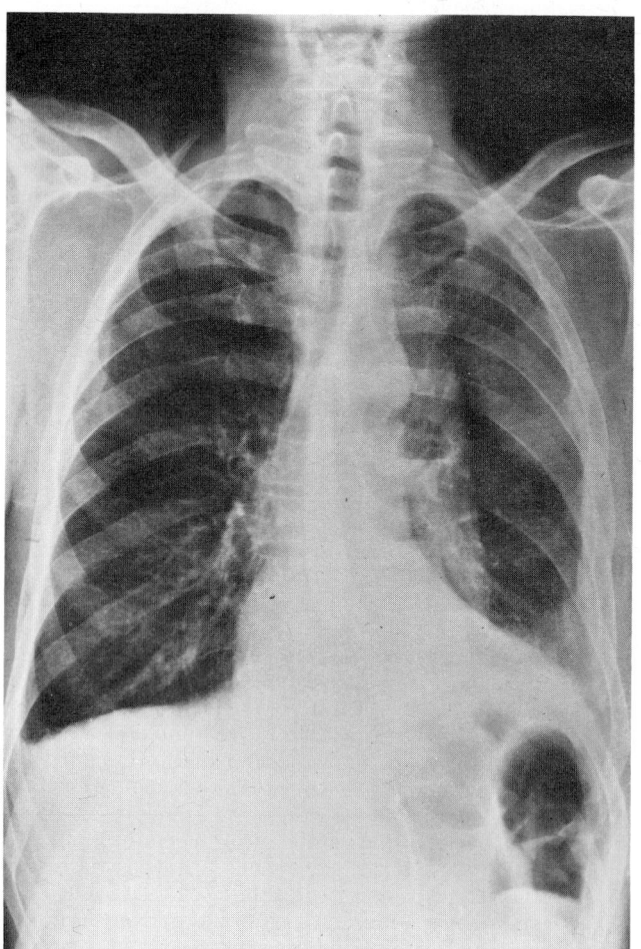

Figure 1. Chest film during a Gastrografin swallow in a patient suffering from spontaneous distal esophageal perforation. Notice the mediastinal widening and air-fluid level with partial collapse and infiltration of the left lower lobe.

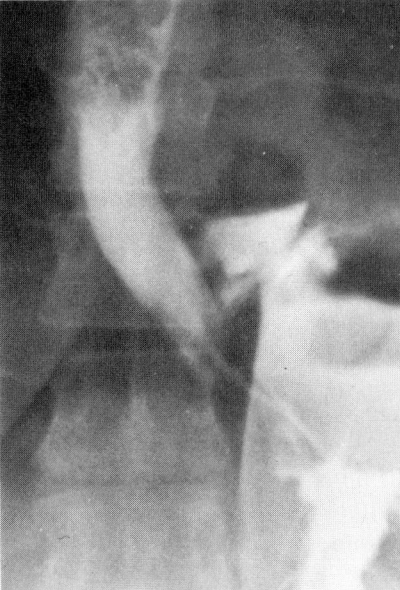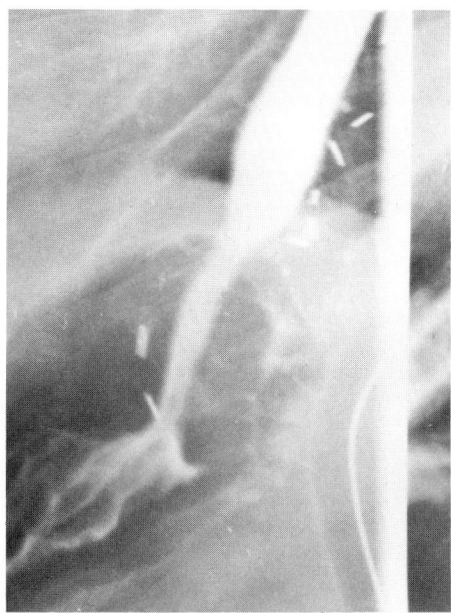

Figure 2. On the left a Gastrografin swallow demonstrates perforation of the distal esophagus following esophagoscopy. On the right, a postoperative barium swallow demonstrates suture closure of the perforation reinforced by a fundoplication around the distal esophagus.

severity of pulmonary dysfunction and the progress of resuscitation. The evaluation of the patient with suspected esophageal rupture should take no more than several hours, so that treatment for the correct diagnosis can be undertaken promptly. Only rarely is esophagoscopy necessary to confirm or establish the level of the perforation. Generally I prefer not to perform this test for fear of enlarging the disruption of the esophagus.

Treatment

In special circumstances, patients treated by nonsurgical methods have survived perforation of the esophagus. Surgical treatment, however, is essential for the successful recovery of most patients suffering from this condition. The operative approach depends upon both the cause of the perforation and the time elapsed between the perforation and surgery.

Cervical Perforation. In patients having perforation of the cervical esophagus, limited extravasation, and no thoracic involvement, intensive antibiotic therapy, eliminating oral feeding, and provision of intravenous alimentation are occasionally sufficient treatment. For perforations of the cervical esophagus causing crepitus and dissection of extravasated material in fascial planes, operative drainage coupled with intensive antibiotic therapy is the minimal procedure necessary. If it is possible technically to close the perforation site this is advantageous. Alternatively, a cervical esophagostomy tube can be inserted through the perforation and led out through a stab wound in the neck to provide drainage and a controlled fistula. With proper treatment, perforations of the cervical esophagus are managed with a low mortality rate.

Thoracic Perforation. Survival following perforation of the thoracic esophagus varies directly with the time interval between perforation and operation. Mortality rates range from 10 to 15 per cent in patients treated in less than 24 hours following injury, whereas the mortality increases to 50 per cent or more for patients with delayed surgical therapy.[3, 10]

For the early treatment of spontaneous or instrumental perforation of the esophagus, suture closure of the opening combined with chest drainage is often successful. If adjacent tissue is available to buttress the closure by an onlay patch, this is recommended. The use of adjacent gastric fundus as described by Thal is especially valuable for lower esophageal ruptures.[11] Flaps of diaphragm or adjacent pleura can be placed over the sutured defect.

If perforation is discovered promptly in a patient with an intrinsic esophageal disease, and surgical treatment is undertaken early, definitive therapy for the disease is desirable. This may necessitate esophagectomy in patients with carcinoma or stricture, myotomy in patients with achalasia, or hiatal hernia repair with an antireflux procedure in patients having reflux esophagitis. Simple closure of a perforation above an obstructing esophageal lesion or in the presence of free acid-peptic reflux cannot be expected to succeed.

When surgical treatment is undertaken late following perforation, operative choices are limited by the dangers of attempting to suture infected and edematous tissues. Extensive drainage of infected secretions is essential in all cases. Simple suture repair of the perforation is unlikely to succeed. In addition to drainage, four approaches to managing the neglected perforation are advocated, indicating that no single method is clearly superior. Abbott and associates describe inserting a T-tube through the opening in the esophagus, closing the perforation as well as possible around the tube, and leading it to the skin surface to facilitate drainage.[6] Placement of the tube away from the aorta is important to avoid secondary infection and rupture of the aorta. Thal and others employ a gastric fundus patch sutured over the lower esophageal perforation to achieve closure.[9, 11] For late perforations of the midthoracic esophagus, esophagectomy with closure of the cardia and a cervical esophagostomy may be necessary to control continuing infection in the mediastinum.[5] At a later stage esophageal reconstruction by substernal colon interposition is undertaken. Urschel and colleagues describe a similar approach but leave the esophagus in place.[12] The cardia is ligated and a lateral cervical esophagostomy is performed with tube drainage of the esophagus until the perforation heals. Thereafter the ligature at the cardia is removed. Unfortunately the ligature at the cardia does not always remain occlusive, as pressure necrosis of the underlying tissue may permit the lumen to reopen. Removal of the ligature embedded in the esophageal wall is not easy. This approach seems less attractive than the others. Results obtained by the several techniques for treating late perforations vary from series to series and appear to be related more to the time interval between perforation and surgery and to the underlying disease than to the specific technique employed.

Following surgical treatment, continuing infection and its complications are a serious threat. Mediastinitis, empyema, lung or mediastinal abscess, subphrenic abscess, and breakdown of the closure or anastomosis must be diagnosed and drained promptly and thoroughly by the appropriate techniques. Other serious complications include pneumonia, pericarditis, aspiration, and hemorrhage from a major vessel such as the aorta weakened by sepsis and eroded by an adjacent drainage tube. Such infectious complications are the major reason why perforation of the esophagus continues to cause high mortality and morbidity.

ACKNOWLEDGMENT

I would like to thank Geoffrey Adkins for his help in preparing this chapter.

SELECTED REFERENCES

Abbott, O. A., Mansour, K. A., Logan, W. D., Jr., Hatcher, C. R., and Symbas, P. N.: Atraumatic so-called "spontaneous" rupture of the esophagus. A review of 47 personal cases with comments on a new method of surgical therapy. J. Thorac. Cardiovasc. Surg., 59:67–83, 1970.
This report of 47 proved cases of atraumatic "spontaneous" rupture of the esophagus provides an excellent analytical description of the symptoms, findings, and cause of this condition. The T-tube method of drainage is presented in detail. An excellent discussion follows.

Meade, R. H.: A History of Thoracic Surgery. Springfield, Ill., Charles C Thomas, Publisher, 1961, pp. 649–655.
The history of rupture of the esophagus is presented — from Boerhaave's first described case to the establishment of successful treatment methods in 1958.

Rosoff, L., and White, E. J.: Perforation of the esophagus. Am. J. Surg., 128:207–218, 1974.
A large experience with 68 patients having perforated esophagus from various causes is presented. A good description is offered of the incidence, findings, and management of perforation due to different etiologies.

Sawyers, J. L., et al: Esophageal perforation. An increasing challenge. Ann. Thorac. Surg., 19:233–238, 1975.
The changing incidence, causes, findings, and management of 64 patients having esophageal perforation from various causes is presented. A somewhat different spectrum of patients is presented than in the preceding reference.

REFERENCES

1. Abbott, O. A., Mansour, K. A., Logan, W. D., Jr., Hatcher, C. R., and Symbas, P. N.: Atraumatic so-called "spontaneous" rupture of the esophagus. A review of 47 personal cases with comments on a new method of surgical therapy. J. Thorac. Cardiovasc. Surg., 59:67–83, 1970.
2. Belsey, R. H. R., and Milligan, F. D.: Esophagoscopy. *In* Skinner, D. B., Belsey, R. H. R., Hendrix, T. R., and Zuidema, G. D. (Eds.): Gastroesophageal Reflux and Hiatal Hernia. Boston, Little, Brown and Company, 1972, pp. 107–120.
3. Berry, B. E., and Ochsner, J. L.: Perforation of the esophagus. A 30 year review. J. Thorac. Cardiovasc. Surg., 65:1–7, 1973.
4. Donner, M. W.: Hemorrhage at the esophagogastric junction (including bleeding esophageal varices). *In* Katz, D., and Hoffman, F. (Eds.): The Esophagogastric Junction. Netherlands, Excerpta Medica, 1971, pp. 76–77.
5. Kerr, W. F.: Emergency oesophagectomy. Thorax, 23:204, 1968.
6. Mallory, G. K., and Weiss, S.: Hemorrhage from lacerations of the cardiac orifice of the stomach due to vomiting. Am. J. Med. Sci., 178:506, 1929.
7. Meade, R. H.: A History of Thoracic Surgery. Springfield, Ill., Charles C Thomas, Publisher, 1961, pp. 649–655.
8. Rea, W. J., Gallivan, G. J., Ecker, R. R., and Sugg, W. L.: Traumatic esophageal perforation. Ann. Thorac. Surg., 14:671, 1972.
9. Rosoff, L., and White, E. J.: Perforation of the esophagus. Am. J. Surg., 128:207–218, 1974.
10. Sawyers, J. L., et al.: Esophageal perforation. An increasing challenge. Ann. Thorac. Surg., 19:233–238, 1975.
11. Thal, A. P., and Hatafuku, T.: Improved operation for esophageal rupture. J.A.M.A., 188:826, 1964.
12. Urschel, H. C., Razzuk, M. A., Wood, R. E., Galbraith, N., Pockey, M., and Paulson, D. L.: Improved management of esophageal perforation: Exclusion and diversion in continuity. Ann. Surg., 179:587–591, 1974.
13. Wirthlin, L. S., and Malt, R. A.: Accidents of vagotomy. Surg. Gynecol. Obstet., 135:913–916, 1972.

VII ———————————————————

HIATUS HERNIA

E. R. Woodward, M.D.

In its course through the thorax, the esophagus traverses the diaphragm through an opening known as the esophageal *hiatus*. This structure is intimately associated with the lower esophageal *sphincter,* the junction between esophagus and stomach and the closure mechanism that exists between these two structures. Pressure within the thorax is *less* than atmospheric, whereas intra-abdominal pressure is *above* atmospheric. This is one of the important factors that tend to promote passage of a portion of the stomach upward through the hiatus, with creation of an esophageal hiatus hernia. There are two types: (1) the relatively common *sliding* hiatal hernia and (2) the less frequent *paraesophageal* hernia.

ANATOMY

The wall of the esophageal hiatus is formed in its entirety of the skeletal muscle composing the diaphragm. There is a separation in the anteroposterior plane of muscle fibers composing the right crus of the diaphragm. This separation forms a sling anterior to the esophagus, but there is a less definite reunion of the muscle fibers posteriorly, creating a V-shaped, tapered defect. The hiatus is normally just large enough to comfortably permit passage of the esophagus, i.e., approximately 2.5 cm. in diameter. The esophagus passes through the crural tunnel obliquely, being directly anterior to the aorta just above the hiatus and lying to the left of the aorta just below the hiatus. Although the esophageal hiatus is generally constituted entirely from the right crus of the diaphragm, 11 variations in the muscular anatomy about the hiatus have been described. In 50 per cent the hiatus is derived solely from the right crus of the diaphragm. In 40 per cent only a minor contribution from the left crus is seen. Both diaphragmatic crura arise from the lateral aspects of the first to the fourth lumbar vertebrae. The esophageal hiatus contracts with inspiration and from stimulation of the phrenic nerve. With inspiration the diaphragm and hiatus descend, increasing the angulation of the esophagus at the hiatus.

Under normal conditions there is a short segment of esophagus below the diaphragm before it unites with the cardia of the stomach. This distance is variable in vivo, but in the dissecting laboratory usually approximates 2 cm. The esophagus enters the stomach obliquely on its right or lesser curvature side. The entire fundus of the stomach is above and to the left of the esophagogastric junction, completely filling the under surface of the diaphragmatic cupula, except for a small portion laterally occupied by the upper pole of the spleen. The acute angle between the left border of the abdominal esophagus and the medial border of the gastric fundus is known as the angle of His. Since a rise in fundic pressure could compress the adjacent esophagus, a valvelike effect has been theorized.

The cardia of the stomach, the tubular portion connecting to the esophagus, is a narrow ring approximately 1 cm. in width. It differs from the body of the stomach in that its glandular structure is much more like that of the pyloric antrum. The glands are simple, the submucosal stroma is abundant, and parietal and chief cells are absent or sparse. The mucosa joins with the stratified squamous epithelium of the esophagus in a clearly visible, irregular line called the *ora serrata*. This mucosal junction is near, but not necessarily directly at, the esophagogastric junction as observed externally.

The lower esophagus and esophagogastric junction are held loosely in the esophageal hiatus by a tethering device known as the phrenoesophageal ligament or membrane (Fig. 1). This structure arises circumferentially around the hiatal margins and is a fibroelastic membrane which is a continuation of the transversalis fascia in the abdomen and the endothoracic fascia in the thorax. The phrenoesophageal ligament inserts circumferentially around the diaphragmatic esophagus close to the squamocolumnar junction. The insertion of the phrenoesophageal ligament is a broad one, measuring 3 to 5 cm. in length. The upper leaf of the phrenoesophageal ligament generally inserts approximately 3 cm. above the squamocolumnar junction. The lower leaf of the phrenoesophageal liga-

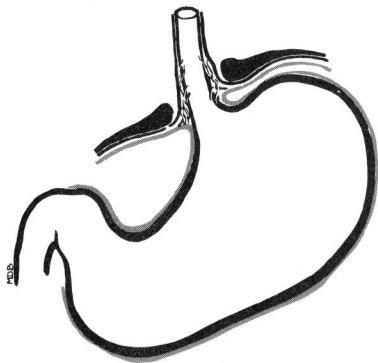

Figure 1. The normal fascial and peritoneal reflections at the diaphragmatic hiatus. The fascia on the deep surface of the diaphragm is reflected onto the esophagus as the phrenoesophageal ligament and fascia propria. Vessels and lymphatics lie between this and peritoneal reflection. (From Allison, P. R.: Surg. Gynecol. Obstet., *92*:419, 1951. By permission of Surgery, Gynecology and Obstetrics.)

ment generally inserts 1.5 cm. below the squamocolumnar junction. This insertion becomes continuous with the fibroelastic tissue of the intermuscular fascia of the esophagus via fine trabeculae piercing the muscle bundles. This tethering device provides for a dynamic relationship between esophagus and diaphragm so that shortening and lengthening of the esophagus associated with peristaltic activity are readily permitted.

PHYSIOLOGY OF THE ESOPHAGOGASTRIC JUNCTION

The closure mechanism at the esophagogastric junction is critically important. The stratified squamous epithelium of the esophagus is exquisitely sensitive to the digestive action of acid gastric juice. The normal pressure relationships favor gastroesophageal reflux, since intragastric pressure is above atmospheric and intraesophageal pressure is negative in relationship to atmospheric pressure. It is only recently that the closure mechanism has been fully understood. Formerly the pinchcock action of the diaphragm was considered important, but experimental studies now indicate clearly that this is not a primary factor. The oblique entrance of the esophagus into the cardia, the *angle of His,* is probably an ancillary factor in maintaining competence of the sphincter mechanism but is certainly not of primary importance.

The absence of an anatomically apparent sphincter was undoubtedly responsible for searches outside the esophagus itself to explain the closure mechanism. Manometric studies have convincingly demonstrated an intrinsic sphincter. The pioneer work of Code[10, 11] and Ingelfinger[19] and their many co-workers has clarified this important physiologic mechanism. Intraluminal pressures were recorded from open-tip catheters attached to transducers and a recorder, or a miniaturized transducer was actually placed within the esophagus. Careful study of the pressures indicated a "high-pressure zone" extending over about 3.5 cm. at

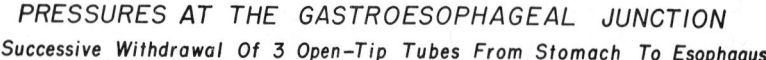

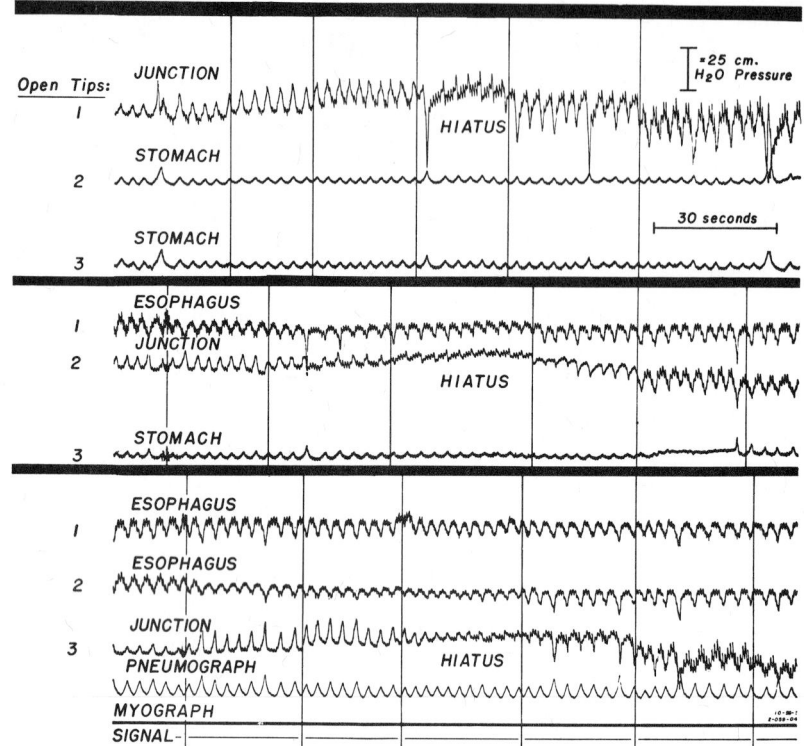

Figure 2. "High-pressure zone" at esophagogastric junction. (From Code, C. F., et al.: An Atlas of Esophageal Motility in Health and Disease. 1958. Courtesy of Charles C Thomas, Publisher, Springfield, Ill.)

the level of the diaphragm (Fig. 2). The diaphragm is located by the pressure inversion point (PIP). Below the diaphragm inspiration causes a rise in pressure, whereas above the diaphragm inspiration causes a fall. In this junctional zone the intraluminal pressure in the esophagus is always higher than that in either stomach below or esophagus above. This is true in all stages of the respiratory cycle and in any position of the body.

This "high-pressure zone" has been shown to be the intrinsic lower esophageal sphincter (Fig. 3).[10] Pressure sensors were placed at 5-cm. intervals in the esophagus, with the lowermost transducer directly in the high-pressure zone. Deglutition initiated a peristaltic wave which was picked up first on the proximal transducer and then on the middle one. As the peristaltic wave passed downward the pressure in the high-pressure zone fell sharply, the classic receptive relaxation of a physiologic sphincter mechanism.

In addition to its autonomic innervation, it appears possible that the lower esophageal sphincter may be under hormonal control. Giles et al.[15] found that both exogenous and endogenous gastrin increased LES pressure. This stimulating effect is blocked by either exogenous or endogenous secretin,[12] glucagon,[20] and cholecystokinin.[29] On the other hand, reduction of pH in the cardia also contracts the LES,[14] and alkalinization of the cardia blocks the LES response to a meat meal despite increased serum gastrin.[21] It remains unclear at present whether the gastrin effect is pharmacologic or mediated through stimulation of gastric acid secretion.

DIAPHRAGMATIC HERNIAS THROUGH THE ESOPHAGEAL HIATUS

These are customarily divided into *sliding* hiatus hernias and *paraesophageal* or parahiatal hernias. Sliding hiatus hernias are much more common and are associated with incompetence of the lower esophageal sphincter and reflux esophagitis. Paraesophageal hernias account for less than 5 per cent of hiatus hernias; the esophagogastric junction remains below the diaphragm and competence of the lower esophageal sphincter is preserved.

PARAESOPHAGEAL HIATUS HERNIA

Pathologic Anatomy

A hernial defect with sharply defined, firm borders is present through the esophageal hiatus to the left of the esophagus. The defect varies widely in size and may be as large as 10 or 12 cm. in diameter. The fundus of the stomach protrudes upward into a well-defined hernial sac composed of thickened and fibrotic diaphragmatic peritoneum. The greater curvature of the stomach literally "rolls" upward as the defect and the hernial sac become larger, so that these are some-

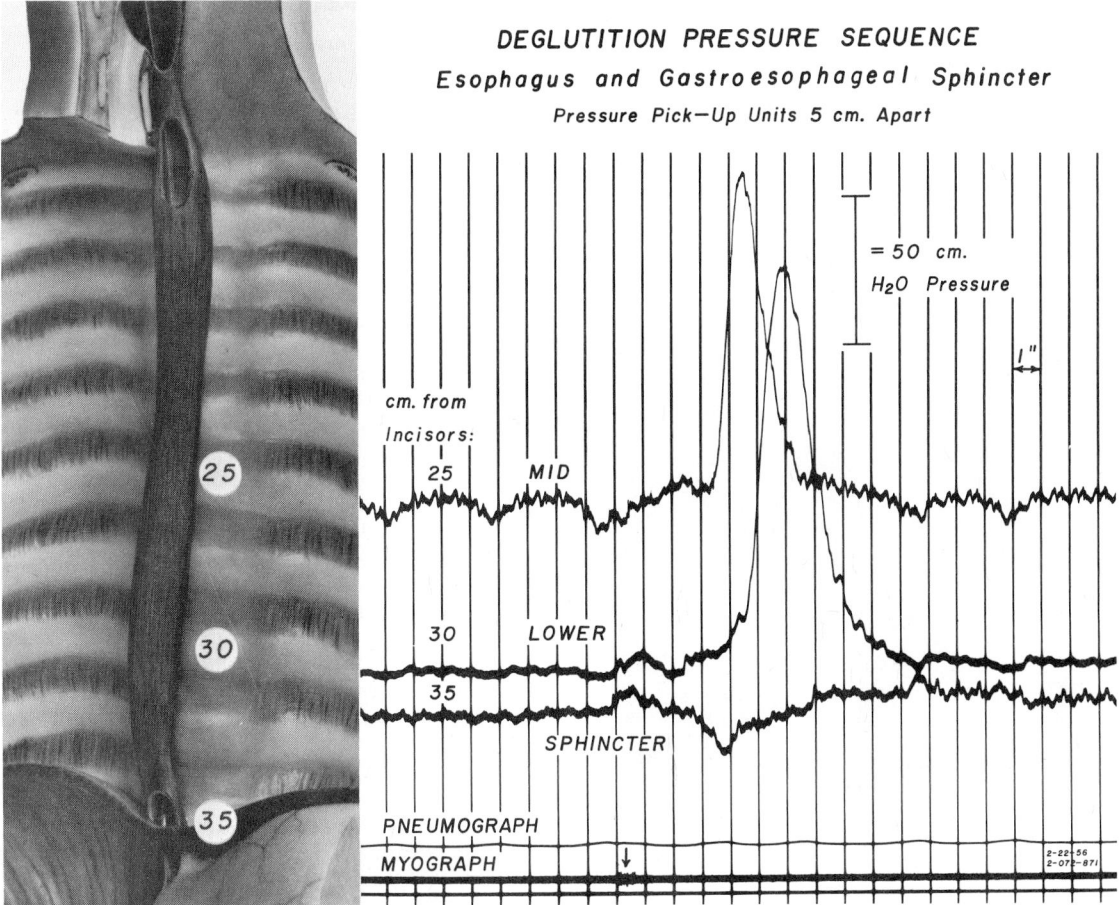

Figure 3. Receptive relaxation of lower esophageal sphincter. (From Code, C. F., et al.: An Atlas of Esophageal Motility in Health and Disease. 1958. Courtesy of Charles C Thomas, Publisher, Springfield, Ill.)

times referred to as "rolling hernias." Almost the entire stomach may rotate upward into the hernial sac so that only the pylorus and antrum remain below the diaphragm, and the cardia and pylorus are close together. This complete herniation gives the radiographic appearance of the so-called "upside-down stomach" (Fig. 4).

Clinical Manifestations

Symptoms from paraesophageal hiatus hernias are largely mechanical in origin. Ingestion of a meal will provide a bolus that enters the thoracic stomach and distends it. This produces pain often described as "crushing" in nature, which frequently can be confused with angina. The pain is so closely associated with eating that the patient often restricts intake of nourishment in order to minimize symptoms. Severe weight loss, even to overt malnutrition, is sometimes seen, particularly in elderly women. Symptoms characteristic of esophagitis are not present except in the occasional case in which there is a sliding as well as a paraesophageal component. Incarceration, increasing distention, pressure necrosis, and rupture can occur in the portion of the stomach herniated through the diaphragm into the mediastinum. Rapidly extending mediastinitis with pain and sepsis followed by rupture into the left pleural space will ensue. Chronic disturbances include the development of peptic ulcer in the thoracic stomach, which drains inadequately through the narrow hernial ring. Both hemorrhage and perforation can occur in association with this lesion.

Diagnosis

The diagnosis of paraesophageal hiatus hernia is usually made from the history and confirmed by radiologic examination. The diagnosis frequently can be made from standard chest films, since the entrapped thoracic stomach retains enough gas to show a radiolucent pocket within the usual cardiac silhouette (Fig. 5). The thoracic stomach fills readily with ingested barium and the diagnosis is easily made (see Fig. 4). It is important for the radiologist to ascertain the location of the esophagogastric junction in order to confirm the type of hernia present. Esophagoscopy is useful only in the negative sense that the subdiaphragmatic location of the esophagogastric junction

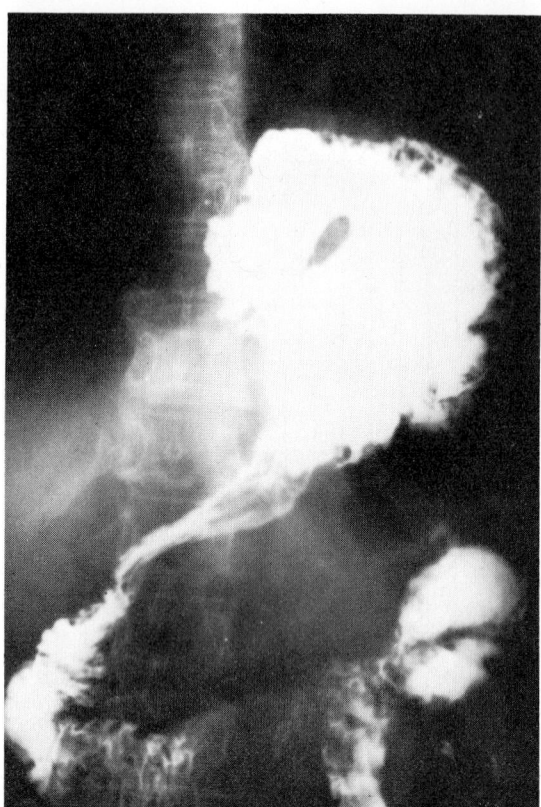

Figure 4. "Upside-down stomach," a large paraesophageal hiatal hernia with almost the entire stomach above the diaphragm and the esophagogastric junction in its normal subdiaphragmatic location.

is confirmed and the absence of esophagitis is ascertained.

Pathogenesis

The etiology of paraesophageal hiatus hernia is completely unknown. It appears to be an acquired lesion, since it is rare before late middle life and is most frequently seen in the elderly.

Management

Treatment of paraesophageal hiatus hernia is exclusively surgical. The lesion can be likened to an indirect inguinal hernia in that there is an anatomic defect that needs surgical correction to alleviate symptoms and to protect against life-threatening complications. The optimal approach is through the abdomen, and the larger the hernia, the more desirable is the abdominal approach. Downward traction on the stomach is required for reduction of the larger hernias, and this permits ready access to the hernial sac. In most cases the sac peels out of the mediastinum with ease; the hernial ring usually is firm and can be approximated rather easily. In order to protect against recurrence the esophagogastric junction is sutured to the median arcuate ligament (see Fig. 9, Hill repair).

The results of operation are extremely good, with prompt relief of symptoms and rapid improvement in nutrition. Recurrence is rare.

SLIDING HIATUS HERNIA

Pathologic Anatomy

A sliding hiatus hernia is in essence a failure of the normal tethering device, the phrenoesophageal ligament, to retain the esophagogastric junction within the esophageal hiatus of the diaphragm. Under these conditions the unfavorable pressure relationships permit the cardiac portion of the stomach to herniate upward in concentric fashion through the esophageal hiatus (Fig. 6). The phrenoesophageal ligament becomes lengthened and thinned; whether this is primary or secondary is unclear. The esophageal hiatus becomes dilated to a variable degree. Under normal conditions it admits only the tip of the index finger; in a patient with a long-standing large sliding hiatus hernia, the hiatus may admit four fingers. The esophagogastric junction slides back and forth readily, depending on body posture, abdominal distention, gastric filling, and contraction of abdominal wall. When the hernia is reduced, it may be difficult indeed for the radiologist to visualize it. The diaphragmatic peritoneum reduces readily along with the cardia, and a well-developed hernial sac is present only in large hernias.

Inflammation and scarring secondary to severe and long-standing reflux esophagitis may remove the "sliding" feature of concentric hiatus hernias. Fixation and contraction of scar tissue may produce acquired short-

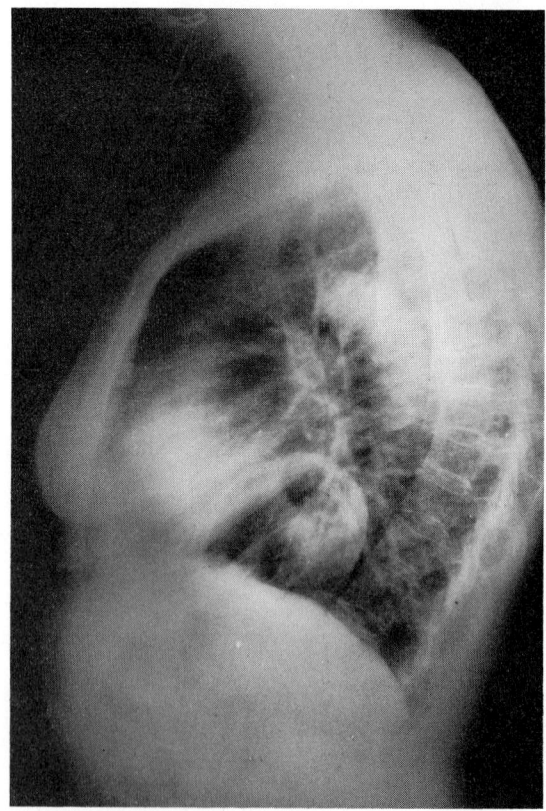

Figure 5. Lateral x-ray of chest shows air-containing fundus of stomach entrapped in a paraesophageal hiatal hernia.

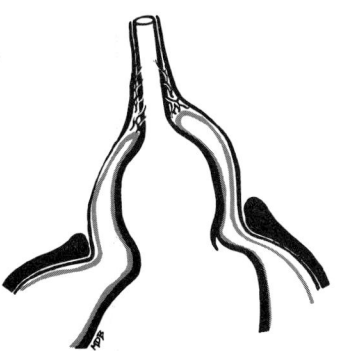

Figure 6. Diagram of the anatomic relations of sliding hiatal hernia. Note the stretching of the peritoneal reflection and the phrenoesophageal ligament. (From Allison, P. R.: Surg. Gynecol. Obstet., *92*:419, 1951. By permission of Surgery, Gynecology & Obstetrics.)

ening of the esophagus and fixation of the esophagogastric junction above the diaphragm. This is a late stage of the disease process and is frequently associated with enough destruction and fibrosis that stenosis of the esophagus is present.

Clinical Manifestations

The majority of patients with sliding esophageal hiatus hernias have no symptoms whatever that are specifically referable to the lesion. Upper gastrointestinal x-ray studies in patients with functional disorders often reveal an incidental sliding hiatus hernia. Physician and patient alike often attribute a wide variety of symptoms to this lesion. We consider that a sliding hiatus hernia in and of itself is totally asymptomatic. It is only when such a lesion is associated with gastroesophageal reflux and reflux esophagitis that symptoms supervene.

The classic symptoms of esophagitis are easily recognized, but variations occur and the unmistakable symptom complex may be difficult to ascertain. The most common symptom of all, described in one manner or another by more than 90 per cent of patients, is substernal burning distress. The patient frequently will spontaneously refer to this as "heartburn." The localization may be subxiphoid, epigastric, or even cervical, and the patient's description of the quality will vary; however, the patient seldom describes the pain as sharp, knifelike, crushing, or bursting. The distress often is postprandial and, unlike the distress of gastric or duodenal ulcer, occurs very early after meals. It often correlates well with the size of the meal and is more bothersome after the customarily large evening meal. Relief is often obtained by swallowing anything from salivary secretions to an antacid mixture. Unlike peptic ulcer of the stomach or duodenum, the relief induced by antacids may be short-lived. The distress is often related to posture; physical activity associated with bending or stooping will induce the burning distress, and under these conditions it may be associated with "waterbrash"—the reflux of irritating fluid into the pharynx and mouth. The characteristic distress often occurs when the patient lies down, particularly after a large evening meal. This distress frequently is relieved by assumption of the upright posi-

tion, and patients will often sleep sitting up to avoid nocturnal distress.

Regurgitation is present much less frequently, probably in not more than half the cases. It is particularly likely to occur after a heavy meal and with a change in posture such as stooping, bending, or lying down. The material regurgitated most often contains little or no food, may or may not be bile-stained, is bitter, and tends to cause a burning sensation in the pharynx. Occasionally regurgitation will be associated with aspiration, and the pulmonary complications of chronic bronchitis, asthma, recurrent pneumonitis, and even lung abscess may develop. In fact, the pulmonary changes sometimes will appear in the complete absence of distress and with no conscious awareness of regurgitation.

Dysphagia ordinarily is a late symptom and is observed in less than 10 per cent of patients. It is often due to spasm of the inflamed distal esophagus and under these conditions tends to be intermittent rather than continuous. As the inflammatory changes progress to stenosis, dysphagia becomes constant and progressive. Whereas the dysphagia due to spasm may occur with liquid foods when they are unusually hot or cold or rapidly ingested, the dysphagia of stenosing esophagitis is related to the physical characteristics of the bolus. The swallowing of meat usually is the most severely disturbed, and beef is more prominently complained of than other meats. The drier foods such as bread also frequently "stick in the throat." The swallowing difficulty in itself is not ordinarily painful but may be associated with the distress of reflux. However, as stenosis progresses and the symptoms of dysphagia increase, reflux often is reduced by the narrowing of the channel so that the symptoms of esophagitis will be reduced and may even disappear.

Hemorrhage is less common and less severe than with gastric or duodenal ulcer. Acute hemorrhage is considerably less frequent than chronic blood loss, when it does occur it is rare for the rate of hemorrhage to be sufficient for the patient to have hematemesis; usually only melena is present. Chronic bleeding is far more common and is especially frequent in elderly females. It is often an extremely trying problem in such patients because other symptoms of esophagitis may be totally absent, and the patient may well present other potential sources of chronic gastrointestinal blood loss such as diverticulosis of the sigmoid colon. It is not uncommon, however, to find blood loss of such a degree that profound anemia develops.

Diagnosis

The diagnosis of sliding hiatus hernia and peptic esophagitis is made from a carefully taken history of the present illness. The diagnosis is confirmed by (1) radiologic examination, (2) esophagoscopy, and occasionally (3) laboratory evaluation.

The *upper gastrointestinal x-ray* study concentrating on the region of the esophagogastric junction is highly successful in revealing the presence of a sliding hiatus hernia. It must be remembered, however, that not all patients with esophagitis have a sliding hiatus hernia. Also, in a small but significant number of patients with typical symptoms of esophagitis, a hiatus hernia cannot be demonstrated by x-ray but will be found to be present at the time of surgical exploration. Obviously these small hernias really do "slide" and in the reduced state may be difficult to visualize. The usual radiologic techniques of putting pressure on this region will generally but not always cause the hernia to protrude into its mediastinal position. Esophagitis usually cannot be visualized by radiologic techniques unless significant spasm or stenosis is present. We consider the so-called Schatzki's ring to be indicative of such a change. For optimal radiologic evaluation of sphincter function and for the demonstration of gastroesophageal reflux, we believe that cineradiologic examination is preferable.

Esophagoscopy is by far the most important test to confirm the presence of peptic esophagitis; this diagnosis may not be considered completely established without positive endoscopy. The traditional rigid hollow tube has been largely replaced by the flexible fiberoptic esophagoscope. The latter instrument has tremendous advantages: (1) The image is clear, in focus, and at a magnification that is readily visualized, in contrast to the small image seen through the small opening in the rigid esophagoscope 50 cm. in length. (2) The flexible characteristic of the instrument renders it easy to pass and reduces the risk of injury to pharynx or esophagus to almost zero. (3) Related to this, the procedure is much less uncomfortable for the patient and is therefore more acceptable. With the fiberoptic instruments, aspiration and inflation as well as biopsy can be performed.

Esophageal mucosa involved in peptic esophagitis is readily identified by esophagoscopy. It is erythematous and friable and bleeds easily. In addition, there are patchy areas covered by a gray-white fibrinous exudate. This peels away to reveal freely bleeding granulations uncovered by epithelium. Isolated punched-out peptic ulcers such as those seen in stomach and duodenum are seen only in the esophagus lined by simple columnar epithelium, the so-called *Barrett's esophagus*.

Not only should the diagnosis of peptic esophagitis not be considered established without esophagoscopy, but surgical therapy should not be undertaken without esophagoscopic confirmation. This will prevent needless surgery in patients with functional disorders erroneously attributed to hiatus hernia. Esophagoscopy will also help prevent the tragic error of missing the early diagnosis of carcinoma at the esophagogastric junction. This lesion may mimic peptic esophagitis very closely.

Laboratory evaluation is frequently unnecessary in studying patients with hiatus hernia and esophagitis with characteristic history and endoscopic findings. Since the precise secretory state of the stomach is unimportant in reflux peptic esophagitis, routine gastric analysis is not indicated. However, it is a useful measure in patients with co-existent duodenal ulcer for which adjunctive surgery is being considered. There is a frequent association between the two disorders, particularly when a complication of peptic esophagitis such as stricture is present. The basal gastric secretory rate is determined by aspiration through a fluoroscopically placed Levin tube for one hour,

followed by a determination of stimulated gastric secretion using Histalog. This information is useful in postoperative determination of the effectiveness of ancillary duodenal ulcer surgery.

The Bernstein test[5] is needed in only a small number of patients but is particularly useful in those with an atypical history or symptoms suggestive of cardiac or biliary tract disease. A Levin tube is placed in the distal esophagus and a 0.1 N solution of hydrochloric acid is infused under circumstances such that the patient cannot identify the infusate. This will reproduce the patient's symptoms with a high degree of accuracy if they are due to esophagitis.

Manometric study will reveal a weak LES, and pH measurements demonstrate gastroesophageal reflux characteristic of an incompetent LES.[11] Successful corrective surgery can be readily evaluated by both methods, but neither is essential in satisfactory clinical management.

Pathogenesis and Pathophysiology

Esophageal hiatus hernia of the sliding type and reflux esophagitis coexist so frequently that a cause-and-effect relationship is suggested. It is attractive to consider that the mediastinal translocation of the esophagogastric junction interferes with the lower esophageal sphincter in some way, thus permitting free gastroesophageal reflux. It is well known that the great majority of patients with sliding hiatus hernia do not develop reflux esophagitis and thus apparently have a physiologically competent lower esophageal sphincter. It seems obvious, therefore, that the mediastinal location of the esophagogastric junction in itself does not cause incompetence of the lower esophageal sphincter. Conversely, a small but significant number of patients with reflux esophagitis do not have a sliding hiatus hernia. Thus, despite the frequent coexistence of sliding esophageal hiatus hernia and reflux esophagitis, we do not believe that there is sufficient evidence to conclude that there is a cause-and-effect relationship. The reason or reasons why the lower esophageal sphincter permits gastroesophageal reflux remain obscure.

The adverse pressure relationships between stomach and esophagus favor reflux when the lower esophageal sphincter is incompetent. The tremendous sensitivity of the esophagus to gastric juice has been demonstrated experimentally.[26] It is not surprising, therefore, that when gastric juice gains access to the esophagus injury results.

Although acid pepsin is the usual cause of reflux esophagitis, duodenal fluids will cause severe esophagitis in the human. This alkaline esophagitis frequently is seen after total gastrectomy when esophagointestinal continuity permits regurgitation of duodenal secretions. It is not known whether bile or pancreatic juice or both are necessary, but succus entericus alone does not cause esophagitis. Alkaline esophagitis occasionally is seen after distal partial gastrectomy, particularly of the Billroth II type. Such patients frequently have so-called "reflux alkaline gastritis"[7, 31] with massive reflux of duodenal fluids from the afferent loop into the empty stomach and through an incompetent lower esophageal sphincter into the esophagus. Alkaline esophagitis is often agonizingly painful. The gross pathologic changes are frequently more severe with more intense inflammatory changes than those seen in peptic esophagitis.

Treatment

The patient with a sliding hiatus hernia without esophagitis needs no therapy. In many patients the esophagitis is so mild and intermittent that again no therapy is indicated. In patients with clinically significant esophagitis an intensive trial on medical therapy should be made before embarking on surgery. It is estimated that, as with duodenal ulcer, such therapy will be successful in approximately 85 per cent of uncomplicated cases. Neutralization of gastric content, the basic principle of medical therapy for gastric and duodenal ulcer, is not quite as successful in reflux peptic esophagitis. Sensitivity of the esophageal mucosa to acid-pepsin is so extreme that intermittent gastric neutralization often fails to control symptoms completely. Weight reduction in obese patients helps by reducing intra-abdominal pressure. Elevating the head of the bed makes gravity an ally in reducing gastroesophageal reflux. A regimen of regular, equal meals with low fat content minimizes gastric retention and thus reduces the bolus available for gastroesophageal reflux. Anticholinergic drugs are contraindicated because they promote gastric retention, permitting increased gastroesophageal reflux. Reduction or abolition of the use of tobacco, coffee, and alcohol has the same favorable influence on esophagitis as that seen in patients with gastric or duodenal ulcer.

Patients whose symptoms of esophagitis do not respond adequately to medical therapy or in whom the complications of hemorrhage or stricture are present require and usually desire operative therapy. Currently available operative methods produce generally good results, but there is still a significant failure rate and a significant morbidity. It is extremely important that functional digestive disorders not be attributed to a sliding hiatus hernia; many operative failures are in this group of patients.

Modern operative therapy for sliding hiatus hernia with reflux esophagitis dates from the classic contribution of Allison in 1951.[1] He first outlined clearly the clinical syndrome and advocated repair of the hernia in order to reduce or abolish gastroesophageal reflux. Allison's technique requires first a left transpleural approach to the esophageal hiatus. The hernia is reduced and the crural structures composing the hiatus are closed snugly posterior to the esophagus. The phrenoesophageal ligament is then reconstructed in an effort to restore its tethering function.

Over the years since the introduction of this method it has been clear that the last maneuver does not prevent recurrence of hernia, because of the inadequate reparative value of the stressed and thinned phrenoesophageal membrane. Crural approximation can be done satisfactorily from the abdominal approach. This has the added advantage that ancillary surgery for coexistent duodenal ulcer or biliary tract disease can be performed at the same time. During the decade 1955 to 1965 this gradually became the preferred procedure in most surgical clinics. Following reduction of the hernia and mobilization of the distal esophagus the diaphragmatic crural structures were approximated posteriorly until the esophageal hiatus was snugly approximated to the esophagus. In addition, the angle of His was often accentuated by suturing the right border of the fundus to the left side of the abdominal esophagus. Vagotomy and pyloroplasty were added in some patients with coexistent duodenal ulcer or gastric hypersecretion, and sometimes as a routine measure to reduce gastric secretory activity.

Results of this method of therapy indicate that within five years there is an anatomic recurrence of sliding hiatus hernia in approximately 40 per cent of patients, with clinical persistence or recurrence of reflux esophagitis in 20 per cent. The addition of vagotomy and pyloroplasty had no influence on the anatomic recurrence rate and caused only an insignificant lowering of the incidence of recurrent esophagitis.[33] Laboratory evaluation also indicated persistent gastroesophageal reflux in approximately 50 per cent of patients. It became clear, therefore, that posterior crural approximation was accompanied by a discouragingly high failure rate uninfluenced by the addition of vagotomy and pyloroplasty. The ancillary surgery also resulted in a significant chronic morbidity from the dumping syndrome and diarrhea; clearly this additive surgery should be utilized only in patients with coexistent severe duodenal ulcer disease.

In the meantime the emphasis gradually shifted from simple anatomic hernia repair to operative procedures *designed to restore competence to the lower esophageal sphincter.* Except in complicated cases, the three methods currently in common use each include repair of the sliding hiatus hernia, but this is not considered the crucial factor.

The "Mark IV" transthoracic reconstruction of the cardia and repair of hiatus hernia was developed by Belsey in 1955 and the results in 632 patients reported in 1966.[28] Two hundred and nineteen cases were followed more than five years, with a recurrence rate of 11 per cent. More recently Orringer et al. have reported on 892 patients operated upon through 1965.[25] There were nine operative deaths (1 per cent). Follow-up was available on 848 cases (95 per cent). Among 776 followed more than three years, 12 per cent had a documented hiatus hernia or recurrent reflux. In 513 patients followed more than seven years, the recurrence rate remained at 12 per cent. Of 98 patients demonstrating recurrent hernia and/or reflux, nine remained asymptomatic. The technique of the Belsey procedure is diagrammed in Figure 7. The distal esophagus and esophagogastric junction are thoroughly mobilized through a left thoracotomy. The hernia is reduced and the fundus approximated to the distal esophagus in a beltlike fashion using three layers of sutures and surrounding approximately two thirds of the distal esophagus. The operation accomplishes the development of intra-abdominal esophagus and at the same time applies positive intrafundic pressure against the lower esophagus. Thus an increase in intragastric pressure tends to compress the lower esophagus. The operation is usually effective in restoring LES competence, but has the disadvantage that it

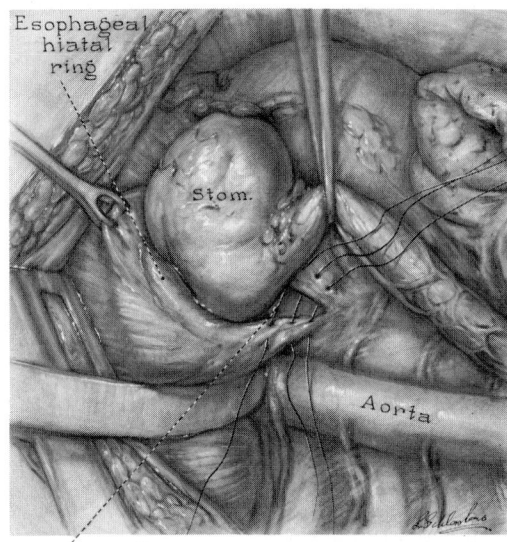

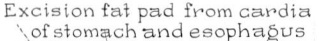

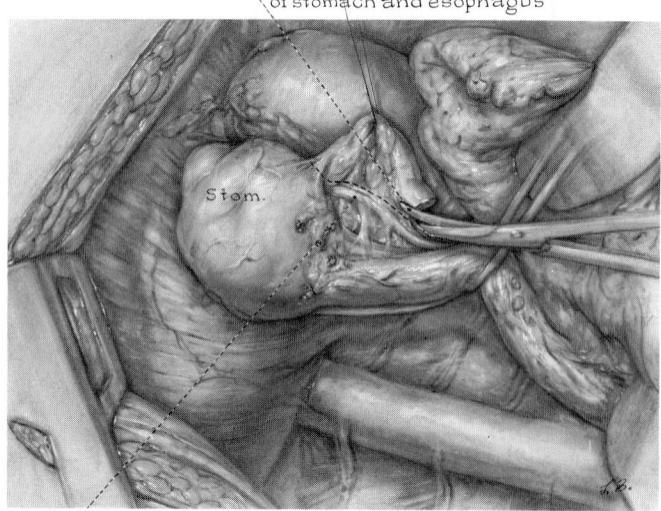

Figure 7. *A,* Mobilization of the distal esophagus and cardia is done through a left sixth interspace lateral thoracotomy. The esophagus with vagus nerves attached is completely freed up to the lung root. After the hernia sac is entered anteriorly, the entire circumference of the cardia is separated from its attachments. This requires division of branches from the left inferior phrenic artery laterally (*illustrated*) and left gastric artery posteriorly (*not shown*).

Figure 7. *Continued. B,* At the start of the repair, sutures are placed in two limbs of the right crus posteriorly, but these are not tied until the completion of the reconstruction. Tension on a clamp applied to the diaphragm anteriorly makes it easier to identify the strong tendinous tissue in the crus where the sutures should be placed.

Figure 7. *Continued. C,* After complete mobilization of the esophagogastric junction, the pad of fibrofatty tissue at the cardia is excised anteriorly and laterally. The vagus nerves, which tend to be elevated off the esophagus during this dissection, are carefully preserved.

Illustration continued on opposite page

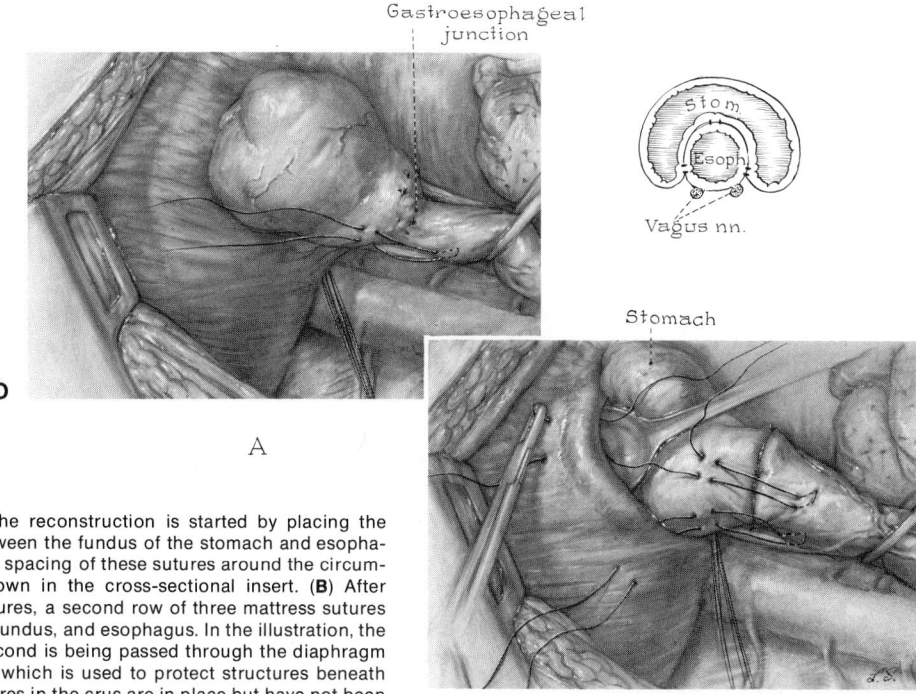

Gastroesophageal junction

Stom

Esoph

Vagus nn.

Stomach

D

A

B

Figure 7. *Continued. D,(A).* The reconstruction is started by placing the first of three mattress sutures between the fundus of the stomach and esophagus 2 cm. above the junction. The spacing of these sutures around the circumference of the esophagus is shown in the cross-sectional insert. **(B)** After completion of the first row of sutures, a second row of three mattress sutures is placed through the diaphragm, fundus, and esophagus. In the illustration, the first suture is in place, and the second is being passed through the diaphragm in the bowl of a spoon retractor, which is used to protect structures beneath the diaphragm. The posterior sutures in the crus are in place but have not been tied.

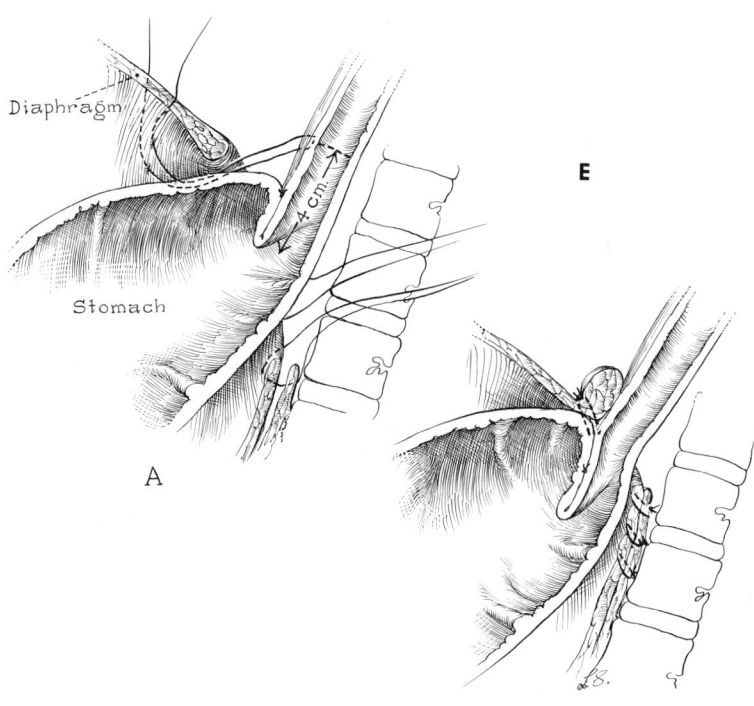

Diaphragm

4 cm.

Stomach

E

A

B

Figure 7. *Continued. E,* Sagittal sections of the repair. **(A)** The sutures in the crus posteriorly have been placed but not yet tied. The first row of mattress sutures between stomach and esophagus have been tied. One of the mattress sutures in the second row is illustrated. **(B)** The completed repair. The posterior sutures in the crus and second row of mattress sutures joining diaphragm, stomach, and esophagus are tied after the reconstruction has been placed beneath the diaphragm. (From Belsey, R. H. R., and Skinner, D. B.: Surgical treatment: Thoracic approach. *In* Skinner, D. B., Belsey, R. H. R., Hendrix, T. R., and Zuidema, G. D. (Eds.): Gastroesophageal Reflux and Hiatal Hernia. Boston, Little, Brown and Company, 1972.)

can be accomplished with ease only by the thoracic approach.

In 1956 Nissen wrote a short note about fundoplication to correct gastroesophageal reflux,[23] and the early results were reported in 1963.[24] In 1973, Rosetti and Allgower[27] reported on 1231 cases of hiatus hernias operated upon, and in patients with uncomplicated reflux esophagitis the operative mortality was 0.6 per cent (7 of 845 patients). The results are presented in 590 patients observed between three and 12 years after surgery. The "postfundoplication syndrome" occurred in 62 cases (10 per cent). We have referred to this as the "gas-bloat syndrome"[33] and have found it to be present in 20 per cent of cases one year following operation. Rosetti and Allgower described seven patients requiring reoperation because of the development of gastric or duodenal ulcers and five patients with recurrence of hernia and reflux esophagitis (1 per cent). Five hundred and sixteen patients (87 per cent) were free of symptoms.

Nissen described his fundoplication as a "valvuloplasty." The fundus of the stomach is wrapped completely around the distal esophagus and sutured on the right or lesser curvature side of the esophagus (Fig. 8). The positive intragastric pressure is, therefore, transmitted to this "jacket" surrounding the lower esophagus and compressing it. When intragastric pressure increases from whatever cause, the pressure within the fundus increases and the esophagus is more firmly compressed. This functions as a one-way valve, permitting antegrade emptying into the stomach and preventing gastroesophageal reflux. The postfundoplication syndrome results from aerophagia with inability of the subject to eructate the excess air. The resultant distention produces a feeling of pressure in the left upper quadrant or epigastrium, particularly postprandially and often to the point of overt pain.

The Nissen fundoplication is performed by the transabdominal approach in the uncomplicated case. It has the added advantage that the procedure is also easily performed by the left transthoracic approach. This is useful in cases of extreme obesity or in patients who have had a previous unsuccessful transabdominal hiatal herniorrhaphy. It is especially useful, however, in patients with brachyesophagus or acquired short esophagus due to extensive scarring and subsequent contracture. In addition to ease of dissection in the frequently observed periesophagitis, the fundus can be brought through the esophageal hiatus, enlarged by a short radial incision, and the fundoplication left above the diaphragm with no tension on the repair or the esophagus.[32] Clinical, cineradiographic, manometric, and pH studies indicate that the endothoracic fundoplication exerts an equally effective valvuloplastic effect and also restores resting pressure in the LES to the normal range.[18]

A new concept in hiatal herniorrhaphy in strengthening of the LES was proposed by Hill et al. in 1961[17] and the results of an eight-year experience presented in 1967.[16] One hundred and forty-nine cases were presented without mortality. In no patient could anatomic recurrence of hernia be demonstrated radiographically. While three patients had gastroesophageal reflux demonstrated by pH measurements, only four (3 per cent) patients had symptoms suggestive of persistent or recurrent esophagitis. Side effects of surgery were negligible, and manometric study revealed return of LES resting pressure to normal or near normal levels in most cases.

The Hill procedure is performed through a transabdominal approach; reducing the hernia and mobilizing the distal esophagus (Fig. 9). The crural structures are approximated posterior to the esophagus, and the esophagogastric junction is sutured to the median arcuate ligament. Hill refers to this as "posterior gastropexy." This maneuver maintains a long segment of intra-abdominal esophagus, thus exposing the LES to the positive intra-abdominal pressure. In addition, the medial border of the gastric fundus is plicated to the left wall of the abdominal esophagus, although not as extensively as in the Belsey procedure.

In summary, three operative procedures are currently employed to repair sliding hiatus hernias and to correct gastroesophageal reflux. These are the Bel-

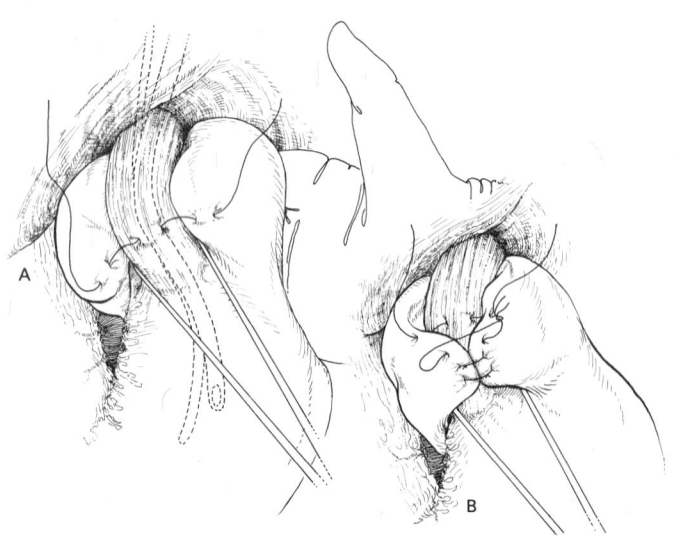

Figure 8. Nissen's "fundoplication" repair of sliding esophageal hiatal hernia, by transabdominal approach.

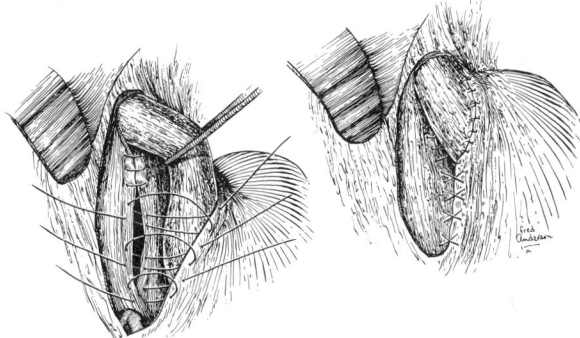

Figure 9. The Hill posterior gastropexy technique for hiatal herniorrhaphy and correction of gastroesophageal reflux.

The crural structures are approximated posterior to the esophagus. The median arcuate ligament is thoroughly sutured to the esophagogastric junction (*left*). The repair is completed by approximating the gastric fundus to the left border of the abdominal esophagus (*right*).

sey cardioplasty, the Nissen fundoplication, and the Hill posterior gastropexy. All are demonstrably effective in restoring LES function in most patients. The Belsey procedure may be slightly less effective than the Nissen operation and can be accomplished only through a thoracic approach. While the postfundoplication syndrome is also seen in this procedure, it occurs less frequently and in a milder form. The Nissen operation appears to be more effective in correcting gastroesophageal reflux,[13] but is also associated with the highest incidence of side effects, i.e., the pathologic retention of intragastric air resulting in the postfundoplication syndrome.[26, 32] The Hill procedure is effective in correcting gastroesophageal reflux and has the advantage of negligible side effects. Its disadvantage is that it can be performed only by the transabdominal route, whereas the Nissen maneuver can be accomplished also by the thoracic approach.

PEPTIC STRICTURES OF THE ESOPHAGUS

Stricture secondary to peptic esophagitis will usually require operative therapy. The simplest operative procedure is dilation; this is accomplished by bougienage, usually with Hurst or Maloney mercury-weighted bougies. This measure will provide dramatic relief of dysphagia; however, dilation of the stricture will often permit recurrent reflux of corrosive gastric fluid into the esophagus with prompt recurrence of the characteristic symptoms of esophagitis. Dilation alone will, therefore, seldom provide long-term relief from peptic stricture of the esophagus unless accompanied by medical therapy or surgical correction of gastroesophageal reflux.

In patients whose stricture is readily dilated, an anatomically satisfactory hiatal herniorrhaphy by either the posterior gastropexy or the fundoplication technique will often provide lasting relief from both stenosis and reflux esophagitis. This method should be

used primarily in all good-risk patients with stenosing esophagitis in whom the stricture is dilatable. In patients with tough, fibrous strictures, however, forceful dilation followed by hiatal herniorrhaphy will usually result in recurring stenosis. In these cases the fundal patch technique described by Thal can be used.[30] The stricture is divided longitudinally and the fundus onlaid into the defect as a patch graft with the serosal surface toward the lumen of the esophagus (Fig. 10). The serosa is rapidly replaced by stratified squamous epithelium and is completely covered within three weeks. When the stricture is large the serosal surface can be faced with a split-thickness skin graft. This hastens healing and reduces the likelihood of contraction and recurrent obstruction. The Thal patch alone will not prevent gastroesophageal reflux,[8] and it is necessary to perform a partial or complete wrap of the fundus about the lower esophagus. The combined procedure will give lasting relief in about 85 per cent of patients.[18] In those patients in whom this procedure fails, resection of the strictured area of esophagus with interposition with a segment of intestine can be used. The jejunum is useful for this purpose, as described by Merendino,[22] or the colon may be utilized.

PEPTIC ULCER IN ESOPHAGUS LINED BY COLUMNAR EPITHELIUM

In 1950, Barrett called attention to a condition in which the lower esophagus is lined with simple columnar epithelium.[3] Deep, penetrating peptic ulcers

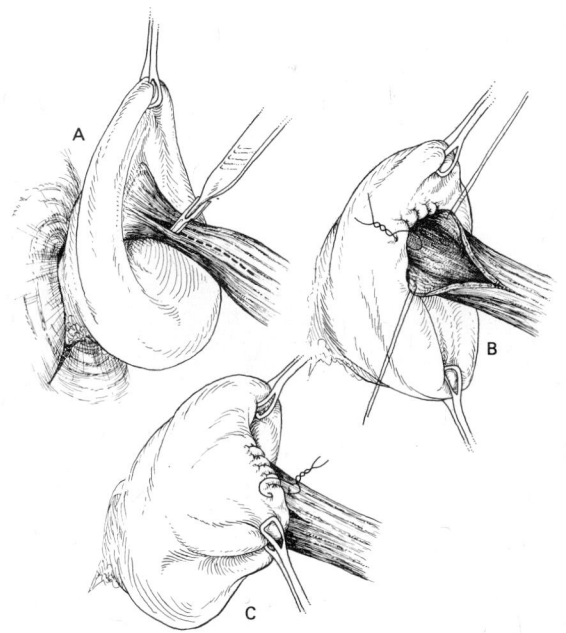

Figure 10. Fundal patch repair of peptic stricture. *A,* Stenotic segment incised longitudinally. *B,* Fundus sutured to esophagogastric junction. *C,* Patch sutured in place, serosa surface in esophageal lumen.

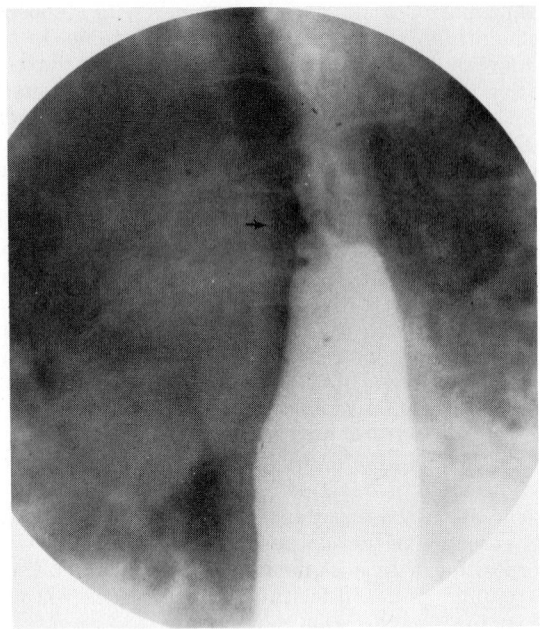

Figure 11. Barrett's ulcer of esophagus, in stricture 21 cm. from incisor teeth.

usually associated with stricture, form in this epithelium, frequently high in the esophagus and often mistaken for carcinoma (Fig. 11). He at first considered that this structure, apparently lined by gastric mucosa, must be tubular stomach. In 1953, Allison and Johnstone[2] stated their reasons for considering this structure to be esophagus, lined with gastric mucous membrane. First, it is a tubular structure resembling esophagus grossly and with no peritoneal covering. Second, the submucosa has mucous glands, and the

muscular coats resemble those of the esophagus. Third, islands of squamous epithelium can be found within the sheet of columnar epithelium. They also pointed out that there were no acid-producing parietal cells in the columnar mucosa that lines this segment of esophagus (Fig. 12). In 1957, Barrett[4] altered his views and suggested that the condition be called "lower esophagus lined by columnar epithelium." It frequently is referred to by the eponym "Barrett's esophagus" and the characteristic deep penetrating peptic ulcer as "Barrett's ulcer."

The esophagus lined by columnar epithelium generally has been considered to represent a congenital anomaly. The embryonic esophagus is first lined by columnar epithelium, and this is thought to be incompletely replaced with squamous epithelium, leaving the fetal columnar layer in the lower esophagus. More recently, however, the theory that this is an acquired condition has been gaining more support. First, it is difficult to understand why symptoms should be so delayed in onset; practically all reported cases have been in persons in the sixth or seventh decades. Second, it is not easy to understand why the columnar epithelium should always occur in the lower esophagus, since the replacement of fetal columnar epithelium begins in the middle and progresses toward each end. The acquired theory interprets the columnar epithelium to be an adaptive change in response to the continued destructive action of acid-pepsin. Bremner et al.[6] have produced a suggestive experimental model in the dog. The distal esophagus is denuded and reflux is produced by making a hiatus hernia and performing a cardioplasty. In this preparation, columnar epithelium grows slowly upward, whereas squamous epithelium grows rapidly downward. The time sequence is reversed when gastric secretion is stimulated with histamine and beeswax, so that the denuded portion of esophagus is covered mainly by columnar epithelium.

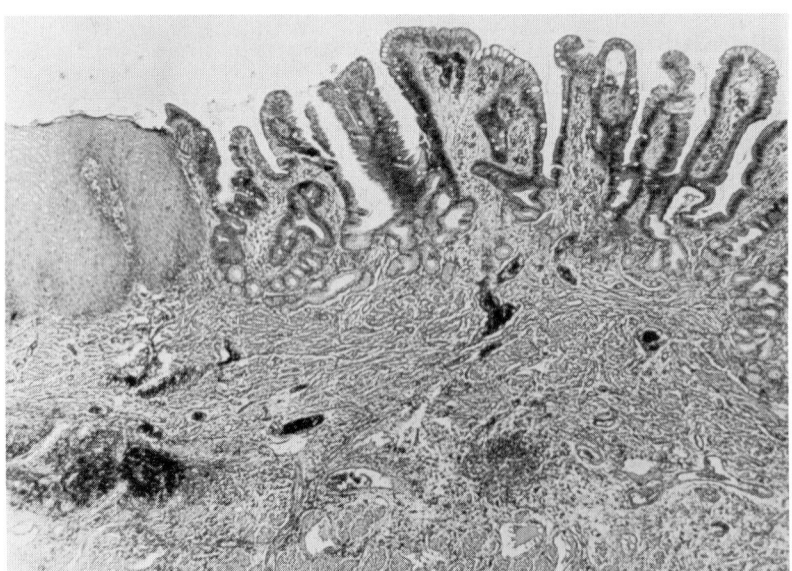

Figure 12. Biopsy from patient in Figure 11 at level of ulcer, showing simple columnar epithelium in esophagus.

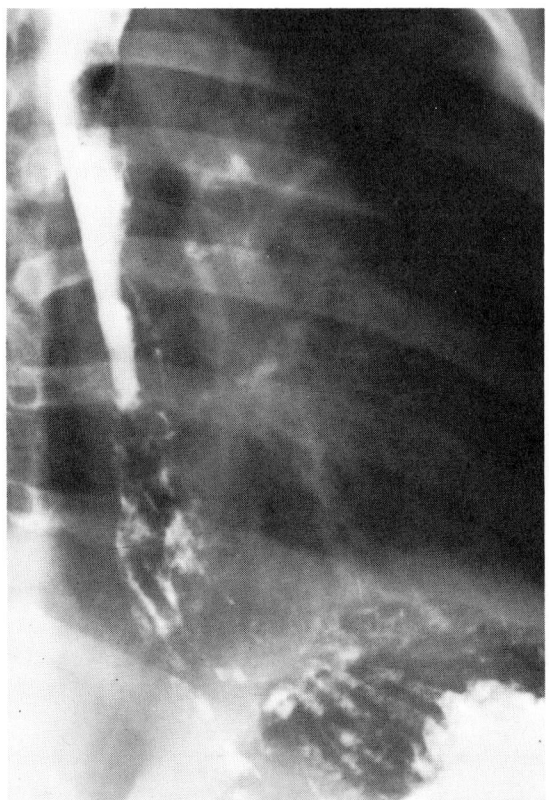

Figure 13. Congenital short esophagus in 31-month-old child presenting with pulmonary infection.

CONGENITAL SHORT ESOPHAGUS

A rare form of hiatus hernia is seen in infancy and childhood and appears to be caused by congenital shortening of the esophagus. A considerable portion of the cardia and fundus of the stomach is mediastinal in location and fixed in position with no hernia sac and no "sliding" (Fig. 13). Although stricture and hemorrhage may occur in these patients, the most common symptoms are those of spontaneous regurgitation when in the reclining position and the pulmonary complications of repeated bouts of pneumonitis and lung abscess. The stomach cannot be reduced below the diaphragm because of the short esophagus. In our experience this condition can be well treated by a transthoracic Nissen fundoplication procedure, leaving the repair entirely within the thorax.[9]

SELECTED REFERENCES

Demeester, T. R., Johnson, L. F., and Kent, A. H.: Evaluation of current operations for the prevention of gastroesophageal reflux. Ann. Surg., *180*:511, 1974.
Forty-five patients with reflux peptic esophagitis were randomized and treated by the Hill, Nissen, or Belsey antireflux procedure. Clinical scoring revealed 47 per cent good results with the Hill method, 80 per cent with the Belsey, and 100 per cent with the Nissen. pH reflux tests indicated the Hill method 80 per cent effective, the Belsey 60 per cent, and the Nissen 100 per cent. The Hill method improved resting LES pressure 4.5 mm. Hg, the Belsey 10.2, and the Nissen 12.9. Only 2 of 15 Nissen patients had "gas-bloat syndrome."

The latter procedure was recommended as the current operation of choice for correcting gastroesophageal reflux.

Giles, G. R., Mason, M. C., Humphries, C., and Clark, C. G.: Action of gastrin on the lower oesophageal sphincter in man. Gut, *10*:730, 1969.
Both hog gastrin and synthetic gastrin stimulate the cardiac sphincter to increase tone and augment the resistance to reflux. Endogenous gastrin has a similar effect, and gastrin also stimulates the secretion of acid, which has also been found to increase the resistance of the sphincter, but the effect of gastrin appears to be independent of the secretory stimulus.

Orringer, M. B., Skinner, D. B., and Belsey, R. H. R.: Long-term results of the Mark IV operation for hiatal hernia and analyses of recurrences and their treatment. J. Thorac. Cardiovasc. Surg., *63*:25, 1972.
Long-term results with the Belsey Mark IV operation are presented in 848 patients. Five hundred and fourteen (60.6 per cent) are entirely symptom free; 181 have no reflux symptoms but mild unrelated complaints (21.3 per cent). Fifty-five (6.5 per cent) have symptoms suggesting reflux, but without objective evidence, and 98 (11.6 per cent) have documented recurrent hiatus hernia or gastroesophageal reflux or both. Operative mortality has been 1 per cent.

Rosetti, M., and Allgower, M.: Fundoplication for treatment of hiatal hernia. Progr. Surg., *12*:1, 1973.
The authors report on 1231 cases of hiatus hernias of all types operated upon by the Nissen fundoplication technique. In patients with reflux esophagitis due to sliding hiatus hernia, the mortality has been 0.6 per cent in 845 patients. Long-term results are reported in 590 patients with simple reflux disease. Five hundred and sixteen or 87 per cent are free of symptoms. Ten per cent suffer from postfundoplication syndrome. Only 12 patients have required reoperation because of recurrence or peptic ulcer disease. Hazards in patients with short esophagus are pointed out.

REFERENCES

1. Allison, P. R.: Reflux esophagitis, sliding hiatal hernia, and the anatomy of repair. Surg. Gynecol. Obstet., *92*:419, 1951.
2. Allison, P. R., and Johnstone, A. S.: The esophagus lined with gastric mucous membrane. Thorax, *8*:87, 1953.
3. Barrett, N. R.: Chronic peptic ulcer of the esophagus and "esophagitis." Br. J. Surg., *38*:175, 1950.
4. Barrett, N. R.: The lower esophagus lined by columnar epithelium. Surgery, *41*:881, 1957.
5. Bernstein, L. M., and Baker, L. A.: A clinical test for esophagitis. Gastroenterology, *34*:760, 1958.
6. Bremner, C. G., Shorter, R. G., Lynhh, V. P., and Ellis, R. H., Jr.: Barrett's esophagus: Congenital or acquired? Experimental study of esophageal mucosal regeneration in the dog. Surgery, *68*:209, 1970.
7. Bushkin, F. L., Wickbom, G., DeFord, J. W., and Woodward, E. R.: Postoperative alkaline reflux gastritis. Surg. Gynecol. Obstet., *138*:933, 1974.
8. Clarke, J. M., Rayl, J. E., and Woodward, E. R.: Experience with the Thal and Nissen operations in the treatment of reflux esophagitis with stricture: A preliminary report. Am. Surg., *35*:89, 1969.
9. Clarke, J. M., and Woodward, E. R.: Transthoracic fundoplication for hiatal hernia and short esophagus in a 3-year-old child: Case report. Surgery, *64*:858, 1968.
10. Code, C. F., Creamer, B., Schlegel, J. F., Olsen, A. M., Donoghue, F. E., and Andersen, H. A.: An atlas of esophageal motility in health and disease. Springfield, Ill., Charles C Thomas, Publisher, 1958.
11. Code, C. F., Kelly, M. I., Jr., Schlegel, J. F., and Olsen, A. M.: Detection of hiatal hernia during esophageal motility tests. Gastroenterology, *43*:521, 1962.
12. Cohen, S., and Lipshutz, W.: Hormonal regulation of human lower esophageal sphincter competence: Interaction of gastrin and secretin. J. Clin. Invest., *50*:449, 1971.
13. Demeester, T. R., Johnson, L. F., and Kent, A. H.: Evaluation of current operations for the prevention of gastroesophageal reflux. Ann. Surg., *180*:511, 1974.
14. Giles, G. R., Humphries, C., Mason, M. C., and Clark, C. G.: Effect of pH changes on the cardiac sphincter. Gut, *10*:852, 1969.
15. Giles, G. R., Mason, M. C., Humphries, C., and Clark, C. G.: Action of gastrin on the lower esophageal sphincter in man. Gut, *10*:730, 1969.
16. Hill, L. D.: An effective operation for hiatal hernia: An eight year appraisal. Ann. Surg., *166*:681, 1967.

17. Hill, L. D., Chapman, K. W., and Morgan, E. H.: Objective evaluation of surgery for hiatus hernia and esophagitis. J. Thorac. Cardiovasc. Surg., *41*:60, 1961.
18. Hollenbeck, J. I., and Woodward, E. R.: The treatment of peptic esophageal stricture with combined fundic patch–fundoplication. Ann. Surg., *182*:472, 1975.
19. Ingelfinger, F. J.: Esophageal motility. Physiol. Rev., *38*:533, 1958.
20. Jennewein, H. M., Woldeck, F., Siewert, R., Weiser, F., and Thimm, R.: The interaction of glucagon and pentagastrin on the lower oesophageal sphincter in man and dog. Gut, *14*:861, 1973.
21. Maher, J. W., Hollenbeck, J. I., Sierakowski, N., Woodward, E. R., and McGuigan, J. E.: The effects of bicarbonate perfusion on lower esophageal sphincter response to feeding. Surg. Forum, *26*:366, 1975.
22. Merendino, K. A., and Dillard, D. H.: The concept of sphincter substitution by an interposed jejunal segment for anatomic and physiologic abnormalities at the esophagogastric junction—with special reference to reflux esophagitis, cardiospasm and esophageal varices. Ann. Surg., *142*:486, 1955.
23. Nissen, R.: Eine einfache Operation zur Beeinflussung der Reflux-oesophagitis. Schweiz. Med. Wochenschr., *86*:590, 1956.
24. Nissen, R., and Rosetti, M.: Surgery of the cardia ventriculi. CIBA Sympos., *11*:195, 1963.
25. Orringer, M. B., Skinner, D. B., and Belsey, R. H. R.: Long-term results of the Mark IV operation for hiatal hernia and analyses of recurrences and their treatment. J. Thorac. Cardiovasc. Surg., *63*:25, 1972.
26. Plzak, L. F., Jr., Fried, W., and Woodward, E. R.: Relative susceptibility of the gastrointestinal tract to experimental acute peptic ulceration. Surg. Forum, 7:389, 1957.
27. Rosetti, M., and Allgower, M.: Fundoplication for treatment of hiatal hernia. Progr. Surg., *12*:1, 1973.
28. Skinner, D. B., and Belsey, R. H. R.: Surgical management of esophageal reflux and hiatus hernia. J. Thorac. Cardiovasc. Surg., *53*:33, 1967.
29. Studevant, R. A. L., and Kun, T.: Interaction of pentagastrin and the octapeptide of cholecystokinin on the human lower oesophageal sphincter. Gut, *15*:700, 1974.
30. Thal, A. P., Hatafuku, T., and Kurtzman, R.: New operation for distal esophageal stricture. Arch. Surg., *90*:464, 1965.
31. Wickbom, G., Bushkin, F. L., and Woodward, E. R.: Alkaline reflux esophagitis. Surg. Gynecol. Obstet., *139*:267, 1974.
32. Woodward, E. R.: Hiatal herniorrhaphy. Surg. Tech. Illus., *1*:43–50, 1976.
33. Woodward, E. R., Thomas, H. F., and McAlhany, J. C.: Comparison of crural repair and Nissen fundoplication in the treatment of esophageal hiatus hernia with peptic esophagitis. Ann. Surg., *173*:782, 1971.

VIII

CORROSIVE STRICTURES OF THE ESOPHAGUS

James L. Talbert, M.D.

Corrosive strictures of the esophagus result from the ingestion of solid or liquid caustic substances. The most frequent victims are children between one and five years of age, who all too often are tragically enticed by chemical solutions that have been carelessly placed in familiar soft drink containers or by crystalline caustics that resemble sugar or candy when exposed in jars or cans (Fig. 1).[3] Each year in the United States approximately 5000 children under the age of five accidentally swallow strong alkaline preparations, usually one of the commonly available drain cleaners.[22] Instances of caustic ingestion in adults usually represent attempted suicide in emotionally disturbed or psychotic persons.[5]

ETIOLOGY

The most common chemicals implicated in corrosive burns of the esophagus include the alkaline caustics, acid or acid-like corrosives, and household bleaches. The alkaline caustics consist of sodium hydroxide (the active ingredient of household lye and drain cleaners such as Drano or Liquid Plumr), sodium carbonate (washing soda), sodium metasilicate (dishwashing detergent), and ammonia water (household cleaners). In the 40 years preceding 1965 most of the caustics ingested in the United States were flakes or solid pellets of sodium hydroxide. The introduction of liquid drain cleaning products on the American market in 1967, however, added another means by which children may be easily and frequently injured in household accidents.[19] In concentrated solutions, these caustics can produce liquefaction necrosis of the mucosa and underlying tissues. The extent of the resultant tissue injury is directly proportional to the concentration of chemical agent and the duration of tissue contact. Acids produce a coagulation necrosis that appears to impede deep penetration and usually do not result in as serious an esophageal injury as lye ingestion.[15] Caustic burns from common household bleaches such as Clorox are encountered with increasing frequency but rarely produce permanent damage.[11] More recently, it has also been noted that esophageal burns can result from the ingestion of Clinitest Tablets, which contain significant amounts of anhydrous sodium hydroxide.[6]

Corrosive burns from ingested caustic agents may involve the oropharynx, larynx, esophagus, stomach, or even intestine and colon. As in the case of external body burns, the resultant injuries can be categorized as superficial or deep on the basis of their gross ap-

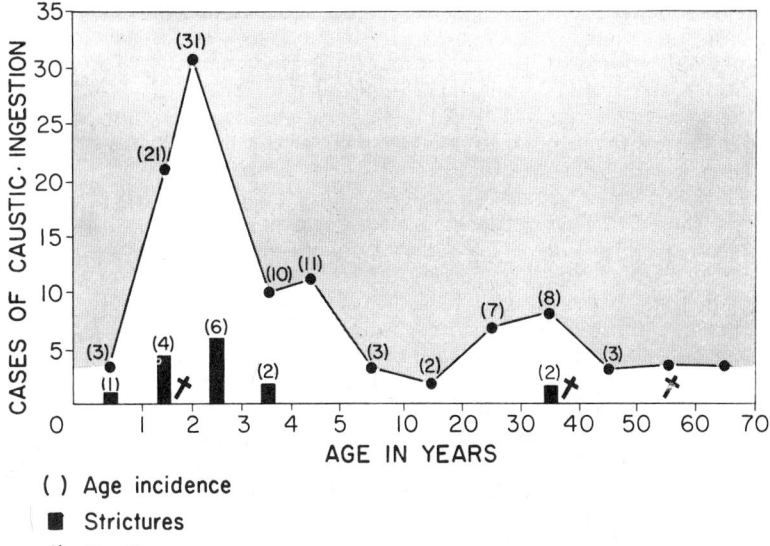

Figure 1. Summary of 22 years' experience (1944–1966) at the University of Cincinnati Medical Center in management of caustic ingestions. The age incidence and frequency of complications in these 105 patients is representative of the overall problem. (From Bikhazi, H. B., et al.: Arch. Otolaryngol., *89*:770, 1969.)

( ) Age incidence
■ Strictures
✗ Deaths

pearance and clinical behavior.[17, 23] Superficial burns are limited to the esophageal wall and are manifested by hyperemia, edema, blister formation, or superficial ulceration. Deep, or third-degree, burns characteristically extend through the full thickness of the esophageal wall into adjacent mediastinal tissues and may even penetrate into the pleural or peritoneal cavities.

In all instances, there is an acute, subacute, and chronic or cicatricial phase of burn wound healing. The acute or inflammatory phase encompasses the first few days following injury and is characterized by tissue destruction, inflammatory reaction, vascular thrombosis, and secondary bacterial infection. During the subsequent subacute phase, which may last as long as two weeks, depending on the severity of the original insult, necrotic tissue is spontaneously debrided and granulation tissue is formed by fibroblast and vascular proliferation. The injured esophageal wall is potentially weakest during this intermediate phase (7 to 14 days post burn). Symptoms of pain and dysphagia will often improve during this period, as healing progresses to the third or final phase of reepithelialization and scarring. The process of epithelial formation is usually complete by the sixth week following injury, but maturation and contracture of the scarred esophageal wall may continue for a period of months.

The advent of the liquid lye substances since 1967 has not only increased the potential for esophageal injury, but has also added an increased risk of damage to the stomach and distal gastrointestinal tract, especially in young children.[24] The ingestion of crystals of lye causes pain, and most children will attempt to spit out the caustic material immediately on tasting it. However, this defense mechanism is absent in the case of the liquid caustics, which are colorless and odorless and may produce serious damage even in concentrations less than 10 per cent.[2] In one recent series only

10 to 25 per cent of patients who ingested granular lye sustained serious esophageal burns, while more than 50 per cent of those who swallowed liquid lye incurred such injuries.[9] In instances of liquid lye ingestion, the patient should be monitored closely for evidence of gastric perforation, bleeding, or pyloric outlet obstruction in addition to esophageal injury.

TREATMENT OF CAUSTIC BURNS

The most important element in successful management of corrosive burns of the esophagus is immediate verification of the etiologic agent and accurate assessment of the depth and extent of injury.[17, 23] It is important always to ask to see the container from which the caustic material is obtained in order to confirm the type. First-aid treatment of these patients by antidotal administration is probably ineffective unless implemented immediately, within a matter of minutes or even seconds following caustic ingestion. Induced vomiting and gastric lavage are contraindicated because of the threat of compounding the original injury. Previous reports have emphasized an increased incidence of severe laryngeal and pharyngeal injury following vomiting of ingested lye.[5]

The mucosa of the lips, tongue, and oropharynx, the skin of the face, hands, and neck, and the clothing of the victim should be carefully inspected for evidence of corrosive burns. Substernal and back discomfort or abdominal pain and rigidity are suggestive of mediastinal or peritoneal perforation. Hoarseness, stridor, and dyspnea characterize laryngeal edema or actual epiglottic and laryngeal destruction through aspiration of the chemical agent. The absence of any visible evidence of oropharyngeal burns does not exclude the possibility of esophageal injury, since in one series 15 per cent of patients with no external evidence of burn were subsequently confirmed by esophagoscopy to have esophageal damage.[1] At the same time, as many as 70 per cent of patients with evidence of oropharyngeal burns will escape without associated esophageal injury.[14] It is essential, therefore, that esophagoscopy be performed within the first 12 to 24 hours to confirm the extent and severity of the burn. The only exceptions to this rule are those patients in whom esophageal or gastric perforation or impending airway obstruction is suspected. Any evidence of significant pharyngeal or laryngeal damage, either as identified by direct laryngoscopy or as suggested by symptoms of hoarseness, stridor, or dyspnea, demands immediate hospitalization and observation since the period of maximal edema and danger may be delayed for 6 to 24 hours. Esophagoscopy is contraindicated in these situations because of its potential for compounding the original injury. Immediate treatment with steroids and antibiotics should be instituted in all such cases. Blood gases should be monitored serially, and tracheostomy should be performed immediately if the airway obstruction or respiratory distress appears progressive. Chest x-rays should be examined for evidence of pulmonary infiltration or free perforation into the mediastinum or pleural or peritoneal cavities.

Since most caustic esophageal burns occur in children, esophagoscopy should be performed only under endotracheal anesthesia, preferably by a physician who is experienced in evaluating and managing this type of injury. The goal of the esophagoscopist is confirmation of the presence or absence of an esophageal burn and estimation of its severity by gross inspection. The hazard of instrumental perforation or damage to the friable esophageal wall is minimized if the operator immediately discontinues the procedure as soon as evidence of a mucosal burn is visualized. It is essential that no attempt be made to pass the esophagoscope beyond the proximal point of injury.[17] The depth of burn, as evaluated on the basis of superficial or deep involvement, has appeared important as a prognostic guide.[23] With appropriate treatment, superficial burns will usually heal without residual deformity, while deep burns are likely to progress to scarring and stricture formation, regardless of the choice of therapy. Since esophagoscopy must be terminated at the proximal point of injury, the status of the distal esophagus must be evaluated subsequently by serial esophagograms. In mild burns, the esophagogram in the acute phase may reveal only minimal abnormalities, including delayed passage of contrast material and a spiral appearance of the mucosal folds.[19] Edematous mucosal folds and linear ulcerations have been noted in patients who have ingested highly concentrated alkaline agents. In severe esophageal injuries the esophagus may appear atonic and dilated, rigid and persistently narrowed, or excessively irritable.[10] If no burns are identified in the esophagus and if local care seems sufficient for management of any limited oropharyngeal lesions, follow-up barium esophagography should be repeated at three weeks, three months, six months, and one year following injury, to exclude those rare instances of esophageal injury and scarring which may escape recognition at the time of initial esophagoscopy.

In cases in which an esophageal burn is definitely identified, two treatment options have been generally advocated: (1) maintenance of an esophageal lumen by mechanical means, or (2) pharmacologic modification of wound healing to prevent stricture formation.

The use of bougienage as a modality of treatment for corrosive esophageal burns was first introduced by Salzer in 1920 and characteristically has been performed blindly, with tapered bougies.[27] A graduated program is established in which esophageal dilation is performed daily for several weeks, then every other day for two to three weeks, and finally once a week for many months. Previously, it was felt that early bougienage prevented intraluminal adhesions within the injured esophagus, but experimental observations have subsequently suggested that this form of treatment may actually enhance cicatrix formation and increase the risk of perforation.[15, 20] Certainly, in young children, the age group most susceptible to caustic burns, esophageal bougienage appears to add potential psychologic and physical hazards which are unwarranted if other, less traumatic, methods of treatment can produce equally satisfactory results. A recent modification of the bougienage technique has been suggested by Reyes and co-workers in which an intraluminal esophageal silicone splint is left in place for three weeks following a caustic burn. Experiments in cats utilizing this technique have suggested that it may be an effective method for preventing esophageal strictures but requires careful monitoring in order to prevent aspiration and pneumonia.[25]

The medical management of esophageal burns has been predicated on the use of steroids to modify the inflammatory response to the burn injury and antibiotics to control secondary bacterial infection. Experimental studies by Spain and colleagues in 1950 first suggested that early administration of cortisone produced an anti-inflammatory effect that would inhibit fibroplasia in wound healing.[28] These findings were subsequently applied to the treatment of experimental esophageal burns in animals, and the beneficial effects of steroids in reducing incidence of postinjury stricture appeared to be confirmed when antibiotic coverage was added to control secondary suppurative complications.[15, 20] These studies also suggested that steroid therapy should be instituted immediately after injury, and most authors have discouraged this form of treatment if the patient is seen later than 48 hours following injury.[20] In patients treated with steroids and antibiotics, self-bougienage through ingestion and swallowing of food is probably an important component of treatment. In small children who are able to swallow without discomfort, this is the simplest method of achieving esophageal dilation. The tendency to early esophageal obstruction secondary to edema and spasm is minimized by steroid administration, so that early institution of oral feedings is facilitated.[15]

Although some disparity in results is evident in reported series, a signficant decrease in the incidence of esophageal stricture has appeared to result in those patients treated with steroids and antibiotic therapy.[17] Alford has reported a 50 per cent incidence of esophageal stricture in humans with esophageal burns who have not received steroids.[1] In patients who have been treated with steroids, the reported stricture rate usually varies between 5 and 17 per cent.[5] Although some reports have recorded a higher incidence, the discrepancies in response probably reflect a lack of conformity between the various series. Animal experiments have also substantiated the clinical impression that steroid and antibiotic treatment is beneficial when applied under standardized conditions.[15, 20]

Steroid treatment is contraindicated in cases of severe caustic burns that are associated with evidence of perforation of the esophagus or necrosis of the stomach. In contrast, patients with signs of dyspnea, hoarseness, or stridor should be treated immediately with steroids and antibiotics, since esophagoscopy is contraindicated in these cases and the probability of associated severe esophageal injury is extremely high. Immediate steroid and antibiotic treatment should also be considered in those cases in which diagnostic esophagoscopy must be delayed for longer than 12 hours. If no esophageal lesion is subsequently identified by an experienced esophagoscopist, this treatment can then be discontinued.

The steroid and antibiotic regimen that has been employed most frequently for treatment of esophageal burns consists of prednisone, administered in divided doses of 2 to 3 mg. per kilogram of body weight every 24 hours, and ampicillin, administered in divided doses of 50 to 100 mg. per kilogram of body weight every 24 hours for a total of three weeks.[23] If the patient is initially unable to take oral alimentation, these medications should be administered intravenously with hydrocortisone or methylprednisolone sodium succinate substituted in equivalent doses. Since the act of swallowing food probably contributes to the success of steroid therapy, oral feedings are instituted as soon as they can be tolerated by the patient, beginning first with a modified Sippy diet for three to four days to prevent acid gastric reflux, then rapidly progressing to soft, regular foods.

Once the initial edema of injury has resolved, after two to three days, the patient should experience gradual improvement in his ability to swallow. If dysphagia reappears, stricture formation should be suspected and an immediate barium esophagogram should be obtained for evaluation. At the end of a full three weeks of treatment, the steroid dosage should be tapered and finally discontinued. The experience of Middelkamp and his associates suggests that further prolongation of treatment simply postpones stricture formation and does not alter the eventual outcome.[23] A complete radiographic evaluation of the esophagus is obtained at the termination of steroid therapy and is repeated again at three months, six months, and one year after injury. If stricture formation is evident at any time during this follow-up, bougienage should be instituted immediately. Continuation of steroid therapy under these circumstances does not appear to alter the eventual course of stricture formation and may unnecessarily expose the patient to the added hazard of an excessively friable esophagus when esophageal dilation is performed.[23]

Recent experimental studies have been directed toward identification of additional pharmacologic agents which may prevent the development of esophageal strictures following caustic injury. The use of beta-aminoproprionitrile (BAPN) has been evaluated in animals and appears especially promising for this purpose.[7, 26] BAPN is a powerful lathyrogen and inhibits the action of lysyl oxidase, thus preventing collagen cross-linking. The collagen thus formed appears histologically normal but yields quite easily to mechanical stretching as a result of a decrease in tensile strength. In the presence of lathyritic scars, ingestion of a soft, solid diet appears to dilate the esophagus and maintain patency. Although agents such as BAPN and penicillamine, or a combination of both, have appeared effective experimentally in the prevention of esophageal stenosis, this experience has not been verified with clinical trials in man.

MANAGEMENT OF CORROSIVE STRICTURES

The most frequent complication of caustic burns of the esophagus is stricture formation. In some instances, these lesions are mild and will immediately respond to dilation without subsequent recurrence. All too often, however, lye burns cause extensive full-thickness damage which eventually produces multiple areas of stricture throughout the extent of the esophagus (Fig. 2). In those cases in which ultimate stenosis can be anticipated on the basis of the severity of the original injury, early passage of a string through the patient's nose into his stomach will facilitate subsequent bougienage.[17] In some instances it may be necessary to utilize a gastrostomy in order to maintain satisfactory gastrointestinal alimentation and to facilitate esophageal dilation. Cases of multiple, tight strictures are probably best handled by this approach, by performing retrograde esophageal

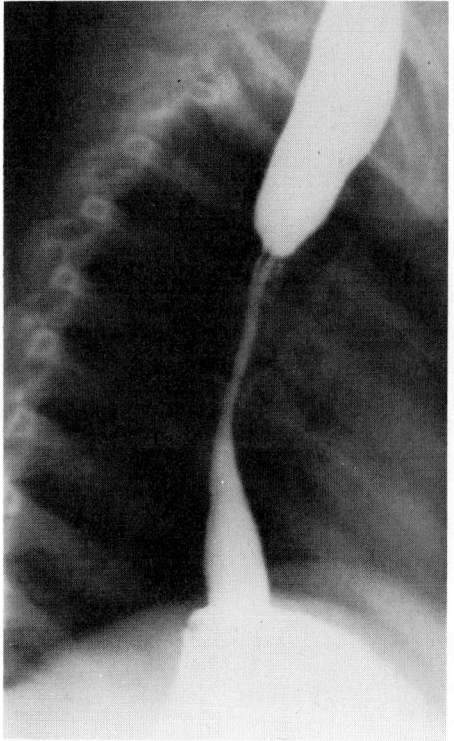

Figure 2. A characteristic extensive esophageal stricture in a child resulting from lye (Liquid Plumr) ingestion.

dilation with rubber tapered-tip Tucker bougies guided by a string previously passed from above.

When a gastrostomy is required for feeding purposes, it should be positioned on the stomach wall so that a gastric tube can be formed subsequently from the greater curvature, in the event this procedure proves necessary for esophageal reconstruction.[8] It is also important that the antrum and pylorus of the stomach be inspected carefully when performing a gastrostomy, since a stricture may not be visible from the serosal side and careful intraluminal palpation may be necessary to identify a circumferential thickening.[12] If destruction by the ingested chemical has involved the stomach and pylorus with extensive necrosis and edema, a feeding jejunostomy may be utilized as an alternate route for alimentation.

Although the safest method of esophageal dilation is probably retrograde through a gastrostomy, this approach is not necessarily required for all cases.[4] Alternate approaches include antegrade dilation by a filiform-guided bougie, which can be inserted under direct vision through an esophagoscope, or by a swallowed Mixter-type bougie, which is inserted over a string guide. Chronic cases with minimal or moderate esophageal strictures can be treated by swallowed mercury-filled Hurst bougies when the patient is cooperative.

In cases of localized strictures that extend less than 1.5 cm. in length and fail to respond to bougienage

alone, an alternate treatment involves direct local injection of steroids into the circumferential scar.[16] This technique was suggested initially by the success reported in management of cutaneous hypertrophic scars and burn contractures by local infiltration of triamcinolone diacetate. In a limited series of clinical patients, 40 mg. of triamcinolone diacetate was injected under direct vision through an esophagoscope into the four quadrants of a circumferential esophageal scar. This treatment was followed by bougienage, and steroid injections were repeated on several occasions when necessary. In some of the cases, previously unresponsive strictures resolved completely with this therapy. Clinitest Tablets appear especially prone to produce localized esophageal strictures at the level of the carina. If these lesions do not respond to dilation, resection and esophageal anastomosis are usually feasible.[6]

A need for surgical reconstruction of the esophagus is indicated by the presence of extensive, persistent strictures, a need for frequent dilation, failure or refusal of the patient to follow a regimen of regular dilation or the presence of high strictures or fistulas between the esophagus and tracheobronchial tree. Prolonged attempts at unsuccessful dilation not only expose the patient, frequently a child, to unnecessary physical and psychologic trauma, but also may impede normal growth and development. Use of the right colon with an attached segment of terminal ileum,

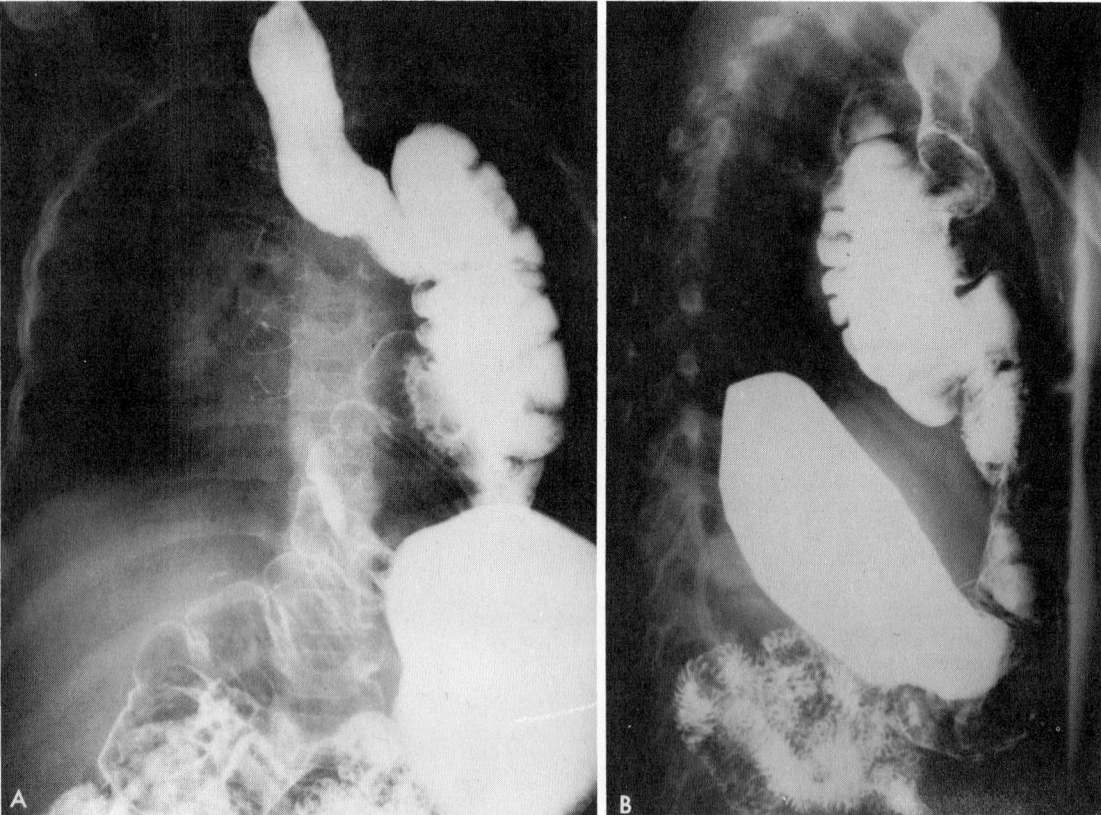

Figure 3. *A,* Anteroposterior, and *B,* lateral view of a retrosternal pull-through of terminal ileum and right colon for bypass of an extensive esophageal lye stricture in a child.

tunneling it through the retrosternal space into the neck, has proved eminently satisfactory in all patients over one year of age with extensive esophageal scarring (Fig. 3). The inclusion of terminal ileum for anastomosis to the proximal esophagus in the neck decreases the bulk of tissue and avoids obstruction at the thoracic inlet, previously a frequent problem in young children undergoing this procedure. Preservation of the ileocecal valve has also appeared to decrease the hazard of regurgitation from the patulous substernal colonic segment. An alternate method for colonic interposition is provided by the technique of Waterston, in which transverse and descending colon is brought through the left pleural cavity in an isoperistaltic position and interposed between the proximal esophagus and the stomach.[13] A final method which is available to the surgeon in instances when the colon proves unsuitable for esophageal substitution because of an aberrant blood supply, colitis, or anatomic abnormality is the gastric tube technique.[8] This procedure most frequently involves the use of a reversed antiperistaltic gastric tube which is based proximally on the greater curvature of the stomach and receives its blood supply from the left gastroepiploic artery. The gastric tube is then passed through a retrosternal tunnel for anastomosis to the cervical esophagus. Early results of the use of this technique in children have proved encouraging, although late postural regurgitation with recurrent esophagitis and stricture may pose a problem.

A late complication of corrosive burns of the esophagus which has not been widely recognized is the development of a hiatus hernia between 25 and 69 years following injury.[18] Apparently, the fibrotic esophagus contracts and pulls the stomach into the chest. The patient then develops esophagitis and peptic stricture in an already narrowed esophagus secondary to gastroesophageal reflux. Dilation of the esophageal stricture in such cases is pointless because it increases the reflux and the fibrotic stricture becomes tighter.

A final long-term complication of esophageal scarring and stricture formation is malignant degeneration. It has been estimated that the incidence of esophageal carcinoma in patients who have previously suffered lye stricture is at least 1000-fold greater than in the general population.[21] Any change in symptoms in a patient with a chronic lye stricture, especially one of greater than 16 years' duration, should immediately suggest the need for radiographic and esophagoscopic examination. Inability to dilate a chronic stricture that has previously responded to treatment or late radiographic evidence of progressive stenosis should strongly suggest malignant change. Biopsies performed through the esophagoscope can easily miss the tumor in such cases, since the carcinoma may be located distal to the area of stenosis and prove inaccessible to the biopsy forceps. Negative biopsies in such cases, therefore, must be considered inconclusive. Fortunately, those carcinomas which do develop in scar tissue of the esophagus appear to be less aggressive in behavior than the usual esophageal cancer, possibly because the surrounding scar tissue limits invasion and the resultant intraluminal proliferation produces early obstructive symptoms.

Resection of a strictured esophageal segment is indicated in any patient with a chronic lye stricture in whom the changes noted above have occurred. Identification of the tumor provides the patient an excellent chance of being cured of a lesion that ordinarily carries a dismal prognosis.

SELECTED REFERENCES

Ashcraft, K. W., and Padula, R. T.: The effect of dilute corrosives on the esophagus. Pediatrics, *53*:226, 1974.
This paper confirms that the dilute corrosive drain cleaners which are currently available to the public are capable of producing severe damage to the esophagus. The authors note that even in the previously allowed, very concentrated forms, most of the liquid drain cleaners were ineffective in cleaning drains. Accordingly, in view of their potential hazard, it would seem logical to ban the sale of these chemical substances to the public.

Holinger, P. H.: Management of esophageal lesions caused by chemical burns. Ann. Otol. Rhinol. Laryngol., *77*:819, 1968.
This excellent paper provides a comprehensive review of all aspects of management of esophageal chemical burns. The presentation is substantiated by the extensive personal experience of the author in treatment of these injuries.

Kirsh, M. M., and Ritter, F.: Caustic ingestion and subsequent damage to the oropharyngeal and digestive passages. Ann. Thorac. Surg., *21*:74, 1976.
This article presents an updated review of the characteristics, diagnosis, and management of oropharyngeal and digestive passage lesions resulting from ingestion of caustic agents. Special attention is directed to the changing spectrum of injuries and treatment regimens which have been required by the introduction of liquid drain cleaning products on the American market.

Middelkamp, J. N., Ferguson, T. B., Roper, C. L., and Hoffman, F. D.: The management and problems of caustic burns in children. J. Thorac. Cardiovasc. Surg., *57*:341, 1969.
The clinical results in a large, well-controlled series of caustic burns treated with a standardized regimen of steroids and antibiotics are summarized in this excellent review. The experience emphasizes the importance of early esophagoscopy in establishing the presence and extent of injury as well as suggesting eventual prognosis.

REFERENCES

1. Alford, B. R., and Harris, H. H.: Chemical burns of the mouth, pharynx and esophagus. Ann. Otol. Rhinol. Laryngol., *68*:122, 1959.
2. Ashcraft, K. W., and Padula, R. T.: The effect of dilute corrosives on the esophagus. Pediatrics, *53*:226, 1974.
3. Bikhazi, H. B., Thompson, E. R., and Shumrick, D. A.: Caustic ingestion: Current status. Arch. Otolaryngol., *89*:770, 1969.
4. Bill, A. J., Jr., Mebust, W. K., and Sauvage, L. R.: Evaluation of techniques of esophageal dilation in relation to danger of perforation. J. Thorac. Cardiovasc. Surg., *45*:510, 1963.
5. Borja, A. R., Ransdell, H. T., Jr., Thomas, T. C., and Johnson, W.: Lye injuries of the esophagus: Analysis of 90 cases of lye ingestion. J. Thorac. Cardiovasc. Surg., *57*:533, 1969.
6. Burrington, J. D.: Clintest burns of the esophagus. Ann. Thorac. Surg., *20*:400, 1975.
7. Davis, W. M., Madden, J. W., and Peacock, E. E.: A new approach to the control of esophageal stenosis. Ann. Surg., *176*:469, 1972.
8. Ein, S. H., Shandling, B., Simpson, J. S., and Stephens, C. A.: A further look at the gastric tube as an esophageal replacement in infants and children. J. Pediatr. Surg., *8*:859, 1973.
9. Feldman, M., Iben, A. B., and Hurley, E. J.: Corrosive injury to oropharynx and esophagus. West. J. Med., *118*:6, 1973.
10. Franken, E. A.: Caustic damage of the gastrointestinal tract: Roentgen features. Am. J. Roentgenol., *118*:77, 1973.
11. French, R. J., Tabb, H. G., and Rutledge, L. J.: Esophageal stenosis produced by ingestion of bleach. South. Med. J., *63*:1140, 1970.
12. Gavriliu, D.: Operative management of caustic strictures of the stomach and duodenum; the jejunostomy. Curr. Probl. Surg., *12*:13, 1975.
13. German, J. C., and Waterston, D. J.: Colon interposition for the

    replacement of the esophagus in children. J. Pediatr. Surg., 11:227, 1976.
14. Haller, J. A., Jr., Andrews, H. G., White, J. J., and Cleveland, W. W.: Pathophysiology and management of acute corrosive burns of the esophagus: Results of treatment in 285 children. J. Pediatr. Surg., 6:579, 1971.
15. Haller, J. A., and Bachman, K.: The comparative effect of current therapy on experimental caustic burns of the esophagus. Pediatrics, 34:236, 1964.
16. Holder, T. M., Ashcraft, K. W., and Leape, L.: The treatment of patients with esophageal strictures by local steroid injections. J. Pediatr. Surg., 4:646, 1969.
17. Holinger, P. H.: Management of esophageal lesions caused by chemical burns. Ann. Otol. Rhinol. Laryngol., 77:819, 1968.
18. Imre, J., and Kopp, M.: Arguments against long-term conservative treatment of oesophageal strictures due to corrosive burns. Thorax, 27:594, 1972.
19. Kirsh, M. M., and Ritter, F.: Caustic injestion and subsequent damage to the oropharyngeal and digestive passages. Ann. Thorac. Surg., 21:74, 1976.
20. Knox, W. G., Scott, J. R., Zintel, H. A., Guthrie, R., and McCabe, R. E.: Bougienage and steroids used singly or in combination in experimental corrosive esophagitis. Ann. Surg., 166:930, 1967.

21. Lansing, P. B., Ferrante, W. A., and Ochsner, J. L.: Carcinoma of the esophagus at the site of the lye stricture. Am. J. Surg., 118:108, 1969.
22. Leape, L. L., Ashcraft, K. W., Scarpelli, D. G., and Holder, T. M.: Hazard to health—liquid lye. N. Engl. J. Med., 284:578, 1971.
23. Middelkamp, J. N., Ferguson, T. B., Roper, C. L., and Hoffman, F. D.: The management and problems of caustic burns in children. J. Thorac. Cardiovasc. Surg., 57:341, 1969.
24. Ray, J. F., III, Myers, W. O., Lawton, B. R., Lee, F. Y., Wenzel, F. J., and Sautter, R. D.: The natural history of liquid lye ingestion: Rationale for aggressive surgical approach. Arch. Surg., 109:436, 1974.
25. Reyes, H. M., Lin, C.-Y., Schlunk, F. F., and Replogle, R. L.: Experimental treatment of corrosive esophageal burns. J. Pediatr. Surg., 9:317, 1974.
26. Saedi, S., Nyhus, L. M., Gabrys, B. F., Kusakari, K., and Bombeck, C. T.: Pharmacological prevention of esophageal stricture: An experimental study in the cat. Am. Surg., 39:465, 1973.
27. Salzer, H.: Early treatment of corrosive esophagitis. Wien. Klin. Wochenschr., 33:307, 1920.
28. Spain, D. M., Malomert, N., and Haber, A.: The effect of cortisone on the formation of granulation tissue in mice. Am. J. Pathol., 26:710, 1950.

IX

TUMORS OF THE ESOPHAGUS

Paul C. Adkins, M.D.

HISTORICAL ASPECTS

The esophagus is a relatively inaccessible structure, and consequently appreciation of disorders of the esophagus including tumors has been relatively recent. The first esophagoscope was designed by Kussmaul in 1863, and since then the development of more sophisticated methods of endoscopy and diagnostic radiology has enabled physicians to diagnose and treat noeplasms of the esophagus ante mortem. In 1877 Czerny[13] reported an operation for a carcinoma of the cervical esophagus. In 1907 the first successful removal of a benign esophageal lesion was accomplished by Chevalier Jackson through an esophagoscope.[21] Torek preformed the first successful resection of the intrathoracic esophagus in 1913.[42] Seo and Oshawa from Japan reported successful intrathoracic resections of the esophagus with esophagogastric reconstruction in 1933. Adams and Phemister reported in 1938 the first successful resection and esophagogastrostomy in this country.[1] At that time they were apparently unaware of the Japanese reports. Subsequently, advances in diagnostic techniques, anesthesiology, and blood replacement and an understanding of the physiologic problems associated with intrathoracic surgery have contributed greatly to the ability of the surgeon to appreciate, diagnose, and treat tumors of the esophagus.

BENIGN TUMORS OF THE ESOPHAGUS

Benign tumors of the esophagus are far less common than their malignant counterparts. In various reported series they have comprised between 0.5 and 0.8 per cent of neoplasms of the esophagus.[43] In general, benign tumors occur at an earlier age than carcinoma of the esophagus, and symptoms, if present, may be of longer duration in those patients who subsequently are found to have a benign obstructing lesion.

Leiomyoma

Leiomyoma is the most common benign tumor of the esophagus. These tumors are found three times more frequently in males than females, and the majority are found in patients under the age of 50. Approximately 90 per cent of these tumors arise in the lower one third of the esophagus. Some may grow to considerable size.

In the overwhelming majority of cases the tumor is solitary and circumscribed. Rare instances of multiple tumors have been reported. Fernandez et al. reported 17 cases from the world literature of diffuse leiomyomatosis of the esophagus. Clinically, these patients had multiple tumors or a more diffuse form without visible nodules. The radiographic appearance of this condition was suggestive of diffuse spasm of the esophagus or achalasia. Symptoms of leiomyoma of the esophagus are primarily dependent upon its size and ability to compress or obstruct the esophagus or its adjacent structures. The predominant complaint is dysphagia, usually due to extrinsic compression of the esophageal lumen. Many of these tumors may be totally asymptomatic and discovered at autopsy or as an incidental finding at radiographic examination for other problems. Bleeding is exceedingly rare. Pain may occasionally be a presenting symptom when the tumor is large, causing a "stretch reflex," or when it causes compression of adjacent mediastinal structures.

The radiographic findings of a leiomyoma are rather characteristic and include a filling defect on esophagogram with an intact esophageal mucosa. This mass may move with deglutition. There may be flattening of the mucosal folds over the tumor with normal folds in the esophageal wall opposite the tumor mass. A shelf may be present where the normal esophageal wall meets the edge of the tumor. The mass itself is usually oval or crescent-shaped with a sharply demarcated outline (Fig. 1). Occasionally calcium may be present in the tumor mass. If the leiomyoma is of sufficient size to cause significant obstruction, there may be proximal dilatation of the esophagus.

The leiomyoma characteristically does not invade the esophageal mucosa and on esophagoscopy there may be extrinsic compression or displacement of the mucosa, but actual mucosal involvement, including ulceration or a tumor mass, should strongly suggest the possibility of a malignant lesion such as a carcinoma or sarcoma. On passing the esophagoscope, the endoscopist frequently may experience the feeling of mobility of the tumor as the instrument is passed through an area of extrinsic compression of the esophageal lumen. If there is no obvious change in the mucosa of the esophagus, biopsy is considered inadvisable. In those patients undergoing biopsy through the esophagoscope, it has been found at subsequent operation that there is a distinct tendency to enter the esophageal lumen at the site of the previous biopsy during enucleation of the tumor.

A leiomyoma arises from the muscular layer or the fibromuscular submucosa of the esophagus.[32] Grossly the tumor usually involves the plane between the circular and longitudinal muscle coats of the esophagus and is well circumscribed. The tumor is frequently multilobulated, smooth, white, and quite mobile (Fig. 2). Microscopically, there are interlacing bundles of smooth muscle cells with uniform nuclei and an absence of mitotic figures.

Sauerbrach performed the best successful partial esophageal resection for a leiomyoma in 1932.[35] However, at that time the true nature of the neoplasm was not appreciated. Oshawa in 1933[43] performed the first enucleation of a leiomyoma, and in 1937 Churchill also enucleated a solid esophageal tumor which at that time was considered a neurofibroma,[12] but was subsequently reclassified by Sweet et al. as a leiomyoma.[39] Since the potential for malignant change of the leiomyoma is relatively insignificant, the tumor can be successfully removed by simply splitting the normal muscle overlying the tumor mass and enucleating the tumor without incising or disturbing the underlying esophageal mucosa. At operation, the tumor mass can be rather easily delineated from the adjacent musculature of the esophagus and removal is a relatively simple process. Since the majority of these tumors are located in the lower third of the esophagus, a left thoracotomy is the preferable approach for that location. Although some of these tumors have been removed by a transabdominal approach, this does not appear to afford the simplest access to the tumor unless there are compelling reasons for avoiding a thoracotomy. Should the tumor occur on the upper thoracic cervical esophagus, a right thoracotomy or cervical approach may be utilized as needed. In those rare patients with diffuse form of disease or leiomyomatosis, esophageal resection or even total esophagectomy may be necessary for cure.

Esophageal Polyp

The fibrovascular polyp (pedunculated or intramural lipoma) represents the second most common type of

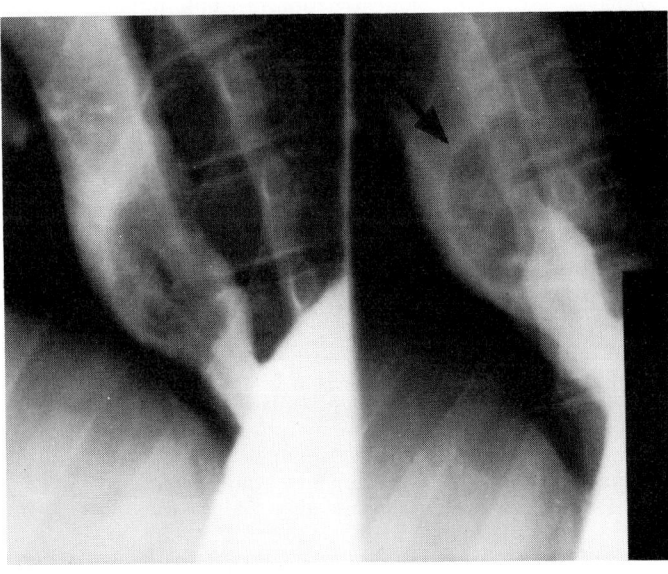

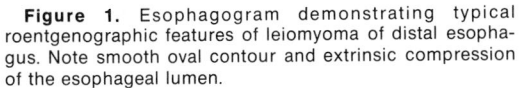
Figure 1. Esophagogram demonstrating typical roentgenographic features of leiomyoma of distal esophagus. Note smooth oval contour and extrinsic compression of the esophageal lumen.

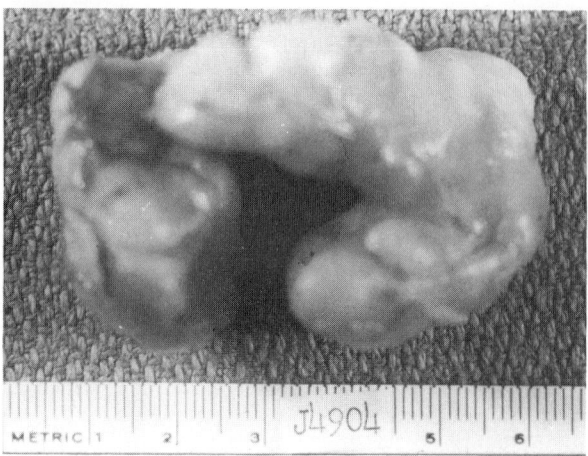

Figure 2. Gross specimen of leiomyoma of lower esophagus removed by enucleation.

benign esophageal tumor. This tumor arises in the mucosa or submucosa and is usually covered by normal esophageal mucosa. It may arise at any level in the esophagus and may cause regurgitation, obstruction, or even asphyxiation as a result of regurgitation of the tumor mass with airway obstruction. It may cause symptoms of dysphagia owing to obstruction, and on esophagogram the diagnosis may be strongly suspected on the basis of a sharply demarcated smooth intraluminal area of radiolucency. Endoscopic examination not only may be helpful in diagnosis or visualization of a smooth mass presenting in the lumen of the esophagus without mucosal ulceration, but also may be therapeutic, since endoscopic resection of an esophageal polyp appears to be quite satisfactory.

Miscellaneous Benign Tumors

Hemangiomas of the esophageal mucosa have been reported infrequently. They may vary in size from a few millimeters to several centimeters. The majority of these are asymptomatic, but may cause hematemesis or symptoms of obstruction. Lymphangiomas are even less frequent, but may present in the esophageal lumen with manifestations of obstruction if they achieve sufficient size.[6] The diagnosis is usually established by esophagoscopy with or without biopsy. If symptoms are present and the true nature of the lesion is established, it would appear that localized resection is the treatment of choice. Irradiation of these lesions has been reported, but with few successful responses.

Even less commonly, esophageal papillomas consisting of a lobulated tumor covered by squamous mucosa with a fibrous core, osteochondromas, and granular cell myoblastomas of the esophagus have been reported. Each of these is sufficiently rare to constitute a pathologic curiosity, but may be suspected by the proper radiographic and endoscopic studies. Papillomas may be removed through the esophagoscope. Granular cell myoblastomas may present in a similar manner to the leiomyoma and diagnosis may be possible only after surgical removal of the tumor mass.[15]

MALIGNANT TUMORS OF THE ESOPHAGUS

Epidermoid carcinoma is by far the most common neoplasm of the esophagus. It is encountered much more frequently than benign tumors, and other malignant tumors of the esophagus are rare in comparison. Although adenocarcinoma involving the lower end of the esophagus is not uncommon, in the majority of cases it originates primarily in the stomach and extends upward into the distal esophagus, and consequently cannot be classified as a primary esophageal neoplasm.

EPIDERMOID CARCINOMA

Incidence

There appears to be marked variation in the incidence of epidermoid carcinoma of the esophagus when analyzed by geographic distribution, race, and socioeconomic status. In our own institution esophageal carcinoma accounted for a little less than 1 per cent of all cases of malignant disease. However, it is extremely frequent in certain parts of South Africa, in China, Japan, and Puerto Rico, in certain areas of Russia, and in the Dutch West Indies. It is uncommon in whites in the United States, but is particularly frequent in Negroes of low socioeconomic level, as evidenced by reports by Parker from the low country of South Carolina.[30] Indeed, in that area it is the most common malignant disease encountered in male Negro patients and is second only to carcinoma of the cervix in the total Negro population. In a study by Davies[14] of the frequency of carcinoma of the esophagus in Africa, it was considered that certain environmental and dietary factors were important in the epidemiology of this malignancy. There has been considerable investigation of the possible dietary factors in other areas such as Japan, China, Russia, and Curaçao. In these areas the use of hot liquids, hot rice, strong alcoholic beverages, and coarse diets has been proposed as a contributory factor in the development of malignant tumors of the esophagus. However, there is little tangible evidence at this time to confirm this thesis unequivocally. Nevertheless, it seems apparent that there is some relation between chronic irritation of the esophagus and the development of carcinoma.

In addition, numerous other benign conditions have been observed to be accompanied by an increase in the incidence of carcinoma. These include achalasia,[10] hiatus hernia,[2] lye burns, and leukoplakia, as well as excessive alcoholic intake and cigarette smoking.

Carcinoma of the esophagus is primarily a disease of the older age group. In a review of over 7500 cases, Postlethwait and Sealy[34] found the peak incidence, 34 per cent, in the seventh decade. It is most commonly seen after the age of 40 and is a great rarity in the first three decades of life. It is predominantly a disease of males, with a ratio of between 2:1 and 5:1 in terms of frequency of carcinoma of the esophagus in males over females. An exception to this is carcinoma of the cervical esophagus, which in some areas is more common in females. This has been pointed out by Jacobson in Sweden and suggests a relationship to the higher incidence of the Plummer-Vinson syndrome occurring in the female population of that country.[30]

Pathology

The esophagus is arbitrarily divided into four portions: cervical, upper thoracic, midthoracic, and lower thoracic. These are generally measured by esophagoscopy with the reference point being the upper alveolar margin. The arbitrary division of the esophagus is of some practical importance, not only in terms of recording the frequency of carcinoma at the various levels, but also in terms of planning a therapeutic approach and determining prognosis. If one considers primary carcinoma of the esophagus and excludes adenocarcinoma of the stomach involving the distal one third, the middle third of the intrathoracic esophagus is the area most frequently involved by carcinoma. The majority of authors report the lower third as next most commonly involved and the upper thoracic and cervical esophagus as least commonly involved (Fig. 3).

Grossly, esophageal carcinoma may present as an ulcerating hard tumor mass on the mucosal surface of the esophagus. It may also present as a polypoid infiltrative process growing in the submucosal layer without obvious ulceration of the mucosal surface. Not infrequently there may be a combination of these two changes, with progression proximally and distally, and in far-advanced stages all layers of the esophagus as well as adjacent structures may be involved.

Microscopically, the lesion may be seen as an epidermoid carcinoma that in some instances may be well differentiated, with keratin and pearl formation. In other patients the lesion may be less well differentiated and show marked antiplasticity. In their fascicle on tumors of the esophagus, Stout and Lattes pointed out that there is no correlation between the degree of cellular differentiation of the esophageal carcinoma and its rate of spread involvement of adjacent structures, or prognosis.[38]

The progressing esophageal carcinoma involves adjacent structures in relation to the level of the neoplasm. Carcinomas of the upper and middle third are prone to involve the trachea or main stem bronchi as well as the aorta. The recurrent laryngeal nerve may be involved by extension of the neoplasm. Carcinomas of the lower third may involve the diaphragm or pericardium or even the cardia and fundus of the stomach.

Clinical Manifestations

The most common symptom associated with esophageal neoplasms is dysphagia. This may be accompanied by a sensation of substernal fullness with or without pain. The dysphagia may first be associated with solid food and later with soft foods and then even liquids. As the obstruction in the lumen becomes complete or nearly complete, the inability to swallow saliva becomes apparent and there may be constant drooling of saliva. In addition to the swallowing difficulty, weight loss almost invariably occurs in the later stages of the disease and may go on to severe emaciation. Other symptoms may be associated with growth of the tumor to involve structures adjacent to

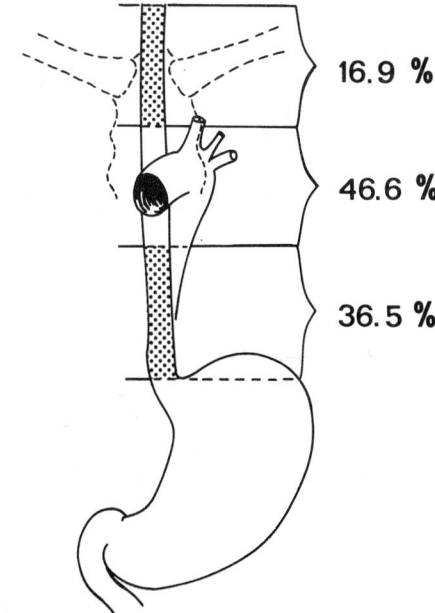

Figure 3. Percentage distribution of carcinoma of the esophagus. (After Postlethwait, R. W., and Sealy, W. C.: Surgery of the Esophagus. 1961. Courtesy of Charles C Thomas, Publisher, Springfield, Ill.)

the esophagus, such as the recurrent laryngeal nerve, the diaphragm, or the trachea or bronchi.

While it is apparent that carcinoma of the esophagus must be strongly suspected in any person over the age of 40 with swallowing difficulty, the majority of cases are relatively far advanced by the time the diagnosis is established. Many of these tumors grow at a rather slow rate and patients tend to minimize or compensate for their difficulty in swallowing. Consequently, a high index of suspicion and appropriate diagnostic studies are essential in order to make an early diagnosis. The two clinical studies most likely to establish a diagnosis are esophagography and esophagoscopy. They are generally performed in that order and, according to Parker,[30] the barium swallow has yielded positive information in 98 per cent of the cases. In some instances the changes may be rather subtle, consisting of interference with normal esophageal peristalsis or minimal irregularity of the esophageal lumen. A gross filling defect in the esophagus, particularly with ulceration or irregularity of the mucosa and narrowing of the lumen, may be present (Figs. 4–6). There may be interference with peristaltic action, proximal to the obvious lesion, due to submucosal infiltration of the esophageal wall. Although some degree of proximal dilatation in the esophagus may be present in the slower-growing carcinomas, this is rarely as prominent as the dilatation associated with a structure or achalasia (Fig. 7).

Esophagoscopy should be performed on all patients in whom the diagnosis of a carcinoma is suspected. With the rigid esophagoscope, a positive biopsy can be obtained in approximately 80 per cent of the patients. There may be edema and obstruction above the gross tumor, preventing the endoscopist from actually ex-

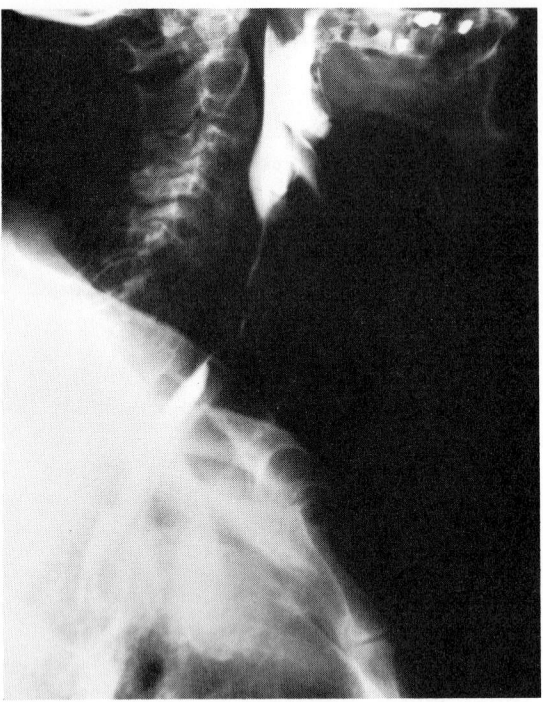

Figure 4. Barium swallow showing marked narrowing of lumen of cervical esophagus due to carcinoma.

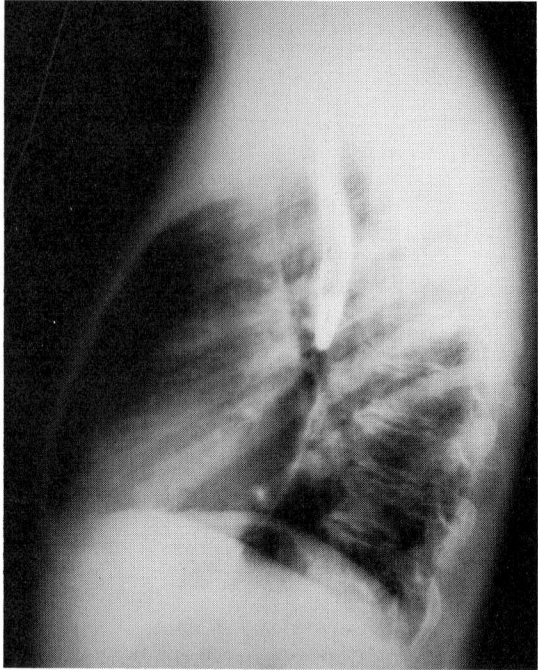

Figure 6. Nearly complete obstruction of distal esophagus demonstrated by esophagogram. Diagnosis of carcinoma was made by endoscopic biopsy. Note absence of proximal dilatation.

posing the intraluminal portion of the carcinoma for a biopsy. With the fiberoptic esophagoscope, the reliability of this examination is much greater. Bruni et al. report a positive histological diagnosis in 96.8 per cent of 73 patients examined with a fiberoptic esophagoscope and using direct biopsy and brush cytology.[7] The fiberoptic scope and a technique of air insufflation of the esophagus to smooth out mucosal folds may also be helpful in establishing a diagnosis in a very early esophageal carcinoma that is not detectable on barium swallow (Fig. 8).[40] Although there may be slight

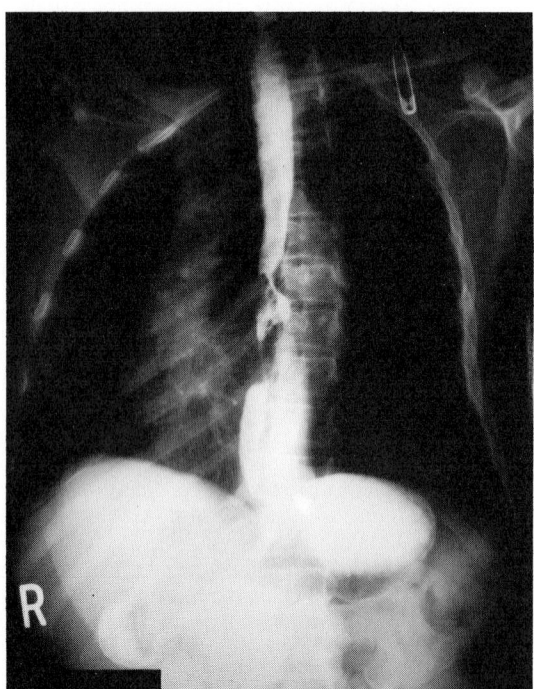

Figure 5. Irregular filling defect of middle third of esophagus due to carcinoma.

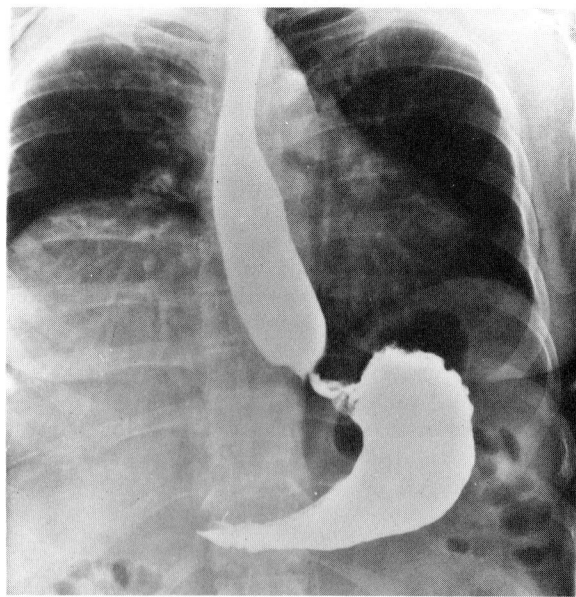

Figure 7. Slowly growing esophageal carcinoma with dilated proximal esophagus. This patient complained of progressive dysphagia for over a year.

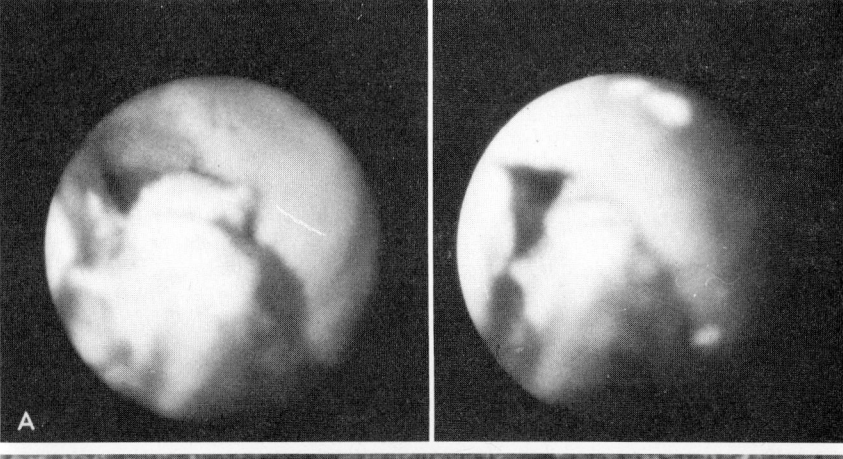

Figure 8. *A*, View of fungating esophageal carcinoma through fiberoptic esophagoscope. *B*, Photograph of gross specimen of same patient demonstrating extensive fungating epidermoid carcinoma of the esophagus.

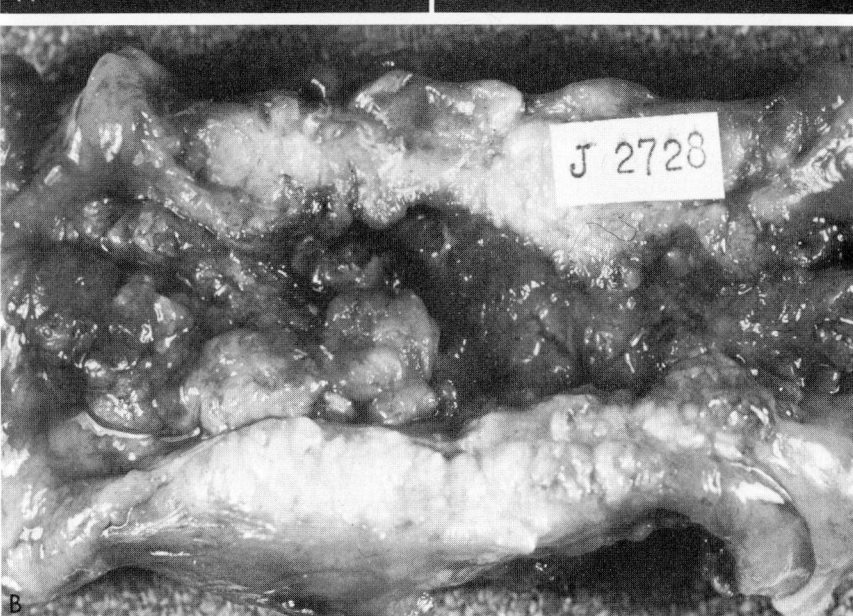

danger of perforation of the esophagus by esophagoscopy and biopsy, the risk is much less when dealing with a carcinoma than it is in a patient with esophagitis alone. In addition to esophagoscopy, bronchoscopy should be performed on those patients who have neoplasms of the middle or upper third of the esophagus, since there may be extension into the trachea or main stem bronchus without obvious clinical signs or symptoms. The vocal cords should be visualized to ascertain whether or not there is paralysis due to involvement of the recurrent laryngeal nerve.

More sophisticated tests for detection of very early esophageal carcinomas have been described. These include the use of a fluorescing hematoporphyrin derivative that is picked up by malignant cells. The material may be given intravenously and can be detected by esophagoscopy.[22] Another study utilizes radioactive phosphorous, which is also taken up by malignant tissues and can be detected by a small Geiger counter passed down the esophagus.[25] Neither of these studies has achieved widespread clinical application.

In the evaluation of a patient with a known carcinoma of the esophagus, other studies should be performed in an attempt to ascertain the degree of spread and the presence or absence of distant metastases. Venous azygography has been used to determine the presence or absence of mediastinal invasion by an esophageal carcinoma as a method of ascertaining operability.[36] The most common sites of metastatic involvement are the regional nodes of the supraclavicular and celiac groups, the liver, and the lungs.

Treatment

Although a carcinoma of the cervical esophagus had been removed by Czerny in 1877,[13] the first successful resection of an intrathoracic esophageal carcinoma was performed by Franz Torek in New York City in 1913.[42] Torek performed a preliminary gastrostomy on a woman with a carcinoma of the middle third of the esophagus. After the patient's nutritional status had improved, a transthoracic resection of the distal two thirds of the intrathoracic esophagus was done. The cardia of the stomach was closed and the proximal end of the esophagus was brought out as an esophagostomy at the skin level just below the left clavicle. The patient survived the procedure and subsequently used a rubber tube to connect the proximal esophagostomy stoma to the gastrostomy. In this way she was able to swallow food, which then passed through the rubber tube into the stomach and thus maintained adequate nutrition. The patient is reported to have survived for more than 11 years.

Although nearly six decades have passed since this historic procedure and many technical advances have been made in thoracic surgery, the results of treatment of carcinoma of the esophagus remain disappointing. A high percentage of the patients have an inoperable lesion when first seen. Many suffer from malnutrition and are poor surgical risks. Consequently a discussion of the treatment of epidermoid carcinoma of the esophagus must be divided into those efforts used to cure the disease and those used to palliate and make the patient more comfortable. At present, there are no chemotherapeutic agents that appear to have any significant beneficial effect on esophageal carcinoma. The two major forms of therapy for carcinoma of the esophagus are irradiation and surgical resection. These may be used alone or combined. In either case, restoration of the ability to swallow is essential, since the constant drooling of saliva and malnutrition associated with total esophageal obstruction combine to make a miserable terminal illness.

Radiation Therapy. The development of supervoltage radiation has allowed the radiotherapist to treat carcinoma of the esophagus with greater efficiency and less skin reaction. In some institutions irradiation is considered the treatment of choice for carcinoma of the upper one third of the intrathoracic esophagus. Contraindications to radiation therapy include mediastinitis, large tracheoesophageal fistulas, and extensive metastatic disease. It is important to maintain the nutrition of the patient with an obstructing esophageal cancer during the course of radiotherapy. To achieve this, it may be necessary to pass a nasogastric tube for feeding, to perform a gastrostomy, or to use intravenous hyperalimentation.

Radiation therapy may be performed with one of three objectives: to cure the malignancy, for palliation alone, or as an adjunct to surgical resection. When the objective is curative irradiation, a total dose of 6000 to 6500 rads is delivered over a period of 6 to 7 weeks. In order to avoid an excessive dose to the spinal cord, the last 2000 rads are given during rotation or through oblique fields. In view of the propensity of esophageal carcinoma to extend along the submucosal lymphatics well beyond the periphery of the lesion, irradiation is delivered to a field that includes the esophagus well above and below visible tumor. In those patients with partial obstruction of the esophageal lumen, a daily dose of 180 to 200 rads may cause edema resulting in complete obstruction of the esophagus. If this occurs, intravenous hyperalimentation is utilized until the edema has subsided.

In patients presenting with advanced disease in whom the objective is palliation and relief of dysphagia,

the total radiation dose is usually limited to 4000 to 4500 rads delivered over a period of $3\frac{1}{2}$ to 4 weeks. With this form of therapy, one may expect approximately 50 per cent of the patients to improve sufficiently to be able to maintain their nutrition by oral feedings.

There is considerable difference of opinion regarding the use of preoperative irradiation in the treatment of the patient with esophageal carcinoma. Recommendations regarding the amount of radiation given preoperatively range from 2500 to 4000 rads, with an interval of 2 to 4 weeks between completion of radiation and surgical resection of the lesion. The opinion of many surgeons who favor this form of combined therapy is that the radiation reduces the bulk of the neoplasm and creates some edema in the mediastinum, rendering dissection somewhat easier.

The complications of radiation therapy include esophagitis, perforation, hemorrhage, esophageal stenosis, and radiation pneumonitis. In addition, excessive doses can cause spinal cord injury. The frequency of these complications can be greatly reduced by limiting the size of the treatment fields, reducing the size of the fields as the treatment progresses, and avoiding excessively high doses of radiation.

Palliative Procedures.   Since in many patients esophageal carcinoma is not amenable to definitive resection, a number of procedures have been devised to maintain nutrition and to make the patient more comfortable. These may be combined with irradiation in an effort to slow down the progression of the neoplasm. The use of a feeding gastrostomy may be helpful in restoring the nutrition of a patient in an inoperable situation or as a preparatory step before a major surgical operation to resect the carcinoma. It has been found that the performance of a gastrostomy does not in itself prolong the life of the patient suffering from this malignancy. If it is possible to pass a nasogastric tube through a partially obstructed esophagus, this may be utilized for maintenance of nutrition instead of a gastrostomy. Diversion of the saliva by means of a cervical esophagostomy has not been particularly helpful in our hands, since it results in a constantly draining neck wound and this does not add to the patient's comfort. A number of procedures have been devised for diverting a bolus of food around an inoperable carcinoma. These include creation of a subcutaneous tube, superficial to the rib cage, connecting the cervical esophagus to the stomach, and creation of a bypass utilizing the somach, small intestine, or colon either in the mediastinum or in a subcutaneous or substernal tunnel to restore continuity of the alimentary tract and bypass the obstructing tumor.

INTUBATION.   Another approach to the palliation of an inoperable carcinoma of the esophagus is the use of a rigid tube that is pushed or pulled through the obstructing neoplasm, thus allowing the patient to swallow. A number of such tubes have been described, the most popular being those of Souttar,[37] Mousseau-Barbin,[23] Celestin,[11] and Fell.[16] These may be divided into two types, those that are pushed through the tumor from above, with the help of the esophagoscope, and those that are pulled from below after performance of a gastrostomy and the passage of a string or guide through the tumor into the stomach. The pulsion or push-through tubes are more applicable for a carcinoma of the middle third of the esophagus where there is a patent esophageal lumen distal to the tumor. The traction or pull-through tubes are more appropriately used for carcinomas of the distal third of the esophagus. Most of these latter tubes have a tongue or extension allowing the surgeon to anchor the tube in place on the anterior wall of the stomach.

It is obvious that there is some danger associated with the introduction of these tubes. In an extensive review of the literature. Girardet and associates found a hospital mortality, up to one month, of 13.9 per cent associated with use of various tubes.[18] Since the esophageal lesion must be dilated in order for the tube to be introduced, and secondly, since the tube must be jammed through the tumor mass into the distal esophagus or stomach below the obstruction, the complications of esophageal perforation with mediastinitis, bleeding, or aspiration pneumonia are significant hazards of this procedure.

Nevertheless, the technique of esophageal intubation does offer palliation, particularly in those patients who have advanced disease and perhaps only a short time to live. It certainly improves the quality of life. Esophageal intubation is of greatest value in the patient with a bronchoesophageal or tracheoesophageal fistula as a result of the tumor. In those instances if the tube can be placed in the proper position, the fistula is blocked off and continuing leakage of esophageal contents into the tracheobronchial tree can be avoided.

Surgical Treatment. The surgical treatment of carcinoma of the esophagus may be divided into procedures that are presumptively curative and those that are purely palliative. The palliative measures are performed in an effort to restore the swallowing mechanism and to allow the patient to exist in greater comfort. Surgical palliation may be combined with irradiation in an effort to slow down the progression of the neoplasm. It is apparent, however, that extensive surgical procedures in the face of an incurable esophageal carcinoma can rarely be justified. Therefore, the simplest procedure or combination of therapeutic modalities that may enable the patient to swallow and restore his comfort are the most appropriate.

Since the majority of patients presenting with an esophageal carcinoma are elderly and frequently nutritionally depleted, the operative morbidity and mortality in the past has been high. The use of a feeding gastrostomy to restore nutrition in those patients unable to swallow has been helpful. In the past five years, intravenous hyperalimentation has been found to be an extremely useful adjunct, replacing the gastrostomy in those patients for whom operative intervention is contemplated. With this technique, 2500 to 4000 calories per day may be delivered with substantial weight gain and increase in tissue turgor. This may be used in conjunction with preoperative irradiation if desired. We believe that this has substantially improved the patient's general condition and significantly reduced the operative mortality and morbidity, particularly reducing anastomotic leaks associated with malnutrition and hypoproteinemia.

Since the first successful resection of a carcinoma of the intrathoracic esophagus in 1913, a number of refinements and modifications have been made in the techniques of esophagectomy and restoration of the continuity of the upper alimentary tract. The basic principle of the operative procedure is excision of the neoplasm, including wide resection of adjacent areas of the esophagus and the regional lymph nodes. One of the limitations of this procedure is the proximity to the tumor mass of vital structures such as the aorta, heart, and trachea. Consequently, there are limitations in the extent of the resection. Some surgeons advocate total esophagectomy regardless of the level of the tumor in the thorax.[30] There has been a certain pessimism regarding carcinomas of the upper third of the intrathoracic esophagus, and at present there are many surgeons who believe that radiation therapy of the tumor at this level is preferable to resection, since the results of operation in terms of prolongation of life are so unsatisfactory and radiation alone offers a reasonable chance of relief of the obstruction and restoration of the swallowing mechanism.

CARCINOMA OF THE LOWER THIRD OF THE ESOPHAGUS. Primary carcinoma of the lower third of the esophagus probably lends itself more favorably to surgical resection than neoplasms at any other level. This tumor tends to spread down to the lymph nodes around the cardia of the stomach and the left gastric artery, although involvement of this group of nodes does not totally preclude successful resection of the tumor. When extensive intra-abdominal metastases are suspected, a preliminary laparotomy may be performed in order to ascertain the degree of involvement and to make a decision whether to proceed with an attempt at curative resection, to resort to palliative measures, or to rely on radiation alone.

Our own preference for resection of carcinomas of the lower third of the esophagus is an approach by a left thoracotomy. This is generally accomplished by subperiosteal resection of the seventh rib or an incision in the seventh intercostal space. The esophagus, including the tumor mass, is then mobilized, and a radial incision is made in the diaphragm from the esophageal hiatus out to the chest wall. Through the incision in the diaphragm, the stomach may be mobilized as much as necessary with division of the vasa brevia and the left gastric artery. The right gastric artery and the gastroepiploic vessels are preserved. The lymph nodes along the lesser curvature of the stomach and the cardia are mobilized and the stomach is divided at the proximal end at least 5 cm. below the cardia. This portion of the stomach is then closed and the esophagogastric junction, the adjacent lymph nodes, and the distal one half of the esophagus are mobilized and transected proximally. The point of transection should be at least 10 cm. above all visible and palpable tumor; a frozen section is usually taken at the proximal end of the esophagus which is resected, in order to be sure that there is no evidence of microscopic involvement by submucosal extension of the tumor. The mobilized stomach is then brought up into the left thorax and a pyloroplasty is performed, since resection of the esophagus includes the vagus nerves and an atonic or poorly emptying gastric pouch should be avoided. A small circular opening is made in the fundus of the stomach and this is anastomosed in one or two layers to the proximal end of the esophagus (Figs. 9 and 10). In recent years we have brought an additional 3 cm. of the fundus up and sutured it above the anastomosis in an effort to create a valvelike action and minimize reflux. At the time of the esophagogastric anastomosis, a nasogastric tube is placed in the stomach and allowed to remain for several days until active peristalsis returns. The diaphragm is closed and the chest is closed with adequate water-seal drainage. The patient is usually allowed water and clear liquids in small amounts once peristalsis has resumed. The greatest immediate danger in the postoperative period is anastomotic leak, which is most likely to occur on the sixth to eight day postoperatively. The initial manifestation is the appearance of a pneumothorax or hydropneumothorax, which requires immediate drainage. Immediate and continued full re-expansion of the lung after resection, and suturing the additional portion of the fundus of the stomach around and above the esophagogastric anastomosis, have been very helpful in the avoidance of postoperative leakage.

CARCINOMA OF THE MIDDLE THIRD OF THE ESOPHAGUS. There is more difference of opinion regarding the approach and technique for resection of carcinoma of the middle third of the esophagus than for neoplasms arising in the distal portion of the esophagus. Either a left or a right thoracotomy may be utilized, and continuity may be restored by the use of the stomach brought up into the thorax or into the neck. Some surgeons advocate the use of a gastric tube formed from the greater curvature of the stomach and the gastroepiploic vessels. Alternatives to these methods are the use of a segment of colon brought up through the mediastinum and the use of a substernal colon transplant as a separate staged operative procedure before or after resection of the neoplasm. At the present time, some authorities advocate the use of preoperative radiation in doses ranging from 2000 R to 5000 R, with an interval of 2 weeks to several months between the radiation therapy and the time of operation.

The advantage of the left thoracotomy or left thoracoabdominal approach is that a single incision is used for the whole operation. One of the major disadvan-

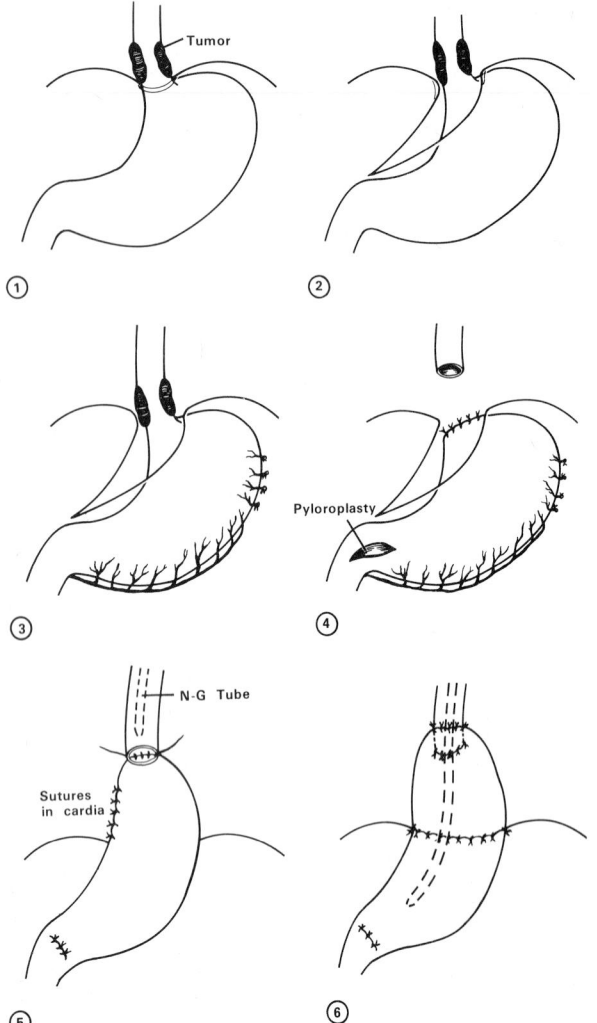

Figure 9. Resection of carcinoma of distal third of the esophagus. The entire procedure may be performed through a left posterolateral thoracotomy. *1*, Tumor and distal esophagus for a distance of 10 cm. above the tumor is mobilized. *2*, Diaphragm is opened radially from esophageal hiatus out to chest wall. *3*, Vasa brevia and left gastric artery are divided through incision in diaphragm. *4*, Distal esophagus including tumor and cardia of stomach are removed. Cardia is closed and a pyloroplasty is performed. *5*, Fundus of stomach is brought up into chest and a single-layer anastomosis is performed. *6*, Additional 3 cm. of fundus is brought up above anastomosis and sutured circumferentially around the esophagus.

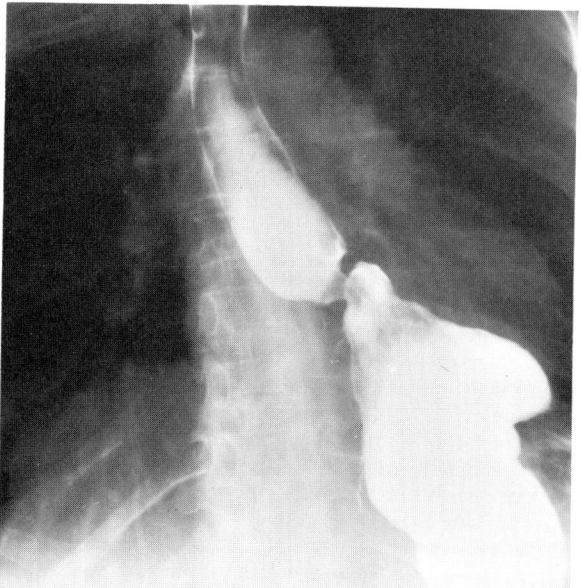

Figure 10. Barium study in a patient after resection of carcinoma of the esophagus and esophagogastrostomy.

tages is that mobilization of the upper portion of the esophagus is more difficult, since it must be taken from under the arch of the aorta.

A right thoracotomy affords easier access to the entire intrathoracic esophagus, since the surgeon does not have to contend with the aortic arch from the right side. The advantage of the right-sided approach is that a separate laparotomy is necessary, since the stomach or colon cannot be mobilized through the right thorax. In using the right-sided approach, most surgeons employ a separate laparotomy for mobilization of the stomach or colon. Belsey and Hiebert described a technique using a right thoracotomy with mobilization of the stomach through the esophageal hiatus, obviating the necessity for an abdominal incision.[5] Our own preference is a right thoracotomy and a separate laparotomy incision (Fig. 11). This can be done by two teams working simultaneously. The entire intrathoracic esophagus is mobilized, as is the stomach; the right gastric and gastroepiploic vessels are preserved. The stomach is transected below the cardia and after removal of the entire esophagus the stomach is delivered

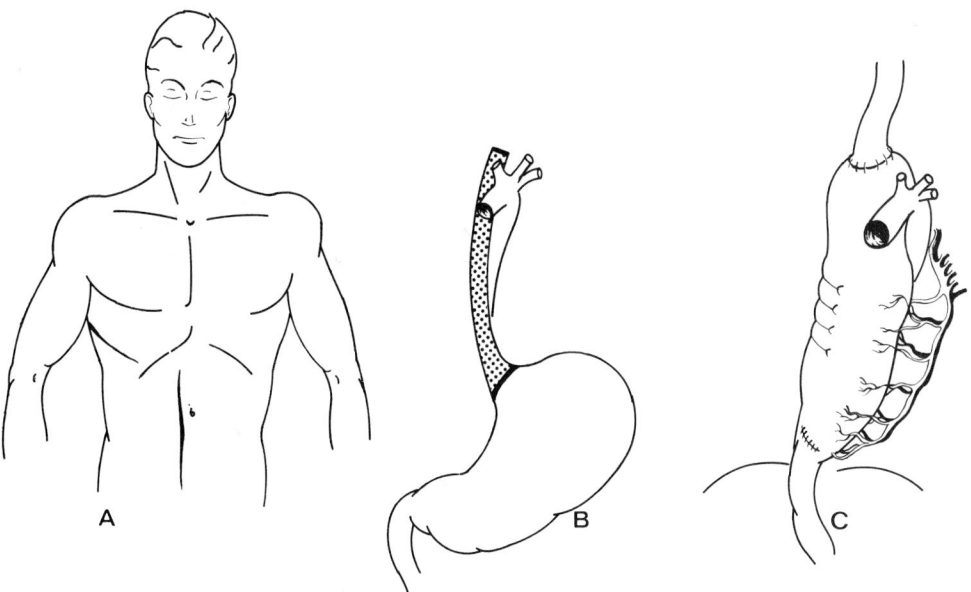

Figure 11. Resection of intrathoracic esophagus with esophagogastrostomy. *A*, Procedure performed through a right thoracotomy and a separate laparotomy incision. *B*, Esophagus and adjacent lymph nodes are resected. *C*, Continuity restored by bringing the stomach up above the aortic arch in the thorax or into the neck. The right gastric and gastroepiploic vessels are preserved. (After Camishion, R. C. *In* Nealon, T. F. (Ed.): Management of the Patient with Cancer. 2nd ed. Philadelphia, W. B. Saunders Company, 1976.)

through the esophageal hiatus into the right mediastinum. The position of the proximal anastomosis between the esophagus and the fundus of the stomach
varies slightly with the level of the lesion. It has been
our own experience that for lesions at the level of the
aortic arch the anastomosis must be made in the apex
of the thorax or in the neck. The latter is preferable,
both from the standpoint of technical facility and
because of the reduced morbidity in the event of an
anastomotic leak or breakdown. There has been no difficulty in maintaining an adequate blood supply to the
stomach even when it is brought up through the
mediastinum into the right side of the neck.

Many surgeons prefer the use of a segment of colon,
usually the splenic flexure and a portion of the descending colon, as an esophageal substitute. This segment of colon is probably preferable to the right colon
because of the more constant blood supply and the
ability to obtain a greater length of the vascular
pedicle. Once the colon and its vascular pedicle have
been mobilized, the bowel is passed posterior to the
stomach through the lesser sac, up through the hiatus,
and into the mediastinum (Fig. 12). An antiperistaltic
anastomosis is made between the proximal segment of
the esophagus in the upper thorax or neck and the
colon. The distal segment of colon is then anastomosed
to the anterior wall of the body of the stomach. A

pyloroplasty is generally performed at this time and a
gastrostomy may be done if desired. In some instances,
when the viability of the upper end of the colon may be
questionable, both the colon and the proximal end of
the esophagus are exteriorized in the neck and left for
an interval of 5 to 7 days until viability of the colon
segment is established unquestionably. If such is the
case, the anastomosis is then done as a separate stage.

An alternative to this technique is a two-stage
procedure in which a segment of colon is mobilized
and passed through a substernal tunnel with anastomosis to the cervical esophagus and to the fundus
of the stomach.[9] At a second stage a total esophagectomy may be performed, with or without intervening
radiation therapy (Fig. 13).[13] The use of a substernal
colon transplant followed by radiation has also been
employed in patients with unresectable lesions of the
intrathoracic esophagus. In general, however, results
of this procedure have not been satisfactory, since few
patients survive for a sufficient period of time to justify this extensive operation.

CARCINOMA OF THE UPPER THIRD OF THE INTRATHO-
RACIC ESOPHAGUS. Carcinomas occurring in the
upper portion of the esophagus are fortunately less
common than those in the middle or lower segments.
There is frequently direct extension to the surrounding structures, including the trachea, superior vena

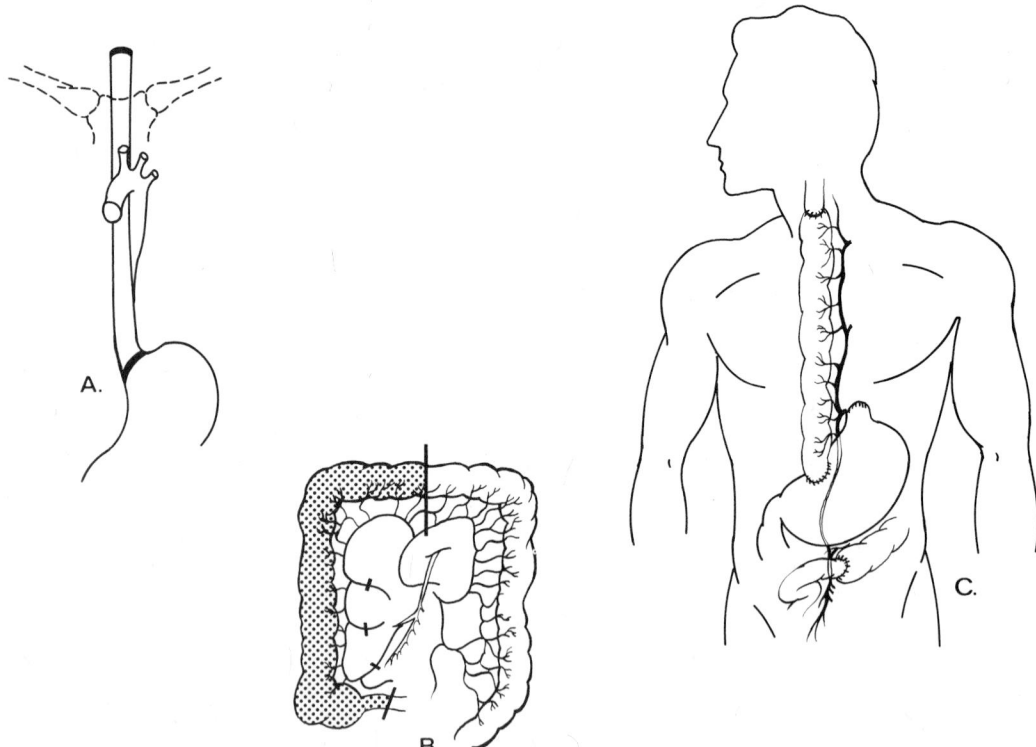

Figure 12.   Use of colon as an esophageal replacement. *A,* Entire esophagus may be resected. *B,* Either right or left colon may be used, with
preservation of its vascular pedicle (see text). *C,* Colon is passed behind stomach and up into neck via the mediastinum or through a substernal
tunnel. Proximal anastomosis is to cervical esophagus or pharynx. Distal anastomosis to anterior wall of stomach. An ileocolostomy or
colocolostomy, pyloroplasty, and gastrostomy are also accomplished. (After Camishion, R. C. *In* Nealon, T. F. (Ed.): Management of the Patient
with Cancer. 2nd ed. Philadelphia, W. B. Saunders Company, 1976.)

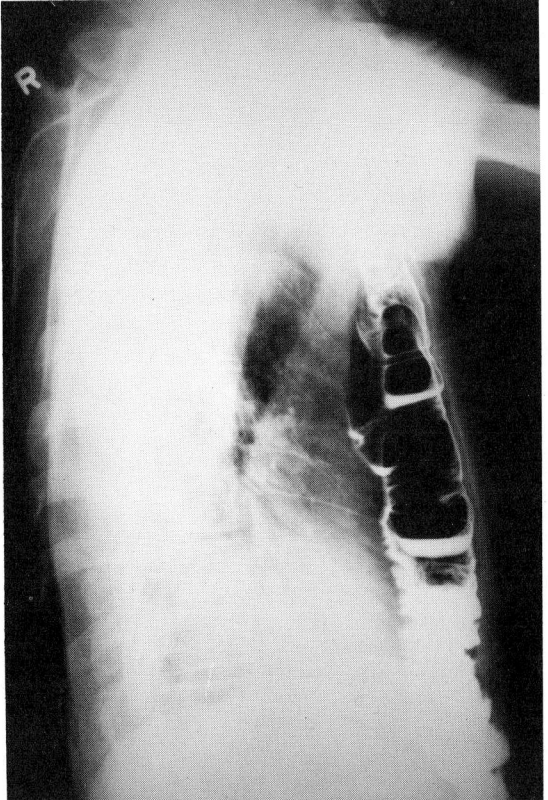

Figure 13. Lateral view of barium swallow after substernal colon transplant for carcinoma of middle third of esophagus. Patient was then irradiated and a total esophagectomy was performed at second operation.

cava, and aorta, rendering curative resection unfeasible. Many believe that the number of cures is so few that operation is hardly justified and radiation alone is the treatment of choice. If the lesion is apparently operable, the technique described for carcinoma of the middle third, including total esophagectomy and anastomosis high in the neck with either stomach or colon, may be utilized.

CERVICAL ESOPHAGUS. Carcinomas occurring in the cervical esophagus present a somewhat different problem in terms of reconstruction than do carcinomas occurring within the intrathoracic esophagus. Carcinoma of the cervical esophagus tends to spread by lymph node metastases and by direct extension into adjacent structures, and a high percentage of these cases may be inoperable when first seen. Wide excision of the carcinoma including laryngectomy, thyroidectomy, and unilateral or bilateral cervical node dissection may be carried out. Restoration of continuity may be accomplished by bringing up into the neck a segment of colon or stomach.[20] An alternative is a staged procedure of creating pedicle skin flaps originally described by Wookey.[44] In this procedure a tubular graft of the skin and platysma is constructed and then anastomosed to the cricopharyngeus or pharynx and to the distal esophagus as it enters the mediastinum. An alternative procedure to restore continuity after resection of the cervical esophagus, described by Bakamjian, utilizes a pectoral flap carried upward and folded over to form a tube.[4] A free graft of a segment of jejunum or ileum, including its vascular

supply, may be brought up to the neck and arterial and venous anastomoses performed between the superior thyroid artery and the facial and internal jugular vein.[26] This latter procedure is technically feasible but has not met with great success.

Recently, Burdette and Jesse[8] have reported experience with carcinoma of the esophagus utilizing radical excision of the primary tumor, reconstruction with an interposed segment of ileocolon followed by subsequent radiation. These authors report a 25 per cent two-year survival. Although systemic chemotherapy for this neoplasm has not been encouraging, Nelson[28] reports a good response with the local injection of cyclophosphamide into the carcinoma in addition to systemic chemotherapy.

OTHER MALIGNANT TUMORS OF THE ESOPHAGUS

Although epidermoid carcinoma is by far the most common primary malignant tumor of the esophagus, occasionally adenocarcinoma may be encountered. Although an adenocarcinoma occurring in the distal one third of the esophagus is generally the result of an upward infiltration from a tumor originating in the stomach, primary adenocarcinomas may arise in the mucous glands of the esophagus or columnar epithelium,[2] possibly as a result of chronic irritation. Naef et al. recently reported a 10 per cent incidence of adenocarcinoma in patients with extensive columnar metaplasia (Barrett's esophagus) and found that surgical

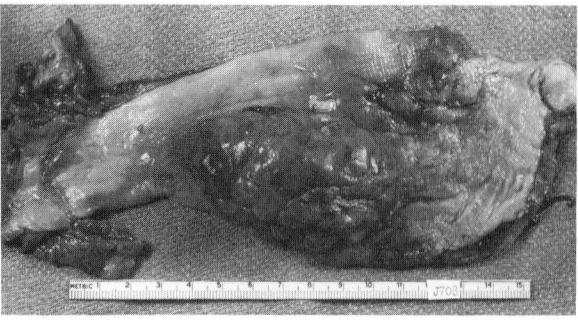

Figure 14. Gross specimen of pseudosarcoma of the esophagus after resection. Note large polypoid tumor and area of infiltrating carcinoma at base.

correction of the reflux did not appear to prevent the development of this malignancy.[24] Adenocarcinoma of the esophagus generally presents in a manner similar to epidermoid carcinoma and is differentiated by biopsy. The management of an adenocarcinoma is similar to that of epidermoid carcinoma in terms of surgical resection.

Leiomyosarcoma is an infrequent malignant neoplasm of the esophagus and rhabdomyosarcoma is even less common. These tumors tend to occur in a younger age group than epidermoid carcinoma and tend to infiltrate adjacent structures. They may be slow-growing and are radioresistant. Wide surgical resection of the involved segment of the esophagus may yield a long-term cure, although late recurrence is not uncommon. Another rare malignant neoplasm of the esophagus is carcinosarcoma, which represents a combination of malignant cells arising from the mucosa and the muscular layer of the esophagus. These tumors grow quite slowly and may reach large proportions.[41] Metastases appear late in the course of the disease. Consequently, surgical resection may be accomplished in a large proportion of these tumors, and a relatively good prognosis may be anticipated. Adenoacanthomas of the distal esophagus, composed of epidermoid and glandular cells, have been reported. They present a clinical picture similar to that of other obstructing neoplasms of the esophageal lumen. A rare but interesting esophageal malignancy is pseudosarcoma. Initially reported by Stout and Lattes,[38] pseudosarcoma of the esophagus occurs within the lumen of the esophagus as a polypoid lesion that microscopically is sarcomatous and is accompanied by an intramucosal or occasionally invasive squamous carcinoma at the base of the polyp (Fig. 14). In most instances if metastases occur, the metastatic deposits are squamous carcinoma. Inasmuch as the squamous portion of the carcinoma may occur not only at the base, but also in the vicinity of the polypoid lesion, radical resection of the esophagus should be performed.[33]

RESULTS

The results of treatment of malignant tumors of the esophagus have been generally unsatisfactory. In most series reporting results of treatment of epidermoid carcinoma, the vast majority of patients were inoperable at the time of initial evaluation. Parker in a recent review found an operability rate of only 34 per cent.[31] These patients were treated with preoperative radiation and subsequently explored. Of those explored, 87 per cent were found to be resectable. Recent reports from Japan are more encouraging. Akakura and associates report a resectability rate of 88 per cent in patients who received preoperative radiation.[3] This undoubtedly represents very strict case selection in those patients who are considered for operation. Another factor that significantly reduces the possibility of long-term survival is the operative mortality. The majority of patients with carcinoma of the esophagus are in an older age group, and most have significant malnutrition as well as degenerative changes of the cardiovascular system. In general, they are poor operative risks and a hospital surgical mortality of 15 to 30 per cent has been reported by various authors. In our own experience, however, the use of preoperative hyperalimentation and modifications in surgical technique have reduced the operative mortality to below 10 per cent.

There is considerable variation in the reports of long-term survival after definitive treatment of carcinoma of the esophagus.[19, 31] Parker states that the average duration of life without treatment for this disease is found to be 7½ months from the onset of symptoms. Consequently, he classifies a survival of two years after completion of treatment as a long-term survival. Using preoperative radiation followed by resection, Parker reports a 27 per cent two-year survival rate, representing a 12 per cent long-term survival of the total number of cases seen. Akakura and associates from Tokyo[3] more recently reported a 25 per cent five-year survival rate following preoperative radiation with a dose of 5000 to 6000 rads followed in two to four weeks by radical resection. Nakayama[27] reports a five-year survival rate of 37.5 per cent utilizing a smaller dose of preoperative irradiation and compares this to a five-year survival rate of 19 per cent in patients treated by resection alone.

The improved survival figures reported from Japan have stimulated many surgeons in this country to follow this general approach, using varying amounts of radiation followed by radical esophageal resection.

Nevertheless, at this time there remains considerable room for improvement in methods of early detection of esophageal carcinoma, reduction in operative mortality, and an achievement of better long-term survivals as well as improvement in the quality of life.

SELECTED REFERENCES

Girardet, R. E., Ransdell, H. T., Jr., and Wheat, M. W., Jr.: Palliative intubation in the management of esophageal carcinoma. Ann. Thorac. Surg., *18*:417, 1974.
This is a collective review outlining the historical background and present use of esophageal intubation. Its comprehensive coverage of the subject should be required reading for anyone contemplating using this method of palliation.

Pack, G. T., and Ariel, I. M.: Treatment of Cancer and Allied Diseases, Volume 4. New York, Hoeber Medical Division, Harper & Row, 1960, Chapters 34–40.
The last seven chapters in this book cover all aspects of the treatment of benign and malignant esophageal neoplasms. A number of different viewpoints are presented, including variations in operative technique as well as palliation and esophageal reconstruction. The last three chapters cover various aspects of the radiation treatment of esophageal cancer using different techniques. These chapters provide an excellent review of the surgical and radiation management of carcinoma of the esophagus.

Parker, E. F., and Gregorie, H. B., Jr.: Carcinoma of the esophagus. Curr. Probl. Surg., April, 1967.
This comprehensive monograph covers all phases of the diagnosis and treatment of esophageal carcinomas. It is based upon the authors' extensive experience in South Carolina and details the evolution of the different methods of treatment leading to their present program of irradiation followed by radical resection. There are excellent illustrations and an extensive bibliography.

Postlethwait, R. W., and Sealy, W. C.: Surgery of the Esophagus. Springfield, Ill., Charles C Thomas, Publisher, 1961.
This scholarly book is recommended, since it covers a large number of cases of esophageal carcinoma from a number of different institutions. The authors' own points of view, as well as differing opinions, are presented in a well-organized fashion, with clarity and logic.

Stout, A. P., and Lattes, R.: Tumors of the Esophagus. Washington, D.C., Armed Forces Institute of Pathology, Fascicle 20, 1957.
This fascicle is the most complete review available of the gross and microscopic pathology of esophageal neoplasms. Although some clinical correlation is presented, this monograph is primarily recommended for its superb review of the wide variations in these tumors encountered by the surgical pathologist.

Watson, R. R., O'Connor, T. M., and Weisel, W.: Solid benign esophageal tumors. Ann. Thorac. Surg., *4*:91, 1967.
This is a collective review with an extensive treatment of the various benign esophageal tumors. Although there are no illustrations, the detailed discussion of these tumors makes this worthwhile reading and an excellent basic reference for this subject.

REFERENCES

1. Adams, W. E., and Phemister, D. B.: Carcinoma of the lower thoracic esophagus: Report of successful resection and esophagogastrostomy. J. Thorac. Surg., 7:621, 1938.
2. Adler, R. H.: The lower esophagus lined by columnar epithelium. Its association with hiatal hernia, ulcer, stricture and tumor. J. Thorac. Cardiovasc. Surg., 45:13, 1963.
3. Akakura, I., Nakamura, Y., Kakegaga, T., Nakayama, R., Watanabe, H., and Yamashita, H.: Surgery of carcinoma of the esophagus with preoperative radiation. Chest, 57:47, 1970.
4. Bakamjian, V. Y.: A two-stage method for pharyngoesophageal reconstruction with a primary pectoral skin flap. Plast. Reconstr. Surg., 36:173, 1965.
5. Belsey, R., and Hiebert, C. A.: An exclusive right thoracic approach for cancer of the middle third of the esophagus. Ann. Thorac. Surg., 18:1, 1974.
6. Brady, P. G., and Mulligan, F. D.: Lymphangioma of the esoph-

agus–diagnosis by endoscopic biopsy. Am. J. Dig. Dis., 18: 423, 1973.
7. Bruni, H. C., and Nelson, R. S.: Carcinoma of esophagus and cardia. J. Thorac. Cardiovasc. Surg., 70:367, 1975.
8. Burdette, W. J., and Jesse, R.: Carcinoma of the cervical esophagus. J. Thorac. Cardiovasc. Surg., 63:41, 1972.
9. Camishion, R. C.: The esophagus. In Nealon, T. (Ed.): Management of the Patient with Cancer. 2nd ed. Philadelphia, W. B. Saunders Company, 1976.
10. Carter, R., and Brewer, L. A.: Achalasia and esophageal carcinoma. Studies in early diagnosis for improved surgical management. Am. J. Surg., 130:114, 1975.
11. Celestin, L. R.: Permanent intubation in inoperable cancer of the oesophagus and cardia: A new tube. Ann. R. Coll. Surg. Engl., 25:165, 1959.
12. Churchill, E. D.: Case records of The Massachusetts General Hospital, No. 23491. N. Engl. J. Med., 217:955, 1937.
13. Czerny: Neue Operationen: Vorlaufige Mittheilung. [A new operation: Preliminary communication.] Zentralbl. Chir., 41:433, 1877.
14. Davies, J. N. P., Elmes, S., Hutt, M. S. R., Mtimavalye, L., Owor, R., and Shaper, L.: Cancer in an African community, 1897–1956. Br. Med. J., 1:336, 1964.
15. De Gouveia, O., Pereira, A. A., Nolte, M. G., Wilhena, A. M., Duta, G., and Bryk, D.: Granular cell myoblastoma of the esophagus. Gastroenterology, 38:805, 1960.
16. Fell, S. C., Yrunwald, R. P., and Hurwitt, E. S.: Palliation of esophageal carcinoma by prosthetic intubation. J. Thorac. Cardiovasc. Surg., 51:272, 1966.
17. Fernandes, J. P., Mascarenhas, M. J., Costa, C. D., and Correia, J. P.: Diffuse leiomyomatosis of the esophagus. A case report and review of the literature. Am. J. Dig. Dis., 20:684, 1975.
18. Girardet, R. E., Ransdell, H. T., Jr., and Wheat, M. W., Jr.: Palliative intubation in the management of esophageal carcinoma. Ann. Thorac. Surg., 18:417, 1974.
19. Gunnlaugsson, G. H., Wychulis, A. R., Roland, C., and Ellis, F. H., Jr.: Analysis of the records of 1,657 patients with carcinoma of the esophagus and cardia of the stomach. Surg. Gynecol. Obstet., 130:997, 1970.
20. Heimlich, H. J.: Carcinoma of the cervical esophagus. J. Thorac. Cardiovasc. Surg., 59:309, 1970.
21. Jackson, C.: Tracheo-Bronchoscopy, Esophagoscopy and Gastroscopy. St. Louis, The Laryngoscope Company, 1904, p. 97.
22. Lipson, R. L., Blades, E. J., and Olsen, A. M.: Hematoporphyrin derivative: A new aid for endoscopic detection of malignant disease. J. Thorac. Cardiovasc. Surg., 42:623, 1961.
23. Mousseau, M., Le Forestier, J., Barbin, J., and Hardy, M.: The indications for permanent intubation in the palliative treatment of carcinoma of the esophagus. Arch. Mal. Appar. Digest, 45:308, 1956.
24. Naef, A. P., Savary, M., and Ozzello, L.: Columnar-lined lower esophagus: An acquired lesion with malignant predisposition. J. Thorac. Cardiovasc. Surg., 70:826, 1975.
25. Nakayama, K.: Diagnostic significance of radioactive isotopes in early cancer of the alimentary tract, especially the esophagus and the cardia. Surgery, 39:736, 1956.
26. Nakayama, K., Yamamoto, K., Tamiya, T., Makino, H., Odaka, M., Ohwada, M., and Takahashi, H.: Experience with free autografts of the bowel with a new venous anastomosis apparatus. Surgery, 55:796, 1964.
27. Nakayama, K., and Kinoshita, Y.: Surgical treatment combined with preoperative concentrated irradiation. J.A.M.A., 227:178, 1974.
28. Nelson, C. S.: In discussion of Burdette et al. J. Thorac. Cardiovasc. Surg., 63:41, 1972.
29. Pack, G. T., and Ariel, I. M.: Treatment of Cancer and Allied Diseases, Vol. 4. New York, Hoeber Medical Division, Harper & Row, 1960, Chapters 34–40.
30. Parker, E. F., and Gregorie, H. B., Jr.: Carcinoma of the esophagus. Curr. Probl. Surg., April, 1967.
31. Parker, E. F., Gregorie, H. B., Jr., Arrants, J. E., and Ravenel, J. M.: Carcinoma of the esophagus. Ann. Surg., 171:746, 1970.
32. Piacentini, L.: Leiomyoma. J. Thorac. Surg., 29:296, 1955.
33. Postlethwait, R. W., Wechsler, A. S., and Shelburne, J. D.: Pseudosarcoma of the esophagus. Ann. Thorac. Surg., 19:198, 1975.
34. Postlethwait, R. W., and Sealy, W. C.: Surgery of the Esophagus. Springfield, Ill., Charles C Thomas, Publisher, 1961.
35. Sauerbrach, F.: Presentations in the field of thoracic surgery. Arch. Klin. Chir., 173:457, 1932.
36. Segarra, M. S., and Cardus, J. C.: The value of azygography in

carcinoma of the esophagus. Surg. Gynecol. Obstet., *141*:248, 1975.

37. Souttar, H. S.: A method of intubating the oesophagus for malignant stricture. Br. Med. J., *1*:782, 1924.

38. Stout, A. P., and Lattes, R.: Tumors of the Esophagus. Washington, D.C., Armed Forces Institute of Pathology, Fascicle 20, 1957.

39. Sweet, R. H., Soutter, L., and Tejada, C.: Muscle wall tumors of the esophagus. J. Thorac. Surg., *27*:13, 1954.

40. Suzuki, H., Kobayashi, S., Endo, M., and Nakayama, K.: Diagnosis of early esophageal cancer. Surgery, *71*:99, 1972.

41. Talbert, J. L., and Cantrell, J. R.: Clinical and pathologic characteristics of carcinosarcoma of the esophagus. J. Thorac. Cardiovasc. Surg., *45*:1, 1963.

42. Torek, F.: The first successful resection of the thoracic portion of the oesophagus for carcinoma. Surg. Gynecol. Obstet., *16*:614, 1913.

43. Watson, R. R., O'Connor, T. M., and Weisel, W.: Solid benign esophageal tumors. Ann. Thorac. Surg., *4*:91, 1967.

44. Wookey, H.: The surgical treatment of carcinoma of the pharynx and upper esophagus. Surg. Gynecol. Obstet., *75*:499, 1942.

29

THE ABDOMINAL WALL, UMBILICUS, PERITONEUM, MESENTERIES, AND RETROPERITONEUM

Robert A. Macbeth, M.D.

A painstaking examination of the abdomen is one of the most rewarding diagnostic procedures available to the physician. Since even minor variations from normal may be of critical diagnostic importance, he must avail himself of every opportunity during his education to examine the abdomens of normal persons, of patients presenting with abdominal complaints, and of postoperative patients.

The physical findings elicited by examination of the abdomen, together with an appreciation of the physiologic mechanisms involved, are the key to the diagnosis of numerous pathologic conditions of the abdominal wall and, more particularly, of the peritoneal cavity. In an acute disease process, abdominal examination is particularly rewarding and yields far more information than laboratory investigations.

The pathology of disease is a continuing process and the clinical findings elicited on abdominal examination vary with the stage of the process present in the abdominal wall or peritoneal cavity. In consequence, repeated abdominal examination enables the physician to follow the course of the pathologic process and detect subtle changes that may have profound prognostic implications.

cal arteries and umbilical vein, and the allantois (*A*), which is a diverticulum of the yolk sac.

By the time the embryo reaches 1.7 mm. in length (Fig. 2), its cephalic and caudal extremities have curled ventrally, pinching off the most dorsal portion of the yolk sac, which now takes a form indicative of its future development into the gastrointestinal tract. The allantois (*A*) arises from that portion of the yolk sac which is taken into the embryo, so that one may now refer to this structure as arising from the primitive hindgut. It is important, for the understanding of future events, to note the depression evident at the neck of the yolk sac (*X*), which, as a result of further development, is to contribute the coelom.

In the 3.5 mm. embryo (Fig. 3) a stage has been reached at which one may describe an umbilical cord. Enlargement of the amniotic cavity has now compressed the elongated body stalk and the elongated yolk sac stalk into a compact structure, the anlage of the umbilical cord. The yolk sac stalk may now properly be referred to as the omphalomesenteric (vitelline) duct (*M*) as it lies free in the extraembryonic coelom, or exocoelom.

The structures in the cord in the 3.5 mm. embryo can be best appreciated by reference to Figure 4, which is a cross section of the cord of the embryo in Figure 3 at *Y*. The patent

THE ABDOMINAL WALL AND UMBILICUS

EMBRYOLOGY

The Umbilical Region

The essential features of the embryology of the umbilical region are illustrated in Figures 1 to 5. Cullen's excellent text should be consulted for more intimate detail.

A human embryo 0.7 mm. long is depicted in Figure 1. The embryo proper is capped dorsally by its amniotic cavity while it sits ventrally on its relatively large yolk sac. This entire structure is attached to the chorion and thence to the uterine wall by its broad body stalk. The body stalk is seen to contain the fetal vascular pedicle (*V*), made up of the paired umbili-

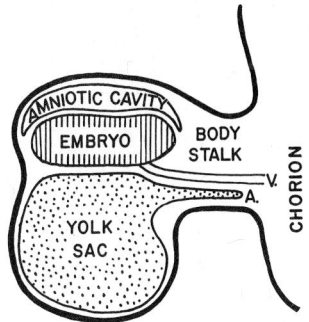

Figure 1. Diagrammatic representation of 0.7 mm. human embryo: *A*, allantois; *V*, vascular pedicle.

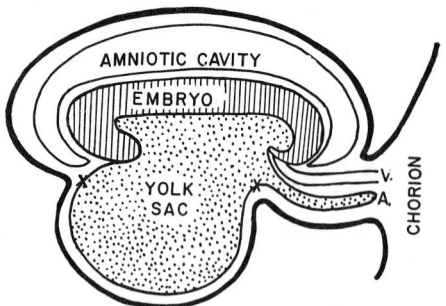

Figure 2. Diagrammatic representation of 1.7 mm. human embryo: *A*, allantois; *V*, vascular pedicle.

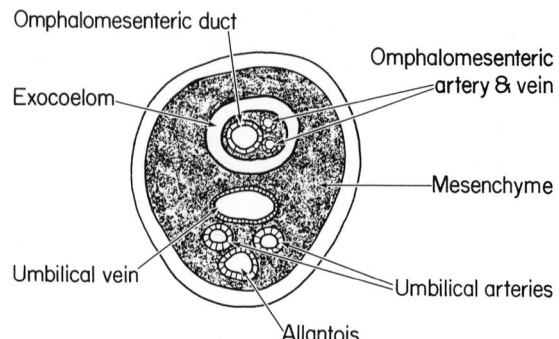

Figure 4. Diagrammatic cross section of umbilical cord of 3.5 mm. human embryo.

omphalomesenteric duct, with the accompanying artery and vein on its surface, lies in the exocoelom and occupies the superior portion of the cord. Inferior to it, embedded in mesenchyme, are, respectively, the umbilical vein, the paired umbilical arteries, and the allantois. The umbilical vein divides, just before entering the embryo, into right and left branches, which pass cephalad to unite with the hepatic circulation.

A diagrammatic sagittal view of a 5.2 cm., approximately 10-week, embryo is shown in Figure 5. The left umbilical vein is now shown superiorly in the cord as it courses toward the porta hepatis. The right umbilical vein disappears before the embryo is 10 mm. long. The left vein remains patent until shortly after birth, at which time physiologic occlusion occurs. It is subsequently designated the ligamentum teres of the liver. It is, however, capable of cannulation and dilatation even in adult life and, by the technique of umbilical vein catheterization, portal venography, portal pressure studies, and portal infusion may be carried out.[16] The paired umbilical arteries are seen inferiorly, just above and on either side of the allantois. On entering the abdomen, they pass inferiorly on the deep surface of the anterior abdominal wall on either side of the bladder to join their parent trunk, the aorta. After birth, the umbilical arteries become occluded as far proximal as that portion which becomes the internal iliac artery. The fibrous cords representing the remains of the impervious portion are referred to as the lateral umbilical ligaments in the adult.

Normally, the omphalomesenteric duct disappears when the embryo is between 4 and 12 mm. in length, though its vessels persist long after this. At 10 weeks the bowel has already entered the extraembryonic coelom, undergone its rotation, and recently re-entered the intraembryonic coelom (peritoneal cavity) and, normally, no vestige of the duct remains. It is depicted in Figure 5 as a patent tube arising from the terminal small bowel, extending to the umbilicus and passing toward the vestigial yolk sac in the extraembryonic coelom. This has been done so that its congenital malformation may be more easily understood.

The allantois, shown in Figure 5, has differentiated in its most caudal portion into the bladder. In the well differentiated embryo, its intra-abdominal portion, extending from the apex of the bladder to the umbilicus, is referred to as the urachus. Even in normal embryos, the obliteration of the allantois and the urachus is an irregular phenomenon, and sections at a wide variety of ages may still demonstrate patent segments.

The Abdominal Wall

Little has been added to our knowledge of the embryology of the abdominal wall since the original researches of Bar-

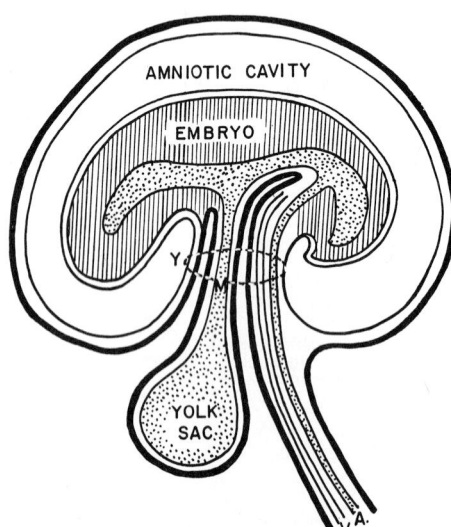

Figure 3. Diagrammatic representation of 3.5 mm. human embryo: *A*, allantois; *M*, omphalomesenteric duct; *V*, vascular pedicle.

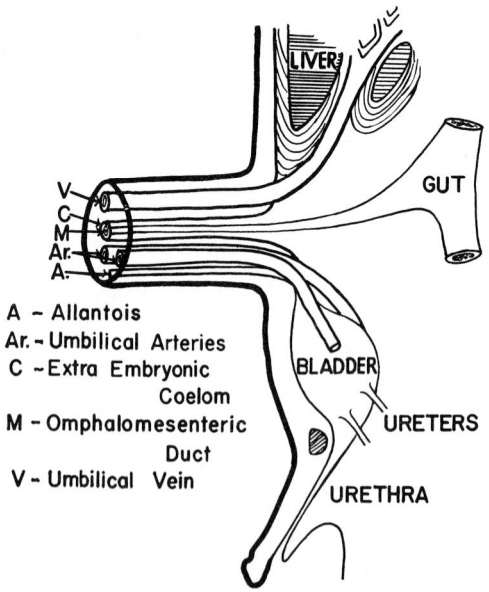

A – Allantois
Ar.– Umbilical Arteries
C – Extra Embryonic
    Coelom
M – Omphalomesenteric
    Duct
V – Umbilical Vein

Figure 5. Diagrammatic sagittal section of 5.2 cm. (approximately 10 week) human embryo.

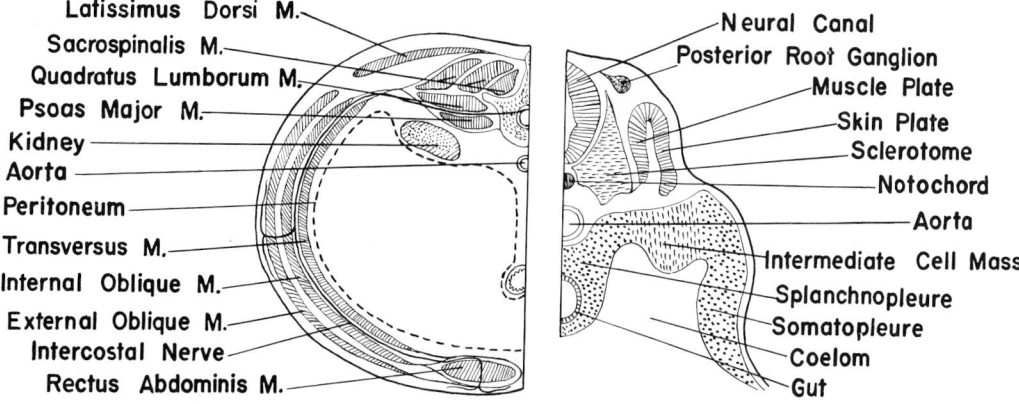

Figure 6. *Left half,* Transverse section showing the structures at the level of the first lumbar segment in the adult. *Right half,* Corresponding section showing diagrammatically the structures of an embryo at 3 weeks.

deen and Lewis, reported in 1901.[1] The muscles of the abdominal wall are segmental in origin, arising from the lower thoracic and upper lumbar somites. They arise by differentiation of cells of the myotome (muscle plate) which multiply and, in the case of the anterolateral abdominal muscles, migrate into the somatopleure. Here, the muscle fibers take a longitudinal direction, extending between the septa that separate the segments. With further development, muscle fibers of adjacent segments fuse and undergo lamination into layers and, finally, the fibers of the various laminae modify their direction to conform with the final pattern as seen in the adult. The final step in this process is the fibrous replacement of certain areas of the muscles with formation of their respective aponeuroses. Reference to Figure 6 indicates the source of these muscle fibers.

The basic vasculature of the abdominal wall, too, is derived from the segmental vessels. The arteries arise in pairs from the aorta, contribute a branch to the epaxial muscles, spine, and skin of that segment, and then course ventrally in the somatopleure to anastomose with the corresponding paired, ventral, longitudinal, superior, and inferior epigastric vessels. The venous pattern is similar, as is, in essence, the pattern of the peripheral nerves, though no ventral longitudinal nerve completes the analogy.

ANATOMY

The anterior abdominal wall may be regarded as a laminated structure, of which the middle or myoaponeurotic layer functions as the essential supporting framework (Fig. 6).[18] This layer is composed of the anteriorly placed rectus abdominis muscles and the laterally situated flat muscles of the abdominal wall, with their aponeuroses. The fibers of the paired recti run longitudinally from the crest of the pubis to their insertion into the cartilages of the fifth, sixth, and seventh ribs. Lateral to the recti, and forming what are commonly referred to as the muscles of the anterolateral abdominal wall, are the external oblique, internal oblique, and transversus muscles, in that order, from without in. The point at which their muscle fibers are replaced by aponeuroses is a feature of some importance. Reference to Figure 7 indicates that the line of transition from muscular to aponeurotic fibers in the case of the external oblique may be represented by a line dropped vertically from the tip of the ninth costal cartilage to join the lateral portion of a line drawn from the anterior superior iliac spine to the umbilicus. In the case of the transversus, the line of transition is indicated by a sigmoid curve, commonly referred to as the linea semilunaris of Spieghel. It is to be noted that in the upper ab-

domen, muscle fibers of the transversus are found medial to the lateral border of the rectus, where they contribute to the posterior rectus sheath.

The formation of the rectus sheath superior to the linea semicircularis of Douglas is depicted diagrammatically in the left-hand portion of Figure 6. It may be seen that the aponeurosis of the internal oblique splits into two lamellae that enclose, respectively, the anterior and posterior surfaces of the rectus and are joined, in the former instance, by the aponeurosis of external oblique and, in the latter, by the transversus abdominis or its aponeurosis. A feature of some importance surgically is the fact that the aponeurosis of the external oblique fuses with the anterior rectus sheath 2 to 3 cm. medial to the lateral margin of the rectus. This fusion allows incision of the deeper of the two leaves of the anterior sheath without disruption of the entire sheath when advancement of portions of the aponeurosis is used in herniorrhaphy. Below the linea semicircularis, which is usually situated about midway between the symphysis pubis and the navel, the aponeuroses of all three anterolateral muscles pass anterior to the rectus muscle, with the result that no posterior sheath exists and the rectus lies on the transversalis fascia. The decussation of the anterior and posterior rectus sheaths in the ventral midline forms the linea alba.

The structures superficial to the myoaponeurotic layer consist of the skin, superficial fascia, and deep fascia, from

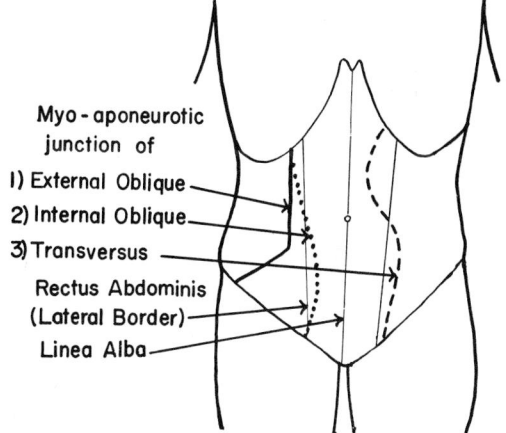

Myo-aponeurotic junction of
1) External Oblique
2) Internal Oblique
3) Transversus
Rectus Abdominis (Lateral Border)
Linea Alba

Figure 7. Myoaponeurotic junctions of the anterolateral abdominal muscles.

without in. The skin of this area requires little special comment. Cosmetic considerations are seldom of paramount importance in the placement of abdominal incisions, but where they are, the long axis of the incision should parallel the tension lines of Langer. The superficial fascia of the anterior abdominal wall has a characteristic feature in that the fibrous stroma that supports the fat cells is condensed, in its inferior portion, to form a rather well-defined fibrous layer. This layer replaces the soft fatty tissue in the deepest portion of the superficial fascia and is referred to as Scarpa's fascia. In children, it has occasionally been mistaken by the uninitiated for the aponeurosis of the external oblique muscle during herniorrhaphy. Many surgeons repair it as a separate layer in lower abdominal wound closure. The deep fascia of the anterior abdominal wall has no peculiar features, save that while it is readily demonstrable over the muscular portion of the external oblique, it becomes fused with and inseparable from the aponeurotic portion of this muscle.

The structures deep to the myoaponeurotic layer consist of the transversalis fascia, the extraperitoneal fat, and the peritoneum, from without in. The transversalis fascia is characterized by its firm attachment medially to the posterior rectus sheath, its loose attachment to the transversus abdominis muscle, and its uninterrupted continuity posterior with the fascia over the quadratus lumborum and psoas muscles. Superiorly, it is continuous with the fascia on the inferior surface of the diaphragm and, inferiorly, with that on the visceral surface of the muscles lining the pelvic cavity.

The distribution of the nerves of the anterior abdominal wall is of importance. The lower five intercostal nerves and subcostal nerve pass downward and medially in the plane between the internal oblique and transversus muscles. They pierce the posterior leaflet of the aponeurosis of the internal oblique muscle at the lateral margin of the rectus sheath, continue their course posterior to the rectus muscle, and terminate by supplying branches to this muscle and the overlying skin. The distribution of the iliohypogastric and ilioinguinal nerves from the first lumbar segment is slightly different. They pierce the internal oblique muscle just medial to the anterior superior spine, and thus lie in the plane between the internal oblique muscle and the aponeurosis of the external oblique, in which situation they are displayed at herniorrhaphy.

The segmental arteries, the posterior intercostal and lumbar branches of the aorta, follow the distribution of the corresponding nerves and terminate in anastomoses deep to the rectus muscle with the superior and inferior epigastric arteries. In their course, they anastomose with the ascending branch of the deep circumflex iliac artery deep to the internal oblique muscle. The veins of the abdominal wall course with their corresponding arteries.

The lymphatic drainage of the abdominal wall is of importance with regard to the spread of infections and malignant disease (Fig. 8). On the right-hand side of the figure, the superficial drainage is shown. A line drawn around the body, from just above the umbilicus to the disc between the second and third lumbar vertebrae, separates the superior from the inferior watershed. The medial portion of the superior watershed drains into the pectoral group and the lateral portion into the subscapular group of the axillary nodes. The inferior watershed, including the integumentum of the umbilicus, drains into the superficial inguinal nodes. There are no significant anastomoses between the superficial lymphatics of the left and right sides of the abdominal wall except at the umbilicus.

The lymphatic drainage of the deep structures of the abdominal wall is shown on the left half of the figure. The lymphatics are seen to course to the internal mammary, the axillary, the abdominal aortic, and the deep femoral nodes from fairly well-defined areas of the wall. Again, the unilaterality of the lymphatic drainage is preserved except for the area immediately around the umbilicus. The umbilical lymphatics

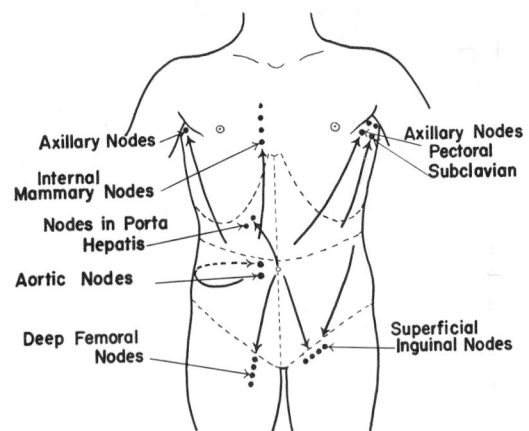

Figure 8. Lymphatic drainage of the abdominal wall. *Right half,* Drainage of superficial structures. *Left half,* Drainage of deep structures.

communicate freely with channels that pass to all four drainage areas bilaterally and also, by means of lymphatics traveling along the round ligament of the liver, drainage may be to nodes in the porta hepatis.

CONGENITAL ABNORMALITIES

Abnormalities of the Muscles of the Abdominal Wall[28]

Agenesis or absence of the muscles of the abdominal wall is a rare abnormality and extreme deficiency rather than absence would appear to be a more appropriate term. It has been noted that the transversus abdominis, the portion of the rectus abdominis below the navel, the internal oblique, the external oblique, and the rectus abdominis above the navel are affected, in decreasing order of frequency. An interesting sex incidence is recorded in that only 2 of 45 acceptable instances occurred in female children. Associated lesions of the urinary tract are very common and considerable discussion centers around which of the two lesions is primary. Congenital malformations of the gastrointestinal tract, mainly in the form of malrotation, occur in at least 20 per cent of such patients. Respiratory and urinary infections have been the most common fatal complications. Treatment consists of external support to the abdominal wall, early surgical correction of associated urinary and gastrointestinal abnormalities, and general measures directed toward the maintenance of an optimal nutritional state and the prevention of complicating infections.

Omphalomesenteric Duct Anomalies[26, 34]

When the omphalomesenteric duct fails to disappear it may persist as a patent structure throughout its entire length (Fig. 9A); may persist only in its peripheral (Fig. 9B₁), its mid (Fig. 9B₂), or its central (Fig. 9B₃) portion as a diverticulum or cyst; or may be represented merely by a rest of ectopic intestinal epithelium at the umbilicus (Fig. 9C) or a fibrous cord (Fig. 9D). Meckel's diverticulum is by far the most common lesion in this class, occurring in 2 to 4 per cent of persons.

Instances of completely patent omphalomesenteric duct (umbilical enteric fistula) are extremely rare.[17, 31] The diagnosis should be suspected in a newborn infant presenting with a reddish, moist, pouting collection of intestinal mucosa at the navel. The intestinal origin of the tissue, as opposed to the more common umbilical granulation, may be suspected by the clinical demonstration of the mucoid nature of its secretion. Intestinal mucosa may, of course, also occur at the navel in association with umbilical polyps and umbilical sinuses, but these three can usually be differentiated by judicious probing and by means of x-ray examination following Lipiodol injection of the sinus, if one exists. The diagnosis is immediately confirmed if, on crying or straining, the infant is observed to pass gas or discharge fecal material from the navel.

Complacency should be avoided in those instances in which normal gastrointestinal tract function appears to exist in the presence of a completely patent omphalomesenteric duct. Ileal prolapse may occur suddenly and rapidly endanger life. The degrees of ileal prolapse are illustrated in Figure 10. The treatment consists of complete excision of the umbilicus and the tract. The ileum is closed transversely following longitudinal excision of the tract from its wall. When the operation is carried out before ileal prolapse with

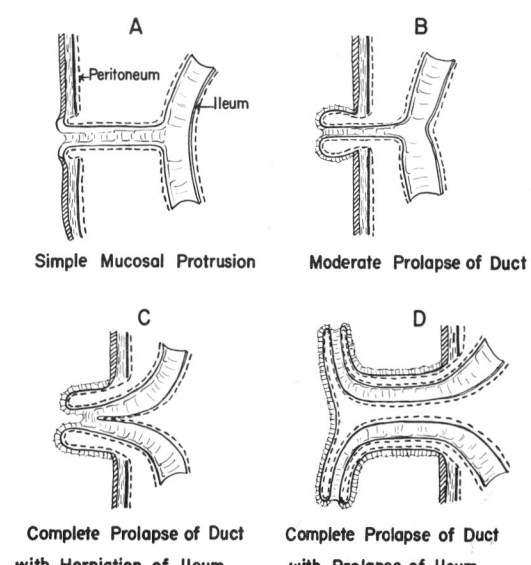

Figure 10. Degrees of prolapse associated with completely patent omphalomesenteric duct.

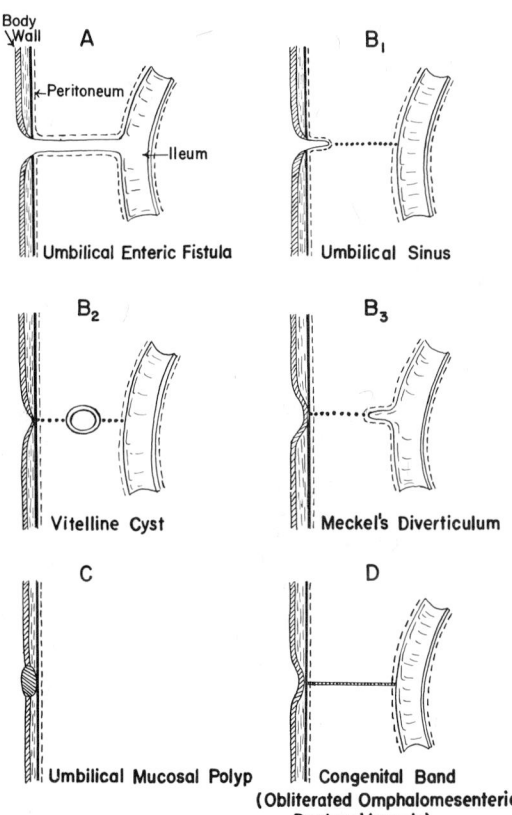

Figure 9. Congenital omphalomesenteric duct anomalies.

vascular embarrassment has occurred, the mortality is minimal.

Umbilical sinuses and polyps are treated by excision. Vitelline cysts are usually asymptomatic unless obstruction occurs around the congenital band that joins them to the ileum or to the navel. Small cysts situated close to the navel or within the abdominal wall, or larger cysts occurring more proximally along the duct, may be palpable. The only satisfactory treatment is excision.

On occasion a large vitelline duct cyst may communicate with the intestinal lumen, in which case it is referred to as either a giant Meckel's diverticulum or a giant communicating vitelline duct cyst.[11] Such cysts may constitute an infrequent cause of neonatal small intestinal obstruction. Classically the infant, after tolerating early feedings and having passed normal amounts of meconium during the first day of life, manifests the delayed onset of abdominal distention and bilious vomiting within the first week. Physical examination confirms the presence of signs of a low small bowel obstruction and of a palpable mass that is deep to the umbilicus or to the anterior abdominal wall to the right of the midline. Plain roentgenograms of the abdomen demonstrate a cystic mass with an air-fluid level or a soap-bubble appearance that, on lateral view, lies anteriorly, immediately behind the umbilicus. Treatment consists of excision of the cyst, including transverse excision of its base from the intestine, along with transverse closure. If the base is too broad for such simplified management, treatment will include concomitant minimal small bowel resection and anastomosis. Additional procedures may, on occasion, be required in the management of the complicating small bowel obstruction.

Congenital bands, of either omphalomesenteric duct or vascular origin, are of importance only as an etiologic factor in intestinal obstruction. Bremer[5] makes the interesting observation that a band derived from the obliterated omphalomesenteric artery corresponds in position to that shown for the congenital band in Figure 9D, while that derived from the corresponding vein runs, not to the antimesenteric border of the bowel, but rather to the base of the mesentery at a more proximal level, or to the porta hepatis.

Urachal Anomalies[26, 34]

Congenital, completely patent urachus (umbilical urinary fistula) is characterized clinically by the intermittent discharge of urine from the navel, the quantity and the frequency depending on the caliber of the fistula and the presence or absence of some degree of obstruction of the lower urinary tract (Fig. 11). A small granular tumor may mark the site of the ostium at the umbilicus, or the navel may appear normal on superficial examination. No symptoms, apart from the discharge, are associated with the anomaly unless infection occurs. Surgical excision is the only satisfactory treatment, but this should be performed only after the patency of the urethra has been confirmed. The entire tract is excised and the site of attachment to the bladder is ligated and inverted with a purse-string suture. In the absence of pre-existing infection, the procedure can usually be accomplished extraperitoneally with minimal risk.

In the so-called acquired type of completely patent urachus, no abnormality is apparent at birth and only at some later date does intermittent discharge of urine occur. This condition is almost invariably associated with lower urinary obstruction, which forces urine through an incompletely obliterated urachal channel. Treatment is excision following correction of the obstructing lesion. The acquired type of anomaly is more common than the congenital type.

Umbilical urachal sinuses present no additional features except that the discharge is minimal and watery and is not urine. Treatment consists of surgical excision.

Urachal cysts are the most common urachal abnormality. If uninfected they are usually asymptomatic and, when small, are recognized only at surgery or autopsy as an incidental finding. Larger cysts may be apparent to the patient as a subumbilical fullness or swelling, or may be discovered incidentally by the surgeon in the course of abdominal examination. Infection is common and this is the usual method of clinical presentation. The symptoms are those of an acute inflammation deep in the subumbilical abdominal wall. In patients in whom the cyst is not infected, extraperitoneal excision is the treatment of choice and usually presents no difficulties unless the cyst is of large size. It is wise in such instances to demonstrate the cord, which almost invariably runs from the cyst to the bladder, and to deal with it as though it were patent. This precaution is also desirable with umbilical urachal sinus. Excision of infected urachal cysts without peritoneal contamination is virtually impossible and treatment should be restricted to incision, drainage, and loose packing of the cavity with gauze. Frequently, as a result of the infection, the transitional epithelium of the wall of the cyst is destroyed and the simple drainage procedure results in permanent cure.

Blichert-Toft and his associates[2] have recently presented a classification of urachal configuration based on anatomical considerations that is helpful in interpreting clinical findings at operation and in determining treatment. In type I (8.5 per cent), the urachal remnant runs from the bladder to the umbilicus in the midline and is completely independent of the lateral umbilical ligaments (i.e., the obliterated umbilical arteries). In type II (12.5 per cent), after a course of some 5 cm., the urachal remnant deviates to one side or other, blends with one of the lateral umbilical ligaments, and continues to the umbilicus as a common ligament. The common ligament is frequently joined by the remaining lateral umbilical ligament before it reaches the umbilical ring. In type III (25 per cent), the urachal remnant and both lateral umbilical ligaments fuse about midway between bladder and umbilicus and continue to the latter as a common ligament. In type IV (54 per cent), the commonest type, after a short course of 2 cm. or less, the urachal remnant ends freely or in a fine fibrous plexus that may or may not receive and blend with the lateral umbilical ligaments. On the basis of these gross anatomical studies, the microscopic demonstration of the occurrence of epithelial rests at various levels in the different anatomical types, and an experience with eight clinical cases, these authors recommend radical excision of the entire urachal remnant, including the apical segment of the bladder, as the treatment of choice for anomalies of the urachus. In the presence of infection the procedure is accomplished in two stages.

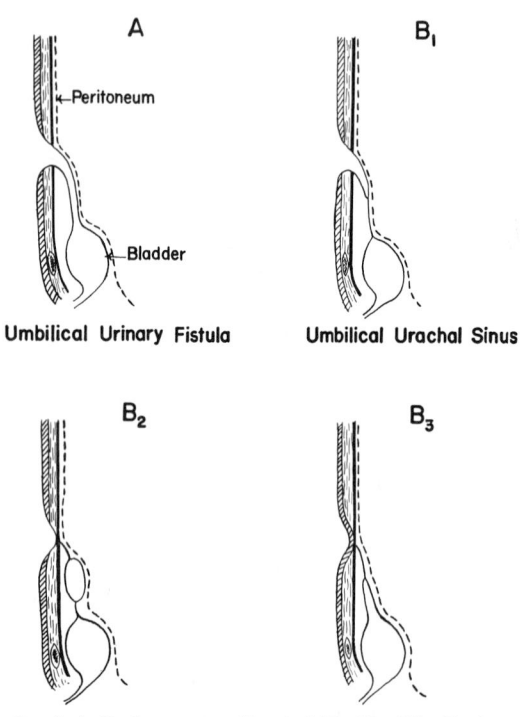

Figure 11. Congenital urachal anomalies.

Vascular Anomalies

Vascular anomalies involving the omphalomesenteric vessels are rare and of little clinical significance. Aberrations in the normal fate of the umbilical vessels are apparently rare if one excludes the possibility that portal vein obstruction may be due to extension into that vessel of the obliterative process that is normally limited to the umbilical vein and ductus venosus. Anomalies of the urachal vessels are apparently of little or no clinical significance.

Somatic Anomalies

Omphalocele, umbilical hernia, and exstrophy of the urinary bladder are somatic anomalies that occur relatively frequently. They are more appropriately dealt with elsewhere.

Endometriosis of the umbilicus is rare. It usually presents as a small mass at the umbilicus that enlarges and becomes tender at the time of the menstrual period. External bleeding may also occur. Treatment is by simple excision. Coexistent pelvic endometriosis will require separate treatment.

INFECTIONS

Infections of the abdominal wall proper are essentially similar to superficial infections occurring elsewhere in the body. Progressive bacterial synergistic gangrene and other relatively rare infections of this area may produce serious postoperative complications.

Omphalitis in the Newborn

While this condition is much less common now than 25 or more years ago, it may be a serious lesion and, therefore, demands prompt recognition and treatment. It usually arises as a result of contamination of the cord at the time of section or during subsequent dressing of the umbilicus. The common organisms are *Staphylococcus aureus* and the hemolytic streptococcus. The widespread lymphatic drainage and the persistence of patent vascular channels in this area account for the rapid dissemination of the infection. Locally, the condition is manifest by redness, heat, swelling, and tenderness, which may spread centrifugally from the navel with alarming rapidity. Usually, pus exudes from the folds of the umbilicus. Occasionally, widespread sloughing of skin occurs. Bloodstream invasion may occur along the incompletely obliterated umbilical vein or umbilical arteries with signs of septicemia. Spread sometimes occurs to the adjacent peritoneum with signs of fulminating peritonitis. Treatment of the omphalitis must be initiated promptly with antibiotics, local hot moist compresses, and surgical incision of any purulent collections. The localized type of omphalitis usually responds rapidly to treatment, but once septicemia or peritonitis has occurred the outlook is grave.

Omphalitis in the Adult

Unlike *neonatal* omphalitis, umbilical infections in the *adult* tend to pursue a relatively benign and chronic course. They are commonly seen in office practice but seldom require hospital care. The one common etiologic factor in almost all patients appears to be neglect of personal hygiene in this area. Congenital aberrations in the depth and configuration of the umbilicus may contribute by making cleansing of the area difficult. The usual complaints are of tenderness in or around the navel and the presence of a seropurulent discharge with an offensive odor. Examination reveals the base of the umbilicus thrown up into a cluster of red, moist, swollen, angry-looking folds that exude the offensive discharge. Extension into periumbilical tissues is uncommon but may occur along with inguinal adenitis. In the acute phase, omphalitis usually responds rapidly to warm, moist saline compresses. Antibiotics are seldom indicated unless systemic manifestations ensue. Once the acute symptoms have subsided, the patient should be instructed to wash the umbilicus carefully while bathing and dry it with equal care afterward. Gentle cleansing with alcohol-dipped absorbent cotton on the end of an applicator is a useful means of eliminating moisture and excoriation in deep clefts.

SPASM OF THE MUSCLES OF THE ABDOMINAL WALL

Spasm of muscles of the abdominal wall, particularly the rectus abdominis, is a common finding on examination. A relatively simple classification of the causes of abdominal wall spasm includes:

1. *Central or cerebral origin,* either organic, as seen in spastic paraplegia, or psychogenic, as seen in the nervous patient, in the patient anticipating some painful experience, and in psychopathic drug addiction.

2. *Spinal cord origin,* as seen in those diseases characterized by irritation of spinal cord neurons, as for example tabes dorsalis.

3. *Thoracic nerve trunk origin,* as seen in pleurisy, infections of the chest wall, chest and spinal column injury, epidemic pleurodynia, and severe alcoholic neuritis.

4. *Reflex origin,* as seen when the peritoneum is irritated by infection, blood, or foreign material or when juxtaperitoneal organs are the origin of extremely painful stimuli, as in renal colic.

5. *Local origin,* as seen in local trauma to, or infection of, the abdominal wall.

While peritonitis, in its broadest sense, is by far the most common cause of true abdominal wall rigidity, the interpretation of this finding after abdominal trauma is of extreme importance. It may arise, on the one hand, from a relatively benign injury to the abdominal wall, or on the other, from a grave intraperitoneal insult that will be rapidly fatal if surgical treatment is withheld. It should be possible in virtually every patient to differentiate these two on a basis of complete and careful abdominal examination.

Abdominal wall rigidity, as an early manifestation of purely thoracic wounds, is now well recognized. Frequently the rigidity, which is usually ipsilateral but may be bilateral, is associated with subcostal tenderness of such intensity, in the early hours after injury, that one is tempted to carry out a laparotomy with a diagnosis of ruptured intra-abdominal viscus. The knowledge that this syndrome may exist, along with the absence of signs of peritoneal contamination, should enable one to avoid needless laparotomy. The abdominal findings rarely persist longer than 48 to 72 hours. The converse situation is also frequently observed, namely, unilateral restriction of movement of the thoracic cage and diminished air entry into the base of the lung on that side, following injury restricted to the abdominal wall. Percussion of the chest along with radiologic examination will quickly clarify the situation.

HEMATOMA OF THE RECTUS SHEATH[6, 7, 9, 23]

In recent years, this uncommon condition has aroused much interest because of the fact that it may mimic acute intra-abdominal disease. It is seldom diagnosed preoperatively because it is not considered. In approximately 90 per cent of instances, the hematoma is situated below the navel; it lies to the right of the midline about twice as often as it does to the left. The frequent occurrence of the hematoma below the semicircular line of Douglas, causing peritoneal irritation, is considered to account for the gastrointestinal manifestations that are often seen. It is seldom possible to demonstrate the exact site of hemorrhage, but the inferior epigastric vein is more commonly the source than the artery. There is general agreement that the condition is more frequent during pregnancy. Even in pregnant patients, it is usually possible to elicit a history of indirect trauma or upper respiratory infection with cough as the immediate cause of the hemorrhage. Apart from pregnancy, the etiology of the lesion may be classified relative to its association with:

1. *Trauma,* either direct or indirect, of which the latter is far more common.

2. *Infections and debilitating diseases,* in which case a severe paroxysm of coughing is often the immediate cause of the hemorrhage.

3. *Degenerative vascular disease, blood dyscrasias, and abnormalities of coagulation,* including an increasing number of cases ascribed to anticoagulant therapy.

4. *The postoperative period,* when the injudicious positioning of rectus muscle retractors or retention sutures is usually considered to be the cause.

5. *Unknown (idiopathic) causes,* implying that the lesion can occur spontaneously without associated disease or injury. This appears most unlikely and it is probably that one of the preceding factors is present, though overlooked, in patients so classified.

The symptomatology is classic. Following trauma, which may be mild or severe, there is usually a rather sudden onset of excruciating abdominal pain. When bleeding occurs slowly, the pain will be more gradual in onset and of less severity. It is usually localized to the site of rupture but may be generalized. Nausea and vomiting are relatively common and constipation may occur. Characteristically, after a period of increased pain, there is a gradual improvement that leaves in its wake a persistent dull ache. Apart from the occasional patient who appears acutely ill and in

shock, the significant findings are limited to the abdomen. A hard, exquisitely tender mass may be palpated in one or the other rectus, which may be misinterpreted as localized muscle spasm. If one demonstrates that the mass is restricted to the confines of the rectus sheath and that tenderness and rigidity in the adjacent lateral abdominal muscles are lacking, the diagnosis is supported. Fothergill[9] described a sign that assists in differentiating abdominal wall masses from those arising within the peritoneal cavity. When the recti are contracted, as when the patient attempts to sit up, a mass situated in the wall may still be felt and is fixed, while an intra-abdominal mass is no longer easily palpable. An additional late sign is the appearance of ecchymosis about the umbilicus. The hematoma is usually accompanied by a mild elevation of temperature and pulse, and moderate polymorphonuclear leukocytosis is common, further simulating acute intra-abdominal disease. The natural history of the disease is usually one of spontaneous recovery, with cessation of pain after a few days and gradual disappearance of the mass in the course of 3 to 4 weeks. Occasionally, the hematoma becomes infected and forms an abscess or persists and calcifies to give rise to continuing pain.

Some surgeons feel that the safest and surest treatment is to confirm the diagnosis by means of a short paramedian incision, evacuate the clot, and ligate the epigastric artery and vein above and below the assumed point of hemorrhage. It is our belief that most of these patients can be successfully managed conservatively. It should be pointed out that some patients will be operated upon in error with a preoperative diagnosis of appendicitis or some other intra-abdominal lesion. In this group, surgical control of the hemorrhage is readily carried out.

TUMORS OF THE ABDOMINAL WALL

Benign Tumors[25]

According to Pack and Ehrlich[25] benign tumors constitute 60 per cent of all neoplasms and 80 per cent of the primary neoplasms of the abdominal wall. In order of frequency, the more common types of benign tumors encountered are lipomas, neuronevi, hemangiomas, epithelial papillomas, fibromas, neurofibromas, keratoses, and desmoid tumors. Lipomas, constituting 20 per cent of the benign neoplasms, are the most common. The treatment of these lesions is similar to that recommended in other situations and presents no special problem. Lipomas, papillomas, fibromas, and keratoses are treated by simple excision. Hemangiomas should be excised when the lesion occurs in the abdominal wall, since cure is rapidly achieved and the resulting scar is of little consequence.

Neurofibromas of the solitary type are easily excised surgically, but in over half of the patients in whom this lesion presents in the abdominal wall it takes the form of the plexiform von Recklinghausen type. This lesion, with its known predisposition to malignant transformation, is often extensive and invasive and requires wide excision, sometimes in stages.

Nevi of the abdominal wall must be treated with considerable respect. A high percentage of melanomas follow chronic irritation of a pre-existing mole. It is obvious that any such lesion should be widely excised surgically, especially if it presents in an area in which irritation from a belt, girdle, or other clothing occurs.

Desmoid tumors are essentially hard, nonencapsulated fibromas arising from the deep fascial and myoaponeurotic layers of the anterior abdominal wall.[4, 25] They are characteristically infiltrative and may attain large size. The etiology is unknown. The preponderance in the female, frequently within a year of parturition, has led to the suggestion that stretching of the abdominal wall during pregnancy, or some gestational endocrine factor, may be important etiologically. However, their occurrence in the male and in the nulliparous female would tend to minimize the etiologic significance of pregnancy. A history of antecedent trauma is also rare, but their occurrence in laparotomy scars is too frequent to be dismissed as incidental.

Clinically, the patient usually presents complaining of the presence of an abdominal mass or a sensation of weight in the abdomen. Less commonly, a vague feeling of pressure on the bladder or bizarre abdominal pains may cause the patient to seek advice. On examination, a mass is usually palpated deep to the skin and unattached to it. Characteristically, it is firm, smooth, and discrete. Bouchacourt's sign, which is similar to that of Fothergill (vide supra) but applies to intramural masses situated anywhere in the anterior abdominal wall, is helpful in localizing the mass to the muscular layer of the abdominal wall. The rectus abdominis is the muscle most commonly affected, but the infiltrative nature of the tumor frequently results in multiple muscle involvement.

The gross pathologic features of the tumor are its denseness and hardness, its glistening white or pinkish color, and its apparent infiltrative character. Microscopically, it varies from an acellular fibroma to a low-grade cellular fibrosarcoma, and the inclusion at its periphery of engulfed and sequestrated degenerating muscle fibers is characteristic. Desmoid tumors are clinically benign and metastases do not occur. Local recurrence and infiltration is the rule, unless excision has been complete. Treatment is by wide surgical resection which, because of the large size of some of these tumors, often results in defects that require plastic procedures for closure. The place of radiation therapy in the management of these tumors is controversial and no opinion as to its value is possible at this time.

Malignant Tumors

Malignant tumors constitute about one third of all neoplasms of the abdominal wall, and secondary malignant tumors are as common as primary malignant growths. This is in marked contrast to other soft tissue areas, where secondary deposits are extremely rare. The initial presentation of malignant lymphoma may be an abdominal wall mass.

Primary Malignant Tumors. Of this group approximately one half are sarcomas. The more common sarcomas, in order of frequency, are neurogenic sarcoma, spindle cell sarcoma, synovioma, and rhabdomyosarcoma. Carcinomas are mainly epidermoid in type, with occasional basal cell lesions and very rarely an adenocarcinoma.

Most sarcomas arise from the deeper layers of the wall and not infrequently give rise to blood-borne metastases, though lymph node involvement does not occur. As a group, these sarcomas tend to be radioresistant and the treatment, if treatment is possible, consists of wide excision of the full thickness of the abdominal wall, including the peritoneum. Synoviomas and rhabdomyosarcomas appear to have a particularly unfavorable prognosis.

Carcinoma of the skin of the abdominal wall is relatively uncommon, as compared with its occurrence elsewhere in the body. It does, however, present some interesting and rather unusual features when it occurs in this situation. Epidermoid carcinoma may arise in an area of pre-existing tissue abnormality, such as an abdominal scar, an abdominal sinus, or an area of radiation dermatitis. Epidermoid carcinoma arising in normal skin has a relatively good prognosis following total surgical removal. Superficial lymphatics are scarce in the abdominal wall and lymph node metastases are unusual. Epidermoid carcinoma arising in laparotomy scars and postoperative draining sinuses is a clinical entity with an extremely grave prognosis, for while lymph node metastases are rare, early extensive involvement of the peritoneum is common.

Melanomas appear to be relatively uncommon in the abdominal wall. These lesions appear to have a predilection for the area about the umbilicus, which is a most undesirable situation from the standpoint of facility of lymphatic and venous spread. Melanoma carries with it a grave prognosis, and since these lesions are rarely radiosensitive, radical surgical excision is the only available treatment that offers any hope of eradication of the disease. Wide local excision of the lesion is mandatory and this, at the umbilicus, includes ample excision of the full thickness of the abdominal wall and the round ligament of the liver. Block dissection of lymphatic glands in areas of apparent spread should be carried out. If the lesion is situated in a quadrant of the abdomen where its lymphatic drainage can be predicted with assurance, then block dissection of the regional lymphatics should be carried out even in the absence of clinically demonstrable metastases. The principle of excision of the primary lesion with dissection of the regional lymphatic nodes in continuity can frequently be effectively employed in the case of the abdominal wall.

Secondary Malignant Tumors. Metastatic spread of malignant tumors to the abdominal wall is a relatively frequent occurrence in contrast to the infrequency of such spread to other soft tissue areas. The source of the metastatic deposit is most commonly a carcinoma. According to Pack and Ehrlich[25] the common sources in order of frequency are the ovary, stomach, uterus, bronchus, kidney, breast, and sigmoid colon. Metastatic carcinoma of the abdominal wall most commonly occurs in the region of the umbilicus.

The presence of secondary malignant deposits in the abdominal wall, with one notable exception, is a sign of advanced disease and inoperability. The one exception is the implantation carcinoma occasionally seen in the scars of operations carried out for malignant disease. These lesions, surprisingly, do not tend to invade the peritoneal cavity and while lymph node metastases may occur, wide surgical excision of the implanted lesion, along with block dissection of involved nodes, may be rewarded by long-term survival.

THE PERITONEUM

EMBRYOLOGY

The primitive coelom is partially divided by the septum transversum, or future diaphragm, into a pericardial cavity and a peritoneal cavity in the fourth week of intrauterine life. For a time, the two cavities communicate over the dorsal edge of the thick septum transversum by the paired pleural canals (Fig. 12). By the seventh week, the peritoneal cavity is completely separated from the pleural cavities by the pleural-peritoneal membranes. Initially, the peritoneal cavity is separated into right and left halves by the primitive gut and its mesentery. The mesentery is designated as ventral or dorsal, according to its relationship to the gut (Fig. 13). The ventral mesentery then disappears, except for the lesser omentum and falciform ligament, its contributions to the diaphragm, and the suspensory ligament of the bladder. With resorption of the greater part of the ventral mesentery, the coelom becomes a single cavity. That portion of the gut that will become the second part of the duodenum gives rise to two evaginations (Fig. 14). Into the ventral mesentery grows the hepatic diverticulum, from which branches the accessory pancreas. Into the dorsal mesentery grows the diverticulum that is to become the main pancreas. In the dorsal mesogastrium, the spleen develops in relation to blood vessels, not the lymphatics, and then bulges into the left leaf of the mesentery (Fig. 15).

The mesenteries of the foregut shift their attachments as the stomach rotates 90 degrees on a long axis and as overgrowth takes place on the greater curvature side (Fig. 16). The ventral mesentery, bearing the hepatic diverticulum, shifts to the right and cranially to become the lesser omentum. The rotation of the foregut is accompanied by a modification in the attachment of its dorsal mesentery. In its cranial portion, in which the spleen is developing, the rotation of the stomach carries the dorsal mesogastrium to the left with its contained spleen. Fusion of a portion of the left leaf of the dorsal mesogastrium with the posterior parietal peritoneum results in the apparent origin of the dorsal mesogastrium (gastrolienal and lienorenal ligaments) from a site well to the left of the midline in this situation. Immediately caudal to the spleen-containing dorsal mesogastrium, the ballooned-out mesogastrium overlaps the transverse colon and its meso-

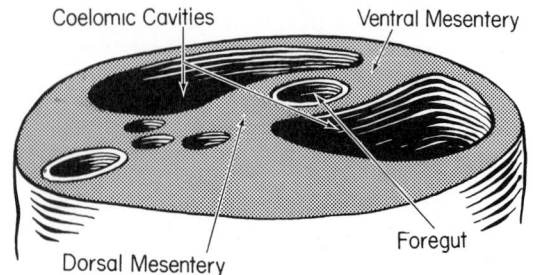

Figure 13. Cross section through the level of the foregut. The peritoneal portion of the coelom is initially divided into two cavities by the gut, the transient ventral mesentery, and the dorsal mesentery.

colon and subsequently fuses with the latter. Its further overgrowth in this situation and the subsequent fusion of its adjacent layers form the greater omentum (Fig. 17), which, therefore, appears to gain attachment to both stomach and transverse colon. More caudal still, the dorsal mesogastrium containing the pancreatic diverticulum is carried to the right as a result of displacement of the duodenum. In this situation, there is extensive fusion of the right leaf of the dorsal mesogastrium with the parietal peritoneum, as a result of which both the pancreas and the second portion of the duodenum assume a retroperitoneal position.

ANATOMY

Gross Anatomy. The peritoneal cavity was mentioned in the Papyrus Ebers some 3500 years ago, but it was not thoroughly described until 1730, when James Douglas of Edinburgh published a lucid account that has not been appreciably improved upon to this day.

The peritoneum is a serous membrane that lines the peritoneal cavity and invests a number of abdominal structures. Except for the openings of the fallopian tubes, the peritoneum is a completely closed sac. In a strict sense, the peritoneal cavity does not contain any organs, since the entire gastrointestinal tract and its derivatives are really retroperitoneal in position. However, it is customary to speak of those structures that are almost completely enfolded by peritoneum, such as stomach, jejunum, ileum, transverse colon, sig-

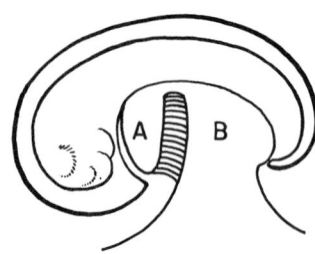

Figure 12. Parasagittal section of an embryo at 4 weeks. The thick septum transversum divides the coelom into the pericardial cavity *(A)* and the peritoneal cavity *(B)*. The two cavities communicate over the dorsal aspect of the septum transversum by means of the pleural canals.

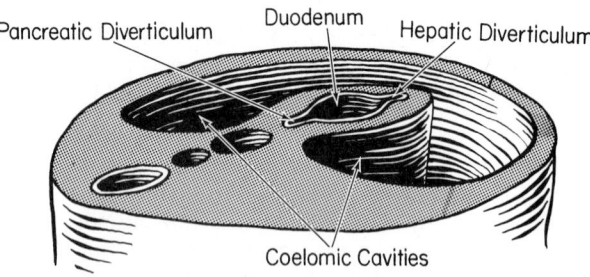

Figure 14. Cross section through that level of the gut destined to become the second part of the duodenum. There is no ventral mesentery at this level and the peritoneal cavity is a continuous space. The hepatic diverticulum arises as a ventral evagination of the gut and will give rise to the ventral contribution to the pancreas and to the biliary tree and liver. The pancreatic diverticulum arises as a dorsal evagination and forms the major portion of the pancreas.

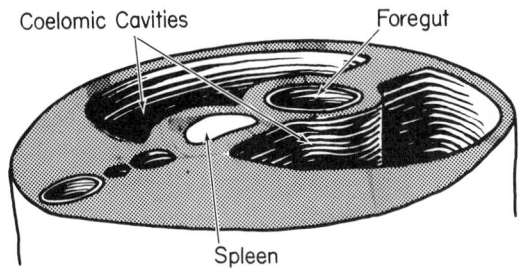

Figure 15. Cross section somewhat cranial to that shown in Figure 14. The peritoneal cavity lies on either side of that portion of the foregut destined to become the stomach. The spleen arises in the dorsal mesogastrium. The hepatic diverticulum, after giving off the ventral pancreas, will grow cranially into the ventral mesogastrium and septum transversum to give rise to the liver. The pancreatic diverticulum will extend cranially in the dorsal mesogastrium and come to lie dorsal to the spleen. Subsequent rotation of the stomach with its mesenteries will cause these structures to lie to the right (liver) and left (spleen) of the stomach.

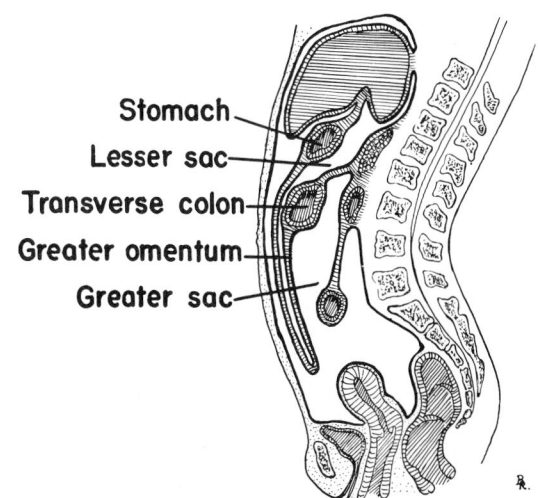

Figure 17. Diagrammatic sagittal section through a fetus, showing the relations of the greater and lesser peritoneal sacs. The two layers of the greater omentum have not yet fused. Basically the greater omentum is the dorsal mesentery of the stomach, which has fused with the transverse mesocolon.

moid colon, appendix, cecum, liver, gallbladder, and spleen, as being intraperitoneal.

That portion of the peritoneum which invests the intraperitoneal organs, and which makes up the coverings of the mesenteries, is the visceral peritoneum. That portion which lines the anterior, lateral, and posterior abdominal walls, the under surface of the diaphragm, and the floor of the pelvis is the parietal peritoneum. Although these are parts of the same membrane, the distinction is of some importance in regard to differences in sensory innervation. The peritoneum of the anterior and lateral abdominal wall is reinforced by the transversalis fascia.

The peritoneal cavity is divided into the general peritoneal cavity, or greater sac, and the lesser sac (Fig. 17). The latter has, as its only natural opening, the foramen of Winslow. The lesser sac is bounded anteriorly by gastrohepatic ligament,

stomach, and gastrocolic ligament and posteriorly by parietal peritoneum. Hanging from the transverse colon, and covering much of the ventral aspect of the lower abdominal viscera, is the greater omentum. This structure has a rich vascular supply and carries a variable amount of fat. The surface area of the peritoneum is about 2 square meters and approximates that of the skin. Unlike skin, however, the peritoneum is a highly permeable membrane. This fact has a number of important physiologic implications. Normally, the peritoneal cavity contains 75 to 100 ml. of clear, straw-colored fluid, which facilitates the normal lubricating function of the membrane.

Microscopic Anatomy. The peritoneum consists of a surface layer of mesothelium and a deeper, loose connective tissue layer containing collagen and elastic fibers, fat cells, reticulum cells, and macrophages. The mesothelium is a simple squamous cell layer. As a result of irritation, these cells may become cuboidal and enclose small cystic spaces, a reaction that the pathologist must distinguish from neoplasia. Normal peritoneal fluid contains 2000 to 2500 cells per cu. mm. The majority of these are macrophages with some desquamated mesothelial cells and lymphocytes. There are few polymorphonuclear neutrophils or eosinophils, but the number of granulocytes is greatly increased in the presence of inflammation. Peritoneal aspiration may be of value, not only to obtain fluid for culture and chemical analysis, but also because immediate study of the cells in the fluid may facilitate the diagnosis of tumors, inflammatory conditions, and intraperitoneal trauma.

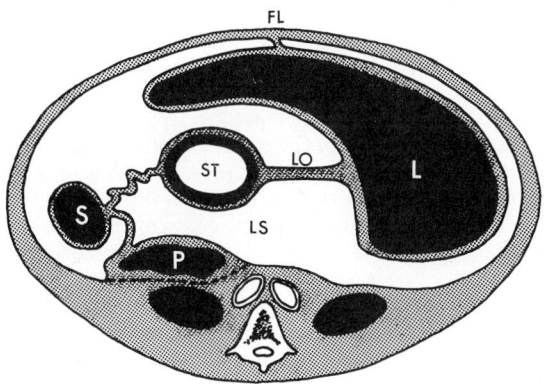

Figure 16. Diagrammatic cross section through a 4-month fetus at approximately the level shown in Figure 15. The liver (L) and pancreas (P) have grown cranially from their points of origin shown in Figure 14. Rotation has converted the right half of the peritoneal cavity shown in Figure 15 into the lesser sac (LS). It can be seen that fundamentally the spleen (S) and pancreas lie in the dorsal mesentery of the stomach (ST). Note the falciform ligament (FL), the lesser omentum (LO), and the broken line that represents the site of fusion of the two layers of the peritoneum.

PHYSIOLOGY

Relation to Extracellular Fluid Compartment.[27] Since the peritoneum is a highly permeable membrane of considerable surface area, peritoneal fluid is a physiologically active collection constituting part of the extracellular fluid. Deuterium oxide placed in the peritoneal cavity very rapidly becomes equilibrated with the plasma and interstitial fluid of the patient. The intraperitoneal route of fluid administration is used in experimental animals. Not only are water, electrolytes, and urea rapidly transported across the peritoneal membrane, but endogenous and exogenous toxic substances are freely absorbed. Rapid absorption of bacterial toxins is one of several reasons for the very high mortality in untreated peritonitis. In bowel obstruction with distention and impairment of circulation, transperitoneal absorption of bacterial toxins, even without peritonitis, is probable. It has been proved by the introduction of antibiotics and iron-dextran into the peritoneal cavity that the peritoneum is an efficient absorbing surface.

In addition to the intimate relation of peritoneum to the circulating blood, there are communications between the peritoneal and pleural cavities that appear to be independent of the bloodstream. In patients with Meigs' syndrome, colloidal radioactive gold (^{198}Au) instilled into one serous sac rapidly appears in the other, probably as a result of transdiaphragmatic lymphatic transport.

Sensory Innervation. The parietal peritoneum is well supplied with somatic afferent nerves and is sensitive to all forms of stimuli. This is particularly true of the anterior parietal peritoneum, which, along with the rest of the anterior abdominal wall, is supplied by the lower six thoracic nerves. The parietal peritoneum posteriorly and in the pelvis is somewhat less sensitive. The ability of the parietal peritoneum of the anterior abdominal wall to initiate the sensation of sharp pain in response to an adjacent inflammatory process and to permit localization of its origin is of the utmost importance in the diagnosis of acute abdominal conditions. In the case of the parietal peritoneum of the diaphragm, irritation of the peripheral portion is perceived in the vicinity of the adjacent body wall, whereas that of the central portion is referred to the shoulder as a result of central misinterpretation. The sharp, well-localized pain of parietal peritoneal irritation is in marked contrast to that which arises from the relatively insensitive visceral peritoneum.

In addition to causing sharp and well-localized pain, stimulation of the parietal peritoneum may cause involuntary rigidity of the abdominal musculature, tenderness, and rebound tenderness, if the stimulus is sufficiently intense. These characteristics identify the parietal peritoneum as the source of the pain, identify the pain stimuli as being inflammatory in origin, and localize the site of the stimuli. Without the pain fibers of the parietal peritoneum, the clinical diagnosis of an acute abdomen would be impossible.

The visceral peritoneum is relatively insensitive, but it does register stimuli if they are sufficiently strong or prolonged, particularly in the presence of pre-existing inflammation. The root of the mesentery is quite sensitive to traction.

Most visceral afferent nerve fibers for pain run in the splanchnic nerves to the same six segments of the cord that receive somatic afferent fibers. The stimulus of visceral sensation is usually tension, whether the result of increased intraluminal pressure or increased tissue pressure from inflammation. Visceral pain is usually dull and vaguely localized to the central portion of the abdomen, although there are some exceptions to this rule, notably visceral pain initiated by the biliary tree.

HEALING OF PERITONEAL DEFECTS[15]

The speed with which intra-abdominal areas denuded of peritoneum rapidly undergo reperitonealization has long been a source of wonder to surgeons. Available evidence suggests that reperitonealization may be accomplished in one of, or a combination of, three ways. First, the denuded area may be seeded by viable mesothelial cells shed from adjacent peritoneal surfaces, which subsequently proliferate to form is-

lands that coalesce. Second, the surface may be covered by ingrowth of mesothelium from intact adjacent peritoneum. Finally, there is evidence that blood monocytes and tissue histiocytes may be capable of migrating to the denuded surface from deeper layers and then differentiating to form mesothelial cells.

INFLAMMATION

Peritonitis is an inflammation of the peritoneum. The process may be acute or chronic, it may be septic or aseptic, and it may be primary or secondary. The most frequently encountered type is an acute bacterial inflammation of the peritoneum secondary to contamination. It is to this disease that the surgeon refers when the designation "peritonitis" is used without qualification. Since acute secondary bacterial peritonitis invariably occurs as a complication of some pre-existing primary disease or operation, it is dealt with elsewhere. However, some of the less common types of peritonitis are appropriately included in this section.

Primary Peritonitis[10, 22]

Primary peritonitis is defined as a diffuse peritoneal infection without an apparent intra-abdominal source. In the early part of the century it contributed approximately 10 per cent of pediatric abdominal emergencies, while more recently, presumably as a result of the availability of more effective antimicrobial agents, the incidence of primary peritonitis had decreased to between 1 and 2 per cent of such cases. However, if one considers only patients with diffuse peritonitis in infancy and childhood, primary peritonitis will account for some 15 per cent of this more selected group. It is therefore a disease that must be considered in the differential diagnosis of diffuse peritoneal sepsis in this age group.[22]

Interestingly, there has been a significant change in the clinical and bacteriological pattern of the disease over the past 10 to 20 years, as well as in its mortality and morbidity. This has occurred without any apparent modification in its frequency relative to age and sex, as recorded in large series.[10] The peak incidence of the disease occurs in childhood between the fifth and ninth years, while a minor peak is apparent in infants in the first year of life. Occasionally the disease occurs in adults. In childhood females predominate over males in a ratio of 4 to 1, whereas in infants this ratio is reversed, with twice as many cases of the disease occurring in the male as in the female. In a more recent series this classic sex distribution has not been observed, and this too may therefore be changing along with the altered pattern of infecting organisms.[22]

Primary peritonitis is unique in that it is almost always due to a single pathogenic organism, whereas secondary peritonitis is classically polymicrobial. In Fowler's[10] initial series of 97 patients with primary peritonitis prior to 1955, the pneumococcus was the offending pathogen in just over 50 per cent of patients, with the hemolytic streptococcus accounting for some 15 per cent. In that era the occurrence of primary peritonitis due to *Escherichia coli* was so rare as to suggest that the diagnosis must be in some doubt and that the possibility of secondary peritonitis, due to contamination from some occult intestinal lesion, need be seriously considered. However, in a subsequent series of 71 patients observed by Fowler[10] between 1956 and 1970, the pneumococcus accounted for only 8.5 per cent of the patients with primary peritonitis; the hemolytic streptococcus, as the etiologic factor in 13 per cent of cases, now became the chief offender. The greatest change was in relation to *E. coli* and the other gram-negative organisms that now accounted for 10 per cent and 7 per cent of cases respectively. Of equal interest is the observation that the number of patients with primary peritonitis in whom no organism could be cultured rose from 20 per cent in the first series to almost 50 per cent in the second. That these changes in the bacteriological aspects of primary peritonitis are not peculiar to Australia, the setting of Fowler's observations, is attested to by the more recent studies of McDougal and associates[22] in Cleveland, in which the *E. coli* was the pathogen in 46 per cent of patients in whom a culture was obtained.

Not unexpectedly, in a disease bearing the designation "primary," there continues to be much debate as to the means by which the infection gains access to the peritoneal cavity. Four possible routes of infection are usually cited: (1) ascending infection via the genital tract, (2) hematogenous spread from some distant focus, either occult or manifest, (3) spread from the pleural cavity by means of transdiaphragmatic lymphatics, and (4) transmural migration through the gut wall. In addition, the frequent demonstration of a urinary tract infection with an organism identical to that causing the peritonitis suggests yet another source of infection in primary peritonitis without explaining the mechanism by which the peritoneal cavity becomes infected. Early in the history of the disease the genital route was the favored explanation, while more recently the demonstration that intestinal transmural spread of bacteria is indeed possible establishes this mechanism as the prime antagonist of the proposal that the spread of bacteria to the peritoneum in primary peritonitis is probably by means of the blood stream.

In childhood, acute appendicitis with perforation is the commonest cause of diffuse peritoneal sepsis and is the disease from which primary peritonitis requires to be differentiated. Unfortunately the symptoms and signs of both conditions are essentially similar, and therefore a precise diagnosis can seldom be made with confidence. One should, however, be suspicious that primary peritonitis is the likely diagnosis when the abdominal findings of diffuse peritonitis occur in less than 24 hours from the onset of symptoms. Rapid onset, with severity of fever and local abdominal signs out of proportion to the short duration of the illness, favors a diagnosis of primary peritonitis. A history of associated nephrotic syndrome[32] or postnecrotic cirrhosis increases the confidence with which the diagnosis of primary peritonitis may be made, since the latter is a well-recognized complication of these diseases.

In infancy, the clinical situation is somewhat different, since spontaneous enteric perforation is the commonest cause of diffuse peritonitis and presents as a catastrophic event that evolves over a period of a few hours.[22] By comparison, primary peritonitis is more gradual in onset and slower in its development. Not infrequently the initial manifestations of primary peritonitis in this age group are merely the nonspecific signs associated with sepsis, such as poor feeding and lethargy. To these, over the course of 24 to 48 hours, is added the localizing sign of a doughy, distended abdomen. Frequently the neonate suffers from a major infection, often pneumonia, which precedes the peritonitis. Characteristically, the plain roentgenogram of the abdomen shows only nonspecific changes in primary peritonitis. Since spontaneous enteric perforation is commonly associated with free intraperitoneal air and other causes of generalized peritoneal sepsis may also present diagnostic features on radiologic examination, the fact that the roentgenogram is nondiagnostic favors a diagnosis of primary peritonitis.

Apart from the all-important bacteriological studies and the assistance that may be indirectly provided by abdominal roentgenograms, the laboratory is usually not of assistance in establishing a diagnosis of primary peritonitis. A significant polymorphonuclear leukocytosis occurs, but the same is true of other conditions from which differentiation is required. In patients with the nephrotic syndrome, severe proteinuria will be a prominent and helpful finding.

The most important single factor in the treatment of primary peritonitis is clearly the administration of the appropriate antibiotic along with the well-recognized supportive management of diffuse intraperitoneal suppuration, including intestinal decompression and parenteral fluid and electrolyte replacement. The role of surgery is restricted to diagnostic exploration whenever other intra-abdominal emergencies cannot be excluded. Theoretically, diagnostic paracentesis with immediate smear and Gram stain of the exudate should be the ideal procedure to establish a diagnosis of primary peritonitis. In such circumstances the presence of gram-positive cocci would constitute a contraindication to operation, while gram-negative organisms would imply that a surgically correctible lesion could not be excluded. In practice, initial diagnostic paracentesis is usually reserved for the two groups at greatest risk—the neonate with a nondiagnostic plain abdominal roentgenogram, and the child with the nephrotic syndrome. In all other circumstances the chances that a surgically correctible lesion exists are sufficiently great and the risk of operation is sufficiently small that diagnostic exploratory laparotomy is usually performed without preliminary paracentesis. However, if a diagnosis of primary peritonitis is being seriously entertained, some authors[22] would obtain sputum, urine, and rectal cultures, and initiate antibiotic therapy on the basis of microscopic examination of stained urine and sputum specimens (on the assumption that the infecting organism within the peritoneal cavity is likely to be identical to that in the urine or sputum) before embarking on diagnostic laparotomy. In any case, while opinions may differ as to the assignment of preoperative priorities, there is now general agreement as to the correct procedure once the abdomen has been opened and the diagnosis confirmed.

It is of prime importance that a specimen of peritoneal exudate be obtained for immediate Gram stain, in order to determine subsequent antibiotic therapy, and for culture. Although once considered to be contraindicated, appendectomy has not been shown to increase morbidity or mortality and is now universally recommended. Likewise, drainage of the peritoneal cavity, which was at one time considered essential, has now been shown to be not only unnecessary but actually harmful in that it increases morbidity.[10] Drainage is best omitted unless specifically indicated for the drainage of a localized abscess. Recently there has been increased advocacy of peritoneal lavage at the time of laparotomy for diffuse septic peritonitis, but this procedure has not yet gained universal acceptance.

Finally, the changing story of primary peritonitis is also mirrored in its markedly reduced morbidity and mortality rates.[10] In the preantibiotic era this condition carried a 50 per cent mortality rate. Now, with improved diagnostic measures and more effective antimicrobial therapy and supportive measures, a survival rate of about 90 per cent should be attainable in these desperately ill infants and children.

Bacterial Peritonitis Due to Hematogenous Spread

This entity is blood-borne from a known infection elsewhere in the body so that it is really a secondary peritonitis. It differs from contamination peritonitis in that it does not arise from a lesion in the vicinity of the peritoneum.

The source of the infection may or may not be apparent. Many surgeons believe that, in most patients, primary peritonitis is actually due to a hidden focus. Thus, it is really hematogenous and so belongs in this group.

The clinical features are identical to those which have been described for primary peritonitis. This disease, like primary peritonitis, should be treated conservatively when the diagnosis can be made.

Tuberculous Peritonitis[29, 30]

Tuberculous peritonitis was at one time fairly common and associated with a mortality of the order of 50 per cent. Fortunately, along with the overall decreased incidence of tuberculosis, it is now rarely seen, and improved chemotherapeutic measures have reduced the mortality to below 5 per cent. It is more common in the female and is most commonly manifest between the ages of 20 and 40 years. The infecting organism is *Mycobacterium tuberculosis*. Tuberculous peritonitis is invariably secondary to tuberculosis elsewhere. In over 97 per cent of subjects in autopsy series, a primary focus of the disease has been demonstrated. In clinical practice, however, the situation is quite different. In one recent series[29] only 6 per cent of patients with tuberculous peritonitis manifested a parenchymal tuberculous focus in the lung on roentgenography of the chest, although 32 per cent did demonstrate a pleural effusion, which was usually minimal. In addition, none of these patients revealed any abnormality on barium examination of the upper or lower intestinal tract, on intravenous urography, or on salpingography in the female.

Classically the disease is classified into acute and chronic forms, although in most patients the disease would more appropriately be referred to as subacute. On rare occasions acute generalized tuberculous peritonitis presents as one of the manifestations of an acute miliary tuberculous infection. More useful is the classification into moist and dry varieties of the disease, of which the former is much the more common.

In the moist form fever and progressive ascites, which may be massive, are the most consistent clinical features and are often accompanied by abdominal pain, anorexia, weight loss, and night sweats. Pain, while common, is usually not severe and tends to be diffuse and poorly localized. Occasionally, in the more acute case, the pain may be of such intensity as to mimic that seen in acute suppurative peritonitis. In the dry form the systemic manifestations are similar, but ascites is absent and masses of nodes and matted bowel frequently present as palpable intra-abdominal masses. An encysted subvariety of the disease is also recognized, which is a combination of both the moist and the dry forms. It presents as localized areas of encysted fluid that may readily be mistaken for other cystic lesions of the peritoneum.

Tubercles are present on the peritoneum in both varieties but may not be immediately apparent on gross examination because of fibrinous or purulent exudate, caseation, or fibrous adhesions. In the dry form, there is usually a dense inflammatory exudate and numerous adhesions matting coils of bowel together. Fecal fistula formation may occur in either type, either spontaneously or, more commonly, following operation, but is more frequent in the dry form. In children the fistula may communicate with the umbilicus. In the moist form the fluid is usually thin, has a green, yellow, or clear color, and may coagulate on standing. Its specific gravity is over 1.018 and its protein content over 4 per cent, which distinguishes it from a transudate. The cell count is variable, ranging from 150 to 2800 cells per cu. mm., with lymphocytes normally constituting over 70 per cent of the cells.

The diagnosis may be established in the moist form by examination of the peritoneal fluid for acid-fast bacilli. Direct smear techniques are seldom helpful and it is desirable to provide the laboratory with up to a liter of ascitic fluid for concentration and subsequent culture or guinea pig inoculation in order to assure positive confirmation. However, such bacteriologic studies are so time-consuming as to be of little assistance in establishing a diagnosis that is to form a basis for rational therapy. If laparotomy is performed the diagnosis may be rapidly established by histologic demonstration of typical caseating granulomas obtained by open peritoneal biopsy. Recently percutaneous peritoneal needle biopsy, without laparotomy, proved effective in establishing the diagnosis in 64 per cent of cases, and this figure was further improved through the use of peritoneoscopy.[29] These techniques are, of course, indicated only in the moist form of the disease. They apparently are associated with little morbidity or mortality if proper technique and surveillance are employed, but at least one fatality has been recorded.[19]

Treatment consists chiefly of general supportive measures for tuberculosis, which should ideally be carried out in a sanatorium. The use of the antituberculous drugs—streptomycin, para-aminosalicylic acid, and isonicotinic acid hydrazide—has dramatically altered the previously unfavorable prognosis, and death due to toxemia, extension of the tuberculous process, and amyloidosis is now rarely seen. Control of the acute manifestations of the ascitic form of the disease by this regimen may, however, enable the patient to survive and subsequently fall heir to intestinal obstruction due to the formation of dense fibrous adhesions. Adjunctive therapy with prednisone during the first 3 months of antituberculous drug therapy has been shown to reduce complicating adhesive intestinal obstruction.[29]

Operation should be avoided in the dry form of the disease except when intervention is made necessary because of intestinal obstruction. Fistula formation is a frequent and often disastrous complication under such circumstances. In the ascitic variety laparotomy, evacuation of fluid and biopsy of the peritoneum carry little risk, and there is some evidence from the predrug era that benefit may be derived from this procedure. However, most authorities would now agree that nonoperative management of both types of the disease is to be preferred when the diagnosis has been established and no specific indications for operation exist. When laparotomy has been carried out in the presence of tuberculous peritonitis, drainage and exteriorization of bowel should be avoided.

Aseptic Peritonitis

Aseptic peritonitis is important for two reasons: (1) a variety of sterile materials that may gain entrance to the peritoneal cavity are irritants and set up aseptic inflammatory reactions that give rise to sequelae and clinical symptoms; and (2) the chemical peritonitis produced by any of these substances may be followed by a superimposed bacterial peritonitis. Foreign bodies may reach the peritoneal cavity as a result of operative procedures, e.g, sponges, suture material, and instruments. They may result from penetrating injuries, with either the missile itself or material carried in with it, e.g., bits of clothing, acting as the irritant. In addition, the gastrointestinal and urinary tracts may be the source of fish bones, wood splinters, needles, pins, and glass. Such foreign bodies usually cause one of three types of reaction: bacterial inflammation in which the foreign body is incidental; aseptic inflammation, which usually results in a localized sterile abscess as the peritoneum walls off the foreign body; and a similar process with formation of a sinus or fistula. The relative amounts of exudation and fibrosis vary greatly with the nature of the foreign body.

The clinical manifestations of a sterile intraperitoneal foreign body are highly variable. A surgical sponge may give rise to an abscess, with a mass, fever, chills, and toxic manifestations; there are also legal implications. This type of foreign body must be removed. Intraperitoneal shrapnel, if sterile, may be simply walled off by fibrous tissue and give rise to few if any manifestations in the emotionally stable patient. The surgeon must guard against being persuaded by the patient to undertake a search for this type of foreign body, on the basis of vague subjective complaints.

Bile may ooze through the wall of a gallbladder that is distended but intact. More commonly, bile reaches the peritoneal cavity as a result of biliary tract rupture or as a sequel to operations on the biliary system. Sterile bile is a mild irritant in its own right, but should it become secondarily infected, it may give rise to a virulent type of peritonitis. To prevent this unfortunate sequel, the adequate routine drainage of Morison's hepatorenal space is recommended after biliary surgery or liver trauma.

Blood is only a mild irritant and it is slowly absorbed. However, blood in the peritoneal cavity may serve as a nidus for bacterial infection. For this reason, it should always be evacuated at the end of an operation. An oozing surface, capable of producing a hematoma, should be drained.

A most interesting entity is meconium or fetal peritonitis, which was first described by Sir James Young Simpson in 1838. The disease results from perforation of the bowel and inflammation of the peritoneal membrane due to sterile meconium. The perforation of the intestine may occur any time from the third fetal month to the neonatal period. It may result from meconium ileus, congenital bands, hernia, volvulus, or intussusception. If the opening is still present at birth or if perforation occurs after birth, secondary bacterial infection is the rule and the outlook in such cases is very poor.

Gastric juice is very irritating and the chemical peritonitis set up by a perforated ulcer is followed, after several hours, by bacterial infection. Sterile urine from traumatic intraperitoneal rupture of the bladder is also an irritating fluid and this chemical insult is frequently followed by secondary infection. These lesions must be diagnosed early and treated by appropriate operation.

Intraperitoneal pancreatic juice usually becomes infected and, in hemorrhagic pancreatitis, superadded bacterial infection should always be anticipated. Intensive antibiotic therapy deals adequately with this infection in most instances, but occasionally an abscess or collection will have to be drained 10 to 14 days after the onset.

Granulomatous Lesions of the Peritoneum

Separation of foreign body granulomas of the peritoneum from aseptic peritonitis due to foreign bodies is somewhat arbitrary. The basic pathologic process is the same—the response of the peritoneum to a noninfected irritant. The varying degrees of exudation and fibrosis distinguish the two reactions.

Some of the substances more commonly reported as causes of granulomatous reaction by the peritoneal membrane are talc, starch, Lycopodium spores, mineral oil, and silica. These etiologic agents are often introduced into the peritoneal cavity by the surgeon. In the past, granulomatous lesions due to talc were often seen, because this substance was widely used as a glove powder. Talc is composed mainly of hydrated magnesium silicate and incites a very intense fibroblastic reaction that may give rise to dense adhesions within a few weeks, or the process may take years. In an attempt to overcome this problem, powdered starch was introduced as a glove powder. The starch is made from either corn or rice and should be relatively innocuous because it is gradually absorbed by the peritoneum. Unfortunately, it has been found that starch may also give rise to a foreign body reaction, although less frequently and to a lesser degree than talc. It appears that soluble starch is the glove powder of choice at the present time. Gloves should be washed or wiped off before hands are put into the peritoneal cavity and care should be taken to avoid spillage of glove powder, should a glove be torn during an operation.

The gross appearance of these granulomatous lesions ranges from a studding of the serous membranes with nodules resembling tubercles or larger masses to the formation of dense fibrous adhesions. Microscopically, the reaction is seen to be the formation of a chronic granuloma. There may be monocytes, epithelioid cells, multinucleated giant cells, lymphocytes, plasma cells, fibroblasts, and sometimes areas of necrosis. Particles of the particular foreign material responsible can often be identified in the monocytes or giant cells by their characteristic appearance.

Recently, Tinker et al.[33] have described a rare but distinctive type of granulomatous peritonitis developing within the first month following operation; it is associated with signs and symptoms suggestive of a low-grade intra-abdominal inflammatory process, including leukocytosis with eosinophilia, and is characterized pathologically by a foreign body granulomatous reaction rich in eosinophils and associated with fragments of cellulose fiber. It appears that the cellulose is derived from surgical fabrics that have recently gained wide acceptance in the manufacture of disposable gowns and drapes for operating room use. Its occurrence is of particular concern, since cellulose is not normally broken down in the human body and therefore the natural history of such lesions is, as yet, undetermined. It would appear that cellulose lint should be added to the growing list of potentially hazardous peritoneal contaminants.

Adhesions and Bands

Adhesions are abnormal attachments between peritoneal surfaces; they may be either fibrinous or fibrous. A band is a long, narrow, fibrous adhesion.

Etiology. Most adhesions are inflammatory in origin and follow either a surgical operation or peritonitis. Some adhesions are thought to be congenital. Others are due to mechanical violence and foreign bodies, but for the most part they may be considered to be inflammatory. The amount of fibrin produced from the inflamed mesothelial surface of the peritoneum varies according to the chemical irritant or the microorganisms involved. If the action of the irritant is of only a few days' duration, the fibrin is usually absorbed. Intact mesothelium is necessary for resorption of fibrin. If the fibrinous adhesions are not absorbed for any reason, they are invaded by fibroblasts and capillaries and organization begins between 5 and 10 days after the initial insult. Factors favoring the development of fibrous adhesions following chemical or bacterial peritonitis include continuing action of the irritant, necrosis of the mesothelium due to intense action of the irritant, and a predisposition in certain persons that is not well understood.

A surgical operation promotes fibrinous exudation by mechanical factors, i.e., handling of viscera, sponges, instruments, foreign bodies, blood, and, in some instances, low-grade and unsuspected infection. Fibrinous adhesions become fibrous in postoperative

patients for the same reasons that they do in patients who have had peritonitis, but in the former there may be an additional factor of denudation of mesothelium—areas that are not adequately reperitonealized at the conclusion of operation. Fortunately, even fibrous adhesions may become attenuated and disappear in time. Formation of adhesions is a protective process, without which irritants could not be localized and abdominal surgery would be impossible. These beneficial effects should be considered before attempts are made to abolish adhesion formation by means of drugs and chemicals.

Pathology. The chief complication of adhesions and bands is intestinal obstruction. At the present time, this lesion has displaced external hernia as the most common single cause of mechanical intestinal obstruction. The adhesions and bands may involve intestine, mesentery, parietes, omentum, or any other abdominal structure. They are usually fibrous by the time they give rise to obstruction. Small bowel is most often obstructed, usually the distal ileum. This is probably because more inflammations and operations occur in the right lower quadrant than in any other location. Adhesions and bands obstruct the bowel by several mechanisms. Adhesions, by contracture of the fibrous tissue, may kink, compress, or otherwise distort the bowel to cause a nonstrangulating obstruction. A pocket may form into which bowel prolapses, or a narrow aperture may be produced through which a loop of bowel may herniate. A band may also serve as a pivot point for a volvulus.

Prior to the availability of antibiotics, a blend of paralytic ileus and mechanical obstruction frequently followed operations for perforated appendicitis with peritonitis. Today, this is a rare complication and when it does occur the extent of the mechanical obstruction can be accurately assessed by the oral administration of sodium diatrizoate solution followed by roentgenographic studies of the small bowel.

Symptoms and Signs. Adhesions may produce symptoms other than those of intestinal obstruction, but this happens rarely, and such a diagnosis should be made with reservations. The great majority of patients present with a mechanical small bowel obstruction and an abdominal scar. The obstruction may be strangulating or nonstrangulating, a differentiation that frequently cannot be made with assurance on clinical grounds.

Prevention. There is no reliable way by which the formation of adhesions can be prevented, even if it were desirable to do so. The most a surgeon can hope to accomplish is the reduction of adhesion formation to a minimum. Of all the methods that have been tried to minimize adhesions, nothing has been shown to be as worthwhile as careful attention to the details of surgical technique.

All denuded areas should be reperitonealized; attention should be paid to hemostasis, and blood should be evacuated from the peritoneal cavity at the end of the operation; tissues should be handled gently; warm, moist sponges and padded retractors should be used; preoperative bowel preparation by mechanical cleansing and enteric antibiotics and sulfonamides before intestinal surgery is helpful; the area about an open viscus should be packed off and spillage should be avoided, and drains should be used when indicated but should be removed as soon as it is safe to do so. Local use of sulfonamides and antibiotics has no advantage over systemic administration and these chemicals may act as foreign bodies and irritants.

Treatment. When a mechanical small bowel obstruction develops within a week or 10 days after operation, or after peritonitis without surgical operation, and one believes that the obstruction is due to fibrinous adhesions, the patient may be treated with supportive measures and introduction of a long intestinal tube. The patient must be watched carefully and, if there is no response to this management, operative intervention may be necessary. As a rule, the tube will pass through the small bowel and the obstruction will be relieved. In cases of mechanical small bowel obstruction due to fibrous adhesions, the patient will require an operation. Supportive measures and the use of the long tube are part of the preoperative preparation and not a substitute for operation. In patients with a predisposition to form adhesions, ordinary methods of prophylaxis and treatment will prove futile. The most satisfactory solution to this problem is to recognize that in a patient of this kind adhesions will inevitably re-form, and to replace haphazard adhesions with an organized pattern of nonobstructing adhesions such as one obtains with the Noble plication procedure.

HEMOPERITONEUM

Hemoperitoneum may be either traumatic or spontaneous. The trauma may be trivial, especially if bleeding comes from a previously diseased organ. Delayed hemorrhage from nonpenetrating trauma to the abdomen may also occur. The lesions that may cause spontaneous hemoperitoneum include ectopic pregnancy; blood dyscrasias; rupture of an artery that is the seat of a degenerative process; torsion of omentum, spleen, fibroid tumor, or ovarian cyst; mesenteric vascular occlusion; and pancreatitis. The most probable source of a large amount of blood in the male is rupture of the spleen. In the female of childbearing age, it is ectopic pregnancy. Hemorrhage should be controlled and the blood evacuated. Blood in the peritoneal cavity is a much greater hazard to the patient than any possible benefit that might accrue from having this blood as a source of iron.

PNEUMOPERITONEUM

Pneumoperitoneum is the presence of gas within the peritoneal cavity. The detection of free intraperitoneal gas is of great value in the diagnosis of a perforated abdominal viscus. There are, however, other important causes of pneumoperitoneum, which are included in the following etiologic classification:

1. From within the Lumen of the Gastrointestinal Tract
    Perforated peptic ulcer
    Other perforative disease
    Blunt and penetrating trauma to the abdomen
    Endoscopic instrumentation
    Infections
    Postanesthetic
2. From outside the Lumen of the Gastrointestinal Tract
    Postoperative
    Diagnostic
      Rubin Test
      Needle
    Therapeutic
    Penetrating trauma
3. Idiopathic

Perforated Viscus. Perforated peptic ulcer is the commonest disease process producing pneumoperitoneum. The demonstration of free intraperitoneal air in a patient with an acute abdomen usually indicates a perforation of the gastrointestinal tract.

Demonstrable pneumoperitoneum occurs in the majority of patients with perforated peptic ulcers. The detection of air depends upon many factors, including the time elapsed since perforation, the location and size of the perforation, the effectiveness of reaction in walling off the perforation, the amount of air in the stomach at the time of perforation, and the amount swallowed subsequently.

Benign and malignant ulcerating lesions and obstructing lesions in which perforation of the gastrointestinal tract occasionally occurs may produce pneumoperitoneum. Diastatic perforation of the cecum typically results in a very extensive degree of pneumoperitoneum.

Free gas in the peritoneal cavity seeks the highest level and, in the upright position, tends to accumulate under the diaphragm. Although absence of liver dullness in the midaxillary line is clinically indicative of pneumoperitoneum, accurate detection requires careful radiologic examination (Fig. 18). A few cubic

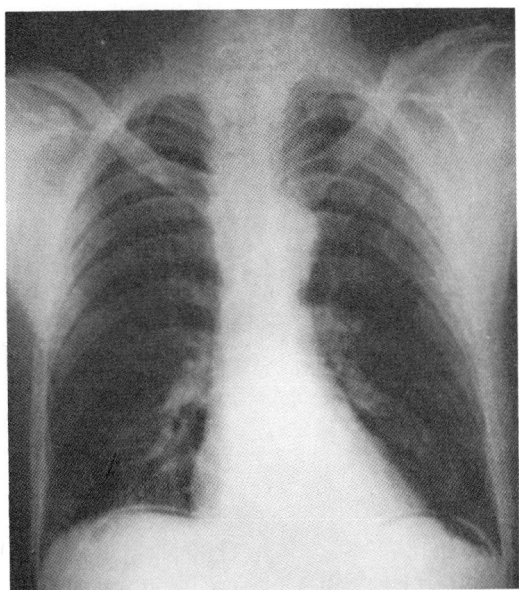

Figure 18. Posteroanterior x-ray of chest, showing a thin rim of free air beneath both leaves of the diaphragm. The patient has a perforated peptic ulcer, the most common cause of pneumoperitoneum other than laparotomy.

centimeters of air may be seen on a scout film of the abdomen if sufficient time is allowed for the gas to collect in whatever part of the cavity is uppermost. Erect and left lateral decubitus views are commonly used.

Traumatic. Pneumoperitoneum following blunt trauma to the abdomen indicates a perforated viscus. Pneumoperitoneum following a penetrating or perforating abdominal wound reveals only peritoneal entrance, since air may enter with the missile. Visceral involvement, however, is common if the peritoneum is entered, and the detection of free intraperitoneal air is a positive indication for laparotomy.

Accidental. Instrumental visualization of abdominal organs, often accompanied by air insufflation, may perforate a normal or diseased viscus and produce pneumoperitoneum. Perforation during sigmoidoscopy under direct vision is rare. Pneumoperitoenum occasionally follows gastroscopy, but usually gross perforation is not found at laparotomy. In the absence of clinical peritonitis, these patients have been successfully treated conservatively.

Bacterial. Certain gas-forming organisms may cause pneumoperitoneum in an intra-abdominal abscess. *Clostridium welchii* and related bacteria are the commonest infecting organisms that produce gas, but *Escherichia coli*, anaerobic streptococci, and Proteus have also occasionally been cultured. The formation of gas in an abdominal abscess may be a valuable aid in diagnosis and localization.

Postanesthetic. Pneumoperitoneum following operation is occasionally related to anesthesia. Excessive airway pressure during assisted respiration, or rapid oxygen flow through a nasal catheter, may produce gastric dilatation and, rarely, gastric perforation. Intraperitoneal gas following anesthesia is not always associated with perforation or peritonitis; the gas may diffuse beneath the mucosa along the vessels of the stomach into the peritoneal cavity.

Postoperative. The most frequent cause of pneumoperitoneum is abdominal surgery. The peritoneal cavity is normally a potential space in which there is a negative pressure. When the peritoneum is opened at operation, an inrush of air may be noted. The duration of postoperative pneumoperitoneum is variable; small quantities of air are usually absorbed within a few days. In the majority of patients, the air has disappeared by 14 days, but rarely it may persist for as long as 6 weeks.

There is no apparent correlation between pneumoperitoneum and postoperative pulmonary complications. The presence of intraperitoneal air following operation may confuse the assessment of postoperative abdominal complications.

Diagnostic. Direct injection of gas into the peritoneal cavity to outline the abdominal and pelvic organs has been used in selected patients as an aid in the radiologic diagnosis. The potential communication between the peritoneal cavity and the exterior existing in the normal female, via the fallopian tubes and the uterine cavity, is utilized in the Rubin test.

Therapeutic. Artificial pneumoperitoneum has been used in the treatment of pulmonary and abdominal tuberculosis for many years. Five hundred to 1000 cc. of air or oxygen is injected directly into the peritoneal cavity with periodic refills. Elevation of the diaphragms with reduction of pulmonary volume tends to promote collapse of tuberculous cavities, particularly if they are located in the base of the lungs. This treatment, often combined with phrenicectomy and chemotherapy, is considered of value in some instances. Another use therapeutically is the preparation for operation of the patient with a very large ventral hernia. The air is introduced into the peritoneal cavity while the hernia is under control with strapping. This has been a very useful procedure in selected cases.

Idiopathic or Undetermined Cause. Spontaneous idiopathic pneumoperitoneum occurs rarely with no demonstrable perforation of a viscus, known exogenous cause, or underlying disease process. It produces few clinical manifestations and usually subsides without ill effect.

TUMORS

The great majority of peritoneal tumors are secondary. Primary tumors of the peritoneum or of any serous membrane are very rare.

Primary Tumors

Neoplasms may arise from any of the fibrous, fatty, vascular, or reticular tissues that lie beneath the peritoneal mesothelium, but such are best regarded as tumors of the viscera, parietes, or retroperitoneum. Although it is very rare, most pathologists agree that the primary peritoneal mesothelioma is a recognizable entity. Both benign and malignant varieties of mesothelioma exist. The lesions may be localized or diffuse and they occur in plaquelike and nodular forms. The tumor may spread over and encompass the viscera, producing fibrous thickening of the peritoneum and shortening of the mesentery. Viscid ascites is the commonest presenting symptom, although intestinal obstruction and total obliteration of the peritoneal cavity have occasionally been reported. Even malignant forms do not invade until late and seldom metastasize.

The neoplasm may have the microscopic appearance of a papillary, fibrous, acinar, or even squamous cell tumor. It is very difficult for the pathologist to establish the diagnosis on the basis of examination of ascitic fluid or a small amount of biopsy material.

The benign form, if localized, can be effectively treated by surgical excision.

Secondary Tumors

Most secondary tumors of the peritoneum are metastatic carcinomas. The malignant tumor reaches the peritoneal surface by permeation through the wall of a viscus, by hematogenous or lymphatic spread, or, occasionally, by inoculation at the time of surgery. Once in the peritoneal cavity, tumor may be widely disseminated over the serosal surface as a result of transperitoneal seeding.

The gross appearance of secondary tumors varies widely, according to the primary lesion and the mode of spread. The main features are ascites and tumor nodules. The ascitic fluid is usually bloody and often contains exfoliated tumor cells. The tumor nodules range from minute deposits, a millimeter or less in diameter, studded diffusely over the peritoneal membrane, to large plaques and masses of neoplastic tissue. As a rule, they are less than a centimeter in diameter. The omentum may be so infiltrated with tumor that it is converted into a hard mass. There may be drop metastases to the cul-de-sac, giving rise to a rectal shelf. Sometimes a reticular pattern of white lymphatics, permeated with tumor, is seen beneath the serosa. It may be difficult to distinguish grossly the nodular lesions of secondary peritoneal tumor from those of tuberculosis, fat necrosis, or foreign body granuloma.

Not all secondary tumors are malignant. One benign secondary lesion is the parasitic fibroid, a leiomyoma that has become detached from the uterus and taken up a new attachment on the peritoneal surface. Similarly, dermoid cysts of the ovary sometimes become secondarily attached to peritoneum.

An interesting form of secondary tumor of the peritoneum is pseudomyxoma peritonei, which arises from rupture of a pseudomucinous cystadenoma of the ovary or rarely of the appendix.[20] A lesion of similar appearance may be produced by rupture of a mucocele of the appendix, in which case the mucus acts as an irritant and produces chemical peritonitis. The mucus-producing cells become implanted on the peritoneum and continue to produce a gelatinous exudate, causing the so-called jelly belly.

The patient with metastases to the peritoneum usually has advanced symptoms of the primary lesion. He may complain of pain, discomfort, or cardiorespiratory symptoms from abdominal distention. Cachexia, pallor, and ascites are often present when the patient is seen for the first time. One may palpate tumor tissue in the form of a primary lesion, a Virchow's node, liver nodules, an omental mass, or a rectal shelf.

If there is no evidence of metastatic malignancy other than the ascites, abdominal fluid may be examined cytologically. This examination is subject to the limitations inherent in the cytologic method.

MESENTERIES AND OMENTUM

ANATOMY AND PHYSIOLOGY

The stomach, jejunoileum, appendix, transverse colon, sigmoid colon, liver, and spleen are attached to the posterior wall of the abdominal cavity by mesenteries, which carry their respective blood vessels, lymphatics, and lymph nodes. The gastrohepatic ligament is the ventral mesentery of the stomach and first part of the duodenum, but it is also, in a sense, a dorsal mesentery of the liver and gallbladder. The gastrocolic ligament is continuous with the anterior layer of the greater omentum. The mesentery of the jejunoileum is described as fan-shaped, averaging 12 to 25 cm. in height. Its junction with parietal peritoneum is only 15 cm. long, whereas its other border, where it enfolds small bowel, is about 700 cm. in length. This marked disparity in the lengths of its two borders can only be reconciled by numerous folds toward the enteric border. All mesenteries consist of two layers of mesothelium enclosing a variable amount of fatty and loose connective tissue, vessels, and lymph nodes.

The mesenteries of the duodenum, pancreas, ascending colon, and descending colon have disappeared in fetal life because of fusion with parietal peritoneum. Fortunately for the surgeon, these planes of fusion can usually be converted into planes of cleavage, restoring the primitive state. The mesentery thus created has only one layer of mesothelium, the posterior parietal peritoneum, but it carries in its fatty areolar tissue the blood vessels, lymphatics, and lymph nodes of the organ in question.

The greater omentum is a double fold of mesentery embryologically. One might expect it to contain four mesothelial layers, but the central two have fused and vanished. The size and fat content of the greater omentum are highly variable. Its role as the "abdominal policeman" seems well supported by experimental and clinical evidence. The areolar tissue of the omentum is rich in macrophages. Bacteria or carbon particles injected into the peritoneal cavity are rapidly removed by the omentum and are subsequently seen to be situated in phagocytes beneath its mesothelium. The ability of the omentum to adhere to sites of inflammation and perforation is well known. Foreign bodies in the peritoneal cavity, such as a bullet or a sponge, are often found completely wrapped in omentum.

The presence of the greater omentum is not always beneficial. Adhesions and bands between the omentum and either parietes or viscera, or openings made in the omentum at surgical operations, may lead to intestinal obstruction. Once a patient has had some such difficulty originating in the omentum, surgical excision of the omentum will circumvent further complications.

MESENTERIC LYMPHADENITIS

Acute Nonspecific Mesenteric Lymphadenitis[8]

Over the past 30 years, this disease has been distinguished from tuberculous lymphadenitis and has gradually gained wide acceptance as a clinical entity. Its chief importance lies in the fact that it produces the picture of an acute abdomen and must be considered in the differential diagnosis of appendicitis.

Acute nonspecific mesenteric lymphadenitis is uncommon and, in our experience, the incidence is diminishing. Most patients are between 5 and 15 years of age, and it is somewhat more frequent in boys.

The etiology is unknown and there may be more than one cause. Cultures from the enlarged mesenteric lymph nodes are usually negative. Associated low-grade inflammatory changes in the appendix and distal ileum have been reported in a large proportion of cases and may have a bearing on the etiology.

The appendix is grossly normal. There is discrete enlargement of the mesenteric lymph nodes in the ileocecal angle, particularly those in the juxtaintestinal group. Lymph nodes in this region are prominent in children, and normal lymph nodes must be distinguished from those which are pathologic. The nodes vary from soft and pink in the early stage of the disease to firm and white later. Microscopically, the lymph nodes show only hyperplasia, edema, and hyperemia.

The child with acute nonspecific mesenteric lymphadenitis usually presents with colicky abdominal pain vaguely situated about the umbilicus, right side, or right lower quadrant. The pain is of variable intensity, but in between the cramps the child feels fairly well. There is often a recent upper respiratory infection, which may still be present. There is a history of previous attacks, separated by intervals of several months, in over half the cases. Malaise, anorexia, nausea, and vomiting are also frequently present or reported in earlier attacks.

The child does not look or act ill. There is fever, usually under 38° C. The patient is flushed and there may be circumoral pallor. The pharynx is often injected and the cervical lymph nodes may be enlarged. Abdominal tenderness is higher, more medial, less well localized, and more variable from one time to another than in appendicitis. A shift in the point of maximal tenderness to the left when the child lies on the left side, due to change in position of the mesentery and nodes, is said to be characteristic but is often absent. The white blood count may be increased to 10,000 to 15,000 per cu. mm.

Indiscriminate appendectomy cannot be condoned. However, if one suspects acute appendicitis the matter should be settled by laparotomy. On the other hand, if one can be reasonably confident of a diagnosis of mesenteric adenitis, a few hours of observation may be confirmatory. The signs and symptoms of this latter disease will subside or improve in less than 24 hours.

If, at laparotomy, one finds a normal appendix and the characteristic lymphadenopathy in the ileocecal angle, appendectomy should be carried out. It is not advisable to remove a lymph node for biopsy, because bowel may become adherent to the site. Postoperative respiratory complications should be anticipated. A small proportion of these patients may have further attacks after appendectomy, but there is an overall tendency toward recovery.

Tuberculous Mesenteric Lymphadenitis

Involvement of mesenteric lymph nodes by tubercle bacilli is now uncommon. The disease may be primary, in which case the organisms, usually bovine, gain entry through intact mucosa of Peyer's patches and then reach the nodes. The disease may be secondary to tuberculosis of lungs or bowel.

Tubercle formation, caseation, and eventually calcification are present as in tuberculous lymphadenitis elsewhere. The disease may be complicated by peritoneal adhesions, tuberculous peritonitis, or secondary pyogenic infection.

The disease is seen in acute and chronic forms and its manifestations are highly variable. The salient features are fever, general ill health, weight loss, diarrhea, and cramping abdominal pain.

X-ray examination of the abdomen in a clinically well person may show calcified lymph nodes in the right iliac fossa — the so-called chalky tombstones of tubercle bacilli, which may or may not be dead.

In general, the treatment should be conservative, with antituberculous drugs and supportive measures.

INFARCTION OF THE OMENTUM

Infarction of the greater omentum may be due to torsion, thrombosis, polyarteritis nodosa, embolism, or trauma or may be of unknown etiology.

Idiopathic segmental infarction of the omentum is rare.[21] It is most often found in well nourished men in the third decade. The cause is obscure, but it is thought to be related to venous engorgement and mild trauma, or increase in intra-abdominal pressure lead-ing to thrombosis. Usually, the right, lower, free margin of the omentum is infarcted.

Patients present with steady, severe right lower quadrant pain, the onset of which may be gradual or sudden. Nausea and vomiting are unusual. On examination, the tenderness is usually higher than one would expect for appendicitis and a mass may be palpable. Cutaneous hyperesthesia is said to be characteristic.

The correct diagnosis is never made preoperatively; most cases are diagnosed as acute appendicitis. The finding of a normal appendix and some serosanguineous fluid in the peritoneal cavity should always direct one's attention to disease elsewhere. The infarcted area forms a firm, red to purplish black mass. Treatment is wide excision of the involved omentum.

TORSION OF THE OMENTUM

Torsion of the omentum may be classified as primary and secondary. Secondary torsion is more common and is subdivided into bipolar and unipolar types, depending on whether or not there is a secondary fixation of the omentum. Among the causes are hernias, adhesions, cysts, and tumors.

In primary torsion of the omentum there is no apparent cause, although vigorous exercise, movement of the omentum by intestinal peristalsis, and hemodynamic forces have been blamed. The torsion is always unipolar and may be either complete or incomplete. In the complete type, there may be up to six full turns. The omentum is usually quite large and fatty with a long pedicle and a narrow attachment. It is often the right, free margin of the omentum that is involved in the torsion.

The clinical symptoms and treatment of torsion of the omentum are similar to those of infarction of the omentum.

APPENDICES EPIPLOICAE

The appendices epiploicae are fat-laden pouches of peritoneum found on the large bowel and, rarely, on the appendix. They are usually arranged in two rows, one medial to the taenia libera and one lateral to the taenia omentalis. These are the sites at which some of the vessels enter the bowel wall. One will recall that diverticula also are situated in these positions.

The appendices epiploicae may be the sites of a number of diseases, the most common of which is epiploic appendicitis. This may be due to torsion or thrombosis and so may be regarded as a miniature counterpart of torsion and infarction of the omentum. Epiploic appendicitis is found chiefly in the sigmoid and cecal regions. Other disease processes in which the appendices epiploicae may be involved include acute and chronic inflammation secondary to diverticulitis, degeneration to form an intraperitoneal loose body, initiation of an intussusception, and incarceration in a hernia.

The presenting symptom of epiploic appendicitis is lower abdominal pain on either the right or left side.

The correct diagnosis is seldom made preoperatively. Treatment is excision with care not to open up a diverticulum.

RETROPERITONEUM

ANATOMY

The retroperitoneal space from the surgeon's viewpoint is a potential space extending from the respiratory diaphragm above to the pelvic diaphragm below. Its posterior boundaries are the vertebral bodies, the psoas and quadratus lumborum muscles, and the origin of the transversus abdominis muscle from the lumbar fascia. Below the iliac crests, it is bounded by the sacrum and the psoas and piriformis muscles posteriorly, and by the iliacus and obturator internus muscles laterally. The anterior boundary of the retroperitoneal space is chiefly the posterior parietal peritoneum, but in addition the anterior boundary is made up of the posterior surface of the liver, the ascending and descending portions of the large intestine, the retroperitoneal portion of the duodenum, and the rectum.

The major organs of the retroperitoneal space are the kidneys and ureters, the adrenals, and the pancreas. The space is also occupied by the great systemic vessels and their branches, veins of the portal system, lymphatic vessels and lymph nodes, somatic nerves, sympathetic chains and autonomic plexuses, and an abundance of fatty and areolar connective tissue.

RETROPERITONEAL FIBROSIS[12, 13, 24]

Retroperitoneal fibrosis is a disease of infrequent occurrence, although recent literature would suggest that either the disease or its recognition is occurring with increased frequency. In most cases the etiology remains obscure. Recent evidence would suggest that it may represent a hypersensitivity angiitis. There is, however, little doubt that methysergide (an ergot derivative) therapy, for migraine headaches, is an etiologic factor in up to 25 per cent of cases.[12]

Grossly, retroperitoneal fibrosis presents as a flat, firm, gray-white fibrous plaque of varying thickness. It most commonly occurs in the region of the sacral promontory but may extend upward to the renal pedicles or even into the mediastinum and downward into the true pelvis. It is usually sharply delineated but not encapsulated. As it extends it envelops and obstructs the structures of the retroperitoneal space but without invasion of their walls. Typically, bilateral ureteral encasement eventually takes place.

The clinical symptoms often include constant dull, aching pain in the low back and lower abdomen, fatigue, malaise, anorexia with nausea and vomiting, and weight loss. They tend to parallel the degree of azotemia. Urinary symptoms may be absent or there may be increased urine output as bilateral hydronephrosis develops. The most dramatic presenting symptom may be anuria. A typical triad of diagnostic features is usually seen on intravenous urography consisting of (1) hydronephrosis with dilated and tortuous upper ureters, (2) medial deviation of the ureters, and (3) evidence of extrinsic ureteral compression.[13]

A trial of nonoperative treatment is warranted in patients with minimal impairment of renal function who have been receiving methysergide. The drug is discontinued and steroid therapy with prednisone initiated. On occasion, obstructive changes resolve rapidly and completely. Most patients will, however, require operative therapy. Usually this takes the form of primary simultaneous transperitoneal bilateral ureterolysis, although some patients will require preliminary nephrostomy when renal damage is advanced and azotemia marked. Nephrectomy is resorted to only when one kidney has been totally destroyed and the other exhibits normal function.

RETROPERITONEAL TUMORS[3]

It is customary to exclude tumors of the kidneys, ureters, adrenals, pancreas, and bowel as well as metastatic tumors to the retroperitoneal lymph nodes from the group of neoplasms designated as retroperitoneal tumors. The classification of Ackerman has been widely adopted in relation to these "primary" retroperitoneal neoplasms. It includes, as major groups, (1) tumors of mesodermal origin, (2) tumors of neurogenous origin, and (3) a miscellaneous group comprising alveolar soft part sarcoma, urogenital ridge tumors, and tumors arising from embryonic remnants. The major groups have multiple subgroups and, in theory at least, most are represented by benign and malignant variants.

In large series, such as that reported by Pack and Tabah, approximately 80 per cent of retroperitoneal tumors prove to be malignant. The most common malignant tumors are of the lymphoma group: lymphosarcoma, Hodgkin's disease, and reticulum cell sarcoma, in order of decreasing frequency. The second most common malignant tumor in most series is the liposarcoma—a noteworthy oddity, since elsewhere in the body benign fatty tumors are quite common while malignant fatty tumors are almost unknown. The series of Braasch and Mon[3] is unusual in that fibrosarcoma proved to be the second commonest malignant tumor. Other relatively common malignant tumors include the leiomyosarcoma, the undifferentiated embryonal carcinomas and mesenchymal sarcomas, and malignant tumors of nervous tissue origin.

Because the retroperitoneum is a distensible space, these tumors may reach very large size before they are diagnosed, and fully one third of the malignant tumors have already metastasized when first seen. About half of the patients present with abdominal pain and one third are aware of the presence of an abdominal mass. Less commonly gastrointestinal symptoms, backache, pain and swelling in the leg, genitourinary symptoms, and fever are early symptoms.

The most common physical finding is a nontender abdominal mass, which may be movable or fixed, and which is usually ballotable from the flank. Varicocele, edema or varicosities of a leg, forward displacement of the liver, lumbar dullness on percussion, and neurologic deficits are occasionally present.

The chief laboratory aid is the roentgenogram, and the most important investigation is usually the intravenous urogram with anteroposterior and lateral views to demonstrate displacement of the kidney and ureter. It is important that the function of each kidney also be assessed, since one kidney may need to be sacrificed at operation in order to encompass the lesion. The next most important radiologic procedure is a gastrointestinal series. Presacral oxygen, or carbon dioxide, insufflation may be useful to outline the contents of the retroperitoneal area. Aortography and venography may be useful, as the great vessels are often displaced.

Surgical intervention is mandatory in virtually every patient to establish a definitive diagnosis by open biopsy and to assess operability. Unfortunately, most retroperitoneal tumors will have surrounded or invaded major organs or vessels by the time operation is performed. Wide excision with hope of cure is possible in only about 20 per cent of patients, and the operative mortality ranges from 10 to 25 per cent.

Malignant lymphomas are radiosensitive and are best treated by this means following biopsy. Virtually all other malignant retroperitoneal tumors are radioresistant, and the only hope for long survival depends on wide surgical excision. Close cooperation between the surgeon and the pathologist is necessary in order to determine the nature and curability of the lesion and the extent of surgical extirpation that is justified. Virtually every patient presents a unique challenge and requires careful individual evaluation once the lesion has been exposed. Total removal not infrequently requires en bloc excision of adjacent organs, most usually the kidney and, on occasion, even the vena cava below the renal veins. Notwithstanding the reported radioresistance of the tumors that are not of the lymphoma class, all patients in whom only biopsy or partial excision can be performed should receive postoperative radiation therapy, since a number of unexpected long-term survivals have been reported.

SELECTED REFERENCES

Ackerman, L. V.: Tumors of the Retroperitoneum, Mesentery and Peritoneum. Atlas of Tumor Pathology, Section VI, Fascicles 23 and 24. Washington, D.C., Armed Forces Institute of Pathology, 1954.

This monograph, although concerned primarily with the pathologic aspects of tumors, constitutes the classic reference on this subject for the clinician. It consists largely of excellent illustrations, some of which are in color, and includes a succinct, very readable text in which the essential clinical aspects of the various new growths occurring in these areas are summarized.

Cullen, T. S.: Embryology, Anatomy and Diseases of the Umbilicus Together with Diseases of the Urachus. Philadelphia, W. B. Saunders Company, 1916.

Although more than 60 years old, Cullen's book continues to be the classic in its field. Doubtless its value and its appeal are much enhanced by the beautiful illustrations by Max Brödel. While the treatment of many of the diseases occurring in this area has changed since Cullen's time, the lucid presentation of the embryology and anatomy of the region has not been surpassed and the descriptions of disease are as timely as when they were written.

Pack, G. T., and Tabah, E. J.: Primary retroperitoneal tumors. A study of 120 cases. Int. Abstr. Surg., 99:209, 313, 1945.

This 47-page collective review with its 261 references is the most exhaustive clinical review of the subject in the English literature. It leads one to virtually every relevant publication on the subject in the world literature up to the time of its publication. In spite of the 32 years since its publication, it continues to be an authoritative source of current practice, since significant contributions to new knowledge in this area are meager indeed.

REFERENCES

1. Bardeen, C. R., and Lewis, W. H.: The development of the limbs, body-wall, and back. Am. J. Anat., 1:1, 1901–1902.
2. Blichert-Toft, M., Koch, F., and Nielsen, O. V.: Anatomic variants of the urachus relating to clinical appearance and surgical treatment of urachal lesions. Surg. Gynecol. Obstet., 137:51, 1973.
3. Braasch, J. W., and Mon, A. B.: Primary retroperitoneal tumors. Surg. Clin. North Am., 47:663, 1967.
4. Brasfield, R. D., and Das Gupta, T. K.: Desmoid tumors of the anterior abdominal wall. Surgery, 65:241, 1969.
5. Bremer, J. L.: Congenital Anomalies of the Viscera: Their Embryological Basis. Cambridge, Mass., Harvard University Press, 1957.
6. Brödel, M.: Lesions of the rectus abdominis muscle simulating an acute intra-abdominal condition. I. Anatomy of the rectus muscle. Bull. Johns Hopkins Hosp., 61:295, 1937.
7. Cullen, T. S.: Lesions of the rectus abdominis muscle simulating an acute intra-abdominal condition. II. Hemorrhage into or beneath the rectus muscle simulating an acute abdominal condition. Bull. Johns Hopkins Hosp., 61:317, 1937.
8. Donhauser, J. L.: Primary acute mesenteric lymphadenitis. Arch. Surg., 74:528, 1957.
9. Fothergill, W. E.: Haematoma in the abdominal wall simulating pelvic new growth. Br. Med. J., 1:941, 1926.
10. Fowler, R.: Primary peritonitis: Changing aspects 1956–1970. Aust. Paediatr. J., 7:73, 1971.
11. Grosfeld, J. L., and Franken, E. A.: Intestinal obstruction in the neonate due to vitelline duct cysts. Surg. Gynecol. Obstet., 138:527, 1974.
12. Hewitt, C. B., Nitz, G. L., Kiser, W. S., Straffon, R. A., and Stewart, B. H.: Surgical treatment of retroperitoneal fibrosis. Ann. Surg., 169:610, 1969.
13. Hoffman, W. W., and Trippel, O. H.: Retroperitoneal fibrosis: Etiological considerations. J. Urol., 86:222, 1961.
14. Jamieson, R. A.: Spontaneous rupture of the muscles of the abdomen. Br. J. Surg., 36:434, 1949.
15. Johnson, F. R., and Whitting, H. W.: Repair of parietal peritoneum. Br. J. Surg., 49:653, 1962.
16. Kessler, R. E., Tice, D. A., and Zimmon, D. S.: Value, complications, and limitations of umbilical vein catheterization. Surg. Gynecol. Obstet., 136:529, 1973.
17. Kling, S.: Patent omphalomesenteric duct—a surgical emergency. Arch. Surg., 96:545, 1968.
18. Lampe, E. W.: Surgical anatomy of the abdominal wall. Surg. Clin. North Am., 32:545, 1952.
19. Levine, H.: Needle biopsy in diagnosis of tuberculous peritonitis. Am. Rev. Resp. Dis., 98:519, 1968.
20. Long, R. T. L., Spratt, J. S., Jr., and Dowling, E.: Pseudomyxoma peritonei: New concepts in management with a report of seventeen patients. Am. J. Surg., 117:162, 1969.
21. MacKenzie, W. C., and Small, J.: Primary idiopathic segmental infarction of the greater omentum. Can. Med. Assoc. J., 55:144, 1946.
22. McDougal, W. S., Izant, R. J., and Zollinger, R. M., Jr.: Primary peritonitis in infancy and childhood. Ann. Surg., 181:310, 1975.
23. Murray, S. D., and Burger, R. E.: Rupture of the inferior epigastric vessels. Ann. Surg., 139:90, 1954.
24. Ormond, J. K.: Bilateral ureteral obstruction due to envelopment and compression by an inflammatory retroperitoneal process. J. Urol., 59:1072, 1948.
25. Pack, G. T., and Ehrlich, H. E.: Neoplasms of the anterior abdominal wall with special consideration of desmoid tumors. Int. Abstr. Surg., 79:177, 1944.
26. Paul, M.: The surgery of the congenital anomalies of the midline ventral abdominal wall. Ann. R. Coll. Surg. Eng., 13:313, 1953.
27. Robinson, S. C.: Observations on the peritoneum as an absorbing surface. Am. J. Obstet. Gynecol., 83:446, 1962.
28. Silverman, F. N., and Huang, N.: Congenital absence of the abdominal muscles. Am. J. Dis. Child., 80:91, 1950.
29. Singh, M. M., Bhargava, A. N., and Jain, K. P.: Tuberculous peritonitis: An evaluation of pathogenic mechanisms, diagnostic procedures and therapeutic measures. N. Engl. J. Med., 281:1091, 1969.
30. Sochocky, S.: Tuberculous peritonitis: A review of 100 cases. Am. Rev. Resp. Dis., 95:398, 1967.

31. Soutar, S. F., Douglas, D. M., and Dennison, W. M.: Patent vi-
    tello-intestinal duct: The risk of obstruction due to prolapse.
    Br. J. Surg., 45:617, 1958.
32. Speck, W. T., Dresdale, S. S., and McMillan, R. W.: Primary peri-
    tonitis and the nephrotic syndrome. Am. J. Surg., 127:267,
    1974.
33. Tinker, M. A., Burdman, D., Deysine, M., Teicher, I., Platt, N.,

    and Aufses, A. H., Jr.: Granulomatous peritonitis due to
    cellulose fibers from disposable surgical fabrics: Laboratory
    investigation and clinical implications. Ann. Surg., 180:831,
    1974.
34. Trimingham, H. L., and McDonald, J. R.: Congenital anomalies in
    the region of the umbilicus. Surg. Gynecol. Obstet., 80:152,
    1945.

MESENTERIC CYSTS

Frank T. Kurzweg, M.D.

Mesenteric cysts are uncommon enough to excite interest but common enough to come within the experience of most general surgeons. They were first recognized when an autopsy case was recorded in 1507 by a Florentine anatomist, Benevieni. In 1842, Rokitansky described a chylous cyst, but until 1850, all cases reported were only found at postmortem examination. From 1850 to 1880, cysts of the mesentery were operated upon occasionally but always after a mistaken diagnosis.[2] In 1880, the first successful excision was performed by Tillaux.[2, 8]

Reports of the incidence of mesenteric cysts vary from one case in 30,000 hospital admissions to one in 250,000 admissions.[5] There appears to be a slight preponderance of females to males. Over half of the cysts recorded occur in adult patients, with only 25 per cent in patients under the age of 10 years.

The mesentery consists of two layers of closely approximated peritoneum extending from the posterior wall of the abdomen to the intestines. Between the two layers of mesentery are connective tissue, fat, lymphatic vessels, lymph glands, blood vessels, muscle fibers, and remnants of the müllerian, wolffian, or vitelline ducts. A variety of cysts may arise from these structures. The following forms of cysts have been described: (1) serous cyst, (2) chylous cyst, (3) hydatid cyst, (4) hemorrhagic cyst, (5) dermoid cyst, and (6) cystic malignant disease.

Mesenteric cysts may occur in almost any location within the abdomen from the second portion of the duodenum to the rectum.[5, 13] Approximately half of them occur in the mesentery of the ileum. The mesocolon of the sigmoid, transverse colon, and cecum are frequent sites.[13]

CLASSIFICATION

The classification of Beahrs et al.[1] is widely accepted. They suggest that cysts should be classified not according to contents, location, or size, but according to the basic cytology of the cyst wall, known history, and etiology. These cysts are divided into four groups:

1. *Embryonic and developmental cysts.* Most of the cysts are of developmental origin and arise from the continued growth of congenitally malformed and malpositioned lymphatic tissue. This group also includes the enteric, urogenital, lymphoid and dermoid cysts.

2. *Traumatic or acquired cysts.* It appears that in some cases forceful rupture of lacteals with extravasation of chyle and subsequent encystment occurs. Approximately 78 cases of chylous cysts have been reported in patients who had undergone pelvic surgery. Many of these are reported from Japan and follow pelvic lymphadenectomy.[9]

3. *Neoplastic cysts.* Both benign and malignant variants have been reported.

4. *Infective and degenerative cysts.* Lymph node degeneration associated with tuberculosis or mycotic infections are found. Parasitic cysts also occur.

CLINICAL MANIFESTATIONS

The manner of presentation of mesenteric cysts is quite variable. Usually the patient complains of abdominal pain. The pain may be colicky in nature, suggestive of intestinal obstruction, or it may be associated simply with the enlarging cyst. In some it is probably due to traction on the mesentery or to intermittent entrapment of the cyst in the pelvis. Some patients may present with slow painless enlargement of the abdomen. Often, the clinical manifestations are related to complications of the cyst, such as intestinal obstruction, volvulus, hemorrhage, rupture, or torsion of the cyst and the associated bowel. Hematochezia may be due to actual erosion or invasion of the bowel wall by the cyst. Inflammatory reaction as a complication of pregnancy is reported.[6] A mesenteric cyst may produce urinary tract obstruction, which may or may not be symptomatic. On occasion the cyst may be found incidentally at abdominal laparotomy.

Most authors[5, 11, 13] recognize that a palpable mass is the most common physical finding. Warfield[13] emphasized that the mobility of the mass, particularly lateral motion, should suggest a mesentery cyst (Fig. 19). When demonstrable, this physical finding aids in

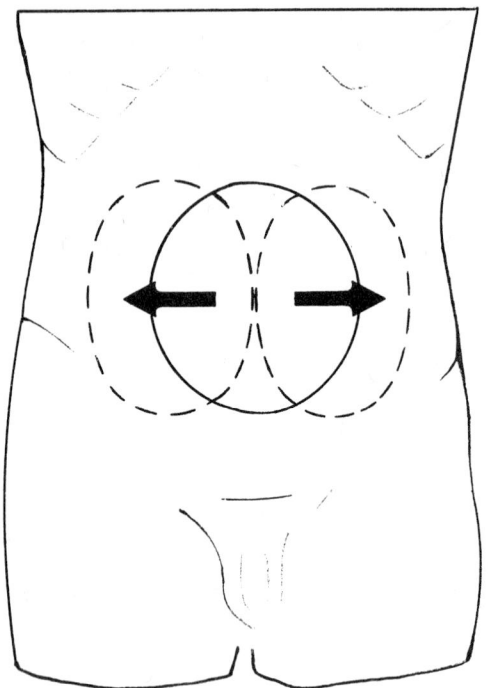

Figure 19. Lateral mobility of a cystic abdominal mass suggests a mesenteric cyst. (From Kurzweg, F. T., et al.: Mesenteric cysts. Am. Surg., *40*:464, 1974.)

localizing the cyst in the mesentery of the small bowel.

LABORATORY

Laboratory examinations are not specific. The blood count is not altered significantly unless there is hemorrhage or infection. X-ray films of the abdomen sometimes reveal displacement of normal gas shadows indicative of a mass or show evidence of intestinal obstruction. Occasionally, calcification that points to the site of pathology is seen. Gastrointestinal series, barium enema, and intravenous pyelography are usually not diagnostic but frequently show displacement of normal structures by the mass. Lymphangiography does not visualize the cyst because lymphangiomas ordinarily do not communicate with neighboring lymphatics and also because the intestinal lymphatics are not visualized by lower extremity injection. Often the patients are operated upon as an emergency and do not undergo extensive study. X-ray examination is of value in that it tends to confirm what is found on physical examination, but more importantly, it may rule out other entities, such as tumor involvement of the bowel, which might require different management.

In addition to mesenteric cyst, the differential diagnosis includes such entities as omental cyst, ovarian cyst, pancreatic cyst, pedunculated uterine fibroid, hydronephrosis, hydrops of the gallbladder, retroperi-

toneal tumor, movable kidney, and splenic cyst or tumor.

PATHOLOGY

Cysts have been reported varying in size from 3 to 25 cm. in diameter,[3] and some may fill the entire abdomen (up to 8000 ml. of fluid) (Fig. 20). Most of the cysts are multilocular with loculi of varying sizes and shapes. The chambers may communicate or may be independent. An occasional one may be dumbbell-shaped, with large masses on either side of the mesentery connected by a constricted portion. Multiple cysts have been recorded.

Although the majority of the cysts are lymphangiomas, a variety of cell types are found. Of the cysts showing a histological picture of lymphangioma, only an occasional one contains chyle. Most of them contain clear or bloody fluid. Usually the cyst wall is composed mainly of connective tissue with occasional fibers of smooth muscle. Cholesterol clefts, foam cells, and fatty degeneration may be present. Occasionally, evidence of hemorrhage and inflammation is seen. Lymph follicles may be present. The cyst lining may consist of endothelial cells or in many areas only a fibrous tissue wall. Malignant mesenteric cysts are uncommon. The usual malignant form is a sarcoma, but adenocarcinoma arising in a cyst has been reported.[12]

Chylous fluid shows a remarkable property of resisting putrefaction, fermentation, and bacterial growth.[11, 14] It has been reported that, with no effort to control bacterial contamination other than ordinary refrigeration, fluid from a chylous cyst was kept in the laboratory for two months. This protein-rich material did not putrefy or ferment, and there was no bacterial growth in it except for a few saprophytic organisms.

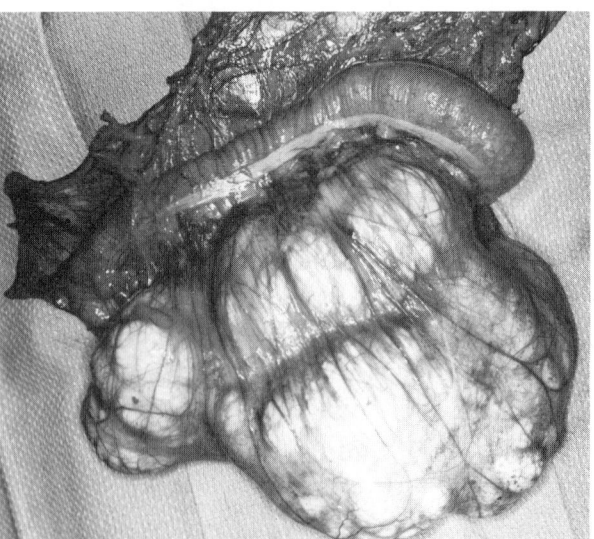

Figure 20. Chylous cyst in situ. Transverse mesocolon with omentum reflected cephalad. (From Kurzweg, F. T., et al.: Mesenteric cysts. Am. Surg., *40*:464, 1974.)

The nature of the bacteriostatic action has not been explained.

TREATMENT

Because the cysts tend to grow and cause complications, they should be removed.[4] Enucleation of the cyst without damage to the blood supply of the bowel is the treatment of choice. However, resection of the intestine may be necessary because of involvement of the cyst with the mesenteric vessels and adjacent gut. This, too, usually produces good results but is more hazardous. Simple aspiration of the cyst is not recommended because the fluid usually reaccumulates and the risk of contamination is engendered. External marsupialization of the cyst was often done in the past but has lost favor to resectional therapy. Where complicating adherence to vital structures makes resection impossible or unduly hazardous, internal drainage into the free peritoneal cavity may be necessary.[5]

One problem sometimes encountered at operation is the differentiation of a mesenteric cyst from duplication of the bowel. The latter is usually thick-walled and lined by intestinal mucosa. Duplication shares a common blood supply with the adjacent normal bowel and simple excision cannot be performed. Attempted dissection often injures the blood supply and leads to infarction of the bowel.

The previously high mortality rate has been reduced in recent years by the advances in surgery and the ancillary supportive services. Today, mortality rates of 0 to 8 per cent following enucleation of the cyst and of 3 to 15 per cent if bowel resection is necessary might be expected.[7, 10]

SELECTED REFERENCES

Beahrs, O. H., Judd, E. S., Jr., and Dockerty, M. B.: Chylous cysts of the abdomen. Surg. Clin. North Am., *30*:1081, 1950.
This is an excellent review of the subject. The authors propose a classification of mesenteric cysts that is presently the one most widely accepted.

Caropreso, P.: Mesenteric cysts. A review. Arch. Surg., *180*:242, 1974.
This is a comprehensive, current review of mesenteric cysts.

Moynihan, B.: Mesenteric cysts. Ann. Surg., *26*:1, 1897.
This article is of historical interest. It is an early review of mesenteric cysts in the English language.

Slocum, M. A.: Surgical treatment of chylous mesenteric cyst by marsupialization. Am. J. Surg., *129*:709, 1975.
The author reports his study of the bacteriostatic powers of chylous fluid. He corroborates this observation, which was originally made by Wells.

Warfield, J. O.: A study of mesenteric cysts with a report of two recent cases. Ann. Surg., *96*:329, 1932.
This author emphasizes that lateral mobility of an abdominal cystic mass suggests the probability of a mesenteric cyst. If present, this physical finding is pathognomonic of a cyst in the mesentery of the small bowel.

REFERENCES

1. Beahrs, O. H., Judd, E. S., Jr., and Dockerty, M. B.: Chylous cysts of the abdomen. Surg. Clin. North Am., *30*:1081, 1950.
2. Braquehaye, J.: Des kystes du mesentery. Arch. Gen. Med. Paris, *170*:291, 1892.
3. Burnett, W. E., Rosemond, G. P., and Bucher, R. M.: Mesenteric cysts. Arch. Surg., *60*:699, 1950.
4. Caropreso, P. R.: Mesenteric cysts: A review. Arch. Surg., *108*:242, 1974.
5. Hardin, W. J., and Hardy, J. D.: Mesenteric cysts. Am. J. Surg., *119*:640, 1970.
6. Hill, W. L., Jr., and Woomer, D. F.: Retroperitoneal cyst complicating pregnancy: Report of a recent case. Obstet. Gynecol., *25*:858, 1965.
7. Kurzweg, F. T., Daron, P. B., Williamson, J. W., Danna, S. J., and Johnson, J. F.: Mesenteric cysts. Am. Surg., *40*:462, 1974.
8. Moynihan, B. G. A.: Mesenteric cysts. Ann. Surg., *26*:1, 1897.
9. Nelson, J. H., and Huston, J. W.: Lymphocyst formation following pelvic lymphadenectomy. Am. J. Obstet. Gynecol., *78*:1298, 1959.
10. Sanchez, R. E., Gordon, H. E., and Passard, E., Jr.: Mesenteric cysts. Am. Surg., *36*:378, 1970.
11. Slocum, M. A.: Surgical treatment of chylous mesenteric cyst by marsupialization. Am. J. Surg., *41*:464, 1938.
12. Tykka, H., and Koivieniemi, A.: Carcinoma arising in a mesenteric cyst. Am. J. Surg., *129*:709, 1975.
13. Warfield, J. O.: A study of mesenteric cysts with a report of two recent cases. Ann. Surg., *96*:329, 1932.
14. Wells, H. C.: Chem. Pathol., *5*:404, 1925.

30

THE ACUTE ABDOMEN

John M. Beal, M.D.

HISTORICAL ASPECTS

The catastrophic potential of abdominal problems that currently are included in the category of the "acute abdomen" has been recognized since the era of Hippocrates. In the past, a variety of terms were given to acute abdominal problems, among which were "iliac passion" and "ileus." Both of these latter terms were familiar to Celsus, Hippocrates, and Caelius Aurelianus. The term "volvulus" has been found also in the works of Celsus but throughout ancient times was used loosely. Iliac passion, which can be considered synonymous with acute abdomen, was recognized by Paracelsus (1493–1541) and by Sydenham (1624–1689).

The boldness of early surgeons who performed trephination of the skull and advocated drainage of empyema cavities was not evident in the treatment of acute abdominal diseases. For many years, the reluctance to enter the peritoneal cavity was related to the absence of postmortem examinations to correlate clinical findings with pathologic changes and to the lack of diagnostic techniques other than physical examination. The emergence of pathology, the development of anesthesia, and the introduction of antiseptic techniques prepared the path for advancement of abdominal surgery.

The courage of a few surgeons and the remarkable endurance of certain hardy patients in the days preceding anesthesia and antisepsis are impressive. Inguinal hernia attracted the attention of physicians many years ago, probably because its external manifestations could be observed and examined. As early as 1556, operation was recommended by Pierre Franco, a French Huguenot and barber-surgeon. His publication, *Petit Traite,* proposed surgical intervention in the treatment of strangulated inguinal hernia when efforts at manual reduction were unsuccessful. He suggested that removal of the testicle facilitated the procedure in some cases.

Only sporadic reports of operation appeared for many years. In 1709, Jean-Louis Petit reported that he operated upon patients with strangulated hernia and used a method that did not require entry into the peritoneal cavity. It was not until 1836 that Johann Friedrich Dieffenbach reported the first successful account of resection of the small intestine in a patient found to have a segment of gangrenous bowel in a strangulated inguinal hernia. There was similar reluctance to intervene in acute obstruction of the large intestine. In 1710, Littré suggested that the colon should be opened when obstruction occurred; however, it was not until 1776 that Pillore of Rouen performed the first cecostomy. The performance of the first transverse colostomy seems to have been inadvertent. In 1797, Fine of Montpellier, who operated upon a patient with intestinal obstruction, had planned to open a segment of small bowel. When the transverse colon presented in the abdominal incision, he decided to open this portion of the bowel instead. Jean-Zuléma Amussat developed the use of the lumbar colostomy (1839), and this method of large bowel decompression was utilized for many years because it avoided the peritoneal cavity.

Confusion between disease of the cecum and that of the appendix lasted for a long time. In 1886, Reginald Fitz, Shattuck Professor of Pathological Anatomy at Harvard Medical School, read his paper, "Perforating Inflammation of the Vermiform Appendix," before the Association of American Physicians. He clearly outlined the main symptoms and employed the term "appendicitis" to describe the disease.

INTRODUCTION

The clinical picture generally referred to as the *acute abdomen* is a frequent problem. Acute abdominal pain requires prompt investigation and often presents an intriguing diagnostic challenge to the physician. In the majority of patients, a proper diagnosis may be reached by means of careful history and complete physical examination, supplemented by a few simple laboratory tests.

The objective of the physician who is confronted with a patient with an acute abdominal problem is to reach an early and accurate working diagnosis so that a correct plan of treatment may be instituted promptly. The physician frequently must exercise careful judgment to determine when evaluation of the patient must be curtailed in order that treatment may be started. In some instances, minutes may be critical if the patient is suffering from intra-abdominal hemorrhage, while in other patients, a few hours of conservative management may be advantageous, even though operation is indicated.

Accurate diagnosis and appropriate treatment depend upon knowledge of the anatomy and physiology of the peritoneum and the intra-abdominal viscera. Differentiation between disease entities is based upon applied anatomy and physiology. The separation of problems that arise outside the abdominal cavity and yet produce abdominal pain requires careful consideration of the anatomic pathways of pain and the functional effects of disease processes.

ANATOMIC CONSIDERATIONS

Under normal conditions, the peritoneal cavity is a potential space that has a lining consisting of a mesothelial layer, the serosal surface, and the subserosal layer, which contains blood vessels and lymphatics. There are two major divisions of the peritoneal cavity: the general peritoneal cavity, which contains the intra-abdominal viscera, and the lesser peritoneal cavity, or lesser omental bursa. The foramen of Winslow is the opening through which these cavities communicate. For descriptive purposes, the anterior abdominal wall is divided into four quadrants, with imaginary horizontal and vertical lines crossing at the umbilicus. This permits the examiner to indicate that the patient complained of pain in the right upper quadrant or that tenderness was felt in the left lower quadrant. The use of the quadrants of the abdomen for topographic location of pain, tenderness, or masses is helpful for the clinician; but it is important to recall that this external division of the abdominal wall has little anatomic basis.

The anatomic relationships of the abdominal viscera and the visceral attachments have a significant influence upon the localization of signs and symptoms of acute abdominal diseases. The visceral attachments influence the location and spread of blood, purulent material, and intra-abdominal fluid within the peritoneal cavity.

Pain sensations from the abdomen are mediated through both the spinal nerves and the autonomic nervous system. The individual abdominal organs and the visceral peritoneum are innervated by the autonomic system. The parietal peritoneum, which invests the abdominal walls and the diaphragmatic and pelvic surfaces, is innervated by the intercostal branches of the spinal nerves that arise from the fifth to the eleventh thoracic spinal cord segments. In addition, the phrenic nerves innervate the diaphragm and its peritoneal surface. The innervation of the abdomen by these two systems of nerves has influence upon the localization of pain by the patient with acute abdominal problems.

Painful stimuli that originate in the stomach and proximal duodenum are felt in the epigastrium because these structures are derived from the foregut and receive splanchnic innervation that localizes painful sensations to this area (Fig. 1). Midgut pain is felt in the periumbilical region and is characteristic of small bowel pain. Hindgut pain is felt in the hypogastrium and is typical of colonic involvement beyond the midtransverse colon. In each instance, the pain is not as well localized as that experienced with somatic nerves. However, if the disease process extends to involve the parietal peritoneum, more precise localization of pain occurs because of the involvement of the branches of the spinal nerves.

CLINICAL CONSIDERATIONS

THE HISTORY

Pain

"The general rule can be laid down that the majority of cases of severe abdominal pain which ensue in patients who have been previously fairly well, and which last as long as six hours, are caused by conditions of surgical import."[4]

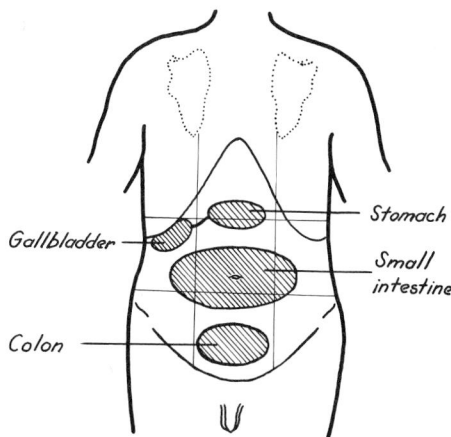

Figure 1. The shaded areas indicate the location of pain, according to site of origin.

Both the site and the character of the pain felt by the patient should be determined carefully. Cramping or colicky pain is characteristic of obstruction of a hollow viscus. Obstruction of the stomach, large or small bowel, or biliary or renal tract will result in the production of cramping pain. Colic is usually intermittent, and the interval of freedom from pain may at times be helpful. For example, in obstruction of the intestinal tract, the interval between episodes of abdominal cramping pain is longer the more distal is the site of obstruction in the intestinal tract. The characteristics of the pain pattern in patients with acute abdominal disease are understood better when the mechanisms of pain are reviewed (Table 1).

Other characteristics of painful sensations must be sought. Steady pain implies a disease process that does not cause obstruction of the lumen of the abdominal viscera. Burning pain is often applied to the sensation of active peptic ulceration. The pain associated with pancreatitis has been described as prostrating. The pain associated with a dissecting aneurysm, as well as with rupture of the esophagus, has been described as tearing.

The time of onset of pain has diagnostic importance. Pain that awakens a patient from sleep at night is usually serious. Relation of pain to meals or other activity may be a clue in diagnosis. The patient is usually able to describe the onset of pain as being gradual or sudden at the inception. Further interrogation is needed to determine if there has been a change in the character or location of the pain during the development of the patient's illness.

Other symptoms may be associated with or in-

TABLE 1. Pathogenesis of Acute Abdominal Pain

Mechanisms of Pain	Underlying Causes
Perforation	Neoplasm
Obstruction	Trauma
Ischemia	Infection
Inflammation	Neurogenic
Hemorrhage	Vascular

fluenced by the pain. Flank pain, associated with burning on urination, suggests renal calculi. Pain on inspiration is often found in patients with acute cholecystitis or an inflammatory process that involves the surface of the diaphragm. In some instances, the patient may notice that the assumption of the recumbent position is associated with shoulder pain. This is occasionally encountered in patients with blunt abdominal injury who have suffered rupture of the spleen and who have free blood in the peritoneal cavity.

Vomiting

Vomiting is an important symptom that frequently is associated with acute abdominal crises. A careful history will include the following aspects concerning vomiting: the relationship of vomiting to the onset of pain, the character of the vomitus, and the frequency and volume of vomiting. In the majority of acute abdominal problems, pain precedes vomiting. In patients with biliary colic, renal colic, or upper small bowel obstruction, vomiting occurs soon after the onset of pain. Distal small bowel obstruction may be manifested by cramping pain for 2 to 4 hours before vomiting occurs, while vomiting is a late complication of large bowel obstruction, if it occurs at all.

Most patients are able to describe the character of the vomitus, and many will have residual vomitus about the face or on their clothing. Patients with gastric lesions, particularly if there is some obstruction to the outlet of the stomach, have relatively clear vomitus that contains little if any bile. The vomitus that occurs in patients with renal colic, biliary colic, and early small bowel obstruction is a green, bile-containing liquid. Distal obstruction of the small bowel often results in the development of vomitus that is first green, later yellowish, and finally fecal in character.

The volume of gastrointestinal fluid is greatest when there is obstruction of the upper gastrointestinal tract. While the volume can be assessed accurately only by measurement after a nasogastric tube has been inserted, some patients are capable of giving information that the vomitus filled a cup, a small emesis basin, or some similar container. Small bowel obstruction also produces frequent vomiting, emesis occurring shortly after or in association with episodes of cramping abdominal pain. Emesis is a prominent symptom in biliary colic but subsides as the colicky pain diminishes.

A number of serious acute intra-abdominal diseases are not associated with vomiting. Vomiting is not an important symptom of perforated duodenal ulcer. Although nausea and retching may occur after the acute perforation has developed, vomiting is infrequent. Vomiting may not occur in patients with large bowel obstruction or in many patients with appendicitis. The latter problem is associated with loss of appetite and frequent nausea, even though emesis has not occurred. Vomiting may be infrequent or absent in intra-abdominal hemorrhage, whether from an ectopic pregnancy or from rupture of the spleen.

Syncope

Fainting may occur in patients as a result of sudden pain at the time of perforation of a peptic ulcer. This must be differentiated from the hypotension that occurs in patients who have suffered from intra-abdominal hemorrhage. Syncope may occur in ectopic pregnancy, rupture of the spleen, or rupture of an aneurysm of the splenic or mesenteric vessels, as a result of reduction in circulating blood volume.

Bowel Function

Evaluation of the status of the patient must include an appraisal of bowel function. This is often more difficult to assess than other gastrointestinal functions. While diarrhea may suggest the presence of gastroenteritis in a patient with abdominal pain, appendicitis may be present. In some patients with acute inflammation of the appendix, diarrhea is a significant symptom. The finding of obstipation in association with abdominal distention supports the diagnosis of large bowel obstruction in patients who have the other signs and symptoms of this problem. However, in patients with pancreatitis, cholecystitis, and inflammatory problems of the abdominal viscera, ileus may develop, with distention and failure to pass flatus or stool. Thus, bowel function must be considered in conjunction with other findings in the history and physical examination.

The character of stools must be noted. The presence of blood, dark or fresh, tarry stools, and other abnormalities should be sought for, as well as the presence or absence of diarrhea. Inquiry concerning tenesmus and decreased caliber of stools should be made in patients in whom a lesion of the large bowel is suspected.

Menstrual History

History-taking in a woman is incomplete without a review of the menstrual history. The date of the last period and a statement of the patient's menstrual cycle must be included in the history of each female patient with abdominal pain. The patient should be asked whether the last period was normal, both in character and in time in the cycle, particularly if ectopic pregnancy is likely. The relation of abdominal pain to the menstrual cycle should be stated.

Urinary Symptoms

Urinary frequency and dysuria often are associated with renal colic and serve to confirm the presence of suspected calculi. Patients with renal stones often give a history of previous attacks, the passage of "sand" or "gravel," and hematuria.

Abdominal pain is sometimes increased with voiding in patients with ureteral calculi, acute appendicitis, and diverticulitis. It should be emphasized that a distended bladder is a cause of abdominal pain in elderly men with prostatism, and voiding brings relief in such patients. The color of urine should be noted, and inquiry made concerning blood.

PHYSICAL EXAMINATION

The general condition of the patient with acute abdominal pain must be assessed carefully. The customary vital signs—temperature, pulse, respiratory rate, and blood pressure—are essential in the appraisal of a patient who complains of abdominal distress. While the examiner is obtaining the history of the illness from the patient, he should be observing the patient's position, color, respiratory effort, and other actions to detect any abnormalities. The physical examination should begin with careful inspection of the entire body for possible change in color of skin, cyanosis of lips or mucous membranes, distention of veins on the neck or trunk, respiratory effort, position of limbs, and contour of the abdomen.

Although the patient's temperature, respiratory rate, and pulse rate are essential in the evaluation of the status of the patient, there are limitations to the value of these observations and they must be considered in relation to other findings. The patient's temperature should be obtained by rectum, rather than the oral route. Fever is particularly difficult to evaluate as a diagnostic finding in children with abdominal pain. Some children with acute pharyngitis complain of abdominal pain and are febrile. The differentiation between acute gastroenteritis and appendicitis in children is notoriously difficult, and fever is often present in both conditions.

Similarly, a normal pulse rate is of limited value. Generally, emphasis is placed upon the elevation of the pulse rate in the presence of shock and of peritonitis. However, early in the development of common acute abdominal diseases, such as acute appendicitis, acute cholecystitis, and perforated peptic ulcer, the pulse rate may be within normal limits.

Both the respiratory rate and the character of respiratory effort should be observed. Patients with severe abdominal pain associated with perforation of peptic ulcer and with acute pancreatitis often have shallow respiratory excursions. Marked abdominal distention also interferes with respiration.

The respiratory rate has an important role in the differentiation between abdominal and pulmonary problems. Lobar pneumonia is noted for sudden onset and is associated with abdominal pain. A number of patients with this disease have been subjected to laparotomy, with the mistaken diagnosis of perforated duodenal ulcer. Pneumonitis is usually associated with fever, cough, splinting of the chest, and a rapid respiratory rate, often with cyanosis, and frequently with flaring of the nares with respiration. Chest pain is also present.

The position of the patient may provide a clue. The patient with renal or biliary colic is restless and has been described as "climbing the wall with pain." In contrast, the patient who has peritoneal irritation from pancreatitis, or perforation of a viscus, prefers to be immobile because movement tends to increase the abdominal discomfort. Small bowel obstruction produces intermittent cramping pain, and the patient will "double up" at intervals when episodes of cramping pain occur. Similarly, a child with intussusception will draw up the legs and cry from time to time with pain, as a result of the peristaltic activity of the obstructed bowel.

Abdominal Examination

Following inspection of the abdomen, the patient should be asked to indicate the site of pain and to lo-calize the site with one finger, if possible. Palpation of the abdomen is then in order and should begin in an area remote from the indicated site of maximal discomfort. Warm hands, patience, and gentleness are required for an adequate examination of the abdomen, particularly if the patient is apprehensive or in severe distress. Pressure should be light when palpation is started, and the degree of muscular resistance should be assessed. Palpation is accomplished by pressure with the fingertips and with the fingers extended fully.

The examiner should attempt to determine whether the liver and spleen are palpable and, if so, whether enlarged or otherwise abnormal. Masses, if present, should be noted, the size measured, and the shape and contour accurately described. Evidence of fluid may be detected by determination of shifting dullness or the presence of a fluid wave.

There are a few areas of the abdominal wall that require special attention. In patients in whom intestinal obstruction is suspected, the presence of a scar from a previous operation suggests that the small intestinal obstruction may be due to an adhesion or intraperitoneal band. It is equally important to examine the inguinal rings and femoral triangles for possible inguinal or femoral hernias in patients with signs or symptoms of small bowel obstruction.

Rebound tenderness is an important sign of peritoneal irritation and signifies that the peritoneal surfaces are involved by an inflammatory reaction. Rebound tenderness is detected by the sudden removal of the palpating hand from the abdomen and should be done without warning, so that it is not expected by the patient.

Percussion of the abdomen is often omitted, unfortunately, although this portion of the examination may yield valuable information. Percussion should be performed gently. One can determine promptly whether distention of the abdomen is the result of gas or fluid. The presence of a distended urinary bladder can often be detected by percussion of the lower abdomen. One may determine whether abnormal liver dullness is present, an important finding if free air in the peritoneal cavity is suspected. Estimation of liver dullness has limitations in patients with marked abdominal distention, because the intestines may become interposed between the liver and the anterior abdominal and thoracic wall in such circumstances.

Auscultation of the abdomen is omitted often, and yet, in the patient with an acute abdominal problem, it is as important to listen to the abdomen as it is to listen to the heart and lungs. Bowel sounds are normally present, and experience is valuable in differentiating between normal and abnormal sounds, because these sounds may become either absent or increased in abdominal disease. In peritonitis, for example, bowel sounds are usually absent. Conversely, in patients with small bowel obstruction, the sounds occur with increased frequency and become high-pitched in character. In some conditions, bowel sounds may be present in the early stages of the disease process and later disappear. Early mesenteric arterial occlusion is associated with increased peristaltic activity, and bowel sounds are loud and active. Within a few hours, the ischemic bowel loses peristaltic function, and the bowel sounds disappear.

When listening to the abdomen, it is important to spend as long as 1 minute with the stethoscope to the abdominal wall. Often, it is advantageous to listen before palpation of the abdomen and again following percussion and palpation before concluding that the bowel sounds are absent.

Examination is incomplete unless a rectal examination is performed and, in the female patient, a pelvic examination as well. The person responsible for the management of the patient should do these examinations personally. Rectal examination is performed most satisfactorily in the patient with an acute abdomen with the patient supine and with the legs flexed. This position permits tactile appraisal of the prostate, the seminal vesicles, and the cul-de-sac, as well as an opportunity to determine whether the tenderness is more prominent on either side. It is necessary to distinguish between the anal discomfort that the patient may experience and internal pain, if present.

In the female patient, the pelvic examination should be performed bimanually in order to detect tenderness or masses in the adnexal areas, as well as to estimate the size and position of the uterus, if present. Pelvic examination must also be accomplished gently. Rough manipulation of the cervix will be uncomfortable in most patients, whether disease is present or not. In most patients the expression on the face will tell the examiner if gentle pressure on the cervix or in the adnexa is painful.

When rectal examination has been completed, the gloved fingers should be inspected to note the presence of blood or the character of any stool. Stool should be tested for occult blood.

Supplementary Physical Findings

Hyperesthesia of the skin of the abdominal wall has been stated to be an important diagnostic physical finding in patients with acute abdominal diseases. Pin-prick is recommended or light stroking with pin point of the abdominal skin. Hyperesthesia of the skin of the abdominal wall is an indication of parietal peritoneal inflammation and may be included in the examination of patients with suspected inflammatory intra-abdominal disease, especially acute appendicitis. It is a helpful sign when present but is not present in many patients, particularly during the early stages.

Iliopsoas test: this test is often positive in patients who have an inflammatory process that is in contact with the psoas muscle and should be performed in patients who are suspected of having appendicitis. With the patient supine, and with the legs fully extended, the patient is requested to elevate the right leg. Pain is experienced if the inflammatory process involves the psoas muscle.

Obturator test: this test is performed by flexing the thigh at right angles to the trunk and then rotating the leg externally. The test may elicit pain in the hypogastrium if there is an inflammatory process in contact with the obturator internus muscle, such as a pelvic abscess or acutely inflamed appendix extending into the pelvis.

Murphy's sign: the examiner exerts pressure against the abdominal wall in the right upper quadrant of the abdomen, in the region of the gallbladder, and asks the patient to inhale deeply. Deep inspiration causes the liver to descend and, if the gallbladder is large and inflamed, it strikes the examining fingers. The patient then experiences pain, and the inspiratory effort halts. This is a useful maneuver in patients who are suspected of having acute cholecystitis.

Cullen's sign is bluish or purplish discoloration in the region of the umbilicus and is present in extensive hemoperitoneum. Reliable when present, it is frequently not evident in the presence of serious intraperitoneal hemorrhage.

Peritoneal aspiration, or "tap," is a valuable diagnostic aid, particularly if intraperitoneal bleeding is suspected. This procedure is simple, safe, and easily performed. Several methods have been recommended and are useful if the limitations are understood. The simplest type of peritoneal tap is accomplished by gently inserting an 18-gauge needle through the abdominal wall, after infiltrating the site of puncture with a small amount of local anesthetic. If the syringe contains approximately 10 ml. of saline solution, blood or purulent material is more easily detected when the needle enters the peritoneal cavity. The failure to find blood or pus does not mean that such is *not* present, but a *positive* "tap" is a valuable discovery that may speed appropriate treatment.

Somewhat more complicated is the insertion of a small plastic catheter through a small incision in the midline just below the umbilicus. This permits irrigation of the peritoneal cavity with as much as 300 ml. of saline solution. The results of study of the irrigation fluid that is retrieved through this method have yielded a higher correlation with the presence or absence of infection or hemorrhage in the peritoneal cavity.

LABORATORY AIDS

A working diagnosis may be achieved in the majority of patients with acute abdominal problems after a history of the illness has been taken, a physical examination performed, and a blood count and urinalysis obtained. Despite the development of a large number of sophisticated laboratory tests that have aided the clinician in the diagnosis of a wide variety of diseases under elective circumstances, a few standard laboratory procedures are adequate to provide appropriate confirmation of the clinical impression in the common abdominal emergencies. Time is a factor in the management of patients with acute abdominal illnesses, and laboratory tests and roentgen examinations must be selected that will yield significant information in a short time, so that prompt and proper therapy can be instituted.

Hemogram

A sample of blood should be obtained as soon as practical after a patient with abdominal pain has been examined. The blood specimen should be obtained by venipuncture when possible and analyzed for hematocrit, red blood cell count, white blood cell count, and differential count. The hematocrit is more valuable than the red blood cell count and is preferable to a hemoglobin determination. The initial blood study is often of relative importance and frequently forms a baseline for later comparative evaluation. In the presence of hemorrhage, the hematocrit is little changed early in the course of bleeding and does not decrease until transcapillary filling of the intravascular space has occurred. The value of the white blood cell count varies greatly among the different causes of acute abdominal pain, and discussion of this determination will be seen in the sections devoted to the specific problems.

Urinalysis

Diagnostic studies are incomplete without urinalysis. Before specific therapy is instituted, particularly operation, a specimen of urine must be obtained, even if catheterization of the patient is required. The specific gravity of the urine may be helpful in the assessment of hydration of the patient. Analysis for the presence of albumin, reducing substances, and bile may give significant insight into the nature of the patient's disease. Microscopic study of the urine for white and red blood cells and detection of bacteriuria may have profound influence on the treatment of the patient. A properly performed urinalysis must be carried out before operation under general anesthesia is performed.

Special Blood Tests

Few laboratory tests are required in most patients with acute abdominal distress. When acute pancreatitis is suspected, serum amylase values should be determined. In patients with severe pancreatitis, determinations of serum calcium and phosphorus levels are indicated and may also be helpful in patients with duodenal ulcer and other patients with pancreatitis, if hyperparathyroidism is suspected.

Serum bilirubin values are sometimes valuable in patients with acute cholecystitis or with acute pancreatitis. Serum electrolyte determinations are seldom of diagnostic significance but serve to aid the physician who must manage the serious fluid and electrolyte derangements in patients with intestinal obstruction or perforated peptic ulcer.

ROENTGENOGRAPHIC STUDIES

Roentgenograms are among our most valuable diagnostic tools when properly used. Roentgenologic study should be used for specific reasons after the history and physical examination have been completed. The examining physician should have a specific indication for requesting roentgenograms and, once the films have been obtained, he should review them with the radiologist. This is particularly helpful when the differential diagnosis is difficult and it assures the physician that he has the most accurate and complete information that the radiologic study may provide.

It is unnecessary to obtain a film of the abdomen in every case of acute abdominal distress. In some instances, a trip to the x-ray department will delay operation unduly and will constitute a hazard to the patient. This includes patients with hemorrhage from an ectopic pregnancy or from a ruptured aortic aneurysm who may require immediate operation in order to prevent exsanguination. There seems little reason to obtain films of the abdomen in patients in whom the diagnosis of acute appendicitis is well established on clinical grounds.

When roentgenograms are obtained, the study ordered should be appropriate, and the films must be of a technical quality to permit adequate interpretation. If a patient has abdominal findings that require radiologic study, it is well to request an x-ray of the chest at the same time. Not only does the chest roentgenogram provide information concerning the diaphragm as well as the lung fields, but often it prevents further delay in emergency operations if this becomes the treatment of choice later.

Plain Film of the Abdomen

This study, often referred to as a "scout film" or "survey film," is requested more often than any other radiologic study in the diagnosis of patients with acute abdominal problems (Fig. 2). Films of good quality will provide much information concerning the position and configuration of normal organs, as well as detecting abnormalities. In most instances, the study is

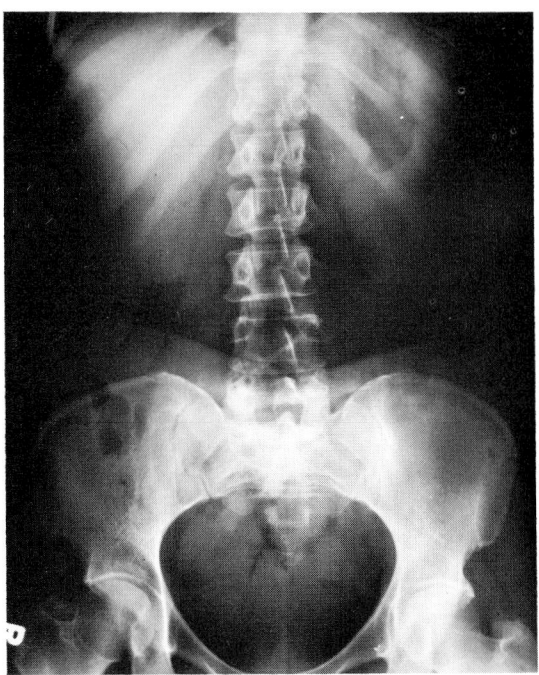

Figure 2. Normal plain film of abdomen demonstrates small amount of air in stomach and colon, well-defined margins of psoas muscles, and outline of right and left kidneys.

requested to determine whether there is evidence of abnormal gas patterns, both intraluminally and extraluminally. Abnormal calcifications and masses may be sought, and evidence of collection of fluid appears in some patients. The skeletal structures must be examined, particularly if a history of trauma is elicited. Fracture of a rib in the lower chest cage on the left in a patient with evidence of intraperitoneal hemorrhage after injury is supporting evidence that rupture of the spleen is likely.

Gas patterns in the abdomen usually provide the most striking findings. Small amounts of gas are detected commonly in the stomach and colon, with smaller amounts being found in the small intestine. Abnormal gas patterns in the gastrointestinal tract occur when there are motor disturbances, such as adynamic, or "paralytic," ileus, or when obstruction is present. In general, ileus is characterized by gas being seen throughout the gastrointestinal tract. Ileus follows such diverse problems as operation, injury without intra-abdominal disorder, and fractures of the lumbar spine. The differentiation between obstruction and ileus may be very difficult at times. Obstruction is characterized by dilatation of the intestine proximal to the point of obstruction. Thus, if the obstruction is present in the sigmoid colon, the colon proximal to this point will appear distended, as will the small bowel if the ileocecal valve is incompetent. When the small intestine is obstructed by an adhesion or band, small bowel dilatation will be seen without evidence of gas in the large intestine.

Small intestine may be distinguished from the colon on x-rays by the presence of the circular valvulae conniventes, or plicae circulares (valves of Kerckring), which extend completely across the shadow of distended small bowel. The haustral folds of the large bowel are usually recognized without difficulty.

Abnormal gas patterns are found in other conditions. Gas may be detected in the biliary tract when there are fistulous connections between the intestinal tract and the common duct or gallbladder. Collections of gas are detected in the retroperitoneal tissues in certain infections. Gas may be seen in the bowel wall and in the portal vein in advanced mesenteric infarction.

Free air in the peritoneal cavity may develop in association with perforation of a hollow viscus. The most common cause of free air is perforation of a duodenal ulcer, but free air is also seen with perforation of diverticulitis and of the small bowel. Pneumoperitoneum is unusual in acute appendicitis.

Free air is detected most satisfactorily by a roentgenogram taken with the patient in an upright position. The film must include the diaphragm to be satisfactory, and often free air is detected when the chest film is obtained. The upright position should be maintained for at least 5 minutes for a satisfactory study to be obtained. If the patient is too ill to maintain an upright position for 5 minutes or longer, he may be placed in a lateral position, that is, lying with one flank up, and the roentgenogram obtained as a lateral view of the abdomen.

In addition to gas patterns, the intra-abdominal organs should be inspected to assess their size, shape, and position. Enlargement of the spleen may be sought as evidence of portal hypertension in patients with cirrhosis of the liver. The kidneys are visible in many studies, and their size and position can be ascertained. The psoas shadows should be sought. Loss of the psoas shadow is evidence of retroperitoneal disease and occurs in abscess formation in the retroperitoneal area. The commonest large lower abdominal mass in a man is a distended bladder.

Calcific deposits may be seen in some patients. A calcific deposit in the right upper quadrant of the abdomen that has concentric rings may be a gallstone, and its location can be determined from a lateral view of the abdomen. Gallstones are located anterior to the vertebral column when viewed from the side, while renal calculi are located posteriorly. Calcific deposits may be seen in the vascular tree as well. Abdominal aortic aneurysms are often detected by means of plain films of the abdomen and have a typical shell of calcium along the margin of the aneurysm. Gallstone ileus is characterized by air in the biliary tree, dilatation of the small bowel, and a concentric ring of calcium, the gallstone, in the right lower quadrant, where the gallstone has become lodged in the terminal ileum.

When renal calculi are suspected, calcified stones may be detected along the course of the ureters (Fig. 3). Phleboliths in the pelvis may make identification of ureteral calculi difficult if they are lodged in the lower portion of the ureter. Other calcifications seen in the pelvis include prostatic calculi, calcifications in dermoid cysts, and uterine fibromyomas. Their presence should be noted, although it is unlikely that this

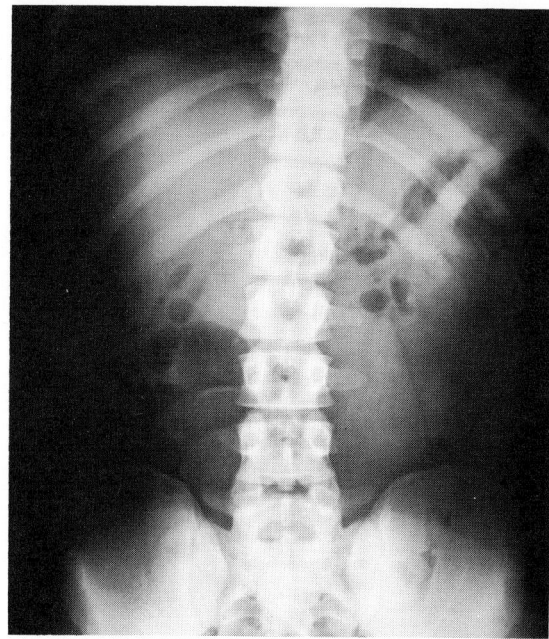

Figure 3. Ureteral calculus may be seen adjacent to the lower margin of the second lumbar vertebral body on the right side.

last group would contribute to the symptomatology of the acute abdomen.

Other Radiologic Studies

Although in the majority of patients, a working diagnosis can be reached after the clinical picture has been assessed with the aid of a chest x-ray and plain films of the abdomen, in some patients the diagnosis can be confirmed or a more accurate impression reached by the use of special radiologic studies. Occasionally, the application of appropriate x-ray studies is essential if proper treatment is to be instituted.

One of the frequently employed special studies is intravenous pyelography. This is particularly useful if renal disease, such as a renal or ureteral calculus, is suspected or if injury to the kidney is likely in association with trauma. Although the diagnosis of a ureteral calculus may be made by means of urinalysis and plain abdominal film, if the patient has a more complex and uncertain clinical picture including flank pain, an intravenous pyelogram will help in differential diagnosis of the pain.

Intravenous cholangiography may be employed in patients who are suspected of having acute cholecystitis or in whom the status of the biliary tract is important in the differential diagnosis. This procedure is valuable when the common duct is visualized but does not contribute to the diagnosis when the biliary tract is not seen. If contrast studies, such as intravenous cholangiography or pyelography, are undertaken, they should be performed before barium is administered either orally or rectally. The presence of barium in the gastrointestinal tract obscures visualization of the biliary and urinary tract.

The oral route is seldom used for administration of

contrast media in the radiologic investigation of patients with acute abdominal problems because of the possibility that the ingested barium or other material might enter the peritoneal cavity or interfere with evacuation of the upper gastrointestinal tract if operation is undertaken. Barium enema is often useful, however, if patients are suspected of having intestinal obstruction. This study is particularly helpful if the differentiation of the site of obstruction between the large and small intestine is difficult. When the large bowel is the site of obstruction, the location of the obstruction and, often, the nature of the obstructing lesion may be determined by barium enema.

Angiography has attracted attention for its ability to localize gastrointestinal bleeding, as well as to detect organ injury following abdominal trauma. While aortography is seldom needed or advisable in patients with leaking or ruptured abdominal aortic aneurysm, angiographic studies are useful in the management of dissecting aneurysms and of renal and mesenteric aneurysms.

THE PERITONEUM AND PERITONITIS

The peritoneal cavity, lined by a serous membrane, a single layer of mesothelial cells, is a closed sac, except for the openings of the fallopian tubes in the female. Normally, the peritoneal cavity contains less than 100 ml. of straw-colored fluid that has a lubricating function. When an abnormal amount of fluid is present, its distribution is influenced by the bowel, the mesenteric attachments of the intestine, and the division of the peritoneal cavity into the greater and lesser sacs (Fig. 4). For example, a duodenal ulcer may perforate, and the irritating, highly acid fluid that escapes may continue along the lateral gutter, lateral to the mesenteric attachment of the ascending colon, so

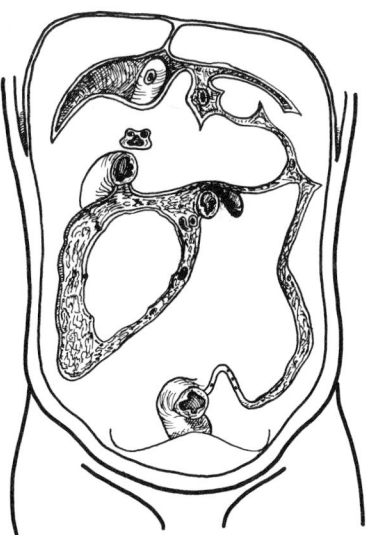

Figure 4. Diagram of the mesenteric attachments in the posterior portion of the abdomen.

that the patient experiences the maximal pain in the right lower abdomen.

Primary Peritonitis

Peritonitis is defined as an inflammation of the peritoneum and is customarily divided into primary and secondary peritonitis. Primary peritonitis implies that the inflammatory process is primary within the abdominal cavity and is not secondary to a primary focus of disease elsewhere. This is not strictly true in many patients but does serve to distinguish two forms, of which one is obviously secondary to other disease processes or to the introduction of infection from external sources. The organisms most commonly found in patients with primary peritonitis are pneumococcus and hemolytic streptococcus.

The typical patient is a girl, 5 to 6 years of age, with evidence of a recent respiratory infection, in whom restlessness and irritability, chills, and vomiting develop abruptly and who complains of diffuse abdominal pain. Diarrhea may be present. The child is found to have a fever of 104 to 105° F. and appears acutely ill, toxic, and dehydrated. The abdomen is diffusely tender and moderately distended, with fluid present. It should be noted that pneumococcal peritonitis may occur as a complication in children with nephrosis. If bowel sounds are present, they soon become diminished or absent. The abdominal wall varies from being rigid to having a soft, doughy consistency.

The white blood cell count is markedly elevated, often with counts of 30,000 to 50,000 cells per cu. mm. The diagnosis may be made by aspiration of the abdomen. A smear of the fluid should be stained and examined. Culture of the fluid is essential.

The most important consideration in the differential diagnosis is the possibility that the peritonitis is secondary to a source in the gastrointestinal tract, particularly perforation of acute appendicitis. The history of the onset and course of the illness differs from that in acute appendicitis, and the absence of enteric organisms does much to exclude acute appendicitis or diverticulitis.

Secondary Peritonitis

General inflammation of the peritoneal cavity is usually caused by bacterial invasion, either secondary to a defect in the gastrointestinal tract, the biliary system, or pelvic organs or through a wound of the abdominal wall. The majority of cases of peritonitis involve organisms that are residents of the gastrointestinal tract. Perforation of a hollow viscus is frequently the source of entry of these organisms (Table 2).

From a review of Table 2, it is apparent that the onset of peritonitis varies widely, depending in large part upon the organ involved and the nature of the primary process. Perforation of a duodenal ulcer occurs suddenly and dramatically, and the initial insult is primarily a chemical peritonitis due to the acid gastric juice. Bacterial invasion occurs late, usually in patients in whom treatment has been delayed. Perforation of the acutely inflamed gallbladder is more insidious and may occur with few, if any, changes in the clinical picture in a patient with acute cholecystitis.

TABLE 2. Secondary Peritonitis:
Source of Infection

Perforation of Viscus:
    Acute appendicitis
    Gastric or duodenal ulcer
    Diverticulum of colon
    Acute cholecystitis
Ischemia of Intra-abdominal Organ:
    Strangulation of small bowel
    Mesenteric vascular occlusion
    Volvulus of colon
Extension of Infection from Abdominal Organs:
    Liver abscess
    Pyosalpinx
    Pyometrium

When the origin of the peritonitis lies within the pelvis, the patient may report that the pain began in the hypogastrium and spread upward.

Physical findings vary widely. Temperature and pulse are elevated in most patients with peritonitis. However, temperature and pulse rate may remain normal in the early stages, notably in perforation of a duodenal ulcer. Pain is the most important symptom and is present in most patients with peritonitis. It is most difficult to evaluate in the very young or very old. Pain is often most severe in the area of origin of the peritoneal contamination, for example, in the right upper portion of the abdomen when the gallbladder has perforated, or in the left lower quadrant following perforation of sigmoid diverticulitis. Spreading of the pain to involve more of the abdomen is a significant finding in patients who are suspected of having acute intra-abdominal infection and is strong evidence that peritonitis is developing. Pain in the shoulders indicates involvement of the diaphragmatic surfaces by the inflammatory process but does not assist materially in localizing the site of origin.

Vomiting is a commonly associated symptom. Unless the primary process has produced obstruction of the gastrointestinal tract, the vomiting is largely reflex in nature or is a result of the paralytic ileus that develops as the peritoneal irritation progresses.

When examined, the patient usually lies still, with thighs flexed to relax the abdominal musculature. Respirations are shallow. A careful physical examination must be conducted to detect associated disease processes that may be a factor in the development or influence the management of the patient. Following inspection of the abdomen, palpation must be performed gently. Rebound tenderness must be sought after attempts to localize maximal tenderness or to detect masses. Auscultation will usually detect decrease or absence of bowel sounds. Rectal examination and pelvic examination in women are as important as the abdominal examination.

The diagnosis of acute peritonitis usually is not difficult. It is of great importance to determine the problems that preceded the development of peritonitis. In patients who have not been operated upon or are not the victims of injury, the most commonly encountered diseases that lead to peritonitis, when not treated early, are acute appendicitis, acute cholecystitis, perforated peptic ulcer, and acute diverticulitis (Fig. 5). There are a variety of other conditions that may result in the development of peritonitis, such as perforation of the colon following obstruction, perforation of the small bowel from foreign bodies, and inflammatory lesions of the intestine, but these are encountered less frequently.

In each, a careful history and physical examination is the basis of a proper diagnosis, and more detail is provided in subsequent portions of this chapter. Acute appendicitis almost always includes a history of right lower quadrant pain and tenderness, although this may be of short duration, before perforation occurs. Often, perforation is followed by a period of diminished pain before signs and symptoms of peritonitis develop. Acute cholecystitis usually develops in patients with earlier symptoms suggestive of gallbladder disease. Perforation of the gallbladder should be contemplated as a possibility in patients whose symptoms do not improve with the institution of nasogastric intubation and suction, intravenous fluids, and bed rest. Perforation is more likely to occur in the elderly patient.

Perforation of peptic ulcer is usually encountered in patients with a history of ulcer distress who have recently had an exacerbation of their disease. Acute diverticulitis is more common in the sigmoid colon and is characterized by episodes of left lower quadrant pain. The patient usually will report a history of recurring left lower pain before perforation will occur.

Perforation of the bowel and subsequent peritonitis may be encountered in a number of other diseases. Chronic nonspecific ulcerative colitis is a disease with exacerbations and remissions, occurs in young persons, and is characterized by diarrhea, with 10 to 20 stools a day containing blood and mucus, weight loss, and debility. Perforation is one of the most serious complications of the disease and usually occurs during an exacerbation of the illness. Regional enteritis, or Crohn's disease, a chronic granulomatous disease of the intestinal tract that most commonly involves the distal small bowel, is characterized by its chronicity, diarrhea, blood in the stools, and weight loss. Free perforation is rare, although fistula formation and obstruction are common.

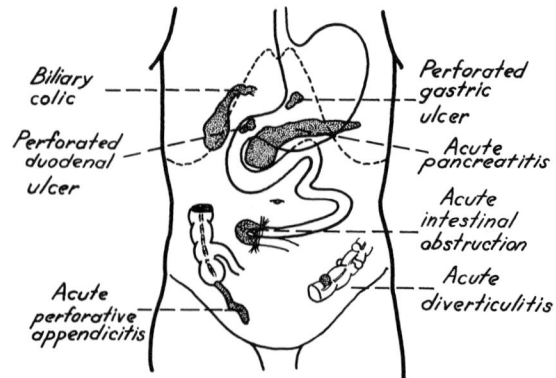

Figure 5. Common causes of the acute abdomen.

Strangulation obstruction of the small bowel may lead to perforation. Also, involvement of the small bowel by primary or metastatic neoplasms may occasionally be followed by perforation. Ingested foreign bodies, such as toothpicks, also have been found to be the cause of perforation of the wall of the intestine. Carcinoma of the colon is associated with perforation more frequently than is disease of the small bowel. Obstruction of the large intestine is more common in the sigmoid colon than elsewhere in the large bowel, and the distended colon may perforate in the cecal area or in a diverticulum proximal to the site of obstruction. Perforation of the neoplasm itself may occur in any portion of the colon. These patients usually have had symptoms of change in bowel habits or blood in the stool. The perforation is heralded by the appearance of signs of peritoneal irritation and by the findings of fever, tachycardia, rebound tenderness, and absence of peristalsis.

Differential Diagnosis

A variety of systemic diseases are accompanied by abdominal pain. In some, pain is intermittent or episodic, may be severe, and may be confused with that of acute abdominal disease, including peritonitis. The pain of acute intermittent porphyria may mimic that of appendicitis or intestinal obstruction. Acute porphyria is associated with severe abdominal pain and vomiting. The pain is usually centrally located but may radiate to the back. The attacks of pain usually are precipitated by the ingestion of barbiturates, sulfonamides, or alcohol. The pain is out of proportion to the objective findings when the abdomen is examined. The absence of muscle guarding, distention, and significant tenderness and the presence of muscle weakness and mental symptoms are important leads to the diagnosis. The diagnosis can be established by the detection of porphobilinogen in the urine.

Hemolytic crises in patients with hereditary spherocytosis may be accompanied by abdominal pain and fever that suggest the presence of primary intra-abdominal disease. Signs of peritoneal irritation are absent, and the spleen is usually enlarged. Anemia is present, and often the patient is icteric, without bile in the urine (acholuric jaundice). Increased amounts of urobilinogen may be detected in the urine.

A number of metabolic and neurologic problems are associated with abdominal pain that may cause diagnostic difficulties. Patients with diabetes mellitus with ketosis and impending coma may complain of abdominal pain. Urinalysis is the key to the correct diagnosis in such patients. The gastric crises of tabes dorsalis produce severe abdominal pain. The presence of a soft abdomen at the time of examination, abnormality of pupillary reactions, and the absence of knee jerks should suggest the diagnosis.

SPECIFIC TYPES OF ACUTE ABDOMINAL DISEASE

The assignment of acute abdominal diseases to categories is difficult and often arbitrary. However, there are certain disease processes that are manifested primarily by signs and symptoms involving the upper abdomen and others that are primarily situated in the lower abdomen. Some produce primarily obstruction of the gastrointestinal tract, and others are basically vascular in origin. Acute upper abdominal pain is caused most frequently by peptic ulcer, gallbladder disease, and pancreatitis. Lower abdominal pain is seen in association with acute inflammation of the appendix, colon, and rectum, or the female internal genital organs. Obstruction of the small bowel is the result of benign processes in the majority of patients, while carcinoma is the most common cause of large bowel obstruction. For these reasons, the specific problems that lead to the development of the acute abdomen appear in these general categories.

PERFORATED PEPTIC ULCER

Perforation of a peptic ulcer, usually duodenal ulcer, is one of the important causes of the development of sudden severe abdominal pain. Men are more often the victims of perforation than are women, and the peak incidence is between the ages of 20 and 40 years, although perforation is encountered in newborns and in the very elderly.

The typical history involves a male who has had episodes of epigastric distress that has been relieved by milk or antacids. For several days, he has had an exacerbation of ulcer symptoms. The onset of perforation is usually dramatic and often occurs 3 to 4 hours after a heavy meal or at night. In a small group of patients, the perforation occurs without a preceding ulcer history.

The pain is sudden, severe, and midepigastric in location. It spreads rapidly to involve the entire abdomen. The patient lies quietly and resists efforts to move. The patient often complains of pain in either or both shoulders. After the appearance of the pain, the patient may retch or vomit once or twice. However, vomiting is not a prominent feature of perforated ulcer, unless there has been associated obstruction of the stomach. The pain is so severe that the paient may suffer a syncopal episode at the time of the perforation but recovers upon assuming the recumbent position.

At the time of examination, the patient usually is lying in a supine position. The temperature remains within the normal range for a few hours after the perforation and then rises. The patient appears ill and in distress and has a moderate tachycardia. The blood pressure, however, remains within normal limits for the first several hours. Respirations are shallow as the patient avoids taking a breath deep enough to disturb the abdomen. Palpation of the abdomen demonstrates diffuse tenderness, and the rigidity of the musculature has been described appropriately as "boardlike." Percussion of the abdomen may disclose a tympanitic note over the area of the lower right chest cage and upper abdomen where a dull note is normally found because of the liver; this loss of liver dullness is evidence that free air is present in the abdomen and lies over the liver when the patient is supine. Auscultation of the abdomen reveals the bowel sounds to be absent or markedly diminished. Rectal examination is usually

**TABLE 3. Summary of Signs and Symptoms
of Perforated Peptic Ulcer**

Sudden onset, severe abdominal pain
Abdominal rigidity—"boardlike"
Free air in peritoneal cavity

unremarkable, although when large amounts of gastric juice have escaped through the perforation, tenderness in the cul-de-sac may be detected.

The white blood cell count increases quickly, and a leukocytosis of 15,000 white cells per cu. mm. is found within a few hours. The hematocrit may become increased early because of the marked shift of plasma into the peritoneal cavity. Although the serum amylase is normal in most instances, elevated serum amylase levels are encountered but not to the levels usually found in acute pancreatitis.

Chest and abdominal roentgenograms are valuable diagnostic aids. To demonstrate free air under the diaphragm, the patient should be in an upright position for at least 5 minutes before the x-ray is taken (Fig. 6). A chest film should be obtained to demonstrate the diaphragm, which is often better seen with this study than with films of the abdomen. If the patient cannot tolerate the upright position, a lateral film, with the patient lying on one side, is satisfactory (Fig. 7).

Differential Diagnosis. Acute pancreatitis may be difficult to distinguish from a perforated ulcer. The

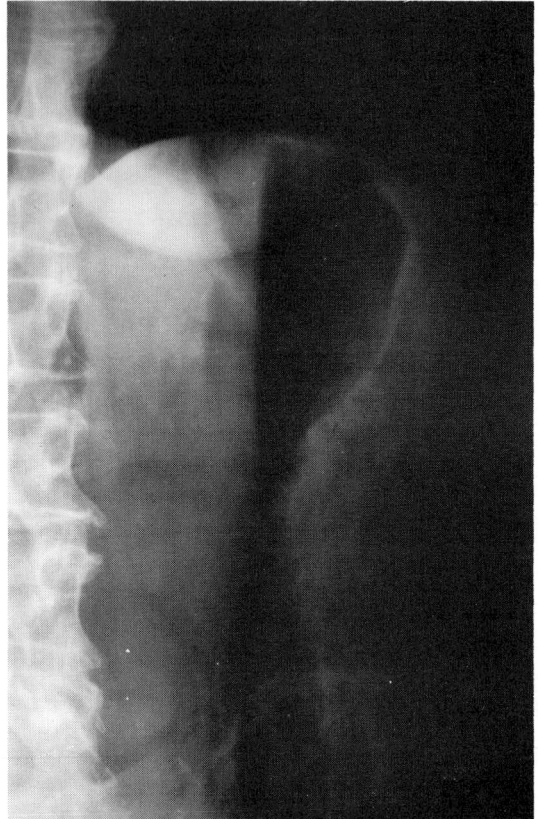

Figure 7. Roentgenogram obtained in a patient with a perforated duodenal ulcer. The patient was lying with the left side up, and free air may be seen within the peritoneal cavity.

onset of pancreatitis is more gradual, and is associated with prodromal episodes of pain that differ from the usual pattern of ulcer distress. Many patients with pancreatitis have either a history of alcoholism or gallstone disease. The abdomen is less rigid in acute pancreatitis, and muscle guarding may be limited to or more marked in the upper abdomen. Back pain is often a prominent feature in pancreatitis. The serum amylase level is often markedly elevated in inflammatory disease of the pancreas, and free air is not found on x-ray examination.

Acute cholecystitis must be considered in the differential diagnosis. The age incidence differs, with the peak incidence of acute cholecystitis in persons over 50 years. Acute cholecystitis begins with episodes of biliary colic in contrast to the burning pain of ulcer distress and the steady severe pain after perforation. Gallbladder pain is localized more laterally in the right upper quadrant, and the tenderness is less diffuse. Muscular guarding is confined to the right hypochondrium.

Gravitation of fluid from a perforated duodenal ulcer along the right gutter into the right lower quadrant may lead to a mistaken diagnosis of acute appendicitis. The history of ulcer distress, the absence of fever, and the presence of free air should suggest the proper diagnosis.

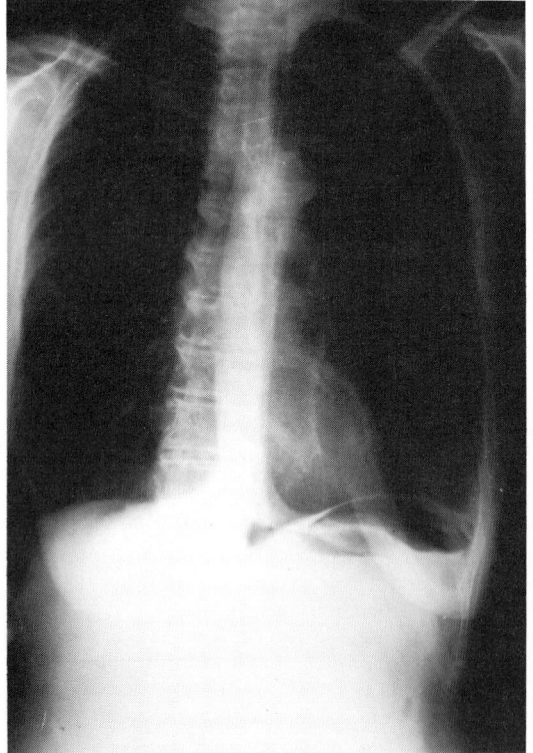

Figure 6. Roentgenogram, taken with the patient erect, demonstrates free air beneath the diaphragm on the left.

Lobar pneumonia and other types of acute pneumonitis involving the right lower lung fields may lead to a mistaken diagnosis of subdiaphragmatic disease. A careful history and examination of the patient should provide a clue to the pulmonary disease. Rapid respirations with cyanosis or flaring of the alae nasi, cough, fever, and lack of free air may be helpful signs in establishing a correct diagnosis.

Rupture of an abdominal aneurysm may produce sudden pain, but the picture of blood loss predominates quickly, suggesting the true nature of the catastrophe.

ACUTE CHOLECYSTITIS

Acute cholecystitis is essentially a disease of adulthood. Patients usually have previous episodes of biliary colic over a period of months or years preceding the attack of acute cholecystitis. This disease is more common in women than in men and reflects the incidence of gallstones. More than 90 per cent of patients with acute cholecystitis have gallstones.

The acute attack begins with an episode of biliary colic. The onset is acute with a rapid increase in pain. Initially, the patient is restless and moves about during the early stages of the episode. The pain is followed by nausea and vomiting. The vomitus is usually green and bitter-tasting, and emesis may initially provide partial relief. After a period of 2 to 6 hours, the pain becomes continuous and localizes in the right upper quadrant of the abdomen. It may radiate to the right scapular region, around both costal margins, or occasionally to the subxiphoid or substernal region. The pain is accentuated by deep inspiration, and the patient usually breathes shallowly to decrease the distress.

Elevation of temperature is not a prominent feature during the early stages. Within 24 to 48 hours after the onset of pain, a febrile response of 101 to 102° F. is common, and chills may occur. The pulse rate is proportional to the fever.

The significant physical findings are found on palpation of the abdomen. There is tenderness throughout the upper abdomen, most marked in the right upper quadrant. There is usually marked guarding and rebound tenderness. In approximately 20 per cent, an enlarged tender gallbladder may be felt; this facilitates establishment of the proper diagnosis. There are varying degrees of abdominal distention. In some patients a moderate paralytic ileus develops, and in most patients bowel sounds are diminished and are hypoactive. Rectal examination does not contribute to the diagnosis.

TABLE 4. Characteristics of Acute Cholecystitis

History of biliary colic
More frequent in women
Severe right upper quadrant abdominal pain,
    associated with nausea and vomiting
Right upper quadrant tenderness
    and guarding

Urinalysis is unremarkable in the uncomplicated case. However, many patients with acute cholecystitis have associated illnesses, among which diabetes mellitus occurs with significant frequency. The presence of reducing substances in the urine may be the initial clue to the presence of diabetes in patients with an acute illness, such as acute cholecystitis. The white blood cell count is often within the normal range, although elevation of the leukocyte count to 15,000 per cu. mm. is not uncommon and is compatible with the diagnosis. If the white count exceeds 20,000, complications of the disease are likely.

Serum amylase levels may be elevated in acute cholecystitis. Because pancreatitis and cholecystitis may be present at the same time, evaluation of this laboratory finding is often difficult. Serum bilirubin levels are elevated in some patients with acute cholecystitis, even though a common duct stone is not demonstrated. If the bilirubin level is greater than 3 mg. per 100 ml., choledocholithiasis is likely.

Roentgenograms may contribute significantly to the diagnosis. Plain films of the abdomen demonstrate radiopaque calculi in less than 10 per cent of patients (Fig. 8). Oral cholecystography is usually not performed in patients with acute cholecystitis, either because the clinical state prevents the oral administration of the contrast agent, or because the emergency nature of the problem requires a decision earlier than can be obtained with this method. Intravenous cholangiography may be a valuable procedure in establishing the nature of the right upper quadrant pain, because the common duct may be visualized by this method in approximately 60 per

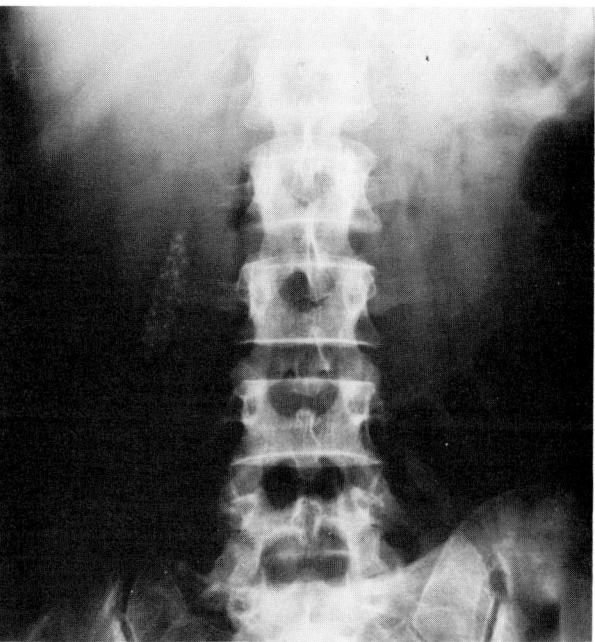

Figure 8. Plain film of abdomen from a 57-year-old woman with acute upper abdomen pain in whom a diagnosis of acute cholecystitis was made. Radiopaque stones are visible on the right side, which have the appearance of cholelithiasis.

cent of patients with acute cholecystitis. If the gall-bladder is seen, the patient does not have acute chole-cystitis. If the common duct is visualized and the gallbladder is not visualized this is supporting evidence for the diagnosis of acute cholecystitis.

The principal diseases that must be considered in the differential diagnosis include perforating or perforated duodenal ulcer, acute pancreatitis, acute appendicitis, hepatitis, and pneumonitis involving the right lower lobe of the lung. When the findings are atypical, each of these may be difficult to distinguish. In general, the history is most important in determining the correct diagnosis.

Duodenal ulcer disease is characterized by pain that occurs 1 to 2 hours after meals and is relieved by milk or antacids. Heartburn and sour "acid" eructations are frequent, in contrast to the bitter bilious regurgitation of biliary tract disease. The character of the pain at the onset is perhaps most distinctive. Ulcer pain is burning in nature, and perforation is associated with the sudden exacerbation of abdominal pain. This is in contrast to the colicky nature of biliary paroxysm.

When the gallbladder extends lower than usual, the differentiation between an inflamed gallbladder and acute appendicitis may be quite difficult, particularly in obese persons. A history of previous distress that suggests gallbladder disease and colicky pain may be a clue to the presence of acute cholecystitis.

Hepatitis has a more gradual onset than acute cholecystitis. The pain in hepatitis is the result of distention and stretching of Glisson's capsule, so that the entire margin of the liver is tender to palpation. Occasionally, liver metastases cause pain in the right upper portion of the abdomen. In these patients, evidence of the existence of a primary neoplasm elsewhere and the presence of a nodular liver at the time of examination may be revealing.

ACUTE PANCREATITIS

The majority of patients with acute pancreatitis have associated gallstone disease or alcoholism. Pancreatitis is more frequent in men, and the majority of patients are between 30 and 50 years of age. The severity of acute pancreatitis varies. A severe case may have rapid onset, with prostration within 2 to 3 hours.

The pain of pancreatitis is epigastric in location, usually deep and unrelenting, and is associated with radiation through to the back or bilaterally around the costal margins. Prodromal episodes of pain are common, and the patient may report the occurrence of vague dull epigastric distress for several days before severe pain occurs. A severe case may have rapid onset, with prostration within two to three hours. The pain is associated with anorexia, nausea, and vomiting. In occasional patients, the pain is colicky in na-

TABLE 5. Characteristics of Acute Pancreatitis

History of alcoholism or cholelithiasis
Diffuse epigastric pain and tenderness
Elevation of serum amylase levels

ture, apparently due to obstruction of the pancreatic ductal system. The pain may be more severe in the left upper quadrant in some patients. In hemorrhagic pancreatitis, the pain may be very severe, and the patient appears much more ill.

Temperature and pulse may be moderately elevated in acute pancreatitis, and blood pressure is usually within normal limits. In hemorrhagic or necrotizing pancreatitis, evidence of shock develops, and the patient may have a rapid, thready pulse with hypotension.

When examined, the patient lies quietly, although some patients may find relief by sitting and bending forward. Tenderness is usually diffuse over the upper abdomen, and varying degrees of muscular resistance and rebound tenderness are found. Rigidity is less prominent than with perforated peptic ulcer, and less localized than with acute cholecystitis. Peristalsis is diminished and may become absent. Ileus may become pronounced at times. Rectal examination is not of diagnostic aid.

Although uncommon, the presence of ecchymosis in the flanks (Grey-Turner sign) or in the periumbilical region (Cullen's sign) is associated with severe hemorrhagic pancreatitis and is the result of retroperitoneal hemorrhage.

The white blood cell count is usually moderately elevated, 12,000 to 18,000, and the hematocrit is within normal limits in uncomplicated cases. A white blood count of over 20,000 is an unfavorable finding and is associated with the more severe forms of the disease. In severe cases, the hematocrit level may rise as a result of the extravasation of plasma-rich fluid into the retroperitoneal areas, fluid that is also rich in pancreatic enzymes.

Among laboratory tests, the serum amylase is the most important in acute pancreatitis and is increased in approximately two thirds of patients with this problem. While elevation of the serum amylase occurs in other diseases, the greatest elevations are found in pancreatitis. In mild acute forms, the increase in serum amylase may be transient and present for only 24 hours. In such instances, urinary diastase levels are increased for approximately 24 hours longer, and serum lipase may be elevated for several more days. Amylase values should be determined as early in the illness as possible when pancreatitis is suspected.

Serum bilirubin levels may be increased in some patients because of obstruction of the common bile duct, thus complicating the problems of differential diagnosis. The serum calcium level may be depressed in the more severe forms of pancreatitis, such as hemorrhagic pancreatitis. Blood samples for calcium, phosphorus, and alkaline phosphatase determinations should be obtained in patients with pancreatitis and the tests should be repeated if the values are elevated, because of the occasional association of hyperparathyroidism.

X-rays often do not contribute to the diagnosis of this disease. A small segment of dilated small bowel is frequently demonstrated in the left upper abdomen, when plain abdominal films are obtained, and this is supporting evidence for the presence of pancreatitis. In addition, multiple calcific deposits in the upper abdomen may be detected in some patients who have had previous episodes of pancreatitis.

The differential diagnosis of acute pancreatitis includes acute cholecystitis, perforated peptic ulcer, and high small bowel obstruction. Frequently, the diagnosis is established by exclusion of other problems. "Pancreatitis is difficult to diagnose with complete assurance. The patient is presumed to have the disease on the basis of clinical findings and laboratory studies, none of which are specific. A number of other catastrophic intra-abdominal problems, including perforated ulcer, strangulation obstruction, gangrenous cholecystitis, and perforated appendicitis, may be confused with severe pancreatitis on the basis of physical findings and elevated enzyme levels."[1]

Pancreatitis may be distinguished from perforated ulcer usually by careful history and examination. Abdominal rigidity is less marked and is not as diffuse in pancreatitis. The serum amylase elevation is not as great in perforated ulcer, and free air in the peritoneal cavity is not associated with pancreatitis. It is often difficult to distinguish between acute cholecystitis and pancreatitis, particularly because they may coexist. Acute cholecystitis is typically an acute inflammatory process localized to the right hypochondrium and is preceded by episodes of biliary colic, two findings of importance in the differential diagnosis.

ACUTE APPENDICITIS

Although the incidence seems to be decreasing, acute appendicitis remains a common cause of abdominal pain. Early diagnosis of appendicitis continues to be important. Uncomplicated acute appendicitis, when treated by appendectomy, is associated with few complications, and recovery is prompt. When perforation occurs, a variety of serious complications are encountered, including abscess formation, intestinal obstruction, wound infection, and fecal fistula, and recovery may be prolonged. Deaths from appendicitis are confined almost entirely to patients with perforation.

Pain is typically the first symptom of acute appendicitis. Often, acute appendicitis has an insidious onset, with rather vague midabdominal pain that slowly increases in severity. In other instances, the onset may be sudden, and the symptoms severe from the start. In many patients, there is a history of previous episodes of pain in the lower part of the abdomen, more on the right side, that disappeared spontaneously. A history of "indigestion" of a vague nature for a few days before the acute episode of appendicitis

TABLE 6. Acute Appendicitis: Signs and Symptoms

Pain—first symptom to appear; begins in epigastrium, shifts to right lower quadrant
Loss of appetite—appears early
Vomiting—variable
Tenderness in right lower quadrant—most significant finding

occurs is often elicited. Frequently, the initial pain is diffuse and not well localized. Some patients experience a dull pain in the periumbilical region. After a period of a few hours, the pain shifts to the right lower quadrant of the abdomen. However, the first symptom in some may be right lower quadrant pain.

Acute appendicitis usually develops without relation to the ingestion of food, despite the patient's attempt to correlate the onset of symptoms with some dietary indiscretion. Absence of definite bowel dysfunction characterizes the onset of appendicitis, although children commonly have diarrhea preceding the onset of abdominal pain. The differentiation between acute gastroenteritis and acute appendicitis may be very difficult in children.

Acute appendicitis may occur at any age but is most common in persons between 20 and 50 years of age. The diagnosis is most difficult in children under the age of 2 years and in the elderly patient. There is no predilection for either sex.

Anorexia is an important symptom in patients with appendicitis. Nausea and vomiting are variable in frequency and intensity, but the majority of patients lose the desire to eat or drink and may actually have an aversion to food.

The location of the appendix influences the clinical picture when the organ becomes acutely inflamed. When the appendix is located in the retrocecal area, the pain may become localized in the right flank and mimic renal disease. The appendix may extend into the pelvis in other instances and become adherent to the bladder, rectum, or tubes and ovary. In such instances, voiding or defecation may actually cause an exacerbation of pain.

Temperature, pulse, and respiratory rate are within normal limits early in the disease. Later, the temperature may be elevated, but seldom exceeds 101° F., unless perforation has occurred. A pulse rate in excess of 100 beats per minute and temperature of 101° F. or greater suggests perforated appendix.

At the onset, the patient with colicky pain may be somewhat restless. However, when the pain has become localized to the right lower quadrant, the patient usually prefers to lie on the right side, with the thigh flexed slightly on the trunk. If the patient walks, he usually walks bent to the right side and without fully extending the right thigh.

Tenderness in the right lower quadrant is the single most important finding in acute appendicitis. Acute appendicitis should be included in the differential diagnosis in any patient who is tender to palpation in the right lower portion of the abdomen. The degree of muscle guarding varies considerably. Rebound tenderness, direct and referred, depends upon the degree of involvement of the surface of the appendix and upon the location of the appendix.

Hyperesthesia of the skin is frequently present in the right lower portion of the abdomen. If the appendix is situated medially and is in contact with the psoas musculature, a positive psoas sign may be present. When the tip of the inflamed appendix lies against the wall of the pelvis, the obturator test may be positive.

Rectal examination is essential in the examination

of patients suspected of having appendicitis, and pelvic examination should be performed in women. At times, the appendix may be inflamed but covered by omentum and intestine, so that the abdominal findings are not impressive, but when it extends into the pelvis, vaginal or rectal examination may elicit marked tenderness.

The customary laboratory determinations are of limited value. The white blood cell count may be normal or slightly elevated. Approximately 90 per cent of patients with appendicitis will have a white blood cell count in excess of 10,000 per cu. mm., and approximately three fourths will have a neutrophil count over 75 per cent. However, there is a considerable overlap in these findings when a comparison is made with healthy persons. There is a tendency for the degree of leukocytosis to increase in patients with perforation of the appendix.

Urinalysis must include microscopic examination of the urinary sediment. While red cells are suggestive of the presence of renal disease, the inflammatory process from an appendix that is adjacent to the right ureter may result in the appearance of both red and white blood cells in the urine. However, the cellular content of urine under this condition is much less than that seen in urinary tract infections or renal disease.

Complications of Appendicitis. The chief complications of acute appendicitis are abscess formation and diffuse peritonitis, the result of perforation of the appendix. Abscess formation may be suspected in a patient who has had right lower quadrant pain, anorexia, and fever for 5 to 7 days, or longer, and is found to have a tender mass in the right lower quadrant. This clinical picture is encountered more often in elderly patients than in the young.

The temperature usually ranges from 2 to 4° F. above normal, is irregularly elevated, and is accompanied by a proportional increase in the pulse rate. Varying degrees of abdominal distention are present, although usually the patient does not have the findings of intestinal obstruction. The tender mass in the right lower quadrant may also be detected by rectal or pelvic examination. The white blood cell count is usually elevated.

Free perforation of the actually inflamed appendix is a serious complication that still results in significant morbidity and mortality. In patients in whom the acute suppurative process has resulted from obstruction of the lumen of the appendix with a fecalith, perforation may occur within a few hours of the onset of pain. Often, the severe right lower quadrant pain subsides promptly at the time of perforation, and the patient is relieved of the acute symptoms for a brief period. Steady pain develops that spreads to involve the remainder of the abdomen. Then the clinical picture associated with diffuse peritonitis develops.

Differential Diagnosis of Acute Appendicitis. A wide variety of problems may mimic acute appendicitis. Because the specific treatment of appendicitis is appendectomy, a short period of observation of 2 to 4 hours may be helpful in patients who have relatively mild symptoms and in whom the clinical picture is equivocal. This period of observation should include repeated examination and determination of tempera-

ture, pulse, and respiratory rate at intervals, as well as repeated white blood cell counts.

Ruptured graafian follicle may simulate appendicitis. This is a common cause of right lower abdominal pain of ovarian origin and typically occurs in the midportion of the menstrual cycle. Blood escapes from the ruptured follicle in the ovary and causes peritoneal irritation, which may closely resemble pain of appendiceal origin. Often the diagnosis remains obscure until operation is performed and the only finding is the ovarian follicle and a small amount of blood in the lower abdomen. Occasionally, an ovarian cyst may undergo ischemic changes as a result of torsion on its attachment. This can usually be detected by careful pelvic examination.

Pelvic inflammatory disease is a frequent consideration in the diagnosis of pain in the right lower quadrant. The differentiation between this disease and acute appendicitis may be very difficult. The relation of the onset of symptoms to the menstrual cycle is pertinent. If the symptoms have their onset during the menstrual period, it is more likely that pelvic inflammatory disease is the cause. Gastrointestinal symptoms are less pronounced in patients with pelvic inflammatory disease. Vomiting is a more prominent early symptom in appendicitis. In addition, fever and tachycardia are seldom present early in the course of appendicitis, while an elevated temperature and pulse rate are usually present in women with pelvic inflammatory disease, even during the first 24 hours. Pain and tenderness are usually bilateral and low in the hypogastrium in women with adnexal infections. Pelvic examination may disclose a vaginal discharge and tenderness or masses in the adnexal regions.

Ectopic pregnancy may be confused with acute appendicitis. The history of a missed period in a young woman should raise the question of ectopic pregnancy. On pelvic examination a mass may be detected in the adnexal region.

The age of the patient influences the conditions that may be considered in the differential diagnosis. In young children, the differentiation between acute nonspecific gastroenteritis and appendicitis may tax the clinician. Mesenteric lymphadenitis is also associated with abdominal pain in young children. It often follows upper respiratory infections and may be indistinguishable from acute appendicitis before operation. The pain and tenderness tend not to be as well localized as those of acute appendicitis, and an increase in the lymphocyte count may be found. Acute inflammation of a Meckel's diverticulum is an uncommon cause of right lower quadrant pain but should be sought in patients who are found to have a normal appendix at the time of operation.

Right renal or ureteral calculi may cause right-sided abdominal pain. Radiation of pain into the flank, or into the right groin or testicle, associated with costovertebral angle tenderness and microscopic hematuria, may lead to the proper diagnosis. Right hydronephrosis in a young person causes right-sided pain, but the history and physical findings should elicit sufficient differences to result in the performance of appropriate tests, including intravenous pyelography.

The differentiation between acute ileitis involving the terminal ileum and acute appendicitis is seldom made before operation. In some, a history of earlier attacks of cramping pain and diarrhea may suggest the possibility of ileitis, but operation is usually required to determine the specific diagnosis.

In older patients, other problems should be considered. Acute cholecystitis may occasionally pose a problem in differential diagnosis. Carcinoma of the ascending colon or cecum will occasionally produce acute symptoms that resemble those of appendicitis. In others, the presence of a right lower quadrant mass may be of either neoplastic or inflammatory origin.

Diverticulitis must be considered in patients beyond the age of 50 years. Cecal diverticulitis is usually indistinguishable from acute appendicitis until operation is performed. Occasionally, the sigmoid colon is involved in diverticulitis and is sufficiently redundant to be present in the right side of the abdomen.

Perforation of a duodenal ulcer may be followed by the development of physical findings that suggest acute appendicitis. This occurs when the irritating gastric fluid that escapes through the perforation follows the peritoneal reflection along the right "gutter" into the right lower portion of the abdomen. A history of peptic ulcer symptomatology, the suddenness of onset, and the absence of significant fever in the presence of marked abdominal findings may indicate the correct diagnosis.

ACUTE DIVERTICULITIS

Acute diverticulitis is produced by inflammatory changes of diverticula of the large intestine and occurs most frequently in the sigmoid colon. The incidence of diverticula in the colon increases with age; approximately 40 per cent of patients over the age of 40 years have diverticulosis. It has been estimated that 80 per cent of colon diverticula are in the sigmoid and descending colon. When this is considered and it is noted that diverticulitis develops in approximately 20 per cent of patients over the age of 40 years with diverticulosis, it is not surprising that the disease is more prevalent in the sigmoid colon in patients beyond the age of 40.

Abdominal pain is the most common complaint in patients with diverticulitis. A history of previous episodes of intermittent left lower abdominal pain of varying severity is often obtained. This is usually described as cramping and may be associated with a history of constipation. The acute episode of sigmoid diverticulitis often begins with a rather sudden onset

of left lower quadrant pain or a sudden increase in mild pain already present in the same region. Vomiting is not a reliable sign and may not be present. When vomiting does occur, it appears after the pain and is usually not a prominent feature of the clinical picture.

The most common picture is one of localized peritonitis. The patient is moderately febrile, with temperatures commonly in the range of 102 to 103° F. Tenderness is present in the lower abdomen and is most marked in the left lower quadrant. Muscle guarding is often present, and in many a tender mass may be felt in the left iliac fossa. The extent of tenderness and guarding varies considerably. When the peritoneal signs extend across the lower abdomen or into the upper abdomen, the possibility of generalized peritonitis must be considered. Rectal examination frequently discloses tenderness in the cul-de-sac and in the left vault. Sigmoidoscopy may be performed, and one may observe edema of the mucosa of the rectosigmoid, as well as a purulent mucoid discharge in the lumen. However, this examination is seldom diagnostic.

Plain films of the abdomen usually yield rather nonspecific findings, unless there is free air or obstruction of the bowel. Perforation from diverticulitis is second only to perforated gastroduodenal ulcer as a cause of free air in the peritoneal cavity, excluding operation or injury. Barium enema examination should be postponed and not performed during the acute period.

Treatment during the initial phase is conservative and consists of either withholding oral fluids or nasogastric intubation and suction, intravenous fluid therapy, and systemic antibiotic therapy. The response to this regimen will contribute to the decision as to the diagnosis. Failure to respond promptly indicates that the inflammatory process has extended beyond the bowel wall and that more generalized infection is present, such as a pericolic abscess.

Free perforation of a sigmoid diverticulum may be the first manifestation of diverticulitis. This occurs with sudden onset, usually with the initial pain being felt in the left lower quadrant of the abdomen. The pain spreads rapidly to involve the entire abdomen. The patient is found to have the signs of generalized peritonitis, with a rigid abdomen and with the signs of a severe intraperitoneal infection. The maximal signs usually are present in the lower abdomen. The bowel sounds are absent, and the abdomen is moderately distended in a short time. The finding of maximal tenderness in the lower portion of the abdomen with the onset of pain in the left lower quadrant should suggest that the process has evolved from perforation of diverticulitis rather than from peptic ulceration of the gastroduodenal area.

TABLE 7. Characteristics of Diverticulitis
of the Sigmoid Colon

Left lower abdominal pain
Majority of patients 50 years of age
   or older
Tenderness in left lower abdomen
Left lower quadrant, tender mass
   often felt

ACUTE GYNECOLOGIC DISEASE

Ectopic Pregnancy

The diagnosis of tubal pregnancy usually is made when extratubal rupture occurs, and this catastrophe constitutes one of the major emergency conditions within the abdomen. Rupture commonly occurs 6 to 12 weeks after the onset of pregnancy, and tubal pregnancy is usually not detected until rupture has taken place.

Typically, lower abdominal pain develops suddenly; it may be continuous and is usually described as tearing or stabbing in nature at its inception. Although the acute episode may occur at the time of coughing or straining, it is often a spontaneous event. The pain is typically felt throughout the lower abdomen but may at times be unilateral. Nausea may occur, and the patient may vomit and have a desire to defecate. The patient actually may take a laxative or an enema because of the desire to evacuate the bowels.

A careful history will disclose that the patient has missed a period or has had abnormal or scanty menses at the time of the last period. However, amenorrhea is not reported in approximately 25 per cent, and some patients ignore an abnormal menstrual flow unless carefully questioned.

The patient's symptoms are related to the blood loss in the abdomen, and the severity of the symptoms depends upon the amount and rate of hemorrhage. Approximately one third of patients are admitted with evidence of hemorrhagic shock. The patient usually appears pale. Temperature may be normal or subnormal. The pulse and blood pressure changes are related to the amount of blood loss. Examination of the abdomen discloses tenderness in the lower abdomen, usually with mild to moderate muscle guarding and rebound.

Pelvic examination is essential. Manipulation of the cervix produces pain. A boggy, tender mass can be felt in the adnexal area on one side.

Soon after rupture, the hematocrit is little changed, although the white blood cell count may be as high as 15,000 per cu. mm.

This problem is one of the serious emergencies that require immediate preparation for operation. When blood is drawn for blood counts and crossmatching, an intravenous route should be established for the administration of Ringer's lactate until whole blood can be obtained. The patient should be taken to the operating room without delay.

Differential Diagnosis. Acute appendicitis can be differentiated on the basis of history in most instances. The onset of pain in appendicitis is seldom as dramatic as that in ectopic pregnancy. Gastrointestinal symptoms are more prominent in acute appendicitis, particularly when nausea, vomiting, and fever are present. The signs and symptoms of pregnancy are absent in appendicitis. The pain and tenderness of ruptured tubal pregnancy are lower in the hypogastrium than McBurney's point. Pelvic examination is essential in differentiating these two problems.

Pelvic inflammatory disease may at times be considered. Patients with inflammatory disease do not have amenorrhea and often give a history of previous episodes of pelvic pain. Bilateral pain and tenderness is typical of pelvic inflammatory disease, and fever is often present during an acute episode.

Ovarian cysts may give acute pain when hemorrhage or torsion occurs. However, this occurs with a normal menstrual history, and the uterus is of normal consistency. The ovarian cyst is discrete and smooth, in contrast to the boggy, tender, often ill defined mass in ectopic or tubal pregnancy.

Complications of Ovarian Cysts

Ovarian cysts may undergo torsion, which causes sudden pain in the hypogastrium. The pain may begin in either lower abdominal quadrant but usually involves the entire lower abdomen. Gastrointestinal symptoms are not prominent, although the patient may vomit with the onset of pain. Examination of the patient reveals tenderness and rigidity in the lower abdomen. Bowel sounds are not present or are hypoactive. Temperature and pulse may be moderately elevated. Pelvic examination is most important and often leads to the correct diagnosis. Acute appendicitis and acute diverticulitis may be entertained in the differential diagnosis in some patients.

Ovarian cysts may rupture or cause intraperitoneal bleeding. These complications produce signs of peritonitis in the pelvis, with abdominal and pelvic tenderness when the patient is examined. If the cyst or tumor can be felt at the time of pelvic examination, the diagnosis is easy.

Acute Salpingitis

This disease is usually caused by gonococcal infection, although the history of sexual exposure may be difficult to elicit. The peak incidence is between the ages of 15 and 30 years. The pain begins as bilateral lower abdominal pain and tends to spread upward. It may be felt more on one side than the other and is moderately severe. The onset is gradual, and gastrointestinal symptoms are not prominent. Pain with voiding is common.

The patient is usually febrile, with oral temperatures of 100 to 101° F. commonly found. Abdominal examination reveals tenderness in both lower quadrants, which may be more marked on either side or in the suprapubic region. Bowel sounds are normal. Pelvic and rectal examination cause marked pain with manipulation of the cervix. There is tenderness in the adnexal regions bilaterally. There is usually an obvious cervical discharge, which should be smeared and stained to detect the intracellular gram-negative diplococci.

**TABLE 8.   Cardinal Features of
Ruptured Tubal Pregnancy**

Amenorrhea—missed period or abnormal scant
    period
Abdominal and pelvic pain—sudden onset
Unilateral, tender adnexal mass
Signs of blood loss

ACUTE SMALL INTESTINAL OBSTRUCTION

Acute obstruction of the small bowel is caused most commonly either by hernia or adhesions and bands within the peritoneal cavity. Age has a significant influence upon the cause of small bowel obstruction. In neonates, congenital problems, such as atresia, and meconium ileus, are important causes of obstruction; and in children, intussusception is encountered with frequency. In general, the higher the site of obstruction within the intestinal tract, the more severe are the symptoms.

The pain of intestinal obstruction is relatively sudden in onset, severe, and intermittent. Small bowel pain is felt in the epigastrium and periumbilical region, while colonic pain is felt in the hypogastrium. The pain is spasmodic in nature because it results from the vigorous peristaltic activity of the bowel as it attempts to propel the intestinal contents through the site of obstruction.

Vomiting is more copious in upper gastrointestinal obstruction and occurs early in obstruction that involves the proximal portion of the small bowel. Gastric contents appear in the vomitus initially, followed by small intestinal contents, usually bile-colored. Later, if persistent vomiting occurs and if the obstruction is in the lower portion of small bowel, the vomitus may become feculent in character.

The typical patient with established intestinal obstruction is unable to pass flatus or stool spontaneously. However, this symptom varies in reliability. For example, the initial response to acute obstruction may be an attempt on the part of the bowel to expel contents acutely beyond the point of obstruction. In children with intussusception, the expulsion, shortly after the beginning of abdominal pain, of a "currant jelly" stool is a finding of considerable diagnostic value. Other patients use self-administered enemas in an effort to obtain relief of symptoms.

Temperature, pulse rate, and respiratory rate are normal in the early stages of intestinal obstruction and become altered when there are significant fluid shifts or permeability of the bowel wall is altered. Observation of the patient will usually demonstrate that he "doubles up" with pain during cramping distress and then has a brief period of freedom from distress.

In an adult patient, inspection of the abdomen must be performed with care and note made of the presence or absence of scars of an earlier operation or injury. The inguinal and femoral areas must be examined for the presence of hernia. Palpation of the abdomen early in the course of the disease is not revealing. As distention progresses, and if impairment of the blood supply of the bowel develops, tenderness becomes apparent. Tenderness and muscular rigidity in the presence of intestinal obstruction are suggestive of peritoneal inflammation and may be signs of strangulation obstruction.

Abdominal distention is variable and is not a feature of early obstruction. When the upper small bowel is the site of obstruction, distention may not become

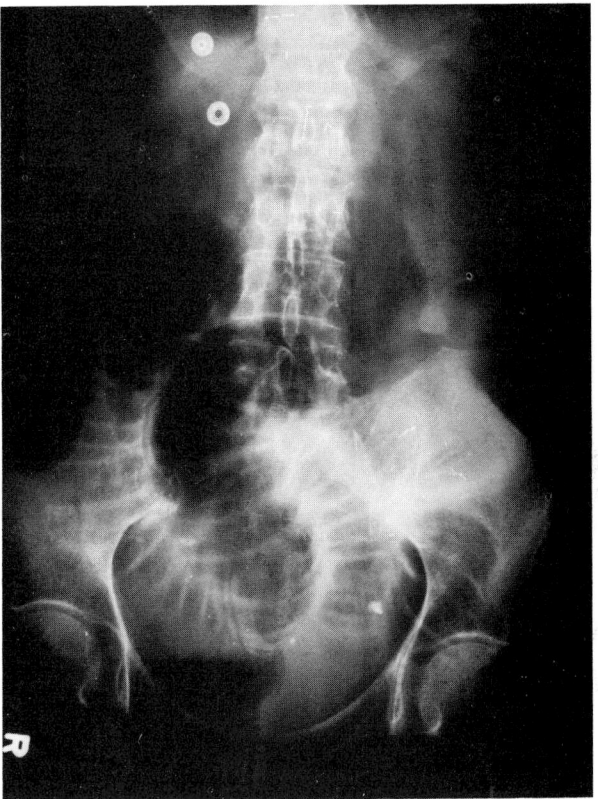

Figure 9. A dilated segment of small bowel is visible in the abdomen of a patient with small bowel obstruction caused by a femoral hernia.

apparent. When obstruction has been present for several hours, and particularly if the distal portion of the ileum is obstructed, increasing evidence of distention appears with tympany and, in thin individuals, peristaltic waves may become visible.

Auscultation of the abdomen will reveal increased bowel sounds. During episodes of pain, the examiner will detect augmented bowel sounds as the peristaltic waves attempt to push the intraluminal gas and fluid beyond the site of obstruction. Rectal examination is seldom of diagnostic value. An empty rectum supports the diagnosis, and tenderness in the cul-de-sac is suggestive of strangulation of the bowel.

The white blood cell count is normal in uncomplicated intestinal obstruction. An elevated or increasing white count is suggestive that strangulation obstruction is developing. The serum amylase may be elevated in intestinal obstruction but is seldom more than twice the normal value. The hematocrit may increase when vomiting has led to significant loss of extracellular fluid. The urine may have an increased specific gravity, and acetonuria may be present.

Roentgenographic study of the abdomen is an important diagnostic aid in the diagnosis of intestinal obstruction. The plain film of the abdomen will demonstrate an abnormal pattern of gas within the small bowel (Fig. 9), and fluid levels may often be demonstrated when the patient is examined in an upright position. The absence of gas in the large bowel helps to confirm the impression of small bowel obstruction.

TABLE 9. Characteristics of Acute Intestinal Obstruction

Peristaltic pain
Nausea and vomiting
Failure to expel flatus
Previous abdominal operation or presence of hernia

The problems that are most commonly considered in the differential diagnosis of small bowel obstruction are paralytic ileus, mesenteric vascular occlusion, and large bowel obstruction. Ileus is usually associated with some other disease or injury. Examination of the abdomen with the stethoscope is most helpful. Bowel sounds in paralytic ileus are hypoactive or absent, in contrast to hyperactive sounds associated with obstruction. X-ray examination in ileus demonstrates gas in both large and small bowel. Mesenteric vascular occlusion from an embolus should be suspected in patients with recent myocardial infarction or with atrial fibrillation in whom sudden severe abdominal pain develops. Large bowel obstruction is typified by the development of marked abdominal distention before significant symptoms appear.

LARGE BOWEL OBSTRUCTION

Obstruction of the large intestine is caused in most patients by carcinoma of the distal portion of the colon. Sigmoid diverticulitis and volvulus of the colon may cause acute obstruction also. The development of the clinical picture is slower than in small bowel obstruction, and the patients do not appear as ill in comparable stages.

Because the underlying causes of large bowel obstruction occur later in life, most patients with this problem are over 50 years of age. In the majority, the acute episode of obstruction is superimposed on progressive change of bowel habits, although occasionally it may be the first symptom.

When lesions are located beyond the midtransverse colon and produce obstruction, the pain is felt in the hypogastrium, a characteristic of hindgut pain. Obstruction of the large bowel is most commonly caused by neoplasms arising in the sigmoid or rectosigmoid colon, and the patient gives a history of progressive constipation. After a few days of failure to have stools, the patient complains of distention, "bloating," gaseous eructations, and occasional cramping pain.

When diverticulitis is the cause of obstruction, the patient may have suffered from previous episodes of diverticulitis, and obstruction may be superimposed upon an acute attack. In many instances, however, the clinical picture is indistinguishable from that associated with carcinoma. Sigmoid volvulus presents a more acute problem. It is a problem seen among elderly persons and often occurs in patients who have long-standing constipation and poor bowel habits. The acute attack is characterized by acute and marked abdominal distention, failure to pass either gas or stool, and acute lower abdominal pain.

Nausea and vomiting are present in patients with large bowel obstruction but are less prominent than in small bowel obstruction, unless the proximal portion of the colon is the site of obstruction and the ileocecal valve is incompetent.

The chief feature of examination of the patient is distention of the abdomen. There is a tympanitic note to percussion, and auscultation of the abdomen leads to the detection of peristaltic rushes. Tenderness is

TABLE 10.   Clinical Characteristics of Large Bowel Obstruction

Majority of patients are over 50 years of age
Gradual onset of lower abdominal cramping pain
Abdominal distention prominent feature
Sigmoidoscopy and barium enema important

usually not present, and an abdominal mass is seldom felt.

Rectal examination is important, and a mass may be felt in the rectum or rectosigmoid in some patients. In addition, if stool is present in the rectum, a specimen should be obtained and tested for occult blood, the presence of which supports the diagnosis of carcinoma.

Sigmoidoscopy should be performed early in patients thought to have large bowel obstruction. This examination may lead to the detection of the obstructing neoplasm because approximately two thirds of colonic and rectal carcinomas are within reach of the sigmoidoscope. The diagnosis of volvulus may also be made with the sigmoidoscope. The point of the torsion usually lies approximately 15 cm. above the anus.

Roentgenograms of the abdomen show distention of the colon proximal to the site of obstruction (Fig. 10), or in the case of volvulus (Fig. 11) demonstrate a massively distended portion of large bowel that is centrally located. Barium enema examination will clarify

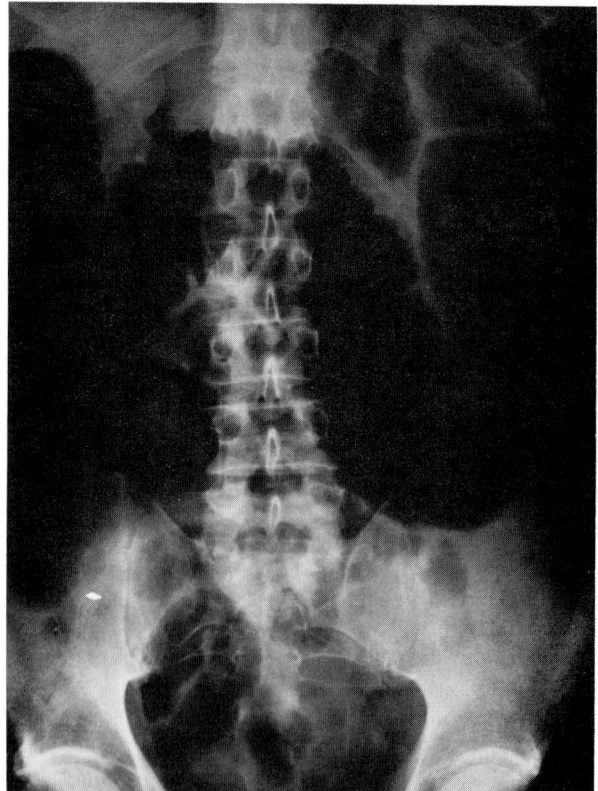

Figure 10. Plain film of the abdomen demonstrates marked dilatation of the colon, caused by carcinoma of the sigmoid colon with obstruction.

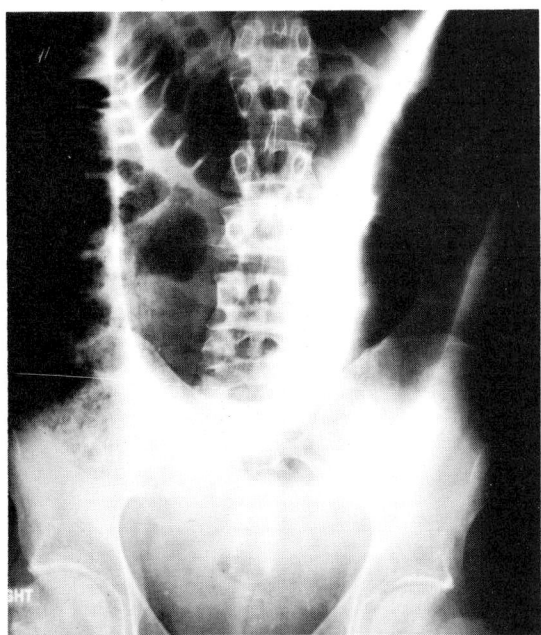

Figure 11. The centrally located, markedly dilated portion of colon in this film is typical of sigmoid volvulus.

the site of obstruction and usually will determine the cause of the obstruction. However, in patients with obstruction caused by diverticulitis, the clinical picture and radiologic study may not distinguish between carcinoma and diverticulitis.

There are other less common causes of large bowel obstruction. Metastatic carcinoma, fecal impaction, endometriosis, and chronic nonspecific ulcerative colitis are problems that are encountered occasionally. Evidence of coexisting or previous carcinoma should arouse suspicions that metastatic carcinoma is the cause of obstruction, particularly when an irregular extraluminal mass is felt in the cul-de-sac by rectal examination. Fecal impaction is more common in chronically ill, bed-ridden, or debilitated patients and can be detected by rectal examination. Endometriosis usually does not produce complete obstruction, and the symptoms and signs are associated with the menstrual cycle. The history of diarrhea associated with mucus and blood and weight loss in a young patient is found in most patients with ulcerative colitis. In doubtful cases, the diagnosis can be confirmed by sigmoidoscopic examination. The most serious complications of an acute attack of ulcerative colitis are hemorrhage, perforation, and toxic dilatation. The last is characterized by fever, as high as 105° F., bloody diarrhea, abdominal cramps, anorexia, and recent weight loss. Abdominal distention is present but is usually not marked. Bowel sounds are hypoactive, and there is mild to moderate abdominal tenderness.

There is often disparity between the marked distention of the colon shown by x-ray and the rather moderate or minimal distention of the abdomen at the time of physical examination. The plain abdominal x-ray film is a considerable assistance. Not only is the

degree of dilatation determined, but the possibility of impending perforation is suggested by presence of air within the wall of the colon.

VASCULAR LESIONS

Superior Mesenteric Artery Embolism

The majority of patients with embolism involving the superior mesenteric artery have a cardiac lesion that is capable of thrombus formation and embolization. Recent myocardial infarction and atrial fibrillation are the two cardiac problems that give rise to mesenteric emboli most often. Occlusion of the superior mesenteric artery may also result from an atheromatous fragment or clot from the aorta, but this is rare.

Periumbilical or generalized abdominal pain develops which is usually sudden in onset. The pain increases in severity after onset and may be colicky in nature. It is steady and without radiation. Typically, the pain is out of proportion to the physical findings. Vomiting usually follows the onset of pain. The patient usually has a desire to defecate, and diarrhea, including bloody stools, may occur. The patient may report that the pain has gradually subsided after a period of 2 to 4 hours. If not treated, signs of peritonitis appear.

Physical findings often are not helpful in the early stages. Abdominal tenderness is present but often is poorly localized, although it is often more pronounced in the upper abdomen. Initially, peristalsis is hyperactive, then gradually diminished. When peristalsis is absent, the bowel wall is usually not viable.

Temperature elevation is not present until late changes have occurred. The white blood cell count usually is elevated, and in most patients there is a progressive increase in the count until the treatment is undertaken. The stool usually contains occult blood, and gross blood may be detected in many. The plain abdominal roentgenogram shows a normal pattern or a nonspecific distribution of gas.

Rupture of Abdominal Aortic Aneurysm

Abdominal aortic aneurysms that rupture are almost always more than 5 cm. in diameter. Rupture may result in extravasation of blood into the free abdominal cavity or into the retroperitoneal area. The patient complains of abdominal or back pain, often with syncope, and is found to have a tender pulsatile abdominal mass. If a patient is known to have an abdominal aortic aneurysm and develops abdominal or back pain, impending rupture of the aneurysm should be suspected.

Abdominal Apoplexy

Spontaneous intra-abdominal hemorrhage, often called abdominal apoplexy, is rare, but life-threatening when it occurs. The onset is sudden, with severe abdominal pain, followed by signs of shock. The evidence of intra-abdominal involvement is indicated by peritoneal irritation and abdominal pain, often associated with nausea and vomiting. Peritoneal tap will be helpful, unless the bleeding is confined to the retroperitoneal space. Selective angiography has been useful in localization of the site of bleeding, which is usually from an aneurysm or area weakened by arteriosclerosis in an artery in the splanchnic bed.

ACUTE ABDOMINAL PAIN OF UROLOGIC ORIGIN

Renal Colic

Acute abdominal pain from urolithiasis is important because of its frequency and occasional consideration in the differential diagnosis. The pain of renal or ureteral colic is usually sudden in onset and may vary from mild discomfort to severe pain. Renal colic affects both sexes but is more common in men. The typical pain begins in the flank and radiates toward the groin, often reaching the scrotum or vulva. The pain, colicky in nature, is often associated with frequency of urination, nausea, vomiting, and sweating. Urination may be painful.

The patient is seldom febrile unless a urinary tract infection is present. During the attack, the patient is found to have tenderness in the flank, particularly in the costovertebral angle. Abdominal tenderness is present on the affected side, but muscular guarding is often less than would be expected from the degree of pain. Abdominal distention is frequent, particularly when the pain is severe. Bowel sounds are diminished.

Red blood cells are found on urinalysis. White blood cells and bacteria are present when the urinary tract is infected. Calculi may be visualized in approximately 75 per cent by plain abdominal roentgenograms. Intravenous pyelography is useful in the localization of stones and to determine whether the ureter is obstructed.

Torsion of the Testicle

The rotation of the testis on the spermatic cord may result in occlusion of the blood supply to the testis. This emergency occurs in active young males, often in infancy, and if not treated promptly may result in infarction of the testis. The pain begins suddenly and is located in the inguinal region, in the testis, and in the hypogastrium. Nausea and vomiting usually occur. The scrotum on the affected side becomes swollen, and the testis is enlarged and tender. The differential diagnosis is usually not difficult, but acute epididymitis and strangulated inguinal hernia must be considered.

SELECTED REFERENCES

Barbee, C. L., and Gilsdorf, R. B.: Diagnostic peritoneal lavage in evaluating acute abdominal pain. Ann. Surg., *181*:853–856, 1975.
The value of peritoneal lavage in patients with acute abdominal problems not related to trauma was studied. It was concluded that peritoneal lavage can be a useful adjunct and should be considered in difficult diagnostic problems but not routinely employed.

Cope, Z.: The Early Diagnosis of the Acute Abdomen. New York, Oxford University Press, 1963.
This concise monograph has for many years been an international reference in the diagnosis of the acute abdomen. Succinctly written, it places much emphasis upon the clinical signs that characterize the various conditions that may present as an acute abdomen. It is a delightful text and is highly recommended.

Friday, R. O., Barriga, P., and Crummy, A. B.: Detection and localization of intra-abdominal abscesses by diagnostic ultrasound. Arch. Surg., *110*:335–337, 1975.
Detection of intra-abdominal abscesses may be difficult. Their development is often insidious, and diagnosis and localization are often difficult. Intra-abdominal abscesses were identified by ultrasonic technique in patients with right lower quadrant abscess formation in Crohn's disease, pyogenic liver abscess, pelvic abscess, and perinephric abscess.

Lewis, F. R., Holcroft, J. W., Boey, J., and Dunphy, J. E.: Appendicitis. A critical review of diagnosis and treatment in 1,000 cases. Arch. Surg., *110*:677–684, 1975.
One thousand cases of appendicitis from 1963 to 1973 were analyzed. Major errors in diagnosis were made most often in young female patients.

McDougal, W. S., Izant, R. J., and Zollinger, R. M., Jr.: Primary peritonitis in infancy and childhood. Ann. Surg., *181*:310–313, 1975.
Primary peritonitis, rarely diagnosed preoperatively, is an uncommon disease accounting for 2.1 per cent of all pediatric abdominal emergencies. It is often associated with urinary or hepatic pathology. In this series, gram-negative bacteria accounted for 69 per cent of organisms.

REFERENCES

1. Anderson, M. C.: Surgical intervention in acute pancreatitis. Surg. Gynecol. Obstet., *120*:1301, 1965.
2. Botsford, T. W., and Zollinger, R. M., Jr. Diverticulitis of the colon. Surg. Gynecol. Obstet., *128*:1209, 1969.
3. Carson, H. W.: The iliac passion. Ann. Med. Hist., *3*:638, 1931.
4. Glenn, F.: Pain in biliary tract disease. Surg. Gynecol. Obstet., *122*:495, 1966.
5. Kerry, R. L., and Ransom, H. K.: Volvulus of the colon. Arch. Surg., *99*:215, 1969.
6. Kleinsasser, L. J.: Abdominal apoplexy. Am. J. Surg., *120*:623, 1970.
7. Lo, A. M., Evans, W. E., and Carey, L. C.: Review of small bowel obstruction at Milwaukee County General Hospital. Am. J. Surg., *111*:884, 1966.
8. Mannick, J. A.: Diagnosis of ruptured aneurysm of the abdominal aorta. N. Engl. J. Med., *276*:1305, 1967.

31

THE STOMACH AND DUODENUM

James C. Thompson, M.D., M.A.

The stomach and duodenum may be considered logically as a unit, since many physiologic mechanisms and certain diseases are either shared by or interact between these two segments of the gut. They are both affected by peptic ulcer, which is the most common serious inflammatory condition of the gastrointestinal tract. Fortunately, peptic ulceration has a relatively low mortality rate, but it does have a high rate of disability and is responsible for great costs to society in loss of productive time and in medical care.

Carcinoma of the stomach, which has undergone a dramatic and unexplained diminution in incidence, is discussed in the following chapter, and congenital hypertrophic pyloric stenosis is covered in Chapter 40. The major attention in this section will be devoted to the physiology of the stomach and duodenum and to peptic ulceration. Other conditions will be discussed separately at the end of the chapter.

ANATOMY

The stomach arises as a spindle-shaped dilatation of the foregut during the fourth week of embryonic life. With later growth it undergoes a rotation so that the previous left side of the stomach becomes the anterior wall and the previous right side comes to lie posteriorly (mnemonic—LARP). The duodenum, which was initially suspended between dorsal and ventral mesenteries, also rotates so that the second portion of the duodenum becomes retroperitoneal and encompasses the head of the pancreas in its C loop.

The fully developed stomach is the largest dilatation of the gut and lies between the esophagus and the duodenum (Fig. 1). The topographic anatomy of the stomach is quite simple, although it has been confused by the application of various terms by anatomists, surgeons, endoscopists, and radiologists. For gross description, the stomach can be divided into fundus, body, and antrum. The fundus is the dome of the stomach, to the left of and superior to the esophagogastric junction. An angulation at about the midline of the body, approximately 5 to 6 cm. proximal to the pylorus on the lesser curvature, is called the incisura angu-

laris (at *A* on lesser curvature, Fig. 1). The area between the fundus and a line drawn from the incisura angularis to the greater curvature of the stomach (in approximately the position of a line from *A* to *A′* in Figure 1) is the body of the stomach; the area distal to that line and proximal to the pylorus is the gastric antrum. The pylorus may be palpated as a thick ring of muscle and is externally marked by the prominent veins of Mayo.

In terms of *function*, the stomach may be divided into fundus (oxyntic gland area) and antrum (pyloric gland area). The fundus secretes acid peptic juice, and the antrum, the distal segment, secretes a thick, viscid, relatively alkaline mucus and the hormone gastrin. The division between the functional area of the fundus and the antrum is a line from A to A′.

The esophagogastric junction, the cardia, is located just to the left of the tenth thoracic vertebra, and the gastroduodenal junction, the pylorus, is located to the right of the midline at about the interspace between the first and second lumbar vertebrae. The superior margin of the stomach between the cardia and pylorus (a distance of about 12 to 14 cm.) is the lesser curvature of the stomach. It is suspended from the liver by the gastrohepatic ligament, which forms the superior portion of the anterior wall of the lesser omental bursa. The inferior and lateral convex border of the stomach is the greater curvature, which is about three times as long as the lesser. From the major portion of the greater curvature is suspended the gastrocolic ligament, which forms the lower portion of the anterior wall of the lesser omental bursa.

The *blood supply of the stomach* is particularly rich. There are innumerable variations in the arrangement of blood vessels, and the schema shown in Figure 1 is only one of many variations. Six vessels provide the main blood supply: the left and right gastric arteries supply the area of the lesser curvature, the right and left gastroepiploic arteries supply the greater curvature, the splenic artery supplies the area of the fundus by way of the short gastric arteries, and the gastroduodenal artery sends branches to the area of the pylorus. The arteries of secondary importance are numbered *7* through *12* in Figure 1. For comparison, the radiologic appearance of the blood supply to the stomach in man,

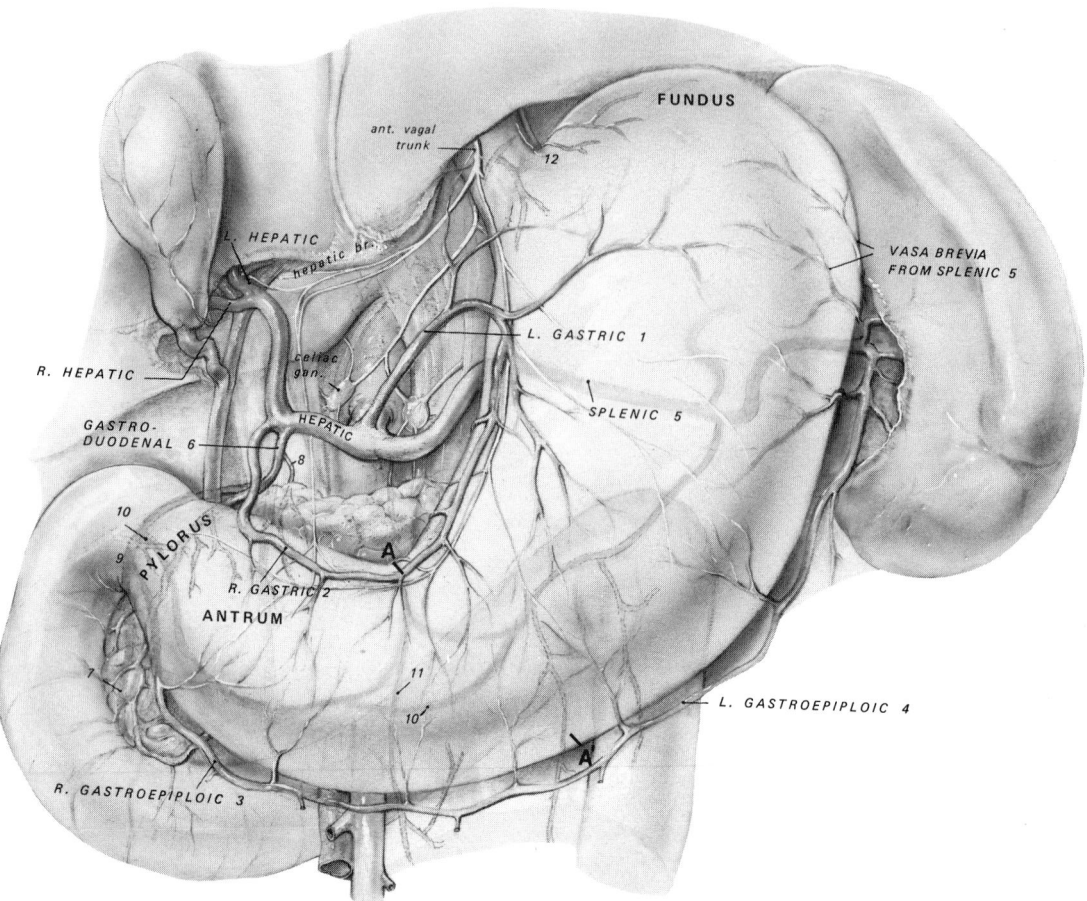

Figure 1. Anatomy of the stomach and duodenum. Grossly, the stomach is divided into fundus (the area superior to the gastroesophageal junction), body, and antrum. The antrum begins proximally at about a line drawn from A on the lesser curvature to A' on the greater curvature and extends distally to the pylorus. There are only two important physiologic divisions, the fundic gland (parietal cell) area and the pyloric gland (antral) area. The junction of these two histologic zones is again roughly at a line between A and A'. The blood supply to the stomach is carried by six major vessels and by six other vessels of lesser consequence.[125] The most important vessels are: *1*, left gastric artery; *2*, right gastric artery; *3*, right gastroepiploic artery; *4*, left gastroepiploic artery; *5*, splenic artery via the vasa brevia; and *6*, gastroduodenal artery. The remaining vessels are indicated by number only in the illustration: *7*, superior pancreaticoduodenal artery; *8*, supraduodenal artery of Wilkie; *9*, retro-duodenal artery; *10*, transverse pancreatic artery; *11*, dorsal pancreatic artery; and *12*, left inferior phrenic artery. The anterior (left) vagus is shown dividing into a gastric and a hepatic branch. Just behind it is also shown the posterior (right) vagus dividing into a gastric and a celiac branch. The duodenal-jejunal flexure is shown here behind the stomach. Its position is variable and may often be seen on x-ray protruding above the lesser curvature of the stomach just to the left of the midline.

as demonstrated by selective celiac angiography, is shown in Figure 2. A rich anastomotic network is evident and no area is served by end-arteries. Michels[125] studied the blood supply of the stomach in a meticulous fashion and called attention to possible surgical hazards (e.g., in more than 20 per cent of patients, the primary or secondary blood supply of the left lobe of the liver would be lost if the left gastric artery were divided at its origin).

The *blood supply of the duodenum* is carried by the supraduodenal and retroduodenal arteries, by the superior pancreaticoduodenal artery, which arises from the gastroduodenal, and by the inferior pancreaticoduodenal artery, which arises from the superior mesenteric artery.

The *parasympathetic nerve supply* to the stomach is from the vagus nerves, which stimulate motility of the stomach and the secretion of acid, pepsin, and gastrin. The left and right vagal trunks give off numerous branches and are somewhat inconstant in their relations at the diaphragm (Figs. 1 and 29). The left or anterior vagus nerve gives off a hepatic branch, which also sends fibers to the area of the pylorus. The remaining portion of the left nerve innervates the anterior wall of the stomach. The posterior vagus nerve gives off a large branch to the celiac plexus, and the remaining nerve goes to the posterior wall of the stomach.

The wall of the stomach is composed of four layers: mucosa, submucosa, muscle, and serosa. Mucosal ar-

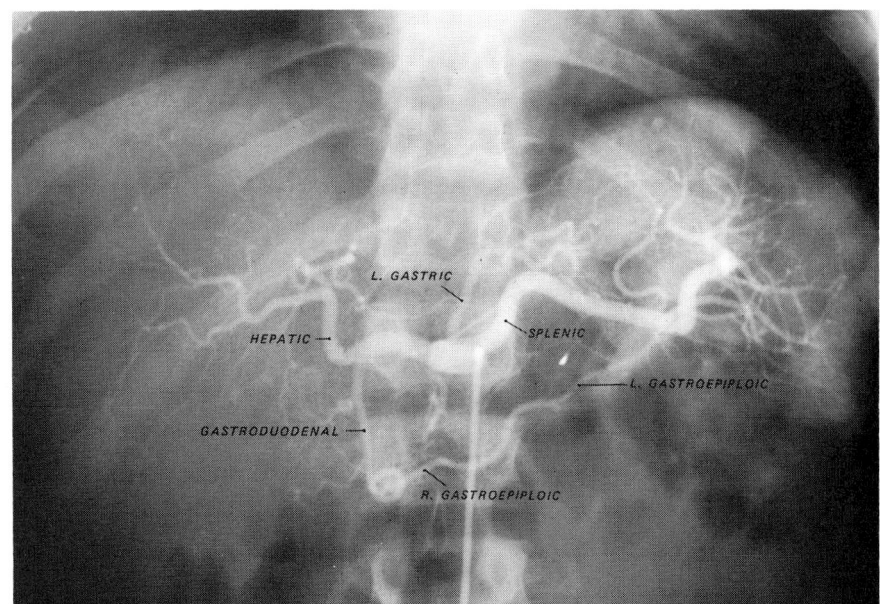

Figure 2. The blood supply of the stomach demonstrated by selective celiac angiography. The angiographic catheter is shown hooked into the orifice of the celiac artery and injection of radiopaque material outlines the major vessels supplying the stomach (see Fig. 1).

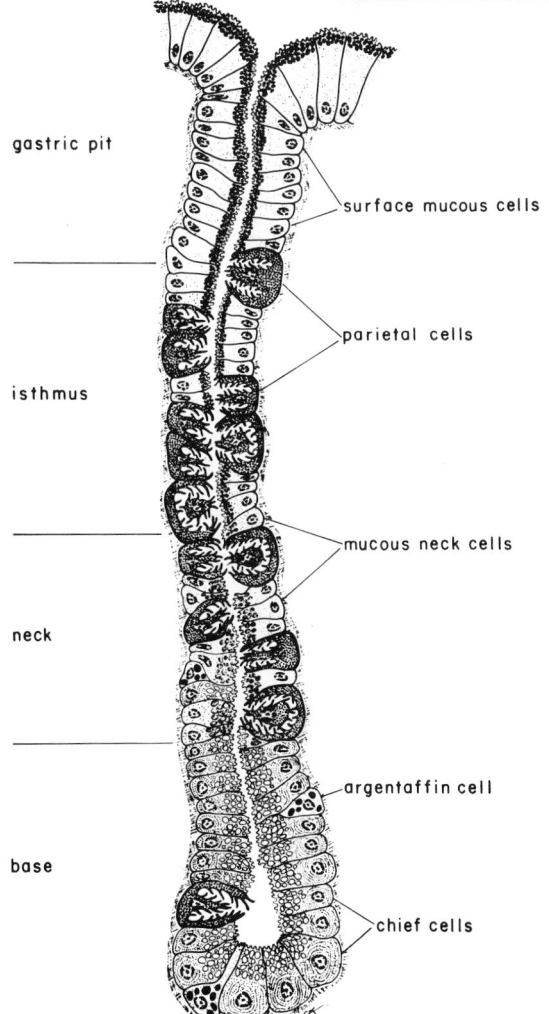

GASTRIC GLAND

Figure 3. Diagram of a simple tubular gastric gland from fundic mucosa. (From Ito, S., and Winchester, R. J., J. Cell Biol., *16*:541, 1963.)

chitecture varies with the area of the stomach. Several types of cells in the stomach have specific functions: parietal cells manufacture and secrete hydrochloric acid and gastric intrinsic factor, chief cells make and secrete pepsinogen, goblet cells secrete mucus, epithelial cells probably secrete extracellular fluid (nonparietal secretion), and specialized cells (gastrin cells or G cells) within the antral gland synthesize (presumably), store, and secrete gastrin. Mast cells store heparin, histamine, and other vasoactive substances within granules. The functions of the fundic argentaffin cell are unknown; they may synthesize or store enteroglucagon or other peptide hormones. Fundic mucosa consists of deep tubular glands (Fig. 3) lined superficially with epithelial cells and containing, in the deeper portions, characteristic parietal cells and chief cells with occasional argentaffin cells. Light and electron micrographs of resting and active fundic tubular cells are shown in Figure 4. The histologic appearance of the mucosa immediately adjacent to the cardia is similar to that of the antrum, except that G cells are lacking. Pyloric glands consist of branching tubules lined predominantly with mucous cells. Some of these epithelial cells, located chiefly in the middle third of the glands, react immunochemically with antigastrin antibodies[19] and are presumably the locus of gastrin synthesis and storage. An electron micrograph of a gastrin cell is shown in Figure 5.

The junction between antral and fundic mucosa cannot be differentiated on gross inspection, but application of a pH indicator to the mucosal surface after the stimulation of gastric secretion will quickly and clearly differentiate the proximal acid-secreting mucosa from the distal neutral antrum.

The duodenum begins at the pylorus and ends at the duodenal-jejunal junction just to the left of the second lumbar vertebra (Fig. 6). The duodenum is divided into four portions: superior, descending, transverse, and ascending. The majority of the first portion is occupied by the slightly dilated duodenal bulb whose

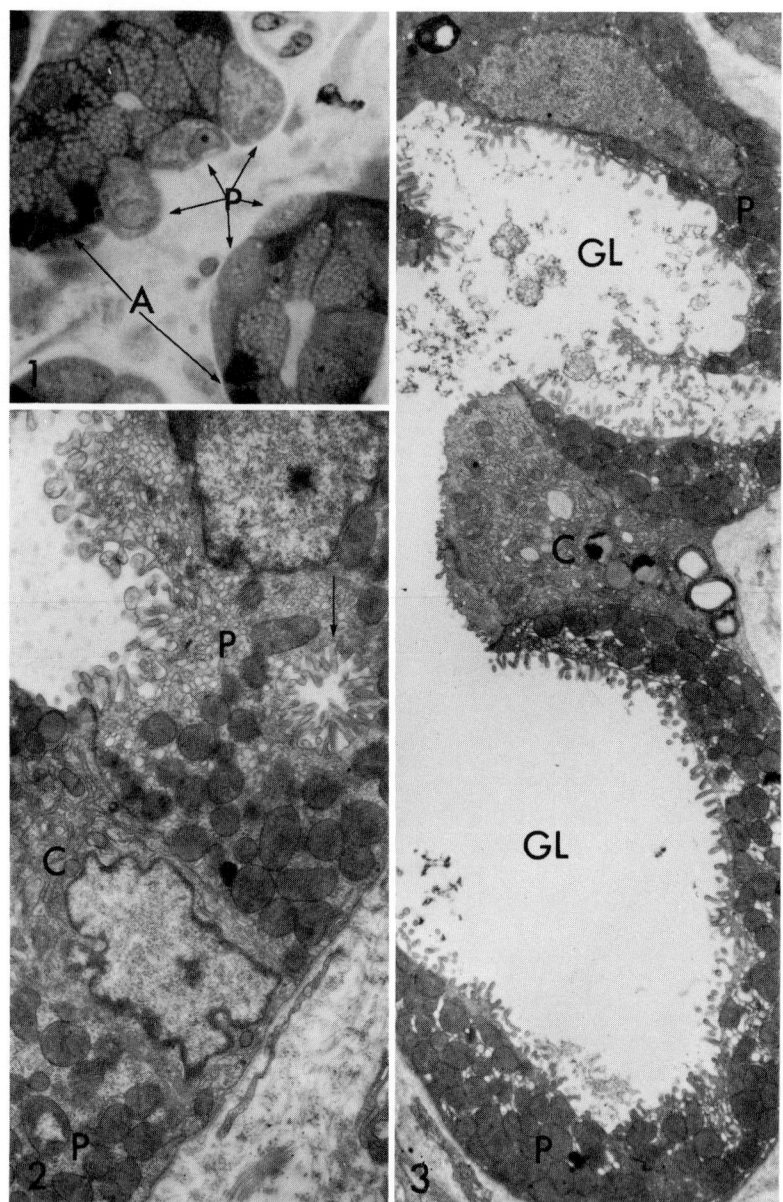

Figure 4.   Light and electron micrographs of fundic glands. *1,* Light micrograph in which the chief cells are easily recognized by the presence of numerous secretory granules. *P,* Parietal cells; *A,* argentaffin cells. ×600 (approximate). *2,* Electron micrograph of resting parietal cells (*P*), and chief cells (*C*) of fundic gland. The arrow points to an intracellular canaliculus. ×10,800. *3,* Electron micrograph of two parietal cells (*P*) of a fundic gland. The cells are at their maximal secretory activity and are in the process of discharging the contents of the intracellular canaliculi into the gland lumen (*GL*). Comparison with the resting parietal cell indicates that the active cell opens out into the gland lumen to expose the entire surface of the intracellular canaliculi into the lumen of the gland. A chief cell (*C*) is located between the two secreting parietal cells. ×6000. (Courtesy of Luciano Zamboni, M.D.)

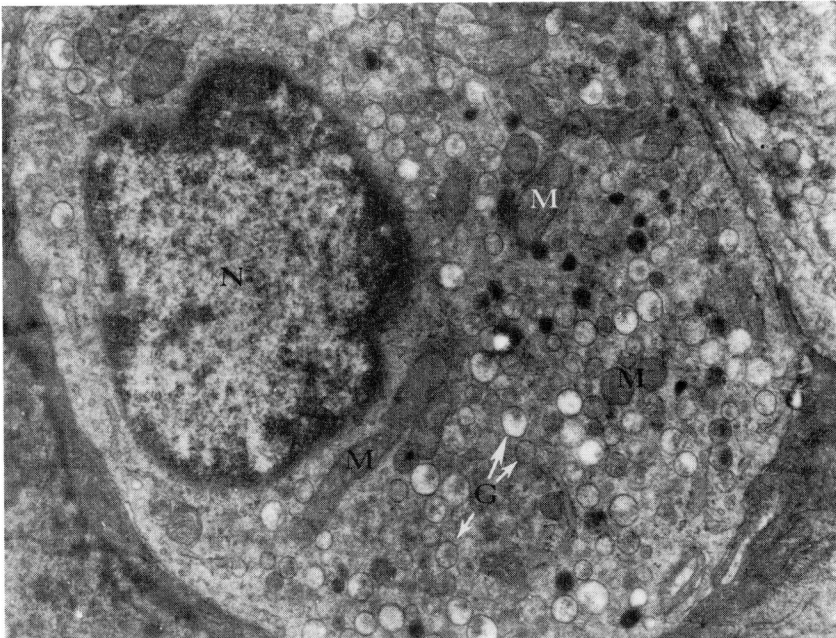

Figure 5. Electron micrograph of a G (gastrin) cell from a pyloric gland. The secretory granules (G), some of which are nearly empty, contain gastrin.

mucosa is characterized by lack of plicae circulares. The common bile duct enters the pancreas immediately posterior to the duodenal bulb and lies within the head of the pancreas. It and the main pancreatic duct open onto the medial wall of the midportion of the second part of the duodenum at the duodenal papilla (ampulla of Vater). The superior mesenteric vessels emerge from behind the pancreas to cross over the third part of the duodenum. The fourth part ascends to the duodenal-jejunal flexure, which is suspended from the posterior body wall by the ligament of Treitz.

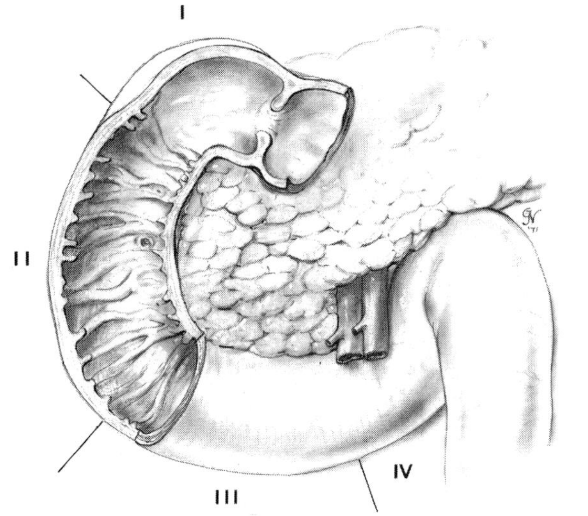

PHYSIOLOGY

The normal flow and ebb of acid gastric secretion in response to a meal provides clear evidence of regulatory mechanisms designed initially to stimulate and later to curtail gastric secretion. Swallowed food enters the stomach where it is mixed with gastric juice and changed to a more liquid form. The viscid, pulpy chyme undergoes only a small amount of digestion in the stomach, mostly proteolysis, before being passed in small boluses into the duodenum, where it is further mixed with bile and pancreatic juice and where major digestion and absorption begin. The mucosa of the small bowel carries out the function of absorption of food, which is the raison d'être of the gut. The main function of the stomach is to mix and churn the food so that it is delivered slowly, as small particles, into the duodenum. Within the duodenum, the delivered acidic gastric contents are neutralized and are mixed with pancreatic digestive juices, bile, and enzymes from the duodenal mucosa.

Since *pepsin* is active only in an acid environment (pH <5), no peptic ulceration can occur in the absence of acid, and in one sense, the goal of all ulcer therapy is to maintain intragastric pH above that level required for activation of pepsin. Because of the important role of acid in digestion and in ulcerogenesis, major attention in gastric physiology has been placed on the study of acid secretion by the stomach.

The parietal cells concentrate hydrogen ions more

Figure 6. Detailed anatomy of the duodenum. The duodenum is divided into four parts. The first part is occupied almost entirely by the bulb of the duodenum, which has flattened mucosa free of the circular folds (plicae circulares of Kerckring) of mucosa that are characteristic of the rest of the small intestine. The major duodenal papilla is seen in the mid part of the second (descending) portion of the duodenum; the minor duodenal papilla is located about 1 cm. proximally. The third, or transverse, portion of the duodenum extends to the superior mesenteric vessels, and the fourth part from the vessels to the duodenal-jejunal flexure.

than one million times. Grossman[71] has suggested that the parietal cell is probably stimulated by five chemical agents: *acetylcholine* released from cholinergic nerve endings; *gastrin* from G cells of the antrum and duodenum; *entero-oxyntin,* the proposed hormone of the intestinal phase;[135] *digested protein,* which apparently stimulates the parietal cell without intermediaries; and *histamine* from fundic mast cells.

STIMULATION OF GASTRIC SECRETION

Gastric juice is composed of parietal and nonparietal components. Pure parietal cell secretion contains between 150 and 170 mEq. H^+ per liter, between 165 and 170 mEq. Cl^- per liter, and 7 mEq. K^+ per liter and is free of sodium.[85,87] In nonparietal secretion, which is virtually identical with extracellular fluid, the chief cation is sodium (about 150 mEq. per liter), and H^+ is virtually absent. Concentration of acid in gastric juice is dependent therefore on the rate of parietal cell secretion and on the degree of admixture with nonparietal secretion.[115] Jacobson and associates[96,159] have shown that there is a direct relation between the rate of gastric secretion and the blood flow to the mucosa of the stomach. It is not clear whether secretory stimulants directly influence the flow of blood to mucosa.

Gastric secretion has been classified as spontaneous (or interdigestive) and stimulated (or prandial). Spontaneous gastric secretion occurs without intentional stimulation in man and in certain other species and may reflect a background secretion of gastrin and acetylcholine. Pavlov[132] observed that food stimulation of gastric secretion could be effected by a stimulus from the head or the stomach, and later it was found that stimuli might arise in the intestine. The *cephalic phase* is stimulated by the sight or smell or chewing of food; the *gastric phase* is stimulated by the presence of food in the stomach; and the *intestinal phase* is stimulated by the presence of food in the small intestine. The phases of gastric secretion were originally thought to be separate and distinct and to bring about stimulation of secretion at different times. It is now known that the hormone gastrin is released by the vagus and that gastric distention causes vagal stimulation, that gastrin and acetylocholine (and probably the intestinal stimulant) potentiate one another, and furthermore, that, with minor variations, the periods of secretion stimulated by each of the phases overlap extensively.

Grossman[71] has proposed that the parietal cell has receptor sites for acetylcholine, gastrin, and histamine and that maximal stimulation of the cell is achieved only when each of these sites is occupied. This hypothesis would explain why blockade of the receptors for any one of these agents (for example, blockade of the receptors for acetylcholine by atropine, or of those for histamine by an H_2-blocking agent) will depress the response to the other stimulants.

Cephalic Phase

Cephalic phase stimuli presumably activate the vagal nuclei in the medulla. Impulses traverse the pe-

ripheral vagi and terminate in the gastric mucosa with the release of acetylcholine from vagal nerve endings. Release of acetylcholine in the fundic mucosa directly stimulates acid secretion by the parietal cell and release of pepsinogen by chief cells. Acetylcholine release in the antral mucosa causes discharge of the antral hormone, gastrin, which also stimulates the parietal cell. In addition, the stimulatory effect of gastrin in the presence of acetylcholine is greater than the sum of either stimulus alone, so that true potentiation is achieved.[66]

Stimulation of the vagus occurs with the sight or smell of food. In addition, distention of the stomach excites a vagovagal reflex that also results in the release of acetylcholine in fundic and antral mucosa.

Gastric Phase

The gastric phase of secretion is stimulated by food in the stomach, which by direct contact and by distention brings about gastric secretion. The humoral mediator of the gastric phase is the hormone gastrin, discovered by Edkins in 1905.[44, 45] Gastrin is liberated from the antral mucosa by acetylcholine (released by local reflexes upon antral distention), upon contact with certain substances (for example, 2-carbon alcohols, small peptides, and amino acids), and by the vagus itself.

One of the most important aspects of the mechanism for gastrin release is its acid sensitivity. When in the course of gastric secretion the surface pH of the antral mucosa reaches 3.5, gastrin output is diminished; when it reaches about 1.5, further gastrin secretion is halted. As is true with other endocrine organs, there seems to be a closed-loop inverse relation between the concentration of the hormone and the output of the end organ, in this case between gastrin and H^+.[16]

Gastrin.[136, 174] Although stimulation of acid secretion by extracts from antral mucosa was reported by Edkins in 1905, it was not until 1964 that the biochemical era in the study of gastrin was initiated when Gregory and Tracy began the experiments that eventuated in the isolation, purification, and synthesis of gastrin.[61, 62, 64] The initial form of gastrin (later to be known as *little* gastrin) was composed of 17 linearly arranged L-amino acids with a molecular weight of around 2100 (Table 1). The C-terminal four amino acids of the gastrin molecule (Trp-Met-Asp-Phe-NH$_2$) have been shown to possess the full physiologic range of action of the parent molecule. This material is now available (with a prosthetic β alanine group attached to the N-terminus) as pentagastrin (Table 1).

Gastrin has been shown to exist in a variety of sizes; all the larger sizes apparently contain the smaller forms (Table 1).[136, 174] Minigastrin (14 amino acids, G-14) consists of the 14 C-terminal amino acid residues of G-17. G-34 (big gastrin) has been found to be the predominant form in circulation; little gastrin can be split enzymatically from big gastrin, which separates it from the apparently inactive N-terminal 17-amino acid tryptic residue. Two larger forms (Rehfeld's Component I and big-big gastrin) have been identified by chromatography, but their molecular structure and their physiologic functions are unknown.

Cholecystokinin, the duodenal hormone that acts to

TABLE 1. The Gastrin-Cholecystokinin Family*

Gastrin[a]	Approximate Molecular Weight		Sequence
	I	II	

Positions: 1 2 3 4 5 6 7 8 9 10 11 12 13 14 15 16 17

Little gastrin (G-17)

	I	II	
			SO$_3$H (on position 12)
Man	2098	2178	Glp^b-Gly-Pro-Trp-Leu-Glu-Glu-Glu-Glu-Ala-Tyr^c-Gly-Trp-Met-Asp-Phe-NH$_2$
Hog	2116	2196	-Met-
Dog	2058	2138	-Met- -Ala-
Cow and sheep	2026	2106	-Val- -Ala-
Cat	2040	2120	-Ala-

Minigastrin (G-14-I, 5-17)

	I	
Man	1833	Trp-Leu-Glu-Glu-Glu-Glu-Glu-Ala-Tyr-Gly-Trp-Met-Asp-Phe-NH$_2$

Big gastrin (G-34-I)

Man	3839	Glp^b-Leu-Gly-Pro-Gln-Gly-His-Pro-Ser-Leu-Val-Ala-Asp-Pro-Ser-Lys-Lys^d- Gln-Gly-Pro-Trp-Leu-Glu-Glu-Glu-Glu-Glu-Ala-Tyr-Gly-Trp-Met-Asp-Phe-NH$_2$
Hog	3883	Glp^b-Leu-Gly-*Leu*-Gln-Gly-His-Pro-*Pro*-Leu-Val-Ala-Asp-*Leu-Ala*-Lys-Lys^d- Gln-Gly-Pro-Trp-*Met*-Glu-Glu-Glu-Glu-Glu-Ala-Tyr-Gly-Trp-Met-Asp-Phe-NH$_2$

Pentagastrin

	768	N-t-butyloxycarbonyl-β-Ala-Trp-Met-Asp-Phe-NH$_2$

Cholecystokinin (CCK-33)^e

	3918	Lys-Ala-Pro-Ser-Gly-Arg-Val- Ser-Met-Ile-Lys-Asn-Leu-Gln-Ser- SO$_3$H (on Tyr) Leu-Asp-Pro-Ser-His-Arg-Ile-Ser-Asp-Arg-Asp-Tyr-Met-Gly-Trp-Met-Asp-Phe-NH$_2$

*Modified from Thompson, J. C. (Ed.): *Gastrointestinal Hormones.* Austin, University of Texas Press, 1975, Appendix p. 653.
[a]Except where noted, the amino acid sequences for gastrins of different species are identical.
[b]Glp = Pyroglutamyl.
[c]Gastrin of each species exists in forms I and II; in form I, there is no SO$_3$H attached to Tyr in position 12.
[d]Points of cleavage by trypsin.
[e]Another form of CCK with 39 amino acid residues [CCK-39] has been isolated; the two forms are equally potent. The larger form is not yet chemically characterized.

stimulate secretion of pancreatic enzymes and to stimulate contraction of the gallbladder, has a C-terminal group of seven amino acids that is remarkably similar to that of gastrin (Table 1). It shares many physiologic activities with gastrin.[135]

The metabolic functions of gastrin have been recently reviewed.[136, 174] The most remarkable action of gastrin is its ability to stimulate gastric acid secretion; it is 30 times more potent than histamine by weight and 500 times more potent on a molar basis. In pharmacologic quantities, gastrin seems to have many motor and secretory actions on various target organs in the gut, liver, and pancreas. In addition to its effect on acid secretion, the only other actions of gastrin that have been shown to be physiologic are stimulation of pepsin secretion and of gastric mucosal blood flow. Gastrin does have a pronounced trophic effect on the stomach and pancreas, and it has been shown to stimulate pancreatic enzyme secretion in man. These actions may also prove to be physiologic.

Gastrin appears to be synthesized and stored by G cells in the pyloric glands of antral mucosa[120] and in the mucosa of the proximal small intestine.[176] Gastrin is present in fundic mucosa in concentrations of 1×10^{-12} by weight, whereas in antral mucosa the concentration is more than 1000 times greater.[94] The duodenum in man contains 10 to 20 per cent as much gastrin as does the antrum.[141]

Gastrin is released from G cells and is carried by the blood to effector sites in various organs of the gut. Gastrin and cholecystokinin and secretin act on the same target organs, and because of their structural similarity (Table 1), cholecystokinin and gastrin probably act on the same receptor site.[67] Secretin,[169] as well as other members of the secretin family of hormones (glucagon, gastric inhibitory polypeptide [GIP], and vasoactive intestinal polypeptide [VIP]), has been shown to block the action of gastrin on the parietal cell and, in addition, to block food-stimulated release of gastrin.[135] Calcium, given intravenously[137] or orally,[138] stimulates gastric secretion by releasing gastrin. Cyclic AMP may be involved as an intraparietal cell second messenger, but the evidence that gastrin works by this pathway is at best inconclusive.[95]

Gastrin has been shown to disappear rapidly from circulation[139] and the kidney is the main organ of catabolism.[168] Gastrin is also taken up by the small bowel and the secreting gastric fundus, but not, apparently, by the liver, lung, or skeletal muscle.[170]

The Zollinger-Ellison syndrome[188] of massive gastric hypersecretion and peptic ulceration was shown by Gregory and colleagues[63, 65] to be caused by high levels of circulating gastrin elaborated by gastrinomas of the pancreas or duodenum. Hypergastrinemia is also seen in patients with pernicious anemia (due to loss of acid inhibition of antral gastrin release), in patients with the antral exclusion operation (which results in permanent sequestration of antral mucosa in the alkaline environment of the duodenum), in chronic renal failure (presumably caused by loss of normal renal catabolism),[77] and occasionally in patients with pyloric obstruction.

Detailed studies on the metabolism of gastrin have been made possible by the development of specific and sensitive radioimmunoassay methods.[26, 118, 187] Normal values for the concentration of gastrin in serum vary according to technique; the upper limit of normal in our assay is 200 picograms (pg.) per milliliter of serum. Many patients with the Zollinger-Ellison syndrome have serum gastrin levels greater than 1000 pg. per ml. and some have values as high as 100,000 pg. per ml.

Since gastrin stimulates secretion of gastric acid and since the duodenal ulcer diathesis is associated with hypersecretion of acid, it was common (before the days of radioimmunoassay) to assume that patients with duodenal ulcer would have high levels of circulating gastrin. Such is not the case. Only in the Zollinger-Ellison syndrome (and in rare patients with antral exclusion) is acid hypersecretion caused by excess gastrin; basal gastrin levels in duodenal ulcer patients are normal. Duodenal ulcer patients do release more gastrin in a more rapid fashion in response to a standard meal than does normal man (Fig. 7).[140]

Because duodenal ulcer patients seem to release more gastrin in spite of acid hypersecretion, these patients may have a defect in the normal feedback mechanism for inhibition of gastrin release.[16]

After truncal vagotomy and a drainage procedure, gastric acid secretion is diminished but gastrin values increase, presumably because of loss of acid inhibition. In fact, recent evidence indicates that all types of vagotomy cause an increase of basal and postprandial serum gastrin levels.[166]

Serum gastrin concentrations are higher in patients with gastric ulcer than in patients with duodenal ulcer,[171] probably because of lower acid output; in patients with gastric achlorhydria, serum gastrin levels are apt to be very high and instillation of acid into the stomach causes an abrupt decrease in serum gastrin.

It is now possible in many hospitals to obtain radioimmunoassay measurement of serum gastrin concentrations. Serum gastrin measurements are indicated in any patient in whom the Zollinger-Ellison syndrome is suspected and specifically under the following conditions:

1. Patients with recurrent peptic ulcers or with recurrent peptic ulcer symptoms after an acid-reducing operation

2. Patients with a duodenal ulcer and massive hypersecretion of acid (greater than 15 mEq per hr. basal)

3. Patients with duodenal ulcer and diarrhea

4. Patients with duodenal ulcer and hypercalcemia

5. Patients with relatives who have the Zollinger-Ellison syndrome or the multiple endocrine adenoma I syndrome

6. Patients who have postbulbar or jejunal ulceration

7. Patients whose upper gastrointestinal radiologic studies are suggestive of the Zollinger-Ellison syndrome

8. Duodenal ulcer patients under 20 years of age

9. Postoperative patients in whom antral exclusion is suspected

Intestinal Phase

There is clear evidence that various stimulants applied to the mid-small bowel can bring about secretion of acid from a denervated gastric pouch.[164] The intestinal phase can be stimulated by the instillation of food, particularly proteins, or acid into the proximal jejunum. Distention of the jejunum will also stimulate secretion.

The nature of the humoral agent of intestinal stimulation of gastric secretion has not been fully identified, but it does not appear to be either cholecystokinin or extra-antral gastrin (agents which themselves can produce acid secretion).[135] Portacaval shunting is known to augment gastric secretory response to a meal; this increase is thought to be caused by an "unmasking" of the intestinal phase secretagogue that is normally inactivated by the liver.[164] Orlaff and colleagues[130, 131] have shown that postportacaval shunt hypersecretion exists in man as well as in dogs, and they provide strong evidence that the agent is a hormone arising from the jejunum. Grossman has proposed the name "entero-oxyntin" for the intestinal phase secretagogue.[70]

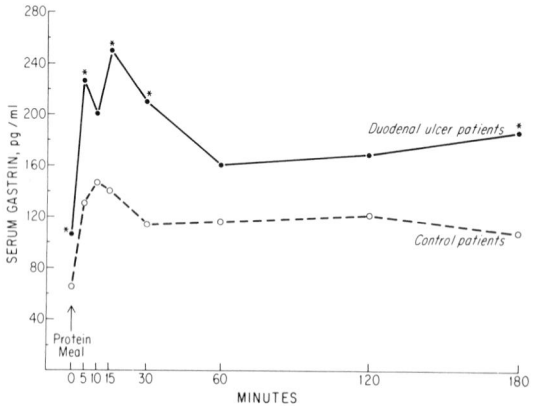

Figure 7. Fasting and postprandial serum gastrin concentrations in six duodenal ulcer patients and five control patients. Significant differences in gastrin levels between ulcer and control patients are indicated by asterisks. (From Reeder, D. D., Jackson, B. M., Ban, J. L., Davidson, W. D., and Thompson, J. C.: Surg. Forum, *21*:290, 1970.)

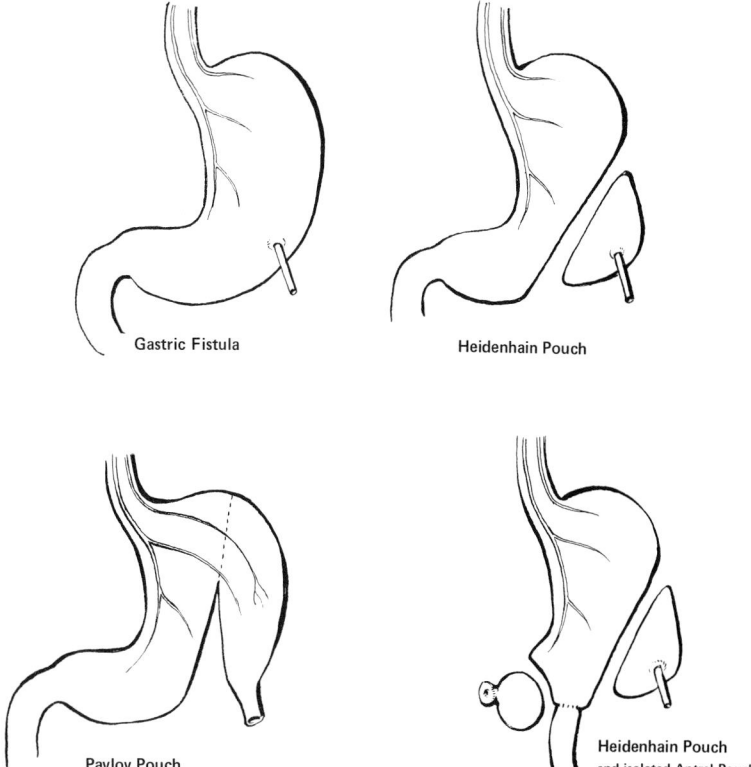

Figure 8. Experimental gastric pouches in common use (classic experimental preparations used in the study of gastric secretion). The gastric fistula is simply a cannula placed into the intact innervated stomach. The Heidenhain pouch is a denervated segment of fundic mucosa drained with a cannula. The Pavlov pouch is an innervated fundic pouch separated from the main stomach by an internal mucosal septum. Pouches of the antrum may be innervated or denervated. They allow study of the mechanisms for stimulation and suppression of gastrin release. The isolated antral pouch may be constructed in association with a Heidenhain pouch, as shown on the lower right, or with a Pavlov pouch or a gastric fistula.

Gastric Fistula

Heidenhain Pouch

Pavlov Pouch

Heidenhain Pouch
and isolated Antral Pouch

The contribution of the intestinal phase to total secretory output is difficult to estimate. In order to study one aspect of gastric secretion it is often necessary to curtail or alter normally coexisting stimuli. It now appears that the contribution of the intestinal phase to the total stimulation of acid secretion may be far more important than we formerly suspected.

MEASUREMENT OF GASTRIC SECRETION

Studies on gastric secretion have been made in dogs with experimental pouches (Fig. 8) and in man. The most common experimental preparations in use today are denervated pouches of fundic mucosa (Heidenhain) or simple gastric fistulas draining the entire stomach. Pavlov pouches have the advantage of providing juice from innervated pouches free of contamination of food, but construction of Pavlov pouches is difficult and leaks are common. Gastric fistulas suffice for the study of all stimuli except food. Antral pouches provide means for the study of the stimulation and inhibition of gastrin release.

Although the obvious usefulness of a gastric pouch is to serve as a mirror of what is happening in the main stomach, it is not always an exact mirror, since for example, the secretion from a Heidenhain pouch is responsive only to humoral stimulation.

Gastric secretion in man is measured by collecting gastric juice with a nasogastric tube from fasting subjects. Fluoroscopic control for placement of the tip has been recommended, but this is probably not neces-

sary.[79] Gastric juice is collected for fixed periods, usually 15 or 30 minutes, and each sample is titrated to pH 7 and the results are expressed in terms of volume for a given period (usually 1 hour), in acid concentration (milliequivalents per liter) and in acid output (milliequivalents per 30 minutes or per hour). Acid secretion may be collected overnight, but the vagaries of collection over 12 hours are so great that shorter collecting periods are preferable. The terms free acid, combined acid, degrees of acidity, and clinical units are obsolete and should be abandoned.

The first 30-minute specimen is usually discarded and the second 30-minute specimen is kept for basal output, after which a secretory stimulant is administered. The dose of a stimulant that yields a maximal secretory output is commonly used, since the maximal dose has been found to give more reliable and reproducible results. Standard secretory stimulants in the doses employed for maximal acid output are shown in Table 2. Although various studies give different results, it is useful to assign arbitrary values for the upper limit of normal of gastric secretion; these values are also given in Table 2.

Pentagastrin has recently been approved by the Food and Drug Administration for routine use in this country. Pentagastrin (and probably gastrin as well) has far fewer side effects than the other three standard agents and should become the standard secretory stimulant. Secretory responses to pentagastrin in man are almost identical with the maximal response to histamine and are reproducible.[1]

Grossman and colleagues [72] studied basal and His-

TABLE 2. Acid Secretory Studies in Man

Dosages of Stimulants for Maximal Acid Output	
Stimulant	Dose
Histamine acid phosphate	40 μg./kg. subcutaneously (40 μg./kg. intravenously)
Histalog (betazole)	1.5 to 2.0 mg./kg. subcutaneously
Insulin (crystalline)	0.2 U./kg. intravenously
Pentagastrin	6 μg./kg. subcutaneously (6 μg./kg./hr. intravenously)
Gastrin (synthetic human gastrin, Imperial Chemical Industries)	2 μg./kg. subcutaneously (1 μg./kg./hr. intravenously)

Upper Limit of Normal for Acid Output (mEq./hr.)		
	Basal Acid Output (BAO)	Maximal Acid Output (MAO)
Women	4	30
Men	6	40

talog-stimulated gastric secretion in more than 2500 patients. They concluded that (1) males secrete more acid than females; (2) after the age of 50 gastric secretion begins to fall; (3) the mean rate of gastric secretion in duodenal ulcer patients is twice that of controls, although more than 60 per cent of duodenal ulcer patients had secretory rates within the normal range; (4) 27 per cent of duodenal ulcer patients exceed the upper limit of normal for basal gastric secretion and 35 per cent exceed the upper limit of normal of stimulated acid secretion; and (5) patients with gastric ulcers secrete less acid than controls.

The value of the study of the basal acid output is that it allows an estimation of the amount of acid present during the interdigestive phases when the stomach is empty. Use of the maximal acid output allows assessment of the secretory capacity of the stomach, which in turn is a function of the parietal cell mass. In addition, use of the maximal dose is the only way to prove true achlorhydria. There does seem to be some correlation between the severity of clinical problems (both before and after operation) and the degree of acid hypersecretion in duodenal ulcer patients.[104, 105]

The explanation for the relationship of the number of parietal cells to acid secretion is unknown. They vary directly, but it is unknown whether this means that patients with hypersecretion have a genetically larger mass of parietal cells, or whether (which seems far more probable) the parietal cell mass increases in response to chronic stimulation. Patients with the Zollinger-Ellison syndrome have a greatly enlarged parietal cell mass, probably as a result of the trophic action of gastrin on parietal cells.

The amount of acid secreted by patients with gastric ulcers is normal or often less than normal. Since pepsinogen requires an acid environment for activation, any ulcer existing in a truly achlorhydric stomach cannot be peptic and must be malignant, and the dictum "no acid, no ulcer" is a true one.

INHIBITION OF GASTRIC SECRETION

Once secretion is stimulated by a meal, what halts the flow of acid? Vagal activity is decreased because cephalic stimulation is removed, but most important, the secretion of acid itself acts to block further release of gastrin and to bring about active duodenal suppression of gastric secretion.

Antral acidification has been clearly demonstrated to suppress the release of gastrin.[185] Significant diminution in acid stimulation may occur with an antral pH as high as 5, and at about pH 1.5 there is no release of gastrin.

For years the mode of action of antral acidification in suppressing gastric secretion was a subject of controversy: does it suppress secretion simply by halting gastrin release, or is a separate inhibitory hormone elaborated? The evidence for a separate antral chalone has been reviewed,[163] and the weight of evidence seems to be against a separate agent. The evidence for inhibition of gastric secretion by the duodenum is much more clear.[3, 164] Gastric secretion is inhibited by the presence of acid or fat or hypertonic solutions in the duodenum. Gastric inhibitory polypeptide (GIP) is probably responsible for this humoral inhibition, which formerly was ascribed to enterogastrone.[22, 135] Whether nervous reflexes play a primary or a permissive role in duodenal inhibition has not been clarified.

Acidification of the duodenum inhibits gastric secretion; it also releases secretin and secretin is known to inhibit gastrin-stimulated gastric secretion. Secretin has been proposed as the enterogastrone from the duodenum, but Andersson[4] has demurred and has proposed that a specific inhibitory hormone is released from the acidified duodenal bulb.[5] The suppressive effect of acidification of the duodenum has been confirmed in man, although the suppression is somewhat less effective in patients with duodenal ulcer than in normal man.[97] Acid-stimulated release of secretin is apparently not altered in duodenal ulcer patients.[24]

Fat in the duodenum in an absorbable form is a highly effective inhibitor of postprandial gastric secretion. GIP is released by fat and probably mediates this inhibition. Hypertonic solutions of sugars, salts, and peptone inhibit gastric secretion, apparently by stimulating a duodenal osmoreceptor that releases a humoral inhibitor, as yet unidentified.

PEPTIC ULCER AND OTHER SYNDROMES OF MUCOSAL INJURY

Peptic ulcer of the stomach and the duodenum afflicts more than 10 million citizens of the United States according to our best statistics, and probably only one half of the cases are recognized.[2] The condition is most common in men between the ages of 20 and 60 and the cost to our society is in excess of $1 billion per year. Recent evidence indicates that the incidence of duodenal ulcer is decreasing.[121]

Peptic ulcers may occur wherever mucosa is bathed by fundic secretion and are found in the esophagus, stomach, and duodenum, adjacent to Meckel's diverticula with ectopic gastric mucosa (rarely), and in any segment of bowel that may be surgically anastomosed to the gastric fundus. Acute ulcers are commonly shallow and multiple, whereas chronic ulcers are apt to be single and deep and scirrhous.

PATHOGENESIS

Abundant information is available from many studies,[73, 151] but the pathogenesis of gastroduodenal ulcers is still not fully understood. No single theory explains all types of lesions. Duodenal ulcers tend to be associated with hypersecretion of acid, but not all patients with duodenal ulcers hypersecrete. Gastric ulcers and the ulcerations associated with acute mucosal injury are not associated with the hypersecretion of acid. Nonetheless, the presence of acid is necessary in order for all peptic ulcers to occur.

It is perhaps worthwhile to use a simplistic model in considering the genesis of ulcers (Table 3). Several factors might be listed that tend to attack the mucosa and others might properly be thought of as defense mechanisms against mucosal ulceration. Peptic ulcers are caused by acid peptic digestion, and pepsin is inactive above a pH of 5.4 to 6 and has an optimal pH of around 1.5 to 2.5. Acid peptic digestion is certainly the most potent agent attacking the mucosa. Recent studies have shown that antiinflammatory drugs such as salicylates may injure the mucosa and allow back-diffusion of acid. The consumption of aspirin has increased enormously in this country and the incidence of aspirin-induced gastric bleeding has increased concomitantly. Direct trauma to the mucosa from instrumentation or foreign bodies and mucosal ischemia are rare causes of ulceration.

The mechanisms of mucosal defense are not well understood. The greater the fraction of nonparietal cell secretion in gastric juice, the lower will be the concentration of H^+, but the mechanisms governing the relative stimulation of the parietal and nonparietal components of gastric secretion are unknown. Emptying of

TABLE 3. Factors Involved in the Pathogenesis
of Peptic Ulceration

| Enzymatic Digestion of Mucous Membrane | |
Attack	Defense
Acid peptic digestion (pH <4)	Dilution (nonparietal secretion)
Drugs (salicylates, steroids)	Emptying
Trauma	Neutralization (HCO_3^- from bile and pancreas)
Ischemia	Mucosal barrier
	Rich blood supply
No acid — no ulcer	

the acid gastric chyme into the crucible of the duodenal bulb where it is neutralized by HCO_3^- from bile and pancreatic juice is certainly one of the most important defenses. The surface epithelium of the stomach and duodenum constitutes a barrier to the backdiffusion of H^+. The integrity of the mucosal barrier is enhanced by the rich blood supply of the mucosa of the stomach and duodenum.

Duodenal Ulcer

The association of duodenal ulcer with acid hypersecretion is firmly established. In most collected series, the mean basal and maximal acid output of duodenal ulcer patients is one and one-half to two times as great as that of control patients, and Cox[31] has shown that the stomachs of patients with duodenal ulcer have almost twice the number of parietal cells as do normal stomachs. Samloff and colleagues[146] have shown increased levels of serum group I pepsinogen in duodenal ulcer patients and have suggested that the acid secretory potential of the stomach may be reflected by the level of serum group I pepsinogens. Ulcer patients show increased acid response to stimulation with the gastrin analogue, pentagastrin.[92] In addition, evidence is available that duodenal ulcer patients show a decreased inhibition of gastrin release at low antral pH, an increased rate of gastric emptying, and an increased acid load delivered to the duodenum.[73] There is as yet no evidence that duodenal defense mechanisms are faulty in patients who develop duodenal ulcer.

Strong public opinion holds that emotional factors play an important role in the development of peptic ulcer. The possibility of this association has been reviewed by Fordtran,[50] who concluded that the evidence favors a role for anxiety in the etiology of peptic ulcer.

Gastric Ulcer

Whereas doudenal ulcers appear to be caused by increased potency of the acid peptic forces attacking the mucosa, gastric ulcers may be related primarily to injury of the gastric mucosa, which renders it more susceptible to acid peptic damage. Most studies report that gastric ulcer patients secrete either low normal or below normal amounts of acid, and only 5 per cent of patients with gastric ulcer demonstrate acid hypersecretion.[72] The evidence is now abundant that reflux of bile and pancreatic juice (and, possibly, pyloric dysfunction) is involved in the pathogenesis of gastric ulcer.[151] Gastric reflux of bile after meals is increased in patients with gastric ulcer,[43, 142] which may be caused, at least in part, by dysfunction of the pyloric sphincter.[48] Bile salts apparently damage the mucosa, which is then attacked by acid peptic digestion.[36, 43] Gastric ulcers invariably occur in areas of gastritis.[36, 43] Since the gastritis progresses proximally from the pylorus, patients with gastric ulcer have a larger distal area of alkaline mucosa, and gastric ulcers lie in achlorhydric zones of mucosa.[25]

Oi and colleagues[129] observed that the vast majority of gastric ulcers occur in an area of 5 per cent of the gastric mucosal surface in the proximal antrum near the site of the incisura angularis. They suggested that all peptic ulcers occur adjacent to boundaries between different types of mucosa and on the side *away* from the acid-secreting mucosa. In addition, they suggested that the location of ulcers is influenced by the motility of underlying muscle bundles.

Acute Mucosal Erosions

Acute superficial ulcerative lesions of the gastroduodenal area have been variously called acute mucosal erosions, stress ulcer, acute peptic ulcer, erosive gastritis, hemorrhagic gastritis, and Curling's or Cushing's ulcers. The latter two eponymic lesions have specific causes; the other terms are roughly synonymous and are often used interchangeably. None of the terms is satisfactory.

The mechanism whereby stress results in mucosal ulceration is poorly understood. If a rat is restrained for 24 hours, it will develop many superficial gastric erosions.[20] In stress ulceration, the stomach appears to be the target organ for metabolic alterations caused by a variety of diseases that in the past progressed rapidly to a fatal outcome. With improved techniques for resuscitation and intensive care, patients now survive these diseases long enough to fall prey to a sequential series of organ failures: gastrointestinal, pulmonary, renal, hepatic, and cardiac. After long periods of hypotension or sepsis or pulmonary insufficiency, the patients become so debilitated that they may be the victim of whichever organ system fails first. The high concentration of acid and digested enzymes in the stomach and duodenum renders this area especially vulnerable to autolysis. Much attention has been given to the study of the gastric mucosal barrier, which prevents the back-diffusion of H^+, and to the luminal diffusion of Na^+ ion.[33, 82, 179] Hollander[86] defined the gastric mucosal barrier as a two-component system consisting of a layer of mucus covering the luminal surface of the stomach and a layer of columnar epithelial cells beneath it. Mucus is no longer thought to play an important protective role, but the apical membrane of the epithelial cells is apparently essential. Aspirin has been shown to damage these membranes,[33] and shock and sepsis as well as other metabolic disturbances may also compromise the function of the barrier, but this has never been proved. Once acid does enter the cell, damage occurs that may allow further back-diffusion of acid with resultant release of histamine, which causes vasodilatation and bleeding[32] (Fig. 9). An episode of shock almost invariably precedes acute mucosal bleeding in man. Many critically ill patients have small bowel ileus with consequent bile reflux, which contributes, along with shock, to mucosal injury. A strong correlation between increased gastric mucosal permeability and the incidence of sepsis, hypotension, and respiratory and renal failure has been reported.[60]

Experimental evidence, summarized by Menguy,[123] suggests that the initial event leading to the development of acute mucosal erosions is a severe and sudden decrease in mucosal energy metabolism. The degree of shock-induced energy deficit is correlated with the frequency of mucosal lesions (high in fundus, low in antrum).

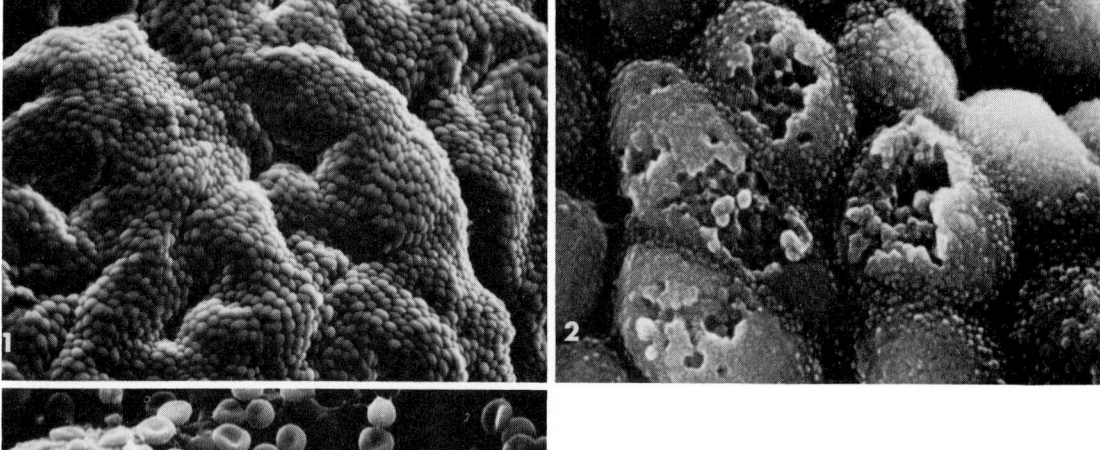

Figure 9. Scanning electron micrographs of gastric mucosa. *1,* Normal surface topography showing folds, gastric pits, and numerous epithelial cells. ×375. *2,* High magnification showing damage to four surface epithelial cells demonstrating disruption of apical membrane. ×8000. *3,* Section taken from area of hemorrhagic gastritis. Surface of epithelial cells covered with network of fibrin containing many erythrocytes. ×2000. (From Lucas, C. E., et al.: Arch. Surg., *102:*266, 1971.)

The pathogenesis of the acute mucosal lesions that occur in neurosurgical patients (Cushing's ulcer) almost certainly is different from the pathogenesis of other stress-induced lesions. Patients with acute gastric hemorrhage associated with injury to the central nervous system tend to have higher acid secretory levels than do other patients with acute mucosal lesions.[60, 158] In a study of 39 U.S. servicemen injured in Viet Nam, Bowen and colleagues[18] found the levels of serum gastrin in patients with CNS injury to be higher than in patients with injuries not involving the central nervous system. The higher rate of acid secretion and higher gastrin levels strongly suggest that patients with head injury may have increased vagal activity.

Certain factors seem to be required for the development of acute mucosal erosions: ischemia, the presence of even small amounts of acid, and disruption of the gastric mucosal barrier, which leads to increased back-diffusion of H^+.[151]

DUODENAL ULCER

Duodenal ulcer is a chronic disease that occurs four times more often in men than in women. It may appear at any age but occurs most frequently between the ages of 20 and 60 and has a peak incidence in the fourth decade of life. The clinical course is characterized by long periods of remission and periods of exacerbation that may last from days to months. The chief symptom is pain, which classically is perceived in the epigastrium in, or just to the right of the midline. The pain is often relieved by food or milk or antacid and the most important differential characteristic of the pain is that it often awakens the patient two or three hours after he goes to sleep. After relieving the pain with food or antacid, the patient goes to sleep again and awakens in the morning without pain. Heartburn, a burning substernal discomfort, is common in patients with duodenal ulcer and apparently is due to regurgitation of acid into the esophagus (it may be a symptom of hiatal hernia). Early satiety, anorexia, and nausea are common and are often experienced by patients in the early phases of the development of the ulcer. Even during exacerbation, the pain usually lasts for only a few hours at a time. A change in the pattern of pain so that it becomes continuous and no longer is relieved by antacid usually signifies a posterior penetration of the ulcer crater. Atypical pain patterns are often seen in children and in patients with ulcers at the pylorus or distal to the duodenal bulb. Pain is frequently absent in postbulbar ulcers. When present, however, it often has bizarre characteristics and is often unresponsive to antacid therapy.

ASSOCIATED CONDITIONS

It is difficult to prove true statistical relationship between diseases. Increased incidences of duodenal ulcer have been reported in hyperparathyroidism, polycythemia rubra vera, chronic liver disease, uremia, chronic respiratory insufficiency, and certain central nervous system lesions, and after burns and portacaval shunting. One difficulty in establishing statistical relationships is the disparity between the incidence of peptic ulcer in clinical and in autopsy series and the uncertainty as to whether an appropriate control series would consist of chronically ill patients or of patients who are well.[108] The incidence of peptic ulcer in the general population has been variously estimated at between 5 and 15 per cent. In order to be meaningful, any series purporting to demonstrate a slight to moderate increase in the incidence of peptic ulcer would have to be compared to a local control series.

Evidence for an etiologic relationship with peptic ulcer disease appears to be strongest for hyperparathyroidism,[14] chronic respiratory insufficiency,[54, 180] cirrhosis, and nonhypertensive cardiovascular disease.[108] In no instance, however, is the evidence compelling; the purported relationship of cirrhosis and portacaval shunt with peptic ulcer has been reviewed[161] and the evidence found to be insufficient.

DIAGNOSIS

A presumption of the presence of a duodenal ulcer may be made from a patient's history, but definitive diagnosis depends upon either endoscopy or radiology. Although radiologic diagnosis will be given precedence in this discussion, within a very few years, fiberoptic endoscopy will almost certainly become the standard by which all diagnostic procedures are graded.

History

Most important in the history is the character of the pain. It may take various forms and be interpreted in various ways. Care should be taken to avoid misunderstanding because of different connotations given to the word "pain." It is often necessary to use several synonyms, "discomfort," "ache," "pressure," or even "hunger pain," in order to be sure that disavowal of pain is valid. The pain is often exacerbated by certain foods, such as tomato sauce, hot spices, fried food, onions, or alcohol. Patients may inadvertently exacerbate their difficulties by taking antacids that contain aspirin (Alka-Seltzer). Ingelfinger[89] has concluded that any patient who has periodic epigastric pain that is relieved by antacids, who is being awakened by this pain at 1 to 2 A.M., who can go back to sleep following relief of this pain and awakens in the morning without pain, and who does not have pain during meals, has an 80 per cent chance of having a duodenal ulcer and should probably be treated for the disease. There are many persons, however, who have frequent bouts of epigastric pain and heartburn for years and who get relief with antacids but in whom a duodenal ulcer is never demonstrated. About 15 to 20 per cent of patients who require treatment for perforation or bleeding will not have an antecedent history of ulcer pain.

Radiology

The radiologic diagnosis of duodenal ulcer is 75 to 80 per cent accurate. The patient may show an actual crater deformity indicative of active disease, or he may merely demonstrate scarring of the duodenal bulb caused by previous ulceration. About 95 per cent

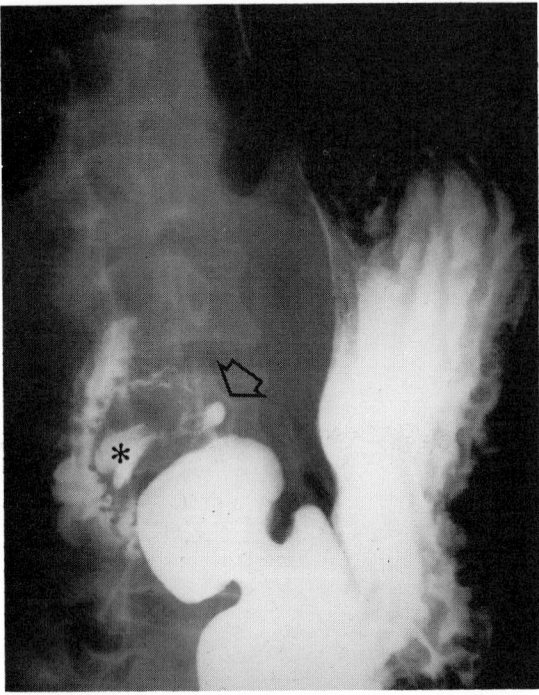

Figure 10. Radiograph of the stomach and duodenum. The arrow points to an ulcer crater of the bulb shown tangentially. The asterisk lies within a pseudodiverticulum produced by scarring. Irritability and scarring prevent filling of the duodenal bulb with barium. (This and subsequent radiographs are from the teaching files of the Department of Radiology, University of Texas Medical Branch, Galveston. They were selected in consultation with Melvyn H. Schreiber, M.D.)

of duodenal ulcers occur in the duodenal bulb (see Fig. 6) and 5 per cent are postbulbar. An indeterminate number occur in the pyloric canal and are often called channel ulcers.

The normal duodenal bulb is rounded and full. Ulcer disease usually causes irritability and the bulb becomes difficult to fill with contrast material (Fig. 10).

The most important sign in the diagnosis of duodenal ulcer is the demonstration of the ulcer crater itself. Since ulcer craters are much more commonly located on the anterior or posterior wall of the duodenal bulb, the crater is more likely to be seen en face (Figs. 11 and 12). Since the crater has no mucosa, barium sticks to the bottom of the crater and compression films (Fig. 12) will show barium displaced from the other areas of the bulb while it remains adherent to the crater itself. Less commonly, the crater may appear tangentially as a niche or burrowed excavation on the lateral wall of the duodenum (Figs. 13 and 14).

Secondary radiologic signs that are indicative of active duodenal ulcer are mucosal edema and spasm. Edema results in widening of the radiolucent folds (Fig. 11, upper right, and Fig. 12), clearly demarcated by barium lying in the crevices between the thickened folds. These folds often radiate toward the margin of the ulcer. The edema may also take the form of a radiolucent halo about the ulcer crater (Fig. 13). Edema of the mucosa may extend for several centimeters distal to the site of the crater.

An ulcer in the bulb frequently gives rise to spasm of the pylorus, which may result in poor emptying of the stomach, seen radiologically as a granular dilution of barium in the stomach and perhaps an air-fluid level in pictures taken in the erect position before the administration of barium. Spasm in the presence of an

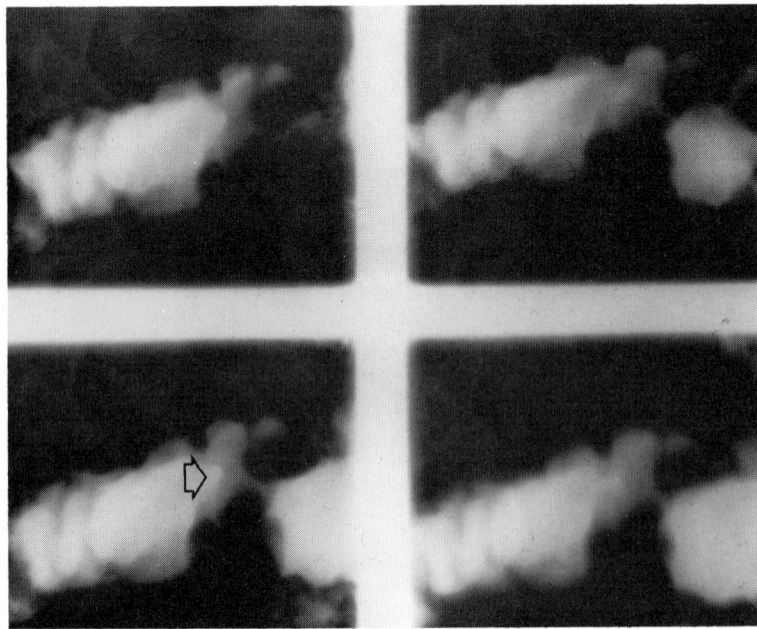

Figure 11. Radiograph of the distal stomach, pylorus, and proximal duodenum. These four views show the ulcer crater (arrow) of the bulb en face. There is an incisura just above the crater in each film and in the upper right picture an edematous fold of mucosa is shown just distal to the ulcer crater.

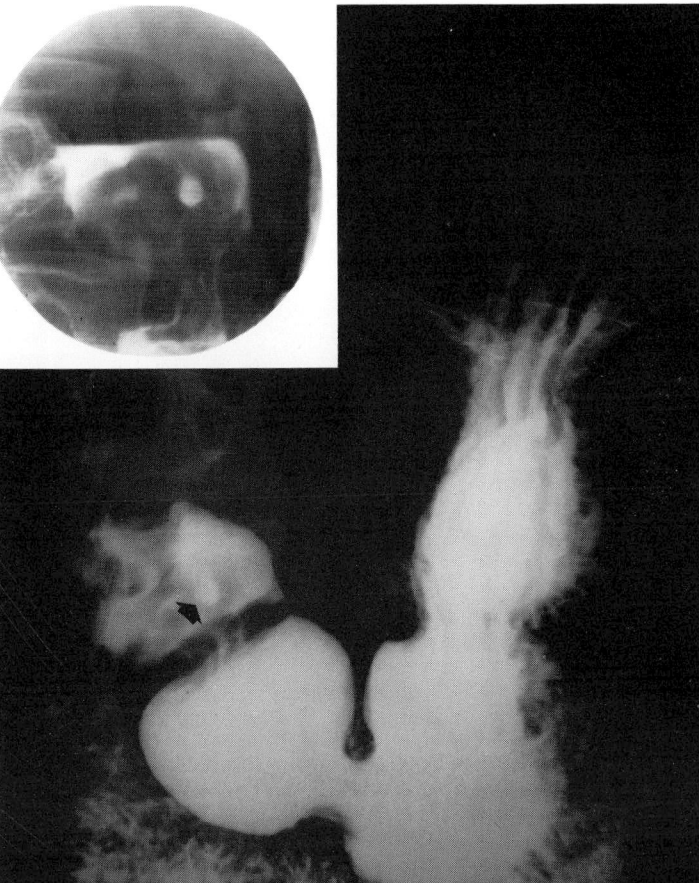

Figure 12. Radiograph of the stomach and duodenum showing a large ulcer crater of the duodenal bulb en face (arrow). The mucosal fold just distal to the ulcer crater is thickened and edematous. The compression film (inset) shows displacement of barium by pressure from all areas of the bulb except the ulcer crater to which the barium remains adherent.

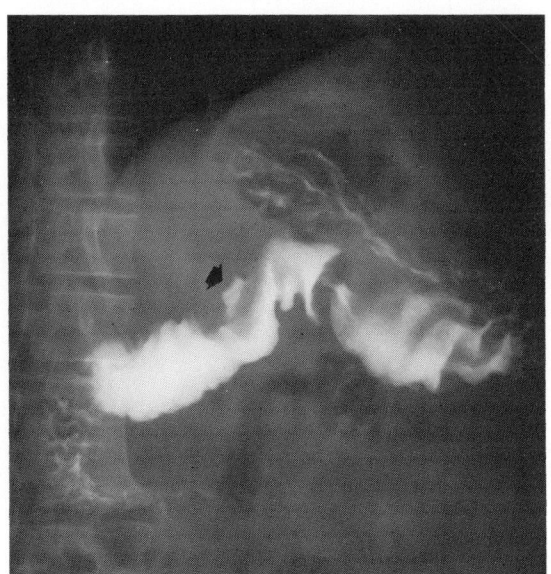

Figure 13. Tangenital view of large postbulbar ulcer (arrow) with ring of edematous mucosa around the base of the ulcer.

active ulcer crater in the duodenum may take the form of niches or incisurae owing to asymmetrical muscle contraction, which produces radiolucent finger-like indentations into the wall of the duodenum (Figs. 11 and 14). These incisurae point toward the ulcer crater. Between the incusurae, normal areas of duodenum will often appear as pouch-like protrusions, called pseudodiverticula, which contain barium and may easily be mistaken for the ulcer crater (Fig. 10). Spasm also results in extremely rapid emptying so that the radiologist is unable to obtain pictures of the filled bulb (Fig. 10).

Although postbulbar ulcers (Figs. 13 and 14) may occur anywhere in the duodenum distal to the bulb, 75 per cent of postbulbar ulcers occur proximal to the duodenal papilla.[128] They are often small and buried in folds. Because of this and perhaps because of their relative rarity, they are often missed. About 15 per cent of patients with postbulbar ulcers also have an ulcer located in the bulb.[28] Figures 11 and 14 are x-ray pictures of bulbar and postbulbar ulcers obtained from the same patient at the same time.

With healing, the duodenal ulcer becomes smaller and may finally disappear altogether. At other times

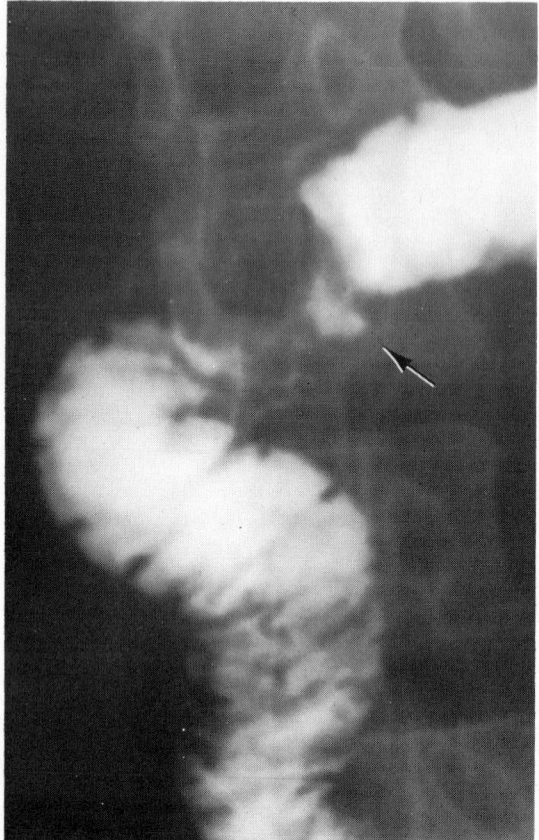

Figure 14. Tangential view of postbulbar ulcer (arrow) with large incisura indenting the opposite wall of the duodenum.

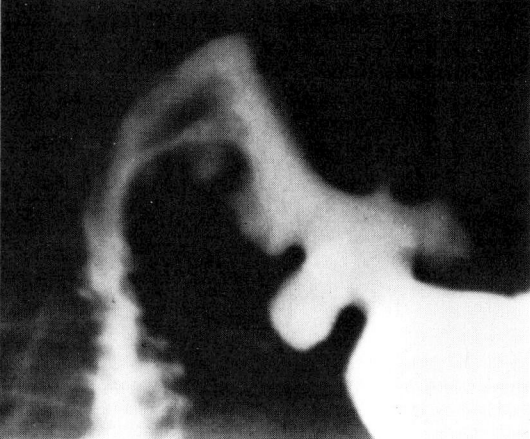

Figure 15. Radiograph of the distal stomach and proximal duodenum showing cloverleaf deformity of the duodenal bulb caused by scarring which makes permanent the indentations and intervening pseudodiverticula.

It is important that multiple films be taken in order to obtain more than one view of the area of possible ulcer disease. Radiologic findings of an active ulcer are often quite subtle and it is often necessary to see the abnormalities repeated in multiple views in order to be sure that they are due to an organic lesion (see Fig. 11) and are not caused simply by an infortuitous pattern of the distribution of barium.

Fiberoptic Endoscopy

The development of the flexible fiberoptic panendoscope has greatly facilitated diagnosis of peptic ulcer disease (Fig. 16A). By use of the side- and forward-viewing scopes, diagnostic accuracy of 95 per cent or even greater may be achieved, and the evidence is clear that endoscopy is superior to radiography in defining the presence of lesions of the esophagus, stomach, and duodenum. In as many as one fourth of patients examined, the side-viewing fiberoptic endoscope will be required to correctly visualize the duodenal ulceration.[145] In addition to demonstrating the

the ulcer may heal as a pitted scar and a tiny excavation may remain, which may erroneously be interpreted as an active ulcer. The cloverleaf deformity of the duodenal bulb (Fig. 15) seen in healed ulcer disease is the consequence of fibrosis in the wake of inflammation. This scarring will often make the incisurae and pseudodiverticula permanent.

Figure 16. Photographs of eight upper gastrointestinal lesions obtained by fiberoptic endoscopy: *A,* Chronic duodenal ulcer. A sharply inscribed crater in the duodenal bulb viewed from the pylorus. *B,* Bleeding duodenal ulcer. This ulcer was on the posterior wall of the duodenal bulb and had previously been bleeding massively. *C,* Bleeding esophageal varix. Close-up view of actual jet of blood under pressure from distended esophageal varix. (Courtesy of Hugo V. Villar, M.D., and Osvaldo L. Llanos, M.D.). *D,* Benign gastric ulcer. The view is from the proximal stomach into the antrum with the lesser curvature on right. The sharply defined ulcer crater is on the incisura, which projects into the lumen on the right. Note the large rugal fold in the foreground. *E,* Channel ulcer. This view is from the gastric antrum looking into the pyloric canal with a triangular benign gastric ulcer situated in the pyloric channel. *F,* Ulcerating carcinoma. The patient had previously undergone a Billroth I resection for carcinoma of the distal antrum. This tumor has recurred at the anastomotic line. Black filaments in the photograph are silk sutures. *G,* Stress ulcers. View from proximal stomach looking into lumen of body of stomach with lesser curvature on the right. A superficial bleeding ulcer appears in the right foreground on the anterior wall of the stomach. There are two more superficial gastric erosions located distally on the incisura, which projects into the lumen from the right. *H,* Marginal ulcer. This view is from the gastric remnant (following a Billroth II gastric resection) looking into the gastrojejunal anastomosis. The ulcerated area in the foreground is a benign ulcer on the gastric side of the anastomotic stoma. (Courtesy of Marcel Patterson, M.D.).

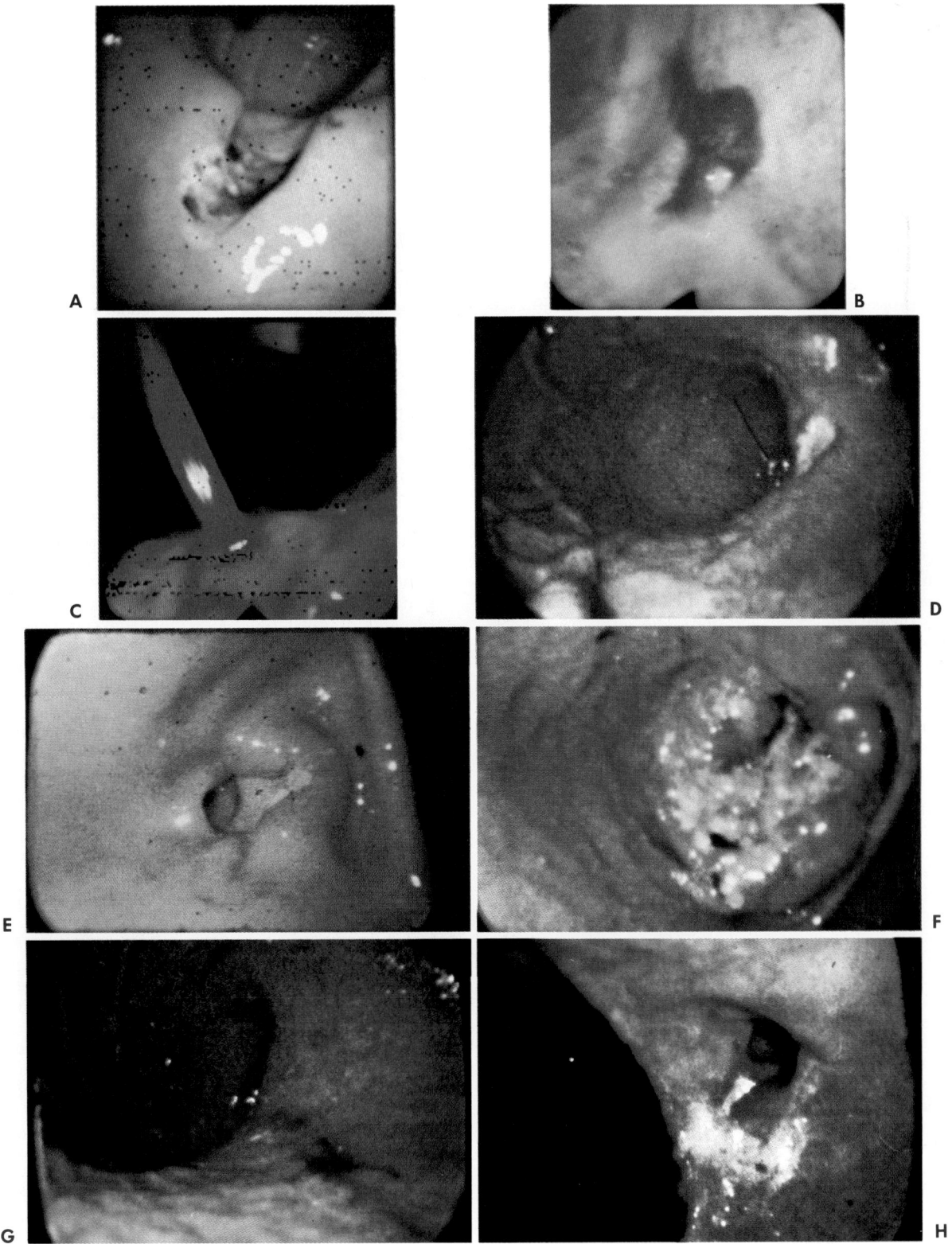

actual presence of the lesions, endoscopy allows further information to be collected: the operator can biopsy the lesion, he can touch it with his scope to determine its consistency, and most important, he can tell whether or not it is bleeding. Endoscopy is of greatest value in bleeding patients. Roentgenograms may show an ulcer or esophageal varices, but they do not tell us the site of bleeding. In addition to providing information on whether varices or ulcers are bleeding, endoscopy has its greatest value in demonstrating Mallory-Weiss tears of the gastroesophageal junction, acute mucosal erosions, gastritis, duodenitis, and marginal ulcers, all of which are not well demonstrated by barium contrast radiologic studies (Fig. 16).

Gastric Analysis

The clinical value of gastric secretory tests has been recently reviewed.[90, 107] It is not possible to make a diagnosis of duodenal ulcer by means of gastric analysis alone (we recently studied a 70-year-old woman who had a basal acid secretion of 40 mEq. per hr. who did not have a peptic ulcer), but very low secretory values (a maximal acid output of less than 12 mEq. per hr., for example) make the diagnosis of duodenal ulcer unlikely. Baron[12] found that in duodenal ulcer patients over 30 years of age, half of the men and all of the women had a maximal acid output above the upper limit of normal, whereas in a companion series of control subjects, 44 per cent of the men and all of the women had a maximal acid output less than the least value of the duodenal ulcer patients.

Is prognosis in a duodenal ulcer patient related to the severity of hypersecretion? The data are not entirely clear, but Krag[104] followed a series of ulcer patients for several years and concluded that those patients with a higher acid output had a significantly more serious clinical course and required operation more often than those with low gastric secretory levels. In some ulcer patients there is a sharp decrease in acid secretory rates when the ulcer heals.[111] Measurements of the pH in situ within the duodenal bulb in normal and duodenal ulcer subjects have shown an average bulbar pH of 2.9 in duodenal ulcer patients and 4.5 in controls.[7] The antrum was uniformly more acid than the duodenum, but antral pH was equal in both control and duodenal ulcer patients. The pH in the antrum and in the postbulbar duodenum was much more stable than the pH within the bulb.

Gastric analysis has fallen into disfavor because it lacks precise correlation with disease. The test is uncomfortable for the patient, and the physician is often unsure of the role of gastric analysis in planning treatment for the patient. The great importance of gastric analysis for the surgeon who performs acid-reducing procedures for ulcer disease is that pre- and postoperative measurement of gastric acid secretion allows the best current means for evaluation of the success of the operation. In addition, we believe that gastric analysis may play an important role in all patients in whom the Zollinger-Ellison syndrome is suspected and in patients with gastric ulcer to determine whether the patient has achlorhydria, which would strongly point to carcinoma.

TREATMENT

A large percentage of patients, perhaps most with duodenal ulcer, never have any formal treatment. These patients may handle their difficulties quite well with the occasional administration of a solution of bicarbonate of soda or with proprietary antacid tablets (Tums or Rolaids). Of patients whose ulcer diathesis is sufficiently severe to require medical attention, fully 80 per cent may be managed successfully by medical therapy.

Medical Treatment

A legitimate aim of all ulcer therapy is to keep the intraluminal pH above about 5.5 so that pepsinogen is not activated. The mainstay of this effort is antacid therapy. Baking soda ($NaHCO_3$) should be avoided on a long-term basis because its use leads to a metabolic alkalosis and if it is coupled with an increased intake of calcium (usually taken in the form of milk), the milk-alkali syndrome of hypercalcemia, nephrocalcinosis, and eventual renal failure may develop.

Calcium carbonate has long been a mainstay of antacid therapy because it allegedly is not absorbed and acts within the lumen of the gut without changing the acid-base balance in the blood. Calcium carbonate may actually stimulate acid secretion,[13] and a study from our laboratory[138] shows that the administration of oral calcium carbonate caused a release of gastrin, which may be the agent responsible for the stimulation of acid secretion.

Antacids are the current cornerstone of medical treatment of duodenal ulcer, and the commercially available medications vary significantly in their buffering capacity; mixtures of the hydroxides of aluminum and magnesium appear to be the agents of choice.[51] Since oral antacids are effective for only about 30 minutes, they should be taken frequently. If patients are having pain at night, it is important that antacids be taken just before bedtime. It may be advantageous to have the patient set an alarm clock so that he can take antacids about one hour before he is usually awakened with pain. Liquid antacid preparations are probably more effective, but an important advantage of the proprietary tablet form is that patients will carry them and take them throughout the day.

Beyond antacids, the rest of medical therapy becomes somewhat controversial. The most common other medication used in day-to-day maintenance of ambulatory ulcer patient is an anticholinergic drug. In order to be effective, the dosage must be at a level near that which causes side effects (dryness of the mouth, tachycardia, constipation, and, in patients with incipient obstruction of the neck of the urinary bladder, possible urinary obstruction). It is our feeling that anticholinergic drugs do not have a place in the routine management of duodenal ulcer and should be reserved for those hospitalized patients who are troubled with severe hypersecretion of acid.

A new group of potent antisecretory drugs, H_2-receptor antagonists, have excited a great deal of clinical interest.[91] Standard antihistaminics (H_1-receptor antagonists) do not inhibit histamine stimulation of acid secretion. The new agents (e.g., metiamide and cimetidine) are potent inhibitors of acid secretion. Because a few patients who were taking metiamide developed transient agranulocytosis, studies on this drug have been discontinued, but cimetidine is now undergoing extensive clinical testing, and preliminary results suggest that it is as effective as metiamide. Other antisecretory agents that may become clinically useful are the prostaglandins and gastrointestinal inhibitory polypeptide and related hormones.

In the past, duodenal ulcer patients were almost routinely admonished to control their diet in a rigid fashion, and the hallmark of having an ulcer was the grueling necessity of adhering to an unpalatable white diet. It is now generally recognized that diet plays little role in the treatment of ulcers. If a patient notices that he has an exacerbation of pain on eating pizza or onions or fried foods, he obviously should avoid them. It is probably not a good idea for the patient to eat just before going to bed, but he should, instead, take a dose of antacid medication. Milk is widely used in the treatment of ulcer disease, but there is little data to support its efficacy and, in fact, it may stimulate acid secretion by releasing gastrin.

Many physicians use tranquilizers in managing hyperkinetic, anxious patients who have symptomatic ulcers. Mild sedation with small doses of phenobarbital may be helpful during periods of acute exacerbation. Routine use of sedation should be rigorously avoided.

During acute bouts of pain, it is often worthwhile to hospitalize the patient and thereby remove him from the stresses that may precipitate ulcer activity. At this time the patient should receive hourly antacid therapy while awake, sedatives, and perhaps anticholinergic drugs. If relief of pain does not occur after one day on this regimen, it may be necessary to resort to nasogastric suction to aspirate acid peptic secretion. If suction does not relieve pain, the ulcer has probably penetrated through the posterior wall of the duodenum and the patient is a likely candidate for surgical treatment.

Indications for Surgical Treatment

Only one of five patients whose duodenal ulcer is sufficiently severe for him to seek medical help will require operation. Surgical techniques in operations on the stomach will be discussed in a subsequent section. The complications of duodenal ulcer that require surgical management are hemorrhage, perforation, obstruction, and intractability.

Hemorrhage. Bleeding is the most serious complication of peptic ulcer and accounts for about 40 per cent of deaths due to the disease. Bleeding may be chronic and insidious or brisk and life-threatening. Even when large vessels are eroded by enzymatic digestion, bleeding is usually periodic and it is rare for a patient to begin to bleed and bleed continuously to death. Spontaneous remission of the hemorrhage occurs when the blood pressure falls because of hypovolemic shock and a clot then forms. Bleeding may be heralded by several days of exacerbation of pain or may arise de novo in a patient who has never had ulcer symptoms. Bleeding from duodenal ulcer is usually manifested by passage of black tarry stools (melena), but with rapid

bleeding, bright red blood may appear per rectum and blood may also regurgitate into the stomach and be vomited. Hematemesis usually connotes much more rapid and serious loss of blood than melena alone, although some patients with bleeding ulcer may have sufficient pyloric stenosis that they will not regurgitate blood regardless of the briskness of the hemorrhage.

Mortality rates for operations on patients during acute bleeding episodes are several times greater than for elective operations.[52] Everything possible must be done to stop the bleeding so that the patient may be resuscitated and evaluated for elective operation. Obviously, however, if the patient starts to bleed and bleeds without stopping, as about 10 per cent of patients do, he must be operated upon as an emergency in order to save his life.

A patient who comes in with signs and symptoms of significant bleeding should receive vigorous blood replacement. Blood should be drawn at once for hematocrit measurement and for blood typing and cross-matching. A large-bore plastic catheter for estimation of central venous blood pressure and for rapid blood replacement should be inserted into the superior vena cava through a vein in the upper arm. A nasogastric tube should be placed into the stomach and connected to suction. Presence of gross blood in the aspirate indicates that the source of bleeding is proximal to the ligament of Treitz. A urinary catheter should be inserted for measurement of hourly urinary output; a urinary output of more than 30 ml. per hour should be maintained if possible.

The availability of fiberoptic endoscopy has revolutionized the emergency management of patients with massive upper gastrointestinal bleeding. The procedure is safe and accurate and provides critical information quickly (Fig. 16). In a series of 195 consecutive patients admitted to our hospital with massive gastrointestinal hemorrhage (Table 4),[173] 14 were later found to be bleeding from lesions distal to the ligament of Treitz. In three others, no diagnosis was made and the patients stopped bleeding spontaneously. Only five diagnostic errors were made in this series (2.6 per

TABLE 4. Final Diagnosis in 195 Consecutive Patients with Gastrointestinal Bleeding*

Diagnosis	Number of Patients	Per Cent
Duodenal ulcer	50	25.6
Hemorrhagic gastritis	35	17.9
Bleeding esophageal varices	29	14.9
Mallory-Weiss tears	15	7.7
Gastric ulcer	20	10.3
Esophagitis	7	3.6
Carcinoma	7	3.6
Miscellaneous	15	7.7
Normal (lesions below the ligament of Treitz)	14	7.2
No diagnosis	3	1.5
Total	195	

*Modified from Villar et al., in press.

cent). Of the 50 bleeding patients in whom the final diagnosis was duodenal ulcer, a correct endoscopic diagnosis was made in 49 (for example, see Fig. 16B). Radiologic examination of the upper gastrointestinal tract was performed in 37 patients and was reported as normal in nine (that is, the false-negative rate was 24 per cent). Yajko and colleagues[186] reported correct endoscopic diagnosis of the cause of bleeding in 80 per cent of 200 patients with massive upper gastrointestinal bleeding.

What are the criteria for deciding which bleeding patients should be operated upon? Any patient who has suffered a massive blood loss, by any of the following criteria, should be considered a *candidate* for operation: (1) loss of 1500 to 2000 ml. of blood; (2) blood loss that causes an acute fall in the hematocrit to 25 or below; (3) acute blood loss resulting in syncope; (4) blood loss that, after the patient's vital signs have been stablized, requires more than 1000 ml. of blood per 24 hours to maintain a stable hematocrit and stable blood pressure.

If a patient comes into the hospital bleeding massively, stops bleeding spontaneously and is completely resuscitated, and then has another massive hemorrhage while in the hospital, he should be operated upon. There are other factors that may influence a decision to operate. Usually, the older a patient is, the more dangerous will be hemorrhagic shock, and older patients should be operated upon earlier. When massive hemorrhage intervenes in a patient who is already seriously ill with another disease, the added stress of bleeding may result in an intolerable risk and early operation may be indicated. Patients who have had a long history of difficulty with their ulcer, previous hemorrhages, severe pain, or previous perforation, should be operated upon sooner than patients in whom hemorrhage is the initial ulcer symptom. Another practical consideration may influence the decision: if the patient has a rare blood type or if there is a shortage of his specific type for any reason, a decision to operate may be precipitated.

Once the decision has been made to operate on the patient, efforts should be made to empty the stomach. Great care should be taken to prevent vomiting and aspiration of gastric contents during induction of anesthesia. The most certain way of preventing this is to insert the endotracheal tube and to inflate the balloon cuff around the tube while the patient is still awake. This usually can be accomplished with facility by skilled anesthesiologists and is a most important maneuver. The sequelae of aspiration are often fatal.

At operation the surgeon should proceed quickly to identify and suture the point of bleeding. After this, the choice of procedures usually lies between vagotomy and a drainage procedure (pyloroplasty or gastroenterostomy), and vagotomy with distal gastric resection. An argument for early operative approach in upper gastrointestinal bleeding is provided in a recent retrospective study[149] of more than 2100 patients admitted to the emergency hospital at Oxford for a 15-year period which reported that 81 per cent of the patients had a previous history of gastric symptoms and one third had bled previously. There was a steady decline in surgical mortality over the 15 years, but the overall mortality showed little change. It was suggested that more patients should be treated by immediate or early operation in order to achieve an overall reduction in the mortality rate.

Hemorrhage occurs when a posterior penetrating ulcer erodes into a blood vessel. Another quite rare complication of posterior penetration of an ulcer is erosion into the common bile duct. Fistulas between the gallbladder and gastrointestinal tract are usually caused by erosion of gallstones, but fistulas between the duodenum and common bile duct are almost always caused by peptic ulcers.[39]

Perforation. Perforation of a duodenal ulcer brings about a remarkable series of dramatic changes. Immediately prior to perforation, the patient may feel entirely well, within a few minutes be in great pain, and within an hour desperately ill. As already noted, hemorrhage is associated with *posterior* erosion of an ulcer; perforation occurs when an anteriorly or laterally placed ulcer erodes through the full thickness of the wall of the duodenum into the free peritoneal cavity, spilling acid peptic juice, bile, and pancreatic juice into the peritoneal cavity. These chemically active ferments cause havoc; the resultant chemical injury has been aptly compared to a burn of the peritoneum. Within a short time massive amounts of extracellular fluid may be sequestered in the area of peritoneal injury, and this loss of fluid may bring about hypovolemic shock.

Diagnosis in most cases is not difficult, but in atypical instances may be extraordinarily so. Other conditions to be considered are acute pancreatitis, acute appendicitis, acute cholecystitis, and less commonly, diverticulitis or acute pyelonephritis.

The patient usually gives a typical history of the sudden development of severe epigastric and later generalized abdominal pain. Movement is painful and the patient lies still. By the time he gets to the hospital he may be in shock.

Examination of the abdomen usually reveals considerable guarding and often boardlike rigidity of the abdominal musculature. With free air in the peritoneal cavity there is often a loss of the normal dullness on percussion over the liver. If gastric contents have flowed into the right lower quadrant guided by the attachment of the small bowel mesentery, the patient may have signs and symptoms of peritonitis in the right lower quadrant, which may confuse the picture and suggest appendicitis.

About 75 per cent of patients will show free air under the diaphragm on an upright chest x-ray film (Fig. 17), or on a lateral decubitus film if the patient is unable to sit. Conversely, this means that about one in four patients with a perforated duodenal ulcer will not show free air, and that it is perfectly proper, if other evidence warrants, to make the diagnosis of perforation without the demonstration of free intraperitoneal air on upright chest film or on lateral abdominal decubitus films.

Although there have been repeated flurries of interest in the nonoperative management of perforated duodenal ulcer, the overwhelming consensus of surgeons in the United States would be that this catastrophic event should be treated by surgical re-

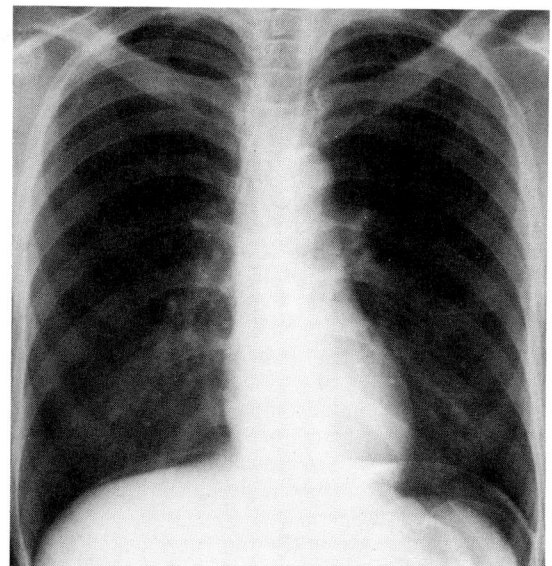

Figure 17. Chest x-ray film taken with the patient in the upright position. Free air is clearly visible under both the right and left leaves of the diaphragm. This patient had a perforated duodenal ulcer.

pair. Mortality rates for early operation are low, but the risk increases with delay. The leak in the duodenum must be closed rapidly in order to reduce the extent of peritoneal contamination.

At operation the site of perforation should be located and the hole either closed with an omental patch (Graham closure) or incorporated into a pyloroplasty, which, when coupled with a vagotomy, will not only repair the perforation but will also serve as definitive treatment for the duodenal ulcer itself. When vagotomy and pyloroplasty were first advocated in the treatment of perforated ulcer more than two decades ago, the suggestion represented such a radical departure from conventional thinking that it was necessary to satisfy stringent criteria to justify its use. In spite of expectations, opening the peritoneum around the esophagus in order to perform a vagotomy has not led to any significant increase in morbidity or mortality. Since vagotomy and pyloroplasty provide definitive treatment for the ulcer diathesis, and since definitive treatment will be required eventually by a large percentage of patients treated initially by simple closure, it seems proper now to advocate vagotomy and pyloroplasty in the treatment of perforated duodenal ulcer *except* in instances in which the risk is high. This means that simple closure of the perforation would be reserved for fragile patients in whom prolongation of the operative procedure is contraindicated or in whom massive contamination of the peritoneal cavity appears certain to cause future complications. Patients without prodromal difficulties or whose ulcer arises from a temporary stressful situation may be candidates for simple closure of the perforation. There is a close correlation between pre- and postperforation symptomatology. A group of patients were studied for the presence of ulcer symptoms after simple closure of a perforation; of those who had no symptoms before,

72 per cent were asymptomatic after operation; of those with previous ulcer symptoms, only 23 per cent were asymptomatic.[148]

After management of the perforation itself, great care should be taken to wash the peritoneal cavity many, many times with warm Ringer's lactate solution to dilute and wash out contamination.

Obstruction. Obstruction of the gastric outlet may occur at two different times in the history of the duodenal ulcer. There will occasionally be sufficient edema associated with an acute ulcer to obstruct the lumen of the bowel and cause vomiting. This obstruction is transient and usually self-limited and responds to conservative treatment with nasogastric suction for two or three days. Second and more important, obstruction may be caused by chronic cicatrization in which scar contracture gradually narrows the lumen of the duodenum to the point of obstruction. In the latter instance, patients with a massively dilated stomach may seek help after months of intermittent obstruction or they may suddenly undergo complete obstruction of the pylorus and vomit perniciously for several days. Because of the massive loss of H^+ and Cl^-, the patient may have a severe hypochloremic alkalosis along with hypokalemia. The potassium deficiency is due to a moderate loss from vomiting (gastric juice has about 10 mEq. K^+ per liter) and to an important renal loss caused by substitution of K^+ for H^+. It is necessary to correct the hypokalemia as well as the hypochloremic alkalosis. Administration of sodium chloride and potassium chloride solutions usually suffices; rarely, however, it may be necessary to administer hydrochloric acid intravenously to achieve correction of the metabolic alkalosis.[78]

When a patient with gastric outlet obstruction is admitted to the hospital any significant acid-base and electrolyte abnormalities must be corrected and fluid deficiences must be restored. In addition, it is important to empty the stomach of retained food. This may require prolonged irrigation and aspiration with a large-bore tube. Evacuation should be accomplished in order to allow the walls of the stomach to return to their original size and to permit the edema of obstruction to subside.

The degree of outlet obstruction can be estimated by means of the saline load test.[55] This test should be conducted in a fasting patient whose stomach has been emptied completely. A No. 18 sump-type nasogastric tube is placed in the stomach and 750 ml. of 0.9 per cent sodium chloride solution is instilled at room temperature. The tube should then be clamped for 30 minutes after which the stomach should be aspirated. If more than 400 ml. is retained, obstruction is certain (retention of more than 200 ml. is abnormal). If the results of the test are abnormal after three days of nasogastric suction, operative therapy is indicated.

The operative procedure usually recommended is either truncal vagotomy with antrectomy or with gastroenterostomy. Because the obstructed stomach is edematous and because edematous tissue heals poorly, the stomach should be decompressed for two or three days before operation. Several days may be required after operation for the stomach to regain its tone and empty normally.

Intractability. Although it is the least clearly defined of the indications for operation for duodenal ulcer, intractability necessitates surgical treatment for duodenal ulcer more often than any of the other complications. An ulcer may be intractable because the ulcer disease is so severe that the patient does not secure relief from antacid therapy and because he is disabled from work or any gainful life. Other patients may elect operation because they do not want to put up with the problems of the medical treatment of peptic ulcer disease or with the vicissitudes of recurrent attacks of pain. Patients operated upon for intractability often have had active recurrent ulcer disease for many years, often with previous episodes of bleeding or perforation, and they may finally decide that living with the disease is too difficult and too complex and too time-consuming and may choose surgical treatment in hopes of being able to lead a more simple and pain-free life. Conversations with other patients who have had operations for peptic ulcer often convince a long-standing sufferer from ulcer disease that operation can greatly improve his lot. As risks diminish with the increased use of conservative operative procedures, criteria for operation may, in many instances, be liberalized.

Physicians often deal with patients who are addicted to alcohol or to aspirin or who have such a wildly disorganized style of living that they can never adhere to any sort of medical treatment of duodenal ulcer. In these instances, the patient may be considered intractable and surgical treatment may be advisable to prevent serious later complications of the ulcer.

Either a vagotomy plus a drainage procedure or vagotomy plus distal gastric resection is the usual elective operation performed for intractability.

GASTRIC ULCER

Gastric ulcers generally occur later in life than duodenal ulcers and have a peak incidence in the fifth decade. They affect about twice as many men as women, and although variously estimated as only one third to one fifth as common as duodenal ulcers in this country, they are responsible for almost half of the deaths due to peptic ulcer disease.[122]

DIAGNOSIS

History

Although the clinical findings in a patient with gastric ulcer may be quite similar to those in a patient with duodenal ulcer, there are often important differences. The pain pattern is not nearly so clear-cut; pain usually appears just at or slightly to the left of the midline. Although the pain is often relieved by food, many patients with gastric ulcer report an exacerbation on eating, or particularly on drinking warm liquids or alcohol. Early satiety, nausea, and vomiting are often troublesome, and postprandial discomfort may be of such consequence that the patient may decide not to eat in order to relieve the pain. Chronicity is common and patients often do not seek help from a physician for years. There does seem to be some difference in the socioeconomic classes of patients with duodenal and gastric ulcers, since patients with gastric ulcer are more common among the poor.

Whereas most patients with duodenal ulcer disease do well on medical management, patients with gastric ulcers have a higher rate of recurrence and of complications, and the complications tend to be more serious than in patients with duodenal ulcer.

Radiology

As with duodenal ulcer disease, the diagnosis of gastric ulcer is still made chiefly by radiology in this country, although the use of the fiberoptic gastroscope is becoming more and more common. In Japan, techniques of gastroscopy are sufficiently advanced that as many gastric ulcers are diagnosed by gastroscopy as by x-ray.

An important consideration in the diagnosis of gastric ulcer is the possibility of malignancy. Much has been written about the differentiation between benign and malignant ulcers. In most patients with carcinoma of the stomach, there is no confusion with gastric ulcer. Only in those instances in which the patient with carcinoma has an ulcerating lesion does confusion arise. The most important differentiating characteristic is whether the ulcer crater penetrates beyond the projected line of the wall of the stomach, which benign ulcers tend to do (Fig. 18), whereas malignant ulcers more often represent an erosion into a filling defect that protrudes into the stomach (Fig. 19). The differentiation of benign from malignant ulcers by x-ray is about 95 per cent accurate,[106] but this statistic reflects in large part the preponderance of benign over malignant ulcers and the classic morphology of most benign ulcers. In atypical cases, differentiation between benign and malignant gastric ulceration can still be a most difficult problem. Widely respected opinions to the contrary, there seems to be no tendency for malignant ulcers to occur more frequently on the greater curvature of the stomach than elsewhere.[68, 106]

About 95 per cent of gastric ulcers are located on or near the lesser curvature, and a majority have been reported in the region of the incisura[129] (Fig. 20).

Gastroscopy

Fiberoptic gastroscopy examination allows the endoscopist to look directly at the gastric ulcer, to take a picture of it, and to obtain with a biopsy forceps small fragments of the edges of the ulcer for histologic examination. These techniques are available in almost all centers in this country and within a few years will allow even greater accuracy in the differentiation between benign and malignant gastric ulcers (see Fig. 16 *D, E* and *F*).

TREATMENT

Whereas most patients with duodenal ulcer do well on antacid therapy, there is a much higher rate of recurrence with gastric ulcers. Because of this and be-

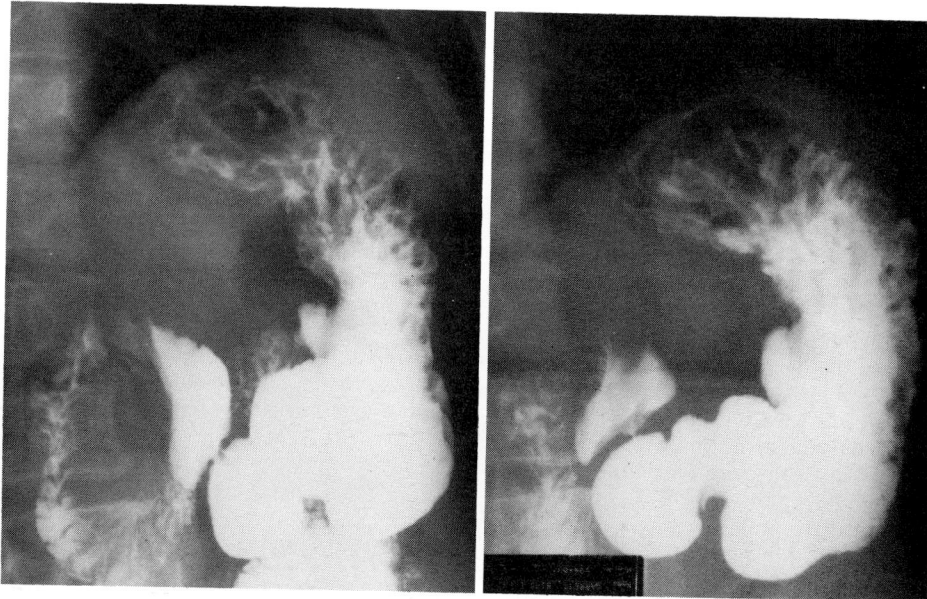

Figure 18. Two views of a benign gastric ulcer located on the lesser curvature of the stomach just proximal to the incisura angularis. After the film on the left was obtained, the patient was placed on a strict antacid regimen for 1 month, after which time the picture on the right was taken, which demonstrates enlargement of the crater in spite of the treatment program. Both pictures show that the ulcer crater penetrates beyond the projected line of the wall of the stomach, and there is a ring of radiolucent edematous mucosa about the base of the ulcer.

cause of the frequency (as high as 63 per cent[6]) and the serious consequences of complications, many surgeons have suggested that patients with benign gastric ulcer be operated upon earlier in the course of their disease.

The basic aim of medical therapy of gastric ulcer is the same as that for duodenal ulcer, namely the maintenance of the pH of the gastric lumen above pH 5.5. The mainstay of the program is repeated antacid ther-

apy. If patients are in symptomatic difficulty, they should be hospitalized and treated with sedation and with antacid therapy at regularly specified intervals. The role of anticholinergic drugs is again controver-

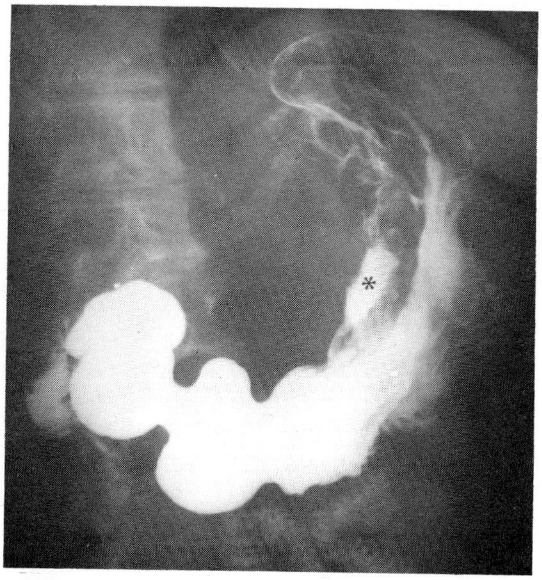

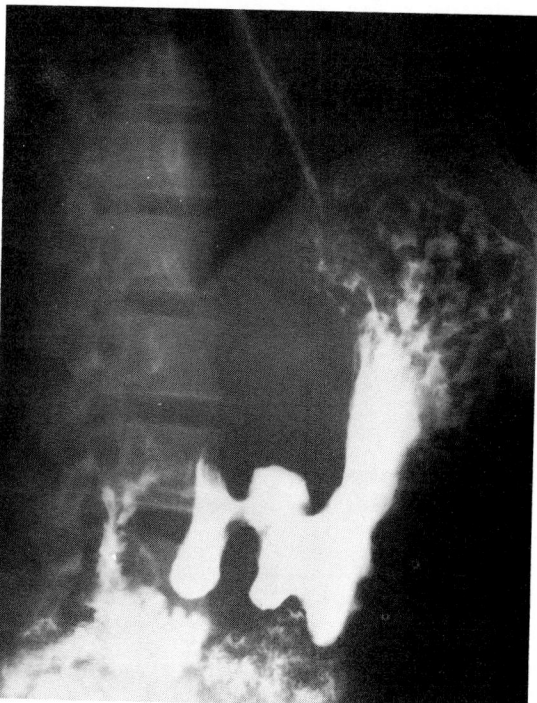

Figure 19. Ulcerating carcinoma of the lesser curvature of the stomach. There is a large filling defect of the lesser curvature protruding into the lumen of the stomach in the center of which there is an ulcer crater marked with an asterisk.

Figure 20. Large gastric ulcer of the lesser curvature just distal to the incisura angularis. The large incisura on the greater curvature is caused by contraction due to the ulcer itself. Lesions such as this often must be seen in multiple views in order to be certain that they are not caused by waves of contraction.

sial, and they should be used only in hospitalized patients who are in difficulty because of the hypersecretion of gastric acid.

The indications for operation in patients with gastric ulcer are hemorrhage, perforation, obstruction, intractability, and the need to rule out the possibility of carcinoma of the stomach. Since malignancy is a possibility in all gastric ulcers, it is important at operation either to remove the entire ulcer and obtain pathologic examination by frozen section technique or to obtain biopsy specimens from four quadrants of the ulcer and examine them by frozen section.

The signs and symptoms of bleeding from gastric ulcers are similar to those of bleeding duodenal ulcers. Since patients with gastric ulcers are apt to be older and since bleeding is apt to be more persistent, the outlook is more serious and operation should be undertaken earlier in gastric ulcer patients than in patients with duodenal ulcer.

At operation the ulcer should be excised if possible and included in a distal gastrectomy. If the bleeding ulcer is located high in the stomach, the surgeon may place sutures at the site of bleeding after obtaining a biopsy of the ulcer, or (preferably) he may excise the ulcer locally, repair the defect, and then perform a distal gastrectomy.

Patients with perforation of the stomach due to a gastric ulcer manifest the same signs and symptoms as do patients with perforated duodenal ulcer. There is usually free air under the diaphragm, although if the ulcer has perforated into the lesser omental bursa, the air may collect in that bursa and show a characteristic rectangular pattern on x-ray.

Perforated gastric ulcer may be treated either by simple closure of the perforation after biopsy of the ulcer or by gastric resection. The choice is influenced by the status of the patient.

Patients with obstructing benign gastric ulcers usually have a large dilated stomach filled with accumulated food. Their preoperative management should be identical with that of patients with obstructing duodenal ulcers. The operative treatment is either a distal gastrectomy or a simple bypass of the obstructed distal stomach, depending upon whether the patient is a suitable candidate for a resective procedure.

The main problem in dealing with patients with gastric ulcer who do not have a complication requiring operation is when to advocate surgical intervention. In the past, the specter of carcinoma was often raised in these arguments, and although the risk is still real, many surgeons and some internists now feel that the recurrence rate of gastric ulcer is sufficiently high and the surgical risk with conservative operative approaches is sufficiently low that many gastric ulcer patients should be operated upon earlier, before hemorrhage, perforation, obstruction, or intractable pain develops.

The standard program is to submit the patient to a specified period of intense medical treatment and to utilize this as a test of healing. If the ulcer heals, the patient should be examined at intervals, and probably at the time of the first and certainly upon the second recurrence, he should have an operation.

A recent cooperative 7-year study[68] of 638 male gastric ulcer patients from 16 Veterans Administration Hospitals compared the results of medical and surgical treatment of gastric ulcer. The patients were initially placed on a regimen of antacids and diet in a protocol that defined satisfactory healing as a decrease in crater size of 50 per cent or more at 3 weeks, 90 per cent or more at 6 weeks, and 100 per cent at 12 weeks. Seventy per cent of the ulcers were healed completely at 6 weeks and 76 per cent were healed at 12 weeks. Patients whose ulcers did not heal at the defined satisfactory rate were randomly assigned to operation or to continuation of medical treatment up to a total of 12 weeks.

Among those patients whose ulcer healed in the initial 12 weeks of medical therapy there was a 42 per cent recurrence rate within two years. Of those patients whose rate of healing was slower than defined as satisfactory but whose ulcers did heal completely at 12 weeks, the recurrence rate in two years was 62 per cent. Of 42 patients randomly assigned to operation, six had carcinoma. There was one postoperative death and there were no recurrences following operation. In other series[6, 106] the respective mortality rates for medical and surgical treatment were similar (about 5 per cent), whereas the incidence of satisfactory results following surgery was 90 to 95 per cent, versus 38 to 48 per cent for medical treatment.

In summary, it would appear proper to subject patients with gastric ulcers that do not have the characteristics of malignancy on x-ray or gastroscopy to a rigidly prescribed 6-week test of healing (Fig. 21). Those patients whose ulcers fail to heal completely should be operated upon. The patients whose ulcers do heal should be operated upon at the first recurrence. It should be recognized that as many as 16 per cent of patients with gastric carcinoma may pass a 12-week test of healing,[68] and that benign ulcers may enlarge during a test of healing (see Fig. 18).

In a significant percentage of patients with duodenal ulcer, gastric ulceration will develop. In the absence of a specific complication of the gastric ulcer, the patient should be treated as though he had a duodenal ulcer alone.

ZOLLINGER-ELLISON SYNDROME[93, 167]

Zollinger and Ellison[188] in 1955 described a clinical syndrome that is now recognized to consist of massive gastric hypersecretion, peptic ulceration (often multiple, often jejunal, and frequently fatal), and a non-beta cell islet tumor of the pancreas that produces gastrin. The gastrinoma metastasizes to the liver and regional lymph nodes in more than 50 per cent of cases.[75] Diarrhea and malabsorption are frequently associated and may precede the development of peptic ulcers.

Patients with the Zollinger-Ellison syndrome usually have a basal acid secretion of greater than 15 mEq. per hr; in 12 patients with the Zollinger-Ellison syndrome, we found a range of basal acid output of between 15 and 76 mEq. per hr. with a mean of 34.3.[167] Hypergastrinemia measured by radioimmunoassay is a nearly constant finding, although gastrin values (as well as acid secretory output) vary greatly from time

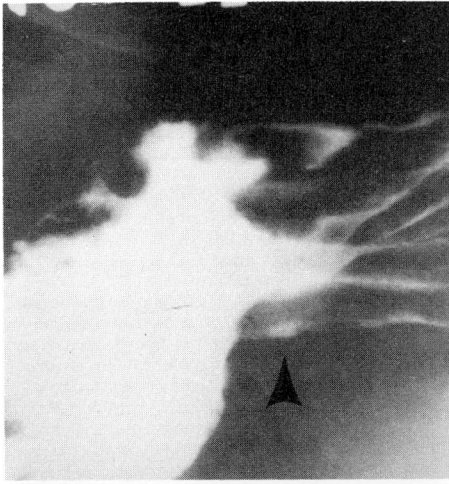
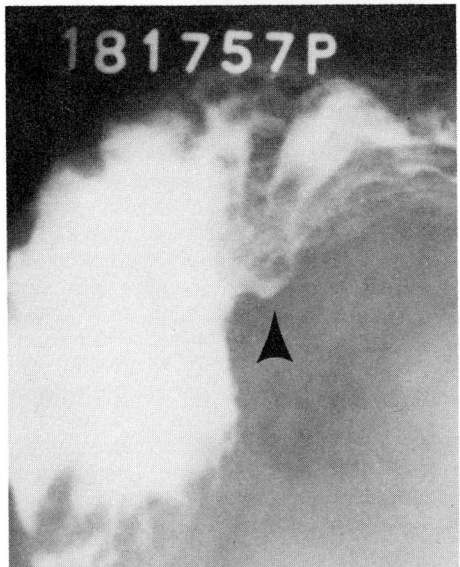
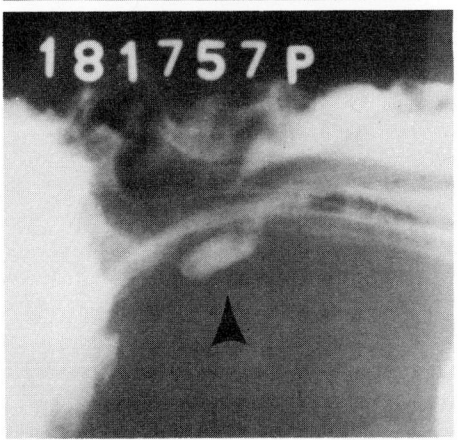

Figure 21. Three views of a gastric ulcer that healed on a strict antacid regimen. Arrows point to benign gastric ulcer on proximal lesser curvature. After the upper radiograph was obtained, the patient was placed on a strict antacid regimen for 10 days, after which the radiograph shown in the center was taken. After six more weeks on the same program, the lower picture was obtained, which shows nearly complete healing of the ulcer.

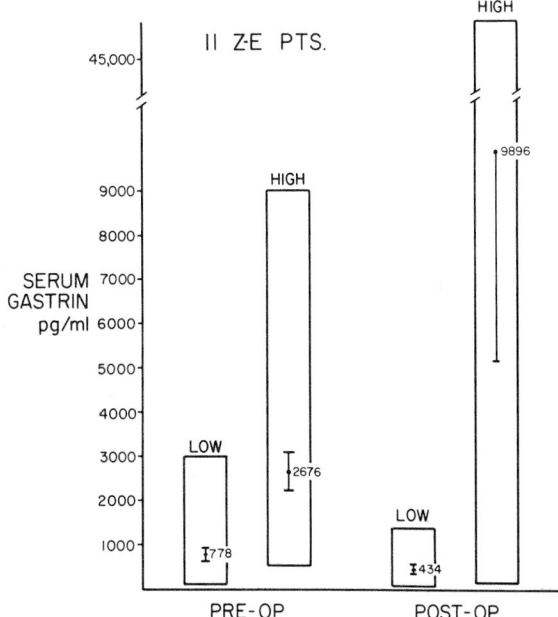

Figure 22. Basal serum gastrin levels before and after total gastrectomy in 10 patients with the Zollinger-Ellison syndrome. Several values were available for each patient; they are grouped into the lowest and highest values available for each patient. Low preoperative values ranged between 100 and 2997 pg. per ml., with a mean of 778 pg. per ml. High values ranged between 383 and 8833 pg. per ml., with a mean of 2676 pg. per ml. Postoperatively, low values ranged between 86 and 1367 pg. per ml., with a mean of 434 pg. per ml.; high values after operation ranged between 174 and 4580 pg. per ml., with a mean of 9896 pg. per ml. (From Thompson, J. C., et al.: Surg. Gynecol. Obstet., *140*:721, 1975.)

to time, and multiple samples may be required for diagnosis (Fig. 22). Release of gastrin by calcium and secretin infusion has proved to be a valuable diagnostic test in patients with gastrinomas (Fig. 23).

The diagnosis of the Zollinger-Ellison syndrome is usually not difficult. Most patients have severe symptoms of peptic ulcer, although rarely patients will seek help who have diarrhea without ulcer symptoms. The diarrhea is apparently caused by the massive acid hypersecretion and is not caused by any intrinsic action of gastrin itself. It is always completely alleviated by total gastrectomy. The most important factor in diagnosis is demonstration of elevated levels of serum gastrin (basal or after calcium or secretin challenge) along with gastric hypersecretion. Occasional patients with pyloric obstruction will show some elevation of serum gastrin, but these patients, as well as those with retained antral mucosa, should demonstrate a *fall* in gastrin levels after secretin.

Radiologic studies may be quite helpful. On upper gastrointestinal barium study, the stomach is often seen to be enlarged with thickened edematous mucosa thrown into great folds (Fig. 24). The barium in the stomach is often diluted by the large secretory output, and when the barium column reaches the small intestine there are often signs of mucosal edema and hypermotility, along with puddling and clumping of the barium. The pancreatic tumor itself may be demon-

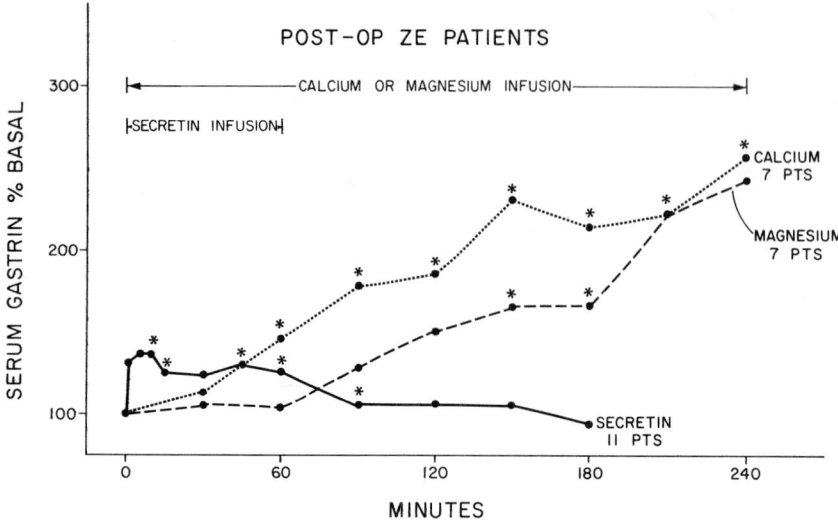

Figure 23. Release of tumor gastrin (in patients with the Zollinger-Ellison syndrome) caused by calcium, magnesium, or secretin. Note that the gastrin release after secretin challenge is almost immediate; the incremental rise after both calcium and magnesium is much greater than after secretin, but the rate of release is slower. Calcium (and to a lesser extent magnesium) released gastrin in both normal individuals and duodenal ulcer patients. The important discriminatory value of secretin is that it causes *suppression* of gastrin release (with few exceptions) in all individuals except those with the Zollinger-Ellison syndrome. (From Thompson, J. C., et al.: Surg. Gynecol. Obstet., *140*:721, 1975.)

strated on selective abdominal angiography in about 30 per cent of cases; the neoplasms often exhibit a characteristic tumor blush that denotes increased vascularity (Fig. 25).

About one out of four patients with a gastrinoma will be found to have the familial multiple endocrine adenoma syndrome, type I (that is multiple endocrine neoplasms involving the parathyroid, pancreas, pituitary, adrenal, and thyroid). Any patients with duodenal ulcer and hypercalcemia should be suspected of having the MEA I syndrome with a parathyroid adenoma and a gastrinoma. The gastrinomas are frequently multiple within the pancreas and may arise ectopically in the duodenum.

Although the full-blown syndrome is a fulminant one, many patients have been troubled with peptic ulcer symptoms and diarrhea for 5 to 10 years before the syndrome is recognized. With the availability of gastrin radioimmunoassay, the diagnosis will be made earlier and more atypical forms will be found.

Patients with the Zollinger-Ellison syndrome and severe hypersecretion should be operated upon as soon as possible after the restoration of fluid and electrolyte balance, a task that may be facilitated by temporary suppression of the massive gastric output with large doses of cholinergic drugs, or when they become available, the H$_2$-blocking agents.[143] At operation, the diagnosis can be confirmed by demonstrating the characteristic tumor in the pancreas or in the wall of the duodenum. These tumors are often multiple and often have occult metastasis and the recommended treatment is total gastrectomy, which excises the gastrin end-organ, the mass of parietal cells. Since it is never possible to be sure whether all gastrinoma tissue has been excised, the entire mass of parietal cells must be removed. If the diagnosis is secure by clinical and laboratory criteria, total gastrectomy should be performed even if the primary tumor is not found, or even if large hepatic metastases are present. Every attempt should be made to locate the tumor and to excise as much of it as possible.

For reasons that are not clear but that may be related to the trophic actions of gastrin, patients with the Zollinger-Ellison syndrome have an unexpectedly low mortality rate for total gastrectomy and they tolerate the procedure surprisingly well. Although cautious trials of medical management with anticholinergics[93] or H$_2$-receptor antagonists[143] have been reported, the arguments for operation are compelling, even if the hypersecretion can be quelled by drugs. These patients have tumors that should be considered malignant; three of our original 12 patients are now dead with hepatic metastases. The patients may tolerate their hepatic metastases for long periods, in a manner similar to patients with the carcinoid syn-

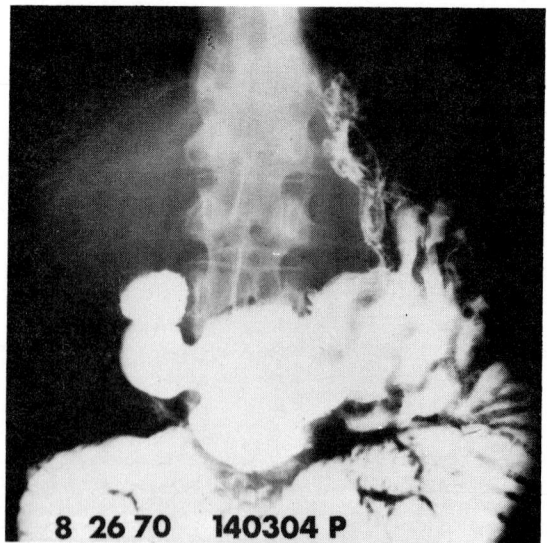

Figure 24. Upper gastrointestinal x-ray study in a patient with the Zollinger-Ellison syndrome. Note the greatly enlarged thickened folds of mucosa in the stomach and in the jejunum, striking representations of mucosal edema.

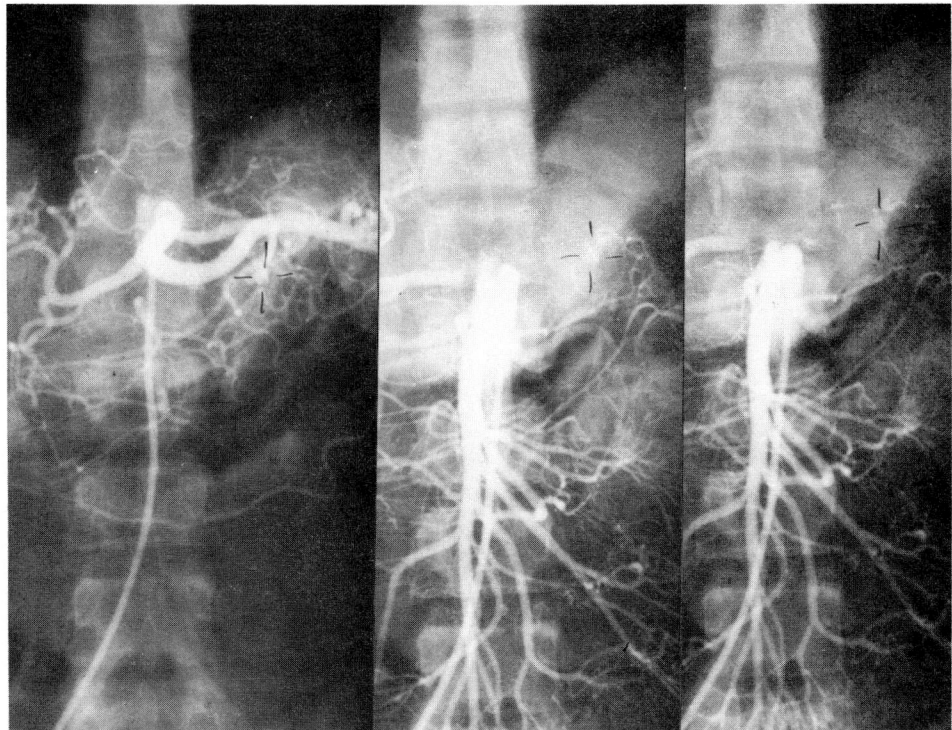

Figure 25. Selective arteriographic demonstration of gastrinoma in a patient with the Zollinger-Ellison syndrome. *Left,* A selective celiac arteriogram. *Center and right,* Superior mesenteric arteriograms. All three views show the small isolated tumor that was found at operation in the midportion of the tail of the pancreas. (From Thompson, J. C., et al.: Surg. Gynecol. Obstet., *140*:721, 1975.)

drome, but the tumors have a clear potential of killing their hosts, and we have not seen any spontaneous resolution of the tumor. An aggressive combined approach with surgery and chemotherapy offers hope of success.[155, 167, 189]

PEPTIC ULCER IN CHILDREN

Although it is relatively rare, peptic ulcer in patients under the age of 15 often has a complicated and serious clinical course. Whenever children develop peptic ulcer, gastrin levels should be measured and the patient evaluated for the Zollinger-Ellison syndrome. Spontaneous perforations of the gastrointestinal tract in the newborn are apparently due to ischemia induced by remote circulatory disturbances initiated by shock,[112] although stress ulceration may be implicated in a few cases.[27]

There appear to be four distinct clinical patterns of peptic ulceration in childhood.[98] In the first two weeks of life perforation or hemorrhage may occur without premonitory signs and often with few findings, or none at all, on abdominal examination. If the ulcer has perforated, plain x-ray films of the abdomen will usually show free air. Barium studies of the upper gastrointestinal tract in infants who are bleeding often demonstrate a duodenal ulcer.

From the second week of life until the age of two,

peptic ulceration may be manifested by bleeding or by poor feeding and frequent vomiting. Perforation and massive bleeding are again the principal complications but usually occur with antecedent symptoms of abdominal pain or anorexia or vomiting and the radiologist is usually able to demonstrate a distinct ulcer of the duodenum. In the first two weeks of life, complications in peptic ulcer have a frightening mortality rate and early operation is mandatory. In these infants it is usually sufficient to close the perforation or to ligate the bleeding point, since they do not seem to have an ulcer diathesis and will not later suffer from ulcer disease.[134] After the second week of life, vagotomy and pyloroplasty appear to be the best treatment for complications of peptic ulcer.[98]

From the age of two until the age of seven, the incidence of peptic ulceration is the lowest in childhood and is often associated with lesions of the central nervous system or sepsis or other causes of stress ulceration.

After the age of seven to eight, the pathogenesis and clinical course of peptic ulcer disease become more and more like the typical syndrome seen in adults. Hemorrhage, perforation, obstruction of the gastric outlet, and intractable pain are relatively common. Early in the course of the disease the radiologic studies are often difficult to interpret, and in the absence of an ulcer crater, the most important findings may be evidence of increased gastric secretion and persistent pylorospasm. The appearance of a duodenal ulcer in a child suggests either a diminished resistance of the mucosa or an especially virulent form of the ulcer diathesis; complications are common and serious. Because of this and because the results with conservative operative approaches (vagotomy and drainage) are good and have few detectable later sequelae, early operative treatment of complications of peptic ulcer in childhood is advisable.

ACUTE MUCOSAL EROSIONS

Perhaps the most important point to make about the treatment of acute mucosal lesions of the upper GI tract (stress ulcers or hemorrhagic gastritis) is that they should be anticipated in patients who are chronically ill with sepsis and hypotension (see section on Pathogenesis). Since the occurrence of these lesions has been demystified, surgeons who work with patients in intensive care units know to anticipate bleeding from acute mucosal erosions in patients who are critically ill for long periods, especially those with sepsis and hypotension.

Production of gastric acid by patients bleeding from acute mucosal lesions has been reported variously to be low or normal or high. Patients with Cushing's ulcers (associated with lesions of the central nervous system) appear to have higher levels of acid secretion[60, 158] than do patients without CNS trauma, in whom low levels of acid secretion may reflect the severe nature of associated diseases or may be due to back-diffusion of acid through the damaged mucosal barrier. Acid output has been found to be low during hypotension caused by hypovolemia or sepsis but often has been found to increase in a striking fashion after correction of the fluid losses and hemodynamic abnormalities.[114]

DIAGNOSIS

Acute mucosal lesions should be considered whenever acute upper gastrointestinal bleeding or perforation occurs after a major injury or during the course of an important metabolic insult. Bleeding may begin insidiously, making its initial appearance as coffee-ground flecks in the nasogastric aspirate of postoperative patients, changing during the course of hours or days to brisk bleeding. On the other hand, major bleeding may supervene dramatically. If the blood first appears by rectum, and if the patient has not vomited, a nasogastric tube should be inserted for diagnosis. Bleeding may be continuous but is usually episodic.

Gastroscopy is the most important diagnostic technique available (Fig. 16G).[114, 173, 186] It is usually possible to demonstrate acute, superficial, bleeding gastric lesions when the patients are examined during gastric hemorrhage. Upper gastrointestinal x-ray series obtained during bleeding episodes are rarely helpful because the erosions are quite superficial. Gastric mucosal changes were seen consistently in all patients in whom gastroscopy was performed within 24 hours of severe trauma by Lucas and associates,[114] and it

was possible to follow the progression of the erosions from petechiae to superficial ulceration. The lesions appeared first in the proximal stomach on the greater curvature and then spread distally to the antrofundic junction, but rarely beyond. Menguy et al.[124] have emphasized that the acute erosions are superficial rather than deep, multiple rather than singular, gastric rather than duodenal, fundic rather than antral, and usually bleed and do not perforate. It is often possible to demonstrate the point of bleeding by selective celiac arteriography (Fig. 26).

TREATMENT

Since bleeding from stress ulceration may vary from minor oozing of blood from a small area of injured mucosa to a brisk, life-threatening hemorrhage, therapeutic programs have varied from iced saline lavage to total gastrectomy.

Regardless of the initial mechanisms of mucosal damage, acid is required for mucosal destruction and bleeding, and *antacid therapy* is therefore a logical prophylaxis for all patients who are at risk of stress ulceration.[19, 109, 153] At the first sign of bleeding, antacid therapy may be combined or alternated with iced saline lavage. This regimen is often successful in halting further hemorrhage.[152] Since we initiated antacid treatment in patients at risk for the development of acute mucosal ulceration, operative intervention has rarely been required. If too much reliance is placed on antacids, however, it is likely that they may be used in excessive quantities, resulting in severe metabolic alkalosis, small bowel ileus, and diarrhea.[113] Spontaneous cessation of bleeding is common, but hemorrhage may recur. Of more than 300 patients at the Detroit General Hospital who required transfusion for bleeding from acute mucosal erosions, only 38 required operation.[114]

Selective arterial infusion of Pitressin into the exact area of bleeding by means of an angiographically placed catheter has been used in the treatment of acute mucosal bleeding. Even in the best of hands, however, this is associated with a failure rate of nearly 50 per cent.[8] (The injection of a vasoconstrictor into an area of mucosa which presumably is already ischemic is a source of concern to some surgeons.)

Decision to operate is difficult because the patients are often extremely ill. Unless they are moribund, however, they can usually withstand a well-timed and well-executed operation far better than they can withstand continued bleeding, recurrent shock, and progressive deterioration of cardiac, pulmonary, and renal function. It is often necessary to set an arbitrary limit to the amount of blood that will be replaced. When that limit is reached, the patient is operated upon.

At operation, the choice of procedure presents difficult problems. If the bleeding is found to be caused by a discrete ulcer in the duodenum or proximal stomach, the lesion should be sutured and a vagotomy and drainage procedure performed. If bleeding is coming from the distal stomach, a distal gastrectomy, preferably combined with vagotomy, is the best procedure. Since recurrent bleeding is common after vagotomy

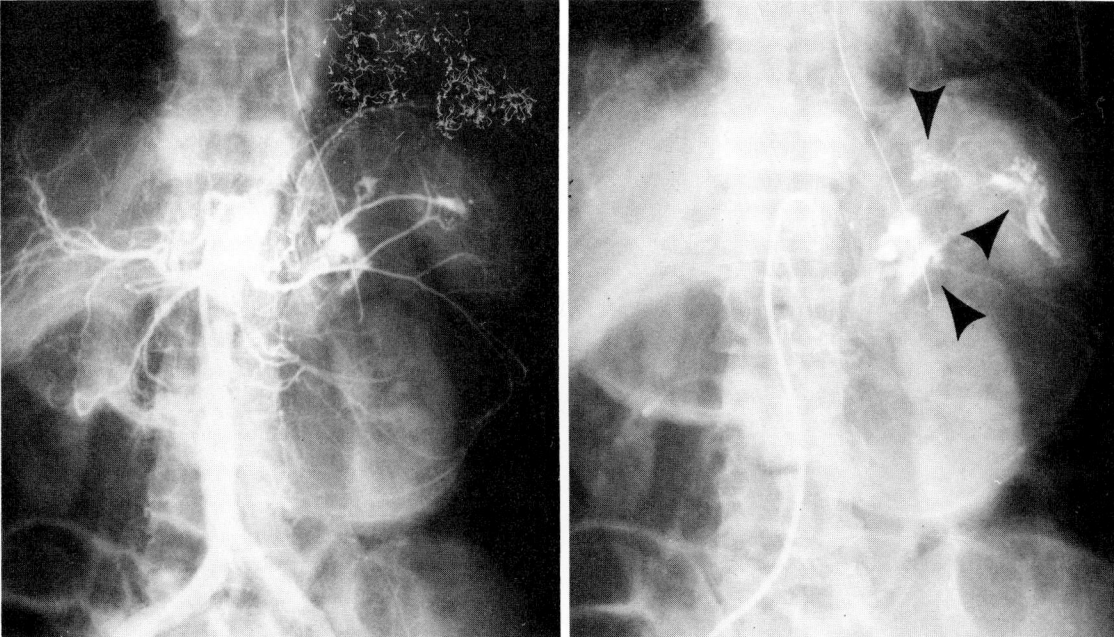

Figure 26. Arteriographic demonstration of acute superficial gastric mucosal lesions. Injection of the celiac axis (and aorta) show extravasation of dye into the lumen of the stomach at the site of acute gastric mucosal erosions. *Right,* After the injection, there is residual dye within the stomach at the point of the superficial gastric erosions.

and drainage, and since the mortality rate for repeated operations is very high, Menguy[123] has advocated total gastrectomy. Spontaneous remission is common, however, and bleeding frequently stops after vagotomy, so that it seems unlikely that total gastrectomy will be widely applied as a primary procedure except in those patients with diffuse hemorrhagic involvement of massive areas of the gastric mucosa. It does seem logical to advocate total gastrectomy after the initial recurrence of bleeding if the bleeding sites cannot be completely excised by a lesser procedure.

Operative mortality rates range from 35 to 80 per cent and largely reflect the severity of the associated diseases. Survival rate will depend largely upon control of the process that initiated the stress; most often this requires correction of sepsis. The generally poor results following operation give impetus to widespread application of prophylactic antacid therapy in severely ill patients in whom stress ulcer is likely to develop.

SURGICAL PROCEDURES ON THE STOMACH

HISTORICAL ASPECTS

The initial development of surgical procedures for peptic ulcer was empirical. The subsequent evolution has been guided by demonstration of physiologic mechanisms controlling gastric secretion.[165]

The first operation for peptic ulcer that gained wide-spread acceptance and one of the most simple operations ever devised for the lesion is gastroenterostomy, an anastomosis between the stomach and the jejunum. The procedure was first described in 1881 by Wölfler, a colleague of Billroth, who used it to bypass a carcinomatous obstruction of the pylorus. Because of the simplicity of the procedure and its relative safety, it was quickly adopted by surgeons in Europe and America. By the turn of the century, however, increasing incidence of marginal ulceration (recurrent peptic ulcer at the margin of the anastomosis) were observed. In 1925, a long-term postoperative study of patients with gastroenterostomy reported a 34 per cent incidence of gastrojejunal ulcer.[110] The operation was gradually abandoned, although it was still in use until the mid-1950s.

The first successful gastric resection was performed by Theodor Billroth in Vienna in 1881 when he excised an obstructing carcinoma of the pylorus and performed a gastroduodenostomy. In 1882, von Rydigier performed the first gastric resection for ulcer disease. The first partial gastrectomies were hardly more than pylorectomies, but as operative techniques improved, surgeons became more radical and by 1940 the term subtotal gastric resection was interpreted as denoting removal of the distal 66 to 75 per cent of the stomach. After resection, the continuity of the gut can be restored by anastomosis of the remaining portion of the fundus to the duodenum (gastroduodenostomy or Billroth I anastomosis) or alternatively by closure of the duodenal stump and by anastomosis of the fundic remnant to the first part of the jejunum (gastrojejunos-

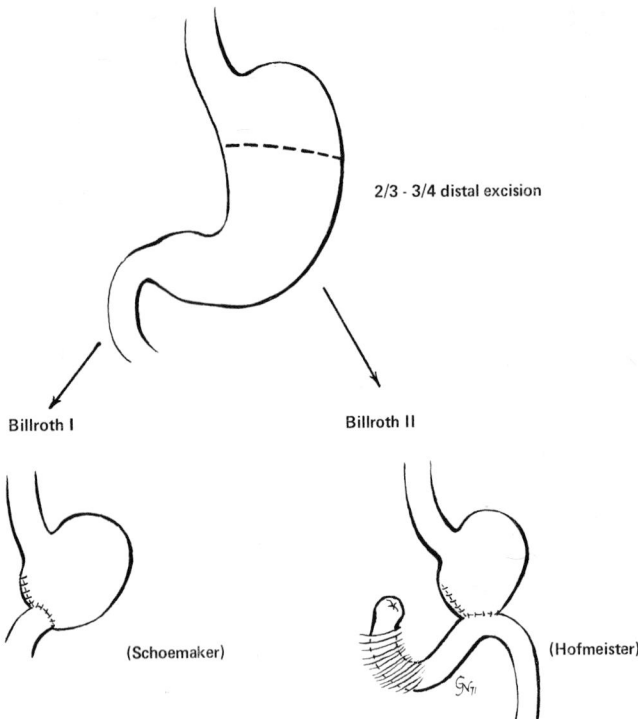

2/3 - 3/4 distal excision

Billroth I

Billroth II

(Schoemaker)

(Hofmeister)

Figure 27. Types of reconstruction after subtotal gastric resection. Resection removes 66 to 75 per cent of the distal stomach, thereby excising the entire antral-gastrin mechanism as well as a large portion of the parietal cell mass. Reconstruction of continuity of the gastrointestinal tract may be performed either with a gastroduodenostomy (Billroth I) anastomosis or with a gastrojejunostomy (Billroth II) anastomosis. The Schoemaker modification of the Billroth I anastomosis includes partial closure of the lesser curvature of the stomach, as does the Hofmeister modification of the Billroth II anastomosis.

tomy or Billroth II anastomosis) (Fig. 27). Subtotal gastrectomy, especially with the Billroth II anastomosis, became very popular in this country by the 1930s, was for two decades the standard treatment for peptic ulcer disease, and is still in wide use. The objections to the procedure are the relatively high mortality rate, especially in patients with severe scarring of the duodenum, and the high incidence of postoperative complications.

Dragstedt reasoned that duodenal ulcer disease was associated usually with an increased secretion of acid and that the success of surgical procedures in the stomach probably was related to reduction of the acid-secreting potential. Since the vagus was known to stimulate acid secretion, he concluded that vagus section would be beneficial in the treatment of ulcer. His first reports[40, 41] of operations in man substantiated this idea.

Gastric emptying is brought about in large part by contraction of the antral musculature; truncal vagotomy denervates the antral pump, resulting in delayed gastric emptying. Dragstedt later added a drainage procedure (posterior gastroenterostomy) as an adjunct. Weinberg[178] substituted a modification of the Heineke-Mikulicz pyloroplasty (a procedure in which an incision is made longitudinally through the distal stomach, pylorus, and proximal duodenum and is then closed vertically) as the drainage procedure. There was great initial resistance to the adoption of vagotomy and drainage, but the simplicity of the procedure and low mortality rate won many converts. Subsequently, the relatively high incidence of recurrence and of postoperative diarrhea has shown clearly that the ideal procedure is not yet available.

OPERATIONS CURRENTLY IN USE

All procedures now used for inflammatory ulcerating lesions of the stomach or duodenum bring about a reduction in the acid-secreting potential of the stomach. The rationale for this is straightforward in duodenal ulcer patients whose disease is clearly related to acid hypersecretion. Although peptic ulcers of the stomach and stress ulcers are not associated with acid hypersecretion, acid does play at least a permissive role in the pathogenesis of these lesions, and if the stomach is achlorhydric, the ulcers will not develop. Although abolition of acid production will probably prevent the development of stress ulcers, once they are present abolition of acid production does not, unfortunately, guarantee cessation of bleeding.

Total gastrectomy with esophagojejunostomy (Fig. 28) is used for treatment of the Zollinger-Ellison syndrome or occasionally for hemorrhagic gastritis or for gastric carcinoma. The procedure has a high mortality rate (10 to 20 per cent) and a high rate of complications. For reasons that are not well understood but that may be related to the trophic role of gastrin, the mortality rate and incidence of complications seem to be greatly diminished in patients with the Zollinger-Ellison syndrome.

The three operations in general use for peptic ulcer are gastric resection without vagotomy, truncal vagotomy and drainage (either gastroenterostomy or pyloroplasty), and truncal vagotomy plus antrectomy. A new operation, consisting of highly selective denervation of the acid-secreting portion of the fundus with preservation of innervation to the antrum and to the rest of the abdominal viscera, is still considered exper-

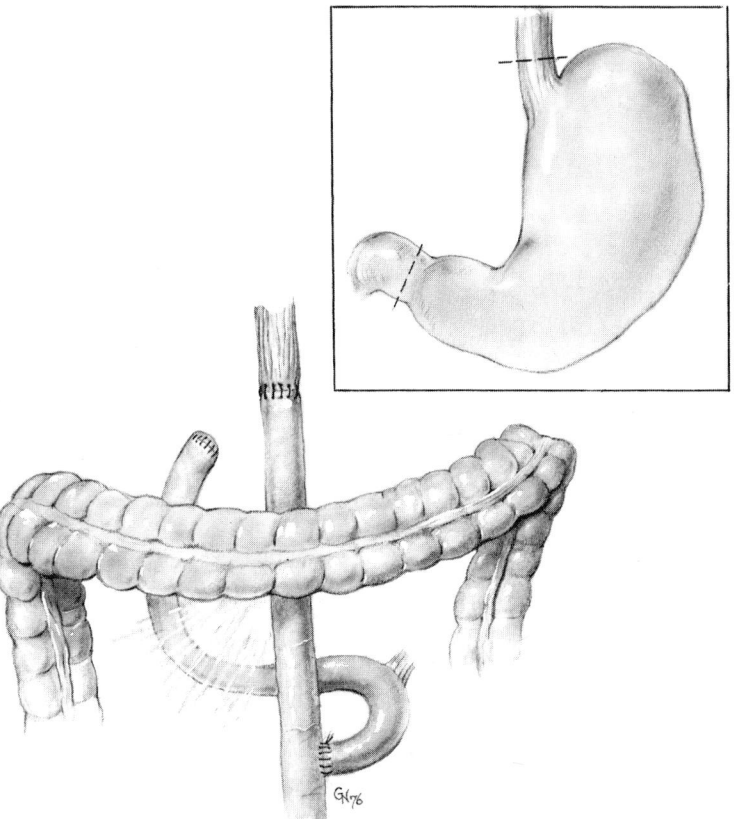

Figure 28. Technique for total gastrectomy. The lesser curvature of the stomach is mobilized by dividing the gastrohepatic omentum and the branches of the left and right gastric vessels. The greater curvature is mobilized by dividing the gastrocolic ligament and the right and left gastroepiploic vessels. A splenectomy is performed. The esophagus is divided proximal to the cardia, and frozen section is obtained to be sure that no gastric mucosa remains with the esophagus. The duodenum is divided just distal to the pylorus and is closed. Gastrointestinal continuity is restored with an end-to-end esophagojejunostomy Roux-en-Y.

imental in this country. The four procedures will be discussed individually.

Subtotal Gastric Resection

Resection of the distal 66 to 75 per cent of the stomach acts to reduce acid production by abolishing the gastrin mechanism and by excision of part of the parietal cell mass. Depending upon the extent of parietal cell resection, subtotal gastrectomy will diminish the postoperative maximal gastric secretory response to histamine by 60 to 80 per cent. It is important that the line of resection be distal to the junction of antral and duodenal mucosa. Planned or inadvertent exclusion of antral mucosa with the duodenal stump in a Billroth II anastomosis leads to sequestration of antral mucosa in a permanently alkaline environment. Since acid suppression of gastrin release is abolished, a syndrome of hypergastrinemia mimicking the Zollinger-Ellison syndrome results. These patients have a high incidence of recurrent marginal ulceration.[150, 172] Excision of the retained antral tissue results in cure.

There have been numerous studies in patients with subtotal gastrectomy on the relative superiority of gastroduodenostomy versus gastrojejunostomy. The picture is somewhat confused because gastroduodenostomy seems to be a clearly superior procedure in dogs. In man, however, the incidence of recurrence of peptic ulcer following subtotal gastrectomy without vagotomy is twice as high with a Billroth I anastomosis as it is with a Billroth II.[175]

Reported mortality rates with subtotal gastrectomy for duodenal ulcer vary between 0.4 and 8.9 per cent;[165] mortality rates of 3 to 4 per cent are usually quoted.

Truncal Vagotomy and Drainage Procedure

Vagotomy causes a great reduction in gastric secretion, but it also greatly suppresses gastric motility. More than half of the patients who have truncal vagotomy alone will later require some procedure to enhance emptying of the stomach. There is great likelihood that poor emptying results in antral stasis and distention, which in turn results in the release of gastrin.

The relatively high incidence of incomplete vagotomy has led to great emphasis on technique. It was initially assumed that with careful attention to detail a complete vagotomy would invariably be possible. Variations in the anatomy of the vagi at the esophageal hiatus and adjacent to the abdominal esophagus and on the stomach make complete interruption of all vagal fibers very difficult indeed in some patients. A common arrangement of the anatomy of the vagi below the diaphragm is shown in Figure 29. Just above the diaphragm, the vagal fibers around the esophagus usually coalesce to form a discrete right and left trunk as they come through the diaphragm; accessory trunks are not uncommon. The right vagus nerve lies posteriorly and slightly to the right along the circumference of the esophagus. A few centimeters superior to the esophagogastric junction, the right

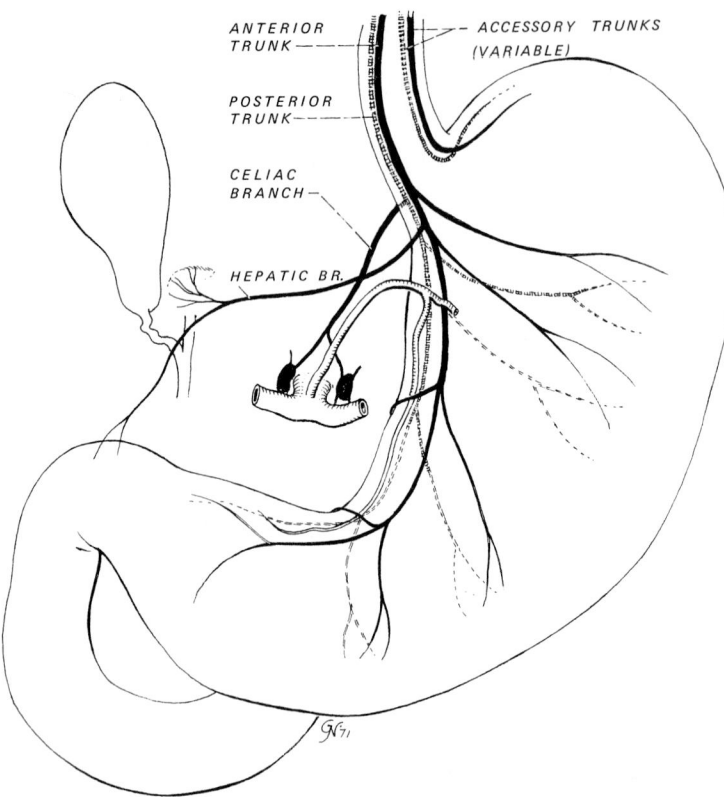

Figure 29. Anatomy of the vagus nerves in relation to the stomach. Both anterior (left) and posterior (right) vagi give off gastric branches. The anterior vagus has a hepatic branch that may send fibers to the region of the pylorus; the posterior vagus has a celiac branch that goes to the celiac ganglia and plexus and from there goes to contribute to the innervation of other abdominal viscera.

vagus divides into celiac and gastric branches. The celiac branch usually follows the left gastric artery and joins the celiac plexus, from which it sends branches to the rest of the abdominal viscera; the gastric branch supplies the posterior wall of the stomach. The left vagus lies anteriorly and again often to the right of the center of the esophageal circumference. It also divides just above the cardia into a hepatic and a gastric branch. The hepatic division runs within the gastrohepatic omentum to the porta hepatis where it joins the hepatic plexus. There is usually a branch that goes from the hepatic division to the distal stomach and proximal duodenum. The gastric division of the left or anterior vagus supplies the anterior wall of the stomach. The right vagus is often located more dorsally and may be found applied to the adventitia covering the anterior surface of the aorta. This is the trunk most often missed when vagotomy is incomplete, and at revagotomy, the surgeon should initially search in the adventitia behind the esophagus for persistent vagal trunks. Rarely, only one large nerve trunk will be present; as many as nine separate discrete trunks have been excised. Demonstration of two (or three or four) nerve trunks by frozen section at operation, therefore, does not guarantee completeness of vagotomy. A transthoracic approach to vagotomy is often used after failure of an earlier abdominal vagotomy. Unfortunately, the results offer little more promise than with the conventional abdominal approach.[30]

When gastroenterostomy was first added to vagot-

omy, the anastomosis was usually placed at the most dependent part of the greater curvature of the stomach. Later, in efforts to avoid antral stasis, the anastomosis was performed in the distal antrum, immediately proximal to the pylorus; this placement of the anastomosis is in current use. Pyloroplasty was introduced by Heineke (1886) and Mikulicz (1888) for treatment of peptic ulcer. Weinberg[178] slightly modified the technique to provide a larger outlet and advocated its use as superior to gastroenterostomy on the grounds that it preserved the normal physiologic pathway of food and that it minimized alkaline regurgitation and possible excitation of the gastrin mechanism. There are multiple techniques for pyloroplasty; of these, the Heinke-Mikulicz and the Finney (Fig. 30) are most commonly in use today. Failure of vagotomy and drainage procedures has frequently been ascribed to inadequate caliber of the recreated gastric outlet. It is imperative that the pyloroplasty or the gastroenterostomy be sufficiently large to allow good drainage from a hypotonic stomach. The gastroenterostomy should be placed just proximal to the pylorus to prevent antral distention.

Selective Proximal Vagotomy. Since only the stomach need be denervated for the treatment of peptic ulcer disease and since vagal denervation of the rest of the abdominal viscera has been blamed for diarrhea and for an increased incidence of gallstones, techniques were developed for selective vagal denervation of the stomach with preservation of the hepatic branch of the anterior vagus and the celiac branch of the pos-

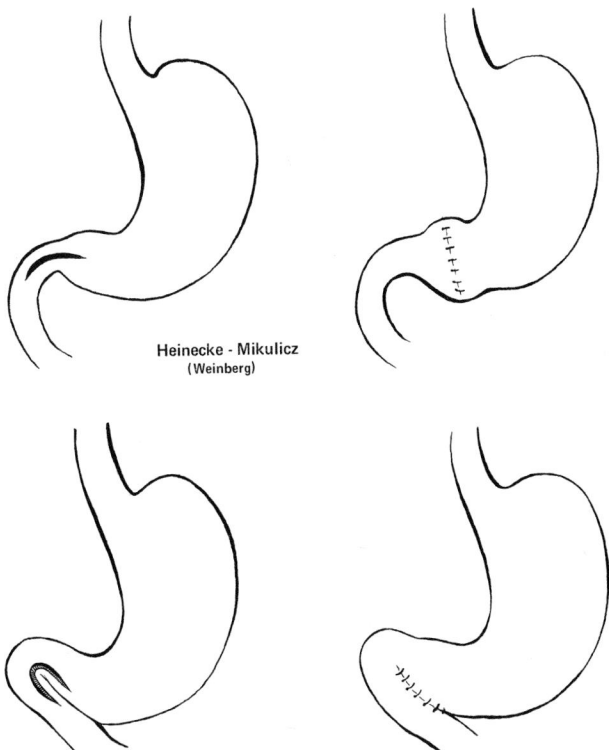

Figure 30. Two types of pyloroplasties in common use. In the Heinecke-Mikulicz pyloroplasty, a longitudinal incision is made through the distal stomach, pylorus, and proximal duodenum. This incision is then closed in the vertical fashion, which destroys the sphincteric mechanism. The Weinberg modification is a one-layer closure. In the Finney pyloroplasty, a two-layer anastomosis is made between the stomach and duodenum utilizing a U-shaped incision through the distal stomach, pylorus, and proximal duodenum. It is important that both procedures be performed in such a manner as to insure a large lumen for gastric drainage.

terior. Evaluation of results of this operation (selective gastric vagotomy) have shown no superiority over the conventional operation of truncal vagotomy plus an emptying procedure,[162] and the newer operation has not achieved popularity. A further extension of the concept of selective vagotomy suggested that denervation should be limited to only the proximal stomach (roughly to the mass of parietal cells) with preservation of the innervation of the antrum (Fig. 31). In this method (variously called selective proximal vagotomy, proximal gastric vagotomy, parietal cell vagotomy, supra- or highly selective vagotomy, *inter alia*), the anterior and posterior leaves of the gastrohepatic omentum are divided at their attachment to the stomach, starting at the incisura angularis distally and proceeding proximally to the esophagogastric junction. All of the gastric branches of the vagi should be meticulously severed; the distal antral branches of the nerves of Latarjet should be preserved. Completeness of denervation of the proximal stomach is possible only with meticulous dissection of the distal esophagus to divide all communications between the vagal trunks

and the proximal stomach.[56, 76] Fear of gastric retention with this procedure led Holle[88] to add an emptying procedure routinely, but analysis of postoperative results suggests that recurrences are a consequence of incomplete denervation of the proximal stomach and not of delayed gastric emptying.

The great appeal of selective proximal vagotomy is that it offers the potential of acid reduction without opening the gastrointestinal tract and without denervating the remainder of the abdominal viscera. Currently, there is great enthusiasm about the procedure; its role in future operative control of duodenal ulcer will depend upon evaluation of long-term results.

Evaluation of Completeness of Vagotomy. Hollander[83] observed that hypoglycemia stimulated vagal activity, which resulted in acid secretion by gastric parietal cells, and suggested that insulin hypoglycemia could be used to test for the presence of intact vagal fibers after vagotomy for peptic ulcer. His criterion for a positive test for persistent vagal innervation[84] was an increase in acidity of at least 20 mEq. per liter over the mean resting value within two hours after the in-

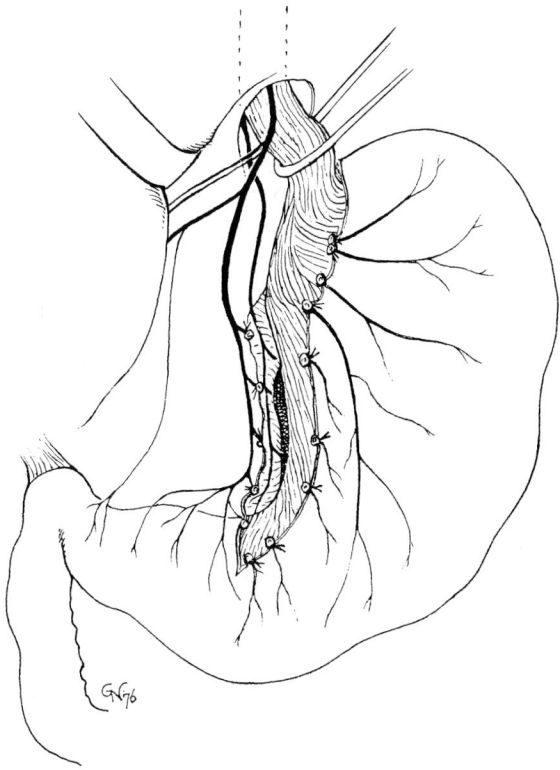

Figure 31. Technique for selective proximal vagotomy. Fundic branches of the gastric divisions of the anterior and posterior vagi are severed and ligated at the attachment of the gastrohepatic ligament to the lesser curvature of the stomach as well as around the circumference of the fundoesophageal junction. The antral branches of the descending nerves of Latarjet are preserved. As stressed by Goligher[56] and by Hallenbeck and colleagues,[76] it is important that the lower esophagus be completely skeletonized so as to divide any vagal fibers which might reach the fundus by way of the distal esophagus. The hepatic branches of the anterior vagus and the celiac branch of the posterior vagus are preserved.

travenous injection of 15 units of regular insulin. If the resting gastric juice was anacidic, an increase of 10 mEq. per liter should be regarded as positive. Provided that an adequate level of hypoglycemia (blood sugar less than 45 mg. per 100 ml.) is achieved, any lesser acid response should be regarded as negative and indicative of complete vagal section. By these criteria, about one of three patients has evidence of persistent vagal innervation of the stomach on insulin testing after vagotomy. Use of the test should be limited to patients under 55 years of age who do not have evidence of cardiovascular disease. The arbitrary criteria for interpretation of the test have proved disappointing and many alternatives have been proposed,[9, 157] including the use of multiple criteria,[10, 53] although none has emerged that is superior to those of Hollander.

Much dissatisfaction has been expressed about the Hollander test. Induction of insulin hypoglycemia in older patients with cardiovascular disease may be dangerous, and several deaths associated with insulin testing have been reported. We have used the Hollander test in the past but are no longer using it routinely. The reasons for this change in attitude have been summarized;[69, 166] gastric secretory tests are of little value in diagnosing recurrent ulcer, insulin tests are no better than other secretory tests in separating patients with recurrence from those without recurrence, and the notion that insulin-stimulated acid secretion is mediated only by the vagus is unproved. Since antrectomy alone may result in a negative Hollander test, the entire anatomic significance of insulin testing must be reassessed. Although insulin tests probably detect most incomplete vagotomies, as few as 60 per cent of patients with recurrent ulcer will have a positive response; 10 per cent of patients with positive Hollander tests and 2 per cent with negative Hollander tests develop recurrence. Because the insulin test is difficult to interpret and is dangerous, and because it provides no better discrimination than does any other secretory test, we have replaced it with determination of maximal acid output using Histalog or pentagastrin. It should also be noted that neither serum gastrin levels nor acid secretory values appear to have any predictive value for ulcer recurrence in any individual patient.[166]

Truncal Vagotomy and Antrectomy

After the introduction of vagotomy and the demonstration that it diminished the capacity of the stomach for acid production, it was inevitable that it should be combined with gastric resection. Initially it was merely added to the standard two thirds to three fourths distal gastric resection but as the physiologic mechanisms became better understood, efforts were made to limit resection, when combined with vagotomy to the antrum itself (usually resulting, in practical application, in a 40 per cent distal gastrectomy). Excision of the antrum and destruction of the vagi remove the major stimulants to acid secretion and leave the entire mass of parietal cells subject to stimulation, as far as we know, by only the intestinal phase secretagogue.

The external landmark for the antrofundic junction on the lesser curvature of the stomach is the incisura angularis. A line drawn inferiorly and 45 degrees to the left down to the greater curvature (Fig. 1, *A–A'*) will roughly approximate the junction of antrum and fundus. It is possible to delineate the junction more precisely by demonstrating the differences in surface pH of the two mucosal zones. At operation, 50 mg. of Histalog may be administered subcutaneously to the patient, and after the stomach is opened and the mucosa sponged dry, strips of pH-sensitive paper placed transversely across the presumed antrofundic junction will clearly delineate the site of pH change. Experimental studies have shown that neutral pH of the mucosa is well correlated with high gastrin content of the mucosa.[94] The stomach should be divided 2 cm. proximal to the line of pH change. There is no great hazard in leaving a small amount of antral tissue adjacent to acid-producing fundic mucosa.

The addition of vagotomy alters the relative superiority of the Billroth II anastomosis following resection without vagotomy. Experience in patients with vagotomy and antrectomy has indicated that if there is any superiority, the technique of gastroduodenostomy is preferable to that of gastrojejunostomy.

Since the aim of all operative procedures for duodenal ulcer is to diminish acid production by the stomach and since vagotomy acts to diminish acid production by abolishing (1) direct stimulation of the parietal cell by acetylcholine, (2) vagal release of gastrin, and (3) synergism of acetylcholine with gastrin at the parietal cell, vagotomy has a place in all operations for duodenal ulcer. Simply stated, in our current state of knowledge, if there is no contraindication because of the frailty of the patient, all operations for duodenal ulcer disease should include vagotomy (Fig. 32).

POSTOPERATIVE COMPLICATIONS

Early Complications

Hemorrhage in the immediate postoperative period may be due to failure to control bleeding from an ulcer or may be due to bleeding at the suture line. The use of gastrostomy tubes for postoperative gastric decompression is attended with a small but definite incidence of complications, including bleeding, leaking of gastric juice into the peritoneal cavity, and rarely, persistent gastrocutaneous fistulas. Gastrostomy tubes for postoperative gastric decompression have been in wide use for more than a decade. The number of complications probably does not justify the purported benefit of gastrostomy tubes in diminishing the incidence of postoperative respiratory complications and aspiration, and many surgeons have abandoned their use. We use gastrostomy tubes only in patients in whom anatomic obstruction prohibits placement of a nasogastric tube and in infants and small children.

The scarified duodenum is the bête noire of gastric resection for duodenal ulcer. The most serious common complication following resection is leakage from the duodenal stump (Billroth II) or leakage at the gastroduodenostomy (Billroth I). Both result in peritoneal

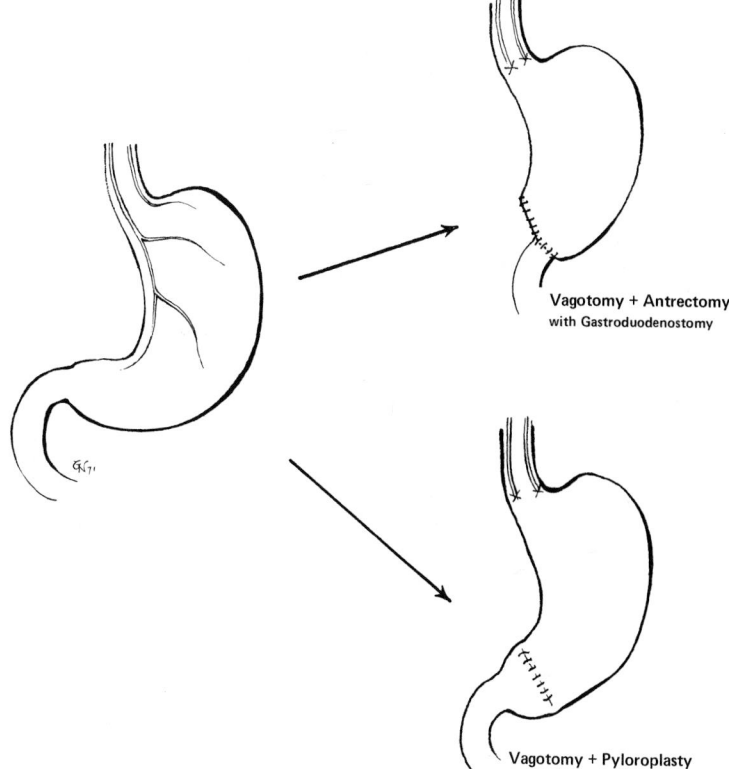

Figure 32. Acceptable operations for duodenal ulcer disease. Since the aim of any surgical procedure for duodenal ulcer is the diminution of acid output, vagotomy should be a part of any such operation if there is no specific contraindication. The choice, therefore, lies between vagotomy plus antrectomy and vagotomy plus drainage. Current information would indicate that gastroenterostomy (with gastric stomach immediately proximal to pylorus) is equally as good a drainage procedure as is pyloroplasty.

Vagotomy + Antrectomy
with Gastroduodenostomy

Vagotomy + Pyloroplasty

soilage with gastroduodenal contents and are associated with peritonitis, ileus, sepsis, and a significant (10 to 15 per cent) mortality rate. Resection is associated with a higher incidence of breakdown of the suture line than are drainage procedures, because dissection is carried out in areas of ulcer scarring and the blood supply to the remaining structures is often compromised. Leakage of the suture line is most commonly caused by ischemia. Another factor that may contribute to leakage of a duodenal stump is obstruction of the afferent limb of the gastrojejunostomy. This obstruction, caused by a kink in the bowel, results in distention of the obstructed loop with bile and pancreatic juice; the increased pressure may cause perforation of the suture line.

A rare complication seen in patients with selective proximal vagotomy procedures is necrosis of the lesser curvature of the stomach caused by devascularization achieved incidentally in the process of denervating the lesser curvature. The collateral circulation of the stomach is usually excellent, and necrosis of the lesser curvature probably occurs only in very rare cases of anomalous blood supply or in those patients in whom splenectomy has interfered with the collateral supply. When there is any suspicion of this complication, a prompt diagnosis can be made by means of fiberoptic gastroscopy. Reoperation and excision of the devascularized stomach is indicated immediately.

Late Complications

Dumping Syndrome. The stomach functions as an osmoregulator by diluting foods and mixing them with gastric juice and by allowing only small amounts of chyme to pass into the duodenum at any one time. Any operative procedure that destroys or bypasses the pylorus may result in the sudden emptying of hyperosmolar material into the jejunum, and this may bring about a large inflow of extracellular fluid into the jejunum. This rapid fluid shift may result clinically in abdominal colic, nausea, vomiting, diarrhea, faintness, sweating, and pallor. There is a transient but often pronounced fall in the serum concentration of potassium, which may be associated with alterations in the T and S-T segments of the electrocardiogram. There is an early increase in blood sugar which is often followed by severe hypoglycemia with its characteristic entourage of symptoms.

The early symptoms of abdominal pain and hypermotility of the gut usually occur within 15 to 20 minutes of eating and seem to be most common after a carbohydrate meal; ice cream is a good provocative test. Many patients find they can obtain relief by lying down. Late symptoms associated with hypoglycemia may occur two hours after a meal.

The etiology of the dumping syndrome is not well understood. Serotonin is apparently released, but concentrations of serotonin do not correlate with the severity of symptoms. Moreover, the anatomic requirements for dumping are met in all patients who have had a gastric resection, and at one time or another almost all postgastrectomy patients will have minor dumping symptoms. Why is it that only about 5 per cent of patients have symptoms severe enough to seek attention and only about one in five of these is disabled? Many physicians have observed a correlation of the severity of the dumping syndrome with symptoms of emotional instability. Kellner and Mellinkoff have proposed that patients who are chronically unhappy and who complain often about minor problems may lack the motivation necessary to shrug off or adapt to minor symptoms of the dumping syndrome.[101] In such patients, it would be wise to avoid operation (and certainly to avoid extensive resection), if this personality could be recognized prior to operation.

The dumping syndrome is often relieved by eating small dry meals and restricting all intake of fluid during meals. There is no standard operative treatment for the dumping syndrome; good results have been reported following conversion of Billroth I to Billroth II anastomoses (and vice versa) and with the use of a small segment of reversed jejunum to impede gastric emptying. It is usually wise to delay in reoperating on patients with the dumping syndrome and to treat them with alterations of diet and mild sedation and small doses of anticholinergic drugs in order to avoid operation. Reassurance and supportive therapy will often enable patients to cope with their symptoms.

Although the dumping syndrome may occur in any patient in whom the pylorus has been destroyed or bypassed, it is in fact quite rare in patients who have not had a gastric resection and seems to be more common in patients who have had a radical subtotal gastrectomy than in patients who have had an excision of the antrum only.

Nutritional Disturbances. Megaloblastic anemia, iron-deficiency anemia, calcium deficiency, and steatorrhea are seen occasionally after gastric resection. Megaloblastic anemia is due to a deficiency of the intrinsic factor, which may result from excision of parietal cells or atrophy of parietal cells as a consequence of postoperative gastritis or of loss of stimuli. Anemia may also be caused by vitamin B_{12} deficiency brought about by stasis in the blind loop of the duodenum and proliferation of bacteria. The deficiencies of iron and of calcium after gastric resection are not well understood but occur in 30 to 50 per cent of patients who are studied carefully. Iron deficiency may be caused by hypochlorhydria and bypass of the duodenum in patients with Billroth II anastomosis. Another factor contributing to anemia may be minute blood loss from areas of inflammation around the gastroenterostomy site.

Steatorrhea, which is the loss in the stool of more than 7 per cent of the total amount of fat ingested, is occasionally seen after Billroth II gastrectomy and probably results from bypass of the duodenum, which may interfere with mixing of bile salts-and pancreatic lipase with ingested fat. Steatorrhea may be intensified by the development of the blind loop syndrome.

The various nutritional problems are manifested in loss of weight by some patients following resection. Except in instances of radical subtotal gastrectomy or total gastrectomy or in occasional patients with disabling dumping syndrome, loss of weight is rarely an important consideration and in fact, many patients may gain weight postoperatively.[100] Postoperative problems with nutrition appear to be more severe in Great Britain; a survey of 204 patients 15 to 20 years after vagotomy and gastroenterostomy reported that more than half of the patients were anemic and one third had undergone significant loss of weight, which was correlated with diminished food intake and with gastrointestinal symptoms.[182]

Diarrhea. The foregoing complications are all more common after resection than after vagotomy and drainage procedures. Vagotomy itself seems to be associated with two complications. One, an alleged increased incidence of gallstones, is difficult to prove statistically and is therefore of questionable importance.

The increased incidence of diarrhea after vagotomy is important. The number of patients with severe diarrhea is small, but symptoms may be disabling for them. Although about 70 per cent of patients report an increase in the frequency of daily bowel movements after vagotomy,[30] this often serves to relieve preoperative constipation, and may be an unexpected bonus of the operation. The incidence of significant postoperative diarrhea varies from about 5 to 20 per cent in various series;[30, 46, 100, 133] it fortunately seems to diminish significantly with time.[100]

Diarrhea may occur two or three times every week or may be episodic, coming once or twice a month and lasting one to three days at a time. It may be mild or of explosive severity, resulting in soiling of clothing.

Most careful studies on postvagotomy diarrhea come from England.[11] The incidence of diarrhea does not seem to be as high in Sweden[21] or in this country,[46, 133, 183] and some American surgeons believe that postvagotomy diarrhea, for unexplained reasons, is not as important a problem in the United States as in Great Britain. Some British colleagues have replied that the incidence will be similar if patients are questioned carefully. A recent study[100] reporting 19 per cent incidence of significant diarrhea one year after vagotomy and drainage gives some support to this concept. Nonetheless, it seems likely that the seeming preoccupation of British surgeons and physicians with the bowel habits of their patients arose because their patients complained of trouble (and not vice versa). Why the incidence of diarrhea should be different, if it is different, in this country remains unexplained. It *is* apparent that patients who have undergone operation for peptic ulcer have been followed more carefully and their postoperative problems chronicled with far greater zeal in Great Britain than in America. Most information of value comes from British studies.[184]

The etiology of the diarrhea after vagotomy is not understood. It might be predicted that excision of the parasympathetic innervation to the small bowel would mimic the effect of atropine and cause the bowels to be sluggish, but such is not the case. Suggested etiologies such as the loss of the protective action of the hyperacidic stomach with resultant increase in gastroenteritis or an alteration of the growth rate and composition of the small bowel mucosa are of interest but do not explain the phenomenon.

The treatment of diarrhea should be symptomatic. The patient should be assured that it will usually improve with time. Only in extremely rare instances is an attempt at operative treatment (by interposition of a small segment of reversed jejunum) justified.

Alkaline Reflux Gastritis.[42] Occasional postoperative patients will be troubled with severe continuous burning epigastric pain, usually aggravated by meals. The pain is usually not relieved by vomiting, and in fact, bilious vomiting may be absent. The condition is diagnosed by gastroscopy, which reveals bile reflux in the stomach and a beefy red, generally inflamed gastric mucosa, often with multiple superficial gastric erosions. Significant blood loss is rare. Although retention and vomiting may occur, there is no organic obstruction of the gastric outlet.

Medical treatment with cholestyramine to bind bile salts has been advocated. Surgical treatment consists of reoperation to divert bile away from the stomach; if the primary anastomosis had been a gastroduodenostomy, a Henley loop is preferred, whereas after a Billroth II anastomosis, a Roux-en-Y reconstruction is preferable.

Although there is great current enthusiasm about this condition and although the diagnosis has achieved considerable popularity in a very short period, restraint should be exercised in planning reoperation. These unfortunate patients have been around for a long time before this label was available to tag them with. Many were miserable for years, but the vast majority of them survived and improved without operation. Caution is necessary until the benefit of reoperation can be clearly demonstrated.

Marginal Ulcer. From 1 to 5 per cent of patients operated upon for peptic ulcer may be expected to develop recurrent peptic ulceration.[154] Recurrent ulcers after gastric resection and Billroth II anastomosis occur classically on the jejunal side of the margin of the anastomosis. The ulcer may give rise to periodic bouts of midabdominal pain or it may make its first appearance with massive hemorrhage or it may erode into the free peritoneal cavity, or into the colon, creating a gastrojejunocolic fistula. Any patient in whom

ulcer-type pain or occult bleeding from the rectum develops after a subtotal gastric resection should be suspected of having a marginal ulcer. Diagnosis may be confirmed by x-ray (Fig. 33) or by gastroscopy (Fig. 16H). The diagnostic superiority of endoscopy in patients with marginal ulcer is clearly established. Recent studies suggest that measurement of serum group I pepsinogens may be of value in the diagnosis of recurrent ulcer.[147]

In a study of 41 patients in whom stomal ulceration developed over a 15-year period, duodenal ulcer was found to be the original lesion in all but one patient.[17] The average duration of freedom from symptoms after operation was 10 months for gastrectomy and 3 years for gastroenterostomy alone. Pain was the most common symptom (36 of 41 patients had pain as their chief complaint), followed by bleeding (17 of 41 patients). The x-ray diagnosis was positive in 30 of 41 patients. The possibility of the Zollinger-Ellison syndrome should be considered in any patient with a marginal ulcer. Any patient suspected of having a recurrent ulcer should have a serum gastrin determination.

Marginal ulcers are notoriously difficult to treat medically. The patient may have a long period of quiescence on a regimen of antacid therapy, only to be suddenly afflicted with a massive hemorrhage. In the absence of a life-threatening bleeding episode, a trial of antacid therapy may be justified. With the first sign of recurrence of pain or bleeding, however, the patient should be operated upon.

If the initial operation did not include vagotomy, the appropriate elective operation for marginal ulcer is vagotomy. If a patient has had a vagotomy and drainage procedure, the second operation should be revagotomy and antrectomy. If the patient has had a vagotomy

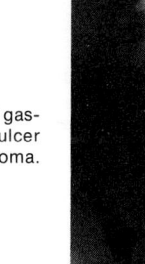

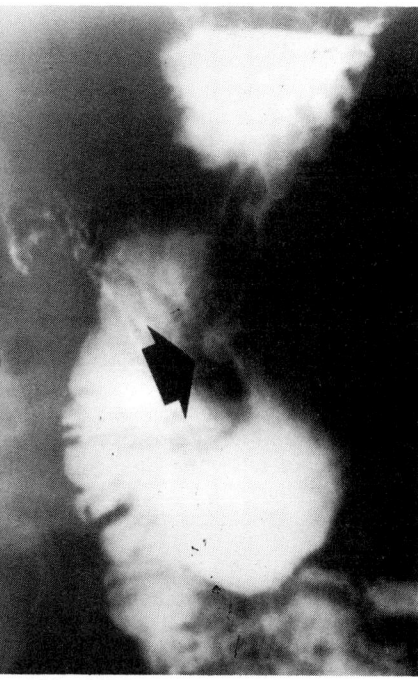

Figure 33. Barium contrast x-ray study of gastrojejunal anastomosis showing marginal ulcer (arrows) on jejunal side of the anastomotic stoma.

and antrectomy, the second operation should be re-vagotomy and reresection and reanastomosis (revagotomy alone may suffice). Transthoracic vagotomy does not have a high success rate after initial failure of vagotomy.[30] Reoperation is successful in between 70[154] and 94 per cent[156] of cases. Any patients with a recurrent marginal ulcer should, of course, be considered most carefully for the Zollinger-Ellison syndrome.

EVALUATION OF OPERATIONS

Although operations for peptic ulcer disease have been performed regularly for more than 70 years, valid data on the comparative effects of different operations have become available only in the last decade. Choice of operative procedures has been dictated by the surgeon's training or experience or prejudice. The priority of aims in operative procedures for peptic ulcer should be first to preserve the life of the patient, second to avoid bad side effects, and third to prevent recurrent ulcer. The best result is an asymptomatic patient. It has been assumed generally that the risk of mortality is less in vagotomy and drainage operations than for resection and that the recurrence rate is lowest with vagotomy and antrectomy, probably intermediate with subtotal gastrectomy alone, and highest with vagotomy plus drainage procedure. Study of disparate series clearly reveals that different criteria are used for the selection of patients, that poor-risk patients are often excluded, and that variability exists in the testing of postoperative gastric secretory potential as well as in the vigor with which the study of complications or unfavorable side effects is pursued.

Carefully planned prospective studies with random assignment of surgical procedures to consecutive ulcer patients are necessary in order to obtain valid data for comparison. Three such studies have been reported recently.[59, 100, 133] The postoperative results of these and many other studies are summarized in Table 5 (clinical ratings on this table are given on the Visick rating scale; I and II correspond to excellent and good results). Goligher and colleagues[59] in Leeds and York in England followed 342 male duodenal ulcer patients for five to eight years following either a standard subtotal gastrectomy, vagotomy and antrectomy, or vagotomy and gastroenterostomy. There were no deaths, but high-risk patients were excluded initially. The recurrence rate (proved plus suspected) was 10 per cent for vagotomy and gastroenterostomy, 6 per cent for vagotomy and antrectomy, and 5 per cent for subtotal gastrectomy. Most postgastrectomy syndromes occurred with equal frequency with all three procedures. Early dumping syndrome was slightly more common following subtotal gastrectomy, and diarrhea was more common following vagotomy, but only rarely was either complication a source of disability. In a companion study,[58] the results of 175 duodenal ulcer patients treated with vagotomy and pyloroplasty and followed for only two years were compared with those in the previous series. The rate of ulcer recurrence in patients with vagotomy and pyloroplasty was 6.3 per cent, compared with 3.6 per cent for vagotomy and gastroenterostomy at two years. Sixty-four per cent of

patients with vagotomy and pyloroplasty were rated as having an excellent to good clinical result versus 73 per cent for vagotomy and gastroenterostomy, 83 per cent for subtotal gastrectomy, and 84 per cent for vagotomy and antrectomy.

The results from a cooperative study involving 1358 male duodenal ulcer patients in Veterans Administration Hospitals[133] were remarkably similar, except that the mortality rate was 2.7 per cent for vagotomy and antrectomy, 2.0 per cent for subtotal gastrectomy, and 1.2 per cent for vagotomy and drainage. The recurrence rate was almost 9 per cent after vagotomy and drainage, 3.9 per cent after vagotomy and antrectomy, and 5.4 per cent after subtotal gastrectomy. The incidence of complications related to operation was almost 10 per cent with the two resective procedures and 6.2 per cent with vagotomy and drainage. It was concluded that the severity of postgastrectomy symptoms was related in a linear fashion to the amount of stomach removed.

Two hundred consecutive male duodenal ulcer patients at the Houston Veterans Administration Hospital were randomly assigned to either vagotomy and drainage or vagotomy and antrectomy with the proviso that any patient who had a badly scarred duodenum would be treated by vagotomy and drainage.[100] There were no deaths and the recurrence rate (known plus suspected) was 10 per cent for vagotomy and drainage and none for vagotomy and antrectomy. Fifty per cent of patients with vagotomy and drainage procedure had a positive Hollander test, as compared to 13 per cent with vagotomy and resection. The lower incidence of the positive Hollander test in patients with antrectomy was thought to be due to the loss of antral potentiation of the remaining vagal fibers. It is clearly apparent that one important advantage of vagotomy and antrectomy over vagotomy plus drainage is the protection offered for incomplete vagotomy.

Several points need to be considered in interpreting these studies. As Goligher[57] has cautioned, gastric resection is followed by more metabolic ill effects, such as weight loss and anemia, than is vagotomy and drainage. Further, the fact that there were no deaths in the original series should be interpreted in view of the selection of cases to avoid patients with high operative risks. It would seem fair to assume that widespread usage of the procedures by the general population of surgeons would be associated with a mortality rate of about 1 per cent in vagotomy plus drainage procedures and of at least 2 per cent in vagotomy and antrectomy.[30] This, then, returns the problem of evaluation to the metaphysical and ultimately unanswerable question: how many ulcer recurrences are equal to one death? It has been suggested[100] that the greater protection offered by vagotomy and resection may be conferred with relatively small risk to 90 per cent of patients if the remaining 10 per cent of patients, who are more serious operative risks because of anatomic distortion of the duodenum, are treated by vagotomy and drainage procedure.

Although experience is not uniform, there appear to be specific indications for vagotomy and drainage procedures. It seems warranted to advocate this procedure in uncomplicated instances of perforated duo-

TABLE 5. Postoperative Results of Operations for Duodenal Ulcer*

Procedure	Investigators	No. of Patients	Duration of Study	Per Cent Mortality	Per Cent Recurrence	Per Cent Neg Hollander	Per Cent Dumping	Per Cent Diarrhea	Per Cent Visick I & II
Subtotal gastrectomy	Goligher et al.	107	5–8 yr.	0	(5);2	–	–	–	94
	Howard et al.	80	>2 yr.	0	5	–	26	15	–
	Postlethwait	346	5 yr.	1.8	3.7	–	12	17.1	89.7
Truncal vagotomy and drainage	Eisenberg et al.	455	1–10 yr.	1;1.85	3.6	–	–	–	–
	Goligher et al.	119	5–8 yr.	0	(10);7	–	–	–	89
	Howard et al.	70	2 yr.	0	10	–	8.5	14	–
	Jordan and Condon	108	2–5 yr.	2	(3);8	50	–	19;5	–
	Kennedy et al.	547	–	0.5	3.3	80	2	27	92
	Postlethwait	337	5 yr.	0.6	6.2	–	12	20.7	83
Truncal vagotomy and antrectomy	Goligher et al.	116	5–8 yr.	0	(6);2	–	–	–	92
	Herrington et al.	3584	1–25 yr.	1.6	0.6	–	25	1	94
	Howard et al.	51	>2 yr.	0	4	–	27	22	–
	Jordan and Condon	92	2–5 yr.	0	0	87	–	16;5	–
	Postlethwait	331	5 yr.	0.9	0.7	–	17.2	21.5	89.2
Selective vagotomy and drainage	Amdrup and Jensen	100	5 yr.	0	6	79	34	1	85
	Humphrey and Wilkinson	67	1–2 yr.	–	–	–	25	19	64
Selective proximal vagotomy	Amdrup and Jensen	108	2 yr.	–	0	–	5	5	86
	Burge	130	3 yr.	1	0	–	–	–	–
	Clarke and Williams	18	3–12 mo.	0	0	89	0	0	100
	Grassi et al.	79	2–4 yr.	1.2	0	97	0	0	97
	Hedenstedt et al.	131	0.5–3 yr.	2.3	0	94	0	0	–
	Holle et al.	732	1–7 yr.	0.7	0.7	70	–	–	89
	Humphrey and Wilkinson	62	1–2 yr.	0	0	–	–	–	86
	Imperati et al.	62	3–10 mo.	–	0	80	0	–	97
	Johnston	400	<66 mo.	0	0	10–20	6	3	88
	Jordan	35	0.3–1 yr.	0	0	59	10	3	97
	Kronborg and Madsen	50	>1 yr.	22	0	–	6	8	78
	Miller et al.	25	2/3–2 1/2 yr.	0	0	–	0	0	–
	Wastell et al.	78	>6 mo.	4	0	28	8	–	70

*Modified from Thompson, J. C.: Texas Med., 70:51, 1974, where references to individual investigators are available.

denal ulcer. More importantly, it is probable that widespread adoption of vagotomy, pyloroplasty, and suture ligation of bleeding duodenal ulcer would lead to a diminution in the frightening mortality rate associated with emergency operations for bleeding. Foster and associates[52] reported a mortality rate of 30 per cent for gastric resection in the emergency treatment of bleeding gastroduodenal ulcers; after adoption of vagotomy and pyloroplasty for bleeding peptic ulcers, the mortality rate fell to 9 per cent; the higher mortality rate associated with resection was especially evident in older patients. It was, therefore, suggested that gastric resection be abandoned for the emergency control of massively bleeding gastric and duodenal ulcers in elderly or poor-risk patients. Analysis of mortality rates following vagotomy, pyloroplasty, and suture ligation for the treatment of bleeding duodenal ulcer reveals some reports as low as 2 and 3 per cent and others as high as 12 per cent, coupled with incidences of rebleeding as high as 25 per cent. Adoption of the "U" suture-ligation technique[15] for bleeding duodenal ulcers would control bleeding from the transverse pancreatic artery and might well diminish the incidence of rebleeding.

The incidence of recurrent ulceration following vagotomy and drainage seems to be inextricably linked to failure of complete vagus section. Recurrence of ulceration in a patient with great reduction of acid output is extremely rare.

Several attempts have been made to select between vagotomy plus antrectomy and vagotomy plus pyloroplasty on the basis of preoperative secretory studies; patients with severe hypersecretion were treated by vagotomy and antrectomy and those with milder hypersecretion were treated by vagotomy and drainage. These studies seem doomed until the technique for vagotomy is improved. Ulcer recurrence is much more closely linked to persistence of vagal innervation than to preoperative secretory activity.

Selective proximal vagotomy is a new procedure, and it is impossible to make any definitive statement about the ultimate place of this operation in the treatment of peptic ulcer disease. Nonetheless, inspection of results (Table 5) shows that the mortality rates are extremely low and that dumping and diarrhea have been nearly eliminated. The large series without any recurrences is exciting, but it must be evaluated along with the report of an early recurrence rate of 22 per cent. There is strong evidence that recurrences are caused by technical failures and that careful attention to the complete denervation of the esophagus will result in substantial improvement.[76]

OTHER SURGICAL DISEASES OF THE STOMACH

MALLORY-WEISS SYNDROME

In 1929, Mallory and Weiss[116] described clinical and autopsy findings in four alcoholic patients who had bled from the upper gastrointestinal tract. These patients had longitudinal tears of the esophagogastric mucosa through which the bleeding has occurred; it was suggested that the tears were caused by forceful vomiting. The first case to be diagnosed preoperatively and treated successfully by operation was reported 26 years later. A review of 229 cases[177] revealed an association with alcohol in 60 per cent of cases and with vomiting in 90 per cent of cases. Other etiologic conditions besides vomiting were closed-chest massage, or bouts of severe coughing, or other severe increases in intra-abdominal pressure. Three of four patients operated upon in this series had mucosal lacerations that were confined to gastric mucosa, only 5 per cent had lacerations confined to the esophageal mucosa, and the remainder had tears across the esophagogastric junction. Several patients had two or more mucosal tears that required repair.

Routine application of fiberoptic endoscopy in patients with upper gastrointestinal hemorrhage will almost certainly uncover a much larger incidence of the Mallory-Weiss syndrome than previously suspected. We found an incidence of 7.7 per cent in 195 consecutive patients admitted with massive upper gastrointestinal hemorrhage.[173]

Most patients with the Mallory-Weiss syndrome will stop bleeding spontaneously. Success may also be achieved with judicious use of the Sengstaken-Blakemore tube. Cautious application of endoscopic cautery techniques offers promise. If bleeding persists, it may be necessary to repair the lesion at operation. A long gastrotomy incision high in the stomach is required for visualization of the tear, which may then best be oversewn from below upward. This laceration should be considered whenever a patient is bleeding vigorously from the upper gastrointestinal tract and there is no obvious diagnosis. There seems to be no indication for performing vagotomy. The mortality rate is fairly high because of delay in diagnosis and because of the metabolic abnormalities associated with alcoholism.

ACUTE GASTRIC DILATATION

Acute dilatation of the stomach is a rare complication seen in patients who are severely ill, often comatose, and who have ileus. The condition develops insidiously and may come to medical attention with symptoms of hypovolemia or of cardiac failure or of pulmonary edema (after the patient vomits and aspirates massive amounts of gastric juice). The condition develops occasionally in patients with bowel obstruction who are being treated with a long intestinal (Miller-Abbott) tube, and the presence of the tube often contributes to the delay in diagnosis as attending physicians are apt to assume mistakenly that the tube is acting to keep the stomach decompressed. Emergency resuscitative measures in patients who have respiratory arrests often result in introduction of massive quantities of air into the stomach.

The vomiting of small amounts of brackish, coffee-ground gastric juice, often associated with hiccups (overflow vomiting), should serve as an immediate clue to the possibility of gastric dilatation. The treatment is introduction of a nasogastric tube and aspiration of gastric contents. With accumulation of air and distention of the stomach there is an outpouring of gastric juice and as distention increases there may be bleeding. Large amounts of air and 3 to 4 liters of gastric juice may be recovered from the stomach by aspiration. Massive hemorrhage or rupture of the stomach may occur, requiring immediate operative repair.

The most important treatment is prophylaxis. Any patient who has ileus should have a functioning nasogastric tube. If a nasogastric tube is removed from a postoperative debilitated or elderly patient whose bowel function is still questionable, it is wise to check the gastric residual in 6 to 8 hours to be sure that the stomach has not dilated. Acute gastric dilatation may be fatal in a short time if not recognized and corrected.

NONPEPTIC SURGICAL DISEASES OF THE DUODENUM

Those conditions of surgical interest that affect the entire small bowel are discussed in the chapter on the small intestine and will be mentioned here only briefly. The duodenum, and even more rarely the stomach, is infrequently involved with Crohn's disease.[23, 47] The symptoms are usually those of upper gastrointestinal obstruction caused by duodenal stenosis. The diagnosis can be made radiographically if the disease involves the rest of the small bowel, but isolated lesions in the duodenum are often difficult to interpret and the diagnosis is commonly made at operation. The symptoms of obstruction are relieved by simple bypass of the stenotic area by gastrojejunostomy or by duodenojejunostomy.

Tumors of the duodenum are classified according to their anatomic relation to the duodenal papilla: 20 per cent are proximal to the papilla, 60 per cent are peripapillary, and 20 per cent are distal.[102] Malignant duodenal tumors may be divided according to the symptoms they produce: obstructing lesions produce vomiting, ulcerating lesions cause bleeding, penetrating lesions may produce refractory pain, and periampullary lesions may produce jaundice and mimic carcinoma of the head of the pancreas. In a study of 24 patients seen at the Mayo Clinic with malignant infrapapillary tumors of the duodenum,[81] the diagnosis was made in 22 cases by x-ray but only half of the patients had tumors that were resectable, and of those patients whose tumors were resected, only one-third were alive five years after operation.

Intramural hematomas of the duodenum may occasionally mimic neoplasms by producing partial obstruction of the duodenum or the common bile duct. There is usually a clear association of the lesion with trauma, but occasionally duodenal hematomas may arise spontaneously in patients who have blood dyscrasias or who are on anticoagulant medication. The hematoma will usually subside in time, but because of persistent obstruction or bleeding, or error in diagnosis, the patient may be operated upon and, rarely, may require resection of the involved segment.[126]

TRAUMATIC RUPTURE

The duodenum is situated deep in the abdominal cavity and is well protected. Trauma to the duodenum usually involves injury to other organs and these associated injuries, especially to the pancreas, liver, and inferior vena cava, are a major factor in the prognosis. The injury may be caused by penetrating wounds from knives or gunshot or may be caused by blunt trauma, especially in automobile accidents or falls. Morton and Jordan[127] have reported 131 patients with duodenal injuries of whom 117 had penetrating wounds and 14 had blunt trauma to the abdomen. Lacerations involved less than half of the circumference of the duodenum in 80 per cent of cases and 3 per cent had complete transection. Associated injuries to all structures of the upper abdomen were common; the liver was involved in 38 per cent of cases, the pancreas in 28 per cent of cases, and the inferior vena cava in 17 per cent.

Diagnosis prior to operation is unusual, but it may be suspected because of the magnitude of the injury. It is particularly difficult to make the diagnosis of retroperitoneal duodenal rupture after blunt trauma, since symptoms may not occur for 24 to 36 hours. Plain x-ray films of the abdomen may reveal free air with penetrating wounds or may show gas in the retroperitoneal tissue around the duodenum and may occasionally outline the kidney. The oral administration of a water-soluble contrast agent may be of help in making the radiologic diagnosis of a duodenal rupture.

Diagnosis of retroperitoneal rupture following blunt trauma may be difficult at laparotomy. Important clues to the diagnosis are bile staining of the peritoneum of the posterior wall of the abdomen, emphysema of the retroperitoneum or of the mesocolon, and boggy crepitance inferior to the curve of the duodenum.[37]

If the site of injury is not apparent, the duodenum should be mobilized by dividing the ligament of Treitz, dividing the lateral peritoneal reflection of the second and third part of the duodenum, and freeing the hepatic flexure of the colon. It was possible to treat 85 per cent of patients by débridement and simple closure of the laceration; the serosal patch technique[103] of using an onlay cover of small bowel sutured to the margins of the laceration may be helpful in closing large defects. In severe injuries, defunctionalization of the repaired duodenal laceration has been advocated.[29] This may be accomplished by internal decompression with an afferent jejunostomy, and distal feeding jejunostomy and gastrostomy, along with external drainage of the repair.

In patients who have an associated rupture of the pancreas, vagotomy and antrectomy with gastrojejunostomy and catheter duodenostomy may offer the best protection against the development of massive pancreatitis, or pancreatic fistula, or bleeding.[38] Although radical pancreaticoduodenectomy (Whipple resection) has been performed for duodenal trauma, it should obviously be reserved for the most extreme degree of destructive injury. Reported mortality rates for duodenal rupture vary between 14 and 50 per cent and depend largely upon the severity of the associated injuries and upon delay in diagnosis, especially with retroperitoneal rupture after blunt trauma. Death is due either to sepsis or to hemorrhage.

The most common postoperative complications are

peritonitis, sepsis associated with intraperitoneal abscesses, and fistulas from the duodenum and pancreas.

DIVERTICULITIS

After the colon, the duodenum is the most common site for diverticula. They are fairly rare in patients under the age of 40 and are slightly more common in women than in men. Diverticula usually arise in the second or third portion of the duodenum on the concave medial wall but may appear posterior to the pancreas. Inflammation of the diverticula may give rise to pain, perforation, hemorrhage, pancreatitis, or obstruction of the common bile duct.[99] Gallstones are common in patients with duodenal diverticula, and the biliary tract should be studied in patients who are thought to have symptomatic duodenal diverticulitis. Vague symptoms of upper abdominal discomfort are common and duodenal diverticula are relatively common, but symptomatic duodenal diverticulitis is rare. The decision to operate on duodenal diverticula should be made with great caution except when there is clear evidence of perforation, bleeding, or obstruction. Rarely, duodenal obstruction will be caused by intraluminal protrusion of the duodenal diverticulum.[49]

At operation, the duodenum should be mobilized by dividing the lateral peritoneal attachments and reflecting the duodenum medialward to expose the posterior surface. The diverticulum will usually protrude between the duodenum and pancreas and may be excised and the defect oversewn.

The mortality rates for operations on duodenal diverticula vary between 5 and 10 per cent, and postoperative complications, particularly duodenal fistula, are common.

OBSTRUCTION

The duodenum may be obstructed by scarring caused by peptic ulcer, by duodenal diverticula, by tumors, rarely by diaphragmatic webs,[144] and uncommonly by the pancreas or the superior mesenteric artery.

Annular Pancreas

The envelopment of the second part of the duodenum with a ring of pancreatic tissue is thought to be due to a failure of the ventral anlage of the pancreas to rotate with the duodenum, an event that normally occurs in the sixth and seventh weeks of gestation. The course of the pancreatic duct in patients with annular pancreas suggests that the ventral anlage is fixed anteriorly and the duodenum in rotating leaves a ring of pancreatic tissue. The age of onset of symptoms depends upon the severity of constriction and on whether or not there is an associated stenosis or atresia of the duodenum. Nearly half of children and 15 per cent of adults with annular pancreas have associated duodenal stenosis. Complications seen with annular pancreas are obstruction of the duodenum, peptic ulcer of the stomach or duodenum seen in one third of patients (probably due to prolonged antral stasis), acute or chronic pancreatitis of the annulus itself (16 per cent),

and rare associated biliary obstruction.[181] Infants with neonatal obstruction of the duodenum caused by annular pancreas often are the product of pregnancies that have been complicated by polyhydramnios. Associated anomalies are common (mongolism, tracheoesophageal fistula, malrotation of the colon, duodenal atresia, and others).[80]

Diagnosis is often made on x-ray, which may show two gas shadows with air-fluid levels *(the double-bubble sign)* or a dumbbell-shaped shadow. In adults, the diagnosis is often made by the radiologic demonstration of a hugely dilated first portion of the duodenum.

Some patients with annular pancreas may live their entire lives without symptoms. For those patients who have obstruction of the duodenum, the proper treatment is bypass of the area of obstruction by anastomosis of the proximal duodenum with the first part of the jejunum.

SELECTED REFERENCES

Barreras, R. F.: Calcium and gastric secretion. Gastroenterology, *64*:1168, 1973.

Davenport, H. W.: Salicylate damage to the gastric mucosal barrier. N. Engl. J. Med., *276*:1307, 1967.

DeBakey, M., and Ochsner, A.: Recent advances in surgery. Bezoars and concretions. A comprehensive review of the literature with an analysis of 303 collected cases and a presentation of 8 additional cases. Surgery, *4*:934, 1938; *5*:132, 1939.

Dragstedt, L. R.: The physiology of the gastric antrum. Arch. Surg., *75*:552, 1957.

DuPlessis, D. J.: Pathogenesis of gastric ulceration. Lancet, *1*:974, 1965.

Goligher, J. C.: A technique for highly selective (parietal cell or proximal gastric) vagotomy for duodenal ulcer. Br. J. Surg., *61*:337, 1974.

Goligher, J. C., Pulvertaft, C. N., DeDombal, F. T., Conyers, J. H., Duthie, H. L., Feather, D. B., Latchmore, A. J. C., Shoesmith, J. H., Smiddy, F. G., and Willson-Pepper, J.: Five- to eight-year results of Leeds-York controlled trial of elective surgery for duodenal ulcer. Br. Med. J., *2*:781, 1968.

Gregory, R. A.: Memorial Lecture: The isolation and chemistry of gastrin. Gastroenterology, *51*:953, 1966.

Gregory, R. A., and Tracy, H. J.: The constitution and properties of two gastrins extracted from hog antral mucosa. Gut, *5*:103, 1964.

Grossman, M. I.: Gastrin and its activities. Nature, *228*:1147, 1970.

Grossman, M. I., Guth, P. H., Isenberg, J. I., Passaro, E. P., Jr., Roth, B. E., Sturdevant, R. A. L., and Walsh, J. H.: A new look at peptic ulcer. Ann. Intern. Med., *84*:57, 1976.

Hinchey, E. J., Hreno, A., Benoit, P. R., Hewson, J. R., and Gurd, F. N.: The stress ulcer syndrome. Adv. Surg., *4*:325, 1970.

Isenberg, J. I., Grossman, M. I., Maxwell, V., and Walsh, J. H.: Increased sensitivity to stimulation of acid secretion by pentagastrin in duodenal ulcer. J. Clin. Invest., *55*:330, 1975.

Kukral, J. C.: Gastric ulcers: An appraisal. Surgery, *63*:1024, 1968.

Littman, A. (Ed.): The Veterans' Administration Cooperative Study on Gastric Ulcer. Gastroenterology,*61*:567, 1971.

Menguy, R.: Surgery of Peptic Ulcer. Philadelphia, W. B. Saunders Company, 1976.

Michels, N. A.: Blood supply of the stomach and the esophagus. *In* Blood Supply and Anatomy of the Upper Abdominal Organs. Philadelphia, J. B. Lippincott Company, 1955, p. 248.

Morton, J. R., and Jordan, G. L.: Traumatic duodenal injuries. Review of 131 cases. J. Trauma, *8*:127, 1968.

Rayford, P. L., Miller, T. A., and Thompson, J. C.: Secretin, cholecystokinin and newer gastrointestinal hormones. N. Engl. J. Med., *294*:1093; 1157, 1976.

Rayford, P. L., and Thompson, J. C.: Gastrin. Surg. Gynecol. Obstet., in press.

Skillman, J. J.: Pathogenesis of peptic ulcer: A selective review. Surgery, *76*:515, 1974.

Stabile, B. E., and Passaro, E., Jr.: Recurrent peptic ulcer. Gastroenterology, *70*:124, 1976.

Thompson, J. C.: Gastrin and gastric secretion. Ann. Rev. Med., 20:291, 1969.

Thompson, J. C.: Standard versus experimental surgical procedures in the treatment of duodenal ulcer. Texas Med., 70:51, 1974.

Thompson, J. C. (Ed.). Gastrointestinal Hormones. Austin, University of Texas Press, 1975.

Thompson, J. C., Fender, H. R., Watson, L. C., and Villar, H. V.: The effects on gastrin and gastric secretion of five current operations for duodenal ulcer. Ann. Surg., 183:599, 1976.

Thompson, J. C., Reeder, D. D., Villar, H. V., and Fender, H. R.: Natural history and experience with diagnosis and treatment of the Zollinger-Ellison syndrome. Surg. Gynecol. Obstet., 140:721, 1975.

Walsh, J. H., and Grossman, M. I..: Gastrin. N. Engl. J. Med., 202:1324; 1377, 1975.

Williams, J. A., and Cox, A. G., (Eds.): After Vagotomy. London, Butterworth & Company, 1969.

Zollinger, R. M., and Ellison, R. H.: Primary peptic ulcerations of the jejunum associated with islet cell tumor of pancreas. Ann. Surg., 142:709, 1955.

REFERENCES

1. Abernethy, R. M., Gillespie, I. E., Lawrie, J. H., Forrest, A. P. M., Payne, R. A., Barabaras, A., Johnston, I. D. A., Burns, G. P., Hobbs, K. E. F., Clegg, R. T., Duthie, H. L., and Fitzgerald, J. D.: Pentagastrin as a stimulant of maximal gastric acid response in man. A multicentre pilot study. Lancet, 1:291, 1967.

2. Almy, T. P.: Digestive disease as a national problem. II. A white paper by the American Gastroenterological Association, 1967. Gastroenterology, 53:821, 1967.

3. Andersson, S.: Gastric and duodenal mechanisms inhibiting gastric secretion of acid. In Code, C. F. (Ed.): American Physiological Society: Handbook of Physiology, Section 6, Alimentary Canal. Baltimore, Williams & Wilkins Company, 1967, Volume 2, pp. 865–877.

4. Andersson, S.: Inhibitory mechanisms in duodenal control of gastric acid secretion. Gastroenterology, 61:778–780, 1971.

5. Andersson, S.: Bulbogastrone. In Thompson, J. C. (Ed.): Gastrointestinal Hormones. Austin, University of Texas Press, 1975, p. 555.

6. Angel, R. T., Giacobine, J. W., and Jordan, G. L., Jr.: A current evaluation of the problem of gastric ulcers. Am. J. Surg., 114:730, 1967.

7. Archambault, A. P., Rovelstad, R. A., and Carlson, H. C.: In situ pH of duodenal bulb contents in normal and duodenal ulcer subjects. Gastroenterology, 52:940, 1967.

8. Athanasoulis, C. A., Baum, S., Waltman, A. C., Ring, E. J., Imbembo, A., and Salm, T. J.: Control of acute gastric mucosal hemorrhage: Intra-arterial infusion of posterior pituitary extracts. N. Engl. J. Med., 290:597, 1974.

9. Bachrach, W. H., and Bachrach, L. B.: Reevaluation of the Hollander test. Ann. N.Y. Acad. Sci., 140:915, 1967.

10. Bank, S., Marks, I. N., and Louw, J. H.: Histamine- and insulin-stimulated gastric secretion after selective and truncal vagotomy. Gut, 8:36, 1968.

11. Barnes, A. D., and Cox, A. G.: Diarrhea. In Williams, J. A., and Cox, A. G. (Eds.): After Vagotomy. London, Butterworth & Company, 1969, p. 211.

12. Baron, J. H.: An assessment of the augmented histamine test in the diagnosis of peptic ulcer. Gut, 4:243, 1963.

13. Barreras, R. F.: Acid secretion after calcium carbonate in patients with duodenal ulcer. N. Engl. J. Med., 282:1402, 1970.

14. Barreras, R. F.: Calcium and gastric secretion. Gastroenterology, 64:1168, 1973.

15. Berne, C. J., and Rosoff, L.: Peptic ulcer perforation of the gastroduodenal artery complex. Ann. Surg., 169:141, 1969.

16. Berson, S. A., and Yalow, R. S.: Gastrin in duodenal ulcers. N. Engl. J. Med., 284:445, 1971.

17. Bondar, G. F., Yakimets, W. W., Williams, T. G., and MacKenzie, W. C.: Diagnosis and management of stomal ulcer. Can. J. Surg., 7:383, 1964.

18. Bowen, J. C., Fleming, W. H., and Thompson, J. C.: Increased gastrin release following penetrating central nervous system injury. Surgery, 75:720, 1974.

19. Breckenridge, I. M., Walton, E. W., and Walker, W. F.: Stress ulcers in the stomach. Br. Med. J., 2:1362, 1959.

20. Brodie, D. A., and Hanson, H. M.: A study of the factors involved in the production of gastric ulcers by the restraint technique. Gastroenterology, 38:353, 1960.

21. Broome, A., and Bergstrom, H.: Selective surgery for duodenal ulcer based on preoperative acid production. Acta Chir. Scand., 132:170, 1966.

22. Brown, J. C., Dryburgh, J. R., Moccia, P., and Pederson, R. A.: The current status of GIP. In Thompson, J. C. (Ed.): Gastrointestinal Hormones. Austin, University of Texas Press, 1975, p. 537.

23. Burgess, J. N., Legge, D. A., and Judd, E. S.: Surgical treatment of regional enteritis of the stomach and duodenum. Surg. Gynecol. Obstet., 132:628, 1971.

24. Cano, R., Bloom, S. R., and Isenberg, J. I.: Pancreatic bicarbonate secretion in serum secretin in response to graded amounts of duodenal acidification in duodenal ulcer and normal subjects. Gastroenterology, 68:870, 1975.

25. Capper, W. M., Butler, T. J., Buckler, K. G., and Hallett, C. P.: Variation in size of the gastric antrum: Measurement of alkaline area associated with ulceration and pyloric stenosis. Ann. Surg., 163:281, 1966.

26. Charters, A. C., Odell, W. D., Davidson, W. D., and Thompson, J. C.: Gastrin: Immunochemical properties and measurement by radioimmunoassay. Surgery, 66:104, 1969.

27. Chenoweth, A. I., and Dimick, A. R.: Stress ulcer in infants and children. Ann. Surg., 161:977, 1965.

28. Cook, L., and Hutton, C. F.: Postbulbar duodenal ulceration. Lancet, 1:754, 1958.

29. Corley, R. D., Norcross, W. J., and Shoemaker, W. C.: Traumatic injuries to the duodenum. Ann. Surg., 181:92, 1975.

30. Cox, A. G.: Vagotomy and drainage procedures. The present position. Progr. Surg., 8:45, 1970.

31. Cox, A. J., Jr.: Stomach size and its relation to chronic peptic ulcer. Arch. Pathol., 54:407, 1952.

32. Davenport, H. W.: Physiologic structure of the gastric mucosa. In Code, C. F. (Ed.): American Physiological Society: Handbook of Physiology, Section 6, Alimentary Canal. Baltimore, Williams & Wilkins Company, 1967, Volume 2, pp. 759–779.

33. Davenport, H. W.: Salicylate damage to the gastric mucosal barrier. N. Engl. J. Med., 276:1307, 1967.

34. Davis, R. C., and Faruqui, A. M. A.: Endoscopic enzymatic dissolution. Nonsurgical therapy for gastric phytobezoars. J.A.M.A., 229:1332, 1974.

35. DeBakey, M., and Ochsner, A.: Recent advances in surgery. Bezoars and concretions. A comprehensive review of the literature with an analysis of 303 collected cases and a presentation of 8 additional cases. Surgery, 4:934, 1938; 5:132, 1939.

36. Delaney, J. P., Cheng, J. W. B., Butler, B. A., and Ritchie, W. P., Jr.: Gastric ulcer and regurgitation gastritis. Gut, 11:715, 1970.

37. Deodhar, M. C., Duleep, K. S., Gill, S. S., and Eggleston, F. C.: Retroperitoneal rupture of the duodenum following blunt trauma. Arch. Surg., 96:963, 1968.

38. Donovan, A. J., and Hagen, W. E.: Traumatic perforation of the duodenum. Am. J. Surg., 111:341, 1966.

39. Dowse, J. L. A.: Spontaneous internal biliary fistulae. Gut, 5:429, 1964.

40. Dragstedt, L. R.: Vagotomy for gastroduodenal ulcer. Ann. Surg., 122:973, 1949.

41. Dragstedt, L. R., and Owens, F. M., Jr.: Supradiaphragmatic section of vagus nerves in treatment of duodenal ulcer. Proc. Soc. Exp. Biol. Med., 53:152, 1943.

42. Drapanas, T., and Bethia, M.: Reflux gastritis following gastric surgery. Ann. Surg., 179:618, 1974.

43. Du Plessis, D. J.: Pathogenesis of gastric ulceration. Lancet, 1:974, 1965.

44. Edkins, J. S.: On the chemical mechanism of gastric secretion. Proc. R. Soc. London, 76:376, 1905.

45. Edkins, J. S.: The chemical mechanism of gastric secretion. J. Physiol., 34:133, 1906.

46. Eisenberg, M. D., Woodward, E. R., Carson, T. J., and Dragstedt, L. R.: Vagotomy and drainage procedure for duodenal ulcer: The results of ten years' experience. Ann. Surg., 170:317, 1969.

47. Fielding, J. F., Toye, D. K. M., Beton, D. C., and Cooke, W. T.: Crohn's disease of the stomach and duodenum. Gut, 11:1001, 1970.

48. Fisher, R. S., and Cohen, S.: Pyloric-sphincter dysfunction in patients with gastric ulcer. N. Engl. J. Med., 288:273, 1973.

49. Fleming, C. R., Newcomer, A. D., Stephens, D. H., and Carlson,

H. C.: Intraluminal duodenal diverticulum. Mayo Clin. Proc., *50*:244, 1975.

50. Fordtran, J. S.: The psychosomatic theory of peptic ulcer. *In* Sleisenger, M. H., and Fordtran, J. S. (Eds.): Gastrointestinal Disease. Pathophysiology, Diagnosis, Management. Philadelphia, W. B. Saunders Company, 1973, p. 163.

51. Fordtran, J. S., Morawski, F. G., and Richardson, C. T.: In vivo and in vitro evaluation of liquid antacids. N. Engl. J. Med., *288*:923, 1973.

52. Foster, J. H., Hickok, D. F., and Dunphy, J. E.: Factors influencing mortality following emergency operation for massive upper gastrointestinal hemorrhage. Surg. Gynecol. Obstet., *117*:257, 1963.

53. Gillespie, G., Gillespie, I. E., and Kay, A. W.: An analysis of the insulin test after vagotomy using single and multiple criteria. Gut, *9*:470, 1968.

54. Glick, D. L., and Kern, F., Jr.: Peptic ulcer and chronic obstructive bronchopulmonary disease. A prospective clinical study of prevalence. Gastroenterology, *47*:153, 1964.

55. Goldstein, H., and Boyle, J. D.: The saline load test — a bedside evaluation of gastric retention. Gastroenterology, *49*:375, 1965.

56. Goligher, J. C.: A technique for highly selective (parietal cell or proximal gastric) vagotomy for duodenal ulcer. Br. J. Surg., *61*:337, 1974.

57. Goligher, J. C., and Pulvertaft, C. M.: Comparison of different operations. *In* Williams, J. A., and Cox, A. G. (Eds.): After Vagotomy. London, Butterworth & Company, 1969, p. 93.

58. Goligher, J. C., Pulvertaft, C. N., De Dombal, F. T., Clark, C. G., Conyers, J. H., Duthie, H. L., Feather, D. B., Latchmore, A. J. C., Matheson, T. S., Shoesmith, J. H., Smiddy, F. G., and Willson-Pepper, J.: Clinical comparison of vagotomy and pyloroplasty with other forms of elective surgery for duodenal ulcer. Br. Med. J., *2*:787, 1968.

59. Goligher, J. C., Pulvertaft, C. N., De Dombal, F. T., Conyers, J. H., Duthie, H. L., Feather, D. B., Latchmore, A. J. C., Shoesmith, J. H., Smiddy, F. G., and Willson-Pepper, J.: Five- to eight-year results of Leeds-York controlled trial of elective surgery for duodenal ulcer. Br. Med. J., *2*:781, 1968.

60. Gordon, M. J., Skillman, J. J., Zervas, N. T., and Silen, W.: Divergent nature of gastric mucosal permeability and gastric acid secretion in sick patients with general surgical and neurosurgical disease. Ann. Surg., *178*:285, 1973.

61. Gregory, R. A.: Memorial lecture: The isolation and chemistry of gastrin. Gastroenterology, *51*:953, 1966.

62. Gregory, R. A.: Isolation and chemistry of gastrin. *In* Code, C. F. (Ed.): American Physiological Society: Handbook of Physiology, Section 6, Alimentary Canal. Baltimore, Williams & Wilkins Company, 1967, Vol. 2, p. 827.

63. Gregory, R. A., Grossman, M. I., Tracy, H. J., and Bentley, P. H.: Nature of the gastric secretagogue in Zollinger-Ellison tumors. Lancet, *2*:543, 1967.

64. Gregory, R. A., and Tracy, H. J.: The constitution and properties of two gastrins extracted from hog antral mucosa. Gut, *5*:103, 1964.

65. Gregory, R. A., and Tracy, H. J.: A note on the nature of the gastrin-like stimulant present in Zollinger-Ellison tumours. Gut, *5*:115, 1964.

66. Grossman, M. I.: Neural and hormonal stimulation of gastric secretion of acid. *In* Code, C. F. (Ed.): American Physiological Society: Handbook of Physiology, Section 6, Alimentary Canal. Baltimore, Williams & Wilkins Company, 1967, Vol. 2, p. 835.

67. Grossman, M. I.: Gastrin and its activities. Nature, *228*:1147, 1970.

68. Grossman, M. I.: Résumé and comment. *In* The Veterans Administration Cooperative Study on Gastric Ulcer. Gastroenterology, *61*:635–638, 1971.

69. Grossman, M. I.: Some minor heresies about vagotomy. Gastroenterology, *67*:1016, 1974.

70. Grossman, M. I.: Candidate hormones of the gut. I. Introduction. Gastroenterology, *67*:730, 1974.

71. Grossman, M. I.: The chemical that activates the "on" switches of the oxyntic cell. Mayo Clin. Proc., *50*:515, 1975.

72. Grossman, M. I., Kirsner, J. B., and Gillespie, I. E.: Basal and histalog-stimulated gastric secretion in control subjects and in patients with peptic ulcer or gastric cancer. Gastroenterology, *45*:14, 1963.

73. Grossman, M. I., Guth, P. H., Isenberg, J. I., Passaro, E. P. Jr.,

Roth, B. E., Sturdevant, R. A. L., and Walsh, J. H.: A new look at peptic ulcer. Ann. Intern. Med., *84*:57, 1976.

74. Haley, A. E.: Bezoars. Ann. Intern. Med., *46*:30, 1957.

75. Hallenbeck, G. A.: The Zollinger-Ellison syndrome. Gastroenterology, *54*:426, 1968.

76. Hallenbeck, G. A., Gleysteen, J. J., Aldrete, J. S., and Slaughter, R. L.: Proximal gastric vagotomy: Effects of two operative techniques on clinical and gastric secretory results. Ann. Surg., *184*:435–442, 1976.

77. Hansky, J., King, R. W., and Holdsworth, S.: Serum gastrin in chronic renal failure. *In* Thompson, J. C. (Ed.): Gastrointestinal Hormones. Austin, University of Texas Press, 1975, p. 115.

78. Harken, A. H., Gabel, R. A., Fencl, V., and Moore, F. D.: Hydrochloric acid in the correction of metabolic alkalosis. Arch. Surg., *110*:819, 1975.

79. Hassan, M. A., and Hobsley, M.: Positioning of subject and of nasogastric tube during a gastric secretion study. Br. Med. J., *1*:458, 1970.

80. Hays, D. M., Greaney, E. M., Jr., and Hill, J. T.: Annular pancreas as a cause of acute neonatal duodenal obstruction. Ann. Surg., *153*:103, 1961.

81. Higgins, D. C., Judd, E. S., and Dockerty, M. B.: Surgical aspects of infrapapillary duodenal tumors. Surgery, *49*:149, 1961.

82. Hinchey, E. J., Hreno, A., Benoit, P. R., Hewson, J. R., and Gurd, F. N.: The stress ulcer syndrome. Adv. Surg., *4*:325, 1970.

83. Hollander, F.: The insulin test for the presence of intact nerve fibers after vagal operations for peptic ulcer. Gastroenterology, *7*:607, 1946.

84. Hollander, F.: Laboratory procedures in the study of vagotomy. Gastroenterology, *11*:419, 1948.

85. Hollander, F.: Gastric secretion of electrolytes. Fed. Proc., *11*:706, 1952.

86. Hollander, F.: Two-component mucous barrier: Its activity in protecting gastroduodenal mucosa against peptic ulceration. Arch. Intern. Med., *93*:107, 1954.

87. Hollander, F.: The significance of sodium and potassium in gastric secretion: A review. Gastroenterology, *40*:477, 1961.

88. Holle, F.: Surgery of gastroduodenal ulcer based on form and function. Importance, reasoning, technique and results in 580 cases, 300 of them postexamined. Chir. Orthop., *54*:1, 1970.

89. Ingelfinger, F. J., and Ochsner, A.: Medical and surgical aspects of duodenal ulcer. Postgrad. Med., *40*:429, 1966.

90. Isenberg, J. I.: Gastric secretory testing. *In* Sleisenger, M. H., and Fordtran, J. S. (Eds.): Gastrointestinal Disease, Pathophysiology, Diagnosis, Management. Philadelphia, W. B. Saunders Company, 1973, p. 536.

91. Isenberg, J. I.: H_2-receptor antagonists in the treatment of peptic ulcer. Ann. Intern. Med., *84*:212, 1976.

92. Isenberg, J. I., Grossman, M. I., Maxwell, V., and Walsh, J. H.: Increased sensitivity to stimulation of acid secretion by pentagastrin in duodenal ulcer. J. Clin. Invest., *55*:330, 1975.

93. Isenberg, J. I., Walsh, J. H., and Grossman, M. I.: Zollinger-Ellison syndrome. Gastroenterology, *65*:140, 1973.

94. Jackson, B. M., Reeder, D. D., Hirose, F., and Thompson, J. C.: Correlation of the surface pH, histology, and gastrin concentration of gastric mucosa. Ann. Surg., *176*:727–731, 1972.

95. Jacobson, E. D., and Thompson, W. J.: Cyclic AMP and gastric secretion: The illusive second messenger. *In* Advances in Cyclic Nucleotide Research. In press.

96. Jacobson, E. D., Linford, R.H., and Grossman, M. I.: Gastric secretion in relation to mucosal blood flow studied by a clearance technique. J. Clin. Invest., *45*:1, 1966.

97. Johnston, D., and Duthie, H. L.: Inhibition of gastrin secretion in the human stomach. Effect of acid in the duodenum. Lancet, *2*:1032, 1965.

98. Johnston, P. W., and Snyder, W. H.: Vagotomy and pyloroplasty in infancy and childhood. J. Pediatr. Surg., *3*:228, 1968.

99. Jones, T. W., and Merendino, K. A.: The perplexing duodenal diverticulum. Surgery, *48*:1068, 1960.

100. Jordan, P. H., and Condon, R. E.: A prospective evaluation of vagotomy-pyloroplasty and vagotomy-antrectomy for treatment of duodenal ulcer. Ann. Surg., *172*:547, 1970.

101. Kellner, H. C., and Mellinkoff, S. M.: The dumping syndrome: An interpretation. Gastroenterology, *44*:424, 1963.

102. Kleinerman, J., Yardumian, K., and Tamaki, H. T.: Primary carcinoma of the duodenum. Ann. Intern. Med., *32*:451, 1950.

103. Kobold, E. E., and Thal, A. P.: A simple method for the manage-

ment of experimental wounds of the duodenum. Surg. Gynecol. Obstet., *118*:340, 1963.

104. Krag, E.: Gastric acid secretion related to prognosis in peptic ulcer. A long-term follow-up study. Acta Med. Scand., *180*:461, 1966.

105. Kronborg, O.: Gastric acid secretion and risk of recurrence of duodenal ulcer within six to eight years after truncal vagotomy and drainage. Gut, *15*:714, 1974.

106. Kukral, J. C.: Gastric ulcers: An appraisal. Surgery, *63*:1024, 1968.

107. Landor, J. H.: Gastric secretory tests and their relevance to surgeons. Surgery, *65*:523, 1969.

108. Langman, M. J. S., and Cooke, A. R.: Gastric and duodenal ulcer and their associated diseases. Lancet, *1*:680, 1976.

109. Levine, R. J., and Senay, E. C.: Studies on the role of acid in the pathogenesis of experimental stress ulcers. Psychosom. Med., *32*:61, 1970.

110. Lewisohn, R.: The frequency of gastrojejunal ulcers. Surg. Gynecol. Obstet., *40*:70, 1925.

111. Littman, A.: Basal gastric secretion in patients with duodenal ulcer: A long-term study of variations in relation to ulcer activity. Gastroenterology, *43*:166, 1962.

112. Lloyd, J. R., Bernstein, J., and Espiasse, E.: The etiology of gastrointestinal perforations in the newborn. Harper Hosp. Bull., *22*:224, 1960.

113. Lucas, C. E., and Wilson, R. F.: Gastrointestinal complications following trauma. *In* Walt, A. J., and Wilson, R. F. (Eds.): Management of Trauma. Philadelphia, Lea & Febiger, 1975, p. 545.

114. Lucas, C. E., Sugawa, C., Riddle, J., Rector, F., Rosenberg, B., and Walt, A. J.: Natural history and surgical dilemma of "stress" gastric bleeding. Arch. Surg., *102*:266, 1971.

115. Makhlouf, G. M., McManus, J. P. A., and Card, W. I.: A quantitative statement of the two-component hypothesis of gastric secretion. Gastroenterology, *51*:149, 1966.

116. Mallory, G. K., and Weiss, S.: Hemorrhages from lacerations of cardiac orifice of the stomach due to vomiting. Am. J. Med. Sci., *178*:506, 1929.

117. Mansberger, A. R., Jr., Hearn, J. B., Byers, R. M., Fleisig, N., and Buxton, R. W.: Vascular compression of the duodenum. Emphasis on accurate diagnosis. Am. J. Surg., *115*:89, 1968.

118. McGuigan, J. E.: Immunochemical studies with antibodies to human gastrin. Gastroenterology, *54*:1256, 1968.

119. McGuigan, J. E.: Gastric mucosal intracellular localization of gastrin by immunofluorescence. Gastroenterology, *55*:315, 1968.

120. McGuigan, J. E., and Greider, M. H.: Correlative immunochemical and light microscopic studies of the gastric cell of the antral mucosa. Gastroenterology, *60*:223, 1971.

121. Mendeloff, A. I.: What has been happening to duodenal ulcer? Gastroenterology, *67*:1020, 1974.

122. Menguy, R.: Stomach. *In* Schwartz, S. I., (Ed.): Principles of Surgery. New York, McGraw-Hill Book Company, 1969, pp. 907–939.

123. Menguy, R.: Surgery of Peptic Ulcer. Philadelphia, W. B. Saunders Company, 1976.

124. Menguy, R., Gadacz, T., and Zajtchuk, R.: The surgical management of acute gastric mucosal bleeding. Stress ulcer, acute erosive gastritis, and acute hemorrhagic gastritis. Arch. Surg., *99*:198, 1969.

125. Michels, N. A.: Blood supply of the stomach and the esophagus. *In* Blood Supply and Anatomy of the Upper Abdominal Organs. Philadelphia, J. B. Lippincott Company, 1955, pp. 248–274.

126. Moore, S. W., and Erlandson, M. E.: Intramural hematoma of the duodenum. Ann. Surg., *157*:798, 1963.

127. Morton, J. R., and Jordan, G. L.: Traumatic duodenal injuries. Review of 131 cases. J. Trauma, *8*:127, 1968.

128. Mullens, J. E., and Bird, G. S.: Peptic ulceration of the postbulbar portion of the duodenum. Can. J. Surg., *12*:27, 1969.

129. Oi, M., Ito, Y., Kumagai, F., Yoshida, K., Tanaka, Y., Yoshikawa, K., Muto, O., and Kijima, M.: A possible dual control mechanism in the origin of peptic ulcer. A study on ulcer location as affected by mucosa and musculature. Gastroenterology, *57*:280, 1969.

130. Orloff, M. J., Abbott, A. G., and Rosen, H.: Nature of the humoral agent responsible for portacaval shunt-related gastric hypersecretion in man. Am. J. Surg., *120*:237, 1970.

131. Orloff, M. J., Villar-Valdez, H., Rosen, H., Thompson, A. G., and Chandler, J. G.: Humoral mediation of the intestinal phase of gastric secretion and of hypersecretion associated with portacaval shunts. Surgery, *66*:118, 1969.

132. Pavlov, I. D.: Lectures on the Work of the Digestive Glands. London, Charles Griffin and Company, 1902.

133. Price, W. E., Grizzle, J. E., Postlethwait, R. W., Johnson, W. D., and Grabicki, P.: Results of operation for duodenal ulcer. Surg. Gynecol. Obstet., *131*:233, 1970.

134. Ravitch, M. D., and Duremdes, G. D.: Operative treatment of chronic duodenal ulcer in childhood. Ann. Surg., *171*:641, 1970.

135. Rayford, P. L., Miller, T. A., and Thompson, J. C.: Secretin, cholecystokinin and newer gastrointestinal hormones. N. Engl. J. Med., *294*:1093; 1157, 1976.

136. Rayford, P. L., and Thompson, J. C.: Gastrin. Surg. Gynecol. Obstet., in press.

137. Reeder, D. D., Becker, H. D., and Thompson, J. C.: Effect of intravenously administered calcium on serum gastrin and gastric secretion in man. Surg. Gynecol. Obstet., *138*:847, 1974.

138. Reeder, D. D., Conlee, J. L., and Thompson, J. C.: Effect of calcium carbonate antacid on serum gastrin concentrations in duodenal ulcer patients. Surg. Forum, *22*:308, 1971.

139. Reeder, D. D., Jackson, B. M., Brandt, E. N., Jr., and Thompson, J. C.: Rate and pattern of disappearance of exogenous gastrin in dogs. Am. J. Physiol., *222*:1571, 1972.

140. Reeder, D. D., Jackson, B. M., Ban, J. L., Davidson, W. D., and Thompson, J. C.: Effect of food on serum gastrin concentrations in duodenal ulcer and control patients. Surg. Forum, *21*:290, 1970.

141. Rehfeld, J. F., Stadil, F., Malmström, J., and Miyata, M.: Gastrin heterogeneity in serum and tissue: A progress report. *In* Thompson, J. C. (Ed.): Gastrointestinal Hormones. Austin, University of Texas Press, 1975, p. 43.

142. Rhodes, J., Barnardo, D. E., Phillips, S. F., Rovelstad, R. A., and Hofman, A. F.: Increased reflux of bile into the stomach in patients with gastric ulcer. Gastroenterology, *57*:241, 1969.

143. Richardson, C. T., and Walsh, J. H.: The value of a histamine H_2-receptor antagonist in the management of patients with the Zollinger-Ellison syndrome. N. Engl. J. Med., *294*:133, 1976.

144. Rowe, M. I., Buckner, D., and Clatworthy, H. W., Jr.: Wind sock web of the duodenum. Am. J. Surg., *116*:444, 1968.

145. Salmon, P. R., Brown, P., Htut, T., and Read, A. E.: Endoscopic examination of the duodenal bulb: Clinical evaluation of forward- and side-viewing fiberoptic systems in 200 cases. Gut, *13*:170–175, 1972.

146. Samloff, I. M., Liebman, W. M., and Panitch, N. M.: Serum group I pepsinogens by radioimmunoassay in control subjects and patients with peptic ulcer. Gastroenterology, *69*:83, 1975.

147. Samloff, I. M., Secrist, D. M., and Passaro, E., Jr.: The effect of Betazole on serum group I pepsinogen levels: Studies in symptomatic patients with and without recurrent ulcer after vagotomy and gastric resection or drainage. Gastroenterology, *70*:1007, 1976.

148. Sawyers, J. L., Herrington, J. L., Jr., Mulherin, J. O., Whitehead, W. A., Mody, B., and Marsh, J.: Acute perforated duodenal ulcer. An evaluation of surgical management. Arch. Surg., *110*:527, 1975.

149. Schiller, K., Truelove, S. C., and Williams, D. G.: Haematemesis and melaena with special reference to factors influencing the outcome. Br. Med. J., *2*:7, 1970.

150. Scobie, B. A., McGill, D. B., Priestley, J. T., and Rovelstad, R. A.: Excluded gastric antrum stimulating the Zollinger-Ellison syndrome. Gastroenterology, *47*:184, 1964.

151. Skillman, J. J.: Pathogenesis of peptic ulcer: A selective review. Surgery, *76*:515, 1974.

152. Skillman, J. J., Bushnell, L. S., Goldman, H., and Silen, W.: Respiratory failure, hypotension, sepsis and jaundice: A clinical syndrome associated with lethal hemorrhage from acute ulceration of the stomach. Am. J. Surg., *117*:523, 1969.

153. Skillman, J. J., Gould, S. A., Chung, R. S. K., and Silen, W.: The gastric mucosal barrier: Clinical and experimental studies in critically ill and normal man, and in the rabbit. Ann. Surg., *172*:564, 1970.

154. Stabile, B. E., and Passaro, E., Jr.: Recurrent peptic ulcer. Gastroenterology, *70*:124, 1976.

155. Stadil, F., Stage, G., Rehfeld, J. F., Efsen, F., and Fischerman, K.: Treatment of Zollinger-Ellison syndrome with streptozotocin. N. Engl. J. Med., *294*:1440, 1976.

156. Steinberg, D. M., Masselink, B. A., and Alexander-Williams, J.: Assessment and treatment of recurrent peptic ulceration. Ann. R. Coll. Surg. Engl., *56*:135–140, 1975.

157. Stempien, S. J., Lee, E. R., and Dagradi, A. E.: Clinical appraisal of insulin gastric analysis. Am. J. Dig. Dis., 13:21, 1968.
158. Stremple, J. F., Molot, M. D., McNamara, J., Mori, H., and Jerzy Glass, G. B.: Posttraumatic gastric bleeding. Prospective gastric secretion composition. Arch. Surg., 105:177, 1972.
159. Swan, K. G., and Jacobson, E. D.: Gastric blood flow and secretion in conscious dogs. Am. J. Physiol., 212:891, 1967.
160. Thieme, E. T., and Postmus, R.: Superior mesenteric artery syndrome. Ann. Surg., 154:139, 1961.
161. Thompson, J. C.: Alterations in gastric secretion after portacaval shunting. Am. J. Surg., 117:854, 1969.
162. Thompson, J. C.: Standard versus experimental surgical procedures in the treatment of duodenal ulcer. Texas Med., 70:51, 1974.
163. Thompson, J. C.: Antral chalone. In Grossman, M. I., et al.: Candidate hormones of the gut. Gastroenterology, 67:730, 1974.
164. Thompson, J. C., and Peskin, G. W.: The intestinal phase of gastric secretion. Am. J. Med. Sci., 241:253, 1961.
165. Thompson, J. C., and Peskin, G. W.: Collective review. The gastric antrum in the operative treatment of duodenal ulcer. Surg. Gynecol. Obstet., 112:205, 1961.
166. Thompson, J. C., Fender, H. R., Watson, L. C., and Villar, H. V.: The effects on gastrin and gastric secretion of five current operations for duodenal ulcer. Ann. Surg., 183:599, 1976.
167. Thompson, J. C., Reeder, D. D., Villar, H. V., and Fender, H. R.: Natural history and experience with diagnosis and treatment of the Zollinger-Ellison syndrome. Surg. Gynecol. Obstet., 140:721, 1975.
168. Thompson, J. C., Rayford, P. L., Ramus, N. I., Fender, H. R., and Villar, H. V.: Patterns of release and uptake of heterogeneous forms of gastrin. In Thompson, J. C. (Ed.): Gastrointestinal Hormones. Austin, University of Texas Press, 1975, p. 125.
169. Thompson, J. C., Reeder, D. D., Bunchman, H. H., Becker, H. D., and Brandt, E. N., Jr.: Effect of secretin on circulating gastrin. Ann. Surg., 176:384, 1972.
170. Thompson, J. C., Becker, H. D., Evans, J. C. W., Hjelmquist, U. B. E., Brandt, E. N., and Reeder, D. D.: Studies on the catabolism of gastrin. In Chey, W. Y., and Brooks, F. P., (Eds.): Endocrinology of the Gut. Thorofare, N. J., Charles B. Slack, Inc., 1974, p. 327.
171. Trudeau, W. L., and McGuigan, J. E.: Relations between serum gastrin levels and rates of gastric hydrochloric acid secretion. N. Engl. J. Med., 284:408, 1971.
172. Van Heerden, J. A., Bernatz, P. E., and Rovelstad, R. A.: The retained gastric antrum: Clinical considerations. Mayo Clin. Proc., 46:25, 1971.
173. Villar, H. V., Fender, H. R., Watson, L. C., and Thompson, J. C.: Emergency diagnosis of upper gastrointestinal bleeding by fiberoptic endoscopy. Ann. Surg., in press.
174. Walsh, J. H., and Grossman, M. I.: Gastrin. N. Engl. J. Med., 202:1324; 1377, 1975.
175. Walters, W., and Lynn, T. E.: Billroth I and Billroth II operations. Arch. Surg., 74:680, 1957.
176. Watson, L. C., Reeder, D. D., Becker, H. D., LaGrone, L., and Thompson, J. C.: Gastrin concentrations in upper gastrointestinal mucosa in dogs. Surgery, 76:419, 1974.
177. Weaver, D. H., Maxwell, J. G., and Castleton, K. B.: Mallory-Weiss syndrome. Am. J. Surg., 118:887, 1969.
178. Weinberg, J. A.: Vagotomy and pyloroplasty in the treatment of duodenal ulcer. Am. J. Surg., 105:347, 1963.
179. Werther, J. L.: The gastric mucosal barrier: Physiological and clinical considerations. Mt. Sinai J. Med. N.Y., 37:482, 1970.
180. West, W. O., Burns, R. O., Daniel, J. M., and Jackson, H. A.: The syndrome of chronic pulmonary disease and gastroduodenal ulceration. Arch. Intern. Med., 103:897, 1959.
181. Whelan, T. J., Jr., and Hamilton, G. B.: Annular pancreas. Ann. Surg., 146:252, 1957.
182. Wheldon, E. J., Venables, C. W., and Johnston, I. D. A.: The nutritional effects of vagotomy and gastro-enterostomy 15–20 years after surgery. Br. J. Surg., 56:706, 1969.
183. Whittaker, L. D., Judd, E. S., and Stauffer, M. H.: Analysis of use of vagotomy with drainage procedure in surgical management of duodenal ulcer. Surg. Gynecol. Obstet., 125:1018, 1967.
184. Williams, J. A., and Cox, A. G. (Eds.): After Vagotomy. London, Butterworth & Company, 1969.
185. Woodward, E. R.: The role of the gastric antrum in the regulation of gastric secretion. Gastroenterology, 38:7, 1960.
186. Yajko, R. D., Norton, L. W., and Eiseman, B.: Current management of upper gastrointestinal bleeding. Ann. Surg., 181:474, 1975.
187. Yalow, R. S., and Berson, S. A.: Radioimmunoassay of gastrin. Gastroenterology, 58:1, 1970.
188. Zollinger, R. M., and Ellison, R. H.: Primary peptic ulcerations of the jejunum associated with islet cell tumor of pancreas. Ann. Surg., 142:709, 1955.
189. Zollinger, R. M., Martin, E. W., Jr., and Carey, L. C.: Observations on the postoperative tumor growth behavior of certain islet cell tumors. Ann. Surg., 184:525–530, 1976.

I

BENIGN TUMORS OF THE STOMACH

Arthur J. Donovan, M.D.

Historical Aspects

Amatus Lusitanus is credited with the recognition of a gastric polyp in 1557,[10] while Quain made an antemortem diagnosis of gastric polyp in 1857.[18] This diagnosis was based on examination of fragments of tissue vomited by a 19-year-old girl. In 1867 Virchow described the pathology of leiomyoma with precision.[24] The report of Menetrier in 1888 has received particular attention.[13] He introduced the terms *polyadenoma polypeux* for the lesion of diffuse polyposis and *polyadenoma en nappe* for giant hyperrugosity.

Incidence

Among tumors of the stomach identified prior to death, 7 per cent are benign.[14] These benign tumors include both neoplasms and space-occupying lesions that may be confused with neoplastic growth. A classification of benign tumors of the stomach is depicted in Table 1. Approximately 40 per cent of these tumors will be polyps and another 40 per cent smooth muscle neoplasms. None of the other tumors individually reaches an incidence of 5 per cent of all benign tumors, indicative of their rarity.[14]

Clinical Syndrome

The benign gastric tumors possess several characteristics in common. Diagnosis is made predominantly in the middle decades of life. They are located most frequently in the antrum or body of the stomach, less frequently in the fundic region, and rarely in the cardiac or pyloric areas. All have a propensity for ulceration of their endogastric surface. Occult loss of blood may ensue with development of iron deficiency anemia and its attendant symptomatology. Deep ulceration of intramural tumors may lead to overt and major hemorrhage. Ulceration may result in a pain complex indistinguishable from that due to peptic ulcer. An ill-defined sense of epigastric distress and fullness may be noted. Mesodermal tumors may reach such size as to be palpable on abdominal examination. If the tumor is located near the cardiac or pyloric orifice, partial obstruction may occur that can progress to complete and unremitting obstruction. Alternatively, if pedunculated, the tumor may prolapse through the orifice, usually pyloric. Intermittent obstruction due to a ball-valve type of action may ensue.

Neither the radiologist nor the endoscopist can distinguish with assurance the precise nature of the benign gastric tumors. Gross characteristics that can distinguish between the various types of polyps do not exist. Gastric varices in patients with portal hypertension should be correctly identified, but instances will occur in which they masquerade radiologically and endoscopically as polyps. The mesodermal derived tumors and heterotopic pancreas are all intramural lesions with quite similar gross features. They may encroach on the lumen of the stomach, or conversely,

protrude exogastrically. The various types of benign hypertrophic gastropathy each result in hyperrugosity.

When a diagnosis of gastric tumor is established by radiological or endoscopic visualization, the question of benignity or malignancy inevitably arises. Absolute radiologic criteria for this differentiation do not exist. Absence of thickening of the gastric wall surrounding the tumor and pliability of the walls as observed fluoroscopically suggest a diagnosis of benignity. An intramural mass with endogastric component and without mucosal ulceration strongly suggests a benign tumor. Gastric washings for exfoliative cytology will be of questionable value. Absence of malignant cells will not exclude malignancy. Biopsy through the fiberoptic gastroscope can be diagnostic. The specific type of polyp may be established. The precise nature of hyperplastic gastropathy may be defined. Biopsy in the case of intramural tumors will usually not be adequate. The biopsy forceps employed with the fiberoptic gastroscope will not be able to penetrate deeply enough to obtain an adequate sample of the tumor for histological examination.

In general, the treatment of benign gastric tumors is extirpative. The indications for extirpation are elimination of the maleffects of the tumor and the necessity to exclude a diagnosis of malignancy. Specific aspects of treatment of the more important benign tumors will be considered separately.

POLYPS

The word polyp, derived from the Greek *polypus*, means many-footed and refers to any growth from a mucous membrane, neoplastic or non-neoplastic. Gastric polyps may be neoplastic, inflammatory, possibly regenerative, or hamartomatous. The terminology employed for gastric polyps is incredibly confusing, reflecting at the least a lack of precise knowledge regarding the pathogenesis of these lesions. Unanimity of opinion on terminology is nonexistant.

Ming and Goldman, acknowledged authorities, in 1964 classified the two most frequent types of gastric polyps as regenerative and adenomatous.[15] They did not consider the more common regenerative polyp to be a neoplasm. In 1973, Ming redesignated the regenerative polyp as hyperplastic adenomatous polyp and the adenomatous polyp as papillary adenoma.[14] With respect to the regenerative nature of the hyperplastic adenomatous polyp, he states that "this aspect is by no means certain."[14] Monaco and associates in discussing "adenomatous polyp" include both the lesion designated as hyperplastic adenomatous polyp by Ming and polyps with a papillary character.[16] In this chapter the terms *hyperplastic adenomatous polyp* and *papillary adenoma* will be employed to distinguish the two principal types of benign epithelial polyps that occur in the stomach. These tumors of epithelial derivation should be distinguished from the inflammatory fibroid polyp, the hamartomatous polyp of Peutz-Jeghers syndrome, the adenoma of familial polyposis, or Gardner's syndrome and islands of residual mucosa that may exist in the presence of otherwise diffuse atrophic gastritis.

Hyperplastic Adenomatous Polyp

Hyperplastic adenomatous polyps comprise between one third and one half of all benign tumors and as many as 90 per cent of all benign polyps of the stomach.[14] Most often solitary, these tumors may be sessile or pedunculated. They are the result of glandular proliferation, are lined by columnar mucous-secreting cells, possess an abundant stroma, and may contain areas of cystic degeneration. Their size varies from a few millimeters to several centimeters. The majority are less than 2 cm. in diameter. Pedunculation occurs predominantly in larger polyps. Atrophic gastritis, pernicious anemia, and intestinalization of the gastric mucosa are each associated with hyperplastic adenomatous polyp of the stomach. Achlorhydria is present in more than 90 per cent of cases.[11, 16] Whether these polyps are regenerative or neoplastic has not been established.

The antrum is the site of predeliction for solitary hyperplastic adenomatous polyp. Multiple polyps may occur randomly distributed throughout the stomach, or a myriad of polyps may be closely aligned in one portion of the stomach. When innumerable polyps are present throughout the stomach, the term polyposis is usually employed. Figure 1 is a reproduction of a radiogram of a solitary pedunculated polyp. Figure 2A depicts the radiological appearance of multiple hyperplastic adenomatous polyps and Figure 2B, the gross characteristics of such polyps.

Intense interest has existed and conflicting opinions have been expressed regarding the malignant potential of hyperplastic adenomatous polyp of the stomach. Approximately one third coexist in stomachs that are the site of invasive carcinoma.[22] These observations suggest that the mucosa of the achlorhydric patient with intestinalization of gastric mucosa is fertile soil for the development of both frank cancer and hyperplastic adenomatous polyp. This is consistent with the increased incidence of gastric cancer in the achlorhydric patient.[19]

Monaco and associates in 153 cases observed focal atypia in the tip of 10 per cent of "adenomatous polyps."[16] One case of microinvasive carcinoma was documented. Metastatic disease, including lymph node metastases, was not identified in any instance in which "adenomatous polyp" was the only gastric neoplasm present. Their cases included only three polyps with a papillary character.

The evolving evidence would not support the concept that hyperplastic adenomatous polyp is in itself a premalignant lesion. Reports that include cases of hyperplastic adenomatous polyps alone and hyperplastic adenomatous polyp associated with invasive cancer have undoubtedly contributed to the confusion surrounding this issue. A diagnosis of hyperplastic adenomatous polyp should arouse a high index of suspicion of concurrent or subsequent independent adenocarcinoma.

Papillary (Villous) Adenoma

Papillary adenoma of the stomach is sessile or pedunculated, composed of multiple frondlike processes, and is a potentially malignant lesion. A photomicrograph of a papillary adenoma of the stomach is depicted in Figure 3, as contrasted with a photomicrograph of a hyperplastic adenomatous polyp. The papillary adenoma most frequently develops in the achlorhydric patient with atrophic gastritis and intestinalization of the gastric mucosa. Ten of 49 "polyps" reported by Ming and Goldman were of the papillary type. Invasive carcinoma was present in 2 of these 10 cases.[15] The similarity with current concepts regarding villous adenoma of the colon is remarkable.[2] Papillary adenoma, hyperplastic adenomatous polyp, and the inflammatory fibroid polyp, which will be discussed subsequently, may all coexist in the same stomach.

Inflammatory Fibroid Polyp

Inflammatory fibroid polyp is probably a localized form of eosinophilic gastritis. It may occur as a single or as multiple polyps and is predominantly antral in location. The polyp may be sessile or possess a short stalk.

The histological pattern of the inflammatory fibroid polyp is one of fibrous tissue, thin-walled blood vessels, and dense infiltration with eosinophils, lymphocytes, histiocytes, and plasma cells. Located predominantly in the submucosa, the lesion projects into the gastric lumen.

Helwig and Rainer prefer the term *inflammatory fibroid polyp* for this lesion,[8] and Ming concurs.[14] This term is selected in preference to eosinophilic granu-

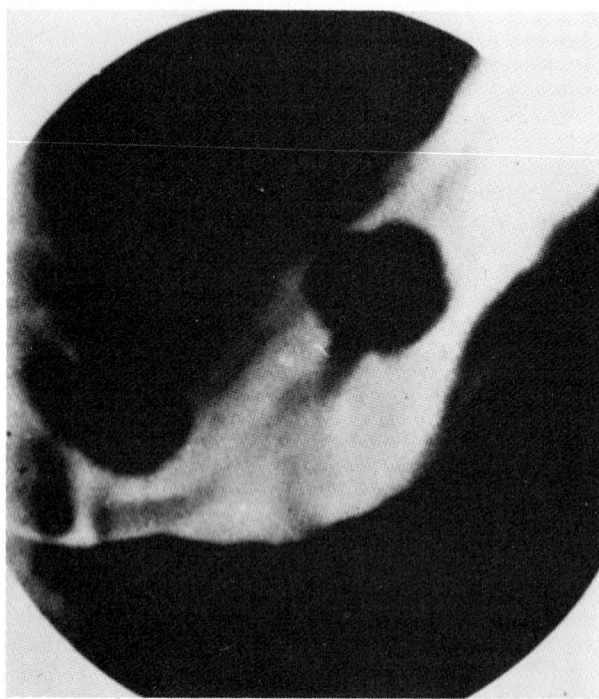

Figure 1. A pedunculated polyp located in the gastric antrum. The radiological image does not permit a precise diagnosis as to type of polyp. (From Frik, W.: Neoplastic diseases of the stomach. *In* Margulis, A. R., and Burhenne, H. J. (Eds.): Alimentary Tract Roentgenology, 2nd ed., St. Louis, The C. V. Mosby Co., 1973, p. 699.)

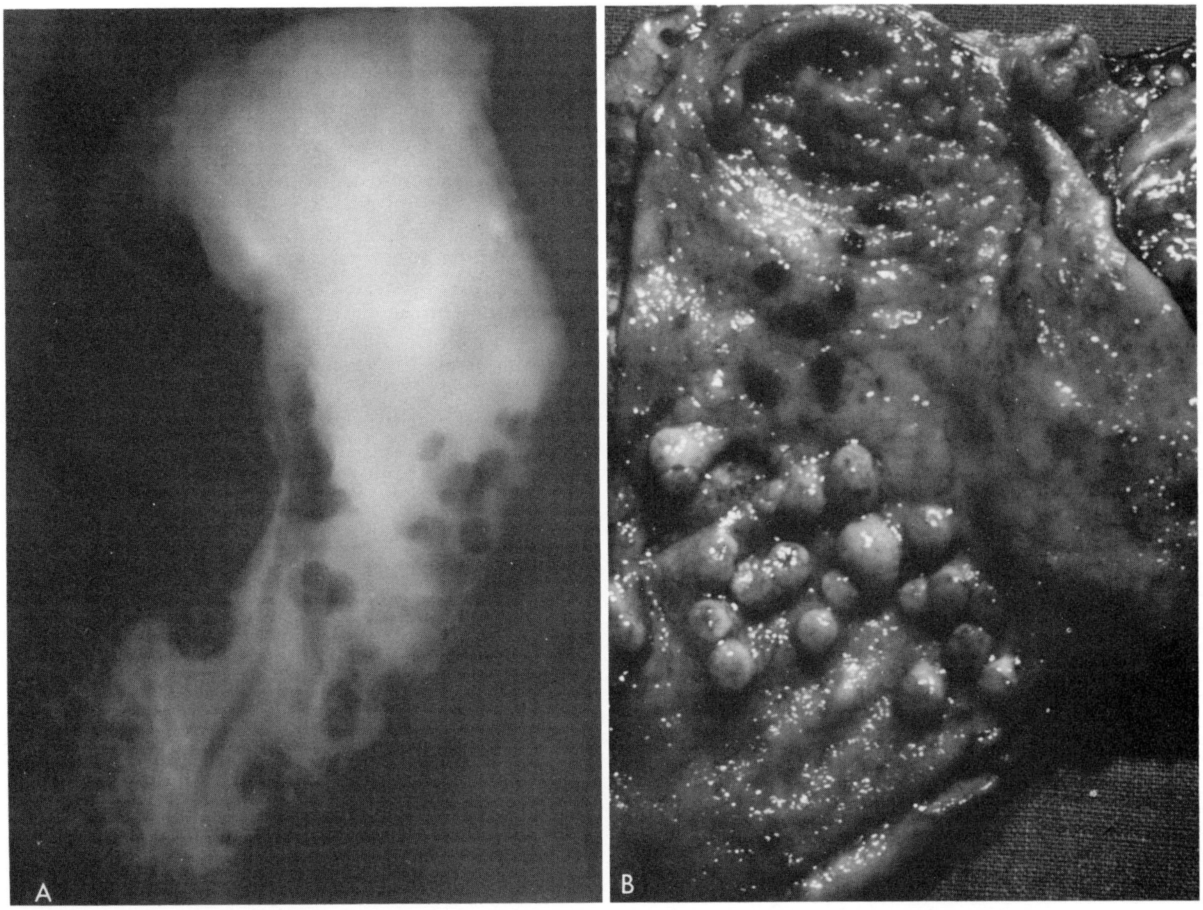

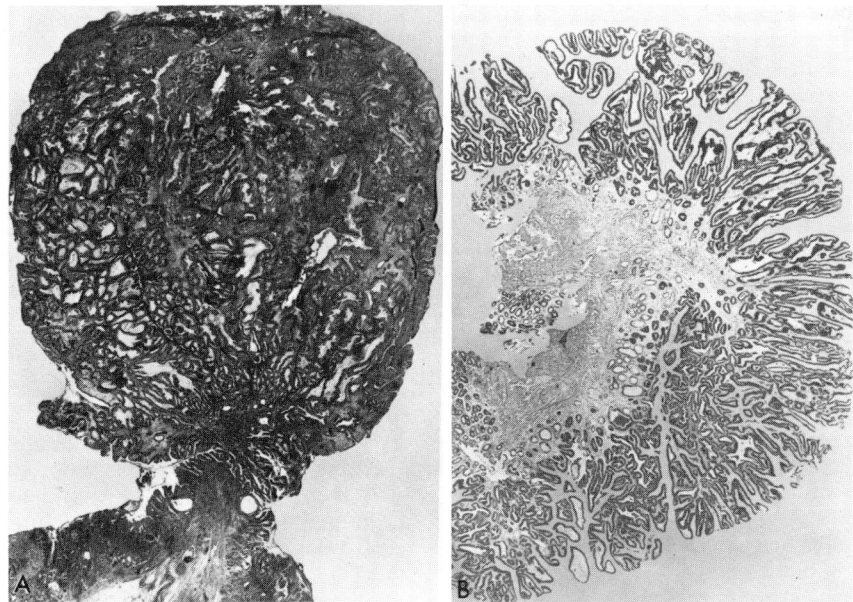

Figure 2. *A,* The radiological image of multiple polyps located in the distal stomach. *B,* The gross characteristics of multiple hyperplastic, adenomatous polyps located in the distal stomach. The polyp at 11 o'clock possesses a short pedicle.

Figure 3. *A,* The microscopic appearance of the hyperplastic, adenomatous polyp and (*B*) the microscopic appearance of a papillary (villous) adenoma. The latter lesion is potentially malignant. (From Ming, S.-C.: Tumors of the esophagus and stomach, 2nd series. Washington, D.C., Armed Forces Institute of Pathology, 1973, pp. 120 and 135.)

loma, polypoid fibroma, or fibrinous polyp. The pathogenesis of the inflammatory fibroid polyp is unknown, but the term in itself denotes an inflammatory process. An allergic cause for inflammatory fibroid polyp has not been established, and peripheral eosinophilia usually is not present. This is in contradistinction to diffuse eosinophilic gastritis, in which peripheral eosinophilia is usually present and which probably has an allergic basis.

On occasion seen in association with pernicious anemia, a dominant relationship of inflammatory fibroid polyp to this disease or its associated atrophic gastritis has not been established. Helwig and Rainer provide arguments against a vascular or neurogenic origin of the tumor.[8]

Treatment

A polyp less than 2 cm. in diameter can be observed.[11] The lesion can be studied by serial radiological upper gastrointestinal examinations for evidence of growth. When a polyp exceeds 2 cm. in diameter, a histological diagnosis must be established. The radiologist cannot distinguish the innocuous hyperplastic adenomatous polyp or inflammatory fibroid polyp from the potentially lethal papillary adenoma or a polypoid carcinoma.

Modern techniques of endoscopy will facilitate the diagnosis and treatment of gastric polyps. By the combination of direct visualization and biopsy, the precise nature of the lesion may be established. Pedunculated lesions can be totally excised by use of the snare and cautery and can be submitted for histological examination.

Further surgical treatment is indicated (1) when the benignity of all pedunculated polyps greater than 2 cm. in diameter has not been established and definitive treatment completed by endoscopic methods; (2) when examination of the tissue removed endoscopically arouses a question of malignancy; or (3) when a sessile lesion is present that exceeds 2 cm. in diameter.

Individual judgment is necessary regarding the specific surgical procedure that is indicated for gastric polyp(s). A solitary sessile lesion is best removed by wedge excision with a margin of surrounding gastric wall and submitted for frozen section examination. The further surgical procedure will be dictated by the nature of the lesion. If multiple polyps involve the distal stomach, a subtotal gastrectomy is advisable. Should a few polyps remain in the proximal pouch, these are removed by endogastric amputation and submitted for frozen section examination. Admittedly, frozen section diagnosis may be difficult in these circumstances, but to perform a total gastrectomy for benign polyp(s) would be a serious surgical error. When 4 to 6 polyps are randomly located in the stomach, a gastrotomy is indicated, with endogastric amputation, frozen section, and further treatment dictated by the nature of the lesions. A group of closely aligned polyps in the body of the stomach can be excised by wide local excision. In cases of diffuse polyposis that includes the fundus of the stomach, a total gastrectomy is usually indicated. Detection of coexisting adenocarcinoma is almost impossible in diffuse gastric polyposis.

INTRAMURAL TUMORS

Smooth Muscle Neoplasms

Among benign gastric neoplasms of mesodermal origin, those derived from smooth muscle are the most common, representing over 90 per cent of such tumors. A distinction must be made between the incidence of leiomyoma identified by assiduous examination of the stomach at autopsy and the number of such neoplasms that reach a size sufficient to produce clinical symptoms. Meissner in an autopsy study identified a smooth muscle neoplasm in the gastric wall in 46 per cent of cases, the overwhelming majority less than 1 cm. in diameter.[12] Conversely, considerably less than 2 per cent of gastric neoplasms that are resected surgically will be of smooth muscle origin.

At an early stage of growth the leiomyoma is intramural. With expansion the tumor may protrude into the gastric lumen as a submucosal mass or alternatively develop as an exogastric mass. These types of presentation were described by Virchow as inneren (submucosal) or ausseren (subserosal).[24] Submucosal expansion is by far the more common mode of growth. On rare occasion a dumbbell tumor will occur with both submucosal and subserosal components. The tumor may be smooth or lobulated.

Central mucosal ulceration occurs in approximately one half of submucosal leiomyomas that are diagnosed ante mortem. This ulceration does not appear to be totally a factor of necrosis of tumor that has outgrown its blood supply. Ulceration may be present in smaller tumors and absent in very large tumors. Areas of necrosis and cavitation may occur within the tumor. Focal calcification may develop. Large subserosal leiomyomas with necrosis may communicate with the gastric lumen through one or more sinuses. Alternatively, rupture into the peritoneal cavity may occur. In Figure 4A is depicted the gross appearance of leiomyoma with deep central ulceration and in Figure 4B, the radiological image of such a lesion.

Gastric leiomyomas are not encapsulated, and tumor cells at the margin may intermingle with cells of the surrounding gastric wall. This is one factor that has led to confusion in the distinction of benign from malignant leiomyoma. On microscopic examination the leiomyoma is found to be composed of spindle cells that, in contradistinction to uterine leiomyoma, lack myofibrils. Pallisading may occur, which leads to confusion between leiomyoma and neurilemoma. The neurilemoma is always encapsulated.

The histological picture in benign smooth muscle tumors may be bizarre. Stout has reported 69 cases of smooth muscle tumor in which the cells are polyhedral and rounded rather than elongated and are without trace of smooth muscle fibers. A clear zone surrounds the nucleus. Only two of these tumors manifested malignant behavior.[23] The term leiomyoblastoma has been applied to these particular tumors.

Histologic criteria that sharply separate smooth muscle tumors into benign and malignant variants do not exist. Pleomorphism and presence of mitoses suggest malignancy, but metastases can occur in the case of a leiomyoma that is benign by all histologic

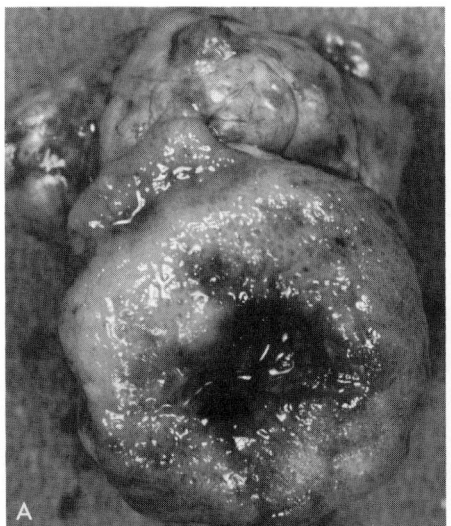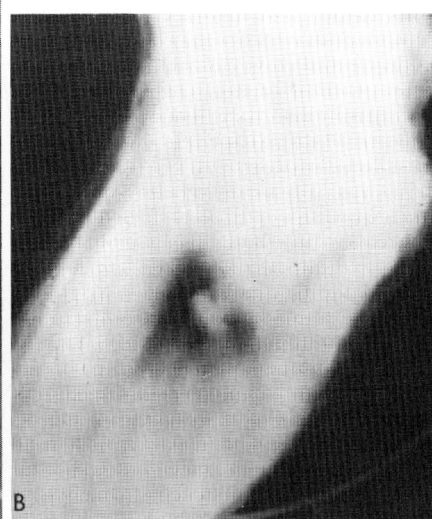

Figure 4. *A*, A leiomyoma of the stomach with central mucosal ulceration. The tumor has been removed with a rim of surrounding gastric wall. The radiogram (*B*) depicts the filling defect created on the upper gastrointestinal series by a leiomyoma. The barium-filled central ulcer is apparent. This characteristic image can be compared to a "doughnut," with the tumor the "doughnut" and the barium-filled ulcer crater the "hole." (From Frik, W.: Neoplastic diseases of the stomach. *In* Margulis, A. R., and Burhenne, H. J. (Eds.): Alimentary Tract Roentgenology, 2nd ed. St. Louis, The C. V. Mosby Co., 1973, p. 702.)

criteria. Misclassification has undoubtedly occurred in some reported cases.

Golden and Stout state that "if two or more mitoses per high power field are present, one can feel fairly secure in predicting malignancy."[7] On this basis they classified two thirds of their cases as malignant. Giberson and associates identified metastases at the time of surgery in only six of forty cases classified histologically as malignant leiomyoma.[5] Twelve additional cases subsequently manifested metastases. In the remaining twenty-two cases with a histological diagnosis of malignancy, behavior confirmatory of this diagnosis was never observed. Thus, the aggressiveness of even those tumors reported as malignant is low. As a consequence, the term malignant leiomyoma is usually employed rather than the more ominous leiomyosarcoma.

In the final analysis the only conclusive evidence of malignancy is metastasis of the tumor or invasive intragastric growth, which is noted either during a surgical procedure or in the natural course of the disease following surgical resection. The malignant variant of leiomyoma may invade adjacent organs, rarely invade lymph nodes by direct extension, be seeded in the peritoneal cavity, and metastasize to the liver or on an unusual occasion to the lung. All smooth muscle tumors of the stomach should be considered malignant until time and the demonstrated behavior of the tumor provide proof to the contrary.

The basic principle in surgical treatment of smooth muscle tumors of the stomach is local excision with a 2- to 3-cm. margin of surrounding gastric wall. Enucleation is an inappropriate method of treatment. The excised specimen should be submitted to the pathologist. Should a histological diagnosis of malignancy be made on the basis of examination of frozen section, an additional margin of gastric wall may be excised.

In the instance of very large tumors or a prepyloric tumor, a standard gastric resection may be the most expeditious form of excision. With tumors in the body of the stomach, local excision is feasible. The more difficult decision is required when the tumor encroaches on the esophagogastric junction. Resection of the esophagogastric junction for a benign leiomyoma would be a surgical misadventure, and a conservative approach is indicated.

Regional lymphadenectomy is not indicated. Even if malignant, metastasis to lymph nodes is rare.

Heterotopic Pancreas

A mass of pancreatic tissue may be present within the wall of the stomach, almost invariably in the antrum or the prepyloric area. Usually less than 3 cm. in diameter, the tumor may project into the lumen of the stomach and will on occasion cause pyloric obstruction.

Technically a hamartoma, the mass of heterotopic pancreas is composed of glands and intervening connective tissue. Islets of Langerhans may be absent. If present, their number is generally less than in normal pancreas. Ductal dilatation may be present and cyst formation may occur. The heterotopic pancreas characteristically has a large central duct that may fill with contrast media and be demonstrable on radiograms obtained during an upper gastrointestinal series.[17]

Brunner's Gland Adenoma

Brunner's gland adenoma may occur in the antrum or juxtapyloric region representing heterotopic location of a hamartomatous lesion, usually occurring in the duodenum. The Brunner's gland adenoma is composed of intermingled glands and bands of smooth muscle fibers. Islands of pancreatic tissue may be present. Certain of these lesions may be referred to as adenomyoma.[6]

HYPERPLASTIC GASTROPATHY

The general term hyperplastic gastropathy refers to a condition in which there is an enlargement of rugal folds in the stomach. The etiology of the hyperplastic process is varied.

Menetrier in 1888 described two processes in the stomach—one designated as polyadenoma polypeux and the other polyadenoma en nappe.[13] The term Menetrier's disease is by general agreement now limited to one specific form of polyadenoma en nappe or giant rugosity.[21]

Menetrier's Disease

Menetrier's disease is a process in which there is a marked proliferation of mucous-secreting cells in the stomach with atrophy of the chief and parietal cells. Intramural cysts may form. Edema is prominent. The gastric wall is thickened and the mucosa thrown into folds that resemble cerebral convolutions. Nodular areas on these folds may resemble sessile polyps. The cardia, fundus, and body of the stomach are usually diffusely involved and the antrum spared. A localized form may occur. Patients with Menetrier's disease are usually achlorhydric. Carcinoma of the stomach may occur. The gross features of Menetrier's disease are depicted in Figure 5A and radiologic image of hyper-rugosity in Figure 5B.

An essential component of Menetrier's disease is a protein-losing enteropathy and marked hypoproteinemia.[3] Weight loss, edema, and malnutrition are common. Epigastric distress, nausea, vomiting, and gastrointestinal bleeding may occur.

Menetrier's disease may be diagnosed at any age. The etiology is unknown. Spontaneous resolution with development of atrophic gastritis has been reported.[1, 4]

Treatment of Menetrier's disease is importantly related to the debilitating effects of the protein-losing enteropathy. In view of reports of spontaneous resolution, nutritional support and a period of observation are justified if a deep biopsy of the stomach has established the precise diagnosis based on the demonstration of the typical histological pattern of the disease. Surgical treatment is usually necessary, and total gastrectomy most often is the indicated form of therapy.

Pseudolymphoma

Extensive lymphocytic infiltration of a segment of the stomach may occur, dominantly in association with benign gastric ulcer. A large segment of the stomach may be involved. Submucosal nodules, diffuse thickening, or enlarged rugal folds may be present. The infiltrate has a follicular pattern leading to confusion with follicular lymphoma. In fact, review of series of gastric lymphoma invariably has resulted in reclassification of cases previously diagnosed as lymphoma into the category of pseudolymphoma. The converse may also be true. The distinction between lymphoma and pseudolymphoma can be extraordinarily difficult.[9] The reasonably favorable prognosis reported for gastric lymphoma may reflect inclusion in some series of a number of cases of pseudolymphoma.

Other Causes

Hyperrugosity may occur in association with gastric cancer and malignant lymphoma. Another very dis-

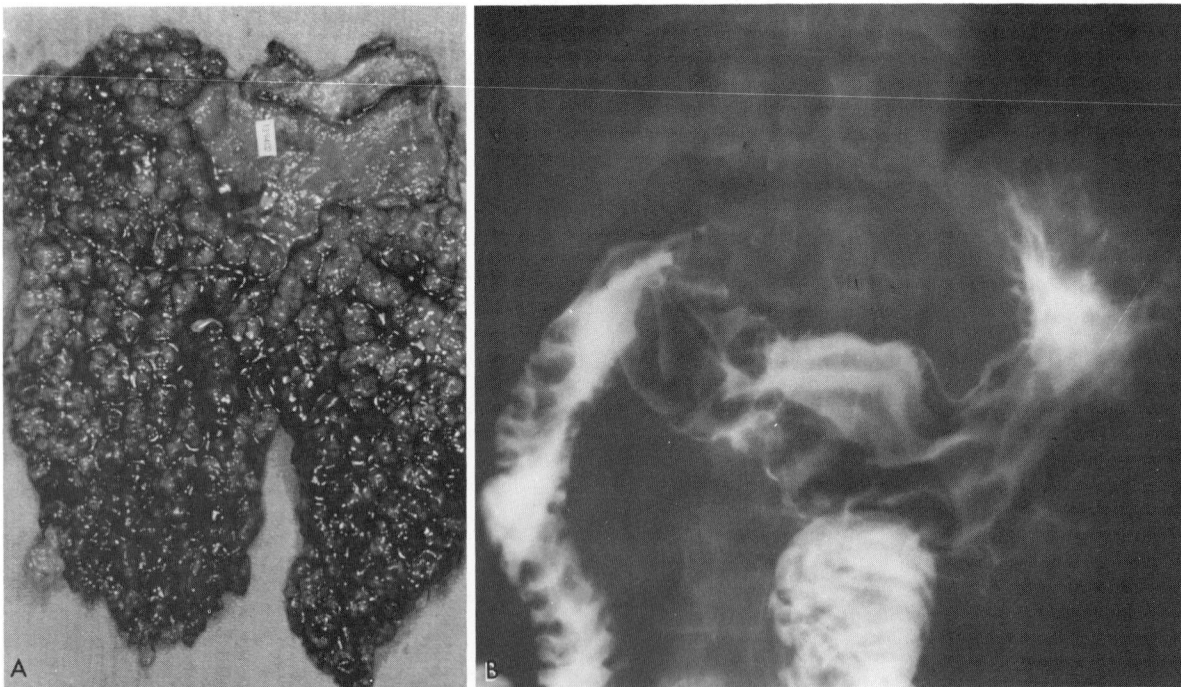

Figure 5. A gross appearance of the giant hyperrugosity of the gastric mucosa in a case of Menetrier's disease. The relative sparing of the antrum is apparent at the top of the specimen. B, The radiological appearance of hyperrugosity in Menetrier's disease. This radiological image is similar to that visualized in other types of hyperrugosity.

tinct form of hyperrugosity is that in which there is non-neoplastic proliferation of all epithelial elements—mucus-secreting cells as in Menetrier's disease but also parietal cells and chief cells. This was referred to by Schindler as the glandular type of "chronic hypertrophic gastritis."[20] The lesion is not inflammatory, and thus the term *gastropathy* is preferred to gastritis.

Subsequent study has revealed that at least certain cases with this glandular form of hyperplastic gastropathy represent instances of stimulation of the gastric epithelium by gastrin produced by a non-beta islet cell tumor of the pancreas—the Zollinger-Ellison syndrome.[25] In cases of glandular hyperplastic gastropathy in which a diagnosis of gastrin-secreting tumor is not established, one must question whether the stomach is responding to yet another unrecognized humoral stimulant.

CYSTIC TUMORS

Obstruction of a mucous-secreting gland can result in a mucocele in the gastric wall. The more important cystic lesion is a reduplication cyst. Usually encountered in the distal stomach, it may or may not communicate with the gastric lumen.

SELECTED REFERENCES

Ming, S.-C.: Tumors of the Esophagus and Stomach, 2nd series. Washington D.C., Armed Forces Institute of Pathology, 1973.
This fascicle from the excellent series on tumor pathology published by the Armed Forces Institute of Pathology is a compendium of information on the pathology of all types of benign tumors of the stomach. Both neoplastic and non-neoplastic tumors are reviewed. References are provided that facilitate access to the important original papers on various subjects. The confusing subject of gastric polyp is presented clearly and differing viewpoints discussed.

Monaco, A. P., Roth, S. I., Castleman, B., and Welch, C. E.: Adenomatous polyps of the stomach. Cancer, 15:456, 1962.
This is a review of experience at the Massachusetts General Hospital with gastric polyps. Data is presented to support the contention that the adenomatous polyp is in itself not a premalignant lesion. Confusion that has existed regarding this matter is clarified. Specific therapeutic recommendations are included.

Palmer, E. D.: Benign intramural tumors of the stomach with special reference to gross pathology. Medicine, 30:81, 1951.
This is an exhaustive review of all benign intramural tumors of the stomach, neoplastic and non-neoplastic. The data collected on incidence and pathology are encyclopedic. Options in therapy are not considered in detail.

Stout, A. P.: (A) Smooth muscle tumors of the gastrointestinal tract and retroperitoneal tissues. Surg. Gynecol. Obstet., 73:784, 1941. (B) Bizarre smooth muscle tumors of the stomach. Cancer, 15:400, 1962.
These two articles by Dr. Arthur Purdy Stout are derived from experience in the Laboratory of Surgical Pathology at Columbia University. They provide excellent descriptions of smooth muscle tumors of the stomach. Clinical and pathological considerations

with respect to benignity or malignancy of the smooth muscle tumors are particularly well discussed.

REFERENCES

1. Burns, B., and Gay, B. B.: Menetrier's disease of the stomach in children. Am. J. Roentgenol., 103:300, 1968.
2. Castleman, B., and Erickstein, H. L.: Do adenomatous polyps of the stomach become malignant? N. Engl. J. Med., 267:469, 1962.
3. Citrin, Y., Sterling, K., and Halstead, J. A.: The mechanism of hypoproteinemia associated with giant hypertrophy of the gastric mucosa. N. Engl. J. Med., 257:906, 1957.
4. Frank, B. W., and Kern, F.: Menetrier's disease: Spontaneous metamorphosis of giant hypertrophy of the gastric mucosa to atrophic gastritis. Gastroenterology, 53:953, 1967.
5. Giberson, R., Dockerty, M. B., and Gray, H. K.: Leiomyosarcoma of the stomach; clinicopathologic study of 40 cases. Surg. Gynecol. Obstet., 98:186, 1954.
6. Goldberg, H. I., and Margulis, A. R.: Adenomyoma of the stomach; report of a case. Am. J. Roentgenol., 96:382, 1966.
7. Golden, T., and Stout, A. P.: Smooth muscle tumors of the gastrointestinal tract and retroperitoneal tissues. Surg. Gynecol. Obstet., 73:784, 1941.
8. Helwig, E., and Rainer, A.: Inflammatory fibroid polyps of the stomach. Surg. Gynecol Obstet., 96:355, 1953.
9. Jacobs, D. S.: Primary gastric malignant lymphoma and pseudolymphoma. Am. J. Clin. Pathol., 40:379, 1963.
10. Lusitanus, A.: Curatorium medicinalium centuria septima, curatio 23, p. 58: Venet, 1653 (Originally published 1557) cited by Marshak.[11]
11. Marshak, R., and Feldman, F.: Gastric polyps. Am. J. Dig. Dis., 10:909, 1965.
12. Meissner, W. A.: Leiomyoma of the stomach. Arch. Pathol., 38:207, 1944.
13. Menetrier, P.: Des polyadenomes gastriques et de leurs rapport avec la cancer de l'estomac. Arch. Physiol. Norm. Pathol., 1:32, 1888.
14. Ming, S.-C.: Tumors of the esophagus and stomach, 2nd series. Washington, D.C., Armed Forces Institute of Pathology, 1973, pp. 82, 101, 125, and 127.
15. Ming, S. C., and Goldman, H.: Gastric polyps, a histogenetic classification and its relation to carcinoma. Cancer, 18:721, 1965.
16. Monaco, A. P., Roth, S. I., Castleman, B., and Welch, C. E.: Adenomatous polyps of the stomach. Cancer, 15:456, 1962.
17. Palmer, E.: Benign intramural tumors of the stomach; a review with special reference to gross pathology. Medicine, 30:81, 1951.
18. Quain, R.: Case of polypus ejected from stomach. Trans. Pathol. Soc. London, 8:219, 1957.
19. Rigler, L. G., and Kaplan, H. A.: Pernicious anemia and tumors of the stomach. J. Natl. Cancer Inst., 7:327, 1947.
20. Schindler, R.: Gastric carcinoma and gastritis with reference to coexistence of carcinoma and chronic hypertrophic glandular gastritis. Am. J. Dig. Dis., 10:607, 1965.
21. Scott, W. H., Shull, H. J., Law, D., IV, Burko, H., and Page, D.: Surgical management of Menetrier's disease with protein-losing gastropathy. Ann. Surg., 181:765, 1975.
22. Stewart, M. J.: Observations on the relation of malignant disease to benign tumors of the gastrointestinal tract. Br. Med. J., 2:567, 1929.
23. Stout, A. P.: Bizarre smooth muscle tumors of the stomach. Cancer, 15:400, 1962.
24. Virchow, R. L. K.: Die krankhaften Geschwulste. Berlin, A. Hirschwald, 1867.
25. Zollinger, R. M., and Moore, F. T.: Zollinger-Ellison syndrome comes of age; recognition of the complete clinical spectrum and its management. J.A.M.A., 204:361, 1968.

II ———————————————————————————————

LYMPHOMAS OF THE STOMACH

Richard C. Karl, M.D.

Malignant lymphomas may involve the stomach as a localized primary lesion or more commonly as part of a generalized disease. Postmortem examination of 251 adults dying of generalized lymphoma revealed secondary gastric involvement by the tumor in 29.4 per cent.[10] Primary lymphomas of the stomach compose a small but significant proportion of all malignant gastric tumors, constituting 4.5 per cent of all gastric neoplasms[13] and approximately 60 per cent of all sarcomas of the stomach.[8] Clinically, primary lymphomas usually cannot be differentiated from the more frequently occurring gastric carcinomas. Because a more favorable response to treatment of gastric lymphomas may be anticipated than with carcinoma, it is essential that these lesions be identified and appropriate therapy instituted. Criteria for establishing the diagnosis of primary lymphoma require that the patient's symptoms be exclusively or predominantly gastrointestinal and that the lesion be limited to the stomach or originate there. The possibility of secondary involvement of the stomach by a more generalized disease must be ruled out by appropriate evaluation.

PATHOLOGY

Gross Findings

Primary gastric lymphomas may occur in any portion of the stomach. The distal part of the stomach appears to be involved more frequently. The lesions may extend into the adjacent duodenum or esophagus. Although the tumors may be small and confined to the submucosa and mucosa, often they are large and occasionally multicentric. They may extend contiguously into adjacent viscera. Perigastric lymph node metastases are common. However, pronounced regional adenopathy due to reactive hyperplasia may be present.

Friedman[4] has classified the gross morphological characteristics of primary gastric lymphoma as follows:

1. Infiltrative—a localized or diffusely infiltrative lesion with thickened rugal folds. Occasionally this form may appear as a flat, annular, rubbery mass.

2. Ulcerative—a shallow ulcerating lesion characterizes this form. The ulcers vary from 3 to 18 cm. in diameter. The necrotic base of the ulcer, accompanied by raised indurated edges, makes this lesion similar to carcinoma in appearance. This was the most common type of gross appearance noted in Friedman's series.

3. Nodular—characterized by multiple nodules 0.5 to 4 cm. in diameter scattered in the submucosa. The nodules often extend to the mucosal or serosal surface. Superficial or deep ulceration is common.

4. Polypoid—a large polypoid, predominantly extraluminal mass, spongy in consistency and often deeply ulcerated. This type often involves adjacent structures.

5. Combined—a form in which 2 or 3 of the previously mentioned types occur in one specimen.

Histological Findings

When strict criteria are used, the incidence of primary Hodgkin's disease of the stomach in all series is low. The terminology applied to the histopathological classification of non-Hodgkin's lymphomas has been variable and confusing. The histological classification that currently is accepted is based on the identification of cell types, their degree of differentiation, and their patterns of proliferation (diffuse or nodular).[11] The cytologic types are as follows:

1. Malignant lymphoma, well-differentiated lymphocytic type—the proliferation of mature lymphocytes that do not possess the usual cytologic characteristics of malignant cells.

2. Malignant lymphoma, poorly differentiated, lymphocytic type—the lymphocytes show varying degrees of immaturity. This type roughly corresponds with what many have previously been referred to as large-cell or lymphoblastic lymphosarcoma.

3. Malignant lymphoma, mixed-cell type—a neoplastic proliferation of both lymphocytes and histiocytes without appreciable preponderance of either cell type. These tumors usually have a nodular pattern.

4. Malignant lymphoma, histiocytic type—a proliferation of neoplastic histiocytes in various stages of maturation and differentiation.

5. Malignant lymphoma, undifferentiated type—a neoplastic proliferation of primitive reticular cells without appreciable differentiation along histiocytic or lymphocytic lines.

Each of these cytologic types is followed by the term "nodular" or "diffuse," depending on the pattern of proliferation of the cells. The employment of this histological classification will undoubtedly improve the clinicopathological correlation, which has heretofore been unsatisfactory.

CLINICAL FEATURES

In many reported series there has been a remarkable consistency in the clinical features of the disorder. The average age of onset is about 56 years. In most series the age range has been 28 to 78 years, with greatest incidence in the sixth decade. There are isolated instances of children and patients over 90 years of age presenting with primary lymphoma of the stomach. In all series males predominate with a ratio of about 1.7:1.

Symptoms

No distinctive clinical features have been observed. Usually symptoms have been present for a matter of months, occasionally longer. The most common complaint is abdominal pain. This is usually epigastric or periumbilical in location. In some instances it is similar to the pain characteristic of peptic ulcer, aggravated by hunger and relieved by food and antacids. Weight loss is another frequently encountered symptom. In most instances it is moderate in amount, but in some it may be pronounced. Anorexia, nausea, and vomiting occur in about half the patients. Dysphagia is occasionally experienced in association with lesions in the cardia of the stomach. Gastrointestinal hemorrhage may be severe enough to produce hematemesis or melena. Symptoms due to spontaneous perforation of the tumor into the general peritoneal cavity or into adjacent colon or small intestine are occasionally encountered.

Physical Examination

In contrast to patients with carcinoma of the stomach, those with primary gastric lymphoma often present in good physical condition without the stigmata of anemia and cachexia. An upper abdominal mass, which may be large, has been noted in about 25 per cent of patients with primary lymphoma of the stomach. Abdominal tenderness, hepatomegaly, and splenomegaly may be observed separately or in combination.

Laboratory Examination

Routine laboratory studies generally are unremarkable. Stools often contain occult blood. Anemia may be present and in some patients severe. Gastric analysis may reveal anacidity or normal and even high values of free hydrochloric acid.

X-Ray Studies

The roentgenologic findings are usually nonspecific and may suggest gastric carcinoma, benign gastric ulcer, and, in cases with the diffuse infiltrative lesions, hypertrophic gastritis, Menetrier's disease, and granulomatous diseases. On occasion no abnormality may be demonstrated. In most instances the findings are those of a malignant tumor that may or may not be ulcerated. Extension of the tumor across the pylorus to involve the duodenum suggests malignant lymphoma.[7]

Endoscopy

Endoscopy is being employed with increasing frequency in an attempt to establish a diagnosis of lymphoma of the stomach preoperatively. The reported experiences with occasional exceptions have been disappointing. The gross appearances of these tumors are frequently not diagnostic, and when the lesion is submucosal, positive biopsies of the underlying neoplasm may be difficult to obtain. When the lymphoma presents as an ulcerating lesion, brush cytology and biopsy may be positive.

Exfoliative Cytology

The cytologic diagnosis of lymphoma of the stomach utilizing gastric washings has not been accurate. When special care is taken in obtaining specimens, some investigators have been able to attain success rates on the order of 65 per cent.[9] Experience with newer endoscopic techniques for obtaining cytologic washings directly from the tumor site in gastric lymphoma has not been extensive enough to evaluate. It would appear to be a promising approach.

TREATMENT

The treatment of primary gastric lymphoma is surgical resection whenever this is technically feasible. Usually a precise diagnosis has not been established preoperatively. Often the gross appearance of a lymphomatous lesion as noted at surgical exploration is undistinguishable from that of carcinoma of the stomach. Because the therapeutic response to treatment of primary gastric lymphoma is so much more favorable than for carcinoma of the stomach, it is essential that all apparent unresectable gastric malignancies be biopsied. If the lesion proves to be an extensive primary lymphoma, surgical extirpation may be warranted and certainly irradiation therapy should be given postoperatively. In some cases of diffusely infiltrating lymphomatous lesions, palpation of the stomach may not reveal any obvious tumor mass. In such instances, gastrotomy and full-thickness biopsy of hypertrophic gastric rugae may provide the diagnosis.

The principles in the surgical management of primary lymphoma of the stomach are essentially those employed in management of gastric carcinoma. Often these lesions metastasize to regional lymph nodes, and not infrequently the tumors involve adjacent structures or extend beyond the stomach into the duodenum or esophagus. The margins of localized lymphomas may be indistinct. The tumors often extend microscopically for some distance beyond the gross limits of the lesions. For this reason it is essential to obtain frozen section biopsies of the distal and proximal margins of the removed specimens. If tumor is present in these biopsies, a wider resection should be performed.

An aggressive surgical approach is warranted for lesions limited to the stomach and adjacent lymph nodes. In a series of 66 patients[1] who underwent surgical exploration for this disorder, the resectability rate was 57 per cent. The perigastric lymph nodes contained metastases in 52 per cent of the patients undergoing resection. There was a 5-year survival rate of 40 per cent in those patients undergoing gastrectomy, 10 of whom had total gastrectomies. When the tumor extends beyond the confines of the stomach into the adjacent viscera, however, the increased mortality associated with extended resections designed to remove all tumor-bearing tissue has raised the question of the validity of performing such procedures. Such lesions may be better treated with radiotherapy.

Opinion varies regarding the value of postoperative irradiation. Some recommend that radiation therapy be used only when the lesion is unresectable, when there are known remnants of unresected tumor, or when recurrence develops. Others feel strongly that all patients should receive postoperative irradiation whether or not tumor has been left behind or the perigastric nodes contained tumor. Crile[2] stressed that it was not possible for the surgeon to estimate accurately the presence or extent of lymph node metastases. Loehr[6] reported that the longest survivals occurred in those undergoing definitive resection of the lymphoma followed by a "curative" tumor dose (3000 to 4000 rads) of x-ray. It is probable that the combined therapy will achieve better results.

The results obtainable with irradiation alone are difficult to assess. It is usually employed adjunctively following resection, or it is offered as the primary modality of treatment in those with advanced nonresectable disease. Lack of information concerning results in comparative patient groups makes it difficult to evaluate the efficacy of radiotherapy as the primary approach to the treatment of gastric lymphomas at all clinical stages, including those which also are amenable to resection. There are isolated reports of long-term survival in patients with unresectable lesions following radiotherapy only. In those lesions too diffuse for effective x-ray therapy, some combination of chemotherapeutic agents may be effective.

Factors that influence a favorable therapeutic outcome generally are dependent upon the extent of the tumor when initially treated and the histological character of the tumor. Lesions confined to the stomach and those with the greatest cellular differentiation have the most favorable prognosis. The range of 5-year survival reported in various series is between 20 and 60 per cent. A small but significant number of patients who survive for 5 years succumb or present with metastatic disease before the tenth year. It is possible that the variation in survival rate reported may in part be related to the inclusion of patients with pseudolymphoma of the stomach in some of the series reporting high survival rates.

PSEUDOLYMPHOMA

Smith and Helwig[12] reviewed 131 tumors classified as gastric lymphoma and compared these with lesions felt to be benign gastric reactive lymphoid hyperplasia. From this study they concluded that it is possible that some of the localized lesions which appear histologically malignant but behave in a benign fashion are actually instances of reactive hyperplasia. The histologic features of this benign condition are not always readily distinguished from those observed in malignant lymphoma of the stomach. The term "pseudolymphoma" has been given to such lesions. The hyperplastic lesions seen are believed to be a reaction to inflammation associated with chronic gastric ulcer or gastritis. Jacobs[5] stated that patients who have pseudolymphoma are more likely to have a prolonged history of gastric ulcer and are less likely to have a palpable abdominal mass.

The histological criteria for the diagnosis of pseudolymphoma as listed by Helwig include a polymorphous cellular infiltrate, the presence of reaction centers, and a fibroblastic reaction. The regional lymph nodes must be free of lymphoma. Faris and Saltzstein[3] reviewed 21 patients suspected on reappraisal of having pseudolymphoma instead of malignant lymphoma and confirmed the findings of Jacobs. It is probable that some of the favorable results reported in the treatment of malignant lymphomas of the stomach have included some patients who indeed had pseudolymphoma. It is also possible that some lesions diagnosed as pseudolymphoma will, in time, prove to be malignant. The pathologic differential diagnosis between the two lesions may be very difficult in some instances.

SELECTED REFERENCES

Friedman, A. I.: Primary lymphosarcoma of the stomach. Am. J. Med., 26:783, 1959.
In this careful study of 75 cases of primary lymphoma of the stomach, the author has written an excellent description of the gross morphology of these lesions. This information is very useful to surgeons, radiologists, and endoscopists. Understanding the morphology of these tumors should result in more accurate preoperative diagnosis of gastric lymphomas and better intraoperative management.

Jacobs, D. S.: Primary gastric malignant lymphoma and pseudolymphoma. Am. J. Clin. Pathol., 40:379, 1963.
The author has carefully reviewed 27 lymphomas of the stomach and identified 12 of these as meeting the criteria of Smith and Helwig for pseudolymphoma. This work confirmed the observations of Smith and Helwig and more firmly established the concept of pseudolymphoma.

Sheehan, W. W., and Rappaport, H.: Morphological criteria in the classification of malignant lymphomas. *In* Proceedings of the Sixth National Cancer Conference. Philadelphia, J. B. Lippincott Company, 1968, p. 59.
The histological classification developed by these authors of non-Hodgkin's disease malignant lymphomas has proved to be of great value in understanding and managing patients with generalized malignant lymphoma. It will prove equally valuable in localized lymphomas. Using this classification should result in a better selection of patients for different modalities of therapy.

Smith, J. L., Jr., and Helwig, E. B.: Malignant lymphoma of the stomach; its diagnosis, distinction and biologic behavior. Am. J. Pathol., 34:553, 1958.
These investigators raised the possibility that some lesions felt to be primary gastric lymphomas are indeed not malignant tumors at all but instead represent a benign reactive lymphoid hyperplasia. The differentiation between the two lesions has obvious therapeutic importance.

REFERENCES

1. Connors, J., and Wise, L.: Management of gastric lymphomas. Am. J. Surg., 127:102, 1974.
2. Crile, G., Jr., Hazard, J. B., and Allen, K. L.: Primary lymphosarcoma of the stomach. Ann. Surg., 135:39, 1952.
3. Faris, T. D., and Saltzstein, S. L.: Gastric lymphoid hyperplasia: A lesion confused with lymphosarcoma. Cancer, 17:207, 1964.
4. Friedman, A. I.: Primary lymphosarcoma of the stomach. Am. J. Med., 26:783, 1959.
5. Jacobs, D. S.: Primary gastric malignant lymphoma and pseudolymphoma. Am. J. Clin. Pathol., 40:379, 1963.
6. Loehr, W. J., Mujahed, Z., Zahn, F. D., Gray, G. F., and Thorbjarnarson, B.: Primary lymphoma of the gastrointestinal tract, a review of 100 cases. Ann. Surg., 170:232, 1969.
7. Meyers, M. A., Katzen, B., and Alonso, D. R.: Transpyloric extension to duodenal bulb in gastric lymphoma. Radiology, 115:575, 1975.
8. Palmer, E. D.: The sarcomas of the stomach: A review with reference to gross pathology and gastroscopic manifestations. Am. J. Dig. Dis., 17:186, 1950.

9. Prolla, J. C., Kobayashi, S., and Kirsner, J. B.: Cytology of malignant lymphomas of the stomach. Acta Cytol., *14*:291, 1970.
10. Rosenberg, S. A., Diamond, H. D., Jaslowitz, B., and Craver, L. F.: Lymphosarcoma: A review of 1269 cases. Medicine, *40*:31, 1961.
11. Sheehan, W. W., and Rappaport, H.: Morphological criteria in the classification of malignant lymphomas. *In* Proceedings of the Sixth National Cancer Conference. Philadelphia, J. B. Lippincott Company, 1969, p. 59.
12. Smith, J. L., Jr., and Helwig, E. B.: Malignant lymphoma of the stomach; its diagnosis, distinction and biologic behavior. Am. J. Pathol., *34*:553, 1958.
13. Third National Cancer Survey: Incidence data. National Cancer Institute Monograph 41, March, 1975.

III

EROSIVE GASTRITIS

Alexander J. Walt, M.B., Ch.B.

Acute erosive gastritis (AEG) is not a new disease. Well described at the turn of the century, AEG claimed the life of Halsted in 1922 when he developed terminal hematemesis on the sixteenth day after removal of a common duct stone in the presence of dehydration, jaundice, and cholangitis, classic precursors of the characteristic erosive lesions.

The term erosive gastritis is a generic term embracing many entities variously described as "stress ulceration," "hemorrhagic gastritis," "alkaline gastritis," and "reflux gastritis." The normal stomach is the site of a remarkable hourly shedding and renewal of approximately 30 million cells in an environment characterized by frequent changes in pH and muscular motility. Preservation of the integrity of the gastric wall against the corrosive potential of hydrochloric acid is the primary function of the gastric mucosal barrier, which in addition to its specific anatomic architecture possesses vital intracellular physiologic, biochemical, and dynamic energy resources that are essential contributors to its defenses. The appearance of AEG is evidence of failure of this protective barrier and may occur under a wide variety of clinical circumstances. In the intensely depleted patient, AEG has been aptly described as "the bedsore of the gut."

Grossly, AEG is manifested by a wide range of superficial lesions primarily affecting the gastric lining superficial to the muscularis mucosa. As this level is seldom transgressed to any substantial degree, perforation is extremely rare. The extent of the lesion may vary from small and widely separated punctate erosive areas to almost universal sloughing of the mucosa. The topographical variation of the lesions is striking and often reflects the precipitating cause. In the AEG of sepsis, the acid-producing proximal segment of the stomach bears the brunt of the lesion, with the antrum affected only in severe cases; in alkaline reflux gastritis, the antrum is primarily involved, with the body and fundus affected in only the more florid syndrome; in the AEG of burns, the entire stomach and duodenum are frequently damaged.

The advent of the gastrocamera and later the flexible gastroscope greatly changed the understanding of AEG. The speed with which lesions may appear and regress, and the spectrum of edema, ecchymoses, erosions, superficial ulcerations, and finally diffuse mucosal sloughing had not been sufficiently appreciated.[10, 11] Furthermore, the fact that the clinical picture may not reflect the degree of mucosal damage was not previously recognized. Today, it is known that marked mucosal changes may be present in the asymptomatic patient; conversely, bleeding may occur in individuals who have relatively few lesions.

Mechanisms

The nature of the mucosal barrier and the mechanisms which cause its disruption remain in dispute.[3] Speculation abounds on the biochemical, vascular, and cellular mechanisms that produce the erosive changes. Substances such as urea, bile, ethanol, eugenol, and aspirin produce differing cellular ultrastructural changes. However, they share in common the fact that the tight intercellular junctions remain intact in the early stages (Figs. 1 to 6). It is probable that the tissue changes are the result of many contributory factors. In severe cases, lesions similar to those in the stomach may be found in the small intestine and the colon.[11] The theories advanced to account for the gastric lesions may be considered under the following headings.

Ischemia. In both the experimental animal and the shocked human, patchy areas of pallor adjacent to areas of congestion are clearly visible on gastroscopy within 12 hours of the insult. While the assumption that these changes reflect a local redistribution of blood seems obvious and accurate, measurement of gastric mucosal blood flow in humans cannot yet be accurately made. Nevertheless, it seems reasonable that ischemia may initiate a series of cellular changes culminating in superficial infarction.

Disruption of the Mucosal Barrier and Back Diffusion of H^+. It has been thought that, in both man and animals, disruption of the mucosal barrier may be crudely indicated by measurement of the loss of H^+ from the lumen, passage of Na^+ into the lumen, increased lithium ion absorption, a fall in the electropotential difference, and the appearance of serum proteins in the gastric lumen.[17] Recently the validity of these indications as estimates of the integrity of the mucosal

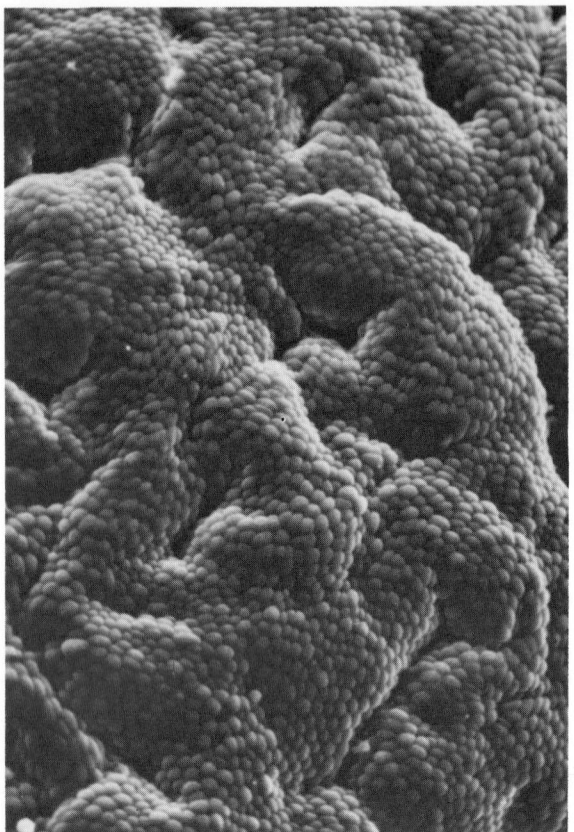

Figure 1. The surface topography of the near-normal stomach exhibits a continuous sheet of epithelial cells. (×540). (Courtesy of Dr. Jeanne Riddle.)

the main precipitating cause. The entity of alkaline erosive gastritis is well recognized, and the potential deleterious effects of bile salts have been shown experimentally. In animal models, binding of the bile by cholestyramine prevents ulcerogenesis. It would seem that the ability of the bile salts to produce their damaging effects is influenced by the pk' of the individual salts and by the pH of the gastric juice. Where the pK' of bile salt is not exceeded, the salts precipitate as the bile acid becomes insoluble. It may well be significant that frank bleeding in humans with acute erosive gastritis is often preceded by the presence of bile in the gastric content for 24 to 48 hours.

The most striking data on hyperacidity in humans have been derived from studies on patients with head injuries, although similar but less consistent measurements have been obtained in patients with sepsis. Gastric secretory measurements made from the time of injury to the beginning of hemorrhage, often 7 to 14 days later, may reflect an increased acidity only a day or two before bleeding occurs. Once acid diffuses into the mucosal wall, a number of changes may occur. These changes include disruption of capillaries with increase of fluid in the interstitium producing edema, the passage of plasma proteins and red cells into the gastric content, and stimulation of mast cells to produce histamine, which further stimulates acid produc-

barrier has been seriously challenged.[6] Experimentally, neither the infusion of vasoconstrictor agents for a few hours[5] nor the production of local hypovolemic hypotension has been shown to cause an invariable increase in permeability of the gastric mucosa in selected models.[16] This observation has been further strengthened in humans by McAlhany et al., who have shown that AEG may occur with no demonstrable back-diffusion.[13] Nevertheless, where unequivocal back-diffusion is present, frank superficial ulcerations are far more likely to develop. Not surprisingly, then, it would seem that the absolute amount of acid that diffuses does not necessarily reflect the degree of damage inflicted and that other factors affecting the barrier function assume a vital role.

Blood Flow, Intracellular pH, and Availability of Energy Substrates. It has been widely accepted that at least some degree of acidity in the stomach is necessary to produce or potentiate the erosive changes. While a small amount of H^+ diffuses into the gastric mucosa normally, this quantity is liable to be greatly increased in conditions of stress. The efficiency of the microcirculation may be important in helping to clear or neutralize any increased acid. It is also speculated that an actively secreting mucosa with a consequent alkaline tide may protect against the destructive local effects of acid. Acid alone, however, is not necessarily

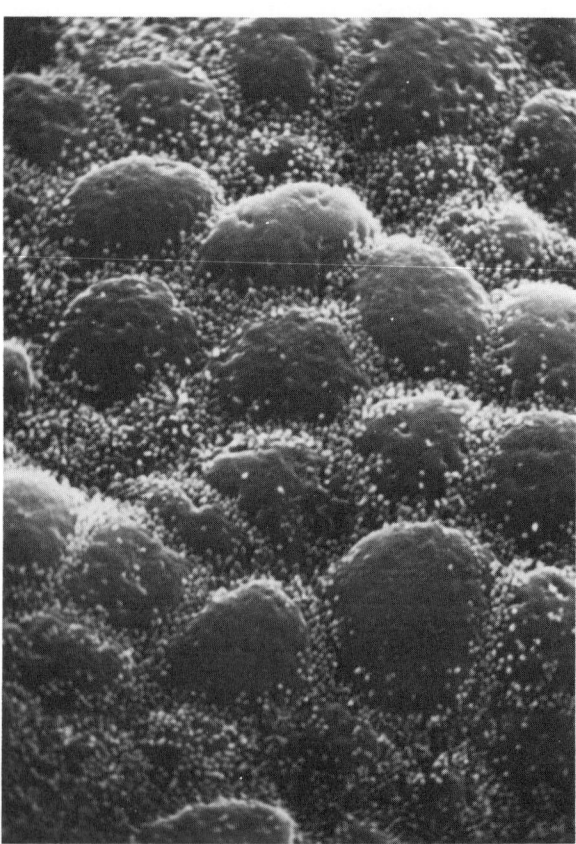

Figure 2. Numerous microvilli project from the exterior of individual epithelial cells on the surface of the near-normal stomach (×7900). (Courtesy of Dr. Jeanne Riddle.)

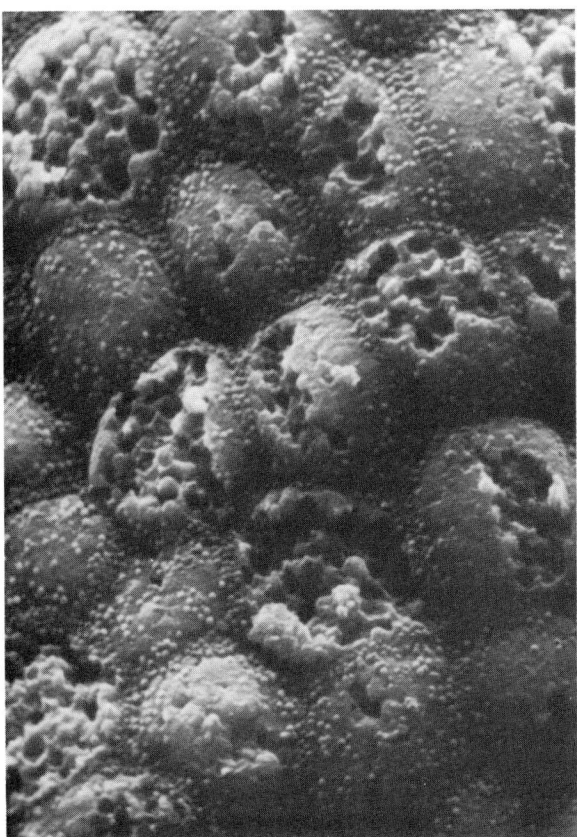

Figure 3. Epithelial cells showing a partial loss of cellular contents in a patient with AEG. Cell walls still intact (×5400). (Courtesy of Dr. Jeanne Riddle.)

permeable to back-diffusion and so more susceptible to destruction.

Clinical Picture

In many institutions, AEG (poorly termed "stress ulceration") became the most common cause of upper gastrointestinal hemorrhage in the 1960s. The increase in incidence appears to coincide with the establishment of sophisticated intensive care units where the lives of severely ill patients are significantly prolonged. The lesion occurs most commonly in patients who have undergone episodes of shock or sepsis but also appears to be a nonspecific end result of a wide variety of insults such as (a) drugs, e.g., alcohol, aspirin, indomethacin, phenylbutazole; (b) head injuries; (c) burns, often associated with an element of sepsis; (d) cardiac surgery; (e) uremia (and hence occurs in patients undergoing renal transplantation); and (g) general debility and malnutrition. In the past few years, the incidence seems to have fallen markedly, which may perhaps reflect in part the vigorous therapeutic measures that have been instituted now that the syndrome is better understood.

While the bleeding usually begins about 7 to 10 days after the initial insult, it may appear within the first few days. Sequential gastroscopy in humans has shown that the lesions characteristically appear first

tion. In this manner, a self-perpetuating destructive process which ultimately results in increasing hypoxia and infarction of the gastric wall may be initiated.

Changes in energy substrates in the mucosa have been postulated to play an important role in the preservation of mucosal integrity. Menguy[14] has devised models in which multiple insults are combined and has concluded that the final mucosal necrosis results from a mucosal energy deficit. This thesis incorporates the concepts of a greatly increased energy requirement in the body of the stomach as compared to the antrum. Fasting animals were strikingly more susceptible to the development of erosions. These observations have relevance to the adverse clinical effects of inadequate nutrition in the severely stressed patient in whom intravenous hyperalimentation seems to reduce the incidence of gastric erosions.

Sepsis is the central feature in many patients with AEG, but its role is difficult to define precisely. The stomach in these patients seems to be a target organ and hypersecretion is a frequent concomitant of sepsis. Attempts to study the problem in animal models suggest that sepsis may produce a hyperdynamic state in the stomach, as it has been shown to do in the kidneys and elsewhere. It seems probable that sepsis affects cellular membranes adversely, rendering these

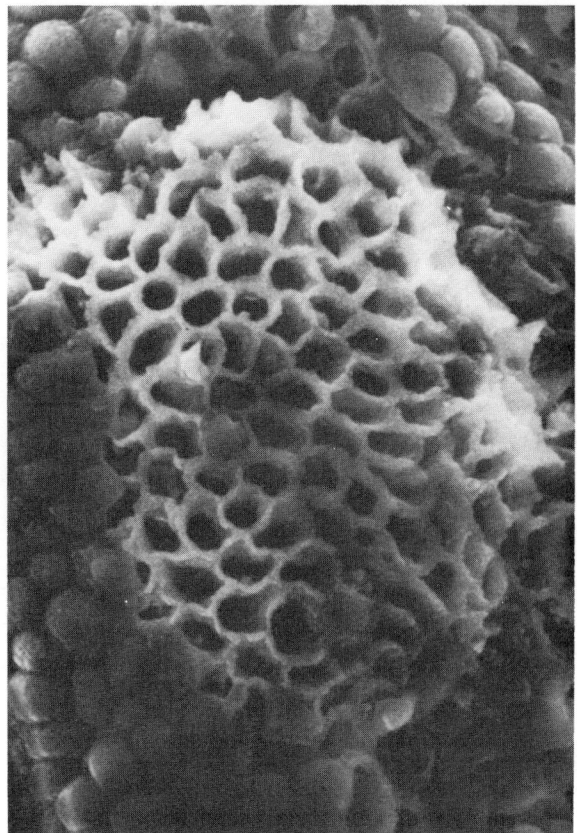

Figure 4. Focal groups of gastric epithelial cells demonstrate extensive loss of internal contents (×1900). (Courtesy of Dr. Jeanne Riddle.)

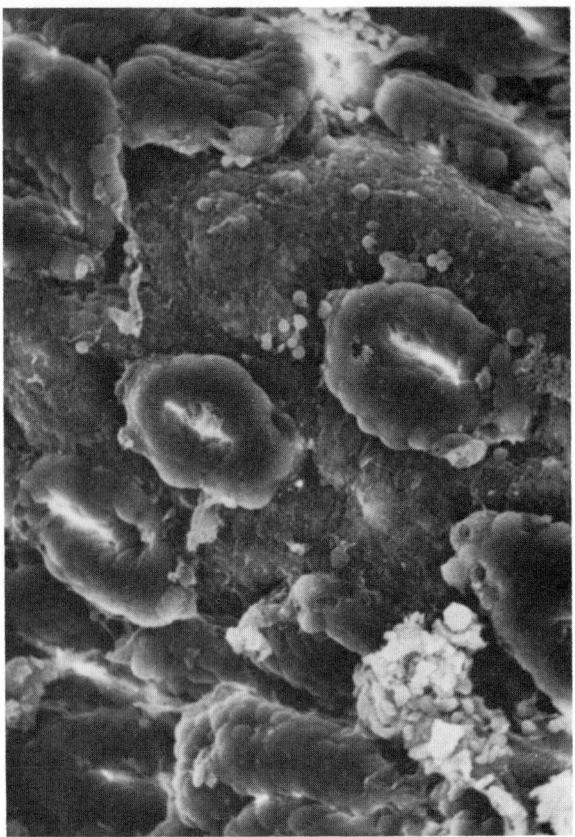

Figure 5. A partial loss of gastric epithelial cells from a patient with AEG (×1000). (Courtesy of Dr. Jeanne Riddle.)

quantity to maintain an intraluminal pH of 6 to 7, at which level it neutralizes the acid, inactivates pepsin, and possibly enhances the coagulation mechanism by inducing an alkaline microenvironment on the surface of the gastric mucosa. A more fundamental concept involves the prevention of acid production in the first place. Metiamide, an H^2 receptor blocking agent, administered by mouth or through a nasogastric tube, has a very rapid action. Metiamide stops acid production for about two hours and reduces it considerably for another four hours. Used in 11 patients with erosive gastritis, metiamide effectively stopped bleeding in all.[12] The newer and hematologically safer H^2 blocker, Cimetadine, deserves a clinical trial.

Once bleeding has begun, the stomach is thoroughly and repeatedly lavaged with iced water or iced saline. When necessary, the freshest blood available, with or without fresh frozen plasma, is given to restore blood volume and reduce coagulation abnormalities.

Other nonsurgical methods that have been advocated with varying degrees of enthusiasm include (a) use of an intragastric hypothermic balloon, but in the hands of most teams, this has proven clumsy, prone to cause aspiration, and often ineffective; (b) intragastric adrenaline, the success of which is largely anecdotal; (c) selective catheterization of the left gastric artery for continuous infusion of vasopressin—a 61 per cent

in the fundus and progress to the junction of the body and antrum, which is relatively seldom involved to any marked degree except in very severe cases. Often, the bleeding is heralded by 24 to 48 hours of ileus and the appearance of bile in the nasogastric suction. Flecks of blood first appear, and these are followed by steady bleeding. Occasionally, hemorrhage is catastrophic from the start. About 90 per cent of patients stop bleeding in response to active nonsurgical treatment; less than 10 per cent require surgical intervention. Of those who require an operation, 30 to 50 per cent die. Mortality is highest in patients over 60 years of age and in those with sepsis.

Treatment

Nonsurgical. Ideally, prophylaxis may prevent the development of AEG by prompt attention to sepsis, pulmonary ventilation, intravascular volume, nutrition, impending ileus, and excessive gastric acidity.

In that acid may be harmful where barrier function is inefficient, prophylactic administration of antacids appears to be effective in obviating or at least in reducing the incidence of gastritis. While no controlled prospective randomized clinical trials have been reported as yet, many observations support the validity of the concept. The antacid must be given in sufficient

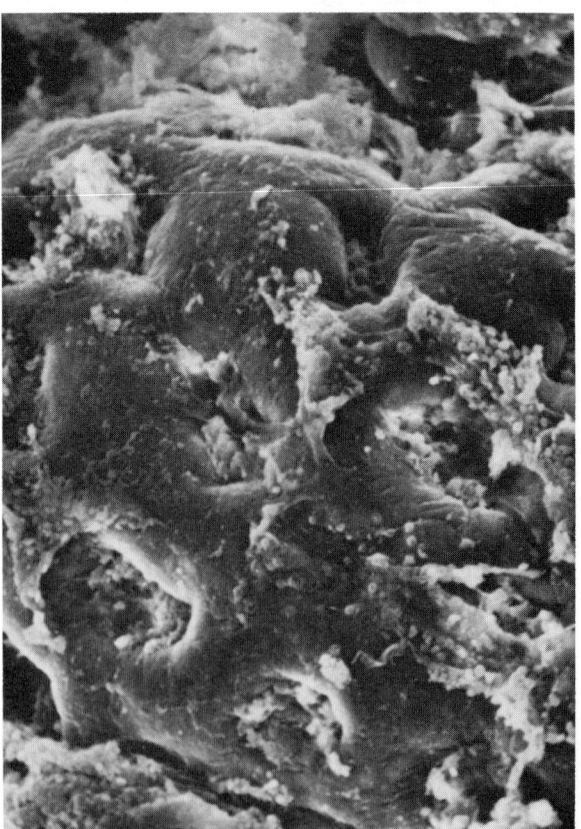

Figure 6. Total denudation of the gastric epithelium from a patient with AEG (×540). (Courtesy of Dr. Jeanne Riddle.)

overall success rate in the control of AEG and and 84 per cent success rate where catheterization was technically feasible has been reported by Baum's group,[1] but these results have not been achieved by others; (d) embolization of autologous clots, muscle, or gelfoam, which may achieve occasional dramatic results; (e) external counterpressure to the abdomen by a G suit, which is largely impractical and ultimately ineffective; (f) direct electrocoagulation of individual bleeding points as described by Sugawa[18] and Katon,[8] an innovation that in skilled and practical hands may be completely successful and that is very useful in the depleted, jaundiced patient in whom general anesthesia promises to constitute a death warrant; (g) the laser beam, recently used in a small number of humans, is highly promising but is still in the investigative stage. As the mucosal cells have the capacity to renew the gastric lining within two to four days, a successful therapeutic holding action may enable complete regeneration to occur.

Surgical

It is not surprising that no prospective randomized study of the ideal operation for AEG has been reported. The clinical setting and accurate categorization of subsets of etiologic factors and the mucosal changes provide almost insuperable difficulties. Operation is embarked upon whenever nonsurgical therapy, as measured by continuing or uncontrollable bleeding, has failed. The procedure selected should reflect the cause and stage of the gastric lesions. Most AEG caused by aspirin or alcohol may be treated by vagotomy, pyloroplasty, and undersewing of individual lesions, whether or not these are bleeding at the time of operation. In more florid cases, and in patients in whom continuing sepsis may be predicted, vagotomy and high subtotal gastrectomy are advisable. The extent of gastric corpus resected should depend on the site(s) of bleeding and the state of the fundic mucosa. Not infrequently, the proximal mucosa, which was affected earliest, will show signs of substantial healing by the time of operation. Paradoxically, as recurrent bleeding (not necessarily of a degree to warrant reoperation) occurs in approximately 40 per cent of patients who have vagotomy and pyloroplasty and about 15 per cent of those who have vagotomy and subtotal gastrectomy, the older and sicker patient should have the larger initial operation, as his margin of reserve is diminished. Total gastrectomy is necessary in the patient whose entire mucosa is bleeding and who is unresponsive to vagotomy or who has bled severely following a lesser surgical procedure. These constitute about 10 per cent of patients who require operation. Whatever operation is done, vigorous supportive measures, including parenteral hyperalimentation, are essential to improved results.

Alkaline Erosive Gastritis

Alkaline erosive gastritis is characterized by persistent dyspepsia, epigastric pain, nausea, heartburn, vomiting of bile, substantial loss of weight, and slow anemia. Food will frequently aggravate the pain, and vomiting gives little relief.

While reflux gastritis may frequently occur with an anatomically intact pylorus in patients who have never undergone a gastric operation, it is very much more common in individuals who have had a Billroth I, Billroth II, pyloroplasty, or gastric jejunostomy.[9] In this postoperative group, the majority of patients develop their symptoms more than a year after the initial operation, but symptoms may appear any time from within a few weeks to 10 or more years.

The wide variability of mucosal change, the severity of symptomatology not necessarily reflecting the gross mucosal appearance, and the clinical factors responsible for the mucosal destruction are not completely understood. While extrapolation of animal studies to the human stomach is fraught with pitfalls, it is noteworthy that pure pancreatic juice will not produce more than minor gastric changes in dogs but that a combination with bile is synergistic and made much more potent by the addition of jejunal content. The factors influencing the efficient functioning of the antropyloroduodenal pump are complex. Experiments in humans have suggested that smoking may encourage regurgitation of duodenal content.[15] It has been estimated that more than 50 per cent of patients with gastric or duodenal ulcer can be demonstrated to have reflux of bile and pancreatic juice into the stomch, particularly at night when supine. Not all of these patients will show gastritis. This individual variation may be partially explained by differences in gastric motility, which, when sluggish, permits the refluxed material to maintain contact with the mucosa for an appreciable period of time in contrast to the situation in those patients in whom the stomach empties rapidly. Where stasis and an alkaline pH occur, whether due to the refluxed fluid or to reduction of the parietal cell mass by inflammatory change, aerobic and anaerobic microorganisms may appear in the stomach.[4] These organisms may further deconjugate bile salts, increasing the inflammatory reaction.

In reflux gastritis, the mucosal changes are concentrated in the antrum, but in severe cases may also affect the body and even the esophagus. Inflammation of the parietal cell mass may produce hypochlorhydria or achlorhydria, which is often temporarily histamine-fast. This reduction in secretion of gastric acid may be deceptive in that the parietal cells may regenerate once the reflux gastritis is surgically cured. It is therefore essential that provision be made to counter this potential return of acids by the addition of vagotomy to any remedial operation if subsequent stomal ulceration is to be avoided.

Definitive diagnosis is best made by direct gastroscopic visualization and biopsy. Sampling of gastric content for bile[2] or reliance on the radiologic demonstration of mucosal change is of much less value. In less severe cases, superficial ulcerations may cause occult bleeding, but on occasion marked hemorrhage may occur. In more severe cases, the gastric mucosa may be intensely involved and appears edematous, beefy, friable, and hemorrhagic. The presence of limited mucosal change around gastroenterostomy stomas or close to gastroduodenal anastomoses is very common and should not be categorized as significant alkaline gastritis.

Treatment

Medical. In patients who have had no previous operation, cessation of smoking and using alcohol, regular doses of aluminum hydroxide, and a bland diet may be sufficient to produce healing. In cases that fail to respond, cholestyramine may be helpful. When gastric stasis is marked, metoclopramide has been advocated to produce relief of symptoms by enhancing a gastric emptying. Where severe reflux gastritis occurs following operation, however, medical measures of this kind seldom produce permanent comfort. A remedial operation is required in the presence of persistent symptoms, anemia, or frank bleeding once other possible causes of the clinical picture have been excluded.

Surgical. Herrington et al.[7] and van Heerden et al.[19] have reported on 48 and 49 surgically treated patients respectively. In the past, interposition of a 20 to 25 cm. isoperistaltic loop of jejunum between the stomach and the duodenum was popular, but the results achieved were not dependable. In recent years, a Roux-en-Y jejunal limb separating the gastric remnant from the entrance of the rerouted bile by about 40 to 60 cm. has gained acceptance. Both these operations share a similar basic principle, which holds that the diversion of duodenal, pancreatic, and jejunal content from the stomach eliminates the precipitating cause of the gastritis. When a Roux-en-Y procedure with vagotomy is used, approximately 70 per cent of patients have excellent results, 20 per cent have good results, and 10 per cent have relatively poor results.

SELECTED REFERENCES

Bushkin, F. L., Wickbom, G., DeFord, J. W., and Woodward, E. R.: Postoperative alkaline reflux gastritis. Surg. Gynecol. Obstet., 138:933–939, 1974.
The authors review the many etiologic factors—anatomic, physiologic, and biochemical—that have been advanced to account for alkaline gastritis, and they also provide a useful bibliography.

Desmond, A. M., and Reynolds, K. W.: Erosive gastritis: Its diagnosis, management, and surgical treatment. Br. J. Surg., 59:5–13, 1972.
Members of the surgical unit at St. James Hospital, London, under the direction of Mr. Norman Tanner and subsequently of Mr. Andrew Desmond, have long enjoyed a great reputation for their thoughtful studies and excellent results in the therapy of upper gastrointestinal bleeding. This analysis of 331 patients operated upon for acute erosive gastritis and representing almost 10 per cent of 3938 patients with severe gastroduodenal hemorrhage serves as a yardstick against which other approaches may be measured. Allowance should be made, however, for the fact that these data precede the use of the flexible gastroduodenoscope (although the rigid gastroscope was used with great expertise in this institution for many years) and for the difference in etiologic factors that precipitated acute erosive gastritis on the south bank of the Thames.

Herrington, J. L., Jr., Sawyers, J. L., and Whitehead, W. A.: Surgical management of reflux gastritis. Ann. Surg., 180:526–537, 1974.
Many papers are written which review the wide variety of complications that may follow the operative disruption of gastric physiologic mechanisms. Few have dealt with the specific problem of alkaline gastritis in as comprehensive a manner as the authors of this article. Dr. Herrington and his colleagues have a possibly unparalleled personal experience in dealing with symptomatic alkaline gastritis, and this paper established the current standard approach to this problem.

Lucas, C. E., Sugawa, C., Friend, W., and Walt, A. J.: Therapeutic indications of disturbed gastric physiology in patients with stress ulcerations. Am. J. Surg., 123:25–34, 1972.
The sequential mapping of the evolution and natural history of acute erosive gastritis in critically ill patients became possible only with the advent of the flexible gastroscope. This paper illustrates the gross mucosal changes in humans and correlates these with the histologic picture obtained by biopsy. Practical aspects of management are presented.

Schrager, J.: The chemical composition and function of gastrointestinal mucus. Gut, 11:450–456, 1970.
Over the past decade, the physiologic role of gastric mucus as a protective mechansim has been much discussed. This progress report summarizes succinctly and attractively the properties and function of gastric mucus.

Silen, W., and Skillen, J. J.: Stress ulcer, acute erosive gastritis and the gastric mucosal barrier. Adv. Intern. Med., 19:195–212, 1974.
These two authors, who have contributed as much as anyone both in the laboratory and on the wards to our understanding of erosive gastritis, summarize current beliefs in an extremely lucid manner. This relatively brief article provides an excellent perspective on the problem and a reading list which is an intelligent guide to individual facets of the broader problem.

Simonian, S. J., and Curtis, L. E.: Treatment of hemorrhagic gastritis by antacid. Ann. Surg., 184:429–434, 1976.
This paper serves as a reminder that acid is the usual villain in acute erosive gastritis and discusses the likely benefits to be derived from the administration of antacids therapeutically. The discussion which follows expresses certain important caveats and poses many relevant questions. Above all, speculation on the role of histamine H_2 receptor blocking agents in the future is introduced.

Stremple, J. F., Mori, H., Lev, R., and Glass, G. B. J.: The stress ulcer syndrome. Curr. Probl. Surg., April, 1973.
This monograph, based largely on work done in the Army Surgical Research Unit during the Vietnam conflict but ranging widely to include concepts derived from laboratories and patients in quieter settings, provides a detailed examination of the entity of the "stress ulcer syndrome." The 281 references constitute an easily available source of information.

REFERENCES

1. Athanasoulis, C. A., Baum, S., Waltman, A. C., Ring, E. J., Imbembo, A., and Vander Salm, T. J.: Control of acute gastric mucosal hemorrhage. N. Engl. J. Med., 290:597, 1974.
2. Brooks, W. S., Wenger, J., and Hersh, T.: Bile reflux gastritis. Am. J. Gastroenterol., 64:286, 1975.
3. Davenport, H. W.: The gastric mucosal barrier. Mayo Clin. Proc., 50:507, 1975.
4. Davidson, E. D., and Hersh, T.: Bile reflux gastritis: Contribution of inadequate gastric emptying. Am. J. Surg., 130:514, 1975.
5. Dorricott, N. J., Isenberg, J. I., and Silen, W.: Effect of intraarterial vasopressin on canine gastric mucosal permeability. Gastroenterology, 65:625, 1973.
6. Fisher, R. P., Jelense, S., and Fulton, R. L.: The maintenance of gastric mucosal barrier during the early erosive gastritis component of stress ulceration. Surgery, 80:40, 1976.
7. Herrington, J. L., Sawyers, J. L., and Whitehead, W. A.: Surgical management of reflux gastritis. Ann. Surg., 180:526, 1974.
8. Kanton, R. M.: Experimental control of gastrointestinal hemorrhage via the endoscope: A new era dawns. Gastroenterology, 70:272, 1976.
9. Keighley, M. R. B., Asquith, P., Edwards, J. A. C., and Williams, J. A.: The importance of an innervated and intact antrum and pylorus in preventing postoperative duodenogastric reflux and gastritis. Br. J. Surg., 62:845, 1975.
10. Lucas, C. E., Sugawa, C., Riddle, J., Rector, F., Rosenberg, B., and Walt, A. J.: The natural history and surgical dilemma of "stress" gastric bleeding. Arch. Surg., 102:266, 1971.
11. Lucas, C. E., Sugawa, C., Friend, W., Riddle, J., and Walt, A. J.: Therapeutic implications of the gastric defense mechanism in stress patients. Am. J. Surg., 123:25, 1972.
12. MacDonald, A. S., Steele, B. J., and Bottomley, M. G.: Treatment of stress-induced upper gastrointestinal haemorrhage with metiamide. Lancet, 1:68, 1976.
13. McAlhany, J. C., Czaja, A. J., and Pruitt, B. A.: Antacid control of complications from acute gastroduodenal disease after burns. J. Trauma, 16:645, 1976.
14. Menguy, R., and Masters, Y. F.: Gastric mucosal energy metabolism and "stress ulceration." Ann. Surg., 180:538, 1974.
15. Read, N. W., and Grech, P.: Effect of cigarette smoking on competence of the pylorus: Preliminary study. Br. Med. J., 3:313, 1973.
16. Ritchie, W. P.: Ischemia and the gastric mucosal barrier: A note of caution. Surgery, 76:363, 1974.

17. Silen, W., and Skillman, J. J.: Stress ulcer, acute erosive gastritis and the gastric mucosal barrier. Adv. Intern. Med., *19*:195, 1974.
18. Sugawa, C., Shier, M., Lucas, C. E., and Walt, A. J.: Electrocoagulation of bleeding in the upper part of the gastrointestinal tract: A preliminary experimental clinical report. Arch. Surg., *110*:975, 1975.
19. van Heerden, J. A., Phillipps, S. F., Adson, M. A., and McIlrath, D. C.: Postoperative reflux gastritis. Am. J. Surg., *129*:82, 1975.

IV

ANGIOGRAPHY IN DIAGNOSIS AND TREATMENT OF GASTROINTESTINAL BLEEDING

William S. Blakemore, M.D.,
and William R. Schiller, M.D.

Although gastrointestinal bleeding often is self-limited, some seriously ill patients develop massive bleeding, often from undiagnosed sites. The bleeding site remains undiscovered in some 20 per cent of the patients with gastrointestinal bleeding even after barium studies and endoscopy.[1] This problem is especially frustrating in patients who are *poor risks* for surgical treatment. Intraoperative angiography is recognized as an effective method of localizing sites of bleeding.[2, 3] Development of the percutaneous catheter insertion technique by Seldinger in 1953[4] has made more practical the nonoperative intra-arterial catheterization for diagnosis and control of gastrointestinal bleeding. Nusbaum and Baum[5] compared the results of several possible methods of detecting the source of experimental gastrointestinal bleeding. Neither injected ^{32}P nor ^{131}I tagged serum albumin produced meaningful localization of bleeding sites nor did flush aortography. Operative segmental mesenteric angiography gave good localization and demonstrated sites with bleeding rates in the range of 0.5 ml. per minute. Percutaneous selective arteriography of the celiac, superior, and inferior mesenteric arteries was also successful, and with further development has allowed for diagnosis of a variety of lesions[6] and, in many patients, nonoperative therapy to control the bleeding sites. Control of bleeding esophageal varices by infusion of vasopressin into the superior mesenteric artery was reported by the same group in 1968.[7]

TECHNIQUES

The technique of percutaneous selective angiography is standardized using the methods described by Seldinger for introduction of the catheter and selective catheterization as reported by Odman.[8, 9] Although the femoral vessels are generally used, the axillary vessels are suitable if the femoral vessels cannot be used.

Following preparation of the skin, a small wheal of local anesthetic is raised at the puncture site. A Seldinger needle, consisting of an outer blunt cannula and an inner sharp needle and stylet, is then inserted into the artery indicated by a jet of blood ejected from the needle after removal of the stylet. A flexible steel guidewire is inserted through the needle via the femoral artery into the aorta; the needle is then withdrawn and compression applied temporarily at the puncture site. Next the flexible angiography catheter is introduced into the artery over the guidewire, which is then withdrawn after successful intra-aortic catheter placement. A variety of curved catheters are available for selective catheterization of vessels originating from the aorta, the procedure being facilitated by image intensification fluoroscopy. Position of the catheter can be ascertained by injection of small amounts of meglumine diatrizoate (Renografin). After satisfactory positioning, contrast material can be injected rapidly into the selected artery using a high-pressure injector and multiple films taken to include arterial, capillary, and venous phases of vascular visualization by means of a rapid film changer. In some cases magnification angiography for improved vascular detail may be performed by using an x-ray tube with a very small focal spot (0.3 mm.) and by positioning the organs under study farther from the x-ray film, usually about 20 inches.[10] Further improvements in x-rays, tables, tubes, and injection devices have allowed for more patient comfort and safety in performance of these tests.[11]

USE OF INTRA-ARTERIAL VASOCONSTRICTORS

The ability to catheterize selectively more distal arteries and accurately visualize sites of bleeding has stimulated development of nonoperative methods to achieve control of bleeding. Foremost in these efforts has been the use of intra-arterial vasoconstrictors to allow for locally reduced blood flow and cessation of bleeding by clot formation. Vasoactive agents most widely proposed have been either vasopressin[12] or epinephrine with or without propranolol, a beta-adrenergic blocking agent.[13]

In 1911, the vasoconstrictive properties of vasopressin were reported by Wiggers.[14] However, very little clinical use was made of this finding with the exception of an attempt by Rist in 1913 to control hemoptysis by intravenous injection of vasopressin.[15] Several studies in the mid 1950s stimulated the idea that vasopressin might be useful in controlling gastrointestinal bleeding. Animal studies showing the arterial constrictive and portal vein pressure lowering effects of vasopressin were performed and are summarized in a paper by Hoffbauer and associates.[16] Subsequently, two additional reports were published describing the effects of vasopressin in humans. Davis and co-workers[17] studied vasopressin-induced reduction of portal pressure in humans, and Kehne, Hughes, and Gompertz used it intravenously in two humans to control bleeding from esophageal varices in 1956.[18] Intravenous use of vasopressin for control of bleeding from esophageal varices was subsequently reported by other investigators[19, 20] who reported a high rate of success in acute bleeding episodes. Both groups, however, mentioned the development of tachyphylaxis by this method and commented that 20 units diluted in 100 to 200 ml. of dextrose in water should be given rapidly over 10 to 30 minutes for best results. Although no definite intestinal ischemic complication could be proved following this regimen, unpleasant side effects such as colicky abdominal pains were frequently observed. Fortunately, these side effects subsided within 30 minutes after stopping the infusion of the drug. No cardiac complications were seen by these investigators, although vasopressin is known to be a potent constrictor of the coronary arteries. In an experimental study, Drapanas and associates demonstrated a 58 per cent decrease in cardiac output and a similar decrease in coronary blood flow at the same time that a decrease in blood flow in the mesenteric artery and portal vein was observed.[21] As a consequence of these undesirable side effects, peripheral intravenous use of vasopressin has not met with wide acceptance or clinical use for controlling acute variceal hemorrhage. However, an alternative use which is now receiving some attention is intravenous infusion during portacaval shunt operations to control excessive bleeding commonly observed during these procedures. Intravenous or selective intra-arterial infusion has been used intraoperatively to decrease the portal pressure and thereby the bleeding.[22, 23] Development of techniques for catheterization of the major splanchnic arteries has stimulated additional methods for delivering vasoconstrictive medications to control bleeding plus a search for other compounds for this purpose.

Nusbaum and associates published data in 1967 in which the pharmacologic effects of vasopressin, epinephrine, norepinephrine, and angiotensin were studied when delivered into the mesenteric artery of dogs. They found that intra-arterial infusion of vasopressin at a dose of 0.2 unit per minute produced more than 50 per cent reduction in mesenteric arterial blood flow, significant reduction of portal venous pressure, and no change in cardiac output. In addition, they did not observe tachyphylaxis when the vasopressin was given in this manner. While the remaining three drugs under study produced a decrease in mesenteric artery blood flow, portal vein pressures were only briefly decreased, then became elevated.[24] These investigators concluded that vasopressin was the optimal drug for use as an intra-arterial vasoconstrictor, and indeed it remains the most popular material in clinical use at present.

Further inquiry into the physiology of mesenteric artery blood flow and the effects of intravenous epinephrine and norepinephrine by Ross in 1967 revealed a biphasic response of blood flow to these agents.[25] He reported that, although an initial vasoconstrictive effect was observed, this was soon followed by a sustained period of vasodilatation and concluded that the mechanism of this phenomenon was stimulation of beta-adrenergic receptor sites in the splanchnic vasculature. Ross and his associates were able to block the vasodilator response of both drugs by pretreatment with propranolol, a beta-adrenergic blocking agent. The effects of this procedure were to produce a vasoconstrictor effect without the subsequent period of vasodilatation, as shown by a series of angiograms which they included in one of their reports.[26] A clinical trial of intra-arterial infusion of a combination of epinephrine and propranolol was subsequently published by Rosch and colleagues in which they reported success in stopping bleeding in five patients with a variety of bleeding gastrointestinal lesions.[27] Further communications from this group indicate success with epinephrine combined with propranolol for treating arterial bleeders, while bleeding from esophageal varices was best treated with intra-arterial vasopressin.[28] They had some concerns about the effects of stopping the epinephrine infusions which, at least experimentally, resulted in a rebound increase in blood flow above the control levels, while a similar effect was not seen with vasopressin (Fig. 1). They were also concerned with potential ill effects on myocardial contraction by propranolol, especially in older patients.[29] Potential effects of vasopressin on the liver stimulated a report published in 1975 which demonstrated that at least in dogs celiac infusions of vasopressin resulted in a biphasic response of initial constriction followed by subsequent increase in flow in the hepatic artery. They concluded that such infusions were not harmful to the liver if given over brief periods of time.[30] Further studies of prolonged infusions are needed.

Other methods of using vasoconstrictor drugs for control of gastrointestinal bleeding have included intragastric or intraperitoneal instillation of norepinephrine, which resulted in cessation of bleeding in 54 per cent of patients in one series[31] and 66 per cent in another.[32] Predictable success has not been obtained in most clinics.

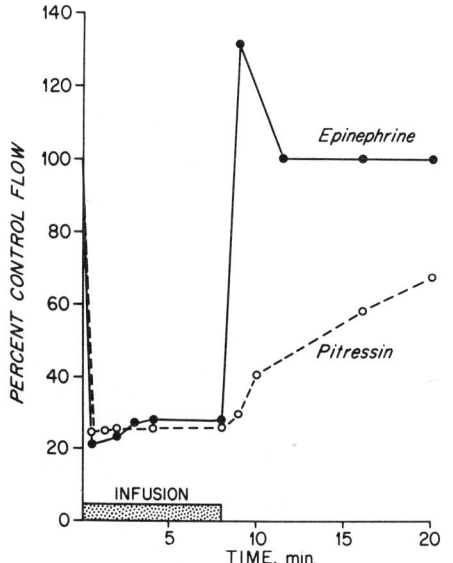

Figure 1. Comparison of effects of epinephrine and Pitressin (vasopressin) on superior mesenteric arterial blood flow in the dog. Both agents were infused directly into the superior mesenteric artery. Each point is the mean of experiments in three dogs. The epinephrine dose was 3.8 μg. per minute and was preceded by intramesenteric arterial infusion of propranolol, 3 mg. The Pitressin dose was 0.19 unit per minute. The shaded horizontal bar indicates the duration of infusion. (From Brant, B., et al.: Ann. Surg., *176*:419, 1972.)

CLINICAL USE OF ANGIOGRAPHY AND VASOCONSTRICTOR THERAPY

Widespread use of selective splanchnic angiography for massive gastrointestinal bleeding has occurred in the recent past. A recent publication by Nusbaum and associates summarizes their experience with diagnosis and control of bleeding esophageal varices.[33] Angiographic findings suggestive of portal hypertension are corkscrew appearance of intrahepatic arteries and presence of retrograde portal flow in addition to direct visualization of varices and collateral venous circulation.

Following diagnosis of varices as the site of hemorrhage, the arterial catheter is placed in the superior mesenteric artery for perfusion with vasopressin, since the largest fraction of portal blood is derived from the mesenteric circulation. Perfusion is begun at a rate of 0.2 unit per minute, and after approximately 15 minutes a repeat mesenteric angiogram is performed to evaluate the degree of vasoconstriction achieved. Constriction of branches of the mesenteric artery without reflux of contrast material into the aorta is a sign of adequate vasoconstriction. They have achieved approximately 50 per cent decrease in mesenteric artery blood flow and portal vein pressures with no change in systemic arterial pressure using this technique (Fig. 2). In their series of 41 patients with bleeding esophageal varices, only one failed to stop bleeding. When compared to a series of 69 patients treated before availability of vasopressin infusion, the newer technique seemed to increase the elective shunt rate from 36 to 44 per cent and has lowered the overall mortality from 74 to 61 per cent.

These authors have also used vasopressin infusion into the superior mesenteric artery as a surgical adjunct during operations to construct portal-systemic shunts. This technique resulted in greatly diminished blood loss and increased ease of dissection. One disadvantage that they noted, however, was difficulty in

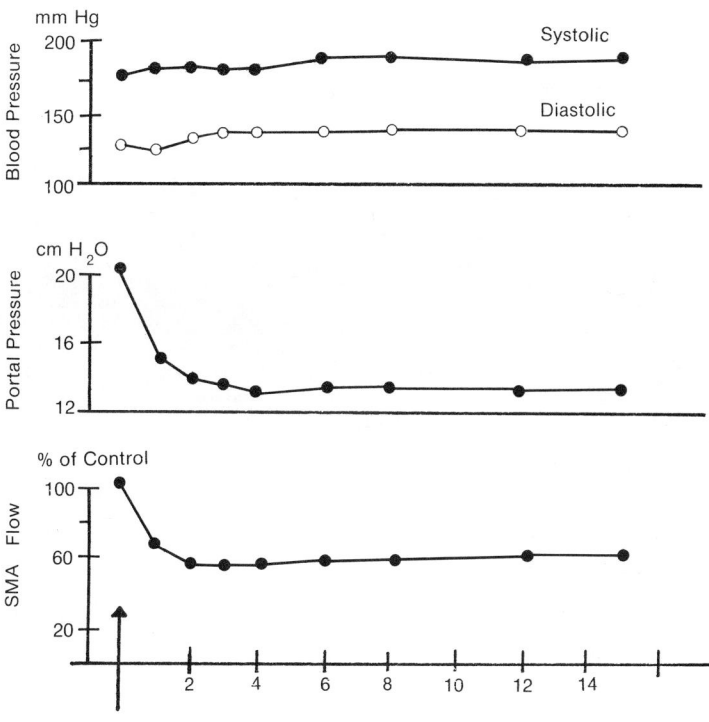

Figure 2. Concomitant fall in superior mesenteric arterial flow and portal pressure with infusion of vasopressin derivative into superior mesenteric artery. Note small dose used and prompt response. (From Nusbaum, M., et al.: Arch. Surg., *108*:342, 1974. Copyright 1974, American Medical Association.)

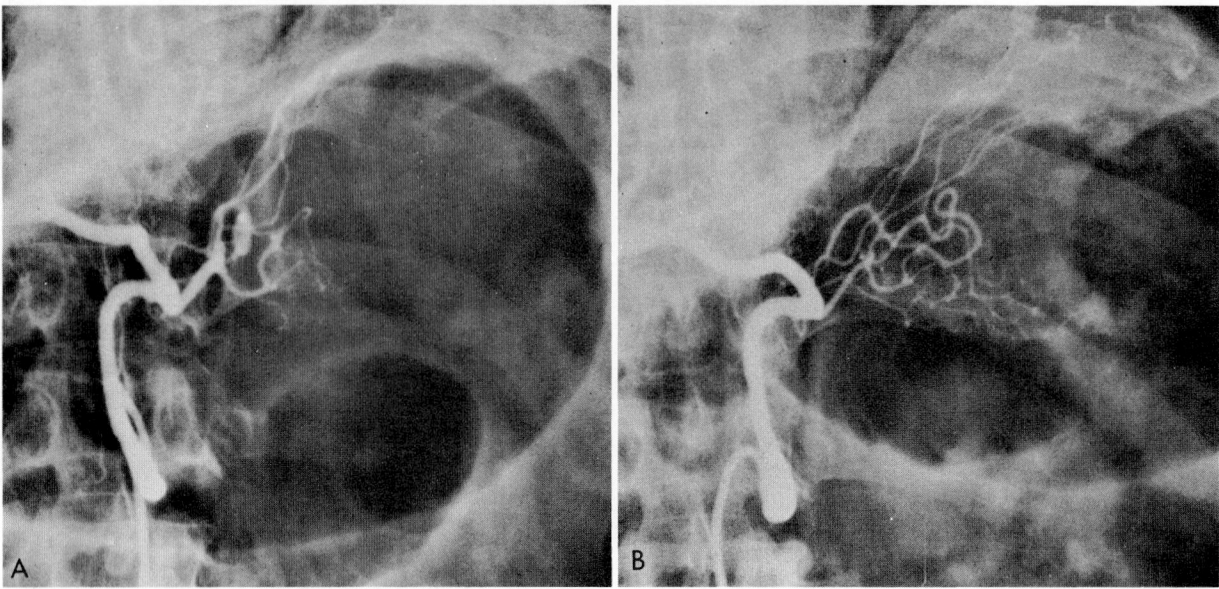

Figure 3. *A*, Bleeding gastric ulcer. Selective celiac injection shows extravasation of contrast material from branch of left gastric artery. (From Rau, R. M., et al.: Am. J. Surg., *128*:160, 1974.) *B*, Bleeding gastric ulcer. No further extravasation of contrast material and vasoconstriction after a 30-minute infusion of Pitressin in left gastric artery.

assessment of portal hemodynamics after completing the shunt.[34]

Not all bleeding patients with portal hypertension will be found to have variceal bleeding. Ring and co-workers reported 49 patients with portal hypertension evaluated for gastrointestinal bleeding and in 13 of these, bleeding was found to be arterial in origin from the esophagus, stomach, or duodenum. Bleeding was controlled by infusion of vasopressin into the appropri-

ate artery in 11 of the 13, and 7 of the 13 survived to be discharged from the hospital.[35]

Visceral angiography has been helpful in situations involving gastrointestinal bleeding from a wide spectrum of pathologic lesions. Several investigators have now published their experience with this procedure for treating nonvariceal bleeding.[35-37] Success in stopping the bleeding from a wide range of lesions such as gastric and duodenal ulcers, gastritis, esophagitis, and a

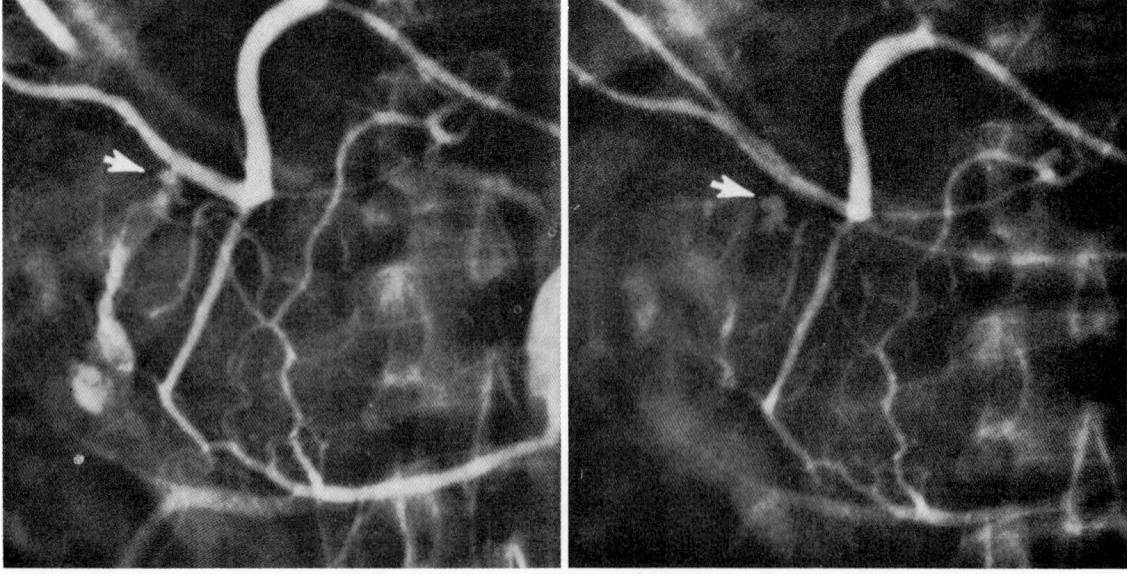

Figure 4. *A*, Bleeding duodenal ulcer. Selective celiac injection reveals extravasation from gastroduodenal artery into duodenum. (From Rau, R. M., et al.: Am. J. Surg., *128*:160, 1974.) *B*, Bleeding duodenal ulcer. Extravasation of contrast material has stopped after 15-minute infusion of Pitressin in the gastroduodenal artery.

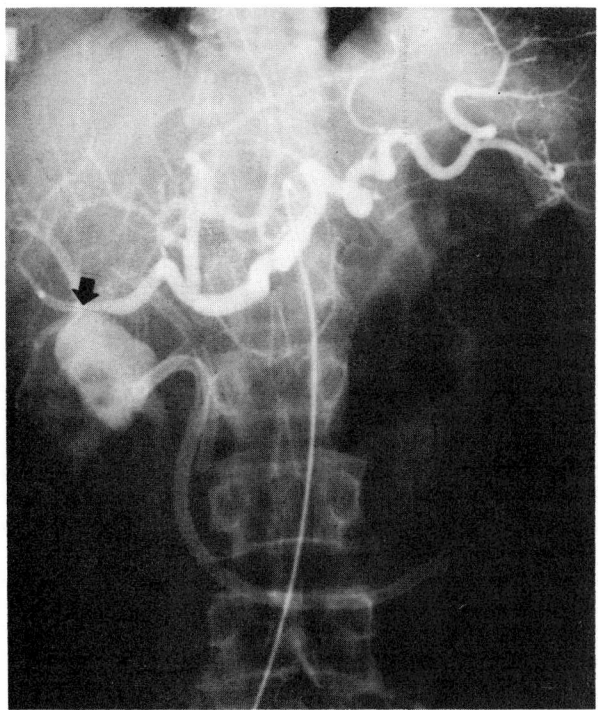

Figure 5. Celiac arteriogram from a patient in whom bleeding from the right upper quadrant drain site developed after cholecystectomy. The bleeding is seen to originate from the cystic artery, from which the ligature had loosened (arrow).

tigation of intra-arterial vasopressin infusion into the stomachs of dogs failed to show evidence of back-diffusion.[40]

Other lesions, such as Mallory-Weiss tears and esophagitis, also may be successfully treated using these techniques. We have also found angiography to be useful in treatment of hemobilia. One patient who was referred to us with hemobilia following a difficult cholecystectomy was found to have a bleeding cystic artery on angiography that was controlled by prompt surgical intervention (Fig. 5). Another patient with an hepatic artery aneurysm which had eroded into the common bile duct entered the hospital with upper gastrointestinal bleeding and the angiograms revealed the nature of the pathology (Fig. 6). Ligation of the hepatic artery was followed by an uneventful recovery.

Hereditary hemorrhagic telangiectasia, although a rare lesion, may cause gastrointestinal bleeding which is very difficult to manage because of the diffuse nature of intestinal involvement by the multiple telangiectasias. Precise localization is, however, possible by selective angiography, and constrictive therapy may obviate the necessity for an operation in this group of patients who tend to require multiple operations for complications of hereditary telangiectasia. A summary of management of this disease is included in a monograph by Baum and coworkers reviewing

variety of intestinal bleeding sites ranged from 65 to 80 per cent.

Superselective arterial catheterization has been of further help in diagnosis and control of bleeding exemplified by the bleeding gastric ulcer seen in Figure 3A. Advancement of the catheter into the left gastric artery allowed for infusion of vasopressin, constriction of the vessel, and cessation of the bleeding (Fig. 3B). The technique for this procedure as described by Waltman and associates and some newly developed catheters have greatly facilitated performance of left gastric cannulation.[38] Similarly, bleeding duodenal ulcers may be visualized and controlled by celiac artery injections showing extravasation from the gastroduodenal artery followed by intra-arterial vasopressin infusion (Fig. 4).

Recent experience indicates that acute gastric mucosal hemorrhages secondary to stress or ingestion of noxious materials such as alcohol may be evaluated by this technique. According to a publication by Athanasoulis and associates, bleeding may be seen as one or more discrete points superimposed upon either an otherwise normal-appearing stomach or upon an intensely hypervascular stomach.[39] They were able to control this type of bleeding in 31 of 37 patients (84 per cent). In 29 of these, the left gastric artery was selected for intra-arterial infusion of vasopressin. Some concern has been expressed over whether vasopressin infusion might worsen the mucosal injury by causing an increase in hydrogen ion back-diffusion secondary to mucosal ischemia. However, an inves-

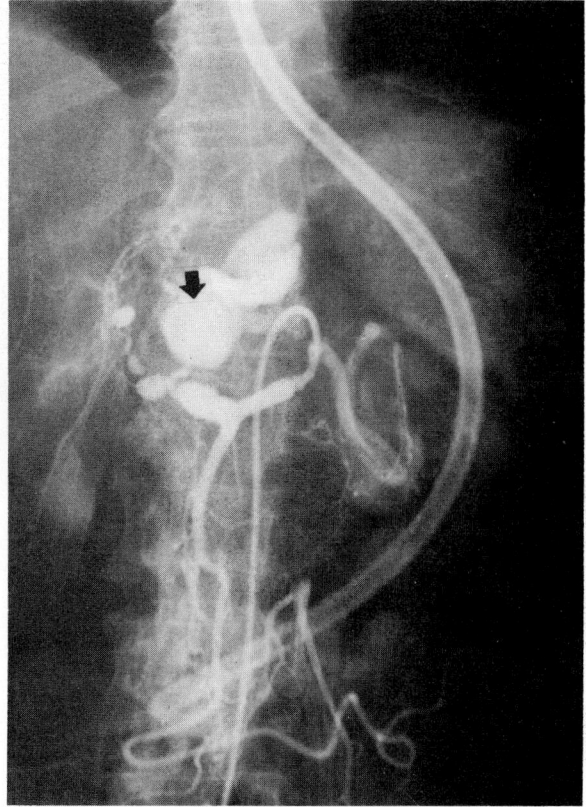

Figure 6. A hepatic artery aneurysm (arrow) was observed as the source of bleeding in this celiac angiogram from a patient with upper gastrointestinal bleeding.

angiography for diagnosis and management of gastrointestinal bleeding.[41]

Severe colonic bleeding not only may be difficult to localize but tends to occur in elderly, poor-risk patients who tolerate it poorly, and in whom an alternative to operation is often desirable. Such bleeding commonly arises from colonic diverticulosis, but when the colon is extensively involved, localization may be difficult, resulting in a widespread advocacy of colectomy. However, localization by angiography may allow for less formidable procedures or, if vasoconstrictive therapy is feasible, operation often may be avoided. In a review of 24 patients from two separate institutions treated for colonic hemorrhage by intraarterial vasopressin infusion, control of bleeding was observed in 22 patients. Twelve of these required no further treatment and were subsequently discharged from the hospital. Ten patients underwent elective colon resection following initial control without any operative mortality. Both patients who failed to respond to the vasopressin underwent emergency colectomy, and one died postoperatively.[42]

Other types of colonic lesions are now being recognized as the cause of intestinal bleeding from seemingly obscure sources not apparent on conventional types of gastrointestinal roentgenograms. One such group of lesions is the angiodysplasia, especially prevalent in the right side of the colon. On angiography these may appear as gross bleeding points or, more frequently, as areas with dilated, tortuous arteries with dense capillary filling and early opacification of the veins draining the area (Fig. 7A). Guided by angiography, surgical treatment by excision of the involved intestine can be directed confidently and effectively in relieving the problem. Postoperatively, it may be difficult to identify the lesion, and use of a silicone rubber injection technique has been very useful in identifying the lesion.[43] One such lesion has been clearly identified in a publication by Baum in 1974[44] (Fig. 7B). The etiology of these lesions is not entirely clear, but they may represent some form of chronic ischemic bowel disease rather than a congenital defect. These submucosal ectatic formations which contain both arteries and veins apparently develop small areas of ulceration in the overlying mucosa and subsequent bleeding.

We have recently observed another variant of the obscure bleeding lesion in the right colon in an elderly woman. This bleeding was identified angiographically and then controlled by selective arterial infusion of

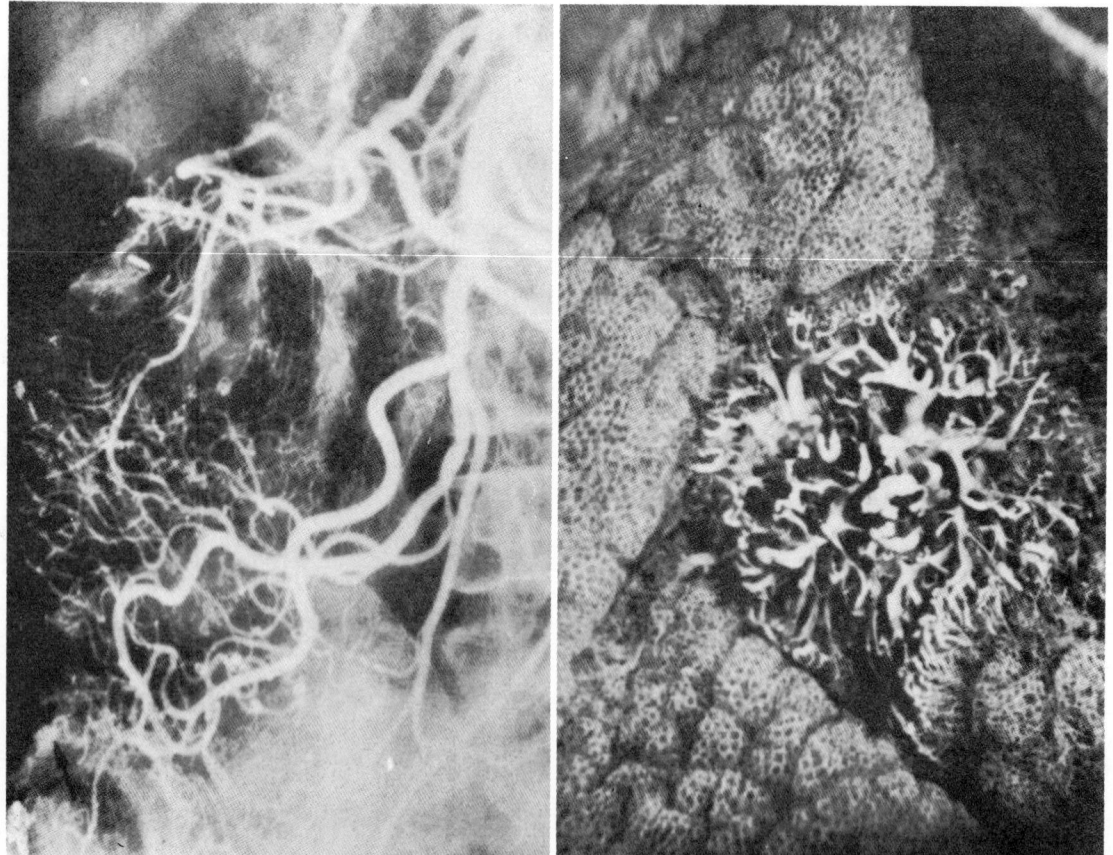

Figure 7. *A,* Selective superior mesenteric arteriogram, early arterial phase, showing a cluster of abnormally dilated arteries (arrow) in the cecum. *B,* Section of the operative specimen after silicone rubber injection and clearing, demonstrating a cluster of tortuous vessels surrounded by otherwise normal mucosal vasculature (×20). (From Baum, S., et al.: N. Engl. J. Med., *291:*569, 1974.)

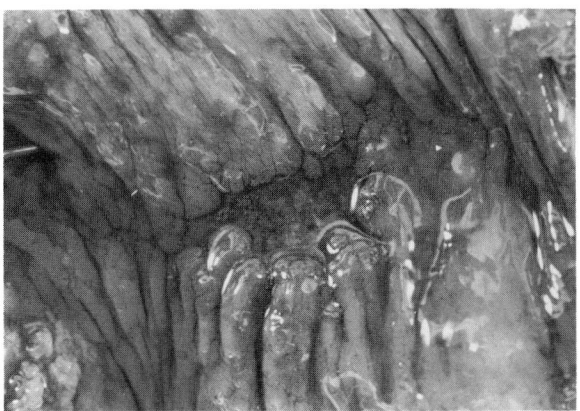

Figure 8. The right colon specimen from an elderly female with severe gastrointestinal hemorrhage shows areas of ulceration as the source of bleeding.

vasopressin, allowing for elective resection of the right colon. Study of the specimen revealed the source of bleeding to be several discrete ulcerated areas which, however, did not contain the typically tortuous, dilated blood vessels (Fig. 8). Similar experiences with angiography as a diagnostic and therapeutic aid have been reported with bleeding from inflammatory bowel disease and with carcinoma of the colon.

RECENT TECHNICAL REFINEMENTS

Visualization of splanchnic vasculature is significantly improved by administration of vasodilating agents prior to injection of contrast material. Agents which have been used include tolazoline, isoproterenol with or without phentolamine, bradykinin, glucagon, prostaglandin E, and contrast material itself.[45] Both arterial and venous visualization are enhanced by this technique, although compensation for the increased flow by increase in the amount of contrast material injected must be borne in mind or the vascular opacification may be of poor quality.

Some investigators have been developing other methods of hemostasis as an alternative to the use of vasoconstrictors. Embolization of materials such as autogenous blood clot or small bits of Gelfoam via catheters introduced into arterial branches in as close proximity to the bleeding site as possible has been successfully performed.[46] A variety of bleeding lesions have been controlled using this technique. Another potentially useful development involves transjugular catheterization of the portal vein. Retrograde advancement of the catheter into the gastric coronary vein is technically feasible, allowing for either embolization therapy, occlusion of the vein by inflation of a balloon at the catheter tip, or possibly injection of a tissue adhesive such as isobutyl-2-cyanoacrylate.[47] Further refinements of these methods may provide additional options in diagnosis and treatment of gastrointestinal bleeding in the future.

COMPLICATIONS

With careful attention to the details of insertion and manipulation of the arterial catheters, few complications occur. Some patients will develop small, self-limited hematomas at the site of catheter insertion. A few reports of major arterial complications are available, although most occurred in very ill patients or as a result of prolonged time of the catheter within the vessel. Nusbaum and co-workers reported one false aneurysm of the common femoral artery and another patient who developed thrombosis at the insertion site which required thrombectomy. Each had the catheter in place for more than a week.[32] Femoral artery thrombosis at the time of angiography on a patient in shock secondary to bleeding hypertrophic gastritis was reported by one investigator.[48] Although she recovered following a gastric resection, a major amputation was necessary due to ischemia of the limb.

Complications may also occur secondary to the infusion of vasopressin. A publication by Conn and associates divides the complications of this technique into infections and undesirable cardiorespiratory and vascular effects.[36] Bacteremias seem to be most prevalent in cirrhotic patients, and while the association with angiography was apparent, the exact causal relationship was not clear. Bradycardia was the most common of the cardiorespiratory problems, and vascular complications included arterial bleeding, catheter clotting or migration, embolism, and intestinal necrosis in one case. Antidiuretic effect of vasopressin may also be encountered in some patients, which can be managed by dose adjustment and attention to fluid balance.

Gastrointestinal complications have been reported and, although few in number, may be of considerable severity. Renert and associates[49] reported a case where exsanguination from bleeding esophageal varices unresponsive to balloon tamponade was controlled by superior mesenteric artery infusion of vasopressin. However, the patient died 26 hours later and autopsy revealed thrombosis of the mesenteric veins and segmental intestinal infarction. It should be noted, however, that this patient received three sizable doses of intravenous vasopressin prior to the intra-arterial therapy in an unsuccessful attempt to stop the bleeding.

Chait and Dann[50] reported the case of a man with nonbleeding duodenal ulcers who underwent selective angiography for evaluation of a possible nonbeta islet cell pancreatic tumor. During the procedure massive bleeding from the ulcers occurred, necessitating immediate surgery. In addition, Prochaska et al.[51] reported the case of a man in whom an autogenous blood clot was embolized into the left gastric artery for control of a massively bleeding lesser curvature gastric ulcer. This was performed after vasopressin had failed to stop the bleeding. The bleeding stopped following embolization, but the patient died the next day because of cardiorespiratory arrest. At autopsy, an area of full-thickness necrosis of the lesser curvature was observed. The patient also had severe atherosclerosis involving all arteries to the stomach, and the authors believed that collateral circulation, usually profuse in the stomach, was severely compromised in this patient, causing the gastric necrosis.

REFERENCES

1. Atik, M., and Simeone, F. A.: Massive gastrointestinal bleeding. Arch. Surg., 69:355–365, 1954.
2. Schobinger, R., Blackman, G., and Lin, R. K.: Operative intestinal arteriography. Acta. Radiol., 48:330, 1957.
3. Margulis, A. R., Heinbecker, P., and Bernard, H. R.: Operative mesenteric arteriography in the search for the site of the bleeding in unexplained gastrointestinal hemorrhage. A preliminary report. Surgery, 48:534, 1960.
4. Seldinger, S. I.: Catheter replacement of needle in percutaneous arteriography; new technique. Acta. Radiol., 39:369, 1953.
5. Nusbaum, M., and Baum, S.: Roentgenographic demonstrations of the unknown sites of gastrointestinal bleeding. Surg. Forum, 14:374, 1963.
6. Nusbaum, M., Baum, S., Blakemore, W. S., and Finklestein, A.: Demonstration of intra-abdominal bleeding by selective arteriography: Visualization of celiac and superior mesenteric arteries. J.A.M.A., 191:389, 1965.
7. Nusbaum, M., Baum, S., Kuroda, K., and Blakemore, W. S.: Control of portal hypertension by selective mesenteric drug infusion. Arch. Surg., 97:1005, 1968.
8. Odman, P.: Percutaneous selective angiography of the main branches of the aorta (preliminary report). Acta. Radiol., 45:1, 1956.
9. Odman, P.: Percutaneous selective angiography of the celiac artery. Acta. Radiol., Suppl. 159, 1958.
10. Greenspan, R. H., Simon, A. L., Ricketts, H. J., Rojas, R. H., and Watson, J. C.: In vivo magnification angiography. Invest. Radiol., 2:419, 1967.
11. Kuroda, K., and Baum, S.: New advances in abdominal angiography. Surg. Ann., 2:113–143, 1970.
12. Nusbaum, M., Baum, S., Blakemore, W. S., and Tumen, H.: Clinical experience with selective intra-arterial infusion of vasopressin in the control of gastrointestinal bleeding from arterial sources. Am. J. Surg., 123:165–172, 1972.
13. Rösch, J., Gray, R. K., Grollman, J. H., Ross, G., Steckel, R. J., and Weiner, M.: Selective arterial drug infusions in the treatment of acute gastrointestinal bleeding. Gastroenterology, 59:341–349, 1970.
14. Wiggers, C. J.: The physiology of the pituitary gland and the action of its extract. Am. J. Med. Sci., 141:502, 1911.
15. Rist, E.: Treatment of hemoptysis by intravenous injection of pituitrin. Bull. Mem. Hosp. Paris, 1:776, 1913.
16. Hoffbauer, F. W., Bollman, J. L., and Grindlay, J. L.: Factors influencing pressure in portal vein as studied in intact animal. Gastroenterology, 16:194–210, 1950.
17. Davis, W. D., Jr., Gorlin, R., Reichman, S., and Storaasli, J. P.: Effect of pituitrin in reducing portal pressure in the human being. N. Engl. J. Med., 256:108, 1957.
18. Kehne, J. H., Hughes, F. A., and Gompertz, M. L.: Use of surgical pituitrin in control of esophageal varix bleeding: Experimental study and report of two cases. Surgery, 39:917–925, 1956.
19. Shaldon, S., and Sherlock, S.: The use of vasopressin (Pitressin) in the control of bleeding from oesophageal varices. Lancet, 2:222, 1960.
20. Schwartz, S. I., Bales, H. W., Emerson, G. L., and Mahoney, E. B.: The use of intravenous pituitrin in treatment of bleeding esophageal varices. Surgery, 45:72–80, 1959.
21. Drapanas, T., Crowe, C. P., Shim, W. K. T., and Schenk, W. G., Jr.: The effect of pitressin on cardiac output and coronary, hepatic, and intestinal blood flow. Surg. Gynecol. Obstet., 113:484–489, 1961.
22. Sirinek, K. R., Martin, E. W., and Thomford, N. R.: Peripheral vasopressin provides safe and adequate control of portal hypertension during shunt operations. Am. J. Surg., 131:103–107, 1976.
23. Nusbaum, M., Baum, S., and Blakemore, W. S.: Clinical experience with the diagnosis and management of gastrointestinal hemorrhage by selective mesenteric catheterization. Ann. Surg., 170:506–514, 1969.
24. Nusbaum, M., Baum, S., Sakiyalak, P., and Blakemore, W. S.: Pharmacologic control of portal hypertension. Surgery, 62:299–310, 1967.
25. Ross, G.: Effects of epinephrine and norepinephrine on the mesenteric circulation of the cat. Am. J. Physiol., 212:1037–1042, 1967.
26. Steckel, R. J., Ross, G., and Grollman, J. H., Jr.: A potent drug combination for producing constriction of the superior mesenteric artery and its branches. Radiology, 91:579–581, 1968.
27. Rösch, J., Gray, R. K., Grollman, J. H., Jr., Ross, G., Steckel, R. J., and Weiner, M.: Selective arterial drug infusions in the treatment of acute gastrointestinal bleeding. Gastroenterology, 59:341–349, 1970.
28. Rösch, J., Dotter, C. T., and Rose, R. W.: Selective arterial infusions of vasoconstrictors in acute gastrointestinal bleeding. Radiology, 99:27–36, 1971.
29. Brant, B., Rösch, J., and Krippaehne, W. W.: Experience with angiography in diagnosis and treatment of acute gastrointestinal bleeding of various etiologies. Ann. Surg., 176:419–434, 1972.
30. Barr, J. W., Lakin, R. C., and Rösch, J.: Vasopressin and hepatic artery. Effect of selective celiac infusion of vasopressin on the hepatic artery flow. Invest. Radiol., 10:200–205, 1975.
31. Kiselow, M. C., and Wagner, M.: Intragastric instillation of levarternol. Arch. Surg., 107:387–389, 1973.
32. LeVeen, H. H., Falk, G., Diaz, C., Wynkoop, B., Piccone, V. A., Yarnoz, M. D., Langsam, A. A., Nelson, J. H., Pedowitz, W. J., and Belfasky, R. B.: Control of gastrointestinal bleeding. Am. J. Surg., 123:154–159, 1972.
33. Nusbaum, M., Younis, M. T., Baum, S., and Blakemore, W. S.: Control of portal hypertension. Arch. Surg., 108:342–347, 1974.
34. Nusbaum, M., Younis, M. T., Baum, S., and Blakemore, W. S.: Selective superior mesenteric arterial infusion of vasopressin during portosystemic shunt operations. Am. J. Surg., 127:35–39, 1974.
35. Ring, E. J., Baum, S., Athanasoulis, C., and Waltman, A. C.: Angiography in the diagnosis and treatment of nonvariceal bleeding in patients with portal hypertension. Surg. Gynecol. Obstet., 139:205–207, 1974.
36. Conn, H. O., Ramsby, G. R., and Storer, E. H.: Selective intra-arterial vasopressin in the treatment of upper gastrointestinal hemorrhage. Gastroenterology, 63:634–645, 1972.
37. Rau, R. M., II, Thompson, R. J., Simmons, C. R., Hinshaw, D. B., and Branson, B.: Selective visceral angiography in the diagnosis and treatment of gastrointestinal hemorrhage. Am. J. Surg., 128:160–167, 1974.
38. Waltman, A. C., Courey, W. R., Athanasoulis, C., and Baum, S.: Technique for left gastric artery catheterization. Radiology, 109:732–734, 1973.
39. Athanasoulis, C. A., Baum, S., Waltman, A. C., Ring, E. J., Imbembo, A., and Vander Salm, T. J.: Control of acute gastric mucosal hemorrhage. N. Engl. J. Med., 290:597–603, 1974.
40. Dorricott, N. J., Eisenberg, H., and Silen, W.: Effect of intraarterial vasopressin on canine gastric mucosal permeability. Gastroenterology, 65:625–629, 1973.
41. Baum, S., Athanasoulis, C. A., Waltman, A. C., and Ring, E. J.: Gastrointestinal hemorrhage. Angiographic diagnosis and control. Adv. Surg., 7:149–198, 1973.
42. Athanasoulis, C. A., Baum, S., Rösch, J., Waltman, A. C., Ring, E. J., Smith, J. C., Jr., Sugarbaker, E., and Wood, W.: Mesenteric arterial infusions of vasopressin for hemorrhage from colonic diverticulosis. Am. J. Surg., 129:212–216, 1975.
43. Sobin, S. S.: Vascular Injection Methods. Methods Med. Res., 11:233, 1965.
44. Case Records of the Massachusetts General Hospital (Case 36-1974). N. Engl. J. Med., 291:569–575, 1974.
45. Davis, L. J., Anderson, J. H., Wallace, S., Gianturco, C., and Jacobson, E. D.: The use of prostaglandin E to enhance the angiographic visualization of the splanchnic circulation. Radiology, 114:281–286, 1975.
46. Rösch, J., Dotter, C. T., and Brown, M. J.: Selective arterial embolization: a new method for control of acute gastrointestinal bleeding. Radiology, 102:303–306, 1972.
47. Rösch, J., Goldman, M. L., and Dotter, C. T.: Experimental catheter obstruction of the gastric coronary vein. Invest. Radiol., 10:206–211, 1975.
48. Reuter, S. R., and Bookstein, J. J.: Angiographic localization of gastrointestinal bleeding. Gastroenterology, 54:876–883, 1968.
49. Renert, W. A., Button, K. F., Field, S. L., and Casarella, W. J.: Mesenteric venous thrombosis and small bowel infarction following infusion of vasopressin into the superior and mesenteric artery. Radiology, 102:299–302, 1972.
50. Chait, A., and Dann, R. H.: G-I bleeding after angiography. N. Engl. J. Med., 286:1418–1419, 1972.
51. Prochaska, J. M., Flye, M. W., and Johnstrude, I. S.: Left gastric artery embolization for control of gastric bleeding: A complication. Radiology, 107:521–522, 1973.

V

TUMORS OF THE DUODENUM AND SMALL INTESTINE

G. Robert Mason, M.D., Ph.D.

Tumors of the small intestine are medical curiosities from several points of view. For example, the small intestine is estimated to have a surface area of 4500 m.[2]. An average adult has 2 m.[2] of body surface area, yet skin tumors are the most common site of malignancy and intestinal tumors are a clinical rarity. Anatomically, at autopsy, small intestinal tumors are relatively common, having been found in 225 of 28,750 postmortem examinations (1/127)[8, 42] as opposed to 1 in 3,000 surgical admissions or 1 in 9,000 general hospital admissions.[12] Clearly, lack of visibility is a problem; lack of symptoms of a specific nature may be another; difficulty in diagnosis a third; and perhaps most important, in view of the autopsy series, is a low index of suspicion on the part of the attending physician. It may be helpful to recall that 5 per cent of gastrointestinal malignancies and 25 per cent of benign gastrointestinal lesions are to be found in the small intestine.[37]

Benign Tumors of the Small Intestine (Table 1)

Epithelial Lesions. These tumors may be adenomatous or hamartomatous polyps or may derive from the argentaffin (Kulchitsky) or argyrophil cells of the mucosa. Adenomatous polyps may form at the ampulla of Vater and cause obstructive symptoms.[17] In general these polyps are benign. Although the inflammatory changes may make frozen section diagnosis difficult, permanent sections may be more helpful. The intestinal mucosa may be ectopically located and form cysts that may be within the intestinal wall or may be attached to it. Similarly, there may be a complete duplication of the intestine that may or may not be in continuity with the alimentary tract and may present as a tumor. Polyps are most commonly adenomatous and in the adult may

have a relationship to malignancy. In children, however, so called "juvenile polyps" may occur, most commonly in association with large intestinal manifestations. These polyps do not have a relationship to malignant change. Hamartomatous polyps have contributions from all tissues of the intestinal wall and are usually manifestations of the Peutz-Jeghers syndrome (see below). Hamartomatous polyps of Brunner's glands are found in the first and second portions of the duodenum and are similar to Peutz-Jeghers polyps but are not associated with oral pigmentation or family incidence. The Cronkhite-Canada syndrome is a variant on polypoid growths characterized by diffuse mucosal polyposis with edematous lamina propria containing dilated cystic glands. The argentaffin cells contain 5-hydroxytryptamine and may form carcinoid tumors. The argyrophil cells are similar to pancreatic islet cells and the medullary cells of the thyroid that produce calcitonin. These amino precursor uptake and decarboxylation (APUD) cells may produce tumors that in turn produce hormones such as gastrin, glucagon, and parathormone.

Lymphatic Lesions. Lymphoid tissue tumors may derive from the intestinal wall and seem to be more common distally than proximally. These tumors may be part of a generalized systemic disease but also may be primary in the intestine. The benign form includes polypoid lymphoid hyperplasia and is most commonly found in the distal ileum. This condition may be an inflammatory response and is not related to malignancy. In some cases there may be an associated hypogammaglobulinemia. Abnormalities of the lymph channels may also exist and may produce lymphatic cysts, lymphangiomas or chylangiomas, and lymphangiectasis.

Connective Tissue Tumors. Connective tissue may also produce benign tumors. As a collective group these are the most common tumors of the gastrointestinal tract and the most common of these are leiomyomas (Table 2). However, lipomas, fibromas, fibromyxomas, ganglioneuromas, neurilemomas, and hemangiomas may also be found. Lipid deposits at the ileocecal valve may be in the form of lipoma or may be diffusely localized as ileocecal lipomatosis. Although lipomas may occur throughout the small intestine, they are most common in the ileum.[33]

Congenital Abnormalities. Ectopic tissue, particularly from the pancreas, may be found in the wall of the stomach and small bowel or in Meckel's diverticula. This tissue is not active in an endocrine fashion as are the APUD cells. Diverticula may be found throughout the small intestine. They are usually found on the mesenteric surface of the gut and have been related to muscular weakness at the site of vascular penetration. These diverticula may be single but are more often multiple. Traction diverticula may also form secon-

TABLE 1. Benign Lesions of the Small Intestine*

Site	Type of Lesion	Number
Mucosa	Adenoma, adenomatous polyp, Peutz-Jeghers polyp	456
Fibrous tissue	Fibroma, myoma, fibromyoma, myofibroma, fibroadenoma, fibromyxoma, myxoma	484
Vascular	Angioma, hemangiopericytoma, lymphangioma	146
Neurogenic	Neurofibroma, neurinoma, ganglioneuroma	90
Fat	Lipoma	219
Other		4
Total		1399

*Adapted from River, L., Silverstein, J., and Tope, J. W.: Benign neoplasms of the small intestine: A critical comprehensive review with reports of 20 new cases. Int. Abstr. Surg., *102*:1–38, 1956.

TABLE 2.   Tumors of the Small Intestine: Combined Results of Eight Studies*

	Duodenum	Jejunum	Ileum	Total
Malignant				
Adenocarcinoma	92	90	28	210
Lymphoma	3	57	69	129
Sarcoma	15	23	33	71
Miscellaneous	1	4	4	9
	111	174	134	419
Carcinoid	15	19	229	263
Benign				
Leiomyoma	31	77	54	162
Adenoma	39	38	38	115
Lipoma	25	11	42	78
Miscellaneous	33	18	23	74
Hemangioma	3	39	21	63
Neurofibroma	2	6	3	11
Lymphangioma	0	2	4	6
Fibroma	0	2	2	4
Fibromyoma	0	1	0	1
	133	194	187	514
				1196

*See references 12, 16, 20, 24, 28, 42, 49, and 51.

dary to adhesions and are usually single. Diverticula may give symptoms from bleeding, diverticulitis, or the blind loop syndrome.

Inflammatory Diseases. Various inflammatory diseases or responses to disease may be considered as small intestinal tumors. These include eosinophilic granulomatous polyps and eosinophilic enteritis. The former are usually single and unassociated with systemic manifestations, and present as the cause of obstruction and/or intussusception. The latter is more commonly a thickening of a segment of gut associated with systemic blood eosinophilia and may be associated with malabsorption or protein-losing enteropathy. Here again, the presentation is usually acute obstruction. In both cases, the tissue is edematous with eosinophilic infiltration. Amyloid deposits rarely may occur in the intestine either as primary amyloid or secondary to disease such as ulcerative colitis. Mural thickening, partial obstruction, and malabsorption may be presenting symptoms. Crohn's disease per se can also cause similar symptoms and will be discussed elsewhere. Connective tissue disorders such as scleroderma are known for their association with esophageal thickening and loss of motility; however, such findings may also be present in the small intestine. Rarely, endometriosis may also present with obstructive symptoms or bleeding. Historically, the relationship may be established with menstrual periods. In the recent past, ulcers and strictures of the small intestine were associated with enteric-coated medications such as KCl. Since these products have no longer been commercially available, these lesions seem to be less common; however, a careful history of medication ingestion should be elicited in all patients.

Radiation Damage. Radiation damage to the intestine after therapy for malignancy may cause malab-

sorption, blood loss, and protein loss, as well as scarring and stenosis that may be mistaken for recurrent malignancy.[32]

Malignant Tumors of the Small Intestine

Adenocarcinoma. Adenocarcinoma of the small intestine is said to form less than 1 per cent of all intestinal carcinomas but is the most common small intestinal malignancy. In the Mayo Clinic series, 55 cases of small intestinal cancer were found relative to 4597 colon carcinomas and 4315 gastric carcinomas.[42] The duodenum was the most common site for primary carcinoma in Rochlin's review (1961), with numbers decreasing distally.[46] Within the duodenum, the most common site appears to be the periampullary region, with otherwise even distribution.

Lymphomas. Lymphomas appear to be the most common small intestinal sarcoma (Table 2). As previously noted, these may be primary or part of a more general disease pattern. Dawson[10] has suggested four criteria for the diagnosis of primary bowel lymphoma: (1) no generalized, superficial, or mediastinal lymphadenopathy; (2) normal white cell total and differential count; (3) at laparotomy or autopsy, the bowel lesion and drainage nodes should be the only ones obviously affected; and (4) the liver and spleen should be free of tumor.

The various manifestations of lymphoma, reticulum cell sarcoma, Hodgkin's disease, etc., may all be primary in the intestine. Patterns of association exist with gluten-sensitive enteropathy and idiopathic steatorrhea. A specific pattern also has been reported of duodenal lymphoma in young people in the Middle East.[39]

Leiomyomas and other fibrous tumors form approximately 20 per cent of the benign tumors of the small intestine. These lesions have a wide variety of histological characteristics relating to cellularity, nuclear patterns, etc. In many cases metastatic lesions may be found, clearly establishing the malignant nature of the tumor.[50] There is not always a clear diagnosis with solitary lesions. Other sarcomas are relatively rare, i.e., fibromyxosarcomas, liposarcomas, etc.

Secondary Malignancies. Rarely, the small intestine may be a site for metastases from the lung, stomach, colon, adrenal gland, kidney, ovary, uterine corpus, and cervix and from malignant melanoma, plasmacytomas, and leukemia.

Carcinoid and APUD Tumors. Carcinoid tumors are most common in the more distal intestine, particularly the appendix, but are found wherever argentaffin cells are located. APUDomas are most common in stomach and rectum, but are also found in the small intestine, most commonly the duodenum. Both these tumors are well differentiated and slow growing. Criteria of malignancy are invasion of lymph nodes, blood vessels, and nerve sheath, or the presence of distant (hepatic) metastasis. Their ill effects are primarily endocrine in nature.[55]

Relationship to Other Neoplastic Growth. Alexander and Altemeier have reported 83 of 112 patients with primary neoplasms of the small intestine as having another independent neoplasm at death. Of those with benign intestinal neoplasms, 57 per cent had benign neoplasms elsewhere from the small intestine and 23 per cent had a second primary malignancy elsewhere.[1]

Syndromes Associated with Small Intestinal Neoplasms

Peutz-Jeghers syndrome is characterized by hamartomatous polyps of the gastrointestinal tract (stomach, small bowel, colon), which are associated with mucocutaneous pigmentation (lips, oral mucosa, fingers, forearm, toes, umbilical area). The skin pigmentation may fade after puberty, but that of the mucous membrane is retained.[23, 41] Although there is said to be no relation of this syndrome to development of cancer, River reported 10 of 51 cases (19.6 per cent) in which carcinomatous changes were observed in the polyps. The syndrome is probably transmitted as a dominant trait. Peak presentation age in River's series was in the 10- to 29-year-old group.[45] The polyps usually develop later than the pigmentation.

The *Cronkhite-Canada syndrome* is characterized by generalized gastrointestinal polyposis and ectodermal defects such as alopecia, excessive skin pigmentation, and nail atrophy. In the intestinal polyps, dilated cystic glands are found in an edematous lamina propria. Loss of protein from the gut with calcium, magnesium, and potassium deficiencies may occur.[6, 25]

Gordon's disease is a protein-losing gastroenteropathy, usually manifested as Menetrier's disease, which involves mucosal hypertrophy, hyperplasia of the superficial epithelium, degeneration in the glandular layer, and hypoproteinemia due to leakage of proteins through the mucous membranes. A diffuse gastrointestinal polyposis associated with protein loss has also been reported.[15]

Juvenile polyposis is most commonly found in the colon and rectum; however, isolated examples of generalized gastrointestinal polyposis are reported with and without family history or other congenital abnormalities. The polyps have normal mucosa but have cysts and increased thickness in the lamina propria.[48] No apparent relationship to malignancy is known.

Gardner's syndrome is generally characterized by rectal and colonic polyposis; however, generalized polyposis has been recorded. These polyps have a relationship to the development of adenocarcinoma. The syndrome also includes cysts of the skin, osteomas, fibrous and fatty tumors of the skin and mesentery, follicular odontomas, and dentigerous cysts and changes in the bony structures of the jaws. This syndrome is familial and is transmitted as an autosomal dominant trait.[13]

Rendu-Osler-Weber disease is described as telangiectasia of the nasopharynx or gastrointestinal tract. The disease is characterized by a familial incidence and also by lesions of the palmar surface of the hands and of the nail beds.[31]

Turner's syndrome. Intestinal telangiectasia has been noted in 4 of 55 patients in one series.[18]

Pseudoxanthoma elasticum. Benign vascular lesions of the intestinal tract have been reported in association with this disease.[31]

Carter-Horsley-Hughes syndrome. Diffuse polyposis of the small and large intestine was noted in one family.[5]

Bessauds-Hillmand-Augier syndrome. Sexual infantilism is associated with intestinal polyposis.[44]

von Recklinghausen's disease. Generalized neurofibromatosis with café au lait skin pigmentation may also include neurofibromas of the gastrointestinal tract.[14]

Familial polyposis of the colon. This syndrome is customarily associated with polyps of the colon; however, several cases of generalized polyposis have been recorded with associated malignancy.[47]

Symptoms and Complications

The numbers and variety of small bowel tumors found at autopsy suggest that many such tumors are asymptomatic. When symptoms do arise they are usually related to either obstructive phenomena or bleeding. Because the content of the small intestine is largely liquid, the degree of obstruction must be almost complete before symptoms are noted. Epigastric discomfort or cramping pain associated with nausea or nausea and vomiting will slowly increase in severity as the lesion occludes the intestinal lumen. Obstruction is the most common complication (50 per cent), with benign tumors and intussusception as its most common presentation. Bleeding is associated with angiomatous lesions and also with myomas, fibromas, fibromyomas, fibroadenomas and metastatic tumors. The rate of bleeding may be quite variable, from occult blood loss causing marginal anemia to exsanguinating hemorrhage.

Other complications such as volvulus, necrosis, and peritonitis are less common. Malignant lesions more commonly present with symptoms of pain, anorexia, weight loss, and occult bleeding, whereas benign lesions may bleed more briskly and may have less anorexia and weight loss. Periampullary duodenal tumors are distinguished by their association with painless jaundice, which is said to vary in degree as the tumor undergoes central necrosis, sloughs, and again allows free passage of bile. The presence of a palpable gallbladder in these cases further supports the diagnosis of neoplasm (Courvoisier's Law).

Diagnosis

The specific diagnosis of small intestinal neoplasms is now theoretically possible by direct visualization and biopsy through various fiberoptic endoscopes capable of traversing the entire small bowel from either end. Radiologic contrast studies utilizing various forms of barium are thought to be the best technique for demonstration of lesions in the mid range of small intestine. Hypotonic duodenography involves use of drugs such as glucagon to render the duodenum flaccid and relatively immobile, allowing for more accurate delineation of mucosal abnormalities. Lesions that are bleeding at the time of investigation may be identified by arteriography if the bleeding rate is greater than 1 to 2 ml. per minute. Laparotomy often is chosen as the diagnostic technique of choice, particularly for bleeding lesions. However, few experiences are more frustrating for the surgeon than the search for a poorly localized bleeding point that ceases its activity with induction of anesthesia.

Management

The majority of small intestinal lesions can be treated successfully by resection and by end-to-end anastomosis of the residual bowel. These operations were developed by numerous surgeons during the latter part of the last century and are relatively unchanged to this date.

The technical development of surgery for lesions of the duodenum began with Billroth's successful resection of the entire pancreas as early as 1884.[38] In 1898, Halsted described a carcinoma of the ampulla of Vater and removed it with a V-shaped wedge of duodenum and reimplanted the biliary and pancreatic ducts.[19] Although the patient eventually died from her neoplasm, she recovered from her original procedure, and a second exploration in which a cholecystoduodenostomy was done. During the next 42 years an emphasis was made on the importance of biliary decompression as a preliminary procedure for definitive therapy, which was almost always a transduodenal wedge resection of ampullary tumor. Moynihan stated in 1905 that "the mechanical difficulties of the operation are well nigh insuperable, and that if boldness and good fortune are the operator's gifts, the result to the patient hardly justifies the means."[38]

It was thought for a time that the duodenum and its secretions and the external secretions of the pancreas were necessary to life. The observations of Dragstedt et al. in 1918 were important in demonstrating that neither circumstance was true.[11] Reimplantation of the biliary and pancreatic ducts into the GI tract was then, as now, the basis of major complications of operations on these structures. Several possibilities may account for this. The pancreas and duodenum are only peritonealized on their ventral surface and thus provide a less secure base for sutures. In addition, the

activation of pancreatic enzymes by bile and duodenal secretions promotes digestion of absorbable sutures as well as tissue. Also, multiple suture lines multiply chances for leakage with possible development of fistula, abscess, and hemorrhage. The mortality is greater in the jaundiced patient with compromised liver function. Whipple et al. in 1935 described only four known successful cases of reimplantation of the pancreatic head or duct following resection for carcinoma of the ampulla of Vater.[59] In their report, they followed the common practice by advising a primary biliary decompression procedure in such cases but made a major contribution by utilizing pancreatic duct ligation as the second stage, combined with an en bloc dissection of pancreatic head and duodenum. Their initial success was soon reinforced by Brunschwig[3] and then again by single stage "Whipple procedures" by Whipple, Trimble et al.,[52] and Brunschwig[4] (Figs. 1 and 2).

Although fat absorption was said to be 85 to 90 per cent of normal and steatorrhea absent in such patients with ligated pancreatic ducts, it was found that the incidence of fistula was still higher following ligation than with intestinal anastomosis.[26, 34] Numerous techniques have evolved, which include end-to-end pancreatojejunostomy, end-to-side pancreatojejunostomy with meticulous mucosal anastomosis, the use of various stents, and pancreatogastrostomy (Fig. 3). A recent report by Mackie et al. gives credit to this last procedure for reduction of operative mortality from more than 25 per cent to 8 per cent.[30] A fully peritonealized stomach plus relative fixation of both stomach and pancreas has persuaded this author of its value, and in the last three cases in which it was used, no pancreatic complications have been observed. Total pancreatectomy has also been advised, but it seems more appropriate for adenocarcinoma of the pancreas than for that arising from the ampulla of Vater or the bile ducts because of the mode of spread of pancreatic cancer as well as its threat of multicentricity. In general, current practice seems to include an anastomosis of pancreas and common bile duct, end-to-end and end-to-side, respectively, to an antecolic jejunal loop proximal to the gastroenterostomy in order to neutralize the effect of acid gastric juice on the jejunal anastomosis. Although vagotomy and antrectomy might reduce this insult and the common complication of hemorrhage at the anastomosis, they do not seem to be customary adjuncts to the procedure. These procedures have been done at the University of Maryland without apparent adverse effect.

It has been our preference to remove the gallbladder if the common duct is anastomosed to the intestine, because we are concerned about stasis and infection in the gallbladder. Also, we have divided the duodenum beyond the ligament of Treitz and brought the jejunum up antecolic for the various anastomoses to avoid constriction under the mesenteric vessels.

The gallbladder was used in the early series for both decompression in the first stage and for definitive diversion with major resections. Because of a high incidence of biliary fistula in the latter case, direct bile duct–jejunal anastomoses are recommended for diversion with major resections. Depending on bile duct size

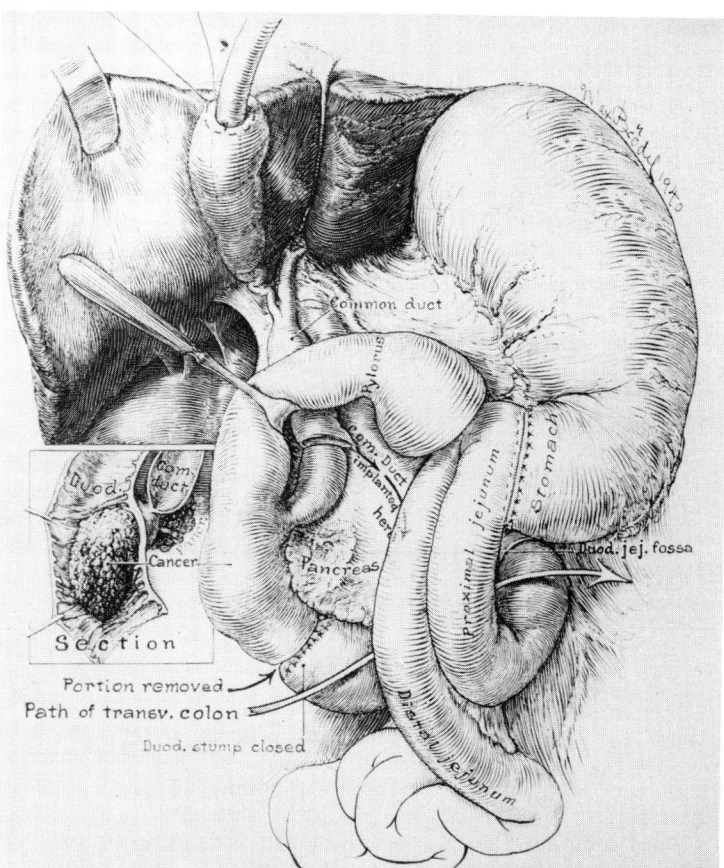

Figure 1. Resection of the duodenum, common duct, gastric antrum, and pancreatic head as described by Trimble et al. Insert shows the opened specimen with ampullary malignancy. (From Trimble, J. R., Parsons, J. W., and Sherman, C. P.: Surg. Gynecol. Obstet., *73*:711, 1941.)

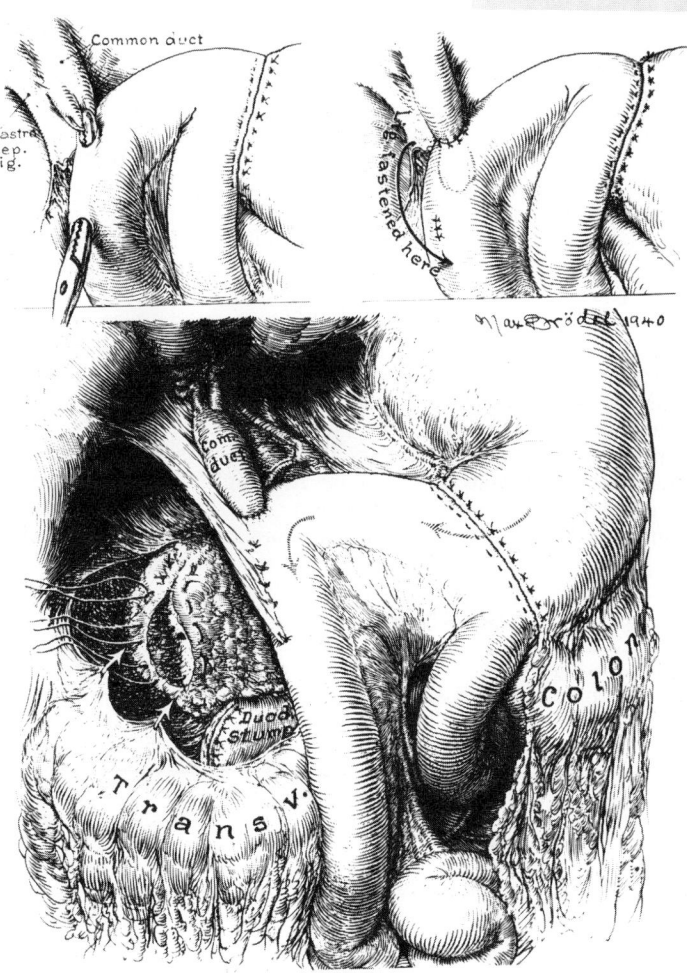

Figure 2. Reconstruction of gastrointestinal continuity with anterior Polya anastomosis, choledochojejunostomy, and suture ligation of the pancreatic stump. (From Trimble, I. R., Parsons, J. W., and Sherman, C. P.: Surg. Gynecol. Obstet., *73*:711, 1941.)

973

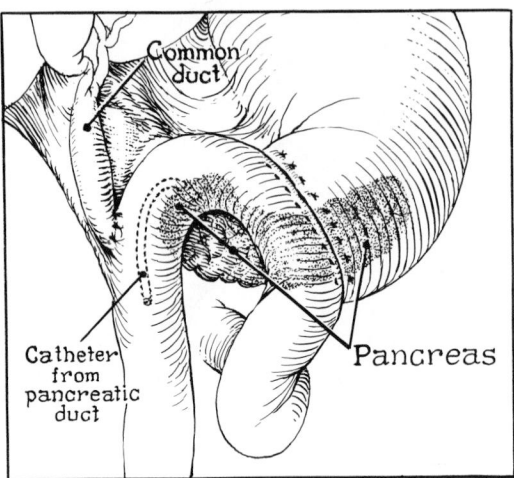

Figure 3. Alternative method of reconstruction utilizing end-to-side pancreatojejunosomy. Note the use of a stent in the pancreatic duct. (From Trimble, I. R., Parsons, J. W., and Sherman, C. P.: Surg. Gynecol. Obstet., 73:711, 1941.)

these may be end to end, but are most commonly end to side, with careful mucosal suture. Late stenosis of this anastomosis may be confused with recurrent malignancy. In major centers a mortality rate of 8 to 10 per cent may be expected, although one author has reported a large series (41 cases) with no mortality.[21, 35, 53]

Determination of Resectability

Carcinoma of the duodenum and ampulla should be diagnosed preoperatively by radiologic and endoscopic procedures with biopsy. The lesion may be approached through an upper abdominal vertical or transverse incision, depending on patient habitus. The presence of liver or nodal metastases or peritoneal seeding from such a lesion carries an ominous prognosis and indicates bypass of the lesion as described above. Gastroenterostomy may be advisable in some cases, depending on the size and location of the lesion. Barring obvious metastases, and if the middle colic artery is free at its base, the gastroduodenal artery is divided and ligated. If the operator's fingers can be passed between the pancreatic neck and the superior mesenteric vessels, resection can usually be accomplished. Several published reports describe ligation or resection of the portal vein and superior mesenteric

artery, when involved with tumor, with graft replacement of the artery and survival of the patient.[22, 36] A high operative mortality and probable high recurrence rate for such advanced tumors should not be unexpected.

Results of Surgical Management

In determination of results of therapy for carcinoma of the duodenum, a careful analysis is needed regarding tumor type, particularly at the ampulla of Vater. Here duodenal mucosa and mucosa of the ducts of Wirsung and Santorini and the common bile duct merge in or near the head of the pancreas. Characteristics of pancreatic tumors include perineural invasion, multicentricity, and local nodal metastases. Ampullary and duodenal lesions are more often of a lower grade of malignancy, spread more locally, and do not as commonly invade bile duct, perineural lymphatics, or local nodes. As noted earlier in this chapter, small bowel tumors are relatively rare, and malignant tumors are rarer than benign tumors. Hence, any evaluation of overall success at resection must depend on comparison of small numbers of cases done by various surgeons with varying degrees of skill as well as on an accurate histological identification of tumor source. Two of the largest series of pancreatoduodenectomies reported are summarized in Table 3.

Because of the liquid content of the small intestine, symptoms are often a late manifestation of adenocarcinoma of the small intestine. Tumor has frequently spread through the wall and into regional lymph nodes and mesentery by the time laparotomy is performed. A five-year survival rate from en bloc resection has been reported by various authors as ranging from 14 to 22 per cent.[10, 40]

Localized *lymphomas* of the gastrointestinal tract treated by curative resection and 3000 to 4000 rads have had five-year survival rates as high as 85 per cent (11/13).[27] With recent advances in combined therapy, the overall outlook for this disease should be better in future reports.

Leiomyosarcoma and fibrosarcoma are said to be the most common lesions in the sarcoma group. Starr and Dockerty reported 38 per cent of 26 patients with these lesions, treated by resection, to be well five years later.[50]

Carcinoid tumors are extremely slow growing, well-differentiated lesions. Although their name implies that the lesion is not a true cancer, some authors believe that all such tumors are malignant. MacDon-

TABLE 3. Incidence and Survival of Cancer by Anatomic Site*

Anatomic Site	Mayo Clinic (1964)		Lahey Clinic (1975)	
	No. of Cases	5-Yr. Survivals (%)	No. of Cases	5-Yr. Survivals (%)
Head of pancreas	119	18.2	104	12.5
Ampulla	77	39.1	112	32.0
Duodenum	25	38.5	47	25.0
Common bile duct	18	11.1	39	41.3

*See references 35 and 53.

TABLE 4. Malignant Tumors of the Small Intestine: Combined Results of 12 Studies*

	Cases	Per Cent
Adenocarcinoma	446	36
Carcinoid	392	31
Sarcoma	179	14
Lymphoma	233	19
Total	1250	

*See references 2, 7, 9, 12, 16, 20, 24, 28, 40, 42, 49, and 51.

ald collected 356 gastrointestinal carcinoid tumors, which showed an incidence of 31 per cent nodal metastases and 11 per cent hepatic metastases at operation.[29] Darling and Welch have reported a series of 12 patients treated by en bloc resection. Of the nine operative survivals, eight lived five or more years.[8] Because of the slow rate of growth of carcinoid tumors, a five-year span is probably inadequate to predict cures. As noted earlier, carcinoid tumors synthesize 5-hydroxytryptamine (serotonin) as well as kallikrein and bradykinin. Metastatic carcinoid tumors in the liver may release these and perhaps other substances into the blood to produce episodic symptoms of cutaneous flushing, diarrhea, asthma, and right-sided valvular heart disease. Treatment of the "carcinoid syndrome" may include resection of hepatic masses and oral administration of methysergide and antihistamines. Radiotherapy and chemotherapy have not been beneficial,[55] except for some preliminary reports of efficacy of streptazotocin.

SELECTED REFERENCES

Good, C. A.: Tumors of the small intestine. Am. J. Roentgenol., 89:685, 1963.
The Mayo Clinic experience with small intestinal tumors is described from the radiologist's point of view. The illustrations are excellent and cover the many variations in radiographic appearance of these tumors.

Morson, B. C., and Dawson, I. M. P.: Gastrointestinal Pathology. Oxford, Blackwell Scientific Publications, Ltd., 1972.
The authors of this text have had an unusually broad experience with gastrointestinal pathology. Their text can be recommended for its clarity and completeness.

River, L., Silverstein, J., and Tope, J. W.: Benign neoplasms of the small intestine: A critical comprehensive review with reports of 20 new cases. Int. Abstr. Surg., 102:1–38, 1956.
Although published over twenty years ago, this is still the most extensive study available concerning benign small intestinal tumors.

Trimble, I. R., Parsons, J. W., and Sherman, C. P.: A one stage operation for the cure of carcinomas of the ampulla of Vater and of the head of the pancreas. Surg. Gynecol. Obstet., 73:711–722, 1941.
The historical development of en bloc resection of the pancreatic head and duodenum is superbly covered in this first published description of the single-stage "Whipple procedure."

REFERENCES

1. Alexander, J. W., and Altemeier, W. A.: Association of primary neoplasms of the small intestine with other neoplastic growths. Ann. Surg., 167:958–964, 1968.
2. Brooks, V. S., Waterhouse, J. A. H., and Powell, D. J.: Malignant lesions of the small intestine. Br. J. Surg., 55:405–410, 1968.
3. Brunschwig, A.: Resection of head of pancreas and duodenum for carcinoma-pancreatoduodenectomy. Surg. Gynecol. Obstet., 65:681–684, 1937.
4. Brunschwig, A.: One stage pancreato-duodenectomy. Surg. Gynecol. Obstet., 77:581, 1943.
5. Carter, B. N., Horsley, G. W., Horsley, J. J., and Hughes, R. D.: A new form of diffuse familial polyposis: A probable genetic explanation. Ann. Surg., 167:942–948, 1968.
6. Cronkhite, L. W., and Canada, W. J.: Generalized gastrointestinal polyposis: An unusual syndrome of polyposis, pigmentation, alopecia and onychotrophia. N. Engl. J. Med., 252:1011, 1955.
7. Croome, R. D., III, and Newsome, J. F.: Benign and malignant tumors of the small intestine. South. Med. J., 61:271–274, 1968.
8. Darling, R. C., and Welch, C. E.: Tumors of the small intestine. N. Engl. J. Med., 260:408, 1959.
9. Darman, J. E., Floyd, E., and Cohn, I., Jr.: Malignant neoplasms of the small bowel. Am. J. Surg., 113:131, 1967.
10. Dawson, I. M. P., Cornes, J. J., and Morson, B. C.: Primary malignant lymphoid tumors of the intestinal tract. Report of 37 cases with a study of factors influencing prognosis. Br. J. Surg., 49:80, 1961.
11. Dragstedt, L. R., Dragstedt, C. A., McClintoch, J. T., and Chase, C. S.: Extirpation of the duodenum. Am. J. Physiol., 46:584–590, 1918.
12. Dundon, C. C.: Primary tumors of the small intestine. Am. J. Roentgenol., 59:492–504, 1948.
13. Gardner, E. J.: Genetic and clinical study of intestinal polyposis. Predisposing factor for carcinoma of colon and rectum. Am. J. Hum. Genet., 3:167–176, 1951.
14. Ghrist, T. D.: Gastrointestinal involvement in neurofibromatosis. Arch. Int. Med., 112:357–362, 1963.
15. Gill, W. J., and Wilken, B. J.: Diffuse gastrointestinal polyposis associated with hypoproteinemia. J. R. Coll. Surg. Edin., 12:149–156, 1967.
16. Good, C. A.: Tumors of the small intestine. Am. J. Roentgenol., 89:685, 1963.
17. Griffen, W. O., Jr., Schaefer, J. W., Schindler, S., Hyde, G., and Bryant, L. R.: Ampullary obstruction by benign duodenal polyps. Arch. Surg., 97:444–449, 1968.
18. Haddad, H. M., and Wilkins, L.: Congenital anomalies associated with gonadal aplasia. Review of 55 cases. Pediatrics, 23:885–902, 1959.
19. Halsted, W. S.: Contributions to surgery of the bile passages, especially of the common bile duct. Johns Hopkins Med. Bull., 11:1–11, 1900 (Surgical papers by William Stewart Halsted, Baltimore, The Johns Hopkins Press, 1924).
20. Hancock, R. J.: An 11 year review of primary tumors of the small bowel including the duodenum. Can. Med. Assoc. J., 103:1177–1179, 1970.
21. Howard, J. M.: Pancreatoduodenectomy. Forty-one consecutive Whipple resections without an operative mortality. Ann. Surg., 168:629, 1968.
22. Hubbard, T. B., Jr.: Carcinoma of the head of the pancreas: Resection of the portal vein and porta caval shunt. Am. Surg., 147:935, 1958.
23. Jegher, H., McKusick, V. A., and Katz, K. H.: Generalized intestinal polyposis and melanin spots of oral mucosa, lips and digits. N. Engl. J. Med., 241:993, 1949.
24. Jenkinson, E. L., Pfisterer, W. H., and Seitz, E. R.: Primary tumors of the small intestine. Radiology, 55:12, 1950.
25. Johnson, M. M., Vosburgh, J. W., Weins, A. T., and Walsh, G. C.: Gastrointestinal polyposis associated with alopecia, pigmentation and atrophy of the fingernails and toenails. Ann. Int. Med., 56:935, 1962.
26. Kaufman, L. W., and Wilson, G. W.: Carcinoma of the head of the pancreas and periampullary region. Am. J. Med. Sci., 230:200–212, 1955.
27. Loehr, W. J., Mujahed, Z., Zahn, F. D., Gray, G. F., and Thorbjarnarson, B.: Primary lymphoma of the gastrointestinal tract: A review of 100 cases. Ann. Surg., 170:232–238, 1969.
28. Macbeth, W. A. A. G., and Gwynne, J. F.: Tumours of the small bowel. Aust. N. Z. J. Surg., 38:206–215, 1969.
29. Macdonald, R. A.: Study of 356 carcinoids of gastrointestinal tract: Report of four new cases of carcinoid syndrome. Am. J. Med., 21:867–878, 1956.
30. Mackie, J. A., Rhoads J. E., and Park C. D.: Pancreaticogastrostomy: A further evaluation. Ann. Surg., 181:541–545, 1975.
31. Manley, K. A., and Skyring, A. P.: Some heritable causes of gastrointestinal disease. Arch. Int. Med., 107:182–203, 1961.
32. Mason, G. R., Guernsey, J. M., Hanks, G. E., and Nelsen, T. S.:

Surgical therapy for radiation enteritis. Oncology, 22:251–257, 1968.

33. Mayo, C. W., Pagtalunan, R. J. G., and Brown, D. J.: Lipoma of the alimentary tract. Surgery, 53:598–603, 1963.

34. Miller, E. M., Dockerty, M. B., Wollaeger, E. E., and Waugh, J. M.: Carcinoma in the region of the ampulla of Vater. Surg. Gynecol. Obstet., 92:172–182, 1951.

35. Monge, J. J., Judd, E. S., and Gage, R. P.: Radical pancreatoduodenectomy: A 22-year experience with the complications, mortality rate, and survival rate. Ann. Surg., 160:711–722, 1964.

36. Moore, G. E., and Ure, B.: One stage pancreatectomy with resection of the superior mesenteric vein. Surgery, 35:734, 1954.

37. Morson, B. C., and Dawson, I. M. P.: Gastrointestinal Pathology. Oxford, Blackwell Scientific Publications, Ltd., 1972.

38. Moynihan, B.: Abdominal Operations, 4th ed. Philadelphia, W. B. Saunders Company, 1926, p. 521.

39. Nasr, K., Haghighi, P., Bakhshanden, K., and Haghshenas, M.: Primary lymphoma of the upper small intestine. Gut, 11:673, 1970.

40. Pagtalunan, R. J. G., Mayo, C. W., and Dockerty, M. B.: Primary malignant tumors of the small intestine. Am. J. Surg., 108:13–18, 1964.

41. Peutz, J. L. A.: Very remarkable case of familial polyposis of mucous membrane of the intestinal tract and nasal pharynx accompanied by peculiar pigmentation of skin and mucous membrane. Ned. M. Aandschr. Geneeskd., 10:134, 1921.

42. Raiford, T. S.: Tumors of small intestine. Arch. Surg., 25:122–321, 1932.

43. Rankin, F. W., and Mayo, C.: Carcinoma of the small bowel. Surg. Gynecol. Obstet., 50:939, 1930.

44. Ravitch, M. M.: Discussion of "A New Form of Diffuse Familial Polyposis" by Carter, B. N., Horsley, G. W., Horsley, J. J., and Hughes, R. D. Ann. Surg., 167:942–948, 1968.

45. River, L., Silverstein, J., and Tope, J. W.: Benign neoplasms of the small intestine: A critical comprehensive review with reports of 20 new cases. Int. Abstr. Surg., 102:1–38, 1956.

46. Rochlin, D. B., and Longmire, W. P., Jr.: Primary tumors of the small intestine. Surgery, 50:586–592, 1961.

47. Ross, J. E., and Mara, J. E.: Small bowel polyps and carcinoma in multiple intestinal polyposis. Arch. Surg., 108:736–738, 1974.

48. Sachatello, C. R., Pickren, J. W., and Grace, J. T., Jr.: Generalized juvenile gastrointestinal polyposis: A hereditary syndrome. Gastroenterology, 58:699–708, 1970.

49. Schmutzer, K. J., Holleran, W. M., and Regan, J. F.: Tumors of the small bowel. Am. J. Surg., 108:270–276, 1964.

50. Starr, G. F., and Dockerty, M. B.: Leiomyomas and leiomyosarcomas of the small intestine. Cancer, 8:101–111, 1955.

51. Thomas, D.: Primary tumors of the small intestine. Aust. N. Z. J. Surg., 37:359–362, 1968.

52. Trimble, I. R., Parsons, J. W., and Sherman, C. P.: A one stage operation for the cure of carcinomas of the ampulla of Vater and of the head of the pancreas. Surg. Gynecol. Obstet., 73:711–722, 1941.

53. Warren, K. W., Choe, D. S., Plaza, J., and Relihan, J.: Results of radical resection for periampullary cancer. Ann. Surg., 181:534–540, 1975.

54. Whipple, A. O., Parsons, W. B., and Mullins, C. R.: Treatment of carcinoma of the ampulla of Vater. Ann. Surg., 102:763, 1935.

55. Wilson, H., Cheek, R. C., Sherman, R. T., and Storer, E. H.: Carcinoid tumors. Curr. Probl. Surg., November, 1970.

VI

VASCULAR COMPRESSION OF THE DUODENUM

Arlie R. Mansberger, Jr., M.D.

HISTORICAL ASPECTS

In 1752 Boernerus[5] described the symptoms and postmortem findings of a patient with chronic duodenal obstruction. One hundred years later, Rokitanksy[30] first recognized and described vascular compression of the duodenum as an etiologic factor in obstruction of the transverse portion of the duodenum. Kundrat[21] in 1891 suggested that persistent incomplete obstruction of the duodenum was the result of compression by the root of the mesentery. In 1900, Robinson[29] described his impressions from a study of 30 autopsies in which the superior mesenteric vessels had caused compression of the duodenum with dilatation of the duodenum proximal to the level of compression.

At the turn of the century, much was written regarding this entity as a cause of acute gastric dilatation in the postoperative period.[4] Barker, discussing Finney's observations[12] regarding the relationship of dilatation of the duodenum to postoperative gastric disturbances, suggested duodenojejunostomy as a method of operative management: "I am wondering, too, since gastroenterostomy seems to be of no avail in these cases, whether or not a duodenojejunostomy connecting the lowermost part of the dilated duodenum with the closest part of the jejunum, would be of any service. It is conceivable that, by permitting the normal flow of bile, pancreatic juice, and duodenal secretion, as well as chyme, some benefit might result." Bloodgood,[3] one year later, apparently unaware of Dr. Barker's comments, also suggested duodenojejunostomy as an operative approach to the problem. In 1908, Stavely[31] of the Johns Hopkins Hospital reported the first successful duodenojejunostomy for vascular compression of the duodenum. The opening comments of his successful case report were very concise: "Author's first case. Chronic gastromesenteric ileus. Operation, duodenojenunostomy. Result cured."

Synonyms for vascular compression of the duodenum include chronic duodenal ileus, superior mesenteric artery syndrome, arteriomesenteric duodenal compression, Wilke's syndrome, "cast" syndrome, and chronic duodenal stasis.

Between 1920 and 1930 more than 100 such operations were reported and much enthusiasm was evidenced for the surgical management of vascular compression of the duodenum, but the indications and diagnostic criteria were not clearly defined and the results of therapy were poor. As a result, many physicians became skeptical of the existence of the entity and from 1934 to 1954 only *seven* operative cases were reported.[2]

Recent resurgence of interest in vascular compression[6, 11, 13, 19, 23, 25, 28, 33, 35, 37, 39] has, in part, resulted from further definition of diagnostic criteria originally suggested by Pool and associates in 1933.[24] Arteriographic studies combined with upper gastrointestinal examination with barium have allowed better definition of the point of obstruction and visualization of the pathologic anatomy of the point of obstruction and visualization of the pathologic anatomy of the superior mesenteric artery.[17, 23, 39]

ANATOMIC CONSIDERATIONS

The transverse and ascending segment of the duodenum is the most fixed portion of the alimentary canal. During the development of the small intestine in fetal life, a rotation occurs which causes the descending, transverse, and ascending portions to assume a retroperitoneal position. The duodenum is limited in its distal extreme by the ligament of Treitz and is bound posteriorly by the vena cava, vertebral bodies, and abdominal aorta and crossed anteriorly by the radix mesenterii containing the superior mesenteric neurovascular bundle.

Since the descending portion of the duodenum lies in the right paravertebral gutter somewhat posterior to the bodies of the vertebrae, the transverse and ascending portion of the duodenum must move anteriorly as well as transversely to cross the retroperitoneal unyielding structures.

In normal individuals, fat in the retroperitoneal space tends to hold the root of the mesentery and the superior mesenteric artery away from the aorta. Perinephric and retroperitoneal fat in normal persons displaces the descending portion of the duodenum anteriorly and partially out of the right paravertebral gutter so that the anterior angulation of the transverse duodenum is less acute as it rises to cross the vertebral bodies.

The superior mesenteric artery normally leaves the aorta at an average angle of 30 to 42 degrees opposite the first lumbar vertebra. Derrick and Fadhli,[9] in a study of the surgical anatomy of the superior mesenteric artery from the dissection of 63 specimens, re-

ported an average angle of "take-off" of 41.65 degrees, with a range of 20 to 70 degrees and a standard deviation of 10.65 degrees. In another series of anatomic dissections, the author[23] found the average aortomesenteric artery angle to be 30 degrees, with variations from 18 to 60 degrees. The average distance from this angle to the midpoint of the duodenum at the vertebral aortic fissure was 10 cm. The shortest duodenal midpoint was 4.5 cm. and the longest 16 cm. In the patient whose duodenal midpoint was only 4.5 cm., the arterial angle of "take-off" measured 56 degrees (Table 1).

The usual anatomic description of the superior mesenteric artery directs it from its point of origin on the aorta toward the right lower quadrant so that it lies directly over the aorta and vertebral bodies only in its most proximal portion. Thus, it is apparent that although the superior mesenteric artery–aortic angle may be quite acute in the sagittal plane, the same angle in the frontal plane might allow ample room for the duodenum to pass behind the superior mesenteric artery and anterior to the vena cava.

Furthermore, in spite of the fact that rapid significant weight loss would tend to decrease the aortomesenteric angle and drop the descending duodenum deeper into the right paravertebral gutter, the majority of persons with weight loss do not exhibit symptoms of duodenal obstruction from vascular compression.

It becomes apparent that for duodenal obstruction to be caused by vascular compression, either the duodenum must be fixed high in a narrow angle of superior mesenteric arterial origin by a firm and unyielding ligament of Treitz, as described by Strong,[32] or a narrow angled artery must continue its course abnormally and directly over the posterior structures capable of trapping the duodenum to a point beyond the duodenovertebral or duodenoaortic crossing.

The important mechanical obstructing factors, then, are a combination of a narrow angle of origin with either an abnormally highly positioned but fixed duodenum or an anomalous arterial course directly over the posterior unyielding vertebral bodies and/or aorta to a point beyond the position at which the duodenum traverses one or both of these structures.

INCIDENCE

The true incidence of this disease is unknown. In fact, there are those who deny its existence.[7, 8] Goin

TABLE 1.   Measurements Determined by Anatomic Dissection

Authors	No. of Dissections	Average Superior Mesenteric Artery–Aorta Take-off Angle	Range	Distance from Angle to Duodenal Midpoint	Range
Derrick and Fadhli	64	41.65°	20°–70°		
Byers and Mansberger	31	30°	18°–60°	10 cm.	4.5 cm.–16 cm.

and Wilk[13] reported that in 1500 consecutive upper gastrointestinal series, five (0.33 per cent) showed definite vascular duodenal compression and 450 showed some gross abnormality of the superior mesenteric artery–duodenal crossing. They also cited a similar series of 480 examinations from Harbor General Hospital in Torrance, California, which showed some gross abnormality in 173 and definite vascular compression of the duodenum in two (0.42 per cent).

Thus, although the true incidence is difficult to estimate, it is fair to assume that in its mildest form the disease occurs occasionally but in its severe form, only rarely.

CLINICAL MANIFESTATIONS

Two distinct forms of duodenal obstruction from vascular compression have been described, acute and chronic. The acute variety often occurs in patients without antecedent gastrointestinal symptoms and follows trauma,[39] burns,[27, 37] the application of body casts,[16] traction,[11] and positioning on hyperextension frames, and has been reported following a variety of operative procedures. Characteristically, the patient is immobilized for variable periods of time in the supine position. Weight loss becomes progressive and contributes to a greater degree of obstruction, with complaints of postprandial fullness, anorexia, and epigastric discomfort. Nausea and vomiting of bile-stained material follows. Emotional overlay of the serious illness may suggest no cause for the symptoms.

When external compression factors associated with hyperextension compound the situation, as with the application of a body cast, the onset of symptoms may begin immediately following cast application. In the more chronic forms, a variety of factors has been reported which may enhance tightening of the "pincer mechanism" and trigger the obstruction, including prolonged bed rest, a variety of systemic diseases, previous surgical procedures, increased lordosis, loss of muscle tone of the anterior abdominal wall leading to visceroptosis, and rapid growth in children.

Typically the patient has an asthenic habitus. A long history of episodic epigastric distress with or without periodic vomiting dating to childhood may be elicited. A history of weight loss is usual. The patient complains of postprandial pain and bloating associated with nausea and vomiting of bile-stained material. Often food ingested 24 hours previously may be noted in the vomitus. The patient soon learns to limit his intake so that vomiting may become less frequent. His symptoms then become bloating, eructation, and epigastric pain. The patient may learn that assumption of the left lateral decubitus or the prone position may afford relief of symptoms.

Frequently the picture is not as clear-cut as described. The patient's complaints may be episodic, with cyclic vomiting intermingled with intervals that are relatively symptom-free. On the other hand, vague and ill-defined epigastric discomfort, anorexia, and bloating associated with food intake may be the only gastrointestinal complaints. These symptoms may be associated with easy fatigability, malaise, nervousness, anorexia, and emotional instability.

DIAGNOSIS

A flat film may suggest the diagnosis (particularly in the acute form) when it demonstrates gross gastric and duodenal distention with minimal air in the small bowel. A "double bubble" sign is occasionally present, especially in children.[6]

With the introduction of barium into the upper gastrointestinal tract, dilatation of the first and second portion of the duodenum is seen at, or just to the right of, the midline where an oblique or straight line extrinsic pressure defect can be visualized (Fig. 1). The duodenum distal to that point is normal in size. Reverse and "to-and-fro" peristaltic waves are apparent by fluoroscopic examination. It is noteworthy that with the patient supine it is often difficult to obtain a film which shows the exact point of obstruction in the transverse or ascending portion of the duodenum. Because the proximal duodenum is dilated, the barium tends to fall back into the more dependent portions of the obstructed duodenum and will only intermittently be propelled against the site of obstruction.[17] Cinefluorography demonstrates this point to great advantage. Disappearance of duodenal retention when the patient is placed in the prone or left lateral decubitus position enhances the radiologic diagnosis.

Biplanar aortography performed simultaneously with barium studies will demonstrate the point of ob-

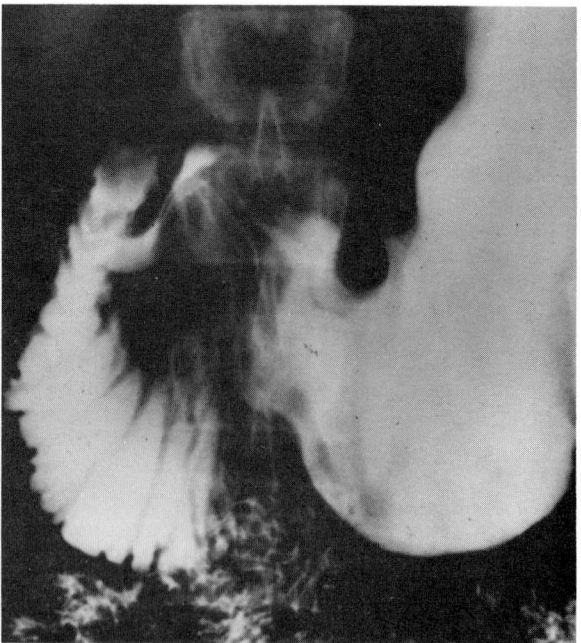

Figure 1. Gastrointestinal series of patient with vascular compression demonstrating sharp and slightly oblique cut-off at the point of compression by the superior mesenteric artery.

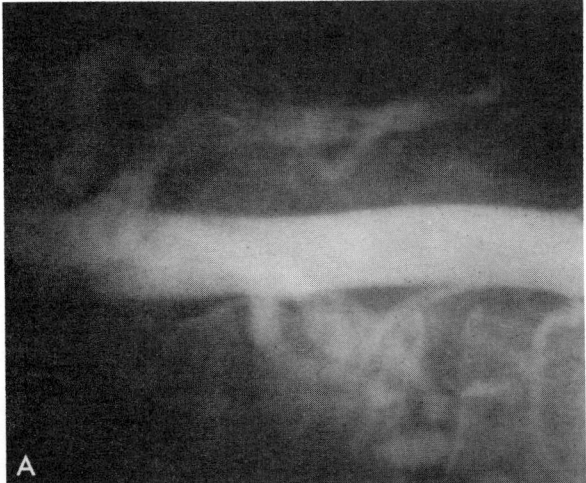

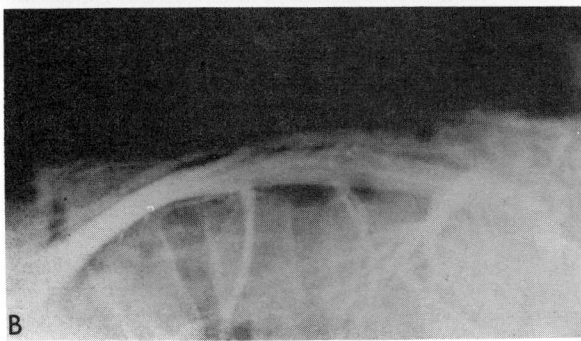

Figure 2. Lateral aortograms showing (A) normal "take-off" angle and normal "space" at site of duodenal crossing and (B) narrow angle and compromised space in vascular compression syndrome.

narrow aorto- or vertebromesenteric artery space at the site of duodenal crossing (Figs. 2 and 3 and Table 2).[17, 23, 39] Arteriographic techniques, however, are rarely necessary for radiologic diagnosis.

Because of the variability of symptoms and because the so-called "classic" radiologic signs are apparently not always present (dilatation, delay in barium passage, to-and-fro peristalsis, and oblique extrinsic pressure defects occur singly or in combination as normal variants in patients without symptoms and in patients with duodenal obstruction from a variety of causes), other causes of duodenal obstruction must be ruled out. Obstructing lesions such as tumors and duodenal webs can be visualized by fiberoptic endoscopy, and the use of this technique is to be encouraged in differential diagnosis.[36]

The frequent association with other diseases that cause similar symptoms, including gastric and duodenal ulcer, cholelithiasis, cholecystitis, pancreatitis, duodenitis, and irritable colon has not enhanced the clarity of diagnosis. Each of these must be painstakingly eliminated as the cause of symptoms. Even more distressing is the fact that one or more of the diseases mentioned above can occur concomitantly with vascular compression.

As early as 1921, Kellogg and Kellogg[20] suggested that there might be an increased incidence of peptic ulcer associated with this disease. A comprehensive analysis of 291 cases described in 65 reports since 1960[35] revealed that 31.8 per cent of 182 patients with chronic vascular compression of the duodenum had peptic ulcers. In that group, duodenal ulcers were present in 44 patients, gastric ulcers in 11 patients, and both types of ulcers in two patients. Ulcer disease was not described among patients with the acute form of the disease (109 patients), except for stress ulcers occurring in 8 of 28 patients described recently with severe injuries, including thermal burns. Dreiling et al.[10] reported several cases of pancreatitis associated with chronic duodenal obstruction from a variety of causes, including vascular compression from the superior mesenteric artery.

struction to be the site of duodenal crossing by the superior mesenteric artery, the narrow aortomesenteric angle, the abnormal anatomic course of the superior mesenteric artery, and, in the lateral view, the very

Figure 3. Combined gastrointestinal barium and aortography study revealing point of compression and abnormal course of the superior mesenteric artery.

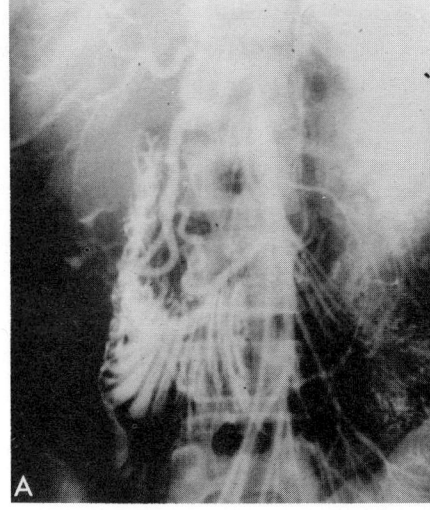

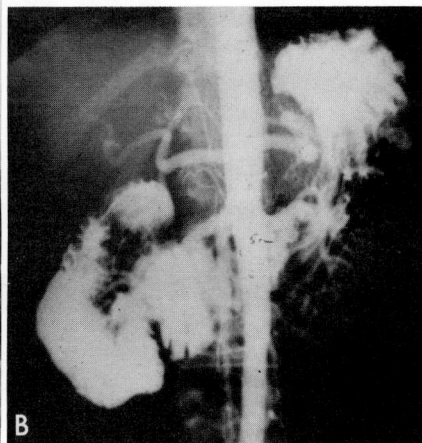

TABLE 2.   Arteriographic Relationship Between Superior Mesenteric Artery and Aorta (in vivo)

Patient	SMA-to-Aorta Angle	Distance from SMA to Aorta at Duodenal Crossing
Normal		
1	55°	7 mm.
2	60°	16 mm.
3	65°	16 mm.
4	55°	20 mm.
5	45°	20 mm.
Vascular Compression of Duodenum		
1	12°	3 mm.
2	10°	2 mm.
3	22°	2 mm.
4	10°	3 mm.
5	17°	2 mm.

TREATMENT

Each patient diagnosed as having symptomatic vascular compression of the duodenum should be given a trial of conservative management. Weight gain leading to deposition of fat in the retroperitoneal space leads to amelioration of symptoms. Increasing numbers of patients successfully treated by medical management have been reported. Medical therapy includes lying in the prone or left lateral decubitus position following meals or dependent postprandial positioning on a Stryker frame[39] or circoelectric bed. Treatment with hyperalimentation is worthy of a therapeutic trial.

If operation is deemed necessary, intraduodenal insufflation of air via an indwelling nasogastric tube helps to substantiate the diagnosis by demonstrating the point of obstruction.[18]

Methods of operative management include (1) division of the ligament of Treitz, (2) duodenojejunostomy, or (3) repositioning of the duodenum. The first method of surgical therapy has met with only limited success. Duodenojejunostomy has had widespread acceptance as an operative method of management leading to good results (Fig. 4).

Recently, however, total mobilization of the duodenum has gained some popularity, especially in the management of patients in the pediatric age group.[6] This method includes mobilization of the right colon and entire "C" loop of the duodenum to the level of constriction under the mesenteric vessels. The ligament of Treitz is lysed and the entire retroperitoneal (third and fourth) portion of the duodenum is mobilized. The duodenum and jejunum are then passed under the mesenteric vessels until most of the small bowel is positioned to the right of the midline (Fig. 5). This method has the advantage of being noninvasive with regard to the gastrointestinal tract and of restoring the proximal small bowel to the embryonic position it assumed before bowel rotation began. The concern of some regarding duodenal viability related to division of blood vessels required to gain total duodenal mobility has not been a limiting factor.

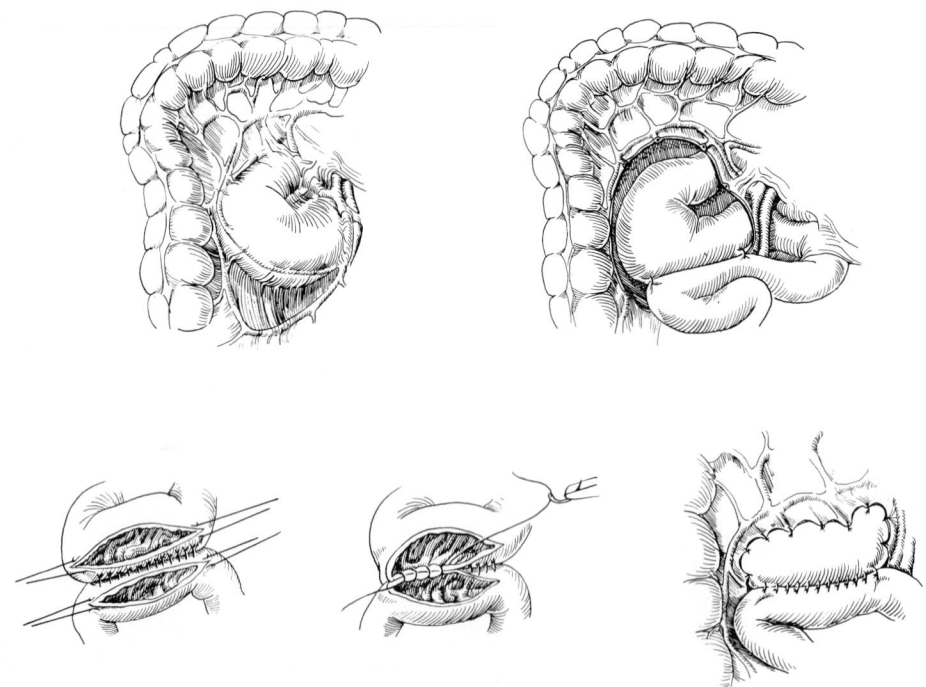

Figure 4.   Duodenojejunostomy for vascular compression of the duodenum.

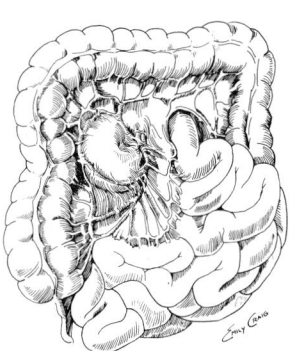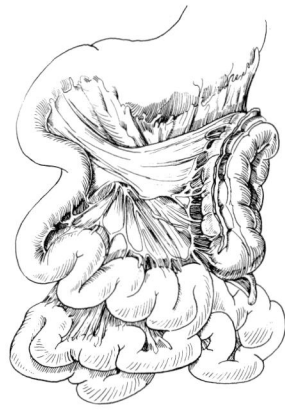

Figure 5. Operation to straighten duodenum and return it to its prerotation position.

SELECTED REFERENCES

Burrington, J. D., and Wayne, E. R.: Obstruction of the duodenum by the superior mesenteric artery—Does it exist in children? J. Ped. Surg., 9:733, 1974.
The largest single experience in the diagnosis and management of this disease in children. The authors challenge some traditional concepts and describe and defend total duodenal repositioning as the operation of choice for duodenal obstruction secondary to vascular compression.

Cimmino, C. V.: Arteriomesenteric occlusion of the duodenum: An entity? Radiology, 76:828, 1961.
Although less so in recent years, the subject of vascular compression and duodenal obstruction remains controversial. This treatise challenges the very existence of this entity.

Evarts, C. M., Winter, R. B., and Hall, J. E.: Vascular compression of the duodenum associated with the treatment of scoliosis. J. Bone Joint Surg., 53A:431, 1971.
A good comprehensive review of this disease and its association with operations on the vertebral column is of value especially to the orthopedic student and surgeon.

Hearn, J. B.: Duodenal ileus with special reference to superior mesenteric artery compression. Radiology, 86:305, 1966.
An excellent article which reports the original in vivo investigation of arteriographic techniques in the diagnosis of vascular compression of the duodenum.

Jones, S. A., Carter, R., Smith, L. L., and Joergensen, E. J.: Arteriomesenteric duodenal compression. Am. J. Surg., 100:262, 1960.
A comprehensive treatise on the subject of vascular compression. The intra-operative technique of air insufflation is described and its value as a diagnostic aid emphasized.

Thompson, N. W., and Stanley, J. C.: Vascular compression of the duodenum and peptic ulcer disease. Arch. Surg., 108:674, 1974.
An excellent article which reviews the subject of the association of peptic ulcer disease with vascular compression of the duodenum. The authors suggest methods of surgical management when confronted with synchronous occurrence of these diseases.

Wayne, E., Miller, R. E., and Eiseman, B.: Duodenal obstruction by the superior mesenteric artery in bedridden combat casualties. Ann. Surg., 174:339, 1971.
A brief and concise article which stresses nonoperative management in the acute form of vascular duodenal compression.

REFERENCES

1. Anderson, W. C., Vinet, R., Kirsh, I. E., and Greenlee, H. B.: Arteriomesenteric duodenal compression syndrome—Its association with peptic ulcer. Am. J. Surg., 125:681, 1973.
2. Berley, F. V., and Brown, R. B.: Arteriomesenteric obstruction of the duodenum. U.S. Armed Forces Med. J., 5:1044, 1954.
3. Bloodgood, J. C.: Acute dilatation of the stomach—gastromesenteric ileus. Ann. Surg., 46:736, 1907.
4. Bloodgood, J. C.: Dilatation of the duodenum in relation to surgery of the stomach and colon. J.A.M.A., 59:117–121, 1912.
5. Boernerus, F.: DeTabe Lethale A Mirabili Duodeni et Praeternaturali Plane Ventriculi, Situ, Disquisitio Anatomico-Medico-practica, Academiae Caesariae Naturae Curiosorum pevsi Ordinarii Loco oblati. Acta. Acad. Nat. Curios, 1752, pp. 225.
6. Burrington, J. D., and Wayne, E. R.: Obstruction of the duodenum by the superior mesenteric artery—Does it exist in children? J. Ped. Surg., 9:733–741, 1974.
7. Cimmino, C. V.: The status of the syndrome of arteriomesenteric occlusion of the duodenum. Va. Med. Month., 88:192, 1961.
8. Cimmino, C. V.: Arteriomesenteric occlusion of the duodenum: An entity? Radiology, 76:828, 1961.
9. Derrick, T. R., and Fadhli, H. A.: Surgical anatomy of the superior mesenteric artery. Am. Surg., 31:545, 1965.
10. Dreiling, D. A., Kirschner, P. A., and Nemser, H.: Chronic duodenal obstruction: A mechano-vascular etiology of pancreatitis. Am. J. Dig. Dis., 5:991, 1960.
11. Evarts, C. M., Winter, R. B., and Hall, J. E.: Vascular compression of the duodenum associated with the treatment of scoliosis. J. Bone Joint Surg., 53A:431, 1971.
12. Finney, J. M. T.: The relation of the duodenum to gastric disturbances. Bull. Johns Hopkins Hosp., 17:37, 1906.
13. Goin, L. S., and Wilk, S. P.: Intermittent arteriomesenteric occlusion of the duodenum. Radiology, 67:729, 1956.
14. Guthrie, R. H., Jr.: Wilkie's syndrome. Ann. Surg., 173:290, 1971.
15. Gwinn, J. L., and Lee, F. A.: Radiological case of the month. Am. J. Dis. Child., 129:617, 1975.
16. Hall, L. W.: The cast syndrome incognito. Am. J. Surg., 127:371, 1974.
17. Hearne, J. B.: Duodenal ileus with special reference to superior mesenteric artery compression. Radiology, 86:305, 1966.
18. Jones, S. A., Carter, R., Smith, L. L., and Joergensen, E. J.: Arteriomesenteric duodenal compression. Am. J. Surg., 100:262, 1960.
19. Kaiser, G. C., McKain, J. M., and Shumacker, H. B., Jr. The superior mesenteric artery syndrome. Surg. Gynecol. Obstet., 110:133, 1960.
20. Kellogg, E. L., and Kellogg, W. A.: Chronic duodenal obstruction with duodenojejunostomy as a method of treatment. Ann. Surg., 73:578, 1921.
21. Kundrat: Uber sine seltene Form der inneren Incarceration. Weiner Med. Wochenschr., 41:352, 353, 1891.
22. Louw, J. H., Sender, B., and Shandling, B.: A rational approach to the surgical treatment of duodenal ileus. South Afr. J. Lab. Clin. Med., 3:249, 1957.
23. Mansberger, A. R., Jr., Hearn, J. B., Byers, R. M., Fleisig, N., and Buxton, R. W.: Vascular compression of the duodenum, emphasis on accurate diagnosis. Am. J. Surg., 115:89, 1968.
24. Pool, E. H., Niles, W. L., and Martin, K. A.: Duodenal stasis; duodeno-jejunostomy. Ann. Surg., 98:587, 1933.
25. Puranik, S. R., Keiser, R. P., and Gilbert, M. D.: Arteriomesenteric duodenal compression in children. Am. J. Surg., 124:334, 1972.

26. Ray, J. F., III, Lawton, B. R., Myers, W. O., and Sautter, R. D.: Wilkie's syndrome. A true clinical disease entity. Wis. Med. J., 73:71, 1974.

27. Reckler, J. M., Bruck, H. M., Munster, A. M., Curreri, P. W., and Pruitt, B. A.: Superior mesenteric artery syndrome as a consequence of burn injury. J. Trauma, 12:979, 1972.

28. Reid, R. L., and Gamon, R. S.: The cast syndrome. Clin. Orthop., 79:85, 1971.

29. Robinson, B.: Dilatation of the stomach from pressure of the superior mesenteric artery, vein and nerve on the transverse segment of the duodenum. Cincinnati Lan. Clin., 45:577–586, 1900.

30. Rokitansky, C.: Lehrbuch der Pathologicochen Anatomie. Vol. III. Wein, W. Barumuller, 1842, p. 187.

31. Stavely, A. L.: Chronic gastromesenteric ileus. Surg. Gynecol. Obstet., 11:288–297, 1910.

32. Strong, E. K.: Mechanics of arteriomesenteric duodenal obstruction. Ann. Surg., 148:725, 1958.

33. Sutherland, D. E. R., Miller, I. D., and Najarian, J. S.: Occurrence of both congenital duodenal diaphragm and vascular compression of the duodenum in an elderly patient. Am. J. Surg., 123:351, 1972.

34. Thomas, T. V.: Arteriomesenteric compression of the duodenum. Intern. Surg., 56:304, 1971.

35. Thompson, N. W., and Stanley, J. C.: Vascular compression of the duodenum and peptic ulcer disease. Arch. Surg., 108:674, 1974.

36. Wald, A., and Milligan, F. D.: The role of fiberoptic endoscopy in the diagnosis and management of duodenal neoplasms. Am. J. Dig. Dis., 20:499, 1975.

37. Wallace, R. G., and Howard, W. B.: Acute superior mesenteric artery syndrome in the severely burned patient. Radiology, 94:307, 1970.

38. Wayne, E. R., and Burrington, J. D.: Duodenal obstruction by the superior mesenteric artery in children. Surgery, 72:762, 1972.

39. Wayne, E., Miller, R. E., and Eiseman, B.: Duodenal obstruction by the superior mesenteric artery in bedridden combat casualties. Am. Surg., 174:339, 1971.

32

CARCINOMA OF THE STOMACH

William P. Longmire, Jr., M.D.

HISTORICAL ASPECTS

"You were the first to tell the truth," wrote Nikolai Ivanovich Pirogoff, the great nineteenth century Russian surgeon, to Theodor Billroth of Vienna when commenting on Billroth's introduction of a statistical method of study of clinical material and his rigidly honest practice of reporting failures as fearlessly as successes.[6] Another of Billroth's great contributions was in the field of surgery of the stomach and, in a way, the story of gastric cancer may be said to start with his first successful gastric resection for cancer in 1881,[1] although descriptions of what were probably gastric cancer specimens date as far back as the millennium between 500 B.C. and A.D. 500. In 1830, Cruveilhier had attempted to distinguish between benign and malignant gastric ulceration, and Bayle had published a book as early as 1839 describing the symptoms and lesions of gastric malignant disease; yet the general medical profession was largely ignorant of the signs, symptoms, and pathologic anatomy of this disease until anesthesia became available and techniques of abdominal operations were perfected.

Advances in diagnosis of gastric cancer included a demonstration of the value of gastric analysis by von den Velden in 1879[26] and the development of gastric roentgenography (largely by the German school) in about 1910. The latter technique, with subsequent refinements, has given us the single most useful diagnostic method available today.

Among recent developments that have substantially improved the accuracy of diagnosing malignant lesions of the stomach are the flexible gastroscope (refined in Japan and adapted both to photography and biopsy of the stomach lining) and the cytologic studies of gastric washings.

As the extent of gastric resection has been increased, other methods of gastrointestinal anastomosis have evolved in addition to the Billroth I (end-to-end gastroduodenostomy) and Billroth II (side-to-side gastrojejunostomy) procedures. Of these, the most frequently employed reconstructive procedures after subtotal gastric resection for cancer have been the Hofmeister type of gastrojejunostomy (first performed by Von Eiselsberg in 1888), in which the lesser curvature portion of the cut end of the stomach is closed and only the greater curvature portion anastomosed to the jejunum, and the Polya end-to-side gastrojejunostomy popularized by Polya's report in 1911.

Total gastrectomy, first successfully performed by Schlatter in 1897, was attended by an almost prohibitive operative mortality until the 1940s, when the introduction of antibiotics and blood replacement, together with improved anesthetic and surgical techniques, helped to reduce the immediate surgical death rate to about 10 per cent. During this period total gastrectomy was proposed as a routine treatment for all resectable cancers of the stomach; after a relatively brief clinical trial, however, the idea was abandoned, since improved follow-up survival rates could not be demonstrated and immediate operative mortality and adverse side-effects continued to be greater than after subtotal resection.

Extended total gastrectomy, proposed by McNeer and Pack in 1954, included, in addition to excision of the stomach, an en bloc resection of omenta, spleen, and tail of the pancreas. Reported mortality rates ranged from 15.4 to 26.3 per cent and, on the basis of experience from limited clinical trials, use of the procedure currently is restricted to carefully selected cases.

At present, total gastrectomy is used infrequently, and extended total gastrectomy is performed only in rare and highly selected cases. Total resection may be considered when almost the entire stomach is involved with tumor and there is no evidence of lymph node involvement or distant spread.

INCIDENCE

One of the most fascinating aspects of malignant disease is the marked reduction in the incidence of carcinoma of the stomach in the United States during the past 40 years (Fig. 1).[22] For example, when the age-adjusted death rate from cancer of the stomach per 100,000 population during the period of 1950 to 1952 is compared to that during the period 1965 to 1967, the following dramatic decrease is noted:*

---

*Trends in Age-Adjusted Cancer Death Rates per 100,000 Population 1950–52 to 1965–67. Washington, D.C., National Vital Statistics Division and Bureau of the Census.

Sex	Site	1950–52	1965–67	Per cent change
Male	Stomach	17.9	9.7	−46
Female	Stomach	9.4	4.8	−49

This striking change in the national incidence has been reflected as well in carefully collected statistics from certain state registries. The Connecticut Tumor Registry,[4] for example, has been collecting statistical information from virtually all its cancer patients for more than 30 years on the incidence of disease and the mortality rate. This survey has disclosed interesting relationships among the three major sites of cancer of the gastric intestinal tract. In that group of gastrointestinal cancer classified as *rectal* cancer, little variation in incidence has occurred within either sex, whereas the incidence of proportion classified as *colonic* cancer increased over the 30-year period from 21 to 33 per cent for men and 31 to 46 per cent for women, establishing the colon as the most frequent site of cancer of the gastrointestinal tract today. Conversely, in this series, the incidence of that proportion classified as *stomach* cancer decreased steadily from 37 to 21 per cent for men and from 28 to 14 per cent for women.

In 1935 to 1939, there were 17 men with cancer of the stomach for every 10 men with cancer of the colon. Colonic cancer increased steadily over the next 30 years as stomach cancer declined, so that by 1960 to 1964, there were only six men with stomach cancer for every 10 men with colonic cancer.

The cause of this dramatic decline in stomach cancer has provoked a great deal of speculation but remains an enigma.

ETIOLOGY

The relationships of gastric cancer to a variety of possible etiologic factors, such as the composition of

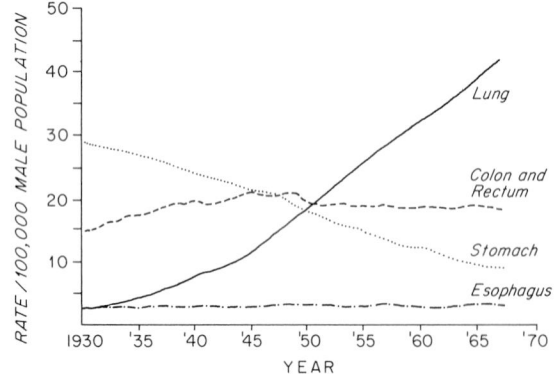

Figure 1. Declining death rate from cancer of the stomach (1930 to 1967) compared to death rates from other malignant tumors in the male population. (Redrawn from Silverberg, E., and Holleb, A. I.: CA, *21*:13, 1971; source of data: National Vital Statistics Division and Bureau of the Census, United States.)

soil or air in a particular region, diet, or the influence of race or other hereditary factors, have been investigated. Although correlations have been suggested in some areas, firm relationships have not been established for any specific agent.

Environment

Noting that deaths from cancer of the stomach were twice as high in certain rural counties of Wales as compared to the national average, Stocks and Davies proposed a relationship between the amount of organic material found in soil samples from a particular region and the gastric cancer mortality rate of that region. The increased mortality rate of the disease in certain urban areas of England led Stocks also to propose that a carcinogen or carcinogenic substance that might be ingested or inhaled was an important etiologic factor in carcinoma of the stomach.

Diet

A number of authors have commented on the hot rice, rice wine, raw fish, and pickled vegetable diet of the Japanese and the relationship of this diet to the fact that Japan has the highest incidence of gastric cancer in the world. Dangal noted that in Iceland the distribution of gastric cancer corresponded roughly with the consumption of smoked salmon and smoked trout. On the other hand, in the United States, Moore failed to find any significant dietary factor other than cabbage in gastric cancer patients and concluded that the disease must be associated with environmental factors.

Race and Heredity

Evidence for a racial factor is suggested by a comparison of the age-adjusted death rate per 100,000 population, 1964 to 1965, for males with cancer of the stomach in the United States (10.45) with that in Japan during the same period (68.57). Gastric cancer has been reported to occur more frequently in Hawaiian males and among Negroes in the United States than among the Caucasian population. In 1958, after analyzing six genetic studies of gastric cancer in humans, Graham and Lilienfeld concluded that, despite the limitations of all studies reviewed, the results suggested that cancer of the stomach is more concentrated in some families than in others.

While recognizing the importance of ethnic and racial factors, it is probable that the specific etiologic agent is as yet an undefined environmental or dietary factor.

PRECURSORS OF GASTRIC CANCER

Adenomatous Polyps

Adenomatous gastric polyps are uncommon but could possibly be the precursor of cancer in a small percentage of gastric tumors. They occur most frequently between the fifth and seventh decades and do not have characteristic symptoms or physical findings. The diagnosis of a polyp or polyps usually is made on roentgenologic examination, but one cannot rely entirely on such an examination to differentiate between benign and malignant lesions. The incidence of cancer is increased in polyps larger than 2 cm. in diameter. Huppler and associates[9] reviewed the records of 465 patients with gastric polyps seen at the Mayo Clinic. In approximately 20 per cent of the patients operated upon, the polyp was malignant. The high incidence of gastric achlorhydria in association with gastric polyps was confirmed in this study, 80 per cent of the patients examined having no free gastric acid. Twenty-five patients had zones of adenocarcinoma at the tip of the polyp without invasion of the stalk. On the basis of these findings, it was recommended that when a roentgenologic diagnosis of gastric polyp is made, the possibility of a malignant tumor is sufficiently great to warrant surgical intervention, provided the patient is in reasonably good general condition. Whether or not one accepts the theory that adenomatous gastric polyps can undergo malignant change, it seems clear that the possibility of malignancy cannot be completely excluded without removal and pathologic examination of the specimen. Endoscopic excisional biopsy of gastric polyps is indicated today, followed by appropriate gastric resection if malignancy is present.

Achlorhydria

As the absence of free gastric acid is noted in two thirds of patients with gastric cancer, it is assumed that there must be some relationship between this abnormal function of the gastric mucosa and the development of cancer. A threefold increase in the incidence of gastric cancer in patients with pernicious anemia has been established. These patients, who invariably have achlorhydria, should be observed periodically for evidence of gastric cancer.

Atrophic Gastritis

The relationship of atrophic gastritis to cancer has been debated, since the frequency of both conditions increases with advancing age, and it has been difficult to demonstrate any characteristic change in the gastritis that accompanies the development of cancer. Stout[24] contends that it is also difficult to prove that carcinomas have developed from gastric glands exhibiting intestinal metaplasia.

Giant Hypertrophic Gastritis

Both the clinical and roentgenologic findings in this condition may closely resemble those of multiple gastric polyps or gastric cancer, and gastric cancer has been reported to occur in such cases. Strode[25] noted in 1961 that both hypertrophic gastritis and gastric carcinoma were unusually prevalent in Japanese men in Hawaii and that hypochlorhydria was common in both conditions, suggesting a relationship between the two lesions. However, he recommended a rather conservative surgical approach, suggesting that total gastrectomy or even extensive proximal gastric resection was not indicated but that distal gastrectomy might be utilized if the antrum in uncharacteristic fashion was extensively involved.

Blood Group A

The correlation of gastric cancer with blood group A, as proposed by Aird and associates in 1953, has been the subject of conflicting studies. This relationship remains an unsettled, controversial matter at the present time.

PATHOLOGY

Carcinoma of the stomach, uncommon before the fifth decade of life, reaches its peak incidence in the sixth and seventh decades, with a predominance of three to two in males over females. Although such malignant tumors may develop from the mucus-secreting cells anywhere in the stomach from the cardia to the pylorus, the majority develop in the pyloric and antral regions, particularly along the lesser curvature. Benign gastric ulcer also occurs most frequently in the antrum and pylorus but rarely on the greater curvature. This difference in location may be helpful in the differential diagnosis.

Grossly, most carcinomas of the stomach may be classified as one of four types, as proposed by Borrmann in 1926.[3] Listed in order of a supposedly increasing degree of malignancy, they are: Group I—circumscribed, solitary, polypoid carcinomas without important ulceration; Group II—ulcerated carcinomas with wall-like marginal elevation and sharply defined borders; Group III—partially ulcerated carcinomas with marginal elevation and partial diffuse spread; and Group IV—diffuse carcinomas.

Regarding the importance of the histologic type of the carcinoma, Stout[24] pointed out: "Since almost all gastric carcinomas are derived from the mucus-secreting cells of the gastric pits or gastric glands, it is not surprising to find that almost all of them show some differentiation by forming more or less atypical tubes and by secreting mucus. The most distinctive feature characterizing the majority is their extreme degree of variability of differentiation. A very small number are almost exclusively glandular, and another tiny group may consist entirely of undifferentiated cells; but the vast majority show both of these features in different parts of the same tumor. It is this fact which makes the histological classification so hopeless and unrewarding."

Gross or microscopic evidence of involvement of regional lymph nodes, on the other hand, significantly alters the prognosis. In the study by Kennedy,[12] spread to the perigastric lymph nodes in the immediate vicinity of the tumor was associated with a reduction in 5-year survival from 48 to 21 per cent.

Unfortunately, 60 to 75 per cent of patients undergoing palliative or curative gastric resections have been found to have positive lymph nodes at the time of operation because the diagnosis is usually made so late in the course of the disease.

In addition to the spread of cancer cells within the gastric wall and into the lymphatics, three other methods of extension from the primary tumor have been identified: (1) direct extension into adjacent organs, i.e., liver, pancreas, transverse colon, or mesocolon; (2) bloodstream spread via the portal vein to the liver or into the systemic circulation to the lungs, bones, and elsewhere; and (3) peritoneal seeding from tumor emboli arising from the involved serosa of the stomach wall and spreading to the omentum, parietal peritoneum, the ovary (Krukenberg's tumor), and other sites including the pelvic cul-de-sac. This may produce a firm metastatic mass referred to as a rectal or Blumer's shelf and is an indication of advanced carcinomatosis.

Although the gross and histologic characteristics of stomach cancers are regularly recorded in routine patient records and pathology reports, clinicians have become increasingly dissatisfied with the prognostic significance of these descriptive analyses alone.

The task force on carcinoma of the stomach of the American Joint Committee for Cancer Staging and End Results Reporting[23] has proposed a staging system for carcinoma of the stomach that, it is hoped, will provide more meaningful methods of assessing the extent of malignancy, determining prognosis, and aiding in selection of treatment. If widely adopted, meaning-ful comparisons of end results from different sources should be possible.

This staging scheme, which was tested on an analysis of 1241 patients, proposes that in carcinoma of the stomach the prognosis is dependent upon the degree of penetration into the stomach wall by the primary lesion, the involvement of regional lymph nodes, and the presence of distant metastasis. The size or location of the primary tumor is of less significance. The histologic classification of carcinoma is not considered helpful in assessing prognosis.

The extent of disease is defined in terms of three components: (1) the primary tumor designated by the letter "T" and expressed in terms of the degree of penetration by the cancer through the stomach wall; (2) the regional lymph nodes designated by the letter "N"; and (3) distant metastasis designated by the letter "M."

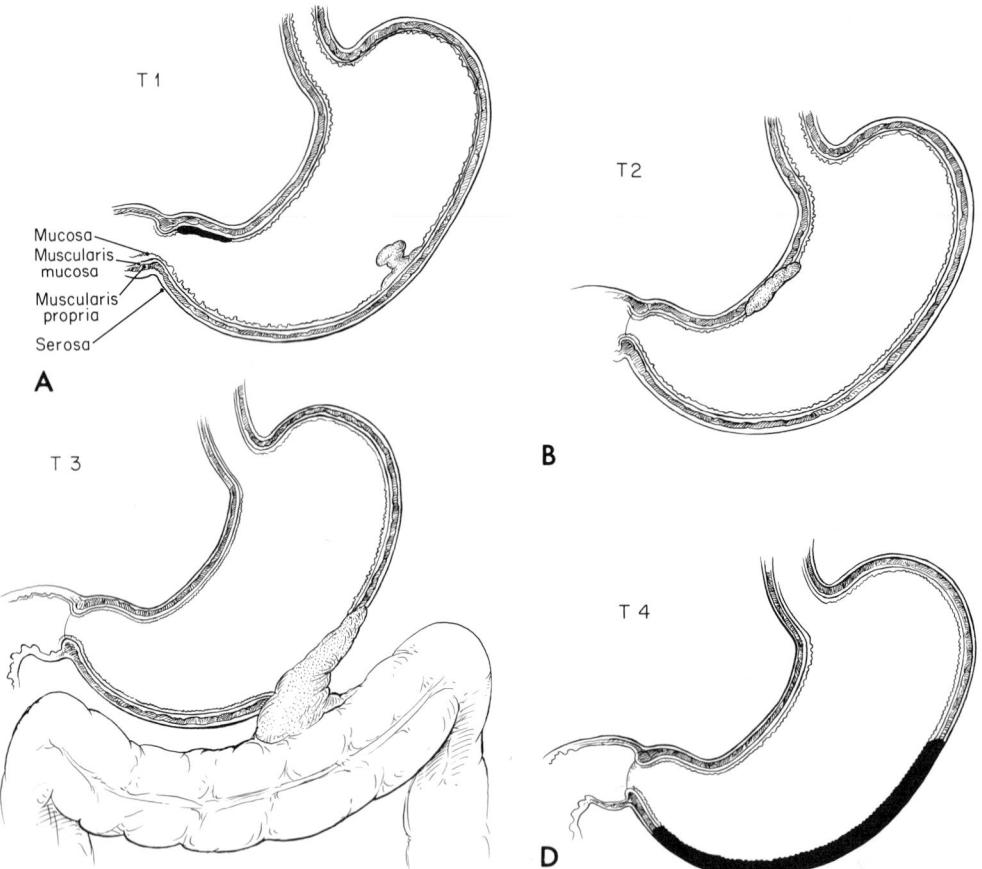

Figure 2.   TNM categories. Primary tumor penetration of stomach wall. *A*, T1 – Primary tumor confined to the mucosa including muscularis mucosae but not involving the submucosa. Two examples of T1 lesion are given, one on the lesser curvature and one on the greater curvature. *B*, T2 – Primary tumor involving the mucosa and the submucosa, including the muscularis propria and extending to but not penetrating through the serosa. *C*, T3 – Primary tumor penetrating through the serosa with or without invasion of the contiguous structures. *D*, T4 – Primary lesion involving the entire thickness of the stomach wall without obvious boundaries (including linitis plastica). (Redrawn from Staging System for Carcinoma of the Stomach – 1971. Chicago, American Joint Committee for Cancer Staging and End Results Reporting, 1971.)

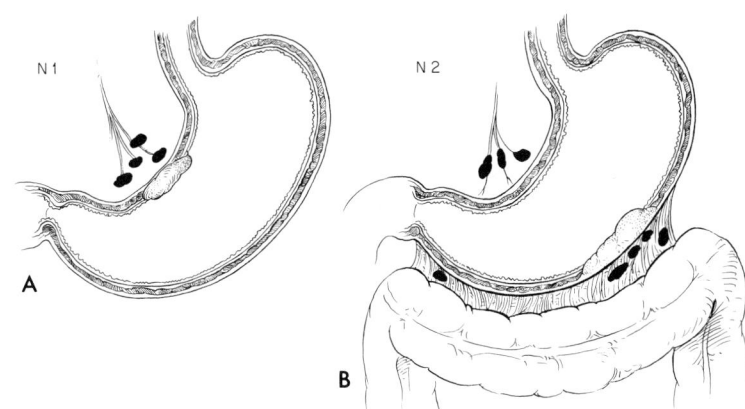

Figure 3. TNM categories. Lymph node involvement. *A,* N1—Involvement of the perigastric lymph nodes in the immediate vicinity of the primary tumor. *B,* N2—Involvement of the perigastric lymph nodes at a distance from the primary tumor or on both curvatures of the stomach. (Redrawn from Staging System for Carcinoma of the Stomach—1971. Chicago, American Joint Committee for Cancer Staging and End Results Reporting, 1971.)

DEFINITIONS OF THE TNM CATEGORIES AS APPLIED TO CARCINOMA OF THE STOMACH

T—Primary tumor. The principal factor is the degree of penetration of the stomach wall by the carcinoma

T1   Confined to the mucosa (Fig. 2*A*)

T2   Involves the mucosa and the submucosa, including the muscularis propria, and extends to or into the serosa but does not penetrate through the serosa (Fig. 2*B*)

T3   Penetrates through the serosa with or without invasion of contiguous structures (Fig. 2*C*)

T4   Diffusely involves the entire thickness of the stomach wall without obvious boundaries (including linitis plastica) (Fig. 2*D*)

TX   Degree of penetration of stomach wall not determined

N—Regional lymph nodes

N0   No metastasis to nodes

N1   Metastasis to the perigastric lymph nodes in the immediate vicinity of the primary tumor (Fig. 3*A*)

N2   Metastasis to the perigastric lymph nodes at a distance from the primary tumor or on both curvatures of the stomach (Fig. 3*B*)

NX   Metastasis of nodes not determined (i.e., laparotomy not done)

M—Distant metastasis

M0   No distant metastasis

M1   Clinical, radiographic, or exploratory evidence of distant metastasis, including nodes beyond the regional lymph nodes but excluding direct extension in continuity by the primary tumor

Classification of a tumor is based on the anatomic extent of disease as determined by all diagnostic methods, including physical examination, radiographic and endoscopic studies, cytopathologic examination, findings observed at surgical exploration, and findings obtained on gross and histopathologic study of operative specimens.

With the widespread use of gastric endoscopy in Japan, visualization and recognition of a superficial type of gastric cancer led Takasu, President of the Japan Society for Gastroenterological Endoscopy in 1962, to propose a classification of "early gastric cancer" (Figs. 4*A* and *B*).[20] Although there have been

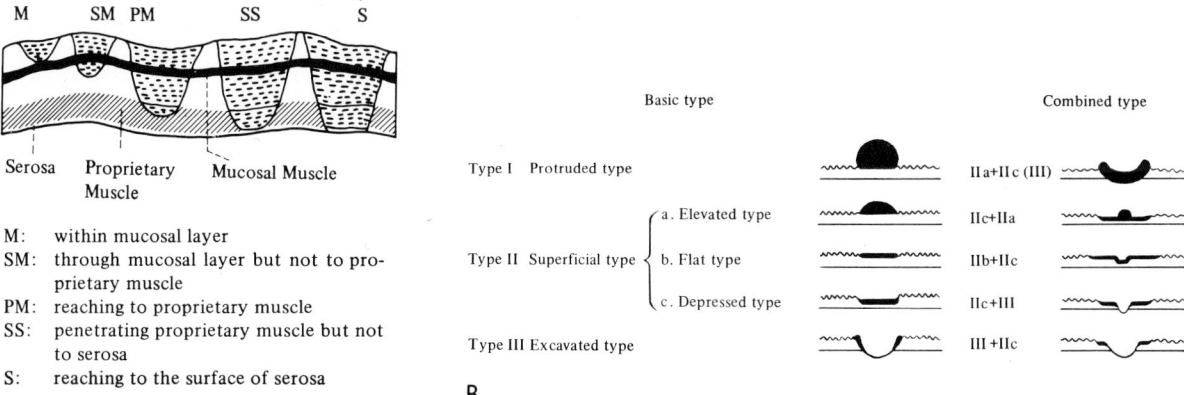

Figure 4. *A,* Schematic drawing of classification of carcinoma of the stomach based on depth of penetration of the stomach wall. *B,* Further detailed classification of "early" gastric cancer based on gross and microscopic presentation of tumor in relation to surrounding gastric wall. Classification proposed by Japanese Endoscopic Society. (From Sakita, T., Oguro, Y., Takasu, S., Fukutomi, H., and Miwa, T.: The development of endoscopic diagnosis of early carcinoma of the stomach. Jap. J. Clin. Oncol., *1:*118, 1971.)

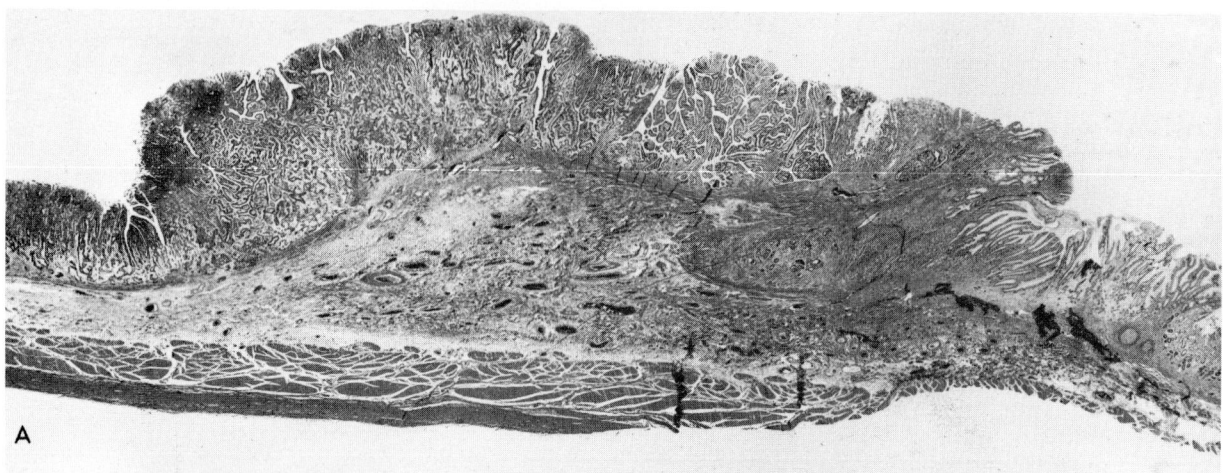

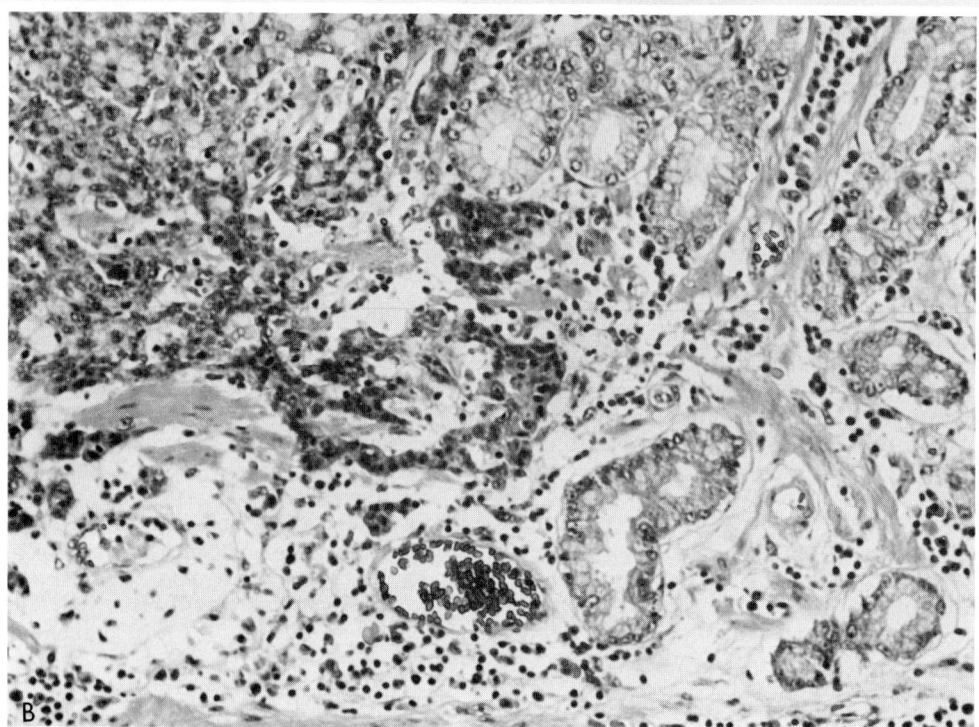

Figure 5. *A*, Photomicrograph of early gastric adenocarcinoma, Type IIa (superficial elevated type). *B*, Higher magnification of section from same patient, showing junction of normal and neoplastic mucosa. (Courtesy of Professor Walter F. Coulson, Department of Pathology, UCLA School of Medicine.)

objections that such a classification offers no special advantage over the TNM classification, and that the TNM system provides greater prognostic significance, the Japanese classification seems to have stimulated recognition of this type of carcinoma by both the endoscopist and the radiologist. Kodokoro[11] reported that the incidence of "early carcinoma" in resectable cases of gastric cancer at the University of Tokyo Branch Hospital had increased from 5.7 per cent in 1961 to 34 per cent in 1969 (Figs. 5*A* and *B*).

DIAGNOSIS

Symptoms

Unfortunately, there are no symptoms of "early" carcinoma of the stomach. Symptoms are generally not produced unless the tumor is of sufficient size to interfere with (1) the motor activity of a significant segment of the gastric wall or (2) the normal passageway in the lumen of the stomach. When these circumstances develop, indigestion, fullness after meals, eructation, loss of appetite, and heartburn may ensue. Vomiting is a late sign and usually occurs with pronounced dilatation and thickening of the stomach wall. Obstructive symptoms appear earlier with tumors located near the pylorus than with fundic lesions. Weakness may be associated with anorexia and weight loss. Anemia occurring with chronic blood loss from an ulcerated lesion also contributes to weakness.

Pain has been reported as a common first symptom and has been observed in as many as 85 per cent of patients by the time a diagnosis of carcinoma of the stomach is made. The type of pain may be similar to that of a benign peptic ulcer and may be relieved by food or antacids. More or less continuous abdominal pain generally suggests tumor involvement outside of the stomach wall. Substernal or precordial pain may be associated with tumors at the cardia.

Free perforation into the peritoneal cavity with signs of peritonitis or gross bloody vomitus are rare but occasional initial manifestations of the disease.

Symptoms of fatigue, dyspepsia, weight loss, or anemia in a patient over 40 require diligent examination to rule out a gastric cancer. At present there are no adequate mass screening tests to detect gastric neoplasms in the early stages before onset of such symptoms.

Physical Examination

There are no special findings in early cases of gastric cancer. Evidence of anemia and weight loss almost certainly appear at some stage in the course of the unattended patient but are rarely present in the early stages of the disease. A firm, nontender, movable epigastric mass separate from the liver may suggest cancer of the stomach; however, the size of the mass alone is not an accurate indicator of the operability of the lesion. A mass in the cul-de-sac on rectal examination (Blumer's shelf) or enlarged left supraclavicular lymph nodes (Virchow's node) are manifestations of advanced disease.

Laboratory Examination

Routine laboratory tests of particular interest are hematocrit, hemoglobin, and erythrocyte determinations, and stool examinations for occult blood. In the examination of the early suspect case, determination of gastric acidity to detect achlorhydria or hypochlorhydria is important.

X-Ray Studies

Roentgenographic examination of the stomach after ingestion of barium remains the basic diagnostic aid. Visualization of a large polypoid mass protruding into the lumen of the stomach generally leaves little doubt as to the presence of polypoid carcinoma. Lesions less than 2 cm. in diameter may be benign, but their true nature can best be identified by endoscopy.

Demonstration of an ulcer crater presents a difficult differential diagnostic problem. As seen on x-ray examination, the characteristic malignant ulcer crater lies in a mass and does not extend outside the boundary of the gastric wall. The mucosal folds do not radiate toward the center of the crater but maintain instead their usual contour up to and beyond the ulcer. Malignant ulcers are usually larger than 1 cm. and, on fluoroscopy, the surrounding gastric wall is rigid. Benign ulcers, on the other hand, penetrate beyond the limit of the stomach wall; there is no surrounding tumor, although edema may cause prominence of the mucosal borders, and the rugal folds radiate outward from the center of the crater. Benign ulcers may be of any size.

The double contrast technique, which enhances the details of a thin layer of barium on the mucosal surface of the stomach by simultaneously introducing air and a barium solution into the stomach, has been utilized widely to detect "early" gastric cancer in Japan.[10] In 1968 more than 1,500,000 persons were studied by mass roentgenologic screening techniques in Japan. Of the 0.1 to 0.2 per cent who were found to have gastric cancer, 30 to 50 per cent were considered to be in an "early stage."

Gastroscopy

Following the introduction of the flexible fiberoptic gastroscope by Hirschowitz in 1958,[7] as well as the technical innovations and advances of the art emanating from Japan, endoscopy has become an important complemental procedure to the radiologic examination in the diagnosis and management of gastric cancer and other gastrointestinal diseases. Instruments currently available possess sufficient flexibility to permit a U-turn in the stomach and to provide a good view of the cardia (including all other areas of the interior of the stomach), so that there are no longer any "blind spots" in the gastric mucosa. Current instruments are equipped for photography and have channels for irrigation and for biopsy. Skilled endoscopists can regularly inspect the duodenum and, when indicated, cannulate the ampulla of Vater and inject solutions for the x-ray examination of the biliary and pancreatic ductal system in approximately 85 per cent of cases.

Biopsies can be taken under direct vision from any point in the stomach, and brush specimens and washings can be obtained for cytologic examination. With the widespread use of gastric endoscopy, small early gastric cancers still confined to the gastric mucosa are being detected; these are lesions that cannot be readily diagnosed with the usual radiologic examination.

Differentiating the benign gastric ulcer from the ulcerated carcinoma, long one of the most troublesome gastric diagnostic problems, can be accomplished with a diagnostic accuracy of 97 per cent by combining multiple endoscopic biopsies and gastric cytology.[13]

Exfoliative Cytology

Naylor[17] proposed that gastric cytologic study should complement clinical or radiologic findings that suggest cancer and that its results should be assessed by the clinician in light of all the available data. Used as a routine screening test even in patients with pernicious anemia or chronic gastritis, cytologic examination would be an expensive and time-consuming procedure. Blendis and his colleagues[2] compared the diagnostic accuracy of radiology, gastric photography, and cytology in 100 patients in whom gastric cancer was suspected clinically. Radiologic studies rendered the correct diagnosis in 83 patients, cytologic studies were correct in 81, and gastric photography was correct in 70. They emphasized that these three methods were complementary. Although a number of special techniques have been developed for the collection of gastric cells, such as abrasive brushes or balloons, mucolytic enzyme lavage, and fluorescent staining, the majority of hospitals utilize the simpler technique of saline lavage of the stomach. However, as endoscopy and direct vision biopsy become more widely used, and as the skills and techniques of these procedures are perfected, it seems likely that endoscopic biopsy and brush cytology will be relied upon for cellular diagnosis more frequently in the future than will the cytologic examination of gastric saline lavage solutions.

TREATMENT

It is true today, as it was in Billroth's time, that the only method offering hope of curing cancer of the stomach is surgical excision of the involved portion of the stomach. The results of such therapy, however, are profoundly affected by the growth rate of the cancer cells, a process that in turn is controlled by both the aggressiveness of the malignant cell and the degree of host resistance. Neither of these factors can, at present, be identified or measured. In more than 50 per cent of patients, the tumor is no longer localized when first identified, and gastric resection will be only moderately beneficial in most cases of this type. On the other hand, for patients who do have a high degree of resistance to the growth of their tumor, an operation sufficiently extensive to remove all viable tumor cells in the stomach wall and the immediately adjacent lymph nodes does have considerable significance. One could logically assume, then, that gastric resection with an 8 cm. margin would provide a greater chance of removing all microscopic intramural extensions and locally involved lymph nodes than would resection of a 0.5 cm. margin of gastric wall.

Zinninger's[28] studies suggested proximal extensions of tumor cells in the gastric wall 6 cm. from the primary tumor, mainly in the submucous lymphatics in the upper stomach or esophagus. Spread toward the duodenum usually occurred by way of serosal lymphatics and by direct muscular infiltration. The farthest duodenal extension was 3 cm. beyond the pylorus. Unfortunately, there seems to be an ill-defined upper boundary to limit to the extent of the resection beyond which more radical excisions no longer contribute to improved survival rates. Total gastrectomy, for example, has thus far failed to yield any better 5-year survival rates than does subtotal gastrectomy; indeed, the immediate mortality rate and side-effects are greater. It also has been demonstrated that routine use of extended gastric resections with removal of lymph nodes about the pancreas and celiac axis and perigastric organs increases operative mortality without improving the 5-year survival rate.[5] The type and extent of gastric resection must be suited to the individual patient and will be influenced largely by the location and extent of the gross primary tumor and

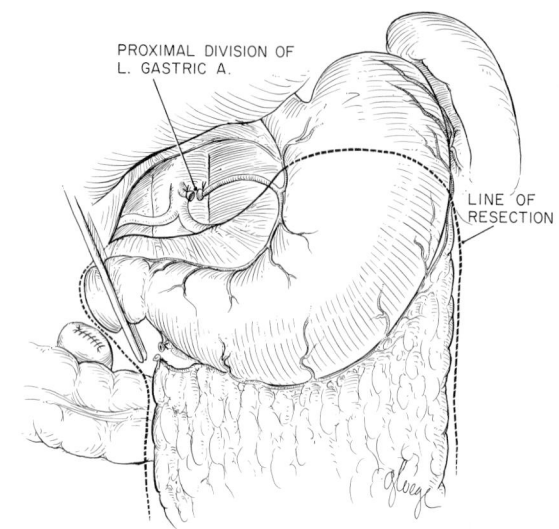

Figure 6. "Standard" subtotal gastric resection for cancer of the distal portion of stomach.

dectectable lymph nodes. In general, it would seem that the "standard" resection for the distal gastric cancer should include the greater and lesser omenta, division of the duodenum 2 or 3 cm. distal to the pylorus but with an adequate cuff for a secure duodenal closure, ligation of the left gastric artery at the celiac axis, and division of the lesser curvature adjacent to the esophagogastric junction. Division of the greater curvature at the level of the vasa brevia just distal to the spleen completes the resection (Fig. 6). Within such limits, a maximal resection of gastric wall and primary lymphatic drainage areas is performed without making the duodenal stump closure or gastrointestinal anastomosis unduly difficult and thereby potentially hazardous. Minimal trauma occurs to adjacent organs, and widespread secondary lymphatics are not laid bare.[8] More extensive subtotal resection may require removal of the spleen. When the blood supply from the left gastric and splenic arteries is interrupted, the chief blood supply to the gastric remnant is abolished, and the remaining blood supply is precarious. Alimentary continuity following subtotal resection is restored by a gastroduodenostomy (Billroth I) if the ends of the stomach and duodenum can be approximated without tension, or by gastrojejunostomy either anterior or posterior to the transverse colon.

Total gastrectomy was given a brief trial 20 to 25 years ago in a few clinics as a routine method of treatment for cancer of the stomach. Despite a marked improvement in operative mortality over previous years, the procedure continued to be more risky than subtotal resection, the postoperative complications were more frequent and serious, and the survival rate was not improved.[21]

In recent years total gastrectomy has been employed rather infrequently and its use restricted to those gastric tumors without evidence of distant spread that involved practically the entire stomach wall, making resection by any other means virtually impossible.[18] Moreover, in such cases gross involvement should be restricted to the lymph nodes in the primary drainage area that will be removed with total extirpation. Although remarkably good operative mortality rates have been reported in selected series of total gastrectomies, the usual mortality rate for this procedure in most hospitals is 15 to 18 per cent. The 5-year survival depends almost entirely on the selection of cases; the best reported series give 10 to 15 per cent.

Kock and associates[14] pointed out that none of their patients with carcinoma of the gastric cardia survived 5 years after proximal subtotal gastric resection, whereas 10 of 29 patients lived more than 5 years after treatment by total gastrectomy. They proposed total resection as the treatment of choice for cancer of the gastric cardia.

RESULTS

If 100 patients with cancer of the stomach were selected at random at the time of initial diagnosis by the techniques and methods currently employed in the United States and followed for a period of 5 years, approximately 15 would be alive at the end of the observation period. Although survival rates have improved in recent years as a result of better diagnostic methods, more advanced operative techniques, and greater public awareness of cancer, the gains in this country have been disappointingly small.[16] In two consecutive 10-year periods reported from the Mayo Clinic, there was an improvement in the overall 5-year survival rate from 14 per cent in the period from 1940 to 1949 to 15 per cent during the time between 1950 and 1959.[19] The fate of patients with cancer of the stomach seen at the Mayo Clinic during these two periods is shown in Figure 7.

One of the most comprehensive analyses of the results of surgical treatment for carcinoma of the stomach has resulted from the cooperative adjuvant chemotherapy studies conducted by the Veterans Administration Hospitals and the Cooperative University Hospital Group supported by the National Cancer Institute, United States Public Health Service.[15] The survival curves are identical both for the patients receiving chemotherapy and for the control group, suggesting that the chemotherapy utilized was ineffective; however, the study does provide follow-up data of up to 10 years from an initial group of 616 patients treated in 27 different hospitals. At the time of the first 5-year report, only 1.0 per cent of the patients were lost to follow-up. The cases were divided into three categories: Category I—subtotal gastrectomy for cure; Category II—total gastrectomy for cure; and Category III—all palliative procedures including both total and subtotal resections. Operative mortality as usually calculated was included in the report of deaths occurring during the first 30 days after operation. These 30-day mortality figures are, therefore, higher than the usual reports comprising more immediate postoperative mortality rates. Considering all cases, including those in which resection was done for palliation as well as those in which it was done for cure, the 30-day postoperative mortality was 20 per cent for total gastrectomy and 12 per cent for subtotal resection. For survival analysis, the patients in Categories I, II, and III were divided into Stages 0, 1, 2, and 3 according to the following criteria:

Stage 0: No positive lymph nodes, serosal involvement, or tumor cells at the lines of resection

Stage 1: Any one descriptor present and the other two not present or not reported

Stage 2: Any two descriptors present and the other one not present or not reported

Stage 3: All three descriptors present

The survival rate of patients after curative resections (Categories I and II) for the different stages over a 9- or 10-year period is shown in Figure 8A, and of patients after palliative resection in Figure 8B. Survival rates by indication for operation and type of operation are seen in Figure 9.

The 5-year survival rate of patients without lymph node or serosal involvement after total or subtotal resection was 47 per cent. With either lymph node or serosal involvement, survival dropped to 39 per cent; with both lymph node and serosal involvement, survival declined to 20 per cent.

The survival rate of palliative cases was generally poor, with over 87 per cent of the patients dead within 3 years of operation. Relief of pyloric obstruction and arrest of persistent bleeding may, however, make palliative operations worthwhile. Subtotal resection, when technically feasible, gives more satisfactory palliation than does gastroenterostomy.

These average figures obtained by pooling results from 27 hospitals are less favorable than the reported results from single institutions but may be more indicative of the achievements of the "average" hospital.[27]

The most hopeful aspects of gastric cancer are (1) the marked decline (although the exact cause of this dramatic improvement still eludes us) in the incidence of this disease in the United States during the last 35 years, and (2) the demonstration by Japanese endos-

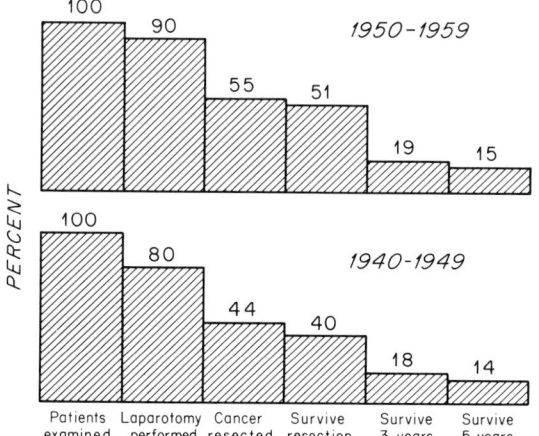

Figure 7. Comparison of ultimate survival rates for original patients diagnosed in 1940 to 1949 and 1950 to 1959. (Redrawn from ReMine, W. H., Priestley, J. T., and Berkson, J.: Cancer of the Stomach. Philadelphia, W. B. Saunders Company, 1964.)

copists and surgeons that superficial "early" gastric cancer can be diagnosed with increasing frequency and with excellent 5-year survival rates. Kidokoro,[11] who reported the collective data from 22 institutions in Japan, stated that during the 6-year period from 1962 to 1968, 2364 cases of "early" gastric carcinoma were operated upon. Of the 368 cases treated in 1962 and 1963, more than 5 years before the review, 5 (who were considered operative deaths) died within 30 days; of the remaining 363 cases, 336 survived longer than 5 years (92.5 per cent). Twenty-seven patients died within the 5-year period, 9 of apparent recurrent cancer, 15 of apparently unrelated diseases, and 3 of unknown causes. Two cases could not be followed. Such excellent results obtained when gastric cancer is diagnosed and treated in its early course again emphasize the urgent need for a practical mass diagnostic screening technique for gastric cancer.

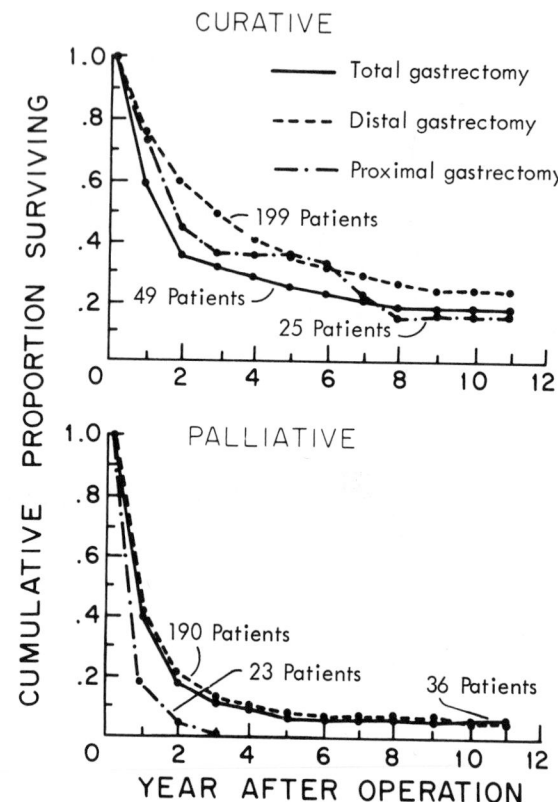

Figure 9.   Survival curves for gastric cancer patients by category and type of operation (excluding 30-day deaths). (Redrawn from Dixon, W. J., Longmire, W. P., Jr., and Holden, W. D.: Ann. Surg., *173*: 33, 1971.)

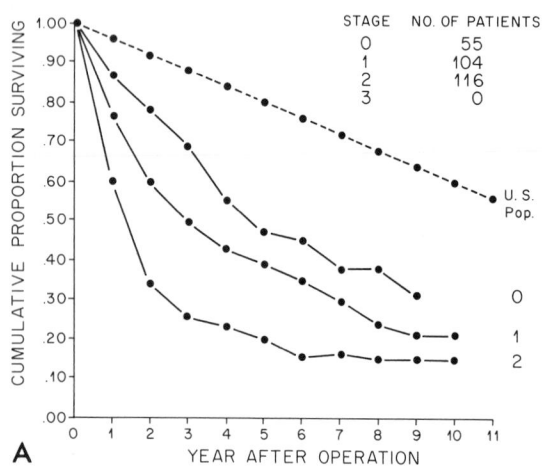

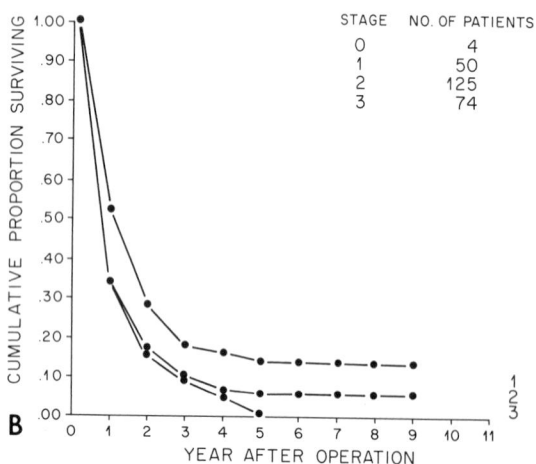

Figure 8.   *A,* Survival curves for patients treated by curative gastric resection by operative staging (excluding 30-day deaths). *B,* Survival curves for patients treated by palliative gastric resection by operative staging (excluding 30-day deaths). (Redrawn from Dixon, W. J., Longmire, W. P., Jr., and Holden, W. D.: Ann. Surg., *173*:36, 1971.)

SELECTED REFERENCES

Gilbertsen, V. A.: Results of treatment of stomach cancer. An appraisal of efforts for more extensive surgery and a report of 1,983 cases. Cancer, *23*:1305, 1969.
   This study of 1983 cases of carcinoma of the stomach seen at the University of Minnesota Hospitals between 1936 and 1963 emphasizes a critical analysis of the 227 patients seen during the years from 1958 to 1963, when efforts were being made for widespread employment of more extensive surgical excision procedures. Follow-up studies of patients seen during this period indicated that this practice was associated with a substantial increase in operative mortality and a significant decrease in overall rates of survival as well as in survival of those who underwent gastrectomy. The most favorable results were obtained during the first part of the 1950s when less extensive excisional procedures were utilized.

Early Gastric Cancer. Japanese Cancer Association, Gann Monograph on Cancer Research No. 11, edited by T. Murakami. Baltimore, University Park Press, 1972.
   This monograph reviews the advances made during the past two decades in the diagnosis and treatment of gastric cancer in Japan, where the incidence of the disease is among the highest in the world. The pathology of "early gastric cancer" is presented, and the two techniques (gastroscopy and double contrast barium x-ray examination) that have contributed so greatly to identifying early gastric cancer in Japan are discussed in detail.

Hoerr, S. O.: Carcinoma of the stomach. Am. J. Surg., *101*:284, 1961.
   From a review of 254 personally treated cases of carcinoma of the stomach, Hoerr presents three cardinal therapeutic principles that are today basically sound: (1) Every patient with suspected malignant disease of the stomach should have surgical exploration unless there is histologic proof of distant metastasis or the patient is physically unable to withstand an operation. (2) At operation, when a careful search for distant metastasis proves to be negative,

the primary lesion is excised widely and without biopsy; the adjacent nonessential structures are included in an en bloc resection if they are invaded upon by the primary tumor. However, neither routine total gastrectomy nor ultraradical lymphadenectomy is advocated. (3) If the lesion is incurable by reason of distant metastasis or local extension, one should think carefully before performing a palliative resection. Mortality is high and palliation often fails. Obstruction should be the chief indication for palliation.

Scott, H. W., Jr., and Longmire, W. P., Jr.: Total gastrectomy. Report of sixty-three cases. Surgery, 26:488, 1949.

This study was of one of the earliest reported series of total gastrectomies with an operative mortality of 9.5 per cent and offered the suggestion, on the basis of early results and theoretical considerations, that total gastrectomy was a more effective treatment for gastric cancer than was subtotal resection. On the basis of subsequent 5-year survival rates, such a concept has not been supported; however, an accurate statistical evaluation of a comparable series of patients with similar cancers treated by total versus subtotal gastrectomy has never been conducted. This study did support the concept that total gastrectomy could be performed with an acceptable operative mortality rate and that an adequate nutritional state could be maintained in the absence of the stomach.

Staging System for Carcinoma of the Stomach — 1971. Chicago, American Joint Committee for Cancer Staging and End Results Reporting, 1971.

This report describes the purpose, method, and summary of a field trial of the TNM Staging or Classification System for carcinoma of the stomach. The system is in keeping with the results of a number of large retrospective studies of the life history of carcinoma of the stomach. The results of the field trial have been reported in the following reference: Kennedy, B. J.: TNM classification for stomach cancer. Cancer, 26:971, 1960. A uniform system for classification of stomach cancer was developed after a review of 1241 case records from seven participating institutions. Clinical, radiographic, or gastroscopic studies and biopsies of the primary tumor or metastasis provided the information necessary to stage a stomach cancer. Survival was dependent upon the extent of the penetration of the gastric wall of the tumor. As the depth of penetration increased, the rate of survival decreased. Once the neoplasm involved the regional lymph nodes, a marked reduction in survival rate was demonstrated. With distant metastasis, there was seldom survival beyond 3 years.

REFERENCES

1. Billroth, T.: Uber einen neuen Fall von gelungener Resektion des Carcinomatosen Pylorus. Wein. Med. Woschenschr., 31:1427, 1881.
2. Blendis, L. M., Beilby, J. O. W., Wilson, J. P., Coles, M. J., and Hadley, G. D.: Carcinoma of the stomach: Evaluation of individual and combined diagnostic accuracy of radiology, cytology and gastrophotography. Br. Med. J., 1:656, 1967.
3. Borrmann, R.: Geschwülste des Magens und Duodenums. In Henke, F., und Lubarsch, O.: Handbuch der speziellen pathologischen Anatomie und Histologie. Berlin, J. Springer, 1926, Volume IV, Part 1, pp. 812–1054.
4. Eisenberg, H., and Shambaugh, E.: Cancer of the gastrointestinal tract: Trends in incidence and mortality rates. In Proceedings of the Sixth National Cancer Conference. Philadelphia, J. B. Lippincott Company, 1968, p. 417.
5. Gilbertsen, V. A.: Results of treatment of stomach cancer. An appraisal of efforts for more extensive surgery and a report of 1,983 cases. Cancer, 23:1305, 1969.
6. Halperin, G.: Theodor Billroth. Surg. Gynecol. Obstet., 107:539, 1958.
7. Hirschowitz, B. I., Curtiss, L. E., Peters, C. W., and Pollard, H. M.: Demonstration of a new gastroscopy — the fiberscope. Gastroenterology, 35:50, 1958.
8. Hoerr, S. O.: Carcinoma of the stomach. Am. J. Surg., 101:284, 1961.
9. Huppler, E. G., Priestley, J. T., Morlock, C. G., and Gage, R. P.: Diagnosis and results of treatment of gastric polyps. Surg. Gynecol. Obstet., 110:390, 1960.
10. Ichikawa, H., Yamada, T., Horikoshi, H., Doi, H., Matsue, H., Tobayashi, K., Sasagawa, M., and Higa, A.: X-ray diagnosis of early gastric cancer. Jap. J. Clin. Oncol., 1:1, 1970.
11. Kidokoro, T.: Frequency of Resection Metastasis and Five-year Survival Rate of Early Gastric Carcinoma in a Surgical Clinic: Early Gastric Cancer. Japanese Cancer Assoc., Gann Monograph on Cancer Research No. 11, edited by T. Murakami. Baltimore, University Park Press, 1972.
12. Kennedy, B. J.: TNM classification for stomach cancer. Cancer, 26:971, 1960.
13. Kobayashi, S., Prolla, J. C., Winns, C. S., and Kirsner, J. B.: Improved endoscopic diagnosis of gastroesophageal malignancy: Combined use of direct vision cytology and biopsy. J.A.M.A., 212:2086, 1970.
14. Kock, N. G., Lewin, E., and Pettersson, S.: Partial or total gastrectomy for adenocarcinoma of the cardia. Acta Chir. Scand., 135:340, 1969.
15. Longmire, W. P., Jr., Kuzma, J. W., and Dixon, W. J.: The use of triethylenethiophosphoramide as an adjuvant to the surgical treatment of gastric carcinoma. Ann. Surg., 167:293, 1968.
16. Lumpkin, W. M., Crow, R. L., Jr., Hernandez, C. M., and Cohn, I., Jr.: Carcinoma of the stomach: Review of 1035 cases. Ann. Surg., 159:919, 1964.
17. Naylor, B.: The place of cytology in the diagnosis of lesions of the gastrointestinal tract and contiguous organs. In Proceedings of the Sixth National Cancer Conference. Philadelphia, J. B. Lippincott Company, 1968, p. 429.
18. Paulino, F., and Roselli, A.: Carcinoma of the stomach, with special reference to total gastrectomy. In Ravitch, M. M. (Ed.): Current Problems in Surgery. Chicago, Year Book Medical Publishers, 1973.
19. ReMine, W. H., Priestley, J. T., and Berkson, J.: Cancer of the Stomach. Philadelphia, W. B. Saunders Company, 1964.
20. Sakita, T., Oguro, Y., Takasu, S., Fukutomi, H., and Miwa, T.: The development of endoscopic diagnosis of early carcinoma of the stomach. Jap. J. Clin. Oncol., 1:113, 1971.
21. Scott, H. W., Jr., and Longmire, W. P., Jr.: Total gastrectomy. Report of sixty-three cases. Surgery, 26:488, 1949.
22. Silverberg, E., and Holleb, A. I.: Cancer statistics, 1971. CA, 21:13, 1971.
23. Staging System for Carcinoma of the Stomach — 1971. Chicago, American Joint Committee for Cancer Staging and End Results Reporting, 1971.
24. Stout, A. P.: Tumors of the stomach. Atlas of Tumor Pathology, Section VI, Fascicle 21. Washington, D.C., Armed Forces Institute of Pathology, 1953.
25. Strode, J. E.: Malignant lesions of the stomach in Hawaii: Experiences with 350 patients. Surgery, 49:573, 1961.
26. von den Velden, R.: Ueber Vorkommen und Mangel der freien Salzsauer im Magensaft bei Gastrektasie. Dtsch. Arch. Klin. Med., 23:396, 1878–79.
27. Welch, C. E., and Wilkins, E. W., Jr.: Carcinoma of the stomach. Ann. Surg., 148:666, 1958.
28. Zinninger, M. M.: Extension of gastric cancer in the intramural lymphatics and its relations to gastrectomy. Am. Surg., 20:920, 1954.

33

THE SMALL INTESTINE

I

ANATOMY

R. Scott Jones, M.D.

The small intestine is that portion of the alimentary tract which extends from the pylorus to the cecum. Its major function is absorption, which depends upon amazingly complex integration of structural, physiologic, and chemical factors. The neurohormonal regulation of gastric, biliary, pancreatic, and intestinal secretion and of motor function provides the appropriate luminal milieu for complete digestion of foodstuffs and presentation of the products of digestion to the specialized intestinal epithelium for absorption.[3] The following material will deal with the structure and functions of this segment of the gut.

An essential anatomic characteristic of the small intestine is its large surface area, which it provides for absorption. The gross, microscopic, and ultrastructural features of the small intestine that account for this remarkable arrangement are: (1) intestinal length, (2) mucosal folds, (3) villi, and (4) microvilli. The effectiveness of digestion and absorption is also greatly influenced by various types of intestinal movements.

GROSS ANATOMY

General Description

The length of the alimentary tract in normal humans is best estimated by means of small polyethylene catheters passed through the intestine via the nose. The average distance from the nose to the anus is 453 cm. The duodenum is approximately 21 cm. long and the colon is approximately 109 cm. long. The combined length of the jejunum and ileum is 261 cm. or about three fifths of the entire canal, or eight fifths of body height.[9] The duodenum is described in Chapter 31. The jejunum begins at the duodenojejunal angle, which is supported by the ligament of Treitz. The proximal two fifths of the small intestine is called the jejunum and the distal three fifths is the ileum; however, this distinction is arbitrary, since there is no clear demarcation between jejunum and ileum. The small intestinal tube, which decreases in luminal diameter as it proceeds distally, is convoluted or folded upon itself and occupies the central and lower part of the abdominal cavity; it is enclosed laterally and superiorly by the colon.[6]

The Mesentery

The small intestine is suspended from the posterior abdominal wall by a large fold of peritoneum, the mesentery, which is attached to the posterior abdominal wall to the left of the second lumbar vertebra, passing obliquely to the right and inferiorly to the right sacroiliac joint. The mesentery contains blood vessels, nerves, lymphatics, and lymph nodes, as well as considerable fat. It is attached to the small intestine along the length of one side, the mesenteric border, leaving the remainder of the surface of the bowel covered by its visceral peritoneum, the serosa. The relationship of the mesentery to the small bowel is important, since the broad-based attachment of the mesenteric root stabilizes the small bowel and prevents it from twisting upon its blood supply. This relationship of the bowel to the mesentery is an important consideration in surgery of the intestine.

Blood Supply

The small intestine receives its blood supply from the superior mesenteric artery, the second large branch of the abdominal aorta. The superior mesenteric artery courses anterior to the uncinate process of the pancreas and the third portion of the duodenum where it divides to supply the pancreas, duodenum, and entire small intestine, as well as the ascending and transverse colon. The intestinal arteries branch within the mesentery to unite with adjacent arteries to form a series of arterial arcades before sending small straight arteries to the small intestine. The intestinal arteries contact the small intestine on the mesenteric border where they pass toward the antemesenteric border, sending small branches into the layers of the intestine. The veins of the small intestine drain into the superior mesenteric vein, a major tributary to the portal vein. The unique relationship of the small intestine and its blood supply enables surgical mobilization of long segments of intestine. For example, small intestine may be used to replace the esophagus.

Lymphatics

There are aggregated lymphatic nodules, Peyer's patches, in the submucosa of the small intestine. These lymphatic nodules are most abundant in the ileum, but are present in the jejunum. The lymphatic drainage from the small intestine passes into three sets of mesenteric nodes: the first set is close to the wall of the small intestine, the second set is adjacent to the mesenteric arcades, and the third set is along the trunk of the superior mesenteric artery. The superior mesenteric preaortic group drains into the intestinal trunk, which drains into the cisterna chyli. The lymphatic drainage of the small intestine is the major route by which absorbed lipid is transported into the circulation.

Mucosa

The mucosal surface of the small intestine contains numerous circular mucosal folds called the *plicae circulares* (valvulae conniventes, or valves of Kerckring). These folds are 3 to 10 mm. in height, taller and more numerous in the distal duodenum and proximal jejunum, becoming shorter and fewer distally. Barely visible to the naked eye are the intestinal villi, tiny finger-like processes projecting into the intestinal lumen.

Innervation

The efferent nerve supply to the small intestine is from the parasympathetic and sympathetic divisions of the autonomic nervous system. The parasympathetic innervation is via preganglionic fibers passing through the vagus nerves to synapse with neurons of the intrinsic plexuses of the intestine. The sympathetic innervation of the small intestine is from preganglionic fibers arising from the ninth and tenth thoracic segments of the spinal cord, passing to synapse in the superior mesenteric ganglion. The postganglionic sympathetic fibers pass along the branches of the superior mesenteric artery to the intestine. Pain from the intestine is mediated through thoracic visceral afferents and not vagal afferents, although the vagus does contain large numbers of afferent fibers.[1]

MICROSCOPIC ANATOMY

The small intestine is made up of four layers, which, from the lumen outward, are the mucosa, the submucosa, the muscularis, and the adventitia or serosa.

MUCOSA

The mucosa of the small intestine is composed of (1) the epithelium, (2) the lamina propria, and (3) the muscularis mucosa. The mucosal surface has two important structural features: the villi and the crypts of Lieberkühn (Fig. 1). The villi are finger-like luminal projections having a columnar epithelial surface and a cellular connective tissue core of lamina propria. Each villus contains a central lymphatic vessel called a lacteal, a small artery, vein, and capillary network. Human jejunal villi are approximately 0.5 to 1.0 mm. high and there are 10 to 40 villi per square millimeter of mucosal surface. In addition to the vessels, the villi contain smooth muscle fibers extending from the muscularis mucosa, providing contractility to each villus. The crypts of Lieberkühn, or intestinal glands, are adjacent to the bases of the villi and extend down to, but not through, the muscularis mucosae.

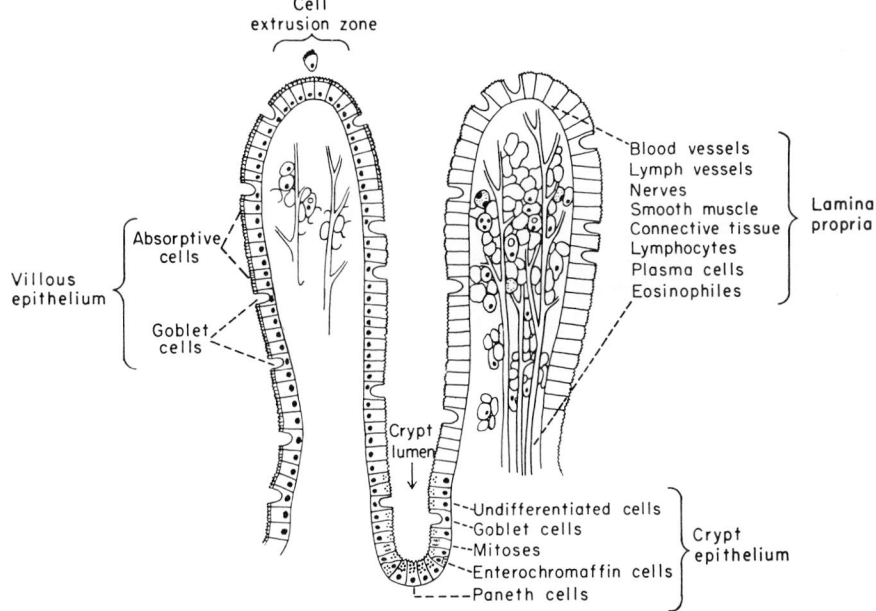

Figure 1. Schematic diagram of two sectioned villi and a crypt to illustrate the histologic organization of the small intestinal mucosa. (From Trier, J. S.: Morphology of epithelium of small intestine. In: American Physiological Society: Handbook of Physiology, Section 6, Alimentary Canal. C. F. Code, ed. Baltimore, Williams & Wilkins Company, 1968.)

The lamina propria is between the intestinal epithelium and the muscularis mucosa and contains blood and lymph vessels, nerve fibers, smooth muscle fibers, fibroblasts, macrophages, plasma cells, lymphocytes, eosinophils, and mast cells, as well as connective tissue elements.[2]

Recent studies with the scanning electron microscope have provided new information on the topography of the mucosal surface. Scanning electron micrographs provide an in-depth perspective of the mucosa with excellent resolution (Fig. 2). The villi vary in shape from circular to flattened or finger-shaped. The finger-shaped villi are 0.1 to 0.25 mm. in diameter. The villi are corrugated by deep horizontal clefts and there are holes 3 to 8 μ across on the surface of the villi representing the openings of the goblet cells.[12] The muscularis mucosa is a thin layer of smooth muscle separating the mucosa from the submucosa.

Cells of the Epithelium

Cells of the Villi. The columnar epithelial cells are responsible for absorption. These cells are about 22 to 26 μ tall and are characterized by a striated luminal border (brush border) and a basally placed nucleus (Fig. 3). The striated or brush border appearance is due to the microvilli, which are projections 1 μ tall and 0.1 μ wide produced by numerous folds in the apical plasma membrane. The microvilli greatly increase the absorptive surface of the epithelial cell. The plasma membranes of the epithelial cells have a three-layered or trilamellar appearance and are somewhat thicker over the microvilli than in the lateral and basal portion of the cell. The membrane of the microvillus is continuous without fenestrations discernible by electron microscopic techniques and separates the lumen of the gut from the interior of the epithelial cell. Presumably any absorbed substance must pass through the apical plasma membrane of absorptive cells. A coat of fine filaments called the "fuzz" or glycocalyx is closely applied to the luminal surface of the micro-

villus membrane (Fig. 4). High concentrations of digestive enzymes, particularly disaccharidases, are present in the brush border. The plasma membrane contains 80 to 90 per cent of the disaccharidase activity of the intestinal cell. These findings indicate that the microvilli, in addition to providing increased absorptive surface, play a very important digestive function.[1]

Three specialized areas of the lateral plasma membrane deserve comment. The "tight junctions" are fusions of the lateral plasma membranes between the terminal web and the intestinal lumen. This tight junction is present about the circumference of the cell and prevents communication of the lumen with the intracellular space so that all exchange between the absorptive cell and the lumen takes place through the apical plasma membrane. Immediately below the tight junction is an intermediate junction that has an intracellular space of approximately 200 A. At intervals along the lateral plasma membranes are very close attachments of adjacent membranes called *desmosomes*. The intermediate junction and desmosomes bind adjacent cells together.[1]

The nuclei and mitochondria of absorptive cells are not particularly distinctive. The absorptive cells contain granular and agranular endoplasmic reticulum, which has an important synthetic function in the cell. It is likely that the endoplasmic reticulum synthesizes the protein component of the chylomicron during fat absorption. This organelle has also been shown to be capable of triglyceride synthesis, which is an important step in fat absorption. The endoplasmic reticulum may synthesize the cytoplasmic enzymes of the absorptive cell.

The Golgi material probably stores or modifies substances absorbed or synthesized by the cell. Lysosomes contain lytic enzymes and eliminate waste materials by either lysing them or segregating the noxious substance for extrusion.

Goblet Cells. Goblet cells are present in both the

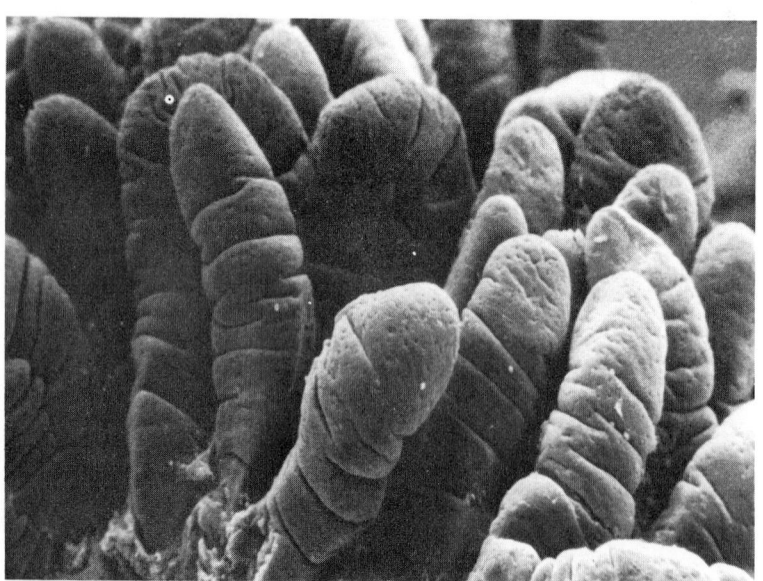

Figure 2. Scanning electron mcirograph of human jejunal mucosa. × 42. The villi are finger-shaped and are indented with numerous transverse grooves. The pitlike impressions on the villi are the openings of goblet cells. (Courtesy of A. L. Jones, M.D., Professor of Anatomy and Medicine, University of California, San Francisco.)

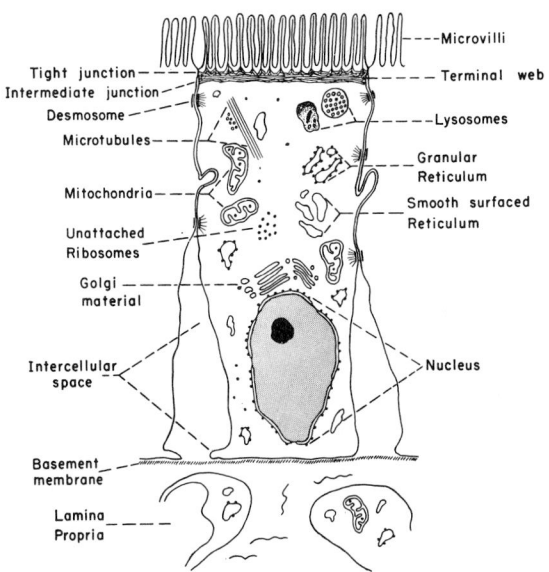

Figure 3. Schematic diagram of an intestinal absorptive cell. (From Trier, J. S., and Rubin, C. E.: Gastroenterology, *49*:574, 1965.)

villi and the crypts. These cells are characterized by a cytoplasm filled with mucus granules between the nucleus and the apical brush border. Electron microscopic studies suggest that intestinal goblet cells secrete their mucus by merocrine secretion.[1]

Cells of the Crypts

Enterochromaffin Cells. Enterochromaffin cells are found in the crypts of the small intestine, but are in other parts of the gastrointestinal system as well, including the esophagus, stomach, colon, gallbladder, and pancreas. These cells are usually not in contact with the intestinal lumen and their secretory granules are usually below the nuclei away from the lumen, suggesting secretion into the blood rather than the lumen.

Serotonin has been identified in enterochromaffin cells, but the significance of this observation is unknown. The structure of enterochromaffin cells has suggested an endocrine function. A recent study using immunocytochemical and radioimmunoassay techniques showed that duodenal acidification caused depletion of secretin from intestinal endocrine cells associated with increased concentrations of secretin in serum.[1]

Paneth Cells. Paneth cells occur in the base of the crypts and are structurally similar to cells known to secrete large amounts of protein, such as pancreatic or parotid acinar cells. The function of Paneth cells is unknown.

Undifferentiated Cells. Undifferentiated cells are found only in the crypts, particularly at the bases, where they are the most frequent cell type. These cells exhibit mitoses, since they multiply and differentiate to replace lost absorptive cells.

Epithelial Renewal

The epithelium of the small intestine is a dynamic, rapidly proliferating tissue in which old dying cells are constantly replaced by newly formed cells, thus maintaining the structural integrity of the mucosa. Mitotic division of undifferentiated cells occurs in the crypts. An undifferentiated cell may do one of three things: (1) differentiate into an absorptive cell and migrate into the villus, (2) remain in the crypt and continue mitotic activity, or (3) remain in the crypt in a resting stage. The cells entering the villi migrate to the villus tips, where they are shed into the lumen. This process has been studied by observing the fate of injected tritiated thymidine and by means of radioautography on serial biopsies. In the human duodenum and jejunum, cells labeled in this fashion are in the crypts for 12 hours following ^{3}H-thymidine injection, appearing at the villus base in 24 hours and the villus tip in 5 to 7 days. In the ileum, labeled cells reach the villus tips in 3 days. These findings indicate that the population of intestinal epithelial cells is replaced every 3 to 7 days.[1]

SUBMUCOSA

The submucosa is a strong fibroelastic and areolar connective tissue layer containing vessels, nerves, and lymph nodules. This layer provides much of the strength for sutures of the intestinal wall, and indeed any method of intestinal suturing should include stitches through the submucosa.

MUSCULAR LAYER AND INTRAMURAL NEURAL STRUCTURES

The muscular portion of the small intestine is formed by two distinct layers of smooth or nonstriated muscle, an outer longitudinal coat and an inner circular coat. Intestinal smooth muscle fibers are spindle-shaped structures about 250 μ long. In the past it was thought that intestinal smooth muscle was a syncytium, but recent electron microscopic studies show intestinal smooth muscle cells to be discrete structures.

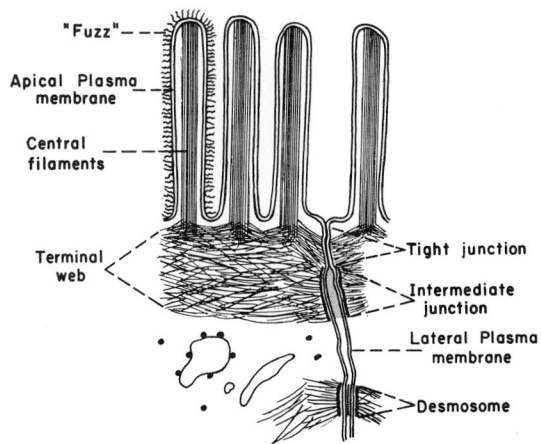

Figure 4. Schematic illustration of the specialization of the apical cytoplasm of the plasma membrane of intestinal absorption cells. (From Trier, J. S., and Rubin, C. E.: Gastroenterology, *49*:574, 1965.)

However, there are points at which the plasma membrane of adjacent cells is approximated, forming structures called nexuses. It is believed that the nexuses allow electrical continuity between smooth muscle cells and permit conduction through the muscle layer.

There are four identifiable neural plexuses in the small intestine: (1) the subserous plexus is most noticeable on the mesenteric attachment and forms the transition between the mesenteric nerve fibers and the myenteric plexus. Ganglia can be found in the sub-serous plexus. (2) The myenteric plexus is located between the longitudinal and circular muscle layers and consists of three networks linking various ganglia and ramifying within the muscle layers. (3) The submucosal plexus is a network of nerve fibers and ganglia in the submucosa. (4) The mucous plexus consists of fibers from the submucosal plexus extending into the mucosa. This plexus does not contain nerve cell bodies.[1]

For references, see page 1010.

II

PHYSIOLOGY

R. Scott Jones, M.D.

DIGESTION AND ABSORPTION

Carbohydrate[1] (Fig. 1)

An adult may ingest daily about 350 gm. of carbohydrate, consisting of starch, sucrose, and lactose. Dietary starch comprises two glucose polymers, amylopectin and amylose. Amylopectin, the most abundant constituent (80 per cent) of starch, comprises a 1–4 linked straight chain of glucose molecules. In addition, amylopectin possesses a 1–6 branching side chain at approximately every 25 glucose units along the straight chain. Amylose, the other constituent of starch, is made up only of 1–4 linkages of glucose molecules in a straight chain.

Pancreatic and salivary amylases break the interior 1–4 glucose linkages and for that reason the end product of amylose digestion by amylase is maltose (glucose-glucose) and maltotriose (glucose-glucose-glucose), which cannot be digested further by amylase because the only linkages present between glucose molecules in this circumstance are terminal bonds.

Because amylopectin contains 1–6 as well as 1–4 glucose linkages, the end products of amylase digestion of amylopectin are maltose, maltotriose, and the residual branched saccharides, the dextrins. The digestion of starch by amylase probably occurs predominantly in the lumen of the alimentary tract. The finding of high concentrations of digestive enzymes in isolated brush border preparations suggests that maltose, maltotriose, and dextrin, as well as the dietary disaccharides, lactose (glucose-galactose) and sucrose (glucose-fructose), are completely broken down to the

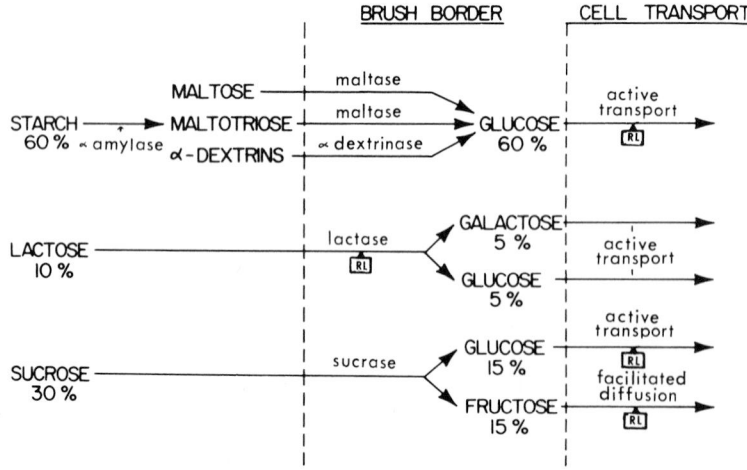

Figure 1. Outline of carbohydrate digestion and absorption in man. Percentages refer to proportion of total carbohydrate in diet; RL locates the rate-limiting step in the overall digestion-absorption process for each carbohydrate ingested. (From Gray, G. M.: Gastroenterology, 58:96, 1970.)

constituent monosaccharides by the microvilli, probably at the level of the glycocalyx (fuzz coat). It is possible that some disaccharides may be absorbed intact, possibly facilitated by monosaccharide transport, but the significance of that event is not known.

Glucose and galactose are actively transported into the intestinal cells against a concentration gradient. Such transport of these sugars has been demonstrated in vivo as well as in vitro. Glucose and galactose compete for transport in a manner similar to competitive inhibition in other enzyme substrate systems. The active transport of sugars requires metabolic energy as well as oxygen. Sodium ion plays a role in the transport of glucose and galactose; however, only very small concentrations appear to be required. Glucose and galactose are, therefore, probably absorbed by carrier-mediated active transport. Fructose, the other significant monosaccharide, is not absorbed by active transport, but probably enters the intestinal cells by a process called facilitated diffusion.[1]

Protein

Protein digestion is initiated in the stomach by two factors: (1) the acidic gastric environment favors denaturation of protein, and (2) pepsin hydrolyzes protein to polypeptides. Protein digestion is far from complete when gastric chyme enters the duodenum where pepsin is inactivated by the higher pH.

Pancreatic proteolytic enzyme precursors are secreted into the duodenum. Trypsinogen is converted to trypsin by the intestinal enzyme enterokinase. The activation of trypsinogen is autocatalytic; i.e., trypsin also activates trypsinogen. Trypsin likewise activates the other pancreatic proteolytic enzyme precursors. Trypsin, chymotrypsin, and elastase are pancreatic endopeptidases that split peptide bonds in the central portion of protein molecules, while carboxypeptidases are pancreatic exopeptidases that remove amino acids from the C-terminal position of protein molecules. Aminopeptidases are intestinal exopeptidases that split amino acids from the N-terminal position of protein molecules. Amino acids are the final product of protein digestion and are the molecules that are absorbed. That some dipeptides are absorbed by adult man is likely, and certain in the human neonate for a brief period. The nutritional significance of this phenomenon is undetermined.

Amino acids are absorbed from the intestinal lumen by a process of carrier-mediated active transport.[1] The active transport of amino acids against a concentration gradient has been demonstrated in vitro by everted intestinal sacs and tissue accumulation methods in animals and man, and in vivo with intestinal perfusion methods. The transport of amino acids requires oxygen and sodium. Carrier-mediated active transport is supported by evidence that suggests that certain amino acids exhibit mutual competitive inhibition. Experiments on competitive inhibition of various L-amino acids have suggested several distinct pathways for absorption of amino acids determined by the chemical structure of the amino acids. In normal man, digestion and absorption of protein is usually 80 to 90 per cent completed in the jejunum.

Fat

Although fat emulsification occurs in the stomach, little or no fat digestion occurs outside the small intestine. The entry of gastric chyme into the duodenum is regulated in part by a negative feedback system in which fat in the duodenum inhibits gastric emptying. In the duodenum the dietary fat in the form of triglycerides is mixed with biliary and pancreatic secretions, the important constituents of which are bile salts, pancreatic lipase, and bicarbonate ion.

The naturally occurring bile salts in man are glycine or taurine conjugates of cholic acid, deoxycholic acid, or chenodeoxycholic acid. Bile salts are detergents, being water-soluble at one portion of the molecule and fat-soluble at the other. Such substances tend to produce polymolecular aggregates called micelles. Bile salt molecules in micelles in biologic solutions are thought to be arranged with the fat-soluble portion of the molecule toward the center of the aggregate, and with the water-soluble portion toward the periphery of the aggregate. This phenomenon permits solubilization of lipid in an aqueous environment and results in a micellar solution. Bile salts allow further emulsification to occur, providing optimal physicochemical environment for the action of pancreatic lipase (Fig. 2).

Pancreatic lipase catalyzes the hydrolysis of dietary triglyceride into 2-monoglyceride and fatty acids. The 2-monoglyceride and fatty acids then enter the micelles and are held in micellar solution. The bile salt, monoglyceride, fatty acid micelle can also solubilize other lipids such as cholesterol, phospholipid, and fat-soluble vitamins. Pancreatic bicarbonate is important in regulating the pH of the intestinal lumen to allow lipase to function optimally. An alkaline pH favors ionization of fatty acids and bile salts, which increases their solubility in micelles.[10] Alkaline pH also increases the solubility of bile salts. When the micelles encounter the microvilli of the intestinal epithelial cells, the fatty acids and 2-monoglycerides pass into the epithelial cells by a process not requiring energy, probably diffusion.

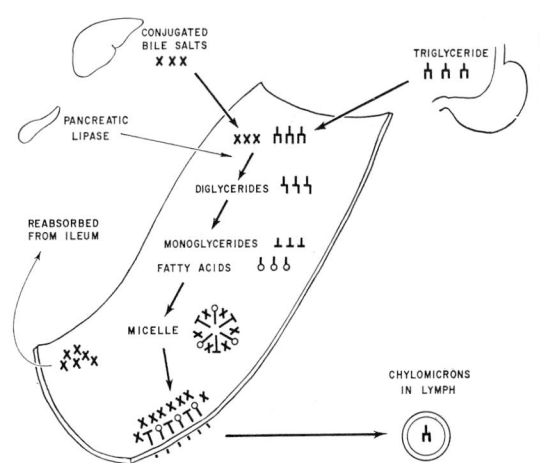

Figure 2. Diagram depicting the intraluminal events in fat absorption. (From Isselbacher, K. J.: Fed. Proc., 26:1420, 1967.)

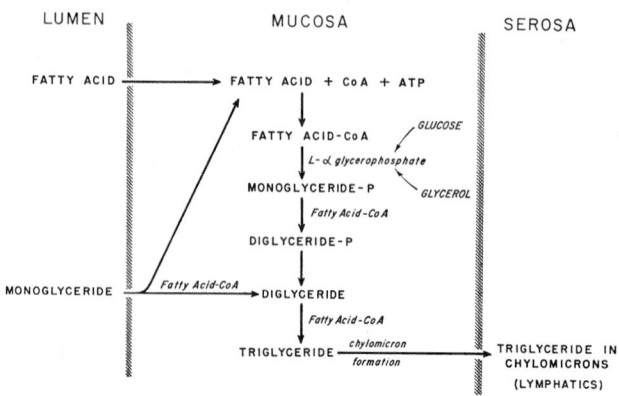

Figure 3. Major biochemical reactions in the transport of long-chain fatty acids and monoglycerides. (From Isselbacher, K. J.: Fed. Proc., *26*:1420, 1967.)

After entering the epithelial cell, 2-monoglyceride and fatty acids are synthesized into triglyceride in the endoplasmic reticulum. The biosynthesis of triglyceride in the gut may occur by two pathways: (1) the α-glycerophosphate pathway, in which the triglyceride is synthesized from glycerol and fatty acids; and (2) the monoglyceride pathway, in which the triglyceride is formed by the addition of fatty acids to the 1 positions of the 2-monoglyceride. The monoglyceride pathway is probably the more important in man (Fig. 3).

After triglyceride synthesis, chylomicrons are formed by triglycerides, phospholipid, cholesterol, cholesterol esters, and protein. Lipoprotein synthesis is necessary for chylomicron formation. Chylomicrons pass from the epithelial cells into the lacteals where they pass through the lymphatics into the venous system (Fig. 4). All long-chain fat is absorbed in the manner just described; however, medium-chain triglyceride (C_8 to C_{10}) may be absorbed without hydrolysis and pass into portal blood rather than into lymph via chylomicron formation.[1]

Fat is absorbed mainly in the jejunum. Although unconjugated bile acids are absorbed in the jejunum by passive diffusion, the conjugated bile acids that form micelles are absorbed in the ileum by an active transport process. There they are almost completely absorbed and pass via the portal venous blood to the liver, where they are secreted into the bile. Only a small fraction of the total bile salt pool, about 500 to 600 mg., escapes the enterohepatic circulation daily, and this small loss is replaced by hepatic synthesis of bile salts from cholesterol. In a normal adult, the bile acid pool of about 4 to 5 gm. circulates six to eight times daily. Normally, all dietary fat is absorbed and the 5 gm. of fat excreted in the feces daily comes from desquamated cells and bacteria.

Water and Electrolytes

Large quantities of water are presented to the small intestine. Some water is ingested, but a larger amount is secreted by the digestive glands to provide the appropriate luminal environment for digestion and absorption. It has been estimated that 5 to 10 liters of water enters the small bowel daily, while only about 500 ml. or less leaves the ileum entering the colon. The small intestine, therefore, absorbs large quanti-

ties of water. Experiments with isotopes reveal that there are simultaneous movements of large quantities of water from lumen to blood as well as from blood to intestinal lumen. Intestinal absorption is the result of two large oppositely directed fluxes.[23] The net lumen-to-blood flux of water from an isotonic sodium chloride solution containing glucose in the human small intestine is estimated to be 12.7 and 12.1 ml. per hour per centimeter in jejunum and ileum, respectively.[4]

The important factors in the movement of water across the intestinal mucosa are diffusion and osmotic filtration caused by osmotic or hydrostatic pressure differences across the membrane. In other words, water absorption results from osmotic gradients established by the active transport of solutes such as sodium ion, glucose, or amino acids into the cells. According to Fordtran the intestinal mucosa behaves as if the absorptive cell plasma membrane were penetrated by aqueous channels called pores.[1] These pores allow the transfer of water and water-soluble substances across the lipoidal cell membrane by a process of simple diffusion. The effective pore radii of the jejunum and ileum are estimated to be 7.5 and 3.4 Å,

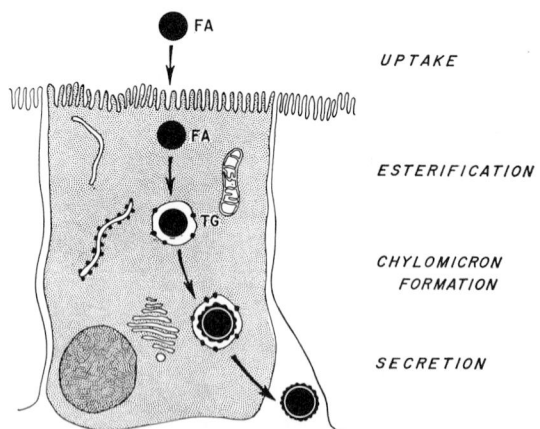

Figure 4. The major steps in the absorption of fat. This diagram depicts the role of the smooth endoplasmic reticulum in esterification and of the rough endoplasmic reticulum in protein synthesis, which is necessary for chylomicron formation. (From Isselbacher, K. J.: Fed. Proc., *26*:1420, 1967.)

respectively. The small size of these hypothetical pores prevents their identification by electron microscopy.

In the human jejunum, sodium ion absorption (net transfer from lumen to blood): (1) occurs against a modest concentration gradient, (2) is dramatically influenced by the rate and direction of water flux, and (3) is stimulated by glucose, galactose, and bicarbonate ions. It appears that in the jejunum a small portion of sodium absorption is mediated by active transport, while the major part of jejunal sodium absorption occurs by bulk flow along osmotic gradients. In the jejunum, bicarbonate is effectively absorbed against steep electrochemical gradients. One explanation for this process is that bicarbonate absorption is mediated by H^+ secretion and the relationship between Na and HCO_3^- transport is explained by a Na^+-H^+ exchange.[22]

The human ileum absorbs Na against steep electrochemical gradients; this absorption is unaffected by water flow and is not stimulated by glucose, galactose, or HCO_3^-. These observations suggest a very efficient Na^+ transport in the ileum. The human ileum also absorbs Cl^- against steep electrochemical gradients. When net ileal Na^+ movement is zero, there is an equimolar exchange of Cl^- and HCO_3^-. Regardless of the rate or direction of fluid movement, ileal content becomes more alkaline, either by water absorption, causing HCO_3^- concentration, or by HCO_3^- secretion.[21] It appears that potassium is passively absorbed from the intestine according to its electrochemical gradients.

Calcium is absorbed, particularly in the proximal small intestine (duodenum and jejunum), by a process of active transport. This ion is absorbed better from an acid than an alkaline environment, which may explain the better absorption in the proximal intestine. Vitamin D and parathyroid hormone enhance calcium absorption.[1]

An important electrolyte absorbed by the small intestine is iron. One of the important functions of the small intestine is the regulation of the body pool of iron. In the person with normal iron stores there is only a slight transfer of iron from intestinal absorptive cells to plasma, and only a small amount of iron enters the mucosal cell from the lumen. In iron deficiency there is no effective block to transfer of iron from absorption cell to plasma and no block to the entry of luminal iron into the mucosal cell.[1]

MOTILITY

There are several types of visible small intestinal muscular activity. The *segmenting contraction* is a localized circumferential contraction of the circular muscle over a length of about 1 cm. of the small intestine. Segmenting contractions divide the luminal content within the area of contraction. Their rhythmic segmenting activity occurs in the proximal small intestine at a rate of approximately 11 contractions per minute and in the distal small intestine at about eight contractions per minute. Segmenting contractions occurring regularly and rhythmically in adjacent portions of the small intestine divide and subdivide the intestinal content, mixing it and exposing it to larger areas of mucosa, which facilitates digestion and absorption. *Pendular movements* are probably the same or are a minor modification of rhythmic segmentation.

Peristalsis consists of intestinal contraction passing aborally at a rate of 1 to 2 cm. per second through several centimeters of intestine. Peristalsis is somewhat slower in the distal than in the proximal small bowel. The major function of peristalsis is the distal movement of intestinal chyme. Under abnormal circumstances *peristaltic rushes* may occur. Peristaltic rushes usually begin in the proximal small bowel or duodenum and rapidly traverse the entire length of the small intestine. When the peristaltic rush ends, there may be a quiescent period of no motor activity.

The small bowel basal intraluminal pressures are about 8 to 9 cm. H_2O. There are several types of intestinal pressure waves. The type 1 wave is less than $7\frac{1}{2}$ seconds long with an amplitude of 15 to 60 cm. H_2O, and is the most common pressure wave observed in man. Type 1 pressure waves generally correlate with segmenting motor activity. The other type of small intestinal pressure wave is the type 3 wave, which is defined as an elevation of baseline pressures with superimposed type 1 waves. Type 3 waves last from 10 seconds up to 8 minutes and have an amplitude of 5 to 30 cm. H_2O. Type 3 waves have usually been correlated with peristaltic motion.[1]

Regulation of Small Intestinal Motility

Myogenic Factors. Two types of electrical activity can be recorded from the small intestine. Slow-wave electrical activity begins in the longitudinal muscle layer of the duodenum and is propagated distally. In human adults this activity occurs at 11.7 ± 0.5 (SEM) cycles per minute. This phenomenon, called the *basic electrical rhythm* (BER), is independent of the intrinsic neural plexuses, and is unrelated to motor activity. Intestinal *spike potential* may occur spontaneously during depolarization, or from stretching of the bowel, and is associated with motor activity.

Neurogenic Factors. Intrinsic neural regulation is initiated by stimulation of the mucosa, or particularly by distention, which causes contraction of longitudinal and circular muscle, propelling luminal content distally. The intrinsic nerve supply regulates rather than initiates motor action. In general, sympathetic activity inhibits while parasympathetic activity stimulates motor function. Epinephrine inhibits small intestinal motor activity while acetylcholine stimulates it. Distention of the small intestine can inhibit small intestinal motility by what is called the intestinointestinal inhibitory reflex. Distention of the ureter, renal pelvis, or biliary system or peritoneal irritation may inhibit intestinal movements.[1]

Hormonal Factors. Gastrointestinal hormones may play an important role in regulating intestinal motility. Gastrin stimulates gastric and intestinal motility and relaxes the ileocecal sphincter. Cholecystokinin-pancreozymin (CCK-PZ) also stimulates intestinal motility and may decrease intestinal transit time. Secretin and chemically similar glucagon inhibit intestinal motility. The role of the hormones in regulating intestinal motility is poorly understood.

ENDOCRINE FUNCTION OF THE SMALL INTESTINE

The mucosa of the small intestine is an important source of peptide hormones whose main function is regulation of the gastrointestinal tract.[7] *Secretin* was the first gastrointestinal hormone to be described. This hormone, a helical polypeptide with 27 amino acid residues, is released from duodenal and jejunal mucosa in response to H^+. Secretin promotes digestion by stimulating copious water and bicarbonate secretion from the pancreas. This action facilitates entry of pancreatic enzymes into the intestinal lumen and provides a pH favoring digestion of fat. Secretin is also a choleretic, stimulating increased water and electrolyte secretion from the liver. Secretion inhibits gastric acid secretion and gastrointestinal motility.

Cholecystokinin-Pancreozymin (CCK-PZ)

Cholecystokinin and pancreozymin are the same substance which is released from intestinal mucosa bathed by amino acids or fatty acids. This substance facilitates digestion and absorption by stimulating emptying of the gallbladder as well as by increasing bile flow and relaxing the sphincter of Oddi. Another important action of CCK-PZ is stimulation of pancreatic enzyme secretion. CCK-PZ is a linear polypeptide having 33 residues. The C-terminal tetrapeptide of CCK-PZ is identical to that of another gastrointestinal hormone, gastrin, and this fragment posseses the actions of both intact hormones. In general CCK-PZ and gastrin share actions and differ mainly in potency for a given action.

Each of these hormones acts on the same target organs and may be stimulatory or inhibitory for a given action. When administered in combination the gastrointestinal hormones may augment or inhibit each other.

Fat introduced into the duodenum or small intestine inhibits gastric acid secretion. This phenomenon has suggested the existence of a hormone, enterogastrone, that inhibits gastric secretion and motility. At the present time it is not clear whether gastric inhibition by fat in the intestine is due to CCK-PZ and secretin or to another as yet unidentified substance.

IMMUNOLOGIC FUNCTION OF THE INTESTINE

Recently it was found that the intestine is a source of immunoglobulin, particularly IgA.[20] It is believed that this immunoglobulin arises from plasma cells in the lamina propria and after linkage with a protein synthesized by epithelial cells is secreted into the lumen. Secretory IgA contains antibody activities, the exact roles of which are not yet known.

For references, see page 1010.

III ——————————————————————————————

INTESTINAL OBSTRUCTION

R. Scott Jones, M.D.

HISTORY

Intestinal obstruction was observed and treated by Hippocrates. The earliest recorded operation for intestinal obstruction was probably performed by Praxagoras (350 B.C.), who created an enterocutaneous fistula to relieve the obstruction. However, nonoperative treatment remained the general rule, including reduction of hernias, opium for pain, orally administered mercury or lead shot in an endeavor to open the occluded bowel, electrical stimulation, and gastric lavage.

In the nineteenth century, amid considerable debate, surgery became used more frequently for intestinal obstruction. Most of the significant advances in the management of this disorder were made after the turn of the twentieth century. Hartwell and Houget[8] observed in 1912 that parenteral administration of saline solution prolonged the lives of dogs with intestinal obstruction, and this has become a cardinal principle of the management of intestinal obstruction today.

The second decade of the twentieth century saw the development of radiographic techniques in the diagnosis of intestinal obstruction. In the 1930s nasogastric or intestinal tubes were employed to prevent or relieve intestinal distention in patients with intestinal obstruction. Antibiotics were added to the therapy of bowel obstruction in the 1940s and 1950s. Fluid replacement, intestinal decompression, antibiotics, and improvements in surgical and anesthetic techniques have reduced the mortality rate in simple intestinal obstruction; however, the recognition and treatment of strangulating intestinal obstruction remain important problems for surgeons today.[25]

ETIOLOGY

When gastrointestinal luminal content is pathologically prevented from passing distally, intestinal obstruction exists. Intestinal obstruction may be caused by mechanical occlusion of the bowel lumen, called *mechanical obstruction,* or by paralysis of the intestinal muscle, called *paralytic ileus.*

Mechanical Obstruction

Three types of abnormalities may produce mechanical obstruction:[15, 18]

1. *Obturation of the intestinal lumen* may be caused by several kinds of disease, such as polypoid tumors of the bowel. Intussusception is an invagination of the bowel lumen with the invaginated portion (the intussusceptum) passing distally into the ensheathing outer portion (the intussuscipiens) by peristalsis. This process will occlude the blood supply of the intussusceptum. In adults intussusception is usually caused by an abnormality of the bowel wall, such as a tumor or Meckel's diverticulum; however, in infants and children intussusception may occur without apparent anatomic cause. Obturation obstruction may be caused by large gallstones, which can enter the intestinal lumen via a cholecystoenteric fistula. This causes a rare condition called gallstone ileus.

Feces, meconium, or bezoars may obstruct the intestine. Bezoars occur more frequently in children, the mentally retarded, and the toothless, and in patients after gastrectomy.

2. *Intrinsic bowel lesions* producing intestinal obstruction are often congenital (atresia, stenosis, duplication), are seen most commonly in infants and small children, and are described in Chapter 40, Pediatric Surgery. Strictures of the intestine may result from neoplasm, as in carcinoma of the sigmoid colon, or from inflammation, as in Crohn's disease. Rarely, one encounters iatrogenic strictures following intestinal anastomosis, after radiation therapy, or after treatment with enteric-coated potassium chloride tablets.

3. *Lesions extrinsic to the bowel* are important causes of intestinal obstruction. Occlusion of the intestine by adhesions from previous surgery or inflammation is the leading cause of small intestinal obstruction. Adhesions may produce obstruction by kinking or angulation, or by creating bands of tissue that compress the bowel. External hernias are second only to adhesions as a cause of mechanical small intestinal obstruction. Inguinal, femoral, umbilical, and incisional hernias are important causes of bowel obstruction. The risk of intestinal obstruction is the principal reason for the elective repair of hernias. Internal hernias due to congenital abnormalities of the mesentery, or to surgical defects in the mesentery, occasionally cause bowel obstruction. Extrinsic masses such as neoplasms and abscesses may cause mechanical bowel obstruction. A volvulus is an extrinsic abnormality in which a portion of the alimentary canal rotates or twists about itself, the twist usually involving the blood supply of the twisted portion of the bowel. This abnormality results in kinking of the gut, producing mechanical obstruction, frequently with occlusion of the blood supply to the bowel. A volvulus is usually associated with some underlying abnormality; for example, midgut volvulus is caused by the mesenteric abnormality of malrotation. Cecal volvulus occurs when the cecum or right colon is on a mesentery, rather than retroperitoneal. Sigmoid volvulus develops when the sigmoid colon is abnormally long or redundant. Another type of volvulus occurs when adhesions fix the intestine to a point that acts as a pivot for the volvulus. The most common causes of intestinal obstruction in adults are adhesions, usually resulting from previous surgery, hernias, and neoplasms. Neoplasms are the commonest cause of colon obstruction.

Paralytic Ileus

Paralytic ileus is a common disorder, occurring to some extent in most patients undergoing abdominal surgery. This abnormality is caused by several neural, humoral, and metabolic factors. There are reflexes that inhibit intestinal motility, such as the intestinointestinal reflex resulting from prolonged intestinal distention. Distention of other organs, such as the ureter, can inhibit intestinal motility. Spine fracture, retroperitoneal hemorrhage, or trauma may also be associated with paralytic ileus. A humoral factor in paralytic ileus is suggested by experiments in dogs in which motility of transplanted (denervated) intestinal loops was inhibited during experimental peritonitis.[11] The substances responsible for this phenomenon are unknown. Clinically, peritonitis is associated with paralytic ileus. Electrolyte imbalances, particularly hypokalemia, contribute to paralytic ileus by interfering with the normal ionic movements during smooth muscle contraction. Finally, ischemia of the intestine rapidly inhibits motility.

PATHOGENESIS

Simple Mechanical Small Intestinal Obstruction

Mechanical obstruction of the small intestine results in accumulation of fluid and gas proximal to the obstruction, producing *distention* of the intestine. Distention is initiated by ingested fluid, digestive secretions, and intestinal gas. As mentioned previously, large volumes of saliva, gastric secretion, bile, and pancreatic juice enter the gut daily. The stomach has a very small capacity for fluid absorption, so most alimentary fluid is absorbed by the small intestine.

Intestinal gas normally is propelled aborally by peristalsis and is expelled from the rectum as flatus. Gas accumulating in the intestine proximal to an obstruction originates from: (1) swallowed air, (2) carbon dioxide from neutralization of bicarbonate, and (3) organic gases from bacterial fermentation. Swallowed air is the most important source of gas in intestinal obstruction because its nitrogen content is very high and nitrogen is not absorbed by the intestinal mucosa. As a result the intestinal gas is predominantly (70 per cent) nitrogen. Large quantities of carbon dioxide are produced in the lumen of the gut, but this gas is readily absorbed and therefore contributes little to the distention of intestinal obstruction.

One of the most important events during simple mechanical small bowel obstruction is loss of water and electrolytes from the body, caused mainly by intestinal distention. First, reflex vomiting may result from intestinal distention. In addition, intestinal distention is self-perpetuating in the obstructed small bowel, since distention increases intestinal secretion. Experiments on dogs show that intestinal distention initially causes decreased absorption (decreased lumen-to-blood flux of water) and may subsequently cause increased secretion (increased blood-to-lumen flux of water) in the obstructed segment, but not in the intestine distal to the obstruction.[19] This phenomenon results in increased fluid accumulation in the bowel proximal to the obstruction, which may further accentuate dehydration and cause further intestinal distention, which proceeds proximally. Increased secretion of obstructed bowel has also been demonstrated in man.[26]

The metabolic results of fluid loss in simple mechanical obstruction of the small bowel depend upon the site and the duration of the obstruction. Proximal small bowel obstruction causes relatively greater vomiting and less intestinal distention than distal obstruction. Proximal obstruction causes losses of water, Na^+, Cl^-, H^+, and K^+, producing dehydration with hypochloremia, hypokalemia, and metabolic alkalosis. Distal small bowel obstruction may entail loss of large quantities of fluid into the bowel; however, the abnormalities of serum electrolyte values are usually less dramatic, probably because hydrochloric acid losses are less.[13]

Accompanying dehydration are oliguria, azotemia, and hemoconcentration. If dehydration persists, circulatory changes such as tachycardia, low central venous pressure, and reduced cardiac output may lead to hypotension and hypovolemic shock. Other sequelae of intestinal distention may be increased intra-abdominal pressure, impeding venous return from the legs, and elevation of the diaphragm sufficient to impair ventilation.

Also taking place during intestinal obstruction is rapid proliferation of intestinal bacteria. Normally the small intestine contains very small quantities of bacteria and may be almost sterile. There may be several causes for the sparse bacterial population of the small intestine, but normal peristalsis with continued aboral progression of luminal content is important in minimizing the small intestinal flora. During small intestinal stasis, whatever the cause, bacteria proliferate rapidly and this phenomenon is particularly notable in intestinal obstruction. The small intestinal contents will thus become "feculent" during obstruction because of large quantities of bacteria. Normally the colon, an organ functioning as a reservoir, contains large numbers of bacteria.

The bacteria in the small intestine probably play no role in the ill effects of simple mechanical small intestinal obstruction, since the bacteria or bacterial toxins do not cross the normal intestinal mucosa.

Strangulation Obstruction

Strangulation develops when the circulation to the obstructed intestine is impaired. The circulation to the bowel may be impaired by sustained increased intraluminal pressure. Closed-loop obstruction occurs when the bowel lumen is occluded at two points along its length. This type of obstruction may proceed more rapidly to strangulation than simple obstruction. Pressure necrosis can develop if the obstructed distending bowel is held by unyielding adhesive bands or hernial rings. The mesenteric vessels can be occluded by deformity or twisting of the mesentery, as in volvulus or intussusception. In strangulation obstruction the patient may suffer all of the ill effects of simple obstruction in addition to the effects of strangulation. Strangulation causes loss of blood and plasma from the strangulated segment, which may be particularly severe if the vascular obstruction is predominantly venous. This loss of blood and plasma will cause shock, particularly if the patient is already dehydrated. If strangulation produces gangrene, peritonitis with its sequelae will occur. Rupture or perforation of a strangulated segment is possible and is a devastating complication.

In addition to the loss of blood and plasma, another important factor in strangulation obstruction is the toxic material from the strangulated loop. The luminal fluid from a strangulated intestinal loop and the bloody, malodorous peritoneal fluid are lethal when administered to normal animals. Bacteria and necrotic tissue appear to be necessary for the development of the toxic fluid. Apparently this lethal factor is formed in the lumen of the strangulated intestine and passes through the intestinal wall when the gut is injured by distention, vascular compromise, and bacteria. The toxic material is absorbed from the peritoneal cavity, producing systemic effects.[13] Animal experiments show that antibiotics prolong the lives of animals with experimentally induced strangulation obstruction. The efficacy of antibiotics in humans with intestinal obstruction has not been demonstrated as clearly.

Colon Obstruction

In general, colon obstruction produces less fluid and electrolyte disturbance than mechanical small bowel obstruction. If the patient has a "competent" ileocecal valve there may be little or no small bowel distention, but in this instance the colon will behave as a closed loop. When the colon is massively distended by gas, it may perforate and in this situation, because of its spherical shape and large diameter, the cecum is the most likely site for perforation. In patients with "incompetent" ileocecal valves, signs of small bowel distention may accompany colon obstruction. The colon, of course, is also subject to strangulation when obstruction compromises the blood supply.

DIAGNOSIS OF INTESTINAL OBSTRUCTION

The questions to ask in evaluating a patient suspected of having intestinal obstruction are as follows: (1) Does the patient have bowel obstruction? (2) If so, where is it? (3) What is the anatomic and pathologic nature of the obstructing lesions? (4) Has strangulation occurred? (5) What is the general condition of the patient (fluid-electrolyte balance, other systemic disease, and so forth)?

The syndrome of intestinal obstruction is characterized by abdominal pain, vomiting, obstipation, abdominal distention, and failure to pass flatus. The pain in intestinal obstruction is typically crampy, with paroxysms occurring at 4- to 5-minute intervals in proximal obstruction and less frequently in distal obstruction. After a longer period of mechanical obstruction the crampy pain may subside because motility may be inhibited by bowel distention. When crampy abdominal pain is succeeded by continuous severe abdominal pain, strangulation with peritonitis should be suspected.

In patients with proximal intestinal obstruction, vomiting may be profuse, and unassociated with abdominal distention. In distal obstruction, the vomiting will be less frequent and may be "feculent" because of the large bacterial population of intestinal contents. Obstipation and failure to pass gas from the rectum are characteristic of complete obstruction, but are evident only after the bowel distal to the obstruction has been evacuated. Increase in abdominal girth, due to accumulation of fluid and gas in the intestine, is often noted by patients with distal small bowel obstruction, colon obstruction, or paralytic ileus.

A complete physical examination is indicated, but particular attention should be given to certain points. Tachycardia and hypotension may indicate severe dehydration, peritonitis, or both. Fever suggests the possibility of strangulation. The status of hydration should be estimated by examination of skin turgor and moisture of the mucous membrane. The abdomen is usually distended. Occasionally the examiner must determine whether abdominal distention is due to bowel obstruction or ascites. Ascites is characterized by a fluid wave, shifting dullness, and fullness in the flanks. Peristaltic waves characteristic of small bowel obstruction are sometimes visible through the abdominal wall of thin patients with longer-standing obstruction. Surgical scars should be noted because of the etiologic implication of previous surgery; for example, the presence of adhesions or cancer. Incarcerated hernias may be obscure, particularly in obese patients. Abdominal masses (neoplasm, intussusception, abscess) should be sought. Abdominal tenderness is a characteristic finding in patients with intestinal obstruction; however, localized tenderness, rebound tenderness, and guarding suggest peritonitis and the likelihood of strangulation.

Abdominal auscultation in patients with mechanical intestinal obstruction will usually reveal periods of increasing or crescendoing bowel sounds separated by relatively quiet periods. The quality of bowel sounds in intestinal obstruction is usually high-pitched, tinkling, or musical in character.

Rectal examination should be done to detect luminal masses. The presence or absence of feces should be noted, and if feces are present, examination for occult blood should be done. Blood in the feces suggests an alimentary mucosal lesion as may occur with cancer, intussusception, or infarction. Sigmoidoscopic examination should be done if colon obstruction is suspected.

Acute intestinal obstruction can usually be diagnosed on the basis of history and physical examination. Any patient having crampy abdominal pain, vomiting, obstipation, abdominal distention, abdominal tenderness, and peristaltic rushes should be considered to have intestinal obstruction until that diagnosis can be confidently excluded.

Radiologic Examination

X-rays are essential to confirm the clinical diagnosis and to define more accurately the site of obstruction.[5] Abdominal x-ray examination of patients with intestinal obstruction usually reveals abnormally large quantities of gas in the bowel. One can usually determine whether small intestine, colon, or both are distended (Fig. 1). Gas in the small bowel outlines the valvulae conniventes, which usually occupy the entire transverse diameter of the bowel image. Colonic haustral markings, on the other hand, occupy only a portion of the transverse diameter of the bowel. Typically, the small bowel pattern occupies the more central portion of the abdomen (Fig. 2), while the colon shadow is on the periphery of the abdominal film or in the pelvis. Patients with mechanical small intestinal obstruction usually have minimal or no colonic gas. Radiographs of patients who have colon obstruction with a competent ileocecal valve will show colon distention but little small bowel gas. Patients with colon obstruction and incompetent ileocecal valves usually have radiographic evidence of small bowel and colon distention. Films taken in the upright or lateral decubitus position in patients with mechanical small bowel obstruction usually show multiple gas-fluid levels, with distended bowel resembling an inverted U (Fig. 3). Occasionally, ordinary x-ray films fail to distinguish colonic from small intestinal obstruction and it may be valuable to administer a radiographic contrast agent. Probably the safest and quickest way to distinguish colonic from small bowel obstruction preoperatively is by a carefully performed barium enema.

It is often difficult on x-rays to distinguish paralytic ileus from mechanical obstruction. One radiographic feature of paralytic ileus is that gaseous distention occurs somewhat uniformly in stomach, small bowel, and colon (Fig. 4). Gas-fluid levels may be seen in paralytic ileus. Examination after a barium meal may assist in distinguishing between paralytic ileus and mechanical obstruction, but should be avoided if colon obstruction cannot be excluded.

Laboratory Tests

Any patient with vomiting or evidence of intra-abdominal fluid loss who is suspected of having intestinal obstruction should have laboratory measurements of serum, sodium, chloride, potassium, bicarbonate, and creatinine. The hematocrit, white blood cell count, and serum electrolytes should be measured serially to assess adequacy of therapy and to detect the earliest evidence of tissue necrosis.

TREATMENT OF INTESTINAL OBSTRUCTION

With few exceptions, the appropriate treatment for intestinal obstruction is surgical relief of the obstruction.[16] Since severe metabolic derangements may accompany bowel obstruction, the decision of when to operate requires careful judgment. The overlapping sequence of events in managing patients with intestinal obstruction should be investigation, resuscitation, and operation. The timing of operation depends upon

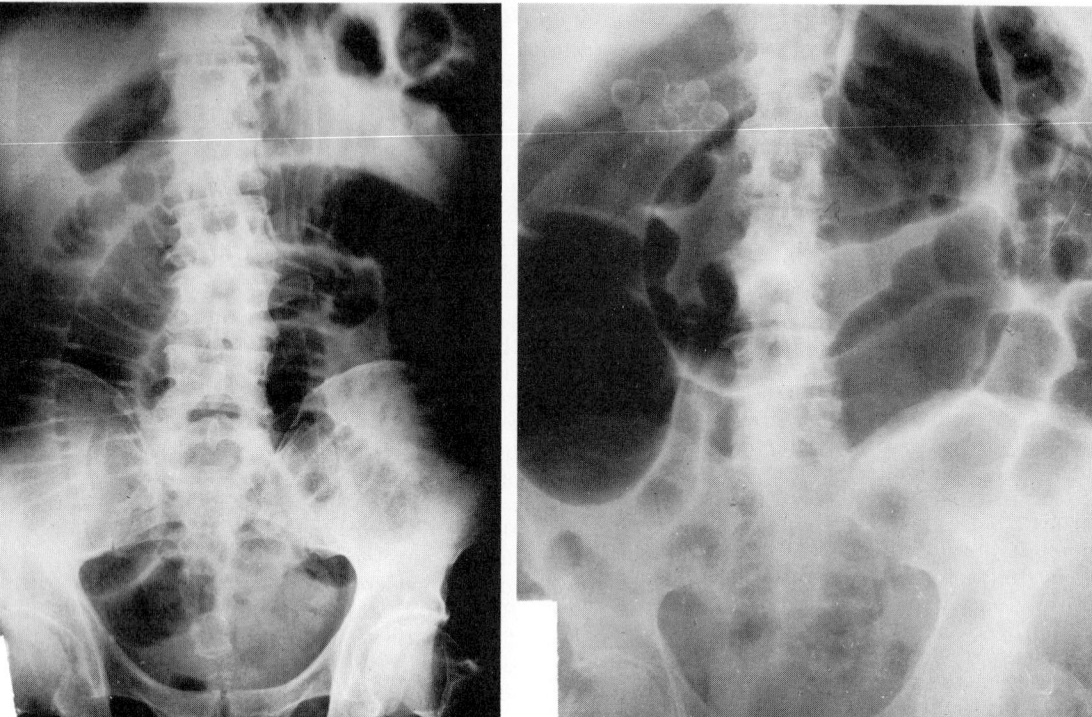

Figure 1.   The picture on the left shows the centrally located loops and clearly depicts the valvulae conniventes, both of which are typical of distended small intestine. On the right the haustral markings and the tendency toward peripheral gas accumulation typical of colon distention are seen. This patient incidentally had multiple radiopaque gallstones. (This and the subsequent radiographs were selected with the assistance of John Amberg, M.D., Professor of Radiology, University of California, San Francisco.)

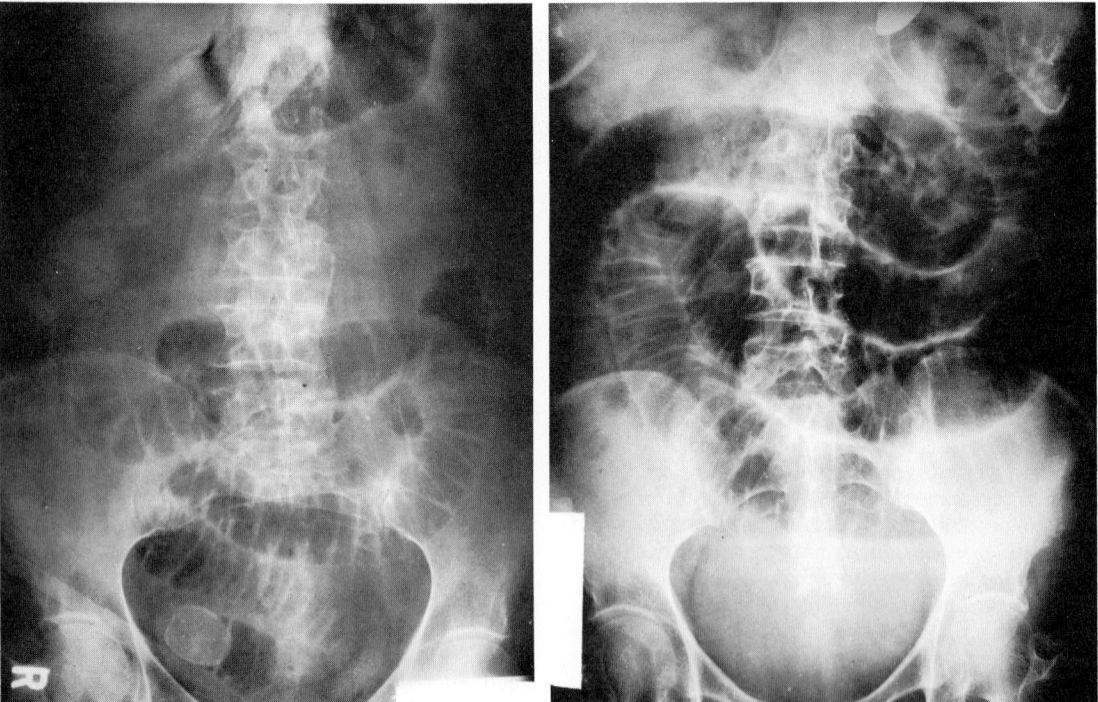

Figure 2.   Gallstone ileus is an uncommon cause of intestinal obstruction, but often can be diagnosed from plain films when present. The film on the left shows complete mechanical small bowel obstruction caused by a radiopaque gallstone in the right lower abdomen. The film on the right is from another patient with gallstone ileus due to a radiolucent gallstone. The diagnosis was suggested by the presence of gas in the biliary tract.

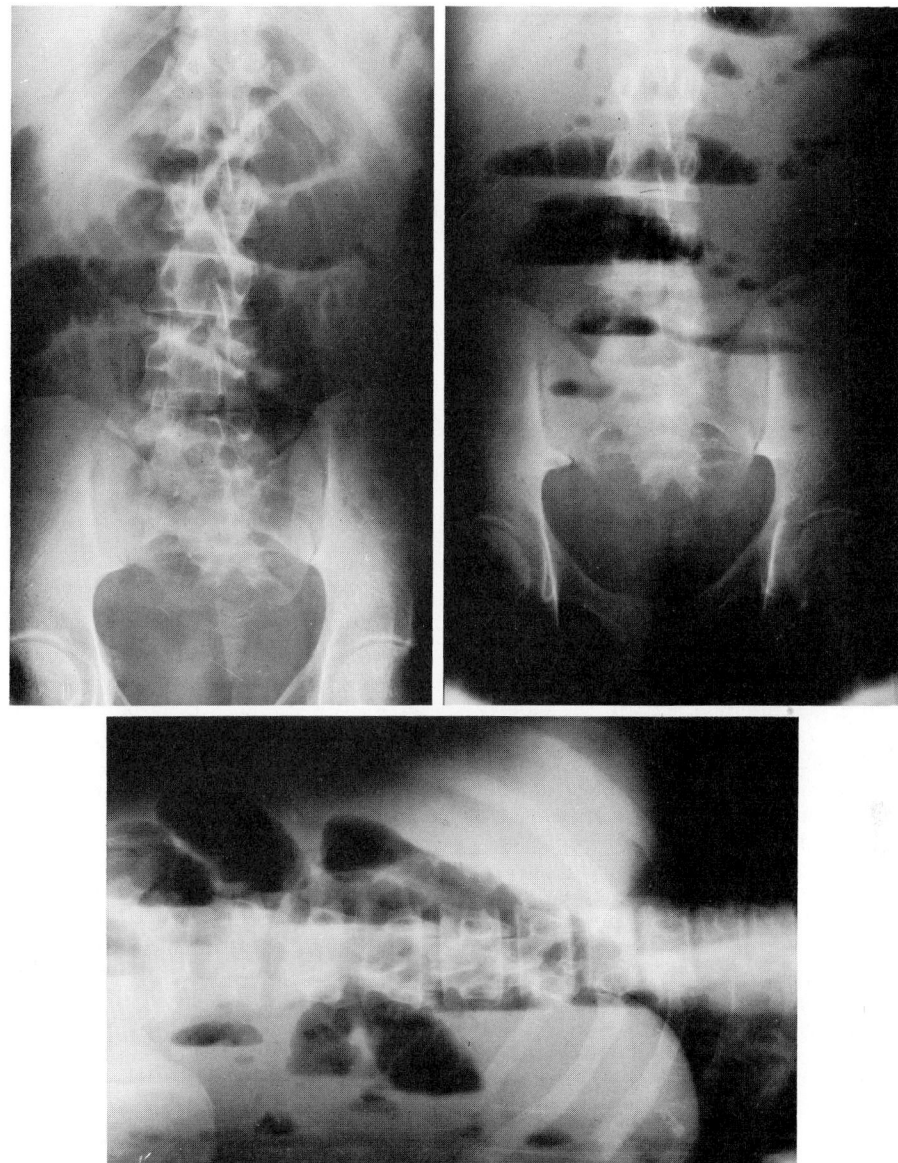

Figure 3. Supine (left upper), upright (right upper), and occasionally lateral decubitus (lower) films usually confirm the diagnosis of acute complete mechanical small bowel obstruction by revealing distended small bowel loops, gas-fluid levels, inverted U-shaped loops, and the absence of gas in the colon or rectum.

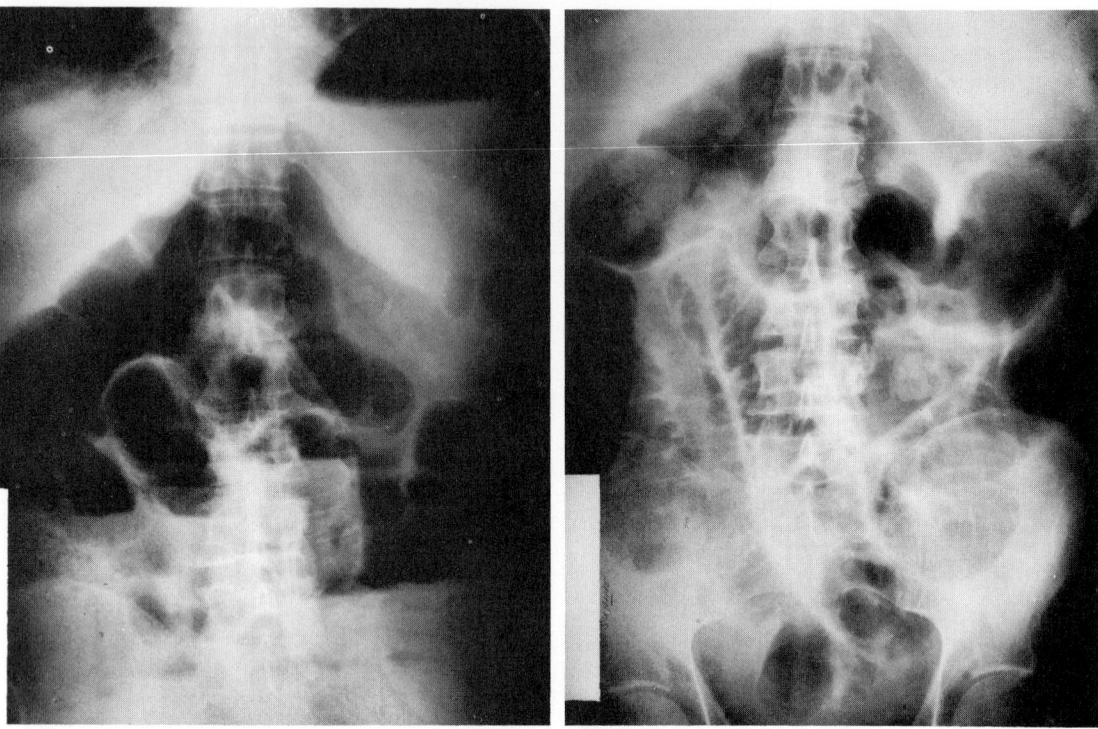

Figure 4. Paralytic ileus is usually difficult to distinguish from mechanical obstruction. The presence of gas in stomach, small bowel, and colon suggests ileus, as shown in these films.

three factors (1) duration of obstruction, i.e., severity of fluid, electrolyte, and acid-base abnormalities; (2) improvement of vital organ function, e.g., in the elderly patient with cardiac disease, rapid preoperative digitalization may be helpful; (3) consideration of the risk of strangulation.[14] The mortality from intestinal obstruction with intestinal gangrene is 31 per cent,[16] while in simple mechanical obstruction when operation is done within 24 hours the mortality rate is about 1 per cent.[18] Since there is no reliable way to detect strangulation preoperatively, operation should be performed as soon as is reasonable.

A patient with symptoms of short duration, 24 to 30 hours, with minimal metabolic disturbance and no pre-existing pulmonary, cardiac, or renal disease, can be operated upon when the diagnosis is made. An elderly patient in whom fluid and electrolyte imbalance develops after several days of illness may benefit from 18 to 24 hours of preoperative preparation.

Patients with bowel obstruction are likely to be depleted of water, sodium, chloride, and potassium, so that intravenous therapy should usually begin with intravenous isotonic sodium chloride solution. After adequate urine formation is observed, potassium chloride should be added to the infusion. Sufficient fluid should be given to elevate and maintain the central venous pressure to between 5 and 10 cm. of saline. Administration of blood, plasma, or both should be considered if the patient is in shock and if strangulation is suspected. After pulse, blood pressure, central venous pressure, and urinary output are normal, surgery

may be considered. If marked hemoconcentration and severe electrolyte imbalance were present initially, laboratory studies should be repeated, and if the values are returning to normal the patient should be operated upon. Antibiotics should be given during the period of resuscitation, particularly if strangulation is suspected.

In addition to fluid therapy another important adjunct to the supportive care of patients with intestinal obstruction is nasogastric or intestinal suction.[24] Nasogastric suction with a Levin tube will empty the stomach, reducing the hazard of pulmonary aspiration of vomitus, as well as minimizing further intestinal distention from swallowed air during the preoperative period. A nasogastric tube is not effective in decompressing distended intestine and for that reason long intestinal tubes, such as the Miller-Abbott tube, are often passed through the nostril with the tip of the tube being placed in the pyloric antrum. It is usually necessary to position the tube fluoroscopically and in some patients intubation of the small intestine may be very difficult. When the small bowel is successfully intubated the tube should be allowed to pass distally, on suction, to deflate the bowel. The principal hazard of the use of long intestinal tubes in small bowel obstruction is that it may delay operative treatment in patients with unsuspected strangulation obstruction. Operation for intestinal obstruction should generally not be delayed if the bowel is not successfully intubated or decompressed preoperatively.

Operation may be delayed under the following circumstances: (1) In patients with pyloric obstruction, operation can be postponed safely until the fluid and electrolyte imbalance is completely corrected. (2) The patient in whom intestinal obstruction develops in the immediate postoperative period following an abdominal operation initially may be treated conservatively with a Miller-Abbott tube. Overlooked strangulation is, however, a risk in this instance. (3) The patient with obstruction due to documented disseminated intra-abdominal cancer may be treated with passage of a Miller-Abbott tube. (4) Infants with ileocecal intussusception may be managed by hydrostatic reduction of the intussusception, which avoids operation entirely. Adults with intussception (Fig. 5) should be operated upon because of the high frequency of underlying causes for the intussusception. (5) In patients with sigmoid volvulus, decompression can be performed with a sigmoidoscope, but elective operation should be performed later to prevent recurrent volvulus. (6) In patients with intestinal obstruction due to an acute exacerbation of Crohn's disease, a period of conservative treatment may permit resolution of the obstruction. (7) Patients with chronic partial obstruction may be managed by less urgent operative treatment than patients with acute mechanical obstruction.

Operative Treatment of Intestinal Obstruction

In general the four commonly used approaches to management of intestinal obstruction are determined by the nature of the problem: (1) In simple obstruction, i.e., an incarcerated inguinal hernia, reduction of the hernia suffices; or obstruction caused by peritoneal adhesions can be relieved by division of these structures. (2) A second approach to obstructing lesions is the creation of an intestinal bypass. An example of this therapy is the treatment of obstructing Crohn's disease of the ileum by ileotransverse colon anastomoses. (3) The placement of an enterocutaneous fistula such as a colostomy proximal to an obstruction is a standard form of therapy. (4) Excision of a lesion with restoration of intestinal continuity is used frequently. An example of this approach is the excision of the right colon with ileotransverse colostomy for obstructing carcinoma of the cecum.

With few exceptions, operation for intestinal obstruction should be performed under general anesthesia administered with an endotracheal tube. One of the risks in operating on patients with intestinal obstruction is vomiting and tracheobronchial aspiration of the feculent vomitus.

In the absence of external hernia in patients with small bowel obstruction, abdominal exploration should

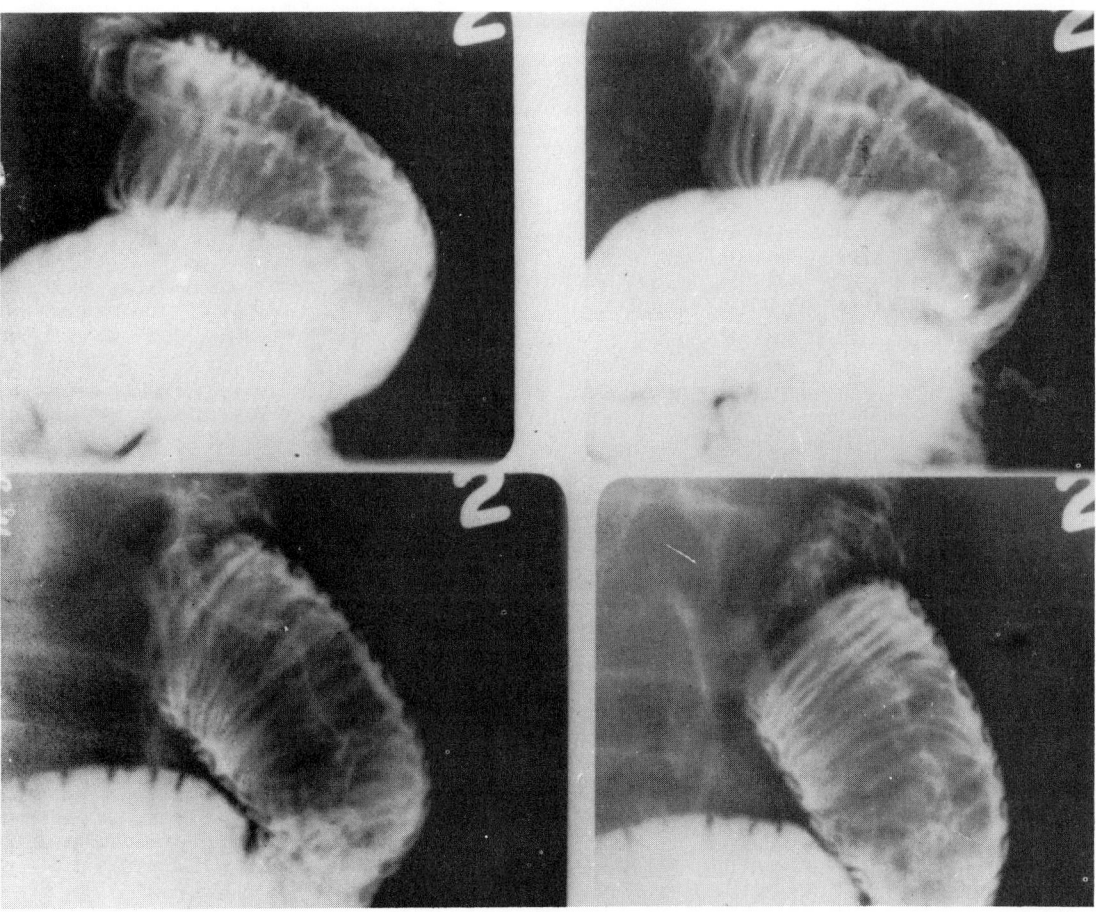

Figure 5. This series of spot films reveals an ileoileal intussusception in an adult.

be performed through a midline vertical incision. The obstructed point can be located by following distended bowel distally until collapsed intestine is found. The operative manipulation of obstructed intestine is easier if the intestine has been decompressed preoperatively. It may be desirable to empty the distended bowel during the operation. This can frequently be accomplished by passing an intestinal tube into the intestine at operation.

In operating on patients with multiple intra-abdominal adhesions the surgeon should be certain that there are no additional sites of obstruction distal to that which is clinically obvious. One may want to express manually the luminal contents into the cecum to rule out other possible distal obstructing points.

It is often difficult to determine whether a segment of bowel is viable. The criteria generally used in determining bowel viability are (1) color, (2) motility, and (3) arterial pulsation. If intestinal viability is questionable, the bowel segment should be completely released and placed in a saline-moistened sponge for 15 to 20 minutes, and then re-examined. If normal color has returned and peristalsis is evident, it is safe to retain the bowel. If there is reasonable doubt of the bowel's viability, it should be resected.

The approach to colon obstruction is somewhat different from that to small bowel obstruction. The classic method of treating obstruction of the left colon entails three separate operative steps: (1) relief of gaseous distention by colostomy proximal to the obstruction; (2) removal of the diseased segment of colon and anastomosis, leaving the colostomy intact; and (3) closure of the colostomy when healing of the anastomosis is complete. The staged procedure is performed because: (1) Intestinal obstruction and its sequelae are a significant and immediate threat to life that should be eliminated as simply as possible. Colon resection may be a formidable operation and is more safely performed electively. (2) Surgical anastomosis of distended colon is hazardous. A technically excellent colon anastomosis cannot be made with distended, thin-walled bowel filled with fluid and feces. Colostomies can be performed where the colon is mobile with a mesentery such as in sigmoid or transverse colon. In most instances transverse colostomy is the best choice in treating left-sided colon obstruction. In elderly poor-risk patients with extensive colon distention a tube cecostomy inserted with local anesthesia may be the procedure of choice.[14]

Obstructive lesions of the cecum and right colon are managed differently. In treating cecal or right colon obstruction due to cancer one must usually choose between right colectomy with ileotransverse colostomy and a bypassing operation, ileotransverse colostomy, to relieve the obstruction, with later elective resection of the right colon. The bypass operation should be reserved for poor-risk patients. Right colectomy can be done safely in patients with obstruction because the obstructed colon can be removed and the dilated small bowel can usually be sutured safely to normal colon. The treatment of volvulus of the cecum depends upon the viability of the cecum. If it is nonviable, right colectomy should be done. If it is viable, detorsion and fixation of the cecum is appropriate.

Treatment of Paralytic Ileus

Paralytic ileus is treated by nasogastric suction and intravenous fluid administration. Correction of electrolyte imbalance, especially hypokalemia, is particularly important in managing this disorder.[14] In some cases of paralytic ileus, particularly with extreme distention, passage of a Miller-Abbott tube into the intestine should be tried, since this method of suction provides superior intestinal decompression. If it is clear that mechanical obstruction or intra-abdominal sepsis is not present, parasympathomimetic drugs, such as neostigmine (Prostigmin), may be of value.

Most often, ileus develops after abdominal surgery and is transient, lasting 2 to 3 days. When ileus persists or occurs without obvious etiology, one should endeavor to rule out mechanical obstruction or intra-abdominal sepsis and a laparotomy may be necessary to exclude confidently those factors.

Occasionally bowel distention secondary to ileus will be so great as to threaten viability of bowel.

SELECTED REFERENCES

American Physiological Society: Handbook of Physiology, Section 6, Alimentary Canal. C. F. Code (Ed.). Baltimore, Williams & Wilkins Company, 1967–1968.
The five volumes of this publication sponsored by the American Physiological Society provide the best reference source on gastrointestinal function available at the present time. The authors, all of whom are pre-eminent authorities on their subject, provide a comprehensive, detailed, critical description of current fact and hypothesis concerning food intake, gastrointestinal secretion, digestion, absorption, and gastrointestinal motility. The references in these chapters represent complete review of the pertinent literature through 1966.

Davenport, H. W.: Physiology of the Digestive Tract, 2nd ed. Chicago, Year Book Medical Publishers, 1966.
This book is an excellent starting point for reading about gastrointestinal physiology. All aspects of intestinal function are discussed clearly, authoritatively, and succinctly.

Hartwell, J. A., and Hoguet, J. P.: Experimental intestinal obstruction in dogs with especial reference to the cause of death and the treatment by large amounts of normal saline solution. J.A.M.A., 59:82, 1912.
The authors emphasize the importance of fluid loss in the pathogenesis of intestinal obstruction and show that the administration of saline solutions prevented death from high intestinal obstruction in dogs. This paper was presented before the Annual Session of the American Medical Association in June, 1912, and the authors' observations have stood the test of time.

Moore, F. D.: Metabolic Care of the Surgical Patient. Philadelphia, W. B. Saunders Company, 1959.
This excellent reference describes the analysis and repair of the metabolic derangements in patients with intestinal obstruction. Small bowel obstruction is classified on the basis of duration or severity of fluid and electrolyte imbalance to assist in planning therapy. This book also provides guides for planning the timing of operation to relieve obstruction. The sections on ileus and postoperative ileus-obstruction are particularly helpful.

REFERENCES

1. American Physiological Society: Handbook of Physiology, Section 6, Alimentary Canal. C. F. Code (Ed.). Baltimore, Williams & Wilkins Company, 1967–1968.
2. Bloom, W., and Fawcett, D. W.: A Textbook of Histology, 9th ed. Philadelphia, W. B. Saunders Company, 1968, pp. 560–581.
3. Brooks, F. P.: Control of Gastrointestinal Function. New York, Macmillan Co., 1970.
4. Davenport, H. W.: Physiology of the Digestive Tract, 2nd ed. Chicago, Year Book Medical Publishers, 1966.
5. Frimann-Dahl, J.: The acute abdomen. *In* Margulis, A. R., and

Burhenne, J. J. (Eds.): Alimentary Tract Roentgenology. St. Louis, The C. V. Mosby Company, 1967, Volume 1, pp. 141–196.

6. Gray, H.: Anatomy of the Human Body, 28th ed. C. M. Goss (Ed.). Philadelphia, Lea & Febiger, 1966.

7. Grossman, M. I.: Spectrum of biological actions of gastrointestinal hormones. *In* Andersson, S. (Ed.): Nobel Symposium XVI: Frontiers in Gastrointestinal Hormone Research. Stockholm, Almqvist & Wiksell/Gebers Forlag, 1973.

8. Hartwell, J. A., and Hoguet, J. P.: Experimental intestinal obstruction in dogs with especial reference to the cause of death and the treatment by large amounts of normal saline solution. J.A.M.A., *59*:82, 1912.

9. Hirsch, J. E., Arhens, E. H., Jr., and Blankenhorn, D. H.: Measurement of the human intestinal length in vivo and some causes of variation. Gastroenterology, *31*:274, 1956.

10. Hoffman, A. F.: A physicochemical approach to the intraluminal phase of fat absorption. Gastroenterology, 50:56, 1966.

11. Landman, M. D., and Longmire, W. P., Jr.: Neural and hormonal influence of peritonitis on paralytic ileus. Am. Surg., *33*:756, 1967.

12. Marsh, M. N., and Swift, J. A.: A study of the small intestinal mucosa using the scanning electron microscope. Gut, *10*:940, 1969.

13. Miller, L. D., Mackie, J. A., and Rhoads, J. E.: The pathophysiology and management of intestinal obstruction. Surg. Clin. North Am., *42*:1285, 1962.

14. Moore, F. D.: Metabolic Care of the Surgical Patient. Philadelphia, W. B. Saunders Company, 1959.

15. Moyer, C. A., Rhoads, J. E., Allen, J. G., and Harkins, H. N.: Surgery, Principles and Practice, 3rd ed. Philadelphia, J. B. Lippincott Company, 1965.

16. Nemir, P., Jr.: Intestinal obstruction; 10-year statistical survey at Hospital of University of Pennsylvania. Ann. Surg., *135*:367, 1952.

17. Polak, J. M., Pearse, A. G. E., Joffe, S. N., and Bloom, S. R.: Quantification of secretin release by acid using immunocytochemistry and radioimmunoassay. Experientia, *31*:462, 1975.

18. Schwartz, S. I., et al. (Eds.): Principles of Surgery. New York, McGraw-Hill Book Company, 1969, pp. 843–855.

19. Shields, R.: The absorption and secretion of fluid and electrolytes by the obstructed bowel. Br. J. Surg., *52*:774, 1965.

20. Tomasi, T. B., Jr.: Human immunoglobulin A. N. Engl. J. Med., *279*:1327, 1968.

21. Turnberg, L. A., Bieberdorf, F. A., Morawski, S. G., and Fordtran, J. S.: Interrelationships of chloride, bicarbonate, sodium, and hydrogen transport in human ileum. J. Clin. Invest., *49*:557, 1970.

22. Turnberg, L. A., Fordtran, J. S., Carter, N. W., and Rector, F. C., Jr.: Mechanism of bicarbonate absorption and its relation to sodium transport in the human jejunum. J. Clin. Invest., *49*:548, 1970.

23. Visscher, M. B., Fetcher, E. S., Jr., Carr, C. W., Gregore, H. P., Bushey, M. S., and Barker, D. E.: Isotopic tracer studies on the movement of water and ions between intestinal lumen and blood. Am. J. Physiol., *142*:550, 1944.

24. Wangensteen, O. H.: Intestinal Obstructions, 3rd ed. Springfield, Ill., Charles C Thomas, Publisher, 1955.

25. Wangensteen, O. H.: Historical aspects of the management of acute intestinal obstruction. Surgery, 65:363, 1969.

26. Wright, H. K., O'Brien, J. J., and Tilson, M. D.: Water absorption in experimental closed segment obstruction of the ileum in man. Am. J. Surg., *121*:96, 1971.

IV

REGIONAL ENTERITIS (CROHN'S DISEASE)

William R. Drucker, M.D.

CLINICAL AND PATHOLOGIC ASPECTS

Crohn's disease is an active, chronic inflammatory disorder of unknown cause and uncertain natural history occurring in any portion of the gastrointestinal tract with occasional systemic manifestations. The disease is a heterogeneous entity with multiple manifestations, various sites of involvement, and unequal incidence among populations. The patient suffers a lifelong affliction, which fortunately is rarely fatal and, with consistent medical surveillance, is compatible with a long, productive life. There is no known definitive therapy for total irradiation, nor, perhaps, even to influence the natural course of the disease. Medical and surgical therapy can effectively palliate most acute episodes, but the hallmark of the disease is a chronic course of remissions and exacerbations.

Characteristically a patient with Crohn's disease consults a physician for crampy abdominal pain and diarrhea indicating partial obstruction of intestine thickened by a chronic inflammatory process. Being an inflammatory disease, it is associated with malaise, fever, and weight loss. There may be a palpable abdominal mass, some form of anal pathology, and occasionally visible changes in the rectal mucosa. But sometimes advanced disease is completely asymptomatic, or no abdominal signs may be found in a patient with chronic disabling symptoms.[17] Appendicitis is often mimicked because the terminal ileum is involved earlier and more often than other areas of bowel.[12] While the mean age of onset of the disease is 25 years, children and the aged are not exempt. By the time most patients seek medical attention, the process has advanced to granulomatous inflammation of all layers of the diseased segment of bowel. When surgery becomes necessary, as it does in most patients,[14] the bowel lesions are readily identified by mesenteric fat creeping over a granular, engorged, serosal surface of thickened bowel with a thick mesentery containing enlarged lymph nodes (Figs. 1 and 2). Loops of bowel may be matted together or connected by fistulae, and segments of diseased bowel ("skip lesions") may be separated by apparently normal bowel (Figs. 2 and 3). The mucosal surface of involved areas is fissured

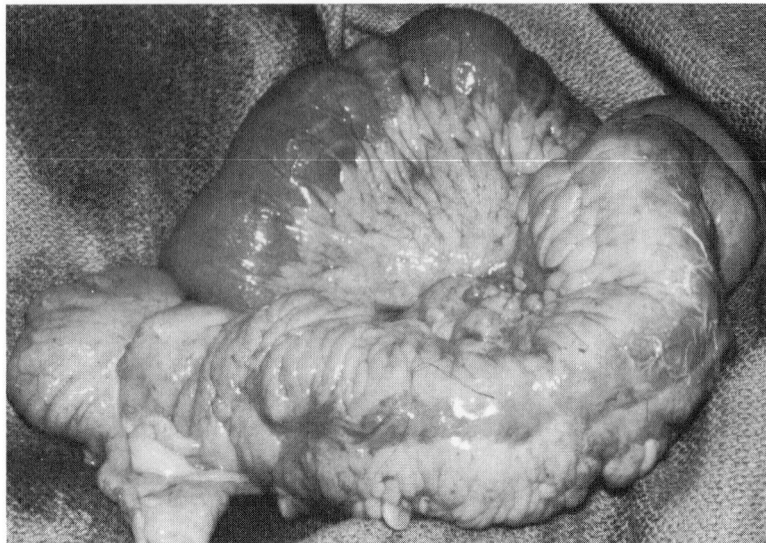

Figure 1. Crohn's disease of the ileum with mesenteric fat "creeping" over the surface of involved segments.

and covers an edematous submucosa to produce a "cobblestone" appearance (Figs. 2 and 4). Marked relief follows resection of the diseased areas, but there is a high rate of recurrence following surgery.[14, 21]

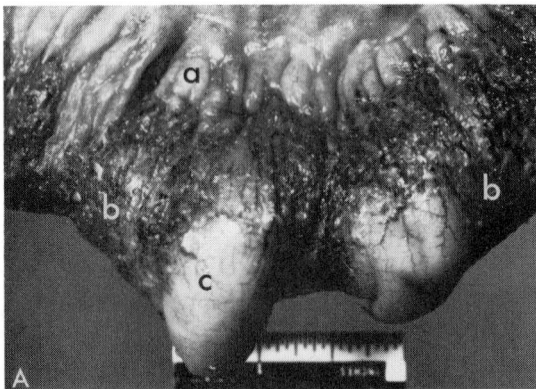

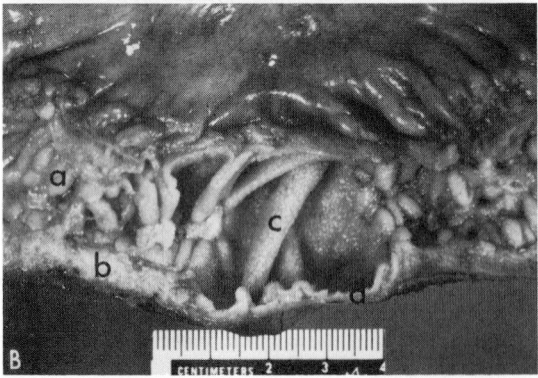

Figure 2. *A,* Segment of diseased and normal bowel showing: (a) edematous mesentery; (b) granular engorged serosal surface; and (c) short segments of normal bowel. *B,* Opened segment of bowel illustrated in *A* showing: (a) "cobblestone" mucosa; (b) thickened bowel wall; (c) normal mucosa; and (d) normal bowel wall.

HISTORY

The original clinicopathologic description by Crohn et al.[7] of the Mount Sinai Hospital in New York in 1932, supplemented by the detailed account of pathologic changes by Blackburn et al.[1] in 1939, has stood the test of time. Many excellent reviews of the history of this disorder are available.[12, 16, 19, 25] Students who credit Morgagni with initiating the study of pathologic anatomy have been able to find a report suggestive of "Crohn's disease" included among his many classic descriptions of gross pathology in *De Sedibus et Causis Morborum* published in 1769. Almost half a century later, in 1813, Saunders and Combe described the autopsy of a young man who had inflammatory thickening of the terminal ileum with three additional constrictions at intervals along the colon. Wilks and Moran, in their book on *Pathological Anatomy* published in 1875, noted "severe local acute ileitis in the shape of a thickening of the whole of the coats . . . found in a circumscribed patch of from six inches to two to three feet." Moynihan in 1907 and Mayo-Robson in 1908 described mimicry of malignant disease in the large and small bowel.[12] Dalziel wrote an apt gross description of diseased bowel when he noted in 1913 that "bowel gives the consistency and smoothness of an eel in a state of rigor mortis." Moschcowitz and Wilenski in 1923 provided an excellent microscopic description of nonspecific granulomata of the intestine quite distinct from tuberculosis. But it was Crohn, in 1932, with a strong background in pathology supplemented by careful extensive clinical observation, who was able to recognize and correlate the clinical and pathologic changes and thereby delineate the entity which is now widely known by his name.

Authors with an aversion to the use of eponyms subsequently proposed a variety of synonyms for this illness. In this original description, Crohn described a disease limited to the terminal ileum, a terminal ileitis. Soon, however, it became apparent that this disease could occur anywhere in the intestinal tract

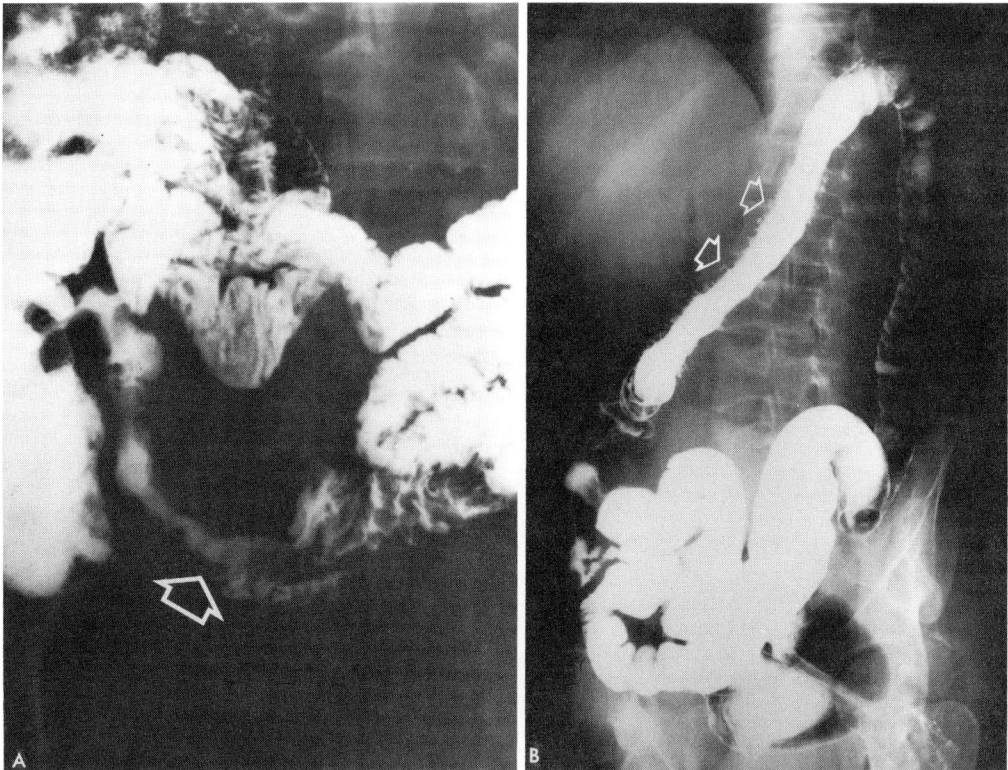

Figure 3. Barium studies showing: *A*, marked disease of terminal ileum (arrow); *B*, "spicules" (arrows) in rigid narrow transverse colon.

from the esophagus to the anus; in fact, a regional enteritis. Since granulomas are frequently found, it is a granulomatous enteritis. The characteristic "skip lesions," in which diseases areas of bowel are separated by segments of normal bowel, were described more than a century ago in 1828 by Abercrombie and indicate that the disease is a segmental enteritis. Wells found the disorder occasionally confined to the colon as a segmental or granulomatous colitis.[16] Since the pathologic process extends through and causes thickening of the bowel wall with scarring, it has been referred to as a transmural or cicatrizing enteritis. In view of these many incomplete designations, perhaps the disorder should more properly be known as

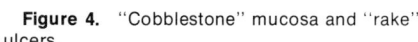

Figure 4. "Cobblestone" mucosa and "rake" ulcers.

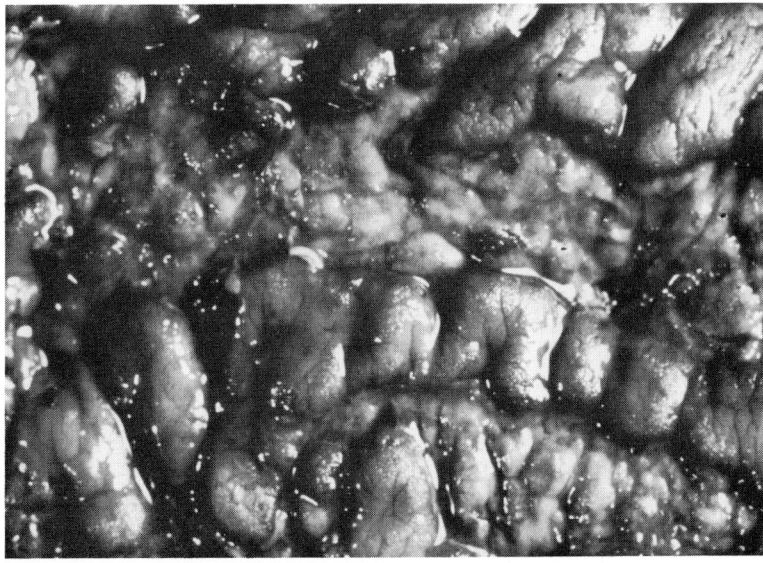

"Crohn's disease"; this denotes a specific clinical and pathologic inflammatory disease of the intestine, albeit one of unknown etiology.

ETIOLOGY

Consideration of the etiology of this disease is hampered by a distressing paucity of factual information from controlled research; a satisfactory animal model is not available for study. Numerous theories have been advanced, but the specific etiology remains unknown.

Tuberculosis, Sarcoidosis, and Other Granulomatous Diseases

Initially Crohn's disease was confused with other chronic inflammatory diseases of the intestine, particularly tuberculosis. Moschcowitz and Wilenski[19] showed 10 years before the classic description by Crohn that the granulomata are noncaseating. While the debate regarding an altered sensitivity to tuberculin is not settled, extensive bacteriologic studies have been singularly unsuccessful in culturing the mycobacterium.[16, 17] In view of the marked similarity of the granulomas, the disease has been considered a variant of sarcoidosis. Longcope and Fryman, however, noted that patients with sarcoid rarely have evidence of intestinal involvement.[23] In contrast, patients with Crohn's disease do not develop systemic manifestations of sarcoidosis. The reaction to the Kvein antigen no longer is considered definitive in differentiating these diseases.[23] It is clear, however, that the noncaseating tubercle-like granuloma is a characteristic but not a pathognomonic feature of Crohn's disease.[20, 25] Similar "sarcoid" granulomatous lesions in the bowel are found with infections, foreign bodies, lymph nodes draining areas of malignancy, and other diseases of unknown etiology. The Schauman bodies found within the giant cells of the sarcoid reaction in 10 per cent of patients with Crohn's disease are also found in sarcoidosis, beryllium disease, and tuberculosis.[17]

Altered Immune Mechanisms

There is considerable evidence that Crohn's disease is associated with immunologic disturbances. At issue is whether these alterations are etiologically important. Is Crohn's disease an immunologic disorder due either to deficient immunologic defenses or to altered reactivity of immune mechanisms? The conflicting reports of defective in vivo and in vitro indices of hypersensitivity describe relatively nonspecific phenomena without convincing evidence that they have a key role in the pathogenesis of the disease.[1, 20] Recent studies indicate no alteration in the immune competence of patients with inflammatory bowel disease,[3] and in patients with Crohn's disease antibody production is not impaired.[4]

A number of pathologic, clinical, and experimental observations, however, suggest that Crohn's disease may result from altered reactivity of immune mechanisms. Histologically, the sarcoid-like noncaseating epithelioid granuloma containing multinucleated Langerhan's giant cells is suggestive of an immunopathologic reaction. Recent detailed studies of ultrastructure of these granuloma form the basis for the hypothesis that episodic passage of exogenous antigens (dietary) from the gut lumen into the bowel tissues stimulates cell-mediated hypersensitivity reactions.[6] Findings of an abnormal secretion of the immunoglobulin system in diseased areas of the bowel suggest that irrespective of the mechanisms responsible for the focal decrease in IgA, the resulting deficiency in the "mucosal block" permits penetration of antigenic material and stimulation of antibody production.[11] The protean nature of the inflammatory response of Crohn's disease could be explained by the diverse responses of the bowel to deep penetration of the wall by a variety of antigens.[13]

In man the alimentary tract participates in hypersensitivity reactions. In Crohn's disease several systemic manifestations of hypersensitivity, such as elevation of gamma globulin, erythema nodosum, uveitis, iritis, eczema, or migratory arthritis, may be encountered.[16] Two of the drugs most widely used to control the disease, corticosteroids and azathioprine, are known to modify immune reactions.

Attempts to distinguish Crohn's disease from ulcerative colitis on an immunologic basis have been unrewarding. The findings in patients of lymphocyte toxicity to colonic epithelium, antibodies against intestinal epithelium, cross-reactive enterobacterial antigens, and circulatory antibodies to bovine albumin suggest only a state of altered immunologic activity and do not indicate a fundamental role in the pathogenesis of either disease.[11, 20, 21]

Thus, while immunologic studies have advanced our understanding of the pathogenesis of Crohn's disease, unfortunately none of the observations solves the basic problem of which comes first, Crohn's disease or a state of altered immunologic activity. This question remains a stimulus for further investigation.

Bacteria and Viruses

For several years after Crohn clearly separated the entity of tuberculosis enteritis from terminal ileal inflammation, granulomatosis, stenosis, and fistulization, an intensive search was undertaken for an infectious cause of the disease. Acute terminal ileitis due to infection with the newly discovered organism, Yersinia enterocolitica (Yersenia pseucotuberculosis), is regarded as a distinct, self-limited disease that does not progress to a chronic course.[16, 21] Frustrated in efforts to identify a causative organism for Crohn's disease, current research has centered largely on the search for an immunologic etiology.[6, 11, 13, 16] Now perhaps the most promising clue to etiology is the observation of Mitchell and Cave that granulomatous changes can be induced in the footpads of CBA mice and in the gastrointestinal tract of rabbits by inoculation of tissue homogenates obtained from patients with Crohn's disease.[5] While these findings have not been confirmed in rats, guinea pigs, or TO strain mice[2] and certainly do not establish that a virus is being transmitted, Aronson notes the isolation of an agent, possibly a small RNA virus, from the tissues of patients with Crohn's disease.[5] The specificity of these findings may be questioned in view of the recent reports of the transmission of granulomas by homogenates obtained from the colon of a patient with ulcerative colitis and from a normal colon interposed into the esophagus for two years.[22] The viral agent also has been isolated from patients with other intestinal disorders.[5]

It is clearly premature, therefore, to conclude that a virus is responsible for Crohn's disease or even that transmission of a granulomatous inflammatory tissue reaction indicates transmission of this disease.

Other Etiologies

Diseases with morphologic features similar to those of Crohn's disease have been identified in cocker spaniel and boxer dogs and in swine.[16, 19, 25] There is some resemblance to Crohn's disease, but also many different features, in Johne's disease (paratuberculosis) of domestic animals, goats, deer, sheep, and cattle caused by an acid-fast mycobacterium.[25] Additional suggestions for etiologic agents have included such widely disparate entities as trauma to the intestine, absorption of toxic substances from food, an inherited metabolic defect, predisposing congenital abnormalities, and an imbalance between sympathetic and parasympathetic nerve activity. It is inevitable that a psychosomatic cause will be suggested for any disease of unknown etiology, but few data support this consideration in Crohn's disease.

EPIDEMIOLOGY

Crohn's is a relatively uncommon disease, with reported average annual incidence rates varying from 0.8 to 3.5 per 100,000 of the population, an overall prevalence rate of 30 to 40 patients per 100,000 and a death rate of approximately 10 per cent.[16, 21, 25] There has been an apparent increased incidence of the disease in recent years, but it is difficult to determine whether this is due to a real increase in numbers or to improved diagnostic and epidemiologic techniques.[12, 24] The disease seems to afflict populations in northwestern Europe and the northeastern United States more often than those in other areas of the globe.[16] Janowitz found a low rate in blacks, American Indians, and Spanish Americans, but a rate in Jews six times that of other distinct patient populations.[21] However, in Sephardic Jews, who constitute approximately half the population of Israel, this rate is not confirmed.[19] While sexes are affected equally, colonic involvement is more frequent in patients over age 50, and this involvement occurs more frequently in females.[24] It is, however, chiefly a disease of youth, with the age-specific incidence rates showing a peak in the third decade.[16, 25] There is a distinct tendency for the disease to occur among families. Ten per cent of patients have blood relatives with either Crohn's disease or ulcerative colitis. Whatever basis of genetic susceptibility there may be, the predisposing factor might be polygenic, with both diseases sharing some of the same genes.[21]

PATHOGENESIS

Unknown Natural History

All considerations of pathogenesis are hampered by poor understanding of the natural history of the chronic disease process and ignorance of etiology. Presumably early changes have been described, but they are rarely seen because the chronic pathologic process does not produce sufficient functional disturbance early in the illness to make patients seek assistance. The late pathologic changes, however, are reasonably well defined.[20]

Obstructed Lymph Drainage

The disease may begin as an inflammation in the mucosa and submucosa of the bowel, where numerous thin-walled lymphatic vessels originate to drain into mesenteric nodes. Alternatively, the granulomatous inflammation may be initiated by minute crypt abscesses. As the submucosal granulomas increase in size, lymphedema develops owing to obstruction to lymph flow. A similar process would develop if, as Warren and Sommers suggest, the initial obstruction to lymph flow originates in a site remote from the gut wall.[12] Hodgkins disease, associated with enlargement and disorganization of mesenteric lymph nodes, may obstruct lymph flow sufficiently to cause changes in the bowel wall similar to those found in Crohn's disease. Richet and Mathes found similar changes in bowel following experimental chronic mesenteric lymphedema.[23] The sequence of events, if this concept is valid, would not differ; only the primary site of obstruction, submucosal or mesenteric, is disputed.

Granulomatous Inflammation

As lymph extravasates into tissues and stagnates due to obstructed lymph drainage, a protein- and lipid-rich edema fluid accumulates. Such protein- and lipid-rich fluid triggers a granulomatous inflammation, which may compound and aggravate the very process that initiated the lymph stagnation. Aggregates of lymphoid cells and edema spread to all layers of the bowel. The lesions become confluent as they spread laterally, and edema of the bowel wall becomes generalized, leading to narrowing of the lumen. The mesentery becomes grossly thickened, and lymph nodes become prominent. The productive inflammation may so impair venous drainage at this stage that the bowel becomes intensely congested and gives a gross appearance of an acute inflammatory reaction (Fig. 2). This is a deceptive impression because on microscopic examination polymorphonuclear cells are usually not prominent.

The inflammatory reaction of Crohn's disease initially consists of diffuse aggregates of lymphoid cells and more circumscribed granulomas. Lymphocytes and plasma cells predominate and the granulomas are composed of epithelioid and multinucleated giant cells. In advanced disease, the pathologic picture is similar to the tuberculoid hypersensitivity reaction that occurs characteristically after the subcutaneous injection of tuberculin. But there is no caseation and the histologic pattern is reminiscent of the granulomatous lesion found with sarcoidosis, although the etiology of these conditions may be quite different. A useful diagnostic feature of Crohn's disease, found in 75 per cent of patients, is the sarcoid-like reaction, a noncaseating granuloma, which can be seen in any layer of the bowel wall and in the regional lymph nodes.[1, 19]

Bowel Adhesions, Fistulae, and Abscess Formation

When the chronic inflammatory process ultimately reaches the peritoneal surface of the bowel, fluid extravasates from the capillaries and lymphatics of the serous membrane. At first this exudate is serous, but in time it becomes more fibrinous. Adhesions of adjacent loops of bowel and organization of the exudate ensue. A mass of contorted bowel bound together by fibrinous adhesions is the end result. In 7 to 21 per cent of patients, fistulae develop as a late complication at sites where the inflammatory process causes adherence of adjacent loops of bowel.[8, 21] Communications also occur with other viscera, particularly the urinary tract.[21] The transmural ulceration of an intramural abscess may initiate the fistula. Surgical intervention is usually responsible for external fistulae.[8, 21] An intraperitoneal abscess may result from an insidious perforation of the bowel. Once formed, the abscess can produce pelvic osteomyelitis or septic hip arthritis, or lead to portal pyemia.[17] Rarely the abscess perforates freely to cause peritonitis.

Ulcers or Fissures, Cobblestone Mucosa

Extension of the inflammatory process in the bowel causes the rugae of the mucosa to become ironed out and the crypts to disappear. The entire mucosal surface becomes tense, and in time it develops a "cobblestone" appearance due to the bulging produced by focal accumulation of lymphedema in the submucosa (Figs. 2 and 4). This appearance is accentuated by extensive longitudinal ulcers with relatively normal intervening mucosa, intersected at intervals by short, transverse ulcers. These long ulcers give the appearance of a rake's having been drawn along the length of the involved segment (rake ulcers) (Fig. 4). The ulcers may be superficial but often extend deeply into the bowel wall to produce fissures (Fig. 5), which appear radiologically as "spicules" and later as deep ulcers when barium fills the bowel lumen (see Fig. 3). The cause of these ulcers is quite unknown, and they frequently have no relation to the most grossly diseased areas of the bowel. Stasis of stercoral material, disturbed peristalsis, and altered perfusion in the diseased gut may contribute to their development.

Fibrosis, Partial Intestinal Obstruction

Both granulomatous inflammation and persisting lymphedema, as found in elephantiasis, lead to fibrosis. It is notable that the extent of fibrosis in Crohn's disease is in excess of the usual reparative fibrosis.[19] When the disease becomes advanced, the granulomas may be replaced completely by dense fibrous tissue and nonspecific inflammatory changes.[1, 8] This may explain why not all resected specimens of bowel exhibit granulomas on microscopic examination. The combination of chronic inflammation and

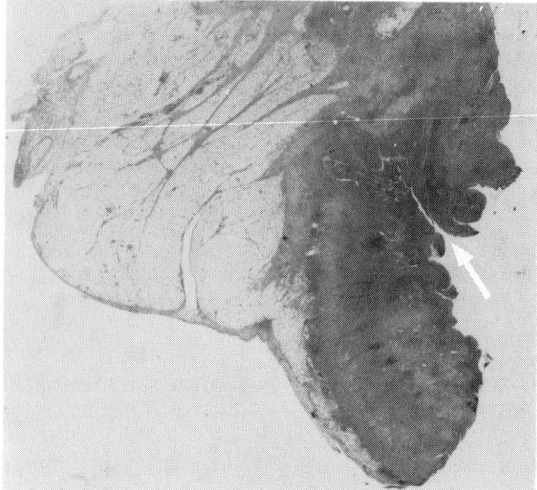

Figure 5. Photomicrograph showing narrow fissure penetrating deep into thickened bowel wall, lymphoid infiltration, and a layer of mesenteric fat adherent to serosal surface of diseased bowel.

fibrosis which involves and thickens all layers of the bowel wall leads to the most serious late pathologic alteration of this illness, stenosis of the intestinal lumen. The consequent partial intestinal obstruction is primarily responsible for the distressing symptoms of this disease.

Stagnant Bowel Contents

When bowel contents are not evacuated completely through a partially obstructed lumen or when a loop of normal bowel is bypassed by an intestinal fistula, bacteria may proliferate in the stagnant bowel (Fig. 6). Similar stagnation occurs in the "blind loop" occasionally created by surgical procedures for Crohn's disease (Figs. 6C and 7B). Serious nutritional alterations result from the multifaceted effect of bacteria on digestion and absorption.

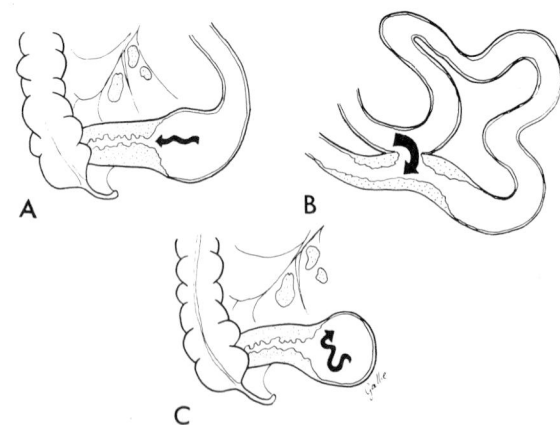

Figure 6. Structural deformities causing the stagnant loop syndrome: (A) partial obstruction; (B) fistula bypassing a loop of bowel; and (C) bowel excluded by surgical bypass. (Drawing by Dr. B. Gallie.)

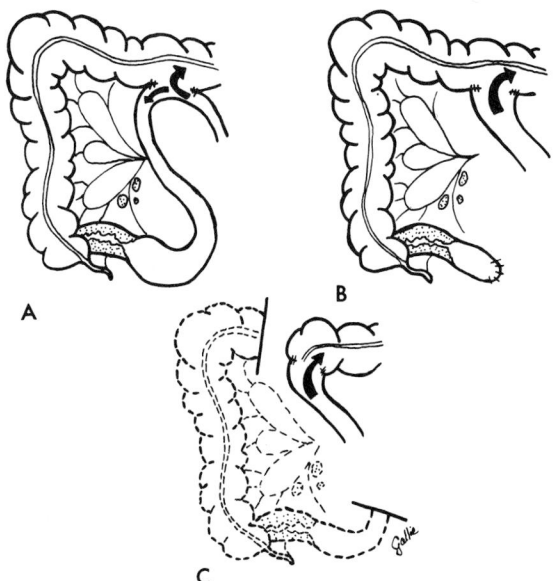

Figure 7. Operations for Crohn's disease: (*A*) bypass of diseased bowel; (*B*) bypass with exclusion of diseased segment; and (*C*) resection of diseased segment. (Drawing by Dr. B. Gallie.)

Healing

Healing in the true sense is never completed in Crohn's disease; residual inflammation is constant. Remission of chronic inflammation can be induced and fibrosis can be hastened by diversion of the fecal stream in order to put the involved bowel at rest. But restoration of bowel continuity quickly reactivates a relatively dormant inflammatory process in the bowel wall.

CLINICAL MANIFESTATIONS

Pain

The most frequent clinical symptom of this disease is intermittent abdominal pain. By the time patients seek medical attention, the segmental diseased areas of the bowel are thickened sufficiently to cause partial obstruction of the lumen. An increase in motility proximal to the site of obstruction is an adaptive physiologic response to promote progress of intestinal contents.[10] If drainage is inadequate, distention develops in the proximal nondiseased bowel. A combination of more vigorous motility and distended bowel stimulates activity in the afferent visceral nervous system, producing a sensation of discomfort or cramping pain along the midline of the abdomen. This sensation is most likely to occur when bowel motility is increased by eating. When the inflammatory process extends through the bowel wall, as it frequently does in the terminal ileum, the sensation of pain becomes localized by involvement of the somatic nervous system in the parietal peritoneum. Pain localized in the right lower quadrant, often indistinguishable from acute appendicitis, is the presenting symptom in over 25 per

cent of patients.[12, 16] Constant pain is usually associated with a tender, palpable abdominal mass and suggests the presence of thickened adherent intestine, an abscess, or a bowel fistula.

Diarrhea

Most patients with Crohn's disease complain of an increased frequency of stools with a marked tendency to watery or unformed stools. Pus, mucus, and gross blood are not usually seen in the stools. Frothy, foul-smelling stools, characteristic of steatorrhea, represent a more advanced stage of illness. The watery diarrhea reflects any one or a combination of the following factors.

Partial Intestinal Obstruction. Episodes of diarrhea frequently occur with partial gastrointestinal obstruction from any cause and at any level of the intestine.[10] Ordinarily the large volume of fluid secreted each day into the intestinal lumen, which greatly exceeds the conventional figure of eight liters, is reabsorbed in the upper small intestine.[10] In the presence of either an increased hydrostatic pressure or increased motility consequent to partial intestinal obstruction, absorption is inhibited but secretion continues unchanged until hydrostatic pressure is markedly increased. The net result is a load of fluid transported into the colon in excess of its capacity for absorption. Even with normal absorptive function, the colon cannot compensate fully for the loss of the absorptive function of the small bowel.[10]

Impaired Absorption. If the inflammatory process in the bowel is extensive or if intestinal fistulae bypass long segments of bowel with normal absorptive capacity, an increased volume of fluid moves into the colon.

Bile Salts. Failure of the diseased terminal ileum to perform its normal function of absorbing bile salts permits their passage into the ascending colon. Forth demonstrated that in this site bile salts inhibit the absorption of water and salt, promoting watery diarrhea.[25] If the loss of bile salts from the enterohepatic circulation is not replaced by hepatic synthesis, the total bile salt pool is depleted and malabsorption of fat ensues, changing watery diarrhea to steatorrhea.[8]

Bacterial Proliferation. In stagnant bowel contents bacterial growth can accentuate diarrhea and produce steatorrhea by deconjugating bile salts to bile acids. Hydroxylation of fatty acids by bacteria forms compounds such as ricinoleic acid, similar in structure to a component of castor oil.

Lactose Intolerance. A disaccharidase deficiency has been reported in Crohn's disease.[25] This deficiency impairs lactose digestion, and the unabsorbed sugars exert a cathartic effect.

Loss of the Right Colon. Most of the 500 to 700 ml. of fluid normally discharged into the colon daily is absorbed in the ascending colon.[10] Without this segment of bowel there is a notable increase in fecal water loss.

Fever

Most patients develop fever during the course of their illness, and it may precede the onset of intestinal manifestations by several years. Crohn and Yarnis emphasized that granulomatous enteritis must always be considered in patients with pyrexia of unknown origin.[21] Fever can reflect the development of intramural or abdominal abscesses or perianal disease, or may be a systemic sign produced by unknown "toxins."

Nutrition

The persistent chronic diarrhea, decreased absorptive capacity of diseased or bypassed small bowel, and the stagnant loop syndrome all contribute to disturbances in nutrition such as weight loss, anemia, hypoproteinemia, and vitamin and mineral deficiency.

Stagnant Loop Syndrome. Many of the nutritional complications of Crohn's disease are aggravated by the intestinal lesions that produce stasis within the lumen of the bowel (see Fig. 6). Bacterial proliferation in stagnant intestinal contents impairs digestion and absorption, resulting in loss of weight, diarrhea with steatorrhea, multiple vitamin deficiencies, and macrocytic anemia. Under the influence of bacteria, bile salts are deconjugated to bile acids with consequent impairment of fat absorption. Once steatorrhea is manifest, fat-soluble vitamins A, D, E, and K become deficient. Change in bacterial flora can inhibit the synthesis by the normal bacterial inhabitants of the bowel of biotin, folic acid, and vitamins B_1, B_2, and K. Bacteria in stagnant bowel consume dietary vitamin B_{12} and may impair its absorption in the terminal ileum, resulting in a megaloblastic anemia.

Weight Loss. Weight loss is characteristic of the acute stage of illness. This is due to fever, anorexia, and inadequate dietary intake, self imposed in fear of the abdominal pain and diarrhea that occur with eating. In our study of fat absorption, all patients exhibited a measurable increase in fecal fat, insufficient, however, to account for the decline in body weight.[9]

Anemia. Anemia is common and may be either microcytic or macrocytic. There may be a toxic depression of bone marrow activity by as yet unidentified mechanisms.[8] In contrast to ulcerative colitis, voluminous bright red rectal bleeding rarely occurs, but there is usually a chronic persistent loss of blood with the diarrheal stool. This course of blood loss is not overt and therefore is not usually compensated for by an oral intake of iron. A macrocytic anemia results from a deficiency of vitamin B_{12} or folic acid or both.[23] Folic acid deficiency can develop in patients who, in an effort to reduce dietary fiber intake, restrict their oral intake of fresh vegetables, rich in folic acid. The chronic inflammatory disease may impose an increased requirement for folic acid,[8] but it is unlikely that folate malabsorption occurs, since the jejunum, believed to be the anatomic site for folate absorpton, is rarely involved in Crohn's disease.

Hypoproteinemia. Hypoproteinemia may not be readily apparent in Crohn's disease, although most patients have an excessive loss of protein through the inflamed bowel.[8, 21] In common with many other gastrointestinal disorders, protein lost into the bowel is digested and rapidly reabsorbed if the loss is in the upper small intestine.[8] The limiting factor for return of the extruded protein to body economy is not the rate of absorption but the rate by which protein can be degraded to amino acids in preparation for absorption. Most patients with Crohn's disease have a protein-losing enteropathy not manifest by analysis of fecal con-

tent unless the loss of protein occurs too distal in the bowel to allow time for reabsorption, or hypermotility induced by partial obstruction removes the protein before it can be digested sufficiently to allow reabsorption to occur. The liver can compensate by increased synthesis of albumin if dietary intake is adequate. When the appetite fails, or when dietary intake is curtailed to minimize abdominal discomfort, or if the extent of inflamed bowel causes malabsorption, a generalized protein deficiency and hypoalbuminemia ensues. Quantitative assessment of increased protein loss into the bowel may be performed by the intravenous injection of a protein or another polymer with a high molecular weight which will not be reabsorbed from the intestinal lumen.[8] Such a substance is polyvinyl pyrrolidine (PVP) labelled with [131]I. Albumin labelled with ^{51}Cr injected intravenously can also be used to indicate protein loss into the bowel, since the chromium label will not be reabsorbed from the bowel.[8]

Vitamin Deficiencies. All fat-soluble vitamins (A, D, E, and K) can become deficient if steatorrhea is a significant feature of Crohn's disease. Bacteria proliferating in stagnant bowel may inhibit the synthesis of vitamins by normal bowel bacteria. Vitamin B_{12} deficiency may result from the stagnant loop syndrome, or it can develop when the terminal ileum is excised.[23]

Mineral Depletion. When one recalls that as potassium is secreted sodium is absorbed in the bowel, it is clear why significant quantities of potassium can be lost in watery stools. Fecal concentration of potassium can be 6 to 15 times that of the extracellular fluid. With severe diarrhea, 10 gm. of potassium may be lost daily; with only 1 to 3 stools a day, as much as 5 to 7 gm. may be lost.[10] Total body potassium deficiency may develop insidiously and undetected by analysis of serum concentration. Calcium may be lost in insoluble soaps with steatorrhea, but the serum concentration is protected by rapid mobilization of this mineral from bone. With severe steatorrhea, loss of vitamin D can be sufficiently great to impair calcium absorption and result in a fall of the concentration of calcium in the serum. If hypoproteinemia develops, the calcium level in the serum will be further reduced by the low level of calcium-binding albumin. Magnesium depletion also occurs with chronic diarrhea if there is a large loss of fat and insoluble magnesium soaps.[8] A deficiency of calcium, magnesium, or potassium contributes to the complaints of malaise and lethargy manifested by patients with Crohn's disease.

Colitis

Within two years after Crohn's original description, it was recognized that the large bowel can be affected by the inflammatory process. The colon may contain the solitary manifestation of the disease,[12, 20] or may be associated with small bowel disease as a direct extension or separated by a segment of normal colon as a "skip lesion" (see Fig. 3). Pathophysiologic alterations in the colon do not differ in any respect from changes observed in the small bowel.[17, 20] Most patients present for examination complaining of diarrhea and abdominal pain with well-established anal ulceration or other forms of anal pathology.[12] In contrast to patients with small bowel enteritis, these patients are more likely to have recognizable rectal bleeding and to have reached an older age at the onset of their disease. Weight loss is common. Recently it has been found that these patients may develop toxic magacolon[21] or have a massive intestinal hemorrhage.[21, 25] Perforation of the bowel into the peritoneal cavity is rare, but at least 100 cases of this complication have been reported and the incidence may be as high as 3 per cent.[25] Sigmoidoscopic examination reveals a completely normal rectal mucosa in 50 per cent of patients; in the other patients sigmoidoscopy reveals scattered ulcers with islands of normal intervening mucosa or "cobblestone" appearance characteristic of Crohn's disease. Frank pus in the lumen is a frequent finding. Biopsy of the anal lesions or of the edge of the ulcerated areas in the rectum often reveals sarcoid foci, especially when the submucosa is included in the biopsy specimen.[17]

Anal Lesions

Anal lesions may herald the onset of the disease by many years.[17] They are almost invariably present when the large bowel is involved but occur much less frequently with disease in the small bowel.[12] The most common lesion, an anal fissure, differs in several ways from the usual anal fissure. It is a broad, shallow ulcer rather than a crack, it may occur anteriorly and laterally as often as posteriorly, and it causes discomfort rather than severe pain. Anal ulcers are indolent and extend from the anal verge both outward and up the anal canal. In advanced disease the ulceration may involve perianal skin, external genitalia, and the groin. It may destroy the anal sphincter and, in females, produce a rectovaginal fistula. Frequently multiple ulcers occur. Fistula in ano, ischiorectal abscess, and a simple fissure are also common anal lesions. The anal pathology may be considered a form of "skip lesion" because the proximal rectal mucosa is normal in 50 per cent of the patients. Biopsy of the anal lesions usually reveals a granulomatous process.[20] These lesions frequently remain active despite local therapy until the diseased segments of more proximal bowel have been resected.[20, 21]

Extraintestinal Manifestations

The usual systemic signs of Crohn's disease are erythema nodosum and arthritis. Two forms of arthritis occur: an ankylosing spondylitis which may be asymptomatic or badly crippling, and a migratory polyarthritis.[25] A negative Rose-Waller test differentiates rheumatoid arthritis. Resection of the inflamed bowel usually causes complete regression of the polyarthritis, but it has no discernible effect on spondylitis. Acute uveitis, iritis, episcleritis, vasculitis, pyoderma gangrenosum, and an increased sensitivity to blood transfusions have all been reported with granulomatous enteritis, suggesting a hypersensitivity reaction.[16, 25]

Peptic ulcer and many hepatobiliary disorders occur with increased frequency unrelated to the duration or severity of the bowel lesion.[16, 23] Recurrent portal bacteremia secondary to loss of the barrier function of the bowel or prolonged marginal nutritional disturbances, particularly in bile metabolism, may be responsible for these lesions. Granulating obliterative arteritis and phlebitis are now recognized as nonspecific alterations that occur in association with both Crohn's disease and ulcerative colitis.[25] Both renal calculi, a complication of longstanding diarrhea, and amyloidosis, which develops in chronic granulomatous disease, may be found in Crohn's disease.[8, 21] When children are affected, growth may be retarded if there is a delay in instituting medical or surgical therapy. Resection of the diseased areas of bowel in some way ameliorates the toxic depression of growth.[25]

Malignancy

The risk of cancer in Crohn's colitis is greater than in the general population.[17, 21, 25] Because malignant lesions of the small bowel are rare, an increase of cancer with Crohn's disease has not been recognized until recently. Most of the reports involve patients with longstanding ileitis with the cancer developing in bypassed loops of ileum or in other areas of diseased bowel.[21]

RADIOLOGIC FEATURES

Barium study of the bowel is vital to the diagnosis of Crohn's disease, as the distinctive radiologic features reflect the gross pathologic alterations of this disease (see Fig. 3).[18] Because it is a low-grade inflammatory process with episodes of acute exacerbation, it is difficult to identify clear-cut patterns indicative of the state of disease. For example, the "string sign," Kantor's classic description of the narrow lumen of the terminal ileum, is usually the result of acute transmural inflammation and edema with spasm but could be the end result of fibrosis leading to stricture.

The diseased bowel is, as a rule, sharply delimited and for descriptive purposes is characterized as either nonstenotic or stenotic. The earliest radiologic changes are blunting, flattening, thickening, and distortion of the mucosa, followed by contour irregularities that are often asymmetrical. Both longitudinal and transverse mucosal ulcers or fissures present as "spicules" in profile and as linear streaks en face. The irregular network of intersecting ulcers combines with the submucosal edema to result in a coarse nodularity or "cobblestone" pattern. The mucosa may become completely denuded, giving the radiologic appearance of a nonpliable, nondistensible, rigid, castlike tube (see Fig. 3). Because there is a manifold increase in wall thickness, the involved loops of small bowel tend to be separated from each other. When stenosis has caused partial intestinal obstruction, stagnation of pus and mucus and inflammatory edema proximal to the obstruction cause a hazy, ill-defined, reticular pattern as barium fills the gut. Bowel proximal to an area of stenosis may dilate to such an extent that it obscures a short stenotic segment. Fistulae can track from any area of the bowel but are usually found in the terminal ileum. Mass lesions extrinsic to bowel can be abscesses with or without demonstrable fistulae but are more often indurated mesentery. A hallmark of the disease is the presence of "skip lesions," with apparently normal intervening bowel that may measure a few inches to several feet in length.

DIFFERENTIAL DIAGNOSIS

The differential diagnosis of Crohn's disease is primarily a radiologic exercise[18] coupled with a keen appreciation of the pathophysiology of the disease. The major pathologic features are transmural inflammation with narrowing of the bowel lumen, asymmetric mucosal involvement, confluent linear ulceration, and deep transverse fissure formation, producing a cobblestone appearance of the mucosa, fistula formation, segmental distribution, and noncaseating epithelioid granulomas.

Functional

"Irritable bowel syndrome" or "spastic colon" presents one of the most common diagnostic problems. Adequate radiologic study of the small and large intestine should delineate Crohn's disease from a functional disorder.

Appendicitis

Acute appendicitis so closely simulates an acute exacerbation of Crohn's disease that as a rule surgery must be performed to establish the proper diagnosis.[12] Almost invariably diarrhea precedes the acute attack of Crohn's disease. If a tender mass is palpable with Crohn's ileitis, it is more likely to be oval rather than round, slightly movable rather than fixed, and unlikely to regress with continued observation. At the time of laparotomy the diagnosis of Crohn's disease may be supported by biopsy of a mesenteric lymph node if resection of the inflammatory lesion is contraindicated.

Partial Intestinal Obstruction

The clinical history, radiologic examination, and rectal biopsy may not distinguish Crohn's disease from other partially obstructing lesions such as tuberculosis, actinomycosis, amoebic granuloma, carcinoma, and lymphoma.[8] The finding at laparotomy of thickened mesentery with growth of mesenteric fat around the circumference of an engorged bowel is almost pathognomonic of Crohn's disease (see Figs. 1 and 2). Biopsy of a lymph node may be confirming evidence.

The systemic signs of Whipple's disease are initially similar to those of Crohn's disease, but it eventually becomes a recognizable clinical entity with a distinctive pathology.

Ileocecal Tuberculosis

Perhaps the disease most likely to mimic Crohn's enteritis is tuberculosis. The strictures in tuberculosis are usually multiple and the ulceration circumferential rather than linear and serpiginous. Granulomas tend to be confluent and may appear in regional nodes, although absent from the bowel wall. Caseation in granulomas or identification of acid-fast bacilli confirm the diagnosis.[20]

Colon Lesions

When Crohn's disease is confined to the colon there are a number of conditions with which it can be confused:

Ischemia of the Colon. Arterial disease or resection of an abdominal aortic aneurysm can result in a localized ischemic stricture in the splenic flexure or descending colon. This condition, previously described as nonspecific colitis, has the characteristic radiologic features of "thumb printing," "saw tooth irregularity" of bowel contour, tubular narrowing and sacculation, and distinctive angiography. Laparotomy and biopsy may be necessary for diagnosis. Marston considers macrophages laden with hemosiderin to be the characteristic histopathologic feature of ischemic stricture.[16]

Diverticular Disease and Carcinoma. Both of these diseases can coexist with Crohn's disease; they may be detected radiologically or only when the diseased colon is removed.

Ulcerative Colitis. A need for this differential rarely arises, since the colon is involved in only half of all patients with Crohn's disease and in only 20 per cent of these is the involvement confined to the colon. Within this group, comprising approximately 10 per cent of all patients with Crohn's disease, the differential diagnosis between Crohn's colitis and ulcerative colitis utilizing the clinical, radiologic, and pathologic criteria so clearly defined by Lockhart, Mummery, and Morson is a relatively straightforward matter for approximately 80 per cent of patients.[16, 17, 19, 20] It is the remaining small and highly select group of patients for whom differentiation of the disease involving the colon may be extraordinarily difficult. Up to 10 per cent of colectomy specimens that are sufficiently atypical to deny differentiation of Crohn's colitis and ulcerative colitis at the time of laparotomy cannot be classified by histologic criteria.[20] On the basis of these findings, Morson now postulates the existence of a variant of colitis in which the classic pathology of Crohn's disease and ulcerative colitis is modified to become common to both.[20]

Ordinarily, differentiation of the two intestinal inflammatory diseases is simple because, in contrast to Crohn's disease, ulcerative colitis is confined to the colon, abdominal pain is rare, there is no palpable abdominal mass, and gross bleeding occurs in most patients.[16, 17, 20, 21] The rectum is uniformly and almost invariably involved, but anal lesions are relatively infrequent. Sigmoidoscopy reveals islands of mucosa (pseudopolyps) surrounded by granular denuded areas.

Barium studies in ulcerative colitis usually reveal disease in continuity extending proximally from the rectum and involving the bowel circumferentially. Spasm and mucosal edema precede minute superficial ulcerations. The spicules characteristic of deep ulceration in Crohn's disease are not seen. Ulcers may escape detection by radiologic methods early in the course of the disease even in view of an abdominal sigmoidoscopic examination. The ileocecal valve and terminal ileum are usually dilated rather than stenosed. "Back-wash ileitis" refers to insignificant mucosal edema associated with total colonic involvement; otherwise the terminal ileum is not altered with ulcerative colitis.

At laparotomy the colon can appear grossly normal, since the basic pathologic change in ulcerative colitis is extensive ulceration of the mucosa and superficial submucosa rather than a transmural inflammation of all bowel layers. In advanced disease the colon becomes markedly shortened due to contraction of muscle rather than to fibrosis.[17] The bowel walls are not thickened and partial obstruction of the lumen, so characteristic of Crohn's disease, does not occur. Spontaneous internal fistulae other than rectovaginal communications are not present.[17] Perhaps the most distinctive lesion for differentiation is the sarcoid-like granuloma which is found in 60 to 70 per cent of patients with Crohn's disease but does not occur with ulcerative colitis.[19, 20] It is important to distinguish these diseases, since total colectomy will cure ulcerative colitis but not Crohn's disease.[16]

THERAPY

Therapy for Crohn's disease is at best symptomatic; no known treatment alters the natural history of the disorder. Patients should be informed regarding the anticipated course of exacerbations and remissions throughout their illness and reassured that with their cooperation significant palliation can be obtained. Little accurate information is available regarding the response to various forms of therapy because Crohn's is an uncommon entity with an unpredictable course, and most of the therapeutic agents used have not been studied in a controlled trial. The overall mortality is about 10 per cent.[21]

Supportive

Although no definitive therapy exists, many supportive measures do have merit. The principal complaints of diarrhea and abdominal pain can be modified by use of analgesics, codeine, belladonna compounds, and diphenoxylate (Lomotil). Rationale for the use of salicylazosulfapyridene (azulfidine) remains uncertain; it is less useful in Crohn's disease than in ulcerative colitis, although it has not received a properly controlled trial. Cholestyramine, by binding the bile salts not absorbed in the terminal ileum, can effectively reduce fecal water loss if the right colon remains intact. Use of cholestyramine should be combined with a low-fat diet to minimize the steatorrhea that results from a decrease in the total body pool of bile salts. Proliferation of bacteria in stagnant bowel contents can be managed successfully by administration of broad-spectrum antibiotics; but unless the abnormal segment of bowel is removed, the problem will recur when antibiotics are discontinued. Therapy for anemia in Crohn's disease may require both iron and vitamin B_{12} or folic acid.

The most important goals of dietary management are to avoid stimulating the bowel and to restore nutritional losses, since malnutrition is common during an exacerbation of the disease. Many dietary fads have been tried with little success. Milk should be withheld in the occasional patient unable to absorb lactose. A low-residue diet (such as Vivonex or W-T Low Residue Food) is valuable only insofar as it contains reduced fiber content, since it is the fiber bulk which may cause bolus colic when the bowel lumen is narrowed by the disease. When steatorrhea is marked, patients should be placed on a low-fat diet with a high caloric intake provided by carbohydrate and protein supplemented by synthetic medium-chain triglycerides which are readily absorbed (Portagen, Flexical), vitamins D and K, and calcium. To avoid colic it is important to introduce the medium-chain triglycerides to the diet slowly. For patients unwilling to eat, or with an acute exacerbation of severe disease or the shortened bowel syndrome, parenteral "hyperalimentation" will improve nitrogen balance for a prolonged period. Increased attention to nutrition has resulted in healing of intestinal fistulae, gain in body weight, and improved general well-being.

Anti-inflammatory and Antimetabolic Agents

Various anti-inflammatory and antimetabolic agents have been tried, since this inflammatory disease may have an immunologic basis.

Steroids. Adrenal corticosteroids will induce a remission in most patients, but all too frequently these drugs are overused in an endeavor to maintain the initial beneficial response; no controlled study attests to their value in long-term therapy. Chronic administration of these compounds may produce a Cushingoid state with the potential hazards of hypokalemia, retention of sodium and water, hypertension, diabetes, osteoporosis, and psychotic behavior. Many physicians, therefore, confine the use of the steroids to patients with recurrent disease in an attempt to avoid surgery. Strictures, fistulae, and abdominal masses, however, do not respond to steroid therapy, and there are no convincing data to indicate the high recurrence rate following surgery can be mitigated by the routine postoperative use of adrenal steroids.[21]

Azathioprine. Introduced some years ago by Brooke and his colleagues, azathioprine has now been evaluated by several controlled trials.[15] The conflicting results of these studies are eloquent testimony to the lack of homogeneity among patients with this disease. The consensus of many studies is that while azathioprine is not a wonder drug, it has a valuable role in the therapy of some patients with Crohn's disease, particularly those who have a serious therapeutic problem not amenable to surgery. The drug may reduce the dose of steroids required to maintain a remission of the disease, but it seems unlikely that its action is secondary to immunosuppression. Given in the dose of 2 mg. per kg. of body weight, hematologic complications are almost unknown. Even with this slightly greater dose than that employed in our original studies,[9] the onset of discernible improvement does not occur until 3 to 9 weeks after the initiation of therapy. Although neither corticosteroids nor azathioprine will reverse fibrotic changes, when surgical intervention becomes necessary, the extent of the procedure may be modified by prior therapy with these agents. Currently, efforts are underway to develop criteria for the selection of patients who benefit from azathioprine therapy.

Surgery

Almost 90 per cent of patients with Crohn's disease will ultimately require an operation. Surgery must be regarded as palliative therapy, because it does not in any demonstrable way alter the course of the underlying disease. However, most of the debilitating complications of the disease are amenable to surgical correction, often with dramatic improvement. The primary indication for surgery is symptomatic disease associated with partial intestinal obstruction. Less common but compelling reasons for surgery are the development of internal or external intestinal fistulae, the stagnant bowel syndrome, anal lesions unresponsive to local therapy, an abdominal mass or abscess, perforation of the bowel, and massive rectal hemorrhage. Various operative procedures have been employed (Fig. 7). A simple bypass procedure (Fig. 7A) is rarely used today except when a more extensive procedure is not warranted. A short-circuiting procedure such as an ileotransverse colostomy (Fig. 7B) with closure of the proximal end of the bypassed loop alleviates the obstruction without extensive resection of the bowel. The patient does not profit by preserving the bypassed segment, and three major complications can result from this operation: (a) the inflammatory process may continue, thereby causing a closed loop obstruction susceptible to perforation; (b) the excluded loop may promote the overgrowth of bacteria, with development of the stagnant loop syndrome; and (c) there is a risk of carcinoma developing in the bypassed bowel.[21] Therefore, most surgeons prefer to resect the involved segments of bowel whenever possible (Fig. 7C). Furthermore, the systemic signs of the disease frequently will not regress unless the bowel is removed. Unless the cecum is also involved with terminal ileitis, it is wiser to restrict resection to the involved ileum, since recurrence is almost always proximal to the diseased area rather than in the ascending colon. Resection is ill-advised, however, when acute terminal ileitis is found during an emergency operation, since the etiology may be other than Crohn's disease. In the rare patient with Crohn's disease of the duodenum a gastroenterostomy and vagotomy are preferable to the more formidable procedure of resecting the duodenum.

Special Surgical Problems

APPENDICITIS. When Crohn's disease is discovered during a laparotomy for suspected appendicitis, most surgeons favor a prophylactic appendectomy unless the appendix is directly involved. The risk of postoperative enterocutaneous fistulae secondary to appendectomy in the presence of Crohn's disease is less than the risk of differentiating right lower quadrant pain.[16] When a fistula does develop, it is more likely to originate from the involved bowel than from the stump of the appendix.

EXTRAINTESTINAL MANIFESTATIONS. Many of the extraintestinal manifestations of Crohn's disease will not subside until the area of diseased bowel is resected. Also, surgery for anal lesions is rarely successful unless the area of diseased bowel is removed.[16]

ILEOSTOMY. Occasionally, the extent of the anal or colon disease necessitates a proctocolectomy and ileostomy. In contrast to ulcerative colitis, where the colon is extensively involved and resection curative, a more conservative segmental resection with preservation of the anus may be indicated in Crohn's colitis.[21] If an ileostomy is required an obstructing serositis at the orifice can be prevented by everting mucosa over the exposed ileum as advocated by Brooke.[16] Constructed in this manner, an ileostomy rarely discharges more than a liter of fluid per day, clearly indicating that the major site for reabsorption of the voluminous gastrointestinal secretions is the proximal small bowel rather than the colon.[10] Should the volume of ileostomy discharge increase, it is more likely due to a newly developed partial obstruction from Crohn's disease in proximal ileum than to "ileostomy dysfunction."[16] Resection of the lesion may be curative without revision of the ileostomy. Enthusiasm for creation of a Kock pouch to reduce ileostomy effluent is tempered by the possibility that recurrence of disease in any portion would require resection of the entire pouch.[21]

Results of Surgery

MORTALITY. Today, the operative mortality is in the range of 1 to 3 per cent, rising to 5 per cent when surgery is performed on debilitated patients on prolonged steroid therapy and to 25 per cent for the rare patients who suffer perforation of the bowel.[12, 16]

COMPLICATIONS. The predominant surgical complications are the results of the short bowel syndrome, the creation of an ileostomy, occasional fluid and electrolyte imbalance, or the complications of any major abdominal procedure.

RECURRENCE. The exceptionally high rate of postoperative recurrence (50 to 80 per cent) reported by Van Patter and his colleagues at the Mayo Clinic almost a quarter of a century ago[21] was interpreted by many as indicating that surgery might promote the spontaneous spread of the disease and should be withheld as long as possible.[21] Owing to the inexorable course of the disease, it has now become apparent that 80 to 90 per cent of all patients eventually will need surgery.[14] Therefore, the view has developed that palliative benefits afforded by surgery with a relatively low operative risk justify an earlier intervention. However, long-term analysis of patients with ileocolitis or colitis, using actuarial methods which take into account the postoperative time factor, indicate the overall recurrence rate of symptomatic disease may be as high as 90 per cent, with the yearly rate for operation or reoperation roughly constant at 15 per cent.[14] Less discouraging results are reported in previous studies utilizing crude recurrence data.[12, 17, 25] However, by failing to correct for differing lengths of patient follow-up time, it is difficult to ascertain the influence on recurrence of many factors such as age, sex, previous operations, the extent or site of disease, extent of resection, or the removal of lymph nodes.[12, 16]

PROGNOSIS. At any given time 70 per cent of all patients with Crohn's disease are living and well with their disease.[12] Not all recurrences necessitate surgery, owing to modern nutrition and drug therapy. It is encouraging to know that the patients who do require further surgery may enjoy complete relief of symptoms and restoration of normal activity for another considerable period.

Thus, while the natural course of the disease is probably not altered, modern palliative medical and surgical therapy has greatly improved both the life expectancy and the quality of life for patients with Crohn's disease.

SELECTED REFERENCES

Drucker, W. R., and Wright, H. K.: Physiology and pathophysiology of gastrointestinal fluids. Current Problems in Surgery, Chicago, Year Book Medical Publisher, 1964.
This monograph presents studies that have contributed to a better understanding of disorders of fluid physiology produced by diseases of the gastrointestinal tract.

Goligher, J. C., de Dombal, F. T., and Burton, I.: Crohn's disease with special reference to surgical management. Progr. Surg., 10:1–23, 1972.
A comprehensive presentation of the surgical therapy for Crohn's disease, including its results, complications, and limitations, with an authoritative evaluation of various surgical procedures.

Kyle, J.: Crohn's Disease. New York, Appleton-Century-Crofts, 1972.
This monograph is a thorough, lucid, well-balanced review of all aspects of Crohn's disease from the historical introduction to the discussion of various features of etiology, therapy, and prognosis for the disease.

Marshak, R. H., and Lindner, A. E.: Radiology of the Small Intestine, 2nd ed. Philadelphia, W. B. Saunders Company, 1976.
This textbook contains many excellent illustrations of x-rays. The authors, from Mount Sinai Hospital in New York, wrote the classic description of the radiologic changes which are fundamental in the clinical diagnosis of Crohn's disease.

Mottett, N. K.: Histopathologic Spectrum of Regional Enteritis and Ulcerative Colitis. Philadelphia, W. B. Saunders Company, 1971.
This book by a pathologist with a long-standing interest in intestinal diseases differentiates between Crohn's disease and ulcerative colitis on the basis of pathophysiologic alterations. Selected aspects of the natural history and clinical management of the disease and many illustrations are included to make the observations of morphology more meaningful. A review of the massive literature on the subject has been condensed to numerous key references.

Price, A. B., and Morson, B. C.: Inflammatory bowel disease. Hum. Pathol., 6:7–29, 1975.
The most up-to-date description of the surgical pathology of Crohn's disease and ulcerative colitis presented clearly and as a sequel to the original differentiaton between these two diseases published in 1960 and 1964.

REFERENCES

1. Blackburn, G., Hadfield, G., and Hunt, A. H.: Regional ileitis. St. Barth. Hosp. Rev., 72:181, 1939.
2. Bolton, P. M., Heatley, R. V., Owen, E., Williams, W. J., and Hughes, L. E.: Aetiology of Crohn's disease. Lancet, 2:951, 1974.
3. Bolton, P. M., James, S. L., Newcombe, R. G., Whitehead, R. H., and Hughes, L. E.: The immune competence of patients with inflammatory bowel disease. Gut, 15:213–219, 1974.
4. Bucknall, R. C., Jones, J. V., and Peacock, D. B.: The immune response to $\phi \times 174$ in man. II. Primary and secondary antibody production in patients with Crohn's disease. Am. J. Dig. Dis., 20:430–436, 1975.
5. Cave, D. R., Mitchell, D. N., and Brooke, B. N.: Experimental animal studies of the etiology and pathogenesis of Crohn's disease. Gastroenterology, 69:618–624, 1975.
6. Cook, M. G., and Turnbull, G. J.: A hypothesis for the pathogenesis of Crohn's disease based on an ultrastructural study. Virchows Arch., 365:327–336, 1975.
7. Crohn, B. B., Ginzburg, L., and Oppenheimer, G. D.: Regional ileitis: A pathologic and clinical entity. J.A.M.A., 99:1323, 1932.
8. Dawson, A. M.: Crohn's disease. *In* Maingot, R.: Abdominal Operations, 5th ed. Volume 2. New York, Appleton-Century-Crofts, 1969, p. 1445.
9. Drucker, W. R., and Jeejeebhoy, K. N.: Azathioprine: An adjunct to surgical therapy of granulomatous enteritis. Ann. Surg., 172:618, 1970.
10. Drucker, W. R., and Wright, H. K.: Physiology and pathophysiology of gastrointestinal fluids. Curr. Probl. Surg., May, 1964.
11. Falchuk, K. R., and Isselbacher, K. J.: Alimentary tract: Circulating antibodies to bovine albumin in ulcerative colitis and Crohn's disease. Gastroenterology, 70:5–8, 1976.
12. Goligher, J. C., de Dombal, F. T., and Burton, I.: Crohn's disease, with special reference to surgical management. Progr. Surg., 10:1–23, 1972.
13. Green, F. H. Y., and Fox, H.: The distribution of mucosal antibodies in the bowel of patients with Crohn's disease. Gut, 16:125–131, 1975.
14. Greenstein, A. J., Sachar, D. B., Pasternack, B. S., and Janowitz, H. D.: Reoperation and recurrence in Crohn's colitis and ileocolitis, N. Engl. J. Med., 293:685–690, 1975.
15. Klein, M., Binder, H. J., Mitchell, M., Aaronson, R., and Spiro, H.: Treatment of Crohn's disease with azathioprine: A controlled evaluation. Gastroenterology, 66:916–922, 1974.
16. Kyle, J.: Crohn's Disease. New York, Appleton-Century-Crofts, 1972.
17. Lennard-Jones, J. E., and Morson, B. C.: Changing concepts in Crohn's disease. Disease-a-Month, Aug., 1969.
18. Marshak, R. H., and Lindner, A. E.: Radiology of the Small Intestine, 2nd ed. Philadelphia, W. B. Saunders Company, 1976.
19. Mottet, N. K.: Histopathologic Spectrum of Regional Enteritis and Ulcerative Colitis. Philadelphia, W. B. Saunders Company, 1971.
20. Price, A. B., and Morson, B. C.: Inflammatory bowel disease. Hum. Pathol., 6:7–29, 1975.
21. Sachar, D. B., and Janowitz, H. D.: Inflammatory bowel disease. Disease-a-Month, July, 1974.
22. Sachar, D. B., Taub, R. N., and Janowitz, H. D.: A transmissible agent in Crohn's disease? New pursuit of an old concept. N. Engl. J. Med., 293:354–355, 1975.
23. Schofield, P. F.: The natural history and treatment of Crohn's disease. Ann. R. Coll. Surg. Engl., 36:258, 1965.
24. Smith, I. S., Young, S., Gillespie, G., O'Connor, J., and Bell, J. R.: Epidemiological aspects of Crohn's disease in Clydesdale 1961–1970. Gut, 16:62–67, 1975.
25. Thayer, W. R.: Crohn's disease (regional enteritis). A look at the last four years. Scand. J. Gastroenterol., (Suppl. 6), 5:165, 1970.

V

INTESTINAL BYPASS PROCEDURES FOR HYPERLIPIDEMIA AND FOR MORBID OBESITY

Henry Buchwald, M.D., Ph.D., Richard B. Moore, M.D., and Richard L. Varco, M.D., Ph.D.

It is the purpose of this chapter to discuss two surgical procedures designed specifically for the management of two medical problems: the partial ileal bypass for hyperlipidemia and the jejunoileal bypass for morbid obesity. These operations are the results of careful assessment of the respective problems, appreciation of the great need for effective therapy, and application of laboratory investigation of basic metabolic mechanisms. Partial ileal bypass and jejunoileal bypass are representative of the field of metabolic surgery – the operative manipulation of normal organs to achieve a biological result for a potential health gain.

Although both procedures are metabolic in intent and consist of a small intestinal bypass, the two operations vary in technical aspects, postoperative course, expected side effects, potential complications, results, and, of course, rationale and purpose. We will review the pertinent aspects of both procedures, as well as the more interesting historical aspects and basic science antecedents.

PARTIAL ILEAL BYPASS

HISTORICAL APPRAISAL

Atherosclerosis is an ancient disease. An autopsy performed by G. Elliot Smith[146] on the mummy of the Pharoah Memephtah, the nemesis of Moses in the Bible, revealed a piece of atherosclerotic aorta which remained after the preparative evisceration. Retrospective and prospective studies of atherosclerotic risk in man over the past 40 years have incriminated certain atherosclerotic risk factors[53, 87]: family history, hyperlipidemia (hypercholesterolemia and hypertriglyceridemia), hypertension, cigarette smoking, and, to a lesser degree, obesity and other independent variables. We will, in this chapter, identify the role of the hyperlipidemias. Cornfield[50] showed that the risk of a definitive atherosclerotic event (e.g., myocardial infarction) is an exponential function of the plasma cholesterol concentration, with these exponents ranging from three to six. Thus, a doubling of the circulating cholesterol content increases the atherosclerotic risk rate from 8- to 64-fold.

Today's generally accepted tenet that the level of circulating cholesterol is a major indicator of atherosclerotic risk has evolved from epidemiologic studies of the past 40 years. In 1934 Rosenthal[128] concluded that

"in no race for which a high cholesterol intake (in the form of eggs, butter and milk) and fat intake are recorded is atherosclerosis absent ... where the neutral fat intake is low, atherosclerosis is not prevalent." After reviewing 787 articles on the subject, Katz et al.[87] concluded that in addition to the dietary neutral fat content and the presence of atherosclerosis, a third component in this computation of correlation is the circulating cholesterol concentration. These retrospective analyses have been confirmed by prospective data from population studies at Framingham,[53] Albany,[56] and Los Angeles.[45]

Since increases in the circulating concentration of cholesterol and/or triglyceride are associated with a greater incidence of atherosclerosis, it is logical to postulate that lowering the circulating cholesterol and/or triglyceride level will reduce atherosclerotic risk. Unfortunately, the converse of a true statement of association is not necessarily true as well. To fulfill the Koch's postulate formulation for risk factor modification, attempts are currently underway in national clinical trials to test the efficacy of prolonged lipid lowering. One of these tests will utilize the partial ileal bypass operation for maximum lipid reduction. It seeks to evaluate realistically the lipid hypothesis of atherogenesis.

Should we set aside our efforts at modifying circulating lipid levels until the benefits of this modification are statistically demonstrable? This must be answered individually. The majority of physicians, however, have adopted the concept that it is prudent to attempt atherosclerotic risk modification by lipid reduction, at this time, while we await the results of the national trials (at least 8 to 10 years in the future), as long as the means utilized for lipid lowering are effective and acceptably safe.

We performed the first human partial ileal bypass operation specifically for cholesterol reduction on May 29, 1963. Currently, other institutions in the United States and in Europe have programs testing this method of cholesterol lowering.[3, 48, 67, 79, 100, 108, 129, 147, 158]* The effectiveness and safety of this operative approach can only be properly judged in comparison to nonoperative management.

After an extensive review of the literature on cholesterol modification by diet, we summarized the 16 most widely referred-to studies.[9, 54, 62, 73, 85, 97, 112, 125, 127,]

---

*Streuter; Morgan and Moore; Personal communications.

[154, 161] These studies examined 2516 patients, nearly evenly divided into 1370 free-living and 1146 confined individuals. This distinction is relevant, since adherence, and possibly response, to a dietary program is often a function of whether food selection, preparation, and availability are institutionalized or occur in the community at large.[22, 101] The range of mean percentage circulating cholesterol level change from the pretreatment baseline varied from +6.0 per cent to −22.0 per cent for the free-living subjects and from −8.1 per cent to −18.4 per cent for the confined subjects.

The average follow-up period was 32.44 months in these 16 studies, or 81,619 patient-months experience. The average circulating cholesterol level reduction in these studies was 12.68 per cent. In those studies with control groups, a universal decrease of about 6 per cent occurred in the plasma cholesterol of the controls. This finding implies that inclusion in a study program of at-risk individuals, especially those having had a myocardial infarction, induces some voluntary life pattern changes, possibly dietary, in all individuals, both those who are given specific therapeutic recommendations and those who are not. If we subtract the control group plasma cholesterol reduction from the gross test group average cholesterol reduction (12.68 per cent −6 per cent), a net cholesterol lowering of 6 to 7 per cent resulted from these dietary programs.

No comparable studies exist from which we can derive an equivalent appraisal of dietary influence on triglyceride reduction. We have also recently reviewed the literature on drugs currently utilized for lipid modification. From our study we conclude that data on long-term triglyceride lowering are sketchy.

The mean reduction of circulating cholesterol levels for the more common drugs utilized in hyperlipidemia management includes 22 per cent for cholestyramine.[7, 14, 20, 44, 49, 63, 72, 74, 77, 80, 84, 91, 98] Cholestyramine is not absorbed from the gut, and no adverse systemic side effects have been reported. Its bile acid binding action can cause constipation when the resin is given in therapeutic amounts. To date, this powdered substance is available only for suspension in a liquid medium.

The average range of the plasma cholesterol response to clofibrate has been reported to be a lowering of 15 to 20 per cent.[8, 64, 78, 82, 84, 85, 93, 99, 115, 126] In the recently terminated Coronary Drug Project, a large and well-controlled drug intervention trial, the mean cholesterol reduction achieved by clofibrate was only 6.5 per cent.[51]

For clofibrate the evidence is quite explicit that escape from effective therapy can occur in the face of adequate drug dosage.[82] Also, lipid level rebound well above the pretreatment baseline after discontinuation of clofibrate management has been documented.[99] The side effects and complications of clofibrate therapy are significant and include liver dysfunction, myositis, coagulation difficulties, cholelithiasis, breast tenderness, and diminished libido.[51, 95, 159] The manufacturer warns that clofibrate can potentiate Coumadin anticoagulants and causes nausea in about 5 per cent of individuals taking this medication.

For nicotinic acid, effective therapeutic dosage yielded, on the average, a 23 per cent plasma cholesterol level reduction in the studies of Berge et al.,[6] Parsons,[118, 119] Heffernan et al.,[78] Nordøy and Gjone,[115] Vikrot et al.,[164] and Charman et al.[47] However, the far larger Coronary Drug Project showed only a 9.9 per cent cholesterol lowering under placebo and controlled test conditions.[51] The mechanisms by which nicotinic acid affects circulating cholesterol levels are not fully understood. The use of nicotinic acid has been limited by its predictable and rather potent side effects. Flushing of the skin occurs initially in nearly all patients started on therapy and persists in 10 to 15 per cent of all individuals who remain on this agent.[60] Other known side effects of nicotinic acid include erythematous rash, pruritis, hyperpigmentation, gastrointestinal disturbances, hyperglycemia, and postural hypotension. More serious reactions are induced hyperuricemia and impairment of liver function, including jaundice.[6, 57, 60, 118, 119]

New drugs are continuously being proposed for the management of the hyperlipidemias. Clinicians should be wary of ready recourse to agents before their actions are well studied and their reactions characterized. Estrogen therapy has now been abandoned; it caused feminization in men[131] and intravascular clotting,[83] and its use was associated with an increased frequency of sudden death.[151] Though the early reports on the use of dextrothyroxine were promising, other effects of this agent have argued against its greater usage. Dextrothyroxine can potentiate angina pectoris and arrhythmias, induce hypermetabolism, and lead to functional hyperthyroidism.[18, 60, 61, 109, 153] Indeed, because of these consequences, the code in the Coronary Drug Project was broken for dextrothyroxine, and it was removed from the protocol.[149, 150]

Some knowledge of the current classification of the hyperlipoproteinemias is essential for all clinicians. The reader is referred to the publications of Fredrickson and his associates.[5, 65] We previously published a brief summary of this classification.[40]

METABOLIC STUDIES AND CHOLESTEROL DYNAMICS

From 1962 to 1964, the first experiments designed to develop the rationale for partial ileal bypass management of the hyperlipidemias were carried out at the University of Minnesota.[24-26, 32-34, 69] Studies in white New Zealand rabbits, in pigs and, by retrospective analysis, in patients who had undergone ileal resections for causes other than carcinoma (e.g., incarcerated hernia) showed that both the cholesterol absorption from the intestinal tract and the whole blood cholesterol concentration were markedly and significantly (statistically) reduced, without concomitant weight loss, following diversion or loss of substantial lengths of bowel. Additional studies demonstrated that, although the entire small intestine is capable of cholesterol absorption, with normal bowel continuity, preferential cholesterol uptake occurs in the distal half of the small bowel. Transit time in the small intestine strongly influences quantitative cholesterol absorption.

The data with respect to absorption sites for bile acids are not as clear as the experimental findings for cholesterol absorption, and often they have been contradictory. We have demonstrated that bypass of the distal third of the small bowel interferes with the enterohepatic bile acid cycle and results in a loss of bile acids in the feces at a rate at least threefold that of normal.[33] Thus, the partial ileal bypass operation alters body cholesterol homeostasis by (1) a direct drain on the body cholesterol pool, and (2) an indirect drain on the cholesterol pool through forced conversion of cholesterol to its metabolic end-product bile acids, in order to maintain the stressed bile acid reservoir (Fig. 1).

An animal model of a reproducible 50 per cent myocardial infarction attack rate has been developed in the rabbit by feeding a high cholesterol content diet for prolonged periods of time.[28] Using this model, it has been demonstrated for both adult[29] and infant[35] rabbits that partial ileal bypass will prevent hypercholesterolemia and atherosclerosis despite consumption of a severely atherogenic (2 per cent cholesterol) diet for four months. The operation in rabbits with established hypercholesterolemia and atherosclerosis returns their whole blood cholesterol values to below normal and reduces cholesterol xanthomata accumulations, even though they remain on the 2 per cent cholesterol diet. In addition, partial ileal bypass will arrest and reverse their atherosclerotic process. The plaque lesions evolve from a proliferative to a scarring or healing phase with quantitatively less cholesterol content. For the infant rabbit, loss of absorption from

the bypassed segment does not interfere with structural growth or normal body weight gain. Finally, adaptive mechanisms do not, in time, lead to increased cholesterol or bile salt absorption.

Investigators have confirmed these findings in other animal species: Scott et al.[140] in the dog and Shepard et al.[141] in the Rhesus monkey. Scott et al. have also shown that partial ileal bypass achieved twice the circulating cholesterol reduction that cholestyramine (1.5 mg./kg. daily) did in the rhesus monkey.[141] With all animals on the same atherogenic regimen, the average serum cholesterol concentration for the non-treated monkeys was 803 mg. per 100 ml., the cholestyramine treated animals 418 mg. per 100 ml., and the partial ileal bypass animals 175 mg. per 100 ml. In addition, a significant difference in the protection afforded against the development of atherosclerotic plaque lesions, by comparison of the aortas of the partial ileal bypass treated monkeys, the cholestyramine treated animals, and the nontreated hypercholesterolemic animals was demonstrated (Fig. 2). In studies with the white Carneau pigeon,[71] birds with naturally occurring atherosclerosis, partial bypass decreased the aortic atherosclerosis involvement, without interfering with avian growth and weight gain. This study also demonstrated atherosclerotic plaque regression following partial ileal bypass.

These laboratory experiments have been complemented by human cholesterol dynamics studies utilizing radioisotope methods.[110, 111] Cholesterol absorption

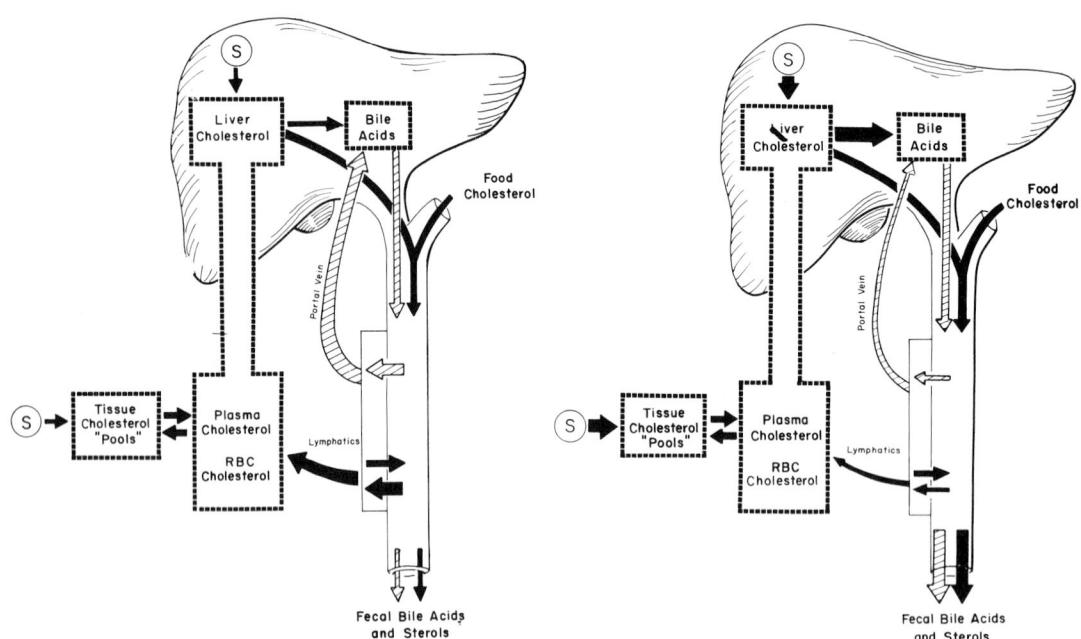

Figure 1. Prior to partial ileal bypass (diagram on the left), the major portion of the exogenous, and bile- and mucosal-secreted, cholesterol is absorbed from the distal small intestine; similarly, the majority of secreted bile acids are reabsorbed by the ileum. After the operation (diagram on the right), there is a marked decrease in intestinal absorption and an increase in fecal excretion of both cholesterol and bile acids. There is also an increase in cholesterol synthesis (S). The net effect is a reduction in the circulating cholesterol concentration and the miscible body cholesterol pool. (Reproduced from Buchwald et al. *In* Sabiston, D. C., Jr., and Spencer, F. C. (Eds.): Gibbon's Surgery of the Chest, 3rd ed. Philadelphia, W. B. Saunders Company, 1976.)

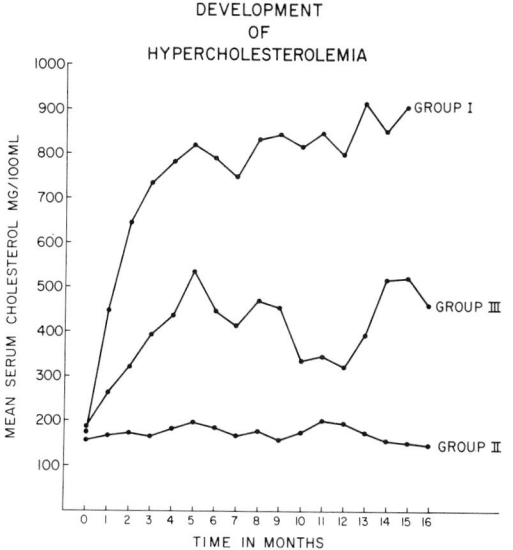

Figure 2. Graph of mean serum cholesterol concentrations for three groups of Rhesus monkeys on the identical atherogenic regimen and no therapy (Group I), cholestyramine therapy (Group III), and following partial ileal bypass (Group II). (From Younger et al.: Comparison of the protective effects of cholestyramine and ileal bypass in Rhesus monkeys on an atherogenic regimen. Surg. Forum, 20:101, 1969.)

is reduced 60 per cent following partial ileal bypass. This state of reduced absorption capacity has been maintained for at least 10 years. Complementary data in human subjects show a 3.8-fold increase in total fecal steroid excretion, with a much greater increase in bile acids (4.9-fold) than in neutral steroids (2.7-fold). This state of increased steroid excretion has also been maintained for years of follow-up. Compensatory cholesterol and bile acid absorptive adaptation by the functioning small intestine apparently does not occur. Thus, the effect of partial ileal bypass on the choles-

terol and the bile acid enterohepatic cycles appears to endure.

Other homeostatic mechanisms in man do respond to the increased loss of cholesterol and bile acids by increasing cholesterol synthesis. Indeed, a 5.7-fold increase in cholesterol synthesis rate has been shown to occur following partial ileal bypass, and this effect, too, has been maintained. Concomitantly, the cholesterol turnover rate has been demonstrated to increase markedly. The total exchangeable cholesterol pool, on the other hand, is reduced by about one third at one year after partial ileal bypass. This lowering is reflected in both the freely miscible cholesterol pool (plasma, red blood cells, liver, intestinal mucosa) and the less freely miscible cholesterol pool (depot fat, muscle, organs). The less freely miscible cholesterol pool includes cholesterol in the arterial walls. Therefore, loss of cholesterol from this pool can reflect a loss of cholesterol from atherosclerotic plaques.

Human cholesterol dynamics are graphically summarized in Figure 3.

OPERATIVE TECHNIQUE (Fig. 4)

Usually, the abdomen is entered through a right lower quadrant transverse incision about 2 cm. below the umbilicus. When an additional procedure (e.g., cholecystectomy) is planned, we prefer a right paramedian or upper transverse abdominal incision. After abdominal exploration, the entire small intestine is measured along the mesenteric border with a piece of calibrated umbilical tape. This intestinal length as measured between the ileocecal valve and the ligament of Treitz, and under general anesthesia, will vary from 400 to 650 cm. The bowel is then transected at a site 200 cm. or one third the length of the small bowel (whichever is longer) from the ileocecal valve.*

_____

*In small children it has seemed wiser to bypass less than the distal 200 cm. of small intestine.

Figure 3. Summary of changes in cholesterol dynamics following partial ileal bypass (NS = neutral steroids; BA = bile acids; P_2 = less freely miscible cholesterol pool). (From Buchwald et al.: Surgical treatment of the hyperlipidemias. Circulation, 49 (Suppl. 1):1, 1974. By permission of the American Heart Association, Inc.)

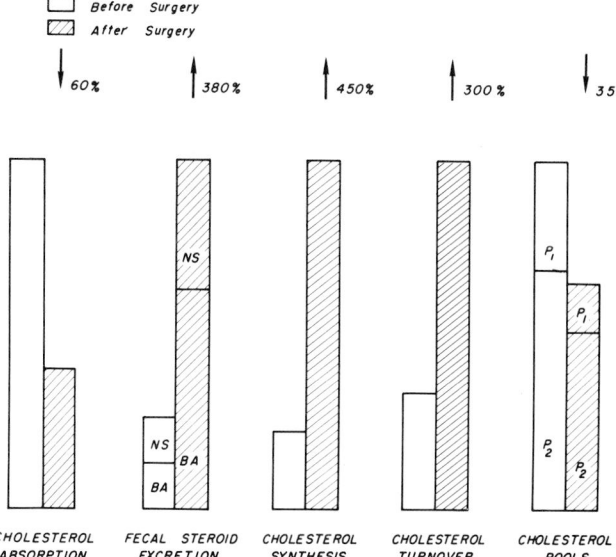

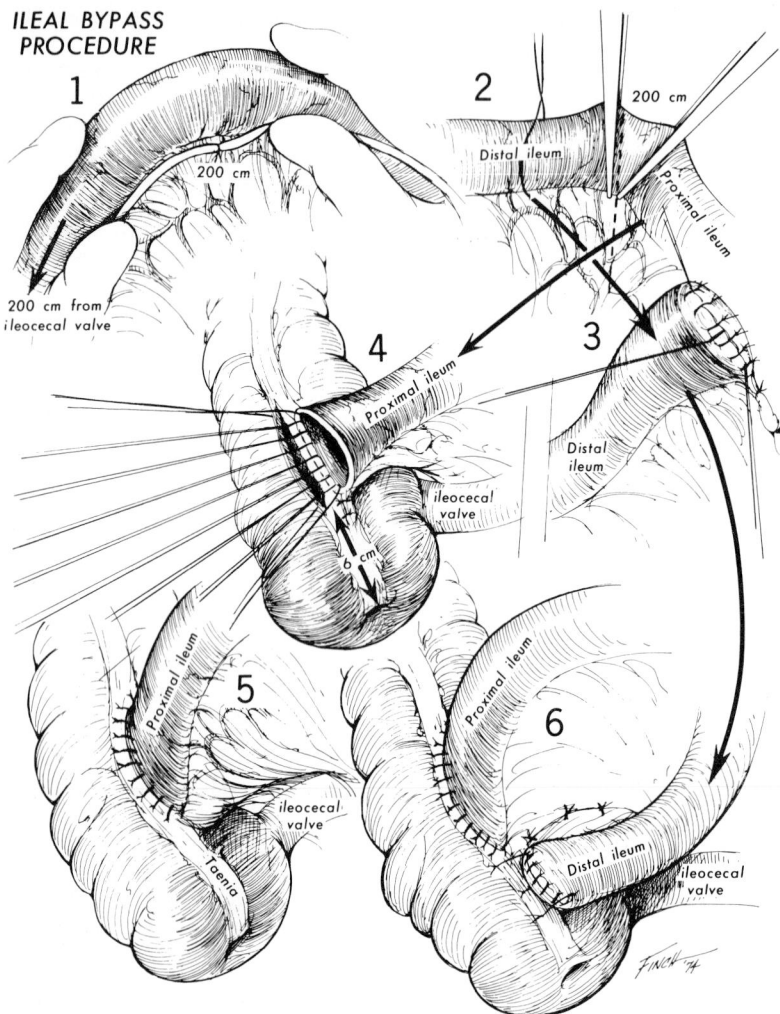

ILEAL BYPASS
PROCEDURE

Figure 4. Operative technique of partial ileal bypass: (1) measurement of the bowel along the mesenteric border; (2) division of bowel between marking sutures; (3) closure of distal end of the division, with the middle and the two corner sutures left uncut; (4) anastomosis of proximal bowel, end-to-side, to the anterior taenia of the cecum; (5) completion of anastomosis; and (6) suturing of closed end of bypassed segment, utilizing the uncut sutures, to the anterior taenia and closure of mesenteric defects. From Buchwald et al. *In* Sabiston, D. C., Jr., and Spencer, F. C. (Eds.): Gibbon's Surgery of the Chest, 3rd ed. Philadelphia, W. B. Saunders Company, 1976.)

The distal end of the divided ileum is closed. The proximal end is anastomosed, end-to-side, to the cecum into the anterior taenia some 6 cm. above the inverted appendiceal stump (the appendix if present is removed). The cecum has been retained to maximize the colonic water-absorbing surface. The anastomosis is distal to the ileocecal valve to minimize ileal absorption of cholesterol and bile acids. The closed end of the bypassed distal bowel is sutured to the anterior taenia of the cecum, between the anastomosis and the appendiceal stump, to prevent intussusception. The small divisional mesenteric defect and the large rotational mesenteric defect are carefully closed to prevent internal herniation. The abdomen is thoroughly irrigated and closed in layers, using nonabsorbable sutures for the fascia. No drains are used. Postoperative, in-hospital convalescence averages about six days.

EFFECT ON PLASMA LIPIDS AND LIPOPROTEINS

Cholesterol Concentration

The plasma cholesterol content is a fraction of the freely miscible cholesterol pool and represents a small

percentage of the total exchangeable pool. It is, nevertheless, indicative of body cholesterol balance. The plasma cholesterol content is also the cholesterol environment of the arteries and the source most accessible to easy measurement.

In our experience, the circulating cholesterol concentration is reduced an average of 41 per cent from the preoperative and postdietary baseline after partial ileal bypass.[38, 39] In combination with type-specific dietary management, a 53 per cent cholesterol level lowering, on the average, has been achieved in type IIA individuals (Fig. 5).[37] Parenthetically, certain type IIA patients are likely to be refractory to solely dietary therapy or to drugs, singly or in combination. Partial ileal bypass, in addition to its effectiveness in the type IIA individual, lowers the cholesterol concentration in all of the hyperlipidemia types. These results have not been compromised by effect escape in our 13 years of experience.

The cholesterol lowering effect of the operation is neither uniform nor is it precisely predictable for each person. The lowering of cholesterol from the preoperative postdietary baseline has varied from 5 to 79 per

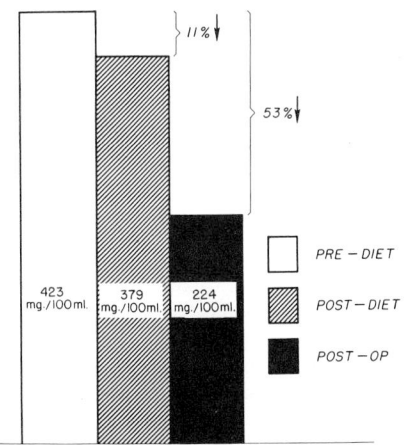

Figure 5. Lowering of circulating cholesterol level following type-specific diet and partial ileal bypass management, in 24 type IIA individuals. (From Buchwald et al.: Surgical treatment of the hyperlipidemias. Circulation, *49* (Suppl. 1):1, 1974. By permission of The American Heart Association, Inc.)

cent. But in the series reported by investigative groups elsewhere in the United States and Europe, the mean cholesterol concentration reduction after dietary therapy has been virtually identical to our finding of 40 per cent.[48, 67, 79, 100, 108, 129, 147, 154, 158] *

To date, the least impressive responders have been the type IIA homozygous young people. Yet, Balfour and Kim[3] reported two homozygous children followed for three years, with sustained cholesterol reductions of 42 and 33 per cent.

Let us examine more closely the cholesterol response as a function of lipoprotein typing carried out prior to operation. We will employ "mixed type" to describe those individuals with electrophoretic staining patterns characteristic for both type II and IV, and for IIX for those imprecisely classifiable because they were operated upon prior to the publication of the Fredrickson classification system. One year postoperatively the plasma cholesterol reductions from the postdietary preoperative baseline were as follows: type IIA – 34.8 per cent, type IIB – 41.3 per cent, type IIX – 32.0 per cent, type III – 47.5 per cent, type IV – 45.6 per cent, and mixed type – 41.1 per cent.

The average cholesterol concentration of middle-aged men in the United States is about 250 mg. per 100 ml.; the average preoperative cholesterol concentration reported for individuals who have undergone partial ileal bypass has been over 330 mg. per 100 ml. Following partial ileal bypass, more than 80 per cent of these subjects have circulating cholesterol levels below 250 mg. per 100 ml., and more than 50 per cent have levels below 200 mg. per 100 ml.

Triglyceride Concentration

Published data on the effect of partial ileal bypass upon triglyceride levels are not as extensive as for cholesterol. Partial ileal bypass, however, has demonstrated effectiveness in lowering triglyceride levels following maximum type-specific dietary therapy.[38, 39] The largest reductions have been achieved in the type IV individuals (those with primary hypertriglyceridemia). For the type IV, the average triglyceride concentration reduction by partial ileal bypass from the postdietary preoperative baseline has been 53 per cent in our experience. A small paradoxical increase in triglyceride levels has been noted in the type IIA patients, those hypercholesterolemic individuals with low or normal preoperative triglyceride concentrations. Nevertheless, despite this increase, the average triglyceride level has remained within the accepted normal range. A satisfactory explanation for this phenomenon in the type IIA patients is currently unavailable, but it may be related to the bile acid loss engendered by the bypass operation. A similar finding has been reported following the use of cholestyramine.[74]

Lipoprotein Concentrations

The information is meager with respect to changes in the circulating lipoprotein concentrations and the synthesis of lipoproteins following partial ileal bypass. Reports have indicated a reduction in circulating low-density lipoproteins following this operation.[100, 155] It will be extremely pertinent to document the effect of this lipid lowering procedure on the protein moiety of the circulating lipoprotein complex. If a secondary effect in carrier globulin synthesis is achieved by a reduction in the transported lipid substances, this finding can influence our fundamental concept of the hyperlipoproteinemias.

IN-HOSPITAL STATISTICS, MORTALITY, AND COMPLICATIONS

We believe that the partial ileal bypass procedure can be performed with an in-hospital, or operative, mortality of about 1 per cent, the presence of co-existing coronary artery disease in many of these patients notwithstanding. Wound infections, pulmonary emboli, or other serious postoperative complications that resulted in prolonging hospitalization beyond a week have occurred in 2 per cent of these patients.[38, 39] Bowel obstruction requiring reoperation, early or late, developed in four of our total of 175 cases.

To date, in the Minnesota series no instance of intussusception of the proximal end of the bypassed segment or obstruction secondary to an internal hernia created by inadequate closure of the rotational mesenteric defect has occurred. These complications seem to be avoidable.

SIDE EFFECTS OF THIS PROCEDURE

Diarrhea is the one annoying side effect experienced by the majority of individuals after partial ileal bypass.[38, 39, 79, 147, 154, 158] * Commonly, it is not persistent. Within a year or so, approximately 90 per cent of patients have less than five bowel movements

---

*Streuter; Morgan and Moore; personal communication.

*Streuter; Miettinen; Brown; personal communications.

daily, while taking no bowel control medications. Patients generally also report an increase in the firmness and consistency of stools with time. Only one patient (out of 175) in our experience has requested operative restoration of bowel continuity because of intractable diarrhea.

It has been stated that the terminal ileum is uniquely capable of absorbing vitamin B_{12} (combination of intrinsic and extrinsic factors) and that only vitamin B_{12} has the distinction of a single site for absorption from the gut.[16] Following partial ileal bypass, vitamin B_{12} absorption is either severely impaired or totally lost.[27] However, after several years, we, as well as others,[116] have found that absorptive adaptation for vitamin B_{12} occurs in about half of these patients. Nevertheless, we believe it prudent to prescribe parenteral vitamin B_{12} supplementation, 1000 micrograms intramuscularly every two months, for all partial ileal bypass patients. We continue this regimen indefinitely.

We have had a longstanding interest in the effect of partial ileal bypass on gastric secretion. We have demonstrated no clinically significant increase in gastric volume or acid content, and no increase in serum gastrin, following partial ileal bypass.[31, 42, 52]

Contrary to the often encountered experience with jejunoileal bypass for obesity is the fact that no change in the serum electrolytes follows partial ileal bypass. Specifically, the serum potassium, calcium, and magnesium values remain within normal limits.[36] We have found no recorded need for electrolyte supplements following partial ileal bypass. Nutrient malabsorption has not been described following partial ileal bypass; no essential long-term weight change occurs.[38]

Arthritic phenomena or an increased rate of nephrolithiasis, as described following jejunoileal bypass, has not been found after partial ileal bypass. Lithogenic bile and the formation of gall stones have not been causatively related to partial ileal bypass in our experience. Finally, and of considerable importance in distinguishing partial ileal bypass from jejunoileal bypass for obesity, hepatic fatty infiltration or decompensation has not occurred following partial ileal bypass, either clinically or experimentally.[134]

CLINICAL OBSERVATIONS
Xanthomata

Various investigators have reported a postoperative decrease in size, or even disappearance, of periorbital xanthelasma, subcutaneous xanthomata (Fig. 6), and tendon xanthomata, especially of the plantar extensor tendons.[30, 38, 39, 79] By analogy, a reduction in size of xanthomatous lesions should indicate that other tissue stores of lipid have been mobilized and excreted from the body. During a period of rapid mobilization, lipid transport may occur at the expense of a reduction in circulating lipid concentrations.

Angina Pectoris

Many individuals afflicted with angina pectoris have testified to a reduction in the frequency of their attacks or the complete disappearance of these symptoms during comparable effort after partial ileal bypass.[38, 67, 147, 158]* A survey[39] of 101 patients, by personal interviews, showed that of the 41 individuals who were angina pectoris negative prior to the partial ileal bypass operation, none developed these symptoms subsequently. Of the 60 preoperative angina positive patients, 7 per cent stated that they were worse, 27 per cent had no change, 23 per cent reported moderate improvement as determined by a reduction in their use of nitroglycerine, 18 per cent stated that they had marked improvement as determined by their reduced use of nitroglycerine and their increased exercise

---

*Streuter, personal communication.

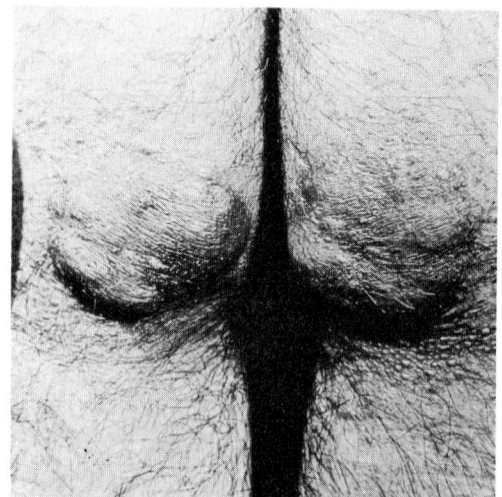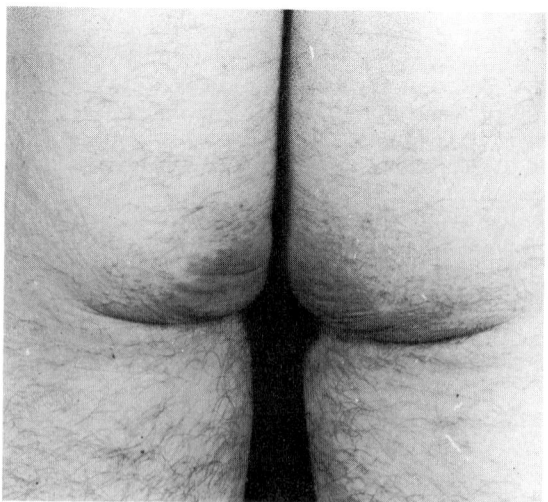

Figure 6. Disappearance of lipid contents from buttock xanthomata one year after partial ileal bypass (left—preoperative, right—postoperative). (Reproduced from Buchwald et al. *In* Sabiston, D. C., Jr., and Spencer, F. C. (Eds.): Gibbon's Surgery of the Chest, 3rd ed. Philadelphia, W. B. Saunders Company, 1976.)

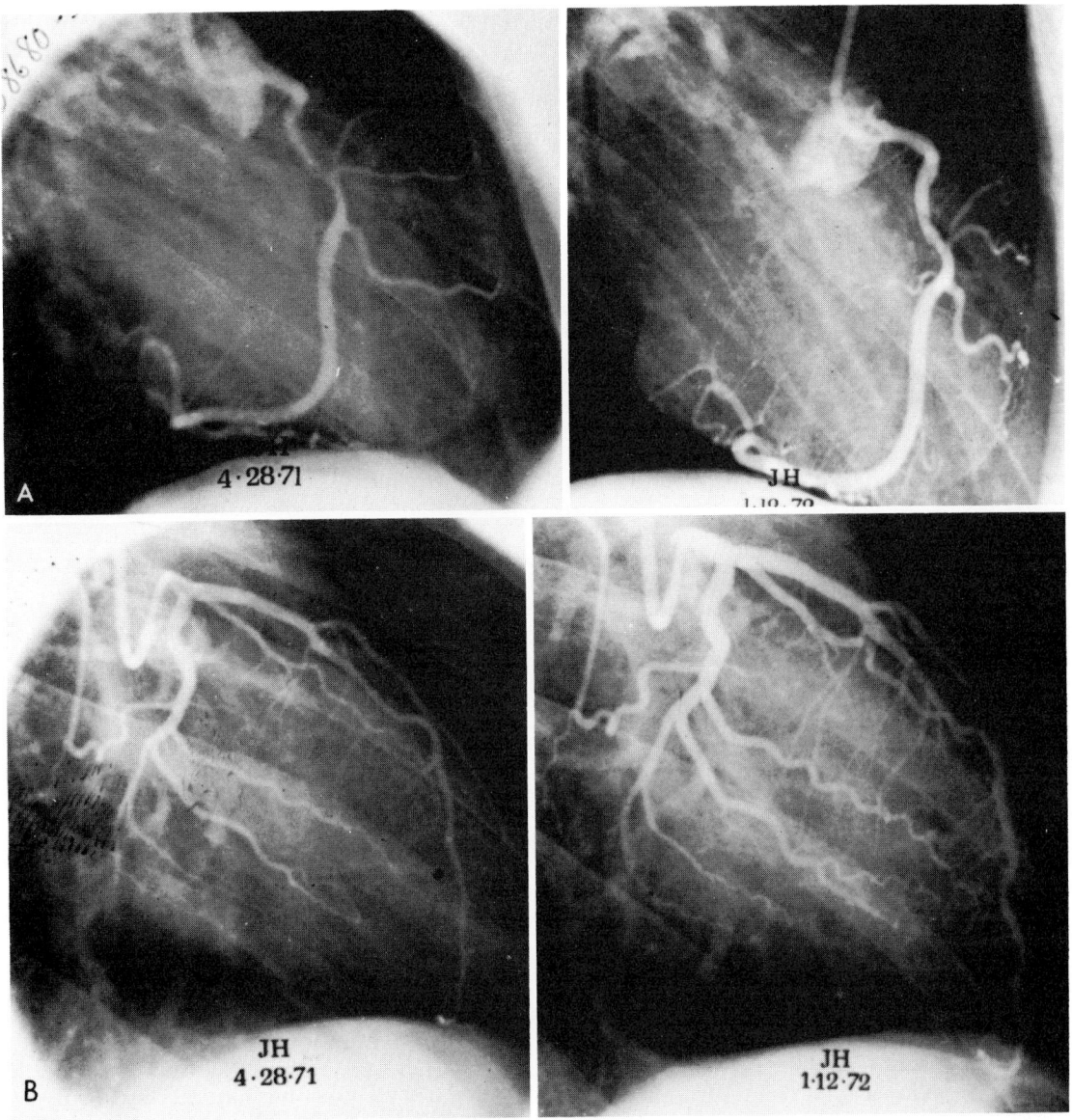

Figure 7. *A*, Right coronary arteriogram showing plaque regression following partial ileal bypass (preoperative x-ray on the left, one year postoperative on the right. *B*, Preoperative (left) and one year postoperative (right) left coronary arteriograms of the same patient shown in *A*. (Reproduced from Buchwald et al. *In* Sabiston, D. C., Jr., and Spencer, F. C. (Eds.): Gibbon's Surgery of the Chest, 3rd ed. Philadelphia, W. B. Saunders Company, 1976.)

capacity, and 25 per cent stated that they had complete remission of angina. Thus, 66 per cent of the patients with angina pectoris present prior to operation experienced improvement postoperatively. In certain of these patients, though not in all, there has been a concomitant improvement in exercise tolerance, free of the development of ischemic ST-T changes, on the time- and grade-controlled treadmill exercise electrocardiogram. Although difficult to quantify, these findings may be indicative of an improvement in circulatory hemodynamics and/or tissue oxygen availability.

In vitro experiments utilizing rabbit blood demonstrate that oxygen extraction from blood with a high cholesterol content is significantly less than from blood with a low cholesterol content.[152] Seemingly, a barrier to oxygen diffusion resides within the red blood cell membrane when its cholesterol content is increased sufficiently owing to hypercholesterolemia. The effect of this diffusion block is to shift the oxygen hemoglobin dissociation curve to the left.

Serial Arteriography

Serial evaluation of coronary atherosclerotic plaque changes by serial arteriography yields data that are inconclusive.[4, 92, 129] A randomized control population for objective statistical comparison has not been available. One study[92] indicates an apparent nonprogression rate of coronary artery disease in 55 per cent of patients followed for up to three years. Apparent coronary arteriographic evidence of plaque regression has been noted in three partial ileal bypass patients at one to two years (Fig. 7).

CONCLUSION

Atherosclerosis is not equivalent to arterial aging. It is a disease and it is the most common major health problem in industrialized countries today.[89] It is endemic in the United States, with approximately 600,000 coronary deaths yearly. Cardiac, cerebral, and peripheral vascular disease in the United States accounts for 53 per cent of the national deaths. This incidence, obviously, exceeds the combined death rate for cancer, accidents, and all other causes.[162] Since only about one of every four myocardial infarctions results in death, and only end-stage peripheral vascular disease results in death, clearly the pain, incapacitation, emotional impact, and economic and career deprivation from atherosclerotic cardiovascular diseases create problems of substantial magnitude for both those who suffer from and those who treat these afflictions. The surgeon's efforts today are primarily directed toward management of the complications of atherosclerosis. These procedures are, at best, palliative. It is time that the surgeon direct his efforts toward the amelioration of the basic disease problem.

Partial ileal bypass is not proposed as a treatment of choice for that segment of the population with hyperlipidemic disease. It may be the treatment of choice for certain patients with hyperlipidemia. The available data clearly show that diet and drug therapy, singly or in combination, rarely achieve the lipid reductions reached by partial ileal bypass. Contrary to the results of drug therapy, the cholesterol lowering effect of partial ileal bypass is lasting. Patients may or may not adhere to diet and may or may not take pills, but once the operation is performed, its therapeutic effects are obligatory.

JEJUNOILEAL BYPASS

HISTORICAL APPRAISAL

"... that bolting-hutch of beastliness, that swollen parcel of dropsies, that huge bombard of sack, that stuffed cloak-bag of guts, that roasted Manningtree ox with the pudding in his belly ..."

—Shakespeare, Henry IV, Act II: Scene IV

The above description of Falstaff fits an unfortunately large number of Americans. We have the impression that our affluent society is an overweight society. Yet we have no national statistics on the incidence of morbid obesity.

Scott et al.[139] have defined the morbidly obese individual as "one who has reached two to three or more times his ideal weight and who has maintained this level for five years or more despite efforts by himself, his family and his physician to bring about effective and sustained reduction of weight to acceptable medical standards." Others have defined morbid obesity simply as greater than 100 pounds over insurance table "ideal weight."[19, 121]

The treatment of choice for obesity is, of course, a dietary program of caloric restriction. When caloric intake is less than energy expenditure, depot fat (potential energy) is mobilized and utilized as kinetic energy in body processes. Unfortunately, most morbidly obese individuals will not maintain a dietary program of caloric restrictions or will intermittently diet successfully and then rapidly regain their weight. Morbidly obese patients hospitalized and under close medical supervision have lost up to 100 pounds over the course of a year, only to regain that weight rapidly upon returning to a free-living environment.[59, 120] Equally unsuccessful has been the management of these individuals by psychotherapy. Hypnosis and group therapy, including the private commercial organizations that specialize in group enforcement and shaming the dietary offender, also fail frequently. Stunkard and McLaren-Hume[156] reviewed the literature for the failure rate for nonsurgical management of the grossly obese and found that only 25 per cent of the individuals in their cumulative series lost as much as 20 pounds and only 5 per cent lost 40 pounds. In their own clinic, out of 100 consecutive obese patients, only 12 per cent lost 20 pounds and only one lost 40 pounds. Furthermore, 28 per cent never returned after the first visit.

Several drugs, notably thyroid preparations and amphetamines, have been advocated in the management of obesity. The popularity of these preparations has recently diminished, and few physicians today prescribe them. Indeed, the Federal Food and Drug Administration has banned the use of amphetamines for weight reduction purposes.

The impetus for a surgical approach to the treatment of obesity evolved from the general failure of available methods of nonsurgical therapy. Bypass of a sufficient length of small intestine creates an absorptive caloric deficit. This forces conversion of body depot fat to energy with a concomitant weight loss. This process continues until caloric absorption reaches equilibrium with the energy requirements of the smaller body mass. Intestinal absorptive compensation also contributes to weight adjustment, which occurs between one and three years after jejunoileal bypass.

In 1954, Kremen,[94] in a discussion of certain nutritional aspects of the small intestine, described a patient upon whom he had performed an end-to-end jejunoileostomy for the reduction of body weight. Payne in 1956 initiated the first clinical program of massive small intestinal bypass for the management of morbid obesity.[120] He sought rapid and marked weight reduction through bypass of nearly the entire small intestine, the right colon, and half of the transverse colon. Bowel continuity was restored by end-to-side anastomosis of the proximal 15 inches of jejunum to the midtransverse colon. He presented his initial results in 11 patients in 1963.[120] Weight loss from this procedure was dramatic, but the morbidity (uncontrolled diarrhea, electrolyte imbalance, and liver failure) was prohibitive, and one death was reported. Payne originally conceived a need for a second operation to restore additional bowel length when ideal weight was obtained.

An operation similar to the original Payne procedure was adopted at the Cleveland Clinic,[102] but it rapidly gave way to utilization of an end-to-side jejunocecostomy.[103] Sherman and associates,[143] as well as Payne,[121] then proposed restoration of bowel continuity proximal to the ileocecal valve by an end-to-side jejunoileostomy. The aim of these somewhat less radical bypass operations was to achieve an eventual balance between caloric intake and body caloric needs, with elimination of a second operation.

With greater experience, plus the successful anticipatory management of electrolyte abnormalities, diarrhea, and operative complications, the general results improved. Slowly, massive jejunoileal bypass for morbid obesity found a place in the management of these unfortunate individuals. The end-to-side jejunoileostomy became the most commonly used procedure. This is the so-called "14+4" operation, with the proximal 14 inches of jejunum anastomosed end to side to the terminal ileum four inches proximal to the ileocecal valve. This is the procedure that continues to be used by Payne and DeWind[121] with satisfactory results.

Yet several modifications of the "14+4" jejunoileostomy have been advanced by other investigators. These modifications consist primarily of conversion of the end-to-side anastomosis to an obligatory end-to-end restoration of bowel continuity.[41] Such a procedure requires a second anastomosis of the distal end of the bypassed segment to a portion of the functioning gastrointestinal tract. We have shown that the reflux demonstrable by barium swallow after an end-to-side anastomosis would permit additional caloric absorption and interfere with the primary purpose of the operative intervention. All end-to-end procedures preserve the ileocecal valve as a means of diminishing postoperative diarrhea. We drain the bypassed segment, end to side, into the cecum near the ileocecal valve. Salmon[132, 133] drains the bypassed segment into the transverse colon, and Scott[136] originally preferred the sigmoid colon. The relative lengths of jejunum and ileum in functional continuity vary in the hands of different investigators. No available data indicate the preferential ratio for jejunum to ileum.

METABOLIC BASIS FOR MORBID OBESITY

Obesity results when caloric intake exceeds expenditure. The excess is stored as fat. Thus, obesity is the result of overeating, and massive obesity is the product of food "addiction." There remains the essential question: Why does the obese individual overeat?

It has been postulated that obesity in infancy or early childhood results in the formation of an excess number of fat cells and that although these lipocytes can vary their fat content during life, they do not diminish in number.[12, 13, 21] Obese individuals may have inefficient caloric utilization or, possibly, carry a "humoral" factor that triggers overeating. The theory has been advocated that, without chemical evidence of hypothyroidism, the morbidly obese have impaired thyroid utilization at the cellular level.[124] In discussing possible causative endocrine mechanisms, we exclude from consideration known disease states that have obesity as a characteristic, e.g., Cushing's syndrome and myxedema.

The obese individual has been subjected to extensive metabolic evaluation to determine the etiology of this pathologic state and/or the metabolic consequences of morbid obesity. It has been shown that the obese, in a fed and steady-weight state, have increased fat utilization, a relative decrease in fat formation, lowered glucose utilization, and increased glucose formation. This is the precise metabolic situation found in the lean individual during a state of starvation.[17] It would appear that the obese person is primed for starvation while in the fed state. This may have survival value to a person subjected to famine or cold but, in the current environment confronting most obese individuals, such characteristics are more of a liability than a benefit.

Bjorntorp,[11] in a review article, presents evidence for decreased physical activity in the obese resulting in decreased muscle insulin sensitivity. This, in turn, leads to increased insulin release, secondary hypoglycemia, and stimulation of the central nervous system trigger for eating. Physical activity analyses have shown that the obese sleep more and exercise less than the nonobese.[15] An obvious area for metabolic exploration has been intestinal absorption; no absorptive capacity abnormality has been found in the obese.[10] Furthermore, excessive intestinal length in the obese has not been documented.[75]

Genetic and induced hypothalamic, other central nervous system, and endocrine obesity models have been developed in mice, rats, dogs, monkeys, pigs, fowl, and cattle. These are reviewed by Mayer.[106, 107] No systematized study of jejunoileal bypass in chronic obesity preparations has been published.

It has been demonstrated that obesity runs in families. The correlation between identical twins for weight has been found to be extremely high (r = 0.973).[113] Withers[167] found a significant positive correlation between the weights of natural children and their parents, whereas there was no correlation between the weights of adopted children and their parents.

Certainly, psychological or emotional factors must be considered in a discussion of the etiology of obesity. Nisbet[114] concludes that there are distinct differences in the types of cues which govern the eating behavior of obese and nonobese humans and that the peculiarities observed in eating behavior of the obese human are displayed by several animal obesity preparations. A psychiatric appraisal of morbidly obese individuals at our hospital has led to the conclusion that these persons equate food with love and that their emotional attachment is to the act of eating and the consumption of large amounts of food, but not to the product of this activity. Indeed, their own body image is anything but complimentary.

COMPLICATIONS OF MORBID OBESITY

The concept of obesity as a causative agent for certain related disease states was proposed as early as 1819 by Wadd:[165] "Corpulancy is not only a disease itself but an harbinger of others." Because of these associated conditions, the mortality of obesity rises geometrically as a function of the per cent of increase in weight over the "ideal." It has also been documented that the increased risk of death for the obese individual diminishes as the weight approaches the "ideal"; indeed, the obese patient who reduces to his "ideal" weight before the complications of obesity have supervened becomes a standard insurance risk.[58]

The complications of obesity affect nearly every organ system and are both structural (bulk-related) and functional. In the cardiovascular system there is a statistically positive correlation of obesity with the complications of atherosclerotic cardiovascular disease, e.g., myocardial infarctions and strokes.[2, 58] Due to the requirement for a greater cardiac output, at a cost of an increased heart rate and/or stroke volume, the obese individual with atherosclerotic or hypertensive heart disease has a greater risk of developing congestive heart failure.[2, 46, 90] In addition, obesity per se results in cardiac hypertrophy, predominantly left ventricular hypertrophy, and can be responsible for heart failure without evidence of other heart disease.[1] Furthermore, the incidence of hypertension is higher in an obese population than in a nonobese.[142, 160] Venous insufficiency and thrombophlebitis are more prevalent in the obese. The obese individual has, as a rule, impairment of ventilation parameters with a diminished P_{O_2}.[55, 104] Chest wall bulk can be responsible for alveolar hypoventilation, resulting in drowsiness and episodic involuntary sleep—the pickwickian syndrome.[43, 157]

Chronic cholelithiasis and cholecystitis have been observed in 30 to 40 per cent of morbidly obese individuals.[105] It has been suggested that obesity may be correlated with carcinoma of the stomach.[169] Altered liver function has been described in the presence of marked obesity,[130, 163, 170] and many of the morbidly obese have some degree of fatty metamorphosis of the liver.[96, 120, 130, 132, 163, 170] The incidence of cirrhosis of the liver has been reported to be two and one half times greater in the obese male and one and one half times greater in the obese female.[170] Diabetes mellitus of adult onset is three to four times more prevalent in the obese.[58, 81] Orthopedic problems are more frequent in the markedly obese and include osteoarthritis of the lumbar spine, herniated intervertebral discs, and osteoarthritic changes in the knees.[88] The obese female is often subject to infertility problems,[70] and birth complications are higher.[66, 122] There is an increased incidence of carcinoma of the endometrium in association with excess body weight.[123] Intertriginous dermatitis and stasis dermatitis are two of the cutaneous problems encountered in obese individuals.[68]

Obesity is not only a medical problem. It is also a social, psychological, and economic problem. Though many people in western society are obese, obesity is not considered a desirable social attribute. The obese can experience great difficulty in interpersonal relationships, courtship, marriage, employment, and community acceptance. Obese individuals tend to isolate themselves and withdraw from exposure to ridicule. They become increasingly less active, and they avoid sports and physical activities. In addition, the obese have great difficulty in finding employment and often are sustained by welfare. Employers may believe that they are unable to cope with a job, unsightly to customers, and, most important, too expensive to insure.

PATIENT SELECTION CRITERIA

Criteria for selecting jejunoileal bypass patients vary from surgeon to surgeon. The following are our patient selection criteria: (1) greater than 100 pounds over insurance table "ideal weight" for age and sex; (2) a minimum five-year effort at weight reduction by dietary means; (3) no known causative correctable metabolic or endocrine dysfunction; (4) willingness to undergo the procedure after having the postoperative side effects, potential complications, and chances of success fully explained; (5) mental capacity and emotional stability to tolerate the operation and postoperative sequelae; and (6) no history of alcoholism and patient commitment to avoid alcoholic beverages for a minimum of three years after the operation (see section on hepatic complications).

SURGICAL TECHNIQUE (Fig. 8)

There are a number of articles in the medical literature explaining the different techniques for end-to-end or end-to-side jejunoileal bypass. We will discuss only our current operative approach, not because it is necessarily the best, but because we are most familiar with it and because our data are based on its utilization.

We enter the abdomen through a transverse incision made 4 cm. above the umbilicus, dividing both recti but not the oblique muscles. Following abdominal exploration and positioning of the nasogastric tube, a needle biopsy of the liver is obtained. If cholelithiasis is present, the gallbladder is removed. If the appendix is present, it is removed. The entire small intestinal length is carefully measured along the mesenteric border, using a marked umbilical tape (in our experience of more than 700 jejunoileal and partial ileal bypass operations, the small intestinal length has generally measured between 400 and 650 cm.). At a point 40 cm. from the ligament of Treitz, the bowel is divided between marking sutures. The distal end of the divided bowel (proximal end of the bypassed segment) is closed in two layers. The two corner sutures and the middle suture of the outer row are left long. The mesentery and bowel just proximal to the ileocecal valve are divided, leaving a distal segment of no more than 4 cm. of terminal ileum. A two-layer open anastomosis is made between the proximal jejunum and terminal ileum with interrupted nonabsorbable 5-0 sutures for the outer row and an inner running layer of 4-0 absorbable material. The distal end of the bypassed bowel is then united to the cecum by end-to-

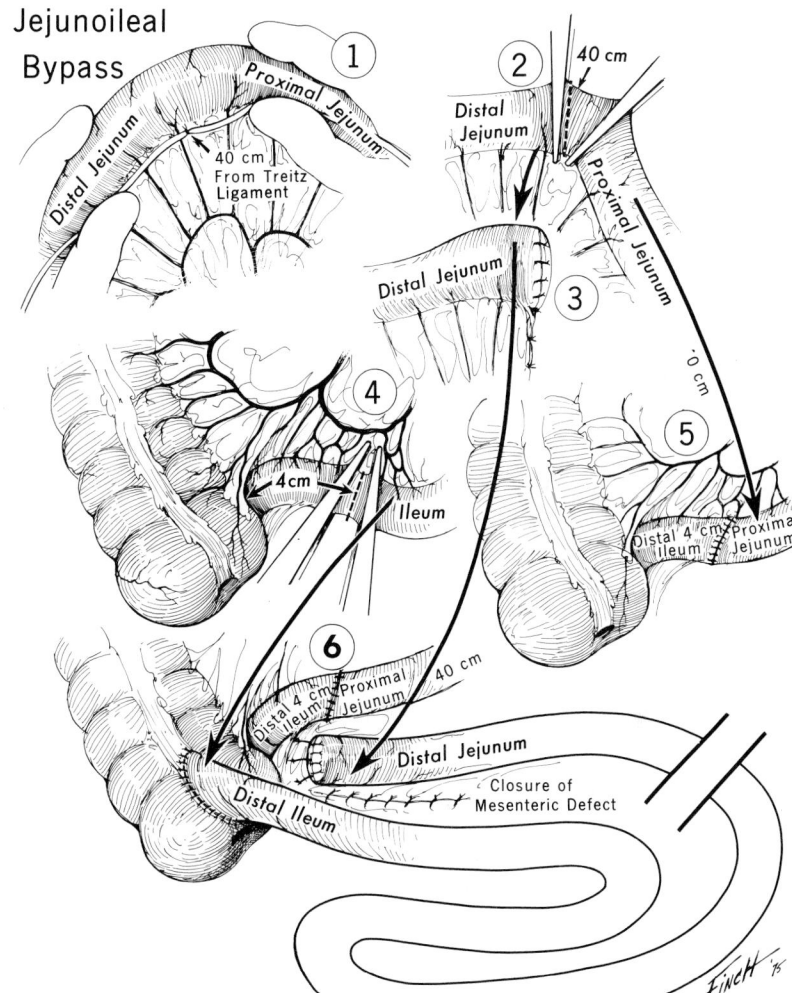

Jejunoileal Bypass

Figure 8. Operative technique of jejuno-ileal bypass: (1) measurement of the bowel along the mesenteric border to determine the point of proximal division, 40 cm. from the ligament of Treitz; (2) division of bowel between marking sutures; (3) closure of distal end of the division, with the middle and the two corner sutures left uncut; (4) distal division of the bowel 4 cm. from the ileocecal valve; (5) end-to-end anastomosis of the proximal 40 cm. of jejunum to the distal 4 cm. of ileum; and (6) completion of the procedure with suturing of the closed end of the by-passed segment, utilizing the uncut sutures, to the adjacent mesentery and closure of all mesenteric defects.

side anastomosis utilizing a two-layer open technique. Next, the small and large mesenteric defects secondary to bowel division and the wide rotational mesenteric defect are closed with interrupted 5-0 permanent sutures. The three sutures previously retained at the closure of the proximal end of the bypass intestine are attached to an adjacent viscus or mesentery to prevent future intussusception.

Surgeons and scrub nurses change gloves and gowns prior to closure, and a separate set of instruments is utilized for the closure. We irrigate the abdominal cavity with both saline and 0.25 per cent neomycin solution and close in the following manner: The posterior and the anterior rectus fasciae are closed separately with interrupted sutures of 0 nonabsorbable material. A large hemovac drain is placed along the anterior fascial closure and led out through a separate stab wound. The deeper half of the panniculus is closed with interrupted absorbable sutures (a depth closure of 5 to 10 cm.). A second hemovac drain is placed at the midpanniculus, generally coinciding with Scarpa's fascia, and it is brought out through a

separate stab wound at the other corner. The rest of the fat is closed (another 5 to 10 cm.) with interrupted absorbable monofilament material and fine skin approximation is carried out with a nonabsorbable monofilament material.

IN-HOSPITAL STATISTICS AND MORTALITY

There are few, if any, detailed appraisals in the literature of the immediate postoperative mortality and morbidity following jejunoileal bypass in a large patient series. Many reports give anecdotal accounts of difficulties or present an unusually high incidence of complications. In 1973, we cited a consecutive series of 94 patients[135] and our current postoperative data, in nearly 600 patients, remain essentially unchanged.

The average postoperative hospitalization has been 10.5 days, though the majority of patients were discharged on the sixth or seventh postoperative day. Serolipid wound drainage longer than seven days, delaying removal of the hemovac drains, has occurred in

11 per cent of our patients. The wound infection rate has been only 2 per cent. We have had a single case of wound dehiscense. Thrombophlebitis has been documented in less than 4 per cent of our patients, and pulmonary embolization has occurred in 2 per cent. Less than 1 per cent have developed pneumonitis.

With respect to late operative complications, we have never seen a case of intussusception of the closed end of the bypassed loop nor a bowel obstruction secondary to an internal hernia through the rotational mesenteric defect (carefully closed at operation). As with partial ileal bypass surgery, these problems are avoidable.

The in-hospital mortality has been relatively low at most institutions. Payne and DeWind[121] in a series of 80 patients, which included ten jejunocolic bypass patients, reported two in-hospital deaths following myocardial infarction. Salmon[132] reported five deaths in a series of 120 patients; four died as a result of wound complications and the fifth succumbed to a pulmonary embolus. In our current series, we have had four deaths within 30 days of operation, an incidence of less than 1 per cent. One patient ruptured an intracranial aneurysm; another died of the complications of a perforated stress ulcer of the descending colon; the third of urinary retention, sepsis, shock, and bowel infarction; and the fourth of sudden death, unexplained at autopsy.

LONG-TERM SIDE EFFECTS AND METABOLIC CHANGES

The predictable long-term side effects of jejunoileal bypass consist of diarrhea, electrolyte imbalance and, as a rule, impaired vitamin B_{12} absorption. In nearly all patients following jejunoileal bypass these manifestations will, to a certain degree, be present. It is preferable to anticipate these events and to initiate prophylactic management prior to discharge from the hospital, rather than to wait for patient distress or overt clinical symptoms. Payne,[120, 121] Weismann,[166] Salmon,[132] and we have noted a downward drift in serum calcium and potassium levels in nearly all post-jejunoileal bypass patients; therefore, routine oral supplementation therapy is recommended. Approximately 90 per cent of our patients can be taken off electrolyte supplements between six months and one year after operation.

Following jejunoileal bypass, serum protein levels will fall, in our experience and in that of others.[120, 121, 137, 138, 144, 166] This fall occurs primarily in the albumin fraction, at times accompanied by a rise in the serum gamma globulin. We stress the necessity for a high-protein diet postoperatively and, on occasion, we will prescribe commercially available protein supplements. In addition to at least a transitory postoperative malabsorption of proteins, there is impaired carbohydrate absorption and a significant and lasting inability to absorb the fat load present in the average American diet.

Diarrhea is the universally most annoying problem to the patient. Salmon defines diarrhea as three or more liquid stools per day or the need to maintain the use of diarrhea-controllong agents. He[132] reported that 39 per cent of his postoperative patients had diarrhea at six months, 25 per cent after one year, and 13 per cent after two years. Payne[121] does not cite a specific incidence for diarrhea but states that "gastrointestinal problems were merely an annoyance and easily controlled by diet or medications." We agree with this statement for the majority of patients; at one year the average daily number of bowel movements was 4 (range 1 to 10) in our patient population.[76] What does one do, however, with those few individuals with persistent diarrhea or those with episodic diarrhea? Dietary advice is likely to be ignored or heeded transiently; nevertheless, we find nearly all patients can be regulated if they follow a diet of only cottage cheese, cheddar cheese, skim milk, peanut butter, and bananas. If this program does not control an episode of diarrhea, we tend to employ judicious doses of paregoric. For anticipatory bowel control we use agents to retard bowel motility, add bulk, and saponify fatty acids. If the diarrhea is intolerable to the patient, bowel continuity may have to be restored. To this date, we have restored bowel continuity in only one patient (out of 600) for this complaint.

UNIQUE COMPLICATIONS OF JEJUNOILEAL BYPASS

Certain long-term complications are uniquely associated with jejunoileal bypass. They include hair loss, polyarthralgia or polyarthritis, urinary calculi, and hepatic decompensation. It has been predicted that intestinal bypass will inevitably cause cholelithiasis.[145] This theory has not been supported by the factual experience of investigators actively working in this field.

Hair loss following jejunoileal bypass has been reported,[120] and we have documented this phenomenon in about 10 per cent of our patients. We attribute this finding to a diffuse protein deficiency; analysis of hair follicles reveals a lack of keratin. The alopecia has never been more than a thinning out of hair, and full recovery has taken place. In management, we encourage the patient to follow a high-protein diet.

A migratory polyarthralgia without swelling or erythema, lasting up to three months, has been observed in approximately 5 per cent of our patients. Rarely, we have also observed a true arthritic syndrome; Buchanan and Wilkins[23] have reported this finding as well. These patients manifest symptoms and signs indistinguishable from rheumatoid arthritis; however, rheumatoid factor and antinuclear antibody studies have been negative. Patients with polyarthralgia or polyarthritis are treated symptomatically with analgesics, antiinflammatory agents, and physiotherapy.

The formation of urinary calculi to a degree that cannot be expected in the general population has been found by O'Leary and Woodward,[117] who report an incidence as high as 23 per cent (7 of 31 patients followed 6 months to 5.5 years). No one else has reported a similar percentage. We are seeing an increase over the general population mean in the rate of calculi formation following jejunoileal bypass; however, our incidence is currently about 10 per cent.

It has been shown in several reports that approximately 75 per cent of morbidly obese individuals at the time of jejunoileal bypass exhibit some degree of fatty metamorphosis of the liver.[86, 96, 121, 132] We have now performed intraoperative liver biopsies on about 400 successive jejunoileal bypass patients, and we concur with this finding. We have also seen at the time of operation pericentral fibrosis, periportal fibrosis, focal necrosis, and lymphocytic infiltration. These changes may prove to be more indicative of hepatic degeneration than fatty infiltration.

We see liver failure in about 5 per cent of our jejunoileal bypass patients, usually between 8 and 16 months following the procedure. Half of these patients can be successfully managed by a high-protein diet and commercially available oral protein supplements. The remainder require hospitalization and may need intravenous amino acids, establishment of a feeding jejunostomy for amino acid infusion into the proximal end of the bypassed segment, or take-down of the shunt and re-establishment of bowel continuity. To this writing, we have restored bowel continuity in four patients for intractable liver failure (<1 per cent). A death from sepsis following a staphlococcus infection of a catheter site occurred nine months after bypass in a patient in liver failure.

Clinically, we make the diagnosis of hepatic failure on the basis of a low serum albumin concentration (<3 gm. per 100 ml), abnormalities in the coagulation parameters, and development of peripheral edema, in addition to anorexia and easy fatiguability. One should not have to wait for a massive derangement in liver function tests, anasarca, further symptomatic decompensation, or the presence of jaundice.

Considerable work has been done to attempt to understand the cause, or causes, of hepatic derangement in obesity and after jejunoileal bypass. The laboratory and clinical literature in this area is rapidly growing. It is, however, not within the scope of this chapter to analyze these theories of causation.

RESULTS—WEIGHT REDUCTION

The end result of jejunoileal bypass surgery is measured in the weight response and the amelioration of obesity-related conditions. The literature reveals that jejunoileal bypass results in an average 35 per cent weight loss.[86, 102, 120, 121, 132, 139, 143, 144] Weight reduction occurs primarily within the first year following the procedure.[137] The amount of weight loss has been noted to be related to the degree of excess weight present prior to the operation[76, 166] and the intraoperative bowel length.[76] Payne reported an average weight loss at one year of 123 pounds.[121] Salmon[132] reported that two thirds of his patients were within 20 pounds of their "ideal weight" one to three years after operation. Using the end-to-end bypass, we have achieved a mean weight reduction of 90.6 pounds (70 per cent of mean "ideal weight") at one year, 106.7 pounds (81.7 per cent of "ideal weight") at two years, and 100 pounds (78.4 per cent of "ideal weight") at

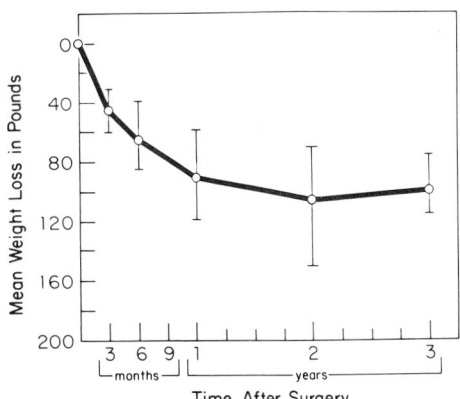

Figure 9. Three-year plot of the mean ± standard deviation weight loss in pounds following jejunoileal bypass surgery.

three years (Fig. 9). Ninety per cent of our patients have lost to within 50 pounds of their "ideal weight," and no individual's weight has dropped below "ideal weight." An excellent result of the jejunoileal bypass procedure is illustrated in Figure 10.

ASSOCIATED BENEFITS

Lewis et al. in 1962[102] reported two patients who, following jejunocolic bypass, had a decrease in the serum cholesterol level to less than 50 per cent of their preoperative values. Payne,[120, 121] Weismann,[166] Shibata,[144] and Scott[137] have made similar observa-

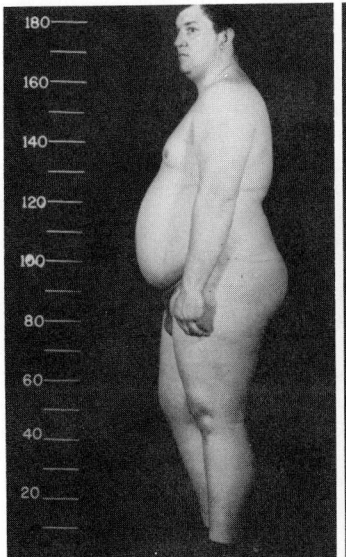
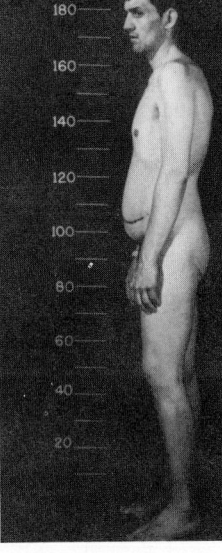

Figure 10. Patient immediately preceding his jejunoileal bypass, weighing 343 pounds (left) and the same patient one year later, weighing 193 pounds (right). (From Buchwald, H., et al.: Intestinal Bypass Procedures in Ravitch, M. M. (eds.): CURRENT PROBLEMS IN SURGERY, April, 1975. Copyright © 1975 by Year Book Medical Publishers, Inc., Chicago. Used by permission.)

tions. Weismann has also noted a significant reduction in the serum triglyceride level,[66] as has Scott.[137] All patients in our series have had a marked reduction in both serum cholesterol (average reduction, 40 per cent) and serum triglyceride (average reduction, 35 per cent) levels. The cholesterol reduction seems to be independent of the preoperative cholesterol concentration. An equivalent percentage of cholesterol lowering has been observed in individuals with initial values below 200 mg. per 100 ml. and those with higher preoperative concentrations, including the truly hypercholesterolemic patients. A significant number of our patients have a postoperative cholesterol value below 100 mg. per 100 ml. In distinction, the serum triglyceride response appears to be directly related to the initial triglyceride level.

A common finding in the obese is hypertension. Many of our hypertensive patients have significant blood pressure reductions after bypass. This correlation between weight reduction and a fall in blood pressure has been reported by others.[120, 166] Payne has noted reversal of cardiovascular decompensation accompanying postbypass weight reduction.[120]

With progressive weight loss, we have seen insulin-dependent diabetics convert to only dietary control or exhibit a marked reduction in their insulin requirements. Shibata[144] noted conversion from a diabetic oral glucose tolerance curve preoperatively to a normal curve one year following operation in four patients. Weismann[166] has made a similar observation.

We have noted, as have others,[137] a definite decrease in the symptoms of lower extremity varicosities after substantial weight loss. Relief of symptomatic osteoarthritic spine and hip pathology has been reported by Weismann.[166] We have had several individuals referred to us by orthopedic surgeons for weight reduction to precede remedial reconstructive surgery. Relief of respiratory distress symptoms and disappearance of a pickwickian state can be expected after significant postoperative weight loss. Six of our patients have given birth to normal children one year or longer after their bypass operations. As previously stated, the long-term effect of jejunoileal bypass on the liver remains unclear.

A long-term beneficial effect on longevity following substantial weight reduction has been documented.[58] Currently, our determination of cardiovascular disease risk is based on the presence of certain factors, including obesity, hyperlipidemia, hypertension, and diabetes. Since the jejunoileal bypass operation has been shown to reverse or mitigate these risk factors, it seems reasonable to assume that the procedure will be demonstrated to prolong life.

Certainly, the quality of life can be improved after marked weight reduction in the morbidly obese. As a rule, they are well satisfied with the results of the operation and can make better social adjustments. Many return to school and plan a more productive future. The rate of gainful employment has increased in the jejunoileal bypass population after weight reduction. Improvement in self-image and interpersonal relationships is difficult to assess except by a compilation of anecdotal experiences, which in our patient series tend to be largely positive and appear to have been responsible for beneficial alterations in personality. A more stringent psychiatric analysis of the personality changes in the post jejunoileal bypass patient has been published by Solow and associates,[148] who conclude that patients following bypass, on the whole, exhibit greater maturity and increased emotional stability in response to personal and external stresses.

CONCLUSION

Although the pathophysiologic state of obesity has been investigated thoroughly and the associated morbidity has been well demonstrated, clinicians tend to ignore the obese. The lack of an effective and simple method of treatment has surely been a deterrent. Diet, drugs, and psychiatric therapy have had too little lasting influence on the food addict. Treatment of this disease by massive small bowel bypass has been available for nearly two decades but, until recently, this procedure has been slow to find acceptance by the medical community, not because of its inability to effect weight loss but because of the potential acute and long-term complications, as well as the side effects, associated with the procedure.

It has now been demonstrated that the short-term complications of jejunoileal bypass can be kept to a minimum if a trained team of surgical personnel adheres to a well-conceived protocol and gives close attention to certain details before, during, and after the operative procedure. The long-term complications and side effects can, with some understanding of the problems involved, also be minimized. Yet we are still ignorant of the specific etiology of the long-term problems, as well as the best treatment and/or prevention of these hazards. We have yet to come to definitive grips with the unknowns, e.g., liver degeneration. The 10- and 20-year follow-up data for this therapeutic approach must still be developed.

SELECTED REFERENCES

Buchwald, H., Moore, R. B., and Varco, R. L.: Surgical treatment of hyperlipidemia. Circulation, 49(I):1, 1974.
 This is the one reference of ours that we will annotate. This three-part monograph, subtitled, "Apologia, The Laboratory Experience, and Clinical Status of the Partial Ileal Bypass Operation," summarizes our thoughts and work in this field over a 10-year period. It offers the reader the only appraisal of diet and drug therapy of the hyperlipidemias written by surgeons, as well as an overview of the world experimental and clinical partial ileal bypass literature. It details our methodology and offers tabulations of the data. The references provided therein include all of our publications on this subject through 1974, as well as the related publications of others. It may be useful to the student interested in the laboratory experiments and the study of clinical cholesterol dynamics.

Cornfield, J.: Joint dependence of risk of coronary heart disease on serum cholesterol and systolic blood pressure: Discriminant function analysis. Fed. Proc., 21:58, 1962.
 One of the original publications from the prospective Framingham study establishing the correlation of atherosclerotic risk with an exponential function of the cholesterol concentration.

Payne, J. H., and DeWind, L. T.: Surgical treatment of obesity. Am. J. Surg., 118:414, 1969.
 A review by one of the pioneers in this field of their very large series of end-to-side jejunoileal bypass procedures. A first-hand account of the early days in the development of this operative approach to the management of morbid obesity.

Scott, H. W., Jr., Dean, R., Shull, H. J., Abram, H. S., Webb, W., and Younger, R. K.: New considerations in use of jejuno-ileal bypass in patients with morbid obesity. Ann. Surg., *177*:723, 1973.

An exploration by a talented and innovative group of different types of end-to-end jejunoileal bypass operations. A critical analysis of their results with these various procedures and an exposition of their effort to tailor the operation to the patient's needs. Ileal preservation as a means to preserve vitamin B_{12} absorptive capacity is also discussed.

Solow, C., Silberfarb, P. M., and Swift, K.: Psychosocial effects of intestinal bypass surgery for severe obesity. N. Engl. J. Med., *290*:300, 1974.

The surgeon, and the student of surgery, is advised to read this excellent psychosocial appraisal of the obese patient and the response of the patient to jejunoileal bypass surgery. In summary, the authors conclude that the psychological, social, and economic benefits of postjejunoileal bypass weight reduction far outweigh the detrimental emotional effects of this operation.

Younger, R. K., Shepard, G. H., Butts, W. H., and Scott, H. W., Jr.: Comparison of the protective effects of cholestyramine and ileal bypass in Rhesus monkeys on an atherogenic regimen. Surg. Forum, *20*:101, 1969.

The only published experiment comparing the relative efficacy of cholestyramine and the partial ileal bypass operation in the reduction of circulating cholesterol levels and the development of atherosclerotic plauqe lesions. This paper clearly demonstrates that partial ileal bypass is twice as effective as cholestyramine in accomplishing these ends.

REFERENCES

1. Amad, K. H., Brennan, J. C., and Alexander, J. K.: The cardiac pathology of chronic exogenous obesity. Circulation, *32*:740, 1963.
2. Baird, I. M.: Obesity and coronary heart disease. Postgrad. Med. J., *47*:30, 1971.
3. Balfour, J. F., and Kim, R.: Homozygous type II hyperlipoproteinemia treatment, partial ileal bypass in two children. J.A.M.A., *227*:1145, 1974.
4. Baltaxe, H., Amplatz, K., Varco, R. L., and Buchwald, H.: Coronary arteriography in hypercholesterolemic patients. Am. J. Roentgenol., *105*:784, 1969.
5. Beaumont, J. L., Carlson, L. A., Cooper, G. R., Fejfar, Z., Fredrickson, D. S., and Strasser, T.: Classification of hyperlipidemias and hyperlipoproteinemias. Bull. WHO, *43*:891, 1970.
6. Berge, K. G., Achor, R. W. P., Christensen, N. A., Mason, H. L., and Barker, N. W.: Hypercholesteremia and nicotinic acid: A long-term study. Am. J. Med., *31*:24, 1961.
7. Berkowitz, D.: Selective blood lipid reductions by newer pharmacological agents. Am. J. Cardiol., *12*:834, 1963.
8. Best, M. M., and Duncan, C. H.: Effects of clofibrate and dextrothyroxine singly and in combination on serum lipids. Arch. Intern. Med., *118*:97, 1966.
9. Bierenbaum, M. L., Fleischman, A. I., Green, D. P., Raichelson, R. I., Hayton, T., Watson, P. B., and Caldwell, A. B.: The five-year experience of modified fat diets on younger men with coronary heart disease. Circulation, *42*:943, 1970.
10. Billich, C., Brag, G. A., Gallagher, T. F., Jr., Hoffbrand, A. V., and Levitan, R.: Absorptive capacity of the jejunum of obese and lean subjects. Arch. Intern. Med., *130*:377, 1972.
11. Bjorntorp, P.: Disturbances in the regulation of food intake. Adv. Psychosom. Med., 7:116, 1972.
12. Bjorntorp, P., Gustafson, A., and Persson, B.: Adipose tissue fat cell size and number in relation to metabolism in endogenous hypertriglyceridemia. Acta. Med. Scand., *190*:363, 1971.
13. Bjorntorp, P., and Sjostrom, L.: Number size of adipose tissue fat cells in relation to metabolism in human obesity. Metabolism, *20*:703, 1971.
14. Blacket, R. B., Woodhill, J., and Brown, W. D.: The effect of cholestyramine ("MK 135") on the serum cholesterol level in man. Med. J. Austr., 2:15, 1964.
15. Bloom, W. L., and Eidex, M. F.: Inactivity as a major factor in adult obesity. Metabolism, *16*:679, 1967.
16. Booth, C. C., and Mollin, D. L.: The site of absorption of B_{12} in man. Lancet, 1:18, 1959.
17. Bortz, W. M.: Metabolic consequences of obesity. Ann. Intern. Med., *71*:833, 1969.
18. Boyd, G. S., and Oliver, M. F.: Effect of certain thyroxine analogues on the serum lipids in human subjects. J. Endocrinol., *21*:33, 1960.
19. Braasch, J.: The surgical treatment of obesity: A study in applied physiology. Surg. Clin. North Am., *51*:667, 1971.
20. Bressler, R., Nowlin, J., and Bogdonoff, M. D.: Treatment of hypercholesterolemia and hypertriglyceridemia by anion exchange resin. South. Med. J., *59*:1097, 1966.
21. Brook, C. G. D., Lloyd, J. K., and Wolf, O. H.: Relation between age and onset of obesity and size and number of adipose cells. Br. Med. J., *2*:25, 1972.
22. Brown, H. B., and Green, J. G.: Diets suitable for reduction of serum cholesterol levels. The Cleveland Clinic Dietary Research Project. Cleveland Clin. Q., *29*:101, 1962.
23. Buchanan, R. F., and Wilkens, R. F.: Arthritis after jejunoileostomy. Arthritis Rheum., *15*:644, 1972.
24. Buchwald, H.: Localization of cholesterol absorption. Circulation, *28*(II):649, 1963.
25. Buchwald, H.: Surgical operation to lower circulating cholesterol. Circulation, *28*(II):649, 1963.
26. Buchwald, H.: Lowering of cholesterol absorption and blood levels by ileal exclusion: Experimental basis and preliminary clinical report. Circulation, *29*:713, 1964.
27. Buchwald, H.: Vitamin B_{12} absorption deficiency following bypass of the ileum. Am. J. Dig. Dis., *9*:755, 1964.
28. Buchwald, H.: Myocardial infarction in rabbits induced solely by a hypercholesterolemic diet. J. Atheroscler. Res., *5*:407, 1965.
29. Buchwald, H.: The effect of ileal bypass on atherosclerosis and hypercholesterolemia in the rabbit. Surgery, *58*:22, 1965.
30. Buchwald, H.: Alterations in the cutaneous lesions of the hyperlipidemias following partial ileal bypass. Derm. Dig., *9*:65, 1970.
31. Buchwald, H., Coyle, J. J., and Varco, R. L.: Effect of small bowel bypass on gastric secretory function: Post-intestinal exclusion hypersecretion, a phenomenon in search of a syndrome. Surgery, *75*:821, 1974.
32. Buchwald, H., and Gebhard, R. L.: Effect of intestinal bypass on cholesterol absorption and blood levels in the rabbit. Am. J. Physiol., *207*:567, 1964.
33. Buchwald, H., and Gebhard, R. L.: Localization of bile salt absorption in-vivo in the rabbit. Ann. Surg., *167*:191, 1968.
34. Buchwald, H., and Gebhard, R. L.: Relative secretion of cholesterol-4-^{14}C in the bile and upper and lower small intestinal washings of the bile fistula rabbit. Surgery, *75*:266, 1974.
35. Buchwald, H., Moore, R. B., Bertish, J., and Varco, R. L.: Effect of ileal bypass on cholesterol levels, atherosclerosis and growth in the infant rabbit. Ann. Surg., *175*:311, 1972.
36. Buchwald, H., Moore, R. B., and Frantz, I. D., Jr.: Serum uric acid, carotene and vitamin A, proteins, sugar, and electrolytes before and after partial ileal bypass for hyperlipidemia. Circulation, *40*(III):4, 1969.
37. Buchwald, H., Moore, R. B., Lee, G. B., Frantz, I. D., Jr., and Varco, R. L.: Combined dietary, surgical, and bile salt binding resin therapy in the treatment of hypercholesterolemia. Arch. Surg., *97*:275, 1968.
38. Buchwald, H., Moore, R. B., and Varco, R. L.: Surgical treatment of hyperlipidemia. Circulation, *49*(I): 1, 1974.
39. Buchwald, H., Moore, R. B., and Varco, R. L.: Ten years clinical experience with partial ileal bypass in management of the hyperlipidemias. Ann. Surg., *180*:384, 1974.
40. Buchwald, H., Moore, R. B., and Varco, R. L.: Partial ileal bypass operation for control of hyperlipidemia and atherosclerosis. *In* Sabiston, D. C., Jr., and Spencer, F. C. (Eds.): Gibbon's Surgery of the Chest, 3rd ed. Philadelphia, W. B. Saunders Company, 1976.
41. Buchwald, H., and Varco, R. L.: A bypass operation for obese hyperlipidemics. Surgery, *70*:62, 1970.
42. Buchwald, H., and Varco, R. L.: Human gastric secretory studies following distal small bowel bypass. Curr. Top. Surg. Res., *3*:409, 1971.
43. Burwell, C. S., Robin, E. D., Whaley, R. D., and Bickelmann, A. G.: Extreme obesity associated with alveolar hypoventilation – A Pickwickian syndrome. Am. J. Med., *21*:811, 1956.
44. Casdorph, H. R.: Hypercholesterolemia – treatment with cholestyramine, a bile acid sequestering resin. Calif. Med., *106*:293, 1967.

45. Chapman, J. M., Goerke, L. S., Dixon, W., Loveland, D. B., and Phillips, E.: The clinical status of a population group in Los Angeles under observation for two to three years. Am. J. Pub. Health, 47(II):33, 1957.

46. Chapman, J. M., and Mossey, F. J.: The interrelationship of serum cholesterol, hypertension, body weight and risk of coronary disease: Results of the first ten year follow-up in the Los Angeles Heart Study. J. Chron. Dis., 17:933, 1964.

47. Charman, R. C., Matthews, L. B., and Braeuler, C.: Nicotinic acid in the treatment of hypercholesterolemia. Angiology, 23:29, 1972.

48. Clot, J. P., Rouffy, J., Loeper, J., and Mercadier, M.: Derivation ileale, therapeutique, chirurgicale des hypercholesterolemies pures majeures á propose de deux observations). Chirurgie, 97:57, 1971.

49. Connor, W. E.: Measures to reduce the serum lipid levels in coronary heart disease. Med. Clin. North Am., 52:1249, 1968.

50. Cornfield, J.: Joint dependence of risk of coronary heart disease on serum cholesterol and systolic blood pressure: Discriminant function analysis. Fed. Proc., 21:58, 1962.

51. Coronary Drug Project: Clofibrate and niacin in coronary heart disease. J.A.M.A., 231:360, 1975.

52. Coyle, J. J., Varco, R. L., and Buchwald, H.: Gastric secretion and serum gastrin in human small bowel bypass. Arch. Surg., 110:1036, 1975.

53. Dawber, T. R., Moore, F. E., and Mann, G. V.: Coronary heart disease in the Framingham study. Am. J. Pub. Health, 47(II):4, 1957.

54. Dayton, S., and Bierce, M. L.: Diet high in unsaturated fat. Minn. Med., 52:1237, 1969.

55. Dinda, P., Riding, W. D., and Chatterjee, S. S.: Obesity with cardiorespiratory failure. Postgrad. Med. J., 47:158, 1971.

56. Doyle, J. T., Heslin, A. S., Hilleboe, H. E., Formel, P. F., and Korns, R. F.: A prospective study of degenerative cardiovascular disease in Albany: Report of three years' experience—I. Ischemic heart disease. Am. J. Pub. Health, 47(II):25, 1957.

57. Drugs which lower the blood lipids. Met. Lett. Drugs Ther., 5:81, 1963.

58. Dublin, L. I., and Marks, H. H.: Mortality among insured overweights in recent years. In Transactions of the Association of Life Insurance Medical Directors of America: Sixtieth Annual Meeting, Vol. 35. New York, Press of Recording and Statistical Corporation, 1951, p. 235.

59. Duncan, G. G., Jensen, W. K., Fraser, R. I., and Cristofori, F. C.: Correction and control of intractable obesity. J.A.M.A., 181:309, 1962.

60. Eder, H. A.: Drugs used in the prevention and treatment of atherosclerosis. In Goodman, L. S., and Gilman, A. (Eds.): The Pharmacological Basis of Therapeutics, 3rd ed. New York, Macmillan Company, 1965, p. 754.

61. Eisalo, A., Ahrenberg, P., and Nikkila, E. A.: Treatment of hyperlipidemia with d-thyroxine. Acta Med. Scand., 173:639, 1963.

62. Evans, D. W., Turner, S. M., and Ghosh, P.: Feasibility of long-term plasma-cholesterol reduction by diet. Lancet, 1:172, 1972.

63. Fallon, H. J., and Woods, J. W.: Response of hyperlipoproteinemia to cholestyramine resin. J.A.M.A., 204:1161, 1968.

64. Five-year study by a group of physicians of the Newcastle upon Tyne Region: Trial of clofibrate in the treatment of ischaemic heart disease. Brit. Med. J., 4:767, 1971.

65. Fredrickson, D. S., Levy, R. I., and Lees, R. S.: Fat transport in lipoproteins: An integrated approach to mechanisms and disorders. N. Engl. J. Med., 276:32, 1967.

66. Freedman, M. A., Wilds, P. L., and George, W. M.: Grotesque obesity: A serious complication of labor and delivery. South. Med. J., 65:732, 1972.

67. Fritz, S. H., and Walker, W. J.: Ileal bypass in the control of intractable hypercholesterolemia. Am. Surg., 32:691, 1966.

68. Canor, S., and Even-Paz, Z.: Fragilitas cutis inguinalis: A phenomenon associated with obesity. Dermatologica, 134:113, 1967.

69. Gebhard, R. L., and Buchwald, H.: Cholesterol absorption after reversal of the upper and lower halves of the small intestine. Surgery, 67:474, 1970.

70. Geogate, A. N.: Symposium on obesity endocrine aspects. J. Assoc. Phys. India, 16:245, 1968.

71. Gomes, M. M., Kottke, B. A., Bernatz, P., and Titus, J. L.: Effect of ileal bypass on aortic atherosclerosis of white Carneau pigeons. Surgery, 70:353, 1971.

72. Goodman, D. S., and Nobel, R. P.: Turnover of plasma cholesterol in man. J. Clin. Invest., 47:231, 1968.

73. Green, J. G., Brown, H. B., Meredith, A. P., and Page, I. H.: Use of fat-modified foods for serum cholesterol reduction. J.A.M.A., 183:5, 1963.

74. Grundy, S. M., Ahrens, E. H., Jr., and Salen, G.: Interruption of the enterohepatic circulation of bile acids in man: Comparative effects of cholestyramine and ileal exclusion on cholesterol metabolism. J. Lab. Clin. Med., 78:94, 1971.

75. Guzman, I. J., Fitch, L. L., Varco, R. L., and Buchwald, H.: Small bowel length in hyperlipidemia and massive obesity. Submitted for publication, 1976.

76. Guzman, I. J., Varco, R. L., and Buchwald, H.: Factors determining weight loss following jejuno-ileal bypass for obesity. J. Surg. Res., 18:399, 1975.

77. Hashim, S. A., and Van Itallie, T. B.: Cholestyramine resin therapy for hypercholesterolemia. J.A.M.A., 192:289, 1965.

78. Heffernan, A., Hickey, N., Mulcahy, R., and Fitzgerald, O.: The chemotherapy of hypercholesterolaemia. Acta Cardiol., 24:47, 1969.

79. Helsinger, N., Jr., and Rootwelt, K.: Partial ileal bypass for surgical treatment of hypercholesterolemia. Nord. Med., 82:1409, 1969.

80. Howard, A. N., and Hyams, D. E.: Combined use of clofibrate and cholestyramine or DEAE sephadex in hypercholesterolemia. Br. Med. J., 3:25, 1971.

81. Hundley, J. M.: Diabetes—overweight: U.S. Problems. J. Am. Dietet. Assoc., 32:417, 1956.

82. Hunninghake, D. B., Tucker, D. R., and Azarnoff, D. L.: Long-term effects of clofibrate (Atromid-S) on serum lipids in man. Circulation, 39:675, 1969.

83. Jeffcoate, T. N. A., Miller, J., Roos, R. F., and Tindall, V. R.: Puerperal thromboembolism in relation to the inhibition of lactation by oestrogen therapy. Br. Med. J., 4:19, 1968.

84. Jepson, E. M., Fahmy, M. F. I., Torrens, P. E., and Billimoria, J. D.: Treatment of essential hyperlipidaemia. Lancet, 2:1315, 1969.

85. Jolliffe, N., Maslansky, E., Rudensey, F., Simon, M., and Faulkner, A.: Dietary control of serum cholesterol in clinical practice. Circulation, 24:1415, 1961.

86. Juhl, E., Christoffersen, P., Baden, H., and Quaade, F.: Liver morphology and biochemistry in eight obese patients treated with jejuno-ileal anastomosis. N. Engl. J. Med., 285:543, 1971.

87. Katz, L. N., Stamler, J., and Pick, R.: Nutrition and atherosclerosis. Philadelphia, Lea and Febiger, 1958.

88. Keck, C.: Obesity and orthopedics. J.A.M.A., 19:759, 1964.

89. Keys, A.: Coronary heart disease in seven countries. Circulation, 41(I):1, 1970.

90. Keys, A., Aravanis, C., Blackburn, H., VanBuchem, F. S. P., Buzina, R., et al.: Coronary heart disease: Overweight and obesity as risk factors. Ann. Intern. Med., 77:15, 1972.

91. Khachadurian, A. K., and Demirjian, Z. N.: Cholestyramine therapy in patients homozygous for familial hypercholesterolemia. J. Atheroscler. Res., 8:177, 1968.

92. Knight, L., Scheibel, R., Amplatz, K., Varco, R. L., and Buchwald, H.: Radiographic appraisal of the Minnesota partial ileal bypass study. Surg. Forum, 23:141, 1972.

93. Krasno, L. R., and Kidera, G. J.: Clofibrate in coronary heart disease: Effect on morbidity and mortality. J.A.M.A., 219:845, 1972.

94. Kremen, A. J., Linner, J. H., and Nelson, C.: An experimental evaluation of the nutritional importance of proximal and distal small intestine. Ann. Surg., 140:439, 1954.

95. Langer, T., and Levy, R. I.: Acute muscular syndrome associated with administration of clofibrate. N. Engl. J. Med., 279:856, 1968.

96. Leevy, C.: Fatty liver: A study of 270 patients with biopsy proven fatty liver. Medicine, 41:249, 1962.

97. Leren, P.: The effect of plasma-cholesterol-lowering diet in male survivors of myocardial infarction. Bull. N.Y. Acad. Med., 44:1012, 1968.

98. Levy, R. L.: Dietary and drug treatment of primary hyperlipoproteinemia. Ann. Intern. Med., 77:267, 1972.

99. Levy, R. L., Quarfardt, S. H., and Brown, W. V.: The efficacy of clofibrate (CPIB) in familial hyperlipoproteinemias. Adv. Exper. Med. Biol., 4:377, 1969.

100. Lewis, L. A., Brown, H. B., and Page, I. H.: Ten years' treatment of hyperlipidemia. Circulation, 38(6):128, 1968.

101. Lewis, L. A., Brown, H. B., and Page, I. H.: Ten years' dietary treatment of primary hyperlipidemia. Geriatrics, 25:64, 1970.

102. Lewis, L. A., Turnbull, R. B., and Page, I. H.: "Short-circuiting" of the small intestine. J.A.M.A., 182:77, 1962.

103. Lewis, L. A., Turnbull, R. B., and Page, I. H.: Effects of jejunocolic shunt on obesity, serum liporpoteins, lipids and electrolytes. Arch. Intern. Med., 117:4, 1966.

104. Lillington, G. A., Anderson, M. W., and Brandenburg, R. O.: The cardiorespiratory syndrome of obesity. Dis. Chest, 32:1, 1957.

105. Marks, H. H.: Influence of obesity on morbidity and mortality. Bull. N.Y. Acad. Med., 36:296, 1960.

106. Mayer, J.: Some aspects of the problem of regulation of food intake and obesity. N. Engl. J. Med., 274:662, 1966.

107. Mayer, J., Monello, L. F., and Selzer, C. C.: Hunger and satiety sensations in man. Postgrad. Med., 37:A-97, 1965.

108. Miettinen, T.: Commentary. In Jones, R. J. (Ed.): Proceedings of the Second International Symposium on Atherosclerosis. New York, Springer-Verlag, 1970, p. 304.

109. Mishkel, M. A.: Diagnosis and management of the patient with xanthomatosis: An experience with thirty-five cases. Q. J. Med., 36:107, 1967.

110. Moore, R. B., Frantz, I. D., Jr., and Buchwald, H.: Changes in cholesterol pool size, turnover rate, and fecal bile acid and sterol excretion after partial ileal bypass in hypercholesterolemic patients. Surgery, 65:98, 1969.

111. Moore, R. B., Frantz, I. D., Jr., Varco, R. L., and Buchwald, H.: Cholesterol dynamics after partial ileal bypass. In Jones, R. J. (Ed.): Proceedings of the Second International Symposium on Atherosclerosis. New York, Springer-Verlag, 1970, p. 295.

112. National Diet Heart Study. Circulation, 37(I), 1968.

113. Newman, H. H., Freeman, F. N., and Holzinger, K. J.: Twins: A study of heredity and environment. Chicago, University of Chicago Press, 1937, p. 369.

114. Nisbett, R. E.: Eating behavior and obesity in men and animals. Adv. Psychosom. Med., 7:173, 1972.

115. Nordøy, A., and Gjone, E.: Treatment of essential hypercholesterolemia with clofibrate and nicotinic acid. Acta Med. Scand., 188:487, 1970.

116. Nygaard, K., Helsinger, N., and Rootwelt, K.: Adaptation of vitamin B_{12} absorption after ileal bypass. Scand. J. Gastroenterol., 5:349, 1970.

117. O'Leary, J. P., Thomas, W. C., Jr., and Woodward, E. R.: Urinary tract stone after small bowel bypass for morbid obesity. Am. J. Surg., 127:142, 1974.

118. Parsons, W. B., Jr.: Treatment of hypercholesterolemia by nicotinic acid: Progress report with review of studies regarding mechanism of action. Arch. Intern. Med., 107:639, 1961.

119. Parsons, W. B., Jr.: Studies of nicotinic acid use in hypercholesteremia: Changes in hepatic function, carbohydrate tolerance, and uric acid metabolism. Arch. Intern. Med., 107:653, 1961.

120. Payne, J. H.: Metabolic observations in patients with jejuno-colic shunts. Am. J. Surg., 106:273, 1963.

121. Payne, J. H., and DeWind, L. T.: Surgical treatment of obesity. Am. J. Surg., 118:141, 1969.

122. Peckham, C. H., and Christianson, R. E.: The relationship between prepregnancy weight and certain obstetric factors. Am. J. Obstet. Gynecol., 111:1, 1971.

123. Prem, K. A., Menshehad, N. M., and McKelvey, J. L.: Operative treatment of adenocarcinoma of the endometrium in obese women. Am. J. Obstet. Gynecol., 92:16, 1965.

124. Premachandra, B. N., Perlstein, I. B., and Blumenthal, H. T.: Thyroid autoimmunity, thyroxine transport and angiopathy in human obesity. In Vogue, J. (Ed.): Physiopathology of Adipose Tissue: Third International Meeting of Endocrinologists. Amsterdam, Exerpta Medica, 1969, p. 289.

125. Report of a Research Committee to the Medical Research Council: Controlled trial of soya-bean oil in myocardial infarction. Lancet, 2:693, 1968.

126. Report by a Research Committee of the Scottish Society of Physicians: Ischaemic heart disease: A secondary prevention trial using clofibrate. Br. Med. J., 4:775, 1971.

127. Rinzler, S. H.: Primary prevention of coronary heart disease by diet. Bull. N.Y. Acad. Med., 44:936, 1968.

128. Rosenthal, S. R.: Studies in atherosclerosis: Chemical, experimental and morphological; roles of cholesterol metabolism, blood pressure and structure of aorta; fat angle of aorta (F.A.A.), and infiltration-expression theory of lipoid deposit. Arch. Pathol., 18:473, 1934.

129. Rowe, G. G., Young, W., and Wasserburger, R. H.: The effect of reduced serum cholesterol on human coronary atherosclerosis. Circulation, 40(II):22, 1969.

130. Rozenthal, P., Biava, C., Spencer, H., and Zimmerman, H. L.: Liver morphology and function tests in obesity and during total starvation. Am. J. Digest. Dis., 12:198, 1967.

131. Russ, E. M., Eder, H. A., and Barr, D. P.: Influence on gonadal hormones on protein-lipid relationships in human plasma. Am. J. Med., 19:4, 1955.

132. Salmon, P. A.: The results of small intestinal bypass operations for the treatment of obesity. Surg. Gynecol. Obstet., 132:965, 1971.

133. Salmon, P. A.: Treatment of massive obesity by intestinal bypass. Bull. Soc. Intern. Chir., 31:206, 1972.

134. Schwartz, M. Z., Varco, R. L., and Buchwald, H.: Liver function and morphology following distal ileal excision in the rabbit. Surg. Forum, 22:355, 1971.

135. Schwartz, M. Z., Varco, R. L., and Buchwald, H.: Preoperative preparation, operative technique and postoperative care of patients undergoing jejunoileal bypass for massive exogenous obesity. J. Surg. Res., 14:147, 1973.

136. Scott, H. W., Jr.: Intestinal bypass operations in treatment of massive obesity. Hosp. Pract., 7:104, 1972.

137. Scott, H. W., Dean, R., Shull, H. J., Abram, H. S., Webb, W., and Younger, R. K.: New considerations in use of jejuno-ileal bypass in patients with morbid obesity. Ann. Surg., 177:723, 1973.

138. Scott, H. W., Jr., and Law, D. H., IV: Clinical appraisal of jejunoileal shunt in patients with morbid obesity. Am. J. Surg., 171:246, 1969.

139. Scott, H. W., Jr., Law, D. H., IV, Sandstead, H. H., Lanier, V. C., Jr., and Younger, R. K.: Jejuno-ileal shunt in surgical treatment of morbid obesity. Ann. Surg., 171:770, 1970.

140. Scott, H. W., Jr., Stephenson, S. E., Jr., Younger, R., Carlisle, R. B., and Turney, S. W.: Prevention of experimental atherosclerosis by ileal bypass: Twenty-percent cholesterol diet and I^{131} induced hypothyroidism in dogs. Ann. Surg., 163:795, 1966.

141. Shepard, G. H., Wimberly, J. E., Younger, R. K., Stephenson, S. E., Jr., and Scott, H. W., Jr.: Effects of bypass of the distal third of the small intestinal on experimental hypercholesterolemia and atherosclerosis in rhesus monkeys. Surg. Forum, 19:302, 1968.

142. Sheridan, J. T., and McC.Peck, J.: Overweight as a contributing factor in the development of hypertension. In Transactions of the Association of Life Insurance Medical Directors of America: Sixtieth Annual Meeting, Vol. 35. New York, Press of Recording and Statistical Corporation, 1951, p. 291.

143. Sherman, C. D., Jr., May, A. G., Nye, W., and Waterhourse, C.: Clinical and metabolic studies following bowel bypassing for obesity. Ann. N. Y. Acad. Sci., 131:614, 1965.

144. Shibata, H. R., MacKenzie, J. R., and Long, R. C.: Metabolic effects of controlled jejuno-colic bypass. Arch. Surg., 95:413, 1967.

145. Small, D. M., Downling, R. H., and Redinger, R.: The enterohepatic circulation of bile salts. Arch. Intern. Med., 130:552, 1972.

146. Smith, G. E. Cited by Long, E. R.: The development of our knowledge of arteriosclerosis. In Cowdry, E. V. (Ed.): Arteriosclerosis. New York, Macmillan Co., 1933, p. 21.

147. Sodal, G., Gjertsen, K. T., and Schrumpf, A.: Surgical treatment of hypercholesterolemia. Acta Chir. Scand., 136:671, 1970.

148. Solow, C., Silberfarb, P. M., and Swift, K.: Psychosocial effects of intestinal bypass surgery for severe obesity. N. Engl. J. Med., 290:300, 1974.

149. Special Communication: Coronary Drug Project. Initial findings leading to modifications of its research protocol. J.A.M.A., 214:1303, 1970.

150. Special Communication: Coronary Drug Project. Findings leading to further modifications of its protocol with respect to d-thyroxine. J.A.M.A., 220:996, 1972.

151. Stamler, J., Pick, R., Katz, L. N., Pick, A., Kaplan, B. M., Berkson, D. M., and Century, D.: Effectiveness of estrogens for therapy of myocardial infarction in middle-age men. J.A.M.A., 183:632, 1963.

152. Steinbach, J. H., Blackshear, P. L., Jr., Varco, R. L., and Buch-

wald, H.: High blood cholesterol reduces in-vitro blood oxygen delivery. J. Surg. Res., *16*:134, 1974.

153. Steinberg, D.: Chemotherapeutic control of serum lipid levels. Trans. N. Y. Acad. Sci., *24*:704, 1962.

154. Strisower, E. H., Adamson, G., and Strisower, B.: Treatment of hyperlipidemias. Am. J. Med., *45*:488, 1968.

155. Strisower, E. H., Kradjian, R., Nichols, A. V., Coggiola, E., and Tasai, J.: Effect of ileal bypass on serum lipoproteins in essential hypercholesterolemia. J. Atheroscl. Res., *8*:525, 1968.

156. Stunkard, A., and McLaren-Hume, M.: The results of treatment for obesity. Arch. Intern. Med., *103*:79, 1959.

157. Suzuki, M.: Picwickian syndrome and endocardial fibroelastosis: A possible pathogenetic correlation. Am. J. Med., *53*:123, 1972.

158. Swan, D. M., and McGowan, J. M.: Ileal bypass in hypercholesterolemia associated with heart disease. Am. J. Surg., *116*:81, 1968.

159. Symposium on Atromid: Proceedings of a conference held in Buxton (England), June 5–6, 1963. J. Atheroscler. Res., *3*:341, 1963.

160. Thomson, K. J.: Some observations on the development and course of hypertensive vascular disease. Proc. Med. Sec. Am. Life Conv., p. 85, June, 1950.

161. Turpeinen, O., Miettinen, M., Karovenen, M. J., Roine, P., Pekkarinen, M., Lehtosuo, E. J., and Alivirta, P.: Blood lipids and primary coronary events. Minn. Med., *52*:1247, 1969.

162. United States Department of Health, Education, and Welfare, National Center for Health Statistics. Vital Statistics of the United States: 1968. Rockville, Maryland, Government Printing Office, 1971, p. 7.

163. Verdy, M.: BSP retention during total fasting. Metabolism, *15*:769, 1966.

164. Vikrot, O., Beslin, R., and Oldfelt, C. O.: Influence of nicotinic acid on individual plasma phospholipids in hypercholesterolemia. Acta Med. Scand., *190*:133, 1971.

165. Wadd, W.: Cursory remarks on corpulence; or obesity considered as a disease: With a critical examination of ancient and modern opinions, relative to its causes and cure: Containing a reference to the most remarkable cases that have occurred in this country. London, J. Callow, 1816.

166. Weisman, R. E.: Surgical palliation of massive and severe obesity. Am. J. Surg., *125*:437, 1973.

167. Withers, R. F. J.: Problems in genetics of human obesity. Eugen. Rev., *56*:81, 1964.

168. Younger, R. K., Shepard, G. H., Butts, W., and Scott, H. W., Jr.: Comparison of the protective effects of cholestyramine and ileal bypass in rhesus monkeys on an atherogenic regimen. Surg. Forum, *20*:101, 1969.

169. Zacho, A., Larsen, V., and Christiansen, J.: Body weight and cancer of the stomach. Acta Chir. Scand., *130*:125, 1965.

170. Zellman, S.: The liver in obesity. Arch. Intern. Med., *90*:141, 1952.

VI

MECKEL'S DIVERTICULUM

Ward O. Griffen, Jr., M.D., Ph.D.

The most frequently encountered diverticulum of the small intestine was first described completely by Johann Meckel in 1809. Meckel's diverticulum occurs in the terminal ileum 45 to 90 cm. proximal to the ileocecal valve. Almost invariably the diverticulum arises from the antimesenteric border of the ileum and is a true diverticulum, since it contains all layers of the intestinal wall (Fig. 1). It varies in length and diameter from 1 to 10 or 12 cm. In autopsy studies the incidence of Meckel's diverticulum is 0.3 per cent but may be placed as high as 2 per cent when surgical cases are reviewed.

The *embryologic origin* and usual location of Meckel's diverticulum are explained by the development of the midgut. During the first few weeks of fetal life the primitive yolk sac divides into two portions, the larger becoming the primitive gut, the smaller continuing as a yolk sac near the placenta. These two portions remain connected by a tube contained within the umbilical cord. This tube, the *omphalomesenteric* or *vitelline duct,* ordinarily is obliterated by the seventh week. Persistence of this duct may lead to: (1) a fistula between the umbilicus and the ileum when the entire duct remains patent; (2) Meckel's diverticulum due to failure of closure of the intestinal end of the duct; (3) an umbilical sinus when the umbilical side of the duct is not obliterated; (4) a fibrous cord between the umbilicus and ileum representing the obliterated duct and its vessels; or (5) any combination of these four entities, the most frequent being Meckel's diverticulum connected to the umbilicus by a fibrous strand.

Dr. Charles W. Mayo is credited with having stated: "Meckel's diverticulum is frequently suspected, often looked for, and seldom found." The clinical manifestations are most common in the pediatric age group, but the diverticulum can produce symptoms at all ages. The average mortality of Meckel's diverticulum as reported in several surgical series is 6 per cent, with a large proportion of the deaths occurring in the elderly. As with many other less common intra-abdominal conditions, death frequently occurs because of delay in diagnosis and proper therapy. For this reason, techniques aimed at detecting a Meckel's diverticulum have been evaluated recently. The use of technetium scanning seems to hold the greatest promise as a diagnostic aid. ^{99m}Tc-pertechnetate is taken up by gastric mucosa, and, therefore, in patients who have ectopic gastric mucosa in a Meckel's diverticulum (about 50 per cent), this may be a helpful diagnostic maneuver. Administration of potassium perchlorate prior to injecting the technetium may reduce the uptake of the isotope by the ectopic gastric mucosa. The accuracy of this technique has yet to be determined, but instances of both

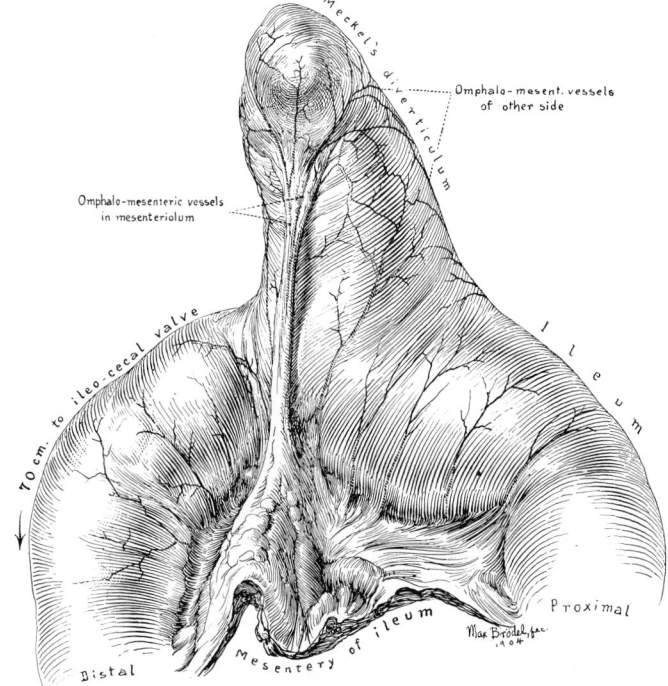

Figure 1. Typical anatomic example of a Meckel's diverticulum. Note the separate blood supply and gross appearance. (From Kelly, H. A., and Huron, E.: The Vermiform Appendix and Its Diseases. Philadelphia, W. B. Saunders Company, 1905.)

false negative and false positive results have been reported. Because of the continuing difficulty in making a diagnosis and the significant mortality and morbidity associated with the treatment of complicated Meckel's diverticulum, prophylactic removal of the diverticulum, found incidentally, is indicated whenever feasible. Simple inversion of the diverticulum to avoid opening the bowel is condemned because it may lead to intestinal absorption.

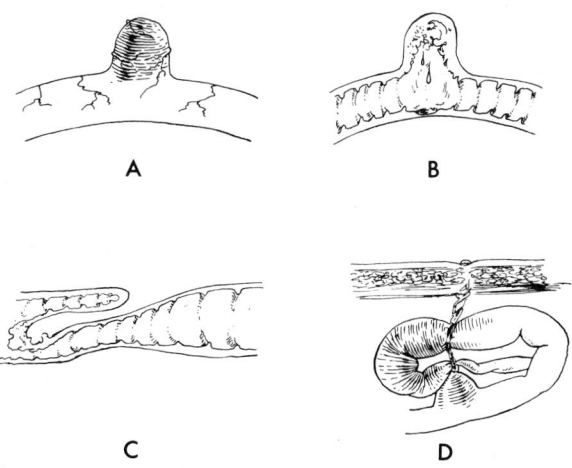

Figure 2. Presenting clinical manifestations of Meckel's diverticulum. *A,* Diverticulitis. *B,* Peptic ulcer secondary to heterotopic gastric mucosa within the diverticulum. *C,* Intussusception with the diverticulum acting as the leading portion of the intussusceptum. *D,* Volvulus of a segment of small bowel about a fibrous strand connecting the diverticulum to the umbilicus.

The important mechanisms of the clinical presentation of a Meckel's diverticulum are depicted in Figure 2. The most common clinical problem associated with Meckel's diverticulum is *bleeding,* which usually presents as melena or bright red blood per rectum. Classically the stool is burgundy red rather than tarry, but exsanguinating hemorrhages have been reported. The usual source of the bleeding is a chronic peptic ulcer in normal ileal mucosa, and this is associated with heterotopic gastric tissue within the diverticulum. Approximately 50 per cent of patients with Meckel's diverticulum have heterotopic tissue, usually gastric but occasionally pancreatic mucosa. Owing to a high index of suspicion, bleeding from this source is usually treated during childhood. However, it is not unusual to encounter an adult with a history of three or more isolated episodes of intestinal bleeding before a laparotomy was advised. In collected series this complication of Meckel's diverticulum occurs in half of the patients.

The second most common symptom associated with a Meckel's diverticulum is *intestinal obstruction.* The cause of this obstruction may be either volvulus of the small bowel around a diverticulum that is attached to the anterior abdominal wall, intussusception, or rarely incarceration of the diverticulum in a hernia (Littre). In the first instance acute mechanical obstruction is the usual picture and if allowed to progress long enough may result in strangulation of the involved bowel. The intussusception may be ileoileal or ileocolic and presents as acute obstruction associated with an urge to defecate and the passage of the classic currant jelly stool. This complication occurs in about 25 per cent of patients reported in surgical series. Barium enema reduction of an intussusception secondary to a Meckel's diverticulum can be performed. However, if the diverticulum is identified at the time of the barium enema, the patient should undergo surgery for resection of the diverticulum. Rarely will a Meckel's diverticulum be the site of a malignant lesion, and often this presents as an obstruction or acute diverticulitis.

Finally, the next most common complication, occurring in about 20 per cent of patients, is *diverticulitis*. It often presents as the picture of acute appendicitis except for the location of the pain, and may or may not be associated with enteroliths within the diverticulum. Failure to establish a prompt diagnosis may lead to perforation of the diverticulum, peritonitis, and death. As a corollary to prompt intervention in patients with Meckel's diverticulitis, when a patient is operated upon for acute appendicitis and the appendix is found to be normal, it is imperative that the distal three feet of terminal ileum be inspected for the presence of a Meckel's diverticulum. Inflamed or not, a diverticulum, if present, should be resected.

Occasionally a Meckel's diverticulum may be detected on small bowel follow-through x-rays or barium enema (Fig. 3). In an entirely asymptomatic patient it should be left alone. However, if the patient has any abdominal complaints that may be related to the presence of the diverticulum its removal should be advised. The mortality and morbidity for resection of an uncomplicated Meckel's diverticulum should be and are negligible. Usually the diverticulum can be excised by clamping its base, cutting it free, and closing the defect so that the suture line is diagonal or transverse.

Surgical treatment of a complicated Meckel's diverticulum does not have such favorable results. The postoperative mortality rate is between 5 and 10 per cent; the morbidity of wound infection, intra-abdominal sepsis, pneumonia, urinary tract infection, and pulmonary embolus has been reported as high as 25 per cent. Better anesthetic management should improve these figures. The only technical controversy concerns the choice between diverticulectomy and segmental resection. Since bleeding associated with a Meckel's diverticulum comes from a peptic ulcer of the adjacent ileal mucosa, simple diverticulectomy usually will not remove the ulcer. Postoperative bleeding may occur, and for this reason most surgeons prefer wider excision of the diverticulum or segmental resection of the portion of ileum containing the lesion.

SUMMARY

Meckel's diverticulum is an uncommon clinical disorder. Only a high index of suspicion will lead to proper diagnosis by use of further radiologic studies. Bleeding and obstruction are the most common manifestations of this lesion. Earlier diagnosis will enhance the surgical statistics.

SELECTED REFERENCES

DeBartolo, H. M., Jr., and van Heerden, J. A.: Meckel's diverticulum. Ann.. Surg., *183*:30, 1976.
  This is an updated review of the wide experience of the Mayo Clinic with Meckel's diverticulum. One hundred and ninety cases of patients are presented in this important and detailed review.

Moses, W. R.: Meckel's diverticulum, a report of 2 unusual cases. N. Engl. J. Med., *237*:118, 1947.
  The largest collected series of Meckel's diverticulum, 1605 cases. This short article reports the complications in tabular form with hemorrhage occurring in 30.9 per cent and obstruction in 23.8 per cent of the cases. One of the two cases reported is a leiomyosarcoma in a Meckel's diverticulum, a rare occurrence, seen in only 24 cases of the 1605 reviewed.

Soderlund, S.: Meckel's diverticulum. A clinical and histologic study. Acta Chir. Scand., Suppl. 248, 1959.
  A detailed report including a histologic review, a clinical review of 413 cases of Meckel's diverticulum, and a complete histologic survey. Included in the discussion is the embryologic explanation for heterotopic tissue in a Meckel's diverticulum and the physiologic reason for peptic ulceration occurring when there is gastric mucosa in the diverticulum; i.e., a critical amount of gastric mucosa must be present to induce ulceration.

REFERENCES

1. Berman, E. J., Schneider, A., and Potts, W. J.: Importance of gastric mucosa in Meckel's diverticulum. J.A.M.A., *156*:6, 1954.
2. DeBartolo, H. M., Jr., and van Herrden, J. A.: Meckel's diverticulum. Ann. Surg., *183*:30, 1976.
3. Enge, I., and Frimann-Dahl, J.: Radiology in acute abdominal disorders due to Meckel's diverticulum. Br. J. Radiol., *37*:775, 1964.
4. Jewett, T. C., Jr., and Butsch, W. L.: Meckel's diverticulum. The abdominal masquerader. Surgery, *46*:440, 1959.
5. Kiewsetter, W. B.: Meckel's diverticulum in children. Arch. Surg., *75*:914, 1957.
6. Passaro, E., Jr., Richmond, D., and Gordon, H. E.: Surgery for Meckel's diverticulum in the adult: Factors in morbidity and mortality. Arch. Surg., *93*:315, 1966.
7. Rutherford, R. B., and Akers, D. R.: Meckel's diverticulum: A review of 148 pediatric patients with special reference to the

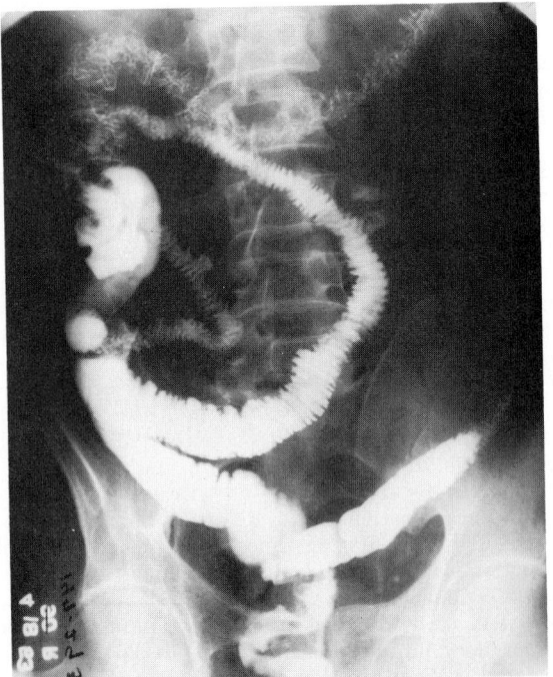

Figure 3. Meckel's diverticulum noted on a small bowel follow-through x-ray examination.

pattern of bleeding and to mesodiverticular bands. Surgery, *59*:618, 1966.

8. Sharma, G., and Benson, C. K.: Enteroliths in Meckel's diverticulum: Report of a case and review of the literature. Can. J. Surg., *13*:54, 1970.

9. Weinstein, E. C.: Meckel's diverticulum. J. Am. Geriatr. Soc., *13*:903, 1965.

10. Wine, C. R., Nahrwold, D. L., and Waldhausen, J. A.: Role of the technetium scan in the diagnosis of Meckel's diverticulum. J. Pediatr. Surg., *9*:88, 1974.

VII

CARCINOID TUMORS AND THE CARCINOID SYNDROME

William G. Anlyan, M.D.

HISTORY

Whereas Merling[20] in 1838 provided the first gross description of a tumor of the appendix, and Lubarsch[15] in 1888 provided the first complete description of the tumor in the autopsy findings from two patients with multiple tumors of the ileum, which he distinguished microscopically from adenocarcinoma, it remained for Oberndorfer[23] in 1907 to introduce the term "karzinoide" to differentiate it from carcinoma and yet show its resemblance to carcinoma of the intestine. Since 1907 carcinoids have been described throughout the gastrointestinal tract, its appendages, and the tracheobronchial tree.

The cells involved in the carcinoid tumor were shown by Gosset and Masson[9] to be granular cells in the crypts of Lieberkühn, first described in 1897 by Kultschitzky.[14] Because of the affinity of the cells for silver stain, the terms "argentaffin tumors" and "argentaffinomas" were introduced as synonyms for carcinoid tumors. It should be emphasized, however, that the cells of bronchial carcinoids do not have the same affinity for silver stain.

Knowledge of the humoral aspects of carcinoid tumors was derived from two independent sources of investigation. Erspamer[3] described the identification of a substance extracted from the intestine causing the contraction of smooth muscle and presumed to be derived from the Kultschitzky cells; he named the substance "enteramine." In a different arena of research, Rapport, Page, and Green,[26] seeking a humoral factor in hypertension, isolated a "nuisance" vasoconstrictor substance in serum that interfered with their studies; they named it "serotonin" and subsequently identified it chemically as 5-hydroxytryptamine. In 1952, Erspamer[4] found the chemical composition of enteramine to be identical to that of 5-hydroxytryptamine. Thus, a chemical substance, 5-hydroxytryptamine, had been discovered to be a serum vasoconstrictor and a humoral factor released from the Kultschitzky (or argentaffin) cells of the intestine. The name "serotonin" gained wider acceptance than "enteramine,"

and the association of serotonin with one or more diseases was not long in coming.

Lembeck[15] in 1953 isolated 5-hydroxytryptamine from carcinoid tumors. In 1954 Pernow and Waldenstrom[24] described paroxysmal flushing and other symptoms of the "functioning syndrome" in two patients with carcinoid tumors; they reported the symptoms to be due to elevated levels of serotonin in the blood and urine. Independently, in 1953 and 1954, Rosenbaum et al.[27] in the United States, Isler and Hedinger[11] in Switzerland, and Thorson[28] in Sweden described the elements of the composite of manifestations and findings that has been recognized as the *malignant carcinoid syndrome*. Since then, the association between gastrointestinal carcinoids, and bronchial carcinoids, with or without metastases, and serotonin and related constrictor amines has evolved in the world literature

GASTROINTESTINAL CARCINOID TUMORS

Incidence

Carcinoid tumors of the gastrointestinal tract may occur anywhere between the esophagus and the rectum. Wilson and Cheek[30] have tabulated and illustrated the site of incidence, average percentage of metastases, and cases of malignant carcinoid syndrome in the reported series in the literature.

As noted in Figure 1, only one case of carcinoid tumor of the esophagus has been reported, at the cardioesophageal junction. The commonest site of carcinoid tumors is the appendix; metastases and the functioning syndrome originating from an appendiceal primary tumor are extremely rare. In contrast, the second most frequent site of carcinoid tumors, the jejunum and ileum, is associated with a high incidence of metastases and the functioning syndrome. The rectum is the third most common site of carcinoid tumors, but the overwhelming majority are benign and the functioning syndrome has been reported only once. The most malignant site of carcinoid tumors appears to be in the colon.

SITE	CASES	AVERAGE % METASTASIS	CASES OF CARCINOID SYNDROME
Esophagus	1	—	0
Stomach	93	23	8
Duodenum	135	20	4
Jejuno-ileum	1,032	34	91
Meckel's diverticulum	42	19	3
Appendix	1,686	2	6
Colon	91	60	5
Rectum	592	18	1
Ovary	34	6	17
Biliary tract	10	30	0
Pancreas	2	—	1
	3,718		136

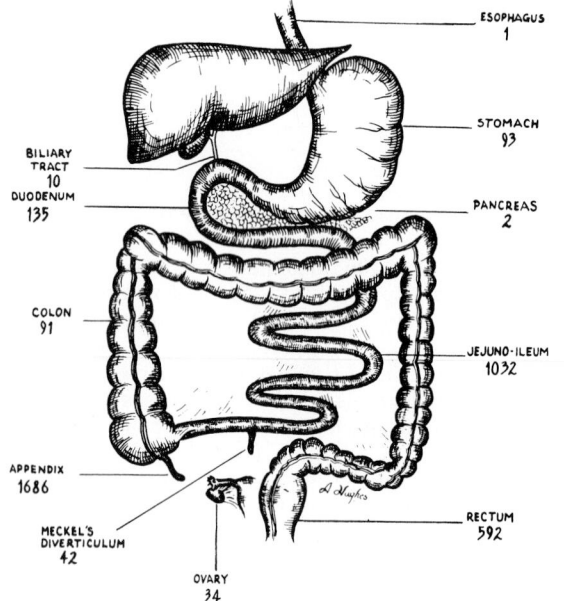

Figure 1. Total collected series of carcinoid tumors. (From Wilson, H., Cheek, R. C., Sherman, R. T., and Storer, E. H.: Curr Pobl. Surg. Nov. 1970. Copyright © 1970, Year Book Medical Publishers. Used by permission.)

Pathologic Characteristics

Benign tumors are usually small and 75 per cent of them are less than 1 cm. in diameter. They are well circumscribed and vary in color from yellow to tan or gray. As expected from the cell of origin (Kultschitzky), they originate in the submucosa and, in the process of slow growth, bulge into the lumen of the intestine.

The *malignant tumors* are presumed to evolve from previous benign tumors that initially invade the surrounding structures such as the muscularis and serosa and subsequently spread through the lymphatic system to the regional nodes and the liver. The metastases, in particular those in the liver, may become considerably larger than the primary tumor. From the liver, the spread may eventually involve the lung. In very advanced cases, metastases have been reported in most organs. The gross characteristics of an ileal carcinoid tumor growing submucosally and bulging sufficiently into the lumen to cause objective symptoms

are shown in Figure 2. The microscopic features are shown in Figure 3. The cells occur in irregular-shaped islands with a tendency for the peripheral cells to be radially arranged. The individual cells and nuclei are relatively uniform in size. In spite of the uniform appearance of these cells, metastasis has occurred. It is not always possible on the basis of microscopic appearance alone to differentiate between benign and malignant tumors, but rather this distinction is made on the basis of biologic behavior.

Special Clinical Features According to Site of Carcinoid Tumor in Gastrointestinal Tract

The patient with a carcinoid tumor in the stomach may present with symptoms not unlike those of a malignant, ulcerated adenocarcinoma, which mimic peptic ulcer complaints but are unrelieved by an antacid regimen. This may be due to the higher incidence of mucosal ulceration of gastric carcinoids. The gastroscopic and radiologic features may be indistinguishable from those of malignant adenocarcinoma.

Duodenal carcinoids cause symptoms in the majority of patients; the complaints resemble those of peptic ulcers. Radiologic examination should reveal a polypoid lesion in the lumen of the duodenum.

Carcinoids are the most common tumor of the *jejunum and ileum* and are progressively more frequent as one proceeds from the proximal jejunum to the distant ileum. In over 20 per cent of cases, the tumors may be multiple. In reported series there has been an associated unrelated malignant disease in over 30 per cent of cases. A fibrous tissue reaction to serosal invasion may cause a secondary intestinal obstruction by binding adjacent loops of bowel. The spectrum of clinical symptomatology may vary from total absence of symptoms to vague gastrointestinal symptoms or intestinal obstruction. With the paucity of mucosal ulceration, gastrointestinal bleeding is rare. In exceptional cases, the presenting picture may be that of an acute abdominal catastrophe due to gangrene of the intestine secondary to obstruction, perforation, intussusception, or an acute segmental necrosing enteritis (Jouanneau et al.[12]). Physical examination and radiologic evaluation are usually indeterminate.

Appendiceal carcinoids are discovered incidentally or in association with acute appendicitis. In the latter instance, the tumor may or may not be the etiologic factor precipitating obstruction of the appendiceal lumen and subsequent acute inflammation. Metastases and the functioning syndrome are extremely rare.

Colonic carcinoids tend to be the most virulent in terms of the high percentage of malignancy. They are commonest in the cecum. Symptoms, signs, and radiologic findings are indistinguishable from those of adenocarcinoma of the colon.

Rectal carcinoids are preponderantly benign, though the malignant lesions metastasize rapidly and widely. Rectal carcinoids may occur at any level in the rectum. The benign lesions usually present a gross picture similar to that of a benign polyp without a stalk; since mucosal ulceration and subsequent bleeding are rare, they are usually found as incidental findings on

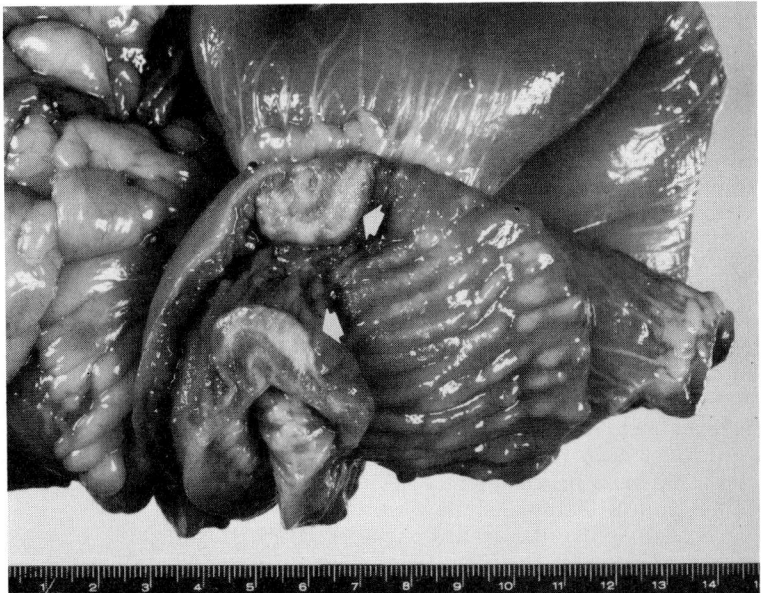

Figure 2. Gross characteristics of an ileal carcinoid tumor growing submucosally and bulging into the lumen.

rectal or proctoscopic examination. The malignant tumors may be similar in appearance to an ulcerated adenocarcinoma of the rectum with bleeding and possible obstruction; metastases may occur in the absence of mucosal ulceration.

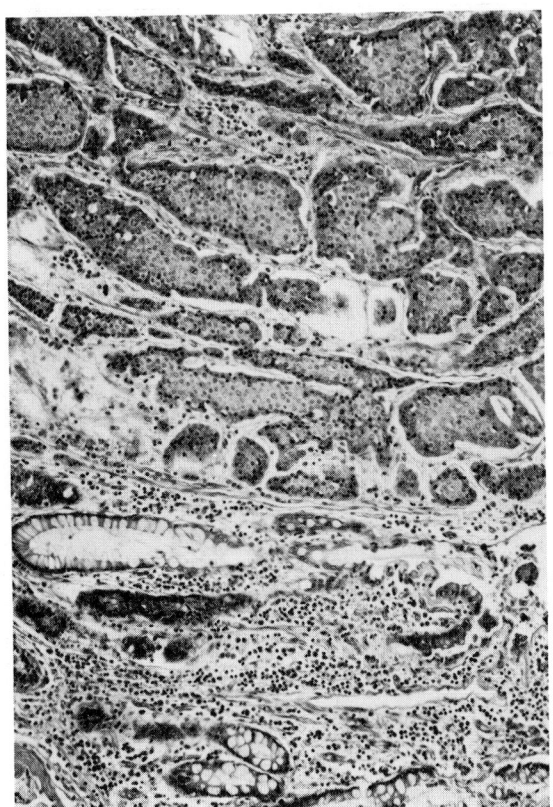

Figure 3. Microscopic characteristics of an ileal carcinoid tumor.

Carcinoid tumors have also been reported in (1) the biliary tract as incidental findings; and (2) the pancreas, either as an autopsy finding or with metastases and the functioning syndrome. More recent reports indicate the incidence of carcinoid tumors in the ovary,[29] in the thymus gland,[10] in association with other endocrine tumors, as a familial trait,[21] and as part of a neoplastic diathesis present concomitantly with other primary nonendocrine tumors.[2]

Treatment

With few exceptions, the prevailing surgical treatment of benign and malignant tumors of the gastrointestinal tract applies to carcinoid tumors. Local resection and reconstitution of the continuity of the gut are sufficient for benign tumors. Wide resection to include the lymphatic drainage of the involved segment in a manner similar to the treatment of adenocarcinomas of the gastrointestinal tract is recommended for the malignant carcinoids.

Unlike the approach to *hepatic metastases* of adenocarcinomas of the gastrointestinal tract, in which beyond biopsy confirmation no further surgical intervention is recommended, every effort should be made to excise isolated, large, well-circumscribed hepatic metastases from carcinoid tumors, especially in patients with the malignant functioning syndrome. In more fortunate cases, large, isolated metastases have been removed, for example, by left hepatic lobectomy (if only the left lobe is involved); complete relief from the functioning syndrome may ensue for a number of years.

Beyond surgical extirpation, radiation therapy has been of no avail in palliation of unresectable carcinoid tumors or their metastases. Mengel[18] has reported some success, with transient improvement, with parenteral administration of the chemotherapeutic agent methotrexate, alone or in combination with oral cyclophosphamide.

THE FUNCTIONING CARCINOID SYNDROME

The clinical manifestations of the functioning carcinoid syndrome are as follows: *vasomotor*—cutaneous purple-red flushing, mainly of the upper half of the body, precipitated by food or alcohol ingestion or emotional upset: *gastrointestinal*—abdominal cramping pain and diarrhea; *cardiopulmonary*—quite similar to asthma, with wheezing and dyspnea. In the late stages of the disease, right-sided heart failure may develop, with subendothelial fibrosis of the heart and secondary valvular incompetence; carcinoid pericarditis with effusion may present as a dominant clinical feature. These symptoms have been reported in one degree or another with carcinoid tumors in all locations. Whereas initially it was felt that hepatic metastases were a sine qua non to the development of symptoms, it has now been recognized that milder forms of the syndrome exist in the absence of metastatic disease. Other clinical features of the carcinoid syndrome include scleroderma-like lesions of the skin, arthralgia and arthropathy of the hands, and plastic induration of the penis (Peyronie's disease).[1, 8, 25] Metabolic and endocrine abnormalities noted in the carcinoid syndrome include (a) a high incidence of glucose intolerance and impaired insulin secretion;[7] (b) elevated plasma growth hormone and serum luteinizing hormone levels;[5, 6] (c) carcinoid tumors and medullary carcinomas of the thyroid may contain and secrete or cause secretion of calcitonin and prostaglandin E, as well as serotonin.[13] The functioning syndrome has also been described in noncarcinoid tumors such as cystic ovarian teratomas, tumors of bile ducts and the pancreas, and oat cell bronchogenic tumors.

The chemical causation of the syndrome was once thought to be due to the overproduction of serotonin by the tumor, measurable by the elevated blood levels of serotonin or of its degradation product, 5-hydroxyindoleacetic acid (5-HIAA), in the urine. It is now apparent that at least five active substances may be involved in the functioning carcinoid syndrome: serotonin (5-hydroxytryptamine), 5-hydroxytryptophan, kallikrein, histamine, and ACTH. The metabolic interrelationships of these substances and their relative importance in the production of the functioning syndrome remain as problems to be solved.

The formation of serotonin and its principal degradation pathway is as follows:

```
                     tryptophan
                     5-hydroxylase
Dietary tryptophan→5-Hydroxytryptophan
                         |
                         |        aromatic
                         |        L-amino acid
     monoamine           |        decarboxylase
     oxidase             |
5-Hydroxyindole←——— 5-Hydroxytryptamine
 acetaldehyde
       |
       |  aldehyde
       |  dehydrogenase
       └————————————→5-Hydroxyindoleacetic acid
```

Whereas normally about 1 per cent of dietary tryptophan goes through this metabolic cycle, carcinoid tumors may consume up to 60 per cent of dietary tryptophan. There is no constant relationship between the individual symptoms of the syndrome and blood levels of serotonin or urinary levels of 5-HIAA. Some patients with markedly elevated levels of both serotonin and 5-HIAA never experience symptoms of the syndrome. During flushes, vasodilating kinins have been found in hepatic venous blood draining carcinoid metastases.[22] In addition, kallikrein, a bradykinin-releasing enzyme, has been demonstrated in some hepatic metastases of carcinoid tumors.[17]

Antihumoral therapy with the antiserotonin agents methysergide, cyproheptadine, and *p*-chlorophenylalanine has been ineffective except for some alleviation of gastrointestinal symptoms. Mengel[19] has reported some limited success with higher doses given during the period of the day when patients experience their maximal symptoms.

SELECTED REFERENCES

Sandler, M.: The role of 5-hydroxyindoles in the carcinoid syndrome. Adv. Pharmacol., 6:(Suppl.) 127, 1968.
   This is a very comprehensive review of the pertinent literature on 5-hydroxyindole in the relationship of the carcinoid syndrome, with approximately 240 references of the pertinent literature up to 1967.

Wilson, H., Cheek, R. C., Sherman, R. T., and Storer, E. H.: Carcinoid tumors. Curr. Probl. Surg., Nov., 1970.
   This excellent, up-to-date monograph on carcinoid tumors gives a complete overview of the subject, especially for postdoctoral students and practicing surgeons. The section by Storer on the pharmacologic and biochemical nature of carcinoid tumors is highly commended. The 290 references listed cover the spectrum from the historic past to the current contributions.

REFERENCES

1. Bivens, C. H., Marecek, R. L., and Feldman, J. M.: Peyronie's disease—presenting complaint of carcinoid syndrome. N. Engl. J. Med., 288:844, 1973.
2. Brown, N. K., and Smith, M. P.: Neoplastic diathesis of patients with carcinoid. Cancer, 32:216, 1973.
3. Erspamer, V., and Asero, B.: Ricerche farmacologiche sull'enteramina. VII. Enteramina e indolalchilamine del veleno di rospo. Arch. Sci. Biol., 31:86, 1946.
4. Erspamer, V., and Asero, B.: Identification of enteramine, the specific hormone of the enterochromaffin cell system, as 5-hydroxytryptamine. Nature, 169:800, 1952.
5. Feldman, J. M., Plonk, J. W., and Bivens, C. E.: Alterations of pituitary-gonadal function in the carcinoid syndrome. Am. J. Med. Sci., 268:215, 1974.
6. Feldman, J. M., Plonk, J. W., Bivens, C. H., Lebovitz, H. E., and Handwerger, S.: Growth hormone and prolactin secretion in the carcinoid syndrome. J. Med. Sci., 269:333, 1975.
7. Feldman, J. M., Plonk, J. W., Bivens, C. H., and Lebovitz, H. E.: Glucose intolerance in the carcinoid syndrome. J. Am. Diabetes Assoc., 24:664–671, 1975.
8. Fries, J. F., Lindgren, J. A., and Bull, J. M.: Scleroderma-like lesions and the carcinoid syndrome. Arch. Intern. Med., 131:550–553, 1973.
9. Gosset, A., and Masson, P.: Tumeurs endocrines de l'appendice. Presse Méd., 22:237, 1914.
10. Hughes, J. P., Ancalmo, N., Leonard, G. L., and Oschsner, J. L.: Carcinoid tumour of the thymus gland: Report of a case. Thorax, 30:470, 1975.
11. Isler, P., and Hedinger, C.: Mestastasierendes Dünndarmcarcinoid mit schweren, vorwiegend das rechte Herz Betreffenden Klappenfehlern und Pulmonalstenose—ein eigenartiger Symptomenkomplex? Schweiz. Med. Wochenschr., 83:4, 1953.
12. Jouanneau, P., Melafosser, N., Bourreille, J., and Hemet, J.: Segmental necrosing enteritis and carcinoid tumor: The arterial lesions. Chirurgie, 96:756, 1970.
13. Kaplan, E. L., Sizemore, G. W., Peskin, G. W., and Jaffe, B. M.:

Humoral similarities of carcinoid tumors and medullary carcinomas of the thyroid. Surgery, 74:21–29, 1973.

14. Kultschitzky, N.: Zur Frage über den Bau des Darmkanals. Arch. Mikr. Anat., 49:7, 1897.

15. Lembeck, F.: 5-Hydroxytryptamine in carcinoid tumors. Nature, 172:910, 1953.

16. Lubarsch, O.: Uber den primaren Krebs des Ileum nebst Bemerkungen über das gleichzeitige vorkommen von Krebs und Tuberculose. Virchows Arch. Path., 111:281, 1888.

17. Melmon, K., Lovenberg, W., and Sjoersdma, A.: Identification of lysylbradykinin as the peptide formed in vitro by carcinoid tumour kallikrein. Clin. Chim. Acta, 12:292, 1965.

18. Mengel, C. E.: Malignant carcinoid: Effect of parenteral methotrexate (NSC-740) therapy alone and in combination with cyclophosphamide (NSC-26271) orally. Cancer Chemother. Rep., 51:239, 1967.

19. Mengel, C. E., and Lotito, C. A.: A new antiserotonin in the carcinoid syndrome. Arch. Intern. Med., 121:507, 1968.

20. Merling, F.: Anatomie pathologipue de l'appendice due caecum. Expérience, 1:337, 1838.

21. Moertel, C. G., and Dockerty, M. B.: Familial occurrence of metastasizing carcinoid tumors. Ann. Intern. Med., 78:3, 1975.

22. Oates, J. A., and Butler, T. C.: Pharmacologic and endocrine aspects of carcinoid syndrome. Adv. Pharmacol., 5:109, 1967.

23. Oberndorfer, S.: Karzinoide Tumoren des Dunndarms. Frankfurt Z. Path., 1:426, 1907.

24. Pernow, B., and Wladenström, J.: Paroxysmal flushing and other symptoms caused by 5-hydroxytryptamine and histamine in patients with malignant tumours. Lancet, 2:951, 1954.

25. Plonk, J. W., and Feldman, J. M.: Carcinoid arthropathy. Arch. Intern. Med., 134:651, 1974.

26. Rapport, M. M., Green, A. A., and Page, I. H.: Partial purification of the vasoconstrictor in beef serum. J. Biol. Chem., 174:735, 1948.

27. Rosenbaum, F. F., Santer, D. G., and Claudon, D. B.: Essential telangiectasia, pulmonary stenosis and neoplastic liver disease, a possible new clinical syndrome. J. Lab. Clin. Med., 42:941, 1953.

28. Thorson, A. H.: Studies on carcinoid disease. Acta Med. Scand. (Suppl. 334), 161:1, 1958.

29. Trevenen, C., Banerjee, R., and Laughlan, S. C.: The ovarian carcinoid. Cancer, 31:1482, 1973.

30. Wilson, H., Cheek, R. C., Sherman, R. T., and Storer, E. H.: Carcinoid tumors. Curr. Probl. Surg., Nov., 1970.

VIII

MALABSORPTION SYNDROMES

William W. Shingleton, M.D.

Malabsorption may be defined as any disorder with impaired absorption of fat, carbohydrate, protein, vitamins, electrolytes, minerals, and water. This abnormal physiologic state is seen in a wide variety of diseases involving various portions of the gastrointestinal tract.

Kirschner[48] states that knowledge of malabsorption dates to antiquity and he cites pertinent references. Such problems apparently were mentioned in the Ebers Papyrus dating back before the time of Christ. Aretaeus of Cappadocia (A.D. 120–220) may be credited with the earliest account of sprue. William Hillary (1722–1762), a pupil of Boerhaave, published the first account of sprue in the English language. The term "steatorrhea" apparently was first used in 1824 by Kunzmann. Modern understanding of absorption and malabsorption actually dates only to recent decades, as a result of advances in knowledge concerning physicochemical and biochemical processes involved in intestinal absorption and transport. The advent of the electron microscope, the use of radioisotopes, and intestinal biopsy procedures have greatly increased knowledge in the field. The addition of intravenous hyperalimentation to the treatment program of severely malnourished patients has been a notable recent advance.[18] Intestinal digestion and absorption have been discussed previously in the section on small intestinal physiology.

DETECTION OF MALABSORPTION

The major manifestations of malabsorption are weight loss, steatorrhea and diarrhea, anemia, tetany, bone pain and pathologic fractures, bleeding, edema, neuropathy, and glossitis. Though there may be malabsorption of carbohydrate and protein, there is generally a selectively greater defect in fat absorption. Iron-deficiency anemia is quite common in postgastrectomy states and in diffuse disease of the small bowel. Megaloblastic anemia due to vitamin B_{12} malabsorption occurs after gastrectomy, in diffuse small bowel disease, localized to the ileum (regional enteritis, ileal resection), when there is overgrowth of intestinal bacteria (blind loops, diverticula), and in the presence of fish tapeworm *(Diphyllobothrium latum)* infestation.[74] In postgastrectomy states, folic acid deficiency is due more often to decreased intake than to malabsorption. Malabsorption of calcium and vitamin D may lead to the particularly difficult problems of osteomalacia and tetany. Magnesium deficiency may occur and its correction may be necessary in order to permit correction of hypocalcemia. Vitamin K malabsorption leads to hypoprothrombinemia and, when severe, may result in generalized hemorrhagic phenomena. As body protein stores are depleted, hypoalbuminemia develops and may be manifested by peripheral edema and ascites. Peripheral neuropathies are related to folate and vitamin B_{12} malabsorption, while cheilosis and glossitis are related to malabsorption of nicotinic acid and riboflavin. Skin changes may be seen secondary to vitamin A deficiency.

Tests for Malabsorption

Tests for malabsorption are designed to detect the deficiencies that have been outlined. Laboratory tests may be grouped as follows:[74]

1. Screening tests.
   a. Gross inspection of the stool.
   b. Microscopic examination of the stool for fat.

c. Determination of lipid-soluble materials to total dry weight in random stool.

d Serum carotene.

e. Lipiodol absorption test.

f. d-Xylose and other sugar absorption tests.

2. Intake-output balance tests.

a. Fat balance tests.

b. Radioactive tracer balance tests.

c. Nitrogen balance tests.

3. Tests for specific compounds.

a. Schilling test—vitamin B_{12} absorption.

b. Other radioactive compounds—vitamin D, folic acid, iron, calcium, amino acids.

Screening tests will detect the more clinically significant degrees of malabsorption. Microscopic examination of the stool for excessive fat is effective in detecting moderate and severe degrees of steatorrhea. The serum carotene serves as a convenient screening test for malabsorption.[64] Serum carotene levels below 70 μg. usually indicate fat malabsorption or decreased dietary intake.

Lipiodol absorption has been found to be an effective screening test for malabsorption in pediatric patients.[46] Lipiodol, containing 40 per cent iodine, consists of poppyseed oil with the addition of hydriotic acid. The iodine is firmly bound to the unsaturated double bonds of the fat of poppyseed oil and remains bound until after absorption. Then the iodine is split off and excreted in the urine and the degree of recovery of iodine in urine reflects the percentage of fat absorption.

Quantitation of a 5-hour urine collection following oral administration of a 25 gm. dose of d-xylose is a useful screening test for diffuse small bowel disease.[65] Normally, 5 gm. or more should be excreted in the 5-hour collection period.

Intake-output balance tests are the most accurate means available for the diagnosis of malabsorption.[74] Balance tests are useful in confirming malabsorption detected by screening methods and are necessary to establish milder degrees of malabsorption. Chemical measurement of fecal fatty acids in 3- to 5-day stool collections taken while the patient is ingesting a relatively constant intake of mixed fat is a very reliable procedure.

Radioiodinated triolein has been used to investigate intestinal absorption of neutral fat; however, recent studies have emphasized the limitations of these tests utilizing ^{131}I-labeled fats, due to the poor stability of the commercial preparations available.[74]

Several techniques using radioactive macromolecules are available for the quantification of gastrointestinal protein loss. These labeled macromolecules include ^{131}I albumin, ^{131}I PVP, chromium-51 albumin, and copper-67 ceruloplasmin. Techniques utilizing these macromolecules are adequate as screening procedures for detection of protein loss.[82]

Procedures are available to test specifically for malabsorption of iron, calcium, vitamin B_{12}, amino acids, folic acid, pyridoxine, vitamin D, and virtually all compounds that are easily labeled with radioisotopes.[42] Except for the Schilling test (cobalt-57-labeled vitamin B_{12} absorption), these tests are rarely clinically useful.

Radiologic examination of the small intestine following a barium meal is useful in the detection of localized lesions, but it is of limited value as a screening test for diffuse disease.[53] Small bowel biopsy by the peroral route is utilized to investigate malabsorption in selected patients.[65] This procedure has greatly added to the understanding of structural changes associated with malabsorptive states.

DISORDERS ASSOCIATED WITH MALABSORPTION

Many classifications of malabsorption syndromes have been suggested. A useful classification is that of Johnson shown in Table 1. It is seen that malabsorption can be explained by abnormalities in the intestinal lumen, in the mucosal epithelium, or in the intestinal lymphatics. A review of the list of disorders shown in Table 1 indicates that a significant number of the conditions occur in the surgeon's domain, some being cured by operation, others being the sequel to operative removal or rearrangement of parts of the gastrointestinal tract. In the discussion to follow, emphasis will be placed on the disorders seen in surgical patients.

Esophagectomy and Esophagogastrectomy

Absorption studies on patients undergoing esophagectomy or esophagogastrectomy for either benign or malignant disease have been infrequently reported. Two independent studies,[61, 72] involving 30 patients, in which absorption studies were done after esophagogastrectomy, revealed the presence of fat malabsorption of moderate degree. The amount of nitrogen excreted in the stool was only slightly abnormal. Both d-xylose and vitamin B_{12} absorption and a small bowel biopsy were within normal limits. The suggestion was made that the malabsorption of fat seen in patients after esophagectomy or esophagogastrectomy is most likely related to the vagotomy performed as a part of the esophageal resection. The most effective treatment in these patients is the substitution of medium-chain triglycerides for the longer-chain fats ordinarily present in regular food.

Total Gastrectomy

Total gastrectomy commonly leads to rather severe nutritional abnormality as a consequence of loss of gastric storage capacity, inadequate mixing of food with digestive enzymes, loss of intrinsic factor, and interference with iron absorption, resulting in weight loss, steatorrhea, and anemia. Everson[22] collected results of all reported metabolic studies on patients who had undergone total gastric resection from 1897 to 1952, and found that 21 showed defective fat absorption and 14 showed impairment of protein absorption. Special emphasis has been placed on lack of caloric intake in patients after total gastrectomy, related to pain associated with peptic esophagitis or an inadequate food reservoir, or both. Scott and Weidner[69] suggested that the use of a Roux-en-Y esophagojejunostomy would eliminate the esophagitis if the isoperistaltic limb of the jejunum between esophageal and en-

TABLE 1. Classification of Malabsorption Syndromes*

Intraluminal factors	Tropical sprue
Decrease in effective length	Disaccharidase deficiency
Resection of stomach or small bowel	Radiation enteritis
Intestinal fistulization	Drug-induced (neomycin, etc.)
Hypermotility (hyperthyroidism)	Triglyceride enzyme deficiency
Decreased digestive activity	Ground substance
Pancreatic juice	Lymphoma, leukemia
Pancreatitis	Whipple's disease
Carcinoma of pancreas	Regional enteritis
Pancreatectomy	Systemic mast cell disease
Cystic fibrosis	Amyloidosis
Pancreatic duct lithiasis with obstruction	Tuberculosis
Pancreaticocutaneous fistula	Carcinoma, sarcoma
Bile	
Hepatitis	Abnormalities in blood or lymphatic channels
Cirrhosis	Blood
T tube drainage	Arterial or venous insufficiency
Biliary obstruction	Congestive heart failure
Inadequate resorption of bile salts	Vasculitis
Congenital absence of bile salts	Lymphatics
Changes in microorganism population	Intestinal lymphangiectasis
Blind loop	Lymphatic obstruction
Small intestinal diverticula	
Intestinal stasis	Indeterminate
Visceral neuropathy (diabetes mellitus)	Zollinger-Ellison syndrome
Primary neurologic diseases	Malignant carcinoid
Scleroderma	A-beta-lipoproteinemia
Partial obstruction	Protein-losing enteropathy
Oral antibiotics (neomycin)	Pernicious anemia
Giardiasis (also hookworm, whipworm)	Hyperthyroidism
Acute infectious diarrhea	Hypoparathyroidism
Gastric achlorhydria	Pneumatosis cystoides intestinalis
	Hemochromatosis
Changes in intestinal wall	Kwashiorkor
Mucosal epithelial cell	Hypogammaglobulinemia
Celiac disease of childhood	Adrenal-pituitary insufficiency
Glutein-induced enteropathy	Tabes mesenterica

*From Johnson, C. F.: Postgrad. Med., *37*:667, 1965. Copyright © McGraw-Hill, Inc.

teric anastomoses is 16 to 18 cm. in length. Longmire and Beal[4, 54] found that interpolation of an isoperistaltic segment of jejunum between the esophagus and the duodenum accomplished the same purpose. The most popular method of gastrointestinal reconstruction after total gastrectomy, namely, end-to-side gastrojejunostomy with an enteroenterostomy between the ascending and descending limbs, apparently does not protect adequately against the development of esophagitis.

Techniques for construction of pouches for reservoirs as gastric substitutes have been described by various investigators in the past 40 years (Fig. 1). Hoffman,[38] in 1922, suggested the creation of a reservoir by the production of a long enteroenterostomy between the afferent and efferent limbs of the jejunum below the end-to-side esophagojejunostomy. More recently, Hunnicutt[41] has advocated the interposition of an ileocolic segment of the intestine between the esophagus and the duodenum. Interposition of a segment of transverse colon has been used by State and his associates,[75] by Moroney,[60] and by McCorkle and Harper.[58] Experience with most of these procedures has been quite limited, and the results of the procedures are difficult to assess. A procedure for creation of a gastric

substitute pouch, first described by Hunt in 1952, modified by Lawrence, and recently evaluated by Scott, has been advocated (Fig. 2). In this procedure a pouch is created from a double loop of jejunum which is anastomosed side to side just below the esophagojejunostomy stoma. Scott has studied the nutritional state of eight patients in whom this procedure was used, reporting that all are in a good state of nutrition 10 months to 3 years postoperatively. None of these patients, however, has had balance studies of fat and protein absorption.

The incidence of pernicious anemia in persons subjected to total gastrectomy has been recorded as considerably less than the theoretical 100 per cent because of the normally large hepatic reserve of intrinsic factor and the relatively poor survival record (perhaps 3 or 4 years) of most patients. It should be emphasized that a minimum of as little as 1 to 2 cm. of normal fundic mucosa (left behind in cases described as total gastrectomy) could provide sufficient intrinsic factor in man to prevent development of pernicious anemia.[86] Hypochromic anemia has been observed in both humans and dogs following total gastrectomy. Such an anemia usually responds favorably to iron therapy.

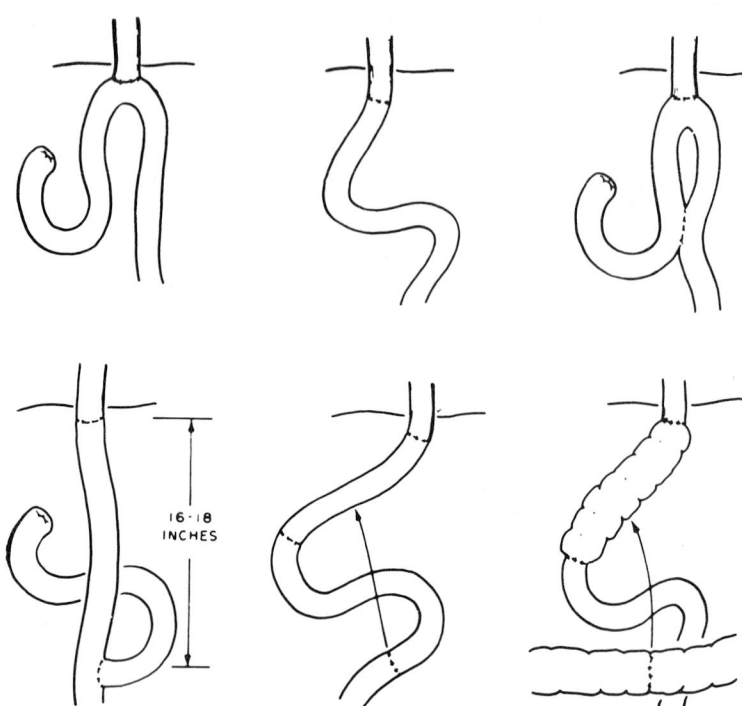

Figure 1. Methods of alimentary tract reconstruction most frequently used after total gastrectomy. (From Scott, H. W., Jr., Gobbel, W. G., Jr., and Law, D. H., IV: Clinical experience with a jejunal pouch [Hunt-Lawrence] as a substitute stomach after total gastrectomy. Surg. Gynecol. Obstet., *121*:1231, Dec., 1965. By permission of Surgery, Gynecology & Obstetrics.)

Partial Gastrectomy

Since the introduction of partial resection of the stomach for control of complicated peptic ulcer disease and gastric carcinoma, there has been a continually growing literature on nutritional disorders seen after these procedures. These operations are generally carried out as partial or subtotal gastrectomy, and the continuity after the gastrectomy is restored by means of anastomosis of the stomach with the duodenum (Billroth I) or with a loop of jejunum (Billroth II). In the Billroth I anastomosis the food passes through the duodenum; in the Billroth II anastomosis the duodenum and part of the jejunum are bypassed by the food, which enters the jejunum directly.

Opinions recorded in the literature are divided on the question of the nutritional state of patients after these two types of anastomoses. All the studies agree that the most common sign of nutritional impairment is loss of weight. In 1954, Zollinger and Ellison[88] reported that of 203 patients studied after various types of partial gastrectomies, 127 were underweight. Two thirds of the Billroth II patients were underweight, as compared with 33 per cent of Billroth I patients. Harkins and Nyhus[34] reported that 74 per cent of patients with Billroth II anastomosis had lost weight, as compared with 42 per cent of those with Billroth I anastomosis.

There has been much debate in the literature concerning the relative importance of inadequate caloric intake versus impaired digestion or absorption (or both) of ingested food in patients after partial gastrectomy. Clinical evidence has been presented that substantiates both points of view. The fact that a variable number of patients remain poorly nourished in spite of an adequate diet suggests the possibility of malabsorption. Metabolic balance studies have shown that patients after partial gastrectomy may show variable degrees of fat and protein loss, above normal, in the stool.[6, 87] Experimental and clinical studies suggest that the degree of malabsorption of fat is greater in patients who have had a Billroth II than in those with a Billroth I type of anastomosis.[21, 45] Several factors that appear significant in the development of malabsorption after gastric surgery are: (1) insufficient gastric digestion, (2) defective stimulation of biliary and

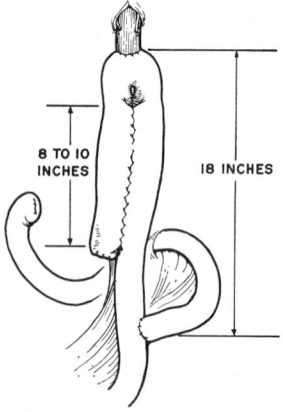

Figure 2. Alimentary reconstruction after total gastrectomy by Hunt-Lawrence jejunal pouch and Roux-en-Y esophagojejunostomy. (From Scott, H. W., Jr., Law, D. H., IV, Gobbel, W. G., Jr., and Sawyers, J. L: Clinical and metabolic studies after total gastrectomy with a Hunt-Lawrence jejunal pouch. Am. J. Surg., *115*:148, Feb., 1968.)

pancreatic secretion, (3) incoordination of gastric emptying with biliary and pancreatic secretion, and (4) rapid intestinal passage. Small bowel biopsy studies carried out by several investigators have shown inconstant and nonspecific histologic changes in mucosa not adequate to explain the changes in function seen in these patients.[42]

The treatment of patients with malnutrition secondary to gastrectomy consists of the administration of a diet high in calories, fat, and protein. The administration of anabolic agents such as testosterone propionate is of value in some patients, since this drug increases appetite as well as bringing about a decrease in protein catabolism. Rare patients in whom severe malnutrition with hypoalbuminemia develops after partial gastrectomy are treated best by intravenous administration of serum albumin. Since the anemia most commonly present in postgastrectomy patients is due to iron deficiency, oral administration of inorganic iron salts is helpful. Refractory cases may require intramuscular iron administration or blood transfusion.

There has been some interest in the use of operative procedures for improvement of the nutrition of patients following subtotal gastrectomy. Conversion of a Billroth II to a Billroth I anastomosis by interposition of a jejunal segment between stomach and duodenum has been the procedure most widely employed (Fig. 3). Except on rare occasions, surgical intervention for

postgastrectomy malnutrition does not appear warranted.

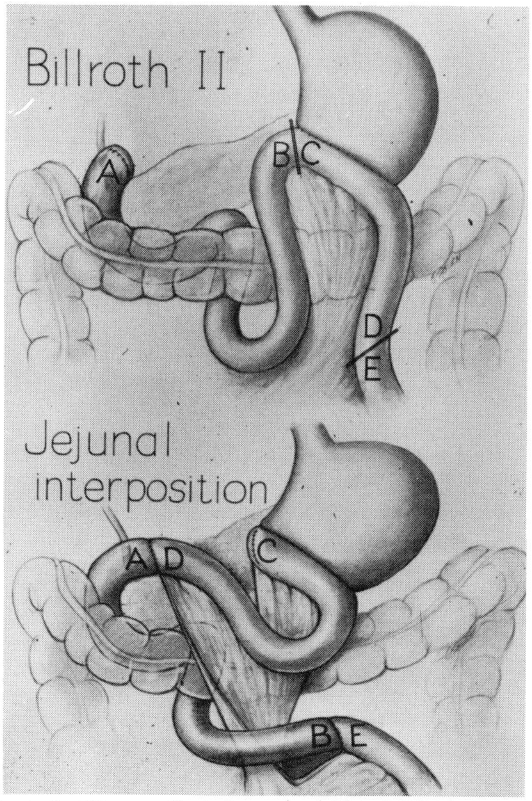

Vagotomy

Vagotomy with a drainage procedure, either pyloroplasty or gastrojejunostomy, is an operation commonly employed at present in the surgical management of patients with peptic ulcer. An operative procedure that employs vagotomy with limited gastric resection (antrectomy) is also being used in the treatment of peptic ulcer disease. Another variant is the use of selective vagotomy rather than truncal vagotomy, combined with a gastric drainage procedure.

When vagotomy is combined with a drainage procedure, or with partial resection of the stomach, it becomes very difficult to determine which particular aspect of the operation contributes most to the nutritional problems that may occur after this type of surgery. Experimental studies have indicated that vagal denervation alters to some degree the normal physiology of the stomach, pancreas, biliary system, and small bowel.[2, 3, 32, 36] Pyloroplasty or gastroenterostomy may also cause some disturbance in these organs. When one combines vagotomy with resection of a part of the stomach, then the derangement may be a combination of vagal denervation, decrease in storage capacity of the stomach, and the creation of gastroenterostomy.

The cause of the diarrhea occurring after vagotomy has not been established; some relate it to increased stasis of food in the stomach and small bowel, resulting in periodic bacterial overgrowth. The reported incidence of diarrhea following vagotomy varies from 28 to 68 per cent.[7, 24, 35, 49] Fox and Grimson[29] reported fecal fat studies in nine patients following vagus resection without a drainage procedure. Eight of the nine patients showed excess excretion of fat. Shingleton[73] reported that the amount of excess fat excreted in the stool was less after vagotomy and drainage than after partial gastrectomy with Billroth II anastomosis. Further, weight loss following vagotomy with gastroenterostomy was found to be less severe than that following partial gastrectomy. There seems to be no difference between fecal fat levels after truncal vagotomy and selective vagotomy.[55] To date, there are insufficient clinical observations and metabolic studies to assess accurately the nutritional effects of the combined procedure of truncal vagotomy with antrectomy, although Scott[68] has reported that 604 of 715 patients who have undergone antrectomy with truncal vagotomy have maintained their ideal weight as determined by a standard height, age, and weight chart.

Pancreatic Insufficiency

The pancreas, like the liver, is an organ with a large functional reserve. In many patients with various types of pancreatic disease, malabsorption may not be present. However, advanced inflammatory pancreatic disease is a well-established cause of malabsorption. Chronic pancreatic insufficiency may be the end result of chronic relapsing pancreatitis, cystic fibrosis of the pancreas, and tumors, either primary or metastatic. Pancreatic insufficiency also may be associated with pancreatic fistulas resulting from disease or trauma.

Figure 3. Diagram illustrating conversion of Billroth II anastomosis to the jejunal interposition of Henley. (From Wirts, C. W., et al.: Gastroenterology, 49:141, 1965.)

Resection of a major portion of the pancreas or ligation of its duct in conjunction with partial pancreatectomy may result in pancreatic insufficiency.

The diagnosis of pancreatic insufficiency is usually not difficult. Diabetes, pancreatic calcification, and a normal d-xylose absorption test in the presence of steatorrhea suggest pancreatic insufficiency. Patients may give a history of trauma to or operations on the pancreas. Demonstration of depressed pancreatic secretion provides evidence for some form of pancreatic disease. The "secretin test" is the most reliable of these procedures. This method utilizes intravenous secretin as a stimulus, and a timed sample of duodenal juice is obtained through an indwelling gastroduodenal tube, before and after stimulation. The alteration of the secretin response in pancreatic tumors depends upon the degree and site of pancreatic duct obstruction. The greatest abnormalities are seen in the advanced, diffuse lesions, and in tumors that involve the head of the pancreas. Serum calcium determination is indicated in pancreatic disease, since calcium metabolism may be disturbed.

In general, the treatment regimen for patients with various disorders of the pancreas leading to malabsorption and malnutrition will depend upon the nature of the underlying disease process. In the case of children with cystic fibrosis of the pancreas, replacement therapy with pancreatic enzymes offers the most helpful type of management. Patients who have chronic relapsing pancreatitis with severe malabsorption are also greatly benefited by the proper administration of a pancreatic enzyme preparation, such as Viokase or Cotazym.[52] However, if the patient with chronic relapsing pancreatitis is having recurring attacks of pain that may require surgical intervention, the performance of a procedure to decompress the dilated obstructed pancreatic duct may result in improvement of absorption, since pancreatic enzymes can be rerouted into a segment of the intestinal tract. In those patients in whom there is loss of pancreatic juice by external pancreatic fistula, malabsorption will improve following implantation of the fistulous tract into a segment of the intestine. For patients who have a tumor in the head of the pancreas that occludes the major pancreatic duct, resection of the tumor with reimplantation of the pancreatic duct into the upper small bowel may result in satisfactory digestion and absorption of protein and fat. In case of islet cell tumors producing hypersecretion of acid (Zollinger-Ellison syndrome) with malnutrition and diarrhea, excision of the tumor and total gastrectomy is the current procedure of choice.

Total pancreatectomy, although an infrequently used procedure for advanced inflammatory neoplastic disease of the pancreas, produces both diabetes and malabsorption. Although insulin requirements are not high in these patients, control of the diabetes may be difficult. Steatorrhea and malnutrition are best managed by use of pancreatic enzyme substitution therapy.

Biliary Tract Disease

Hepatobiliary diseases may cause malabsorptive states through two mechanisms: (1) the absence of adequate amounts of bile in the intestinal tract, and (2) the hepatic disease itself.[70] Thus, steatorrhea has been described in patients suffering from acute bile hepatitis,[33] chronic intrahepatic cholestasis,[71] chronic extrahepatic obstructive jaundice,[1] and cirrhosis of the liver.[76] Physiologic and biochemical studies have shown that fat absorption requires conjugated bile salts.[42] This is true not only for micelle formation in the intestinal lumen but also for the activation of pancreatic lipase and the normal metabolism of intestinal epithelial cells.[39, 40] Thus, the steatorrhea resulting from liver or biliary tract disease may be due to a decrease in bile acid secretion, either through impaired synthesis or through abnormalities in which normal bile salt conjugates are not excreted. The frequency of bone disease in patients with chronic intrahepatic cholestasis indicates a disturbance of calcium metabolism.[76] Bone changes may be those of both osteoporosis and osteomalacia.[1] It is presumed that the clinical abnormalities result from both malabsorption of vitamin D and calcium loss in the stools.

Treatment of patients with obstructive jaundice, whether it is caused by bile duct obstruction or acute cholestasis, often calls for parenteral administration of vitamin K. In patients with chronic cholestasis, prophylactic therapy with fat-soluble vitamins A, D, and K and calcium salts is advocated.[71] Diarrhea may be controlled by reduction in fat intake, which may also reduce the losses of fat-soluble vitamins and calcium in the stools. Whenever obstructive jaundice is present, surgical intervention is indicated in order to re-establish bile flow into the intestinal tract. In patients with biliary fistulas, bile collected from the fistula can be placed back into the gastrointestinal tract through a stomach tube as a temporary measure until the fistula closes spontaneously or is closed operatively.

Small Bowel Resection

Small bowel resection is commonly employed in treatment of small bowel diseases, including regional enteritis, small bowel tumors, gangrene of bowel due to intestinal obstruction or vascular occlusion, ulceration, and infiltrating lesions.

Experimental studies on dogs have revealed that animals can be deprived of 50 to 70 per cent of their small intestine and maintain a near-normal nutritional state.[50] Clatworthy et al.[11] have reported on the effect of extensive intestinal resection on growth of newborn dogs and found that there was no difference in subsequent growth with sacrifice of comparable lengths of proximal, middle, or distal small intestine. Ileal resection in man often leads to diarrhea with or without steatorrhea, due to failure of reabsorption of bile salts in the small bowel. Cholestyramine, which binds the bile salts, may be very effective treatment.[53]

There have been several reports suggesting that man may survive the sacrifice of large segments of small intestine.[9, 37, 59, 79, 83] Most massive resections are performed as emergency or semiemergency procedures on critically ill patients, and the operative mortality is high. The morbidity in those surviving the initial operation is likewise high; the primary problem is maintenance of adequate nutrition. One of the interesting side-effects of massive small bowel resection is the experimental and clinical observation that a marked gastric hypersecretion of acid may develop in these patients.[30] This complication of massive small bowel resection may require a surgical procedure such as vagotomy to control the gastric hypersecretion.

The treatment of patients with extensive resection of the small intestine requires careful observation and management. Since large quantities of calories are lost by failure of absorption, these patients are given a diet high in calories, protein, fat, and carbohydrate and supplements of iron and vitamins. One of the most beneficial recent advances in management of patients with malnutrition secondary to massive bowel resection has been the use of long-term intravenous alimentation to allow the residual intestine to hypertrophy and gain greater absorptive surface.[83]

The major surgical effort in management of patients with massive resection of the small intestine has been an attempt to slow down transit time by reversing short loops of remaining small bowel in an antiperistaltic fashion. It has been used only occasionally in patients.[31, 78] The procedure requires further evaluation before its clinical usefulness can be determined.

Blind Loop Syndrome

Although the term "blind loop syndrome" was originally used to describe the complications of blind loops of the small intestine that resulted from surgery, there are many other conditions that give rise to this symptom complex, such as stricture of the intestine, diverticula, and other types of blind pouch formation, all of which have in common stasis and subsequent infection. This disorder is uncommon and is becoming even less common. The syndrome is characterized by diarrhea, steatorrhea, anemia, loss of weight, abdominal pain, and multiple vitamin deficiencies. Involvement of the central nervous system may also occur.

The diagnosis of the syndrome should be confirmed by a Schilling test, which should reveal a pernicious anemia-like urinary excretion of vitamin B_{12} (0 to 6 per cent compared to the normal 7 to 25 per cent).[63] When the test is repeated with the addition of intrinsic factor, there is no increase in uptake, as will occur in true pernicious anemia. Tetracycline is then given in a dosage of 2 gm. daily for 3 to 5 days; in the blind loop syndrome the Schilling test should return to normal or near-normal levels.

The hematologic aspect of the intestinal stagnation syndrome revolves chiefly around the picture of vitamin B_{12} deficiency, although it is possible that folic acid deficiency may be a complicating factor. There are two main hypotheses that attempt to explain the development of the vitamin B_{12} deficiency.[20] One school of thought supports the contention that the bacteria in the stagnant area utilize vitamin B_{12} and render it unavailable for absorption.[83, 85] The other school suggests that the bacteria produce a toxin that inhibits the absorptive process by interfering with enzymatic transfer across the small bowel mucosa.[17, 23]

The importance of steatorrhea in patients with blind loop syndrome has been the subject of a good deal of discussion. Recent evidence has been presented to suggest that the bacteria present in the small intestine in the blind loop syndrome bring about structural alterations of bile salts that interfere with absorption of fat.[47]

Treatment of patients with blind loop syndrome involves two principles of therapy. First, the symptoms of the condition can be controlled temporarily by the administration of antibiotics; second, the cure of the condition requires surgical correction of the cause of the underlying small intestinal stasis.

Miscellaneous Small Bowel Lesions of Surgical Interest

Regional enteritis and granulomatous ileocolitis often cause a multiplicity of absorptive defects, including malabsorption of protein, fat, vitamin B_{12}, and iron.[5]

Radiation enteritis, and tuberculosis may cause malabsorption as a result of intrinsic involvement of bowel wall or lymphatics or stasis due to partial obstruction. Resection of involved segments may be required. Vascular occlusive lesions (atherosclerosis, periarteritis, lupus erythematosus) may rarely lead to malabsorption and may require surgical therapy. Intravenous or oral hyperalimentation in the pre- and postoperative period in these patients is a most helpful therapeutic measure. Intestinal lymphangiectasis and intestinal lymphatic obstruction due to tumor or infection are rare causes of malabsorption.

Other Diseases and Disorders Producing Malabsorption

A variety of primary and secondary medical diseases may be associated with malabsorption, as shown in Table 1. The reader is referred to one of the several excellent review articles on malabsorption for a discussion of these disorders.[27, 43, 48]

SELECTED REFERENCES

Floch, M. H.: Recent contributions in intestinal absorption and malabsorption. Am. J. Clin. Nutr., 22:327, 1969.
This is a review article in depth by a gastroenterologist who concentrates his attention on new areas of research in the wide field of absorption and malabsorption. The article has 205 references, thus presenting the reader with an extensive bibliography for review of all aspects of the problem of malabsorption. This is an excellent review by one who has had a long-standing interest in this field of gastrointestinal disease.

French, A. B., Cook, H. B., and Pollard, H. M.: Nutritional problems after gastrointestinal surgery. Med. Clin. North Am., 53:1389, 1969.
This article, written by gastroenterologists, presents a more detailed analysis of the nutritional problems seen after operations on the gastrointestinal tract. The authors classify various disorders, discuss the multiple etiologic factors and pathophysiologic mechanisms leading to malnutrition after surgery, and recommend therapeutic management based on a careful analysis of the problems presented by each individual patient.

Kirschner, J. B.: Clinical observations on malabsorption. Med. Clin. North Am., 53:1169, 1969.
This is a review article in the general field of malabsorption, both medical and surgical, presented by one of the leaders in the field of gastroenterology. The author presents observations on the wide variety of clinical problems encountered in patients. The article contains an excellent section on the differential diagnosis of the various malabsorption disorders and includes up-to-date information on the latest methods of management.

Losowsky, M. S., Walker, B. E., and Kelleher, J.: Malabsorption in Clinical Practice. London, Churchill-Livingstone, 1974.
This monograph is an extensive review of basic and clinical features of the commonly recognized malabsorption syndromes. There

are excellent references included for each syndrome described. The volume is an in-depth review as well as a practical guide in patient management.

Shingleton, W. W., and Dobbins, W. O.: Malabsorption Syndromes. Springfield, Ill., Charles C Thomas, Publisher, 1968.
This monograph is written by a surgeon and a gastroenterologist. It provides information regarding the anatomy, biochemistry, and physiology of absorption, followed by a discussion of the digestion and absorption of the various constituents in the diet. The methods of the demonstration of malabsorption of nutrients are well described. The emphasis of the monograph is on fat absorption and malabsorption; the authors review the world literature on the problem.

REFERENCES

1. Atkinson, M., Nordin, B. E. C., and Sherlock, S.: Malabsorption and bone disease in prolonged obstructive jaundice. J. Med., 25:299, 1956.
2. Baldwin, J. N., Albo, R., Jaffe, B., and Silen, W.: Metabolic effects of selective and total vagotomy. Surg. Gynecol. Obstet., 120:777, 1965.
3. Ballinger, W. F., II, Christy, M. G., and Ashby, W. B.: Autotransplantation of the small intestine; the effect of denervation. Surgery, 52:151, 1962.
4. Beal, J. M., Briggs, J. D., and Longmire, W. P., Jr.: Use of a jejunal segment to replace the stomach after total gastrectomy. Am. J. Surg., 88:194, 1954.
5. Beeken, W. L.: Remedial defects in Crohn's disease. Arch. Int. Med., 135:686–690, 1975.
6. Bohmansson, G.: Studien über die chirurgische Behandlung von Gastroduodenalschwuren mit besonderer Berucksichtigung der Operationsanatomie und der postoperativen Digestionsphysiologie nebst einem Beitrag dur Frage der chirurgischen Behandlung akuter Ulcusblutungen. Acta Chir. Scand., 7, 1926.
7. Burge, C. E., Hutchison, J. S. F., Longland, C. J., McLennan, I., and Miln, D. C.: Selective vagotomy in the prevention of postvagotomy diarrhea. Lancet, 2:897, 1961.
8. Carter, C. W., Coxon, R. V., Parsons, D. S., and Thompson, R. H. S.: Biochemistry in Relation to Medicine. London, Longmans, Green and Co., 1959.
9. Cattel, R. B.: Massive resection of the small intestine. Lahey Clin. Bull., 4:167, 1945.
10. Clarkson, T. W., Rothstein, A., and Cross, A.: Transport of monovalent anions by isolated small intestine in the rat. Am. J. Physiol., 200:781, 1961.
11. Clatworthy, H. W., Jr., Saleeby, R., and Lovinggood, C.: Extensive small bowel resection in young dogs: Its effect on growth and development. An experimental study. Surgery, 32:341, 1952.
12. Davenport, H. W.: Physiology of the Digestive Tract, 2nd ed. Chicago, Year Book Medical Publishers, 1966.
13. Dobbins, W. O., III: The intestinal mucosal lymphatic in man. A light and electron microscopic study. Gastroenterology, 51:994, 1966.
14. Dobbins, W. O., III: Electron microscopy of intestinal fat absorption under normal conditions and in malabsorptive states. In Glass, G. B. J. (Ed.): Progress in Gastroenterology. New York, Grune & Stratton, 1967.
15. Doig, A., and Girdwood, R. H.: The absorption of folic acid and labelled cyanocobalamin in intestinal malabsorption. Q. J. Med., 29:333, 1960.
16. Donaldson, R. M., Jr.: Malabsorption of CO 60-labeled cyanocobalamin in rats with intestinal diverticula. I. Evaluation of possible mechanisms. Gastroenterology, 43:271, 1962.
17. Drexler, J.: Effect of indole compounds on vitamin B_{12} utilization. Blood, 13:239, 1958.
18. Dudrick, S. J.: Historical perspectives in intravenous hyperalimentation. In Winters, R. W., and Hasselmeyer, E. G. (Eds.): Intravenous Nutrition in the High Risk Infant. New York, John Wiley and Sons, 1975, pp. 7–31.
19. Eichholz, A., and Crane, R. K.: Studies on the organization of the brush border in intestinal epithelial cells. J. Cell Biol., 26:687, 1965.
20. Ellis, H., and Smith, A. D. M.: The blind loop syndrome. Westminster Hosp. Bull. (London). Monographs in Surgical Sciences, 4:193, 1967.

21. Ellison, E. H.: Nutritional problems following gastrectomy. Surg. Clin. North Am., 35:1683, 1955.
22. Everson, T. C.: Nutrition following total gastrectomy with particular reference to fat and protein assimilation. Surg. Gynecol. Obstet., 95:209, 1952.
23. Faber, K. I.: Perniciose anamie bei Dundarmstricturen. Lin. Wochenschr., 34:643, 1897.
24. Farris, J. M., and Smith, G. K.: Vagotomy and pyloroplasty for bleeding duodenal ulcer. Am. J. Surg., 105:388, 1963.
25. Fletcher, R. F., Henly, A. A., Sammons, H. G., and Squire, J. R.: Case of magnesium deficiency following massive intestinal resection. Lancet, 1:522, 1960.
26. Flink, E. B., McCollister, R., Prasad, A. S., Melby, J. C., and Doe, R. P.: Evidences for clinical magnesium deficiency. Ann. Intern. Med., 47:956, 1957.
27. Floch, M. H.: Recent contributions in intestinal absorption and malabsorption. Am. J. Clin. Nutr., 22:327, 1969.
28. Fordtran, J. S., and Dietschy, J.: Water and electrolyte movement in the intestine. Gastroenterology, 50:263, 1966.
29. Fox, J., and Grimson, K. S.: Defective fat absorption following vagotomy. J. Lab. Clin. Med., 35:362, 1950.
30. Frederick, P. L., Sizer, J. S., and Osborne, M. P.: Relation of massive bowel resection to gastric secretion. N. Engl. J. Med., 272:509, 1965.
31. Gibson, L. D., Carter, R., and Hinshaw, D. B.: Segmental reversal of small intestine after massive bowel resection. J.A.M.A., 182:952, 1962.
32. Griffith, C. A., and Harkins, H. N.: Partial gastric vagotomy; an experimental study. Gastroenterology, 32:96, 1957.
33. Gross, J. B., Comfort, M. W., Wollaeger, E. E., and Power, M. H.: Total solids, fat, and nitrogen in the feces. V. A study of patients with primary parenchymatous hepatic disease. Gastroenterology, 16:140, 1950.
34. Harkins, H. N., and Nyhus, L. M.: A comparison of the Billroth I and Billroth II procedures; clinical and experimental studies. Bull. Soc. Int. Chir., 15:111, 1956.
35. Harkins, H. N., Stavney, L. S., Griffith, C. A., Savage, L. E., Kato, T., and Nyhus, L. M.: Selective gastric vagotomy. Ann. Surg., 158:448, 1963.
36. Hayama, T., Magee, D. F., and White, T. T.: Influence of autonomic nerves on the daily secretion of pancreatic juice in dogs. Ann. Surg., 158:290, 1963.
37. Haymond, H. E.: Massive resection of the small intestine: An analysis of 257 collected cases. Surg. Gynecol. Obstet., 61:693, 1935.
38. Hoffman, V.: Eine methode des plastischen magenersatzes. Z. Chir., 49:1477, 1922.
39. Hofman, A. F., and Borgstrom, B.: Physico-chemical state of lipids in intestinal content during their digestion and absorption. Fed. Proc., 21:43, 1962.
40. Holt, P. R., Haessler, H. A., and Isselbacher, K. J.: Effects of bile salts on glucose metabolism by slices of hamster small intestine. J. Clin. Invest., 42:777, 1963.
41. Hunnicutt, A. J.: Total gastrectomy for Ca; a new procedure. Bull. Alameida County Med. Assoc., 5:16, 1949.
42. Jefferies, G. H., Weser, E., and Sleisenger, M. H.: Malabsorption. Gastroenterology, 46:434, 1964.
43. Jeffries, G. H., Weser, E., and Sleisenger, M. H.: Progress in gastroenterology. Gastroenterology, 56:777, 1969.
44. Jenenius, H.: Results of experimental resections of the small intestine in dogs. Copenhagen, NYT Nordisk Forlag, Arnold Busck, 1945.
45. Johnson, A. H., Goldman, P., Davis, C., Harper, H. A., McCorkle, H. J., and Gardner, R. E.: An experimental study of the nutrition of animals following gastrectomy. Surg. Forum, 1952, p. 40.
46. Jones, W. O., and Di Sant'Agnese, P. A.: Laboratory aids in the diagnosis of malabsorption in pediatrics. J. Pediatr., 62:44, 1963.
47. Kim, Y. S., Spritz, N., Blum, M., Terz, J., and Sherlock, P.: The role of altered bile and metabolism in the steatorrhea of experimental blind loop. J. Clin. Invest., 45:956, 1966.
48. Kirschner, J. B.: Clinical observations on malabsorption. Med. Clin. North Am., 53:1169, 1969.
49. Kraft, R. O., Fry, W. J., and Ransom, H. K.: Selective gastric vagotomy. Arch. Surg., 85:687, 1962.
50. Kremen, A. J., Linner, J. H., and Nelson, C. H.: An experimental evaluation of the nutritional importance of proximal and distal small intestine. Ann. Surg., 140:439, 1954.

51. Laster, L., and Inglefinger, F. J.: Intestinal absorption—aspects of structure, function, and diseases of the small-intestine mucosa. N. Engl. J. Med., 264:1138, 1192, 1246, 1961.

52. Law, D. H.: Medium chain triglyceride therapy of malabsorption. Clin. Res., 14:48, 1966.

53. Laws, J. W., Shawdon, H., Booth, C. C., and Stewart, J. S.: Correlation of radiological and histological findings in idiopathic steatorrhea. Br. Med. J., 1:1311, 1963.

54. Longmire, W. P., Jr., and Beal, J. M.: Construction of a substitute gastric reservoir following total gastrectomy. Ann. Surg., 135:637, 1952.

55. Losowsky, M. S., Walker, B. E., and Kelleher, J.: Malabsorption in Clinical Practice. London, Churchill-Livingstone, 1974, p. 191.

56. Lubran, M., and McAllen, P. M.: Potassium deficiency in ulcerative colitis. Q. J. Med., 20:221, 1951.

57. MacIntyre, I., Hanna, S., Booth, C. C., and Read, A. E.: Intracellular magnesium deficiency in man. Clin. Sci., 20:07, 1961.

58. McCorkle, H. J., and Harper, H. A.: The problem of nutrition following complete gastrectomy. Ann. Surg., 140:467, 1954.

59. Meyer, H. W.: Acute superior artery thrombosis: Recovery following extensive resection of the large and small intestine. Arch. Surg., 53:298, 1946.

60. Moroney, J.: Colonic replacement and restoration of the human stomach. Ann. R. Coll. Surg. Eng., 12:328, 1953.

61. Phillips, D. F., Wollaeger, E. E., Ellis, F. H., Jr., and Power, M. H.: Fecal excretion of fat and nitrogen after esophagogastrectomy in man. Surgery, 49:433, 1961.

62. Reifenstein, E. C., Jr.: Disease of the parathyroid glands. In Williams, R. H. (Ed.): Textbook of Endocrinology, 2nd ed. Philadelphia, W. B. Saunders Company, 1955.

63. Reilly, R. W., and Kirsner, B.: The blind loop syndrome. Gastroenterology, 37:491, 1959.

64. Ross, G., and Parker, J. G.: Serum carotene concentration in normal individuals and its clinical interpretation. N.Y. J. Med., 62:3584, 1962.

65. Rubin, C. E., and Dobbins, W. O., III: Peroral biopsy of the small intestine. A review of its diagnostic usefulness. Gastroenterology, 49:676, 1965.

66. Schachter, D., and Rosen, S. M.: Active transport of Ca 45 by the small intestine and its dependence on vitamin D. Am. J. Physiol., 196:357, 1959.

67. Schultz, S. G., and Zolusky, R.: Inter-actions between sodium transport and active amino acid transport in isolated rabbit ileum. Nature, 205:292, 19659

68. Scott, H. W., Jr., Herrington, J. L., Jr., Edwards, L. W., Shull, H. J., Stephenson, S. E., Jr., Sawyers, J. L., and Classen, K. L.: Results of vagotomy and antral resection in surgical treatment of duodenal ulcer. Gastroenterology, 39:590, 1960.

69. Scott, H. W., Jr., and Weidner, M. G.: Total gastrectomy with Roux-en-Y esophagojejunostomy in treatment of gastric cancer. Ann. Surg., 143:682, 1956.

70. Sheehy, T. W., and Floch, M. H.: The Small Intestine: Its Function and Disease. New York, Hoeber Medical Division, Harper & Row, 1964.

71. Sherlock, S.: Primary biliary cirrhosis (chronic intrahepatic obstructive jaundice). Gastroenterology, 37:574, 1959.

72. Shils, M. E., and Gilat, T.: The effect of esophagectomy on absorption in man: Clinical and metabolic observations. Gastroenterology, 50:347, 1966.

73. Shingleton, W. W., Baylin, G. J., Isley, J. K., Sanders, A. P., and Ruffin, J. M.: A study of fat absorption after gastric surgery using I-131 labeled fat. Ann. Surg., 144:433, 1956.

74. Shingleton, W. W., and Dobbins, W. O., III: Malabsorption Syndromes. Springfield, Ill., Charles C Thomas, Publisher, 1968.

75. State, D., Barclay, T., and Kelley, W. D.: Total gastrectomy with utilization of a segment of transverse colon to replace the excised stomach. Ann. Surg., 134:1035, 1951.

76. Summerskill, W. H. J., and Moertel, C. G.: Malabsorption syndrome associated with anicteric liver disease. Gastroenterology, 43:380, 1962.

77. Thomas, J. E.: Secretion and absorption in the intestine. In Best, C. H., and Taylor, N. B., (Eds.): The Physiological Basis of Medical Practice, 7th ed. Baltimore, Williams & Wilkins, 1961.

78. Thomas, J. E., and Jordan, G. L., Jr.: Massive resection of small bowel and total colectomy: Use of reversed segment. Arch. Surg., 90:781, 1965.

79. Todd, W. R., Ditterbrandt, M., Montague, J. R., and West, E. I.: Digestion and absorption in a man with all but three feet of small intestine removed surgically. Am. J. Dig. Dis., 7:295, 1940.

80. Tuna, N., Mangold, H. K., and Mosser, D. G.: Re-evaluation of the I-131 triolein absorption test. J. Lab. Clin. Med., 61:620, 1963.

81. Verzar, F., and McDougall, E. J.: Absorption from the Intestine. New York, Longmans, Green and Co., 1936.

82. Waldmann, T. A.: Protein-losing enteropathy. Gastroenterology, 50:422, 1966.

83. Wecklesser, E. C., Chinn, A. B., Scott, M. W., and Price, J. W.: Extensive resection of the small intestine. Am. J. Surg., 78:706, 1949.

84. Williams, D. W., and Dudrick, S. J.: Growth and development of an infant receiving nutrients exclusively by vein. J.A.M.A., 203:860, 1968.

85. Wilson, T. H.: Intestinal Absorption. Philadelphia, W. B. Saunders Company, 1962.

86. Wiseman, G.: Absorption from the Intestine. New York, Academic Press, 1964.

87. Wollaeger, E. E., Comfort, M. W., Weier, J. F., and Osterberg, A. E.: The total solids, fat and nitrogen in the feces. 2. A study of persons who had undergone partial gastrectomy with anastomosis of the entire cut end of the stomach and the jejunum (Polya anastomosis). Gastroenterology, 6:93, 1946.

88. Zollinger, R. M., and Ellison, E. H.: Nutrition after gastric operations. J.A.M.A., 154:811, 1954.

IX

RADIATION INJURY TO THE INTESTINE

Jerome J. DeCosse, M.D., Ph.D.

THE BIOLOGIC BASIS OF RADIATION INJURY

The fundamental biologic effect of radiation begins by excitation and ionization of molecules within cells. In terms of energy deposited within the cell, ionizing radiation is by far the most potent of all chemical or physical agents. For example, a total-body radiation dose of 500 rads would be lethal to most humans and yet the heat input would result in a temperature rise of only 0.001° C. Since discovery of x-rays by Röntgen in 1895, various types of ionizing radiation have evolved (Table 1). Forms of direct external ionizing radiation in use today include alpha (α) particles result-

TABLE 1.   Types of Ionizing Radiation

Type	Description
Alpha particle	Helium nucleus
Beta particle	Negative electron
Positron	Positive electron
Proton	Hydrogen nuclei
Neutron	Neutron
Gamma rays	Electromagnetic radiation
X-rays	Electromagnetic radiation

ing from radioactive decay of heavy atoms, beta (β) particles produced by radioactive decay and betatrons, protons from van de Graaff generators and cyclotrons, heavy nuclei, and neutrons. In addition, gamma rays and x-rays, which have neither mass nor charge, indirectly delivery photons or quantums of energy to the cell. Ionizing radiation may be administered by a variety of external sources, by direct application to the tumor as with radium, and by intravenous or intracavitary insertion as with radioisotopes.

Different amounts of energy are lost by various types of ionizing radiations as they pass through a given tissue over a fixed distance; that is, they are different in their linear energy transfer (LET).[6] Highly penetrating radiations such as gamma rays have a relatively low LET; that is, energy dissipation occurs over a long distance. In the case of radiation of relatively low penetration, such as alpha particles, the LET and ion concentration are relatively high at the end of their path. Beta particles and x-rays are intermediate in this respect.

The LET describes the energy liberated or released along the path of ionizing radiation. It is only the energy absorbed in a biologic system that will produce an effect. The absorbed dose is measured by the rad, which is defined as 100 ergs, or 10^{12} primary ionizations, per gram of absorbed energy in any medium from any type of ionizing radiation. The rad is less restrictive and more meaningful than the roentgen (R), which is a unit of exposure dose for x-rays and gamma rays only and is defined as the amount of radiation required to liberate 1 electrostatic unit in 0.001293 gm. of air. The important measurement is not the ionizing radiation delivered in air but the amount absorbed in the tumor-bearing target tissue. Different kinds of radiation have different biologic effectiveness, which depends not only upon the LET but also upon the dose rate and upon whether the dose is given all at once or in fractions. In addition, the continued development of electrical generators, dosimetry, filtration devices, field rotations, and other modern innovations further enhances the flexibility as well as the precision of therapeutic irradiation.

Regardless of variable physical factors for different kinds of ionizing radiation, the primary cellular effect can be regarded as identical. Energy is transferred by random collision within the cell, generating a series of biochemical events. Either directly or indirectly, through formation of free radicals derived from cellular water, macromolecular damage occurs. Probably

DNA is the critical molecule most sensitive to injury. Sublethal injury may generate repair mechanisms that lead to recovery. Lethal injury usually results in prompt death from mitotic arrest, or death may be preceded by a temporary nonmitotic period of cellular growth; hence the clinical experience that a tumor may not show a favorable response until a week or two has passed after radiation therapy was initiated.

In addition to acute cellular effects, the classic work of Muller demonstrated clearly that any kind of ionizing radiation can induce true point mutations with breakage and rearrangement of chromosomes[3] (Fig. 1). These effects of radiation, a linear function of dose, are persistent and cumulative over long periods of time.

There is considerable variation in the sensitivity of different kinds of cells to ionizing radiation. In general, those normal cells that have renewal systems, that is, proliferating cells, have the greatest sensitivity. Hence hematopoietic cells, the epithelium of the gastrointestinal tract, and reproductive cells have the greatest sensitivity to radiation and, accordingly, the greatest risk for injury. Static cell populations, such as nerve cells, are relatively resistant to radiation. Curiously, cells with renewal systems are the site of most human cancers.

Tissue and whole-organ effects depend upon age, sex, temperature, oxygenation, metabolic activity, weight, stress, species variation, and other variables. The effect on tissues results primarily from cellular injury, but radiation damage to the fine vasculature and interstitial connective tissue and resulting progressive changes are probably instrumental in the production of chronic or delayed lesions in tissues of all kinds. A result of ionizing radiation is a vasculitis that may be unrelenting and independent of the relative radiosensitivity of parenchymal cells. Blood supply to the irradiated tissue may be progressively depleted by subendothelial proliferation and by medial thickening[1] (Fig. 2). In addition, interstitial collagen deposition may result in severe scarring and further obliterate blood flow. Tissue hypoxia and, sometimes, necrosis are the consequences. Infection or diffuse trauma of irradiated organs is often a precipitating factor in de-

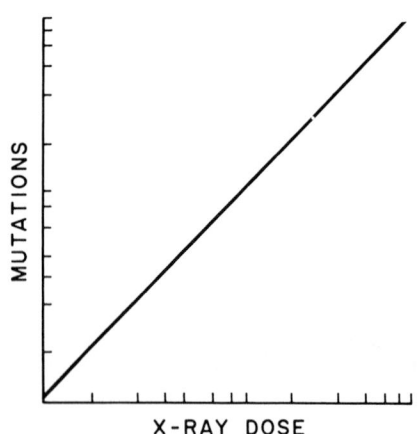

Figure 1. The frequency of mutations in Drosophila spermatozoa relates directly to the intensity of radiation administered.

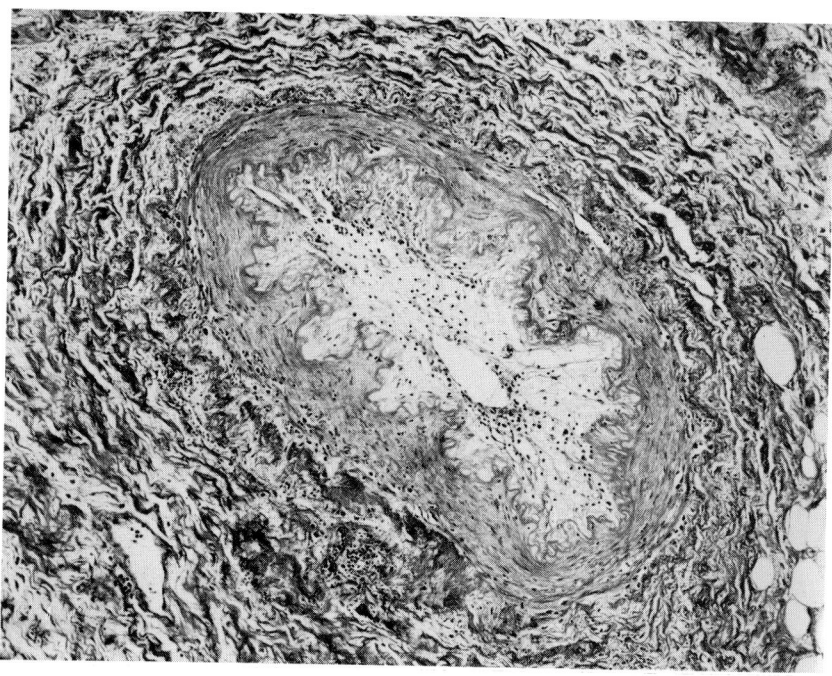

Figure 2. Photomicrograph ($\times$ 80) of an ileal arteriole demonstrating occlusive radiation vasculitis and surrounding perivascular fibrosis, findings characteristic of chronic radiation injury.

layed radiation necrosis of such organs. Repair is inhibited by a fibrotic barrier to revascularization.

Radiation therapy is the primary method of management in some forms of curable cancer such as squamous carcinoma of the cervix, lymphoma, Hodgkin's disease, carcinoma of the intrinsic larynx, and seminoma of the testis. Radiation therapy complements surgery or is an alternative form of therapy in curable tumors at other sites, such as squamous carcinoma of the oral cavity, adenocarcinoma of the endometrium, and carcinoma of the breast. Radiation therapy is used frequently in the palliative management of incurable cancer at many sites. The result has been emergence of an increasing number of patients cured of cancer by radiation, of whom a few have persistent damage to normal tissues as a result of curative therapy.

ACUTE INTESTINAL INJURY

An important fact about the intestinal villus is that its population of epithelial cells normally remain in a dynamic equilibrium. Intestinal epithelial cells are in a steady state; production of new cells in the intestinal crypt is matched by loss of differentiated epithelial or mucous cells being shed at the tip of the intestinal villus. Complete replacement of the epithelium in the small intestine, as measured by migration of tritiated thymidine-labeled crypt cells, occurs within 4 to 6 days.

The acute intestinal effects of ionizing radiation are related closely to the field size in which the radiation is delivered; that is, with small portals, other physical factors being equal, large amounts of radiation may be given safely, whereas with total-body radiation, approximately 400 rads constitutes an L.D.$_{50}$ in man. In this latter kind of injury, which has resulted from atomic disasters and accidental radiation overexposure, intestinal mucosal sloughing and intestinal hemorrhage are prominent effects, associated with hematopoietic depression and destruction of gonadal tissues.[7] The earliest critical effect of intestinal radiation injury is the cessation of production of viable cells in the generative zone within the crypts of the intestinal epithelium.[5] Production of new cells is blocked until the epithelial cells vanish and active transport processes are damaged. Severe diarrhea and intestinal hemorrhage result. Bacteria are probably not absorbed, but with loss of intestinal barrier function, poorly understood malabsorption contributes to systemic toxemia. These gastrointestinal pathophysiologic alterations, together with the pancytopenia that ensues from hematopoietic depression, may progress inexorably to death. Following lesser amounts of total-body radiation, survival may be achieved by prolonged and vigorous water and electrolyte replacement, antibiotic protection, and possibly use of bone marrow transfusions.

Far more common are the intestinal alterations that follow therapeutic irradiation. The basic pathophysiologic mechanisms for injury of the intestinal epithelium are the same but are ordinarily transient, self-limited, and localized. Epithelial changes include decreased mitoses in the intestinal crypts, necrosis of crypt epithelial cells, and decreased height of crypts and villi. Despite development of a mucosal lesion, gastrointestinal symptoms may be minimal or absent.

However, some asymptomatic patients with small intestinal injury may have malabsorption demonstrable biochemically.

Intensive radiation is often administered to the pelvis for carcinoma of the cervix, endometrium, ovary, or bladder—hence the risk for a radiation-induced or factitial proctitis—or to the paraortic area for lymphosarcoma or testicular tumors, with a risk for symptomatology related to transient small intestinal injury. Diarrhea or rectal bleeding is the usual manner of presentation in patients with proctitis. Nausea is common and crampy abdominal pain may be present after small intestinal radiation. Ordinarily, these symptoms subside shortly after completion of radiation therapy, and patients require only supportive therapy with antinausea and antidiarrheal medications.

LATE INTESTINAL INJURY

In some patients, gastrointestinal symptoms persist after radiation therapy; weeks, months, or even years later, overt and severe radiation injury to the intestine may become evident clinically. Late radiation injury is the result of a progressive vasculitis and diffuse collagen deposition and fibrosis, not of altered epithelial proliferative kinetics. The vasculitis may result in tissue hypoxia, which progresses to necrosis, ulceration, and perforation. If collagen deposition dominates the injury, as it may inexplicably, resultant fibrosis may lead to obstruction of the intestine. Acute injury may progress to chronic injury with a continuous display of intestinal symptomatology, or a long symptom-free period may intervene before chronic radiation injury becomes evident. There is evidence that subclinical injury may become overt when low-flow states such as congestive heart failure or vascular narrowing from hypertension and arteriosclerosis worsen the hypoxia from radiation vasculitis until, finally, cellular oxygenation and nutrition are reduced below critical levels (Fig. 3).

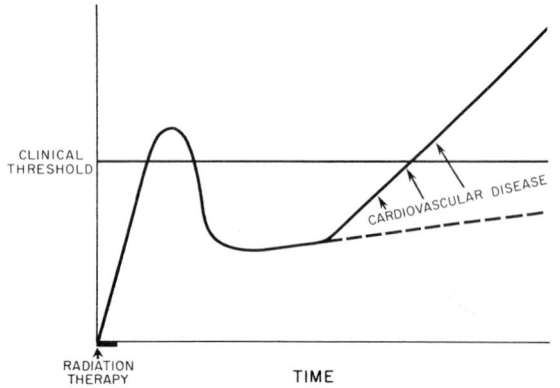

Figure 3. A model, after Rubin and Cassarett,[6] suggesting a pattern for radiation injury: early transient symptoms, a latent period of subclinical activity, and precipitation of clinical symptoms, often by onset of cardiovascular disease.

In some instances injury may be attributed to the physical factors inherent in the administered radiation. It should be remembered that curative radiation therapy is being directed against life-threatening abdominal or pelvic cancer; therapeutic ranges, of necessity, are close to amounts injurious to adjacent tissues. Prior surgery or prior intra-abdominal infection is associated with a greater risk for injury because loops of small or large intestine adhere to the tissue being irradiated. The presence of persisting vascular disease from diabetes mellitus, arteriosclerosis, or hypertension also increases the risk for injury. Some chemotherapeutic drugs, such as actinomycin or adriamycin, enhance the effects of radiation.[4]

A second long-term risk from abdominal irradiation is possible development of intestinal neoplasia. Although an unequivocal cause-and-effect relationship has not been documented in man, a nonrandom relationship appears evident from animal investigations, probably a result of the well-documented mutogenic effect of ionizing radiation.

Chronic radiation injury of the intestine is frequently associated with injury to cutaneous, bony, and other visceral structures encompassed by the radiation portals. The radiation portal may be demarcated by a chronic dermatitis with capillary telangiectasia, epidermal atrophy, hyperkeratosis, and indolent ulceration. Injury of the pelvic bones has followed pelvic radiation. Sterility and amenorrhea may be evident. There is a close relationship between gastrointestinal and genitourinary injury and the latter may be more life-threatening; investigation of intestinal injury should include assessment by intravenous pyelography and cystoscopy for cystitis or urethral injury. Radiation nephritis may also occur.

Radiation injury of the small intestine or colon may result in malabsorption, acute or chronic obstruction, ulceration, perforation, abscess formation, and fistulization. Radiation-induced enteritis should be regarded as a possible cause for abdominal pain after abdominal or pelvic irradiation. Appearance of symptoms ranges from a few weeks after irradiation therapy to several decades after the inciting physical injury. A patient who appears well and maintains his body weight but continues to have crampy, abdominal pain often has a radiation injury, not residual or recurrent cancer. Identification of steatorrhea and other effects of malabsorption, such as hypocalcemia, is helpful in making a diagnosis of small intestinal injury.

Jejunal or ileal injury is suggested by crampy, periumbilical pain, nausea, vomiting, abdominal distention, and obstipation. Diarrhea may be caused by malabsorption but usually suggests distal colonic or rectal injury. Symptoms of partial obstruction may be quite insidious, with limited nausea, no vomiting, and only slight crampy pain and modest distention. If obstruction is complete, conventional abdominal x-rays taken in the flat and upright, or decubitus, positions will demonstrate dilated loops of bowel, air-fluid levels, and minimal or no gas in the colon. In the presence of symptoms and findings of partial obstruction, both a barium enema and a small intestinal barium examination should be obtained. Partial small intestinal obstruction need not preclude oral adminis-

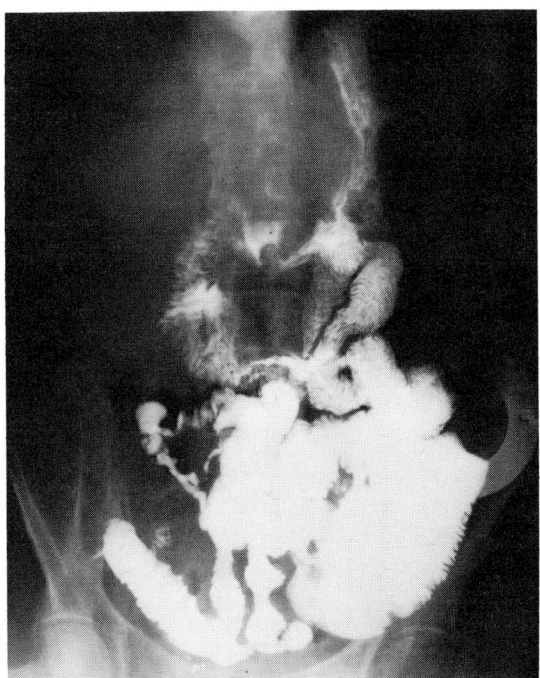

Figure 4. The relatively normal, feathery appearance of the upper jejunum can be contrasted with stenosis, loss of valvular markings, and puddling evident in the distal radiation-injured small intestine.

tration of barium. Small intestine barium examinations are difficult to interpret; considerable pathologic change may be hidden by apparently negative x-rays. Constricted, narrow loops of intestine or puddling of barium is indicative of partial obstruction[2] (Fig. 4).

In examining patients with obstruction, it is extremely important not only to determine the completeness of obstruction but also to establish whether or not vascular compromise is present. The findings in patients who have vascular compromise include continuous abdominal pain between cramps, presence of back pain suggesting torsion on the mesentery, involuntary guarding, localized and persistent tenderness to percussion or palpation or on rebound, reduced or absent peristaltic sounds, a rectal temperature above 38° C., and a white blood cell count in excess of 12,000 cells per cu. mm.

In the presence of vascular compromise or complete obstruction, surgical exploration is necessary; in the former, it is urgent, and in the latter it should be done after a longer period of preparation by nasointestinal intubation and decompression and fluid and electrolyte replacement. At laparotomy, radiation-injured bowel is stenotic and thick-walled; the serosal surface is gray and opaque from serositis. Loose fibrinous adhesions congeal loops of small intestine together and to adjacent surfaces. Wide resection of the diseased bowel, or occasionally a bypass, is the treatment of choice. The important objective is that normal unirradiated intestine be used for the enteroenterostomy.

Partial obstruction from radiation-induced stenosis

of the small intestine can be managed initially by conservative intestinal decompression and water and electrolyte replacement. Obstructive symptoms will sometimes relent without necessity for surgery. Oral steroids, sulfasalazine, and a low-residue diet may reduce symptoms to a tolerable subclinical level.

Perforation of the intestine usually follows prodromal obstructive symptoms and is a consequence of vascular occlusion leading to hypoxia and then necrosis. Perforation will result in a diffuse peritonitis if the perforated loop has free access to the peritoneal cavity, a localized abscess if matted loops of intestine and adjacent structures preclude free egress into the peritoneal cavity, or fistulization if perforation occurs into bladder, ureter, vagina, intestine, or an operative wound agglutinated to the injured intestine.

Free perforation produces precipitant abdominal pain and acute peritoneal signs. Abdominal findings of spreading tenderness to percussion and palpation and on rebound, involuntary guarding, and reduced or absent peristaltic sounds, physical or x-ray findings of free intraperitoneal air, and the systemic findings of fever, leukocytosis, and hypovolemia all herald a catastrophic event requiring urgent surgery. An abscess has a somewhat more insidious course with findings of localized tenderness and guarding that persist and may be associated with a mass. Roentgen studies of the abdomen may show displacement of normal viscera. Simple drainage of an abscess will result in an intestinal fistula to the wound. Wide resection of involved intestine should be performed for both perforation and abscess resulting from radiation injury.

Occasionally, continued progression of the intestinal injury will result in fistulization. Because patients have often had both surgery and radiation therapy for carcinoma of the cervix or carcinoma of the endometrium, fistulization commonly occurs into the vaginal vault. In the usual event of pelvic fistulization, a prodromal period of pelvic inflammation precedes by hours or days the emergence of bowel contents in the vagina. Fistulization may develop between loops of bowel, thereby excluding a segment of intestine and causing diarrhea or a blind loop syndrome with vitamin B_{12} deficiency. Fistulization into the bladder or ureter is often heralded by a urinary tract infection and then pneumaturia, or passage of air in the urine. Although the site of intestinal injury may seem readily apparent, it is important to localize the site of injury as accurately as possible by sigmoidoscopy, barium enema examination, small bowel barium examination, and fistulograms, the latter by instillation of iodinated water-soluble dyes. Recurrent cancer must be excluded.

These patients are usually severely ill; they are calorically depleted, dehydrated, and toxic from chronic infection. Radiation-induced small intestinal fistulas rarely heal and excision is necessary. However, a preliminary program of gastrointestinal decompression, resolution of pelvic sepsis, and nutritional replacement, often requiring hyperalimentation, reduces operative risk and improves the likelihood of healing.

Since the rectum is apposed to the uterine cervix and body, most patients receiving irradiation therapy for cancers at these sites will have transient and self-limited diarrhea managed effectively by simple supportive measures. In some instances, proctitis is persistent, lasting for months or years. Pelvic pain, pain on defecation, and rectal bleeding may be severe. Persistence of these symptoms after radiation therapy merits assessment by proctosigmoidoscopy and barium enema examination, the latter to exclude more cephalad colonic injury. Generally, patients with proctitis are managed successfully by a low-residue diet, stool softeners, sedation, antispasmodics, and general supportive measures. Oral steroids, sulfasalazine, and rectal steroid enemas are beneficial in more severe injuries. Occasionally, a proximal defunctionalizing colostomy will be required for severe rectal bleeding or intractable pain; relief of symptoms does not always follow.

Proctitis may progress to ulceration. In such patients, proctoscopy will show the ulcer to be located anteriorly, opposed to the level of the cervix or uterus, and to have a gray, shaggy, friable base without the elevated perimeter suggestive of carcinoma. A rectal ulcer may ultimately heal, or it may progress to perforation or formation of a rectovaginal fistula. Since a rectovaginal fistula may be associated with recurrent carcinoma, biopsy is necessary.

A rectovaginal fistula from radiation injury is rarely self-healing; defunctionalization of the rectum by colostomy is required. The extent of adjacent rectal and vaginal injury is so severe that it is uncommon for the fistula to be ultimately repaired and gastrointestinal continuity restored; a sigmoid colon or descending colon colostomy is usually permanent. Occasionally, an exenteration is warranted for radiation necrosis of the vagina and rectum.

Continued proctitis may lead to rectal stenosis. Little is known about why radiation injury should prompt a fibrotic response in some patients and an ulcerative response in others. Both genitourinary and rectal obstruction may occur from radiation injury. Radiation fibrosis in the pelvis closely simulates recurrent cancer; biopsy is essential. Usually, rectal stenosis can be managed effectively by conservative measures, including instrumental or digital dilations.

Occasionally, a sigmoid or descending colon colostomy will be necessary to defunctionalize the rectum.

REFERENCES

1. DeCosse, J. J., Rhodes, R. S., Wentz, W. B., Reagan, J. W., Dworken, H. J., and Holden, W. D.: The natural history and management of radiation induced injury of the gastrointestinal tract. Ann. Surg., 170:369, 1970.
   The course of 100 patients with intestinal injury from radiation is reviewed. The long interval from radiation to onset of clinical symptoms is documented. In patients with small intestinal damage, an average of 2 years elapsed before definitive symptoms became evident. The authors also develop the clinical evidence for a relationship between cardiovascular disease and radiation injury.

2. Mason, G. R., Dietrich, P., Friedland, G. W., and Hanks, G. E.: The radiological findings in radiation-induced enteritis and colitis. Clin. Radiol., 21:232, 1970.
   An excellent review of the difficult diagnostic criteria for radiation damage to small and large bowel.

3. Muller, H. J.: Radiation damage to the genetic material. Am. Sci., 38:33, 1950.
   The author reviews his Nobel Prize–winning work on mutation frequency. Although his publications about this subject began in 1927, the cited report summarizes his many important contributions.

4. Phillips, T. L., Wharam, M. D., and Margolis, L. W.: Modification of radiation injury to normal tissues by chemotherapeutic agents. Cancer, 35:1678, 1975.
   As modern multimodality treatment of patients with cancer expands, other interactions of chemotherapeutic drugs with radiation therapy will be demonstrated.

5. Quastler, H.: The nature of intestinal radiation death. Radiat. Res., 4:303, 1956.
   The cell kinetic evidence for radiation injury to the proliferative epithelium of the intestine is developed by a man who made outstanding contributions in the field of cell cycle studies.

6. Rubin, P., and Casarett, G. W.: Clinical Radiation Pathology. Philadelphia, W. B. Saunders Company, 1968.
   This two-volume set is probably the outstanding current resource about pathophysiologic mechanisms of radiation effects. These prolific writers and educators from the University of Rochester have collated the literature and their own extensive experience into a thorough, well-written, and well-indexed text.

7. Warren, S. L., and Whipple, G. H.: Roentgen ray intoxication. I. Unit dose over thorax negative—over abdomen lethal—epithelium of small intestine—sensitive to x-rays. J. Exp. Med., 35:187, 1922.
   In a classic paper by two distinguished investigators and leaders of American medicine, intestinal epithelial necrosis after radiation is carefully described. In this and subsequent papers by these authors the pathology of acute and chronic radiation injury was developed.

X

APPENDICITIS

Robert E. Condon, M.D.

Acute appendicitis always should be considered in any patient who complains of abdominal pain or who presents with minimal symptoms suggestive of peritoneal irritation. Acute appendicitis is the most frequent cause of persisting, progressive abdominal pain in teenagers, and is a common, sometimes confusing, and often treacherous cause of an acute abdomen at all ages. There is no way to prevent the development of appendicitis. The only way to reduce morbidity and to prevent mortality is to perform appendectomy before perforation or gangrene has occurred.

INCIDENCE

The incidence of acute appendicitis decreased from 10 per cent of all surgical procedures in 1941 to only 2 per cent in 1956.[4, 23] Over the past decade the incidence of appendicitis has remained more or less constant.[17, 20, 29] The decreased incidence of appendicitis may be an effect of the widespread use of antibiotics.

Every fifteenth person is destined to develop acute appendicitis sometime during life. Appendicitis is rare in infants, becomes increasingly common throughout childhood, and reaches its maximal incidence in the early teen years. Thereafter the incidence declines, though appendicitis remains relatively common throughout adulthood and into old age.

Prior to puberty, appendicitis develops in boys about as frequently as in girls. Among teenagers and young adults, the male-female ratio is about 3:2. After age 25, the excess male incidence gradually declines until the sex ratio is again equal.

HISTORICAL ASPECTS

Curiously, a condition as common as appendicitis was not recorded in medical literature until about 500 years ago.[19] When first recognized as a distinct disease entity in the sixteenth century, appendicitis was called "perityphlitis" because the inflammatory process that brought about death of the patient was thought to have originated in the cecum. It now seems obvious that what was so described was perforative appendicitis.

Appendectomy was first performed by Claudius Amyand, sergeant-surgeon to King George II, in a 12-year-old boy whose scrotal hernia was complicated by a fecal fistula. Amyand discovered a pin perforating the appendix, which was in the hernia. He removed the appendix and repaired the hernia. Following his report, appendectomy was performed occasionally, but intervention typically was late and mortality high.

Although Melier, in 1827, correctly ascribed the origin of purulent "iliac tumor" to inflammation of the appendix, it was not until 1886 that Fitz clearly defined appendicitis as the initial process in cases previously diagnosed as "perityphlitis." Fitz suggested that appendectomy would be essential to cure.

The first surgeon to correctly diagnose acute appendicitis prior to rupture, perform appendectomy, have the patient recover, and report his experience was Senn.[27] Groves, practicing in rural Canada, apparently had done a successful appendectomy six years earlier, but his case was not reported until 1961. Also in 1889, McBurney described the clinical findings of acute appendicitis prior to rupture, including description of the point of maximal abdominal tenderness that now bears his name. The gridiron incision commonly attributed to McBurney actually was devised by McArthur.

Over the relatively short span of somewhat less than a century, acceptance of prompt appendectomy as the treatment of appendicitis has improved the prognosis from that of a usually fatal disease to one in which, however complicated, death is uncommon.

ANATOMY

Embryologically, the appendix is a continuation of the cecum, arising from its inferior tip. Suppression of the development of the apical segment of the cecum is followed by appendicular hypoplasia or agenesis. During infancy, more rapid growth of the right and anterior portions of the cecum results in rotation of the appendix posteriorly and medially to its adult position, about 2.5 cm. below the ileocecal valve (Fig. 1).

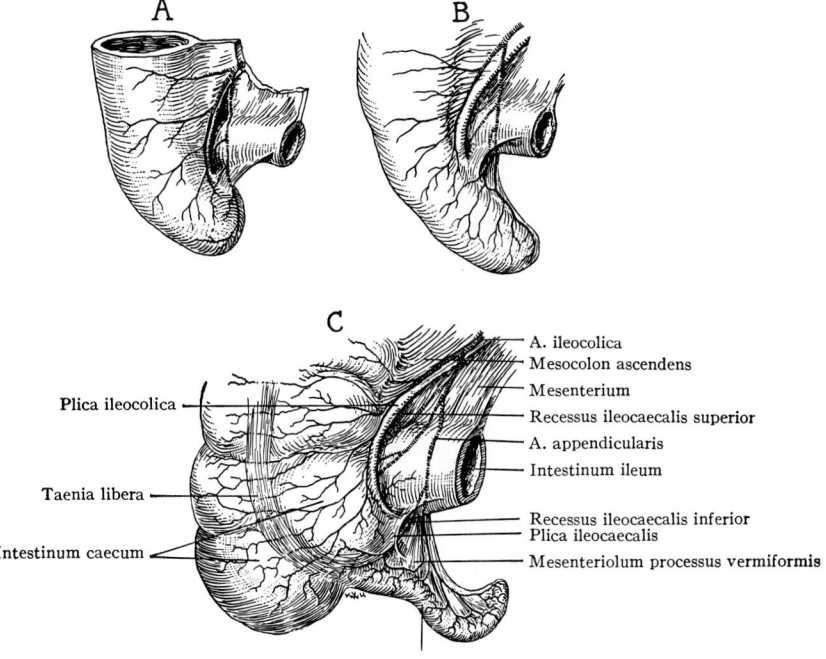

Figure 1. Development of the appendix. Lagging growth of the inferior tip of the cecum during early intrauterine development (*A*) produces the infantile appendix (*B*). Continued differential growth of the lateral cecal wall leads to the posteromedial position (*C*) of the appendix in older children and adults. (From Anson, B., and McVay, C. B.: Surgical Anatomy, 5th ed. Philadelphia, W. B. Saunders Company, 1971.)

Plica ileocolica

Taenia libera

Intestinum caecum

A. ileocolica
Mesocolon ascendens
Mesenterium
Recessus ileocaecalis superior
A. appendicularis
Intestinum ileum
Recessus ileocaecalis inferior
Plica ileocaecalis
Mesenteriolum processus vermiformis

Processus vermiformis

The appendix averages 10 cm. in length in adults, although it is not uncommon to find an appendix more than twice that long. The narrow lumen of the appendix is lined by colonic epithelium. There are a few submucosal lymphoid follicles present at birth; these gradually increase in number to a peak of approximately 200 follicles between the ages of 12 and 20. After age 30, there is an abrupt reduction to less than half that number, and, subsequently, to a trace or a total absence of lymphoid tissue after age 60.

The walls of the appendix are muscular; the inner circular layer is a continuation of the same muscle in the cecum. The outer longitudinal muscle coat is formed by coalescence of the three taeniae coli at the junction of the cecum and appendix. Thus the taeniae, particularly the anterior taenia, may be used as a landmark to locate an elusive appendix. The mesentery of the appendix passes behind the terminal ileum to join the mesentery of the small intestine. The appendicular artery runs in the free border of the mesoappendix and is a branch of the ileocolic artery. In many patients, in addition, an accessory appendicular branch from the posterior cecal artery supplies the base of the appendix at its junction with the cecum.

The relation of the base of the appendix to the cecum is constant, but the tip of the appendix may be found in a variety of locations. Most commonly, the appendix lies behind the cecum although still in an intraperitoneal location.[32] This low retrocecal position is found in 65 per cent of patients (Fig. 2) and is due to the fact that several inches of the cecum usually remain in an intraperitoneal position, since the reflection of the peritoneum to the parieties from the cecum occurs opposite the ileocecal junction. The second most common position of the tip of the appendix, found in about 30 per cent of patients, is at the brim of or in the pelvis. In about 5 per cent of patients, the tip of the appendix lies extraperitoneally, either behind the cecum and ascending colon or passing behind the distal ileum along the right margin of the ascending colon.

Malrotation or maldescent of the cecum is associated with abnormal locations of the appendix, which may be found anywhere between the right iliac fossa and the left infrasplenic area. In cases of transposition of the viscera, the appendix is in the left lower quadrant. Abnormal positions of the cecum are important because they introduce difficulties in diagnosis should appendicitis supervene.

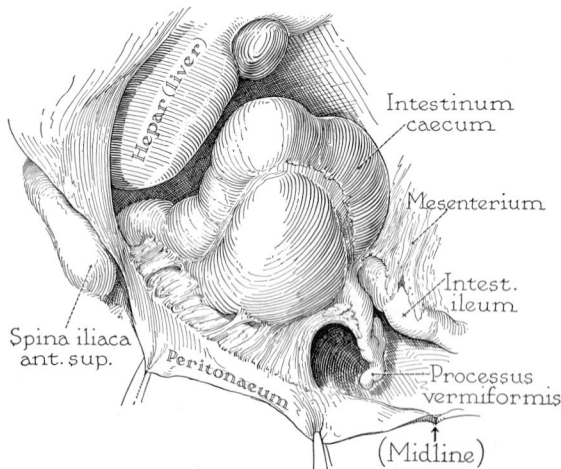

Figure 2. The most common position of the appendix is behind the cecum. (From Anson, B., and McVay, C. B.: Surgical Anatomy, 5th ed. Philadelphia, W. B. Saunders Company, 1971.)

PATHOPHYSIOLOGY

Appendicitis results from obstruction followed by infection. Approximately 60 per cent of cases are related to hyperplasia of submucosal lymphoid follicles, 35 per cent to the presence of fecal stasis or a fecalith, 4 per cent to the presence of other foreign bodies, and 1 per cent to strictures or tumors of the wall of the appendix or the cecum. Lymphatic hyperplasia leading to obstruction is most frequent in children; obstruction due to a fecalith is more frequent in older adults. Fecalith formation may be promoted by the relatively tenacious feces of those, particularly urbanized Westerners, who consume a low fiber, high carbohydrate diet.

The amount of lymphoid tissue in the appendix parallels the incidence of acute appendicitis, the peak for both occurring in the early teens. Hyperplastic follicles may partially obstruct the lumen, setting the stage for development of appendicitis. Hyperplasia of lymphoid tissue may be a response to an acute respiratory infection, measles, mononucleosis, or other diseases producing a generalized reaction of lymphatic tissue. The follicles of the appendix also respond to infections in the gut; appendicitis has been reported, for example, in association with salmonella and shigella enterocolitis.

Formation of an appendiceal fecalith begins with entrapment of a bit of vegetable fiber in the lumen of the appendix, stimulating the secretion and deposition of calcium-rich mucus. The mucus subsequently becomes inspissated around the bit of fiber; this sets up a second round of irritation and deposition of mucus. Eventually, concretions reach a diameter of about a centimeter, at which point, if not expelled, they may obstruct the lumen; appendicitis ensues.

Among other intraluminal objects that may precipitate an attack of appendicitis, pinworms *(Enterobius vermicularis)* are the commonest parasites reported in this country, but Taenia and Ascaris also have caused appendicitis. Other foreign bodies include vegetable seeds, cherry stones, and inspissated barium. In older patients, obstruction by a cecal carcinoma, and in younger adults, carcinoid tumors, are occasional causes of appendicitis. Metastases to the appendix, particularly from carcinoma of the breast, also may cause appendicitis.

The events that follow obstruction of the appendix depend upon interactions among four factors: the content in the lumen, the degree of obstruction, continued secretion by the mucosa, and the inelastic character of the appendiceal serosa. The sequence following obstruction of the appendix probably is as follows: Mucus accumulates in the lumen, and pressure within the organ begins to increase. Virulent bacteria convert the accumulating mucus into pus. Continued secretion combined with the relative inelasticity of the serosa leads to a further rise in pressure within the lumen. Obstruction of lymphatic drainage ensues, leading to edema of the appendix, beginning diapedesis of bacteria, and the appearance of mucosal ulcers. This is the stage of *acute focal appendicitis.*

The inflammation and increased pressure in the lumen present at this stage are perceived by the patient as poorly localized visceral pain tending to be periumbilical or epigastric in location, accompanied by anorexia, nausea, and occasional vomiting. It is because the appendix and the small bowel have the same nerve supply that visceral pain is first perceived in the epigastrium or periumbilical area.

Relentless secretion causes a further rise in intraluminal pressure, which brings about venous obstruction and thrombosis, producing, in turn, further edema and ischemia in the appendix. Bacterial invasion spreads through the wall of the appendix. This stage is called *acute suppurative appendicitis*. The inflamed serosa of the appendix contacts the parietal peritoneum. Somatic pain, arising from the peritoneum as a result of contact with the inflamed appendix, is perceived as the classic shift and localization of pain in the right lower quadrant.

Continuation of this pathologic process eventually leads to compromise of the arterial blood supply. The area of the appendix with the poorest blood supply, the midportion of the antimesenteric border, undergoes gangrene with the appearance of ellipsoidal infarcts. The development of *gangrenous appendicitis* is the first stage of complicated appendicitis; morbidity increases, since these infarcts functionally act as perforations, permitting escape of bacteria from the lumen of the appendix and contamination of the peritoneal cavity.

Continued secretion from viable portions of the appendiceal mucosa and continued high intraluminal pressure finally lead to perforation through the gangrenous infarct, spilling accumulated pus. *Perforative appendicitis* is now present; morbidity and mortality increase. Fortunately, in most cases, the obstruction that initially led to appendicitis blocks continued spillage of feces from the cecum through the perforated appendix. If appendicitis has not progressed too rapidly, inflammatory adhesions have formed between loops of bowel, peritoneum, and omentum to hem in the appendix. Perforation then leads to localized peritonitis; a periappendiceal abscess forms eventually if untreated. In 1 to 2 per cent of patients, particularly the very young and the very old, rapidity of progression of the disease is such that defense mechanisms are not fully effective and generalized peritonitis ensues.

PROGNOSIS

Fifty years ago, 15 of every 100,000 persons in this country could expect to die each year of appendicitis. Today, mortality has decreased to less than 1 in 100,000 persons annually. The mortality risk of an individual patient with acute but not gangrenous appendicitis is less than 0.1 per cent. In gangrenous appendicitis mortality rises to about 0.6 per cent. The mortality rate of perforative appendicitis today is approximately 5 per cent, down from over 50 per cent a half century ago and over 25 per cent just 25 years ago. Although the mortality of appendicitis has declined progressively, morbidity from appendicitis continues to be high. Overall, morbidity currently occurs in 10 per cent of all patients with appendicitis. Wound infections account for one third of all morbidity. The presence of gangrene or perforation increases the morbidity risk four- or fivefold, wound infection rates of 40 to 50 per cent being commonly reported.[17, 20, 29]

The role that delay in diagnosis and treatment plays in mortality and serious morbidity cannot be overemphasized. Delay in carrying out appendectomy is often due to uncertainty of diagnosis or to trial of antibiotic therapy. The use of antibiotics in an attempt to avoid or postpone appendectomy ignores the fact that acute appendicitis begins as an obstruction. Observation until typical or definite symptoms appear is dangerous and ill-advised. Exploration to discover the cause of minimal symptoms, even in poor-risk patients, is safer than waiting.[11]

CLINICAL DIAGNOSIS

The diagnosis of acute appendicitis is the classic example of the application of clinical skills. Ancillary laboratory and radiologic tests are not essential in making the diagnosis. Although symptoms and signs in many cases are atypical, it is a tribute to the clinical acumen of medical students and physicians that the findings at operation usually confirm the clinical diagnosis.

Symptomatic History

The sequence of symptoms in acute appendicitis usually begins with diffuse abdominal pain, felt most prominently in the epigastrium or around the umbilicus; this is followed, in turn, by anorexia and some nausea. Vomiting, if it is to occur, appears next. After a variable time, pain shifts toward the right side and then into the right lower quadrant and becomes localized. Anorexia of some degree always accompanies appendicitis and is so constant a complaint that the diagnosis should be questioned if the appetite is retained.

Abdominal pain is present in all patients with appendicitis except those with transverse myelitis or similar disabilities. Pain may be characterized as either typical or atypical. Typical pain consists of initial diffuse, central, not very severe visceral pain, followed by somatic pain that is more severe and well localized in the right lower quadrant. This classic pain sequence is found in 55 per cent of patients with appendicitis but also may occur in one fourth of patients with other intra-abdominal conditions.

Atypical abdominal pain is common in acute appendicitis, occurring in 45 per cent of patients who prove to have appendicitis and 75 per cent of patients in whom appendicitis initially is suspected but who prove to have some other disease. Atypical pain is defined as pain that fails to follow the classic visceral-somatic sequence. Pain may be entirely somatic, often well localized in the right lower quadrant, from the beginning. Conversely, pain may never become localized and may remain diffuse throughout the preoperative course of acute appendicitis. Atypical pain is found more frequently in older patients, in whom pain is always less intense and characteristically localizes much later, and in patients receiving chronic antibiotic therapy for some unrelated condition, such as acne.

Nausea, at least of some degree, is present in 9 of 10 patients with appendicitis. Vomiting is more variable; children and teenagers frequently vomit; vomiting may be entirely absent in older adults. Vomiting in appendicitis is not persistent or prolonged; most patients vomit only once or twice. Vomiting appears after the onset of pain. If vomiting precedes pain, the diagnosis should be questioned. The character of bowel function is of little diagnostic value. Many patients admit to constipation; a few voluntarily state that defecation might relieve their pain. Diarrhea occurs in some patients, especially young children, and can be a confusing sign.

The pain of appendicitis is said to be relieved immediately after perforation, remaining diminished in severity for a short time, until pain due to diffuse peritonitis supervenes. Relief of pain is attributed to decreased pressure in the appendix. In fact, relief of pain following perforation occurs rarely. In most patients, pain continues or increases in severity. The characteristic feature of pain following perforation is that it is no longer so discretely localized. In addition, the patient obviously is more ill and abdominal distention begins to develop.

Any patient with an abnormally located appendix is likely to have an atypical history, particularly of pain. A high retrocecal appendicitis commonly causes nothing more than diffuse pain in the right flank and loin. An inflamed appendix entirely within the true pelvis may never produce somatic pain involving the anterior abdominal wall but may instead cause tenesmus and only vague discomfort in the suprapubic area.

Physical Examination

The traditional physical signs of appendicitis are local tenderness, rebound tenderness, muscle guarding, cutaneous hyperesthesia, pelvic tenderness on the right side on rectal examination. and the presence of the psoas and obturator signs. Appendicitis may cause a rise in temperature up to 38°C, but higher fever is unusual; a normal temperature often is present even with advanced appendicitis. The pulse rate usually remains normal. In fact, all physical diagnostic signs are fallible. Remember: prior to gangrene and rupture, symptoms are more reliable diagnostically than are physical signs.

If symptoms have been present for more than a few hours, inspection may disclose some limitation of respiratory movement in the lower half of the abdomen. Systematic gentle palpation will detect an area of maximal tenderness that corresponds to the position of the appendix and usually is located in the right lower quadrant at or near McBurney's point (Fig. 3).

The presence of peritoneal inflammation can be suspected if a cough or percussion of the abdominal wall elicits pain. The classic method of demonstrating peritoneal inflammation is rebound tenderness following release of abdominal palpation pressure. The finding of rebound tenderness may be of occasional help in doubtful cases, but it is unnecessary to distress a patient with clear signs of appendicitis by eliciting rebound tenderness as a routine maneuver. Rovsing's sign, pain in the right lower quadrant when palpation pressure is exerted in the left lower quadrant, is a

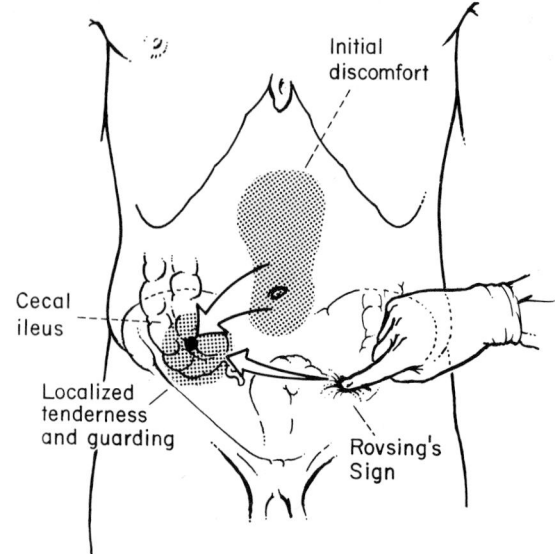

Figure 3. Some physical signs of appendicitis prior to rupture. McBurney's point is indicated by the black dot in the right lower quadrant. (From Gelin, L.-E, Nyhus, L. M., and Condon, R. E.: Abdominal Pain: A Guide to Rapid Diagnosis, Philadelphia, J. B. Lippincott Company, 1969.)

manifestation of referred rebound tenderness and is sometimes helpful in supporting a diagnosis of appendicitis.

Muscular guarding, or resistance to palpation, roughly parallels the severity of the inflammatory process, particularly in younger patients. As peritoneal irritation progresses, voluntary muscle guarding increases and eventually is replaced by reflex involuntary rigidity. True rigidity does not diminish during expiration, a finding that allows it to be differentiated by palpation from voluntary guarding.

If symptoms have been present for two days or more, the presence of a palpable right lower quadrant mass may be detected. The mass results from adherent coils of small bowel and omentum about the inflamed appendix. Cutaneous hyperesthesia will be reported by an occasional patient able to distinguish the difference in sensation elicited by light stroking of the skin on the right and left sides of the abdomen. This sign, although classic, is unreliable, since the degree of discrimination required is beyond the capacities of most patients ill with appendicitis.

Once appendicitis is sufficiently advanced so that inflammation involves the anterior abdominal wall, the posture of the patient becomes a useful corroborative sign. Movement is avoided. If asked to turn or sit up, the patient does so gingerly to avoid pain caused by sudden movement of the abdominal wall. The right hip often is slightly flexed. Further active flexion against resistance or passive extension of the hip stretches the iliopsoas muscle; the patient may complain of increased pain. This is a positive psoas sign, said to indicate irritation of the psoas muscle by the inflamed appendix. A psoas sign rarely is present early in appendicitis; whenever it can be elicited, other clinical signs of appendicitis are clear. The obturator sign, hypogastric or adductor pain elicited by passive internal rotation of the flexed thigh, is said to indicate an inflamed appendix lying against the internal obturator muscle. This sign is positive less often than is the psoas sign.

Rectal examination is essential in every patient suspected of having appendicitis. Its primary purpose is to exclude pelvic lesions such as ovarian cyst or tubal abscess. A secondary purpose is to elicit tenderness in cases of pelvic appendicitis. Tenderness of the pelvic peritoneum must be distinguished from the general discomfort commonly felt during rectal examination. There rarely is any acute disorder posterior to the rectum so that a useful baseline of discomfort can be established by first palpating the coccyx. In about one patient in three, in whom the inflamed appendix lies in or adjacent to the pelvis, the presence of a mass or tenderness specifically localized to the right side may be elicited. In those few cases in which the inflamed appendix lies wholly within the pelvis, tenderness on rectal examination may be the only positive physical sign.

Following rupture, physical signs usually become much more definite. If the rupture is contained in the right lower quadrant, a boggy, tender mass usually can be felt. Tenderness, which classically is finger-point with simple acute appendicitis, now encompasses the whole right lower quadrant. Rebound tenderness and muscular rigidity are more marked. The temperature may rise to 39°C, and there is a corresponding rise in the pulse rate.

If the rupture fails to localize, signs of spreading peritonitis ensue. Tenderness becomes diffuse and there is more generalized rigidity of the abdominal muscles. The temperature usually is above 38°C, with spikes to 40°C quite common; the pulse rate rises to over 100 per minute.

Complicated appendicitis mimicking or associated with mechanical small bowel obstruction is particularly prevalent in elderly patients. Inflammatory adhesive bands secondary to appendicitis cause the obstruction. The clinical history typically is of two to five days of diffuse abdominal pain; there are signs of peritoneal irritation on physical examination in addition to signs of mechanical small bowel obstruction.

Laboratory Examinations

Far too much stress has been laid upon the alleged value of laboratory work in the diagnosis of acute appendicitis. The differential white cell count and the total leukocyte count usually are abnormal in appendicitis, but the degree of abnormality does not correlate with degree of abnormality in the appendix. Up to one third of patients, particularly older adults and blacks,[13] will have a normal total leukocyte count in the presence of acute appendicitis. Most patients, however, will have a shift to the left in the differential white count, even when the total count is normal.[26] Fewer than 4 per cent of patients with acute appendicitis have both a normal differential count and a normal total white count. In cases of suspected appendicitis, whenever the clinical findings are at variance with the white cell count, clinical findings should take precedence. The hematocrit is normal in appendicitis. If an older patient presents with symptoms suggesting

appendicitis and has a significant anemia, carcinoma of the cecum should be suspected.

Minimal albuminuria and some white blood cells in the urine are present in 20 per cent of male patients with appendicitis. Identification of significant numbers of microorganisms in the urinary sediment confirms the presence of a urinary tract infection but does not exclude the diagnosis of appendicitis. The finding of a few red blood cells in the urine of a patient with appendicitis also is not unusual. It is not necessary for the appendix to be in contact with the ureter or bladder for an occasional red cell to be found. However, patients with more than 30 red cells or more than 20 white cells in a centrifuged specimen of voided urine should be suspected of having primary urinary tract pathology.[15]

X-ray Examination

X-ray examination of the abdomen does not show any pathognomonic signs in early acute appendicitis with the exception of demonstration of an appendiceal fecalith.[14] Plain films may show a distended cecum with fluid levels (cecal ileus) early in appendicitis. However, if x-rays demonstrate more positive signs of appendicitis, such as gas in the lumen of the appendix or a mass extrinsic to the cecum, the appendix nearly always is gangrenous and often perforated. In late complicated acute appendicitis, x-rays may reveal scoliosis to the right, absence of the right psoas shadow, absence of small bowel gas in the right lower quadrant though abundantly present elsewhere, edema of the abdominal wall, or interruption of the properitoneal fat line in the flank. Barium enema usually is contraindicated in patients with suspected appendicitis who have positive abdominal physical signs because of the danger of rupturing the inflamed appendix or adjacent cecum. The possible utility of ultrasonography or computerized tomographic scanning in establishing a diagnosis in obscure cases of appendicitis remains to be established.

DISTINCTIVE CLINICAL SETTINGS OF APPENDICITIS

Appendicitis In Infants and Young Children

Accurate diagnosis of appendicitis in infants and young children is very difficult. First, the patient is, for obvious reasons, unable to give a history of the illness; second, acute nonspecific abdominal pains are common in infants and young children; and third, appendicitis is infrequent in infants. These features serve to decrease the level of diagnostic suspicion. Because the diagnosis frequently is difficult to establish, treatment is delayed, complications develop, and subsequent management becomes more involved.

Appendicitis is uncommon in infants, probably because the conical configuration of the appendix makes obstruction of the lumen unlikely. Before differential growth of the cecum occurs, the lumen of the appendix is larger at its junction with the cecum than at the tip (see Fig. 1). Perforative appendicitis in the first month of life often is associated with Hirschsprung's disease.[18]

Despite the fact that every child with appendicitis has abdominal pain, the picture can be so like that of nonspecific gastroenteritis that suspicion of appendicitis may not be aroused. Not until after rupture has occurred and the child is obviously ill is a diagnosis of appendicitis seriously entertained. Two thirds of young children with appendicitis have had symptoms for more than three days preceding appendectomy.[30]

The unavoidable fact that a young child cannot give a history means that other clinical aspects of appendicitis become the diagnostic features. The diagnosis can be missed easily if the classic picture of appendicitis is expected. Vomiting, fever, irritability, flexing of the thighs, and diarrhea are likely to be early complaints. "Beware of diarrhea in a child whose illness begins with abdominal pain" is good advice. The most consistent finding on physical examination is abdominal distention. Leukocyte counts are not reliable. The presence of a fecalith noted on a plain abdominal x-ray in a child with suspicious symptoms is sufficient evidence to consider the diagnosis of appendicitis as established.[8]

The incidence of perforation in acute appendicitis approaches 100 per cent in infants less than a year of age, is between 70 and 80 per cent in infants under two years of age, and remains above 50 per cent up to the age of five years. Because of the high incidence of perforation, the mortality of acute appendicitis in this age group remains at about 10 per cent. The higher mortality that occurs in young patients often has been attributed to the absence of a fully developed omentum, with consequent widespread peritonitis following rupture of the appendix. While the omentum is undoubtedly a factor, the most important element is failure of the physician to consider the diagnosis. In one recently reported series, nearly 40 per cent of children with gangrenous or perforative appendicitis previously had been seen by a physician who failed to appreciate the nature of the disease process.[30]

It should be a universal rule that any child with abdominal pain, unexplained after consideration of the history and a careful physical examination, should be assumed to have appendicitis. Exploratory laparotomy in this age group is well tolerated, provided that appropriate attention is paid to adequate fluid and antibiotic therapy, and should be undertaken on the same minimal indications as obtain for older children and adults.

Appendicitis in the Elderly

The incidence of appendicitis in older patients is rising, in contrast to the incidence in the population generally. The increase is due almost entirely to improved longevity among the aged. As is true of infants, acute appendicitis among older patients has a mortality rate many times that of appendicitis in younger adults.[31] The high mortality is due chiefly to delay in definitive treatment, although the concomitant presence of other diseases that lower physiologic reserve plays a role.

The classic symptoms of pain, anorexia, and nausea are present in most older patients but are less pronounced than in younger adults.[25] Pain in the right lower quadrant is the most frequent complaint but often is mild and causes little initial concern. Localization occurs much later than in younger patients.

Physical examination in elderly patients with appendicitis differs mainly by the paucity of findings in the presence of severe disease. The initial examination may reveal nothing abnormal, although tenderness in the right lower quadrant will be elicited eventually in most patients. Distention of the abdomen, as is also true of infants, is prominent in elderly patients, even in the absence of perforation. Symptoms and signs mimicking mechanical small bowel obstruction are not uncommonly present. Subnormal temperatures are more frequently encountered in the aged, especially with an abscess or generalized peritonitis. An occasional older patient will enter the hospital with a painless right lower quadrant mass, denying any previous history suggestive of appendicitis. Conversely, some elderly patients present with generalized peritonitis of obscure etiology; they, too, deny previous acute symptoms.

More than 30 per cent of elderly patients have a ruptured appendix at the time of operation. Impaired blood supply and structural weakness of the appendix are said to produce earlier perforation in older patients. Although such factors may play a role, it is delay in getting the patient to the operating room that really accounts for the high incidence of perforation. If it is probable that an aged patient has acute appendicitis, an urgent operation should be advised. More elderly patients die because surgeons do not operate in doubtful cases than die from misdiagnosis and removal of a normal appendix.[11]

Appendicitis During Pregnancy

The incidence of appendicitis during pregnancy parallels that in nonpregnant women of the same age. Appendicitis occurs once in every one thousand pregnancies and is the most common extrauterine condition requiring an abdominal operation during pregnancy. The mortality rate in the last trimester is five times as high as during the first six months. Frequency of appendicitis during the first two trimesters is greater than during the third trimester. During the first six months of pregnancy, symptoms of appendicitis do not differ from those in the nonpregnant woman. This fact needs emphasis, since the manifestations of appendicitis often are assumed to be markedly different, even during early pregnancy.

Appendectomy should be performed upon suspicion of the presence of appendicitis, just as if the pregnancy were not present. If performed before the appendix ruptures, appendectomy usually does not disturb the pregnancy. Furthermore, the effects of a negative laparotomy are sufficiently minor that early operation for acute appendicitis should be carried out whenever the diagnosis is entertained.[7]

During the third trimester, the clinical picture is slightly altered; displacement of the cecum and appendix by the enlarged uterus leads to localization of pain higher in the abdomen or in the right flank. In addition, appendicitis during the final trimester tends to be more serious if less frequent. The displaced omentum often is unable to reach the area of the inflamed appendix to help contain the infection. In addition, contractions of the nearby uterus serve to impair localization. If the appendicitis proceeds to rupture, it is often followed by diffuse peritonitis.

Premature labor occurs in about half of women who develop appendicitis during the third trimester; the prognosis for the infant in cases of uncomplicated appendicitis is directly related to the infant's birth weight. In cases of appendicitis with peritonitis and other septic complications, fetal loss is much higher and is due not only to prematurity but also to the effects of sepsis in the fetus.

Acute pyelitis of pregnancy and torsion of an ovarian cyst, when they occur during pregnancy, can be difficult to distinguish from appendicitis. However confusing differential diagnosis may be, one fact must be kept in mind: the mortality of appendicitis in pregnancy is due to delayed diagnosis and operation. Early appendectomy is the treatment of choice for appendicitis at all stages of a pregnancy.

DIFFERENTIAL DIAGNOSIS

Differential diagnosis of abdominal pain is one of the fascinating exercises of clinical surgery. This is particularly true in a patient with suspected appendicitis. But before too much time and effort are expended in diagnostic investigation, it must be remembered that most of the entities that enter into the differential diagnosis of appendicitis require operative therapy in any case. If they do not, at least they usually are not made worse by an exploratory operation. The essential differential diagnostic maneuver then is to eliminate those entities that do not need operative therapy, for example, myocardial infarction, basilar pneumonia, and acute pancreatitis.

In young children, the diseases most frequently mistaken for appendicitis are acute gastroenteritis, mesenteric lymphadenitis, pyelitis, Meckel's diverticulitis, intussusception, enteric duplication, Henoch-Schönlein purpura, and primary peritonitis. In this age group, basal pneumonia (even on the left side) may mimic appendicitis and should be particularly looked for. Acute gastroenteritis is usually associated with cramping abdominal pain and watery diarrhea. In mesenteric adenitis, an upper respiratory infection is present or has recently subsided.

It is important to differentiate intussusception from acute appendicitis. Appendicitis is uncommon under age two, whereas most attacks of idiopathic intussusception occur in that age group. A sausage-shaped mass may be palpable in the right lower quadrant. The preferred treatment of intussusception is reduction by gentle barium enema, but treatment of acute appendicitis by barium enema might well be catastrophic.

Children with acute lymphocytic leukemia may develop inflammation progressing to necrosis and perforation of the appendix or the adjacent ileum or cecum.[28] This entity is called the "leukemic ileocecal syndrome." It is of importance not only because of its clinical similarity to acute appendicitis but also because, despite a high mortality risk, surgical intervention is not helpful.

In teenagers and young adults, differential diagnosis is directed by the patient's sex. In young women, diseases of the ovary and tube commonly mimic appendicitis; ruptured ectopic pregnancy, mittelschmerz, endometriosis, and salpingitis (pelvic inflammatory disease) must be differentiated.

Ruptured ectopic pregnancy may produce right lower quadrant pain, but in most patients there will be a palpable tubal mass on pelvic examination, and culdocentesis will yield nonclotting blood. Mittelschmerz is distinguished by its characteristic onset in mid menstrual cycle; symptoms spontaneously subside in a few hours. Endometriosis can be differentiated by the repetitive recurrence of pain with each menses. Salpingitis may cause the greatest diagnostic difficulty, but usually the pain is bilateral, low in the abdomen, and symptoms occur at the end of a menstrual period. Women taking "the pill" sometimes report right lower abdominal discomfort at the end of the second week of each pill cycle; pain is diffuse, and leukocytosis and fever are absent. Regional enteritis can be confusing; cramps and diarrhea are more frequent than with appendicitis.

In a young man, the list of alternative diagnoses is quite small: acute regional enteritis, right renal or ureteral calculus, torsion of a testis, and acute epididymitis. The frequent presence of cramps and diarrhea and the infrequency of anorexia are hints that the process is regional enteritis. Renal or ureteral calculi characteristically cause severe pain, more severe than that of acute appendicitis, but the pain does not persist or progress, since it is related to movement of the calculus; there will be associated microscopic hematuria. Torsion of a testis and acute epididymitis are easily diagnosed by examination of the external genitalia.

In adults, diseases that must be considered in differential diagnosis of acute appendicitis are diverticulitis, perforated duodenal or gastric ulcer, acute cholecystitis, pancreatitis, intestinal obstruction, perforating cecal carcinoma, torsion of an ovarian cyst, perforated ileal diverticulum, mesenteric vascular occlusion, rupturing aortic aneurysm, and idiopathic infarction of an epiploic appendage or the omentum.

TREATMENT

Preoperative Preparation

No patient with acute appendicitis needs to be rushed directly to the operating room immediately after admission to the hospital. All patients, but especially those in whom perforation and peritonitis are suspected, should receive intensive preoperative preparation. This rarely requires more than three or four hours and often can be accomplished in an hour or less.

Fluid replacement should be carried out as rapidly as possible, with the objective of establishing a good urinary output. Nasogastric suction is helpful in all patients with appendicitis but particularly in those with peritonitis. Hyperpyrexia often is a problem in children and should be treated with salicylates in addition to hydration and antibiotics. If fever does not subside, a cooling mattress may be required. Anesthesia should not be induced in patients whose temperature is over 39°C until appropriate measures have been initiated to reduce the fever.

Single intravenous doses of kanamycin and clindamycin are administered sequentially in the preoperative period. The objective of administering these antibiotics is to help control any local or generalized sepsis which may be present and to reduce the incidence of postoperative wound infection. Although prophylactic administration of antibiotics continues to be a matter of controversy, the evidence that has accumulated over the past decade is clearly in favor of antibiotic administration.[6] While antibiotics may not be necessary unless the appendix is gangrenous or has perforated, that fact cannot be determined until after the appendix is exposed during operation. On the other hand, it has been clearly established that if antibiotics are to have any favorable effect at all in reducing the incidence of wound infection, they must be started preoperatively. Hence, we administer antibiotics to all patients suspected of having appendicitis but continue administration intraoperatively and postoperatively only in those patients demonstrated to have complicated appendicitis.

Examination under Anesthesia

After the patient has been anesthetized, the abdomen should be carefully and systematically palpated once more. On occasion, such examination will show the gallbladder to be the real cause of the patient's symptoms. If an appendiceal mass is detected, it should be determined whether the mass is mobile or firmly fixed. The mass may be due to a periappendiceal phlegmon without perforation, to a collection of fluid and pus associated with localized perforation of the appendix, or to a frank periappendiceal abscess.

Management of the Patient without a Palpable Mass (Presumed Uncomplicated Appendicitis)

There is no question about what operation needs to be done: the patient needs appendectomy. The questions to be considered concern choice of incision, the handling of the appendiceal stump, whether or not to employ drains, and the method of wound closure.

Transverse Incision. This incision (Fowler-Weir; Davis-Rockey) is made at a level 1 to 3 cm. below the umbilicus and is centered on the midclavicular-midinguinal line. The length of the incision is a centimeter or so longer than the breadth of the surgeon's hand. The aponeurosis and muscles of the abdominal wall are split or incised in the direction of the skin wound (Fig. 4). The incision lies in the direction of skin wrinkle lines and yields a cosmetically superior scar even if of necessity it is not sutured.

Exposure of the appendix through this approach is better, particularly in patients with a retrocecal appendix and in those who are obese. After the peritoneum is opened, the appendix is identified by following the anterior cecal taenia, and the inflamed appendix is coaxed into the wound, cupped in the palm of the hand. If this maneuver is done properly, the cecum will lie within the wound at the level of the abdominal musculature and the appendix will be above the level of the anterior abdominal wall. It will be unnecessary for vigorous retraction to be maintained throughout the operation.

The disadvantage of the transverse incision is that the rectus sheath is opened; the medial end of the wound is closer to the midline, so if pus is present and spills, there is a theoretical danger of dissemination and peritonitis. Despite this disadvantage, there is no substitute for good exposure in any operation and for this reason the transverse incision is preferred.

Gridiron Incision. The muscle-splitting incision (McArthur-McBurney) is a time-honored approach and one widely used today (Figs. 5 to 7). Its advantage is that separation of muscles in the line of their fibers produces a wound that does not depend entirely upon sutures for restoration of tissue continuity. The skin incision is made obliquely in the right lower quadrant. As in all incisions across skin wrinkle lines, the scar widens with time and the cosmetic result is less than optimal. Exposure of the appendix, especially a retrocecal appendix, through a gridiron incision can be awkward unless the appendix lies immediately below the incision. The gridiron incision can be extended medially, partially transecting the rectus sheath, which usually provides the additional exposure required to approach a pelvic appendix but often does not improve exposure of a retrocecal appendix. Under desperate circumstances, a gridiron incision can be extended vertically; this destroys the rationale of this incision but is occasionally necessary to expose a retrocecal appendix.

Other Incisions. Some surgeons use a vertical right paramedian incision or a pararectus (Battle) incision. Neither provides access to the appendix that is as good as that achieved through a transverse or gridiron incision. In addition, the Battle incision is particularly prone to disruption or development of a ventral hernia should wound infection occur.

If there is doubt about the diagnosis, so that general exploration of the abdomen is indicated, a vertical midline incision centered on the umbilicus is preferred. Appendectomy usually can be done through such an incision, though exposure is not ideal. If a gangrenous or perforated appendicitis is encountered, the midline incision can be closed and a lateral approach made to the appendix.

The Appendiceal Stump. The mesoappendix is transected beginning at its free border by taking small bits of tissue between pairs of hemostats placed approximately a centimeter from and parallel to the appendix. A suture should be passed through the mesoappendix and into the wall of the cecum close to the base of the appendix in order to secure the intramural accessory branch of the posterior cecal artery. If exposure of a long appendix is difficult, the mesoappendix can be transected retrogradely beginning at the base of the appendix.

In most cases of appendicitis, inversion of the unligated stump using a Z stitch, rather than the more conventional purse-string suture, is preferred (Fig. 8). This maneuver accomplishes inversion of the appendiceal stump without spillage of cecal content. The appendix that is to be inverted should not be ligated,

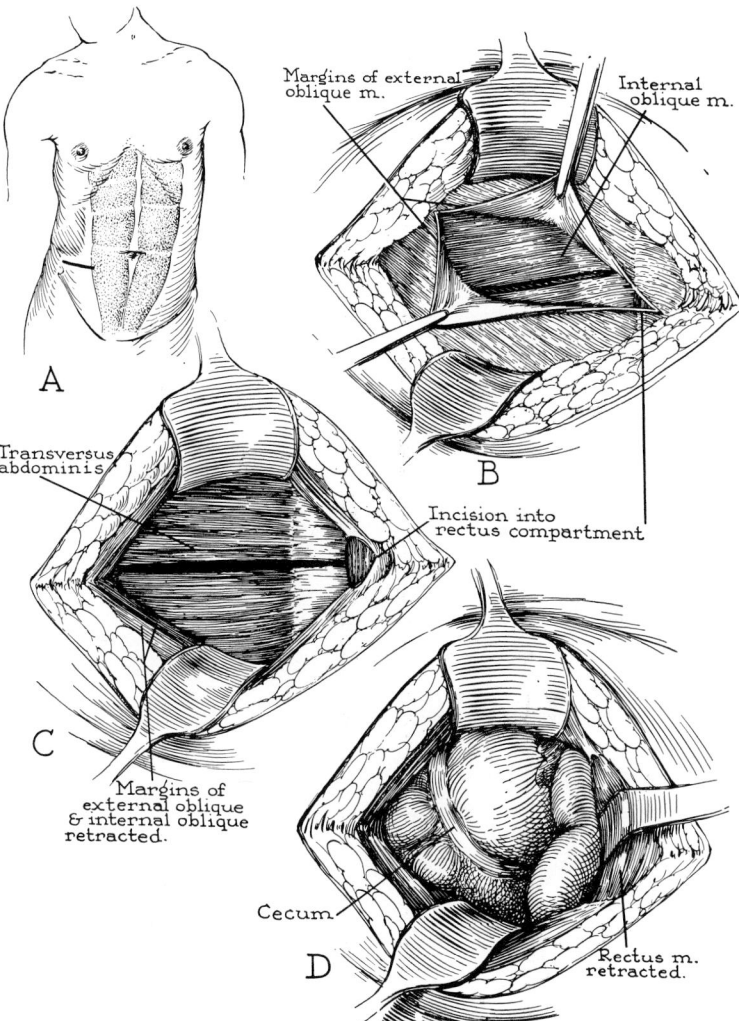

Figure 4. Transverse incision for appendectomy. Placement of skin incision (*A*). External oblique may be split, as illustrated (*B*), or incised transversely. The internal oblique and transversus abdominis are split and the rectus sheath, but not the rectus muscle, is incised (*B* and *C*). Retraction exposes the cecum (*D*), which is rotated into the wound. (From Shackelford, R. T.: Surgery of the Alimentary Tract, Philadelphia, W. B. Saunders Company, 1977.)

since ligation plus inversion creates conditions conducive to development of an intramural abscess or mucocele (Fig. 9). In addition, the ligated plus inverted appendiceal stump may later appear as a cecal tumor and be a vexing source of diagnostic difficulties.[22]

If the appendix is edematous, turgid, or otherwise unsuitable for inversion, it should be doubly ligated at its base, the distal ligature being placed as a suture ligature. It is unnecessary to paint the appendiceal stump with alcohol or iodophor, or to suture the mesoappendix or omentum over the base of the cecum.

Erroneous Diagnosis. While every surgeon feels somewhat chagrined at removing a "lily-white" appendix, the diagnosis of appendicitis is not always clear, and a finite number of normal appendices always are going to be excised in appropriate clinical circumstances. As Ravitch has said, "there is only one way to have a 100 per cent accurate diagnostic record for acute appendicitis, and that is to wait until they all rupture." Recently, recommendations by some surgeons have indicated that intensive in-hospital observation may reduce the incidence of removal of a

normal appendix. In this context, the unfortunate term "unnecessary appendectomy" has been used, a pejorative phrase which only serves to confuse the real issues. A judgment that appendectomy was "unnecessary" can only be made in retrospect. The removal of a normal appendix in appropriate clinical circumstances never constitutes an unnecessary appendectomy. A policy of active surgical intervention on the basis of minimal clinical suspicion has been demonstrated to reduce both the morbidity and the mortality of appendicitis.[10, 12] Watchful waiting, however careful it may be, runs the risk of increasing both morbidity and mortality. In addition, cost-benefit analysis supports a policy of early appendectomy with a low threshold of suspicion.[24]

If exploration reveals a normal appendix, orderly investigation for the cause of the patient's symptoms must be carried out. The first maneuver is to obtain a specimen of any peritoneal fluid or exudate for Gram stain to determine whether bacteria are present; this specimen also should be cultured for aerobes and anaerobes. Next, the cecum should be inspected; in 3 per cent of patients older than age 40, the symptoms

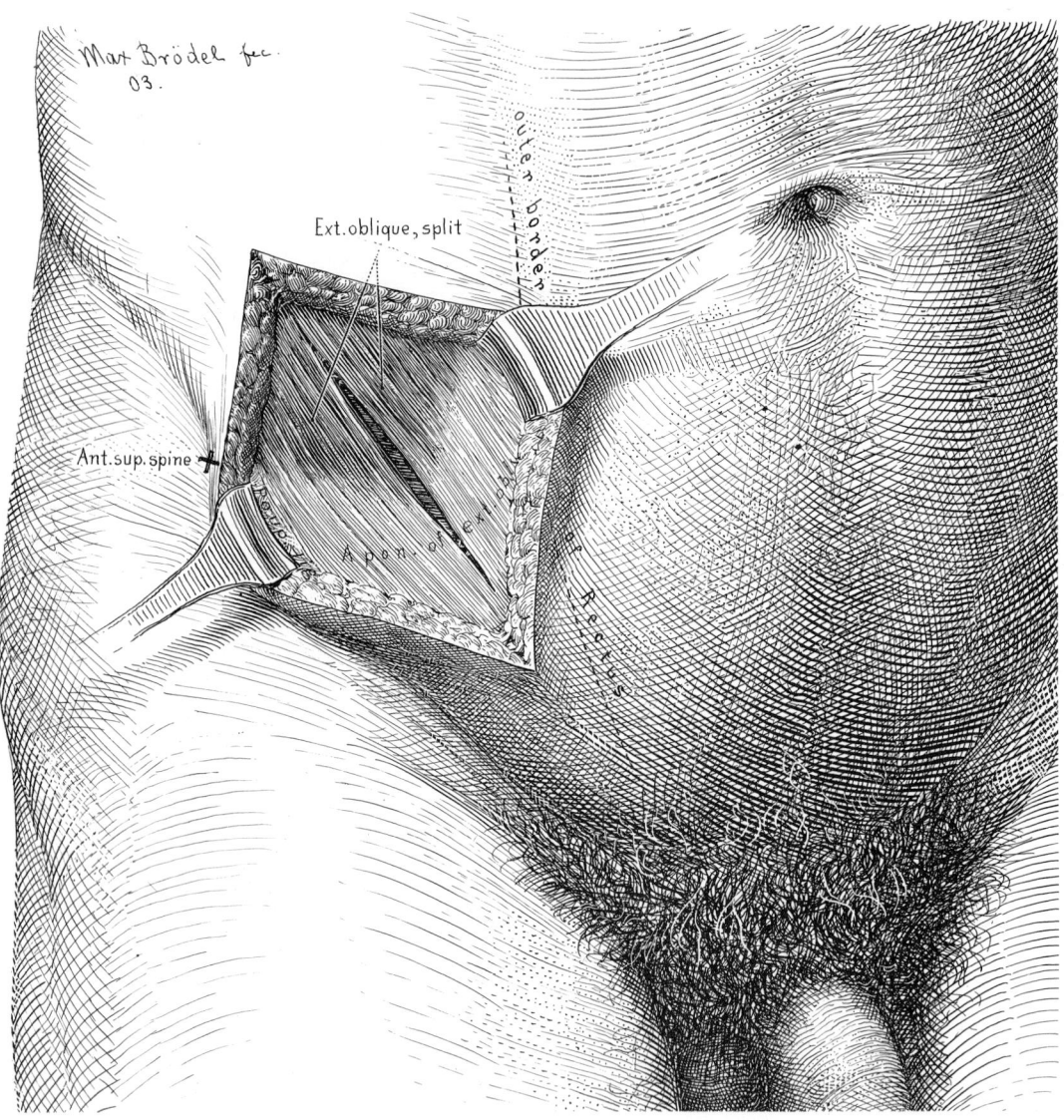

Figure 5. Gridiron incision. Skin has been incised and retracted; separation of the external oblique muscle and aponeurosis in the line of its fibers is indicated. (From Kelly, H. A., and Hurdon, E.: The Vermiform Appendix and Its Diseases. Philadelphia, W. B. Saunders Company, 1905.)

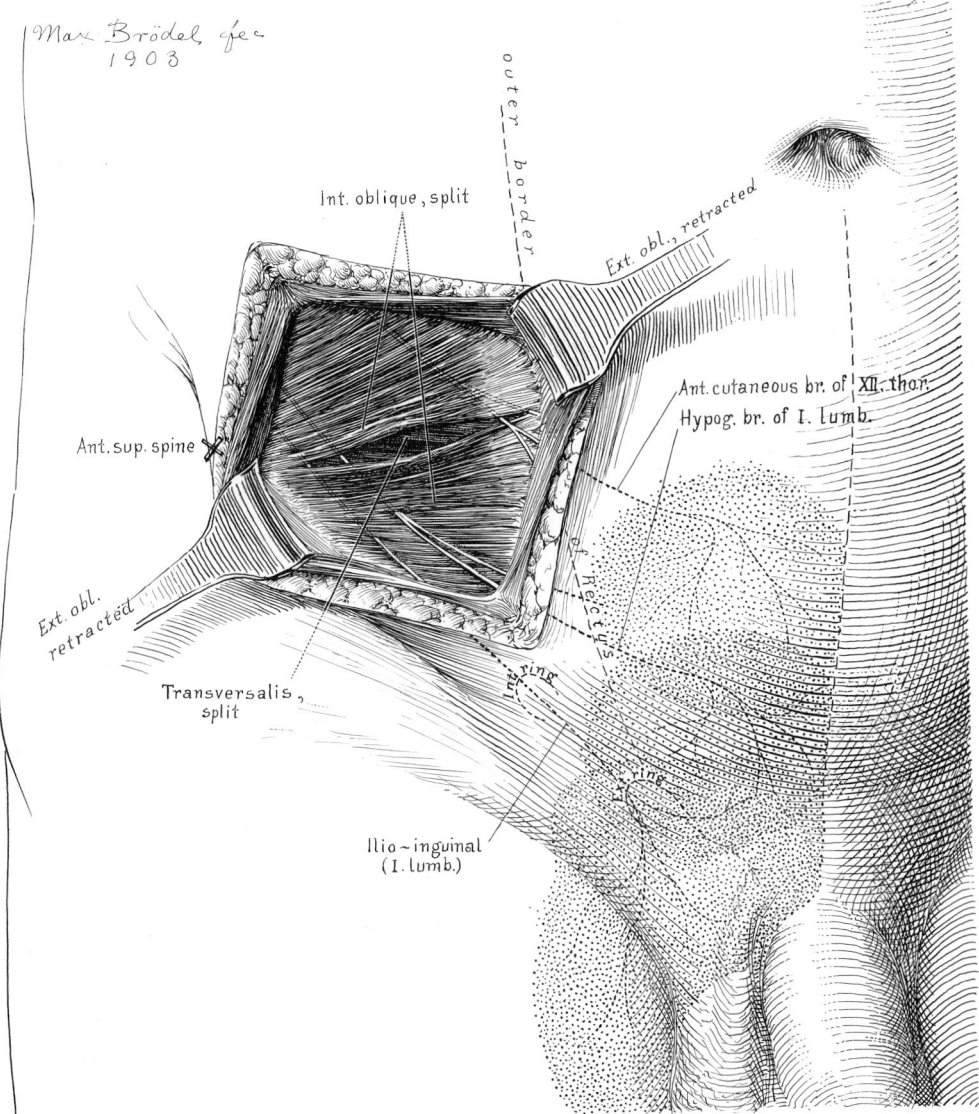

Figure 6. Gridiron incision. External oblique retracted, separation of the internal oblique muscle indicated. (From Kelly, H. A., and Hurdon, E.: The Vermiform Appendix and Its Diseases. Philadelphia, W. B. Saunders Company, 1905.)

mimicking appendicitis are secondary to malignant disease of the colon. The small intestine is examined in retrograde fashion for evidence of regional enteritis or a Meckel's diverticulum; the pelvic organs are palpated and inspected, seeking disease in that area. The intra-abdominal colon should be palpated next, after which the gallbladder and the duodenum should be sought in the right upper quadrant. If enlarged lymph nodes are present in the small bowel mesentery, a representative node should be excised and sent for culture. The presence of infection by Yersinia organisms recently has been recognized in several cases which clinically appeared to be mesenteric adenitis. Explora-

tion should not cease until the cause of the acute abdominal symptoms has been identified or the surgeon is certain that no remediable lesion is present within the abdominal cavity.

Wound Closure. The area of the cecum, the right iliac fossa, and the margins of the wound are irrigated prior to closure with dilute antibiotic solution: 500 mg. kanamycin and 50,000 units bacitracin dissolved in 500 ml. sterile normal saline. Irrigation should be repeated after the muscles and aponeuroses have been sutured.

Closure of the peritoneum is not necessary and may promote formation of adhesions. Each fascia layer is

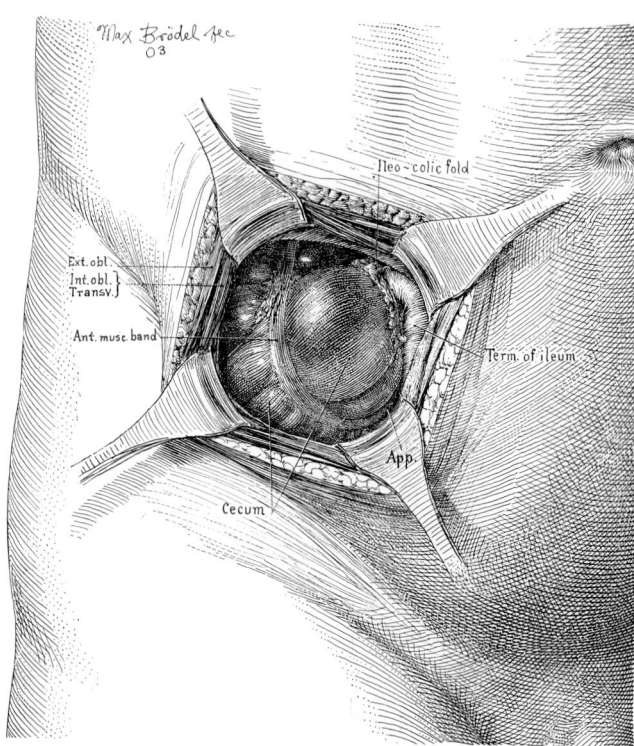

Figure 7. Gridiron incision. All musculoaponeurotic layers have been split, the peritoneum opened transversely, and the wound margins retracted. (From Kelly, H. A., and Hurdon, E.: The Vermiform Appendix and Its Diseases. Philadelphia, W. B. Saunders Company, 1905.)

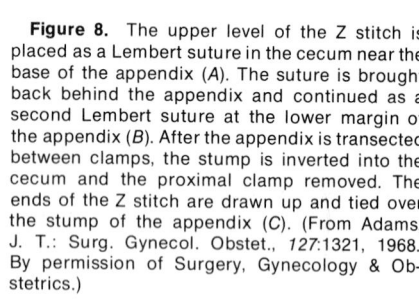

Figure 8. The upper level of the Z stitch is placed as a Lembert suture in the cecum near the base of the appendix (*A*). The suture is brought back behind the appendix and continued as a second Lembert suture at the lower margin of the appendix (*B*). After the appendix is transected between clamps, the stump is inverted into the cecum and the proximal clamp removed. The ends of the Z stitch are drawn up and tied over the stump of the appendix (*C*). (From Adams, J. T.: Surg. Gynecol. Obstet., *127*:1321, 1968. By permission of Surgery, Gynecology & Obstetrics.)

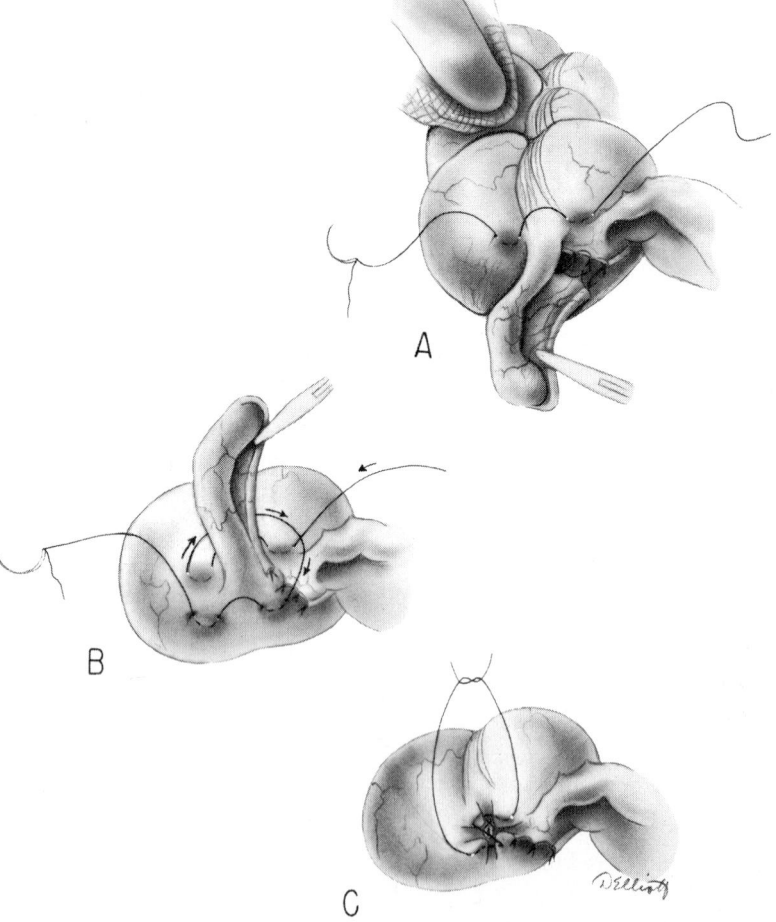

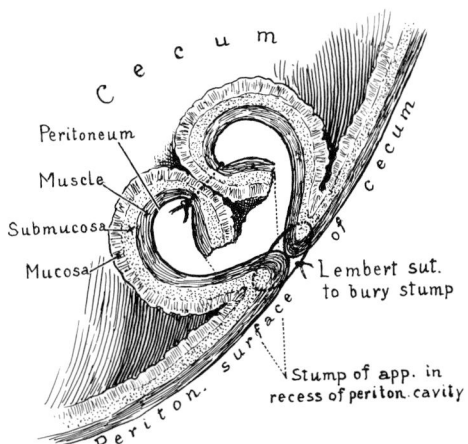

Figure 9. Ligation plus inversion of an appendix stump leads to a closed space and sets the stage for future trouble. (From Kelly, H. A., and Hurdon, E.: The Vermiform Appendix and Its Diseases. Philadelphia, W. B. Saunders Company, 1905.)

closed with nonabsorbable sutures. It is preferable not to place sutures in subcutaneous fat, since they have a distressing tendency to "spit out" weeks or months postoperatively. Instead, a locking mattress suture is used to accomplish obliteration of dead space in the subcutaneous portion of the wound.[5]

Drainage of either the deep or subcutaneous portions of the wound is unnecessary, and possibly harmful, when an unperforated appendix has been removed intact. If there has been contamination of the subcutaneous tissue by periappendiceal pus, it is preferable to pack the subcutaneous portion of the wound loosely open for 24 to 48 hours; the pack is then removed, but the skin is not reapproximated with paper tape until the fifth postoperative day.

Antibiotic therapy should not be continued postoperatively unless the appendix is gangrenous or perforated. The patient may be discharged as early as the third postoperative day provided there is no undue wound tenderness or fever and antibiotics have not been administered for 48 hours prior to discharge.

Management of the Patient with a Mobile Periappendiceal Mass (Presumed Gangrenous or Locally Perforated Appendicitis)

Appendectomy is the treatment of choice for patients with a nonfixed mass whose symptoms are of less than five days' duration. Operation always should be advised in children, pregnant women, elderly patients, and patients in whom the duration of symptoms is in doubt. The incision should be made transversely over the most prominent portion of the mass and the muscles and aponeuroses split using the gridiron principle. The medial aspect of the wound should be packed to prevent contamination of the peritoneal cavity by spillage from the periappendiceal phlegmon.

Fluid and pus, if present, are aspirated after a specimen has been obtained for culture and sensitivity tests. The tissues are dissected sufficiently to expose the appendix. Care should be taken not to disturb adherent coils of intestine or omentum on the medial side of the mass when accomplishing appendectomy. More often than not, the base of the appendix will be quite turgid and the surgeon will have to settle for double ligation of the stump, inversion being impossible. The question of whether to drain in these cases has been debated for years. In most patients with a gangrenous but unperforated appendix and without a collection of periappendiceal pus, closure without subfascial drainage is preferred. If a periappendiceal abscess is present or the tissues are so turgid as to create a dead space, the cavity should be drained with a soft rubber drain brought out through a separate stab incision to avoid incisional hernia.

As in uncomplicated appendicitis, the right iliac fossa and the wound should be liberally irrigated with dilute antibiotic solution prior to layer closure of the muscles with interrupted nonabsorbable sutures. Although some surgeons close the skin incision in these cases, leaving a drain in the subcutaneous tissues, it is preferable to leave the skin and subcutaneous tissues unsutured. Gauze soaked in antibiotic irrigating solution is placed within the wound and a dressing is applied. After 24 to 48 hours, the dressing and gauze pack are removed and the wound covered with a dry dressing. If needed, the skin may be loosely approximated on the fifth or sixth postoperative day with paper tape. If the wound does not appear clean and healthy at this time, it should not be closed; granulation occurs rapidly and the wound will heal spontaneously in three to six weeks.

Systemic antibiotics should be continued for four to five days after operation. A rectal examination is conducted daily to detect development of pelvic abscess. Discharge from the hospital is delayed until the patient has been afebrile for two days, has not had antibiotics for 72 hours, and has no evidence of wound infection or intraperitoneal or pelvic abscess.

Management of the Patient with a Fixed Periappendiceal Mass (Presumed Appendiceal Abscess)

If a patient is first seen when symptoms are subsiding and a well-localized periappendiceal mass is found by physical examination, it is reasonable in most adults to start sytemic antibiotics and to continue expectant treatment. However, all children, pregnant women, and most elderly patients should not be managed by expectant treatment of the appendix mass; drainage of the appendiceal abscess should be carried out as soon as the patient can be prepared for operation. In two out of three adults in whom expectant treatment of the appendix mass is indicated, symptoms will continue to subside and a subsequent interval appendectomy can be accomplished. In one out of three such patients, however, symptoms do not continue to subside, and prompt appendectomy or drainage of the appendiceal abscess should be performed.

In infants, an appendectomy always should be accomplished in addition to draining the abscess. The reason is that the conical shape and broad lumen of the infant appendix promotes continued drainage of feces from the cecum through the perforation. In adults, appendectomy also should be accomplished if it can be done without breaking down adhesions that have walled off the abscess. Accomplishment of appendectomy at the time of draining the abscess is less important in adults, since the narrow obstructed lumen of the adult appendix usually prevents retrograde cecal drainage of feces. If the appendix is not removed when the abscess is drained, interval appendectomy should be done six to eight weeks after drainage from the abscess has ceased and the wound is healed.

The location of an appendiceal abscess corresponds exactly with the anatomic location of the tip of the appendix: about two thirds are situated behind the cecum, 30 per cent form in the pelvis, and 4 per cent are found behind the terminal ileum or extraperitoneally behind the ascending colon.

The incision for drainage is made just medial to the crest of the ilium at the level of the most prominent portion of the periappendiceal mass. The muscles are split and the lateral edge of the peritoneum is exposed and stripped medially so that the mass surrounding the appendix is approached from its lateral retroperitoneal aspect. If pus is present under pressure, the abscess may rupture spontaneously. If not, a finger should be slowly introduced into the abscess and its loculations broken down by blunt dissection. Care is taken not to break down adhesions walling off the medial aspect of the abscess mass. If the appendix is readily accessible, appendectomy can be performed.

A sump drainage tube should be inserted into the abscess cavity and extracted through a stab wound in the flank. The wound is irrigated with dilute antibiotic solution, the muscular layers are closed, and the subcutaneous tissues and skin incision are packed open as described above for patients with a mobile periappendiceal mass. The sump tube should be left undisturbed for at least 72 hours. If it is then draining less than 100 ml. per day, it may be rotated and slowly removed an inch each day.

Systemic antibiotics should be continued for at least five days postoperatively, and longer if clinically indicated. A daily rectal examination is made to detect a developing pelvic abscess. The head of the bed should be elevated 15 to 30 degrees (semi-Fowler position); while this position will not prevent the development of a subphrenic abscess, it will promote drainage toward the pelvis and is more comfortable for the patient.

If, after a week or so, the patient is afebrile and shows no signs of complications secondary to the drained appendiceal abscess, continued treatment in a hospital is not strictly necessary, although it often will be found to be more convenient. Criteria for discharge are the same as those noted above for patients with a mobile periappendiceal mass.

Management of Patients with Diffuse Peritonitis due to Appendicitis

Spreading peritonitis is the principal cause of continuing mortality from appendicitis and requires careful and energetic treatment. It is generally agreed that appendectomy must be performed in children whether peritonitis is diffuse or not, since any other course is associated with a higher mortality.

There is continuing controversy about the management of adults. The patient with perforative appendicitis in whom diffuse peritonitis develops, and whose tissues have failed to wall off the process so that the perforated appendix is a continuing source of peritoneal contamination, will benefit from appendectomy. On the other hand, a patient whose perforation initially leads to diffuse peritonitis, but in whom the perforated appendix is subsequently walled off as an appendiceal abscess, is best managed by operation limited to drainage of the abscess. In both types of patients, general principles governing the management of bacterial peritonitis apply.

The question of if and what to drain in patients with diffuse appendiceal peritonitis also has been an issue of controversy for years. While drainage of each localized collection of pus by means of soft rubber drains is certainly indicated, prophylactic placement of multiple drains within the abdominal cavity is an unwarranted practice.[9] Such prophylactic intra-abdominal drains are rapidly walled off and do not succeed in draining the peritoneal cavity except for a few hours. They may be detrimental rather than helpful, since they perpetuate inflammation by the presence of an unnecessary foreign body and lead to formation of adhesions that may later cause intestinal obstruction.

The principles of wound management in these cases are irrigation of the wound with dilute antibiotic solution, subfascial drains only to localized collections of pus, closure of musculoaponeurotic layers, skin and subcutaneous tissues packed open rather than sutured and drained, daily rectal examination to detect development of pelvic abscess, and nursing the patient in a semiupright position for the initial postoperative week. Systemic administration of antibiotics should be continued for as long as clinically indicated.

Recurrent, Subacute, and Chronic Appendicitis

There are a few patients in whom an initial attack of acute appendicitis subsides spontaneously. If the initial diagnosis is clear, the risk of a recurrent episode of appendicitis is about 50 per cent;[1] elective appendectomy within six to eight weeks therefore should be advised.

Even if a full-blown appendicitis does not ensue, the appendix thereafter may become, in Maingot's phrase, a "grumbler," precipitating recurrent attacks, usually milder than the initial attack, of right lower quadrant pain. Characteristically, patients are symptom-free between attacks; physical examination is normal unless the patient is examined while symptoms are present. If abdominal x-rays demonstrate the presence of a fecalith, a barium enema shows nonfilling of the obstructed appendix, or observation of repeated attacks provides evidence that the patient is suffering from recurrent subacute appendicitis, elective appendectomy should be undertaken.

The presence of retained barium in the appendix or of an asymptomatic fecalith, noted on investigation of the patient for other symptoms, should probably lead to elective interval appendectomy, as appendicitis is likely to develop in such patients within two to three years.

In order to sustain a diagnosis of chronic appendicitis, the resected appendix must show fibrosis throughout the appendiceal wall, partial to complete obstruction of the lumen with evidence of old mucosal ulceration and scarring, and infiltration by chronic inflammatory cells. It is not sufficient to diagnose chronic appendicitis on the basis of a few polymorphonuclear leukocytes found within the wall of an excised appendix. This latter degree of "inflammatory response" can be elicited by the manipulations required for excision of a normal appendix.

Incidental Appendectomy

Opinion regarding the advisability of incidental appendectomy as a routine during other intra-abdominal operations is not settled, but most surgeons would agree that removal of the appendix is a worthwhile procedure, particularly during gynecologic operations and, in the opinion of some surgeons, during right inguinal hernia repair and cholecystectomy.

Incidental appendectomy serves to obviate the future development of appendicitis and its attendant mortality risk. Such risk, although quite small, is probably greater than any risk associated with incidental appendectomy. Several studies have shown that the removal of the appendix *en passant* does not increase total operative time, length of hospital stay, or the incidence of infectious postoperative complications. One curious finding noted in nearly every series reported concerning incidental appendectomy is that between 10 and 15 per cent of incidentally excised appendices show evidence of concurrent or antecedent appendicitis.

Several conditions must be present if incidental appendectomy is to be conducted with minimal risk. The possibility of performing appendectomy needs to be discussed with the patient and appropriate consent obtained. The appendectomy must be conducted with adequate exposure, without undue dissection, and using the incision already made without further extension. In addition, the patient must have tolerated the main operative procedure well and there should be no existing complications expected to result from the main procedure.

Appendectomy and Cancer Risk

A decade ago it was suggested, on the basis of epidemiologic evidence, that removal of the appendix, particularly after age 40, was associated with an increased expectation of the development of a malignancy.[3] The evidence was largely deduced by noting at autopsy the incidence of absence of the appendix in relation to the presence or absence of cancer.

A major difficulty in attempting to elucidate or settle questions of this kind based on epidemiologic autopsy data is that the subjects being investigated are usually hospitalized patients, and they differ in various ways from the general population. Comparisons are thus inherently biased. Such extraneous considerations as socioeconomic status influence the incidence of appendectomy; educated, economically well-off persons tend to overutilize medical resources and also have an excess incidence of appendectomy.

When the possible association of neoplasia and appendectomy is approached by means of large prospective patient population studies, no excess cancer risk can be discerned.[2, 21] In one study it was noted that hospitalized patients had three times the incidence of appendectomy of the population as a whole, but no connection between previous appendectomy and the future development of a cancer could be discerned.

COMPLICATIONS OF APPENDECTOMY

Postoperative complications occur in only 5 per cent of patients if an unperforated appendix is removed intact, but in over 30 per cent of patients with gangrenous or perforated appendicitis. The incidence of perforation is less than 20 per cent in the first 24 hours of symptoms, but rapidly climbs to over 70 per cent after 48 hours. There is considerable urgency in making a correct diagnosis and accomplishing appendectomy within 24 hours after the onset of symptoms in order to reduce the incidence of complications. The more frequent complications of appendectomy include wound infection, pelvic, subphrenic, and intraperitoneal abscesses, fecal fistula, pylephlebitis, and intestinal obstruction. Infection of the subcutaneous tissues is the most common complication following appendectomy. The organisms recovered from the appendiceal fossa in cases of acute appendicitis are most frequently anaerobic Bacteroides species, followed by the aerobes Klebsiella, Enterobacter, and *Escherichia coli.*[16] Since wound infections in cases of appendicitis are caused by fecal organisms, the classic signs of infection (calor, dolor, rubor, tumor) may not be present. The early signs of a fecal wound infection are undue pain and modest edema around the wound. If such signs are present, the skin and subcutaneous tissue should be opened. A rush of pus should not be expected. Fecal infections induce necrosis of subcutaneous fat, often of considerable extent, but only as damaged fat liquefies does much pus form.

Pelvic, subphrenic, or intra-abdominal abscess occurs in up to 20 per cent of patients with gangrenous or perforative appendicitis. Such abscesses usually are due to preoperative contamination of the peritoneal cavity by organisms leaking from a gangrenous or perforated appendix. Less often, contamination ensues from intraoperative spillage. Occasionally, an abscess forms around a retained fecalith or other foreign body. The presence of an abscess is manifested by recurrent fever, malaise, and anorexia, usually beginning about one week after appendectomy. A pelvic abscess may cause diarrhea and can be palpated on vaginal or rectal examination. Subphrenic abscess can be diagnosed by the classic signs of effusion in the overlying thorax and immobility of the involved diaphragm. Confirmation of the presence of an intra-abdominal abscess may require an exploratory laparotomy. All abscesses must be drained.

Fecal fistula is not usually a dangerous complication of appendectomy. Fistulas may be due to retained foreign body, such as a sponge, or to a purse-string suture tied too tightly, a ligature slipping from a tied but noninverted appendiceal stump, necrosis from a periappendiceal abscess encroaching on the cecum, erosion of the wall of the cecum by a drain, regional enteritis, colon obstruction by an undetected neoplasm, or retention of a mucus-producing tip of the appendix.

Most fecal fistulas close spontaneously; all that is

required is to insure that the track remains open until drainage ceases. Fecal fistulas will not close spontaneously if the tip of the appendix or a foreign body is present, if the bowel beyond the fistula is obstructed, or if the mucous membrane of the gut is continuous with the skin. In such cases, closure of the fistula requires an operation.

Pylephlebitis, or portal pyemia, is a serious illness characterized by jaundice, chills, and high fever. It is due to septicemia of the portal venous system, leading to development of multiple liver abscesses. Pylephlebitis is associated with gangrenous or perforated appendicitis and may appear either preoperatively or postoperatively. The infecting organism is usually *Escherichia coli*. Fortunately, now that antibiotics are utilized both before and after appendectomy, this complication has become rare.

Intestinal obstruction, initially paralytic but occasionally going on to true mechanical obstruction, may occur with slowly resolving peritonitis in complicated appendicitis. Late mechanical obstruction following appendicitis is uncommon. The development of a mechanical bowel obstruction usually requires operative relief.

SELECTED REFERENCES

Fitz, R. H.: Perforating inflammation of the vermiform appendix, with special reference to its early diagnosis and treatment. Trans. Assoc. Am. Phys., *1*:107, 1886.
In this paper, Reginald Fitz describes 25 patients, correlating pathologic findings with clinical symptoms to demonstrate conclusively that "perityphlitis" begins with inflammation of the appendix. Fitz was the first physician to use the term "appendicitis." This classic study marks the beginning of modern operative treatment of acute appendicitis.

McBurney, C.: Experience with early operative interference in cases of disease of the vermiform appendix. N.Y. Med. J., *50*:676, 1889.
The purpose of this paper was to report successful treatment by appendectomy of appendicitis prior to perforation. In describing the early clinical symptoms of his patients, McBurney said, "The seat of greatest pain, determined by the pressure of one finger, has been very exactly between an inch and a half and two inches from the anterior spinous process of the ilium on a straight line drawn from the process to the umbilicus." This is now known as McBurney's point. He also recommended the gridiron incision which had been described earlier by McArthur. Despite McArthur's priority, this incision is universally known today as the McBurney incision.

Wangensteen, O. H., and Dennis, C.: Experimental proof of obstructive origin of appendicitis in man. Ann. Surg., *110*:629, 1939.
In a group of patients with carcinoma of the colon but normal appendix who were undergoing decompressive colostomy, the appendix was exteriorized and ligated at its base to produce obstruction, and the tip was cannulated and connected to a recording manometer. Intraluminal pressures up to 126 cm. H₂O (93 mm. Hg) developed in less than 24 hours. Despite the very high pressure in the lumen, the appendiceal mucosa continued to secrete mucus. This paper clearly established obstruction-secretion as the fundamental process in acute appendicitis.

Worcester, A.: Early operations for appendicitis. N. Engl. J. Med., *218*:651, 1938.
A delightfully candid account of the first group of patients in the United States to have an appendectomy. The year was 1886. Dr. Worcester himself was one of the patients.

Zwalenburg, C. V.: The relation of mechanical distention to the etiology of appendicitis. Ann. Surg., *41*:437, 1905.
This is a remarkably prescient paper by a turn-of-the-century surgeon practicing in California. In this paper, Dr. Zwalenburg first proposed, based on his clinical observations of cases of appendicitis, that obstruction was the basic pathophysiologic process in this disease. His hypothesis was later supported by the work of Wangensteen and Dennis, cited above.

REFERENCES

1. Befeler, D.: Recurrent appendicitis: Incidence and prophylaxis. Arch. Surg., *89*:666, 1964.
2. Berndt, H.: Is appendectomy followed by increased cancer risk? Digestion, *3*:187, 1970.
3. Bierman, H. R.: Human appendix and neoplasia. Cancer, *21*:109, 1968.
4. Castleton, K. B., Puestow, C. B., and Sauer, D.: Is appendicitis decreasing in frequency? Arch. Surg., *78*:794, 1959.
5. Condon, R. E.: Locked vertical mattress stitch for skin closure. Surg. Gynecol. Obstet., *127*:839, 1968.
6. Condon, R. E.: Rational use of prophylactic antibiotics in gastrointestinal surgery. Surg. Clin. North Am., *55*:1309, 1975.
7. Cunningham, F. G., and McCubbin, J. H.: Appendicitis complicating pregnancy. Obstet. Gynecol., *45*:415, 1975.
8. Gill, B., and Cudmore, R. E.: Significance of faecoliths in the diagnosis of acute appendicitis. Br. J. Surg., *62*:535, 1975.
9. Haller, J. A., Jr., Shaker, I. J., Donahoo, J. S., Schnaufer, L., and White, J. J.: Peritoneal drainage versus non-drainage for generalized peritonitis from ruptured appendicitis in children. Ann. Surg., *177*:595, 1973.
10. Hobson, T., and Rosenman, L. D.: Acute appendicitis—when is it right to be wrong? Am. J. Surg., *108*:306, 1964.
11. Howie, J. G. R.: Death from appendicitis and appendicectomy. Lancet, *2*:1334, 1966.
12. Howie, J. G. R.: The place of appendicectomy in the treatment of young adult patients with possible appendicitis. Lancet, *1*:1365, 1968.
13. Hyman, P., and Westring, D. W.: Leukocytosis in acute appendicitis: Observed racial difference. J.A.M.A., *229*:1630, 1974.
14. Jenkins, D., and Lee, P.: Radiology in acute appendicitis. J. R. Coll. Surg. Edinb., *15*:34, 1970.
15. Kretchmar, L. H., and McDonald, D. F.: The urine sediment in
16. Leigh, D. A., Simmons, K., and Norman, E.: Bacterial flora of the appendix fossa in appendicitis and postoperative wound infection. J. Clin. Pathol., *27*:997, 1974.
17. Lewis, F. R., Holcroft, J. W., Boey, J., and Dunphy, J. E.: Appendicitis: A critical review of diagnosis and treatment in 1,000 cases. Arch. Surg., *110*:677, 1975.
18. Martin, L. W., and Perrin, E. V.: Neonatal perforation of the appendix in association with Hirschsprung's disease. Ann. Surg., *166*:799, 1967.
19. Meade, R. H.: The evolution of surgery for appendicitis. Surgery, *55*:741, 1964.
20. Mittelpunkt, A., and Nora, P. F.: Current features in the treatment of acute appendicitis: An analysis of 1,000 consecutive cases. Surgery, *60*:971, 1966.
21. Moertel, C. G., Nobrega, F. T., Elveback, L. R., and Wentz, J. R.: A prospective study of appendectomy and predisposition to cancer. Surg. Gynecol. Obstet., *138*:549, 1974.
22. Myllarniemi, H., Perttala, Y., and Peltokallio, P.: Tumor-like lesions of the cecum following inversion of the appendix. Am. J. Dig. Dis., *19*:547, 1974.
23. Noer, T.: Decreasing incidence of acute appendicitis. Acta Chir. Scand., *141*:431, 1975.
24. Parker, S. G., and Kassirer, J. P.: Therapeutic decision making: A cost-benefit analysis. N. Engl. J. Med., *293*:229, 1975.
25. Peltokallio, P., and Janhiainen, K.: Acute appendicitis in the aged patient: Study of 300 cases after the age of 60. Arch. Surg., *100*:140, 1970.
26. Sasso, R. D., Hanna, E. A., and Moore, D. L.: Leukocytic and neutrophilic counts in acute appendicitis. Am. J. Surg., *120*:563, 1970.
27. Senn, N.: A plea in favor of early laparotomy for catarrhal and ulcerative appendicitis, with the report of two cases. J.A.M.A., *12*:630, 1889.
28. Sherman, N. J., and Woolley, M. M.: The ileocecal syndrome in acute childhood leukemia. Arch. Surg., *107*:39, 1973.
29. Spitz, L.: Acute appendicitis: An analysis of six hundred and sixty-six appendicectomies in adults 1959–1968. South Afr. J. Surg., *7*:129, 1969.
30. Stone, H. H., Sanders, S. L., and Martin, J. D., Jr.: Perforated appendicitis in children. Surgery, *69*:673, 1971.
31. Thorbjarnarson, B., and Loehr, W. J.: Acute appendicitis in patients over the age of sixty. Surg. Gynecol. Obstet., *125*:1277, 1967.
32. Wakeley, C. P. G.: Position of vermiform appendix as ascertained by analysis of 10,000 cases. J. Anat., *67*:277, 1933.

34

THE COLON AND RECTUM

I _____

ANATOMY AND SURGICAL PROCEDURES

Isidore Cohn, Jr., M.D.,
and Francis C. Nance, M.D.

The colon, rectum, and anus compose all of the gastrointestinal tract distal to the ileocecal valve. Surgical problems of this area fall into the congenital, inflammatory, traumatic, mechanical, vascular, and neoplastic categories. Proper care of these problems requires knowledge of the anatomy, physiology, pathology, microbiology, and prior surgical approaches to the colon. Review of these basic areas will be integrated with the necessary clinical knowledge as a means of providing appropriate background for the understanding of the surgical problems of the large intestine.

ANATOMY

The large intestine extends about 1.5 meters from the ileocecal valve to the anus, and is approximately one fifth the length of the entire gastrointestinal tract. Since it comes into contact with almost every organ in the peritoneal and retroperitoneal spaces, its diseases and complications may be manifested by symptoms related to any of these organs or areas. Detailed knowledge of its anatomy, embryology, and blood and lymphatic supply is essential to any surgeon interested in the operative care of diseases of the colon.

The internal diameter of the colon is largest in the cecum, where it averages from 7.5 to 8.5 cm., and it diminishes in size progressively to an average of 2.5 cm. in the sigmoid. The narrow lumen of the sigmoid, with its bulky and more solid contents, explains how relatively small lesions can create significant amounts of obstruction, while lesions of the same size in the cecum—with its large diameter and liquid contents—often produce no symptoms detectable by the patient or even by the unwary clinician. The large size of the cecum also explains why it is the first part of the bowel to rupture in the presence of unrelieved distal obstruction, since Laplace's law relates tension in the wall of the bowel to the radius of the tube and its internal pressure ($T = PR$).

Certain gross characteristics help distinguish the colon. (1) The *taeniae coli* are the three strips of longitudinal muscle distributed around the circumference of colon. Thus the outer longitudinal muscle layer of the gut is incomplete in the colon. The three bands converge on the appendix and may be used as a means of locating it in difficult cases. (2) The *haustra* are sacculations about the bowel that are the result of the outpouchings of bowel wall between the taeniae. The haustra are separated by the plicae semilunares or crescentic folds of bowel wall, which give the colon its characteristic x-ray appearance when filled with either barium or air. (3) The *appendices epiploicae*, or fatty appendages along the bowel, have no function but are often useful in helping to protect a suture line or closure of a perforation in the colon. (4) The relative fixation of most of the colon is related to the retroperitoneal location of the ascending and descending portions of the bowel. The intraperitoneal transverse colon is comparatively free but it is marked by a relatively constant location and by the attachment of the omentum to its anterior superior edge. The fixation of the ascending and descending colon in the lateral peritoneal gutters eliminates these areas from the problem of volvulus, which is most commonly seen in the mobile sigmoid and less commonly seen in the cecum or transverse colon.

As the sigmoid colon goes through the peritoneal reflections and the pelvic diaphragm, it becomes the rectum, which is completely extraperitoneal and therefore has no serosal covering, an important consideration in the management of its surgical problems. The level of the peritoneal reflection is of particular importance in decisions regarding the management of malignant lesions, since this is a "fixed" point in any given patient, while the distance from the rectum to the lesion may vary depending on the position in which the patient is examined, the state of contraction or relaxation of the bowel, and other factors.

The arterial blood supply to the ascending colon, hepatic flexure, and transverse colon comes from the superior mesenteric artery via the ileocolic, right colic, and middle colic arteries. The blood supply to the left colon and proximal rectum is derived from the inferior mesenteric artery via its left colic, sigmoid, and superior hemorrhoidal branches. There are almost always good collaterals between adjacent major vessels through a marginal arterial arcade that parallels the course of the colon. The viability of long segments of colon, such as are used for esophageal replacement, is dependent on the collateral circulation and the functional integrity of this marginal vessel. The paired middle and inferior hemorrhoidal arteries supply the rectum below the peritoneal reflection. Detailed anatomic studies of the blood supply of the colon are available for those interested in studying this further.[23] The veins of the colon generally parallel the course of the arteries. The lymphatics are intertwined with the two vascular trees.

OPERATIVE PROCEDURES

The need for a detailed knowedge of the anatomy and embryology in the surgical therapy of diseases of the colon is best illustrated in connection with the selection of an operation for cancer of any part of the colon.

The modern concept of proper cancer surgery requires that a curative operation should: (1) remove all the malignant tissue, (2) remove all or most of the organ in which the cancer originates, (3) eliminate the primary route of lymphatic spread, and (4) provide early control of the venous supply to prevent tumor cell embolization during manipulation of the tumor. When one applies these principles to the surgery of cancer of the large bowel, proper removal of the lymphatics necessitates ligation of the vascular supply as

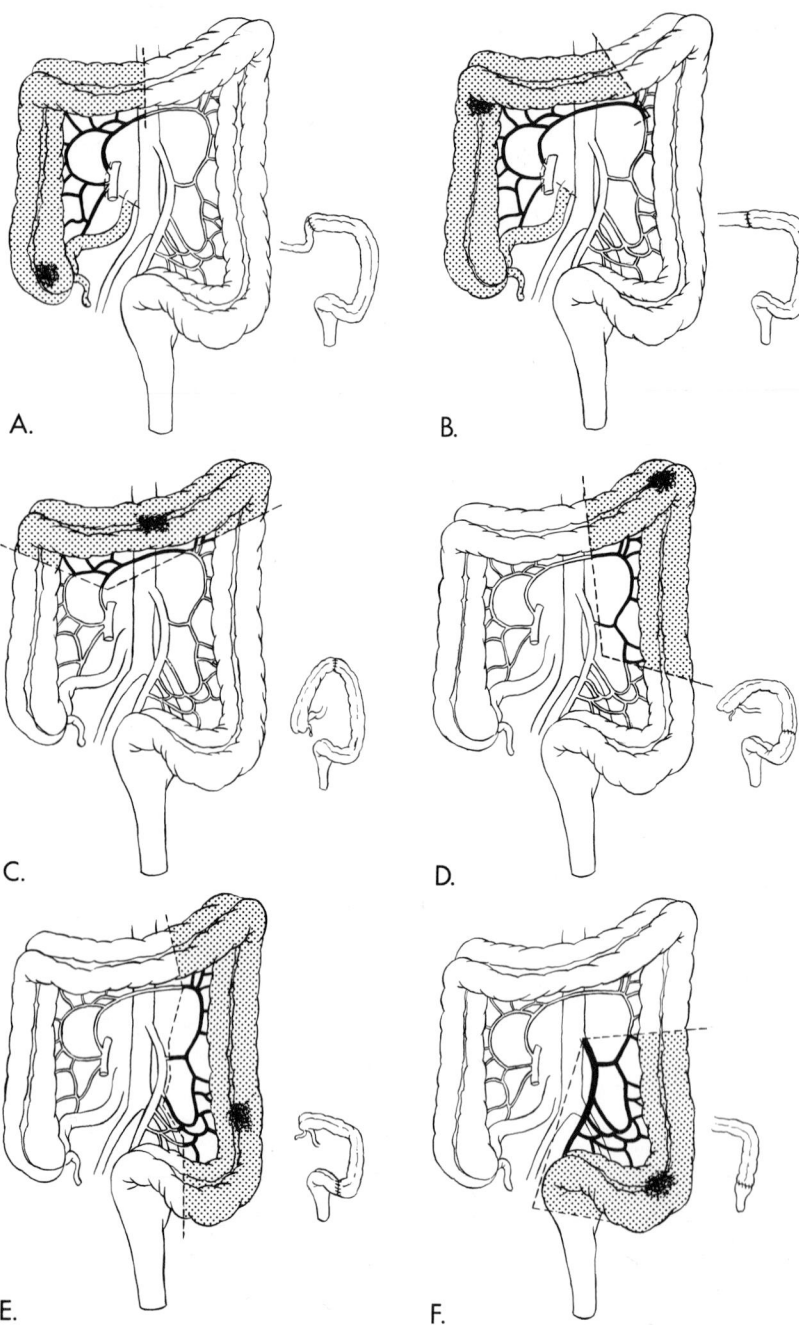

Figure 1. Sections of the colon along with blood vessels that should be resected for cancers in various locations. The method of restoration of continuity is indicated in each case. *A,* Cecum and lower ascending colon, *B,* Upper ascending colon and hepatic flexure. *C,* Transverse colon. *D,* Splenic flexure. *E,* Descending colon and upper sigmoid. *F,* Low sigmoid and upper rectum. (Modified from Coller, F. A.: Cancer of the Colon and Rectum. New York, American Cancer Society, Inc., 1956.)

A.

B.

C.

D.

E.

F.

close to its origin from the aorta as possible; on the left side this means ligation of the inferior mesenteric artery flush with the aorta, while on the right side it means ligation flush with the origin of the vessels from the superior mesenteric. Ligation of the lymphatic channels and of the blood supply at this high level necessitates the removal of more of the colon than might otherwise seem necessary, but is dictated by the elimination of its blood supply. The accompanying drawings (Fig. 1) indicate the proper levels of resection for malignant lesions in various portions of the colon. There is considerable discussion regarding the advisability of a total left colectomy for all lesions in the left colon. Most surgeons have agreed that there is an increased morbidity and mortality associated with a complete left colectomy, and that most of this increased risk is associated with mobilizing the splenic flexure, particularly for lesions lying in the lower sigmoid. However, some contend that the better control of cancer justifies the additional risk. Until more documentation is available, each surgeon should temper his decision in this regard with consideration of the requirements of an individual case, his own capabilities, and the training he obtained.

If a colon resection is performed for a benign lesion, then totally different considerations become pertinent. It is no longer necessary to seek out all the lymphatics, and therefore only that segment of colon involved by the disease process need be resected. Furthermore it is possible to reduce operative risk by carrying the resection close to the bowel rather than attempting to remove so much of the mesentery. Thus resections for ulcerative colitis, diverticulitis, volvulus, trauma, and other benign conditions do not require "high ligation" of the lymphatics or vessels, and the blood supply to the involved bowel can be ligated at a point of convenience in relation to the disease.

Since the arrangement of intramural vessels in the colon is so different from that in the small bowel, and since there are other features that make a colon anastomosis more hazardous than a similar anatomosis in the small intestine, it is important to be sure that any colonic anastomosis is made in bowel that has an optimal blood supply. This is best assured by ascertaining that the divided ends of the bowel bleed actively before any colonic anastomosis is made. It is equally important to see that there is no tension on any anastomosis in the colon in order to minimize the chances for anastomotic breakdown. Other specific dangers in colonic anastomoses include the tremendous bacterial flora normally present in the large bowel and the relatively solid character of colonic contents. These features tend to increase the risk of any colonic procedure when it is compared with a similar procedure in the small bowel.

Colostomy

As one means of decreasing the risk of colonic procedures it is often desirable or necessary to provide proximal decompression for an anastomosis, an obstructing lesion in the bowel, a perforation, or any other lesion that increases the risk of completing the procedure in a single stage (Fig. 2). This is accomplished by a "colostomy."

A colostomy is an opening in the colon serving some or all of the functions of the anus. Since colostomy may be an integral part of the surgical treatment of colonic disease, it is necessary to understand thoroughly the uses and types of colostomies. A colostomy is used for one of three purposes. (1) It may *replace* the anus as the distal opening of the gastrointestinal tract. (2) It may *divert* the fecal stream from some more distal pathologic process (such as a colonic perforation). (3) It may *decompress* the obstructed colon. A colostomy is most often placed on the anterior abdominal wall. The type of colostomy employed by the surgeon should be based on a consideration of its specific purpose. A glossary of terms may aid the understanding of colostomy.

A *permanent colostomy* is intended to replace the anus when the anus and rectum must be removed. The ideal permanent colostomy should have a single stoma (for easy care), pass formed feces, be in a location easily accessible to the patient for irrigation, function satisfactorily without a bag, and be comfortable. These criteria are met best by an end colostomy in the left colon located in the left iliac fossa.

A *temporary colostomy* is intended only as a temporary measure, pending restoration of colonic continuity after the acute condition prompting colostomy has resolved. The ideal temporary colostomy should be easily performed, should permit definitive resection without disturbing the colostomy, and should allow easy, safe restoration of bowel continuity. A right

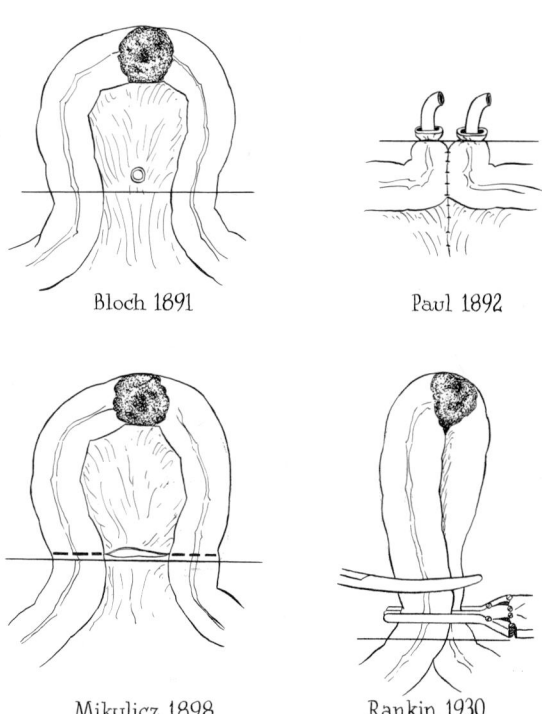

Bloch 1891   Paul 1892

Mikulicz 1898   Rankin 1930

Figure 2. Schematic representation of the operations described by Bloch, Paul, Mikulicz, and Rankin for management of obstructing carcinoma in mobile parts of the colon. (Modified from McKittrick, L. S.: Surg. Gynecol. Obstet., *87*:15, 1948.)

transverse loop colostomy meets most of these criteria when the disease is in the sigmoid colon (as it usually is).

Loop colostomy, exteriorization colostomy, resective colostomy, and Mikulicz colostomy are almost synonymous. The colon is exteriorized as a loop, with proximal and distal portions brought through the same incision. This type of colostomy may be quickly performed and is particularly useful when decompression of the obstructed colon is desired along with ex-

teriorization of the area of disease. An example is the exteriorization of a perforated carcinoma of the sigmoid colon.

An end colostomy is a single-stoma colostomy. Only the proximal limb of the colon is exteriorized.

In a Hartmann colostomy, the colonic lesion is excised, the proximal colonic limb is brought out as an end colostomy, and the distal limb (rectum) is oversewn and left within the abdomen. This has the advantage of removing the pathologic lesion, but the

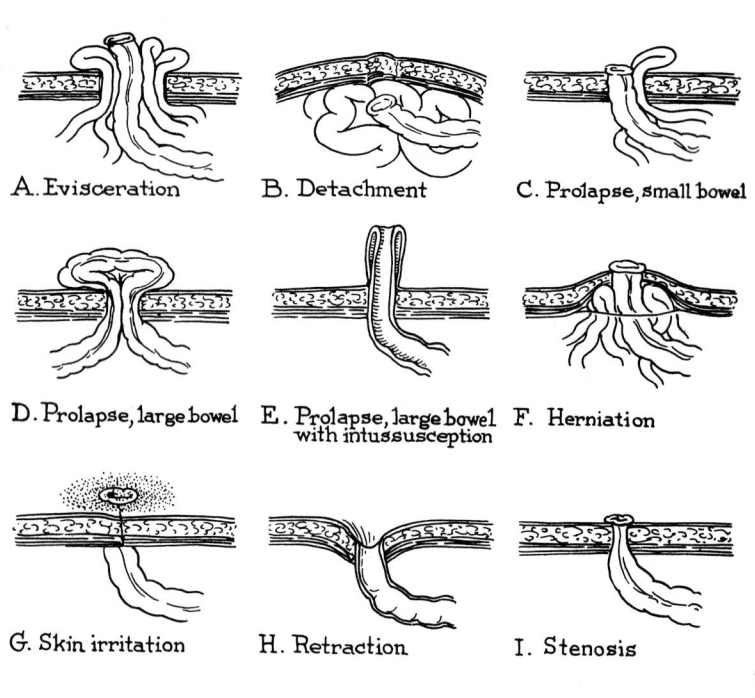

Figure 3. Complications and sequelae of colostomy. (From Lichtenstein, M. R.: Surg. Clin. North Am., *35*:1347, 1955.)

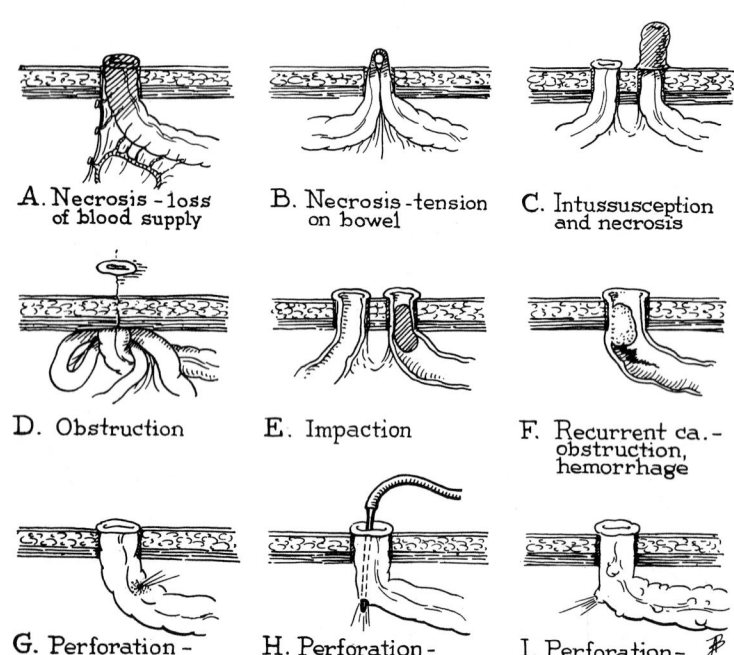

disadvantage of making restoration of bowel continuity difficult.

A divided-stoma colostomy or Devine colostomy is the most effective method of completely diverting the fecal stream from a distal lesion. The two limbs of the colon are brought out through separate skin incisions. The proximal stoma is thus an end colostomy. The distal stoma is called a mucous fistula. This colostomy assures complete, temporary diversion of feces but restoration of bowel continuity is more difficult.

A cecostomy may consist of exteriorization of the cecum or placement of a tube in the cecum. Tube cecostomy was once widely used for decompression of an obstructed colon but most surgeons have abandoned this practice.

As previously stated, the surgeon should have clearly in mind the purpose for which the colostomy is to be used. Thus, in the care of a patient with carcinoma of the rectum, the main consideration should be provision of a long-term substitute for the rectum. A single-barreled end colostomy satisfies this requirement. In treating an emergency condition of the colon, survival of the patient should be the primary consideration. Therefore, an easily performed colostomy that allows subsequent removal of the lesion or restoration of bowel continuity or both should be used. Thus for an obstructing sigmoid cancer without liver metastases, a right transverse colostomy provides adequate rapid decompression, allows the surgeon to resect the left colon subsequently without disturbing the colostomy, and permits safe restoration of bowel continuity after recovery from the resection. This is not a good permanent colostomy. When complete and long-term (but not permanent) diversion of the fecal stream is desired (such as for rectovaginal fistula) it is best to use a divided-stoma colostomy, accepting the greater difficulty in restoration of bowel continuity in exchange for more complete diversion. Familiarity with some of the complications of colostomy may prevent or minimize them (Fig. 3).

For references, see page 1108.

II

PHYSIOLOGY

Isidore Cohn, Jr., M.D.,
and Francis C. Nance, M.D.

The colon serves three primary functions in the normal person: it is a site for absorption of water and some electrolytes, it serves as a convenient temporary storage compartment for feces, and it is an effective excretory organ. The colon is separated from the small bowel by the ileocecal valve, which prevents the contents of the ileum from passing into the cecum before the digestive process has been completed and serves as a barrier preventing reflux of colonic contents. The valve and the relative immobility of colonic contents have been used to explain the marked difference in bacterial ecology between colon and small bowel, but these observations may be open to question. The bacterial flora of the small bowel seldom exceeds 10^5 organisms per milliliter, in contrast to colonic counts up to 10^{10} organisms. In the colon one third of the fecal mass is bacteria.

The absorptive function of the colon dries the fecal mass. The ileum discharges 500 to 600 ml. of water into the cecum daily, but only 180 ml. is excreted in the feces. Most of the remaining water is absorbed in the cecum and ascending colon. The colon normally secretes small quantities of mucus. In pathologic states, or when irritated mechanically, mucous secretion increases markedly.

Two motility patterns are observed in the colon. Agitating or segmenting contractions knead and mix the fecal mass primarily in the right and transverse colon. These movements appear to aid in water absorption. A second type of contraction, "mass movement" propels the colonic contents distally. These contraction waves are not true peristalsis, since there is a simultaneous constriction of long segments of colon. The mass movements empty the contents of the right colon into the sigmoid and upper rectum. Mass movements of the colon can be initiated by filling the stomach with food—the gastrocolic reflex. True peristalsis, similar to that seen in the small bowel, occurs only rarely in the human colon except in association with the act of defecation.

Colonic motility may be altered by a number of stimuli. The colon appears to be particularly sensitive to paralytic ileus from trauma, infection, or handling at surgery. Motility patterns demonstrate an increase in intraluminal pressures in chronically constipated persons and in patients with diverticulosis. Morphine and codeine markedly increase muscle tone of the large bowel and reduce propulsive action. Anticholinergics are potent inhibitors of colonic motility while parasympathomimetic drugs such as neostigmine increase colonic motor activity.

The act of defecation results in expulsion of feces. It is a controlled reflex which may be inhibited by the adult until it is convenient (medical students facing a surgery test may dispute this). The rectum is normally empty, but when mass movements propel feces into the rectum or when intraluminal pressure rises to 20 to 25 cm. H$_2$O, the desire to defecate will be experienced. The receptors within the wall of the rectum are normally able to discriminate between solids, liquids, and gas. The normal person finds this discrimination important in discreetly eliminating the 500 ml. of gas usually passed during the day.

The act of defecation is preceded by assumption of appropriate posture, voluntary relaxation of the external sphincter, and a substantial increase in intra-abdominal pressure by the Valsalva mechanism. A mass contraction of the colon results and the internal sphincter relaxes. The entire distal colon from the splenic flexure may be emptied. Considerable shortening of the colon and rectum during contraction aids in expelling feces.

Other than bacteria, the 75 to 180 gm. of feces excreted daily contain 70 per cent water, undigested cellulose, proteins, and fats. Only a small amount of food residue is excreted in the normal person. Ammonia is produced and absorbed in the colon, principally as a result of bacterial degradation of urea, and is of no clinical significance in normal persons, since the ammonia in portal blood is rapidly detoxified by the liver. In the presence of cirrhosis, portal hypertension, and portasystemic shunts, ammonia absorption from the colon may play a significant role in the pathogenesis of hepatic coma.

Gas in the colon comes primarily from swallowed air. Most is nitrogen (carbon dioxide and oxygen are rapidly absorbed). Methane and hydrogen are present in small (but noninflammable) quantities, and result from bacterial putrefaction. The propulsion of gas and the passage of flatus are among the earliest signs of returning bowel function in the postoperative patient.

The act of defecation requires adequate sensation within the rectum, control of sphincteric relaxation and contraction, motility within the colon, and an intact innervation. In planning colon resections these factors must be considered in order to preserve continence.

Changes in colonic function are important in the diagnosis of surgical disease of the colon. Any change in bowel function that persists more than a few weeks should be investigated.

For references, see page 1108.

III

DIAGNOSTIC STUDIES

Isidore Cohn, Jr., M.D.,
and Francis C. Nance, M.D.

A careful and complete history and physical examination are the starting point for evaluation of any patient with suspected disease of the colon. This statement seems so obvious as to be trite. Unfortunately, both history and physical examination are frequently inadequate, even in good institutions. Visual examination of the anus and a careful digital rectal examination are essential parts of *any* complete physical examination, and whenever this is "deferred" one can make certain assumptions about the adequacy of the remainder of the examination. In addition to the information from a visual inspection of the perirectal area, from the digital rectal examination, and from the presence or absence of any intrinsic lesion within reach of the palpating finger, there is the additional information that may be determined from the appearance of the stool on the examining finger. If there is anemia or other reason to suspect bleeding and gross examination of the stool does not confirm this, then a chemical examination of the stool should be made to determine the presence of occult blood. Bleeding from the right colon is particularly likely to be occult, since the blood will be well mixed with the stool, and thus the physician may miss a lesion at a time when it would be amenable to surgical removal.

The biochemical tests that should be performed in any patient with known or suspected disease of the colon will be determined by the specific problems presented by the patient. In a patient who is being prepared for major colonic surgery, some information about the hematologic, cardiac, respiratory, and renal status should be part of the general information obtained preoperatively. For the patient with severe diarrhea, or marked obstruction, knowledge of the electrolyte status is important. In the patient who has metastatic disease, knowledge of the functional capacity of the organ with metastases may be desirable. Thus liver function tests may be helpful, but it must be recognized that there can be extensive malignant involvement of the liver with little or no alteration in any of the commonly available biochemical tests of liver function. An elevated alkaline phosphatase level is a particularly ominous sign of liver metastases.

A new and promising approach to the diagnosis of cancer of the colon is the use of the Gold antigen, or carcinoembryonic antigen (CEA). This is a tumor-specific antigen found in adenocarcinomas of the digestive epithelium that is identical with an antigen in embryonic and fetal digestive organs during the first two trimesters of gestation. The circulating antigen in patients with cancer of the digestive system can be detected by radioimmunoassay. Unfortunately the lack of specificity and sensitivity of the examination has not permitted the use of CEA as a screening test for occult carcinomas, but it has proved useful for detecting *recurrence* in patients following resection of colon cancers.

Sigmoidoscopy

Sigmoidoscopy is the most important single diagnostic study for the patient with colonic disease. The importance of this test is demonstrated by the observation that 75 per cent of all colonic cancers are within reach of the sigmoidoscope. If all patients with suspected colonic lesions were subjected to sigmoidoscopy on their first physician visit, the earlier diagnosis of these lesions would almost certainly improve the long-term outlook for colonic cancer. In addition to its obvious value in cancer, sigmoidoscopic examination permits identification of a large number of benign diseases. All physicians should be familiar with the technique of sigmoidoscopy. The standard sigmoidoscope is a 25-cm. tube with a light source, a magnifying eyepiece, and provisions for aspiration, biopsy, electrodesiccation, and swabbing of the mucosa. The anoscope is shorter (8 cm.) and larger in diameter. It is useful for diagnosis and treatment of lesions at or near the anal verge, such as hemorrhoids and fissures.

Sigmoidoscopy may be performed at any time, but elective examination will be more productive if the patient has been properly prepared. The patient should fast on the morning of the examination. The distal colon is cleansed by administration of two successive nonirritating enemas. This is most conveniently carried out with ready-to-use disposable enema units.

The examination should be conducted with the patient in the jackknife or knee-chest position. Careful visual inspection of the anus and digital rectal examination should precede the introduction of the instrument. The sigmoidoscope, with the obturator in place, is gently inserted into the rectum and then passed under direct vision to its full length. Introduction of the first 15 cm. will cause little discomfort, but at this point angulation of the bowel occurs and further insertion of the sigmoidoscope must be done carefully and gently.

Lesions seen during insertion of the sigmoidoscope are noted, but careful examination is performed during its withdrawal. After complete insertion (aided by occasional air insufflation), the instrument is withdrawn slowly and rotated so that every inch of mucosa is seen. Small lesions may successfully hide on a valve of Houston or in the posterior rectal vault if the endoscopist is not scrupulously careful.

Polypoid lesions less than 1 cm. usually can be removed for pathologic examination. For benign lesions this is also therapeutic. All lesions seen should be biopsied. Diffuse disease such as radiation colitis or ulcerative colitis may be identified grossly and by biopsy. If infectious disease such as amebic colitis is suspected, mucosal swab for trophozoites and culture may be obtained.

All physicians should be equipped to perform proctosigmoidoscopy. The technique is easily learned and is an important screening procedure. If electrocautery and the aid of a pathologist are not available, biopsy or removal of lesions should not be performed. Instead, their location should be carefully described and the patient referred for definitive diagnosis.

Colonoscopy

Fiberoptic instruments that range in length from 85 to 200 cm. permit examination of the entire colon. This procedure requires meticulous preparation of the bowel, but it has proved invaluable in evaluating and treating lesions beyond the reach of the conventional sigmoidoscope.[37]

Indications for colonoscopy include (1) abnormalities on barium x-ray (filling defects, segmental colonic narrowing, and polyps); (2) chronic gastrointestinal bleeding; (3) anastomotic abnormalities following colonic surgery; and (4) selected patients with chronic inflammatory bowel disease. Colonoscopy permits diagnostic biopsy of proximal lesions. In the case of pedunculated polyps, removal for biopsy or definitive therapy may be accomplished, avoiding, in some cases, the need for laparotomy and resection.[29, 38]

Radiologic Studies

The most valuable screening examination for identifying colonic disease is roentgen examination of the colon. A barium enema should be preceded by digital examination of the rectum and by sigmoidoscopy in almost all cases, since this sequence of procedures will give the greatest amount of information in the shortest time and with the least distortion of the normal colonic appearance. A barium enema is advisable in almost everyone with suspected disease of the colon with the exception of those who are known to have a perforation of the colon. Some surgeons would not recommend a barium enema in the presence of obstruction if the plain film of the abdomen is diagnostic. The radiologist should be forewarned if the patient is thought to have any inflammatory disease of the colon in order to minimize the dangers of perforation. The radiologist also should be informed if there is partial or complete obstruction of the colon, to prevent his using undue pressure to force barium past the obstruction, with the possible attendant difficulties in removing the barium after the examination. If a polyp is demonstrated by barium studies, colonoscopy should be performed. In the presence of an obstructive lesion in the colon, a barium enema may be most helpful in locating the exact site and the extent of obstruction. In a partially obstructing lesion, it may be determined whether there are additional lesions located elsewhere in the colon. Plain films of the abdomen may reveal a closed-loop obstruction of the colon due to a competent ileocecal valve, or a volvulus with its tremendous dilatation and characteristic distribution of air. Contrast examinations may establish the presence of a fistulous tract and its location.

While barium enema is most helpful, it is not infallible, and the most expert radiologist will have difficulty on occasion in distinguishing between a carcinoma and an area of constriction resulting from diverticulitis. When critical studies are required, it is important to remember that the radiologist is a consultant and should be given the benefit of all available clinical information.

Selective angiography has been useful in locating sites of bleeding within the colon and in identifying vascular lesions of the bowel. The technique requires selective catheterization of the superior or inferior mesenteric arteries. In some cases, infusion of vasopressin or epinephrine has stopped bleeding in patients who might otherwise have required emergency surgery for massive colonic hemorrhage.[2] Radioisotope scanning of the liver may provide additional information regarding the amount of metastatic involvement of the liver.

Other Diagnostic Tests

Lymphogranuloma venereum can be diagnosed by identification of the virus in the lesion or in involved lymph nodes, by the Frei skin test, or by complement fixation with a titer of 1 to 32 or higher, or with a rising antibody titer during the active stage.

Additional studies are indicated preoperatively to minimize the enhanced risk to other viscera that results from their anatomic proximity to the colon. Because of the very close relationship between the right colon and the retroperitoneal duodenum, there is always the risk of injury to the duodenum when the colon is being mobilized. An upper gastrointestinal series is advisable except in patients with any degree of large bowel obstruction.

Resections of either the right or left colon bring the surgeon into such close proximity to the ureters that a knowledge of their location and of any abnormalities in their course is paramount to the safe conduct of the operation. Thus, any planned procedure on the colon should be preceded by either an intravenous or a retrograde pyelogram to forewarn the surgeon about displacement of the ureter secondary to disease in the colon. When difficulty locating the ureter can be anticipated, particularly in an abdominoperineal resection in an obese patient or one with significant displacement of the left ureter, preoperative insertion of ureteral catheters will aid localization of the ureter during the operative procedure. While this can be most helpful in the difficult case, it is not recommended as a routine measure because of the additional risk of urinary tract infection.

Various newer modifications of older ideas have been employed to assist in the detection of gastrointestinal bleeding. One involves the use of isotopes injected intravenously with subsequent monitoring of the stool. Another involves a simple chemical reaction performed on a stool specimen swabbed on a slide that the patient can mail in to the physician. This test may become a valuable screening measure for the early detection of any gastrointestinal pathologic lesion.

For references, see page 1108.

IV

INTESTINAL ANTISEPSIS AND PERITONITIS FROM PERFORATION

Isidore Cohn, Jr., M.D.,
and Francis C. Nance, M.D.

INTESTINAL ANTISEPSIS*

Intestinal antisepsis involves the use of antibacterial agents to control the bacterial flora of the colon. An "ideal" intestinal antiseptic should have: (1) rapid, highly bactericidal activity against pathogenic organisms in the gastrointestinal tract; (2) ability to prevent development or overgrowth of pathogenic organisms; and (3) low toxicity (local as well as systemic) and limited absorption from the intestine.

---

*A more detailed exposition may be found in Cohn, I., Jr.: Intestinal Antisepsis. Springfield, Ill., Charles C Thomas, Publisher, 1968.

Since intestinal antisepsis was introduced in 1938 there has been considerable discussion of its values and dangers. The following are undisputed facts. The colon is the largest normal reservoir of bacteria in man. Whenever the colon is opened by operation, by trauma, or by disease, the potential exists for peritonitis, wound infection, or other bacterial complication. Historically, the development of the operative approach to lesions of the colon has been dictated by the fear of infection, and each new approach to diseases of the colon has been based on methods for improved control of infection. The risk of infection in elective operations upon the colon is as high as, or higher than, that for almost any organ system in the body.

ORGANISMS IN FECES
200 CONSECUTIVE UNSELECTED PATIENTS

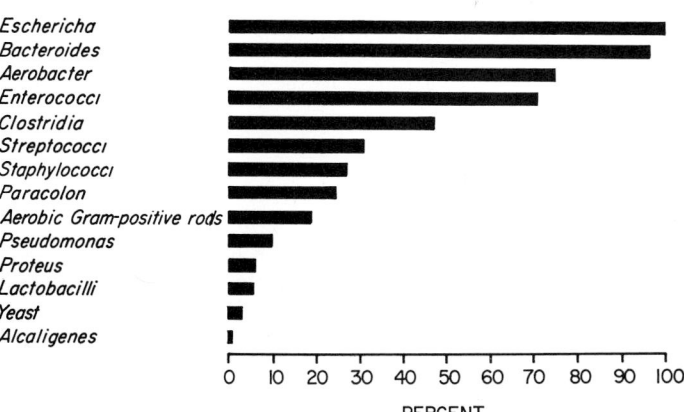

Figure 1. Incidence of various microorganisms in the flora of 200 consecutive hospitalized patients. (From Cohn, I., Jr.: Intestinal Antisepsis. 1968. Courtesy of Charles C Thomas, Publisher, Springfield, Ill.)

The more rational objections to the use of intestinal antisepsis include the following ideas. Intestinal antisepsis may produce complications by upsetting the normal intestinal ecologic balance and permit the overgrowth of pathogenic organisms. The misguided use of antibiotics will encourage the adoption of unsound surgical practices. Sterilization of the bowel contents will increase the risk of tumor implantation during operative procedures for colonic cancer. "Controlled clinical studies" have failed to demonstrate the value of intestinal antiseptics.

It is our contention, based upon both experimental and clinical data, that none of these objections has sufficient validity to contraindicate the use of intestinal antisepsis. There is objective evidence that these agents are beneficial. There is scientific information upon which to base a choice of agents for intestinal antisepsis. The dangers cited by the opponents of intestinal antisepsis are more potential than real. Clinical experience has demonstrated the value of these agents.

As a preliminary to any form of antibiotic therapy, it is necessary to know the normal flora of the large bowel, and this has been determined by studies of the fecal flora in 200 hospitalized patients who were not being treated with antibiotics and did not have any known disease of the large bowel. The large size and variety of the flora are obvious from the results (Figs. 1 and 2).

The routine preparation of patients for elective surgery of the colon includes antibiotics and mechanical preparation. *Preoperative preparation of the colon for elective colon surgery should always include adequate mechanical preparation* (Table 1). Preparation of the bowel should begin in the hospital 3 days prior to the scheduled operation and should include mechanical cleansing and drug therapy.

Mechanical cleansing is the *sine qua non* of intestinal antisepsis, but it is not a substitute for antibacterial therapy. At least two recent studies have shown that mechanical cleansing does not produce a significant quantitative change in the fecal flora (Fig. 3).

RANGE OF BACTERIAL COUNTS
HUMAN FECES

Figure 2. Range of bacterial counts in the feces of the 200 patients indicated in the preceding figure. The right and left limits of each bar represent, respectively, the maximal and minimal counts observed for each organism. The circles indicate the median values. The portions of the bar and the circles in the area of "No Growth" indicate actual samples in which no growth was obtained for that particular organism. (From Cohn, I., Jr.: Intestinal Antisepsis. 1968. Courtesy of Charles C Thomas, Publisher, Springfield, Ill.)

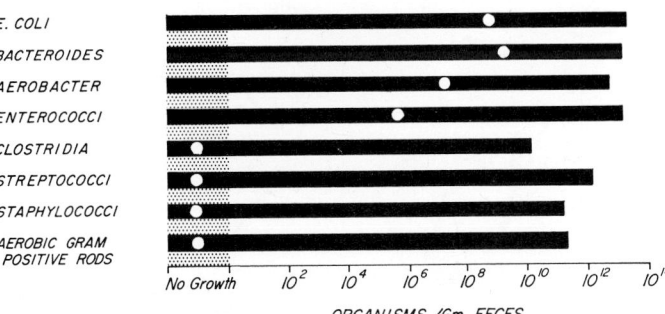

TABLE 1. Routine for Bowel Preparation

On the first day the patient is given a laxative.

A clear liquid diet is begun and continued throughout the period of preparation.

Enemas are given twice daily throughout the period of preparation.

The antibiotic of choice is started on the first day after the laxative has been administered.

The period of preparation is 72 hours.

The first criterion for the evaluation of a potential intestinal antiseptic is whether it controls the bacterial flora of the colon. On the basis of carefully controlled studies of 50 different drugs, only seven agents can be recommended for intestinal antisepsis (Table 2). All of the recommended drugs provide superior control of the intestinal flora, and almost all are poorly absorbed from the gastrointestinal tract and are rarely administered by the oral route for other indications. Antifungal agents in two of the combinations are not a necessary component of intestinal antiseptics, except in infants, who are so much more susceptible to yeast overgrowth.

Kanamycin has been the drug of choice on our service since 1959 because: it is a single drug rather than a combination; it is almost quantitatively excreted in the stool; blood levels are too low to measure after oral administration; a long clinical experience has shown it to be thoroughly acceptable to patients with a minimum of reactions; it provides superior control of the fecal flora; and it can be administered intraperitone-

ally with a greater margin of safety than any of the other agents.

Every potent therapeutic agent has some risk, and intestinal antiseptics are no exception (Table 3). However, most of the dangers are more imagined than real, and some have disappeared with increasing experience. Probably the most important danger is overreliance on antibiotics. If surgeons are tempted to ignore basic surgical principles because they can obtain "antibiotic protection," then the antibiotics are being used erroneously, and their failure to achieve miraculous results should be charged against the surgeon's conscience and not against the agents. Two of the systemic effects of intestinal antiseptics are of considerable importance. Since colonic operations are associated so frequently with spillage of intestinal contents into the peritoneal cavity, it would be desirable to place drugs in the peritoneal cavity that would effectively combat bacterial contamination. Extensive experimental studies, plus clinical experience with well over 1000 patients, have documented the safety of kanamycin in the peritoneal cavity. Sterilization of the intestinal tract increases the incidence of tumor implantation at a suture line in the colon. Almost everyone interested in this problem has agreed that the advantages of antibiotic control of the bacterial complications of colonic operations outweigh the potential disadvantages of a slightly increased incidence of tumor implantation.

During the 10-year period ending in December, 1964, 967 patients received some type of intestinal antisepsis in our institution. Kanamycin was used in over half these patients. Only three of the patients had any side effects from the drug, and in none of

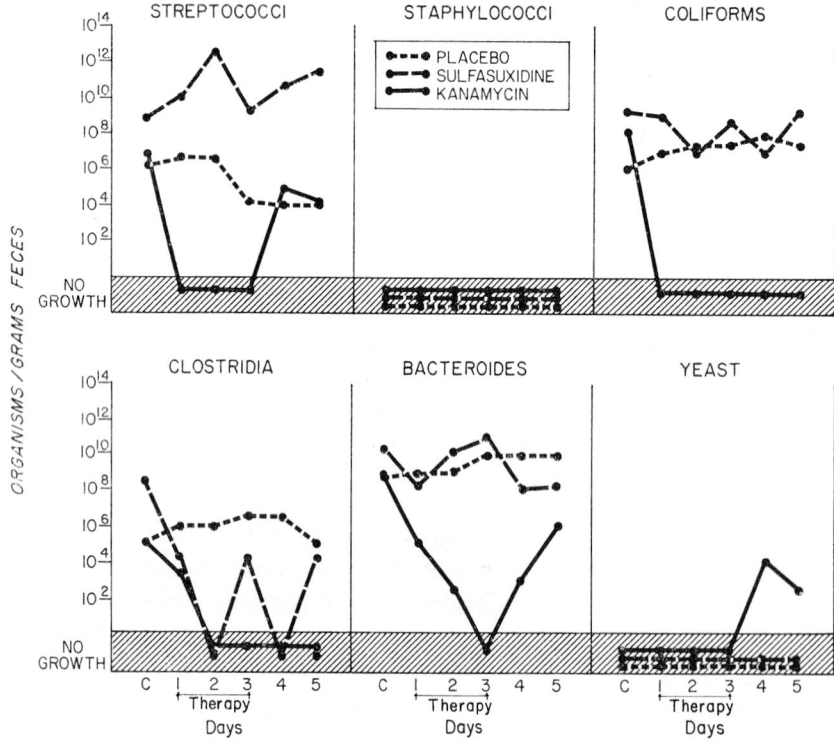

Figure 3. Median counts of organisms in stools of patients treated with three different types of intestinal preparation, each as an example of one of the means of intestinal antisepsis. The placebo shows that mechanical preparation alone does not reduce the bacterial flora of the stool. Sulfasuxidine is an example of the drugs that cannot be recommended for intestinal antisepsis, and kanamycin is an example of the recommended group. (From Cohn, I., Jr.: Surg. Gynecol. Obstet., 130:1006, 1970. By permission of Surgery, Gynecology & Obstetrics.)

TABLE 2.   Recommended Drugs*

Drug	Dosage
Amphotericin-neomycin Amphotericin 50 mg. Neomycin 1 gm.	In combination, every hour for 4 hours, then every 6 hours for a total of 72 hours
Bacitracin-neomycin Bacitracin 40,000 units Neomycin 400 mg.	In combination, every 6 hours for 72 hours
Kanamycin 1 gm.	Every hour for 4 hours, then every 6 hours for a total of 72 hours
Nystatin-neomycin Nystatin 250,000 units Neomycin 1 gm.	In combination, every hour for 4 hours, then every 4 hours for a total of 72 hours
Polymyxin B-neomycin Polymyxin B 50 mg. Neomycin 1 gm. Polymyxin B 100 mg. Neomycin 1 gm.	In combination, every hour for 4 hours Then in combination, every 6 hours for a total of 72 hours
Sulfathalidine-neomycin Sulfathalidine 1.5 gm. Neomycin 1 gm.	In combination, every hour for 4 hours, then every 4 hours for a total of 72 hours
Thiostrepton-neomycin Thiostrepton 500,000 units	Every 6 hours for 72 hours
Neomycin 1 gm.	Every hour for 4 hours, then every 6 hours for a total of 72 hours

*From Cohn, I., Jr.: Surg. Gynecol. Obstet., *130*:1006, 1970. By permission of Surgery, Gynecology & Obstetrics.

these was it necessary to discontinue therapy. The total incidence of wound infections was 11 per cent, or 9.5 per cent in the 652 subjected to some procedure upon the colon. This is less than the 12.9 per cent reported in the 550 patients subjected to operations upon the colon from five major university centers participating in a study of infection. It is a significant improvement over the conclusion from a study in Edinburgh for the 10 years ending in 1956, in which it was

TABLE 3.   Dangers of Intestinal Antisepsis

Improper use
    Poor selection of agent
    Too rapid preparation
    Transient antibiotic activity
    Overreliance
Normal flora imbalance
    Yeast complications
    Pseudomembranous enterocolitis
Systemic effects
    Hypoprothrombinemia
    Intraperitoneal use
    Spread of tumors

TABLE 4.   Comparative Incidence of Major Bacterial Complications in Five Large Series of Colon Cases with and without Intestinal Antisepsis*

Institution	No. of Patients	Wound Infections, Per Cent	Peritonitis Leak, Fistula, Per Cent	Combined Per Cent
L.S.U.	372	12.1	1.6	13.7
Columbia				
Prepared	724	8.1	10.1	18.2
Not prepared	318	10.7	14.2	24.9
Pittsburgh				
Prepared	414			17.9
Not prepared	31			35.4
U.C.L.A.—V.A.				
Prepared	75	26.6	2.7	29.3
Not prepared	17	11.8	11.8	23.6
Melbourne				
Prepared	77	31.1	2.6	33.7
Not prepared	40	47.5	12.5	60.0

*From Cohn, I., Jr.: Surg. Gynecol. Obstet., *130*:1006, 1970. By permission of Surgery, Gynecology & Obstetrics.

shown that infection was responsible for 40 per cent of the mortality and 70 per cent of the morbidity in the surgical treatment of carcinoma of the colon. The figures belie claims that antibiotics have had no effect on the incidence of infection and complications in colon surgery (Table 4). In only one of these studies was the infection rate lower in those patients who did not receive antibiotics. These studies should leave little doubt that intestinal antisepsis has justified its clinical use as a valuable addition to surgical therapy.[33]

PERITONITIS FROM PERFORATION

Perforation of the colon from any of its major causes (Table 5) may be expected to produce a more virulent form of peritonitis than perforation of any other part of the gastrointestinal tract. This is true because of the normally large bacterial population of the colon in relation to that of the rest of the abdominal viscera.

Prior to the development of antibiotics, colonic perforations led to an extremely high mortality, and the surgical approach to such a problem was concerned chiefly with the most rapid possible exteriorization or elimination of the site of perforation. Antibiotics have changed the mortality from perforations and have permitted the development of some newer approaches to the therapy of colonic perforations.

The basic surgical principle in the management of a perforation of the colon includes the earliest possible elimination of the site of drainage. A single contamination with bacteria and feces is not so damaging, but continuing soilage of the peritoneal cavity is the real danger in colonic perforations. The current controversy is over exteriorization, proximal decompression, or resection. At the moment the majority opinion

TABLE 5.   Causes of Perforation of the Colon

Trauma
    Blunt
    Penetrating
        Incised "clean" wounds, as knife wounds
        Ragged or bullet wounds

Inflammatory
    Diverticulitis
    Ulcerative colitis

Vascular
    Ischemic colitis
    Volvulus
    Vascular occlusion

Mechanical
    Volvulus
    Obstruction
        Band
        Malignant—proximal perforation

Malignant disease
    Perforation at site of lesion

favors exteriorization of the lesion if possible, or, if it cannot be exteriorized, closure of the perforation combined with a proximal colostomy to prevent further fecal spill from the perforation. This should be accompanied by copious irrigation of the peritoneal cavity to remove as much of the fecal material as possible.

On the basis of a large experimental and clinical experience we have advocated irrigation of the peritoneal cavity with kanamycin during the operative procedure. Experimental evidence demonstrated the safety of this procedure. A 12-year clinical experience with a large number of patients has solidified our thinking about both the safety and the value of this form of therapy. Irrigation of the peritoneal cavity with other antibiotics has been either unsatisfactory, unsafe, or both, but we have not had difficulty with kanamycin in well over 1000 patients. For those who are hesitant to use kanamycin in the operating room, the insertion of a small intravenous-type catheter into the peritonal cavity for the instillation of kanamycin in the postoperative period has demonstrated its value and can be recommended as a satisfactory alternative.[12]

Almost all of the comments in this section deal with perforations of the left colon. Similar lesions of the right colon can be handled with immediate definitive therapy because resection or closure of the perforation on the right side is not associated with the same problems as in left-sided lesions for reasons described in detail elsewhere in this chapter.

Perforation due to a malignant lesion probably should be handled in a slightly different fashion, because of the added hazard from spillage of malignant cells, and the poor prognosis associated with colonic cancers that perforate. Under these circumstances a more aggressive approach is probably justified.[11]

Within the past few years, a number of surgeons have advocated a definitive operative approach regardless of the etiology of the perforation, regardless of the complicating intraperitoneal lesion, and regardless of the site of perforation. These men have suggested that primary resection in the presence of peritonitis from perforated diverticulitis or obstruction is justifiable, and their reports would seem to vindicate their proposal.[21, 25] We believe this approach should be further evaluated before it is accorded widespread acceptance.

For references, see page 1108.

V

MECHANICAL, INFLAMMATORY, VASCULAR, AND MISCELLANEOUS BENIGN LESIONS

Isidore Cohn, Jr., M.D.,
and Francis C. Nance, M.D.

MECHANICAL LESIONS

Volvulus

Volvulus is defined as an abnormal twisting of a segment of bowel on itself along its longitudinal axis. This results in compromised circulation and partial or complete occlusion of the lumen at each end of the segment to produce a closed-loop obstruction.

Volvulus of the colon accounts for 1 to 4 per cent of all intestinal obstruction in the United States. In Eastern Europe and parts of Africa and Asia, volvulus accounts for 30 to 50 per cent of colon obstructions (85 per cent in Northern Iran). Volvulus is primarily a disease of the older age groups, with the greatest incidence occurring in the sixth and seventh decades.

Two factors are necessary for the development of

volvulus. (1) There must be a redundant segment of the colon that is freely movable within the peritoneal cavity. (2) There must be close approximation of the points of fixation of the segment to serve as a focus about which the volvulus can occur.

The sigmoid flexure, with its redundant loop and the close proximity of its points of fixation, is the most frequent site of volvulus of the colon. Most patients have a long history of disordered bowel habits, usually chronic constipation with excess laxative use. The disease is more common in psychiatric or senile patients in nursing homes. The high-residue diets of Eastern Europe, Africa, and Asia probably account for the increased incidence of volvulus in these geographic areas.

Acute sigmoid volvulus presents with sudden onset of nausea, vomiting, colicky abdominal pain, and obstipation. Gross distention of the abdomen, usually asymmetric, develops rapidly, along with progressive dehydration and fever. The twisted sigmoid fills with gas because the volvulus produces a check-valve that allows entry of feces and air but prevents their egress. Physical examination reveals marked abdominal tenderness, localized or generalized, frequently with a palpable tympanitic mass. Bowel sounds are usually present but may be either decreased or hyperactive. Rectal examination commonly shows absence of feces within the ampulla. If gangrenous changes have occurred, tachycardia, toxicity, and signs of generalized peritonitis may be present. Plain x-ray films of the abdomen reveal markedly dilated loops of large bowel forming the so-called "bent inner tube" or "omega loop" sign with the convexity of the loop lying away from the site of obstruction. Pointing toward the obstruction is the so-called "bird's beak," a narrowing of the air-filled colon. Two air-fluid levels are almost always seen within the sigmoid loop. Barium enema characteristically shows a narrowing at the site of torsion with "spiraling" of the mucosal folds and the pathognomonic "bird's beak" or "ace of spades" deformity. Barium enema is contraindicated when gangrene is suspected, because of the danger of perforation of the necrotic segment.

Since the overall mortality for sigmoid volvulus approaches 35 per cent, treatment should be prompt. The high mortality usually occurs in patients with gangrenous changes or in elderly patients with concomitant disease of the cardiovascular, respiratory, and renal systems.

Initial treatment should include an attempt to reduce the volvulus by proctoscopy and insertion of a rectal tube. The prudent surgeon is well advised to wear a waterproof apron. A well-lubricated rectal tube can be passed through the proctoscope and eased past the area of torsion. Once the proctoscope or rectal tube enters the twisted segment, there is often a very satisfying explosive passage of gas and liquid feces through the tube. After decompression, the involved segment usually undergoes spontaneous detorsion. The rectal tube should be left in place to prevent recurrence. If proctoscopic reduction is successful, further treatment should be considered because of the extremely high recurrence rate (33 to 60 per cent). Elective resection of the redundant sigmoid with primary anastomosis, fol-

lowing adequate preparation of the bowel, should be performed in good-risk patients. If proctoscopic decompression is unsuccessful, barium enema or saline enema may be tried. Nonoperative reduction was successful in 76 per cent of patients in a large series of patients at Charity Hospital, New Orleans (Table 1).

If nonoperative reduction fails or clinical evidence of gangrene is present, immediate laparotomy is mandatory. If the segment is viable at exploration simple detorsion should be performed. If gangrene is present, immediate resection of the involved area is indicated. The resection may be accompanied by primary anastomosis in carefully selected cases, Mickulicz exteriorization, or a Hartmann procedure. Recently a few authors have advocated primary resection and anastomosis for all patients with volvulus who require emergency laparotomy. Following successful nonoperative reduction, good-risk patients should probably undergo elective resection, since the risk of recurrence is very high (55 per cent). However, an operative mortality of 15 per cent for elective resection in this elderly patient population dictates careful selection of patients. Poor-risk patients may be followed until they have a recurrence, since their operative risk may exceed their risk of dying from a recurrent episode of volvulus.[1]

Cecal volvulus accounts for approximately 15 per cent of cases of volvulus of the colon. Poor fixation of the cecum, usually the result of malrotation of the colon during embryologic development, sets the stage for torsion to occur, commonly around the pedicle of the ileocolic artery.

The symptoms of cecal volvulus are those of small bowel obstruction. With progression of the disease, abdominal distention usually occurs, with the development of a tympanitic mass extending from the right lower to the right upper quadrant.

The pertinent radiologic features of cecal volvulus include (1) massive distention of the cecum; (2) evidence of small bowel obstruction; (3) visualization of the gas-outlined ileocecal valve on the right side of the cecum; and (4) single air-fluid level in the cecum. The filling of the entire left and transverse colon on barium enema can be used to differentiate sigmoid volvulus from cecal volvulus.

Attempts at conservative reduction of cecal volvulus

TABLE 1. Sigmoid Volvulus at Charity Hospital, New Orleans, 1960–1971*

	Nonoperative Reduction		
Method	Number Attempts	Number Successful	Per Cent Successful
Proctoscopy	114	87	77
Barium enema	18	12	67
Saline enema	8	6	75
Rectal tube	5	5	100
Total	145	110	76

*From Arnold, G. J., and Nance, F. C.: Ann. Surg., *177*:527, 1973.

are useless and immediate surgical reduction after resuscitation is required. If no gangrene is found, the recommended approach is detorsion with fixation of the cecum by cecopexy or cecostomy. The presence of gangrene necessitates immediate resection of the right colon, usually with ileotransverse colostomy.

Intussusception

Intussusception is the invagination of one segment of intestine into another. It is a common cause of intestinal obstruction in infants and children, and a relatively uncommon cause in adults (Fig. 1). At Charity Hospital in New Orleans there were 287 cases in children (84 per cent) and only 55 cases in adults (16 per cent) from 1904 to 1959. In children there is usually no detectable organic lesion leading the intussusception, and therefore the cause cannot be determined. In contrast, a leading cause is usually found in adults and is always to be sought.

Intussusception is usually subdivided into four types: (1) enteric—small bowel into small bowel; (2) ileocecal—ileocecal valve leads intussusception into colon; (3) ileocolic—terminal ileum intussuscepts into colon; and (4) colocolic—colon into colon. The second and third types are the most common. In adults the organic lesions that lead the intussusception are usually malignant in the large bowel and benign in the small bowel.

The symptoms are fairly classic in the infant, in whom the diagnosis should be missed only rarely. The sudden onset of cramping abdominal pain in a previously well infant, and the alternation between episodes of normalcy and recurrent attacks of severe cramping, should almost establish the diagnosis. Passage of bloody mucus per rectum should further strengthen the diagnostic impression. The presence of vomiting and a palpable abdominal mass should clinch the diagnosis.

Similar symptoms may occur in the older child or adult, but usually they are not so dramatic, and the symptom-free interval may be days to months so that the diagnosis may be obscure. In spite of the presence of an organic lesion in most adults, it is frequently missed because of the tendency of the intussusception to reduce itself and leave little evidence on x-ray. Lesions in the large bowel are much easier to detect, and are not so likely to be perplexing diagnostic problems.

X-ray is helpful for diagnostic and for therapeutic purposes in infants. In an institution that is properly staffed, and where the surgeon and roentgenologist work in close cooperation with mutual understanding of the problems involved, barium enema reduction of intussusception in the infant should be given a trial, unless it is obvious that complications have already occurred, or the intussusception has been present for over 24 hours when the patient is first seen. X-rays may not be helpful in the adult, depending on whether the condition has temporarily resolved itself, and on its location. Plain films of the abdomen should give some indication of the degree of obstruction, and this might give a clue as to the chance of finding some more specific lesion on barium contrast studies.

Simple operative reduction of the intussusception should be sufficient in the infant who is treated surgically. If reduction is not possible, if gangrene has already occurred, or if some organic lesion is found, then resection with primary anastomosis should be done. In the adult, since an organic lesion is usually present, resection probably will be necessary. If intussusception involves the left colon, then serious consideration must be given to exteriorization and colostomy be-

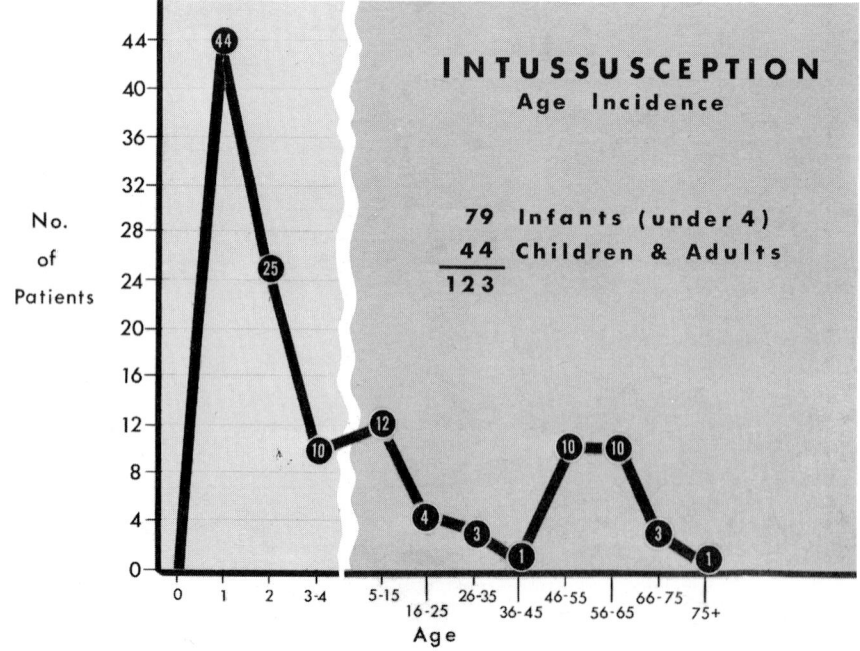

Figure 1. Age incidence of intussusception in 79 infants under 4 years old and 44 children and adults. The high incidence is shown to be in infants under the age of 2 years. During adulthood and into middle age benign and malignant tumors cause the next highest incidence of intestinal invagination. (From Ponka, J. L.: Surg. Gynecol. Obstet., 124:99, 1967. By permission of Surgery, Gynecology & Obstetrics.)

cause of the danger of large bowel anastomoses in an edematous and unprepared bowel. The incidence of cancer in the large bowel is high enough to warrant serious consideration of a cancer resection in all such cases. If the intussusception involves only the right colon, then a primary resection and anastomosis is in order.

Intussusception rarely recurs following operative correction and the outlook is good, except for the patient whose lesion was etiologically related to a primary gastrointestinal cancer.

Large Bowel Obstruction

The commonest cause of large bowel obstruction is cancer of the colon, and it is so far ahead of all other causes that it should be considered first whenever a patient with obstruction is seen. The next most common causes are volvulus, hernia, intussusception, and diverticulitis (Table 2). In contrast to obstruction of the small bowel, in which adhesions are common, adhesive obstruction is almost nonexistent in the large bowel.

The diagnosis often can be made on the basis of history and physical examination. Progressive constipation, abdominal pain, and distention are the dominant findings. X-rays of the abdomen may be diagnostic. Specific findings in patients with volvulus or diverticulitis are discussed in their respective sections. In any patient suspected of having large bowel obstruction, particularly when there is further suggestion on plain films of the abdomen, the next x-ray study should be a barium enema. This should be performed by a radiologist who has been given full information about the clinical impression, so that he will not force barium past a partially obstructing lesion and possibly

TABLE 2. Large Bowel Obstruction

Etiology of Obstruction	Becker[4]		Byrne[6]	
	Number of Cases	Number of Deaths	Number of Cases	Number of Deaths
Carcinoma	100	42	129	39
Volvulus	51	12	22	5
Hernia	25	4	2	1
Intussusception	12	4		
Diverticulitis	5	0	14	3
Adhesions	5	1	1	0
Extrinsic pressure	7	4		
Other			29	15
Total	205	67	197	63

convert it to a completely obstructing one. Radiologic demonstration of the lesion, its location, and its characteristics will do much to guide further therapy.

If the ileocecal valve is competent, the patient will have a closed-loop obstruction of the large bowel. If the ileocecal valve is incompetent, there will be continuous distention of large and small bowel. The danger of perforation of the cecum is always present in the closed loop. Decompression of the large bowel is urgent, and should be the primary consideration in the therapy of all these patients (Fig. 2).

The mortality for large bowel obstruction has remained in the range of 30 per cent in contrast to that for small bowel obstruction, which has decreased. Explanations for this difference are related to the primary disease causing the obstruction, the age of the patients, the duration of the obstruction, and its site

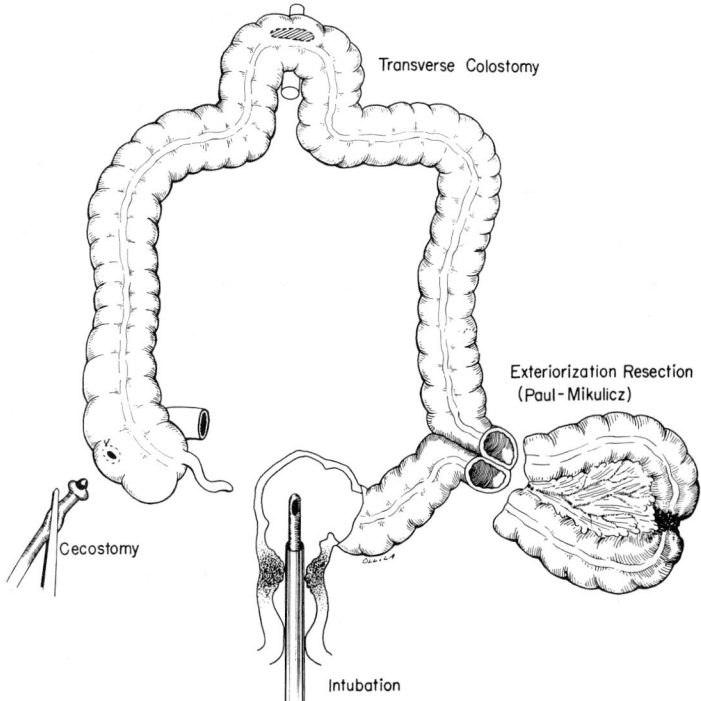

Figure 2. The alternative methods of treating large bowel obstruction. (From Zollinger, R. M., and Howe, C. T. *In* Davis, L. (Ed.): Christopher's Textbook of Surgery, 9th ed. Philadelphia, W. B. Saunders Company 1968.)

and type. When strangulation has occurred, the mortality may exceed 60 per cent.

Since the vast majority of patients with large bowel obstruction have cancer of the large bowel, any discussion of management must revolve around the combined management of cancer and large bowel obstruction. Decompression is the urgent need, and the methods for obtaining adequate decompression form the basis for any further discussion.

If the obstructing lesion is in the right colon, then an immediate primary resection with restoration of intestinal continuity and without any proximal vent will provide proper therapy. This assumes that the lesion is resectable, and that the patient is in proper condition for such an operative procedure, or else can be prepared for operation in a period of time short enough not to further endanger his long-term outlook. Proper preparation means rehydration, establishment of urine output, restoration of electrolyte balance, and tranfusion if necessary. Upper intestinal decompression by intubation should be accomplished as rapidly as possible, but operation should *not* be delayed until complete decompression has been achieved, regardless of whether the ileocecal valve is open or closed. Preoperative intestinal antisepsis is not possible for these patients, and there should be no delay based on the hope of controlling the bacterial flora of the bowel.

If the obstructing lesion is on the left side, decompression should be accomplished by a proximal colostomy, preferably a transverse colostomy. The colostomy should be placed in a location that will not interfere with the subsequent excision of the primary lesion, nor compromise an adequate cancer operation when that is undertaken. Both limbs of the colostomy should be opened as soon as possible, but the primary consideration should be to open the proximal side to prevent perforation of the cecum.

After the colon has been decompressed, further studies can be instituted by x-ray and whatever other means are desirable. Prior to the definitive operation, it is possible to cleanse the colon completely by enema and antibiotic administration into both limbs of the colostomy and per rectum, and thus provide a clean field in which to do the necessary surgery. The colostomy can be closed at the time of the second operation, or at a third stage, depending on conditions found at that time.

As indicated elsewhere, some surgeons believe definitive operative procedures can be carried out in the presence of obstruction of the left colon, but most believe the dangers associated with large bowel resection and anastomosis in the presence of obstruction contraindicate this approach.

Fecal Impaction

Fecal impaction is a nonsurgical disease of old age, occurring in two primary clinical settings. The most common type occurs in the postsurgical patient at bed rest. Typically, the diagnosis is made by the attending staff after the resident has been assured by the patient that nothing is wrong. Fecal impaction should be searched for in any postsurgical patient in whom diarrhea (the most common symptom) or constipation develops. The rectum often contains hard stool mixed with barium from preoperative diagnostic studies. The

treatment is manual removal of the scabrous stool, followed by oil retention enemas. Prevention by enema before impaction develops is better treatment.

A second clinical picture is seen in senile or psychotic persons, particularly those housed in nursing homes or institutions. These patients may forget to defecate for weeks or months. They become progressively distended and finally manifest signs of intestinal obstruction, with nausea and vomiting. The major clinical problem is to make the correct diagnosis (ruling out organic obstruction or volvulus) and to avoid operation. The mass of feces may usually be identified on the plain film of the abdomen. Treatment includes nasogastric intubation, fluid resuscitation, and persistent enemas until the colon is cleansed, which may take a week or more. A high-bulk diet accompanied by hydrophilic colloids may help avoid recurrences, which are common.

Trauma

Colon injuries may occur following blunt or penetrating trauma, but blunt injuries are uncommon. Improperly placed seat belts around the waist instead of across the lap are the most common cause of blunt injury. A bursting injury or hematoma occurs usually at the points of fixation of the colon.

Penetrating injuries are far more frequent. The colon is the second most commonly injured intra-abdominal organ (after the liver). The types of injury include serosal tears, simple lacerations produced by stab wounds, through-and-through perforations with a bullet, and blast injuries associated with shotgun wounds or high-velocity missiles.

The treatment of colonic injuries has been profoundly influenced by military experience. In World War I when the practice was to avoid operation in penetrating injuries or to suture colon injuries when they were encountered, the mortality from colon injury was 59 per cent. During World War II decompressive colostomy was made mandatory in all patients with left-sided colon injuries. The mortality dropped to 31 per cent. During the Korean conflict, the mortality decreased further to 15 per cent. The Vietnam mortality rate was about 12 per cent.[15] Almost all deaths are associated with serious injury to other organ systems.

Present practice for management of colonic injuries, which has tended to incorporate principles gleaned from military experience, includes:

1. Exteriorization or proximal colostomy for wounds of the left colon. If proximal colostomy is employed, débridement and suture of the colon wound may be accomplished.

2. For rectal injuries, proximal colostomy accompanied by débridement, suture, distal wash-out of the rectum, and adequate drainage in the retrorectal space.

3. For injuries of the right colon, suture of small, relatively clean wounds and right colectomy with primary ileocolic anatomosis for larger lesions.

There are several cogent reasons for proximal colostomy or exteriorization for military wounds of the *left* colon:

1. The wounding missile is of high velocity, producing widespread tissue damage.

2. Patients frequently have other intra-abdominal wounds.

3. Operation is performed under difficult conditions and often in a mass casualty situation.

4. Early evacuation to another center is commonly practiced. The operating surgeon seldom has an opportunity to follow the patients.

In recent years it has been recognized that civilian injuries to the colon may be significantly different from war wounds. This has prompted some surgeons to adopt débridement and primary suture *without* colostomy as a method of treating left-sided civilian injuries. In selected patients with small wounds, without excessive fecal contamination, suture closure may give better results than exteriorization or proximal colostomy.[3] Further evidence would be desirable before this policy can be wholeheartedly endorsed.

INFLAMMATORY LESIONS

Diverticulitis

Diverticula of the colon may be acquired or congenital. The acquired variety are by far the more common. The development of diverticula, particularly in the left colon, is an almost normal part of the aging process. The incidence of diverticulosis in the population rises precipitously from age 35, when the incidence is virtually zero, to age 80, when almost 60 per cent of the population may have diverticula. Diverticula of the colon per se seldom give trouble, but when the diverticula become inflamed diverticulitis results.

Several recent studies have suggested likely mechanisms for the development of diverticula. It has been shown clearly that diverticula develop at the points where blood vessels penetrate the colonic wall. Even in very early disease these weak points in the wall of the colon appear to be the starting point for formation of diverticula. Recent manometric studies have demonstrated that very high intraluminal pressure may be developed along short segments of the colon, particularly in the sigmoid colon. This is another application of Laplace's law of pressures within a cylinder ($P = T/R$). Thus, intraluminal pressures within the colon are greatest at its narrowest point: the descending colon and sigmoid. The pressures are enough to insinuate mucosa through the lattice-like framework of the colonic musculature to form diverticula. It has been demonstrated that patients harboring diverticula have hypertrophied smooth muscle bundles in the sigmoid and that the hypertrophy precedes the development of diverticula. The diverticula seldom develop along the taeniae but are found within the appendices epiploicae and at the mesenteric border. A lack of bulk in modern American and Western European diets has also been implicated as a factor in the development of diverticula.

Uncomplicated diverticulosis seldom produces symptoms. When the orifice of a diverticulum becomes obstructed, inflammation occurs within the diverticulum and adjacent bowel. The resulting edema occludes the orifices of neighboring diverticula, with spread of the process along the colon. The symptoms of diverticulitis are abdominal pain, constipation or diarrhea, rectal bleeding, fever, nausea and vomiting, and pneumaturia.

Pain connected with diverticulitis is usually located in the left lower quadrant, but it may occur anywhere there are diverticula. The pain is usually episodic, lasting for a few hours or days and then subsiding. It is commonly associated with tenderness over the colon in the left lower quadrant. In severe attacks the pain may become very pronounced and give signs of peritonitis. Usually the patients have a history of constipation, often associated with excessive laxative use. With the onset of diverticulitis, alternating diarrhea and constipation may be encountered. Nausea and vomiting occur during severe bouts of diverticulitis. Rectal bleeding is common but usually of the occult type. Massive rectal bleeding, if it occurs, usually appears in patients with diverticulosis, without clinical evidence of diverticulitis. Massive bleeding is the indication for surgery in 6 to 10 per cent of patients with diverticular disease.

Physical findings are usually limited to the abdomen and rectum. In some patients there may be no findings at all. Tenderness over the sigmoid colon, peritoneal signs, a left lower quadrant or pelvic mass, and pelvic tenderness may all be found in attacks of diverticulitis.

Sigmoidoscopy and barium enema are of great importance in the diagnosis of this disease. Occasionally one may visualize diverticula through the proctoscope but more commonly seen are narrowing of the colon, spasm, fixation, and angulation. Barium enema shows segmental spasm with serrations (sawtoothing) of the bowel in the area of the disease. Mucosal edema, fixation of the bowel, and narrowing of the lumen may be present. On x-ray diverticulitis may be difficult to differentiate from cancer, but the following features are suggestive of it: (1) involvement of a long segment of bowel, (2) spasm, (3) presence of diverticula elsewhere in the bowel, and (4) tapered or conical ends in the bowel segment involved. Occasionally the barium enema will show a leak into an abscess cavity or a fistula into an adjacent organ. Other diagnostic studies useful in diverticulosis include tests for occult blood, selective angiography, flat films of the abdomen, intravenous pyelography, cystography (in cases of suspected fistula), and cystoscopy.

The usual therapy of diverticulitis is medical and consists of antispasmodics, meperidine, an intestinal antibiotic such as salicylazosulfapyridine (Azulfidine), and diet. Dietary therapy once consisted of low-residue foods, but the presence of bulk in the stool is thought to reduce intraluminal pressure so that a high-residue diet supplemented by hydrophilic colloids is often prescribed. For patients with signs of peritoneal irritation and fever, one should add nasogastric intubation, intravenous fluids, and systemic antibiotics. Most episodes of diverticulitis respond readily to these measures. After an attack, some internists maintain patients on oral antispasmodics and nonabsorbable antibiotics for weeks or months.

Surgical therapy of diverticulitis is reserved for complications and for those patients with recurrent attacks who fail to respond to medical therapy.[7, 10] About half the surgical patients require operation because of repeated attacks that do not respond to medical therapy. These patients may undergo elective resection of the involved segment of colon with very low operative risk. The remaining 50 to 60 per cent of patients require surgical intervention, frequently as an emergency procedure, for one of the complications: perforation (30 to 35 per cent), fistula (10 to 15 per cent), obstruction (10 per cent), or bleeding (6 to 10 per cent). The difference in mortality between elective and emergency surgery in patients with diverticulitis has led many gastroenterologic surgeons to urge earlier elective resection in patients who have repeated episodes of local tenderness in the left lower quadrant, a persistent mass, marked narrowing on roentgenologic examination, or lesions difficult to differentiate from cancer.

Elective colectomy is curative and may be carried out with minimal risk to the patient. The operative technique differs from resections for cancer in that only the involved segment of colon need be removed. Anastomotic complications are somewhat more common than after operations for cancer because edema and thickening of the bowel may be present. A one-stage resection is the usual procedure.

The complications of diverticulitis often require emergency surgical treatment and carry a high morbidity and mortality rate (Fig. 3). The most common complication is perforation with peritonitis or abscess formation. The seriousness of this complication is illustrated by a mortality of 47 per cent in one recently reported series of 267 patients. The perforation may be into the free peritoneal cavity or it may be walled off by omentum and adjacent small bowel to form an abscess. An occasional patient has a perforation into the mesentery of the colon. Patients with perforated diverticulitis usually have signs of peritonitis with pain, direct tenderness, rebound tenderness, ab-

sence of bowel sounds, fever, leukocytosis, dehydration, tachycardia, tachypnea, and an abdominal mass.

Patients with the clinical picture of perforation need early surgical intervention. A transverse colostomy is appropriate for a perforation or abscess. Most surgeons would also drain the abscess. Following a recovery period of 3 to 6 months, definitive resection of the involved segment should be accomplished. The colostomy may be closed later. This is known as a three-stage resection and is the most widely practiced approach to this serious complication. Recently several studies have made it clear that most of the major complications of three-stage resections occur after the *first* stage, i.e., after the colostomy. This has led several surgeons to consider removal of the primary disease at the first operation. A few have suggested primary resection and anastomosis even in the presence of abscesses or peritonitis.

The next most common complication of diverticulitis is fistula formation. The usual types are colocutaneous and colovesical fistulas, with colovaginal fistula a distant third. The diagnosis of colocutaneous fistula may be established by a barium enema showing diverticula and by injecting the cutaneous sinus with contrast material to show communication with the colon.

Colovesical fistula presents with the rather spectacular symptom of pneumaturia or fecaluria or both. Females appear to be partially protected from this complication by the interposition of the uterus. Barium enema will confirm the presence of diverticula but seldom shows the fistula. The fistula may be visualized at cystoscopy, by a cystogram, or by an intravenous pyelogram. Some patients may be managed by one-stage elective resection and anastomosis.

Obstruction occurs much less frequently in diverticulitis than in cancer and is the sole indication for surgery in only 5 to 10 per cent of patients. A decompressive colostomy should be performed, followed later by resection of the diseased colon. The mortality remains high, as it does for all patients who require emergency surgery.

Massive hemorrhage seldom occurs as a complication of diverticulitis and is in fact seen primarily in patients with diverticulosis. Dark red to black stools are seen. Proctoscopy is useful to demonstrate that bleeding is coming from the more proximal colon and to rule out other causes of colonic bleeding. A barium enema will help locate the diverticula. Selective mesenteric arteriography may help in the difficult task of pinpointing the area of bleeding.

Adequate blood replacement and the usual medical measures should be employed initially. Bleeding usually stops and elective resection may be carried out. If bleeding continues, emergency resection must be performed. If the specific bleeding site has been identified preoperatively by selective arteriography or if the diverticula are limited to one area of the colon, limited colonic resection with anastomosis is acceptable, but most patients requiring emergency resection for continued bleeding are best managed by total colectomy with ileoproctostomy.[13, 19]

Diverticulitis is a disease that must not be underestimated. Early and elective surgery is safe and curative, with an anticipated mortality of considerably less

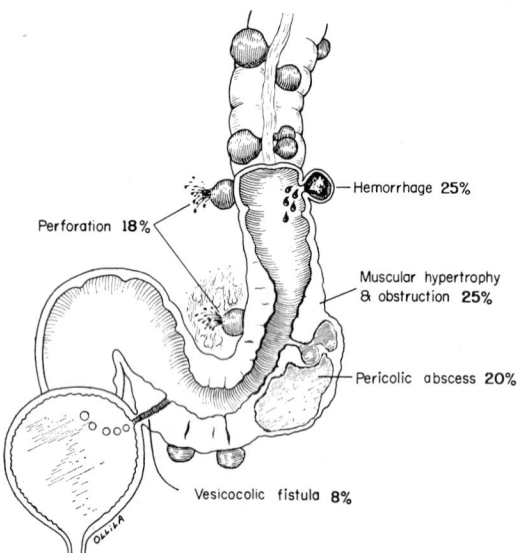

Perforation 18%

Hemorrhage 25%

Muscular hypertrophy & obstruction 25%

Pericolic abscess 20%

Vesicocolic fistula 8%

Figure 3. The complications of diverticulitis. (From Zollinger, R. M., and Howe, C. T. *In* Davis, L. (Ed.): Christopher's Textbook of Surgery, 9th ed. Philadelphia, W. B. Saunders Company, 1968.)

than 5 per cent. Emergency surgery related to one of the complications may be lethal. The surgical mortality for complications usually exceeds the mortality for similar complications of cancer of the colon.

Pseudomembranous Enterocolitis

Pseudomembranous enterocolitis or staphylococcal enterocolitis is an infrequent but serious problem that can be fatal with an alarming rapidity. It varies from mild forms with some diarrhea and abdominal discomfort all the way to the fatal case that may be associated with severe diarrhea, shock due to fluid and electrolyte loss, sudden rise in temperature, abdominal pain and distention, nausea and vomiting, lethargy, and the development of a pseudomembrane visible by sigmoidoscopy. Smear and culture of the stool may reveal massive overgrowth of staphylococci, but it must be noted that the disease can occur in the absence of stool findings, and the presence of staphylococci in the stool is not diagnostic per se of pseudomembranous enterocolitis.

Although this complication has occasionally occurred following the use of intestinal antiseptics, it is very seldom seen and does not constitute a contraindication to preoperative antibiotic bowel preparation.

When the problem does develop—either before or after an operative procedure, and whether the patient has been given antibiotics or not—urgent therapy is indicated. Gram stains of the stool may confirm staphylococcal overgrowth. Cultures and sensitivity tests should be done on stool organisms, and specific therapy should be instituted as soon as possible. In the interim, antistaphylococcal antibiotics should be administered in large doses and other antibiotic therapy should be discontinued. Vigorous intravenous therapy should be instituted to combat the shock and fluid and electrolyte loss. Blood should be administered as indicated. All oral intake should be discontinued. Steroids probably should be administered.

The mild cases usually respond without much difficulty. The severe cases may respond if therapy is begun soon enough. The very severe case, or the unrecognized case, may proceed to a rapid death in spite of vigorous therapy.

Lymphogranuloma Venereum

This venereal disease is fortunately rare in the United States. When the disease affects the colon, ulceration, proctitis, rectal strictures, cutaneous sinus tracts, and rectovaginal fistulas may result. The anorectal complications occur most frequently in women. The most serious complications are obstructive in nature, usually from a long tubular stricture. The diagnosis can be established by the Frei intracutaneous test.

In the prestricture stage, tetracycline is specifically curative. Some physicians include steroids with the antibiotic regimen. Once a stricture has occurred, restoration of bowel continuity is extremely difficult. Simple colostomy is of no value except for acute obstruction, since it has no effect on the primary pathologic condition. Because of the very definite risk of developing adenocarcinoma in the rectosigmoid area or epidermoid cancer in the fistulous tracts, most surgeons would perform an abdominoperineal resection of the anorectum during a quiescent period in patients who have an obstructing stricture of the rectum.

Amebic Colitis

Amebic colitis is usually a relatively mild disease that responds to medical therapy. Although hepatic abscess remains the most common complication of amebiasis requiring an operative approach, occasional patients require surgical intervention for specific colonic complications. The most lethal complication is fulminating colitis. These patients present with marked bloody and mucoid diarrhea, followed by signs of an intraperitoneal disaster. Sloughing of the mucosa may be seen on proctoscopic examination. Early exploration is mandatory, since multiple perforations of the bowel may be present. Subtotal colectomy with colostomy or ileostomy should be performed. It is necessary to begin antiamebic therapy in the early postoperative period. This should consist of metronidazole and tetracycline. Emetine hydrochloride or chloroquine diphosphate also may be required. Other colonic complications listed by Rives[28] are localized perforation, hemorrhage, amebic appendicitis, and perianal abscess. Ameboma or amebic granuloma may occasionally simulate carcinoma, but these are extremely rare. Surgical intervention in amebic colitis carries a high mortality if the disease is not recognized and the patient is not protected by chemotherapeutic agents.

VASCULAR LESIONS

The vascular lesions of the bowel may be classified into three general groups: (1) gradual occlusion of a major splanchnic vessel; (2) embolic obstruction of a major vessel; and (3) mesenteric vascular occlusion not involving a major vessel.

Gradual occlusion of a major vessel usually is secondary to atherosclerosis. Initial symptoms consist of cramplike pains coming on after a large meal. Weight loss may occur, associated with malabsorption or diarrhea. The symptoms have been called "intestinal angina" and the term seems apt, since the symptoms are produced by splanchnic effort. A bruit may be heard in the epigastrium. Arteriography may confirm the presence of stenosis of one or more of the major vessels (celiac artery, superior mesenteric artery, or the inferior mesenteric artery). This lesion characteristically occurs in patients with other manifestations of atherosclerosis. In occasional patients sudden thrombosis may develop in an atherosclerotic vessel. The clinical picture here is similar to that for embolic occlusion.

Embolic occlusion of the splanchnic vessels produces sudden onset of vague abdominal pain. Typically pain is diffuse over the entire abdomen. As necrosis of the bowel supervenes, signs of an intraperitoneal disaster may become manifest with rapid pulse, fever, marked leukocytosis (20,000 to 40,000 per cu. mm.), and signs of peripheral vascular collapse. The typical patient is recovering from a recent myocardial infarct. On initial examination hyperactive bowel sounds may be present, but as necrosis of the bowel progresses, the abdomen becomes silent. Early surgery is mandatory as soon as the diagnosis is made and the patient resuscitated. Unfortunately, the early symptoms are so vague that exploration frequently is delayed until massive gangrene of the bowel is present.

Treatment of major splanchnic vessel occlusion consists of restoration of blood flow if possible and resection of obviously necrotic bowel.

Mesenteric vascular occlusion *without* major vessel involvement may be further subdivided into generalized vascular occlusion and localized ischemia. In the first, the patient presents with massive necrosis of the large and small bowel. Most patients are already receiving therapy for recent myocardial infarction or hemorrhagic or septic shock, and have received vasopressors, steroids, or digitalis alone or in combination. The profound effect of digitalis in reducing splanchnic blood flow has been shown, and the routine administration of this agent to patients in shock may constitute a significant and unacceptable risk. The outlook for this complication is dismal, with a mortality exceeding 80 per cent. Therapy often requires the resection of most of the large and small bowel.

Ischemic Colitis

Localized ischemia of the bowel occurs most often in the colon and has been termed ischemic colitis. Despite the fact that this lesion has been defined adequately only recently,[5] it is not rare. The syndrome usually occurs in older patients but we have seen it in a 26-year-old woman. Mild lower abdominal pain and rectal bleeding of bright red blood are the most prominent symptoms. Previous attacks are not characteristic and precipitating causes such as shock are not present. Physical examination usually reveals only mild tenderness. Proctosigmoidoscopy shows only bleeding from above. Although any portion of the colon may be involved, the splenic flexure and descending colon appear to be most vulnerable.[35]

The pathogenesis of this lesion is not well understood. Some patients have had subintimal thickening of the smaller arterioles within the bowel wall. Ischemic colitis has occasionally developed in patients with thromboangiitis obliterans, as well as in patients with periarteritis nodosa or other collagen diseases. In the majority of patients, no specific vascular disease has been found.

The gross appearance of the bowel may be normal from the serosal surface or it may be obviously ischemic. The mucosal surface shows edema, darkening, and patchy ulceration. In far advanced or chronic cases, tubular stenosis of the bowel may occur. The microscopic feature of resolving colitis is full-thickness loss of mucosa. In the ulcerated areas, patchy atrophy of remaining mucosa, widening of the submucosa with a marked inflammatory response, and hemorrhagic necrosis are found.

The diagnosis can be made radiographically. The most common finding is "thumb printing" of the bowel. This consists of a polypoid radiolucency producing a scalloped margin of the bowel wall on the filled phase of the barium enema. Other radiographic manifestations have been ragged sawtooth irregularity of the small bowel, sacculation of the bowel, and tubular narrowing. This last finding is seen later and results from scarring. Arteriography usually does not demonstrate any abnormalities, giving further emphasis to the fact that this is a disease of the small arterioles, not visible by present arteriographic techniques.

Therapy depends on the severity of the symptoms. Patients with mild symptoms, minimal leukocytosis, fever, and the typical thumb printing may simply be observed. The episode usually will subside with no sequelae. Other patients may present with more prominent symptoms. If the typical roentgenologic findings of thumb printing are present, careful observation is appropriate. These patients must be followed carefully, since their disease may progress to frank gangrene of the bowel. In patients with severe symptoms ischemic stricture may develop, which later will require elective resection. A small number of patients will have signs of bowel necrosis or perforation and indications for surgery from the beginning. These patients will require exteriorization or resection of the involved segment of bowel.

Recognition of this syndrome as a specific clinical entity has permitted a much more rational approach to therapy. In most cases the symptoms will subside. Surgery will be required only for bowel necrosis and for late ischemic strictures.

Radiation Injury

Radiation injury to the colon is most commonly the result of irradiation of the cervix and uterus. A smaller number of injuries have occurred in patients irradiated for bladder and ovarian lesions. Serious radiation injuries of the colon may be expected in 1 to 2 per cent of women treated for cervical carcinoma, although the incidence may increase with the recent trend to doses exceeding 6600 R. Important etiologic factors other than radiation dose are individual idiosyncrasies, previous surgery, pelvic inflammation, and extensive tumors.

Three major clinical manifestations are seen: proctitis, rectal stenosis, and rectovaginal fistula. Proctitis is common in patients undergoing pelvic radiation therapy, but is seldom serious. The symptoms of tenesmus, pain, rectal bleeding, and diarrhea may be controlled by low-residue diet, stool softener, sedation, antispasmodics, and nonabsorbable sulfonamides. Occasionally steroid enemas may be required. Symptoms usually subside after completion of radiation therapy.

Rectal stenosis occurs 6 to 18 months after irradiation. Bleeding and diarrhea signal the onset of symptoms. The lesion is almost always in the high rectum at 10 to 14 cm. Ulceration of the mucosa at the site of obstruction is common. Initial therapy may consist of intermittent dilation, which may relieve symptoms. Progressive obstruction may require diverting colostomy. If biopsy and clinical evaluation fail to show recurrence of the primary tumor, the stenotic area should be treated by resection and anastomosis, with a protecting proximal colostomy. Radiation injury results in endarteritis and thrombosis of small vessels within the bowel, and healing of anastomoses is tenuous. Diversion of the fecal stream is mandatory until healing is complete.

Rectovaginal fistula is most commonly the result of tumor necrosis in patients with recurrent carcinoma of the cervix, but this disabling complication does develop in some patients otherwise cured of their tumor. Virtually all the lesions are located 4 to 10 cm. from the anus. The development of the fistula usually is preceded by bleeding from the rectum or vagina 6 to 18 months after completion of radiation therapy. An immediate colostomy at this point may prevent actual development of the fistula. Once the fistula has occurred, vaginal discharge of feces begins. In occasional patients vesicovaginal fistula may develop to add to their discomfort. Diverting colostomy is necessary. In patients with biopsy-proven recurrent tumors, this palliative procedure may be sufficient. In patients without recurrent tumor, an attempt should be made to repair the fistula. Under protection of the colostomy, local excision of the fistula is feasible. If the lesion is high enough, anterior resection occasionally can be attempted.

Unfortunately, too many patients with radiation injuries are left untreated because their symptoms are assumed to be due to recurrent tumor.[26] An aggressive approach to the therapy of these injuries is justified if clinical evaluation fails to show evidence of recurrent tumor.

MISCELLANEOUS BENIGN LESIONS

Endometriosis

Endometriosis of the colon is an unusual condition, since it represents an invasion of previously normal bowel by hormone-dependent nonmalignant cells from another organ of the same patient. While uterine endometrial cells implant almost anywhere in the peritoneal cavity, the rectum and sigmoid are the most commonly involved parts of the gastrointestinal tract, one study showing that 26 per cent of patients had involvement of the rectosigmoid.[18]

Symptoms related to bowel involvement may vary from none to complete intestinal obstruction. The diagnosis should be suspected when bowel symptoms supervene in a woman in the reproductive years with the typical picture of endometriosis. The intestinal symptoms, which may include cramping pain, diarrhea, constipation, or radiation of pain to the rectum, tend to be exaggerated during the menstrual period, when the endometrial implants become engorged as does all other endometrial tissue. Since the lesions do not ulcerate the intestinal mucosa, bleeding is uncommon.

Barium enema may show constriction of the lumen, and the absence of mucosal involvement may be of significant help in distinguishing this lesion from a carcinoma. The greater length of bowel involved by endometriosis and the possible detection of any inflammatory response to the endometrial implants are additional aids in the differential diagnosis.

The treatment of intestinal endometriosis is the treatment of the primary problem of endometriosis. Once the diagnosis of carcinoma can be excluded, the treatment of the intestinal lesion should be conservative because the lesions will disappear with proper hormone management. In some instances direct biopsy of the lesion may be required, but the history, vaginal findings, sigmoidoscopic and roentgenologic observations, and presence of implants elsewhere in the peritoneal cavity should lead one to the proper diagnosis. Bowel should be removed only when the lesions so completely involve a segment that it cannot be saved. Permanent colostomy should be avoided, but a temporary colostomy may be necessary for relief of severe obstruction due to low-lying lesions. Primary therapy should be directed to the ovarian tissue, with only a partial resection of the ovaries in a young patient still desirous of having children. The colonic lesion will usually disappear after either castration or hormone therapy, unless extreme fibrosis has occurred.

Lipoma

Lipoma is the second most common benign tumor of the colon after adenomas (see Polyps of the Colon and Rectum, p. 1124). Lipomas are usually sessile and located in the submucosa of the bowel. The right colon is affected most commonly. Pain is the most common symptom. Half the patients have rectal bleeding. In 20 per cent the tumor is the lead point of an intussusception. An intramural filling defect can be demonstrated by barium enema. An alert radiologist can make the diagnosis from the characteristic radiolucent appearance of the tumor.

Lipomas should be excised if they cause symptoms. They can often be identified as lipomas at surgery by their submucosal location and their very soft consistency. If the diagnosis is certain, enucleation is sufficient treatment. If the diagnosis is in doubt, the surgeon should perform a segmental resection.

Carcinoid Tumors

Carcinoid tumors of the rectum appear to differ in several respects from carcinoid tumors elsewhere in the gastrointestinal tract. They are almost never associated with the carcinoid syndrome, even when metastatic. They often do not have the silver-staining characteristic of other carcinoid tumors, and they do not produce vasoactive substances.

Most rectal carcinoids are found on routine rectal or sigmoidoscopic examination at 5 to 8 cm. Their gross appearance is that of a pale yellow, submucosal nodule covered by an intact epithelium. About one third of rectal carcinoids are malignant. The most reliable histologic criterion for malignancy is evidence of extension into and beyond the muscular coat of the bowel. The most reliable gross indication of malignancy is the size of the tumor. Peskin and Orloff[27] found that only 7 per cent of tumors less than 2 cm. were malignant, whereas 90 per cent of lesions greater than 2 cm. showed evidence of invasion and lymph node metastases.

Small rectal carcinoids should be completely removed by full-thickness excision. A tumor greater than 1.5 cm. should be treated as a malignant lesion. The prognosis is poor if smooth muscle invasion has occurred.

Carcinoid tumors of the right colon and cecum are quite rare and highly malignant. Two thirds of the tumors have metastasized at the time of resection. Colonic symptoms are similar to those produced by adenocarcinoma. Patients with hepatic metastases may exhibit the carcinoid syndrome. The treatment of colonic carcinoids is the same as that for other malignant tumors of the colon.

Colitis Cystica Profunda

This lesion appears as a plaquelike polypoid mass in the rectum. Microscopically, the lesion consists of small cystic mucous lakes lined with normal epithelium beneath the mucosa. The most important symptoms are rectal bleeding, mucorrhea, and diarrhea. The lesion is rare but important because occasionally it has been confused with rectal cancer. This benign lesion can be treated by local excision.

For references, see page 1108.

VI

INTERMEDIATE OR PRECANCEROUS LESIONS AND MALIGNANT LESIONS

Isidore Cohn, Jr., M.D.,
and Francis C. Nance, M.D.

INTERMEDIATE OR PRECANCEROUS LESIONS

Villous Adenoma

This is a dangerous, treacherous lesion that should be treated with respect for its malignant potential. Villous tumors were studied in 1899, but the 1948 report by Sunderland and Binkley[31] first adequately separated these tumors from other adenomatous polyps.

Sunderland and Binkley reported an incidence for villous adenoma of about 1.5 per cent of all colon tumors (48 villous adenomas among 3356 tumors of the large intestine). In recent reports the incidence has ranged from 4 to 8 per cent. The tumors occur with equal frequency in males and females. Villous adenomas are unusual in young patients. The highest incidence is in the age range of 60 to 79, and the average age of patients is 65.

Villous adenomas are soft, velvety, sessile neoplasms, reddish gray in color with numerous finger-like projections. The lesions are usually covered by thick viscid mucus. Their size ranges from 0. 5 cm. to a huge 14 cm. and they may occupy the entire circumference of the bowel. The experienced endoscopist can usually recognize these lesions grossly through the proctoscope. The tumors are so soft that more than one clinician has missed the lesion on routine digital rectal examination (including the authors). Microscopically these tumors arise abruptly from normal mucosa and spread along the surface of the bowel. There are numerous frondlike villi covered by a single layer of columnar epithelial cells (Fig. 1).

The most common symptoms are a change in bowel habit and rectal bleeding, but many patients have no symptoms. Constipation, mucus in the stool, diarrhea, and mucorrhea all may be associated with the tumors. Rectal bleeding in small amounts occurs in about half the patients. A few patients have had tenesmus or protrusion of the tumor through the rectum.

The diagnosis is best made by proctoscopy and by careful digital examination of the rectum. One third of the tumors are within reach of the finger and 80 to 90 per cent are within view of a 25-cm. proctoscope. Barium enema always should be done to visualize more proximal lesions and to rule out other tumors in the colon. The radiologist may make a specific diagnosis from the characteristic reticulated pattern of a villous tumor.

Villous adenomas have a high malignant potential. Thus, Wheat and Ackerman[34] reported that in 76 per cent of the tumors reviewed by them there were atypical changes, focal carcinoma, or frankly invasive carcinoma. The reported incidence of invasive carcinoma ranges from 12 to 40 per cent. In 483 collected cases, 23 per cent of the patients had invasive carcinoma, 46 per cent had benign tumors, and 22 per cent had focal atypia or carcinoma-in-situ. Unfortunately, a single biopsy does not assure adequate identification of malignant areas within these tumors. Biopsy is helpful in confirming the diagnosis of villous adenoma, but cannot be relied upon to rule out a carcinoma.

Gross characteristics of the tumor may be helpful in suggesting the presence of malignancy. A soft velvety tumor with no areas of ulceration or firmness may be

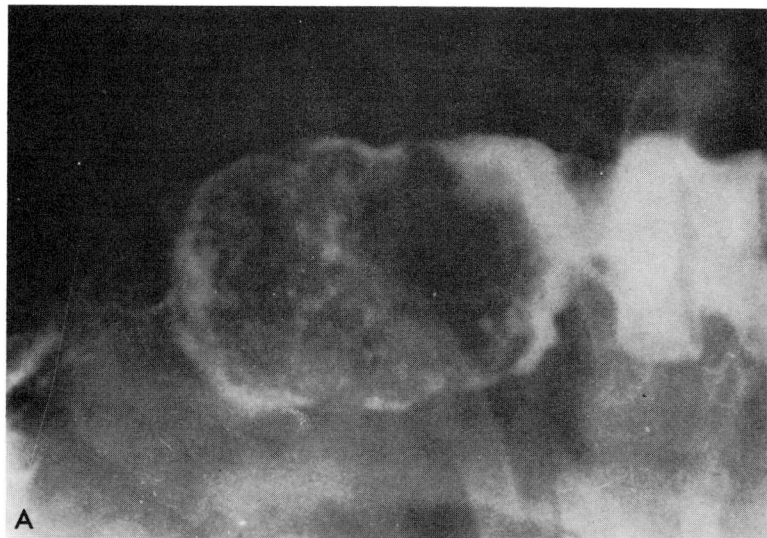

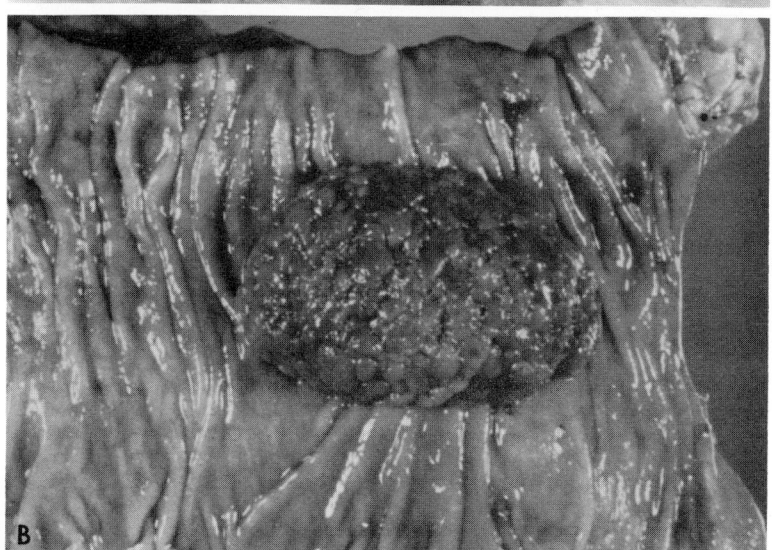

Figure 1. Villous adenoma of transverse colon. *A,* X-ray shows typical reticulated pattern of a villous adenoma. Segmental resection performed. *B,* Pathologic specimen shows sessile 2-cm. polyp with no areas of cancer present. Note soft frondlike villous projections.

benign. The presence of firm areas within the tumor and ulceration of the surface are ominous signs of malignancy. Gross evaluation is no substitute for providing the pathologist with a completely excised tumor.

The treatment is surgical resection. For the 20 to 30 per cent of villous adenomas located proximal to the peritoneal reflection (15 cm.), most surgeons would perform a segmental resection of the involved colon.

The majority of villous adenomas are located within the rectum and a considerable controversy exists over proper therapy. When biopsy or gross characteristics suggest the presence of malignancy, the appropriate cancer operation should be performed. If careful gross examination suggests the tumor is benign, it should be completely excised. This can usually be done through a proctoscope or by delivering the tumor through the anus. For larger tumors of the midrectum complete excision may require a posterior procto-

tomy, as in a Kraske or David procedure. If pathologic examination of the complete tumor shows invasive carcinoma, the appropriate cancer operation should be performed.

Some authors advocate piecemeal excision and fulguration of these tumors. We do not believe this approach should be used, since recurrence is common (multiple fulgurations may be required) and the entire specimen is not available for examination by the pathologist.

Adequate local excision of benign villous adenoma is curative, but it should be borne in mind that these patients have a demonstrated propensity for development of another tumor in the same area. Inadequately excised tumors have a tendency to recur, as vividly described in the report of Wheat and Ackerman.[34] If invasive cancer is present, the prognosis in most reported series has been somewhat worse than for ordinary colonic cancer.

Hypersecreting Villous Adenoma

A spectacular syndrome, first reported by McKittrick and Wheelock,[20] is seen occasionally in patients with villous adenoma. These patients have massive mucorrhea with rectal discharge of 1 to 3 liters per day of a clear viscid mucus. Since the fluid contains large amounts of potassium (25 to 35 mEq. per liter) and sodium (100 to 150 mEq. per liter), dehydration, hypokalemia, hyponatremia, hypochloremia, and renal failure may occur rapidly, particularly in elderly patients. The patient may present in vascular collapse or coma, but earlier symptoms are diarrhea and weakness. Since the villous adenoma is so soft, the tumor may be missed on digital examination.

Treatment must begin with vigorous fluid resuscitation, preferably with monitoring of central venous pressure. As much as 200 mEq. of K^+ per day may be required to restore and maintain serum potassium levels. As soon as fluid resuscitation has been accomplished, the tumor should be completely excised. Temporizing colostomy is of no value, since the mucorrhea does not abate following diversion of the fecal stream.

Although this syndrome is associated with large villous adenomas, most patients have had benign tumors.

MALIGNANT LESIONS

Cancer of the Colon and Rectum

It was predicted that cancer of the colorectal area would afflict 99,000 new patients and cause 49,000 deaths in the United States in 1976 (Fig. 2). This makes the colon and rectum the leading site of cancer in this country (exclusive of skin, cancers of which are rarely associated with any mortality) and the second most fatal of all sites of cancer (Table 1). At least 10 other countries have an even higher incidence of colonic cancer than the United States (Fig. 3). The very frequency with which cancer of the colon occurs makes some knowledge of its course and therapy mandatory for all physicians.

The ease with which the proper diagnosis can be

TABLE 1. Cancer in the United States—1976. Estimated New Cases and Deaths*

Site	New Cases	Deaths
Colon and rectum	99,000	49,000
Lung	93,000	84,000
Breast	89,000	33,000
Uterus	47,000	11,000

*From '76 Cancer Facts and Figures. New York, American Cancer Society, 1975.

made in most instances and the significant effect such early diagnosis should have on mortality emphasize even further the importance to every physician of being on the lookout for this disease. A digital examination of the rectum and a sigmoidoscopic examination on all patients—both of which should be available to all patients from all physicians—would do more to aid the diagnosis of colonic cancer than any other test. The distribution of cancers in our own series (Fig. 4), along with the comparable statistics from almost all studies, showing that approximately 75 per cent of all colonic cancers are within reach of the sigmoidoscope, underscores the importance of this simple study.

The 5-year survival rate for patients treated for colonic cancer is good when compared with the rates for patients with cancer at other common sites, and

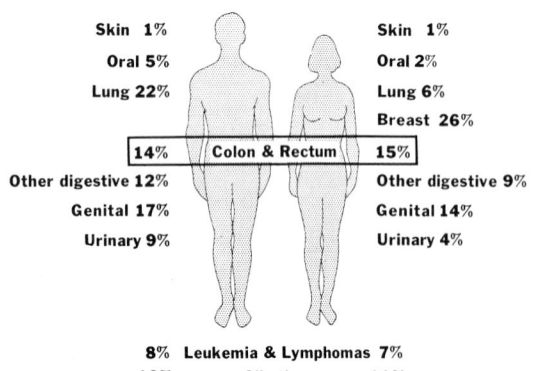

Figure 2. Cancer incidence by site and sex as predicted for 1976. (Modified from data in '76 Cancer Facts and Figures. New York, American Cancer Society, 1975.)

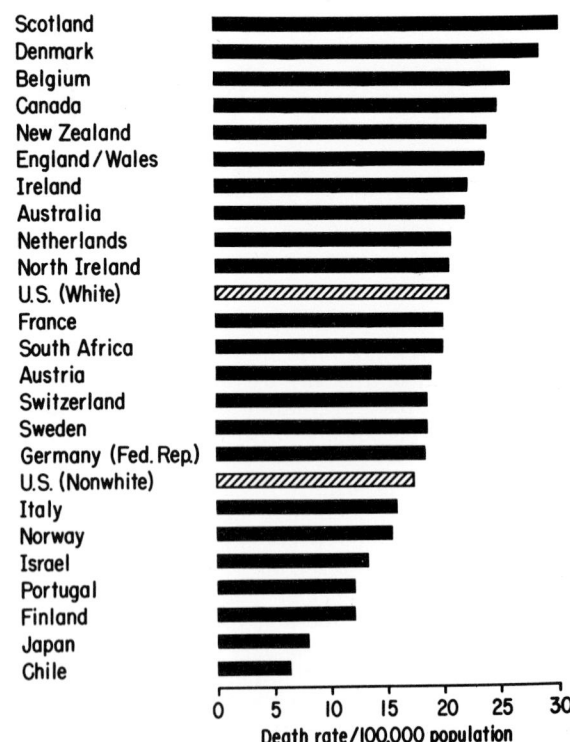

Figure 3. Comparative death rate from intestinal cancer in various geographic areas. (Modified from Progress Against Cancer. Washington, D.C., U.S. Department of Health, Education and Welfare, Public Health Service, National Institutes of Health, 1970.)

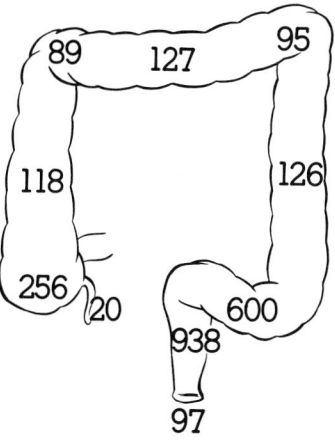

Figure 4. Anatomical location of 2466 colorectal cancers in 2313 patients at Charity Hospital in New Orleans. (From Falterman, K. W., Hill, C. B., Markey, J. C., Fox, J. W., and Cohn, I., Jr.: Cancer, *34*:951, 1974.)

TABLE 2. Qualitative Differences in Symptoms and Signs of Right and Left Colorectal Carcinoma

	Right	Left
Occult blood in stools	+	−
Anemia	+	−
Gallbladder disease-like symptoms	+	−
"Sentinel polyps"	+	+
Bright blood in stools	−	+
Obstructive signs	−	+
"Sentinel hemorrhoids"	−	+
Small caliber of stools	−	+

the results are significantly improved when the lesion is resected in its early stages (see the further discussion of prognosis later in this section).

Much of the following data is based on a study at Charity Hospital, New Orleans, of 2313 patients with histologically confirmed cancer of the colon, rectum, and anus.[14] Publications from other institutions with large patient populations have tended to confirm these observations.

Cancer of the colon is predominantly a disease of older persons but does occur at all ages (Fig. 5).

The distinction between various features of carcinoma of the left and right colon has been noted (Table 2). Separating the two halves of the colon at the distal transverse colon, these differences relate to embryologic origin, blood supply, function, fecal content, type of lesion to be found, clinical symptomatology, diagnostic consideration, and type of therapy (Fig. 6).

The right colon has its embryologic origin from the midgut and the same source for its blood supply as the midgut. The contents are mainly liquid, and water absorption is one of its major functions.

The left colon has its embryologic origin from the hindgut and the same source for its blood supply as

the hindgut. The contents are more solid and storage and excretion are its major functions.

The surgical approach to any malignant lesion of the colon is totally dependent on a knowledge of the arterial, venous, and lymphatic supply of the colon. Removal of part or all of the colon may change a person's daily routine but should not alter his life span in any way.

Malignant lesions of the right colon are typically bulky, fungating, ulcerating lesions that project into the lumen of the bowel. They are commonly the cause of significant anemia because of the large surface area that bleeds freely. The blood is not noticed by the patient because it is mixed with the rest of the stool. These lesions rarely cause obstruction. The common triad of findings for right-sided lesions is anemia, weakness, and a mass in the right lower quadrant.

The common lesion of the left colon is an annular, napkin-ring tumor that encircles the bowel and often causes obstruction. Constipation, diarrhea, or alternating periods of constipation and diarrhea may be the first symptom noted by the patient. A change in bowel habit, obstructive symptoms, and gross blood in the stool are commonly seen. Small-caliber "pencil" stools are of considerable importance when noted. The circumferential character of the lesion and the solid state of the feces lead to the obstructive symptoms. Obstruction may be minor, progressive, or total and acute when the patient first becomes aware of the lesion. The occurrence of obstruction significantly alters prognosis.

Key features to be observed are change in bowel habits, blood in the stools, pain, and anemia. A cardinal rule for all physicians should be: *any change in bowel habit in a person over 40 demands investigation.*

The value of simple studies has been emphasized by everyone who has studied colon cancer (Table 3). Any lesion that can be felt by digital examination or seen by sigmoidoscopy should be biopsied immediately, and therapeutic plans based upon the histologic information. Sigmoidoscopy can be performed on the patient's first visit to the physician without the need for prior enemas. The improved visualization of the colonic mucosa following cleansing is not essential. Palpation of an abdominal mass or an enlarged liver suggests late disease, but does not preclude further study or exploration. Hemorrhoids should not be accepted as the only cause of the patient's symptoms until complete study has excluded the presence of other disease. The

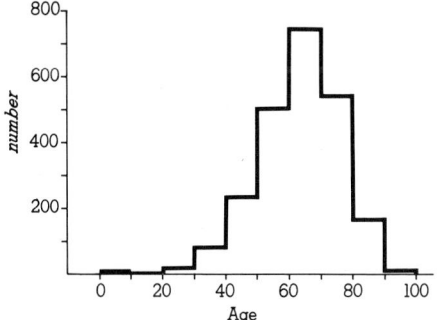

Figure 5. Age range for 2313 patients with cancer of the colon. (From Falterman, K. W., Hill, C. B., Markey, J. C., Fox, J. W., and Cohn, I., Jr.: Cancer, *34*:951, 1974.)

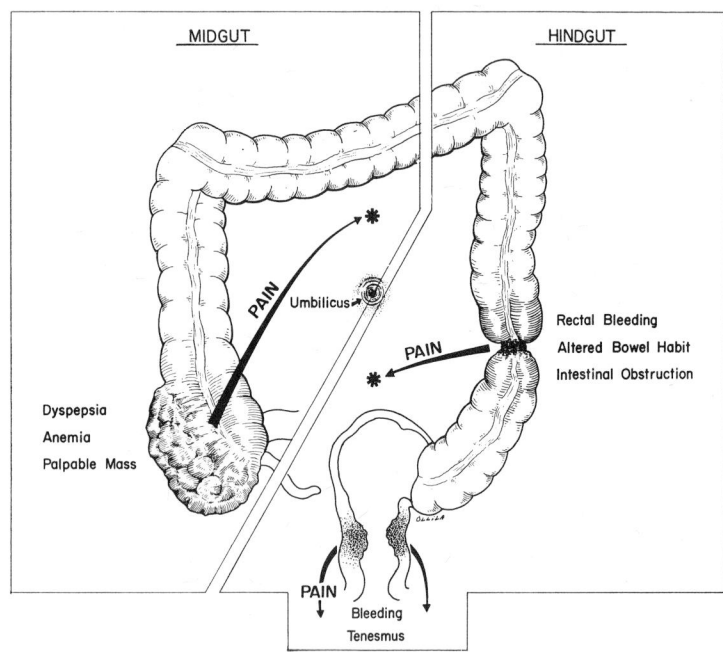

Figure 6. The symptoms of carcinoma of the colon. The symptoms of a tumor of the right colon are different from those of a tumor of the left colon, owing to different embryologic derivation. (From Zollinger, R. M., and Howe, C. T. *In* Davis, L. (Ed.): Christopher's Textbook of Surgery, 9th ed. Philadelphia, W. B. Saunders Company, 1968.)

failure to seek another more important lesion often has led to fatal delay.

Obstruction of the colon as a result of cancer is a relatively common accompaniment of colonic cancer.

Perforation and cancer coexistent in the same patient present that patient with a dual threat to life. The perforation is the more immediate danger, since it leads to fecal peritonitis and is therefore the lesion that demands first attention. Because of the poor long-term results when only the perforation is handled, it has been suggested that the more radical approach of immediate resection may be desirable.[11, 21]

In the differential diagnosis one should consider diverticulitis, lymphogranuloma venereum, tuberculosis, endometriosis, appendicitis, ulcerative colitis, simple ulcer of the colon, and benign polyps. Sometimes the differentiation is quite easy, and on other occasions it may be very difficult. Biopsy of the lesion is the surest and only way to make the differential diagnosis whenever the lesion can be seen. X-ray will often be diagnostic, but there will be times when even an expert radiologist will have difficulty. Whenever the diagnosis of cancer cannot be excluded, surgical exploration is required.

Surgical removal is the only acceptable curative therapy for colonic cancer. Excision should follow

TABLE 3.   Positive Diagnostic Studies in 2313 Patients with Cancer of the Colon*

X-ray	1504
Proctoscopy or sigmoidoscopy	1091
Rectal examination	929

*Modified from Falterman, K. W., Hill, C. B., Markey, J. C., Fox, J. W., and Cohn, I., Jr.: Cancer, *34*:951, 1974.

diagnosis as quickly as possible. If the lesion causes obstruction, it may be necessary to relieve the obstruction before a definitive operative procedure is performed, depending on the location of the lesion and other factors discussed elsewhere.

Removal of the primary lesion is not necessarily contraindicated by the presence of metastases, since there are cogent reasons for removal of the primary even when a curative procedure is not possible. Removal of the primary eliminates or diminishes the possibility of obstruction, bleeding, perforation, fistulization, infection, and the continuous discharge of foul material per rectum, which so often accompany colonic lesions. Visible or palpable metastases in the liver sometimes may be removed along with the primary, rather than serving as a contraindication to its therapy. If the lesion has spread outside the confines of the colon and has invaded adjacent structures, it is often possible and desirable to remove these simultaneously with the primary in the colon rather than leave any tumor behind.

Cancer chemotherapy is recommended by some for the patient who has inoperable, recurrent, or metastatic colonic cancer. The agent used most frequently has been 5-fluorouracil, and some are enthusiastic about its value. Chemotherapy is not accepted by all, mainly because the ideal drug has not been found.

For rectal lesions, two other approaches have elicited varying degrees of interest at different times. Electrocoagulation was originally proposed by Strauss et al.[30] for the poor-risk patient, but the results were so striking that they soon recommended it for all patients. The same approach has been advocated more recently by Madden.[22] Most other surgeons have not accepted this as a primary mode of therapy when the lesion can be resected, but all are watching with interest because of the obvious advantages of a nonresective approach, *provided* the results are as good as those obtained by other techniques. Irradiation of rectal lesions prior to their surgical removal has been championed by the group at Memorial Hospital in New York, and has been advocated by others, but once again there is no general acceptance of this form of therapy.

Immunotherapy is the newest approach to the treatment of patients with cancer, and there are some promising reports based on early experience with this form of therapy. As the technique of producing immunity develops, and as experience increases, it should be possible to involve a larger number of patients and a larger number of institutions for a better evaluation of immunotherapy.

Definitive surgical resection involves a consideration of at least six factors in the spread of the tumor (Fig. 7).

1. Intramural spread. Any curative resection should be performed with sufficient margin on each side of the lesion to provide a cut edge of the specimen free of tumor.

2. Lymphatic metastases. The direction and extent of lymphatic spread determine the scope of the operation that will be required. First metastases occur in pericolic nodes. The process extends up to the chain of nodes that parallel closely the blood vessels to the affected segment of colon. Adequate resection should include wide removal of the proximal lymphatic channels. Lymphatic involvement alone will reduce the 5-year survival figures by approximately 50 per cent.[16]

3. Venous spread. The demonstration of tumor cells in the venous effluent from tumor-bearing segments of colon, particularly during the manipulation of these areas, has emphasized the importance of this route of spread. This information has been employed clinically by Turnbull[32] to emphasize the advantages of early ligation of the venous supply to a segment of colon before any other approach to the tumor is made. How-

ever, the significance of tumor cells in the venous effluent is not clear. The presence of tumor cells in portal blood has not been correlated directly with survival.

4. Implantation in the anastomosis. Our own experimental and clinical studies,[9] as well as those of a number of others, have shown quite clearly that this route of spread can and does account for a number of "recurrences" and has been ignored for too long. Experimental data (Fig. 8) show that there are relatively few techniques that are effective in controlling this form of spread.

5. Direct extension. Tumors of the colon may break through the serosa and invade any organ in contact with the colon. Spread to the prostate may produce difficulty in the male, and spread can also occur in the reverse direction. Often the involved organ can be removed at the same time as the primary, and the presence of extension to another organ is not necessarily a reason for abandoning the operative approach.

6. Transperitoneal spread. Spread by this route usually means widespread involvement and in general indicates an incurable lesion.

A good cancer operation, as discussed earlier in this chapter, removes the tumor, as much of the organ in which the tumor arises as is necessary or practical, and all the vascular and lymphatic pathways that are appropriate to the particular lesion. Surgical procedures for colonic cancers should follow these principles just as should cancer operations for lesions elsewhere. For lesions of the anus and low rectum, the Miles abdominoperineal resection is the treatment of choice.

Ernest Miles, subsequently knighted for his work, described the operation in 1908. The original article[24] should be read by everyone interested in colon surgery because it includes so much that is vital to rectal surgery, and does so in the remarkably brief space of only one and a half pages. Since no one has described his principles better, it is best to let him speak for himself:

> The study of the spread of cancer from the rectum has led me to formulate certain essentials in the technique of the operation...(1) that an abdominal anus is a necessity; (2) that the whole of the pelvic colon, with the exception of the part from which the colostomy is made, must be removed because its blood-supply is contained in the zone of upward spread; (3) that the whole of the pelvic mesocolon below the point where it crosses the common iliac artery, together with a strip of peritoneum at least an inch wide on either side of it, must be cleared away; (4) that the group of lymph nodes situated over the bifurcation of the common iliac artery are in all instances to be removed; and lastly (5), that the perineal portion of the operation should be carried out as widely as possible so that the lateral and downward zones of spread may be effectively extirpated.

The Miles abdominoperineal resection remains the measuring rod against which all procedures for rectal lesions must be compared for mortality, morbidity, long-term results, and patient satisfaction. The last criterion is the one that the abdominoperineal resection most often fails to meet, since patients often are

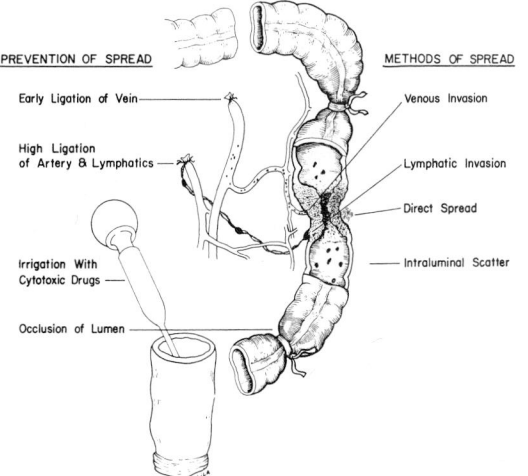

PREVENTION OF SPREAD   METHODS OF SPREAD

Early Ligation of Vein — — Venous Invasion

High Ligation of Artery & Lymphatics — — Lymphatic Invasion

— Direct Spread

Irrigation With Cytotoxic Drugs — — Intraluminal Scatter

Occlusion of Lumen —

Figure 7. The principles of surgical treatment of cancer of the colon to prevent spread by various routes. (From Zollinger, R. M., and Howe, C. T. *In* Davis, L. (Ed.): Christopher's Textbook of Surgery, 9th ed. Philadelphia, W. B. Saunders Company, 1968.)

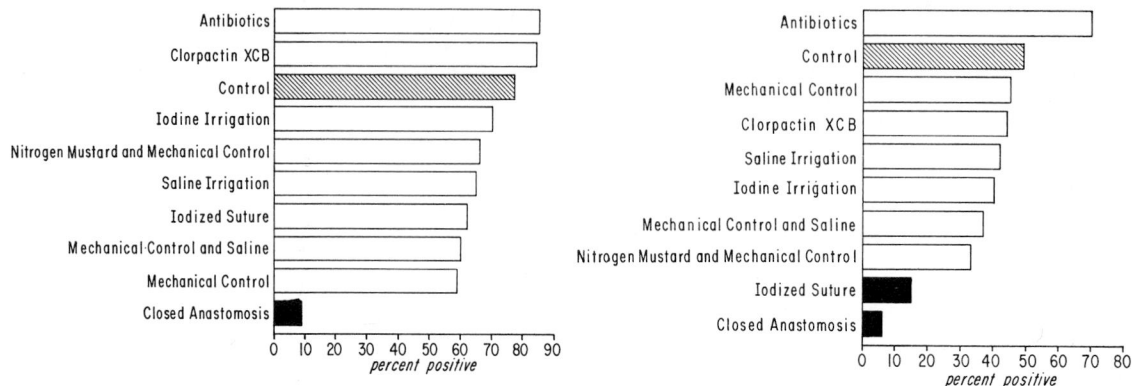

Figure 8. Incidence of tumor implantation *(A)* anywhere in the peritoneal cavity and *(B)* at the anastomosis in various types of experiments. The cross-hatched bars represent the incidence in the control series of experiments, with increase in tumor implantation in only two experiments. The solid black bars are the only ones with a statistically significant decrease in the incidence of tumor implantation. (From Cohn, I., Jr.: Surg. Gynecol. Obstet., *124*:501, 1967. By permission of Surgery, Gynecology & Obstetrics.)

dissatisfied with the prospect of an abdominal colostomy. However, the improved long-term result is the factor that must be explained most carefully to patients.

For more proximal colon cancers, "anterior resection" is appropriate. This operation removes the tumor and associated lymphatic channels and permits re-establishment of bowel continuity (and thus normal bowel function) by anastomosis.

For lesions proximal to 15 cm. from the anal verge, anterior resection should be performed in most cases. For lesions distal to 8 cm. from the anal verge, the Miles abdominoperineal resection is appropriate. For lesions located between 8 and 15 cm., the operation chosen will depend on local conditions (extent of tumor, size of pelvis, etc.) and the experience and preference of the surgeon.[36]

Leading the list of complications of colonic operations should be the danger of a leak at the anastomosis, which is significantly more important in colonic operations than in other gastrointestinal operations. This is related to the large bacterial and fecal content of any spillage in colonic operations, as compared with the relatively lesser bacterial population involved in operations on the small bowel. The various techniques to prevent leakage and disruption of a colonic anastomosis have been pointed out earlier.

Operations that involve dissection in the pelvis are frequently associated with some degree of urinary and sexual difficulties. Almost all patients undergoing such operations have some degree of voiding disturbance in the immediate postoperative period, and the extent and duration of the distress vary. Some men never completely recover from their voiding problems, and a prostatectomy is not an unusual secondary operation. If an abdominoperineal resection has been done with an adequate pelvic dissection, then difficulty with erection, ejaculation, or both, is a common accompaniment in male patients. All male patients should be forewarned about this, and the problem should be clearly discussed in advance of the operation, particularly with the younger patients.

Colostomy difficulties, such as retraction, devascu-

larization, and stenosis should also be considered, and these have been noted earlier.

The possibility of wound infection is ever present with colonic surgery, and the dangers of anastomoses below the peritoneal floor need to be mentioned because of their greater frequency.

The most important single distinguishing factor in long-term results is the histologic status of the lymph nodes. Cancer in the nodes reduces the 5- and 10-year survival figures to half their values in the absence of lymph node metastases. This is evident from our own studies[14] as well as from the figures reported for a compilation of over 14,000 cases in the *Cancer Prognosis Manual* (Table 4).[17] Some of the other factors that must be considered are location of the tumor in the colon, extent of the lesion, operative procedure utilized, some recognized and some not well-recognized geographic factors, and a list of other factors about which there is insufficient information.

Our own experience[14] provided a sufficient data base to evaluate some factors related to prognosis (Figs. 9 and 10). There is a marked mortality during the first year after the diagnosis is made, regardless of how the patient is managed during this period. Even cursory observation of the survival figures shows tremendous differences in survival depending on whether the operative procedure was curative, palliative, or decompressive. These differences emphasize the extent of disease as evaluated by the surgeon and they also emphasize the extremely poor outlook for a patient who does not seek medical attention until the disease has progressed too far.

Survival studies based on the extent of the lesion histologically show the same marked decrease in survival as the lesion is traced from its beginning to the obvious areas of spread. Thus, a single study has emphasized the relation of ultimate prognosis to the surgeon's evaluation of his operation and the histologic extent of the lesion. A combined evaluation leads to a fairly accurate prognosis.

These studies also show that the outlook can be quite good when the lesion is found and operated upon early, and that there is a good outlook for those patients

TABLE 4. The Influence of Extent of Disease on Survival in Cancer of the Colon and Anus*

		No. Cases Eval.	5 Year Survival	No. Cases Eval.	10 Year Survival
Colon	I. Absolute survival rates	14,865	34.0%	1,187	30.1%
	II. Determinant survival rates	12,525	39.8%	888	35.7%
	Stages				
	Stage I	838	80.3%	141	68.8%
	Disease strictly confined to bowel wall No evidence of metastases				
	Stage II	1,202	70.6%	220	55.9%
	Extension into the pericolonic tissues but not involving other organs. No evidence of metastases				
	Stage III	1,934	31.9%	297	21.5%
	Regional lymph node metastases				
	Stage IV	577	1.2%	0	
	Extension into other organs or with distant metastases				
Anus	I. Absolute survival rates	357	38.7%	101	21.8%
	II. Determinant survival rates	344	40.1%	96	22.9%

*From James, A. G.: Cancer Prognosis Manual. New York, American Cancer Society, 1970.

who have survived 5 years without evidence of recurrence.

The Dukes classification (Fig. 11) of the extent of cancer in malignant disease of the colon is one of the commonly employed methods of staging cancer. The figures just quoted show the correlation between the extent of the disease based on this classification and the prognosis.

Cancer of the Anus

Cancer arising in the anal canal is most likely to be of squamous cell origin. It is relatively uncommon in comparison with all the cancers found in the colon and rectum. The pure squamous cell variety is more common in males than in females. The diagnosis may be suspected on the basis of history, inspection, and palpation, but should always be confirmed by biopsy. A significant danger with these lesions is that they will be thought to be benign and mishandled accordingly.

Treatment is an abdominoperineal resection that varies from the standard operation only in that the perianal excision should be wider than usual because of the spread of these lesions through the skin lymphatics surrounding the anus. Because of this route of

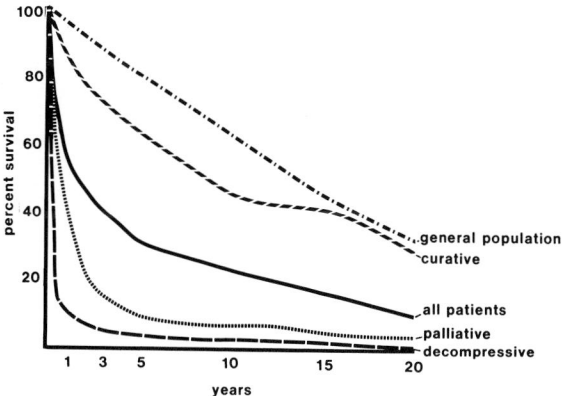

Figure 9. Survival after diagnosis of cancer of the colon, rectum, and anus computed by life-table method for 2313 patients reviewed at Charity Hospital. The curves are based upon all patients and the various surgical procedures upon judgments made by the surgeon at the time of operation. (Modified from data in Falterman, K. W., Hill, C. B., Markey, J. C., Fox, J. W., and Cohn, I., Jr.: Cancer, 34:951, 1974.)

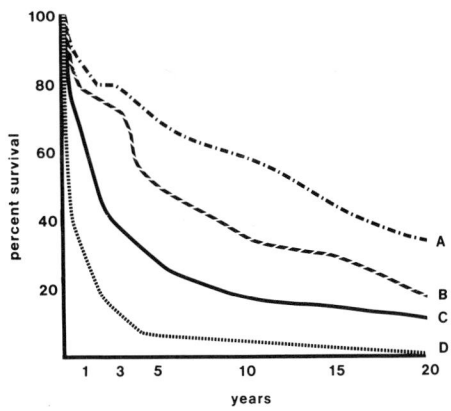

Figure 10. Survival curve based upon Dukes classification computed by the same technique as in Figure 9 and using the same data. (Modified from data in Falterman, K. W., Hill, C. B., Markey, J. C., Fox, J. W., and Cohn, I., Jr.: Cancer, 34:951, 1974.)

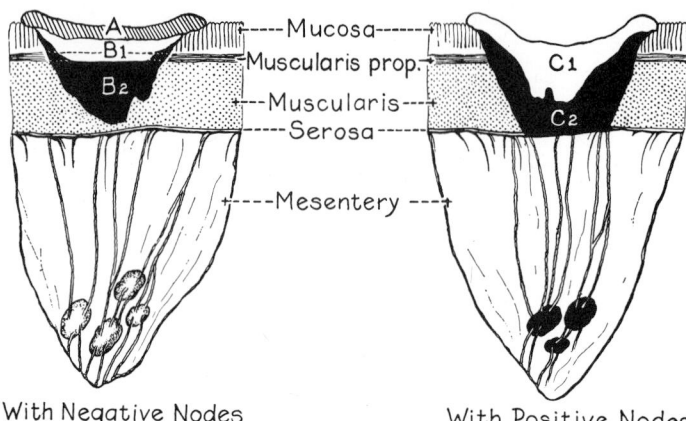

With Negative Nodes   With Positive Nodes

Figure 11. Diagram illustrating the modified Dukes classification: In Type A the lesion is confined to the mucosa; B_1, the lesion extends into the muscularis mucosae, but not through it with negative nodes; B_2, the lesion extends through the muscularis mucosae without involved nodes; C_1, the lesion is Type B_1 or B_2 limited to the wall with involved nodes; C_2, the lesion extends through the wall layers with positive nodes. (From Turell, R. (Ed.): Diseases of the Colon and Anorectum, 2nd ed. Philadelphia, W. B. Saunders Comapny, 1969.)

spread, the condition of the inguinal lymphatics is of particular importance in the treatment of these lesions. In the absence of clinical involvement of lymph nodes, the abdominoperineal resection will suffice. Careful follow-up is essential to determine if the inguinal nodes become palpable. Whenever the inguinal nodes are positive, then inguinal node dissection should be performed as soon as the patient has recuperated from the primary operation. Combining the two operations is usually too extensive a procedure for the patient, and increases the risk of slough of the inguinal skin flaps because of the proximity to the new colostomy.

The prognosis for cancer of the anus usually is considered to be poorer than that for cancer of the colon, but review of collected experience demonstrates this is not correct (Table 4), and these patients do appear to have an acceptable prognosis. Once inguinal nodes become positive, the outlook is poor.

Even rarer lesions of this area include melanoma, basal cell carcinoma, carcinoma of the perianal apocrine glands, carcinoma arising in an old fistula, and transitional cell or cloacogenic cancer. Cancer arising in the skin adjacent to the anus may be handled by the excision appropriate to skin cancer elsewhere.

SELECTED REFERENCES

Bockus, H. L.: Gastroenterology, Volume II, The Small Intestine and Colon. 3rd ed. Philadelphia, W. B. Saunders Company, 1976, pp. 781–1149.
This is the standard reference work in gastroenterology and contains the most detailed descriptions to be found in any single text for most of the conditions. There are numerous illustrations and good bibliographic references at the end of each section. For a medically oriented text, there is a surprising surgical leaning in many of the sections, and this is a valuable text as a starting point for further information in most of the areas covered.

Cohn, I., Jr.: Intestinal Antisepsis. Springfield, Ill., Charles C Thomas, Publisher, 1968.
This is a detailed description of the author's experimental and clinical experience to document the value of intestinal antisepsis, the background for the use of antibacterial agents, the experimental basis for their use, the bacteriologic studies involved in the selection of proper agents, and the clinical evaluation of a large series of patients. There is an extensive bibliography.

Goligher, J. C.: Surgery of the Anus, Rectum and Colon. Springfield, Ill., Charles C Thomas, Publisher, 1967.
This is an excellent example of the British approach to the surgical problems of the colon. The discussions, references, and illustrations are all excellent. The author has drawn heavily on articles from other places, for both content and illustrations, and thus does not present a one-sided approach to any of the problems, though he does add from his own extensive experience.

Pack, G. T., and Ariel, I. M. (Eds.): Treatment of Cancer and Allied Diseases. Volume 5, Tumors of the Gastrointestinal Tract, Pancreas, Biliary System and Liver. 2nd ed. New York, Hoeber Medical Division, Harper & Row, 1962, pp. 523–766.
This is an extensive discussion of the various neoplastic lesions of the colon, rectum, and anus, their classification, surgical management, and prognosis, and the problems involved in distinguishing between benign and malignant lesions. The various sections are written by experts in their field, and the volume contains much that is of value to both the beginner and the more advanced surgeon.

Proceedings of the First and Second National Conference on Cancer of the Colon and Rectum. Cancer, 28:1, 1971; Cancer, Suppl. 34:799, 1974.
A condensation of current information.

Turell, R. (Ed.): Diseases of the Colon and Anorectum. 2nd ed. Philadelphia, W. B. Saunders Company, 1969.
This is an extensive two-volume coverage of the surgical – and some nonsurgical – problems of the colon. There is complete coverage of a number of different aspects of colon surgery, from the basic anatomy through the detailed surgical approaches, with good illustrations, good references, and a variety of authors who present different viewpoints.

REFERENCES

1. Arnold, G. J., and Nance, F. C.: Volvulus of the sigmoid colon. Ann. Surg., 177:527–537, 1973.
2. Athanasoulis, C. A., Baum, S., Rosch, J., Waltman, A. C., Ring, E. J., Smith, J. C., Jr., Sugarbaker, E., and Wood, W.: Mesenteric arterial infusions of vasopressin for hemorrhage from colonic diverticulosis. Am. J. Surg., 129:212–216, 1975.
3. Axelrod, A. J., and Hanley, P. H.: Treatment of perforating wounds of the colon and rectum: A reevaluation. Southern Med. J., 60:811, 1967.
4. Becker, W. F.: Acute obstruction of the colon. An analysis of 205 cases. Surg. Gynecol. Obstet., 96:677, 1953.
5. Boley, S. J., Schwartz, S., Lash, J., and Sternhill, V.: Reversible vascular occlusion of the colon. Surg. Gynecol. Obstet., 116:53, 1963.
6. Byrne, J. J.: Large bowel obstruction. Am. J. Surg., 99:168, 1960.
7. Byrne, J. J., and Garick, E. I.: Surgical treatment of diverticulitis. Am. J. Surg., 121:379, 1971.
8. Cady, B.: Preoperative radiation. Surg. Gynecol. Obstet., 126:851, 1091, 1968.

9. Cohn, I., Jr.: Cause and prevention of recurrence following surgery for colon cancer. Cancer, 28:183, 1971.
10. Colcock, B. P.: Surgical treatment of diverticulitis. Twenty years' experience. Am. J. Surg., 115:264, 1968.
11. Crowder, V. H., Jr., and Cohn, I., Jr.: Perforation in cancer of the colon and rectum. Dis. Colon Rectum, 10:415, 1967.
12. DiVincenti, F. C., and Cohn, I., Jr.: Prolonged administration of intraperitoneal kanamycin in the treatment of peritonitis. Am. Surg., 37:177, 1971.
13. Drapanas, T., Pennington, D. G., Kappelman, M., and Lindsey, E. S.: Emergency subtotal colectomy: Preferred approach to management of massively bleeding diverticular disease. Ann. Surg., 177:519–526, 1973.
14. Falterman, K. W., Hill, C. B., Markey, J. C., Fox, J. W., and Cohn, I., Jr.: Cancer of the colon, rectum, and anus: A review of 2313 cases. Cancer, 34:951–959, 1974.
15. Ganchrow, M. I., Lavenson, G. S., Jr., and McNamara, J. J.: Surgical management of traumatic injuries of the colon and rectum. Arch. Surg., 100:515, 1970.
16. Gilchrist, R. K., and David, V. C.: Lymphatic spread of carcinoma of the rectum. Ann. Surg., 108:621, 1938.
17. James, A. G.: Cancer Prognosis Manual. New York, American Cancer Society, 1970.
18. Jenkinson, E. L., and Brown, W. H.: Endometriosis. A study of one hundred and seventeen cases with special reference to constricting lesions of the rectum and sigmoid colon. J.A.M.A., 122:349, 1943.
19. McGuire, H. H., Jr., and Haynes, B. W., Jr.: Massive hemorrhage from diverticulosis of the colon: Guidelines for therapy based on bleeding patterns observed in fifty cases. Ann. Surg., 175:847–855, 1972.
20. McKittrick, L. S., and Wheelock, F. C., Jr.: Carcinoma of the Colon. Springfield, Ill., Charles C Thomas, Publisher, 1954.
21. Madden, J. L.: Primary resection and anastomosis in the treatment of perforated lesions of the colon. Am. Surg., 31:781, 1965.
22. Madden, J. L., and Kandalaft, S.: Electrocoagulation in the treatment of cancer of the rectum. A continuing study. Ann. Surg., 174:530, 1971.
23. Michels, N. A., Siddharth, P., Kornblith, P. L., and Parke, W. W.: The variant blood supply to the descending colon, rectosigmoid and rectum based on 400 dissections. Its importance in regional resections: A review of medical literature. Dis. Colon Rectum, 8:251, 1965.
24. Miles, W. E.: A method of performing abdominoperineal excision for carcinoma of the rectum and of the terminal portion of the pelvic colon. Lancet, 2:1812, 1908.
25. Miller, L. D., Boruchow, I. B., and Fitts, W. T., Jr.: An analysis of 284 patients with perforative carcinoma of the colon. Surg. Gynecol. Obstet., 123:1212, 1966.
26. Nance, F. C., Persson, A. V., and Piker, J. F.: Radiation injuries to the lower gastrointestinal tract. Am. Surg., 34:21, 1968.
27. Peskin, G. W., and Orloff, M. J.: A clinical study of 25 patients with carcinoid tumors of the rectum. Surg. Gynecol. Obstet., 109:673, 1959.
28. Rives, J. D., Heibner, W. C., and Powell, J. L.: The surgical complications of amebiasis of the colon (exclusive of liver abscess). Surg. Clin. North Am., 45:1421, 1965.
29. Schmitt, M. G., Jr., Wu, W. C., Geenen, J. E., and Hogan, W. J.: Diagnostic colonoscopy. An assessment of the clinical indications. Gastroenterology, 69:765–769, 1975.
30. Strauss, A. A., Strauss, S. F., Crawford, R. A., and Strauss, H. A.: Surgical diathermy of carcinoma of the rectum. Its clinical end results. J.A.M.A., 104:1480, 1935.
31. Sunderland, D. A., and Binkley, G. E.: Papillary adenomas of the large intestine. A clinical and morphological study of forty-eight cases. Cancer, 1:184, 1948.
32. Turnbull, R. B., Jr., Kyle, K., Watson, F. R., and Spratt, J.: Cancer of the colon: The influence of the no-touch isolation technic on survival rates. Ann. Surg., 166:420, 1967.
33. Washington, J. A., II, Dearing, W. H., Judd, E. S., and Elveback, L. R.: Effect of preoperative antibiotic regimen on development of infection after intestinal surgery: Prospective, randomized, double-blind study. Ann. Surg., 180:567–572, 1974.
34. Wheat, M. W., Jr., and Ackerman, L. V.: Villous adenomas of the large intestine. Clinicopathologic evaluation of 50 cases of villous adenomas with emphasis on treatment. Ann. Surg., 147:476, 1958.
35. Williams, L. F., Jr., Bosniak, M. A., Wittenberg, J., Manuel, B., Grimes, E. T., and Byrne, J. J.: Ischemic colitis. Am. J. Surg., 117:254, 1969.
36. Wilson, S. M., and Beahrs, O. H.: The curative treatment of colonic carcinoma of the sigmoid, rectosigmoid and rectum. Ann. Surg., 183:556, 1976.
37. Wolff, W. I., and Shinya, H.: A new approach to colonic polyps. Ann. Surg., 178:367–378, 1973.
38. Wolff, W. I., and Shinya, H.: Definitive treatment of "malignant" polyps of the colon. Ann. Surg., 182:516–525, 1975.

VII

GARDNER'S SYNDROME

Alvin L. Watne, M.D.

Historical Aspects

In a series of papers in the 1950's, Elden J. Gardner and associates described a disease syndrome that bears his name.[15, 17-20, 31] The syndrome, inherited as a Mendelian dominant characteristic, includes connective tissue lesions (fibromas), skin lesions (sebaceous cysts), bony tumors (osteomas), and multiple polyps of the lower digestive tract, and the patients are at high risk to develop cancer of the large bowel. The association of visible and palpable soft tissue and bony tumors with the development of polyps of the colon was recognized in 1912 by Devic and Bussy,[10] and a few similar patients were reported before 1950.[4, 14] By 1967 MacDonald et al.[26] reported that 118 cases had appeared in the literature and since then numerous patients, manifesting part or all of the syndrome, have been reported.

Anatomical and Histological Aspects

The diagnostic features of the syndrome show a great variation among the patients. In a classic article giving the follow-up study for the 112 family members of Kindred 109, Gardner reported 9 patients with the entire syndrome, 16 with colonic polyposis, 21 with sebaceous cysts, 13 with fibromas, 13 with osteomas, and 9 deaths from colon cancer.[16] Table 1 shows the occurrence of the syndrome characteristics in members of 11 families with the syndrome. The Mendelian dominant trait is apparent, with 126 of the 280 patients or

TABLE 1. Characteristics of Gardner's Syndrome*

Number	Characteristic
75	Soft tissue tumors
40	Osteomatosis
85	Polyposis
41	Bowel cancer

6 alive; 21 dead of CA; 14 dead of other causes

*11 families, 280 patients
126 with syndrome
154 without syndrome

45 per cent of the patients at risk exhibiting some part of the syndrome. There is no known consanguinity within or between the 11 families. Soft tissue tumors were seen in 75 or 60 per cent of these patients. Cabot,[4] Gardner and Richards,[19] and Oldfield[30] all emphasized the relation of sebaceous cysts and polyps of the colon. The presence of large cysts around the face and extremities is characteristic of the syndrome (Fig. 1). The cysts have been observed on a 14-day-old infant, but have generally appeared before puberty and have continued to increase in size, even after colectomy for the polyposis. Gardner's original patients had fibromas as well as cysts, and his follow-up

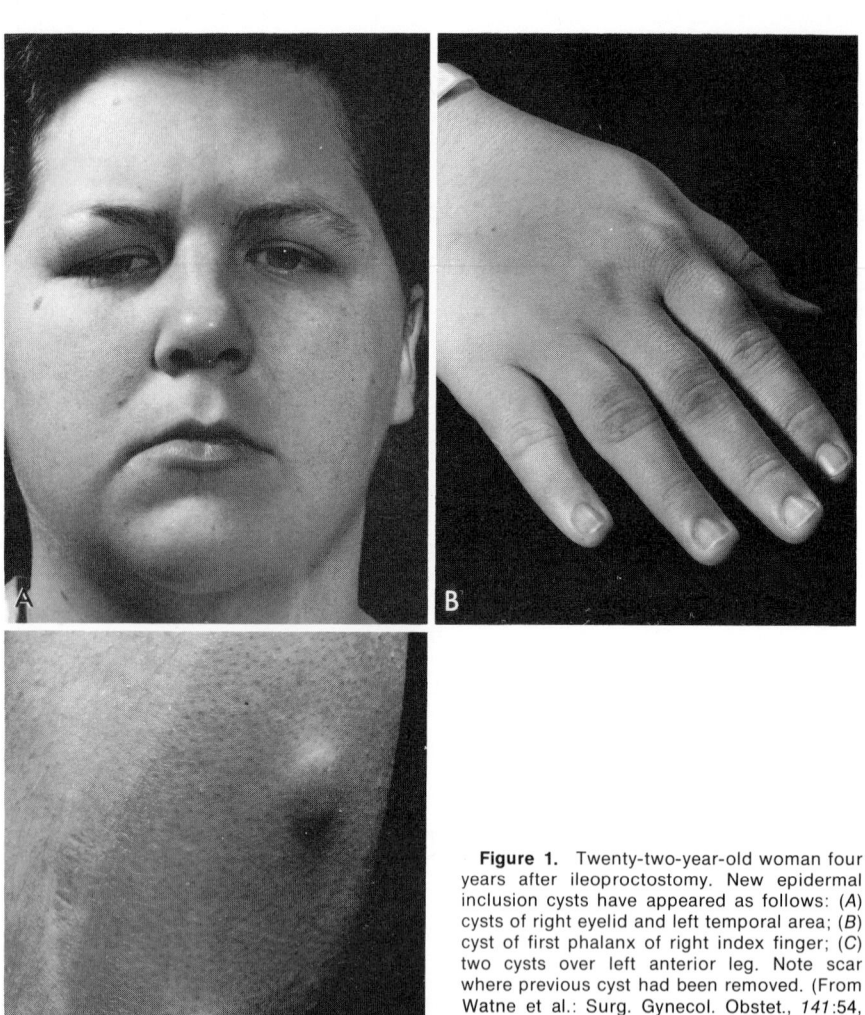

Figure 1. Twenty-two-year-old woman four years after ileoproctostomy. New epidermal inclusion cysts have appeared as follows: (A) cysts of right eyelid and left temporal area; (B) cyst of first phalanx of right index finger; (C) two cysts over left anterior leg. Note scar where previous cyst had been removed. (From Watne et al.: Surg. Gynecol. Obstet., *141*:54, 1975.)

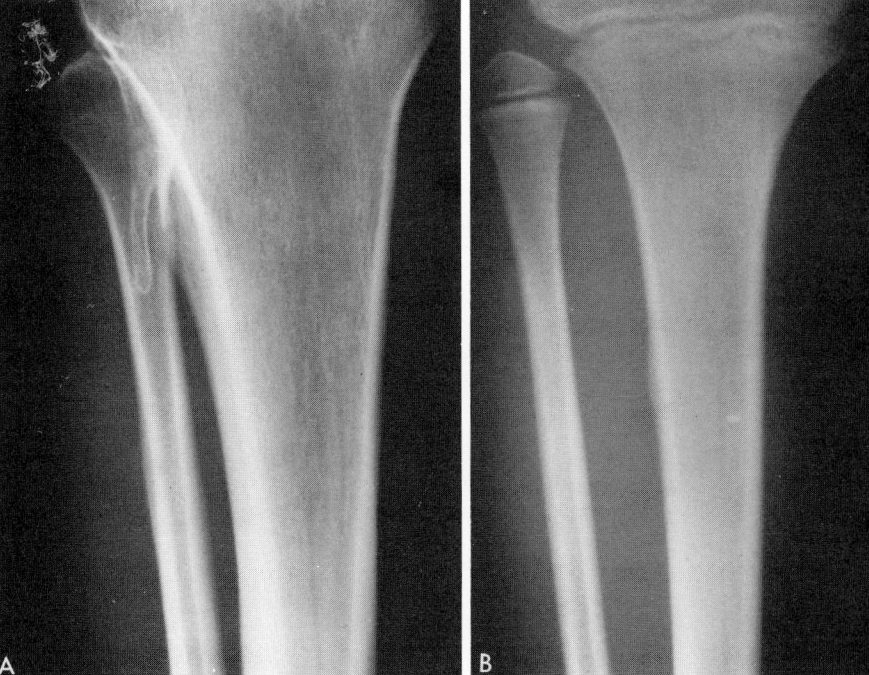

Figure 2. *A*, Exostosis of proximal part of tibial epiphysis in 18-year-old man with Gardner's syndrome. *B*, Cortical thickening of proximal part of tibial metaphysis in 14-year-old boy with Gardner's syndrome. These cortical thickenings have not progressed to a classic bony exostosis. (From Watne et al.: Surg. Gynecol. Obstet., *141*:54, 1975.)

report included two patients with fibrosarcomas. The association of desmoid tumors with familial polyposis was reported by Miller and Sweet in 1937.[28] Smith[32] reported a 26-year-old woman who died as a result of a desmoid tumor that arose "de novo" in her neck. He stated that desmoid tumors occurred in 3.5 per cent of the patients with familial polyposis, compared to 0.03 per cent for the general population. Patients have been reported with lipomas[7, 25] or liposarcoma.[12]

The bony tumors seen most often with Gardner's syndrome are benign osteomatosis, which have appeared in 40 patients. They may involve almost all parts of the skeletal system, and vary from slight cortical thickenings (Fig. 2*A*) to large bony proliferations (Fig. 2*B*). Mandibular osteomas or central enostosis and dental abnormalities were frequently seen. Localized cortical thickening of the long and short tubular bones was the most common abnormality in a survey of our patients.[5] The frontal bone was the most frequent site of osteoma in the skull. Fitzgerald's[14] original patient had multiple compound odontoma, torus palatinus, carious teeth, and 37 rudimentary and 2 permanent teeth embedded in the alveolar process. Fader et al.[13] associated multiple impacted supernumerary and permanent teeth with the syndrome. We have seen supernumerary teeth and unerupted teeth in 8 patients. Two patients with Gardner's syndrome and bone sarcoma have been reported.[22] One of our patients underwent an above-the-knee amputation at age 15 for osteogenic sarcoma. She did not develop colonic polyposis until the age of 34.

Polyps of the colon were diagnosed by proctosigmoidoscopy, biopsy, and air-contrast barium enema in 85 patients (Fig. 3). The polyps appear to arise first in the rectum. We have never diagnosed colonic polyposis by

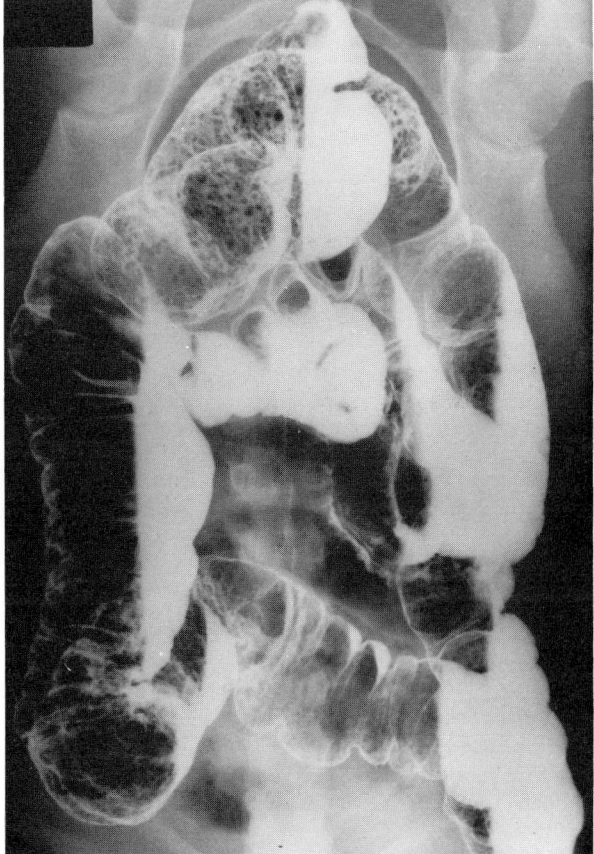

Figure 3. Air-contrast barium enema of a 16-year-old girl with Gardner's syndrome. Meticulous cleansing of the bowel is required for accurate air-contrast study.

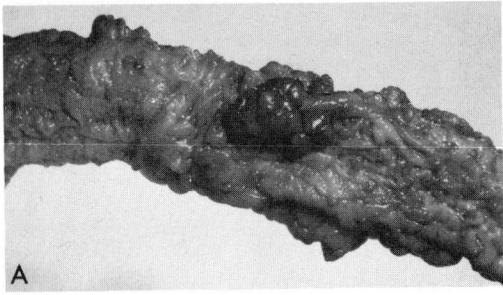
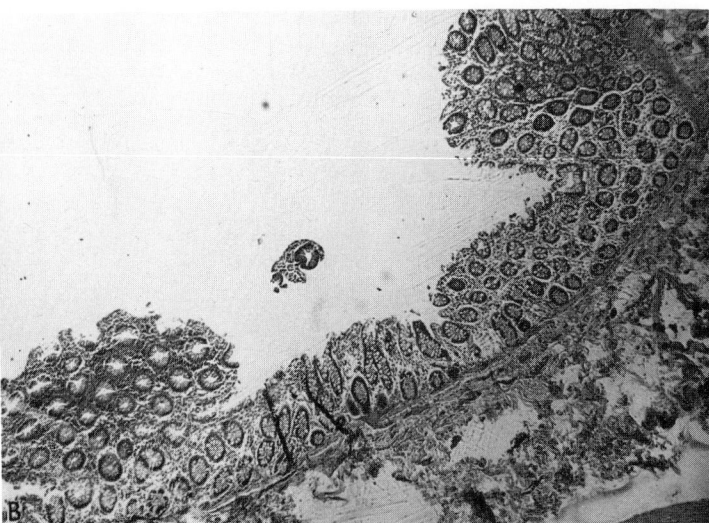

Figure 4. *A*, Colonic polyposis associated with Gardner's syndrome in 34-year-old woman. Pedunculated lesion was an adenomatous polyp; no cancer was present. (From Watne et al.: Surg. Gynecol. Obstet., *141*:54, 1975.)

B, Adenomatous polyps from the colon of a 34-year-old woman with Gardner's syndrome. Note that the mucosal cell changes occur on the surface as seen in the polyp on the left, H & E. ×40.

air-contrast barium enema when the polyps were not readily visible by the proctoscope. We must emphasize the importance of confirmation of adenomatous polyps by biopsy. The polypoid lesions of infants and children may be inflammatory polyps, lymphoid hyperplasia, or juvenile polyps, which are hamartomas and are not premalignant. We have seen adenomatous polyps in a 10-year-old boy and have demonstrated colonic polyps in 16 patients less than 15 years of age. The adenomatous polyps begin as mucosal excrescences, eventually covering the entire rectum and colon like cobblestones (Fig. 4). As described by Gardner,[16] we have observed the polyps always to be progressive in both size and number in these young patients.

Twenty-five patients had the complete triad of soft tissue tumors, bony tumors, and colonic polyposis. Two patients had colonic polyposis without soft tissue or bony tumors, and one 54-year-old man had extensive soft tissue and bony lesions with an absolutely normal colonic mucosa. Colorectal carcinoma developed in 41 patients. Thirty are dead, 21 with known cancer—a 27 per cent crude survival rate. The average age of death was 41 years, which is virtually identical with that reported by Dukes for patients with familial polyposis.[11] In one family we found colon cancer appearing at an earlier age for each successive generation, being 66, 43, 40, 30, and 24 years, respectively.[36]

The causes of death of 38 patients with the syndrome and 24 patients without the syndrome are shown in Table 2. In addition to the 30 patients dying of bowel cancer, two patients with the syndrome developed carcinoma of the ampulla of Vater. Bussey has reported 17 such patients from the literature.[2] Additional deaths for patients with the syndrome included liver cancer (possibly metastatic), ovarian cancer, heart disease, GI hemorrhage, and ulcerative colitis. The 24 patients without the syndrome died of cardiovascular disease, leukemia, metastatic cancer, pancreatic cancer, GI hemorrhage, chronic emphysema, pneumonia, Bright's disease, tuberculosis, and accidents.

The associated diseases not necessarily fatal to the

patients with Gardner's syndrome are listed in Table 3. Fibrous dysplasia was seen in 10, or 8 per cent of the patients with the syndrome, and in 2 patients it caused bowel obstruction and death.[24] The patients frequently had surgery for appendicitis and hemorrhoids, the symptoms of which may be manifestations of the colonic polyposis. There was a significant increase in the incidence of peptic ulcer in patients with the syndrome. Pigmented nevi requiring excision were frequently seen, and ulcerative colitis was diagnosed in patients with and without the syndrome. Cancer of other organs was seen in patients with and without the syndrome. Cancer of the ampulla of Vater was seen in 2 patients with the syndrome, and cancer of the pancreas was seen in a patient without the syndrome. Congenital defects were seen in both groups and 2 patients with the syndrome had an ectopic kidney. No associated endocrine adenopathy was seen with the syndrome patients; only one patient developed a nontoxic nodular goiter. No other frequently associated diseases were found.

Genetic Aspects

Gardner's original reports and follow-up data suggest that the syndrome results from a single defec-

TABLE 2. Gardner's Syndrome: Cause of Death

With Syndrome (N = 126)	Without Syndrome (N = 154)
30 cancer of bowel	4 stroke
2 cancer of ampulla of Vater	3 heart disease
1 cancer of liver	2 leukemia
1 cancer of ovary	2 cancer (site unknown)
2 heart disease	2 hemorrhage
1 hemorrhage	2 lung disease
1 ulcerative colitis	1 cancer of pancreas
	8 other
38	24

TABLE 3. Gardner's Syndrome: Associated Diseases

With Syndrome (N = 126)	Disease	Without Syndrome (N = 154)
10	Fibrosis, desmoid, fibrosarcoma	0
9	Appendicitis	5
9	Peptic ulcer	1
6	Hemorrhoids	3
4	Pigmented nevi	1
3	Ulcerative colitis	1
3	Cancer, other organs	1
2	Cancer, ampulla of Vater of pancreas	1
2	Ectopic kidney	0
2	Congenital defect	4
1	Osteogenic sarcoma	0
1	Diverticular disease	0
1	Varicose veins	0
1	Diabetes	0
1	Endocrine adenopathy	2
0	Leukemia	2
0	Melanoma	1

tive gene or several separate but closely linked genes. McKusick[27] gave evidence that this syndrome resulted from a single gene, different from that responsible for familial polyposis. Smith[33] believed that Gardner's syndrome represented a manifestation of a number of possible changes that might be present in any patient with multiple polyposis. Within the families with Gardner's syndrome we have seen two patients with only colonic polyposis without skin or bony tumors, and one 54-year-old patient had skin cysts and bony tumors without colon involvement. With the variation in the occurrence of the different characteristics of the syndrome, we would agree with Smith. Bussey, in his excellent monograph,[3] states that "the idea that all adenomatous polyposis may be Gardner's syndrome with different degrees of manifestation of the subsidiary lesions is interesting. Certainly, the more these are looked for the more they are found."

Altered cell replication in the colonic mucosa of patients with polyposis coli was demonstrated by Cole et al.[6] Using the colon mucosa incubation technique by Deschner et al.,[9] we have demonstrated an increased formation of DNA, RNA, and protein in the superficial cells of the crypts of Lieberkuhn in patients with Gardner's syndrome (Fig. 5). While the role of a genetic factor in Gardner's syndrome is well established, this trait may manifest itself by some increased susceptibility to an environmental carcinogen resulting in the altered mucosal cell growth.

Burkitt[1] pointed out that diet and slow bowel transit time may increase exposure to colon carcinogens. However, the bowel transit time in patients with Gardner's syndrome is three times as rapid as in control subjects.[37] Hill et al.[21] pointed out the importance of the fecal flora and fecal steroids as related to the incidence of colon cancer. Gas chromatography of fecal steroids and anaerobic bacterial culture have shown a higher concentration of fecal cholesterol and primary bile acids in the Gardner's syndrome patients, associated with a relative increase in Clostridia and Bifi-

dobacteria. The original observation by Hubbard[23] that the polyps may regress in the rectal segment after colectomy and ileorectal anastomosis has been confirmed many times, including our own clinical observations (Table 4). After ileorectostomy, the Gardner's syndrome patients' stool transit times dropped from 19.4 hours to 14.2 hours.[38] The bacterial metabolite coprostanol disappeared completely from the feces, and three years postoperatively the patients were still unable to hydrogenate cholesterol. Chenodeoxycholic and cholic acids were also significantly higher in the ileorectostomy patients, while lithocholic and deoxycholic acids were significantly lower.[35] The recent observations by De Cosse[8] that oral vitamin C, acting as an antioxidant, enhances the regression of polyps from the rectal stump, gives added stimulus to further observations on the mechanism of action following ileorectostomy in these patients.

In conclusion, the surgical implications of Gardner's syndrome present the surgeon with a challenge in cancer prevention, since the recognition of any part of the syndrome in the patient should alert the physician to examine the rectum and colon. The definite familial inheritance pattern should stimulate the physician to investigate all of the family members. Recognition and biopsy confirmation of adenomatous polyps of the colon is an indication for prophylactic colectomy and ileorectostomy. It is important that the ileum be anastomosed to the rectum and not to the sigmoid.[34] To assure this we insert and secure a rectal tube to the 12-cm. level preoperatively and perform an open two-layer anastomosis at this level, which is roughly at or just below the peritoneal reflection. We do not fulgurate any rectal polyps preoperatively or for one year postoperatively. We proctoscope the patients at 3- to 6-month intervals; as shown in Table 4, 12 of our 16 patients have had regression of their rectal polyps, 3 of which have been complete. Moertel et al.[29] advo-

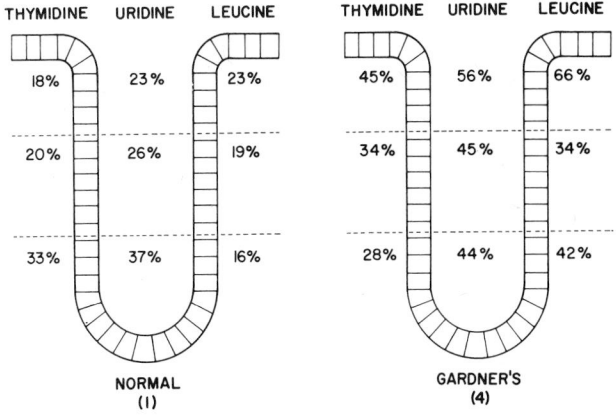

COLON MUCOSA INCUBATION 4 HOURS

Figure 5. Radioautographs of colon mucosa incubated with tritiated thymidine, leucine, and uridine demonstrate the variation in production of DNA, RNA, and protein of cells at various levels of the crypts of Lieberkühn.

TABLE 4. Gardner's Syndrome: Ileorectal Anastomosis Polyp Regression (1- to 8-year follow-up)

16 Patients, 10 to 35 years of age
9 Partial regression
3 Complete regression

cated total proctocolectomy for multiple polyposis because of a 5 to 59 per cent incidence of subsequent rectal cancer. These observations are not supported by Bussey's results from the polyposes register at St. Mark's, where the cumulative risk for developing rectal cancer after ileorectal anastomoses was only 3.6 per cent.[3] Many surgeons feel that the morbidity of a permanent ileostomy outweighs this 3.6 per cent risk. However, the patient must be cooperative and sophisticated enough to realize the importance of lifelong attention to the disease, necessitating regular physical and proctoscopic examinations, which after all are advocated for all adults over the age of 40.

SELECTED REFERENCES

Bussey, H. J. R.: Familial Polyposis Coli. Baltimore. Johns Hopkins University Press, 1975
This elegant and concise monograph represents the cumulative experience of Dr. Bussey and his many fine colleagues at St. Mark's Hospital. The St. Mark's Hospital Polyposis Register begun in 1925 now includes 200 families with 1958 members at risk. Their studies document the genetic and epidemiologic aspects of the disease, as well as the pathology and natural history of the disease, its relationship to cancer, the differential diagnosis, and recommended treatment. The section on associated lesions includes their experience with Gardner's syndrome and Turcot's syndrome and associated polypoid conditions.

Gardner, E. J.: Follow-up study of a family group exhibiting dominant inheritance for a syndrome including intestinal polyps, osteomas, fibromas, and epidermal cysts. Am. J. Hum. Genet., *14*:376, 1962.
This report represents Dr. Gardner's scientific description and follow-up of 112 members of his Kindred 109. He discusses each manifestation of the syndrome, its occurrence and natural history, and correlates the development of cysts, fibrous tumors, bony tumors, polyps, and cancers within the patient growth patterns from 1948 through 1962. This establishes an outstanding three-dimensional concept of the syndrome and its inheritance pattern.

Smith, W. G.: Familial multiple polyposis: Research tool for investigating the etiology of carcinoma of the colon. Dis. Colon Rectum, *11*:17, 1968.
Dr. Smith puts together his vast experience in treating patients with familial multiple polyposis, and shows the overlapping nature of the syndrome. He shows the wide variations possible with multiple polyposis and brings his thoughts together with a unified concept of familial multiple polyposis. His conclusions then are challenging in outlining broad avenues of approach to better understand the syndrome and its etiology. These projects are now being addressed by various groups around the world.

REFERENCES

1. Burkitt, D. P.: Epidemiology of cancer of the colon and rectum. Cancer, *28*:3, 1971.
2. Bussey, H. J. R.: Extracolonic lesions associated with polyposis coli. Proc. R. Soc. Med., *65*:294, 1972.
3. Bussey, H. F. R.: Familial polyposis coli. Baltimore, Johns Hopkins University Press, 1975, p. 63.
4. Cabot, R. C.: Case records of the Massachusetts General Hospital. Case No. 21061. N. Engl. J. Med., *22*:263, 1935.
5. Chang, C. H., Piatt, E. D., Thomas, K. E., and Watne, A. L.: Bone abnormalities in Gardner's syndrome. Am. J. Roentgenol., *103*:645, 1968.
6. Cole, J. W., and McKalen, A.: Studies on the morphognesis of adenomatous polyps in the human colon. Cancer, *16*:998, 1963.
7. Collins, D. C.: The frequent association of other body tumors with familial polyps. Am. J. Gastroenterol., *31*:376, 1959.
8. De Cosse, J. J., Adams, M. B., Kuzma, J. F., Lo Gerfo, P., and Condon, R. E.: Effect of ascorbic acid on rectal polyps in patients with familial polyposis. Am. J. Surg., *78*:608, 1975.
9. Deschner, E. E., Lipkin, M., and Solomon, D.: Study of human rectal epithelial cells in vitro. II. H³-thymidine incorporation into polyps and adjacent mucosa. J. Natl. Cancer Inst., *36*:849, 1966.
10. Devic, A., and Bussy: Un cas de polypose adenomateuse generalisee a tout de l'intestin. Arch. Mal. App. Digest., *6*:278, 1912.
11. Dukes, C. E.: Familial intestinal polyposis. Am. Eugenics, *17*:1, 1952.
12. Enterline, H. T., Culberson, J. D., Rocklin, D. B., and Brady, L. W.: Liposarcoma. Cancer, *13*:932, 1960.
13. Fader, M., Kline, S. N., Spatz, S. S., and Zubrow, H. J.: Gardner's syndrome (intestinal polyposis, osteomas, sebaceous cysts) and a new dental discovery. Oral Surg., *15*:153, 1962.
14. Fitzgerald, G. M.: Multiple composite odontomas coincidental with other tumourous conditions. Report of case. J. Am. Dent. Assoc., *30*:1408, 1943.
15. Gardner, E. J.: A genetic and clinical study of familial polyposis, a predisposing factor for carcinoma of the colon and rectum. Am. J. Hum. Genet., *3*:167, 1951.
16. Gardner, E. J.: Follow-up study of a family group exhibiting dominant inheritance for a syndrome including intestinal polyps, osteomas, fibromas, and epidermal cysts. Am. J. Hum. Genet., *14*:376, 1962.
17. Gardner, E. J.: Mendelian pattern of dominant inheritance for a syndrome including intestinal polyposis, osteomas, fibromas and sebaceous cysts in a human family group. Novant anni delle Leggi, Mendelione. L. Gedda (Ed.). 1955, pp. 321–329.
18. Gardner, E. J., and Plenk, H. P.: Hereditary pattern for multiple osteomas in a family group. Am. J. Hum. Genet., *4*:31, 1952.
19. Gardner, E. J., and Richards, R. C.: Multiple cutaneous and subcutaneous lesions occurring simultaneously with hereditary intestinal polyposis and osteomas. Am. J. Hum. Genet., *5*:139, 1953.
20. Gardner, E. J., and Stephens, F. E.: Cancer of the lower digestive tract in one family group. Am. J. Hum. Genet., *2*:41, 1950.
21. Hill, M. J., Drasar, B. S., Aries, V. C., Crowther, J. D., Hawksworth, G. M., and Williams, R. E. O.: Bacteria and aetiology of cancer of large bowel. Lancet, *1*:95, 1971.
22. Hoffman, D. C., and Brooke, B. N.: Familial sarcoma of bone in a polyposis coli family. Dis. Colon Rectum, *13*:119, 1970.
23. Hubbard, T. B.: Familial polyposis of the colon: The fate of the retained rectum after colectomy in children. Am. Surg., *23*:577, 1957.
24. Johnson, J. G., Gilbert, E., Zimmermann, B., and Watne, A. L.: Gardner's syndrome, colon cancer, and sarcoma. J. Surg. Oncol., *4*:354, 1972.
25. Laberge, M. Y., Sauer, W. G., and Mayo, C. W.: Soft-tissue tumors associated with familial polyposis. Mayo Clin. Proc., *32*:749, 1957.
26. MacDonald, J. M., Davis, W. C., Crago, H. R., and Beck, A. O.: Gardner's syndrome and periampullary malignancy. Am. J. Surg., *113*:425–430, 1967.
27. McKusick, V. A.: Genetic factors in intestinal polyposis. J.A.M.A., *182*:271, 1962.
28. Miller, R. H., and Sweet, R. H.: Multiple polyposis of the colon: A familial disease. Ann. Surg., *105*:511, 1937.
29. Moertel, C. G., Hill, J. R., and Adson, M. A.: Surgical management of multiple polyposis. Arch. Surg., *100*:521, 1970.
30. Oldfield, M. C.: Association of familial polyposis of colon with multiple sebaceous cysts. Br. J. Surg., *41*:534, 1954.
31. Plenk, H. P., and Gardner, E. J.: Osteomatosis (Leontiasis Ossea) hereditary disease of membranous bone formation associated in one family with polyposis of the colon. Radiology, *62*:830, 1954.
32. Smith, W. G.: Desmoid tumors in familial multiple polyposis. Mayo Clin. Proc., *34*:31, 1959.
33. Smith, W. G.: Familial multiple polyposis: Research tool for investigating the etiology of carcinoma of the colon. Dis. Colon Rectum, *11*:17, 1968.
34. Turnbull, R. B.: Discussion of McLachlin, A. D.: Familial intestinal polyposis. Arch. Surg., *79*:393, 1959.

35. Watne, A. L., and Core, S. K.: Fecal steroids in polyposis coli and ileorectostomy patients. J. Surg. Res., *19*:157, 1975.
36. Watne, A. L., Johnson, J. G., and Chang, C. H.: The challenge of Gardner's syndrome. Cancer, *19*:268, 1969.
37. Watne, A. L., and Johnson, R.: Bowel transit time in patients with Gardner's syndrome. Dis. Colon Rectum, *17*:52, 1974.
38. Watne, A. L., Lai, H., Mance, T., and Core, S.: Fecal steroids and bacterial flora in polyposis coli patients. Am. J. Surg., in press.

VIII

ULCERATIVE COLITIS

Frank G. Moody, M.D.

Ulcerative colitis, a diffuse inflammatory disease of the mucosal lining of colon and rectum, is characterized by bloody diarrhea and by remissions and exacerbations without apparent cause. It is difficult to imagine that a disease so devastating remains without an identified etiology or specific medical therapy. Fortunately, total removal of the affected organ, the colon and rectum, provides a complete cure, but at a price, since patients so treated must learn to tolerate an external abdominal stoma (an ileostomy) for the remainder of their lives. Since the disease has its peak onset in early and middle adulthood, for most patients it represents a long time span.

HISTORICAL BACKGROUND

While diarrheal illnesses have been described since the early medical writings of Hippocrates (circa 400 B.C.),[1] there is little evidence that they were distinguished from the all too common infectious enteritides until the court testimony on the appearance of the colon of a Mrs. Banks by Wilkes in 1859. This case was more formally documented in 1875, but by that time the pathologic anatomy of the disease had been described in a study of over 200 cases which occurred in the Union Army during the Civil War (Fig. 1).[9] By the turn of the century, the disease was fully characterized as to its nonspecific nature and distinguishable from the infectious diarrheas by clinical as well as pathologic criteria.

Goligher and his colleagues have traced the evolution of surgical approaches to the disease in an authoritative manner.[16] The following description has been paraphrased from their delightful chapter on this topic. Sigmoid colostomy, curiously enough, was the first well-documented surgical procedure for inflammatory bowel disease as performed by Pennel in 1850. During the remainder of the nineteenth century, a variety of diverting procedures were accomplished, but without success. Appendicostomy, first performed in 1902 for ulcerative colitis, represented a major advance. It soon, however, was displaced by a completely diverting ileostomy (1913). Ileostomy was accompanied by piecemeal resection of the diseased colon over the ensuing 20 to 30 years. By the mid 1940s, however, the extirpative procedures were reduced to three,

and shortly thereafter a single-stage ileostomy with subtotal colectomy or coloproctectomy was adopted by most surgical clinics. The first such procedure was performed by Miller of Montreal in 1959 on a patient in whom only ileostomy was planned.[24] The bowel, however, was close to perforation at several points; therefore, partial colectomy was carried out, with recovery of the patient. The subsequent rapid development of an effective and relatively safe surgical approach to the disease is a testimonial to the large number of well-trained surgeons who emerged following World War II.

ETIOLOGY

The etiology of ulcerative colitis remains unknown in spite of intensive work by many investigators.[23] A bacterial origin has been reasonably well excluded and a viral etiology also appears unlikely, since the disease cannot be transmitted and viral particles have not been identified by transmission electron microscopy. While serum lysozymes are elevated in patients with Crohn's disease, they are normal in ulcerative colitis.[13] Genetic factors may, indeed, play a role, since it is known that ulcerative colitis is two to four times more common in Jewish versus non-Jewish Caucasians and is probably about 50 per cent less frequent in the nonwhite population.[3, 19] Gilat and his colleagues,[14] in a recent study of Jews in Tel Aviv, reported a remarkably decreased incidence of ulcerative colitis (3.8 per 100,000 population), compared to

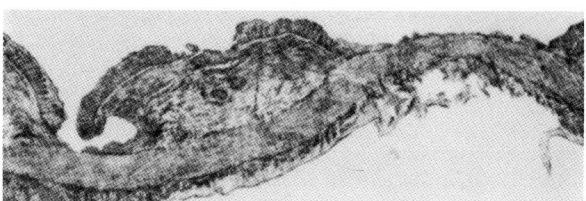

Figure 1. This classic photomicrograph of ulcerative colitis taken during the Civil War reveals the mucosal ulceration so characteristic of the disease. (From Chrohn, B. B.: Letters to the Editor. Gastroenterology, *42*:366, 1962. © 1962 The Williams & Wilkins Co., Baltimore.)

the incidences reported from Copenhagen (7.3 per 100,000), Oxford, England (7.3 per 100,000), and Rochester, Minnesota (7.2 per 100,000). In addition, the female-to-male ratio was only 0.8 as compared to 1.3 for the other studies. Obviously, geographic as well as racial differences influence the occurrence of the disease.

Psychologic factors have long been thought to play a critical role in exacerbations of the disease.[12] It is now clear, however, that patients with ulcerative colitis have no unusual predisposing factors in the onset of their disease, when compared to matched controls.[25] Furthermore, colectomy is usually followed by a marked improvement in pre-existing morbid psychologic states such as depression or social estrangement.

There has been considerable speculation that ulcerative colitis is an autoimmune disease.[21] For example, many patients with the disease have circulating antibodies to normal colon epithelium which crossreact with specific enterobacterial lipopolysaccharide antigens.[26] This raises the possibility that the bacterial wall constituents of common enteric bacteria such as *Escherichia coli* may play an etiologic role. The cell-mediated immune system (delayed hypersensitivity) may also be involved, since lymphocytes from patients with inflammatory bowel disease are cytotoxic to normal colonic epithelial cells.[35] Furthermore, lymphocytes may be rendered cytotoxic to colon epithelium by incubation with serum from patients with colitis. Patients with colitis have also been found to have alteration of their T and B cell lymphocyte populations. These interesting aberrations have been reviewed by a special group with emphasis on the fact that these changes may not necessarily contribute to the pathogenesis of the disease, but may, indeed, be a consequence of its activity.[8] In fact, Brandtzaeg and his colleagues[6] have demonstrated quite clearly that, rather than there being a defect in immunoglobulin activity at the tissue level in the remaining glands of patients with ulcerative colitis, IgA transport is normal, while IgG immunocyte response is five times that of control patients. It is, therefore, possible that IgG antibodies play a role in the chronicity of the disease but may not be involved in its onset.

A decided drawback to accumulation of knowledge regarding the etiology of ulcerative colitis is the lack of an appropriate animal model. The ingestion of amylopectin, a substance found in high concentrations in seaweed, a potent antipepsin agent, leads in several species to pathologic changes in the colon similar to those observed in ulcerative colitis in man.[9] Gibbons also develop a pathologic entity analogous to human ulcerative colitis.[32] Possibly further detailed study of this model may yield important clues toward an understanding of the etiology of this curious, almost mysterious, disease entity.

PATHOLOGY

Ulcerative colitis is generally a disease confined to the mucosal and submucosal layers of the colonic wall. This is in contradistinction to the intramural inflam-

matory changes found in Crohn's disease of the colon, where all layers may be involved in a granulomatous inflammatory process. The pathologic changes observed in ulcerative colitis, however, are nonspecific and can be seen in shigellosis, amebiasis, and gonorrheal colitis.

The typical lesion in its earliest stage consists of infiltration of round cells and polymorphonuclear leukocytes into the crypts of Lieberkühn at the base of the mucosa, forming crypt abscesses. Light microscopy reveals poor staining and vacuolization of overlying epithelial cells. There is swelling of mitochondria, widening of intercellular spaces, and broadening of the endoplasmic reticulum observed by transmission electron microscopy.

As the lesions progress, there is a coalescence of crypt abscesses and desquamation of overlying cells to form an ulcer. This is associated with undermining of adjacent relatively normal mucosa, which becomes edematous and assumes a polypoid configuration as it becomes isolated between adjacent ulcers. Collagen and a luxurious growth of granulation tissue occupy the areas of ulceration which extend down to, but rarely through, the muscularis. The histologic features of a typical ulcer and pseudopolyp are shown in Figure 2. In fulminating ulcerative colitis and toxic megacolon, such lesions may penetrate through the full thickness of the bowel wall and lead to perforation into the peritoneal cavity. Fortunately, these forms of the disease are infrequent (15 per cent and 3 per cent, respectively).

The pathologic changes described above, therefore, offer a very clear explanation of the clinical manifestations of the disease. It is little wonder that a colon, as shown in Figure 3, allows almost constant passage of twenty or more bloody bowel movements per day. The denuded, remarkably distorted mucosal lining provides little opportunity for absorption of sodium or water. Each bowel action milks large volumes of blood from the exposed hullocks of granulation tissue. Loss of haustral markings, an early roentgenographic finding in the disease, is thought to be due to paralysis of the muscularis mucosa. The foreshortening of the colon and its rigid stovepipe appearance on barium roentgenogram are consequences of repeated injury and the scar which forms with repair (Fig. 4).

There is little knowledge as to why some patients have involvement of the rectum only, while others may develop changes throughout the colon. Furthermore, there is little understanding of what determines the severity and time course of the disease. Possibly these factors relate to the extent of immunologic disturbance engendered by the initial attack. Smith and MacPhee[30] suggest such a possibility, from their observation that patients with extensive ulcerative colitis have significant increases in serum immunoproteins, while patients with ulcerative proctitis retain normal levels.

CLINICAL MANIFESTATIONS

The initial presentation of ulcerative colitis may take many forms. While bloody diarrhea is the most

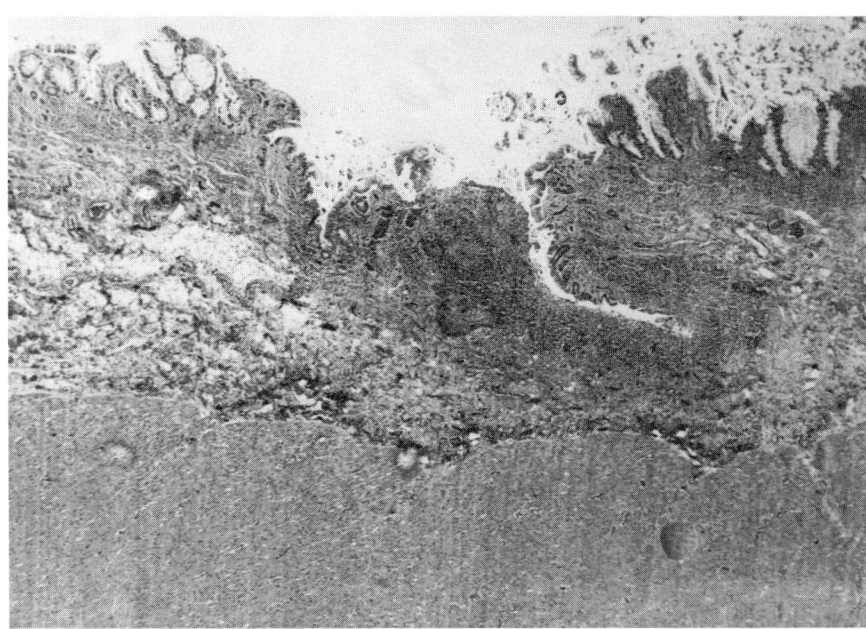

Figure 2. This low-power photomicrograph reveals the details of a chronic mucosal ulceration of the colon in ulcerative colitis. Note the round cell infiltration and granulation tissue at its base. The mucosa at its margins is edematous and hypertrophic, providing a pseudopolypoid appearance. The poor staining of the mucosal cells is a characteristic finding. (From Goligher, J. C., de Dombal, F. T., Watts, J. McK., and Watkinson, G.: Ulcerative Colitis. Baltimore, Williams and Wilkins Co., 1968.)

common early symptom, occasionally extracolonic manifestations such as arthritis, iritis, hepatic dysfunction, and skin lesions may be paramount. The most common clinical manifestations of the disease are enumerated in Table 1.[27] You will note, and will probably be surprised to find, that fever is a relatively uncommon sign. This is consistent with the fact that the disease presents as a chronic, relatively low-grade illness in most patients. Furthermore, it is a disease of exacerbations and remissions. Patients defer medical attention and at the time of diagnosis may already have far advanced pathologic changes within their colon. In a small number of cases, the disease has an acute and catastrophic fulminating course (15 per cent). Such patients present with frequent bloody bowel movements (up to 30 per day), high fever, and abdominal pain. The disease, therefore, offers a wide spectrum of clinical manifestations from a mild diarrheal illness to an overwhelming, life-threatening event of short duration which demands immediate medical attention.

Physical findings are directly related to the duration and presentation of the disease. Weight loss and pallor are usually present, and in the active phase of the disease, the abdomen in the region of the colon is usually tender to palpation. There may be signs of an acute abdomen (see Chapter 30), accompanied by fever and decreased bowel sounds. This is especially true during acute attacks or in the fulminating form of the disease. Abdominal distention is unusual, except in patients who have toxic megacolon, and in this instance the patient is usually febrile and reveals the signs of an acute abdomen. The perianal area may be excoriated from the numerous wipings associated with

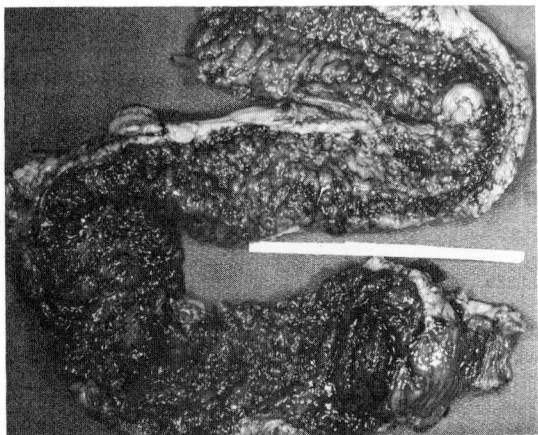

Figure 3. As shown in this photograph, the mucosal lining of the colon in ulcerative colitis is remarkably disturbed. Islands of edematous mucosa are isolated by ulcerations which are contiguous throughout the entire colon in this case. Note that the process stops abruptly at the ileocecal valve.

TABLE 1.   Principal Symptoms of Ulcerative Colitis (525 Cases)*

Diarrhea	79%
Abdominal pain	71%
Rectal bleeding	55%
Weight Loss	18%
Tenesmus	16%
Vomiting	14%
Fever	11%
Constipation	5%
Arthralgia	2%

*From Peete, W. P. J., and Sabiston, D. C., Jr.: Ulcerative colitis. *In* Sabiston, D. C., Jr. (Ed.): Davis-Christopher Textbook of Surgery, 10th ed. Philadelphia, W. B. Saunders Company, 1972.

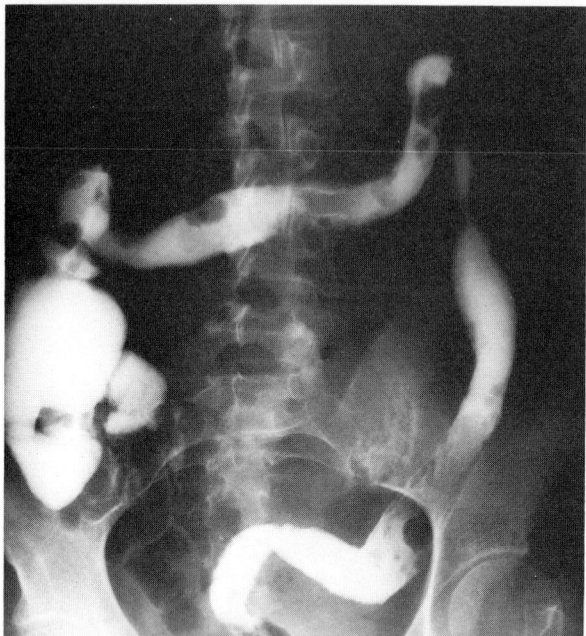

Figure 4. The contracted, "stove pipe" appearance of this colon, as viewed by barium roentgenogram, is typical of advanced ulcerative colitis in its chronic phase. The large lucent areas in the barium column probably represent fecal matter, while the smaller, more subtle shadows along the left colon are most likely pseudopolyps.

the disease called toxic megacolon, in which there may be free air within the peritoneal cavity from perforation of the colon. A more common sign is a remarkable dilatation of the transverse colon as shown in Figure 5. Several fairly large pseudopolyps within this remarkably dilated organ can be identified. Barium enema can be performed safely in most cases, and it is extremely helpful in identifying the extent and severity of the disease. Barium roentgenographic signs include loss of haustral markings and irregularities of the colon wall, which represent small ulcerations. These are well demonstrated in Figure 6, which contrasts the appearance of the left side of the splenic flexure with that of the right. As the disease progresses, pseudopolyps become a prominent roentgenographic sign (Fig. 7). In advanced disease, the colon assumes the appearance of a rigid contracted tube, as seen in Figure 4. While useful information can be obtained from the barium roentgenogram, it should be used with discretion.

Preparation of the colon should be omitted, since it may initiate an exacerbation of the disease. When diarrhea is not present, it is best to prepare the patient by placing him on a liquid diet three days prior to examination. While perforation is rare, it can occur, especially in the presence of toxic megacolon and, on occasion, it may initiate the latter. Therefore, when the clinical signs of toxic megacolon are present, barium roentgenogram should be omitted. With these admonitions in mind, a barium view of the colon should be obtained in all patients with ulcerative

bowel movements. There may be evidence of perianal inflammation in the form of a fissure or fistula in ano, although the latter is more common in patients with Crohn's disease. Rectal examination is almost always painful and should be done gently in the presence of perianal inflammation. Examination of the integument, tongue, joints, and eyes is important, since the presence of pathology in these areas may help to direct your attention to ulcerative colitis as a likely cause of the diarrheal illness.

Proctosigmoidoscopy is a most helpful and specific diagnostic aid, since ulcerative colitis involves the distal colon in 90 to 95 per cent of the cases. In fact the mucosa of the rectum, as well as the sigmoid, is usually erythematous, granular, and bleeds easily when touched by the endoscope or rubbed with a cotton swab. In advanced disease, ulcers may be present, surrounded by heaped up areas of granulation tissue and edematous mucosa, which may assume a polypoid appearance (pseudopolyps). In chronic advanced disease, the lumen of the rectosigmoid may be remarkably contracted. Multiple rectal biopsies are helpful in differentiating ulcerative colitis from Crohn's disease of the colon but may yield granulomata even when the latter are present. The role of colonoscopic examination has not yet been fully assessed. It is of value in cases in which the rectosigmoid does not reveal the nature of the disease and of extreme importance in long-standing disease in which cancer may be suspect. In addition, it allows identification of skip areas characteristic of Crohn's disease.

The plain abdominal film may reveal a variant of

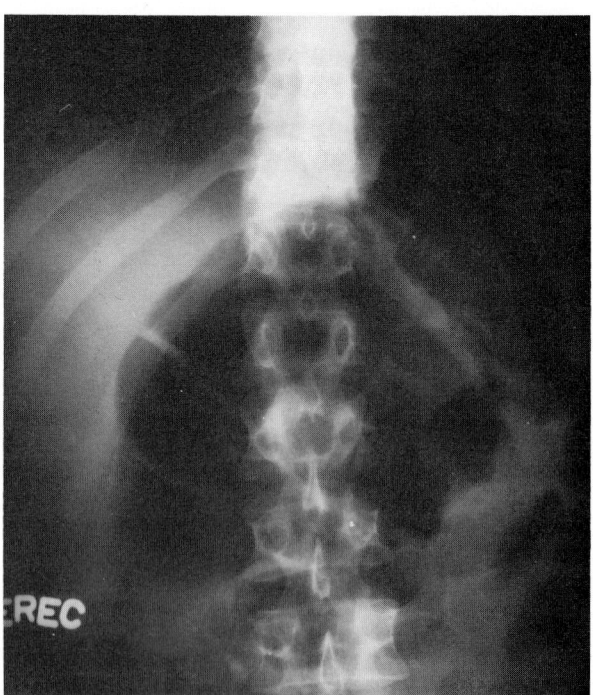

Figure 5. Toxic megacolon is characterized by massive distention of the right colon by air as shown in this upright roentgenogram of the abdomen. Distention of the cecum in excess of 12 to 14 cm. is felt to represent a sign of impending perforation. The irregularities in the air column represent pseudopolyps within the lumen of the colon.

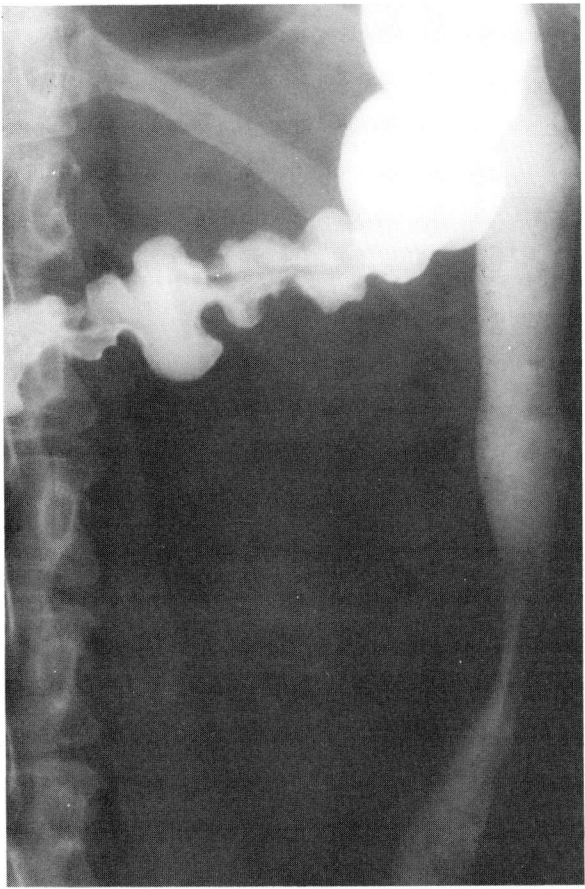

Figure 6. This barium roentgenogram of the splenic flexure of the colon reveals loss of haustral markings in the descending colon in contrast to their presence in the transverse. The irregular appearance of the barium column in the descending colon is indicative of the inflammation and ulceration of its mucosal lining.

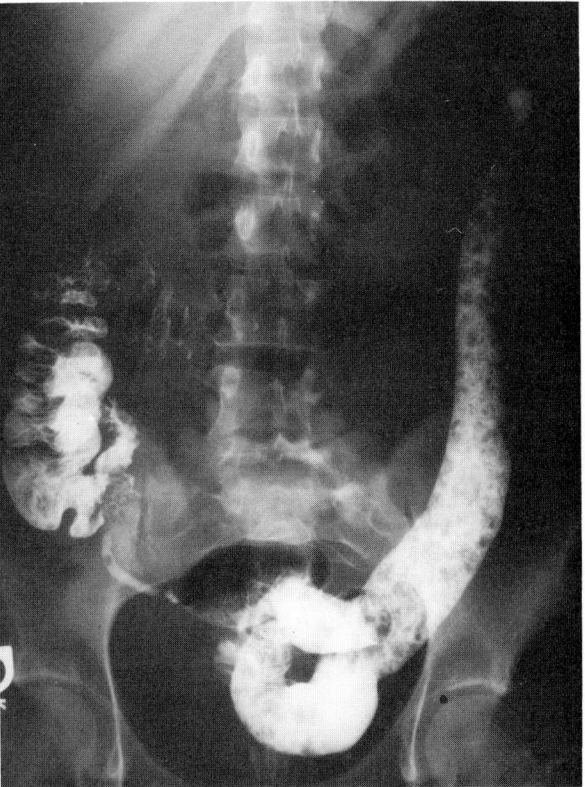

Figure 7. Mucosal pseudopolyp formation is well demonstrated in the descending colon in this barium roentgenogram. The right colon appears relatively spared.

colitis at a convenient time in the disease, in order to exclude the presence of cancer. How often to repeat the examination in the course of the illness, which is lifelong in many patients, remains an open question. Since the incidence of malignancy is strikingly high, especially after 10 years of the disease, it is appropriate to obtain a yearly barium examination alternating at six-month intervals with colonoscopy. An upper barium gastrointestinal study, to include the small bowel, should be obtained in order to aid in differentiating Crohn's disease of the bowel from ulcerative colitis, since only the former involves the small intestine.

The above clinical manifestations and simple diagnostic tests usually help to identify the presence of ulcerative colitis. It is necessary, however, to obtain stool smears and cultures to rule out amebic colitis. Meyer and Sleisenger[23] have provided a useful schema for distinguishing ulcerative colitis from granulomatous colitis (Table 2). Note, however, the low frequency of discriminating clinical characteristics except for associated small bowel disease or skip areas within the colon when the etiology is Crohn's disease.

TABLE 2. Clinical Features Distinguishing Ulcerative Colitis from Granulomatous Colitis*

	Incidence	
	Ulcerative Colitis (per cent)	Granulomatous Colitis (per cent)
Pathognomonic for ulcerative colitis:		
Pseudopolyps	15	0
Disease limited to rectosigmoid	10	0
Free colonic perforation	3	<0.2
Pathognomonic for granulomatous colitis:		
Associated small bowel disease	5	80
Skip areas of colitis	0	50
Enteric fistula	<0.5	10
Nondistinguishing:		
Diarrhea	80	70
Hematochezia	90	50
Rectal involvement	95	50
Rectal sparing	5	50
Perianal disease	25	70
Deep ulcers	25	60
Colonic stricture	11	23
Toxic megacolon	3	0.5
Colonic carcinoma†	3.5	1.2

*From Meyer, J. H., and Sleisenger, M. H.: Granulomatous disease of the colon. *In* Sleisenger, M. H., and Fordtran, J. S. (Eds.): Gastrointestinal Disease. Philadelphia, W. B. Saunders Company, 1973.

†Observed incidence in all cases of ulcerative colitis (segmental or universal) and all cases of granulomatous disease of the colon (with or without associated regional enteritis of the small bowel).

The issue of the high incidence of cancer of the colon in ulcerative colitis bears emphasis. For example, two of five patients with total colonic involvement may die of cancer if they survive their disease and the colon is left in place.[22] Three per cent of children with ulcerative colitis will develop cancer of the colon at 10 years; 20 per cent will develop cancer during each ensuing decade.[10] These startling figures demand close medical management of such patients, and surgical intervention on this basis alone when chronicity is well established.

MEDICAL MANAGEMENT

The outcome from an acute attack of ulcerative colitis relates to the severity of the disease as manifested by systemic symptoms. Duration of the disease or extent of involvement of the colon does not appear to be a determinant of survival, if ulcerative proctitis is excluded from consideration. Medical therapy, therefore, is based upon familiar signs of illness. Those who present with advanced signs of an acute illness require hospitalization and supportive as well as specific therapy for associated metabolic and hematologic derangements. Because of massive fluid and electrolyte loss per rectum, such patients usually present with a metabolic acidosis, contracted extravascular volume, and prerenal azotemia. Usually the potassium is low because of excessive loss in stool and urine. Intravenous administration of balanced salt solutions in amounts sufficient to replace these losses is an initial step in management. It must also be kept in mind that patients with long-standing disease may have lost considerable protein and probably are in a depleted nutritional state. Steroids remain the primary basis of therapy for an acute attack. The controversy of intravenous steroids versus intravenous ACTH has now been resolved by a randomized trial that reveals a similar response to equipotent doses of either.[18] The usual doses recommended are in the range of 300 milligrams of hydrocortisone or 40 units of ACTH per day. Occasionally massive doses of steroids (over a gram per day) are required. The usual response is rapid, and within a few days acute signs of inflammation subside. Proctoscopic examination is a useful method to follow response to therapy. There is still controversy as to whether maintenance steroid therapy will reduce recurrence of the disease. The consensus favors the view that they do not help and should not be used in view of their side effects when given over a long time span.

Milder forms of the disease may be treated with rectal steroids (100 milligrams of hydrocortisone per rectum at bedtime) when the disease is localized to the left colon and rectum. Salicylazosulfapyridine (Azulfidine) has also had widespread usage in the chronic phases of the disease. Its mode of action is unknown, but it appears to be associated with fewer exacerbations as assessed by controlled randomized trials.[11] A third approach has been through immunosuppression by Azathioprine. Rosenberg and his colleagues[28] have recently concluded from a well-controlled study that Azathioprine allows reduction of the use of steroids in chronic cases but does not, in itself, control exacerbations of the disease.

The major therapeutic problem between acute attacks is control of diarrhea and maintenance of nutrition. Diet therapy is now out of vogue and patients are encouraged to eat a substantial diet of their choice. Milk products should be avoided only if they cause problems such as increasing diarrhea or cramps, as they may in about half of the patients with the disease. The reason for this is not clear but relates to something specific in cow's milk rather than to the lactase deficiency that exists in many patients with ulcerative colitis. As regards bowel control, opiates such as codeine or paregoric should be avoided. They are not very effective in colonic diarrhea and can precipitate an attack of toxic megacolon. Nocturnal diarrhea can be controlled by anticholinergics or Lomotil. Stool bulk formers such as Metamucil are also helpful in this regard. Finally, the importance of rest and peace of mind cannot be overemphasized. Patients are well advised to remain home from work when exacerbations occur.

SURGICAL MANAGEMENT

Since total removal of the colon and rectum (coloproctectomy) cures ulcerative colitis, one might reasonably ask why all patients with established chronicity are not so treated. It appears that the incidence of surgical intervention relates to the availability of highly skilled and knowledgeable gastrointestinal surgeons and enlightened physicians. For example, the clinic at Leeds offers surgical care to approximately half of their patient population,[16] while in other series the operative rate is below 10 per cent.[15] There are several well-identified complications which require urgent operation for survival. These include (1) massive, unrelenting hemorrhage; (2) toxic megacolon with impending or frank perforation; (3) fulminating acute ulcerative colitis without response to steroid therapy; (4) obstruction from stricture formation; and (5) suspicion or demonstration of colonic cancer. Surgical therapy is also recommended in children who fail to mature at an acceptable rate. The largest number of colectomies for ulcerative colitis are performed for less dramatic indications, as the disease enters an intractable chronic phase and becomes both a physical and social burden to patients so afflicted.

The historic development of surgical procedures for ulcerative colitis has been reviewed above, and at present single-stage total coloproctectomy is the procedure of choice when complications of the disease are treated electively. This procedure is performed through either a midline or a left paramedian incision (Fig. 8). The rectum may be excised from the abdomen by division at the level of the anal verge or by circumferential incision from the perineum. When cancer is not suspected, excision is performed rapidly with division of the mesentery close to the bowel wall. This principle is especially important in the pelvic colon and rectum, where injury to the sacral parasympathetics may lead to bladder and sexual dysfunction. Management of the perianal wound may be a problem,

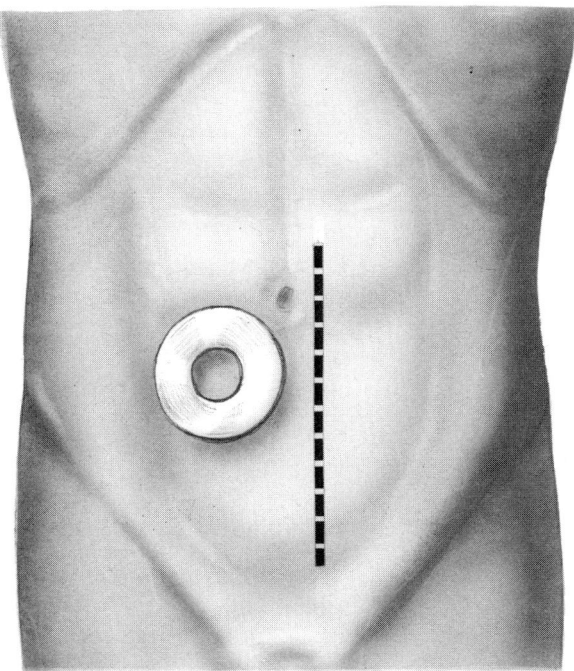

Figure 8. The abdominal portion of a coloproctectomy is best performed through a left paramedian incision, as shown in this drawing. This incision allows for the convenient placement of an ileostomy appliance. (From Turnbull, R. B., Jr., Weakley, F. L., and Farmer, R. G.: Ileitis after colectomy and ileostomy for nonspecific ulcerative colitis: Report of 35 cases. Dis. Colon Rectum, 7:427–435, 1964.)

since chronic infection and poor healing may provide a lingering sinus tract between the buttocks. The author's preference is to provide soft rubber drains to this area for three to five days following surgery. An active sump drain is included at operation if the residual space is large. Gauze packing of the perineum should be avoided, since this technique appears to encourage the development of chronic inflammation in this space. Irwin and Goligher[17] have provided strong evidence for primary closure with suprapubic drainage, a technique that may help to resolve this problem.

A critical part of the operation as far as the long term is concerned is construction of the ileostomy. The importance of providing the patient with a well-functioning, trouble-free ileostomy cannot be overemphasized. Most surgeons have accepted the technique of Brooke,[7] so well illustrated in Turnbull and Weakley's *Atlas of Intestinal Stomas*[34] and shown in Figure 9. The principles include passing the end of the ileum through an opening in the mid aspect of the right rectus muscle at a point below the umbilicus that will allow convenient placement of the forepiece of an ileostomy bag. Placement too low or too laterally may offer serious problems to ileostomy care and function. The length of the stoma is important, and approximately four inches should be withdrawn above the skin so that when the tip is folded back upon itself, two inches protrude from the surface. The folding back

(called "maturing") serves to prevent the development of an inflammatory response in the serosa and provides more substance to the protruding ileal nipple which, in turn, allows ejection of ileal contents into the ileostomy appliance without soiling of the skin. Unfortunately, ileal contents are quite corrosive. It is, indeed, fortunate that simple and easily applied receptacles are now available, such as shown in Figure 10. Note the karaya gum ring, which provides a firm seal to the ileostomy stoma. The application of such an appliance to an ileostomy at the completion of surgery, helps to avoid skin problems in the early postoperative period and assures the patient of a relatively easy adjustment to a new way of life. In the final analysis, it is the need for an external stoma that limits the more general use of colectomy for patients with established chronic ulcerative colitis. Kock[20] of Sweden has pioneered an attempt to overcome this problem by providing reservoir function for the ileostomy. This technique has recently been evaluated and refined by Beahrs,[5] who concludes that a reservoir provides an improved quality of life for such patients. It is likely, therefore, that this approach will gain wider use in the ensuing decade.

When emergent or urgent surgery is required for the more devastating complications of ulcerative colitis, less than total coloproctectomy may be a wise decision.[29] For example, subtotal colectomy with ileostomy with exteriorization of the distal end of the rectosigmoid onto the anterior abdominal wall provides a means for avoiding rectal excision in a sick patient. This procedure is known to be effective when acute fulminating disease or toxic megacolon is the indication for surgery. When operating for massive hemorrhage, total coloproctectomy should be carried out, since the incidence of rebleeding from the rectal stump is high. While ileostomy alone for acute complications has been abandoned, it is currently used by Turnbull in combination with skin level transverse and sigmoid colostomies for toxic megacolon, with good success.[33] This is a relatively simple procedure that spares such desperately ill patients a major operative intervention until a later date when the acute illness has subsided. Attempts to preserve the rectal segment have not been successful in the hands of most surgeons, since the incidence of persistence or recurrence of the disease when the fecal stream is returned to such segments is high, as is the risk for cancer.[2] Aylett,[4] however, has had a unique experience with 300 patients in England, where he has performed an ileoproctostomy with a proximal loop ileostomy. Following re-establishment of the fecal stream by ileostomy closure, only 15 patients required reileostomy and only 10 to 15 per cent revealed evidence of a leak at their anastomosis. Since few other surgeons have been able to achieve this level of success, it is likely that total excision of the involved gut will remain the procedure of choice for the immediate future.

The remaining question, therefore, relates to the immediate and late burden of surgical therapy beyond the inconvenience of abdominal stoma. Mortality for elective surgery is in the range of 3 per cent and for emergent surgery 10 to 15 per cent. These are remarkable statistics when one considers the debili-

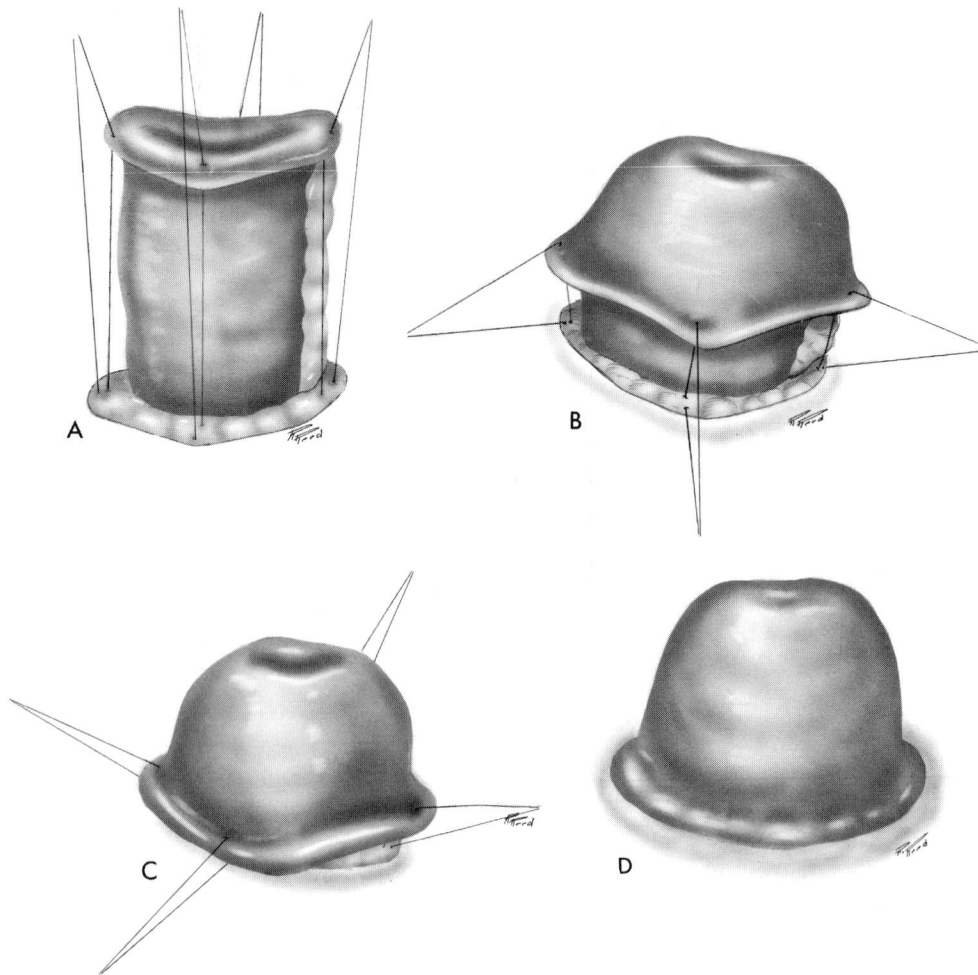

Figure 9. In construction of an ileostomy, the terminal ileum is brought out through a circular opening in the anterior abdominal wall. A convenient point is selected below the umbilicus in the mid aspect of the rectus abdominus muscle. The cut edge of the ileum is secured to the skin, so that a stoma of approximately two inches protrudes from the surface of the anterior abdominal wall. (From Turnbull, R. B., Jr., Weakley, F. L., and Farmer, R. G.: Ileitis after colectomy and ileostomy for nonspecific ulcerative colitis, a report of 35. Dis. Colon Rectum, 7: 427–435, 1964.)

Figure 10. Light, secure, disposable ileostomy appliances have greatly simplified ileostomy care (A). The placement of a karaya gum ring over the undersurface of the plastic foreplate reduces the chance of seepage and skin irritation. Most patients tape this to their skin, and change it every several days as needed. Note the opening at the lower end for purposes of emptying the bag.

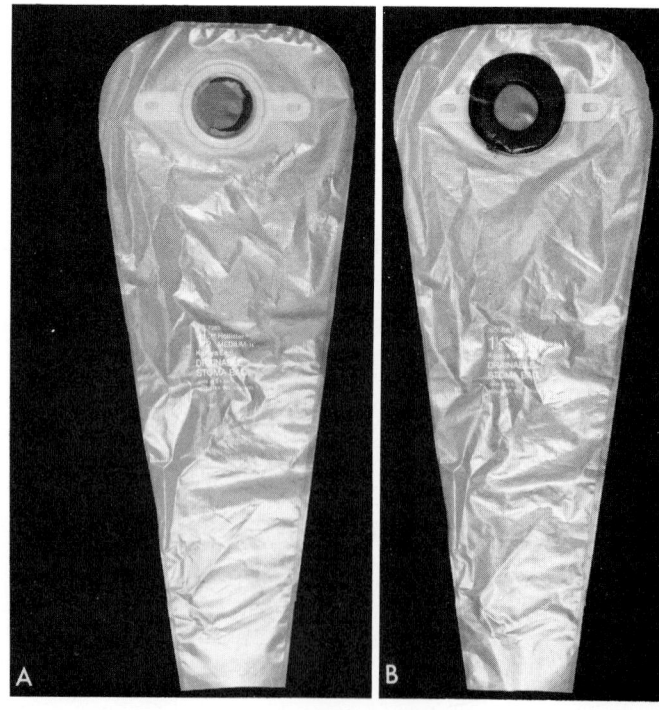

tating nature of the disease and the fact that many patients have had long-term steroid therapy. The relatively low mortality relates to early intervention when medical therapy fails, and an ability to treat the numerous complications which attend such surgery. Watts and his colleagues in Leeds, for example, encountered 40 major complications in 30 patients operated upon as an emergency.[36] The major complication in all reported cases is sepsis, either in the wound or in the abdominal cavity. The detection and management of sepsis in these patients is made difficult by the use of high doses of steroids and the altered resistance of the host as a consequence of protracted disease. There is little evidence that the development of more potent and specific antibiotics has significantly reduced the incidence of this complication, and details of operative management continue to be the most secure way to insure a smooth postoperative course. The most common late complication of resectional therapy is intestinal obstruction, which occurs in about 10 per cent of cases. While the causes are many, most relate to adhesions formed at the site of colon resection, or herniation through an opening in the closure of the pelvic floor. An additional site is at the recess created by suspension of the ileal segment to the anterior abdominal wall. Other bothersome but nonlethal complications include delay in perineal closure (25 per cent), sexual dysfunction (10 per cent), and renal stones (10 per cent). Ileostomy dysfunction as a consequence of stenosis has been reduced to a range of 2 per cent by the Brooke-Turnbull ileostomy. Additional uncommon complications include prolapse, herniation, and ulceration of the stoma. The latter is usually a sign of the development of Crohn's disease within the ileal stoma. Whether, in fact, the outcome following surgery for Crohn's disease of the colon is as favorable as for ulcerative colitis continues to be a source of controversy.[31]

The association of patients with ileostomies into social groups (ileostomy clubs) has provided an important mechanism for education and adjustment of patients with abdominal stomata. Preparation of a patient for surgical therapy of his ulcerative colitis should include one or more visits with a patient who has mastered the techniques of ileostomy management. Ileostomy clubs offer this service in most urban communities. Some hospitals have enterostomal therapists. These professionals are individuals with ostomies who are highly skilled in dealing with the physical and emotional problems of stoma management. Institutions that perform a large number of colectomies for inflammatory bowel disease find these individuals to be indispensable to their patient care team.

These are extraordinary advances for patients who suffer from this complicated, poorly understood disease. It is conceivable that further refinement in surgical therapy may make an operative approach even more attractive to the ulcerative colitis patient. The cumulative mortality, as revealed by Goligher[16] in his excellent monograph on the subject, would suggest that operative therapy should be applied quite liberally in the chronic or acutely fatal forms of the disease. Fortunately, for most patients, ulcerative colitis will be only episodic and mild in its clinical presentation. Unfortunately, the high incidence of cancer in the presence of persistent disease (especially after 10 years' duration) does not allow even these fortunate patients a life without undue concern.

SELECTED REFERENCES

Beahrs, O. H.: Use of ileal reservoir following proctocolectomy. Surg. Gynecol. Obstet., *141*:363, 1975.
The Kock ileal pouch, as modified by Beahrs, offers an alternative to the patient who may find an external abdominal stoma an impossible compromise. It is possible that further refinement of this technique will allow the application of surgical therapy to an increasing number of patients with ulcerative colitis in an earlier phase of their disease.

Goligher, J. D., De Dombal, F. T., Watts, J. M., and Watkinson, G.: Ulcerative Colitis. Baltimore, Williams and Wilkins Company, 1968.
This remains the single best reference source for students interested in an in-depth study of the surgical implications of ulcerative colitis. Indications for surgery and surgical results are clearly described and carefully documented. Much of what is contained in this monograph has not been superseded by the intervening nine years since its publication.

Lukash, W. M., and Johnson, R. B. (Eds.): The Systemic Manifestations of Inflammatory Bowel Disease. Springfield, Ill., Charles C Thomas, Publisher, 1975.
This monograph describes in detail the various colonic as well as extracolonic manifestations of ulcerative colitis. I recommend it because of the latter, where associated liver, eye, shin, joint, blood, metabolic, and endocrine problems are discussed in detail.

Meyer, J. B., and Sleisenger, M. H.: Granulomatous disease of the colon. In Sleisenger, M. H., and Fordtran, J. D.(Eds.): Gastrointestinal Disease. Philadelphia, W. B. Saunders Company, 1973.
The authors provide a very readable, authoritative text on the various facets of ulcerative colitis that relate to diagnosis, medical management, and the natural history of the disease. Their discussion of new concepts of etiology places the numerous variables in a contemporary perspective. A subsequent chapter on Crohn's disease allows comparison to the clinical and pathologic characteristics of ulcerative colitis.

Turnbull, R. B., Jr., and Weakley, F. L.: Atlas of Intestinal Stomas. St. Louis, The C. V. Mosby Company, 1967.
Turnbull and Weakley provide a step-by-step, foolproof way of constructing an ileostomy. The technical features offered by them cannot be overemphasized and, if adhered to, will minimize ileostomy problems.

REFERENCES

1. Adams, F.: The Genuine Works of Hippocrates. Baltimore, Williams and Wilkins Company, 1939.
2. Adson, M. A., Cooperman, A. M., and Farrow, G. M.: Ileorectostomy for ulcerative disease of the colon. Arch. Surg., *104*:424, 1972.
3. Almy, T. P., and Sherlock, P.: Genetic aspects of ulcerative colitis and regional enteritis. Gastroenterology, *51*:757, 1966.
4. Aylett, S. O.: Three hundred cases of diffuse ulcerative colitis treated by total colectomy and ileo-rectal anastomosis. Br. Med. J., *1*:1001, 1966.
5. Beahrs, O. H.: Use of ileal reservoir following proctocolectomy. Surg. Gynecol. Obstet., *141*:363, 1975.
6. Brandtzaeg, P., Baklien, K., Fausa, O., and Hoel, P. S.: Immunohistochemical characterization of local immunoglobulin formation in ulcerative colitis. Gastroenterology, *66*:1123, 1974.
7. Brooke, B. N.: The management of ileostomy including its complications. Lancet, *2*:102, 1952.
8. Colonic and inflammatory bowel disease. Work Group VII. Gastroenterology, *69*:1140, 1975.
9. Crohn, B. B.: An historic note on ulcerative colitis. Letters to the Editor. Gastroenterology, *42*:366, 1962.
10. Devroede, G. J., Taylor, W. F., Sauer, W. G., et al.: Cancer risk and life expectance of children with ulcerative colitis. N. Engl. J. Med., *285*:17, 1971.
11. Dick, A. P., Grayson, M. J., Carpenter, R. G., and Petrie, A.: Controlled trial of sulphasalazine in the treatment of ulcerative colitis. Gut, *5*:437, 1964.
12. Engle, G. L.: Studies of ulcerative colitis III: The nature of the physiological process. Am. J. Med., *19*:231, 1955.

13. Falchuk, K. R., Perrotto, J. L., and Isselbacher, K. J.: Serum lysozyme in Crohn's disease and ulcerative colitis. N. Engl. J. Med., *292*:395, 1975.

14. Gilat, T., Ribak, J., Benaroya, Y., Zemishlany, Z., and Weissman, I.: Ulcerative colitis in the Jewish population of Tel-Aviv Yafo. Gastroenterology, *66*:335, 1974.

15. Gilat, T., Lilos, P., Zemishlany, Z., et al.: Ulcerative colitis in the Jewish population of Tel-Aviv Yafo III. Gastroenterology, *70*:14, 1976.

16. Goligher, J. C., De Dombal, F. T., Watts, J. M., and Watkinson, G.: Ulcerative Colitis. Baltimore, Williams and Wilkins Company, 1968.

17. Irvin, T. T., and Goligher, J. C.: A controlled trial of three different methods of perineal wound management following excision of the rectum. Br. J. Surg., *62*:287, 1975.

18. Kaplan, H. P., Portnoy, B., Binder, H. J., et al.: A controlled evaluation of intravenous adrenocorticotropic hormone and hydrocortisone in the treatment of acute colitis. Gastroenterology, *69*:91, 1975.

19. Kirsner, J. B.: Genetic aspects of inflammatory bowel disease. Clin. Gastroenterol., *2*:557, 1973.

20. Kock, N. G.: Intra-abdominal "reservoir" in patients with permanent ileostomy. Arch. Surg., *99*:223, 1969.

21. Kraft, S. C., and Kirsner, J. B.: Present status of immunological mechanisms in ulcerative colitis. Gastroenterology, *51*:788, 1966.

22. MacDougall, I. P. M.: The cancer risk in ulcerative colitis. Lancet, *2*:655, 1964.

23. Meyer, J. H., and Sleisenger, M. H.: Granulomatous disease of the colon. *In* Sleisenger, M. H., and Fordtran, J. S. (Eds.): Gastrointestinal Disease. Philadelphia, W. B. Saunders Company, 1973.

24. Miller, C. G., Gardiner, C. McG., and Ripstein, C. B.: Primary resection of the colon in ulcerative colitis. J. Can. Med. Assoc., *60*:584, 1949.

25. Monk, M., Mendeloff, A. I., Siegel, C. I., and Lilienfeld, A.: An epidemiological study of ulcerative colitis and regional enteritis among adults in Baltimore—III. J. Chron. Dis., *22*:565, 1970.

26. Montiero, E., Fossey, J., Shiner, M., Drasar, B., and Allison, A.: Antibacterial antibodies in rectal and colonic mucosa in ulcerative colitis. Lancet, *1*:249, 1971.

27. Peete, W. P. J., and Sabiston, D. C., Jr.: Ulcerative colitis. *In* Sabiston, D. C., Jr. (Ed.): Davis-Christopher Textbook of Surgery, 10th ed. Philadelphia, W. B. Saunders Company, 1972.

28. Rosenberg, J. L., Wall, A. J., et al.: A controlled trial of Azathioprine in the management of chronic ulcerative colitis. Gastroenterology, *69*:96, 1975.

29. Scott, H. W., Jr., Sawyers, J. L., et al.: Surgical management of toxic dilatation of the colon in ulcerative colitis. Ann. Surg., *179*:647, 1974.

30. Smith, A. H., and MacPhee, I. W.: A clinico-immunological study of ulcerative colitis and ulcerative proctitis. Gut, *12*:20, 1971.

31. Steinberg, D. M., Allan, R. D., Brooke, B. N., et al.: Sequelae of colectomy and ileostomy: Comparison between Crohn's colitis and ulcerative colitis. Gastroenterology, *68*:33, 1975.

32. Stout, C., and Synder, R. L.: Ulcerative colitis-like lesion in Siamang Gibbons. Gastroenterology, *57*:256, 1969.

33. Turnbull, R. B., Jr., Hawk, W. A., and Weakley, F. L.: Surgical treatment of toxic megacolon: Ileostomy and colostomy to prepare patient for colectomy. Am. J. Surg., *122*:325, 1971.

34. Turnbull, R. B., Jr., and Weakley, F. L.: Atlas of Intestinal Stomas. St. Louis, The C. V. Mosby Company, 1967.

35. Watson, D. W., Quigley, A., and Bolt, R. J.: Effect of lymphocytes from patients with ulcerative colitis on human adult colon epithelial cells. Gastroenterology, *51*:985, 1966.

36. Watts, J. M., De Dombal, F. T., and Goligher, J. C.: The early results of surgery for ulcerative colitis. Br. J. Surg., *53*:1005, 1966.

IX

POLYPS OF THE COLON AND RECTUM

Jack W. Cole, M.D.

DEFINITION

Polyp is a nonspecific term indicating a tumor within the lumen of the colon or rectum. Polyps may be neoplastic, arising from various parent cell types, the result of an inflammatory process, or hamartomas. They may occur singly or be multiple. They may be pedunculated or sessile (Table 1).

ADENOMAS

Incidence

The most common neoplastic polyp is the adenoma. The true incidence of adenomatous polyps of the colon and rectum has been difficult to determine in the general population, and marked differences in the incidence may be found in various reports. These discrep-

ancies are explained in part by the fact that the data have been derived from different patient populations using different investigative techniques, but perhaps the greatest error has been the inclusion in the study of polypoid lesions designated as adenomas without histologic confirmation.

Adenomas occur most commonly in the sigmoid colon and rectum but may be found throughout the entire large bowel. They are multiple in approximately 30 per cent of patients and have an equal incidence in males and females. Adenomas are uncommon before the age of 20 and show a progressive increase in incidence until the eighth decade of life, when they may be found in 50 per cent of the population. Autopsy studies might be expected to provide the most accurate estimate of the incidence; however, review of the literature discloses variations from 7 per cent to 51 per cent.

TABLE 1. Polypoid Lesions of Colon and Rectum*

	Solitary	Multiple
Neoplastic	Epithelial origin	
	Adenomas	
	Villous adenomas	
	Papillary adenomas	Familial polyposis
	Others	Gardner's syndrome
	Leiomyoma	
	Lipoma	
	Neurofibroma	
Inflammatory	Pseudopolyposis	
	(ulcerative colitis,	
	Crohn's disease)	
	Juvenile polyp	Juvenile polyposis
	Benign lymphoid	Benign lymphoid
		polyposis
Hamartomas	Peutz-Jegher polyp	Peutz-Jegher syndrome
	Juvenile polyp	Juvenile polyposis
	Hemangioma	Multiple hemangiomas
Unclassified	Cystic pneumatosis	
	intestinalis	Hyperplastic polyposis
	Hyperplastic polyp	
	(metaplastic)	

*Modified from Morson, B. C., and Bussey, H. J. R.: Curr. Probl. Surg., Feb. 1970.

Etiology

Attempts to establish an etiology for adenomatous polyps or carcinoma of the large bowel have been unsuccessful. Nevertheless, there is increasing evidence to suggest that some factor or combination of factors in the environment plays an important role in the induction of neoplastic growth. Recent investigations, stemming from recognized demographic differences in the incidence of colon tumors, have implicated various dietary constituents.[20] Other studies in animals and man suggest that bacteria interacting with certain bile acids may be significant etiological factors.[14]

Morphogenesis

Precisely how adenomatous polyps are formed is not known at present. The epithelium of the colon and rectum is one of the most prolific cell populations in the body. In vivo studies of turnover rates in human colonic epithelium by means of radioactive labeling of cells have established that the epithelium is renewed every 3 to 4 days.[4] Under normal conditions the colonic epithelium is in steady-state equilibrium wherein new cells are being formed at the base of the crypts at a rate equivalent to that of loss of cells from the surface of the epithelium into the lumen of the bowel. It is not known whether, in the course of polyp formation, there is an increase in cell production or a reduction in the rate of cell loss of some combination of these two mechanisms.

Some studies suggest that the basic cellular abnormality begins in the surface cells of the colorectal mucosa. Ordinarily these cells are not engaged in cell division. However, in a careful search of routine microscopic sections of apparently normal mucosa from adenoma-bearing epithelium, one can find foci of cells near the surface epithelium showing early neoplastic alterations such as reduction in mucus formation, hyperchromatic nuclei, decreased nucleocytoplasmic ratio, and increased numbers of cells. By means of the subcutaneous administration of chemical carcinogens, 3,2-dimethyl-4-aminobiphenyl and 3-2 dimethylhydrazine, in experimental animals, investigators have been able to produce all stages of tumor formation in the rat colon from focal hyperplasia to adenocarcinoma. The earliest changes observed were confined in the main to the more superficial portions of the epithelium.[22] Additional evidence for the thesis that neoplastic growth begins in the surface cells can be found in the in vitro studies of Deschner and Lipkin,[8] who found that human colonic epithelium with a known propensity for adenoma formation incorporated tritiated thymidine, a deoxyribonucleic acid precursor, when grown in culture, and that when this occurred it was characteristic of more superficial cells. Finally, in chemically induced colonic tumors in rats, there is evidence that the tumor-inducing agent acts directly on the superficial cells, inasmuch as diversion of the fecal stream prevents tumor formation in the bypassed segment of bowel.[3] Most investigators are of the opinion that the morphologic variations observed clinically and histologically in adenomatous tumors are simply different expressions of the same fundamental process[1] and related in part to the amount of surface area involved in the abnormal growth.

Adenomas may be pedunuclated or sessile (Figs. 1 and 2) and microscopically may be predominantly glandular, villous, or papillary. The latter term is frequently considered to be synonymous with villous; however, several authors use the term to describe an adenomatous polyp whose histologic appearance rests somewhere between that of the classic adenoma and that of the villous adenoma by having characteristics of both, with somewhat blunter villous projections of the surface. Although these various growth patterns have somewhat different implications with respect to their malignant potential and hence their clinical management, there is considerable evidence to suggest that they have a common etiologic basis. First, it is not uncommon for different histologic pat-

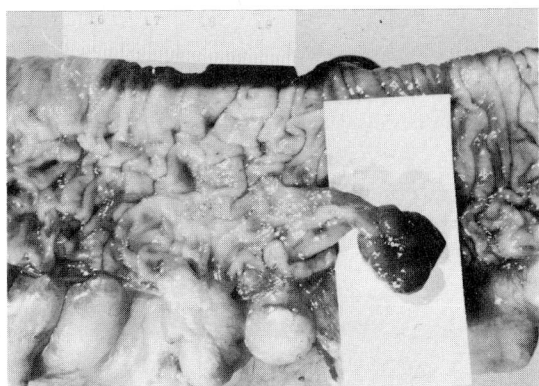

Figure 1. A benign pedunculated adenoma. (From Welch, C. E., and Hedberg, S. E.: Polypoid Lesions of the Gastrointestinal Tract, Philadelphia, W. B. Saunders Company, 1975.

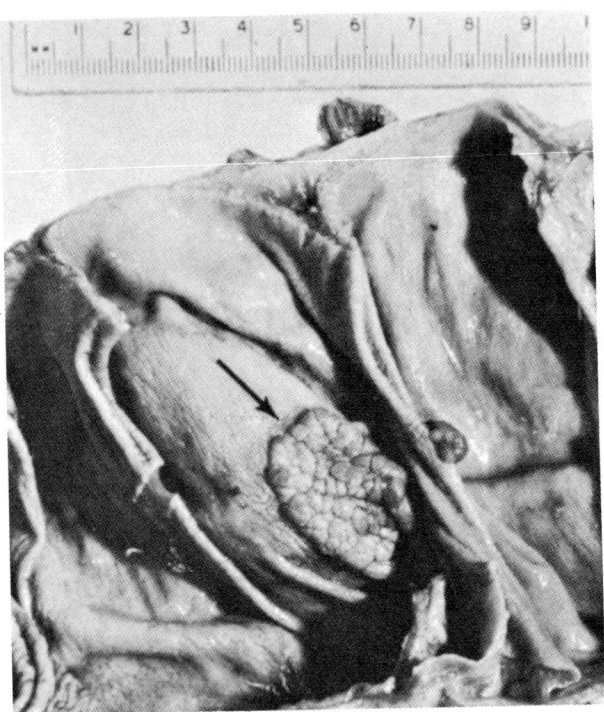

Figure 2. A sessile adenomatous polyp. (From Predisposing causes of intestinal cancer, by Morson, B. C., and Bussey, H. J. R., in Current Problems in Surgery, edited by Ravitch, M. M., et al. Copyright © 1970, Year Book Medical Publishers. Used by permission.)

terns to be found within a single tumor. Second, the different growth variations may be present simultaneously within the same bowel. Third, in experimental animals all variations may be produced in the same bowel by the administration of a single tumorigenic agent.

Malignant Potential of Adenomas

The malignant potential of adenomas remains controversial and as yet the issue is unsettled. There is a growing body of evidence, albeit circumstantial, that benign adenomatous tumors may with the passage of time and under certain, as yet unknown, conditions undergo malignant transformation. The evidence supporting this concept may be summarized as follows: (1) It is not uncommon to identify foci of malignant cells in otherwise benign adenomatous polyps by careful microscopic examination of these lesions. Such terms as carcinoma-in-situ, atypism, and focal dysplasia have been used to describe this finding. Occasionally, malignant cells may be seen penetrating the muscularis mucosae. (2) Benign adenomatous remnants may be found microscopically in about 10 per cent of the cases of frank carcinomas of the colon and rectum, according to Morson.[19] (3) It is well established that the risk of development of colon cancer is greater in patients with adenomatous polyps of the bowel than in nonadenoma-bearing persons, and the more adenomas the greater the risk. Furthermore, according to studies at London's St. Mark's Hospital for anorectal diseases,

patients from whom colon cancers with coexisting adenomas were removed were twice as likely to have a subsequent recurrence of cancer as those patients in whom no adenomas were found at the time of initial surgery.[19] (4) Karyotyping studies of adenomatous polyps and colonic cancer have revealed similar chromosomal abnormalities to be present in both the benign and malignant lesion.[10] (5) Histochemical studies of various intracellular oxidative enzymes in adenomas and adenocarcinomas tend to support the concept of the adenoma-carcinoma sequence by demonstrating enzymatic transition from normal to carcinomatous colonic epithelium.[7] (6) Early carcinomas of the bowel commonly present as polypoid lesions. (7) The incidence of "invasive" cancer in villous adenomas in some series may be as high as 30 per cent.

One cannot infer from these and other available data that *all* adenomatous polyps become malignant, but Morson's data suggest that approximately one half of colon cancers arise in an antecedent adenoma.[19] Presumably, the other 50 per cent of colon cancers arise "de novo." However, this phenomenon, if indeed it occurs, has not been well documented clinically or histologically, although recent studies support the theory.[5-13, 15] Very small adenocarcinomas apparently arising "de novo" are rare in the experience of most clinicans and pathologists.

In our present state of knowledge, Morson's assessment of the situation seems to be most consistent with the facts, namely, that "a malignant polyp is only a stage in a progressive neoplastic hyperplasia of a few epithelial tubules to a frank carcinoma."[19]

Diagnosis

Adenomas are usually detected in the course of routine sigmoidoscopy and barium enemas, although the growing use of the fiberoptic colonoscope in evaluating patients with large bowel complaints is playing an ever increasing role in finding occult adenomas in the large bowel. Adenomas seldom produce symptoms until they reach considerable size, when bleeding may occur. The bleeding is often occult but may be bright red and noted by the patient. It is uncommon for these tumors to produce symptoms of abdominal distress or pain. When this does occur it is probably due to traction on the lesion by peristaltic action of the bowel. Villous adenomas when large may produce copious amounts of mucus and diarrhea. This may on rare occasion be of such magnitude as to result in hypokalemia due to severe loss of electrolytes.[21]

Treatment

Treatment of patients with adenomatous polyps is based on two premises. First, in the absence of histologic examination one cannot say unequivocally that the lesion is not malignant and a period of watchful waiting with repeated barium enema examinations may compromise the chances for cure should the lesion prove to be a polypoid carcinoma. Second, in the opinion of many, adenomas may with the passage of time increase in size and become malignant. For these reasons most surgeons recommend removal of polypoid lesions of the colon and rectum, provided the risk of laparotomy is not considered unduly high.

Therapy of adenomatous polyps is conveniently divided into those lesions within the reach of the conventional sigmoidoscope, and those above, which require laparotomy. In the first instance, all tumors should be removed for histologic examination. When the adenoma is pedunculated, this can usually be accomplished by a cautery snare, with care to remove as much of the pedicle as possible and cauterization of the base. For small sessile tumors, excisional biopsy is preferred, with cauterization of the base for hemostasis. In removing tumors situated above 10 cm. from the anal verge, caution must be exercised to avoid perforation of the bowel, which will result in peritoneal contamination and require a laparotomy for repair.

Adenomas above the reach of the conventional sigmoidoscope may be removed in one of two ways. The first method, and the one that is increasingly preferred, is removal by means of the flexible colonoscope. If proper instruments and personnel skilled in their use are available, most adenomas can now be removed from any portion of the large bowel by this method. In a clean, well-prepared bowel, when the procedure is carried out by an experienced endoscopist, the risk of hemorrhage, perforation, or other complications is negligible. This method has the additional advantage over surgery in reducing the need for lengthy hospitalization. Indeed, many patients can be managed on an ambulatory basis, although this is still reserved for the simpler cases. It is still viewed as essential that complete surgical facilities be immediately available in the event that complications do occur and that patients undergoing colonoscopy for removal of adenomatous polyps have the same preparation required for major abdominal surgery.

The actual removal of the adenoma is usually by means of the cautery snare. The reader should consult the growing body of literature on this subject for refinements in technique.[24, 25]

If colonoscopy is not available or if it is attempted and proves unsuccessful, the second method for the removal of adenomas above the reach of the standard sigmoidoscope is laparotomy, which has an increased risk to the patient.

Prior to surgery the bowel should be thoroughly cleansed to minimize the likelihood of peritoneal soilage at the time of surgery. This is best accomplished by placing the patient on a low-residue diet several days prior to surgery, followed by mild cathartics and cleansing enemas the day before operation. Intestinal antibiotics are considered by many surgeons to be an important adjunct to preparation of the bowel but are not a substitute for careful mechanical cleansing.

Pedunculated adenomas less than 2 cm. in greatest diameter may be removed by colotomy and polypectomy. It is important to remove the entire pedicle for histologic examination. Frozen section of the lesion is advocated to determine the presence or absence of malignant change. If a focus of malignant change is found in the body of the tumor, it is necessary to determine whether or not the stalk has been invaded by malignant cells. If cancer is found to be invading the stalk, resection of the bowel will be required. If there is no evidence of stalk invasion, polypectomy will usually suffice.

Pedunculated adenomas larger than 2 cm. in diameter are best managed by resection of the bowel, including sufficient margins on either side of the lesion and adequate mesocolon, because of the increased risk of malignancy in tumors of this size.[11, 13]

Sessile adenomas, irrespective of size, should be managed, in the author's opinion, by segmental resection of the bowel because of the likelihood of the lesion being malignant.

Not infrequently, several adenomatous polyps may be present in a single segment of the bowel, in which case resection may be preferable to multiple colotomies and polypectomies with their risk of peritoneal soilage. In some patients in whom adenomas are scattered randomly throughout the large colon, a subtotal colectomy with ileorectal anastomosis may be the procedure of choice. This therapy is based on the high incidence of recurrent adenomas developing in a colonic mucosa with a propensity for tumor formation, as well as the limitations of barium enemas in detecting small early lesions.

Colonoscopy at the time of surgery may be used to detect additional lesions. However, because of the added risk of infection by peritoneal contamination, great care must be exercised if this technique is used. Opinions vary as to the wisdom of colonoscopy because of the increased morbidity with its use, but there is little doubt of its efficacy in detecting unsuspected lesions at laparotomy and it may be of great help when lesions are difficult to locate by palpation or transillumination of the bowel.

Villous tumors generally involve somewhat larger areas of the colonic epithelium, are most often sessile, but may be pedunculated in 10 per cent of the cases. When they occur above the level of the sigmoidoscope they usually require colon resection for complete removal. Furthermore, they often have very ill-defined borders so that adequate margins of normal tissue must be removed to reduce the chances of local recurrence. Frequently, villous tumors occur in the lower sigmoid and rectum and will have attained considerable size when first seen by the surgeon (Fig. 3). Efforts must be made to determine whether or not any portion of the lesion is malignant. This is best accomplished by multiple biopsies, particularly of any "suspicious" areas as evidenced by ulceration or increased firmness.

In the absence of a histologic diagnosis of cancer, local excision and fulguration, particularly of the smaller lesions, is the preferred treatment, although a more aggressive approach such as combined abdominoperineal resection has been advocated because of the added risk of cancer.

Local excision of small villous adenomas can frequently be performed through the anal canal. Occasionally, a posterior proctotomy may be required to insure adequate removal. In either case repeated postoperative examinations will be required to make certain that total removal has been accomplished. In those cases in which the lesion is so large as to preclude local removal or in which carcinoma has been found, a total proctectomy will be required. Pull-through procedures as a means of maintaining intestinal continuity and fecal continence in the benign

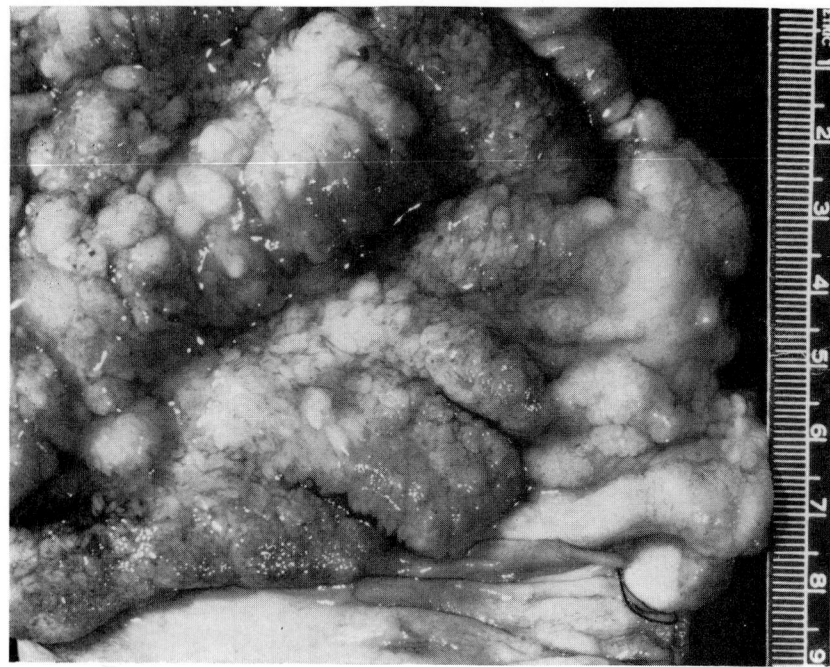

Figure 3. Villous adenoma. (From Welch, C. E., and Hedberg, S. E.: Polypoid Lesions of the Gastrointestinal Tract, Philadelphia, W. B. Saunders Company, 1975.)

lesions may be utilized in carefully selected cases. Depending somewhat on the level of the villous adenoma above the anal verge, anterior resection of the rectum may be feasible.

JUVENILE POLYPS

Juvenile polyps are non-neoplastic lesions that usually occur in the colon and rectum of infants and adolescents. On rare occasions they may be found in adults. These lesions have a characteristic histologic appearance consisting of large, dilated, mucus-filled glands with an abundance of supporting stroma and frequently devoid of an epithelial cover. The epithelial cells give no evidence of neoplastic growth and are uniform in appearance with minimal mitotic activity (Fig. 4).

Opinion remains divided as to the cause of these tumors. In the minds of some, they are considered to develop in response to some inflammatory stimulus; others feel that they are more likely hamartomas. During the past few years, several cases of multiple juvenile polyposis have been reported within families, which establishes a genetic basis for these tumors.[17]

In most instances, attention is drawn to the presence of juvenile polyps by the passage of blood per rectum. This finding occurs in approximately 95 per cent of the cases. Occasionally, the polyps can be the cause of abdominal pain owing to intussusception or traction on the polyp by peristaltic activity.

Because they are not premalignant tumors, therapy should be conservative unless the symptoms are of such magnitude as to jeopardize the patient's general health. Frequently, juvenile polyps will undergo au-

toamputation. It should be borne in mind, however, that other polypoid lesions are known to occur in the colon and rectum of children, including polypoid carcinoma. Hence, careful observation is required and good judgment must be exercised in determining how long these lesions can be safely treated expectantly.

HYPERPLASTIC (METAPLASTIC) POLYPS

Hyperplastic polyps are very common and generally appear as small mucosal excrescences arising in the colon and rectal epithelium (Fig. 5).

Microscopically they show cystic dilatation of the tubules of the mucosa, with a characteristic "sawtooth" appearance of the glands near the surface. There is a reduction in the number of goblet cells and varying degrees of hyperplastic activity. These polyps are not associated with the development of adenomas or carcinoma and clinical observation suggests that they may be a transient lesion.

Lane et al.[16] found, in a detailed histologic examination of polypoid lesions of the colon and rectum measuring less than 3 mm. in diameter, that well over 90 per cent of the polyps were hyperplastic. When larger polyps were studied, the incidence of hyperplastic polyps decreased and the incidence of adenomatous polyps increased. Lane and his colleagues are of the opinion that the greater frequency of small hyperplastic polyps reflects a restricted growth potential of hyperplastic epithelium. Furthermore, they point out that true adenomatous polyps of a very small size are by no means rare and that one need not postulate that hyperplastic polyps are necessarily precursors of true adenomatous polyps. Other cytologic and histologic

The hereditary nature of the disease was first reported by Cripps[5] in 1882 when he noted the presence of adenomatous polyps of the rectum in a brother and sister. Earlier accounts of "polyposis coli" may be found in the literature, but the exact histologic features of the lesions described are obscure. Lockhart-Mummery in 1925 clearly established the hereditary nature of the disease, described its clinical manifestations, and drew attention to its malignant potential through his study of three families at St. Mark's Hospital in London. Subsequent reports by Dukes[9] provided the modern-day basis for our understanding and management of disease.

Pathology

In an affected person the adenomas may vary in numbers from a few scattered lesions to so many that they almost obliterate the mucosa. The lesions vary in size from small mucosal excrescences a few millimeters in greatest dimension to individual lesions so large that they may partially occlude the lumen of the bowel. The adenoma may be sessile or pedunculated (Fig. 6). In most patients the majority of the adenomas occur in the sigmoid colon and rectum; however, the distribution pattern may be quite varied. The disease does not affect the small intestine.

In a study of 143 patients at St. Mark's Hospital, Bussey[2] found that although a difference in the density of adenomas in different segments of the bowel may occur, in no instance was the rectum ever free of tumors.

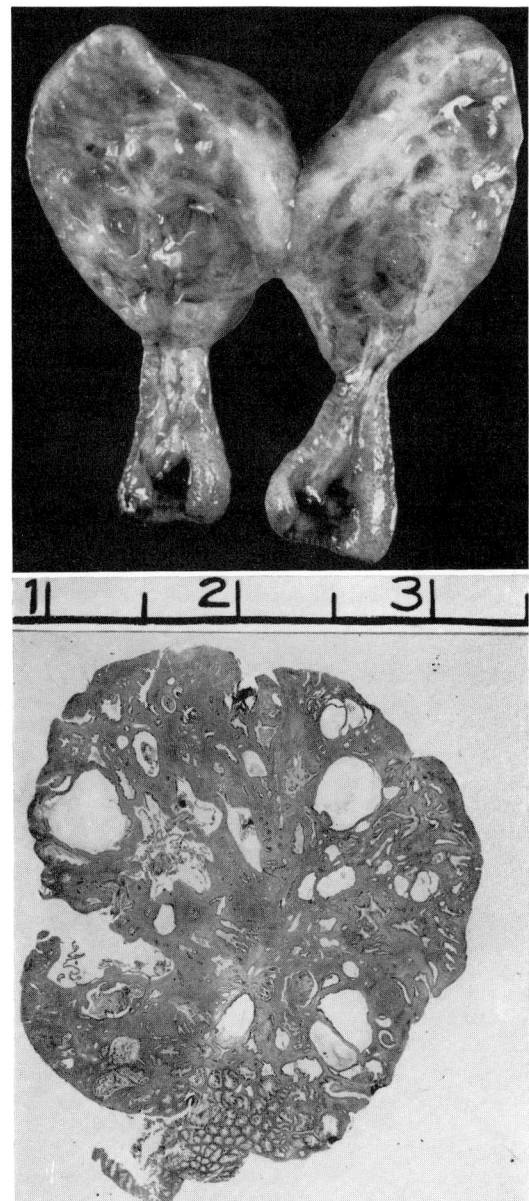

Figure 4. Juvenile polyps. (From Welch, C. E., and Hedberg, S. E.: Polypoid Lesions of the Gastrointestinal Tract. Philadelphia, W. B. Saunders Company, 1975.)

differences were noted which clearly established these very common polyps as being quite distinct from the small neoplastic adenoma.

FAMILIAL POLYPOSIS

Familial polyposis is an uncommon *hereditary* disease characterized by the presence of large numbers of adenomatous polyps in the colon and rectum, and, if untreated, will almost certainly eventuate in adenocarcinoma of the large bowel. The lesions seldom appear before puberty.

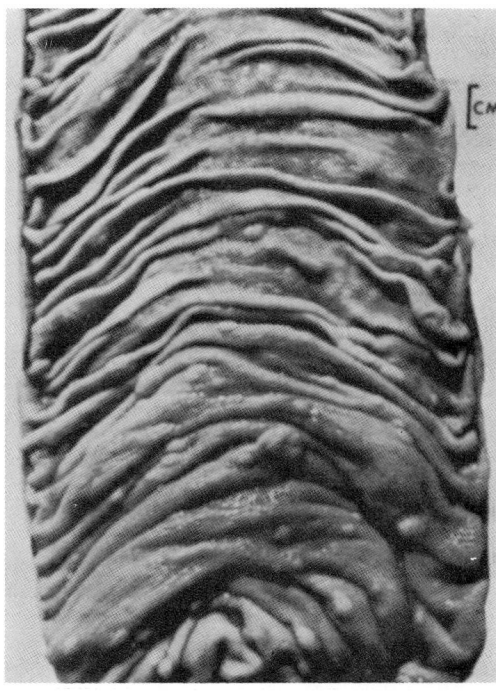

Figure 5. Hyperplastic polyps—multiple mucosal excrescences. (From Predisposing causes of intestinal cancer, by Morson, B. C., and Bussey, H. J. R., in Current Problems in Surgery, edited by Ravitch, M. M., et al. Copyright © 1970, Year Book Medical Publishers. Used by permission.)

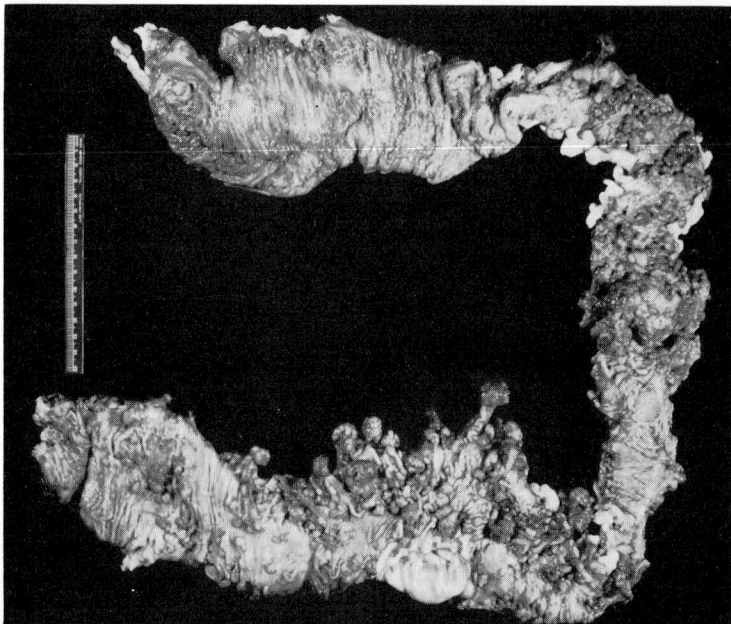

Figure 6. Multiple adenomas in familial polyposis. (From Welch, C. E., and Hedberg, S. E.: Polypoid Lesions of the Gastrointestinal Tract. Philadelphia, W. B. Saunders Company, 1975.)

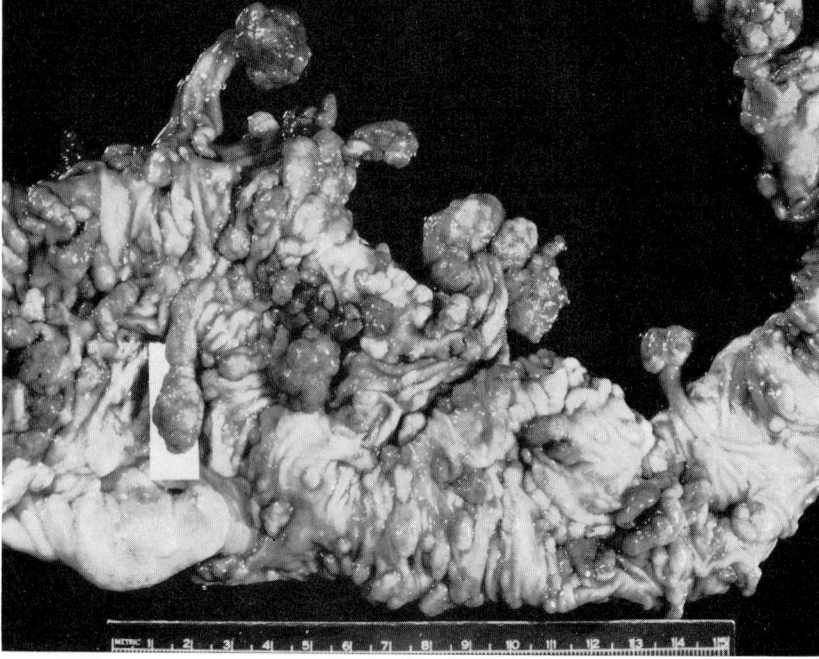

The surface of the lesion on gross inspection may vary from the more common smooth lobulated appearance to one that is somewhat irregular and ragged. Microscopically, the polyps are neoplastic lesions of epithelial origin. While the majority are composed of hyperplastic mucus-secreting cells, forming a tortuous and distorted glandular configuration, villous elements with finger-like projections are not uncommon. All stages of adenoma developed are usually found within the diseased colon, from a solitary hyperplastic gland not visible on gross inspection to the fully developed glandular tumor with different degrees of cellu-

lar differentiation. In late or untreated cases, adenocarcinoma is a common finding.

Genetics

Familial polyposis is transmitted as a mendelian dominant, non-sex-linked trait with a high degree of penetrance. Theoretically, one half of the offspring of a parent harboring the abnormal gene may be expected to manifest the disease (Fig. 7).

Occasionally, no familial history can be elicited in some patients with multiple adenomatous polyps of the colon at an early age. Under these circumstances,

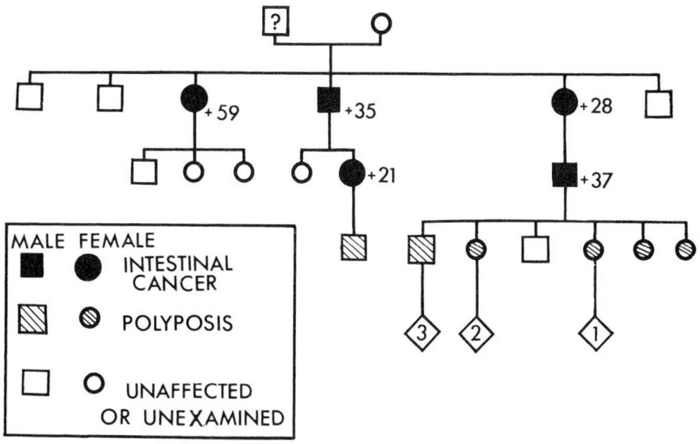

Figure 7. Family pedigree in a case of familial polyposis. (From Predisposing causes of intestinal cancer, by Morson, B. C., and Bussey, H. J. R., in Current Problems in Surgery, edited by Ravitch, M. M., et al. Copyright © 1970, Year Book Medical Publishers. Used by permission.)

it is generally assumed that a new mutation has occurred, since subsequent generations are found to be at risk.

Veale[23] has proposed that two genes may be involved in adenoma formation, one dominant (P) and one recessive (p), the former relating to familial polyposis and the latter involved in formation of the more common solitary adenomas of adult life. According to Veale's theory, the genotype Pp results in early expression of polyposis, whereas the genotype Px is manifested in familial polyposis at a somewhat older age. The genotype Pp would explain multiple polyps in the older age groups without the evidence of the familial trait. Further evidence for this theory is required. It does, however, help to explain the variations that are seen in the numbers of adenomas noted in the population as well as the early and late appearance of the lesions in patients with the inherited form of the disease. Efforts to predict, by studying such genetic markers as blood groups, which offspring of a parent having familial polyposis will inherit the disease have thus far been to no avail.

It is well established that familial polyposis is a precancerous condition and if patients with the disease are untreated for a sufficiently long time, adenocarcinomas will almost certainly develop. In the St. Mark's series, 63.1 per cent of the patients presenting with symptoms had adenocarcinomas of the colon *at the time of the initial examination.* The cancers associated with familial polyposis tend to appear at a much earlier age than in nonpolyposis patients. Furthermore, the incidence of multiple cancers is 12 times greater in polyposis patients than in the general population with colorectal cancer.

The distribution of colonic cancer in polyposis patients does not differ significantly from that seen in the general population; however, there is some evidence to suggest that adenocarcinoma arising in polyposis patients is more likely to be well differentiated histologically.

Clinical Manifestations

Although patients who have inherited the disease may show evidence of polyp formation in the prepubertal period, it is uncommon for patients to have symptoms before early adult life. Polyps may appear at any time, but on the average they will be noted during the second and third decades of life. For this reason, relatives of affected persons should be examined annually for evidence of the disease.

The commonest sign is rectal bleeding, which occurs in over three fourths of the patients with the disease. Occasionally, bleeding may be of such magnitude as to result in anemia. Diarrhea is the next most common finding noted in over one half of the patients. Abdominal pain may occur. When it does, it is intermittent, rarely severe, and seldom the reason that the patient seeks medical care. Mucous discharge, with or without blood, has been noted in less than half of the patients with the disease. In those patients in whom adenocarcinoma has developed, other symptoms may be present, such as obstruction and, in the very advanced case, perforation with associated peritonitis.

Diagnosis

The diagnosis of familial polyposis can usually be made by proctosigmoidoscopy, biopsy of the tumors, and barium enema, and by eliciting a family history of the disease. Histologic confirmation by biopsy is mandatory to avoid an erroneous diagnosis that may lead to inappropriate therapy. There are several diseases that have to be distinguished from familial adenomatous polyposis.

The most common is to be found in patients having multiple adenomas in the large bowel but for whom no hereditary background can be identified. Distinguishing these patients from those with true familial polyposis may be difficult in those instances in which family health records are unavailable. Histologic examination of biopsy specimen alone is of no help, since the tumors are identical. In general, one may say that the multiple adenomas in the nonfamilial group are fewer in number, appear later in life, and tend to be confined to the sigmoid colon and rectum. With our present state of knowledge, the differences between classic familial polyposis coli and multiple adenomas are somewhat contrived. However, the distinction does have practical significance in genetic counseling of the affected persons.

The next most common disease to be differentiated in the *pseudopolyposis* seen in chronic inflammatory disease of the large bowel, such as idiopathic ulcerative colitis and Crohn's disease. These polyps are hyperplastic mucosal remnants that grossly may look like neoplastic growth, but their true character is revealed upon microscopic examination.

Multiple juvenile polyposis is a rare condition described originally by McColl et al.[17] in 1964 and is easily distinguished from familial adenomatous polyposis on microscopic examination of the lesions. These lesions are not neoplastic. They are characterized by the presence of normal epithelial elements, mucus-filled cystic spaces, and an abundance of supporting stroma. The lesions appear at a much earlier age, may occur in areas of the gastrointestinal tract other than the colon, and are not premalignant. There are 22 affected families now recorded in the files of St. Mark's Hospital. Other congenital defects such as hydrocephalus, cardiac abnormalities, and intestinal malformation may also be present.

The so-called *Peutz-Jeghers syndrome* seldom poses difficulty in a differential diagnosis. Although it is an inherited disease, the polyps are present throughout the gastrointestinal tract and are associated with melanin spots on the lips and buccal mucosa. Histologically, the tumors are considered hamartomas consisting of normal intestinal epithelium and smooth muscle. They are not disposed to malignant change (Fig. 8). However, several cases of adenocarcinoma occurring in patients with Peutz-Jeghers syndrome have been reported.

Gardner's syndrome,[12] as originally described, consists of adenomatous polyps of the colon, osteomas of the mandible and skull, multiple epidermoid cysts, and soft tissue tumors of the skin. Since the risk of cancer occurring in the colon is high in this syndrome, the management of these patients for practical purposes is identical to that for those with familial polyposis. (For further discussion, see Section VII of this chapter, page 1109).

Other still less common diseases that must be differentiated from familial polyposis of the colon include multiple neurofibromatosis, cystic pneumatosis intestinalis, multiple benign lymphoid polyps, leukemic polyposis, multiple metaplastic (hyperplastic) polyps, and lipomatous polyposis. In all these diseases a careful family history and histologic examination of the lesions should establish the correct diagnosis.

Management

The proper management of patients with familial polyposis may be difficult. There is general agreement that once the diagnosis has been established, the colon should be removed as soon as feasible to reduce the risk of cancer developing in the bowel. A difference of opinion continues to exist, however, with respect to whether or not the rectum should be retained. There is

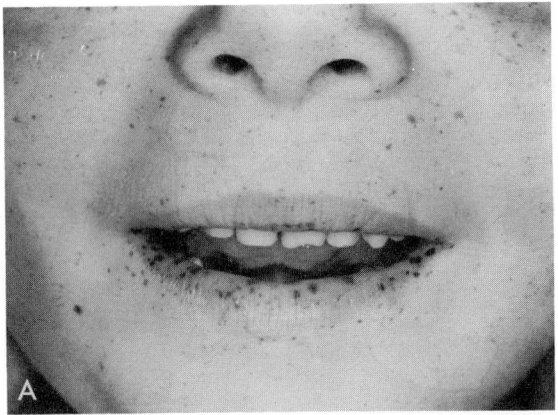

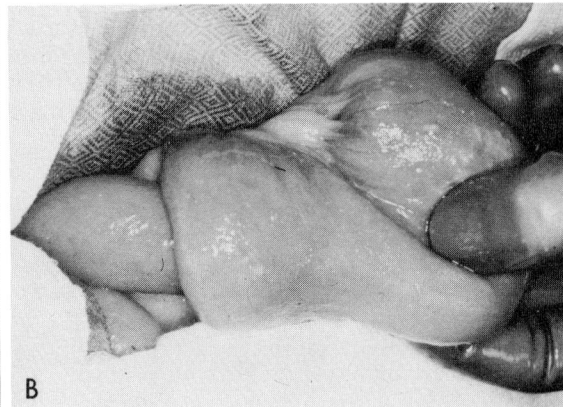

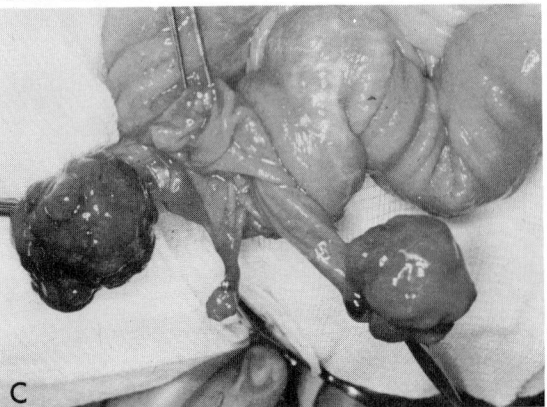

Figure 8. Peutz-Jeghers syndrome. (From Welch, C. E., and Hedberg, S. E.: Polypoid Lesions of the Gastrointestinal Tract. Philadelphia, W. B. Saunders Company, 1975.)

no disagreement that the rectum should be removed if cancer is present there or if the patient is unlikely to return for proctoscopic examinations. However, in those circumstances in which there is no cancer and the patient is willing and able to submit to repeated examinations for the remainder of his life, many clinicians feel that the rectum may be spared.

There is little doubt that in those patients in whom the rectum is preserved, the risk of cancer at some future time is a real and ever present threat. Nonetheless, the advocates of this procedure maintain that the risk is outweighed by certain advantages. The maintenance of intestinal continuity with its social and psychologic significance is of the utmost importance, particularly in the young patients. If patients are spared the inconvenience and morbidity associated with a permanent abdominal ileostomy, afflicted families are frequently more cooperative in calling up family members with and without symptoms for examination. Lastly, in patients kept under close surveillance, the development of a cancer in the retained rectum at some future time does not preclude a cure.

At St. Mark's Hospital, 73 patients with the diagnosis of familial polyposis underwent total colectomy and ileoproctostomy; a carcinoma in the retained rectal segment subsequently developed in three patients, at intervals of 2, 6, and 21 years following surgery, an incidence of 4 per cent. Patients in this series had been followed for periods up to 20 years, with an average follow-up of 10 years.

In Moertel's report of the experience of the Mayo Clinic,[18] cancer developed in the retained rectum in 59 per cent of those patients followed for 23 years. Moertel believes that colectomy and ileorectal anastomosis is inadequate treatment for diffuse multiple polyposis involving the colon and rectum. Not all of the patients in this study gave positive family histories for polyposis.

There are alternative surgical procedures such as pull-through operations and ileoanal anastomosis with removal of the diseased rectal epithelium so that intestinal continuity may be maintained, but they have not gained wide acceptance.

Occasionally following colectomy and ileorectal anastomosis, the adenomas in the retained rectum may spontaneously regress. In most patients, however, excision and repeated fulguration will be required to rid the rectum of existing adenomas or to destroy new adenomas that may appear during the postoperative period. Repeated fulguration of the rectum is not devoid of risk, and care must be taken to prevent strictures, perforations of the bowel, and hemorrhage. Total colectomy and ileorectal anastomosis is well tolerated. Although these patients have frequent, loose bowel movements for several months, they are continent. Normal growth and development is not impaired when the procedure is found necessary in the very young.

SELECTED REFERENCES

Bussey, H. J. R.: Familial Polyposis Coli. Baltimore, Johns Hopkins University Press, 1975.
This comprehensive review of familial polyposis coli, based on a detailed study of the disease begun at St. Mark's Hospital in 1925, is the most definitive work available on the subject.

Morson, B. C., and Bussey, H. J. R.: Predisposing causes of intestinal cancer. Curr. Probl. Surg., Feb., 1970.
This well-illustrated monograph gives a comprehensive review of premalignant lesions of the colon and rectum based on the extensive experience at St. Mark's Hospital in London. All aspects of colonic neoplasia are covered from a pathologist's point of view with a discussion of their clinical implications. This authoritative publication with an up-to-date list of references is highly recommended for students of this disease.

Welch, C. E., and Hedberg, S.: Polypoid Lesions of the Gastrointestinal Tract, 2nd ed. Philadelphia, W. B. Saunders Company, 1975.
Although portions of this book are devoted to a discussion of polypoid lesions of the stomach and small intestine, most of it deals with a consideration of polypoid lesions of the colon and rectum. The discussion of the histopathology of colorectal lesions and their management is extremely well done by an experienced clinician. All sides of controversial issues in therapy are carefully considered and the authors' rationale for their approach to clinical problems is set forth in a most lucid manner.

REFERENCES

1. Behringer, G.: Changing concepts in the histopathologic diagnosis of polypoid lesions of the colon. Dis. Colon Rectum, 13:116, 1970.
2. Bussey, H. J. R.: The Pathology of Familial Polyposis Coli (Multiple Adenomatosis). Ph.D. thesis, London, 1970.
3. Cleveland, J. C., Litvak, S. F., and Cole, J. W.: Identification of the route of action of the carcinogen 3:2-dimethyl-4-aminobiphenyl in the induction of intestinal neoplasia. Cancer Res., 27:708, 1967.
4. Cole, J. W., and McKalen, A.: Observations of cell renewal in human rectal mucosa in vivo with thymidine-H³. Gastroenterology, 41:122, 1961.
5. Cripps, W. H.: Two cases of disseminated polypus of the rectum. Trans. Path. Soc. London, 33:165, 1882.
6. Crocker, D., and Veith, F. J.: Focal primary mucosal hyperplasia of the colon. Ann. Surg., 160:215, 1964.
7. Czernobilsky, B., and Tsou, K. C.: Adenocarcinomas, adenomas and polyps of the colon. Histochemical study. Cancer, 21:165, 1968.
8. Deschner, E. E., Lipkin, M., and Solomon, C.: Study of human rectal epithelial cells in vitro. II. H³-thymidine incorporation into polyps and adjacent mucosa. J. Natl. Cancer Inst., 36:849, 1966.
9. Dukes, C. E.: Familial intestinal polyposis. Ann. Eugenics, 17:1, 1952.
10. Enterline, H. T., and Arvan, D. A.: Carcinomas, adenomatous polyps. Cancer, 20:1746, 1967.
11. Enterline, H. T., Evans, G. W., Mercado-Lugo, R., Miller, L., and Fitts, W. T.: Malignant potential of adenomas of the colon and rectum. J.A.M.A., 179:322, 1962.
12. Gardner, E. S.: Gardner's syndrome (1951). Am. J. Hum. Genet., p. 5, 1967.
13. Grinnell, R. S., and Lane, N.: Benign and malignant adenomatous polyps and papillary adenomas of the colon and rectum. Surg. Gynecol. Obstet., 106:519, 1958.
14. Hill, M. J., Crowther, J. H., Drasar, B. S., Hawksworth, G., Aries, V., and Williams, R. E. O.: Bacteria and etiology of cancer of the large bowel. Lancet, 1:95–100, 1971.
15. Kjeldsberg, C., and Altschuler, J. H.: Carcinoma in situ of the colon. Dis. Colon Rectum, 13:376, 1970.
16. Lane, N., Kaplan, H., and Pascal, R. R.: Minute adenomatous and hyperplastic polyps of the colon: Divergent patterns of epithelial growth with specific associated mesenchymal changes. Gastroenterology, 60:537, 1971.
17. McColl, I., Bussey, H. J. R., Veale, A. M. O., and Morson, B. C.: Familial polyposis. Proc. R. Soc. Med., 57:896, 1964.
18. Moertel, C. G., Hill, J. R., and Adson, M. A.: Surgical management of multiple polyposis. The problems of cancer in the retained bowel segment. Arch. Surg., 100:521, 1970.
19. Morson, B. C., and Bussey, H. J. R.: Predisposing causes of intestinal cancer. Curr. Probl. Surg., Feb., 1970.
20. Reddy, B. S., Dhar, A. K., Weisburger, J. H., and Wynder, E. L.: Effect of high risk and low risk diets for colon carcinogenesis on fecal bile acids and neutral steroids in main. Fed. Proc., 33:663, 1974.
21. Shnitka, T. K., Friedman, M. H. W., Kidd, E. G., and MacKenzie, W. C.: Villous tumors of the rectum and colon characterized by

severe fluid and electrolyte loss. Surg. Gynecol. Obstet., *112*: 609, 1961.

22. Spjut, H. J., and Spratt, J. S., Jr.: Endemic and morphologic similarities existing between spontaneous colon neoplasms in man and 3:2-dimethyl-4-aminobiphenyl induced colonic neoplasms in rats. Ann. Surg., *161*:309, 1965.

23. Veale, A. M. O.: Intestinal Polyposis. London, Cambridge University Press, 1965.

24. Wolff, W., and Shinya, H.: Modern endoscopy of the alimentary tract. Curr. Probl. Surg., Jan., 1974.

25. Wolff, W., and Shinya, H.: Polypectomy via the fiber colonoscope. N. Engl. J. Med., *288*:329, 1973.

X

THE RECTUM AND ANAL CANAL

Alan G. Parks, M.D., and James P. S. Thomson, M.S.

ANATOMY AND PHYSIOLOGY

It has become apparent in recent years that physiologic considerations are of great importance both in the etiology of many anorectal disorders and in the production of symptoms. The anorectal mechanism is made up of two parts, both of which have a tubular shape, one ensheathing the other. The innermost structure is the termination of the alimentary viscus and is surrounded by the skeletal muscles of the pelvic floor, the lower part of which form the external anal sphincters (Figs. 1 and 2). The viscus, that is, the lower rectum and anal canal, is innervated by the autonomic nervous system and is therefore not subject to voluntary control. It is the surrounding skeletal muscle sphincter that is largely responsible for establishing normal continence. The visceral component is lined in its upper part by unstratified, mucus-secreting columnar epithelium which is almost devoid of sensory receptors. Fortunately, in the process of embryologic development, squamous mucosa migrates into the anal canal for about 2 cm. This mucosa does not secrete mucus; hence, the perineum is not continuously soiled by mucous discharge. It is supplied with many sensory nerve endings of a specialized type which supply information to the spinal centers, and is a valuable part of the mechanism of continence.[3] The terminal part of the circular muscle of the viscus is greatly enlarged to form the internal sphincter muscle. Its visceral tone is the most important factor in maintaining a closed anal canal; it is maximal in normal circumstances and relaxes when distention of the rectum takes place. The muscles of the rectum and the internal sphincter are linked by the intramural autonomic network of nerves. Outside this there is a relatively thin layer of longitudinal muscle that has no significant function in this area.

The gut tube is surrounded by the external sphincter muscles, which also have the form of a tube. Between them is an embryonic fusion layer called the intersphincteric plane. Infection tends to spread in this plane. The external sphincter muscles maintain control over the visceral outlet. In addition to their sphincter action they have an antigravity function in maintaining a closed pelvic outlet against the forces of abdominal pressure. These muscles have an unusual physiologic tone maintained even at rest and during sleep by a spinal reflex centered in the cauda equina[5] (Fig. 3). It is maintained by stretch receptors in the muscles themselves. Several factors influence this basal resting tone, some of them increasing it, others inhibiting it altogether. A rise in intra-abdominal pressure will cause an immediate reflex rise in the tone of the pelvic floor muscles. This will tend to counteract stress incontinence liable to occur at such a time and will also prevent any tendency to prolapse on the part

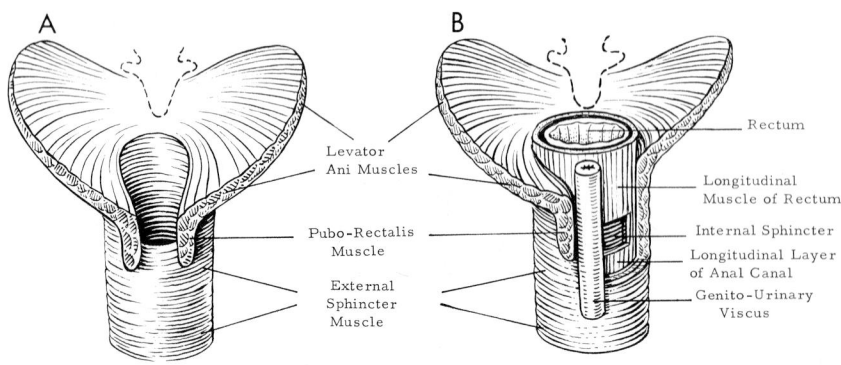

A

B

Levator Ani Muscles

Pubo-Rectalis Muscle

External Sphincter Muscle

Rectum

Longitudinal Muscle of Rectum

Internal Sphincter

Longitudinal Layer of Anal Canal

Genito-Urinary Viscus

Figure 1. The anal mechanism comprises two components, visceral and somatic, each of which is tubular. The visceral tube is enclosed by a skeletal muscle tube by means of which continence is maintained. *A,* Diagrammatic representation of the skeletal muscle component. *B,* Composite arrangement after insertion of the simple visceral component. (From Hemorrhoidectomy, by Alan G. Parks, in Advances in Surgery, edited by C. E. Welch. Copyright © 1971, Year Book Medical Publishers. Used by permission.)

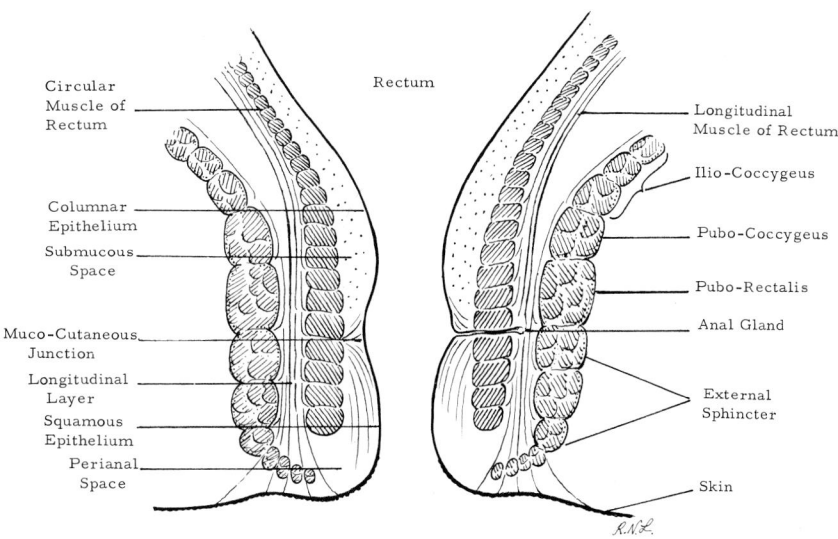

Figure 2. Diagrammatic section through the pelvic floor. The visceral and skeletal muscle components are apparent, separated by the interphincteric plane. Squamous mucosa lines the lower half of the anal canal, up to the level of the anal crypts. (From Hemorrhoidectomy, by Alan G. Parks, in Advances in Surgery, edited by C. E. Welch. Copyright © 1971, Year Book Medical Publishers. Used by permission.)

of the pelvic viscera. Distention of the rectum also activates sphincter tone and so contributes to the preservation of continence.[15]

Several factors decrease the resting tone of the external sphincters, defecation straining being one of the most potent. This is probably part of the normal physiologic mechanism, but excessive straining produces abnormalities that will be discussed later. Micturition also induces total cessation of anal sphincter activity. Extreme distention of the rectum, such as occurs in impaction of feces, will totally abolish sphincter tone, and this accounts for the incontinence such patients suffer.

The direct effect of sphincter activity is not the only

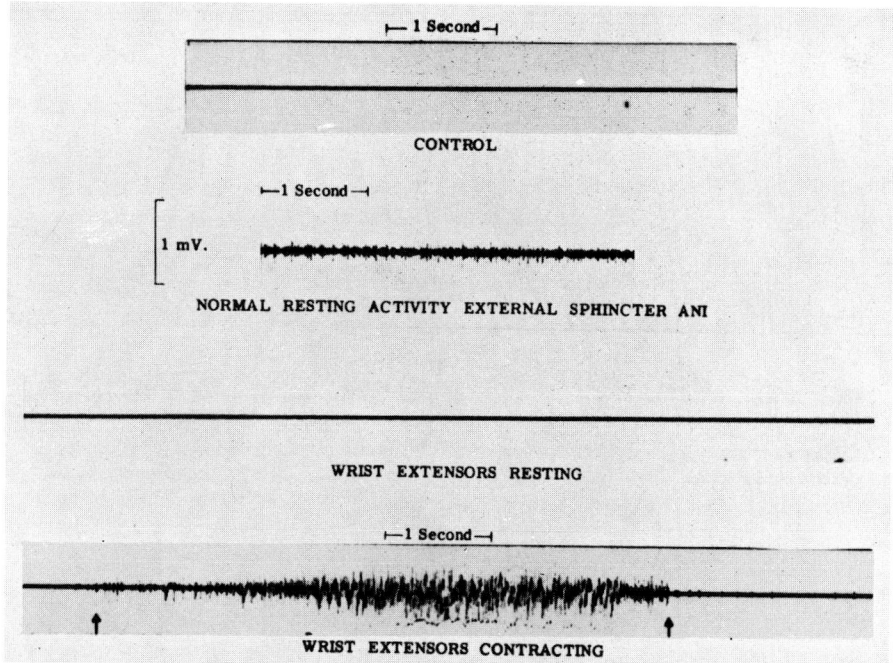

Figure 3. An electromyogram comparing the extensors of the wrist and the anal sphincters. There is no electrical activity in the wrist muscles at rest, in contrast with the continuous reflex activity of the anal sphincters. (From Parks, A. G., Porter, N. H., and Melzak, J.: Dis. Colon Rectum, 5:407, 1962.)

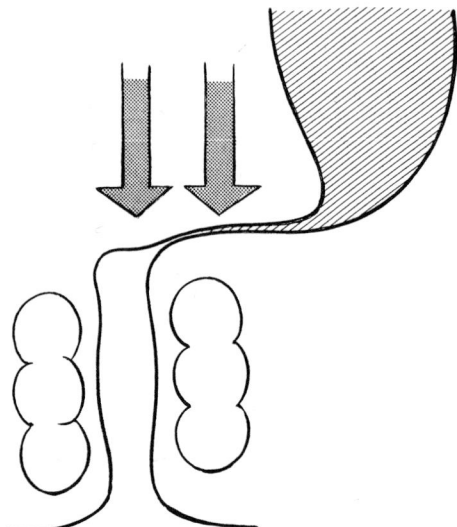

Figure 4. The gut makes two right angles in its course through the anorectal region. This arrangement is mostly maintained by the contraction of the puborectalis muscle. The lowermost part of the anterior rectal wall is opposed to the closed anal canal, thereby forming a valve. Increase in abdominal pressure will automatically increase the firmness of closure of the valve. (From Hemorrhoidectomy, by Alan G. Parks, in Advances in Surgery, edited by C. E. Welch. Copyright © 1971, Year Book Medical Publishers. Used by permission.)

factor, nor is is it the most important one, in establishing anorectal control. The structural arrangements of the anorectal region are certainly of equal importance, though these are, indeed, maintained by muscle action.[16] The lower rectum makes a right angle with the axis of the anal canal; as a result the mucosa of the anterior wall of the lower rectum is firmly opposed to the top of the closed anal canal. The force of abdominal pressure is transmitted directly through the anterior rectal wall, thus pressing it firmly into the anal canal and effectively closing it (Fig. 4). The greater the force of abdominal pressure, the more secure the closure, thus counteracting the tendency for stress in-

continence to occur.[13] This valvelike action is similar to the one present at the esophagogastric junction and indeed is found at most sites where a viscus passes from a cavity of high pressure to one of low pressure. A rise of pressure in the high-pressure system will make the valve more secure; the most potent force unlocking the valve will be a rise in pressure in the viscus itself.

The upper parts of the external sphincters are continuous with the levator ani muscles; they form a unified muscle mass and contract as one. The lowest muscle of the levator group is the puborectalis, which in fact has a strong sphincteric action as it passes as a sling behind the upper anal canal. The upper parts of the levator muscle, the pubococcygeus and iliococcygeus, close off the pelvic hiatus on either side of the visceral outlet. They divide the pelvic cavity from the perineum. Below them on either side of the anal canal is the ischiorectal fossa containing mostly fat; above is the fat of the pararectal space. These arrangements are especially important in relation to the anatomy of fistula in ano.

As mentioned previously, the lower anal canal is lined by squamous epithelium, the upper by mucus-secreting columnar epithelium. Where these two join is a short transitional zone of hybrid character. Small glands of unusual character arise from this transitional zone[2] (Fig. 5). They pass through the submucosa and thence, in most cases, actually into the internal sphincter (see Fig. 3). In about two thirds of cases they terminate in small glandular structures in the connective tissue between the internal and external sphincters (the intersphincteric plane). Here there is often a condensation of lymphoid tissue around them. Evidence indicates that infection in these glands is the common cause of anal fistula.[9, 11]

PRINCIPLES OF DIAGNOSIS

The steps taken to assess a patient with anorectal disease are essentially the same as those for any other system. These are an accurate history, a careful examination, and the use of special investigations.

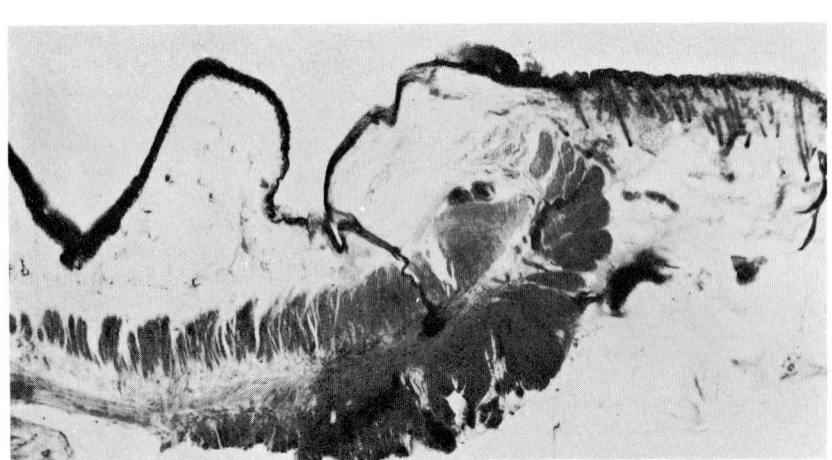

Figure 5. Photograph of a thick section through the anal canal showing an anal gland situated in the plane between the internal and external sphincters. Its duct passes through the internal sphincter and discharges into the anal canal at the base of an anal crypt. (From Hemorrhoidectomy, by Alan G. Parks, in Advances in Surgery, edited by C. E. Welch. Copyright © 1971, Year Book Medical Publishers. Used by permission.)

HISTORY

There are two symptoms that may occur with reference to this region which are of special importance, as they may suggest the presence of neoplastic or inflammatory disease. These symptoms are anorectal bleeding and an alteration in bowel habit. *Anorectal bleeding* is a very common symptom, but only approximately 10 per cent of patients with this symptom have serious bowel disease, the majority of the others having hemorrhoids or an anal fissure. Further inquiry will then give more information as to the time of bleeding (for instance with defecation or on other occasions), the quantity of blood, its site (that is, whether it is merely on the paper or mixed together with the stool), and its character (clotted, dark, or bright red).

To determine whether there has been an *alteration in bowel habit* it is necessary to establish the previous pattern. Careful inquiry will enable the surgeon to understand exactly what a patient means when he complains of diarrhea or constipation. Furthermore, the use of, or any change in the use of laxatives should be noted, as this may indicate a change in bowel function. Other symptoms may include *anal discharge* (purulent or mucoid), *perianal swelling, prolapse, pain, or pruritus* (irritation or soreness).

EXAMINATION

A general assessment of the patient should be made, but the main areas of the examination are the abdomen and lower alimentary tract.

The *abdomen* is carefully examined for the presence of tenderness, a mass which might indicate a carcinoma of the colon, enlargement of the liver, or ascites. At this time the opportunity should be taken to examine the inguinal regions for lymph node enlargement, as this may occur with diseases of the perianal skin or lower anal canal such as a primary chancre or carcinoma.

Prior to the examination of the lower part of the alimentary tract the patient must be suitably placed. The knee-elbow position is perhaps the best for the physician, but it may be an ordeal for the patient. The left lateral position is widely used, since it is more comfortable for the patient, though somewhat less convenient for the doctor. Other positions used include the jack-knife and the lithotomy. Preparation for this examination is, again, the subject of dispute; any interference causes some abnormality of the epithelial appearance, and some reddening of the mucosa with loss of vascular pattern is not uncommon after administration of an enema or evacuant suppository. Mucus also is produced, which may raise unnecessary suspicions of a lesion higher in the colon. However, an empty rectum is much easier to examine. A compromise therefore is to perform a proctoscopy first without preparation; if this is unsatisfactory a repeat examination after administration of a disposable enema will enable satisfactory visualization of the rectum and lower colon.

Inspection

With the aid of good illumination, the perianal area is inspected. It is often not possible to diagnose a suspected fissure without gently parting the folds of perianal skin. Another maneuver which is helpful is to ask the patient to strain as at defecation, as this will enable the diagnosis of the descending perineum syndrome or varying degrees of prolapse to be made.

Palpation

The index finger, covered with a soft thin lubricated fingerstall, first palpates the perianal area to detect any possible induration or tenderness. The anal canal is then examined. In addition to palpating for lumps and induration, some assessment of the muscle tone should be made. Within the rectum attention should be paid to the lumen, the wall, and the extrarectal tissues. The presence of large quantities of feces in the rectum may be responsible for or aggravate some conditions, such as hemorrhoids, and this should therefore be determined so that steps may be taken to correct it.

The rectal wall is carefully palpated for granularity, which may indicate inflammatory disease or proliferative lesions suggestive of neoplastic disease. The extrarectal structures which ought to receive attention are the prostate in the male and the uterus and ovaries in the female.

Proctoscopy

After palpation the proctoscope should be passed if possible to 25 cm. However, if it is not possible to pass this instrument further than the rectosigmoid junction at 15 cm. then it should not be forced, as it may cause the patient unnecessary discomfort and indeed possible damage. Gross lesions such as carcinoma or polyps will be seen with ease. The mucosa is carefully scanned for signs of inflammation. The earliest sign is the loss of the typical pattern of submucosal vessels; this is followed by reddening of the mucosa, granular change, and occasionally frank ulceration. If the mucosa is normal, care is taken to note the presence of blood, mucus, or pus in the lumen, which may indicate the presence of a lesion above reach of the instrument. Finally, any suspicious area should be biopsied so that a precise pathologic diagnosis can be made.

Anoscopy

Finally, the anoscope is passed; this instrument is used to examine the anal canal, but it is of little value in the examination of the rectum. It enables anterior mucosal prolapse, hemorrhoids, anal polyps, and internal openings of fistulas to be seen.

The above clinical assessment should be done without exception in all patients with anorectal symptoms. It is possible to perform these parts of the examination on an ambulant patient.

Special Investigations

Radiology. A plain film of the abdomen is useful for determining the fecal distribution and also if there is any abnormal dilatation of the large intestine. The most commonly performed investigation, though, is a barium enema. This requires careful preparation of the patient to empty the large intestine of fecal matter and, taken with proctoscopy, allows an opinion on the state of the whole large intestine to be made in most patients.

Endoscopy. It is now possible to examine the whole of the large intestine by means of the fiberoptic colonoscope. Not only is this a valuable diagnostic aid, but it can be used to remove polyps from any part of the colon.

Microbiology. Examination of the feces for pathogenic bacteria and parasites is an important part of the assessment of patients with diarrhea. In patients with pruritus a fungus infection may be present and perianal skin scrapings may be examined in the mycology laboratory. In patients with sexually transmitted disease a rectal swab may be examined for gonorrhea, and dark-ground examination of a smear taken from a perianal ulcer may show spirochetes.

Histopathology. The histopathologic examination of a biopsy is a most valuable method in determining the different types of inflammatory bowel disease and is essential in the assessment of patients with neoplastic disease.

Electromyography and Pressure Manometry. The electromyography of the pelvic floor and anal sphincters, together with rectal and anal manometry, will give valuable help in assessing patients with rectal prolapse, incontinence, and certain cases of megacolon.

RECTAL PROLAPSE

A condition caused chiefly by disorder of anorectal physiology is complete rectal prolapse (or procidentia). The rectal wall, including its muscle layer, literally turns inside out like a glove. The rectum prolapses 3 or more inches, its outer surface now being mucus-secreting epithelium. Not only is the presence of the prolapse itself unpleasant, but the mucosa secretes quantities of mucus, which causes soiling and perineal excoriation. At first the prolapse occurs only with defecation and is relatively easily replaced. Later it occurs with any rise of intra-abdominal pressure such as coughing, lifting, and even walking.

The condition occurs most commonly at the extremes of life, in children below the age of 5 and in elderly females. It is occasionally seen from the third decade onward but again almost always in women. In children it usually disappears spontaneously by the age of 5. Why it occurs in this age group is unknown; defecation straining in children can be excessive and this is possibly the cause. Seldom is operative treatment indicated in children; simple bowel training advice is usually sufficient. In adults the most obvious abnormality to be found, apart from the prolapse itself, is laxity of the anal sphincters. Usually, the anal canal gapes because of the lack of sphincter tone, but even if this is not apparent on inspection it can be readily induced by asking the patient to strain. Sphincteric response to voluntary contraction is also poor and may be absent. Seldom, however, is there any frank neurologic defect, and the preponderance of cases in women points to some anatomic cause for the

functional abnormality. However, oddly enough, the condition is commoner in women who have not borne children; it is not possible therefore to ascribe it to birth trauma. The deficient sphincter function leads to a symptom that is the most distressing of all. About two thirds of patients with rectal prolapse are frankly incontinent of feces.[17] They regard themselves as social outcasts and are usually unwilling to leave their homes. This symptom is usually elicited only on direct questioning, as the patient is too ashamed to mention it spontaneously.

Treatment depends on the severity of the symptoms and the age and general condition of the patient. There has been a trend in recent years to perform major surgery at an earlier stage than was previously considered desirable. This is partly because lesser procedures are so often ineffectual, and also because patients tolerate the abdominal repairs very well indeed, no matter how old they may be. The operation performed is one of the several types of abdominal rectopexy currently practiced. Through a lower abdominal incision the rectum is mobilized and some procedure performed that will cause adherence of the rectum to the sacrum, thus preventing it from prolapsing.[6, 19, 23] One effective way of doing this is to surround the rectum partially with polyvinyl sponge. The success rate from the point of view of correction of the prolapse is high and the incidence of incontinence is reduced; even so, one third of the patients will still be incontinent to some degree.

If the patient is such a bad operative risk that an abdominal procedure is considered unjustified, then a local anal operation may be helpful. This usually takes the form of some modification of the Thiersch wire operation. A ring of silver (or nylon) wire is inserted into the tissues around the canal through two small puncture wounds in the perineum, one in front and one behind the anus. The ring is made about 3 cm. in diameter, just large enough to allow the passage of stool but not large enough to allow the prolapse to appear. This is effective provided the patient clears her rectum adequately; if not, fecal impaction rapidly develops. It has no beneficial effect whatsoever on incontinence.

INCONTINENCE

The distressing nature of rectal incontinence has already been emphasized. It is usually found accompanying quite severe degrees of rectal prolapse. However, it occasionally occurs without any obvious degree of prolapse. It has the same female preponderance. In most cases no cause can be found; there is no neurologic defect or evidence of trauma to the sphincter muscles. This idiopathic variety is probably due to stretching of the anal sphincters over many years. In those under 65 years of age it can be treated by a muscle-tightening procedure performed *behind* the anal canal. The levator ani muscles, the puborectalis muscle, and the external sphincter muscles are apposed behind the anorectal junction. The effect of this is to thrust the anal canal forward, to restore the anorectal angle, and to shorten the muscles, making their action more efficient. A more physiologic approach has recently been suggested. Electrodes can be implanted into the muscles themselves and activated by a buried induction coil; or stimulation can be achieved by two electrodes inserted into the anal canal in the form of a plug. Unfortunately, the results of this method in the treatment of idiopathic incontinence have been uniformly disappointing.

Incontinence may be secondary to organic disease or abnormality in the colon or anal canal. A person with a normal pelvic sphincter mechanism may nevertheless lose control if he has severe diarrhea, and this is the state in which many colitic patients find themselves. If there is a mild sphincter weakness, diarrhea may cause frank incontinence. This is a state of affairs quite commonly found in the elderly patient whose pelvic floor muscles have lost their tone and who has diverticulitis in addition. Elimination of the factor causing diarrhea will restore normal continence.

Trauma or abnormality of the sphincters may cause incontinence. In anorectal agenesis the external sphincter muscle is often grossly deficient and such as is left may be inadequate to restore the rectal lumen. Childbirth may result in total severance of the muscle ring anteriorly, causing varying degrees of incontinence. Total section of the sphincters may occur as the result of fistula surgery or direct trauma. Fortunately this situation can be remedied by sphincteroplasty, though a temporary colostomy is required in the process.[13]

IMPACTION OF FECES

This is a condition caused by disordered anorectal physiology. The rectum becomes overloaded and filled with a hard mass of feces that cannot be spontaneously evacuated. It may be secondary to idiopathic megacolon ("lazy colon") which is found in children and young adults. It occurs spontaneously in the aged and may complicate the convalescence after orthopedic, pelvic, or abdominal operations. If a patient has a painful anal fissure, this sometimes results in such an inhibition to defecation that rectal overloading occurs. This tendency is increased if codeine-containing tablets for pain relief are taken. The large fecal mass causes reflex relaxation of the external anal sphincter. Liquid stool passes around the impaction and then leaks out in a totally uncontrolled fashion. The patient will complain of diarrhea and incontinence. Manual disimpaction under anesthesia is often necessary, followed by a brief enema regimen to allow the rectal wall to recover its tone.

PROCTITIS

Proctitis is a general term covering any inflammation in the rectal ampulla. There are four main groups; that due to nonspecific inflammation, that caused by specific organisms, that due to trauma, and that caused by irradiation.

Nonspecific Proctitis

Granular Proctitis. This is the commonest cause of inflammation of the rectal mucosa in Western countries. It is in fact a localized form of ulcerative colitis;

indeed, it is the commonest form of this disease. It is much commoner in women than in men and is one of the most frequent causes of bleeding in women of the third decade.

The usual symptoms are bleeding and the production of mucus; the blood may be coating the stool or mixed with mucus. If the inflammation has spread into the sigmoid colon diarrhea may occur, but in the strictly localized form the patient may even complain of constipation.

The diagnosis can be made only on proctoscopy. The mucosa is granular, bleeds readily on touch, and has lost its pattern of submucosal blood vessels. Mucus and blood can be seen in the rectal lumen. A biopsy of the mucosa should be taken in all cases. Pathologic examination reveals superficial inflammation of the mucosa with the presence of crypt abscesses. Microbiologic investigation is essential in all such cases to eliminate confusion with one of the forms of infective proctitis mentioned below.

This is a cyclic condition, the acute phase lasting a few months, followed by remission of months or years. It is important to explain this to the patient so that he does not become discouraged with the onset of a new attack. Usually the disease gets milder and ceases altogether after some years. However, in a small percentage (5 to 10 per cent) of cases it will occur higher in the colon and may progress to florid ulcerative colitis.

Treatment in the localized form is often not indicated. Explanation of the situation to the patient is enough; the symptoms are so mild that no therapy is needed. When symptoms are more severe, however, they can be readily relieved by oral salicylazosulfapyridine (Azulfidine) and local prednisolone suppositories. Malignant degeneration in this type of the disease is almost unknown.

Granulomatous Proctitis (Crohn's Disease). This form of rectal inflammation is becoming increasingly common, or perhaps it is more frequently being recognized as a distinct entity separate from granular proctitis. It can resemble the latter in every way (except histologically) but usually causes a more patchy inflammation with intervening areas of normal epithelium. Granulomatous infiltration of the submucosa can cause nodular areas readily detectable with the examining finger. Frank ulceration, rather than the diffuse granular change of granular proctitis, is not uncommon. In about 80 per cent of cases there is an associated anal fissure or fistula, a useful diagnostic point. The diagnosis is again established by the proctoscopic appearances and the histologic changes seen on biopsy. Dense lymphocytic infiltration of the submucosa occurs, with occasional giant cell—containing granulomas.

The course of this disease is not such a benign one as that of granular proctitis. Simultaneous occurrence in the ileum and colon is common. The fibrotic changes, so characteristic of granulomatous enteritis, cause narrowing and stenosis of the rectum. Quite severe anal lesions are very likely to coexist with rectal disease. Unlike ulcerative colitis, this is a progressive disease and it is not characterized by long phases of remission.

Treatment is conservative in the first instance and the same regimen is used. If severe stenosis or fistulation occurs, it may be justified to give oral prednisone in adequate doses. Recently, some good reports have appeared on the use of immunosuppressive drugs, but as yet there is conflicting evidence and opinion on the desirability of this mode of therapy. Occasionally the disease can progress to such a degree that excision of the rectum is the only possible course. In any case where excision of the rectum has to be performed for benign disease such as this, it is essential that it be carried out in a manner quite different from excision for carcinoma. The dissection is performed as close to the rectal muscle as possible to avoid damage to other pelvic structures and in particular the nervi erigentes. Failure to observe this precaution in young people (and this disease affects the young predominantly) may lead to severe bladder or sexual dysfunction.

See Section IV of Chapter 33 for more extensive discussion of Crohn's disease.

Infective Proctitis

Amebiasis. This disease usually affects the whole colon in the acute phase but in the chronic state can be localized to the rectum. Acute amebiasis resembles acute ulcerative colitis when seen through a proctoscope, but the chronic situation resembles granulomatous proctitis quite closely. Deep, punched-out ulcers with areas of normal mucosa between them are seen. The diagnosis is made by examining fresh scrapings of the rectal wall under the microscope at about 37° C. Of equal value is histologic examination of biopsy material. This disease must be considered in nonendemic areas or it is liable to be overlooked, with most unfortunate consequences.

Bacillary Infections. Infections of the colon with several of the types of Shigella or Salmonella organisms can produce erythematous changes in the rectum visible on proctoscopy. Microbiologic examination of the stool will confirm this diagnosis.

Gonococcal Proctitis. Infection of the rectum can be either direct or secondary to gynecologic disease. In all phases it is difficult to differentiate it from nonspecific granular proctitis as the rectoscopic appearances are so similar. Symptoms are often minimal, mucous discharge being the commonest. The diagnosis is, however, readily made by bacteriologic examination of rectal mucus, the specimen taken being plunged straight into Stuart's medium.

Lymphopathia Venereum. This disease not infrequently affects the rectum, giving rise to an acute proctitis indistinguishable from that of granular proctitis. Infection usually occurs directly in the male but by transference from the gynecologic tract in the female. In the acute phase diagnosis is difficult unless the possibility is considered. Serologic examination will confirm the presence of the disease. The chronic phase is characterized by the development of a long, indurated stricture. Treatment of this is difficult but should be conservative if possible, repeated bougienage under anesthesia may be necessary. After many years malignant change may supervene.

Traumatic Proctitis

The trauma may be of several kinds. The commonest is that due to repeated prolapse. Proctitis is almost always present in some degree in patients with complete prolapse, but lesser degrees of prolapse also cause it. Some patients regularly evacuate the rectum by digital means, a not uncommon practice, and this causes localized rectal inflammation, usually on the anterior rectal wall. These various factors cause an inflammatory change, often localized to the anterior rectal wall mucosa, which may be so severe as to result in frank ulceration. The lesion so produced is called "solitary ulcer" of the rectum. It is shallow with a yellowish sloughing base. It may be large, up to 5 cm. in diameter. Bleeding and mucous discharge are the usual symptoms. Diagnosis is made on the typical proctoscopic appearance and nonspecific histologic findings.[10] One of the most important aspects of this condition is that it may be mistaken for a carcinoma and an excision of the rectum performed. This latter procedure must never be performed without a positive biopsy for malignancy.

Radiation Proctitis

The rectum and vagina are separated by a few millimeters of areolar tissues. It is not surprising therefore that radium inserted for treatment of carcinoma of the cervix should also affect the rectal mucosa. This it does to varying degrees; in most cases an acute proctitis subsides completely. However, in other cases a chronic inflammation may persist for many years. In these chronic forms stenosis of the rectum is relatively common, as is the development of ulceration on the anterior wall at the level of the cervix. The symptoms produced by these changes are often minimal, bleeding and mucous discharge being the commonest. The differential diagnosis is often difficult, since the bleeding is colonic in type and the possibility of a neoplastic lesion above the rectum must always be borne in mind. The diagnosis is established by the history, proctoscopic appearance, nonspecific histologic appearance, and negative barium enema. Treatment is seldom required; occasionally a stricture requires dilatation or a rectovaginal fistula needs operative intervention, the latter being a difficult but not insuperable problem.

HEMORRHOIDS

The condition generally called hemorrhoids can be divided into three components as follows: abnormal prolapse of upper anal and lower rectal mucosa, venous engorgement in the submucosa of the upper anal canal, and protuberances at the anal margin commonly called skin tags or external hemorrhoids. These can exist independently of each other but all three are usually found together. Some degree of physiologic prolapse of the anal mucosa occurs during normal defecation, and there is partial eversion of the anal canal. Abnormal mucosal prolapse is merely an exaggeration of the normal; why this should happen is unknown. Perhaps it is due to the constipating habits induced by the dietary and physical limitations of our civilization. The first symptom is bleeding; the veins in the submucosa of the prolapsing tissue contain blood at high pressure, as they communicate directly with the abdominal cavity. During prolapse this region is exposed to atmospheric pressure, and the pressure gradient causes bleeding which is characteristically arterial in type. The arterial nature of the venous blood may be due to the presence of arteriovenous fistulas in this region.[22]

In the course of time there is further downward descent of the anal mucosa. Rectal mucosa passes into the anal canal, forcing the squamous mucosa of the lower anal canal downward and outward so that it comes to lie at the anal margin. The columnar, goblet cell mucosa of the upper anal canal is intermittently exteriorized and, owing to the minor trauma it receives, secretes mucus. The mucus is produced below the level of effective sphincter action, so that leakage occurs. Mucous soiling of the perineum causes excoriation of the perianal skin, soreness, and pruritus. Later mucus production may be somewhat diminished by squamous metaplasia which occurs in the columnar mucosa of the upper anal canal as a result of repeated prolapse.

The squamous mucosa of the lower anal canal is forced out altogether, and it forms bulging excrescences which are called either external hemorrhoids or anal skin tags. This is particularly likely to happen in women after delivery. The squamous mucosa is highly sensitive and when exposed can cause considerable soreness and pruritic symptoms. An understanding of the nature of the descent of the anal mucosa in hemorrhoidal change is essential for proper treatment.

In some cases the veins in the submucosa of the upper anal canal become greatly dilated and varicose. In this case bleeding is particularly likely to occur in considerable quantity. The protrusion of the hemorrhoidal tissue into the anal canal exaggerates any tendency to mucosal prolapse as it is forcibly exteriorized during defecation. The prolapsed mass may return spontaneously after defecation or it may require manual replacement. Some patients have an associated laxness of the external sphincters; now large internal hemorrhoids will tend to prolapse with any transitory rise in intra-abdominal pressure such as occurs during coughing or even walking. When this stage has been reached (which is sometimes called third degree hemorrhoidal change) the patient is liable to acute anal discomfort at any time. The prolapsed hemorrhoidal mass causes perineal aching and the mucous discharge previously mentioned. Once this state of affairs has been reached conservative treatment is usually of little avail.

There are two main complications of hemorrhoids, *anemia* due to continued and excessive bleeding and *acute thrombosis*. So uncommon is anemia as the result of hemorrhoidal bleeding that other causes of this condition should be sought, such as carcinoma of the stomach or cecum, before making a firm diagnosis. Thrombosis is a common event and can occur either in the external anal plexus under the squamous mucosa, in the main hemorrhoidal plexus of the submucosa of the upper anal canal, or in both. External anal thrombosis is common and is often seen in patients who have no other stigmata of hemorrhoids. The cause is unknown, but it is possibly due to the high venous pressures that develop during excessive straining efforts and that cause distention and stasis in the veins. The patient notices an acute swelling that may be intensely painful; it is situated at the anal verge. Pain may continue for several days and then gradually subside spontaneously. The swelling itself may take 3 to 4 weeks to disappear. Occasionally the clot wears through the overlying mucosa and is extruded, causing soiling of the clothing with dark clotted blood. Treatment is usually symptomatic only, as the condition clears up in a relatively short while. However, if pain is severe it may be justified to incise the hemorrhoid and enucleate the clot under local anesthesia.

Acute thrombosis of the internal hemorrhoidal plexus is a much more unpleasant situation. The patient experiences sudden severe anal pain followed by protrusion of the thrombosed area. The pain can be extremely severe and may last for as long as a week. Gradually the edema subsides and the thrombus is absorbed. Occasionally this process has a therapeutic effect, entirely relieving the patient of his previous hemorrhoidal symptoms. Treatment is conservative in the first instance, consisting of analgesics to relieve the pain and a mild laxative to avoid constipation. Various local applications are used, but it is doubtful whether any of them have any specific effect. If symptoms continue to be severe after several days have passed, surgical treatment may be considered but this is not a light undertaking. The surgical technique is not particularly difficult despite the presence of the thrombosis, but the postoperative course is more prone to pain and complication than that after an ordinary hemorrhoidectomy.

Conservative Treatment of Hemorrhoids

In many patients hemorrhoidal symptoms can be relieved by attention to hygiene and by avoiding excessive defecation straining. Such is the artificiality of our dietary and other habits that constipation with consequent defecation straining is often the rule rather than the exception. Straining causes descent of the pelvic floor, weakening of the sphincter muscles, and both rectal and gynecologic prolapse. It would seem sensible, therefore, that a person with these tendencies should compensate by taking sufficient fruit and bran in the diet; failing this a hydrophilic laxative taken as often as necessary is usually effective and quite harmless. Injection therapy has been practiced for about 100 years and gives considerable relief for varying periods of time. Many different substances have been used, such as sterilized arachis oil containing a small percentage (5 per cent) of phenol, or a mixture of quinine and urea. The injection is placed in the submucosa of the upper anal canal well above the sensitive squamous mucosa. It is quite simply performed through an anoscope and if properly done gives rise to very little pain. There is no direct effect on the veins themselves, as is commonly thought, but a fibrous tissue reaction is induced in the submucosa of the upper anal canal and lower rectum, thereby drawing the dropped mucosa upward toward its normal site. It is particularly valuable in early cases when it prevents the excessive mucosal prolapse from occurring at defecation and so stops bleeding. It is less successful for the more advanced type of hemorrhoid but even so can be sometimes most helpful in the elderly or others in whom there is a contraindication to operative treatment. More recently another conservative method has been advocated. Each hemorrhoid is visualized through a proctoscope; the upper part above the mucocutaneous line is grasped by an instrument and a small rubber band is slipped over it. A special intrument has been designed to perform this maneuver.[1] The tissue distal to the rubber band undergoes necrosis and excess mucosa in the upper anal canal is removed. The lower anal mucosa is drawn up by the ensuing fibrosis which also causes adherence of the mucosa to the underlying muscle. This method accomplishes its task satisfactorily, but it is associated with pain in some cases and secondary hemorrhage in others. A new form of therapy has come into vogue recently which involves freezing the tissues of the hemorrhoid for a sufficient time to cause necrosis.[8] If carefully used and applied only to the upper part of the hemorrhoidal area at the anorectal junction, it

achieves a similar result to elastic banding but there is no pain associated with it. The effectiveness of this form of cryosurgery is at present being evaluated. Both these methods may well come to occupy a midposition between injection therapy and surgical excision. In the advanced case they do little to correct the anal mucosal descent, nor do they remove the external anal tags that are the result of this descent. They are therefore unlikely to replace surgery for this type of case but may nevertheless be a valuable addition to our conservative armamentarium.

After a time such a degree of permanent mucosal descent of the whole anal mucosa occurs that, coupled with more gross hemorrhoidal protrusion at defecation, it is unlikely that any conservative treatment will be of avail. The aim of surgical correction should be to remove all the vascular hemorrhoidal tissue in the submucosa and to correct the deformities due to mucosal prolapse (Fig. 6). Excision of unwanted tissue must be coupled with a reconstruction of the deformed mucosa of the anal canal. It is highly desirable that

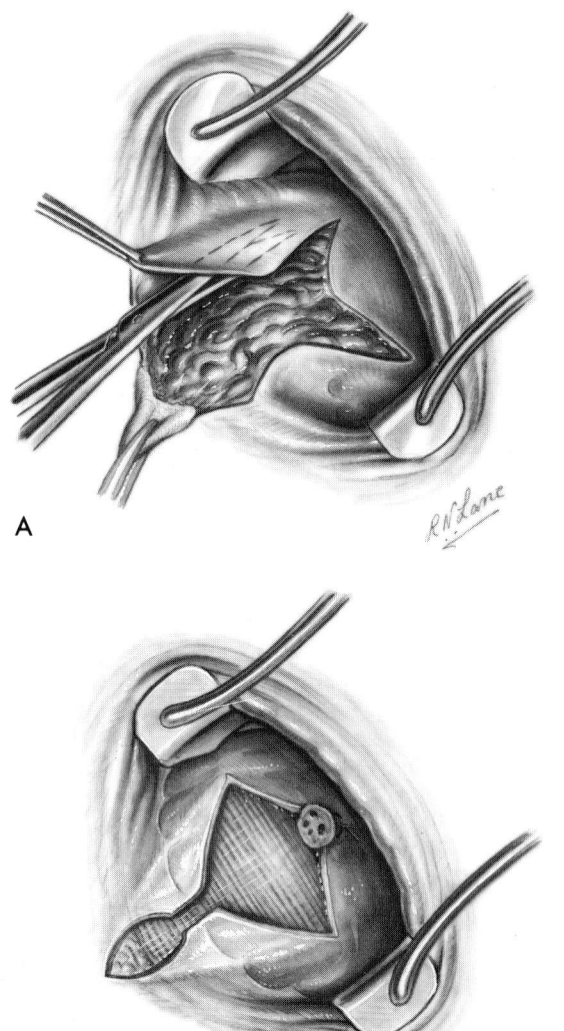

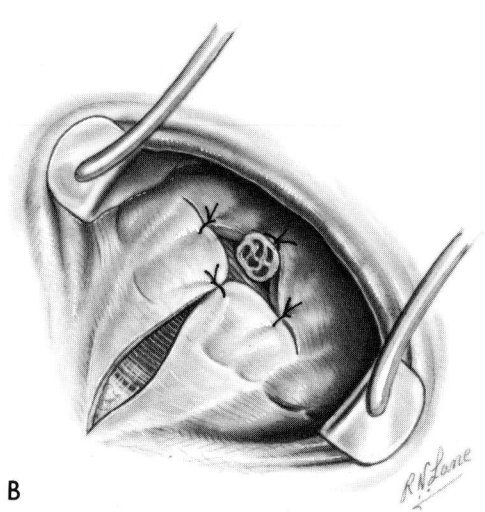

A

B

C

Figure 6. A technique of hemorrhoidectomy. *A,* The mucosa of the anal canal is dissected off the vascular submucosa. The submucosa is then itself stripped off the internal sphincter. *B,* The vascular hemorrhoidal tissue has been removed, leaving the floor of the wound formed by the internal sphincter. The two mucosal flaps are demonstrated. *C,* Mucosal anatomy is reconstituted. Squamous mucosa is fixed at the correct level in the anal canal.

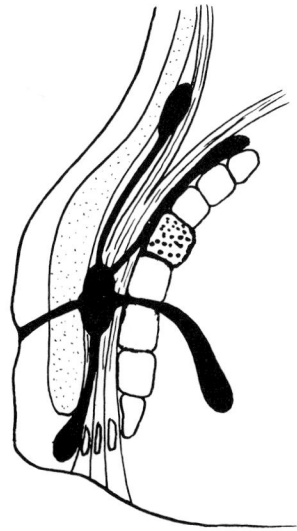

Figure 7. A diagrammatic representation of the various directions in which infection can spread from a primary focus in the intersphincteric plane of the mid anal canal.

the squamous mucosa that has been driven out of the anal margin by mucosal descent should be replaced to its original position. However, in most operative techniques it is excised as unwanted tissue, liable to form tags unless removed in some quantity. This is a major disadvantage of most hemorrhoidectomy techniques, as it leads to the lower anal canals being lined by secondary epithelium that has spread in from the skin edges in the course of healing; it lacks the sensitivity of the original anal squamous mucosa. To avoid this, the prolapsed squamous mucosa of the anal canal can be mobilized and resutured to a point about 2 cm. within the lumen. In this way the canal is lined once more by dry, squamous, highly sensitive epithelium. In order to allow for this advancement it will be necessary to excise some of the upper anal and lower rectal

mucosa that has migrated lower into the anal canal. However, this is no loss, as it is quite insensitive and therefore of no physiologic value, and it is also mucus-secreting, a cause of symptoms if left in the lower anal canal. For details regarding operative techniques standard textbooks of operative surgery should be consulted.[3, 12, 20]

ANORECTAL INFECTION

Abscess and Fistula

The pathogenesis of these two apparently separate conditions is often the same. Infection commences in the intersphincteric plane of the midanal canal, probably in one of the anal glands previously described. From here it can spread, generally speaking, in three directions to give three rather different types of presentation (Fig. 7).

ACUTE PHASE: ABSCESS

Abscesses in this area can be simple or complex, but generally can be classified into one of the following groups.

Intersphincteric Abscess. Infection is very occasionally limited to the primary site. It may be symptomless but it can cause severe, throbbing pain which resembles that of a fissure in that it is initiated by defecation and goes on for many hours afterward. It may be so severe as to prevent sleep. No fissure is present and the diagnosis may be overlooked. Chronic infection may persist in this site to give intermittent anal pain.

Perianal Abscess. Infection here has spread directly downward in the intersphincteric plane to present at the anal margin (Fig. 8). It is seen as a swelling which may be misdiagnosed in the early stages as an external anal thrombosis.

Figure 8. Infection commences in the intersphincteric plane of the mid zone of the anal canal. It passes downward to reach the skin of the anal margin and there forms a perianal abscess. In the chronic phase, seen on the right-hand side of the diagram, it forms an intersphincteric fistula. (From Cooper, P., ed.: Craft of Surgery. 2nd ed. Boston, Little, Brown and Company, 1970.)

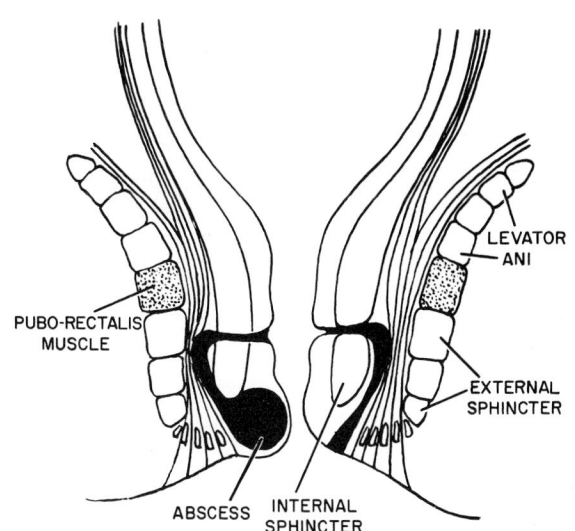

LEVATOR ANI

PUBO-RECTALIS MUSCLE

EXTERNAL SPHINCTER

ABSCESS INTERNAL SPHINCTER

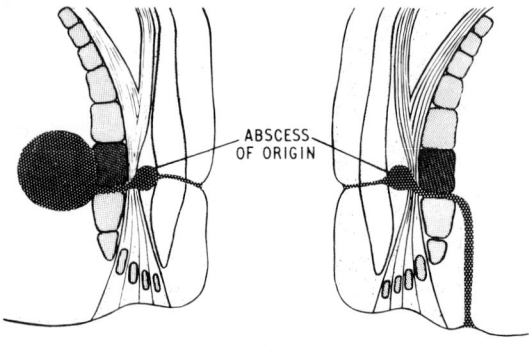

Figure 9. Infection from the mid zone of the anal canal passes through the external sphincter into the ischiorectal fossa. If the infection becomes chronic it will form a transsphincteric fistula (seen on the right-hand side). (From Cooper, P., ed.: Craft of Surgery. 2nd ed. Boston, Little, Brown and Company, 1970).

Ischiorectal Abscess. In this case infection has spread across the external sphincter into the ischiorectal fossa (Fig. 9). Here it may form quite a large abscess extending upward to the top of the fossa as well as downward to the perineal skin. The patient may complain of pain and fever before a swelling is visible. Induration then occurs under the skin over the ischiorectal fossa and finally a typically red fluctuant abscess is seen.

Rectal Wall Abscess. Infection spreads upward in this case, unlike the two previous examples. The patient will experience a vague pelvic pain and will probably have a fever. An abscess can be detected only by a rectal examination, when a tender, boggy swelling is palpable in the rectal wall. If untreated this type will usually discharge into the rectum.

Treatment

The management of abscesses in this area is relatively straightforward: they should all be drained as soon as diagnosed. A perianal abscess needs only a simple incision; an ischiorectal abscess will often require removal of a circle of skin over the ischiorectal fossa to give it adequate drainage. As it may extend quite high in the fat of the fossa and also may spread circumferentially, it is wise to explore the cavity digitally and breakdown any locules that may be present, but great care must be exercised.

Chronic Phase: Fistula in Ano

A fistula is by definition an abnormal communication between any two epithelial surfaces. Fistula in ano is indeed such a communication but the situation is not quite a straightforward one. The external opening of the fistula onto the perineal skin is a sinus leading down to a small chronic abscess in the intersphincteric plane. However, this abscess is usually due to infection in an anal gland or the surrounding lymphoid tissue, and only a minute duct communicates between it and the anal canal at the level of the mucocutaneous junction (see Fig. 5). In about half the cases the intersphincteric abscess discharges into the anal canal also, so that there is now a larger sinus entering the canal.

Clinical Presentation

Fistula may present as an acute abscess or in a number of less dramatic ways. The patient may notice a small discharging sinus and the discharge from the sinus may cause skin excoriation and pruritus.

On examination subcutaneous induration can often be traced from the external opening to the anal margin, and this is indicative of an underlying track. On digital examination there may be a nodule palpable in the wall of the anal canal which gives away the site of the primary abscess. A probe is classically used in the diagnosis of fistula, but it can be a dangerous instrument in inexperienced hands. It is possible to create false openings into the anal canal or even into the rectum by injudicious probing. A probe passed into the external sinus will usually demonstrate the site in the anal canal where the fistula is coming from. If there is an internal opening of reasonable size then the probe will pass into the canal itself. Under no circumstances should force be used in this maneuver as false tracks may result.

The Anatomy of Fistula

The path that fistulas follow is largely determined by the anatomy of the region. They tend to run in fascial or fatty planes, the most usual being the intersphincteric plane between the two groups of sphincters, and the fat of the ischiorectal fossa. In most cases the arrangement is a straightforward one, the track passing directly to the perineal skin. However, much more complex situations occasionally occur. In particular, circumferential spread is not uncommon; this usually occurs in the ischiorectal fossa and the track may pass from one fossa to the other behind the rectum, constituting what is known as a horseshoe fistula.

The classic treatment of fistula in ano consists of passing a probe through it and then cutting down onto it with a knife, dividing all the tissue below the probe. In this way the fistula track is thrown open into the anal canal. It will be readily appreciated that this may involve cutting a significant amount of sphincter muscle in certain cases. A knowledge of the course taken by these tracks is essential for the surgeon; without this he may divide too much of the sphincter mass and render the patient incontinent. It is therefore highly desirable to know the general pattern that fistulas may pursue.

From the chronic intersphincteric abscess in the midanal canal, infection can spread in a number of directions.[21] In practice it is usually found to conform to one of four main anatomic types, which will now be briefly considered (Fig. 10).

Intersphincteric Fistula. This is by far the most common type, constituting about 70 per cent of all cases. The infection passes directly downward to the anal margin (see Fig. 8). There are some less common and more complicated variants of this fistula; for instance, a track may pass upward into the rectal wall and discharge into the rectal ampulla. This high intersphincteric fistula, frequently and erroneously called a submucous fistula, may cause intermittent rectal wall abscesses but is still quite easy to treat.

Transsphincteric Fistula. In this type the track crosses the external sphincter and enters the ischiorectal fossa en route to the skin (see Fig. 9). If it passes through musle at a low level it is an easy situation to treat. However, it may pass through the upper part of the sphincter mass and constitute a more difficult therapeutic problem. A further complication of this type of fistula is the presence of a high extension in the ischiorectal fossa. The fistula is now the shape of a T on its side and the high extension causes induration which can be felt on digital examination through the rectal wall. A probe passes directly into the high extension and thus may mislead the surgeon into thinking that the fistula has a much higher connection with the rectum itself. Overenthusiastic probing may produce an artificial connection between the high part of the fistula and the rectum, with disastrous results for the patient. Transphincteric fistulas constitute about 25 per cent of all fistulas and are, generally speaking, not difficult to treat.

Suprasphincteric Fistula. The remaining 5 per cent of fistulas are made up of two rare types in which treatment is difficult, and hazardous when done by the in-experienced. The first of these is called a suprasphincteric fistula because the track passes first upward in the intersphincteric plane, then laterally over the top of the puborectalis muscle, and finally downward into the ischiorectal fossa to the skin (see Fig. 10, 3). It passes above all the muscles of continence before pursuing a downward course to the perineal skin. Clearly, division of all the external sphincter muscles will make the patient incontinent, so that this fistula constitutes a therapeutic challenge. This fistula may also have a high extension but this time it is in the pelvis and runs pararectally. It produces high induration that can be felt per rectum.

Extrasphincteric Fistula. The final type is fortunately the rarest and constitutes perhaps 1 per cent of all fistulas. It passes from the skin of the perineum up through the ischiorectal fat, through the levator ani muscles, and then communicates with the rectum (see Fig. 10, 4). The track of this fistula passes outside all the muscles of continence. It is therefore called extrasphincteric. If treated in the classic manner, incontinence would be inevitable. There are a variety of causes, some of them gross disease such as Crohn's disease or carcinoma. Trauma, either direct external or internal, as for example a swallowed fish bone penetrating the rectal wall, is another cause. Then there is the type already mentioned, a transsphincteric fistula with a high extension passing upward that may burst spontaneously into the rectum or a communication forcibly produced by exuberant probing. Whatever the cause, this type of fistula has an additional cause for its persistence: high rectal pressures cause mucus and feces to enter into the internal opening. Treatment entails abolishing these pressure changes by means of a temporary colostomy. Whatever the cause of extrasphincteric fistula, treatment is difficult and usually a long, drawn-out affair lasting several months.

Horseshoe Fistula. Another mode of extension of fistula is in the circumferential plane. A transsphincteric fistula penetrates the external sphincter,

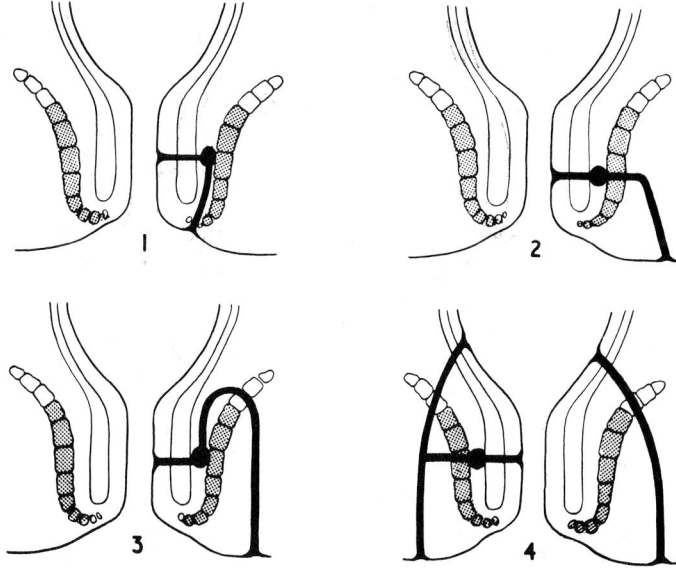

Figure 10. Illustration to show the four main types of fistula: (*1*) intersphincteric, (*2*) trans-sphincteric, (*3*) suprasphincteric, and (*4*) extrasphincteric. It will be seen that the important factor in each case is the relationship of the track to the external sphincter muscles, which are shaded. The uppermost shaded portion is the puborectalis muscle. (From Cooper, P., ed.: Craft of Surgery. 2nd ed. Boston, Little, Brown and Company, 1970.)

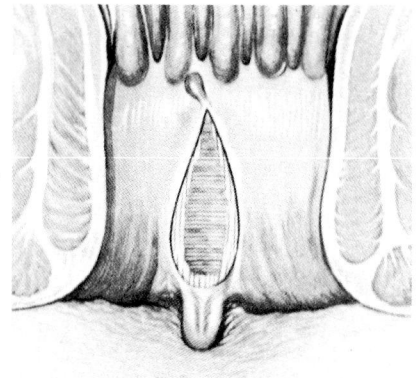

Figure 11. The typical appearance of a posterior fissure-in-ano showing the sentinel tag and the circular muscle fibers in the floor of the ulcer. (From Morgan, C. N., and Thompson, H. R.: Ann R. Coll. Surg. Engl., *19*:88, 1956.)

usually in the posterior position, and then spreads into both ischiorectal fossae. These extensions are, in fact, less difficult to treat than might appear, though quite a large wound may be necessary to drain them.

Treatment

The general principles of treatment are the same for all but the rarest extrasphincteric fistula. The primary source of the fistula in the intersphincteric plane must be opened and given free drainage; this applies to a chronic intersphincteric abscess as well as to the difficult suprasphincteric fistula. Secondly, the ramifications in the ischiorectal fossa (and sometimes above) must be given free drainage. These aims are usually achieved by the ancient method known as the lay-open. A probe is passed through the external sinus, along the tract, and finally on through the internal opening. All structures below this are divided, including muscle. The muscle retracts, leaving a guttered wound which is packed and allowed to heal from the edges. This simple maneuver will deal satisfactorily with 80 per cent of fistulas. The remainder require more sophisticated techniques that depend on the same basic principles but enable part of the sphincter mass to be conserved.

ANAL FISSURE

The squamous mucosa of the lower half of the anal canal is prone to superficial ulceration, which presents clinically as an anal fissure. It is a linear ulcer, usually situated in the posterior commissure of the canal (Fig. 11). Because it involves the highly sensitive squamous epithelium it is often a painful condition. With each act of defecation the ulcer is stretched, causing pain which may last several hours and also bleeding which is characteristically anal in type. The natural sequel of anal pain is for the patient to avoid defecation, with

the resultant formation of a hard, constipated stool. When the event can be delayed no longer, pain may be excruciating. The condition tends to be cyclic, pain lasting for 1 to 2 months followed by a remission. Should the patient become constipated the healed fissure will split open and another episode is initiated. Though the cause of fissure is unknown, once it has occurred it is readily reactivated by constipation. It is very common in women just before and after childbirth and is frequently misdiagnosed as hemorrhoids at this time. Oddly enough, over one third of all patients with Crohn's disease have an anal fissure, though the latter is far too common for this disease to be responsible in more than a small fraction of cases.

Patients learn to keep the stool soft by the use of laxatives but this, coupled with the fibrous tissue response to the ulceration, results in a contracted anal canal. The internal sphincter ring becomes narrower than normal and the submucosa infiltrated with scar tissue. Return to an even normally formed stool may cause immediate recurrence of the condition. It is not uncommon for patients to take laxatives regularly for 20 or more years before seeking advice; yet the situation is susceptible to rapid and complete cure.

The history of pain during and after defecation is typical. On examination the fissure can usually be seen situated posteriorly (see Fig. 11). There may be a skin tag protruding from the anal margin, the so-called *sentinel pile*. The fissure is usually situated just within the anus and may be overlooked; it can readily be revealed by traction on the anal skin that partially everts the canal. Pain may cause an exaggerated anal reflex so that any attempt at digital examination is impossible because of intense external sphincter spasm. Rectal examination is usually possible, however, and the fissure can again be detected by local tenderness.

There are several important conditions to bear in mind in the differential diagnosis. Crohn's disease will cause a fissure exactly like the nonspecific variety; other symptoms will alert one to the possibility. Primary syphilis may cause a fissure-like lesion, but it does not have the same predilection for the commissures and is often laterally situated. The inguinal lymph nodes are usually enlarged. Carcinoma of the anal canal sometimes causes symptoms entirely compatible with fissure and indeed in the early stages may give the same appearance on examination. It is a useful axiom to be suspicious of any fissure-like lesion that is not in the posterior or anterior commissure or that does not rapidly respond to therapy.

Treatment is usually entirely satisfactory. In about two-thirds of the cases the fissure will heal with conservative measures, the remainder requiring a minor surgical procedure for cure. There are many types of local treatment. A local anesthetic application will diminish pain, and abolish the exaggerated anal reflex. Healing is even more rapid if the anesthetic is combined with a steroid. Avoidance of constipation by the use of a bland laxative is essential. If these measures fail, stretching of the anal sphincter ring under anesthesia will cure 85 per cent permanently. Even more effective is the division of the lower half of the internal sphincter.[4, 7, 18] Either of these maneuvers causes enlargement of the lower anal canal and eliminates defecation trauma.

PERIANAL DISORDERS

There are a number of conditions that affect the perianal skin which should be borne in mind when assessing patients with anorectal symptoms. The most common symptoms are of itching (pruritus) or soreness in the region, but other symptoms outlined previously may occur.

Infections

Bacterial. Although most septic conditions occurring in this region are in association with fistula in ano or pilonidal infection, occasionally a simple staphylococcal boil may occur. There is another infection which affects the perianal skin ducts, *Corynebacteria minutissimum,* and which is called erythrasma. This can be readily diagnosed by the salmon-pink fluorescence in ultraviolet light and is treated with erythromycin.

The apocrine sweat glands of the area may be involved in an inflammatory process which is probably bacterial, known as hidradenitis suppurativa. This produces a purulent discharge and the treatment is essentially operative. The infected areas are laid open and allowed to heal by second intention. If there is extensive involvement, the skin may have to be excised and the defect covered with a split skin graft.

Infection with *Treponema pallidum* (syphillis) may result in a chancre or in condylomata lata. The former should always be considered when a fissure in ano is diagnosed, and the latter when viral condylomata accuminata are being considered.

Fungal. Fungal infection of the perianal skin occurs in association with diabetes mellitus, the use of oral antibiotics, the use of perianal topical steroids, or a mucus leak from the anus.

It is diagnosed by direct examination of a smear of perianal skin scrapings or by culture. Treatment is directed to some predisposing condition, such as hemorrhoids if present, and an appropriate antifungal application.

Viral. Perianal warts (condylomata accuminata) are caused by the papova virus and may cover the perianal skin extensively. They may also be present on the male external genitalia and on the vulva, vagina, and cervix. In addition, warts may be present in the anal canal and even in the lower rectum. While a proportion of patients may practice anal intercourse, this is by no means the rule. When a few perianal warts are present the local application of podophyllin is usually effective, but when the warts are extensive both in the perianal area and in the anal canal excisional treatment under general anesthesia is required. These warts are probably sexually transmitted and so other forms of sexually transmitted disease should be excluded.

Parasitic. Patients with a threadworm infestation of the gastrointestinal tract may complain of pruritus; it can be treated with piperazine.

Neoplasms

The most usual neoplasm to occur in the perianal region is a squamous cell carcinoma. This may occur in association with leukoplakia or Bowen's disease. Other tumors include basal cell carcinoma, melanoma, and Paget's disease. In order to establish the appropriate diagnoses, a biopsy is required.

Miscellaneous

There are a variety of other disorders that may occur, and these include psoriasis, contact dermatitis, lichen sclerosis, and multiple small sebaceous cysts.

Pruritus

This is a symptom which may be caused by any of the disorders previously mentioned, by poor hygiene, or as the result of certain anorectal conditions such as hemorrhoids, fissure, anal polyps, proctitis, rectal prolapse, and neoplasms. The investigation of a patient with pruritus should follow the usual pattern with a thorough examination of the perianal skin, anal canal, and rectum with a proctoscope. The special investigations performed might include (a) urine testing for glycosuria; (b) perianal skin scrapings for mycological examination. These should be taken before lubricant is placed on the skin; (c) examination of the perianal skin under ultraviolet light; and (d) biopsy.

Treatment consists of dealing with any underlying or aggravating cause. However, in a large proportion of patients the situation can be relieved by simple attention to anal hygiene. This involves not only cleanliness but the avoidance of rubbing and scratching. It is virtually impossible to cure a patient who persists in the latter habits.

REFERENCES

1. Barron, J.: Office ligation of internal hemorrhoids. Am. J. Surg., *105*:563, 1963.
2. Chiari, H.: Ueber die analen Divertikel der Rectumsschleimhaut und ihre Beziehung zu den Analfistelen. Med. Jahrb., Wein, 1878, pp. 419–427.
3. Duthie, H. L., and Gairns, F. W.: Sensory nerve endings and sensation in the anal region of man. Br. J. Surg., *47*:585, 1960.
4. Eisenhammer, S.: Internal anal sphincter: Its surgical importance. S. Afr. Med. J., *27*:266, 1953.
5. Floyd, W. F., and Walls, E. W.: Electromyography of the sphincter ani externus in man. J. Physiol., *122*:599, 1953.
6. Graham, R. R.: The operative repair of massive rectal prolapse. Ann. Surg., *115*:1007, 1942.
7. Hoffman, D. C., and Goligher, J. C.: Lateral subcutaneous internal sphincterotomy in treatment of anal fissure. Br. Med. J., *3*:673, 1970.
8. Lewis, M. D.: Cryosurgical hemorrhoidectomy. Dis. Colon Rectum, *15*:128, 1972.
9. Lilius, H. G.: Fistula-in-ano. An investigation on human foetal anal ducts and intramuscular glands and a study on 150 patients. Acta Chir. Scand., Supp. 383, 1968.
10. Madigan, M. R., and Morson, B. C.: Solitary ulcer of the rectum. Gut, *10*:871, 1969.
11. Parks, A. G.: Pathogenesis and treatment of fistula-in-ano. Br. Med. J., *1*:463, 1961.
12. Parks, A. G.: Hemorrhoidectomy. *In* Welch, C. E. (Ed.): Advances in Surgery. Chicago, Year Book Medical Publishers, 1971.
13. Parks, A. G., and McPartlin, J. F.: Proc. R. Soc. Med., *64*:1187, 1971.
14. Parks, A. G., Porter, N. H., and Hardcastle, J. D.: The syndrome of the descending perineum. Proc. R. Soc. Med., *59*:477, 1966.
15. Parks, A. G., Porter, N. H., and Melzak, J.: Experimental study of

the reflex mechanism controlling the muscles of the pelvic floor. Dis. Colon Rectum, 5:407, 1962.

16. Phillips, S. F., and Edwards, D. A. W.: Some aspects of anal continence and defecation. Gut, 6:396, 1965.

17. Porter, N. H.: A physiological study of the pelvic floor in rectal prolapse. Ann. R. Coll. Surg. Engl., 31:379, 1962.

18. Ray, J. E., Penfold, J. C. B., Gathright, J. B., and Roberson, S. H.: Lateral subcutaneous internal anal sphincterotomy for anal fissure. Dis. Colon Rectum, 17:139, 1974.

19. Ripstein, C. B.: Surgical care of massive rectal prolapse. Dis. Colon Rectum, 8:34, 1965.

20. Shackelford, R. T.: Hemorrhoids and their surgical treatment. In Turell, R. (Ed.): Diseases of the Colon and Anorectum, 2nd ed. Philadelphia, W. B. Saunders Company, 1969.

21. Stelzner, F.: Hemorrhoids and other diseases of the corpus cavernosum recti and the anal canal. German Med. Monthly, 8:177, 1963.

22. Stelzer, F., Staubesand, J., and Machleidt, H.: Das Corpus Cavernosum rect—die Grundlage der inneren Hamorrhoiden. Langenbecks Arch. Klin. Chir., 299:302, 1962.

23. Wells, C. A.: Polyvinyl alcohol sponge prosthesis. Proc. R. Soc. Med., 55:1083, 1962.

35

THE LIVER

Marshall J. Orloff, M.D.

ANATOMY

Embryology

The liver arises from the entoderm of the foregut and the mesoderm of the septum transversum (Fig. 1). In the 2.5-mm. embryo, approximately 4 weeks old, a diverticulum develops from the ventral floor of the foregut at the level of the future duodenum and extends into the septum transversum in close association with a capillary plexus that connects to the vitelline veins from the yolk sac. The caudal portion of the diverticulum develops into the cystic duct and gallbladder, and the cranial portion becomes the liver. In the early embryo, the two vitelline veins pass through the hepatic anlage to enter the sinus venosus of the heart in conjunction with the paired umbilical veins from the placenta. At a later stage, the vitelline veins form the portal vein and the hepatic veins, whereas the left umbilical vein becomes the ductus venosus which largely bypasses the liver and shunts oxygenated placental blood directly into the inferior vena cava. At birth, the ductus venosus closes and along with the re-

mainder of the obliterated left umbilical vein becomes the ligamentum venosum and its continuation, the ligamentum teres hepatis, in the caudal free border of the falciform ligament, which connects the liver to the umbilicus and anterior body wall. In the adult, it is possible to catheterize the portal vein for diagnostic studies by surgically reopening the obliterated left umbilical vein through a small incision adjacent to the umbilicus. The other ligamentous attachments of the liver are derived from the two layers of the ventral mesentery between which the hepatic anlage develops. Table 1 shows the adult structures derived from the embryonic blood vessels and mesentery.

Microscopic Anatomy

The liver is covered by a thick capsule of collagen and elastic tissue, called Glisson's capsule, which extends into the parenchyma along the blood vessels and bile ducts. The capsule encases a spongelike mass of cells arranged in plates through which passes an intricate system of capillaries called sinusoids (Fig. 2). The sinusoids differ from ordinary capil-

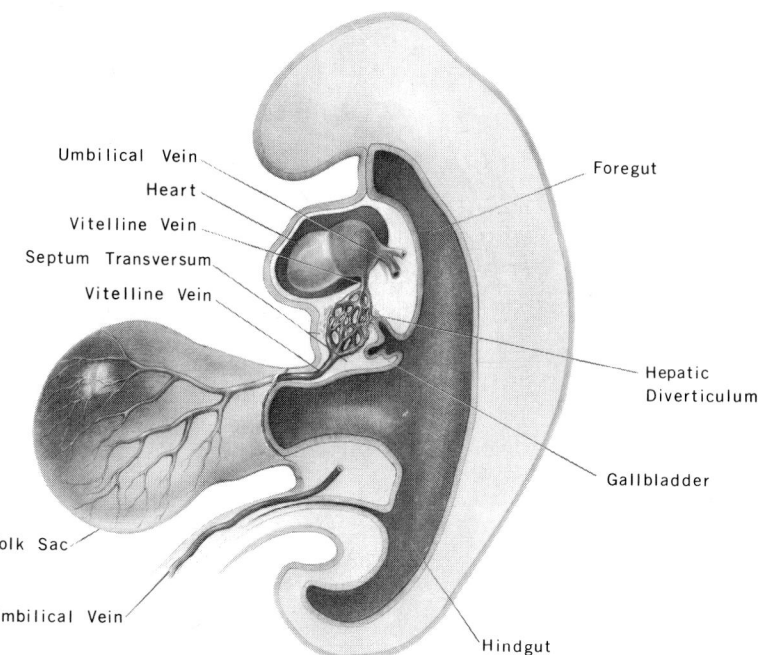

Figure 1. Embryology of the liver shown in an embryo of approximately 4 mm.

Umbilical Vein

Heart

Vitelline Vein

Septum Transversum

Vitelline Vein

Foregut

Hepatic Diverticulum

Gallbladder

Yolk Sac

Umbilical Vein

Hindgut

TABLE 1. Adult Liver Structures Derived from Embryonic Blood Vessels and Mesentery

Embryo	Adult
Right and left vitelline veins	Portal vein Hepatic veins
Left umbilical vein, ductus venosus	Ligamentum venosum and ligamentum teres hepatis
Anterior portion of ventral mesentery	Falciform ligament Right and left anterior coronary ligaments Right and left triangular ligaments
Posterior portion of ventral mesentery	Gastrohepatic ligament Hepatoduodenal ligament Right and left posterior coronary ligaments Right and left triangular ligaments

laries in that their endothelial lining is made up of specialized phagocytic cells, the *Kupffer cells,* and they are more permeable to macromolecules than are systemic capillaries. The liver cell plates are one cell thick and have an intimate association with the sinusoids to facilitate maximal exchange of nutrients and products of metabolism. On microscopic examination the hepatic parenchyma appears to be distributed in poorly defined lobules (Fig. 3). At the center of each lobule is a central vein, a tributary of the hepatic venous outflow system that carries blood from the liver toward the heart. The central veins drain into progressively enlarging sublobular veins and intrahepatic veins until connections are made with the major hepatic veins that enter the inferior vena cava. At the periphery, between several lobules, is a collection of connective tissue called a portal tract or triad which contains branches of the portal veins, the hepatic artery, and the bile duct (Fig. 3). The branches of both the portal vein and hepatic artery empty directly into the sinusoids after a series of divisions and ramifications. In addition, the branches of the hepatic artery nourish the structures in the portal tracts. The bile duct system originates as fine bile canaliculi located between the hepatic cells and forming a part of the cell membrane. Bile is secreted by the hepatocytes into the canaliculi. These bile capillaries drain into intralobular ductules and then into large bile ducts in the portal tracts.

Gross Anatomy

Topography. The liver is the largest organ in the body with a weight of from 1200 to 1600 gm. It occupies the right hypochondrium and much of the epigastrium and extends into the left hypochondrium. Its superior surface conforms to the under surface of the diaphragm and its inferior surface rests on the viscera in the upper abdomen. It is held in position mainly by intra-abdominal pressure. Except in the epigastrium, the organ is largely surrounded by the thoracic cage and in normal subjects usually cannot be palpated on physical examination. When the body is supine, the upper border of the liver is located between the levels of the fourth and fifth ribs anteriorly on the right, and at the level of the sixth rib anteriorly on the left. In the midaxillary line, the right lobe of the liver is covered by lung, pleura, and diaphragm down to the level of the eighth rib (dullness to percussion), and by the pleura and diaphragm alone between the eighth and tenth ribs (flatness to percussion). The under surface of the liver is in contact with the duodenum, colon, kidney, and adrenal gland on the right, and with the esophagus and stomach on the left (see Fig. 5). The liver is covered by peritoneum except for an area on the posterior superior surface adjacent to the inferior vena cava which is in direct contact with the diaphragm and is called the bare area.

Ligaments. The peritoneal reflections from the anterior ab-

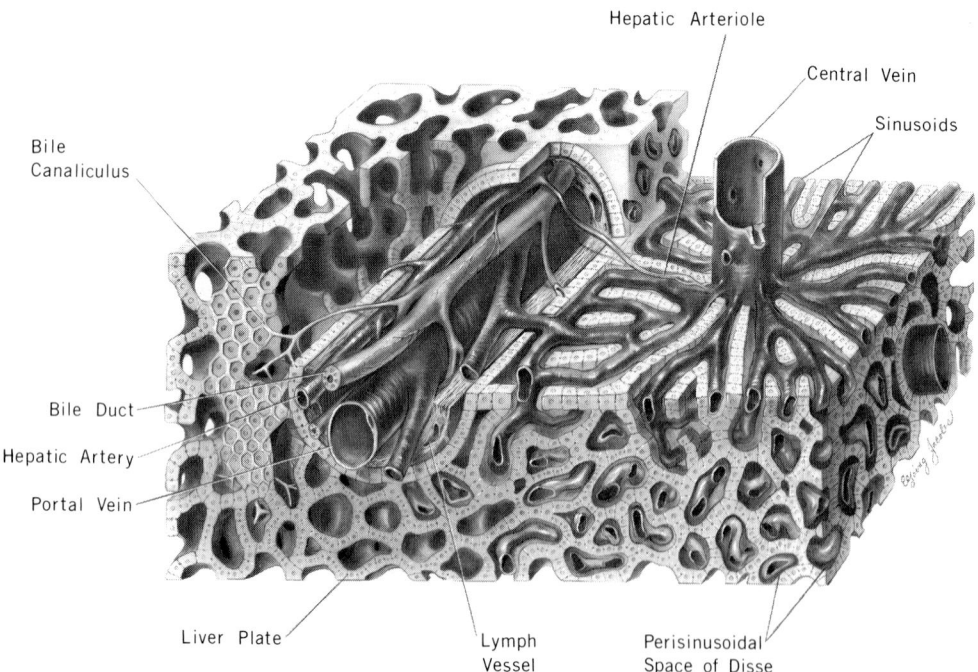

Figure 2.   Three-dimensional model of liver. (After Elias, H., and Sherrick, J. C.: Morphology of the Liver. New York, Academic Press, 1969.)

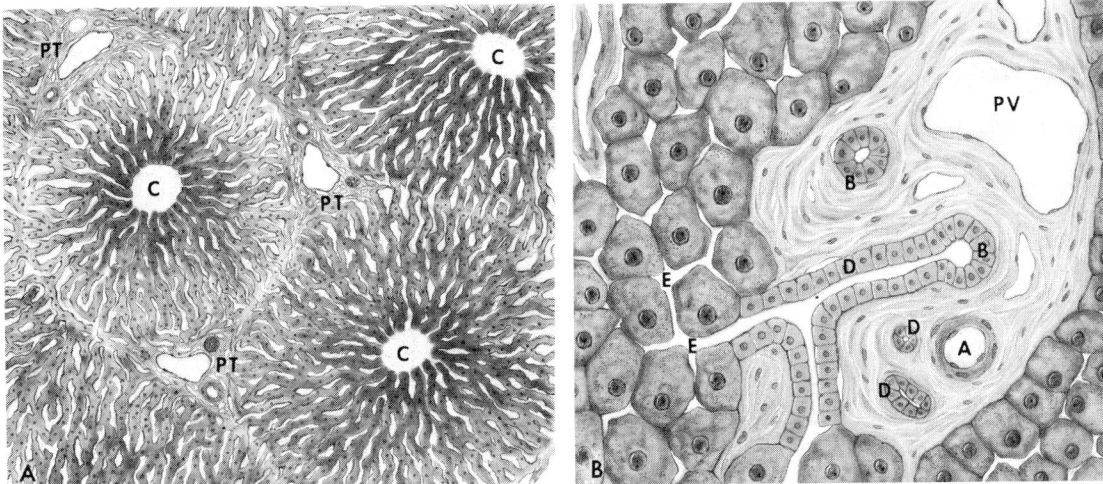

Figure 3. Microscopic appearance of normal liver, showing (*A*) lobular pattern and (*B*) components of portal triad. A, Hepatic artery; B, bile duct; C, central vein; D, bile ductule; E, bile canaliculi; PT, portal triad; PV, portal vein.

dominal wall, diaphragm, and abdominal viscera to the liver form 10 distinct ligaments (Fig. 4). These are:

1. The falciform ligament, which attaches the liver to the anterior abdominal wall between the diaphragm and umbilicus.

2. The ligamentum teres hepatis, which occupies the lower free border of the falciform ligament and represents the obliterated left umbilical vein.

3 and 4. The gastrohepatic ligament and hepatoduodenal ligament, which are the portions of the lesser omentum extending to the liver from the lesser curvature of the stomach and the proximal duodenum. These ligaments contain the hepatic artery, portal vein, and common bile duct. The hepatoduodenal ligament forms the anterior boundary of the epiploic foramen of Winslow.

5, 6, 7, and 8. The right and left anterior coronary ligaments and the right and left posterior coronary ligaments, which represent the peritoneal reflections from the diaphragm onto the liver.

9 and 10. The right and left triangular ligaments, which are produced by fusion of the anterior and posterior coronary ligaments at the right and left lateral borders of the liver.

Lobes and Segments. The falciform ligament divides the liver topographically, but not anatomically or functionally, into a large right lobe and a smaller left lobe. In addition, on the visceral surface several fissures and fossae arranged in the shape of an H demarcate two additional small lobes, the quadrate and caudate. The cross-bar of the H is the porta hepatis in which are found the hepatic artery, portal vein, bile duct branches, lymphatics, nerves, and attachment of the

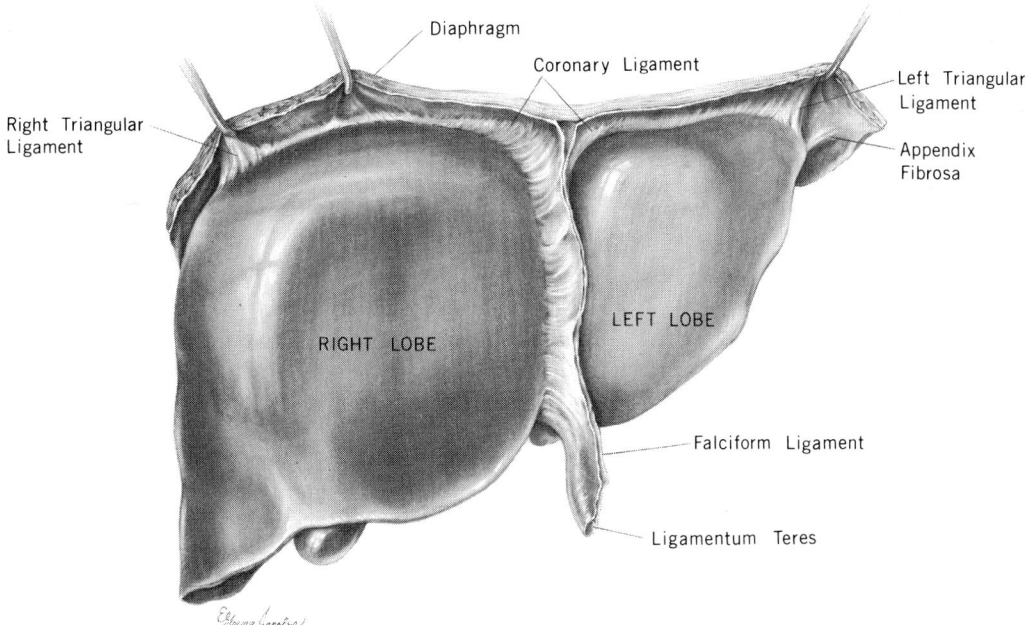

Figure 4. Ligaments of the liver.

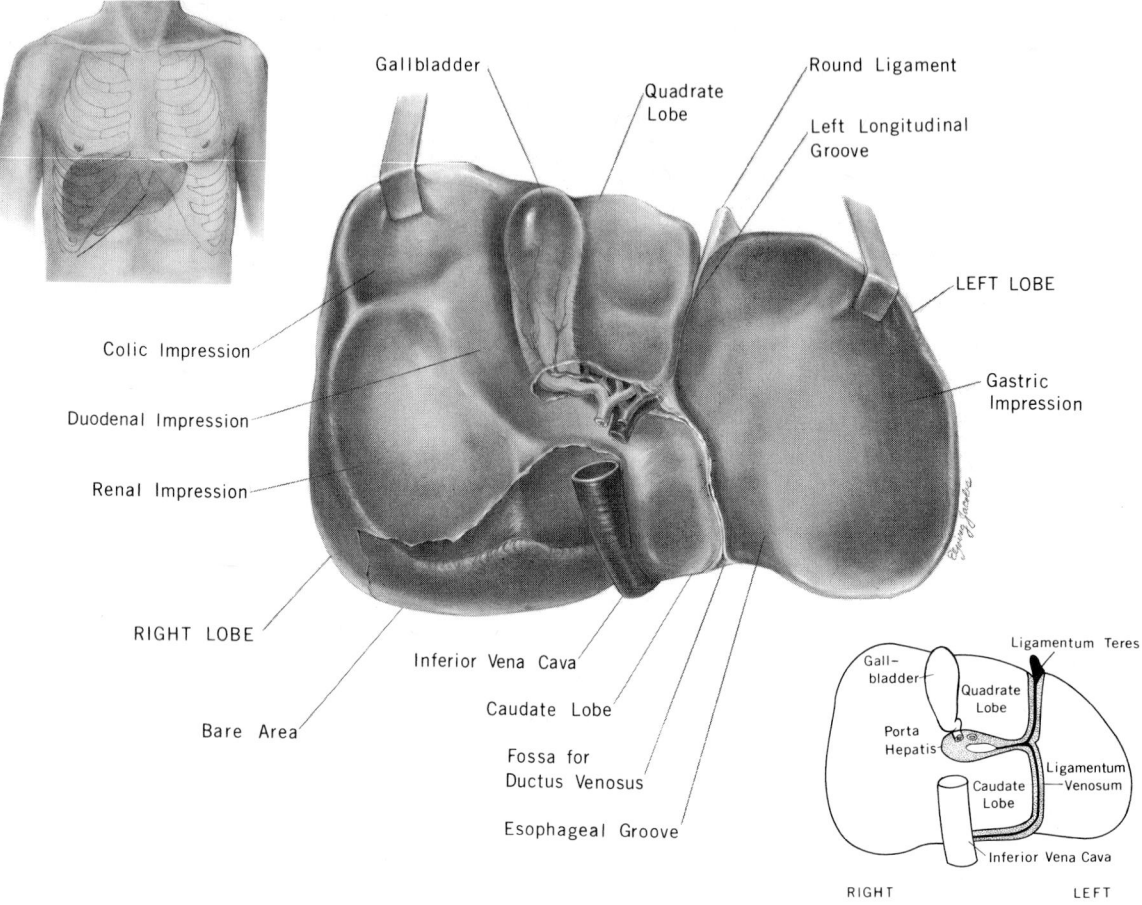

Figure 5. Topographic lobes and impressions of the liver.

lesser omentum (Fig. 5). Recent interest in and success with resection of portions of the liver have served to re-emphasize the fact that the classic topographic division of the liver into right and left lobes is not anatomically or functionally correct. The liver is similar to the lung in that it can be divided into anatomic segments on the basis of the pattern of branching of the hepatic artery, portal vein, and bile duct (Fig. 6). Accordingly, the true anatomic left lobe consists of a medial segment that lies to the right of the falciform ligament and a lateral segment made up of the classic topographic left lobe. The topographic quadrate lobe is part of the anatomic left lobe. The true anatomic right lobe consists of anterior and posterior segments. The line of division between the anatomic right and left lobes is not marked on the surface but follows a line from the gallbladder fossa below to the inferior vena cava fossa above. The topographic caudate lobe is divided, according to its blood supply and bile duct drainage, between the anatomic right and left lobes. The hepatic veins have an interlobar distribution between the liver segments.

Blood Supply, Lymphatics, and Nerves. The liver is unique among the abdominal viscera in having a dual blood supply. The common hepatic artery arises from the celiac axis along with the left gastric artery and splenic artery, and courses to the liver in the lesser omentum to the left of the common bile duct and anterior to the portal vein (Fig. 7). It gives off three major branches, the gastroduodenal artery, supraduodenal artery, and right gastric artery, after which it divides into a right and left ramus. The right ramus passes behind the com-

mon hepatic duct and gives off the cystic artery before entering the liver. In over 40 per cent of subjects, variations from the classic pattern occur (Fig. 8). The surgeon must be aware of these variations if he is to avoid serious operative accidents.

The valveless portal vein carries blood to the liver from the stomach, small intestine, large intestine, pancreas, and spleen. It is formed from the junction of the superior mesenteric vein and splenic vein behind the head of the pancreas, and passes posterior to the first part of the duodenum, through the hepatoduodenal ligament, to the porta hepatis where it divides into right and left branches. The hepatic artery and common bile duct lie anterior to it. The inferior mesenteric vein usually drains into the splenic vein. The tributaries of the portal vein connect with the systemic venous system in several areas (Fig. 9). In normal subjects these communications are of little importance, but in patients with portal hypertension they may assume great clinical significance. Portal-systemic anastomoses occur at the following sites:

1. The left gastric (coronary) vein, a tributary of the portal vein, connects with the esophageal plexus of veins and, in turn, with the azygos vein, hemiazygos vein, and other tributaries of the superior vena cava. Esophageal varices develop in the esophageal plexus as a result of portal hypertension.

2. The short gastric veins and left gastroepiploic vein, tributaries of the splenic vein, connect with the esophageal plexus.

3. The paraumbilical veins, tributaries of the portal vein, and occasionally a persistent umbilical vein anastomose with the inferior and superior epigastric veins of the systemic system. These connections are the site of the caput medusae and the Cruveilhier-Baumgarten syndrome in patients with portal hypertension.

4. The superior hemorrhoidal vein, a tributory of the inferior mesenteric vein, communicates with the middle and inferior hemorrhoidal veins of the systemic circulation and may form large hemorrhoids in the presence of portal hypertension.

5. Retroperitoneal veins form communications between the portal vein, superior mesenteric vein, inferior mesenteric vein, pancreatic veins, and the tributaries of the inferior vena cava. In portal hypertension these communications produce striking "staining" of the peritoneum similar to a port-wine stain and familiar to surgeons, particularly because they cause troublesome bleeding during operations in patients with cirrhosis.

The venous outflow from the liver is carried by the valveless hepatic veins which enter the inferior vena cava just below the diaphragm (Fig. 10). Beginning with the central veins in the liver lobules, the venous effluent passes through progressively larger sublobular veins and collecting veins into the major right, middle, and left hepatic veins. The middle and left hepatic veins usually join and enter the vena cava as one vessel. Several smaller hepatic veins from the caudate lobe and other parts of the liver are consistently found. Because of their interlobar distribution the hepatic veins may be accidentally entered during resections of segments or lobes of the liver.

Recent interest in the role of the hepatic lymph in cirrhosis has focused attention on the lymphatic drainage of the liver. Between the liver cell plates and the sinusoids, tissue spaces called the perisinusoidal spaces of Disse are found, through which fluid exchange between the blood and the hepatocyte takes place. Fluid from these spaces drains into small lymphatic vessels in the portal tracts and then into major lymphatics, which leave the liver in the porta hepatis and empty into the cisterna chyli from which the lymph drains into the thoracic duct. In addition, lymphatic vessels are found around the hepatic veins, in Glisson's capsule, and around the bile ducts. Many of these pass through the diaphragm and empty into the thoracic duct in the thorax. The lymph nodes to which the hepatic lymphatics connect are located in the porta hepatis, and these, in turn, connect with the celiac nodes and nodes around the termination of the inferior vena cava, along the left gastric artery, and near the pylorus.

Text continued on page 1157

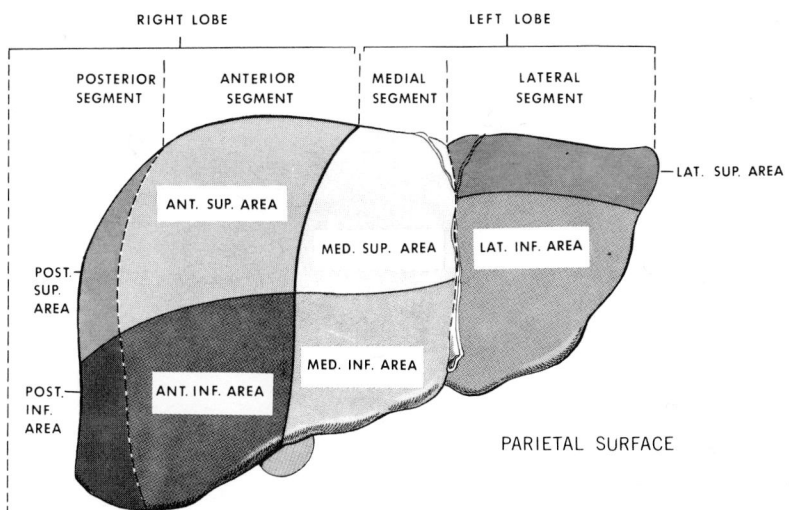

Figure 6. Anatomic lobes and segments of the liver.

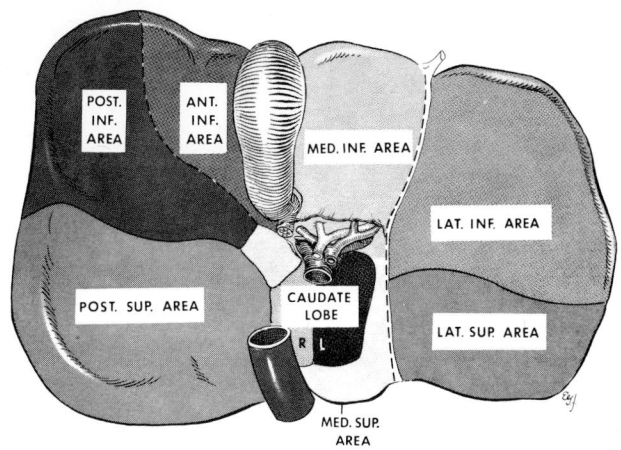

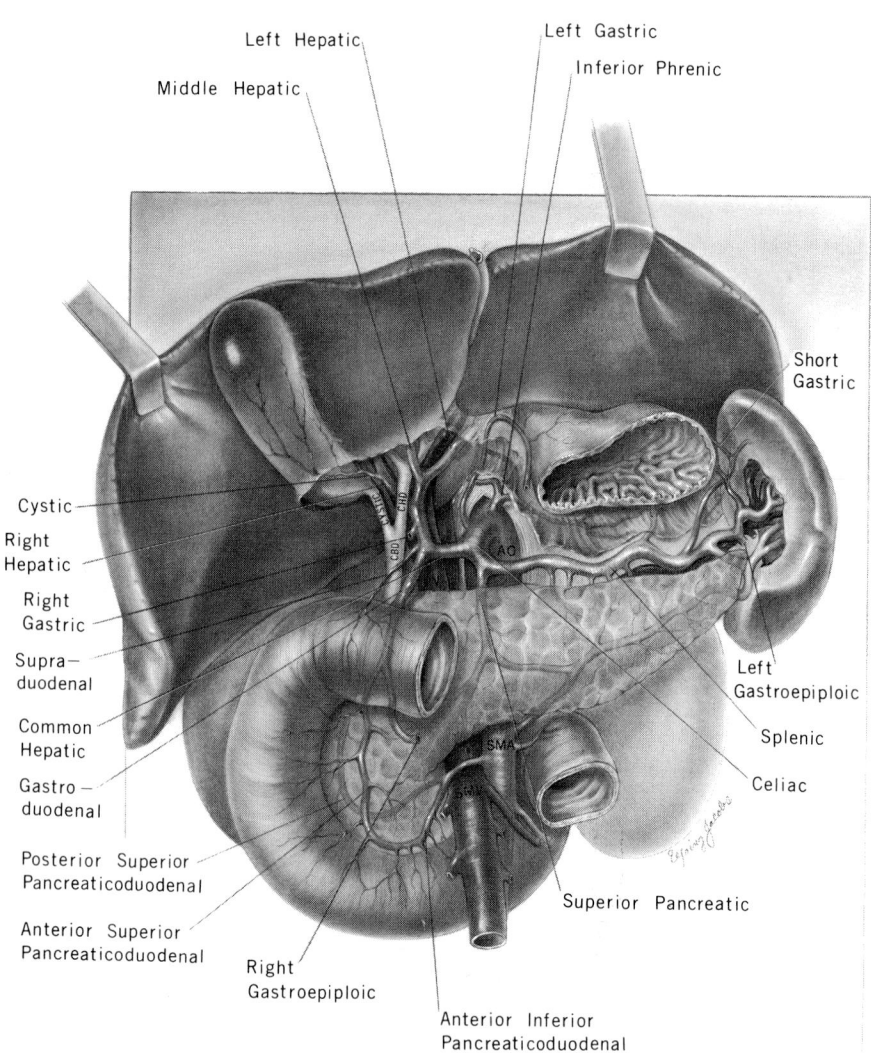

Left Hepatic

Middle Hepatic

Left Gastric

Inferior Phrenic

Short Gastric

Cystic

Right Hepatic

Right Gastric

Supra-duodenal

Common Hepatic

Gastro-duodenal

Posterior Superior Pancreaticoduodenal

Anterior Superior Pancreaticoduodenal

Right Gastroepiploic

Anterior Inferior Pancreaticoduodenal

Left Gastroepiploic

Splenic

Celiac

Superior Pancreatic

Figure 7.   Arterial blood supply of the liver and biliary system.

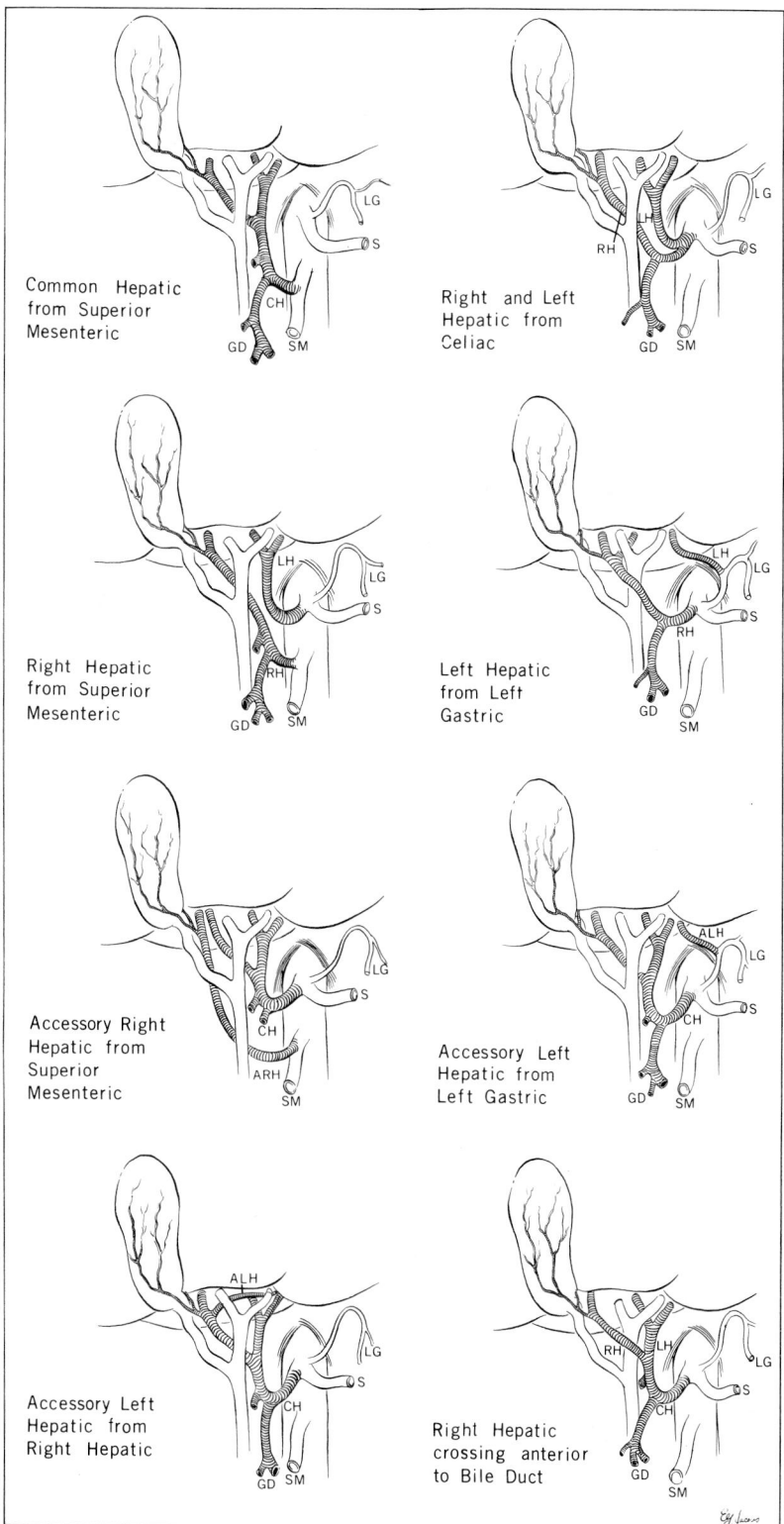

Figure 8. Common variations in the anatomy of the hepatic artery. CH, Common hepatic artery; RH, right hepatic artery; LH, left hepatic artery; ARH, accessory right hepatic artery; ALH, accessory left hepatic artery; LG, left gastric artery; S, splenic artery; SM, superior mesenteric artery; GD, gastroduodenal artery.

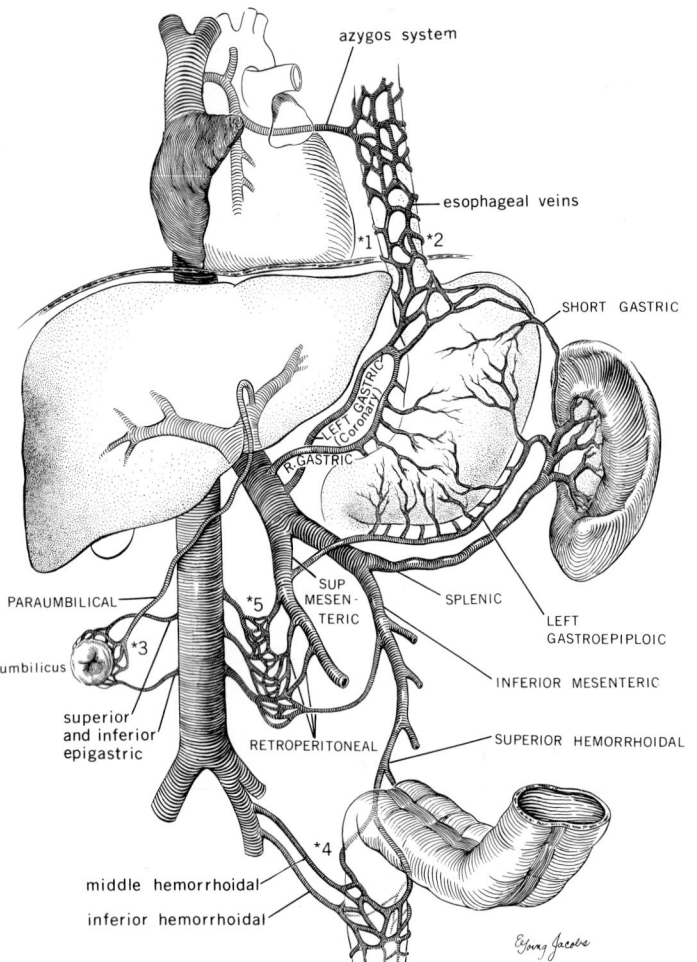

Figure 9. The portal venous system, showing sites of portal-systemic anastomoses labeled 1 to 5. See text for description of these collateral communications.

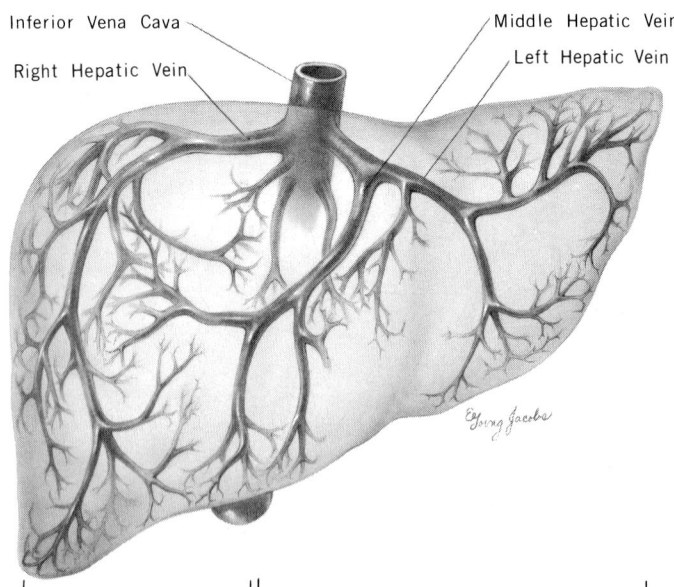

Figure 10. The hepatic venous outflow system.

The nerve supply to the liver consists of sympathetic fibers from the seventh to the tenth thoracic segments of the spinal cord and parasympathetic fibers carried in the right and left vagus nerves. The sympathetic nerves pass through the celiac ganglia. The nerves form an anterior and posterior hepatic plexus in the porta hepatis and are distributed throughout the liver along the blood vessels and bile ducts. The afferent innervation is carried in the sympathetic splanchnic nerves and in the right phrenic nerve. Hepatic pain is dull and is distributed over the area occupied by the liver, with occasional radiation to the right shoulder.

Biliary System. The extrahepatic biliary system is described in detail in the next chapter. The intrahepatic biliary system originates in the tiny bile canaliculi located between the hepatic cells, into which bile is secreted. The canaliculi drain into progressively enlarging intralobular and segmental bile ducts which, in turn, drain into the main right and left hepatic ducts. In the porta hepatis, the right and left hepatic ducts unite to form the common hepatic duct which, in its descent toward the duodenum, is joined by the cystic duct to form the common bile duct.

PHYSIOLOGY

Functions of the Liver

Just as the heart is the focal organ in the circulatory system, and the brain is the hub of integrative activity, the liver is the center of metabolism in the body. The synthesis, modification, storage, breakdown, and excretion of many of the substances upon which life depends occur in the liver. The functions of the liver exceed those of all other organs in number and complexity. Although much remains to be learned about the many vital activities of the liver, the known functions can be divided into eight categories.

Bile Formation and Excretion. Bile is a complex aqueous solution composed of bile pigments (mainly conjugated bilirubin), the conjugated salts of bile acids, phospholipids (mainly lecithin), cholesterol, small quantities of protein (mainly albumin), inorganic electrolytes, mucin, water and a host of metabolites. Its osmolality is about 300 mOsm. per kg., similar to that of plasma. It is secreted at the rate of 600 to 1000 ml. per day. The liver synthesizes bile acids from cholesterol, and bile represents the main route by which cholesterol is eliminated from the body. Substantial evidence indicates that the bile acids and organic compounds in bile are secreted by an active process that involves independent transport mechanisms for the various components. Almost all of the bile acid load that enters the intestine is reabsorbed, mainly in the distal ileum, and undergoes enterohepatic circulation from six to ten times each day.

Bilirubin is formed mainly from the breakdown of hemoglobin in the reticuloendothelial system at various sites in the body, but particularly in the bone marrow and spleen. A small amount of bilirubin originates as a byproduct of hemoglobin synthesis in the bone marrow and from heme proteins other than hemoglobin, mechanisms that become significant only in certain rare diseases that produce "shunt hyperbilirubinemia." The first step in the process of hemoglobin breakdown involves the opening of the tetrapyrrole ring in the heme radical to form biliverdin-iron-globin. Next, the iron and globin components are separated to form biliverdin. Reduction of the biliverdin produces unconjugated bilirubin. This compound is largely insoluble in water and does not react with diazotized sulfanilic acid in the van den Bergh reaction unless it is first treated with alcohol to make it water-soluble. The unconjugated bilirubin is carried to the liver cell in the blood, bound mainly to albumin. In the liver, bilirubin is conjugated with glucuronic acid to form mainly bilirubin diglucuronide and a small amount of bilirubin monoglucuronide. Conjugation with other compounds, such as sulfate and acidic disaccharides, also occurs to a very limited extent. A microsomal enzyme, bilirubin UDP-glucuronyl transferase, catalyzes conjugation with glucuronic acid. The conjugated compounds are water-soluble and give the van den Bergh reaction without pretreatment with alcohol. Conjugated bilirubin is secreted into the bile canaliculi and is excreted via the bile ducts into the intestine, where it is reduced by bacteria to colorless compounds, mesobilirubinogen and stercobilinogen, collectively called urobilinogen. Much of the urobilinogen is excreted in the stool, where part of it is oxidized to the colored pigment urobilin. However, about one third to one half of the urobilinogen is reabsorbed from the intestine in what is called the enterohepatic circulation, and is carried to the liver, where it is again excreted or is transformed back to bilirubin. A small amount of the reabsorbed urobilinogen escapes processing by the liver and is excreted in the urine. Figure 11 summarizes the steps in the breakdown of hemoglobin.

Carbohydrate Metabolism. Hepatic synthesis, transformation, and breakdown of carbohydrates, fats, and proteins are so intimately related that the liver has been referred to as a metabolic pool. The liver is capable of forming these major substances from each other so that separation of the metabolic processes is done mainly for discussion purposes. The liver converts pentoses and hexoses absorbed from the intestine to glycogen, the major form of carbohydrate storage in the body, by enzymatic mechanisms called glycogenesis. In reverse, the liver breaks down glycogen by glycogenolysis, and, thereby, serves as a primary source of glucose for the body. The liver converts glucose, via the hexose monophosphate shunt, to pentoses, which have several uses. They are metabolized to provide energy. They are used in the biosynthesis of nucleotides, nucleic acids, and adenosine triphosphate. They are used to produce 3-carbon compounds, such as pyruvic acid, which serve as precursors for active acetate, a compound that forms a link between carbohydrate, fat, and protein metabolism and plays a central role in the tricarboxylic acid cycle.

Fat Metabolism. The liver both synthesizes and catabolizes fatty acids and neutral fats. Fatty acids are transformed into 4-carbon compounds, the ketone bodies, and into 2-carbon compounds such as active acetate. Similarly, glycerol is broken down into active acetate. The liver is the predominant site of cholesterol synthesis and esterification, and it plays a major role in the synthesis and breakdown of phospholipids and lipoproteins.

Protein Metabolism. The liver synthesizes a large

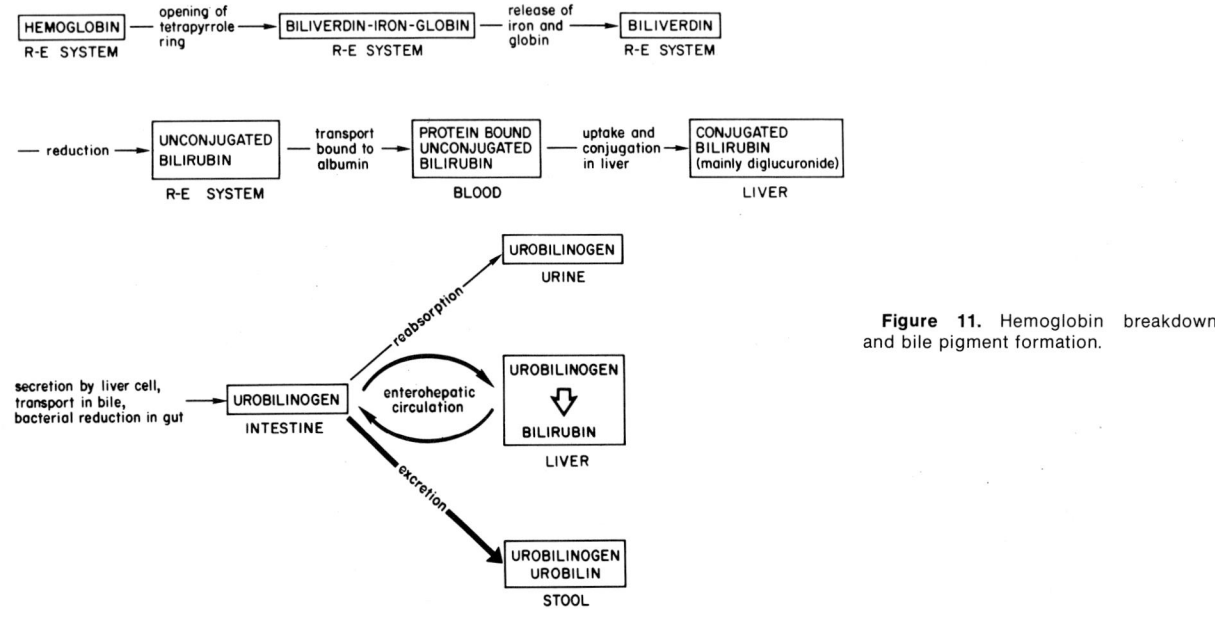

Figure 11. Hemoglobin breakdown and bile pigment formation.

variety of proteins from amino acids. By deamination the liver forms sugars and fatty acids from amino acids, and by transamination it produces amino acids from non-nitrogenous compounds. The liver is the only organ that produces plasma albumin and alpha globulin, and it is the major site for the production of urea, the end product of protein metabolism. Beta and gamma globulins are also formed in the liver.

Blood Coagulation. The liver is the primary center for the synthesis of most of the proteins involved in blood coagulation. It manufactures fibrinogen, prothrombin, and factors, V, VII, VIII, IX, X, XI, and XII. Vitamin K is required for the formation of prothrombin and factors VII, IX, and X. In addition, the normal liver removes plasminogen activators from the blood and thereby prevents uncontrolled fibrinolysis.

Vitamin Metabolism. All the vitamins are stored in and utilized by the liver. It is the primary site for the storage of vitamins A, D, E, K, and B_{12}.

Detoxification. The liver is the detoxification center of the body. By oxidation, reduction, methylation, acetylation, esterification, and conjugation the liver degrades or modifies a great variety of endogenous substances such as the steroid hormones and exogenous drugs and chemicals.

Phagocytosis and Immunity. Through the Kupffer cells of its reticuloendothelial system, the liver serves as a large filter where bacteria, pigments, and other debris are removed from the blood by phagocytosis. Furthermore, the Kupffer cells are an important source of gamma globulin, which is involved in immune defense mechanisms.

Hepatic Hemodynamics

Measurements of hepatic blood flow by indirect and direct methods have shown that the liver receives about one fourth of the cardiac output. Liver blood flow in normal subjects averages 1500 ml. per minute (1000 ml. per minute per kilogram of liver), with a range of from 1000 to 1800 ml. per minute. The hepatic artery contributes about one fourth of the blood flowing to the liver, and the portal vein contributes about three fourths (Fig. 12). The pressure in the portal vein ranges from approximately 7 to 10 mm. Hg (100 to 140 mm. saline), whereas the pressure in the hepatic artery is the same as the systemic arterial pressure. In the hepatic sinusoids, where the two systems join, the pressure is reduced to 4 to 8 mm. Hg. The pressure in the hepatic veins ranges from 3 to 6 mm. Hg and in the inferior vena cava at the level of the diaphragm it is about 2 to 5 mm. Hg. The consecutive pressure gradients assure movement of blood toward the heart.

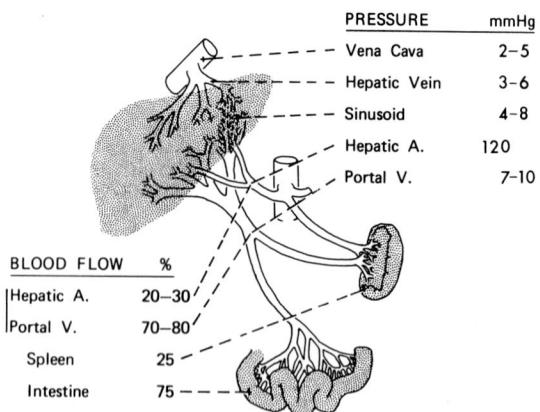

PRESSURE	mmHg
Vena Cava	2–5
Hepatic Vein	3–6
Sinusoid	4–8
Hepatic A.	120
Portal V.	7–10

BLOOD FLOW	%
Hepatic A.	20–30
Portal V.	70–80
Spleen	25
Intestine	75

Figure 12. Pressures in the hepatic circulation and the percentage of contribution to hepatic blood flow made by the various components.

The oxygen content of portal vein blood is higher than that of systemic blood, averaging approximately 80 per cent saturation. The flow of blood to the liver is controlled by mechanical, neural, and humoral mechanisms. Rapid and striking changes in hepatic blood flow occur under various conditions such as exercise, fever, and shock. Thus, the liver is important in maintaining circulatory homeostasis.

Effects of Hepatectomy

Studies in hepatectomized dogs have provided important information about liver function and have raised a number of questions not yet answered. Immediately following complete removal of the liver the animals awake from anesthesia and appear normal. After several hours, however, muscular weakness and depression of reflexes develop, followed in a short time by convulsions and death. These abnormalities are due to hypoglycemia and can be prevented by the administration of glucose. The animal treated with glucose survives in good health for up to 48 hours. However, despite the continued provision of sugar, restlessness, vomiting, and tachypnea ultimately develop, followed by ataxia, spasticity, coma, and death. The cause of death is unknown. A number of biochemical abnormalities have been observed, but none has been proved to be responsible for the terminal events. These include a mild increase in blood ammonia, a rise in the amino acid content of blood, cerebrospinal fluid, and brain, an elevation of blood uric acid, an increase in serum bilirubin and the appearance of bilirubin in the urine, a decrease in the proteins involved in blood coagulation, and a fall in blood urea.

The Eck Fistula Dog

Performance of a portacaval shunt (Eck fistula) in normal animals results in a number of serious disturbances that suggest that sudden diversion of portal blood from the normal liver is incompatible with good hepatic function. In such animals a syndrome of central nervous system symptoms develops following the ingestion of meat which has come to be known as meat intoxication. In addition, animals with an Eck fistula have a decreased capacity to synthesize proteins, impaired bile formation, decreased hepatic storage of glycogen, a fall in serum cholesterol and fatty acids, a progressive rise in blood and urine uric acid, and a hypochromic anemia. The liver undergoes atrophy and accumulates fat, and polydipsia, polyuria, anorexia, weight loss, and lassitude develop. Unless care is meticulous, the animals do not survive for more than a few months. In dogs with experimental cirrhosis, construction of an Eck fistula does not produce the abnormalities observed in animals with an initially normal liver; this fact suggests that the liver can compensate for a gradual reduction in portal blood flow. Similarly, in humans with extrahepatic obstruction of the portal vein due to thrombosis or atresia marked disturbances of hepatic function are not usually observed. One of the important unsettled issues regarding the therapeutic use of portacaval shunt in patients with cirrhosis is the question of whether or not diversion of portal blood away from a liver with an already reduced portal blood flow adversely affects liver function.

Liver Regeneration

Liver regeneration is a phenomenon of fundamental biologic significance and of importance in the understanding and treatment of hepatic disease. The normal adult mammalian hepatocyte shows little turnover of nuclear DNA, rarely undergoes mitosis, and has a life span commensurate with the adult life of the organism, be it the rat or man. However, destruction or removal of part of the liver gives rise to mitotic activity and cell division of such intensity that the organ is reconstituted within days or weeks, depending upon the species. All of the mitotic activity involves mature cells, and there is no evidence of progenitor stem cells. Following removal of two thirds of the liver, complete restoration requires 10 to 14 days in the rat, 6 to 8 weeks in the dog, and 4 to 6 months in man.

Extensive research has been directed at identifying the factors responsible for initiating and regulating the remarkable chain of events involved in liver regeneration. It has been suggested that liver injury or loss causes release of a humoral stimulant of hepatic origin, that partial hepatectomy removes an inhibitor of cell division that is normally present, and that total liver blood flow controls regeneration. None of these suggestions has received solid scientific support. Recently, however, it has been demonstrated that portal blood is essential for restoration of the liver, and convincing evidence indicates that there is a hepatotrophic portal blood factor (HPBF) or factors that regulate hepatic regneration. Furthermore, recent evidence indicates that the HPBF comes from the pancreas. The nature of the HPBF remains to be determined.

DIAGNOSIS OF LIVER DISEASE

HISTORY

Diseases of the liver produce a variety of symptoms depending on the etiology and nature of the underlying disturbance, and upon the rapidity with which liver damage occurs. Many of the symptoms are nonspecific. Nevertheless, certain symptoms occur with sufficient frequency in various hepatic diseases to alert the physician to the possibility that a liver disorder is the cause of the patient's illness (Table 2).

Jaundice is a common symptom of many liver diseases and is perhaps the complaint that most frequently leads the patient to seek medical attention. Jaundice is often accompanied by dark urine and sometimes by light stools. The investigation of a patient with jaundice should include a search for a history of transfusions of blood or blood products, injections, contact with jaundiced persons, occurrence of jaundice in the family, exposure to chemicals at work or in the home, and a record of travel. The possibility that jaundice is due to biliary obstruction requires questioning about fatty food intolerance, attacks of colic, bloating, and belching. Pruritus sometimes accompanies jaundice and may be the patient's predominant complaint.

Fatigue, malaise, headache, myalgia, arthralgia, and fever are frequent symptoms associated with

TABLE 2. Common Symptoms and Signs of Liver Disease

Symptoms

Jaundice, dark urine, pruritus
Fatigue, malaise, myalgia, headache
Anorexia and nausea
Pain in right upper quadrant of abdomen
Fever
Hematemesis and melena
Pedal edema and abdominal enlargement (ascites)
Mental changes, forgetfulness, confusion
Weight loss
Purpura and epistaxis

Signs

Jaundice
Hepatomegaly and liver tenderness
Splenomegaly
Fever
Ascites (with shifting dullness) and edema
Spider angiomas
Palmar erythema
Collateral veins in abdominal wall
Tremor, asterixis, mental confusion
Muscle wasting (shoulder girdles, extremities)
Xanthomas
Gynecomastia, testicular atrophy, loss of axillary and pubic hair
Hematemesis, melena, hematochezia
Purpura

acute hepatic inflammation and necrosis. Anorexia and nausea are striking manifestations of hepatitis, but are also found in chronic liver disease. Pain in the right hypochondrium may occur in most liver diseases as well as in disturbances of the biliary system. The distinction between continuous dull hepatic pain and biliary colic is of diagnostic importance.

Hematemesis and melena are complications of chronic liver disturbances, and particularly of cirrhosis. Liver disease must be considered, at least initially, in every patient with upper gastrointestinal bleeding. Similarly, ascites, dependent edema, weight loss, and a bleeding tendency are manifestations of severe and usually long-standing liver damage. Mental abnormalities such as forgetfulness, confusion, inability to concentrate, and personality changes are common symptoms of advanced cirrhosis. A history of alcohol intake and a dietary history are of great importance.

PHYSICAL EXAMINATION

The findings on physical examination again depend on the type of liver disease and its chronicity. Jaundice, seen best in the sclerae, is an important sign. Hepatomegaly and liver tenderness are found frequently in both acute and chronic liver disease, whereas splenomegaly is a common finding in long-standing hepatic disorders. Fever occurs most often in acute inflammation and necrosis of the liver. Circulatory disturbances, such as spider angiomas seen

usually on the face, neck, upper trunk, and arms, telangiectasis over the nose and cheeks, palmar erythema, and collateral veins beneath the skin of the abdomen are characteristic signs of chronic hepatic dysfunction. Similarly, ascites with shifting dullness, dependent edema, gynecomastia, testicular atrophy, loss of axillary and pubic hair, and muscle wasting are classic manifestations of cirrhosis. Neurologic disturbances such as tremor, asterixis, peripheral neuritis, and disorders of consciousness varying from confusion to coma are associated with severe destruction of the hepatic parenchyma. Xanthomas, which occur most often in the skin of the eyelids, extremities, and upper trunk, are found in liver diseases associated with chronic biliary obstruction. An interesting but uncommon sign of advanced liver disease is a sweet, musty odor of the breath called fetor hepaticus.

LIVER FUNCTION TESTS

A large number of laboratory procedures are used to detect the presence of liver disease. Some of these measure functions of the liver, some measure activities that the liver shares with other organs and systems, and many measure biochemical changes that are associated with hepatic injury but have nothing to do with the known functions of the liver. Collectively, these studies are called liver function tests. Normal adult values for these tests are listed in Table 3.

Bilirubin Metabolism

Serum Bilirubin. The liver conjugates and excretes bilirubin carried to it in the unconjugated form by the blood. Conjugated bilirubin is water-soluble and gives the prompt, direct red diazo reaction of van den Bergh. Unconjugated bilirubin is largely water-insoluble and must be pretreated with alcohol to give the van den Bergh reaction. The total concentration of bilirubin in normal serum is less than 1.2 mg. per 100 ml. and almost all of it is in the unconjugated form. A rise in unconjugated bilirubin in the blood occurs when there is an increased breakdown of hemoglobin and in certain liver disorders in which there is impaired uptake of bilirubin or a deficiency of the enzymes involved in bilirubin conjugation. Jaundice due mainly to an increase in conjugated bilirubin in the blood is found in intrahepatic and extrahepatic bile duct obstruction, in hepatocellular damage, and in certain rare diseases in which the transport of bilirubin after conjugation is disturbed.

Urine Bilirubin. Normally, bilirubin is not present in the urine because the kidney is capable of excreting only the conjugated form of the pigment. Bilirubin appears in the urine in diseases in which there is an elevated level of conjugated bilirubin in the blood.

Urine Urobilinogen. The bilirubin excreted into the intestines is transformed into urobilinogen by intestinal bacteria. A substantial amount of the urobilinogen is reabsorbed, and a small portion of that which is reabsorbed is excreted in the urine (0.2 to 3.3 mg. per day). If renal function is normal, absence of urobilinogen in the urine occurs in obstruction to bile flow and when the intestines are sterilized with antibiotics.

**TABLE 3. Normal Adult Values for
Liver Function Tests**

Serum bilirubin, total	0.3–1.2 mg./100 ml.
Serum bilirubin, direct	0–0.25 mg./100 ml.
Serum bilirubin, indirect	0.2–0.8 mg./100 ml.
Urine bilirubin	0
Urine urobilinogen	0.2–3.3 mg./day
Fecal urobilinogen	40–280 mg./day
Serum alkaline phosphatase	
International	21–85 units
Bodansky	1.5–4.0 units
King-Armstrong	3–13 units
Bessey-Lowry	0.8–3.0 units
Shinowara-Jones-Reinhart	2.8–8.6 units
SGOT	8–40 units
SGPT	5–35 units
Serum 5′-nucleotidase	0.3–3.2 units
Serum leucine aminopeptidase	
(LAP)	50–220 units
Serum lactic dehydrogenase	
(LDH)	200–450 units
Prothrombin time	80–100% of control
Fibrinogen	200–400 mg./100 ml.
Bromsulphalein retention	
(45 min. after 5 mg./kg.)	0–6%
Indocyanine green plasma	
clearance (after 5 mg./kg.)	18–28%/min.
Serum albumin	4.7–5.7 gm./100 ml.
Serum globulins	1.3–2.5 gm./100 ml.
Serum proteins, total	6.5–7.9 gm./100 ml.
Serum alpha fetoprotein	0
Cephalin-cholesterol flocculation	0
Thymol turbidity	0–4 units
Zinc sulfate turbidity	0–4 units
Serum cholesterol	140–280 mg./100 ml.
Serum cholesterol esters, fraction	
of total cholesterol	66–72%
Arterial blood ammonia	20–60 μg./100 ml.

Increased urine urobilinogen is found in hepatocellular disease because the liver is unable to dispose of the reabsorbed pigment, and in conditions that produce an increase in hemoglobin breakdown. The pH of the urine influences renal excretion of urobilinogen.

Fecal Urobilinogen. Normally, fecal urobilinogen excretion ranges from 40 to 280 mg. per day. The excretion rate decreases markedly in biliary obstruction and increases in association with increased bilirubin production. Excretion rates in hepatocellular disease are variable.

Serum Enzymes

Alkaline Phosphatase. These are a group of isoenzymes that hydrolyze phosphate esters in an alkaline medium. They occur in a number of tissues, including, the liver, biliary system, bone, intestine, kidney, and placenta. Alkaline phosphatase in serum originates mainly from the bones (40 to 75 per cent), hepatobiliary system, and intestines. Recently, it has become possible to separate the isoenzymes of serum alkaline phosphatase according to their sites of origin, although the electrophoretic techniques are not yet available as routine laboratory procedures. Alkaline phosphatase is excreted from the body in bile. Elevations of serum alkaline phosphatase occur in a number

of hepatobiliary disorders, as well as in osteoblastic diseases of bone, in pregnancy, and during normal growth. Among the hepatobiliary disorders, the most striking increases are observed in conditions that produce bile duct obstruction. In fact, the finding of a normal level of serum alkaline phosphatase is strong evidence against extrahepatic obstructive disease. Elevations of serum alkaline phosphatase occur also in metastatic neoplasms to the liver (in over 90 per cent of the cases with hepatomegaly), and in primary liver cancer, hepatic abscess, cholangitis, and diffuse liver damage. For many years, elevation of serum alkaline phosphatase was attributed solely to mechanical obstruction of the excretory pathway. Although biliary obstruction is a major cause of regurgitation of the enzyme into the blood, recent evidence suggests that overproduction of alkaline phosphatase by the liver occurs in response to a variety of noxious stimuli, in the absence of impairment of bile flow.

Glutamic Oxalacetic Transaminase (SGOT). This enzyme facilitates the transfer of an amino group from glutamic acid to oxalacetic acid. It is found in skeletal muscle, kidney, brain, and pancreas but the highest levels occur in liver and heart. When tissues containing the enzyme are injured, it is released into the bloodstream. Neither the biliary system nor the kidney is an important route of GOT excretion. Normal serum contains up to 40 units of GOT. SGOT elevations are found in association with severe damage of cardiac and skeletal muscle, as well as in a variety of hepatic disorders. Marked elevations in excess of 300 units suggest the presence of acute hepatic inflammation or necrosis, and are most commonly observed in viral hepatitis.

Glutamic Pyruvic Transaminase (SGPT). This enzyme promotes the transfer of an amino group from glutamic acid to pyruvic acid. Its concentration in liver greatly exceeds that in other tissues or organs. Normal serum contains 35 units or less. Although it has been suggested that a rise in GPT is a more specific indicator of liver damage than an elevation of GOT, both enzymes increase similarly in various liver diseases.

Other Enzymes. Abnormal serum levels of lactic dehydrogenase (LDH), leucine aminopeptidase (LAP), isocitric dehydrogenase (ICD), cholinesterase, 5′-nucleotidase, gamma-glutamyl transpeptidase (GGT), and a number of other enzymes have been observed in various hepatic disorders as well as in diseases of other organs. While determinations of these enzymes may be of value, they have not displaced the other liver function tests and do not appear to significantly enhance the differential diagnosis of liver disease.

Blood Coagulation Factors

The liver is the primary site for synthesis of most of the proteins involved in blood coagulation. Methods have been devised for measuring individual factors, such as fibrinogen, factor V, factor VII, and prothrombin, but they are seldom used. Rather, a composite test is employed that depends on the presence of all the factors in the prothrombin complex and is a useful indicator of liver disease. This test is called the prothrombin time, and the one-stage clotting method of Quick is most commonly used. The test is influenced by the levels of fibrinogen, prothrombin, and factors V, VII, and X. Normally, the prothrombin time is at least 80 per cent of the time obtained with control plasma. The prothrombin time is prolonged or, in other terms, the percentage of normal is decreased in hepatocellular disease because of depressed protein synthesis, and in obstructive jaundice because of impaired absorption of vitamin K, which is required for synthesis of the prothrombin complex. Normalization of the prothrombin test (30 per cent or greater increase within 24 hours) occurs in biliary obstruction following parenteral administration of vitamin K, but does not occur when the coagulation deficiency is due to liver damage. The prothrombin response to parenteral vitamin K is a useful method of distinguishing between hepatocellular and biliary disease.

Dye Excretion

Bromsulphalein Excretion (BSP). Sodium phenoltetrabromphthalein disulfonate, or Bromsulphalein, is a synthetic dye that is removed from the blood mainly by the liver. Following intravenous injection, the dye is carried to the liver bound to albumin and alpha lipoprotein, is taken up by the hepatic cells by an active transport mechanism, is conjugated mainly with glutathione, and is excreted into the biliary canaliculi in both the free and conjugated forms by an active, carrier-mediated transport process. The dye is removed from the body in bile and is not reabsorbed from the intestines. In normal subjects, less than 6 per cent of an injected dose of 5 mg. per kilogram body weight is present in the blood 45 minutes after administration. The BSP test is a very sensitive measure of hepatic functional reserve, and retention of the dye is found consistently in patients with significant liver damage. It is the test that is most frequently abnormal in cirrhosis. Bilirubin competes with BSP for both the hepatic uptake and excretion transport mechanisms, and therefore the BSP test is not valid in the presence of a serum bilirubin greater than 5 mg. per 100 ml., or in obstruction of the bile ducts. Similarly, dyes used for radiographic visualization of the gallbladder compete with BSP for hepatic uptake, and the test should not be done for several days after biliary radiography. BSP retention regularly occurs in very obese patients, and occasionally occurs in the presence of significant fever. In shock, BSP may be retained because of impaired hepatic blood flow.

Indocyanine Green Excretion (ICG). Indocyanine green is a synthetic dye that is removed from the blood almost exclusively by the liver. It is excreted in the bile in an unconjugated form, and is not reabsorbed from the intestines. Evidence indicates that ICG and BSP utilize the same uptake and excretion transport mechanisms, and that agents that compete with BSP also compete with ICG. Experience with the ICG test suggests that it is similar to the BSP test in both sensitivity and limitations.

Iodine-131–Rose Bengal Excretion. Rose bengal is a synthetic phthalein dye that is removed from the blood almost entirely by the liver parenchymal cells and excreted in the bile. The dye can be labeled with ^{131}I, and by positioning detectors over the head, liver, and abdomen, its disappearance from the blood, its hepatic uptake, and its excretion into the intestines can be determined. It has been suggested that the radioactive rose bengal test makes possible a differentiation between hepatocellular and obstructive jaundice, but the results have not been consistent. Rose bengal and Bromsulphalein are retained under similar circumstances.

Protein Metabolism

Serum Albumin. The liver is the sole source of serum albumin. In normal subjects, the serum albumin concentration averages 5.2 gm. per 100 ml. by the commonly used salting out method, and 4.3 gm. per 100 ml. by the more accurate paper electrophoresis method. Serum albumin levels decline in hepatocellular damage, particularly when albumin is lost into the peritoneal cavity in ascites. Normal levels are not infrequently found in advanced liver disease, so that measurements of serum albumin do not serve as a sensitive test of liver function. Moreover, serum albumin changes are not specific for liver disease and are of little value in differential diagnosis.

Serum Globulins. Hyperglobulinemia occurs in acute and chronic liver disease, as well as in a number of nonhepatic illnesses. The elevations are due mainly to augmented gamma globulin production, although increases in alpha and beta globulins are sometimes found. Because gamma globulin is produced by the hepatic and extrahepatic reticuloendothelial system, it is not certain that the liver is completely responsible for a rise in gamma globulin. Changes in various serum protein fractions are detected by serum electrophoresis.

Turbidity and Flocculation Tests. There are a number of tests that do not measure liver function, but reflect qualitative and quantitative changes in serum proteins and are frequently positive in the presence of hepatocellular damage. The most frequently used studies in this category are the cephalin-cholesterol flocculation, the thymol turbidity, and the zinc sulfate turbidity. Flocculation of a cephalin-cholesterol suspension occurs upon the addition of serum containing decreased or altered albumin, increased or altered gamma globulin, altered alpha and beta globulins, or reduced alpha lipoproteins. Turbidity of a thymolbarbital buffer solution occurs upon exposure to serum containing increased gamma globulin, increased beta globulin, an increase of certain lipoproteins, or decreased or altered albumin. Turbidity of a zinc sulfate solution develops upon addition of serum containing an increase in gamma globulin. In all these tests, the degree of turbidity or flocculation is quantitated in terms of arbitrary units. None of the tests are abnormal in uncomplicated obstructive jaundice in the absence of liver injury. Unfortunately, the tests are often negative in the presence of advanced chronic hepatic disease and are sometimes positive in disorders unrelated to the liver. Moreover, the tests do not indicate the severity of liver damage.

Serum Alpha Fetoprotein. Embryonic liver and yolk sac produce alpha fetoprotein, a globulin that is a normal constituent of fetal serum. Alpha fetoprotein is present in small quantities in serum at birth, but it disappears early in life and is not normally present in adult human serum. Initially, the only adults in whom alpha fetoprotein was found were patients with primary hepatocellular carcinoma of the liver and with embryonic neoplasms of the ovary and testes. Recently, however, alpha fetoprotein has been detected in a small number of patients with neoplasms that metastasized to the liver, cirrhosis, hepatitis, and gastric carcinoma. Serum alpha fetoprotein is becoming widely used as a test for primary liver cancer in areas where this disease is common. Its presence can be detected by a screening test that employs Ouchterlony immunodiffusion, or by a more precise quantitative immunoassay. A positive test has been obtained in from 46 to 82 per cent of patients with hepatoma, and no definite false-positive tests have been reported.

Carbohydrate Metabolism

Although the liver plays a central role in carbohydrate metabolism, tests of this hepatic function are of limited value. The standard glucose tolerance test often produces a diabetic curve and glycosuria in patients with severe hepatocellular damage. The intravenous galactose tolerance test measures the specific capacity of the liver to convert galactose to glucose. Impaired clearance of galactose from the blood and its appearance in increased quantities in the urine indicate liver dysfunction.

Lipid Metabolism

The liver is the major site of cholesterol synthesis and esterification, and the bile is the primary avenue of cholesterol elimination from the body. Serum cholesterol levels decrease, as does the esterified fraction, in severe liver damage. Intrahepatic or extrahepatic biliary obstruction, in the absence of severe hepatocellular injury, causes an increase in serum cholesterol. Cholesterol and cholesterol ester determinations are of limited value in the diagnosis of liver disease.

Ammonia Metabolism

Ammonia is formed from nitrogenous substances in the intestines by the action of bacterial enzymes. Ammonia absorbed into portal blood is largely converted to urea by a highly efficient enzyme system in the liver, involving arginine, ornithine, and citrulline. In the presence of severe hepatic damage or portal-systemic venous connections, ammonia levels in peripheral arterial blood may rise above the normal concentration of less than 100 μg. per 100 ml. Although theoretically attractive, determinations of blood ammonia show no consistent correlation with the type or extent of hepatic damage and are of limited diagnostic value. The only circumstance in which measurement of blood ammonia is consistently helpful is in the patient with protein-related portal-systemic encephalopathy.

LIVER BIOPSY

Biopsy of the liver is valuable in the diagnosis of liver disease as well as in the assessment of therapy. It is not a routine procedure, but is indicated in a variety of situations when there is doubt about the diag-

nosis or uncertainty about the activity of a pathologic process. If necessary, biopsy can be performed under direct vision through an abdominal incision or during peritoneoscopy. Usually, however, a percutaneous liver biopsy is possible, in which a cutting or aspirating needle is inserted through the right eighth or ninth intercostal space between the anterior and posterior axillary lines. When the liver is large, a subcostal approach may be used. Serious complications of the procedure have been reported to occur in only 0.3 to 0.4 per cent of the cases and consist mainly of bleeding and bile peritonitis. The mortality rate has been reported to be between 0.1 and 0.2 per cent. Use of the one-second biopsy technique of Menghini has substantially reduced the incidence of complications. In patients with a prothrombin time less than 50 per cent, platelet count below 100,000, or with obstructive jaundice, the risk of needle biopsy is increased. Liver biopsy provides accurate information in patients with diffuse hepatic disease. Focal lesions in the liver may be missed.

ROENTGENOGRAPHIC STUDIES

Barium Contrast Upper Gastrointestinal Series

In our experience, the upper gastrointestinal series is a simple and accurate method of making the diagnosis of esophageal varices (Fig. 13). In a large series, this procedure provided accurate information in more

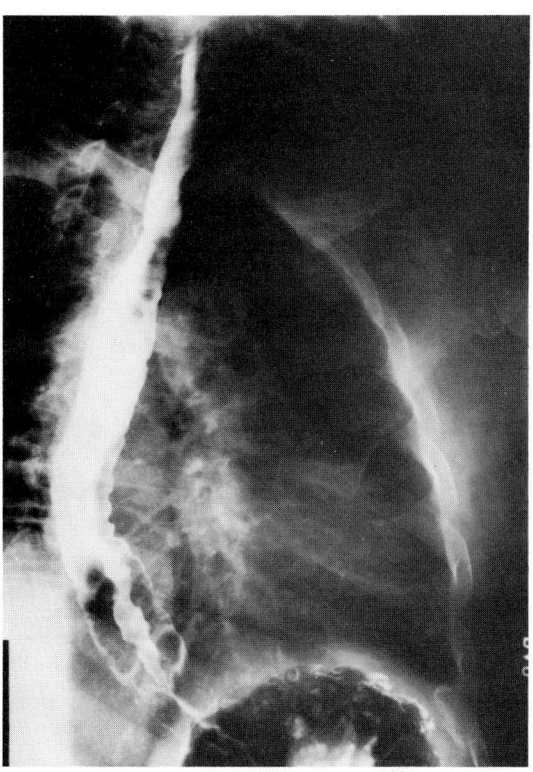

Figure 13. Barium contrast upper gastrointestinal x-rays showing large esophageal varices.

than 90 per cent of the patients. Barium contrast x-rays of the esophagus, stomach, and duodenum have proved particularly helpful in the differential diagnosis of upper gastrointestinal hemorrhage because they demonstrate the presence or absence of lesions other than varices that may be responsible for bleeding, such as duodenal and gastric ulcers. This valuable diagnostic study can be performed safely at the time of bleeding in almost all patients.

Portal Venography

Visualization of the portal venous system by the injection of contrast media is most valuable in the diagnosis and evaluation of portal hypertension, and occasionally may be helpful in the diagnosis of space-occupying lesions within the liver. Portal venography provides important information about the site of venous obstruction, the type and extent of portal-systemic collaterals, the size of the major components of the portal system, and, with appropriate timing, the rate of portal venous blood flow. Several methods are available for demonstrating the portal vasculature. The most frequently used technique is that of percutaneous splenoportography, which involves injection of a radiopaque dye into the spleen through a needle inserted through the left ninth or tenth intercostal space between the midaxillary and posterior axillary lines (Fig. 14). Bleeding from laceration of the spleen is an occasional serious complication of this procedure. Another technique is that of operative portal venography, in which a tributary of the portal vein is catheterized under direct vision at laparotomy. Catheterization of the umbilical vein through a small incision in the abdominal wall permits transumbilical portal venography, a technique that is particularly useful in splenectomized patients. Direct percutaneous needle puncture of the portal vein has been used to perform transhepatic portal venography. Finally, splenic and superior mesenteric arteriography performed by percutaneous catheterization of the splenic or superior mesenteric arteries via the femoral artery permits delayed visualization of the portal venous system by appropriately timed x-rays. None of these techniques is a routine procedure that is required in all patients. All of them are associated with risks which must be weighed against the information to be obtained. However, usually they can be performed safely and often they are extremely useful.

Hepatic Venography

Percutaneous catheterization of the hepatic veins via either the basilic vein in the arm or the femoral vein is a relatively simple procedure. Visualization of the inferior vena cava (vena cavography) may be combined with wedged hepatic venography. Injection of contrast medium into the hepatic veins may be used to determine retrograde blood flow in cirrhosis by showing filling of the portal vein, and to demonstrate hepatic vein occlusion in the Budd-Chiari syndrome and in veno-occlusive disease of the liver. Both hepatic venography and inferior vena cavography may be helpful in demonstrating space-occupying lesions situated in the posterior segments of the liver. Figure 15 shows a hepatic venogram.

Hepatic, Celiac, and Superior Mesenteric Arteriography

Percutaneous selective catheterization of the hepatic, celiac, and superior mesenteric arteries for visualization of the splanchnic vasculature is a safe procedure that has become very valuable in the diagnosis of liver disease (Fig. 16). It is particularly useful for demonstrating space-occupying lesions, hepatic vascular lesions, the status of the arterial tree in cirrhosis, hemobilia, and injury to the liver associated with blunt trauma. With proper timing, superior mesenteric arteriography may be used to visualize the portal venous system and to demonstrate patency of portacaval shunts. We have found that selective injection of contrast medium into the left gastric artery is an excellent technique for delayed visualization of esophageal varices.

Cholecystography and Cholangiography

Techniques for oral, intravenous, and direct percutaneous visualization of the biliary system are important in the diagnosis of biliary disease, and may be of help in the differential diagnosis of jaundice. They are discussed in detail in the next chapter.

ESOPHAGOGASTRODUODENOSCOPY

Esophagogastroduodenoscopy is the best means of determining the presence of esophageal varices, of demonstrating varix hemorrhage, and of identifying other lesions that might be responsible for upper gastrointestinal bleeding, such as gastric ulcer and duodenal ulcer. It is the only reliable means of making

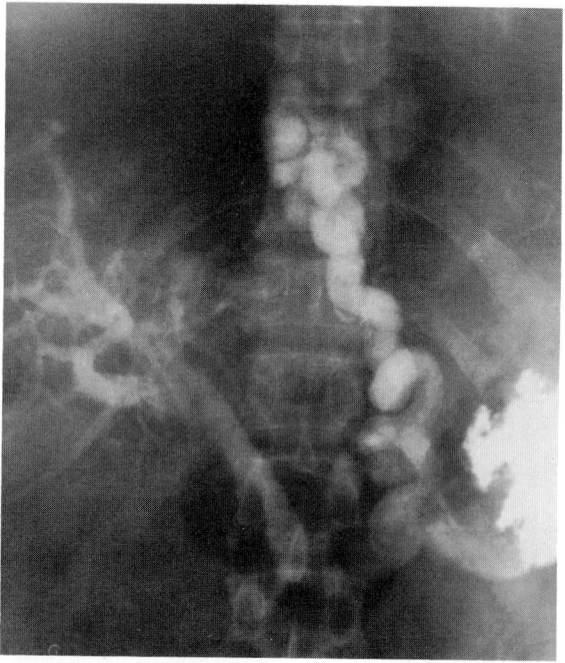

Figure 14. Splenoportogram in a patient with cirrhosis showing large gastroesophageal varices.

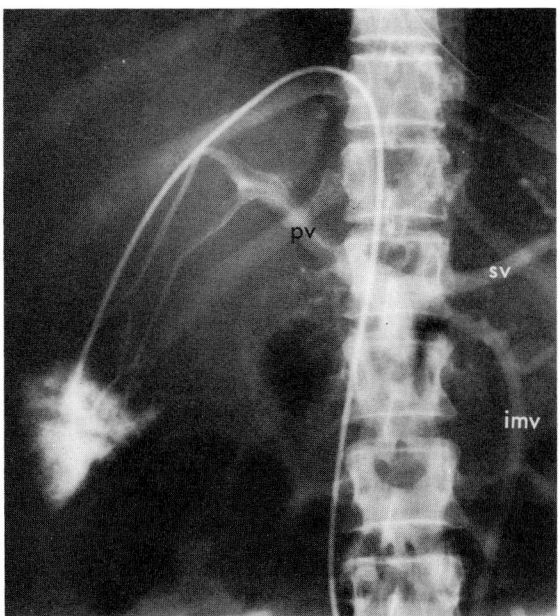

Figure 15. Hepatic venogram in a patient with cirrhosis showing retrograde filling of portal vein indicative of reversal of portal blood flow. pv, Portal vein; sv, splenic vein; imv, inferior mesenteric vein.

the diagnosis of hemorrhagic gastritis. The development of the flexible fiberoptic endoscope has revolutionized the field of endoscopy and made it a relatively simple bedside procedure that is usually well tolerated by patients. Endoscopy should not be considered to be in competition with barium contrast roentgenography as a means of identifying the cause of upper gastrointestinal hemorrhage. Rather, the two procedures complement each other and together they improve diagnostic accuracy substantially. Endoscopy should always precede barium contrast studies because barium retained in the stomach obscures endoscopic visualization.

PORTAL PRESSURE MEASUREMENTS

Wedged Hepatic Vein Pressure (WHVP)

Measurements of portal venous pressure are helpful in the diagnosis of portal hypertension and in the selection of appropriate surgical therapy. Under most circumstances the portal pressure can be determined indirectly by percutaneous hepatic vein catheterization via an arm vein or the femoral vein, and this procedure is used routinely in many clinics. The catheter tip is wedged in a hepatic venule and produces a static column of blood that extends back to the sinusoid. The pressures in the sinusoid, and in portal blood entering the sinusoid, are transmitted through the static blood to the catheter. The correlation between measurements of WHVP and portal pressure are extremely good under most conditions. When there is sinusoidal or postsinusoidal obstruction to portal blood flow, as occurs in the common forms of cirrhosis, portal pressure rises and WHVP increases correspondingly. In portal hypertension due to an extrahepatic block (presinusoidal), WHVP is normal and does not reflect

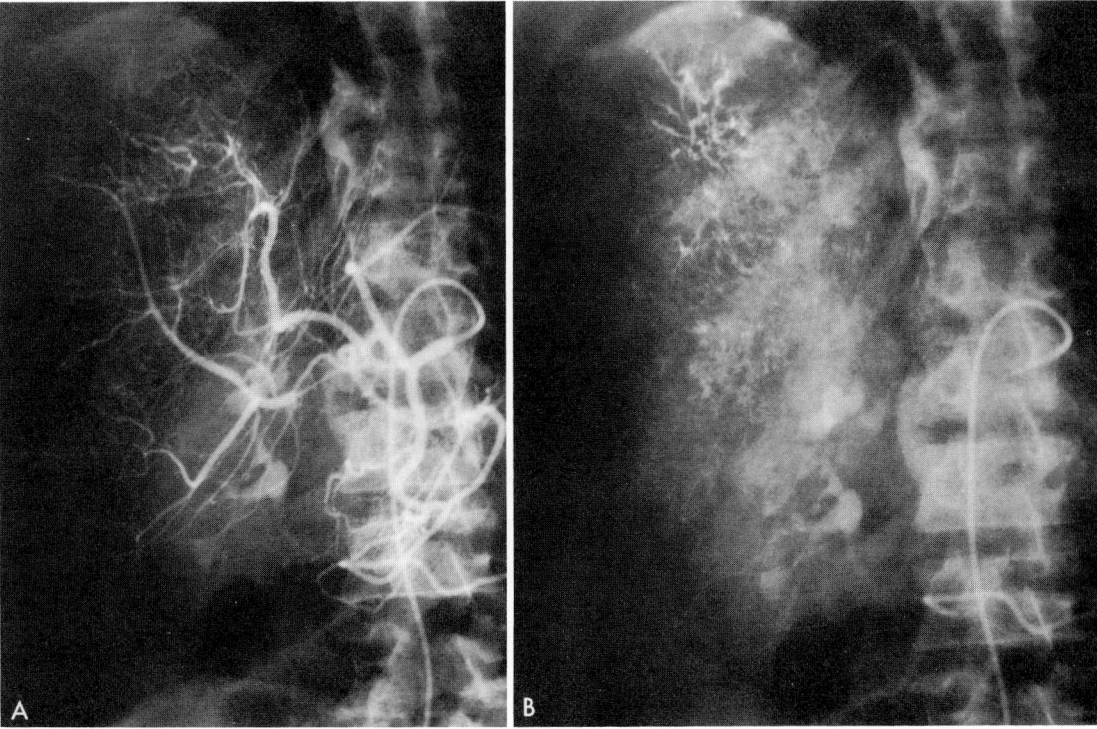

Figure 16. Hepatic arteriogram showing a large malignant neoplasm in the right lobe of the liver. *A,* Distortion of the arterial tree by the neoplasm. *B,* Extensive "tumor staining" during the venous phase of the study.

portal pressure. During hepatic vein catheterization, the free hepatic vein and inferior vena cava pressures are always determined also, and the WHVP is usually expressed in terms of its difference from vena cava pressure.

Splenic Pulp Pressure

The splenic pulp pressure reflects the pressure in the valveless portal venous system, and it can be measured by the same percutaneous technique as that used for splenoportography. Often the two procedures are combined. If necessary, splenic pulp pressure can be determined at the bedside.

Umbilical Vein Catheterization

As described previously, the portal vein can be catheterized for direct pressure measurements through the umbilical vein, which is isolated through a small paraumbilical incision and forcefully reopened.

Intraoperative Pressure Measurements

Direct pressure measurements are always made at operations for portal hypertension, both before and after a portacaval shunt is performed. These include the inferior vena cava pressure (IVCP), the free portal pressure (FPP), and the pressures on the hepatic and splanchnic sides of a clamp temporarily occluding the portal vein. The latter determinations are called the hepatic occluded portal pressure (HOPP) and the splanchnic occluded portal pressure, (SOPP), respectively. When the liver is normal, HOPP is markedly lower than FPP. In cirrhosis with hepatic outflow obstruction, HOPP rises progressively and occasionally exceeds FPP, a finding which indicates that hepatic outflow obstruction is severe and which may reflect reversal of portal blood flow (although pressure and flow are distinctly different parameters that do not have a direct relationship to each other in the portal circulation). Pressure measurements following construction of a portacaval shunt are essential, and provide the only reliable means of determining that the anastomosis is functioning satisfactorily.

Postoperative Pressure Measurements Following Portacaval Shunt

The patency of a portacaval shunt is readily determined by percutaneous catheterization via the femoral vein and performance of both angiography and measurements of portal and vena caval pressures.

RADIOISOTOPE STUDIES

Hepatic Blood Flow

Estimation of hepatic blood flow may be helpful in the assessment of portal hypertension and in the selection of appropriate therapy. Indirect methods for measuring liver blood flow involve the infusion of a tracer substance that is removed mainly, and preferably completely, by the liver. Bromsulphalein was the first tracer used for this purpose, and the technique consisted of simultaneous measurements of concentrations in arterial and hepatic venous blood during a

continuous intravenous infusion of the dye. Indocyanine green may be used instead of BSP. More recently, simple methods have been developed for measuring the blood disappearance rate of a radioactive tracer that is removed mainly by the liver. Either external monitoring or analysis of radioactivity in serial blood samples is used to measure removal of the injected tracer from the peripheral blood. Radioactive colloidal gold (^{198}Au), colloidal human serum albumin (^{131}I or ^{125}I), colloidal technetium sulfide (^{99m}Tc), and colloidal chromic phosphate (^{32}P) have been used as tracers. All of the methods of estimating hepatic blood flow have several inherent sources of error which become magnified in the presence of liver disease. When liver damage is marked, hepatic uptake of the tracer is reduced regardless of changes in blood flow, and extrahepatic removal of the test substance increases, leading to unreliable results. A portacaval shunt further complicates the measurements.

Liver Scanning

Scintillation scanning following the administration of a radioisotope that selectively localizes in the liver is helpful in determining liver size and shape and in detecting lesions that occupy space within the hepatic parenchyma or compress the liver from without. Isotopically labeled colloidal gold (^{198}Au), colloidal human serum albumin (^{131}I or ^{125}I), colloidal technetium sulfide (^{99m}Tc), rose bengal (^{131}I), and ammonium molybdate (^{99}Mo) are employed. Figure 17 shows typical scans.

ULTRASONIC SCANNING

Ultrasonic scanning is a harmless, noninvasive procedure that has proved to be useful in the diagnosis of mass lesions in and around the liver. It involves the recording on an oscilloscope of the pattern of reflections or echoes that are produced by passing high-frequency ultrasonic waves into the body. Echoes are produced at interfaces between materials of different density. Normal liver parenchyma is homogeneous and produces no reflections (Fig. 18A). Tumors or abscesses within the liver produce abnormal echoes (Fig. 18B).

HEMATOLOGIC STUDIES

Hematologic abnormalities are common in chronic liver disease. Gastrointestinal bleeding, of course, is a major complication of cirrhosis. In addition, chronic anemia is frequently found as a result of a decreased red blood cell survival time and poor nutrition. Hypersplenism, with a depression of any or all of the formed elements of the blood, is often associated with portal hypertension. In particular, thrombocytopenia occurs frequently in advanced cirrhosis. Appropriate hematologic studies, including the usual complete blood count, platelet count, determinations of red cell indices, measurements of serum iron, and determinations of red blood cell survival time and splenic trap-

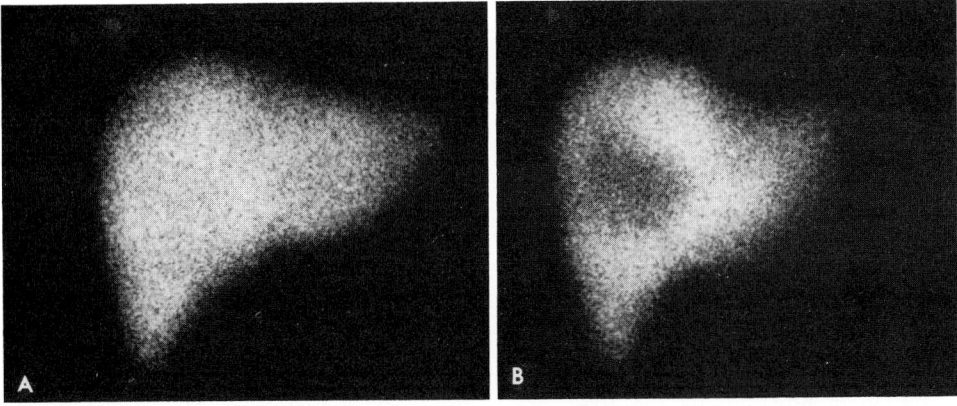

Figure 17. Scintillation scans following administration of colloidal technetium sulfide (^{99m}Tc), showing (A) normal liver and (B) large area of reduced radioactivity in right lobe of liver due to a metastasis from carcinoma of the colon.

ping of red cells, may be important components of the diagnostic work-up.

BALLOON TAMPONADE CONTROL OF BLEEDING

Control of upper gastrointestinal hemorrhage by esophageal or gastric balloon tamponade has been interpreted as evidence that the bleeding is coming from esophageal varices. This diagnostic procedure has been accurate in approximately 75 per cent of patients. It is infrequently indicated as a diagnostic procedure.

JAUNDICE

Jaundice or icterus is a yellow discoloration of the tissues that results from staining with bilirubin. It is best observed in sites containing elastic tissue such as the sclerae and skin of the face and neck. Jaundice is easily recognizable when the conjugated bilirubin concentration in the serum reaches 2 to 3 mg. per 100 ml., or the unconjugated bilirubin level is 3 to 4 mg. per 100 ml. With experience jaundice can be detected at lower levels of serum bilirubin. Jaundice occurs in a substantial number of diseases, and determination of the precise cause can be one of the more difficult problems in clinical medicine.

There is no satisfactory classification of jaundice that accounts for all conditions. The classic separation of jaundice into hemolytic, hepatocellular, and obstructive types is useful but does not explain all the pathophysiologic mechanisms that recent studies have clarified. Classification on the basis of the type of bilirubin, conjugated or unconjugated, that predominates in the blood is of limited clinical validity because of the frequent occurrence of mixed forms of hyperbilirubinemia. An understanding of bilirubin metabolism and of the stages at which it may be disturbed by disease provides the soundest approach to the differential diagnosis of icterus.

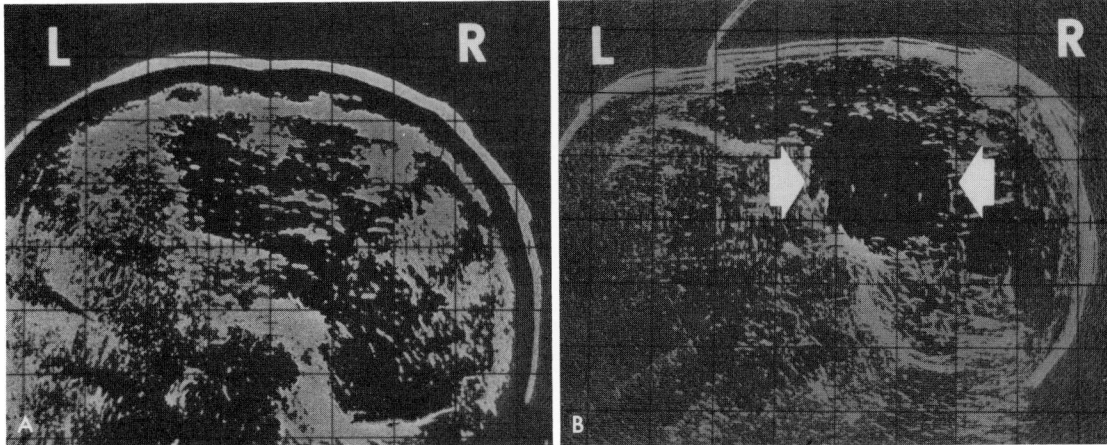

Figure 18. Ultrasonic scans showing (A) normal liver and (B) large amebic abscess in right lobe of liver.

The metabolism and excretion of bilirubin involve the formation of free bilirubin mainly from the breakdown of hemoglobin in the reticuloendothelial system; transport of the unconjugated bilirubin to the liver; uptake and conjugation of the bilirubin by the hepatic cell; excretion of the conjugated bilirubin by the hepatic cell into the bile; excretion of the bile along the biliary ducts into the intestines, where conjugated bilirubin is converted to urobilinogen. A classification of jaundice according to the stage at which bilirubin metabolism is disturbed is presented in Table 4 and Figure 19.

Increased production of bilirubin from hemolysis of red blood cells or during erythropoiesis, impaired transport of bilirubin to the liver, and impaired uptake and conjugation of bilirubin by the liver cell result in icterus due to unconjugated hyperbilirubinemia. The term "retention jaundice" has been used to describe this type, and it is not accompanied by impairment of bile flow. The jaundice in most of these disorders is mild, there is no bilirubin in the urine, urine urobilinogen is not increased, and the liver function tests are usually normal.

Impaired transport and excretion of conjugated bilirubin by the hepatic cell produces jaundice with a substantial amount of conjugated bilirubin in the blood. The term "regurgitation jaundice" has been applied to this type. Most of the common liver diseases fall into this category. Because the damaged hepatic cells are unable to conjugate all the bilirubin resulting from normal hemoglobin breakdown, an increase in unconjugated bilirubin develops along with the regurgitated conjugated pigment in the blood. Bilirubin appears in the urine, urine urobilinogen levels rise, and liver function tests are usually abnormal. One group of disorders that produce impaired cellular excretion of conjugated bilirubin does not conform to the usual pattern of liver disease and presents problems in the differential diagnosis of obstructive jaundice. The terms intrahepatic cholestasis and cholestatic hepatitis have been used to describe these conditions. They are characterized by a clinical and biochemical picture similar to that of bile duct obstruction, normal or mildly abnormal liver function tests, and a histologic picture of bile stasis without mechanical obstruction. A growing number of drugs, including phenothiazine compounds, certain diuretics, testosterone derivatives, oral contraceptives, oral antidiabetes agents, and arsenicals, are known to injure the cellular excretion mechanism and cause intrahepatic cholestasis. A sensitization reaction to the drug is usually responsible. A similar picture has been observed during pregnancy and, as a transient phenomenon, during viral hepatitis. In some instances, no etiologic agent can be identified.

Mechanical bile duct obstruction results in conjugated hyperbilirubinemia, along with an increase in unconjugated pigment in the blood. The mechanism is similar to that which occurs in primary liver disease, and the jaundice is of the regurgitation type. Bilirubin appears in the urine but, if the obstruction is complete, urobilinogen is absent from the urine and stool, and the stools are light- or clay-colored. The serum alkaline phosphatase levels are significantly elevated, but the other liver function tests are usually normal early in the course of obstruction. However, repeated or longstanding obstruction or infection results in substantial liver damage and makes it difficult to distinguish the symptoms and findings from those of primary hepatic disease. Prolonged absence of bile from the intestine impairs the absorption of fat-soluble vitamin K and produces a decrease in prothrombin activity that can be corrected by parenteral administration of the vitamin. The prothrombin response to vitamin K is helpful in differentiating liver disease from biliary obstruction.

The first steps in the diagnostic approach to the patient with jaundice are the taking of a thorough history and the performance of a careful physical examination. These routine aspects of every work-up often provide crucial information that points to the diagnosis. Taking of the history should include pointed questions about rapidity of onset and course of the jaundice, color of the urine and stools, pruritus, weight loss, abdominal pain, digestive symptoms, malaise, anorexia, occupation, travel, jaundice in the family, contact with jaundiced persons, exposure to hepatotoxins, alcohol consumption, ingestion of drugs, transfusions, injections, and previous operations. The physical examination should include particularly careful palpation of the liver, gallbladder, and spleen, a search for the stigmata of cirrhosis, gross determination of stool color, and chemical examination of the stool for blood. After the history and physical exami-

TABLE 4. Classification of Jaundice

I. *Excessive bilirubin production usually due to hemolysis ("hemolytic jaundice")*
  A. Inherited hemolytic anemias
  B. Acquired hemolytic disorders
    1. Hemolytic anemias
    2. Sepsis
    3. Hemolysins (snake venom, mushrooms)
    4. Absorption of sequestered blood (hematomas, hemothorax, hemoperitoneum, infarcts)
    5. Burns
    6. Mismatched blood transfusions
    7. Massive blood transfusions
  C. Shunt hyperbilirubinemia
II. *Impaired transport of bilirubin to liver*
  Some types of Gilbert's syndrome
III. *Impaired hepatic conjugation of bilirubin*
  A. Inborn errors
    1. Crigler-Najjar syndrome
    2. Some types of Gilbert's syndrome
  B. Immaturity of enzyme systems
    1. Physiologic jaundice of newborn
    2. Jaundice of prematurity
IV. *Impaired hepatic transport and excretion of bilirubin after conjugation ("hepatocellular jaundice")*
  A. Acquired liver diseases (e.g., hepatitis, cirrhosis, neoplasms)
  B. Dubin-Johnson syndrome and Rotor syndrome
  C. Intrahepatic cholestasis (drug-induced, disease-related, and idiopathic)
V. *Mechanical bile duct obstruction ("obstructive jaundice")*
  A. Extrahepatic (stone, neoplasm, stricture, atresia, etc.)
  B. Intrahepatic

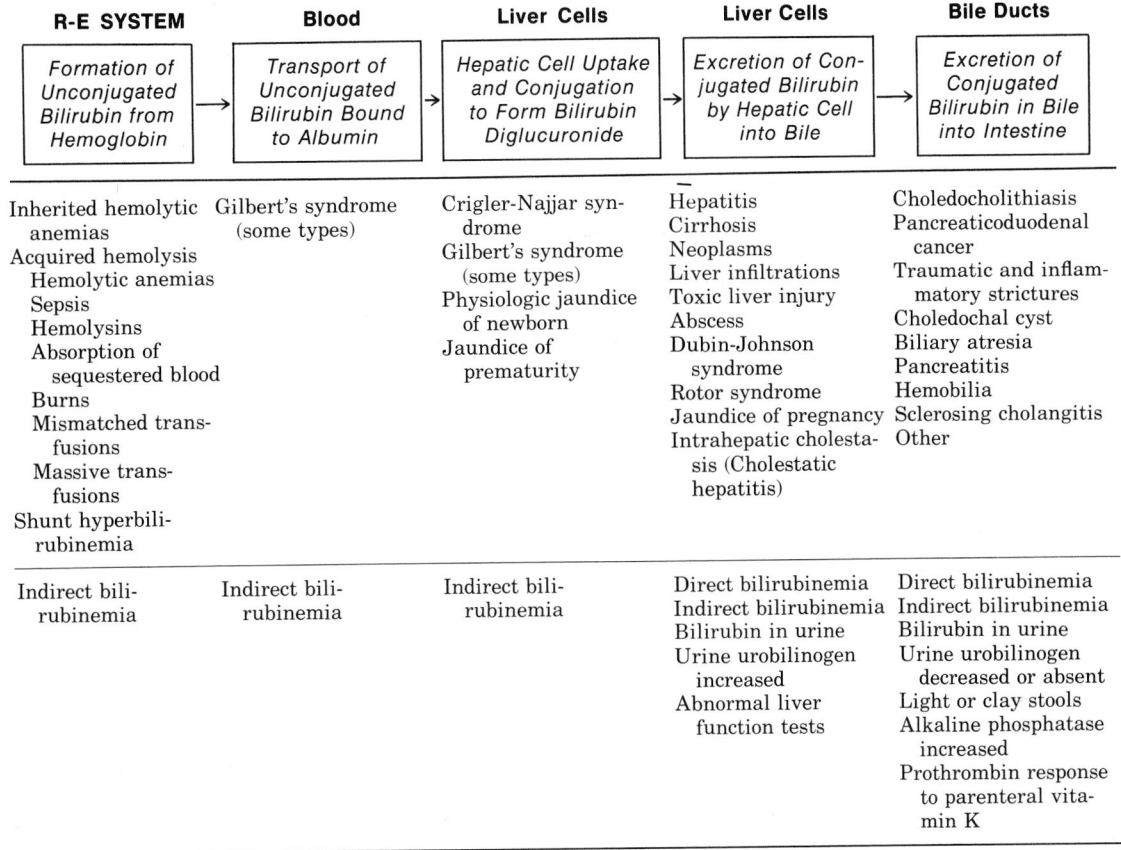

R-E SYSTEM	Blood	Liver Cells	Liver Cells	Bile Ducts
Formation of Unconjugated Bilirubin from Hemoglobin	Transport of Unconjugated Bilirubin Bound to Albumin	Hepatic Cell Uptake and Conjugation to Form Bilirubin Diglucuronide	Excretion of Conjugated Bilirubin by Hepatic Cell into Bile	Excretion of Conjugated Bilirubin in Bile into Intestine
Inherited hemolytic anemias Acquired hemolysis 　Hemolytic anemias 　Sepsis 　Hemolysins 　Absorption of 　　sequestered blood 　Burns 　Mismatched trans- 　　fusions 　Massive trans- 　　fusions Shunt hyperbili- 　rubinemia	Gilbert's syndrome (some types)	Crigler-Najjar syndrome Gilbert's syndrome (some types) Physiologic jaundice of newborn Jaundice of prematurity	Hepatitis Cirrhosis Neoplasms Liver infiltrations Toxic liver injury Abscess Dubin-Johnson syndrome Rotor syndrome Jaundice of pregnancy Intrahepatic cholestasis (Cholestatic hepatitis)	Choledocholithiasis Pancreaticoduodenal cancer Traumatic and inflammatory strictures Choledochal cyst Biliary atresia Pancreatitis Hemobilia Sclerosing cholangitis Other
Indirect bilirubinemia	Indirect bilirubinemia	Indirect bilirubinemia	Direct bilirubinemia Indirect bilirubinemia Bilirubin in urine Urine urobilinogen increased Abnormal liver function tests	Direct bilirubinemia Indirect bilirubinemia Bilirubin in urine Urine urobilinogen decreased or absent Light or clay stools Alkaline phosphatase increased Prothrombin response to parenteral vitamin K

Figure 19. Stages of bilirubin metabolism at which diseases produce jaundice, and the types of jaundice that result.

nation, the next steps involve determinations of the levels of direct-reacting and indirect-reacting bilirubin in the blood, and the amounts of bilirubin and urobilinogen in the urine. Hyperbilirubinemia that is mainly of the unconjugated pigment, combined with the absence of bilirubin in the urine, indicates that the icterus is of the retention type. In an adult patient, the odds are overwhelming that the cause is hemolysis of red blood cells. The liver function tests under these circumstances will be normal, and appropriate hematologic studies and other tests should be performed to identify the underlying disease.

If a substantial portion of the bilirubin in the blood is of the direct-reacting variety, as is commonly the case, and there is bilirubin in the urine, the jaundice is of the regurgitation type and the problem is usually one of distinguishing between liver disease and bile duct obstruction. Liver function tests, stool color examination, and urobilinogen measurements should be performed. Normal liver function tests except for a depressed prothrombin activity and an elevated serum alkaline phosphatase, light- or clay-colored stools, absence of urobilinogen in the urine, a good prothrombin response to parenteral vitamin K, and a history and physical examination that are compatible indicate clearly that the jaundice is due to biliary obstruction that requires surgical relief. On the other hand, ab-

normal liver function tests, a normal-colored stool, increased urobilinogen in the urine, a negative or incomplete prothrombin response to parenteral vitamin K, an enlarged liver, and the absence of symptoms of biliary tract disease such as abdominal colic and fatty food intolerance indicate that the jaundice should be treated by nonsurgical measures. Needless to say, the history and physical findings are of great importance in arriving at the correct diagnosis.

In a number of patients, perhaps 10 to 15 per cent, a diagnosis will not be possible on the basis of the initial work-up. Additional studies, repeated tests, and a period of observation will be required to determine the etiology of the jaundice. In some patients liver scan, liver biopsy, upper gastrointestinal x-rays, cholangiography, arteriography, peritoneoscopy, and duodenal drainage must be performed. Occasionally, laparotomy must be done for diagnostic as well as therapeutic purposes.

PORTAL HYPERTENSION

Portal hypertension is a manifestation of various diseases of the liver and its circulation. It is the complication of hepatic disease that most frequently requires surgical treatment. Although the portal pressure in normal subjects varies considerably with activity, at rest it ranges from about 100 to 140 mm. saline (7 to 10 mm. Hg). In terms of pressure measurements, portal hypertension may be defined as a portal vein pressure of 250 mm. saline (18 mm. Hg) or greater in the presence of a normal pressure in the inferior vena cava. Stated in other terms, portal hypertension exists when the difference between portal and inferior vena cava pressure exceeds 150 mm. saline. More important, portal hypertension may be defined in terms of the pathologic disturbances it produces that compromise health and threaten life. Some of these disorders, such as bleeding esophageal varices and hypersplenism, are a direct reflection of the high pressure in the portal circulation and its collateral communications. Others, such as ascites, hepatic coma, peptic ulcers, and renal failure, are complicated manifestations of a number of factors including the portal hypertension, the underlying liver disease, and the required treatment.

ETIOLOGY OF PORTAL HYPERTENSION

Table 5 lists the causes of portal hypertension. From both clinical and pathologic standpoints these may be divided into diseases within the liver and diseases of the blood vessels outside the liver. With the exception of the rare splanchnic arteriovenous fistulas, all the conditions cause portal hypertension by producing obstruction to portal blood flow.

Intrahepatic obstructive diseases account for more than 90 per cent of the patients with portal hypertension. Of these, portal cirrhosis associated with chronic alcoholism is by far the most common etiology in the United States. Postnecrotic cirrhosis due to viral hepa-

TABLE 5.   Etiology of Portal Hypertension

I. *Intrahepatic obstructive disease*
   A. Portal cirrhosis (alcoholic, nutritional, Laennec's)
   B. Postnecrotic cirrhosis (posthepatitic, idiopathic)
   C. Biliary cirrhosis
   D. Uncommon forms of cirrhosis and fibrosis (hemochromatosis, Wilson's disease)
   E. Alcoholic hepatitis
   F. Neoplasms and granulomas
   G. Schistosomiasis
   H. Veno-occlusive disease
   I. Congenital hepatic fibrosis
   J. Hepatoportal sclerosis
II. *Extrahepatic disease*
   A. Portal vein obstruction
      1. Congenital atresia or stenosis
      2. Thrombosis due to infection or trauma
      3. Cavernomatous transformation
      4. Extrinsic compression
   B. Hepatic vein (outflow) obstruction
      1. Budd-Chiari syndrome
      2. Constrictive pericarditis
   C. Excessive portal blood flow
      1. Arteriovenous fistula between hepatic artery and portal vein
      2. Arteriovenous fistula between splenic artery and vein

titis is a fairly common cause of portal hypertension, whereas the incidence of biliary cirrhosis due to extrahepatic bile duct obstruction or primary intrahepatic disease is low. The other forms of intrahepatic obstruction are uncommon. Because cirrhosis is largely a disease of adulthood and, particularly in alcoholic cirrhosis, develops slowly over many years, patients with portal hypertension of the intrahepatic type are most often in the fifth or sixth decades of life. Morover, they are usually in poor health because of the underlying liver disease, and the risk of operative treatment is significant.

Extrahepatic obstruction of the portal vein is most often due to thrombosis. Neonatal omphalitis is a relatively frequent cause, but often the etiology of the thrombosis cannot be determined. Cavernomatous transformation is most likely the end result of thrombosis and recanalization of the portal vein. Congenital atresia of the portal vein and extrinsic compression are rare causes of portal hypertension. Extrahepatic portal hypertension usually develops in childhood or early adult life. Furthermore, the patients usually do not have liver damage, are otherwise in good health, and usually tolerate both the complications of their circulatory disorder and the required surgical therapy quite well.

Extrahepatic obstruction of the hepatic venous outflow system occurs in a group of rare conditions called the Budd-Chiari syndrome. The obstruction is usually due to inflammatory or neoplastic thrombosis or fibrosis of the hepatic veins and, sometimes, of the adjacent inferior vena cava. The etiology of the process is often obscure, although some cases are associated with polycythemia vera and with neoplasms. Marked hepatomegaly and massive ascites are the most striking clinical findings. The condition has been relieved by construction of a side-to-side portacaval shunt.

PORTAL HYPERTENSION DUE TO CIRRHOSIS

PATHOPHYSIOLOGY

The widespread destruction of the hepatic parenchyma in cirrhosis leads to overgrowth of fibrous tissue and the formation of regenerative nodules in a pathologic rearrangement of liver architecture. As a result, the hepatic blood vessels are compressed and distorted. The branches of the hepatic vein, because of their low pressure and thin protective coat of connective tissue, are affected more than the other components of the vasculature, and hepatic venous outflow obstruction develops. This postsinusoidal obstruction is the fundamental hemodynamic lesion in the common forms of cirrhosis. Outflow obstruction leads to an increase in sinusoidal pressure which, in turn, is reflected in an elevation of portal pressure and a decrease in portal blood flow to the liver. In extreme stages of postsinusoidal obstruction, the valveless portal vein may become an outflow tract and conduct blood in a retrograde manner away from the liver, leaving the hepatic artery alone to nourish the parenchyma. An additional consequence of the disruption of hepatic integrity is the development of communications between the intrahepatic branches of the hepatic artery and portal vein, and between the tributaries of the portal vein and hepatic vein. The arteriovenous shunts contribute to the portal hypertension. Moreover, both types of shunts divert blood away from the hepatic parenchyma and compromise the nutrition of the liver cells. In an unsuccessful attempt to compensate for the reduction in portal flow to the liver, hepatic artery flow increases and the liver becomes dependent upon the hepatic artery for a major portion of its blood supply.

The elevated pressure in the portal vein leads to an enlargement of all the collateral venous connections between the portal and systemic circulations, and development of varicosities (see Fig. 9). In addition, splenomegaly develops. Blood flow through the collaterals is away from the liver, which further impairs hepatic nutrition. Despite their large size, the portal-systemic anastomoses are insufficient to accommodate the volume flow of portal blood and to overcome portal hypertension. Most prominent among the collaterals are those in the submucosa of the lower esophagus and upper stomach, and those around the umbilicus and anterior abdominal wall. Rupture of the esophageal varices often causes massive hemorrhage and is associated with a high mortality rate.

NATURAL HISTORY OF CIRRHOSIS

Cirrhosis of the liver is a common and highly lethal disease. Currently in the United States it is the eighth leading cause of death and ranks ninth in economic cost among the major illnesses. In subjects older than 40 years it is the fourth ranking cause of mortality. Furthermore, during the past two decades the death rate of cirrhosis increased more than that of any of the other common causes of death. Chronic alcoholism, the most frequent etiologic factor in cirrhosis, has been estimated to involve 9 million people in the United States. During the past decade there has been an increase of 3 million chronic alcoholics, so that alcoholism is now one of the largest social, economic, and public health problems in our country. The social cost of alcoholism has been estimated to amount to 25 billion dollars per year.

The survival rates of patients admitted to general hospitals because of cirrhosis are shown in Table 6. In the classic study of Ratnoff and Patek, who examined in retrospect the histories of 386 patients admitted to five New York hospitals between 1916 and 1938, only one third of the patients with ascites were alive after 1 year and only a few survived for 5 years. Survival rates for patients with jaundice and hematemesis were similar. In the more recent prospective study of the Boston Inter-Hospital Liver Group, 79 per cent of the patients who bled from esophageal varices were dead within 1 year of bleeding, and in the entire group of 467 patients, with and without bleeding, only 26 lived for 5 years. The exact mortality rate of alcoholic cirrhosis in the United States today is difficult to determine because studies of this matter have involved different populations of patients, but there is no question that it is a highly lethal disease. The results of the two sutdies shown in Table 6 indicate that once a patient entered the hospital for treatment of cirrhosis, his chances of living for 1 year were similar to those of a patient with acute lymphocytic leukemia, and his chances of surviving 5 years were about the same as those observed in most untreated cancers.

The causes of death in patients with cirrhosis and varices were tabulated by the Boston Group (Table 7). Hemorrhage from esophageal varices was responsible for one third of the deaths, hepatic failure accounted for one third, renal shutdown for 11 per cent, infection for 9 per cent, and miscellaneous causes for the remainder. These figures, which are similar to those obtained in other studies, clearly show that varix bleeding is a major cause of death in cirrhosis. This complication in particular has occupied the attention of surgeons and serves as the major indication for surgical therapy.

BLEEDING ESOPHAGEAL VARICES

The most frequent cause of death from upper gastrointestinal bleeding is *rupture* of an esophageal varix with hemorrhage. Until recently, approximately three out of four cirrhotic patients who entered the hospital with their first episode of bleeding varices failed to leave the hospital alive. Table 8, which shows the results of a number of studies conducted during the past 40 years, indicates that as of 1962 the immediate mortality rate of the first variceal hemorrhage averaged 73 per cent. From these statistics, it is apparent that the emergency treatment of bleeding esophageal varices is the single most important aspect of the therapy of portal hypertension.

TABLE 6. Natural History of Cirrhosis

Authors	Cases	Complications	Survival (%)		
			1 Year	2 Years	5 Years
Ratnoff and Patek (five	296	Ascites	32	17	7
New York Hospitals,	245	Jaundice	26	23	5
1916–1938)	106	Hematemesis	28	25	20
Boston Inter-Hospital Liver	467	Varices	34	21	5.5
Group (seven Boston	288	Varices without bleeding	43	25	8
Hospitals, 1959–1961)	179	Varices with bleeding	21	14	1.5

**TABLE 7. Causes of Death in 235 Patients
with Cirrhosis and Varices
(Boston Inter-Hospital Liver Group, 1959–1961)[94]**

	% of Deaths
Hemorrhage	34
Hepatic failure	32
Renal shutdown	11
Infection	9
Indeterminate and other	14

The precipitating cause of rupture of esophageal varices is uncertain. It has been proposed that erosion of the mucosa by reflux acid-peptic esophagitis is involved. However, in a gross and microscopic study of the distal esophagus in 20 patients at the time of bleeding we found esophagitis in only one patient. Moreover, bleeding from esophageal varices has been reported in patients with proven gastric achlorhydria. The evidence strongly suggests that increased hydrostatic pressure is responsible for "blowout" rupture of esophageal varices.

Emergency Diagnosis

In most patients who enter the hospital with upper gastrointestinal hemorrhage, the diagnosis of bleeding esophageal varices depends on affirmative answers to three questions. Does the patient have cirrhosis? Does the patient have portal hypertension and esophageal varices? Are the varices the site of the bleeding, rather than some other lesion such as duodenal or gastric ulcer, gastritis, or hiatus hernia? Information sufficient to answer these questions usually can be obtained within a few hours of the patient's admission to the hospital by means of an organized diagnostic plan that includes some, and if necessary all, of the following steps:

1. History and Physical Examination. A history of chronic alcoholism, hepatitis, jaundice, previous bleeding episodes, melena, abdominal swelling, edema, and mental abnormalities, and the absence of symptoms of peptic ulcer suggest the diagnosis of cirrhosis. The most important physical findings are hepatosplenomegaly, spider angiomas, palmar erythema, collateral abdominal veins, muscle wasting, jaundice, ascites, edema, and neurologic signs such as tremor and asterixis. In many patients, not all these classic signs are present. Confirmation of gastrointestinal bleeding by aspiration of the stomach through a nasogastric tube and by gross and chemical examination of the stool is an essential early measure and should really be considered part of the physical examination. A nasogastric tube is inserted in all patients.

2. Blood Studies. Blood samples for typing and crossmatching and for studies are drawn immediately on admission. The initial studies include a complete blood count, liver function tests (Bromsulphalein excretion, prothrombin, bilirubin, alkaline phosphatase, albumin, globulin, glutamic oxalacetic transaminase, glutamic pyruvic transaminase), urea nitrogen, electrolytes, pH, blood gases, and blood alcohol. The liver tests that are most consistently abnormal and of greatest value are the BSP excretion, if performed in the absence of marked jaundice and after hypovolemic shock has been corrected, and the prothrombin and serum bilirubin. It is not unusual for the other liver function tests to be normal in the presence of advanced cirrhosis.

3. Esophagogastroduodenoscopy. With the development of the flexible fiberoptic esophagogastroscope, endoscopy has become a well-tolerated, relatively simple procedure that can be performed rapidly at the bedside in the emergency room. It is the best diagnostic measure for determining with certainty the presence or absence of gastritis and of the uncommon Mallory-Weiss syndrome, and, in combination with roentgenographic studies, it makes possible the diagnosis of esophageal varices with a high degree of confidence.

4. Upper Gastrointestinal X-rays. As soon as shock has been corrected and the patient's condition stabilized, a barium contrast upper gastrointestinal series is obtained. Parenteral fluid therapy and monitoring should continue throughout this procedure, and the physician in charge of treatment should accompany the patient to the radiology department and remain in constant attendance. When this is done, x-ray studies can be performed safely in almost all patients. It is to be emphasized that roentgenographic studies are directed at determining the presence or absence not only of esophageal varices, but also of other lesions such as a duodenal ulcer, gastric ulcer, or hiatus hernia. The literature contains many statements that

TABLE 8. Mortality of First Variceal Hemorrhage in Cirrhosis

Authors	Year Reported	Type of Hospital	Number of Patients	Mortality (%)
Ratnoff and Patek	1942	Five private-teaching	106	40
Higgins	1947	City indigent	45	76
Atik and Simeone	1954	City indigent	59	83
Nachlas, O'Neal, and Campbell	1955	City indigent	102	59
Cohn and Blaisdell	1958	City indigent	456	74
Taylor and Jontz	1959	Veterans	102	45
Merigan, Hollister, Gryska, Starkey, and Davidson	1960	City indigent	74	76
Orloff	1962	City indigent	87	84
		Total	1031	Mean 73

suggest that esophageal varices are demonstrated in only 50 to 60 per cent of patients who have them. Our experience indicates that a skillful and interested radiologist can accurately demonstrate varices at the time of bleeding in more than 90 per cent of cirrhotic patients (see Fig. 13).

5. Hepatic Vein Catheterization. This relatively simple procedure has become a routine diagnostic measure in our institution. It is used to determine wedged hepatic vein pressure, free hepatic vein pressure, and inferior vena cava pressure. Hepatic venography is usually added to the studies, although it is not essential and does not yield information that is as important as that obtained from the pressure measurements. The main purpose of venography is to determine the direction of flow in the portal vein (see Fig. 15). WHVP accurately reflects portal pressure in the common forms of cirrhosis and establishes the diagnosis of portal hypertension with certainty.

The emergency diagnosis of bleeding esophageal varices has been made accurately from information obtained in these first five steps in more than 95 per cent of our patients. It has been regularly possible to complete these diagnostic measures within 6 hours of the patient's admission to the emergency room.

6. Splenoportography and Splenic Manometry. Visualization of the portal venous system is not usually required for emergency diagnosis of varix hemorrhage in patients with cirrhosis. In the small number of patients with normal liver function who are suspected of having extrahepatic portal obstruction, splenoportography provides crucial information about the site of obstruction and patency of the portal venous system. Until recently, we regularly performed splenoportography as part of the emergency diagnostic work-up in all patients (see Fig. 14). However, we have discontinued use of the procedure in most patients with cirrhosis because it has failed to yield information not provided by other, less invasive diagnostic tests. Splenic manometry is usually combined with splenoportography and offers an alternative to hepatic vein catheterization. If desired, the splenic pulp pressure can be determined readily at the bedside by percutaneous puncture of the spleen under local anesthesia. Although this procedure does not determine the site of bleeding, it indicates the presence or absence of portal hypertension. Bleeding from esophageal varices infrequently occurs with a splenic pulp pressure below 300 mm. saline and rarely occurs with a pressure below 250 mm.

7. Splenic, Hepatic, Celiac, Left Gastric, and Superior Mesenteric Arteriography. Percutaneous selective catheterization and visualization of the splanchnic arteries provide interesting hemodynamic information about the status of the circulation in cirrhosis. With proper timing, injection of contrast media into the splenic artery or superior mesenteric artery provides delayed visualization of the portal vein and its collateral connections, a technique known as indirect portography. Arteriography and indirect portography have largely replaced splenoportography as the initial approach to visualization of the portal system because the risk and incidence of complications are somewhat lower. It is particularly useful in patients whose spleen has been

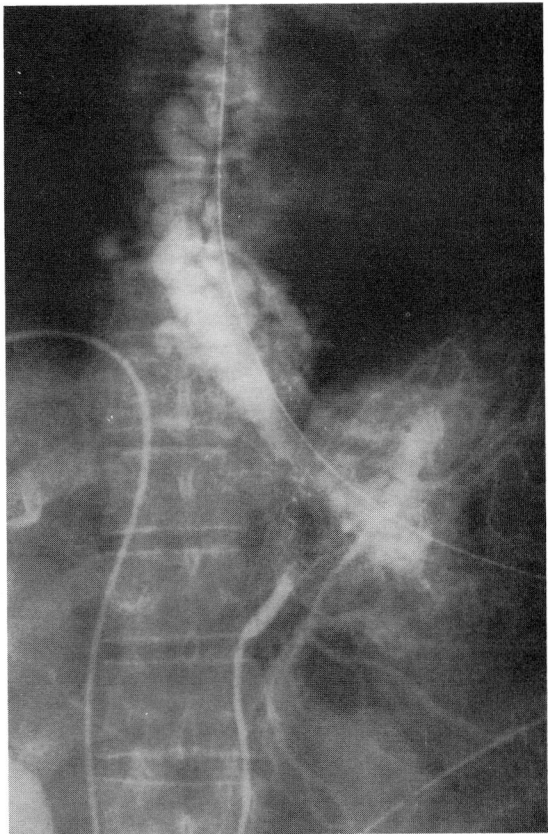

Figure 20. Selective left gastric arteriogram with delayed visualization of large esophageal varices during the venous phase.

removed previously. We have found that selective injection of the left gastric artery frequently produces excellent delayed visualization of esophageal varices (Fig. 20). It should be emphasized that selective arteriography is not an essential or routine emergency diagnostic procedure in cirrhotic patients with varix hemorrhage. After performing the procedure as a regular part of the emergency diagnostic work-up in all patients over a period of seven years, we have discontinued its routine use because it did not provide essential information.

8. Radioisotope Hepatic Blood Flow. For many years there has been a search for methods of evaluating the hepatic circulation that would provide information of value in selecting and assessing therapy of bleeding esophageal varices. In the hope that measurements of hepatic blood flow would provide useful hemodynamic information, we routinely performed such measurements as part of our emergency diagnostic work-up over a period of seven years. However, the results have failed to yield data that are helpful in predicting survival or selecting one or another form of treatment. The most commonly used technique involves injection of a radionuclide and external monitoring of its disappearance rate from the blood. Radioactive colloidal technetium sulfide (^{99m}Tc), colloidal gold (^{198}Au), colloidal human serum albumin (^{131}I or ^{125}I), and colloidal chromic phosphate (^{32}P) are used as tracers.

9. Balloon Tamponade Control of Bleeding. Control of bleeding by esophageal balloon tamponade is presumptive evidence that an esophageal varix is the site of bleeding. The balloon tamponade test is accurate in approximately three fourths of patients. The development of new and better diagnostic measures has made this indirect diagnostic procedure almost obsolete.

Several years ago we evaluated the use of a vigorous emergency diagnostic approach in 89 consecutive adult patients in whom cirrhosis and varix hemorrhage were suspected on admission to our emergency room. In all of the patients a history was taken, and physical examination, blood studies, and barium contrast upper gastrointestinal x-ray examinations were done. Splenic manometry and esophagoscopy with the rigid esophagoscope were performed only if the other measures failed to reveal the diagnosis. Table 9 summarizes the results of this diagnostic approach. Upper gastrointestinal x-rays correctly demonstrated the presence or absence of varices in 96 per cent of the patients. Roentgenography gave false-negative results in 4 per cent of the patients. Splenic manometry was performed in 11 patients in whom x-rays failed to show varices; in two patients, portal hypertension was found and bleeding varices were demonstrated subsequently at operation, whereas in nine patients the finding of a normal portal pressure corresponded to the absence of varices on x-ray. Esophagoscopy was performed in six patients in whom no varices were demonstrated by roentgenography; in two patients bleeding varices were observed and subsequently proved at operation, whereas in the other four patients the absence of varices was confirmed by endoscopy. In 97 per cent of the patients, the diagnostic work-up was completed within 6 hours of admission to the hospital. Fifty-nine of the 89 patients were subjected to emergency operations with the preoperative diagnosis of cirrhosis and bleeding esophageal varices, and in each instance this diagnosis proved to be correct. Since this study was completed, we have added esophagogastroduodenoscopy with the flexible fiberoptic instrument and hepatic vein catheterization to the routine diagnostic work-up done in all patients. Our experience has shown that the diagnosis of varix hemorrhage in cirrhosis can be made rapidly and with a high degree of accuracy.

The differential diagnosis of upper gastrointestinal bleeding in 99 per cent of cirrhotic patients is confined to a consideration of six lesions in addition to ruptured varices. Three of these lesions, hemorrhagic gastritis, duodenal ulcer, and gastric ulcer, are common. The other three lesions, gastric cancer, hiatus hernia, and the Mallory-Weiss syndrome (a tear of the esophagogastric mucosa produced by forceful vomiting), are infrequent causes of bleeding. Each of these conditions produces characteristic symptoms, and each can be ruled in or out by the combination of esophagogastroduodenoscopy and barium contrast upper gastrointestinal x-rays. It is general experience that bleeding in cirrhotic patients originates from lesions other than esophageal varices in 20 to 25 per cent of cases. While this statistic should serve to alert the clinician to a spectrum of etiologic considerations, it should not be interpreted as an indication that the diagnosis of varix hemorrhage is particularly complicated or cannot be made with accuracy. In point of fact, once esophageal varices have been demonstrated, the chances that another lesion is responsible for the bleeding are not more than 10 per cent. Furthermore, if instances of mild bleeding in cirrhotic patients with proven varices are eliminated, gastrointestinal hemorrhage will be found to arise from rupture of the varices in over 95 per cent of patients. Thus, demonstration of esophageal varices in a cirrhotic patient with significant upper gastrointestinal bleeding provides overwhelming odds that the varices are the source of the hemorrhage.

Emergency Treatment

In view of the high mortality rate associated with varix hemorrhage in patients with cirrhosis, it is clear that the efforts of physicians must be concentrated on the prompt and definitive control of the first bleeding episode if the survival rate of these patients is to be improved. Emergency treatment of bleeding esophageal varices can be categorized into general meas-

TABLE 9. Diagnostic Findings in 89 Consecutive Cirrhotic Patients Suspected of Bleeding from Esophageal Varices*

Final Diagnosis	Number of Cases	History Compatible with Cirrhosis	Physical Exam Compatible with Cirrhosis	Liver Function Tests Compatible with Cirrhosis	Varices on Upper GI X-ray	Other Lesion on Upper GI X-ray	Portal Hypertension on Splenic Manometry	Varices on Esophagoscopy
Bleeding varices	74	74	74	74	70/74	4/74	2/2	2/2
Peptic ulcer	6	6	6	6	0/6	6/6	–	0/2
Gastritis	9	9	9	9	0/9	0/9	0/9	0/2

*From Emergency treatment of bleeding esophageal varices in cirrhosis, by Orloff, M. J. in Portal Hypertension, edited by Longmire, W. P., Jr., Current Problems in Surgery, edited by Ravitch, M. M., et al. Copyright © 1966, Year Book Medical Publishers. Used by permission.

ures of therapy, specific medical treatment aimed at stopping the bleeding, and specific surgical procedures for controlling the hemorrhage.

General Measures of Emergency Therapy. Cirrhosis of the liver is a severe, debilitating disease with remote manifestations, only one of which is bleeding from esophageal varices. Death after varix rupture is frequently due to hepatic decompensation, renal failure, or infection, rather than to exsanguination. Although control of bleeding is of primary importance, the effectiveness of therapy of the underlying liver disease often determines the outcome. Therefore, there are certain general principles of treatment that apply to all patients, regardless of the specific therapeutic measures used to stop the hemorrhage.

1. PROMPT RESTORATION OF THE BLOOD VOLUME. Vigorous replacement of blood loss with whole blood transfusions is essential. Large-bore intravenous catheters should be inserted in each arm at the start of therapy. Every effort is made to obtain fresh blood less than 12 hours old for administration because of the serious defects in coagulation associated with liver disease plus those superimposed by multiple transfusions. Bleeding cirrhotic patients usually have thrombocytopenia in addition to abnormalities of the protein blood clotting factors. In addition, recent evidence indicates that the red blood cells of cirrhotic patients are deficient in 2,3-diphosphoglyceric acid, a substance that mediates the dissociation of oxygen from hemoglobin. It has been proposed that this deficiency impairs the delivery of oxygen to the tissues. Since there is a progressive decline in 2,3-DPG levels in blood during storage, the use of fresh blood has been recommended to correct the abnormality in oxygen transport.

2. PREVENTION OF HEPATIC COMA. Although the nervous disorders associated with liver disease are diverse and poorly understood, the encephalopathy observed in patients with bleeding esophageal varices sometimes appears to be due to the absorption of large quantities of ammonia directly into the systemic circulation via portal-systemic collaterals. For this reason, measures directed at destroying ammonia-forming bacteria and eliminating all nitrogen from the gastrointestinal tract are initiated promptly. These include removal of blood from the stomach by lavage with iced saline through a nasogastric tube, instillation of cathartics (60 ml. magnesium sulfate) and neomycin (4 gm.) into the stomach, and thorough and repeated cleansing of the colon with enemas containing neomycin (4 gm. per liter of water). The fear that insertion of a nasogastric tube will perforate the varices is unfounded, and such a tube should be placed at the start of the diagnostic work-up. Although ammonia-binding agents, such as sodium glutamate and arginine, and ion exchange resins have been used, we have obtained no evidence that agents of this sort have been of value.

3. SUPPORT OF THE FAILING LIVER. Parenterally administered hypertonic glucose solutions containing therapeutic doses of vitamins K, B, and C are included in the initial treatment regimen. Appropriate amounts of electrolytes are added to the parenteral fluids. In general, administration of sodium is avoided

because patients with advanced cirrhosis usually have an increase in total-body sodium and a tendency to retain salt and water.

4. CORRECTION OF HYPOKALEMIA AND METABOLIC ALKALOSIS. The vast majority of the many bleeding cirrhotic patients that we have studied have been found to have significant hypokalemia and a metabolic alkalosis preoperatively or immediately postoperatively. The deleterious effects of hypokalemia are well known. In addition, alkalosis has a number of harmful consequences that include: (1) interference with the release of oxygen to the tissues by shifting the oxyhemoglobin dissociation curve to the left; (2) in combination with hypokalemia, precipitation of cardiac arrhythmias, particularly in patients taking digitalis; (3) potentiation of ammonia toxicity by elevating the tissue concentration of ammonia, and increasing the passage of ammonia across the blood-brain barrier; and (4) production of tetany by lowering the level of ionized calcium in extracellular fluid. Correction of hypokalemia and metabolic alkalosis is undertaken soon after admission to the hospital and consists of parenteral administration of large quantities of potassium chloride supplemented, occasionally, by infusion of an acidifying agent such as arginine hydrochloride, hydrochloric acid, or ammonium chloride. Administration of potassium is usually required for several days in amounts occasionally as high as 500 mEq. per day.

5. FREQUENT MONITORING OF VITAL FUNCTIONS. The usual techniques are used to determine the magnitude of bleeding and adequacy of blood volume replacement. These include measurements of vital signs, of urine output by way of an indwelling catheter, of central venous pressure via a polyethylene catheter threaded through an arm cutdown into the superior vena cava, of hematocrit, and of rate of blood loss by continuous suction through a nasogastric tube. Serial measurements of arterial pH and blood gases are facilitated by insertion of an indwelling catheter into the radial artery, which also makes possible continuous recordings of blood pressure. Because of the systemic circulatory abnormalities and hyperdynamic state that frequently exist in bleeding cirrhotic patients, we have added serial determinations of cardiac output by the dye dilution technique, using indocyanine green, to our monitoring regimen, and often perform measurements of pulmonary artery wedge pressure by percutaneous insertion of a Swan-Ganz pulmonary artery catheter.

Specific Emergency Medical Therapy. Emergency medical treatment used specifically to stop varix bleeding includes esophageal balloon tamponade, systemic intravenous administration of vasopressin (posterior pituitary extract), selective mesenteric intra-arterial administration of vasopressin, and gastroesophageal hypothermia. Although each of these measures is capable of temporarily controlling bleeding esophageal varices, it has been our experience, as well as that reported by many other workers, that they have not significantly influenced the mortality rate of varix hemorrhage in cirrhotic patients.

1. ESOPHAGEAL BALLOON TAMPONADE. The most widely used nonoperative method of treatment has been esophageal balloon tamponade (Fig. 21). Since its

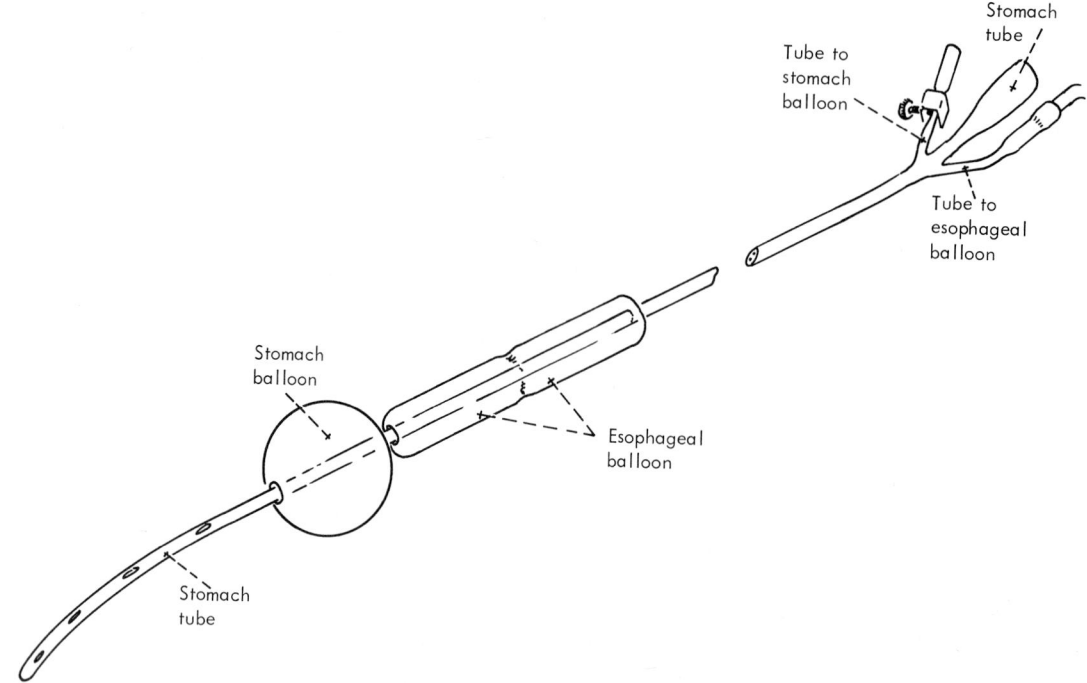

Figure 21. The Sengstaken-Blakemore triple-lumen, double-balloon tube used to tamponade esophageal varices. The gastric balloon is inflated first and pulled up against the cardiac sphincter by continuous mild traction. The esophageal balloon directly compresses the varices in the lower esophagus. The third lumen is used for irrigation of the stomach and removal of blood and gastric contents.

introduction in 1930 by Westphal, and its popularization in 1950 by Sengstaken and Blakemore, balloon tamponade has been adopted by many hospitals in the world as standard treatment for bleeding esophageal varices. As shown in Table 10, there is no doubt that this popular mode of therapy has initially stopped varix bleeding in many patients. The disheartening aspect of this form of management has been that many of the patients have resumed bleeding when the balloons were deflated. Moreover, we and others have observed frequent and sometimes lethal complications of balloon tamponade, which include perforation of the esophagus, asphyxiation from regurgitation of the

balloon into the pharynx, and aspiration pneumonia. Most important, data from a number of institutions clearly indicate that balloon tamponade has failed to influence measurably the mortality rate of bleeding esophageal varices during a trial of 25 years. For these reasons, we have abandoned the use of balloon tamponade as a definitive form of treatment and use it only on infrequent occasions as a temporary measure to prepare patients for operation when massive bleeding cannot be initially controlled by other means.

2. SYSTEMIC INTRAVENOUS VASOPRESSIN (POSTERIOR PITUITARY EXTRACT). It has been shown in both experimental animals and man that vasopressin reduces

TABLE 10.   Results of Esophageal Balloon Tamponade in Cirrhotic Patients with Bleeding Varices

Authors	Year Reported	Number of Patients	Initial Control (%)	Ultimate Control (%)	Mortality (%)
Reynolds, Freedman, and Winsor	1952	32	66	50	47
Hamilton	1955	20	45	—	75
Ludington	1958	58	75	43	—
Conn	1958	50	70	—	82
Read, Dawson, Kerr, Turner, and Sherlock	1960	38	84	24	74
Merigan, Hollister, Gryska, Starkey, and Davidson	1960	68	—	—	80
Orloff	1962	45	56	20	82
		Total 311			Mean 74

TABLE 11. Results of Systemic Intravenous Vasopressin in Cirrhotic Patients with Bleeding Varices

Authors	Number of Patients	Number of Trials	Initial Success (%)	Rebled (%)	Mortality (%)
Schwartz, Bales, Emerson, and Mahoney	11	27	89	Frequent	—
Merigan, Plotkin, and Davidson	15	22	73	Frequent	93
Shaldon and Sherlock	8	25	100	63	75
Orloff	138	138	94	Immediate operation	—
	18	18	88	83	—

portal pressure and blood flow by constricting the splanchnic arterioles. The response is directly related to the dose and rapidity of injection, and in the usual clinical dosage range has a duration of 1 hour or less. However, as shown in Table 11, the transient reduction of portal pressure has been sufficient to stop varix hemorrhage temporarily in a large percentage of patients. Unfortunately, most of the patients have bled again unless operation was performed within 8 hours of treatment, and subsequent administration of the drug has been much less effective in stopping bleeding. Recently, continuous rather than bolus intravenous infusion of vasopressin in low doses has been tried in an attempt to lengthen the period of hemostasis. It is apparent, however, that vasopressin alone is not a definitive form of treatment but may be of considerable immediate value while other measures are being readied or the patient is being prepared for operation. Every patient with bleeding esophageal varices is given vasopressin soon after admission to our institution. The agent is administered intravenously over a 15- to 20-minute period in a dose of 20 units of Pituitrin diluted in 200 ml. of solution. We have not observed any cardiac abnormalities related to single-dose infusion of Pituitrin, but prolonged infusion may be hazardous in patients with coronary artery disease. Posterior pituitary extract (Pituitrin) is as effective in controlling bleeding as pure vasopressin. This measure of therapy has largely replaced esophageal balloon tamponade as our means of obtaining immediate control of hemorrhage.

3. SELECTIVE MESENTERIC INTRA-ARTERIAL VASOPRESSIN. Continuous infusion of vasopressin into an indwelling catheter inserted in the superior mesenteric artery was introduced by Nusbaum et al. in 1967 for the control of bleeding esophageal varices. Since that time, the technique has been widely used and rather uncritically accepted. The objective of the method is to obtain prolonged effects of vasopressin on the splanchnic circulation without systemic hemodynamic effects. However, a number of recent studies have shown that continuous selective mesenteric intra-arterial infusion of vasopressin often is accompanied by a decrease in cardiac output, a fall in femoral arterial Po_2 and a rise in arterial blood pressure, so that the systemic effects of the drug clearly are not avoided. Moreover, portal venous Po_2 regularly falls during infusion, an undesirable side effect. Initial control of varix bleeding has

been good, but it has not been superior to that obtained with the much simpler and less invasive systemic intravenous administration of vasopressin. Most important, in the only prospective, controlled clinical trial that has been performed to date, Conn et al. found that mesenteric intra-arterial infusion of vasopressin failed to influence significantly the mortality of varix hemorrhage when compared to conventional therapy. When the potential and actual complications of indwelling catheterization of the superior mesenteric artery are added to these recent findings, there is little to indicate that the selective intra-arterial technique is worthwhile.

4. GASTROESOPHAGEAL HYPOTHERMIA. Use of gastroesophageal hypothermia to stop varix bleeding is based on the demonstration that lowering the temperature of the stomach to 10 to 14° C. abolishes the digestive activity of gastric juice and produces a significant reduction of blood flow in the stomach. Cooling is accomplished with balloons in the stomach and esophagus through which a cold alcohol-water solution is circulated. The rationale of gastroesophageal cooling in part hinges on the theory that rupture of esophageal varices is the result of reflux acid-peptic esophagitis. However, our studies have cast considerable doubt on the acid-peptic hypothesis. Experience with gastroesophageal hypothermia has been small but reports indicate that this technique, although often effective in temporarily stopping bleeding, has failed to lower the mortality rate of varix hemorrhage and probably does not warrant serious consideration.

5. OTHER NONSURGICAL MEASURES. Over the years, numerous nonsurgical methods of controlling bleeding from esophageal varices have been tried, all of them without success. Injection of sclerosing solutions directly into bleeding varices through the esophagoscope has been advocated intermittently since its initial description 37 years ago, but it has failed to receive general acceptance as a safe and effective procedure. The most recent nonsurgical approach, still in the experimental stage, involves percutaneous transhepatic catheterization of the portal vein and its branches, and injection of blood clots or sclerosing solutions into the coronary vein and the varices. While opinion may differ on the likelihood that this technique will succeed, it is important to emphasize that it is an invasive and potentially dangerous measure that should not be widely attempted until careful trials are

conducted in a few centers. The ultimate and essential test of any new therapeutic modality is its influence on the high mortality rate of the disease.

Specific Emergency Surgical Therapy. During the past quarter century, the widely accepted approach to the treatment of bleeding varices in patients with cirrhosis has involved the use of temporary nonsurgical emergency measures directed at stopping the hemorrhage so as to permit deliberate and methodical preparation of the patients for an elective portacaval shunt. This approach has been based on the belief that, on the one hand, it is often possible to stabilize and improve the underlying liver disease and, on the other hand, cirrhotic patients will not tolerate major operations performed under emergency circumstances in the face of hemorrhage. A wealth of evidence indicates that this approach has not substantially influenced survival of the bleeding cirrhotic population, since two thirds to three fourths of the patients have died during the initial bleeding episode and only 10 to 20 per cent have become eligible for elective therapy. Because of the failure of the "traditional" approach there has been considerable recent interest in emergency surgical management. Results obtained during the past 10 years have been encouraging and suggest that immediate operation is the treatment of choice in most patients. Experience is insufficient as yet to establish definite criteria for selection of patients for operation. Although it is clear that the risk of operation is great in patients with decompensated cirrhosis, it is also certain that such patients have little chance of surviving with nonoperative therapy. Currently, emergency operative treatment is largely confined to the use of two operations, transesophageal varix ligation and the emergency portacaval shunt. Both procedures stop varix bleeding in almost all patients, and the problem associated with them is mainly that of hepatic decompensation which may result when a critically ill patient with a severely damaged liver is subjected to anesthesia and major trauma, in addition to hemorrhage.

1. TRANSESOPHAGEAL VARIX LIGATION (Fig. 22). Since Boerema first described transesophageal ligation of esophageal varices in 1949, the reported experience with this procedure has not been large. Moreover, the cases have varied so greatly as to etiology, severity of the underlying disease, prior treatment, and time lapse between onset of bleeding and ligation, that accurate assessment of the results is difficult. The mortality rate has ranged from 15 to 86 per cent. The largest reported series has involved 72 selected patients with an operative mortality rate of 50 per cent. Because the value of this procedure was not clearly established, several years ago we undertook a prospective comparison of emergency transesophageal varix ligation and medical therapy. Every cirrhotic patient admitted to the hospital with varix bleeding was included in the study with no attempt at selection. The diagnostic work-up was completed within 6 hours and, in the surgical group, operation was performed within 8 hours of admission to the hospital. The study was conducted in comparable groups of chronic alcoholics with moderate to advanced cirrhosis and massive varix hemorrhage. Approximately half the pa-

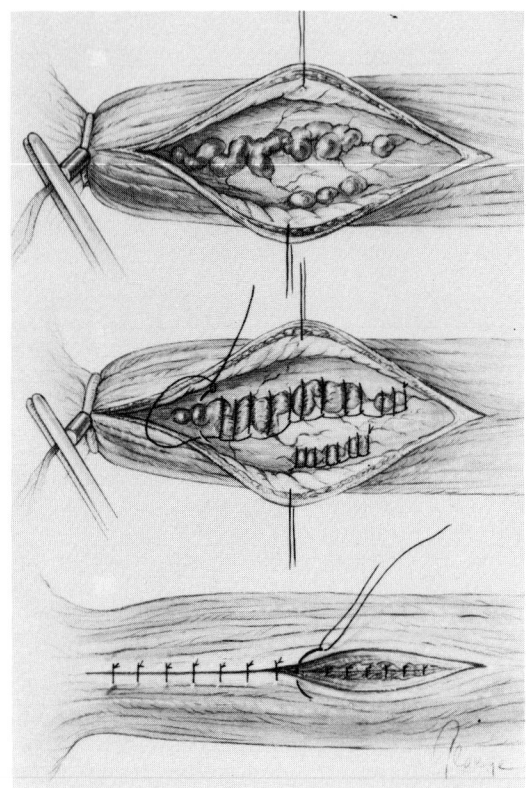

Figure 22. Technique of transesophageal varix ligation. (From Orloff, M. J.: Surgery, 52:103, 1962.)

tients in each group had jaundice and ascites, and one fourth had hepatic encephalopathy. When feasible, the patients who survived emergency surgical or medical therapy were prepared for and underwent an elective portacaval shunt at a later date.

The results of this study are included in the summary presented in Table 12. Emergency transesophageal varix ligation consistently controlled bleeding. The early survival rate was 54 per cent following operative ligation compared to 14 per cent in the medically treated patients. The five-year survival rate was 21 per cent in the surgical group and 3 per cent in the medical group, and the ten-year survival rates were 11 per cent and 0, respectively. Our experience showed that varix ligation is not a definitive procedure, but must be considered the first of two stages in treatment, the second stage of which is an elective portacaval shunt. The refusal of some patients to undergo an elective shunt was invariably associated with rebleeding and played a major role in the declining survival rate. Moreover, in evaluating the long-term results of both varix ligation and medical therapy, the mortality rate of the subsequent elective portacaval shunt must be considered.

A major reason for considering transesophageal varix ligation as emergency treatment for bleeding varices is the belief that it is an effective procedure of lesser magnitude than other emergency operations. Our experience has shown that such is not the case.

TABLE 12.   Comparison of Results of Emergency Portacaval Shunt, Transesophageal Varix Ligation, and Medical Treatment in Unselected Patients with Cirrhosis and Bleeding Varices

	Medical Treatment*	Varix Ligation*	Emergency Shunt
Number of patients	59	28	146
Jaundice on admission	42%	57%	47%
Ascites on admission	41%	50%	53%
Encephalopathy on admission	25%	25%	20%
Mean liver index	2.8	2.8	2.4
Admission hemoglobin 11 gm./100 ml. or less	70%	71%	69%
Varices demonstrated	95%	100%	100%
Mean volume of blood transfused – liters	7.2	4.2	5.2
Early survival (30 days)	17%	54%	53%
Ten-year survival	0%	11%	30%

*Followed by elective portacaval shunt when possible.

The time required to perform the operation, the magnitude of the trauma, the metabolic response, and the effects on liver function are similar to those associated with emergency portacaval shunt. While varix ligation appears to have distinct advantages over medical therapy, it does not appear to be the best emergency surgical procedure available.

2. EMERGENCY PORTACAVAL SHUNT. Portal-systemic shunt is the only available definitive treatment for portal hypertension and esophageal varices. Numerous studies have shown that a technically satisfactory portacaval shunt will permanently solve the problem of bleeding varices in the vast majority of patients. The obvious potential advantage of performing this procedure under emergency circumstances is that, unlike other forms of treatment, it can be expected to provide both immediate and prolonged control of varix hemorrhage. The question is, can cirrhotic patients tolerate an operation of this magnitude when it is performed as an emergency in the face of bleeding? To answer this question, we have been conducting a prospective study of emergency portacaval shunt, similar to our comparative evaluation of varix ligation and medical therapy. The study is distinguished from all other reported studies of emergency treatment in that it has involved *every* cirrhotic patient admitted with varix bleeding, regardless of his or her condition on admission. Between 1962 and 1975, 146 consecutive, unselected patients underwent emergency portacaval shunt within 8 hours of admission to the emergency room. Follow-up study has been conducted in a special clinic, and the current status of 97.3 per cent of the patients is known. The results are shown in the comparative summary in Table 12 and Figure 23. The early survival rate was 53 per cent, compared to 54 per cent for varix ligation and 17 per cent for medical therapy. The ten-year survival rate, calculated according to the actuarial method, was 30 per cent, compared to 11 per cent for varix ligation and 0 for medical treatment. The actual ten-year survival rate for the patients operated upon ten or more years ago was 37 per cent. Portacaval shunt controlled the bleeding promptly and permanently in 97 per cent of the patients. Encephalopathy of any degree requiring temporary or prolonged dietary protein restriction

developed at some time in 26 per cent of the survivors. Fifty-nine per cent of the survivors abstained from alcohol permanently, and 57 per cent resumed gainful employment or full-time housekeeping.

Since our study involved unselected patients, a careful analysis was performed of all of the factors present on admission that might have influenced survival in the hope of identifying criteria for future selection of patients for operation. The results of this analysis, shown in Table 13, indicated that there were two factors which increased the mortality rate, but that a substantial number of patients survived the shunt procedure despite the presence. The two preoperative clinical features that significantly affected survival were ascites and a SGOT level of 100 units or higher. Severe muscle wasting and the presence of encephalopathy were each associated with a higher mortality rate, but the association was not statistically signifi-

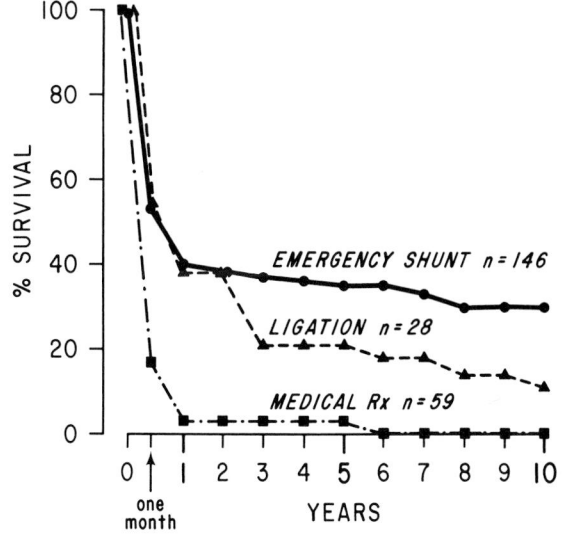

Figure 23. Cumulative 5-year survival rates of patients with cirrhosis and varix hemorrhage following emergency portacaval shunt, transesophageal varix ligation, and medical treatment.

TABLE 13.   Influence on Operative Survival of Clinical and Laboratory Findings on Admission in 146 Bleeding Cirrhotic Patients

	Per Cent of Group	Survival Rate (%)	Significant Influence on Survival
Ascites			
Present	53	40	P < 0.01
Absent	47	68	
SGOT			
≥ 100 units	34	40	P < 0.05
< 100 units	66	64	
Muscle wasting			
Severe	27	42	None
Moderate to mild	73	58	
Liver size			
Small	16	46	None
Enlarged	84	54	
Jaundice			
Present	47	54	None
Absent	53	53	
Encephalopathy			
Present	20	41	None
Past history only	11	41	
Absent at admission and in past	69	59	
Splenomegaly			
Present	43	52	None
Absent	57	48	
Hypokalemic alkalosis			
pH 7.5 or > and K^+ < 3.5	17	38	None
pH < 7.5 and/or K^+ > 3.5	83	57	
Liver function index (0–4.0)			
> 3.4	8	10	P < 0.01
3.0–3.4	26	55 ⎫	
2.0–2.9	44	55 ⎬	None
< 2.0	22	78 ⎭	

cant. Jaundice and encephalopathy together did not adversely affect the mortality rate. Similarly, there was no statistically significant correlation between the results of liver function tests (considered individually or together as a liver index) and survival, except at the extreme of hepatic dysfunction. Interestingly, fourteen patients had concurrent jaundice, ascites, encephalopathy, and severe muscle wasting on admis-

sion, and 36 per cent survived the shunt. However, all 14 died within one year of operation.

The experience of others with emergency portacaval shunt is shown in Table 14. All but one of these studies were retrospective in nature, and all involved selected patients; therefore, they cannot be compared with our experience in an unselected population.

The results of our studies indicate that emergency

TABLE 14.   Overall Immediate Results of Emergency Portacaval Shunt in the Therapy of Bleeding Esophageal Varices in Cirrhotic Patients

Authors	Year	Number of Patients	Type of Evaluation	Operative Survival (%)
Orloff	1975	146	Prospective—Unselected patients	53
VA Cooperative Study	1971	50	Prospective—Selected patients	52
Mikkelsen	1962	37	Retrospective—Selected patients	65
Wantz and Payne	1961	34	Retrospective—Selected patients	59
Ekman and Sandblom	1964	30	Retrospective—Selected patients	83
Balasegaram and Damodaran	1970	30	Retrospective—Selected patients	70
Megevand	1970	30	Retrospective—Selected patients	70
Adson	1967	30	Retrospective—Selected patients	73
Weinberger	1965	29	Retrospective—Selected patients	72
Preston and Trippel	1965	25	Retrospective—Selected patients	56
Hoffman, Jepson, and Harris	1969	20	Retrospective—Selected patients	55

portacaval shunt has produced a significant improvement in immediate and long-term survival of cirrhotic patients with bleeding esophageal varices. As is true of survival statistics for cancer and other lethal disorders, the absolute survival rate is of limited meaning unless it is viewed in the context of the natural history of the disease. The 10-year survival rate in our experience to date is many times greater than that associated with emergency medical therapy followed by elective portacaval shunt in the few patients who survive. Undoubtedly, some patients with advanced cirrhosis will not survive with any form of therapy currently available. The problem is that criteria for identifying such patients are not yet known. Thus far, we have been able to identify only one type of patient who does not stand a better chance of survival with emergency shunt than with other forms of therapy, namely, the patient who presents with concurrent ascites, jaundice, encephalopathy and severe muscle wasting. The development of additional sound criteria for selection of patients for various forms of treatment unquestionably will improve the results of operative management. Until such additional guidelines are developed by well-controlled, prospective studies or until alternative effective therapy is devised, it would appear that emergency portacaval shunt is the therapy of choice for most cirrhotic patients who bleed from esophageal varices.

3. OTHER EMERGENCY OPERATIONS. A host of other operative procedures have been used as emergency treatment of bleeding esophageal varices. Included among these are gastric or esophageal transection, sometimes combined with extensive ligation of the veins around the distal esophagus and upper stomach; esophagogastrectomy with or without interposition of a segment of colon or jejunum; splenectomy alone or with coronary vein ligation; combination of splenectomy, resection of the proximal two thirds of the greater curvature of the stomach, ligation of gastric and esophageal varices, ligation of the left gastric artery, and, sometimes, vagotomy and pyloroplasty; ligation of the hepatic, left gastric, and splenic arteries; external drainage of the thoracic duct; and an extracorporeal or subcutaneous shunt between the umbilical and saphenous veins. Although some success has been obtained with each of these procedures, often in a small number of cases, general experience with them has not been good for a variety of reasons, and they do not warrant serious consideration.

Postoperative Care Following Emergency Portacaval Shunt. Cirrhotic patients who bleed from esophageal varices are among the most seriously ill patients in any hospital, regardless of the specific therapy used to control the bleeding. In those who undergo emergency portacaval shunt, the expertness of the postoperative care is a major factor in determining survival. All such patients should be admitted to an intensive care unit with equipment and personnel geared to managing the complicated problems associated with this disease. Specific prophylactic and therapeutic aspects of postoperative care are as follows:

1. MONITORING. Careful monitoring of vital signs, central venous pressure, urine output, arterial pH, arterial and alveolar gases, fluid balance, body weight, and abdominal girth are essential. Serial electrocardiograms and determinations of cardiac output, peripheral resistance, and pulmonary artery wedge pressure with a Swan-Ganz catheter often are very helpful. Serial measurements of liver function, of the formed elements in the blood, including platelets, of blood coagulation, of serum electrolytes, and of renal function must be done.

2. PARENTERAL FLUID THERAPY. Patients with cirrhosis are often water-logged even before the onset of bleeding from varices, and they have a markedly impaired capacity to excrete water loads. The bleeding episode and the operation intensify renal sodium and water retention and exaggerate the already existing fluid intolerance. Parenteral fluid therapy should be calculated to maintain such patients on the dry side. Fluid losses are replaced by a solution of 10 per cent dextrose in water containing vitamins B, C, and K. The total volume usually amounts to 1500 to 2000 ml. per day, based on daily losses of 500 ml. of nasogastric aspirate, 500 to 1000 ml. of urine, 800 to 1000 ml. of insensible water, and a *gain* of 250 to 500 ml. from endogenous water formation. Sodium is given only to replace nasogastric losses, which rarely exceed 30 to 40 mEq. per day. Parenteral potassium therapy is started as soon as the urine output is adequate, and is given in whatever amounts are necessary to maintain the serum potassium concentration between 4 and 5 mEq. per liter. Usually, the requirement is 150 to 200 mEq. per day, but doses as high as 500 mEq. per day may be necessary. If a metabolic alkalosis develops, as is often the case, it usually responds to repletion of potassium with large quantities of parenteral potassium chloride. If the alkalosis fails to respond, an acidifying agent such as arginine hydrochloride, hydrochloric acid, or ammonium chloride, should be administered slowly so as to lower the arterial blood pH below 7.50. In addition to crystalloid fluid therapy, it is often necessary to add colloid therapy to replace continuing losses of blood and plasma. Transfusions of fresh blood are given for blood loss or a hematocrit below 30 per cent. Type-specific, single-donor plasma, fresh-frozen plasma, or salt-poor concentrated albumin is given for losses of fluid into the operation site and peritoneal cavity (acute ascites), as determined by the combined measurements of abdominal girth, central venous pressure, urine output, body weight, and a hematocrit showing hemoconcentration.

A major shortcoming of current parenteral fluid therapy is its caloric deficiency. It is estimated that a patient who has undergone an emergency portacaval shunt for varix hemorrhage has a metabolic response that consumes 4000 to 5000 calories per day for the first few postoperative days. Two liters of 10 per cent dextrose in water provides a total of only 800 calories. There is little doubt that postoperative cirrhotic patients would derive benefit from early nutritional therapy. For this reason, during the past several years we have been involved in a trial of parenteral hyperalimentation with a concentrated glucose-amino acid solution starting on the first day postoperatively. However, it is not certain that the potential benefits of such treatment outweigh the complications and difficulties associated with its use.

3. Pulmonary Therapy. Pulmonary complications, particularly infection and wet lung, are a major cause of morbidity and mortality in patients with cirrhosis and bleeding varices. In about 10 per cent of our cases it has been necessary to maintain the patient on a respirator for several days postoperatively. In such cases, mechanical ventilatory support usually can be provided through an endotracheal tube that may be left indwelling for 48 to 72 hours. Occasionally it is necessary to perform a tracheostomy for ventilation and tracheobronchial toilet, but it should be recognized that complications of tracheostomy, particularly bleeding, are more frequent in cirrhotic patients. Portable chest x-rays are obtained daily in patients on respirators or those having pulmonary problems. The decision to taper off and then discontinue mechanical ventilatory support is based on measurements of arterial blood and alveolar gases, ventilatory volumes, chest x-rays, and physical findings.

All patients not on a respirator are given continuous oxygen therapy by nasal catheter, nasal prongs, or mask for 5 to 7 days postoperatively because of the frequent cardiovascular abnormalities and arteriovenous shunting that exist in cirrhosis. From the start, all patients receive intensive respiratory therapy that consists of intermittent tracheobronchial aspiration, postural drainage, chest physiotherapy, intermittent positive-pressure respiration, frequent turning, encouragement to cough and breathe deeply, and the use of blow bottles and a humidifier. Diuretics may be of value in the treatment of pulmonary edema due to left heart failure or infection.

4. Hyperdynamic Circulation. Numerous studies have shown that patients with cirrhosis and portal hypertension frequently have a hyperdynamic state that consists of a decrease in vascular tone and peripheral resistance, an increase in cardiac index, an increase in venous oxygen saturation with widespread peripheral arteriovenous shunting and marked pulmonary arteriovenous admixture. These abnormalities are sometimes intensified by bleeding from esophageal varices or performance of a portacaval shunt, and high-output cardiac failure may develop, particularly in older patients and those with far advanced liver disease. It is for this reason that we perform serial measurements of cardiac output in all patients both preoperatively and postoperatively. Patients with a hyperdynamic state are digitalized immediately postoperatively, before there are any signs of cardiac failure. Vigorous correction of hypovolemia is undertaken simultaneously. Once blood volume is restored, fluids are restricted to avoid circulatory overload, and diuretics are used if there are any signs of overhydration. Positive inotropic drugs are used when appropriate.

5. Delirium Tremens. Alcoholic cirrhotic patients frequently have delirium tremens following hemorrhage alone or in combination with a portacaval shunt or other operation. There is not always a close temporal correlation between alcohol withdrawal and the development of this serious disorder; we have observed postoperative delirium tremens weeks and months after ingestion of alcohol was stopped. Delirium tremens by itself, in the absence of bleeding or an operation, is associated with a mortality rate of 15 to 35 per cent. When added to the stress of hemorrhage or major surgery, the mortality rate climbs to 50 to 60 per cent. Initial treatment consists of administration of a central nervous system depressant. We prefer intramuscular magnesium sulfate in doses of 5 gm. every 2 to 4 hours. If magnesium sulfate therapy is not rapidly effective, chlordiazepoxide hydrochloride (Librium) is added in a dose of 25 to 50 mg. intramuscularly every 4 hours. Supportive treatment in the form of adequate parenteral fluids containing concentrated glucose and vitamins, antipyretic agents, and pulmonary therapy is important. This hyperactive, hypermetabolic disorder must not be confused with hepatic encephalopathy, since the use of a central nervous system depressant in hepatic encephalopathy may be lethal. Intravenous alcohol is a severe hepatotoxin, and there is no basis for its use in cirrhotic patients with postoperative delirium tremens. Parenteral paraldehyde has no advantages over other hypnotic drugs and, in the author's opinion, should not be used because of the frequent soft tissue abscesses and noxious odor it produces.

6. Hepatic Failure. The majority of patients appear to be in surprisingly good condition immediately following an emergency portacaval shunt. However, by the second or third postoperative day there is evidence of some deterioration of liver function in almost all patients. In many patients the liver dysfunction stabilizes and then improves, but in some it progresses to hepatic coma and the full syndrome of hepatic failure, with jaundice, severe abnormalities of blood coagulation, ascites, and renal insufficiency. Liver failure is the most frequent cause of death in cirrhotic patients who bleed from esophageal varices, whether or not they have had a portacaval shunt.

The subject of hepatic coma is discussed in detail later in this chapter. It should be emphasized that the hepatic coma that occurs during the immediate postoperative period is due to liver cell failure, and is *not* related to ammonia intoxication or systemic shunting of nitrogenous substances absorbed from the intestines. Unfortunately, there is no specific therapy for hepatic failure, and all that can be done is to provide parenteral nutritional support and symptomatic therapy of the individual abnormalities that arise. There is no evidence that exchange transfusion, hemodialysis, or extracorporal perfusion of the blood through a pig, baboon, or human liver are of value in this situation. Spontaneous recovery sometimes occurs.

Because it is rarely possible to remove all of the blood from the gastrointestinal tract preoperatively, neomycin therapy (1 gm. every 6 hours via the nasogastric tube), cathartics (60 ml. magnesium sulfate per day via the nasogastric tube), and a daily neomycin enema (4 gm. in 1 quart of water) are continued for 3 days postoperatively. If continued beyond 3 days, troublesome diarrhea usually follows. With this regimen, significantly elevated blood ammonia levels or signs of nitrogen-related encephalopathy rarely occur within the first postoperative week.

7. Gastric Acid Hypersecretion. The subjects of gastric acid hypersecretion and peptic ulcer following portacaval shunt are discussed in detail later in this chapter. To protect against this potential complica-

tion, nasogastric suction is continued for 3 or 4 days postoperatively. As soon as the nasogastric tube is removed, the patient is started on hourly antacid therapy until his oral dietary intake is good, and then the antacid schedule is changed to between meals and at bedtime. An antacid that does not contain sodium is used. Antacid therapy and avoidance of ulcerogenic foods are continued for life.

8. RENAL FAILURE. The subject of renal failure is discussed in detail later in this chapter. There are two common forms of renal dysfunction following varix hemorrhage and portacaval shunt. The first is acute tubular necrosis which results from a period of hypotension and consequent renal ischemia. It is manifested by oliguria, azotemia, hyperkalemia, a low fixed urine specific gravity and osmolality, substantial quantities of sodium in the urine, and a urine sediment containing casts and red blood cells. Treatment consists of stringent fluid restriction, measures to reduce serum potassium, and, if necessary, hemodialysis. The second renal disorder is spontaneous renal failure associated with hepatic decompensation, the so-called "hepatorenal syndrome." It is more insidious in onset than acute tubular necrosis and is manifested initially by progressive azotemia without striking oliguria. In contrast to acute tubular necrosis, the urine specific gravity is variable and ranges up to 1.020, there is almost no sodium in the urine, the osmolality of the urine is high, and the urine sediment is normal. There is no specific treatment for spontaneous renal failure, and therapy is directed at reversing the hepatic decompensation, minimizing dilutional hyponatremia, and correcting problems as they appear. There is no indication for the use of diuretics and, in fact, they may intensify the renal abnormality. Numerous vasoactive agents have been used for the purpose of improving renal blood flow, but none have influenced the outcome significantly. Hemodialysis has created more problems than it has solved. The mortality rate of the combined syndrome of hepatic and renal decompensation is very high.

9. INFECTION. Substantial evidence indicates that patients with cirrhosis have a high incidence of infection, perhaps because of their debilitated general condition. Surprisingly, wound and intraperitoneal infections following emergency portacaval shunt have been uncommon in our experience. However, pulmonary infections have been common and urinary tract infections not infrequent. The value of prophylactic antibiotic therapy in this condition has not been establi.hed. Appropriate antibiotics are given for proven infections, always on the basis of bacterial cultures and antibiotic sensitivity tests. We routinely obtain cultures of tracheal aspirates and urine during the early postoperative period to avoid delays in therapy should infection develop.

10. NUTRITION. Nutritional therapy is very important in liver disease. Oral diet is started as soon as the patient tolerates removal of the nasogastric tube for 24 hours, usually on the fifth or sixth postoperative day. Initially, a 200 mg. sodium, 4000 calorie, high carbohydrate, regular fat, 20 gm. protein, bland diet is introduced. There is no basis for restricting fat, and doing so only serves to make the diet unpalatable. The

TABLE 15. Influence of Resumption of Alcoholism Following Emergency Portacaval Shunt on Five-year Survival

	Survivors of Shunt		Five-year Survival (%)
	No.	Per Cent of Group	
Resumption of alcohol	27	41	52
Abstinence from alcohol	39	59	80

protein content of the diet is increased in 20 gm. increments every 3 days up to 80 gm., and the patient is carefully observed for signs of encephalopathy. If the patient tolerates 80 gm. of protein per day, he is discharged on a 60 gm. protein diet after having received a diet list and specific instructions from a dietician. Rigorous sodium restriction is continued for several months and, even after a year has elapsed, sodium intake is not allowed to advance above 2.5 gm. per day. Daily therapeutic doses of vitamins B and C are added to the diet.

11. ALCOHOLISM. Perhaps the major factor that determines long-term survival following portacaval shunt is abstinence or failure to abstain from alcohol. Table 15 shows the difference in survival between patients who consumed alcohol at any time following emergency portacaval shunt and patients who abstained from alcohol. If the group that resumed alcohol consumption were restricted to those who returned to chronic drinking, the difference in survival would be even more striking. It is vitally important that a frank discussion be held with the patient regarding the extremely serious dangers of further ingestion of alcohol. The help of psychiatrists and social workers should be obtained while the patient is in the hospital and continued after discharge. It is incumbent upon the surgeon to exploit his special relationship with the patient in a long-term effort to cure the underlying cause of the patient's liver disease.

12. FOLLOW-UP. A lifelong program of follow-up evaluation and treatment is a crucial part of the care of cirrhotic patients who have undergone portacaval shunt. The liver disease cannot be cured, but it can be stabilized to the point of permitting a long and productive life in reasonable comfort. After discharge from the hospital, out-patient visits are scheduled weekly for the first 8 weeks, monthly for the remainder of the first postoperative year, and every 3 months thereafter for the remainder of the patient's life.

Elective Treatment

In patients who have not undergone an emergency portacaval shunt and have recovered from an episode of bleeding esophageal varices, there is general agreement that elective surgical treatment directed at overcoming portal hypertension is indicated, provided there is a reasonable likelihood that the patient will survive the elective operation. Our study of 27 patients who recovered from their first bleeding episode and qualified for surgical therapy but were deliberately not operated upon showed that 93 per cent bled again, 74 per cent died from the subsequent hemorrhage, and all were dead within 5 years. The only consistently effective treatment for portal hypertension is the portal-systemic shunt, which, when performed properly, will protect more than 90 per cent of patients against subsequent varix hemorrhage. Therefore, one episode of varix bleeding is an indication for elective shunt therapy in all cirrhotic patients, unless they have hepatic decompensation. Unfortunately, only 10 to 20 per cent of bleeding cirrhotic patients survive nonsurgical emergency therapy and recover sufficient hepatic function to become eligible for elective shunt.

What criteria can be used to predict the likelihood of a patient's surviving an elective shunt procedure without serious sequelae? The answer to this question is not known with any degree of certainty and is particularly difficult because the decision not to operate is tantamount to accepting a lethal outcome. The criteria for selection of patients for operation have been undergoing progressive change as knowledge regarding the underlying liver disease and its management has accumulated. The results of liver function tests such as the level of serum albumin, the amount of BSP retention, or the magnitude of prothrombin deficiency do not correlate well with the response to shunt except at the extremes. In the final analysis, the decision concerning operation is based on a composite of many features of a patient's disease, determined during a period of intensive medical treatment in the hospital. Certain features are ominous; thus, the presence of persistent jaundice, of ascites that cannot be stabilized, of repeated bouts of encephalopathy, of advanced muscle wasting, and of a poor appetite indicate that operation should not be undertaken. If these general criteria have been followed, the operative mortality rate has been in the acceptable range of 10 per cent. It should be emphasized that, whenever possible, patients are prepared for an elective operation during a 3- to 6-week period in the hospital with a regimen directed at improving nutrition, slowly restoring blood volume and red cell mass, correcting electrolyte and acid-base abnormalities, and unloading excess fluid.

There are several untoward sequelae of the portal-systemic anastomosis. The most important of these is postshunt encephalopathy, which presumably is due to shunting of ammonia, or some nitrogenous substance absorbed from the intestine, directly into the systemic circulation. The reported incidence of this disturbing complication has varied considerably, but has been in the range of 15 to 30 per cent of patients. Because ammonia is formed by the action of bacteria on nitrogenous substances in the terminal ileum and colon, encephalopathy usually can be controlled by limiting the protein content of the diet and by the use of intestinal antibiotics such as neomycin. If these measures fail, operative exclusion of the colon by ileostomy or ileosigmoidostomy may be effective. The central nervous system disorders associated with liver disease are discussed in greater detail later in this chapter.

The development of peptic ulcer is another potential complication of portal-systemic shunt. Hepatic bypass of a potent intestinal hormone that stimulates gastric acid hypersecretion is a regular consequence of a por-

tacaval anastomosis. This phenomenon is discussed in detail later in this chapter. It would seem prudent to institute antacid therapy and a dietary ulcer regimen following shunt operations.

Venous shunt therapy, of course, represents treatment of the complications of cirrhosis and has no direct beneficial effect on the liver disease itself. In contrast to the effects of portacaval shunt in experimental animals with normal livers, the influence of the operation on liver function in humans with cirrhosis and portal hypertension is variable. In our studies, hepatic function did not change or improved moderately in the majority of patients following operation. Deterioration of hepatic function has been related more closely to whether or not the patient resumed the ingestion of alcohol than to any other factor. Beyond any doubt, the portal-systemic shunt prevents subsequent varix bleeding in the vast majority of patients. Moreover, 39 to 70 per cent of the patients subjected to elective treatment have survived 5 years (Table 16).

The crucial question regarding the value of elective, therapeutic portal-systemic shunt concerns whether a comparable, selected group of patients who were treated medically rather than surgically would survive as long or as well. Unfortunately, despite use of the shunt operation for 30 years, this question has not yet been answered. Three prospective clinical trials of this important matter have been reported recently, two of them showing an advantage of shunt surgery and one of them showing no advantage. However, all three trials have involved small numbers of highly selected patients and have had a number of shortcomings in design and conduct, so that the results do not warrant a conclusive answer. Figure 24 shows the results of a prospective study of elective, therapeutic portacaval shunt recently reported by Mikkelsen and his colleagues. The study was restricted to 75 good risk patients who were randomized into portacaval shunt (37 patients) and medical treatment (38 patients) groups. The 5-year survival rates, calculated by the actuarial method, were 60 per cent for the shunted patients and 10 per cent for the patients treated medically. On the basis of our current knowledge, and until conclusive information to the contrary is available, the elective portacaval shunt is indicated in patients who have bled one or more times from esophageal varices.

Choice of Portal-Systemic Shunt. Because the portal venous system contains no valves, it is possible to decompress it at various points, provided the anastomosis with the low-pressure systemic venous system is of sufficient size to accommodate a large flow of blood. Several types of portal-systemic shunts are available for relief of portal hypertension (Fig. 25). The most commonly used procedures are the end-to-side and side-to-side anastomoses between the portal vein and inferior vena cava, and the end-to-side splenorenal shunt. The *end-to-side portacaval* shunt accomplishes splanchnic decompression by shunting all splanchnic venous blood into the inferior vena cava and, at the same time, it decompresses the liver sinusoid by eliminating the contribution of portal venous blood to hepatic inflow and pressure. However, it

TABLE 16. **Results of Elective Portal-Systemic Shunt in Patients with Cirrhosis**

Authors	No. of Patients	Type of Shunt	Operative Mortality (%)	Varix Rebleeding (%)	5 Year Survival (%)
Voorhees, Price, and Britton	404	324 portacaval 80 splenorenal & other	12	7	51
McDermott, Palazzi, Nardi, and Mondet	237	166 splenorenal 71 portacaval	23	15	54
Barnes et al.	173	103 portacaval 70 splenorenal	13	14	39
Mikkelsen, Turrill, and Pattison	173	All portacaval	12	7	44
Linton, Ellis, and Geary	169	129 splenorenal 47 portacaval	12	19	50
Bismuth, Franco, and Hepp	120	72 central splenorenal 48 portacaval	2	3	66
Wantz and Payne	97	All portacaval	11	5	68 (4 year)
Walker	50	All portacaval	6	12	70
Orloff	82	All portacaval	3	2	60

rarely lowers hepatic sinusoidal pressure to normal, and sinusoidal hypertension often persists because hepatic arterial blood continues to encounter difficulty in leaving the liver through the obstructed hepatic venous outflow system. The *side-to-side portacaval* shunt produces splanchnic decompression equivalent to the end-to-side anastomosis, but it accomplishes significantly greater hepatic decompression by allowing egress of liver blood in a retrograde direction through the portal vein into the low-pressure vena cava. The side-to-side shunt converts the portal vein into an outflow tract, and portal blood does not continue to perfuse the liver. An important question about the side-to-side anastomosis concerns the theoretical possibility that it creates an intrahepatic arteriovenous fistula in which hepatic arterial blood leaves the liver via the portal vein without having made contact with

the hepatic cells and having contributed to hepatic nutrition and metabolism. Studies in experimental animals suggest that arteriovenous shunting occurs to some degree but is compensated for by an increase in afferent hepatic arterial blood flow so that hepatic nutrition is not compromised.

Although the two types of direct portacaval shunt produce similar splanchnic decompression and are equally effective in relieving and preventing varix hemorrhage, the overall hemodynamic effects of the two procedures are distinctly different. Hence, there has been a continuing controversy regarding the comparative advantages and disadvantages of the end-to-side and side-to-side anastomoses. In a series of studies, we have compared the effects of the two types of shunt on hepatic blood flow, liver function, liver morphology, and ammonia tolerance in dogs with experimental cirrhosis, and on hepatic function, ammonia tolerance, the 5-year incidence of encephalopathy, and the 5-year survival rate in cirrhotic humans who were operated on for bleeding esophageal varices. The results are shown in Table 17. There were no significant differences between end-to-side and side-to-side portacaval shunt in any of the parameters that were evaluated. We have concluded that there is no demonstrable advantage of one type of direct portacaval shunt over the other under most circumstances. The one exception may be the unusual patient with severe hepatic outflow obstruction manifested by a pressure on the hepatic side of a clamp occluding the portal vein (HOPP) that is higher than the free portal pressure (FPP). Such patients may have reversal of portal flow, and they have been known to develop intractable ascites following an end-to-side portacaval shunt, which eliminates the portal vein as an outflow tract and, thereby, may increase sinusoidal hypertension. Although clear documentation of this phenomenon does not exist, a side-to-side portacaval shunt would seem to be the procedure of choice in such cases.

The *splenorenal anastomosis* is a variant of the side-to-side, in-continuity shunt. It utilizes tributaries of the portal vein and vena cava which, obviously, are of

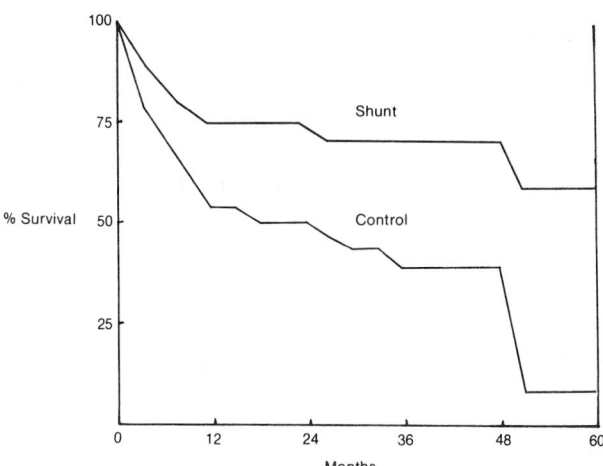

Figure 24. Results of a prospective, randomized clinical comparison of elective therapeutic portacaval shunt and medical treatment in good-risk cirrhotic patients. (From Mikkelsen, W. P.: Therapeutic portacaval shunt. Arch. Surg., *108*:302, 1974.)

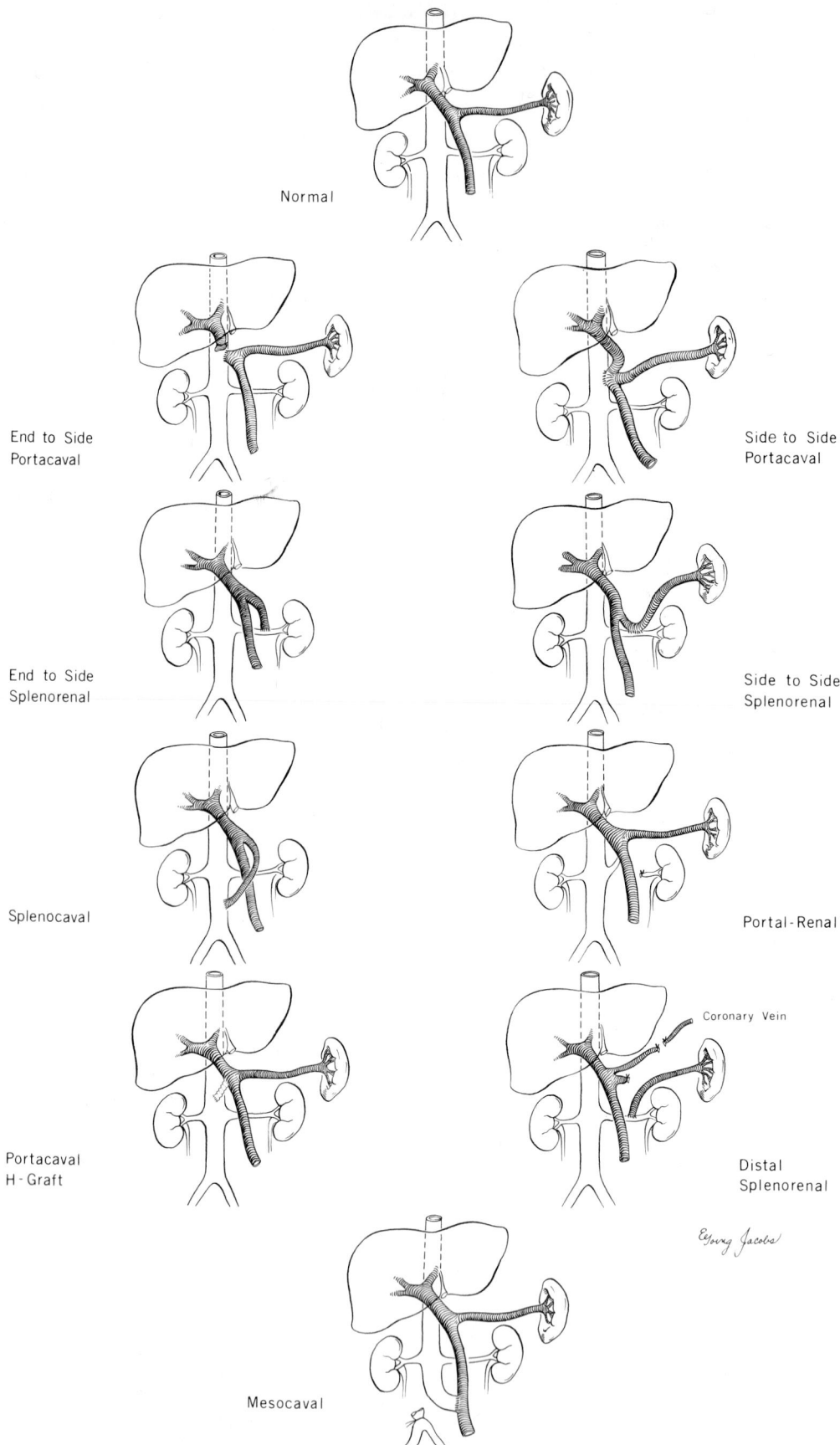

Normal

End to Side
Portacaval

Side to Side
Portacaval

End to Side
Splenorenal

Side to Side
Splenorenal

Splenocaval

Portal-Renal

Portacaval
H-Graft

Coronary Vein

Distal
Splenorenal

Mesocaval

Figure 25. Types of portal-systemic venous shunts used to relieve portal hypertension.

TABLE 17. Comparison of End-to-side and Side-to-side Portacaval Shunt in Dogs with Experimental Cirrhosis and in Cirrhotic Humans Who Were Treated for Bleeding Esophageal Varices

	End-to-side Shunt	Side-to-side Shunt
Cirrhotic dogs		
Hepatic blood flow (mean decrease)	17%	18%
Ammonia tolerance (mean peak blood NH₃)	881 μg./100 ml.	884 μg./100 ml.
Effect on liver function	Same	
Effect on liver morphology	Same	

	Elective Shunt		Emergency Shunt	
	End-to-side	*Side-to-side*	*End-to-side*	*Side-to-side*
Cirrhotic humans				
Number of patients	25	35	26	117
Ammonia tolerance (mean peak blood NH₃)	543 μg./100 ml.	532 μg./100 ml.	–	–
Liver function index at 1 year	1.6	1.7	2.4	2.3
Encephalopathy	25%	23%	27%	25%
Early survival	64%	69%	54%	55%
Five-year survival	48%	57%	29%	36%
Shunt patency at 5 years	100%	100%	92%	100%

smaller size than the parent vessels. It is followed by a lower incidence of protein-related portal-systemic encephalopathy than the direct portacaval anastomosis because it shunts a small volume of nitrogen-containing portal blood into the systemic circulation. At the same time, it does not decompress the portal bed as effectively as the direct portacaval shunt, is associated with a significant incidence of varix rebleeding, and has a high incidence of thrombosis. In the author's opinion it is the procedure of choice only in rare instances when severe and intractable hypersplenism complicates portal hypertension and requires splenectomy. The most commonly used type of splenorenal shunt involves removal of the spleen and anastomosis of the end of the splenic vein to the side of the left renal vein. However, a central side-to-side splenorenal shunt can be done in continuity, without splenectomy. It has been proposed that the latter operation permits continued portal venous perfusion of the liver, but it is doubtful that such is the case since the principles that govern the hemodynamics of a valveless system dictate that flow is in the direction of the area of lowest pressure, i.e., the splenorenal anastomosis.

The *mesocaval shunt* is an anastomosis between the upper end of the divided inferior vena cava and the side of the superior mesenteric vein. In principle, it is hemodynamically similar to the side-to-side portacaval shunt. In patients with extrahepatic portal hypertension due to occlusion of the portal vein, this type of shunt is very effective. However, in adult cirrhotic patients it is doubtful that this procedure represents a first choice. Cirrhotic patients have a tendency to retain salt and water, and division of the inferior vena cava may lead to intractable edema of the lower extremities.

The use of H grafts between the intact portal or superior mesenteric vein and inferior vena cava, introduced 25 years ago, recently has attracted renewed interest. Synthetic prostheses of Dacron and Teflon,

autogenous jugular vein, and homologous vena cava have been used for this purpose. *The interposition mesocaval or portacaval H graft* is a relatively minor technical variation of the direct side-to-side portacaval shunt and, despite claims to the contrary, the two procedures are hemodynamically identical. The major advantage claimed for the H-graft procedure is that it is technically less difficult to perform than conventional shunts. The major potential disadvantage is the possibility of thrombosis, particularly of the synthetic prostheses. In general, the use of grafts in the venous system has had a long history of failure, so that there is justifiable skepticism about the possibility of consistent long-term patency of the H graft. Short-term results of interposition shunts involving a collective total of some 240 patients have been reported from 10 centers. The operative mortality rate in this heterogeneous collection of patients has been about 15 per cent, which is not different from that associated with conventional portacaval shunts. The short-term incidence of thrombosis has ranged from 5 to 20 per cent, which if it continues or increases with prolonged observation, will be unacceptable when compared to the less than 2 per cent long-term occlusion rate of direct portacaval anastomoses in experienced hands. The incidence of post-shunt encephalopathy has been similar to that following direct portacaval shunt, as expected. It is essential that long-term studies of graft patency be performed in a substantial number of carefully observed patients before the H-graft procedure receives general acceptance as an alternative to direct portacaval shunt.

An unsettled issue of great importance regarding the use of portacaval shunt concerns its effects both on liver cell function (presumably related to liver blood flow) and on portal-systemic encephalopathy (presumably related to hepatic bypass of nitrogenous substances absorbed from the intestines). When portal blood is completely shunted away from the liver, further liver damage might be anticipated unless there is a compensatory increase in hepatic arterial blood flow. It is not possible by any currently available, practical method to predict the adequacy of hepatic arterial compensation prior to performance of a portacaval shunt. It has been proposed that a worsening of liver function or outright hepatic failure following portacaval shunt is due to sudden diversion of needed blood away from the liver. The familiar hepatic dysfunction that follows creation of a portacaval shunt (Eck fistula) in the dog with a normal liver is cited as evidence for this proposal. The fact that patients with extrahepatic occlusion of the portal vein do not usually have significant hepatic dysfunction, either before or after portal-systemic anastomosis, has been interpreted as resulting from the combination of a long period of adaptation to diminished portal flow and an initially normal hepatic parenchyma. On the basis of preoperative and intraoperative measurements made in a small group of subjects, it has been proposed that cirrhotic patients with normal or near-normal portal blood flow, who often appear to be the best-risk patients with the least severe liver disease, are intolerant of sudden shunting of portal blood, and often die of progressive hepatic failure. On the other hand, it has been proposed that patients with substantially reduced portal blood flow tolerate a portacaval shunt well, since the bypass produces little further reduction in the blood supply to the liver. Finally, it has been suggested that calculations of maximal portal perfusion pressure from intraoperative pressure measurements accurately reflect portal blood flow and permit a prediction of the response to portacaval shunt. The logic of this simple hypothesis is attractive, even though it ignores the vital role of the hepatic arterial blood supply in compensating for portal diversion and the complex nature of the hepatic circulation. However, a wealth of recent data obtained by four separate groups from preoperative and intraoperative measurements of both pressure and blood flow in the portal vein in large numbers of patients has failed to show a correlation between any hemodynamic measurements performed prior to portacaval shunt and survival, hepatic function, or development of encephalopathy after shunt. The results of one such study that we have performed are shown in Table 18. There was no statistically significant correlation between preshunt maximum perfusion pressure and postshunt survival, liver function, hepatic failure, or development of encephalopathy. Contrary to the hypothesis, patients with the lowest preshunt maximum perfusion

pressure had the lowest survival rate and the highest incidence of encephalopathy, whereas patients with the highest preshunt maximum perfusion pressure had the highest survival rate and the lowest incidence of encephalopathy following portacaval shunt. The only hemodynamic parameter that has been shown to correlate with the response to portacaval shunt is the magnitude of compensatory increase in hepatic artery flow, determined in retrospect after performance of the shunt. In a recent study, Burchell et al. demonstrated, by direct intraoperative blood flow measurements immediately after portacaval shunt, that survival and incidence of encephalopathy were directly related to the amount of increase in hepatic artery flow. Unfortunately, there is no currently available method of predicting this increase preoperatively.

On the presumption that portacaval shunt injures the liver and increases portal-systemic encephalopathy in patients with a large hepatopetal portal flow, Warren and his associates proposed in 1967 a modified shunting procedure that is believed to selectively decompress esophageal varices while, at the same time, preserving blood flow to the liver and avoiding systemic shunting of intestinal blood. The operation consists of a *distal splenorenal shunt* in which the splenic side of the divided splenic vein is anastomosed to the intact left renal vein, and *gastrosplenic isolation* aimed at diverting the gastroesophageal venous flow through the shunt (Fig. 26). Gastrosplenic isolation is accomplished by ligation of the coronary vein, the right gastric vein, and the right gastroepiploic vein and division of the gastrohepatic, gastrocolic, and splenocolic ligaments. The most recent report of Warren et al. indicates that over a 7-year period the operation was performed electively in 55 patients with various forms of mild to moderate liver disease, good liver function, and excellent liver blood flow. It is important to recognize that this highly selected group of good risk subjects who survived one or more episodes of varix hemorrhage is not representative of the spectrum of bleeding cirrhotics admitted to a general hospital. Ascites was considered a contraindication to the operation. The overall operative mortality was 17 per cent, but it has been lower in the patients operated on recently. Long-term survival statistics have not yet been reported. In short-term studies, the incidence of rebleeding and of encephalopathy has been low. In fact, the frequency of encephalopathy has been lower than that encountered in a general population of unoperated cirrhotics, which reflects the highly selected nature of the patients subjected to the proce-

TABLE 18.   Relationship of Maximum Portal Perfusion Pressure before Portacaval Shunt
to Survival and Encephalopathy after Shunt

Maximum Portal Perfusion Pressure (mm. saline)	Number of Patients	Overall Survival (%)	Encephalopathy in Survivors (%)
≤ 100	65	46	30
101–200	35	63	23
201–300	23	52	17
> 300	17	71	17

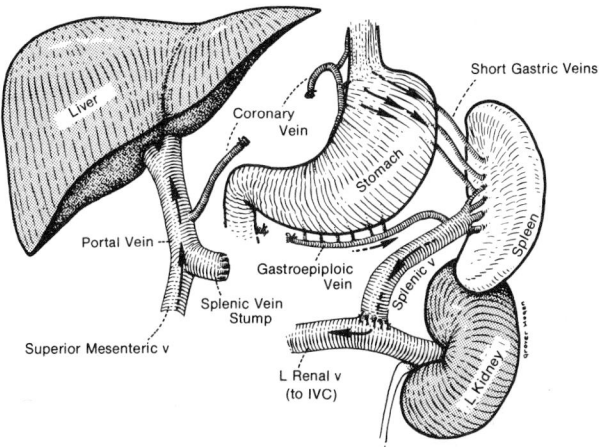

Figure 26. Selective distal splenorenal shunt and gastrosplenic isolation. (From Salam, A. A., Warren, W. D., LePage, R., Jr., Viamonte, M. R., Hutson, D., and Zeppa, R.: Hemodynamic contrasts between selective and total portal-systemic decompression. Ann. Surg., 173:827, 1971.)

dure. The theoretical attractiveness of the distal splenorenal shunt for a selected segment of the bleeding cirrhotic population is undeniable, and the short-term results have been encouraging. However, the operation is technically the most difficult of all of the shunt procedures. Moreover, its value remains to be established by long-term studies of survival, incidence of shunt thrombosis, frequency of rebleeding, and incidence of liver failure and encephalopathy.

In the hope of improving liver blood flow after end-to-side portacaval shunt, in 1968 Maillard et al. proposed a procedure that *combined portacaval shunt with arterialization of the hepatic stump of the portal vein.* Recently, Maillard et al. summarized the experience of others using this approach in 46 patients, and described in detail their own experience with 36 patients. Maillard et al. used the splenic artery to arterialize the hepatic stump of the portal vein, and performed the procedure electively in good risk patients (Child's groups A and B). The operative mortality was 17 per cent, and one month postoperatively 30 per cent of the arteriovenous anastomoses had thrombosed. After one year, the majority of the patients studied had developed thromboses of either the anastomosis or the intrahepatic branches of the portal vein. The incidence of encephalopathy in the patients with patent anastomoses was 17 per cent. On the basis of these results, there is little to recommend serious consideration of this operation.

Prophylactic Portacaval Shunt. Because of the very high mortality rate associated with varix bleeding, some workers have advocated prophylactic performance of portacaval shunt in patients with demonstrable varices who have never bled. Although once a patient has bled from esophageal varices he is almost certain to bleed again, there is nothing to suggest that the mere demonstration of varices in a patient with no history of bleeding permits a prediction regarding the likelihood of varix rupture. In fact, recent statistics indicate that only one fourth to one third of patients with esophageal varices who have no history of bleed-

ing will subsequently have varix hemorrhage. Thus, two thirds to three fourths of the patients subjected to prophylactic portacaval shunt would undergo an operation to prevent a complication that would not have developed had they not received surgical therapy. Herein lies the fallacy of prophylactic shunt.

Recently, prophylactic portacaval shunt was compared with medical therapy in three prospective studies that were performed in selected cirrhotic patients with esophageal varices that had not bled. All three studies showed that prophylactic shunt, while protecting the patients against bleeding, had no influence on survival of selected patients. These results are not surprising. When a major operation is performed in seriously ill patients to prevent a complication that might develop in only one fourth of the patients if they did not have the operation, the results can hardly be expected to be good! Therefore, there is no indication for the prophylactic operation. However, it is important to emphasize that the results of prophylactic portacaval shunt are in no way applicable to the treatment of bleeding esophageal varices by therapeutic portacaval shunt, since, in the therapeutic situation, the patients already have developed the complication of bleeding and it is almost certain to recur unless the portal hypertension is relieved.

ASCITES

Ascites is a serious complication of cirrhosis. In many patients, it develops suddenly in association with severe hepatocellular damage and is a manifestation of hepatic decompensation. In others, it develops gradually and persists as a chronic disturbance that leads to progressive discomfort, nutritional depletion, and debilitation.

The pathogenesis of ascites is best explained by Starling's hypothesis, which states that the exchange of fluid across capillary membranes is a result of the hydrostatic pressure and osmotic pressure on each side of the membrane. Although several factors may be involved in the pathogenesis of ascites, including abnormalities of the serum albumin concentration, the sodium ion, and hormones such as aldosterone, results of recent studies indicate that increased pressure within the liver plays a major role in ascites formation and is the primary mechanism responsible for transudation of ascitic fluid. Moreover, substantial evidence suggests that the intrahepatic hypertension in cirrhosis is a result of hepatic venous outflow obstruction.

Experimentally, ascites is produced by any procedure that obstructs hepatic venous outflow but does not result from obstruction of portal venous or hepatic arterial inflow. Furthermore, in experimental ascites the fluid leaks into the peritoneal cavity from the surface and hilum of the liver, a finding that suggests that it originates from some intrahepatic disturbance. Under experimental circumstances, therefore, hepatic outflow obstruction is the sine qua non for ascites formation. In man, a similar striking difference is seen in the ascites-producing effects of outflow and inflow obstruction. In the Budd-Chiari syndrome, a condition resulting from occlusion of the hepatic veins, massive ascites is an invariable complication. In contrast, ascites rarely accompanies extrahepatic obstruction of the portal vein. Comparative observations such as these, both experimental and clinical, plus substantial supporting evidence obtained from hemodynamic and histopathologic studies in man, have led to the conclusion that hepatic outflow block is involved in the pathogenesis of ascites in cirrhosis.

A number of studies have demonstrated a marked increase in the flow of lymph in the hepatic hilar lymphatics and thoracic duct in association with experimental ascites, hepatic outflow obstruction, or experimental cirrhosis. A similar increase in lymph flow in the thoracic duct has been observed in humans with cirrhosis and with congestive heart failure, and the marked enlargement of the lymphatics in the hilum of the cirrhotic liver, so familiar to surgeons who have performed operations for portal hypertension, has been documented by careful histopathologic studies. The bulk of evidence indicates that the augmented production of hepatic lymph is in large part a mechanical phenomenon resulting from obstruction to the outflow of blood from the liver sinusoids and the consequent spillover of the plasma portion of the blood into the perisinusoidal spaces and lymphatics. Ascites, in turn, has been attributed to the inability of the lymphatic system to accommodate the excessive formation of lymph, with resultant leakage of fluid into the peritoneal cavity from the overburdened hepatic lymphatics. This chain of events in ascites formation is depicted in Figure 27.

Humans with cirrhosis and ascites present a characteristic picture of marked salt and water retention, secondary hyperaldosteronism, hypervolemia, and dilutional hyponatremia. It is generally believed, although not proved by scientific data, that ascites precedes the hyperaldosteronism and sodium retention, and that a decrease in nonsplanchnic or "effective blood volume" is the stimulus to aldosterone hypersecretion. However, studies by Lieberman and his colleagues indicate that sodium retention antedates ascites formation and probably plays a role in its pathogenesis. Furthermore, studies in our laboratory

have uncovered an aldosterone-regulating mechanism in the liver which is activated by increased intrahepatic pressure, and have shown that aldosterone hypersecretion and renal sodium retention precede the appearance of experimental ascites. Thus, it appears possible that increased intrahepatic pressure sets in motion a sequence of events that includes leakage of fluid, increased secretion of aldosterone, and retention of sodium by the kidney, all of which contribute to the formation and persistence of ascites.

In the vast majority of cirrhotic patients, ascites disappears in response to a regimen consisting of abstinence from alcohol, a nourishing diet, salt restriction, and one or more of a variety of diuretic and antialdosterone drugs. Nevertheless, in a small but disturbing group of patients, ascites is refractory to these measures. It is for this group that the surgeon has attempted to devise operative measures of relief. If it is assumed, on the basis of substantial evidence, that increased hydrostatic pressure within the liver is important in the pathogenesis of ascites, it should be possible to relieve ascites by reducing the intrahepatic pressure. Theoretically, decompression of the obstructed hepatic vascular bed may be accomplished, to a greater or lesser degree, by reducing the inflow of blood to the liver or by improving the outflow of blood from the liver. Inflow-reducing procedures include ligation of the hepatic artery and the end-to-side portacaval shunt, both of which have been used in the treatment of cirrhotic ascites. Hepatic artery ligation no longer merits serious consideration, because it is an unpredictable operation that is associated with a high mortality rate. Improving the outflow of blood from the liver by a direct attack on the hepatic veins is not possible. However, numerous studies have demonstrated that the valveless portal vein is capable of serving as an outflow tract and that the objective of hepatic decompression is realized by a side-to-side portacaval shunt.

In a series of experiments, we evaluated the effects of portacaval shunts on ascites. These studies showed that the side-to-side portacaval shunt was effective in relieving ascites, overcoming intrahepatic hypertension, eliminating the hypersecretion of aldosterone that follows hepatic outflow occlusion, and reducing the markedly augmented thoracic duct lymph flow to normal. The end-to-side portacaval anastomosis was much less effective than the lateral anastomosis in relieving the sequelae of increased pressure in the liver.

On the basis of these experimental observations, we have performed side-to-side portacaval shunt in 16 selected patients with alcoholic cirrhosis and truly intractable ascites. All of our patients failed to respond to prolonged and intensive medical treatment for ascites before operation was considered. Fourteen of the 16 patients (88 per cent) survived the operation, and all the survivors have been relieved of ascites, salt retention, and hyperaldosteronism for periods ranging from 3 to 11 years (Fig. 28). The most notable feature of the response to operation, other than relief of ascites, has been a striking improvement in nutrition and vigor accompanied by substantial gains in lean tissue mass and body fat. Figure 29 shows the effects

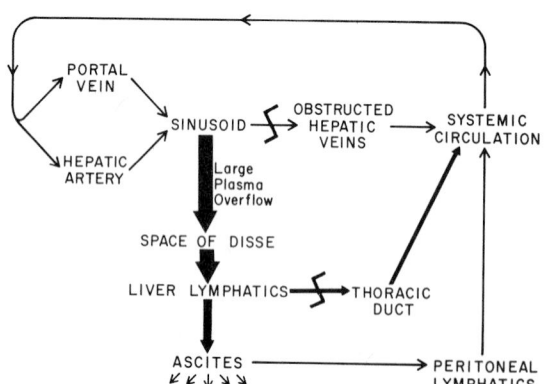

Figure 27. The chain of events in ascites formation. Hepatic venous outflow obstruction and the resultant intrahepatic hypertension play a primary role in causing transudation of ascitic fluid. (From Orloff, M. J., et al.: Arch. Surg., *93*:119, 1966.)

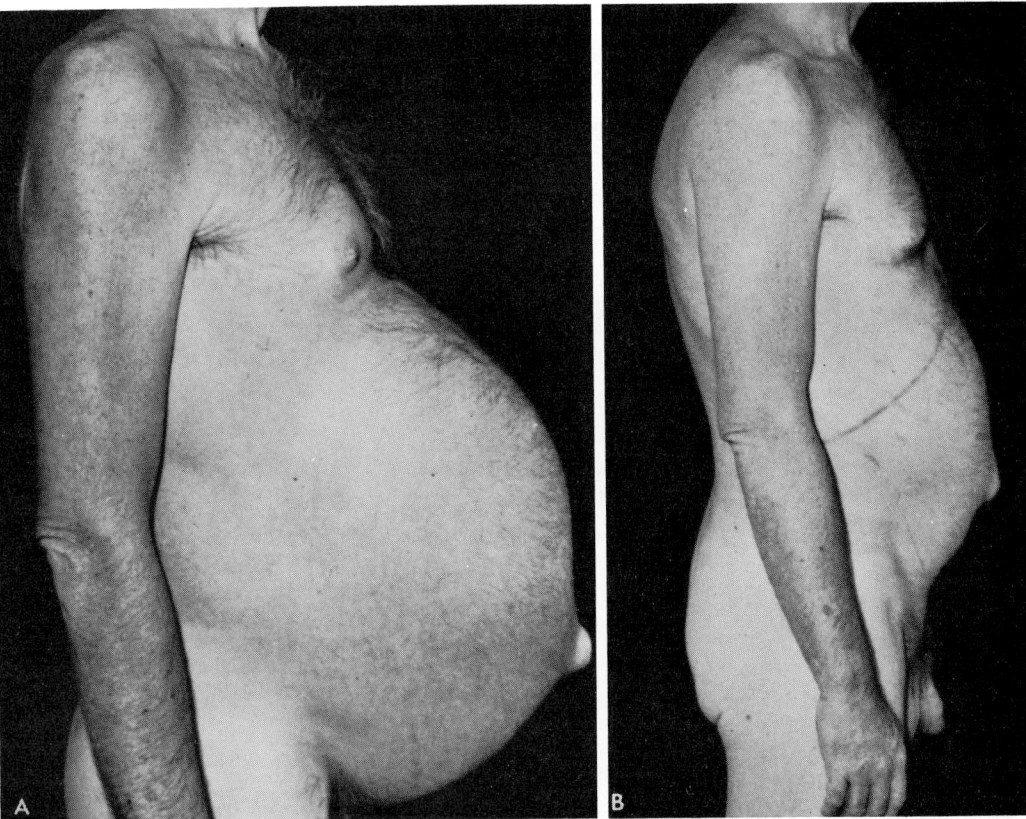

Figure 28. Photographs of a patient with cirrhosis and intractable ascites taken before and after side-to-side portacaval shunt. *A*, Preoperatively, when ascites was massive. *B*, Six weeks after side-to-side portacaval shunt. (From Orloff, M. J.: Am. J. Surg., *112:287, 1966.)

of the shunt on water and electrolyte balance and on aldosterone excretion in one of our patients. Our small but consistent experience has led to the conclusion that side-to-side portacaval shunt is of lasting benefit when used in carefully selected cirrhotic patients with truly intractable ascites who have failed to respond to vigorous and expert medical management. It must be emphasized that the number of such patients is small.

HEPATIC ENCEPHALOPATHY

The central nervous system disorders associated with hepatic cell failure and portal-systemic shunting are included under the umbrella of the terms "hepatic encephalopathy" or "hepatic coma" and represent the most common terminal event in cirrhosis. The etiology and pathogenesis of most of these disturbances are unknown. It appears likely that these disorders have a multifactorial etiology, and that toxic substances acting alone or together are responsible. Among the many toxic agents that have been proposed, evidence is strongest, although by no means conclusive, for involvement of ammonia or some similar product of nitrogen metabolism, of fatty acids, and of mercaptans. In a small percentage of patients, hepatic encephalopathy appears to be due to ammonia intoxication resulting from hepatic bypass through spontaneous or surgical portacaval shunts of ammonia absorbed from

the intestines, or to the inability of the damaged liver to transform ammonia to urea. The symptoms are related to the amount of nitrogen in the intestine and to the level of blood ammonia, and are described by the terms "portal-systemic encephalopathy" and "exogenous hepatic coma." Ammonia is believed to produce central nervous system depression by interfering with aerobic glycolysis in the brain. The level of spinal fluid glutamine, the primary product of ammonia metabolism in the brain, correlates more closely with this form of hepatic encephalopathy than does the level of blood ammonia. In most patients with hepatic encephalopathy, the neurologic abnormalities are unrelated to intestinal ammonia absorption but appear to be a mysterious manifestation of hepatic failure.

Hepatic encephalopathy occurs under a variety of circumstances in patients with advanced liver damage. Often, it is an aspect of progressive clinical deterioration. Not infrequently it occurs following an episode of varix bleeding or after major operations of any type in cirrhotic patients. It may be precipitated by infection, disorders of fluid and electrolyte balance, certain diuretics such as chlorothiazide, sedatives and analgesics, a bout of alcohol ingestion, or paracentesis.

The incidence of portal-systemic encephalopathy due to shunting of ammonia absorbed from the intestine in patients with a portacaval shunt is not known. Hepatic encephalopathy has been reported to occur in

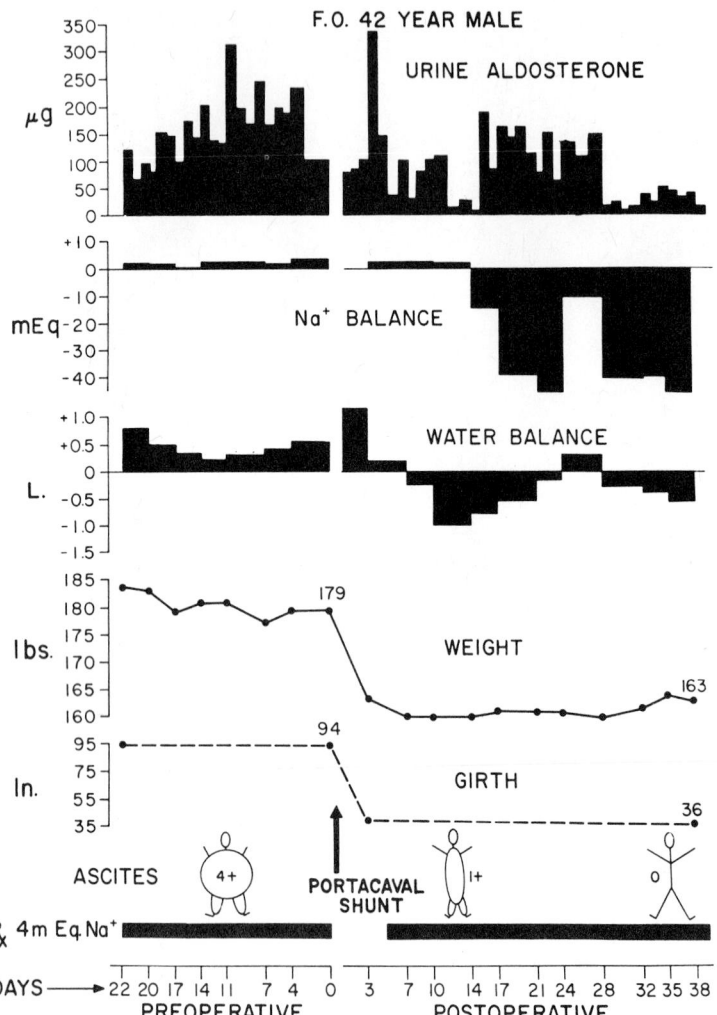

Figure 29. Results of a metabolic balance study of the patient shown in Figure 28, conducted before and after treatment of intractable ascites by side-to-side shunt. (From Orloff, M. J.: Am. J. Surg., *112*: 287, 1966.)

15 to 30 per cent of shunted patients but, unfortunately, most reports combine all neurologic sequelae under the term encephalopathy, including instances of central nervous system disturbance due to liver cell failure as well as the chronic or recurring disorders due to systemic shunting of nitrogenous substances. In our experience with 279 patients with portacaval shunts who were followed closely for life, the incidence of protein-related portal-systemic encephalopathy of any degree of severity and occurring at any time postoperatively was 20 per cent. The incidence of chronic, recurrent portal-systemic encephalopathy was 7 per cent.

The symptoms and signs of hepatic encephalopathy from any cause are nonspecific and run the gamut of alterations of consciousness. In the early stage, called "hepatic precoma," a variety of personality changes occur, including euphoria, untidiness, inability to concentrate, insomnia, and mild confusion. Later, depression and disorientation progressing to stupor and unconsciousness develop. Occasionally, convulsions occur. Asterixis or "liver flap" is a characteristic sign

which consists of a flapping, rough tremor best demonstrated by having the patient extend the arms, dorsiflex the hands, and spread the fingers. The electroencephalogram shows paroxysms of bilaterally synchronous, high-voltage, slow waves. Fluctuations of the symptoms and level of consciousness are usual.

The treatment of hepatic encephalopathy is generally supportive and nonspecific. In the most common form, which is related to liver cell failure, there is no correlation between the level of blood ammonia and the severity of symptoms, and measures directed at lowering blood ammonia are of little benefit. In patients with portal-systemic encephalopathy related to intestinal ammonia absorption, elimination of protein from the diet, removal of nitrogen from the gastrointestinal tract by cathartics and enemas, and administration of intestinal antibiotics such as neomycin may be helpful. In chronic intractable encephalopathy, bypass of the colon by ileostomy or ileosigmoidostomy may be indicated if other measures have failed. The use of ammonia-binding agents, such as glutamic acid and arginine, of levodopa, and of ion exchange resins has met with inconsistent success. The use of oral lactulose, a nonabsorbable synthetic disaccharide composed of galactose and fructose that is believed to diminish ammonia absorption by lowering colonic pH and inducing mild diarrhea, has been reported to be as effective as neomycin. Treatment of abnormalities known to precipitate hepatic encephalopathy and support of liver failure with parenteral glucose and vitamins are of value. Spontaneous recovery from hepatic encephalopathy occurs with sufficient frequency to make evaluation of the efficacy of therapy difficult.

In recent years, numerous attempts have been made to treat hepatic encephalopathy associated with liver failure by exchange transfusion, hemodialysis, peritoneal dialysis, cross circulation with a human or baboon donor, and extracorporal perfusion of the patient's blood through an isolated liver obtained from a pig, baboon, or human cadaver. Although several of these techniques have produced dramatic improvement in consciousness for brief periods, they have not influenced the mortality rate of the disease. Exchange transfusion is the simplest of these procedures and it has been used most widely. However, the results have not been significantly different from those obtained with noninvasive measures of therapy. The most recent of these extracorporeal dialysis methods, coated charcoal hemoperfusion, is in the early stages of evaluation.

GASTRIC ACID HYPERSECRETION AND PEPTIC ULCER

The association of peptic ulcer and cirrhosis of the liver has been the subject of numerous studies. The diagnosis of the two diseases has been based on clinical information in some investigations, and on autopsy findings in others. All of the studies have been retrospective in nature, and all of them have suffered from a lack of suitable controls. The reported incidence of peptic ulcer in patients with cirrhosis has ranged from 2.6 to 24 per cent. Depending upon the references cited, it is possible to conclude that ulcer disease is either more frequent or less frequent in cirrhotic patients than in a comparable noncirrhotic population. Neither conclusion is valid, and the facts remain to be determined by a careful prospective clinical evaluation.

Studies in humans concerning the influence of cirrhosis on gastric acid secretion have almost all demonstrated a depression of basal and histamine-stimulated acid production or no change from the normal. Our studies of the intestinal phase of gastric secretion in cirrhotic patients showed a secretory response within the normal range. Thus, there is no evidence that liver disease per se stimulates the gastric parietal cells.

In contrast to the studies in cirrhosis, it has been observed repeatedly in experimental animals that portacaval shunt produces profound gastric acid hypersecretion. The nature and cause of this excessive acid production associated with portacaval shunt has been determined only recently. Studies in our laboratory have demonstrated conclusively that it is due to unmasking of the intestinal phase of gastric secretion by

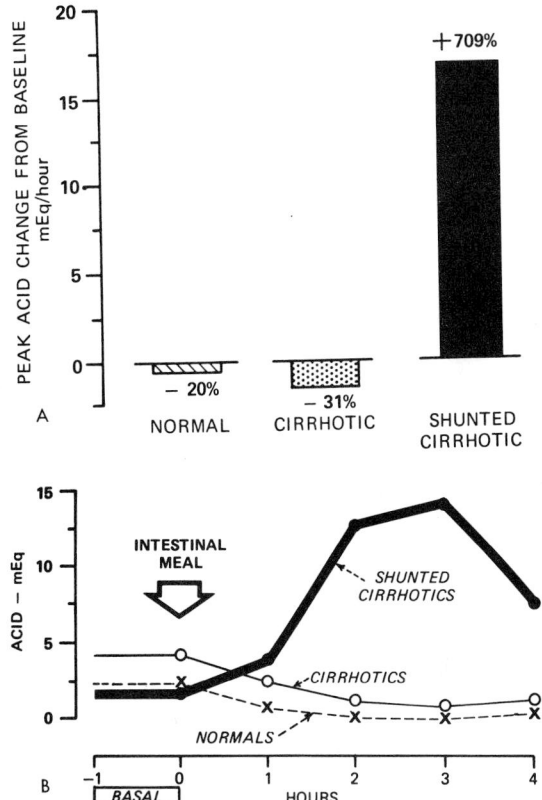

Figure 30. Gastric acid hypersecretion in humans with portacaval shunts due to hepatic bypass of an intestinal hormone. A shows mean peak gastric acid response and B shows mean 4-hour gastric acid response to an intestinal meal in normal, cirrhotic, and shunted cirrhotic humans. (From Orloff, M. J., et al.: Ann. Surg., 170:515, 1969.)

hepatic bypass of an intestinal hormone that is normally almost totally degraded by the liver (Fig. 30). The hormone has been shown to originate from the jejunum in both dogs and humans and to be released by the entry of any type of food into the intestine or by intestinal distention. The hormone has been extracted in crude form from hog intestinal mucosa and has been found to be a peptide of low molecular weight. The acid hypersecretion is confined to the intestinal phase of gastric secretion and does not involve the cephalic or gastric phases.

The relationship of the exaggerated intestinal phase of gastric secretion to the development of peptic ulcer in patients with a portacaval shunt is uncertain. It is generally believed that there is an abnormally high incidence of peptic ulcer in shunted cirrhotic patients, and that ulcer disease runs an unusually virulent course in these patients. At least 15 studies of this matter, all retrospective and without suitable controls, have been performed. The frequency of peptic ulcer has ranged from 1.6 to 23 per cent, and the results have been equally divided between those suggesting a causal relationship between shunt and ulcer, and those showing only a coincidental association between the two diseases. In a recent prospective study of a selected population, Phillips et al. observed the frequent development of peptic ulcer in both un-shunted cirrhotics (8.7 per cent) and shunted cirrhotics (11.8 per cent) after inclusion in the study, but no statistically significant difference in ulcer incidence between the two groups. Our prospective study currently in progress has revealed a 9 per cent chronic ulcer incidence in a group of 66 shunted patients followed for 5 or more years. The true relationship of portacaval shunt to peptic ulcer requires further investigation. In view of the invariable gastric acid hypersecretion following shunt operations, it would seem prudent to institute antacid therapy and a dietary ulcer regimen postoperatively.

RENAL FAILURE

Between 10 and 15 per cent of patients who die from advanced liver disease have renal failure. In some instances the renal disorder can be attributed to a specific kidney injury such as acute tubular necrosis resulting from shock associated with bleeding esophageal varices, or nephropathy secondary to sodium or potassium depletion produced by excessive use of diuretics in the treatment of ascites. In many cases, however, azotemia and oliguric renal failure develop spontaneously from no discernible cause. Such cases are commonly referred to as the "hepatorenal syndrome," although some workers object to the use of this term because the exact relationship of the liver disease to the associated renal dysfunction has not been identified.

There is no specific kidney lesion in the spontaneous renal failure associated with hepatic decompensation and, in fact, microscopic examination of the kidney usually reveals normal architecture or only trivial abnormalities. Cadaver kidney allografts obtained from cirrhotic donors who died of renal failure have been reported to have functioned promptly and normally when transplanted into living recipients. The evidence indicates that the renal dysfunction is caused by a disturbance in the blood flow to the kidney resulting from an underlying systemic circulatory abnormality. A number of studies have shown a decrease in renal plasma flow and glomerular filtration rate, an increase in renal vascular resistance, and a redistribution of flow within the kidney such that a disproportionate amount of blood is routed to the medulla. Since these changes frequently occur in the presence of an increased cardiac output and increased blood volume, it is apparent that some systemic mechanism produces a diversion of blood flow from the kidneys to other parts of the body. There is reason to believe that the disturbance in renal blood flow is a manifestation of the hyperdynamic circulatory abnormality found in advanced liver disease in which there is a loss of peripheral vascular tone and widespread arteriovenous shunting.

Spontaneous renal failure is most commonly observed in patients with advanced cirrhosis whose hepatic function is deteriorating. Many of the patients have ascites that is progressively refractory to treatment. During the early stages oliguria is not striking and the physician usually first becomes aware of the renal disorder when he finds elevated levels of urea and creatinine in the blood which increase progressively. Unlike acute tubular necrosis due to hypotension and renal ischemia, the urine in spontaneous renal failure is moderately concentrated (1.016 to 1.020), contains almost no sodium, has substantial quantities of potassium, has an osmolality that often exceeds that of plasma, and is free of protein, casts, and red blood cells. As the renal disorder progresses, dilutional hyponatremia and water retention become marked, and oliguria develops. Toward the end, hyperkalemia may become prominent. In most instances, there should be no difficulty in distinguishing this syndrome from acute tubular necrosis, since the latter is usually characterized by early oliguria, a fixed urine specific gravity around 1.010, an increase in sodium and decrease in potassium in the urine, a low urine osmolality, and a highly abnormal urine sediment. Terminally, patients with spontaneous renal failure often show the combined effects of loss of liver and kidney function such as hepatic coma, severe azotemia, hypotension, ascites, edema, and defects in blood coagulation.

The mortality rate of spontaneous renal failure associated with decompensated cirrhosis exceeds 70 per cent, and in some reports has approached 100 per cent. There is no specific treatment for the condition, and therapy is focused on improving liver function. A search should be made for specific causes of renal dysfunction, since they may be amenable to treatment. Because of the marked sodium and water retention and the consequent dilutional hyponatremia and waterlogging, intakes of sodium and fluids are restricted. Diuretic therapy is of no value in this disorder, and may be harmful. Attempts have been made to improve renal blood flow by the use of mannitol, colloid infusions, norepinephrine, metaraminol, aminophylline, dopamine, octapressin, and other vasoactive substances, but there is no solid evidence that these agents have significantly influenced the course of the renal disease or survival. Hemodialysis has been unsuccessful in the treatment of spontaneous renal failure and, because of the multisystem abnormalities that occur in decompensated cirrhosis, has been associated with serious complications.

PORTAL HYPERTENSION DUE TO EXTRAHEPATIC PORTAL OBSTRUCTION

Portal hypertension due to extrahepatic portal obstruction is a strikingly different condition from intrahepatic portal hypertension. The patients are usually much younger and most often are children. They do not have liver disease and, consequently, have a much greater tolerance for bleeding and for operations. Except in infancy, they rarely have ascites, and hepatic coma due to liver cell failure does not develop. Because the portal vein is usually obliterated, a direct portal vein to vena cava anastomosis cannot be performed for portal decompression. Finally, age and the related technical matter of adequate vessel size influence treatment. Patients with extrahepatic portal obstruction come to the attention of the surgeon usually because of bleeding from esophageal varices or splenomegaly. Although hematemesis is the most common symptom, the bleeding sometimes presents as melena. Exsanguinating hemorrhage does not occur nearly as often as in cirrhosis. On physical examination, splenomegaly is almost always found, but the liver is not palpable. Dilated collateral veins in the abdominal wall may be striking. The liver function tests usually are normal, but hematologic studies often reveal peripheral cytopenia that reflects hypersplenism. The hypersplenism is infrequently severe. Upper gastrointestinal x-rays and esophagogastroscopy demonstrate varices. Because the obstruction is presinusoidal, hepatic vein catheterization shows a normal wedged hepatic vein pressure. Splenic or superior mesenteric arteriography, with indirect portography, provides crucial information about the site of the portal obstruction and the size of the vessels available for portal decompression. Splenoportography with manometry is equally and sometimes more effective in demonstrating the obstruction but is a diagnostic procedure of second choice because of the small risk of bleeding from the spleen that might require a precipitant and premature operation.

The definitive treatment of extrahepatic portal obstruction is the portal-systemic venous shunt. However, for technical reasons related to the size of the vessels required for the shunt, temporizing hemostatic measures may have to be used in infants and young children until they have grown to the point where an adequate anastomosis is feasible. The mesocaval shunt usually should not be performed before the age of 4, and splenorenal shunt is often not feasible before the age of 7 or 8. We have preferred to delay operation until the age of 10 if at all possible. Consequently, the emergency treatment of varix bleeding in infants and young children consists of blood transfusions and, when necessary, medical measures such as esophageal balloon tamponade and intravenous vasopressin. Failure to control bleeding is an indication for transesophageal varix ligation. Rebleeding following these temporizing measures is the rule, but it is usually well tolerated and controllable until the child reaches a suitable age.

The types of portal-systemic anastomoses used in patients with an obliterated portal vein are the superior mesenteric vein–inferior vena cava shunt and the splenorenal shunt. The mesocaval shunt has been followed by a lower incidence of rebleeding and is clearly the procedure of choice. Both operations have been associated with operative mortality rates below 5 per cent. Other operative procedures, such as esophagogastrectomy with intestinal interposition, are associated with a high mortality rate and incidence of failure, and are indicated only when a portal-systemic shunt is impossible, and the patient has severe and recurrent bleeding.

Portacaval Shunt in the Budd-Chiari Syndrome, Glycogen Storage Disease, and Hyperlipemia

In addition to its well-established use in the usual forms of portal hypertension, portacaval shunt has

recently been used in three rare and unrelated conditions. These are the Budd-Chiari syndrome, glycogen storage disease, and type II hyperlipoproteinemia. The Budd-Chiari syndrome consists of obstruction to hepatic venous outflow as a result of occlusion of the hepatic veins and/or the adjacent inferior vena cava. The syndrome has been associated with, and presumably caused by, a wide variety of diseases, including myeloproliferative disorders (particularly polycythemia vera), malignant neoplasms, paroxysmal nocturnal hemoglobinuria, pregnancy, use of oral contraceptives and, particularly in the Orient, a fibrous vena caval web believed to be congenital in origin. In over half of the cases, the etiology has not been known. The obstruction produces severe congestion and swelling of the liver and portal hypertension. The clinical picture consists of ascites, hepatomegaly, abdominal pain, and, if the vena cava is involved, swelling of the lower extremities. The diagnosis is made by inferior vena cava and hepatic vein venography, supplemented by pressure measurements. The syndrome is almost invariably fatal, often in a matter of weeks or months. The Budd-Chiari syndrome has been produced experimentally in dogs by hepatic vein ligation, and has been consistently and permanently relieved by side-to-side portacaval shunt, which decompresses the obstructed hepatic vascular bed. Treatment of the Budd-Chiari syndrome by side-to-side portacaval shunt or one of its variations has been reported in 14 patients, some of whom were in a terminal condition. Six patients have survived the operation and have experienced dramatic relief of ascites and clinical symptoms. The shunt operation is indicated only if the obstruction is confined to the hepatic veins and inferior vena caval hypertension is absent.

Hepatic glycogen storage diseases are inborn errors of carbohydrate metabolism caused by deficiencies of enzymes involved in the conversion of glycogen to glucose. Eight types have been described, each due to a specific enzyme defect, and all characterized by excessive deposition of glycogen in the liver as well as diverse other abnormalities. Among the many clinical features of these disorders, those believed to be due to the inability of the liver to convert glycogen to glucose include chronic hypoglycemia and acidosis, hyperlipidemia, hyperuricemia, seizures, hepatomegaly and liver damage, and retarded growth and development. Portacaval shunt has been performed in 15 children with severe glycogen storage diseases, of whom 10 had type I, 4 had type III, and 1 had type VI disease. There have been one operative and two late deaths. The survivors have experienced an increase in growth rate, partial relief of hypoglycemia and acidosis, marked lowering of hyperlipidemia, and variable decreases in serum uric acid levels and liver size. The rationale for performance of the portacaval shunt is to deliver glucose absorbed from the intestines and pancreatic hormones directly to the peripheral tissues before they reach the liver.

Homozygous type IIa hyperlipoproteinemia is a rare and lethal genetic disorder that is characterized by high blood levels of cholesterol and low-density lipoprotein, widespread deposition of lipids in tissues, premature atherosclerosis, resistance to medical therapy, and death before the end of the second decade, usually from cardiovascular disease. Two children with this disorder have undergone portacaval shunt by Starzl and his colleagues. The operation was followed by prompt and sustained lowering of hypercholesterolemia and hyperlipoproteinemia, and a striking objective improvement in the condition of the patients. The shunt procedure was undertaken on the basis of the observation that it markedly reduced the hyperlipidemia in patients with glycogen storage disease. The mechanism remains to be determined.

LIVER TRAUMA

Because of its size, the liver is the solid viscus most frequently injured by penetrating wounds of the abdomen; it is involved in approximately 20 to 25 per cent of patients who have received penetrating trauma. In blunt injuries to the abdomen, liver damage occurs in 5 to 10 per cent of the patients. As a result of the marked increase in automobile accidents, blunt liver trauma has become a common clinical entity.

Liver wounds vary greatly in direct relationship to the type and magnitude of the trauma. Stab wounds often cause relatively simple lacerations, while gunshot injuries frequently traverse the full depth of the liver and may produce widespread destruction of hepatic tissue. Blunt injuries range from simple subcapsular hematomas to complicated stellate fractures and, occasionally, central rupture of the liver parenchyma. Direct damage to the hilar structures and avulsion of hepatic veins may occur with both penetrating and blunt injuries, and present complicated problems that are often lethal.

Because the liver is highly vascular, tolerates anoxia poorly, and is an unpaired organ upon which life depends, hepatic injuries generally are more difficult to treat than other forms of abdominal trauma. Moreover, as a result of its location, injuries to certain parts of the liver are not easily accessible to rapid surgical repair. Consequently, liver trauma carries a higher mortality rate than injury to any other abdominal viscus. Furthermore, liver wounds are often associated with injuries to other organs and systems which complicate treatment and significantly increase the mortality rate. It is common for a patient with liver trauma to have concomitant extra-abdominal injuries of the head, thorax, or long bones, as well as intra-abdominal wounds of the spleen, pancreas, kidney, duodenum, or colon. Table 19 shows the direct relationship of the mortality rate of liver trauma to the number of other organs injured.

Diagnosis

Since it is general policy to perform exploratory laparotomy in all gunshot wounds of the abdomen, the diagnosis of liver injury under such circumstances is made by direct inspection at operation and does not present any diagnostic difficulties. However, in stab wounds and blunt trauma to the abdomen, the decision regarding whether or not to operate is based on obtaining diagnostic evidence of intraperitoneal organ

TABLE 19.   Relationship of Number of Organs Injured to Mortality Rate in 134 Cases of Liver Trauma

Number of Organs Injured	Cases	Deaths	Mortality (%)
Gunshot Wounds			
Liver alone	9	1	11
Liver + 1	15	2	13
Liver + 2	10	3	30
Blunt Trauma			
Liver alone	6	0	0
Liver + 1	60	8	13
Liver + 2	20	7	35
Liver + 3 or more	14	9	64

damage. As a result of its rich blood supply, hemorrhage and shock dominate the clinical picture of liver trauma in many patients. In addition, the patient with a liver injury usually complains of pain in the right upper quadrant of the abdomen and on physical examination there are distinct signs of peritoneal irritation such as tenderness and rigidity in the right hypochondrium and hypoactive or absent bowel sounds. Occasionally, pain in the right shoulder from diaphragmatic irritation is a prominent feature. Laboratory studies reveal an elevated white blood cell count and a fall in the hematocrit and hemoglobin concentration, although early in the course hematocrit and hemoglobin determinations may be of no value. Liver function tests rarely provide useful information during the initial 12 hours following injury, when the diagnosis must be made. Abdominal and chest x-rays are of limited value, but may demonstrate signs of blood in the peritoneal cavity, an elevated right hemidiaphragm, and telltale fractures of the right lower ribs. Sometimes, evidence on abdominal x-rays of injury to other organs such as the spleen, duodenum, or colon, an abnormal intravenous pyelogram, or an elevated serum amylase from pancreatic injury provides the indications for performing a laparotomy at which liver damage is discovered.

The most helpful diagnostic procedures in our experience are the abdominal tap and hepatic arteriography. Although a negative tap does not rule out serious intra-abdominal organ damage, a tap productive of free blood is obtained in over 80 per cent of patients with liver injury. Several techniques of abdominal paracentesis are used, including aspiration from an 18-gauge spinal needle inserted into each of the four abdominal quadrants, aspiration from a plastic catheter inserted into the peritoneal cavity through a needle, and aspiration from a plastic catheter following irrigation of the peritoneal cavity with 1 or 2 liters of saline. In our experience, the technique of peritoneal lavage is most accurate, and we use it whenever initial aspiration is negative. Selective hepatic, splenic, and superior mesenteric arteriography is a safe and extremely valuable procedure in the diagnosis of abdominal injury. Hepatic arteriography is used in our clinic whenever there is a question about the diagnosis of liver trauma, and it has proved to be highly accurate and very helpful (Fig. 31). Finally, the radioisotope liver scan is sometimes of value in the diagnosis of liver wounds, although it infrequently yields information not provided by other diagnostic meauures.

Treatment

Preoperative Preparation. Liver trauma requires emergency surgical therapy. In some hepatic injuries, hemorrhage is so massive that operative control of bleeding is the only possible means of resuscitation, and operation should be undertaken promptly without preoperative preparation. In most liver wounds, however, several hours of preoperative treatment facilitate the operation and improve the chances of survival. Usually preoperative therapy is undertaken simultaneously with the diagnostic work-up. The following are important preoperative preparatory measures used in all but minor liver wounds:

1. Shock is corrected by restoration of the blood volume with whole blood transfusions administered through two large-bore plastic catheters inserted via a cutdown in each arm. Because of the potential coagulation defects associated with liver damage, liver resection, and multiple transfusions of stored blood, correction of hypovolemia involves as much fresh blood (less than 12 hours old) as can be obtained.

2. Assurance of adequate ventilation is a matter of first priority along with the treatment of shock. This involves the administration of oxygen, and may require insertion of a thoracostomy catheter to evacuate blood or air, insertion of an endotracheal tube, and mechanical ventilatory support.

3. Vital functions are monitored by insertion of a central venous pressure catheter through an arm cutdown into the superior vena cava, a radial artery catheter for arterial pressure recordings, an indwelling bladder catheter for hourly measurements of urine output, and a rectal or esophageal probe for temperature recordings. The patient is connected by body surface leads to an electrocardiograph for continuous recordings of the electrocardiogram. Arterial pH and blood gases, blood urea nitrogen, and serum electrolytes are determined.

4. Both the chest and the abdomen are shaved and prepared with antiseptic soap for operation.

5. A hypothermia blanket is placed on the operating table so that total-body cooling can be initiated as soon as anesthesia is induced.

6. Equipment for intraoperative cholangiography and visceral angiography is brought to the operating room, if not already present, and appropriate scout x-rays are taken before induction of anesthesia. The surgeon should not find himself in the position of needing these studies and discovering after the abdomen has been entered that he has failed to provide for the necessary equipment.

Operative Treatment. The operative treatment of liver wounds is based on three important principles: (1) excision of devitalized liver tissue; (2) securing liver hemostasis; and (3) drainage of the peritoneal cavity to prevent bile collections. Excision of devitalized liver tissue is essential to prevent the often lethal sequelae of delayed necrosis, infection, and late hemorrhage. Unroofing of deep missile tracts, segmental liver resection, or hepatic lobectomy in extensive injuries may be necessary to accomplish this important objective. Securing liver hemostasis is accomplished by direct suture, but the use of hemostatic agents or resection of the liver may be required. Through-and-through perforating injuries with bleeding in the depths of the liver should never be treated by simply suturing closed the surface openings of the wound, since such a maneuver often leads to an expanding intrahepatic hematoma with serious consequences. Instead, the wound should be laid open throughout its length and the bleeding points should be controlled by direct suture. Drainage of the peritoneal cavity is necessary to remove the bile that invariably leaks from the hepatic wound. If the bile is not evacuated, infected bile collections or bile peritonitis may develop. Drainage is accomplished by the combined use of Penrose drains and sump drains that are placed on suction. In addition, in recent years some workers have advocated deliberate T tube drainage of the common bile duct or cholecystostomy on the assumption that controlled extrahepatic biliary drainage will prevent bile leakage from the liver wound. While theoretically attractive, there is no solid evidence to indicate that controlled drainage of the common bile duct accomplishes the objective for which it was proposed. To the contrary, Lucas et al. have demonstrated in extensive experimental and clinical studies that drainage of the common bile duct does not

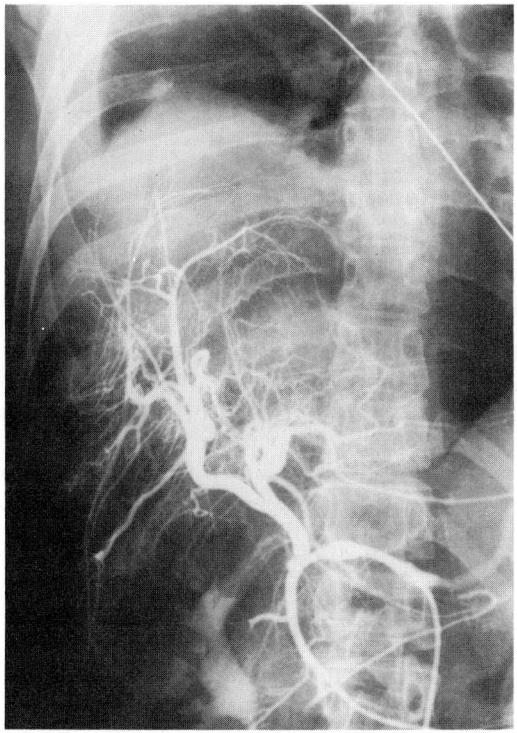

Figure 31. Hepatic arteriogram in a patient with blunt abdominal trauma showing distortion of the vasculature due to herniation of the liver into the thorax through a ruptured right diaphragm.

reduce intrahepatic biliary pressure, does not diminish bile drainage from the liver wound, and is associated with increased morbidity, mortality, and stress ulceration in patients with liver trauma. Furthermore, Lucas et al. have emphasized that insertion of a T tube into a small common bile duct may damage the duct. For these reasons, we do not advocate the routine use of controlled extrahepatic biliary drainage in liver trauma.

In extensive liver injury, there are certain technical maneuvers of which the surgeon must be aware if he is to control bleeding. Reflection of the duodenum by a Kocher maneuver so as to gain fingertip control of the afferent blood supply to the liver is a simple first step in the approach to serious hepatic injuries. Occlusion of the hepatic artery and portal vein by cross-clamping the porta hepatis with a vascular clamp (Pringle maneuver) is helpful in controlling and repairing extensive liver wounds, and in performing hepatic resections. Vascular inflow occlusion is tolerated for 20 minutes when body temperature is normal and for 60 minutes under hypothermia of 30°C. The time period can be extended by releasing the occluding vascular clamp for several minutes at appropriate intervals so as to produce intermittent vascular occlusion. Division of the falciform, coronary, and triangular ligaments provides access to all parts of the liver except the bare area and major hepatic veins, and should be done early in operations for wounds of the posterior and superior segments. Deliberate ligation of the main hepatic artery or its major branches is sometimes necessary to control hemorrhage. The safety of hepatic artery ligation, provided portal venous blood flow is maintained, has been only recently recognized.

Liver wounds that involve the major hepatic veins are the most difficult to repair and have the highest mortality rate because of their inaccessibility and the danger of both exsanguination and air embolism. Such injuries must be recognized promptly and approached rapidly by extending the usual midline abdominal incision into the thorax through the seventh or eighth right intercostal space or through a sternum-splitting extension. The diaphragm is divided down to the orifice of the inferior vena cava. In addition to occlusion of hepatic vascular inflow, occlusion of the inferior vena cava below the liver and above the liver in the pericardial cavity is used to isolate and repair the injured hepatic veins. Clamping of the inferior vena cava for more than 15 to 20 minutes produces severe hypotension, so the use of intermittent occlusion may be required. Additional techniques for isolating the large hepatic veins involve combined occlusion of the inferior vena cava and aorta above the celiac axis so as to avoid hypotension from pooling of blood in the lower half of the body, unroofing of the inferior vena cava within the liver from a posterior approach, and insertion of an internal shunt into the vena cava through the right atrium or infrahepatic vena cava.

The methods of operative treatment used in 204 cases of penetrating and blunt liver trauma are listed in Table 20.

Postoperative Complications. Table 21 shows the postoperative complications in 100 cases of blunt liver trauma. Infection is the most frequent problem following liver injury. Subphrenic, subhepatic, and intrahepatic abscesses, peritonitis, wound infection, and wound dehiscence occur with disturbing frequency. The importance of thoroughly irrigating the peritoneal cavity and wound with antibiotic solutions at the time of operation, and of closing the abdominal incision with retention sutures, cannot be overemphasized.

Respiratory complications such as pneumonia, atelectasis, pulmonary edema, and "shock lung" are common in all types of major trauma. The use of mechanical ventilatory assistance delivered through an endotracheal tube or tracheostomy, an intensive program of tracheobronchial toilet, and careful monitoring of arterial pH and blood gases, pulmonary function, and radiographic changes in the lungs are essential aspects of postoperative care.

Secondary hemorrhage from necrosis and infection of hepatic tissue is a major cause of delayed death following liver trauma. Moreover, it is not uncommon for serious coagulopathies to develop in patients with liver injuries as a result of the combination of hepatic dysfunction and replacement of the blood volume with banked blood. To the extent possible, fresh blood transfusions should be used to restore platelets, replenish the protein blood clotting factors, and provide 2,3-DPG for delivery of oxygen to the tissues.

Renal failure associated with hepatic trauma is almost always due to acute tubular necrosis resulting from a period of hypotension and renal ischemia. Although this complication cannot be prevented in all cases, it can be minimized by a vigorous program of resuscitation starting when the patient first enters the emergency room. The development of stress ulceration with gastrointestinal hemorrhage is not uncommon in patients with massive trauma of any type. Prophy-

TABLE 20. Methods of Operative Treatment Used in 204 Cases of Penetrating and Blunt Liver Trauma

	Number of Cases
Suture of liver	104
Suture and hemostatic agents	43
Resection of liver	24
Laparotomy alone	22
Died without operation	7

TABLE 21. Postoperative Complications in 100 Cases of Blunt Liver Trauma

	Incidence (%)
Infection—intra-abdominal and wound	22
Respiratory problems	19
Hemorrhage	14
Renal failure	9
Stress ulcer	6
Pancreatitis	5
Other	14

TABLE 22.   Causes of 151 Deaths from Liver Trauma from 1960 to 1970

	Per Cent of Deaths
Liver hemorrhage — intraoperative and postoperative	53
Respiratory failure	14
Infection — intra-abdominal and wound	12
Pancreatitis	8
Stress ulcer bleeding	6
Other	7

laxis against this complication includes continuous nasogastric suction during the first several days postoperatively, followed by hourly oral antacid therapy beginning immediately upon removal of the nasogastric tube. Finally, liver failure rarely develops as a direct result of an uncomplicated hepatic injury or from resection of hepatic tissue, but frequently occurs when other complications, such as sepsis or pulmonary failure, are added to the liver trauma. There is no specific treatment for hepatic failure, but the use of parenteral hyperalimentation may be helpful and has become a regularly used measure in our management of serious liver wounds.

Traumatic Hemobilia. An unusual but interesting complication of liver trauma is hemobilia. This disorder usually follows central rupture of the liver, or suture of lacerations on the liver surface without obliteration of dead space in the depths of the hepatic substance. The communication between the vasculature and the biliary tract develops as a result of necrosis of a portion of liver parenchyma within a closed space. Symptoms may occur at any time, but commonly they appear 3 to 4 weeks after injury and consist of episodes of biliary colic due to passage of blood clots down the bile ducts, mild jaundice, and gastrointestinal bleeding that presents as melena or, less often, hematemesis. Elevations of the serum alkaline phosphatase and bilirubin usually accompany the attacks, and sometimes the SGOT is increased. Hepatic arteriography is particularly useful in establishing the diagnosis, and splenoportography, cholangiography, and radioisotope liver scanning may be helpful. Although many different operations have been used, definitive treatment consists of either resection of the lesion or ligation of the ends of the contributing blood vessels.

Intraoperative angiography and cholangiography are helpful in localizing the involved part of the liver.

Mortality

A significant number of patients with liver trauma die before reaching the hospital. Moreover, hepatic injury is often associated with trauma to other organs and systems, and death is sometimes due to associated injuries. Patients who die as a direct result of the liver wound usually succumb from hepatic hemorrhage, respiratory complications, or infection in the peritoneal cavity or wound (Table 22).

The mortality rate of penetrating liver injuries has been reduced from more than 60 per cent prior to 1940 to approximately 10 per cent at present (Table 23). Stab wounds of the liver are associated with a mortality rate of only 2 to 3 per cent, while gunshot injuries are more often lethal because of the magnitude of liver damage and the frequent involvement of other organs. The mortality rate of blunt trauma to the liver has been reduced significantly to about 30 per cent during the past decade as a result of better organized emergency care and more effective operative treatment (Table 24). Nevertheless, blunt liver injury remains the most lethal form of trauma to the abdominal viscera.

ECHINOCOCCUS CYST

Hydatid disease is common in many parts of the world, but it is a rare condition in the United States and is found mainly in immigrants who bring the disease to this country. Two forms of the echinococcus tapeworm produce disease in man, *Echinococcus granulosus* and *Echinococcus multilocularis*. The adult tapeworm lives in the intestine of the dog, wolf, or fox, from which ova are passed in the stool. The ova are ingested by an intermediate host, usually sheep, cattle, and pigs but occasionally man, and hatch into embryos in the duodenum. The embryos pass into the portal venous system and are filtered out by the liver, although occasionally they escape to the lung or other organs. In the liver, the embryos reproduce asexually and form multiloculated cysts. The cyst in the liver usually has a well-defined wall with an inner germinative layer and a thick outer laminated layer which often calcifies. The cyst fluid contains numerous embryonal scolices called "hydatid sand." The cycle is

TABLE 23.   Mortality Rate of Penetrating Liver Trauma

Author and Year Reported	Cases	Mortality (%)	Stab Wounds No.	Mortality (%)	Gunshot Wounds No.	Mortality (%)
Amerson and Blair, 1959	167	13	68	0	99	21
Crosthwait et al., 1962	297	12	—	—	—	—
Shafton et al., 1963	73	12	61	8	12	33
McClelland and Shires, 1965	228	9	—	—	—	—
Lucas and Walt, 1970	539	10	290	2	249	18
Lim et al., 1972	182	12	83	4	99	18
Trunkey et al., 1974	638	11	206	—	432	—

TABLE 24. Mortality Rate of Blunt Liver Trauma

Authors and Year Reported	Cases	Mortality (%)
Edler, 1887	96	78
O'Neill, 1940	100	81
Mikesky et al., 1956	24	71
Crosthwait et al., 1962	43	30
Orloff et al., 1967	100	24
Lucas and Walt, 1970	65	28
Fry et al., 1973	139	26
Trunkey et al., 1974	173	21

completed when a dog feeds on the infected tissues of an intermediate host, and the scolices develop into mature tapeworms in the dog's intestines.

Hydatid cysts frequently are present for many years without producing symptoms. Often, the discovery of a liver mass on physical examination or the pathognomonic finding of a calcified, round mass in the liver on x-ray leads to the diagnosis (Fig. 30). Liver scans, ultrasonography, and hepatic arteriography may be helpful in defining the lesion. Eosinophilia occurs in one fourth to one half of the cases. A complement fixation test and the response to intradermal injection of cyst fluid (Casoni test) are positive in the vast majority of patients. Several serologic tests that indicate hydatid infection are also available, such as the indirect hemagglutination test and the recently developed immunoelectrophoretic assay.

The major cause of morbidity and mortality associated with echinococcus cyst of the liver is rupture of the cyst. Rupture into the bile ducts produces a syndrome of biliary colic, jaundice, urticaria, and fever. Rupture into the peritoneal cavity results in abdominal pain, urticaria, sometimes anaphylactic shock, and the development of multiple intra-abdominal cysts. Rupture into the pleural cavity causes pain, cough, fever, and the development of empyema. Rarely, hydatid cysts rupture into the gastrointestinal tract. Secondary infection of liver cysts with pyogenic bacteria occurs sometimes and produces the signs and symptoms of pyogenic liver abscess.

The treatment of hydatid cyst is surgical removal, since there are no effective scolicidal drugs. Usually the cyst can be removed by shelling out, but occasionally hepatic resection is required. In order to prevent seeding of the cyst contents, preliminary aspiration and instillation of hydrogen peroxide, absolute alcohol, or formalin are done. Care must be taken to avoid spilling viable scolices into the peritoneal cavity. The defect in the liver that remains after removal of the cyst should be closed, covered with omentum or, if necessary, marsupialized. The mortality rate for treatment of uncomplicated cysts is less than 5 per cent.

BENIGN NEOPLASMS AND CYSTS

Usually, benign neoplasms of the liver are of clinical significance only in that they pose problems in differential diagnosis from more serious lesions. The most common benign tumor is the hemangioma, a lesion of blood vessels that presents the microscopic appearance of endothelium-lined cystic spaces filled with blood. The liver is the parenchymatous organ in which hemangiomas are most frequently found. The tumors vary greatly in size. They are usually asymptomatic, although they may grow so large as to compress adjacent viscera. When clinically significant, they present as an abdominal mass and produce x-ray, angiographic, and liver scan abnormalities. The most serious complication of the hepatic hemangioma is rupture with massive intraperitoneal hemorrhage, an event that has been reported with some frequency. Treatment is required when the tumors become clinically significant and consists of excision or hepatic lobectomy. Radiation therapy may be effective and is indicated in inoperable lesions.

Hepatic adenomas are rare tumors of liver cells or bile duct epithelium. They are usually asymptomatic and when discovered at laparotomy may be mistaken for primary or metastatic cancers. They require excision only when large.

Hamartomas are congenital collections of normal hepatic cell plates, bile ducts, blood vessels, and fibrous tissue in an abnormal arrangement. They are developmental disturbances and are not true neoplasms. They may be single or multiple and vary

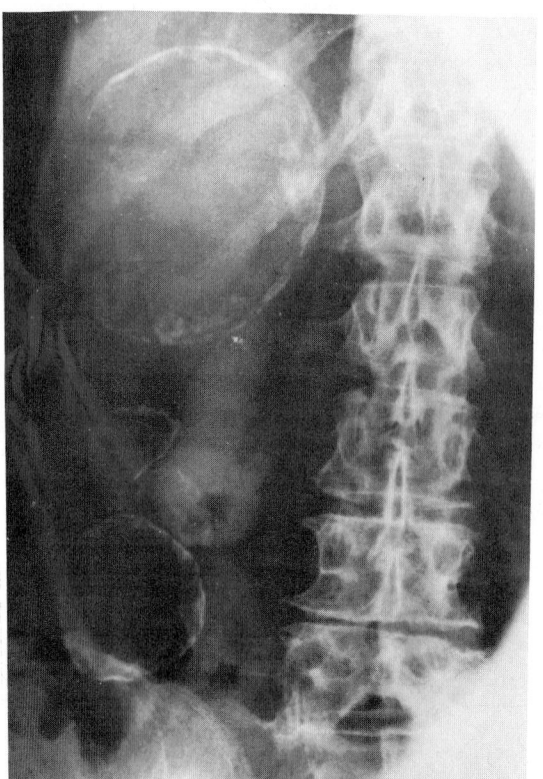

Figure 32. Calcified masses in the right upper quadrant indicative of echinococcus cysts in the liver, discovered during an oral cholecystogram performed for right upper quadrant abdominal pain.

greatly in size. Some are quite large and are palpable on physical examination. Usually, they are asymptomatic. No treatment is necessary unless they are very large. Hamartomas are of clinical significance mainly because of the difficulty in distinguishing them from malignant tumors on gross examination.

Cysts of the liver are uncommon. Most of the solitary cysts are congenital lesions caused by arrest in the development of the bile ducts. Some single cysts originate from trauma, and in rare instances true neoplastic cystadenomas are found. Multiple cysts of the liver, or polycystic disease, represent congenital bile duct anomalies; associated polycystic disease of the kidneys is found in half of the patients and accompanying cystic disease of other organs has been reported. Other congenital anomalies are often found in patients with polycystic disease. Both solitary cysts and polycystic disease are usually not discovered until adulthood.

Cysts of the liver are usually asymptomatic and come to the attention of a physician because of the finding of an enlarged liver or a mass in the abdomen. Liver function is normal. X-rays of the abdomen, liver scans, and hepatic arteriography are helpful in demonstrating the presence of a liver mass. Treatment consists of excision of the cyst, hepatic resection, or external drainage with packing. Polycystic disease requires no treatment and is compatible with long life if serious associated anomalies are absent.

MALIGNANT NEOPLASMS

Primary Cancer

Primary cancer of the liver is uncommon in the United States, but in Africa and Asia it is one of the most frequent malignant neoplasms. Only the Caucasian race is relatively free of liver cancer. The disease occurs in infants, and in parts of Africa and Asia it is common in children and young adults, but in North America it predominates in the fifth and sixth decades of life. Two thirds to three fourths of hepatic cancers in the United States develop in patients with cirrhosis, particularly cirrhosis of the postnecrotic type. The incidence of liver cancer among cirrhotic patients is approximately 5 per cent. Patients with hemochromatosis also have a high incidence of hepatic carcinoma. In Africa and Asia, a number of carcinogenic substances in food and infestation of the liver with certain parasites have been implicated in the etiology of liver cancer. In particular, there is suggestive evidence that aflatoxin, a potent hepatocarcinogen from the plant *Aspergillus flavus* that is contained in food, plays an etiologic role in the frequent occurrence of cancer of the liver.

There are two major forms of liver cancer. These are liver cell carcinoma (hepatocellular carcinoma, hepatoma) and bile duct carcinoma (cholangiocarcinoma). A third type that represents a mixture of the other two and is called hepatobiliary carcinoma or cholangiohepatoma is infrequent compared to the two major malignant neoplasms. An uncommon variant of liver cell carcinoma seen most often in infants, hepa-

toblastoma, is the most amenable of the hepatic malignant tumors to cure by resection. Liver cell carcinomas outnumber bile duct cancers five to one. Other primary liver cancers are rare. Carcinoma of the liver metastasizes widely, but the most frequent sites are the lungs and regional lymph nodes.

The clinical features of liver carcinoma in the United States most often consist of a rapid increase of signs and symptoms in a patient with cirrhosis and include the appearance of ascites, edema, jaundice, anemia, weakness, and weight loss. Occasionally, hepatic carcinoma is responsible for the first episode of bleeding varices. In noncirrhotic patients, the common symptoms are weakness, weight loss, dull pain in the hypochondrium, abdominal swelling, edema, and fever. The usual signs are nodular hepatomegaly and ascites. Jaundice is found in about one third of the patients when first seen. Hemorrhage into the peritoneal cavity is an occasional terminal event.

All the liver function tests may be abnormal, but elevation of the serum alkaline phosphatase and SGOT and Bromsulphalein retention are the most consistent biochemical abnormalities. The appearance of alpha fetoprotein in the serum shows a high correlation with the presence of liver cell carcinoma and strongly suggests the diagnosis. Hepatic arteriography, radioisotope liver scanning, ultrasonic liver scanning, splenoportography, and needle liver biopsy alone or under direct vision during peritoneoscopy may provide the diagnosis.

The treatment of primary carcinoma of the liver is hepatic resection when the lesion is solitary and there are no regional or distant metastases. Unfortunately, these circumstances rarely occur and cure of the disease by resection, while possible and definitely worth considering, is infrequent. Orthotopic liver allotransplantation has been attempted in a number of cases of hepatic cancer but, to date, has not resulted in cure of the disease. Radiation therapy is of no value. Infusion of chemotherapeutic agents, such as methotrexate and 5-fluorouracil, into the hepatic artery has provided brief palliation in occasional patients. Duration of life after discovery of hepatic cancer averages only 3 to 4 months.

Metastatic Cancer

Because of its rich and unique blood supply, the liver is the most common organ to be involved by metastatic cancer. One half to two thirds of the patients who die of cancer of the gastrointestinal tract, pancreas, breast, and ovary, and one third of the patients who die of lung and kidney cancers have liver metastases. Neoplasms spread to the liver by way of the portal vein, hepatic artery, and lymphatics and by direct extension. Right upper quadrant abdominal pain, anorexia, weight loss, nodular hepatomegaly, and ascites are the most common clinical features. Jaundice occurs in one fourth of the cases. Bromsulphalein retention and elevation of serum alkaline phosphatase are consistent findings, and SGOT is frequently increased. Hepatic arteriography, liver scans, portography, and needle liver biopsy help to make the diagnosis. The yield of liver biopsy is increased by performing the procedure under direct vision during peritoneoscopy. Although rare cases of metastatic carcinoma have been cured by hepatic resections performed after control of the primary neoplasm, the vast majority of hepatic metastases are incurable. Chemotherapy by hepatic arterial infusion has resulted in palliation in occasional cases. Duration of life following discovery of liver metastases varies according to the nature of the primary neoplasms, but it rarely exceeds 1 year.

REFERENCES

General

1. Popper, H., and Schaffner, F.: Liver: Structure and Function. New York, McGraw-Hill Book Company, 1957.
2. Popper, H., and Schaffner, F.: Progress in Liver Diseases. Volume 4. New York, Grune and Stratton, 1972.
3. Schiff, L.: Diseases of the Liver, 4th ed. Philadelphia, J. B. Lippincott Company, 1975.
4. Sherlock, S.: Diseases of the Liver and Biliary System, 4th ed. Oxford, Blackwell Scientific Publications, 1975.

Anatomy

5. Douglass, B. E., Baggenstoss, A. H., and Hollenshead, W. H.: The anatomy of the portal vein and its tributaries. Surg. Gynecol. Obstet., 91:562, 1950.
6. Elias, H., and Sherrick, J. C.: Morphology of the Liver. New York, Academic Press, 1969.
7. Gilfillan, R. S.: Anatomic study of the portal vein and its main branches. Arch. Surg., 61:449, 1950.
8. Michels, N.: The hepatic cystic and retroduodenal arteries and their relations to the biliary ducts. Ann. Surg., 133:503, 1951.

Physiology

Bile Formation

9. Brauer, R. W.: Hepatic blood supply and the secretion of bile. In Taylor, W. (Ed.): The Biliary System. Oxford, Blackwell Scientific Publications, 1965, pp. 41–67.

Bilirubin Metabolism

10. Arias, I. M.: The excretion of conjugated bilirubin by the liver cell. Medicine, 45:513, 1966.
11. Arias, I. M.: Bilirubin metabolism. II. Excretion of bilirubin. In Schaffner, F., Sherlock, S., and Leevy, C. M. (Eds.): The Liver and Its Diseases. New York, Intercontinental Medical Book Corp., 1974, pp. 97–104.
12. Klatskin, G.: Bile pigment metabolism. Ann. Rev. Med., 12:211, 1961.
13. Lester, R., and Schmid, R.: Bilirubin metabolism. N. Engl. J. Med., 270:779, 1964.
14. Schmid, R.: Bilirubin metabolism. I. Formation of bilirubin. In Schaffner, F., Sherlock, S., and Leevy, C. M. (Eds.): The Liver and Its Diseases. New York, Intercontinental Medical Book Corp., 1974, pp. 85–96.

Protein Metabolism

15. Miller, L. L., and Bale, W. F.: Synthesis of all plasma protein fractions except gamma globulin by the liver. J. Exp. Med., 99:125, 1954.

Blood Coagulation

16. Spector, I., and Corn, M.: Laboratory tests of hemostasis. The relation to hemorrhage in liver disease. Arch. Intern. Med., 119:577, 1967.
17. Walls, W. D., and Losowsky, M. S.: The hemostatic defect of liver disease. Gastroenterology, 60:108, 1971.

Hepatic Hemodynamics

18. Brauer, R. W.: Liver circulation and function. Physiol. Rev., 43:115, 1963.
19. Grayson, J., and Mendel, D.: Physiology of the Splanchnic Circulation. Monographs of the Physiological Society. London, Arnold, 1965.
20. Greenway, C. V., and Stark, R. D.: Hepatic vascular bed. Physiol. Rev., 51:23, 1971.
21. Reynolds, T. B., and Redeker, A. G.: Hepatic hemodynamics and portal hypertension. In Popper, H., and Schaffner, F. (Eds.):

Progress in Liver Diseases. Volume 2. New York, Grune & Stratton, Inc., 1965.
22. Shoemaker, W. C., and Elwyn, D. H.: Liver: Functional interactions within the intact animal. Ann. Rev. Physiol., 31:227, 1969.

Hepatectomy

23. Bollman, J. L., and Mann, F. C.: Studies on the physiology of the liver. XVIII: The effect of removal of the liver on the formation of ammonia. Am. J. Physiol., 92:92, 1930.
24. Bollman, J. L., Mann, F. C., and Magath, T. B.: Studies on the physiology of the liver. Effect of total removal of the liver on formation of urea. Am. J. Physiol., 69:371, 1924.
25. Bollman, J. L., Mann, F. C., and Magath, T. B.: Studies on the physiology of the liver. The effect of total removal of the liver on deaminization. Am. J. Physiol., 78:258, 1926.
26. Mann, F. C.: Studies in the physiology of the liver. I. Technic and general effects of removal. Am. J. Physiol., 55:285, 1921.
27. Mann, F. C.: The effects of complete and partial removal of the liver. Medicine, 6:419, 1927.

Eck Fistula

28. Harper, H. A., Gardner, R. E., Johansen, R., Galante, M., and McCorkle, H. J.: Amino acid tolerance in experimental portacaval anastomosis. Surgery, 29:210, 1951.
29. McDermott, W. V., Jr., and Adams, R. D.: Episodic stupor associated with an Eck fistula in the human with particular reference to the metabolism of ammonia. J. Clin. Invest., 33:1, 1954.
30. Silen, W., Mawdsley, D. L., Weirich, W. L., and Harper, H. A.: Studies of hepatic function in dogs with Eck fistula or portacaval transposition. Arch. Surg., 74:964, 1957.
31. Whipple, G. H., Robscheit-Robbins, F. S., and Hawkins, W. B.: Eck fistula liver subnormal in producing hemoglobin and plasma proteins on diets rich in liver and iron. J. Exp. Med., 81:171, 1945.

Liver Regeneration

32. Becker, F. F.: The normal hepatocyte in division: Regeneration of the mammalian liver. In Popper, H., and Schaffner, F. (Eds.): Progress in Liver Disease. Volume 3. New York, Grune & Stratton, Inc., 1970, p. 60.
33. Bucher, N. L. R.: Experimental aspects of hepatic regeneration. N. Engl. J. Med., 277:686, 738, 1967.
34. Broelsch, C. E., Lee, S., Charters, A. C., Chandler, J. G., Grambort, D. E., and Orloff, M. J.: Regeneration of liver isografts transplanted in continuity with splanchnic organs. Surg. Forum, 25:394, 1974.
35. Chandler, J. G., Lee, S., Krubel, R., Rosen, H., and Orloff, M. J.: The roles of inter-liver competition and portal blood in regeneration of auxiliary liver transplants. Surg. Forum, 22:341, 1971.
36. Duguay, L. R., Charters, A. C., Lee, S., Sviokla, S. C., and Orloff, M. J.: Time course of liver regeneration after splanchnic organ ablation. Surg. Forum, 26:408, 1975.
37. Fisher, B., Szuch, P., and Fisher, E. R.: Evaluation of a humoral factor in liver regeneration utilizing liver transplants. Cancer Res., 31:322, 1971.
38. Lee, S., Edgington, T. S., and Orloff, M. J.: The role of afferent blood supply in regeneration of liver isografts in rats. Surg. Forum, 19:360, 1968.
39. Lee, S., Keiter, J. E., Rosen, H., Chandler, J. G., and Orloff, M. J.: Influence of blood supply on regeneration of liver transplants. Surg. Forum, 20:369, 1969.
40. Lee, S., Broelsch, C. E., Flamant, Y. M., Chandler, J. G., Charters, A. C., and Orloff, M. J.: Liver regeneration after portacaval transposition in rats. Surgery, 77:144, 1975.
41. Moolten, F. L., and Bucher, N. L. R.: Regneration of rat liver: Transfer of humoral agent by cross circulation. Science, 158:272, 1967.
42. Sgro, J-C., Charters, A. C., Chandler, J. G., Grambort, D. E., and Orloff, M. J.: Studies of the site of origin of the hepatotrophic portal blood factor involved in liver regeneration. Surg. Forum, 24:377, 1973.
43. Starzl, T. E., Francavilla, A., Halgrimson, C. G., Francavilla, F. R., Porter, K. A., Brown, T. H., and Putnam, C. W.: The origin, hormonal nature, and action of hepatotrophic substances in portal venous blood. Surg. Gynecol. Obstet., 137:179, 1973.
44. Starzl, T. E., Porter, K. A., Kashiwagi, N., and Putnam, C. W.: Portal hepatotrophic factors, diabetes mellitus and acute liver atrophy, hypertrophy and regeneration. Surg. Gynecol. Obstet., 141:843, 1975.

Diagnosis of Liver Disease

Liver Function Tests

45. Clermont, R. J., and Chalmers, T. C.: The transaminase tests in liver disease. Medicine, *46*:197, 1967.

46. Combes, B.: The importance of conjugation with glutathione for sulfobromophthalein sodium (BSP) transfer from blood to bile. J. Clin. Invest., *44*:1214, 1965.

47. Combes, B., Wheeler, H. O., Childs, R. W., and Bradley, S. E.: The mechanisms of Bromsulphalein removal from the blood. Trans. Assoc. Am. Physicians, *69*:276, 1956.

48. Goresky, C. A.: Initial distribution and rate of uptake of sulfobromophthalein in the liver. Am. J. Physiol., *207*:13, 1964.

49. Leevy, C. M., Smith, F., Longueville, J., Paumgartner, G., and Howard, M. M.: Indocyanine green clearance as a test for hepatic function. J.A.M.A., *200*:236, 1967.

50. Muting, D., and Reikowski, H.: Protein metabolism in liver disease. *In* Popper, H., and Schaffner, F. (Eds.): Progress in Liver Diseases. Volume 2. New York, Grune & Stratton, Inc., 1965, p. 84.

51. Newton, M. A.: The clinical application of alkaline phosphatase electrophoresis. Q. J. Med., *36*:17, 1967.

52. Owen, J. A., and Robertson, R. F.: Paper electrophoresis of serum proteins in hepatobiliary disease. Lancet, *2*:1125, 1956.

53. Posen, S.: Alkaline phosphatase. Ann. Intern. Med., *67*:183, 1967.

54. Quick, A. J.: Hemorrhagic Diseases and Thrombosis, 2nd ed. Philadelphia, Lea & Febiger, 1966, p. 391.

55. Rappaport, S. F., Ames, S. B., Mikkelsen, S., and Goodman, J. R.: Plasma clotting factors in chronic hepatocellular disease. N. Engl. J. Med., *263*:278, 1960.

56. Ratnoff, O. D.: Hemostatic mechanisms in liver disease. Med. Clin. North Am., *47*:721, 1963.

57. Reinhold, J. G.: Flocculation tests and their application to the study of liver disease. *In* Sobotka, H., and Stewart, E. P. (Eds.): Advances in Clinical Chemistry. Volume 3. New York, Academic Press, 1960, p. 83.

58. Watson, C. J.: The importance of the fractional serum bilirubin determination in clinical medicine. Ann. Intern. Med., *45*:351, 1956.

59. Wheeler, H. O., Meltzer, J. I., and Bradler, S. E.: Biliary transport and hepatic storage of sulfobromophthalein sodium in unanaesthetized dog, in normal man, and in patients with hepatic disease J. Clin. Invest., *39*:1131, 1960.

60. Zieve, L., Hill, E., Hanson, M., Falcone, A. B., and Watson, C. J.: Normal and abnormal variations and clinical significance of the one-minute and total serum bilirubin determinations. J. Lab. Clin. Med., *38*:446, 1951.

61. Zimmerman, H. J., and West, M.: Serum enzyme levels in the diagnosis of hepatic disease. Am. J. Gastroenterol., *40*:387, 1963.

Liver Biopsy

62. Linder, H.: Limitations and dangers in percutaneous liver biopsies with the Menghini needle. Proceedings of the Third World Congress of Gastroenterology, *3*:373, 1966.

63. Menghini, G.: One-second needle biopsy of the liver. Gastroenterology, *35*:190, 1958.

64. Nelson, R. S.: The development and function of a liver biopsy program: Training of personnel, description of a modified Vim-Silverman needle and clinical value of 500 biopsies. Am. J. Med. Sci., *227*:152, 1951.

65. Zamcheck, N., and Klausenstock, O.: Needle biopsy of the liver. II. The risk of needle biopsy. N. Engl. J. Med., *249*:1062, 1953.

66. Zamcheck, N., and Sideman, R. L.: Needle biopsy of the liver. I. Its use in clinical and investigative medicine. N. Engl. J. Med., *249*:1020, 1953.

Roentgenography

67. Boijsen, E., Eckman, C. A., and Olin, T.: Coeliac and superior mesenteric angiography in portal hypertension. Acta Chir. Scand., *126*:315, 1963.

68. Kahn, P. C., and Alexander, F. K.: Total hepatic angiography and vascular dynamics in liver disease. Am. J. Gastroenterol., *52*:317, 1969.

69. Kirsh, I. E., Blackwell, C. C., and Bennett, H. D.: Roentgen diagnosis of esophageal varices: Comparison of roentgen and esophagoscopic findings in 502 cases. Am. J. Roentgenol., *74*:477, 1955.

70. Kreel, L., Jones, E. A., and Tavill, A. S.: A comparative study of

71. Lavoie, P., Jacob, M., Leduc, J., Legare, A., and Viallet, A.: The umbilicoportal approach for the study of splanchnic circulation: Technical, radiological and hemodynamic considerations. Can. J. Surg., *9*:338, 1968.

72. Leger, L. H.: Splenoportography: Diagnostic Phlebography of the Portal Venous System. Springfield, Ill., Charles C Thomas, Publisher, 1966.

73. Viamonte, M., Jr., Warren, W. D., and Foman, J. J.: Liver panangiography in the assessment of portal hypertension in liver cirrhosis. Radiol. Clin. North Am., *8*:147, 1970.

74. Wise, R. E., and Scholz, F. J.: Radiology of the liver and biliary tract. Gastroenterology, *65*:967, 1973.

Esophagogastroscopy

75. Conn, H. O., Binder, H., and Brodoff, M.: Fiberoptic and conventional esophagoscopy in the diagnosis of esophageal varices. Gastroenterology, *52*:810, 1967.

76. Conn, H. O., Smith, H. W., and Brodoff, M.: Observer variation in the endoscopic diagnosis of esophageal varices. N. Engl. J. Med., *272*:830, 1965.

Portal Pressure Measurements

77. Leevy, C. M., and Gliedman, M. L.: Practical and research value of hepatic vein catheterization. N. Engl. J. Med., *258*:738, 1958.

78. Reynolds, T. B., Ito, S., and Iwatsuki, S.: Measurement of portal pressure and its clinical application. Am. J. Med., *49*:649, 1970.

79. Reynolds, T. B.: The role of hemodynamic measurements in portosystemic shunt. Arch. Surg., *108*:276, 1974.

80. Viallet, A., Legare, A., and Lavoie, P.: Hepatic and umbilico-portal catheterization in portal hypertension. Ann. N. Y. Acad. Sci., *170*:177, 1970.

81. Warren, W. D., and Muller, W. H.: Clarification of some hemodynamic changes in cirrhosis and their surgical significance. Ann. Surg., *150*:413, 1959.

Radioisotope Liver Blood Flow

82. Restrepo, J. E., Warren, W. D., Nolan, S., and Muller, W. H., Jr.: Radioactive gold technique for the estimation of liver blood flow: Normal values and technical considerations. Surgery, *48*:748, 1960.

83. Shaldon, S., Chiandussi, L., Guevara, I., Caesar, J., and Sherlock, S.: The estimation of hepatic blood flow and intrahepatic shunted blood flow by colloidal heat-denatured human serum albumin labeled with I^{131}. J. Clin. Invest., *40*:1346, 1961.

84. Warren, W. D., Fomon, J. J., Viamonte, M., and Zeppa, R.: Preoperative assessment of portal hypertension. Ann. Surg., *165*:999, 1967.

Radioisotope Liver Scanning

85. McAfee, J. G., Ause, R. G., and Wagner, H. N., Jr.: Diagnostic value of scintillation scanning of the liver. Arch. Intern. Med., *116*:95, 1965.

Ultrasonic Scanning

86. Lehman, J. S.: Ultrasound in the diagnosis of hepatobiliary disease. Radiol. Clin. North Am., *4*:605, 1966.

87. McCarthy, C. F., Davies, E. R., Wells, P. N. T., Ross, F. G. M., Follet, D. H., Muir, K. M., and Read, A. E.: A comparison of ultrasonic and isotope scanning in the diagnosis of liver disease. Br. J. Radiol., *43*:100, 1970.

arteriography and scintillation scanning in space-occupying lesions of the liver. Br. J. Radiol., *41*:401, 1968.

Jaundice

88. Hanger, F. M.: Diagnostic problems of jaundice. Arch. Intern. Med., *86*:169, 1950.

89. Hoffman, H. N., II, Whitcomb, F. F., Jr., Butt, H. R., and Bollman, J. L.: Bile pigments of jaundice. J. Clin. Invest., *39*:132, 1960.

90. Ingelfinger, F.: Differential diagnosis of jaundice. Disease-a-Month, November, 1958.

91. Schenker, S., Balent, J., and Schiff, L.: Differential diagnosis of jaundice: A report of a prospective study of 61 proved cases. Am. J. Dig. Dis., *7*:449, 1962.

92. Schiff, L.: The differential diagnosis of jaundice. Postgrad. Med., *41*:39, 1967.

93. With, T. K.: Bile Pigments: Chemical, Biological and Clinical Aspects. New York, Academic Press, 1968.

Natural History of Cirrhosis

94. Garceau, A. J., and the Boston Inter-Hospital Liver Group: The

natural history of cirrhosis. I. Survival with esophageal varices. N. Engl. J. Med., *268*:469, 1963.

95. Popper, H., Davidson, C. S., Leevy, C. M., and Schaffner, F.: The social impact of liver disease. N. Engl. J. Med., *281*:1455, 1969.

96. Powell, W. J., Jr., and Klatskin, G.: Duration of survival in patients with Laennec's cirrhosis: Influence of alcohol withdrawal, and possible effects of recent changes in general management of the disease. Am. J. Med., *44*:406, 1968.

97. Ratnoff, O. D., and Patek, A. J., Jr.: Natural history of Laennec's cirrhosis of the liver: Analysis of 386 cases. Medicine, *21*:207, 1942.

98. Mortality from cirrhosis of the liver—United States, Canada, and Western Europe. Stat. Bull. Metropolitan Life Ins. Co., *54*:5, 1973.

Bleeding Esophageal Varices

Natural Hisotry

99. Atik, M., and Simeone, F.: Massive gastrointestinal bleeding: A study of 296 patients at City Hospital of Cleveland. Arch. Surg., *69*:355, 1954.

100. Baker, L. A., Smith, C., and Lieberman, G.: The natural history of esophageal varices. Am. J. Med., *26*:228, 1959.

101. Cohn, R., and Blaisdell, F. W.: The natural history of the patient with cirrhosis of the liver with esophageal varices following the first massive hemorrhage. Surg. Gynecol. Obstet., *106*:699, 1958.

102. Higgins, W. H., Jr.: The esophageal varix: A report of one hundred and fifteen cases. Am. J. Med. Sci., *214*:436, 1947.

103. Liebowitz, H. R.: Pathogenesis of esophageal varix rupture. J.A.M.A., *175*:874, 1961.

104. Merigan, T. C., Jr., Hollister, R. M., Gryska, P. F., Starkey, G. W. G., and Davidson, C. S.: Gastrointestinal bleeding with cirrhosis: Study of 172 episodes in 158 patients. N. Engl. J. Med., *263*:579, 1960.

105. Nachlas, M. M., O'Neil, J. E., and Campbell, A. J. A.: The life history of patients with cirrhosis of the liver and bleeding esophageal varices. Ann. Surg., *141*:10, 1955.

106. Olsson, R.: The natural history of esophageal varices. A retrospective study of 224 cases with liver cirrhosis. Digestion, *6*:65, 1972.

107. Orloff, M. J., and Thomas, H. S.: Pathogenesis of esophageal varix rupture: A study based on gross and microscopic examination of the esophagus at the time of bleeding. Arch. Surg., *87*:301, 1963.

108. Taylor, F. W., and Jontz, J. G.: Cirrhosis with hemorrhage. Arch. Surg., *78*:786, 1959.

Emergency Diagnosis

109. Orloff, M. J.: Emergency treatment of bleeding esophageal varices in cirrhosis. *In* Longmire, W. P., Jr. (Ed.): Portal hypertension. Curr. Probl. Surg., July, 1966.

110. Viamonte, M., Jr., Warren, W. D., Fomon, J. J., and Martinez, L. O.: Angiographic investigations in portal hypertension. Surg. Gynecol. Obstet., *130*:37, 1970.

Emergency Medical Therapy

ESOPHAGEAL BALLOON TAMPONADE

111. Conn, H. O.: Hazards attending the use of esophageal tamponade. N. Engl. J. Med., *259*:701, 1958.

112. Conn, H. O., and Simpson, J. A.: Excessive mortality associated with balloon tamponade of bleeding varices. J.A.M.A., *202*:587, 1967.

113. Hamilton, J. E.: Management of bleeding esophageal varices associated with cirrhosis of liver. Ann. Surg., *141*:637, 1955.

114. Ludington, A. G.: A study of 158 cases of esophageal varices. Surg. Gynecol. Obstet., *106*:519, 1958.

115. Orloff, M. J., Halasz, N. A., Lipman, C., Schwabe, A. D., Thompson, J. C., and Weidner, W. A.: The complications of cirrhosis of the liver. Ann. Intern. Med., *66*:165, 1967.

116. Read, A. E., Dawson, A. M., Kerr, D. N. S., Turner, M. D., and Sherlock, S.: Bleeding oesophageal varices treated by oesophageal compression tube. Br. Med. J., *1*:227, 1960.

117. Reynolds, T. B., Freedman, T., and Winsor, W.: Results of the treatment of bleeding esophageal varices with balloon tamponade. Am. J. Med. Sci., *224*:500, 1952.

SYSTEMIC INTRAVENOUS VASOPRESSIN

118. Merigan, T. C., Plotkin, G. R., and Davidson, C. S.: Effect of intravenously administered posterior pituitary extract on hemorrhage from bleeding varices. N. Engl. J. Med., *266*:134, 1962.

119. Schwartz, S. I., Bales, H. W., Emerson, G. L., and Mahoney, E.

B.: Use of intravenous Pituitrin in treatment of bleeding esophageal varices. Surgery, *45*:72, 1959.

120. Shaldon, S., and Sherlock, S.: The use of vasopressin (Pitressin) in the control of bleeding from oesophageal varices. Lancet, *2*:222, 1960.

SELECTIVE MESENTERIC INTRA-ARTERIAL VASOPRESSIN

121. Barr, J. W., Lakin, R. C., and Rösch, J.: Similarity of arterial and intravenous vasopressin on portal and systemic hemodynamics. Gastroenterology, *69*:13, 1975.

122. Conn, H. O., Ramsby, G. R., Storer, E. H., et al.: Intra-arterial vasopressin in the treatment of upper gastrointestinal hemorrhage: A prospective, controlled clinical trial. Gastroenterology, *68*:211, 1975.

123. Millette, B., Huet, P-M., Lavoie, P., and Viallet, A.: Portal and systemic effects of selective infusion of vasopressin into the superior mesenteric artery in cirrhotic patients. Gastroenterology, *69*:6, 1975.

124. Nusbaum, M., Younis, M. T., Baum, S., and Blakemore, W. S.: Control of portal hypertension. Selective mesenteric arterial infusion of vasopressin. Arch. Surg., *108*:342, 1974.

GASTROESOPHAGEAL HYPOTHERMIA

125. Wangensteen, S. L., and Smith, R. S., III: Intragastric cooling for upper gastrointestinal bleeding. Ann. N. Y. Acad. Sci., *115*:328, 1964.

OTHER NONSURGICAL MEASURES

126. Johnston, G. W., and Rodgers, H. W.: A review of 15 years' experience in the use of sclerotherapy in the control of acute haemorrhage from oesophageal varices. Br. J. Surg., *60*:797, 1973.

127. Lunderquist, A., and Vang, J.: Transhepatic catheterization and obliteration of the coronary vein in patients with portal hypertension and esophageal varices. N. Engl. J. Med., *291*:646, 1974.

Emergency Transesophageal Varix Ligation

128. Orloff, M. J.: A comparative study of emergency transesophageal ligation and nonsurgical treatment of bleeding esophageal varices in unselected patients with cirrhosis. Surgery, *52*:103, 1962.

129. Ottinger, L. W., and Moncure, A. C.: Transthoracic ligation of bleeding esophageal varices in patients with intrahepatic portal obstruction. Ann. Surg., *179*:35, 1974.

130. Rothwell-Jackson, R. L., and Hunt, A. G.: The results obtained with emergency surgery in the treatment of persistent haemorrhage from gastro-oesophageal varices in the cirrhotic patient. Br. J. Surg., *58*:205, 1971.

131. Wirthlin, L. S., Linton, R. R., and Ellis, D. S.: Transthoracoesophageal ligation of bleeding esophageal varices. A reappraisal. Arch. Surg., *109*:688, 1974.

Emergency Portacaval Shunt

132. Adson, M. A.: Emergency portal–systemic shunts, Surg. Clin. North Am., *47*:887, 1967.

133. Balasegaram, M., and Damodaran, A.: Emergency shunt surgery for bleeding oesophagogastric varices. Aust. N. Z. J. Surg., *40*:152, 1970.

134. Edmonson, H. T., Jackson, F. C., Juler, G. L., Siegel, B., and Perrin, E. B.: Clinical investigation of the portacaval shunt. IV. A report of early survival from the emergency operation. Ann. Surg., *173*:372, 1971.

135. Ekman, C. A., and Sandblom, P.: Shunt-operation in acute bleeding from esophageal varices. Ann. Surg., *160*:531, 1964.

136. Hoffman, D. C., Jepson, R. P., and Harris, J. D.: Experiences with emergency porta-caval shunt. Aust. Ann. Med., *18*:238, 1969.

137. Mikkelsen, W. P.: Emergency portacaval shunt. Rev. Surg., *19*:141, 1962.

138. Orloff, M. J.: Emergency portacaval shunt: A comparative study of shunt, varix ligation and nonsurgical treatment of bleeding esophageal varices in unselected patients with cirrhosis. Ann. Surg., *166*:456, 1967.

139. Orloff, M. J.: Emergency treatment of bleeding esophageal varices. *In* Markoff, N. G. (Ed.): The Therapy of Portal Hypertension. Stuttgart, Georg Thieme Verlag, 1968, p. 211.

140. Orloff, M. J.: Emergency treatment of bleeding esophageal varices in alcoholic cirrhosis. *In* Sardesai, V. M. (Ed.): Biochemical and Clinical Aspects of Alcohol Metabolism. Springfield, Ill., Charles C Thomas, Publisher, 1969, p. 288.

141. Orloff, M. J., Chandler, J. G., Charters, A. C., Condon, J. K., Grambort, D. E., Modafferi, T. R., and Levin, S. E.: Emergency portacaval shunt for bleeding esophageal varices.

Prospective study in unselected patients with alcoholic cirrhosis. Arch. Surg., *108*:293, 1974.

142. Orloff, M. J., Charters, A. C., Chandler, J. G., Condon, J. K., Grambort, D. E., Modafferi, T. R., Levin, S. E., Brown, N. B., Sviokla, S. C., and Knox, D. G.: Portacaval shunt as emergency procedure in unselected patients with alcoholic cirrhosis. Surg. Gynecol. Obstet., *141*:59, 1975.

143. Peskin, G. W., Chrichlow, R. W., Berggren, R. B., and Miller, L. D.: Portacaval shunt in the emergency treatment of variceal bleeding. Surgery, *56*:800, 1964.

144. Preston, F. W., and Trippel, O. H.: Emergency portacaval shunt. Arch. Surg., *90*:770, 1965.

145. Rousselot, L. M., Gilbertson, F. E., and Panke, W. F.: Severe hemorrhage from esophagogastric varices. Its emergency management with particular reference to portacaval anastomsosis. N. Engl. J. Med., *262*:269, 1960.

146. Wantz, G. E., and Payne, M. A.: Experience with portacaval shunt for portal hypertension. N. Engl. J. Med., *265*:721, 1961.

147. Weinberger, H. A.: Emergency portacaval shunt for esophagogastric hemorrhage. Arch. Surg., *91*:333, 1965.

Postoperative Care Following Emergency Portacaval Shunt

148. Del Guercio, L. R. M., Coommaraswamy, R. P., Feins, N. R., Woolman, S. B., and State, D.: Pulmonary arteriovenous admixture and the hyperdynamic cardiovascular state in surgery for portal hypertension. Surgery, *56*:74, 1964.

149. Gabuzda, G. J.: Nutrition and liver disease. Practical considerations. Med. Clin. North Am., *54*:1455, 1970.

150. Glickman, L., and Herbsman, H.: Delirium tremens in surgical patients. Surgery, *64*:882, 1968.

151. Isbell, H., Fraser, H. F., Wikler, A., Belleville, R. E., and Eisenman, A. J.: An experimental study of the etiology of "rum fits" and delirium tremens. Q. J. Stud. Alcohol, *16*:1, 1955.

152. Nielson, J.: An intensive one year study of delirium tremens in Copenhagen. Acta Psychiatr. Scand. (Suppl. 187), *41*:32, 1965.

153. Siegel, J. H., Greenspan, M., Cohn, J. D., and Del Guercio, L. R.M.: The prognostic implications of altered physiology in operations for portal hypertension. Surg. Gynecol. Obstet., *126*:249, 1968.

154. Siegel, J. H., and Williams, J. B.: A computer based index for the prediction of operative survival in patients with cirrhosis and portal hypertension. Ann. Surg., *169*:191, 1969.

155. Siegel, J. H., Goldwyn, R. M., Farrell, E. J., Gallin, P., and Friedman, H. P.: Hyperdynamic states and the physiologic determinants of survival. In patients with cirrhosis and portal hypertension. Arch. Surg., *108*:282, 1974.

156. Sloop, R. D., and Orloff, M. J.: An important syndrome of metabolic alkalosis in patients with cirrhosis, bleeding varices, and portacaval shunt. Surg. Forum, *17*:37, 1966.

Elective Portacaval Shunt

157. Barnes, B. A., Ackroyd, F. W., Battit, G. E., Kantrowitz, P. A., Schapiro, R. H., Strole, W. E., Jr., Todd, D. P., and McDermott, W. V., Jr.: Elective portosystemic shunts: Morbidity and survival data. Ann. Surg., *174*:76, 1971.

158. Bismuth, H., Franco, D., and Hepp, J.: Portal-systemic shunt in hepatic cirrhosis. Does the type of shunt decisively influence the clinical result. Ann. Surg., *179*:209, 1974.

159. Child, C. G., III: The Shattuck lecture: The portal circulation. N. Engl. J. Med., *262*:837, 1955.

160. Conn, H. O.: Therapeutic portacaval anastomosis: To shunt or not to shunt. Gastroenterology, *67*:1065, 1974.

161. Eckman, C. A.: Portal hypertension. Acta Chir. Scand., *113*:1, 1957.

162. Grace, N. D., Muench, H., and Chalmers, T. C.: The present status of shunts for portal hypertension in cirrhosis. Gastroenterology, *50*:684, 1966.

163. Hallenbeck, G. A., Wollaeger, E. E., Adson, M. A., and Gage, R. P.: Results after portal-systemic shunts in 120 patients with cirrhosis of liver. Surg. Gynecol. Obstet., *116*:435, 1963.

164. Jackson, F. C., Perrin, E. D., Felix, W. R., and Smith, A. G.: A clinical investigation of the portacaval shunt: V. Survival analyses of the therapeutic operation. Ann. Surg., *174*:672, 1971.

165. Linton, R. R., Ellis, D. S., and Geary, J. E.: Critical comparative analysis of early and late results of splenorenal and direct portacaval shunts performed in 169 patients with portal cirrhosis. Ann. Surg., *154*:446, 1961.

166. McDermott, W. V., Palazzi, H., Nardi, G. L., and Mondet, A.: Elective portal systemic shunt. N. Engl. J. Med., *264*:419, 1961.

167. Mikkelson, W. P., Turrill, F. R., and Pattison, A. C.: Portacaval shunt in cirrhosis of the liver. Clinical and hemodynamic aspects. Am. J. Surg., *104*:204, 1962.

168. Mikkelson, W. P.: Therapeutic portacaval shunt. Preliminary data on controlled trial and morbid effects of acute hyaline necrosis. Arch. Surg., *108*:302, 1974.

169. Resnick, R. H., Iber, F. L., Ishihara, A. M., Chalmers, T. C., and Zimmerman, H.: A controlled study of the therapeutic portacaval shunt. Gastroenterology, *67*:843, 1974.

170. Rousselot, L. M., Panke, W. F., Bono, R. F., and Moreno, A. H.: Experiences with portacaval anastomosis: Analysis of 104 elective end-to-side shunts for prevention of recurrent hemorrhage from esophagogastric varices (1952 through 1961). Am. J. Med., *34*:297, 1963.

171. Schapiro, R. H., Strole, W. E., Jr., Todd, D. P., and McDermott, W. V., Jr.: Elective portosystemic shunts: Morbidity and survival data. Ann. Surg., *174*:76, 1971.

172. Sedgwick, C. E., Poulantzas, J. K., and Miller, W. H.: Portasystemic shunts in 102 patients with portal hypertension. N. Engl. J. Med., *274*:1290, 1966.

173. Voorhees, A. B., Jr., Price, J. B., Jr., and Britton, R. C.: Portasystemic shunting procedures for portal hypertension. Twenty-six year experience in adults with cirrhosis of the liver. Ann. Surg., *119*:501, 1970.

174. Walker, R. M., Shaldon, C., and Vowles, K. D.: Late results of portacaval anastomosis. Lancet, *2*:727, 1961.

Choice of Portal-Systemic Shunt
DIRECT PORTACAVAL SHUNT

175. Bernstein, J. E., Nutting, R. O., and Orloff, M. J.: Comparison of the effects of end-to-side and side-to-side portacaval shunts on liver function, liver blood flow, and ammonia metabolism in dogs and man. Surg. Forum, *19*:328, 1968.

176. Britton, R. C., Voorhees, A. B., Jr., and Price, J. B., Jr.: Perfusion of the liver following a side-to-side portacaval shunt. Surgery, *62*:181, 1967.

177. Charters, A. C., Chandler, J. G., Condon, J. K., Grambort, D. E., Levin, S. E., Modafferi, T. R., and Orloff, M. J.: Spontaneous reversal of portal flow in patients with bleeding varices treated by emergency portacaval shunt. Am. J. Surg., *127*:25, 1974.

178. Iwatsuki, S., Mikkelsen, W. P., Redeker, A. G., Reynolds, T. B., and Turrill, F. L.: Clinical comparison of the end-to-side and side-to-side portacaval shunt: Ten year follow-up. Ann. Surg., *178*:65, 1973.

179. Orloff, M. J., Chandler, J. G., Charters, A. C., Condon, J. K., Grambort, D. E., Modafferi, T. R., and Levin, S. E.: Comparison of end-to-side and side-to-side portacaval shunt in dogs and human subjects with cirrhosis and portal hypertension. Am. J. Surg., *128*:195, 1974.

180. Panke, W. F., Rousselot, L. M., and Burchell, A. R.: A sixteen-year experience with end-to-side portacaval shunt for variceal hemorrhage: Analysis of data and comparison with other types of portasystemic anastomoses. Ann. Surg., *168*:957, 1968.

181. Reynolds, T. B., Hudson, N. M., Mikkelsen, W. P., Turrill, F. L., and Redeker, A. G.: Clinical comparison of end-to-side and side-to-side portacaval shunt. N. Engl. J. Med., *274*:706, 1966.

182. Tamaki, A., Golby, M., and Orloff, M. J.: Effects of side-to-side portacaval shunt on hepatic hemodynamics and metabolism. Surg. Forum, *19*:324, 1968.

183. Turcotte, J. G., Wallin, V. W., Jr., and Child, C. G., II: End-to-side versus side-to-side portacaval shunts in patients with hepatic cirrhosis. Am. J. Surg., *117*:108, 1969.

184. Warren, W. D., and Muller, W. H., Jr.: Clarification of some hemodynamic changes in cirrhosis and their surgical significance. Ann. Surg., *150*:413, 1959.

INTERPOSITION MESOCAVAL H GRAFT SHUNT

185. Drapanas, T.: Interposition mesocaval shunt for treatment of portal hypertension. Ann. Surg., *176*:435, 1972.

186. Drapanas, T., Lo Cicero, J., III, and Dowling, J. B.: Hemodynamics of the interposition mesocaval shunt. Ann. Surg., *181*:523, 1975.

187. Graziano, J. L., and Sullivan, H. J.: Portal decompression: Clinical experience with the "H" graft. Ann. Surg., *178*:209, 1973.

188. Thompson, B. W., and Read, R. C.: Interposition "H" grafting for portal hypertension. Arch. Surg., *108*:502, 1974.

SELECTIVE DISTAL SPLENORENAL SHUNT

189. Britton, R. C., and Voorhees, A. B., Jr.: Selective portal decompression. Surgery, 67:104, 1970.
190. Salam, A. A., Warren,W. D., LePage, J. R., Viamonte, M. R., Hutson, D., and Zeppa, R.: Hemodynamic contrasts between selective and total portal-systemic decompression. Ann. Surg., 173:827, 1971.
191. Warren, W. D., Salam, A. A., Hutson, D., and Zeppa, R.: Selective distal splenorenal shunt. Technique and results of operation. Arch. Surg., 108:306, 1974.
192. Warren, W. D., and Salam, A. A.: Surgery for the portal hypertension of cirrhosis: The need for change. Major Problems in Clinical Surgery, 14:127, 1974.

ARTERIALIZATION OF THE LIVER WITH PORTACAVAL SHUNT

193. Maillard, J. N., Benhamou, J. P., and Rueff, B.: Arterialization of the liver with portacaval shunt in the treatment of portal hypertension due to intrahepatic block. Surgery, 67:883, 1970.
194. Maillard, J. N., Rueff, B., Prandi, D., and Sicot, C.: Hepatic arterialization and portacaval shunt in hepatic cirrhosis. An assessment. Arch. Surg., 108:315, 1974.

HEMODYNAMIC CRITERIA FOR SELECTING SHUNT

195. Burchell, A. R., Moreno, A. H., Panke, W. F., and Nealon, T. F.: Hemodynamic variables and prognosis following portacaval shunt. Surg. Gynecol. Obstet., 138:359, 1974.
196. Charters, A. C., Brown, B. N., Sviokla, S. C., Knox, D. G., and Orloff, M. J.: The influence of portal perfusion on the response to portacaval shunt. Am. J. Surg., 130:226, 1975.
197. Price, J. B., Jr., Britton, R. C., and Voorhees, A. B., Jr.: The significance and limitations of operative hemodynamics in portal hypertension. Arch. Surg., 95:843, 1967.
198. Smith, G. W.: Use of hemodynamic selection criteria in the management of cirrhotic patients with portal hypertension. Ann. Surg., 179:782, 1974.

Prophylactic Portacaval Shunt

199. Conn, H. O.: Prophylactic portacaval shunts. Ann. Intern. Med., 70:859, 1969.
200. Conn, H. O., and Lindenmuth, W. W.: Prophylactic portacaval anastomosis in cirrhotic patients with esophageal varices. Interim results with suggestions for subsequent investigations. N. Engl. J. Med., 279:725, 1968.
201. Jackson, F. C., Perrin, E. B., Smith, A. G., Dagradi, A. E., and Nadal, H. M.: A clinical investigation of the portacaval shunt. II. Survival analysis of the prophylactic operation. Am. J. Surg., 115:22, 1967.
202. Resnick, R. H., Chalmers, T. C., Ishihara, A. M., Garceau, A. J., Callow, A. D., Schimmel, E. M., O'Hara, E. T., and the Boston Inter-Hospital Liver Group: A controlled study of the prophylactic portacaval shunt. A final report. Ann. Intern. Med., 70:675, 1969.

Cirrhotic Ascites

203. Hyatt, R. E., and Smith, J. R.: The mechanism of ascites. Am. J. Med., 16:434, 1954.
204. Lieberman, F. L., Denison, E. K., and Reynolds, T. B.: The relationship of plasma volume, portal hypertension, ascites, and renal sodium retention in cirrhosis. The overflow theory of ascites formation. Ann. N. Y. Acad. Sci., 170:202, 1970.
205. Madden, J. L., Lore, J. M., Jr., Gerold, F. P., and Ravid, J. M.: The pathogenesis of ascites and a consideration of its treatment. Surg. Gynecol. Obstet., 99:385, 1954.
206. Orloff, M. J.: Surgical treatment of intractable cirrhotic ascites. In Longmire, W. P., Jr. (Ed.): Portal hypertension. Curr. Probl. Surg., July, 1966, p. 28.
207. Orloff, M. J.: Effect of side-to-side portacaval shunt on intractable ascites, sodium excretion, and aldosterone metabolism in man. Am. J. Surg., 112:297, 1966.
208. Orloff, M. J.: Pathogenesis and surgical treatment of intractable ascites associated with alcoholic cirrhosis. Ann. N. Y. Acad. Sci., 170:273, 1970.
209. Orloff, M. J., Ross, T. H., Baddeley, R. M., Nutting, R. O., Spitz, B. R., Sloop, R. D., Neesby, T., and Halasz, N. A.: Experimental ascites. VI. The effects of hepatic venous outflow obstruction and ascites on aldosterone secretion. Surgery, 56:83, 1964.
210. Orloff, M. J., Spitz, B. R., Wall, M. H., Thomas, H. S., and Halasz, N. A.: Experimental ascites. IV. A comparison of the effects of end-to-side and side-to-side portacaval shunts on intractable ascites. Surgery, 56:784, 1964.
211. Orloff, M. J., Wright, P. W., DeBenedetti, M. J., Halasz, N. A.,

212. Annetts, D. L., Musicant, M. E., and Goodhead, B.: Experimental ascites. VII. The effects of external drainage of the thoracic duct on ascites and hepatic hemodynamics. Arch. Surg., 93:119, 1966.
213. Parker, R. G. F.: Occlusion of the hepatic veins in man. Medicine, 38:369, 1959.
214. Sherlock, S., and Shaldon, S.: The aetiology and management of ascites in patients with hepatic cirrhosis. A review. Gut, 4:95, 1963.
215. Welch, C. S., Welch, H. F., and Carter, J. H.: The treatment of ascites by side-to-side portacaval shunt. Ann. Surg., 150:428, 1959.
216. Witte, M. H., Witte, C. L., and Dumont, A. E.: Progress in liver disease: Physiological factors involved in the causation of cirrhotic ascites. Gastroenterology, 61:742, 1971.

Hepatic Encephalopathy

216. Fischer, J. E.: Hepatic coma in cirrhosis, portal hypertension, and following portacaval shunt. Its etiologies and the current status of its treatment. Arch. Surg., 108:325, 1974.
217. Gabuzda, G. J.: Hepatic coma: Clinical considerations, pathogenesis, and management. Adv. Intern. Med., 11:11, 1962.
218. McDermott, W. V., Jr.: Metabolism and toxicity of ammonia. N. Engl. J. Med., 257:1076, 1957.
219. McDermott, W. V., Jr., Barnes, B. A., Nardi, G. L., and Ackroyd, F. W.: Postshunt encephalopathy. Surg. Gynecol. Obstet., 126:585, 1968.
220. Orloff, M. J., Wall, M. H., Hickman, E. B., and Neesby, T.: The influence of the stomal size of portacaval shunts on peripheral blood ammonia levels. Ann. Surg., 158:172, 1963.
221. Read, A. E.: The medical treatment of hepatic coma. In Read, A. E. (Ed.): The Liver. Colston Papers, Volume 19. London, Butterworths, 1967, p. 191.
222. Resnick, R. H., Ishihara, A., Shimmel, A., and Chalmers, T. C.: A controlled trial of colon by-pass in chronic hepatic encephalopathy. Gastroenterology, 54:1057, 1968.
223. Schenker, S., Breen, K. J., and Hoyumpa, A. M., Jr.: Hepatic encephalopathy: Current status. Gastroenterology, 66:121, 1974.
224. Trey, C., and Davidson, C. S.: The management of fulminant hepatic failure. In Popper, H., and Schaffner, F. (Eds.): Progress in Liver Diseases. Volume 3. New York, Grune & Stratton, Inc., 1970, p. 282.
225. Zieve, L.: Pathogenesis of hepatic coma. Arch. Intern. Med., 118:211, 1966.
226. Zieve, L., and Nicoloff, D. M.: Pathogenesis of hepatic coma. Ann. Rev. Med., 26:143, 1975.

Gastric Acid Hypersecretion and Peptic Ulcer Associated with Liver Disease and Portacaval Shunt

227. Clarke, J. S., Ozeran, R. S., Hart, J. C., Cruze, K., and Crevling, V.: Peptic ulcer following portacaval shunt. Ann. Surg., 148:551, 1958.
228. Orloff, M. J., Abbott, A. G., and Rosen, H.: Nature of the humoral agent responsible for portacaval shunt-related gastric hypersecretion in man. Am. J. Surg., 120:237, 1970.
229. Orloff, M. J., Chandler, J. G., Alderman, S. J., Keiter, J. E., and Rosen, H.: Gastric secretion and peptic ulcer following portacaval shunt in man. Ann. Surg., 170:515, 1969.
230. Orloff, M. J., Villar-Valdes, H., Abbott, A. G., Williams, R. J., and Rosen, H.: Site of origin of the hormone responsible for gastric hypersecretion associated with portacaval shunt. Surgery, 68:202, 1970.
231. Orloff, M. J., Villar-Valdes, H., Rosen, H., Thompson, A. G., and Chandler, J. G.: Humoral mediation of the intestinal phase of gastric secretion and of acid hypersecretion associated with portacaval shunts. Surgery, 66:118, 1969.
232. Ostrow, J. D., Timmerman, R. J., and Gray, S. J.: Gastric secretion in human hepatic cirrhosis. Gastroenterology, 38:303, 1960.
233. Phillips, M. M., Ramsby, G. A., and Conn, H. O.: Portacaval anastomosis and peptic ulcer: A nonassociation. Gastroenterology, 68:121, 1975.
234. Thompson, J. C.: Alterations in gastric secretion after portacaval shunting. Am. J. Surg., 117:854, 1969.

Renal Failure Associated with Liver Disease

235. Baldus, W. P., and Summerskill, W. H. J.: The kidney in hepatic disease. In Foulk, W. T. (Ed.): Diseases of the Liver. New York. McGraw-Hill Book Company, 1968, p. 107.

236. Conn, H. O.: A rational approach to the hepatorenal syndrome. Gastroenterology, 65:321, 1973.
237. Goresky, C. A., and Kummer, G.: Renal failure in cirrhosis of the liver. Can. Med. Assoc. J., 90:353, 1964.
238. Papper, S.: The role of the kidney in Laennec's cirrhosis of the liver. Medicine, 37:299, 1958.
239. Papper, S.: The kidney in liver disease. In Strauss, M. B., and Welt, L. G. (Eds.): Diseases of the Kidney. Boston, Little, Brown & Company, 1963, p. 841.
240. Papper, S.: The hepatorenal syndrome. Clin. Nephrol., 4:41, 1975.
241. Shear, L., Hall, P. W., III, and Gabuzada, G. J.: Renal failure in patients with cirrhosis of the liver. II. Factors influencing maximal urinary flow rate. Am. J. Med., 39:199, 1965.
242. Shear, L., Kleinerman, J., and Gabuzda, G. J.: Renal failure in patients with cirrhosis of the liver. I. Clinical and pathologic characteristics. Am. J. Med., 39:184, 1965.

Portal Hypertension Due to Extrahepatic Portal Obstruction

243. Clatworthy, H. W., Jr., and Boles, E. T., Jr.: Extrahepatic portal bed block in children: Pathogenesis and treatment. Ann. Surg., 150:371, 1959.
244. Clatworthy, H. W., Jr., and DeLorimer, A. A.: Portal decompression procedures in children. Am. J. Surg., 107:447, 1964.
245. Mikkelsen, W. P.: Extrahepatic portal hypertension in children. Am. J. Surg., 111:333, 1966.
246. Voorhees, A. B., Jr., Harris, R. C., Britton, R. C., Price, J. B., and Santulli, T. V.: Portal hypertension in children: 98 cases. Surgery, 58:540, 1965.
247. Voorhees, A. B., Jr., and Price, J. B., Jr.: Extrahepatic portal hypertension. A retrospective analysis of 127 cases and associated clinical implications. Arch. Surg., 108:338, 1974.
248. Walker, R. M.: Treatment of portal hypertension in children. Proc. R. Soc. Med., 55:770, 1962.

Portacaval Shunt in the Budd-Chiari Syndrome, Glycogen Storage Disease and Hyperlipidemia

249. Ahrens, E. H., Jr.: Homozygous hypercholesterolemia and the portacaval shunt. Lancet, 2:449, 1974.
250. Clain, D., Freston, J., Dreel, L., and Sherlock, S.: Clinical diagnosis of the Budd-Chiari syndrome. Am. J. Med., 43:544, 1967.
251. Erlik, D., Shramek, A., Brandstaetter, S., and Bason, H.: Surgical cure of primary hepatic vein occlusion syndrome by side-to-side portacaval shunt. Surg. Gynecol. Obstet., 114:368, 1962.
252. Folkman, J., Philipport, A., Tze, W-J., and Crigler, J., Jr.: Portacaval shunt for glycogen storage disease: Value of prolonged intravenous hyperalimentation before surgery. Surgery, 72:306, 1972.
253. Parker, R. G. F.: Occlusion of the hepatic veins in man. Medicine, 38:369, 1959.
254. Prondi, D., Rueff, B., and Benhamou, J. P.: Side-to-side portacaval shunt in the treatment of Budd-Chiari syndrome. Gastroenterology, 68:137, 1975.
255. Starzl, T. E., Putnam, C. W., Porter, K. A., Halgrimson, C. G., Corman, J., Brown, B. I., Gotlin, R. W., Rodgerson, D. O., and Greene, H. I.: Portal diversion for the treatment of glycogen storage disease in humans. Ann. Surg., 178:525, 1973.
256. Starzl, T. E., Putnam, C. W., Chase, H. P., and Porter, K. A.: Portacaval shunt in hyperlipoproteinaemia. Lancet, 2:940, 1973.

Liver Trauma

257. Crosthwait, R. W., Allen, J. E., Murga, F., Beall, A. C., Jr., and DeBakey, M. E.: The surgical management of 640 consecutive liver injuries in civilian practice. Surg. Gynecol. Obstet., 144:650, 1962.
258. Donovan, A. J., Turrill, F. L., and Facey, F. L.: Hepatic trauma. Surg. Clin. North Am., 48:1313, 1968.
259. Frey, C. F., Trollope, M., Harpster, W., and Snyder, R.: A fifteen-year experience with automotive hepatic trauma. J. Trauma, 13:1039, 1973.
260. Kindling, P. H., Wilson, R. F., and Walt, A. J.: Hepatic trauma with particular reference to blunt injury. J. Trauma, 9:17, 1969.
261. Lewis, F. R., Lim, R. C., Jr., and Blaisdell, F. W.: Hepatic artery ligation: Adjunct in the management of massive hemorrhage from the liver. J. Trauma, 14:743, 1974.
262. Lim, R. C., Jr., Knudson, J., and Steele, M.: Liver trauma. Current method of management. Arch. Surg., 104:544, 1972.
263. Lucas, C. E., and Walt, A. J.: Critical decisions in liver trauma. Arch. Surg., 101:277, 1970.
264. Madding, G. F., and Kennedy, P. A.: Trauma to the liver, 2nd ed. Philadelphia, W. B. Saunders Company, 1971.
265. Trunkey, D. D., Shires, G. T., and McClelland, R.: Management of liver trauma in 811 consecutive patients. Ann. Surg., 179:722, 1974.
266. Whelan, T. J., and Gillespie, J. T.: Treatment of traumatic hemobilia. Ann. Surg., 162:920, 1965.
267. Wright, P. N., and Orloff, M. J.: Traumatic hemobilia. Ann. Surg., 160:42, 1964.

Echinococcus Cyst

268. Hankins, J. R.: Management of complicated hepatic hydatid cysts. Ann. Surg., 158:1020, 1963.
269. Katz, A. M., and Pan, C.: Echinococcus disease in the United States. Am. J. Med., 25:759, 1958.
270. Lewis, J. W., Koss, N., and Kerstein, M. D.: A review of echinococcal disease. Ann. Surg., 181:390, 1975.

I
PYOGENIC LIVER ABSCESS

Arthur S. McFee, M.D., Ph.D.,
Morris E. Franklin, Jr., M.D.,
and J. Bradley Aust, M.D., Ph.D.

Pyogenic liver abscess has been described in the literature since 1836, when Richard Bright[8] included it in a discussion on jaundice. In 1898, Dieulafoy[13] noted the incidence of liver abscess in association with appendicitis and coined the term "le foie appendiculaire" to denote hepatic abscess following appendicitis, an event with a uniformly fatal outcome. In 1938, an extensive literature review and presentation of collected cases from the Charity Hospital and Touro Infirmary, New Orleans, was made by Ochsner et al.[31] In the intervening years, there have been several more such reviews and collected series published.* No one institution can present a large number of cases from its own files. Many of the clinical aspects of liver abscess have changed markedly or improved in the past four decades; unfortunately, many others have not.

The classic concept of the development of hepatic pyogenic abscess has been direct contamination of the liver by bacteria through any one of several routes:

1. From a source within the biliary tree.

2. From a source within the venous drainage of the portal system.

3. From an outside infectious focus causing blood-borne contamination through the hepatic artery.

4. From an adjacent septic focus such as a subphrenic or perinephric abscess.

5. From a direct injury and contamination of the liver as with a laceration. In a surprisingly high number of patients, the abscess is said to be "cryptogenic," inasmuch as no primary infective focus can be identified.

Since the 1938 report of Ochsner, changes in the disease process have been recorded in bacteriology, etiology, clinical presentation, and, in selected groups, mortality. The changes reflect a wide use of antibiotics, better diagnostic techniques, and a more alert appreciation of incidence. Some other aspects of hepatic pyogenic abscess have remained stable.

INCIDENCE

A true estimate of the incidence of hepatic abscess cannot be made. In autopsy studies dating to 1875, the incidence has remained stable at 0.57 per cent (0.45 to 1.47 per cent).[48] The incidence with regard to numbers of hospital admissions has similarly not changed, ranging from 0.004 to 0.016 per cent.[1, 31, 35, 48] While no significant change has been observed in the last 50 years, some authors speculate that the reported incidence should be higher.

In many early studies, a preponderance of abscesses was noted in the male. More recently, the male:female distribution has become more nearly equal, reflecting the fact that more hepatic abscesses are associated with primary biliary tract disease.[35] There is no identifiable racial predilection for the development of the process.

The age range of patients is broad, from several days to 90 or more years at the extremes. In many series, an increased incidence of abscess and of multiple abscesses is seen at the two extremes.[2] Overall, the age of incidence of hepatic pyogenic abscess has been increasing, and it is now seen most frequently in the sixth and seventh decades.[31, 35]

ETIOLOGY

Bacterial contamination of the liver is the source of development of hepatic pyogenic abscess. The predom-

---

*See references 1, 2, 9–11, 23, 24, 28, 35, 42, 44, and 48.

inant route of contamination has, however, changed. Benign and malignant biliary tract disease and subsequent obstruction of the common bile duct with associated cholangitis have supplanted infection within the portal venous bed as the principal source for hepatic abscess.[9, 11, 31, 35, 48] Specific direct contamination of the liver through rupture or laceration of the organ, hematogenous infection through the hepatic artery, and direct extension of an abscess from a neighboring focus have each contributed a relatively small percentage to the overall incidence of the disease.

An attractive thesis of the pathogenesis of the cryptogenic hepatic abscess for which no prior infective focus can be found was advanced by Lee and Block.[24] Secondary infection of hepatic infarcts based on microthromboembolic processes from the splanchnic venous bed was cited as the source of these abscesses. Experimental and clinical support can be adduced for this theory, but it is not yet widely accepted.

Unquestionably, a change has occurred in the bacterial culture results of abscesses diagnosed or treated. It is likely that this finding does not represent a true alteration in the specific microbiologic etiology of the abscess, but rather a reflection of more fastidious means of culturing samples taken. The freer use of antimicrobial therapy and a more effective host immunomechanism have both been cited as reasons for the observed changes in cultured organisms.[34] In early studies, the commonest organism cultured from pyogenic hepatic abscesses was *Escherichia coli*.[2, 10, 31, 48] With the advent of the use of proper transport media and better culture techniques, anaerobic bacteria are more frequently seen;[5, 23, 45] however, *E. coli* remains the preponderant overall organism. In the last two years, some series have reported only anaerobic organisms in cultures from hepatic abscesses which heretofore would have been labeled sterile.[45] The incidence of sterile abscesses has shown a corresponding decline. Microaerophilic strains of streptococci follow *E. coli* in frequency of cultures; and, indeed, some of the rarer strains of streptococci are now being isolated from these patients.[5, 10]

MORTALITY

Untreated hepatic pyogenic abscess carries a 100 per cent mortality. The death rate is now directly related to the multiplicity of abscesses, the multiplicity of organisms, the age of the patient, and the treatment given. Mortality rates as low as 5 per cent have been reported for single hepatic abscesses containing one kind of bacteria, treated with extensive drainage and appropriate antibiotics.[45] An overall mortality rate of 79.6 per cent was reported in Ochsner's 1938 review.[31] Brodine and Schwartz[9] reported an overall mortality rate of 68.3 per cent in 1973. Pitt and Zuidema[35] in 1975 related mortality principally to the age of the patient and then to multiplicity of abscesses and associated malignant disease. In their series an overall death rate of 65 per cent was partitioned between 57 per cent for patients under the age of 70 and 81 per cent for patients over.

TABLE 25.   Hepatic Pyogenic Abscess: Spectrum of Changes

Review	Publication Date	Average Age of Patients	Number of Patients	Diagnosis	Principal Organisms	Principal Etiology	Treatment	Overall Mortality
Ochsner et al.	1938	4th decade	47 (authors') 518 (collected)	Physical signs; plain chest and abdominal films	*Escherichia coli*; streptococci	Portal suppuration; cryptogenic	Extraserous drainage	79.6%
Sherman and Robbins	1960	61.2 years (17 days to 91 years)	21,945 (autopsy studies) 31 cases	Physical signs	*E. coli; Staphylococcus aureus* (generally resistant to antibacterial agents)	Bilary tract suppuration	Not recorded	Autopsy series
Butler and McCarthy	1969	50% over 60 years	48 (authors')	Physical signs; serum vitamin B_{12} levels	*E. coli*; anaerobic streptococci	Cryptogenic; biliary tract suppuration	Open drainage; antibiotics	53% (100% undrained)
Altemeier et al.	1970	47.2 years (12 days to 90 years); multiple abscesses at extremes	65 (authors')	Isotopic hepatic photoscans; leukocytosis; mild elevation of alkaline phosphatase and BSP	*E. coli*; anaerobic species (last cases all anaerobic organisms)	Biliary tract suppuration	Transabdominal drainage; antibiotics	28% (in most recently treated group)
Lee and Block	1972	36.5 years	36 (authors')	Isotopic hepatic photoscans (mortality decline related to scans said to be 98.6% reliable)	*E. coli*; anaerobic species	Biliary tract suppuration; cryptogenic	Drainage; antibiotics	83% pre-scan; 23% post-scan
Brodine and Schwartz	1973	6th to 8th decades	10 (authors') 200 (collected)	Isotopic hepatic photoscans; ultrasound; angiography	Bacteroides; *E. coli*; streptococci; staphylococci	Biliary tract suppuration; cryptogenic	Percutaneous or transabdominal drainage	68.3%
Pitt and Zuidema	1975	60 years (5 weeks to 92 years)	80 (authors')	Isotopic hepatic photoscans	*E. coli*; anaerobic species	Biliary tract suppuration	Transabdominal exploration	65%

DIAGNOSIS

The diagnosis of pyogenic hepatic abscess can be extremely simple or very complex. It may be suggested from the clinical course of the patient during recovery from an intra-abdominal operation or from the initial clinical symptomatology. The older picture of drenching sweats, a hectic fever, and sepsis, together with right upper quadrant pain and subcostal or intercostal tenderness, is now rarely seen.[34] Clinical presentation may be very obscure and, indeed, an occasional abscess is reported without any significant antecedent symptomatology. Diagnosis occasionally can be determined only by specific related studies or a surgical procedure.

A careful review of the history of recent illnesses, abdominal trauma, recent or distant abdominal operations, ongoing chronic disease, or malignancy may produce some important clues in diagnosing a suspected liver abscess. Similarly, if a patient reports a recent or distant visit to an area of the world where hepatic parasitic disease is endemic, the possibility should be investigated. Ordinarily, one cannot make the diagnosis of liver abscess on history alone.

The physical examination may or may not be helpful. Frequently a temperature elevation is noted, but it is not a universal finding. Temperature may range from 100° F to 108° F, depending on the severity of the abscess and the organisms involved. Other important physical findings include tenderness over the liver, an elevated right hemidiaphragm, atelectasis of the right lung base, and ileus. The gallbladder or liver abscess itself may be palpable; again, this is not a uniform finding. There may be evidence of marked wasting, particularly if the abscess has been present for a prolonged period of time.

Laboratory studies for the most part are not diagnostic but may add important reproducible supporting evidence. Generally, leukocytosis is present and platelet count may be abnormal, either with thrombocytopenia or thrombocytosis. There may be an elevation of the serum glutamic oxaloacetic transaminase and alkaline phosphatase; more frequently, hypoalbuminemia and hypocholesterolemia are noted.[2, 9, 10, 23, 31, 35] Clinical or laboratory evidence of jaundice may be present, but it is an unusual finding. One group of reporters indicated the utility of serum vitamin B_{12} levels as an indication of parenchymal damage.[10] Levels of 2000 to 4000 $\mu\mu$ gm per 100 ml. were noted in 83 per cent of these patients tested and were taken to indicate hepatocellular destruction and release of the compound.

The bacteriologic studies may give a hint to the diagnosis specifically in instances of positive blood cultures. They most commonly reveal fusiform bacteria, microaerophilic streptococci, *Escherichia coli*, enterobacter, or other specific anaerobic organisms. Serum amoebic titers may be positive in instances of amoebic abscesses, but this is not a routine finding. A positive amoebic titer, however, in the presence of an hepatic mass, palpable or found on liver scan, is considered diagnostic for an amoebic abscess.

Plain Radiography

Routine x-rays of the liver, right upper quadrant, chest, and abdomen usually supply only supportive ev-idence or raise the suspicion of an hepatic abscess. Basal atelectasis, elevation of the right hemi-diaphragm, pleural reaction, or the presence of pleural fluid in the costophrenic angle exist as a result of the subdiaphragmatic inflammatory process. On occasion the upright chest films show no lesion at all. Frequently, fluoroscopy of the diaphragm may help in detecting disproportionate movement of the right hemi-diaphragm. Upright abdominal films may show an air-fluid level in the liver itself or displacement of the colon or stomach. The liver may be enlarged. Barium contrast studies can reveal displacement of adjacent hollow viscera and give some clue to the presence and extent of the process.[16, 46]

Liver Scanning

In the face of the multiple diagnostic possibilities for fever of unknown origin, refined examinations of the liver often help in the specific diagnosis of an hepatic abscess. At the present time, the most frequently done and most consistently reliable examination is the liver scan using Technetium-99 sulfur colloid.[2, 12, 22, 26, 41, 46] Many radioactive-tagged substances have been employed for liver scanning, including rose bengal and colloidal gold. The technetium-tagged sulfur colloid has produced the highest degree of accuracy on the scans. Pyogenic hepatic abscess appears as a cold area in the scan. A proper scan includes anterior, oblique, and lateral views in order to determine the exact location and extent of a cold area within the liver substance. Lesions under 2 cm.[2, 45] in diameter rarely appear on liver scanning (Fig. 33).

Ultrasound

The widespread use of liver scanning has been credited by many authors as the direct cause of markedly improved mortality statistics. It must be emphasized that a liver scan can only reveal to the examiner the presence or absence of an area within the liver not capable of picking up the radioactive substance. It does not determine whether this area is an abscess or a metastatic lesion. The differentiation between these two lesions has been attempted with varying success using an ultrasound technique. In general, ultrasound, based on the recording of an echo from a fluid-tissue or fluid-air interface, is felt to be valuable in determining a liquid-filled cold area as opposed to a solid cold spot seen with metastatic disease (Fig. 33).[14, 29, 40]

Angiography

Arteriography through hepatic artery cannulation has also helped differentiation between metastatic lesions and liver abscesses. The abscess itself is avascular, with a rim of tissue made up of fairly dense blood vessels.[30, 41, 46] Metastatic lesions tend to have decreased blood supply within the lesions themselves, reflecting central tumor necrosis.

Venography as a diagnostic aid in determining the nature of the space-occupying lesion in the liver has been minimally useful.[10, 42] It has been stated that this technique can be employed particularly with posterior lesions when there is access to the portal system. Portal venography can delineate the size and number of space-occupying lesions in the liver. Reliability and

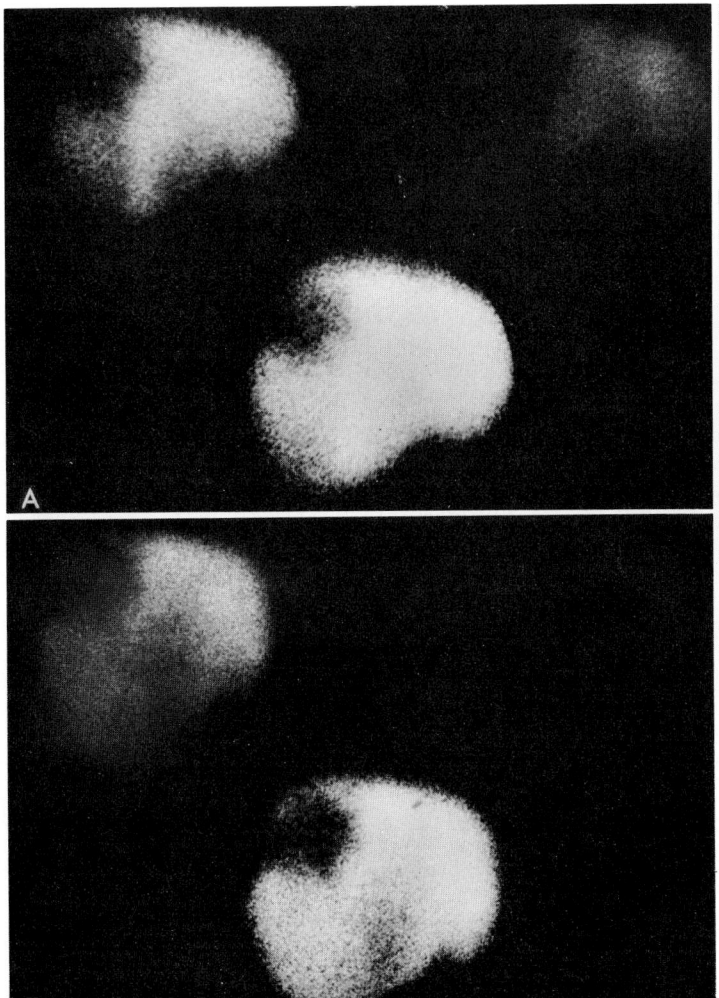

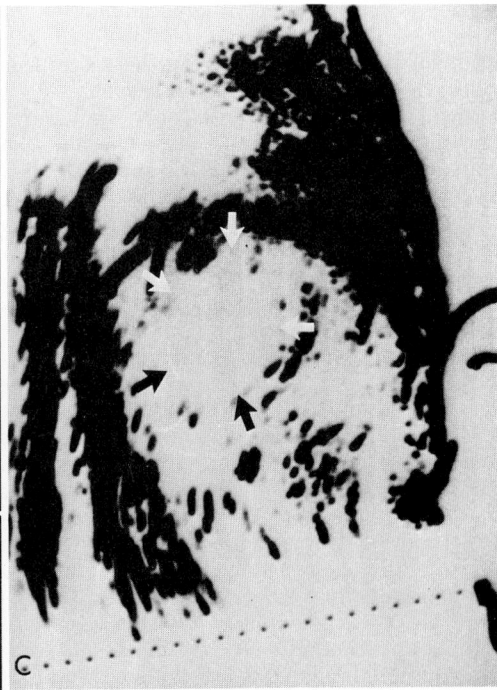

Figure 33. *A*, Patient D. M. (Bexar County Hospital). This patient sustained a gunshot wound through the lung and the right lobe of the liver on 3/18/76. On 3/25/76, the RAO (right anterior oblique) projection of the ⁹⁹Tc liver scan reveals a right lobar defect consistent with the wound sustained seven days previously. *B*, The same patient: The RAO projection of the ⁹⁹Tc liver scan on 4/2/76 shows a marked enlargement of the defect seen earlier. *C*, The same patient: The ultrasound scan in a sagittal plane 6 cm. to the right of the midline reveals a cystic area (arrows) denoted by the lack of the normal echoic pattern from liver substance. This study was done on 4/1/76. A large quantity of infected hematoma fluid was drained on 4/2/76.

diagnostic accuracy of the technique are, however, not consistent.

Cholangiography, either intravenously, through a T-tube, percutaneously, or as a retrograde study through duodenal cannulation, many times can reveal a large intrahepatic cavity or solid mass outlined by displaced biliary radicals. The technique is not diagnostic but may aid in the localization of a lesion.[2, 35]

Frequently the diagnosis of a liver abscess cannot be made with any of these techniques, and exploration of the liver must be carried out. At exploration, a single abscess may be palpated or multiple small abscesses may be noted. Cholangiography at the operating table may aid in the localization of an abscess. The presence of multiple small abscesses presents the most difficult problem in regard to specific diagnostic techniques. A blind needle biopsy of the liver and blind needle probings have, on occasion, both proved helpful in the identification and localization of abscesses. In general, however, these procedures are not recommended.

At the present time, the cornerstone of the diagnosis of pyogenic hepatic abscess is the hepatic scan. Confirmatory studies may include examinations of the

serum, the plain roentgenogram, ultrasound examinations, and cannulation of hepatic artery, portal vein, or biliary ducts.

TREATMENT

The sine qua non of treatment for pyogenic liver abscess is adequate surgical drainage combined with use of long-term systemic antimicrobial agents chosen through appropriate culture and sensitivity testing. A number of specific operative approaches have been entertained.

An extraserous approach to the liver avoiding the general peritoneal cavity has been advocated since Ochsner's review.[31] Its use is based on the fact that the abscess frequently causes adhesion between the surface of the liver and the overlying parietal peritoneum. If an abscess can be accurately localized preoperatively and identified as a single lesion, this approach may be employed without the risk of further contaminating the peritoneal cavity. Use of the extraserous approach is largely limited to single abscesses of the posterior right lobe, which may be drained through an incision in the bed of the twelfth rib or the very rare single anterior abscess which has formed a strong adhesion with the adjacent parietal peritoneum.[15] Extraserous drainage has been associated with excellent results in many series where it has been reported.

Most authors currently favor a transperitoneal exploration of the liver for a number of reasons.[2, 15, 17] Hepatic abscesses frequently are not solitary, and secondary or tertiary abscesses cannot be drained easily through an extraserous approach. A multiloculated abscess requires division of intracavitary septa, which is facilitated by the widest approach to the liver possible. The patient in whom multiple small hepatic abscesses are suspected is similarly not a candidate for a localized drainage procedure. In all these instances, complete exposure of the liver is a necessary condition for treatment. Proper use of antibiotics, aspiration of the abscess with a needle once it has been localized, and careful packing of abdominal contents away from the operative field have all allowed the routine use of the transperitoneal approach with a minimum risk to the patient of additional contamination. A transperitoneal approach is regarded now as the procedure of choice for draining these abscesses.

In the patient with the multiloculated large abscess, a transperitoneal approach allows the operator an opportunity to identify the abscess and manually to break the septa within the cavity.[17] Several techniques are described. For the abscess deep within the hepatic substance a bimanual examination of the liver may be required for its identification. If the divisions are not broken, a residual pocket can act as a retained untreated abscess and result in a poor result for the incompletely drained patient.

At least one review and other case reports have been presented advocating the use of systemic antibiotic therapy and percutaneous needle or trocar drainage of hepatic pyogenic abscesses.[10, 28, 30, 50] Other authors have not been equally successful using this regimen. Theoretically, contamination along the needle or trocar tract should occur; but it has not appeared to be a significant factor in the hands of proponents of the technique. Additionally, however, material contained within an hepatic abscess may have a wide range of consistencies. It is sometimes necessary to introduce a large drain through a trocar tract to aspirate thick pus contained within a cavity.[50] In this particular adaptation, irrigation is maintained for several days or until the irrigant fluid returns without purulent characteristics.[17]

No good treatment exists for the patient with multiple small hepatic pyogenic abscesses. They are more frequently seen at the extremes of the age spectrum and are not amenable to operative drainage.

Many techniques of actual drainage of the cavity have been described, ranging from the placement of large numbers of Penrose drains to the use of soft large sump tubes maintained on suction or continuously irrigated. As long as adequate dependent drainage is instituted, the choice of technique is not pertinent.

The use of systemic antimicrobial agents in these patients is mandatory. The choice of agent should be dictated by the culture and sensitivity results from material aspirated from the abscess itself. Long-term treatment should be anticipated, and therapy ought to be maintained until an insignificant cavity or complete healing can be demonstrated. In the absence of appropriate culture results, more recent studies indicate that treatment ought to be directed toward the anaerobic spectrum of microbial organisms.

SELECTED REFERENCES

Altemeier, W. A., Schowengerdt, C. G., and Whitely, D. H.: Abscesses of the liver: Surgical considerations. Arch. Surg., 101:258, 1970.
From a group long interested in surgical bacteriologic disease, this article details experience over 15 years with pyogenic abscess of the liver at a major medical center in the United States. The patients are logically divided into three groups reflecting changing diagnostic and therapeutic techniques. A marked change in mortality was seen as diagnostic accuracy increased. Transabdominal exploration of the liver is felt to be the cornerstone of appropriate operative therapy.

Lee, J. F., and Block, G. E.: The changing clinical pattern of hepatic abscesses. Arch. Surg., 104:465, 1972.
Of particular interest in this review is a statement of the authors explaining the etiology and pathogenesis of the "cryptogenic" hepatic abscess. Microembolic phenomena, resulting in multiple microscopic infarctions in the liver subject to postoperative secondary infection, are felt to be the source of this somewhat puzzling phenomenon.

Ochsner, A., DeBakey, M., and Murray, S.: Pyogenic abscess of the liver. Am. J. Surg., 40:292, 1938.
This is a classic study from which much of the work describing the pathogenesis and treatment of hepatic pyogenic abscess in the United States can be dated. It is one of the series of extensive review articles carried out by these authors in the late 1930s and early 1940s and is an exhaustive statement of the knowledge concerning pyogenic hepatic abscess at that time.

Pitt, H. A., and Zuidema, G. D.: Factors influencing mortality in the treatment of pyogenic hepatic abscess. Surg. Gynecol. Obstet., 140:228, 1975.
The authors, in an extremely well-written article, demonstrate that almost 40 years after the exhaustive review of Ochsner and DeBakey, there has been no significant change in the incidence, age, race, location, number of abscesses, symptoms, physical findings, laboratory data, or routine roentgenograms of patients with hepatic pyogenic abscesses. They were able to show that relatively more women were developing hepatic abscesses and that the cause of the abscesses had shifted specifically from appendicitis as the principal etiologic factor to biliary suppuration. Escherichia coli remained the most commonly isolated single organism. A significant increase in the number of gram-negative organisms isolated from these abscesses was also shown. Factors associated with a poor prognosis were identified by the authors; and a significant mortality associated with the increased age of the patient was noted. Unfortunately, the authors were unable to demonstrate an overall decreased mortality in their series.

Sanders, R. C.: Radiological and radioisotopic diagnosis of perihepatic abscess. CRC Crit. Rev. Clin. Radiol. Nucl. Med., 5:165, 1974.
An exhaustive review article describing virtually every radiologic and ultrasound technique available currently is presented. There are excellent diagrams of the anatomy of the liver and the perihepatic spaces. The diagrams are related to ultrasonographic and scan images. An extensive bibliography is appended.

REFERENCES

1. Abbruzzese, A. A., and Khaja, N.: Pyogenic abscess of the liver. Am. J. Gastroenterol., 58:288, 1972.
2. Altemeier, W. A., Schowengerdt, C. G., and Whiteley, D. H.: Abscesses of the liver: Surgical considerations. Arch. Surg., 101:258, 1970.
3. Andrews, J. T., Steven, L. W., Arkles, L. B., Sephton, R. G., and

Martin, J. J.: Reticulo-endothelial and blood-pool scanning in the diagnosis and differentiation of space-occupying lesions of the liver. Aust. N. Z. J. Surg., 43:14, 1973.

4. Bahk, Y. W.: Half-clearance time of Au colloid as a discriminant of liver abscess and malignancy. Br. J. Radiology, 47:857, 1974.

5. Bateman, N. T., Eykyn, S. J., and Phillips, I.: Pyogenic liver abscess caused by streptococcus milleri. Lancet, 1:657, 1975.

6. Block, M. A.: Surgery of liver abscesses. Arch. Surg., 88:602, 1964.

7. Bockus, H. L.: Gastroenterology. Philadelphia, W. B. Saunders Company, 1975.

8. Bright, R.: Observations on jaundice. Guys Hosp. Rep., 1:630, 1836.

9. Brodine, W. N., and Schwartz, S. I.: Pyogenic hepatic abscess. N.Y. State J. Med., 73:1657, 1973.

10. Butler, T. J., and McCarthy, C. F.: Pyogenic liver abscess. Gut, 10:389, 1969.

11. de la Maza, L. M., Naeim, F., and Berman, L. D.: The changing etiology of liver abscess. Further observations. J.A.M.A., 227:161, 1974.

12. DeNardo, G. L., Stadainik, R. C., DeNardo, S. J., and Raventos, A.: Hepatic scintiangiographic patterns. Radiology, 111:135, 1974.

13. Dieulafoy: Le foie appendiculaire: Abcès du foie consecutifs à l'appendicite. Sem. Med. (Paris), 18:449, 1898.

14. Friday, R. O., Barriga, P., and Crummy, A. B.: Detection and localization of intra-abdominal abscesses by diagnostic ultrasound. Arch. Surg., 110:335, 1975.

15. Gaisford, W. D., and Mark, J. B. D.: Surgical management of hepatic abscess. Am. J. Surg., 118:317, 1969.

16. Gelfand, D. W.: The liver: Plain film diagnosis. Sem. Roentgenol., 10:177, 1975.

17. Goldsmith, H. S., and Chen, W.: Management of a pyogenic abscess of the liver. Surg. Clin. North Am., 53:711, 1973.

18. Gottschalk, A.: Liver scanning. J.A.M.A., 200:630, 1967.

19. Grant, R. N., Morgan, L. R., and Cohen, A.: Hepatic abscesses. Am. J. Surg., 118:15, 1969.

20. Hupe, C., Maroske, D., Nitschke, J., Stender, M., Dombrowski, H., and Joseph, K.: Diagnostik und therapie umschriebener lebererkrankungen. Bruns. Beitr. Klin. Chir., 219:289, 1972.

21. Johnston, G. S., and Jones, A. E.: Sequential liver scanning. J. Surg. Oncol., 1:205, 1969.

22. Kaude, J. V., and DeLand, F.: Hepatomegaly. Med. Clin. North Am., 59:145, 1975.

23. Lazarchick, J., deSouza e Silva, N. A., Nichols, D. R., and Washington, J. A., II: Pyogenic liver abscess. Mayo Clin. Proc., 48:349, 1973.

24. Lee, J. F., and Block, G. E.: The changing clinical pattern of hepatic abscesses. Arch. Surg., 104:465, 1972.

25. Longmire, W. P.: Hepatic surgery: Trauma, tumors and cysts. Ann. Surg., 161:1, 1965.

26. McConnell, V. A., Saunders, S. J., Werner, I. D., LeRoux, P. L. M., and Weir, H.: Liver scanning, with special reference to 99mTechnetium. S. Afr. Med. J., 42:1259, 1968.

27. McCort, J. J.: Acute hepatobiliary disease. Sem. Roentgenol. 8:389, 1973.

28. McFadzean, A. J. S., Chang, K. P. S., and Wong, C. C.: Solitary pyogenic abscess of the liver treated by closed aspiration and antibiotics. Br. J. Surg., 41:141, 1953.

29. Monroe, L. S., Leopold, G. R., Brown, J. W., and Smith, J. L.: The ultrasonic scan in the management of amebic hepatic abscess. Dig. Dis., 16:523, 1971.

30. Novy, S. B., Wallace, S., Goldman, A. M., and Ben-Menachem, Y.: Pyogenic liver abscess: Angiographic diagnosis and treatment by closed aspiration. Am. J. Roentgenol., 121:388, 1974.

31. Ochsner, A., DeBakey, M., and Murray, S.: Pyogenic abscess of the liver. Am. J. Surg., 40:292, 1938.

32. Ostermiller, W., Jr., and Carter, R.: Hepatic abscess. Arch. Surg., 94:353, 1967.

33. Pai, S. T., and Bakk, Y. W.: Radioisotope scanning in the diagnosis of liver abscess. Am. J. Surg., 119:330, 1970.

34. Palmer, E. D.: The changing manifestations of pyogenic liver abscess. J.A.M.A., 231:2:192, 1975.

35. Pitt, H. A., and Zuidema, G. D.: Factors influencing mortality in the treatment of pyogenic hepatic abscess. Surg. Gynecol. Obstet., 140:228, 1975.

36. Powell, S. J.: The treatment of intestinal and hepatic amoebiasis. S. Afr. Med. J., 47:452, 1973.

37. Pyrtek, L. J., and Bartus, S. A.: Hepatic pyemia. N. Engl. J. Med., 272:551, 1965.

38. Ramanathan, P., Ganatra, R. D., and Blau, M.: Dynamic blood flow studies of space-occupying lesions in the liver. J. Nucl. Med., 15:1021, 1974.

39. Rambo, W. M., and Black, H. C.: Intrahepatic abscess. Am. Surg., 35:144, 1969.

40. Rasmussen, S. N., Holm, H. H., Kristensen, J. D., Pedersen, J. F., and Hancke, S.: Ultrasound in the diagnosis of liver disease. J. Clin. Ultrasound, 1:220, 1973.

41. Ranson, J. H. C., Madayag, M. A., Localio, S. A., and Spencer, F. C.: New diagnostic and therapeutic techniques in the management of pyogenic liver abscesses. Ann. Surg., 181:508, 1975.

42. Ribaudo, J. M., and Ochsner, A.: Intrahepatic abscesses: Amebic and pyogenic. Am. J. Surg., 125:570, 1973.

43. Ross, F. G. M.: Ultrasound in the diagnosis of liver disease. Proc. R. Soc. Med., 67:211, 1974.

44. Rubin, R. H., Swartz, M. N., and Malt, R.: Hepatic abscess: Changes in clinical, bacteriologic and therapeutic aspects. Am. J. Med., 57:601, 1974.

45. Sabbaj, J., Sutter, V. L., and Finegold, S. M.: Anaerobic pyogenic liver abscess. Ann. Intern. Med., 77:629, 1972.

46. Sanders, R. C.: Radiologic and radioisotopic diagnosis of perihepatic abscess. CRC Crit. Rev. Clin. Radiol. Nucl. Med., 5:165, 1974.

47. Schiff, L.: Diseases of the Liver, 4th ed. Philadelphia, J. B. Lippincott Company, 1975.

48. Sherman, J. D., and Robbins, S. L.: Changing trends in the casuistics of hepatic abscess. Am. J. Med., 28:943, 1960.

49. Stanford, W., and Nielson, A. A.: The use of the liver scan in the treatment of hepatic abscess. Milit. Med., 134:43, 1969.

50. Tetz, E. M., Reeves, C. D., and Longerbeam, J. K.: Treatment of liver abscesses. Am. J. Surg., 126:263, 1973.

51. Todd, D. W.: Pyogenic liver abscess: A case report. Milit. Med., 136:154, 1971.

52. Top, S. F., Jr., and Wehrle, P. F.: Communicable and Infectious Disease. St. Louis, The C. V. Mosby Co., 1972.

53. Yeh, S. H., Shih, W. J., and Liang, J. C.: Intravenous radionuclide hepatography in the differential diagnosis of intrahepatic mass lesions. J. Nucl. Med., 14:565, 1973.

II

AMEBIC ABSCESS OF THE LIVER

Leonard Rosoff, Sr., M.D.

Amebic abscess of the liver frequently presents with the clinical manifestations of an acute abdominal catastrophy requiring an emergency operation. This may be avoided and complications of the lesion aborted by early suspicion of the diagnosis and prompt institution of appropriate therapy. If an amebic abscess of the liver is first observed at celiotomy, prompt recognition and appropriate treatment will have a salutary effect on the significant morbidity and mortality associated with this lesion.

HISTORICAL ASPECTS

Abscesses of the liver associated with dysenteric disorders are described in the earliest medical records. According to Kean,[24] James Bontius, in 1629, possibly attempting to differentiate bacillary from amebic dysentery, wrote that "the hepatic flux of the belly, though no less dangerous than the dysentery, is however not attended with symptoms equally severe: there never having been an excoriation of the intestines nearly as considerably and sometimes none at all."[3] In this textbook, Bontius also described in detail the technique of draining a liver abscess.

Although observation of amebae in the feces of man had been described in 1860 by Lambl,[31] the first description of *Entamoeba histolytica* is ascribed to Losch, of St. Petersburg, Russia, in 1875.[33] In a classical historical review, Wilmot[63] indicates that Losch not only gave an excellent description of amebae in the stools of a patient with severe dysentery, but also established amebae as the causative organisms by administering fecal material orally and rectally to dogs, producing dysentery and evidence of amebae in the stools of the experimental animals. In 1882, Koch[29] demonstrated the pathogenic relationship of amebae to tropical dysentery and two years later described amebae in the wall of a liver abscess.[63] Kartulis[22] in 1886 identified amebae in the pus from liver abscesses as well as in the stools of patients with dysentery. In 1891, Councilman and Lafleur[9] gave a detailed and classic description of the clinical and pathologic features of amebiasis, using the terms *amebic dysentery* and *amebic abscess of the liver.* Faust[13] credits Strong for differentiating the pathogenic *E. histolytica* from the common and harmless *Escherichia coli* in 1901,[57] also asserted by Schaudinn in 1903.[53]

Much of our present understanding of the etiology, diagnosis, and treatment of amebic liver abscess is based on the work of Sir Leonard Rogers, initiated at the beginning of the twentieth century and summarized in his monumental report, the *Lettsomian Lecture,* delivered before the Medical Society of London in 1922.[49]

INCIDENCE

The protozoan parasite *Entamoeba histolytica* is frequently found in the human intestine of peoples throughout the world. Although it is hyperendemic in tropical regions, surveys have disclosed that a significant percentage of the world's population harbors the parasite, which has been found in native populations of virtually all parts of the world from the Arctic to the Antarctic circles.[13]

Although the incidence of infestation with *E. histolytica* is extremely high in tropical zones, estimates of the incidence in temperate zones vary from 10 to 20 per cent. Sanford[51] in 1916 reported that in a study of 5000 patients at the Mayo Clinic, 10 per cent of the patients from northern United States and Canada had evidence of infection with *E. histolytica,* with an overall incidence of 18 per cent. In 1951, Craig and Faust[10] summarized the results of surveys of different groups of the population in various geographic areas of the United States. The incidence of *E. histolytica* infections varied from 1.4 per cent in New England college students to 36.4 per cent in rural Tennessee and from 40 to 55 per cent in charity institutions. The average incidence was 8.1 per cent. As these figures were for the most part based on a single examination, they suggested the probability of twice this incidence if multiple examinations had been done, and an overall incidence of 20 per cent or greater in the United States.

Epidemics of amebic dysentery have occurred in temperate zones as a result of contaminated water supplies. Over 900 cases of amebic dysentery with 52 deaths occurred in the United States in 1933, all traced to a contaminated water supply in a Chicago hotel.[5]

Current figures of the incidence of amebiasis in the United States are unavailable. Figures from the Center for Disease Control in Atlanta, Georgia,[7] indicate that there were 1.3 cases of amebiasis reported per 100,000 population in 1975. Obviously this does not include the vast group of "carriers," nor even all patients with symptomatic amebiasis in this country who are not reported. The incidence in the United States is higher in areas in which there is significant migration from hyperendemic areas, and it is increasing yearly, as indicated in Table 26.

The incidence of amebiasis is much greater in areas of poor sanitation, and the frequency with which amebic dysentery and amebic abscess of the liver are encountered in such areas, especially in hot, humid climes gave rise to the names "tropical dysentery" and "tropical abscess." However, these are encountered with increasing frequency in the United States and other temperate zones because of introduction and spread of the disease as a result of the significant migration of permanent residents of hyperendemic

TABLE 26. Cases of Amebiasis Reported to the Community Health Services in the County of Los Angeles during a Period of 10 Years

Year	Cases	Year	Cases
1966	96	1971	244
1967	121	1972	160
1968	140	1973	172
1969	127	1974	279
1970	197	1975	461

areas and the marked increase of travel to and from such areas by civilian visitors and military personnel.

There is no substantive evidence that there is a difference in racial susceptibility to amebiasis, and it is the consensus that the variations reported in different racial groups permanently residing in various countries are essentially due to socioeconomic factors affecting water pollution, contamination of food, other problems of sanitation, and, possibly, the state of nutrition.

The actual incidence of liver involvement in patients with intestinal amebiasis is difficult to ascertain. Reported figures vary greatly. Payne[45] reported an incidence of 2.8 per cent of hepatic abscess in his review of 1000 cases of amebiasis, but in his report indicated a 50 per cent incidence of "mild amebic hepatitis," plus a 3.9 per cent incidence of "acute amebic hepatitis." It is extremely likely that the latter two entities represented multiple small areas of necrosis or miliary abscesses of the liver, which responded to treatment before a large single abscess or large multiple abscesses developed. The actual incidence then would be 56.7 per cent, which is considerably higher than that of most other reported series.

In a collective review of 6886 cases of hepatic amebiasis by DeBakey and Ochsner[11] in 1951, the incidence of hepatic abscess in clinical cases was found to range from less than 1 per cent to more than 25 per cent, with an average incidence of 13.2 per cent. This closely approached the incidence of 11.1 per cent of hepatic involvement in their own series of cases. The incidence of hepatic involvement established by postmortem examination in the collected series averaged 36.6 per cent, with wide variation depending on the stage of the disease at which treatment was started and the general characteristics of the population from which the reports originated.

Amebic abscess of the liver is encountered predominantly in the third, fourth, and fifth decades; however, it may occur in infants and children, as well as in the elderly. For some reason not yet explained, amebic abscess of the liver occurs more frequently in males than in females, with a ratio of approximately 10:1 or greater, in almost all reported series from various parts of the world. It has been suggested that an endocrine factor may be the cause, because in series of cases of amebic abscess of the liver in prepubertal children there is an equal incidence in males and females.[4]

PATHOGENESIS

The life cycle of *E. histolytica* consists of trophozoite, precystic, cystic, and metacystic stages. Cysts are passed in the stools of the host and may survive for prolonged periods in moist surroundings. Cysts ingested with fecally contaminated water and food transmit the infection to the new host. The actively motile trophozoites are released from the cysts during passage through the distal small intestine and large bowel, where they survive and multiply by feeding on bacteria and other bowel contents (Fig. 34). Lesions in man are caused by the trophozoites, apparently the only form of the parasite found in the tissues. The exact mode of entry into the tissues by the trophozoites remains in dispute, and it is not known definitely whether a small area of disruption of the mucosa of the bowel is a prerequisite to invasion by the amebae. Cytolytic enzyme production, mechanical extension by pseudopodia, or both, have been suggested as the mechanisms of penetration of the colonic mucosa. Although various enzymes have been identified with amebae, a specific cytolytic enzyme or enzymes have not yet been demonstrated. A gelatinase, glutaminase, and casease have been described, but no protease capable of acting on undenatured protease. A hyaluronidase has been identified, which may be the

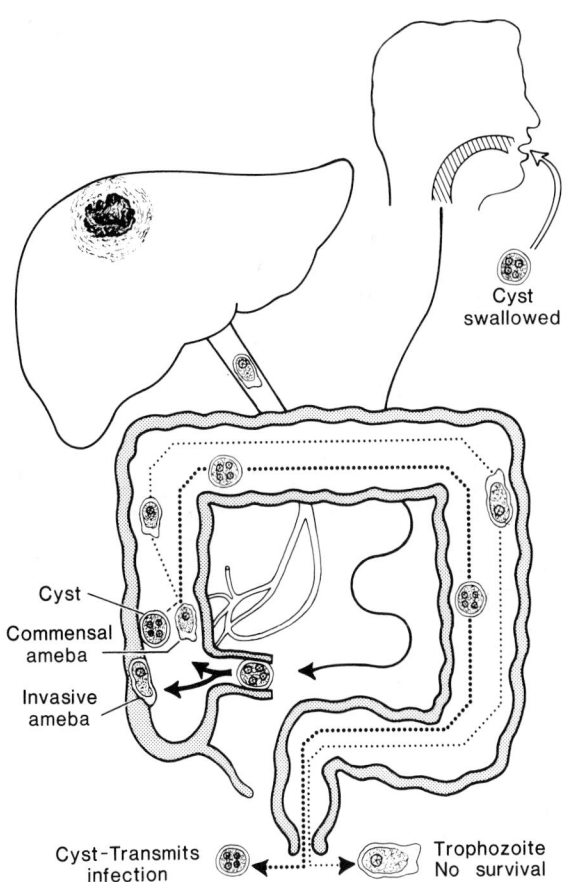

Figure 34. Diagram of colonization of the human host by *Entamoeba histolytica*.

source of the general enzymatic activity of the parasite.[4]

It is currently widely accepted that trophozoites may live commensally in the lumen of the bowel, without invading tissue or producing symptoms. Commensal amebae are usually smaller in size than trophozoites invading tissues. The increased size is attributed to ingested red blood cells. Trophozoites do not transmit the disease, as they do not survive when extruded in feces or other exudates.

PATHOLOGY

The most common site of metastatic amebiasis in man is the liver. The abscess usually is located in the dome or near the inferior surface of the right lobe, which is involved much more frequently than the left, with a ratio of approximately 10:1.

Amebae have been identified in capillaries in the gut and in thrombi in small interlobular branches of the portal vein. It is generally accepted that amebae reach the liver by the portal bloodstream from an ulcerated lesion in the bowel wall, rather than by the lymphatics or by traversing the peritoneal cavity. Amebae reaching the liver undergo degeneration in the interlobular veins and usually do not survive. If they survived, one would expect multiple hepatic lesions in the majority of patients suffering from ulcerative intestinal amebiasis, and the reverse is the case. Tissue sensitization may affect survival of the amebae in the liver. Malgraith and Harinasuta[35] demonstrated that amebae injected into the portal vein in guinea pigs do not usually produce hepatic abscesses unless the animals have a persistent or chronic intestinal infection or have been previously sensitized by injection of specially prepared amebic antigens.

As the result of lytic action of the amebae at the site of the thrombotic occlusion of the small intrahepatic branches of the portal veins, necrosis of the wall of the veins occurs and some of the amebae migrate into the periportal sinusoids, with subsequent lysis and liquefaction of small areas of liver tissue. In the early stages, a single site or numerous sites may be involved.[4, 6, 43] The clinically characteristic large single abscess (Fig. 35) results from the coalescence of multiple small areas of necrosis associated with infarction due to thrombosis of contiguous portal radicals. In series based on postmortem examination, however, multiple abscesses are found in approximately one third of the cases.[11] This may be an indication of an advanced stage of the disease in fatal cases.

An amebic abscess of the liver is usually a large spherical lesion with a very thin wall of granulation tissue only a few millimeters thick, and with little if any fibrosis. On microscopic examination, the lesion is composed of granular and eosinophilic necrotic material with much nuclear debris. Amebae are rarely seen in the center of the necrotic material but are found at the periphery. There is an abrupt transition from necrotic hepatic cells to hepatic tissue essentially normal in appearance without evidence of amebae or cellular infiltration.[4, 44] The absence of polymorphonuclear leukocytes is striking and at variance with the

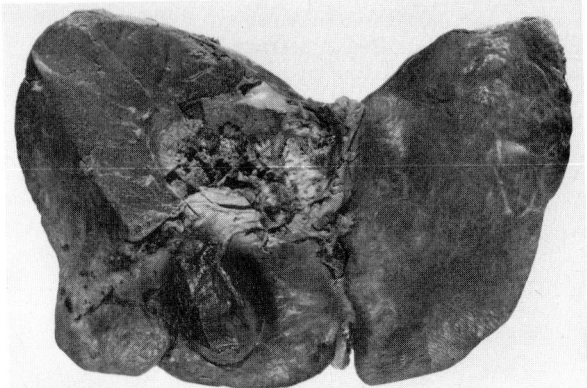

Figure 35. Characteristic appearance at postmortem examination of a large solitary amebic abscess of the liver.

commonly accepted histologic description of an abscess. For this reason some authors question the identification of this lesion as a true abscess[6] and have suggested the phrase "amebic necrosis of the liver."[4] Although there is no inflammatory reaction in early lesions, as the necrosis becomes extensive, infiltration with large numbers of neutrophilic leukocytes may occur, possibly in response to the necrotic tissue.[6]

As a result of the minimal inflammatory response and fibrotic reaction to amebae in tissues, amebic lesions heal with little or no scarring. Even extremely large abscesses of the liver, which respond to amebicidal therapy, heal by regeneration of liver tissue, frequently with little or no significant scarring and with no evidence of functional disturbances of the liver.

The abscess cavity contains liquefied and necrotic liver cells in addition to crenated and intact red blood cells. Polymorphonuclear leukocytes are frequently present. Amebae may be found in the fluid, but this occurs in less than one third of the cases. This material is usually thick and gelatinous and frequently pinkish to reddish-brown in color. According to Paul,[44] the reddish-brown color is essentially due to red blood cells, which can be identified in the contents, as a result of hemorrhage in the margins of the abscess, and not due to the lysis of liver cells, as "a liver drained of blood is white, not brown." Although such material, having the appearance of "anchovy paste" or "chocolate sauce," is considered to be characteristic of amebic abscess of the liver, there is a significant variation in the color and consistency of the contents. The color may be yellow, green, or white, and the consistency may vary from a very thin fluid to a thick, gelatinous material. In the series reported by Berne,[2] the abscess contents in one third of the cases were creamy, white fluid with no evidence of secondary infection.

Characteristically, amebic pus is bacteriologically sterile, and it is exceptionally rare to find bacteria in the original contents of the abscess. Infection is usually secondary to open drainage or aspiration. In extremely rare instances, bacteria may be found in the pus at the time of initial aspiration. In such cases, it is possible that the bacteria have entered the abscess via the portal bloodstream from ulcerations in the colon. It has been postulated also that the trophozoites, which contain colonic bacteria, carry such bacteria to the liver where they are usually destroyed, but in rare instances may persist to produce secondary infection.

There is considerable controversy regarding the existence of amebic hepatitis consisting of a diffuse inflammation due to colonization of the liver with amebae as a presuppurative lesion.[13] Some use the term to describe the stage of abscess formation in which there are small areas of infarction and necrosis of liver cells as the result of intrahepatic portal thrombosis by amebae without actual abscess formation.[11, 43] Amebic hepatitis has been described as the sudden appearance of hepatomegaly associated with tenderness and fever in patients with intestinal amebiasis and the decrease in size and tenderness of such livers in response to amebicidal therapy, frequently luminal amebicides, which are otherwise ineffective in the treatment of liver abscess. In some series, amebic hepatitis has been reported to be present in 50 per cent of patients with intestinal amebiasis.

Except for a single report of the presence of amebae in liver biopsy material obtained from a case of "chronic diffuse nonsuppurative hepatitis,"[12] amebae have not been identified in livers of this description in specimens obtained by liver biopsy or postmortem examination.

Parenchymal changes not detected with light microscopy have been reported with electron microscopy in liver biopsies of patients with intestinal amebiasis,[58] and Kean[23, 24] suggests that possibly tender hepatomegaly accompanying symptomatic intestinal amebiasis may be due to the presence of bacteria and the products of destruction of tissue secondary to the ulcerative processes in the large bowel. Others believe that it is more likely due to one or many small intrahepatic abscesses.

It is currently the consensus that diffuse amebic hepatitis cannot be accepted as a definite pathologic entity and that "the only proved amebic lesion of the liver is the abscess."[24] A tender, enlarged liver in a patient in whom amebiasis is suspected should be considered to be the seat of an abscess and treated accordingly.

CLINICAL MANIFESTATIONS

The onset of symptoms of amebic abscess of the liver may be sudden or insidious, with considerable variation in the intensity, duration, and manifestations of the disease process. In some instances the illness is acute and of less than a week's duration, and, in others, symptoms may be present for several months preceding the diagnosis. Although the liver abscess is always secondary to intestinal amebiasis, the diagnosis frequently has to be made without evidence of the primary disease process. It is unusual to have coexisting amebic dysentery in its usual connotation, and even diarrhea is not frequently encountered concurrently or by history. Cysts or trophozoites are demonstrated in the stools in less than 15 per cent of cases.

The clinical manifestations of amebic abscess of the

liver are related to the site of the abscess in the liver and duration of the disease.

Continuous *pain* in the hypochondriac and epigastric regions is the single most common and striking symptom and is present in approximately 90 per cent of patients. In over 75 per cent of patients, the pain is in the right hypochondrium, owing to the frequency with which the abscess involves the dome of the right lobe of the liver. The pain in the hypochondrium may appear to be essentially pulmonary in nature and related to respiration rather than a manifestation of intra-abdominal disease, which is usually associated with an abscess in the inferior portion of the lobe.

The pain may be severe and made worse by movement, percussion, or respiration. Pain may be present in the right shoulder top and right side of the neck with or without pain in the hypochrondriac region. An abscess involving the left lobe tends to produce pain most frequently in the epigastrium or to the left of the xiphoid, and, on occasion, in the left hypochondrium. Left shoulder top pain may be associated with a left lobe abscess.

Cough, usually nonproductive, is a common symptom and found in approximately 50 per cent of patients with liver abscess. It is not necessarily indicative of rupture of a liver abscess into the pleural cavity or lung, and may be the result of a transdiaphragmatic inflammatory reaction.

Fever, usually sustained and up to 104°F (40° C), is commonly present, although reported to be absent in 10 to 25 per cent of patients in some series. *Chills* may be a predominant finding in acute cases of considerable severity, and suggestive of pyelonephritis or malaria. In chronic cases, *night sweats* are frequent and chills rarely encountered. Nausea and vomiting occur in about 15 per cent of patients. With a gradual onset of symptoms, loss of weight and weakness become prominent symptoms.

The most commonly encountered and important physical finding is tenderness to palpation over the liver, which is palpable abdominally in over 50 per cent of patients.[8] Intercostal tenderness is one of the cardinal signs of hepatic abscess. Careful and gentle palpation with the tips of the fingers between the ribs in the lateral chest wall overlying the liver and, if necessary, more firm pressure with the ulnar aspect of the hand, discloses this important finding. This is also an important factor in determining the most suitable site for aspiration when necessary.

Some patients may present with a visible or palpable mass, usually in the right subcostal or epigastric area, or, occasionally, as a bulge over the ribs in the lateral chest wall. Such masses are tender and may be firm to palpation, or, if seen late, fluctuant.

In over 50 per cent of cases of amebic abscess of the right lobe of the liver, changes are produced at the base of the right lung apart from the findings due to rupture of the abscess through the diaphragm. These findings are due primarily to elevation and immobility of the diaphragm and compression of the lower lobe of the lung, and manifest by dullness on percussion, diminished breath sounds and rales at the right base. Less commonly, a pleural friction rub may be heard.

Although infrequent, jaundice may be present as a

result of obstruction of the porta hepatis by a large centrally and inferiorly located abscess.[8] In acute cases, suppurative cholangitis is usually suspected if the patient is jaundiced.

On the basis of the variation in duration of symptoms and clinical manifestations, Berne[2] in 1942 described four clinical syndromes associated with amebic abscess of the right lobe of the liver.

The *acute costal margin syndrome* is frequently misdiagnosed as acute cholecystitis, perforated peptic ulcer, or acute alcoholic hepatitis. The *chronic costal margin syndrome* must be differentiated from malignancy of the liver, biliary tract, colon, or stomach, as well as ecchinococcus cyst of the liver, cirrhosis, and pancreatic pseudocyst. The *acute pulmonary syndrome* may be mistaken for primary pneumonitis, acute pleurisy with effusion, or empyema, and the *chronic pulmonary syndrome* may simulate chronic lung disease, malignancy, or tuberculosis. Findings of the pulmonary and costal syndromes frequently coexist.

Involvement of the left lobe of the liver, which also may be acute or chronic, is usually manifest by symptoms and signs in the epigastrium. In addition to the pleuropulmonary manifestations, as on the right, cardiac manifestation may also occur.

The usual laboratory studies are of little help in establishing the diagnosis. Leukocytosis is present in 75 per cent of the patients, and a shift to the left on differential count is a constant finding. In approximately 50 per cent of the patients, anemia will be found. In the majority of cases there is a significant increase in the blood sedimentation rate, and repeated determinations may be of aid in assessing the efficacy of treatment of the infection. In approximately 50 per cent of patients, the serum albumin is reduced to less than 3.5 grams per 100 ml.

Liver indicia are not significant or diagnostic, and no distinctive pattern exists. Serum alkaline phosphatase appears to be most commonly affected and is increased in approximately 25 per cent of cases. The serum bilirubin is elevated in 10 per cent of cases and the serum transaminases are only rarely altered.

In nonendemic areas, acute abscess of the right lobe of the liver is frequently misdiagnosed as acute cholecystitis.[61] It is important to note that frequently in patients with amebic abscess of the liver, the gallbladder and common duct cannot be visualized with cholecystography or cholangiography. This occurred in 85 per cent of the patients with hepatic abscess in the series reported by Cohen and Reynolds.[8]

LABORATORY AIDS IN DIAGNOSIS

Coprologic Studies

A careful examination of properly collected stool specimens should be done in any patient suspected of having an amebic abscess of the liver. Cysts or trophozoites, or both, are reported to be found in the stools in less than 15 per cent of cases of liver abscess. However, even in the absence of diarrhea, careful examination of the stools may reveal the presence of the parasites. Repeated examinations may be necessary, and saline catharsis may increase the incidence of positive findings.

Radiologic Studies

Posteroanterior and lateral roentgenograms of the chest provide important diagnostic information. With an abscess of the liver, the adjacent diaphragm is elevated, with evidence of restricted motion or immobility on fluoroscopic examination. Patchy pneumonitis in the contiguous lung base, atelectasis, and most frequently pleural effusion are also seen. One or more of these findings can be demonstrated in over 80 per cent of patients with amebic abscess of the right lobe of the liver. However, such changes also occur in patients with pyogenic liver abscess, subphrenic abscess, and many other entities. The demonstration of elevation of the medial portion of the right leaf of the diaphragm with obliteration of the cardiophrenic angle on the posteroanterior view, and elevation of the diaphragm anteriorly with obliteration of the anterior costophrenic angle on lateral views may be helpful in differentiating amebic infections of the liver and subphrenic space from primary pyogenic lesions in these areas, which most frequently affect the lateral and posterior aspects of the diaphragm.[42] Such distinctive roentgenograms are rarely encountered, and there are no roentgenographic findings specifically diagnostic of amebic abscess of the liver. The majority of cases when first seen at the hospital have evidence of pleural effusion, which, in association with an enlarged liver, is highly suggestive of a liver abscess (Fig. 36).

Similar roentgenologic pleuropulmonary changes may be seen with abscess of the left lobe of the liver. In many instances, a left lobe abscess extends into the abdomen and may produce characteristic pressure deformities visualized with barium studies of the gastrointestinal tract. Displacement of the gastric cardia, lesser curvature, and duodenal cap, with a crescentic deformity of the lesser curvature of the stomach and downward displacement of the splenic flexure, are frequently found with abscess of the left lobe.[42]

Computerized Axial Tomography

The recent introduction of means of obtaining rapid radiologic scans of the body without motion artifacts should prove to be of great value in the localization and definition of abscesses in the liver.[53, 54] This technique is capable of defining smaller lesions than currently possible with other scanning procedures.

Radionuclide Images

Anterior, posterior, and lateral images of the liver using technetium-99m sulfur colloid provide an excellent method of demonstrating space-occupying lesions in the liver (Fig. 37). The scintiphoto obtained does not differentiate an abscess from hepatoma or metastatic malignancy. The radionuclide image is especially useful in confirming the diagnosis of suspected liver abscess, and particularly in identifying lesions in the left lobe, which are difficult to diagnose by other measures.

Images of amebic abscess of the liver obtained with gallium-67 citrate are considered to be less useful than the colloid image. Gallium may reveal increased activity near the periphery of the lesion, which is also characteristic of a large neoplasm with central ne-

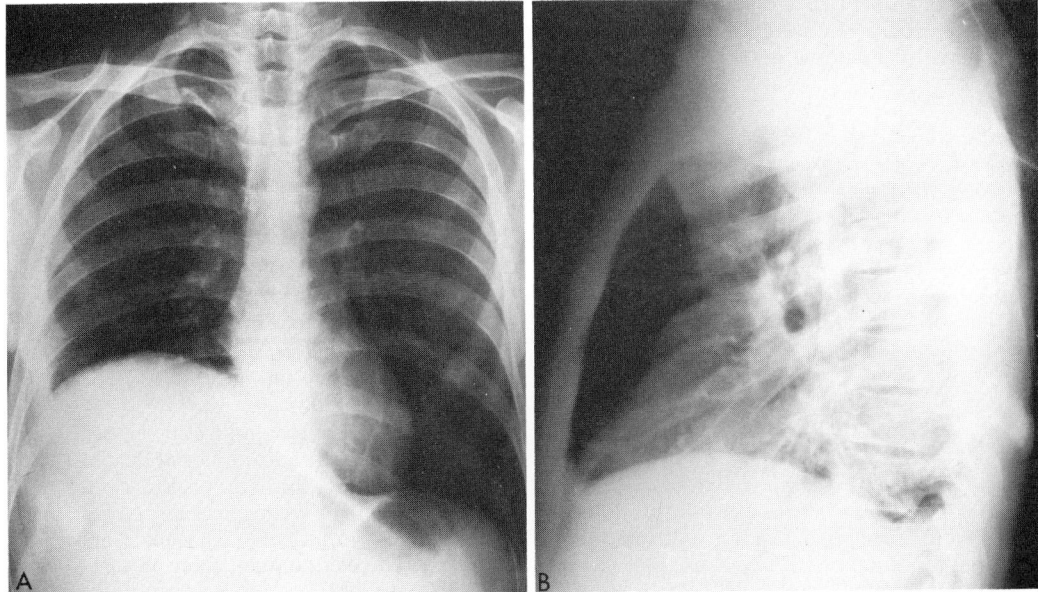

Figure 36. Usual roentgenologic changes associated with amebic abscess of the right lobe of the liver. *A*, Posteroanterior view. Right pleural effusion with presumed elevation of right diaphragm. *B*, Lateral view. Same findings, with blunting of anterior and posterior costophrenic angles.

crosis.[14, 38] It has been suggested that the addition of a gallium study of a liver abscess may possibly provide additional information in assessing the size and resolution of the abscess in response to specific therapy.

A recent report indicates that labeled metronidazoles have been prepared as possible agents for imaging hepatic amebic abscesses by selective accumulation of these agents in the abscess contents.[59] This may provide a method of specifically identifying an amebic abscess and differentiating such an abscess from other space-occupying lesions of the liver. No clinical results are available as yet. However, the

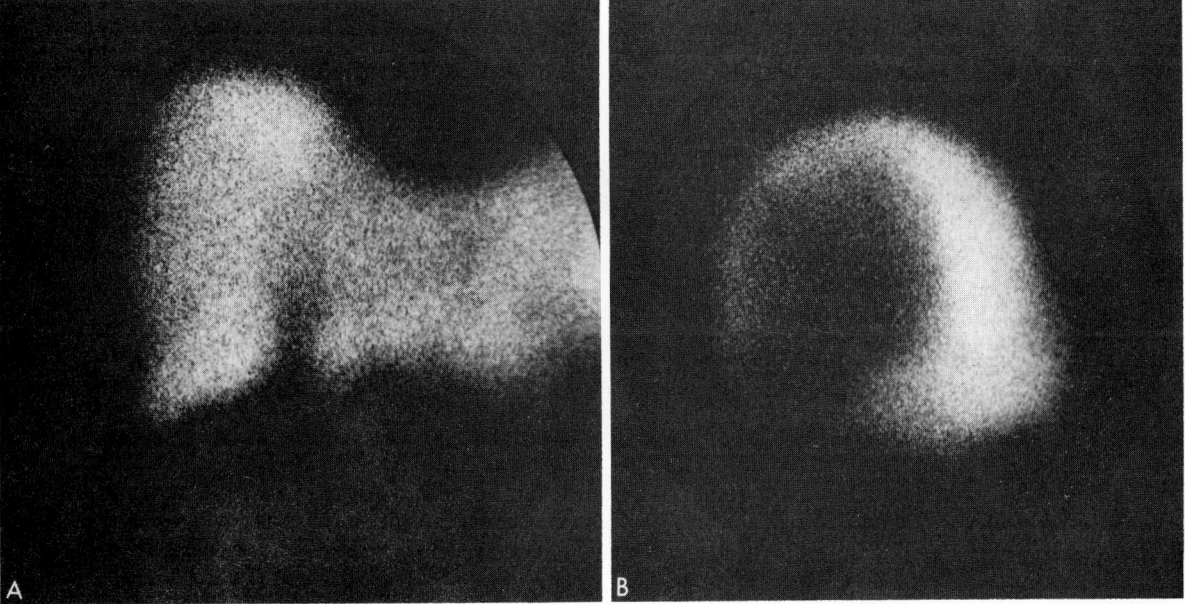

Figure 37. Radionuclide image of the liver using 99m-Technetium sulfur colloid. *A*, Anterior view. No gross defect evident. *B*, Lateral view. Large filling defect in posterior portion of right lobe due to an amebic abscess.

agents are being evaluated in a cooperative study by nuclear medicine groups in a number of countries where amebiasis is hyperendemic.

Ultrasonic Scanning

Early reports indicate that ultrasonic scanning has not been as accurate as scintiscanning in detecting a localized lesion in the liver, but it has a high degree of accuracy in determining whether the lesion located is fluid-filled or solid.[36] With improved technology and methodology, ultrasonic scanning appears to be increasingly reliable in detecting and localizing lesions in the liver. The addition of a B-mode ultrasonograph to the radionuclide image is extremely helpful in establishing a diagnosis of amebic abscess of the liver (Fig. 38).

Serologic Tests

Indirect hemagglutination, complement fixation, and *gel-diffusion precipitation tests* are all useful in detecting antibodies of *E. histolytica* in man. All are more strongly positive in patients with liver abscess than in intestinal amebiasis, symptomatic or asymptomatic. Negative serologic tests are helpful in excluding an amebic abscess of the liver as a diagnostic possibility. Intradermal hypersensitivity tests have not proved to be as valuable as serologic tests in the differential diagnosis of amebic abscess of the liver.[34]

The indirect hemagglutination test introduced by Kessel and Lewis,[26] with the use of axenically grown *E. histolytica* as antigen, has been shown to be a highly sensitive and specific test, and more sensitive in invasive amebiasis than the complement fixation and gel-diffusion tests.[21] It has been found to be positive with high titers in over 98 per cent of cases with proved abscess of the liver.[8, 27, 37] As with the other tests, it is not helpful in differentiating intestinal from invasive amebiasis, and titers tend to remain positive for months or years after cure, which presents a problem in the diagnosis of acute invasive disease in hyperendemic areas. In nonendemic areas the test is extremely useful for patients in whom an amebic abscess of the liver is suspected. Although false-positives may occur, a negative test appears to be quite reliable in excluding amebic abscess as a diagnosis in such patients, and especially helpful in differentiating an amebic abscess from a pyogenic abscess and other space-occupying lesions of the liver. A positive reaction in a titer of 1:128 is regarded as suspicious, and 1:512 characteristic of tissue-invasive amebiasis, past or present.[8] In some patients with amebic abscess of the liver, low titers obtained initially may be found to be more strongly positive on repeat testing. Additionally, titers may vary in tests run in different laboratories, possibly due to a difference in antigens[8] and the method of preparation and type of red cells used in the test.[17]

The indirect hemagglutination test is currently available in a limited number of hospital and commercial laboratories throughout the country. When not available locally, serum may be sent for testing to the National Communicable Disease Center in Atlanta, Georgia. The complement fixation test is also a highly technical laboratory procedure and even more time consuming, and the gel-diffusion test, although simpler to perform, is usually slower and less sensitive.[21]

Counterimmunoelectrophoresis, the technique used for the detection of hepatitis-associated antigen, has recently been advocated as a test for amebic disease. The advantages are the ease in setting up the test, simplicity of reagents, and relative rapidity of obtaining results. The specificity of the test has been found to compare favorably with indirect hemagglutination; however, the latter currently remains the serologic test of choice because of its greater sensitivity to lower levels of antibodies of *E. histolytica.*[30]

Parasitologic Studies

Identification of amebae in pus obtained by aspiration of a liver abscess (Fig. 39) or pleural fluid, or in material coughed up is the only method of positively establishing a diagnosis of amebic abscess of the liver.

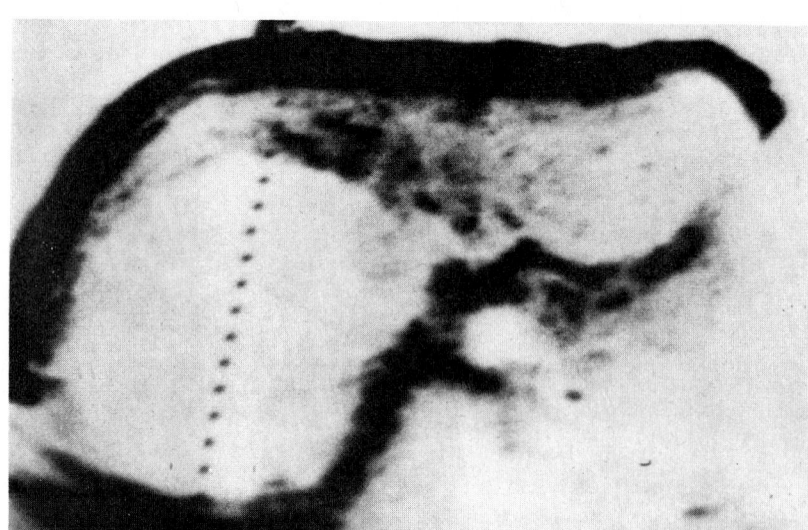

Figure 38. B-mode sonar scan: Large amebic abscess of the right lobe of the liver. The range marker, indicated by broken lines 1 cm. apart, passes through the center of the abscess.

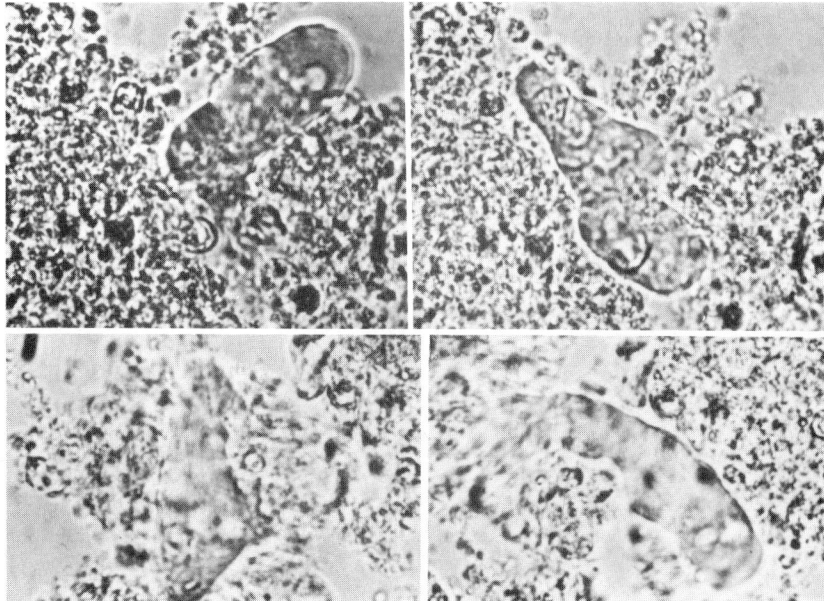

Figure 39. *Entamoeba histolytica* trophozoites in "anchovy-paste" pus from an amebic abscess of the liver.

In the majority of cases, trophozoites are not identified in the pus obtained by aspiration. It has been suggested that proper preparation of the specimen and a careful search should significantly increase the number of positive identifications.[52] Aspiration of "anchovy paste" or "chocolate sauce" material containing no bacteria is considered to be pathognomonic of amebic abscess of the liver, even if no amebae are demonstrated. However, in many cases, the color of the bacteriologically sterile aspirate is creamy white, yellow, or green.

COMPLICATIONS

With earlier recognition and prompt treatment of amebic abscess of the liver, there has been a significant decrease in the incidence of complications of this lesion, which are frequently associated with a high mortality.

An untreated amebic abscess of the liver continues to destroy tissue concentrically until the surface of the liver is reached and the process progresses by direct extension into other structures or organs or by rupture into adjacent serous cavities or hollow viscera (Fig. 40).

Figure 40. Complications of amebic abscess of the liver, the most common source of extraintestinal amebiasis in the human.

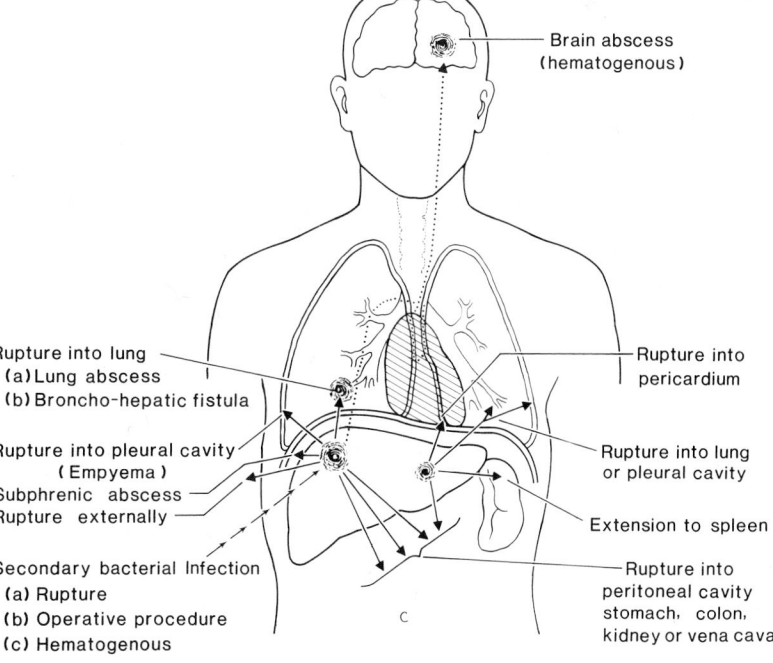

Brain abscess (hematogenous)

Rupture into lung
(a) Lung abscess
(b) Broncho-hepatic fistula

Rupture into pleural cavity (Empyema)
Subphrenic abscess
Rupture externally

Secondary bacterial Infection
(a) Rupture
(b) Operative procedure
(c) Hematogenous

Rupture into pericardium

Rupture into lung or pleural cavity

Extension to spleen

Rupture into peritoneal cavity stomach, colon, kidney or vena cava

Most commonly, this is manifested by pleuropulmonary complications on the right as a result of transdiaphragmatic rupture of an abscess in the dome of the right lobe of the liver. In acute and rapidly progressive cases, the abscess may rupture into the unobliterated pleural cavity without extension into the lung. More commonly, with a gradually enlarging abscess, the inflammatory reaction may obliterate the pleural cavity, permitting the abscess to rupture directly into the base of the lung.

With the onset of these complications, there is a sudden appearance of or increase in the pulmonary findings that may have been present owing to transphrenic inflammatory changes from a contiguous intrahepatic abscess. Increased pain in the lower chest, increased cough which may become productive, increased dyspnea associated with findings of consolidation or cavitation in the lower lobe of the lung, and evidence of a pleural empyema are manifestations of such complications.

A cough productive of large quantities of purulent material with "chocolate sauce" appearance indicates that an hepatic abscess communicates with a bronchus, establishing a bronchohepatic fistula. This occurs in approximately 50 per cent of cases in which a liver abscess ruptures into the lung.[11] Owing to the spontaneous evacuation of the liver abscess, an acute bronchohepatic fistula had been noted in early reports to have a good prognosis, even without specific amebicidal therapy,[32, 41] and now has an excellent prognosis.[2, 8, 60]

Rupture of an amebic abscess of the liver into the peritoneal cavity may occur suddenly, with the signs and symptoms of severe shock and evidence of severe spreading peritonitis, or the leak may be gradual, with the development of a localized abscess. Free perforation is highly lethal and difficult to distinguish clinically from perforation of a hollow viscus from other causes.

Rupture more commonly occurs with abscesses in the left lobe of the liver, probably because of its smaller size and more complete peritoneal cover. This, together with delayed diagnosis of abscesses of the left lobe because of its relatively hidden location, considerably increases the mortality from these abscesses.[1]

Rupture into the duodenum, stomach, or colon occurs relatively infrequently and often does not produce any significant change in symptoms. The spontaneous drainage of the abscess appears to be beneficial, and the lesions heal rapidly with amebicidal therapy.

Purulent pericarditis from perforation of an amebic abscess of the liver is relatively uncommon and usually associated with an abscess involving the left lobe. This highly lethal complication may be manifested by the sudden onset of substernal pain, severe shock, and evidence of cardiac tamponade. More commonly the manifestations are gradual in onset, with substernal pain, discomfort, and respiratory distress superimposed on the symptoms of the hepatic abscess and the clinical and laboratory evidence of pericardial effusion.

Brain abscess, usually the result of hematogenous spread from a liver abscess, occurs rarely but is highly lethal. There may be a single abscess or multiple abscesses, which do not respond readily to standard amebicidal drugs. There are no distinctive symptoms, and in many of the cases reported the lesion has been encountered unexpectedly at postmortem examination. Any symptoms of possible cerebral origin in a patient with amebic abscess of the liver should be investigated promptly with appropriate brain studies to facilitate early aspiration, which may improve the prognosis.[19]

Other rare complications have been reported, such as extension of an amebic abscess of the liver to the spleen, kidney, bile ducts, and other adjacent structures.

DIAGNOSIS

The diagnosis of amebic abscess of the liver in nonendemic areas must be considered in any patient with acute symptoms and findings referable to the right upper quadrant of the abdomen or the lower right chest who has resided in or visited areas in which amebiasis is prevalent. In such cases, a filling defect on hepatic scan, a positive serologic test for antibody to *E. histolytica,* and response to amebicidal medication are considered diagnostic.

TREATMENT

In 1935, on the basis of a study of 4484 collected and personal cases of amebic abscess of the liver, Ochsner and DeBakey[4] advocated the following three principles of treatment, which were re-emphasized in their subsequent reports.[11, 42] These principles remain the basis of treatment today. (1) Every case of suspected amebic abscess should be given a course of amebicidal drug therapy before any other procedure is used, unless rupture of the abscess appears imminent. (2) In cases in which evacuation of the abscess becomes necessary, aspiration and preliminary administration of amebicidal drugs are the procedures of choice. (3) Open drainage of the abscess should be reserved for the relatively few cases of secondarily infected abscesses.[40]

It is important to note that the authors carefully differentiated "closed drainage" with a needle, even though done at the time of celiotomy, from "open drainage" by unroofing or incising the abscess and inserting drains into it.

In a study utilizing serial hepatoscan, it was shown that amebic abscesses of the liver healed gradually over a period of two to four months after emetine therapy, and that occasionally resolution did not take place for as long as a year. The addition of open surgical drainage, or needle aspiration, or both, did not significantly alter the resolution time in this study.[55]

Metronidazole (Flagyl), introduced by Powell in 1966 for the treatment of amebiasis, is currently the drug of choice, with a dosage of 750 to 800 mg. orally, three times daily for 10 days. It is highly effective in curing intrahepatic amebic abscess as well as in eradicating intestinal amebiasis.[8, 46] In some cases, a second course of treatment is required, and failures of treatment have been reported.[15, 16, 18] The use of an intravenous preparation was reported recently,[39] and a parenteral form of metronidazole is currently undergoing investigation in this country. As yet, however, only the oral form is available for general use.

Metronidazole appears to be pharmacologically inert and nontoxic. Infrequent side effects of nausea, vomiting, drowsiness, skin eruptions, and pruritis have been reported. It is easily administered, rapidly acting, effective in courses of relatively short duration, and appears to approximate most closely the ideal amebicide. In the acutely ill patient suspected of having an amebic abscess of the liver, blood should be drawn for serologic studies and metronidazole therapy started while proceeding with the confirmation of the diagnosis with hepatic scans and parasitologic and serologic studies.

Chloraquine has also been found to be extremely efficacious in the treatment of amebic abscess of the liver, although less effective than metronidazole as a luminal antibiotic and not as rapidly acting. High relapse or failure rates have been reported;[31] however, in a dosage of 500 mg. daily for 10 weeks, relapses appear to be effectively controlled.[8, 60]

Ipecacuanha had been used in the treatment of dysentery since 1658, but the parenteral injection of its principal alkaloid, emetine hydrochloride, as first reported by Rogers in 1912,[48] was one of the most significant advances in the treatment of invasive amebiasis.

The remarkable efficacy of emetine in the treatment of amebic abscess of the liver was recognized early, with a curative effect reported to be nearly 100 per cent.[46] Emetine is ineffective as a luminal amebicide, which must be given with it to avoid recurrence. In an excellent study by Klatskin,[28] the local, cardiovascular, gastrointestinal, and neuromuscular toxic properties of emetine, which had been of concern for many years, were evaluated relative to duration and dosage. The reversibility of most of these effects after cessation of emetine therapy was noted, which has been also stressed by others.[25, 62] Its use has been deprecated by some authors. However, Wilmot[63] and Powell[46] make strong pleas not to abandon the use of emetine entirely, and indicate that in the most severe cases of invasive amebiasis when peritonitis is imminent or already present, parenteral therapy is mandatory and the life-saving properties of emetine preparations should be borne in mind. This also applies to patients with extremely large abscesses of the liver that prove to be refractory to oral therapy or have ruptured into the peritoneal cavity. A daily dosage of 65 mg. (1 grain) subcutaneously or intramuscularly for 10 days has been found to be highly effective in the treatment of abscess of the liver. Metronidazole should be given in conjunction with emetine as soon as oral medication can be tolerated. Although electrocardiographic changes are commonly encountered, no significant cardiac complications have been noted with a dosage no greater than 0.65 gm. and with strict adherence to the proper precautions. The patient must be at absolute bed rest and observed closely, and the medication must be discontinued on the appearance of a progressive tachycardia, evidence of conduction defects, or other manifestations of severe toxicity. Toxic effects

may become manifest several days after the medication is discontinued. Because of the toxic effects, emetine should not be used unless absolutely necessary and only if the probable benefit outweighs the possible hazard. Establishment of the safety and efficacy of an intravenous metronidazole preparation may eventually eliminate this highly effective but potentially dangerous drug.

The tetracyclines and other antibiotics have been used for the treatment of intestinal amebiasis. However, relapse is not infrequent, and these agents are not effective in treating hepatic amebic abscess.[46] Broad-spectrum antibiotics used in conjunction with amebicidal agents are of value in the treatment of a secondarily infected amebic abscess of the liver, and in some of the complications due to rupture of the abscess.

Percutaneous aspiration of a liver abscess with a large-bore spinal needle is a safe procedure if done with meticulous attention to aseptic technique. However, it is not necessary in all cases to assure recovery[8, 16, 60] and does not appear to affect resolution time. Its use should be reserved for patients with large abscesses who do not show a satisfactory clinical response after 48 to 72 hours of treatment with metronidazole, or earlier if the collection is extremely large and rupture appears to be imminent. When necessary, needle aspiration of an abscess of the right lobe of the liver is done at the site of local evidence of an underlying abscess, or in the absence of such evidence, through the ninth or tenth interspace in the right midaxillary line, guided by the physical and radiographic findings. Every attempt should be made to avoid traversing the pleural or peritoneal cavities. It is also important to aspirate an abscess of the left lobe early to prevent rupture into the pericardium, which is highly lethal.

It is not necessary to inject amebicides into the abscess cavity after it has been evacuated. However, whenever possible, aspiration should be preceded by the administration of amebicidal medication. The contents of the abscess should be examined by direct smear and culture as well as in wet mounts.

On occasion, an unsuspected intrahepatic amebic abscess is found at an operation undertaken for some other diagnosis. An abscess encountered under such circumstances should be evacuated by needle aspiration; a ventriculogram needle with stylet is highly desirable for aspiration under such circumstances. A direct smear of the contents should be examined immediately, and, if no bacteria are seen and the appearance of the contents is consistent with an amebic abscess, open drainage should be avoided, despite the improved outlook of such a procedure since the advent of antibiotic therapy.[20, 52]

In some instances, celiotomy may be necessary for closed drainage by needle aspiration of an abscess not safely accessible to a needle introduced through the skin. This is not often required for an abscess of the right lobe of the liver, but more often for lesions in the left lobe, which have an extremely high rate of complications and a poor prognosis.[1] It is also required more frequently in infants and children because of the frequency of multiple abscesses that are inaccessible for percutaneous aspiration.[54]

The sole indication for open drainage of an amebic

abscess of the liver is secondary infection which fails to respond to appropriate antibiotic therapy in addition to amebicidal therapy and aspiration. Open drainage may be instituted in cases of rupture of the liver abscess with peritonitis or for pleural empyema which fails to respond to aspiration and amebicidal drug therapy. Rupture into the lung with abscess formation rarely requires operation, as most will respond to amebicides or will drain spontaneously by erosion through a bronchus with establishment of a bronchohepatic fistula. Occasionally, a thoracotomy is necessary for decortication of fibrotic lung tissue. Rupture of an abscess into the pericardium requires repeated aspiration. Open transpleural drainage may be necessary in some cases for secondary infection or failure of the symptoms of cardiac tamponade to respond to aspiration. Brain abscess, which is highly lethal, appears to be nonresponsive to amebicidal therapy and probably is best treated by early drainage, preferably by aspiration.[19]

PROGNOSIS

The response of amebic abscess of the liver to similar therapeutic regimens varies greatly in reports emanating from different parts of the world. Results appear to be dependent upon the stage of the disease when the patient is first seen, the nutritional state and general health of the patient, and the presence of complications. With current therapy, the mortality from amebic abscess of the liver in all parts of the world has been dramatically reduced, even in patients in hyperendemic areas with complications of the disease.[47] In this country, the mortality from treated amebic abscess of the liver is currently less than 4 per cent.

SELECTED REFERENCES

Berne, C. J.: Diagnosis and treatment of amebic liver abscess. Surg. Gynecol. Obstet., 75:235, 1942.
An extremely well written and perspicacious analysis of the ambiguous clinical manifestations of amebic abscess of the liver and its treatment, based on the personal observations and extensive experience of the author. This relatively brief report remains as pertinent today as when first written.

Ochsner, A., and DeBakey, M.: Amebic hepatitis and hepatic abscess. Surgery, 13:460, 612, 1943.
This is a monumental presentation of the subject of amebic disease of the liver based on the extensive personal experience of the authors and an encyclopedic review of the world literature. The publications of Dr. Ochsner and Dr. DeBakey, beginning in 1935, relative to the diagnosis, complications, and treatment of hepatic amebiasis, are among the foremost in the world's literature, and the basis of current management. This two-part review is one of their most comprehensive and summarizes the material appearing in their previous publications. A classic.

Powell, S. J.: Latest developments in the treatment of amebiasis. Adv. Pharmacol. Chemother., 10:91, 1972.
An excellent summary and evaluation of chemotherapeutic agents currently used for the treatment of amebiasis, based on the author's extensive experience and clinical trials of these agents in a hyperendemic area. The late Dr. Powell achieved world-wide recognition for his numerous publications on the subject of amebic disease, and especially for introducing metronidazole in 1966 for its treatment.

Wilmot, A. J.: Clinical amoebiasis. Oxford, Blackwell Scientific Publications, 1962.

A highly readable and enjoyable presentation covering all aspects of amebiasis. This authoritative monograph is based on the extensive experience of the author and his scholarly review of the world's pertinent literature. The entire text is of great interest and value to the surgeon as well as the physician, especially the sections on diagnosis, complications, and treatment.

REFERENCES

1. Alkan, W. J., Kalmi, B., and Kalderon, M.: The clinical syndrome of amebic abscess of the left lobe of the liver. Ann. Intern. Med., 55:800, 1961.
2. Berne, C. J.: Diagnosis and treatment of amebic liver abscess. Surg. Gynecol. Obstet., 75:235, 1942.
3. Bontius, J. (1629): An account of the diseases, natural history and medicine of East Indies. London, T. Noteman. Translated from the Latin, 1769 (cited by Kean[24]).
4. Brandt, H., and Tamayo, R. P.: Pathology of human amebiasis. Hum. Pathol., 1:351, 1970.
5. Bundesen, H. N.: The Chicago epidemic of amoebic dysentery in 1933. Publ. Health Rep., 49:1266, 1934.
6. Carrera, G. M.: Pathology of early amebic hepatitis. Arch. Pathol., 50:440, 1950.
7. Center for Disease Control: Morbidity and mortality weekly report. Ann. Suppl., 1975.
8. Cohen, H. G., and Reynolds, T. B.: Comparison of metronidazole and chloroquine for the treatment of amoebic liver abscess. Gastroenterology, 69:35, 1975.
9. Councilman, W. T., and Lafleur, H. A.: Amoebic dysentery. Johns Hopkins Hosp. Rep., 2:395, 1891 (cited by Wilmot[63]).
10. Craig, C. F., and Faust, E. C.: Clinical parasitology, 5th ed. Philadelphia, 1951.
11. DeBakey, M. E., and Ochsner, A.: Hepatic amebiasis: A 20 year experience and analysis of 263 cases. Int. Abstr. Surg., 92:209, 1951.
12. Doxiades, J., Candreviotis, N., Tiliakos, M., and Polymeropoulos, I.: Chronic diffuse non-suppurative amoebic hepatitis. Br. Med. J., 1:460, 1961.
13. Faust, E. C.: Amebiasis. Springfield, Ill., Charles C Thomas, Publisher, 1954.
14. Geslien, G. E., Thrall, J. H., and Johnson, M. C.: Gallium scanning in acute hepatic amebic abscess. J. Nucl. Med., 15:561, 1974.
15. Griffin, F. M., Jr.: Failure of metronidazole to cure hepatic amebic abscess. N. Engl. J. Med., 288:1397, 1973.
16. Griffin, F. M., Jr.: Treatment of amebic abscess. N. Engl. J. Med., 289:869, 1973.
17. Farshy, D. C., and Healy, G. R.: Use of stable, sensitized cells in indirect micro hemagglutination test for amebiasis. Appl. Microbiol., 27:11, 1974.
18. Henn, R. M., and Collin, D. B.: Amebic abscess of the liver. J.A.M.A., 224:1394, 1973.
19. Hughes, F. B., Faehnle, S. T., and Simon, J. L.: Multiple cerebral abscesses complicating hepatopulmonary amebiasis. J. Pediatr., 86:95, 1975.
20. Jordan, P. H., Jr.: Treatment of amebic abscess of the liver by open surgical drainage. Ann. Surg., 141:70, 1955.
21. Juniper, K., Jr., Worrell, C. L., Minshew, M. C., Roth, L. S., Cypert, H., and Lloyd, R. E.: Serologic diagnosis of amebiasis. Am. J. Trop. Med., 21:157, 1972.
22. Kartulis, S.: Zur aetiologie der dysenterie in aegypten. Virchows Arch. Pathol. Anat., 105:521, 1886 (cited by Wilmot[63]).
23. Kean, B. H.: Amebic hepatitis. Arch. Intern. Med., 96:667, 1955.
24. Kean, B. H.: The nature of diffuse amebic hepatitis. Am. J. Dig. Dis., 2:342, 1957.
25. Kent, L., and Kingsland, R. C.: Effects of emetine hydrochloride on the electrocardiogram in man. Am. Heart J., 39:576, 1950.
26. Kessel, J. F., Lewis, W. P., Ma, S., and Kim, H.: Preliminary report on a hemagglutination test for entamoebae. Proc. Soc. Exp. Biol. Med., 106:409, 1961.
27. Kessel, J. F., Lewis, W. P., Pasquel, C. M., and Turner, J. A.: Indirect hemagglutination and complement fixation tests in amebiasis. Am. J. Trop. Med., 14:540, 1965.
28. Klatskin, G., and Friedman, H.: Emetine toxicity in man: Studies on the nature of early toxic manifestations, their relation to the dose level, and their significance in determining safe dosage. Ann. Intern. Med., 28:892, 1948.
29. Koch, R.: Zur untersuchung von pathogenen organismen. Mitth. k. Besundh.-Amte, 1:48, 1881 (cited by Faust[13]).

30. Krupp, I. M.: Comparison of counterimmunoelectrophoresis with other serologic tests in the diagnosis of amebiasis. Am. J. Trop. Med., 23:27, 1974.

31. Lambl, W. D.: Studien aus dem Franz-Josef-Kinder-Spitale. *In* Prag., 1:362, 1860 (cited by Wilmot[63]).

32. Lamont, N. M., and Pooler, N. R.: Hepatic amoebiasis. Q. J. Med., 27:389, 1958.

33. Losch, F.: Massenhafte entwickelung von amoben im dickdarm. Virchows Arch. Pathol. Anat., 65:196, 1875 (cited by Wilmot[63]).

34. Maddison, S. E., Kagan, I. G., and Elsdon-Dew, R.: Comparison of intradermal and serologic tests for the diagnosis of amebiasis. Am. J. Trop. Med., 17:540, 1968.

35. Maegraith, B. G., and Harinasuta, C.: Experimental amoebic infection of the liver in guinea pigs. Ann. Trop. Med. Parasitol., 48:421, 434, 1954.

36. Matthews, A. W., Gough, K. R., Rhys Davies, E., Ross, F. G. M., and Hinchliffe, A.: The use of combined ultrasonic and isotope scanning in the diagnosis of amoebic liver disease. Gut, 14:50, 1973.

37. Milgram, E. A., Healy, G. R., and Kagan, I. G.: Studies on the use of the indirect hemagglutination tests in the diagnosis of amebiasis. Gastroenterology, 50:645, 1966.

38. Miyamoto, A. T., Thadepalli, H., and Mishkin, F. S.: [67]Gallium images of amebic liver abscesses. N. Engl. J. Med., 291:1363, 1974.

39. Nair, K. G., Kothari, N. N., and Sheth, U. K.: Intravenous metronidazole in amoebic liver abscess. Lancet, 1:1238, 1974.

40. Ochsner, A., and DeBakey, M.: Diagnosis and treatment of amebic abscess of the liver. Am. J. Dig. Dis., 2:47, 1935.

41. Ochsner, A., and DeBakey, M.: Pleuropulmonary complications of amebiasis. J. Thorac. Surg., 5:225, 1936.

42. Ochsner, A., and DeBakey, M.: Amebic hepatitis and hepatic abscess. Surgery, 13:460, 612, 1943.

43. Palmer, R. B.: Changes in the liver in amebic dysentery. Arch. Pathol., 25:327, 1938.

44. Paul, M.: New concepts in amoebic abscess of the liver. Br. J. Surg., 47:502, 1960.

45. Payne, A. M. M.: Amoebic dysentery in Eastern India. Lancet, 248:206, 1945.

46. Powell, S. J.: Latest developments in the treatment of amebiasis. Adv. Pharmacol. Chemother., 10:91, 1972.

47. Rasaretnam, R., Paul, A. T. S., and Yoganathan, M.: Pleural empyema due to ruptured amoebic liver abscess. Br. J. Surg., 61:713, 1974.

48. Rogers, L.: The rapid cure of amoebic dysentery and hepatitis by hypodermic injections of soluble salts of emetine. Br. Med. J., 1:1424, 1912.

49. Rogers, L.: Lettsomian lectures on amoebic liver abscess. Lancet, 202:463, 569, 677, 1922.

50. Sagel, S., Stanley, R. J., and Evens, R. G.: Early clinical experience with motionless whole-body computed tomography. Radiology, 119:321, 1976.

51. Sanford, A. H.: The geographic distribution of amebiasis. J.A.M.A., 67:1923, 1916.

52. Schapiro, M. M.: Open surgical drainage for hepatic amebic abscess. Arch. Surg., 73:780, 1956.

53. Schaudinn, F.: Untersuchungen uber die fortpflanzung einiger rhizopoden. Arb. GesundhAmte (Berl.), 19:547, 1903 (cited by Wilmot[63]).

54. Scragg, J. N., and Powell, S. J.: Metronidazole in treatment of children with amoebic liver abscess. Arch. Dis. Child., 48:911, 1973.

55. Sheehy, T. W., Parmley, L. F., Jr., Johnston, G. S., and Boyce, H. W.: Resolution time of an amebic liver abscess. Gastroenterology, 55:26, 1968.

56. Stephens, D. H., Hattery, R. R., and Sheedy, P. F., II: Computed tomography of the abdomen. Radiology, 119:331, 1976.

57. Strong, R. P.: The etiology of the dysenteries of the Philippine Islands. Circ. Trop. Dis., Manila, 1901 (cited by Faust[13]).

58. Tandon, B. N., Tandon, H. D., and Puri, B. K.: An electron microscopic study of liver in hepatomegaly presumably caused by amebiasis. Exp. Mol. Pathol., 22:118, 1975.

59. Tubis, M., Krishnamurthy, G. T., Endow, J. S., Stein, R. A., Suwanik, R., and Blahd, W. H.: Labeled metronidazoles as potential new agents for amebic hepatic abscess imaging. Nuclearmedizin, 14:164, 1975.

60. Turrill, F. L., and Burnham, J. R.: Hepatic amebiasis. Am. J. Surg., 111:424, 1966.

61. Wagner, V. P., Smale, L. E., and Lischke, J. H.: Amebic abscess of the liver and spleen in pregnancy and the puerperium. Obstet. Gynecol., 45:562, 1975.

62. Welchman, J. M.: The cardiac toxicity of emetine. J. Trop. Med. Hyg., 60:296, 1957.

63. Wilmot, A. J.: Clinical amoebiasis. Oxford, Blackwell Scientific Publications, 1962.

III

NEOPLASMS OF THE LIVER

George L. Jordan, Jr., M.D.

Primary tumors of the liver are uncommon neoplasms, but the liver is the organ most frequently involved with metastatic disease.

BENIGN TUMORS

Benign tumors may arise from any of the cells found in the liver. These include hepatic parenchymal cells, the epithelium of the bile ducts, vascular structures, and any mesenchymal tissue. Benign neoplasms of clinical significance are rare. A modification of the classification by Henson, Gray, and Dockerty is as follows:[12, 13]

   I. Parenchymal tumors
      A. Hepatic cell adenomas (hepatoadenomas)
      B. Bile duct adenomas (cholangioadenomas)
      C. Mixed hepatic cell and bile duct adenomas (cholangiohepatoadenomas)
         1. Hamartomas
   II. Vascular tumors
      A. Hemangiomas
      B. Lymphangiomas

III. Neoplastic cysts
   A. Cystadenomas
   B. Dermoids
   C. Cystic teratomas
IV. Mesenchymal tumors
   A. Fibromas
   B. Lipomas
   C. Leiomyomas

Adenomas

Adenomas of the liver are rare but, among the benign tumors, occur second in frequency to hemangioma. There are three pathologic types. One arises from liver cells, the hepatic cell adenoma (hepatoadenoma). Bile duct adenoma (cholangioadenoma) arises from bile duct epithelium, and a third type is composed of mixed hepatic and bile duct cells. Some of these may be classified as *hamartomas,* representing normal tissue which has developed in a pattern at variance with normal histology. The tumors are usually asymptomatic but on occasion may produce nausea and vomiting, epigastric discomfort, or a sensation of weight in the abdomen. If the tumor is large the liver will become palpable and nodularity may be appreciated. The majority do not need surgical therapy. When treatment is indicated for relief of symptoms, or when a lesion is found at the time of operation and the exact nature cannot be determined, surgical excision should be performed. The primary purpose of excision of small tumors may be histologic examination to eliminate the possibility of a malignant lesion.

Vascular Tumors

Hemangioma is a benign tumor arising from blood vessels and is the benign tumor most frequently encountered in the liver. The microscopic appearance is that of endothelial lined spaces filled with blood. Both capillary and cavernous types occur, although the latter is the more common. Small subcapsular hemangiomas are found not infrequently at the time of abdominal exploration for lesions in other organs and at autopsy. These tumors do not cause symptoms and need no therapy. Hemangiomas of the cavernous type, however, may involve large portions of the organ, and such neoplasms are potential threats to life. Although occurring at all ages, the majority of symptomatic lesions are in children and are more frequent in males than in females. Clinical findings are those of a palpable mass that may present in the right upper quadrant, the epigastrium, or the left upper quadrant, since either lobe may be involved. Symptoms of congestive failure may also appear. Rupture with severe hemorrhage is the most frequent complication, and the mortality rate associated with this complication is high. Treatment consists of resection of large cavernous hemangiomas, particularly in children, because of the possibility of rupture. Hepatic artery ligation has been utilized in the management of some patients exhibiting congestive failure. Radiation therapy has been used for those patients in whom surgical therapy cannot be applied. This may result in some shrinking of the neoplasm and a decrease in symptoms.[4, 6, 17]

MALIGNANT TUMORS

Malignant tumors may be classified according to the following outline.
I. Carcinoma
   A. Primary
      1. Hepatoma
      2. Cholangioma
      3. Mixed and anaplastic
   B. Metastatic
II. Sarcoma
   A. Hemangioendothelioma
   B. Rhabdomyosarcoma
   C. Leiomyosarcoma
   D. Lymphoma
III. Malignant teratoma

Etiology

The etiology of primary hepatoma is unknown. There is, however, a significant variation in the distribution of this tumor in diverse parts of the world. In the United States this tumor is relatively uncommon, being found in less than 1 per cent of necropsies and constituting about $2\frac{1}{2}$ per cent of all malignancies. On the other hand, this tumor is quite prevalent in Malaysia, Asia, and Africa, particularly in the Bantu tribe, where it appears to be the most common malignant neoplasm. The incidence ranges as high as 55 per cent of all cancers among Bantu men.[1, 3, 18]

It has been suggested that cirrhosis is an etiologic factor, and at one time it was believed that a majority of patients having cancer of the liver had cirrhosis. There is an increased incidence of cancer of the liver among cirrhotics, as approximately 60 to 70 per cent of patients having this neoplasm have concomitant cirrhosis. Furthermore, primary cancer of the liver has been reported in 3.4 to 8.5 per cent of all cases of cirrhosis in the United States, most frequently in the postnecrotic type.[1, 21]

Parasitic infections, nutritional deficiencies, hemachromatosis, hepatotoxic agents, and other factors have been incriminated, but precise documentation of the role of these agents has not been forthcoming.[3]

In the experimental animal, carcinomas of the liver can be produced by a variety of carcinogenic agents, including *p*-dimenthyl-amino-azobenzene (butter yellow). The incidence of this experimental tumor is increased by a high-fat, low-protein diet or a diet deficient in cystine and methionine.[23] There are a number of other carcinogens used in experimental animals, including thiourea and safrole.[3]

Pathology

A single tumor may encompass a large portion of the liver or a significant portion of a single lobe. More common, however, is the multinodular or diffuse form, in which there are multiple nodules of tumor throughout both lobes of the liver (Fig. 41). In some instances, the liver is markedly enlarged, whereas in others the liver is normal in size or even contracted.

The liver is one of the few organs in which multiple gross tumors are commonly seen at the time that the disease is diagnosed. Cancer in other organs usually presents as a single gross tumor, even though micro-

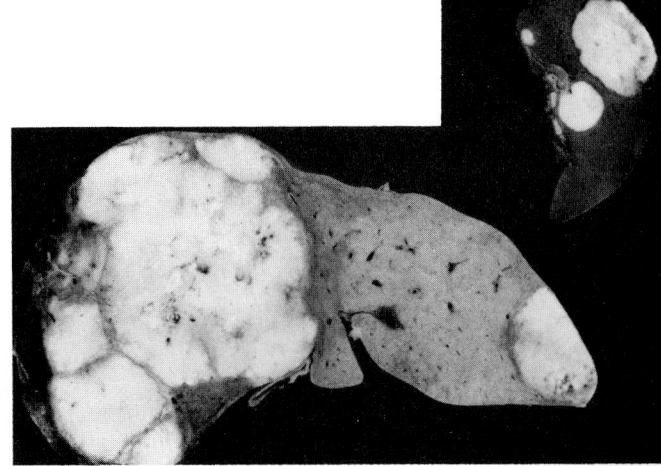

Figure 41. Gross appearance of primary carcinoma of the liver demonstrating multiple nodules involving both lobes.

scopic foci may be found elsewhere. Whether these multiple nodules represent metastases from a primary focus or whether there is simultaneous multifocal origin of the tumor is unknown.

Malignant hepatoma is more common than malignant cholangioma by a ratio of approximately 5 to 1. Histologically, the microscopic appearance may be similar to that of the normal liver, and malignant hepatomas may secrete bile.

Metastases to regional lymph nodes are frequent. Pulmonary, pleural, and peritoneal metastases also occur but are less common. Involvement of veins with secondary thrombosis is common, and tumor emboli may pass through the right heart into the pulmonary artery, resulting in pulmonary infarction. Other extra-abdominal sites such as the brain or bone are occasionally involved. In rare patients, there are widespread extra-abdominal metastases.

Clinical Features

Primary carcinoma of the liver is most frequent in the sixth decade, though it may occur at any age. It is more common in males by a ratio of four to one. Anorexia, loss of weight and strength, and abdominal pain are the most common symptoms, with such symptoms developing gradually, but over a relatively short period of time. Although hematemesis and melena may occur as a result of this disease, these manifestations may be caused by underlying cirrhosis. Hypoglycemia may result from inadequate hepatic function or from secretion of abnormal hormonal substances. Hepatomas may release polypeptide hormones or other abnormal proteins which produce systemic effects. Those reported include erythrocytosis, hypercalcemia, and hyperlipidemia. Rare syndromes include porphyria cutanea tarda, dysfibrinogenemia, and osteoporosis.[22] The most significant physical abnormality is hepatomegaly, which is present in approximately three fourths of the patients. The liver may become tremendously enlarged, and nodularity of the liver may be palpated. As a rule there is little or no tenderness. Splenomegaly is observed in approximately one third of patients. Ascites may develop.

The tumors tend to rupture spontaneously, and the symptoms of intra-abdominal hemorrhage with the development of shock may be the terminal episode.

Laboratory Findings

The most frequent laboratory finding is a rise in the serum alkaline phosphatase concentration, which may become markedly elevated. A rapid rise in this enzyme concentration in a patient with cirrhosis should suggest the possibility of malignant degeneration. Some increase in the serum bilirubin concentration frequently occurs, but this is often relatively modest. All of the other liver function tests may show some abnormality, but these findings are inconsistent. In recent years the development of the measurement of alpha fetoprotein has aided in detection of hepatic malignancy, and an abnormality in this test is highly significant. Unfortunately, it is positive in only 30 per cent of patients in the United States, though it is more frequently positive in patients in other geographic areas. This test becomes negative after successful surgical removal of the tumor and is useful in the follow-up evaluation of surgically treated patients, for conversion of this test from negative to positive suggests recurrent disease.[5, 20]

Roentgenographic Studies

A variety of roentgenographic studies may give clues to the presence of hepatic tumor, including changes in the elevation of the diaphragm seen on simple roentgenograms, and displacement of the stomach or colon documented by barium studies. The diagnostic procedure most commonly used to demonstrate liver tumors is scan of the liver after administration of radioactive materials. Single or multiple nodules may be visualized. A number of radioactive substances have been used, including radioactive gold and radioactive rose bengal dye. In recent years, radioactive technetium has been the agent of choice. Currently, abnormalities of the intrahepatic vessels demonstrated on selective hepatic angiography provide the correct diagnosis in 75 per cent of patients. This study typically reveals displacement and distortion of the vessels in the hepatic arterial tree with the presence of a "tumor stain."[16, 21]

Specific Procedures

When the liver is extensively involved or when single lesions are large, the diagnosis may be made on needle biopsy of the liver. There is a certain hazard in performing this test, however, as these tumors are quite vascular and hemorrhage into the liver or into the peritoneal cavity may result.

Peritoneoscopy has been utilized with varying degrees of success in the diagnosis of hepatic tumors. The majority of surgeons do not utilize this technique, although some have reported excellent results.[15]

Treatment

The treatment of choice is surgical removal of the tumor with an appropriate amount of surrounding normal tissue. Although this can occasionally be accomplished by a segmental resection, it will usually require a total hepatic lobectomy or even an extended hepatic lobectomy.[9, 19]

In a review of a large number of tumors found at surgery and at necropsy, surgical excision could be considered technically in less than 10 per cent. Furthermore, the fact that many of these patients have cirrhosis limits the role of surgery in treatment of this tumor, because in such patients sacrifice of a large volume of hepatic tissue is not compatible with survival. Although applicable in only a limited number of cases, hepatic resection will yield a small percentage of five-year survivals. The best five-year survival rate reported in the literature for the United States is 36 per cent survival following major hepatic resection.[11] For those patients subjected to major hepatic resection, however, most reports do not document results as good as these.[2, 21]

In addition to planned surgical attack for cure, emergency surgical procedures are occasionally required to treat complications such as hemorrhage.

Other treatments have included hepatic artery ligation, ligation of branches of the portal vein, systemic chemotherapy, infusion of chemotherapeutic agents into the hepatic artery with or without arterial ligation, radiation, and, most recently, immunotherapy. There are reports of regression of the tumor mass and apparent prolongation of survival time with each of these techniques. None of these techniques, however, cures the disease, and there is no consensus on the precise indication for their use or the results that may be obtained.[2, 10, 14, 26]

The ideal treatment would appear to be a total hepatectomy and hepatic transplantation. This treatment has been tried, and a few long-term survivals have been reported. Most patients who survive the operative procedure develop recurrence of disease within two years, however. It is possible that the immunosuppressants used for prevention of rejection contribute to the rapid growth of metastases. Thus, this technique is considered experimental at this time.[25]

Prognosis

The prognosis for patients with this tumor is extremely poor. The disease progresses rapidly, and death occurs, on an average, within four to six months after the onset of the first symptom. Since even those patients undergoing surgical therapy are rarely salvaged, the overall five-year survival rate for cancer of the liver is less than 5 per cent.[1, 21]

METASTATIC CARCINOMA

The liver is the organ most often involved with secondary deposits of carcinoma. Metastases may reach the liver through the lymphatics, but are often blood-borne, and the high incidence of metastases may be due in part to the fact that the liver has a double blood supply, being supplied through the systemic arterial system and the portal vein. Metastases to the liver occur in over 50 per cent of patients dying with carcinoma of the intra-abdominal organs, including stomach, pancreas, colon, and kidney. In addition, however, it is a common site of metastasis for tumors outside of the abdominal cavity, particularly those of the lung and breast and melanomas. The liver may also be involved by direct extension of tumors in the stomach.

Metastases to the liver may occur without producing significant clinical symptoms before death. An elevation of the serum alkaline phosphatase concentration suggests the possibility of hepatic involvement, and jaundice may appear. Death from liver failure occurs in the minority of patients, when extensive replacement with tumor occurs. Ascites is common, and the spleen may be palpable. The carcinoid tumor, discussed elsewhere, produces the carcinoid syndrome only after metastasis to the liver has occurred.

On physical examination the liver may be normal in size, even in the presence of numerous metastatic implants. More typically the liver does become enlarged and is palpable and nodular.

Roentgenographic studies for metastatic disease are similar to those used in diagnosis of primary malignancy. Hepatic angiography is useful, though not as diagnostic in this disease as in primary hepatoma. Studies with these radioactive agents will be positive if the nodules are sufficiently large to produce filling defects.

Final diagnosis requires histologic confirmation, and material for examination may be obtained by needle biopsy in some patients. At other times a biopsy may be obtained at laparotomy. The histologic pattern may at times be sufficiently characteristic to allow the pathologist to suspect the site of origin, while highly anaplastic neoplasms give no clue to the original site.

MALIGNANT TUMORS IN CHILDHOOD

Some malignant tumors occurring in childhood are biologically different from those in the adult. A number of special types of malignant tumors occur, including malignant teratoma, embryonal hepatoma, and hepatoblastoma.[7] These tumors seem to grow more slowly than hepatomas in the adult and are more often resectable. In a review by Fish and McCary of 130 malignant tumors occurring in childhood, 70 patients had a tumor localized to one lobe and in only five was cirrhosis present, in contradistinction to the high incidence of cirrhosis in the adult.[8] Surgical resection, therefore, can be performed in a much higher percentage of children than adults and the operation accomplished with greater technical facility. Malignant tumors in childhood, therefore, should be approached aggressively.

The liver has great capacity for regeneration, and following major hepatic resection both in children and in adults regrowth of the liver occurs to a size similar to that of the normal organ. Thus, resections in children do not produce a permanent physiologic handicap.[9, 24]

SARCOMAS OF THE LIVER

Sarcomas of the liver and malignant teratomas are rare lesions. Their clinical features do not differ significantly from those of primary hepatoma, and the diagnosis is made only on histologic examination.

LEUKEMIC INFILTRATION AND LYMPHOMA

The liver is frequently involved by leukemic infiltration or by lymphoma in patients with these diseases. Currently, patients found to have Hodgkin's disease are often submitted to abdominal exploration to evaluate the extent of this type of lymphoma, and a biopsy of the liver with histologic examination is a standard part of a so called "staging laparotomy."

SELECTED REFERENCES

Balasegaram, M.: Management of primary liver cell carcinoma. Am. J. Surg., 130:33, 1975.
Tumors of the liver are more common in some of the Asian countries, and this report of 352 patients with primary liver cell carcinoma is one of the largest in the current literature. The author reports treatment by resection, hepatic artery ligation, chemotherapy, and an early investigation of immunotherapy.

Burdette, W. J.: Neoplasms of the liver. In Schiff, L. (Ed.): Diseases of the Liver, 4th ed. Philadelphia, J. B. Lippincott Co., 1975, pp. 1051–1070.
This is one of the most authoritative publications concerning the liver. The section on neoplasms provides a detailed discussion of this problem by a recognized authority on the subject.

Fish, J. C., and McCary, R. G.: Primary cancer of the liver in childhood. Arch. Surg., 93:355, 1966.
These authors report a collected review of 130 patients with malignant tumors diagnosed in childhood. A detailed evaluation of methods of treatment and results is presented.

Fortner, J. G., et al.: Surgery in liver tumors. Curr. Probl. Surg., June, 1972.
This publication presents a detailed discussion of the problems of liver tumors based upon the extensive experience of the problems at Memorial Hospital in New York, which is one of the largest cancer institutions in the United States.

Henson, F. W., Jr., Gray, H. K., and Dockerty, M. B.: Benign tumors of the liver. I. Adenomas. Surg. Gynecol. Obstet., 103:23, 1956; II. Hemangiomas. 103:27, 1956.
Although this article was written several years ago, it is one of the largest studies of benign tumors of the liver from one institution.

Margolis, S., and Homcy, D.: Systemic manifestations of hepatoma. Medicine, 51:381, 1972.

This is an extensive review article directing attention to some of the less common manifestations of hepatoma. The recognition of these abnormalities, however, will increase the likelihood of diagnosis of this neoplasm.

REFERENCES

1. Al-Sarraf, M., Go, T. S., Kitnior, K., and Vaitkevicius, V. K.: Primary liver cancer. Cancer, 33:574, 1974.
2. Balasegaram, M.: Management of primary liver cell carcinoma. Am. J. Surg., 130:33, 1975.
3. Burdette, W. J.: Neoplasms of the liver. In Schiff, L. (Ed.): Diseases of the Liver, 4th ed. Philadelphia, J. B. Lippincott Co., 1975, pp. 1051–1070.
4. Clatworthy, H. W., Jr., Schiller, M., and Grosfeld, J. L.: Primary liver tumors in infancy and childhood: 41 cases variously treated. Arch. Surg., 109:143, 1974.
5. Curutchet, H. P., Turz, J. J., Kay, S., and Lawrence, W., Jr.: Primary liver cancer. Surgery, 70:467, 1971.
6. Dehner, L. P., and Ishak, K. G.: Vascular tumors of the liver in infants and children: Study of 30 cases and review of the literature. Arch. Pathol., 92:101, 1971.
7. Ein, S. H., and Stephens, C. A.: Malignant liver tumors in children. J. Pediatr. Surg., 9:491, 1974.
8. Fish, J. C., and McCary, R. G.: Primary cancer of the liver in childhood. Arch. Surg., 93:355, 1966.
9. Fortner, J. G., et al.: Surgery in liver tumors. Curr. Probl. Surg., June, 1972.
10. Fortner, J. G., Mulcare, R. J., Solis, A., Watson, R. C., and Golbey, R. B.: Treatment of primary and secondary liver cancer by hepatic artery ligation and infusion chemotherapy. Ann. Surg., 178:161, 1973.
11. Foster, J. H.: Survival after liver resection for cancer. Cancer, 26:493, 1970.
12. Henson, F. W., Jr., Gray, H. K., and Dockerty, M. B.: Benign tumors of the liver. I. Adenomas. Surg. Gynecol. Obstet., 103:23, 1956.
13. Henson, F. W., Jr., Gray, H. K. and Dockerty, M. B.: Benign tumors of the liver. II. Hemangiomas. Surg. Gynecol. Obstet., 103:27, 1956.
14. Honjo, I., Suzuki, T., Ozawa, K., Takasan, H., Kitamura, O., and Ishikawa, T.: Ligation of a branch of the portal vein for carcinoma of the liver. Ann. J. Surg., 130:296, 1975.
15. Kato, M., Sugawara, I., Okada, A., Kuwata, K., Satani, M., Okamoto, E., and Manabe, H.: Hemangioma of the liver: Diagnosis with combined use of laparoscopy and hepatic arteriography. Am. J. Surg., 129:698, 1975.
16. Kim, D. K., McSweeney, J., Yeh, S. D. J., and Fortner, J. G.: Tumors of the liver as demonstrated by angiography, scan and laparotomy. Surg. Gynecol. Obstet., 141:409, 1975.
17. Leonidas, J. C., Strauss, L., and Beck, A. R.: Vascular tumors of the liver in newborns: Pediatric emergency. Am. J. Dis. Child., 125:507, 1973.
18. Lin, T. Y.: Primary cancer of the liver. Scand. J. Gastroenterol. (Supple.), 6:223, 1970.
19. Lin, T. Y.: Results of 107 hepatic lobectomies with preliminary report on the use of a clamp to reduce blood loss. Ann. Surg., 177:413, 1973.
20. Lin, T. Y., Chu, S. H., Chen, M. F., and Chen, C. H.: Serum alpha fetaglobulin and primary cancer of the liver in Taiwan. Cancer, 30:435, 1972.
21. Linder, G. T., Crook, J. N., and Cohn, I., Jr.: Primary liver carcinoma. Cancer, 33:1624, 1974.
22. Margolis, S., and Homcy, C.: Systemic manifestations of hepatoma. Medicine, 51:381, 1972.
23. Opie, E. L.: Influence of diet on the production of tumors of the liver by butter yellow. J. Exp. Med., 80:219, 1944.
24. Price, J. B., Takeshige, K., Max, M. H., and Voorhees, A. B., Jr.: Glucagon as a portal factor modifying hepatic regeneration. Surgery, 72:74, 1972.
25. Starzl, T. E., Putnam, C. W., and Corman, J. L.: Transplantation of the liver. In Schiff L. (Ed.): Diseases of the Liver, 4th ed. Philadelphia, J. B. Lippincott Co., 1975, pp. 1147–1172.
26. Tandon, R. N., Bunnell, I. L., and Cooper, R. G.: The treatment of metastatic carcinoma of the liver by the percutaneous selective hepatic artery infusion of 5-fluorouracil. Surgery, 73:118, 1973.

IV

HEMOBILIA

Thomas J. Whelan, Jr., M.D.

Hemobilia, defined by Sandblom in 1948, is manifested by upper gastrointestinal bleeding. The origin of the bleeding is in the intra- or extrahepatic biliary tract or, rarely, in the pancreas. Classically, hemobilia refers only to significant, sometimes massive bleeding, producing a recognizable symptom complex, consisting of a triad of colicky right upper quadrant pain, hematemesis and/or melena, and jaundice. These symptoms most commonly are intermittent, recurring repeatedly, until successfully treated. Usually there are several days to weeks between episodes. The patient often is able to predict the gastrointestinal hemorrhage because of its temporal relationship to the abdominal colic, occurring shortly after the latter. A lesser degree of biliary tract bleeding may cause chronic anemia without development of the clinical triad.

Blood may enter the biliary tract from either a point within the liver, the extrahepatic bile ducts, the gallbladder, or the pancreas. The incidence of the origin of hemobilia is:

Liver	53 per cent
Gallbladder	23 per cent
Extrahepatic bile ducts	22 per cent
Pancreas	2 per cent

The cause of hemobilia is trauma in about half the cases, and inflammation, calculi, tumor, or hepatic artery aneurysm in the other half. Of 545 cases collected by Sandblom in 1973, the etiology of hemobilia is as follows:

Inflammation	153
Gall stone	55
Tumor	28
Aneurysm	40
Traffic accidents	100
Other accidents	82
Operative trauma	78
Unknown	9

PATHOLOGY AND PATHOGENESIS

The lesion is basically an arteriobiliary fistula, although venobiliary fistula has been reported. The fistula may be by direct communication, via an aneurysm, or across a cavity in the liver in the wall of which is located an open artery and an open bile duct.

Although the erosion of an extrahepatic hepatic artery aneurysm, either true or false, into the bile ducts is easy to understand, the pathogenesis of an arteriobiliary fistula inside the liver secondary to trauma or inflammation may be more obscure. The segmental anatomy of the liver is pertinent in this regard, since the hepatic artery and the hepatic ducts within the liver accompany each other. The fistula may be produced initially by simultaneous laceration of a branch of the hepatic artery and a branch of a bile duct at the time of trauma, establishing an early communication between the two. It may also occur later, owing to secondary erosion of a vessel and a duct in the peripheral zone of necrosis in the wall of an expanding liver cavity. The late development of an intrahepatic false aneurysm secondary to an injury to the arterial wall, which initially is nondisruptive, is another mechanism which, when it expands and produces pressure necrosis of an intrahepatic bile duct, eventuates in hemobilia, which is delayed in appearance.

In addition, the lytic action of bile is important in the perpetuation of the lesion. This accounts for the unlikely occurrence of spontaneous healing by thrombosis of the arterial defect.

CLINICAL MANIFESTATIONS

Despite the causative factor, all cases have similar symptoms and signs when hemobilia supervenes. There is usually a background of discomfort or dull pain in the right upper quadrant of the abdomen or in the epigastrium. There may or may not be an enlarged liver or mass within the liver. The gallbladder may become transiently palpable but need not be. The classic symptoms of the entity may occur de novo or against the preceding background. These consist of sudden onset of severe colicky right upper quadrant pain, followed within a matter of minutes to hours by hematemesis and melena when bleeding is severe, or melena alone with lesser bleeding. The vomited clots on rare occasions have resembled the cast of the biliary tree, with slender, sometimes bifurcated shapes. The severe colicky pain is relieved soon after the overt appearance of gastrointestinal bleeding. Jaundice is variably present, depending upon the degree of common duct obstruction from clots and sequestered liver tissue. Such acute episodes are usually repeated again and again until surgical treatment is instituted. Sandblom described a female patient who had repeated episodes of hemobilia for 36 years. Most cases, however, have such massive bleeding that surgical therapy becomes mandatory much earlier.

DIAGNOSIS

There are several procedures that are available preoperatively to substantiate the presumptive clinical diagnosis of hemobilia. By far the most accurate and most helpful in surgical management is hepatic or celiac angiography. Contrast material escaping from a

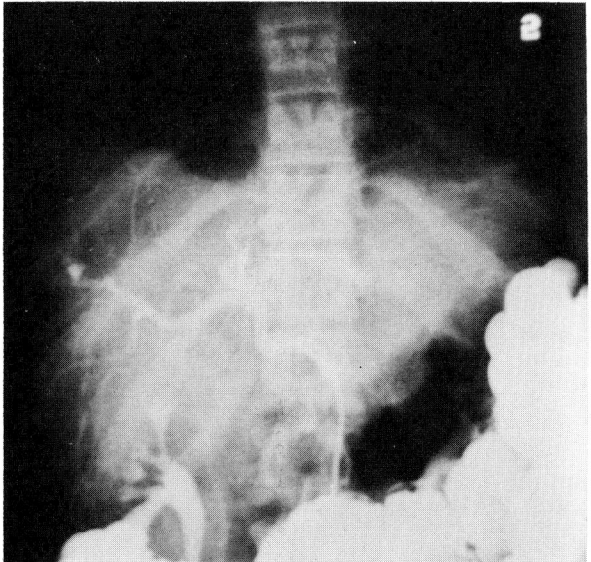

Figure 42. Hepatic angiography demonstrates extravasation from a peripheral branch of the right hepatic artery within the liver. This study is diagnostic of an arteriobiliary fistula in the clinical setting of hemobilia.

branch of the hepatic artery and collecting either in an aneurysm sac or in an hepatic cavity is demonstrated in most cases of hemobilia (Fig. 42).

Liver scintiscan may demonstrate a filling defect, respresenting a liver cavity containing necrotic tissue, clots, and bile (Fig. 43). This is of particular value in hemobilia secondary to trauma, tumor, or inflammation.

The third study, of use in some cases, is cholangiography, either intravenous (if the patient is not jaundiced), transampullary retrograde, or percutaneous transhepatic. The latter procedure, however, has actually been incriminated in producing hemobilia, even though it is sometimes helpful in the diagnosis. The retrograde technique has the additional advantage of visualizing bleeding from the ampulla if hemobilia is present at the time. There are two possible cholangiographic findings that aid in the diagnosis: (1) radiolucent irregular filling defects in the bile ducts and/or gallbladder, representing clots, or (2) an hepatic cavity in communication with the bile ducts (Fig. 44).

An upper gastrointestinal series is important for its failure to demonstrate other lesions in the upper gastrointestinal tract. On occasion, a characteristic extrinsic filling defect is noted impinging upon the first portion of the duodenum and the postbulbar region by a gallbladder and/or common duct distended by clots. Esophagogastroduodenoscopy is indispensable in ruling out other more frequent sources of upper gastrointestinal bleeding.

Despite the accuracy of preoperative diagnosis with the above measures, there will continue to be cases which are operated upon without hemobilia having been considered. At operation, the diagnosis may be made by palpation of a liver mass, demonstration of a liver cavity in communication with the bile ducts by operative cholangiography (Fig. 45), and aspiration of old, liquid blood and small particulate fragments of

Figure 43. Liver scintiscan demonstrates in this case a large filling defect, the site of a liver cavity containing necrotic liver tissue, and old blood and bile. This finding, although suggestive of the diagnosis in the proper clinical setting, is not diagnostic.

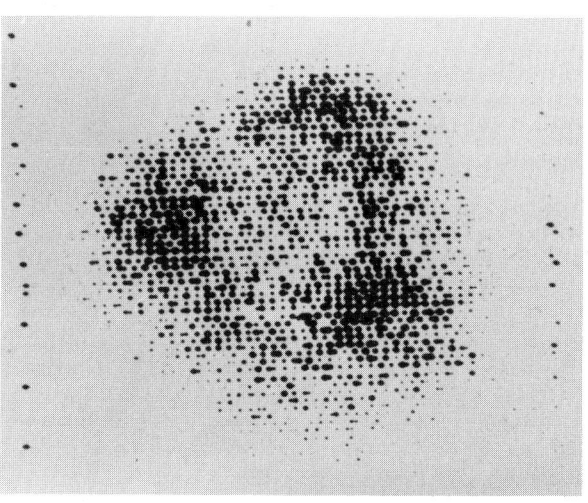

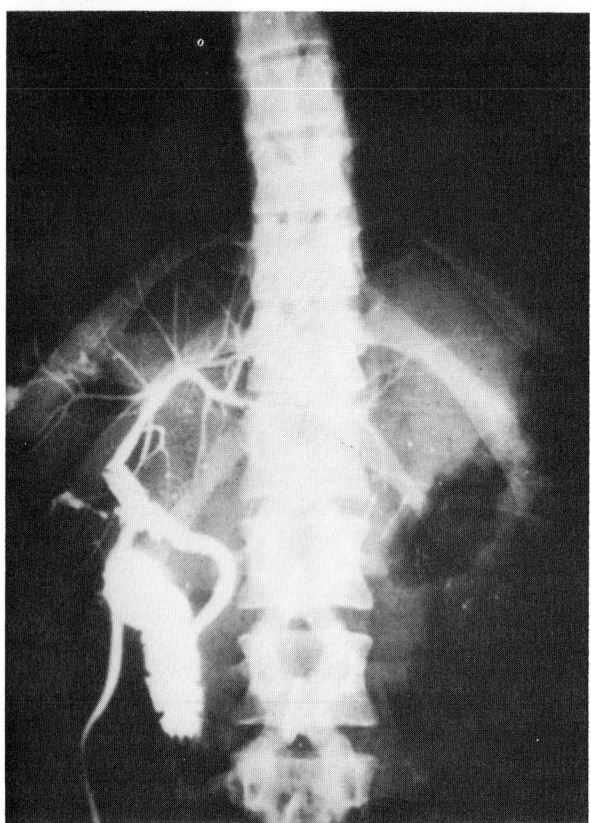

Figure 44. T-tube cholangiogram demonstrates the defect in the peripheral bile duct at the same site as the arterial defect shown in Figure 42.

Figure 45. Operative cholangiogram demonstrates a large cavity within the left lobe of the liver in communication with the left hepatic duct. A vascular clamp occludes the distal common duct, allowing better filling of the proximal ducts.

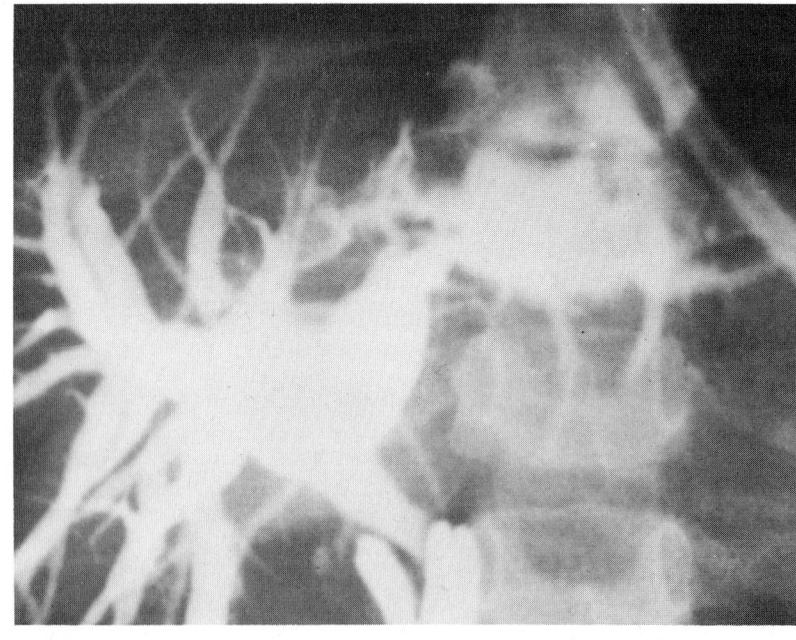

liver from such a cavity. Intraoperative hepatic angiography, although dangerous because of friability of the artery, may sometimes, if other measures fail, aid in the diagnosis at operation. Finally, if bleeding is occurring actively, exploration of the common duct may indicate not only the blood within the ducts but also the hepatic duct from which it arises. Temporary clamping of either of the hepatic artery branches may assess whether active bleeding is controllable by ligation.

ETIOLOGY

Trauma

Over half the cases of hemobilia are due to trauma, and blunt trauma is the usual mechanism.

Blunt trauma may produce the lesion causing hemobilia by either (1) central liver rupture, or (2) deep liver rupture, including rupture of Glissen's capsule. Approximately one third of the cases are secondary to central rupture. In cases of central rupture, the initial clinical picture is one of mild to moderate upper abdominal discomfort that may gradually increase in severity. At no time in these early days to weeks is laparotomy necessary. After a latent period of six days to four months, overt hemobilia with its attendant dramatic and classic symptomatology supervenes. Two thirds of the cases due to blunt trauma, however, have had an earlier laparotomy because of intraperitoneal bleeding from a liver laceration involving the deep liver tissue and the capsule. The setting for hemobilia has been produced in these cases by the surgeon when he has not controlled bleeding in the depths of the liver and has sutured the liver laceration superficially, thus creating a deep cavity within the liver filled with contused, disrupted, and bleeding liver tissue. A lacerated liver with capsular involvement may also spontaneously heal superficially by sealing of the capsule by the diaphragm or other surrounding tissue, leaving unhealed the depths of the laceration. It is probably remarkable that hemobilia is not more often produced, but it is most rare after liver injury despite the fact that trauma most frequently produces it.

Penetrating trauma, either gunshot wounds, shell fragment wounds, or stab wounds, may also cause hemobilia. The lesion so produced may be intrahepatic and similar to that produced by blunt trauma, but frequently it may produce a false aneurysm owing to an injury to the hepatic artery or one of its branches. A special type of injury is that produced by needle biopsy. In the reported cases, hemobilia occurred early, within three days of needle biopsy. This has occurred regardless of the type of biopsy needle used.

Finally, surgical trauma has accounted for 17 per cent of all reported cases of hemobilia. This has usually followed cholecystectomy with or without common duct exploration, although operations upon liver, stomach, duodenum, and pancreas have also caused the lesion. The most vulnerable area during operations on the biliary tract is the porta hepatis. The hepatic artery, and particularly the right hepatic artery when it lies anterior to the common duct, are susceptible to injury. This injury may be incisional trauma with partial thickness injury of the artery, or, more frequently, a suture plunged through it at the time of choledochotomy closure or when attempting to control troublesome bleeding. The result is an aneurysm that later ruptures either intraperitoneally or into the common duct, producing hemobilia. Seven deaths occurred among 19 cases of hemobilia due to surgically produced arterial lesions. The diagnosis may be obvious if a T-tube is still in place within the common duct.

A second region that is vulnerable to injury is the ductal system within the liver. In exploring for and extracting intrahepatic biliary tract calculi, disruptive injury to the duct may occur and, since extrahepatic arterial branches accompany the ducts, concomitant injury to the artery is likely. Often the T-tube is blamed for causing an erosion of the common duct in such a case, whereas the lesion is more proximal at the hepatic duct level within the liver. Proper localization of the lesion with angiography and T-tube cholangiography is necessary.

Aneurysm

There are causes other than trauma for development of aneurysms of the hepatic artery or its branches. In a series of 227 cases of hepatic artery aneurysm, the following causes were noted: arteriosclerosis (34 per cent), trauma (18 per cent), mycosis (16 per cent), and other causes (21 per cent).

Rare cases of aneurysm due to idiopathic arteritis, fibromuscular hyperplasia, and congenital weakness have been reported. More recently, some drug abusers have been noted to have multiple visceral artery aneurysms. Methamphetamine given intravenously has been suspect in this regard. The location of hepatic artery aneurysms are:

Extrahepatic	75 per cent
Intrahepatic	12.5 per cent
Combined	12.5 per cent

In another report of 176 hepatic artery aneurysms, 103 became evident upon rupture. Of these 103 ruptured hepatic artery aneurysms, 45 bled intraperitoneally, 43 bled into the biliary ducts or gallbladder, and 15 ruptured into the stomach, duodenum, portal vein, or a combination of the above.

In cases presenting with hemobilia due to hepatic artery aneurysm, findings of an upper abdominal mass and a systolic bruit in the epigastrium or right upper quadrant are highly suggestive but require confirmation with angiography to establish the diagnosis and the surgical management.

Before 1950 only three of 87 patients with hepatic artery aneurysm survived. Since 1950, 41 of 92 patients have been salvaged by operation.

Inflammation

In the Orient, chronic cholangitis and pericholangiolar abscesses secondary to parasites (ascaris and *Clonorchis sinensis*) have produced hemobilia. The frequency in these countries is such that, with more adequate reporting, this would probably prove to be the leading cause of hemobilia worldwide. This cause, however, is relatively unknown in North America and

Europe. Amebic abscess and tuberculosis of the liver have also produced hemobilia.

Gallstones may erode the gallbladder wall or the common duct wall, producing hemobilia. When bleeding is confined to the gallbladder alone, the term more properly is hemocholecyst and the triad of hemobilia is lacking. Only 50 cases of hemobilia due to calculi have been reported, and these are cases in which the stones eroded into the cystic artery or into another viscus.

Cholecystitis glandularis proliferans or hemorrhagic cholecystitis may cause bleeding into the biliary tract but is a very rare cause of hemobilia, only 24 cases having been reported.

Pseudocysts of the pancreas may erode into a significant artery, such as the splenic or gastroduodenal artery. This complication is highly lethal. When this blood enters the pancreatic duct and common bile duct, hemobilia occurs.

Tumors

Twenty-eight cases of tumor producing hemobilia have been reported by Sandblom. Hemobilia does not occur with metastatic tumors to the liver. It may occur with metastases to the gallbladder, cholangiocarcinoma, hepatoma, angioma, and diffuse polyposis of the bile ducts with hepatoma secondary to cirrhosis being most significant in this regard.

MANAGEMENT

The management of hemobilia is primarily surgical. There are three procedures used to control hemobilia of hepatic origin:

1. Resection of that portion of the liver containing the arteriobiliary fistula if localized to one lobe or segment.

2. Opening of the liver cavity, with suture ligation of the involved artery and bile duct within the cavity and drainage of the cavity in centrally located lesions.

3. Ligation of the common hepatic artery or of the right or left hepatic artery in centrally located lesions or when resection is hazardous.

Although mortality with hepatic resection has been higher than with the other methods, there has been surer control of hemobilia with the method. Rebleeding has occurred more frequently with hepatic artery ligation, either within the intrahepatic cavity or in the extrahepatic location. In the most extensive review, the following results were obtained with each method:

	Cases	Rebled	Died
Vessels sutured in liver cavity	50	25	12
Ligation of hepatic artery (most of these were right or left branch)	30	10	4
Hepatic resection	30	2	6

If hemobilia is due to an hepatic artery aneurysm, proximal and distal ligation and resection of the aneurysm are preferable if the lesion is proximal to the gastroduodenal artery or if the aneurysm arises in either the right or left branch of the hepatic artery. Col-

lateral circulation maintains an adequate blood supply to the liver when sites of ligation are as noted above. That portion of the hepatic artery between the origin of the gastroduodenal artery and the bifurcation into right and left branches is the most vulnerable site in causing liver necrosis when ligation is employed. In this location reconstruction of the artery should be attempted. In all such cases careful repair of the eroded common bile duct over a T-tube should accompany the arterial surgery.

In the rare patient with hemobilia arising in the gallbladder, cholecystectomy is curative; and in the even rarer case arising in a pseudocyst of the pancreas, the cyst is opened, the offending artery suture ligated, and the cyst decompressed to the outside or into a defunctionalized loop of jejunum or adjacent viscus.

Rarely, nonoperative management has been successful in children, but it must be used only if bleeding is not life-threatening and careful monitoring with repeated angiography is performed. In earlier reported cases, this possiblity was suggested when, despite the use of nondefinitive procedures, i.e., gastrectomy, cholecystectomy with or without choledochotomy, for managing hemobilia of liver origin, the patient recovered. It was noted at that time that recovery was more likely in children.

SELECTED REFERENCES

Bismuth, H.: Hemobilia. N. Engl. J. Med., *288*:617, 1973.
This paper is an excellent review of hemobilia, with clarification of terms, sites of bleeding, and various causes of hemobilia. Clinical manifestations, methods of diagnosis, and treatment are described. Most specifically, the paper emphasizes three unanswered questions: (1) Which forms of hemobilia, if any, do not require surgical therapy? (2) Is ligation of the hepatic artery adequate therapy to control hemobilia? (3) What are the respective indications for hepatic artery ligation versus liver resection?

Hendren, W. H., Warshaw, A. L., Fleischli, D. J., and Bartlett, M.: Traumatic hemobilia: Non-operative management with healing documented by serial angiography. Ann. Surg., *174*:991, 1971.
This paper for the first time emphasizes nonsurgical treatment in childhood cases, provided that serial angiography monitors progressive healing. Two such cases are reported. These were treated with transfusions only, one five-year-old child requiring 1000 ml. whole blood replacement and the other, a six-year-old child, requiring 2500 ml. Serial angiography demonstrated spontaneous healing of an offending lesion in the right hepatic lobe over a two-month period in the first case and healing within three weeks in the second.

Sandblom, P.: Hemobilia (Biliary Tract Hemorrhage): History, Pathology, Diagnosis, Treatment. Springfield, Ill., Charles C Thomas, Publisher, 1972.
This is a classic monograph written by the master surgeon who first described hemobilia.

Sandblom, P.: Hemobilia. Surg. Clin. North Am., *53*:1191, 1973.
In this paper the author, who first described and used the term "hemobilia" in 1948, analyzes 545 cases of hemobilia reported since 1654. Data presented shows that the condition is not only described more frequently but also is more often successfully treated by operation. This source has more hard data regarding etiology and results of various methods of treatment than any other. Mortality is reported to be under 20 per cent when adequate operation is performed following angiographic localization of the lesion.

Seel, D. J., Jehoom, Y., and Lee, K. Y.: Inflammatory hemobilia. Surgery, *66*:821, 1969.
This is a report from Korea on left hepatic duct cholangitis and pericholangiolar abscesses with secondary erosion of arteries and

*ducts producing hemobilia. This is the most recent report empha-
sizing the importance of ascariasis in producing hemobilia due to
inflammatory lesions. This type of lesion is infrequently reported in
the English literature, yet it is a frequent lesion in the Orient.*

REFERENCES

1. Ball, T. J., Mutchnik, M. G., Cohen, G. M., and Burrel, M.: Hemobilia following percutaneous liver biopsy. Gastroenterology, *68*:1297, 1975.
2. Berenson, M. M., and Freston, J. W.: Intrahepatic artery aneurysm associated with hemobilia. Gastroenterology, *66*:254, 1974.
3. Butterfield, W. C., and Chou, U.: Hemobilia associated with hemorrhagic cholecystitis in a patient with alcoholic cirrhosis. Conn. Med., *35*:295, 1971.
4. Hughes, J. H., Guzman, J. G., and Roberts, S. S.: Massive hemobilia from ruptured hepatic artery aneurysm. J.A.M.A., *214*:913, 1970.
5. Levinson, J. D., Olsen, G., Terman, J. W., Cleaveland, C. R., Graham, C. P., Jr., and Breen, K. J.: Hemobilia secondary to percutaneous liver biopsy. A.M.A. Arch. Intern. Med., *130*:396, 1972.
6. Powell, S. J., Sutton, J. B., and Lautre, G.: Haemobilia in amoebic liver abscess. South Afr. Med. J., *47*:1555, 1973.
7. Sandblom, P.: Hemorrhage into biliary tract following trauma: "Traumatic hemobilia." Surgery, *42*:571, 1948.
8. Sparkman, R. S.: Massive hemobilia following traumatic rupture of the liver. Report of a case and review of the literature. Ann. Surg., *138*:899, 1953.
9. Stratoudakis, A. C., Kittle, C. F., and Anagnostopoulos, C. E.: Haemobilia from ruptured hepatic artery aneurysm. A complication after aortic valve replacement. J. R. Coll. Surg. Edinb., *19*:305, 1974.
10. Whelan, T. J., and Gillespie, J. T.: Treatment of traumatic hemobilia. Ann. Surg., *162*:920, 1966.
11. Wilkinson, G. M., Mikkelson, W. P., and Berne, C. J.: The treatment of post-traumatic hemobilia by ligation of the common hepatic artery. Surg. Clin. North Am., *48*:1337, 1968.
12. Winchester, D. P., Seed, R. W., Bergan, J. J., and Conn, J., Jr.: Jaundice, hemobilia and hemoperitoneum. Consequences of rupture of hepatic artery aneurysm. Am. J. Surg., *120*:384, 1970.

36

THE BILIARY SYSTEM

Marshall J. Orloff, M.D.

ANATOMY

The biliary system and liver develop together from a diverticulum that arises in the embryo from the ventral floor of the foregut and extends into the septum transversum. The caudal portion of this diverticulum becomes the gallbladder, cystic duct, and common bile duct, whereas the cranial portion develops into the liver and hepatic bile ducts.

The gallbladder is a thin-walled, pear-shaped organ covered by peritoneum and attached to the the inferior surfaces of the right and quadrate lobes of the liver. Normally, it is 7 to 10 cm. long and 3 to 5 cm. in diameter and has a capacity of 30 to 60 ml. Anatomically, it is divided into a fundus or tip, which protrudes from the anterior edge of the liver, a corpus or body, an infundibulum called Hartmann's pouch, and a narrow neck that leads into the cystic duct (Fig. 1). Topographically, the fundus of the gallbladder is located behind the ninth right costal cartilage at the junction of the costal margin with the right border of the rectus abdominis muscle.

The cystic duct from the gallbladder is about 2 to 4 cm. long and contains prominent mucosal folds called spiral folds or valves of Heister. It is questionable whether these folds have any valvular function in regulating bile flow. The cystic duct joins the right lateral aspect of the common hepatic duct to form the common bile duct (Fig. 1).

The extrahepatic bile duct system orginates from the liver as the right and left hepatic ducts, each of which is 1 to 2 cm. long and drains the respective lobe of the liver. The two ducts join to form the common hepatic duct, a 2- to 4-cm.-long structure in the porta hepatis. The union of the common hepatic duct with the cystic duct gives rise to the common bile duct, which is 8 to 15 cm. long and 5 to 10 mm. in outside diameter. The common bile duct descends in the hepatoduodenal ligament to the right of the hepatic artery and anterior to the portal vein, passes behind the first part of the duodenum and through the pancreas, and enters the descending duodenum on its posteromedial aspect about 10 cm. distal to the pylorus at the papilla of Vater. The choledochoduodenal junction is an oblique passageway through the duodenal wall occupied by the common bile duct and the main pancreatic duct of Wirsung. These two ducts usually join in a common channel, the ampulla of Vater, which opens into the duodenum at the papilla of Vater; however, the two ducts may join before entering the duodenal wall or may empty into the duodenum through separate openings. The muscle of the choledochoduodenal junction, called the sphincter of Oddi, regulates the flow of bile and consists of several components. The two major components are the sphincter ductus choledochi, which surrounds the common bile duct within the duodenal wall proximal to its junction with the pancreatic duct, and the sphincter ampullae, which surrounds the common ampulla of Vater (Fig. 2).

The arterial blood supply to the common bile duct comes mainly from the retroduodenal artery, a branch of the gastroduodenal artery. The gallbladder is nourished by the cystic artery, which originates from the right hepatic artery, to the right of and behind the common hepatic duct, and divides into anterior and posterior branches. During cholecystectomy, the cystic artery is usually found in the cystic triangle of Calot, a space bounded by the liver, the common hepatic duct, and the cystic duct. The triangle contains the right hepatic artery with its cystic artery branch, a large lymph node, and, in its depths, the right branch of the portal vein. Venous drainage from the extrahepatic biliary system is into the portal vein. Lymphatic vessels from the gallbladder join those from the liver to empty into the cisterna chyli and thoracic duct. Lymph nodes at the neck of the gallbladder, at the junction of the cystic duct and hepatic ducts, and at the end of the common duct play a prominent role in the lymphatic drainage and are regularly enlarged in cholecystitis. The innervation of the biliary system is similar to that of the liver. Vagal stimulation causes contraction of the gallbladder, whereas sympathetic stimulation produces the reverse actions. The effect of vagal stimulation on the sphincter of Oddi is variable.

Histologically, the gallbladder consists of a mucosa of columnar epithelium, a muscularis, a subserosa, and a serosa. Mucous glands are found only in the neck. Gallbladder inflammation characteristically pro-

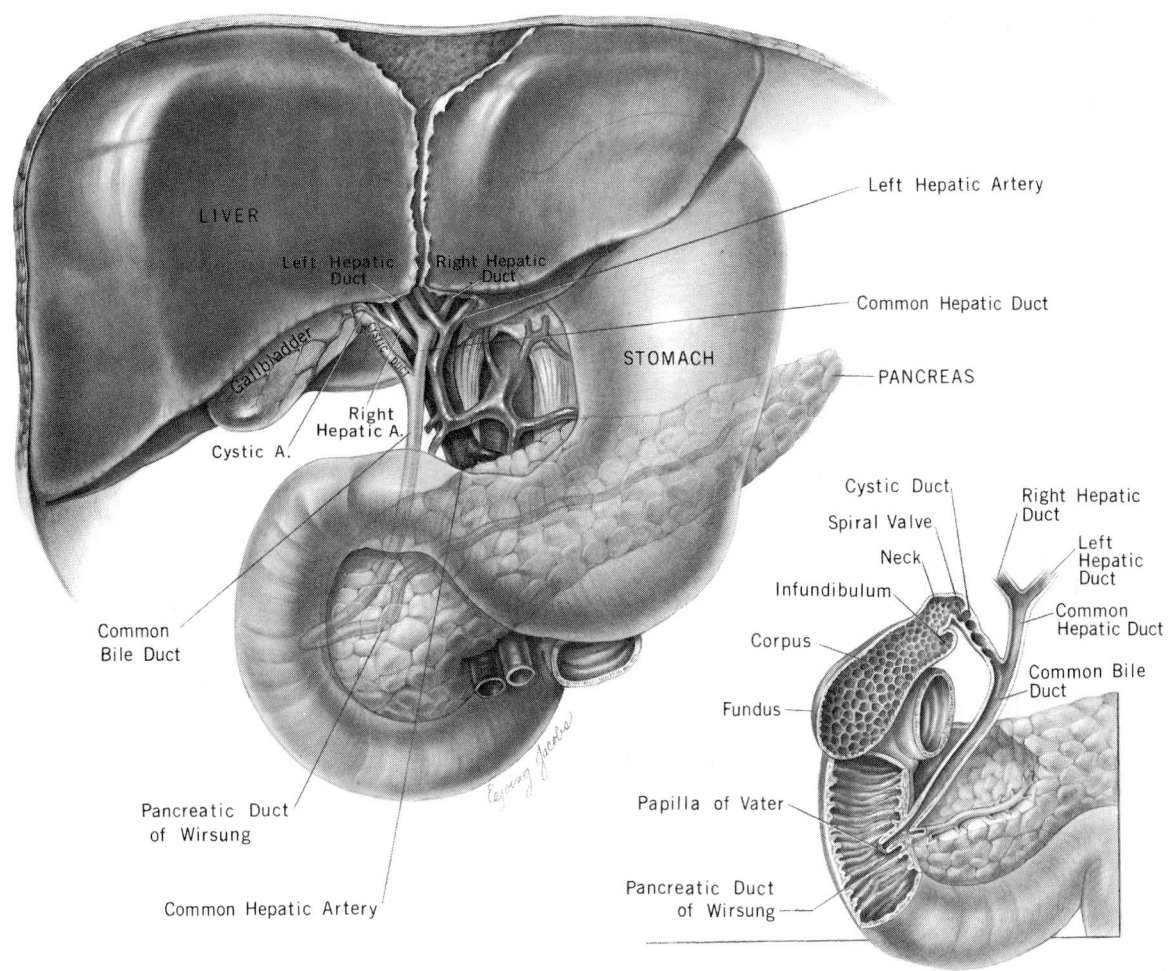

Figure 1. Anatomy of the biliary system.

duces invaginations of the mucosa into the muscularis called Rokitansky-Aschoff sinuses. The bile ducts are lined by columnar epithelium and contain mucous glands.

A most striking and, for the surgeon, dangerous feature of the anatomy of the extrahepatic biliary system is its *variability*. Variations in the bile ducts, cystic artery, and hepatic artery are very common. For this reason, biliary operations require extremely careful technique. Anomalies of the gallbladder are rare and include congenital absence, duplications, left-sided gallbladder with the cystic duct entering the left side of the common bile duct or left hepatic duct, and location of the gallbladder partially or completely within the liver. "Floating gallbladder," in which the vesicle is suspended from the liver by a peritoneal mesentery, is the most common anomaly and occasionally results in acute torsion of the organ.

Anomalies of the cystic duct are shown in Figure 3. Some of these variations are common and the surgeon must be aware of them in performing cholecystectomy. Variations in the other extrahepatic bile ducts are of less surgical significance, although they occur in one of 10 humans. The most important common anomaly of the bile ducts consists of one or more accessory hepatic ducts, which enter the gallbladder directly from the liver. If such ducts are overlooked during excision of the gallbladder, persistent leakage of bile into the peritoneal cavity may result. This possibility constitutes one reason for draining the gallbladder bed following cholecystectomy.

Anomalies of the hepatic arteries were discussed in the previous chapter, and those of the cystic artery are shown in Figure 4. Variations in the origin and location of the arterial blood supply to the gallbladder are very common.

Injuries to the bile ducts during cholecystectomy usually result from failure to recognize anatomic variations in the biliary tree and its blood supply. The consequences of such injuries are often very serious, and they underscore the importance to surgeons of a thorough knowledge of anatomy. The mechanisms whereby some of these injuries occur are illustrated in Figure 5.

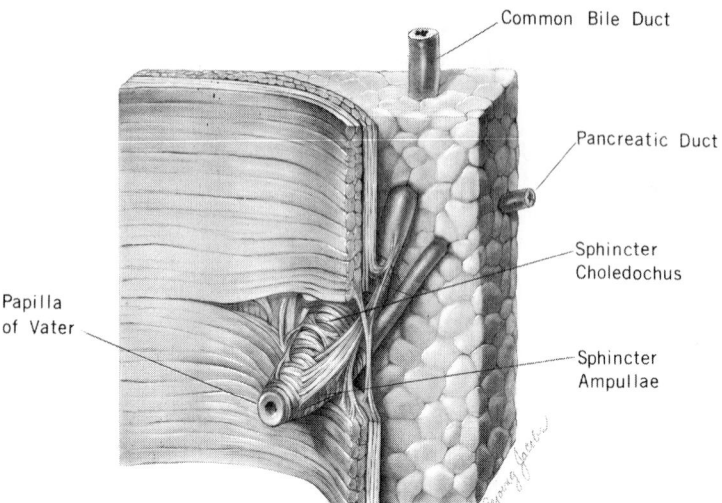

Common Bile Duct

Pancreatic Duct

Sphincter Choledochus

Sphincter Ampullae

Papilla of Vater

Figure 2. Choledochoduodenal junction.

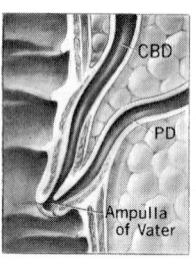
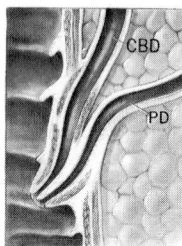
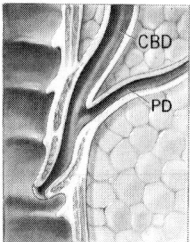

Figure 3. Anomalies of the cystic duct.

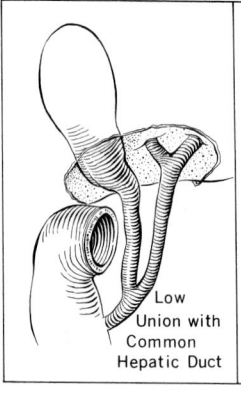

Low Union with Common Hepatic Duct

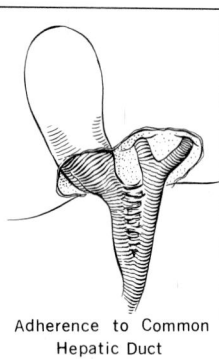

Adherence to Common Hepatic Duct

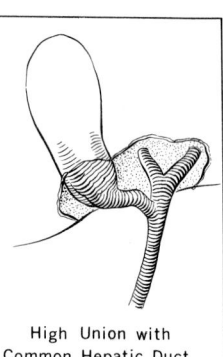

High Union with Common Hepatic Duct

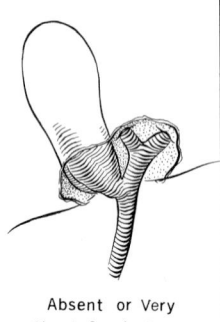

Absent or Very Short Cystic Duct

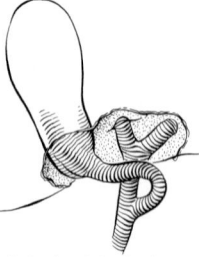

Anterior Spiral with Union on Left Side of Common Hepatic Duct

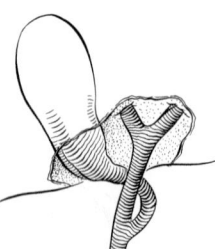

Posterior Spiral with Union on Left Side of Common Hepatic Duct

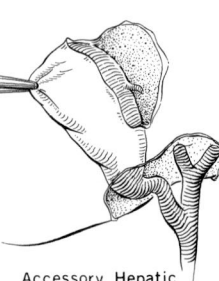

Accessory Hepatic Duct Entering the Gallbladder

E. G. JACOBS

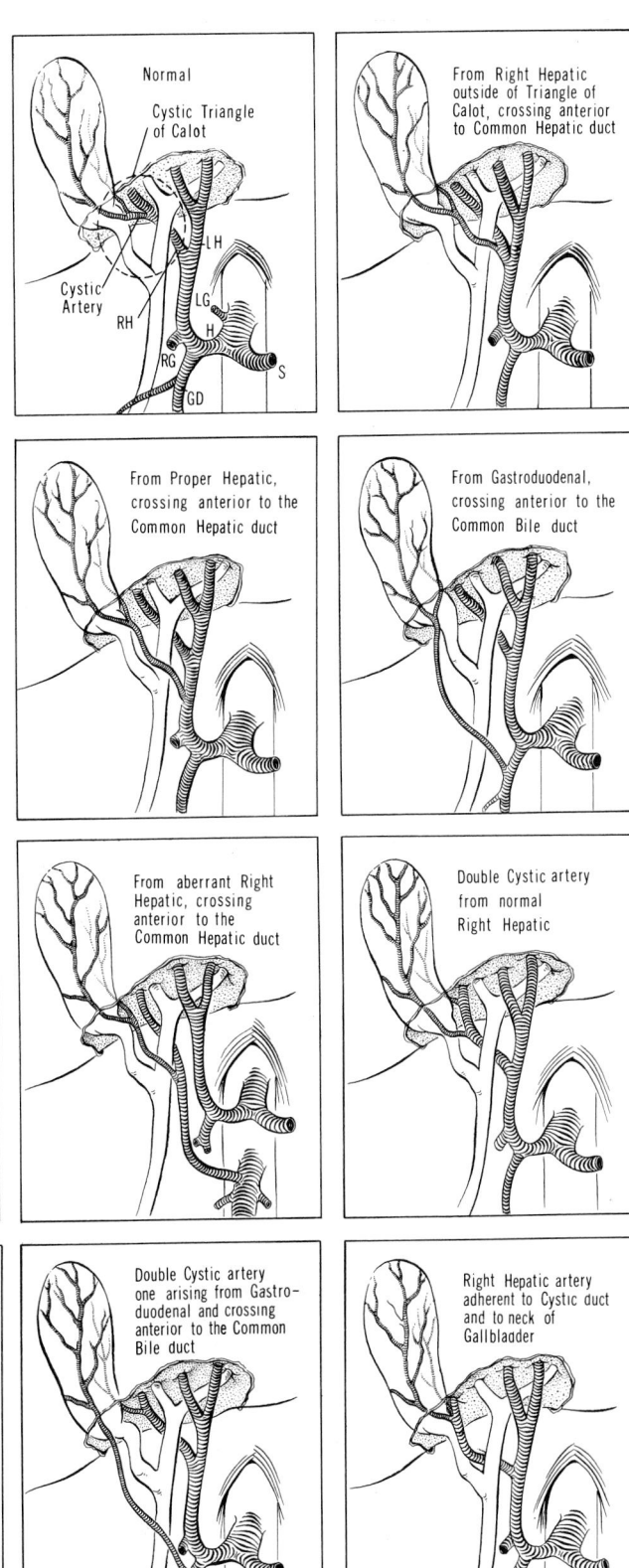

Figure 4. Anomalies of the cystic artery.

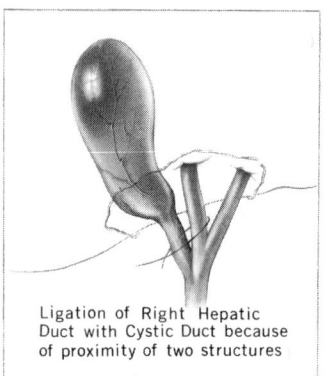

Ligation of Right Hepatic Duct with Cystic Duct because of proximity of two structures

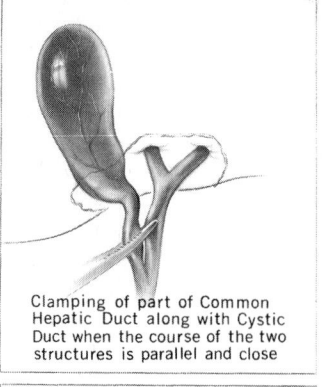

Clamping of part of Common Hepatic Duct along with Cystic Duct when the course of the two structures is parallel and close

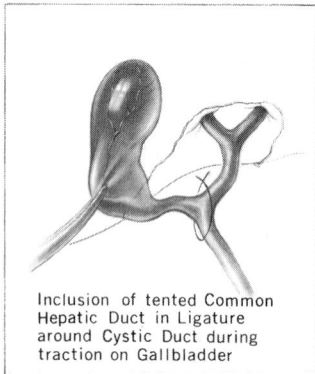

Inclusion of tented Common Hepatic Duct in Ligature around Cystic Duct during traction on Gallbladder

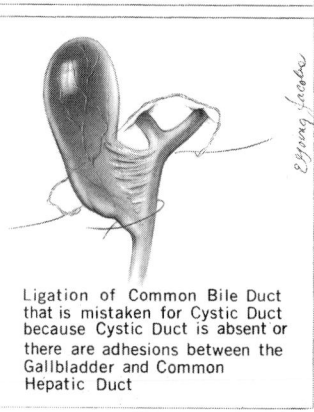

Ligation of Common Bile Duct that is mistaken for Cystic Duct because Cystic Duct is absent or there are adhesions between the Gallbladder and Common Hepatic Duct

Figure 5. Mechanisms whereby injuries to the bile ducts may occur during cholecystectomy.

PHYSIOLOGY

Bile secreted by the liver into the biliary canaliculi is an aqueous solution of conjugated salts of bile acids, bile pigments, cholesterol, lecithin, small quantities of fatty acids and protein, inorganic electrolytes, water, and a large number and variety of products of hepatic metabolism. The bile salts are glycine and taurine conjugates of cholic and chenodeoxycholic acid, which are synthesized in the liver from cholesterol and then conjugated in the hepatocyte. Added to these two primary bile acids are two derivatives, deoxycholic acid and lithocholic acid, which are formed in the intestine by the action of bacterial enzymes on the primary acids. All of the bile acids except lithocholic acid are readily reabsorbed, mainly in the terminal ileum, and resecreted continuously throughout the day in an enterohepatic circulation. The total bile salt pool is about 3 to 5 gm., and only 200 to 600 mg. are lost in the feces each day. In hepatobiliary diseases, secretion of bile acids and their enterohepatic circulation are disturbed and they accumulate in the blood and tissues. The pruritis associated with obstructive jaundice is due to the deposition of bile acids in the skin. The bile acids behave as anions and are balanced by the cations sodium and potassium to form salts. The active transport of bile salts by the liver is the major factor regulating the volume of bile secreted. Hepatic synthesis of bile acids is regulated by the rate at which they are returned to the liver by the enterohepatic circulation. Bile salts, lecithin, cholesterol, and bilirubin make up over 90 per cent of the total

solids in bile, with the first two solutes contributing the major fraction. The bile pigments are mainly conjugated bilirubin diglucuronide and a small amount of urobilinogen. Electrolytes are present in concentrations similar to those found in plasma and consist mainly of the cations sodium, potassium, calcium, and magnesium, and the anions chloride and bicarbonate. The pH of bile normally ranges from 6.0 to 8.8, and the osmolality is about 300 mOsm. per kg., close to that of plasma.

Bile has a number of important functions. It plays a role in the hydrolysis and absorption of lipids through a complex mechanism of emulsification. It is involved in the absorption of minerals such as calcium, iron, and copper, of cholesterol, and of the fat-soluble vitamins, A, D, K, and E. It activates and stimulates secretion of certain digestive enzymes, such as pancreatic lipase. It provides alkali for the neutralization of gastric acid in the duodenum. Finally, bile serves as a vehicle for the excretion of numerous compounds metabolized by the liver.

The functions of the extrahepatic biliary system consist of the transport of bile secreted by the liver to the intestines, the regulation of bile flow, and the storage and concentration of bile. The liver secretes 600 to 1000 ml. of bile per day. Liver bile has a specific gravity of 1.011, and 97 per cent of its content is water. The gallbladder concentrates the bile at least 5 to 10 times by absorbing water and electrolytes, mainly sodium, chloride, and bicarbonate, and excretes a product with a specific gravity of 1.040. The absorptive capacity of the gallbladder mucosa is greater than that of the small intestine per unit of surface. Normally, the gallbladder does not absorb bile pigments, bile salts, proteins, or lipids to any substantial extent. In addition to its absorptive function, the mucosa secretes a thick mucus, and it is this substance that constitutes the so-called white bile in hydrops of the gallbladder associated with cystic duct obstruction. The bile ducts are not simply conduits, but have a profound influence on the flow and composition of bile. The bile duct walls are highly permeable to sodium and potassium so that the ducts are involved in absorption of bile. Furthermore, the bile ducts actively secrete water and electrolyte, and the choleretic action of many stimulants, such as secretin, is mainly on the bile ducts rather than on the canaliculi.

In the absence of food in the intestine, bile secreted continuously by the liver is retained within the bile ducts as a result of steady contraction of the sphincter of Oddi. As the biliary pressure rises, the bile refluxes into the gallbladder where it is concentrated and stored. Entrance of food into the duodenum causes the release of *cholecystokinin,* an intestinal hormone that produces contraction of the gallbladder, relaxation of the sphincter of Oddi and duodenum, and free flow of bile into the intestine. Cholecystokinin was isolated and purified in 1968 by Jorpes and Mutt. It has been found to be identical to pancreozymin, a substance that stimulates the pancreas to secrete an enzyme-rich fluid, and the two agents are now known to be a single hormone, sometimes called CCK-PZ. Cholecystokinin is a peptide hormone that consists of 33 amino acid residues and has a molecular weight of approximately 4300. Of great interest, the C-terminal pentapeptide amide is identical to that of the hormone gastrin. It is believed that nervous stimuli, mediated by the vagus nerves, participate in the process of gallbladder emptying, although motor function is normal after vagotomy and hormonal stimulation is the most important mechanism that regulates the flow of bile into the duodenum. Fats and proteins are strong stimuli to gallbladder contraction, whereas carbohydrates have litte effect on motor activity. Following cholecystectomy, regulation of bile flow is dependent entirely on the sphincter of Oddi.

The bile secretory pressure of the liver varies throughout the day but averages 300 mm. saline. At rest, the pressure within the gallbladder averages only 100 mm., so that with the sphincter of Oddi contracted bile is directed into the gallbladder for storage and concentration, and the gallbladder dilates. When the gallbladder contracts in response to a meal, the pressure rises to 200 to 300 mm., and this hydrostatic force plus inhibition of the sphincter of Oddi by cholecystokinin and nervous impulses causes the sphincter to open completely and bile to flow into the duodenum. Pressures in the bile ducts greater than 350 mm. cause suppression of hepatic bile secretion.

In addition to its actions on the motor functions of the biliary system, cholecystokinin is a choleretic, increasing the flow of bile by stimulating the output of water and electrolyte. Moreover, other digestive system hormones affect the motor and secretory activities of the biliary system. Secretin potentiates the action of cholecystokinin on gallbladder contraction and sphincter relaxation and, in addition, produces an increase in bile flow by stimulating water and electrolyte secretion. It is likely that these actions are physiologic. Gastrin produces similar motor and secretory effects, but only in pharmacologic doses, and it probably does not play a physiologic role in biliary function. Glucagon relaxes the gallbladder and choledochal sphincter but, like gastrin, it is active only at pharmacologic levels.

Pain from the gallbladder and bile ducts is produced by stretching or distention of the biliary tree, or by abnormal tension of the biliary musculature (spasm). It is often accompanied by nausea and vomiting. Such pain is transmitted by visceral sensory fibers in the splanchnic nerves connected to the seventh to tenth thoracic segments, and is perceived in the epigastrium. As a result of the motor activity in the biliary system and the related changes in pressure, biliary pain often has an intermittent component. Inflammation of the gallbladder causes referral of the visceral sensory impulses to somatic segments, giving rise to pain in the right hypochondrium, infrascapular area, substernal area, and, occasionally, as a result of connections with the phrenic nerve, the right shoulder tip. If inflammation of the gallbladder spreads to the adjacent parietal peritoneum, such as occurs in acute cholecystitis, well-localized somatic sensory pain develops. Most of the common analgesics used to relieve biliary tract pain, such as morphine and meperidine, unfortunately produce spasm of the sphincter of Oddi and duodenum and actually increase the pressure in the biliary tree. Distention of the gallbladder or bile ducts may cause a reflex decrease in coronary blood flow and cardiac arrhythmias, and is believed to explain the association of biliary tract disease and cardiac abnormalities.

DIAGNOSIS

History and Physical Examination

The history and physical examination play important roles in the diagnosis of biliary diseases. Biliary symptoms fall into three major categories, namely, pain, jaundice, and digestive disturbances sometimes called dyspepsia. Several varieties of pain are produced by diseases of the biliary system, but the most common type is colic in the right upper quadrant of the abdomen with radiation to the back or tip of the scapula. Biliary colic is, in fact, a continuous pain that waxes and wanes in intensity. Jaundice has been discussed at length in the previous chapter. The jaundice associated with extrahepatic biliary obstruction is of the *regurgitation* type, with light or clay-colored stools, dark urine, mixed bilirubinemia with a predominance of the conjugated, direct-reacting fraction, bilirubin in the urine, and, sometimes, pruritus. Jaundice due to a stone in the common bile duct often is intermittent, while jaundice caused by neoplastic obstruction of the biliary tree is usually relentless and progressive. The term "dyspepsia" refers to a number of vague and nonspecific symptoms that are commonly associated with biliary disease. It includes excessive belching, flatulence, bloating, nausea, constipation, and intolerance for fried and fatty foods, onions, cabbage, and tomatoes.

Physical findings produced by biliary diseases include jaundice, light or clay-colored stools, and tenderness in the right upper quadrant and epigastrium of the abdomen. When the gallbladder is acutely inflamed, signs of parietal peritoneal irritation such as muscle guarding or rigidity appear, fever develops as a systemic manifestation of the inflammation, and the gallbladder sometimes can be palpated as a tender mass in the upper abdomen. In obstructive jaundice due to a periampullary neoplasm, a distended, nontender gallbladder can be palpated in about one fourth of the cases.

Roentgenographic Studies

The diagnosis of biliary tract disease is in large part dependent on roentgenographic studies.

Plain X-rays of the Abdomen. Plain x-rays of the abdomen may be helpful in directing attention to or making the diagnosis of biliary disease. Between 10 and 15 per cent of gallstones contain sufficient calcium to be seen on plain abdominal films (Fig. 6). An uncommon condition called "milk of calcium" bile, which consists of a collection of calcified debris, may cause opacification of the dependent portion of the gallbladder or of the entire organ (Fig. 7). This sediment of calcium carbonate is associated with obstruction of the cystic duct and chronic gallbladder inflammation. Gas in the bile ducts is a diagnostic sign of an abnormal communication between the biliary system and gastrointestinal tract (Fig. 8). Emphysematous cholecys-

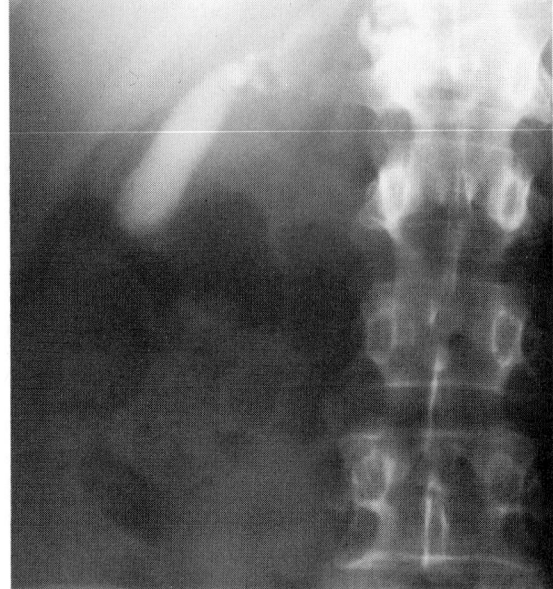

Figure 7. Plain x-ray of abdomen showing gallbladder opacified by "milk of calcium" bile.

titis is an unusual inflammation of the gallbladder due to gas-producing bacteria that results in gas in the wall and lumen of the gallbladder (Fig. 9). Intestinal obstruction due to a gallstone that has eroded through the biliary tree and into the intestine, called gallstone

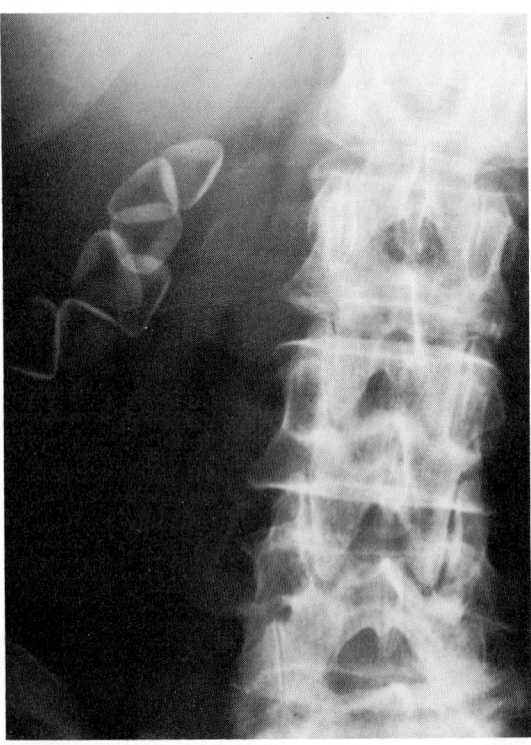

Figure 6. Plain x-ray of abdomen showing radiopaque calculi in gallbladder.

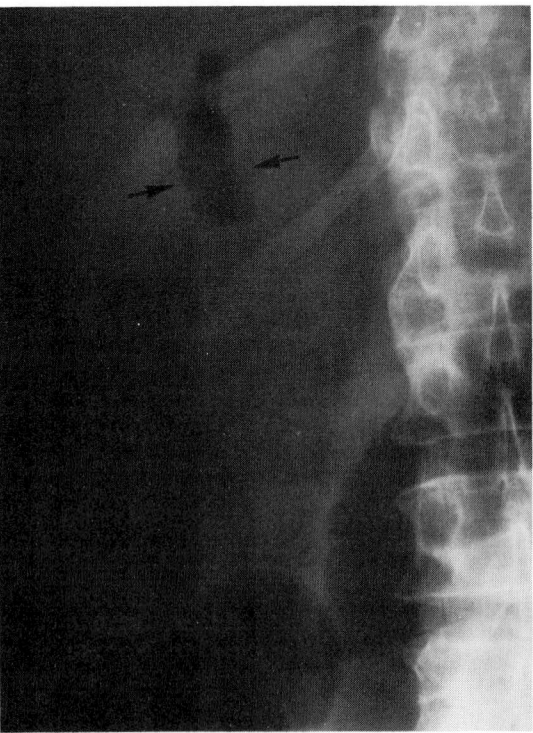

Figure 8. Plain x-ray of abdomen showing gas in the biliary tree from a biliary-enteric fistula.

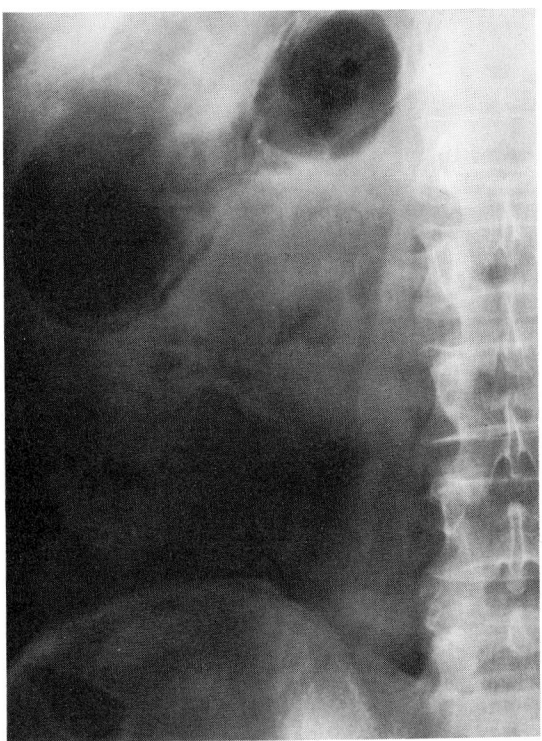

Figure 9. Plain x-ray of abdomen showing gas in the lumen and wall of the gallbladder due to emphysematous cholecystitis.

cholecystography are radiolucent shadows in the opaque dye and failure of visualization of the gallbladder. The radiolucent shadows are almost always due to gallstones and are diagnostic of disease (Fig. 11). Failure of visualization, however, should be interpreted cautiously and requires a careful consideration of the patient's history, physical findings, and results of other studies. Approximately 5 per cent of nonvisualized gallbladders prove to be normal and no cause for nonvisualization can be identified. As a minimum, oral cholecystography should be repeated before failure of visualization is accepted as an indicator of gallbladder pathology.

Intravenous Cholecystography and Cholangiography. The development of dyes such as sodium iodipamide that do not require concentration in the gallbladder for visualization of the biliary system is the basis for intravenous cholangiography. Although this procedure was originally aimed at demonstrating the extrahepatic bile ducts, it can be employed to visualize the gallbladder. Intravenous cholangiography and cholecystography are used in patients who cannot take the dye orally, in patients who have had a cholecystectomy, and when demonstration of the extrahepatic bile ducts is desired. The procedure is of particular value in patients suspected of having acute cholecystitis, which is usually associated with obstruction of the cystic duct (Fig. 12). Such patients have nausea and vomiting and cannot tolerate oral administration of dye. Visualization of the gallbladder by intravenous

ileus, is a well-known complication of cholecystitis and produces the characteristic roentgenographic signs of dilatation of the bowel (Fig. 10). Finally, a dilated loop of small intestine adjacent to an inflamed gallbladder, the so-called sentinel loop, represents a localized ileus and may be of diagnostic significance.

Oral Cholecystography. In 1924, Graham and Cole produced radiographic opacification of the gallbladder by the oral administration of an organic iodide-containing dye and initiated a new era in x-ray diagnosis. A wide variety of iodinated organic agents that are absorbed from the intestine, excreted by the liver in the bile, and concentrated in the gallbladder are now available for visualization of the biliary system. Failure of visualization of the gallbladder usually indicates obstruction of the bile ducts or inability of the gallbladder to concentrate the dye. However, other causes of failure must be ruled out and include inadequate dose of dye, failure of intestinal absorption, inadequate hepatic excretion due to liver disease, and, rarely, a full gallbladder or improper radiographic technique. Administration of a double dose of dye or administration of dye daily for 4 days sometimes demonstrates a gallbladder that could not be visualized with the standard technique. Visualization of the gallbladder rarely occurs when the serum bilirubin is above 4 mg. per 100 ml., and does not usually occur when the serum bilirubin exceeds 3 mg. per 100 ml. The contrast media and bilirubin compete for the same excretion pathway in the liver.

The two most important diagnostic findings of oral

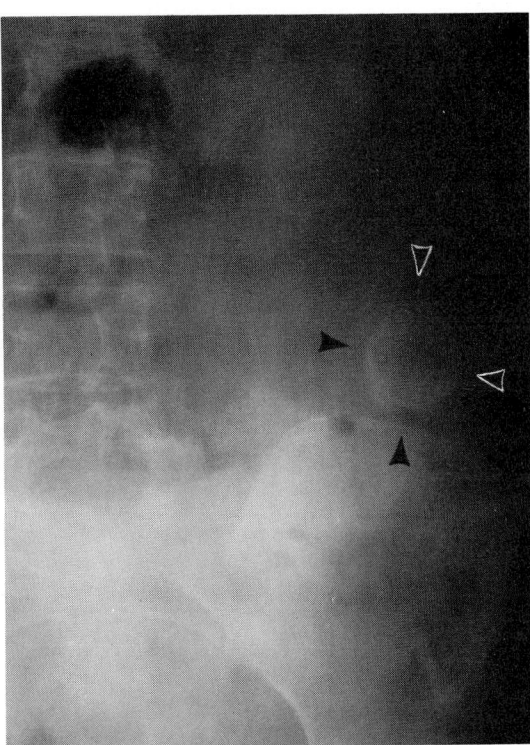

Figure 10. Plain x-ray of abdomen of patient with intestinal obstruction due to gallstone ileus, showing calculus in an ectopic location.

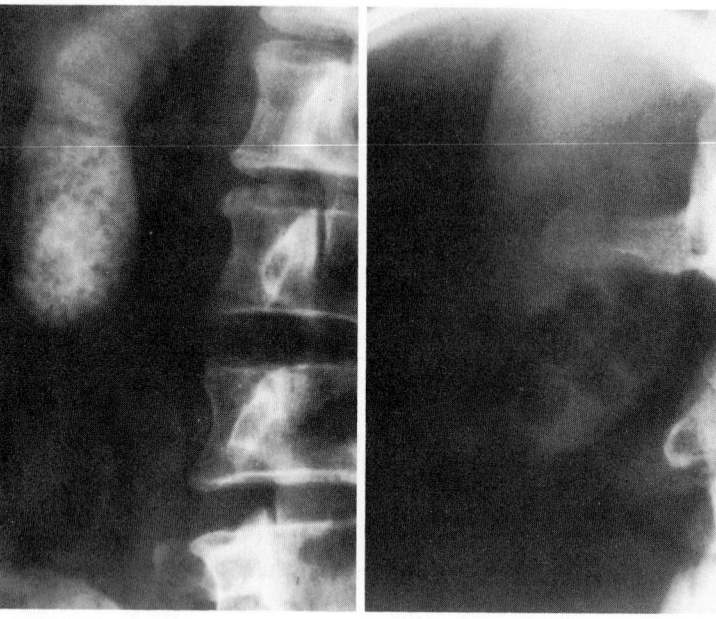

Figure 11. Radiolucent calculi demonstrated by oral cholecystography in two patients with symptoms of chronic cholecystitis.

cholecystography eliminates the diagnosis of acute cholecystitis. Dilatation or stricture of the bile ducts, choledocholithiasis, choledochal cysts, and cystic duct remnants may be demonstrated by intravenous cholangiography (Fig. 13). A successful study is unusual in the presence of a serum bilirubin greater than 4 mg. per 100 ml. Intravenous cholangiography should not be performed without clear indications because rare hypersensitivity reactions to the dye resulting in circulatory collapse and death have been reported.

Percutaneous Transhepatic Cholangiography. Instillation of opaque media into the biliary system by percu-

taneous needle puncture of a bile duct has been used primarily in jaundiced patients to determine whether biliary obstruction is extrahepatic or intrahepatic (Fig. 14). Leakage of bile, bleeding, and accidental perforation of other viscera are significant hazards of this technique, and it is generally performed when determination of the site of obstruction may make possible a lifesaving operation. When surgical therapy is indicated, operation is usually undertaken immediately after the cholangiographic study. Failure to visualize the biliary tree after repeated attempts usually means that the obstruction is intrahepatic and that the extrahepatic biliary system is small in cali-

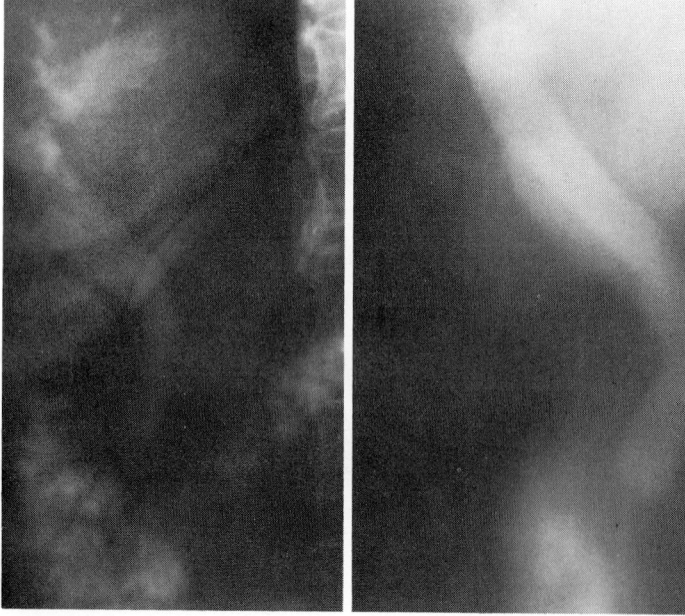

Figure 12. Intravenous cholangiogram from patient with acute cholecystitis showing good visualization of the bile ducts, but nonvisualization of the gallbladder. As is usual, at operation a stone was found blocking the cystic duct. The x-ray on the right is a tomogram, which is used to show the common bile duct in greater detail.

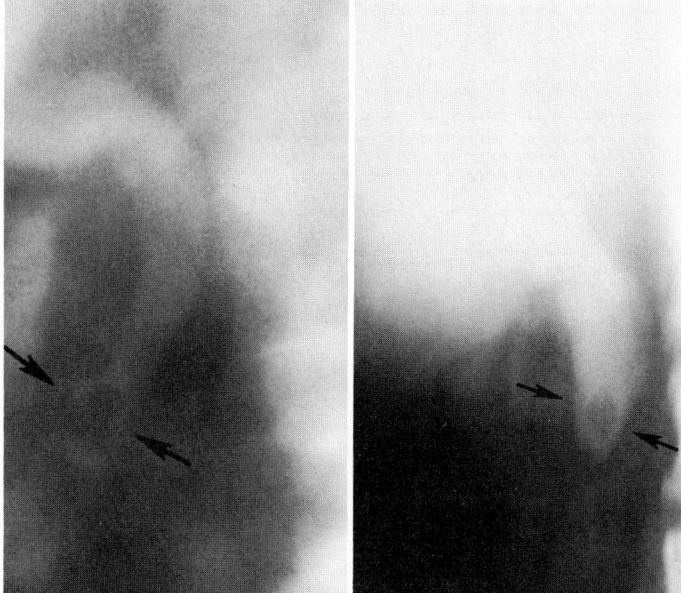

Figure 13. Intravenous cholangiograms showing calculi in the common bile ducts of two patients who had had cholecystectomy several years previously.

ber. In carefully selected cases, transhepatic cholangiography may provide valuable information about the nature and site of biliary obstruction, and may make it possible to avoid unnecessary operations. Recently, an improved technique of percutaneous transhepatic cholangiography has been introduced, in-

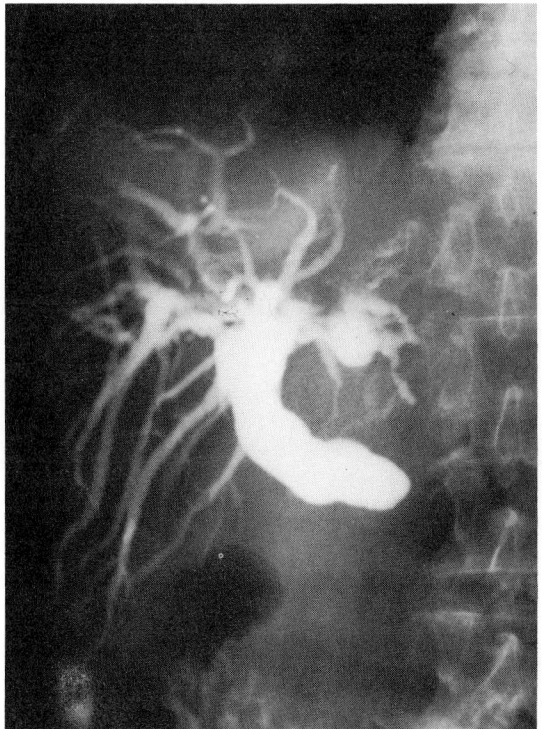

Figure 14. Percutaneous transhepatic cholangiogram from a patient with obstruction of the common bile duct due to carcinoma of the head of the pancreas.

volving the use of a thin (2.7 mm. in diameter) steel needle developed at Chiba University in Japan. It is reported that the "skinny needle" technique is much safer than the standard method and, accordingly, does not require preparation of the patient for surgery in advance, or immediate performance of operation upon demonstration of bile duct obstruction.

Transjugular Cholangiography. Another direct percutaneous method of visualizing the biliary system in selected jaundiced patients involves catheterization of an hepatic vein via the internal jugular vein in the neck, and entry into a bile duct by puncture across the wall of the hepatic vein (Fig. 15). The method has been successful in visualizing the bile ducts in about three fourths of the trials. Because the peritoneal cavity is not entered and the liver capsule is not punctured, the transjugular technique has the advantages over transhepatic cholangiography of avoiding the dangers of bile peritonitis and bleeding and, therefore, of not requiring an immediate operation when extrahepatic biliary obstruction is found. However, transjugular cholangiography has been associated with a disturbing incidence of septicemia and fever due to entry of infected bile directly into the venous outflow from the liver. Consequently, the procedure is contraindicated in patients with a history of cholangitis. Recently, the transjugular approach has been used for liver biopsy as well as for cholangiography, and the two diagnostic procedures have been combined in a single technique.

Endoscopic Retrograde Cholangiopancreatography (ERCP). The recent development of flexible fiberoptic endoscopes has made it possible to cannulate the common bile duct and pancreatic duct through the papilla of Vater under direct vision and to visualize these ductal systems radiographically by retrograde injection of radiopaque contrast media (Fig. 16). The technique requires substantial skill and practice, but it has the great advantage of avoiding blind needle puncture of

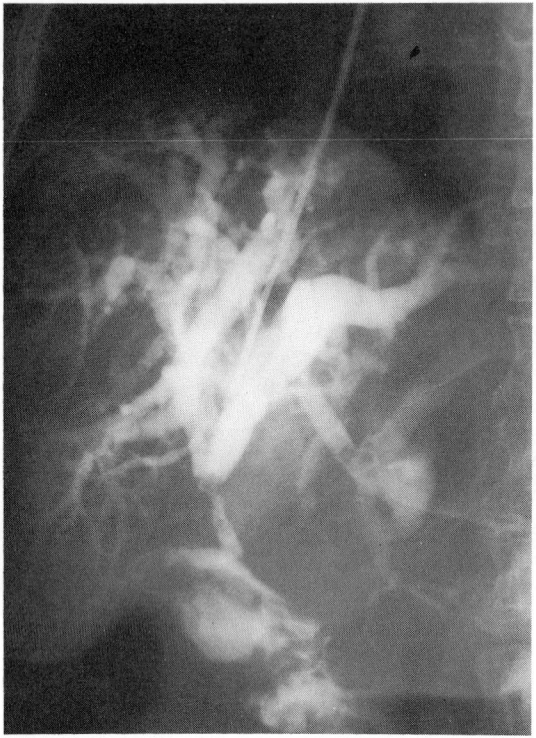

Figure 15. Transjugular cholangiogram from a patient with a stricture of the common bile duct produced by injury during cholecystectomy.

bile duct during operations on the biliary system has become an important method for identifying stones and other abnormalities. During cholecystectomy, many surgeons perform operative cholangiography via the cystic duct routinely to help decide whether or not to explore the common bile duct for stones, and to plan the strategy of common duct exploration. Following exploration of the common bile duct, almost all surgeons obtain a completion tube cholangiogram before terminating the operation to be certain that stones or strictures have not been overlooked (Fig. 17). For similar reasons, tube cholangiograms are regularly obtained postoperatively before biliary drainage is discontinued.

Barium Contrast Upper Gastrointestinal X-rays. The upper gastrointestinal series is an important study in the investigation of patients suspected of having biliary disease. Because the symptoms of gastrointestinal diseases such as peptic ulcer and hiatus hernia often mimic those of biliary disorders, it is important to establish the presence or absence of extrabiliary disturbances that may account for symptoms. The upper gastrointestinal x-rays may be helpful in the differential diagnosis of obstructive jaundice, and particularly in distinguishing between neoplastic and calculus obstruction. Widening of the duodenal sweep, the "reverse 3" sign of Frostberg, distortion of the duodenal mucosa, and displacement of the stomach are important radiographic signs of carcinoma of the head of the pancreas.

A valuable adjunct to the routine upper gastrointestinal series is *hypotonic duodenography*. The technique involves relaxation of the duodenum by the intramuscular administration of a blocking agent such as propantheline during the instillation of barium and air into the duodenum by mouth or via a properly positioned tube. The method is particularly useful in demonstrating pancreaticoduodenal neoplasms in patients with obstructive jaundice (Fig. 18).

Splanchnic Arteriography. Splanchnic arteriography is of value mainly in the differential diagnosis of jaundice. As described in the previous chapter, hepatic arteriography is useful in demonstrating various liver diseases that produce jaundice. Furthermore, celiac arteriography is becoming increasingly accurate in demonstrating pancreatic disease, particularly cancer of the head of the pancreas.

viscera. ERCP is not a routine diagnostic procedure, but it has become an attractive alternative to transhepatic cholangiography for differentiating between intrahepatic and extrahepatic jaundice, and for distinguishing between stones and neoplasms obstructing the common bile duct in difficult diagnostic cases in which the cause of jaundice cannot be determined by simple tests. Pancreatitis associated with injection of the pancreatic duct and sepsis in patients with cholangitis have been occasional complications of ERCP.

Operative and Postoperative Direct Cholangiography. Visualization of the extrahepatic bile ducts by instillation of dye via a catheter in the cystic duct or common

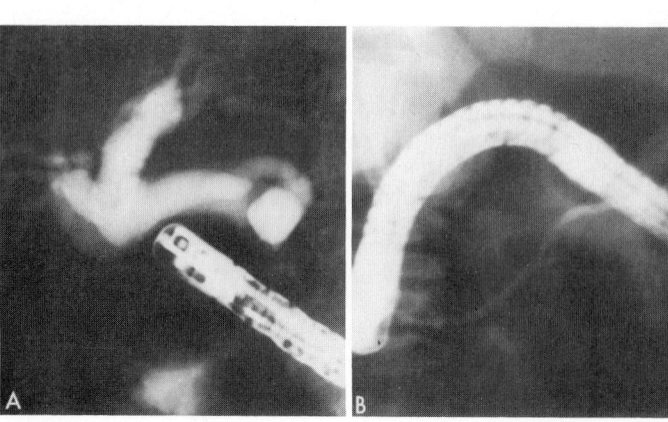

Figure 16. Transduodenal cholangiograms showing *(A)* dilatation of the common bile duct caused by stenosis of the sphincter of Oddi, and *(B)* a normal pancreatic duct.

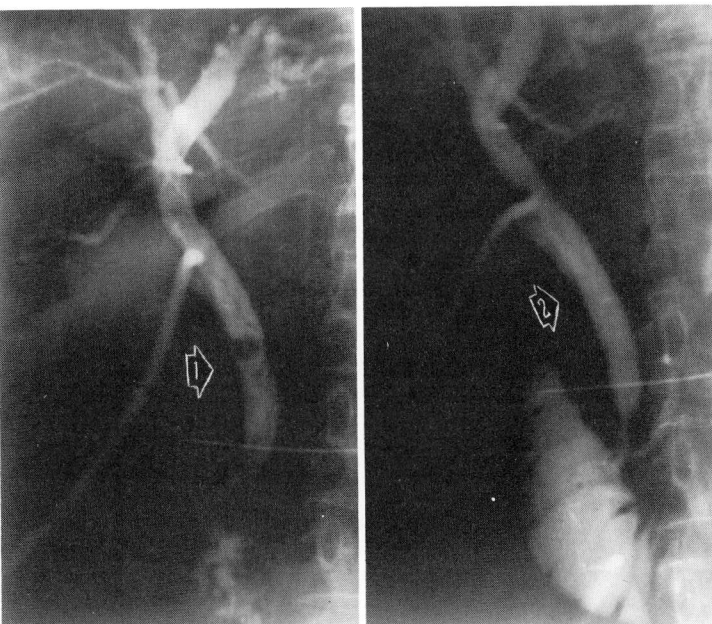

Figure 17. Intraoperative T tube cholangiograms taken after exploration of the common bile duct showing (1) a calculus that had been overlooked, and (2) appearance on a repeat cholangiogram following removal of the stone.

Ultrasonography

Ultrasonic scanning is a relatively new diagnostic technique. It has undergone considerable technical development in the past few years and has become a useful tool in the diagnosis of biliary disease. Its major advantages are that it is rapid, inexpensive, noninvasive and free of risk, and applicable to patients with and without jaundice alike. The recently developed gray scale scanner and television scan converter have improved the quality of ultrasonic cholecystography remarkably. The principle involves recording reflected pulses or "echoes" that are produced by passing ultrasonic pulses into the body. Figure 19 is an ultrasonic

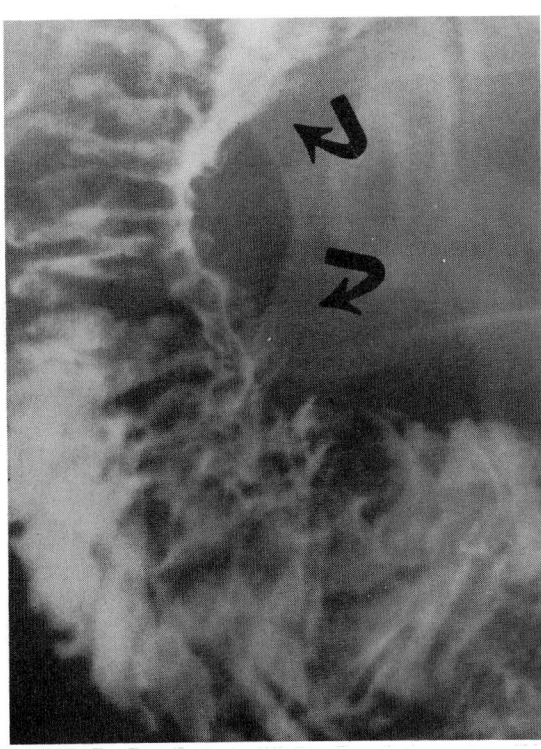

Figure 18. Hypotonic duodenography with barium in a patient with carcinoma of the head of the pancreas.

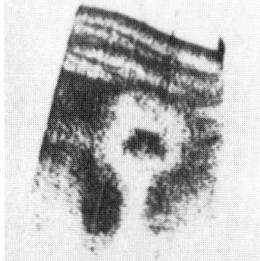

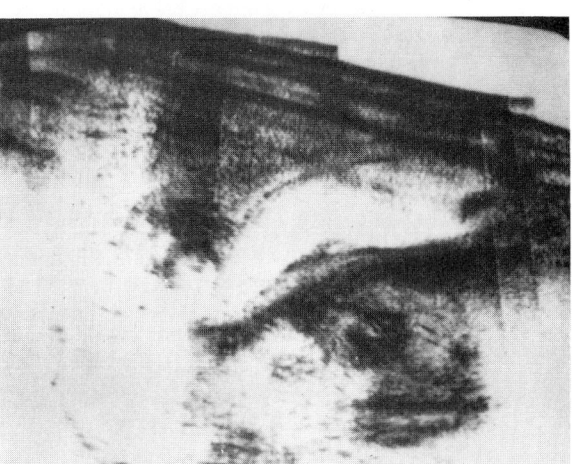

Figure 19. Ultrasonic scans showing a calculus in the gallbladder of a patient with chronic cholecystitis and obstructive jaundice (Courtesy of Dr. George Leopold, UCSD).

scan that shows a gallbladder containing stones in a patient with chronic cholecystitis and obstructive jaundice. Recently, Leopold and his associates at our institution conducted a prospective comparison of ultrasonic cholecystography and repeat oral cholecystography in 75 patients in whom the gallbladder failed to visualize on an initial oral cholecystogram (Table 1). Of 38 patients proven to have gallstones at subsequent operations, ultrasonic scanning demonstrated the calculi in 26, whereas the repeat oral cholecystogram showed them in only 19. Ultrasonic cholecystography produced 6 false-negative and one false-positive diagnoses, a diagnostic error rate of 9 per cent. Ultrasonography has not replaced oral cholecystography, but it is a valuable diagnostic adjunct, particularly in patients who have nonvisualizing oral cholecystograms and in jaundiced patients.

Biochemical Studies

The use of liver function tests in the differential diagnosis of jaundice is discussed in detail in the preceding chapter. The hallmarks of extrahepatic bile duct obstruction are an elevation of serum bilirubin, with a preponderance of the direct-reacting, conjugated fraction, and a parallel rise in serum alkaline phosphatase. A rise in the serum 5'-nucleotidase level, similar to that of alkaline phosphatase, also occurs. Depression of prothrombin activity that can be corrected by parenteral administration of vitamin K is characteristic of prolonged obstructive jaundice. Appearance of bilirubin in the urine and, if obstruction is complete, disappearance of urobilinogen from the urine and stool are regular biochemical abnormalities produced by biliary obstruction. In uncomplicated obstructive jaundice of short duration, the other liver function tests are usually normal. However, in longstanding bile duct obstruction, or in biliary infection such as cholangitis, abnormalities of all of the common liver function tests and particularly of the enzyme levels may develop.

Because of the intimate association of diseases of the biliary system and pancreas, determinations of serum amylase and lipase and of urinary diastase are frequently indicated. Elevations of these enzymes are often found in patients with acute biliary inflammations in the absence of gross disease of the pancreas. Recently, the renal clearance of amylase, expressed as a percentage of creatinine clearance, has been reported to differentiate pancreatitis from biliary disease without pancreatitis in patients who have an elevated serum amylase level. An amylase-creatinine clearance ratio of greater than 5.5 per cent indicated the presence of clinically important pancreatitis. The frequent occurrence of biliary disorders in patients with diabetes requires determinations of blood and urine sugar.

Liver Biopsy

The role of percutaneous needle biopsy of the liver in the diagnosis of jaundice is discussed in the previous chapter. It may be of help in distinguishing between jaundice due to liver disease and extrahepatic obstructive jaundice. Percutaneous liver biopsy usually has been avoided in jaundiced patients suspected of having extrahepatic bile duct obstruction because of the fear of causing a biliary leak and bile peritonitis. However, recent experience indicates that biopsy by the Menghini one-second technique is associated with a low incidence of complications so that it is not contraindicated in circumstances where the liver biopsy is likely to provide valuable information. Use of the "skinny needle" for liver biopsy may reduce the dangers even further.

Duodenal Drainage

Aspiration of bile from a tube inserted via the nose or mouth into the duodenum may provide valuable information in the diagnosis of biliary disease and in the differential diagnosis of jaundice. Instillation of magnesium sulfate or olive oil into the duodenum or administration of cholecystokinin causes contraction of the gallbladder and permits collection of bile emanating from the gallbladder. By proper timing of specimens, bile from the extrahepatic ducts and fresh liver bile may be obtained. The finding of cholesterol and calcium bilirubinate crystals on microscopic examination of the duodenal aspirate strongly suggests the presence of gallstones. Cytologic studies for cancer cells may provide evidence of carcinoma of the biliary ducts or duodenum. Duodenal drainage is indicated when other diagnostic studies fail to yield positive results in patients with symptoms suggestive of biliary disease. In the future, it may become a valuable tool for detection of lithogenic bile in asymptomatic patients.

Peritoneoscopy

Peritoneoscopy or laparoscopy is occasionally of value in the differential diagnosis of jaundice. Direct visualization of the peritoneal cavity may reveal the dilated normal gallbladder associated with malignant

TABLE 1. Prospective Comparison of Ultrasonic Cholecystography and Repeat Oral Cholecystography in 75 Patients Who Had an Initial Nonvisualizing Oral Cholecystogram*

Results of Repeat Oral Cholecystogram		Results of Ultrasonic Cholecystogram			Stones Proven at Surgery	False Positive or Negative Ultrasonography
		Normal	Stones	Nonvisualization		
Normal	32	31	1	0	—	3% false positive
Stones	19	3	16	0	19	16% false negative
Nonvisualization	24	8	10	6	19	13% false negative

*From Leopold, G. R., Amberg, J., Gosink, B. B., and Mittelstaedt, C.: Radiology, 1976.

biliary obstruction, peritoneal and hepatic metastases from a pancreaticoduodenal cancer, the shrunken, diseased gallbladder of chronic cholecystitis, or the "pearls" of fat necrosis associated with acute pancreatitis. Needle biopsy of suspicious lesions in the liver can be done under direct vision during peritoneoscopy. Such lesions may be missed by blind percutaneous needle biopsy of the liver.

GALLSTONES

Approximately 16 million people in the United States have gallstones, and about 800,000 new cases are discovered yearly. Approximately 400,000 gallbladders are removed surgically each year because of calculi, and the annual medical expenditures for gallstone disease in our country approximates 1.5 billion dollars. Gallstone disease occurs in approximately 10 per cent of the adult population of the United States and in about 20 per cent of persons over the age of 40. Thus, cholelithiasis is one of the most common health disorders of adult life. The incidence of gallstones increases progressively with age; approximately one third of persons in their eighth decade of life have biliary calculi. At the same time, the occurrence of gallstones in children with hemolytic anemias is by no means rare, and the finding of cholelithiasis in young adults, particularly women who are or have been pregnant, is not usual. Biliary calculi develop about four times more frequently in women than in men, although with age the incidence among males progressively approaches that among females.

The pathogenesis of gallstones is not completely understood and it is likely that several mechanisms are involved. For more than a century, three major factors have been considered to be of etiologic importance: (1) a primary physiochemical disorder of bile, (2) stasis of bile, and (3) infection or inflammation of the biliary system. In recent years, substantial evidence has been obtained to indicate that a primary abnormality in the physicochemical composition of bile is the most important factor in gallstone formation.

Types of Gallstones

Gallstones are formed from the constituents of bile. In the United States three major types of calculi are found (Fig. 20). Two of the three types contain cholesterol as the predominant component, and together constitute approximately 90 per cent of stones. The three types are as follows:

1. *Mixed cholesterol stones* are the most common type, accounting for about 80 per cent of the calculi in this country. Cholesterol makes up at least 70 per cent of the content of these stones. In addition, they contain variable amounts of calcium salts, bilirubin, protein, bile acids, and debris. They may be round or faceted, smooth or rough. They are usually multiple and not often larger than 2 cm. in diameter.

2. *Pure cholesterol stones* constitute approximately 10 per cent of calculi. They are often solitary and large with a round configuration.

3. *Pigment stones* make up the remaining 10 per cent of calculi. They are composed of unconjugated bilirubin, calcium, and variable amounts of organic material, and do not contain cholesterol. They are multiple, small, black or dark green, irregular, and hard. The pathogenesis of pigment stones is clearly different from that of cholesterol stones. They form when excess unconjugated bilirubin is present in bile and precipitates as a complex with calcium or copper. In the Unites States, they are found mainly in patients with diseases that cause increased bilirubin production, such as hemolytic anemias. In the Orient they occur commonly in association with *Ascaris lumbricoides* or *Escherichia coli* infection of the biliary system. It is believed that the infectious organisms produce B-glucuronidase, which hydrolyses water-soluble bilirubin diglucuronide to form insoluble free bilirubin. The liberated bilirubin precipitates as calcium bilirubinate.

Physiochemical Characteristics of Bile

More than 90 per cent of the dry weight of bile is made up of three constituents. These are (1) the salts of three bile acids, namely, the two primary bile acids formed in the liver (cholate and chenodeoxycholate), and one of the two secondary bile acids absorbed from the intestine in the enterohepatic circulation (deoxycholate); (2) phospholipid, 90 per cent of which is lecithin; and (3) cholesterol. The bile acids and their salts are water soluble and have the unique capacity to form highly charged polymolecular aggregates called *micelles.* Lecithin and cholesterol are insoluble in aqueous systems, but they become soluble by incorporation into a bile salt–lecithin–cholesterol mixed micelle. The capacity of these mixed micelles to keep cholesterol in solution is related to the relative concentrations of bile salts, lecithin, and cholesterol in bile. This important relationship can be expressed on triangular coordinates in a phase diagram devised by Admirand and Small and shown in Figure 21. The limits of cholesterol solubility at various relative concentrations of bile salt, lecithin, and cholesterol in solutions of various dilutions are defined by such a diagram. The line ABC represents the maximal solubility of cholesterol in varying mixtures of bile salt and lecithin. Mixtures falling below the ABC line are in a single aqueous phase and are not completely saturated with cholesterol (i.e., cholesterol is completely solubilized), while those above the ABC line are oversaturated with cholesterol and, therefore, contain insoluble cholesterol crystals. Further studies of cholesterol solubility, particularly by Holzbach et al., indicate that the limit of the cholesterol solubility zone is smaller than initially proposed and that the true equilibrium line is DBC in Figure 21. Other workers have devised a variety of other methods for expressing cholesterol solubility in bile and for defining a "lithogenic index" to indicate the likelihood of cholesterol crystal formation. Substantial evidence indicates that bile containing excess cholesterol relative to bile salts and lecithin is prerequisite for gallstone formation.

Stages of Cholesterol Gallstone Formation

It has been proposed that the formation of cholesterol gallstones occurs in three stages: saturation, crystallization, and growth.

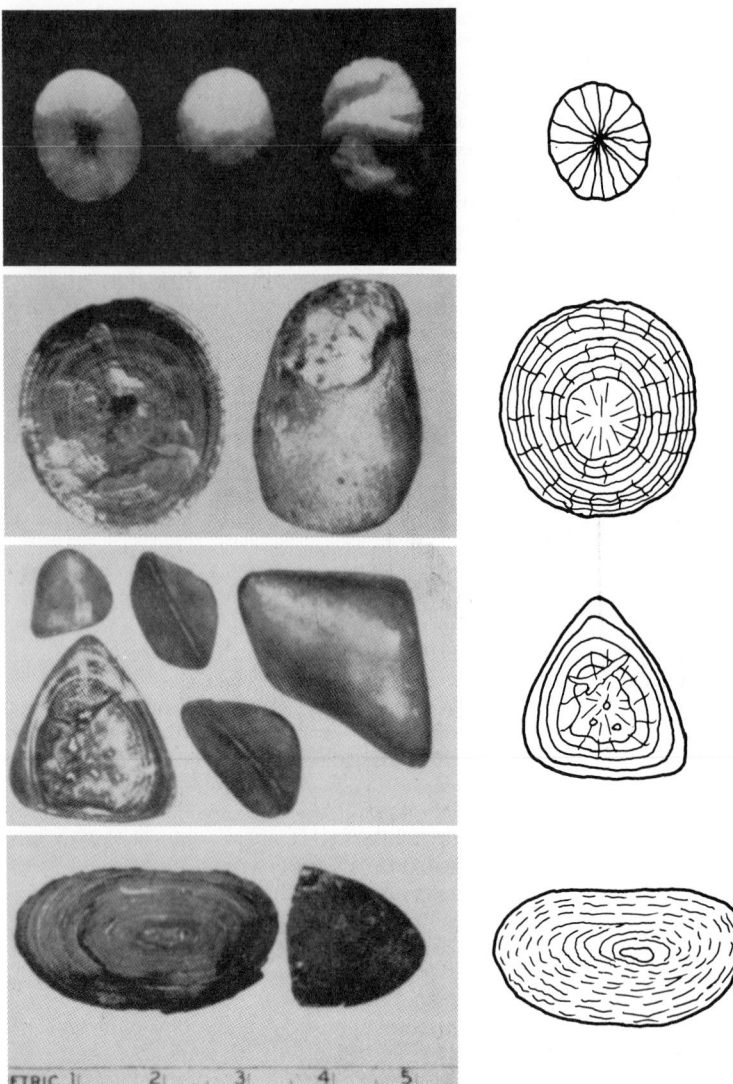

Figure 20. Various types of gallstones. *Top* shows "pure" cholesterol stone; *upper middle* shows laminated mixed stone; *lower middle* shows faceted mixed stone; *bottom* shows pigment stone. (From Juniper, K., Jr. *In* Paulson, M. (Ed.): Gastroenterologic Medicine. Philadelphia, Lea & Febiger, 1969; upper middle photo from Juniper, K., Jr.: Mod. Treat., *5*:480, 1968.)

Saturation. This initial stage involves an alteration of the relative concentrations of cholesterol, bile salt, and lecithin to form an abnormal bile that is supersaturated with cholesterol. Supersaturated bile is thermodynamically unstable and has the potential to precipitate. Although the correlation is not precise, studies of patients with gallstones have shown that their bile is usually saturated or supersaturated. Moreover, studies of high-risk groups which did not have demonstrable gallstones, such as American Indian women and siblings of young patients with gallstones, have shown a significantly higher incidence of saturated bile than was found in controls.

Crystallization. This stage involves a change in the state of bile from a single aqueous phase that is supersaturated with cholesterol to a system with two or more phases, one of which is solid and contains cholesterol crystals. The change involves the processes of nucleation, flocculation, and precipitation of cholesterol from the supersaturated bile. This chain of events may be initiated by a nidus that triggers cholesterol crystallization, such as refluxed intestinal contents, bacteria, epithelial debris, mucoproteins, or precipitated bile pigments.

Growth. This stage involves the growth of the tiny crystals into macroscopic stones by aggregation or by coalescence around a nidus. Since this stage usually takes place in the gallbladder, where bile is stored for hours, stasis may play a role.

Sources of Supersaturated Bile

The source of the abnormal lithogenic bile is uncertain. It could be formed in the liver, or it could result from alterations that occur in the gallbladder and bile ducts. The weight of evidence from studies in animals and humans indicates that the liver is the source of the abnormal bile, so that cholesterol gallstone formation is probably a primary hepatic disease. The excessive concentration of cholesterol relative to the concentrations of bile salt and lecithin could result from

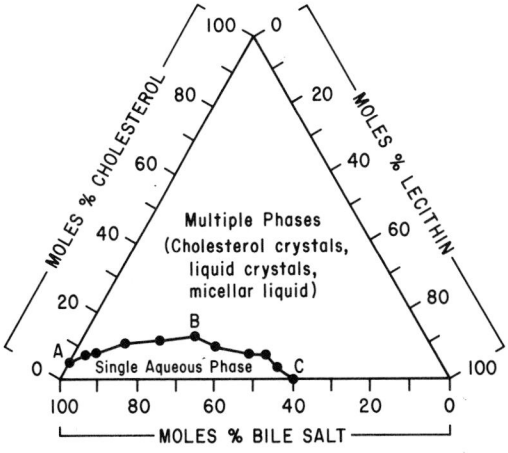

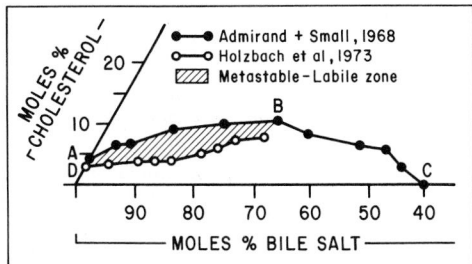

Figure 21. Admirand and Small's phase diagram in which the three components of bile are plotted on triangular coordinates. Any combination of bile salt, lecithin, and cholesterol may be expressed as a single point within the triangle. Line ABC represents the maximal effective solubility of cholesterol in varying mixtures of bile salt and lecithin, as originally determined by Admirand and Small in 1968. Line DBC represents the true equilibrium solubility line determined by Holzbach et al. in 1973. Between the two lines is a metastable-labile zone in which bile might require specific nucleating factors to initiate stone formation.

decreased secretion of bile acids (or lecithin) or from increased secretion of cholesterol. Available evidence indicates that both of these mechanisms, acting separately in some cases and together in others, are involved. A decrease in the size of the bile acid pool and in the secretion of bile acids has been demonstrated in patients with gallstones and in American Indians without cholelithiasis. Moreover, in certain conditions associated with an increased incidence of cholesterol gallstones, particularly those involving disease, resection, or bypass of the distal ileum, there is a decrease in the bile acid pool as a result of excessive fecal loss of bile acids without a corresponding increase in hepatic bile acid synthesis. On the other hand, increased secretion of cholesterol in bile has been demonstrated in both Caucasian and American Indian women with cholelithiasis and in obese patients with saturated bile.

Role of the Gallbladder

Some evidence suggests that alteration of hepatic bile by the gallbladder may play a role in stone formation. While the normal gallbladder absorbs mainly water and electrolytes, it has been known for many years that the inflamed gallbladder can absorb bile

salts and thereby change the physiochemical composition of bile. Moreover, recent studies in mice fed a cholesterogenic diet indicate that absorption of bile salts by a damaged gallbladder mucosa is responsible for gallstone formation in these animals. Stasis of bile in the gallbladder and the presence of a variety of nucleating substances such as desquamated cells, mucus, bacteria, and bile pigments undoubtedly contribute to gallstone formation in many instances. Finally, the possibility that the gallbladder plays a primary role in the development of calculi has received support from some studies that have shown normalization of lithogenic bile following cholecystectomy. It has been proposed that the gallbladder, by interrupting enterohepatic recycling or by altering the pressure in the biliary system, in some way suppresses hepatic synthesis of bile acids. However, contradictory studies showing persistence of supersaturated bile following cholecystectomy also have been reported.

Role of Infection

The role of infection in the pathogenesis of cholelithiasis is uncertain. Although bacteria are commonly found in inflamed gallbladders and in stones, substantial evidence indicates that normal bile is usually sterile. As mentioned above, the inflamed gallbladder mucosa has a markedly altered permeability, which permits the absorption of bile acids and the movement of inorganic salts into the gallbladder lumen. It is possible that these changes alter the distribution of the constituents of bile and cause precipitation of cholesterol. Equally important may be the role of excessive cellular debris and increased protein secretion, which occur in response to inflammation and may form a nidus for gallstones. Finally, the effects of bacterial enzymes on the constituents of bile may alter solubility conditions and lead to precipitation of cholesterol or bilirubin.

Medical Therapy of Gallstones

The recent progress in identifying the physiochemical abnormalities in gallstone formation has led to attempts to dissolve gallstones in vivo. Some years ago it was shown that human gallstones dissolved when placed in the gallbladder of dogs, pigs, sheep, and goats. Subsequent studies demonstrated that human cholesterol calculi could be dissolved in vitro by an appropriate lecithin–bile salt mixture. Finally, Danzinger et al. in 1972 reported the disappearance or reduction in size of gallstones in four of seven patients given chenodeoxycholic acid orally for periods of 6 to 22 months. Since then, a number of clinical trials of chenodeoxycholic acid therapy have been initiated and over 200 patients have been or are being treated. The results to date indicate that chenodeoxycholic acid therapy given over periods of six months to two years frequently reduces the lithogenicity of bile and causes a reduction in size or dissolution of gallstones, particularly radiolucent calculi in patients with a functioning gallbladder. Adverse reactions to the drug have consisted mainly of diarrhea due to irritation of the colon by the bile acid, and mild elevations in liver enzymes such as SGOT. Administration of chenodeoxycholic acid to monkeys has produced liver damage, and the question of hepatotoxicity in humans has not yet been answered, although liver biopsies have not shown hepatic injury to date. Interestingly, administration of the other primary bile acid, cholic acid, is ineffective in dissolving gallstones. The action of chenodeoxycholic acid is clearly not attributable to expansion of the bile acid pool. Rather, the mechanism appears to be that of inhibition of cholesterol synthesis and secretion associated with conversion of over 90 per cent of the bile acid pool to chenodeoxycholic acid. The concept of dissolution of gallstones by bile acids is exciting, but the future of this form of therapy is uncertain. In addition to potential side effects, such as hepatotoxicity, and expense related to daily therapy, it appears likely that lifelong treatment will be necessary. Within three months after therapy has been discontinued bile again becomes saturated with cholesterol, and within one year a 10 per cent recurrence rate of gallstones has been reported.

Phenobarbital induces the production of hepatic microsomal enzymes, and in monkeys it facilitates the conversion of cholesterol to bile acids so that cholesterol secretion decreases and bile acid secretion increases. In human trials, phenobarbital decreased the lithogenicity of bile but failed to dissolve gallstones over a one-year period. It has been proposed that therapy with a combination of phenobarbital and chenodeoxycholic acid may have potential.

It should be emphasized that the medical treatment of gallstones is an experimental undertaking and that, as of the present, surgical therapy constitutes the only highly effective, safe, and practical therapeutic measure available.

CHOLEDOCHOLITHIASIS

Calculi in the extrahepatic bile ducts usually originate in the gallbladder, although they may form in the biliary ducts. Choledocholithiasis develops in 10 to 15 per cent of patients with gallbladder stones. Although stones in the bile ducts may be silent, they usually produce biliary obstruction, which is often incomplete and intermittent. In addition, they may be associated with bile duct infection and, if present for long periods, may be responsible for significant liver damage and occasionally for secondary biliary cirrhosis.

Diagnosis

Choledocholithiasis in its classic form produces a syndrome of jaundice, biliary colic, and fever. However, in a substantial number of patients one or more symptoms of this triad are absent. Jaundice occurs in about 80 per cent of the patients and is characteristically fluctuating in nature. Progressive, relentless jaundice is unusual and suggests the presence of neoplastic obstruction rather than stones. The jaundice is accompanied by dark urine and light stools, but clay-colored stools lasting for a significant length of time do not usually occur. Biliary colic due to distention of the bile ducts is a common early symptom of choledocholithiasis. The pain is similar in nature and location to

gallbladder colic and is often accompanied by restlessness, nausea, and vomiting. Fever and chills occur in only one third of the patients with bile duct stones. A past history of the dyspeptic symptoms of chronic cholecystitis is common.

Physical findings include tenderness and rigidity in the epigastrium and right hypochondrium in proportion to the existence and severity of infection. The liver is often palpable and tender if cholangitis is present. The gallbladder usually is not palpable, even in the presence of severe biliary obstruction. According to the autopsy studies of Courvoisier in the late nineteenth century, the gallbladder was normal and usually distended in obstructive jaundice due to neoplasm, but was seldom distended in obstructive jaundice due to calculi because of pre-existing cholecystitis and fibrosis. These observations have become known as *Courvoisier's law*.

The diagnosis of choledocholithiasis usually, although by no means invariably, involves the differential diagnosis of jaundice. The hyperbilirubinemia shows a predominance of conjugated bilirubin, there is bilirubin in the urine, and, if the obstruction is complete, urine and stool urobilinogen are decreased. Serum alkaline phosphatase is consistently elevated, even in the absence of jaundice. The enzyme, turbidity, and flocculation liver function tests are usually normal except in longstanding obstruction or when cholangitis is present. Intravenous cholangiography may show calculi, or dilatation of the common bile duct greater than 15 mm. if performed in the absence of marked jaundice. The finding of crystals in the duodenal aspirate is suggestive of biliary stones.

In patients with jaundice, the most important diagnostic considerations include obstructive jaundice due to neoplasm, intrahepatic cholestasis, and regurgitation jaundice due to primary liver disease. Neoplastic obstruction of the bile ducts is usually complete and relentless, and occurs in a patient with debilitating manifestations of cancer and no history of dyspeptic symptoms; stone obstruction is usually incomplete and fluctuating. Intrahepatic cholestasis usually does not produce pain, a history of ingestion of one of the causative agents may be obtained, and a history of dyspeptic symptoms is usually absent. Jaundice due to hepatic cell damage is regularly associated with typical liver function test abnormalities and the absence of colicky pain. Occasionally, cholangiography by the percutaneous transhepatic, transjugular, or transduodenal technique may be required to differentiate these three forms of jaundice.

Other diagnostic possibilities, particularly in patients without jaundice, include renal or intestinal colic, acute congestive heart failure, acute hepatitis, and the numerous diseases that may produce acute abdominal pain.

Primary Treatment

The treatment of choledocholithiasis involves surgical exploration of the common bile duct and removal of the calculi after preparation of the patient for operation, which may require parenteral vitamin K therapy in patients with prolonged jaundice. Usually, this is combined with treatment of the associated gallbladder disease by cholecystectomy. Occasionally, choledochotomy is required for newly formed or overlooked calculi in patients who have previously undergone cholecystectomy.

Indications for Common Bile Duct Exploration. In every operation on the gallbladder, the surgeon must decide whether or not to explore the common bile duct. Such explorations are not performed routinely because of the increased morbidity and slightly increased mortality associated with them. Common bile duct exploration is performed in 20 to 30 per cent of cholecystectomies. Table 2 lists the absolute and relative indications for exploring the common bile duct as a supplement to cholecystectomy. The absolute indications are associated with a high yield of bile duct calculi, and the presence of any one of them demands choledochotomy. The relative indications, when existing as solitary findings, have a low yield of bile duct stones and their use as a basis for common duct exploration requires the judgment of the surgeon. Coexistence of two or more relative indications may add up to an absolute indication. The absolute and relative indications are as follows:

1. *Palpable stones* in the bile ducts provide the most reliable indication for exploration. Therefore, it is important that the surgeon expose the common duct to an extent that permits easy palpation of its entire length. This is best accomplished by the routine mobilization and medial reflection of the duodenum in a Kocher maneuver at the beginning of every cholecystectomy operation.

2. *Obstructive jaundice with cholangitis,* manifested by fever, chills, and parallel elevations of serum bilirubin and alkaline phsophatase, is a second highly reliable and therefore absolute indication for choledochotomy.

3. *Demonstration of bile duct calculi by cholangiography,* usually at the time of operation but sometimes preoperatively, is an absolute and reliable indication for common duct exploration.

4. *Dilatation of the common bile duct* to a diameter greater than 12 mm. is an absolute indication for choledochotomy, even though the yield of positive results is only about 35 per cent because there is an overlap between the upper limits of normal diameter and pathologic enlargement. The larger the diameter

of the duct, the greater is the chance that it contains stones. Measurement of the diameter of the common duct with calipers is much more accurate than estimating the size with the naked eye, and should be a routine procedure.

5. *Recent or current obstructive jaundice without cholangitis* is associated with a variable incidence of positive common duct explorations, depending on the severity of the jaundice. When mild jaundice is the sole indication for choledochotomy, the yield of calculi is very low. On the other hand, the incidence of bile duct stones is high in patients with substantial elevations of serum bilirubin and alkaline phosphatase.

6. *Biliary-enteric fistula* is an indication for common duct exploration if the abnormal communication involves the bile duct, but not if it is confined to the gallbladder.

7. *Small stones in the gallbladder* that are smaller than the diameter of the cystic duct are associated with choledocholithiasis in only about 10 per cent of the cases in which this finding serves as the sole indication for common duct exploration. In this situation, operative cholangiography is very helpful in determining whether or not to explore the common duct.

8. *A single faceted stone in the gallbladder* is a rare indication for common duct exploration. Since stones become faceted only by rubbing against other stones, this finding indicates that a second stone was present at some time and, presumably, has passed into the common duct.

9. *Pancreatitis* is a weak indication for choledochotomy. Substantial data show that the incidence of choledocholithiasis is only 12 per cent in pancreatitis associated with biliary disease, which is no higher than the incidence of bile duct stones in biliary disease unassociated with pancreatitis.

Technical Aspects of Common Bile Duct Exploration. The technique of common bile duct exploration has been standardized by widespread usage over many years. However, there are several technical aspects of the procedure that warrant emphasis or comment because they have not been adopted uniformly. These are (1) routine pre-exploratory operative cholangiography; (2) use of the balloon-tipped catheter; (3) routine completion cholangiography through the T tube; and (4) operative biliary endoscopy. Many surgeons, including the author, routinely perform operative cholangiography through a catheter inserted via the cystic duct into the common bile duct during all cholecystectomy operations. There are several reasons for routinely performing operative cholangiography regardless of whether there exist clear indications for common duct exploration. The first is to establish the absence of choledocholithiasis when there are none of the usual indications for exploring the common bile duct or when the indications are relative. The second reason is to reveal occult stones when none are suspected, a finding that occurs in 4 to 5 per cent of cases. A third reason is to demonstrate the number and location of bile duct calculi when there are absolute indications for choledochotomy so that the surgeon will not perform an incomplete choledocholithotomy. The final reason is to demonstrate the anatomy of the bile ducts before manipulation, so that post-

---

TABLE 2. Indications for Common Bile Duct Exploration

Absolute Indications

Palpable stones (99% reliable)
Jaundice with cholangitis (97% reliable)
Demonstration of stones by cholangiography (85% reliable)
Dilatation of common bile duct > 12 mm. (35% reliable)

Relative Indications

Obstructive jaundice, recent or current
Biliary fistula
Small stones in gallbladder
Single faceted stone in gallbladder
Pancreatitis

exploratory completion cholangiograms are not misleading. For operative cholangiography to be of value it is essential that the established procedure be followed carefully and that high resolution radiographic equipment be used.

The balloon-tipped catheter is an important recent addition to the instruments available for common duct exploration (Fig. 22). This device, introduced initially by Fogarty for vascular surgery, is now used by many surgeons in preference to metal scoops and forceps for extracting biliary calculi. It is particularly useful for removing stones for the intrahepatic bile ducts. Although the balloon-tipped catheter is potentially less traumatic than metal instruments, it must be used gently, since it is possible to rupture intrahepatic ducts by overinflating the balloon and using excessive traction.

Upon completion of the choledocholithotomy, it is important to drain the common bile duct with a T tube or catheter and to obtain a postexploratory completion cholangiogram through the T tube. In view of the significant incidence of overlooked bile duct stones, closure of the choledochotomy without drainage or completion cholangiography is not advisable. Before the operation is concluded, it is essential that the completion cholangiogram demonstrate absence of stones, complete filling of the bile ducts, and flow of the contrast medium into the duodenum. Seven to 10 days postoperatively, a second T tube cholangiogram is obtained to be certain that the bile ducts are free of stones before the T tube is removed. With the recent development of an effective technique for mechanically extracting overlooked bile duct stones (see below), the common duct should be drained with a large caliber T tube (at least No. 16 French, with the back wall of the intraluminal portion cut off), and the tube should be brought out of the abdomen in a straight line at right angles to the common duct.

Operative endoscopy has been used by some surgeons as an aid to locating and removing bile duct stones. Both a flexible fiberoptic choledochoscope and a rigid choledochoscope have been developed for use in the operating room. The instrument is inserted through the standard choledochotomy. Although biliary endoscopy has not been adopted widely, some impressive results have been reported recently.

Treatment of Retained or Recurrent Choledocholithiasis

Despite enormous surgical experience with choledocholithiasis and a large amount of information about the indications for and technique of common bile duct exploration, a small but extremely troublesome group of patients is found to have retained or recurrent bile duct stones after the initial biliary operation. The incidence of residual calculi is highest among patients who have had an initial choledocholithotomy, in whom it averages about 10 per cent (Table 3). There are several sources of residual bile duct calculi. The majority are *retained* stones that were overlooked at the initial operation. These are often discovered on the tube cholangiogram obtained 7 to 10 days postoperatively (Fig. 23). A second but uncommon source of *retained* stones consists of calculi that were recognized at the initial operation but could not be extracted for technical reasons, such as intrahepatic stones. Finally, there are true *recurrent* calculi that reform in the bile ducts months or years after the gallbladder has been removed and a complete choledocholithotomy has been done. These primary bile duct stones, sometimes called "stasis" or "earthy" stones, have a high content

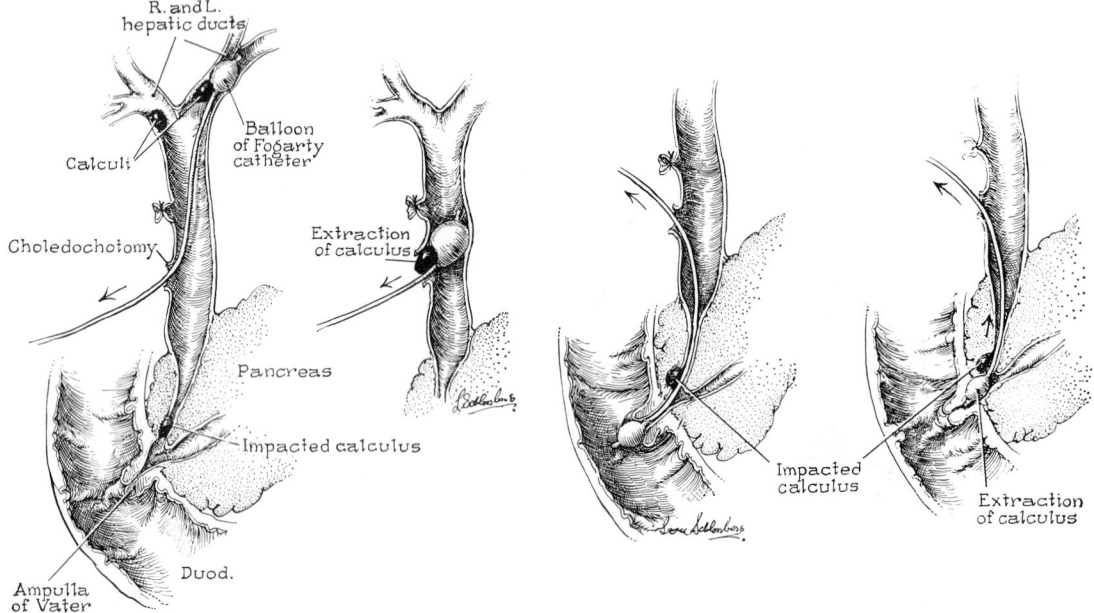

Figure 22. Use of balloon-tipped catheter to extract intrahepatic bile duct calculi and to extract an impacted calculus from the distal common duct. (From Anderson, R. P., Leand, P. M., and Zuidema, G. D.: Uses of the balloon-tipped catheter in biliary tract surgery. Am. J. Surg., *117*:55, 1969.)

TABLE 3.   Incidence of Retained or Recurrent Bile Duct Stones

Authors	Year of Report	Number of Cholecyst-ectomies	Choledochotomies No.	Per Cent	Stones Found At Choledochotomy No.	Per Cent	No. Cases	Retained or Recurrent Stones Per Cent of Cho-ledo-choto-mies	Per Cent of Cho-ledocho-lithoto-mies
Hicken and McAllister	1964	— —	2200	—	1293	59	152	—	12
Colcock and Perey	1964	1754	503	29	139	28	8	2	4
Hampson and Petrie	1964	2090	327	16	156	48	23	7	12
Jolly et al.	1968	1460	309	21	192	62	25	8	13
Way et al.	1972	952	200	21	137	69	14	7	10

of cholesterol and form in bile that is highly litho-genic. Moreover, they have a characteristic appear-ance that permits their easy identification at the operating table. They are ovoid, their shape conforms to the contour of the common duct, and they are soft and easily crushed with the fingers or instruments to form "biliary mud." Because primary bile duct stones are likely to reform despite their repeated removal, their surgical significance is quite different from that of the more common calculi that drop into the bile duct from the gallbladder.

The treatment of residual bile duct stones depends on when they are discovered. Those that are discov-ered on the tube cholangiogram in the immediate post-operative period are managed quite differently from those that produce symptoms months or years after the initial operation.

Treatment of Retained Stones Discovered in the Immedi-ate Postoperative Period. Until recently, most pa-tients with retained stones discovered on the post-operative tube cholangiogram required a second operation to remove the calculi. Today, reoperation is infrequently necessary as a result of the development of nonoperative methods of removing such retained bile duct stones. The most successful method involves instrument extraction under fluoroscopic control with the Dormia ureteral stone basket or Mondet forceps. The extraction is an outpatient procedure performed without premedication or analgesia five or more weeks after the initial operation in order to permit sufficient time for formation of a firm tract along the T tube. The T tube is removed, a "steerable" catheter is inserted through the T tube tract into the common duct, the stone basket is inserted through the "steerable" catheter, and the stone is captured and extracted (Fig. 24). The reason why it is important for surgeons to routinely use a large caliber T tube to drain the common duct, and to bring the tube out of the abdomen in a straight line at right angles to the common duct, is to form a large, straight tract that will accommodate the extrac-tion instruments should stone extraction become nec-essary. Table 4 shows recently reported results of in-

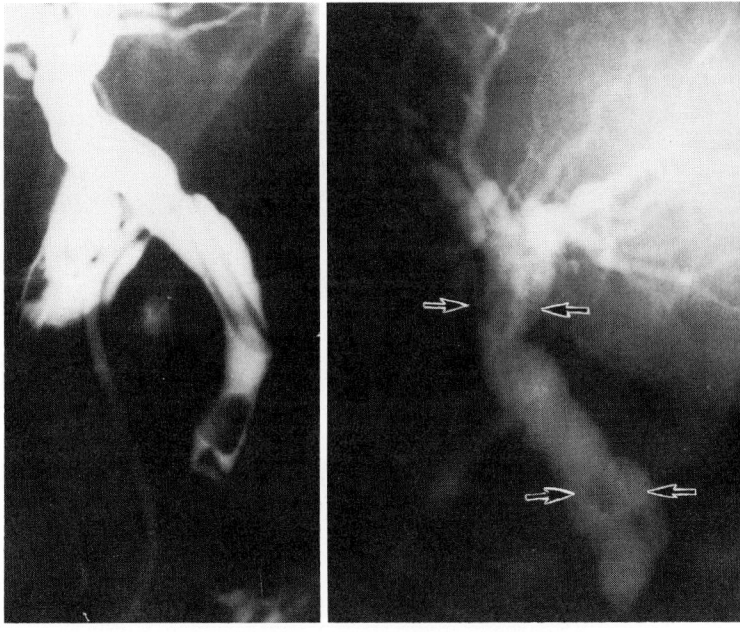

Figure 23.   Retained stones in the common bile duct demonstrated by postoperative T tube cholangiograms in two patients who had undergone cholecystectomy and choledoch-otomy.

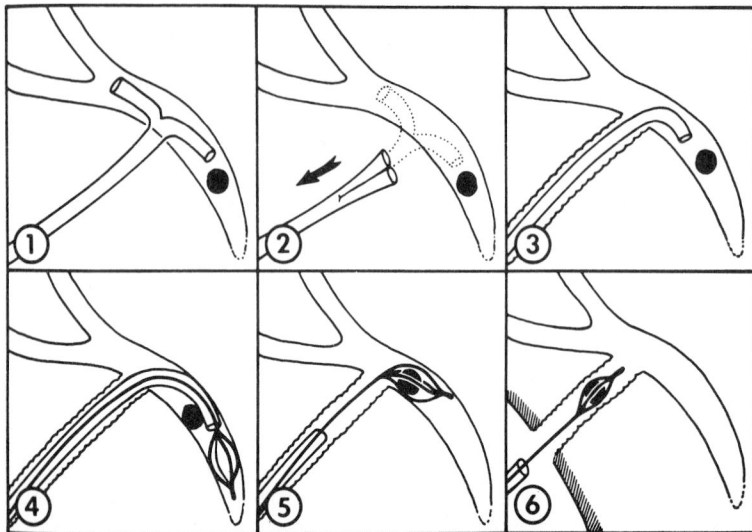

Figure 24. Steps in instrument extraction of retained common duct stone.

1. Repeat T tube cholangiogram is obtained on the day of stone extraction 4 to 5 weeks after choledochotomy.

2. After the location of the retained stone has been ascertained, the T tube is withdrawn.

3. Using the sinus tract of the T tube, the steerable catheter is guided into the bile duct, and its movable tip is advanced beyond the retained stone.

4. The basket is inserted through the steerable catheter, the catheter is withdrawn and the basket opened.

5. The open basket is withdrawn in order to engage the stone. The basket is only retracted, never advanced, outside the enclosure of the steerable catheter.

6. The stone is extracted through the drain tract.

(From Burhenne, H. J.: Nonoperative retained biliary tract stone extraction. A new roentgenologic technique. Am. J. Roentgenol., *117*:388, 1973.)

strument extraction of retained bile duct stones. A success rate exceeding 90 per cent can be expected. The complications of the technique have been few, and no deaths have been reported to date.

Over the years, a variety of chemical agents have been introduced into the common bile duct to dissolve retained calculi, with little success. However, two chemical agents, heparin and the sodium salt of cholic acid, have been used recently with some good results. On the basis of experiments in vitro and in animals, Gardner proposed that heparin increases the negative surface charge of the bile salt–lecithin–cholesterol micelle and thereby leads to the dispersion of the micelles. Administration of heparin as a continuous infusion into the T tube in a dose of 25,000 units in 250 ml. saline every 8 hours for approximately one week has resulted in dissolution of retained stones in 31 of 43 patients treated by Gardner et al. Other workers have not yet obtained similar success, and failure of heparin to dissolve gallstones in vitro has been reported recently.

The rationale for the use of sodium cholate to dissolve retained gallstones is based on the previously described important role of bile salts in solublizing cholesterol. In this regard, both chenodeoxycholic acid and deoxycholic acid have been shown to be more effective than cholic acid in dissolving gallstones in vitro, but these agents have not been used in patients because of toxicity and expense. Way and Admirand have infused a solution of sodium cholate into the T tube at the rate of 30 ml. per hour under manometric control for up to 10 days and have reported dissolution of retained bile duct stones in about one half of the 22 patients so treated. The bile salt irrigation regularly produces diarrhea, and occasional hypotensive reactions and septicemia have been observed.

If the nonoperative methods of extracting or dissolving retained bile duct stones are not successful, and if the calculi fail to pass spontaneously into the intestine, operative removal is usually indicated. Hicken and McAllister reported that 60 per cent of 152 patients discharged from the hospital with retained stones developed symptoms requiring reoperation within 18 months, and 96 per cent required surgical treatment within five years.

Treatment of Retained or Recurrent Stones Discovered Months or Years Postoperatively. When retained or recurrent bile duct stones become symptomatic months or years after the initial biliary operation, they should be removed by choledocholithotomy unless there are strong contraindications related to increased operative risk. The question is: should anything else be done surgically to prevent another recurrence of choledocholithiasis? This is a particularly pertinent question, since approximately 25 per cent of patients who have undergone reoperation for residual stones, whether early or late, have developed choledocholithiasis again. Currently, two adjunctive biliary drainage procedures, sphincteroplasty and choledochoduodenostomy, have been used under some circumstances. Sphincteroplasty (or transduodenal choledochoduodenostomy) involves total ablation of the terminal common bile duct sphincters and creation of an internal opening between the common duct and duodenum that is equal to the largest diameter of the common duct. It should not be confused with sphincterotomy, a much less effective operation that consists of transection of only the distal portion of the sphincter of Oddi. When used for treatment of choledocholithiasis, sphincteroplasty has been associated with a mortality rate of 1 to

TABLE 4.   Instrument Extraction of Retained Bile Duct Stones Discovered in the Immediate Postoperative Period

Authors	Year Reported	Number of Cases	Successful Stone Extraction (Per Cent)
Mazzariello	1974	330	96
Burhenne	1974	126	96
Bean et al.	1974	44	75

TABLE 5. Indications for Sphincteroplasty or Choledochoduodenostomy in Patients with Choledocholithiasis

1. Recurrent primary bile duct stones
2. Bile duct stones that cannot be extracted (e.g., intrahepatic stones)
3. Third operations for bile duct stones of any type
4. First operation on biliary tree "packed" with stones
5. ? Bile duct stones with stenosis of the papilla of Vater

4 per cent, and with a less than 2 per cent recurrence rate of bile duct calculi. Choledochoduodenostomy is a lateral anastomosis between the side of the common bile duct and the side of the duodenum. It should be done only if the common duct is dilated to a diameter of 15 mm. or greater, and the size of the anastomosis should be at least 2 cm. in diameter. The mortality and stone recurrence rates are not significantly different from those of sphincteroplasty. Given a dilated common bile duct, either of the two operations is satisfactory under most circumstances. If the common duct is not substantially dilated or if a stone is impacted in the ampulla of Vater, sphincteroplasty is clearly the procedure of choice.

The indications for performance of an adjunctive biliary drainage procedure are listed in Table 5. Sphincteroplasty or choledochoduodenostomy should be done whenever reoperation is required for primary bile duct stones because the chances of another recurrence are high. Biliary drainage should be performed whenever it is impossible to extract bile duct calculi, such as sometimes occurs when the stones are in the intrahepatic ducts. A biliary drainage procedure is indicated in all third operations for choledocholithiasis of any type. In patients with a biliary tree that is "packed" with many stones, a biliary drainage procedure should be added to the initial choledocholithotomy because of the likelihood that some calculi will be left behind. Finally, some surgeons advocate a biliary drainage procedure when bile duct stones are associated with stenosis of the papilla of Vater. However, this is an uncertain indication because of the difficulty in distinguishing true stenosis from muscle spasm.

PRIMARY SCLEROSING CHOLANGITIS

Primary sclerosing cholangitis, known also as "stenosing cholangitis," "fibrosing cholangitis," and "obliterative cholangitis," is a rare, diffuse, chronic inflammation of unknown etiology that involves the extrahepatic bile ducts. It occurs at least three times more commonly in males than in females, and has been reported in patients ranging in age from 20 to 67 years. It is characterized by marked thickening of the common bile duct and sometimes the hepatic ducts, with extreme narrowing of the lumen due to inflammation and edema of the submucosa and subserosa. Adjacent lymph nodes are often enlarged, but the gallbladder is usually normal and free of calculi.

There is no specific microscopic lesion. Involvement of the liver invariably occurs as a result of the chronic extrahepatic biliary obstruction, and may progress to the development of secondary biliary cirrhosis and portal hypertension.

Etiology

The cause of this unusual disorder is unknown. Bacterial, viral, and autoimmune etiologies have been proposed, but there is no objective evidence to support any of these factors. Cultures of the bile and biliary tissue are often sterile. The condition has been found in association with a number of other diseases, including chronic ulcerative colitis, Riedel's struma, scleroderma, regional enteritis, thrombocytopenic purpura, orbital pseudotumor, and fibrous retroperitonitis and mediastinitis. Of these, chronic ulcerative colitis is by far the most common associated disorder, and involvement of the intrahepatic bile ducts as well as the extrahepatic biliary system in these cases is not uncommon. Several authors have proposed that the term primary sclerosing cholangitis be reserved for cases in which there are no associated diseases, and that all other cases be classified as "secondary sclerosing cholangitis." A number of patients originally thought to have primary sclerosing cholangitis have proved on follow-up to have sclerosing bile duct carcinoma, and this neoplasm must always be considered in the differential diagnosis. As experience with primary sclerosing cholangitis has increased, the following criteria have been established for the diagnosis: (1) absence of gallstones; (2) absence of previous biliary surgery; (3) absence of biliary tract malignant disease on long-term follow-up; (4) absence of primary biliary cirrhosis on biopsy; (5) absence of associated diseases such as ulcerative colitis or retroperitoneal fibrosis; (6) generalized thickening and stenosis of the extrahepatic bile ducts; and (7) progressive obstructive jaundice. With application of these criteria, fewer than 50 cases have been reported in the literature.

Diagnosis

The clinical manifestations of primary sclerosing cholangitis are variable, but obstructive jaundice is the key feature of the picture. The jaundice may be intermittent initially, but ultimately it becomes continuous and progressive and may be accompanied by pruritus. Intermittent low-grade fever, chills, malaise, weakness, weight loss, nausea and vomiting, and dull abdominal pain in the right upper quadrant and epigastrium are frequent symptoms. The liver is often palpable and tender on physical examination, and the usual stigmata of portal hypertension may be present. Liver function studies show hyperbilirubinemia, with a preponderance of the direct-reacting pigment, and an elevation of the serum alkaline phosphatase. Other abnormalities of liver function are variable, depending on the stage of the disease. Oral and intravenous cholangiography are seldom possible because of the jaundice, and attempts at percutaneous transhepatic cholangiography usually fail because the lumen of the bile ducts is so tiny. Endoscopic retrograde cholangiography and transjugular cholangiography may be informative. Operative cholangiograms are characteristic and show a common bile duct irregularly narrowed to threadlike size, with beading of the intrahepatic ducts and a "pruned-tree" appearance. The diagnosis can be made only by surgical exploration of the biliary tract.

Treatment

Prolonged T tube drainage of the common bile duct and long-term adrenal steroid therapy are the essential elements of treatment. Forceful dilatation of the common duct may be required for insertion of the T tube. Although beneficial effects of biliary decompression have been documented, the mechanism by which this procedure influences the disease is not clear. The T tube should be left in place until cholangiograms show satisfactory dilatation of the biliary tree and free flow of dye into the duodenum. The undiseased gallbladder should not be removed at the time of the initial exploration because, in cases in which the disease is confined to the common bile duct, it may be used at a later time for biliary decompression via a cholecystoduodenostomy. Biopsies of the liver and bile ducts should always be obtained at the time of operation. Antibiotic therapy is indicated when positive cultures of bile are obtained, and attempts to decrease the viscosity of bile by the administration of bile salt cholegogues may have some limited value. On the presumption that the disease has an autoimmune etiology, treatment with the immunosuppressive agent azathioprine has been attempted, but experience is insufficient to judge the merits of such therapy. In the secondary form of the disease associated with chronic ulcerative colitis, total colectomy may be of benefit.

The mortality rate of primary sclerosing cholangitis is uncertain. Until the past decade, almost all of the patients died, usually of liver damage or the complications of portal hypertension. However, with proper therapy, a number of patients have recovered and remained asymptomatic for prolonged periods of time. The specter of bile duct carcinoma dictates a guarded prognosis for at least five years after the onset of symptoms.

STENOSIS OF THE SPHINCTER OF ODDI AND STENOSING PAPILLITIS

Stenosis of the sphincter of Oddi, from spasm or fibrosis, and inflammatory stenosis of the papilla of Vater are conditions that may cause the clinical manifestations of common bile duct obstruction and pancreatitis. However, their clinical importance is uncertain and a matter of controversy. The vast majority of cases are associated with calculi in the common bile duct or gallbladder and are believed to result from the inflammatory response to the choledocholithiasis and cholecystitis. A small number of primary cases without biliary calculi have been reported, and the etiology of these is unknown.

Stenosis of the sphincter or the papilla is believed to be responsible for some cases of persistence of symptoms following cholecystectomy, the *postcholecystectomy syndrome,* for some forms of recurrent pancreatitis, and for some cases of obstructive jaundice in the absence of choledocholithiasis or other demonstrable etiologic processes. The most frequent clinical manifestation is pain, usually in the form of attacks of biliary colic. Some patients have intermittent clinical or subclinical jaundice, with increased serum bilirubin and alkaline phosphatase, and attacks of pancreatitis with elevations of serum amylase and lipase. Cholangiographic demonstration of dilatation of the common bile duct above 1.5 cm., unusual narrowing of the terminal portion of the duct, and delay in emptying of the contrast medium into the duodenum are helpful in making the diagnosis preoperatively.

Operations for stenosis of the sphincter or the papilla in the absence of gallstones should be undertaken only after other causes of the symptoms have been excluded by a thorough diagnostic investigation. At operation, the stenosis should be demonstrated by inability to pass a 3-mm. probe into the duodenum through a choledochotomy, by operative cholangiography, or by radiomanometry. The latter technique involves pressure and flow measurements in the common bile duct and is used frequently in Europe but not in the United States. The operation of choice is transduodenal sphincteroplasty in which the terminal common bile duct sphincters are ablated and a large internal opening between the common duct and duodenum is created. Addition of sphincteroplasty of the duct of Wirsung to the standard Oddi sphincteroplasty has been advocated by some workers. Some surgeons have reported comparable benefits from choledochoduodenostomy. In all initial explorations of the common bile duct during operations for calculous disease, calibration of the sphincter of Oddi with a probe or dilator is an integral part of the surgical procedure. A number of surgeons have advocated the performance of a sphincteroplasty whenever evidence of terminal duct stenosis is obtained during a routine exploration. However, the added potential morbidity and mortality of this procedure must be weighed against its potential benefits in routine initial choledochotomies.

HYPERPLASTIC CHOLECYSTOSES

The hyperplastic cholecystoses are a group of benign, degenerative lesions in which there is excessive proliferation of gallbladder tissue. Unlike true papillomas of the gallbladder, they are not neoplasms. According to Jutras et al., included among these uncommon conditions are cholesterolosis, adenomyomatosis, neuromatosis, lipomatosis, fibromatosis, and hyalinocalcinosis (calcified gallbladder). In cholecystograms, they often appear as filling defects in an otherwise normal gallbladder. Most of these lesions are discovered at operations or in roentgenograms in patients who do not have symptoms of biliary disease. However, occasionally they are associated with symptoms similar to those of chronic calculous cholecystitis. Cholecystectomy is recommended only for patients with well-documented symptoms that cannot be accounted for by other diseases after a thorough investigation. Relief of symptoms following removal of the gallbladder has been reported.

ACALCULOUS CHOLECYSTITIS

Acalculous cholecystitis is not a single disease entity or syndrome but rather is a term used to describe the approximately 5 per cent of cases of gallbladder inflammation in which no calculi are demonstrable in the biliary system. Some of the cases of acalculous cholecystitis are attributable to specific causes such as bacterial infections, congenital anomalies, pancreatitis, obstruction of the cystic duct by neoplasm, fibrosis, or kinking, thrombosis of the blood supply to the gallbladder, and stenosis of the sphincter of Oddi or papilla of Vater. However, in the majority of cases, the etiology is unclear. Three clinical syndromes associated with acalculous cholecystitis have received considerable recent attention. These are acute post-traumatic cholecystitis, acute postoperative cholecystitis, and acute cholecystitis in children.

Acute post-traumatic cholecystitis develops in patients who have had severe trauma, sepsis, or burns and is part of the multiple system and organ failure syndrome associated with severe stress. Most of the reported cases have involved young males who sustained life-threatening injuries and underwent multiple operations. The clinical features of the disease are identical to those of ordinary acute calculous cholecystitis, but they are clouded by the disturbances in other organs that have been injured. The key to successful treatment is awareness that this disease entity may occur so that in an injured patient who develops signs and symptoms in the right hypochondrium, the necessary diagnostic studies are performed and surgical therapy is undertaken promptly. The mortality rate of acute post-traumatic cholecystitis has been substantial, in part due to the severe associated injuries.

Acute postoperative cholecystitis develops in the postoperative period following operations for unrelated disease. Over 200 cases have been reported. Most of the patients have been elderly males and the majority have not had gallstones. The etiology is unknown, although it has been proposed that the inflammation is caused by bile stasis resulting from dehydration, fasting, and narcotic analgesics. It is likely that acute acalculous postoperative cholecystitis and acute acalculous post-traumatic cholecystitis are one and the same entity. The major problem with the condition is its recognition. Although the symptoms and signs are the same as those produced by ordinary acute calculous cholecystitis, attributing them to gallbladder inflammation in a postoperative patient may be difficult. Consequently, the incidence of gallbladder perforation and the mortality rate have been high. Awareness of the existence of this disease entity is the key to its recognition. Operative treatment is almost always indicated.

Acute cholecystitis in children other than those who have hemolytic anemias is a third form of usually acalculous inflammation of the gallbladder that develops as a complication of unrelated acute systemic illness and severe stress. Most of the reported cases have occurred during the course of an acute febrile disease and have presented difficult problems in diagnosis because physicians are not in the habit of thinking of cholecystitis in children. The treatment is removal or drainage of the gallbladder, which is lifesaving.

SYMPTOMS AFTER CHOLECYSTECTOMY

Ninety to ninety-five per cent of patients subjected to cholecystectomy for chronic cholecystitis have complete or substantial relief of symptoms. However, in a small number of patients, symptoms continue or new complaints develop after operation. The causes of these disturbances are several, and they have been lumped together under the term "postcholecystectomy syndrome." The conditions responsible for symptoms after cholecystectomy may be categorized as follows:

1. *Diseases of other systems.* Included in this category are functional disorders and conditions such as peptic ulcer, pancreatitis, hiatus hernia, and coronary insufficiency. The discovery of these diseases does not necessarily indicate an error in initial diagnosis, although this is often the case. This group represents the most frequent cause of the postcholecystectomy syndrome.

2. *Organic biliary tract disease.* This category includes overlooked cholelithiasis, a large cystic duct stump in which calculi may develop, stenosis of the sphincter of Oddi, and injuries to the biliary ducts. These disorders require surgical correction.

3. *Biliary dyskinesia.* This is presumed to be a functional disorder of the bile ducts that causes abnormal elevations of pressure and disturbances of bile flow in the biliary system. The existence of this condition as a demonstrable clinical entity has been questioned.

A significant reduction in the incidence of symptoms after cholecystectomy will occur if every patient is evaluated thoroughly before biliary surgery is undertaken.

INJURIES TO THE EXTRAHEPATIC BILIARY SYSTEM

EXTERNAL TRAUMA

Because of the protected location of the extrahepatic biliary system, injuries to the gallbladder and bile ducts from external trauma are uncommon. Moreover, biliary wounds are usually associated with injuries to adjacent viscera, particularly the liver, colon, small intestine, and pancreas, and the symptoms and signs of the associated organ damage frequently dominate the clinical picture. Penetrating trauma due to gunshot wounds, stab wounds, and needle lacerations during liver biopsy and percutaneous cholangiography make up the bulk of biliary injuries. Wounds caused by blunt trauma are rare, and are usually the result of automobile accidents.

The clinical manifestations of biliary wounds are initially caused by leakage of bile and bleeding. Although bile in the peritoneal cavity of experimental animals has been found to cause a severe peritonitis and a high mortality rate, human bile is usually sterile and produces only a mild inflammatory reaction. However, if bile leakage continues for several days, large fluid losses, loculated collections, and secondary infection are common sequelae. Pain in the right upper abdomen, abdominal tenderness and rigidity, absence of bowel sounds, fever, and leukocytosis are the usual clinical findings. If the blood vessels to the biliary tract or liver are damaged, shock from bleeding may occur. A positive abdominal tap productive of bile or blood is often obtained. Since isolated biliary injuries are rare, the clinical manifestations are frequently those of associated wounds of the liver or intestinal tract.

The treatment of biliary tract injuries consists of prompt operation and surgical repair of the damage. In the case of gallbladder wounds, cholecystectomy is usually necessary. Wounds of the bile ducts are repaired by direct reconstruction when possible, or by a bypass anastomosis between the biliary system (bile duct or gallbladder) and intestine (duodenum or jejunum). Catheter drainage of the biliary tree is an essential adjunct. In cases involving common bile duct injury or retroperitoneal hematomas in the right upper quadrant of the abdomen, it is important to examine thoroughly the retroduodenal portion of the common duct by reflecting the duodenum medially by means of a Kocher maneuver. The mortality rate of biliary wounds is almost entirely related to associated injuries of other viscera.

ACQUIRED STRICTURES DUE TO OPERATIVE INJURY

Etiology

Almost all of the acquired strictures of the bile ducts are due to accidental injury during operations, and this condition is one of several very serious complications of biliary surgery. In the large experience of the Lahey Clinic with the treatment of 958 patients with bile duct strictures, 97 per cent of the strictures were due to surgical trauma. While a few cases were associated with gastroduodenal and pancreatic operations, 96 per cent of the injuries occurred during the course of operations on the biliary tract. In 3 per cent of the cases, the strictures were due to nonsurgical causes such as erosion by gallstones, inflammatory conditions, and blunt external trauma. The mechanism of surgical injury was identifiable in only one third of the cases and consisted of recognized direct damage to the bile duct, ligation of the bile duct, massive bleeding managed by blind clamping of the blood vessels, and difficulties in dissection due to adhesions and inflammation. There is no doubt that almost all surgical injuries to the bile ducts can be avoided if the surgeon has a thorough knowledge of the frequent anatomic variations in the porta hepatis, performs a careful dissection of the hepatic artery, cystic artery, and junction of the cystic duct with the common hepatic duct, is familiar with the principles that govern the management of bleeding in the right upper quadrant, and is aware of the occasional necessity of identifying and intubating the common bile duct during difficult operations for penetrating duodenal ulcer.

As might be expected from the age and sex incidence of calculous cholecystitis, biliary strictures occur most commonly in middle-aged women. The site of the stricture is usually around the level of the junction between the cystic duct and common hepatic duct. In the Lahey Clinic series, 40 per cent of the strictures were confined to the common hepatic duct, 28 per cent involved both the common hepatic and common bile ducts, and 23 per cent occurred in the common bile duct alone. Fortunately, only 10 per cent of the injuries occurred at a level above the common hepatic duct.

Diagnosis

When injuries to the bile ducts are recognized at the time of their occurrence during cholecystectomy, substantial morbidity and mortality can be prevented. Immediate repair by plastic reconstruction, end-to-end duct anastomosis, or biliary-intestinal anastomosis provides an excellent chance of normal biliary function. Unfortunately, the initial damage is frequently overlooked. The most common clinical manifestations of bile duct injury are the onset of obstructive jaundice within 48 hours after operation and the appearance of bile in sizable quantities from an external drain site or from the wound during the first postoperative week. These two telltale signs may be accompanied by fever and chills and light or clay-colored stools. Laboratory studies show hyperbilirubinemia, with substantial conjugated pigment, and an elevated serum alkaline phosphatase. If a drain is in place, x-rays following instillation of a contrast medium may demonstrate the fistula.

In some patients, the early manifestations abate, go unheeded, or do not occur. In such cases, the patient may present weeks, months, and occasionally years after operation with a history of intermittent jaundice and attacks of cholangitis consisting of fever, chills, clay-colored stools, and continuous dull pain in the right hypochondrium. Tender hepatomegaly and sometimes splenomegaly are found on examination, and laboratory studies show leukocytosis, hyperbilirubinemia, elevated serum alkaline phosphatase, and, depending on the timing in relation to infection, elevations of SGOT and SGPT. Prothrombin activity may be depressed. In time, liver damage may progress to biliary cirrhosis. Portal hypertension and hypersplenism develop in 15 to 20 per cent of patients because of liver disease resulting from continuing biliary obstruction and infection. Hepatic failure, bleeding from esophageal varices, and systemic infection are common complications.

In most cases, the diagnosis is clear-cut. However, in some instances, radiographic visualization of the bile duct stricture by transhepatic, transjugular, or endoscopic retrograde cholangiography may be necessary for diagnosis.

Treatment

Biliary strictures are fatal if uncorrected. Therefore, attempts at surgical correction are indicated, even if repeated operations are required. However, the greatest chances for success, other than those associated with immediate repair at the time of injury, are provided by the first reconstructive operation. It should be planned carefully and undertaken by a surgeon with experience in such procedures. The patient should be prepared for operation, if indicated, with antibiotics to control infection, parenteral nutritional therapy, and parenteral vitamin K. If the patient has portal hypertension and hypersplenism and has bled from esophageal varices, a splenorenal shunt should be performed prior to the biliary reconstruction. Dissection of the porta hepatis may be associated with significant bleeding in the presence of portal hypertension.

The most important determinants of the outcome of biliary reconstruction are the site of the stricture and the condition of the proximal bile duct. Other factors

that bear on the outcome are the amount of inflammation and scarring, the number of previous attempts at correction, and the extent of liver damage. An important initial step in operations for biliary strictures is identification of the proximal duct by needle aspiration and assessment of the biliary tree by operative cholangiography through a needle or a catheter inserted in the duct.

The operations used for correction of biliary strictures are illustrated in Figure 25. Plastic repair by vertical excision of the stricture and horizontal closure of the duct can be used in minor strictures of the common bile duct but is infrequently possible. End-to-end anastomosis of the bile duct after excision of the stricture is the procedure of choice, provided there is an ad-

Figure 25. Operations for correction of acquired traumatic strictures of the bile ducts.

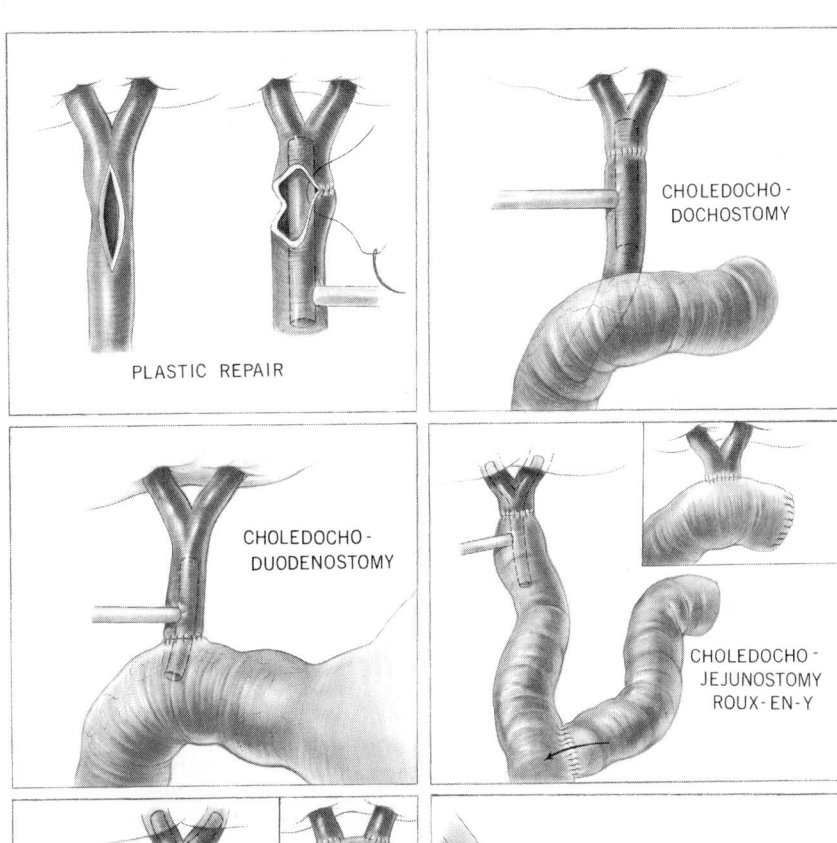

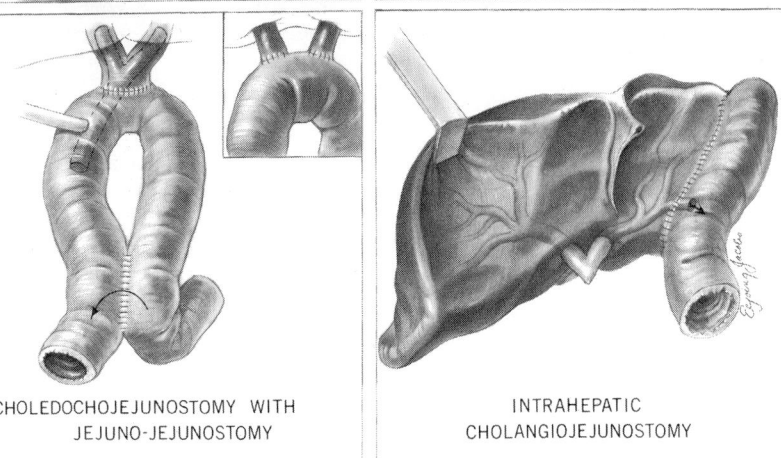

equate length of vascularized distal duct, and the anastomosis can be performed *without tension.* It is important to resist the temptation to perform a duct-to-duct anastomosis under any tension, since such repairs invariably fail. Anastomoses of the bile duct to the duodenum, a loop of jejunum combined with a jejunojejunostomy, or a defunctionalized segment of jejunum by the Roux-en-Y technique give comparable results. Again, it is important to avoid tension at the anastomosis, and this consideration sometimes limits the use of duodenum. The jejunal segment or loop should be at least 16 inches removed from the stream of intestinal contents to minimize reflux into the biliary tree, although substantial evidence indicates that such reflux is harmless in the absence of obstruction. Recently, Smith has reported good results with a sutureless anastomosis between the jejunal mucosa and the bile duct mucosa in a Roux-en-Y choledochojejunostomy, using a rubber tube inserted through the liver parenchyma as a stent. Finally, resection of the left lobe of the liver and anastomosis of an intrahepatic bile duct to the jejunum may be attempted if no other procedure is feasible. Use of this procedure is predicated on the demonstration that the selected duct communicates freely with the ductal system in the right lobe of the liver, so that it is essential to obtain a cholangiogram through the duct to be used for the anastomosis before proceeding with the definitive operation. The success of intrahepatic cholangiojejunostomy has been limited.

There is controversy regarding the use of rubber stents across the anastomosis, and no controlled studes of this matter have been done. At one time, internal stents were regularly inserted and allowed to pass spontaneously or were removed at a second operation, but these are rarely used today. At present, it is general practice to insert a T tube or Y tube stent that exits to the outside and can be easily removed at a later time. The external limb of the stent must always be brought out through a site at a distance from the biliary anastomosis (proximal or distal bile duct, or intestine), since bringing it out through the anastomosis results in a high incidence of recurrence of stricture. Many surgeons leave the stent in place for months and even years. However, when these long-indwelling tubes are removed, they are invariably plugged and covered with biliary sludge and debris; this finding suggests that they have stimulated a reaction within the duct and have been an impediment to biliary

drainage. Experimental evidence indicates that a rubber tube in the common bile duct stimulates a foreign body inflammation that increases with time. There is reason to doubt that a stent will prevent formation of scar tissue, and it is possible that the foreign body may increase fibrosis. Cole et al. reported 29 successful operations without the use of internal drainage. It is our practice to use rubber stents in biliary reconstructions, but to remove them after obtaining a cholangiogram within a few weeks of operation.

Some results of reconstructive operations for biliary stricture are shown in Table 6. An operative mortality rate of 5 to 10 per cent and an overall mortality rate of 15 to 20 per cent have been observed in patients treated by experienced surgeons. With long-term follow-up it is likely that the mortality increases to 25 or 30 per cent. Hepatic failure, hemorrhage from esophageal varices or during operation, and infection are the most frequent causes of death. Operations for biliary stricture are associated with significant morbidity in about one-fourth of the cases. Common complications include wound infections, intraperitoneal abscesses, biliary fistula, a variety of bleeding problems, and various degrees of hepatic insufficiency.

Two thirds to three fourths of patients are cured of their biliary stricture by present surgical techniques. The severity of pre-existing liver damage influences the overall results and provides an impetus for early diagnosis and prompt surgical treatment.

CONGENITAL ANOMALIES OF THE BILE DUCTS

CHOLEDOCHAL CYST

Cystic dilatation of the common bile duct is an uncommon congenital lesion that may produce symptoms in infancy but more often is discovered at some time during the first two decades of life. More than 500 cases have been reported in the literature, 83 per cent of which have been diagnosed in patients below the age of 30. Female patients have outnumbered males 3 or 4 to 1. The lesion is usually characterized by a well circumscribed dilatation of the common duct. The terminal bile duct distal to the lesion may be narrowed or, rarely, obliterated, but the intrahepatic biliary tree is usually normal. The etiology of the condition is unknown, although many theories have been proposed.

TABLE 6.   Results of Operations for Acquired Biliary Stricture

Authors	No. Patients	No. Operations	Results (Per Cent)				
			Excellent	*Good*	*Poor*	*Died*	*Lost*
Warren and Jefferson (1973)	987	1553	52	26	4	13	4
Hertzer, Gray, Hoerr, and Hermann (1973)	100	122	76	8	16	?	
Walters, Nixon, and Hodgins (1959)	191 Survivors	217	30	31	39	?	
Cole, Ireneus, and Reynolds (1955)	122	188	76		7	16	

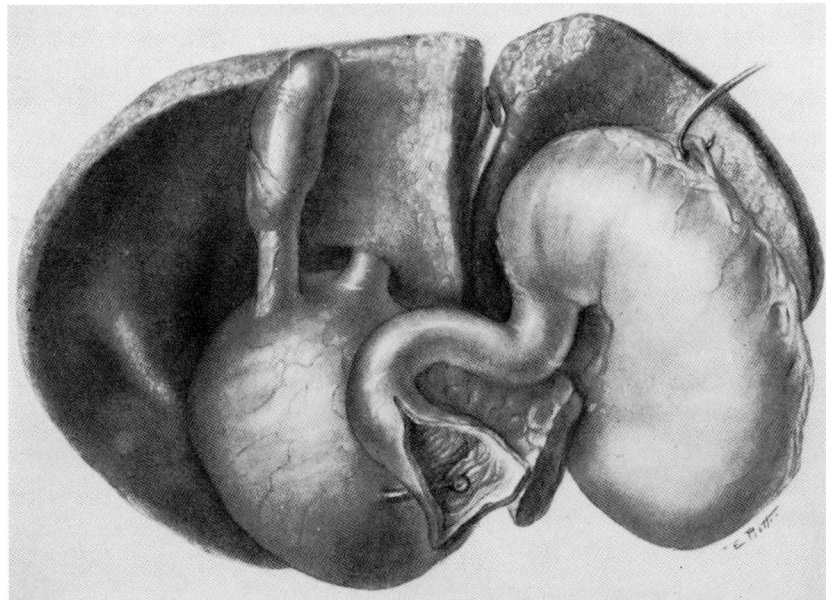

Figure 26. Choledochal cyst. (From Gross, R. E.: The Surgery of Infancy and Childhood. Philadelphia, W. B. Saunders Company, 1953.)

Among these is the theory that the cyst is a congenital malformation that results from an abnormality of epithelial cell proliferation during development of the bile ducts, and the proposal that the cyst results from the combination of a congenital weakness in the bile duct wall and distal duct obstruction.

Pathology

Choledochal cysts have been classified into three anatomic categories. Type I is an aneurysmal dilatation of the common bile duct, and it is by far the most frequent form (Fig. 26). Type II is a diverticulum that arises laterally from the wall of the common bile duct. Only 14 cases of this type have been reported. Type III, of which only nine cases have been reported, arises in the terminal intraduodenal portion of the common bile duct, involves the entrance of the pancreatic duct, and is lined by duodenal mucosa inside and out. It has been called a choledochocele, and it may represent an entergenous cyst rather than a true choledochal cyst. To these three types, Longmire et al. have added a rare fourth type in which the common and hepatic ducts have multiple diverticula. This condition has been called polycystic formation or diverticulosis of the bile ducts. In addition to these extrahepatic choledochal cysts, a variety of rare and presumably congenital cysts and dilatations of the intrahepatic bile ducts have been described. The intrahepatic bile duct abnormalities may occur singly or multiply, with or without associated periportal fibrosis of the hepatic parenchyma, and they may give rise to cholangitis and calculi within the liver. Occasionally, intrahepatic bile duct cysts have been associated with extrahepatic choledochal cysts.

Choledochal cysts have been found to vary in size from 3 to 25 cm. in diameter. The cyst wall is composed of fibrous tissue with interspersed elastic and sparse smooth muscle fibers. The internal lining consists of columnar epithelium, but it is often destroyed by inflammation and the pressure of the distending fluid. Surprisingly, gallstones are only occasionally found in the biliary system or in the cyst. Carcinoma in the cyst or the adjacent bile ducts has been reported in 16 cases, an unusually high incidence.

Diagnosis

The clinical manifestations of choledochal cyst are often intermittent and are due to filling of the cyst with fluid and resultant compression of the biliary tree. A triad of abdominal pain, jaundice, and a palpable abdominal mass in the right hypochondrium has been classically associated with this condition. The pain in the right hypochondrium is usually colicky and most severe during episodes of jaundice, but it may be dull and constant. Jaundice with dark urine and light stools is characteristically intermittent, but, particularly in infants, it may be continuous and raise the possibility of biliary atresia. Laboratory studies confirm the obstructive nature of the jaundice. The abdominal mass is typically cystic and nontender on palpation. In at least one third of the patients, all of the elements of the clinical triad are not present. Additional symptoms in some cases include fever and chills (cholangitis), nausea, vomiting, and anorexia. If untreated, choledochal cyst produces liver damage, which progresses to biliary cirrhosis and portal hypertension with all of its sequelae. In some instances, the portal hypertension results from compression of the portal vein by the cyst. Rupture of the cyst with bile peritonitis has been reported a number of times.

In addition to the usual laboratory tests used in the diagnosis of jaundice, barium contrast upper gastrointestinal x-rays and hypotonic duodenography may be of value in showing displacement and distortion of the duodenum. Intravenous cholangiography in the patient without jaundice, and cholangiography by the endoscopic retrograde, percutaneous transhepatic, or percutaneous transjugular approach may demonstrate the cystic dilatation of the common bile duct. Ultrasonic scanning has been successful in demonstrating the abdominal mass in several instances. In all cases, the precise relationship of the cyst to the biliary tree should be demonstrated by cholangiography at operation.

Treatment

Once a choledochal cyst has produced symptoms, it is almost invariably fatal unless it is treated surgically. Treatment of the rare type II diverticulum consists of simple excision, while the rare type III choledochocele is treated by transduodenal excision of the cyst wall so as to create a wide opening into the duodenum. The common type I fusiform cyst is currently treated either by excision combined with a biliary-intestinal anastomosis or by anastomosis of the cyst to the intestinal tract. Excision of the cyst may be difficult and has seldom been practiced in the United States, although it is popular in Japan. Anastomosis of the cyst to the intestinal tract may take the form of cystoduodenostomy, cystojejunostomy using a loop of intestine, and cystojejunostomy by the Roux-en-Y technique. The Roux-en-Y anastomosis has been associated with somewhat better results than the other two techniques, and there would appear to be some advantage in avoiding reflux of intestinal contents into the cyst by using a defunctionalized limb of intestine. Incidental cholecystectomy should be performed because of the significant postoperative incidence of cholecystitis and gallstones. The current mortality rate of choledochal cyst treated by surgical decompression is 5 to 10 per cent. The long-term results of operative therapy are quite good, although secondary operations to correct stenosis at the biliary-intestinal anastomosis are sometimes necessary.

ATRESIA OF THE BILE DUCTS

Biliary atresia is the most frequent cause of persistent jaundice in newborn infants, although it is by no means a common condition, occurring in only one of 10,000 live births in the United States. The etiology of biliary atresia is not known, but during the past decade concepts regarding its pathogenesis and treatment have changed considerably. Until recently it was believed to be a congenital disease that results from an arrest in development of part or all of the bile ducts at the embryonic stage, when the biliary system consists of solid cords. However, substantial recent evidence suggests that biliary atresia may be an inflammatory disease that is dynamic in nature and may progress after birth. Moreover, some evidence indicates that biliary atresia, the neonatal hepatitis syndrome, and, perhaps, choledochal cyst may be variations or stages of the same disease process.

Although the extent of involvement of the biliary system by the occlusive process varies considerably, biliary atresia occurs in two major anatomic forms. In the first form, represented by 5 to 15 per cent of the cases, the proximal part of the extrahepatic biliary tree is patent and conventional surgical treatment may be possible by means of an anastomosis between the biliary system (common bile duct, gallbladder, or common hepatic duct) and intestine (duodenum or jejunum). This form has been called "extrahepatic" or "correctable" biliary atresia and until recently, has included all of the survivors of the disease (types 1, 2, and 3 in Figure 27). In the second anatomic form, found in the vast majority of patients, the large proximal extrahepatic bile ducts or the entire extrahepatic ductal system are occluded. It has often been concluded, on the basis of autopsy studies performed months after onset of the disease, that the intrahepatic bile ducts are also involved in the atretic process. This form has been called "intrahepatic" or "noncorrectable" biliary atresia (types 4, 5, 6, and 7, Figure 27). However, recent observations have demonstrated that the secondary extrahepatic bile ducts in the hilum of the liver as well as the intrahepatic bile ducts are frequently patent at an early stage in the "noncorrectable" form so that effective surgical treatment may be possible.

Diagnosis

The onset of jaundice in patients with biliary atresia is classically described as occurring during the middle or end of the first week of life, because of clearing of bilirubin in utero across the mother's placenta. However, a significant number of patients are observed to have jaundice at birth, and some patients have been described who did not become icteric until several weeks after birth. The influence of observer error in determining the time of onset of jaundice is difficult to assess. Onset of jaundice after the first month of life is rarely due to biliary atresia. The jaundice is progressive, although there are often small fluctuations, until a high plateau is reached after several weeks. Dark urine and light or clay-colored stools accompany the icterus. Small amounts of pigment may appear in the feces from time to time as a result of desquamation of intestinal epithelial cells and secretion of intestinal mucus stained with bilirubin. During the first month after birth, the infant usually grows normally, has a good appetite, and is alert and active. Subsequently, anorexia develops and the baby becomes irritable. As the disease progresses, the abdomen enlarges owing to hepatomegaly and often splenomegaly and ascites. Ultimately, biliary cirrhosis and portal hypertension develop, with all of the usual manifestations of these conditions. Death is usually due to liver failure, malnutrition, or bleeding from esophageal varices or a coagulopathy. Associated congenital anomalies, particularly of the cardiovascular system, occur in 15 to 30 per cent of cases.

Laboratory studies show a high serum bilirubin with substantial quantities of conjugated pigment, bilirubin in the urine, absence of urobilinogen in the urine and stool, elevated serum alkaline phosphatase, depressed prothrombin, and variable abnormalities of hepatic enzyme and turbidity tests. Rising or sustained high levels of serum bilirubin with a significant direct-reacting fraction on weekly determinations over a period of several weeks are helpful in making the diagnosis early in the course of the disease. The radioactive rose bengal test has been used extensively in Japan to make the diagnosis of bile duct obstruction, but it is employed infrequently in this country because of difficulties in conduct and interpretation.

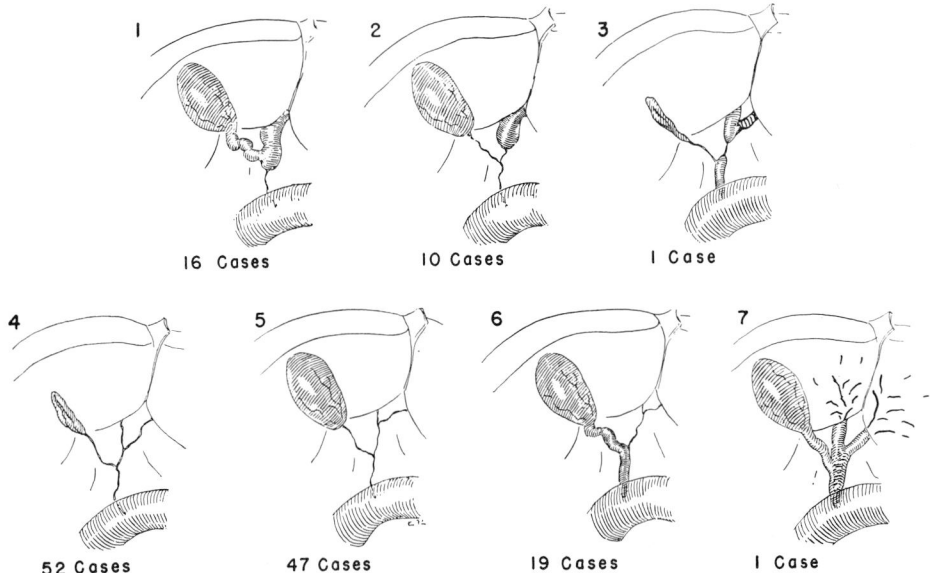

Figure 27. Types of biliary atresia encountered by Gross in 146 patients. The conditions in the upper row are surgically correctable by conventional operations; those in the lower row were considered noncorrectable until recently, but now may be correctable by hepatic portoenterostomy. (From Gross, R. E.: The Surgery of Infancy and Childhood. Philadelphia, W. B. Saunders Company, 1953.)

The diagnosis of biliary atresia may be very difficult. The differential diagnosis of neonatal jaundice includes the neonatal hepatitis syndrome, choledochal cyst, inspissated bile syndrome (the existence of which, as a discrete entity, is now doubtful), physiologic jaundice of the newborn or prematurity, sepsis, hemolytic diseases, galactosemia, cytomegalic inclusion disease, syphilis, the Crigler-Najjar syndrome, and toxoplasmosis. Most of these conditions can be ruled out by appropriate laboratory studies and observations of the course of the disease over a brief period of time. However, differentiation of biliary atresia from the neonatal hepatitis syndrome presents a major problem and may not be possible. The time of onset, progression of jaundice, obstructive pattern, and results of laboratory studies may be identical in the two conditions. The incidence of neonatal hepatitis is similar to that of biliary atresia. On liver biopsy, both conditions may show giant cell transformation of the parenchymal cells, disorganization of the hepatic architecture, bile duct proliferation, and bile stasis, and there is substantial overlapping of the microscopic findings in the two diseases. In a study of diagnostic accuracy, Hays and his associates observed that the differentiation of biliary atresia and the neonatal hepatitis syndrome was erroneous or indeterminate in 40 per cent of needle liver biopsies, 38 per cent of open liver biopsies, and 20 per cent of operative cholangiograms. Herein lies the dilemma in the management of biliary atresia.

Treatment

Biliary atresia is invariably fatal if not relieved by surgery. Survival ranges from 3 to 90 months, with a mean of 19 months. The majority of patients die within two years of birth. It is essential that all patients with biliary atresia undergo laparotomy for de-

termination of the feasibility of surgical correction and for appropriate treatment. However, because of the difficulties in preoperative diagnosis and presumed hazards of operation in jaundiced infants who do not have biliary atresia, there has been considerable controversy about the timing of exploratory laparotomy. Many clinicians have advocated operation during the first month of life on the basis that delay causes irreparable liver damage that may be fatal even if the obstruction is relieved. Others have argued that waiting for two or three months will help to sort out the patients whose jaundice is due to conditions other than biliary atresia and who may recover spontaneously unless they are subjected to the trauma of operation. Recent studies have provided crucial information which should resolve this controversy. It has been shown that the occlusive process in biliary atresia is often progressive unless the obstruction is relieved and that infants subjected to corrective operations after the third month of life have little chance of being cured. Furthermore, it has been demonstrated that the mortality rate of neonatal hepatitis is not increased by exploratory laparotomy. The recent development of a corrective operation that is applicable to the previously "uncorrectable" form of biliary atresia makes it imperative that exploratory laparotomy be undertaken before the tenth week of life in all infants suspected of having the disease.

The operative approach initially is directed at making the diagnosis. A liver biopsy with frozen section examination is obtained for histologic information that may be of value. If the gallbladder can be identified, it is aspirated to determine the presence of bilirubin-stained bile as an indicator of intact cystic and hepatic ducts. Operative cholangiography, if necessary with occlusion of the hepatoduodenal ligament to direct dye into the intrahepatic bile ducts, is then

TABLE 7.   Results of Hepatic Portoenterostomy for "Uncorrectable" Biliary Atresia in Japan (1968 to 1971)*

Infants < 90 Days of Age	Hospital No. 1	Hospital No. 2	Hospital No. 3	Hospital No. 4	Hospital No. 5	Total
Number of patients	8	43	20	19	26	116
Good bile excretion	5	25	5	13	23	71
Cured > 1 year: Number	3	18	5	10	14	50
Per Cent	38	42	25	53	54	43
Infants > 90 Days of Age						
Number of patients	12	37	31	6	23	99
Good bile excretion	9	15	4	1	4	33
Cured > 1 year: Number	0	5	2	0	0	7
Per Cent	0	14	6	0	0	7

*Study conducted by Drs. M. Kasai, S. Kimura, S. Sawaguchi, K. Suruga, and T. Ueda.

performed via the gallbladder. If the cholangiogram shows an intact biliary tree, the diagnosis is not biliary atresia and nothing further is done. If the cholangiogram demonstrates a correctable anomaly, or nonvisualization of the bile ducts, or if no gallbladder can be identified, an extremely careful and meticulous dissection of the hepatoduodenal ligament and porta hepatis is undertaken in the hope of finding an intact proximal ductal system. Cholangiography via intact-appearing ducts may be helpful in assessing the situation. Anastomosis of the gallbladder or proximal common bile or hepatic duct to the duodenum or jejunum by the loop or Roux-en-Y technique is performed in the fortunate circumstance of finding a reparable lesion. This circumstance occurs in only 5 to 15 per cent of the patients and, until recently, the remaining 85 to 95 per cent were considered hopeless.

In 1959, Kasai of Japan described an operation in an infant in whom there were no visible extrahepatic bile ducts. On careful dissection of the hilus of the liver he obtained a flow of bile and then attached a Roux-en-Y loop of jejunum to the tissues surrounding the area where the bile originated. The patient rapidly became free of jaundice and is alive and well today. Kasai called the operation hepatic portoenterostomy. Subsequently, the operation was applied widely in Japan to patients with "noncorrectable" biliary atresia, and recently the procedure has undergone trials in the United States, Europe, and Australia. Because of the frequent development of cholangitis following hepatic portoenterostomy, the original procedure has been modified by various techniques that vent the jejunal loop to the exterior for several months. Some results of the operation reported by Japanese surgeons are shown in Table 7. These results have demonstrated clearly that (1) a substantial number of patients with biliary atresia previously considered uncorrectable have patent bile ducts in the hilus of the liver and proximally; (2) the operation is generally unsuccessful if undertaken after the third month of life; and (3) the number of patients who have derived benefit from the operation is sufficient to warrant its widespread trial in what, until now, has been a hopeless condition.

Transplantation of the liver offers some hope for pa-

tients with biliary atresia that cannot be corrected by the surgical procedures described above. Several patients are now living and well more than five years after orthotopic liver transplantation for otherwise fatal atresia of the bile ducts.

REFERENCES

General

1. Glenn, F.: Atlas of Biliary Tract Surgery. New York, Macmillan Company, 1963.
2. Hess, W.: Surgery of the Biliary Passages and the Pancreas. Princeton, N.J., D. Van Nostrand Company, 1965.
3. Smith, R., and Sherlock, S.: Surgery of the Gallbladder and Bile Ducts. London, Butterworth & Company, 1964.

Anatomy

4. Boyden, E. A.: The anatomy of the choledochoduodenal junction in man. Surg. Gynecol. Obstet., 104:641, 1957.
5. Daseler, E. H., Anson, B. J. Hambley, W. C., and Reimann, A. F.: Cystic artery and constituents of the hepatic pedicle. Surg. Gynecol. Obstet., 85:47, 1947.
6. Flanney, M. G., and Caster, M. P.: Congenital anomalies of the gallbladder. Surg. Gynecol. Obstet., 103:439, 1956.
7. Kune, G. A.: The influence of structure and function in the surgery of the biliary tract. Ann. R. Coll. Surg., 47:78, 1970.
8. Michels, N. A.: Blood Supply and Anatomy of the Upper Abdominal Organs. Philadelphia, J. B. Lippincott Company, 1955.

Physiology

9. Banfield, W. J.: Physiology of the gallbladder. Gastroenterology, 69:770, 1975.
10. Dowling, R. H.: The enterohepatic circulation. Gastroenterology, 62:122, 1972.
11. Hofman, A. F.: The emerging importance of bile acids in human disease. Hormone Metab. Res. (Suppl.), 4:45, 1974.
12. Ivy, A. C., and Goldman, L.: Physiology of biliary tract. J.A.M.A., 113:2413, 1939.
13. Johnson, L. R., and Grossman, M. I.: Intestinal hormones as inhibitors of gastric secretion. Gastroenterology, 60:120, 1971.
14. Jorpes, J. E.: The isolation and chemistry of secretin and cholecystokinin. Gastroenterology, 55:157, 1968.
15. Lin, T-M.: Actions of gastrointestinal hormones and related peptides on the motor function of the biliary tract. Gastroenterology, 69:1006, 1975.
16. Wheeler, H. O.: Concentrating function of the gallbladder. Am. J. Med., 51:588, 1971.

Roentgenographic Studies in Diagnosis

17. Baker, H. L., Jr., and Hodgson, J. R.: Further studies on the accuracy of oral cholecystography. Radiology, 74:239, 1960.

18. Berk, R. N.: Radiology of the gallbladder and bile ducts. Surg. Clin. North Am., *53*:973, 1973.
19. Eaton, S. B., Benedict, K. T., Jr., Ferrucci, J. T., Jr., and Fleischli, D. J.: Hypotonic duodenography. Radiol. Clin. North Am., *8*:125, 1970.
20. Ferrucci, J. T., Jr., and Eaton, S. B., Jr.: Radiologic evaluation of obstructive jaundice. Surg. Clin. North Am., *54*:573, 1974.
21. Kadell, B. M., and Weiner, M.: Current status of the transjugular approach for direct cholangiography. Surg. Clin. North Am., *53*:1019, 1973.
22. Kittredge, R. D., and Finby, M.: Percutaneous transhepatic cholangiography. Am. J. Roentgenol., *101*:592, 1967.
23. Kasugai, T., Kuno, N., Kobayashi, S., and Hattori, K.: Endoscopic pancreatocholangiography (2 parts). Gastroenterology, *63*: 217, 1972.
24. Ogoshi, K., Niwa, M., Hara, Y., and Nebel, O. T.: Endoscopic pancreatocholangiography in the evaluation of pancreatic and biliary disease. Gastroenterology, *64*:210, 1973.
25. Okuda, K., Tanikawa, K., Emura, T., et al.: Nonsurgical, percutaneous transhepatic cholangiography: Diagnostic significance in medical problems of the liver. Dig. Dis., *19*:21, 1974.
26. Redeker, A. G., Karvountzis, G. G., Richman, R. H., and Horisawa, M.: Percutaneous transhepatic cholangiography. An improved method. J.A.M.A., *231*:386, 1975.
27. Rösch, J., Laken, P. C., Antonovic, R., and Dotter, C. T.: Transjugular approach to liver biopsy and transhepatic cholangiography. N. Engl. J. Med., *289*:227, 1973.
28. Seldinger, S. I.: Percutaneous transhepatic cholangiography. Acta Radiol., Suppl. 253, 1966.
29. Shehadi, W. H.: Clinical Radiology of the Biliary Tract. New York, McGraw-Hill Book Company, 1963.
30. Vennes, J. A., Jacobson, J., Jr., and Silbis, S. E.: Endoscopic cholangiography for biliary system diagnosis. Ann. Intern. Med., *80*:61, 1974.
31. Wise, R. E., and Scholz, F. J.: Radiology of the liver and biliary tract. Gastroenterology, *65*:967, 1973.

Ultrasonography in Diagnosis

32. Leopold, G. R., Amberg, J., Gosink, B. B., and Mittelstaedt, C.: Gray scale ultrasonic cholecystography: A comparison with conventional radiographic techniques. Radiology, 1976.
33. Tabrisky, J., Lindstrom, R. R., Herman, M. W., Castagna, J., and Sarti, D.: Value of gallbladder B-scan ultrasonography. Gastroenterology, *68*:1246, 1975.

Liver Biopsy in Diagnosis

34. Conn, H. O.: Liver biopsy in extrahepatic biliary obstruction and in other "contraindicated" disorders. Gastroenterology, *68*:817, 1975.
35. Morris, J. S., Gallo, G. A., Scheuer, P. J., and Sherlock, S.: Percutaneous liver biopsy in patients with large bile duct obstruction. Gastroenterology, *68*:750, 1975.

Gallstones

36. Admirand, W. H., and Small, D. M.: The physicochemical basis of cholesterol gallstone formation in man. J. Clin. Invest., *47*:1043, 1967.
37. Bouchier, I. A. D., and Freston, J. W.: The aetiology of gallstones. Lancet, *1*:340, 1968.
38. Coyne, M. J., Bonorris, G. G., Chung, A., Goldstein, L. I., Lahana, D., and Schoenfield, L. J.: Treatment of gallstones with chenodeoxycholic acid and phenobarbital. N. Engl. J. Med., *292*:604, 1975.
39. Dam, H.: Determinants of cholesterol cholelithiasis in man and animals. Am. J. Med., *51*:596, 1971.
40. Danzinger, R. G., Hofmann, A. F., Schoenfield, L. J., and Thistle, J. L.: Dissolution of cholesterol gallstones by chenodeoxycholic acid. N. Engl. J. Med., *286*:1, 1972.
41. Goldstein, L. I., and Schoenfield, L. J.: Gallstones: Pathogenesis and Medical Treatment. Adv. Intern. Med., *20*:89, 1975.
42. Iser, J. H., Dowling, R. H., Mok, H. Y. I., and Bell, G. D.: Chenodeoxycholic acid treatment of gallstones. A follow-up report and analysis of factors influencing response to therapy. N. Engl. J. Med., *293*:378, 1975.
43. Juniper, K.: Cause of gallstone disease. Mod. Treat., *5*:480, 1968.
44. Sampliner, R., and Bennett, P. H.: Gallbladder disease in Pima Indians demonstrative of high prevalance and early onset by cholecystography. N. Engl. J. Med., *283*:1358, 1970.
45. Small, D. M.: Gallstones. N. Engl. J. Med., *279*:588, 1968.
46. Small, D. M.: The formation of gallstones. Adv. Intern. Med., *16*:243, 1970.

47. Strasberg, S. M., and Fisher, M. M.: Pathogenesis of human cholesterol cholelithiasis. Can. Med. Assoc., J., *112*:484, 1975.
48. Swell, L., Gregory, D. H., and Vlahcevic, Z. R.: Current concepts of the pathogenesis of cholesterol gallstones. Med. Clin. North Am., *58*:1449, 1974.

Choledocholithiasis

49. Bartlett, M. K., and Dreyfuss, J. R.: Residual common duct stones. Surgery, *47*:202, 1960.
50. Bartlett, M. K., and Waddell, W. R.: Indications for common duct exploration. N. Engl. J. Med., *258*:164, 1958.
51. Britton, D. C., Gill, B. S., Taylor, R. M. R., and James, O.: The removal of retained gallstones from the common bile duct: Experience with sodium cholate infusion and the Burhenne catheter. Br. J. Surg., *62*:520, 1975.
52. Burhenne, H. J.: The technique of biliary duct stone extraction. Experience with 126 cases. Radiology, *113*:567, 1974.
53. Colcock, B. P., and Perey, B.: Exploration of the common bile duct. Surg. Gynecol. Obstet., *118*:20, 1964.
54. Gardner, B., Dennis, C. R., and Patti, J.: Current status of heparin dissolution of gallstones. Experimental and clinical observations. Am. J. Surg., *130*:293, 1973.
55. Gardner, B.: Experiences with the use of intracholedochal heparinized saline for the treatment of retained common duct stones. Ann. Surg., *177*:240, 1973.
56. Hall, R. C., Sakiyalak, P., Kim, S. K., Rogers, L. S., and Webb, W. R.: Failure of operative cholangiography to prevent retained common duct stones. Am. J. Surg., *125*:51, 1973.
57. Hampson, L. G., and Petrie, E. A.: The problem of stones in the common bile duct with particular reference to retained stones. Can. J. Surg., *7*:361, 1964.
58. Henzel, J. H., and DeWeese, M. S.: Common duct exploration with and without balloon-tipped biliary catheters. Arch. Surg., *103*:199, 1971.
59. Hiken, N. F., and McAllister, A. J.: Operative cholangiography as an aid in reducing the incidence of "overlooked" common bile duct stones: A study of 1293 choledocholithotomies. Surgery, *55*:753, 1964.
60. Hoerr, S. O., and Hermann, R. E.: Side-to-side choledochoduodenostomy. Surg. Clin. North Am., *53*:1115, 1973.
61. Jolly, P. C., Baker, J. W., Schmidt, H. M., Walker, J. H., and Holm, J. C.: Operative cholangiography: A case for its routine use. Ann. Surg., *168*:551, 1968.
62. Jones, S. A.: Sphincteroplasty (not sphincterotomy) in the treatment of biliary tract disease. Surg. Clin. North Am., *53*:1123, 1973.
63. Longmire, W. P., Jr., and Rangel, D. M.: Difficult problems encountered in the management of biliary obstruction due to stones and other benign conditions. Adv. Surg., *4*:105, 1970.
64. Madden, J. L., Chien, J. Y., Kondaloft, S., and Parekh, M.: Choledochoduodenostomy, an unjustly maligned surgical procedure? Am. J. Surg., *119*:45, 1970.
65. Madden, J. L., Vanderheyden, L., and Kondaloft, S.: The nature and surgical significance of common duct stones. Surg. Gynecol. Obstet., *126*:3, 1968.
66. Madden, J. L.: Common duct stones. Their origin and surgical management. Surg. Clin. North Am., *53*:1095, 1973.
67. Mazzariello, R.: Review of 220 cases of residual biliary tract calculi treated without reoperation: An eight-year study. Surgery, *73*:299, 1973.
68. Shore, J. M., and Shore, E.: Operative biliary endoscopy: Experience with the flexible choledochoscope in 100 consecutive choledocholithotomies. Ann. Surg., *171*:269, 1970.
69. Stefanini, P., Carboni, M., Patrassi, N., DeBernardinis, G., Negro, P., and Loriga, P.: Transduodenal sphincteroplasty. Its use in the treatment of lithiasis and benign obstruction of the common duct. Am. J. Surg., *128*:672, 1974.
70. Thomas, C. G., Nicholson, C. P., and Owen, J.: Effectiveness of choledochoduodenostomy and transduodenal sphincterotomy in the treatment of benign obstruction of the common duct. Ann. Surg., *173*:845, 1971.
71. Way, L. W., Admirand, W. H., and Dunphy, J. E.: Management of choledocholithiasis. Ann. Surg., *176*:347, 1972.

Primary Sclerosing Cholangitis

72. Cutler, B., and Donaldson, G. A.: Primary sclerosing cholangitis and obliterative cholangitis. Am. J. Surg., *117*:502, 1969.
73. Glenn, F., and Whitsell, J. C., II: Primary sclerosing cholangitis. Surg. Gynecol. Obstet., *123*:1037, 1966.
74. Krieger, J., Seaman, W. B., and Porter, M. R.: The roentgenologic appearance of sclerosing cholangitis. Radiology, *95*:369, 1970.

75. Longmire, W. P., Joseph, W. L., Levin, P. M., and Mellinkoff, S. M.: Diagnosis and treatment of cholangiolitic hepatitis (primary biliary cirrhosis). Ann. Surg., 162:356, 1965.

76. Myers, R. N., Cooper, J. H., and Padis, N.: Primary sclerosing cholangitis. Complete gross and histologic reversal after long-term steroid therapy. Am. J. Gastroenterol., 53:527, 1970.

77. Perry, A. W., Djang, E., Katrouni, G., and Ludington, L. G.: Primary sclerosing cholangitis. Am. J. Surg., 121:743, 1971.

78. Schwartz, S. I.: Primary sclerosing cholangitis: A disease revisited. Surg. Clin. North Am., 53:1161, 1973.

79. Sherlock, S.: Chronic cholangitides: Aetiology, diagnosis, and treatment, Br. Med. J., 3:515, 1968.

80. Thorpe, M. E. C., Scheuer P. J., and Sherlock, S.: Primary sclerosing cholangitis, the biliary tree, and ulcerative colitis. Gut, 8:435, 1967.

81. Warren, K. W., Athanassiades, S., and Mange, J. J.: Primary sclerosing cholangitis. Am. J. Surg., 111:23, 1966.

Stenosis of the Sphincter of Oddi and Stenosing Papillitis

82. Bartlett, M. K.: Might gallstones and recurrent pancreatitis have a common cause? Arch. Surg., 95:887, 1967.

83. Cattell, R. B., and Colcock, B. P.: Fibrosis of the sphincter of Oddi. Ann. Surg., 137:797, 1953.

84. Grage, T. B., Lober, P. H., Imamoglu, K., and Wangensteen, O. H.: Stenosis of the Sphincter of Oddi. Surgery, 48:304, 1960.

85. Jones, S. A., Smith, L. L., and Gregory, G.: Sphincteroplasty for recurrent pancreatitis. Ann. Surg., 147:180, 1958.

86. Nardi, G. L., and Acosta, J. M.: Papillitis as a cause of pancreatitis and abdominal pain. Ann. Surg., 164:611, 1966.

87. Nardi, G. L.: Papillitis and stenosis of the sphincter of Oddi. Surg. Clin. North Am., 53:1149, 1973.

Hyperplastic Cholecystoses

88. Jutras, J. A., Longtin, J. M., and Levesque, H. P.: Hyperplastic cholecystoses. Am. J. Roentgenol., 83:795, 1960.

89. Ram, M. D., and Medha, D.: Adenomyomatosis of the gallbladder. Surgery, 78:224, 1975.

Acalculous Cholecystitis

90. Glenn, F., and Mannix, H.: The acalculous gallbladder. Ann. Surg., 114:670, 1956.

91. Hoerr, S. O., and Hazard, J. B.: Acute cholecystitis without gallbladder stones. Am. J. Surg., 111:47, 1966.

92. Lindberg, E. F., Grinnan, G. L. B., and Smith, L.: Acalculous cholecystitis in Viet Nam casualities. Ann. Surg., 171:152, 1970.

93. Munster, A. M., and Brown, J. R.: Acalculous cholecystitis. Am. J. Surg., 113:730, 1967.

94. Pieretti, R., Auldist, A. W., and Stephens, C. A.: Acute cholecystitis in children. Surg. Gynecol. Obstet., 140:16, 1975.

95. Ternberg, J. L., and Keating, J. P.: Acute acalculous cholecystitis. Complication of other illnesses in childhood. Arch. Surg., 110:543, 1975.

96. Thompson, J. W., Ferris, D. O., and Baggenstoss, A. H.: Acute cholecystitis complicating operation for other diseases. Ann. Surg., 155:489, 1962.

97. Winegarner, F. G., and Jackson, G. F.: Posttraumatic acalculous cholecystitis: A highly lethal complication. J. Trauma, 11:567, 1971.

Symptoms after Cholecystectomy

98. Colcock, B. P., and McManus, J. E.: Experience with 1,356 cases of cholecystitis and cholelithiasis. Surg. Gynecol. Obstet., 101:161, 1955.

99. Glenn, F.: A 26 year experience in the surgical treatment of 5,037 patients with nonmalignant biliary tract disease. Surg. Gynecol. Obstet., 109:591, 1959.

100. Womack, N. A., and Crider, R. L.: Persistence of symptoms following cholecystectomy. Ann. Surg., 126:31, 1947.

Injuries to the Extrahepatic Biliary System

101. Diethrich, E. B., Beall, A. C., Jr., Jordon, G. L., Jr., and DeBakey, M. E.: Traumatic injuries to the extrahepatic biliary tract. Am. J. Surg., 112:756, 1966.

102. Cattell, R. B., and Braasch, J. W.: Primary repair of benign strictures of the bile duct. Surg. Gynecol. Obstet., 109:531, 1959.

103. Cole, W. H.: Strictures of the common duct. Surgery, 43:320, 1958.

104. Hertzer, N. R., Gray, H. W., Hoerr, S. O., and Hermann, R. E.: The use of T-tube splints in bile duct repairs. Surg. Gynecol. Obstet., 137:413, 1973.

105. Lary, B. G., and Scheibe, J. R.: Effect of rubber tubing on healing of common duct anastomoses. Surgery, 32:789, 1952.

106. Longmire, W. P., Jr.: Early management of injury to the extrahepatic biliary tract. J.A.M.A., 195:111, 1966.

107. Longmire, W. P., Jr., and Lippman, H. N.: Intrahepatic cholangiojejunostomy. An operation for biliary obstruction. Surg. Clin. North Am., 36:849, 1956.

108. Manlove, C. A., Quattlebaum, F. W., and Ambrus, L.: Nonpenetrating trauma to the biliary tract. Am. J. Surg., 97:113, 1959.

109. Penn, I.: Injuries of the gallbladder. Br. J. Surg., 49:636, 1961–62.

110. ReMine, W. H., and Ferris, D. O.: Surgery for biliary strictures. Surg. Clin. North Am., 47:877, 1967.

111. Walters, W., Nixon, J. W., Jr., Hodgins, T. E., and Ramsdell, J. A.: Strictures of the common and hepatic bile ducts. Arch. Surg., 78:908, 1959.

112. Warren, K. W., and McDonald, W. M.: Facts and fiction regarding strictures of the extrahepatic bile ducts. Ann. Surg., 159:996, 1964.

113. Warren, K. W., and Jefferson, M. F.: Prevention and repair of strictures of the extrahepatic bile ducts. Surg. Clin. North Am., 53:1169, 1973.

114. Wexler, M. J., and Smith, R.: Jejunal mucosal graft. A sutureless technic for repair of high bile duct strictures. Am. J. Surg., 129:204, 1975.

Choledochal Cyst

115. Alonso-Lej, F., Rever, W. B., Jr., and Pessagno, D. J.: Congenital choledochal cyst, with a report of 2, and an analysis of 94 cases. Surg. Gynecol. Obstet., 108:1, 1959.

116. Caroli, J.: Diseases of the intrahepatic biliary tree. Clin. Gastroenterol., 2:147, 1973.

117. Kasai, M., Asakura, Y., and Taira, Y.: Surgical treatment of choledochal cyst. Ann. Surg., 172:844, 1970.

118. Lee, S. S., Min, P. C., Kim, G. S., and Hong, P. W.: Choledochal cyst. A report of nine cases and review of the literature. Arch. Surg., 99:19, 1969.

119. Longmire, W. P., Jr., Mondiola, S. A., and Gordon, H. E.: Congenital cystic disease of the liver and biliary system. Ann. Surg., 174:711, 1971.

120. Saito, S., and Ishida, M.: Congenital choledochol cyst (cystic dilatation of the common bile duct). Progr. Pediatr. Surg., 6:63, 1974.

121. Trout, H. H., and Longmire, W. P., Jr.: Long-term followup study of patients with congenital cystic dilatation of the common bile duct. Am. J. Surg., 121:68, 1971.

122. Tsardakas, E. N., and Robnett, A. H.: Congenital cystic dilatation of common bile duct; report of 3 cases, analysis of 57 cases, and review of literature. Arch. Surg., 72:311, 1956.

Atresia of the Bile Ducts

123. Bennett, D. E.: Problems in neonatal obstructive jaundice. Pediatrics, 33:735, 1964.

124. Bill, A. H.: Treatment of biliary atresia. Adv. Surg., 8:63, 1974.

125. Hays, D. M., and Snyder, W. H.: Life-span in untreated biliary atresia. Surgery, 54:373, 1963.

126. Hays, D. M., Wooley, M. M., Snyder, W. H., Reed, G. B., Bwinn, J. L., and Landing, B. H.: Diagnosis of biliary atresia: Relative accuracy of percutaneous liver biopsy, open liver biopsy, and operative cholangiography. J. Pediatr., 71:598, 1967.

127. Hays, D. M.: Biliary atresia: The current state of confusion. Surg. Clin. North Am., 53:1257, 1973.

128. Holder, T. M.: Atresia of the extrahepatic bile duct. Am. J. Surg., 107:458, 1964.

129. Kasai, M.: Treatment of biliary atresia with special reference to hepatic portoenterostomy and its modifications. Progr. Pediatr. Surg., 6:5, 1974.

130. Kasai, M., Watanabe, I., and Ohi, R.: Follow-up studies of long-term survivors after hepatic portoenterostomy for "noncorrectable" biliary atresia. J. Pediatr. Surg., 10:173, 1975.

131. Krovetz, L. T.: Congenital biliary atresia: I. Analysis of thirty cases with particular reference to diagnosis. Surgery, 47:453, 1960.

132. Krovetz, L. T.: Congenital biliary atresia: II. Analysis of the therapeutic problem. Surgery, 47:468, 1960.
133. Landing, B. H.: Considerations of the pathogenesis of neonatal hepatitis, biliary atresia and choledochal cyst – The concept of infantile obstructive cholangiopathy. Progr. Pediatr. Surg., 6:113, 1974.
134. Lilly, J. R., and Altman, R. P.: Hepatic portoenterostomy (the Kasai operation) for biliary atresia. Surgery, 78:76, 1975.
135. Longmire, W. P., Jr.: Congenital biliary hypoplasia. Ann. Surg., 159:335, 1964.
136. Stowens, D.: Congenital biliary atresia. Ann. N. Y. Acad. Sci., 111:337, 1963.

I

ACUTE CHOLECYSTITIS

Larry C. Carey, M.D., and Philip W. Catalano, M.D.

PATHOGENESIS

Acute cholecystitis is associated with gallstones in 90 to 95 per cent of patients. In more than 85 per cent of those in the United States who have gallstones, the stones are composed of pure cholesterol or a mixture of cholesterol and pigments. Cholesterol is almost completely insoluble in water, requiring critical concentrations of bile salts and phospholipids (lecithin) for solubility, so that lithogenicity of bile is determined mainly by the relative proportions of these three substances in bile. It is significant that as bile is concentrated in the normal gallbladder the absolute relationships of these three substances do not change.

A fixed amount of bile salts recirculates through the enterohepatic system approximately 10 times each day. If emptying of the gallbladder were complete in each cycle, large gallstones would probably not form and even small particles would be removed. However, it has been estimated that the maximum degree of gallbladder emptying is only about 84 per cent, and some studies have shown it to be less in women (65 per cent). The efficiency of gallbladder emptying and the composition of residual "stasis" bile are important factors influencing stone formation.

The gallbladder itself may contribute to the process of gallstone formation by means of modification of bile composition, which provides a favorable environment for cholesterol precipitation, but the mechanism is yet to be determined. In the presence of infection and bacteria, conjugated bile acids can be rapidly absorbed, since any inflammation enhances absorption of bile salts. A decrease in bile salt concentration favors cholesterol precipitation. Another possible explanation is that bacteria or bile pigment may serve as a nidus for crystal formation when the bile is supersaturated. Stones formed in the gallbladder cause inflammation of the mucosa, and localized areas of inflammation are vulnerable to bacterial invasion.

Rejuvenated interest in the role of the gallbladder in the development of cholelithiasis stems from the finding that in some Caucasians, but not in Indians, lithogenic bile is restored toward normal by cholecystectomy. This observation remains unexplained.

In acute cholecystitis the gallbladder is unusually enlarged – to twice its normal size. It appears bright red to violet. Thin fibrinous attachments to adjacent structures, such as the hepatic flexure of the colon and frequently the common bile duct, develop. The surrounding tissues become edematous, friable, and inflamed. The histologic picture is consistent with acute inflammation, which varies in degree from mild leukocyte infiltration to frank gangrene.

EPIDEMIOLOGY

The true incidence of acute cholecystitis is probably uncertain because many patients do not consult a physician. Gallstone disease is encountered two to three times more frequently in women than in men, although difference is not significant before puberty or after the age of 60 years. There is considerable evidence implicating the role of hereditary factors in the occurrence of gallstone disease. Patients with disease of the terminal ileum affecting bile salt reabsorption are at greater risk to form gallstones because of interruption of the enterohepatic circulation of bile salts. Recently it has been recognized that patients with prosthetic heart valves (particularly the aortic valve) tend to develop bile pigment gallstones because of hemolysis. It has long been known that patients with hemolytic anemia have a similar propensity.

The incidence of gallbladder disease seems disproportionately higher in the puerperium. It has been shown that the efficiency of the gallbladder contraction is greatly reduced in the last trimester of pregnancy. The incidence of gallstones is higher in women taking birth control pills during the first 6 to 12 months of ingestion, after which it does not appear to be increased. It is possible that estrogen may alter bile composition, but the mechanism is not known.

DIAGNOSIS

About half the patients with gallstones complain of symptoms referable to the biliary tree. Complaints such as eructation, flatulence, pyrosis, and vague epigastric discomfort occur with equal frequency in patients with or without gallstones. Also, the traditional relationship between ingestion of foods such as cabbage, apples, and onions and biliary tract disease has been disproved.

The typical patient with gallbladder disease is a 40-year-old woman who is obese and fair-skinned. Right upper quadrant pain is present in 85 per cent of the patients, although pain may be midepigastric. Obstruction of the cystic duct usually results in pain of an intermittent nature often described as colic. When there is significant inflammation, the pain is more likely to be constant. As the inflammatory process worsens, the visceral and then the parietal peritoneum becomes irritated, resulting in localization of both pain and physical finding to the right subcostal area. Because the pain usually radiates to the tip of the right scapula via the seventh intercostal nerve, which radiates around the side of the chest wall, it is occasionally perceived in the right shoulder, so that the pain may be difficult to differentiate from that of coronary artery disease. Most patients give a history of previous similar "attacks."

Biliary colic is characterized by a sudden onset of pain 30 to 90 minutes after a meal. The pain is caused by obstruction of the cystic duct and is described as crampy. Nausea and possibly vomiting occur. The location of the pain is similar to that caused by acute cholecystitis in that it is midepigastric or right upper quadrant with some radiation to the right infrascapular area. The pain persists for about four hours in the majority of cases, but less than one hour in about 40 per cent. Pain subsides spontaneously. Jaundice, fever, leukocytosis, and amylase elevation do not usually occur.

Acute cholecystitis is characterized by steady right upper quadrant pain, nausea, and vomiting. The onset is not necessarily precipitated by food. The patients appear more ill than do those with colic. The pain is more generalized because of stimulation of the parietal peritoneum. Unlike the patients with biliary colic who frequently are restless, patients with acute cholecystitis frequently are quiet because associated peritoneal irritation causes sudden movement, cough, or deep inspiration to exacerbate the pain. The temperature is usually only mildly elevated, 99 to 101° F orally. The white blood count is only slightly elevated (10,000 to 13,000), with a predominance of polymorphonuclear cells (see Table 8).

Voluntary and involuntary guarding are frequently encountered on physical examination. Tenderness is usually present in the right upper quadrant along the right costal margin. The gallbladder is located along the right costal margin at the midclavicular line. If the gallbladder is distended, it may be palpable, and palpation is facilitated by use of the flat portion of the examining hand rather than the finger tips. The classic examination for acute gallbladder disease includes demonstration of a positive Murphy's sign. To do this, the examiner's hand is placed gently over the right costal margin, pressure is applied, and the patient is asked to take a deep breath. Gentle pressure as the patient takes a deep breath, pushing the liver and the

TABLE 8. Differential Diagnosis of Biliary Colic and Acute Cholecystitis

	Biliary Colic	Acute Cholecystitis
Pain:	± crampy	± steady
Nausea:	+	+
Vomiting:	±	+
Onset:	30–90 min. postprandial	not necessarily related to meals until treated
Duration:	4 hrs. or less, subsides spontaneously	
Fever:	0	± 99°–101° orally
Leukocytosis:	0	± 10,000–13,000
Amylase:	0	±

gallbladder inferiorly, causes the visceral peritoneum of the gallbladder to come into contact with the parietal peritoneum and a sharp localized somatic efferent pain sensation is perceived. This sign is usually positive in acute cholecystitis. Rebound tenderness frequently is present.

The differential diagnosis in over 95 per cent of cases is limited to six conditions:
1. Peptic ulcer disease
2. Coronary artery disease
3. Pancreatitis
4. Acute appendicitis
5. Renal colic
6. Salpingitis with possible Fitz-Hugh-Curtis syndrome

Pertinent laboratory data to be obtained immediately include complete blood count, amylase, urinalysis, chest and abdominal x-rays, and electrocardiogram when indicated. These laboratory studies along with the history and physical examination will enable the physician to make the correct diagnosis in the majority of patients. If the diagnosis of acute cholecystitis remains only suspected, other more sophisticated studies should be obtained. These include alkaline phosphatase, serum concentration of glutamic pyruvic oxaloacetic transaminase, and serum concentration of glutamic pyruvic transaminase and bilirubin (see Table 9).

"Stones" in the right upper quadrant are demonstrated on plain abdominal x-ray film in 10 to 15 per cent of patients with gallbladder disease. These must be differentiated from renal stones.

Acalculous Cholecystitis

Both acute and chronic cholecystitis may occur in the absence of gallstones. The acute form of the illness has been reported by several observers in trauma victims even when trauma does not involve the biliary tract. An impairment of gallbladder emptying has been incriminated. In the presence of recurrent attacks when the gallbladder is visualized but no stones are seen, diagnosis is aided by a plain film taken 36 hours after cholecystography if the gallbladder is still visible.

TABLE 9. Frequency of Abnormal Laboratory Tests with Acute Cholecystitis

Amylase ↑	15–30%
Alkaline Phosphatase ↑	41%
SGOT ↑	45–75%
SGPT ↑	44%
Bilirubin ↑	8%

TREATMENT

The preferred initial treatment of acute cholecystitis is nonsurgical. The regimen includes restriction of oral intake, nasogastric suction (to avoid stimulating the gallbladder or pancreas), intravenous fluids, and antibiotics. Narcotics are used in doses sufficient to relieve pain but not large enough to mask findings. White blood count is performed every six hours. The choice of antibiotics is based on the most common pathogens of the gallbladder (*Eschericia coli*, Klebsiella, Streptococcus) and their specific sensitivities in each hospital. Therapeutic levels of antibiotics in the biliary system are not achieved if there is obstruction of the common or cystic duct. Consequently, antibiotics are not predictably effective in sterilizing an infected biliary tree or in stopping the local inflammatory process in acute cholecystitis or cholangitis. The objective of antibiotic therapy is to achieve adequate blood levels of the drug to lessen the risk of systemic toxicity.

The most important aspect of nonsurgical treatment is repeated frequent examination by one physician. The critical factor is the changing course of the disease. If pain, tenderness, fever, and leukocytosis are progressing, nonoperative treatment should be abandoned and operation performed (Table 10). If the course is one of improvement, continued observation is safe. Up to 25 per cent of patients admitted with the diagnosis of acute cholecystitis will progress to frank gangrene or perforation of the gallbladder. Careful repeated observation will avert these conditions. It is vital to remember that, particularly in elderly pa-

TABLE 10. Nonoperative Treatment of Acute Cholecystitis

Nonoperative Treatment	Failure of Nonoperative Therapy
Nasogastric suction	↑ Pain
NPO	↑ Pulse
IV fluids	↑ Fever
WBC every 6 hrs.	↑ WBC
Antibiotics	
*Frequent Exams, same physician	*No Improvement in 6 to 12 hrs.

*Using the above criteria, nonoperative treatment is quite safe.

tients, there is frequently little or no correlation between fever or pain and the severity of the disease. Patients with diabetes incur a significantly higher risk of serious complications.

If the patient responds favorably to nonsurgical therapy and pain and tenderness subside, complete x-ray evaluation is mandatory in any patient over 40 years of age. This should include upper gastrointestinal series, barium enema, and oral cholecystogram. The oral cholecystogram should be repeated if the gallbladder is not visualized or if stones are not seen. The frequent coexistence of hiatus hernia, gallstones, and diverticulosis of the colon is the recognized Saint's triad. Even in patients under the age of 40 who have localized symptoms of gallbladder disease, an upper gastrointestinal series and oral cholecystogram should be done.

The oral cholecystogram is 95 per cent accurate, provided certain criteria are followed. Iopanoic acid (Telepaque), the contrast material most frequently used, is water-soluble, requires bile acids for solubilization, and undergoes passive diffusion across the intestinal mucosa. It is conjugated in the liver, excreted in the bile, and concentrated in the gallbladder. The criteria for satisfactory cholecystography include the following:

1. The patient ingests the dye—no vomiting.
2. Dye is absorbed—no gastric stasis, no malabsorption, no diarrhea.
3. Dye is conjugated—no hepatic parenchymal disease, bilirubin is less than 3 mg. per 100 ml. urine.
4. Dye is excreted into the hepatic duct.
5. Dye enters the gallbladder, provided the cystic duct is not occluded.
6. Dye is concentrated by gallbladder, provided gallbladder mucosa is not compromised by chronic disease.

Iodipamide, the contrast material used for intravenous cholangiography, has an iodine base and anaphylactic reactions have occurred (1 in 1600 patients). The substance is excreted by the liver into the bile. When the bilirubin is greater than 3 mg. per 100 ml. urine, visualization is not likely. The intravenous cholangiogram is more helpful than the oral cholecystogram in the study of biliary ducts, but the oral cholecystogram is a more accurate procedure in acute or chronic cholecystitis or cholelithiasis. The intravenous cholangiogram is a useful procedure to exclude extrabiliary causes of nonvisualization, while oral cholecystography is more useful in postcholecystectomy syndromes and occasionally in abdominal pain of unknown etiology. The oral cholecystogram is more accurate than the intravenous cholangiogram in certain instances because the gallbladder does not concentrate iodipamide as well as iopanoic acid so that gallstones may not be identified even though the gallbladder is visualized. Aside from visualization of dilated ducts, four possibilities may be demonstrated by intravenous cholangiography (Fig. 28). Numbers 1 and 2 suggest normal gallbladder; number 3 suggests an obstructed cystic duct (if there has been no previous cholecystectomy); number 4 is not diagnostic.

A radioisotope technique is now being studied to as-

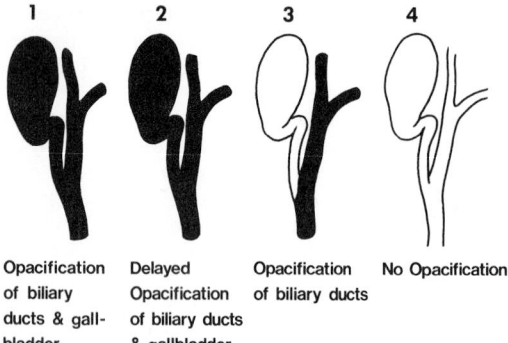

Opacification of biliary ducts & gall-bladder

Delayed Opacification of biliary ducts & gallbladder

Opacification of biliary ducts

No Opacification

Figure 28. The four possibilities with intravenous cholangiogram.

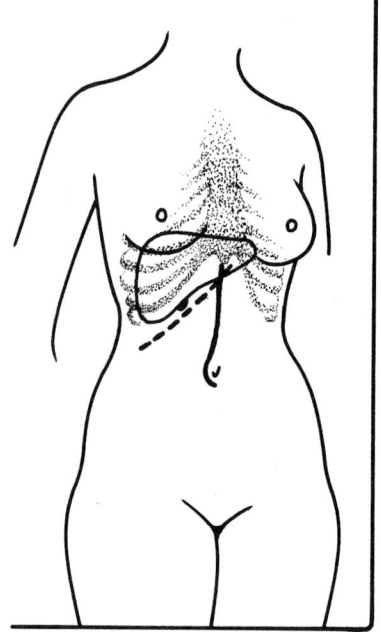

Figure 29. Either vertical or subcostal incision may be used. The determining factor is usually the distance between the costal margins.

sist in the diagnosis of gallbladder disease. Structures of diagnostic importance are monitored by the external gamma-emissions imaging and recording devices. Although scanning techniques are not widely used currently, the improving technology of ultrasound may make this procedure valuable in the future.

Duodenal biliary drainage has been recognized as a method of studying the bile for crystals and/or neoplastic cells and occasionally is a useful adjunct in a patient allergic to dye or in a patient with a normal cholecystogram and a history strongly suggestive of gallbladder disease.

Complications of acute cholecystitis include cholangitis, intra-abdominal sepsis, perforation, and possibly pancreatitis. Perforation can occur locally into a hollow viscus (duodenum, colon, small bowel) with subsequent development of fistula or can occur into the peritoneal cavity. Diabetic patients have increased risk of this complication.

Morbidity and mortality are significantly influenced by the timing of the operation. Elective operation has a morbidity of 6 per cent and mortality of 0.5 per cent, whereas emergency operation has a morbidity of 20 per cent and mortality of 5 per cent.

When cholecystography confirms the presence of gallstones or when the gallbladder is not visualized, operation should be performed if there are no significant medical contraindications. In an 11-year follow-up it has been demonstrated that, if operation is not performed promptly, 35 per cent of the patients will develop severe cholecystitis, icterus or pancreatitis or both, ileus, cancer, or such severe clinical symptoms that surgical intervention will become necessary.

After cholecystectomy the patient should have no recurrent bouts of right upper quadrant abdominal pain and is not restricted in diet. However, other symptoms such as pyrosis, eructation, or flatulence may continue and patient expectations should not be raised inappropriately.

Operative cholangiography should be done at cholecystectomy. In 1896, Halsted, while discussing a paper by Lang, recalled the first operation he performed for gallstones in 1880, when he removed the gallbladder of a young woman who recovered only to die two years later of peritonitis resulting from a retained common duct stone. Ironically, Halsted himself died of post-

operative pneumonia after his second choledochotomy for a retained common duct stone. Operative cholangiography has reduced the number of patients undergoing choledochotomy from 41 to 25 per cent and has strikingly increased the number of positive explorations from 28 to 62 per cent. In addition, it has established the presence of common duct calculi in 4 to 5 per cent of patients in whom they were completely un-

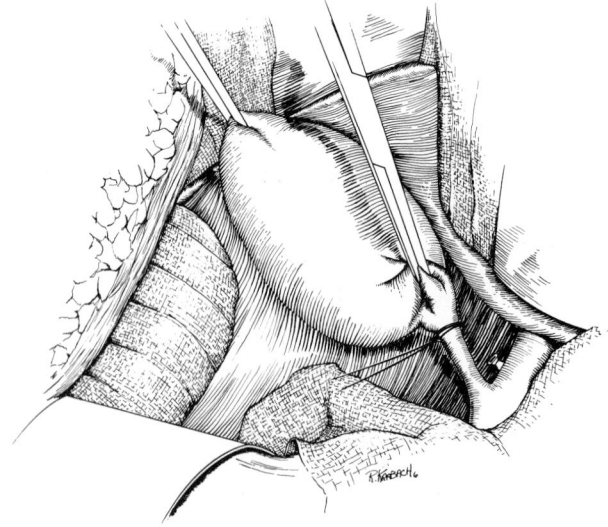

Figure 30. With adequate exposure and the cystic artery divided, the cystic duct is encircled with a ligature to prevent the extrusion of stones into the common duct during the course of the dissection.

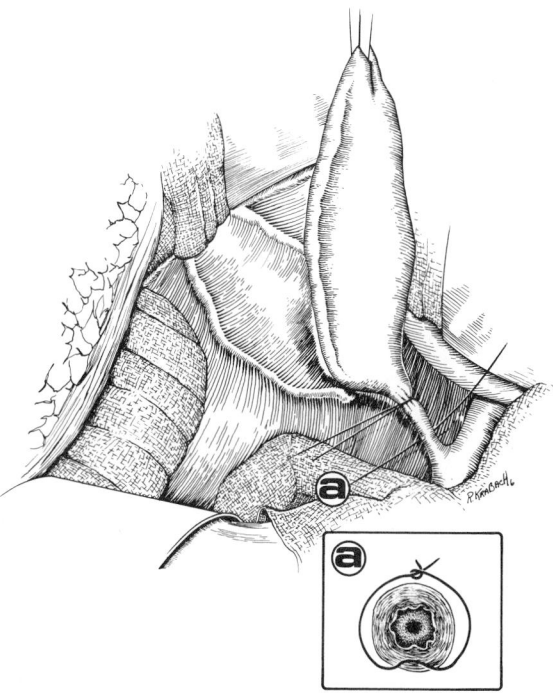

Figure 31. The gallbladder is dissected from above downward. A suture ligature is placed tangentially in the cystic duct to facilitate the operative cholangiogram.

suspected. It is known that about half of the patients who have preoperative clinical indications for common duct exploration will have normal operative cholangiograms and can thus be spared exploration of the common bile duct.

Traditionally, indication for common duct exploration combined with cholecystectomy has been one or more of the following:

1. Palpable common duct stone
2. Presence (or history) of jaundice

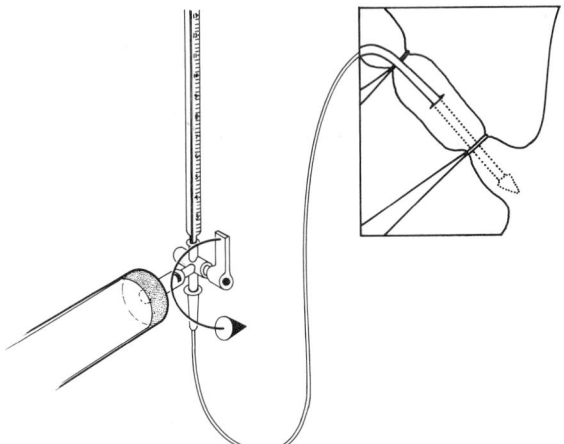

Figure 32. Manometric control of the operative cholangiogram allows detection of common duct hypertension and avoids dangerous forceful injection. The insert shows the previously tangentially placed suture securing the catheter.

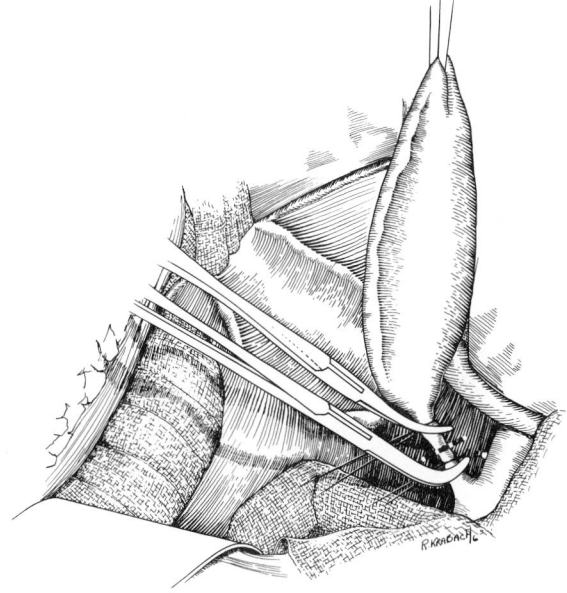

Figure 33. After the cholangiogram, the cystic duct is divided 3 mm. from the common duct and suture ligated. The gallbladder bed is not closed and bleeding is controlled with suture ligatures.

3. Dilated bile duct (12 mm. or more)
4. Associated pancreatitis or cholangitis
5. Small stones or sediment in the gallbladder
6. Small or contracted gallbladder or absence of stones with a history of biliary colic
7. Elevation of serum alkaline phosphatase

Cholecystostomy has a mortality rate five to ten times higher than that reported for cholecystectomy, probably because it is employed in very ill and poor-risk patients, but it has been advocated for patients considered too ill to undergo cholecystectomy or as an alternative for those in whom technical difficulties or deterioration in clinical course develop during operation. Patients deemed too ill for cholecystectomy are usually elderly, with compromised cardiovascular systems, diabetes, or chronic lung disease who have acute gangrenous or perforated cholecystitis.

The cholecystostomy does drain the gallbladder but not the common bile duct when cystic duct obstruction is present. It is of no benefit when used alone for the treatment of cholangitis. In acute cholecystitis, if clear bile is found, one can rely upon cholecystostomy alone without drainage of the common bile duct but, in general, this technique is not satisfactory.

Acute cholecystitis is usually clinically distinguishable from biliary colic. It is most often a complication of gallstones. The acute illness can generally be managed by nonsurgical means but requires diligent observation. When the acute episode has subsided and appropriate diagnostic procedures are completed, cholecystectomy should be done without delay.

SELECTED REFERENCES

Adams, T. W., and Foxley, E. G.: A diagnostic technique for acalculous cholecystitis. Surg. Gynecol. Obstet., *142*:168, 1976.
Routine oral cholecystography with Telepaque frequently will

show normal visualization of the gallbladder in the presence of acalculous cholecystitis and cholesterolosis. Roentgenograms of the abdomen that show persistent opacification of the gallbladder 36 hours after the administration of Telepaque are suggestive of cholecystic disease. Twenty-six patients with previously normal cholecystograms but with continuing symptoms of biliary tract disease were studied with 24-hour delayed films of the gallbladder. All had persistent visualization of the gallbladder, and all had diseased gallbladder verified at operation and by pathologic examinations.

Coyne, M. J., and Schoenfield, L. J.: Gallstone disease. Postgrad. Med., 57:153, 1975.
Factors predisposing to gallstone formation include sex, age, race, childbearing, and possibly diet and obesity. About half of the patients with gallstones have symptoms referable to the biliary tract. Biliary pain lasting longer than 5 or 6 hours is indicative of acute cholecystitis. The reliability of cholecystography is at least 95 per cent. Early operation in patients with acute cholecystitis is advocated.

Glenn, F.: Trends in surgical treatment of calculous disease of the biliary tract. Surg. Gynecol. Obstet., 140:877, 1975.
Dr. Glenn notes that there are five distinct trends in operations for biliary tract disease. There is less delay in operation following diagnosis. Diagnosis is made early in those with symptoms. Asymptomatic calculi are being found more frequently because of more complete overall medical evaluations, including cholecystography. Acute obstructive cholecystitis is becoming less frequent in

proportion to the total number of patients admitted to the hospital. The operative mortality rate is concentrated in patients 65 years of age and older.

Kakos, G. S., Tompkins, R. K., Turnipseed, W., and Zollinger, R. M.: Operative cholangiography during routine cholecystectomy. Arch. Surg., 104:484, 1972.
In a review of 3012 patients treated from 1951 through 1970, the overall incidence of common duct calculi was relatively stable at 13 per cent in patients undergoing cholecystectomy. The use of operative cholangiogram rose progressively from 2.9 per cent in the 1951–1955 period to 93 per cent in the 1966–1970 group. This change was associated with a decrease in the number of patients undergoing choledochotomy from 41 to 25 per cent and by a striking increase in the number of positive explorations from 28 to 62 per cent.

Wenckert, A., and Robertson, B.: The natural course of gallstone disease. Gastroenterology, 50:376, 1966.
This paper is concerned with the natural history of gallstone disease in patients diagnosed but not surgically treated. In 1951 and 1952 cholecystography in 1501 patients showed either gallstones or nonfilling of the gallbladder. Of these, 781 patients were not operated upon. They were followed for 11 years. At least 35 per cent developed complications (severe cholecystitis, icterus or pancreatitis or both, ileus, cancer) or such severe symptoms that elective cholecystectomy was eventually performed.

II ———————————————————————————————————

ACUTE SUPPURATIVE CHOLANGITIS

David B. Hinshaw, M.D.

Acute infection and inflammation of the bile ducts or cholangitis has been well recognized since 1877 when Charcot[2] described the associated triad of chills, fever, and jaundice. The bacteria infecting the bile are almost always of enteric origin, and it is postulated that they may reach the bile ducts by hematogenous or lymphatic routes or from direct "regurgitation" in patients with partial obstruction at the ampulla of Vater or at the site of a biliary intestinal anastomosis (so-called ascending cholangitis). While the bacteria most commonly cultured from the bile are *Escherichia coli, Klebsiella aerogenes,* and *Streptococcus faecalis,* the entire gamut of enteric bacteria is occasionally seen, including the not infrequent appearance of anaerobes (usually anaerobic streptococci and *Clostridium welchii*).[11]

Bile in the gallbladder or biliary ducts is basically subject to infection or at least to continuing infection only in the presence of some degree of obstruction. Common duct calculi are by far the most frequent cause of obstruction, but duct strictures, tumors, ampullary fibrosis,[13] congenital anomalies, pancreatitis, and parasites[12] have all been reported in association with cholangitis.

Cholangitis with its chills, fever, and jaundice is usually seen in its recurrent or intermittent form in association with intermittent or incomplete common bile duct obstruction. These symptoms vary in severity

with the degree or persistence of the obstruction, the virulence of the bacterial organisms, and the stamina of the patient. Transient gram-negative bacteremia is an important, probably essential, component in the etiology of the fever and chills of Charcot's triad. It has been suggested that the bacteremia is probably the result of a pressure gradient from the intrahepatic biliary radicles to the liver sinusoids. This would be a feasible route into the bloodstream for particles the size of gram-negative bacteria. When complete obstruction of the common duct occurs under these circumstances, suppuration promptly appears with ominous consequences for the patient. When there is such a transition from cholangitis to *acute obstructive cholangitis*[1, 8, 10, 15] the infected suppurative bile is under ever increasing pressure, causing progressive fulminating septicemia with the rapid development of septic shock. Multiple liver abscesses and pyelophlebitis also become a prominent part of the pathologic process.

In 1903 Rogers,[17] after noting in necropsy studies the relationship between suppurative cholangitis, bile duct obstruction, and liver abscesses, unsuccessfully attempted surgical decompression of the common bile duct in a patient with acute suppurative cholangitis. The need for prompt surgical intervention was stressed in 1940 by Cutler and Zollinger,[4] and in 1945 Grant[7] reported three patients who survived after biliary tract decompression for acute suppurative cholangitis and common duct obstruction secondary to stones. In 1947 Cole[3] described cases of suppurative cholangitis associated with common duct obstruction from calculi, carcinoma of the head of the pancreas, and stricture. Strictures may be secondary to duct injuries or represent the stenosis of previous duct-to-duct or biliary intestinal anastomoses.

In 1959 Reynolds and Dargan[16] fully characterized acute obstructive cholangitis as a distinct clinical entity consisting of right upper abdominal pain, jaundice, chills, fever, central nervous system depression, and septic shock. They particularly emphasized the symptoms of mental confusion, lethargy, and shock as characteristically being present when purulent material rapidly accumulates under pressure in the biliary tree in the presence of complete common duct obstruction. They also re-emphasized the necessity for immediate surgical decompression of the biliary tract in such patients if they are to have any chance for survival. The high-grade common duct obstruction leads to dilatation, thickening, and edema of the entire duct system. The bile becomes thickened, opaque, seropurulent, and sometimes frankly purulent in appearance. The bile is often under sufficient pressure in the obstructed ductal system that it tends to shoot out or erupt when the common duct is opened for decompression. The liver is usually diffusely enlarged and congested, with degrees of liver necrosis varying from centrolobular degeneration to multiple gross liver abscesses. In several subsequent descriptions of this dangerous form of cholangitis the term acute obstructive suppurative cholangitis has been appropriately used.[5, 6, 9, 10]

CLINICAL FEATURES

The clinical features of fully developed acute obstructive cholangitis consist of right upper abdominal pain, jaundice, fever, chills, central nervous system depression, and shock. This clinical picture varies somewhat from patient to patient. The right upper abdominal pain, often severe, with accompanying tenderness is consistently present in responsive patients and seems directly related to rapid, complete obstruction of the common duct resulting from "pus under pressure" in the ductal system. Jaundice may be more or less pronounced depending on how long complete duct obstruction has been present, but the degree of jaundice does not necessarily parallel the severity of the patient's symptoms. Fever is usually high (often 103 or 104° F), tends to be sustained rather than intermittent, and is usually associated with rigorous chills. The chills often diminish, however, as the general toxemia advances.

The central nervous system depression which manifests itself as mental confusion and lethargy leading to coma is an ominous sign, generally indicative of well-established septicemia and impending shock. Shock is of the septic variety secondary to gram-negative bacterial septicemia with endotoxin production. It is, of course, aggravated by fluid loss through vomiting, fever, and inadequate intake.

Laboratory studies show primarily polymorphonuclear leukocytosis (usually 20,000 WBC or above) with an elevated serum bilirubin and alkaline phosphatase. The blood and bile cultures are usually positive. Other tests such as the serum amylase and the serum glutamic oxaloacetic transaminase may be elevated, creating diagnostic confusion. These clinical features are summarized in Figure 34. There are no roentgenographic examinations that are especially diagnostic.

TREATMENT

The treatment of cholangitis in general is basically surgical—the relief of underlying common bile duct obstruction, whether it be intermittent, incomplete, or complete. The vigorous use of the appropriate antibiotics is also of great importance. However, when acute obstructive cholangitis is present (complete obstruction with suppuration) all efforts should be made to facilitate operative intervention as rapidly as possible. Medical treatment *is not an alternative approach;* it is supportive, preparative, and supplementary only. A "trial of medical management" in the fully developed syndrome with complete obstruction is virtually 100 per cent fatal.

Intensive care measures should be immediately instituted, including frequent accurate monitoring of the urinary output and the placement of a central venous catheter. The full range of hematologic, biochemical, and electrolyte determinations should be obtained. Adequate fluid volume replacement is essential and must be based on the urine output, central venous pressure measurements, biochemical determinations,

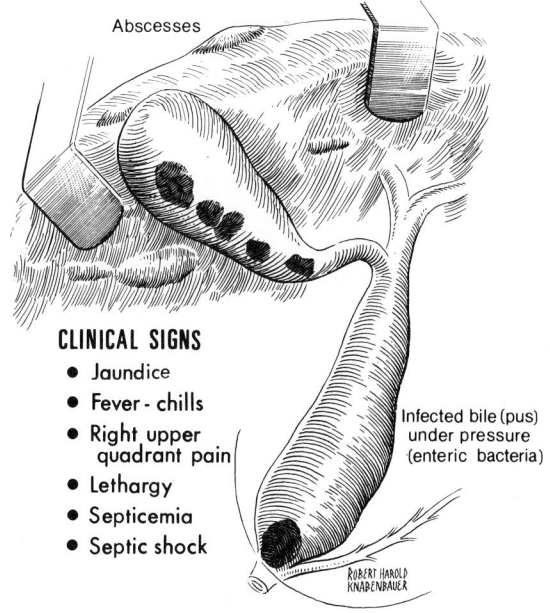

Abscesses

CLINICAL SIGNS
- Jaundice
- Fever - chills
- Right upper quadrant pain
- Lethargy
- Septicemia
- Septic shock

Infected bile (pus) under pressure (enteric bacteria)

ROBERT HAROLD KNABENBAUER

Figure 34. Summary of the clinical and pathologic features of acute suppurative cholangitis.

and the patient's clinical response. The inclusion of fresh blood in the volume replacement is helpful, and liberal quantities of vitamin K oxide should be given intravenously. Intravenous hydrocortisone may be helpful in patients who are particularly refractory to immediate measures.

The patient's bloodstream should be immediately saturated with an antibiotic or combination of antibiotics most likely to be effective against the enteric organisms commonly involved in this entity; these include chloramphenicol, gentamicin, and kanamycin. The primary antibiotic attack in these emergent situations is the septicemia; therefore agents which achieve high effective serum levels are essential. Consequently chloramphenicol, or kanamycin, or gentamicin in combination with ampicillin, are indicated in maximum safe intravenous doses. Although tetracyclines are ordinarily well concentrated in bile, their concentration is relatively insignificant in the presence of complete common duct obstruction and a substantial percentage of the involved organisms are not sensitive to them.[11] Obviously it is extremely important to use antibiotics to which specific sensitivities have been obtained—either from positive blood cultures or from infected bile cultured at operation. However, it is frequently necessary to proceed immediately without the benefit of fully reported bacterial sensitivity studies. Careful monitoring of serum levels of kanamycin and gentamicin are of course essential in view of their nephrotoxic effects.

Surgical intervention should be undertaken as soon as these measures have been instituted and clinical responses noted. If there is not significant improvement in 12 to 24 hours, operation must be immediately performed even in the presence of clinical deterioration. Transitory improvement enticing the surgeon to delay operation is frequently followed by a rapidly fatal outcome. At operation the crucial maneuver is decompression of the common bile duct with T tube drainage. When circumstances permit, the common duct should be fully explored and the obstruction relieved. Cholecystectomy should be performed if appropriate and if the patient's condition permits. In some instances cholecystostomy is preferable. These treatment approaches are summarized in Figure 35.

COMMENT

While patients may initially appear with the full picture of acute obstructive suppurative cholangitis, it more often develops as a complication of more benign forms of choledocholithiasis, particularly those in which signs of intermittent cholangitis have been present. In 1890 Olster[14] pointed out and stressed that Charcot's fever (and triad) was usually irregular, recurrent, and often of short duration. It is in this subtle area of intermittent chills, fever, and jaundice that danger lies, because the intermittent nature of the symptoms constantly suggests a therapeutic course of waiting and compromise. Such cases may escalate rapidly into complete obstruction with entrapment of purulent bile under pressure. It is the subtle variants of this obstructive suppurative complication of chole-

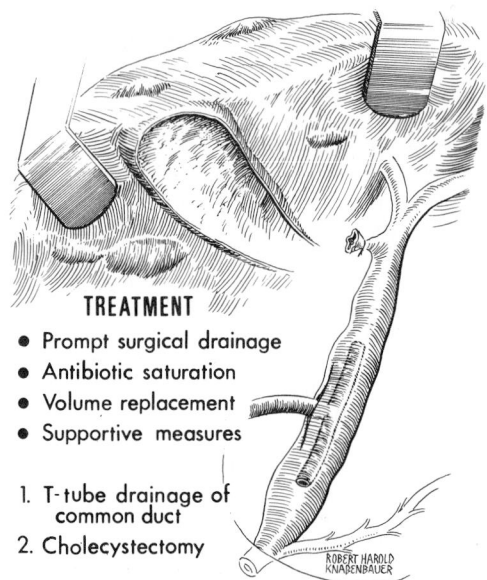

TREATMENT
- Prompt surgical drainage
- Antibiotic saturation
- Volume replacement
- Supportive measures

1. T-tube drainage of common duct
2. Cholecystectomy

Figure 35. Summary of the treatment of acute suppurative cholangitis with emphasis on drainage of the common bile duct.

docholithiasis which are frequently misjudged or poorly managed that ultimately account for a large share of the mortality attributable to gallstones. Early surgical decompression and drainage of the common bile duct is imperative if a mortality rate approaching 100 per cent is to be avoided.

Although this syndrome affects all age groups, the most commonly involved are the elderly who have chronic calculous biliary tract disease. Patients with diabetes mellitus with gallstone disease are likewise prone to develop cholangitis, obstruction, and suppuration. Individuals with biliary duct strictures from whatever cause are also very subject to cholangitis of varying degrees, including the suppurative form.

The cause of central nervous system depression is probably the septicemia with the accompanying endotoxemia; however, hepatic insufficiency may play a significant role. While the shock appears clearly septic in nature due to septicemia and presumably circulating endotoxins, it must be remembered that significant hypovolemia may rapidly develop in severely ill patients with high fever, vomiting, and inadequate fluid intake. The mortality in various reported groups of patients with acute (obstructive) suppurative cholangitis ranges from 30 per cent to nearly 100 per cent, depending upon the criteria used in defining the disease entity and the length of time needed to establish the diagnosis and institute adequate surgical decompression of the bile ducts. Certainly the best treatment is prophylaxis through the surgical correction of chronic calculus biliary tract disease in nonemergent situations. However, if this dangerous form of cholangitis, which is the most fulminating and serious complication of gallstone disease, can be recognized and given prompt appropriate surgical treatment, the majority of these critically ill patients can be expected to recover.

SELECTED REFERENCES

Keighley, M. R. B., Drysdale, R. B., Quoraishi, A. H., Burdon, D. W., and Alexander-Williams, J.: Antibiotic treatment of biliary sepsis. Surg. Clin. North Am., *55*:1379, 1975.

This is an excellent study and review of the bacteria involved in cholangitis and the antibiotics that are best suited to biliary sepsis. Emphasis is placed on serum antibiotic levels and the point is well made that antibiotics are poorly concentrated in bile in the presence of complete common duct obstruction.

Reynolds, B. M., and Dargan, E. L.: Acute obstructive cholangitis. Ann. Surg., *150*:299, 1959.

This is a classic description of acute obstructive (suppurative) cholangitis in which the full entity is developed. Emphasis is placed on the central nervous system depression and septic shock resulting from the entrapped suppuration under obstructive pressure in the biliary tree. The case for prompt surgical decompression of the common bile duct is well made.

REFERENCES

1. Andrew, D. J., and Johnson, S. E.: Acute suppurative cholangitis. A medical and surgical emergency, a review of ten years experience emphasizing early recognition. Am. J. Gastroenterol., *54*:141, 1970.
2. Charcot, J. M.: Leçons sur les maladies du foie des voies filiares et des reins. Paris, Faculté de Medecine de Paris, 1877.
3. Cole, W. H.: Suppurative cholangitis. Surg. Clin. North Am., *27*:23, 1947.
4. Cutler, E., and Zollinger, R.: Surgery of the gallbladder and extrahepatic bile ducts. Am. J. Surg., *47*:185, 1940.
5. Dow, R. W., and Lindenauer, S. M.: Acute obstructive suppurative cholangitis. Ann. Surg., *169*:272, 1969.
6. Glenn, F., and Moody, F. G.: Acute obstructive suppurative cholangitis. Surg. Gynecol. Obstet., *113*:265, 1961.
7. Grant, H. D.: Acute suppurative cholangitis. Permanente Foundation Med. Bull., *3*:175, 1945.
8. Haupert, A. P., Carey, L. C., Evans, W. E., and Ellison, R. H.: Acute suppurative cholangitis, experience with 15 consecutive cases. Arch. Surg., *94*:460, 1966.
9. Hinchey, E. J., and Couper, C. E.: Acute obstructive suppurative cholangitis. Am. J. Surg., *117*:62, 1969.
10. Hinshaw, D. B.: Acute obstructive suppurative cholangitis. Surg. Clin. North Am., *53*:1089, 1973.
11. Keighley, M. R. B., Drysdale, R. B., Quoraishi, A. H., Burdon, D. W., and Alexander-Williams, J.: Antibiotic treatment of biliary sepsis. Surg. Clin. North Am., *55*:1379, 1975.
12. McFadzean, A. J. S., and Young, R. T. T.: Hypoglycemia in suppurative pancholangitis due to clonorchis sinensis. Trans. R. Soc. Trop. Med. Hyg., *59*:180, 1965.
13. Nardi, G. L.: Acute suppurative cholangitis due to ampullary fibrosis. Surg. Clin. North Am., *50*:1137, 1970.
14. Osler, W.: On fever of hepatic origin, particularly intermittent pyrexia association with gallstones. Johns Hopkins Hosp. Rep., *2*:3, 1890–1891.
15. Ostermiller, W., Jr., Thompson, R. J., Jr., Carter, R., and Hinshaw, D. B.: Acute obstructive cholangitis. Arch. Surg., *90*:392, 1965.
16. Reynolds, B. M., and Dargan, E. L.: Acute obstructive cholangitis, a distinct clinical syndrome. Ann. Surg., *150*:299, 1959.
17. Rogers, L.: Biliary abscesses of liver with operation. Br. Med. J., *2*:706, 1903.

III

GALLSTONE ILEUS AND FISTULA

Francis E. Rosato, M.D.

BILIARY FISTULAS

Definition

A biliary fistula is an established and abnormal connection between any portion of the biliary tree and some other area. If this abnormal connection is between the biliary tree and the exterior, it is termed an *external fistula,* while connections between the biliary tree and an internal structure constitute an *internal fistula.* Gallstones, peptic ulcer, trauma, and neoplasia are common causes of such fistulas. In general, external fistulas are most likely due to trauma, particularly operative trauma, while internal fistulas result most often from peptic ulcer, gallstone disease, and cancer.

The mode of presentation varies, depending on the cause and the type of fistula. Most external fistulas occur in a postoperative setting and usually after the formation of an extrabiliary accumulation of bile. Internal biliary fistulas are more insidious in their presentation, since the antecedent neoplastic or inflammatory adherence to another bodily structure occurs over a protracted period of time. Table 11 lists the commonest biliary fistulas and their symptom complex. Cholangitis is a likely associated problem with any biliary fistula. In addition, there also have been reported biliary tract connections made into the kidney, urinary bladder, uterus, vagina, portal vein, inferior vena cava, and pericardial sac.

TABLE 11. Symptoms of Biliary Fistulas

Fistula Type	Symptom Complex
Biliary-cutaneous	Bile peritonitis and/or external bile leakage
Biliary-intestinal	Gallstone ileus
Biliary-pleurobronchial	Bile-tinged coughing

EXTERNAL BILIARY FISTULA

The commonest setting for external biliary fistula is after operation on the biliary tree, particularly when exploration or reconstruction of the common bile duct is included. If bile leakage occurs, a walled-off collection of bile results, producing a chemical peritonitis. This is usually accompanied by a characteristic rise in conjugated serum bilirubin due to absorption from the peritoneal cavity and several days later by an elevation of serum alkaline phosphatase, probably due to pericholangitis.[6] Rarely, bile peritonitis may pursue a more indolent course, producing a mild jaundice and abdominal distention termed "bile ascites."[8] Usually, however, a walled-off bile collection occurs, typically productive of fever and abdominal tenderness, which are persistent until such time as the bile is removed, either operatively by the placement of drains (or reopening drain tracts) or spontaneously.[4] Occasionally, in the absence of any distal bile duct obstruction, such external fistulas may quickly close.

INTERNAL BILIARY FISTULA

Ninety per cent of internal biliary fistulas are from gallstone disease, while 6 per cent are secondary to peptic ulcer. Ulcers on the posterior duodenum invade the common duct; those on the anterior and lateral wall attach and erode into the gallbladder. Gastric ulcers typically erode into the gallbladder also, when they produce fistulas. Tumors of the stomach, gallbladder, pancreas, and common duct erode into contiguous structures, producing a variety of fistulas.[5] After the connection between the biliary tree and adjacent structure has been established, the symptom complex of cholangitis ensues. At times an internal biliary fistula, in the same fashion as an external biliary fistula, may first be a localized bile collection; for example, a choledochobronchial fistula usually follows a bile collection which results in an inflammatory process producing a connection between these two physically disparate structures.

COMPLICATIONS OF FISTULA

There are three important complications of biliary fistula, regardless of the type of fistula or the particular structures involved[7] (Fig. 36). (1) *Hyponatremia.* The sodium content of bile is approximately 150 mEq. per liter and the loss of such bile externally or even internally into the bronchial tree or bladder can produce a severe hyponatremia. (2) *Inanition and weight loss.* The critical role of bile as an emulsifying agent facilitating the absorption of fats and fat-soluble vitamins is well established. The external loss of bile produces a malabsorption problem and the resultant diarrhea may additionally hazard protein and carbohydrate absorption. When internal biliary fistulas have been formed, particularly between the biliary system and the upper reaches of the intestinal tract, this complication is minimized. (3) *Infection.* There are two principal modes by which infection ensues in the biliary

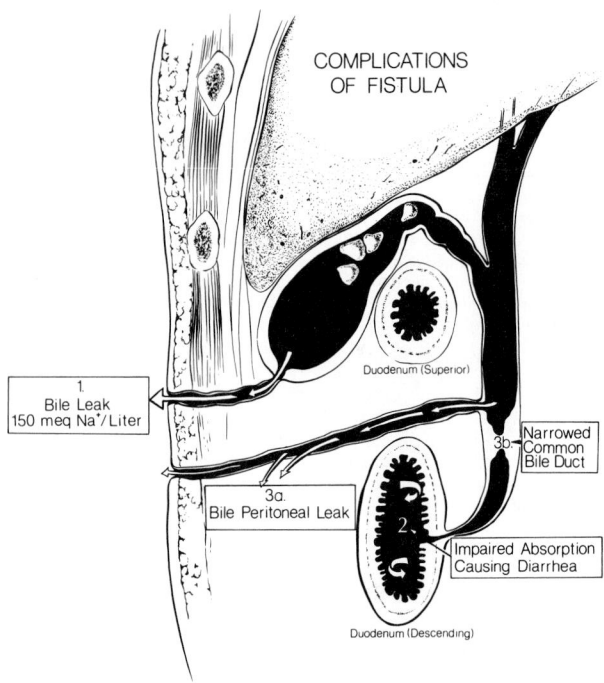

Figure 36. Diagrammatic representation of major biliary fistula complications.

fistula setting. The first is from a transient leakage of bile from the tract, with resultant contamination of the peritoneal space. Bile is not sterile and especially in fistulas contains coliform organisms and occasionally anaerobic Clostridia. Bile leakage into body cavities produces, therefore, transient episodes of bacterial infection, in addition to the anticipated chemical inflammation. The second factor in infection is due to cholangitis, which occurs in about 10 to 15 per cent of cholecystoduodenal fistulas. It is an unusual occurrence in choledochoduodenal fistula. The exact mechanism is not clearly understood, since in general the pressure gradients favor the distal flow of bile; further, cholangitis does not ensue even when reflux has been demonstrated in surgically created biliary-enteric fistulas. Some degree of bile stasis and obstruction seems essential, therefore, in the production of cholangitis. Cholangitis is ushered in with the classic Charcot's triad of jaundice (either appearing or aggravated), fever, and shaking chills.

THERAPY

The management of a biliary fistula should be thought of in sequential steps.

1. Establish the Anatomy of the Fistula

When the fistula is established to the outside, a No. 8 or 10 French red rubber tube can be inserted in the external orifice, snugging it in place with a purse-string suture of 2–0 silk. Injection of contrast material will serve to delineate the site of origin and the fistula

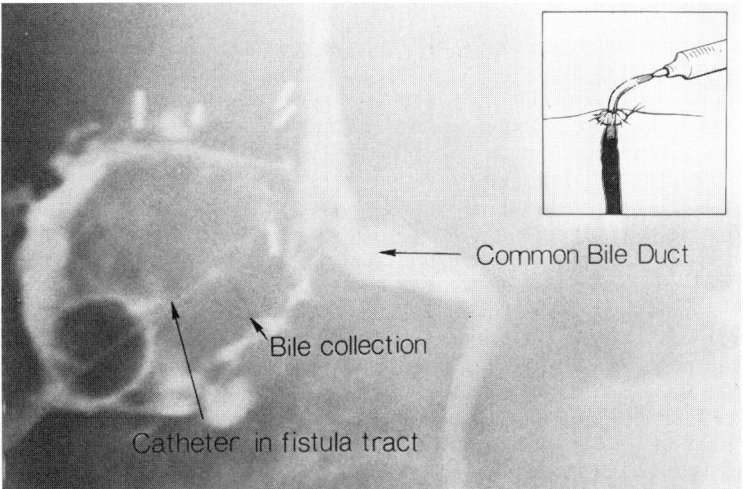

Figure 37. Catheter (insert) introduced into fistula tract and resultant fistulogram demonstrating a choledochocutaneous fistula. The tortuosity of the common bile duct resulted from bile-induced inflammation.

tract as well (Fig. 37). Where internal fistula is present, attempts are made through upper gastrointestinal series, barium enema, cholangiography, bronchoscopy, or cystography to delineate the anatomic extent of the fistula[1] (Fig. 38).

2. Attempt to Establish the Cause of the Fistula

In attempting to localize the fistula, additional information on the underlying cause is often obtained. Studies such as gastroduodenoscopy, radioactive scanning of the liver, sonography (particularly to detect nonopacified gallstones), and cytologic evaluation of a variety of aspirated specimens may be required. The value of surgical exploration for final determination of the cause cannot be overemphasized; very often initial studies will localize the fistula and surgery will delineate its cause. Historically, those 10 per cent of fistulas due to peptic ulcer disease can be suspected when there is a lessening of ulcer symptoms consonant with the appearance of the fistula, presumably due to

alkaline bathing of the ulcer through the choledochoduodenal fistula.

3. Control Infection

Since infection is one of the major complications of fistula, appropriate antibiotics must be chosen to combat such infection. Cultured bile, in the case of external fistula, is often helpful in making the most correct choice of antibiotics. In general, drugs with a high degree of enterohepatic recirculation effective against gram-negative bacilli, at times including those with a spectrum against anaerobes, would be ideal for the preparation of such patients. Ampicillin is an ideal initial agent.

4. Correct Electrolyte Abnormalities

Give particular attention to possible sodium depletion. With the advent of intravenous hyperalimentation, nutritional problems can be corrected during the preparative period while one is studying the type and cause of the fistulas.

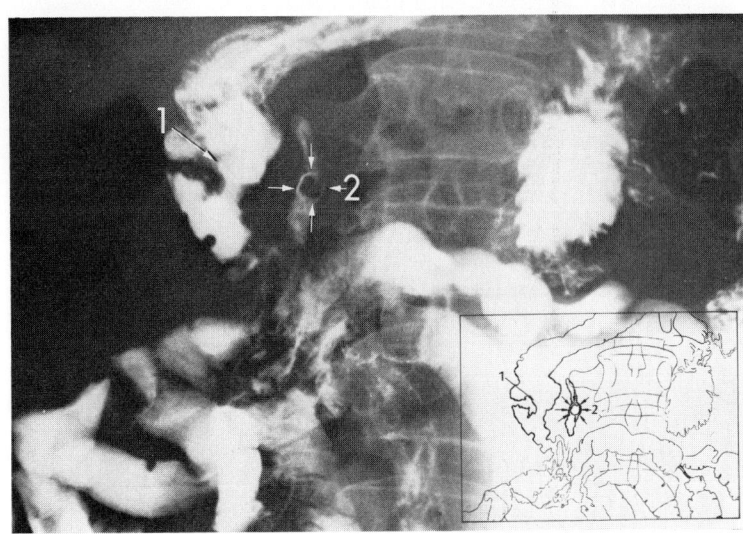

Figure 38. Upper gastrointestinal series showing duodenum (1) and shortly thereafter opacification of common bile duct. This sequence is pathognomonic of choledochoduodenal fistula. Note stone in common bile duct (2).

5. Surgery

Where inflammation is the cause of the fistula, the surgical separation of the partner structures is usually done, with surgical closure of each. Where neoplasia is the underlying problem, separation may not be possible, although, wherever possible, it is obviously urged. Often the relief of distal obstruction to bile flow may be sufficient to result in complete resolution of the fistula without direct operative intervention. An external biliary fistula following common duct exploration may indicate persistent obstruction of the distal common duct, either from a retained stone or from ampullary stenosis. Removal of the distal obstruction (stone or stricture) will usually result in closure of the fistula, obviating any direct approach to the fistula itself. In general, operative cholangiography may be of help in deciding appropriate surgery. Inflammatory fistulas are usually "taken down" and attention given to relief of any attendant biliary obstruction.

Neoplastic fistulas often cannot be closed and in this situation any relief of obstruction to bile flow is recommended. For example, the cholangitis in cholecys-togastric fistulas due to prepyloric tumors often can be controlled by gastrojejunostomy alone.

GALLSTONE ILEUS

This particular complication results from those internal fistulas where a gallbladder or common duct stone, through an internal biliary fistula, gains entrance into the intestinal tract. One would anticipate the usual potential complications attendant on any internal biliary fistula, particularly ascending cholangitis. In addition, in this condition, the presence of a large stone in the intestinal tract produces obstruction at the point where its diameter exceeds that of the intestinal lumen. A typical presentation for gallstone ileus would include frequently previous episodes of partial bowel obstruction, which waxes and wanes as the stone negotiates its way into the narrower region of the intestinal tract. This phenomenon is called "tumbling" obstruction and is predicated on

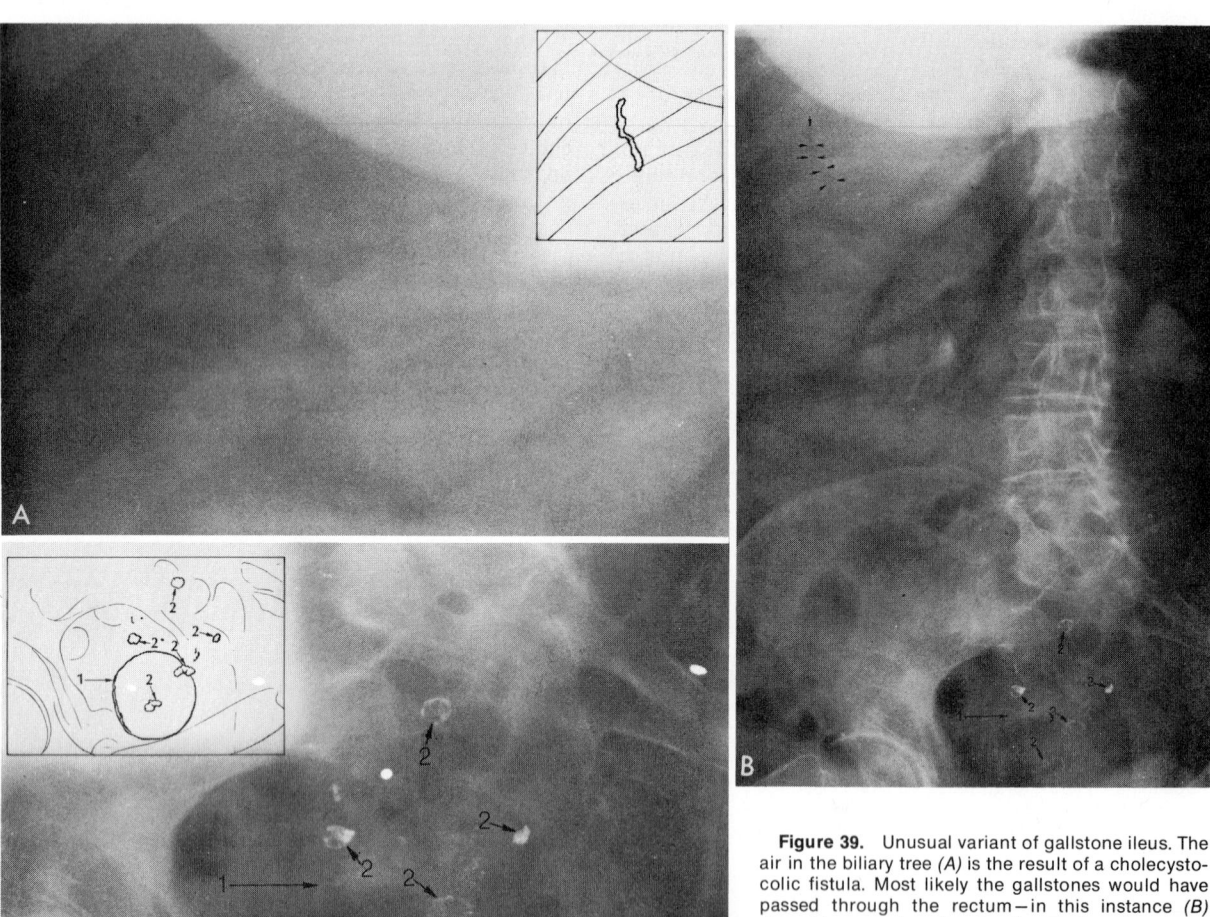

Figure 39. Unusual variant of gallstone ileus. The air in the biliary tree (A) is the result of a cholecystocolic fistula. Most likely the gallstones would have passed through the rectum—in this instance (B) sigmoid narrowing due to diverticular disease resulted in a large gallstone producing a complete large bowel obstruction. Note barium retained in the sigmoid diverticula (2) and the outlines of an obstructing stone in the distal sigmoid (1). A previous colostomy was done so that a large bowel obstructive pattern is not seen (A).

the notion that a stone which obstructs at one point may, with some dilatation of the obstructed gut, proceed aborally with a relief of obstruction, only to have it recur when it has migrated a short distance farther down the intestinal tract.

Three fourths of the spontaneous fistulas underlying gallstone ileus occur between the gallbladder and the duodenum. Most gallstones that enter the gastrointestinal tract are either passed or vomited, but 10 to 15 per cent may result in the condition described above. This disorder accounts for only 1 per cent of all cases of intestinal obstruction, but for 25 per cent of simple obstruction in those over age 70. The commonest site of obstruction, found in two thirds of patients, is the terminal ileum, whereas the proximal jejunum is the least likely.

The diagnosis is easily made if there is the finding of a large mass lesion at the site of bowel obstruction; this "mass" is readily identified if the gallstone is opaque and sometime, even if nonopaque, it can be seen because of surrounding intestinal air. In addition, the finding of air in the biliary tree makes the diagnosis almost certain (Fig. 39).

Treatment

The proper treatment of gallstone ileus is relief of the intestinal obstruction, usually by the performance of an enterotomy and removal of stones. Concomitant definitive correction of the internal fistula is advocated, if the patient is in good condition and has sustained no prolonged preoperative losses or intraoperative complications. Since spontaneous closure of the underlying biliary fistula only rarely occurs, there is a 10 per cent recurrence of gallstone ileus after enterotomy alone. In addition, recurrent cholecystitis, recurrent cholangitis, and a reportedly higher incidence of gallbladder carcinoma in association with biliary enteric fistula all reinforce the recommendation in favor

of complete corrections after enterotomy. This may be delayed as a separate procedure when the patient is judged too ill to withstand the prolonged single operation.[3]

SELECTED REFERENCES

Fox, P. F.: Planning the operation for cholecystoenteric fistula with gallstone ileus. Surg. Clin. North Am., *50*:93–102, 1970.
This reference reviews 13 patients with gallstone ileus but spends considerable effort in detailing surgical operative aspects. This is a fine reference in planning operative intervention and provides some technical detail.

Hicken, N. F., and Coray, Q. B.: Spontaneous gastrointestinal biliary fistulas. Surg. Gynecol. Obstet., *82*:723–730, 1946.
This is one of the most complete references on intraoperative management of biliary-enteric fistula. The author systematically covers most of the fistula types and very specifically lays out treatment plans for those due to tumor, as well as those secondary to benign causes. This is an older reference but still timely, particularly to the surgical house officer.

Safaie-Shirazi, S., Zike, W. L., and Printen, K. J.: Spontaneous enterobiliary fistulas. Surg. Gynecol. Obstet., *137*:769–772, 1973.
This is one of the larger case review series presenting data on 92 patients with spontaneous enterobiliary fistula. It emphasizes clinical presentation, diagnosis, and long-term results of management.

REFERENCES

1. Calonje, M. A., Ozenstark, J. L., and Nice, C. M., Jr.: Internal biliary fistula. J.A.M.A., *179*:112–114, 1962.
2. Constant, E., and Turcotte, J. G.: Choledochoduodenal fistula: The natural history and management of an unusual complication of peptic ulcer disease. Ann. Surg., *167*:220–228, 1968.
3. Cooperman, A. M., Dickson, E. R., and ReMine, W. H.: Changing concepts in the surgical treatment of gallstone ileus: A review of 15 cases with emphasis on diagnosis and treatment. Ann. Surg., *167*:377–383, 1968.
4. Fitchett, C. W.: Spontaneous external biliary fistula. Trans. South. Surg. Assoc., *80*:214–219, 1969.
5. Hicken, N. F., and Coray, Q. B.: Spontaneous gastrointestinal biliary fistulas. Surg. Gynecol. Obstet., *82*:723–730, 1946.
6. McCarthy, J. D., and Picazo, J. G.: Bile peritonitis–diagnosis and course. Am. J. Surg., *116*:664–668, 1968.
7. Norcross, J. W., and Dadey, J. L.: Medical complications of operative bile-duct injuries. N. Engl. J. Med., *257*:1216–1220, 1957.
8. Rosato, E. F., Berkowitz, H. D., and Roberts, B.: Bile ascites. Surg. Gynecol. Obstet., *130*:494–496, 1970.

IV

CARCINOMA OF THE GALLBLADDER

Richard T. Myers, M.D.

Primary carcinoma of the gallbladder is an uncommon tumor, occurring three or more times as frequently in women and most often in the 50 to 70 age group. It accounts for 6500 deaths per year in the United States[1] and for approximately 1 per cent of all carcinomas diagnosed in the United States and Great Britain.[16, 46] Its incidence in patients having cholecystectomy for biliary tract disease is reported to range from 0.3 to 10 per cent, with most estimates below 2

per cent.[1, 6, 9, 16, 17, 47, 51] Gallstones occur frequently in conjunction with carcinoma of the gallbladder and may be related to its development. Their incidence in this disease ranges from 54 to 100 per cent,[1, 5, 7, 9, 13, 17, 33, 35, 42, 52] with most estimates above 60 per cent. Since about 90 per cent of women with cancer of the gallbladder have associated gallstones,[51] it has been suggested that they might be more important in the development of cancer of the gallbladder in women than in men. From another viewpoint, in long-term follow-up of patients with silent gallstones managed without operation, only 0.4 to 0.6 per cent developed carcinoma of the gallbladder.[29, 55]

The incidence of carcinoma in situ in epithelial polyps of the gallbladder has been reported to be from 6 to 22 per cent.[4, 14, 42] Although a causal relationship between these two conditions is unclear, epithelial polyps in the gallbladder appear to predispose to the development of carcinoma.

Most carcinomas of the gallbladder originate in the fundus and spread by local infiltration into the right lobe of the liver and metastasize to regional nodes.[17, 35] Intraperitoneal and intraductal spread is common, and vascular dissemination, distant metastases, and neural spread have also been reported.[1, 17, 52] Most are adenocarcinomas (74 to 87 per cent), with much less frequent occurrence of adenoacanthomas, squamous cell carcinomas, and undifferentiated anaplastic carcinomas.[1, 7, 9, 17, 52]

DIAGNOSIS

The clinical manifestations are primarily those of cholecystitis or acute or chronic cholelithiasis, including right upper abdominal pain, jaundice, weight loss, weakness, and a right upper quadrant mass. Conversion of the classic intermittent pain to a constant pain under the right costal margin may be a sign of far advanced malignant disease.[52]

Plain roentgenograms of the abdomen are usually negative,[17, 52] but occasionally show a mass in the gallbladder or indentation of surrounding structures, particularly in advanced stages of the disease.[7, 24, 51] The gallbladder may not visualize on oral cholecystography[7, 52] but can at times concentrate the dye and demonstrate a filling defect.[52] Procedures such as hypotonic duodenography,[26, 38] percutaneous transhepatic cholangiography,[20, 24, 26] selective visceral angiography,[20, 24, 26] laparoscopy,[37, 42] and ultrasonography[48] have been used and can be of value. Nevertheless, a firm diagnosis of carcinoma of the gallbladder is made preoperatively in only 5 to 10 per cent of patients.[7, 35, 46, 52]

TREATMENT

Most patients with carcinomas of the gallbladder have advanced disease at the time of operation so that the lesions are already nonresectable. Of the very few patients who survive for more than five years, the lesion is usually a localized one and found *incidentally,*

usually a papillary adenocarcinoma and likely one arising in situ. In fact, the diagnosis is often not recognized at the time of operation, but the lesion is discovered in the gallbladder at the time of pathologic evaluation.[7, 9, 22, 33, 35] Some patients who have disease beyond the gallbladder, which involves the gallbladder and its bed in the liver or the lymph nodes, have survived after radical operative procedures such as cholecystectomy followed by en bloc wedge resection of the gallbladder bed and lymphadenectomy (Fig. 40). However, most authors have found that even the most radical operation within acceptable surgical practice does not significantly improve long-term survival.[18, 19, 33, 35, 46] Chemotherapy has been employed and may yield better results in the future with combinations of drugs.[31, 54] In other reports, chemotherapy was not of value.[35] The overall survival is quite low, being about 3.5 per cent, with death usually occurring within six months following operation.

In summary, the following points bear emphasis: (a) early diagnosis is imperative for a cure; (b) the gallbladder should be opened and examined macroscopically, and microscopically when indicated, at operation to allow detection of occult malignancy and an appropriate search for additional involved tissue that should be removed; (c) cholecystectomy followed by en bloc wedge resection of the gallbladder bed and lymphadenectomy should be considered in selected patients when the tumor has spread beyond the gallbladder; and (d) hepatic lobectomy is not apt to enhance survival because the gallbladder lies in the line of division between the right and left lobes, and lobectomy does not greatly extend the resected margin but only removes the bulk of the right lobe distal to the tumor. While extended right hepatic lobectomy theoretically might enhance survival, it would significantly increase the operative risk.

Cholecystectomy for Silent Gallstones

Prophylactic cholecystectomy for patients with silent gallstones has been advocated by many authors to protect the patient from possible later development of carcinoma of the gallbladder. There are other better reasons, however, for doing a cholecystectomy for silent gallstones, since 50 to 75 per cent of these patients will ultimately develop one or more of the complications of cholelithiasis. For these reasons, elective cholecystectomy for silent gallstones is reasonable in patients under 65 years of age who are otherwise in good health, and in patients over 65 years of age if health permits.

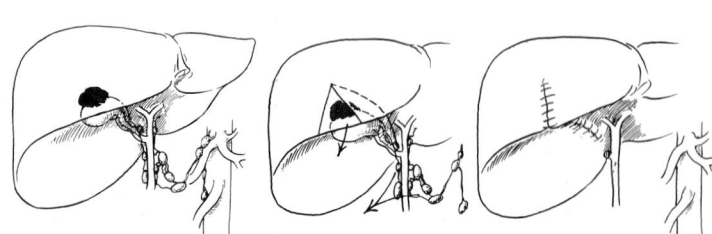

Figure 40. Wedge resection (en bloc) of the gallbladder bed and regional lymphadenectomy for widespread carcinoma of the gallbladder.

CARCINOMA OF THE BILE DUCTS

Primary carcinoma of the extrahepatic bile duct is rare, the incidence in clinical and autopsy series ranging from 0.1 to 0.5 per cent.[2, 32, 41] Unlike carcinoma of the gallbladder, it occurs more commonly in males (ratio of 3:2).[12, 40, 41, 53] The *etiology* of bile duct carcinoma is unknown, but it is frequently associated with two other diseases that may affect its development. Although much less common than in patients with carcinoma of the gallbladder, *gallstones* have been reported in 13 to 57 per cent of patients with biliary duct carcinoma.[12, 32, 40, 53]

The first association of *chronic ulcerative colitis* with carcinoma of the bile ducts was reported in 1954.[34] It has since been confirmed, with an incidence of bile duct tumors from 0.4 to 1.4 per cent.[15, 39] At the Lahey Clinic, 5 per cent of patients with carcinoma of the bile duct had or had had ulcerative colitis. Sclerosing cholangitis is also known to be associated with ulcerative colitis.[44] Two significant features of bile duct carcinoma associated with chronic ulcerative colitis are: (1) the carcinoma in this association appears approximately 30 years earlier than does carcinoma of the bile ducts in the general population; and (2) the extent of severity of colonic disease, surgical removal of the diseased colon, and the mode of medical management of the unresected colon do not appear to be related to subsequent development of the carcinoma.

PATHOLOGIC ASPECTS

Biliary duct tumors are most often circumscribed, firm, nodular lesions that partially or completely occlude the duct. The majority grow slowly and are locally invasive tumors that only rarely metastasize, but neural invasion has been reported in as many as 63 per cent of patients.[12, 28] Most bile duct tumors are adenocarcinomas, but other epithelial tumors such as adenoacanthomas, squamous cell carcinomas, and epidermoid tumors have been reported, as have leiomyosarcomas and melanomas.[11] One distinctive variety is sclerosing carcinoma, peculiarly located at the confluence of the hepatic ducts.[3] This tumor is extremely slow growing, rarely metastasizes, and is often mistaken for benign stricture. Most duct tumors occur in the proximal portion of the extrahepatic biliary tree, the remainder in the distal portion (Fig. 41). In

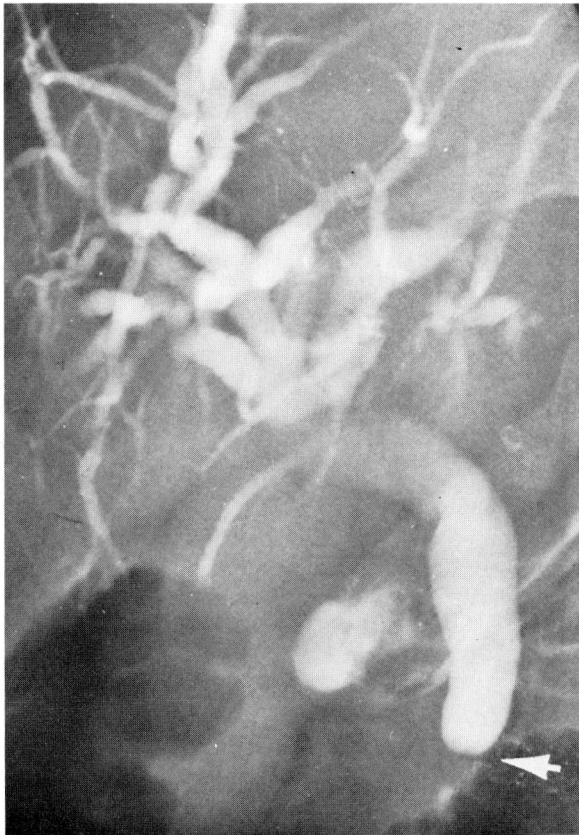

Figure 42. Percutaneous transhepatic cholangiogram showing obstruction of the distal bile duct (arrow) by carcinoma.

addition, some involve the entire duct and cannot be localized to one area.

DIAGNOSIS

The clinical manifestations are those of biliary tract obstruction, including jaundice, upper abdominal pain, pruritis, nausea and vomiting, weight loss, and weakness.[11, 12, 28, 40] There appears to be little correlation between the location of the tumor and the clinical signs and symptoms,[28] and hepatomegaly and portal hypertension may be late manifestations of the disease.[40]

Roentgenographic studies including oral cholecystography, intravenous cholangiography,[28, 40] and transjugular cholangiography[23] may be helpful. Percutaneous transhepatic cholangiography[49, 50] (Fig. 42) is considered by some to be the most useful diagnostic test,[28, 49, 53] particularly when it is combined with selective celiac arteriography.[20, 26] Probably the most helpful technique is endoscopic transduodenal cholangiography,[27] which has yielded positive data in as many as 75 per cent of jaundiced patients.[10]

Despite these procedures, the definitive diagnosis of bile duct carcinoma is rarely made preoperatively and is often difficult to establish at the time of laparotomy,

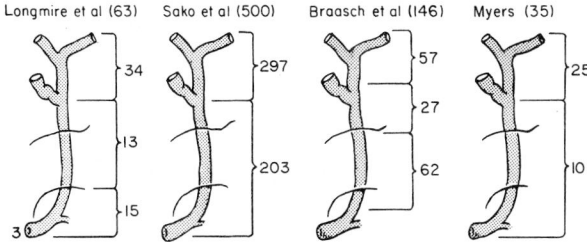

Figure 41. Location of primary carcinoma of the bile duct in four series of patients.

particularly if the lesion lies in the proximal third of the bile duct.[25, 28, 56] If the intraoperative diagnostic rate is to increase, the surgeon must be more alert to the possibility that cancer of the bile duct may be present and his search for a tumor must be vigorous. When the distal bile duct is obstructed, the proximal bile duct and the gallbladder are usually distended. When the proximal duct is obstructed, the bile duct and gallbladder are usually collapsed.[28] Operative cholangiography with complete filling of the duct should be done in all patients. Proper exposure by mobilizing the duodenum, pancreas, and hilar structures in the liver is essential. The duct should be explored with probes and by choledochoscopy to detect areas of induration and ulceration. Probes should be passed into the duodenum and proximally into both main hepatic ducts. When proximal lesions occlude the ducts, ureteral catheters and dilating probes should be passed to reach the dilated portion of the ducts and allow for additional cholangiographic diagnostic procedures. Biopsies should be obtained directly, by curettage or by cytologic studies of washings from the tumor sites, and lymph nodes should be excised for pathologic diagnosis.

TREATMENT

Although biliary duct tumors tend to grow slowly and metastasize infrequently, the ultimate cure rate is extremely low. Nonetheless, their slow growth does permit for extended palliation in some patients when the lesions are nonresectable. Treatment should be

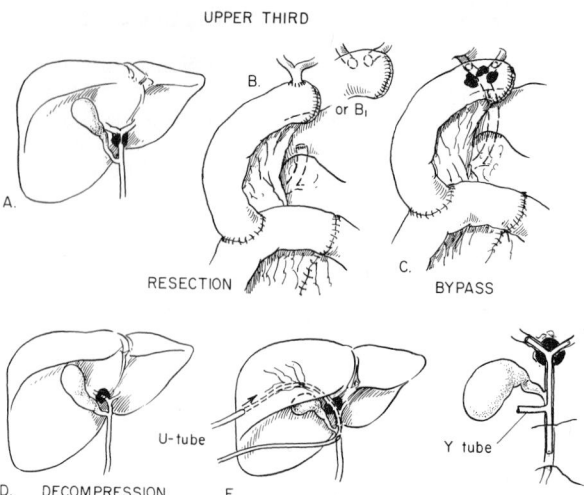

Figure 44. Suggested methods of resection, bypass, and decompression for treatment of carcinoma of the upper third of the bile duct.

directed toward relief of jaundice by curative resection whenever possible or by palliative procedure when the lesion is nonresectable. When in the proximal bile duct at the confluence, or when the lesion is a sclerosing carcinoma, a variety of radical extended resections are available (Figs. 43 and 44).[8, 28, 30, 36, 42, 43, 45] Lesions of the proximal duct are treated with resection and bilateral intrahepatic cholangiojejunostomy. For the palliative management of nonresectable upper-third

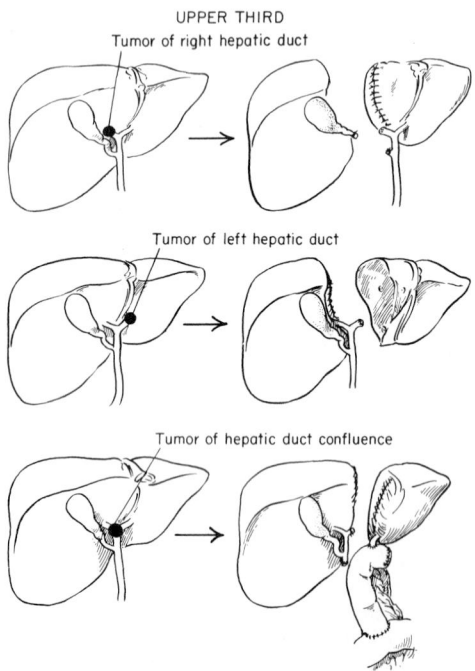

Figure 43. Suggested methods of radical resection and lobectomy for treatment of carcinoma of the upper third of the bile duct.

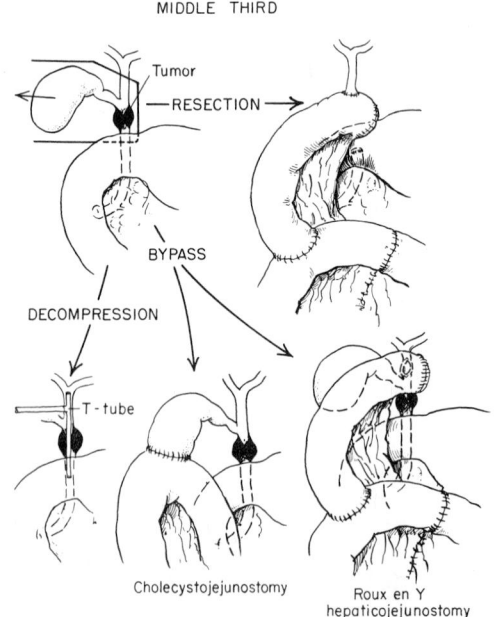

Figure 45. Suggested methods for treatment of carcinoma of the middle third of the bile duct.

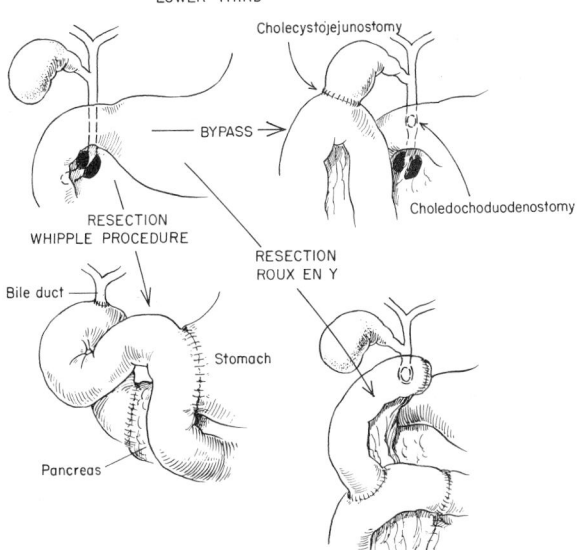

LOWER THIRD

Cholecystojejunostomy

BYPASS

Choledochoduodenostomy

RESECTION
WHIPPLE PROCEDURE

RESECTION
ROUX EN Y

Bile duct

Stomach

Pancreas

Figure 46. Suggested methods for treatment of carcinoma of the distal bile duct.

tumors, forceful dilatation of the proximal ducts and relief of obstructive jaundice by indwelling T tubes, Y tubes, and stents are suggested,[28, 40, 53] as is U tube drainage.[49, 50] Liver transplantation has been recommended for the treatment of carcinoma at the confluence, but the low survival rate and high complication rate do not justify its use at the present time.[50] Lesions in the mid or distal portions are more favorably situated for resection. Those that are nonresectable may be palliated with various procedures, as shown in Figures 45 and 46. Chemotherapy has been reported, but its role is questionable.[12, 28]

Like primary carcinomas of the gallbladder, primary malignant lesions of the bile duct are almost always discovered in the late stages and the prognosis is extremely poor, particularly for lesions of the proximal two thirds of the biliary ductal system. Curative resections of such tumors are rarely possible. In one series of 45 patients, the average survival was 13 months, only one patient being alive after 50 months.[8] In the Lahey Clinic series of 78 operated patients, the resection rate was only 10 per cent. Nine patients survived an average of four and one half years, two of whom lived for nine years.[40] This grim prognosis contrasts with the somewhat better prognosis of 30 per cent survival when lesions are in the distal portion of the bile duct.[12] For example, in the series reported by Longmire,[28] there were 13 distal carcinomas of the bile duct, nine of which were definitively treated by pancreaticoduodenectomy. Five of those patients were alive after one to 15 years. There were 13 mid-duct lesions, only four of which were resectable. Those four patients were alive one, four, five, and 11 years after resection. Again, as with carcinoma of the gallbladder, early diagnosis is probably the factor most important to survival.

SELECTED REFERENCES

Adson, M. A.: Carcinoma of the gallbladder. Surg. Clin. North Am., 53:1203, 1973.
This article commendably reviews the lymphatic and venous drainage of the gallbladder and correlates it with the spread of carcinoma outside the gallbladder. The author reviews methods of surgical treatment and summarizes data from 112 patients with primary carcinoma of the gallbladder seen at the Mayo Clinic from 1960 to 1972.

Beltz, W. R., and Condon, R. E.: Primary carcinoma of the gallbladder. Ann. Surg., 180:180, 1974.
This is an excellent report describing 117 patients with proven carcinoma of the gallbladder. The patients are divided into four groups: (1) localized inapparent disease, (2) localized potentially curable disease, (3) palliative therapy, and (4) late disease. The diagnosis, treatment, and survival are discussed in relation to the position of the lesion within the groups. Even when the tumors were apparently localized and therefore resectable, the survival rate was extremely poor.

Braasch, J. W., Warren, K. W., and Kune, G. A.: Malignant neoplasms of the bile ducts. Surg. Clin. North Am., 47:627, 1967
Ross, A. P., Braasch, J. W., and Warren, K. W.: Carcinoma of the proximal bile ducts. Surg. Gynecol. Obstet., 136:923, 1973.
These papers should be considered jointly, since they involve the same series of patients. The first concentrates on the problems related to the treatment of tumors confined to the proximal section of the biliary tract (103 patients), and the second presents problems related to tumors located in all sections of the biliary tract (173 patients). Of particular value are the discussions of the surgical treatment of these tumors based on their location. Survival after each type of operation is tabulated in the article by Braasch et al. and covered adequately by Ross et al.

Longmire, W. P., Jr., McArthur, M. S., Bastounis, E. A., and Hiatt, J.: Carcinoma of the extrahepatic biliary tract. Ann. Surg., 178:333, 1973.
This is an extremely good review of all aspects of carcinoma of the extrahepatic tract in 63 patients. There is an excellent discussion on the various modifications of the radical hepatic resections and reconstructions of the biliary tract that have been suggested in the treatment of this frequently fatal lesion.

Vaittinen, E.: Carcinoma of the gallbladder: A study of 390 cases diagnosed in Finland, 1953–1967. Ann. Chir. Gynecol. Fenn., 59:(Suppl.)168, 1970.
This is a very comprehensive review with a survey of the world literature (324 references) and a summary of 402 primary malignancies of the gallbladder in Finland from 1953 to 1967.

Wanebo, H. J., and Grimes, O. F.: Cancer of the bile duct: The occult malignancy. Am. J. Surg., 130:262, 1975.
This recent article is short but valuable because of its coverage of the anatomic problems related to the surgical management of malignant tumors in various sections of the bile duct. Simple line drawings are used and illustrate the various degrees of lobectomy and various decompression procedures possible. Some of the difficulties of early diagnosis are summarized, and diagnostic procedures such as percutaneous transhepatic cholangiography and duodenoscopy are evaluated.

REFERENCES

1. Adson, M. A.: Carcinoma of the gallbladder. Surg. Clin. North Am., 53:1203, 1973.
2. Akwari, O. E., Van Heerden, J. A., Foulk, W. T., and Baggenstoss, A. H.: Cancer of the bile ducts associated with ulcerative colitis. Ann. Surg., 181:303, 1975.
3. Altemeier, W. A., and Culbertson, W. R.: Sclerosing carcinoma of the hepatic bile ducts. Surg. Clin. North Am., 53:1229, 1973.
4. Arbab, A. A., and Brasfield, R.: Benign tumors of the gallbladder. Surgery, 61:535, 1967.
5. Arminski, T. C.: Primary carcinoma of the gallbladder. A collective review with addition of twenty-five cases from the Grace Hospital, Detroit, Michigan. Cancer, 2:379, 1949.
6. Balaroutsos, C., Bastounis, E., Karamanakos, P., and Golematis, B.: Primary carcinoma of the gallbladder: Analysis of 22 cases. Am. Surg., 40:605, 1974.
7. Beltz, W. R., and Condon, R. E.: Primary carcinoma of the gallbladder. Ann. Surg., 180:180, 1974.
8. Bismuth, H., and Corlette, M. B.: Intrahepatic cholangioenteric

anastomosis in carcinoma of the hilus of the liver. Surg. Gynecol. Obstet., *140*:170, 1975.

9. Bivins, B. A., Meeker, W. R., Jr., and Griffen, W. O., Jr.: Importance of histologic classification of carcinoma of the gallbladder. Am. Surg., *41*:121, 1975.

10. Blumgart, L. H., Cotton, P. B., Burwood, R., Lawrie, B., Salmon, P., Davies, G. T., Beales, J. S. M., Skirving, A., and Read, A. E.: Endoscopy and retrograde choledochopancreatography in the diagnosis of the jaundiced patient. Lancet, 2:1269, 1972.

11. Braasch, J. W.: Carcinoma of the bile duct. Surg. Clin. North Am., *53*:1217, 1973.

12. Braasch, J. W., Warren, K. W., and Kune, G. A.: Malignant neoplasms of the bile ducts. Surg. Clin. North Am., *47*:627, 1967.

13. Chandler, J. J., and Fletcher, W. S.: A clinical study of primary carcinoma of the gallbladder. Surg., Gynecol. Obstet., *117*:297, 1963.

14. Christensen, S. H., and Ishak, K. G.: Benign tumors and pseudotumors of the gallbladder. Report of 180 cases. Arch. Pathol., *90*:423, 1970.

15. Converse, C. F., Reagan, J. W., and DeCosse, J. J.: Ulcerative colitis and carcinoma of the bile ducts. Am. J. Surg., *121*:39, 1971.

16. Cooke, L., Jones, F. A., and Keech, M. K.: Carcinoma of the gallbladder. A statistical study. Lancet, 2:585, 1953.

17. Donaldson, L. A., and Busuttil, A.: A clinicopathological review of 68 carcinomas of the gallbladder. Br. J. Surg., *62*:26, 1974.

18. Foster, J. H.: Survival after liver resection for cancer. Cancer, *26*:493, 1970.

19. Glenn, F., and Hays, D. M.: The scope of radical surgery in the treatment of malignant tumors of the extrahepatic biliary tract. Surg. Gynecol Obstet., *99*:529, 1954.

20. Gothlin, J., Mansoor, M., and Tranberg, K.-G.: Combined percutaneous transhepatic cholangiography (PTC) and selective visceral angiography (SVA) in obstructive jaundice. Am. J. Roentgenol., *117*:419, 1973.

21. Goldin, A. R.: Percutaneous transhepatic cholangiography. S. Afr. Med. J., *48*:637, 1974.

22. Hardy, M. A., and Volk, H.: Primary carcinoma of the gallbladder. A ten year review. Am. J. Surg., *120*:800, 1970.

23. Kadell, B. M., and Weiner, M.: Current status of the transjugular approach for direct cholangiography. Surg. Clin. North Am., *53*:1019, 1973.

24. Kido, C., and Hibino, K.: Angiography of gallbladder cancer. Nippon Acta Radiol., *34*:1, 1974.

25. Klatskin, G.: Adenocarcinoma of the hepatic duct at its bifurcation within the porta hepatis. An unusual tumor with distinctive clinical and pathological features. Am. J. Med., *38*:241, 1965.

26. Lang, E. K.: Percutaneous transhepatic cholangiography. Radiology, *112*:283, 1974.

27. Loeb, P. M., Wheeler, H. O., and Berk, R. N.: Endoscopic pancreatocholangiography in the diagnosis of biliary tract disease. Surg. Clin. North Am., *53*:1007, 1973.

28. Longmire, W. P., Jr., McArthur, M. S., Bastounis, E. A., and Hiatt, J.: Carcinoma of the extrahepatic biliary tract. Ann. Surg., *178*:333, 1973.

29. Lund, J.: Surgical indications in cholelithiasis: Prophylactic cholecystectomy elucidated on the basis of long-term follow up of 526 nonoperated cases. Ann. Surg., *151*:153, 1960.

30. Mistilis, S., and Schiff, L.: A case of jaundice due to unilateral hepatic duct obstruction with relief after hepatic lobectomy. Gut, *4*:13, 1963.

31. Moertel, C. G.: Clinical management of advanced gastrointestinal cancer. Sem. Drug Treat., *3*:55, 1973.

32. Neibling, H. A., Dockerty, M. B., and Waugh, J. M.: Carcinoma of

the extrahepatic bile ducts. Surg. Gynecol. Obstet., *89*:429, 1949.

33. Ohlsson, E. G., and Aronsen, K. F.: Carcinoma of the gallbladder. A study of 181 cases. Acta Chir. Scand., *140*:475, 1974.

34. Parker, R. G. F., and Kendall, E. J. C.: The liver in ulcerative colitis. Br. Med. J., *2*:1030, 1954.

35. Pemberton, L. B., Diffenbaugh, W. F., and Strohl, E. L.: The surgical significance of carcinoma of the gallbladder. Am. J. Surg., *122*:381, 1971.

36. Ragins, H., Diamond, A., and Meng, C.-H.: Intrahepatic cholangiojejunostomy in the management of malignant biliary obstruction. Surg., Gynecol. Obstet., *136*:27, 1973.

37. Raskin, J. B.: Recent developments in gastrointestinal endoscopy. Postgrad. Med., *57*:85, 1975.

38. Rennell, C. L.: Diagnostic value of hypotonic duodenography. Am. J. Roentgenol., *121*:256, 1974.

39. Roberts-Thomson, I. C., Strickland, R. G., and Mackay, I. R.: Bible duct carcinoma in chronic ulcerative colitis. Aust. N. Z. J. Med., *3*:264, 1973.

40. Ross, A. P., Braasch, J. W., and Warren, K. W.: Carcinoma of the proximal bile ducts. Surg. Gynecol Obstet., *126*:923, 1973.

41. Sako, K., Seitzinger, G. L., and Garside, E.: Carcinoma of the extrahepatic bile ducts. Review of the literature and report of six cases. Surgery, *41*:416, 1957.

42. Sawyer, K. C.: The unrecognized significance of papillomas, polyps and adenomas of the gallbladder. Am. J. Surg., *120*:570, 1970.

43. Schutt, R. P.: Bilateral intrahepatic cholangiojejunostomy. Am. J. Surg., *107*:777, 1964.

44. Schwartz, S. I.: Primary sclerosing cholangitis: A disease revisited. Surg. Clin. North Am., *53*:1161, 1973.

45. Seigert, R. F., Wilson, S. D., and Kauffman, H. M.: Bilateral cholangiojejunostomy for sclerosing carcinoma of the intrahepatic bile ducts. Am. J. Surg., *123*:729, 1972.

46. Solan, M. J., and Jackson, B. T.: Carcinoma of the gall-bladder. A clinical appraisal and review of 57 cases. Br. J. Surg., *58*:593, 1971.

47. Strauch, G. O.: Primary carcinoma of the gall bladder. Presentation of seventy cases from the Rhode Island Hospital and a cumulative review of the last ten years of American literature. Surgery, *47*:368, 1960.

48. Tabrisky, J., Lindstrom, R. R., Herman, M. W., Castagna, J., and Sarti, D.: Value of gallbladder B-scan ultrasonography. Gastroenterology, *68*:1246, 1975.

49. Terblanche, J., and Louw, J. H.: U tube drainage in the palliative therapy of carcinoma of the main hepatic duct junction. Surg. Clin. North Am., *53*:1245, 1973.

50. Terblanche, J.: Is carcinoma of the main hepatic duct junction an indication for liver transplantation or palliative surgery? A plea for the U tube palliative procedure. Surgery, *79*:127, 1976.

51. Thorbjarnarson, B., and Glenn, F.: Carcinoma of the gallbladder. Cancer, *12*:1009, 1959.

52. Vaittinen, E.: Carcinoma of the gallbladder: A study of 390 cases diagnosed in Finland, 1953–1967. Ann. Chir. Gynecol. Fenn., *59*:(Suppl.) 168, 1970.

53. Wanebo, H. J., and Grimes, O. F.: Cancer of the bile duct: The occult malignancy. Am. J. Surg., *130*:262, 1975.

54. Watkins, E., Jr., and Khazei, A. M.: Arterial infusion chemotherapy of liver cancer. Bull. Soc. Int. Chir., *25*:279, 1966.

55. Weckert, E., and Robertson, B.: The natural course of gallstone disease. Eleven-year-review of 781 nonoperated cases. Gastroenterology, *50*:376, 1966.

56. Whelton, M. J., Petrelli, M., George, P., Young, W. B., and Sherlock, S.: Carcinoma at the junction of the main hepatic ducts. Q. J. Med., *38*:211, 1969.

37

THE PANCREAS

Edward L. Bradley, III, M.D.,

Robert Zeppa, M.D.,

and W. Dean Warren, M.D.

ANATOMY

A thorough familiarity with the anatomy of the pancreas is necessary not only for an appreciation of the morphology of those disorders requiring surgical intervention but also for an understanding of the various techniques employed in their treatment.

Fixed Retroperitoneal Position Crossing Abdomen Behind the Lesser Omental Bursa

The pancreas lies transversely in the upper abdomen, extending from the duodenal curve on the right to the hilus of the spleen on the left (Fig. 1). It generally lies in a retroperitoneal, retrogastric position and crosses the vertebral column at the first lumbar vertebra just below the celiac axis. Because of this relatively *fixed* position in close proximity to the vertebral column, the pancreas is susceptible to injury by blunt trauma. The pancreas crosses behind the lesser omental bursa, and, thus much of it is hidden from view by the stomach, transverse colon, and gastrohepatic and gastrocolic ligaments. Consequently, injuries or tumors of the neck, body, and tail of the gland may easily escape casual exploration. Pseudocysts of the pancreas resulting from duct disruption and leakage of pancreatic juice are typically confined to the lesser omental bursa, bounded by the stomach anteriorly, the transverse mesocolon inferiorly, the splenic hilum on the left lateral side, and the foramen of Winslow on the right.

The lack of a mesentery partially explains the low rate of resectability and curability of cancer of the pancreas. This is due not only to the early direct invasion of the posterior abdominal wall, but also to the anatomy of pancreatic lymph drainage. Several groups of nodes, including the celiac, suprapancreatic, subpyloric, subhepatic, superior mesenteric, aortic, and splenic, drain the pancreas. Excision of these nodes is accomplished only with a "node picking" type of procedure rather than an *en bloc* resection with wide surgical margins.

Joint Blood Supply for the Duodenum and Head of the Pancreas

One of the important limitations in pancreatic surgery is the inability to completely excise the pancreas without simultaneous duodenectomy. This is due to the joint blood supply of the head of the pancreas and the second portion of the duodenum. The superior and inferior pancreaticoduodenal arteries course within the pancreatic substance and are necessarily sacrificed during total pancreatectomy. Loss of these vessels markedly impairs the duodenal blood supply, most often leading to ischemic necrosis. The common bile duct also traverses the head of the pancreas immediately before it enters the duodenal wall and poses an additional anatomic hazard in total pancreatectomy. The Whipple operation was designed to overcome the anatomic dangers of total pancreatectomy and also to achieve a wider margin of resection for malignancy. In this procedure the head and varying portions of the body and tail of the pancreas are resected along with the duodenum, the terminal end of the common bile duct, and a portion of the stomach. Recently, the so-called radical distal pancreatectomy (or 95 per cent pancreatectomy) has been designed to resect all of the pancreas except the small crescent necessary to protect the pancreaticoduodenal arteries.[20] This procedure has been employed with success in the treatment of benign pancreatic diseases.

The remainder of the blood supply of the pancreas comes primarily from branches of the splenic and superior mesenteric arteries. In general, the venous drainage of the pancreas follows that of the arterial system. Of clinical significance is the fact that the body and tail of the pancreas are drained by small venous tributaries emptying into the splenic vein. These vessels are fragile and easily torn during dissection. For this reason, resection of the body and tail of the pancreas is frequently combined with splenectomy to minimize dissection and simplify the procedure.

Intimate Association with Vital Vascular Structures

In its transverse course the pancreas passes immediately anterior to the inferior vena cava, the aorta, and the superior mesenteric artery and vein, and lies anterior or slightly inferior to the splenic artery and vein (Fig. 2). One of the great dangers in both penetrating and nonpenetrating injuries of the pancreas is the pos-

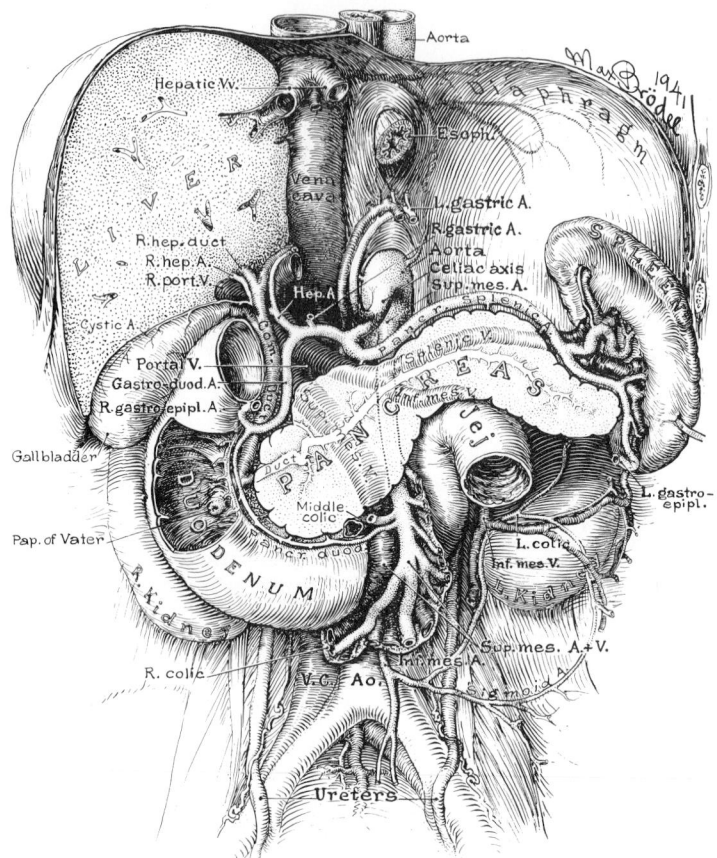

Figure 1. Relationships of the pancreas to other structures in the upper abdomen. (From Trimble, I. R., Parsons, J. W., and Sherman C. P.: Surg. Gynecol. Obstet., *73*:711, 1941.)

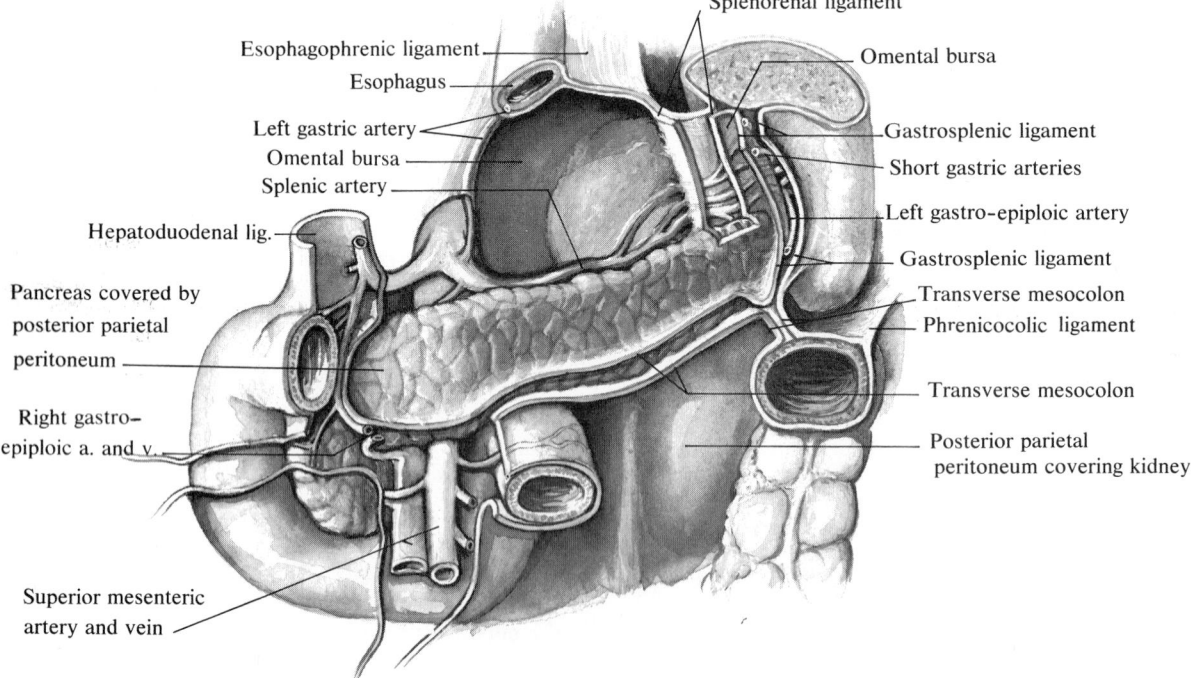

Figure 2. Vascular structures near the pancreas. (From Healey, J. E., Jr.: A Synopsis of Clinical Anatomy. Philadelphia, W. B. Saunders Company, 1969.)

sibility of injury to these large vessels. The pancreas may obscure the site of hemorrhage, and extensive mobilization or even transection of the pancreas may be necessary to control the bleeding vessel. Massive hemorrhage remains the principal cause of death in injuries involving the pancreas. A related problem is the dangerous hemorrhage sometimes seen with necrotizing pancreatitis and pseudocysts of the pancreas. The splenic or superior mesenteric vessels are usually the source of such bleeding.

Relationship of the Pancreatic Duct and Common Bile Duct at the Ampulla of Vater

There are numerous variations in the anatomic relationships between the common bile duct and the pancreatic duct (Fig. 3). At one extreme, each duct terminates in the duodenum through an entirely separate papilla, and at the other end of the spectrum, the two ducts jointly share a conduit, a centimeter or more in length, which terminates at the papilla of Vater. It has been well demonstrated that in patients with chronic pancreatitis some degree of a "common channel" exists between the two ducts. This has been shown both at operation and at autopsy by injection into the common bile duct with reflux into the pancreatic ductal system. From the available data it appears that this relationship is far more common in patients with pancreatitis than in the normal population. This anatomic association is important to help explain the role of biliary tract disease in the development of pancreatitis through obstruction at the ampulla of Vater, induced by either spasm or stones. In addition, papillitis with fibrosis and stenosis is seen in other types of pancreatitis. Enlarging the sphincter

orifice in many instances can decompress both the biliary and pancreatic ductal systems.

Innervation of the Pancreas

Pancreatic secretion is controlled to some extent through vagal innervation. This has led to proposed treatment of acute pancreatitis with vagolytic drugs, and of chronic pancreatitis with bilateral vagectomy combined with gastrojejunostomy. Although such therapeutic proposals are of unproved value, the influence of the vagus on pancreatic secretion is unquestioned. The vagus does not carry sensory fibers, however, and the sensation of pain from the pancreas is mediated by the splanchnic nerves. Procedures to block the splanchnic nerves temporarily, or to divide them, have been utilized in the treatment of various pancreatic disorders. Although the left splanchnic nerve innervates most of the pancreas, failure to control pain after unilateral nerve section in a significant number of cases has necessitated bilateral splanchnicectomy when a maximal effort at pain control is needed. While infrequently performed, splanchnicectomy and splanchnic blocks are important adjuncts in the management of the severe pain of pancreatic cancer and chronic pancreatitis.

Microscopic Anatomy

The pancreas is a complex structure composed of two strikingly different types of tissue having widely disparate functions. The exocrine or digestive portion of the organ is composed of a compound acinar gland divided into lobules clearly demarcated by loose connective tissue septa. In turn, the septa are traversed

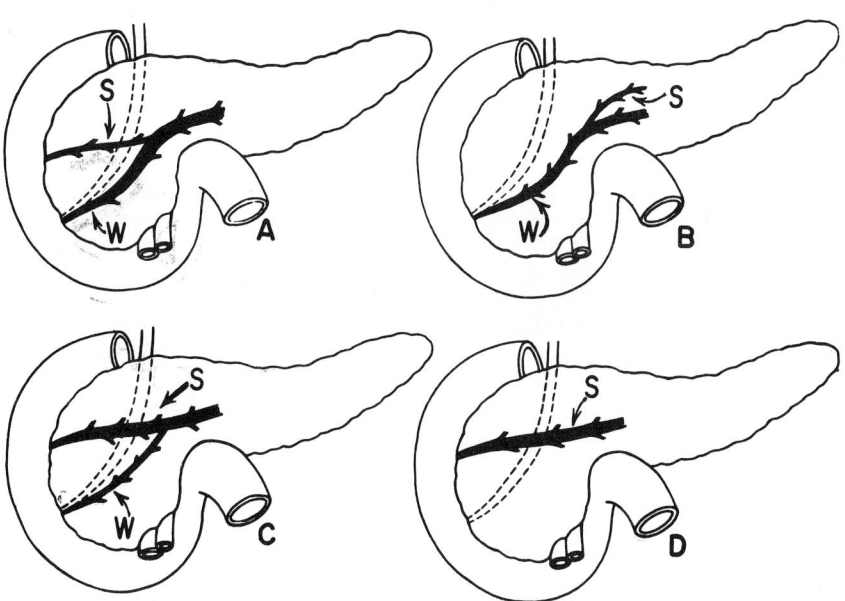

Figure 3. Diagrammatic illustration of several variations in the size and connections of the main duct of Wirsung (W) and the accessory duct of Santorini (S). A, The arrangement reported in the majority of dissections. B, Santorini's duct draining the midportion of the gland and connecting directly into the duct of Wirsung. C and D, The duct of Santorini as the major pancreatic duct. D, Although relatively rare, obliteration of the duct of Wirsung gives the surgeon great difficulty when attempting to catheterize the pancreatic duct preliminary to pancreatogram following sphincterotomy. (From Ellison, E. H., and Carey, L. C. In Davis, L. (Ed.): Christopher's Textbook of Surgery, 9th ed. Philadelphia, W. B. Saunders Company, 1968.)

by nutrient blood vessels, nerves, and lymphatics. The acini are composed of a single row of pyramidal epithelial cells converging toward a central lumen and resting at the opposite pole on a well-demarcated basal lamina (Fig. 4).

The basilar portion of the acinar cells contains the tubular and cisternal elements of the rough endoplasmic reticulum as well as mitochondria appearing in the shape of long rods with well-developed cristae and matrix granules. The Golgi complex is also located in this region of the cells. The free surfaces of the acinar cells forming the interface with the lumen of the acinus contain few short and irregular microvilli. The apical cytoplasm in this area is usually loaded with zymogen droplets. In some preparations these droplets may be seen discharging into the lumen of the acinus. The lumen of each acinus is continuous with the lumen of the terminal duct, which is bounded by centroacinar cells. These cells have been so named because they are surrounded by and appear to extend toward the center of the lumen of the acinus. These are cuboidal to low columnar cells which are pale-staining with hematoxylin and eosin. This terminal portion of the duct system drains proximally into the intralobular or intercalated ducts. The latter are lined by cells that are similar in appearance to the centroacinar cells and are low columnar in variety. In turn, the intercalated ducts are involved in the secretion of water and electrolytes.

Intimately associated with the acinar structure of the exocrine pancreas are small masses of *endocrine* cells composing the islets of Langerhans (Fig. 5). These are scattered throughout the pancreas and are frequently found to number in excess of one million per gland. The islets are clearly demarcated by a thin layer of reticular fibers. Occasionally, the endocrine cells may be found isolated or in smaller groups scattered among the acinar cells. They may be identified by differential staining, since secretory granules cannot be identified within the endocrine cells on routine hematoxylin and eosin staining. However, special techniques have revealed that there are at least three types of endocrine cells which in fact do contain distinctive granules. The alpha cell contains granules that are insoluble in alcohol, while the granules of the other most common type, the beta cell, are soluble in alcohol. Morphologically intermediate between the alpha and beta cells is the delta cell, which contains granules that are usually somewhat larger but less dense than the granules in the alpha cell. While the physiologic significance of the delta cells in the islets is not yet clear, alpha cells have been associated with the production of the hormone glucagon, and the beta cells with insulin.

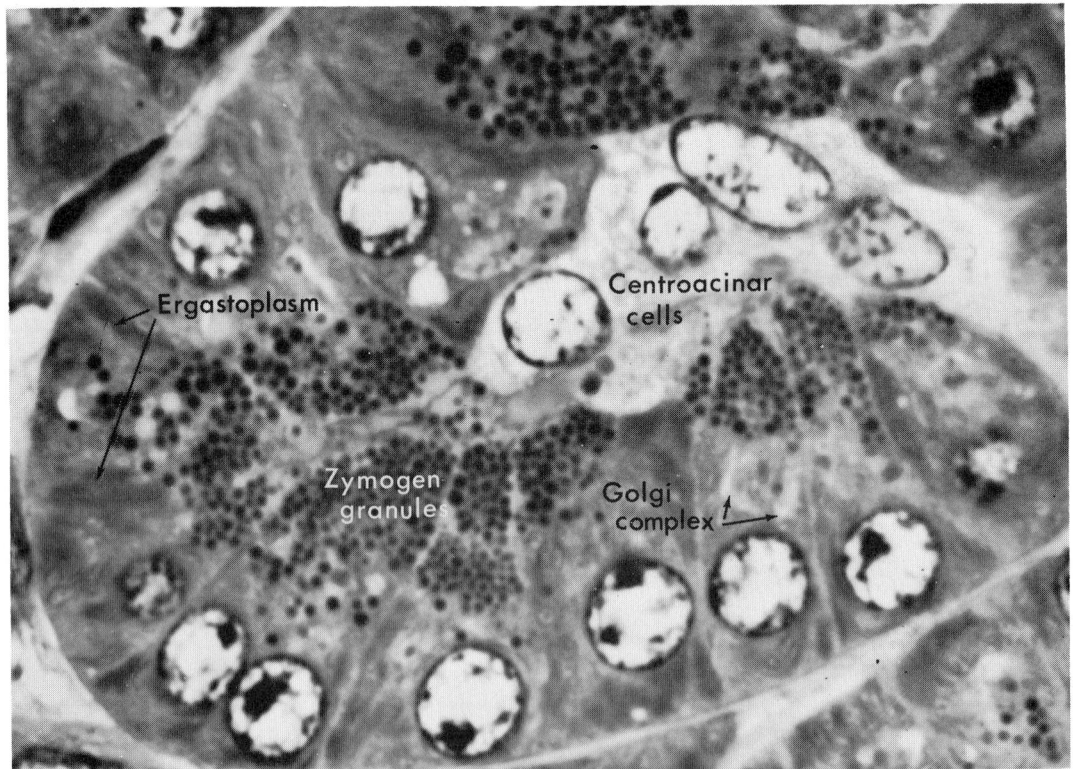

Figure 4. Photomicrograph of human pancreas, showing an acinus and its centroacinar cells. The ergastoplasm, Golgi complex, and zymogen granules of the acinar cells are clearly identifiable. The fixation of the nuclei is less than ideal, but adequate preservation of this organ from postmortem material is difficult. Formalin, osmium fixation, Epon section, stained with toluidine blue, ×3200. (Courtesy of S. Ito. From Bloom, W., and Fawcett, D. W.: A Textbook of Histology, 9th ed. Philadelphia, W. B. Saunders Company, 1968.)

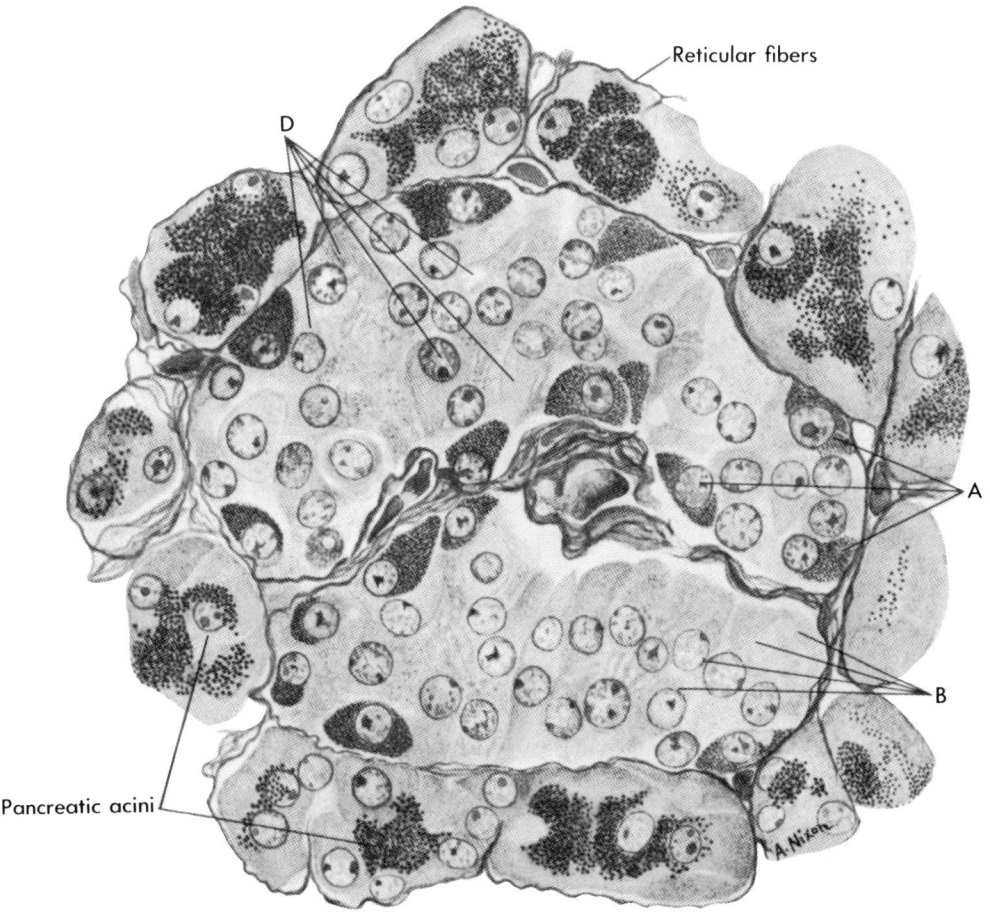

Figure 5. Section of human pancreas. The central part of the figure is an islet of Langerhans with granular cells of types alpha, beta, and delta. Mallory-azan stain, ×960. (After Bloom, 1931. From Bloom, W., and Fawcett, S. W.: A Textbook of Histology, 9th ed. Philadelphia, W. B. Saunders Company, 1968.)

EMBRYOLOGY

An endodermal pouch on the dorsal wall of the duodenum may be seen in the 3-mm. human embryo and identified as the first appearance of the pancreas. Somewhat later, an additional pouch, sometimes two, appears on the inferior portion of an angle formed by the duodenum and the developing hepatic buds. This latter pouch (or pouches) constitutes the ventral pancreas. The dorsal pancreas grows more rapidly than the ventral pancreas, and rotation of the duodenum and common bile duct carries the ventral pancreas to the right. Subsequently, fusion occurs between dorsal and ventral pancreas, the ventral pancreas becoming the uncinate process.

Lobular arrangement within the pancreas becomes evident at about the fourth month of fetal existence, and the lobules are usually small and well separated by connective tissue. Acinus formation may be seen approximately one month earlier, the acini appearing as small groups of cells along the lateral walls and distal ends of the ducts. Continued proliferation of the ducts is associated with formation of new acini. These acini tend to bulge outward, developing small lumina that appear clustered around the ends of the ducts. The duct cells that are surrounded by acinar cells then become known as the centroacinar cells.

Before the acini begin to develop, islets of Langerhans may be discovered in association with the ducts. The first group to be identified undergoes primary degeneration, and a second generation appears sometime during the fourth month of gestation.

Annular pancreas is a relatively rare congenital malformation which occasionally may cause symptoms in the adult. The symptoms may result from obstruction to the duodenum at the site of the annulus or from chronic pancreatitis and peptic ulcer. Jaundice may be the initial presentation, and evaluation of the biliary tract may reveal a dilated common duct with or without stones. While the precise etiology of this abnormality is not clear, two major theories consider the condition to be due to either (1) the failure of the ventral anlage of the pancreas to rotate with the duodenum, or (2) hypertrophy of both the ventral and

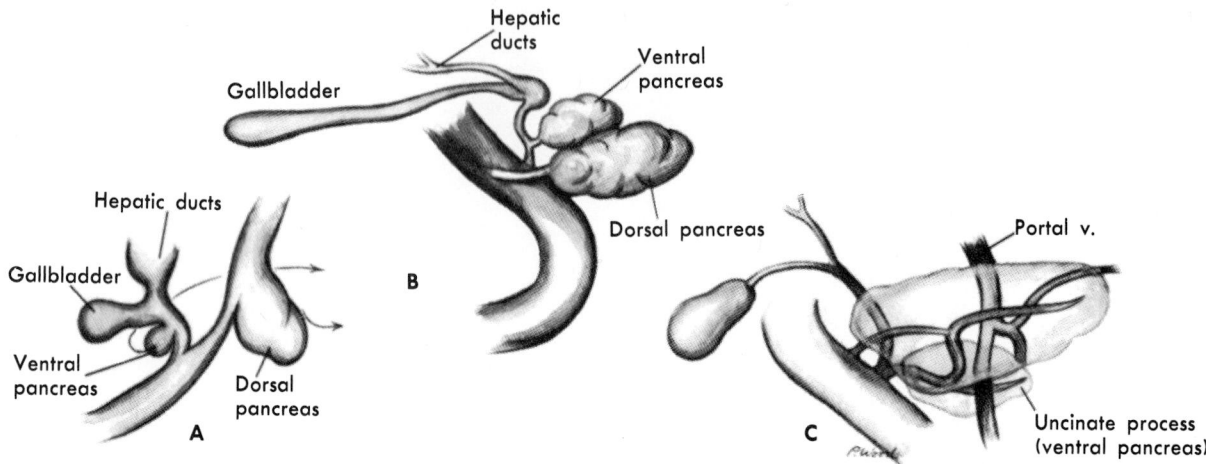

Figure 6. Embryology of the pancreas. *A,* Lateral view of the pancreatic buds in an 8 mm. embryo. The movement of the ventral and dorsal pancreatic anlage is shown by the arrows. *B,* Position of the pancreatic anlage after rotation of the ventral pancreas, also a lateral view (15 mm. embryo). *C,* Anterior view after union showing relationship to both vascular and ductal structures. (From White, T. T.: Surgical anatomy of the pancreas. *In* Carey, L. C. (Ed.): The Pancreas. St. Louis, The C. V. Mosby Co., 1973. Modified from Boyden, E. A.: Am. J. Anat., *38:*177, 1926, with the assistance of Dr. Boyden in April, 1971.)

dorsal pouches. On examination, the annular pancreas contains normal acinar and islet tissue. When the symptoms are primarily those of obstruction, a bypass operation is clearly the procedure of choice, usually a duodenojejunostomy. Although bypass via gastrojejunostomy is also possible, occasional continuing abdominal pain due to the undecompressed duodenum makes this procedure less desirable. Resection or division of the annulus is inadvisable, since the risk of fistula formation and duodenal leakage increases when pancreatic tissue is dispersed throughout the duodenal wall.

Pancreatic heterotopia is a more common congenital malformation.[6] The ectopic pancreas may be found almost anywhere along the gastrointestinal tract. However, in descending order of frequency, it is found in the duodenum, stomach, and jejunum. There is lesser involvement of Meckel's diverticulum and the wall of the ileum. Interestingly, about one fourth of all the reported gastrointestinal diverticula of embryonic origin are found to have ectopic pancreatic tissue within them. The clinical significance of these aberrant foci of pancreatic tissue depends upon the complications they provoke. These complications include ulceration, hemorrhage, and obstruction, either because of the size of the pancreatic mass *per se* or because it serves as the focal point for the development of an intussusception. The differentiation of ectopic pancreas from a primary neoplasm of the organ affected is sometimes difficult and resolved only by excision.

PHYSIOLOGY

The first demonstration of the effect of vagal stimulation on pancreatic secretion was recorded by Heiden-

hain in 1875.[40] These observations were confirmed and further defined by Pavlov and his brilliant group of coworkers.[62] Pavlov's student Babkin was the first to demonstrate that all the secretory nerves to the pancreas are cholinergic, even when derived from the sympathetic nervous system.[3] At the turn of the century, Bayliss and Starling demonstrated the existence of a substance in duodenal mucosa that stimulated pancreatic secretion, to which they gave the name secretin.[7] They demonstrated that the greatest concentration of the hormone was in the duodenum, although it could be found for variable distances in the mucosa farther down the intestinal tract. These contributions were initial milestones in the endeavor to understand pancreatic function, and their validity remains unchallenged today.

EXOCRINE

Despite the accumulation of a wealth of information, a clearly defined schema of integrated exocrine function of the pancreatic gland is not yet clear. Examination of the digestive function of the gland clearly defines two separate components. The first, water and electrolyte secretion, is thought to be located in the centroacinar and intercalated duct cells. Output from these cells results in a stimulated flow rate in man which may reach more than 4.5 ml. per minute. The osmotic pressure of pancreatic juice is isotonic with plasma and responds to changes in plasma osmolality, while the pH of the juice varies from 7 to 8.7 and the specific gravity ranges from 1.007 to 1.042, being primarily dependent upon enzyme concentration. The most important ion in pancreatic juice is bicarbonate, which appears in a concentration range of 25 to 170 mEq. per liter. Bicarbonate concentration varies directly with the rate of flow. Chloride ion varies inversely with bicarbonate, and the sum of bicarbonate and chloride concentrations falls between 154 and 175 mEq. per liter. The sum of the concentrations of sodium and potassium is approximately equal to that found in the plasma and remains independent of the rate of flow of pancreatic secretion.

Secretin, which was defined by Jorpes as a linear polypeptide containing 27 amino acids,[50] stimulates the flow of pancreatic juice, which contains large amounts of bicarbonate. The hormone is released from the duodenal mucosa in the presence of hydrochloric acid, proteolytic byproducts, fatty acids, and amino acids such as glutamic acid. Conversely, the flow of pancreatic juice and the concentration of bicarbonate are reduced by the action of antidiuretic hormone and pancreatic glucagon.

The mechanism of secretion of large volumes of bicarbonate-rich juice is not clear. Two hypotheses are most prevalent. The first, proposed by Janowitz,[46] describes the primary secretion of isotonic bicarbonate with alteration in the final concentrations being due to an exchange for chloride in the collecting system. This scheme favors an increase in the exchange at low flow rates. The alternative hypothesis favors the unicellular concept, which describes the secretion of both bicarbonate and chloride at variable rates. At present there are insufficient data to establish the validity of either concept, although much experimental data supports the exchange hypothesis.

The other component of exocrine function consists of the elaboration and secretion of small volumes of fluid rich in enzymatic activity. Extensive studies on protein synthesis in the acinar cells have revealed that secretory proteins are formed on the ribosomes and then transferred across the membranes of the rough endoplasmic reticulum which appear as cisterns in electron micrographs. Smooth buds develop from the rough vesicles containing newly synthesized secretory protein. These vesicles coalesce, perhaps receiving some membrane from the Golgi apparatus to form immature zymogen granules partially filled with protein. Maturation of these granules occurs during their movement from the basilar portion of the cell toward the free surface and probably involves either the extrusion of water or the internal transport of additional protein (Fig. 7). This protein-rich fluid of high specific gravity contains the inactive forms of the enzymes trypsin, chymotrypsins A and B, carboxypeptidases A and B, and the active forms of ribonuclease, deoxyribonuclease, amylase, and lipase.

Cholecystokin-pancreozymin (CCK-PZ), a peptide hormone released from the mucosa of the duodenum and jejunum by the chemical action of intraluminal food stuffs, is primarily responsible for pancreatic enzyme output. The proteolytic enzymes are released as inactive precursors (trypsinogen, chymotrypsinogen, pro-elastase, and pro-carboxypeptidase), which are activated by contact with enterokinase, a cleaving enzyme present in the intestinal lumen.

In common with secretory function elsewhere in the gastrointestinal tract, the regulation of pancreatic exocrine secretion is bimodal. There are neural secretory effects as well as potent hormonal stimuli. A substantial portion of the secretory innervation to the pancreas enters the gland in the region of the choledocho-duodenal junction. The vagus nerve provides secretory fibers to both acinar and islet cells, and, in addition, distributes motor fibers to the smooth muscles of the major ducts. Both trunks of the vagus nerves appear to be involved. Stimulation of the vagus nerve provokes a secretory response that is characterized by the appearance of pancreatic juice of high specific gravity, rich in enzymes, with only a modest increase in volume. This response may be mimicked by cholinergic drugs and blocked by atropine. Futher, stimulation of the vagus nerve potentiates the actions of the hormones cholecystokinin-pancreozymin and secretin. Both of the hormones are released from the duodenal mucosa in response to similar stimuli. CCK-PZ does not significantly alter the flow of water or electrolytes from the pancreas but profoundly stimulates the output of enzymes. Secretin, as previously mentioned, provokes the secretion of a thin, watery pancreatic juice rich in bicarbonate ions. This information suggests that the integrated control of pancreatic

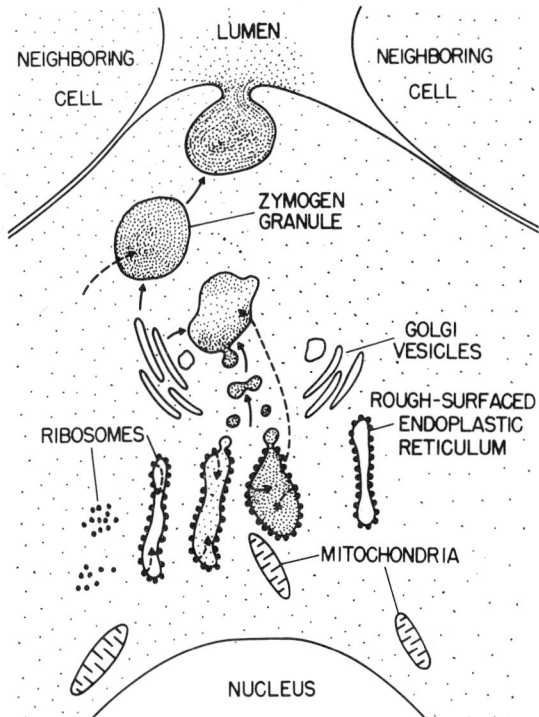

Figure 7. Scheme of intracellular protein transport in the pancreas. After the secretory proteins are formed on the ribosomes they are transferred across the membranes of the rough-surfaced cisternae, where they accumulate. Smooth membranes bud from the ends of the rough-surfaced cisternae in the centrosphere (Golgi) region and form small vesicles containing newly synthesized secretory proteins. Small vesicles coalesce, possibly receiving additional membrane from the Golgi vesicles to form immature zymogen granules, partly filled with secretory protein. Mature zymogen granules are formed by extrusion of water or by transport of additional protein across the membrane of the zymogen vacuoles (or both). *Solid arrows* depict migration of membrane. *Dashed arrows* depict transmembrane transport of protein. Dots depict secretory protein. (From Hokin, L. E. *In* American Physiological Society: Handbook of Physiology. Section 6, Alimentary Canal; Volume II, Secretion. Edited by C. F. Code. Baltimore, Williams & Wilkins, 1968; adapted from Palade, G. E., et al. *In* de Reuck, A. V. S., and Cameron, M. P. (Eds.): Ciba Foundation Symposium, Exocrine Pancreas. London, J. & A. Churchill, 1962, pp. 23–55.)

secretion may be viewed as the action of the two duodenal hormones operating against a background of vagal activity.

In addition to the stimulatory effects of the intestinal hormones secretin and CCK-PZ, there is evidence that suggests that a gastric phase of pancreatic secretion may exist. Pancreatic secretion may be provoked by injecting pure gastrin or by stimulating the antral release of endogenous gastrin by distention or manipulation of intraluminal pH. Conversely, the pancreatic response to a meal may be reduced considerably following partial gastrectomy. The pancreatic response to administered gastrin involves secretion of both bicarbonate and protein.

Pancreatic exocrine contributions to digestion and absorption are covered at length in Chapter 31.

The stimulatory action of secretin forms the basis of the clinically useful test in which the duodenum is intubated, secretin administered, and pancreatic juice aspirated through an indwelling tube. While the normal range of responses must be established for each laboratory, the minimal volume to be expected is approximately 100 ml. per hour, with the secretion of 15 to 20 mEq. of bicarbonate ion and 700 units of amylase.[4, 16, 24, 39, 41]

ENDOCRINE

The relationship between the pancreas and diabetes mellitus was established in 1889 by von Mering and Minkowski, who described diabetes in a dog following removal of the pancreas.[80] However, knowledge that glycosuria was an important factor in the disease has been recognized since ancient times. It was during the seventeenth and eighteenth centuries that diagnosticians had earned the sobriquet "piss prophets," reflecting their observations that the urine of the diabetic patient was "wonderfully sweet as if imbued with honey or sugar." By 1922 Banting and Best[5] had obtained potent pancreatic extracts that were active against hyperglycemia, and by 1926 insulin had been crystallized and found to have a molecular weight of 6000 with two polypeptide chains linked by a disulfide bridge.

Insulin is the product of the beta cell within the islands of Langerhans. The granules of these beta cells represent the storage form of the hormone. Release of insulin from the beta cell is controlled by alterations in the concentration of blood sugar. In isolated, perfused pancreas preparations, an increase in the concentration of sugar was attended by an increase in circulating insulin. Further, after chronic intravenous administration of glucose to animals, an increased amount of islet tissue may be found in the pancreas. The amino acid leucine and some sulfonyl urea compounds are also known to cause the release of stored insulin. In addition, evidence has been obtained from man showing that the hormone secretin causes the release of insulin. Insulin may be measured in the portal venous blood within minutes following intravenous administration of physiologic doses of secretin. This action of secretin may explain the discrepancy between the findings that vagotomy appears to have no effect upon glucose metabolism and, conversely, that stimulation of the vagus nerve has been shown to cause insulin release. Presumably, this action is the result of the effect of vagal stimulation upon acid secretion and, in turn, the stimulation of secretin release by acid in the duodenum. Such studies have more clearly defined the digestive mechanism involved in the homeostasis of blood sugar.

Glucagon is another major pancreatic hormone and is a polypeptide composed of 29 amino acid residues with a molecular weight of 3482. Glucagon stimulates hyperglycemia by promoting the breakdown of liver glycogen with consequent release of glucose into the circulation.[9] This effect upon blood sugar may be the mechanism whereby glucagon provides the release of insulin. The hormone also has exocrine effects which have been noted following administration of exogenous glucagon. Infusion at a dose of 40 mg. per kilogram has resulted in striking reduction in the volume of pancreatic juice secreted through a fistula in man. Other effects of glucagon include (1) inhibition of gastric acid secretion; (2) inhibition of gastric and intestinal motility; (3) stimulation of the flow of bile; and (4) stimulation of Brunner's glands and intestinal secretion.

The physiologic role for the delta cells is unknown; however, it is possible that they are involved in the development of gastrin-secreting tumors of the pancreas, since gastrin has been demonstrated in these cells by immunoassay and immunofluorescence.[18]

PANCREATITIS

The morbid process of pancreatitis includes a broad pathologic spectrum ranging from minimal edema through hemorrhagic necrosis to fibrosis with severe diminution of both endocrine and exocrine function. Because treatment is dictated by the particular stage of the disease process, it has become clinically necessary to distinguish between the various modes of presentation. The Marseilles classification (Table 1) has received general acceptance and will be used here.

ACUTE PANCREATITIS

By definition, acute pancreatitis refers to an acute inflammation superimposed upon a normal gland. Although acute pancreatitis is a relatively common

TABLE 1. Marseilles Classification of Pancreatitis

I. Acute pancreatitis—a single episode of pancreatitis in a previously normal gland.
II. Recurrent acute pancreatitis—recurrent attacks which do not lead to permanent functional damage; clinical and biological normalcy in interval between attacks.
III. Recurrent chronic pancreatitis—progressive functional damage persisting between attacks; frequent pain-free intervals.
IV. Chronic pancreatitis—inexorable and irreversible destruction of pancreatic function; constant pain.

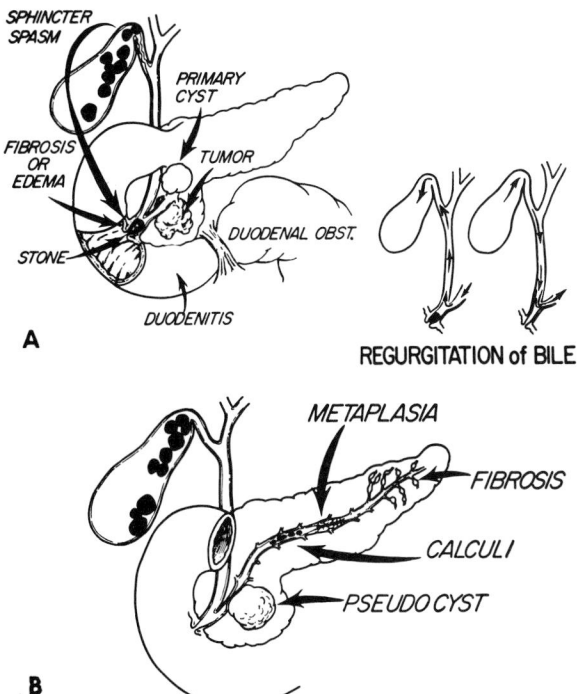

SPHINCTER SPASM

PRIMARY CYST

FIBROSIS OR EDEMA

TUMOR

DUODENAL OBST.

STONE

DUODENITIS

A

REGURGITATION of BILE

METAPLASIA

FIBROSIS

CALCULI

PSEUDOCYST

B

Figure 8. *A,* Conditions associated with and thought to contribute to acute pancreatitis: occlusion of the sphincter of Oddi results in obstruction of the pancreatic duct and permits regurgitation of bile through a common channel; it can result from reflex spasm, stone, fibrosis, or edema. Duodenal obstruction distal to the sphincter may cause reflux of duodenal contents. An enlarging tumor or cyst may result in intrapancreatic obstruction. *B,* Recurrent pancreatitis with fibrosis and metaplasia of the ductal epithelium, calculus formation, or the development of a pancreatic pseudocyst may lead to secondary obstruction of the pancreatic ducts, thus fostering further attacks. (From Ellison, E. H., and Carey, L. C. *In* Davis, L. (Ed.): Christopher's Textbook of Surgery. 9th ed. Philadelphia, W. B. Saunders Company, 1968.)

cause of emergency admission, because of the variability in its presentation, the actual attack rate is unknown. Just as the gross and microscopic manifestations of pancreatitis are variable, so are the concepts concerning the etiology of the disease. Attempts to discover a single precise etiologic factor have occupied medical investigators for more than 100 years. At present, there is general agreement that ductal obstruction, with or without reflux of duodenal or biliary contents combined with vascular insufficiency, and superimposed upon the stimulated exocrine pancreas, is responsible for initiating the process of acute pancreatitis (Fig. 8).

Obstruction and Reflux

Simple obstruction of the major pancreatic ducts, complete or partial, has been considered by some to be the basic cause of this disease. However, the incidence of ductal obstruction in postmortem examinations of fatal pancreatitis does not support this thesis. Autopsies in 100 consecutive patients dying of pancreatitis

in the Los Angeles County General Hospital revealed duct obstruction in only three of the cadavers. Further, deliberate ligation of the major pancreatic duct in treatment of chronic relapsing pancreatitis has not caused the acute disease. These observations do not preclude the possibility of pancreatitis developing as a result of duct obstruction when powerful stimulatory factors simultaneously affect exocrine function. When duct obstruction is imposed in association with stimulation to pancreatic secretion, pancreatitis has been induced in experimental animals.

The role of bile or duodenal reflux into the pancreatic ducts in the etiology of human pancreatitis is equally obscure. After Opie had demonstrated pancreatic duct obstruction by biliary calculi,[59] Halsted proposed that bile reflux into pancreatic ducts was a cause of acute hemorrhagic pancreatitis.[37] The "common channel theory" that he postulated was based on the discovery of a biliary stone lodged in the ampulla of Vater, effectively obstructing both the terminal bile and pancreatic ducts which shared a final common pathway in a patient who died of acute pancreatitis. The theory provided an attractive and easily digestible explanation for the well-recognized association of biliary stones and pancreatitis. The anatomic features required to support a common channel hypothesis appear to exist in two thirds of subjects. However, bidirectional reflux, that is, bile into pancreatic ducts and pancreatic juice into bile ducts, has been observed in humans without pancreatitis. Further, pressures in the pancreatic ductal system are consistently higher than simultaneously recorded pressures in the biliary ductal system. Under these conditions one could not reasonably expect bile to perfuse the pancreatic ducts without postulating some additional mechanism. Active perfusion of pancreatic ducts with normal bile at normal pressures does not cause pancreatitis. Treatment of the bile by incubation with pancreatic juice, trypsin, or bacteria and then injection of this material into the pancreatic ducts at increased pressures (sufficient to injure the finer radicals) is usually effective in provoking acute hemorrhagic pancreatitis. Intensive investigative efforts using animal models have not clarified the reservations concerning the bile reflux hypothesis.

Acute pancreatitis has also been attributed to the reflux of duodenal contents into the pancreatic duct. Such duodenopancreatic reflux has been demonstrated to occur in humans. This concept has the added attraction of describing a mechanism that per se includes activation of proteolytic enzymes via the enterokinase system. Despite such theoretical attractions, it has been shown that continuous perfusion of the pancreatic duct with either duodenal or biliary secretions does not cause pancreatitis in experimental animal models even though intraductal activation of pancreatic enzymes occurs. This is true so long as forceful injection retrograde through the duct is not the mechanism for the introduction of the materials into the pancreatic ductal system. On the other hand, the experimental construction of closed-loop duodenal obstruction with biliary exclusion (Pfeffer preparation) is followed by a most virulent form of acute pancreatitis.[63] The severity of the lesion may be modified by the administration of antibiotics or by pancreatic duct ligation. At present, the clinical significance of these laboratory observations is difficult to assess except to say that the obstructed duodenum may elaborate a factor or factors that may provoke pancreatic inflammation.

Vascular Factors

Interference with the arterial blood supply to the pancreas has been shown to cause pancreatic lesions. The magnitude of the pancreatic injury appears to correlate well with the degree of occlusion of the terminal vascular radicals (Fig. 9). It has been shown recently that gradations in the severity of pancreatic inflammation may be obtained by the injection of microspheres of various sizes into the pancreaticoduodenal arteries of animals. The smallest spheres (8 to 20 μ) provoked the most severe forms of acute pancreatitis. This observation suggests that these smaller particles occlude the terminal arterial supply and effectively preclude the possibility of collateral arterialization which might maintain the viability of the acinar structures. Further studies supporting the importance of a vascular factor in determining the severity of the inflammatory process in the pancreas were done by

Popper.[65] He produced edematous pancreatitis in rats by ligation of the pancreatic ducts in conjunction with the administration of secretin. Subsequent and temporary occlusion of the gastroduodenal artery in this model was followed by the development of full-blown hemorrhagic pancreatitis. Despite these and many other studies, the relative importance of hypoperfusion in the development of clinical disease is unknown.

Clinical Disease

Despite the extensive literature regarding experimental pancreatitis, the etiology of the human disease is unknown. Evidence in favor of ductal obstruction or reflux is meager and seems to apply to a disappointingly small number of patients. In the United States, the majority of persons who present with pancreatitis are chronic alcoholics. Many studies have sought to expose a direct toxic effect of alcohol on the pancreatic acini of experimental animals, but to date these efforts have been singularly unsuccessful. The most prevalent hypothesis concerning the role of alcohol in the production of the disease considers (1) the stimulated production of excessive amounts of highly alkaline juice, leading to alkalinization of the gland which

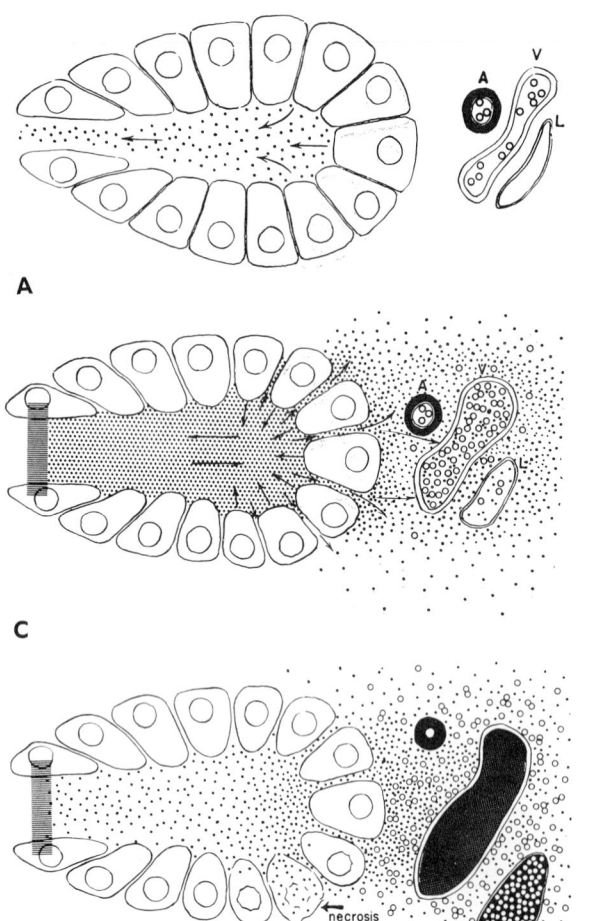

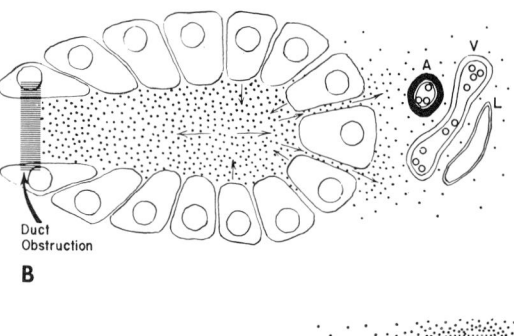

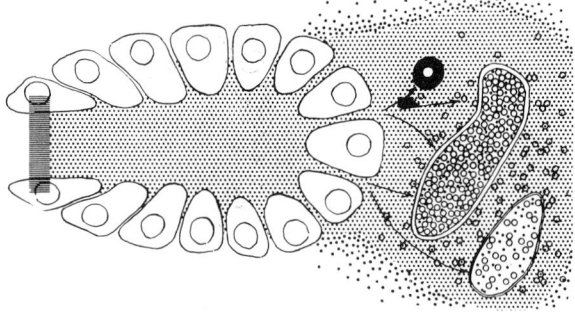

Figure 9. *A*, Normal pancreas. Schematic representation of acinar cell grouping in normal pancreas. Arrows indicate direction of flow of enzymes (stippling) into duct. A, V, and L signify arterial, venous, and lymphatic vessels, respectively, in the interstitial area. *B*, Early pancreatitis: Enzymes enter interstitial area. *C*, Pancreatitis: Enzymes increase vascular permeability. *D*, Pancreatitis: (1) Massive interlobular extravasation, (2) venous dilatation and stasis, (3) red blood cells enter lymphatic circulation, (4) reduced circulating blood volume leading to splanchnic arterial constriction. *E*, Necrotizing pancreatitis: Arterial spasm, venous thrombosis, lymphatics obstructed with red blood cells, progressing to vascular insufficiency and finally cell death. (From Anderson, M. C., et al.: Surg. Clin. North Am., *47*:127, 1967.)

results in instability of the zymogen membranes, *in combination with* (2) spasm of the sphincter of Oddi due to duodenal irritation as a local effect of alcohol. It has also been suggested that alcohol may interfere with the pancreatic production of naturally occurring trypsin inhibitor. However, at this time no data are available to support this concept.

Other significant factors that may have an etiologic role in clinical pancreatitis include biliary tract disease (10 to 20 per cent of patients) and operation (the "postoperative" group, 10 to 15 per cent of patients). About 10 to 15 per cent of patients acquire the disease in the absence of recognized contributory factors (idiopathic group). In addition, a multitude of infrequently cited causes include drug therapy such as corticosteroids and chlorothiazide, hyperparathyroidism, pregnancy, carcinoid disease, hyperlipemia, periarteritis nodosa, trauma, and mumps.

Diagnosis

The signs and symptoms of acute pancreatitis are variable in expression and dependent upon the degree of structural alteration within the gland. In the milder edematous form of the disease, the patient usually complains of penetrating upper abdominal pain, often radiating to the flanks, shoulders, and back. On physical examination there is epigastric tenderness and a low-grade fever. In severe hemorrhagic pancreatitis, the patient may present with a rigid abdomen and signs of shock, including sweating, tachycardia, and hypotension. Nausea, vomiting, and abdominal distention are common, and jaundice may be detected in 20 to 25 per cent of patients. Rarely, discoloration of the skin may be visible in the flanks (Gray-Turner sign) or about the umbilicus (Cullen's sign) (Fig. 10).

The association of high serum amylase activity in pancreatitis was first reported in 1929,[26] with the recommendation for its use as a diagnostic test. Prior to this observation, the recognition of pancreatitis was confined to the operating or autopsy rooms. Usually the serum amylase is elevated within 2 to 12 hours of the onset of symptoms and returns to normal within 3

or 4 days.[87] Hyperamylasemia prolonged beyond a week usually indicates the development of a complication of pancreatitis. At present it is impossible to predict either the certainty of pancreatitis or the severity of the process from the blood level of amylase activity. However, in general, it may be stated that the higher this activity, the greater the probability of acute pancreatitis. Hyperamylasemia may also be found in patients with biliary tract disease, alcoholism in the absence of pancreatitis, perforated peptic ulcer, intestinal obstruction, mesenteric thrombosis, ectopic pregnancy, mumps, and often after the use of drugs such as meperidine (Demerol) or morphine. Fractionation of amylase into its various isoenzymes may permit identification of the tissue of origin in the future.

The rate of urinary amylase excretion has been found to reflect the amount of amylase released from the pancreas into the blood. Quantification of the urinary amylase in addition to serum amylase determination will increase diagnostic accuracy for acute pancreatitis, since urinary amylase remains elevated for longer periods and since lesser rates of amylase excretion are more frequently associated with other diseases (Fig. 11).[32] In particular, calculation of the ratio of amylase clearance to creatinine clearance may prove to be one of the most reliable indicators of the presence of acute pancreatitis.

Recently, it has been recognized that in some individuals amylase will adhere to a large carrier globulin, resulting in reduction of urinary clearance. This condition has been termed *macroamylasemia* and is recognized by an elevated serum amylase without a correspondingly elevated urinary amylase. Although the exact significance of this process is at present unknown, macroamylasemia does not appear to be associated with any known clinical disease.[10]

Elevation in the serum and urinary lipase activities is occasionally associated with acute pancreatitis. However, interpretation of an elevated serum lipase is subject to similar limitations applied to amylase determinations. Hyperlipasemia has also been recorded in patients without pancreatic disease.

In some patients, thoracentesis or paracentesis may be indicated to aid in establishing an accurate diagnosis. Examination of the fluid obtained for both lipase and amylase activity may be helpful, since these enzyme levels are usually increased in patients with hydrothorax or ascites secondary to pancreatitis.

X-ray examinations of the chest and abdomen may be useful in establishing the diagnosis of pancreatitis. Roentgenograms of the abdomen may reveal pancreatic or biliary calcifications that suggest the pancreas as the site of origin for the patient's symptoms. The identification of a single dilated atonic loop of small bowel provides contributory evidence for the diagnosis. When the patient's condition permits, roentgenographic examination of the upper gastrointestinal tract with barium may be helpful. The "C loop" described by the course of the duodenum may be enlarged as a result of swelling of the head of the pancreas. On occasion, the pattern of the duodenal mucosa may be coarse owing to the swelling imposed by lymphatic and venous obstruction. On lateral films the stomach may be displaced anteriorly because of exten-

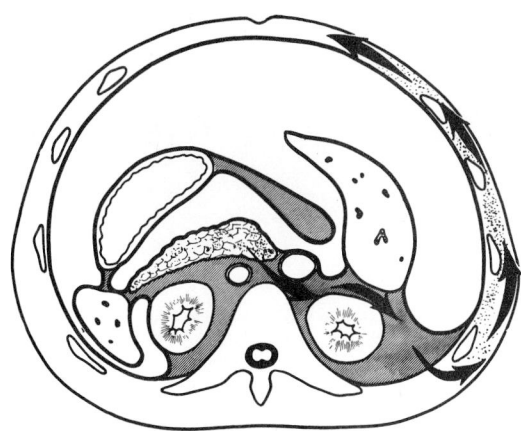

Figure 10. Hemorrhage through the retroperitoneal space into the subcutaneous fat leads to ecchymosis and discoloration in one or both flanks (Gray-Turner sign). A deposit of iron salts may lead to permanent discoloration. (From Ellison, E. H., and Carey, L. C. *In* Davis, L. (Ed.): Christopher's Textbook of Surgery, 9th ed. Philadelphia, W. B. Saunders Company, 1968.)

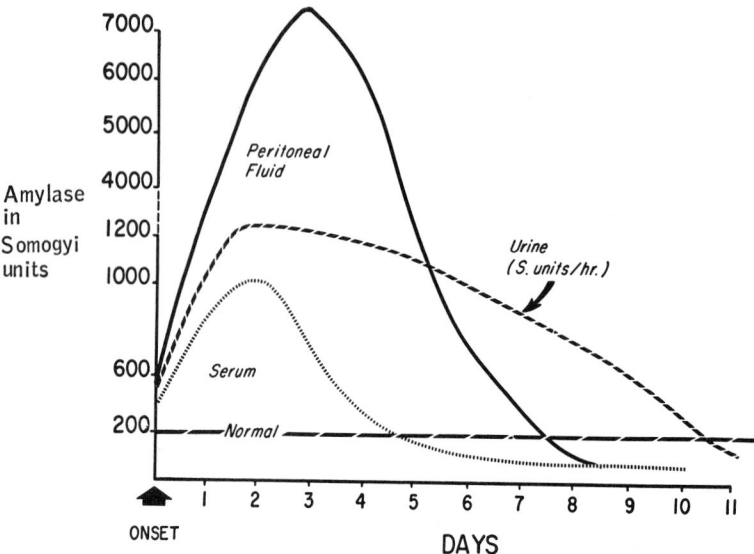

Figure 11. Amylase values in various fluids as a function of time. Note that the urinary amylase remains elevated when serum amylase has returned to normal. (From Ellison, E. H., and Carey, L. C.: *In* Davis, L. (Ed.): Christopher's Textbook of Surgery, 9th ed. Philadelphia, W. B. Saunders Company, 1968.)

sive peripancreatic edema (Fig. 12). Unfortunately, anterior gastric displacement may also signify the accumulation of fluid in the lesser sac or even frank abscess formation. With the conventional indirect diagnostic methods, the necessary therapeutic distinc-

tion between self-limiting peripancreatic edema, early pseudocyst formation, and pancreatic abscess cannot be made. Increasing experience with diagnostic ultrasound has shown that this modality can resolve this clinical dilemma.[13] Patients with a sonic configuration

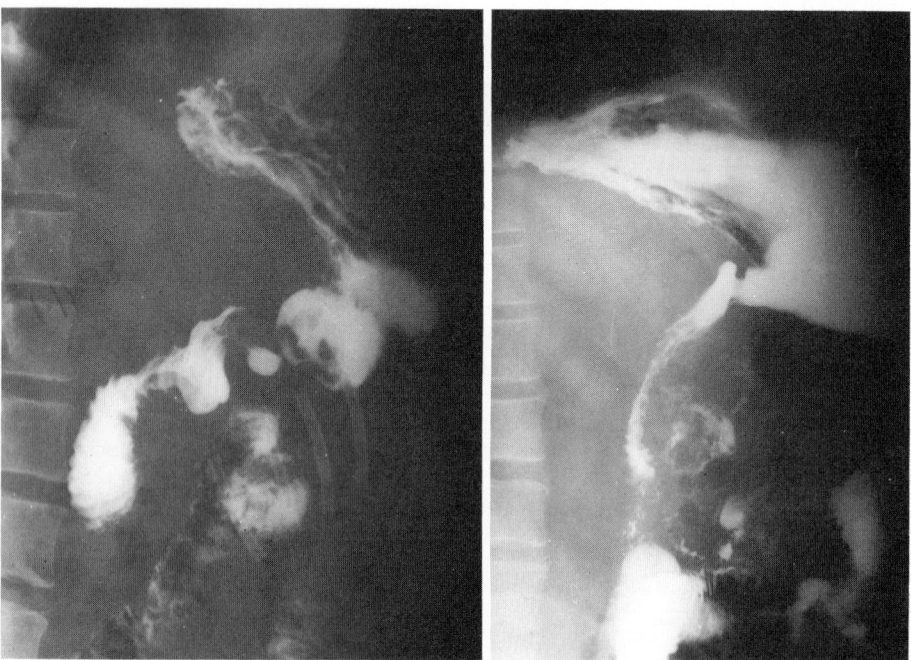

Figure 12. Lateral upper gastrointestinal series in two patients showing marked anterior displacement of the barium-filled stomach. Only extensive peripancreatic edema was found at exploration in both patients. (From Bradley, E. L., III, and Clements, J. L.: Am. J. Surg. *127*:163, 1974.)

suggesting solid (edematous) tissue are managed expectantly, while those with a cystic appearance receive further attention. Since acute lesser sac collections frequently resolve spontaneously,[33] periodic sonic monitoring is advisable. If resolution does occur, the pseudocyst is drained when maturation of the fibrous wall takes place in 4 to 6 weeks. On the other hand, if an acute pseudocyst becomes complicated by regional sepsis, urgent drainage is indicated.

Other laboratory studies have less value as aids in the confirmation of the diagnosis of acute pancreatitis, yet may be of singular importance in guiding therapy. The hematocrit may be followed serially as a guide to the repletion of plasma volume. An elevation in hematocrit is a common finding in patients first seen with severe pancreatitis. Hypocalcemia is a common accompaniment to severe necrotizing pancreatitis, and serum levels below 9 mg. per 100 ml. are common, although frank tetany is rare. The etiology of hypocalcemia in severe acute pancreatitis is unknown, although some evidence exists to implicate excess thyrocalcitonin as a possible mechanism. Hypocalcemia may persist for many days, even after serum amylase activity has returned to normal. Electrocardiographic abnormalities that may attend this electrolyte disturbance include variable prolongation of the Q-T segment, suppression of the S-T segment, and flattening of the T-waves. In an occasional patient a profound hypoalbuminemia appears, requiring exogenous albumin replacement in order to prevent anasarca.

THERAPY

While frequently a benign self-limiting disease, on occasion the pancreatitic process may be so severe as to strain all known supportive measures.[1] Much of the initial therapy is physiologically based.[1] Continuous nasogastric suction is used to decrease hydrogen ion stimulation of secretin and CCK-PZ. In addition, swallowed air is aspirated, preventing increase in the distention that may be present when the patient is first seen. Anticholinergic agents such as propantheline bromide may be administered in an attempt to suppress pancreatic secretion. These agents should be avoided if clinical shock is evident or if the patient has glaucoma.

Perhaps the most challenging aspect of managing acute pancreatitis is the regulation of intravenous fluid therapy.[2, 27] The amount of fluid required is dictated by the degree of severity of any particular episode. Careful monitoring of fluid balance by central venous pressure and urinary output assists accurate replacement. With severe pancreatitis, administration of both crystalloid- and colloid-containing solutions may be superior to administration of crystalloid alone. With early and well-monitored vigorous fluid replacement, shock resulting from pancreatitis should decrease in frequency.

Many patients with pancreatitis present with tachypnea, and about one third of the fatalities due to pancreatitis are associated with respiratory failure. When rapid and shallow respirations are observed, blood gas analysis is indicated, including determination of Po_2, Pco_2, and pH. The finding of abnormal gas exchange should be regarded as an ominous sign indicating the need for respiratory assistance. Ranson and his associates found that 38 per cent of a group of patients with acute pancreatitis exhibited severe arterial oxygen desaturation, as evidenced by a PaO_2 of 66 mm. Hg. The hypoxemia was improved by the administration of albumin and diuretics. The association between severe pancreatitis and pulmonary insufficiency appears to be more than casual, although the mechanism involved is not as yet known.[12, 68]

Relief of severe pain which usually accompanies acute pancreatitis may be difficult. The most effective drugs, morphine and meperidine, both cause spasm of the sphincter of Oddi, resulting in increased intrabiliary pressures. The requirement for large doses of these drugs in the therapy of such pain may be avoided if splanchnic nerve block is successful.

As indicated previously, hypokalemia or hypocalcemia or both may occur and precipitate disturbances in cardiac function. Repletion with intravenous potassium salts must be accomplished by electrocardiographic monitoring, and they must be administered cautiously when any degree of oliguria is present. The intravenous injection of calcium salts is reserved for the therapy of incipient tetany as signaled by the appearance of a positive Chvostek or Trousseau sign, and for the development of previously mentioned electrocardiographic conduction changes.

Theoretically, inhibition of proteolytic activity might affect the course of pancreatitis. The release of trypsin from the affected gland is capable of activating pancreatic kallikrein, another proteolytic ferment, which splits the vasoactive decapeptide kallidin, from a globulin. This peptide is a potent vasodilatory and hypotensive agent. An antitryptic antikallikrein polypeptide (Trasylol) has been extracted from bovine parotid glands. This agent has been shown to inhibit trypsin, chymotrypsin, kallikrein, and plasmin. Despite the demonstration of potent *in vitro* antiproteolytic activity, the efficacy of Trasylol in modifying experimental pancreatitis is still unclear. Although earlier studies had suggested that Trasylol was ineffective in moderating the course of acute pancreatitis, a recent randomized, prospective, double-blind trial came to a different conclusion. Trapnell and his co-workers evaluated mortality in two similar groups of patients with acute pancreatitis associated with biliary calculi and found a significant reduction in mortality in the group treated with Trasylol. Dosages of Trasylol used in this study exceeded previously employed dosages by an order of magnitude.[78] Routine employment of proteolytic inhibitors awaits further confirmation of these data.

Antibiotics are usually given to patients with severe acute pancreatitis. The rationale for this therapy has been based on experimental data showing an improvement with antibiotic therapy in the survival of animals suffering pancreatitis provoked by duodenal obstruction. However, Howes and his co-workers were unable to demonstrate prospectively any significant advantage of routine antibiotic administration in groups of patients with uncomplicated pancreatitis randomized into control and antibiotic groups.[44] Similar results have been reported by others.[71] It is fair to conclude that unequivocal clinical efficacy of antibiotic therapy has not been established, although the institution of such therapy is clearly indicated if sepsis complicates the course of pancreatitis. A lesser sac abscess occasionally develops during the course of this illness and antimicrobial therapy in addition to surgical drainage is mandatory.

Recently, there has been a resurgence of interest regarding indications for surgery in patients with acute pancreatitis.[85] One proposed indication has been a persistently declining course. Total pancreatectomy in patients deteriorating with severe acute pancreatitis has been advocated under these circumstances.[58, 86] but has had little acceptance. Lawson et al. have recommended cholecystostomy, gastrostomy, feeding jejunostomy, and sump drainage in patients with severe acute pancreatitis unresponsive to maximal nonoperative therapy.[53] While representing persuasive viewpoints regarding possible future therapeutic directions, neither these nor any other reported surgical experiences represent controlled evaluations of the efficacy of surgery in acute pancreatitis.

Since the vast majority of patients with acute pancreatitis will improve on supportive therapy alone, the primary difficulty in establishing such controlled trials has been the inability to identify those patients with the more severe form of acute pancreatitis who might reasonably be expected to do poorly on conservative therapy. Ranson and his co-workers evaluated 43 separate parameters in a group of 100 consecutive patients with alcoholic pancreatitis in an effort to provide early identification of those patients with potentially severe disease.[67] Eleven factors were found to be of prognostic significance (Table 2). In 21 patients with three or more of these signs, 13 died and 7 were seriously ill. In contrast, in 79 patients with fewer than three signs, only two patients died and none of the remaining patients was seriously ill. These data would appear to offer a base from which to select patients for randomization into medical and surgical groups, in order to evaluate effectively the potential role of surgery in those patients with severe pancreatitis who appear to be deteriorating.

Since the clinical diagnosis of acute pancreatitis is made by indirect means, many intra-abdominal disorders may simulate pancreatitis—cholecystitis, mesenteric infarction, intestinal obstruction (both simple and strangulated), and duodenal ulcer perforation. Should the diagnosis of pancreatitis be in question and the patient deteriorating, exploration is indicated. Repeated studies have confirmed the observation that simple exploration does not affect mortality rate if the diagnosis of pancreatitis is confirmed.[77] On the contrary, if one of the above life-threatening conditions is found, exploration may be life saving.

A third indication for surgery in patients with acute pancreatitis is a secondary pancreatic abscess which should be drained. Occasionally the abscess will present as a secondarily infected acute pseudocyst. More commonly the abscess will consist primarily of necrotic pancreas. Pancreatic abscess has been said to occur in 4 to 10 per cent of patients with acute pancreatitis and carries a mortality rate ranging from 30 to 50 per cent with drainage and approaching 100 per cent without drainage.[11] In a patient with acute pancreatitis and a prolonged septic course, the appearance of small retrogastric gas bubbles is a finding pathognomonic of pancreatic abscess (Fig. 13). Although the diagnosis may occasionally be difficult, a febrile course not resolving within one week after an episode of acute pancreatitis should alert the clinician to the possibility of abscess formation. Diagnostic ultrasound has been of considerable assistance to us in several patients with pancreatic abscess. If exploration confirms the presence of an abscess, *widespread* drainage, preferably of the sump type, is required.

Since acute pancreatitis is associated with biliary calculi in 10 to 40 per cent of cases, exploration may be indicated in those patients with acute pancreatitis who are known to have biliary tract disease. The timing of surgery in these patients is a matter for considerable surgical judgment. Cholecystectomy and formal common bile duct exploration have been shown to increase both morbidity and mortality in patients with acute pancreatitis, while simple drainage of the gallbladder or common duct has been lifesaving in patients with pancreatitis and biliary calculi with superimposed cholangitis. Under these circumstances, since concomitant biliary surgery is unwarranted, a second procedure for correction of biliary tract disease will be necessary. For this reason, if acute pancreatitis is resolving without complication in a patient with known biliary disease, it is preferable to wait until the pancreatic process is completely resolved and then perform definitive elective biliary surgery.

TABLE 2. Prognostic Factors in Acute Pancreatitis*

On admission:

A. Age greater than 55 years
B. Blood glucose greater than 200 mg. per 100 ml.
C. White blood cell count greater than 16,000 per cu. mm.
D. Lactic dehydrogenasn greater than 700 IU
E. Serum glutamic oxalacetic transaminase greater than 250 Sigma-Frankel units

During the initial 48 hours:

F. Hematocrit decrease greater than 10 percentage points
G. Serum calcium less than 8 mg. per 100 ml.
H. Base deficit greater than 4 mEq. per L.
I. Blood urea nitrogen increase greater than 5 mg. per 100 ml.
J. Estimated fluid sequestration greater than 6 liters
K. Arterial oxygen tension less than 60 mm. Hg.

A combination of three or more factors has been associated with mortality in more than 60 per cent of cases.

*Adapted from Ranson, J. H. C., Rifkind, K. M., Roses, D. F., Fink, S. D., Eng, F., and Spencer, F. C.: Prognostic signs and the role of operative management in acute pancreatitis. Surg. Gynecol. Obstet., *139*:69, 1974.

CHRONIC PANCREATITIS

The term chronic pancreatitis implies active and continuing *irreversible* destruction of the gland, result-

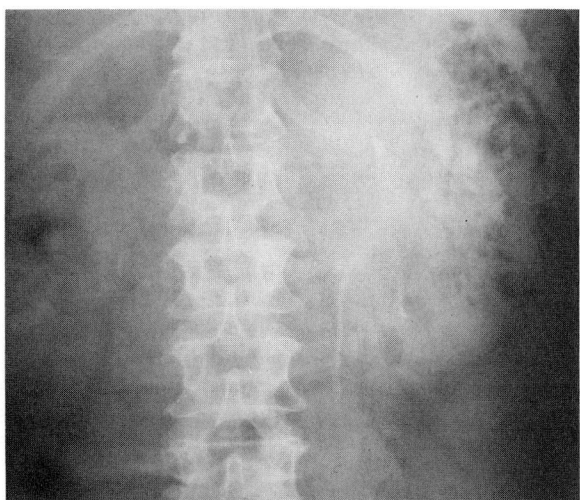

Figure 13. Pancreatic abscess. Note multiple small gas bubbles in left upper quadrant. Multiple views placed these bubbles in a retrogastric position. We refer to these bubbles as the "soap bubble sign." Left kidney function returned following drainage of the abscess.

ing in *progressive* deterioration of anatomic features and physiologic function. The distinction between the terms chronic pancreatitis and chronic relapsing pancreatitis is purely clinical. In chronic relapsing pancreatitis, in spite of progressive destruction of the gland, the patient will have asymptomatic periods of varying duration, while in chronic pancreatitis, abdominal pain is continuous and unrelenting.

The etiology of chronic pancreatitis presumably is as varied as that of acute pancreatitis. Although the term chronic pancreatitis implies a pathophysiologic progression from acute pancreatitis, such a natural progression from acute to chronic has never been established. However, there are well-established relationships with such conditions as biliary tract disease, chronic alcoholism, hyperparathyroidism, and genetic disorders characterized by excessive urinary excretion of certain amino acids, especially cystine and lysine. Nevertheless, the actual pathogenesis of chronic pancreatitis remains unknown. Although there is a direct effect of alcohol on the pancreatic parenchyma, a primary "cirrhosis" type of reaction has not been confirmed. Many believe that obstruction at the ampulla of Vater is a factor common to biliary tract disease and alcoholism. Spasm and edema of the sphincter of Oddi with biliary tract disease is generally accepted, while alcohol presumably causes edema and inflammation of the papilla of Vater by its local effect. Neither of these concepts has been proved, nor, in fact, has the concept of ampullary obstruction been totally accepted. However, intrapancreatic duct obstruction at one or more places can be demonstrated in many instances of advanced chronic pancreatitis. By injection cast studies, Sarles and his co-workers have demonstrated in three dimensions the morphologic ductal changes of concomitant stricture and ectasia in chronic pancreatitis (the so-called "chain of lakes").[56] Precipitated plugs of protein are often found in the ductal system in association with regions of stricture and conceivably could serve as nidi for the formation of ductal calculi.

Clinical Manifestations

Diagnosis can be a difficult task, and a considerable number of patients with "idiopathic" chronic pancreatitis are treated for psychiatric problems before the true nature of their disease is established. Nevertheless, the syndrome is now well known and a high index of suspicion should lead to the correct diagnosis in most instances.

From a practical standpoint, the basic tool of diagnosis is documentation of recurrent attacks of acute pancreatitis with less severe but continuing symptoms between periods of exacerbation. Pathologic confirmation is not always possible, but if the classic triad of *weight loss, diabetes,* and *steatorrhea* has developed, severe pancreatic disease can be assumed to be present.[10]

Laboratory Aids

In addition to the conventional laboratory tests for acute pancreatitis, the diagnosis of chronic pancreatitis relies heavily upon demonstrating changes in the exocrine or endocrine functions of the pancreas. One simple approach is to examine the stool chemically or microscopically for an increase in fat, since steatorrhea is demonstrated in many patients with grossly normal stools. With improved methods for duodenal aspiration, the measurement of pancreatic enzymes following a meal or bicarbonate secretion after secretin stimulation, has added greatly to accuracy in detecting relatively early changes in exocrine function. In similar fashion, a glucose tolerance test will frequently be abnormal in spite of a normal fasting blood sugar. Obstructive jaundice can occur with chronic pancreatitis, and, when it is present, the distinction from tumor can be difficult.

Radiographic Aids to Diagnosis

Pancreatic calcification in combination with the clinical history just presented is presumptive evidence of chronic pancreatitis. Such calcifications may be intraductal or diffusely scattered within the pancreatic parenchyma. Cholecystography is also an important adjunct to diagnosis, and primary biliary tract disease is frequently the key to the diagnosis of associated chronic pancreatitis. An upper gastrointestinal series may occasionally be helpful by demonstrating enlargement of the C loop, and hypotonic duodenography has increased the accuracy of diagnosis by elucidating more subtle changes in pancreaticoduodenal anatomy. But perhaps the most definitive diagnostic tool available at present to define this group of patients is pancreatography. Although originally confined to the operating room by virtue of the inaccessibility of the pancreatic ductal system, recently visualization of the pancreatic ducts has been routinely achieved via per oral fiberoptic endoscopy with cannulation of the ampulla of Vater (Fig. 14). Endoscopic retrograde cholangiopancreatography (ERCP) has proved to be both remarkably safe in experienced hands and informative of the status of the macroscopic pancreatic exocrine system.[22]

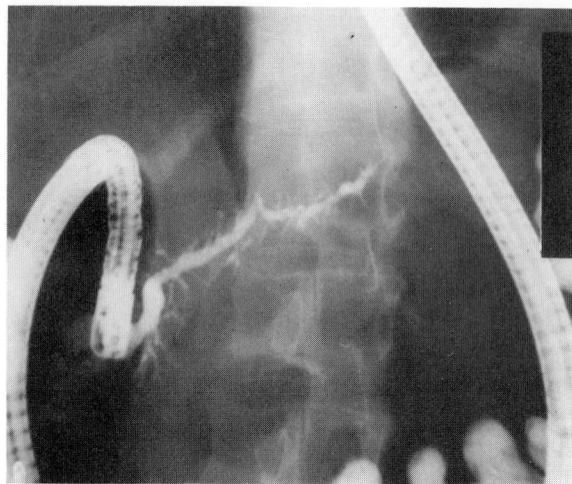

Figure 14. Endoscopic retrograde pancreatogram, showing dilated duct of Wirsung with multiple areas of constriction. Patients with this configuration respond most favorably to pancreatic surgery.

INDICATIONS FOR OPERATIVE INTERVENTION

The one virtually unassailable indication for operative intervention is the diagnosis of primary biliary tract disease as evidenced by gallstones, or by nonvisualization of the gallbladder on repeated examinations. However, it should be emphasized that a "normal" gallbladder may not be visualized for several days after an attack of acute pancreatitis. Apart from this group of patients, the indications for operation are often controversial, although primarily centered on the symptom complex of persistent pain. Because of our inability to ascertain at which point the disease becomes *unresponsive to medical therapy,* fears of mortality and morbidity from an operation, and the uncertainty of obtaining relief of symptoms by the surgical procedure, surgery has been infrequently offered to patients with chronic pancreatitis. Theoretically, it would seem advisable to institute surgical therapy before pancreatic function is irretrievably impaired, but the patient usually seen by the surgical service has had a prolonged history of pancreatitis, frequently complicated, and is found to have far-advanced chronic pancreatitis.

The multiplicity of procedures recommended for the surgical treatment of chronic pancreatitis indicates the failure of any one operation to satisfy the needs of all patients, and emphasizes that different operative procedures may be required at varying stages in the disease. One of the problems in assessment of surgical therapeutics has been the tendency for surgeons to apply one or two operations to virtually all patients with the disease. Each patient must be individually studied and the nature and extent of the disease carefully documented in order to facilitate the rational choice of any particular surgical procedure. The fundamental principles of surgical therapy are as follows:

Correction of Primary Biliary Disease. As the available evidence overwhelmingly supports the concept that primary biliary tract disease can initiate pancreatitis, it follows that correction of the biliary tract disease should be a major priority for surgical therapy.

Relief of Ductal Obstruction. Improvement in pancreatic function is one of the aims of pancreatic ductal decompression. In patients seen fairly soon after onset of the disease, the relief of obstruction is thought to diminish the likelihood of recurrent episodes of acute pancreatitis and thus stop, or at least delay, further pancreatic fibrosis. However, in most cases the pancreatic changes are quite diffuse and significant improvement is hard to document. From an empiric viewpoint the major achievement of successful relief of ductal obstruction has been the control of pain.

Relief of Pain. It is widely believed that the pain of chronic pancreatitis is caused by ductal distention secondary to incomplete ductal obstruction. This concept has been tested by procedures designed to decompress the pancreatic ducts, and successful control of pain has been confirmed by several reliable investigators. Other approaches to control of pain include extirpation of all or a major portion of the pancreas and interruption of the splanchnic nerves, the mediators of visceral pain.

SURGICAL PROCEDURES

Operations on the Biliary Tract. Simple removal of a chronically diseased gallbladder, with or without stones, has successfully controlled the pancreatitis in up to 80 per cent of patients with combined biliary and pancreatic disease. As these are relatively safe procedures without significant metabolic sequelae, there is universal agreement as to their usefulness in the therapy of pancreatitis. However, simple nonvisualization of the gallbladder, as frequently occurs during an acute exacerbation of pancreatitis, should not be misconstrued as primary biliary tract disease. Cholecystectomy frequently has been augmented by sphincteroplasty when multiple common duct stones are present or when symptoms recur after other operative procedures upon the biliary tract.

Sphincteroplasty. It has been shown that simple sphincterotomy will generally close within a few weeks' time with restoration of preoperative common bile duct pressure. However, a properly performed sphincteroplasty remains widely patent and will not result in recurrent obstruction of the common bile duct at the ampulla (Fig. 15). The use of sphincteroplasty in the management of chronic pancreatitis is based upon the theory that ampullary obstruction is a basic mechanism causing pancreatitis in some patients, and that a "common channel" is found in the great majority of patients with chronic pancreatitis.[23] If the intraduodenal portion of the bile duct is widely opened, this should also decompress the pancreatic duct. Several groups of investigators have attested to the success of sphincteroplasty in controlling the symptoms of chronic pancreatitis in some patients.[47, 57] However, correct utilization of this procedure demands that intrapancreatic ductal obstruction must be ruled out by pancreatography. If intrapancreatic obstruction is found, other procedures must be substituted for, or combined with, sphincteroplasty if a successful result is to be anticipated. In the absence of multiple sites of intrapancreatic ductal obstruction, and when general-

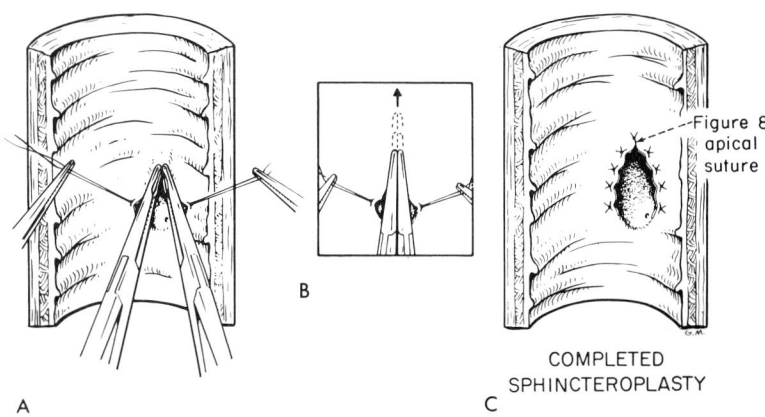

Figure 15. Transduodenal sphincteroplasty. *A,* A pair of mosquito clamps is placed through the ampulla at 11 o'clock and 1 o'clock in order to avoid injury to the pancreatic duct (seen entering at 5 o'clock). *B,* Successive clamping, division, and suture are continued upward for at least 2 cm. *C,* At the upper part of the completed sphincteroplasty, the incision has extended through the duodenal wall and careful suture approximation, particularly at the apex, is mandatory. (From Jones, S. A.: Surg. Clin. North Am., *53*:1123, 1973.)

ized ductal dilatation is present, 50 per cent of patients undergoing sphincteroplasty should have a satisfactory result. The procedure is perhaps best used to obliterate the sphincter in patients with repeated episodes of pancreatitis in whom exploration reveals multiple common duct stones.

Direct Pancreatic Ductal Drainage. The general indication for the use of direct ductal decompression procedures is evidence of pancreatic ductal ectasia with multiple intrapancreatic duct strictures (obviating sphincteroplasty). An important secondary feature is the desire to preserve both exocrine and endocrine functions sufficient to avoid malnutrition and insulin dependency. The initial concept of drainage of the pancreas by anastomosis of the major pancreatic duct to a loop of jejunum was that of DuVal.[25] Subsequent modifications have been developed to increase the efficacy of this operation, the most basic alteration being the one recommended by Puestow and Gillesby[66] and later modified by Partington and Rochelle.[60] In this procedure a long longitudinal incision is made throughout the length of the duct until all strictures have been opened (Fig. 16). A Roux-en-Y loop of jejunum is then anastomosed over this widely opened ductal system, thus affording free drainage to areas obstructed between ductal strictures. Such procedures have in general been successful in controlling pain in up to 80 per cent of patients with dilated ductal systems.[75] Of great importance is preservation of the islet cell mass, as few of these patients are converted to insulin-dependent diabetics. This remains the greatest advantage of such procedures over the use of major pancreatic resections.

Extirpative Procedures. For disease restricted to either the head or tail of the organ, subtotal pancreatic resections (Whipple procedure or caudal pancreatectomy) have proved to be useful.[36, 48] However, disease isolated to either the head or the tail is unusual; more commonly the disease process involves the entire gland. Total and near-total pancreatectomies have been accomplished by a number of investigators, and excellent relief of pain has been achieved, whereas less extensive proximal or distal resections are followed by a significant failure rate. An important addition to the therapy of severe chronic pancreatitis has been the work of Child and his associates[20] in the de-

velopment of the 95 per cent distal pancreatectomy (Fig. 17). This procedure, which leaves the stomach and duodenum in their normal anatomic position, has been quite successful in the relief of pain and is superior to the Whipple procedure and total pancreatectomy in that exocrine replacement and nutritional restoration are more readily accomplished.[83] In addition, the mortality has been surprisingly low, especially in the University of Michigan series.[31] However, in addition to the increased mortality and morbidity of resective procedures, in general, the great deterrent to routine use of these procedures is the conversion of the patient from a non-insulin-dependent status to that of

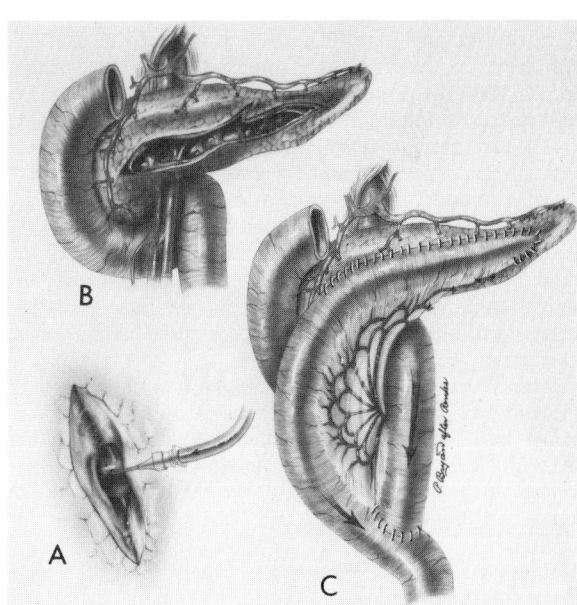

Figure 16. Longitudinal pancreaticojejunostomy via Roux-en-Y, a modification of the Puestow procedure. *A,* Ellipse of pancreas removed from body of gland and needle inserted into duct in order to obtain pancreatogram. *B,* The dilated pancreatic duct is opened extensively in a longitudinal direction. *C,* Opened pancreatic duct is covered by a retrocolic Roux loop of jejunum. (Redrawn from Partington, P. F., and Rochelle, R. E.: Ann. Surg., *152*:1037, 1960.)

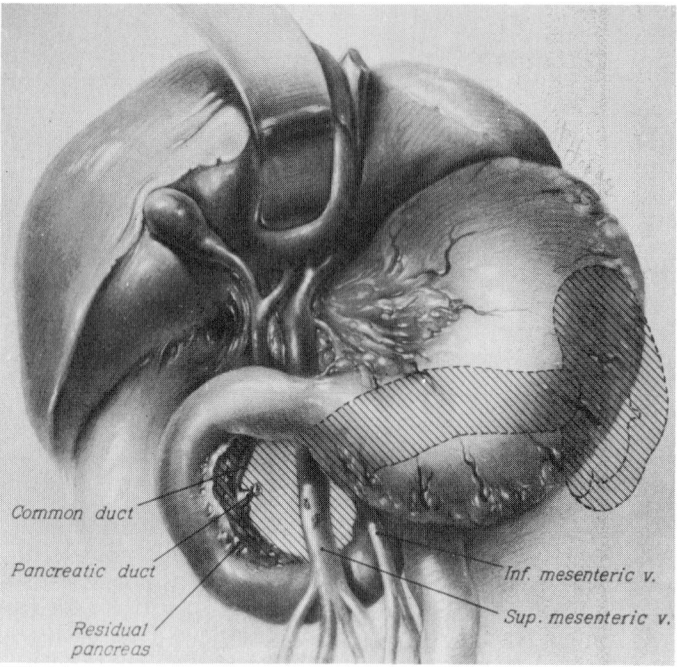

Common duct

Pancreatic duct

Residual
pancreas

Inf. mesenteric v.

Sup. mesenteric v.

Figure 17. General anatomic relationships of the pancreas demonstrated in a diagrammatic illustration of a 95 per cent pancreatectomy. This operation is of great value in the treatment of chronic pancreatitis. Note the small crescent of residual pancreas preserved for the protection of the pancreaticoduodenal arteries and the common bile duct. The superior mesenteric artery is not shown. (From Child, C. G., III, et al.: Surg. Gynecol. Obstet., *129*:49, 1969.)

an insulin-dependent diabetic. The possible long-range complications are significant for any patient, but in the alcoholic there is the added danger of diabetic acidosis or overdosage of insulin during periods of inebriation. The postpancreatectomy diabetic is frequently quite "brittle," requiring meticulous management of diet and insulin dosage. Deaths from diabetic complications are well documented in the literature, and, in the authors' series, at least two patients have died within a few months after operation from failure to follow their prescribed regimen. However, these procedures, especially the 95 per cent pancreatectomy, have provided relief of pain and rehabilitation of patients who have not been helped by one or more of the drainage procedures. In nonalcoholic patients with advanced pancreatitis and alcoholic patients already insulin-dependent preoperatively, serious consideration should be given to such a procedure as the initial operation.

Splanchnicectomy. This procedure has been used by a number of investigators in the treatment of pancreatitis,[92] but the greatest experience has been in European clinics.[54] There is good documentation of initial control of pain in approximately 60 per cent of patients, although the duration of pain control need not necessarily be permanent. In the authors' experience, this operation has been particularly helpful when there has been failure of other operations to control the severe pain of pancreatitis and the patient is not considered a good social or medical candidate for pancreatectomy.

General Operative Approach. The basic principle underlying appropriate surgical treatment of patients with chronic pancreatitis is individualization —selection of the operative procedure best suited

to that particular case. In the authors' opinion, every attempt should be made to conserve pancreatic tissue with the least derangement in physiology. Accordingly, any associated biliary disease is corrected as an initial procedure. In the absence of biliary disease, the choice of a particular procedure is determined by the findings on pancreatography. If generalized enlargement of Wirsung's duct is noted, sphincteroplasty is done. Should the chain-of-lakes configuration be present, an extensive Puestow procedure is indicated. Without pancreatic ductal dilation, we have tended to perform splanchnicectomy rather than extensive pancreatic resections, knowing full well that half of these patients may require resection in the future.

TRAUMA

The majority of pancreatic injuries in large urban centers come from penetrating wounds of the abdomen. The surgical management of isolated pancreatic injuries has been greatly improved in the last decade and should rarely cause death.[49] As the pancreas is closely approximated by several other organs, its involvement in multiple organ injuries is rather common. In addition, the aorta, inferior vena cava, superior mesenteric artery and vein, and the splenic vessels pass along the posterior surface of the pancreas, and associated vascular injuries are frequently seen. Although multiple concomitant organ injury will increase the mortality, by far the major cause of death in wounds involving the pancreas is associated blood vessel injury with massive hemorrhage.

The fixed retroperitoneal position of the pancreas,

particularly where it crosses the vertebral column, makes the pancreas extremely vulnerable to injury in nonpenetrating upper abdominal trauma. A not uncommon finding is laceration of the neck of the gland, which lies anterior to the vertebral column. Occasionally there is complete transection of the gland with exposure of the superior mesenteric vessels. Failure to visualize the injured pancreas during abdominal exploration for trauma has led to fatal complications. This mistake is usually made when there is an obvious injury to another organ, such as deep liver laceration, which seemingly accounts for the patient's clinical findings.

DIAGNOSIS

Of primary concern in the early management of abdominal trauma is whether or not operation is necessary.

The impetus for abdominal exploration under this circumstance comes primarily from progressively developing signs of peritonitis or serious hemorrhage. In some patients, severe injury is first evidenced by signs of abdominal distention, tenderness, or rigidity. In other instances, changes in vital signs, a decrease in hematocrit, and a falling urinary output may be seen with normal abdominal findings. In doubtful circumstances, peritoneal lavage may facilitate early exploration by demonstrating intra-abdominal bleeding or fluid accumulation with a high amylase content.

An isolated injury to the pancreas may produce little early evidence of severe intra-abdominal injury. By far the most frequent cause for immediate operation is evidence of intra-abdominal bleeding. When this is not present the abdominal findings may be minimal for two to three days, after which time tenderness and distention usually occur. An elevated serum amylase when present is most helpful in minimizing the delay in diagnosis, although there is not total agreement that hyperamylasemia, of itself, is an indication for abdominal exploration. With nonpenetrating trauma a patient occasionally may be asymptomatic for weeks or months, until a pseudocyst develops or distal pancreatitis occurs secondary to a ductal stricture.

SURGICAL TREATMENT

There are a variety of surgical techniques that are useful in the management of different types of pancreatic injury. The most useful procedures include the following:

External Drainage of the Injured Tissue

This is a fundamental method and is used in the overwhelming majority of patients with pancreatic injury. When there is contusion or laceration, with no evidence of major duct disruption, external drainage is usually the treatment of choice. Although operative pancreatography has been advocated to demonstrate the presence or absence of ductal injury, its value is unproved, and it is possible that the morbidity of pancreatography under these circumstances may out-weigh the theoretic advantages. Drainage should be of the sump type, as this technique has been shown to be a superior method of drainage. Using drainage for these parenchymal injuries will necessarily result in a significant incidence of pancreatic fistulas. However, this added morbidity is a small price to pay for the intrinsic safety of this procedure, particularly since the management of an isolated pancreatic fistula without an associated enteric fistula is rarely difficult[93] (see also Chapter 20).

Excision

Seldom is there any indication for total pancreatectomy in trauma, but both distal and proximal subtotal pancreatectomy are being utilized with increasing frequency. These are instances in which the experience and judgment of the surgeon are of great importance. An edematous, lacerated, hemorrhagic tail of the pancreas is frequently managed most safely by excision rather than by the more conservative method of external drainage. Although resection of the head of the pancreas is a procedure of considerably greater magnitude than simple distal pancreatectomy, when there is extensive disruption of both the duodenum and the major pancreatic ducts in the head of the pancreas, a Whipple procedure may be the safest method of management. An increasing number of these operations have been done in recent years and with an apparently lowered mortality in these extremely serious injuries.[28] The postoperative morbidity is not as great as that seen following operation for malignant disease, and near-normal nutritional and metabolic status is usually attained.

Re-establishment of Pancreatic Duct Continuity

Following traumatic transection of the gland, reconstruction of the ductal system is frequently considered. Due to technical difficulties, primary anastomosis of the severed ends of the normal-sized duct should not be attempted because of the risk of leak with subsequent abscess formation or stricture.[49] As an alternative, simple closure of both ends of the transected pancreas has been advocated but in our experience has led to death from traumatic pancreatitis of the distal (obstructed) remnant and should be rarely used. Although bidirectional drainage via an interposed Roux-en-Y loop has been proposed in this situation in an effort for maximal preservation of pancreatic tissue, this procedure requires two pancreatic jejunal anastomoses and is therefore subject to anastomotic complications. Since resections of pancreatic tissue up to 80 per cent have been followed by normal endocrine and exocrine function,[56] in the authors' opinion, the safest procedure is closure of the proximal end and resection of that portion of the gland to the left of the traumatic transection.

PANCREATIC CYSTS

A simple classification of cystic lesions of the pancreas is outlined in Table 3. Other than cystadenoma and cystadenocarcinoma, true pancreatic cysts are ei-

TABLE 3. Pancreatic Cysts

A. True Cysts
   1. Congenital
   2. Parasitic
   3. Dermoid
B. Cystic Tumors
   1. Cystadenoma
   2. Cystadenocarcinoma
   3. Cystic lymphoma
C. Pseudocysts

ther quite rare in this country or usually diagnosed as an incidental finding at operation or autopsy. The so-called "retention cysts," which accounted for a significant proportion of the large series reported by Warren et al.,[81] are really obstructed pancreatic ducts and are managed coincidentally with the cause of the obstruction.

Cystadenomas are benign lesions that are considered premalignant and may be difficult to differentiate from cystadenocarcinoma. Characteristically, both of these tumors develop slowly and, unless obstruction of the common bile duct occurs, there are few early symptoms other than vague upper abdominal distress. A palpable mass is frequently discernible and barium studies, angiography, and pancreatic ultrasound will usually give definitive evidence of a cystic pancreatic lesion. In the absence of pre-existing pancreatitis or pancreatic trauma, suggesting pseudocyts, a neoplastic cyst should be considered when a large pancreatic mass can be clearly delineated preoperatively.

Whenever feasible, excision of neoplastic cysts should be accomplished. Five-year survival following resection of a cystadenocarcinoma is not rare, and the premalignant nature of a cystadenoma makes excision desirable. If extirpation is not possible, internal drain-age of the cyst is indicated; external drainage may be followed by persistent fistula or growth of cancer to the abdominal wall.

PANCREATIC PSEUDOCYSTS

Although a few patients may be essentially asymptomatic, in most instances there is upper abdominal pain or discomfort, anorexia, and weight loss. Suspicion of pseudocyst formation should arise in any patient with a history of pancreatitis or pancreatic trauma who remains persistently ill. The serum amylase may or may not be elevated and is generally of little value in establishing a definitive diagnosis of pseudocyst.

The finding of a palpable upper abdominal mass or radiologic evidence of anterior displacement of the stomach offers circumstantial support to the diagnosis. However, abdominal masses are clinically evident in the majority of patients after an episode of severe pancreatitis.[19, 29] In this circumstance, the mass consists of the edematous pancreas and surrounding peripancreatitic swelling of the retroperitoneal tissues. Barring further complications, such retroperitoneal masses can be expected to resolve with time. Diagnostic ultrasound has been of great assistance in distinguishing between acute pseudocyst formation and massive peripancreatic edema (Fig. 18). Serial ultrasonography has proved valuable in identifying those patients with acute pseudocyst formation failing to resolve and progressing to a mature pseudocyst.[13] Although spontaneous resolution of acute pseudocyts occurs in approximately one fifth of patients,[33] similar resolution of a chronic pseudocyst probably occurs only rarely. More commonly an untreated chronic pseudocyst will rupture. Should such rupture take place into the general peritoneal cavity, a prohibitive mortality

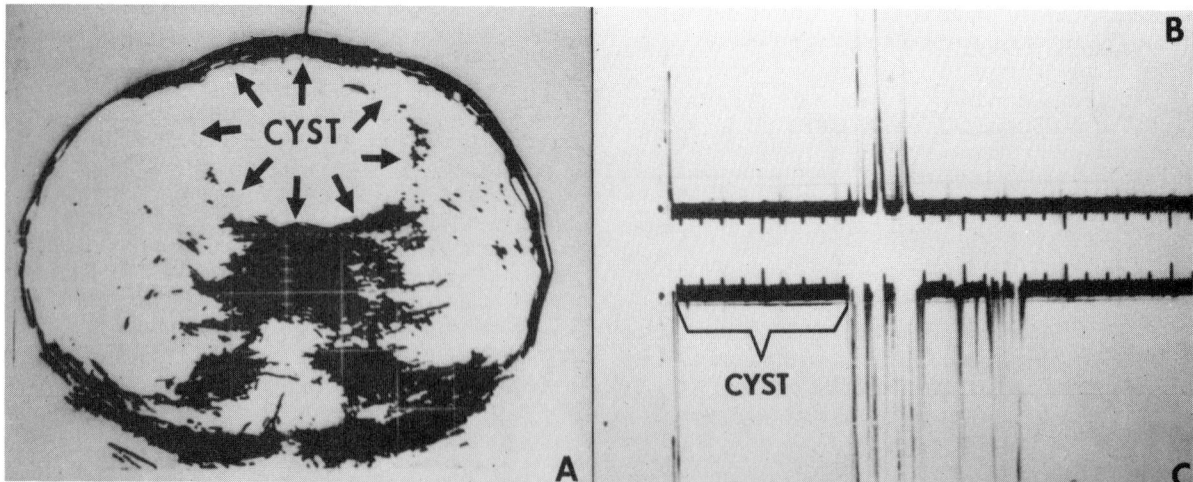

Figure 18.   Pancreatic echography. *A,* Transverse ultrasonic abdominal scan (B-mode) showing transonic clear area (arrows) anterior to the spine. *B,* Longitudinal scan (A-mode) through transonic area at low gain. *C,* High-gain longitudinal scan at same location as *B* confirming the presence of a cystic configuration 10 cm. in diameter. B-mode scans should always be confirmed by high-gain A-mode studies.

ensues.[38] On exceptionally rare occasions, a chronic pseudocyst may spontaneously rupture in the gastrointestinal tract, effectively forming an autoenteric fistula.[14] In general, however, procrastination of definitive surgery in patients with chronic pseudocysts invites spontaneous free perforation with its attendant and inexcusable mortality.

While the advent of ultrasonography has greatly simplified the diagnosis and management of pancreatic pseudocysts, other techniques currently in the investigative stage offer considerable promise with regard to improving resolution of abdominal scans. Foremost among these methods is computerized axial tomography (CAT-scan), a new method of soft tissue radiography.

TREATMENT

A great deal of controversy has surrounded the management of pancreatic pseudocysts. Proposals have ranged from immediate exploration[8] to delaying drainage in order to promote maturation of the fibrous wall.[19] Some confusion exists in this regard because of differences in terminology. An acute lesser sac fluid accumulation, a pancreatic abscess, or a "chronic" pseudocyst could all be included under a definition of pseudocyst of the pancreas. As we have noted, the acute collections frequently resolve spontaneously and an expectant regimen is generally justified. On the other hand, pancreatic abscess demands surgical intervention and external drainage is clearly the treatment of choice.[64] Further, the point at which an "acute" fluid accumulation becomes a "chronic" pseudocyst is a moot question. This is important because it implies both failure of spontaneous resolution and "maturity" of the cyst wall. The latter characteristic has been found to occur in an experimental model at about four weeks,[84] while in the human six weeks might be more appropriate. In both the experimental animal and retrospective patient studies, the mature or solidly formed cyst wall lessened the complications of internal drainage procedures. There is general agreement that the chronic pseudocyst deserves surgical management to control symptoms and, presumably, lessen the incidence of the serious complications of intracystic hemorrhage, secondary infection, or rupture of the cyst.

In the surgical management of chronic pseudocysts there are three primary methods: excision, external drainage, and internal drainage (Fig. 19).

Excision

Although it has several theoretical advantages, excision should be reserved for small cysts of the body or tail of the pancreas with minimal attachments to adjacent organs. Failure to observe this admonition has resulted in an unacceptably high mortality.

External Drainage

Formerly, most pseudocysts were treated by this method. Selection of this procedure was predicated upon the belief that external drainage carried a lower mortality than internal drainage procedures. While it was readily demonstrated that the morbidity of persistent fistula and recurrence of the cyst were greater with external drainage, it was not realized that the mortality (generally due to bleeding or sepsis) was as high as that following internal drainage procedures.[84] However, external drainage is still the preferred technique for infected cysts, pancreatic abscesses, and cysts requiring drainage before the four- to six-week period required for maturation of the cyst wall.

Internal Drainage

The choice of operation and surgical technique employed must be founded upon the following fundamental principles: (1) a suture anastomosis to the fibrous cyst wall cannot be relied upon to prevent leakage; and (2) dependent drainage is highly desirable. Of the several methods of internal drainage, by far the most useful are transgastric cystgastrostomy and cystojejunostomy to a Roux-en-Y loop of jejunum.

The *transgastric cystgastrostomy* has the advantages of speed and ease of performance. If the cyst wall is *densely adherent* to the posterior wall of the stomach, suture anastomosis is unnecessary and, therefore, leakage into the peritoneal cavity can be obviated. The cystgastrostomy is performed by opening the anterior wall of the stomach and then incising through the posterior gastric wall into the cavity of the cyst. Although it had been thought reflux of gastric contents into the cyst cavity might jeopardize the safety of this procedure, subsequent studies have shown that continued gastrocystic reflux does not lead to an increased incidence of complications.[74] Careful hemostasis should be obtained, as gastrointestinal bleeding is a major complication of cystgastrostomy. However, another potential disadvantage of cystgastrostomy is the lack of dependency of the drainage orifice when there is a very large cyst. Postoperatively, cystgastrostomy patients should be maintained on gastric decompression and parenteral fluids for at least several days.

A *cystojejunostomy* with a Roux-en-Y loop is an excellent procedure with the advantage that truly dependent drainage usually can be achieved with this operation. The Roux-en-Y loop, if sufficiently long (at least 30 cm.), protects against reflux of intestinal contents into the cyst and thereby also insures that an enteric fistula will not result should separation of the cystojejunal anastomosis occur. A large drainage orifice is both possible and desirable. This allows for biopsy of the cyst wall and at the same time helps to prevent premature closure of the anastomotic site. In a number of instances the cystojejunostomy anastomosis has separated without resulting in complications. The usual sequence of events in these cases has been successful treatment of the recurrent pseudocyst at a second operation with the same loop of jejunum. Although cystojejunostomy is a somewhat more demanding surgical procedure, it is certainly the choice for very large pancreatic pseudocysts.

The mortality inherent in any type of drainage procedure, whether external or internal, is closely related to two major complications: bleeding and sepsis. The bleeding may come from the area of anastomosis, from the cyst wall, or from erosion of one of

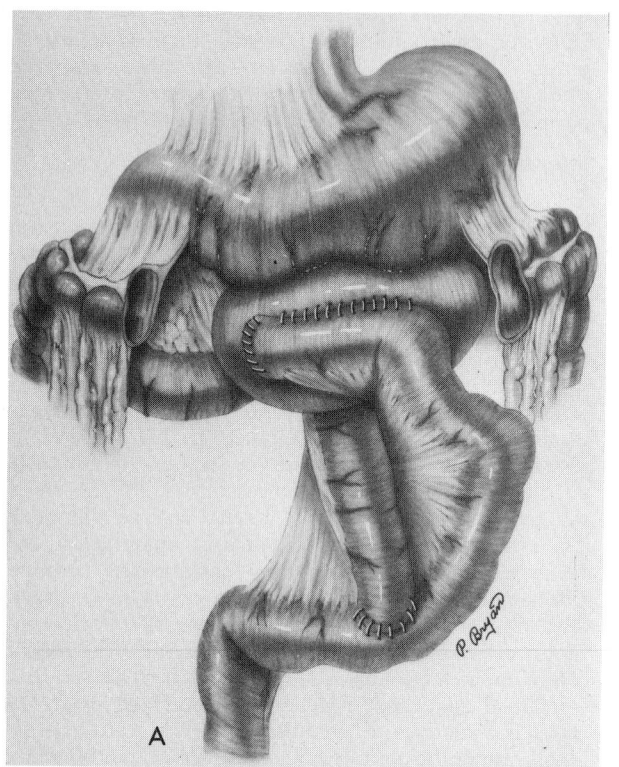

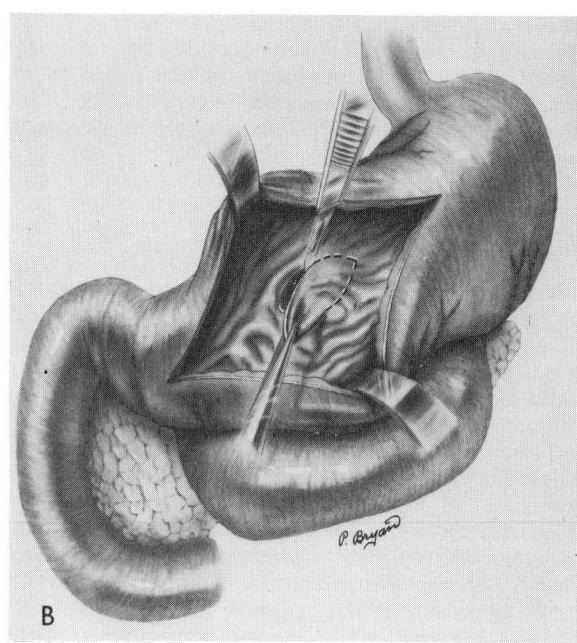

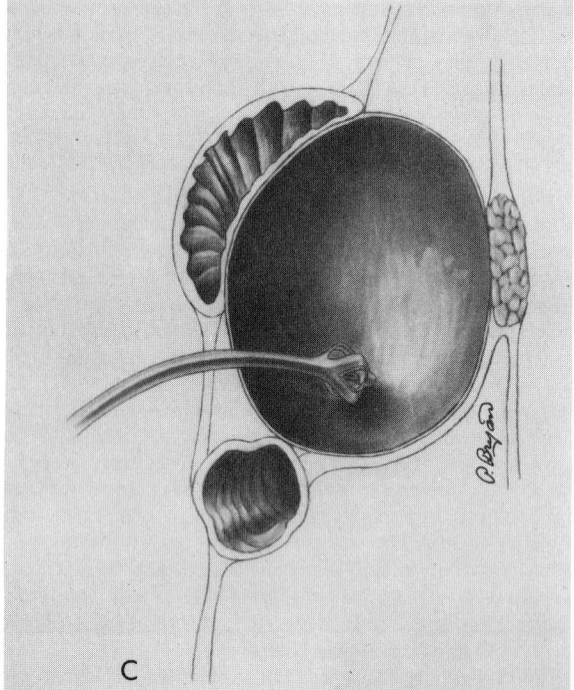

Figure 19. Drainage of pancreatic pseudocysts. *A*, Internal drainage via a Roux-en-Y. Note the retrocolic position of the jejunal limb, and that the cystojejunal anastomosis is made side-to-side rather than end-to-side in order to increase stomal size. *B*, Internal drainage via cystogastrostomy. Note that an ellipse of the common wall is being removed. Gastrocystic reflux has not proved to be as injurious as originally supposed. *C*, Lateral view showing large sump catheter placed in cyst cavity for external drainage. Note the displacement of the stomach superiorly and the transverse colon inferiorly.

the large vessels adjacent to the cyst wall, frequently the splenic artery.[21, 35] Aggressive treatment of hemorrhage will frequently allow a successful outcome, and reoperation should not be delayed unnecessarily.

PANCREATIC ASCITES

Only recently has it been appreciated that the pancreas can occasionally serve as a source of massive ascites.[17, 72] In most of these cases, there has been evidence of communication between the pancreatic ductal system and the free peritoneal cavity, usually a leaking pancreatic pseudocyst (Fig. 20). The diagnosis should be suspected whenever "cirrhotic ascites" is refractory to the usual medical measures and can readily be established by paracentesis and examination of the ascitic fluid. Since the ascitic fluid is in reality pancreatic juice, demonstration of a high peritoneal fluid amylase is a persistent finding. In addition, the ascitic fluid protein content will exceed 2.5 cm. per 100 ml. On the basis of our present knowledge, these combined findings are pathognomonic of pancreatic ascites.

Since the pathophysiology of pancreatic ascites is that of a leaking pancreatic duct, it was natural to assume that surgical correction would be required. However, while several patients with documented pancreatic ascites were being treated with preoperative intravenous hyperalimentation, resolution of the ascitic fluid occurred, suggesting spontaneous closure of the underlying ductal defect.[76] In the authors' opinion, exploration is indicated at present in these patients only if a trial of medical therapy lasting two weeks has been unsuccessful.

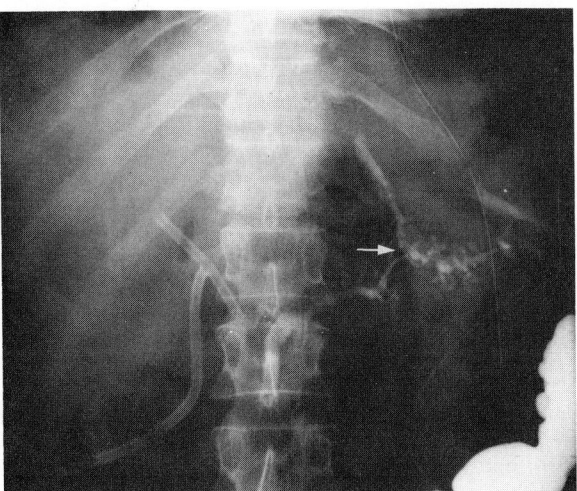

Figure 20. Operative pancreatogram demonstrating a spontaneous leak from the pancreatic ductal system (arrow). This loss of pancreatic juice directly into the free abdominal cavity resulted in pancreatic ascites. Pancreatogram was done by excising a small amount of the tail of the pancreas and inserting a polyethylene tube into the pancreatic duct for contrast injection. Note that pancreatic duct does not communicate with the duodenum. The T-tube is a result of previous common duct exploration.

Surgical therapy is predicated upon demonstration of the specific ductal defect. In those cases due to a leaking pseudocyst, drainage of the cyst, either internally or externally as dictated by local conditions, has proved sufficient. Should a leaking pseudocyst not be found, an operative pancreatogram may be necessary to demonstrate the site of the leak. Once identified, the leak can usually be controlled by performing a jejunal Roux-en-Y anastomosis over the ductal defect.

Results from surgery thus far have indicated an excellent response with little tendency toward reaccumulation of ascites. It is of great importance to have a high index of suspicion of this condition in alcoholics with ascites, since confusion with cirrhotic ascites might easily occur. As medical therapy of pancreatic ascites is frequently unsuccessful and the surgical procedure for resistant cirrhotic ascites (side-to-side portacaval shunt) would be inappropriate and perhaps severely damaging, the necessity for establishing an accurate diagnosis of the type of ascites is obvious.

TUMORS OF THE PANCREAS

Tumors of the pancreas most commonly originate from the two major histologic components of the organ and thus may be classified appropriately into neoplasms of (1) exocrine origin, and (2) endocrine origin.

NEOPLASMS OF THE EXOCRINE GLANDS

The most common tumor of the pancreas is a carcinoma of the exocrine glands.[30] It is a disease of the aged with a peak incidence in the eighth decade; two thirds of its victims are over 60 years of age. During those intervals of time when longevity was increasing at discernible rates, the incidence of pancreatic cancer increased as well, resulting in a trend toward increasing mortality from this disease.

Symptoms

The symptoms of pancreatic cancer depend upon the location of the tumor.[69] Regardless of the anatomic site, pain is the most common initial complaint. Characteristically, the pain is vague in quality but located in the epigastrium with radiation to the back. In tumors of the body and tail, the pain may be described in the left upper quadrant and back. Characteristically, the pain may be less severe in the erect position, and back pain may be eased by bending forward and flexing the left thigh. Rapid weight loss has been reported as the second most frequent complaint. The exact reason for this is not clear but may be related to anorexia due to the abdominal pain and anxiety associated with undiagnosed illness. Frequently abdominal pain due to cancer of the body or tail of the pancreas is not diagnosed until the disease is far advanced. Findings on routine gastrointestinal x-rays are usually negative early in the course of the disease.

Jaundice is frequently an early sign in carcinoma of the head of the pancreas, particularly when the tumor is located in the periampullary area. For this reason, tumors of the head are likely to be less advanced than tumors of the body or tail at the time of surgical exploration.

Diagnosis

The early diagnosis of carcinoma of the body of the pancreas requires a high index of suspicion, leading to early laparotomy. Frequently, patients arrive at near-terminal status as a result of lengthy and often unproductive evaluation in the attempt to find the origin of vague abdominal pain. When jaundice is present, however, completing the triad composed of jaundice, weight loss, and pain, surgical exploration is usually performed with dispatch. Some patients will present with a palpable gallbladder in addition to jaundice. Conventional wisdom describes distention of the gallbladder when the common bile duct is obstructed by cancer, but not when the duct is obstructed by a stone (Courvoisier's law). The rationale is that the gallbladder containing stones is fibrotic and incapable of distention. While theoretically appealing, the clinical usefulness of this concept is limited owing to many apparent exceptions.

Abnormalities of clinical chemical findings may be minimal or absent in this disease. In jaundiced patients with cancer of the head of the pancreas, laboratory tests reveal only those data which are indicative of the extrahepatic biliary obstruction, including elevation of serum alkaline phosphatase activity and high serum bilirubin concentration.

This relative lack of specificity in establishing the diagnosis of carcinoma of the pancreas has served as a stimulus for the study of other diagnostic techniques, primarily physical in nature. Examination of the upper intestinal tract with barium may be helpful, since almost one third of the patients with cancer of the head of the pancreas demonstrate widening of the duodenal C loop and evidence of external pressure or invasion of the duodenum. Percutaneous transjugular or transhepatic cholangiography has been helpful when a tapered obstruction of the common bile duct is discovered (Fig. 21). The recent introduction of the ultrathin Chiba needle has greatly decreased the number of complications of transhepatic cholangiography. Ultrasonic scanning of the pancreas has been useful in some cases; however, there is no unanimity of opinion concerning the accuracy of pancreatic morphology predicted by ultrasound. Selective visceral angiography has received considerable attention as a potentially useful technique. The identification of a "tumor blush," or tumor vessels in the distribution of the pancreatic blood supply, may be diagnostic. Obviously, the degree of vascularization of the neoplasm is the most important factor influencing the accuracy of angiographic diagnosis, and this may vary considerably. Some tumors contain a rich microvascular network, whereas in others the vascularity is poor. Demonstration of vascular irregularity in the region of the tumor ("encasement"), once thought to be pathognomonic of malignancy, may also be seen in chronic pancreatitis and is therefore nonspecific. Occasionally, angiography will reveal invasion of the portal or superior mesenteric veins, a finding generally regarded as a demonstration of surgical irresectability. Pancreatography via endoscopic retrograde cholangiopancrea-

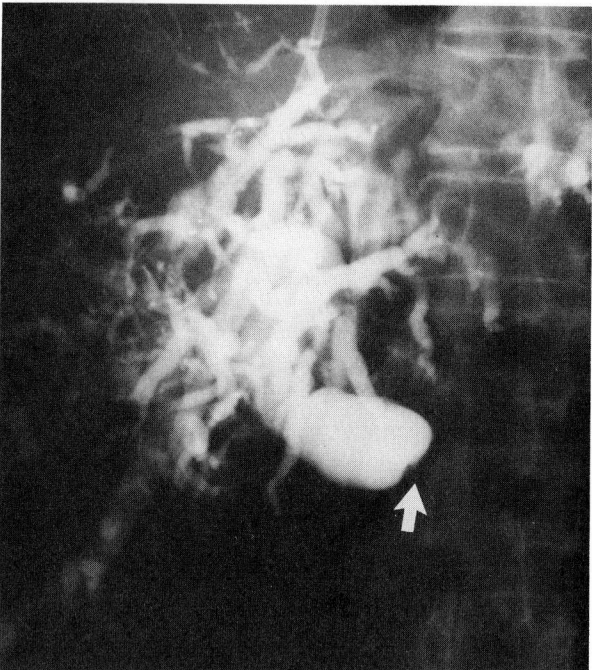

Figure 21. Transjugular cholangiography. The catheter is inserted percutaneously into the jugular vein and advanced downward into a hepatic vein. A specifically designed needle is introduced into the hepatic parenchyma in search of dilated duct. In this particular case, complete obstruction of the hepatic duct is evident (arrow). This procedure is well tolerated, although antibiotic coverage is advisable. The major advantage of this approach over percutaneous transhepatic cholangiography is elimination of the possibility of intraperitoneal bile leakage.

tography (ERCP) will be helpful in those instances when the ductal system is sufficiently displaced, distorted, or interrupted. Unfortunately, even then it will not be possible to be completely certain that the demonstrated changes are due to malignancy.

At present, it is fair to conclude that graphic visualization of the pancreas has not been accomplished satisfactorily, and there is no technique available that has sufficient precision or reproducibility to be of unequivocal diagnostic value. The most precise diagnostic technique remains exploratory celiotomy in the hands of an experienced surgeon.

Therapy

Pancreaticoduodenectomy is the only therapy with proven efficacy for the cure of cancer of the head of the pancreas.[82] Unfortunately, the rate of success is modest, being approximately 10 per cent of patients who have had such resections. However, small tumors in the head of the pancreas and periampullary carcinomas may exhibit survival rates approaching 40 per cent in the absence of lymphatic metastases. More frequently the exploration reveals a neoplasm that is incurable because of (1) metastases to other organs or lymph nodes or (2) invasion of vascular structures such as the portal vein and superior mesenteric vessels. In experienced hands, the operative mortality associated with this procedure has been reduced below 10 per cent, and studies involving as many as 40 patients have been reported with no deaths.[42]

The operative procedure involves resection of the distal stomach, duodenum, and either part or all of the pancreas (Fig. 22).[90] Total pancreatectomy has an advantage of preventing local recurrence of the tumor in the pancreatic remnant.[70] However, the major disadvantage rests in the fact that total pancreatectomy results in varying degrees of exocrine insufficiency and permanent diabetes mellitus with a continuing requirement for insulin therapy. For these reasons, the majority of surgeons prefer to preserve the tail of the pancreas. Reconstruction of the gastrointestinal tract in the Whipple procedure requires anastomosis of the jejunum to the pancreas, the biliary system (usually the common bile duct), and the stomach (Fig. 23). Vagotomy is advocated by some as an ancillary measure to inhibit gastric acid secretion, which in turn reduces the potential for gastrojejunal ulceration. In addition, the reconstruction requires that the inflow of alkaline bile and pancreatic juice be inserted proximal to the gastrojejunostomy to further protect against marginal ulceration.

If pancreaticoduodenectomy is not indicated because of the operative findings of incurability, then some form of biliary decompression to relieve jaundice should be performed (Fig. 24). Cholecystoenterostomy is simple and effective. However, because the gallblad-

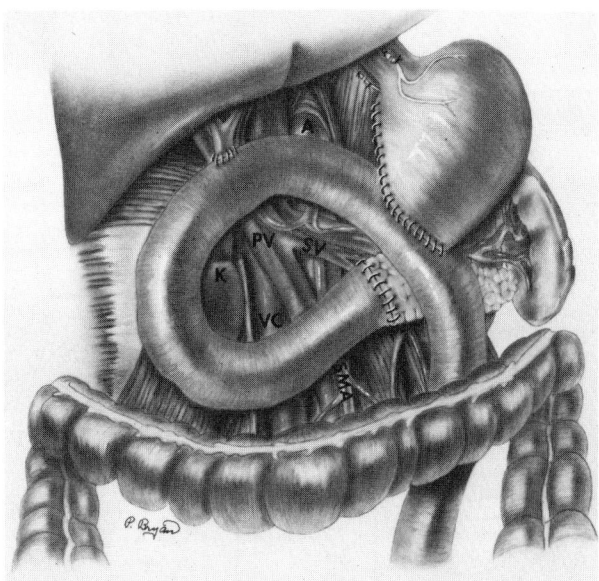

Figure 23. Preferred method of reconstruction after pancreatico-duodenectomy. The pancreatic anastomosis is placed proximal to the biliary anastomosis, which is, in turn, followed by a gastro-jejunostomy of the Hofmeister type. (A, aorta; PV, portal vein; SV, splenic vein; VC, vena cava; K, kidney; SMA, superior mesenteric artery.)

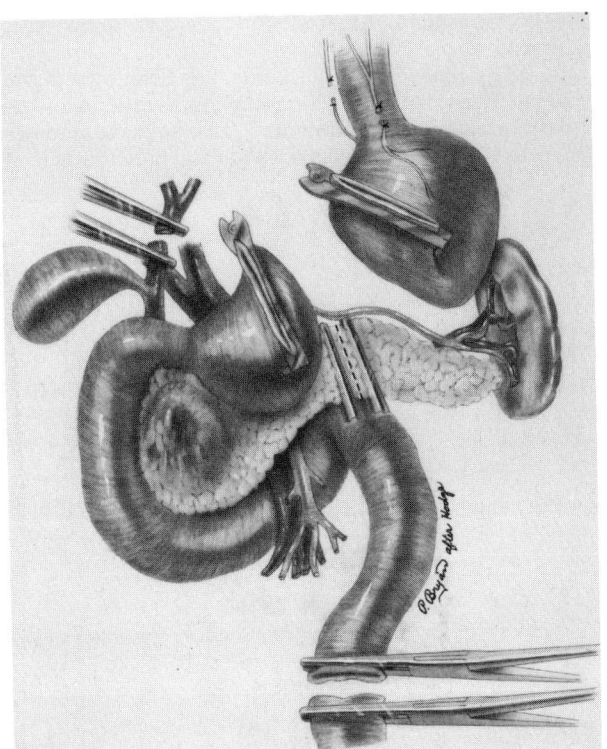

Figure 22. Extent of pancreaticoduodenectomy (Whipple procedure). The distal stomach, duodenum, gallbladder, and right half of the pancreas are removed. A vagotomy is usually added to protect against the development of marginal ulceration.

der is used as a bypass conduit, it is imperative to demonstrate that the tumor is distal to the cystic duct–common duct junction and that the cystic duct is patent. The possibility of impending duodenal obstruction by the tumor mass must also be considered and evaluated. Gastrojejunostomy should be a frequent accompaniment to biliary decompression when continued duodenal patency cannot be reasonably assured. Surgical palliation may possibly be improved by the addition of chemotherapy, although definitive proof of the value of adjunctive therapy in carcinoma of the pancreas is lacking.

NEOPLASMS OF THE ENDOCRINE GLANDS

With increasing recognition of the plenipotentiality of the stem cell of the pancreatic islets, the increasing number of peptide hormones reportedly produced by islet cell tumors is more easily understood (Fig. 25). Patients may present with or without associated endocrine syndromes depending upon whether or not the tumors are hormone producing. In those patients with hormonally active neoplasms, either "pure" or "mixed" endocrine syndromes may be seen reflecting the number and variety of hormones being produced.

Insulinoma

An insulin-producing adenoma of the beta cells is the most common islet cell tumor.[43] Symptoms of an insulinoma are those of spontaneous, episodic hypoglycemia. The complaint may be of "fits" or "spells" which may represent a wide range of nervous system manifestations. Usually the symptom complex has a psy-

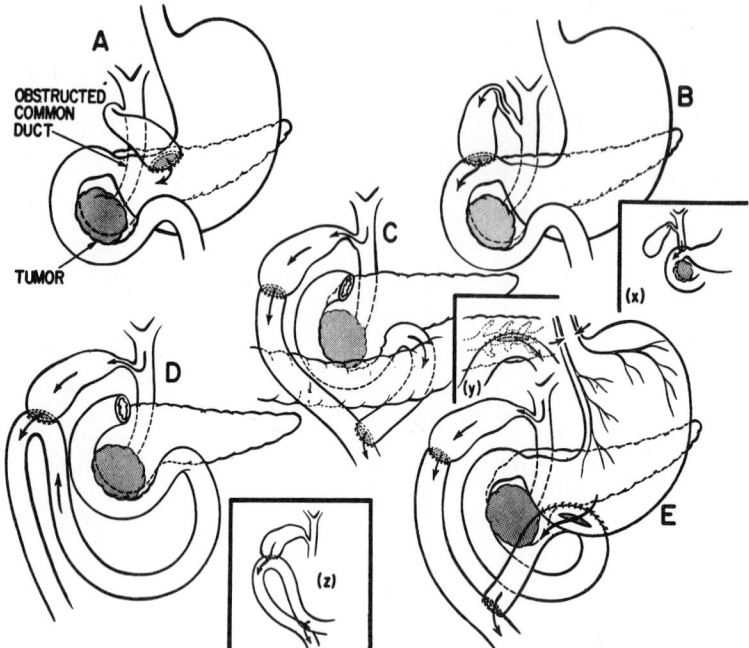

Figure 24. Palliative procedures for nonresectable tumors of the head of the pancreas. *A,* Cholecystoduodenostomy. *B,* Cholecystoduodenostomy and (x), choledochoduodenostomy. *C, D,* and (z), Several modifications of a cholecystojejunostomy. (y), Drainage of an obstructed pancreatic duct into the jejunum. *E,* Gastroenterostomy included to prevent duodenal obstruction. Vagotomy is added as a precaution against peptic ulceration, since the alkaline juices of the biliary tract have been routed away from the gastrojejunostomy. (From Ellison, E. H., and Carey, L. C. *In* Davis, L. (Ed.): Christopher's Textbook of Surgery, 9th ed. Philadelphia, W. B. Saunders Company, 1968.)

chophysiological presentation, with well-regulated time sequences in any given patient. The attacks occur in the fasting state with blood sugar concentrations of less than 50 mg. per 100 ml. and are relieved promptly by the administration of sugar (Whipple's triad).[89]

The simplest test for establishing the diagnosis of insulin-producing tumor consists of withholding food from the patient and confirming the triad sequence. This should be performed only in the hospital environment under continuous observation. It is not without risk, since convulsions, coma, and even death may be precipitated by the resultant hypoglycemia. Other useful tests include measurement of the serum insulin levels, which are the most precise determinant in making the diagnosis and have the virtue of being free of risk. Insulin stimulation tests using tolbutamide or leucine may be helpful but carry a risk of induced hypoglycemia more severe than extended fasting. These tests result in a precipitous fall in blood sugar with delayed return to fasting levels. Localization of suspected adenomas can frequently be obtained if a tumor blush is seen during pancreatic arteriography. Angiographic confirmation and localization can be obtained in 80 per cent of patients.[34]

Surgical therapy for insulin-producing tumors has been complicated by the fact that the neoplasms are usually small and difficult to find. Furthermore, multiple tumors appear in 10 to 15 per cent of cases and heterotopic locations of these adenomas are not uncommon. Such considerations, when associated with imprecise preoperative anatomic localization, have resulted in the necessity for extensive pancreatic resections in some cases in order to insure that the adenoma has been excised. Fortunately, since the overwhelming majority of insulinomas can be localized by preoperative angiography, the necessity for "blind" pancreatic resection has been considerably reduced. At surgery, the majority of tumors can be handled by simple enucleation. However, multiple, locally invasive, or deeply imbedded tumors may require pancreatic resection.

Recently a new drug, diazoxide, has been introduced into the therapeutic armamentarium available for the treatment of hyperinsulinemia.[55] This agent suppresses the release of insulin from both normal pancreatic islet

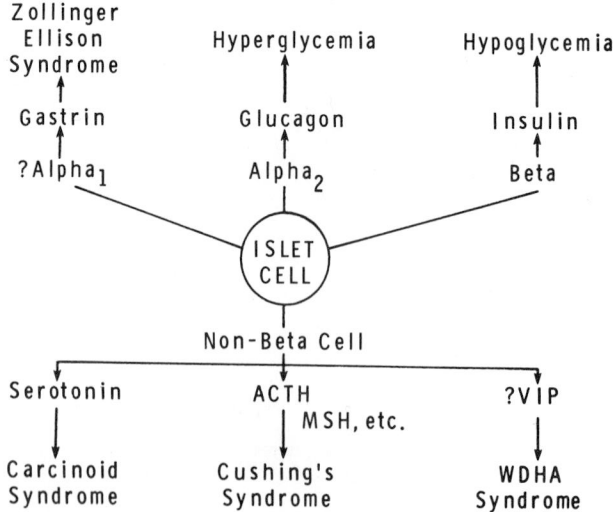

Figure 25. Functioning islet cell tumors. The marked disparity in clinical presentation is thought to be due to the plenipotentiality of the islet stem cell derived from neural crest tissue.

tissue and adenomas and has been used in patients with suspected insulinomas who were regarded as prohibitive surgical risks. Although the magnitude of the effect on the blood sugar is only partially explained by the inhibition of insulin release, clinical results have been good.

Gastrinoma

In 1955, Zollinger and Ellison postulated that a hormone-secreting tumor of the pancreatic islets was responsible for a peculiarly pernicious form of peptic ulceration.[94] Abnormally high levels of gastrin were subsequently demonstrated both in the pancreatic tumor and in the serum of such patients.

It was initially thought that all patients with these tumors pursued a virulent course leading to hemorrhage and perforation. Such presentations are now recognized as only the severe end of this disease spectrum, and that many patients, previously unrecognized because of seemingly uncomplicated "peptic ulcer disease," are being uncovered by more widespread use of gastrin radioimmunoassay.[45]

Typically, such patients have marked gastric hyperchlorhydria almost always exceeding 10 mEq. per hr. When hyperchlorhydria of this magnitude is associated with hypergastrinemia, the diagnosis is established. In borderline cases, considerable diagnostic assistance can be obtained from the calcium infusion[61] and secretin suppression tests.[15] In contrast to the results in other individuals, both intravenous calcium and secretin provoke a marked rise in serum gastrin levels in patients with gastrinoma.

Unfortunately, the surgical therapy of this condition is complicated by the frequent impossibility of precise anatomic localization of these tumors. First, more than 60 per cent are malignant and many have metastasized by the time exploration is undertaken. Second, the benign tumors are most commonly multiple. Because of these factors, pancreatic resection may not include all functioning tumor tissue, thereby subjecting the patient to recurrent peptic ulceration. With regard to patient survival, experience has repeatedly demonstrated the superiority of total gastrectomy when performed as the initial surgical procedure (see also Chapter 31).

WDHA Syndrome

It has become increasingly apparent that certain patients with islet cell tumors experience a diarrhea so severe as to be life threatening.[79] Stool volumes may reach 5 liters daily, and potassium loss frequently may approach 300 mEq. per 24 hrs. In contrast to those patients with gastrinoma who may also suffer severe diarrhea, this group of patients exhibits basal achlorhydria. Characteristically, there is little response to histamine stimulation. The acronym WDHA (watery diarrhea, hypokalemia, achlorhydria) has been proposed to identify this syndrome. Currently, the islet cell hormone responsible for these effects is in debate; secretin, glucagon, CCK-PZ, calcitonin, gastric inhibitory polypeptide (GIP), vasoactive intestinal polypeptide (VIP), and various prostaglandins have been implicated.

At present, almost 100 cases have been reported. Approximately 50 per cent have proved to be malignant, many of which exhibited hepatic and other metastases when initially explored. Thirty per cent have been benign solitary adenomas, most commonly situated in the body and tail, and thus easily curable by partial pancreatectomy. The remaining 20 per cent of cases have represented diffuse islet cell hyperplasia. Under these latter circumstances total pancreatectomy has resulted in cure in 80 per cent. When distant metastases preclude cure, the primary tumor mass should be removed whenever feasible, and the patient treated with intra-arterial streptozotocin. With this regimen, significant palliation consisting of amelioration of diarrhea has resulted in patients with documented metastases.[51] In contrast to other islet cell tumors, this particular neoplasm appears to be particularly susceptible to streptozotocin.

SELECTED REFERENCES

Anderson, G., and Johnson, S. R.: Treatment of acute necrotizing pancreatitis. Acta Chir. Scand., *134*:311, 1968.
This paper emphasizes the potential benefit of early and aggressive surgical therapy in acute necrosis of the pancreas. It reaffirms the concept of early surgery for selected patients proposed earlier by Moynihan.

Banks, P. A., and Janowitz, H. D.: Some metabolic aspects of exocrine pancreatic disease. Gastroenterology, *56*:601, 1969.
This is a well-documented review article from a clinic with extensive experience in the study of normal and abnormal pancreatic function in man and animals. It is concise and well written.

Banting, F. G., and Best, C. H. L.: The internal secretion of the pancreas. J. Lab. Clin. Med., 7:251, 1922.
This paper is a milestone in the efforts of investigators to obtain insulin from pancreatic extracts. Banting and Best induced acinar atrophy by ligation of the pancreatic ducts and subsequently obtained potent hypoglycemic extracts from the residual viable islet tissue.

Barbosa, J. J. de C., Docherty, M. B., and Waugh, J. M.: Pancreatic heterotopia. Review of the literature and report of 41 authenticated surgical uses of which 25 were clinically significant. Surg. Gynecol. Obstet., *82*:527, 1946.
This paper is a valuable reference work, serving as a catalog of pancreatic heterotopia.

Bayliss, W. M., and Starling, E. H.: The mechanism of pancreatic secretion. J. Physiol., *28*:325, 1902.
This is a classic paper, containing the first description of the humoral control of pancreatic secretion by secretin.

Cameron, J. L., Brawley, R. K., Bender, H. W., and Zuidema, G. D.: The treatment of pancreatic ascites. Ann. Surg., *170*:668, 1969.
The authors make an excellent presentation of a large personal experience with chronic pancreatic ascites. Diagnostic methodology is clearly presented; confusion with cirrhotic ascites should be guarded against, as a substantial percentage of cases of both types of ascites occur in alcoholic patients. Operative radiographic examinations clearly establish duct disruption as a primary causative mechanism. Surgical therapy usually requires drainage of a pseudocyst of the pancreas or direct drainage of the leaking pancreatic duct.

Child, C. G., Frey, C. F., and Fry, W. J.: A reappraisal of removal of ninety-five per cent of the distal portion of the pancreas. Surg. Gynecol. Obstet., *129*:49, 1969.

Fry, W. J., and Child, C. G.: Ninety-five per cent distal pancreatectomy for chronic pancreatitis. Ann. Surg., *162*:543, 1965.
These papers announce and confirm the importance of a major new tool for the treatment of chronic pancreatitis, the 95 per cent pancreatectomy. While not performed routinely, this procedure has greatly enhanced the surgical armamentarium with which to combat this difficult disease. In the authors' hands the mortality and morbidity have been surprisingly low and relief of symptoms excellent. The long-term results are influenced chiefly by the continued use of alcohol and drugs and the complications of diabetes.

Dreiling, D. A., Druckerman, L. J., and Hollander, F.: The effect of complete vagisection and vagal stimulation on pancreatic secretion in man. Gastroenterology, *20*:578, 1952.

An important set of observations concerning the quantitative aspects of vagal control of pancreatic secretion in man. The authors demonstrated a lack of effect by vagotomy on secretin-stimulated pancreatic secretion.

Elman, R., Arneson, N., and Graham, E. A.: Value of blood amylase estimations in diagnosis of pancreatic disease: Clinical study. Arch. Surg., 19:943, 1929.

Although he is not often credited, Dr. Elman was the first to demonstrate the elevation of serum amylase in patients with pancreatitis.

Folk, F. A., and Freeark, R. J.: Reoperations for pancreatic pseudocysts. Arch. Surg., 100:430, 1970.

The authors have had extensive experience in pancreatic surgery and utilize case presentations to highlight the various pitfalls associated with the treatment of pancreatic pseudocysts. An analysis of some of the causes of postoperative complications is pertinent, and the general success achieved by reoperation is properly emphasized.

Halsted, W. S.: Retrojection of bile into the pancreas, a cause of acute hemorrhagic pancreatitis. Bull. Johns Hopkins Hosp., 12:179, 1901.

Opie, E. L.: Etiology of acute pancreatitis. Bull. Johns Hopkins Hosp., 12:182, 1901.

These two papers laid the foundation for the "common channel theory" as an etiologic factor in the development of acute pancreatitis. Professor Opie described such an anatomic arrangement from postmortem studies and Professor Halsted demonstrated that the probable cause was the invasion of the pancreatic ducts by bile.

Jones, S. A., Steedman, R. A., Kellen, T. B., and Smith, L. L.: Transduodenal sphincteroplasty (not sphincterotomy) for biliary and pancreatic disease. Am. J. Surg., 118:292, 1969.

This paper, from the originators of the sphincteroplasty technique, is a most illuminating critique of the usefulness and limitations of this operation. The technical details necessary for a successful procedure are clearly outlined and the physiologic differences between sphincteroplasty and sphincterotomy documented. The careful analysis of mortality and immediate morbidity is impressive, as is the study of the long-term results of the operation. This report substantiates the usefulness of the procedure when correctly utilized and confirms the superior results with patients with primary biliary tract disease and other types of nonalcoholic pancreatitis as compared to those with alcoholic pancreatitis.

Kalser, M. H., Leite, C. A., and Warren, W. D.: Fat assimilation after massive distal pancreatectomy. N. Engl. J. Med., 279:570, 1968.

Careful documentation of the exocrine metabolic effects of 95 per cent pancreatectomy is presented. The surprisingly great residual function and ease of clinical management are in contrast to those seen after total pancreatectomy, which required duodenal resection. When 20 to 25 per cent of normal pancreas was preserved, there were no clinical problems with either endocrine or exocrine function.

Pavlov, I. P.: The Works of the Digestive Glands, trans. W. H. Thompson. London, Charles Griffin Company, 1910.

This classic description of the neural influence on pancreatic secretion gives clear demonstration that the vagus is the secretory nerve of the pancreas and describes the first successful chronic pancreatic fistula preparation.

Ranson, J. H. C., Rifkind, K. M., Roses, D. F., Fink, S. D., Eng, F., and Spencer, F. C.: Prognostic signs and the role of operative management in acute pancreatitis. Surg. Gynecol. Obstet., 139:69, 1974.

The authors have established that the clinical course of pancreatitis can be predicted by the presence or absence of certain clinical criteria. Since this relationship permits establishment of degrees of pancreatitis, patients can now be randomized into comparable groups in an effort to confront many of the unanswered questions in acute pancreatitis.

Schein, P. S., DeLellis, R. A., Kahn, C. R., Gorden, P., and Kraft, A. R.: Islet cell tumors: Current concepts and management. Ann. Intern. Med., 79:239, 1973.

In this review article, both functioning and nonfunctioning islet cell tumors are discussed with reference to pathology, clinical symptomatology, diagnosis, and management. Appropriate stress is placed upon the neural crest cell as progenitor, accounting for the myriad clinical syndromes produced by tumors derived from islet cell tissue.

Warren, K. W., Braasch, J. H., and Thum, C. W.: Diagnosis and surgical treatment of carcinoma of the pancreas. Curr. Probl. Surg., June, 1968.

This is an up-to-date and comprehensive treatise on the therapy of pancreatic cancer, and is an excellent reference source.

Warren, W. D., Marsh, W. H., and Sandusky, W. R.: An appraisal of surgical procedures for pancreatic pseudocyst. Ann. Surg., 147:903, 1958.

This study, using an experimental model plus an extensive clinical survey, considers the fundamental principles of treating pancreatic pseudocysts. An understanding of the usefulness of a variety of procedures facilitates the correct choice of operation for a condition in which individual differences are of great importance.

Webster, P. D., and Zieve, L.: Alterations in serum content of pancreatic enzymes. N. Engl. J. Med., 267:604, 1962.

Webster, P. D., and Zieve, L.: Alterations in serum content of pancreatic enzymes. N. Engl. J. Med., 267:654, 1962.

These two articles together are parts of a review of the significance of changes in pancreatic serum enzymes. The papers contain many helpful references and much important information.

Whipple, A. O., and Frantz, V. K.: Adenoma of islet-cells with hyperinsulinism. A review. Ann. Surg., 101:1299, 1935.

This paper records the relationship between islet adenoma and hyperinsulinism. This is one of Dr. Allen Whipple's many contributions.

Whipple, A. O., Parsons, W. W., and Mullins, C. R.: Treatment of carcinoma of the ampulla of Vater. Ann. Surg., 102:763, 1935.

This is the classic description of pancreaticoduodenectomy or Whipple's procedure. This operation continues to be the surgical therapy of choice for carcinoma of the head of the pancreas or tumors of the ampulla of Vater.

White, T. T., and Keith, R. G.: Long term follow-up study of fifty patients with pancreaticojejunostomy. Surg. Gynecol. Obstet., 136:353, 1973.

This paper presents the currently accepted surgical philosophy for patients with chronic pancreatitis in general, and, in particular, reviews the long-term results of lateral pancreaticojejunostomy.

Zollinger, R. M., and Ellison, E. H.: Primary peptic ulcerations of the jejunum associated with islet-cell tumors of the pancreas. Ann. Surg., 142:709, 1955.

This article presents the initial proposal that some cases of peptic ulceration might be due to hormone-secreting tumors of the pancreas.

REFERENCES

1. Anderson, G., and Johnson, S. R.: Treatment of acute necrotizing pancreatitis. Acta Chir. Scand., 134:311, 1968.
2. Anderson, M. C., Schoenfeld, F. B., Iams, W. B., and Suwa, M.: Circulatory changes in acute pancreatitis. Surg. Clin. North Am., 47:127, 1967.
3. Babkin, B. P.: Secretory Mechanisms of the Digestive Glands, 2nd ed. New York, Hoeber Medical Division, Harper & Row, 1950.
4. Banks, P. A., and Janowitz, H. D.: Some metabolic aspects of exocrine pancreatic disease. Gastroenterology, 56:601, 1969.
5. Banting, F. G., and Best, C. H. J.: The internal secretion of the pancreas. J. Lab. Clin. Med., 7:251, 1922.
6. Barbosa, J. J. de C., Docherty, M. B., and Waugh, J. M.: Pancreatic heterotopia. Review of the literature and report of 41 authenticated surgical uses of which 25 were clinically significant. Surg. Gynecol. Obstet., 82:527, 1946.
7. Bayliss, W. M., and Starling, E. H.: The mechanism of pancreatic secretion. J. Physiol., 28:325, 1902.
8. Becker, W. F., Pratt, H. S., and Ganji, H.: Pseudocysts of the pancreas. Surg. Gynecol. Obstet., 127:744, 1968.
9. Behrens, O. K., and Bromer, W. W.: Glucagon, Vitamins and Hormones. Volume 16. New York, Academic Press, 1958.
10. Berk, J. E., Kizu, H., Take, S., and Gridhandler, L.: Macroamylasemia: Clinical and laboratory features. Am. J. Gastroenterol., 53:211, 1970.
11. Bolooki, H., Jaffe, B., and Gliedman, M. L.: Pancreatic abscesses and lesser omental sac collections. Surg. Gynecol. Obstet., 126:1301, 1968.
12. Bolooki, H., Minkowitz, S., Glammona, S. T., and Jude, J. R.: Res-

piratory failure in acute pancreatitis. J. Surg. Oncol., 3:31, 1971.

13. Bradley, E. L., III, and Clements, J. L.: Implications of diagnostic ultrasound in the surgical management of pancreatic pseudocysts. Am. J. Surg., 127:163, 1974.

14. Bradley, E. L., III, and Clements, J. L., Jr.: Trans-enteric rupture of pancreatic pseudocysts: Management of pseudocystenteric fistulae. Am. Surg., 42:827, 1976.

15. Bradley, E. L., III, and Galambos, J. T.: Diagnosis of gastrinoma by the secretin suppression test. Surg. Gynecol. Obstet., 143:784, 1976.

16. Brooks, F. P., and Manfredo, H.: The control of pancreatic secretion and its clinical significance. Am. J. Gastroenterol., 42:42, 1964.

17. Cameron, J. L., Brawley, R. K., Bender, H. W., and Zuidema, G. D.: The treatment of pancreatic ascites. Ann. Surg., 170:668, 1969.

18. Cavellero, C., Solicia, E., and Sampietro, R.: Cytology of islet tumors and hyperplasias associated with Zollinger-Ellison syndrome. Gut, 8:172, 1967.

19. Cerilli, J., and Faris, T. D.: Pancreatic pseudocysts: Delayed versus immediate treatment. Surgery, 615:541, 1971.

20. Child, C. G., Frey, C. F., and Fry, W. J.: A reappraisal of removal of ninety-five per cent of the distal portion of the pancreas. Surg. Gynecol. Obstet., 129:49, 1969.

21. Coghill, C. L.: Hemorrhage in pancreatic pseudocysts. Ann. Surg., 167:112, 1968.

22. Cotton, P. B.: Progress report. Cannulation of the papilla of Vater by endoscopy and retrograde cholangiopancreatography (ERCP). Gut, 13:1014, 1972.

23. Doubilet, H., and Mulholland, J. H.: Eight-year study of pancreatitis and sphincterotomy. J.A.M.A., 160:521, 1956.

24. Dreiling, D. A., Druckerman, L. J., and Hollander, F.: The effect of complete vagisection and vagal stimulation on pancreatic secretion in man. Gastroenterology, 20:578, 1952.

25. DuVal, M. K., Jr.: Caudal pancreaticojejunostomy for chronic relapsing pancreatitis. Ann. Surg., 140:775, 1954.

26. Elman, R., Arneson, N., and Graham, E. A.: Value of blood amylase estimations in diagnosis of pancreatic disease: Clinical Study. Arch. Surg., 19:943, 1929.

27. Facey, F. L., Weill, M. H., and Rosoff, L.: Mechanism and treatment of shock associated with acute pancreatitis. Am. J. Surg., 111:374, 1966.

28. Foley, W. J., Gaines, R. D., and Fry, W. J.: Pancreaticoduodenectomy for severe trauma to the head of the pancreas and associated structures. Ann. Surg., 170:759, 1969.

29. Folk, F. A., and Freeark, R. J.: Reoperations for pancreatic pseudocysts. Arch. Surg., 100:430, 1970.

30. Frantz, V. K.: Tumors of the Pancreas. In Atlas of Tumor Pathology. Section VII. Washington, D.C., Armed Forces Institute of Pathology, 1959.

31. Fry, W. J., and Child, C. G.: Ninety-five per cent distal pancreatectomy for chronic pancreatitis. Ann. Surg., 162:543, 1965.

32. Gambill, E. E., and Mason, H. L.: One hour value for urinary amylase in 96 patients with pancreatitis. Ann. Surg., 162:130, 1963.

33. Gonzalez, A., Bradley, E. L., III, and Clements, J. L., Jr.: Pseudocyst formation in acute pancreatitis: Experience with ultrasonic evaluation of 99 cases. Am. J. Roentgenol., in press.

34. Gray, R. K., Rosch, J., and Grothman, J. H., Jr.: Arteriography in the diagnosis of islet-cell tumors. Radiology, 97:39, 1970.

35. Greenstein, A., De Maio, E. F., and Nabseth, D. C.: Acute hemorrhage associated with pancreatic pseudocysts. Surgery, 69:58, 1971.

36. Guillemin, G., Cuilleret, S., Michel, A., Berard, P., and Feroldi, J.: Chronic relapsing pancreatitis: Surgical management including 63 cases of pancreaticoduodenectomy. Am. J. Surg., 122:802, 1971.

37. Halsted, W. S.: Retrojection of bile into the pancreas, a cause of acute hemorrhagic pancreatitis. Bull. Johns Hopkins Hosp., 12:179, 1901.

38. Hanna, W. A.: Rupture of pancreatic cysts: Report of a case and review of the literature. Br. J. Surg., 47:495, 1963.

39. Harper, A. A.: Physiologic factors regulating pancreatic secretion. Gastroenterology, 36:386, 1959.

40. Heidenhain, R.: Beitrage sur Kenntnis des Pancreas. Arch. Ges. Physiol., 10:557, 1875.

41. Hokin, L. E.: Metabolic aspects and energetics of pancreatic secretion. In Code, C. F. (Ed.): American Physiological Society:

Handbook of Physiology. Section 6, Alimentary Canal, Vol. II, Secretion. Baltimore, Williams & Wilkins, 1967.

42. Howard, J. M.: Pancreatico-duodenectomy: Forty-one consecutive Whipple resections without an operative mortality. Ann. Surg., 168:629, 1968.

43. Howard, J. M., Moss, N. H., and Rhoads, J. E.: Hyperinsulinism and islet-cell tumors of the pancreas with 398 recorded tumors. Surg. Gynecol. Obstet., 90:417, 1950.

44. Howes, R., Zuidema, G., and Cameron, J. L.: Evaluation of prophylactic antibiotics in acute pancreatitis. J. Surg. Res., 18:197, 1975.

45. Isenberg, J. T., Walsh, J. H., and Grossman, M. I.: Zollinger-Ellison syndrome. Gastroenterology, 65:140, 1973.

46. Janowitz, H. D., and Dreiling, D. A.: The Pancreatic Secretion of Fluid and Electrolytes. Ciba Foundation Symposium of the Exocrine Pancreas, Normal and Abnormal Function. London, J. & A. Churchill, 1962.

47. Jones, S. A., Steedman, R. A., Kellen, T. B., and Smith, L. L.: Transduodenal sphincteroplasty (not sphincterotomy) for biliary and pancreatic disease. Am. J. Surg., 118:292, 1969.

48. Jordan, G., and Grossman, M. I.: Pancreaticoduodenectomy in the management of chronic relapsing pancreatitis. Surgery, 41:871, 1957.

49. Jordan, G. L., Overton, R. T., and Werschky, L. R.: Traumatic transections of the pancreas. South. Med. J., 62:90, 1969.

50. Jorpes, J. E., and Mutt, V.: The gastrointestinal hormones, secretin and cholecystokinin-pancreozymin. Ann. Intern. Med., 55:395, 1961.

51. Kahn, R. C., Levy, A. G., Gardner, J. D., Miller, J. V., Gorden, P., and Schein, P. S.: Pancreatic cholera: Beneficial effects of treatment with streptozotocin. N. Engl. J. Med., 292:941, 1975.

52. Kalser, M. H., Leite, C. A., and Warren, W. D.: Fat assimilation after massive distal pancreatectomy. N. Engl. J. Med., 279:570, 1968.

53. Lawson, D. S., Daggett, W. M., Civetta, J. M., Cory, R. J., and Bartlett, M. K.: Surgical treatment of acute necrotizing pancreatitis. Ann. Surg., 172:605, 1970.

54. Mallet-Guy, P., and deBeaujeu, M. J.: Treatment of chronic pancreatitis by unilateral splanchnicectomy. Arch. Surg., 602:33, 1950.

55. Meyer, E. M.: Diazoxide and the treatment of hypoglycemia. Ann. N.Y. Acad. Sci., 150:191, 1968.

56. Nakamura, K., Sarles, H., and Payan, H.: Three dimensional reconstruction of the pancreatic ducts in chronic pancreatitis. Gastroenterology, 62:942, 1972.

57. Nardi, G. L., and Acosta, J. M.: Papillitis as a cause of pancreatitis and abdominal pain: Role of evocative test, operative pancreatography and histologic evaluation. Ann. Surg., 164:611, 1966.

58. Norton, L., and Eiseman, B.: Near total pancreatectomy for hemorrhagic pancreatitis. Am. J. Surg., 127:191, 1974.

59. Opie, E. L.: Etiology of acute pancreatitis. Bull. Johns Hopkins Hosp., 12:182, 1901.

60. Partington, P. F., and Rochelle, R. E. L.: Modified Puestow procedure for retrograde drainage of the pancreatic duct. Ann. Surg., 152:1037, 1960.

61. Passaro, E., Jr., Basso, N., and Walsh, J. H.: Calcium challenge in the Zollinger-Ellison syndrome. Surgery, 72:60, 1972.

62. Pavlov, I. P.: The Work of the Digestive Glands, trans. W. H. Thompson. London, Charles Griffin Company, 1910.

63. Pfeffer, R. B., Lazzarini-Robertson, A., Jr., Safadi, D., Mixter, G., Jr., Secoy, C. F., and Hinton, J. W.: Gradations of pancreatitis, edematous through hemorrhagic, experimentally produced by controlled injection of microspheres into blood vessels in dogs. Surgery, 51:764, 1962.

64. Polk, H. C., Jr., Zeppa, R., and Warren, W. D.: Surgical significance of differentiation between acute and chronic pancreatic collections. Ann. Surg., 169:444, 1969.

65. Popper, H. L., Necheles, H., and Russell, K. C.: Transition of pancreatic edema into pancreatic necrosis. Surg. Gynecol. Obstet., 87:79, 1948.

66. Puestow, C. B., and Gillesby, W. J.: Retrograde surgical drainage of the pancreas for chronic relapsing pancreatitis. Arch. Surg., 76:898, 1958.

67. Ranson, J. H. C., Rifkind, K. M., Roger, D. F., Fink, S. D., Eng, F., and Spencer, F. C.: Prognostic signs and the role of operative management in acute pancreatitis. Surg. Gynecol. Obstet., 138:69, 1974.

68. Ranson, J. H. C., Turner, J. W., Roger, D. F., Rifkind, K. M., and Spencer, F. C.: Respiratory complications in acute pancreatitis. Ann. Surg., *179*:557, 1974.

69. Robertson, G. C., and Eeles, G. H.: Syndrome associated with pancreatic acinar cell carcinoma. Br. Med. J., *2*:708, 1970.

70. Ross, D. E.: Cancer of the pancreas. A plea for total pancreatectomy. Am. J. Surg., *87*:20, 1954.

71. Sawyers, J. L., Finch, W. T., and Schenker, S.: Prospective study to determine the efficacy of antibiotics in acute pancreatitis. Ann. Surg., *183*:667, 1976.

72. Schindler, S. C., Schaefer, J. W., Hull, D., and Griffin, W. O.: Chronic pancreatic ascites. Gastroenterology, *59*:453, 1970.

73. Schein, P. S., DeLellis, R. A., Kahn, C. R., Gorden, P., and Kraft, A. R.: Islet cell tumors: Current concepts and management. Ann. Intern. Med., *79*:239, 1973.

74. Schumer, W., McDonald, G. O., Nichols, R. L., and Miller, B.: Transgastric cystogastrostomy. Surg. Gynecol. Obstet., *137*:48, 1973.

75. Silen, W., Baldwin, J., and Goldman, L.: Treatment of chronic pancreatitis by longitudinal pancreaticojejunostomy. Am. J. Surg., *106*:234, 1963.

76. Smith, R. B., Warren, W. D., Rivard, A. A., and Amerson, J. R.: Pancreatic ascites: Diagnosis and management with particular reference to surgical techniques. Ann. Surg., *177*:538, 1973.

77. Trapnell, J. E., and Anderson, M. C.: Role of early laparotomy in acute pancreatitis. Ann. Surg., *165*:49, 1967.

78. Trapnell, J. E., Rigby, C. C., Talbot, C. H., and Duncan, E. H. L.: A controlled trial of Trasylol in the treatment of acute pancreatitis. Br. J. Surg., *61*:177, 1974.

79. Verner, J. V., and Morrison, A. B.: Endocrine pancreatic islet disease with diarrhea: Report of a case due to diffuse hyperplasia of non-beta islet tissue with a review of 54 additional cases. Arch. Intern. Med., *133*:492, 1974.

80. Von Mering, J., and Minkowski, O.: Diabetes Mellitus nach Pancreasexstirpation. Arch. Exp. Pathol. Pharmakol., *26*:371, 1889.

81. Warren, K. W., Athanassiades, S., Frederick, P., and Kune, G. A.: Surgical treatment of pancreatic pseudocysts: Review of 183 cases. Ann. Surg., *163*:886, 1966.

82. Warren, K. W., Braasch, J. H., and Thum, C. W.: Diagnosis and surgical treatment of carcinoma of the pancreas. Curr. Probl. Surg., June, 1968.

83. Warren, W. D., Leite, C. A., Baumeister, F., Poucher, R. L., and Kalser, M. H.: Clinical and metabolic response to radical distal pancreatectomy for chronic pancreatitis. Am. J. Surg., *113*:77, 1967.

84. Warren, W. D., Marsh, W. H., and Sandusky, W. R.: An appraisal of surgical procedures for pancreatic pseudocyst. Ann. Surg., *147*:903, 1958.

85. Waterman, M. G., Walsky, R., Kasdan, M. L., and Abrams, B. L.: The treatment of acute hemorrhagic pancreatitis by sump drainage. Surg. Gynecol. Obstet., *126*:963, 1968.

86. Watts, G. T.: Total pancreatectomy for fulminant pancreatitis. Lancet, *2*:384, 1963.

87. Webster, P. D., and Zieve, L.: Alterations in serum content of pancreatic enzymes. N. Engl. J. Med., *267*:604, 1962.

88. Webster, P. D., and Zieve, L.: Alterations in serum content of pancreatic enzymes. N. Engl. J. Med., *267*:654, 1962.

89. Whipple, A. O., and Frantz, V. K.: Adenoma of islet-cells with hyperinsulinism. A review. Ann. Surg., *101*:1299, 1935.

90. Whipple, A. O., Parsons, W. W., and Mullins, C. R.: Treatment of carcinoma of the ampulla of Vater. Ann. Surg., *1027*:763, 1935.

91. White, T. T., and Keith, R. G.: Long term follow-up study of fifty patients with pancreaticojejunostomy. Surg. Gynecol. Obstet., *136*:353, 1973.

92. White, T. T., Lawinski, M., Stacher, G., Pangtay Tea, J., Michoulier, J. M., Jr., and Mallet-Guy, P.: The treatment of pancreatitis by left splanchnicectomy and coeliac ganglionectomy. An analysis of 146 cases. Am. J. Surg., *112*:195, 1966.

93. Zinner, M. J., Baker, R. R., and Cameron, J. L.: Pancreatic cutaneous fistulas. Surg. Gynecol. Obstet., *138*:710, 1974.

94. Zollinger, R. M., and Ellison, E. H.: Primary peptic ulcerations of the jejunum associated with islet-cell tumors of the pancreas. Ann. Surg., *142*:709, 1955.

38

THE SPLEEN

Gordon W. Philpott, M.D.,
and Walter F. Ballinger, M.D.

Knowledge of splenic function and splenic disorders has become of increasing importance to the surgeon. Many diseases of the spleen, both primary and secondary, will respond to splenectomy. The operative techniques are seldom a problem for most well-trained surgeons. All too frequently, however, important preoperative and postoperative decisions depend entirely upon the wisdom and judgment of the hematologist. For optimal patient management, the surgeon must evaluate the advisability and proper timing of splenectomy with a clear understanding of the disease process and the risks attendant upon surgical intervention.

HISTORICAL ASPECTS

The spleen has been of interest to many scientific and nonscientific authors for over 2000 years. Galen regarded it as an organ full of mystery, and interesting and imaginative functions such as mirth, anger, and speed in running have been ascribed to the spleen.

A more realistic role of the spleen as a filtering mechanism was suggested by physicians and philosophers such as Plato and Aretaeus, who believed that the spleen "strained black blood or black bile" and helped keep the liver "bright and pure." Aretaeus of Cappadocia (c. A.D. 150) recognized splenic enlargement, which he thought was due to a derangement in this hypothetically important "black bile."

Marcello Malpighi (1659) first described some of the microscopic anatomy of the spleen, including the malpighian corpuscles. He also conclusively demonstrated that the spleen was an organ of the vascular system, located in the splanchnic bed.

Matthis, Barbette, Clark, and Morgagni published some of the earliest studies on the effects of splenectomy in the dog. Each of these investigators clearly showed that the spleen was not necessary for a healthy life, just as Aristotle had suggested centuries before.

Although post-traumatic splenectomies may have been performed by military surgeons earlier, splenectomy for nontraumatic disorders was first performed in the modern era by Quittenbaum (1826) and Wells (1876). Survival, however, was not achieved until 1887, when Spencer Wells removed the spleen of a pa-

tient with hereditary spherocytosis. Plagued by problems with hemorrhage and infection, surgeons for the next 35 years seldom performed the operation, except for trauma, twisted splenic pedicle, or massive tumors. Splenectomy in leukemia was particularly disastrous and the lack of any survivors caused physicians and surgeons to abandon the operation in all patients with leukemia. Only recently has this ban been lifted in carefully selected patients with hypersplenism from leukemic infiltration.[25, 29]

As techniques have improved, splenectomy for the cure or alleviation of hematologic disease once again has become accepted. Since Moynihan (1921) wrote exhaustive reviews on splenectomy, little has been added to the techniques of splenectomy. Important advances have occurred in understanding splenic function and dysfunction and in new methods of diagnosis of hematologic disease. Some of these investigations will be mentioned in the appropriate sections.

ANATOMY

During early embryonic life, the spleen develops from the coalescence of several small subperitoneal swellings. These mesodermal masses arise in the left side of the dorsal mesogastrium, and by 3 months of gestation, they have merged into the adult form of a spleen, occasionally maintaining persistent fetal lobulations. The dorsal mesogastrium becomes the gastrosplenic ligament containing the short gastric vessels. The peritoneal reflections from the splenic capsule to adjacent organs form the surgically important suspensory ligaments of the spleen. These are the splenophrenic, splenorenal, and splenocolic, as well as the gastrosplenic (Fig. 1).

Accessory spleens occur in 14 to 30 per cent of those requiring splenectomy for hematologic diseases. These probably arise from the failure of complete coalescence of normal primordial spleen buds or the formation of spleen buds in unusually distant locations. Another possible explanation is that some splenic tissue becomes pinched off the main mass during development. The most common locations for accessory spleens are in the hilus, in the various suspensory ligaments of the spleen, particularly the gastrosplenic and spleno-

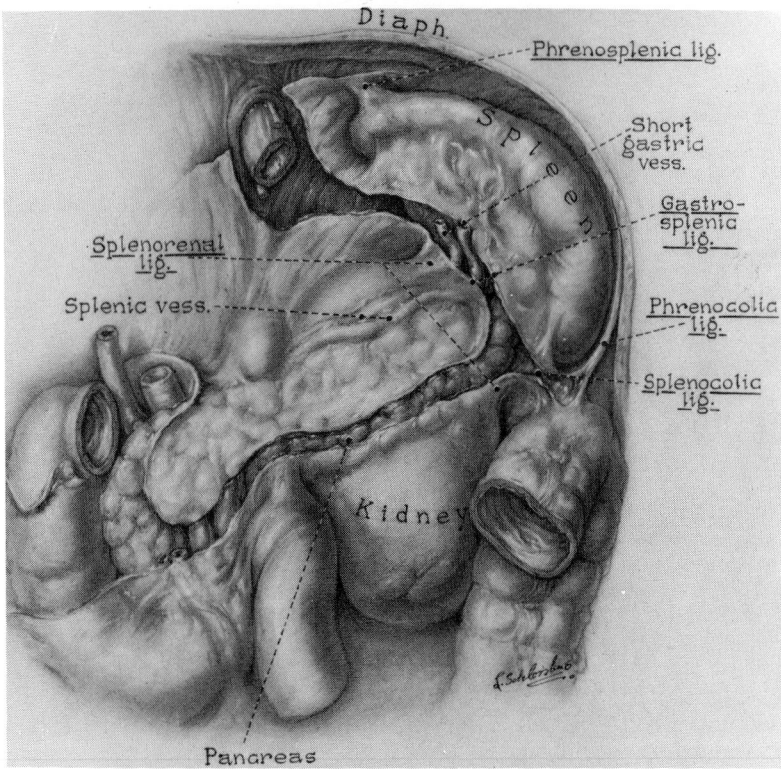

Figure 1. Suspensory ligaments of the spleen. (From Splenectomy, by Ballinger, W. F., and Erslev, A. J., in Current Problems in Surgery, edited by Ravitch, M. M., et al. Copyright © 1965, Year Book Medical Publishers. Used by permission.)

colic ligaments, and in the greater omentum. Accessory splenic tissue also rarely occurs in the mesentery of the gastrointestinal tract, or in the pelvis (Fig. 2).

The spleen is a highly vascular organ composed of a specialized capillary bed between the splenic artery and portal venous system. The normal adult spleen weighs approximately 100 to 225 gm., and is usually not palpable. It is bordered superiorly and laterally by the diaphragm and lower rib cage, inferiorly by the colon, medially by the stomach, and posteriorly by the kidney. The tail of the pancreas extends into the hilus and often is quite close to the spleen. Peritoneal attachments from the surrounding structures to the splenic capsule are of surgical importance. The splenophrenic, splenorenal, and splenocolic ligaments are usually relatively avascular and can be easily transected to bring the spleen and hilus medially and anteriorly into the level of the wound. All of the suspensory ligaments of the spleen, however, contain collaterals, which can be quite large with impairment of the splenic venous or arterial blood flow. The gastrosplenic ligament, containing the short gastric vessels, extends from the greater curvature of the fundus and body of the stomach to the spleen. This ligament is often extremely short in the superior portion and transection must be done carefully. The splenic pedicle, located in the most medial portion of the splenorenal ligament, contains the splenic artery, vein, and lymphatics, and often the tail of the pancreas. The

splenic artery arises from the celiac plexus and follows an irregular course along the superior border of the pancreas. The splenic vein, which is just inferior to the artery, courses posterior to the pancreas before joining the hepatic portal system.

The vessels enter the hilus and branch out along the trabeculae, which form the connective tissue framework, dividing the spleen into smaller and smaller interconnected compartments. Branches of the trabecular arteries pass into both the white pulp and red pulp, proceeding peripherally to communicate through capillaries and sinuses with the venous channels, located in the marginal areas (Fig. 3). The complex microcirculation through the splenic substance is incompletely understood, but the distribution of blood flow is at least partially controlled by an opening and closing of the smaller central arteries and arterioles leading into the splenic sinuses.

The white pulp is composed of lymphatic tissue and lymphoid follicles, or malpighian bodies, that surround the central arteries. They contain predominantly lymphocytes, plasma cells, and macrophages distributed throughout a reticular network.

The marginal zone between the red and white pulp is an ill-defined vascular space that varies in size, depending upon its contents. Sometimes it contains only plasma and, at other times, a variety of cellular elements. Foreign materials are preferentially sequestered in this zone, as well as in the red pulp.

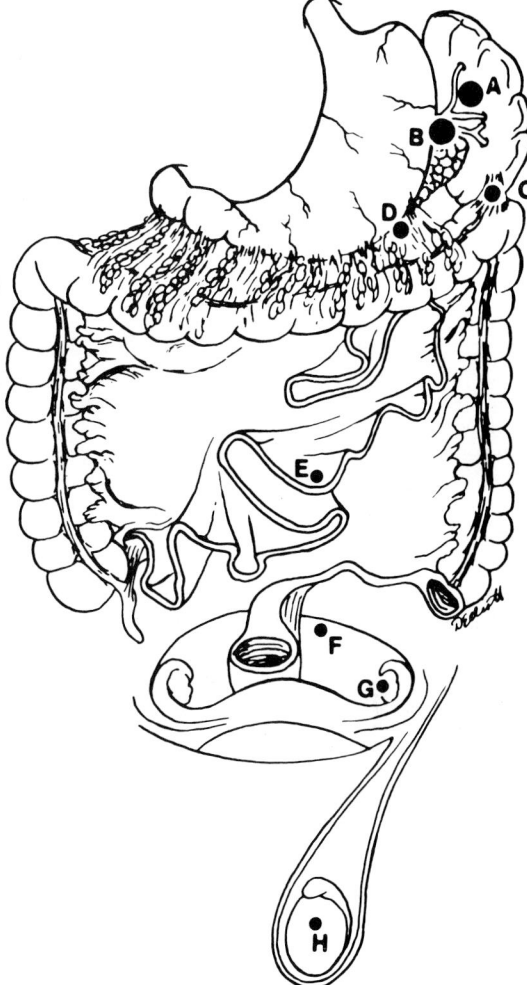

Figure 2. Location of accessory spleens. *A,* Splenic hilus. B, Adjacent to splenic vessels and tail of pancreas. *C,* Splenocolic ligament. *D,* Greater omentum. *E,* Mesentery. *F.* Presacral region. *G,* Adnexal region. *H,* Peritesticular. (From Splenectomy for hematological disorders, by Schwartz, S., et al., in Current Problems in Surgery, edited by Ravitch, M. M., et al. Copyright © 1971, Year Book Medical Publishers. Used by permission.)

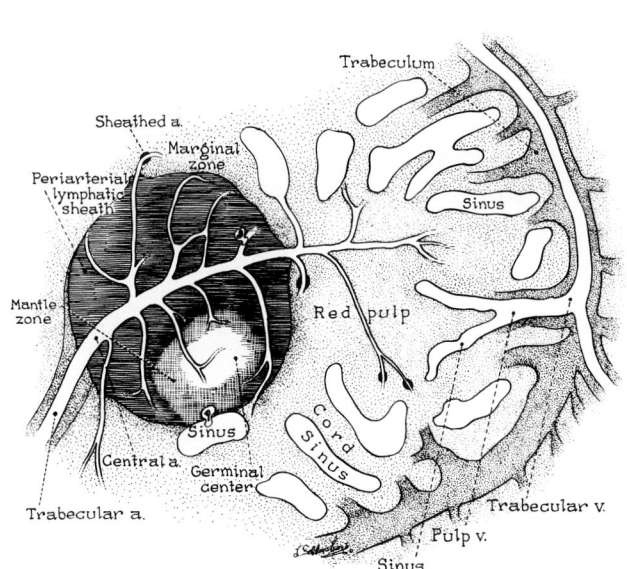

Figure 3. Microcirculation of the spleen. (From Weiss, L. In: Greep, R. O., ed.: Histology. Copyright 1966, McGraw-Hill Book Company. Used with permission of McGraw-Hill Book Company.)

The red pulp is composed of interconnected cords of reticular cells, which form an irregular honeycomb throughout the red pulp. The sinuses lie between the cords and provide meandering channels from the arterial to the venous circulations. There is considerable variation in the size and type of connections between the central arterioles, after they leave the white pulp, and the cords and sinuses. Some end as terminal vessels in the cords. Others empty into the sinuses by tiny openings. Phagocytes line some of the capillaries directly beneath the endothelial membrane, accounting for much of the filtering of foreign material by the spleen. Although the splenic sinuses are 35 to 40 μ in diameter, they have frequent gaps of 2 to 3 μ in their lining membrane, which constrict and impede erythrocytes as they move between the cords and sinuses.

Blood flows through the spleen by a number of these different routes. Normal healthy blood elements pass rapidly through the normal spleen by any number of the various routes. Abnormal or aged elements, on the other hand, are often retarded and entrapped in the normal splenic substance. When the spleen is enlarged, even normal blood elements can be impeded and engulfed, giving rise to a hypersplenic state.

PHYSIOLOGY AND PATHOPHYSIOLOGY

The human spleen has a number of well-known functions, including the filtering of blood elements and foreign material, hematopoiesis, and, in some situations, the production of lymphocytes and antibodies. It may also have an endocrinologic role as a partial regulator of bone marrow function, but available data are inconclusive. The fact that normal health is possible without a spleen indicates that other tissues in the body can assume these duties when the spleen is absent.

Approximately 350 liters of blood flows through a normal spleen daily. Normal blood elements usually pass rapidly through the spleen, while defective and aged cells and foreign material are removed. The mechanisms by which abnormal cells are filtered are not completely defined. The slitlike gaps and narrow channels in the cords and sinuses are undoubtedly one

way that the spleen can retain odd-shaped cells, such as spherocytes and elliptocytes. The methods of filtering normal-shaped cells, with either abnormal particles or membrane coating, are not known. Chromium (^{51}Cr) tagging experiments have shown that normally few cells are filtered in one passage through the spleen, attesting to the efficiency by which the bone marrow produces cells of standard size and shape. The normal bone marrow, however, does make a significant number of cells with abnormal particles, which usually appear in the circulation after splenectomy. These include Howell-Jolly bodies, siderocytes, Pappenheimer bodies, and Heinz bodies (Fig. 4). The spleen can clean out bits of cellular "debris," such as these fragments of nuclear and cytoplasmic material, without necessarily removing the cells. Sequestration of these cells not only allows the spleen to cleanse and filter abnormal cells and particles, but permits a weakening and "aging" of the erythrocytes. Although this process is not well understood, crowding in the pulp probably leads to glucose deprivation, reduction in high-energy phosphates, and deterioration of the sodium pump. With each incident of congestion, this metabolic damage increases, until the aged cell is phagocytized by the reticuloendothelial system. In a normal person, this amounts to 20 ml. of red cells daily. The spleen may also participate in the maturation of erythrocytes, by somehow altering the volume-surface ratio. Target cells (Fig. 4) temporarily appear after splenectomy, suggesting a disproportionate shrinkage in red cell volume, until other tissue in the body takes over the functions of the spleen. After splenectomy in patients without hematologic diseases, anemia and polycythemia do not occur, and red cell survival remains unchanged. These facts suggest that the filtering function of the spleen is quickly assumed by remaining reticuloendothelial tissue and that red cell production must decrease, since a significant vascular component is removed by splenectomy, without ensuing polycythemia.

Normal leukocytes are removed from the circulation by the reticuloendothelial system, including the spleen. When the spleen is removed, a temporary leukocytosis occurs, predominantly a lymphocytosis. This is of no known consequence, except that it can

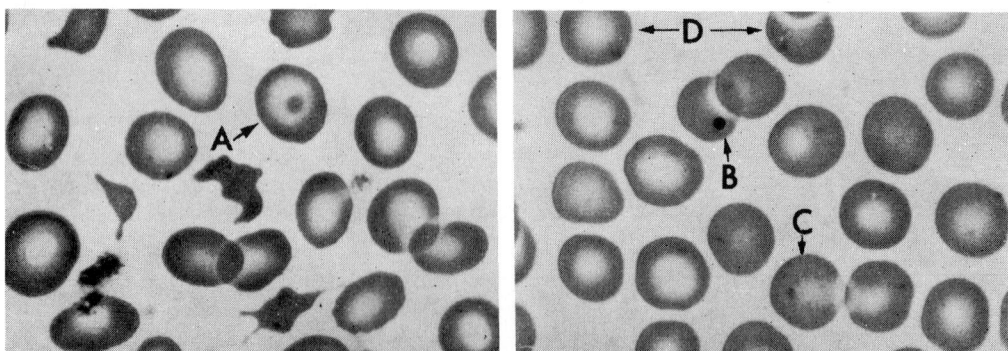

Figure 4. Photomicrograph of blood smears of patients splenectomized because of idiopathic thrombocytopenic purpura. Note the target cell (A), the Howell-Jolly body (B), the stippling (C), and the barely perceptible Pappenheimer bodies (D). (From Wintrobe, M. M.: Clinical Hematology. 6th ed. Philadelphia, Lea & Febiger, 1967.)

confuse the postoperative picture. In the rare disorder splenic neutropenia, leukocytes are preferentially removed by the spleen.

Platelets are also filtered out of the circulation by the spleen. When coated with antibodies, platelets are removed at a much greater rate, giving rise to thrombocytopenia. Following splenectomy, the circulating levels of both the coated and normal platelets rise, sometimes to over 1 million per cubic millimeter. The cause of this thrombocytosis has never been adequately determined. One hypothesis is that it is simply a matter of decreasing sequestration and destruction of platelets. Another hypothesis is that the splenectomy also removes a suppressant of bone marrow platelet production or release; and still another hypothesis is that the bone marrow is geared to regulate the overall platelet mass at a certain size, and when a compartment normally containing a significant portion of the platelet pool is removed, the overall platelet concentration rises.

The reticuloendothelial cells in the adult spleen are involved in the normal production of monocytes, lymphocytes, and plasma cells. Hematopoiesis of the other blood elements occurs in the fetal spleen but normally stops between the sixth and eighth months of gestation. Hematopoietic stem cells then remain in the spleen in a dormant state, but can be reactivated after a prolonged and intense demand for blood cell formation. This extramedullary hematopoiesis apparently is performed in a less favorable environment than in the bone marrow, because there is often cell death in situ and premature release of early erythroid and myeloid cells. The mature cells are characterized by a great deal of anisocytosis and poikilocytosis. Megakaryocyte fragments and giant platelets are often observed. However, it is possible that this dyshematopoiesis is related to the underlying disease process, rather than to the extramedullary hematopoiesis per se. Thus, for example, in myeloid metaplasia, the abnormal proliferation of the primitive mesenchymal precursors from which the hematopoietic system takes origin leads to overgrowth of connective tissue in the bone marrow and reactivation of marrow stem cells in the spleen and liver, and might explain the close association of polycythemia vera, myeloid metaplasia, and myelogenous leukemia.

Antibodies are normally produced by cells within the spleen. Splenectomy can lead to a slight temporary reduction in antibody formation. In acquired hemolytic anemia, splenic neutropenia, and idiopathic thrombocytopenic purpura, antibodies to specific cellular elements are produced. Splenectomy then not only will remove an organ designed to sequester antibody-coated cells, but also will reduce antibody production, at least temporarily.

HYPERSPLENISM

Hypersplenism is the inappropriate sequestration and destruction of blood elements with reduction in circulating red blood cells, white blood cells, or platelets.

Primary hypersplenism includes a group of diseases in which the spleen becomes hypertrophic in response to a sustained and heavy workload (Table 1). In these conditions, the abnormal cells or platelets are removed so efficiently that the resulting cytopenia becomes of greater concern than the presence of the abnormal cells.

Secondary hypersplenism includes a group of diseases (Table 1) in which an enlarged spleen leads to increased destruction of normal or abnormal blood cells or platelets. Secondary hypersplenism can thus be caused by primary hypersplenism, by inflammation, by congestion, by ingestion of macromolecular

TABLE 1. Classification of Potential Hypersplenic Disorders

Primary hypersplenism
  Congenital hemolytic anemia
    Hereditary spherocytosis
    Hereditary elliptocytosis
    Pyruvate kinase deficiency
    Hemoglobinopathies (sickle cell anemia, etc.)
    Thalassemia
    Porphyria hematopoietica
  Acquired hemolytic anemia: "autoimmune"
  Idiopathic thrombocytopenic purpura
  Thrombotic thrombocytopenic purpura
  Primary splenic neutropenia
  Primary splenic pancytopenia
Secondary hypersplenism
  Inflammation
    Acute: typhoid fever, rubella, chickenpox, etc.
    Bacterial subacute endocarditis
    Chronic
      Tuberculosis
      Syphilis
      Boeck's sarcoid
      Beryllium disease
      Rheumatoid arthritis (Felty's syndrome)
      Disseminated lupus erythematosus
      Malaria
      Trypanosomiasis
      Schistosomiasis
      Leishmaniasis
      Echinococcosis
      Histoplasmosis
      Cryptococcosis
  Congestion
    Cirrhosis of liver
    Portal vein obstruction
    Splenic vein obstruction
    Congestive heart failure
  Ingestion
    Gaucher's disease
    Neimann-Pick disease
    Amyloidosis
    Hyperlipemia
  Infiltration
    "Benign": infectious mononucleosis
    "Neoplastic"
      Hodgkin's disease
      Lymphoma
      Leukemia
      Agnogenic myeloid metaplasia
      Histiocytosis (Hand-Schüller-Christian; Letterer-Siwe)
      Polycythemia vera

colloids, or by infiltration of normal or abnormal cells. It must be emphasized that splenomegaly is not necessarily associated wtih hypersplenism (e.g., splenic cysts or some cases of infectious mononucleosis), and conversely, pancytopenia may be associated with splenomegaly without being caused by it (e.g., bone marrow failure with secondary extramedullary hematopoiesis). It is usually necessary in patients with cytopenias to evaluate splenic activity in relation to bone marrow function before splenectomy is considered. Even in some patients with severe hypoplasia of the bone marrow (e.g., aplastic anemia), splenectomy has proved to be of benefit when splenic sequestration exists.[8]

Diagnostic Evaluation of Hypersplenism

The decision to perform a therapeutic splenectomy depends upon an accurate assessment both of the size of the spleen and of the degree of hypersplenism. An enlarged spleen usually can be demonstrated by careful physical examination, roentgenographic examination, or radioisotopic scanning. The spleen normally cannot be palpated or percussed. Splenomegaly can result in significant dullness to percussion at or above the left ninth intercostal space. Bimanual examination, with the left side of the patient tilted upward, will often help in the differentiation between an enlarged spleen (with its typical notch) and the left lobe of the liver, a pancreatic cyst, a large left kidney, or a colonic tumor.

A normal spleen usually can be outlined on a supine x-ray of the abdomen. An enlarged spleen displaces the stomach medially and inferiorly and the splenic flexure of the colon posteriorly and inferiorly. The outline of the spleen can be accentuated by introducing air or contrast material into the stomach or colon. Tomograms may also be of assistance in outlining an atypical spleen, but are seldom necessary.

Two generally available methods for radioisotopic scanning are useful. In the first method, autogenous erythrocytes are heated to 50° C. for 1 hour and tagged with ⁵¹Cr. The heated red blood cells become spheroid and are trapped and destroyed by the spleen, which is then selectively visualized by scintillation scanning. A less selective method, but one giving as good or better results, employs a sulfur colloid linked to indium-113m or to technetium-99m, which is picked up by the reticuloendothelial system, predominantly in the liver and the spleen (Fig. 5). In the future, newer scanning techniques using gallium-67 citrate or computerized axial tomography may prove to be helpful in identifying splenic abnormalities.

The functional abnormalities in hypersplenism may be revealed in the peripheral blood by anemia, leukopenia, or thrombocytopenia. However, the circulating red cells, white cells, or platelets can remain at normal levels indefinitely, because the bone marrow can increase its rate of hematopoiesis by a factor of 6 to 10 times, as long as the metabolic requirements are met. The peripheral blood smear may show characteristic abnormalities such as spherocytes, elliptocytes, target cells, leukoblasts, and megakaryocyte fragments.

The increased destruction of red cells that occurs in hemolytic anemia usually results in a compensatory rise in the rate of erythrocyte production, as evidenced by increases in the reticulocyte count, the erythroid-myeloid ratio in the bone marrow, and the turnover of iron. There are frequently elevations of the serum bilirubin and fecal urobilinogen, and gallstones are common. In acquired hemolytic anemia, the Coombs test is often positive, indicating abnormal protein coating of the red cells that may or may not be due to true "autoantibodies."

Splenic sequestration and destruction of red blood cells can be evaluated indirectly by measuring the rate of cellular destruction or the degree of compensatory production, and directly by measuring splenic sequestration of labeled cells. Transfusion requirements will give a rough, but useful, estimate of the rate of red cell destruction. Since the adult human

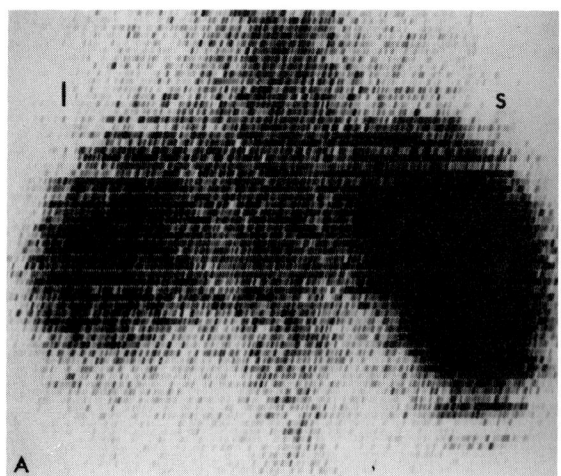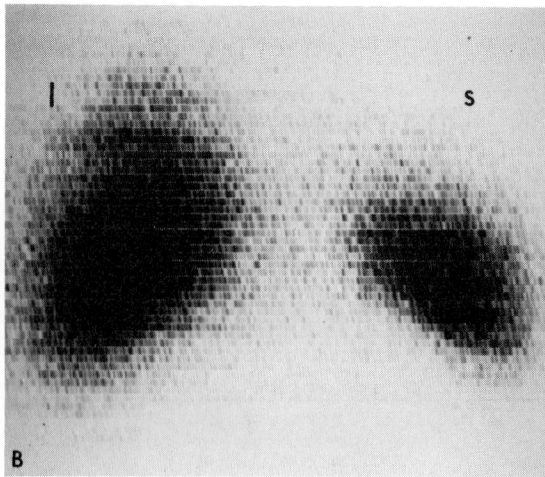

Figure 5. Two technetium-sulfur colloid spleen and liver scans, showing in (A) an enlarged spleen (s) on the right side of the scan, and in (B) a normal-sized spleen (s). Both scintiscans were taken from the posterior, so that the spleen (s) in each is outlined on the right-hand side and the liver (l) on the left. The scan in (A) is from a patient with splenomegaly due to portal hypertension. (Courtesy of Dr. E. J. Potchen, Department of Radiology, Washington University, St. Louis, Missouri.)

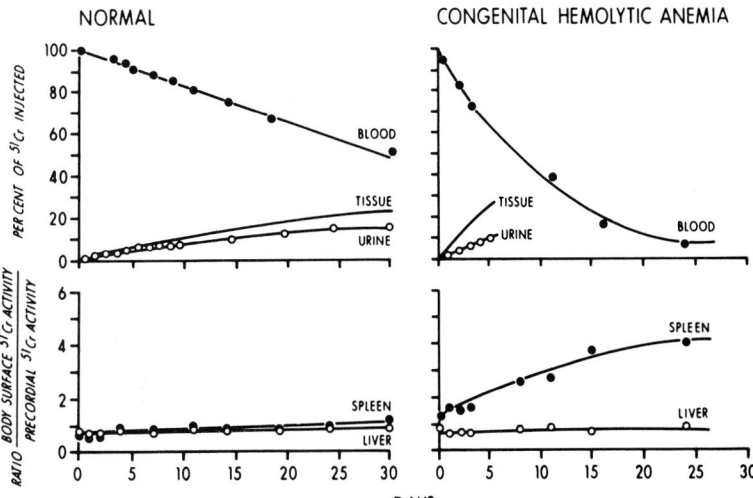

Figure 6. Chromium-51-labeled erythrocyte determinations in normal and hemolytic anemia. In hemolytic anemia, radioactivity disappears from the circulation and accumulates in the tissue much more rapidly than normal, with the spleen taking up more ^{51}Cr than does the liver. (From Splenectomy for hematological disorders, by Schwartz, S., et al., in Current Problems in Surgery, edited by Ravitch, M. M., et al. Copyright © 1971, Year Book Medical Publishers. Used by permission. After Jandl. J., et al., J. Clin. Invest., 35:842, 1956.)

loses approximately 20 ml. of red cells per day, under normal conditions, in 10 days he will have lost approximately 200 ml. of erythrocytes (blood volume × hematocrit × $\frac{1}{RBC\ life\ span}$ or, in a 70 kg. man, 5000 × 48/100 × 1/120 = 20 ml.). Thus, if the transfusion requirements are in excess of one unit of blood every 10 days, it can be assumed that the patient has a shortened red cell life span with accelerated destruction.

A more sophisticated measurement of the rate of disappearance of red cells from the circulation and the sequestration of these cells in the spleen utilizes ^{51}Cr-tagged autologous erythrocytes. A measured half-life of less than 20 to 25 days is considered an accelerated rate of red cell destruction. The relative role of the spleen in this destruction of erythrocytes can be further assessed by daily scanning over the spleen, liver, and precordium (Fig. 6). A selective rise in the ratio of radioactivity in the spleen as compared to the liver or precordium suggests significant splenic sequestration. With this technique, a satisfactory result from splenectomy may be predicted with a degree of accuracy approaching 90 per cent in situations in which the half-life of ^{51}Cr-labeled erythrocytes is below 50 per cent of normal (less than 15 days) and the spleen-liver ratio is greater than two.

The normal half-life of circulating granulocytes is so short (6 to 12 days) that attempts to assess a decreased longevity of leukocytes have not been clinically helpful. Also, there is no satisfactory clinical method of correlating metabolic effects of increased destruction of leukocytes and the relative importance of the spleen in this destruction.

Determination of platelet life span, using ^{51}Cr tagging, has been of some clinical usefulness in evaluating increased destruction of thrombocytes.[3, 29] The normal life span of 7 to 10 days can be significantly reduced in patients with splenomegaly and in many cases of idiopathic thrombocytopenic purpura. When thrombocytopenia is due to increased destruction, the bone marrow will often show a compensatory increase in immature megakaryocytes. Evaluation of the use of surface scanning after injection of ^{51}Cr-labeled platelets is still incomplete. This technique may eventually prove to be a helpful diagnostic test in predicting the value of splenectomy.

POTENTIAL HYPERSPLENIC DISORDERS AMENABLE TO SPLENECTOMY

Table 1 lists a classification of disorders in which splenectomy may be therapeutic. "Primary hypersplenism," as used in this classification, includes the hematologic disorders in which hypersplenism occurs in association with a spleen that is not afflicted with another disease. "Secondary hypersplenism" includes diseases in which hyperactivity results from splenomegaly due secondarily to a variety of other hematologic and nonhematologic disorders. Although this classification is useful in consideration of hypersplenic disorders, it is somewhat arbitrary. A number of authors prefer to limit the term "primary hypersplenism" to primary splenic neutropenia and to primary splenic pancytopenia.[25, 29]

CONGENITAL HEMOLYTIC ANEMIAS

Hereditary Spherocytosis

Spherocytic anemia is also called familial hemolytic anemia, chronic hereditary hemolytic jaundice, and chronic acholuric jaundice. Since Minkowski (1900) first described the familial associations, this disease is now known to be transmitted as an autosomal dominant trait, causing a defect in the red cell membrane. It is characterized by small, dense spheroid erythrocytes that have increased osmotic fragility, as first demonstrated by Chaufford in 1907. As the spherocytes pass into the splenic pulp, they are impeded by the normal gaps and channels, resulting in glucose and ATP deprivation, membrane fragmentation, and cell disruption.

Besides the familial history, the common clinical

manifestations are anemia, jaundice, and spleno-megaly. The anemia is usually not severe, with hemo-globin determinations ranging between 9 and 12 gm. per 100 ml. Anemic "crises" with fever, chills, abdom-inal pain, vomiting, tachycardia, and dyspnea are not uncommon. They are accompanied by jaundice and increased reticulocytosis and occasionally are severe enough to be fatal. Cholelithiasis occurs in 30 to 60 per cent of these patients, but is uncommon before 10 years of age.[3, 25]

Spherocytes can be identified from peripheral blood smears and osmotic fragility tests. Also, spontaneous autohemolysis tests demonstrate an increased lysis of erythrocytes, which is partially corrected by the addi-tion of glucose or adenosine triphosphate (Table 2).

Splenectomy is the treatment of choice and should be performed as soon as the diagnosis is established, even with compensated hemolytic anemia. If gall-stones are present, concomitant cholecystectomy should also be performed. In very young patients, it is probably advisable to delay splenectomy until the third or fourth year. Although there is a difference of opinion among writers, splenectomy before the age of 4 years may predispose to an increased risk of in-fection.

Hereditary Elliptocytosis

This is a familial disease that is usually of little clinical significance. It is characterized by oval and rod-shaped erythrocytes that constitute 50 to 90 per cent of the red cells on peripheral blood smears. Re-ticulocytosis and hyperbilirubinemia respond well to splenectomy in the few patients who do have ane-mia.[3, 25, 29]

Pyruvate-Kinase (P-K) Deficiency

This disorder is one of the nonspherocytic hereditary hemolytic anemias first described by Baty in 1930. It is caused by an autosomal recessive defect in the en-zymatic synthesis of high-energy phosphates (ATP) from glucose utilization. Homozygous patients have a high infant mortality. Those who survive develop

poorly and have a severe macrocytic hemolytic anemia with splenomegaly. Studies with ^{51}Cr-tagged erythro-cytes show that the spleen is a major site for hemol-ysis. Splenectomy can help these patients by reducing the transfusion requirements and improving the anemia.[3, 25] It is important to distinguish between P-K deficiency and the numerous other forms of hereditary nonspherocytic hemolytic anemias caused by glucose-6-phosphate dehydrogenase (G-6-PD) deficiencies. The multiple genetic variants that give rise to G-6-PD-deficient red cells seldom cause splenomegaly and do not require splenectomy. The autohemolysis test will distinguish between these enzyme-deficient patients. The proportion of hemolyzed red cells after incubation at 37° C. for 48 hours, without glucose, is greater than normal with P-K deficiency, but not with G-6-PD deficiency (Table 2). Furthermore, the addition of glucose to the media will not reduce the autohemolysis with P-K deficiency as it does with normal cells, with spherocytes, and to some extent with G-6-PD-deficient cells. The addition of ATP reduces the hemolysis in all the hereditary hemolytic anemias as it does with nor-mal erythrocytes.

Sickle Cell Anemia

This disorder, first described by Herrick in 1910, is the most important disease of the group of hereditary hemoglobinopathies. An abnormality in the beta chain of hemoglobin produces the characteristic crescent-shaped, or sickled, red cells, under appropriate condi-tions of low oxygen tension. As a disease peculiar to Negroes, it is clinically manifested by episodes of acute abdominal pain, jaundice, bone and joint pains, hematuria, priapism, leg ulcers, and a variety of neurologic symptoms. In a few patients, splenic engorgement with hypersplenism and hemolytic crisis occurs early in the course of the disease. Splenectomy is helpful in these patients, to reduce transfusion requirements and to hasten the natural process of "au-tosplenectomy" that occurs in most patients by mul-tiple painful splenic infarctions over a period of years.[3, 25, 29]

Thalassemia Major

This disorder, known also as Cooley's anemia, Medi-terranean anemia, target cell anemia, and erythro-blastic anemia, was first described by Cooley and Lee in 1925. Transmitted as a dominant genetic trait, it is characterized by an ineffective production of abnormal erythrocytes owing to defects in the hemoglobin pep-tide chains. Clinical manifestations include a muddy yellow skin color, retarded growth with a large head and facial bones, cardiac dilatation, leg ulcers, inter-current infections, and hepatosplenomegaly. The hy-pochromic, microcytic anemia may be severe and the peripheral blood smear shows characteristic target cells with decreased osmotic fragility, fragmented forms, stippled cells, and multiple nucleated red blood cells. Reticulocyte and leukocyte counts are high, whereas platelet counts are usually normal. Serum bilirubin is usually only slightly elevated and serum iron is high, with a saturated iron-binding protein. Gallstones occur in about a quarter of the patients. Splenectomy can be palliative to decrease transfusion

TABLE 2. Autohemolysis Test—Per Cent Hemolysis, 37° C., 48 Hours*

Red Cells	Without Glucose	With Glucose	With Adenosine Triphosphate
Normal	2–6%	<1%	
Hereditary spherocytosis	10–20%		
Pyruvate-kinase deficiency	10–20%		
Glucose-6-phosphate dehydrogenase deficiency	2–6%	2–3%	2–3%

*From Splenectomy by Ballinger, W. F., and Erslev, A. J., in Current Problems in Surgery, edited by Ravitch, M. M., et al. Copyright © 1965. Year Book Medical Publishers. Used by permission.

requirements and to eliminate an enlarged uncomfortable spleen.[3, 25, 29]

Porphyria Hematopoietica

This is an extremely rare disorder caused by an intrinsic defect in porphyrin synthesis of red cells, leading to hemolysis and accelerated red cell production. The porphyrins cause excessive photosensitivity and debilitating bullous dermatitis. The hypersplenic condition can be greatly benefited by splenectomy.[3, 25, 29]

ACQUIRED HEMOLYTIC ANEMIA

Nonhereditary hemolytic anemias can be acquired during life by exposure to a variety of chemicals, drugs, bacteria, and physical agents. These can usually be alleviated by removal of the offending agent and temporary support with corticosteroids and transfusions.[8, 29] There is also a type of hemolytic anemia that is of unknown etiology and that is believed to be due to an autoimmune mechanism. This type of acquired hemolytic anemia was first described by Chauffard and Troisier in 1908 and is more common in women over 50 years of age. Clinically, it may be manifested as a chronic and rather mild anemia or as an acute fulminant crisis with chills, fever, backache, jaundice, hemoglobinuria, and uremia. Splenomegaly occurs in over half of the cases, and gallstones are not uncommon. The patient's red cells are coated with abnormal proteins and the serum of these patients contains gamma globulins that agglutinate their own as well as normal erythrocytes. The coated and agglutinated red cells are trapped by the entire reticuloendothelial system, including the spleen. The positive direct and indirect Coombs tests in these patients indicate abnormal protein coating of erythrocytes and antibodies in the serum. They do not prove the presence of a true "autoantibody" to red cells, however, since the tests could be positive because of nonspecific adsorption of various previously formed antigen-antibody complexes.[3, 25, 29]

Corticosteroids and transfusions are relatively successful therapy, with 55 to 90 per cent of the patients showing remission. Only about 25 per cent maintain it, however, and then long-term steroid therapy or splenectomy is needed. Transfusion matching may be extremely difficult, and carefully washed red cells and potent saline-active antisera are often needed to obtain a successful crossmatch. Splenectomy is indicated when corticosteroids cannot be given, or are ineffective after 4 to 6 weeks. The demonstration of splenic sequestration of ^{51}Cr-tagged red cells, with a spleen to liver ratio greater than 2:1, indicates a favorable response to splenectomy. Immediate response occurs in about 50 per cent of unselected cases and in 80 per cent of cases with significant splenic sequestration. Relapses are frequent with all forms of therapy, but tend to be less frequent after a good response to splenectomy.[3, 8, 25, 29]

IDIOPATHIC THROMBOCYTOPENIC PURPURA

This disease, which is also known as purpura hemorrhagica and "immunologic" thrombocytopenic purpura, was first described as a clinical entity by Werlhof in 1735, and was first shown to be due to thrombocytopenia by Brohm in 1883. It is a syndrome characterized by decreased numbers of circulating platelets, abundant megakaryocytes in the bone marrow, and a shortened platelet life span; it probably has an immunologic pathogenesis. Much confusion has resulted from the inclusion of a number of disorders with purpura secondary to drug or toxic reactions, viral and bacterial infections, lymphoproliferative diseases, and disseminated lupus erythematosus in the category of idiopathic thrombocytopenic purpura (ITP). As the name implies, the etiology is unknown, and at present the term should be reserved for cases in which the well-known causes of secondary thrombocytopenia cannot be identified. The acute cases of ITP, which occur mostly in children, may represent responses to inapparent viral infections, but are still included in this syndrome. Chronic cases can occur at any age, but are most common in 15- to 35-year-old women.

A large majority of patients, particularly those with chronic ITP, have platelet-agglutinating and complement-fixing antibodies. A circulating antiplatelet factor, with the characteristics of an antibody, has been demonstrated in a large proportion of these patients, and normal transfused platelets are rapidly destroyed until splenectomy is performed.[8, 13]

The spleen plays an important role in this disease for two, and perhaps three, reasons. First, the spleen contributes to the production of the antiplatelet "antibodies." Whether these are true "autoantibodies" or antibodies directed against foreign antigens with adsorption of the antigen-antibody complex to the platelets is not known. In any case, slight temporary reduction in titers follows splenectomy. Platelet-agglutinating antibodies can be demonstrated in the circulation for some time after splenectomy, even in patients in clinical remission.[3, 25, 29] This attests to the second, and probably the most important, role of the spleen in this disease, namely the sequestration and removal of coated platelets. Harrington and associates demonstrated that blood from ITP patients, transfused into normal matched recipients, could cause rapid thrombocytopenia and that "sensitized" platelets are selectively sequestered in the spleen.[9, 13] The infusion of ^{51}Cr-tagged platelets causes a rise of radioactivity, predominantly in the spleen. The site of platelet removal may depend upon the severity of the disease, with the spleen filtering out "lightly" sensitized platelets and the liver removing the more "heavily" coated ones. Besides these two major roles, the spleen may have some suppressive effect on maturation or release, or both, of platelets from the bone marrow.[8] This, however, is still a controversial theory.

The clinical manifestations of ITP include petechiae, ecchymosis, epistaxis, bleeding gums, vaginal bleeding, gastrointestinal hemorrhage, hematuria, and central nervous system bleeding. The course is sometimes cyclic, with exacerbations occurring during menses. Palpable splenomegaly occurs in 2 to 3 per cent of patients. Laboratory findings include very low platelet counts, often 50,000 or less, prolonged bleeding times, normal clotting times, and increased capillary fragility. Platelet life spans are reduced and the bone marrow contains normal or increased numbers of megakaryocytes. Erythrocyte and leukocyte counts are usually normal.

The treatment of ITP depends upon the age of the patient, the severity of the disease, and the duration of thrombocytopenia. Acute ITP in children under the age of 16 years has an excellent prognosis, with approximately 80 per cent of patients having a complete and permanent spontaneous remission within 3 to 6 months.[25] Corticosteroids may be of use in the acute period to increase platelet levels and avert the danger of severe hemorrhage. The use of steroids, however, has not improved the overall prognosis for recovery, nor has it reduced the incidence of chronic ITP, which occurs in 10 to 20 per cent of these patients.

The proper treatment of chronic ITP and acute ITP in older patients is somewhat more controversial. Both corticosteroids and splenectomy are useful and effective therapy. Corticosteroids will increase circulating platelet levels in as high as 90 per cent of acute cases and in 60 per cent of chronic cases.[8] In most series, however, sustained clinical remissions are much less frequent with corticosteroids (Table 3), ranging from 14 to 38 per cent, depending upon the chronicity of the disease.[5, 6, 7, 9, 18] Furthermore, complications of prolonged administration of corticosteroids, such as nervousness, hyperglycemia, azotemia, and hypertension, are not uncommon.

Splenectomy, which was first advocated for this disease by Kaznelson in 1916, has proved to be a more effective therapy in chronic ITP (Table 3). An increase in platelets is almost always noted within 2 to 3 days of removal of all the splenic tissue, with circulating levels sometimes exceeding 1 to 2 million thrombocytes. Sustained remission occurs in 57 to 90 per cent of patients in reported series, with most "permanent" success rates more than 80 per cent (Table 3). As with corticosteroids, success rates are somewhat better with acute ITP than with the chronic disease. In most series, splenectomy has also proved effective following therapeutic failure with steroids (Table 3). Operative mortality is relatively low (1 to 3 per cent) with most surgical deaths occurring in emergency splenectomies done for uncontrolled hemorrhage.[25] Postoperative

complications occur in about 10 to 15 per cent of patients and are usually correctable. Postoperative thrombocytosis, even as high as 1 to 2 million, is seldom a problem and rarely is prophylactic anticoagulation indicated.

Although some investigators routinely advocate almost immediate splenectomy, most clinicians prefer first to give corticosteroids. With ITP of short duration, it is reasonable to give a trial on steroids for several weeks to a few months. If sustained remission results upon withdrawal of the drug, no further therapy is needed. If a reasonable dosage of corticosteroids does not result in a satisfactory increase in circulating platelets, or if relapse occurs, splenectomy is indicated. In patients with chronic ITP, steroids should be given to effect an increase in circulating platelets, if possible, and splenectomy performed without further delay.

Relapse of ITP following splenectomy, which occurs in 20 to 40 per cent of cases, is seldom due to a "missed" accessory spleen. However, this possibility should be evaluated in these cases by careful isotopic scanning and selective arteriography. Only those patients with positive findings of retained splenic tissue merit re-exploration. Some patients with relapse of ITP after splenectomy have been successfully treated with immunosuppressive drugs such as azathioprine, cyclophosphamide, or vincristine.[8, 29]

THROMBOTIC THROMBOCYTOPENIC PURPURA

In 1925, Moschcowitz described a syndrome of purpura, fever, hemolytic anemia, varied neurologic symptoms, and renal abnormalities. Since then, some 300 cases of thrombotic thrombocytopenic purpura (TTP) have been reported. Some patients with this disease have benefited from splenectomy, which was first successfully performed for TTP in 1951. The syndrome is caused by hyaline thrombosis of terminal arterioles and capillaries, which may be due to an immune mechanism. The course is usually a rapid one, with progression until death. Less than 30 reported patients have had sustained remissions. Adrenocorticosteroids or splenectomy alone seems to give few remissions. The combination of prednisone and splenectomy seems to be more rewarding. It is sometimes

TABLE 3. Sustained Remissions with Corticosteroids and Splenectomy in Patients with Idiopathic Thrombocytopenic Purpura

Authors	No. of Patients	Sustained Remissions (%)		
		Steroids	Splenectomy	Splenectomy after Steroid Failure
Carpenter et al., 1959	50	38	81	73
Doan et al., 1960	167	16	85	78.5
Bunting et al., 1961	134	14	57	—
Myers, 1961	71	14	83	—
Block et al., 1966	67	—	90	100
Washington University Hospitals (unpublished)	148	—	75	75

advantageous to utilize both modalities, so that steroid dosages can be reduced to acceptable levels.[8, 25, 29]

SPLENIC NEUTROPENIA AND SPLENIC PANCYTOPENIA

These two rather rare conditions of unknown etiology were first described by Doan and associates. Some authors prefer to limit the term "primary hypersplenism" to cases classified as splenic neutropenia or splenic pancytopenia.[25, 29] These diseases are characterized by splenomegaly, a normal or hyperplastic bone marrow, and leukopenia, or by varying degrees of pancytopenia. Clinical manifestations may include fever, recurrent infections, purpura, pallor, and pain in the left upper quadrant. Lymph nodes are not enlarged, in spite of the relative lymphoproliferation seen in peripheral blood, which is sometimes marked enough to suggest "premalignant lymphoma." Corticosteroids are occasionally of limited, temporary benefit in these diseases. When the diagnosis is made, splenectomy is indicated and usually curative. In some series, a few patients with initial improvement have been reclassified later as having lymphoma.

SECONDARY HYPERSPLENISM

There are a wide variety of diseases that give rise to splenomegaly and secondary splenic hyperfunction (see Table 1). Inflammation, congestion, ingestion, and infiltration are the major underlying disease processes.

Inflammation

Acute infections can be associated with hemolysis of circulating erythrocytes, as well as with decreased production. This rare state occurs when reticuloendothelial overreactivity leads to splenomegaly. The "acute splenic tumor" can lead to a decrease in other circulating cells as well. Adequate therapy of the acute infection relieves the secondary hypersplenism.

Chronic infections and inflammatory states (see Table 1) may be associated with reticuloendothelial hyperplasia, splenomegaly, and secondary hypersplenism. Worldwide, malaria is probably the most common cause of splenomegaly, which may reach huge proportions and may cause enough symptoms to require splenectomy.[3, 25, 29] In leishmaniasis, Boeck's sarcoid, tuberculosis, and so forth, splenectomy is indicated when clinical manifestations of hyperfunction are significant, or the splenomegaly results in pain and impairment of respiration. Enlarged spleens rupture more easily with minor trauma and prophylactic removal is sometimes advisable.

Rheumatoid arthritis, after several years' duration, may become associated with splenomegaly and neutropenia (Felty's syndrome). Corticosteroids may be of minimal benefit in correcting the neutropenia, but often this is temporary. Splenectomy can be of lasting benefit, not only in correcting the leukopenia, but sometimes in ameliorating the arthritis as well.[21]

Secondary hypersplenism develops in about 5 per cent of patients with sarcoidosis, with thrombocytopenic purpura, hemolytic anemia, leukopenia, or spontaneous splenic rupture. Splenectomy should be considered in these people, since the hematologic deficiencies are usually corrected after removal.

Congestion

Congestive splenomegaly with pancytopenia (Banti's syndrome) can occur with portal hypertension. The spleen is no longer believed to be the primary source of this disorder, but rather it is secondarily involved as a result of increased blood pressure within the splenic or hepatic portal veins.[3, 25, 29] Splenic congestion with sequestration and destruction of circulating blood elements results. Splenectomy will usually correct the cytopenias, but a portal-systemic venous shunt usually is necessary to lower the portal hypertension. Removal of a large spleen can reduce portal hypertension by decreasing the influx of blood into the congested portal system by as much as 40 per cent. However, reduction is usually temporary and a portacaval or splenorenal shunt is preferable to prevent recurrent variceal bleeding. Shunting procedures are seldom indicated for isolated congestive hypersplenism without other symptoms, predominantly variceal bleeding. Successful portal-systemic decompression usually corrects the secondary hypersplenism over a period of several months, although occasionally persistent hypersplenism has required later splenectomy.

Ingestion

In diseases such as Gaucher's disease and Niemann-Pick's disease, the reticuloendothelial system ingests "foreign" macromolecules and undergoes hyperplasia, with splenomegaly and sequestration of blood elements. This eventually results in secondary hypersplenism, which can be corrected by splenectomy. Splenectomy may also be indicated to relieve symptoms, such as respiratory distress or abdominal discomfort, caused by a massively enlarged spleen.

Infiltration

In a number of diseases, abnormal cells infiltrate the splenic parenchyma, which can result in splenomegaly and secondary hypersplenism. For the surgeon, myeloid metaplasia, the lymphomas, and the leukemias are the most important diseases in this category, since splenectomy may become necessary.

Myeloid Metaplasia. This disease is also called agnogenic myeloid metaplasia and chronic nonleukemic myelosis and currently is considered to be a myeloproliferative disorder in which there is an excessive proliferation of primitive mesenchymal elements. Connective tissue proliferates in the bone marrow, spleen, liver, and lymph nodes, with a concomitant proliferation of hematopoietic stem cells in the spleen, liver, and long bones. Overgrowth of fibroblasts eventually obliterates the bone marrow, resulting in myelofibrosis. Although the same fibrotic process can eventually occur in the spleen or liver, the predominant process in these organs is extramedullary hematopoiesis. This current theory of the pathogenesis of the myeloproliferative disorders is more acceptable than the previously held belief that myelofibrosis caused a compensatory extramedullary hematopoiesis. The close association between myeloid metaplasia, polycythemia vera, and myelogenous leukemia is more compatible with the current theory of pathogenesis and even suggests that the mesenchymal stem cells may be altered by a malignant process. Confirmation of these theories, however, is still lacking, even though it is now quite clear that removal of a spleen involved with myeloid metaplasia does not necessarily result in decreased formation of cellular blood elements.[24, 25, 29]

Most patients with myeloid metaplasia are middle-aged to older, and present with anemia, weight loss, and pressure symptoms from splenomegaly. Dyspnea, pallor, edema, bleeding, infections, pruritus, and bone pain are not uncommon during the course of the disease, which ranges from 1 to 20 years. Hematologic findings include anemia, with anisocytosis and poikilocytosis. The white blood count is usually reduced, but can exceed 50,000, with a leukocyte alkaline phosphatase that is usually high. Modest thrombocytopenia is seen in about one third to one half of the patients; normal platelet counts are found in about one fourth of the patients; and thrombocytosis is seen in 5 to 25 per cent of patients with this disease. Splenic scans and erythrocyte survival times are important diagnostic tests to indicate possible benefit from splenectomy. Corticosteroids, testosterone, alkylating agents, and radiotherapy are of some use in myeloid metaplasia. Deterioration in spite of medical therapy is an indication for splenectomy. Even though removal of the spleen does not alter the general course of the disease, it is often palliative by decreasing transfusion requirements, by relieving symptoms of splenomegaly, and by halting bleeding episodes.[24, 25, 29]

Malignant Lymphoma and Leukemia. The spleen can be infiltrated by malignant cells during the various stages of these diseases. This may lead to secondary hypersplenism, or to no clinically detectable abnormality. Splenectomy may be indicated in both of these situations, either as palliative treatment or as a part of a diagnostic staging laparotomy.[1, 3, 8, 12, 15-17, 20, 22-25, 27-29] Palliative therapy can be useful when chemotherapy and radiotherapy fail to prevent splenic infiltration and splenomegaly. This can result in troublesome symptoms from the size or from the hypersplenism.

These diseases can, of course, also affect the marrow, altering the hematologic picture. In deciding on the potential efficacy of splenectomy, it is necessary to establish that reasonable bone marrow function exists as well as splenomegaly and hypersplenism. Red cell survival, transfusion requirements, and splenic scans are helpful. The use of scanning techniques, however, has not been a completely reliable indicator in these situations, because scans show sequestration in only about half of the patients with lymphomas who eventually improve with splenectomy. There is still controversy about the efficacy of splenectomy for palliation in Hodgkin's disease, with some authors favoring it and others much less enthusiastic.[20, 25] Palliative splenectomy for lymphosarcoma and for lymphocytic leukemia has been more uniformly accepted. In chronic myelogenous leukemia, splenectomy is seldom indicated, although some authors feel it can be helpful in permitting further chemotherapy. In reticulum cell sarcoma, results seem to be favorable, but quite short-lived, since operation is usually performed late in the course of the disease. In all of these diseases, it may be better to perform splenectomy when hypersplenism first becomes evident and not to wait until the terminal stages.

Recently, splenectomy has been advocated as part of a diagnostic laparotomy for staging patients with Hodgkin's and non-Hodgkin's lymphomas.[12, 15-17, 23, 27, 28] Although the exact role of surgical staging procedures is still controversial, more precise staging has been of value in defining the patterns of these diseases in untreated patients and in selecting proper therapy for individual patients. Exploratory laparotomy with splenectomy, liver biopsy, and abdominal lymph node biopsies has unquestionably improved the accuracy of staging of malignant lymphomas.

In Hodgkin's disease, most series show an alteration in preoperative evaluation in one fourth to one half of patients. Although there are minor differences in the many reported series, the data in Table 4 are representative. Clinical evaluation of splenic involvement, even at the time of surgery, has been particularly inaccurate except in spleens two to three times normal size. In patients with splenic involvement, more than one third also have or will develop Hodgkin's lymphoma in the liver. Clinical determination of liver involvement is also difficult but might be improved by the use of laparoscopy.[2] Liver involvement does not seem to occur without splenic involvement. The results with lymphangiography in different series have been somewhat more varied, with inaccurate clinical evaluation in 10 to 25 per cent of patients.

Many radiotherapists believe splenectomy is also

TABLE 4. Comparison of Clinical and Histologic Staging for Hodgkin's Disease. Total of 205 Patients*

Preoperative Clinical Status	Histol. + Cases No. Examined	Per Cent Clinically Incorrect
1. Spleen		
a) Clin. involved	33/53	37.7
b) Clin. uninvolved	49/150	32.7
Total	—	34.0
2. Liver		
a) Clin. involved	8/42	81.0
b) Clin. uninvolved	12/163	7.4
Total	—	22.4
3. Para-aortic Lymph Nodes		
a) Clin. involved	45/64	29.7
b) Clin. uninvolved	13/99	13.1
c) Clin. equivocal	6/34	—
Total	—	19.6

*Data from Kadin et al., 1971; Ultmann et al., 1970; Lowenbraun et al., 1970; and Ratkin et al., 1974.

helpful in Hodgkin's disease, particularly when splenomegaly is present, because it makes subsequent radiotherapy easier. The radiotherapy port in the left upper quadrant can be limited to the splenic hilus (marked at laparotomy with metal clips), thus reducing the amount of radiation to the left kidney and lung. Laparotomy also allows bilateral oophoropexy in young women to move the ovaries out of the direct field of radiation. Although this is not completely effective in protecting the ovaries from radiation damage, ovarian function persists after radiotherapy in about half of the patients with oophoropexies.[16] Most reported complication rates for surgical staging procedures are low and mortality is rare. Surgical staging for Hodgkin's disease is, therefore, a worthwhile procedure, but its use should be individualized for each patient depending upon current therapeutic philosophy.

In non-Hodgkin's lymphomas, the role of staging laparotomy is even more uncertain than in Hodgkin's disease. Staging laparotomies have helped to define the extent of disease, with 25 to 50 per cent of patients being restaged after laparotomy and about one third of spleens being misdiagnosed clinically. The major difference compared to Hodgkin's disease has been in the increased degree of mesenteric lymph node and extranodal involvement. Also, the surgical risk and complication rate may be greater in non-Hodgkin's lymphomas because the patients are generally older and more debilitated with extensive disease. Since the classification and definitive treatment of these diseases is still highly controversial, it is not possible to outline any routine approach for the use of surgical staging procedures. This field will continue to change rapidly in the future. At the present time the best general guideline is to consider each patient individually as to whether therapy might be altered by a surgical staging procedure.

RUPTURE OF THE SPLEEN

Splenic rupture is not uncommon, in spite of the fact that the spleen seems well-protected by the ribs and muscular parieties.[14, 19, 26] The spleen is a rather friable, vascular organ, suspended by ligaments that are attached to an adherent capsule, and even relatively minor trauma can result in avulsion of the splenic substance, or tearing of vessels in the suspensory ligaments, causing profuse bleeding. No injury to the spleen should be considered trivial, since delay in diagnosis and institution of the proper therapy can result in serious consequences. The reported mortality of approximately 10 per cent in isolated splenic rupture can be reduced by rapid diagnosis and therapy. Concomitant injuries to other organs are frequent with major trauma and account for a higher mortality and morbidity (15 to 25 per cent) of splenic injury.

The classification of splenic rupture, based on the etiology and the interval between onset and obvious manifestations, is a clinically useful one (Table 5).

Penetrating Trauma. Most penetrating wounds that involve the spleen are obvious and warrant little discussion. Injury from high-speed missiles occasionally

TABLE 5. Classification of Splenic Rupture

1. Penetrating trauma
   a) transabdominal
   b) transthoracic
2. Nonpenetrating trauma
   a) immediate rupture
   b) delayed rupture
3. Operative trauma
4. Spontaneous rupture

can be a diagnostic problem for the unwary physician, particularly if the missile follows an erratic course after entering the skin. Missiles such as bullets quite frequently do not follow a straight trajectory after entering the body, and injury to any organ, including the spleen, should be considered in all such patients. Hemopneumothorax in association with splenic injury indicates penetration of the lung, pleura, and diaphragm, and a transthoracic approach for splenectomy is often preferable to remove clot and repair the damaged thoracic structures. If such an approach is used, careful consideration should be given to abdominal exploration, which usually requires a separate abdominal or a thoracoabdominal incision.

Nonpenetrating Trauma. Automobile accidents are the most common causes of blunt trauma to the spleen, even in children (in whom sledding and bicycle accidents are often the cause of splenic rupture). The spleen can be avulsed from its pedicle, fractured through the capsule and parenchyma, or ruptured beneath an intact capsule to give rise to a subcapsular hematoma. Bleeding is usually profuse with the first two, although a completely avulsed splenic artery can temporarily close with spasm, particularly in children. Delayed exsanguinating hemorrhage can occur when spasm ceases and the thrombus is pushed out. Delayed rupture, which occurs in 15 per cent of nonpenetrating splenic injuries, usually results from a subcapsular hematoma, which becomes manifest any time from a day to several weeks after an injury. Approximately 75 per cent of delayed ruptures are diagnosed within 2 weeks of injury. Delayed rupture not infrequently is heralded by sudden, profuse bleeding and shock, after an episode of minor trauma is forgotten. Delay in diagnosis leads to relatively high mortality rates.

Spontaneous rupture is rare in a normal spleen; it is more often associated with diseased spleens. Rupture with minimal trauma, or spontaneous rupture, has been reported in malaria, mononucleosis (usually in the second to fourth weeks of the disease), sarcoidosis, acute and chronic leukemia, congestive splenomegaly, polycythemia vera, and acquired hemolytic anemia. Rapid, early splenectomy gives an excellent prognosis of survival.

Operative trauma to the spleen necessitating "incidental" splenectomy occurs in a significant number of operations in the left upper quadrant. Such injury is most common in operations involving the stomach and splenic flexure of the colon. Most surgeons recommend splenectomy even for small tears in the capsule because of the very real danger of subsequent hemorrhage.

Clinical Manifestations of Ruptured Spleen

Although some patients, on admission, may be moribund in severe hemorrhagic shock or, at the other extreme, totally asymptomatic, the condition of most patients falls between these two extremes.[14, 19, 26] There is usually some evidence of hypovolemia, particularly tachycardia and orthostatic hypotension. Most patients have varying degrees of generalized abdominal pain, often accompanied by nausea. In only about a third of patients with splenic rupture and no other abdominal injuries is the pain localized to the upper quadrant. Pain radiating into the left shoulder (Kehr's sign) is relatively frequent (15 to 75 per cent of patients, depending upon the series), and can often be elicited by placing the patient in the Trendelenburg position. There is usually tenderness in the left upper quadrant, and often it can be elicited as rebound tenderness.

Occasionally, there is a fixed mass or fixed area of dullness (Ballance's sign) in the left upper quadrant, due to subcapsular or extracapsular hematoma surrounded by omentum. Shifting dullness and a "doughy" feel to the abdomen are uncommon signs of extensive intraperitoneal bleeding. If clinical and laboratory evaluation does not demonstrate the splenic injury, repeated examinations often do. The importance of continued clinical evaluation in suspected splenic injury cannot be overemphasized.

Certain laboratory and radiologic tests can be of help. The white blood cell count often is increased to levels of 15,000 to 20,000. An initial hematocrit is often misleading, but serial determinations usually show a fall. Radiologic examinations are often not conclusive, but occasionally will show an enlarged spleen, without sharp outlines, that compresses the stomach medially and the transverse colon inferiorly. The left kidney and psoas shadows may be indistinct, and sometimes the left diaphragm is elevated. The presence of rib fractures can be helpful in the diagnosis of a splenic rupture, since they are present in about 20 per cent of splenic injuries. Hematuria in association with left rib fractures usually means a damaged spleen as well. An uncommon, but helpful radiographic finding occurs when blood dissects into the gastrosplenic ligament, causing a serrated appearance of the greater curvature of the stomach. Arteriograms of the splenic artery can be diagnostic in difficult cases (Fig. 7), but are seldom needed. Splenic scanning can also be helpful (Fig. 8), and is a procedure that can be done in most institutions.

Paracentesis with an 18- or 20-gauge needle, or a small polyethylene catheter, can be helpful in difficult diagnostic situations. The presence of blood from a four-quadrant tap does much to confirm the diagnosis, and may be expected in as many as 50 per cent of cases with splenic rupture. The procedure, however, is not without some danger, particularly when there are dense peritoneal adhesions or abdominal distention, and a negative tap does not exclude injury to any of the abdominal organs. In the authors' viewpoint, there is little justification for *routine* four-quadrant taps in *all* cases of abdominal trauma, but rather the procedure should be limited to situations with *questionable* indications for abdominal exploration.

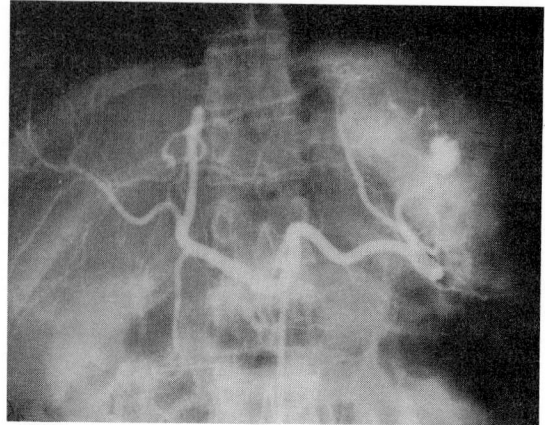

Figure 7. A selective splenic arteriogram showing a subcapsular hematoma following blunt trauma to the abdomen.

Once the diagnosis is made, or even highly suspected, laparotomy usually is indicated. Correction of hypovolemia with whole blood, or lactated Ringer's solution, or plasma expanders until blood is available, should proceed during the evaluation and while transporting the patient to the operating room. Delay for unnecessary diagnostic procedures or "to get the patient in better shape" for operation can be catastrophic. With trauma, a midline incision is preferable, since it allows rapid splenectomy and a complete exploration for injury to other organs, which occurs in about a third of patients with ruptured spleens. Hemorrhage from the spleen can be quickly controlled by clamping the pedicle between two fingers, dividing the lateral attachments, and delivering the spleen into the wound, where careful removal can be easily accomplished. A complete abdominal exploration must then be performed. Isolated splenic rupture treated in this way has a favorable prognosis, with a mortality of 1 per cent or less. The higher

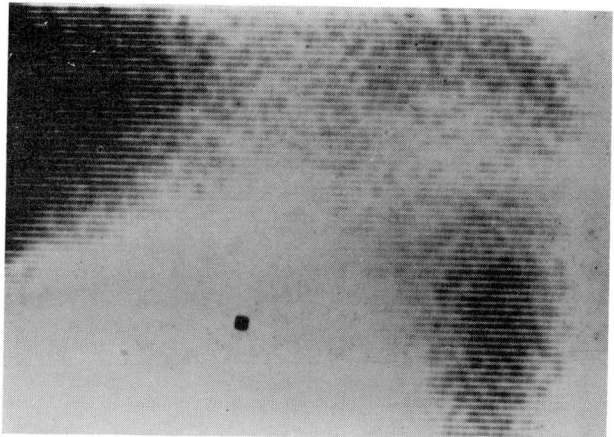

Figure 8. A technetium-sulfur colloid scan done 1 week after minor abdominal trauma. A large subcapsular hematoma can be seen in the midportion of the spleen, which is outlined to the right. A portion of the left lobe of the liver can be seen to the left of the umbilical marker (black square). (Courtesy of Dr. E. J. Potchen.)

reported mortality rates (10 to 25 per cent) are due in large part to associated fatal injuries.[3, 14, 19, 26]

It seems clear that some injuries to the spleen do correct themselves. The occurrence of pseudocysts and old, well-organized hematomas and the fact that splenic puncture usually does not lead to hemorrhage attest to this fact. Recently, some children with traumatic rupture of the spleen have been successfully treated without splenectomy when bleeding was minimal and continued careful observation showed clinical improvement.[10, 14] As these authors emphasize, the nonoperative approach requires careful selection of patients, and splenectomy should be performed if there is any doubt. Experience is still too limited to determine if any late complications might develop.

Splenosis may be one of the late manifestations of previous injury, although the etiology of this condition is still in some doubt. These small bits of splenic tissue scattered throughout the peritoneal cavity probably arise from fragmentation and autotransplantation, and are probably not true accessory spleens. They become of clinical significance if they cause intestinal obstruction, or if they are mistaken for peritoneal nodules due to other causes, such as carcinomatosis.

LESS COMMON SPLENIC DISEASES

Splenic Cysts. Parasitic and nonparasitic cysts rarely occur in the spleen. Echinococcus is the only parasitic infection reported to cause splenic cysts, which occur in less than 2 per cent of people with echinococcal infection. Nonparasitic cysts are either true cysts lined by epithelium or pseudocysts. Pseudocysts probably arise from old hematomas or splenic infarcts. True cysts are exceedingly rare. In the last 30 years, only two of the 11 splenic cysts removed at Barnes Hospital have been lined with epithelium (Fig. 9). Splenectomy, and not aspiration, is the treatment of choice for all cysts.

Neoplasms. Primary tumors of the spleen are also rare. Benign tumors include hamartomas, angiomas, and endotheliomas. Malignant primary tumors are all sarcomas, which grow and spread rapidly before clinical manifestations of a left quadrant mass, cachexia, and ascites occur. Cure is infrequent, but palliation can be achieved with splenectomy. Although metastases to the spleen (other than lymphomas) are felt to be rare, they are not uncommon in autopsy series of advanced lung and breast carcinomas.[3]

Abscesses. Septicemia can rarely result in splenic abscess. Trauma or infarcts in sickle cell disease are the usual antecedent lesions. Splenic scans can be a valuable diagnostic aid. Splenectomy is preferable treatment, but drainage can help if removal is not possible.

Ectopic Spleen. In rare instances, a lengthened splenic pedicle allows for a "wandering spleen," which may present as a mobile mass. It is of clinical significance only in that it can be mistaken for a tumor or a cyst, such as an ovarian cyst, or it can twist on its pedicle. Torsion of the spleen demands emergency splenectomy.

Splenic Artery Aneurysms. Although these are quite

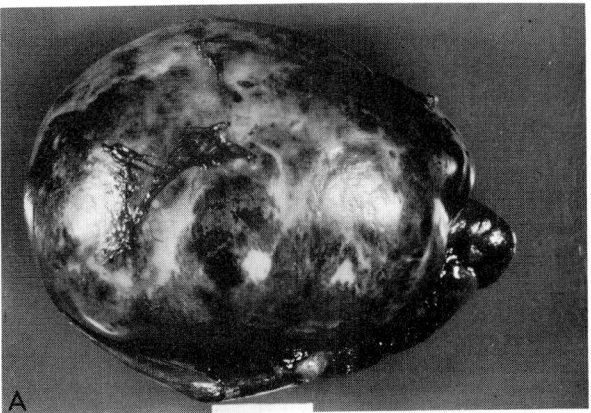

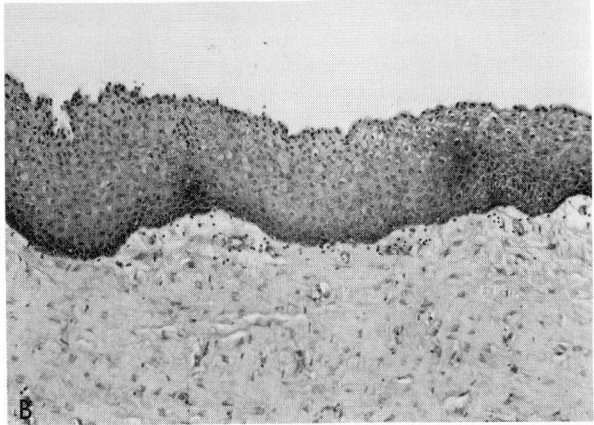

Figure 9. *A*, Anterior view of a spleen containing a large congenital cyst, lined with squamous epithelium *(B)*.

rare, they are clinically important because of occasional rupture. They occur in women more than men, are usually asymptomatic, and may be seen on plain roentgenographs as a thin calcified rim. Excision seems advisable, unless there are complicating factors.

SPLENECTOMY

Preoperative Preparation. Since emergency splenectomy is seldom necessary except for rupture, careful preparation prior to operation is usually possible. With splenic rupture, whole blood should be administered, but operation should not be delayed in the face of continuing hemorrhage. In patients with coagulation disorders that require preoperative transfusions, fresh blood obtained in plastic or siliconized containers is preferable, to preserve platelets as much as possible. Patients with severe thrombocytopenia usually benefit from platelet packs, but it is seldom worthwhile to give them before the splenic pedicle is clamped, since infused platelets are rapidly destroyed by the spleen.[29] In some patients with hematologic disorders, such as acquired hemolytic anemia and lymphomas, the blood bank should be given sufficient warning, since satisfactory matching is often difficult. Patients who have been receiving corticosteroids need adequate coverage during the operative period. Doubling the maintenance dose on the evening prior to operation, and again on the day of operation, is usually satisfactory. Postoperatively, the dose can be slowly tapered back to maintenance levels and, it is hoped, then eventually discontinued. General anesthesia is preferable for splenectomy, with ether a good choice of agent, since it produces a significant decrease in the size of the spleen.

Operative Technique.   After the induction of anesthesia, a nasogastric tube should be passed to decompress the stomach. Left subcostal, upper midline, and left paramedian skin incisions all give adequate exposure. The choice of skin incision is dictated by the indications for operation and the individual preference of the surgeon. For splenectomy alone, a left subcostal incision gives excellent exposure and allows removal of even a massively enlarged spleen if the incision is extended into the flank and across the midline (Fig. 10). Midline and left paramedian incisions are preferable for ruptured spleens, and are often more desirable for severe coagulation disorders, for massively enlarged spleens, and for "staging" operations. Thoracoabdominal incisions are seldom necessary, unless there is an associated pulmonary or diaphragmatic injury (Fig. 11).

The spleen is mobilized by dividing the lateral peritoneal attachments from the colon, left kidney, and diaphragm. These ligaments are usually avascular, but may contain large vessels, especially in portal hypertension or myeloid metaplasia. Adhesions to the diaphragm must be divided and can sometimes cause troublesome hemorrhage. Electrocoagulation can be helpful. The spleen and hilus then can be rotated

forward and medially, and a pack placed in the fossa to help control oozing and to keep the spleen in the wound. The short gastric vessels are divided, with care not to damage the greater curvature of the stomach. After identification of the tail of the pancreas, which extends into the hilus, the splenic artery and vein are ligated and transected. This can often be best accomplished by approaching the hilus posteriorly. Some surgeons prefer to identify and ligate the splenic artery through the gastrosplenic and gastrocolic ligaments before mobilizing the spleen. "Early" ligation of the splenic artery is sometimes difficult with enlarged lymph nodes or with a massively enlarged spleen, but can facilitate dissection by decreasing the size of the spleen and lessening troublesome hemorrhage.

After the spleen is removed, meticulous hemostasis is accomplished; the pancreas and stomach are carefully examined for injury and the splenic fossa is irrigated with saline. Drainage is usually not necessary, unless there has been extensive tissue damage and bleeding from dissection or from injury, or unless the pancreas has been damaged. Sump drains are preferable when the pancreas is injured. Since infection can spread retrograde down a drain from the exterior, attachment of a splenic drain to sterile drainage is preferable.

Accessory spleens, which are often present (14 to 30 per cent of patients), should be found and removed, particularly when the patient has a hematologic disorder. These occur, in the order of decreasing frequency, in the hilus and along the splenic vessels, the gastrosplenic and splenocolic ligaments, the gastrocolic ligament, the splenorenal ligament, the greater omentum, the mesentery of the intestine, and the pelvis (see Fig. 2). When "staging" for lymphoma,

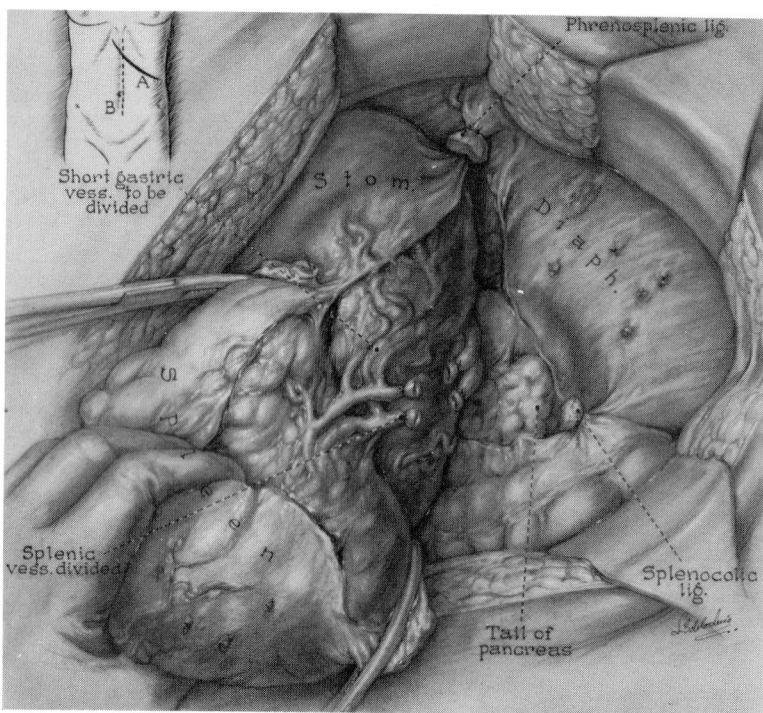

Figure 10.   The spleen just before removal with only a few short gastric vessels still intact. Abdominal incisions for splenectomy are depicted in the upper left insert. (From Splenectomy, By Ballinger, W. F., and Erslev, A. J., in Current Problems in Surgery, edited by Ravitch, M. M., et al. Copyright © 1965, Year Book Medical Publishers. Used by Permission.)

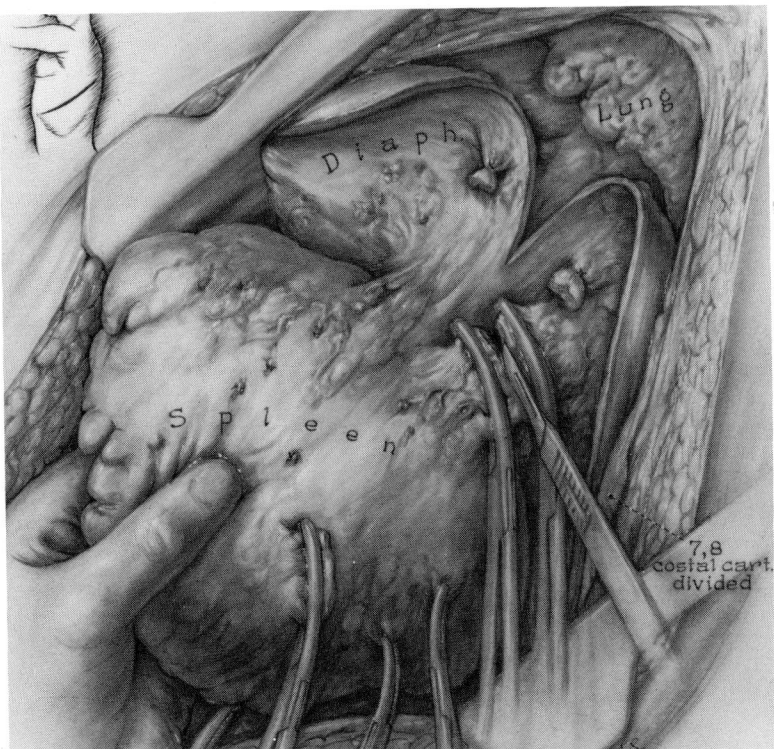

Figure 11. Thoracoabdominal incision with good exposure of dense splenophrenic adhesions. (From Splenectomy, by Ballinger, W. F., and Erslev, A. J., in Current Problems in Surgery, edited by Ravitch, M. M., et al. Copyright © 1965, Year Book Medical Publishers. Used by permission.)

the splenic hilus and areas of lymph node biopsy should be tagged with metal clips. The periaortic lymph nodes in the upper abdomen, as well as along the lower aorta, should be examined and biopsied. The liver is also biopsied, preferably in both lobes.

Postoperative Management. Persistent hemorrhage can occur in the immediate postoperative period. If continued transfusions are required, and the abdominal girth is increasing, re-exploration is mandatory. Often in such situations, intraperitoneal blood and clot are found, but no specific bleeding site is identified. Evacuation of the clot, irrigation with saline, and packing for several minutes will usually control any oozing.

The most common complication of splenectomy is left lower lobe atelectasis. Helpful preventive measures include vigorous deep breathing and coughing, blow bottles, intermittent positive-pressure exercises, and endotracheal suctioning. Rarely bronchoscopy is needed. Pneumonia and pleural effusion can occur. A left pleural effusion may also be due to a left subphrenic abscess. Fluid collections under the left diaphragm may become infected, develop into a subphrenic abscess, and require drainage. Injury to the pancreas or stomach is not common, but does occur. Gastric injury usually results in subphrenic abscess and gastrocutaneous fistula. Pancreatitis, with or without subsequent fistula or pseudocyst, occurs somewhat more frequently.

The proper management of patients with asymptomatic thrombocytosis after splenectomy is still controversial. Although most patients do not have thrombotic complications even with platelet counts greater than a million per cu. mm., a few do.[4, 26] Thrombocytosis in myeloproliferative diseases is particularly prone to thrombotic and bleeding complications.[29] Anticoagulants, antiplatelet drugs (acetylsalicylic acid, dipyridamole), and anticancer agents (e.g., 1-phenylalanine mustard) have been used successfully, but there is no general agreement on routine indications. Currently, most surgeons would agree that some type of prophylactic therapy is indicated in well-hydrated patients without anemia when the platelet count exceeds 1 to 2 million after splenectomy. In any case, patients with definite thrombosis should be treated with anticoagulants, bed rest, and leg wraps, and possibly with antiplatelet and anticancer agents as well.

The risk of infections in children after splenectomy may be higher than in adults,[11] but this remains controversial. This possibility has caused some authors to advocate prophylactic antibiotics after splenectomy in patients under 2 years of age. Actually, this increased risk seems to correlate more with the type of disease process than with the *age* of the patient. Thalassemia, myeloid metaplasia, Wiskott-Aldrich syndrome, and lipoidosis all carry increased risks of infection, regardless of age.

SELECTED REFERENCES

Kaplan, H. S.: Hodgkin's Disease. Cambridge, Mass., Harvard University Press, 1972.
 This comprehensive text covers all aspects of this disease, including current literature through December, 1970. Although the author admittedly presents controversial topics from his own viewpoint, he amply supports his ideas with pertinent data.

Rosenberg, S. A., Dorfman, R. F., and Kaplan, H. S.: The value of sequential bone marrow biopsy and laparotomy and splenectomy in a series of 127 consecutive untreated patients with non-Hodgkin's lymphoma. Br. J. Cancer, 31(Suppl. II):228, 1975.
This thoughtful article is one of the many important series that were presented at the "symposium on non-Hodgkin's Lymphomata" in London in October, 1973, and published in this issue of the British Journal of Cancer.

Schwartz, S. I., Adams, J. T., and Bauman, A. W.: Splenectomy for Hematologic Disorders. Curr. Probl. Surg., May, 1971.
This monograph is an excellent current review of this increasingly important area. The surgically important hematologic disorders are described in detail with a concise presentation of pathophysiology, important diagnostic procedures, therapy, and results. The authors combine an extensive personal experience with a thorough review of the literature to provide a useful reference.

Wintrobe, M. M.: Clinical Hematology. 7th ed. Philadelphia, Lea & Febiger, 1974.
This outstanding text remains the standard hematology reference.

REFERENCES

1. Adler, S., Stutzman, L., Sokol, J. E., and Mittelman, A.: Splenectomy for hematologic depression in lymphocytic lymphoma and leukemia. Cancer, 35:521, 1975.
2. Bagley, C. M., Thomas, L. B., Johnson, R. E., Chretien, P. B., and DeVita, V. T.: Diagnosis of liver involvement by lymphoma: Results in 96 consecutive peritoneoscopies. Cancer, 31:840, 1973.
3. Ballinger, W. F., II, and Erslev, A. J.: Splenectomy. Curr. Probl. Surg., February, 1965.
4. Balz, J., and Minton, J. P.: Mesenteric thrombosis following splenectomy. Ann. Surg., 181:126, 1975.
5. Block, G. E., Evans, R., and Zajtchun, R.: Splenectomy for idiopathic thrombocytopenic purpura. Arch. Surg., 92:484, 1966.
6. Bunting, W. L., Kiely, J. M., and Campbell, D. C.: Idiopathic thrombocytopenic purpura. Arch. Intern. Med., 108:733, 1961.
7. Carpenter, A. F., Wintrobe, M. M., Fuller, E. A., Haut, A., and Cartwright, G. E.: Treatment of idiopathic thrombocytopenic purpura. J.A.M.A., 171:1911, 1959.
8. Dameshek, H. L., and Ellis, L. D.: Hematologic indication for splenectomy. Surg. Clin. North Am., 55:253, 1975.
9. Doan, C. A., Bouroncle, B. A., and Wiseman, B. K.: Idiopathic and secondary thrombocytopenic purpura. Clinical study and evaluation of 381 cases over a period of 28 years. Ann. Intern. Med., 53:861, 1960.
10. Douglas, G. J., and Simpson, J. J.: The conservative management of splenic trauma. J. Pediatr. Surg., 6:565, 1971.
11. Eraklis, A. J., Kevy, S. V., Diamond, L. K., and Gross, R. E.: Hazard of overwhelming infection after splenectomy in childhood. N. Engl. J. Med., 276:1225, 1967.
12. Ferguson, D. J., Allen, L. W., Griem, M. L., Moran, M. E., Rappaport, H., and Ultmann, J. E.: Surgical experience with staging laparotomy in 125 patients with lymphoma. Arch. Intern. Med., 131:356, 1973.
13. Harrington, W. J., Minnick, M., Hollingsworth, J., and Moore, C. V.: Demonstration of a thrombocytopenic factor in the blood of patients with thrombocytopenic purpura. J. Lab. Clin. Med., 38:1, 1951.
14. Hendren, W. H., and Kim, S. H.: Trauma of the spleen and liver in children. Pediatr. Clin. North Am., 22:349, 1975.
15. Kadin, M. E., Glatstein, E., and Dorfman, R. F.: Clinicopathologic studies of 117 untreated patients subjected to laparotomy for the staging of Hodgkin's disease. Cancer, 27:1277, 1971.
16. Kaplan, H. S.: Hodgkin's Disease. Cambridge, Mass., Harvard University Press, 1972.
17. Lowenbraun, S., Ramsey, H., Sutherland, J., and Serpick, A. A.: Diagnostic laparotomy and splenectomy for staging Hodgkin's disease. Ann. Intern. Med., 72:655, 1970.
18. Myers, M. C.: Results of treatment in 71 patients with idiopathic thrombocytopenic purpura. Am. J. Med. Sci., 242:295, 1961.
19. Naylor, R., Cohn, D., and Shires, G. T.: Morbidity and mortality from injuries to the spleen. J. Trauma, 14:773, 1974.
20. O'Brien, P. H., Hartz, W. H., Derlacki, D., and Graulich, K.: Splenectomy for hypersplenism in malignant lymphoma. Arch. Surg., 101:348, 1970.
21. O'Neill, J. A., Jr., Scott, H. W., Jr., Billings, F. T., and Foster, J. H.: The role of splenectomy in Felty's syndrome. Ann. Surg., 167:81, 1968.
22. Ratkin, G. A., Present, C. A., Weinerman, B., and Reinhard, E. H.: Correlation of anemia with infradiaphragmatic involvement in Hodgkin's disease and other malignant lymphomas. Can. Med. Assoc. J., 111:924, 1974.
23. Rosenberg, S. A., Dorfman, R. F., and Kaplan, H. S.: The value of sequential bone marrow biopsy and laparotomy and splenectomy in a series of 127 consecutive untreated patients with non-Hodgkin's lymphoma. Br. J. Cancer, 31(Suppl. II):228, 1975.
24. Schwartz, S. I.: Myeloproliferative disorders. Ann. Surg., 182:464, 1975.
25. Schwartz, S. I., Adams, J. T., and Bauman, A. W.: Splenectomy for hematologic disorders. Curr. Probl. Surg., May, 1971.
26. Steele, M., and Lim, R. C.: Advances in management of splenic injuries. Am. J. Surg., 130:159, 1975.
27. Trueblood, H. W., Guernsey, J. M., and Cohn, R.: Hodgkin's disease and non-Hodgkin's lymphoma—the surgeon's role in therapy. Cur. Probl. Surg., Aug., 1972.
28. Ultmann, J. E.: Current status: The management of lymphoma. Semin. Hematology, 7:441, 1970.
29. Wintrobe, M. M.: Clinical Hematology, 7th ed. Philadelphia, Lea & Febiger, 1974.

39

HERNIAS

Lloyd M. Nyhus, M.D., and C. Thomas Bombeck, M.D.

HISTORICAL ASPECTS

The early history of interest in the problem of hernia is that of the discipline of surgery. The names associated so intimately with the subject of hernia are familiar because of the pioneering thrust these men gave to surgery in general, e.g., Celsus, Henri de Mondeville, Guy de Chauliac, and Ambroïse Paré.[79]

The Egyptian papyri do not contain reference to the operative treatment of hernia, but the Papyrus Ebers (1552 B.C.) recommended diet and externally applied pressure (truss?) for its treatment. The word *barbaric* is frequently used in terms of surgery during the middle ages, and no less so for the treatment of hernia (Fig. 1). Major developments in the knowledge of hernial anatomy and treatment occurred during the eighteenth century. Percival Pott (1714–1788) of London refuted many of the old theories concerning the etiology of hernia and methods of treatment based on these theories.[60] He was probably the first to suggest the congenital origin of hernias.

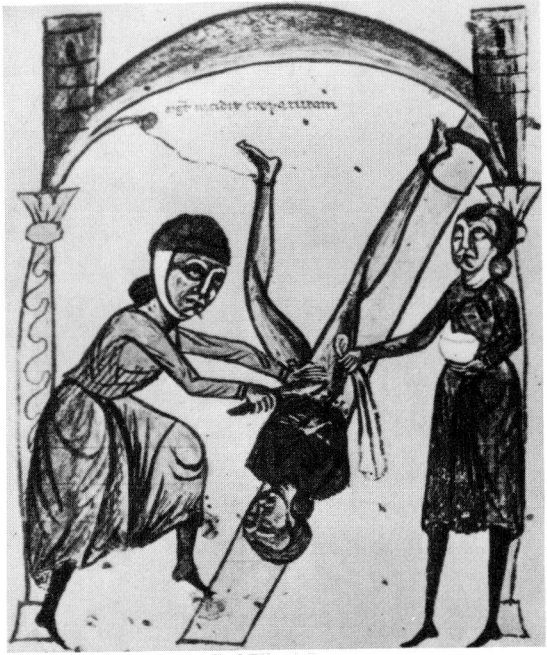

Figure 1. Hernia operation in Trendelenburg position. From a thirteenth century manuscript. (Courtesy of L. M. Zimmerman.)

The Modern Era of Hernial Surgery: Nineteenth and Twentieth Centuries

Early in the nineteenth century, four men contributed significant descriptions of inguinal anatomy: Camper,[12] Cooper,[17] Hesselbach,[35, 36] and Scarpa.[67] In 1801, Pieter Camper published the description of the fascia that bears his name. The skilled anatomist Sir Astley Cooper (1768–1841) published his two-volume work, *The Anatomy and Surgical Treatment of Abdominal Hernia*, in 1804 and 1807. First descriptions credited to Cooper include transversalis fascia, internal ring, inguinal canal, correct formation of femoral sheath by the transversalis fascia, and the complete description of Camper's fascia. He paid little attention to the "ligament of the pubis," now called Cooper's ligament, and he certainly had no idea of how important this structure would become in the modern treatment of hernia. Franz Kaspar Hesselbach (1759–1816) described the triangle that bears his name in 1814 while he was prosector in the anatomic theater of Würzburg. Finally, in this quartet of anatomists must be included Antonio Scarpa (1747–1832), for whom a superficial layer of fascia is named. He is also credited with being the first to describe a sliding hernia (1821).

The nineteenth century brought anesthesia, hemostasis, and antisepsis, which made modern surgery possible. As in every area of surgery, these advances allowed rapid development of the science of hernial surgery. Wide acceptance soon was attained in Europe and America for the operation consisting of ligature and excision of the sac at the external ring and suturing of the pillars around the cord to reduce the size of the ring. This procedure was described in 1877 by Vincenz Czerny (1842–1916).[18] It is to Henry O. Marcy (1837–1924) of Boston that the modern era of hernial surgery is credited.[49, 50] His understanding of the importance of the transversalis fascia and of the anatomic contribution of fascial repair of the internal ring was reported in 1871. Parenthetically, this was 12 years before Bassini did his first operation for hernia, and 16 years before Bassini published his first paper on the subject.

Marcy's writings, however, did not stimulate the imagination of his contemporary surgeons, and further refinements in technique were suggested by Sir William Macewen (1886),[48] Lucas-Championnière (1892),[46] and Alexander H. Ferguson (1899).[23]

It remained for Edoardo Bassini (1844–1924) (Fig. 2) to present a reconstruction technique of the inguinal floor with transposition of the cord.[8] His operation (1884) included high ligation of the sac and reinforcement of the floor of the canal by suturing the conjoined tendon to the inguinal ligament beneath the cord, thus placing the cord under the external oblique aponeurosis. Bassini at this time held the chair of clinical surgery at the University of Padua.

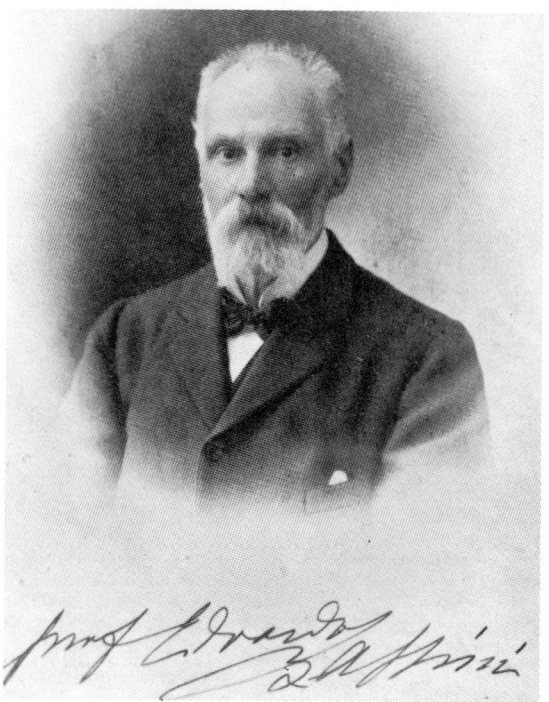

Figure 2. Edoardo Bassini (1844–1924). (Courtesy of L. M. Zimmerman.)

controversy still abounds. The last chapter on the history of groin anatomy and operative repair of hernia defects has not been written.

GROIN HERNIA

ANATOMY OF INGUINAL AND FEMORAL CANALS

As in all areas of the abdomen, the abdominal wall in the groin is composed of multilaminar arrangements of muscle, their aponeuroses, fascia, fat, and either skin or peritoneum. The abdominal wall at the level of the groin may be divided into two groups of laminae, an outer and an inner. These two groups are mirror images of each other and are divided by the inguinal canal and spermatic cord (Table 1; Fig. 5).

Since by definition any hernia is a protrusion of normal cavity contents through the fascial and muscular layers designed to contain them, it is obvious that groin hernias are due to failure of the inner lamina of the abdominal wall, not of the outer.

External Oblique Aponeurosis

The external oblique muscle arises from the lower eight ribs posteriorly and sweeps downward and around the trunk as a broad, flat muscle. The muscle fibers give way to their flat tendon of insertion, the external oblique aponeurosis, at the linea semilunaris, located in approximately the midclavicular line. The

Independently and almost simultaneously, William S. Halsted (1852–1922), Professor of Surgery at Johns Hopkins, developed an operation similar to that of Bassini. The Halsted operation (Halsted I) transposed the cord above the external oblique aponeurosis.[32] This procedure was first mentioned in 1889. The Halsted II operation (1893) did not transpose the cord but added imbrication of the aponeurosis of the external oblique muscle in performing the closure. The first mention of imbrication is credited to E. Wyllys Andrews (1856–1927)[4] of Chicago. The ludicrous overuse of eponyms in this field can be appreciated when we learn that the Halsted II procedure is also known as the Ferguson-Andrews operation, since Ferguson (Fig. 3) left the cord in its normal anatomic position and Andrews stressed the imbrication of the external oblique aponeurosis.

The use of the iliopectineal ligament (Cooper's ligament), or *ligamentum pubicum superius,* B.N.A., to anchor the medial parietal wall in the repair is credited to Georg Lotheissen (1868–1935)[44] of Vienna. The use of this structure as an integral part of hernial repair has been popularized by Chester B. McVay (b. 1911)[53] (Fig. 4) of South Dakota, and the operation is known throughout the United States as the McVay repair.

The importance of the posterior inguinal wall in the etiology as well as repair of hernias was recognized relatively late. One of the strongest advocates of the transversalis fascia layer repair was P. W. Harrison (1883–1962).[34] A thickening in the transversalis fascia layer, the iliopubic tract, has received minimal attention from anatomists and surgeons alike. Depicted by Hesselbach (1814), it was described in detail in 1836 by Thomson.[71] In the past several decades, use of this structure has been recommended by a small number of surgeons interested in the anatomy of the groin (Clark and Hashimoto, 1946,[14] Donald, 1948,[19] Griffith, 1959,[30] and Nyhus, 1964.[56]).

After such a long period of interest in this anatomic area,

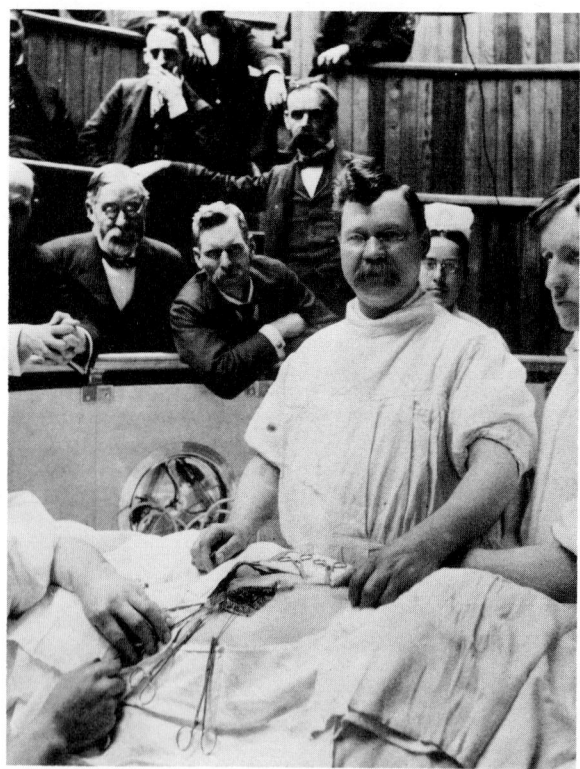

Figure 3. Alexander Hugh Ferguson (1853–1912) in operating theater of Cook County Hospital, Chicago, circa 1900.

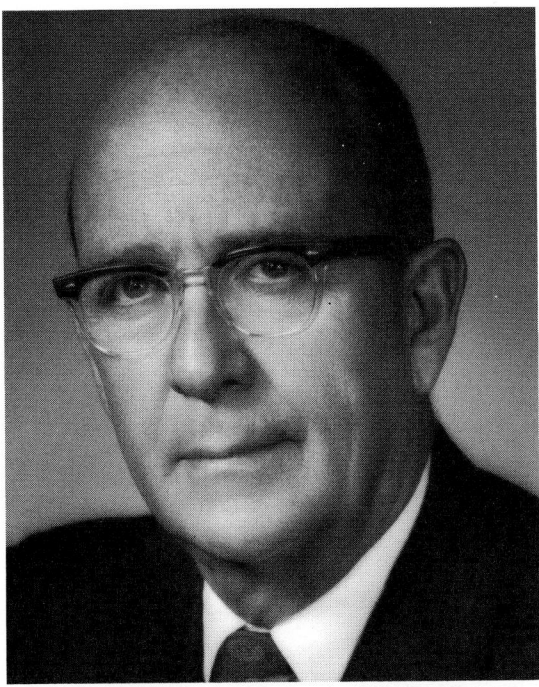

Figure 4. Chester B. McVay (b. 1911).

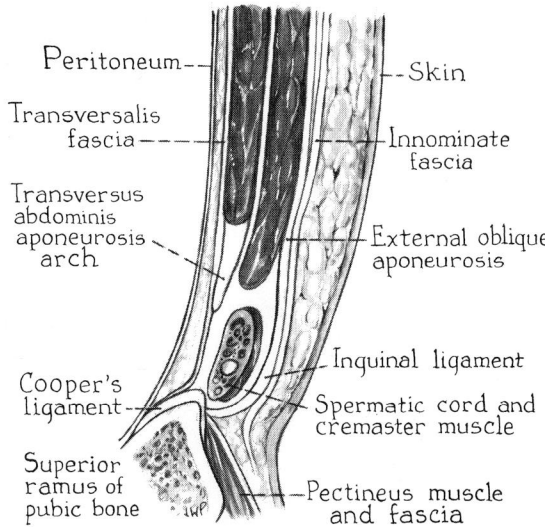

Figure 5. A parasagittal schematic representation of the musculoaponeurotic relationships in the middle of the right inguinal canal, viewed from the lateral aspect of the section. The closer approximation, via their common insertion into the pectineal line of the pubis, of the superficial (external oblique, inguinal ligament) layer to the deep (transversus abdominis, transversalis fascia) musculoaponeurotic layer in the medial portion of the groin is demonstrated. (From Condon, R. E. *In* Nyhus, L. M., and Harkins, H. N.: Hernia. Philadelphia, J. B. Lippincott Company, 1964.)

aponeurosis is attached to the iliac crest and the anterior superior iliac spine laterally (Fig. 6), and inserts rather broadly into the linea alba medially. It makes up a portion of the rectus sheath only very medially and does not attach to the lateral edge of the sheath, that structure being composed of deeper layers. Inferiorly, the aponeurosis is slightly thickened and folded back upon itself to form the inguinal ligament. As such, this structure is not a true ligament, since its function is not to stabilize bone. The lower edge of the inguinal ligament is loosely bound to the fascia lata by the innominate fascia. This fascia also serves to bind together the collagenous fibers of both the aponeurosis and the inguinal ligament. Medially the inguinal ligament inserts on the pubic tubercle and fans downward onto the superior pubic ramus as the lacunar ligament. The medial attachment of the

TABLE 1.   Layers of the Abdominal Wall

Skin	
Fat (abdominal panniculus)	
Fascia (Scarpa's)	
Aponeurosis and muscle (external oblique)	Superficial stratum
Inguinal canal, muscle (internal oblique) and spermatic cord	
Aponeurosis and muscle (transversus abdominis)	
Fascia (transversalis)	Deep stratum
Fat (preperitoneal fat)	
Peritoneum	

inguinal ligament is continuous with the insertion of the aponeurosis into the linea alba.

External Inguinal Ring (Fig. 7)

Just above the inguinal ligament and lateral to its insertion onto the pubic tubercle, the fibers of the external oblique aponeurosis split to form a triangular opening, the external or superficial inguinal ring. The ring serves as the point of egress for the spermatic cord in the male and the round ligament in the female. It has no role in diagnosis, prevention, or treatment of inguinal hernia.

Internal Oblique Muscle

The internal oblique muscle is the central and most muscular layer of the abdominal wall. It originates from the lateral half of the inguinal ligament and the iliac fascia, from the anterior two thirds of the middle lip of iliac crest, and from the lower portion of the lumbar aponeurosis near the crest. The aponeurosis of this muscle proceeds medially to fuse with the aponeurosis of the transversus abdominis muscle to form the anterior and, in the upper abdomen, posterior rectus sheaths. The fused aponeuroses then proceed medially to insert into the linea alba as the rectus sheath. The lowermost portion of the internal oblique, below the semilunar line of Douglas, contributes only to the anterior rectus sheath. In that area, it fuses with the transversus abdominis aponeurosis to form the sheath, but in only 5 per cent of persons does it fuse laterally to the sheath to form a "conjoined tendon." That anatomic structure is more a rarity than a

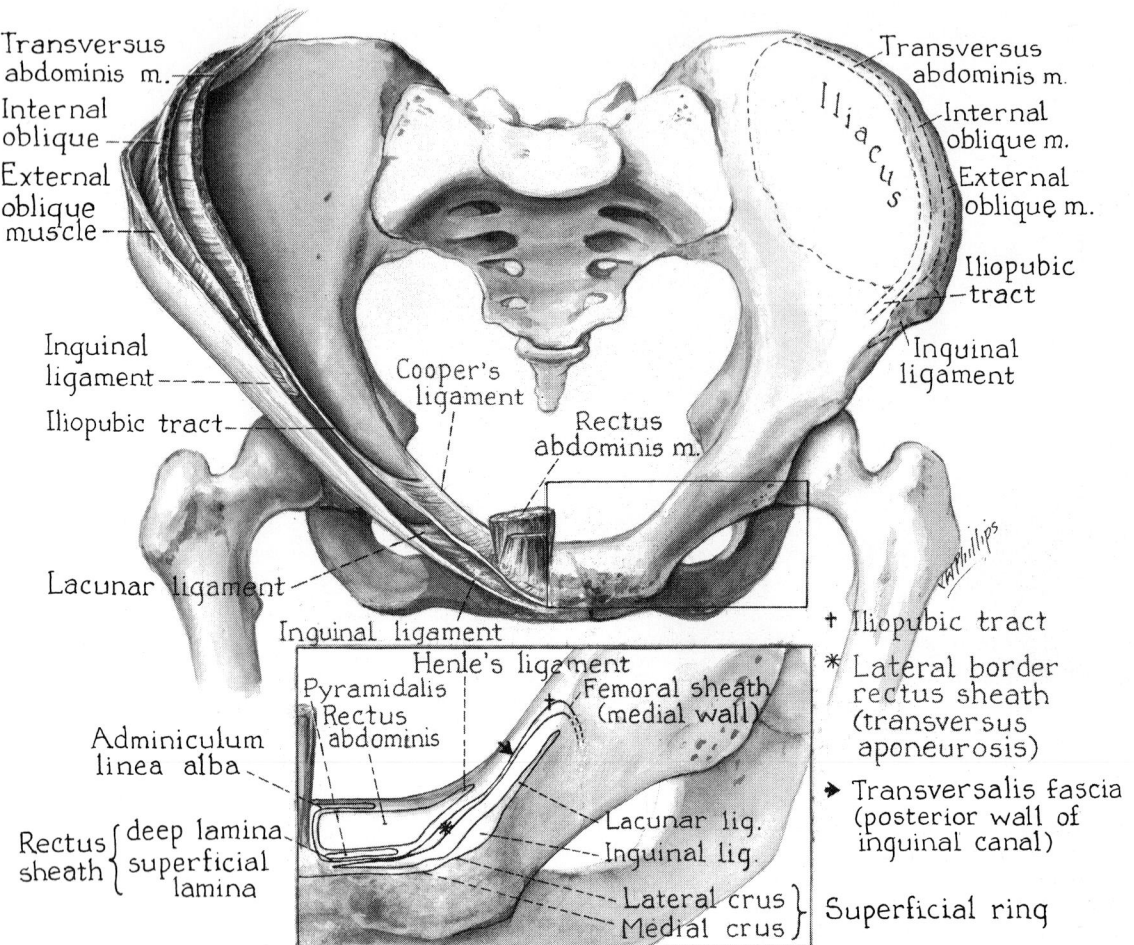

Figure 6. The skeletal origins of the three flat muscles are indicated in the main figure. The origins of the internal oblique and transversus abdominis muscles are not only from the crest of the ilium but also partly from iliacus fascia and the iliopectineal arch (not shown). The complex insertions of the muscle layers of the groin into the body and superior ramus of the pubis are depicted in the inset (left side). The inferior portions of each of the three muscles of the groin have been preserved in this dissection to illustrate the relationships between these layers. The drawing shows well the relationship between the femoral sheath and canal (removed) and the insertions of the iliopubic tract and lacunar ligament. The internal oblique muscle arches above the spermatic cord and across the groin to insert into the deep lamina of the rectus sheath, usually somewhat superior to the line of transection depicted here. (From Condon, R. E. *In* Nyhus, L. M., and Harkins, H. N.: Hernia. Philadelphia, J. B. Lippincott Company, 1964.)

constant finding, and its description should be deleted from the hernia literature.

Inferiorly and laterally the internal oblique originates from the inguinal ligament and the iliac crest and from deeper structures derived from the transversalis fascia. The medial margin of this insertion forms an arch over the internal inguinal ring. From this point fibers of the muscle arch downward and envelop the spermatic cord as it issues from the internal ring (Fig. 8). These fibers form the cremaster muscle. This muscle is important in hernia repair only in that it should be completely removed to expose the internal ring.

Transversus Abdominis

This is the most internal of the three flat muscles of the abdominal wall. It rises by fleshy fibers from the lateral portion of the iliopubic tract, from the inner lip of the iliac crest, the lumbodorsal fascia, and from the inner surfaces of the cartilages of the lower six ribs. It passes medially in a transverse fashion around the lateral aspect of the abdomen onto the anterior abdominal wall. At a point lateral to the rectus sheath, its muscular fibers are replaced by a tendinous aponeurosis, which fuses with the internal oblique aponeurosis to form the rectus sheath. The lower free margin of this muscle arches with the internal oblique from the lateral origin of that muscle over the internal inguinal ring to form a free edge over the ring and above the floor of the inguinal canal medial to the ring (Fig. 9). This arch, called the transversus abdominis aponeurotic arch, occasionally fuses with the arch of the internal oblique aponeurosis to form a "conjoined tendon" or falx inguinalis, but in only 5 per cent of

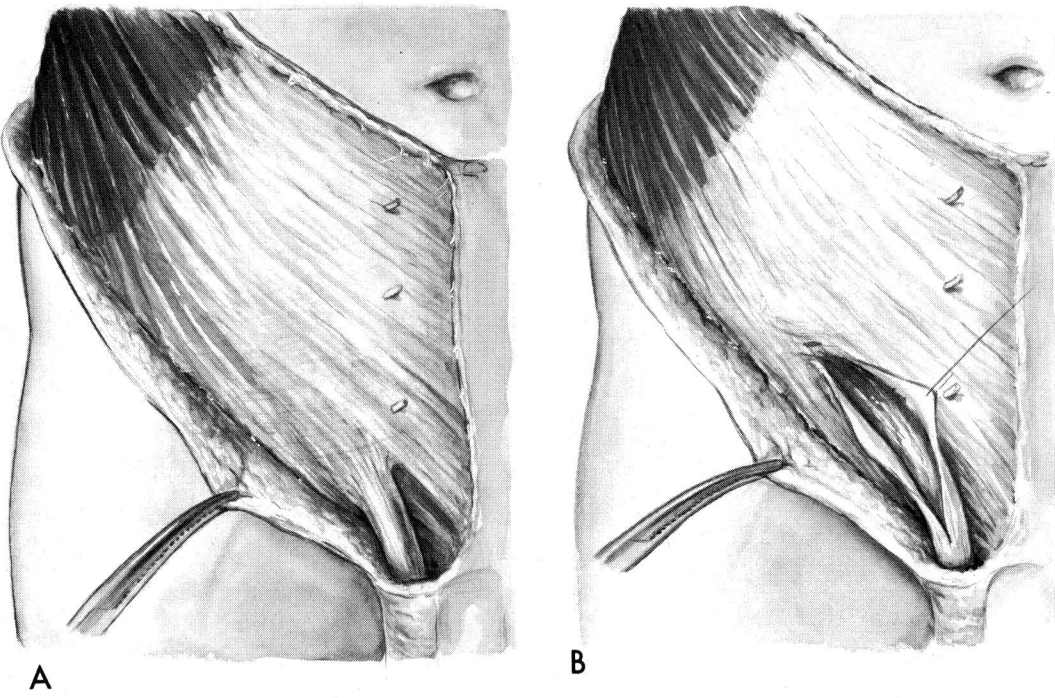

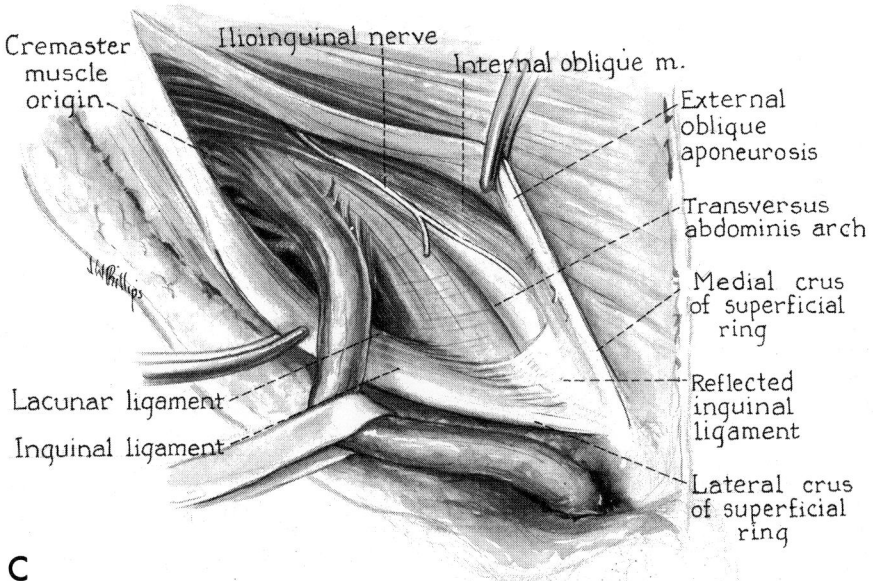

Figure 7. Dissection of the inguinal canal. *A,* The intact external oblique lamina is depicted. *B,* The external spermatic fascia and innominate fascia have been incised through the superficial inguinal ring. *C,* The external oblique aponeurosis has been opened widely and the spermatic cord mobilized by transecting many of its areolar (cremasteric fascia) attachments to the walls of the inguinal canal. (From Condon, R. E. *In* Nyhus, L. M., and Harkins, H. N.: Hernia. Philadelphia, J. B. Lippincott Company, 1964.)

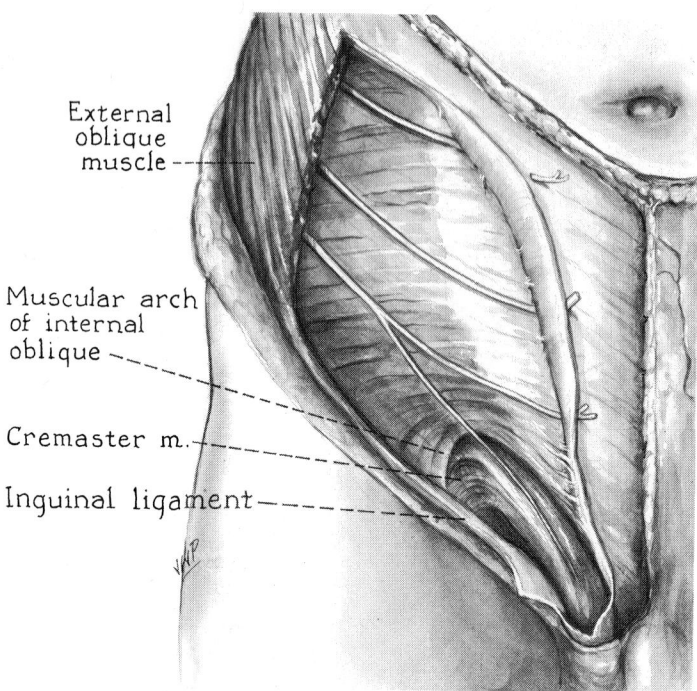

External
oblique
muscle

Muscular arch
of internal
oblique

Cremaster m.

Inguinal ligament

Figure 8. Deeper dissection of the groin (right side) to show the internal oblique muscle layer. The spermatic cord has been left in situ. (From Condon, R. E. *In* Nyhus, L. M., and Harkins, H. N.: Hernia. Philadelphia, J. B. Lippincott Company, 1964.)

cases. The common finding is that the transversus aponeurosis joins the internal oblique at the rectus sheath. The arch forms the upper margin of the area through which inguinal hernias of all types protrude. The arch itself forms a basic component of the anatomic repair of all inguinal hernias.

Endoabdominal Fascia

The endoabdominal or transversalis fascia is the most important layer in the prevention of groin and other abdominal wall hernias. This fascial layer forms a bag that holds the abdominal viscera within, and

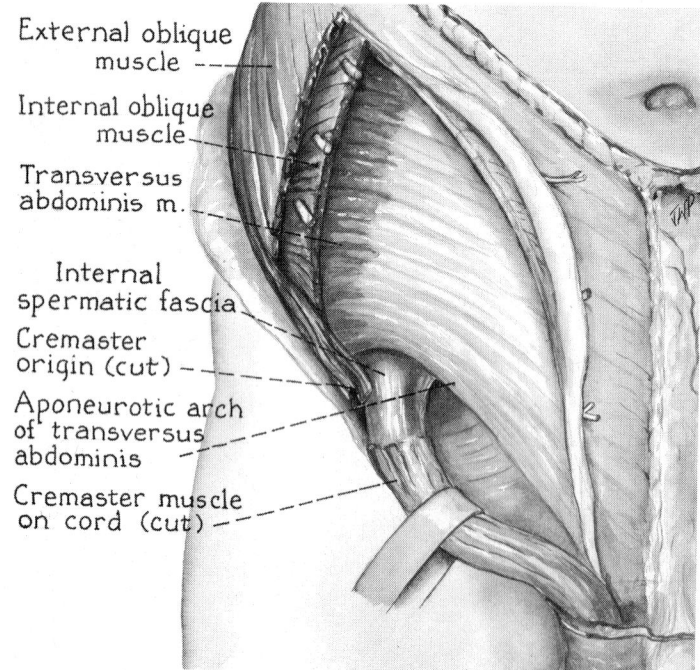

External oblique
muscle

Internal oblique
muscle

Transversus
abdominis m.

Internal
spermatic fascia

Cremaster
origin (cut)

Aponeurotic arch
of transversus
abdominis

Cremaster muscle
on cord (cut)

Figure 9. Dissection to show the deepest of the three muscle layers of the groin. The spermatic cord has been mobilized to show the arching muscular and aponeurotic lower margin of the transversus abdominis (the transversus abdominis arch). Inferior to this arch, the posterior wall of the inguinal canal is formed by transversalis fascia. (From Condon, R. E. *In* Nyhus, L. M., and Harkins, H. N.: Hernia. Philadelphia, J. B. Lippincott Company, 1964.)

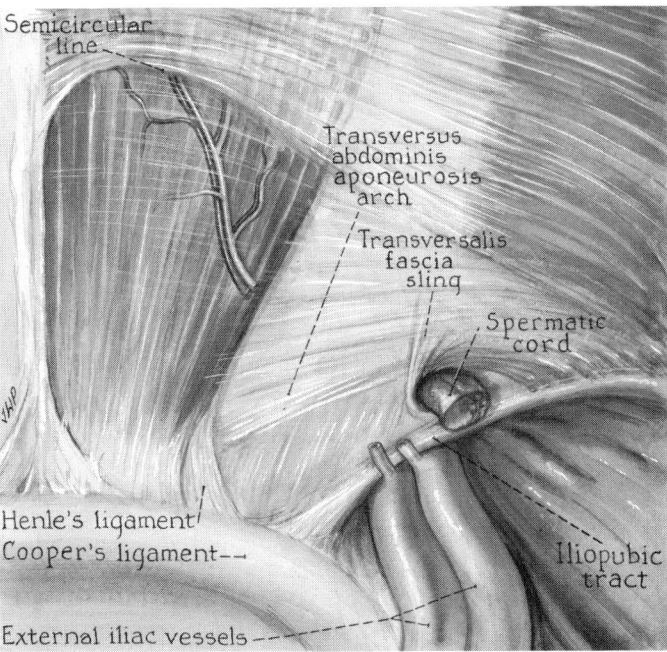

Figure 10. Posterior (internal) view of the right groin following removal of the peritoneum, preperitoneal fat and lymphatics, and the iliacus fascia. The spermatic cord has been transected just internal to the deep inguinal ring. The structures of the transversus abdominis lamina are well shown. The inferior epigastric vein is more frequently a double channel where it lies upon the rectus abdominis, and its junction with the external iliac vein is often a little more proximal.

This drawing is also a good illustration of the difficulties of medical illustration in the groin region, problems similar to those faced by the cartographer in attempting to depict a curved surface on a flat plane. In order to present a drawing with no discontinuities, increasing distortion and exaggeration must be introduced as one proceeds from the central focus to the margins of the picture. The geographic exaggerations of a world map drawn on Mercator's projection are analogous to those of this figure. (From Condon, R. E. *In* Nyhus, L. M., and Harkins, H. N.: Hernia. Philadelphia, J. B. Lippincott Company, 1964.)

separates them from, the muscular and bony layers of the abdomen without. Various portions of the bag are known by different names, depending on the external structure at that point. Thus, the endoabdominal fascia underlying the transversus abdominis muscle and its aponeurosis is known as the transversalis fascia (Fig. 10).

Hesselbach's Triangle

This classic anatomic designation is given to the area bounded superiorly by the falx inguinalis, laterally by the inferior epigastric vessels, and inferiorly by the inguinal ligament. As is already clear, the designation is confusing, since none of the three borders of the triangle is in the same layer of the abdominal wall. The inguinal ligament is superficial to the falx inguinalis (when one exists), and both layers are superficial to the inferior epigastric vessels. Use of this term in the description of hernia repair should be abandoned. More correctly, the boundaries of the floor of the inguinal canal, which is what Hesselbach intended to describe, should be limited to structures within that floor. These comprise the transversalis fascia and its analogs. For a complete understanding of these structures, the most important of the groin structures in hernia surgery, the reader is referred to classic works by Condon[16] and by Anson, Morgan, and McVay.[6] A full understanding of the anatomy and physiology of this layer is basic to a successful treatment of groin hernia.

Transversalis Fascia Analogs

In several locations in the endoabdominal fascial sac, there exist thickenings or condensations of the fascia, which are continuous with and integral to the sac itself (Fig. 11). These condensations, termed transversalis fascial analogs, usually are formed at points of insertion of various muscle groups, or at points of attachment at other fascial or aponeurotic structures into the fascial sac itself. Four important fascial analogs are the transversalis fascial sling, the transversus abdominis aponeurotic arch, the iliopubic tract, and the iliopectineal ligament (Cooper's ligament).

Transversalis Fascial Sling. The transversalis fascial sling reinforces the medial margin of the internal inguinal ring. The internal ring itself is the site of exitus of the spermatic cord from the abdominal cavity. It is located midway between the anterior superior iliac spine and the pubic tubercle, and is 2 cm. above the inguinal ligament. As the cord structures exit through the ring, they turn medially and inferiorly to traverse the inguinal canal. As they perforate the transversalis fascia at the internal ring, they carry a prolongation of the transversalis fascia with them, the internal spermatic fascia. Because of the abrupt inferomedial turn that the cord structures take, this tubular projection of fascia is bent inferomedially, forming a fold at its lower medial margin. This fold has been likened to a monk's hood. The fold itself forms a slinglike thickened condensation in the transversalis fascia at the medial and inferior margin of the ring.

Transversus Abdominis Aponeurotic Arch. The transversus abdominis aponeurotic arch has already been mentioned. It forms the superior border of the floor of the inguinal canal and consists of the fused aponeurosis of the transversus abdominis with the transversalis fascia.

Iliopubic Tract. The iliopubic tract is another fascial condensation wholly integral to the endoabdominal fascial sac (Fig. 12). It arises from the iliopectineal arch, which is a fibrous condensation of endoabdominal fascia, spanning the iliopsoas muscles as they exit from the pelvis. Via this arch, the tract gains in-

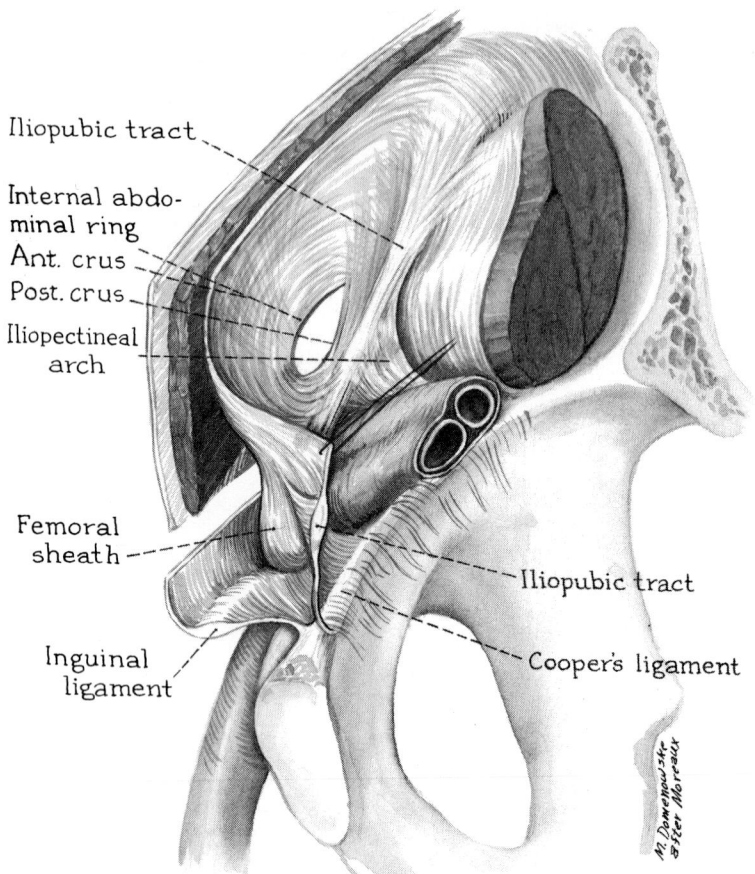

Iliopubic tract

Internal abdo-
minal ring
Ant. crus
Post. crus
Iliopectineal
arch

Femoral
sheath

Inguinal
ligament

Iliopubic tract

Cooper's ligament

Figure 11.   Fasciomusculoaponeurotic components of the lower abdominal wall. Right posterior
oblique view. Note relationship of the transversalis
fascia to the structures in the posterior inguinal
wall. Spermatic cord has been removed and the
iliopubic tract is reflected to demonstrate fascial
continuity with the femoral sheath. The posterior
inguinal wall (transversus abdominis–transversalis
fascia lamina) is firmly "rooted" to the thigh at this
point. The crura of the internal abdominal ring
also are well shown. (From Nyhus, L. M.: Surg.
Clin. North Am., *44*:1305, 1964.)

sertion on the anterior superior iliac spine and inner
lip of the wing of the ilium. From its insertion it extends inferomedially above and slightly behind the
inguinal ligament. Immediately after its origin, it
arches over the femoral vessels forming the anterior
portion of the femoral sheath. It then fans out to insert
along the superior border of the pubic ramus and the
pubic tubercle, and into the body of the pubis. Its lateral, recurved portion, that is, the portion that curves
down to the pubic ramus immediately after the ligament passes over the femoral vessels, forms the medial boundary of the femoral canal. It is this fanlike
recurved portion that ordinarily closes the femoral
canal, and not the lacunar ligament, which is external
to it.

Cooper's Ligament.   On the posterior aspect of the
superior ramus of the pubis and extending posterolaterally from it along the rim of the true pelvis is the
iliopectineal line. Periosteum of the pelvis along the
line is intimately fused with another condensation of
the transversalis fascia and iliopubic tract to form
Cooper's ligament. It is anatomically constant and
always strong in character.

Preperitoneal Space and Preperitoneal Fat

Between the transversalis fascia and peritoneum is
the preperitoneal space, which is loosely filled with fat
and fibrous tissue and is the internal analog of the
abdominal panniculus without. It varies in thickness
and density with the body habitus of the individual

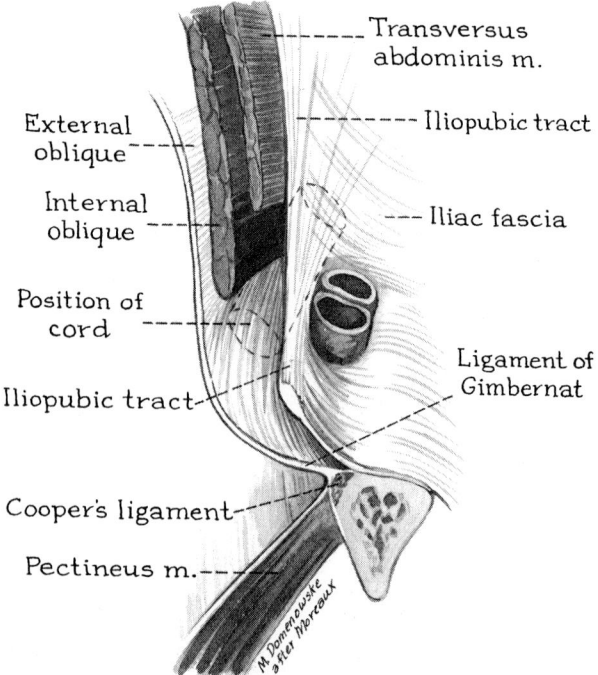

Transversus
abdominis m.

External
oblique

Internal
oblique

Position of
cord

Iliopubic tract

Cooper's ligament

Pectineus m.

Iliopubic tract

Iliac fascia

Ligament of
Gimbernat

Figure 12.   Relation of the iliopubic tract to the femoral vessels
and to Gimbernat's ligament. Medial cross section of right lower
abdominal wall, viewed medial to lateral. (From Nyhus, L. M.: Surg.
Clin. North Am., *44*:1305, 1964.)

and may in the extremely thin person represent only a potential space.

Peritoneum

Deep to the preperitoneal space and forming its innermost boundary is the peritoneum. In the groin, as elsewhere, the peritoneum is a thin elastic membrane, which serves only to provide a lubricating surface for its contained viscera. Because of the elastic character of the peritoneum, it does not act in the prevention of hernia.

Spermatic Cord

The spermatic cord is formed at the internal ring by the confluence of the vas deferens from the testis with the spermatic artery and veins, which are descending into the ring to the testis. In the normal male these structures are also joined by a slip of fibrous tissue, the ligamentum vaginale, which is the remnant of the processus vaginalis of the peritoneum. At the ring the testicular vein is formed by the confluence of the pampiniform plexus of veins, which provide venous drainage of the spermatic cord and testis. As these structures exit through the deeper layers of the abdominal wall, they pursue an oblique downward course for 5 to 7 cm. into the scrotum, through the inguinal canal.

As the cord structures pass through the internal ring, transversalis fascia is reflected onto the cord as the internal spermatic fascia. The internal oblique muscle then contributes muscular fibers, which invest the cord as the cremaster muscle. The cremaster-covered cord then proceeds downward toward the pubic tubercle and the external inguinal ring. As it passes through the external ring, the investing fascia of the external oblique aponeurosis, Gallaudet's fascia,[24] is reflected onto the cord, covering the remaining slips of the cremaster muscle as the external spermatic fascia. The cord then enters the scrotum.

Femoral Canal

This space, the femoral canal, is ordinarily closed by the reflected fibers of the iliopubic tract as they swing around the external iliac vein to attach to Cooper's ligament. It is a common misconception that the medial boundary of this canal is formed by the recurved fibers of the inguinal ligament. Those fibers and indeed that entire fascial layer is within the superficial stratum of the abdominal wall. The next most superficial layer is the inguinal ligament and its recurrent portion, the lacunar ligament. Thus, the hernia sac protrudes through the internal femoral ring lateral to the recurved portion of the iliopubic tract, across Cooper's ligament, which is posterior to the sac, and beneath the inguinal ligament. It protrudes through the fossa ovalis, which is the defect in the fascia lata left for entrance of the greater saphenous vein. The fossa ovalis is loosely closed with the cribriform fascia, which is a prolongation of the innominate fascia from the abdominal wall (Fig. 13).

PHYSIOLOGY OF INGUINAL CANAL STRUCTURES

In the normal person, two mechanisms act to preserve the integrity of the inguinal canal and to prevent protrusion of abdominal contents through the internal ring. The first of these is the sphincter action of the transversus abdominis and internal oblique muscles at the internal ring. The ring is attached to the transversus abdominis muscle via the transversalis fascial sling which reinforces the medial and inferior margin of the ring. When the transversus abdominis contracts it pulls the transversalis fascial sling superiorly and laterally. This serves both to close the internal ring around the cord structures and to pull the internal ring superiorly and laterally, under the buttress formed by the internal oblique. For this action to be effected, the transversalis fascia and its structures must be movable beneath the internal and external obliques. Any operative procedure that fixes the transversalis fascia or internal ring to a more superficial fixed structure, such as the inguinal ligament, destroys the sphincter action of the transversus abdominis.

The second mechanism closing the inguinal canal is the shutter action of the transversus abdominis aponeurotic arch, which normally is upwardly convex at rest, and is straightened and flattened when the transversus abdominis and internal oblique muscles are tensed (Fig. 14). Any tensing action brings the arch in apposition to the inguinal ligament, thereby covering the cord and buttressing the floor of the inguinal canal. It has been postulated that the occurrence of direct inguinal hernia is due primarily to a higher than normal position of this tranversus aponeurotic arch, so that when the abdominal musculature is stimulated and the arch brought down, it does not reach the inguinal ligament and iliopubic tract, thereby leaving a weakened area in the floor of the inguinal canal, which is defended only by the transversalis fascia. The incidence of recurrent hernia following various repairs and, indeed, all direct hernias have been attributed to this "congenital" malformation.

THE BIOLOGY OF INGUINAL HERNIATION

Both indirect and direct inguinal hernias are considered to originate from congenital variants, such as the presence of a preformed sac or processus vaginalis in the former and the failure of the shutter action of the transversus abdominis aponeurotic arch in the latter. The search for other explanations has to await the arrival of sophisticated investigators knowledgeable in the biochemistry of connective tissues. Studies now have been undertaken along these lines in Arkansas[77] and Arizona.[59]

The rectus sheath near inguinal hernias in adults was found to be thinner than normal. Indeed, upon careful analysis, specimens obtained from patients without hernia weighed more than similar specimens in patients with hernia. This decrease in actual weight of the specimens from patients with hernia was found to correlate with a decrease in hydroxyproline and thus collagen content. Fibroblasts were cultured from the anterior rectus sheath of patients with and without hernia. The rate of cell proliferation was less by a factor of 50 per cent in patients with herniation.

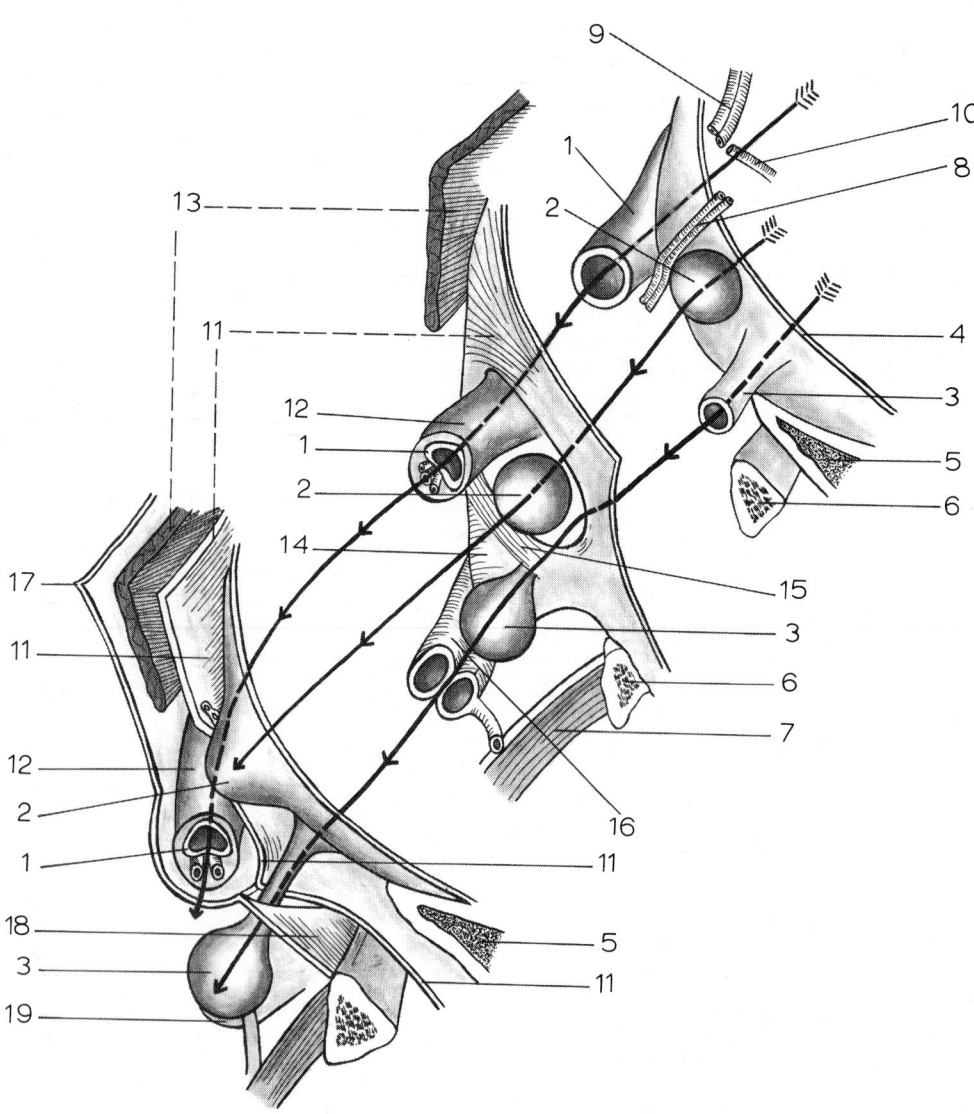

Figure 13. Formation of hernias of the groin.
A, Peritoneal protrusions:
1. Indirect inguinal hernial sac
2. Direct inguinal hernial sac
3. Femoral hernial sac
4. Peritoneum
5. Bladder
6. Pubic bone
7. Pectineus muscle
8. Inferior epigastric vessels
9. Spermatic vessels
10. Vas deferens
(From Gaster, J.: Hernia: One Day Repair. New York, Hafner Publishing Company, 1970.)

B, Transversus musculoaponeurotic fascial lamina:
11. Transversalis aponeurosis and fascia
12. Internal spermatic fascia
13. Internal oblique muscle
14. Femoral sheath
15. Iliopubic tract
16. Femoral vessels
C, Diagrammatic arrangement of groin:
17. External oblique aponeurosis
18. Gimbernat's ligament
19. Fossa ovalis

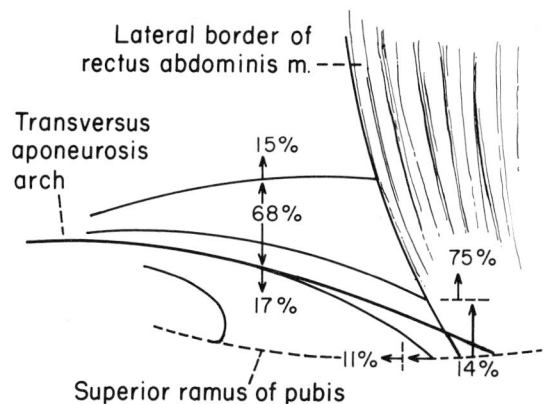

Lateral border of
rectus abdominis m.

Transversus
aponeurosis
arch

15%

68%

17%

75%

11%

14%

Superior ramus of pubis

Figure 14. The relationships of the insertion of the transversus abdominis arch to the lateral border of the rectus abdominis and to the superior ramus of the pubis as found in a group of 135 dissections of the groin. (From Condon, R. E. *In* Nyhus, L. M., and Harkins, H. N.: Hernia. Philadelphia, J. B. Lippincott Company, 1964.)

Other studies were performed and all results seemed to indicate a reduced collagen synthesis as part of the etiologic process in development of herniation in the adult. Peacock[58] has made a strong plea for further studies to elucidate both sides of the collagen equation, i.e., synthesis vs. degradation. These are important and refreshing new approaches to the study of inguinal hernia.

DIAGNOSIS, INCIDENCE, AND PROGNOSIS

Diagnosis

Diagnosis of hernia is made usually on the basis of physical examination rather than history. In children, however, the mother's insistence upon having observed a lump in the groin should alert the examiner to the presence of a groin hernia even if the first examination is negative. Similarly, chronic use of a truss may cause such a degree of scarring that the hernial sac does not readily fill with bowel. A negative examination in this setting should be followed after several days by success if the patient leaves the truss off in the interim. Dragging sensations or pain in the groin suggests the presence of a hernia. Modest pain is common at the outset, but as time progresses, sensations in the area become those of only vague discomfort.

Examination of the groin is best accomplished with the examiner seated on a low chair before the standing patient. The examination consists of the following: (1) observation of the groin area for evidence of a bulge or swelling while the patient coughs or tenses the abdominal musculature, preferably while holding a deep breath; (2) repetition of the preceding step with the index finger invaginated into the external ring for palpation of bulges or significant pressure impulses against the examining finger (note that an enlarged external ring without a palpable mass or impulse does *not* connote the presence of a hernia); and (3) repeti-

tion of steps 1 and 2 while the patient is lying down. At one time it was considered important to differentiate preoperatively between direct and indirect hernias during examination, but this seems less important now when surgeons are able to make an accurate diagnosis and perform an appropriate technical procedure at the operating table. Femoral hernias must be differentiated from inguinal hernias during the examination because their presence often means that a different operative approach is indicated. The common error is to miss a femoral hernia. If, on accurate palpation, the swelling protrudes below the inguinal ligament, it is femoral; if above, it is inguinal. A number of other "lumps and bumps" appear in the groin which must be differentiated from hernial swellings. These include: (1) inguinal adenitis; (2) ectopic testis; (3) hydrocele of the cord; (4) psoas abscess; (5) femoral adenitis; and (6) saphenous varix.

Incidence

Accurate figures for the incidence are difficult to obtain. Statistics available are those from the 1960 survey of the U.S. Department of Health, Education and Welfare,[73] which found that hernia occurred in approximately 15 per 1000 of the population interviewed, i.e., 3 million Americans. The same government agency found that 40 million days of restricted activity per year could be attributed to this problem. Each person with a hernia averaged almost 16 days of restricted activity as a result of the condition. More important, the total amount of work loss by the populace with hernias was 10 million days, a figure that reflects the prevalence of hernias in the male population. The economic aspects of the hernial problem are further revealed by a National Health Survey of 1974.[74] In one year, 1971, 488,000 hernia repairs were performed. Tonsillectomy was the only nongynecologic operative procedure performed with greater frequency.

Approximately 50 per cent of all hernias are indirect inguinal and one quarter are direct inguinal. Incisional and ventral abdominal hernias represent about 10 per cent, followed by femoral, 6 per cent; umbilical, 3 per cent; esophageal hiatus, 1 per cent; and miscellaneous rarer types, 2 per cent. The total balance tips in favor of the groin hernias, roughly 75 per cent of all. Parenthetically, it should be noted that 86 per cent of all groin hernias occur in males, yet 84 per cent of all femoral hernias occur in females. It must be emphasized, however, that the most common groin hernia found in the female is the indirect inguinal, and the incidence of femoral hernia in females is so high only because of the relatively rare incidence of femoral hernia in males.

Prognosis after Treatment

In this modern era of surgery, *recurrence* of the hernia after operative treatment remains a real problem. The poorer results are related to many factors, including: (1) failure of the operating room surgeon to understand the fine nuances of the surgical anatomy within the groin; (2) failure to use meticulous operative technique for the *common* hernia repair; and (3) failure to follow all patients operated upon so that each surgeon is aware of his technical shortcomings.[31] Until this subject is taken seriously, 100,000 patients per year will continue to be disappointed upon the recurrence of what was thought to be a simple problem.

THE DANGER OF HERNIA

Mortality

Morbidity and economic factors have been discussed. Unfortunately, death rates from this potentially curable entity remain high. A 1964 survey of the Department of Health, Education and Welfare showed that 2030 persons died from intestinal obstruction due to hernia. A similar report in 1967 listed hernia associated with intestinal obstruction as one of the 10 leading causes of death in the United States.[26]

Incarceration, Strangulation, and Intestinal Obstruction

The sine qua non of danger is protrusion of a hollow viscus outside its normal environment through a ring of variable size. If the viscus becomes caught by the ring and cannot be replaced it has become incarcerated. If in addition blood flow to or from the protruding viscus is compromised, the process of strangulation begins, with ultimate necrosis of the bowel if left unattended. Incarcerated hernias are difficult to differentiate from those in which the strangulating process has begun and therefore are considered to be surgical emergencies.

Incarcerated hernias may or may not cause intestinal obstruction, but essentially all hernias involving bowel that reach the stage of vascular compromise do cause the signs and symptoms of intestinal obstruction. There are two exceptions, namely, Richter's hernia, i.e., one side of the bowel wall is involved, and Littre's hernia, i.e., the incarceration and strangulation of a Meckel's diverticulum. In all patients with signs and symptoms of intestinal obstruction all potential hernia sites must be visualized and palpated, and contrariwise all patients with incarcerated or strangulated hernia should be carefully reviewed for the presence of intestinal obstruction. Femoral, indirect inguinal, and umbilical hernias are more likely to cause strangulation of bowel because these sacs have smaller necks that tend to be surrounded by rings of rigid tissue. Direct inguinal hernias usually have a broad neck, and incarceration with attendant complications is infrequent.

Recognition of impending or actual strangulation is extremely important, since emergency measures (operation) are indicated. Pain in the region of the hernial swelling and particularly tenderness to palpation are ominous signs. Sudden change from a state of hernial reducibility to irreducibility and discoloration of the tissues over the swelling are additional signs of strangulation.

Without signs of strangulation, an incarcerated hernia of short duration may be carefully reduced by gentle but firm pressure upon the swelling. It is possible to reduce the bowel content from its extracavitary position but not release the bowel from the peritoneal sac, i.e., reduction en masse. Thus, patients must be

observed for a period following reduction to assure restoration of normal bowel activity.

INGUINAL HERNIA IN CHILDHOOD

Infants and children with *inguinal* hernias nearly always have the *indirect* type. The hernias are related to abnormal descent of the testis and failure of normal obliteration of the processus vaginalis. Direct hernias in childhood are quite rare.

Diagnosis

Difficulties may arise in determining the presence of an inguinal hernia in infants; usually the older child presents no problem. A fat pad in infants may obscure the bulge, but careful inspection and palpation will usually suffice to establish the diagnosis. Palpation of the spermatic cord at its entrance into the scrotum may create, when rolling the fingers from side to side, a sensation of silk rubbing on silk if a hernia is present. In female infants, the lack of the spermatic cord may create further difficulties, but again the sensation of gliding silk ("silk glove" test) may be helpful. A definite history from the mother of a lump in the groin plus these suggestive findings is sufficient indication for operative exploration.

Treatment

There is general agreement that once the diagnosis of inguinal hernia is established, elective surgical repair should be performed. In general it is rare to find an infant or child of such poor risk that an operation cannot be done. Further, it is fallacious to believe that hernias in this age group heal spontaneously or that the application of a truss will obliterate the funicular process.

Since the cause of hernia here is failure of the processus vaginalis to become obliterated, and no muscular weakness is present, surgical treatment should include only obliteration of the hernial sac (by high ligation and transection, with or without excision of the distal sac). Thus, operative techniques that reinforce the abdominal wall ordinarily should not be used and the wound is reconstituted but not reconstructed.

INGUINAL HERNIAS IN ADULTS

Hernias may be classified as either funicular or diffuse. The former type protrudes through a tight fibrous ring of some sort, almost always at the site of exitus of some structure from the endoabdominal fascial sac. Indirect inguinal hernias, femoral hernias, and umbilical hernias are all funicular. These hernias tend to incarceration, obstruction, and even strangulation, because of the tight ring through which the herniating viscera protrude. In addition to causing the usual symptoms of dragging discomfort at the site of herniation, these hernias are always potentially disastrous and must be repaired whenever found.

Diffuse hernias, on the other hand, lack the tight constricting ring at the site of exitus from the endoabdominal fascial sac. Most ventral hernias, direct inguinal hernias, and lumbar hernias fit this classification.

In the indirect inguinal hernia the protruding viscus exits from the endoabdominal fascial sac through the internal inguinal ring. The herniating viscus, therefore, always has the same coverings as the investments of the spermatic cord, and does not actually protrude through any layer of the abdominal wall. By its nature, it always requires a preformed or at least a potential sac, which in this instance is the patent processus vaginalis. It is therefore a true congenital defect. Depending on the length of the patent processus vaginalis, the indirect inguinal hernia may protrude into the inguinal canal or through the external ring, or extend into the scrotum.

Indirect Hernia

The processus vaginalis testis is the peritoneal tube through which the fetal testis reaches the scrotum from its intraperitoneal origin in the seventh to eighth month. Normally it obliterates completely to form a fibrous cord, the ligamentum vaginale, which extends from a dimple on the parietal peritoneum deep to the internal ring down through the inguinal canal into the scrotum to the tunica vaginalis and testis. It may only partially obliterate anywhere along the course of its descent. The various anomalies of processus obliteration are frequently associated. An undescended testicle or a testicle in the inguinal canal is always associated with an indirect inguinal hernia. The high association of either testicular or cord hydroceles with inguinal hernias is well known.

Indirect inguinal hernias may be further subdivided with regard to the extent of dilatation of the internal inguinal ring. An infantile or childhood hernia may have a normal or only slightly enlarged internal inguinal ring, with the major defect being only protrusion of bowel into a patent processus vaginalis. It should be emphasized that a simple patent processus vaginalis is not a hernia, but that it possesses a high potential of becoming one.

If the hernia has been present for some time, the internal ring may be enlarged. Such a hernia is frequently found in the young adult. If the ring enlarges sufficiently to begin to push the inferior epigastric vessels medially, a simple adult hernia is present. If the enlargement impinges on the floor of the inguinal canal, a combined indirect-direct hernia is present. Occasionally the ring is dilated sufficiently without displacement of the inferior epigastric vessel to impinge on the floor of the inguinal canal. This condition results in an outpouching of peritoneum around the inferior epigastric vessels, so that both direct and indirect hernial sacs exist, straddling those vessels. This is the pantaloon hernia.

Direct Hernia

In a direct hernia the protruding viscus does not herniate through a preformed ring. The transversalis fascia weakens and bulges outward in front of the hernial mass. In the case of the direct inguinal hernia, the weakness in the wall of the sac is in the floor of the inguinal canal medial to the internal inguinal ring and medial to the inferior epigastric vessels. In the past, the location of the inferior epigastric vessels lateral to the hernia has been considered important. In our experience, these vessels may be anywhere with regard to the location of the direct hernia, and may even be a part of the wall of the hernial sac.

Most recurrent hernias are direct, resulting after the repair of indirect inguinal hernia. A few recurrent hernias will be indirect. In every instance, a recurrent indirect hernia is due to failure of the initial operating surgeon to remove the patent processus vaginalis (hernial sac) from the cord at the internal ring. As long as a peritoneal outpouching is left through the internal ring, hernia is a threat. The sac may be left in the cord if the sac is divided at the internal ring.

INGUINAL HERNIA REPAIR

Currently, controversy exists regarding the proper layers of the abdominal wall to be used for repair of inguinal hernia. On this basis the types of repair have been divided into the posterior (transversalis fascia lamina) and anterior (external-internal oblique lamina). Proponents of the posterior repair insist that the reconstruction of the inguinal canal and of the internal inguinal ring should be accomplished with preservation of deep groin anatomy. Transversalis fascial structures should be sutured to transversalis fascial structures. Layers normally found superficial to the inguinal canal and its content should not be used to reinforce the posterior wall of the inguinal canal. This approach is based on the concept that the basic hernial defect lies within the deep structures of the abdominal wall, that is, those deep to the internal oblique, and therefore the repair should reside within those layers.

On the other hand, proponents of the anterior type of repair do not make the distinction between superficial and deep layers of the abdominal wall, and consequently use superficial structures such as the external oblique aponeurosis and inguinal ligament as either anchoring points or artificial buttresses for repair of the internal ring and floor of the inguinal canal. Surgeons who use the anterior lamina ignore the fact that the superficial stratum of the abdominal wall musculature is movable upon the deep stratum and vice versa. Artificial attachment of the deep layer to the superficial layer results in strain at the suture line or attachment, and this may be the reason for the high incidence of recurrence with this type of hernia repair. Nonetheless, a large fund of experience has been reported with repairs described by Halsted, Bassini, Andrews, and Ferguson. Rarely, the anatomic layers of the deep stratum of the abdominal wall may be insufficient to permit repair strictly within that layer, and the more superficial procedures may be required.

A single operative technique is not appropriate in all patients. The approach must be designed at the operating table to properly handle the following variations: (1) small indirect inguinal; (2) medium indirect inguinal; (3) large indirect and direct inguinal; and (4) femoral hernias.[33]

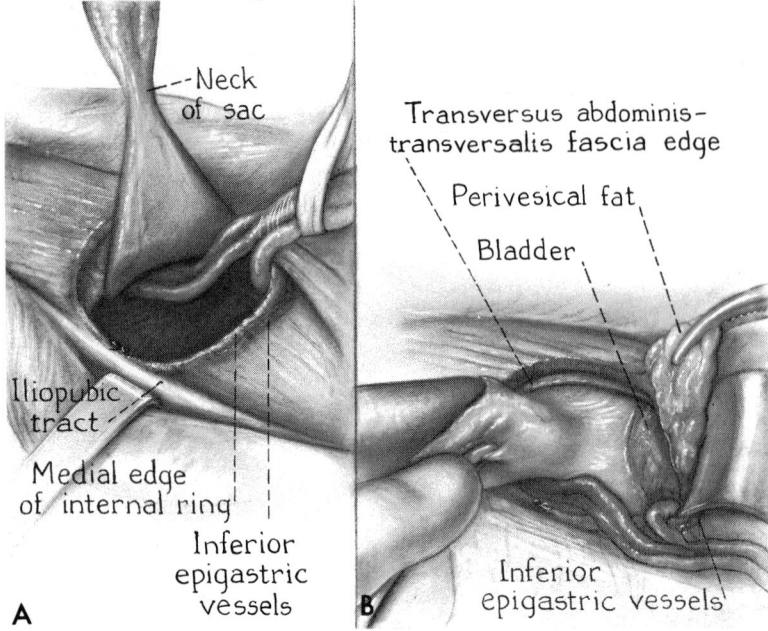

Figure 15. Repair of small indirect inguinal hernia. Identification of the internal ring. *A*, The vas and vessels have been separated from the peritoneum posteriorly. The vas turns medially while the vessels continue upward. Note how the neck of the sac is freed and pulled beyond the internal ring for ligation well above the neck. The medial boundary of the internal ring is now well defined after removal of the internal spermatic fascia. The iliopubic tract is exposed by downward retraction of the inguinal ligament. The iliopubic tract blends with that fascia adjacent to the ligated external spermatic artery. *B*, The retractor inserted into the internal ring pulls the medial edge of the internal ring and inferior epigastric vessels medially. The sac has been opened, and a finger inserted into the sac pulls the peritoneum out. The perivesical fat has been dissected from the peritoneum to expose bladder muscle. This dissection affords high ligation of the sac medially. (From Griffith, C. A.: Surg. Clin. North Am., *39*:531, 1959.)

Small Indirect Inguinal Hernia

The basic pathologic feature here is a patent processus vaginalis with minimal dilatation of the internal abdominal ring. After removal of the hernial sac and high ligation of the neck of the sac, restoration of the transversalis fascia surrounding the spermatic cord at the internal ring will suffice. Since the hernial sac tends to enlarge the ring medially, the sutures are placed medial to the cord structures. Although this is the simplest of all hernial defects to correct, it is also the most common and a meticulous anatomic dissection and repair here gives a great satisfaction. Griffith[30] in 1959 described a technique for this repair (Figs. 15 to 17), an anterior approach to the posterior inguinal wall.

Medium Indirect Inguinal Hernia and Attenuated Posterior Inguinal Floor

Occasionally, the internal ring has expanded (enlarged) further medially, and the posterior inguinal wall appears attenuated. In this instance the sutures are "walked" from the internal ring closure medially between the aponeurotic arch of transversus abdominis and iliopubic tract until the pecten of the pubis is reached. Thus, in addition to the plastic closure of the internal ring, the posterior inguinal floor has been strengthened. Small direct hernias are handled in the same manner except that dissection of the internal ring is unnecessary.

Anterior Inguinal Wall Repairs. It is to the small or medium indirect inguinal hernia that the classic Bassini operation consisting of sutures between the transversus abdominis aponeurotic arch and the lacunar/inguinal ligaments is best suited. The various modifications of Halsted,[32] Lucas-Championnière,[46] Andrews,[4] and Ferguson[23] are well known (Figs. 18 and 19). Literally millions of hernia patients have

been cured by these techniques. Yet an increased risk of recurrence persists (5 to 20 per cent) following the anterior wall repair of all (small and large, direct and indirect) inguinal hernias. If selected for use in repair

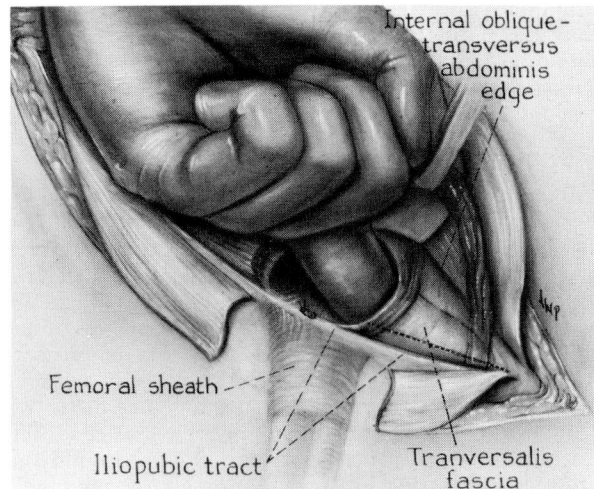

Figure 16. Repair of small indirect inguinal hernia. The hole in transversalis fascia. The sac has been ligated and removed. A finger inserted through the internal ring, behind the transversalis fascia preperitoneally down to the pubic spine, palpates the inguinal floor. A section of inguinal ligament has been diagrammatically removed to show the transversalis fascia comprising the inguinal floor. This diagram demonstrates that the iliopubic tract continues with that fascia adjacent to the ligated external spermatic artery. This fascia is also continuous with the femoral sheath. The stump of the external spermatic artery is therefore a landmark for the fascia comprising the inferior edge of the internal ring. Superiorly, the transversalis fascia continues beneath transversus abdominis aponeurosis. (From Griffith, C. A.: Surg. Clin. North Am., *39*:531, 1959.)

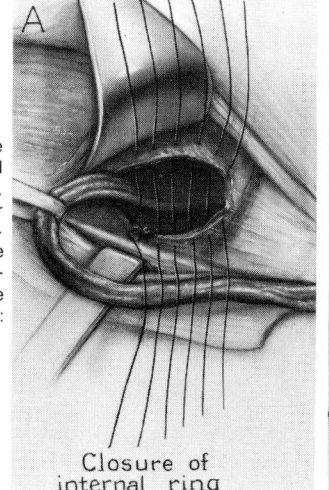

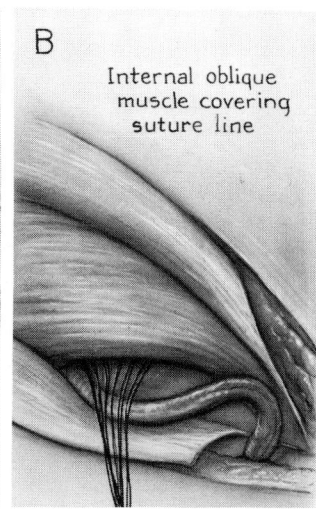

Figure 17. Repair of small indirect inguinal hernia. Repair of the internal ring. *A,* Sutures are placed through transversalis fascia and only transversalis fascia. The cord structures are displaced laterally. The reconstructed ring admits only the tip of a hemostat. The repair has been made possible by removal of cremaster muscle and retraction as illustrated. *B,* Retractors have been removed to allow the inguinal ligament and the internal oblique and transversus abdominis muscles to assume their normal positions at rest. The internal ring is buttressed by overlying muscle. (From Griffith, C. A.: Surg. Clin. North Am., *39*:531, 1959.)

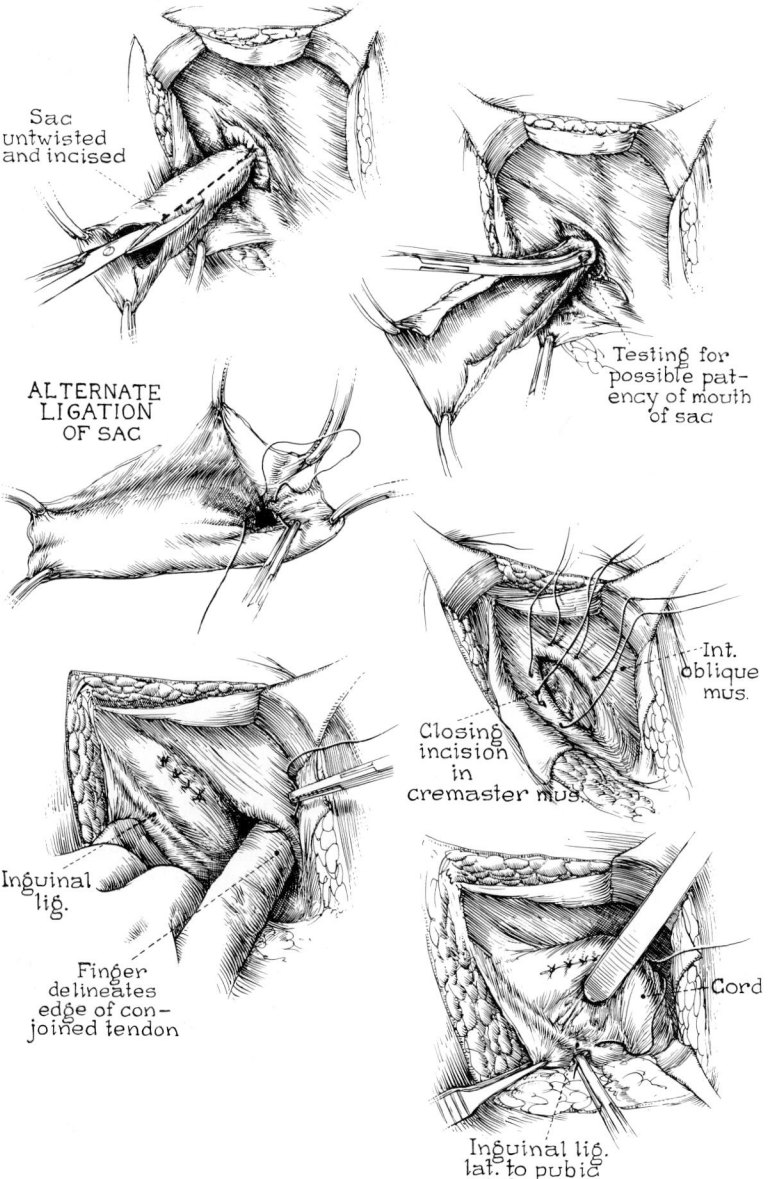

Figure 18. The classic Halsted-Ferguson operation. The anterior approach has reached the stage of high ligation of the peritoneal sac. The arch of transversus abdominis aponeurosis (frequently called conjoined tendon) is delineated as well as the inguinal ligament. (From Ravitch, M. M.: Repair of Hernias. Copyright © 1969 by Year Book Medical Publishers, Inc., Chicago. Used by permission.)

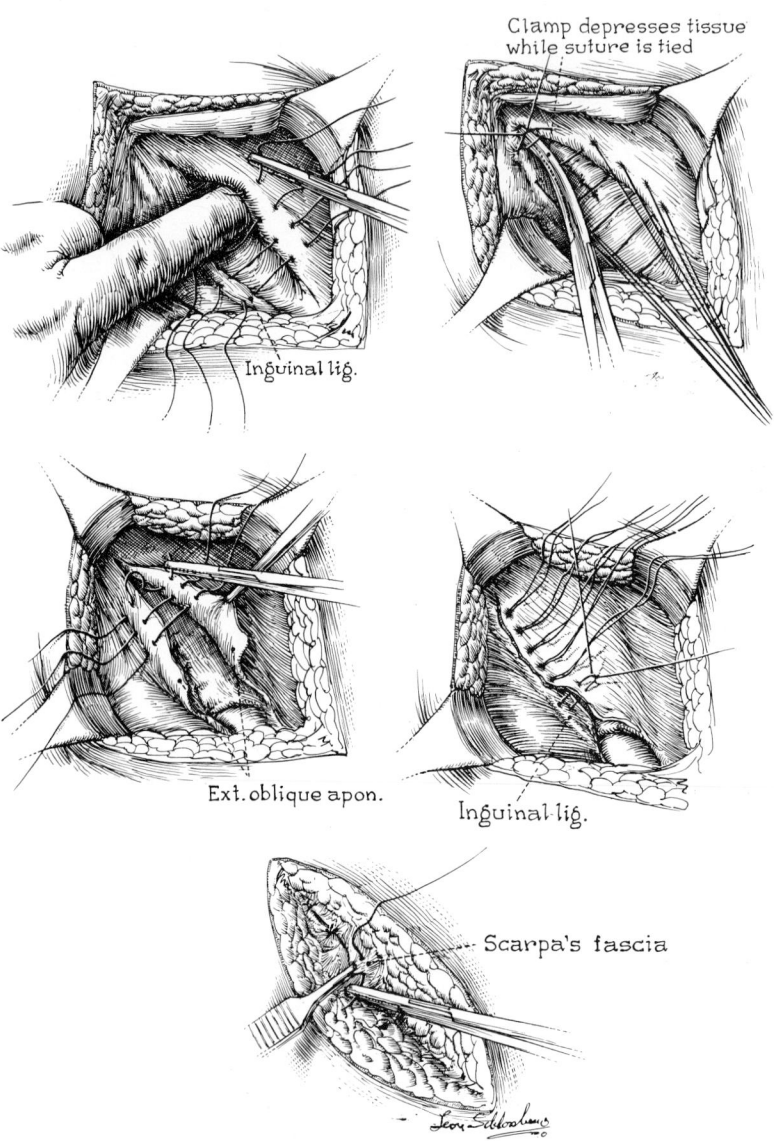

Clamp depresses tissue while suture is tied

Inguinal lig.

Ext. oblique apon.

Inguinal lig.

Scarpa's fascia

Figure 19. The classic Halsted-Ferguson operation. The arch of transversus abdominis is joined to the inguinal ligament from the tubercle of the pubis medially to near the internal ring laterally. Note that the spermatic cord has not been displaced and will lie beneath the joined tissues except for its exit at the superior edge of the pubis. The aponeurosis of the external oblique is imbricated with the medial flap overlapping as demonstrated. The free medial flap of aponeurotic fascia is then sutured to the lateral flap. (From Ravitch, M. M.: Repair of Hernias. Copyright © 1969 by Year Book Medical Publishers, Inc., Chicago. Used by permission.)

of small or medium indirect inguinal hernias, the overall results should be very satisfactory.

Large Indirect and Direct Inguinal Hernia

These are the most difficult problems. As the indirect hernia enlarges, it breaks down the posterior inguinal wall medial to the internal ring, so that in essence the surgeon must reconstruct the entire posterior inguinal wall and form a new internal inguinal ring. McVay has popularized the Cooper's ligament repair for this problem and has reported a 3.6 per cent overall recurrence rate; this result is unexcelled by any other author in the world literature.[33] Because of the importance of this contribution we quote from his description of the technique (Fig. 20).

In addition to the presence of the congenital hernial sac, *a large indirect inguinal hernia*, because of the greatly enlarged abdominal inguinal ring, has destroyed the posterior wall of the inguinal canal. In accomplishing the repair of this type of hernia, one must not only remove the hernial sac and make a snug abdominal inguinal ring, but also reconstruct a new posterior inguinal wall [Fig. 20].

Through the years, innumerable devices have been used to obtain muscular, aponeurotic and fascial material to replace the posterior inguinal wall. Some of them have merit while others are based on false anatomic premises. Any hernioplasty which fastens the new posterior inguinal wall to the inguinal ligament is anatomically unsound. It should be the object of every hernia operation to return the region to the normal anatomic state.

When the posterior inguinal wall is destroyed in part or in toto by a large indirect inguinal hernia, aponeuroticofascial tissue must be borrowed somewhere to close the defect. The simplest device is to use the aponeurosis and fused fasciae of the transversus abdominis immediately above and medial to the defect [Fig. 20]. This aponeuroticofascial plate also contains the lowest aponeurotic fibers of the internal oblique muscle. Where it lies over the rectus abdominis muscle, it is known as the rectus sheath. This layer is the ideal material because it is primarily aponeurotic. The fasciae, of which the

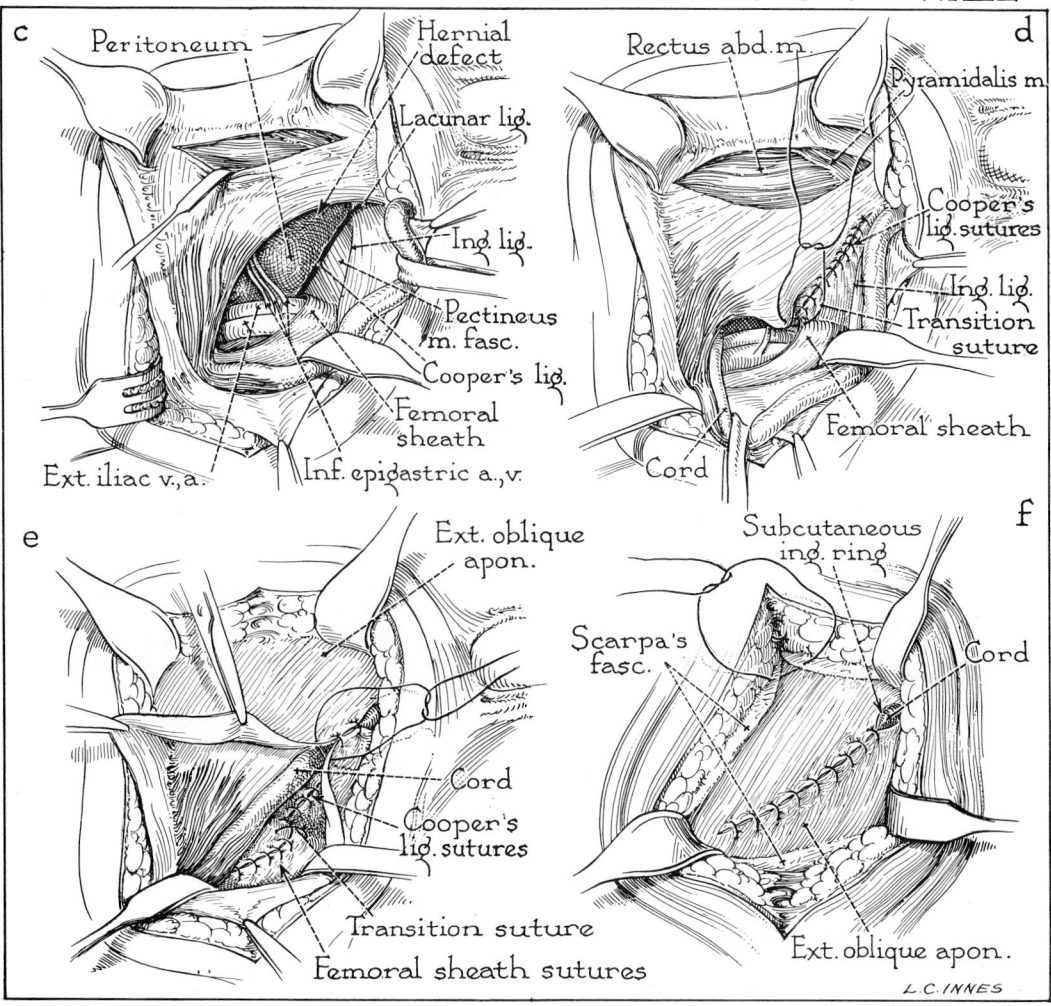

Large Indirect Inguinal Hernia

Direct Inguinal Hernia

RECONSTRUCTION OF THE POSTERIOR INGUINAL WALL

Figure 20. Hernioplasty for large indirect and direct inguinal hernias. *a*, Cutting out the attenuated portion of the posterior inguinal wall in a large indirect inguinal hernia. *b*, Attenuated posterior inguinal wall that is to be removed in a direct inguinal hernia. *c, d, e*, and *f*, Successive steps in the reconstruction of the posterior inguinal wall. Hernioplasty for both large indirect and direct inguinal hernias. (From McVay, C. B. *In* Davis, L.: Christopher's Textbook of Surgery, 9th ed. Philadelphia, W. B. Saunders Company, 1968.)

innermost layer is the transversalis fascia. serve to bind the aponeurotic fibers together into a firm and intact layer. Fascia or muscle does not meet the requirements for a satisfactory layer to close a hernial defect.

Another sound surgical principle is that layers should be approximated without tension. If one sutures the strong edge of the transversus abdominis aponeurosis to Cooper's ligament, there is considerable tension on the suture line. The same difficulty is encountered in the classic herniorrhaphies which use the inguinal ligament as the anchoring structure. To obviate tension, the relaxing incision [Fig. 20] should be used in every instance in which the posterior inguinal wall is reconstructed. A modification of the relaxing incision is the turning downward of a triangular flap of the rectus sheath. The slide of the rectus sheath made possible by the relaxing incision seems more physiologic than the flap method because the normal direction of musculoaponeurotic pull is maintained.

Before the new posterior inguinal wall can be transferred into position, all of the attenuated old posterior inguinal wall and hypertrophied cord fasciae must be excised [Fig. 20]. The peritoneal hernial sac must be dissected out and the neck of the sac ligated as for any indirect inguinal hernia. For an accurate repair of this hernia, one must have an evenly cut margin of transversus abdominis aponeurosis above, from abdominal inguinal ring to Cooper's ligament. Below, the glistening margin of Cooper's ligament must be seen medially and the edge of the anterior femoral sheath laterally. When these margins have been carefully dissected and the peritoneal sac excised, one is then ready to repair the hernia [Fig. 20].

After making the relaxing incision [Fig. 20a and b], the strong cut edge of the transversus abdominis aponeurosis is sutured to Cooper's ligament from the pubic tubercle to within a few millimeters of the external iliac vein [Fig. 20d]. This maneuver not only reconstructs the posterior inguinal wall, but it re-establishes a normally broad insertion into Cooper's ligament and thus obviates the possibility of the development of a femoral hernia. It should be noted that the relaxing incision [Fig. 20d] is now a considerable defect in the rectus sheath, protected behind by the rectus and pyramidalis muscles and their fasciae.

The next suture is the transition suture which approximates the edge of the transversus abdominis aponeurosis to the medial wall of the femoral sheath and pectineus muscle fascia. This suture is necessary to close the angle and permit the line of closure to come up from the level of Cooper's ligament to the more superficial level of the anterior femoral sheath. This distance is represented by the diameter of the external iliac vein.

The remaining defect is closed by suturing the transversus abdominis aponeurosis, or in case the layer is muscular at this point, the transversalis fascia, to the anterior layer of the femoral sheath. This re-establishes the normal continuity of transversalis fascia into the anterior femoral sheath. This line of sutures is continued laterally until a snug abdominal inguinal ring is made just as it is done for the repair of the small- to medium- sized indirect inguinal hernia. The spermatic cord is dropped in against the new posterior inguinal wall and the external oblique aponeurosis closed over it [Fig. 20e and f], thus re-establishing the obliquity of the inguinal canal. The subcutaneous inguinal ring is snugly closed.[54]

Repair of a large direct hernia is performed in a similar manner to replace the destroyed posterior inguinal wall. The only difference in the technique is the management of the peritoneal sac. High ligation of the peritoneal sac is mandatory in the operation for indirect inguinal hernia, but the broad neck of the direct inguinal hernia precludes the necessity of even opening the peritoneum.

Femoral Hernia

By popular usage, femoral hernia has been separated from indirect and direct inguinal hernias because of its exit beneath the inguinal ligament. We believe as others[33] that it should be considered a third variety of inguinal hernia. Its anatomic boundaries are familiar to us after study of the posterior inguinal wall: (1) superior—iliopubic tract (anterior femoral sheath); (2) inferior—Cooper's ligament; (3) lateral—femoral vein; and (4) medial—insertion of iliopubic tract into Cooper's ligament (previously said to be lacunar ligament).

The McVay Cooper's ligament repair is very satisfactory for repair of femoral hernia. Other techniques include the "low approach"[47, 78] and the inguinal approach (Annandale,[5] Moschcowitz,[55] Ruggi[65]). Resurgence of interest in the preperitoneal approach, particularly for femoral hernia, has occurred during the past decade.[56] For safety, for visualization of anatomic structures, and for ease of performance of ancillary procedures, the posterior or preperitoneal approach to the repair of femoral hernia is recommended. It is unquestionably superior to the direct anterior and subinguinal approaches.

Posterior (Preperitoneal) Approach to Femoral Hernia. The skin incision for the preperitoneal approach is different from that employed for the anterior approach (Fig. 21). It is oriented horizontally and is placed approximately three fingerbreadths above the pubic tubercle. One third extends over the rectus muscle and two thirds lateral to it. The edges of the skin incision are retracted and dissection is carried to the preperitoneal space. With blunt dissection the preperitoneal fat is dissected away from the lower abdominal wall.

The hernial sac can readily be seen protruding into the femoral canal medial to the external iliac vein and just lateral to the reflected fibers of the iliopubic tract, and anterior to Cooper's ligament (Fig. 22). The femoral canal is closed by apposition of the iliopubic tract to Cooper's ligament (Fig. 23).

A direct hernia may be repaired through this approach with excellent results.[43, 57, 63] However, since some authors[25, 51] report high recurrence rates following the preperitoneal approach and repair we do not recommend it for general use at this time. A Cooper's ligament repair may be carried out from the same approach. Cooper's ligament is readily identifiable at the inferomedial aspect of the wound as it proceeds posteriorly from the pubic tubercle along the iliopectineal line. As with the anterior approach, sutures are placed through the transversus abdominis aponeurotic arch and Cooper's ligament in the medial aspect of the repair, a transition suture is placed between the transversus arch, iliopubic tract, and Cooper's ligament, and finally the lateral portion of the repair is completed with sutures through the transversus arch and the iliopubic tract.

When Cooper's ligament repair is performed through the posterior approach, the transversus abdominis aponeurosis is seen to be apposed to Cooper's ligament with a deceptive lack of tension. This lack of tension is due to the incision in the transversus abdominis, which was used to enter the preperitoneal space. When the operative wound in the transversus

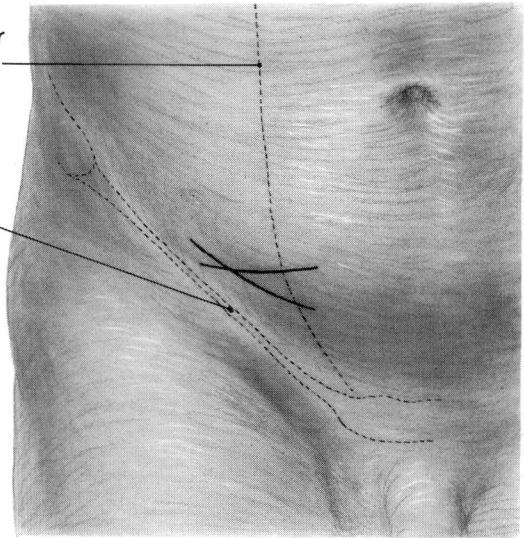

Outer border
of rectus m.

Inguinal lig.

Figure 21. Incisions used in the anterior and preperitoneal approaches. The preperitoneal area is approached through the short, horizontal incision. The direct anterior approach is achieved through the longer incision in the lines of skin tension. (From Nyhus, L. M., and Bombeck, C. T.: GP, *33*:115, 1966.)

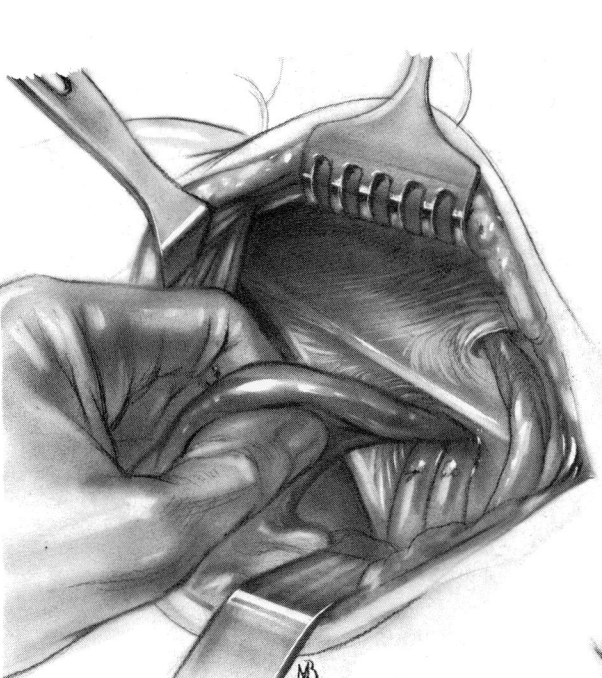

Figure 22. Femoral hernia. The peritoneal sac of the femoral hernia is reduced by traction and blunt dissection. (From Nyhus, L. M. *In* Nyhus, L. M., and Harkins, H. N.: Hernia. Philadelphia, J. B. Lippincott Company, 1964.)

Figure 23. Femoral hernia. The femoral canal is narrowed by sutures placed between the iliopubic tract above and Cooper's ligament below. (From Nyhus, L. M.: *In* Nyhus, L. M., and Harkins, H. N.: Hernia. Philadelphia, J. B. Lippincott Company, 1964.)

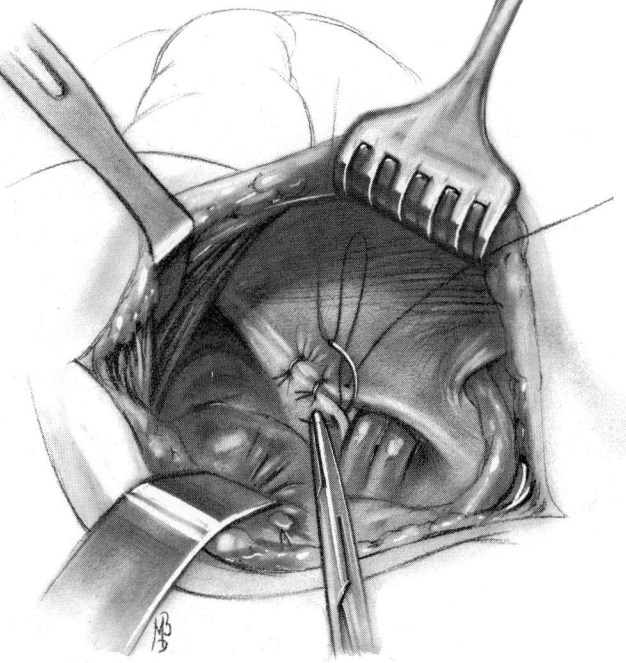

abdominis is closed at the end of the procedure, tension again is placed on this aponeurosis and therefore upon the suture line. Consequently, a relaxing incision must be placed as before.

SPECIAL PROBLEMS, HERNIAS, AND MISCELLANEA

Appendectomy

In the past it was debatable whether the appendix should be removed during repair of a right inguinal hernia. A good rule for the experienced surgeon is to do so if the appendix is adequately exposed and the patient can tolerate the procedure. It is unlikely that any harm will result from removal of the appendix in an otherwise uncomplicated hernia repair,[21] although most surgeons generally do not perform the procedures simultaneously.

Cooper's Hernia

The sac follows the femoral canal but additional tracts pass into the scrotum, toward the labium majus, and toward the obturator foramen.[2]

Division of the Spermatic Cord

Surgical castration, with removal of the testicle on the involved side, division of the spermatic cord at the internal ring, and complete closure of the ring, has been used as a method of treatment of inguinal hernia particularly in aged men and after multiple recurrent hernias. Prior written permission must be obtained if this is contemplated.

If cord division is planned without removal of the testicle, great care must be exercised in dissection of

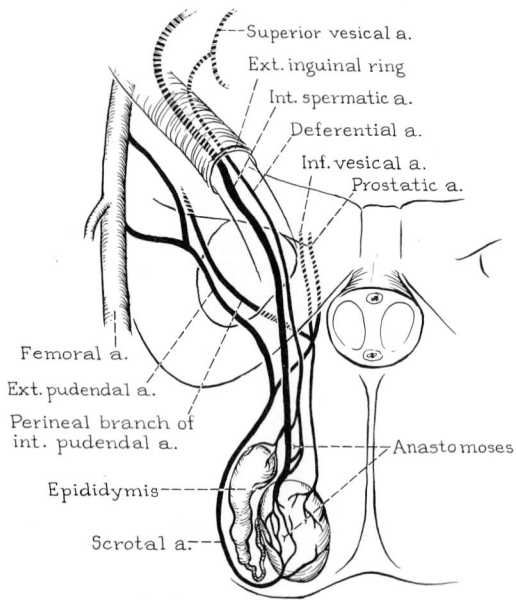

Figure 24. Schematic drawing of both primary and collateral circulation of the testis. (From Nyhus, L. M. *In* Artz, C. P., and Hardy, J. D. (Eds.): Complications in Surgery and Their Management, 2nd ed. Philadelphia, W. B. Saunders Company, 1967.)

Labels in figure: Superior vesical a.; Ext. inguinal ring; Int. spermatic a.; Deferential a.; Inf. vesical a.; Prostatic a.; Femoral a.; Ext. pudendal a.; Perineal branch of int. pudendal a.; Epididymis; Scrotal a.; Anastomoses

the cord to prevent embarrassment of the collateral blood supply of the testicle (Fig. 24).

Exploration of the Opposite Side in Children

Controvery continues whether the opposite groin should be explored in the infant undergoing repair of unilateral inguinal hernia. The incidence of a second hernia appearing on the contralateral side following repair of a clinically unilateral hernia has been reported to be between 3 and 31 per cent. There is an apparent discrepancy between this observation in a series of patients following their first herniorrhaphy, and the findings of other surgeons who report a much higher incidence of patent processus vaginalis on the other side when contralateral exploration is performed at the time of original operation. This has been used as justification for always exploring the contralateral side should conditions permit. Santulli[66] has compared two groups of pediatric patients presenting with unilateral inguinal hernia. In one group the hernia was repaired and nothing further was done; in the second group, the hernia was repaired and contralateral exploration carried out. A 14-year follow-up was conducted on the first group and in 12 per cent a contralateral hernia subsequently developed. In the second group, with contralateral exploration, a patent processus vaginalis was found on the opposite side in 56 per cent. On the basis of this finding, we do not recommend contralateral exploration. Cavanagh and Schnug[13] have stated what appear to be adequate criteria for contralateral exploration.

Given a surgeon familiar with pediatric surgery, an experienced anesthesiologist, an otherwise healthy baby, and an operation that is proceeding rapidly and smoothly, there appears to be little risk associated with bilateral exploration; however, if the baby is premature or has any associated illness, or should the surgeon have any difficulty with his initial repair, or if anesthesia is not being well tolerated, contralateral exploration should not be done. If the baby is being operated on for incarceration, contralateral exploration should not be done. In short, exploration of the opposite side depends to a large extent on the condition of the patient and the experience of the surgeon.

Hesselbach's Hernia (External Femoral Hernia)

This hernial sac passes into the pelvis lateral to the femoral vessels but below the inguinal ligament and iliopubic tract. It is usually associated with an indirect hernia on the same side.

Incarcerated and Strangulated Hernias

An incarcerated hernia is, by definition, simply an irreducible one. Incarceration of itself would not be a particularly emergent condition were it not for the possible supervention of strangulation of the incarcerated viscus. Strangulation of a hernia is a true surgical emergency and must be treated as soon as the diagnosis is made. The most commonly strangulated groin hernia is the femoral, but because it is a rare hernia compared with the inguinal hernia, there are fewer strangulated femoral hernias than there are strangulated inguinal hernias.

The usual vigorous efforts of the surgeon to reduce an incarcerated hernia must be tempered with the awareness of two possible complications. The first of these is "reduction en masse," wherein the hernia, with sac, is reduced within the endoabdominal fascia, so that even though the external bulge is reduced, the hernia remains incarcerated within the sac. Therefore, following reduction of any incarcerated hernia the patient must be carefully observed for signs of continuing intestinal obstruction.

The second possibility is the potentially catastrophic event of reduction of a strangulated, nonviable piece of bowel within the abdominal cavity. At the first sign of strangulation of a hernia all attempts at reduction must be abandoned and the patient operated upon immediately.

Inguinal Hernia in the Female

Indirect inguinal hernia does occur in the female, in which case the sac is adherent to the round ligament, since there is no spermatic cord. Because the round ligament serves no useful function, it can be divided at its exit from the internal ring and, following excision of the sac, the entire internal ring can be closed tightly. Inasmuch as no compromise is required to preserve a spermatic cord, recurrent hernia is almost unknown in the female.

Interparietal and Interstitial Hernias

These hernias represent a subgroup of inguinal hernia. The sac or sacs, in addition to the normal course, burrow within the abdominal wall, i.e., preperitoneally, where the sac lies between the peritoneum and the transversalis fascia; in the abdominal wall, where the sac lies between the transversalis fascia and the transversus abdominis, internal oblique, and external oblique muscles; or superficially, where the sac lies between the external oblique aponeurosis and the skin.[42, 45]

Lacunar Ligament Hernia (Laugier's Hernia or Velpeau's Hernia)

These hernias pass through Gimbernat's ligament. Incision of the ligament may be necessary for reduction of the incarcerated mass.[61]

Lipoma of the Cord

Lobulated preperitoneal fat may project down the cord at the internal ring. Since this fat pad presents as a mass, it may be mistaken for an indirect inguinal hernia. Whenever a lipoma of the cord is identified (usually found at the lateral margin of the cord), it should be excised to prevent confusion as to diagnosis at a later date.

Obturator Hernia

This hernia passes through the obturator foramen or canal in the os innominatum. It is a "hidden" hernia, and diagnosis is difficult. The diagnosis is suggested by a pain that passes down the inner side of the thigh to the knee (Howship-Romberg sign). If the hernial sac content is incarcerated or strangulated, a mass may be felt on rectal examination. These hernias are five times more commonly seen in females than in males. Most of the patients who have this type of hernia are elderly, weak, and often emaciated. Because of

the rigid walls of the orifice, strangulation frequently occurs.

The defect may be approached by the abdominal preperitoneal, inguinal, or obturator routes.[76] Tissue surrounding the defect is of poor quality and it is often necessary to patch the defect with prosthetic material such as Teflon or Marlex.[64]

Pectineal Hernia (Cloquet's Hernia)

This hernia enters the femoral canal and then perforates the aponeurosis of the pectineus muscle. Thus it does not present at the fossa ovalis. This hernia was first described by Callisen[11] and later in more detail by Cloquet.[15]

Perineal Hernia

Defects occur in the muscle floor of the pelvis through which peritoneal sacs project. Fortunately these hernias are usually reducible, and strangulation seldom occurs. There are three types: (1) anterior—protrudes anterior to the transverse perinei muscles and starts as a defect in the levator ani; these hernias usually contain bladder and are found most frequently in females; (2) posterior—similar to anterior but protrudes posteriorly in the levator ani or between this muscle and the coccyx; these sacs contain ileum and are also most commonly found in women; and (3) complete rectal prolapse. These hernias may be approached by the abdominal and perineal route or by synchronous use of both.[9, 28, 41]

Prevascular Hernia

This is a hernia found within the femoral sheath but anterior to the femoral vessels. It is rare, and it may be treated by either the Cooper's ligament or iliopubic tract repair.[10, 72]

Prosthetic Materials

Many artificial aids to hernia repair have been used in past years. These include fascial sutures, fascia lata grafts taken from the thigh, ox fascia, dermal grafts, and all of the various prosthetic meshes such as stainless steel, nylon, tantalum, and finally Marlex or polypropylene.[1, 3, 27, 39, 40, 69, 70] With the currently available methods of repair, these ancillary measures should rarely be required. Nonetheless, should the autogenous tissues be so deficient as to make it impossible to close the defect of a direct inguinal hernia, the newer plastic meshes such as Marlex or polypropylene can be employed.

Retrovascular Hernia (Serafini's Hernia)

This is a hernia that passes within the femoral sheath but exits posterior to the femoral vessels.[68]

Sciatic Hernia

The rarest of all hernias, it makes its exit through the greater or lesser sacrosciatic foramen. The mass presents below the fold in the buttock. It may be approached by the abdominal or sciatic route, but occasionally a synchronous technique is advantageous.[70]

Sliding Inguinal Hernias

Occasionally the cecum on the right or the sigmoid

colon on the left makes up a portion of the sac wall in an indirect inguinal hernia. In that instance, special care must be exercised to avoid opening the bowel or devascularizing it when dealing with the sac. For this reason, since it is difficult to determine whether a sliding hernia is present until the hernial sac is opened, the sac of an indirect hernia is always opened on its anterior medial aspect. The hernia itself is due to failure of fusion of the two leaves of peritoneum as they cover the colon; these leaves are allowed to evert around the colon as it protrudes into a hernial sac. Once the sac has been inverted the repair is carried out as for any other indirect inguinal hernia. In the female, especially the infant and child, the sliding hernia may also contain portions of the female genital tract, but these are dealt with in the same fashion as the colon, with imbrication of the peritoneal sac behind the protruding structure.

Supravesical Hernia

This is another rare hernia first described by Sir Astley Cooper. Keynes[37] has cataloged the types and treatment extensively.

ABDOMINAL WALL HERNIA

Abdominal wall hernia may be defined as any protrusion of the abdominal viscera through the endoabdominal fascial sac. Examples are umbilical, epigastric, lumbar (both superior and inferior), spigelian, and ventral incisional hernia.

Umbilical Hernia

Umbilical hernia is a true congenital defect, occurring through the patent umbilical ring following obliteration of the umbilical vessels after delivery. It is considerably more common in Negro infants than in Caucasian, but the reason for this difference is not clear. True umbilical hernia is to be distinguished from omphalocele, which is due to failure of abdominal wall closure in the midline about the umbilicus, in early intrauterine life.

The hernia is present in 10 per cent of Caucasian infants and in 40 to 90 per cent of Negro infants. In almost all of these, the patent umbilical ring closes spontaneously by the age of 2 years. Opinion is currently divided regarding whether any umbilical hernia in a child ever requires operation except for urgent indication. Some surgeons advise nothing but observation of the hernia until the child is 2 years old, and then surgical correction should a defect greater than 1 cm. persist. Other authors, on the basis of a large series of patients observed for many years, recommend no operation at all on the assumption that all umbilical hernias eventually close.[38]

Incarceration and strangulation of umbilical hernias, although rare, do occur. Rupture of an umbilical hernia may also occur, especially in cases of blunt abdominal trauma. In these instances, the hernia is dealt with in the same way as any strangulated hernia or any external rupture of the abdominal viscera.

In distinction to infantile umbilical hernia, umbilical hernia in the adult must always be treated with the same dispatch used for the treatment of an inguinal hernia, for it is known to be liable to incarceration or strangulation or both. Spontaneous or traumatic rupture of umbilical hernia in pregnancy or in cirrhosis with ascites is not uncommon. Baron[7] has indicated that surgical repair of an umbilical hernia in the cirrhotic patient may precipitate variceal hemorrhage. He attributes this to interruption of collateral venous channels that moderate portal venous pressure.

The Repair. The classic repair for umbilical hernia is that proposed by Mayo[52] in 1907, the "pants-over-vest" method. Farris[22] has proposed that the Mayo repair for umbilical hernia may not be necessary. On the basis of both experimental and human operative experience, he has advocated a simple transverse closure of the defect with good results.

The poor results with umbilical hernia repair prior to the use of the Mayo operation were most likely due to the poor surgical technique and unsuitable suture material that characterized the period. With advances in surgical technique, better suture material, and better anesthesia, simple closure of the defect, whether in the transverse or vertical plane, has become the treatment of choice.

Recurrence of an umbilical hernia is rare, and only isolated reports have appeared in the literature. Should hernia recurrence become a problem in any individual patient, owing to the size of the umbilical hernia, a prosthetic mesh repair may be required.

Epigastric Hernia

All hernias occurring in the midline of the abdomen, with the exception of those of the umbilicus, are collectively referred to as hernias of the linea alba. These hernias are far more common above the umbilicus than below and are termed epigastric hernias. They are much more common than generally realized, occurring in approximately 5 per cent of the general population at autopsy. Most are small and asymptomatic and therefore undiagnosed.

It may be difficult to diagnose a small epigastric hernia consisting only of a tag of omentum herniated through the linea alba. The presence of unexplained upper abdominal symptoms, especially in the obese patient, which are aggravated when the patient reclines on his back, should lead one to suspect this diagnosis. This latter finding, pain on reclining, is thought to be due to traction on the incarcerated tissue.

Pain in the linea alba is also a common presenting finding in other upper abdominal diseases. Therefore, a thorough survey for intra-abdominal disease must be carried out before epigastric hernia is incriminated. The diagnosis is easily made by palpation of a small subcutaneous mass in the linea alba.

Current accepted treatment of epigastric hernia is simple closure of the defect. These hernias are frequently multiple, and a wide exposure of the linea alba through a vertical midline skin incision is indicated.

Ventral (Incisional) Hernia

Incisional hernia is the one true iatrogenic hernia. Principles of treatment of incisional hernia should therefore begin with principles of prevention, that is, principles of proper wound closure. The most common cause of incisional hernia is wound infection, and this should be borne in mind during closure of possibly contaminated wounds. Proper principles of wound closure are dealt with elsewhere in this volume.

Transverse incisions are associated with a significantly lower incidence of wound disruption and incisional hernia than are vertical incisions. Nonetheless, vertical incisions continue to be used for operations on the alimentary tract when transverse incisions would suffice. The anatomic reason for the superiority of transverse incisions is simple. All strata of the abdominal wall, save the rectus abdominis muscle, are collections of fibers, either muscular or fascial, that are oriented in a horizontal direction. The tension exerted by the muscular layers of the abdominal wall is directed horizontally. Vertical incisions are therefore always placed across the lines of force exerted by the abdominal musculature and are always closed under tension. In transverse incisions, tension exerted by the abdominal musculature tends more to appose the edges of the incision than to disrupt them.

More than with any other hernia of the abdominal wall, obesity plays a role in recurrence after ventral hernia repair. Extreme obesity may be regarded as a contraindication to the repair of any incisional hernia, except in the emergent situation.

Incisional hernias, if small, are subject to the same complications as funicular hernias in any other area of the body. They are usually large and diffuse, however. Because of the trauma that has occurred at the operative site, incarceration is relatively common in these hernias, but since they are diffuse, strangulation is rare. One dreaded complication is spontaneous rupture of an incisional hernia with evisceration. Because of the relative fragility of the overlying scar in the superficial layer covering the hernia, this complication is relatively more common with this type of hernia than it is with others.

The treatment of incisional hernia is simple closure of the defect, but this may require a complicated procedure. An incisional hernia is always due to separation of the suture line originally used to close the operative wound. Frequently, the same factors that caused the suture line separation and herniation in the first place will still be operable when a second suture line is placed at the same site. Furthermore, each time a wound disrupts the defect grows larger and more difficult to close. This is especially true of hernias that have occurred through vertical incisions. The surgeon is frequently faced with an ovoid, ever widening defect that is oriented vertically and must be closed under tension.

As might be expected because of the difficult nature of the defect, the absence of suitable contiguous tissues to be used in the repair, and the consequent high recurrence rate, the number of operative procedures proposed for the correction of incisional hernia is high. Prosthetic meshes, autogenous or heterologous fascia, and special suture techniques were first devised for repair of these hernias.

Preoperative treatment of the patient includes correction of any nutritional or metabolic deficits that may be present to contribute to recurrence of the hernia, reduction of weight if the patient is obese, and finally treatment of ancillary systemic conditions which, through augmentation of intra-abdominal pressure, may contribute to recurrence. Some measures to increase intra-abdominal volume may also be necessary in patients with chronic pulmonary dysfunction. Progressive pneumoperitoneum has proved to be very effective.[29] Reinsertion of abdominal content that has been within the hernial sac for an indeterminate length of time may severely limit diaphragmatic excursion in these patients, and possibly result in severe embarrassment of pulmonary function. Very large incisional hernias may even contribute to pulmonary dysfunction by compromise of the efficiency of the cough mechanism in patients with chronic bronchitis and emphysema. Under these circumstances, repair of the hernia is indicated because of respiratory disease, not despite it.

Incisional hernias are treated by three types of operation, varying as to their complexity. In the first, simple closure, nothing is necessary save simple reapproximation of the edges of the fascial defect at the transversalis fascial level and above. This repair is probably sufficient for hernias occurring through transverse incisions and for other small incisional hernias. Special attention must be paid to the ends of the wound created, for it is here that recurrent herniation is most likely to occur.

For larger incisional hernias and those with gaping fascial defects, two relatively complicated types of operation are used, those using autogenous tissues and those using prosthetic devices.

Spigelian Hernia

Spigelian hernia, or spontaneous lateral ventral hernia as it is sometimes called, may be defined as a protrusion through the spigelian fascia. The spigelian fascia is that area of the transversus abdominis aponeurosis lateral to the edge of the rectus sheath, but medial to the spigelian line. The spigelian line is the point of transition of the transversus abdominis muscle to its aponeurotic tendon. The fascia begins at about the level of the eighth or ninth costal cartilage and extends downward to the pubic tubercle. It is widest at a point just below the umbilicus in the region of the semilunar line of Douglas. Most spigelian hernias occur at the widest and therefore weakest area of the spigelian fascia, but they have been reported at the lowermost extent of this fascia, wherein they are easily confused with direct inguinal hernia. The distinction is easily made, since a lower spigelian hernia always protrudes through the transversus abdominis aponeurotic arch, while a direct hernia protrudes below it. Spigelian hernias, being small, are of the funicular type and have a high incidence of incarceration and strangulation.

The treatment is straightforward. A transverse skin incision is made over the defect and carried down through the external oblique aponeurosis, which is opened in the direction of its fibers. The hernial sac is identified, isolated, opened, ligated, and closed in the usual fashion. The transversus abdominis aponeurotic defect can usually be closed with a few interrupted nonabsorbable sutures. Wound closure is carried out in the usual fashion. Cases reported in the literature are too few for assessment of recurrences to be possible.

Lumbar Hernia (Petit's Triangle Hernia and Grynfeltt's Hernia)

These are also relatively rare hernias, only 250 to 300 cases having been reported in the literature. The more common of the two is superior lumbar hernia, or Grynfeltt's. Probably superseding both of these, however, are incisional hernias resulting from nephrectomy or traumatic hernias of the lumbar region.

The inferior lumbar triangle is an anatomic area of weakness, bounded posteriorly by the latissimus dorsi, anteriorly by the external oblique, and inferiorly by the iliac crest. Its floor is formed by the internal oblique and transversus abdominis muscles. The superior triangle or triangle of Grynfeltt-Lesshaft is situated above and anterior to Petit's triangle and is normally covered by the latissimus dorsi and serratus posterior inferior muscle. The boundaries of the triangle are the twelfth rib above, which forms the base, and the anterior border of the internal oblique anteriorly. The floor is ordinarily the quadratus lumborum muscle mass. It is more constant and larger than Petit's triangle, which accounts for the higher incidence of hernia through it. Etiologically, hernias through these triangles are either spontaneous or traumatic. Congenital hernias have also been described in this region. The incidence of strangulation is approximately 10 per cent.

Because of the anatomy of these hernias, treatment is difficult. Until the advent of satisfactory mesh repairs, the basic principle of treatment of Petit's triangle hernia was that advocated by Dowd[20] in 1907, which involved closure of the defect by a pedicle flap of tensor fascia lata and gluteus maximus from below the iliac crest, with side-to-side apposition of the external oblique and latissimus dorsi. Repair of the upper triangle is essentially the same, depending on the development of flaps from adjacent structures. The basic principle of repair of all lumbar hernias is initial closure of the transversalis fascial defect.

With the increasing use of mesh prostheses, it seems likely that the treatment of choice is the employment of one of these aids. If the hernia is small, operative repair by suture of the external oblique to the latissimus dorsi, with or without fascia lata reinforcement, has been successful.

In addition to the aforementioned two varieties of lumbar hernia, there have been isolated reports of hernias occurring through congenital defects or eventrations of other portions of the posterior abdominal wall. Most of these are treated by simple closure of the defect, or by pedicle flap or prosthetic closure should the defect be large. The most common posterior hernia is the postnephrectomy incisional hernia. Its repair is essentially the same as that for incisional hernia in any location.

SELECTED REFERENCES

Anson, B. J., and McVay, C. B.: Surgical Anatomy, 5th ed. Philadelphia, W. B. Saunders Company, 1971.
This two-volume monograph includes the finest review of hernial anatomy available today. The section on the abdominal wall represents a distillate of over 30 years of active study, both in the anatomy laboratory and at the operating room table.

Condon, R. E.: Surgical anatomy of the tranversus abdominis and transversalis fascia. Ann. Surg., *173*:1, 1971.
By reproducing in color a photograph of the posterior inguinal wall, Condon has helped "clear the air" of many anatomic misconceptions of groin anatomy. This report gives a succinct but exceptionally clear description of the posterior inguinal wall.

Fruchaud, H.: Traitement chirurgical des hernies de l'aine chez l'adulte. Paris, G. Doin & Cie, 1956.

Fruchaud, H.: Anatomie chirurgical des hernies de l'aine. Paris, G. Doin & Cie, 1956.
These two monographs are beautifully illustrated. All interested in this subject should review these fine works.

Glassow, F.: Short-stay surgery (Shouldice technique) for repair of inguinal hernia. Ann. R. Col. Surg. Engl., 58:133, 1976.
The Shouldice Hospital in Thornhill, Ontario, is unique because the only operations performed there are related to the problem of hernia. Dr. Glassow reports on his personal 21-year experience with 14,982 consecutive inguinal hernial repairs. He gives an overall recurrence rate of 0.6 per cent using the Shouldice method, which includes a multiple-layer closure of continuous stainless steel wire sutures.

Griffith, C. A.: Inguinal hernia: an anatomic-surgical correlation. Surg. Clin. North Am., *39*:531, 1959.
Crediting H. O. Marcy for original work relating to plastic closure of the internal ring, Griffith shows in this article a fine technique for repair of the small indirect hernia in the adult.

Halvorson, K., and McVay, C. B.: Inguinal and femoral hernioplasty—a 22 year study of the authors' methods. Arch. Surg., *101*:127, 1970.
What is the true recurrence rate after hernial repair? Unfortunately most glowing reports in the world literature fail to assure sufficient follow-up time. These authors after diligent study have suggested a formula by which a more accurate recurrence rate can be assured. The following table represents their method of predicting recurrence up to 25 years after the operation.

All Patients Followed	Multiply Rate
One year	5.0
Two years	2.5
Five years	1.5
Ten years	1.2

When these rates were applied to their own series, an impressive accuracy was noted. Any author reporting results of hernial surgery with follow-up of less than 10 years would be well advised to calculate the 25-year potential for recurrence in his series.

Lytle, W. J.: The deep inguinal ring, development, function, and repair. Br. J. Surg., 57:531, 1970.
The closing mechanism of the internal ring is well described in this short paper. The student of hernial repair should read carefully all the works of Lytle.

McVay, C. B., Read, R. C., and Ravitch, M. M.: Inguinal hernia. Curr. Probl. Surg., Oct., 1967.
This monograph gives a tripartite summary of hernial repair today. McVay presents the complete repair of the posterior inguinal wall which he has popularized so successfully. Read reviews the preperitoneal approach, and Ravitch clearly presents the classic Halsted-Ferguson procedure.

Nyhus, L. M., and Harkins, H. N.: Hernia. Philadelphia, J. B. Lippincott Company, 1964.
Details of all facets of hernial problems are presented. A multiauthor text, it contains diverse views as to the appropriate approach to groin hernias. It also includes sections on diaphragmatic hernia, industrial hernia, muscle hernia, and medicolegal problems related to hernia surgery.

Usher, F. C.: The repair of incisional and inguinal hernia. Surg. Gynecol. Obstet., *131*:525, 1970.
The use of prosthetic material in hernial repair has found a place in the surgical armamentarium largely as a result of the work of Usher. This paper updates the subject and it also includes important references for further reading.

Zimmerman, L. M., and Anson, B. J.: The Anatomy and Surgery of Hernia, 2nd ed. Baltimore, Williams & Wilkins, 1967.
The anatomic genius of Anson is combined here with the fine surgical knowledge of Zimmerman to produce a beautifully illustrated and overall fine text.

REFERENCES

1. Abel, A. L., and Hunt, A. H.: Stainless steel wire for closing abdominal incisions and for the repair of herniae. Br. Med. J., *2*:379, 1948.
2. Aird, I.: A Companion in Surgical Studies, 2nd ed. Baltimore, Williams & Wilkins, 1957.
3. Ali, M.: Cutis strip and patch repair of large inguinal hernias. N. Engl. J. Med., *251*:932, 1954.
4. Andrews, E. W.: Imbrications of lap joint method: A plastic operation for hernia. Chicago Med. Rec., *9*:67, 1895.
5. Annandale, T.: Case in which a reducible oblique and direct inguinal and femoral hernia existed on the same side and were treated by operation. Edinburgh Med. J., *21*:1087, 1876.
6. Anson, B. J., Morgan, E. H., and McVay, C. B.: Surgical anatomy of the inguinal region based upon a study of 500 body-halves. Surg. Gynecol. Obstet., *111*:707, 1960.
7. Baron, H. C.: Umbilical hernia secondary to cirrhosis of the liver—complications of surgical correction. N. Engl. J. Med., *263*:824, 1960.
8. Bassini, E.: Nuovo metodo per la cura radicale dell'ernia. Atti Cong. Ass. Med. Ital. (1887), *2*:179, 1889.
9. Blair, C. R., Nay, H. R., and Rucher, C. M.: Surgical repair of rectal prolapse. Surgery, *53*:625, 1963.
10. Burton, C. C.: Inguinopectineal hernias—a classification and correlation. Int. Abstr. Surg., *97*:419, 1953.
11. Callisen, H.: Herniorum rariorum luga acta societatis medicae hafniae. Hanniae, *2*:321, 1777.
12. Camper, P.: Icones herniarum. Francofurti ad Moenum, Varrentrapp and Wenner, 1801.
13. Cavanagh, C. R., and Schnug, G. E.: Inguinal hernias in infants and children. Northwest Med., *61*:598, 1962.
14. Clark, J. H., and Hashimoto, E. I.: Utilization of Henle's ligament, iliopubic tract, aponeurosis transversus abdominis and Cooper's ligament in inguinal herniorrhaphy. Surg. Gynecol. Obstet., *82*:480, 1946.
15. Cloquet, J.: Recherches anatomiques sur les hernies de l'abdomen. Thèse. Paris, 1817.
16. Condon, R. E.: The anatomy of the inguinal region. *In* Nyhus, L. M., and Harkins, H. N.: Hernia. Philadelphia, J. B. Lippincott Company, 1964.
17. Cooper, A. P.: The Anatomy and Surgical Treatment of Abdominal Hernia. 2 volumes. London, Longman & Co. 1804–1807.
18. Czerny, V.: Studien zur Radikalbehandlung der Hernien. Wein. Med. Wochenschr., *27*:497, 1877.
19. Donald, D. C.: The value derived from utilizing the component parts of the transversalis fascia and Cooper's ligament in the repair of large indirect and direct inguinal hernias. Surgery, *24*:662, 1948.
20. Dowd, C. N.: Congenital lumbar hernia at the triangle of Petit. Ann. Surg., *45*:245, 1907.
21. Eiseman, B., Robinson, R. M., and Brown, J. H.: Simultaneous appendectomy and herniorrhaphy without prophylactic antibiotic therapy. Surgery *51*:578, 1962.
22. Farris, J. M.: Umbilical hernia. *In* Nyhus, L. M., and Harkins, H. N.: Hernia. Philadelphia, J. B. Lippincott Company, 1964.
23. Ferguson, A. H.: The technique of Modern Operations for Hernia. Chicago, Cleveland Press, 1907.
24. Gallaudet, B. B.: A Description of the Planes of Fascia of the Human Body. New York, Columbia University Press, 1931.
25. Gaspar, M. R., and Casberg, M. A.: An appraisal of preperitoneal repair of inguinal hernia. Surg. Gynecol. Obstet., *132*:207, 1971.
26. Gaster, J.: Hernia—One Day Repair. Darien, Conn., Hafner Publishing Co., 1970.
27. Gilsdorf, R. B., and Shea, M. M.: Repair of massive septic abdominal wall defects with marlex mesh. Am. J. Surg., *130*:634, 1975.
28. Goligher, J. C.: Prolapse of the rectum. In Nyhus, L. M., and Harkins, H. N.: Hernia. Philadelphia, J. B. Lippincott Company, 1964.
29. Goñi Moreno, I.: Chronic eventrations and large hernias—preoperative treatment by progressive pneumoperitoneum—original procedure. Surgery, *22*:945, 1947.
30. Griffith, C. A.: Inguinal hernia: An anatomic-surgical correlation. Surg. Clin. North Am., *39*:531, 1959.
31. Guy, C. C., Werelius, C. Y., and Bell, L. B., Jr.: Five years' experience with tantalum mesh in hernia repair. Surg. Clin. North Am., *35*:175, 1955.
32. Halsted, W. S.: The radical cure of hernia. Bull. Johns Hopkins Hosp., *1*:12, 1889.
33. Halverson, K., and McVay, C. B.: Inguinal and femoral hernioplasty. Arch. Surg., *101*:127, 1970.
34. Harrison, P. W.: Inguinal hernia: A study of the principles involved in the surgical treatment. Arch. Surg., *4*:680, 1922.
35. Hesselbach, F. K.: Anatomisch-chirurgische Abhandlung über den Ursprung der Leistenbrücke. Würzburg, Baumgärten, 1806.
36. Hesselbach, F. K.: Nueste anatomisch-pathologische Untersuchungen über den Ursprung und das Fortschreiten der Leisten-und Schenkel-brüche. Würzburg, Baumgartner, 1814.
37. Keynes, W. M.: Supravesical hernia. *In* Nyhus, L. M., and Harkins, H. N.: Hernia. Philadelphia, J. B. Lippincott Company, 1964.
38. Kiesewetter, W. B.: Hernias—inguinal and umbilical. Am. J. Surg., *101*:656, 1961.
39. Koontz, A. R.: Dead (preserved) fascia grafts for hernia repair: Clinical results. J.A.M.A., *89*:1230, 1927.
40. Koontz, A. R.: The use of tantalum mesh in inguinal hernia repair. Surg. Gynecol. Obstet., *92*:101, 1951.
41. Koontz, A. R.: Perineal hernia. *In* Nyhus, L. M., and Harkins, H. N.: Hernia, Philadelphia, J. B. Lippincott Company, 1964.
42. Koontz, A. R., and Stafford, E. S.: Unusual types of interparietal hernia. Arch. Surg., *71*:723, 1955.
43. Lindholm, A., Nilsson, O., and Tholin, B.: Inguinal and femoral hernias. Arch. Surg., *98*:19, 1969.
44. Lotheissen, G.: Zur Radikaloperation der Schenkelhernien. Zentralbl. Chir., *25*:548, 1898.
45. Lower, W. E., and Hicken, N. F.: Interparietal hernias. Ann. Surg., *94*:1070, 1931.
46. Lucas-Championnière, J.: Cure radicale des hernies; avec une étude statistique de deux cents soizante-quinze opérations et cinquante figures intercalées dans le texte. Paris, Rueff et. Cie, 1892.
47. Lytle, W. J.: Femoral hernia. Ann. R. Coll. Surg. Engl., *21*:244, 1957.
48. Macewen, W.: On the radical cure of oblique inguinal hernia by internal abdominal peritoneal pad, and the restoration of the valved form of the inguinal canal. Ann. Surg., *4*:89, 1886.
49. Marcy, H. O.: A new use of carbolized catgut ligatures. Boston Med. Surg. J., *85*:315, 1871.
50. Marcy, H. O.: The radical cure of hernia by the antiseptic use of the carbolized catgut ligature. Trans. A.M.A., *29*:295, 1878.
51. Margoles, J. S., and Braun, R. A.: Preperitoneal versus classical hernioplasty. Am. J. Surg., *121*:641, 1971.
52. Mayo, W. J.: Radical cure of umbilical hernia. J.A.M.A., *48*:1842, 1907.
53. McVay, C. B.: Inguinal and femoral hernioplasty: Anatomic repair. Arch. Surg., *57*:524, 1948.
54. McVay, C. B.: The hernias. In Davis, L. (Ed.): Christopher's Textbook of Surgery, 9th ed. Philadelphia, W. B. Saunders Company, 1968.
55. Moschcowitz, A. V.: Femoral hernia: A new operation for the radical cure. N. Y. J. Med., *7*:396, 1907.
56. Nyhus, L. M.: An anatomic reappraisal of the posterior inguinal wall. Special consideration of the iliopubic tract and its relation to groin hernias. Surg. Clin. North Am., *44*:1305, 1964.
57. Nyhus, L. M.: The preperitoneal approach and iliopubic tract repair of all groin hernias. In Nyhus, L. M., and Harkins, H. N.: Hernia. Philadelphia, J. B. Lippincott Company, 1964.
58. Peacock, E. E., Jr.: Biology of hernia. *In* Nyhus, L. M., and Condon, R. E. (Eds.): Hernia, 2nd ed. Philadelphia, J. B. Lippincott Company, 1977.
59. Peacock, E. E., Jr., and Madden, J. W.: Studies on the biology and treatment of recurrent inguinal hernia: II. Morphological changes. Ann. Surg., *179*:567, 1974.

60. Pott, P. A.: A Treatise on Ruptures. London, C. Hitch and L. Hawes, 1756.

61. Priesching, A.: Laugerische Hernia. Arch. Klin. Chir., *281*:411, 1956.

62. Ravitch, M. M.: Repair of Hernias. Chicago, Year Book Medical Publishers, Inc., 1969.

63. Read, R. C.: Preperitoneal exposure of inguinal herniation. Am. J. Surg., *116*:653, 1968.

64. Rogers, F. A.: Strangulated obturator hernia. *In* Nyhus, L. M., and Harkins, H. N.: Hernia. Philadelphia, J. B. Lippincott Company, 1964.

65. Ruggi, G.: Metodo operative nuovo per la cura radicale dell'ernia crurale. Bull. Sci. Med. Bologna Sev., 7:223, 1892.

66. Santulli, T. V., and Shaw, A.: Inguinal hernia: Infancy and childhood. J.A.M.A., *176*:110, 1961.

67. Scarpa, A.: Sull'ernia del revineo. Pavia, P. Bizzoni, 1821.

68. Serafini, G.: Sulle varieta dell'ernia crurale e particolarmente sull'ernia crurale retrovascolare intravaginale e sull'ernia pettina. Policlinico (Chir.), *24*:230, 1917.

69. Smith, R. S.: Adjuncts in hernial repair: a consideration of basic principles. Arch. Surg., *78*:868, 1959.

70. Thomas, G. I.: Sciatic hernia. *In* Nyhus, L. M., and Harkins, H. N.: Hernia. Philadelphia, J. B. Lippincott Company, 1964.

71. Thomson, A.: Cause anatomique de la hernie inguinale externe. J. Conn. Méd. Prat., *4*:137, 1836.

72. Turner, D. P. B.: Prevascular femoral hernia. Br. J. Surg., *41*:77, 1953.

73. U.S. Department of Health, Education and Welfare: National Health Survey on Hernias. Series B, No. 25, Dec., 1960.

74. U.S. Department of Health, Education and Welfare: National Health Survey—Surgical Operations in Short-stay Hospitals, United States—1971. Series 13, No. 18, Nov., 1974.

75. Usher, F. C.: The repair of incisional and inguinal hernias. Surg. Gynecol. Obstet., *131*:525, 1970.

76. Wakely, C. P. G.: Obturator hernia. Br. J. Surg., *26*:515, 1939.

77. Wagh, P. V., and Read, R. C.: Defective collagen synthesis in inguinal herniation. Am. J. Surg., *124*:819, 1972.

78. Wheeler, M. H.: Femoral hernia: Analysis of the results of surgical treatment. Proc. R. Soc. Med., *68*:177, 1975.

79. Zimmerman, L. M., and Anson, B. J.: Anatomy and Surgery of Hernia, 2nd ed. Baltimore, Williams & Wilkins, 1967.

40

PEDIATRIC SURGERY

Thomas M. Holder, M.D., and Lucian L. Leape, M.D.

Pediatric surgery is that branch of surgery devoted to surgical care and management of infants and children. It bears the same relation to surgery that pediatrics does to internal medicine. The conditions treated surgically in the pediatric age group are usually congenital malformations, neoplasms, or the result of trauma. Most are amenable to definitive treatment and thus offer the deep satisfaction of lifelong cure.

Since the infant's response to disease is quite different from the adult's, it is necessary to be aware of these differences when caring for him.[28] Perhaps the single most important difference is the much greater lability of babies. Because of a higher metabolic rate, the young infant has a more rapid turnover of water and metabolites and a higher oxygen consumption. His body weight usually doubles in the first 6 months. This increased caloric requirement results in an increase in fluid requirement as well. For example, a 5-kg. infant requires about 500 ml. of intravenous fluids per day (100 ml. per kilogram body weight at this size) to meet his metabolic requirement. An equivalent amount for a 70-kg. adult would be 7000 ml. per day, far more than usual needs.

Because of the greater surface area as compared to body mass, the small infant loses heat much more rapidly than an adult. Accordingly, he is much more susceptible to changes in ambient temperature. Temperature control mechanisms are poorly developed in the small infant, especially the premature. If his body temperature is significantly above or below normal, there is a marked increase in oxygen consumption as well. Particularly in the operating room, measures must be taken to conserve body heat or core temperature will drop significantly.

Respiratory problems are common in young infants after operation. There are several reasons for this. First, the neonate is an obligatory nose breather. Accordingly, nasogastric intubation decreases the airway by obstructing one naris. Second, the ribs are soft and horizontal so that intercostal action contributes much less to ventilation than the diaphragm. Third, the infant airway is much more easily compromised by a small amount of edema (such as that caused by an endotracheal tube). One millimeter of edema of the mucosa of a 6-mm. trachea quadruples the airway resistance. Finally, infants mobilize secretions poorly because of inadequate cough reflexes. Assiduous respiratory care is mandatory if these patients are to survive.

Since the diagnostic approach to a patient is usually determined by the predominant symptom or sign, diseases will be grouped by major clinical symptoms. No attempt is made to provide encyclopedic coverage. Rather, major conditions encountered in infancy and childhood requiring surgical treatment are described as part of the differential diagnosis of the major presenting symptom. For more details, the reader is referred to several excellent textbooks of pediatric surgery or to monographs on specific subjects.

RESPIRATORY DISTRESS

Respiratory distress in the newborn is commonly life-threatening, often progressive, and frequently caused by an entity amenable to surgical cure. Whether manifested merely by an increase in respiratory rate, or attended by stridor, retractions, cyanosis, and other signs of oxygen deficiency, the exact cause must be rapidly identified and appropriate treatment instituted. In broad terms the causes of respiratory distress are abnormalities of ventilation, impaired oxygen diffusion, and the shunting of blood from venous to arterial circuits without oxygenation.

Most of the surgically treated problems produce abnormalities of ventilation. These may result from airway obstruction (as in vascular ring compressing the treachea), poorly functioning muscles of respiration (as in phrenic paralysis or central nervous system disorders), or decrease in lung volume (such as from pneumothorax or a diaphragmatic hernia).

Poor oxygen diffusion may result from pneumonia, atelectasis, hyaline membrane disease, or pulmonary congestion and edema due to congestive heart failure. Most of the entities in this category are treated by nonoperative means. Shunting may occur either in the heart or in the lungs. The intrapulmonary shunt is usually the result of blood perfusing unoxygenated alveoli, as in atelectasis. Intracardiac shunting results from septal defects. At times it may be difficult to differentiate pulmonary from cardiac causes of distress. In general, cyanosis due to pulmonary causes improves with oxygen administration, while that due to an intracardiac shunt does not.

In the infant or child with respiratory distress, either with or without cyanosis and retraction, a posteroanterior and lateral chest x-ray film is the most helpful single diagnostic study and should be obtained promptly in any patient with these symptoms. No infant is too sick for a chest x-ray. The cause of the respiratory difficulty is usually apparent. Additional studies may be necessary to further delineate the cause of the symptoms, but at least a provisional diagnosis usually can be made from the chest x-ray.

Further diagnostic studies, if needed, should demonstrate the cause of the respiratory distress with the least risk to the patient. Some patients, particularly neonates or the critically ill, will not tolerate extensive diagnostic evaluation. The choice of specific procedures should be based on the most likely diagnosis in view of the clinical picture; one should not employ all procedures available to exclude every diagnostic possibility. If there is stridor and retraction, upper airway obstruction is likely. Cyanosis and tachypnea without stridor are more suggestive of a pulmonary or cardiac problem. Physical examination may reveal the cause of obstruction, for example, a large cervical mass, cystic hygroma with laryngeal or tongue involvement, or micrognathia. Since the infant is primarily a diaphragmatic breather, marked abdominal distention from any cause will interfere with ventilation.

If there is no obviously visible cause, a reasonable stepwise approach to a patient with respiratory distress is: (1) obtain a chest x-ray; (2) pass a tube through each naris (to detect choanal atresia); (3) obtain an esophagogram (to detect vascular ring or other structure compromising the esophagus and the trachea); (4) look at the larynx and pharynx (to detect a mass, a web, or compression); (5) perform tracheobronchosocpy and obtain a tracheogram to detect subglottic or other narrowing not seen on previous roentgenographic studies. Laryngoscopy should be done first if the patient has severe airway obstruction, and an endotracheal tube is introduced if necessary to relieve the obstruction and perhaps localize the area of narrowing. Recurrent pneumonia, retraction, cyanosis, and even sudden respiratory arrest may occur secondary to gastroesophageal reflux and aspiration. This cause of respiratory distress is often overlooked. Gastroesophageal reflux is discussed in some detail later in this chapter in the section on vomiting.

DIAPHRAGMATIC HERNIA

The Bochdalek diaphragmatic hernia is one of the surgical emergencies of the newborn. While not all infants with the posterolateral diaphragmatic defect have symptoms as newborns, most do, and the risk to these infants is high.

Anatomy and Embryology. The septum transversum forms caudal to the heart at about the eighth week of fetal life and grows posteriorly to meet the dorsal mesentery of the foregut to form the central portion of the diaphragm. Pleuroperitoneal folds develop on each side and progress posteriorly and laterally, dividing the thoracic from the abdominal cavity. Arrest of the process at this time results in a posterolateral

diaphragmatic defect—the persistent pleuroperitoneal canal of Bochdalek. Muscle fibers grow between these folds to form the true diaphragm by about the end of the ninth week. The process is usually complete on the right before the left, partially explaining the 90 per cent predominance of the defect on the left. About this same time the gut returns to the abdomen from the base of the umbilical cord. If the pleuroperitoneal canal is still open, the gut returning to the abdominal cavity will pass through the defect into the chest and not complete the normal process of intestinal rotation. The abdominal viscera in the chest compress the ipsilateral lung and prevent its development to the normal size. The abdominal cavity likewise does not develop to its normal size.

Pathophysiology. With the first breath an infant begins to swallow air, which promptly passes to the small bowel. As the air enters the intestine the volume occupied by the intestine increases. Since the gut is in the chest, and the thoracic volume is relatively fixed, the increase in volume of the intestine occurs at the expense of the most easily compressed of the thoracic contents, the lungs. As pressure increases, there is a shift of the mediastinum with compression of the contralateral lung. The increased intrathoracic pressure and mediastinal shift impede venous return.

The result of this expanding mass is severe hypoxia and respiratory acidosis. These factors have an effect on the labile pulmonary vasculature of the neonate, producing an increase in pulmonary vascular resistance.

Symptoms and Signs. Symptoms and signs vary from severe respiratory difficulty from the time of delivery to no respiratory symptoms at all. Most of these infants do reasonably well initially but have progressive difficulty as the gut fills with air and are in severe respiratory distress within a few hours. On physical examination most patients have a scaphoid abdomen, a barrel-shaped chest, and some degree of cyanosis and respiratory distress. On listening to the chest, the most striking finding is that the heart is best heard well over toward the right anterior axillary line (in the 90 per cent of patients whose defect is on the left). Breath sounds are decreased or absent on the involved side. To the disappointment of the physical diagnosis enthusiast, bowel sounds are seldom heard in the chest.

Some patients have few or no respiratory symptoms but have intermittent or partial intestinal obstruction. These symptoms usually occur after the neonatal period.

Diagnosis. Diagnosis is by chest x-ray. There are loops of air-filled bowel in the chest. Those patients who are in respiratory distress usually show a marked mediastinal shift away from the hernia (Fig. 1).

Treatment. Treatment is prompt reduction and repair of the hernia. The hypoxia and acidosis cannot be corrected until the lung can be expanded. The acidosis can, however, be improved by intravenous sodium bicarbonate, and this should be given empirically. The anesthetic should not be given by mask, as more air will be forced into the intestine. An endotracheal tube is passed in the awake infant, who is then lightly anesthetized.

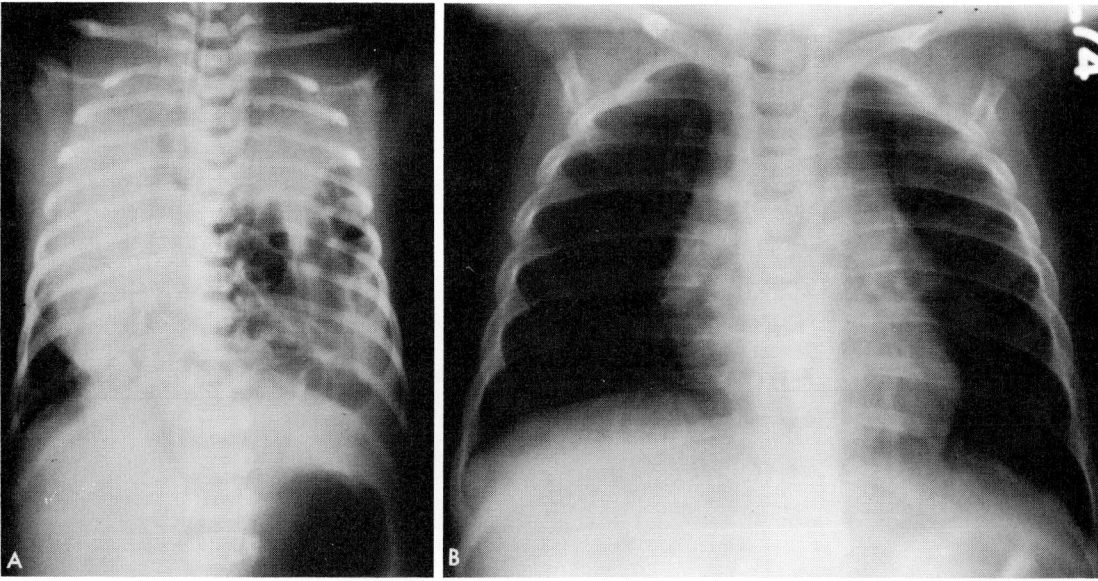

Figure 1. *A*, X-ray appearance of a 12-hour-old male with a Bochdalek diaphragmatic hernia, showing air-filled loops of intestine in the left chest with marked mediastinal shift and compression of the right lung. *B*, Same patient at age 10 months, showing complete expansion of both lungs.

The operative approach is through the abdomen (Fig. 2). The advantages of the abdominal approach as opposed to the thoracic are (1) the diaphragmatic defect is not repaired under the difficult conditions of trying to push the viscera back into the too-small abdominal cavity (hence a more secure closure can be obtained); (2) if there are peritoneal bands obstructing the duodenum or other manifestations of incomplete rotation, they can be readily corrected; and (3) a gastrostomy is easily performed. The viscera are removed from the thorax and the defect in the diaphragm is closed. In the rare instance when there is insufficient diaphragm for a primary closure, it may be closed with a synthetic prosthesis or rotated flap of abdominal wall musculature. A gastrostomy is performed to decompress the stomach and intestinal tract postoperatively. Since the abdominal cavity is small, return of all the viscera that were in the chest to the abdominal cavity may cause a marked increase in intra-abdominal pressure with decreased diaphragmatic excursion and ventilation. Venous return is also impaired. If there is moderate tension in closing the abdomen, a ventral hernia should be left either by closing only the skin or by closing the abdominal wall with a temporary prosthesis, similar to the therapy of omphalocele.[23] If a prosthesis is used, abdominal wall closure can be accomplished 7 to 10 days later without undue tension. A chest tube is left in the pleural space and connected to underwater drainage.

The postoperative care in these infants is critical. Arterial pH, pO_2, and pCO should be closely monitored via an arterial catheter. If these show even moderate acidosis, hypoxia, or hypercarbia, the patient should be given ventilatory assistance.

In patients who survive, the mediastinum shifts back toward the midline, and the ipsilateral lung gradually expands over the next 5 to 10 days to occupy the hemithorax. The lung has the capacity to grow alveoli after birth. On long-term follow-up the lungs are found to be normal by clinical evaluation and x-ray examination.

Results. Survival rate is about 50 per cent for those infants who are in respiratory difficulty during the first 24 hours of life. Many of these babies have a severely hypoplastic lung. The patient who does not have symptoms until after 24 hours of life has a much better outlook, with a mortality of less than 5 per cent. Presumably the lungs in these latter infants are less severely affected.

PNEUMOTHORAX

Pneumothorax is not rare in the neonate. It may occur spontaneously as a result of birth trauma or from a ruptured bleb or cyst. Pneumothorax is a common complication of ventilatory support in infants with hyaline membrane disease. In infants and, less often, children who have elements of bronchiolar obstruction or infection, air may leak back along the bronchi into the mediastinum with subsequent rupture into the pleural space producing a pneumothorax.

In most cases pneumothorax in infants is small, causes no symptoms, and needs no therapy other than observation to see that the air is decreasing rather than increasing in amount. If a tension pneumothorax develops, respiratory distress may be severe. Physical examination reveals a rapid respiratory rate, cyanosis, and retraction. There are no breath sounds on the involved side. Diagnosis is made by chest x-ray. Treatment is by insertion of an intercostal catheter connected to an underwater seal. This is safer than aspiration, since it provides a vent in case of continued or recurrent leak. The tube should remain in place

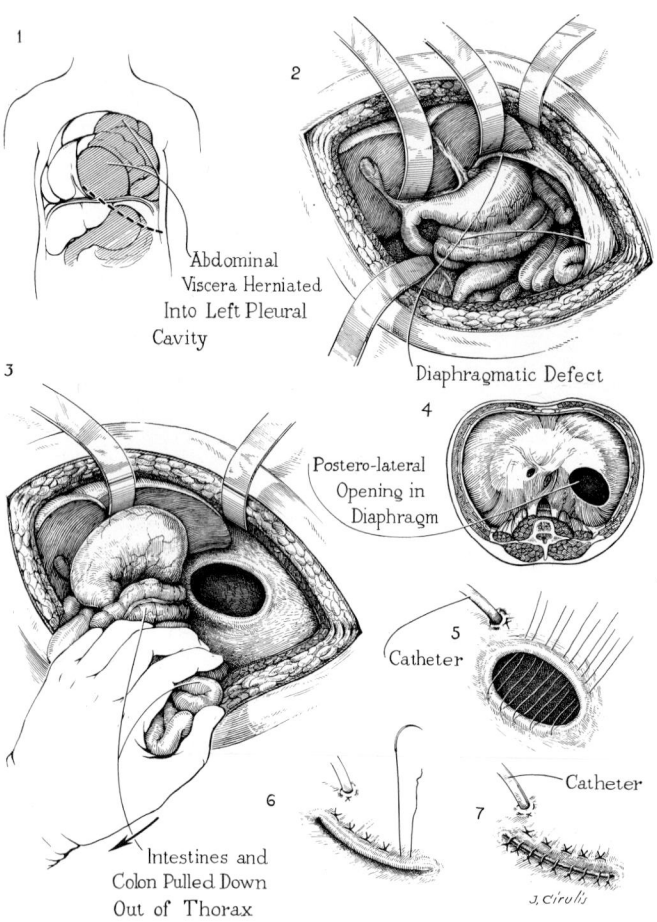

1

Abdominal
Viscera Herniated
Into Left Pleural
Cavity

2

Diaphragmatic Defect

3

4

Postero-lateral
Opening in
Diaphragm

5
Catheter

6
Intestines and
Colon Pulled Down
Out of Thorax

7   Catheter

J. Cirulis

Figure 2. Technique of repair of Bochdalek diaphragmatic defect. An abdominal approach has a decided advantage. A catheter can either be placed through the diaphragm and brought out through a stab wound in the abdomen or brought directly out through the chest wall. In either case it is connected to an underwater seal. Gastrostomy is helpful in preventing postoperative intestinal distention. (From Gross, R. E.: An Atlas of Children's Surgery. Philadelphia, W. B. Saunders Company, 1970.)

until the air leak is well sealed, usually a matter of 3 to 5 days. Premature removal of the tube is apt to be followed by recurrence of the pneumothorax.

Pneumomediastinum may cause caval obstruction. It is more difficult to treat, since there is not a single space that can be easily evacuated. Therapy is usually not necessary, but if the patient is in distress, aspiration of the mediastinum may remove enough air to tide the patient over until the air is absorbed.

INFANTILE LOBAR EMPHYSEMA

Marked overdistention of a single lobe (or segment) of lung may be the cause of respiratory distress in the infant. This condition was first described by Nelson in 1932 and first successfully treated by Gross in 1945.

Pathophysiology. Lobar emphysema may result from partial bronchial obstruction or, less commonly, primary alveolar fibrosis. External bronchial compression may result from an abnormal vessel or lymph node. Intrinsic obstruction can result from bronchomalacia, bronchostenosis, or redundant mucosal fold. In about half the patients, no cause can be found. As the lobe becomes overinflated, the remaining lobes of the ipsilateral lung are compressed and the diaphragm is depressed. As distention progresses, herniation of the

distended lobe across the flexible anterior mediastinum may occur, causing compression of the contralateral lung. The emphysematous lobe acts as any large intrathoracic mass, compressing the normal intrathoracic structures and interfering with ventilation. In addition, the increased intrathoracic pressure produces a shift of the medistinum and may impede venous return to the heart.[21]

Symptoms and Signs. The patient is usually in respiratory distress with tachypnea, dyspnea, and cyanosis. On auscultation, the breath sounds are decreased on the involved side. Hyperinflation and decreased expansions of the affected side may be noted. In some patients symptoms appear shortly after birth and are rapidly progressive. In about half, the onset of symptoms is during the first month of life, and in most of the others, during the first 4 months of age. Rarely the disorder is seen in an older child with congenital heart disease (10 to 15 per cent).

Diagnosis. Diagnosis is by chest x-ray (Fig. 3). The classic findings are (1) radiolucency of the lung field with bronchovascular markings present; (2) wedge-shaped densities adjacent to the affected lobe representing the atelectatic other lobes; (3) depression of the ipsilateral half of the diaphragm; (4) mediastinal shift to the opposite side; and (5) retrosternal radiolucency indicating herniation across the mediastinum.

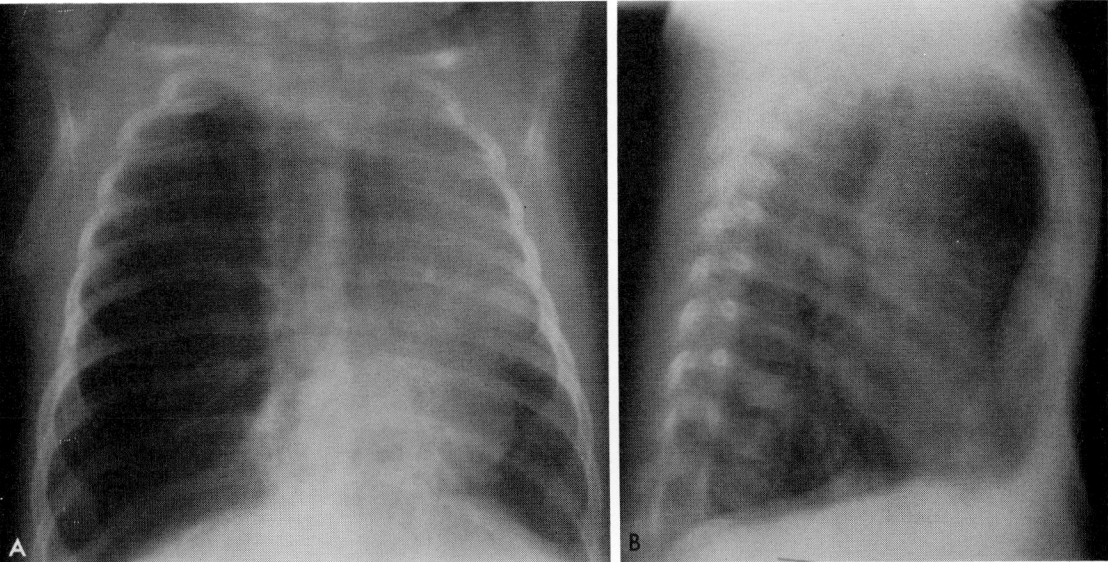

Figure 3. *A,* X-ray appearance of infantile lobar emphysema of the middle lobe. The mediastinum is displaced to the left with herniation of the middle lobe across the midline. The right lower lobe is compressed along the right heart border and the right hemidiaphragm depressed. *B,* The lateral projection shows a large radiolucent area in the upper anterior mediastinum where the middle lobe has expanded across the mediastinum.

Bronchograms are occasionally necessary to demonstrate obstruction in atypical cases.

Treatment. Surgical resection of the diseased lobe is curative and often life-saving.

Results. Operative mortality is low. In rare cases a second lobe will become involved. Long-term follow-up studies have occasionally demonstrated decrease in vital capacity beyond that expected from the volume of the lung removed. This indicates that there may be other residual lung disease.

CYSTIC MALFORMATIONS OF THE LUNG

Congenital cystic disease of the lung is uncommon. Cysts are the result of faulty embryogenesis, are lined by cuboidal or columnar ciliated epithelium, and usually communicate with the tracheobronchial tree. One variety in this spectrum of disease, cystic adenomatoid malformation, consists primarily of the glandular components of the lung and presents as a predominantly solid tumor of the lung in the neonate.

Pathophysiology. The cysts may be single or multiple and are usually segmental or lobar in distribution. Occasionally an entire lung may be involved. In the neonate the cysts are usually large and cause symptoms because of their size. Bronchial communication often permits air to enter more easily than to escape, resulting in a progressive enlargement of the cyst. In older infants and children infection in the cyst is common.

Symptoms. Symptoms are those of an intrathoracic mass or superimposed infection—dyspnea, tachypnea, wheezing, cyanosis, cough, and fever.

Diagnosis. Diagnosis is made by chest x-ray, which shows one or more air-filled cysts varying in size, at times causing a mediastinal shift. Air-fluid levels are more common in infected cysts than in those that are not. Cystic adenomatoid malformation presents as a large, rather homogeneous solid pulmonary mass. Differential diagnosis includes pneumothorax, infantile lobar emphysema, diaphragmatic hernia, acquired cystic disease of the lung secondary to staphylococcal pneumonia, and pulmonary manifestations of cystic fibrosis.

Treatment. Treatment is resection of the involved lobe or lobes. It is not wise to aspirate the cyst except in extreme emergency because of the risk of tension pneumothorax. If necessary as a life-saving measure, aspiration should be followed by immediate thoracotomy and resection of the cyst. The results are good. Infants tolerate pulmonary resection well.

STAPHYLOCOCCAL PNEUMONIA

Staphylococcal pneumonia occurs in persons of all ages, but is most often seen in infants and young children. Peribronchial abscesses occur, with escape of air into the lung parenchyma and development of pneumatoceles. If the abscess is subpleural in location, rupture into the pleural space results in a pneumothorax or empyema or both. Staphylococcal pneumonia in the early phases may be a rapidly progressive, fulminating disease. Close x-ray surveillance is necessary during this phase of the disease to keep abreast of the progression of the disease process. The patients are febrile and have rapid respirations and dyspnea.

Diagnosis. Diagnosis is by chest x-ray showing pneumatoceles and frequently empyema and pneumothorax (Fig. 4). Culture of the Staphylococcus from the nose or throat is suggestive; from a tracheal aspirate or the pleural space it is confirmatory.

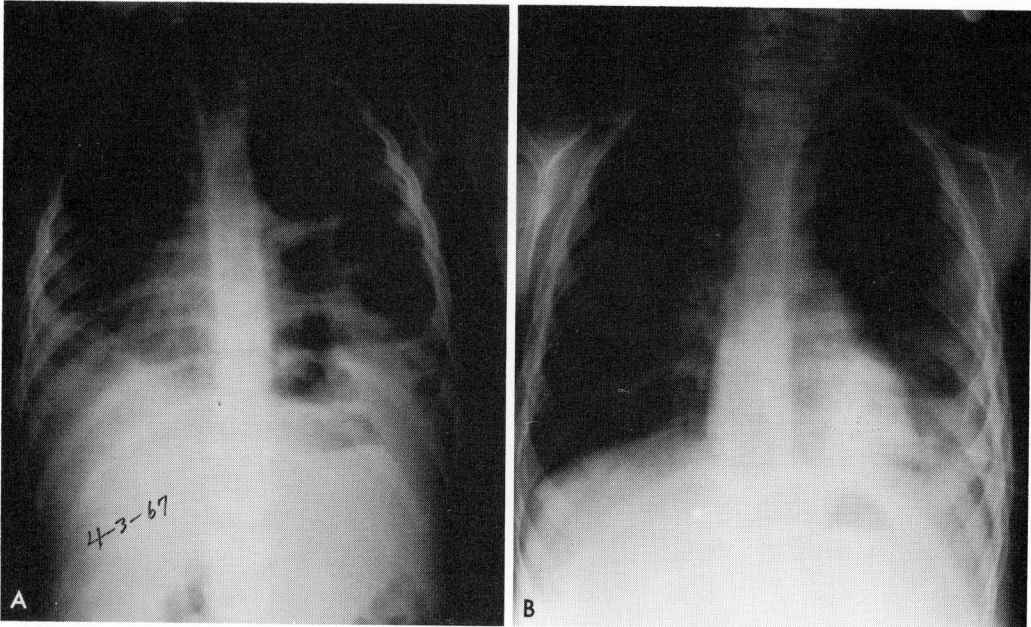

Figure 4. *A,* Staphylococcal pneumonia with pneumatoceles on the left, mediastinal shift to the right, and right empyema, which has been drained by an intercostal catheter. *B,* Four weeks later the right empyema and pleural thickening have subsided. On the left all but one of the pneumatoceles have subsided. A left empyema developed which is being drained by a tube. Over the next 2 months complete resolution occurred.

Treatment. Treatment of the pneumonia is by antibiotics, usually methicillin or cephalothin. Therapy of the complications is surgical. The pneumatoceles rarely become large enough to cause respiratory distress. If they do, tube drainage is safer than aspiration. Pneumothorax, pleural effusion, and empyema are frequent complications, and require tube drainage of the pleural space. Drainage early in the course of empyema is much more efficient than drainage after loculation has occurred.

Once the infection has been controlled by antibiotics, progression of the process ceases. Antibiotics are usually required for several weeks to control the infection. Therapy should be continued until the patient has been afebrile for 10 to 14 days and the white and differential blood counts have returned to the normal range for a similar period of time. The pneumatoceles will regress over a period of weeks or months. If there has been an empyema, there may be marked pleural thickening that restricts ventilation. In spite of the alarming x-ray appearance, the thick pleura will almost always resolve, though it may take several months. Decortication is seldom required.[13]

VASCULAR RING

Vascular rings cause symptoms similar to those of other conditions discussed here and should be considered in the differential diagnosis. The symptoms may be caused by compression of the trachea or compression of the esophagus with resulting aspiration of formula. Diagnosis can usually be made by barium swallow and tracheogram. Treatment is division of the appropriate vessel.

ESOPHAGEAL ATRESIA AND TRACHEOESOPHAGEAL FISTULA

Esophageal atresia and tracheoesophageal fistula (TEF) may occur as separate entities but usually occur in combination. First described in 1697 by Thomas Gibbon, esophageal atresia was not successfully treated until 1939 when Ladd in Boston and Leven in St. Paul obtained the first survivors. These two infants were treated by multiple operations that required months of hospitalization. Two years later Cameron Haight performed the first successful primary repair.

Embryology. Tracheoesophageal fistula is presumably the result of failure of complete midline fusion of the tracheoesophageal septum. Esophageal atresia probably results from epithelial overgrowth in the esophageal lumen along the course of the lateral esophageal grooves.

Classification. The important factors in the pathophysiology, symptoms, and therapy are whether both esophageal atresia and tracheoesophageal fistula are present, and if so, their anatomic relation; i.e., is the fistula proximal or distal to the atresia? The following classification shows the different anomalies (Fig. 5) with their relative frequency (based on 1058 patients, from the survey of the Surgical Section of the American Academy of Pediatrics).

Esophageal atresia with distal TEF	86.5 per cent
Esophageal atresia (without TEF)	7.7 per cent
Isolated TEF (without esophageal atresia)	4.2 per cent
Esophageal atresia with proximal TEF	0.8 per cent

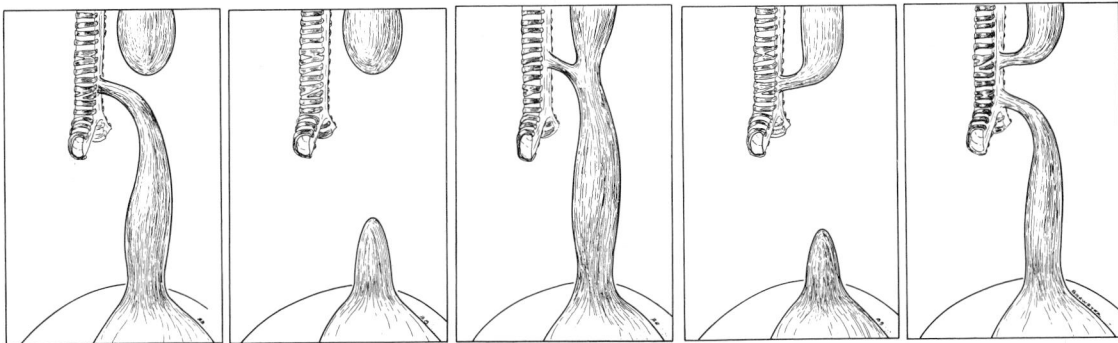

Figure 5. Types of esophageal atresia and tracheoesophageal fistula (TEF) in order of decreasing frequency from left to right: esophageal atresia with distal TEF; esophageal atresia (without TEF); tracheoesophageal fistula (without esophageal atresia); esophageal atresia with proximal TEF; esophageal atresia with proximal and distal TEF.

Esophageal atresia with proximal and distal TEF	0.7 per cent

Esophageal Atresia with Distal Tracheoesophageal Fistula

Anatomy. In this most common form of anomaly the esophagus ends as a dilated, blind pouch in the upper chest at or above the level of the carina. The distal esophagus originates from a small fistulous communication with the membranous portion of the distal trachea.

Pathophysiology and Symptoms. Since esophageal atresia prevents the passage of oral contents to the stomach, the proximal pouch fills with saliva and the infant *drools excessively.* If offered water or formula, he is likely to aspirate it into the trachea, *cough,* and become *cyanotic.*

Crying or coughing increases intratracheal pressure, which in the presence of a tracheoesophageal fistula causes air to pass through the fistula into the esophagus. If there is a distal fistula the stomach and small bowel become distended, causing elevation of the diaphragms. Periodically, the stomach is decompressed back through the fistula, flooding the tracheobronchial tree with gastric secretions, leading to chemical tracheobronchitis, pneumonitis, and atelectasis, which is followed by bacterial pneumonia.

Diagnosis. Since untreated esophageal atresia is a uniformly fatal disease, it is imperative that the diagnosis be confirmed or excluded in any patient in whom it is suspected. The earlier the diagnosis is made, the fewer the pulmonary complications and the better the chance of survival. It is a simple matter to place a small catheter into the upper esophagus, inject 0.5 to 1 ml. of contrast medium, and obtain posteroanterior and lateral x-rays of the chest. If the esophagus ends as a blind pouch, atresia is confirmed. The presence of air in the stomach in this instance indicates a communication of the distal esophagus with the trachea (Fig. 6). The absence of gas in the abdomen usually indicates esophageal atresia without tracheoesophageal fistula. (Occasionally, in the presence of a tracheoesophageal fistula that is very narrow, no gas will have reached the abdomen.)

Esophageal atresia can also be detected by the inability to pass a rather stiff (14 to 16 French) Robinson catheter more than a short distance into the esophagus. Unfortunately, a tube of the size passed through the nose of a neonate can easily coil in the upper esophageal pouch, leading the examiner to the false conclusion that it has been passed into the stomach. The presence of the tube in the stomach must be confirmed by x-ray to exclude esophageal atresia. On this same film the pulmonary status or other causes of respiratory distress can be detected.

Treatment. The principal cause of death in these infants is pulmonary complications. Prior to operation therapy must be directed first toward clearing the pneumonia that is almost always present. Prompt decompressive gastrostomy will prevent reflux of gastric contents into the trachea, and sump catheter decompression of the proximal esophageal pouch will prevent further aspiration. Appropriate antibiotics, high humidity, and frequently endotracheal suction are also indicated. With intravenous fluids the patient can be safely cared for for several days until the lungs clear sufficiently to permit safe thoracotomy.

Surgical correction consists of division of the tracheoesophageal fistula with closure of the tracheal side of the fistula and an anastomosis of the small distal esophageal segment to the dilated proximal pouch. Discrepancy in the size of the segments and tension due to a gap between the two ends lead to a significant number of leaks. A retropleural approach minimizes this hazard, since it results in a localized infection rather than empyema should a leak occur.

Immediate postoperative management is primarily concerned with pulmonary care. High humidity, antibiotics, pharyngeal suction, and often endotracheal suction are necessary.

Results. Two factors that greatly influence survival rate are associated anomalies (present in about half these infants) and the size of the patient (about one third are premature by weight). In the infant over 6 pounds without associated anomalies, the survival rate is over 91 per cent, whereas in the infant weighing less than 4 pounds with associated anomalies, it is less than 20 per cent. Pneumonia, atelectasis, and retained secretions are the major causes of death.[15]

Some small premature infants or infants with associated anomalies benefit from a staged operative

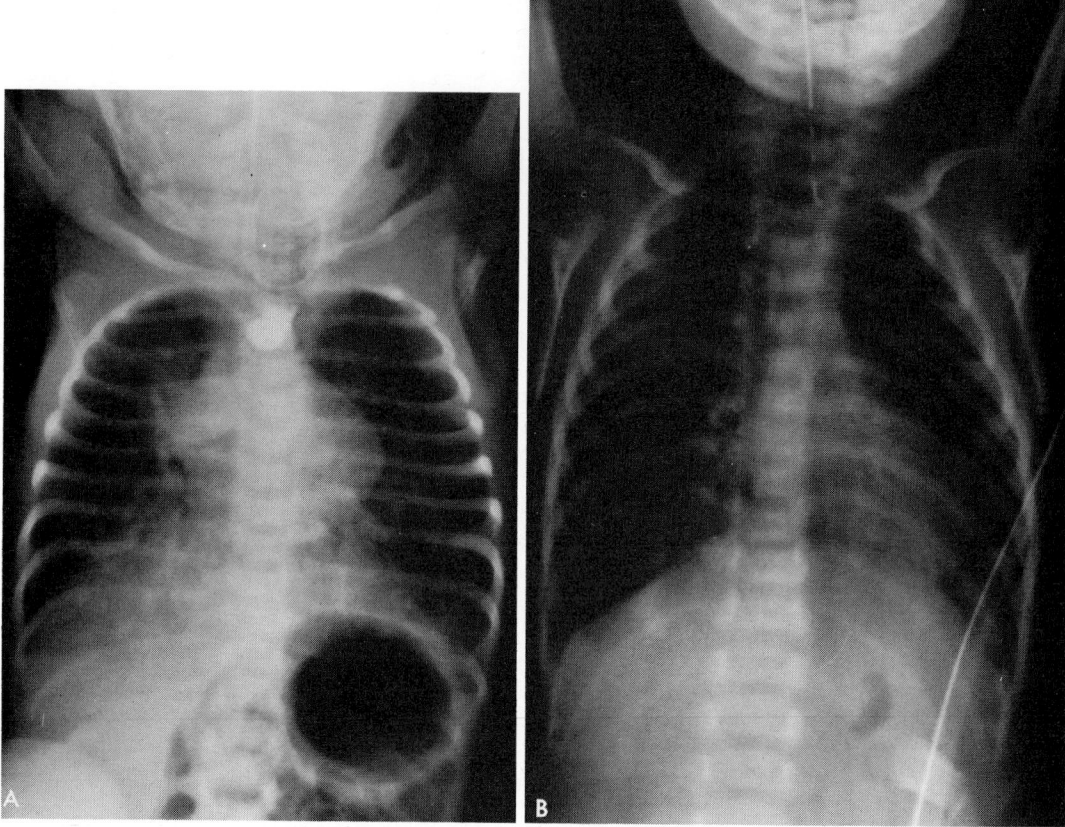

Figure 6. *A,* Esophageal atresia with distal tracheoesophageal fistula is demonstrated in this x-ray by contrast medium in the blind upper esophageal pouch and air in the stomach. Note right upper and lower lung field infiltrates. A gastrostomy was performed shortly after this film. *B,* Same patient 48 hours later showing effect of gastrostomy. The lungs are clear, and the diaphragm is no longer elevated by distended gut. The patient is in a much better condition to tolerate a thoracotomy.

approach in which gastrostomy is done immediately and the upper pouch decompressed with sump suction. Hyperalimentation provides nutrition until the patient is vigorous and gaining weight, when the definitive procedure can be carried out with greater safety.

An anastomotic leak is a major complication. If the prcedure has been done retropleurally and the space is well drained, a small leak is likely to close spontaneously. Recurrent tracheoesophageal fistula is the result of an anastomotic leak and requires division. The most frequent late complication is anastomotic stricture, which usually responds to esophageal dilatation.

Esophageal Atresia without Tracheoesophageal Fistula

Esophageal atresia without tracheoesophageal fistula presents a somewhat different therapeutic problem, since the distal esophageal segment is short and there is a long gap between the two esophageal pouches. Howard has advocated stretching the proximal esophageal pouch with a 12 F mercury-loaded bougie twice daily to make a primary anastomosis possible. This approach has yielded varied results. The other approach is to perform a gastrostomy for feeding and cervical esophagostomy for proximal pouch drain-

age. Later a colon interposition is employed to connect the proximal esophagus and the stomach. Small bowel segments or a gastric tube can also be used for this purpose.

Tracheoesophageal Fistula without Esophageal Atresia

Tracheoesophageal fistula without esophageal atresia often presents a difficult diagnostic problem. These patients have recurrent bouts of pneumonia, they often cough when taking liquids, and they have increased intestinal gas with abdominal distention (from air passing through the fistula). Cine-esophagogram may or may not demonstrate a communication between the esophagus and trachea. It often shows poor peristalsis in the distal esophagus. The fistula is best visualized from the tracheal side in the infant by means of bronchoscopy with fiberoptic light source telescopic insert, and a closed ventilatory system. Another method is to perform esophagoscopy while dye is placed through an endotracheal tube and the patient is forcefully ventilated by the anesthesiologist. This forces air and dye through the fistula, demonstrating the abnormal communication.

Once a fistula has been demonstrated by any means,

it should be divided. Most of the fistulas occur at or above the level of the second thoracic vetebra and can be repaired through a cervical approach.

ESOPHAGEAL STENOSIS

Congenital stenosis of the esophagus is not common. Patients with esophageal stenosis, however, may present with respiratory difficulty secondary to aspiration of formula, recurrent pneumonia, or dysphagia. Diagnosis is by barium swallow and esophagoscopy. Short stenotic segments usually respond to esophageal dilation. A rare one is resistant to dilation and will require resection and esophagoesophagostomy.

VOMITING

Although occasional regurgitation of formula is quite common in infants, persistent vomiting, the vomiting of bile-stained material, or forceful vomiting is abnormal, and its cause should be investigated. In the neonate, bile-stained vomitus is almost always indicative of intestinal obstruction. Nonobstructive causes of vomiting must also be considered, such as increased intracranial pressure (subdural hematoma, hydrocephalus), electrolyte imbalance (adrenogenital syndrome), and, particularly, sepsis.

Abdominal distention is a prominent feature of distal small bowel and colonic obstruction but is absent with obstruction above the proximal jejunum. Most normal infants will pass a meconium stool during the first 24 hours of life. Interestingly, many neonates with small bowel obstruction will pass one or two meconium stools. They simply evacuate the colon of meconium distal to the obstruction. The fact that an infant has passed a stool or does not have abdominal distention therefore does not exclude intestinal obstruction.

After a thorough physical examination to detect extra-abdominal causes of vomiting and evaluation of the abdomen for signs of intra-abdominal sepsis or an abdominal mass, recumbent and upright roentgenograms of the abdomen are of primary diagnostic importance. On plain x-ray of the abdomen it is not possible in the neonate to differentiate colon from small bowel.

Pulmonary complications of vomiting (aspiration and aspiration pneumonia) are a major cause of death for neonates with intestinal obstruction. To avoid this complication the stomach should be promptly aspirated in any infant suspected of having intestinal obstruction and the tube left in the stomach.

An important part of operative correction of neonatal obstruction is a gastrostomy to reduce the chance of postoperative vomiting with the hazard of aspiration. The advantages of a gastrostomy over a nasogastric tube are (1) the larger tube employed does a more efficient job of decompressing the stomach; (2) a tube through the nose and pharynx interferes with the infant's clearing pharyngeal and tracheal secretions, whereas gastrostomy does not; and (3) a gastrostomy can be used for feeding purposes once intestinal

peristalsis has returned to normal in the premature or ill neonate. It is a helpful and safe procedure in pediatric surgery.[16]

Another consideration in neonates with intestinal obstruction is the use of total parenteral nutrition (intravenous hyperalimentation). In many patients it takes a long time for proper gastrointestinal function to be established. It is wise to start parenteral nutrition early in the postoperative period so that the patient does not reach a state of malnutrition and severe negative nitrogen balance before this valuable form of therapy is instituted.

DUODENAL OBSTRUCTION

Duodenal obstruction in the neonate is the result of duodenal atresia or stenosis, annular pancreas (with associated atresia or stenosis), or peritoneal bands secondary to incomplete intestinal rotation.

Embryology. The duodenum is the one portion of the gastrointestinal tract in which a solid phase is known to exist in early fetal life. Lack of recanalization may be the cause of atresia or stenosis. Annular pancreas is thought to be the result of failure of the tip of the ventral pancreatic anlage to rotate with the duodenum. As a consequence, it becomes wrapped around the second portion of the duodenum.

Clinical Findings. The principal symptom is vomiting of bile-stained material. On rare occasions the obstruction is proximal to the ampulla of Vater and the vomitus is not green. With atresia the vomiting usually starts the first day of life. If there has been an asymptomatic period of a few days prior to onset of symptoms, malrotation is more likely. Stenosis causes less severe symptoms, and the patient may have little difficulty until solids are added to the diet. Abdominal distention is not a prominent feature, though there may be fullness in the epigastrium if the stomach is distended. If there is lower distention, malrotation with volvulus should be suspected. The state of hydration depends on how soon after birth the diagnosis is made. About one third of patients with duodenal atresia also have Down's syndrome (mongolism).

Diagnosis. Diagnosis of duodenal obstruction is made by upright x-ray of the abdomen, which shows the typical "double bubble" of stomach and dilated duodenum with no other small bowel gas (Fig. 7). Contrast studies are not necessary unless there is air distal to the duodenum indicating partial obstruction — stenosis or malrotation.

Therapy. Extensive preoperative preparation is not required if the diagnosis has been promptly made. The stomach should be emptied by a nasogastric tube. If the patient is dehydrated, intravenous fluids are given. Since the obstruction is high and the gut proximal to it can be easily decompressed, perforation is not a danger. If there is any question of malrotation with midgut volvulus, a barium study should be obtained.

A right upper transverse incision gives excellent exposure of the duodenum. If there is an intrinsic atresia or stenosis, the duodenum is mobilized by an extensive Kocher maneuver to allow a generous duodenoduoden-

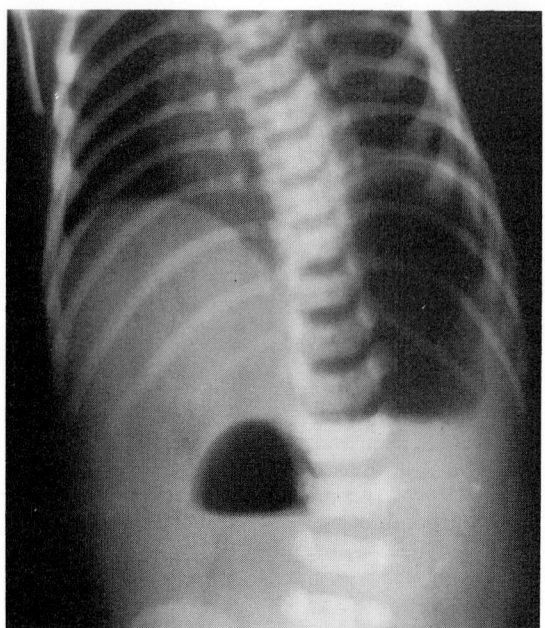

Figure 7. Upright roentgenogram of a neonate with duodenal atresia showing the classic "double bubble" of stomach and dilated duodenum. There is no distal gas.

ostomy without tension. The area of the common bile duct and ampulla of Vater is avoided.

Postoperatively the stomach is decompressed by gastrostomy and the patient is maintained on intravenous fluids until oral feedings can be tolerated. Complications are pneumonia, sepsis, and postoperative intestinal obstruction.

Results. About two thirds of patients with duodenal obstruction survive. Associated anomalies and prematurity significantly influence the mortality rate and are responsible for half the deaths. Respiratory and anastomotic complications cause most of the remaining deaths and are preventable.[11]

Some parents of infants with duodenal atresia and mongolism prefer not to have the infants operated upon. If the diagnosis of mongolism is not definite, the stomach can be safely decompressed by a nasogastric tube for the 48 to 72 hours required to obtain a confirmatory chromosome analysis.

JEJUNOILEAL ATRESIA

In the neonate distal small bowel and colonic obstructions present much the same clinical picture and may be due to atresia or stenosis of the jejunum, ileum (most common), or colon (rare), meconium ileus, malrotation, or Hirschsprung's disease (Fig. 8).

Etiology. Current thinking holds that the etiology of atresia of the small bowel is usually, if not always, the result of an *in utero* vascular accident. Similar lesions can be produced experimentally by ligation of the mesenteric vessels of the fetal dog. Microscopic examination of resected gut distal to an atretic area shows squamous epithelial cells in the lumen, indicating that the gut was patent at some previous time. The gut is often shorter than normal in these infants. Associated intra-abdominal adhesions and calcifications also implicate a previous catastrophic event. The mechanism of the vascular accident is unknown, but it could result from volvulus, thrombosis, embolus, or intussusception.

Clinical Findings. The most prominent symptom is vomiting of bile-stained material from the first day or two of life. The abdomen is distended and may have been so from birth. The infant may be dehydrated both from vomiting and from fluid loss into the dilated loops of intestine.

Diagnosis. X-ray of the abdomen shows dilated loops of gut, usually with air-fluid levels. Barium enema should be performed in all infants with low intestinal obstruction to differentiate atresia from Hirschsprung's disease. In jejunal or ileal atresia it shows a normally rotated, small, unused colon (Fig. 9). (This "microcolon" is actually normal but because of proximal obstruction contains little or no material. It will function normally.)

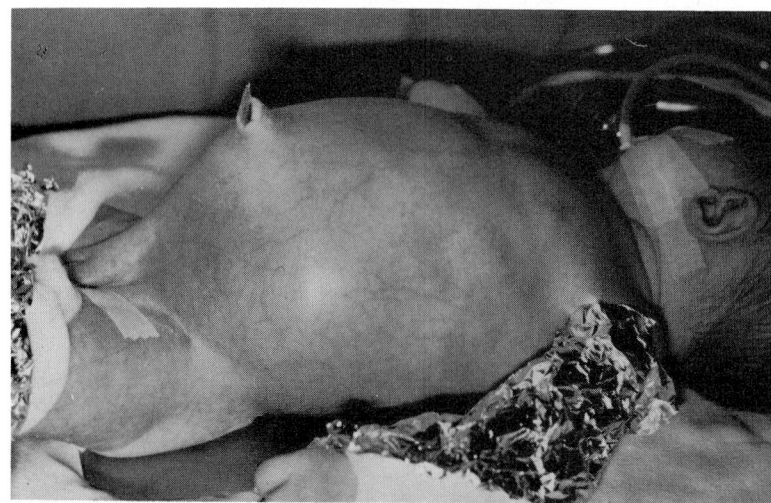

Figure 8. Abdominal distention of this degree in a newborn with symptoms of intestinal obstruction is indicative of distal small bowel or colonic obstruction.

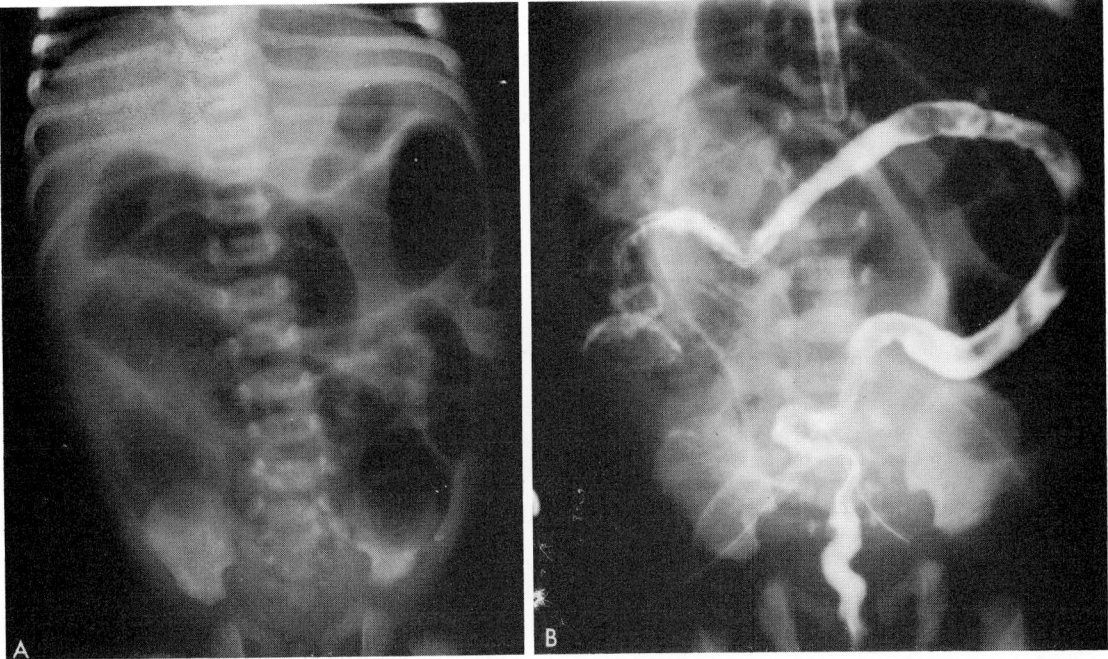

Figure 9. *A*, Typical x-ray of a newborn with distal small bowel or colonic obstruction. It is not possible on a plain film of the abdomen to distinguish large from small bowel gas in patients of this age. *B*, Barium enema in a patient with small bowel obstruction shows a small unused colon.

Treatment. Preoperative preparation consists of gastric decompression, vitamin K administration, and, if the patient's condition warrants, intravenous fluids and plasma. This should not take more than 4 hours. If preoperative chest x-ray shows aspiration pneumonia, antibiotics, usually penicillin and kanamycin, are given.

Operation is through either a transverse incision just above the umbilicus or an upper abdominal midline incision. It is important that the markedly dilated segment of intestine just proximal to the atretic segment be resected (Fig. 10). If the gut is short and an effort is being made to conserve intestinal length, an alternative is to remove a shorter amount of the

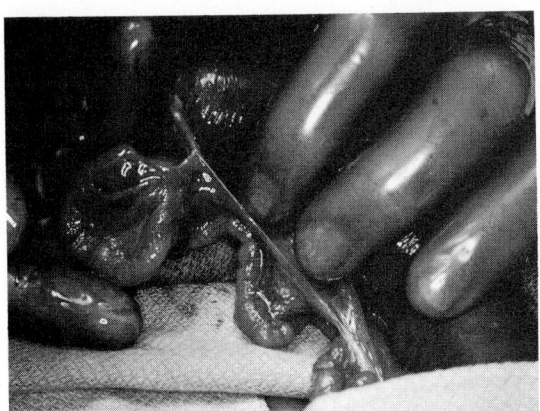

Figure 10. Operative photograph of ileal atresia, showing the proximal bowel to end blindly, a V-shaped mesenteric defect, and the decompressed tiny distal intestine.

dilated atretic segment and do an extensive jejunoplasty. A wedge-shaped segment of the antimesenteric wall of intestine is resected to narrow the proximal limb so that its diameter approximates that of the distal segment.[17] If massively dilated proximal intestine is left, it will not function properly and will result in chronic functional obstruction.[11] Intestinal continuity is established by an end-to-end anastomosis. Bypass operations will lead to later complications associated with the blind loop syndrome. Because of the small caliber of the distal gut the anastomosis must be done with great care. We prefer a single-layer anastomosis using inverting horizontal mattress sutures of 5–0 vascular silk placed from within the lumen. A Stamm gastrostomy provides postoperative gastric decompression.

Since some of these infants have difficulty in the postoperative period with mechanical obstruction or short intestine, parenteral nutrition is of value. If there is less than 12 inches of small intestine, the outlook for survival is bleak.

Results. The overall survival rate is about 75 per cent. Prematurity and associated anomalies are not nearly as frequent as with duodenal atresia. Anastomotic and pulmonary complications account for most of the deaths.

MECONIUM ILEUS

Meconium ileus is the earliest manifestation of cystic fibrosis and is present in approximately 10 to 15 per cent of patients with this disease.

Etiology and Pathology. Cystic fibrosis is a hereditary disease transmitted as an autosomal recessive trait. Cystic fibrosis involves the lungs, pancreas, liver, and skin as well as the gut. The meconium contains an abnormal mucoprotein. There is also a decrease or absence of pancreatic exocrine function.

The terminal ileum is filled with firm, small, gray concretions and is of small caliber. Just proximal to this, the ileum is markedly dilated and filled with a thick, very viscid, and exceedingly sticky meconium which intestinal peristalsis is incapable of propelling. The proximal ileum is less dilated and the meconium is liquid (Fig. 11).

Some patients with meconium ileus have associated atresia, presumably the result of a prenatal volvulus of a segment of the dilated intestine. This may be associated with intra-abdominal calcification.

Diagnosis. Clinical findings are similar to those in patients with intestinal atresia—bilious vomiting and abdominal distention. Dilated meconium-filled loops of ileum may be palpable. A family history of cystic fibrosis provides strong support for a diagnosis of meconium ileus.

X-rays of the abdomen reveal findings similar to those in other forms of neonatal distal intestinal obstruction. There may, however, be fewer fluid levels, a greater variety in the size of intestinal loops, and a granular appearance in some of the dilated loops of gut. The loops may be arranged in concentric circles and change little with upright positioning. Barium enema shows a small, unused, normally positioned colon. If there is reflux of barium into the terminal ileum, the small concretions typical of meconium ileus may be seen. A sweat chloride level over 60 mEq. per liter is diagnostic.

Treatment. Unless the patient has signs of peritonitis or incipient intestinal gangrene, nonoperative treatment should be tried first.[24, 35] After fluid resuscitation and confirmation of the diagnosis by barium enema, the barium is replaced by Gastrografin or Hypaque. The hypertonicity causes fluid to shift into the intestinal lumen, loosening the inspissated stool. It is imperative that intravenous fluid be administered

simultaneously to correct the hypovolemia. A ratio of 6 ml. of intravenous fluid for 1 ml. of contrast material is usually appropriate. If results are inconclusive, the enema may be repeated after 12 hours. If hypertonic enema treatment fails, operation should be carried out promptly. Preoperative preparation is similar to that for neonates with other forms of intestinal obstruction.

Operative therapy consists of resection of the segment of markedly dilated ileum containing the very sticky meconium. The terminal ileum is irrigated with the mucolytic agent N-acetylcysteine in a 2 per cent concentration. (More concentrated solutions are irritating.) If the segment affected is short, it can be evacuated by enterotomy and irrigation and closed. If all of the obstructing meconium cannot be removed from the distal ileum, a T-vented ileostomy is necessary to provide decompression and permit distal irrigation in the postoperative period.

Postoperative care is similar to that in jejunoileal atresia. Special care is taken to avoid pneumonia. If an ileostomy vent has been used, it is closed later. Pancreatic enzyme supplementation must be added to the formula.

Results. While 75 to 80 per cent survive the intestinal obstruction, these patients are still faced with all the pulmonary and nutritional problems of cystic fibrosis. Only about 50 per cent survive the first 6 months.

After the neonatal period obstruction can occur in patients with cystic fibrosis because of inspissated intestinal contents. This is likely to occur if pancreatic supplementation has been deleted from the diet. This condition has been termed meconium ileus equivalent. Nonoperative management by long-tube intestinal decompression plus administration of pancreatic enzymes or N-acetylcysteine through the tube and by enema is usually successful. The inspissated intestinal contents in the cecum or terminal ileum may act as a lead point for an intussusception in the older infant or child. This often requires operative reduction.

MALROTATION OF THE INTESTINE

Malrotation may produce duodenal or distal small bowel obstruction in the neonate as well as in the older child. High obstruction is due to compression of the duodenum by Ladd's bands, and distal obstruction to compression by midgut volvulus. In addition, malrotation may produce chronic malabsorption (celiac-like syndrome).

Embryology. Malrotation or, more accurately, incomplete rotation, results from arrest of the normal rotation of the midgut (that portion of the intestine supplied by the superior mesenteric artery—from the duodenum to the midcolon). About the tenth week of fetal life the midgut returns to the abdominal cavity from the coelomic extension in the base of the umbilical cord. As the gut returns, it rotates in a counterclockwise direction. If the rotational process is arrested when the cecum is in the epigastrium or right upper quadrant, there is no posterior peritoneal attachment of the small bowel mesentery from the ligament of Treitz to the right lower quadrant, nor does the ascending colon have its posterior peritoneal at-

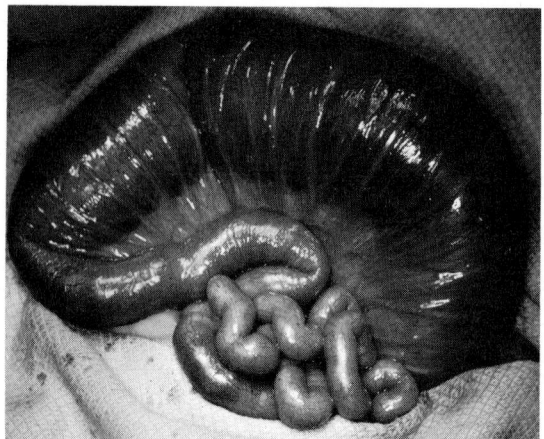

Figure 11. Operative findings in a patient with meconium ileus. The terminal ileum is small and contains small, firm concretions. The portion just proximal to this is dilated and contains exceedingly sticky meconium.

tachments to the right posterior abdomen. Peritoneal bands connect the cecum and proximal colon to the right upper quadrant. In so doing they cross and often obstruct the duodenum. If the duodenum has not rotated inferior to the superior mesenteric vessels, the distal duodenum and jejunum remain on the right side of the spine and there is no ligament of Treitz.[9]

Clinical Findings. Symptoms in the neonate are those of duodenal or low intestinal obstruction. Bile-stained vomitus is present. Abdominal distention may or may not be present. Symptoms may be present from the first day of life. Sometimes there is an asymptomatic period followed by a sudden onset of symptoms due to midgut volvulus. The infant may deteriorate rapidly. Bloody stools can be a prominent feature. This is a catastrophic event and requires prompt treatment.

In the somewhat older infant or child chronic symptoms are likely to result from partial duodenal obstruction. There is recurrent vomiting and poor weight gain. Chronic diarrhea, malnutrition, and abdominal distention may occasionally result from malrotation. The cause of this symptom complex is not clear. It is thought to be the result of partial midgut torsion with venous obstruction, mucosal edema, and malabsorption.

Diagnosis. Diagnosis is by x-ray. Plain films of the abdomen show either duodenal or distal obstruction. Duodenal obstruction is less apt to be as complete as, or to be accompanied by as much duodenal dilatation as, duodenal atresia. With volvulus there are dilated loops of small bowel with air-fluid levels. On occasion when volvulus is associated with a high degree of duodenal obstruction, almost no small bowel gas is present.

Barium upper gastrointestinal examination reveals abnormal position of the duodenojejunal junction and the proximal jejunal loops lying to the right of the midline.[29] Complete obstruction to contrast material is very rare. If the infant has evidence of complete obstruction at the level of the duodenum or signs of volvulus with gangrene, contrast studies are not indicated and serve only to delay definitive therapy.

Treatment. Because of the risk of vascular occlusion, volvulus requires prompt operation. A very short time of preoperative preparation may be required to restore the blood volume if the patient is in shock. On opening the abdomen, the surgeon notes that the colon is not in the right gutter but is wrapped around the root of the small bowel mesentery. The entire small bowel should be delivered onto the abdominal wall and rotated in a counterclockwise direction until the volvulus has been reduced. Nonviable gut must be resected. Unfortunately, that is sometimes the entire midgut. If this extensive resection is required, the wisest course may be to exteriorize only that portion of the gut which is definitely not viable and return any questionable areas to the abdomen. Laparotomy the following day may reveal that some of the remaining intestine is still viable. If not, the patient's chance for survival is nil. Parenteral nutrition is not indicated, since it merely delays the inevitable outcome.

The duodenal obstruction is relieved by division of the peritoneal bands crossing the duodenum. Occasionally intrinsic obstruction of the duodenum is as-

sociated with malrotation, and it should be looked for. The proximal colon is returned to the left side of the abdomen. Intestinal fixation procedures are unnecessary (Fig. 12). Postoperative care usually presents no particular problems unless an extensive resection is required.

Results. Survival exceeds 95 per cent if resection is not required and there is no significant associated anomaly.

AGANGLIONIC MEGACOLON (HIRSCHSPRUNG'S DISEASE)

Hirschsprung, the noted Danish pediatrician, presented his classic description of "Constipation in Newborns Due to Dilatation and Hypertrophy of the Colon" before the Berlin Congress of Children's Disease in 1886. The paper was published in 1888. A true understanding of the nature of the pathology did not come until 60 years later when Swenson and Bill in 1948 described an operative procedure to excise the entire aganglionic segment by an abdominoperineal pull-through technique.

Pathology. The basic defect in Hirschsprung's disease is absence of ganglionic cells of the myenteric plexuses of Auerbach in the involved segment of colon. This absence of ganglion cells extends from the anus proximally for various distances, usually to involve the rectum and a portion of the sigmoid colon. Aganglionosis may, however, on unusual occasions involve the entire colon and, rarely, the entire small bowel as well. Even more rarely, skip areas with intervening normal bowel have been reported. The rectum, however, is not skipped.

Physiology. The absence of parasympathetic innervation leads to lack of peristalsis in the involved portion of colon. Histochemical studies also indicate sympathetic overactivity in the aganglionic segment leading to increased muscle tone. The result is a functional obstruction. The colon just proximal to this area dilates and the musculature becomes hypertrophied as it works to propel the fecal stream through the distal obstruction.

If pressures are measured in the colonic lumen in patients with Hirschsprung's disease, there is no evidence of peristaltic activity in the aganglionic segment. Peristaltic pressures in the proximal colon are higher than normal.

Clinical Findings. Almost all patients with Hirschsprung's disease have some difficulty during the neonatal period. In some the clinical picture is the same as that in other forms of neonatal intestinal obstruction, with green vomitus and abdominal distention. In others the symptoms are less impressive. It is, however, usually possible to obtain a history that the infant was constipated in the neonatal period. Constipation persists and frequent enemas, suppositories, and laxatives are given for relief, even in the infant.

This chronic obstruction leads to enterocolitis in some infants. They may become quite ill with diarrhea, dehydration, and sepsis. The colitis may proceed to perforation. Enterocolitis is the most dangerous

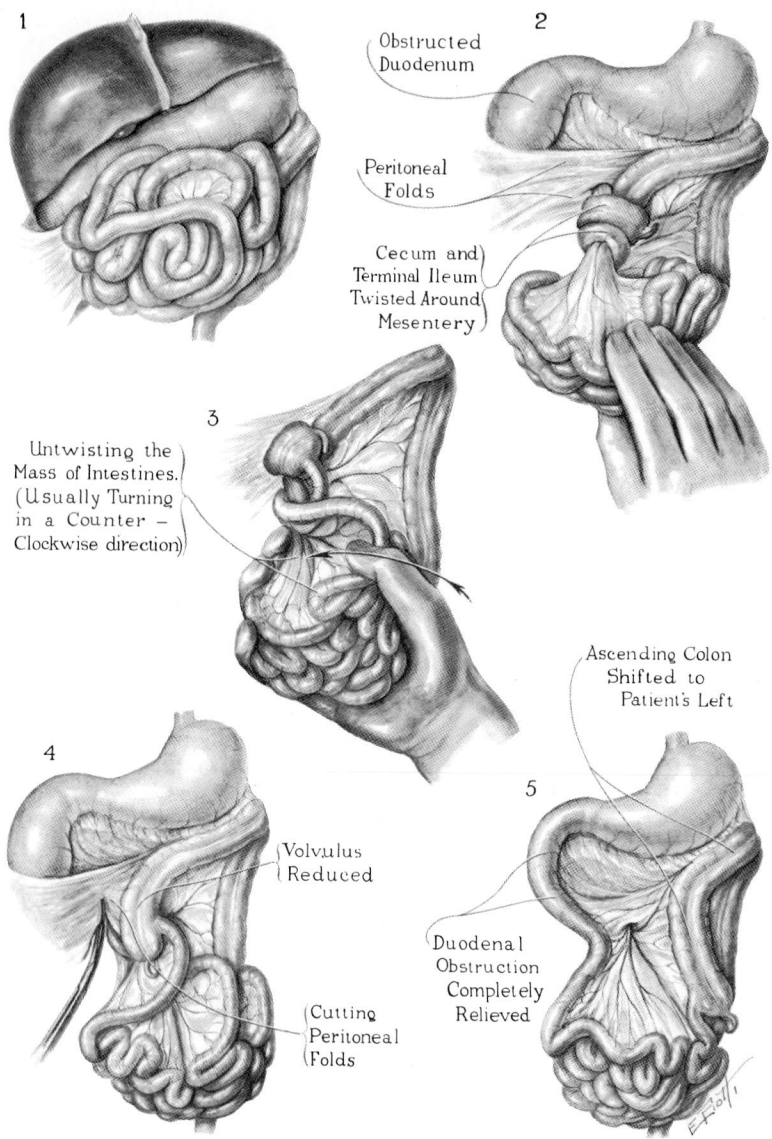

1

2

Obstructed Duodenum

Peritoneal Folds

Cecum and Terminal Ileum Twisted Around Mesentery

3

Untwisting the Mass of Intestines. (Usually Turning in a Counter – Clockwise direction)

Ascending Colon Shifted to Patient's Left

4

5

Volvulus Reduced

Duodenal Obstruction Completely Relieved

Cutting Peritoneal Folds

Figure 12. Operative treatment of malrotation with midgut volvulus and duodenal obstruction. (From Gross, R. E.: An Atlas of Children's Surgery. Philadelphia, W. B. Saunders Company, 1970.)

complication of Hirschsprung's disease and carries a high mortality.

The older child with Hirschsprung's disease must be distinguished from the much larger number of children who are constipated from other causes. The child with Hirschsprung's disease has had symptoms from birth. He seldom soils his underclothing, and on rectal examination the stool is at least 2 to 3 cm. above the sphincter. Stool may be passed after the digital examination. Some of these children go for 2 to 3 weeks without passing stools. In constipation from other causes the onset of symptoms occurs after the neonatal period, the child usually soils his underpants frequently, and rectal examination reveals a large quantity of stool just at the sphincter.

Diagnosis. Diagnosis can usually be made with ease by barium enema in the older infant or child (Fig. 13). There is a relatively normal-sized rectum and rectosigmoid with considerable dilatation of the colon just

proximal to this. The colon empties poorly. In the neonate, plain x-rays of the abdomen may be indistinguishable from those in distal small bowel obstruction. Barium enema, however, will show a relatively normal-appearing colon. The disparity in size has not yet developed. The colon empties poorly, however, and considerable barium will be present in the colon 24 hours later. This retention is highly suggestive of Hirschsprung's disease. A feathered appearance of the colonic mucosa is suggestive of superficial ulceration and is an indication of enterocolitis.

The diagnosis is proved by rectal biopsy, though this is not usually necessary with older infants and children. A full-thickness biopsy of the lateral rectal wall about 2 cm. above the mucocutaneous junction will reveal absence of myenteric ganglion cells if the patient has Hirschsprung's disease. Experienced radiologists and pathologists are most helpful in making the diagnosis of Hirschsprung's disease. Lack of familiarity on their part leads to much confusion in this diagnosis.

Treatment. The treatment of Hirschsprung's disease, as indicated by Swenson, is resection of the entire aganglionic segment with anastomosis at the anus.[33] This is an extensive procedure and is not well tolerated by the sick infant. Preliminary colostomy above the aganglionic segment permits delay of the corrective procedure until the patient can better tolerate it. It should be determined by frozen section that there are ganglion cells present at the colostomy site. Definitive resection is done when the patient is 6 months to a year old. Older patients usually do not require a preliminary colostomy unless the dilated segment is huge and decompression would facilitate anastomosis.

In addition to the Swenson pull-through operation, two modifications of that procedure have gained favor in recent years. In the Duhamel operation the ganglionic proximal colon is brought down posterior to the aganglionic rectum, which is not resected. They are connected by a side-to-side anastomosis. This procedure has particular merit for the patient who has aganglionosis of the entire colon. The small bowel can be connected to a long segment of rectum and sigmoid to provide adequate absorptive surface (colon) while providing a peristaltic segment (small bowel) down to the anus.

In the Soave procedure, the surgeon leaves the aganglionic rectal musculature in place, removes the rectal mucosa, and brings the normal peristaltic ganglionic segment down through the rectal muscular cuff. The advantage of this procedure is that it requires no pelvic dissection outside the rectum.

For patients with a very short aganglionic segment, resection of a strip of the rectal musculature pos-teriorly (in essence, a myotomy of the aganglionic segment) can be accomplished from inside the anus.

Results. The mortality for the older infant and child is 2 to 3 per cent. For the infant with enterocolitis the mortality is as high as 50 per cent. The functional results are quite good in 95 per cent of patients.

NECROTIZING ENTEROCOLITIS

Prior to the advances in neonatology that have made survival of the tiny premature infant possible, necrotizing enterocolitis was seldom recognized. It is truly a "disease of medical progress." In the past few years it has become a major neonatal surgical emergency.

Etiology. A wide variety of stressful circumstances such as exchange transfusion, respiratory distress syndrome, and "shock" have been incriminated as the cause of necrotizing enterocolitis of the newborn. Most are premature infants, not infrequently with birth weights of 1000 to 1500 gm. Many have been "stressed," although not all have overt evidence of this. Almost all patients have been fed, and enteric cultures frequently show Klebsiella species. Intestinal ischemia appears to be the initiating event, whether due to shunting of splanchnic blood to other parts of the body in a pre-shock state or resulting from hypoxia. Bacterial invasion leads to mucosal breakdown and ulceration with the development of intramural gas. Progression of ischemic changes leads to transmural necrosis that may result in perforation, peritonitis, and death.

It is of great interest that breast milk-fed babies seldom develop necrotizing enterocolitis. In an experimental model, it has been demonstrated that it is the macrophages in breast milk that apparently exert a protective effect.[5]

Clinical Findings. A tiny premature infant, usually three days to three weeks of age, typically deteriorates suddenly. Feedings are refused or vomited, abdominal distention develops, and stools may be noted to be guaiac-positive. If prompt treatment is not instituted, hypotension and acidosis occur within a few hours. Even with successful medical therapy, intestinal perforation with abscess formation or pneumoperitoneum may occur. Disseminated intravascular coagulation (DIC) is not uncommon and carries a grave prognosis.

Diagnosis. The diagnosis of necrotizing enterocolitis is confirmed by demonstration of gas in the intestinal wall or portal vein on abdominal x-ray. Prior to this, ileus is noted. Once perforation occurs, pneumoperitoneum is usually readily apparent on upright abdominal examination.

Treatment. Early treatment of necrotizing enterocolitis leads to resolution of the disease in most cases. At the first sign of gastrointestinal malfunction—vomiting, distention, or guaiac-positive stools—feeding should be stopped and the stomach decompressed with a nasogastric tube. Antibiotics are administered intravenously and plasma or blood is given to restore circulating blood volume. Parenteral nutrition should

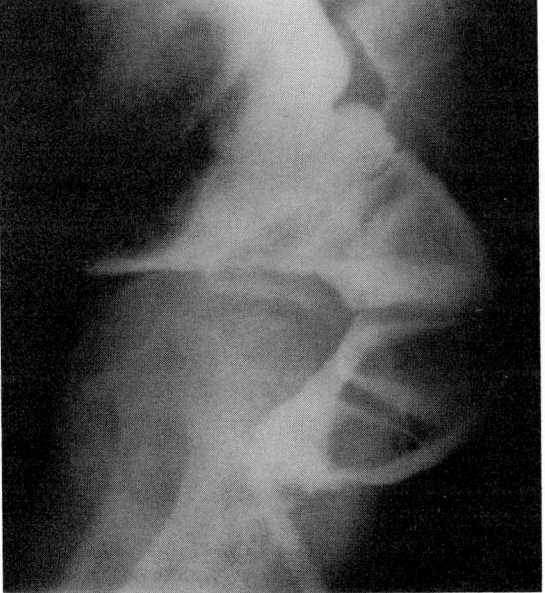

Figure 13. Barium enema in this older boy shows a normal-sized rectum with marked dilatation of the rectosigmoid, which is typical of Hirschsprung's disease.

then be administered for at least 10 days, after which feedings may be cautiously resumed.

If the early symptoms are not promptly treated, cardiovascular collapse may occur within a few hours, together with DIC and subsequent intestinal perforation. Mortality in these infants is very high.

Surgical intervention is clearly necessary if there is evidence of perforation. Prior to this, signs of deterioration, such as the development of abdominal tenderness, progressive acidosis, or DIC should prompt operation.

Operative treatment consists of excision of necrotic bowel and proximal decompressing ileostomy or colostomy, depending on the area affected. The colon is most commonly afflicted, but a considerable amount of ileum may also be involved. Only parts of the intestine that are frankly gangrenous should be removed, since areas of patchy or questionable necrosis will usually heal if the patient survives. Intestinal continuity is re-established 6 to 12 weeks later, after the acute process has subsided and the infant has gained weight to 2000 to 2500 gm.

Results. Medical therapy is usually successful if it is instituted promptly after the onset of the first signs. Once shock, acidosis, or DIC has ensued, failure is the rule. Intestinal resection and ileostomy are successful in 80 per cent or more of patients who have not developed peritonitis and free perforation at the time of operation. In the latter group, mortality is 50 per cent or greater.[32] In a small percentage of patients who have been successfully treated either medically or surgically, colonic stricture develops, requiring resection.

IMPERFORATE ANUS

Imperforate anus is perhaps not the most accurate description of the anorectal malformations under discussion but is the one accepted by general usage. The anatomy in this group of anomalies is complicated. To give some idea of how complicated it is, a classification in outline form recently proposed by an international group of experts requires 30 lines.

Embryology. In the 4-mm. embryo the allantois connects with the hindgut in a terminal cavity, the cloaca. The urorectal septum divides the ventral urogenital portion from the dorsal rectal portion of the 5-mm. embryo down to the pubococcygeal line. Lateral ingrowth of mesenchyma completes the division below this level.

Alterations of this division result in a rectourinary fistula. In the female, müllerian ducts are interposed between the dorsal and ventral portions, so rectourinary fistulas do not occur (except cloacal anomalies). The distal vagina develops from sinovaginal buds that originate from the epithelium of the dorsal wall of the urogenital sinus. (Rectovaginal fistulas are the result of maldevelopment in this area.)

The terminal hindgut forms the upper portion of the anal canal. The lower portion is formed from the proctodeum. The anal sphincter is formed from still another source—mesoderm—and is almost always present.

Pathology. Anatomic conditions that are important in therapy are:

1. The height of the rectal pouch—is it above the pubococcygeal line (high pouch) and hence has not descended through the puborectalis sling?

2. Is there a fistula, and if so, to what? In the male fistulas may connect the rectum to the perineum, urethra, or bladder, and, in the female, to the vulva, vestibule, vagina, or perineum. The large majority of patients have a fistula to one of these locations.

A description of the anomaly should be anatomic and include this information. For example, "low imperforate anus with rectovaginal fistula" is more useful than a complicated system of letters and numbers.

Usually grouped with imperforate anus are rectal atresia (in which there is a normal anus distal to the atretic rectal area), anal stenosis, and anal membrane.

Symptoms. If there is a perineal or vaginal fistula that is large enough to decompress the colon, there may be no symptoms in the neonatal period. In these patients constipation usually develops later as stools become formed. If there is no external fistula or the fistula is small, typical symptoms of low intestinal obstruction appear.

Diagnosis. The diagnosis of imperforate anus is made by inspection of the perineum (Fig. 14). The height of the rectal pouch is determined by lateral x-rays in the upside-down position taken after swallowed air has had ample time to reach the rectum (24 hours of age). An opaque marker is placed on the anus, and the center of the x-ray beam is directed at the greater trochanter. This technique has the limitation that meconium in the pouch may prevent air from reaching the distal end of the pouch, giving a false impression of a high atresia. Conversely, if the baby is crying at the time the film is exposed, the increased intrabdominal pressure may push the pouch down, giving the false impression of a low pouch. In general, the high pouch that has not descended through the puborectalis sling is more than 1.5 cm. above the anus on x-ray and appears above a line drawn from pubis to coccyx. A low pouch is below these points.

The physical findings are more important. If there is a perineal fistula (including ectopic anteriorly displaced anus and fistula opening along the median scrotal raphe) or fistula to the vaginal fourchette or low vagina, the operative approach is from the perineum. A retrograde urethrogram in the male may demonstrate a fistulous communication between the rectum and the posterior urethra or the base of the bladder. These patients, as well as those with no fistula, need a combined abdominoperineal operation.

Imperforate anus is associated with other congenital anomalies about half the time. Some of these are life-threatening, and their recognition is important to the immediate care of the patient. Esophageal atresia is present in about 5 per cent of patients and should be looked for prior to operation in all patients. Urologic anomalies are frequent. A cystourethrogram and intravenous pyelogram should be done to detect these associated anomalies. Congenital heart disease is common. Sacral anomalies are frequent with high imperforate anus.

Treatment. In almost all girls, and in those boys

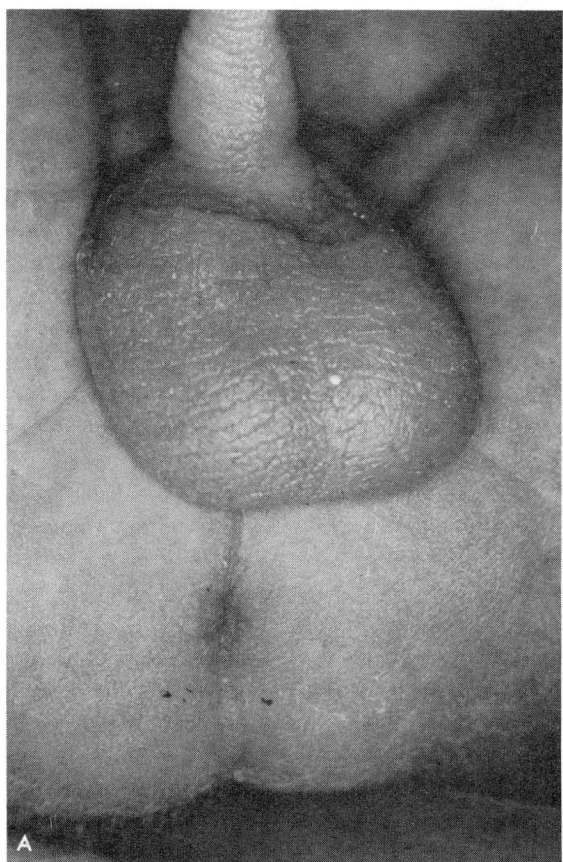
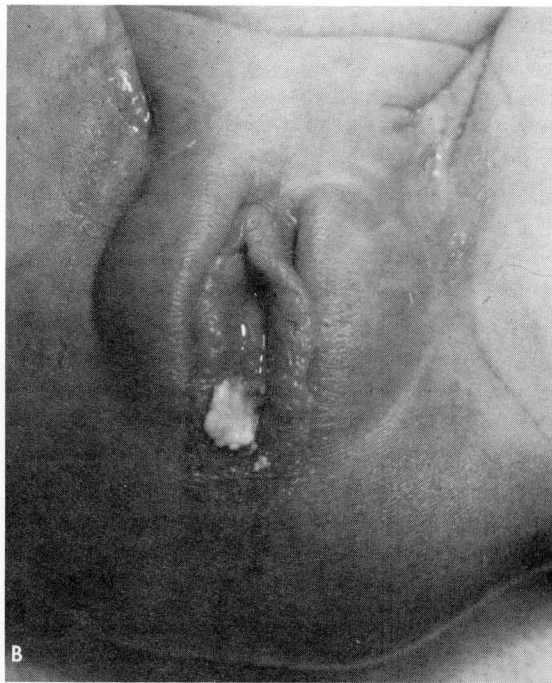

Figure 14. *A,* Imperforate anus in a boy. *B,* Imperforate anus in a girl with rectal fistula to the fourchette.

with perineal fistulas, the condition can be corrected by a perineal anoplasty. In these patients the rectum is normally positioned through the puborectalis sling. The fistulous opening is dissected back to the rectal pouch, which is freed to allow it to be sutured without tension to the anal skin in the normal position. In patients with anteriorly displaced anus this can usually be accomplished by a simple incision posteriorly and suture of the mucous membranes of the perineal skin. This procedure can be safely done in the neonatal period.

For the boy with a high urinary tract fistula and the girl with cloacal anomalies, the best functional results are obtained by definitive operation when the child is older. The initial therapy therefore is creation of a colostomy. With a divided colostomy that completely diverts the fecal stream there are fewer complications, and there is less chance of urinary tract infection in patients with urinary tract fistulas. Either sigmoid or transverse colostomy can be used.

The most important feature of the definitive repair is the accurate placement of the rectum through the puborectalis sling of the levator ani complex just behind the urethra. Stephens advocates a posterior approach just below the sacrum with removal of the coccyx for better visualization of the levator musculature.[31] The colon is mobilized by an abdominal approach, passed through the previously identified puborectalis and external sphincters, and sutured to the

anal skin. Some surgeons feel the posterior approach does not appreciably aid in the identification of the puborectalis and identify this muscle from above. The urinary fistula is divided in the course of the mobilization of the distal rectal pouch and the urethral end is sewn over the catgut.

Results. Mortality is appreciably influenced by associated anomalies. Except for these, operative mortality is about 2 per cent.

Functional results are good for those with a low pouch that can be corrected by a perineal approach. Ninety to 95 per cent of these patients have essentially normal bowel control. Patients with a high pouch have a poorer result. Only about half have good functional control, though most can acquire socially acceptable control with diet, laxatives, and enemas.

GASTROESOPHAGEAL REFLUX

Gastroesophageal reflux is the most common cause of vomiting in infants. Newborns lack a measurable distal esophageal sphincter, so "spitting up" is quite common, though it is not bile-stained if due to reflux. After the first few weeks of life, persistent reflux is abnormal and may require treatment.

Clinical Findings. Vomiting usually occurs shortly after feedings, often when the baby has been returned to the crib and placed in a horizontal position. It may mimic pyloric stenosis and lead to malnutrition and failure to gain weight. In some patients, particularly infants in the first six months of life, gastroesophageal reflux leads to recurrent or refractory aspiration pneumonia. In others, it may cause apneic spells and even cardiac arrest. In the older child, anemia may result from esophagitis, which can also lead to esophageal stricture causing dysphagia. All of the complications of gastroesophageal reflux may occasionally be seen in patients whose reflux is occult, i.e., without vomiting as a symptom.

Diagnosis. The diagnosis of gastroesophageal reflux is made roentgenographically by barium swallow. It is often not easy to demonstrate, and considerable radiologic experience may be necessary to make the diagnosis. If a portion of the cardia is demonstrated above the diaphragm, a true hiatal hernia exists. Esophagitis is detected by esophagoscopy. Strictures may be demonstrated by both these diagnostic approaches.

Treatmemt. For uncomplicated gastroesophageal reflux without esophagitis, the infant is treated by being kept in an infant seat upright at 60 degrees 24 hours a day and given small, frequent, thickened feedings. About two thirds of patients will respond to this therapy. If, however, the patient fails to gain weight or has episodes of aspiration with this treatment, he will benefit from an antireflux operation. The Nissen fundoplication has been most successful. Patients with apneic spells should be treated by operation, since the consequences of medical failure are grave. Patients with esophagitis should be followed closely and operation carried out if it does not subside within 4 to 6 weeks. Older children will benefit from antacids. If stricture is present, repair of the reflux and dilatation may suffice, but esophageal resection with colon or small bowel interposition may be required.

CONGENITAL HYPERTROPHIC PYLORIC STENOSIS

Hypertrophic pyloric stenosis is the most common condition requiring laparotomy in infancy. The operation is the Fredet-Ramstedt procedure. In 1907 Fredet suggested that the circular muscles at the pylorus be divided, with the mucosa left intact. The muscular layer was then closed transversely. In 1912 Ramstedt showed that the muscular closure was not necessary.

Etiology. The cause of pyloric stenosis is obscure. There is an hereditary factor involved. Boys are affected four times as often as girls. Offspring of female patients with pyloric stenosis are, however, more likely to have the disease than descendants of affected males. It seems likely that there is some autonomic nervous imbalance, perhaps due to immature ganglion cells, which leads to muscular hypertrophy.

Pathology. There is marked hypertrophy of the circular musculature at the pylorus. The enlarged musculature encroaches on the pyloric lumen, and there is often edema of the pyloric mucosa. There is disagreement as to whether the ganglion cells of the pylorus are normal or not.

Symptoms. Symptoms are the result of the partial gastric outlet obstruction. Vomiting usually starts at about 1 week of age. Some authorities think this initial asymptomatic period occurs because it takes time for mucosal edema to develop. The edema further narrows the already compromised pyloric canal. Vomiting becomes progressively more frequent and forceful (projectile). Bile is not present in the vomitus, which does occasionally contain coffee-ground material. There is a decrease in the number and volume of stools. The baby is hungry and takes his feedings with vigor. After regaining birth weight and perhaps some additional weight, he begins to lose weight. The loss of hydrogen, chloride, and potassium ions leads to a metabolic alkalosis.

Physical Findings. Physical examination usually reveals a hungry baby of 2 to 6 weeks of age with signs of dehydration. Prominent peristaltic waves may be seen traversing the upper abdomen from left to right as the gastric contractions work against the obstructed pylorus. Although several attempts may be required, it is almost always possible to palpate the hypertrophied pyloric "tumor" characteristically described as an "olive." The "tumor" is best palpated when the stomach is empty—either just after the infant has vomited or after the stomach has been aspirated. Good abdominal relaxation is necessary. With the thighs flexed on the abdomen and the baby pacified with a sugar nipple, deep palpation of the epigastrium usually reveals the typical, firm, transverse mass that can be rolled under the examining fingers.

Diagnosis. Diagnosis is made by palpating the pyloric mass. If the mass is not palpable, roentgenographic visualization of the stomach and duodenum should be done. This will detect pyloric stenosis when present or perhaps other causes of vomiting when it is not present. If pyloric stenosis is demonstrated, the surgeon should persist in his attempt to palpate the tumor before operating because pylorospasm may present a similar x-ray appearance.

Treatment. Preoperative preparation consists of correction of dehydration and alkalosis. If this is not severe, oral electrolyte solutions will usually suffice. The stomach is first emptied of milk curds by saline irrigation through a nasogastric tube. If there is moderate electrolyte imbalance or dehydration, or if the patient cannot retain clear liquids by mouth, intravenous replacement is required. In most cases this is not necessary. In many infants diagnosis is made early in the course of the symptoms and only oral fluids overnight are required preoperatively. Because of the pyloric obstruction there is marked delay in gastric emptying. The stomach should therefore be aspirated before induction of anesthesia to avoid the hazard of vomiting and aspiration.

Operative correction is that described by Ramstedt. A longitudinal incision is made on the anterior superior avascular portion of the pylorus through the entire length of the pyloric canal, and the friable muscle fibers are split with a blunt instrument. The mucosa bulges into the incision, increasing the size of the pyloric lumen (Fig. 15).

Manometric studies after pyloromyotomy have shown that gastric peristalsis does not return for 12 to 18 hours. Clear liquid feedings are started after that time. Feedings are then advanced to full formula over

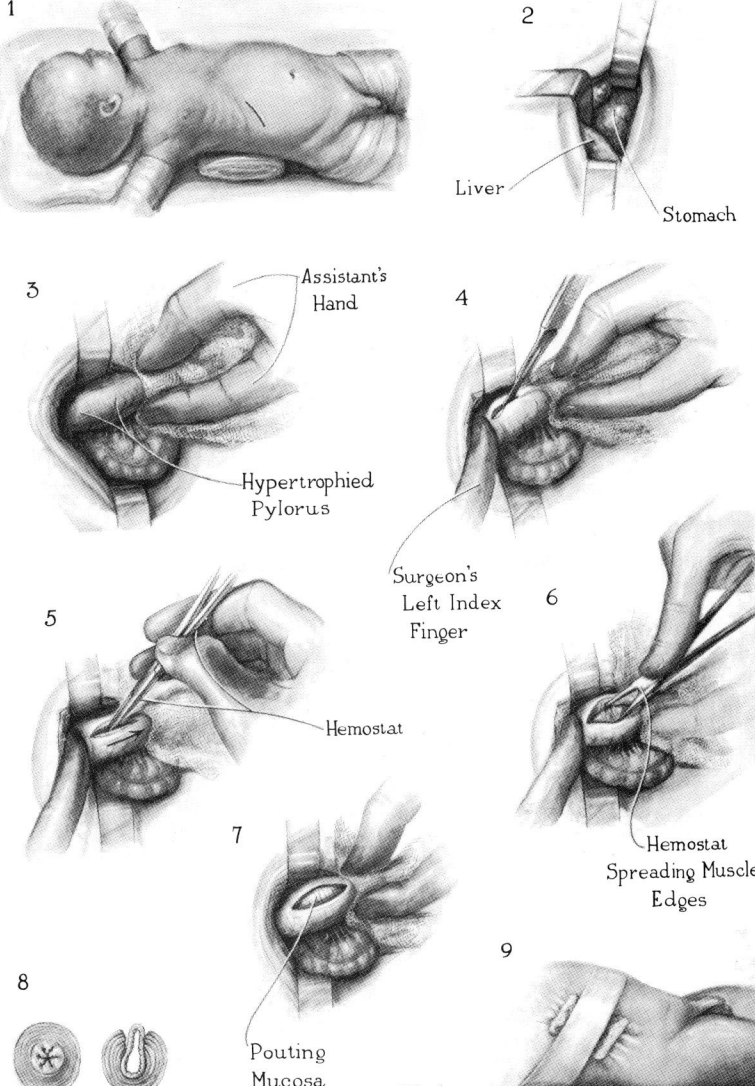

Figure 15. Operative technique for Fredet-Ramstedt pyloromyotomy. An alternate incision that gives excellent exposure in a 3- to 4-cm. transverse skin incision midway between the xiphoid and the umbilicus with longitudinal midline incision through the linea alba. (From Gross, R. E.: An Atlas of Children's Surgery. Philadelphia, W. B. Saunders Company, 1970.)

the next 2 to 3 days, when the patient can be discharged.

Results. Results of operation are excellent. Mortality is currently less than 0.5 per cent. Complications are rare. Inadequate pyloromyotomy is rarely seen if the operation is performed by a competent surgeon. Duodenal perforation at the time of myotomy is not common. If recognized and closed, it carries little risk.[6]

Medical treatment of pyloric stenosis is based on the fact that if the infant can be kept alive the symptoms will usually subside. Antispasmodics, frequent small feedings with refeeding after vomiting, good nursing care, and several weeks of hospitalization are usually required. This form of therapy is not recommended.

GASTROINTESTINAL BLEEDING

Massive gastrointestinal bleeding in the pediatric age group is not common. Small quantities of blood in the stool are. Some of the entities discussed in this section will at times present with symptoms other than bleeding but are discussed here because bleeding is often a prominent feature.

In the diagnostic approach to any patient with bleeding from the gastrointestinal tract it is important to know the color and quantity of blood, whether it is passed in vomitus or by rectum, if there is any evidence of a generalized bleeding disorder, if there are associated symptoms, and if, indeed, the material is blood. When passed in the stool, chocolate, tomato-based foods, red Jello, and some medications may look like blood to both parent and physician. Check it chemically to be sure.

Swallowed blood may be vomited. In the neonate, this may be blood swallowed during delivery. Fetal hemoglobin can be easily distinguished from adult hemoglobin and thus the source of the blood differentiated. In older patients, swallowed blood is usually from a nosebleed.

Vomiting of blood means the bleeding source is

proximal to the ligament of Treitz. Tarry stools imply upper gastrointestinal bleeding, while a bright red color implies bleeding in the left colon or below. Blood from the upper gastrointestinal tract will be passed as red if the transit time is reduced or bleeding is brisk. Blood in the stool is only very rarely the result of malignant disease in the pediatric age group and hence does not cause the same concern as it does in the adult.

Bleeding disorders can usually be detected by a history of easy bruising or excessive bleeding after small cuts. Children have enough incidental trauma that they are repeatedly challenged. A peripheral smear, platelet count, prothrombin time, and partial thromboblastin time will detect most generalized bleeding disorders.

Diagnosis is usually made by upper or lower gastrointestinal x-rays, esophagoscopy, sigmoidoscopy, colonoscopy, or, rarely, celiac arteriography. There are, however, a number of children in whom physical examination and all diagnostic studies are negative, and the diagnosis and therapeutic approach have to be made entirely on clinical grounds. When faced with this problem in a patient bleeding per rectum, it is probably worthwhile to proceed with laparotomy after one massive bleed requiring transfusion. The cause of bleeding will be found and can be corrected in about half these patients. If there is chronic loss of small quantities of blood, the chance of finding and correcting the cause of bleeding is not good. If transfusion has been required on several occasions to maintain hemoglobin, laparotomy is warranted. In upper gastrointestinal bleeding, uncontrolled hemorrhage is the indication for laparotomy.

The neonate is an exception to these guidelines. He should have a laparotomy only as a last resort when blood volume cannot be maintained by transfusion. Only rarely is a surgically correctable lesion present. The usual cause is some form of hemorrhagic disease of the newborn even though the prothrombin time may be normal. These infants should be treated with vitamin K and transfusion.

Massive upper gastrointestinal bleeding in the child, as in the adult, is most likely the result of bleeding from esophageal varices or ulceration in the stomach or duodenum. Both are discussed in detail elsewhere. It is well to remember that the etiology of these entities in the pediatric patient usually differs from that in the adult. Portal hypertension is most likely the result of an extrahepatic block, usually secondary to portal vein thrombosis. There may have been an omphalitis or umbilical vein catheterization in the neonatal period. Since these children have a relatively normal liver, the prognosis is much better than it is for those whose obstruction is the result of liver disease. Intrahepatic block in children is due to postnecrotic cirrhosis, congenital hepatic fibrosis, hepatic changes secondary to cystic fibrosis, Wilson's disease, and congenital cystic disease of the liver (and kidneys).

Ulcers are usually associated with other diseases—burns, central nervous system disease, generalized infection, or steroid therapy. Few in the small child are the result of the usual acid-pepsin disease.

MECKEL'S DIVERTICULUM

Meckel's diverticulum is the most common cause of massive rectal bleeding in the pediatric age group.

Embryology and Pathology. Meckel's diverticulum is the persistence of the communication of the yolk sac with the intestine—a remnant of the vitelline duct. The diverticulum arises on the antimesenteric border of the ileum at about the junction of its middle and distal thirds. Infrequently it is attached to the umbilicus by a fibrous cord and rarely it contains a patent communication with the umbilicus. Ectopic gastric mucosa is often present. Bleeding is usually the result of ulceration of the normal ileal mucosa (of the diverticulum or adjacent ileum) by acid secretion of the ectopic gastric mucosa. Boys are affected three times as frequently as girls.

Symptoms. Meckel's diverticula are present in 1 to 2 per cent of the population. Most are asymptomatic. Those that do cause symptoms usually do so early in life, but symptoms may occur at any age. In the pediatric age symptoms are present in half the cases during the first 2 years of life. Massive rectal bleeding, which is either painless or associated with mild, vague abdominal discomfort, is the most frequent symptom. The blood at first is dark but usually becomes bright. Chronic loss of small quantities of blood is not likely to be caused by Meckel's diverticulum. Since it is almost impossible to demonstrate a Meckel's diverticulum by x-ray, technetium-99m imaging is worthwhile. If gastric mucosa is present in the Meckel's diverticulum, it will be demonstrated in the majority of the patients.[22]

While bleeding is the most common symptom, Meckel's diverticulum may also produce other symptoms. Cramping abdominal pain and vomiting may result from intussusception when the diverticulum acts as a lead point, or obstruction may be secondary to a fibrous band extending to the umbilicus. Pain may also result from perforation of an ulcer or volvulus of the diverticulum with infarction. Symptoms and physical examination may be suggestive of appendicitis.[10]

Treatment. Treatment of Meckel's diverticulum is treatment of its complications. For those who bleed, transfusion is usually necessary prior to operative removal of the diverticulum. This may require resection of the adjacent ileum.

In patients who are operated upon with a tentative diagnosis of appendicitis and do not have an inflamed appendix, the ileum should be explored to detect an inflamed or perforated diverticulum. Patients with intestinal obstruction due to a fibrous band or small bowel intussusception require operation for relief of the obstruction and removal of the diverticulum.

POLYPS

Colonic Polyps

Colonic polyps in children may be solitary, multiple, or diffuse. The juvenile polyp is not a premalignant lesion and is often self-limited. Diffuse polyposis of the colon is often familial and premalignant. Bleeding from polyps is not massive. It is often associated with an urge to defecate, and there may be an excess of mucus in the stool. Blood is usually mixed with the stool. Diagnosis is by digital examination, sigmoidoscopy, colonoscopy, and barium enema. X-ray visualization requires a well-prepared colon devoid of feces. Air contrast studies may be helpful.

Treatment. Approximately 70 per cent of polyps are within the reach of the sigmoidoscope and should be removed. For juvenile polyps beyond the reach of the sigmoidoscope, no therapy is necessary unless symptoms persist. Barium enema a year later will often show that the polyp is no longer present. Diffuse familial polyposis requires a total colectomy or a subtotal colectomy with ileoproctostomy. Subsequent periodic sigmoidoscopic visualization and fulguration of any recurring polyps in the rectum are required.

Rectal bleeding in children is almost never the result of malignant disease. While carcinoma of the colon does occur in children, it is rare. Barium enema shows a sessile or napkin-ring lesion. Treatment is similar to that in the adult.

Small Bowel Polyps

Small bowel polyps may cause bleeding but are more likely to cause symptoms by acting as a lead point for an intussusception. They may be associated with brown pigmented spots around the lips and on the buccal membrane—the Peutz-Jeghers syndrome. There is frequently a family history of intestinal polyps and there are often other polyps in the colon or stomach.

Symptoms. The most frequent symptom is cramping abdominal pain secondary to intussusception (which may spontaneously reduce). Chronic blood loss with anemia is also frequent. Diagnosis is usually on clinical grounds—cramping abdominal pain, palpable abdominal mass, pigmented spots around the lips, and a positive family history. Visualization of small bowel polyps by roentgenography is often difficult. Associated colonic and gastric polyps are demonstrated by upper and lower gastrointestinal roentgenograms, sigmoidoscopy, colonoscopy, or gastroscopy.

Treatment. Small bowel intussusception may require resection. If not, the intussusception is reduced with resection of the polyp or polyps. All palpable polyps should be removed with resection of as little intestine as possible. Although some small bowel polyps have a histologic appearance suggesting malignancy, they do not behave as malignant lesions.

ANAL FISSURE

Anal fissure is the most common cause of blood in the stool in the pediatric age group. Fissures are acute and superficial, are frequently encountered during the first 2 or 3 years of life, and may be single or multiple. They may be located at any part of the anus. They occur at the mucocutaneous junction and are the result of trauma from a hard, bulky, constipated stool or diarrhea. The cardinal symptom is pain on defecation. Blood in the stool is usually scant and streaked on the surface.

Almost all fissures-in-ano in infants will heal with nonoperative treatment. In fact, some will have healed by the time the patient is seen by the physician. Therapy is warm sitz baths, relief of constipation by diet control and laxatives, anesthetic ointment, and rectal dilations. Rarely a chronic fissure will develop that will require operative excision. If pain on defecation persists, it will lead to chronic constipation, which can be a much more difficult problem than the original fissure.

ULCERATIVE COLITIS

Any discussion about gastrointestinal bleeding in the pediatric age group would be incomplete without mention of ulcerative colitis. It is discussed in detail elsewhere. It can occur in infancy but is seen much more frequently in the prepubertal and adolescent child. It should be considered in the differential diagnosis in any child with lower gastrointestinal bleeding.

ABDOMINAL WALL ABNORMALITIES

The most common defect in the abdominal wall in infants and children is indirect inguinal hernia. Umbilical hernias are also common, particularly in Negroes. Both are discussed in detail elsewhere, but a short comment here is warranted.

INGUINAL HERNIA

The diagnosis of inguinal hernia is usually made when the parent notes a groin or scrotal mass (90 per cent are in boys) that is intermittently present, particularly when the patient cries or strains. Incarceration is common, especially in the first year of life. Elective repair should therefore be undertaken when the diagnosis is made. Since the defect in the indirect inguinal hernia of childhood is a persistent patency of the processus vaginalis, treatment consists of high ligation of the sac.

Incarceration, should it occur, can usually be reduced and the hernia repaired as an elective procedure a day or two later when the edema has subsided. There is a higher rate of recurrence in infants who are operated on when the hernia is incarcerated than in those in whom repair is carried out as an elective procedure (less than 1 per cent). If the incarceration cannot be reduced, the patient must, of course, be operated on promptly.

The most common sliding hernia in infancy occurs in the little girl with an indirect inguinal hernia containing a tube and ovary as the sliding component. Hydroceles in infant boys are common and are associated with about 15 per cent of inguinal hernias. Those not associated with hernias will usually regress eventually and hence do not require operation during infancy. Aspiration is ineffective and therefore contraindicated. The communicating hydrocele (i.e., one that fluctuates in size) has a communication with the abdominal cavity by way of a hernia sac. It should be treated like any other pediatric hernia—by repair.

Umbilical hernias in pediatric patients, unlike inguinal hernias in the same age group or umbilical hernias in the adult, seldom become incarcerated and tend spontaneously to close the fascial defect. Umbilical hernias, therefore, need not be repaired during infancy. Those that persist into childhood should be repaired because of the danger of incarceration in later life.

OMPHALOCELE AND GASTROSCHISIS

Omphalocele and gastroschisis are uncommon abdominal wall defects of the newborn. Omphalocele is the herniation of abdominal contents into the base of the umbilical cord. The peritoneal sac is not covered by skin, as in an umbilical hernia, but by Wharton's jelly and amniotic membrane, i.e., the components of the umbilical cord. Gastroschisis is a full-thickness abdominal wall defect lateral to the umbilical cord without any sac or covering for the eviscerated intestines.

Embryology. From the sixth to the tenth week of fetal life the coelomic cavity is too small to accommodate the developing viscera. During this time a portion of the intestine normally occupies a coelomic extension into the base of the umbilical cord. Increase in size of the coelomic cavity is accompanied by return and rotation of the intestine. If this process is arrested, an omphalocele and associated malrotation of the intestine result.

If one side of the lateral somatic fold fails to develop, *gastroschisis* results, with a normally developed cord arising in the midline. Lack of development of the cephalic portion of the somatic fold results in ectopia cordis and pericardial defects, while failure of caudal somatic development results in exstrophy of the bladder—both of which may be associated with omphalocele.

Clinical Findings. Omphalocele varies in size from very small, containing only a knuckle of small bowel, to very large, containing liver, spleen, and most of the gastrointestinal tract. The sac may be quite thin and in danger of rupture or may be rather thick and tough. Rupture of the sac can occur prenatally, during delivery, or after birth. Over half the patients have other congenital anomalies.

In gastroschisis there is no sac. The matted, dusky, edematous gut (usually stomach, small bowel, and a portion of colon) makes an exit from the abdominal wall through a smooth, fibrous defect adjacent to the intact cord. There may be a strip of skin between the cord and defect. The defect is almost always at the right of the cord and usually 3 to 4 cm. in diameter. Frequently the gut is short. Peritonitis is always present.

Treatment. Initial therapy is to protect the intact sac or the intestines if they are exposed. A sterile, moist towel or gauze sponge wrapped around the abdomen is satisfactory. If the intestine is exposed, antibiotics should be given and particular efforts must be taken to combat heat loss. The stomach is decompressed with a nasogastric tube to prevent vomiting and distention of gut, which will hamper subsequent closure.

For the small intact omphalocele the sac is simply excised, the abdominal cavity explored, and the defect closed primarily. If there is a problem from malrotation or other anomalies, it is corrected. The medium-sized omphalocele can be treated in the same fashion if, on manual reduction of its contents, there is no compromise in ventilation in the unanesthetized patient. A gastrostomy should be added to the procedure to insure gastric decompression in the postoperative period.

In the patient with a large omphalocele it is not possible to return the viscera to the small abdominal cavity and close the fascial defect without markedly elevating the intra-abdominal pressure. The result is an elevation of the diaphragm beyond the point where adequate ventilation is possible, as well as compression of the vena cava, impeding venous return to the heart. These infants are best treated by suturing a plastic (Silon) prosthesis to the fascial defect over the intact sac without closure of the skin. The result is a prosthetic cylinder containing the sac and viscera (Fig. 16). The viscera are progressively forced back into the abdominal cavity as the cylinder is shortened daily by placing a row of sutures proximal to the cylinder end. Usually in 7 to 10 days the prosthesis can be removed and a fascial closure obtained. During this time the stomach is decompressed by gastrostomy, and the patient is given total parenteral nutrition and antibiotics. Infection is a hazard.[1]

Nonoperative therapy of omphalocele with intact sac consists of protecting the sac from rupture and allowing it to scar down and become epithelialized. The sac is painted with Mercurochrome or Zephiran. In time a remarkable reduction in the size of the defect occurs. There is probably a place for this approach in the very small premature infant with a large omphalocele or with severe extra-abdominal associated anomalies. Prolonged hospitalization is required.

In the patient with gastroschisis or ruptured omphalocele, the problem is more difficult. If primary closure can be accomplished without significant ventilatory compromise, this should be done. Direct closure is not always possible with gastroschisis in spite of a relatively small fascial defect. These patients are treated in the same manner as those with a large omphalocele except that the prosthesis is in direct contact with the intestine, since there is no sac. Gastrostomy, total parenteral nutrition, and antibiotics are essential supportive measures. Because peritonitis is present before repair, sepsis is a significant hazard.

Results. For the patient with a small omphalocele without associated anomalies, the risk is quite small. For the patient with a large omphalocele, overall mortality is 40 to 50 per cent, and for patients with gastroschisis or ruptured omphalocele the mortality is 50 to 75 per cent. Many of these deaths are related to associated anomalies.

JAUNDICE

Jaundice is common in pediatric patients, but it is not often due to obstruction. In the first few months of

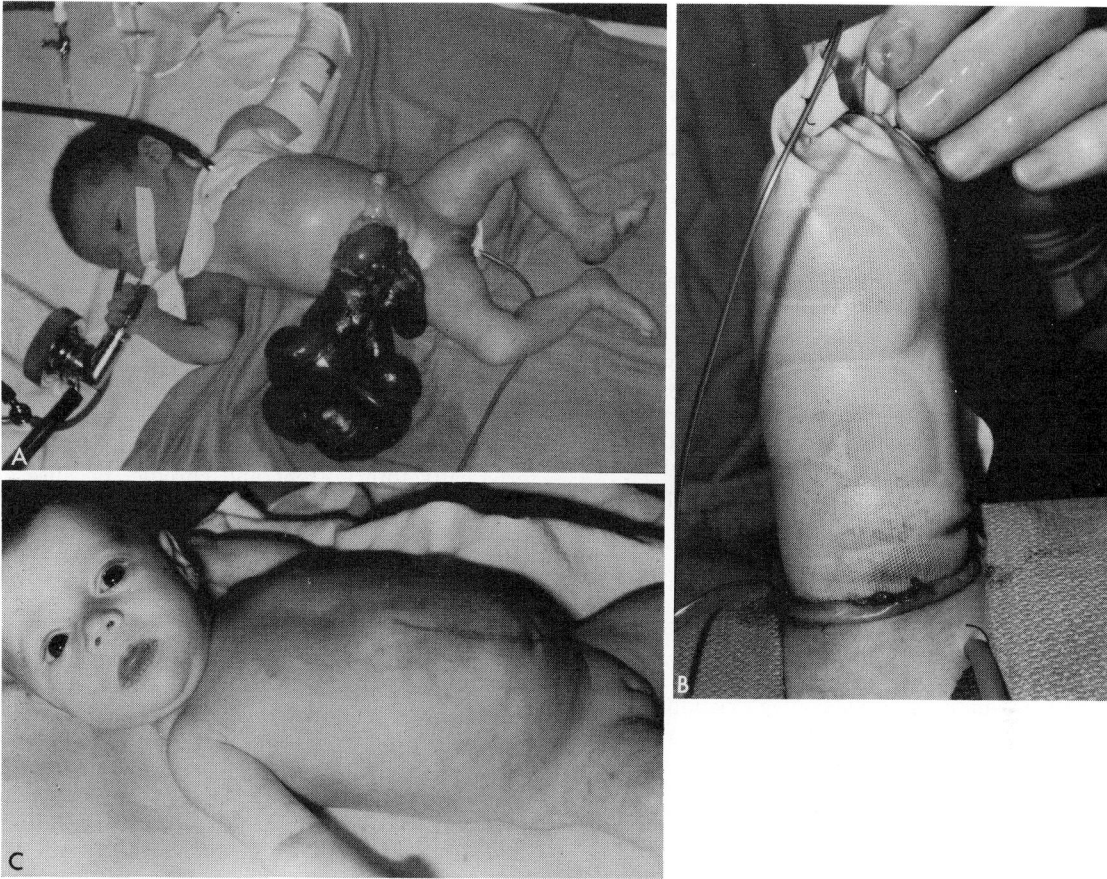

Figure 16. *A,* Gastroschisis with evisceration of stomach, small bowel, and colon just to the right of the umbilical cord. The gut is thickened, matted, and dusky. *B,* A prosthetic cylinder covering the intestine is sutured to the fascia of the defect. The cylinder will be progressively shortened over the next 7 to 10 days, so that the intestine is forced back into the abdominal cavity. *C,* Same patient after removal of prosthesis and closure of defect.

life biliary atresia may cause obstructive jaundice. In the older child, choledochal cysts may cause obstruction. Common duct stones and carcinoma of the head of the pancreas, the common causes of obstructive jaundice in the adult, are rare in children but have been reported.

BILIARY ATRESIA

Biliary atresia is an interesting but poorly understood entity. All or some of the intrahepatic and extrahepatic biliary ducts consist of fibrous cords with little or no lumen. The etiology is not clear. One possibility is faulty embryogenesis. A more likely explanation is that fibrosis of previously normal ducts occurs in fetal life or in the early postnatal period. There is progressive development of biliary cirrhosis, portal hypertension, ascites, and liver failure. Life expectancy is about 18 months, though some children live for several years.[25]

Clinical Findings. The onset of jaundice is usually during the first week of life but may not be noted until 6 to 8 weeks of age. The stools become acholic and the urine dark. Intermittently the stools may be brown or

yellow, presumably because of desquamation of jaundiced mucosal cells. For some time the patient's general condition appears to be good. Then, as liver failure develops, there is a progressive deterioration. The liver is usually enlarged and firm, as is the spleen. Ascites and hemorrhoids may be present later in the course of the disease. Jaundice is unremitting, with total bilirubin in the 10 to 20 mg. per 100 ml. range.

Differential Diagnosis. There are many other causes of jaundice in the neonatal period that must be differentiated from biliary atresia. The most common cause of neonatal jaundice is so-called physiologic jaundice of the newborn, which is a result of an immature glucuronyl transferase enzyme system. Jaundice from this cause is usually cleared by 2 weeks of age. Jaundice beyond that period is pathologic, and therefore its cause should be investigated. Other causes of jaundice include bacterial sepsis, syphilis, cytomegalic inclusion disease, toxoplasmosis, erythroblastosis fetalis or other hemolytic disease, familial nonhemolytic icterus, "enclosed" hemorrhage, pancreatitis, cystic fibrosis, galactosemia, and some drugs. These entities can usually be detected by history or appropriate laboratory tests.

Inspissated bile syndrome and neonatal hepatitis

also cause jaundice at this age and usually cannot be differentiated from biliary atresia by the usual liver function tests. While serum transaminase tends to be high with hepatitis and alkaline phosphatase high with obstruction, these findings are not consistent. The iodine-131 rose bengal test is probably the most helpful test in making a distinction between obstruction and hepatocellular disease in the neonate. Unfortunately, it cannot always be relied upon to give a clear-cut distinction.

Treatment. For those patients in whom biliary atresia cannot be excluded, a limited laparotomy with liver biopsy and operative cholangiogram will provide the diagnosis. This should be carried out by 8 weeks of age, before irreparable liver damage has occurred in patients who otherwise have a surgically correctable lesion. If the extrahepatic ductal system is patent, the procedure is terminated, since the patient does not have extrahepatic biliary atresia. Liver biopsy will probably differentiate between intrahepatic atresia and neonatal hepatitis.

If cholangiogram reveals atresia of the common bile duct, the duct is anastomosed to the intestine. A Roux-en-Y connection to the jejunum is less likely to result in cholangitis than a direct connection of the duct to the duodenum.

If only a small gallbladder is visualized by cholangiography, and none of the ductal system is demonstrated, the proximal extrahepatic biliary tree should be thoroughly explored in search for any patent extrahepatic ducts. If one is present, it is connected to the intestine as with atresia of the common bile duct.

Most patients have no visible bile ducts. For these, Kasai has recommended portoenterostomy in which a Roux loop of jejunum is anastomosed to the porta hepatis after cutting across fibrotic remnants of the hepatic ducts as they leave the liver.[18] If histologic examination of this tissue shows microscopic bile ducts of 200 μ or greater, two thirds of these patients will have remission of jaundice. In fact, these patients do not have true "atresia," since microscopic ducts exist. Most authorities feel that this is the most common form of "biliary atresia" and results from an ascending cholangitis of infective origin. It usually has both intra- and extrahepatic components. It is critical that the operation be performed early, before advanced changes of cirrhosis take place. There have been few successful results in patients over the age of 3 months at the time of operation.

Results. Prior to the Kasai procedure, only approximately 10 per cent of patients with biliary atresia were found to have a surgically correctable lesion, and half of these subsequently died of cirrhosis, portal hypertension, or cholangitis, usually related to advanced disease at the time of correction.

Although initial results with portoenterostomy are very encouraging, with approximately two thirds of the patients demonstrating clearing of jaundice, the long-term results give little cause for optimism. Cirrhosis progresses in all but a few, and long-term disease-free survivors will probably number less than 10 per cent.[3]

Liver transplantation for biliary atresia has proved technically feasible, and there are a small number of long-term survivors. Because of rejection problems, as well as technical difficulties, these are a minor fraction of the group.

CHOLEDOCHAL CYST

Choledochal cyst might more properly be termed aneurysm of the common bile duct. Rarely, a true cystic diverticulum is found. Obstruction results from cystic dilatation and kinking of the distal common duct.

Clinical Findings. The classic "triad" of jaundice, abdominal pain, and a cystic mass is found in only 10 to 20 per cent of patients. The diagnosis is almost always suggested by the appearance of jaundice, which may occur in the first few months of life or later in childhood. Palpation of a cystic mass in the right upper quadrant is highly suggestive. Symptoms are characteristically intermittent and chronic. Because of the vague and nonspecific nature of symptoms, all infants with jaundice should have a definite diagnosis established as soon as possible if this completely curable condition is to be diagnosed and properly treated before the development of cirrhosis.

Diagnosis. The cyst may be demonstrated by barium studies of the duodenum, radioactive rose bengal liver scan (in which the radioactive dye accumulates in the cyst) and, rarely, by oral or intravenous cholangiogram.

Treatment. Although choledochocystojejunostomy has been recommended in the past (and is still appropriate in the treatment of cysts that are acutely inflamed or technically difficult to resect), radical excision is the treatment of choice. Not only does resection with anastomosis of a Roux loop of jejunum to the proximal common duct produce a more satisfactory functional result, it also eliminates the risk of subsequent development of bile duct carcinoma, which occurs in a significant number of patients in whom the cyst is retained.

Results. Operative mortality should be less than 10 per cent. The long-term outlook is determined in large measure by the degree of cirrhosis at the time of operation and by the occurrence of postoperative cholangitis, which is rare in patients in whom choledochocystectomy is performed, but occurs in 15 to 25 per cent of the patients who have only a drainage procedure.

ABDOMINAL MASSES

The presence of a palpable abdominal mass in an infant or child is a cause for alarm and always requires a complete investigation. The outlook for the newborn with an abdominal mass is better than that for the older child. More than half of abdominal masses found in newborns are renal in origin. Multicystic dysplastic kidney is the most common, although hydronephrosis (from a variety of causes) is also common. Intestinal duplications, hydrometrocolpos, and neuroblastoma follow in that order.[9] In the child, neoplasms, particularly Wilms' tumor and neuroblastoma, are more common.

Diagnosis

Physical examination is frequently helpful in determining the etiology of the mass. The location, mobility, and consistency (whether cystic or solid) are important clues. If there are signs or symptoms of intestinal obstruction, duplication, meconium ileus, or malrotation must be considered. Extraintestinal masses rarely cause intestinal obstruction.

Intravenous pyelogram is most likely to give significant information, since the majority of masses in the newborn are renal in origin. The presence of calcium suggests intrauterine intestinal perforation, neuroblastoma, or teratoma. Total-body opacification is frequently helpful in identifying avascular lesions such as cysts, hematomas, and infarcted organs, abscess cavities, and so forth. This entails use of a double dose of contrast medium and early films during the vascular mixing phase of the intravenous pyelogram to show absence of opacification.

If the diagnosis is not clear from these studies, additional radiologic investigation is indicated. Cystogram or sinogram in the case of abnormal external genitalia may be helpful in further delineating the nature of a pelvic or low abdominal mass, as well as defining the presence of massive vesicoureteral reflux that may cause hydronephrosis or hydroureter. Ultrasonic scanning (sonography) can readily distinguish cystic from solid masses. This is particularly helpful in the renal region where the differentiation between hydronephrosis and tumor is of some significance. Computer-assisted tomography is another noninvasive technique that may give valuable information. In the case of a large mass that appears clinically to be malignant, the use of venography or arteriography may be of assistance not only in determining the nature of the mass but also in planning its removal. In most cases this is not necessary and should be used sparingly in infants because of the risk of long-term sequelae from arterial thrombosis secondary to catheterization. Radioisotope scanning of the liver and kidneys may provide additional information. In almost all cases surgical exploration is indicated both to establish the diagnosis and for treatment. From the wide choice of diagnostic procedures available the wise clinician will select the one (or more) most likely to provide the diagnosis with the least risk to the patient. He will also resist the temptation to get additional interesting though unnecessary studies.

MULTICYSTIC KIDNEY

The most common abdominal mass in the neonate, multicystic dysplastic kidney, is also the easiest to treat (Fig. 17). Unlike polycystic kidneys, this lesion is unilateral, nonfamilial, and almost always discovered early in life. There is no associated cystic disease of other organs. Since the opposite kidney is almost always normal, the lesion is no threat to life. These dysplastic kidneys vary greatly in appearance, with multiple cysts of different sizes, some as large as 10 to 20 cm., and usually little in the way of recognizable renal parenchyma. Intravenous urography reveals absence of excretory function of the affected kidney, but

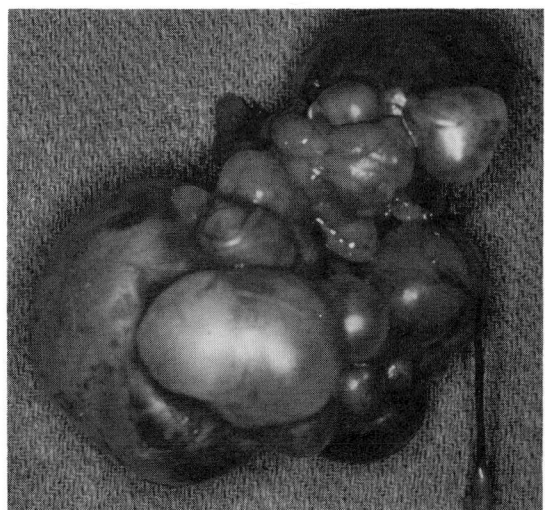

Figure 17. The unilateral multicystic dysplastic kidney is the most common cause of abdominal mass in the newborn. It is often associated with atresia of the upper ureter, as in this specimen.

usually shows a normal pyelogram on the opposite side. Treatment is removal, and the prognosis is excellent.

HYDRONEPHROSIS

Hydronephrosis may be unilateral or bilateral and cause one or two cystic, though at times somewhat firm, flank masses. A hydronephrotic kidney with a good kidney on the opposite side is not associated with impaired renal function.

Bilateral hydronephrosis in the newborn often carries a poor prognosis, since renal function may be severely compromised by the time of diagnosis. The kidneys may not be opacified on intravenous urography. Total-body opacification or sonography will reveal the mass to be cystic. Cystography will reveal vesicoureteral reflux in a large proportion of patients and will thus outline the extent of the pathologic process. If there is severe bilateral involvement the problem can be approached either by high temporary diversion (cutaneous pyelostomy or cutaneous loop ureterostomy) with later reconstruction or by early total reconstruction. Hendren's pioneering experience with early extensive reconstruction has been impressive.[14] With relief of obstruction renal function is often dramatically improved.

URETEROPELVIC OBSTRUCTION

Obstruction at the junction between the kidney pelvis and the ureter may be caused by stenosis or atresia (Fig. 18). Frequently there is an aberrant vessel that may or may not be related to the hypoplastic segment. Adequate drainage is obtained either by a Y-V-plasty to the ureteropelvic junction or by excision of the stenotic segment with anastomosis of the ureter to the kidney pelvis. Part of the dilated redundant pelvis

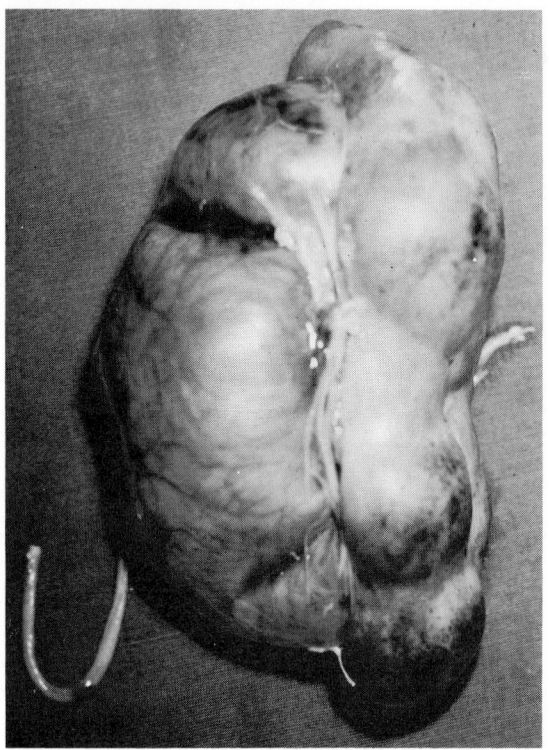

Figure 18. Massive hydronephrosis with destruction of renal parenchyma due to long-standing ureteropelvic obstruction.

should be excised to facilitate urine propulsion. Temporary catheter drainage is essential. In some cases, when the condition is unilateral and when the renal parenchyma is exceedingly thin and unlikely ever to regain significant function, nephrectomy is indicated. In most patients, however, the kidney is well worth saving, and a reconstructive procedure should be performed.

VESICOURETERAL REFLUX

Reflux in the newborn is sometimes the result of an abnormality of the vesicoureteral junction but usually occurs as a consequence of distal obstruction, as from posterior urethral valves. It is also commonly seen in association with massive hydronephrosis and hydroureter in the "prune belly" syndrome with or without urethral obstruction. In the patient with isolated vesicoureteral reflux, reimplantation of the ureters usually produces excellent results (see discussion under Urinary Tract Infection later in this chapter). If there is an obstruction (such as posterior urethral valves), this must be relieved by endoscopic resection, which can be done at the time of reimplantation of the ureters. In patients with a neurogenic bladder, and in most with the "prune belly" syndrome, successful reconstruction cannot be done, so a permanent form of urinary diversion must ultimately be provided. At present the ileal or colon conduit is the most satisfactory method of long-term urinary diversion. The time of permanent diversion depends on the degree of obstruction. For those infants who present with flank masses in infancy, there is usually a high degree of obstruction that will require early diversion.

DUPLICATIONS OF THE ALIMENTARY TRACT

Although they may present at any age, many duplications are first noted in the newborn period. Duplications may occur at any level of the intestinal tract from the mouth to the anus. Absence of an adequate communication between the second lumen and the primary enteric canal leads to accumulation of mucous secretions and cystic dilatation, thus the original term of "enterogenous cysts."

Pathology. Duplications may be cystic or tubular. They are located on the mesenteric side of the involved gut and usually have a common muscular wall with at least a portion of the adjacent intestine. Some connect with the adjacent gut lumen, and some do not. Tubular duplications have a common muscular wall with a long segment of intestine. Others may be separate from the adjacent bowel and on occasion traverse the diaphragm to reside in the posterior mediastinum. The mucosa may be that of the adjacent gut or of any other part of the alimentary tract, including the stomach.[27]

Clinical Findings. Symptoms are *obstruction* due to encroachment of the distended cyst on the adjacent intestine, *pain* from the distention of the cyst wall, or *bleeding,* which may be massive if it is caused by ulceration secondary to ectopic gastric mucosa. Intestinal obstruction and the presence of a mobile *mass* strongly suggest a duplication. Volvulus may also occur, or the patient may be asymptomatic and the mass discovered during a physical examination. This is especially likely to be true with gastric duplications. Pyloric duplications are commonly mistaken for congenital hypertrophic pyloric stenosis because of the symptoms of repeated projectile vomiting of non-bile-stained material. Rectal duplications may cause rectal prolapse. Thoracic duplications may cause dysphagia or tracheal compression.

Diagnosis. Upper gastrointestinal series may show a filling defect in esophageal, gastric, and duodenal duplications. Barium enema is of value in revealing a colonic duplication. Thoracic duplications are usually visible on chest x-ray. The presence of hemivertebrae and a mass suggests a duplication.

Treatment. Since duplication cysts are located on the mesenteric side of the intestinal lumen and have a common wall with the normal channel, simple excision is difficult. With duplications located in the small bowel, segmental excision and end-to-end anastomosis is the procedure of choice. If the duplication is quite long, or is located in an area where resection is not possible, division of the common wall or "windowing" may produce adequate decompression so that the cyst no longer fills. Long tubular duplications that would require an extensive resection are best treated by resection of the mucosa through multiple incisions, with the muscularis of the duplication left in situ.

Results. Although these may be complicated anomalies and, in the case of lower colon and rectal duplications, may be associated with urinary tract anomalies as well, surgical correction is usually possible and a good result is to be expected. Mortality is about 5 per cent overall.

HYDROMETROCOLPOS

Hydrometrocolpos, or fluid accumulation in the vagina and uterus, occurs as the result of prenatal obstruction to the outlet of the vagina with excessive secretion due to circulating maternal estrogens. The most common cause is imperforate hymen, the result of failure of degeneration of the epithelial plate of the müllerian tubercle. Vaginal atresia may result if there is persistence of the solid cord stage of fused müllerian ducts.

Patients present with a suprapubic mass that usually extends up to the umbilicus or higher. It may be mistaken for a distended bladder and the true nature not suspected until the bladder is emptied. Since this condition may assume truly massive proportions, there may be rectal and urinary obstruction. Diagnosis is established by physical examination. When a bulging imperforate hymen is noted, hymenotomy relieves the obstruction as well as any secondary pressure on the urinary or intestinal tracts.

If there is vaginal atresia, a combined abdomino-perineal approach is indicated. After drainage of fluid from above, the atretic end of the vagina is pressed into the perineum where it can be safely incised and drained. In these patients a catheter must be left in the vagina for an extended period of time so that an epithelium-lined tract will be established. Intravenous pyelogram is indicated to assess the extent of damage to the upper urinary tract.

Leakage of fluid from the fallopian tubes, especially if there is a communication between the bladder and the vagina (urogenital sinus) may lead to peritonitis and death. Adequate drainage of both the vagina and the bladder (cutaneous vesicostomy) is required. Many of these patients have a septate vagina and bladder. Imperforate anus is also commonly seen as an associated anomaly. These patients may present very difficult problems in diagnosis and therapy and should not be surgically approached by the inexperienced.

CYSTS

Cystic abdominal masses are typically soft, ballotable, and quite mobile. They are not readily distinguished from duplications except that they seldom, if ever, cause intestinal obstruction. Mesenteric cysts are the most common, but omental cysts, lymphangiomatous cysts (cystic hygroma), and ovarian cysts are also found. Cysts may be small or large, single or multiloculated, and lobulated or smooth, and may contain serous, chylous, or hemorrhagic fluid. True cysts are thin-walled and thus are easily distinguished from duplications, which have a thick wall equal to that of the normal intestine.

Clinical Findings. Most cysts are asymptomatic unless exceedingly large, when they may present as abdominal distention or, rarely, with respiratory distress due to elevation of the diaphragm. In older children abdominal pain may be the presenting symptom, resulting from mesenteric traction in the upright position produced by the weight of the cyst. Physical examination usually reveals a rounded, soft mass that is markedly mobile. X-ray of the abdomen shows an area of absent intestinal gas shadows. Barium studies may help localize the cyst, and excretory urogram occasionally shows ureteral displacement or obstruction. Ultrasonic scanning is of value in differentiating cysts from solid tumors.

Treatment. Since these structures are benign and usually do not involve the wall of the intestine or other vital structures, they usually can be "shelled out." On occasion local intestinal resection may also be necessary. In the treatment of ovarian cysts, an attempt should be made to preserve normal tissue if possible. Lymphangiomatous cysts are typically retroperitoneal. Resection is usually possible, since vital structures are not actually invaded.

Results. The outlook is excellent.

NEUROBLASTOMA

In addition to being the most common solid tumor of childhood, neuroblastoma is among the most interesting because of its occasional capacity for spontaneous regression. Indeed, of *documented* cases of spontaneous disappearance of cancer, approximately one fourth are neuroblastomas. It is, however, a highly malignant tumor that often carries a dim outlook. Recognition of neuroblastoma as a distinct entity occurred during that great age of descriptive pathology, the late nineteenth century. The term "neuroblastoma" was coined by Wright in 1910.

Pathology. Neuroblastoma is the result of malignant proliferation of the primitive precursors of sympathetic ganglion cells and, as such, arises from the areas where these cells are found: the adrenal glands and the sympathetic ganglionic chain. Grossly these tumors are frequently hemorrhagic and multilobulated, and may or may not have a capsule. Soft areas, often the result of necrotic degeneration, alternate with areas of firm nodularity. Histologically the "pure" neuroblastoma is highly cellular, often appearing somewhat lymphoid. Rosettes of dark cell nuclei are frequently seen interspersed with bands of pale fibrillar tissue. With the more differentiated form of the tumor (ganglioneuroma) only ganglion cells and stroma are present and the ganglion cells are mature. In most tumors, both mature and immature cells are present.

Neuroblastoma accounts for 10 to 20 per cent of solid malignant lesions in childhood. Fifty to 80 per cent of neuroblastomas arise within the abdomen, most from the adrenal medulla, but some from paravertebral ganglion cells. Although the mean age is 2½ years at the time of diagnosis, as many as 40 per cent appear within the first year of life.

Clinical Findings. The presence of an abdominal mass is the usual initial finding. Typically the mass is "fixed," irregular in contour, and frequently quite large. It is much less regular and smooth than a Wilms' tumor and tends to be more medially located. Abdominal pain, distention, vomiting, and diarrhea are found, in order of decreasing frequency. Weight loss and weakness are present in approximately 25 per cent of patients. Despite the fact that these tumors arise from sympathetic ganglion precursors and many patients excrete catecholamines and their metabolites in excessive amounts, very few patients have hypertension. An occasional patient presents with neurologic symptoms due to extension of tumor into the spinal canal.

X-rays show calcification in more than 50 per cent of the tumors. Metastases are evident in 60 to 90 per cent of patients at the time of diagnosis. Regional lymph nodes, liver, bones, lungs, subcutaneous tissue, and brain are most commonly affected. Bone marrow biopsy often reveals neuroblastoma cells. The presence of bony metastases carries a particularly poor prognosis. Liver metastases, on the other hand, are quite common in infants, and do not necessarily carry an ominous prognosis.

Diagnosis. In addition to plain films of the abdomen, which should show the mass and often calcification, excretory urogram is always indicated. Unlike Wilms' tumor, neuroblastoma seldom causes evidence of intrarenal distortion, although significant displacement and deformity of the kidney may be seen (Fig. 19). Hydronephrosis occasionally is seen as a result of compression of the ureter or the kidney pelvis. As with Wilms' tumor, the use of inferior vena cavograms may be of value in planning operative extirpation. Bone marrow aspiration is always indicated to determine the extent of metastatic dissemination.

Catecholamines and their breakdown products, including vanillylmandelic acid (VMA), homovanillic acid (HVA), epinephrine, and norepinephrine, can be found in the urine of most patients. The normal values vary with the size and age of the patient. Hence adult values are not applicable to the pediatric patient.[34]

Treatment. Although spontaneous regression does occur, it is rare and should never be considered in planning therapy. Total surgical excision offers the best chance for cure. The use of "triple therapy" further improves survival. If the tumor is large or invading vital structures, total excision may be impossible or hazardous. Biopsy to confirm the diagnosis followed by radiation therapy and later resection has produced cures in many patients in whom the prognosis was initially thought to be hopeless. This course of action should be carried out rather than persisting in a life-threatening surgical procedure. Radiation therapy as a sole form of treatment gives poor results, so surgical excision is still necessary even if the tumor seems to disappear with radiation therapy. The presence of metastatic disease in the liver, skin, and bone marrow does not appear to alter appreciably the survival rate (Stage IV-S), so complete surgical excision of the primary lesion should be carried out on these patients. Even in the presence of proven bony metastases, removal of the primary tumor is indicated, since occasional cures have been reported.

CHEMOTHERAPY. The use of cyclophosphamide (Cytoxan) and vincristine has improved cure rates after surgical therapy. Used alone, these drugs seldom effect cures. As with other uses of chemotherapy, their value is considerably enhanced if the bulk of tumor tissue can be removed surgically so that cancerocidal action is concentrated on a smaller number of cells. Repeat doses over long periods of time appear to give the best results. Metastases may completely disappear with the use of chemotherapy. The use of adriamycin in addition to vincristine and cytoxan has occasionally resulted in survival of patients with widespread metastatic disease.

RADIATION THERAPY. Radiation to the tumor bed, as well as to the liver if it is involved, should be employed routinely in the treatment of neuroblastoma. In young children 1000 to 1500 rads is given in 6 to 10 days. This dose is usually adequate because of the high radiosensitivity of this lesion. In older children doses of 2400 to 4500 rads are used. Results from radiation therapy are also significantly enhanced by surgical removal of the bulk of the tumor when possible. Bony recurrences may be treated effectively with radiation therapy.

Follow-up at frequent intervals is necessary for several years after diagnosis and initial treatment. Repeat chest and bone x-rays, as well as intravenous pyelogram, are indicated during this follow-up. Measurement of catecholamine levels in the follow-up period is a useful and reliable way of detecting recurrences (Fig. 20).

Results. Success in the treatment of neuroblastoma depends on at least five factors: location of the tumor, spread (stage), age of the patient, degree of cellular maturation, and immune mechanisms.

Neuroblastomas arising in the thoracic region carry an excellent prognosis, with long-term survival rates approximating 90 per cent. In contrast, tumors arising in the abdomen have an overall survival of less than 25 per cent. Stage I tumors (localized, no local or distant spread) have a high survival rate, but in most patients the tumor has already spread by the time of diagnosis. Patients with Stage IV disease (metastatic) have a very poor outlook, except for those in whom the

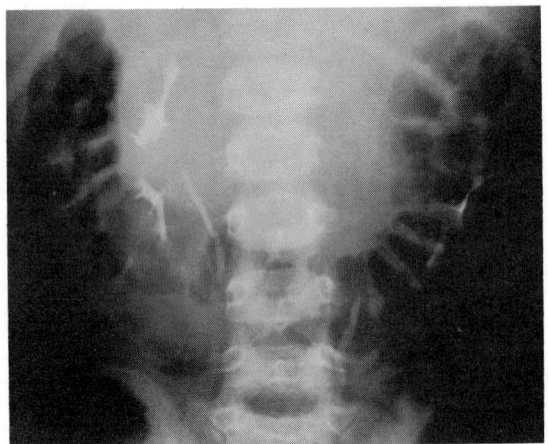

Figure 19. Excretory urogram in a 4-year-old girl with neuroblastoma. There is an upper abdominal midline mass that displaces the left kidney down and laterally without distortion of the collecting system.

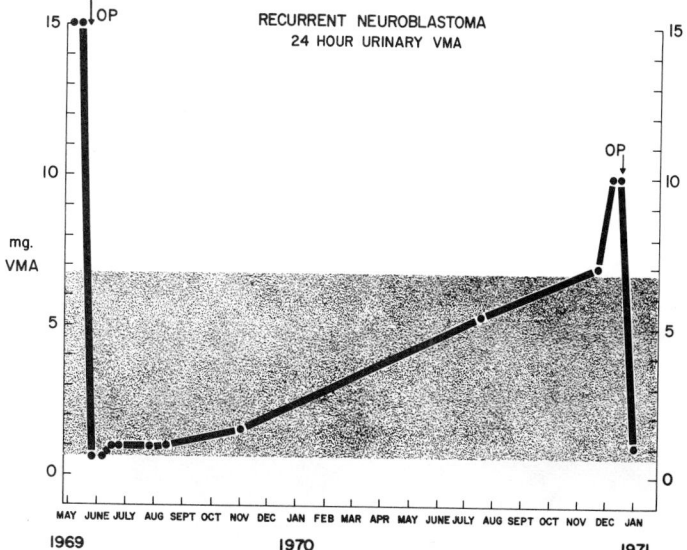

Figure 20. VMA excretion in a 3-year-old with neuroblastoma. He had no symptoms or evidence of mass after the first resection. The second operation was undertaken solely because of the elevated VMA. The shaded area represents normal values for an adult. The value of 5 mg. in July, 1970, was clearly abnormal for a child of this size and should have prompted exploration at that time.

spread is to liver, skin, or bone marrow only (IV-S), in which case the prognosis is not significantly different from those with localized disease.

For all stages, the patient's age at the time of diagnosis exerts a strong influence on the survival. Overall survival in infants under the age of one is approximately 75 per cent, whereas survival of patients over the age of two years is only 10 to 15 per cent. This discrepancy is only partly the result of the frequency of advanced stage disease at the time of diagnosis in the older patient.

Neuroblastoma is one of the few tumors in which histologic evidence of maturation (progression to ganglioneuroma from the undifferentiated "pure" neuroblastoma) correlates well with improved survival. Conversely, if no "mature" cells are seen, few patients survive regardless of age. In general, the more mature tumors also tend to be localized.

Finally, there is strong evidence that host immune factors play a role in the ability of the patient to control residual tumor. Both cellular and humoral factors have been identified, and patients in whom the disease is successfully controlled usually demonstrate lymphocytes with cytotoxic activity against neuroblastoma cells in tissue cultures. Unfortunately, it has not been possible to manipulate these mechanisms to actively control the tumor.

WILMS' TUMOR

The development of effective treatment for Wilms' tumor is one of the important "success stories" in cancer therapy. Above all else, it offers convincing evidence of the value of an aggressive approach to tumors even when metastases have occurred. As the result of combination therapy, employing surgical resection, radiation treatment, and chemotherapy, 80 per cent of affected children are now cured.

Although the classic description of the embryoma of the kidney by Max Wilms, a German surgeon, was

published in 1899, the tumor had been described many times before, and, specifically, the characteristic occurrence of embryonic tubal and connective tissue as the distinguishing characteristic was described by Birch-Hirschfeld in 1898. Because these tumors are found at an early age, and because of their peculiar histologic characteristics, it is generally accepted that they are related to embryologic errors and originate from fetal tissue. The histologic appearance varies from patient to patient, and in different parts of a tumor from a single patient. Abortive tubules or glomeruli may be seen surrounded by hyperchromatic round cells or a mixture of smooth and striated muscle or myxomatous tissue.

Wilms' tumors constitute 15 to 40 per cent of solid tumors of childhood, but undoubtedly carry the best prognosis of any intra-abdominal neoplasm.

Clinical Findings. The average age at time of diagnosis is 3 years, although these tumors may be found at any age from the newborn period to adulthood. The presenting symptom is usually an abdominal mass, noted by either the parent or the examining physician, frequently on a "routine" examination or evaluation for unrelated symptoms. Abdominal pain is present in about 20 per cent of patients; fever and hematuria are found in 15 to 20 per cent. Hypertension may be found in some patients. Secondary infection of the urinary tract is also occasionally seen. Ninety per cent of patients will have a palpable mass in the flank on physical examination. If the mass is large, differentiation from neuroblastoma or hydronephrosis may be difficult.

Diagnosis. Abdominal x-rays will usually show a mass, occasionally (10 per cent) with calcification. Excretory urogram in most patients will show the characteristic findings of Wilms' tumor: distortion of the pelves and calices as they are stretched out over the tumor, rather than displacement or obstruction from an extrarenal mass (Fig. 21). If there is nonfunction of the kidney on excretory urogram, hydro-

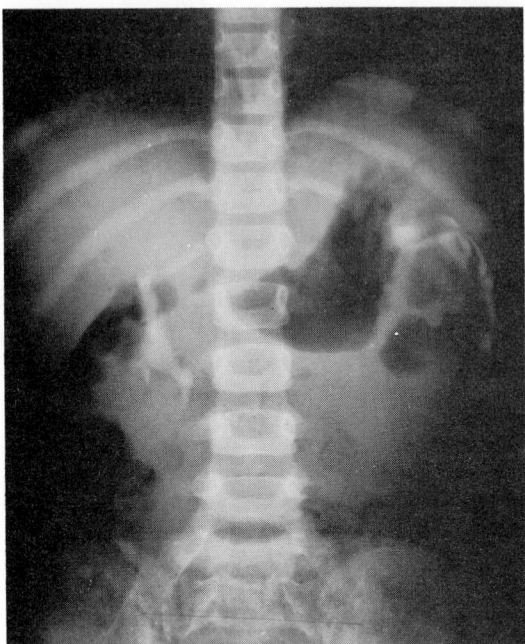

Figure 21. Intravenous pyelogram in a 3-year-old girl with a left Wilms' tumor demonstrating caliceal distortion and lateral displacement. The right kidney is normal.

nephrosis is much more likely than Wilms' tumor. This distinction should be made by retrograde pyelogram. Renal scan and the use of ultrasonic scanning may also be of value. Arteriography is seldom indicated but may be of value in confusing situations.

Chest x-ray must be obtained to determine if pulmonary metastases are present, since these are noted at the time of diagnosis in 20 to 50 per cent of patients. In contrast with neuroblastoma, bony metastases are rare. If the tumor is large or pulmonary metastases are already present, inferior vena cavogram is indicated to assess preoperatively the extent of venous involvement. The excretory urogram of the opposite kidney must be carefully inspected, since approximately 6 per cent of patients with Wilms' tumor have involvement of both kidneys.

Treatment. The history of treatment of Wilms' tumor is one of increasing success as additional modalities were employed. In the 1930s Ladd and Gross demonstrated that the cure rate in Wilms' tumor could be improved by early ligation of the renal pedicle, decreasing metastases secondary to operative manipulation. Postoperative irradiation was added in the 1940s, and cure rates doubled. The addition of actinomycin D at the time of surgery and subsequently has further substantially increased survivals. There is no longer any significant doubt that "triple therapy" gives the best results in the treatment of this tumor.[8]

OPERATIVE TREATMENT. In patients with hematuria or a nonfunctioning kidney, cystoscopy should be performed prior to operation to rule out the presence of distant implants in the bladder. If found, these should be excised and radiation therapy given to the bladder as well as the tumor bed postoperatively.

Radical surgical excision is the most important feature of treatment of Wilms' tumor, and few patients have been cured without removal of the tumor. A long transperitoneal incision is used with a thoracoabdominal extension if additional exposure is desired. Incision of the peritoneum laterally permits reflection of the colon medially so that the renal vessels may be exposed and ligated prior to further tumor manipulation. The entire tumor mass must be removed together with the renal and periaortic lymph nodes. If there is caval invasion, resection may be performed. In massive tumors with extension beyond the capsule, resection of parts of adjacent organs such as the intestine, diaphragm, or liver may also be indicated. Such invasion does not constitute a hopeless situation, and every attempt must be made at complete removal, consistent with safety to the patient. On rare occasions, in truly huge tumors with multiple organ involvement, irradiation after biopsy will usually shrink the tumor to more manageable proportions and permit later total extirpation.

In all cases the opposite kidney must be explored both by palpation and by careful examination because of the high incidence of bilateral disease. When bilateral involvement is present, partial nephrectomy or "shelling out" of the tumor is indicated. In some cases preoperative radiation to both kidneys designed to shrink the tumor is advisable. The "shelling out" operation may then be carried out, leaving a functioning kidney on both sides. At least one patient has been reported in whom bilateral nephrectomy and renal homotransplantation was carried out with long-term survival. Obviously a period of hemodialysis is indicated in such patients to make sure that they will not succumb to metastatic disease.

CHEMOTHERAPY AND RADIATION. There is now ample evidence from well-controlled studies that cyclic therapy with actinomycin D and vincristine substantially improves survival. Repeat courses are administered for 15 months. Supravoltage radiation therapy, 1800 to 4000 rads, depending on the patient's age, is given to the tumor bed in a 2- to 3-week period. Radiation therapy should not be given to children under the age of 2 years with Stage I (localized) disease, since it does not increase the disease-free survival and carries a significant risk of complications.

Although the period of maximal risk of recurrence is the first 2 years after resection, and the great majority of recurrences appear within 6 months, recurrences as late as 29 years later have been reported. Frequent follow-up with chest x-ray and, less frequently, intravenous pyelogram is necessary.

Lung metastases, if they occur, should be treated with the same aggressiveness as the original primary. Irradiation, chemotherapy, and surgery have all been used successfully in the treatment of pulmonary metastases. If the tumor is well localized, surgical resection is safest and carries an equally high cure rate. There are many patients reported who are long-term survivors after treatment of pulmonary metastases.

Congenital renal tumors discovered in the newborn period are almost always both clinically and histologically benign, showing profuse mesenchymal proliferation. These are more properly termed hamartomas or mesoblastic nephromas. Since they are not true Wilms' tumors, surgical excision is sufficient for cure.

Indeed, there is ample evidence that chemotherapy and radiation therapy in this age group carry a higher risk than their omission.

Results. Cure rates of better than 90 per cent can be expected in children in whom there is no evidence of metastatic disease at the time of operation. Even in those with metastases, long-term cure rates of 40 to 50 per cent are to be expected.

TERATOMA

Teratoma may present as an abdominal mass. Most often these tumors occur in the sacrococcygeal area, but they may also be located in the gonads, anterior mediastinum, neck, or nasopharynx.

Pathology. Teratomas are true congenital neoplasms that contain tissue of at least two embryologic germ layers. The origin of these tumors is not clear, but they are thought to arise from pluripotent or totipotent cells that do not respond in the usual way to normal differentiation in the developing embryo. They may be predominantly cystic or solid, often contain calcium, and may contain malignant components. In general, the solid tumors are more likely to be malignant.

Clinical Findings. Most teratomas are detected because a mass is noted. Symptoms usually are the result of encroachment of the tumor on some other adjacent structure.

Approximately half of teratomas are sacrococcygeal and 10 to 20 per cent of these have malignant components. The vast majority present externally (Fig. 22), but many have a sizable internal component and a small percentage are presacral, in which the mass is detected by rectal examination. Presacral teratomas tend to be familial and are inherited as an autosomal dominant characteristic.[4] For this reason, all close relatives of any patient in whom the diagnosis of presacral teratoma is made should be carefully examined for the presence of teratoma that may yet be asymptomatic. Over a third of these tumors are malignant at the time of diagnosis.

Cervical, nasopharyngeal, and mediastinal teratomas may cause airway obstruction. Tumors can grow to quite a large size before symptoms are apparent.

Teratomas of the sacrococcygeal, retroperitoneal, cervical, and nasopharyngeal areas tend to be detected in the first few months of life. Indeed, most are noted in the neonatal period. Those arising in the anterior mediastinum and gonads are most often detected in children or young adults.

Diagnosis. Diagnosis is suspected when a mass is noted in a location where teratomas occur, particularly if it contains calcium. The calcium is often rather coarse or dense. Not all teratomas contain calcium, however, and for these the diagnosis is more difficult.

Treatment. Treatment is excision. Teratomas of the sacrococcygeal region may be quite vascular. The blood supply is from the middle sacral artery, and this should be divided early in the course of the dissection. If there is a presacral extension up to the sacral promontory, a combined abdominosacral approach will be required.

Results. Most teratomas are benign and carry a good prognosis. About 10 per cent of teratomas are malignant. The frequency of malignancy varies with location. In the sacrococcygeal region the outlook is much better for patients who have the teratoma removed in early infancy: less than 10 per cent mortality under one year of age compared to over 55 per cent in patients who are more than two years old at the time of operation. The primary reason for delay in treatment is delay in diagnosis. Sacrococcygeal teratomas are most frequently confused with myelomeningoceles, another reason why the latter should be operated on early in life.

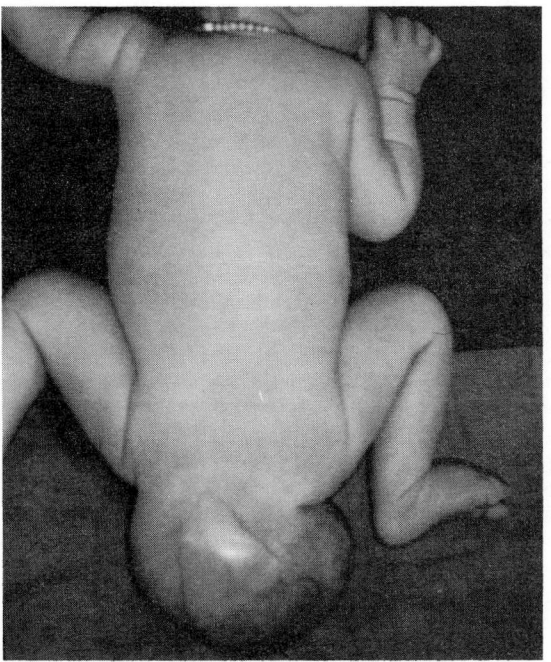

Figure 22. Typical sacrococcygeal teratoma in a newborn infant. Despite its grotesque appearance, this tumor seldom involves vital structures, and complete excision may be accomplished.

ABDOMINAL PAIN

Abdominal pain is a frequent complaint in childhood. The causes are innumerable. Of children whose main symptom is abdominal pain when they see a physician, less than 10 per cent will have a surgical disease. Within this group, however, are most who have a serious, life-threatening illness.

Symptoms of fever, irritability, vomiting, and abdominal pain in children are nonspecific and may be present with most kinds of infection or febrile episodes. They are also the symptoms of appendicitis.

The surgical conditions causing abdominal pain are most often detected by a thorough examination of the abdomen. For this reason it is mandatory than an adequate examination be obtained. Unfortunately, even with almost infinite patience, it is sometimes impossible to gain the cooperation of some ill infants and children. In this circumstance, a satisfactory examination can be obtained by sedating the patient to the point of sleep. (An opiate should not be used since it relieves pain.) Chloral hydrate or a short-acting barbiturate by rectum will produce sleep without masking tenderness. A thorough physical examination is essential to detect the extra-abdominal causes of abdominal pain.

APPENDICITIS

Appendicitis is the most common cause of a surgical abdomen in children. The high incidence of ruptured appendixes in pediatric patients (18 to 45 per cent in reported series) is related to (1) parental delay in seeking medical aid and (2) physician delay in making the diagnosis. Improvement in the former will result only from widespread public education. The latter will improve with the acceptance (1) that abdominal pain should not be treated over the telephone, (2) that in spite of the time consumed, a thorough abdominal examination is essential, and (3) that if it is not possible to make the diagnosis at the time of the original examination the patient should be examined again in 2 to 4 hours.

The other important factor in childhood appendicitis is the recognition and proper preoperative preparation of the very ill child. Almost all deaths and most of the complications from appendicitis occur in patients whose appendix has ruptured. Preoperative preparation of the patient with ruptured appendix and peritonitis should be prompt but adequate and includes expansion of blood volume, hydration, correction of acidosis, treatment of infection with antibiotics, and reduction of fever. Rough guidelines to indicate that the patient is sufficiently prepared for operation include a pulse below 120, rectal temperature below 39° C., and an adequate output of ketone-free urine.

Appendicitis is discussed in detail elsewhere.

INTUSSUSCEPTION

Intussusception is the telescoping of one portion of the bowel into the segment just distal to it. Some intussusceptions reduce spontaneously. Many, however, progress to produce intestinal obstruction and impairment of blood supply with gangrene and perforation.

Etiology. Intussusception may result when a lead point, such as a polyp or Meckel's diverticulum, is carried along downsteam by the intestinal peristalsis, taking its attachment with it. While a lead point is common in adults, it is uncommon in pediatric patients. Gross reported that only 6 per cent of his 702 pediatric patients with intussusception had a lead point.[10]

The idiopathic variety is probably the result of a disturbance in intestinal motility in which there is segmental spasticity and atony. When a peristaltic wave hits a spastic segment just proximal to an atonic segment, the former may be intussuscepted into the latter. Adenovirus, which is known to cause enteric symptoms, has been recovered from the stool in 46 per cent of patients with idiopathic intussusception at a time when 3.6 per cent of the general population harbored the virus. Resulting lymphoid hyperplasia in the bowel wall may act as a lead point. Idiopathic intussusception is decreasing in frequency. Intussusception may also occur a few days after abdominal operation when intestinal peristalsis is returning.

The usual idiopathic intussusception is ileocolic (ileum intussuscepts into colon). Small bowel intussusception is likely to have a lead point and tends to occur in older children.

Clinical Findings. Eighty-five per cent of pediatric intussusceptions occur in patients between 2 months and 2 years of age. The infant has usually been healthy. He exhibits a sudden onset of cramping abdominal pain and crying, often pulls his legs up onto his abdomen with the pains, and frequently vomits. Between episodes, which usually occur at 15- to 30-minute intervals, he is usually completely asymptomatic. Frequently the patient passes bloody mucous (currant jelly) stools. Rectal bleeding may be a prominent feature. If seen between episodes of pain during the asymptomatic period (which may be as long as 2 or 3 hours), the infant looks deceptively healthy. After a number of hours he becomes quite ill.

On physical examination a "sausage-shaped" mass is palpable in 90 per cent of patients, usually in the right upper quadrant. The mass, however, may be difficult to palpate. It is moderately soft, not particularly tender, and somewhat mobile. Sedation of the patient may be necessary for an adequate examination. The stool is usually guaiac-positive, even if not grossly bloody.

Diagnosis. Diagnosis may be made on clinical grounds. Plain x-ray of the abdomen is likely to show more than the usual amount of small bowel gas. The right lower quadrant may be empty of cecal gas and a mass may be seen. Intussusception into the colon can be diagnosed by barium enema. Any infant or child suspected of having an intussusception should have a prompt barium enema—day or night (Fig. 23). Unfortunately, barium enema is of no value in the diagnosis of small bowel intussusception.

Treatment. Reduction may be accomplished by hydrostatic pressure (first advocated by Hirschsprung) or operatively. If the intussusception is irreducible, resection is required. Hydrostatic reduction by barium enema under fluoroscopic control is a safe form of therapy if the following criteria are observed: (1) the surgeon should see the patient and the usual preoperative preparations should be carried out before any attempt is made at reduction; (2) the hydrostatic pressure is not to exceed 3½ feet; (3) no manipulation of the abdomen is attempted (this further increases the intracolonic pressure and risk of bowel rupture); (4) reduction is not considered successful unless there is free reflux of barium into the ileum (if the ileum does not fill freely, operation is required at once); (5) the patient is admitted to the hospital for 24 hours of observation, and if symptoms persist, operation is mandatory; and (6) reduction by barium enema is not attempted in the infant with x-ray evidence of marked intestinal obstruction, with acute toxicity or with clinical signs of strangulated bowel.[26]

Barium enema reduction has the limitations that it

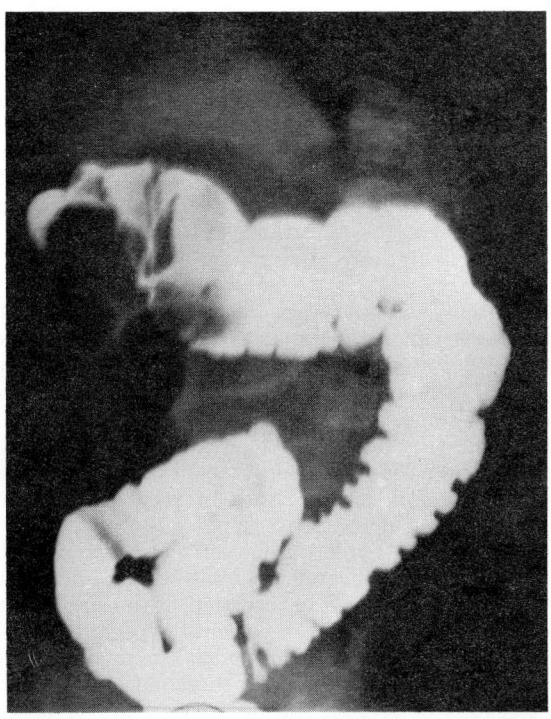

Figure 23. Roentgenogram taken at the time of barium enema reduction of an intussusception. The intussusception can be seen at the hepatic flexure.

is of no value in the patient with small bowel intussusception and usually does not detect any lead point as the cause of the intussusception. The major dangers of barium enema reduction stem from the very factors that make it an appealing form of therapy—its ease and simplicity. The perforations and deaths that have occurred with its use have been in the hands of enthusiasts who have extended the indications or ignored the precautions just listed.

For patients with intussusception who are not candidates for hydrostatic reduction, or in whom it is unsuccessful, operation is performed as soon as adequate preparation has been carried out.

Operative reduction is illustrated in Figure 24. A lead point, if present, should be resected. If the reduction is unsuccessful, if the intestine is not viable, or if the patient is quite sick and toxic, the involved intestine should be resected.

Results. Gross reports no deaths in patients with symptoms of less than 24 hours. With symptoms of over 24 hours' duration, the reported mortality is as high as 40 per cent. The importance of early diagnosis is obvious.

URINARY TRACT INFECTION

Infections of the urinary tract are surprisingly common in preschool and school-age children, even in the

Figure 24. Technique of operative reduction of intussusception. (From Gross, R. E.: An Atlas of Children's Surgery. Philadelphia, W. B. Saunders Company, 1970.)

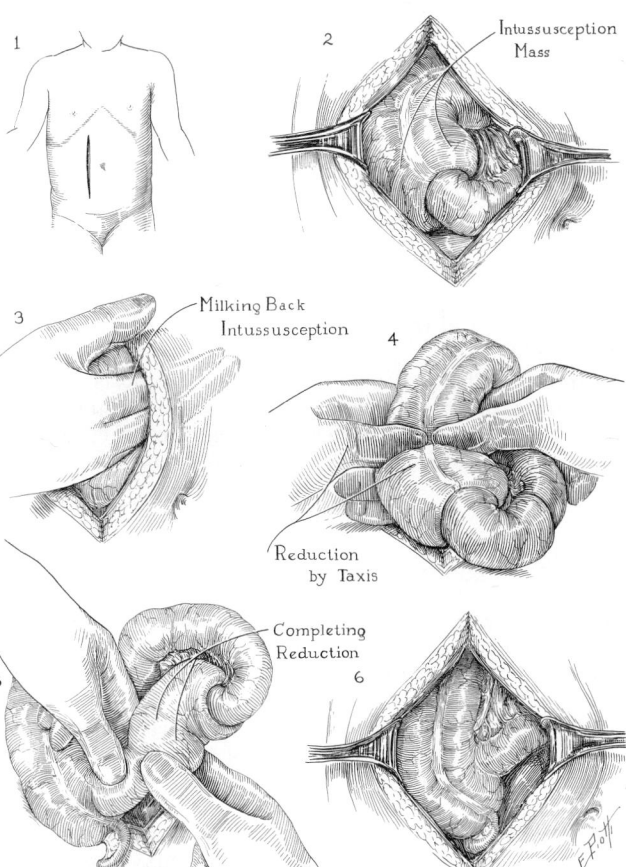

absence of symptoms. Unlike respiratory infections, infections of the urinary tract frequently indicate an underlying organic lesion. It is important that the diagnosis be established by culture of properly obtained clean-voided urine and not by urinalysis. Studies have shown that pyuria is grossly unreliable as an indicator of urinary tract infection. If an infection is diagnosed by culture, not only must it be treated, but the underlying cause must be sought.[2]

Appropriate evaluation consists of a voiding cystourethrogram, excretory urogram, cystoscopy and urethral calibration, and assessment of renal function by creatinine clearance. Occasionally the use of renal scans, retrograde pyelography, and cystometrograms is of value. Most of the time the latter are not necessary, however, and simple x-ray studies and cystoscopy will delineate the disorder. An aggressive diagnostic approach is indicated, for not only is the yield great (approximately 50 per cent) but the chance of permanent cure by surgical methods is quite high.

URETHRAL STENOSIS

A significant percentage of girls with recurring urinary tract infections are found to have marked narrowing of the urethra when it is calibrated at the time of cystoscopy. This narrowing may be present at the meatus or at the midurethral level (Lyon's ring) and is presumably a congenital malformation. The possibility that such narrowing is the result of chronic urethritis (bacterial or otherwise) cannot be excluded.

Diagnosis. In most cases the patient will give few if any symptoms to indicate difficulty in voiding that suggests the degree of obstruction that is found. In girls, the urinary stream is seldom observed by the mother, so this information is usually not available. X-rays also are unreliable and may show a proximal dilatation when no obstruction exists. Urethral calibration with bougies à boule, done with the patient anesthetized at the time of cystoscopy, is the only way of establishing the presence of significant stenosis. Urethral stenosis is sometimes seen in association with vesicoureteral reflux but is rarely the underlying cause of reflux.

Treatment. The treatment of urethral stenosis is urethrotomy or urethral dilatation. If urethral stenosis is the only lesion discovered, the chances of cure of the recurring urinary tract infections by urethrotomy or dilatation are good.

VESICOURETERAL REFLUX

Undoubtedly one of the most controversial subjects of the past decade, vesicoureteral reflux is seen with considerable frequency among girls who are evaluated for recurring urinary tract infections.

Etiology. Reflux occurs when there is a breakdown of the normal one-way valve action of the vesicoureteral junction. There are several causes:

1. Obstruction. The most common form of obstruction in young girls is urethral stenosis (see the preceding section), and relief of this obstruction may bring

about disappearance of the reflux. In boys, posterior urethral valves are the most common cause of lower urinary tract obstruction.

2. Neurogenic bladder. Patients with neurogenic bladder from any cause (myelomeningocele is the most common in the pediatric age group) may have vesicoureteral reflux caused by the inadequacy of the bladder wall itself. In these patients reflux cannot be corrected by the standard methods of reimplantation, and in most some form of urinary diversion will ultimately be necessary.

3. Chronic urinary tract infection. Some have felt that *all* vesicoureteral reflux is a result of changes of the vesicoureteral junction secondary to recurring infections. Although this mechanism undoubtedly accounts for some, many infections are the *result* of the reflux and will not respond to antibacterial treatment until the reflux is corrected. In about one fourth of patients the reflux is the result of recurring urinary tract infections alone.

4. Congenital malformation of the vesicoureteral junction. The most common cause of reflux appears to be a malformation of the insertion of the ureter into the bladder. Some of these patients, especially males, may not have any history or evidence of urinary infection, although most do. It is in these patients that the best results of reimplantation surgery are to be expected.

Pathophysiology. The significance of vesicoureteral reflux is that it may produce renal damage if allowed to persist. Reflux permits a bladder infection to ascend to the kidneys and cause pyelonephritis. There is some evidence that reflux is frequently present when pyelonephritis occurs in the pediatric age group. Even in the absence of infection, reflux can cause significant damage to the kidney, since it exposes this low-pressure system to the high intravesical voiding pressure every time the patient micturates.

Diagnosis. The presence and the extent of reflux can be determined only by instillation of radiopaque contrast medium into the bladder. Although reflux can sometimes be demonstrated in the anesthetized patient, it is its presence during the normal act of voiding that is of significance. For this reason, a voiding cystourethrogram in the awake patient is recommended. The presence of prominent or dilated ureteral orifices at cystoscopy is suggestive, but not diagnostic, of reflux, and may be misleading. Many patients with severe reflux have surprisingly normal-appearing ureteral orifices.

Treatment. In the evaluation of vesicoureteral reflux it is essential that patients with neurogenic bladder be identified, since they will not benefit from a reimplantation operation. Further, it is mandatory that any form of a distal obstruction be corrected prior to (and often instead of) reconstructive reflux surgery. If the patient has no evidence of upper urinary tract damage (hydronephrosis or hydroureter), and if lower urinary obstruction has been ruled out, a trial of antibacterial therapy with one of the usual agents such as sulfisoxazole (Gantrisin), nalidixic acid (NegGram), or nitrofurantoin (Furadantin) is indicated. Six months' antibacterial therapy with frequent urine culture checks to make sure the urine is, in fact, being

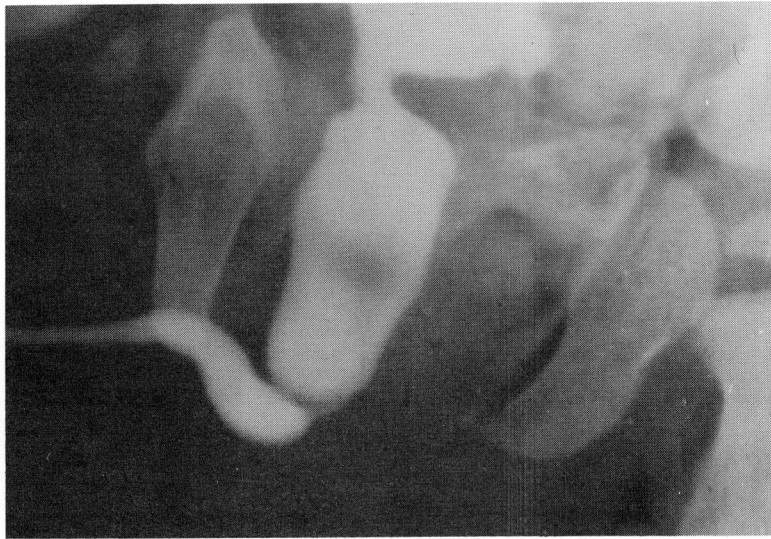

Figure 25. Voiding cystourethrogram in patient with posterior urethral valves. Note massive dilatation of posterior urethra and false impression of bladder neck contracture.

kept sterile will correct the reflux in those patients in whom infection is the sole etiologic basis. If at the end of 6 months the reflux persists, further medicinal therapy is unlikely to be successful, and reconstructive surgery is indicated.

Although many surgical techniques have been suggested, the Leadbetter-Politano method of reimplantation of the ureter, which creates a submucosal tunnel, has received widest acceptance. Properly performed, the operation can be expected to be 95 per cent successful in preventing reflux. Failures are usually in patients with dilated ureters in whom a ureteral-tailoring procedure is indicated. Either obstruction or persistent reflux can occur. Their detection requires periodic follow-up x-ray studies. On the whole, however, the operation has proved eminently satisfactory, and the great majority of patients are cured both of the reflux and of recurring urinary tract infections.[12]

POSTERIOR URETHRAL VALVES

Urinary infection in a newborn male is almost always secondary to urinary tract obstruction or a neurogenic bladder. In this age group urinary obstruction may be due to posterior urethral valves (Fig. 25). Marked degrees of hydronephrosis and hydroureter can result from this obstruction, which clearly is present long before birth. Ureters may be so dilated that they resemble the sigmoid colon, and when filled with radiocontrast material suggest a barium enema study. Severe renal destruction can occur. Especially in patients with severe hydronephrosis, the use of temporary tubeless drainage high in the ureter or at the renal pelvis or early reconstruction is necessary (Fig. 26). This will permit maximal return of renal function. The valves themselves are resected endoscopically at the time of reconstruction. Vesicoureteral reflux is almost always present and requires reimplantation of the ureters. If the ureters are significantly dilated, they will require tailoring of the lower end of

the ureter. For more extensive hydroureter, the entire ureter will need to be narrowed and shortened, which requires a two-stage procedure.

NEUROGENIC BLADDER

Neurogenic bladder is a relatively common condition of infancy, being secondary to myelomeningocele in most patients. At the present time little can be done in the way of reconstructive surgery to permit adequate bladder function. It is essential that these patients receive urinary diversion early enough so that they do not suffer progressive renal damage both from

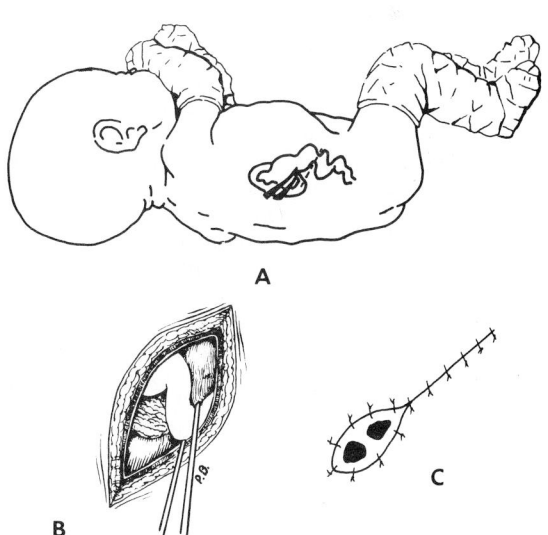

Figure 26. Method of performing in-continuity loop ureterostomies in child with massive hydronephrosis and hydroureter. Kinking of the ureter must be relieved so that the segment brought to the skin readily conducts urine out from the kidney.

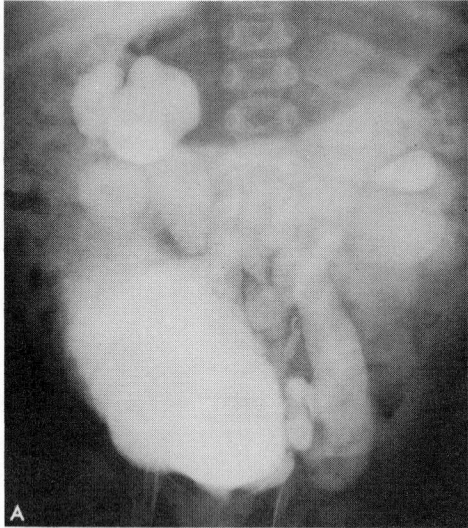
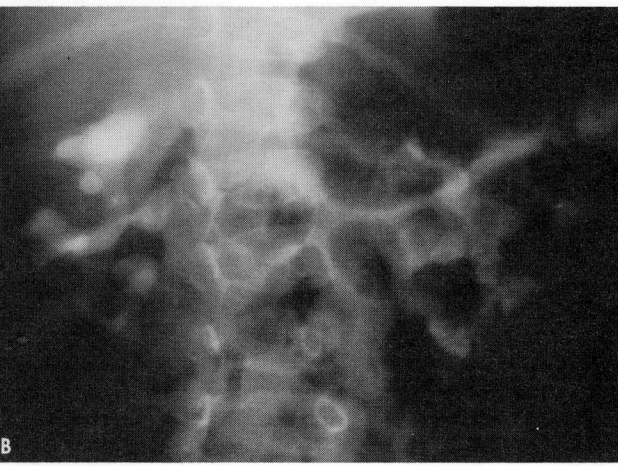

Figure 27. *A,* A cystogram of an 8-month-old child with myelomeningocele, showing bilateral reflux and two massively dilated ureters and kidneys. Note large irregular-shaped bladder. *B,* Intravenous pyelogram of same patient 6 months after bilateral cutaneous ureterostomies. Note marked decrease in hydronephrosis and excellent urine-concentrating ability.

inadequate drainage and from chronic infection (Fig. 27). This may require ileal or colon conduit in the first year or two of life. For more detailed discussion of problems of diagnosis and management of neurogenic bladder, the reader is referred to the section in the chapter on the urinary system.

MISCELLANEOUS CAUSES OF URINARY TRACT INFECTION

There are numerous other urinary tract anomalies that are first brought to the surgeon's attention because of recurring urinary tract infections: ureterocele, ectopic ureters, duplicated collecting systems, vesicoureteral obstruction, and so forth. In general, the diagnosis of these entities is made in the same fashion as that of those that have already been discussed: use of contrast radiography and cystoscopy. Treatment consists of correction of the defect and restoration of a normal urinary tract, which is usually possible. There remain a number of patients, perhaps as many as 40 to 50 per cent, in whom no organic underlying cause for recurring urinary tract infections can be found. These patients are particularly frustrating for the physician and bear witness to the inadequacy of current diagnostic methods. Nevertheless, in the absence of evidence of damage to the upper urinary tract, the long-term prognosis for these patients is good. Many will respond to a prolonged course of antibacterial therapy. The important principle is that they be carefully followed and monitored by periodic cultures so that recurring infections may be promptly detected and treated.

SELECTED REFERENCES

Gross, R. E.: The Surgery of Infancy and Childhood. Philadelphia, W. B. Saunders Company, 1953.
This text is a classic. It is easy to read and contains a vast amount of material based, for the most part, on Dr. Gross' own experience at the Boston Children's Hospital. Despite being published in 1953, it still contains some of the most informative reading in pediatric surgery. The mortality statistics and some forms of therapy are not current.

Gross, R. E.: An Atlas of Children's Surgery. Philadelphia, W. B. Saunders Company, 1970.
This atlas with excellent illustrations by Janis Cirulis and Etta Piotti covers many of the operations in pediatric surgery. A short discussion of operative technique is included. The drawings and text are clear and concise.

Mustard, W. T., Ravitch, M. M., Snyder, W. H., Jr., Welch, K. J., and Benson, C. D.: Pediatric Surgery, 2nd ed. Chicago, Year Book Medical Publishers, 1970.
This two-volume text is the standard reference work in pediatric surgery and provides a comprehensive coverage of virtually all aspects. It is a multiauthor book with 80 contributors, many of them leading authorities on their subjects.

Swenson, O.: Pediatric Surgery, 3rd ed. New York, Appleton-Century-Crofts, 1969.
This two-volume text written by Dr. Swenson and 24 of his colleagues at the Chicago Children's Memorial Hospital and Northwestern University Medical School is unusually well organized for a work with so many authors. The discussion of Hirschsprung's disease, particularly, is outstanding. Most other topics are also very well covered. This is a good and complete text.

Rickham, P. P., and Johnston, J. H.: Neonatal Surgery. New York, Appleton-Century-Crofts, 1970.
The major surgical diseases of the newborn are presented in this compendium which represents the experience of the Alder Hey Children's Hospital. Although various specialists of the staff have contributed to it, the bulk of the book is written by the senior authors and reflects their vast experience in this field. A large segment is devoted to organizational and nonoperative care aspects of neonatal surgery, duly emphasizing the importance these aspects have in determining the overall outcome. Although primarily of interest to the specialist, who will find in here virtually all he needs, it is also a valuable reference for the student seeking more detailed information than is available in the standard texts.

REFERENCES

1. Allen, R. G., and Wrenn, E. L., Jr.: Silon as a sac in the treatment of omphalocele and gastroschisis. J. Pediatr. Surg., *4*:3, 1969.
2. Allen, T. D.: Pathogenesis of urinary tract infection in children. N. Engl. J. Med., 273:1421, 1965.
3. Altman, R. P., Chandra, R., and Lilly, J. R.: Ongoing cirrhosis

after successful porticoenterostomy in infants with biliary atresia. J. Pediatr. Surg., *10*:685, 1975.

4. Ashcraft, K. W., and Holder, T. M.: Hereditary presacral teratoma. J. Pediatr. Surg., *9*:691, 1974.

5. Barlow, B., Santulli, T. V., et al.: An experimental study of acute neonatal enterocolitis—the importance of breast milk. J. Pediatr. Surg., *9*:587, 1974.

6. Benson, C. D., and Loyd, J. R.: Infantile pyloric stenosis. Am. J. Surg., *107*:429, 1964.

7. Bishop, H. C., and Koop, C. E.: Management of meconium ileus: Resection, Roux-en-Y anastomosis and ileostomy irrigation with pancreatic enzymes. Ann. Surg., *145*:410, 1957.

8. Farber, S.: Chemotherapy in the treatment of leukemia and Wilms' tumor. J.A.M.A., *198*:154, 1966.

9. Griscom, T.: The roentgenology of neonatal abdominal masses. Am. J. Roentgen., *93*:447, 1965.

10. Gross, R. E.: The Surgery of Infancy and Childhood. Philadelphia, W. B. Saunders Company, 1953.

11. Hays, D. M.: Intestinal atresia and stenosis. Curr. Probl. Surg., Oct., 1969.

12. Hendren, W. H.: Ureteral reimplantation in children. J. Pediatr. Surg. *3*:649, 1968.

13. Hendren, W. H., and Haggerty, R. J.: Staphylococcic pneumonia in infancy and childhood. J.A.M.A., *168*:6, 1958.

14. Hendren, W. H.: A new approach to infants with severe obstructive uropathy: Early complete reconstruction. J. Pediatr. Surg., *5*:184, 1970.

15. Holder, T. M., and Ashcraft, K. W.: Esophageal atresia and tracheoesophageal fistula. Curr. Probl. Surg., Aug., 1966.

16. Holder, T. M., Leape, L. L., and Ashcraft, K. W.: Gastrostomy: Its use and dangers in pediatric patients. N. Engl. J. Med., *286*:1345, 1972.

17. Howard, E. R., and Othersen, H. B.: Proximal jejunoplasty in the treatment of jejunal atresia. J. Pediatr. Surg., *8*:685, 1973.

18. Kasai, M., Kimura, S., et al.: Surgical treatment of biliary atresia. J. Pediatr. Surg., *3*:665, 1968.

19. Koop, C. E., and Hernandez, J. R.: Neuroblastoma. Experience with 100 cases in children. Surgery, *56*:726, 1964.

20. Leape, L. L., and Holder, T. M.: Temporary tubeless urinary diversion in children. J. Pediatr. Surg., *5*:288, 1970.

21. Leape, L. L., and Longino, L. A.: Infantile lobar emphysema. Pediatrics, *34*:246, 1964.

22. Leonidas, J. C., and Germann, D. R.: Technetium-99m pertechnetate imaging in diagnosis of Meckel's diverticulum. Arch. Dis. Child., *49*:21, 1974.

23. Meeker, I. A., and Kincannon, W. H.: The role of ventral hernia in the correction of diaphragmatic defects in the newborn. Arch. Dis. Child., *40*:146, 1965.

24. Noblett, H. R.: Treatment of uncomplicated meconium ileus by gastrografin enema: A preliminary report. J. Pediatr. Surg., *4*:190, 1969.

25. Pickett, L. K.: Obstructive jaundice. *In* Mustard, W. T., et al. (Eds.): Pediatric Surgery, 2nd ed. Chicago, Year Book Medical Publishers, 1969, p. 732.

26. Ravitch, M. M.: Intussusception in Infants and Children. Springfield, Ill., Charles C Thomas, Publisher, 1959.

27. Ravitch, M. M.: Duplications of the alimentary canal. *In* Mustard, W. T., et al. (Eds.): Pediatric Surgery, 2nd ed. Chicago, Year Book Medical Publishers, 1969, p. 831.

28. Rickman, P. P.: Neonatal physiology and its effect on pre- and postoperative management. *In* Rickham, P. P., and Johnston, J. H. (Eds.): Neontal Surgery. New York, Appleton-Century-Crofts, 1969, p. 33.

29. Simpson, A. J., Leonidas, J. C., et al.: Roentgen diagnosis of midgut malrotation: Value of upper gastrointestinal radiographic study. J. Pediatr. Surg., *7*:243, 1972.

30. Snyder, W. H., Jr., and Chaffen, L.: Malrotation of the intestine. *In* Mustard, W. T., et al. (Eds.): Pediatric Surgery, 2nd ed. Chicago, Year Book Medical Publishers, 1969, p. 808.

31. Stephens, F. D.: Congenital Malformations of the Rectum, Anus and Genitourinary Tract. Edinburgh, E. and S. Livingstone, 1963.

32. Stevenson, J. K., Oliver, T. K., et al.: Aggressive treatment of neonatal necrotizing enterocolitis: 38 patients with 25 survivors. J. Pediatr. Surg., *6*:28, 1971.

33. Swenson, O.: Pediatric Surgery, 3rd ed. New York, Appleton-Century-Crofts, 1969, p. 734.

34. Voorhess, M. L.: Urinary catecholamine excretion by healthy children. Pediatrics, *39*:252, 1967.

35. Wagget, J., Bishop, H. C., and Koop, C. E.: Experience with gastrografin enema in the treatment of meconium ileus. J. Pediatr. Surg., *5*:649, 1970.

36. Waldhausen, J. A., Kilman, J. W., Vellios, F., and Battersby, J. S.: Sacrococcygeal teratoma. Surgery, *54*:933, 1963.

41

SURGICAL DISORDERS OF THE EARS, NOSE, PARANASAL SINUSES, PHARYNX, AND LARYNX

James B. Snow, Jr., M.D.

THE EARS

Progress in surgery of the ear began in 1853 when Sir William Wilde of Dublin, father of Oscar Wilde, advocated a postauricular incision for the drainage of subperiosteal abscesses in acute mastoiditis. The next major advances occurred with Hermann Schwartze's introduction in 1873 of the complete mastoidectomy. This operation gained great popularity because of its effectiveness in resolving acute mastoiditis. Emanuel Zaufal recognized that the operation did not solve the problem in the presence of a cholesteatoma and in 1890 described the radical mastoidectomy, in which the disease process in the middle ear, antrum, and mastoid cell area is exteriorized by removal of the posterior and superior portion of the bony canal wall. Bondy observed that removal of the tympanic membrane remnants and auditory ossicles was not always necessary to exteriorize cholesteatomas and in 1910 introduced the modified radical mastoidectomy in which a cholesteatoma lateral to the ossicles could be exteriorized and the hearing preserved. In the 1930s Lempert popularized endaural incisions. The development of the binocular surgical microscope by Holmgren and improved illumination set the stage for the introduction of tympanoplasty by Wullstein and Zöllner in the early 1950s.[46] The next major advance occurred in 1952 when Rosen mobilized the stapes in a patient with otosclerosis.[34] Shea introduced stapedectomy in 1958 and brought a century of surgery for the middle ear to a dramatic climax.[40] More recently, House has developed endolymphatic-subarachnoid shunt surgery and translabyrinthine and middle cranial fossa approaches for the internal auditory meatus.[15-17] The development of an auditory prosthesis for the profoundly deaf is the new frontier.[24]

ANATOMY OF THE EAR

The external auditory canal makes a slightly S-shaped curve. The outer one third has a cartilaginous skeleton, and the inner two thirds has a bony skeleton. Sebaceous glands and hair are borne in the outer one third. The plane of the tympanic membrane makes an angle of 55 degrees with the long axis of the external auditory canal. The tympanic membrane is divided into the pars tensa and the pars flaccida. The pars tensa is composed of three layers: the outer stratified squamous epithelium, which is continuous with the skin of the canal; the fibrous layer; and the inner mucous membrane, which is continuous with the rest of the mucous membrane of the middle ear. The fibrous layer thickens toward the periphery of the tympanic membrane to form the annulus tympanicus, which rests in the sulcus tympanicus, a groove in the most medial aspect of the canal. The fibrous layer ends at the anterior and posterior malleolar folds. The pars flaccida has only two layers, the stratified squamous epithelium laterally and the mucous membrane medially (Fig. 1). The long process of the malleus is embedded in the fibrous layer of the tympanic membrane, and the short process projects laterally. The head of the malleus articulates with the body of the incus. The lenticular process of the incus

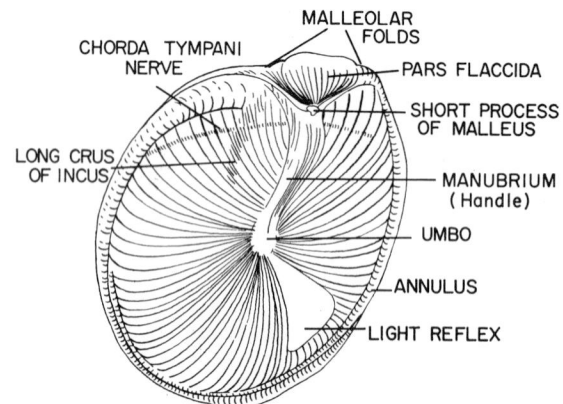

Figure 1. Landmarks of the right tympanic membrane. (From Saunders, W. H. *In* Prior, J. H., and Silberstein, J. S.: Physical Diagnosis. The History and Examination of the Patient. St. Louis, The C. V. Mosby Company, 1963.)

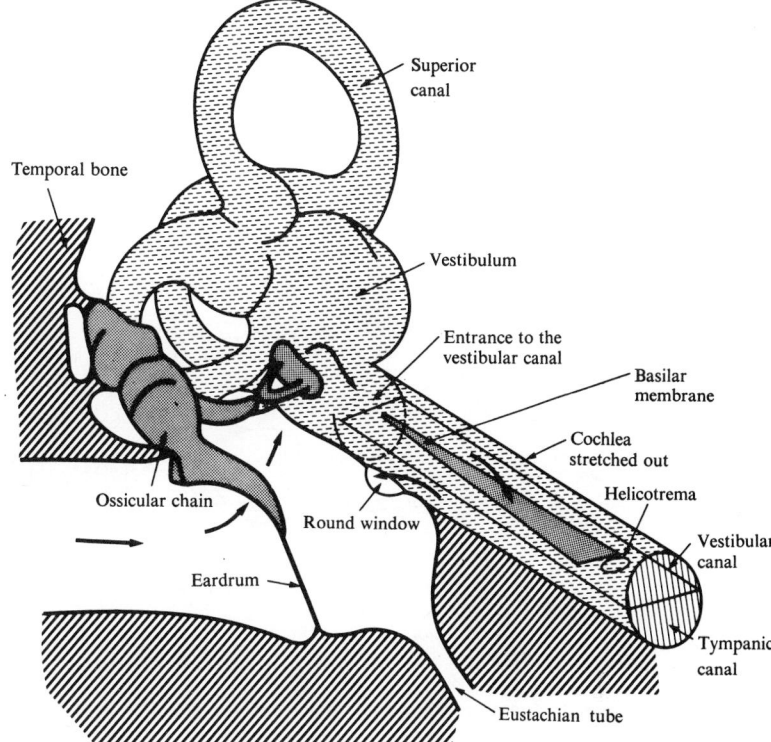

Figure 2. Functional diagram of the external, middle, and inner ear with the cochlea unrolled. (From von Békésy, G. *In* Theoretical and Mathematical Biology, edited by Talbot H. Waterman and Harold J. Morowitz. © 1965, Xerox.)

articulates with the head of the stapes. The footplate of the stapes articulates with the oval window (Fig. 2).

The middle ear space is irregular and compressed laterally. The part superior to the level of the tympanic membrane is the epitympanum or attic. The mesotympanum lies directly medial to the tympanic membrane. The hypotympanum is inferior to the level of the tympanic membrane. The basal turn of the cochlea makes an impression of the medial wall of the middle ear called the promontory. The roof or tegmen of the tympanum is opposite the middle cranial fossa. The tegmen tympani extends posteriorly to become the tegmen of the antrum and mastoid process. The middle ear communicates with the mastoid process through the antrum. All mastoid air cells communicate one through another with the antrum. Pneumatic cells also extend into the petrous pyramid from the antrum, attic, and hypotympanum. The floor of the middle ear is the roof of the jugular fossa.[3]

The cochlea makes two and three-quarters turns in the human. A cross section through the modiolus or central bony framework shows in each turn the scala vestibuli, the scala media, and the scala tympani (Fig. 3). The scala vestibuli is separated from the scala media by Reissner's membrane. The scala media is separated from the scala tympani by the basilar membrane. The organ of Corti with its hair cells and their supporting cells rests on the basilar membrane. The hairs of the hair cells are in contact with the tectorial membrane. Dendrites of the first-order neurons, whose cell bodies are in the spiral canal of Rosenthal in the modiolus, arborize about the base of the hair cells.

The axons terminate in the dorsal and ventral cochlear nuclei in the medulla. The pathway to the auditory cortex consists of at least four orders of neurons and includes the superior olivary complexes, the lateral lemnisci, the inferior colliculi, and the medial geniculate bodies. Crossing of the midline occurs at the level of the brain stem nuclei and the inferior colliculi. In man the auditory cortex lies in the poste-

rior portion of the superior temporal gyrus in the sylvian fissure, which is called Heschl's gyrus.

The saccule is spherical and is connected with the scala media through the canalis reuniens of Hensen (Fig. 4). The saccular duct joins the utricular duct to form the endolymphatic duct. The utricle is larger than the saccule and is ovoid. The utricle has five openings for the three ampullated ends of the semicircular canals, the crus simplex of the horizontal semicircular canal, and the crus commune of the superior and posterior semicircular canals. The endolymphatic duct extends through the vestibular aqueduct to the endolymphatic sac, which is located between sheaves of dura on the posterior surface of the petrous pyramid.

The membranous labyrinth contains endolymph. The space between the bony labyrinth and the membranous labyrinth is filled with perilymph. The perilymphatic space communicates with the subarachnoid space through the cochlear aqueduct which enters the scala tympani. The endolymph is chemically similar to intracellular fluid with a high K^+ concentration and a low Na^+ concentration, whereas the perilymph resembles extracellular fluid with a low K^+ and a high Na^+. There is a resting direct current potential difference of 80 millivolts between the endolymph in the scala media and the perilymph, and the endolymph is positively charged relative to the perilymph.[33]

PHYSIOLOGY OF THE EAR

The external auditory canal maintains the temperature and humidity of the external environment of the tympanic membrane, and this environment varies very little regardless of the ambient temperature or humidity. The canal is self-cleansing. Debris is carried by the migration of a sheet of desquamated epithelial

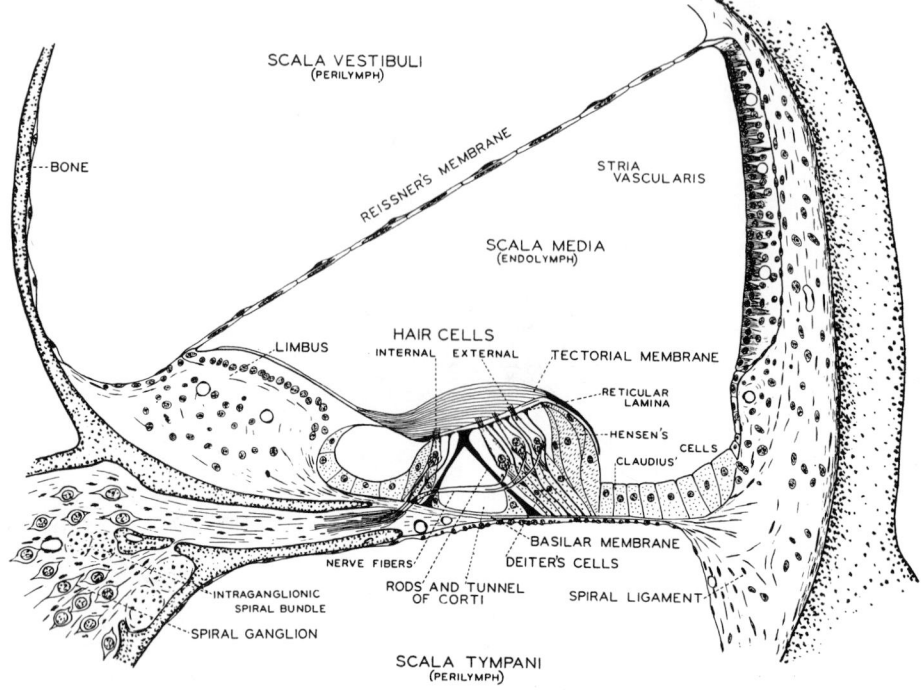

Figure 3.   Cross section of a turn of the cochlea. (From Davis, H., et al.: J. Acoust. Soc. Am., *25*:1180, 1953.)

cells from the center of the tympanic membrane to its periphery and from the medial portion of the canal to its lateral extent.[20]

Auditory Function

Sound waves impinging upon the tympanic membrane set the tympanic membrane in motion. Movement of the tympanic membrane in turn causes movement of the malleus, incus, and stapes. Movement of the stapes results in pressure changes in the fluid in the inner ear. These pressure changes result in deformation of the basilar membrane. A traveling wave is propagated in the basilar membrane from the base to the apex of the cochlea. Along the length of the basilar membrane, a point of maximal displacement occurs with each traveling wave. The location of the point of maximal displacement depends upon the frequency of the stimulating tone. High-frequency tones cause maximal displacement near the base of the cochlea. As the frequency of the stimulating tone is decreased, the point of maximal displacement moves from the base to the apex.

Displacement of the basilar membrane causes movement of the organ of Corti and deformation of the hairs of the hair cells. As the hairs of the hair cells are bent away from the modiolus, a depolarization occurs within the hair cell. An alternating current potential known as the cochlear potential or cochlear microphonic occurs in response to stimulation of the hair cells. The cochlear potential faithfully reproduces the frequency and intensity of the acoustic stimulation through a wide intensity range. A chemical transmitter is released in the region of the end-boutons of the afferent eighth nerve fibers. This chemical transmitter initiates a depolarization of the dendritic terminals of the afferent nerve.

TRAUMA AND FOREIGN BODIES

Blunt trauma to the pinna results in a subperichondrial hematoma. When bleeding occurs between the cartilage and the perichondrium, the pinna becomes a reddish purple, shapeless mass. Since the perichondrium carries the blood supply to the cartilage, the

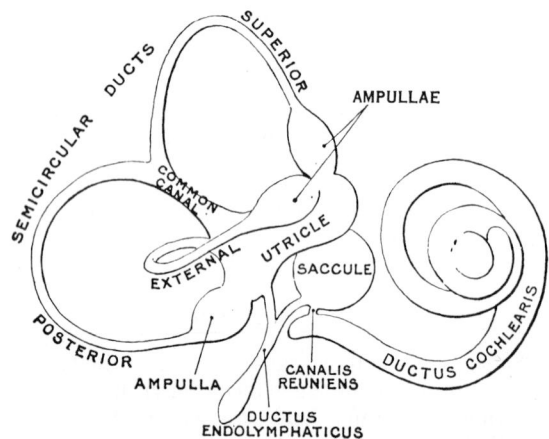

Figure 4.   Membranous labyrinth. (After Goss, C. N. (Ed.): Gray's Anatomy of the Human Body, 27th ed. Philadelphia, Lea & Febiger, 1959.)

cartilage undergoes avascular necrosis if the hematoma is present on both sides of the cartilage, and with time the pinna becomes shriveled. A hematoma may become organized and calcify, resulting in the cauliflower ear characteristic of wrestlers and boxers. Treatment consists of incision for aspiration of the clot, and packing of the skin and perichondrium tightly onto the cartilage by means of a molded splint of cotton soaked in benzoin and a pressure dressing to approximate the cartilage and its blood supply.

Lacerations of the pinna extending through skin, cartilage, and skin are repaired by suturing of the skin margins of the wound, external splinting of the cartilage of the pinna with molded cotton impregnated with benzoin, and protective dressing. Sutures are not placed in the cartilage.

Perichondritis of the pinna results in the accumulation of pus between the perichondrium and the cartilage and leads to avascular and septic necrosis of the cartilage. The infection persists for long periods. The treatment for perichondritis is wide incision for drainage and systemic antibiotic therapy. Often, perichondritis results from a gram-negative rod infection, and culture and sensitivities are of considerable importance. Incisions in the skin of the pinna on its lateral surface for drainage of hematomas and perichondritis should be made just anterior to the antihelix so that the scar will not be visible on the lateral view of the ear.

Incision of superficial infections of the pinna is to be avoided for fear of initiating perichondritis.

Foreign bodies of the external auditory canal are a common problem. Beads, erasers, beans, and other objects may be inserted by children and their siblings into their ears. An insect may find its way into the ear canal and is particularly annoying to the patient until it is killed or removed. Foreign bodies are removed by passing a blunt hook deep to the foreign body and raking it out (Fig. 5). A forceps is likely to push smooth foreign bodies ahead of it. If the foreign body is far medial, it is difficult to remove without injuring the tympanic membrane and ossicular chain. If a child is uncooperative or the mechanical problem is difficult, a general anesthetic is used for the removal of a foreign body. Metal and glass beads may be removed by irrigation, but care is used to be certain that the foreign body is not hygroscopic like a bean, because swelling with the addition of water will complicate its removal. An insect is killed to give the patient immediate relief and facilitate its removal by filling the ear canal with mineral oil. The dead insect is removed with a forceps.

The force of blows to the mandible may be transmitted to the anterior wall of the external auditory canal, which is the posterior wall of the glenoid fossa. In fractures of the anterior wall of the canal, fragments may be displaced to such a degree that stenosis of the canal results. The displaced fragments are excised under general anesthesia.

The tympanic membrane may be perforated with twigs of a tree, cotton applicators, and other objects placed in the ear canal, missiles such as hot slag in welding, and a sudden overpressure in an explosion (acoustic trauma). Perforations of the tympanic membrane may be associated with dislocations of the os-

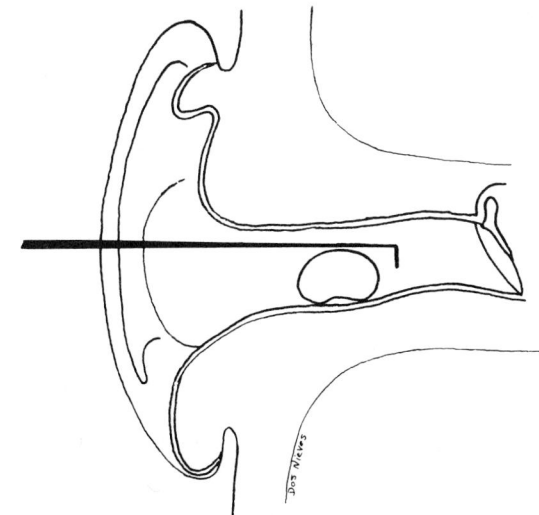

Figure 5. Technique for the removal of foreign bodies of the ear canal. The foreign body is raked out with a blunt Day hook.

sicular chain. Vertigo or a sensorineural hearing loss suggests that a portion of an ossicle or a missile has been driven into the inner ear or that there is a fistula between the perilymphatic space of the vestibule and the middle ear.[38] These conditions require prompt exploration of the middle ear for removal of fragments from the inner ear and repair of the labyrinthine fistula. Most perforations of the tympanic membrane heal spontaneously in 6 weeks. Instrumentation to approximate the wound margins of the tympanic membrane should be carried out under aseptic conditions and microscopic control. It is important to avoid infection during the healing period. The patient must be careful to avoid getting water in the ear. Topical applications carry with them the risk of introducing microorganisms. Prophylactic antibiotic therapy in the form of oral penicillin for the first 7 days is recommended. If the perforation fails to heal or if there is a persisting conductive hearing loss suggesting discontinuity of the ossicular chain, the middle ear is explored and repaired.

Fractures of the Temporal Bone

Basal skull fractures result from blunt trauma to the head, particularly to the occipital area. Basal skull fractures are in essence fractures of the temporal bone, and they are a frequent cause of profound sensorineural hearing loss. Bleeding from the ear following an injury to the skull is pathognomonic of a fracture of the temporal bone whether the bleeding is medial to an intact tympanic membrane, from the middle ear through a rupture of the tympanic membrane, or from a fracture line in the ear canal. Hemotympanum gives the tympanic membrane a blue-black color. Usually, there is a communication with the subarachnoid space through the fracture line. Often there is cerebrospinal fluid otorrhea. Cleaning of the ear canal should be avoided for fear of introducing microorganisms. The immediate danger to the patient is the development of meningitis. Therefore, prophylactic antibiotic therapy is initiated and continued for 7 to 10 days. More fractures of the temporal bone are longitudinal (80 per cent) than transverse (20 per cent) to the long axis of the petrous pyramid. Longitudinal fractures extend through the middle ear into the ear canal and cause rupture of the tympanic membrane. Transverse fractures extend across the cochlea and fallopian canal to produce a profound, permanent sensorineural hearing loss and a facial paralysis.[10] Approximately 35 per cent of longitudinal fractures produce a sensorineural hearing loss, and approximately 15 per cent produce facial paralysis. The fracture extending through the middle ear may result in a dislocation of the ossicular chain that requires subsequent repair. Persistence of a facial paralysis requires decompression of the facial nerve under certain circumstances.

INFECTIOUS DISEASES

External Otitis

Infection of the ear canal occurs in a diffuse form involving the entire canal, called external otitis generalisata, and a localized form due to furunculosis, called external otitis circumscripta. The diffuse form may be caused by a gram-negative rod such as *Escherichia coli, Pseudomonas aeruginosa,* or Proteus or by *Staphylococcus aureus.* Rarely a fungus may play a pathogenic role. Furunculosis is usually due to *Staphylococcus aureus.*

Patients with diffuse external otitis complain of itching, pain, foul-smelling discharge, and loss of hearing if the canal becomes swollen or filled with purulent debris. Tenderness on traction of the pinna and on pressure over the tragus tends to distinguish it from otitis media. The skin of the external auditory canal appears red, swollen, and littered with moist purulent debris.

Treatment with topical antibiotics and corticosteroids is efficacious. Systemic therapy is rarely necessary unless there is a spreading cellulitis about the ear. Furuncles of the canal should be allowed to resolve because incision may lead to perichondritis of the pinna.

Acute Otitis Media

Acute otitis media is an infectious inflammatory process in the middle ear, usually secondary to an upper respiratory tract infection. It is the most common localized infection in children. Most children between 1 and 5 years of age have two or three episodes of acute otitis media each winter. Acute otitis media may be viral or bacterial. Viral otitis media may resolve, or the middle ear may be secondarily invaded by bacteria. Acute suppurative otitis media is caused by group A beta hemolytic streptococcus, *Diplococcus pneumoniae, Staphylococcus aureus,* and *Haemophilus influenzae. H. influenzae* occurs in the age group under 5. In older children and adults, streptococcal infections are most common, followed by pneumococcal and staphylococcal infections. In children under 5 years of age

the same relative frequencies occur, but *Haemophilus influenzae* may predominate or take any place in the ranking. Rarely *Escherichia coli, Klebsiella pneumoniae,* and Bacteroides may produce acute otitis media.

Penicillin is the drug of choice for acute otitis media in patients over 5 years of age. In those under 5 years of age, ampicillin is preferred because of the frequency of *Haemophilus influenzae* infections. The treatment is continued for 12 days to insure resolution and prevention of the sequelae of streptococcal infections.

A myringotomy is indicated if the tympanic membrane is bulging or if the systemic symptoms and signs such as pain, fever, vomiting, and diarrhea are severe. A large curvilinear incision is made parallel to the annulus in the inferior quadrants midway between the umbo and the canal wall (Fig. 6). The appearance and movement of the tympanic membrane and the patient's hearing are followed until there is complete resolution. The management of incomplete resolution is discussed under serous and secretory otitis media.

The infectious complications of acute otitis media are acute mastoiditis, petrositis, labyrinthitis, facial paralysis, conductive and sensorineural hearing loss, epidural abscess, meningitis, brain abscess, lateral sinus thrombosis, subdural empyema, and otitic hydrocephalus. The most common intracranial complication of acute otitis media is meningitis.

Acute Mastoiditis

In acute otitis media, the infection almost invariably extends through the mastoid antrum into the mastoid cells. However, the term acute mastoiditis is not used clinically until destruction of the bony partitions between the mastoid air cells has occurred. Progression of the acute infectious process in the mastoid process is so regularly aborted by antibiotic therapy

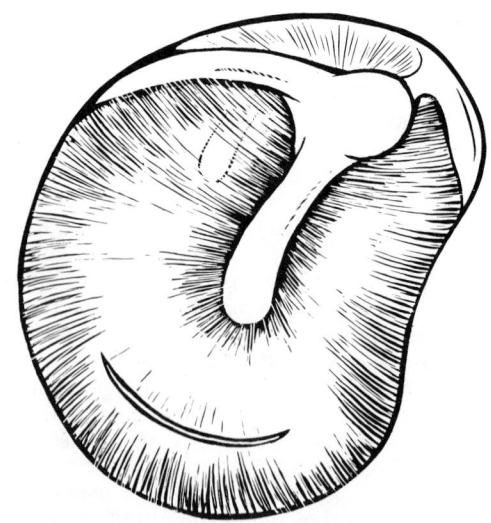

Figure 6. Myringotomy incision that occupies one fourth of the circumference of the tympanic membrane midway between the umbo and the annulus tympanicus. (From Donaldson, J. A. *In* Davis, L. (Ed.): Christopher's Textbook of Surgery, 8th ed. Philadelphia, W. B. Saunders Company, 1964.)

that clinically apparent acute mastoiditis has become a rare condition. The responsible bacteria are the same as those for acute otitis media.

Acute mastoiditis becomes clinically apparent 14 days or more after the onset of acute otitis media as one of the cortices of the mastoid process is destroyed. Usually associated with this destruction of the mastoid cortex is an exacerbation of the aural pain, fever, and otorrhea. The pain tends to be persistent and throbbing, and the discharge is usually creamy and profuse. Increasing hearing loss is characteristic of acute mastoiditis.

The lateral mastoid cortex is most frequently the first to be destroyed, and a postauricular subperiosteal abscess develops. The first signs are thickening of the postauricular tissue, reduced mobility of the skin over the mastoid cortex, and blunting of the postauricular crease. As pus exudes from the mastoid cortex deep to the periosteum, an erythematous, hot, tender, fluctuant postauricular mass develops which displaces the pinna laterally and inferiorly.

In acute otitis media, there is increased radiographic density of the mastoid air cells owing to swollen mucous membrane and purulent fluid in the air cells. In coalescent mastoiditis the air cell partitions become indistinct, and the degree of radiopacity decreases. The individual septa can no longer be seen as one air cell coalesces with another. The resulting radiographic picture suggests the appearance of shattered ice on which hot water has been poured.

In early cases of acute mastoiditis in which there are the postauricular signs of tenderness and edema but no fluctuant subperiosteal abscess, antibiotic therapy may result in complete resolution with spontaneous healing of the tympanic membrane, reventilation of the middle ear, and return of the hearing to the preinfection level.

In the presence of a subperiosteal abscess, complete exenteration of the mastoid air cells (Schwartze operation) should be performed. The operation should include inspection of a small area of the middle and posterior fossa dura to exclude an epidural abscess. The objective of the complete mastoidectomy is to drain the abscess in the mastoid air cells and antrum (Fig. 7). Through-and-through drainage of the middle ear is provided by the myringotomy or perforation anteriorly and through the antrum posteriorly. The goals of this surgery are resolution of the infection, prevention of intracranial infectious complications, spontaneous healing of the perforation of the tympanic membrane, reventilation of the middle ear, and return of the hearing to the preinfection level.

Serous and Secretory Otitis Media

Serous and secretory otitis media are manifested as sterile effusions in the middle ear. Such effusions result from incomplete resolution of acute otitis media or from eustachian tube obstruction due to inflammatory processes in the nasopharynx, allergic manifestations, hypertrophic adenoids, or benign or malignant nasopharyngeal neoplasms. Normally the middle ear is ventilated three to four times per minute as the eustachian tube opens during swallowing. If the patency of the eustachian tube is compromised, oxygen in the middle ear is absorbed by the blood in the vessels of the mucous membrane of the middle ear, and a relative negative pressure develops. At first there is mild retraction of the tympanic membrane. Soon a transudate of fluid occurs from the blood in the vessels in the mucous membrane of the middle ear. The presence of fluid in the middle ear may be recognized by an amber or dark gray color of the tympanic membrane, immobility of the tympanic membrane, and conductive hearing loss. Rarely an air-fluid level or bubbles of air may be seen through the tympanic membrane.

Treatment is directed toward correcting the under-

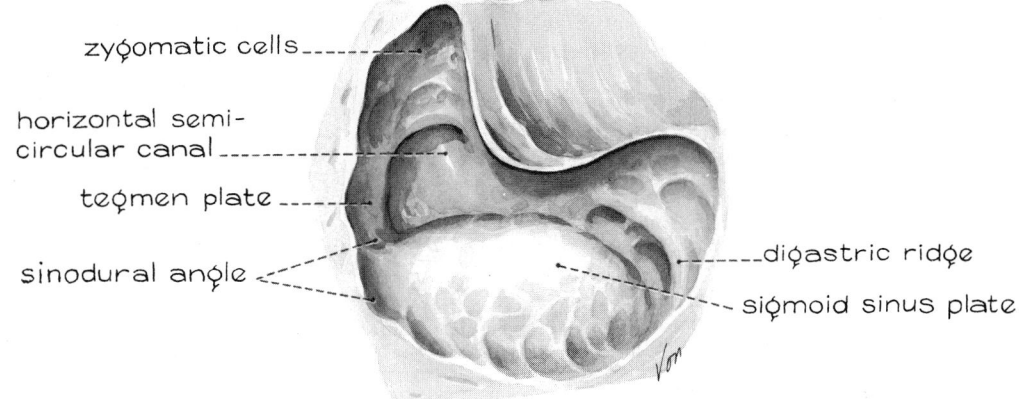

Completed mastoidectomy, moderate pneumatization

Figure 7. Complete mastoidectomy (Schwartze operation) for acute mastoiditis. All pneumatic cells in the mastoid process are removed, and the antrum is drained. The posterior and superior bony canal wall is left in place. (From Shambaugh, G. E., Jr.: Surgery of the Ear, 2nd ed. Philadelphia, W. B. Saunders Company, 1967.)

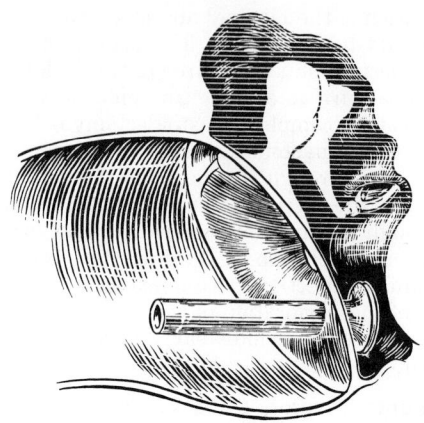

Figure 8. Tympanostomy tube placed through a myringotomy incision for ventilation of the middle ear in serous and secretory otitis media. (From Donaldson, J. A. *In* Davis, L. (Ed.): Christopher's Textbook of Surgery, 8th ed. Philadelphia, W. B. Saunders Company, 1964.)

lying condition in the nasopharynx. Myringotomy for aspiration of the fluid and insertion of a tympanostomy tube for ventilation of the middle ear ameliorate the problem of eustachian tube obstruction regardless of the cause (Fig. 8). In children, thorough adenoidectomy is frequently a necessary part of the treatment. Allergic evaluation and management with either elimination of the allergen from the patient's environment or desensitization therapy is helpful if there is an underlying allergic manifestation. Antibiotic ther-

apy for bacterial rhinitis and sinusitis is similar to that outlined for acute otitis media. Immunologic investigation is occasionally helpful. The Valsalva maneuver and politzerization are employed in the absence of tympanostomy tubes.

Chronic Otitis Media

Chronic otitis media means a permanent perforation of the tympanic membrane. Such perforations result from acute otitis media, mechanical trauma, thermal and chemical burns, and blast injuries. Chronic otitis media can be divided into two major categories depending upon the type of perforation present. There is a benign tubotympanic type, with a central perforation of the tympanic membrane, and a dangerous type, with a pars flaccida or marginal perforation.

A central perforation is one in which there is some substance of the tympanic membrane between the rim of the perforation and the bony sulcus tympanicus. These perforations result most commonly from acute otitis media produced by relatively virulent microorganisms. Exacerbations of the chronic otitis media result in painless, purulent otorrhea which may be foul-smelling and occur secondary to upper respiratory infections and when water gains access to the middle ear in bathing and swimming.

The middle ear can generally be repaired in chronic otitis media with a central perforation. A tympanoplasty provides sound protection for the round window and restores sound-pressure transformation to the oval window.[46] Wullstein categorized tympanoplastic procedures into five types (Fig. 9). The Type I tym-

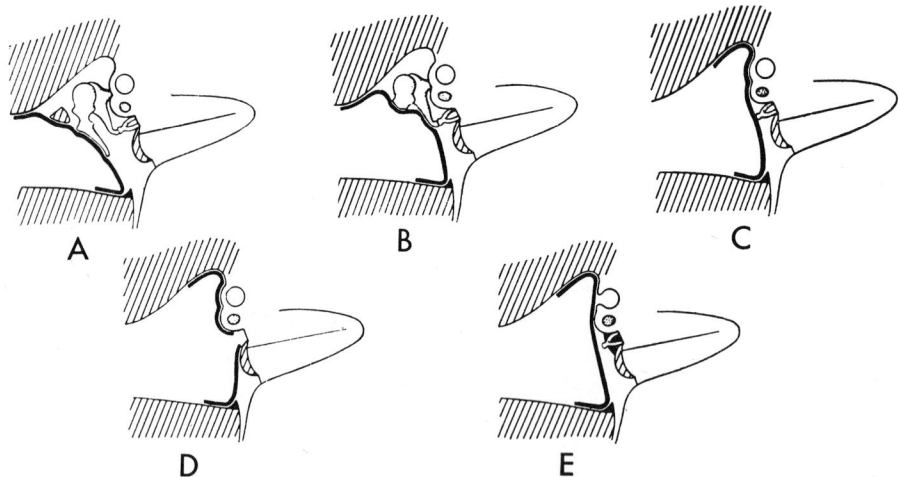

Figure 9. Five types of tympanoplasty: *A,* Type I: Perforation of the tympanic membrane repaired with soft tissue graft to the tympanic membrane remnants. *B,* Type II: Perforation of the tympanic membrane and discontinuity of the ossicular chain repaired by soft tissue graft to the tympanic membrane remnants and by rearrangement of the ossicles, bony graft, or prosthesis. *C,* Type III: Perforation of the tympanic membrane and destruction of the incus and malleus repaired by applying to the tympanic membrane remnants a soft tissue graft which is placed in contact with the head of the stapes (columellar effect). *D,* Type IV: Perforation of the tympanic membrane with destruction of the superstructure (head, neck, and crura) of the stapes repaired by creating an air-filled space between the round window and the eustachian tube to provide sound protection for the round window. *E,* Type V: Perforation of the tympanic membrane with destruction of the stapedial superstructure and fixation of its footplate repaired by protecting the round window from sound and fenestrating the horizontal semicircular canal. (From Shambaugh, G. E., Jr.: Surgery of the Ear, 2nd ed. Philadelphia, W. B. Saunders Company, 1967.)

panoplasty is applicable to the patient with a perforation of the tympanic membrane in which the ossicular chain is intact and mobile. The Type I tympanoplasty, sometimes called a myringoplasty, restores the tympanic membrane by the use of a graft of soft tissue such as temporalis muscle fascia.[14] A Type II tympanoplasty is required if there has been greater damage to the middle ear. Disruption of the ossicular chain, which often occurs as a result of necrosis of the long process of the incus, must be repaired in addition to grafting of the tympanic membrane.[14] Often the remnant of the incus can be remodeled and repositioned to reestablish the continuity of the ossicular chain. A Type III tympanoplasty is required for a still more severely damaged middle ear in which the malleus and incus are not usable and only the stapes remains. Under these circumstances, the graft is placed in contact with the head of the stapes to produce a columellar effect similar to the single middle ear ossicle or columella found in birds. Tympanoplasty Types I, II, and III include sound protection for the round window as well as sound-pressure transformation for the oval window. In more severe degrees of damage to the middle ear in which the superstructure of the stapes has been destroyed, only sound protection of the round window can be achieved by grafting from the promontory to the inferior remnant of the tympanic membrane. This Type IV tympanoplasty creates a small closed space that communicates with the eustachian tube and provides an air-filled cushion over the round window. A Type V tympanoplasty is utilized when the footplate of the stapes is fixed. It provides sound protection for the round window as in a Type IV tympanoplasty and fenestration of the horizontal semicircular canal for the admission of acoustic energy into the inner ear. This type of tympanoplasty is rarely used.

The dangerous type of chronic otitis media occurs with pars flaccida and marginal perforations. Pars flaccida perforations lead into the epitympanum and are called attic perforations. Marginal perforations usually occur in the posterior-superior portion of the pars tensa. There is no substance of tympanic membrane between the periphery of the perforation and the bony sulcus tympanicus. The annulus tympanicus has been destroyed.

Theories of the pathogenesis of perforations of the pars flaccida include progressive retraction of the pars flaccida secondary to eustachian tube obstruction, rupture during acute otitis media, and hyperactivity of the basal layer of the epidermis of the pars flaccida due to long-standing inflammation in the middle ear. Each of these mechanisms may result in an invasive cholesteatoma.[35]

A cholesteatoma occurs when the middle ear is lined with stratified squamous epithelium. The stratified squamous epithelium desquamates in this closed space. The desquamated epithelial debris cannot be cleared and accumulates in ever enlarging concentric layers. This debris serves as a culture medium for microorganisms. Cholesteatomas have the ability to destroy bone, including the tympanic ossicles, probably because of the elaboration of collagenase.[1]

Pars flaccida and marginal perforations are very frequently associated with cholesteatomas. Those cholesteatomas arising in association with pars flaccida perforations are classified as primary acquired cholesteatomas and may develop as an integral part of the development of the perforation or from the migration of stratified squamous epithelium once the perforation has occurred.

Marginal perforations are produced by acute otitis media with an especially virulent bacterium, particularly a group A beta hemolytic streptococcus, or in association with other infectious diseases such as diphtheria, chickenpox, or measles. This necrotizing otitis media destroys large areas of the tympanic membrane, including the annulus tympanicus and the middle ear mucous membrane, as well as the ossicles and their vascular and ligamentous support. During the healing process, the remaining epithelium of the mucous membrane of the middle ear migrates to cover the denuded areas. Likewise, the stratified squamous epithelium of the ear canal migrates into the middle ear to re-epithelialize the denuded areas. Once the stratified squamous epithelium is established in the middle ear, it begins to desquamate and a cholesteatoma results. Cholesteatomas developing by this mechanism are classified as secondary acquired cholesteatomas.

The presence of a cholesteatoma greatly increases the probability of the development of a serious complication such as a purulent labyrinthitis, facial paralysis, or intracranial suppurations.[43] The propensity of cholesteatomas to produce these complications stems from their ability to destroy bone and the persistence of infection in the area bearing cholesteatoma.

Cholesteatomas are usually recognized by the small bits of white, amorphous debris in the middle ear and by the destruction of the external auditory canal bone superior to the pars flaccida or marginal perforation. Cholesteatomas are often associated with aural polyps which may conceal the epithelial debris and bone destruction. Radiography of the temporal bone occasionally demonstrates destruction of bone due to an otherwise unsuspected cholesteatoma. A radiolucency in the area of the antrum measuring greater than 1 cm. in diameter should be considered suspicious of cholesteatoma.

Cholesteatomas require surgical treatment. The objective of the surgery is to exteriorize the cholesteatoma and if possible remove it. In a radical mastoidectomy, the middle ear including the attic, the antrum, and the mastoid air cell area are converted into one cavity that communicates with the exterior through the ear canal (Fig. 10). If the cholesteatoma lies superficial to the remnants of the tympanic membrane and ossicles, a modified radical mastoidectomy can be performed (Fig. 11). The modified radical mastoidectomy spares the tympanic membrane remnants and ossicles and preserves the remaining hearing. Under unusually favorable circumstances, the cholesteatoma can be completely removed and the middle ear reconstructed. Exteriorization or removal of the cholesteatoma greatly reduces the chance of intracranial complications. The primary goal of surgery for cholesteatoma is to make the ear safe, and the secondary goal is to maintain and improve the hearing.

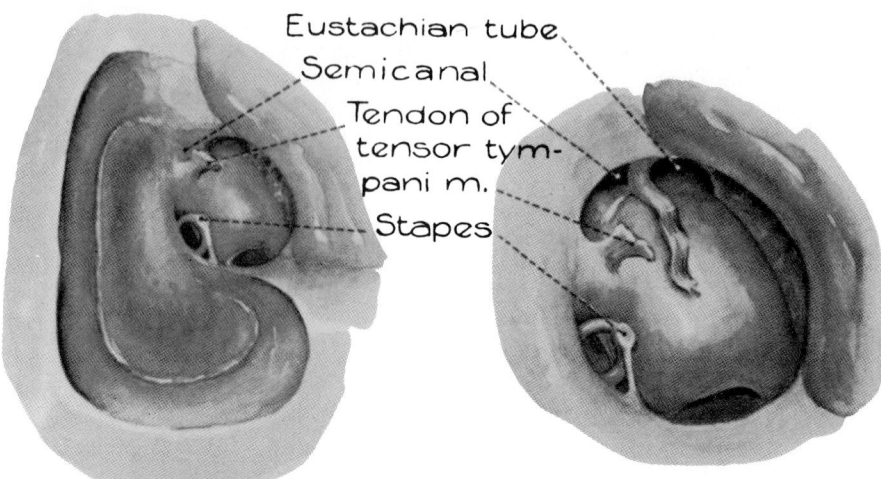

Figure 10.   Radical mastoidectomy for cholesteatoma. The cholesteatoma-bearing area is exteriorized by converting the pneumatic cell area, antrum, and middle ear into one cavity that is accessible through the external auditory canal. (From Shambaugh, G. E., Jr.: Surgery of the Ear, 2nd ed. Philadelphia, W. B. Saunders Company, 1967.)

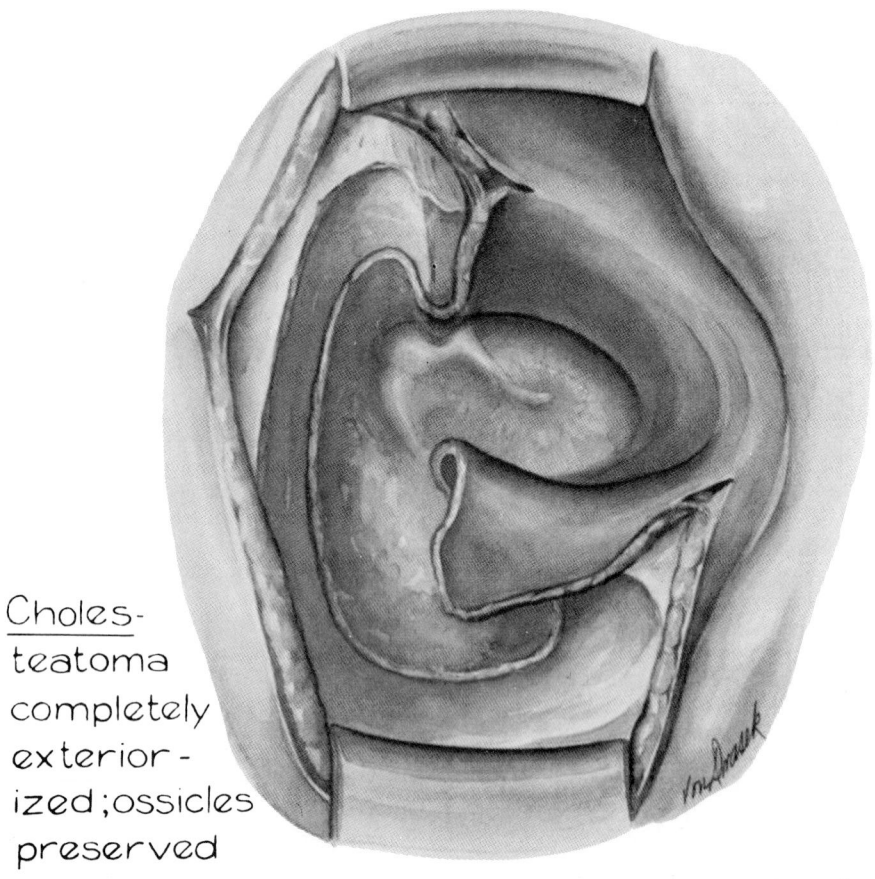

Figure 11.   Modified radical mastoidectomy for exteriorizing cholesteatoma that is superficial to the remnants of the tympanic membrane and ossicles. The remnants of the tympanic membrane and ossicles are preserved. (From Shambaugh, G. E., Jr.: Surgery of the Ear, 2nd ed. Philadelphia, W. B. Saunders Company, 1967.)

CONGENITAL MALFORMATIONS

The auricle may stand out too far from the skull and be termed an outstanding ear, lop ear, or protruding ear. The basic deformity is a lack of development of the antihelix. This deformity can be corrected surgically by weakening the spring of the cartilage of the pinna so that an antihelical fold can be created. This deformity is ideally corrected at age 5 to 6 years.

Preauricular cysts and sinuses are fairly common and may be unilateral or bilateral. They are usually asymptomatic but may become infected and require incision and drainage and later excision. Complete excision is difficult because of the ramification of these sinuses in close proximity to the branches of the facial nerve. Excision is recommended only if recurrent infection has become a problem.

Severe congenital deformities of the ear are spoken of as microtia and are frequently associated with urinary tract malformations. There may be major developmental defects in the pinna resulting in relatively small and misshaped external ears. With absence of a major portion of the auricular cartilage, surgical reconstruction rarely produces a satisfactory cosmetic result. An artistic prosthesis is the best solution to this cosmetic problem. Microtia is often associated with stenosis or atresia of the external auditory canal. These deformities are often associated with developmental abnormalities in the middle ear resulting in profound conductive hearing losses. The course of the facial nerve in the temporal bone may also be abnormal, and surgical repair of the sound-pressure transformation apparatus of the middle ear is hazardous.[37] In unilateral defects with normal hearing in the other ear, middle ear reconstruction is not recommended because of the danger of facial nerve injury. However, if there is a bilateral profound hearing loss, attempts at reconstruction should be made. A bone conduction hearing aid will contribute to the habilitation if surgical reconstruction is not feasible. Congenital malformations of the inner ear resulting in profound sensorineural hearing losses may or may not be associated with abnormalities of the external and middle ear. The evaluation of congenital malformation of the ear is facilitated by radiographic polytomography of the temporal bone.

IDIOPATHIC DISEASES

Otosclerosis

Otosclerosis is the most common cause of a progressive conductive hearing loss in the adult with a normal ear drum. Otosclerosis is a disease of the bone of the otic capsule with predilection for the anterior part of the oval window. Histologically, foci of otosclerosis show irregularly arranged, immature bone interspersed with numerous vascular channels. As the focus of the otosclerotic bone enlarges, it causes ankylosis of the footplate of the stapes and produces a conductive hearing loss. A second site of predilection is the posterior part to the oval window.

Otosclerosis tends to run in families. It is more common in women than in men. Approximately 10 per cent of the adult white population have foci of otosclerosis. Only one in 10 of these, or approximately 1 per cent of the white population, has clinical otosclerosis as evidenced by conductive hearing loss. Otosclerosis is rare in blacks, American Indians, and Japanese. It is common in Asiatic Indians. Otosclerosis also produces a sensorineural hearing loss if the focus is adjacent to the scala media. The conductive hearing loss becomes clinically evident in the late teenage and early adult years. The fixation of the stapes may progress rapidly during pregnancy. The conductive hearing loss can be corrected surgically in the vast majority of instances. With microsurgical techniques, the stapes is removed and replaced by a prosthesis. The most widely used prosthesis is one composed of stainless steel wire and cellulose sponge. The wire, which is shaped like a shepherd's crook, is crimped around the long process of the incus, and the sponge is placed in the oval window (Fig. 12). A membrane forms across the oval window which embeds the stainless steel wire in it. The sound conduction characteristics of this arrangement are excellent. The complication of a profound sensorineural hearing loss occurs in 2 to 4 per cent of patients. If a good initial hearing result is obtained, ordinarily a good result is maintained.

Meniere's Disease

Meniere's disease is characterized by hearing loss, tinnitus, and recurrent prostrating vertigo. The pathologic change in the inner ear is generalized dilatation of the membranous labyrinth, or endolymphatic hydrops. Only one ear is involved in 85 per cent of the patients with Meniere's disease. The sensorineural hearing loss is initially more severe in the lower frequencies than in the higher frequencies. The hearing tends to fluctuate. It is depressed after an attack of vertigo. The tinnitus has a low-pitched, roaring quality and is worse just before, during, and after an attack of vertigo. The attacks of vertigo occur suddenly,

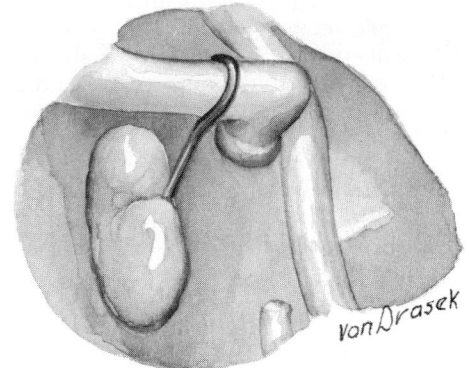

Figure 12. Stapedectomy with replacement of the stapes with a stainless steel wire and cellulose sponge prosthesis. The wire is crimped around the long process of the incus, and the cellulose sponge is in the oval window. (From Shambaugh, G. E., Jr.: Surgery of the Ear, 2nd ed. Philadelphia, W. B. Saunders Company, 1967.)

last from a few to 24 hours, and subside gradually. The attacks are associated with nausea and vomiting. The patient often has a full feeling or a pressure sensation in the affected ear. Over the course of many years, the hearing becomes progressively worse.

Neither medical nor surgical therapy has been demonstrated to be effective in arresting the progression of the hearing disorder or preventing recurrent attacks of vertigo. There are a number of drugs that are effective in suppressing the vertigo and its side effects. Cholinolytic agents such as atropine and scopolamine reduce the autonomic side effects. Phenothiazines, antihistamines, and barbiturates are effective, and diphenhydramine is widely used. Perhaps the most effective agent in suppressing vertigo is diazepam.[23] A number of operations have been advocated for the treatment of the patient who is disabled by the frequency of the recurrent attacks of vertigo. Fick introduced the sacculotomy in which the saccule is ruptured with a pick placed through the footplate of the stapes.[9] Cody has advocated the placement of a stainless steel tack through the footplate of the stapes so that a sacculotomy is performed each time the membranous labyrinth begins to distend.[6] House has advocated the production of an artificial communication between the membranous labyrinth and subarachnoid space.[15] The middle cranial fossa approach for transection of the vestibular division of the eighth nerve is a logical approach to the control of vertigo in Meniere's disease, but it requires further evaluation.[16] A labyrinthectomy can be performed if the vertigo is sufficiently disabling and the hearing has degenerated to a useless level.

Bell's Palsy

Bell's palsy is an idiopathic unilateral facial paralysis that develops suddenly and is accompanied by pain in the postauricular area. All divisions of the nerve are paralyzed; this distinguishes the disease from a supranuclear lesion. The lesion is in the vertical portion of the intratemporal course of the nerve. The initial pathologic changes are hyperemia and edema. The edema compresses the blood supply to the nerve because of the bony confines of the fallopian canal. A conduction block develops without death or degeneration of the axons. Release of the pressure on the nerve results in rapid recovery of function. This type of paralysis is spoken of as neurapraxia. It should be differentiated from axonotmesis in which the pressure on the nerve is sufficiently severe to result in death of the axons distal to the compression within a period of several days. Neurotmesis designates complete transection of the facial nerve. In neurapraxia the flow of axoplasm has been interrupted; with resumption of the flow of axoplasm, the function of the distal axon recovers.

Nerve excitability testing is performed to determine whether neurapraxia or axonotmesis or neurotmesis exists. As long as muscular contraction can be induced at approximately the same direct current stimulus intensity on the affected side as on the normal side, the paralysis is probably a neurapraxia, and complete recovery may be anticipated. Loss of nerve excitability is an indication for decompression of the facial nerve by removing the bone of the fallopian canal through a mastoidectomy approach. Approximately 85 per cent of all patients with idiopathic facial nerve paralysis recover spontaneously. If recovery has not begun at 3 weeks after the onset of the facial paralysis, the chance of spontaneous recovery is greatly reduced. Ordinarily, facial nerve decompression is performed 3 weeks after the onset if there has been no recovery, or at any time when the nerve excitability deteriorates.

NEOPLASMS

Squamous cell and basal cell carcinomas frequently develop on the pinna of those who are exposed to the sun. Early lesions can be successfully treated with irradiation or cautery and curettage. Surgical excision of a V-shaped wedge or larger amounts of the pinna is required in more advanced lesions. Invasion of cartilage usually dictates against radiation therapy and makes surgery the treatment of choice. Squamous cell and basal cell carcinomas also arise in the external auditory canal and under these circumstances require extensive resection in order to offer the best chance of cure. En bloc resection of the external auditory canal with sparing of the facial nerve is performed for lesions that are limited to the ear canal and have not invaded the middle ear.[7] Squamous cell carcinoma may arise in the middle ear. Persistent otorrhea of chronic otitis media predisposes to squamous cell carcinomas arising in the middle ear and the external auditory canal. Squamous cell carcinoma involving the middle ear requires resection of the temporal bone to obtain an adequate margin around the tumor.

Ceruminomas arise in the outer one third of the external auditory canal. Although these tumors appear to be benign histologically, they behave in a malignant manner and should be widely excised.

Chemodectomas arise in the middle ear. These nonchromaffin paragangliomas are called glomus jugulare or glomus tympanicus tumors depending on their site of origin. The glomus tympanicus tumor arises from the area of Jacobson's nerve in the tympanic plexus on the promontory of the middle ear. The glomus jugulare tumor arises from the glomus jugulare body in the jugular bulb. Both tumors consist of rich networks of vascular spaces surrounded by epithelioid cells. Usually the tumors grow slowly, and symptoms may not be evident until the tumor is quite large. Pulsatile tinnitus, facial nerve paralysis, otorrhea, hemorrhage, vertigo, and paralysis of cranial nerves IX, X, XI, and XII are often the presenting symptoms and signs. Characteristically, a red mass that pulsates and blanches with compression with a pneumatic otoscope can be seen in the ear canal or middle ear. There may be x-ray evidence of bone erosion in the mastoid process, middle ear, or petrous pyramid. Treatment consists of excision of the smaller tumors with or without a radical mastoidectomy. With large lesions, radiation therapy is the treatment of choice.

Acoustic neurinomas account for approximately 7 per cent of all intracranial tumors. They arise twice as often from the vestibular division of the eighth nerve as from the auditory division. These tumors are derived from Schwann cells. Initially, they produce tinnitus and a neural hearing loss. The patient complains of unsteadiness or imbalance. True vertigo is not a common complaint. The hearing loss is predominantly a high-tone loss with greater impairment of the speech discrimination than would be expected with a cochlear lesion producing the same amount of pure-tone hearing loss. Békésy audiometry is Type III or IV.[18] Loudness recruitment is absent. Tone decay is present. The short increment sensitivity index is low.[19] Hallpike caloric testing usually shows canal paresis on the involved side.[4] Initially, the tumor is confined to the internal auditory meatus. As it increases in size, it projects into the cerebellopontine angle and begins to compress the cerebellum and brain stem. With the passage of time, the fifth and ultimately the seventh cranial nerves become involved.[42] Papilledema is a late sign of acoustic neurinomas. Early diagnosis is based on auditory findings suggesting a neural loss of hearing, hypoactivity on caloric stimulation, laminagraphy and polytomography of the internal auditory meatus, computerized tomography, and myelography of the posterior fossa. Large acoustic neurinomas are removed through an occipital craniotomy. For the removal of small tumors microsurgical approaches have been developed that utilize a translabyrinthine route if no useful hearing remains and a middle cranial fossa route for the preservation of the

remaining hearing (Fig. 13). Both routes allow preservation of the facial nerve. For very large tumors, the combined occipital and translabyrinthine approach offers the best chance of complete removal.[17]

THE NOSE AND THE PARANASAL SINUSES

In ancient India, adultery was punished by amputation of the nose. Suśruta circa A.D. 1000 described the reconstruction of the nose with a pedicle flap from the cheek. Another ancient Indian method described the forehead flap. Tagliacozzi in Renaissance Italy developed the arm-to-nose pedicle graft. Sir William Fergusion in 1845 introduced an approach for tumors of the nose and paranasal sinuses. It included splitting the lip in the midline as well as a horizontal incision along the inferior orbital rim to reflect the soft tissues of the face laterally. Ingals introduced nasal septal surgery by partial excision of the nasal septum for deviation of the septum in 1882. This operation was later improved by Krieg in 1899 and by Freer in 1902.

In 1903, Killian was the first to operate for an infection in the frontal sinus; and in 1904, he refined the submucous resection of the nasal septum. Joseph, at the turn of the century in Berlin, developed techniques and principles upon which the modern rhinoplasty is based.

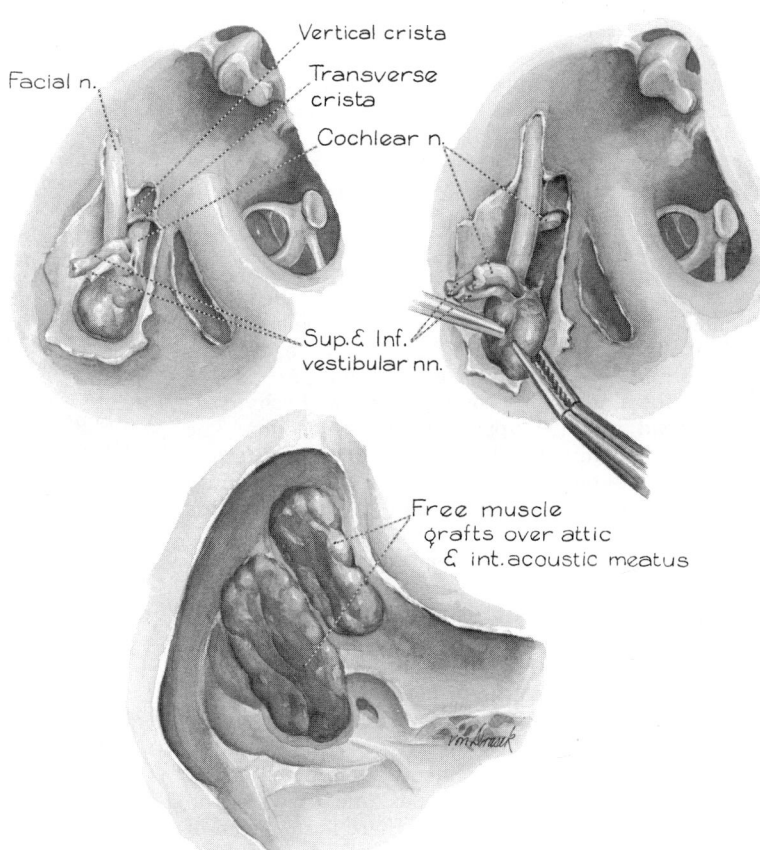

Figure 13. Translabyrinthine approach to the internal auditory canal for acoustic neurinomas. (From Shambaugh, G. E., Jr.: Surgery of the Ear, 2nd ed. Philadelphia, W. B. Saunders Company, 1967.)

ANATOMY OF THE NOSE AND PARANASAL SINUSES

The skeleton of the nose consists of the nasal bones, the ascending processes of the maxilla, the upper lateral cartilages, the lower lateral cartilages, and the septal cartilage. The nasal septum makes up the medial wall of each nasal cavity. The lateral wall of each nasal cavity provides the attachment for the three turbinates. The inferior turbinate is the largest of the three. It extends from far anterior in the nasal cavity to the choana. The middle turbinate is somewhat smaller. Although it extends to the choana, its anterior tip is 2 cm. posterior to the anterior tip of the inferior turbinate. Its attachment to the lateral wall of the nasal cavity is oblique from superior anteriorly to inferior posteriorly. The superior turbinate arises from the far posterior-superior portion of the lateral wall of the nasal cavity. Inferior to the inferior turbinate is the inferior meatus. The nasolacrimal duct opens into the inferior meatus. The middle meatus lies between the middle turbinate and the inferior turbinate. The ostia of the maxillary and anterior ethmoid cells and the nasofrontal duct are in the middle meatus. The superior meatus lies between the superior turbinate and the middle turbinate. The ostia of the posterior ethmoid cells are in the superior meatus. The ostium of the sphenoid sinus is in the posterior part of the superior meatus, the sphenoethmoid recess.

TRAUMA AND FOREIGN BODIES

Nasal Fracture

The nose is a vulnerable leading part. Fractures of the nasal bones are the most common fractures of the facial bones. Fractures of the nose may involve the ascending processes of the maxillas and the nasal processes of the frontal bones as well as the nasal bones. A fracture of the nose is nearly always an open fracture. The skin of the dorsum of the nose may be lacerated, and the mucous membrane in the nasal cavity is nearly always torn. The most common deformity is a deviation of the nasal bones to the right with depression of the nasal bones on the left, characteristically occurring with a right hook. Fractures of the nose may be associated with septal fractures and hematomas.

Fractures of the nasal bones are almost always associated with bleeding from the nose due to the tear of the mucous membrane. A fracture should be suspected if blunt injury causes bleeding from the nose. Soft tissue swelling occurs fairly promptly and may tend to obscure the underlying bony deformity. Ecchymosis may spread into the upper and lower eyelids. The diagnosis can ordinarily be established by gentle palpation of the dorsum of the nose. Any deformity suggests a fracture. At times instability and crepitus may be demonstrated as well as point tenderness. X-rays of the nasal bones will tend to confirm the diagnosis. Linear radiolucencies parallel to the long axis of the nasal bones are usually nutrient vessels. Radiolucencies transverse to the long axis of the nasal bones are usually fractures. Displacement of the bony fragments may be demonstrated; however, the degree of displacement is more readily determined by physical examination.

Fractures of the nasal complex are often associated with fractures of other facial bones, and x-rays of the paranasal sinuses are obtained if there is suspicion of fracture of the other facial bones. Trauma to the facial bones is often associated with a cerebrospinal fluid rhinorrhea. After injury to the central portion of the face, the patient is specifically examined for cerebrospinal fluid rhinorrhea by having him tip his head forward and collecting any drainage from the nose. Cerebrospinal rhinorrhea requires prophylactic antibiotic therapy to prevent meningitis. The patient is instructed to avoid blowing the nose. In most cases cerebrospinal fluid rhinorrhea ceases spontaneously. If the rhinorrhea does not cease within 14 to 21 days, the dural leak is repaired through a frontal craniotomy.

Nasal fractures in adults may be reduced under local anesthesia. General anesthesia is necessary for the reduction of nasal fractures in children. The local anesthesia required is similar to that used for a rhinoplasty. Thorough anesthesia is the key to a satisfactory reduction of the nasal bones. The fracture is manipulated into a good position by internal traction on the fracture fragments with a blunt periosteal elevator in association with external traction with the fingers. The need for internal and external splinting depends on the postreduction stability of the fracture.

If blunt trauma to the nose is neglected, it results in permanent deformity which ultimately requires septal surgery to improve the airway and rhinoplasty to improve the appearance of the nose.

Fractures of the nasal septum may be reduced at the same time as the reduction of the fracture of the nasal bones. Often these fractures are difficult to maintain in a position of good alignment and require a subsequent septoplasty or submucous resection of the nasal septum.

Septal hematomas lie between the quadrilateral cartilage and the perichondrium. If the perichondrium has been elevated from both sides of the septal cartilage, the cartilage will undergo avascular necrosis. Septal hematomas frequently become infected, and abscess formation produces avascular and septic necrosis of the septal cartilage which results in a saddle deformity of the nose. Septal hematomas are incised and drained as soon as the diagnosis is made. An incision in the mucoperichondrium over the anterior part of the hematoma allows access for aspiration. The perichondrium is placed in contact with the septal cartilage by packing the nasal cavity with petrolatum gauze.

Septal abscesses are located between the cartilage and the perichondrium. They may involve both sides of the cartilage. Septal abscesses are incised and drained under general anesthesia as soon as the diagnosis is established. Incisions are made bilaterally if there is pus on both sides of the septum. A small rubber drain is sutured to a lip of the wound until the drainage subsides. Vigorous systemic antibiotic therapy is employed.

Deviations of the Nasal Septum

Deviations of the nasal septum may be caused by trauma or occur as developmental abnormalities, particularly in persons with highly arched palates. The nasal bones and septum are frequently fractured at the time of birth. This injury is of the greenstick type, and often it will correct itself. However, correction is usually simply accomplished by moving the nose digitally back toward the midline. Slight anterior traction is applied to the tip of the nose during this maneuver. No internal or external splinting is required.

Deviations of the nasal septum produce varying degrees of nasal obstruction and predispose the patient to sinusitis, particularly if the deviation tends to obstruct one of the ostia of the paranasal sinuses during acute inflammatory processes, and to epistaxis as a result of drying air currents over the deflected septum. The caudal edge of the nasal septum may be dislocated and produce an external deformity at the columella.

Deviations of the septum are corrected by septoplasty or submucous resection of the nasal septum. In these procedures, the mucoperichondrium is elevated from both sides of the septum. The deviated cartilage and bone are resected or remodeled to straighten the septum.

Perforations of the nasal septum may be secondary to nasal surgery or repeated trauma, as in picking the nose. In the past, perforations due to syphilis and tuberculosis were common. Perforations of the septum produce crusting about their margins and repeated epistaxis. Small perforations whistle. Septal perforations are closed by the development of opposing mucoperichondrial flaps over free grafts of fascia.[8]

Rhinoplasty is performed for physiologic as well as cosmetic purposes. A deformed nose is usually associated with airway obstruction. The aims of rhinoplasty are to eliminate the airway obstruction and to correct the external deformity of the nose. Usually rhinoplasty is performed under local anesthesia. The surgical procedure is directed toward the cartilaginous and bony framework of the nose. The soft tissue of the nose conforms postoperatively to the modification of the bony and cartilaginous framework. As a general rule, modification of each element of the nasal skeleton is necessary in order to achieve aesthetically pleasing results. Saddle deformities of the nose may be corrected by augmentation with autogenous bone or silicone rubber implants.

Foreign Bodies

Children put all manner of objects in their noses. Erasers, beans, buttons, pebbles, wool nap, paper, and sponge rubber are common foreign bodies. A foreign body in the nasal cavity produces a severe inflammatory reaction and causes a foul-smelling, bloody, unilateral discharge. Removal of the foreign body is facilitated by producing vasoconstriction anterior to it with a topical sympathomimetic amine such as phenylephrine. The foreign body is removed by placing a blunt hook posterior to it and raking it anteriorly. Attempts at grasping smooth, firm foreign bodies with forceps tend to push them farther posteriorly. General anesthesia is used if good cooperation from a child cannot be obtained by gentle reassurance.

If a foreign body dwells long in the nose, mineral salts are deposited on it and produce a rhinolith. The rhinolith tends to conform to the contour of the nasal cavity, and its removal is usually difficult.

SINUSITIS

Acute rhinitis is the usual manifestation of a common cold. Acute sinusitis is usually initiated by an acute respiratory tract infection of viral etiology. Nearly all cases of acute sinusitis and most cases of chronic sinusitis respond well to antibiotic therapy. The complications of acute and chronic sinusitis often require surgery, as does unresponsive chronic sinusitis. Complications of maxillary sinusitis are rare. Ethmoid sinusitis is frequently complicated in children by orbital cellulitis and abscess. Eighty per cent of all cases of orbital cellulitis are secondary to ethmoid sinusitis. In the patient who presents with erythema and swelling of the eyelids, proptosis, and displacement of the globe laterally and inferiorly, the source of the infection is sought by inspection of the nose for mucopus in the middle meatus and radiography of the paranasal sinuses for ethmoid sinusitis. Ethmoid sinusitis and its orbital cellulitis respond well to systemic antibiotic therapy. If the proptosis fails to subside or progresses, incision and drainage of the abscess, which is between the lamina papyracea and the orbital periosteum, is performed through a Killian incision that extends from the lateral aspect of the nose to the eyebrow. The orbital periosteum is elevated from the medial wall of the orbit so that the abscess cavity can be reached. The optic nerve tolerates 11 to 14 mm. of proptosis. The point at which extraocular motion is lost is also the limit of stretch of the optic nerve. Therefore, incision and drainage of an orbital abscess is performed prior to complete loss of extraocular motion to prevent permanent blindness.

Frontal sinusitis may cause intracranial complications such as meningitis, epidural abscess, subdural empyema, and brain abscess. In severe acute frontal sinusitis that fails to respond promptly to systemic antibiotic therapy, the anterior wall of the frontal sinus is trephined through an incision in the medial part of the eyebrow. An opening of approximately 7 to 8 mm. is made, and a catheter is placed in the sinus to maintain drainage. Trephination is performed in an attempt to prevent the intracranial complications of frontal sinusitis.

Fractures of the frontal sinus lead to the development of mucoceles. Mucoceles result from duplication of the mucous membrane. They gradually enlarge and destroy the floor of the frontal sinus; and as they expand into the orbital cavity, they produce proptosis and inferior and lateral displacement of the eye. Mucoceles and other other forms of chronic frontal sinusitis that do not respond to medical management can be managed surgically by an osteoplastic flap approach for obliteration of the frontal sinus (Fig. 14). The incision in the bone is made at the periphery of the frontal sinus, and the anterior wall is rotated inferiorly on the hinge of periosteum at the floor of the sinus. Infected mucous membrane is removed with a motor-driven burr under microscopic control, and the cavity of the frontal sinus is obliterated by the implantation of fat taken from the abdominal wall.

Approximately 25 per cent of cases of chronic maxillary sinusitis are secondary to a dental infection. In chronic maxillary sinusitis, radiographs of the apices

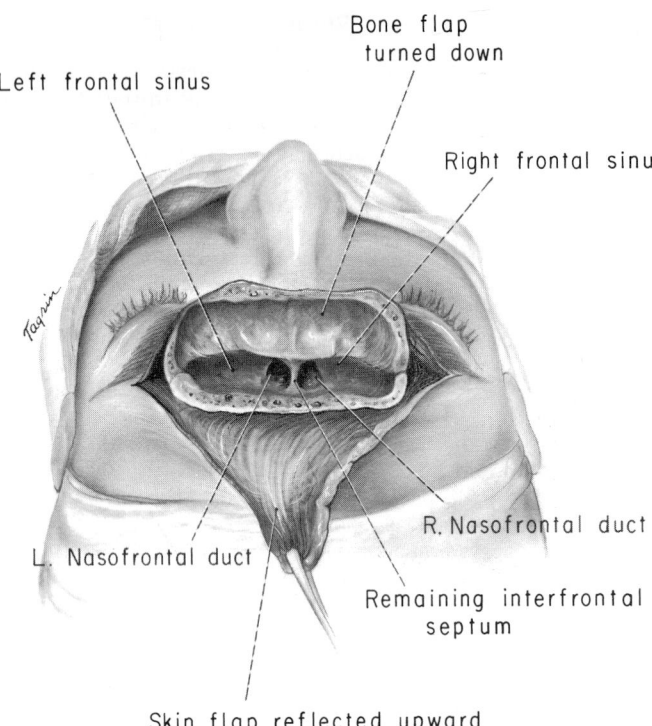

Left frontal sinus

Bone flap
turned down

Right frontal sinus

R. Nasofrontal duct

Remaining interfrontal
septum

L. Nasofrontal duct

Skin flap reflected upward

Figure 14. Approach to the frontal sinuses by the use of an osteoplastic flap for obliteration of the sinuses. (From Goodale, R. L., and Montgomery, W. W.: Arch. Otolaryngol., 79:522, 1964.)

VIEW FROM HEAD OF THE TABLE

of the teeth should be obtained to exclude the possibility of a periapical abscess.

Chronic maxillary sinusitis that does not respond to medical management may be controlled with the Caldwell-Luc operation, which is a maxillary sinusotomy performed through an incision in the canine fossa. The bone of the anterior wall of the maxillary sinus is resected to permit access to the interior of the sinus for removal of infected mucous membrane, cysts, and epithelial debris. Drainage of the maxillary sinus is improved by creating a nasoantral window in the inferior meatus.

Chronic ethmoid sinusitis is usually associated with allergic rhinitis and the formation of nasal polyps. In those persons in whom the formation of nasal polyps and the symptoms of ethmoid sinusitis cannot be controlled adequately by intranasal polypectomy and medical management including desensitization, an ethmoidectomy is indicated. Ethmoidectomy is performed intranasally and through an external approach utilizing a Killian incision. In the external ethmoidectomy, the orbital periosteum is elevated, and the lamina papyracea is removed to give access to the ethmoid air cells. Infected mucous membrane, polypoid tissue, and epithelial debris are removed. The anterior half of the middle turbinate is excised to create a large opening between the ethmoid air cells and the nasal cavity. In essence, an ethmoidectomy incorporates the ethmoid air cell area into the nasal cavity.

Chronic sphenoid sinusitis that does not respond to medical management may be controlled by an operation in which the sphenoid sinus is approached through an external ethmoidectomy. After an external ethmoidectomy has been accomplished, the anterior wall of the sphenoid sinus is resected to remove infected mucous membrane, polypoid tissue, and epithelial debris. The anterior and inferior walls of the sphenoid sinus are removed. In this way, the interior of the sphenoid sinus is incorporated in the posterior part of the nasal cavity and the nasopharynx, and in essence, the sphenoid sinus is eliminated as a separate entity.

Epistaxis

Bleeding from the nose is a common clinical problem. Ninety per cent of the time epistaxis is from a plexus of vessels in the anterior-inferior part of the septum. In the other 10 per cent of cases nasal bleeding occurs from the posterior part of the nose, particularly from far posterior in the inferior meatus at the junction of the inferior meatus and the nasopharynx. It is from this area that persons with arteriosclerosis and hypertension are likely to bleed. This type of bleeding may be difficult to control and is associated with a 4 to 5 per cent mortality. Mild epistaxis from the anterior part of the nasal septum is usually effectively controlled by steady pressure applied by squeezing the mobile portion of the nose between the index finger and thumb for 5 to 10 minutes. Treatment for epistaxis that is not controlled by this simple measure requires visualization of the bleeding point. The bleeding point can be controlled temporarily and anesthesia achieved with pressure applied over a cotton pledget impregnated with a vasoconstrictor and a topically active local anesthetic such as tetracaine (Pontocaine). The bleeding point can be cauterized chemically or with electrocautery. Silver nitrate is preferred as the cauterizing agent, since it produces satisfactory intravascular coagulation without a severe burn of the mucous membrane. If the bleeding cannot be easily controlled with cautery or if the bleeding point cannot be visualized, strips of $1/2$ inch petrolatum gauze are used to apply pressure to the bleeding point. Pressure is applied as atraumatically as possible. This method is preferred in a patient with a bleeding tendency since the periphery of a cauterized area may begin to bleed.

In order to pack the posterior part of the nasal cavity, the choana is obstructed with the balloon of a Foley catheter (Fig. 15) or a postnasal pack (Fig. 16). Although the Foley catheter is easier to insert, the gauze postnasal pack is more secure. The postnasal pack is made by folding and rolling 4 × 4 inch gauze squares into a tight pack and tying the pack with two strands of No. 2 black silk. The ends of one tie are oriented inferiorly, and the ends of the other tie are oriented superiorly. After topical anesthesia of the nose, nasopharynx, and pharynx has been induced, a catheter is introduced through the nasal cavity on the side of the bleeding and brought out through the mouth. The superiorly oriented ends of the tie are tied to the catheter, and the catheter is withdrawn from the nose

as the pack is placed posterior to the soft palate into the nasopharynx. The inferiorly oriented ends of the tie are trimmed below the level of the soft palate so that they can be utilized in removing the pack. The superiorly oriented strands are held taut while the nasal cavity is firmly packed with petrolatum gauze. If the bleeding point is in the inferior meatus, this area is packed tightly. The superiorly oriented strands are tied over a roll of a 4 × 4 inch gauze square. The packing is left in place for 4 days. Prophylactic antibiotic therapy is indicated to prevent sinusitis and otitis media. Patients requiring postnasal packing generally have serious systemic vascular diseases. They have a low arterial pO_2 while the packing is in place and should be given supplemental humidified oxygen by mask.

An alternate method of treatment of patients with severe bleeding from the posterior part of the nose is ligation of the internal maxillary artery (Fig. 17).[5] The artery is reached through the maxillary sinus. An incision is made in the canine fossa, and the anterior wall of the maxillary sinus is removed as in the Caldwell-Luc operation. The bone of the posterior wall of the sinus is removed, and the internal maxillary artery and its branches are gently dissected under microscopic control from the adipose tissue in the pterygomaxillary fossa.[21] Metallic clips are placed on the internal maxillary artery as it enters the fossa and its major branches, the sphenopalatine and descending palatine arteries, as they leave the fossa. This method avoids nasal packing and the problems of hypoxemia associated with it, requires less hospitalization, and involves less discomfort for the patient.[11]

Severe epistaxis is often associated with pre-existing liver disease. Large amounts of blood may have been swallowed prior to the nasal packing. Blood is eliminated from the gastrointestinal tract as promptly as possible by the use of cathartics and enemas. Sterilization of the gastrointestinal tract to prevent the breakdown of blood by microorganisms and the absorption of ammonia is indicated in the presence of liver disease.

Replacement of blood that has been lost as a result of the epistaxis is carried out as indicated by the hemoglobin and hematocrit determinations as well as by the patient's vital signs.

A particularly debilitating form of epistaxis occurs in hereditary hemorrhagic telangiectasia (Rendu-Osler-Weber disease). Patients with this disease have frequent bleeding from the nose and gastrointestinal tract. Often the bleeding from the nose is sufficient to cause a chronic anemia that cannot be overcome by iron supplementation. A septal dermoplasty, in which the mucous membrane of the anterior portions of the nasal cavity is replaced with a split-thickness skin graft, is very effective in reducing the severity and frequency of the epistaxis so that the hemoglobin concentration may be brought to the normal level.[36]

CONGENITAL MALFORMATIONS

Choanal Atresia

Choanal atresia is a malformation in which the opening of the nasal cavity into the nasopharynx is ob-

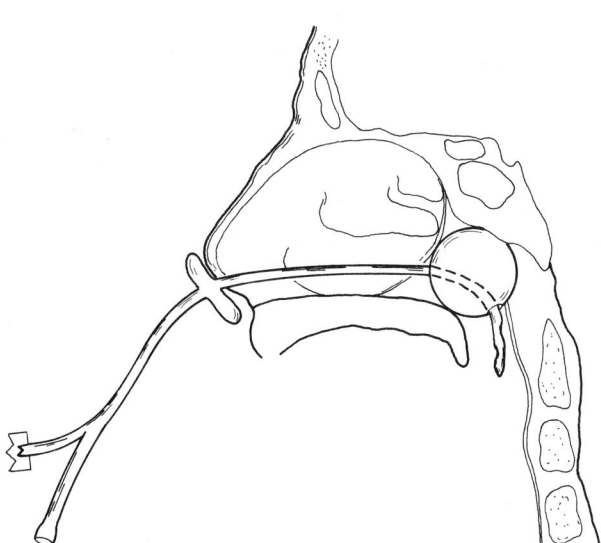

Figure 15. Use of a Foley catheter to obstruct the choana so that petrolatum gauze may be used to pack the nasal cavity tightly without prolapse of the packing in the nasopharynx.

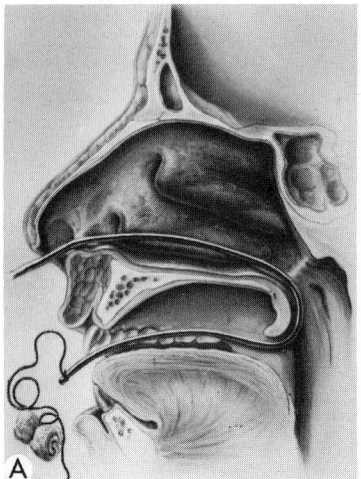
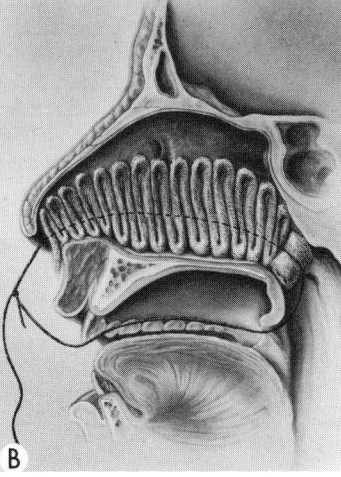

Figure 16. Packing of the nose for epistaxis with a postnasal pack and an anterior nasal pack. (From Boies, L. R., et al.: Fundamentals of Otolaryngology, A Textbook of Ear, Nose and Throat Diseases, 4th ed. Philadelphia, W. B. Saunders Company, 1964.)

structed by a partition of mucous membrane and bone. The malformation may occur unilaterally or bilaterally. If it occurs bilaterally, it produces respiratory distress in the neonate. Newborn infants are obligatory nasal breathers. If there is obstruction to the nasal airway, asphyxia will occur. The newborn presses his tongue against the roof of his mouth during the inspiratory effort. Fortunately, crying with its attendant mouth breathing often allows some ventilatory exchange. This diagnosis should be made in the delivery room. Choanal atresia should be considered in the infant who makes respiratory effort but fails to accomplish ventilatory exchange. The immediate solution to the problem is the insertion of an oral airway. The nursing care of the oral airway during the next 2 to 3 weeks must be extremely meticulous. After 2 to 3

weeks the newborn learns to breathe through his mouth, and the danger abates. Some advocate perforation of the atretic area in the neonatal period for the insertion of polyethylene tubes. This operation often fails to provide permanent improvement, and a better repair can be performed when the child is 4 to 5 years of age through a transpalatal approach (Fig. 18). With careful nursing supervision of the oral airway, a tracheotomy can be avoided in the neonatal period. The diagnosis is made by attempting without success to pass a catheter through the nose into the pharynx. The diagnosis is confirmed by instilling radiopaque dye into the nasal cavity and taking a lateral x-ray of the nasopharynx in the supine position. If choanal atresia is present, the dye pools in the posterior part of the nasal cavity.

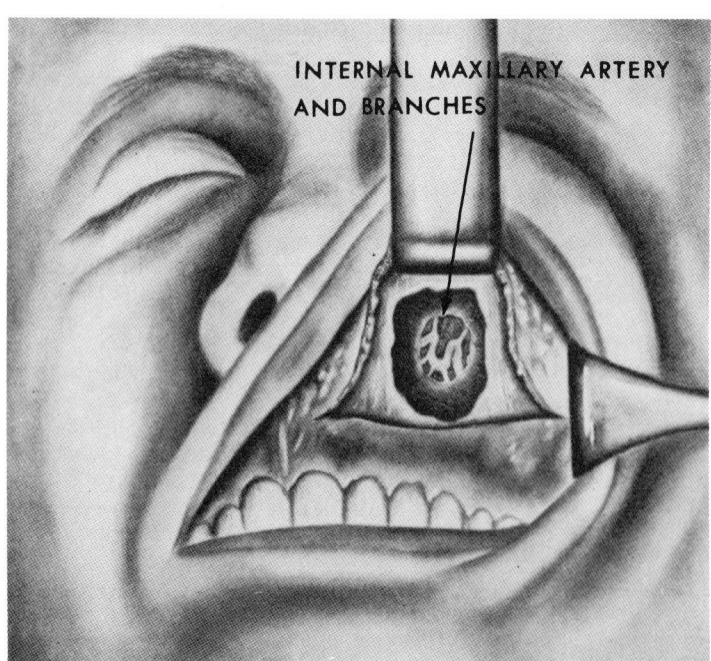

INTERNAL MAXILLARY ARTERY AND BRANCHES

Figure 17. Approach through the canine fossa as in the Caldwell-Luc operation to ligate the internal maxillary artery. The anterior and posterior walls of the maxillary sinus have been removed to expose the artery. (From Chandler, J. R., and Serrins, A. J.: Laryngoscope, 75:1151, 1965.)

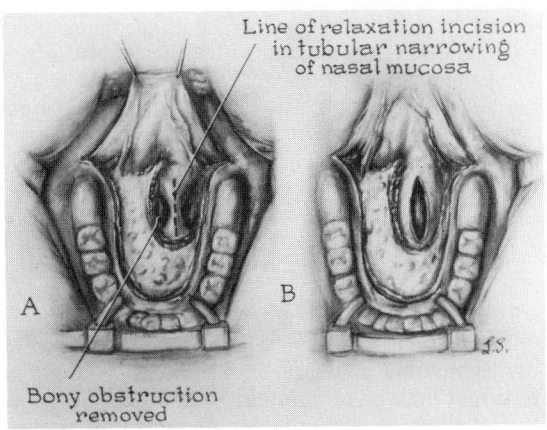

Figure 18. Transpalatal approach for repair of choanal atresia. (From Cherry, J., and Bordley, J. E.: Ann. Otol., 75:911, 1966.)

Nasal Gliomas, Encephaloceles, and Meningoceles

Nasal glioma may present as a malformation of the dorsum of the nose evident at birth or as a mass in the nasal cavity. Nasal gliomas often have intracranial connections. To avoid the development of cerebrospinal fluid rhinorrhea, a frontal craniotomy is performed to exclude the possibility of an intracranial extension prior to the removal of the nasal glioma.[45] Encephaloceles and meningoceles may present in the nasal cavity through defects in the cribriform plate. Clinically they have an appearance similar to that of a nasal polyp. Nasal polyps ordinarily arise from the middle meatus. If what appears to be a nasal polyp does not arise from the middle meatus, thorough investigation to exclude an encephalocele or meningocele is carried out prior to operative intervention. Laminagraphy of the cribriform plate may demonstrate the associated defect in the floor of the anterior cranial fossa.

NEOPLASMS

Benign Tumors of the Nose and Paranasal Sinuses

Squamous cell papillomas occur in the nasal cavity and are thought to be caused by papovaviruses. Exophytic papillomas occasionally recur after excision but have a benign course. Inverted papillomas are invasive and behave in a locally malignant manner. They destroy soft tissue and bone and tend to recur following excision. They require removal with a large margin of normal tissue. Fibromas, hemangiomas, and neurofibromas occur occasionally in the nasal cavity. Fibromas, neurolemmomas, and ossifying fibromas occur in the paranasal sinuses.[2]

Malignant Tumors of the Nose and Paranasal Sinuses

The most common malignant tumor occurring in the nose and paranasal sinuses is the squamous cell car-

cinoma. Adenoid cystic carcinomas, adenocarcinomas (particularly in the ethmoid sinuses), mucoepidermoid carcinomas, malignant mixed tumors, lymphomas, fibrosarcomas, osteosarcomas, chondrosarcomas, and melanomas also occur in the nose and paranasal sinuses.[2] Metastatic tumors may involve the paranasal sinuses, and the most common tumor to metastasize to the paranasal sinuses is the hypernephroma.

Early squamous cell and basal cell carcinomas of the skin of the nose are treated with radiation therapy or cauterization and curettage. Larger carcinomas involving cartilage require excision. Nasal septal carcinomas often require sacrifice of the columella as well as adjacent structures.

A combination of radiation therapy in a tumoricidal dose and radical resection gives the best survival rates in carcinomas and sarcomas of the nasal cavities and paranasal sinuses. Malignant tumors of the lateral wall of the nose require lateral rhinotomy. Malignant tumors of the maxillary sinus require partial or radical maxillectomy.[22] A radical maxillectomy includes exenteration of the orbit. Malignant tumors of the ethmoid sinus require radical resection of the ethmoid complex including exenteration of the orbit and partial maxillectomy. Malignant tumors of the frontal sinus and the sphenoid sinus are not satisfactorily resected and are usually treated with radiation therapy. Lymphomas limited to the nasal cavities or paranasal sinuses are treated with radiation therapy. Disseminated lymphomas require chemotherapy. Melanomas arising in mucous membrane are treated with surgery and radiation therapy, with only rare success.

THE PHARYNX

Celsus is generally recognized as the first to describe tonsillectomy in his first century *De medicina*. However, the Asiatic Indians frequently performed the operation 1000 years earlier.

ANATOMY OF THE PHARYNX

For descriptive purposes the pharynx can be divided into the nasopharynx, oropharynx, and hypopharynx. However, from a functional point of view, the pharynx remains united by the constrictors of the pharynx. They have a common insertion in the median pharyngeal raphe and form a musculomembranous tubular passage from the base of the skull to the opening of the esophagus. The lymphoid structures of the pharynx include the pharyngeal tonsil or adenoid, the palatine tonsils, the lateral bands, and the lingual tonsils.

FOREIGN BODIES

Foreign bodies of the pharynx are likely to be found in four locations: the palatine tonsils, the lingual tonsils, the valleculae, and the pyriform sinuses. Sharp foreign bodies such as fish bones are particularly likely to lodge in the palatine tonsils and the lingual tonsils. Smooth, small, oval foreign bodies such as capsules are likely to come to rest in the valleculae. Irregular sharp foreign bodies are likely to be retained in the pyriform sinuses. Rarely foreign bodies are coughed into the nasopharynx and become trapped there. Radiopaque foreign bodies may be located in a lateral neck x-ray. Foreign bodies in the palatine tonsil are removed by grasping the foreign body with a hemostat. Foreign bodies in the nasopharynx require general anesthesia for their removal. Foreign bodies of the hypopharynx are removed at direct laryngoscopy under local anesthesia.

NASOPHARYNX

The Adenoids

Adenoid hyperplasia in childhood often leads to obstruction of the eustachian tubes and the choanae. This lymphoid hyperplasia may be physiologic or secondary to infectious and allergic manifestations. Obstruction of the eustachian tubes leads to serous or secretory otitis media, recurrent acute otitis media, and exacerbations of chronic otitis media. Obstruction of the choanae produces mouth breathing, a hyponasal voice, and rhinorrhea.

Recurrent serous or secretory otitis media is the most common indication for the removal of the adenoid tissue. A sterile effusion in the middle ear in a child lasting 6 weeks or longer, occurring de novo or following acute otitis media, that does not respond to medical management responds regularly but not invariably to the use of myringotomies with the insertion of tympanostomy tubes. In patients with recurrent or persistent serous or secretory otitis media, adenoidectomy increases the chance of success.

Chronic otitis media in children is another indication for adenoidectomy. The procedure reduces the severity and frequency of exacerbations of chronic otitis media. It prepares the patient for subsequent mastoidectomy and tympanoplasty. Recurrent acute otitis media is a fairly frequent indication for these procedures. Many children between the ages of 1 and 6 years have two or three episodes of acute otitis media per year which completely resolve with antibiotic therapy. On the other hand, the child who is on antibiotic therapy for otitis media half of the time should be considered for this procedure. The duration of the pain, the presence of spontaneous perforation, the regularity with which myringotomy is required, and the associated systemic symptoms deserve consideration. Febrile convulsions with acute otitis media weigh heavily in favor of adenoidectomy, since antibiotic therapy ordinarily is not initiated prior to the convulsion.

Persistent nasal obstruction due to adenoid hyperplasia is a problem in which the age of the patient is considered as well as the severity, since lymphoid tissue reaches a relative and absolute maximum at puberty. Persistent and recurrent purulent rhinorrhea in spite of adequate antibiotic therapy is occasionally encountered in association with adenoid hyperplasia and chronic adenoiditis. Chronic sinusitis in children without an underlying immunologic or other defense mechanism defect such as agammaglobulinemia or hypogammaglobulinemia, pancreatic fibrosis, or Kartagener's syndrome is relatively rare but is rather regularly improved or eliminated by adenoidectomy.

An adenoidectomy is performed under general anesthesia. The adenoid tissue is sheared from the posterior nasopharyngeal wall with a guillotine-type adenotome placed posterior to the soft palate. The lymphoid tissue is removed superficial to the fascia of the superior constrictor of the pharynx without damaging the fascia or the underlying musculature.

Tornwaldt's Cyst

Cysts frequently form in the region of the medial recess of the nasopharynx. These cysts become symptomatic when they become infected. There may be persistent purulent drainage which has a foul taste and odor. Symptoms of eustachian tube obstruction and sore throat may be prominent. Excision or marsupialization of the cyst with an adenotome is the treatment of choice.

Benign Neoplasms of the Nasopharynx

Juvenile angiofibromas are very vascular tumors that occur in pubescent males. They develop in the vault of the nasopharynx from the area of the basisphenoid and grow to large size. Angiofibromas may extend into and obstruct the nasal cavity, and their extensions may develop parasitic attachments distant to their site of origin. They may encroach upon the paranasal sinuses, orbit, and the intracranial cavity. Histologically, these tumors are composed of fibrous tissue and numerous thin-walled vessels without contractile elements. Angiofibromas tend to involute at maturity.

Epistaxis is the major problem with angiofibromas, and the magnitude of the bleeding can be very great. The tumors are red and quite firm. Those portions of the tumor that project into the airway often become ulcerated during upper respiratory tract infections and bleed from the ulcerated surface. Their surgical removal is necessitated by recurrent massive bleeding. The extent of the tumor can be determined radiographically. The pterygomaxillary fissure is often widened on the lateral view of the nasopharynx by the extension of the tumor into the infratemporal fossa. These tumors give a characteristic vascular pattern on angiography, and biopsy is usually not necessary. Usually, they are removed through a transpalatal approach. Often a lateral rhinotomy offers significant advantages. The blood loss during excision is often very great, and rapid blood replacement is required. Treatment with estrogens and embolization of the major vessels found supplying the tumor at angiography have been used to reduce the operative blood loss.[39] These tumors are moderately responsive to radiation therapy. It is often the treatment of choice for the tumor that has invaded the orbit or the intracranial cavity.

Malignant Neoplasms of the Nasopharynx

Malignant tumors of the nasopharynx include squamous cell carcinomas, adenocarcinomas, adenoid cystic carcinomas, mucoepidermoid carcinomas, malignant mixed tumors, melanomas, chordomas, sarcomas including fibrosarcoma, rhabdomyosarcoma, liposarcoma, and myxosarcoma, plasmacytomas, and lymphomas. Among children, the lymphomas and lymphosarcomas are the most common malignant tumors arising from and secondarily involving the nasopharynx. Among the carcinomas, lymphoepithelioma or squamous cell carcinoma is the most common type.

Carcinoma of the nasopharynx occurs at relatively young ages, and there is an unusually high incidence among the Chinese.[25] There are immunologic similarities between patients with Burkitt's lymphoma, carcinoma of the nasopharynx, and infectious mononucleosis. Elevated titers of anti-Epstein-Barr virus antibodies are present in 45 per cent of patients with Stage I carcinoma of the nasopharynx and 100 per cent of patients with Stage V lesions.[13] The majority of patients with carcinoma of the nasopharynx present with nasal or eustachian tube obstruction. Obstruction of the eustachian tube may result in a middle ear effusion. The nasal obstruction may be associated with purulent, blood rhinorrhea and frank epistaxis. The more dramatic symptoms resulting from cranial nerve paralysis and cervical lymph node metastasis are unfortunately common presenting complaints. Metastasis tends to be limited to the neck until the late stages of the disease. A granular mass or ulcer may be seen in the nasopharynx. The palate may be deformed by the bulk of the nasopharyngeal mass, or its mobility may be limited by paralysis of the levator veli palatini. Not infrequently the tumor extends deep to the mucous membrane, appears only as a slight fullness, and produces no abnormality of the mucous membrane. It is this feature of carcinoma of the nasopharynx that makes biopsy through apparently normal mucous membrane occasionally fruitful.

The diagnosis is made by biopsy of the primary tumor. Adequate access to the nasopharynx ordinarily requires general anesthesia. General anesthesia also allows the opportunity to judge the extent of the primary lesion by palpation. Biopsy of the metastasis in the neck should be avoided until the nasopharynx has been inspected and palpated and any suspicious lesion has been biopsied. Biopsy of the cervical metastasis violates the integrity of the block of tissue that is removed in a radical neck dissection. It may result in implantation of the tumor in the skin and subcutaneous tissue. The necessity for demonstrating the tumor in the nasopharynx prior to treatment remains even if a histologic diagnosis is obtained from biopsy of the cervical metastasis.

The treatment of choice for carcinoma of the nasopharynx is irradiation with a supervoltage source. The radiation should be delivered to the primary tumor-bearing area of the nasopharynx and to both sides of the neck whether there is clinically demonstrated metastasis or not. Surgery plays no role in the initial therapy of carcinoma of the nasopharynx. Those cervical metastases that remain clinically palpable following radiation therapy or that subsequently become apparent should be eradicated by radical neck dissection. As a general rule, control of the metastatic lesions should be attempted only after there is evidence that the primary lesion has been controlled. Occasionally, the primary lesion in the nasopharynx persists after radiation therapy without evidence of local or distant metastasis. Under these circumstances, cryosurgery may be applied to the persisting tumor in the nasopharynx. The overall 5-year survival for carcinoma of the nasopharynx is approximately 35 per cent.

OROPHARYNX

Peritonsillar Abscess

Peritonsillar cellulitis and abscess are complications of acute tonsillitis in which the infection has spread deep to the tonsillar capsule. Pus forms between the tonsillar capsule and the superior constrictor of the pharynx, and the tonsil is displaced medially. The uvula becomes tremendously edematous and is displaced to the opposite side. The soft palate is very red and displaced forward. There is marked trismus due to irritation of the pterygoid muscles, and the head is held tilted toward the side of the abscess. It is painful for the patient to talk and to swallow. Swallowing is so painful that the patient drools. The breath is foul-smelling. The temperature is usually 38 to 40° C. Peritonsillar cellulitis or abscess does not occur in children under the age of 10 to 12 years and is usually caused by a group A beta hemolytic streptococcus. If a cellulitis without pus formation exists, it will respond in a matter of 24 to 48 hours to penicillin therapy. If pus is present, it may resolve or require incision and drainage. The pus may be difficult to locate. Incision is performed as the mucous membrane takes on a pale yellow color overlying the pus. The patient is placed in the sitting position to avoid aspiration of the pus. Under topical anesthesia, the incision is made in the anterior pillar parallel to its free edge. The incision need only split the mucous membrane, and the pus is obtained by spreading gently with a hemostat. No drain is required because the abscess cavity is emptied by each swallow.

These abscesses tend to recur and are an indication for tonsillectomy, which is performed 6 weeks after the acute infection. At the time of tonsillectomy, 1 to 2 ml. of pus is usually encountered between the capsule and the tonsillar fossa. This persistent abscess is the apparent reason for the recurrence of these abscesses.

Parapharyngeal Abscess

Parapharyngeal abscess may occur in infants and young children as well as in adults secondary to streptococcal pharyngitis or tonsillitis. Pus forms in the parapharyngeal space secondarily from the breakdown of lymphadenitis. The pus is located lateral to the superior constrictor of the pharynx and adjacent to the carotid sheath. The tonsil and soft palate may be displaced medially, but there may be no inflammatory reaction in the pharynx. There is marked swelling in the anterior cervical triangle. Penicillin is the antibiotic of choice. Once it becomes fluctuant, the abscess is incised and drained. The abscess is not drained through the lateral pharyngeal wall because of the proximity of the internal carotid artery and the internal jugular vein. An incision is made parallel to the skin folds over the anterior border of the sternocleidomastoid muscle. The anterior border of the muscle is identified, and blunt dissection is carried toward the carotid sheath where the pus is encountered. A drain is sewn in place until the drainage subsides.

Retropharyngeal Abscess

Retropharyngeal abscess occurs in infants and young children and is rare after the age of 10 years. These infections are located between the constrictors of the pharynx and the prevertebral fascia. They are secondary to pharyngitis and due to the breakdown of retropharyngeal lymphadenitis. Infants with retropharyngeal abscesses usually present with stridor and hyperextension of the neck. A lumbar puncture is the appropriate diagnostic procedure in a febrile infant who presents in opisthotonos. If the cerebrospinal fluid is normal, the possibility of a retropharyngeal abscess must be excluded. The diagnosis is made by palpating the posterior pharyngeal wall. The infant is held in the prone position for the examination so that if the abscess is ruptured during the examination, the pus will flow out of the infant's mouth and not be aspirated. The abscess has a boggy fluctuant texture, and the bodies of the cervical vertebrae are not palpable. Inspection of the pharynx may not demonstrate the abscess because the whole posterior pharyngeal wall may be displaced forward and there may be no inflammatory reaction in the mucous membrane. In order to maintain the airway the child should be allowed to hyperextend the neck. A tracheotomy is rarely necessary. In addition to penicillin therapy, the posterior pharyngeal wall should be incised under general endotracheal anesthesia with the patient in the Rose position. The mucous membrane at the posterior wall of the pharynx is incised vertically. The incision need only split the mucous membrane. The pus is obtained by gently spreading a hemostat in the wound toward the retropharyngeal space. No drain is necessary because the abscess cavity tends to be emptied on swallowing.

Tonsillectomy

Recurrent acute bacterial tonsillitis due to a group A beta hemolytic streptococcus occurring three to four times during the year in children from 2 to 7 years of age can be adequately managed with penicillin or other appropriate antibiotics if given for 12 days. The rationale for this length of treatment is that a shorter period may not eliminate a streptococcal infection. In addition to inappropriate selection of antibiotics and inadequate duration of therapy, passage of the streptococcus among family members is a cause of failure in the medical management of tonsillitis. This situation requires simultaneous cultures of the whole family and simultaneous treatment of all carriers. In spite of these precautions, in some patients tonsillitis repeatedly develops within a few days after the completion of adequate treatment. When this pattern cannot be altered by medical management, tonsillectomy is indicated.

Chronic tonsillitis with persistent sore throat, either briefly relieved or not at all relieved by antibiotic therapy, constitutes another indication for tonsillectomy. One peritonsillar abscess is an indication for tonsillectomy.

In adults, tonsillectomy is performed under local or general anesthesia. In children, general anesthesia is required. The technique involves an incision in the free edge of the tonsillar pillars. The dissection of the tonsil from the tonsillar fossa is carried out in the plane between the tonsillar capsule and the superior constrictor muscle of the pharynx and is completed by closing a snare placed inferior to the lower pole of the tonsil. The objective is to remove the tonsil and its capsule intact and spare the musculature of the tonsillar fossa.

Carcinoma of the Tonsil

Carcinoma of the tonsil accounts for 1.5 to 3 per cent of all cancers and is second in frequency only to carcinoma of the larynx among malignant tumors of the upper respiratory tract. It is predominantly a disease of males. Squamous cell carcinoma is the predominant histologic type. These carcinomas may be exophytic with superficial ulceration or deeply invasive. At times they present as lobulated submucosal masses. The tumor frequently extends into the base of the tongue. Carcinoma of the tonsil usually remains asymptomatic until it has reached considerable size. Sore throat is the most common presenting complaint, and pain often radiates to the ear on the same side. Not infrequently the patients present with a metastatic mass in the neck as the first symptom. The diagnosis is established by biopsy of the primary lesion. A promising method of treatment consists of radiation therapy and surgery. A tumoricidal dose of radiation is delivered to the tonsillar fossa and to the same side of the neck. Radical resection of the tonsillar fossa, hemimandibulectomy with disarticulation of the temporomandibular joint, and radical neck dissection are carried out 6 weeks after completion of radiation therapy.[26] The 5-year survival for carcinoma of the tonsil treated by irradiation is approximately 25 per cent.

HYPOPHARYNX

Diverticulum of the Hypopharynx

Diverticula of the hypopharynx result from herniation of the mucous membrane of the hypopharynx through weak points in the inferior constrictor muscle; they occur in the older age group. These pulsion diverticula almost always occur on the left side. The sac lies between the prevertebral fascia and the left posterolateral wall of the esophagus. While the origin of the diverticulum is the hypopharynx, the esophagus is compressed by the diverticulum. During deglutition, the diverticulum fills with food and fluid. When the patient lies down, the diverticulum empties into the pharynx, and aspiration of food and fluid into the lower respiratory tract may occur and result in recurrent and debilitating pneumonitis. The diverticulum is demonstrated with a barium swallow. Diverticula are managed surgically by excision through a cervical incision or by endoscopic cautery of the party wall between the cervical esophagus and the diverticulum.

LARYNX

Caelius Aurelianus credits Asclepiades with having first employed tracheotomy in cynanche (probably diphtheria) in the century before the birth of Christ.

In 1778, the French surgeon Pelletan performed a successful laryngofissure for the removal of a bolus of meat that had become entrapped between the vocal cords. In 1854, Manuel Garcia, a Spanish singing teacher, succeeded in observing his own larynx with two mirrors and the sun as a light source. In 1856, Türck and Czermak independently developed the laryngoscope in Vienna. Following the development of the laryngoscope, peroral endolaryngeal surgery flourished in many centers. In the 1870s Bergman performed laryngotomies for removal of parts of the larynx involved with carcinoma. Billroth in 1873 performed the first successful laryngectomy.

ANATOMY OF THE LARYNX

The skeleton of the larynx consists of the thyroid cartilage, the cricoid cartilage, the arytenoid cartilages with the corniculate and cuneiform cartilages, and the epiglottis. Phylogenetically the arytenoid cartilages are the oldest elements of the laryngeal skeleton. This fact emphasizes the primeval role of the larynx as a sphincter rather than a conduit for air. The cricoid cartilage completely encircles the airway and maintains its patency. The arytenoid cartilages articulate with the cricoid cartilage. The true vocal cords are attached to the vocal processes of the arytenoid cartilages and to the isthmus of the thyroid cartilage. The superior surfaces of the true vocal cords are flat, and the inferior surfaces are concave. The inferior surfaces of the false vocal cords are flat, and the superior surfaces of the false vocal cords are convex. The true vocal cords and the false vocal cords make a double-layered sphincter. The configuration of the true vocal cords makes them a good barrier to the ingress of the air and a poor barrier to the egress of air. The configuration of the false vocal cords makes them a poor barrier to the ingress of air and a good barrier to the egress of air. The true vocal cords can be thought of as an inlet valve, and the false vocal cords as an outlet valve.

PHYSIOLOGY OF THE LARYNX

The primary function of the larynx is that of a sphincter. During deglutition both the true vocal cord sphincter and false vocal cord sphincter are closed, and the epiglottis is drawn posterior over the closed sphincters and serves as a watershed deflecting food and fluid into the pyriform sinuses. The larynx also serves as a sphincter during parturition, coughing, and defecation. At these times, it serves primarily as an outlet valve. During the lifting of heavy objects and climbing hand over hand as in climbing a tree, the pull of the shoulder girdles on the thorax tends to expand the thoracic cage. The larynx limits the ingress of air as an inlet valve and thereby stabilizes the thorax.

The larynx serves as the sounding source for speech. A fundamental tone is produced by the movement of the vocal cords which is brought about by the flow of exhaled air past lightly approximated vocal cords. The fundamental tone and its overtones are modified into meaningful symbols or speech by articulators such as the pharynx, palate, tongue, teeth, and lips. Synchrony of the vibration of the two vocal cords exists normally at any given instant, but aperiodicity over time also occurs. The fundamental tone varies with the sex and age of the individual. Adult males produce a fundamental tone of 125 Hz., and adult females produce a fundamental tone of 250 Hz. In the healthy voice, the predominate overtones of these fundamental tones are partial and whole-number multiples of the fundamental tone. The predominance of harmonic overtones gives the voice a musical quality. The distribution of the harmonics gives the voice a timbre which is characteristic of that individual. In the healthy voice there are frequent changes in the frequency of the fundamental tone which provide it with a melodious quality. The normal speaker usually uses changes in frequency rather than changes in intensity for emphasis.

PATHOPHYSIOLOGY OF THE LARYNX

Various pathologic changes in the vocal cords result in the prominence of nonharmonic noise components in the voice. In contrast to the healthy musical voice, overtones that are not partial or whole-number multiples of the fundamental tone produce a noisy voice or hoarseness. Structural changes in the vocal cords result in greater aperiodicity and asynchrony of the vibration of the vocal cords. Aperiodicity and asynchrony disrupt the harmonic relationships of the voice by limiting the possibility of the occurrence of overtones that are partial and whole-number multiples of the fundamental tone. Characteristically, the abnormal voice is monotonous. A monotone may occur because of loss of flexibility in the frequency range of the larynx due to a disease process or it may be acquired as a habit, particularly in speakers who tend to use increases in intensity for emphasis rather than changes in frequency. Structural changes in the vocal cords often interfere with their approximation and result in air wastage which gives the voice a breathy quality.

STRUCTURAL CHANGES IN THE TRUE VOCAL CORDS SECONDARY TO MISUSE AND ABUSE OF THE VOICE

Abuse and misuse of the voice can result in structural changes in the true vocal cords. Using the voice too loudly and too long produces acute and chronic changes in the true vocal cords. Prolonged use of intensity rather than frequency for emphasis, the employment of a monotone, the affectation of a frequency that is too low, and a very abrupt onset of high intensities (sharp glottal attack) produce structural changes in the true vocal cords.

Polyps of the Vocal Cords

Polyps of the true vocal cords develop in response to using the voice too loudly and too long, as in the person who must speak over a great deal of background noise in a factory or who demonstrates wares in a department store or barks at a circus or carnival. Chronic subepithelial edema develops in the lamina propria of the true vocal cords. Similar pathologic changes result from chronic allergic reactions and the chronic inhalation of irritants such as tobacco smoke and industrial fumes. Such polypoid swellings of the free edge of the true vocal cord interfere with the approximation of the true vocal cords and with the maintenance of periodicity and synchrony of the vibration of the vocal cords. They produce hoarseness and give a breathy quality to the voice. To restore the voice, polyps are removed with biting forceps at direct laryngoscopy under local or general anesthesia.

Vocal Nodules

Vocal nodules are caused by using a fundamental frequency that is unnaturally low and using the voice too loudly and too long. Vocal nodules occur in children as well as adults, and are likely to occur in robust, athletic boys 8 to 12 years of age who yell a great deal. Men affect an unnaturally low pitch to give an air of authority; women do it to give an impression of sexiness; and young boys probably do it to identify with older males in the family or community. Vocal nodules are condensations of hyaline connective tissue in the lamina propria at the junction of the anterior one third and the posterior two thirds of the true vocal cord (Fig. 19). These nodules produce hoarseness and give the voice a breathy quality. In adults, these lesions are removed at direct laryngoscopy to restore the voice. However, it is necessary to begin voice therapy prior to the surgery, because if the underlying misuse of the voice is not corrected, the nodules will recur. In children, surgical removal is not usually necessary because the vocal nodules will regress with voice therapy, which consists of voice rest, reduction in intensity and duration of voice production, and elevation of the pitch.

Contact Ulcers

Contact ulcers of the larynx are thought to result from misuse and abuse of the voice, particularly in the

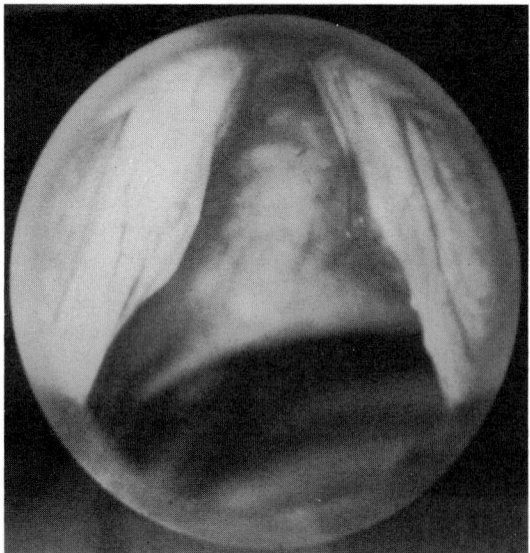

Figure 19. Direct laryngoscopic view of vocal nodules during inspiration. (From the Jacques Holinger Memorial Fund Collection, courtesy of Dr. Paul H. Holinger.)

form of a sharp glottal attack. They occur unilaterally or bilaterally over the vocal process of the arytenoid. The presence of these lesions causes mild pain on phonation and swallowing and varying degrees of hoarseness. The ulcers have a shaggy or granular base. They are biopsied at direct laryngoscopy to exclude the possibility of carcinoma. Voice therapy is important to correct the underlying misuse of the voice. However, prolonged voice rest is required for contact ulcers to heal.

TRAUMA

Trauma has replaced infectious diseases such as diphtheria, streptococcal croup, syphilis, tuberculosis, rhinoscleroma, and typhoid fever as the most common cause of laryngeal stenosis. Automobile accidents in which the patient is thrown forward and the larynx is crushed between the cervical vertebrae and the object against which it decelerates are the single most important cause of laryngeal stenosis. Children may fracture the larynx by falling against the handlebars of a bicycle or riding a horse or bicycle under a taut line. Another cause of laryngeal stenosis is the high tracheotomy in which a perichondritis of the cricoid cartilage results from the pressure of the tube on the cartilage. Prolonged endotracheal intubation frequently results in subglottic stenosis, as do infectious processes.

Fractures of the thyroid cartilage may result in supraglottic, glottic, or transglottic stenosis. Persons with long slender necks are more likely to sustain supraglottic injuries in which the hyoid bone is also fractured. The suprahyoid muscles are disrupted, and the thyrohyoid membrane is ruptured. Fracture of the cricoid cartilage results in subglottic stenosis. Fractures of the cricoid cartilage are more likely to occur in males with short, thick necks and are relatively rare in females. Often a blow to the neck spares the larynx but transects the trachea.

Patients with crush injuries of the larynx complain of pain on swallowing. Hoarseness may progress to aphonia. Hemoptysis is usually present. Progressive dyspnea due to upper respiratory obstruction is to be anticipated. Subcutaneous emphysema is usually present in fractures of the larynx or trachea. The laryngeal cartilages cannot be distinctly palpated, nor can the trachea, owing to soft tissue swelling. On indirect laryngoscopy, the laryngeal lumen appears disrupted or obliterated, and there may be exposed cartilage and lacerated mucous membrane. Vocal cord paralysis may be noted. X-rays of the lateral neck and laminagrams of the larynx may indicate the type and degree of injury. Lateral neck x-rays may demonstrate associated fractures or dislocations of the cervical vertebrae.

In the initial management of the patient with a laryngeal fracture, a tracheotomy is performed and followed by direct laryngoscopy and tracheoscopy. Often, patients with multiple injuries are treated with a tracheotomy because of the upper airway obstruction, and the reason for the need for the tracheotomy is forgotten during the management of the thoracic and abdominal or perhaps intracranial injuries. The laryngeal trauma is rediscovered 10 or so days later when it appears that it would be appropriate to remove the tracheostomy tube. Evaluation of the larynx should be performed early to be certain that there has not been a fracture of the laryngeal cartilages that requires early repair.

The repair of the fracture is done through a transverse incision in the neck. In order to gain access to the interior of the larynx, a laryngofissure is performed by dividing the thyroid cartilage at its isthmus, or the fracture in the thyroid and cricoid cartilage is utilized. Mucous membrane lacerations are repaired, and the cartilages are returned to their normal alignment. Internal splinting is maintained with a solid-core mold for 6 weeks. Failure to reduce a dislocated or fractured cartilage leads to laryngeal stenosis. Late repair of laryngeal stenosis can sometimes be accomplished by an arytenoidectomy. At other times a supraglottic partial laryngectomy is required to restore the airway and the functional integrity of the laryngeal sphincter.[29] A keel is often employed to repair the angle of the anterior commissure. Subglottic stenosis is repaired by excision of the stenotic area and internal splinting for a period of 6 weeks or more.

In addition to external trauma, tracheal stenosis occurs secondary to pressure necrosis of the tracheal walls caused by the inflated cuff in prolonged endotracheal intubation. Tracheal stenosis also occurs secondary to tracheotomy, particularly when the wound becomes infected and there is cicatricial healing of large eroded tracheostomas. Tracheal stenosis may be managed by dilations, excision of the stenotic area with internal splinting for 6 weeks or more, or excision of the stenotic area with end-to-end anastomosis of the trachea. As much as 50 per cent of the length of the trachea can be resected and end-to-end anastomosis performed.[12]

FOREIGN BODIES OF THE LARYNX, TRACHEOBRONCHIAL TREE, AND ESOPHAGUS

Foreign bodies are retained in the larynx as a general rule because they are sharp and stick into the mucous membrane or are irregular and soft and are caught between the two vocal cords in laryngospasm. A frequently fatal laryngeal foreign body is a bolus of meat. The resulting laryngospasm completely occludes the larynx, and death takes place rapidly unless a Pelletan is present and establishes an alternate airway by performance of a prompt tracheotomy. This "café coronary" may be distinguished from a myocardial infarct by the respiratory effort without exchange and the marked suprasternal, intercostal, and subxiphoid retraction. Foreign bodies of the larynx induce a degree of laryngospasm that makes their removal difficult without general anesthesia. Even with a nonobstructing foreign body, a tracheotomy is often the first step in its removal, particularly with subglottic foreign bodies such as sand or grass burrs. The site of the foreign body is exposed with a laryngoscope, and the foreign body is grasped, disengaged, and removed with alligator or other appropriate forceps.

Smooth objects such as nuts, kernels of corn, watermelon seeds, beans, peas, and plastic toys pass through the larynx into the tracheobronchial tree. At the onset, there is severe spasmodic coughing which continues for approximately 30 minutes. During this period of time, the foreign body migrates from one portion of the tracheobronchial tree to another. It more frequently comes to rest in the right bronchus because the right bronchus is larger than the left and makes less of an angle with the long axis of the trachea, and the carina is to the left of the midline of the tracheal lumen. As it finally comes to rest, the coughing subsides, and a latent period begins during which the patient is free of symptoms. The mistaken inference is often made by the family and the physician in attendance that the foreign body has been coughed out. However, careful auscultation of the chest may demonstrate an expiratory wheeze and the signs of obstructive emphysema. The most common mechanism of the bronchial obstruction due to a foreign body is a one-way valve through which air may enter the bronchus distal to the foreign body during inspiration but its egress is limited on expiration. This type of obstruction produces emphysema distal to the foreign body. The obstructive emphysema may become apparent radiographically only on expiration (Fig. 20). The mediastinum shifts away from the obstructed lung, and the obstructed portion of the lung becomes radiolucent compared to the normal lung. This type of partial obstruction of the bronchus is likely to occur with the aspiration of nuts. In the evaluation of a patient with a suspected nonradiopaque foreign body of the bronchus, comparison of inspiratory and expiratory chest x-rays and fluoroscopy of the chest may demonstrate obstructive emphysema that would not be apparent on inspiration x-rays.

A foreign body that completely obstructs the bronchus causes the rapid development of a more serious pathophysiologic state. Complete atelectasis of the obstructed lung occurs as a result of absorption of the remaining air in the lung. The mediastinum shifts toward the atelectatic lung, and the remaining lung undergoes compensatory emphysema (Fig. 21). The atelectatic lung is useless as far as ventilatory exchange is concerned, and the efficiency of the emphysematous lung is greatly reduced. Rapid cardiorespiratory failure occurs unless the foreign body is removed. This type of complete bronchial obstruction is likely to occur with smooth hygroscopic foreign bodies like beans that swell in the bronchus.

Vegetable foreign bodies are very poorly tolerated. Metallic and plastic foreign bodies that cause partial obstruction of the bronchus may be tolerated for long periods. Nuts, particularly peanuts, produce a very severe tracheobronchitis. After the latent period of 24 hours, the patient develops a cough productive of purulent sputum, and a febrile course begins. A long-indwelling foreign body of the bronchus may produce bronchiectasis, recurrent pneumonitis, lung abscess, and empyema. Tracheobronchial foreign bodies are removed under general anesthesia through bronchoscopes with forceps designed specifically for each type of foreign body.

Foreign bodies of the esophagus are likely to lodge just below the cricopharyngeus muscle. Ninety-five per cent of esophageal foreign bodies are found in this location. Other locations are the gastroesophageal

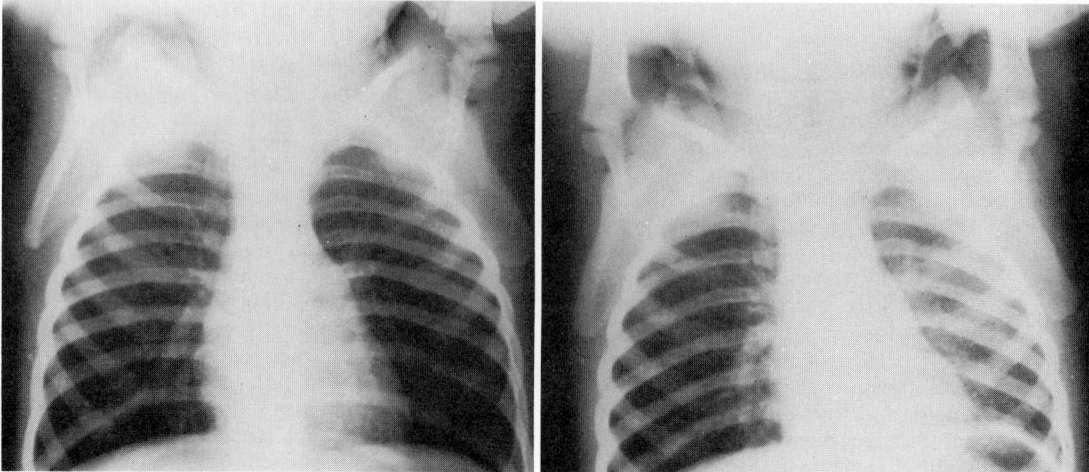

Figure 20. Posterior-anterior radiographs of the chest on inspiration (left) and expiration (right) from a child with a peanut in the right bronchus. The inspiratory film appears normal. On expiration, the obstructive emphysema becomes evident with radiolucency of the right lung compared to the left and shift of the mediastinum to the left.

junction and the indentations of the esophagus caused by the left bronchus and the arch of the aorta. The constrictors of the pharynx are very strong and can propel almost any irregular object through the cricopharyngeus muscle (Fig. 22). Once the foreign body has passed the cricopharyngeus, the muscular activity is very weak, and progress occurs mainly by gravity. Therefore, irregular objects are brought to a very abrupt stop just below the cricopharyngeus muscle.

The symptoms of a foreign body of the esophagus are dysphagia and pain in the suprasternal area on swallowing. Bulky foreign bodies in the cervical esophagus may produce upper airway obstruction by extrinsic pressure through the membranous posterior wall of the trachea. Foreign bodies can be identified on a lateral neck x-ray if they are radiopaque (Fig. 22). If they are radiolucent, evidence of a foreign body may still be obtained, since the foreign body tends to hold the esophageal walls apart and air may be seen in the

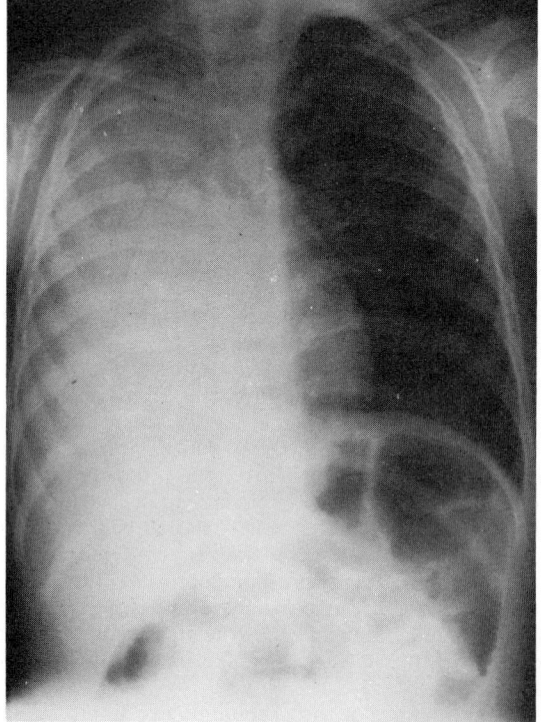

Figure 21. Posterior-anterior radiograph of the chest of a child with a pinto bean in the right bronchus. There is atelectasis of the right lung and compensatory emphysema of the left lung.

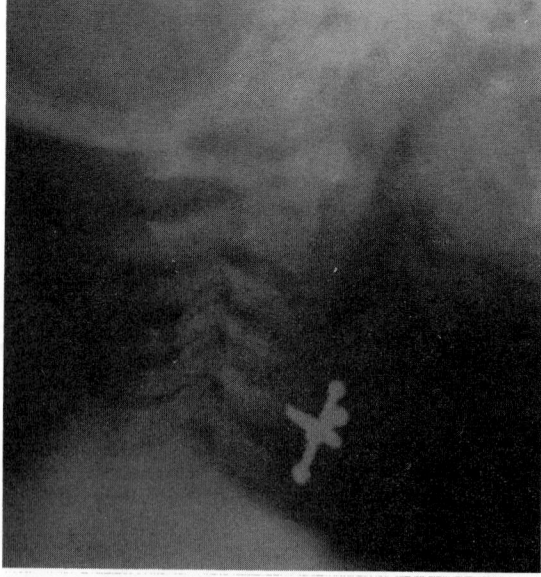

Figure 22. Lateral radiographic view of the neck demonstrating a jack in the cervical esophagus of a child.

cervical esophagus. If the foreign body cannot be located on a lateral neck x-ray, PA and lateral chest x-rays are taken. If the foreign body cannot be located in this manner, an esophagogram may demonstrate it. A small pledget of cotton saturated with a solution of barium sulfate may hang on a sharp foreign body. A foreign body of the esophagus is removed under general anesthesia through an esophagoscope. The foreign body is grasped, disengaged, and removed as a trailing foreign body or through the esophagoscope with a foreign body forceps appropriate to the object. The longer a foreign body remains in the esophagus, the greater the risk of perforation of the esophagus. Perforation of the esophagus results in air and soft tissue swelling in the paraesophageal tissue which may be demonstrated on physical examination and radiographically.

INFECTIOUS DISEASES

Croup

There are two forms of croup, epiglottitis and laryngotracheobronchitis. Croup occurs primarily in children over 1 year and under 5 years of age. It may be viral or bacterial. Parainfluenza Type I is the most frequently isolated agent in viral croup. *Haemophilus influenzae* is the most frequently isolated agent in bacterial croup, but Staphylococcus and Streptococcus may also cause croup.

Haemophilus influenzae type B is the predominant microorganism in epiglottitis and frequently causes a bacteremia. Both epiglottitis and laryngotracheobronchitis may produce the rapid onset of upper respiratory obstruction with inspiratory stridor and suprasternal, supraclavicular, intercostal, and subxiphoid retractions. The voice may be hoarse, and the cough has a brassy quality with subglottic edema. With firm depression of the tongue, the epiglottis in epiglottitis appears as a rounded, red mass like a cherry on the base of the tongue. The supraglottic swelling may be demonstrated on a lateral neck radiograph (Fig. 23).[32] In laryngotracheobronchitis, the major problem is subglottic edema.

Epiglottitis is more likely to cause abrupt and complete airway obstruction. Once the diagnosis of epiglottitis is made, nasotracheal intubation is carried out and maintained for 24 to 48 hours until the supraglottic swelling subsides.[44] In laryngotracheobronchitis, the airway obstruction results in part from edema, but there are also tenacious mucoid secretions. Humidification of the inspired atmosphere liquefies this material, and the patient may cough it out to reduce the degree of airway obstruction. Antibiotic therapy is initiated at the onset of both diseases and ampicillin is the drug of choice since the infection is frequently caused by *Haemophilus influenzae*. Corticosteroid therapy is also initiated in an attempt to reduce the inflammatory swelling. If the degree of airway obstruction becomes severe in laryngotracheobronchitis, a tracheotomy is performed in preference to prolonged endotracheal intubation, because the rate of complications such as laryngeal and subglottic stenosis is quite high with prolonged endotracheal intubation in

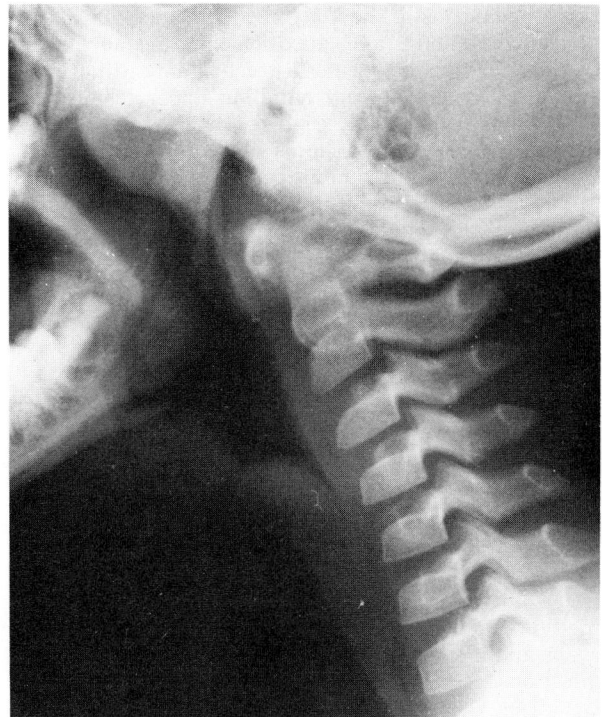

Figure 23. Lateral radiograph of the neck in a child with supraglottic laryngitis. Note the swelling of the epiglottis, aryepiglottic folds, and arytenoids.

laryngotracheobronchitis. The decision regarding a tracheotomy depends on the evaluation of the amount of ventilatory exchange that is taking place, the degree of fatigue of the patient, and the respiratory and pulse rates. Development of cyanosis is a late sign, and the decision to perform a tracheotomy should be made prior to the advent of this ominous sign. Blood gas determinations are not of great value in this particular situation because the clinical situation may change so rapidly. If it appears that the ventilatory exchange is inadequate, the necessary ventilatory effort cannot be maintained, or there is a progressive increase in the pulse rate above 140 per minute, a tracheotomy is performed. The airway emergency is converted to an elective tracheotomy by inserting an endotracheal tube or a bronchoscope. General anesthesia is induced, and the tracheotomy is performed in a relaxed patient under unhurried and ideal circumstances. This approach reduces the incidence of the complications such as pneumothorax.

Tracheotomy

The indications for tracheotomy fall into three broad categories: upper respiratory obstruction, inability to handle upper respiratory secretions, and inability to handle lower respiratory secretions. Among those causes of upper respiratory obstruction that frequently require tracheotomy are congenital malformations of the upper respiratory tract, laryngotracheobronchitis, diphtheria, foreign bodies, bilateral vocal cord paralyses, neoplasms of the larynx, postintubation edema, allergic reactions, and maxillofacial and laryngeal trauma. The importance of a tracheotomy in patients who are having difficulty handling upper respiratory secretions became well recognized during the polio epidemics. Neurologic problems other than infections, such as intracranial trauma and neoplasms, also lead to difficulty in handling upper respiratory secretions. Patients with ineffective respiratory effort on a neurologic or mechanical basis, chronic obstructive pulmonary disease, and parenchymal infections may have difficulty handling lower respiratory secretions.

A tracheotomy has several advantages and disadvantages. It relieves upper respiratory obstruction. It allows more effective access to the lower respiratory tract for suctioning the tracheobronchial tree. It decreases the dead space and reduces the work required for effective ventilation. A tracheotomy can readily be used as a route for the delivery of respiratory assistance. It eliminates the normal warming and humidification of the inspired air by bypassing the upper respiratory tract. A very serious disadvantage of the tracheotomy is the loss of an effective cough. It opens the lower respiratory tract to environmental pathogens and increases the vulnerability to Pseudomonas infections.

Juvenile Papillomas of the Larynx

Papillomas of the larynx are thought to be of viral etiology. Although these lesions may occur as early as 1 year of age, they more commonly make their appearance in the second and third year of life. Papillomas may recur promptly after excision. Exuberant growth from multiple sites in the larynx makes maintenance of an adequate airway difficult. Eventually, most children with laryngeal papillomas require a tracheotomy. The papillomas are periodically removed gingerly at direct laryngoscopy under general anesthesia to maintain the voice and the airway.

CONGENITAL MALFORMATIONS

Congenital malformations of the larynx may produce varying degrees of airway obstruction. Among the well-recognized causes of laryngeal obstruction encountered in the immediate neonatal period are bilateral vocal cord paralyses and subluxation of the arytenoids secondary to traumatic delivery, laryngomalacia or the exaggerated infantile larynx, stenosis and atresia of the larynx, cysts, and subglottic hemangioma.[41] Tracheal obstruction may be due to intrinsic tracheal lesions such as tracheomalacia, absence of tracheal rings, and tracheal stenosis, and to extrinsic tracheal compression from tumors of the thyroid, thymus, esophagus and mediastinum, and the vascular rings. Tetany of the newborn with laryngospasm is usually recognized by other characteristics of this condition. Newborns with tracheoesophageal fistulas certainly have respiratory distress due to aspiration, but usually no true airway obstruction.

In the delivery room, exposure of the vocal cords with a laryngoscope will relieve the obstruction of an exaggerated infantile larynx, in which the flexible epiglottis and arytenoids prolapse into the glottis with inspiration. Inserting a laryngoscope will not relieve obstruction from bilateral vocal cord paralyses, stenosis, or subglottic hemangiomas. Insertion of a 3.5-mm. bronchoscope will improve ventilation in these laryngeal lesions but will not relieve tracheal obstruction until the bronchoscope is passed beyond it. These maneuvers are of the utmost risk to a newborn and should not be undertaken unless the infant's exchange is inadequate for survival. In general, if the exchange is adequate, the infant should be managed expectantly in the neonatal period. Most forms of congenital stridor improve with time. Inappropriate instrumentation may convert a tolerable degree of airway obstruction into one requiring a tracheotomy. A tracheotomy in a newborn is hazardous and difficult to manage.

LARYNGOCELES

Laryngoceles are epithelium-lined diverticula of the laryngeal ventricle and may be located internal or external to the laryngeal skeleton. An internal laryngocele may displace and enlarge the false vocal cord and may result in hoarseness and airway obstruction. External laryngoceles pass through the thyrohyoid membrane and present as a mass in the neck over the thyrohyoid membrane. The mass rises with the larynx on swallowing. Internal and external laryngoceles may coexist. Laryngoceles are more common in glassblowers, wind instruments musicians, and others who develop high intraluminal pressures. Initially, laryngoceles are filled with air and expand and collapse with changes in the intraluminal pressure. They are expanded during the Valsalva maneuver. They appear as a smooth, ovoid, radiolucent mass on x-rays of the neck. Laryngoceles may fill with mucoid fluid and may become infected, under which circumstance the term laryngopyocele is appropriate. External laryngoceles are excised through a transverse cervical incision. The sac is dissected from surrounding tissue to its point of penetration of the thyrohyoid membrane. The sac is transected, and the mucous membrane of the ventricle is repaired. Internal laryngoceles are managed by the same approach but require extension of the dissection into the larynx through a thyrotomy.

NEOPLASMS

Benign neoplasms including papillomas, fibromas, myxomas, chondromas, neurofibromas, hemangiomas, and so forth, may involve any part of the larynx including the true vocal cords. Such lesions can ordinarily be removed at direct laryngoscopy with restoration of the voice, the airway, and the functional integrity of the laryngeal sphincter.

Malignant Neoplasms of the Larynx

The vast majority of malignant neoplasms of the larynx are squamous cell carcinomas. Squamous cell carcinoma of the larynx accounts for approximately 2 per cent of all cancer deaths. It is a disease mainly of males, with a sex ratio of eight to one. The peak incidence of carcinoma of the larynx is in the fifth and sixth decades of life. Laryngeal carcinoma occurs more commonly in persons with a large ethanolic intake. It rarely develops in a person who does not smoke. Leukoplakia results from the inhalation of irritants such as tobacco smoke that contain known potent carcinogens including 3,4-benzpyrene and other polycyclic aromatic hydrocarbons. It is a premalignant condition from which carcinoma may develop after a period of months or years.

Carcinoma may arise from the mucous membrane of any part of the larynx; however, there is a predilection for the true vocal cords, particularly the anterior portions of the true vocal cords. The epiglottis, pyriform sinus, and postcricoid area also are common sites of origin of carcinoma. For purposes of clinical staging and end result reporting, carcinomas of the larynx can be divided into supraglottic, glottic, subglottic, and hypopharyngeal lesions. Supraglottic lesions involve the epiglottis, aryepiglottic fold, and false vocal cords. Glottic lesions are limited to the area of the true vocal cords. Subglottic lesions include the glottic area as well as the subglottic area. Hypopharyngeal lesions may be divided into lesions of the pyriform sinus, postcricoid area, and posterior pharyngeal wall.

The natural history of the carcinoma varies considerably from one location to another. The early symptom of carcinoma of the true vocal cords is hoarseness. In any patient with hoarseness lasting 2 weeks indirect laryngoscopy should be done. Any discrete lesions of the mucous membrane of the larynx should be biopsied. Carcinomas of the true vocal cord limited to the middle one third of the true vocal cord and not impairing the mobility of the cord are treated with radiation therapy or cordectomy with an overall 5-year survival rate of 85 to 95 per cent. Since cordectomy results in permanent hoarseness and irradiation usually results in a return of the voice to normal, radiation therapy is the treatment of choice. Cordectomy is reserved for the 5 to 15 per cent who have persistent carcinoma following radiation therapy. The likelihood of metastasis in early carcinoma of the true vocal cord is very slight.

The mobility of the vocal cord becomes impaired in more advanced carcinomas as a result of invasion of the intrinsic musculature and cartilage. With invasion of the intrinsic musculature, the rate of metastasis increases. With invasion of the thyroid cartilage, the rate of 5-year survival with radiation therapy decreases precipitously. Surgery becomes the treatment of choice for lesions that involve the anterior commissure where cartilage is very early invaded and for larger glottic lesions in which the mobility of the true vocal cord is impaired. Often a vertical hemilaryngectomy can be performed to preserve the phonatory and sphincteric functions of the larynx.[27] In more advanced cases, total laryngectomy is required, and the laryngectomy may be combined with a radical neck dissection if palpable metastases are present. In view of the fact that only 15 to 20 per cent of patients with glottic carcinomas have nonpalpable metastasis present at the time of initial treatment, a radical neck dissection is not performed electively.

Supraglottic carcinomas tend to be asymptomatic until they reach considerable size. They may produce hoarseness by secondary involvement of the vocal cords, or they may produce pain on swallowing as the first symptom. Often the pain radiates to the ears. Not infrequently, a patient with a supraglottic carcinoma presents with the chief complaint of a swelling in the neck which represents a metastasis. The chance of nonpalpable metastasis being present is 35 per cent. The best 5-year survival rates are obtained with a combination of radiation therapy and surgery.[30] In many patients with supraglottic carcinomas, the tumor can be completely removed by performing a supraglottic partial laryngectomy with preservation of the phonatory and sphincteric function of the larynx.[28] If the glottis is involved, a total laryngectomy is usually required. These procedures are usually combined with a radical neck dissection on the same side as the tumor.

Subglottic lesions represent more advanced glottic carcinomas in which the tumor has secondarily invaded the subglottic area as well as the supraglottic area. Metastasis to the same side is present in 50 per cent of patients. Subglottic extension of the carcinoma requires a total laryngectomy and radical neck dissection on the same side. The overall 5 year survival rate for patients with supraglottic, glottic, or subglottic carcinomas treated with total laryngectomy for all stages approximates 65 per cent.

Pyriform sinus carcinomas tend to remain asymptomatic for long periods of time. Often the patient presents with dysphagia and pain on swallowing which may radiate to the ear on the same side. Often the presenting complaint is a mass in the neck which represents a metastasis. A combination of radiation therapy and surgery yields the best 5-year survival rates. Depending on the location of the lesion in the pyriform sinus, a partial laryngectomy can sometimes be accomplished with preservation of the phonatory and sphincteric functions of the larynx. More often, a total laryngectomy is required. Either of these procedures is combined with a radical neck dissection on the same side. The 5-year survival rate for all stages is 30 per cent.

Postcricoid carcinoma has a female predominance of 10 to 1. Women with the Plummer-Vinson syndrome have a predilection for the development of postcricoid carcinoma. The presenting complaint is usually pain on swallowing and dysphagia. Metastasis to both sides of the neck is common. A combination of radiation therapy and surgery is usually employed, and the surgery required is pharyngectomy, total laryngectomy and radical neck dissection on one side followed by radical neck dissection on the other side in approximately 6 weeks. The 5-year survival rate for all stages is 25 per cent.

A total laryngectomy requires the formation of a permanent tracheostomy in which the trachea is transected and anastomosed to the skin of the lower part of the neck. Rehabilitation of the postlaryngectomy patient requires the development of alaryngeal or esophageal speech. In this technique, the patient draws air into the esophagus during inspiration and gradually eructs the air through the cricopharyngeus muscle. The opening of the esophagus vibrates and serves as the sounding source. The sound is articulated by the pharynx, palate, tongue, teeth, and lips into speech. For those persons who, because of age or other physical or emotional reasons, cannot develop alaryngeal speech, an electrolarynx can serve as the sounding source for modification by the articulators. The oscillator of the electrolarynx is placed in the submandibular area, and the sound is articulated into speech. Most persons who require a laryngectomy may return to their former occupation.[31] With proper guidance in their rehabilitation, the laryngectomee may resume all his activities except swimming.

SELECTED REFERENCES

Ballenger, J. J.: Diseases of the Nose, Throat and Ear, 12th ed. Philadelphia, Lea and Febiger, 1977.
Part V provides a comprehensive discussion of peroral endoscopy.

Davis, H., and Silverman, S. R.: Hearing and Deafness, 3rd ed. New York, Holt, Rinehart and Winston, 1970.
This text in audiology is an authoritative introduction to the measurement of hearing.

Jerger, J.: Modern Developments in Audiology, 2nd ed. New York, Academic Press, 1973.
Excellent presentations of diagnostic audiometry, masking, central auditory imperception, evoked response audiometry, and aural rehabilitation.

Maloney, W. H.: Otolaryngology. New York, Harper & Row, 1969.
This is a comprehensive encyclopedia of otology, maxillofacial surgery, bronchoesophagology, and head and neck oncology by many authorities.

Paparella, M. M., and Shumrick, D. A.: Otolaryngology. Philadelphia, W. B. Saunders Company, 1973.
Thorough discussion of numerous important topics in otolaryngology and related basic sciences.

Prior, J. A., and Silberstein, J. S.: Physical Diagnosis, The History and Examination of the Patient. St. Louis, The C. V. Mosby Co., 1963.
The section on physical diagnosis of the ears and upper respiratory tract by William H. Saunders is superb.

Schuknecht, H. F.: Pathology of the Ear. Cambridge, Harvard University Press, 1974.
Comprehensive compendium of otopathology which incorporates much of the author's vast knowledge of otology.

Shambaugh, G. E., Jr.: Surgery of the Ear, 2nd ed. Philadelphia, W. B. Saunders Company, 1967.
This textbook is a comprehensive source of information in operative otology. It is authoritative and well written.

REFERENCES

1. Abramson, M., and Gross, J.: Further studies on a collagenase in middle ear cholesteatoma. Ann. Otol., *80*:177, 1971.
2. Ash, J. E., and Raum, M.: An Atlas of Otolaryngic Pathology. Washington, D.C., Armed Forces Institute of Pathology, 1949.
3. Bast, T. H., and Anson, B. J.: The Temporal Bone and the Ear. Springfield, Ill., Charles C Thomas, Publisher, 1949.
4. Cawthorne, T., Dix, W. R., Hallpike, C. S., and Hood, J. D.: The investigation of vestibular function. Br. Med. Bull., *12*:131, 1956.
5. Chandler, J. R., and Serrins, A. J.: Transantral ligation of the internal maxillary artery for epistaxis. Laryngoscope, *75*:1151, 1965.
6. Cody, D. T. R., Simonton, K. M., and Hallberg, O. E.: Automatic repetitive decompression of the saccule in endolymphatic hydrops (Tack operation). Laryngoscope, *77*:1480, 1967.
7. Conley, J. J., and Novack, A. J.: The surgical treatment of malignant tumors of the ear and temporal bone. Arch. Otol., *71*:635, 1960.
8. Fairbanks, D. N. F.: Closure of large nasal septum perforations. Arch. Otol., *91*:403, 1970.
9. Fick, I. A. van N.: Decompression of the labyrinth. Arch. Otol., *79*:447, 1964.
10. Fredrickson, J. M., Griffith, A. W., and Lindsay, J. R.: Transverse fracture of the temporal bone, a clinical and histopathologic study. Arch. Otol., *78*:770, 1963.
11. Geroulis, A. T., and Powell, W. J.: Internal maxillary artery ligation for posterior epistaxis. Surg. Forum, *26*:531, 1975.
12. Grillo, H. C.: Obstructive lesions of the trachea. Ann. Otol., *82*:770, 1973.
13. Henle, W.: Elevated antibody titers to Epstein-Barr virus in nasopharyngeal carcinoma, other head and neck neoplasms and control groups. J. Natl. Cancer Inst., *44*:225, 1970.
14. Hough, J. V. D.: Tympanoplasty with the interior fascial graft technique and ossicular reconstruction. Laryngoscope, *80*:1385, 1970.
15. House, W. F.: Subarachnoid shunt for drainage of hydrops. Arch. Otol., *79*:328, 1964.
16. House, W. F.: Surgical exposure of internal auditory canal and its contents through middle cranial fossa. Laryngoscope, *71*:1363, 1961.
17. House, W. F.: Transtemporal bone microsurgical removal of acoustic neuromas. Arch. Otol. *80*:601, 1964.
18. Jerger, J.: Békésy audiometry in analyses of auditory disorders. J. Speech Hearing Res., *3*:275, 1960.
19. Jerger, J., Shedd, J. L., and Harford, E.: On detection of extremely small changes in sound intensity. Arch. Otol., *69*:200, 1959.
20. Litton, W. B.: Epithelial migration over tympanic membrane and external canal. Arch. Otol., *77*:254, 1963.
21. Lofgren, R. H.: Surgery of the pterygomaxillary fossa. Arch. Otol., *94*:516, 1971.
22. Martin, H.: Surgery of Head and Neck Tumors. New York, Harper & Row, 1957.
23. McCabe, B. F.: Central aspects of drugs for motion sickness and vertigo. Adv. Otorhinolaryngol., *20*:458, 1973.
24. Michelson, R. P., Merzenich, M. M., Schindler, R. A., and Schindler, D. N.: Present status and future development of the cochlear prosthesis. Ann. Otol., *84*:494, 1975.
25. Muir, C. S., and Shanmugaratnam, L.: Cancer of the Nasopharynx. Flushing, N.Y., Medical Examination Publishing Co., 1967.
26. Neal, L. C., Snow, J. B., and Seda, H. J.: An analysis of therapy for carcinoma of the tonsil. Trans. Am. Acad. Ophthalmol. Otolaryngol., *77*:97, 1973.
27. Ogura, J. H., and Biller, H. F.: Glottic reconstruction following extended frontolateral hemilaryngectomy. Laryngoscope, *75*:2181, 1965.
28. Ogura, J. H., and Dedo, H. H.: Glottic reconstruction following subtotal glottic-supraglottic laryngectomy. Laryngoscope, *75*:865, 1965.
29. Ogura, J. H., and Powers, W. E.: Functional restitution of traumatic stenosis of the larynx and pharynx. Laryngoscope, *74*:1081, 1964.
30. Ogura, J. H., Sessions, D. G., and Spector, G. J.: Conservation surgery for epidermoid carcinoma of the supraglottic larynx. Laryngoscope, *85*:1808, 1975.
31. Ranney, J. L.: Rehabilitation through employment. Laryngoscope, *85*:674, 1975.
32. Rapkin, R. H.: The diagnosis of epiglottitis: Simplicity and reliability of radiographs of the neck in the differential diagnosis of the croup syndrome. J. Pediatr., *80*:96, 1972.
33. Rauch, S., and Rauch, I.: Physio-chemical properties of the inner ear especially ionic transport. *In* Keidel, W. D., and Neff, W. D. (Eds.): Handbook of Sensory Physiology. Vol. 1, Auditory System. New York, Springer-Verlag, 1974.
34. Rosen, S.: Mobilization of the stapes to restore hearing in otosclerosis. N.Y. J. Med., *53*:2650, 1953.
35. Ruedi, L.: Pathogenesis and treatment of cholesteatoma in chronic suppuration of the temporal bone. Ann. Otol., *66*:283, 1957.
36. Saunders, W. H.: Hereditary hemorrhagic telangiectasis. Its familial pattern, clinical characteristics and surgical treatment. Arch. Otol., *76*:245, 1962.
37. Schuknecht, H. F.: Reconstructive procedures for congenital aural atresia. Arch. Otol., *101*:170, 1975.
38. Silverstein, H., Fabian, R. L., Stool, S. E., and Hong, S. W.: Penetrating wounds of the tympanic membrane and ossicular chain. Trans. Am. Acad. Ophthamol. Otolaryngol., *77*:125, 1973.
39. Sessions, R. B., Wills, P. I., Alford, B. R., Harrell, J. E., and Evans, R. A.: Juvenile nasopharyngeal angiofibroma: Radiographic aspects. Laryngoscope, *86*:2, 1976.
40. Shea, J. J., Jr.: Fenestration of the oval window. Ann. Otol., *67*:932, 1958.

41. Snow, J. B.: Clinical evaluation of noisy respiration in infancy. J. Lancet, *85*:504, 1965.

42. Snow, J. B.: Clinical manifestations other than audiologic findings of retrocochlear lesions. Adv. Otorhinolaryngol., *20*:258, 1973.

43. Snow, J. B.: Complications of acute and chronic otitis media. *In* Maloney, W. H. (Ed.): Otolaryngology. Hagerstown, Md., Harper and Row, Publishers, 1974.

44. Tos, M.: Nasotracheal intubation in acute epiglottitis. Arch. Otol., *97*:373, 1973.

45. Walker, E. A., and Resler, D. R.: Nasal gliomas. Laryngoscope, *73*:93, 1963.

46. Wullstein, H.: The restoration of function of the middle ear in chronic otitis media. Ann. Otol., *65*:1020, 1956.

42

THE MOUTH, TONGUE, JAWS, AND SALIVARY GLANDS

Milton T. Edgerton, M.D.,
and Gaylord S. Williams, M.D.

HISTORICAL ASPECTS

There is evidence to indicate that surgery was performed in and about the mouth as early as 3000 B.C.[27] On a wall of the tomb of Hesi-re at Saqqara in Egypt, near the ruins of ancient Memphis, was found a picture of a seated dentist with instruments in his left hand.[38] A Babylonian cuneiform inscription, dating from about 2000 B.C., and now preserved in the British Museum, exorcises the toothworm (believed to be the cause of dental decay until the eighteenth century A.D.). The Edwin Smith Surgical Papyrus, now in the New York Academy of Medicine Library, and dating from the Egypt of 1700 B.C., presents 27 head injury cases with descriptions of fractures and dislocations of the jaw and injuries to the lips and chin, generally with diagnosis, treatment, and prognosis given. From about the sixth century B.C. through the second century of the Christian era, the Greeks developed a system of medicine that was the basis of treatment in Europe until near the end of the fifteenth century A.D. Hippocrates (born about 460 B.C.) is credited with having described a method for reduction of fractures of the lower jaw by binding together the firm teeth on each side of the break with linen thread or gold wire and supporting loose teeth by similar ligatures.[27] Cornelius Celsus, a Roman of the first century A.D., in his multivolume work, *De medicina*, described ulcers of the mouth, which the Greeks called aphthae; small tumors of the gingiva, called parulides by the Greeks; a method for extracting teeth with forceps; treatment for toothache; incision and drainage for abscesses; and reduction of fractures of the jaw very similar to methods of the Egyptians. Galen (A.D. 131–201) wrote voluminously explaining all disease in the light of pure, dogmatic theory, substituting a strict system of medical philosophy for the plain notation and interpretation of facts as taught by Hippocrates. His work was so well accepted as authoritative that "European medicine remained at a dead level for nearly fourteen centuries."[21]

From the death of the Prophet in A.D. 632, the religion of Mohammed spread east to Persia and west along both shores of the Mediterranean to Spain and north through central Europe. Parchments from libraries of overrun provinces traveled by ship and by camel to the various capitals, including Samarkand and Cairo, where they were translated into Arabic. Thus, Islamic and Arabic medicine fell under the influence of Galenic dogma.[27] Medicine in this period of the Dark Ages in Europe and the Mediterranean basin was, for the most part, nonsurgical, because of religious proscriptions against cutting human flesh. Most treatment consisted of ex-

periments in chemistry and pharmacology. Cautery became extremely popular (Fig. 1). In the twelfth century, with the dawning of the Renaissance, medicine again began to move forward. Theodoric, Bishop of Cervia (1205–1298), advocated that wounds should heal by primary intention. William, in his *Praxeox totius medicinae,* in 1275, first described intermaxillary fixation. He advised not only the binding together of firm teeth adjacent to a fracture in the mandible, but also binding of them into contact with the corresponding teeth in the maxilla. Fallopius (1528–1562) adopted the term "hard" and "soft" palate and described the fifth, seventh, and ninth cranial nerves. Eustachius (1520–1574) published in 1563 *Libellus de dentibus*, the first treatise ever written on the anatomy of the teeth and containing the first description of the periodontal membrane.

The celebrated French surgeon, Ambroïse Paré (1510–1590) described methods of transplanting and reimplanting teeth; he used obturators to close cleft or perforated palates; extracted teeth, drained dental abscesses, and set fractured jaws.[27]

In the seventeenth century, the specialties of dentistry and oral surgery began to develop. More than 100 works were published on dentistry.[10] Wilhelm Fabry (1556–1634) reported more than 600 cases, many of which dealt with oral surgical problems running the gamut from toothache to tumor. Anselme Louis Bernard Jourdain-Berchillet (1734–1816) was trained in surgery but specialized in dentistry and oral surgery. In 1778, he published his major work, *Treatise on the Diseases and Essentially Surgical Operations of the Mouth.* In this, he described the treatment of abscesses, caries, and necrosis of the jaws, diseases of salivary glands and ducts, ranuli, calculi, various tumors, hemorrhages, and maxillary sinus problems. He felt that general surgeons needed more special dental knowledge and that dentists "lacked a sufficiently broad surgical view."

The effect of the elevator and depressor muscles on fragments in mandibular fractures was described by F. Chopart and P. J. Desault in 1779.[27]

In the nineteenth and twentieth centuries, because of advances in technology, all forms of surgery advanced exponentially. The rapid developments of asepsis, x-ray diagnosis, blood transfusions, antibiotics, and endotracheal anesthesia made possible what we now know as modern surgical management of lesions about the mouth.

Aseptic technique has been practiced rigorously and generally only in the twentieth century. Understanding of the germ theory of disease and its pragmatic application began in the latter half of the nineteenth century, notably with Lis-

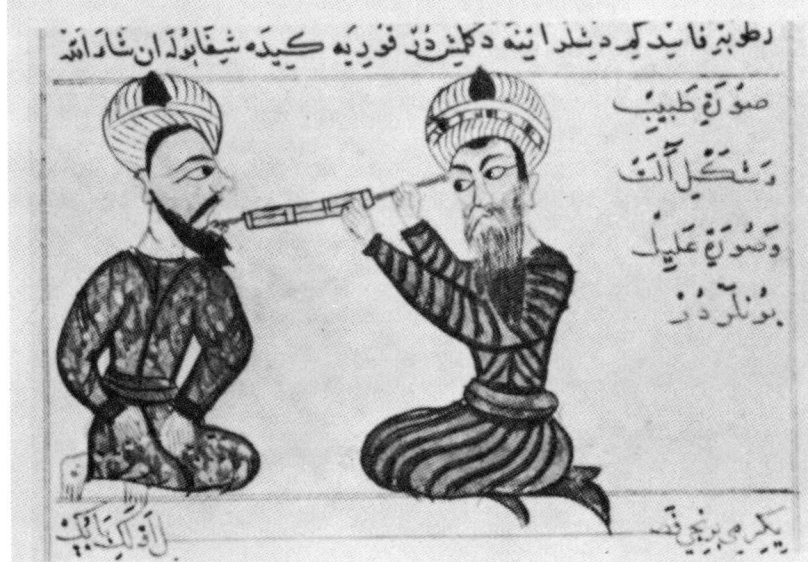

Figure 1. Old Turkish method (C. A.D. 1465) of treating pyorrheic gingivitis by cauterizing the affected area with a hot cautery iron thrust down through a protective sleeve or tube to prevent injury to the surrounding tissues from the heat of the burning iron.

ter (1827–1912) and his antiseptic technique. Principal advocates of the aseptic system were Sir William Macewen (1848–1924), a pupil of Lister, and Ernst von Bergmann (1836–1907), a Berliner, who introduced steam sterilization. Clean, white surgical gowns replaced the handy old frock coat at the operating table only in the 1880s, and rubber gloves were introduced by Halsted in 1890. Infection was so feared that a casual glance through any text on facial fractures antedating World War II reveals that open surgical reductions of mandibular fractures were avoided because of high risk. Antibiotics and chemotherapeutic agents have changed this.

The modern attempt to treat cancer of the head and neck by surgical excision probably began with Billroth's resection of the cervical esophagus and larynx on December 31, 1873.[17] Sir Henry T. Butlin, surgeon to St. Bartholomew's Hospital in London, 1885, published a monograph entitled *Diseases of the Tongue.* Without any of the advantages of modern surgery, Butlin courageously and repeatedly attempted by operation to control cancer of the tongue. He even excised the mandible and portions of the soft tissues and lymphatics of the upper cervical region. He reported more than 100 cases of cancer of the tongue that he had treated personally, performing total glossectomy on many. He noted that in the early nineteenth century, in England alone, more than 750 persons died of cancer of the tongue per year. At a time when American surgeons were making very little effort to cure this type of cancer, Butlin pointed out that "even the smallest, earliest, and most insignificant epithelioma of the tongue could produce cervical lymph node metastases," and, therefore, he concluded, "the surgeon would still be needed for the treatment of the regional metastases even if other methods for controlling the primary lesion should appear."

Röntgen, in 1895, and the Curies, in 1898, introduced the use of the roentgen ray and radium in the treatment of cancer. As is so often true with a new modality, overtreatment and enthusiasm led to discouraging results. Quinby, Janeway, and others contributed importantly to studies in the use of radiation.

In 1906, Crile presented a paper on "Excision of Cancer of the Head and Neck," in which he stated: "The operative treatment is hampered by tradition and conventionality, and the tragic ending of so large a proportion of these cases has held back lay and even professional confidence." He pointed out that less than 1 per cent of patients with head and neck cancer died from metastases to distant tissues, and he became convinced of the necessity of performing wider local excision and radical block dissection of the lymphatics of the neck. Crile was the first to describe staged, bilateral neck dissection. He was able to demonstrate in a personal series that the patient receiving such an en bloc neck dissection had a 25 per cent better chance of living for 3 years without disease than one treated for the primary lesion only.

In 1923, Brewer of New York presented statistics from several New York hospitals that indicated that the results of surgical treatment of cancer of the lip were far superior to those obtained with radium treatment. He felt that the treatment of cancer of the cheek by radium offered more promise. About that time, Sir Harold Gillies in England and Staige Davis and Vilray Blair in this country were pointing out the problems of deformity resulting from the treatment of head and neck cancer and developing techniques for the reconstruction of the face and jaws of these patients once the cancer had been controlled. Reluctance to perform adequate surgical resections led to a disappointing number of cancer recurrences and caused physicians to look again toward radiation therapy. Radium was tried in the form of plaques and molds in the early 1920s and, shortly thereafter, Evans and Cade in Great Britain reported the use of interstitial radium therapy for tongue cancer.

When the 200 kV roentgen ray machine was developed, the therapeutic use of external radium became less popular. Coutard (1937) made an outstanding contribution to head and neck cancer by showing the value of fractionation of x-radiation over a period of approximately 3 weeks, thus greatly reducing damage to overlying normal structures and skin. During the early 1930s, irradiation treatment for oral cancer was very common in America, but gradually physicians began to see increasing numbers of cases of irradiation necrosis and of radioresistant tumors.

Later came the recognition of sarcomas that were indeed *caused* by the irradiation that had been used in the treatment of the primary cancer. Just as surgeons had learned that some tumors appeared to be inoperable, radiotherapists began to appreciate that some of these tumors were not responsive to irradiation. Surgeons such as Hayes Martin, William MacFee, Grant Ward, J. B. Brown, and Louis Byars were obtaining the salvage of many patients previously deemed incurable. Discriminating radiotherapists began to realize that patients with thyroid cancer, salivary gland cancer, and cancers within the jaw or facial bones were *usually not candidates for irradiation treatment.* It was recognized that many squamous cell cancers responded poorly, if at all, to irradiation.[17]

During World War II, striking improvements were made through the use of endotracheal anesthesia, more adequate transfusion with major surgery, and the advent of antibiotics. These changes, and the surgical skills learned by many physicians in dealing with the war wounded, contributed to a marked reduction in the operative mortality in operations on the head and neck. It became increasingly clear that even wider local excisions of oral cavity cancer could be accomplished with low mortality. Many surgeons treating head and neck cancer were trained in the use of modern reconstructive techniques and thus were emboldened to enlarge the reasonable limits of resection. The concept of "excision in continuity" as previously advocated by Halsted in the treatment of cancer of the breast, and by Miles in abdominoperineal resection was regularly applied to oral and laryngeal cancer. As a larger number of patients were cured of their cancers, of necessity more attention was focused on the resulting deformities. Plastic surgeons began to realize that they could contribute much to the rehabilitation of patients with head and neck cancer.[17]

In 1949, Baclesse advocated extending the total treatment time of fractionated external irradiation from 3 to 8 or 10 weeks. In this way, he reduced some of the severe acute irradiation reactions and allowed greater doses to be applied to the tumor. Paterson and Parker had already published, in 1938, their work on the use of low-intensity radium needles. Shortly afterward, the supervoltage machine was developed as a possible improvement in the method of administration. The radiologists of this period began to stress the importance of "knowing the exact site of origin of a tumor rather than the amount of anatomic involvement." Nonetheless, the results with the radiation therapy in almost all clinics in America continued to be disappointing and, after 1945, physicians returned again to modern types of surgery for primary treatment. In 1942, Wookey reported combined therapy by surgery and irradiation for the treatment of intraoral cancer, and Fletcher followed a similar program. Ward and Edgerton and others emphasized the value of preoperative irradiation in reducing exfoliation in many types of oral cavity cancer. Smith and Gehan (1959) at the National Clinical Center, in extensive wound-washing studies, demonstrated that preoperative irradiation does indeed reduce cell viability.

The use of modern methods of reconstructive surgery employed both at the time of tumor resection and shortly afterward has greatly reduced deformity and shortened hospital stay for many patients in recent years. Inevitably, new and complex methods of irradiation are continuously being developed, but each will require some years for adequate evaluation of late effects. Chemotherapy to date has been disappointing in its effect on head and neck cancer and is not sufficiently successful for clinical use, except in conjunction with surgery and irradiation.[17]

Modern treatment of lesions about the mouth, tongue, jaws, and salivary glands demands the attentions of numerous medical, surgical, and paramedical disciplines in order to deliver optimal health care benefits to the patient. General practitioners, dentists, pedodontists, orthodontists, oral surgeons, plastic surgeons, general surgeons, ear, nose, and throat surgeons, radiotherapists, chemotherapists, prosthetists, prosthodontists, speech therapists, social workers, and even cosmeticians may all have a role to play in the diagnosis, operation, reconstruction, and ultimate rehabilitation of patients undergoing treatment for lesions or disease in this area. Because of this, there is a growing tendency in major medical centers for the utilization of a com-

bined cooperative multidisciplinary team approach to the management of complex lesions in the head and neck region.

LIPS

CONGENITAL MALFORMATIONS AND DEVELOPMENTAL ANOMALIES

Clefts

The incidence of cleft lip with or without cleft palate is variously reported as between 1 in 800 and 1 in 1300 live births. This is related to the racial and ethnic composition of the particular community. Cleft lip is eight times as frequent in Caucasians as in Negroes. The usual cleft lip runs vertically upward from the vermilion to the floor of the nose. These clefts may be complete or incomplete and may be unilateral or bilateral. They are caused by a lack of fusion of a single central prolabium with one or both of two lateral mesodermal masses. These units normally come together in the central face of the embryo and fuse between the fourth and seventh weeks of embryonic life. Failure of normal fusion of this tripartite junction of mesodermal masses results in any of the aforementioned types of cleft. Aplasia or hypoplasia of the median mesodermal mass results in the rare central facial cleft of the upper lip.[44] This is the true midline "harelip" seen in rodents. Median clefts of the lower lip are extremely rare but do occur. These represent a failure of the union of the mandibular arch at the ventral midline. They are frequently associated with a cleft in the midline of the mandible in the region of the symphysis and with a bifid tongue. Rare lateral or transverse facial clefts may extend into the cheeks from the commissures of the mouth. These may be unilateral or bilateral and vary in degree. They seldom extend beyond the anterior border of the masseter muscle. Rare oblique facial clefts (meloschisis) extend through the upper lip and toward the eye along an oblique line, passing lateral to both the philtrum and nostril.

The usual type of cleft lip is associated with a cleft palate, and occurs three times as frequently as cleft palate alone. Cleft lip alone is seen predominantly (2:1) with the male sex; cleft palate alone is twice as common in the female. Cleft lip with associated cleft palate occurs with equal frequency in males and females.

Classification. The usual type of vertical paramedian clefts is divided into two main categories: (1) clefts of the primary palate, and (2) clefts of the secondary palate. The primary palate comprises the lip and alveolar ridge and is demarcated posteriorly by the incisive foramen (just behind the upper alveolar ridge). Posterior to the incisive foramen, the hard and soft palates compose the secondary palate. Clefts of the primary palate (lip or alveolus or both) may vary from an incomplete cleft, with only slight notching of the lip, to a complete cleft extending into the floor of the nose. Clefts of the primary palate may be unilateral or bilateral and may or may not be associated with clefts in the secondary palate. Clefts of the secondary palate (the hard and the soft palate behind the incisive foramen) may also be incomplete or complete and may be unilateral or bilateral in the region of the hard palate.[24]

Treatment. Clefts of the lip (primary palate) are usually closed surgically during the first 3 months of life. Some surgeons prefer to close the lip deformity within the first few days after birth in order to take advantage of passively transferred maternal immunity and allow the parents to take home a nearly normal child. Most prefer to delay operation until the child is 2 to 3 months of age, when structures are larger and anesthesia is safer. Some surgeons apply the Rule of Tens—that is, they delay closure of the lip until the child has reached a weight of 10 pounds and has a hemoglobin of 10 gm or greater. This usually occurs when the child is 10 weeks of age or older.

To avoid future deformity, the closure of a cleft lip must be performed with meticulous accuracy, with a fine-layered plastic closure. The defect in a cleft lip deformity involves not only a transverse gap in the soft tissues but also a loss of vertical length of the lip. These two aspects of the deformity must be simultaneously corrected as the defect is surgically closed. In general, lateral lip tissue is brought in by some modification of the Z-plasty principle and used to add tissue to the cleft area, thus increasing the vertical length of the lip on the cleft side to restore symmetry. This is done by one of four basic methods. The first, the straight-line (Rose-Thompson) technique, is occasionally satisfactory for minimal incomplete clefts and notching of the lip.[42, 50] In larger clefts, this procedure sacrifices too much normal tissue and may destroy the shape of the cupid's bow. Straight-line closures tend to contract, producing a notching deformity in the vermilion.[10] If this repair is used, vertical height is gained by curving the lateral borders of the wound with the concavities of the incision toward the cleft after excising the deformed philtrum.

Three modern techniques that are commonly employed all utilize the principle of the Z-plasty. These methods include the quadrilateral flap of Mirault and LeMesurier,[29] and the triangular flap technique first described by Tennison[48] (Fig. 2). All of these may be considered variations of the Z-plasty with the adjacent sides of the cleft as the central limb of the Z-plasty. The techniques vary only in the positioning and lengths of the lateral limbs of the Z-plasty. Vertical height of the repaired side of the lip is provided by transverse incisions across both the lateral and medial lip elements and rotation of the created flap; these transverse incisions correspond to the lateral limbs of the Z-plasty. Rotation or transposition of the flaps lengthens the central limbs at the expense of lip width. Geometrically, the amount of height that is gained depends upon the angle and distance of the transverse incisions. Practically speaking, the height that can be gained also depends upon the extent to which the tissue can be mobilized toward the midline (Fig. 3).

Bilateral clefts of the lip (primary palate) present an even more strikingly grotesque congenital deformity. The problems of surgical repair are frequently compounded by an elevated, protruding prolabium and premaxilla, which usually appears to be suspended from the dome of the nose by a very short columella. The timing of surgical repair for bilateral clefts is essentially the same as for unilateral clefts. As in unilateral cleft repairs, very little or no tissue is discarded or excised in the repair. All of these children suffer from a deficiency of tissue in the region of the upper lips, and great care must be taken to preserve every possible landmark of the normal lip elements. Occasionally, bilateral clefts must be repaired in stages in order to allow muscular action of the repaired side of the lip to mold the premaxilla inward toward the dental arch and thus facilitate closure of the opposite side of the lip. Surgical osteotomy and setback of the premaxilla may on occasion be necessary (Fig. 4).

Congenital Sinuses (Mucous Pits)

These usually appear as a symmetrically placed pair of dimples on the vermilion border of the lower lip, one on each side of the midline. These slitlike pits are the external orifices of blind sinuses, which extend downward through the orbicularis oris muscle, to end blindly just beneath the mucosal surface of the lower lip or gingiva. They are lined with squamous cell epithelium, and numerous mucous glands empty into the lumen of the pits near their blind end. They are usually asymptomatic but cause vermilion deformity and are usually associated with cleft lip or palate. Heredity is the most important factor in their etiology[51] (Fig. 5). The most effective treatment is precise surgical excision of the entire sinus tract after staining of the lumen by filling it with aqueous methylene blue dye. All attached mucous glands whose ducts drain into the sinus must be removed with the tract. Failure to do so may result in the formation of a mucoid cyst.

Retention Cysts

Small retention cysts may involve the mucous glands of the lips. These are mucoceles, caused by plugging of the ducts of the mucous glands. They appear as small, nontender masses that appear to be filled with fluid. They are usually asymptomatic except for their annoying bulk. Treatment consists of surgical extirpation. The defect thereby created can be closed by simple sutures or left to heal by secondary intention.

Microstomia

Children born with extremely small mouths occasionally present problems in feeding. Microstomia is usually associated with a small, retruded jaw (micrognathia). The small mouth opening rarely requires surgical intervention and is best left to enlarge by normal growth and development.

Double Lip

Congenital double lip occurs most frequently in the upper lip. The deformity is not obvious when the mouth is closed; however, with the mouth open a double vermilion is exhibited with a transverse furrow of varying depth between the reduplicated lips. The buccal portion of the double vermilion is rather loose and

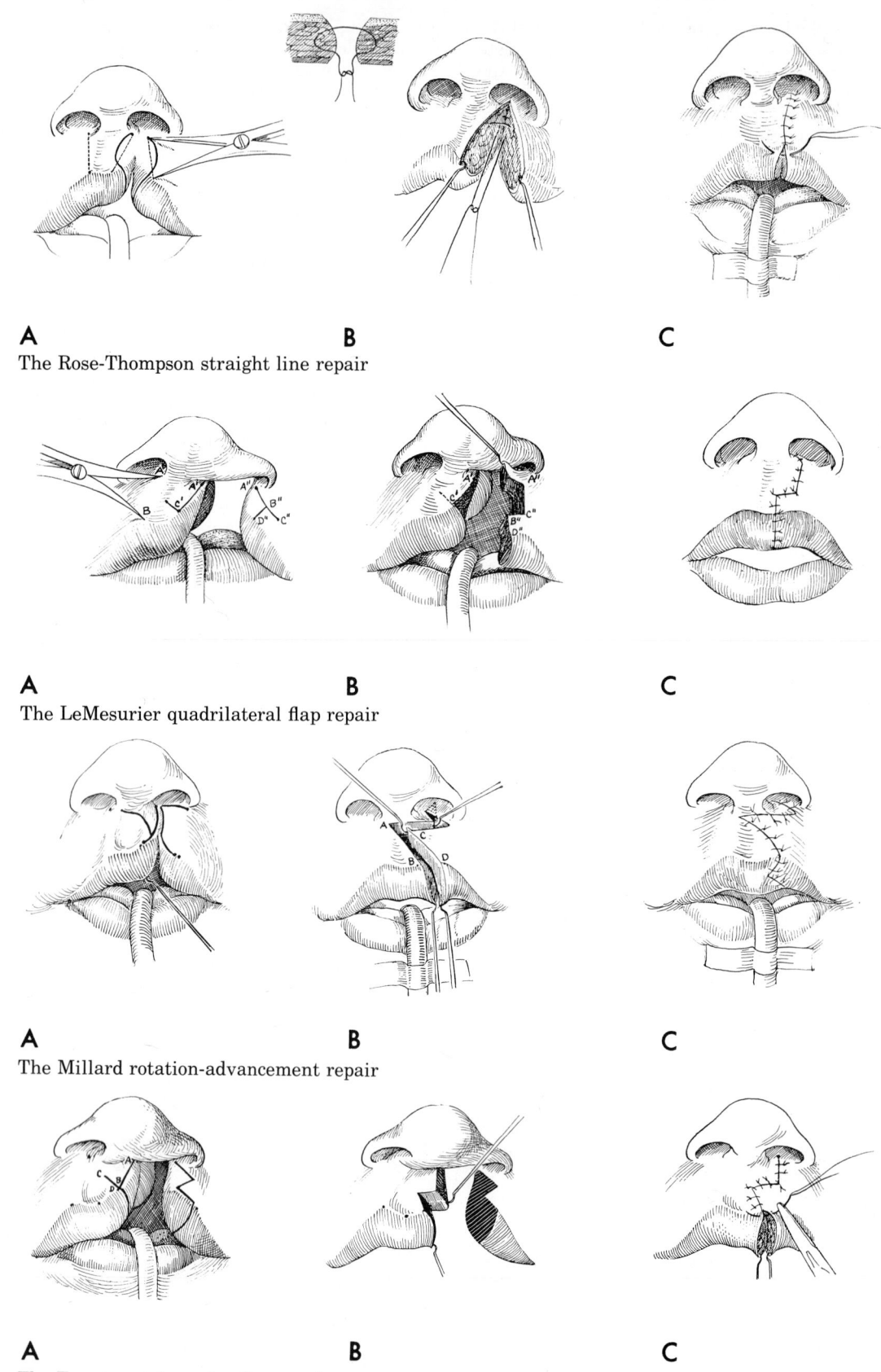

A   B   C

The Rose-Thompson straight line repair

A   B   C

The LeMesurier quadrilateral flap repair

A   B   C

The Millard rotation-advancement repair

A   B   C

The Tennison triangular flap repair.

Figure 2.   *A,* Markings; *B,* incisions; *C,* closure. (From Musgrave, R. H. *In* Converse, J. M. (Ed.): Reconstructive Plastic Surgery. Volume III. Philadelphia, W. B. Saunders Company, 1964.)

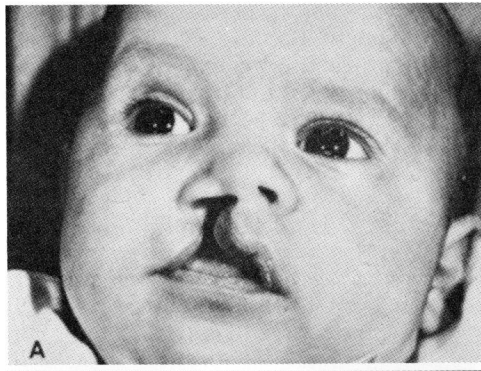

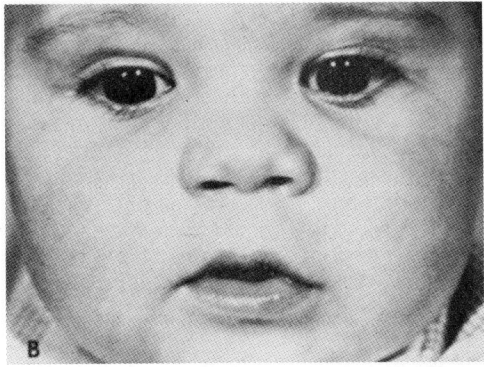

Figure 3. *A,* Complete cleft lip with some nostril distortion. *B,* Seven months after rectangular flap repair (LeMesurier). (From Musgrave, R. H. *In* Converse, J. M. (Ed.): Reconstructive Plastic Surgery, 2nd ed. Volume III. Philadelphia, W. B. Saunders Company, 1977.)

redundant. Treatment consists of transverse excision of the buccal redundancy with primary closure.[51] This is best accomplished by a zigzag (W-plasty) type closure to avoid a bandlike scar in the lip.

Peutz-Jeghers Syndrome

Melanin-like spots of pigmentation on the lips may be associated with multiple intestinal polyposis. This syndrome was first described by Peutz in 1921 and expounded on by Jeghers and associates in 1949. The syndrome is congenital and inherited. The lip (and occasionally buccal) lesions are benign and are significant in calling attention to the possible presence of intestinal polyposis.[37]

INJURIES DUE TO TRAUMA

Lacerations

Lacerations of the lip frequently involve both the mucosal and skin surfaces with division of the intervening musculature. Because of the circular and radial distribution of the perioral musculature, full-thickness lacerations tend to open widely when the muscle is divided. Because of this, inexperienced clinicians may be led to suspect tissue loss when the problem is largely tissue retraction. In closing lacerations of the lip, it is most important to reconstitute accurately the vermilion-cutaneous junction. Even a slight disparity in reconstituting this line will produce an obvious deformity. Therefore, it is most important to repair lip lacerations with good lighting, good assistance, and good anesthesia. It is quite helpful to tattoo temporarily the vermilion-cutaneous junction on either side of a laceration with a 25 gauge needle dipped in aqueous methylene blue, penetrating the skin along the vermilion edge on either side of the laceration prior to the infiltration of local anesthetic. The first skin suture is usually placed at the vermilion-cutaneous junction (Fig. 6). Local anesthetics and vasoconstrictors tend to blanch out the color differentiation between the vermilion and facial skin and, once injected, make the junction line difficult to appreciate. A few needle pricks with methylene blue prior to local

Figure 4. *A* and *B,* Bilateral complete cleft of lip with protruding premaxilla, absence of columella, wide nostril flare, and small prolabium. *C,* The premaxilla has been put back into the alveolar arch and lateral vermilion flaps have been attached to the prolabium for blood supply and cupid's bow. *D, E,* and *F,* Forked flap from prolabium has produced primary columella lengthening. Medial advancement of lateral triangular flaps has narrowed alar flares and incorporated the prolabium as a philtrum. (From Millard, D. R.: Transactions of the International Society of Plastic Surgeons, Second Congress. Edinburgh, E. & S. Livingstone, 1959.)

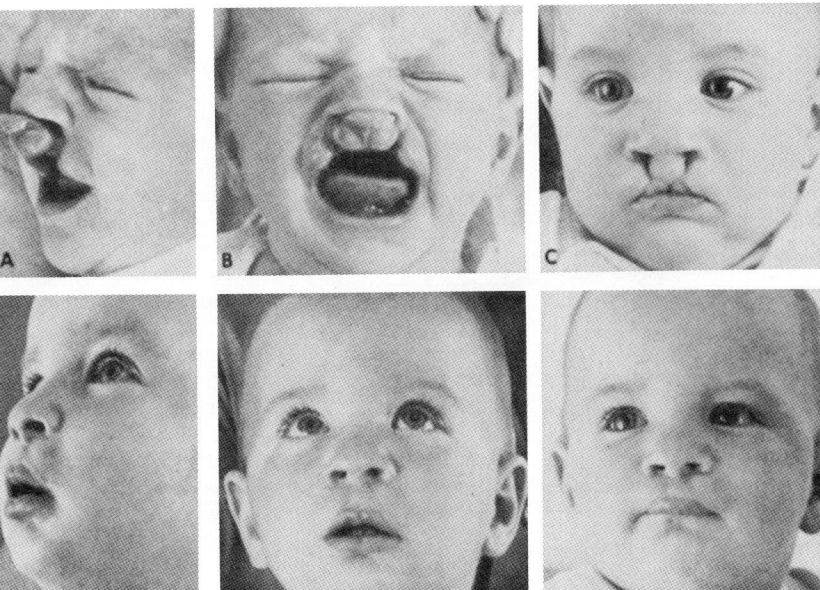

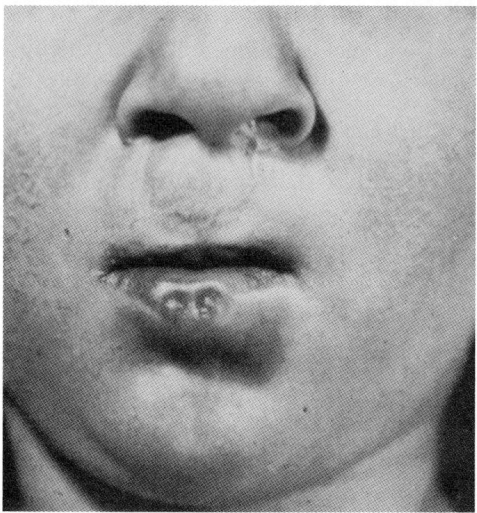

Figure 5. Congenital lip sinuses. The illustration shows bilateral, symmetrically situated sinus openings at the apices of a pair of nipple-like protrusions of the lower lip. Note the associated bilateral cleft lip, shown postoperatively. (From Wang, M. K. H., Macomber, W. B., Converse, J. M., and Wood-Smith, D. *In* Converse, J. M. (Ed.): Reconstructive Plastic Surgery, 2nd ed. Volume II. Philadelphia, W. B. Saunders Company, 1977.)

anesthetic injection can greatly simplify accurate alignment of the vermilion-cutaneous junction.

Through-and-through lacerations should be closed in layers with absorbable suture material in the muscle and subcutaneous tissues. Copious irrigation and complete hemostasis are essential. The skin can be closed with 5-0 or 6-0 silk or nylon. The mucosa is loosely closed with similar-sized silk, polyglycolic acid, or chromic gut.

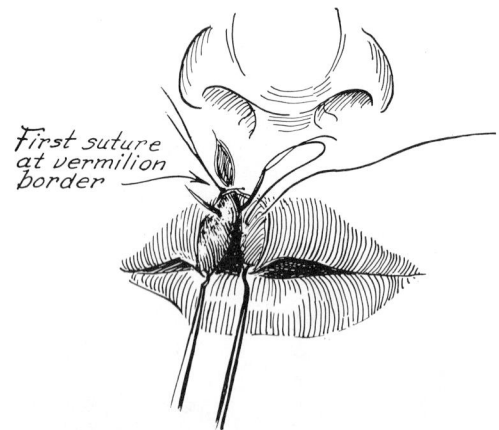

First suture at vermilion border

Figure 6. Repair of vertical lacerations of the vermilion-cutaneous margin. The first skin suture should be used for approximation of the vermilion-cutaneous border. Accurate approximation of this line will avoid conspicuous irregularity of the lip after healing takes place. (From Dingman, R. O. *In* Converse, J. M. (Ed.): Reconstructive Plastic Surgery, Volume II. Philadelphia, W. B. Saunders Company, 1964.)

The lips and most of the face are blessed with an excellent blood supply. Because of this, stellate lacerations with multiple tiny flaps of tissue will usually heal quite well if accurately repaired. Very fine sutures and use of very few buried sutures should be the rule for repairing this type of laceration.

Because of Vincent's spirochetes, fusiform bacilli, and numerous pathogenic anaerobes in the human mouth, it is advisable to give penicillin in therapeutic doses by mouth for several days following closure of lip lacerations involving the oral surface.[37] This is especially true if the tissues have been crushed by the injury.

Burns

Thermal burns of the lips generally involve the exposed skin and mucosal surfaces. They are treated in much the same way as cutaneous burns elsewhere on the body, depending on the depth of burn injury. Topical antibiotic ointment therapy may be applied with care about the mouth and will greatly relieve burn pain. It should be emphasized that the presence of a thermal burn about the mouth or nares should *not* be taken as an absolute indication for a tracheotomy. Certainly, burns in this area should alert the surgeon to the *possible* need for a tracheotomy, but it is becoming increasingly evident that routine tracheotomy for all patients with perioral burns is not only unnecessary but indeed *contra*indicated, unless there are definite signs of upper airway obstruction.[35] Elevation of the head of the patient's bed, croup tent, short courses of anti-inflammatory steroids, and wider use of prolonged endotracheal intubation will serve to further decrease the need for tracheotomy.

Burns of the inner surfaces of the lips, from the accidental ingestion of very hot liquids, are almost never deeper than second-degree. These are usully adequately managed by giving the patient a mild, orally administered analgesic. Alcoholic mouthwashes may be painful and irritating, and topical opiates are unnecessary.

One of the most frequently seen chemical burns of the lips is that due to lye in attempted suicides. This strong alkali penetrates the tissues of the lip, saponifies the fat, and reacts with the proteins to form soluble alkaline proteinate. The combination of lye with fats to form soaps is an exothermic reaction generating sufficient additional heat to damage surrounding tissue. The hygroscopic nature of lye produces cellular dehydration and cell death. The soluble alkaline proteinates formed tend to penetrate deeply into the tissues where they cause delayed further injury and an increase in the depth of the burn wound.

The treatment of lye burns of the mouth should consist of early, copious, and prolonged irrigation with cold tap water. Water dilutes the injurious lye, washes away the noxious agent, and decreases the mass action and exothermic effect of the chemical reaction, thereby diminishing the inflammatory reaction. This is best done with a small rubber hose attached to a water faucet, so that large volumes of fresh, clean water can be used to irrigate the mouth continuously for at least 12 hours. Systemic steroids also are helpful in diminishing the inflammatory reaction, and penicillin should be given as with any other burn. Attempts at chemical neutralization of the lye are fraught with many hazards and have proved to be inferior to simple water irrigation.[53]

Electrical burns of the lips are most frequently seen in small children who are apt to chew on electrical cords or place the ends of extension cords in their mouths. Saliva creates a short circuit across the terminals within the plug, causing an electrical burn. Tissue destruction with electrical burns is sudden and extensive. Extensive, deep coagulation necrosis is instantaneously produced by the extreme temperatures of the electrical arc. If the child is well grounded, the current flow through his body may cause cardiac arrest.

The initial treatment of electrical burns of the lips should be conservative and not unlike the treatment of any other form of burn. Antibiotics should be administered for 5 days. Débridement should be limited to the excision of obviously dead and necrotic tissue, should be done without anesthesia, and should produce no bleeding. The wound should generally be allowed to heal spontaneously, and reconstructive efforts should be reserved until well after healing has occurred, and the scars have softened and matured. Delayed bleeding from the coronary labial arteries of the lips is frequently seen following electrical burns. This is easily controlled with a hemostat and a simple catgut ligature.

INFECTIONS REQUIRING SURGERY

Labial Abscess or Cellulitis

The skin of the lips is well endowed with hair follicles, sweat glands, and sebaceous glands. Minor infections due to blockage of these openings in the skin, producing pustules or small abscesses, are not infrequent. Warm soaks and appropriate surgical drainage are usually adequate therapy. Numerous persistent or recurrent infections should be treated with the appropriate antibiotics following culture. The usual offending organism is the Staphylococcus. Larger abscesses can be drained through the buccal surface of the lips and cheeks to lessen the production of visible external scars. When this is done, a small drain should be sutured in the intraoral wound at two points and left in place for 3 days. Cellulitis of the lips almost always indicates a streptococcal infection and is usually treated with penicillin.

Herpetic Stomatitis

Herpetic stomatitis is a herpes simplex virus infection that presents as yellowish papulovesicular lesions which may be discrete or occur in groups. First, a small vesicle appears and ruptures early. A small ulceration then occurs. Symptoms consist of pain and burning in the region of the ulcer, particularly when the ulcer is touched. After a 10- to 12-day course, the lesion usually clears spontaneously.[3] Topical steroids such as triamcinolone and Orabase may speed symptomatic recovery. Early herpetic lesions may respond to topical 5-fluorouracil cream, but this has no efficacy once an ulcer has developed. Locally recurrent herpetic lesions may respond to subcutaneous injection of small amounts of triamcinolone at the site of recurrence. Chronic cases respond to viral vaccines.

Canker Sores

Canker sores occurring on the buccal surface of the lips are characteristically small, superficial ulcerations, which are exquisitely tender and irritated by acid foods. They are usually surrounded by an inflammatory halo of erythema. These lesions are usually associated with gastrointestinal upsets, dehydration, or nutritional disturbances. They respond well to a bland diet, oral fluids, avoidance of acid foods and juices, and vitamin supplementation. Symptomatic relief may be obtained by holding promethazine (Phenergan) syrup in the mouth in the region of the lesion for 5 to 10 minutes before swallowing. One teaspoon of the syrup every 2 hours during waking hours is sufficient for most adults. The Phenergan acts locally as a topical anesthetic and when swallowed has a systemic sedative effect. Tetracycline syrup, held in the mouth for its topical action and then swallowed, may shorten the course of these lesions.

Noma

Noma is a rapidly progressive gangrenous stomatitis that is rarely seen in well-nourished persons. It occurs in patients with general debility and metabolic dyscrasias (Fig. 7). These lesions rapidly invade and destroy soft tissues about the mouth, may involve

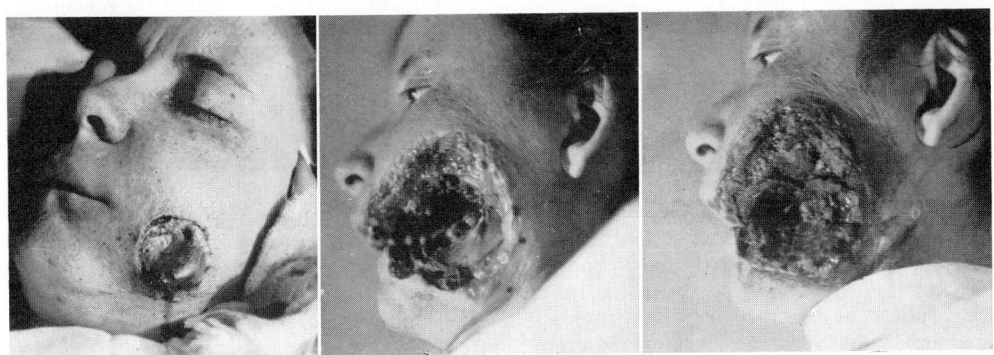

Figure 7. Noma; progressive gangrenous loss of entire cheek. (From Brown, J. B., and Fryer, M. P. *In* Davis, L. (Ed.): Christopher's Textbook of Surgery, 9th ed. Philadelphia, W. B. Saunders Company, 1968.)

bone, and frequently have a fatal termination. They are more common in children and occur after measles and other contagious diseases. They are initiated by anaerobic bacteria, among which are found fusospirochetal organisms.[23]

Moniliasis

Moniliasis (thrush) is the most common fungus disease involving the oral cavity. Its incidence is increased in patients on antibiotic therapy. The acute form produces multiple, white, adherent, curdlike patches, irregularly distributed over the mucosal surfaces. Inflammation and fissuring of the labial commissures and encrustations on the lip frequently accompany the intraoral lesions. The specific treatment agent is nystatin (Mycostatin).[3]

Syphilis

Syphilis, in its primary form, may produce a chancre on the lips. This is a foul, discharging, dirty ulcer without the surrounding characteristic hardness of carcinoma. Treatment is by systemic antisyphilitic therapy.

Other, infrequently encountered infections involving the lips include actinomycosis, histoplasmosis, molluscum contagiosum, and lymphogranuloma venereum.

BENIGN TUMORS OF THE LIPS

Benign tumors may arise from any of the tissues forming the lips. The epithelium, dermis, fibrous tissue, fat, muscle, blood vessels, lymphatics, nerves, or specialized glands may occasionally produce benign tumors. Treatment of these lesions is usually surgical excision and microscopic examination for confirmation of the diagnosis and identification of the margins of the specimen. Larger lesions will require special reconstructive procedures and are best treated by plastic surgery techniques at the time of the initial excision.

Nevi

Nevi may be subdivided microscopically into three groups, based on the depth of penetration of nevus cells across the dermal-epidermal junction: (1) Intradermal nevi have most of the nevus cells within the dermis. They are frequently raised above the skin surface, may contain hair, and show varying degrees of pigmentation. (2) Junctional nevi show the nevus cells to be concentrated at the junction between the dermis and epidermis. They are usually flat, do not contain hair, and may vary in depth of pigmentation. (3) Compound nevi show nevus cells distributed through both the dermis and junctional zones. They may be elevated or sessile and may or may not contain hair. It is generally agreed that intradermal nevi never become malignant and that junctional nevi may become malignant. Compounded nevi have been reported to become malignant, by a few authors. Any nevus of the lip (or elsewhere) that shows change in either size or pigmentation, or in any way appears to be undergoing change, by itching or bleeding for example, should be surgically excised. Similarly, any pigmented nevus that is chronically irritated should be excised.

Papillomas

These are commonly referred to as "skin tags." They are frequently seen about the face and neck and are usually multiple. Microscopically, they appear to be primarily epithelial hyperplasias. The matrix of the skin tag shows a pattern of randomly arranged, delicate fibers that resemble the pattern of normal dermis. They vary in size but are usually less than 1 cm. in diameter. They are usually soft and pedicled on a stalk of soft skin. Surgical excision is the treatment of choice.

Fibromas

These benign tumors arise in the deeper layers of the skin and contain mesodermal or epithelial elements. They may be classified as fibrolipoma, myofibroma, angiofibroma, or neurofibroma. Those with a gelatinous stroma are referred to as fibromyxomas. These tumors are rare but may occur in the lip. Treatment is by local surgical excision.

Lipomas and Myomas

Lipomas and myomas may rarely occur on the lips. These benign tumors are excised surgically for diagnosis and cure.

Hemangiomas

Benign vascular malformations or hamartomas, hyperplasias, and vascular ectasias may occur in the lips. Classification is based on the clinical characteristics and the histology of these angiomas. In general, they can be grouped into three categories: (1) capillary angiomas; (2) cavernous angiomas; and (3) telangiectases.

Capillary Angiomas. Capillary angioma, often called strawberry nevus, is usually present at, or appears shortly after, birth. It tends to be polypoid, raised, and bright red to purple in color, occasionally is bosselated, and involves the dermis and subcutis. Lesions that are superficial are bright red, but those with deep components tend to be darker in color. They may grow rapidly and are occasionally complicated by ulceration and infection. Spontaneous involution usually begins by the age of 2 or 3 years and is first noted by the appearance of patchy, pale areas, usually near the center of the lesion. Gradually, the tumor shrinks and involutes, losing its vascular color. When involution is complete, the site may appear normal or may show loose, wrinkled skin with slight atrophy and occasionally a few telangiectatic vessels.[39]

Treatment of capillary hemangiomas in the past has consisted of cryotherapy, injection of sclerosing agents, surgical excision, and x-ray or radium therapy. Most of these methods have produced cosmetic results that are definitely inferior to those after natural involution. Uncomplicated capillary hemangiomas that are not disturbing function or causing troublesome frequent bleeding are best followed conservatively. Most will undergo natural involution with superior final results. If the hemangioma continues to enlarge alarmingly, the involution can frequently be dramatically stimulated and hastened by the oral administration of prednisolone, given in high doses (40 mg. every 2 days for 10 days), to otherwise healthy babies in whom there is no contraindication to this form of therapy.[15, 54]

X-ray therapy, either as superficial irradiation or in the form of radium implantation, is, unfortunately, still frequently advocated as a method for "inducing regression" of these lesions. This treatment of benign disease is mentioned here only to criticize it. The late sequelae of radiation damage include atrophy, dermatitis, and scarring in surrounding normal tissue, cessation of underlying bony growth and development, radionecrosis, and even late development of malignant neoplastic changes. These complications present problems of much greater magnitude than the original lesion.

Cavernous Angiomas. These are tumor-like aggregates of larger dilated vessels or sinusoidal blood spaces in a fibrous stroma. They are usually not present at birth, but appear during early childhood. They extend into the subcutaneous tissue with poorly defined borders. Histologically, the vessels appear more mature and lack the angioblastic qualities of the capillary hemangioma. Also, unlike capillary hemangiomas, they show no tendency for involution and, indeed, usually show insidious, progressive enlargement. Irradiation is contraindicated and has no more effect on the cavernous hemangioma than on the surrounding normal tissues. Interruption of feeding vessels, by ligation or by injection embolization, has been used with variable success. Usually, surgical resection and reconstruction will give the best results.[39] (Fig. 8).

Telangiectases. *Nevus flammeus* (port-wine stain) is a macular, pink to purple vascular malformation that is frequently distributed along the course of peripheral nerves. Most of these nevi are present at birth and do not tend to grow or involute. They do not respond to irradiation, freezing, or surgical abrasion. Many are managed by the application of cosmetics to hide the discoloration, but this does not relieve the "sense of deformity" and plastic surgeons are now using more "color-matched" skin grafts from the neck or scalp to replace these lesions on the lips and face.

Venous varix (senile hemangioma, venous lake) may appear as a solitary, deep blue nodule on the lips. It resembles a blood blister, but is not tense. It empties easily with pressure. These lesions tend to persist unless excised for cosmetic purposes.[39]

Osler-Rendu-Weber syndrome (hereditary hemorrhagic telangiectasia) is characterized by discrete, red, small, superficial punctate telangiectatic lesions on the skin and oral mucous membranes. They may be flat or slightly raised and are seldom more than a few millimeters in diameter. They are frequently accompanied by lesions on the fingers, face, and nasal mucous membranes. These lesions are prone to ulceration and hemorrhage and are frequently associated with arteriovenous fistulas in the lungs and vascular malformations of the liver. When seen on the lips, they should arouse suspicion of the other facets of the syndrome. The lip lesions can be controlled by cautery or excision.[39]

Lymphangiomas

These are growths of thin-walled, vascular spaces that contain lymph. They may involve the lips and cheeks, producing visible deformity. They show no tendency toward spontaneous involution. They are not radiosensitive. Treatment, if indicated, is surgical, and if incomplete the lesions are likely to recur.[39]

Pyogenic Granulomas

These are localized, superficial polypoid masses of new capillaries within an edematous matrix. They are devoid of epithelium and grossly resemble polyps of granulation tissue. In spite of their name, an infectious etiology for these lesions is not firmly established. These lesions may occur at any age, and symp-

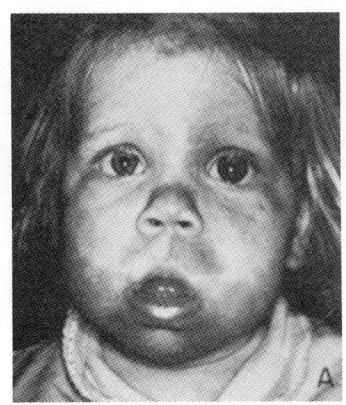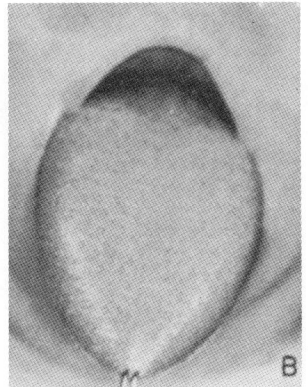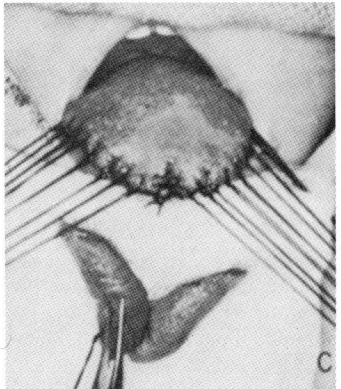

Figure 8. This child was born with a massive facial hemangioma of mixed type. In *A*, the external port-wine stain component is obvious, and her open bite secondary to macroglossia is also apparent. The grossly and diffusely enlarged tongue (*B*) was adequately reduced in size by wedge excision of the tip and lateral margins (*C*). The child can now close her mouth and her dentition has been freed from the distorting forces of a large tongue. (From Edgerton, M. T., and DeVito, R. T. *In* Converse, J. M. (Ed.): Reconstructive Plastic Surgery. Volume III. Philadelphia, W. B. Saunders Company, 1964.)

toms of pain or tenderness are variable. They tend to bleed easily when traumatized. Treatment should be by surgical excision with microscopic confirmation of the diagnosis to rule out the presence of other lesions that may mimic pyogenic granuloma, i.e., Kaposi's disease and metastatic renal cell carcinoma.[39]

Epidermal Inclusion Cysts (Sebaceous Cysts)

These occur commonly on the skin of the lips. They are more common in people with thick, oily skin. They result from occlusion of the drainage pores of the sebaceous glands, and are usually firm and discrete. Palpation of the cyst and moving it about beneath the skin will frequently demonstrate traction umbilication of the skin at the site of the occluded pore. These cysts are best treated by excising a small, elliptical sliver of skin containing the punctum along with the underlying cyst.

Keratoacanthomas

These common benign cutaneous tumors may arise form the hair follicles on the lips. Their rapid growth and histologic appearance may lead the surgeon, and occasionally the pathologist, to make a diagnosis of squamous carcinoma. Keratoacanthoma is, however, a benign tumor that runs a self-limited course. If untreated, it may produce a cicatricial deformity of the lips. This tumor is limited to the white races, and has its highest incidence in persons between the ages of 50 and 70. The etiology of keratoacanthoma is unclear. Actinic rays, chemical carcinogens, trauma, genetic factors, and viral factors may all play a role in its etiology. Clinically, the tumors may appear as dome-shaped buds with a pink to reddish hue. Later in the evolution of the tumor, the epithelium over the center of the dome breaks down to reveal a central keratin plug.. Ultimately the keratin plug detaches, leaving a crater-shaped lesion. Finally, the lesion becomes ulcerated and then regresses completely, healing by scar formation. Treatment is by surgical excision with primary closure. The specimen must be submitted to the pathologist for accurate histopathologic diagnosis. Other methods of treatment such as curettage, cautery, diathermy, or x-ray therapy will usually prove curative for keratoacanthoma but will make accurate pathologic diagnosis difficult or impossible. The excision of large keratoacanthomas may make it advisable for the surgeon to use pedicle flaps or grafts or both to reconstruct the lips.[22]

Keratoses

These rough, scaly, slightly raised lesions occur at the vermilion-cutaneous junction, usually on the lips of elderly patients with fair skin who are chronically exposed to solar radiation. They may give rise to squamous cell carcinomas of the lips. Chronic labial keratoses are best excised by a "lip shave" procedure with mucosal advancement (Fig. 9). The full thickness of the skin should be excised and the tissue should be examined microscopically.[17, 46]

Leukoplakia

This condition commonly presents with slightly elevated, white patches on the buccal mucosa, tongue, palate, or lip vermilion. Treatment should initially consist of the removal of any possible mouth irritant such as tobacco or snuff. General mouth cleanliness and hygiene should be encouraged and any caries or rough teeth should receive prompt dental care. Daily abrasion with a stiff-bristle toothbrush will clear up the superficial varieties. After these conservative measures have been tried, persistent lesions should be excised and examined microscopically, as this condition is definitely precancerous.[4]

SQUAMOUS CANCER OF THE LIPS

Almost all "lip cancer" arises at the skin-vermilion junction. Basal cell cancers and melanomas arising in the skin of the lips are considered elsewhere in this book.

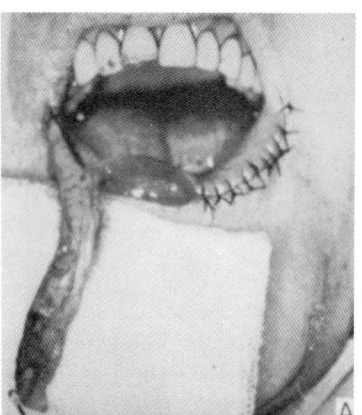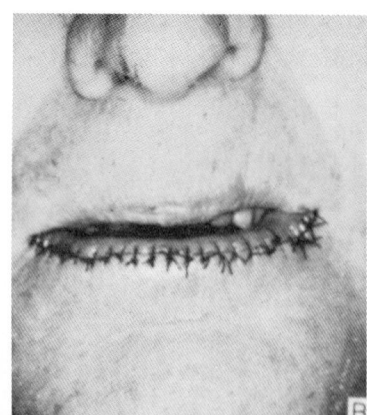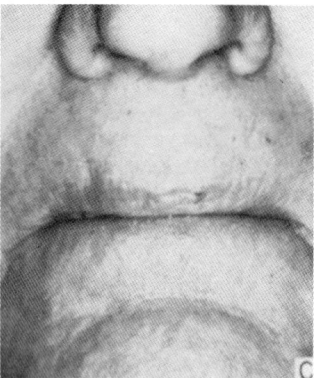

Figure 9. Resection of the vermilion border with mucosal advancement ("lip shave") done for leukoplakia or chronic keratoses of the vermilion is shown in progress *(A)*, at completion *(B)*, and in the late postoperative period *(C)*. (From Edgerton, M. T., and DeVito, R. T. *In* Converse, J. M. (Ed.): Reconstructive Plastic Surgery. Volume III. Philadelphia. W. B. Saunders Company, 1964.)

Lip carcinoma accounts for approximately 15 per cent of all malignant diseases of the head and neck and roughly 1 per cent of all cancers. They almost always occur on the lower lip, and 87 per cent occur in males. They are rarely seen in persons below the age of 40, and there is an increasing incidence with advancing age. Persons with light-colored skin, blue eyes, and light-colored hair who tend to freckle (rather than tan) when exposed to sunlight appear to be highly susceptible. Carcinoma of the lip is rarely seen in blacks. There is a definite correlation between lip cancer and exposure to sunlight.[1] The incidence of these cancers gradually increases in susceptible persons as the equator is approached from the extreme northern or southern latitudes. Persons spending most of their lives out of doors, in higher elevations, where the effects of actinic irradiation are stronger, also are more susceptible to the development of lip cancer. Other factors that frequently turn up in the histories of patients with lip cancer, and that are believed to have some etiologic significance, include syphilis, prior gamma irradiation, excessive use of tobacco (particularly smoking of pipes with clay stems), and heavy alcohol consumption.

Diagnostic work-up with a suspected lip cancer should include biopsy of the lesion. Biopsies are 100 per cent accurate if positive.[6] If negative, they should be repeated. Bidigital examination of the floor of the mouth and the submental and submaxillary triangles for metastatic disease should be carried out. Both sides of the entire neck should be carefully palpated for enlarged lymph nodes. A chest x-ray may reveal metastases.

Classification. Clinically, lip cancer presents as one of two major types: (1) exophytic lesions in which superficial proliferation predominates, or (2) endophytic lesions in which invasion, ulceration, and early involvement of muscle, bone, and skin predominate (Fig. 10). Histologically, epidermoid carcinoma accounts for 99 per cent of all lip cancers.[6] These are usually well differentiated. Basal cell carcinoma occasionally appears on the lips but this can, more often than not, be demonstrated to be associated with basal cell carcinoma arising in the skin surrounding the lips. Melanoma is occasionally seen as a primary lip cancer.

The metastatic behavior of lip cancer is characterized by relatively late spread to regional lymph nodes except in the undifferentiated lesions. The metastatic route is to the facial and submental lymph nodes and the nodes along the anterior portion of the submaxillary gland, and then to the jugular chain. Invasion of the mandible is usually late and occurs via direct soft tissue extension, usually entering the mental foramen to reach the marrow cavity. Distant metastasis to the lungs and liver occurs late and is rare. When death occurs it is usually due to uncontrolled tumor in the neck.

Principles of Treatment. The management of carcinoma of the lip must be individualized in every case. Factors that enter into the decision include:

1. The age of the patient. Younger patients are more likely to have early metastases than older ones.[8]

2. The reliability of the patient and the logistical practicality for close follow-up of the patient. Patients

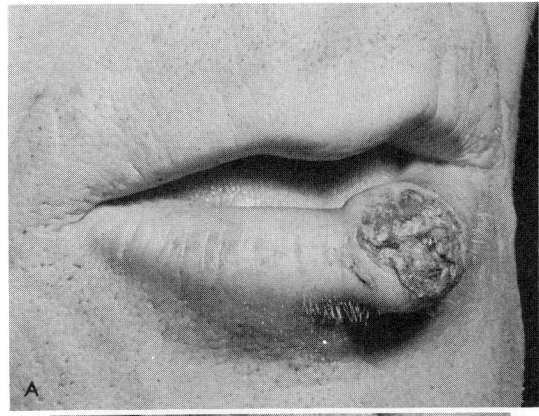

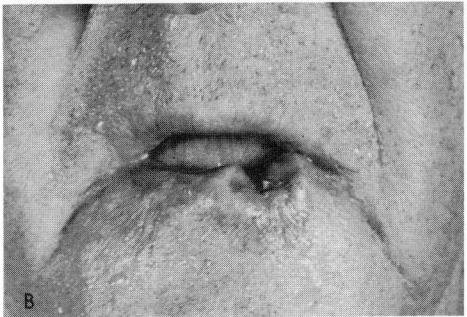

Figure 10. *A*, Exophytic carcinoma of lower lip with central ulceration and raised, rolled borders. *B*, Ulcerating carcinoma of lower lip with diffuse infiltration. (From Ackerman, L. V., and del Regato, J. A.: Cancer: Diagnosis, Treatment, and Prognosis, 4th ed. St. Louis, The C. V. Mosby Company, 1970.)

in whom the potential for close follow-up seems dubious are better served by a diagnostic dissection of the regional lymph nodes at the time of the initial resection of the lip primary. Experience has shown that large recurrences may appear rapidly in the neck, and they are most difficult to treat.

3. The nature of the lesion. The endophytic, invasive type carcinoma tends to metastasize much earlier than the exophytic type.[8]

4. The size of the lesion. Lesions less than 1 cm. in size only rarely will have metastasized to the neck, and these smaller lesions can usually be managed by local lip resection. Lesions larger than 1 cm. in size are much more likely to have spread to the regional nodes. The size of the lesion is usually correlated with its duration on the lip. The longer a lesion has been present, the more likely that metastasis will have occured to the nodes in the neck.[8]

5. The histologic gradation of the cell malignancy. High-grade or undifferentiated carcinoma is more likely to develop early metastasis than are low-grade, well-differentiated tumors.

6. Staging. The presence of palpable enlarged or indurated nodes in the submental area or neck is a definite indication for radical neck dissection to remove regional nodes.

7. Recurrent or persistent lesions. In those lesions which have previously been treated inadequately,

wide re-resection of the lip with in-continuity cervical node dissections should be done.

8. The experience and ability of the surgeon. Those who undertake to treat lip carcinoma should be thoroughly familiar with the techniques of neck dissection, and should be competent in the planning, elevation, mobilization, and transportation of local flap tissue for immediate reconstruction.

Small primary lip cancers of the well-differentiated type are adequately treated by local resection. The "V-excision" is a popular method that facilitates the closure (Fig. 11). Surgical treatment of larger lip lesions, in which adequate resection makes necessary the excision of more than one half of the lip, demands a thorough knowledge of many ingenious local and distant flap techniques that have been designed for lip reconstruction.[5] For the larger lesions, invasive lesions, those with a highly malignant histologic pattern, recurrent lesions, or lip cancers in patients in whom adequate follow-up is doubtful, a "diagnostic" bilateral supraomohyoid neck dissection is recommended at the time of resection of the lip lesion. Depending on microscopic findings, the neck dissection may be extended to include a full neck dissection on one or both sides of the neck (if there is frozen section evidence of nodal metastases on either side).

Radiotherapy still has many advocates as a primary modality in the treatment of lip cancer. A typical course of radiation therapy lasts several weeks with daily treatments five times a week, which is followed by breakdown of the tumor with ulceration and slow healing. In favorable lesions, the cure rate for radiation therapy is 80 to 90 per cent and approaches that of surgery.[20] However, radiation therapy produces considerable morbidity, does not provide pathologic check on the margins of treatment, and usually does not encompass the regional nodes. When cervical nodes are involved, radiation therapy is much less effective than surgical neck dissection. Prior radiotherapy usually increases the problems with wound healing if recurrence develops and surgery is then required.

Melanomas of the lip require wide, radical, surgical resection with in-continuity dissection of the nodal drainage areas in the neck. Radiotherapy is not effective. Chemotherapy for this lesion has thus far been disappointing.

ORAL CAVITY

CONGENITAL MALFORMATIONS AND DEVELOPMENTAL ANOMALIES

Cleft Palate

Clefts of the secondary palate, from the incisive foramen posteriorly to the tip of the uvula, develop during the seventh to twelfth weeks of embryonic life.[44] Normally, two lateral mesodermal shelves develop and fuse in the midline during this time, separating the oral and nasal cavities. Prior to fusion these shelves hang downward alongside the tongue. During the seventh week, as the tongue descends into the oral cavity, they begin to fuse from anterior to posterior. The soft palate is formed by the ninth week; the uvula is completed by the twelfth week. Insults to the developing embryo during this time may produce arrest in the development process, resulting in clefts of the secondary palate.[43] The defect may vary from total, complete, bilateral cleft of the hard and soft palate, with wide communication between the oral and nasal cavities, to a cleft manifested by only slight notching of the tip of the uvula (Fig. 12).

Occult submucosal clefts of the palate occur with an intact mucous membrane, but lack of fusion of the muscle masses in the midline. These are usually associated with a notching of the posterior edge of the bony hard palate and a midline cleft of the uvula. Submucosal clefts quite often cause the child to have rhinolalia aperta or typical "cleft palate speech."

Treatment. Clefts of the palate are repaired surgically when the child is between 1 and 2 years old. This operation requires the use of general endotracheal anesthesia, which is much easier and safer when the child has reached this age. It is desirable to have the palate repair completed by the time the child begins meaningful attempts at speech. If the repair is unduly delayed, the child will develop faulty speech habits which will be difficult, if not impossible, to correct with later speech therapy.[10]

The operations utilized to repair a palatal cleft vary, but most are designed to close the medial cleft with the aid of bilateral relaxing incisions to release the soft tissues of the hard and soft palates. Recent opera-

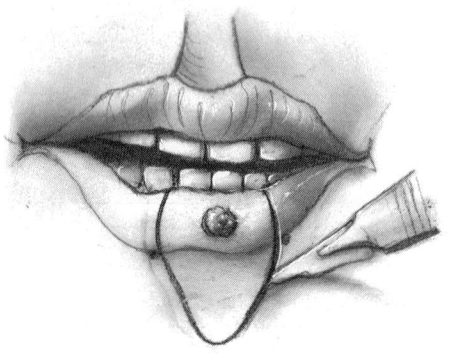
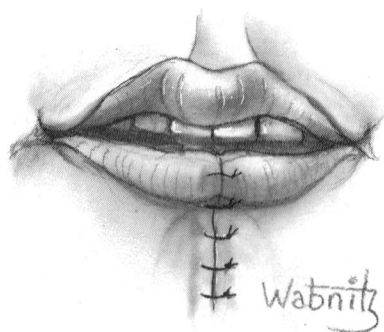

Figure 11. Small squamous carcinoma of lower lip treated by V-excision with direct closure. (From Loré, J. M., Jr.: An Atlas of Head and Neck Surgery, 2nd ed. Philadelphia, W. B. Saunders Company, 1973.)

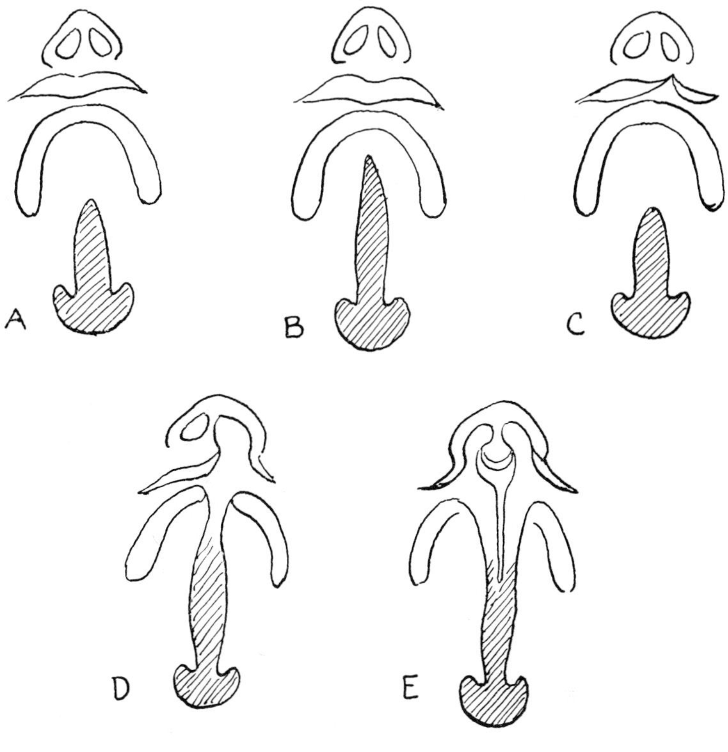

Figure 12. Classification of cleft palate (after Kernahan and Stark, 1958). The division between primary palate (prolabium, premaxilla, and anterior septum) and secondary palate is the incisive foramen. *A*, Incomplete cleft of the secondary palate. *B*, Complete cleft of the secondary palate (extending as far as the incisive foramen). *C*, Incomplete cleft of the primary and secondary palate. *D*, Unilateral complete cleft of the primary and secondary palate. *E*, Bilateral complete cleft of the primary and secondary palate. (From Converse, J. M. *In* Converse, J. M. (Ed.): Reconstructive Plastic Surgery. Volume III. Philadelphia, W. B. Saunders Company, 1964.)

tions also stress lengthening or retrodisplacement of the soft palate by local soft tissue flaps. Elevation and mobilization of mucoperiosteal flaps from the oral surface of the hard palate will allow pushback and lengthening of the soft tissues. Pushback procedures create open defects in the mucous membrane of the floor of the nose, which, if left to heal by cicatrization and epithelialization, will contract and cause postoperative shortening of the palate—partially negating the pushback procedure. Operations incorporating island flaps or the Z-plasty principle have now been designed to close these defects on the nasal surface of the repaired palates.

Flaps of mucosa and muscle may be elevated from the posterior pharyngeal wall and attached to the posterior aspect of the soft palate to form a bridge of tissue that will reduce the velopharyngeal opening and provide a posterior point of fixation for the pushedback palate. This procedure is known as "a posterior pharyngeal flap." More intricate muscle-plasty operations may be used to selectively reposition the levator veli palatinei muscles more posteriorly within the soft palate in order to obtain a better mechanical advantage for elevation of the important dome of the soft palate.[16]

Cleft palate surgery is exacting and demanding. Each patient's repair should be individualized. It should never be attempted by the "occasional palate surgeon."

Pierre Robin Syndrome

This congenital anomaly is characterized by a small mandible, retrodisplacement of the chin, and consequent posterior displacement and ptosis of the tongue into the hypopharynx, producing upper airway obstruction (Fig. 13). It was described in 1923 by the French stomatologist Pierre Robin, who emphasized its frequent fatal termination.[41] Clefts of the secondary palate are found in 40 per cent of the children with this syndrome. The exact etiology is unknown. Many believe the retrognathia is due to intrauterine pressure against the chin caused by sharp flexion of the head downward and forward, delaying forward development of the mandible. The degree of airway obstruction may vary from minimal to quite severe. Infants with greater degrees of airway obstruction expend all of their energy in breathing and cannot eat without choking. Without treatment they rapidly die from exhaustion or sudden respiratory obstruction. Only the very mildest forms should be treated by positioning (the child is kept on his side or in a prone position and is fed with his head held in a vertical, upright position) or by nasoesophageal tube feeding. If the child has an episode of cyanosis, surgical intervention becomes urgent. Tracheotomy may be avoided by several operations that have been described that relieve the obstruction by fixing the tongue forward to the lip, hypoplastic mandible, or hyoid by sutures or strips of fascia.[13, 26, 30, 36] The ultimate growth potential of these hypoplastic mandibles is unpredictable. Most develop to approximately normal size; others may require later secondary corrective surgery.

Torus Palatinus

This relatively common and usually insignificant lesion is an exostosis in the midline of the hard palate (Fig. 14). It is occasionally seen in newborns but is more common after adolescence. Its major significance

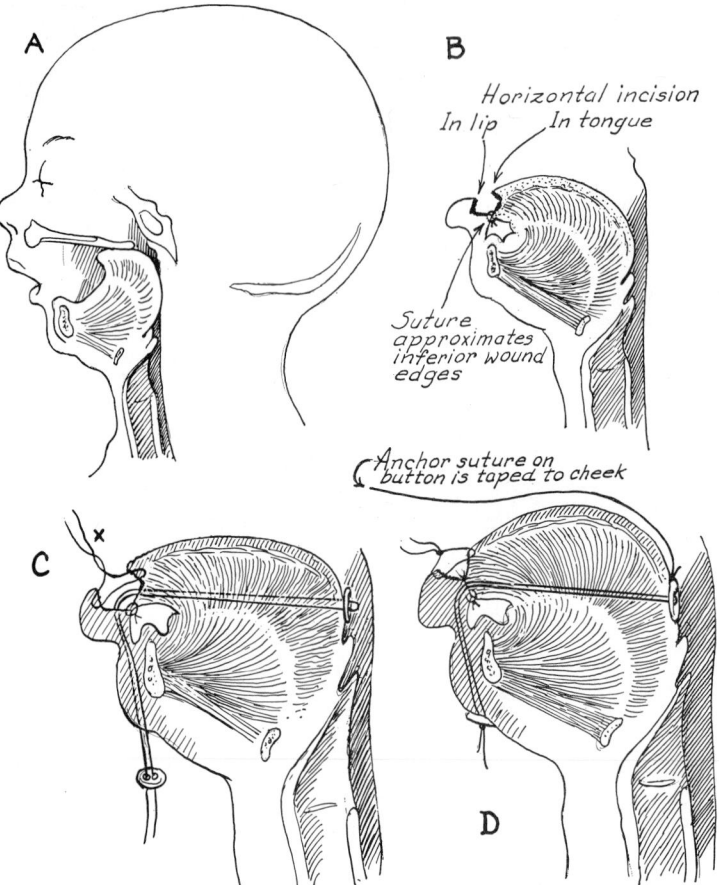

Figure 13. *A*, Cross-section drawing of an infant with micrognathia, glossoptosis, and upper airway obstruction. With the mentum in retroposition the genioglossus muscle is unable to hold the tongue forward. When a cleft palate is also present, the tip of the tongue may be displaced into the nasopharynx. *B*, Cross section showing the horizontal incisions in the tip of the tongue and the labial mucosa with a suture approximating the inferior wound margins. *C*, A heavy tension suture connects a button beneath the chin to one on the posterior surface of the tongue by way of the lip and tongue incisions. A retrieving suture is tied to the tongue button and brought out through the mouth. A suture is placed on either side of the tension suture to approximate the muscle layer of the lip and tongue. *D*, The superior wound margins are approximated. (From Randall, P. *In* Converse, J. M. (Ed.): Reconstructive Plastic Surgery, 2nd ed. Volume III. Philadelphia, W. B. Saunders Company, 1977.)

is that it is occasionally mistaken for a neoplasm. The bone is usually symmetrically distributed on both sides of the midline and is covered with normal mucosa. Excision should be advised if there is chronic irritation of the overlying mucosa or if a full upper denture is to be worn.

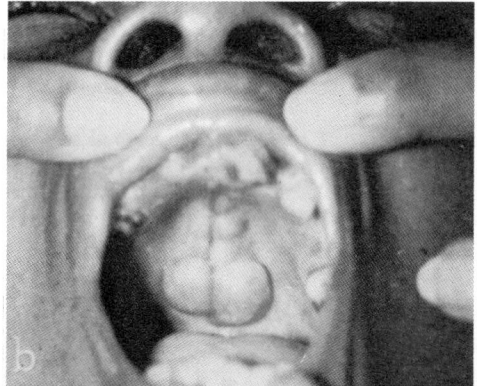

Figure 14. Multilobulated torus palatinus in an adult. (From Ochsner, A. *In* Ochsner, A., and DeBakey, M. E. (Eds.): Christopher's Minor Surgery, 8th ed. Philadelphia, W. B. Saunders Company, 1959.)

Ranula

A ranula is a thin-walled, bluish retention cyst located beneath the tongue in the anterior floor of the oral cavity. It is due to obstruction of a mucous gland or one of the sublingual salivary glands. Ranulas are filled with a thick, crystal-clear, mucoid fluid. They are soft and fluctuant, but not painful. They are usually unilateral and form slowly. They occasionally rupture spontaneously, but usually recur. Treatment consists of marsupialization of the cyst by excision of the anterior, superior wall and suturing of the remaining posterior cyst wall to the mucous membrane of the floor of the surrounding oral cavity. Because of the thinness of the walls of these cysts, excision by enucleation is virtually impossible, and the attempt may result in obstruction of the ipsilateral Wharton's duct.

INJURIES

Burns (Thermal Trauma)

Thermal and electrical burns are rarely seen within the oral cavity beyond the lips and tongue tip. Chemical burns of the oral, palatal, or lingual mucosa due to the accidental or suicidal ingestion of caustics or acids are occasionally seen. These should be immediately treated with copious and prolonged water irrigation, systemic steroids, elevation of the patient's head, nothing by mouth and parenteral alimentation, and pencillin. Rapidly developing edema may necessitate a tracheotomy. Surgery is reserved for late sequelae and contractures. The oral mucous membrane demonstrates a remarkable capacity for rapid healing.

Lacerations

Because of the extreme vascularity of the cheeks, tongue, and mouth, bleeding from lacerations is usually profuse. Hemorrhage is best controlled initially by digital pressure and packing. The application of multiple hemostats in deep lacerations of the cheeks and floor of the mouth to control bleeding in an emergency room is unnecessary and may frequently result in damage to branches of the facial, trigeminal, lingual, or hypoglossal nerve, or to one of the major salivary ducts. Local anesthetic agents containing vasoconstrictor drugs (epinephrine 1:100,000) are recommended for use within the mouth. Adequate lighting, good assistance and anesthesia, and proper instruments are indispensable for efficient repair of intraoral lacerations. After hemostasis is obtained, the membranes are loosely approximated with a proper suture material. Plain catgut sutures will rupture after a few days in the mouth and should not be used. Chromic catgut or polyglycolic acid sutures will last for several weeks, and they do not require later removal. Silk sutures are excellent for repair of intraoral lacerations, but most will require subsequent removal. Monofilament nylon and wire sutures are stiff, bristly, and uncomfortable and should not be used within the mouth.

Dislodged Teeth

Recently dislodged permanent teeth should not be discarded. They can be replaced in an intact alveolar bone socket and wired in place with a high percentage of tooth survival. If the root canal of the tooth is treated and filled prior to replacement or shortly thereafter, the percentage of tooth survival approaches 95 per cent. These free dental grafts are exposed to a traumatized, contaminated oral cavity and should be protected with prophylactic penicillin therapy.

Chronic Trauma

Chronic trauma to the lining tissues of the oral cavity may induce reactive hyperkeratosis or leukoplakia. If prolonged, this may lead to dyskeratosis with dissolution of the epithelial basement membrane and cancer. Irritants such as smoke, snuff, chewing tobacco, strong condiments, alcohol, oral trauma from various dental sources, hot spicy foods, allergy, galvanism, and lesions secondary to avitaminosis A have all been incriminated in the development of oral leukoplakia. Reactive patches appear as grayish white plaques on the epithelial membrane. Initial treatment should consist of identification and elimination of all irritant factors. If the lesion does not disappear within 2 weeks, it should be surgically excised and the defect closed or grafted. Long periods of "watchful waiting" are definitely contraindicated, and may allow the development of invasive carcinoma.

INFECTIONS REQUIRING SURGERY

The greatest number of infections within the oral cavity are odontogenic in origin. Lacerations of the soft tissues or fractures of the maxilla or mandible account for only a small percentage of infections. Extension of infection from an obstructed salivary gland or blood-borne septic emboli from infection elsewhere in the body are unusual. Most oral cavity infections arise from periapical or periodontal infection. They may be associated with cysts, root fragments, or pericoronal pockets.

The bacteria found in infections of the oral cavity are characteristically mixtures of the same organisms that make up the oral flora — unless the flora has been altered by previous antibiotic therapy. Virtually all are penicillin-sensitive. Fungal infections (i.e., actinomycosis) are slow in development and progression and are difficult to diagnose. Biopsies and special culture techniques may be required.

Anatomically, bacterial infections of the oral cavity may extend into the sublingual area, the mental and submental areas, the buccal space, the submandibular or submaxillary areas, the pterygomandibular space, the parapharyngeal space, the zygomaticotemporal space, or the fascial planes of the neck. Massive infections may threaten the airway and necessitate a tracheotomy.

A much feared complication of maxillary or mandibular infection is cavernous sinus thrombophlebitis. Veins of the upper jaw drain via the anterior facial vein or pterygoid plexus into the ophthalmic veins and thence to the cavernous sinus.

Septic phlebitis in the lower jaw may spread along the inferior dental vein into the pterygoid plexus and thence by way of the ophthalmic veins or the vein of Vesalius to the cavernous sinus (Fig. 15). Surprisingly, fatal cavernous sinus thrombosis arising from infections in the *lower* jaw has been reported with twice the frequency of that arising from infections in the *upper* jaw.[4] Treatment is by massive intravenous doses of antibiotics and by anticoagulants. The causative abscess should, of course, be drained.

In general, the treatment of bacterial oral cavity infection should consist initially of large doses of antibiotics. A high circulating antibiotic blood level is desirable prior to manipulation or drainage of the abscess. Relatively small collections such as gumboil or pericoronal abscess may be drained into the mouth. Larger abscess extensions require external incisions through a line of election beneath the mandible in a dependent position. Drainage is maintained by a rubber or gauze drain left in the wound for several days.

BENIGN TUMORS OF THE MOUTH

Nonmalignant tumors or abnormal growths within the soft tissues of the oral cavity arise most frequently from the gingival tissues or the mucoperiosteal membrane of the alveolar processes of the maxilla or mandible. These include fibromas, hyperplasias, pyogenic granulomas, hemangiomas, gingival hyperplasia caused by phenytoin, peripheral giant cell tumors, and

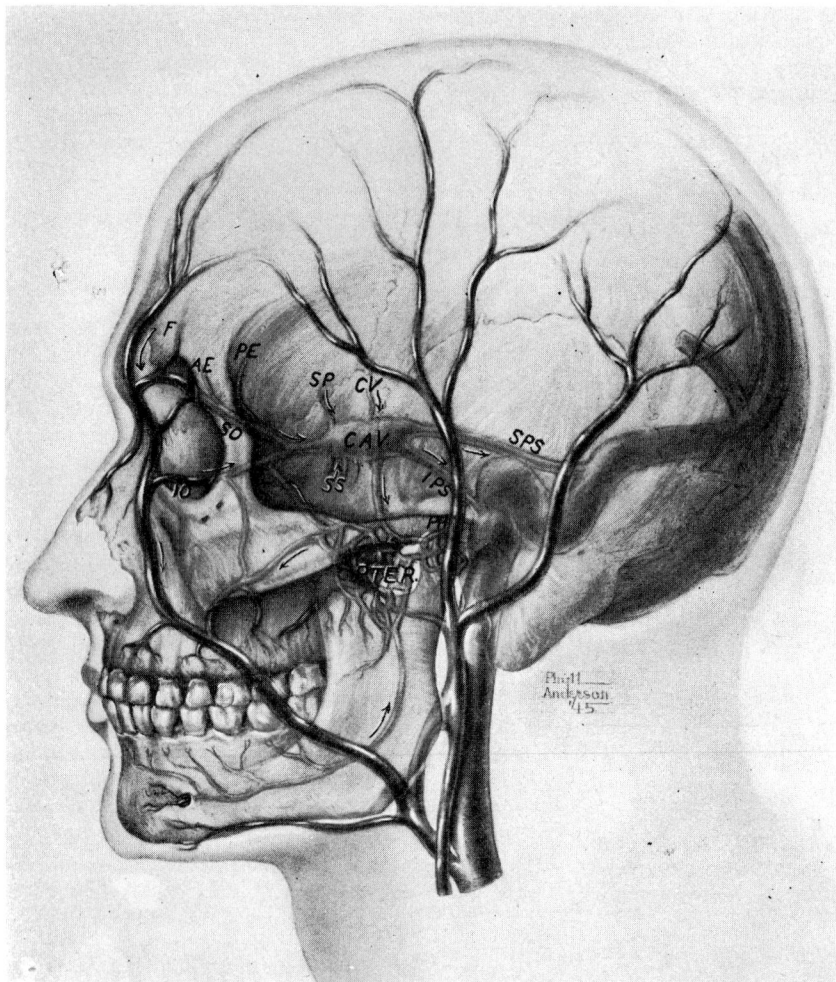

Figure 15. The venous tributaries of the cavernous sinus, including those from the teeth. The arrows indicate the direction of blood flow. (From Archer, W. H.: Oral and Maxillofacial Surgery, 5th ed. Philadelphia, W. B. Saunders Company, 1975.)

neuromas. Second in frequency are the hyperplasias of the lining mucosa of the cheeks and lips from chronic trauma. Third in frequency are benign tumors found on or beneath the mucosa of the cheek. These include fibromas, fibropapillomas, lipomas, hemangiomas, mixed tumors, and traumatic neuromas. Fourth in the order of frequency are benign growths on the palate, including fibromas, fibropapillomas, acute inflammatory papillary hyperplasia, and mixed tumors. The least common site in the oral cavity for the occurrence of nonmalignant tumors is the floor of the mouth. Here may be found mixed tumors, myxofibromas, and dermoid cysts.

Most benign tumors of the oral cavity are readily diagnosed by observation, palpation, and radiographic studies. When the diagnosis is not readily made by these means, biopsy is indicated. Once diagnosed, all benign oral cavity tumors should be treated by simple, total, surgical excision. Radiotherapy has no role in their treatment. Excised surgical specimens should always be examined microscopically by a competent pathologist to confirm the diagnosis.

MALIGNANT NEOPLASMS OF THE SOFT TISSUES OF THE ORAL CAVITY

Sarcoma

This rare neoplasm of the lips and cheeks may mimic a benign tumor. It usually appears as a solid firm growth with an intact mucosal covering. It is frequently seen many years after radiotherapy to the area. Biopsy is usually diagnostic. Treatment is by wide surgical excision. Most sarcomas are resistant to irradiation.

Adenocarcinoma

Adenocarcinomas occur in the mouth more frequently than sarcomas. They arise in minor salivary glands in the soft tissues of the oral cavity, and they often pursue a more malignant course than their counterparts arising from the major salivary glands. Because of their submucosal origin, they exfoliate few cells and cytologic studies are of little help in diagnosis. Adenocystic carcinoma, sometimes referred to as cylindroma, shows a marked invasive tendency and characteristically spreads widely along nerve sheaths.

Epidermoid Carcinoma

By far the most frequent malignant neoplasm of the oral cavity is squamous cell carcinoma. It constitutes 95 to 97 per cent of all malignant lesions in this area. In 1968, carcinoma of the buccal cavity and pharynx accounted for 2 per cent of the mortality from all forms of cancer in the United States. Carcinoma of the oral cavity is best considered anatomically by region.

Floor of the Mouth. Fifteen per cent of oral cavity cancers arise in the crescent-shaped area bounded anteriorly by the inferior dental arch and posteriorly by the inferior surface of the tongue.[1] Squamous cell carcinoma accounts for nearly all lesions. The average age for development of floor of the mouth carcinoma is around 60 years. Ninety-seven per cent of carcinomas in this area occur in males.[6] Carcinoma in this area usually presents as an infiltrative lesion with a fissure-like ulceration. Spread is rapid to involve the contralateral side and the mandible. The tongue may be involved and this may make exact origin of the tumor difficult to determine. Assessment of the extent and staging of the tumor are best done by bimanual palpation. Biopsy is easily accomplished and is always indicated. X-rays of the mandible are indicated to determine bony involvement.

Carcinoma of the floor of the mouth frequently presents with metastases in the submaxillary nodes. These are the primary drainage sites,[1] but subsequent spread to the deep cervical nodes is frequent.

Treatment of carcinoma of the floor of the mouth must be varied according to the size and staging of the primary tumor. Smaller primaries away from the mandible are well controlled with either radiation therapy or surgical excision. Larger primaries that encroach upon or involve the mandible require a composite resection of the floor of the mouth, partial mandibulectomy, and en bloc neck dissection (Fig. 16). Regardless of the treatment of the primary lesion, a neck dissection should be performed on the ipsilateral side of the lesion. If the tumor encroaches the midline, or if positive nodes are found on the ipsilateral side, the neck dissection should be complemented by at least a supraomohyoid dissection of the contralateral side. Studies and experience have shown that in 50 per cent of all patients with carcinoma of the floor of the mouth nodal metastases in the neck will develop within the first year.[32] Thus, a neck dissection is advisable, *even in the absence of clinically suspicious nodes.* The prognosis for 5-year survival is 60 per cent in the absence of palpable nodes in the neck. The presence of clinically positive nodes reduces this figure to 30 per cent.

Buccal Mucosa. The lining of the cheeks extending from the upper to the lower gingivobuccal gutters and from the oral commissures posteriorly to the ascending ramus of the mandible gives rise to 10 per cent of oral cavity cancer. Cancer in this area is more frequent in the older age groups. It is nine times as frequent in males as in females.[6] Certain chronic irritants such as chewing tobacco and betel nut have been

shown to be causative.[1] Carcinoma in this area is preceded by leukoplakia more frequently than carcinoma in any other part of the oral cavity.[6] Squamous cancer in the buccal mucosa tends to be better differentiated and slower-growing and to have a lower rate of nodal metastasis than cancer of the floor of the mouth or tongue. Nodal metastases usually occur first in the submaxillary and upper cervical nodes. The primary lesions are usually painless exophytic growths or ulcerations of the mucosa in areas of leukoplakia or hyperkeratosis. Diagnosis is by direct inspection, bimanual palpation, and biopsy. Treatment for early lesions is surgical excision and reconstruction. Radiation therapy yields a somewhat lower cure rate. The exophytic, verrucous lesions offer a much more favorable prognosis than the ulcerating endophytic type. Adequate surgical resection will almost invariably require excision of the overlying skin of the cheek, so that a through-and-through cheek defect is produced. Immediate flap reconstruction should be performed and will greatly reduce the functional impairment and cosmetic deformity (Fig. 17). The determinate 5-year survival (all methods of treatment) is about 43 per cent.[1]

Gingivae and Hard Palate. Squamous carcinoma is rare in the hard palate, infrequent in the upper gingiva, and fairly common in the lower gingiva, where it accounts for 12 per cent of oral cavity cancer.[6] There is no detectable difference in the incidence between the sexes. The average age of patients with gingival carcinomas is about 60. Characteristically, the tumor is usually a well-differentiated carcinoma in the molar area. Nodal metastases develop in 40 to 65 per cent of these patients.[17] Patients usually complain of difficulty in wearing dentures, pain on mastication, or blood-streaked saliva. Biopsy and mandibular and maxillary x-rays are indispensable diagnostic procedures.

Surgery is the preferred method of treatment for gingival and palatal carcinoma. Since all but the earliest lesions involve bone, which has relatively little resistance to irradiation, this form of therapy is not desirable.[17] Some surgeons precede operation for gingival carcinoma with a course of preoperative irradiation, feeling that this reduces the incidence of exfoliation metastasis.[31] Palatal carcinoma is usually of salivary gland origin and is relatively radioresistant. Since adequate excision of lower gingival carcinoma involves at least a partial mandibulectomy with opening of the tissue planes of the upper portion of the neck, a radical neck dissection should be performed on the ipsilateral side at the time of resection of the primary tumor. In palatal and upper gingival carcinoma, if there are no clinically palpable nodes in the neck, an expectant, careful follow-up without neck dissection is justified. Five-year survival is 25 to 35 per cent.

Oropharynx. This region includes the soft palate, pharyngeal walls, tonsil, lingual tonsil, and posterior one third of the tongue. Carcinoma here occurs predominantly in males with a peak incidence in those about 60 years old. The tonsil is the most common

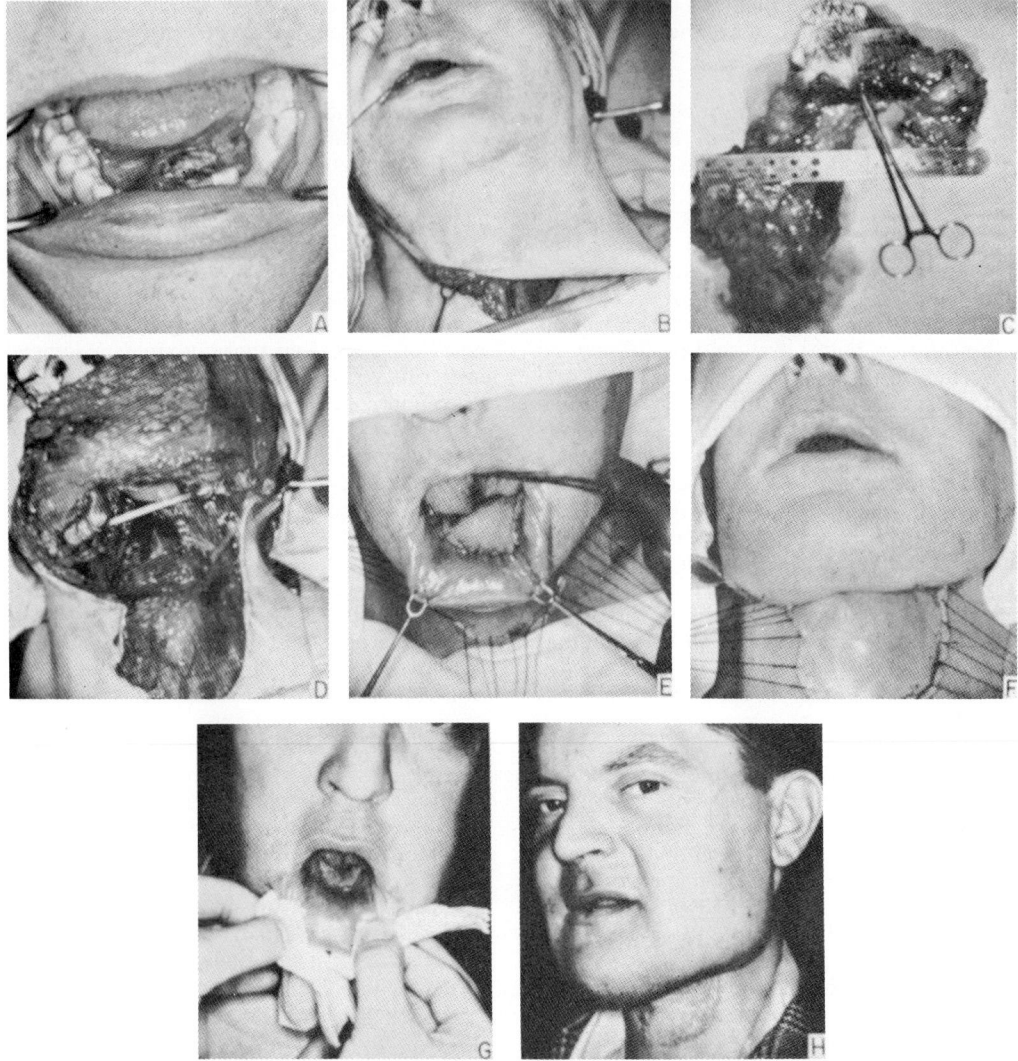

Figure 16. Photographs demonstrating resection of a floor of the mouth carcinoma with a composite resection of the mandible in continuity with a radical neck dissection and repair by an apron flap technique. The lesion is demonstrated preoperatively in *A*. The superiorly based apron flap is shown elevated in *B*. The resected specimen is seen in *C*. The mandibular arch is shown reconstituted with an internal metallic splint in *D*. The apron flap is shown wrapped around the metallic splint and sutured to the labial mucosa in *E*. A split-thickness skin graft covers the flap donor site on the anterior neck in *F*. The final result is shown in *G* and *H*. This technique obviates the need for using tongue tissue to close the defect and also permits immediate restoration of mandibular contour. (From Edgerton, M. T., and DeVito, R. T. *In* Converse, J. M. (Ed.): Reconstructive Plastic Surgery. Volume III. Philadelphia, W. B. Saunders Company, 1964.)

primary site, and carcinoma of the tonsil accounts for 10 per cent of all head and neck cancers.[6] Pain on swallowing, frequently referred to the ear, is a common presenting complaint. An enlarging upper cervical mass beneath the angle of the mandible is frequently noted. In addition to palpation, direct and indirect laryngoscopy is a useful diagnostic tool. Histologically, carcinoma in this region is usually a more undifferentiated variety of squamous cell carcinoma than found elsewhere in the oral cavity.[1] Lymphosarcoma also is frequently seen in this lymphoid-rich area of Waldeyer's ring.

The treatment of oropharyngeal carcinoma is by radical surgical extirpation, with a composite resection including a partial mandibulectomy and en bloc dissection of the neck with flap reconstruction (Fig. 18), or by radiation therapy alone, or by combinations of these modalities. Oropharyngeal carcinomas frequently cross the midline in the soft palate and base of the tongue, making operation less feasible or necessitating bilateral neck dissections to remove the nodal drainage areas. The 5-year survival for patients with carcinoma of the oropharynx, presenting—as they usually do—with stage 3 or stage 4 disease, treated by any form of therapy, is distressingly low and averages approximately 15 to 25 per cent overall.[1]

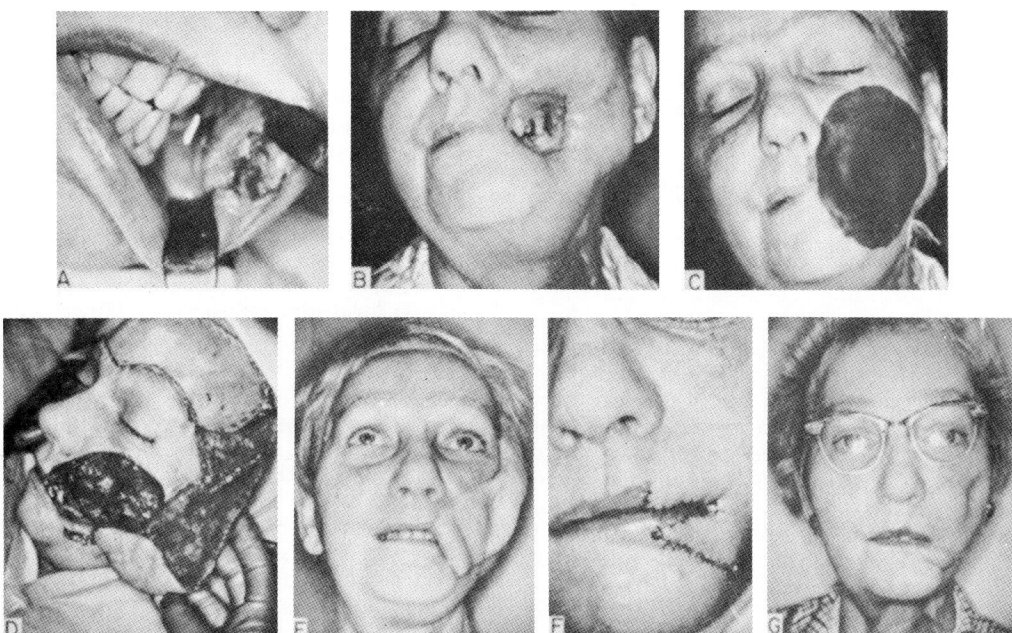

Figure 17.   Middle-aged woman with a massive carcinoma of the buccal mucosa *(A)*. Wide excision with in-continuity lymphatic dissection was performed and a clean oral fistula obtained by suturing skin edges to mucosa *(B)*. Convalescence was facilitated by the use of a rubber-dam "patch" held on the cheek with dermatome cement *(C)*, so that the patient could talk and eat with surprising ease and comfort. Early repair was undertaken using a total forehead flap, pedicled on the side of the defect, with the donor site covered by a split-thickness graft from the infra-clavicular area *(D)*. Note that if the original neck dissection had not been done so as to spare the external carotid artery, reconstruction would have been much more complicated. The distal end of the forehead flap was folded upon itself to provide buccal lining, and the flap sutured into place *(D* and *E)*. Subsequent division of the pedicle and construction of a commissure *(F)* produced a very satisfactory functional and cosmetic result *(G)*. (From Edgerton, M. T., and DeVito, R. T. *In* Converse, J. M. (Ed.): Reconstructive Plastic Surgery. Volume III. Philadelphia, W. B. Saunders Company, 1964.)

Figure 18.   Drawing demonstrating the technique used for large posterior defects. The split-thickness skin graft is mounted on a framework of tantalum mesh and sutured into place. A vascular bed for the graft is provided by adjacent tissue such as a cervical flap or masseter muscle. A tie-on dressing is applied intraorally so that firm contact is maintained between the graft and its bed. (From Edgerton, M. T., and DeVito, R. T. *In* Converse, J. M. (Ed.): Reconstructive Plastic Surgery. Volume III. Philadelphia, W. B. Saunders Company, 1964.)

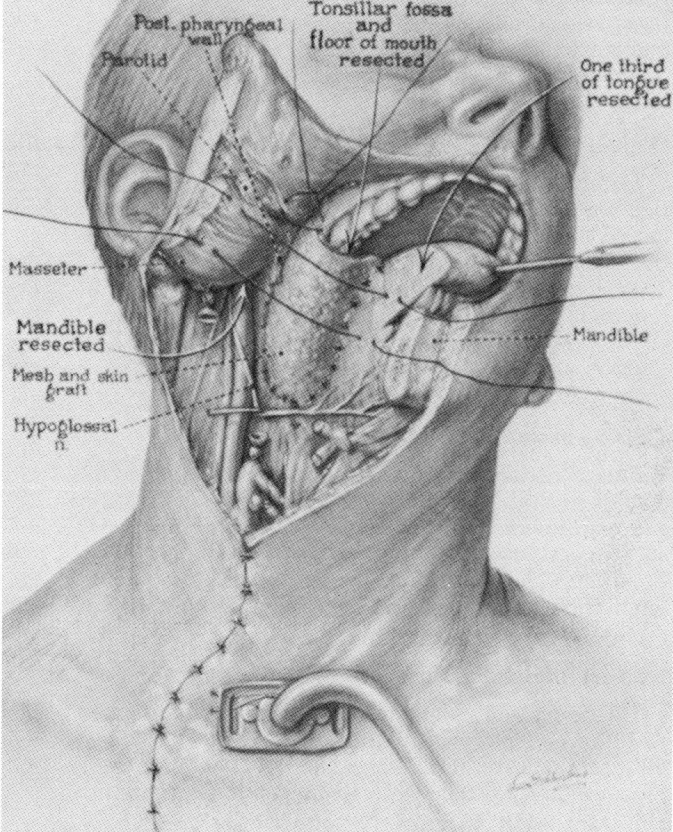

TONGUE

CONGENITAL MALFORMATIONS AND DEVELOPMENTAL ANOMALIES

Thyroglossal Duct Cysts

The pyramidal lobe of the thyroid gland arises from a median pharyngeal diverticulum during embryogenesis. The tongue, which develops later, surrounds the opening of this diverticulum at the foramen cecum. Normally, the diverticulum becomes obliterated and all but the lower portion is resorbed. Failure of obliteration of the diverticulum at any point along its course from the base of the tongue to the thyroid gland may result in the formation of a thyroglossal duct cyst. This situation is very similar to the development of a hydrocele at any level of the spermatic cord and testicle. The hyoid bone develops after the diverticulum is formed and may pass behind, in front of, or around the diverticulum. Clinically, patients present with a midline cystic mass in the neck. The mass may steadily enlarge or fluctuate in size. These cysts usually appear before adulthood, and one third of the cases are seen in children under 10 years of age. The cysts are usually freely movable beneath the strap muscles and are nontender. If spontaneous perforation or previous surgical drainage of the cyst has occurred, a thyroglossal duct fistula may be present. Treatment is by total excision of the cyst and the entire thyroglossal duct tract. This may be facilitated by first injecting the cyst with aqueous methylene blue dye. If infection is present, the cyst should first be drained and several weeks later excised. Complete excision of the tract is essential and this requires resection of the central portion of the hyoid bone. The tract must then be completely removed up through the base of the tongue.

Lingual Thyroid

Failure of descent of the midline pharyngeal diverticulum and the two lateral diverticula from the fourth pharyngeal pouches may result in all of the thyroid tissue remaining in the base of the tongue. This is mentioned only to caution against resection of a mass of reddish brown thyroid tissue from the base of the tongue without first checking to be sure that thyroid is present in its normal position beneath the strap muscles.

Ankyloglossia

Ankyloglossia and "tongue-tie" are terms applied to a short lingual frenulum. If severe, this condition may cause an infant to have difficulty in nursing and may subsequently result in some speech impediment. The condition is readily treated by transverse incision and longitudinal closure of the frenulum, preferably with a Z-plasty, under local anesthesia.

Median Rhomboid Glossitis

This condition, sometimes called grooved tongue, results from embryologic failure of the lateral halves of the tongue to fuse before the tuberculum impar becomes interposed between them, just anterior to the circumvallate papillae. This results in a rhomboid plaque of tissue in the midline of the tongue immediately anterior to the circumvallate papillae. It produces no symptoms and should be recognized to avoid confusion with neoplastic lesions. This condition requires no treatment.

Bifid Tongue

This is an extremely rare congenital anomaly resulting from total lack of fusion of the two halves of the tongue in embryogenesis. This condition should be repaired surgically before the child begins meaningful speech.

INJURIES DUE TO TRAUMA

Lacerations of the tongue bleed freely and may be difficult to expose for repair. Exposure may be facilitated by injection of local anesthetic into the tip of the tongue and passing a suture through the tip to be used for retraction. Lidocaine or procaine, with 1:100,000 epinephrine, gives good anesthesia of adequate duration and hemostasis. Larger bleeding vessels should be carefully grasped with hemostats and ligated with absorbable ligatures. The tongue mucosa should then be carefully approximated with silk or absorbable sutures. If catgut is used, the sutures may be placed in an inverted fashion with the knots buried so that they will have less tendency to untie with the constant motion of the tongue against the palate. The patient should be kept on a liquid diet for several days and advised in the use of a mouthwash. Penicillin should be administered daily for 3 to 4 days.

INJURIES DUE TO INFECTION

Syphilis

Syphilis in the oral cavity is quite likely to involve the tongue and may present as a primary chancre or as a secondary gumma. Syphilitic glossitis is always associated with a positive serologic test for syphilis.[37] Because of numerous varieties of spirochetes normally in the mouth, dark-field examination may be misleading. Syphilitic ulcers of the tongue are frequent in the midline and near the base or tip of the tongue. They should always be biopsied to rule out a malignant neoplasm. Treatment consists of a complete course of antisyphilitic medication.

Lichen Planus

This chronic disease may affect the skin and oral mucous membranes. It characteristically produces hyperkeratotic nodules with associated inflammatory changes. The lesions may appear white or bluish white, and be confused with leukoplakia. The bluish color of these white, often lacelike lesions is helpful in differentiating them from leukoplakia. Lichen planus has not definitely been associated with the development of malignant change. Spontaneous remissions may occur. Vitamin A therapy has been reported to be of value in treatment.

BENIGN TUMORS OF THE TONGUE

Granular Cell Myoblastoma

The myoblastoma is a benign, firm, usually small, spherical mass which may occur in the tongue. While its designation implies origin in muscle tissue, it is not invariably found in relation to striated muscle and is probably not histogenetically derived from muscle cells. Myoblastomas probably arise from perineural fibroblasts; however, their origin remains in debate. They have no malignant potential and are readily cured by local surgical excision. When they occur submucosally, the overlying epithelium may undergo striking hyperplasia, sometimes simulating the development of carcinoma (pseudoepitheliomatous hyperplasia).[40]

Lymphangioma and Cavernous Lymphangioma

These are tumors of the lymph vessels. Many are present at birth as congenital collections of proliferating lymph vessels, quite like cavernous hemangiomas. They have tiny white and red tufts on the surface that are pathognomonic. They may cause great enlargement of the tongue (macroglossia). Surgical excision and debulking of the tumor may be required to establish and maintain an airway, but some tongue should be left, even if it contains residual lymphangioma.

Amyloidosis

This condition may present in the tongue and associated structures of the oral mucosa as submucosal, chiefly perivascular deposits or as solitary multiple nodules. Macroglossia, often to a severe degree, may develop. With enlargement of the tongue, indentations of the teeth along the border become very prominent and impaired mobility may be observed. The upper airway may become obstructed. Ulcerations of the mucosa may also develop. Biopsy will establish the diagnosis. Surgical reduction of the huge tongue may greatly relieve some patients.

MALIGNANT NEOPLASMS OF THE TONGUE

Malignant neoplasms of the tongue usually arise from the mucosa and are mostly epidermoid carcinomas. Those of the posterior one third of the tongue behave like oropharyngeal lesions. Tongue carcinoma accounts for approximately 15 per cent of all cases of malignant disease of the head and neck. Eighty per cent of cases of tongue cancer occur in males.[16] Tongue carcinoma is unusual in persons below age 40 and has a peak incidence in those around age 60. Chronic alcoholism, heavy use of tobacco, poor oral hygiene, syphilis, and the Plummer-Vinson syndrome have all been incriminated as etiologic factors. Premalignant changes of leukoplakia and erythroplasia frequently precede the development of tongue cancer. Clinically, carcinoma of the tongue usually presents as a chronic, nonhealing, painless ulcer. Early involvement of submaxillary and digastric nodes is frequently seen. Biopsy, cultures of the lesion, and x-rays of the mandible and chest are essential diagnostic aides. Ninety-five per cent of all malignant neoplasms of the tongue are epidermoid carcinoma.[1, 6] Adenocarcinoma is occasionally seen. Sarcoma and metastatic carcinoma to the tongue from a distant primary are rare.

In the treatment of carcinoma of the oral tongue, it should be remembered that in half of all patients with nonpalpable nodes in the neck metastasis to these nodes will already have occurred *at the time of diagnosis, regardless of the size of the primary.*[17] Therefore, resection of a tongue carcinoma should always include an en bloc neck dissection at least on the side of the lesion (Fig. 19). For larger primaries or lesions approaching or encroaching upon the midline, a staged, bilateral neck dissection is always indicated. If the mandible is eroded by tumor or adherent to the primary, a composite resection including hemiglossectomy, partial mandibulectomy, and neck dissection is indicated. The treatment of lymph node metastasis in the neck is surgical. The primary reason for surgical failure is too timid a resection of the tongue and failure to adequately clear the nodal drainage areas. The overall 5-year survival rate for carcinoma of the oral tongue is approximately 40 per cent and has improved in recent years with bolder resections of the tongue.

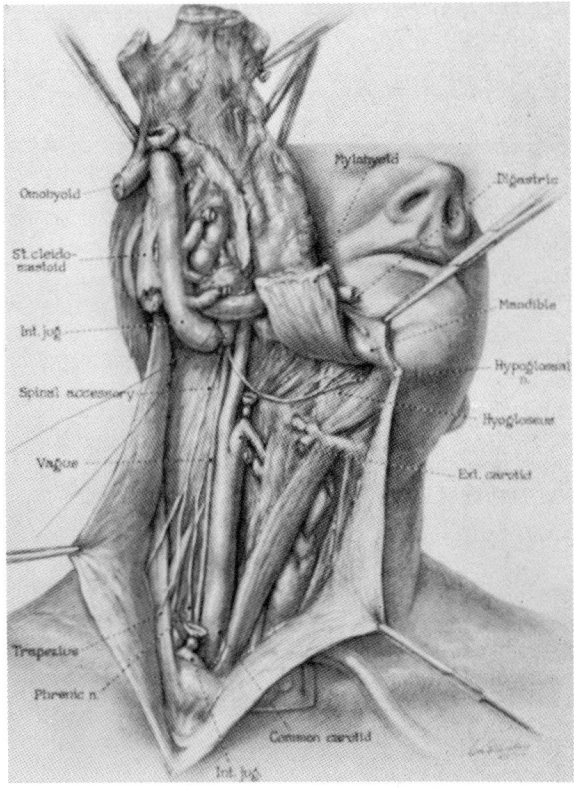

Figure 19. Drawing showing the extent of the usual radical neck dissection. The specimen is retracted superiorly. As is shown, resection of the posterior belly of the digastric muscle permits high ligation of the internal jugular vein and also facilitates dissection around the hypoglossal nerve. (From Edgerton, M. T., and DeVito, R. T. *In* Converse, J. M. (Ed.): Reconstructive Plastic Surgery. Volume III. Philadelphia, W. B. Saunders Company, 1964.)

JAWS

The bony upper and lower jaws in the human are sometimes referred to as the upper maxilla and lower maxilla. Thus, when the two jaws are wired together after injury, the method is called "intermaxillary fixation." More commonly the lower maxilla is known as the mandible. The upper jaw or "maxilla" comprises several membrane bones fused together to form a single functioning unit. This includes two maxillary bones, two palatine bones, and, laterally, the two zygomas which form the bony prominence of each cheek. The upper jaw is thus fixed to the base of the skull and the orbit. The external nose is attached to its anterior surface, the upper teeth emerge from its alveolar process, and the two antral cavities lie within this bony complex on either side of the nasal cavity.

The mandible is composed of heavy cortical bone arising from Meckel's cartilaginous anlage. It articulates with the base of the skull at each glenoid fossa to form the temporomandibular joints. These joints are located just anterior to each bony ear canal. Movements of the mandible are controlled by powerful muscles of mastication and its rigid arch plays a vital role as a base for movements of the tongue and for elevation of the larynx in swallowing and speech. An intact arch of the mandible is critical to maintenance of an adequate air passage into the trachea. Severe deformity of the mandible and chin occasions great psychologic damage to the patient.

Surgical conditions involving the jaws may be conveniently divided on the basis of the etiology of the deformity. Deformities may be thought of as congenital or developmental, traumatic, metabolic, infectious, or neoplastic.

CONGENITAL MALFORMATIONS AND DEVELOPMENTAL ANOMALIES

MAXILLA

More than 100 syndromes involving abnormal development of the jaw have been described. Most may be greatly improved by surgical methods.

Hypoplastic Conditions

These include "dishface" deformities associated with recession of the maxilla, lateral constrictions of the upper arch, and craniofacial dysostoses such as Crouzon's disease or Apert's syndrome (Fig. 20). Maxillary hypoplasias usually result from premature fusion of bony epiphyses and incomplete descent of the midface beneath the skull. There is often associated brachycephaly of the cranial bones and exorbitism, producing a frog-faced appearance of the patient.

Surgical correction is best accomplished by extensive osteotomies of the maxilla to bring the midface and nose forward and re-establish occlusion of the teeth. These techniques are performed in increasingly younger children in order to improve eye function and

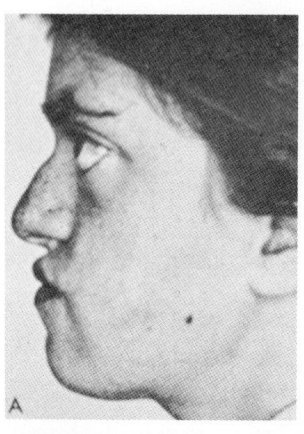
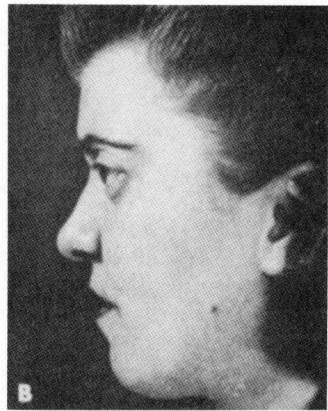
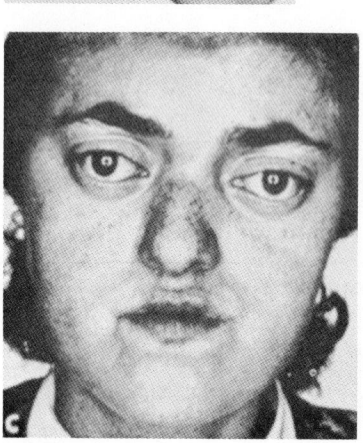
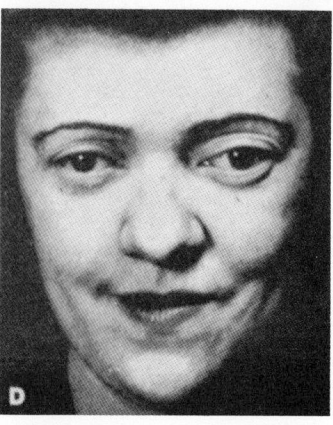

Figure 20. Surgical correction of Crouzon's disease by maxillary osteotomy and forward traction procedures. *A,* Before operation. *B,* After operation. *C,* Before operation. *D,* After operation. (From Gillies, H., and Harrison, S. H.: Br. J. Plast. Surg., *3:*123, 1950.)

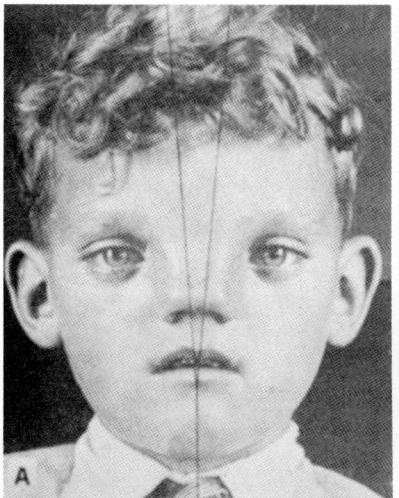
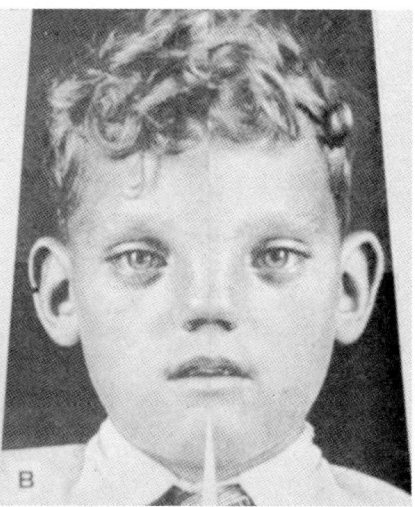

Figure 21. *A,* Hypertelorism and excessive width of the upper portion of the face. *B,* Same photograph as *A* with central wedge removed as marked, showing more normal head and face contour. (From Webster, J. P., and Deming, E. G.: Plast. Reconstr. Surg., *6*:1, 1950.)

overcome deformity before school age. Bone grafting to supplement depressed areas is often required.

Hyperplasias of the Maxilla

Symmetric or asymmetric overgrowths of the upper jaw may occur, producing giantism or hypertrophy of the middle face. This giantism may result from congenital arteriovenous fistulas within the bone or from the presence of plexiform neurofibromatosis associated with von Recklinghausen's syndrome. When the hyperplasia is symmetric and midline, it may be associated with ocular or orbital hypertelorism (Fig. 21). Most of these children have normal intelligence, and surgical correction is effected by geometric osteotomies in association with intracranial exposure in order to protect the brain. This permits resection of excessive bone and translocation of the orbits, upper jaw, and nose, as required.[18, 49]

Enlargement of the peripheral nerve to the affected part is often seen with cases of giantism associated with neurofibromatosis. These patients should receive surgery at an early age, and total resection of the neurofibroma is both unnecessary and undesirable.

Bony Clefts of the Maxilla

In addition to the common clefts of the upper lip and palate, patients may be seen with lateral facial clefts. These usually occupy an oblique position, running from the mouth in a cephalic direction. They may open into the floor of the nose or they may pass lateral to the nose to the midpoint of the floor of the bony orbit. The antrum may be totally absent on one or both sides and little bone is present beneath the eye to provide support. Rarely, one will encounter patients with midline clefts of the upper or lower jaw. Some children are born with complete mandibular agnathia or absence of the premaxillary bone segment. Such patients require complex surgical correction involving bone grafting and, at times, pedicle flap migration.

Other Congenital Syndromes Involving the Maxilla

These include the Byzantine arch of the hard palate with its extremely narrow and high vault obstruction

of the nasal airway. The airway may be opened by surgical division of the bony palate, rapid orthodontic expansion of the upper jaw, and insertion of a stabilizing bone graft.

Children with one of the oro-facial-digital syndromes (OFD I or II) often have constricting mucosal adhesions producing notches in the upper and lower alveolar processes. They also have lobulated tongues, small mandibles, cleft palates, and associated underdevelopment of the maxilla. Multiple reconstructive procedures on tongue, lips, and palate are quite helpful to such children.

THE MANDIBLE

Hypoplasia of the Mandible (Micrognathia)

Micrognathia is probably most commonly seen with the Pierre Robin syndrome, consisting of symmetric underdevelopment of the chin with breathing problems (see Fig. 13) and associated clefts of the soft palate (present in 45 per cent of the patients). Other hypoplasias include asymmetric underdevelopment of one side of the bony face and narrow lower arches with a "pointed chin," owing to lack of development of the symphysis. Lack of development of the mandibular condyles, bilaterally or unilaterally, may produce ankylosis. Very rarely, total absence (agnathia) of the lower jaw has been encountered. All these conditions may be helped by appropriate reconstructive techniques.

Hyperplasia (Prognathism)

Mandibular overgrowth is most commonly symmetric and results in the condition known as prognathism. This deformity usually does not become evident until late childhood or adolescence. With growth of the mandibular body and ramus, the chin and lip are carried forward to produce deformity and associated malocclusion of the teeth. Failure to correct may result in a severe sense of deformity and premature loss of dentition. Correction usually involves appropriate bilateral osteotomies of the ramus or body of the mandible with appropriate retropositioning of the chin

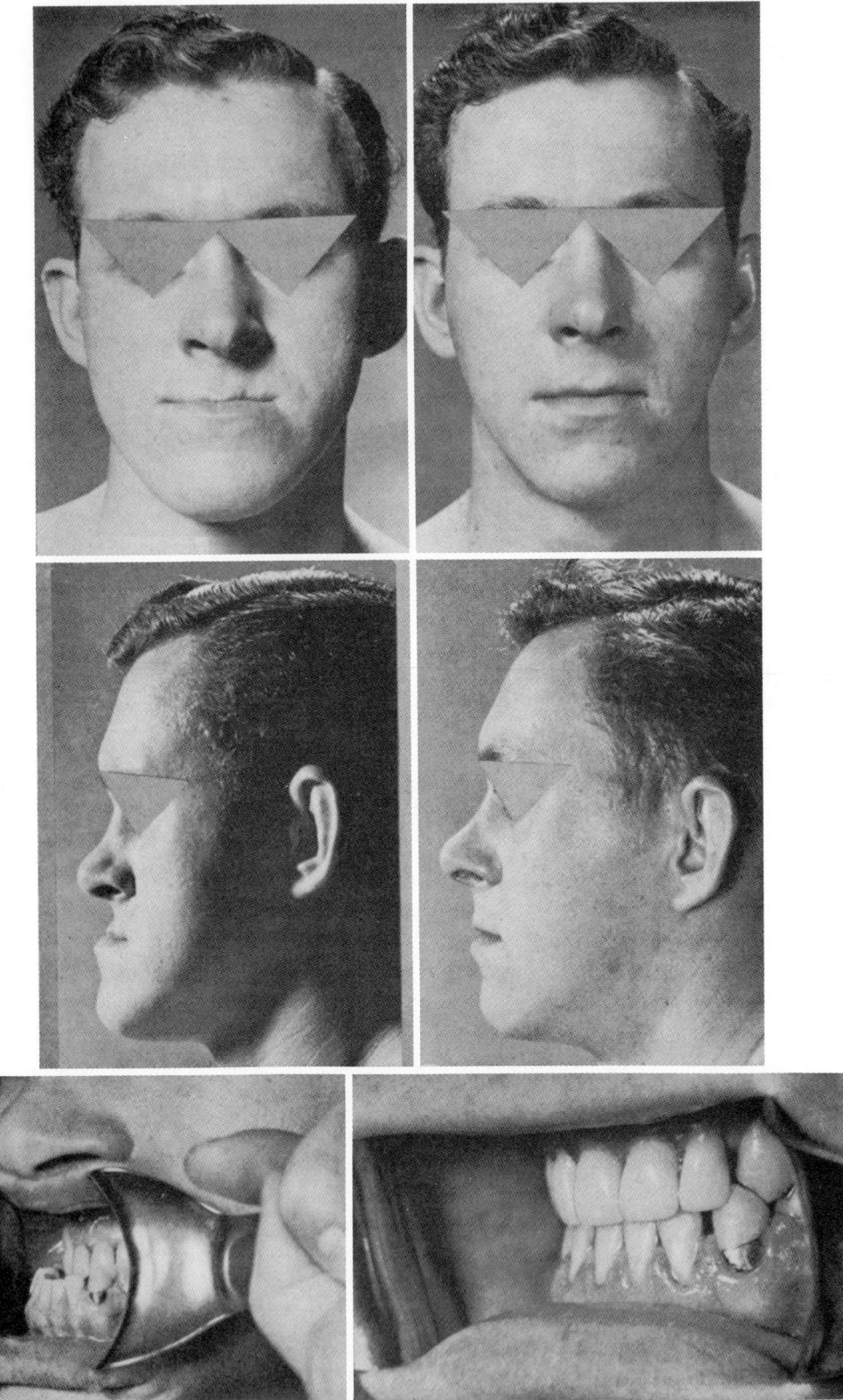

Figure 22. Surgically corrected prognathism. *Top left,* Preoperative frontal view. *Top right,* Postoperative frontal view. *Middle left,* Preoperative lateral view. *Middle right,* Postoperative lateral view. *Bottom left,* Preoperative malocclusion. *Bottom right,* Postoperative balanced occlusion. (From Archer, W. H.: Oral and Maxillofacial Surgery, 5th ed. Philadelphia, W. B. Saunders Company, 1975.)

to improve both appearance and occlusion (Fig. 22). The condition may be unilateral and, if so, the surgical correction is modified appropriately.

Developmental Anomalies of the Second Branchial Arch

These produce characteristic deformities involving the middle and external ear, the mandible, and at times the facial nerve (Fig. 23). Unlike the case in Pierre Robin syndrome, the relative growth rate of the mandible may not be expected to improve with development. Instead, the deformity becomes progressively more severe with increasing age. Such children often require serial augmentation of the affected mandible with bone grafts in order to increase both length and height of the jaw. Many require associated building up of the soft tissues in the overlying parotid region. If reconstruction is performed at an early age, improved dental health and occlusion will be maintained. The associated ear deformities require separate staged reconstructive techniques.

INJURIES

Most injuries to the jaw are secondary to mechanical trauma associated with falls, fights, or automobile ac-

cidents. The membranous bone comprising the support to the upper jaw has great capacity to absorb force with deceleration injuries. This property of energy absorption has saved many lives by protecting the brain from lethal injury when the facial bones crumple from a severe blow.[47]

The muscles attached to the upper jaw are small and lack the strength and leverage of those inserting on the mandible. Consequently, reduction of maxillary fractures does not require strong or prolonged fixation. The fractures usually occur in well-defined patterns located at weak points in the bone.[28] In contrast, fractures of the mandible are often accompanied by severe displacement as a result of the pull of the strong muscles of mastication. Methods of mandibular fixation must thus be more secure and maintained for longer periods than in the case of fractures of the upper jaw.[12]

Mandibular Fractures

Diagnosis of fracture of the mandible is best made by simple physical examination. Point tenderness will usually be found along the lower border of the mandible at the location of the fracture line. Crepitus and movement at this point are usually identified (Fig. 24). The patient will usually complain of some "abnormal" position of his teeth when he attempts to close

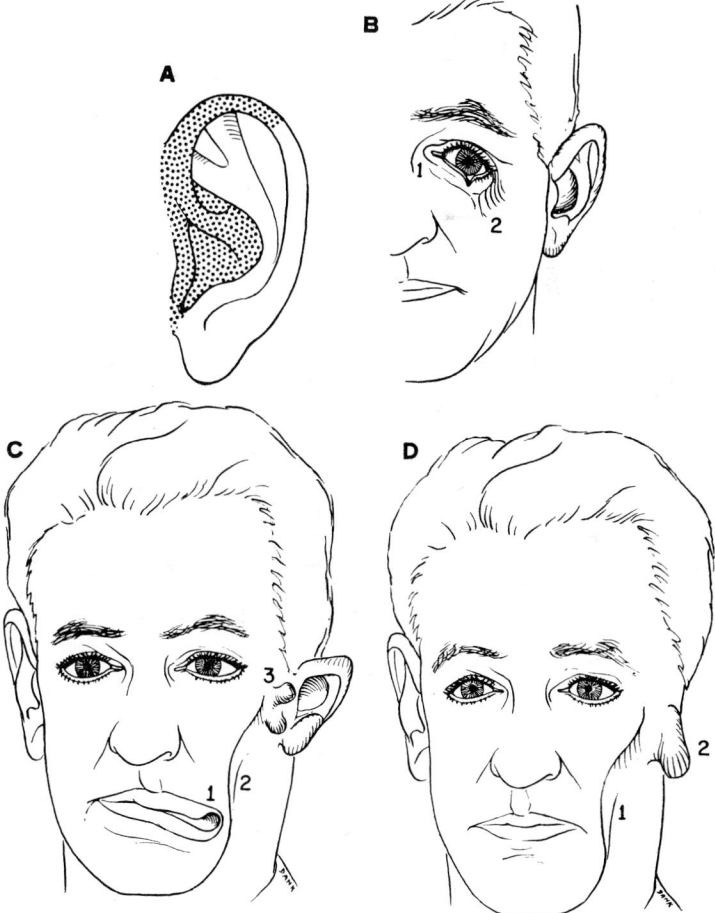

Figure 23. *A,* Representation of contributions by branchial arches 1 (dotted area) and 2 (white area) to normal adult ear. The second branchial arch is represented by antihelix and lower helical crus. *B,* Treacher Collins syndrome (deficient maxillary process). Abnormal palpebral obliquity, coloboma, absence of cilia on medial two thirds of lower lid, lack of malar development, abnormal hair above ear. Deformities are restricted to structures developing from the maxillary process. *C,* First branchial syndrome (mandibular arch). Macrostomia, hemignathia, and abnormalities of the helical crus and tragus (usually associated with preauricular tabs). Deformities are restricted to the first branchial arch derivatives. *D,* First and second branchial arch syndrome. Hemignathia and abnormalities of the entire auricle. Deformities are restricted to derivatives of dorsal part of branchial arches 1 and 2. These two arches normally combine in this area to form auricle, ramus of mandible, and temporomandibular joint. (From Stark, R. B., and Saunders, D. E.: Plast. Reconstr. Surg., 29:229, 1962.)

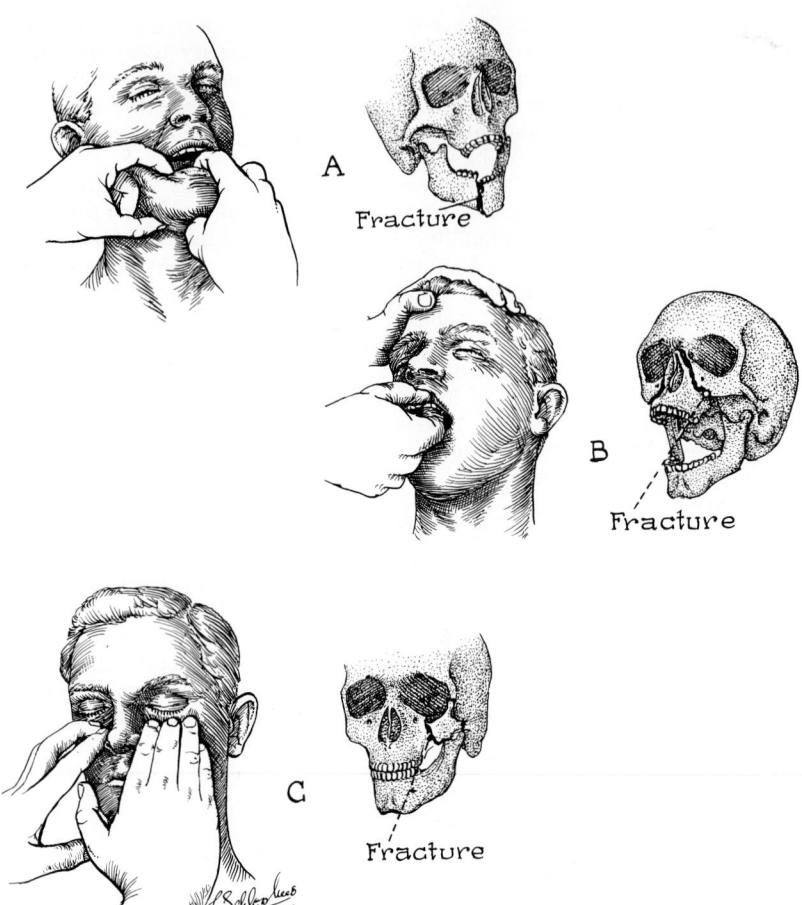

Figure 24. Manual examination for diagnosis of fractured bones of the face and jaws; careful examination with bimanual palpation will reveal the vast majority of facial fractures. In *A*, a gentle rocking motion of the fingers will reveal movement or pain at the site of fractures of the mandibular body or symphysis. In *B*, the top of the head is fixed and an attempt is made to move the hard palate by grasping the upper central incisor teeth. Midface fractures will often reveal slight movement or pain. In *C*, the examiner feels for symmetry of the infraorbital rim, or for a step or "notch" along the normal smooth lateral rim of the orbit. (From Edgerton, M. T. *In* Ballinger, W. F., II, Rutherford, R. B., and Zuidema, G. D. (Eds.): The Management of Trauma, 2nd ed. Philadelphia, W. B. Saunders Company, 1973.)

his mouth. Numbness of the lower lip will be seen if the inferior alveolar nerve has been damaged. Fractures of the body of the mandible are often compounded into the oral cavity.

Treatment of mandibular fractures is most often accomplished by simple intermaxillary wiring or elastic band fixation of the remaining healthy teeth. Soft metallic bars are applied to the remaining teeth in each fracture fragment of the upper and lower jaws, and small elastic bands are used to draw these arch bars and fragments into position so that the teeth will mesh in normal occlusal relationship (Fig. 25). When inadequate teeth remain for this type of stabilization, open reduction may be required. Open reduction may be accomplished through either the intraoral or extraoral route, and a steel wire fixation of the bone in the reduced position is accomplished. This type of fixation is also desirable in patients with displaced fractures when one or more of the fragments do not contain teeth, in children with only deciduous dentition, and in patients with disruption of both maxillary and mandibular arches.

In recent years plastic surgeons have used open reduction increasingly to reduce morbidity with jaw fractures. Such fixation reduces the period of required intermaxillary fixation. If the patient with a jaw fracture has missing teeth that are unaccounted for at the time of initial examination, a chest x-ray should be obtained to be certain that the tooth has not been aspirated. Formerly surgeons recommended the extraction of *all teeth lying within the fracture line of the jaw,* but it is now recognized that many of these teeth may be saved if the fracture is handled conservatively.

Some patients with fractures may be edentulous but may still have an intact denture. This may be used to help align the fragments of the lower jaw by attaching it by circumferential wires to splint the fractured mandible. Circumferential wiring without the aid of a denture as a splint may be used to secure bone fragments with oblique fracture lines. The formerly popular external skeletal pin fixation appliances proved to be cumbersome and unnecessary. They are rarely used for mandibular fractures today. An exception to this is seen in the case of compound injuries such as gunshot wounds of the lower jaw where large segments of bone may be missing and *external* fixation techniques must bridge the bony defect.

Fractures of the Mandibular Condyle

Most condylar neck fractures should be treated conservatively by restoring dental occlusion with simple intermaxillary elastic band fixation for a 3-week period. If the head of the condyle has been badly displaced in a young child, open reduction is probably

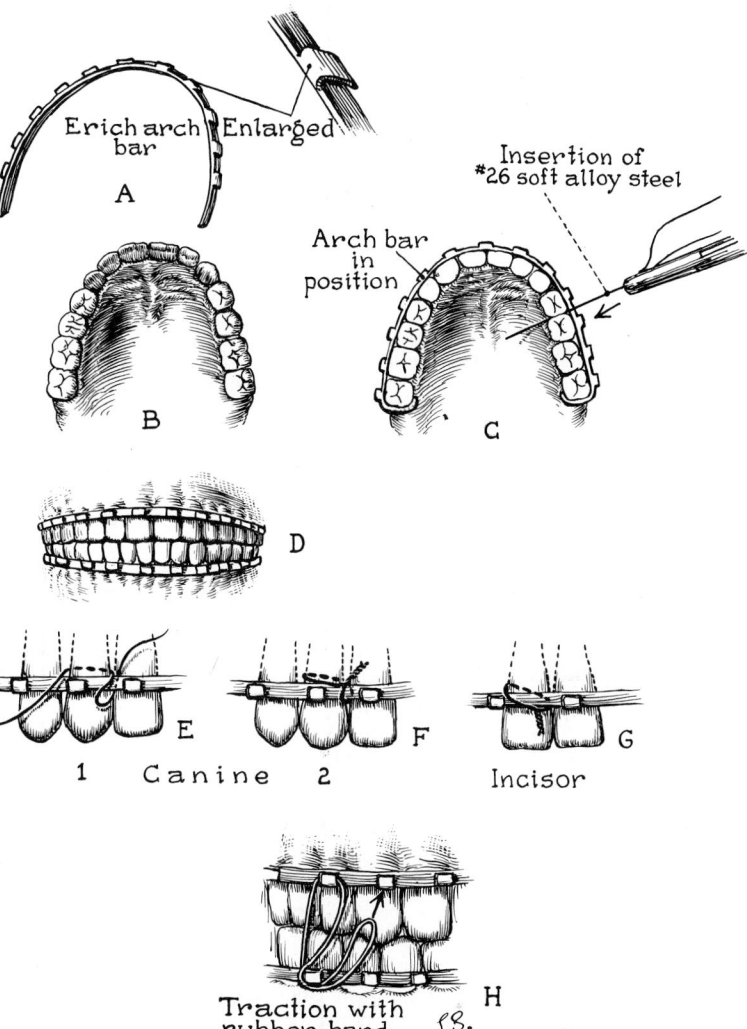

Figure 25. Method of applying soft metallic arch bars to upper or lower jaw in preparation for use of intermaxillary elastic band fixation of a fractured maxilla or mandible: The soft metal Erich bar is bent to fit against the dental arch and allowed to curve about the most posterior tooth. Soft steel wires are then passed about the necks of the molar teeth and about the bar to make the latter secure. *E, F,* and *G* illustrate the variations in applying the wire when it is necessary to use a canine or incisor tooth as one point of fixation. This method prevents the tendency of such forces to slowly extract the anchored tooth. Once the arch bars are properly attached, elastic bands may be applied to the metal hooks, as shown in *H,* to bring the jaw fragments and teeth into satisfactory occlusion. (From Edgerton, M. T. *In* Ballinger, W. F., II, Rutherford, R. B., and Zuidema, G. D. (Eds.): The Management of Trauma, 2nd ed. Philadelphia, W. B. Saunders Company, 1973.)

desirable to reduce the likelihood of progressive unilateral growth arrest of the jaw. With condyle fractures, the external auditory canal should be examined carefully, as it may be fractured by the backward force of the condylar head against the bony ear canal.

Dislocations of the temporomandibular joint usually occur when the head of the condyle comes forward through a tear in the anterior joint capsule. The jaw may be locked in an open-bite position with considerable pain and muscle spasm. Local injection of lidocaine (Xylocaine) and downward traction on the molar teeth will often reduce the dislocation. At times, general anesthesia is required. A history of recurrent dislocation is indication for a reconstruction of the joint capsule by plastic techniques.

Fractures of the Upper Jaw

Middle face fractures usually involve the two maxillas and the paired palatine bones. In 1900 Rene LeFort[28] classified these fractures as follows (Fig. 26).

1. LeFort I fractures (transverse maxillary fractures of Guerin). The fractured segment contains the upper teeth, the palate, lower portions of the pterygoid processes, and a portion of the wall of each maxillary sinus.

2. LeFort II fractures (pyramidal fractures). These fractures also contain the nasal bones and the frontal processes of the maxilla. The malar bones are usually not displaced with this fracture. Significant widening of the inner canthi of the eyes and bridge of the nose usually results with this fracture and there is often destruction of the ethmoid sinus cells.

3. LeFort III fractures (craniofacial disjunction). The maxillas, nasal bones, and zygomatic compound are separated as a unit from the cranial attachments (Fig. 26). Failure to recognize and reduce this type of fracture may result in severe elongation deformity of the central face. Unless it is corrected at the time of primary injury, late repair may be extremely difficult.

Diagnostic features of upper jaw fractures include malocclusion, open-bite deformity, and mobility of the upper jaw and hard palate (when the upper teeth are grasped between the examiner's thumb and index finger). Stereoscopic roentgenograms in the Waters

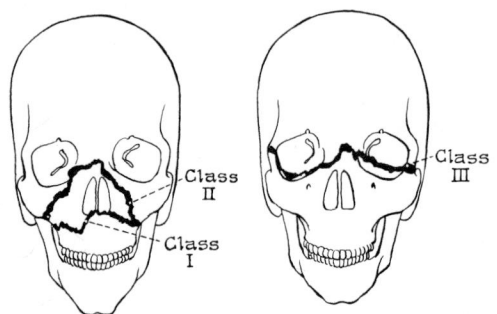

Figure 26. Diagram showing the usual lines of fracture in LeFort's Class I, II, and III fractures. (From Edgerton, M. T. *In* Ballinger, W. F., II, Rutherford, R. B., and Zuidema, G. D. (Eds.): The Management of Trauma, 2nd ed. Philadelphia, W. B. Saunders Company, 1973.)

position (Fig. 27) provide an excellent x-ray view to visualize midface fractures. If the cribriform plate has been fractured, watery cerebrospinal fluid may issue from the nostrils. To the patient this fluid has a salty taste. Treatment of these fractures is best carried out by direct surgical exposure with replacement and wiring together of the pieces of the bony puzzle. A suspension wire sling may be required to draw the maxilla into firm position against the base of the skull. The ends of the wires are allowed to emerge in the space behind the upper lip where they may be fixed to the arch bar, or attached to an upper tooth.

Associated Fractures of the Zygomatic Compound

The malar bone is extremely dense, forming the prominence of each cheek. This bone is commonly fractured with injuries to the upper jaw. Such fractures may or may not involve displacement of the upper teeth or maxilla. The zygoma is often driven into the antrum and beneath the orbit. There are six common types of zygomatic fractures, based on the displacement of the bone and the required method of reduction (Fig. 28). These fractures tear the lining of the maxillary sinus and cause hematoma within the sinus cavity. The floor of the orbit may be displaced, causing injury to the globe or subsequent diplopia. The cheek bone is flattened, the lateral palpebral ligament may be displaced downward. One half of the upper lip is often numb. Irregularity of the bone may be felt by the examining finger when the rim of the orbit is palpated.

Treatment involves closed (Fig. 29) or open reduction to replace the bony parts and fix them with appropriate transosseous wiring. When possible, it is desirable to avoid packing the antral cavity. Existing lacerations or physiologic incisions within the "lines of skin relaxation" are used for exposure. In the case of zygomatic arch fractures, an incision may be made in the temple to allow an elevator to be passed beneath the arch and force the bone laterally into normal position (Gillies maneuver). Head caps with external wire fixation should be avoided whenever possible and are rarely necessary in the reduction of these fractures. If double vision is persistent after healing, it may be cor-

rected by secondary repositioning of the orbit in approximately 80 per cent of the patients.

In approximately 7 per cent of all patients with major fractures in the upper and lower jaws, injuries to the cervical vertebrae may be found. Careful examination and x-rays of the neck are thus indicated in all such patients. It is imperative, on initial examination, to establish the presence of an adequate airway in all patients, and in many cases of displaced fracture of the mandible a tracheotomy is required.

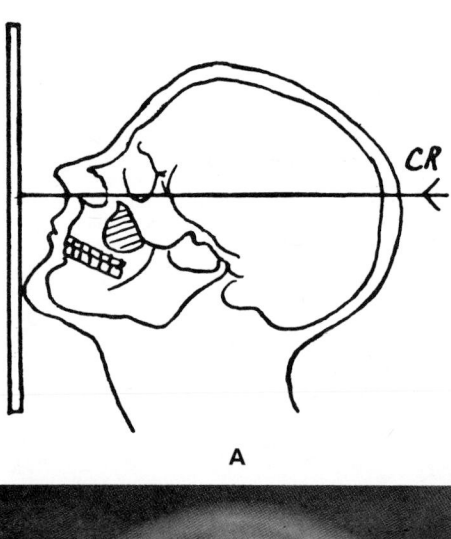

A

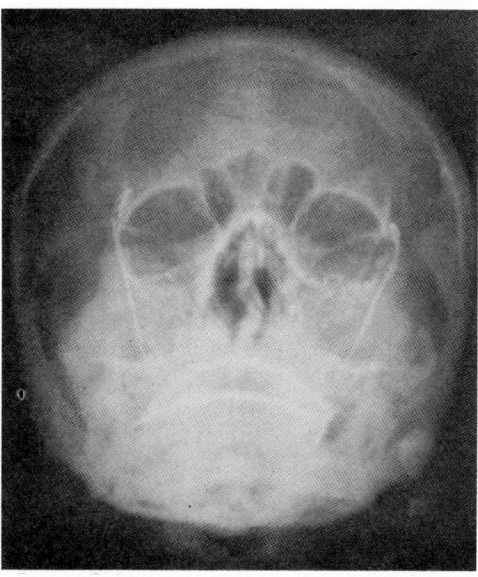

B

Figure 27. Waters position. Posterior-anterior view for maxillary sinuses, maxilla, orbits, and zygomatic arches. This projection also may be helpful in demonstration of fractures of the nasal bones and nasal processes of the maxilla. In this view the petrous ridges are projected just below the floors of the maxillary sinuses. *A,* Position of the patient in relation to the film in the central ray. *B,* Waters view showing internal wire suspension for fixation in fractures of the middle third of the face. (From Dingman, R. O. *In* Converse, J. M. (Ed.): Reconstructive Plastic Surgery, 2nd ed. Volume II. Philadelphia, W. B. Saunders Company, 1977. *A* modified from Zizmor, J. *In* Kazanjian, V. H., and Converse, J. M.: The Surgical Treatment of Facial Injuries, 2nd ed. Baltimore, Williams & Wilkins Company, 1959.)

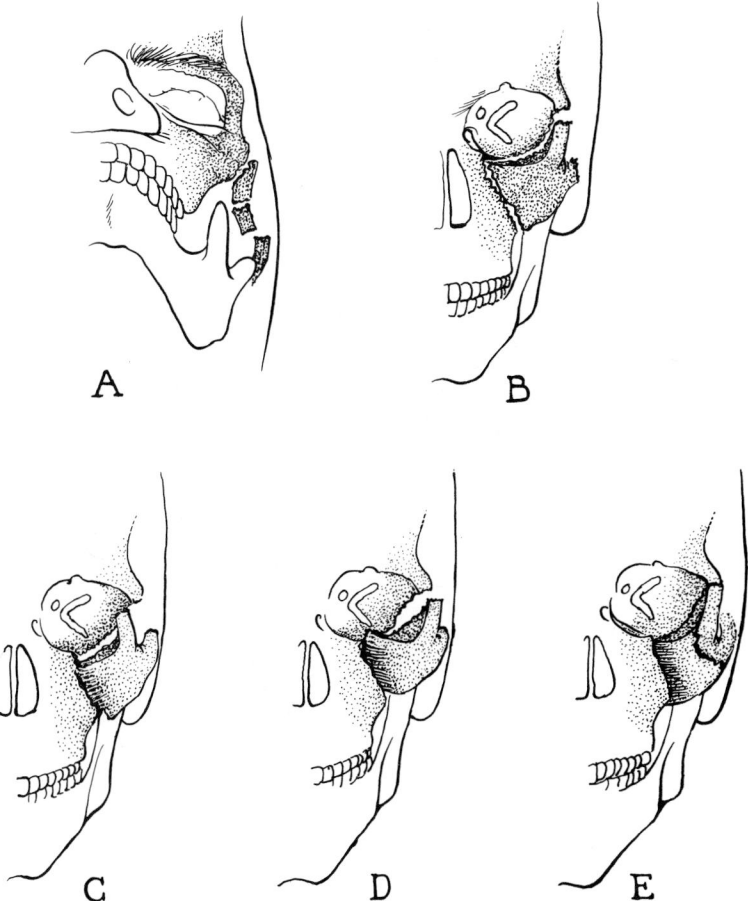

Figure 28. Simple classification of displaced fractures of the zygomatic compound: One in 20 fractures of the malar compound shows no significant displacement, and treatment is not required. One tenth involve the arch only (A), one third show inward or downward displacement without rotation (B), one tenth show medial rotation of the upper part of the zygoma toward the midline (C), one fifth are rotated laterally (D), and one fifth are complicated by additional fractures of the central heavy portion of the malar bone (E). These various types of fracture may be readily determined on examination and x-ray, and their recognition is of considerable help in planning operative reductions. (From Edgerton, M. T. *In* Ballinger, W. F., II, Rutherford, R. B., and Zuidema, G. D. (Eds.): The Management of Trauma, 2nd ed. Philadelphia, W. B. Saunders Company, 1973.)

INFECTIOUS DEFORMITY OF THE JAWS

The most common problem associated with infection in jaw bone results from diseased teeth with root abscesses and secondary osteomyelitis. This may result in chronic draining sinuses with pain, sequestration, and loss of bone. If infection is severe, nonunion of the mandible may result. Treatment usually requires surgical débridement, removal of sequestra, adequate soft tissue closure with drainage, and appropriate antibiotic therapy. If the upper jaw is involved, the infection may enter the antrum and require the surgeon to open and drain the sinus.

Chronic infections such as tuberculosis and actinomycosis must be recognized in patients with low-grade chronic drainage. They may be diagnosed by appropriate stains, cultures, and biopsies of tissue. Syphilis of the jawbone is now quite rare, but should be considered if associated defects in the bone and cartilaginous support of the nose and hard palate are seen.

In recent years, increasing numbers of patients with radio-osteonecrosis of the jaw have been seen following the treatment of cancer. This is sometimes an inevitable complication of adequate treatment of malignant disease; however, a characteristic of this type of bone infection is the severe pain that accompanies it, *even in the absence of significant change on x-ray examination of the bone.* Treatment usually requires wide removal of the damaged bone, as spontaneous recovery is almost always prolonged and unpleasant. Spontaneous sequestration of dead bone is so delayed in such patients that surgical intervention at an early date is indicated.

DEFICIENCY STATES AND METABOLIC DERANGEMENTS INVOLVING THE JAWS

Surgical treatment is of considerable value in many patients with metabolic disorders of bone. This includes young patients with fibrous dysplasia involving, commonly, the maxilla or mandible. Such patients may have associated disorders involving the long bones of the extremities and some will have a sensorineural hearing loss. The extensive facial deformities may be corrected by surgical sculpturing of the involved bones. X-ray therapy should be avoided for such conditions.

Other patients may suffer from ossifying fibromas with localized enlargement of the upper or lower jaw, or they may experience a cyst formation associated with parathyroid adenomas, producing giant cell tumors within the bones. In the mandible, such a condition may result in pathologic fractures. Bone grafting and cyst removal may be required.

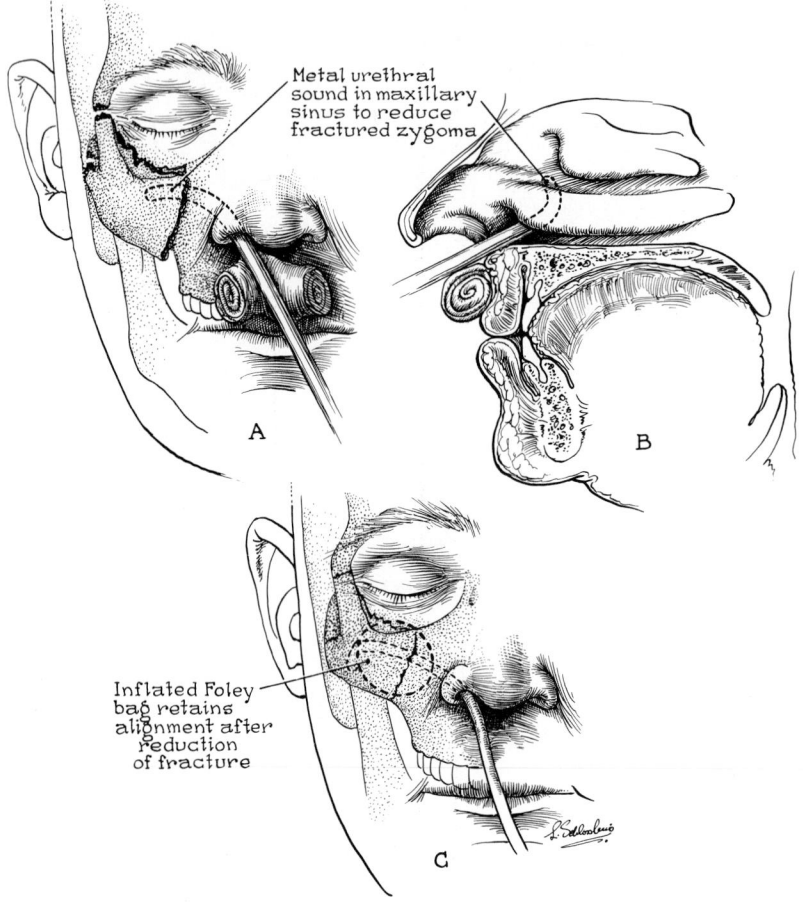

Metal urethral sound in maxillary sinus to reduce fractured zygoma

A

B

Inflated Foley bag retains alignment after reduction of fracture

C

Figure 29. Early nonrotated fractures of the zygoma may at times be effectively reduced by the simple insertion of a metal urethral sound through the thin medial wall of the antrum by means of the nasal cavity. The tip of the sound may then be directed up beneath the solid central portion of the malar bone and a leverage action brought to bear against the bone from within. The roll of gauze acts as a fulcrum to protect the upper lip, and strong outward force can then be brought to bear on the zygoma. At times, the bone will actually be heard to "click" back into place. If the zygoma does not remain stable in the reduced position, a Foley bag catheter can be inserted by the same route and the bag inflated until the bone receives adequate support. (From Edgerton, M. T. *In* Ballinger, W. F., II, Rutherford, R. B., and Zuidema, G. D. (Eds.): The Management of Trauma, 2nd ed. Philadelphia, W. B. Saunders Company, 1973.)

BENIGN TUMORS OF THE JAWS

Most benign tumors of the upper and lower jaw may be readily excised surgically once the diagnosis is established. Radiolucent lesions on x-ray often prove to be dental or root cysts. Radicular dentigerous cysts may cause considerable expansion of the alveolar cortex. Radiopaque benign tumors such as cementomas, osteomas, odontomas, and torus palatinus tumors are also quite common.

Fibromas and osteofibromas are frequently encountered. Most of the these benign lesions may be removed by straightforward intraoral surgical techniques. If the resulting cavities are large and the mandibular bone has been weakened, the cavity may be filled with iliac crest bone chips to accelerate healing and provide strength.

MALIGNANT TUMORS OF THE JAWS

Adamantinoma (Ameloblastoma)

This interesting tumor appears to arise from the embryonic enamel organ of teeth and may be found in either the upper or the lower jaw. It is a slow-growing, low-grade malignant tumor that is known to metastasize to the bones or lungs at times. The histologic appearance is characteristic on biopsy, but local removal by curettement is commonly followed by recurrence. Wide excision of the lesion with bone grafting is the treatment of choice with larger lesions. Smaller lesions may be excised without grafting. The x-ray picture of these lesions shows a characteristic radiolucent "soap bubble" appearance.

Osteogenic Sarcoma

Osteogenic sarcoma may involve either the mandible or the upper jaw. The condition carries a very grave prognosis, but may occasionally be cured by extremely wide resection. Reconstruction of the jaw should be deferred for a reasonable period because of the high incidence of early local recurrence. Postoperative radiation therapy should be used if the surgical margins are in doubt after resection.

Osteochondrosarcoma

This type of cancer may be seen to develop after a history of repeated removal of bony tumors diagnosed as osteochondromas. With each successive recurrence, there may be change in the histologic appearance of the tumor. Wide removal of this lesion at the first opportunity may prevent this progressive and ominous change in clinical character. This tumor is sometimes encountered in children.

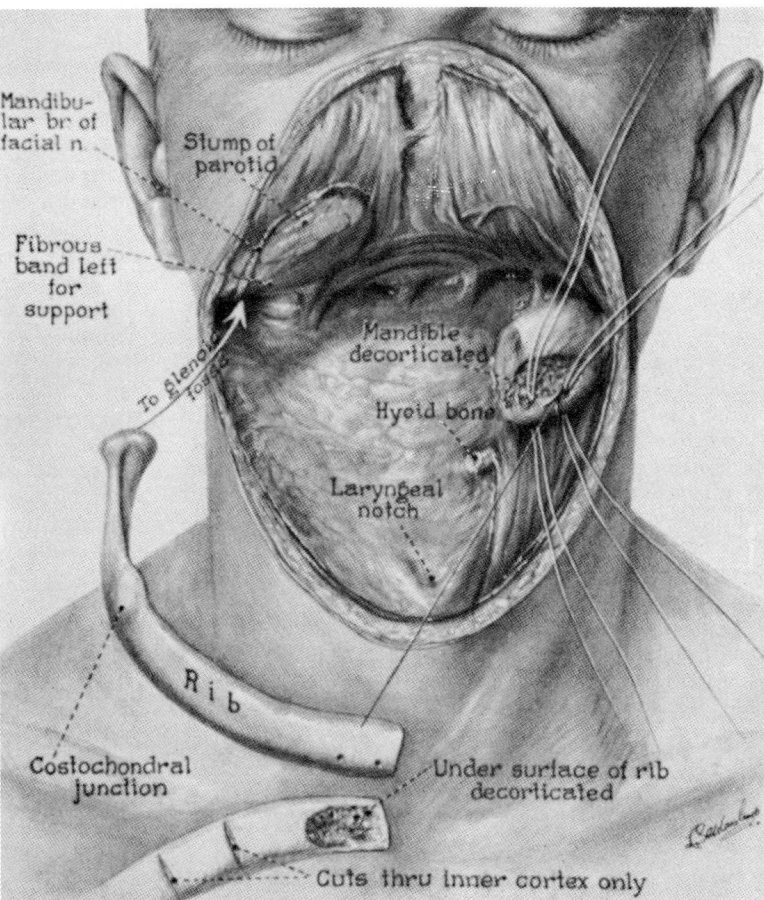

Figure 30. Diagram showing late repair of a mandibular defect after hemimandibulectomy. The osteochondral graft of rib is taken from the opposite side of the chest so that the natural curve of the rib will match that of the mandibular angle. Small cuts through the inner cortex permit further shaping of the rib at the time of implantation. (From Edgerton, M. T., and DeVito, R. T. *In* Converse, J. M. (Ed.): Reconstructive Plastic Surgery. Volume III. Philadelphia, W. B. Saunders Company, 1964.)

Metastatic Carcinoma

The mandible, and less commonly the upper jaw, may be the seat of occasional metastatic tumors. Most commonly, these arise from the breast, thyroid, or prostate. In some instances, the metastasis to the mandible may produce the first symptoms of the patient's disease. Biopsy usually provides the diagnosis.

Bone Grafting for Jaw Reconstruction

Bone grafting to the jaw is most commonly required to reconstruct the mandibular arch. Autogenous bone taken from the patient's iliac crest or rib cage provides the most suitable donor material (Fig. 30). Studies using radioactive material to label the cells of the bone graft would suggest that some of these cells remain viable after transplantation to the jaw region. If bony union is established with the recipient bone, creeping replacement of the cells within the bone graft appears to occur. A period of demineralization of the bone graft develops and reaches its peak about 6 months after surgery. After this, the healthy bone graft develops increased density and strength, manifested by greater density on radiologic examination. It would appear that normal mechanical stresses must be placed on the grafted bone if optimal strength and mineralization are to develop. The transplantation of bone that contains a growing epiphysis to the jaw in

children has been followed by only very limited and clinically insignificant growth. Such bone grafts, utilizing a metatarsal bone, the head of the fibula, or a rib with contained epiphysis, have not produced growth sufficient to match the growth of the normal mandible on the opposite side of the child's face.

Successful bone grafting is correlated with the richness of vascularity of the soft tissue pocket into which the bone is placed, with the degree of bone contact against adequately bleeding recipient bone, with the absence of dead space and hematoma about the graft in the immediate postoperative period, and with the adequacy of fixation of the bone to its recipient site in the immediate weeks following transplantation. Within these guidelines of good technical bone grafting, reconstruction of the upper or lower jaw has proved to be quite successful.

SALIVARY GLANDS

The salivary glands are tubuloacinar glands arising from ectodermal and entodermal invaginations. They may be described as major and minor glands. There are six major salivary glands consisting of three pairs, namely, the parotid, submaxillary, and sublingual glands. Just beneath the mucosa of the oral cavity and pharynx, there are numerous minor salivary glands. All of these minor glands give mucous or mixed secretions except for von Ebner's posterior lingual gland. This produces a pure serous secretion.

Samuel White of Hudson, New York, is credited with the first successful surgical removal of the parotid gland, in 1808. Since that time, surgery has been increasingly useful in treating problems of the salivary glands.

TRAUMA

Mechanical injury to the face may result in the division of parotid glandular tissue or Stensen's duct. When the duct is divided, the two ends should be carefully identified and, after appropriate wound débridement, repaired over a small plastic catheter that is allowed to emerge into the oral cavity (Fig. 31). Closure of the skin over the injured glandular tissue will usually be followed by satisfactory healing. Late complications of injury to the parotid may include the development of salivary-cutaneous fistulas or obstruction to the duct with resulting acute enlargement of the gland. Chronic salivary fistulas that persist for more than 3 months may require reconstruction; a pedicled strip of facial skin is used to redirect the

secretions into the oral cavity. Acute obstruction or ligation of the duct may result in atrophy of the entire parotid gland on that side of the face. Contour reconstruction of the face by dermal grafts or synthetic implant may be required after such an event.

Children suffering from cerebral palsy or patients with damage to the tongue and lips following surgical procedures for cancer may be troubled by chronic drooling (ptyalism). Considerable help can be provided for such patients by transplantation of Stensen's ducts so that they enter the pharynx posteriorly. Further help for drooling may be provided by excision of the submaxillary glands to reduce salivary production.[9, 52]

INFECTIONS OF SALIVARY GLANDS (SIALADENITIS)

Isolated abscesses in the salivary glands are uncommon but may require incision and drainage if they develop. Low-grade infection is probably the most common cause of obstruction within the major salivary ducts and may be associated with the production of calculi.

Acute suppurative sialadenitis (parotid or submaxillary) may develop as a postoperative complication in patients who receive poor mouth care or when secretions are below the normal level. This condition causes

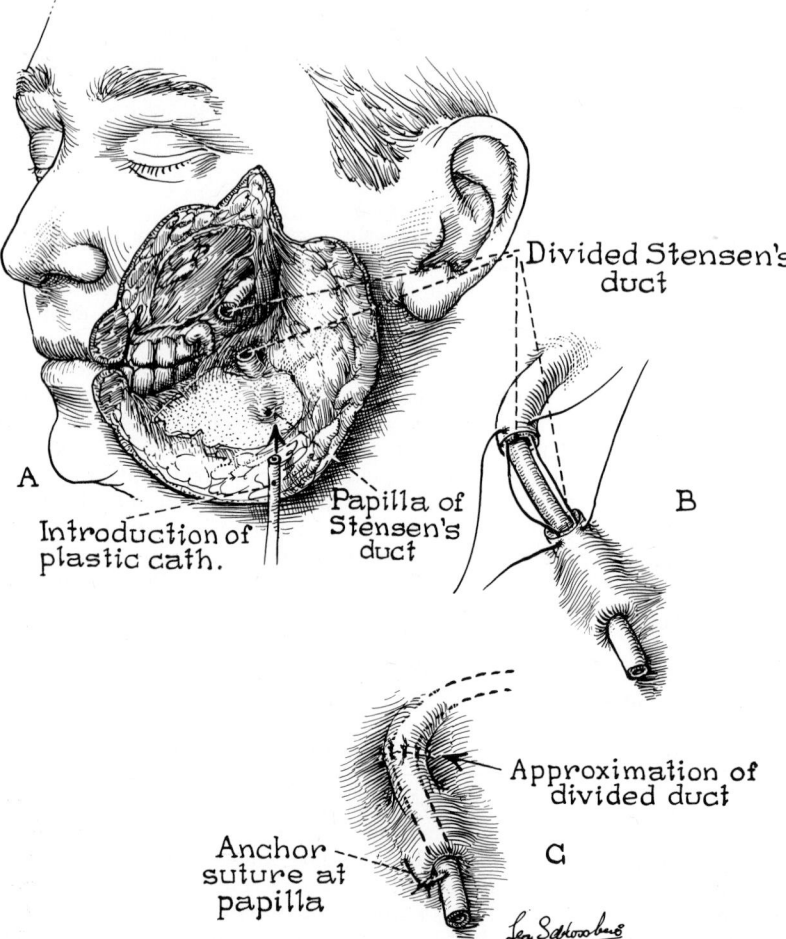

Figure 31. Explosion injury to the cheek resulted in multiple fractures with division of the parotid duct approximately 1½ inches before its entrance into the oral cavity. The proximal end of the duct was found at operation and identified by the slow discharge of serous parotid secretion. The distal cut end was found by a retrograde threading of a polyethylene catheter from the duct papilla on the oral mucosa. Six-zero silk sutures were then placed in the submucosa of the duct to carry out fine closure of the divided duct with interrupted sutures. The catheter is anchored to the oral mucosa to prevent its slipping out in the postoperative period and is removed 2 weeks later. (From Edgerton, M. T. *In* Ballinger, W. F., II, Rutherford, R. B., and Zuidema, G. D. (Eds.): The Management of Trauma, 2nd ed. Philadelphia, W. B. Saunders Company, 1977.)

severe sepsis and high fever and is dangerous to life. Such patients respond poorly to antibiotics and often require radical surgical excision of the necrotic gland. The condition is also seen postoperatively in children, but the prognosis is better in this group.

Recurrent acute sialadentis may develop in some patients with reduced secretions. It is believed that these infections often ascend from the oral cavity by means of the major ducts. Ligation of the ducts produces relief of symptoms and good results in about 65 per cent of the patients. Those who do not respond to this method may require parotidectomy or removal of the submaxillary gland.[11]

METABOLIC DISORDERS

Calculi may form in the sublingual, submaxillary, or parotid ducts. Most commonly they are found near the duct orifice. They are thought to result from improper diet and abnormal salivary pH within the oral cavity, but prevention of further stone formation in such patients is difficult. Infection is present with many calculi but in some instances may be secondary to the obstruction itself. Diagnosis is readily made by palpating the stone with the aid of a small lacrimal duct probe and the use of an intraoral radiograph of the duct in question. Once located, stones may usually be removed by incising the duct directly over the stone by the intraoral route. In some instances, residual infection of the gland after stone removal may make it necessary to carry out total sialoadenectomy.

Sialosis with chronic enlargement of the salivary glands may result from a variety of conditions. These include chronic states of malnutrition such as beriberi, sarcoidosis, and Mikulicz's syndrome. Elderly patients will frequently show a reduction in salivary gland secretion with paradoxical secondary gland enlargement and symptoms of xerostomia (dryness of the mouth). These conditions usually do not require surgical intervention but may be relieved by the use of lemon juice to stimulate secretions and by the administration of a sialogenous agent such as pilocarpine (1 mg. twice a day). In certain collagen disorders such as Sjögren's syndrome, the lack of tear formation by the lacrimal glands may be relieved by transplantation of the distal ends of the parotid ducts into the conjunctival sacs.

SALIVARY TUMORS

Neoplasms of the salivary glands constitute approximately 5 per cent of all head and neck tumors. They provide the major cause for salivary gland surgery. Approximately 70 per cent of salivary gland tumors occur in the parotid gland and approximately 70 per cent of this group are benign. Roughly 60 per cent of submaxillary gland tumors are malignant.[19] The following classification of salivary tumors is useful:

A. Benign Tumors
1. Mixed tumors (pleomorphic adenomas)
2. Warthin's tumors (papillary cystadenoma lymphomatosum)
3. Lymphoepithelial tumors (Mikulicz's disease and Sjögren's syndrome)
4. Hemangiomas (capillary, cavernous, arteriovenous fistulas)
5. Lymphangiomas (including hygroma)
6. Oncocytic adenomas
7. Miscellaneous benign conditions (including epidermoid cysts, lipomas, and branchial cleft cysts)

B. Malignant Tumors
1. Mucoepidermoids (low-grade and high-grade types)
2. Adenocarcinomas
   a. Adenoid-cystic (cylindromatous) type
   b. Acinic cell type
3. Malignant mixed tumors
4. Squamous cell carcinomas
5. Undifferentiated carcinomas
6. Salivary sarcomas
7. Melanomas
8. Metastatic cancers to the salivary gland or contained lymph nodes

Diagnosis of Parotid Tumors

Most parotid tumors arise as slow-growing, firm, nodular masses that are sometimes mistaken for lymph nodes in the upper neck. They are usually painless, and less than 30 per cent of those that are malignant will have produced paralysis of one or more branches of the facial nerve. Sialography with duct injection and x-ray is of interest but only rarely aids with treatment planning. X-ray of the chest and examination of the cervical lymph nodes may give evidence of metastatic spread. *Biopsy is required before final commitment to a surgical plan is made.*

Although needle biopsy has been popular in recent years, Ackerman and others have demonstrated that withdrawal of the needles will drag viable tumor cells outward into the skin. These microscopic nests of cells will implant and grow along the tract and thus complicate later treatment or lead to recurrence (Fig. 32). If the skin overlying the tumor is adherent or ulcerated, it will obviously be sacrificed at operation, and a direct biopsy may be taken directly through this skin at the initial examination. If the skin is uninvolved, it should be reflected from the surface of the tumor as the initial step at operation. The surgeon may then take a direct scalpel biopsy of the most prominent portion of the tumor, and send it to the pathology laboratory for frozen section. The modern cryostat now makes it possible for a competent pathologist to give a reliable frozen section diagnosis of most salivary tumors. The surgeon may then determine accurately whether the facial nerve should be saved or sacrificed in the ensuing dissection. By this approach, he avoids the danger of doing a simple lobectomy for an unsuspected parotid cancer.

Some surgeons prefer to perform a superficial lobectomy of the parotid gland if they suspect the lesion to be a mixed tumor. This approach is troublesome when the frozen section reveals a cancer of a histologically aggressive type.

In all benign parotid tumors and, indeed, with many

A

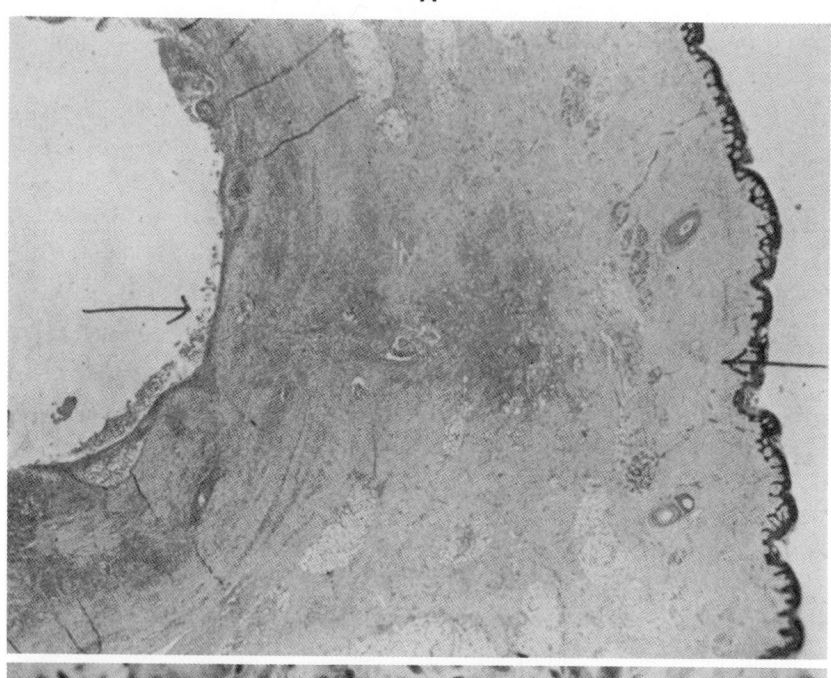

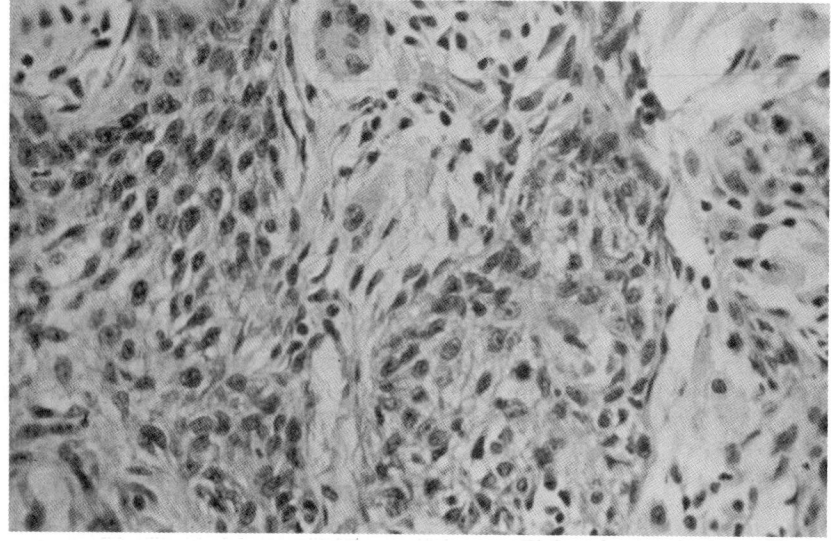

B

Figure 32. *A,* Photomicrograph of excised skin and portion of a node. The arrows point to a needle tract made 16 days previously. *B,* Undifferentiated squamous carcinoma in the needle tract, demonstrated in *A.* (From Ackerman, L. V., and Wheat, M. W., Jr.: Surgery, *37*:342, 1955.)

of the smaller malignant tumors, great care should be taken to preserve the branches of the facial nerve. The patient's lips and eyelids should be left exposed during the operation so that any stimulation of the nerve can be detected (Fig. 33). We do not recommend the use of faradic current nerve stimulators, as the method is less localizing than simple mechanical stimulation and may fatigue the nerve more readily. Most surgeons prefer to find the facial nerve by first exposing the proximal part of the nerve at the stylomastoid foramen. The tumor and parotid gland are rolled forward as the branches of the nerve are exposed. Some surgeons inject the parotid duct with methylene blue at the beginning of the operation to help outline the nerve branches and ducts. Others find the result-

ant staining of the gland undesirable. The operation is tedious and should be undertaken only by those very familiar with the anatomy of the region. Even with great gentleness transient paralysis of the face will sometimes be present after removal of a benign tumor. The patient should be warned of this possibility in advance and told that several months may be required for recovery of facial movements. Any surgical injury to a major branch of the facial nerve should be repaired immediately by suture or nerve grafting (Fig. 34). Following parotid resection with preservation of the facial nerve, about 50 per cent of the patients will have abnormal sweating of the skin overlying the parotid region in response to eating and other stimulation. This condition is known as gustatory sweating or

Frey's syndrome. It is believed to be due to injury of the branches of the auriculotemporal nerve with subsequent crossed regeneration of fibers following surgery. It usually appears within 3 to 9 months after operation. Many such patients will find that these symptoms spontaneously improve. Frey's syndrome is rarely, if ever, seen in patients who have had *total* resection of the facial nerve along with the removal of malignant parotid tumors.

The mixed tumor of the parotid will recur in progressively more malignant forms if any attempt is made to remove it by simple "enucleation" techniques. The tiny nests of tumor cells may be seen extending through and beyond the gross capsule of these tumors.

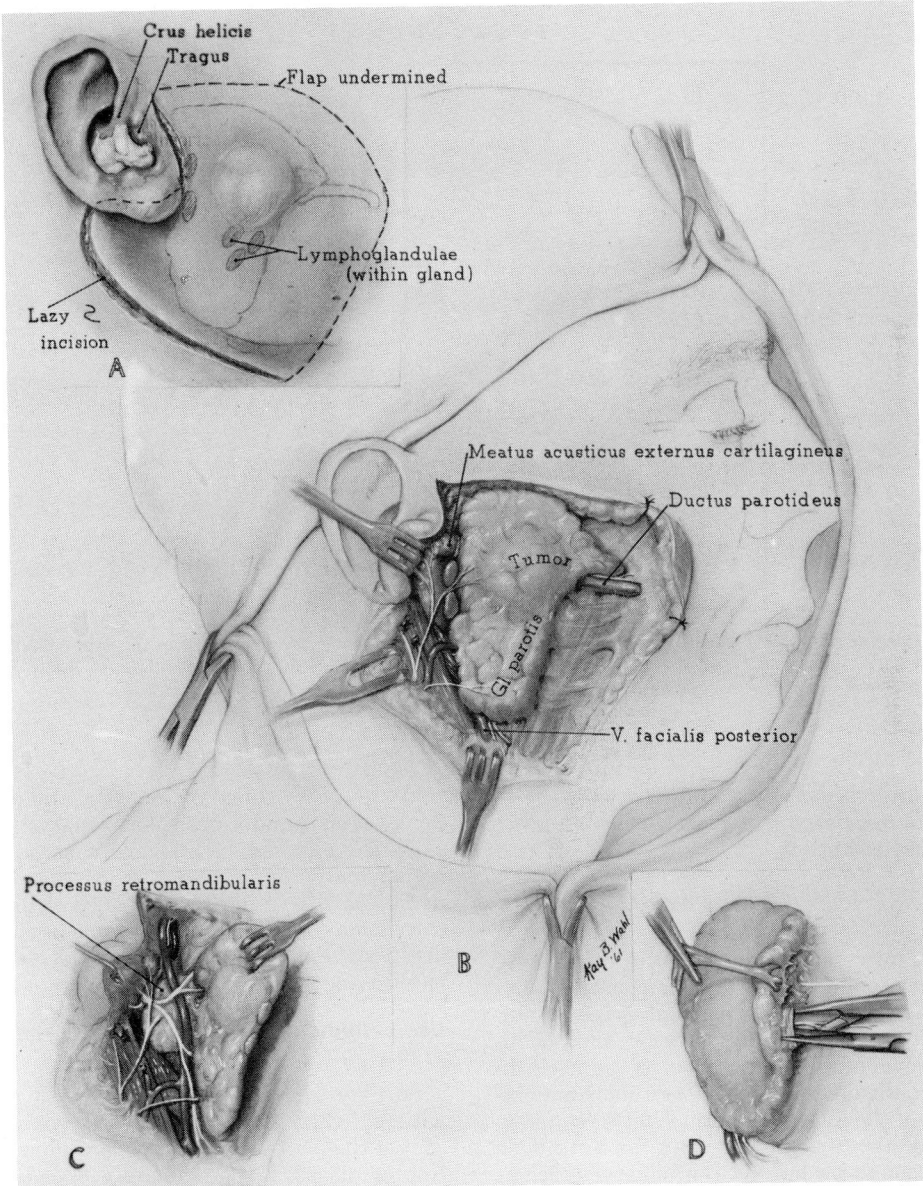

Figure 33. *A*, The incision is made long enough to facilitate complete exposure of the gland. The lower segment often need not extend quite so far posteriorly. *B*, The field exposed with the elevated flap sutured to the cheek. Note the common facial vein and marginal mandibular nerve at the lower pole of the parotid gland. *C*, Posterior approach to the facial nerve with the superficial lobe partly dissected from the nerve, and the retromandibular lobe still partly attached. This is the best approach for tumors located anteriorly. Note the greater auricular nerve with a small severed branch to the parotid capsule. *D*, Anterior approach, dissecting the anterior margin and elevating the gland from the facial nerve branches. Stensen's duct can be used as a tractor. This is the best approach for tumors located posteriorly or in the deep lobe. (From Robinson, D. W., and Masters, F. W. *In* Converse, J. M. (Ed.): Reconstructive Plastic Surgery. Volume III. Philadelphia, W. B. Saunders Company, 1964.)

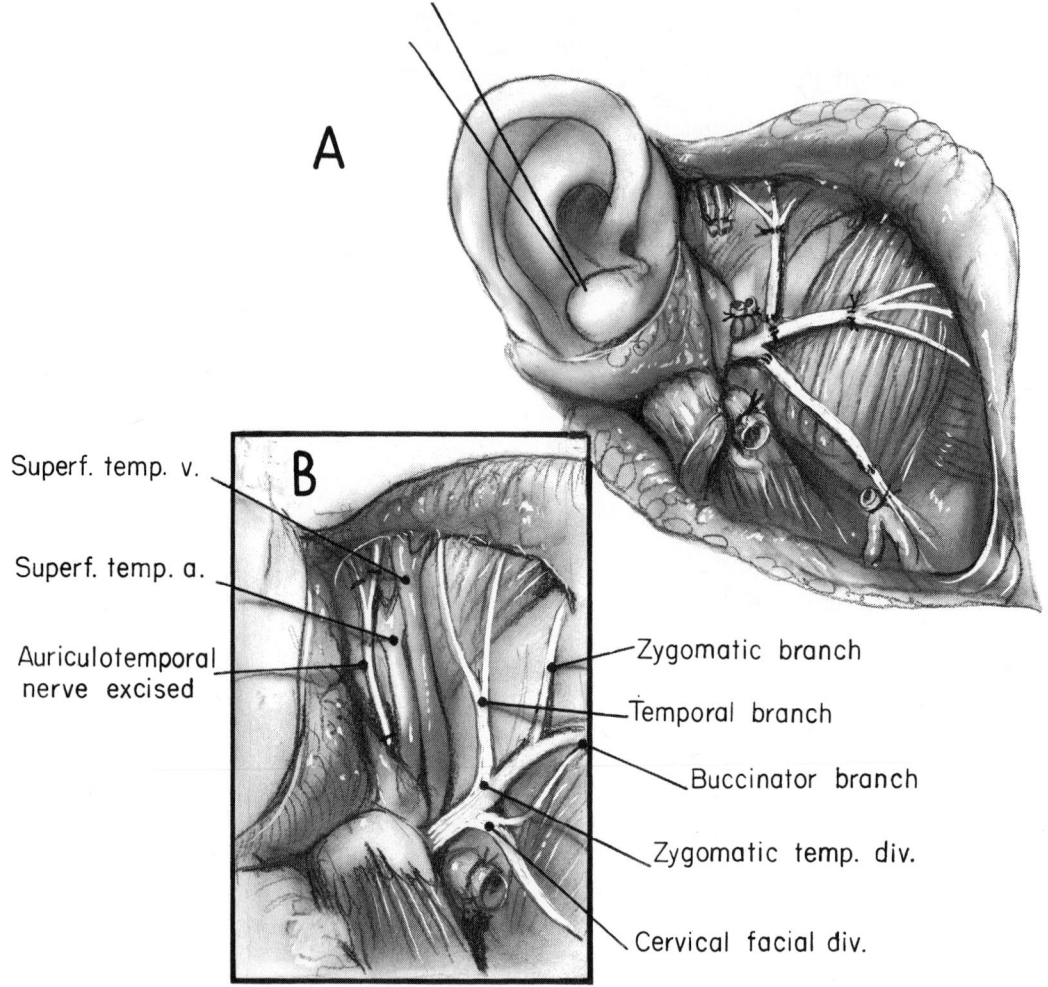

A

B

Superf. temp. v.

Superf. temp. a.

Auriculotemporal
nerve excised

Zygomatic branch

Temporal branch

Buccinator branch

Zygomatic temp. div.

Cervical facial div.

Figure 34. The inset *(B)* shows the usual anatomy of the facial nerve with its branches. *A* demonstrates repair of multiple branches of the facial nerve by free nerve grafts from the greater auricular nerve. (From Loré, J. M., Jr.: An Atlas of Head and Neck Surgery. Philadelphia, W. B. Saunders Company, 1962.)

An abundant layer of normal parotid tissue must be removed around the margins of mixed tumors in order to produce a consistent cure.

Surgical Treatment of Malignant Salivary Tumors

Malignant parotid tumors may require, because of their size or location, removal of portions of the facial nerve, overlying adherent skin, portions of the mandible, or segments of the external auditory canal, or in-continuity removal of the lymph nodes of the neck. In some instances, the deep surface of the tumor may involve the wall of the internal carotid artery, requiring its resection and the use of a vein graft to re-establish carotid circulation to the brain. Cranial nerves such as the vagus or hypoglossal may be involved, and if the patient has a history of pain in the face, the auriculo-temporal nerve should be traced to the gasserian ganglion and resected with biopsy at that point.

Radical neck dissection of the regional cervical lymph nodes should be reserved for salivary tumors that are accompanied by enlarged and palpable nodes, for large or rapidly growing primary tumors, and for tumors diagnosed histologically as squamous carci-noma, malignant mixed tumor, adenoid-cystic carci-noma, or the high-grade variety of mucoepidermoid carcinoma. Lymph node metastasis to the neck is distinctly less common in the other types of malignant parotid and submaxillary tumors.

Use of Immediate Reconstructive Techniques at the Time of Tumor Removal

Surgery continues to offer the best chance of cure with salivary gland tumors. Approximately 50 per cent of the patients receiving parotid resection remain free of disease. Approximately 800 deaths per year from salivary gland cancer are recorded in the United States. The most dramatic improvement in the treat-ment of salivary gland cancer in the past decade has been the increased use of immediate reconstructive techniques that make radical excisional surgery more acceptable to the patient.[25] These techniques include immediate transfer of the masseter muscle to the paralyzed corner of the mouth when the facial nerve must be removed; use of dermal ligaments and modified tarsorrhaphy to support paralyzed eyelids;[14] primary nerve grafts to the facial nerve (when distal and proximal nerve segments remain available);[33] free skin grafts and rotation flaps from neck or forehead to replace cutaneous defects; and occasionally primary bone grafting to replace the mandible. It is now inexcusable to leave any patient with an uncorrected facial nerve paralysis whose prognosis for remaining life exceeds even 1 or 2 years.

Submaxillary Gland Tumors

Because of the deep location of the submaxillary gland and the high incidence of malignancy, lymph node dissection should be performed more often than in parotid cancer. Often the mylohyoid muscle and portions of the mandible must be resected to give adequate local tumor margins. At times, tumors of the submaxillary gland will also require removal of the lingual and hypoglossal nerves to provide adequate margins.

Minor Salivary Gland Tumors

The most frequent tumors of the minor salivary glands occur in the palate and the majority of these are mixed tumors. When mixed tumors lie over the bony hard palate, it is sometimes wise to remove this bone en bloc with the tumor and immediately apply a split-thickness skin graft to the subjacent mucosa of the nasal floor. *Almost 75 per cent of the salivary gland tumors in the palate prove to be malignant.* Patients with such tumor require full-thickness resections of portions of the hard and the soft palate. Although hard palate defects may be managed by the use of a dental prosthesis, defects involving the posterior border of the soft palate are often best managed by an immediate reconstruction, using a flap of mucosa and muscle from the posterior pharynx (Fig. 35). When a prosthesis is to be used, a preoperative dental impression of the palate and upper jaw should be made. Many patients who remain well after resection of a malignant tumor of the palate will benefit from a subsequent pedicle flap reconstruction of the palate. Once the palate is reconstructed, they will not have to rely on a dental prosthesis for the remainder of their lives.

Use of Radiation Therapy for Salivary Gland Tumors

Surgical excision offers the best method for cure of most salivary tumors other than lymphomas or metastatic tumors. However, in certain circumstances postoperative radiation therapy appears to improve the cure rate. Such treatment is indicated if the surgeon feels that there is residual cancer after radical resection, or if the pathologist reports "cancer extending to the margins of the resection." In such instances, postoperative cobalt therapy should be initiated as soon as satisfactory wound healing has been obtained. Other advanced parotid cancers that are clearly nonresectable may be controlled for many months by appropriate x-ray therapy.[7, 45]

Chemotherapy for Salivary Tumors

In occasional circumstances, methotrexate or 5-fluorouracil therapy may produce limited regression of malignant neoplasms of the parotid or submaxillary gland. Such treatment, however, is often disappointing and serves primarily as late palliation rather than for improved cure rate. Infusion of the advanced parotid tumor with cyclophosphamide (Cytoxan) administered by retrograde catheter in the superficial temporal artery has produced marked regression in a few special tumors.

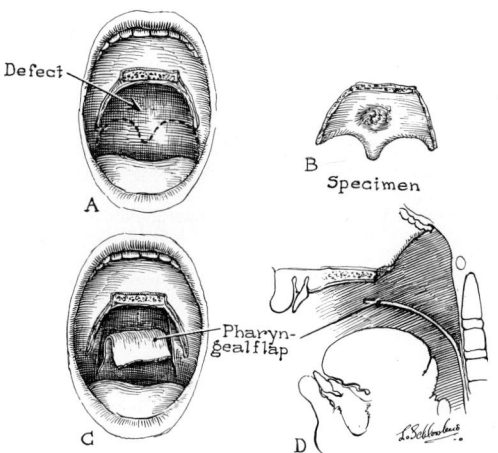

Figure 35. Drawings showing the defect *(A)* is produced with adequate excision of soft palate tumors *(B)*. To restore velopharyngeal competency, a large posterior pharyngeal flap is elevated at the time of resection *(C and D)* and sutured into place. (From Edgerton, M. T., and DeVito, R. T. *In* Converse, J. M. (Ed.): Reconstructive Plastic Surgery. Volume III. Philadelphia, W. B. Saunders Company, 1964.)

SELECTED REFERENCES

Anderson, R., and Hoopes, J. E.: Symposium on Malignancies of the Head and Neck. St. Louis, The C. V. Mosby Co., 1975.
A series of enlightening discussions of current thinking in the management of cancer in this area.

Bardwil, J. M., Luna, M. A., and Healey, J. E.: Salivary glands. *In* MacComb, W. S., and Fletcher, G. H.: Cancer of the Head and Neck. Baltimore, The Williams & Wilkins Co., 1967, p. 357.
A concise review of anatomy and more recent pathologic classifications of parotid tumors. The results reported with postoperative radiotherapy in selected cases are of interest.

Converse, J. M.: Kazanjian & Converse's Surgical Treatment of Facial Injuries, 3rd ed. Baltimore, The Williams & Wilkins Co., 1974.
A thorough and detailed compendium of treatment of all types of facial injuries, early and late, with clear, beautiful illustrations supporting an authoritative text.

Converse, J. M. (Ed.): Reconstructive Plastic Surgery, 2nd ed. Philadelphia, W. B. Saunders Company, 1977.
A very thorough treatise covering the basic aspects of cleft lip and palate surgery. It is well illustrated and referenced and provides a lucid introduction to this subject in full.

Foote, F. W., Jr., and Frazelle, E. L.: Tumors of the major salivary glands. *In* Atlas of Tumor Pathology. Section IV, Fascicle II. Washington, D.C., Armed Forces Institute of Pathology, 1954.
A classic paper on the classification, histology and prognosis of salivary gland tumors.

Hanna, D. C.: Salivary gland tumors. *In* Gaisford, J. C. (Ed.): Symposium on Cancer of the Head and Neck. Volume 2. St. Louis, The C. V. Mosby Co., 1969, p. 352.

A sound review of the practical surgical management of parotid tumors, with emphasis on reconstructive techniques.

REFERENCES

1. Ackerman, L. V., and del Regato, J. A.: Cancer: Diagnosis, Treatment and Prognosis, 4th ed. St. Louis, The C. V. Mosby Co., 1970, pp. 183–354 and 276–296.
2. Ackerman, L. V., and Wheat, M. W., Jr.: The implantation of cancer—an avoidable surgical risk? Surgery, 37:341, 1955.
3. Archard, H. O.: Biology of the human oral integument. *In* Fitzgerald, T. B., et al. (Eds.): Dermatology in General Medicine. New York, McGraw-Hill Book Company, 1971, pp. 804–808.
4. Archer, W. H.: Oral and Maxillofacial Surgery, 5th ed. Philadelphia, W. B. Saunders Company, 1975, pp. 510–514 and 899–917.
5. Bakamjian, V. Y.: Reconstructive use of flaps in cancer surgery of the head and neck. *In* Reviews in Plastic Surgery, General and Reconstructive. Amsterdam, Excerpta Medica, 1974.
6. Bales, H. W.: Head and neck tumors. *In* Clinical Oncology for Medical Students and Physicians. A Multidisciplinary Approach, 3rd ed. New York, American Cancer Society, 1970–1971, pp. 228–261.
7. Bardwil, J. M., Luna, M. A., and Healey, J. E.: Salivary glands. *In* MacComb, W. S., and Fletcher, G. H.: Cancer of the Head and Neck. Baltimore, The Williams & Wilkins Co., 1967, p. 357.
8. Brown, J. B., and Fryer, M. P.: The Mouth, Tongue, Jaws and Salivary Glands. *In* Davis, L. (Ed.): Christopher's Textbook of Surgery, 9th ed. Philadelphia, W. B. Saunders Company, 1968, pp. 323–357.
9. Cohen, I. K., Holmes, E. C., and Edgerton, M. T.: Parotid duct transplantation for correction of drooling in patients with cancer of the head and neck. Surg. Gynecol. Obstet., 133:663, 1971.
10. Converse, J. M. (Ed.): Reconstructive Plastic Surgery, 2nd ed. Philadelphia, W. B. Saunders Company, 1977, Chapters 38–53.
11. Diamant, H., and Salen, B.: Akut varig parotid opusc. Med. (Stockholm), 9:56, 1964.
12. Dingman, R. O., and Natvig, P.: Surgery of Facial Fractures. Philadelphia, W. B. Saunders Company, 1964.
13. Douglas, B.: The treatment of micrognathia associated with obstruction by a plastic procedure. Plast. Reconstr. Surg., 1:300, 1946.
14. Edgerton, M. T.: Surgical correction of facial paralysis—a plea for better reconstruction. Trans. Southern Surg. Assoc., 1966, p. 341.
15. Edgerton, M. T.: The treatment of hemangiomas (with special reference to the role of steroid therapy). Ann. Surg., 183:517, 1976.
16. Edgerton, M. T., and Dellon, A. L.: Surgical retrodisplacement of the levator veli palatini muscle. Plast. Reconstr. Surg., 47:154, 1971.
17. Edgerton, M. T., and Bull, J. C.: Surgery in head and neck tumors: Introduction. *In* Converse, J. M. (Ed.): Reconstructive Plastic Surgery, 2nd ed. Philadelphia, W. B. Saunders Company, 1977.
18. Edgerton, M. T., Udvarhelyi, G. B., and Knox, D. L.: The surgical correction of ocular hypertelorism. Ann. Surg., 172:473, 1970.
19. Foote, F. W., Jr., and Frazelle, E. L.: Tumors of the major salivary glands. *In* Atlas of Tumor Pathology. Section IV, Fascicle II. Washington, D.C., Armed Forces Institute of Pathology, 1954.
20. Freund, R. H.: Principles of Head and Neck Surgery. New York, Appleton-Century-Crofts, 1967, p. 291.
21. Garrison, F. H.: An Introduction to the History of Medicine, 4th ed. Philadelphia, W. B. Saunders Company, 1929.
22. Ghadially, F. N.: Keratoacanthoma. *In* Fitzgerald, T. B., et al. (Eds.): Dermatology in General Medicine. New York, McGraw-Hill Book Company, 1971, pp. 425–435.
23. Glickman, I.: The oral cavity. *In* Robbins, S. L.: Textbook of Pathology, 3rd ed. Philadelphia, W. B. Saunders Company, 1967.
24. Grabb, W. C., Rosenstein, S. W., and Bzoach, K. R.: Cleft Lip and Palate. Boston, Little, Brown and Company, 1971.
25. Hanna, D. C.: Salivary gland tumors. *In* Gaisford, J. E. (Ed.):

Symposium of Cancer of the Head and Neck. Volume 2. St. Louis, The C. V. Mosby Co., 1969, p. 352.
26. Lapidot, A., and Ben-Hur, N.: Fastening the base of the tongue forward to the hyoid for relief of respiratory distress in Pierre Robin syndrome. Plast. Reconstr. Surg., 56:89, 1975.
27. Leake, D.: History of oral surgery. *In* Guralnick, W. C. (Ed.): Textbook of Oral Surgery. Boston, Little, Brown and Company, 1968, pp. 1–8.
28. LeFort, R.: Fractures de la machoire supérieure. Cong. Intern. Med., Paris, 1900, pp. 275–278.
29. LeMesurier, A. B.: The quadrilateral Mirault flap operation for harelip. Plast. Reconstr. Surg., 33:26, 1964.
30. Lewis, S. R., Lynch, J. B., and Blocker, T. G., Jr.: The use of facial slings for tongue stabilization in the Pierre Robin syndrome. Plast. Reconstr. Surg., 42:237, 1968.
31. MacComb, W. S., Fletcher, G. H., and Healey, J. E., Jr.: Intraoral cavity. *In* MacComb, W. S., and Fletcher, G. H.: Cancer of the Head and Neck. Baltimore, The Williams & Wilkins Co., 1967, pp. 89–151.
32. MacFee, W. F.: Carcinoma of the floor of the mouth; clinical observations and surgical treatment. Ann. Surg., 149:172, 1959.
33. Miehlke, A.: Nerve grafting for restoration of lost facial expression. *In* Conley, J.: Cancer of the Head and Neck. Washington, Butterworths, 1967, p. 550.
34. Millard, D. R.: Refinements in rotation-advancement cleft lip technique. Plast. Reconstr. Surg., 33:26, 1964.
35. Moncrief, J. A.: Burns. *In* Schwartz, S. I., et al. (Eds.): Principles of Surgery. New York, McGraw-Hill Book Company, 1969, pp. 211–212.
36. Monroe, C. W., and Ogo, K.: Treatment of micrognathia in the neonatal period. Plast. Reconstr. Surg., 50:317, 1972.
37. Ochsner, A.: Diseases of the mouth. *In* Ochsner, A., and DeBakey, M. E. (Eds.): Christopher's Minor Surgery, 8th ed. Philadelphia, W. B. Saunders Company, 1959, pp. 270–283.
38. Proskauer, C., and Witt, F. H.: Bildgeschichte der Zahnheilkunde. Colonge, Dumont, 1962.
39. Reed, R. J., and O'Quinn, S. E.: Vascular neoplasms. *In* Fitzgerald, T. B., et al. (Eds.): Dermatology in General Medicine. New York, McGraw-Hill Book Company, 1971, pp. 533–547.
40. Robbins, S. L.: Textbook of Pathology, 3rd ed. Philadelphia, W. B. Saunders Company, 1967, pp. 1313–1367.
41. Robin, P.: Backward lowering of the root of the tongue causing respiratory disturbances. Bull. Acad. Natl. Med., 89:38, 1923.
42. Rose, W.: Harelip and Cleft Palate. London, H. K. Lewis and Company, 1891.
43. Stark, R. B.: Pathogenesis of harelip and cleft palate. Plast. Reconstr. Surg., 13:20, 1954.
44. Stark, R. B.: Embryology of cleft lip and palate. *In* Converse, J. M. (Ed.): Reconstructive Plastic Surgery, 2nd ed. Philadelphia, W. B. Saunders Company, 1977.
45. Stewart, J. B., Jackson, A. W., and Chew, M. K.: The role of radiotherapy in the management of malignant tumors of the salivary glands. Am. J. Roentgenol., 102:100, 1968.
46. Stoll, H. L.: Squamous cell carcinoma. *In* Fitzgerald, T. B., et al. (Eds.): Dermatology in General Medicine. New York, McGraw-Hill Book Company, 1971, pp. 407–422.
47. Swearingen, J. J.: Tolerances of the Human Face to Crash Impact. Report from the Office of Aviation Medicine. Washington, D.C., Federal Aviation Agency, July, 1965.
48. Tennison, C. W.: The repair of unilateral cleft lip by the stencil method. Plast. Reconstr. Surg., 9:115, 1952.
49. Tennison, P., Guiot, G., Rougerie, J., Delbet, P., and Pastoriza, J.: Ostéotomies cranio-naso-faciales. Hypertélorisme. Ann. Chir. Plast., 12:103, 1967.
50. Thompson, J. E.: An artistic and mathematically accurate method of repairing the defect in cases of harelip. Surg. Gynecol. Obstet., 14:498, 1912.
51. Wang, M. K. H., and Macomber, W. B.: Deformities of the lips and cheeks. *In* Converse, J. M. (Ed.): Reconstructive Plastic Surgery, 2nd ed. Philadelphia, W. B. Saunders Company, 1977.
52. Wilkie, T. F.: Surgical treatment of drooling. Follow-up report of five years' experience. Plast. Reconstr. Surg., 45:549, 1970.
53. Wolfort, F. G., DeMeester, F., Knorr, N., and Edgerton, M. T.: Surgical management of cutaneous lye burns. Surg. Gynecol. Obstet., 131:873, 1970.
54. Zarem, H. A., and Edgerton, M. T.: Induced resolution of cavernous hemangiomas following prednisolone therapy. J. Plast. Reconstr. Surg., 39:76, 1967.

43

NEUROSURGERY

Guy L. Odom, M.D., and Associates

I

HISTORICAL ASPECTS

Robert H. Wilkins, M.D.

The American student who is interested in the history of neurosurgery has a unique advantage. This specialty is of relatively recent origin and has been developed mainly in the English-speaking countries. For this reason, classic works in neurosurgery are usually obtainable and understandable.[3, 8] In addition, there are several excellent reviews of neurosurgical history that are written in English.[2, 5, 7]

These reviews all point out the fact that although the great majority of neurosurgical procedures have been developed recently, the history of trepanation dates back to the Neolithic Period. In widely separated geographic locations, archeologists have discovered human skulls containing craniectomy defects. Furthermore, in many of these skulls there are evidences of healing along the bony edges, indicating that the "patient" survived the operation. The rationale for these procedures is not known, since there are no written records from this era, but it is conceivable that seizures, headaches, or mental changes might have been the symptoms that led to this drastic form of treatment.

The oldest known writing dealing with surgical topics, the Edwin Smith Papyrus, is of special interest to the neurosurgeon. This treatise dates back to the seventeenth century B.C. and contains the first descriptions of the cranial sutures, the meninges, the external surface of the brain, the cerebrospinal fluid, and the intracranial pulsations. Brain injuries are related to changes in the function of other parts of the body, and hemiplegic contractures are well described. In addition, quadriplegia, urinary incontinence, and priapism are noted to occur in association with cervical vertebral dislocation. The Egyptian physicians of that period had a surprising knowledge of rudimentary neuroanatomy and neurophysiology, but their treatment of injuries of the central nervous system was only supportive. Significantly, trepanation is not mentioned in the Edwin Smith Papyrus.

The writings of Hippocrates contain the first recorded descriptions of trepanation, and his instruments and methods were very similar to their modern counterparts. In addition, Hippocrates dealt with other subjects of neurosurgical interest. He discussed epilepsy, the coexistence of spinal deformity with pulmonary tubercles, and the functional effects of compression of the spinal cord. He devised a method for reducing vertebral dislocations, and described permanent and transient facial paralyses, sciatica, and the complex of headache, visual disturbance, and vomiting. The ability of Hippocrates as an observer is well demonstrated by his descriptions of aphasia, unconsciousness, respiratory and cardiac irregularity, carphologia, pupillary inequality, and ophthalmoplegia associated with cerebral disease. He realized that a blow on one side of the head occasionally is followed by convulsions or paralysis of the contralateral side of the body, and he recognized the poor prognosis of the patient with a head injury complicated by a dural laceration. These and other observations made the works of Hippocrates a beacon to surgeons for over 2000 years, until the development of anesthesia, asepsis, and cerebral localization in the nineteenth century established the foundation of modern neurosurgery.

The introduction of anesthesia and asepsis vastly increased the scope of surgery in general and made brain surgery feasible. Such operations were not performed often, however, because there was no way to locate lesions that did not involve the skull. The problem was solved when it was discovered by Jean Bouillaud, Paul Broca, Gustav Fritsch, Eduard Hitzig, David Ferrier, and others that there is focal representation of bodily function in the brain. This third fundamental concept—cerebral localization—became an important part of the foundation upon which modern neurosurgery was built.

Another vital advancement made during the late nineteenth century was the development of the technique of osteoplastic craniotomy by Wilhelm Wagner, which was later facilitated by the use of Leonardo Gigli's wire saw. The introduction of this technique permitted the exploration of relatively large areas of cortex, and in so doing significantly extended the limits of brain surgery.

British surgeons were among the first to take advantage of these new developments, and they guided neurosurgery through its infancy in the last two decades of the nineteenth century. William Macewen, professor of surgery at the University of Glasgow, and a powerful figure in international surgical circles, was a pioneer in surgery of the central nervous system. Macewen was a pupil of Joseph Lister, and he strongly believed in Lister's principles of antisepsis. His phenomenal success in treating intracranial abscesses rarely has been equaled since that time, despite the subsequent introduction of antibiotics.

Rickman Godlee also applied Lister's principles of antisepsis to neurosurgery in 1884, when he became the first surgeon to attack an intracranial tumor that had been localized solely by neurologic means. William Bennett was another of these pioneering British surgeons. In 1888 he introduced the operation of posterior rhizotomy for the relief of pain.

The most outstanding surgeon in this field at that time, however, was Victor Horsley of London. He devoted the majority of his efforts to clinical and experimental neurosurgery, with exceptional results. Although he made myriad contributions, Horsley is best remembered today as the first surgeon to remove a neoplasm from the spinal canal (1887), and the first to attempt retrogasserian neurotomy for tic douloureux (1890). He also introduced bone wax (1892), and described a stereotactic apparatus for intracranial procedures in 1908, with Robert Clarke.

During the early development of neurosurgery, it was common for neurologists to diagnose the disease, devise the operation, and direct the surgeon in its performance. For example, Hughes Bennett localized the brain tumor that was removed in 1884 by Rickman Godlee, and William Gowers diagnosed the spinal cord tumor that was removed by Victor Horsley in 1887. In the United States, similar situations were encountered frequently. William Spiller, at the University of Pennsylvania, directed Charles Frazier in the performance of a successful retrogasserian neurotomy in 1901, and 10 years later directed Edward Martin in the performance of the first cordotomy. Similarly, Charles Dana at the Cornell University Medical College proposed posterior rhizotomy as performed a short time later by William Bennett in London and Robert Abbe in New York. Two outstanding neurologists of a later generation, Otfrid Foerster in Germany and Clovis Vincent in France, actually became neurosurgeons to facilitate the procedures they devised. Foerster, for example, independently devised the operation of cordotomy and performed classic studies of cortical function and peripheral sensory innervation.

A host of general surgeons tried their hands at neurosurgery during its formative years at the turn of the century. Most were soon discouraged by the innumerable difficulties accompanying this type of surgery. Between 1886 and 1896, for example, more than 500 different general surgeons reported brain operations they had performed, but between 1896 and 1906 the number fell below 80.

Fortunately, during this time a young surgeon at Johns Hopkins University took an interest in neurosurgery and decided to devote his full attention to it. With little help, Harvey Cushing advanced neurosurgery from its infancy through its childhood.[1] He standardized operating technique, and by applying the rigid principles of William Halsted to neurosurgical procedures, Cushing was able to make major reductions in operative morbidity and mortality. Before Cushing's time hemorrhage had presented an almost insurmountable problem during brain surgery. In his typically thorough manner, Cushing mastered the techniques of others for compressing the scalp, waxing the diploë, and so forth, and then he introduced the vessel clips and electrocautery that have become virtually indispensable for the control of intracranial and intraspinal bleeding.

Brain tumors also attracted Cushing's attention, and during the course of his career more than 2000 patients with brain tumors were seen in his clinic. With the aid of several brilliant assistants, such as Percival Bailey, Louise Eisenhardt, and Paul Bucy, Dr. Cushing classified these tumors morphologically, described their biologic behavior, and formulated their surgical treatment. The standardization of technique and the classification of brain tumors were only two of Harvey Cushing's many contributions. There are few areas of modern neurosurgical interest that are not based to some extent on the important investigations of this one man. Another such giant was Walter Dandy. Dandy worked with

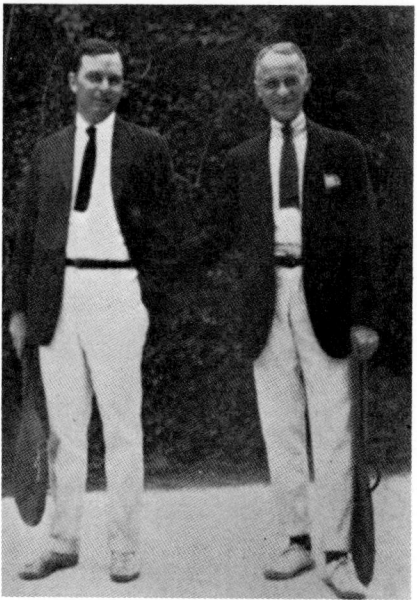

Figure 1. Walter Dandy (left) and Harvey Cushing (right) after a game of tennis in 1921. (From Fulton, J. F.: Harvey Cushing. A Biography: 1946. Courtesy of Charles C Thomas, Publisher, Springfield, Ill.)

Cushing for a short time at the Johns Hopkins Hospital before Cushing moved on to the Peter Bent Brigham Hospital. Dandy stayed at Johns Hopkins, and before he had finished his residency in surgery, he made two very important discoveries. In association with Kenneth Blackfan, he established the modern concept of hydrocephalus and developed the operations of choroid plexectomy and third ventriculostomy for the relief of communicating and obstructive hydrocephalus. A few years later, in 1918 and 1919, he introduced pneumoventriculography and pneumoencephalography, which have proved to be of inestimable diagnostic value to neurosurgeons since that time. As was true of Cushing, Dandy's contributions to neurosurgery were legion and his many pupils have influenced profoundly the subsequent course of modern neurosurgery (Fig. 1).

A third such contributor was the Portuguese neurologist, Antonio Caetano de Abreu Freire Egas Moniz. Moniz was unusually talented in a number of fields other than medicine, but he still found time to produce more than 300 medical publications. With neurosurgeon Pedro Manuel de Almeida Lima, he introduced the diagnostic technique of carotid arteriography in 1927 and initiated prefrontal lobotomy for psychiatric illnesses in 1936. For the latter work, Egas Moniz received a Nobel Prize in 1949.

Despite the outstanding work of Cushing, Dandy, and Moniz, most advancements in neurosurgery have been made slowly by the patient efforts of many pioneers. The subsequent developments in the various areas of neurosurgery are outlined in the remainder of this chapter.

SELECTED REFERENCES

Walker, A. E.: History of Neurological Surgery. Baltimore, Williams & Wilkins Company, 1951.
   This book is the standard history of neurosurgery, with 18 chapters on various aspects of the specialty by 12 contributors. It also contains 14 biographic sketches of pioneering neurosurgeons, and a bibliography containing 2371 references.

Wilkins, R. H.: Neurosurgical Classics. New York, Johnson Reprint Corp., 1965.

This is a collection of 52 of the most outstanding written contributions in the field of neurologic surgery. These have been compiled into 38 groups, each of which is accompanied by a commentary and a list of related references. The 15 works originally printed in other languages have been translated into English.

REFERENCES

1. Fulton, J. F.: Harvey Cushing. A Biography. Springfield, Ill., Charles C Thomas, Publisher, 1946.
2. Horrax, G.: Neurosurgery: An Historical Sketch. Springfield, Ill., Charles C Thomas, Publisher, 1952.
3. Morton, L. T.: A Medical Bibliography (Garrison and Morton): An Annotated Check-list of Texts Illustrating the History of Medicine, 3rd ed. Philadelphia, J. B. Lippincott Company, 1970.
4. Penfield, W.: Neurosurgery, yesterday, today and tomorrow. J. Neurosurg., 6:6, 1949.
5. Sachs, E.: History and Development of Neurological Surgery. New York, Paul B. Hoeber, Inc., 1952.
6. Scarff, J. E.: Fifty years of neurosurgery, 1905–1955. Int. Abstr. Surg., 101:417, 1955.
7. Walker, A. E.: History of Neurological Surgery. Baltimore, Williams & Wilkins Company, 1951.
8. Wilkins, R. H.: Neurosurgical Classics. New York, Johnson Reprint Corp., 1965.

II

DIAGNOSTIC STUDIES

M. Stephen Mahaley, Jr., M.D.

Skull X-rays

Plain film roentgenographic examination of the neurosurgical patient remains an extremely valuable though often underemphasized aid in diagnosis.[5, 19] In instances of cranial trauma, skull films are used in outlining linear, comminuted, or depressed skull fractures; foreign bodies such as missile or bone fragments; pneumocephalus; and air-fluid levels in the sphenoid sinus. With intracranial mass lesions, a shift of the calcified pineal gland may indicate the side of a lesion. Separation of the cranial suture lines and presence of a "hammered silver" appearance of the calvarium characterize chronically increased intracranial pressure in children. Pathologic calcification may be visible in lesions such as tumors, toxoplasmosis, tuberous sclerosis, and vascular structures. Certain congenital abnormalities such as hydrocephalus, platybasia, craniosynostosis, encephalocele, and microcephaly often require skull x-rays for accurate evaluation. In postoperative cases, skull films may be quite helpful in evaluating obliteration of the subdural space when tantalum dust and silver clips have been used as markers,[21] in determining tumor recurrence when such markers have been placed in the tumor bed at the time of original surgery (Fig. 2), and in searching for retained foreign bodies following trauma surgery. It is recommended that a routine chest x-ray be obtained for all neurosurgical patients suspected of having an intracranial or intraspinal mass lesion. It is not uncommon for a patient with signs and symptoms of a nervous system mass to harbor an asymptomatic pulmonary lesion such as a carcinoma.

Spine X-rays

Plain spine x-rays are secured whenever a pathologic process is suspected in the cervical, dorsal, or lumbosacral area.[19] In instances of trauma, fractures and dislocations may be apparent, and subsequent films become essential as one attempts reduction and realignment. Congenital spine problems, such as spondylolisthesis, kyphoscoliosis, spina bifida, and diastematomyelia, can be evaluated. Views of the interspace area may reveal degenerative disc disease or infection while changes (lytic or blastic) in the bony structure may suggest a neoplastic process. Erosion of the bony pedicles often indicates the site of an expanding mass within the spinal canal. Transaxial tomograms permit more accurate assessment of the spinal canal shape and size.[8]

Lumbar Puncture

The diagnostic lumbar puncture is essential to the establishment of the diagnosis of meningitis or subarachnoid hemorrhage and is valuable in other diagnoses. However, particularly as regards the neurosurgical patient, one must be aware of the possible rapid neurologic deterioration of a patient with a focal mass lesion such as a brain abscess, tumor, or hematoma when cerebrospinal fluid is removed from the spinal route. As part of the routine of a lumbar puncture, cerebrospinal fluid pressure should be noted, with the patient as relaxed as possible and without any compressive force upon the neck or abdominal areas. The cerebrospinal fluid should be compared with water, as a control, for color and clarity. Cerebrospinal fluid should be examined for protein and sugar content, cells, reactivity with syphilis, and colloidal gold. Protein electrophoretic patterns, when available, are used instead of colloidal gold reactions, and Millipore cerebrospinal fluid cytology may be an added diagnostic aid.[10, 22] Several special techniques are *not* part of a routine diagnostic lumbar puncture: the Queckenstedt maneuver to determine the patency of the spinal canal,[16] the Tobey-Ayer maneuver for testing the patency of the transverse venous sinuses,[20] and isotope cisternography, in which radioactive materials are injected intrathecally in an attempt to clarify diagnostic problems such as cerebrospinal fluid rhin-

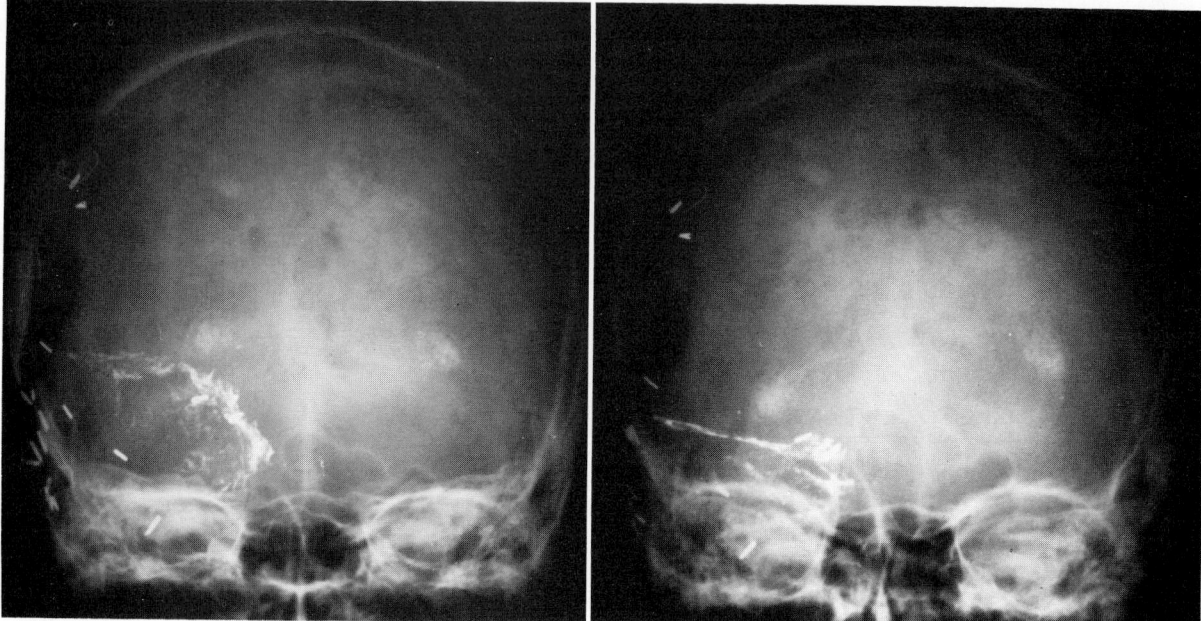

Figure 2. *Left,* Tantalum dust is shown in the area of tumor resection in the right temporal lobe, soon after surgery. *Right,* Several months later, the dust, as well as the calcified glomus, is seen to be displaced inferiorly into the floor of the middle fossa, indicating expansion of tumor recurrence above the marker material.

orrhea,[4] hydrocephalus, including normal-pressure hydrocephalus,[13, 15] and shunt tube patency. The most convenient site for lumbar puncture, under local anesthesia, is between the laminal arches of L4 and L5 or of L5 and the sacrum.

Subdural Tap

Diagnostic tapping of the subdural space represents a technique useful primarily in children with non-fused cranial sutures.[14] A lumbar puncture or special subdural tap needle containing a solid stylus is passed through the scalp at an angle and then perpendicularly through the coronal suture line just lateral to the anterior fontanelle. The stylus is withdrawn after the needle tip passes through the dura, and any fluid issuing forth is collected. This technique serves not only to establish the diagnosis of the subdural hematoma or effusion but also may effectively treat such lesions. The volume and color of the fluid should always be noted and the fluid cultured when indicated.

Myelography

Myelography is a radiographic means of outlining the contents of the spinal canal, utilizing positive (Pantopaque) or negative (air) contrast media. As regards Pantopaque myelography, this technique has been adequately described[17] and has proved invaluable as a diagnostic aid with disorders such as ruptured discs, osteoarthritic ridges and spurs, spinal tumors, angiomatous malformations on the surface of the cord, and spinal extradural hematomas. When the Queckenstedt maneuver is positive (sluggish or nonreactive), indicating probable block in the continuity of the cerebrospinal fluid pathway, a small amount of in-

trathecal Pantopaque usually suffices to delineate the location and configuration of the lesion. A lateral spinal tap at C2 is sometimes desirable for introduction of a small quantity of Pantopaque to delineate the upper level of a spinal block. Air myelography[9, 18] is the procedure of choice in outlining lesions of the upper cervical cord and foramen magnum: meningiomas, neurinomas, Arnold-Chiari malformations, syringomyelia,[2] and hydromyelia.

Pneumoencephalography

Pneumoencephalography is used less frequently now to localize brain tumors because of its possible deleterious effect on intracranial hydrodynamics in the presence of a mass lesion. However, it remains the definitive diagnostic procedure for cortical atrophy, hydrocephalus, porencephaly, focal cicatrix, and seizure disorders not accompanied by localizing signs of increased intracranial pressure.[19] Fractional pneumoencephalography permits the identification of cerebellar tonsillar location early in the study, gives exquisite detail of posterior fossa structures without confusing overlying supratentorial air, and allows control of the movement of air during the study.

Ventriculography

Ventriculography with oxygen or air is utilized in cases of hydrocephalus either in the newborn or in older patients with evidence of increased intracranial pressure, when an air study from the spinal route might be complicated by tissue herniation at the tentorial notch or foramen magnum. The transcoronal suture approach can be used in children, and in adults a twist drill opening in the skull or a burr hole is used to permit passage of the ventricular needle. Positive contrast materials such as Pantopaque may be needed to outline small acoustic neurinomas and anatomic structures in the posterior third ventricle and aqueduct areas.[12]

Angiography

Cerebral angiography is possible by several approaches—carotid, brachial, or femoral artery catheterization—depending largely upon the disease suspected. Angiography has to a great degree supplanted air study as the definitive diagnostic study for supratentorial tumors (neoplasms, abscesses, and hematomas) and, of course, is the definitive study in the diagnosis of aneurysms, arteriovenous malformations, and arterial occlusive disease.

Electroencephalography

Electroencephalography is most useful in the diagnosis of seizure disorders, metabolic disturbances, and certain encephalitides.[6] It is used as an indicator of brain death. The brain surface corticogram is used extensively in surgery for epileptic disorders. It should be remembered, however, that the neurologic examination, brain scan, or angiography may provide a more definitive localization of intracranial pathologic change than the electroencephalogram, which may be completely normal in extracerebral lesions, such as meningiomas.

Isotopic Brain Scanning

Isotopic brain scanning has proved useful in the localization of neoplasms, abscesses, subdural hematomas, and cerebral infarctions, and as a study of relative cerebral blood flow.[3, 7]

Computerized Axial Tomography (CAT)

The revolutionary concept of this diagnostic tool as applied to the head was conceived and developed by Godfrey N. Hounsfield, Senior Research Scientist of EMI Central Research Laboratories at Hayes, Middlesex, England.[1, 4] A narrow beam of conventional x-ray scans the head with an axial plane from many different angles at 1-degree intervals. By repeating this process 180 times, differential x-ray absorption coefficients (μ values) are calculated across the head and displayed on a cathode ray tube, which is photographed for permanent recording. Anatomic structures such as the pineal gland when calcified, the bone of the cranium, cerebral ventricles, and the calcified choroid plexi can be identified in various axial planes. Pathologic processes such as intracerebral hematomas, infarctions, brain tumors (Fig. 3), aneurysms (Fig. 4), intracranial foreign bodies, fluid in the subdural space, and edema around pathologic processes may be visualized.[3, 5] As a diagnostic tool, this method finds usefulness through identification and localization of areas of abnormal absorption standing out from the background absorption, which for cerebrospinal fluid is 0 to 13 μ, white matter 12 to 20 μ, gray matter 18 to 33 μ, and bone 300 to 500 μ. Thus, the specific absorption values for abnormal areas can be calculated. In addition, deformation of normal structures such as the ventricles, pineal gland, or choroid plexi is used to localize the presence of a focal mass effect. The use of enhancement by intravenous injection of contrast media has improved the incidence of tumor localization. In experienced hands, this new diagnostic tool presently has a diagnostic error of slightly greater than 3.5 per cent and is second only to pneumoencephalography in accuracy of diagnosis.[2]

Electromyography

Electromyography, combined with nerve conduction studies, has proved valuable in the initial evaluation and subsequent following of peripheral nerve inju-

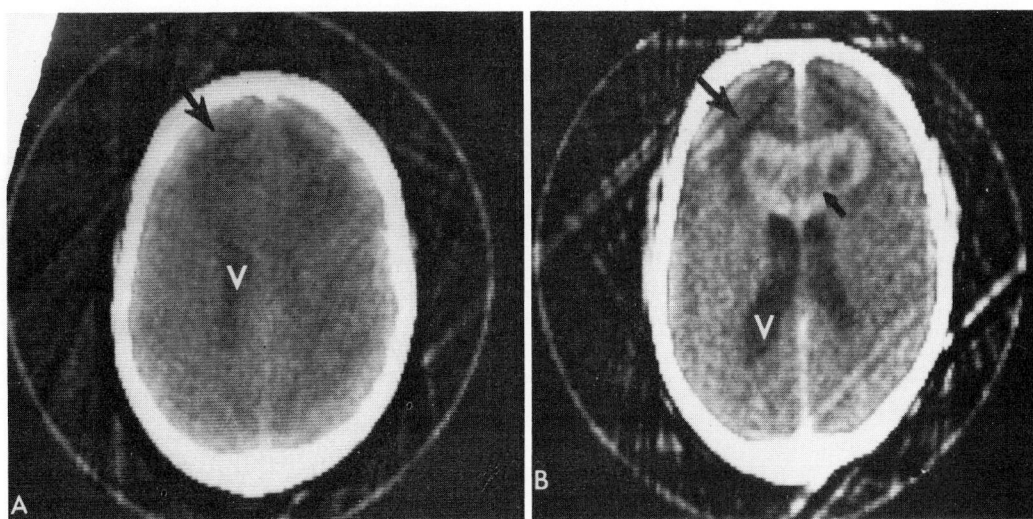

Figure 3. CAT scan of glioma of corpus callosum: *A*, without injection of contrast material, showing (arrow) only area of decreased density (edema) around the neoplasm; *B*, after contrast injection, showing tumor with low density, necrotic center (large arrow) and the surrounding area of low density edema (small arrow). The lateral ventricles (V) are seen on both photos. (Courtesy of Dr. George M. McCord, Jr., Department of Radiology, Methodist Hospital, Indianapolis, Indiana.)

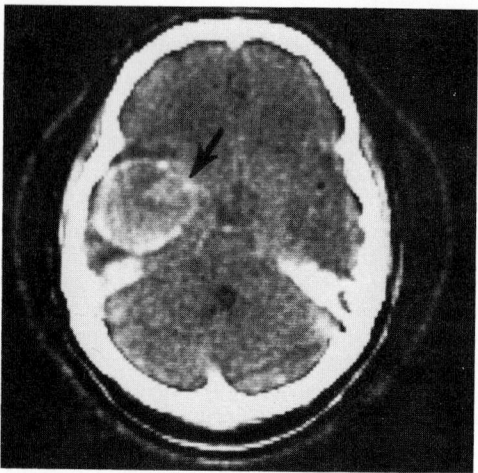

Figure 4. CAT scan of large congenital aneurysm (arrow) of middle cerebral artery in left middle fossa. (Courtesy of Dr. George M. McCord, Jr., Department of Radiology, Methodist Hospital, Indianapolis, Indiana.)

ries.[11] When the neurologic signs and myelography are not conclusive, the electromyogram may aid in localization of spinal root lesions.

SELECTED REFERENCES

Ambrose, J.: Computerized transverse axial scanning (tomography): Part 2. Clinical application. Br. J. Radiol., 46:1023, 1973.
The newest and one of the most promising diagnostic aids for evaluation of neurologic disturbances is the x-ray scanner, and this article is written by one of the developers of this instrumentation. It describes technique and results of scanning various intracranial problems.

Ojemann, R. G., Fisher, C. M., Adams, R. D., Sweet, W. H., and New, P. F. J.: Further experiences with the syndrome of "normal" pressure hydrocephalus. J. Neurosurg., 31:279, 1969.
The definition of this interesting syndrome is discussed, as well as the perplexing dilemma of diagnosis and treatment of these cases.

ADDITIONAL REFERENCES

Baker, H. L., Campbell, J. K., Houser, O. W., et al.: Computer assisted tomography of the head. An early evaluation. Mayo Clin. Proc., 49:17, 1974.

Cornell, S. H., Christie, J. H., Chiu, C. L., et al.: Computerized axial tomography of the cerebral ventricles and subarachnoid spaces. Am. J. Roentgenol., 124:186, 1975.

Hounsfield, G. N.: Computerized transverse axial scanning (tomography): Part 1. Description of system. Br. J. Radiol., 46:1016–1022, 1973.

Kistler, J. P., Hochberg, F. H., Brooks, B. R., et al.: Computerized

axial tomography: Clinicopathologic correlation. Neurology, 25:201, 1975.

REFERENCES

1. Ambrose, J.: Computerized x-ray scanning of the brain. J. Neurosurg., 40:679, 1974.
2. Conway, W. L.: Hydrodynamic studies in syringomyelia. J. Neurosurg., 27:501, 1967.
3. Davis, C. H., Jr., Alexander, E. J., Witcofski, R. L., and Maynard, C. D.: Brain scanning with 99m technetium. J. Neurosurg., 24:987, 1966.
4. DiChiro, G., Ommaya, A. K., Ashburn, W. L., and Briner, W. H.: Isotope cisternography in the diagnosis and follow-up of cerebrospinal fluid rhinorrhea. J. Neurosurg., 28:522, 1968.
5. Du Boulay, G. H.: Principles of X-ray Diagnosis of the Skull. London, Butterworth & Co., 1965.
6. Gibbs, F. A., and Gibbs, E. L.: Atlas of Electroencephalography, 2nd ed. Reading, Mass., Addison-Wesley Publishing Company, Volumes I, II, III, 1950, 1952, 1964.
7. Gilson, A. J., and Smoak, W. M., III: Central Nervous System Investigation with Radionuclides. Springfield, Ill., Charles C Thomas, Publisher, 1971.
8. Jacobson, R. E., Gargano, F. P., and Rosomoff, H. L.: Transverse axial tomography of the spine. Parts 1 and 2. J. Neurosurg., 42:406, 1975.
9. Jirout, J.: Pneumomyelography. Springfield, Ill., Charles C Thomas, Publisher, 1969.
10. Koss, L. G.: Diagnostic Cytology and Its Histopathologic Basis, 2nd ed. Philadelphia, J. B. Lippincott Company, 1968.
11. Krusen, F. H. (Ed.): Handbook of Physical Medicine and Rehabilitation, 2nd ed. Philadelphia, W. B. Saunders Company, 1971.
12. Lang, E. K., and Russell, J. R.: Pantopaque ventriculography: Demonstration and assessment of lesions of the third ventricle and posterior fossa. J. Neurosurg., 32:5, 1970.
13. Mahaley, M. S., Jr., Wilkinson, R. H., Jr., Sivalingham, S., Friedman, H., Tyson, W., and Goodrich, J. K.: Radionuclide blood levels during cisternography of patients with normal-pressure hydrocephalus or Alzheimer's disease. J. Neurosurg., 41:471, 1974.
14. Matson, D. D.: Neurosurgery of Infancy and Childhood, 2nd ed. Springfield, Ill., Charles C Thomas, Publisher, 1969.
15. Ojemann, R. G., Fisher, C. M., Adams, R. D., Sweet, W. H., and New, P. F. J.: Further experience with the syndrome of "normal" pressure hydrocephalus. J. Neurosurg., 31:279, 1969.
16. Queckenstedt, M. E.: Zur Diagnose der rückenmarks Kompression. Dtsch. Z. Nervenheilkd., 55:316, 1916.
17. Shapiro, R.: Myelography. Chicago, Year Book Medical Publishers, 1975.
18. Southworth, L. E., Jimenez, J. P., and Goree, J. A.: A practical approach to cervical air myelography. Am. J. Roentgenol., 107:486, 1969.
19. Taveras, J. M., and Wood, E. H.: Diagnostic Neuroradiology. Baltimore, Williams & Wilkins Company, 1964.
20. Tobey, G. L., Jr., and Ayer, J. B.: Dynamic studies of cerebrospinal fluid in differential diagnosis of lateral sinus thrombosis. Arch. Otolaryngol., 2:50, 1925.
21. Vieth, R. G., Tindall, G. T., and Odom, G. L.: The use of tantalum dust as an adjunct in the postoperative management of subdural hematomas. J. Neurosurg., 24:514, 1966.
22. Wilkins, R. H., and Odom, G. L.: Cytological changes in cerebrospinal fluid associated with resections of intracranial neoplasms. J. Neurosurg., 25:24, 1966.

III

INTRACRANIAL TUMORS

M. Stephen Mahaley, Jr., M.D.

The brain may host malignant or nonmalignant neoplasms, and brain tumors have been recognized to possess several rather unique features: a broad spectrum of cell types participating in neoplasms of different histologic patterns and a variety of growth characteristics; the rarity of metastasis of malignant gliomas despite rapid local growth and invasiveness; a peculiar vascular proliferation as part of the neoplastic process in many malignant gliomas;[13] and a difference in predominant tumor type and tumor location between children and adults. Brain tumors are usually classified according to tissue of origin and cell type. Table 1 lists the incidence of various intracranial neoplasms operated upon at Duke University Medical Center over a span of approximately 10 years. The biologic behavior of intracranial tumors varies as much as the methods of classification.[6] In any evaluation of the treatment of intracranial tumors, the exact neuropathologic classification of each case represents the foundation upon which other statistical studies must be based.[15]

The most common brain tumors are the gliomas, and in adults the most frequent glioma is unfortunately the most malignant—the glioblastoma multiforme, characterized histologically by pleomorphism of cell types, invasiveness, mitotic figures, hemorrhage, necrosis, and vascular wall proliferation.[3, 14] Other gliomas (astrocytomas, oligodendrogliomas, spongioblastomas, and ependymomas) show lesser degrees of malignancy or are totally benign in growth characteristics. Extracerebral neoplasms include such tumors as the pituitary adenoma, meningioma, acoustic neurinoma, and cholesteatoma. In children, the most common brain tumor is the medulloblastoma, a malignant neoplasm of the cerebellar vermis.[11] Other posterior fossa neoplasms (ependymoma, cerebellar astrocytoma, and pontine glioma) make up the majority of the childhood tumors.

Symptoms and Signs

Symptoms that may arise from a brain tumor include headache, nausea and vomiting due to increased intracranial pressure, and seizures and progressive focal neurologic deficits due to the local effects of tumor growth. A seizure without obvious cause commencing in adult life should be considered a symptom of brain tumor until proved otherwise; childhood seizures, on the other hand, less often indicate the presence of an intracranial neoplasm. Tumors of the pituitary gland often present with endocrine disturbances, the first symptom frequently being loss of menses in women and impotence in men; later, visual field defects characteristic of optic nerve or chiasmal compression may occur as the tumor enlarges above the sella turcica. Tumors of the eighth cranial nerve usually present with tinnitus and unilateral hearing loss.

On examination, signs of increased intracranial pressure may be evidenced as papilledema or an alteration in the state of consciousness. A focal neurologic deficit, such as weakness, sensory loss, or visual field defect, may be seen with supratentorial tumors, as brain tissue is compressed or infiltrated by tumor. Acoustic neurinomas usually cause neurosensory hearing loss and decreased or absent caloric responses on the side of the tumor. Posterior fossa tumors may cause dystaxia due to the local tumor effect and generalized increased intracranial pressure signs due to blockage of the fourth ventricle and resulting noncommunicating hydrocephalus. A pontine glioma should be suspected whenever a child presents with bilateral sixth nerve palsies or progressive cranial nerve palsies or both and long tract signs, usually without hydrocephalus. A child with a cerebellar astrocytoma frequently has a rather insidious onset of ipsilateral dystaxia and may show a head tilt toward the side of the

TABLE 1. 705 Intracranial Neoplasms—Duke Series*

Neoplasm	No.	%
Glioblastoma multiforme	150	21.3
Ependymoblastoma	23	3.3
Ependymal spongioblastoma	11	1.6
Astroblastoma	6	.9
Medulloblastoma	23	3.3
Mixed glioma	19	2.7
Neuroblastoma	3	.4
Astrocytoma	96	13.6
Oligodendroglioma	17	2.4
Ependymoma	40	5.7
Spongioblastoma	11	1.6
Ganglioneuroma	6	.9
Pinealoma	5	.7
Microglioma	1	.1
Neuroepithelioma	1	.1
Acoustic neurinoma	39	5.5
Neurinoma, V	2	.3
Neurofibroma	2	.3
Meningioma	89	12.6
Hemangioblastoma	9	1.3
Hemangioma	3	.4
Hemangiopericytoma	1	.1
Osteoma	2	.3
Chondroma	1	.1
Pituitary tumor	28	4.0
Craniopharyngioma	17	2.4
Cholesteatoma	8	1.1
Metastases	90	12.8
Teratoma	2	.3

*Data compiled by Information Science Division, Community Health Sciences Department, Duke University Medical Center.

tumor. Optic nerve gliomas, also occurring most frequently in children, usually cause visual loss with optic atrophy; large tumors of the chiasm cause signs of increased intracranial pressure from blockage of the third ventricle.

Diagnosis

Studies such as brain scanning (isotopic and/or computerized x-ray), electroencephalography, arteriography, and pneumoencephalography are used in tumor diagnosis and localization. Most tumor suspects are screened first with plain skull x-rays, electroencephalogram, and brain scan. Ependymomas, oligodendrogliomas, and meningiomas most frequently cause pathologic intracranial calcification visible on plain skull x-rays. Meningiomas may cause hyperostosis or erosion of the adjacent calvarium near their dural attachments. A pineal shift may be the only clue on plain skull x-rays as to the side of the tumor. If a focal area of abnormality is seen on these studies, angiography is generally the next study performed. The neoplasm may show up as an avascular area with displacement of normal vessels or as a "tumor stain" with radiographic filling of vessels within the tumor or its capsule (Fig. 5). Although computerized x-ray scanning with contrast material injection appears to have great accuracy, pneumoencephalography still offers the surest screen of the entire intracranial cavity for tumor and is the diagnostic tool most likely to reveal small neoplasms, whether they be within the brain parenchyma or in the subarachnoid or cisternal spaces.

Treatment

Whether benign or malignant, any enlarging intracranial mass ultimately threatens survival. Whenever possible, surgical resection of an intracerebral tumor remains the therapy of choice. However, it is well recognized that it is almost never possible to surgically cure a patient of a glioblastoma multiforme.[5] Sometimes the tumor, though histologically benign, is in a vital area such as the motor strip, brain stem, or speech region, so that total surgical extirpation is precluded. A benign meningioma may present in a "malignant" location, such as the clivus or the tuberculum sellae, so that complete removal without sacrifice of essential central nervous system structures is very difficult. In cases of tumors of the third ventricle, hypothalamus, or pineal region, where noncommunicating hydrocephalus plays an important role in the illness, a palliative shunt procedure for rerouting of the cerebrospinal fluid may produce dramatic relief of many of the symptoms and signs secondary to the tumor, although the lesion itself may not be surgically resectable. High-voltage radiation therapy is utilized in many cases when surgical resection seems unwise or when incomplete resection is necessary.[12] Tumors such as medulloblastomas and ependymomas in children, and perhaps craniopharyngiomas,[7] have shown radiosensitivity. In adults, the chromophobe adenoma of the pituitary gland and some gliomas appear radiosensitive. Cooperative studies are currently under way to determine more precisely the effectiveness of radiation therapy (cobalt-60) and chemotherapy in the management of malignant gliomas.[1] These studies thus far have shown a three-fold increase in survival time of patients with anaplastic gliomas treated following surgery with cobalt therapy (6000 r., whole brain, over 6 weeks) and intravenous bis-chloroethyl-nitrosourea. With longer survival times, patients treated with radiotherapy are more likely to suffer radiation necrosis of the brain.[2] The isotopic brain scan has proved

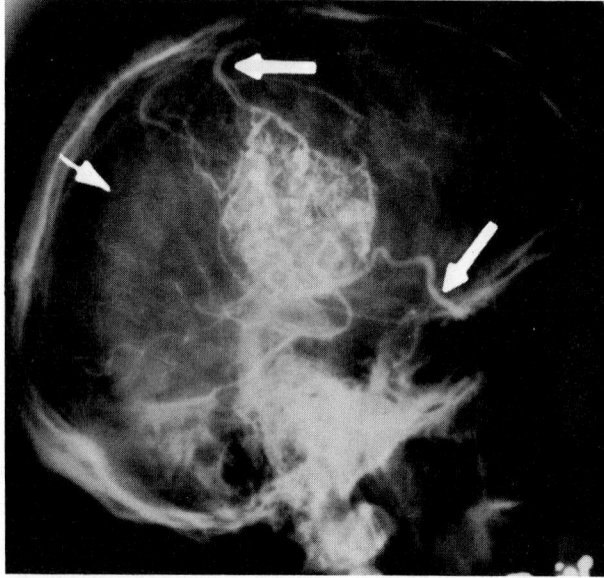
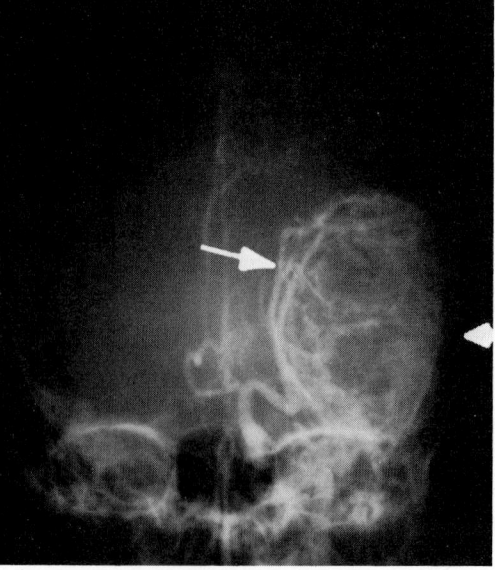

Figure 5. Angiograms, showing vascular stain of a malignant glioma (*left,* lateral view) and a benign meningioma (*right,* anteroposterior view). *Left,* The characteristic early venous filling (broad arrows) due to neoplastic arteriovenous shunting seen in malignant gliomas during the capillary phase (thin arrow) of the brain circulation. *Right,* The lateral meningeal attachment and origin (broad arrow) of the meningioma, with medial displacement of the middle cerebral artery (thin arrow).

to be a useful method for evaluation of tumor recurrence following diagnosis and therapy.[8] Investigational studies have just begun to explore the immune status of brain tumor patients,[9] and the role of immunotherapy in the treatment of brain tumors remains uncertain.[10, 16]

Surgery for metastatic tumors merits special consideration, pertaining to one's philosophy regarding management of these often difficult cases, particularly when a primary lesion is known to exist elsewhere in the body. The lung represents the most common primary site in the male, and the breast in the female. Unfortunately, surgery for the most common metastases to the brain offers little as regards prolongation of survival time,[17] although the prognosis following intracranial surgery for metastases from other primary sites such as the gastrointestinal and genitourinary tract is sometimes quite good. Since the period of *useful* survival may be lengthened by removal of an intracranial metastasis, it is our general practice to consider surgical resection of a likely intracranial metastasis when it represents the only intracranial lesion as judged by all diagnostic criteria, when the general medical condition of the patient permits surgery, when the tumor is surgically approachable, and when the patient or his family realize the uniqueness of the situation. It is occasionally discovered that a tumor stain seen by angiography in a patient known to have had a previous malignant disease elsewhere in the body is, in fact, a meningioma and not a metastasis at all. In such instances, surgery may be the only way to establish the true diagnosis and may rescue what otherwise might be considered a hopeless case.

SELECTED REFERENCES

Hoshino, T., and Wilson, C. B.: Review of basic concepts of cell kinetics as applied to brain tumors. J. Neurosurg., *42*:123, 1975.
As the title implies, this article reviews cell kinetics and attempts to relate brain tumor cellular metabolism to the rationale of chemotherapy.
Mahaley, M. S., Jr.: Immunotherapy of brain tumors. Sem. Oncol., *2*:75, 1975.
The current status of immunological investigations of brain tumor
patients is reviewed and the possible future role of immunotherapy is discussed.
Rubinstein, L. J.: Tumors of the Central Nervous System. Washington, D.C., Armed Forces Institute of Pathology, 1972.
This text is a classic organized review of the various types of brain tumors, with neuropathological description and illustrations from the extensive files of the AFIP.

REFERENCES

1. Brain Tumor Study Group, National Cancer Institute, National Institutes of Health, Bethesda, Md.
2. Eyster, E. F., Nielsen, S. L., Sheline, G. E., and Wilson, C. B.: Cerebral radiation necrosis simulating a brain tumor. Case report. J. Neurosurg., *39*:267, 1974.
3. Frankel, S. A., and Serman, W. J.: Glioblastoma multiforme. J. Neurosurg., *15*:489, 1958.
4. Hoshino, T., and Wilson, C. B.: Review of basic concepts of cell kinetics as applied to brain tumors. J. Neurosurg., *42*:123, 1975.
5. Jelsma, R., and Bucy, P. C.: Glioblastoma multiforme. Its treatment and some factors affecting survival. Arch. Neurol., *20*:161, 1969.
6. Kirsch, W. M., Paoletti, E. G., and Paoletti, P.: The Experimental Biology of Brain Tumors. Springfield, Ill., Charles C Thomas, Publisher, 1972.
7. Kramer, S., McKissock, W., and Cancannon, J. P.: Craniopharyngiomas. Treatment by combined surgery and radiation therapy. J. Neurosurg., *18*:217, 1961.
8. Leonard, J. R., Witherspoon, L. R., Mahaley, M. S., Jr., and Goodrich, J. K.: Value of sequential postoperative brain scans in patients with anaplastic gliomas. J. Neurosurg., *42*:551, 1975.
9. Mahaley, M. S., Jr.: Immunological investigations on human brain tumor patients. 7th Natl. Cancer Conf. Proc., 811–815, 1973.
10. Mahaley, M. S., Jr.: Immunotherapy of brain tumors. Sem. Oncol., *2*:75, 1975.
11. Matson, D. D.: Neurosurgery of Infancy and Childhood, 2nd ed. Springfield, Ill., Charles C Thomas, Publisher, 1969.
12. Moss, W. T.: Therapeutic Radiology. St. Louis, The C. V. Mosby Company, 1959.
13. Nystrom, S.: Pathological changes in blood vessels of human glioblastoma multiforme. Acta Pathol. Microbiol. Scand., *49*:1, 1960.
14. Roth, J. G., and Elvidge, A. R.: Glioblastoma multiforme: A clinical survey. J. Neurosurg., *17*:736, 1960.
15. Rubinstein, L. J.: Tumors of the Central Nervous System. Washington, D.C., Armed Forces Institute of Pathology, 1972.
16. Trouillas, P., and Lapras, C.: Immunothérapie active des tumeurs cérébrales. Neurochirurgie, *16*:143, 1970.
17. Vieth, R. G., and Odom, G. L.: Intracranial metastases and their neurosurgical treatment. J. Neurosurg., *23*:375, 1965.

IV

SPONTANEOUS INTRACRANIAL HEMORRHAGE

Robert H. Wilkins, M.D.

When intracranial bleeding occurs in the absence of head trauma, it usually happens within the subarachnoid space or within the substance of the brain.

SPONTANEOUS SUBARACHNOID HEMORRHAGE AND INTRACRANIAL ANEURYSMS[8, 11, 15, 16, 18]

Subarachnoid Hemorrhage

Characteristically, this type of bleeding has an explosive onset, causing severe headache, nausea, vomiting, and perhaps loss of consciousness, with or without a concomitant seizure.[6] These symptoms are most likely due to the sudden increase in intracranial pressure caused by a jet of arterial blood at a mean pressure of perhaps 100 to 150 mm. Hg squirting into a space filled with cerebrospinal fluid having a pressure of about 10 to 15 mm. Hg. Fortunately, the bleeding ceases after about 10 to 20 ml. or so of blood has escaped, perhaps as a result of a transient muscular spasm in the walls of the arteries adjacent to the site of bleeding. Then, as the blood induces a sterile meningitis over the ensuing hours, stiff neck, minor fever, and photophobia develop. Occasionally, headaches may precede the dramatic onset of subarachnoid hemorrhage, and there may be one or two "small leaks," but these events usually go unrecognized.

The ictal event itself may be precipitated by physical stress, but more than a third of patients sustain the subarachnoid hemorrhage during sleep. An unusually high number of patients who have experienced a subarachnoid hemorrhage are noted to be hypertensive when they are brought to the hospital. However, in many instances this systemic arterial hypertension simply reflects a physiologic response (the Cushing reflex) to increased intracranial pressure. It has not been possible to obtain accurate information on a large group of these patients as to their previous blood pressure, especially during the hours just preceding the ictus.

Retinal hemorrhages may develop, because the blood in the subarachnoid spaces about each optic nerve compresses the central retinal vein at its exit from the nerve, thus causing retrograde venous distention back to the eye itself. Changes in the electrocardiogram, primarily involving altered and delayed ventricular repolarization, may also occur in association with subarachnoid hemorrhage, but the etiology of these electrocardiographic changes is obscure.

Roughly 10 per cent of the patients will die within 24 hours of their first major subarachnoid hemorrhage, largely as a result of the damage done to the brain by concomitant intracerebral hemorrhage, by herniation of the uncus of one or both temporal lobes over the tentorial edge against the midbrain, or by infarcts and hemorrhages within the midbrain and pons that are secondary to downward displacement of the brain stem by the acute increase in the supratentorial pressure just described.

The survivors frequently recover within a few days with little or no neurologic deficit, only to face two more serious threats: cerebral arterial spasm and recurrent subarachnoid hemorrhage.

Cerebral Arterial Spasm. Cerebral arterial spasm is demonstrated in cerebral arteriograms as a narrowing of previously normal arteries.[19] This phenomenon is encountered in the arteriograms of about 40 per cent of patients with subarachnoid hemorrhage. It characteristically does not appear until a few days after the bleeding episode, and then it lasts for a few weeks. In a large proportion of these patients, cerebral arterial spasm appears to be simply an epiphenomenon,[10] but in some it is associated with decreased blood flow through the involved arteries, and cerebral ischemia and infarction in the area they supply. Therefore, under the latter circumstances, such arterial spasm can increase both the morbidity and mortality associated with subarachnoid hemorrhage.

After the first bleeding episode, the patient's subsequent course depends a great deal on whether an aneurysm, arteriovenous malformation, or some other detectable lesion was responsible. In an extensive cooperative study involving 19 medical centers, the causes of spontaneous (i.e., nontraumatic) subarach-

noid hemorrhage in 5834 cases were found to be intracranial aneurysm in 51 per cent, cerebral angiomatous malformation in 6 per cent, and both in 0.7 per cent.[16] A small number of additional patients had hypertensive intracerebral hemorrhages, primary or metastatic brain tumors, cerebral emboli, blood dyscrasias, anticoagulation therapy, eclampsia, intracranial infections, spinal angiomatous malformations, and so forth. In the remainder, the etiology of the hemorrhage was never satisfactorily explained.

Recurrent Bleeding. The patients in whom arteriography of both carotid and both vertebral circulations is normal seldom have any recurrence of bleeding, and their prognosis is very good. On the other hand, an untreated aneurysm is likely to rupture again within 2 weeks, and the second rupture has a higher morbidity and mortality than the first. Often the original blood in the subarachnoid spaces about the aneurysm will organize into an imperfect barrier of fibrous tissue. It is usually not adequate to prevent a recurrent rupture of the aneurysm, but may be dense enough to deflect the recurrent bleeding into the cerebral substance, with devastating results. This points up the necessity for early cerebral arteriography in these patients in order to detect those with treatable lesions.

Occasionally, an aneurysm will compress adjacent structures, such as the third cranial nerve, as it enlarges.[13] Under these circumstances, the aneurysm may be detected before it ruptures. It is extremely important that these cases be identified promptly, since the treatment of an unruptured aneurysm is not complicated by intracranial hemorrhage or cerebral arterial spasm and therefore it has a much better prognosis.

Similarly, a small percentage of the aneurysms of the internal carotid artery occur within the cavernous sinus. Such an aneurysm may compress the adjacent ipsilateral third, fourth, fifth, and sixth cranial nerves as it enlarges, but if it ruptures it will cause a carotid-cavernous fistula rather than a subarachnoid hemorrhage.[13] Though this does not involve a serious threat to the patient's life, it may cause a series of disabling complications from an annoying bruit to bilateral blindness. Here again, it is important to recognize and treat this type of aneurysm before it ruptures.

Cerebral Aneurysms

As stated earlier, congenital cerebral arterial aneurysms (called berry aneurysms because of their resemblance to berries) account for slightly more than half of all cases of spontaneous subarachnoid hemorrhage. These typically develop at vessel forks, and may be etiologically related to congenital deficiencies in the muscular arterial media that occur at these locations. As the aneurysm enlarges, its internal elastic lamina frays apart, and its dome consists primarily of the remaining adventitial connective tissue. The turbulent and irregular flow of the blood entering the aneurysm through its relatively narrow neck contributes to its enlargement, and also to the laminations of thrombus that are frequently laid down within its sac. These thrombi may be looked upon as the body's attempts to obliterate the aneurysm. As such, they are usually inadequate to prevent rupture of the aneurysm, especially after it becomes larger than 1 cm. in diameter. However, this process may be aided by certain therapeutic measures to be described, with the result of successful obliteration of the aneurysm.

Although they seem to be due to a congenital weakness of the arterial wall, cerebral aneurysms seldom rupture or otherwise make their presence known during childhood. Instead, they are one of the causes of "stroke" or "cerebrovascular accident" in the adult. Atherosclerosis, inflammation, and other pathologic processes may also involve the walls of a congenital aneurysm. Furthermore, several other types of aneurysms may occur on the larger cerebral arteries, and may be demonstrated angiographically. These include: (1) fusiform atherosclerotic aneurysms or ectasias involving mainly the proximal internal carotid arteries or the vertebrobasilar complex; (2) mycotic aneurysms, usually involving the distal branches of the middle cerebral arteries; (3) dissecting aneurysms; (4) traumatic aneurysms; and (5) luetic aneurysms. But these are unusual or rare forms of intracranial aneurysms, and a discussion of their pathogenesis and treatment is beyond the scope of this chapter.

Congenital berry aneurysms occur almost anywhere along the components and larger branches of the arterial circle of Willis, but especially at a few specific locations. Most of these aneurysms are located at the junction of the posterior communicating artery with the internal carotid artery (Figs. 6 and 7), at the junction of the anterior communicating artery with one of the anterior cerebral arteries (Fig. 8), or at the first major branching of the middle cerebral artery (Fig. 9). Another, less common site is the terminal bifurcation of the basilar artery. Approximately 20 per cent of patients with intracranial aneurysms have more than one, and this of course complicates their management.

Management of Subarachnoid Hemorrhage

In a patient with a spontaneous subarachnoid hemorrhage the diagnosis should be verified by lumbar

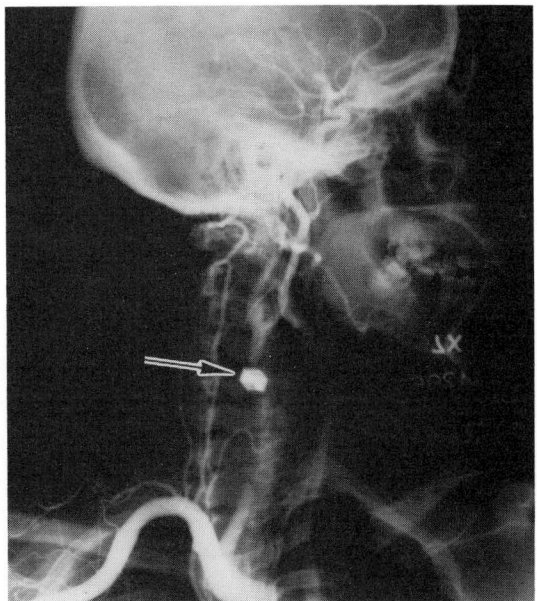

Figure 7. Arteriogram from same case as shown in Figure 6, after gradual occlusion of the right common carotid artery with a metal clamp (arrow). The arteries distal to the clamp fill via collaterals. The aneurysm is no longer visualized, and is presumably filled with an organizing thrombus.

puncture at the first opportunity. A few milliliters of the bloody cerebrospinal fluid should be centrifuged, and the appearance of the supernatant fluid noted. Oxyhemoglobin will appear in the cerebrospinal fluid a few hours after the hemorrhage and then bilirubin will appear and will persist for 2 to 3 weeks.[1]

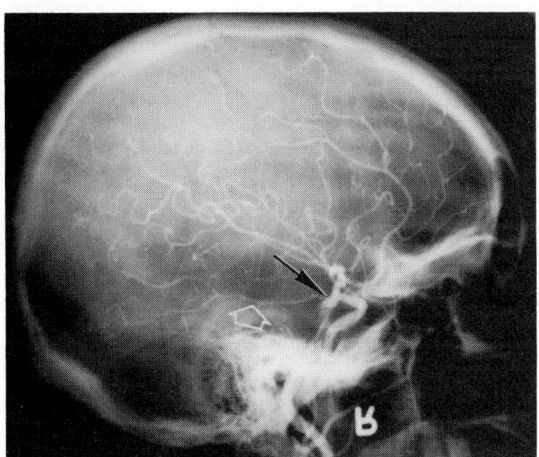

Figure 6. Arteriographic demonstration of an aneurysm (dark arrow) on the right internal carotid artery at the origin of the posterior communicating artery (just below tip of dark arrow). The white arrow points to the posterior cerebral artery.

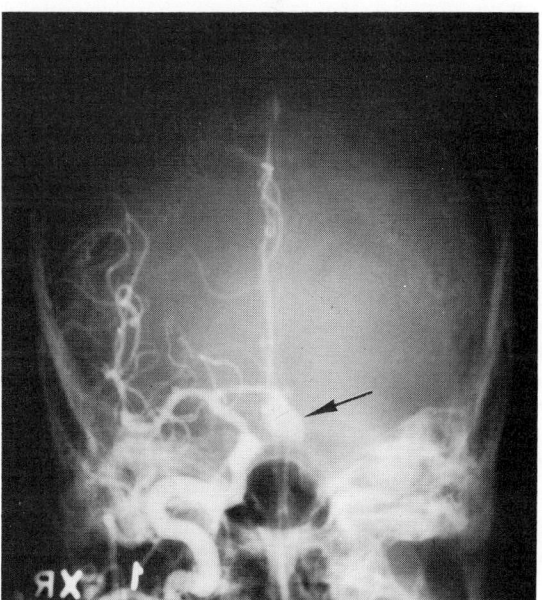

Figure 8. Anteroposterior view of a right carotid arteriogram, demonstrating an aneurysm (arrow) originating from the junction of the right anterior cerebral and anterior communicating arteries.

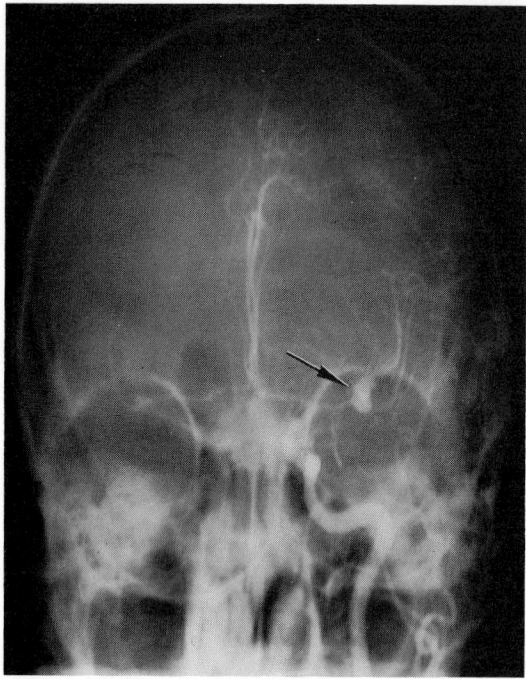

Figure 9. Anteroposterior view of a left carotid arteriogram, showing an aneurysm (arrow) of the left middle cerebral artery, and marked spasm of the intracranial arteries.

Therefore, during the first few days after the hemorrhage, the presence of xanthochromia in the supernatant will establish that bleeding has occurred and that the bloody cerebrospinal fluid is not the result of a traumatic lumbar puncture. Similarly, when cerebrospinal fluid is obtained 1 to 3 weeks after hemorrhage, the red blood cells are usually not present and xanthochromia may be the only proof that bleeding did occur. There may also be an abnormally low cerebrospinal fluid sugar value, probably because of the obstruction by the blood of routes of entry of sugar from the bloodstream into the cerebrospinal fluid.

The patient should then be transferred as soon as possible to a neurosurgical center equipped to treat intracranial aneurysms. He is maintained at strict bed rest in peaceful surroundings to minimize the danger of rebleeding, and cerebral angiography is performed within 24 hours to visualize the cerebral arteries. If this is normal, the patient is kept at bed rest for 1 month from the time of his hemorrhage and is then allowed to resume all of his previous activities. For the doctor, it is intellectually unsatisfying that the source of the subarachnoid hemorrhage cannot be demonstrated in such patients. But it is far better for the patient, since he seldom has either a residual neurologic deficit or a recurrence of this problem.

Surgical Treatment of Aneurysm

If an aneurysm is demonstrated arteriographically, the neurosurgeon must then decide whether, when, and how to treat it. The location and size of the aneurysm play an important role. A small percentage of aneurysms can be considered inoperable from the

start, and others, such as those originating at the basilar bifurcation, carry a prohibitive operative mortality except in the hands of a few neurosurgeons who have become especially skilled in their treatment.[4]

Another important factor is the condition of the patient. If he is alert and neurologically normal, the surgeon may wish to operate immediately, taking the risk that cerebral arterial spasm may then develop in its usual delayed fashion and complicate the patient's postoperative course. On the other hand, if the patient is comatose and hemiplegic, surgery is ordinarily delayed unless there is arteriographic evidence of a significant intracerebral hematoma. In that unusual situation, the immediate evacuation of the hematoma via craniotomy is sometimes worthwhile.

Usually, though, the patient is somewhere between these extremes, and the surgeon decides to delay surgical treatment. By the judicious use of bed rest, controlled hypotension to reduce the blood pressure within the aneurysm, and antifibrinolytic agents to try to retard the rate of lysis of blood clots on both sides of the aneurysmal wall, the surgeon is often able to delay operating on an intracranial aneurysm until the initial intracranial hypertension and the delayed cerebral arterial spasm have subsided and conditions are more favorable for a good result. This regimen exposes the patient to the risk of a devastating recurrent hemorrhage, but at present this is the lesser of two evils.[11]

Surgical therapy of intracranial aneurysms is aimed at the prevention of rebleeding by encouraging the development of clotting within the aneurysm, by strengthening its walls, or by removing it entirely from the cerebral circulation (Table 2). A variety of

TABLE 2. Surgical Treatment of Aneurysms

1. Exclusion of the aneurysm from the circulation
   a. With maintenance of flow through the parent artery—clip or suture ligation of the neck of the aneurysm
   b. Sacrificing the parent artery—clip or suture ligation of the parent artery on each side of the aneurysm ("trap" ligation)
2. Reinforcement of the aneurysm wall
   a. Muscle, fascia, or other biologic materials
   b. Muslin, or other types of cloth
   c. Acrylic resins, or other types of plastic
3. Reduction of blood pressure and flow within the aneurysm, and promotion of intra-aneurysmal thrombosis
   a. Systemic hypotension
   b. Systemic administration of antifibrinolytic agents
   c. Carotid ligation—common vs. internal carotid, rapid vs. gradual ligation. Vertebral ligation.
   d. Carotid ligation combined with ligation of the proximal portion of the contralateral anterior cerebral artery
   e. Ligation of the parent artery proximal to the aneurysm
   f. Electric thrombosis of the aneurysm, or the injection or insertion of foreign materials, such as wires or iron particles, into the aneurysm, either stereotactically or after operative exposure of the aneurysm

agents and techniques have been used for many years, and new ones are being developed constantly. Their very number attests to their deficits.

Theoretically, an aneurysm is best treated by removing it from the cerebral circulation, while keeping the arteries from which it arises intact. If the aneurysm is accessible surgically and has a narrow neck that involves only a short segment of its parent artery, this goal can be accomplished by placing a metal clip or ligature about its neck. Though it leads to the best theoretical result, such a procedure is attended by various hazards, such as the possible rupture of the aneurysm while it is being exposed. In experienced hands, with use of the most modern equipment such as the operating microscope, the operative mortality should be less than 5 per cent.[20]

These same hazards also apply to the reinforcement of the aneurysm by wrapping it with strips of muscle, fascia, cloth, or other material or by coating it with plastic. But, unlike the cases in which just the neck of the aneurysm must be exposed to accept a clip or ligature, in these cases the entire aneurysm, including its previous point of rupture, must be dissected free of the surrounding tissue before it can be adequately reinforced.

The last technique, involving the reduction of pressure and promotion of thrombosis within the aneurysm, carries with it the danger of distal cerebral ischemia and infarction, especially if such treatment is complicated by cerebral arterial spasm. Gradual occlusion of the common carotid artery over 7 to 10 days has been found to be safer than rapid occlusion of the common or internal carotid artery or than gradual occlusion of the internal carotid artery, since it allows for the development of collateral circulation through the external carotid system. Such carotid ligation, usually performed with a specially designed metal clamp, will result in significant long-term reduction in the pressure within the proximal components of the circle of Willis, but it has less effect on more distal pressures.

Despite the dangers implicit in the surgical treatment of intracranial aneurysms, most neurosurgeons proceed anyway because of the poor prognosis of most untreated aneurysms. Each case must be individualized for treatment, but some generalizations may be made. Aneurysms of the internal carotid artery may be treated by common carotid ligation, or may be clipped intracranially if they are accessible and have a small neck. Aneurysms of the anterior communicating—anterior cerebral complex may be clipped intracranially, but there are sizable technical difficulties associated with this procedure. Carotid ligation is of value when the aneurysm is supplied by only one carotid tree, i.e., when the proximal portion of the contralateral anterior cerebral artery is developmentally hypoplastic or has been purposely ligated via a craniotomy. Aneurysms of the middle cerebral artery seldom have a narrow neck that can be easily ligated, and they may be too far distal to be helped by carotid ligation. Many are therefore treated by reinforcement. Aneurysms of the vertebral and basilar arteries usually either are considered inoperable or are attacked directly. Prox-

imal ligation of the vertebral artery is hazardous, but may be used on occasion.[4]

Blood within the subarachnoid space from any cause will obliterate the arachnoidal villi and other arachnoidal channels that are important in the normal absorption of cerebrospinal fluid. This frequently results in mild hydrocephalus for a few days or weeks until the blood has been absorbed. However, in some cases the communicating hydrocephalus will persist, and some type of shunt operation (e.g., ventriculo- or lumbo-peritoneal) may then be required.

SPONTANEOUS INTRACEREBRAL HEMORRHAGE, CEREBRAL MICROANEURYSMS, AND ANGIOMATOUS MALFORMATIONS

Whereas congenital berry aneurysms bleed primarily into the subarachnoid space, and only at times bleed into the cerebral substance, the intracranial bleeding associated with hypertension and with angiomatous malformations is just the reverse. It occurs mainly within the substance of the brain, and extends into the subarachnoid space or ventricular system in only a portion of the patients.

Hypertensive Hemorrhage

By hypertensive intracerebral hemorrhage is meant the spontaneous development in the previously hypertensive patient of bleeding within the basal ganglia on one side (most common site), or within the pons, cerebellum, or other sites.

A century ago, Charcot and Bouchard grossly dissected the brains of persons dying of intracerebral hemorrhages and found objects a few millimeters in size that they assumed to be intracerebral microaneurysms. Later investigators raised the possibility that Charcot and Bouchard had actually seen small blood clots rather than tiny aneurysms. More recent studies, using postmortem arterial injections and special histologic techniques, have established the presence of miliary microaneurysms measuring 300 to 900 μ in diameter, especially along the lenticulostriate arterial branches in elderly hypertensive subjects. It is assumed that these are the weak points from which intracerebral hemorrhages arise in hypertensive patients.[5]

If the hemorrhage occurs in the pons, the patient usually loses consciousness quickly. The pupils are characteristically small and there are bilateral pyramidal signs and various abnormalities of conjugate eye movements. Ordinarily this type of hemorrhage is fatal.[6]

If the hemorrhage originates in the cerebellar hemisphere, its prompt recognition on clinical grounds is imperative to permit evacuation of the clot before the condition ends fatally. The typical picture consists of progressive neurologic deterioration from intracranial bleeding in the presence of hypertension, with vomiting, early inability to walk, vertigo, headache, paresis of conjugate lateral gaze, and so forth, combined with

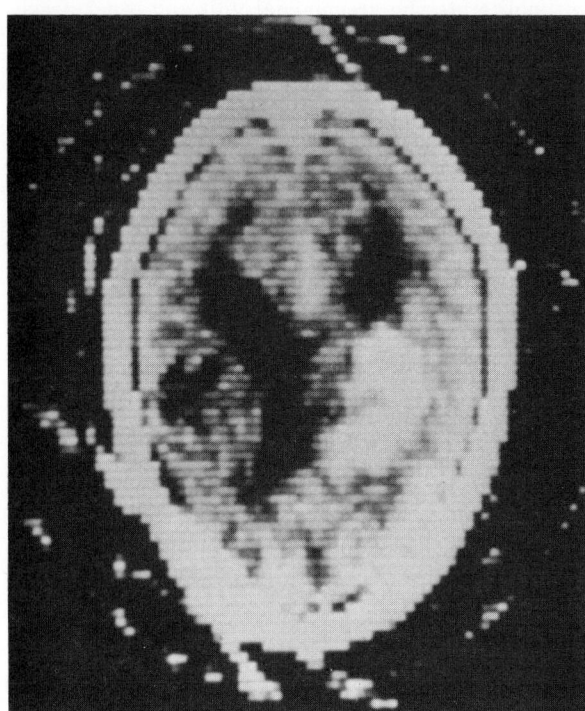
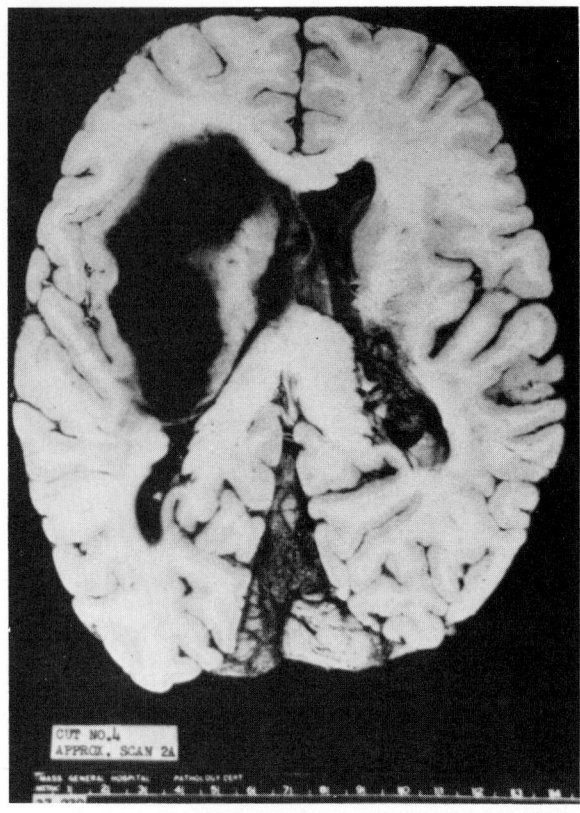

Figures 10 and 11. Computerized axial tomogram (Fig. 10) and corresponding horizontal brain section (Fig. 11) from a hypertensive patient who died of a spontaneous intracerebral hemorrhage in the left basal ganglia. (From Scott, W. R., New, P. F. J., Davis, K. R., and Schnur, J. A.: Computerized axial tomography of intracerebral and intraventricular hemorrhage. Radiology, *112*:73, 1974.)

the lack of hemiparesis, sensory deficit, homonymous field defect, or aphasia. Since the clot is quite tenacious, it cannot be simply evacuated through a burr hole with a needle and syringe. A suboccipital craniectomy and surgical evacuation of the hematoma with suction are required.

Similarly, a craniotomy is required if a hematoma is to be evacuated from the region of the basal ganglia.[14] This operation is not performed often, however, because of the devastating effects of the hemorrhage. The patient typically experiences a headache and then, over minutes to hours, develops hemiplegia, aphasia (if the hemorrhage is in the dominant hemisphere), and loss of consciousness.[6] The hemorrhage is frequently extensive, and it may break into the ventricular system. It is associated with a high mortality rate, even when the clot is evacuated soon after onset, and the few survivors usually retain their severe neurologic deficit. Therefore, most neurosurgeons simply verify the diagnosis by computerized axial tomography[17] (Figs. 10 and 11), lumbar puncture (often bloody cerebrospinal fluid), and carotid arteriography (an avascular mass in the region of the basal ganglia on one side, with no evidence of aneurysm, angiomatous malformation, or other cause), and give the patient supportive care. If he survives, a rehabilitation program is then of value.

Angiomatous Malformations[7, 8, 9, 15, 16, 18]

The exact classification of intracranial angiomatous malformations is still a debated subject, but for this discussion, three varieties are important. Telangiectasias (capillary angiomas) and cavernous angiomas are typically solitary developmental malformations within the brain substance that are too small to be visualized by angiography. They may serve as the site of origin of a large spontaneous intracerebral or intracerebellar hemorrhage, with the lesion itself being destroyed by the hemorrhage. This type of hematoma is frequently accessible surgically, and the diagnosis can at times be verified by microscopic examination of a biopsy from the walls of the hematoma. The prognosis of the treated case depends on the exact location and extent of the hemorrhage, but in general it is good.

Arteriovenous malformations are usually much larger, and most often can be visualized angiographically in the distribution of the middle cerebral artery (Fig. 12). The superficial portions of the malformation may cover part of the cerebral surface, but the lesion frequently extends like a cone down to the ventricular surface (Figs. 13 and 14). Therefore, the intracerebral hemorrhage that may occur from these lesions may spill into the subarachnoid space or ventricular system.

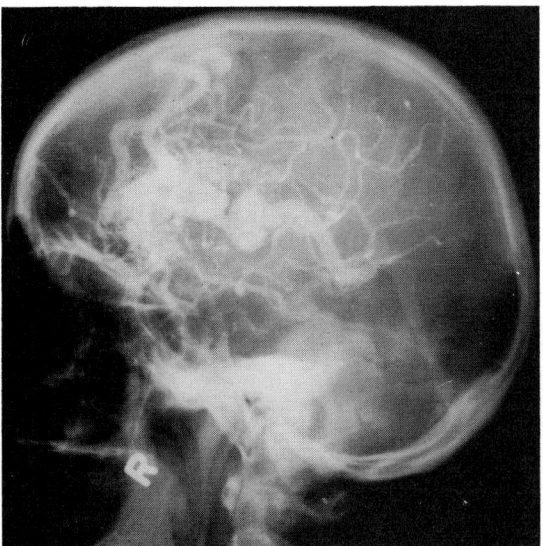

Figure 12. Arteriographic demonstration of an intracranial arteriovenous malformation.

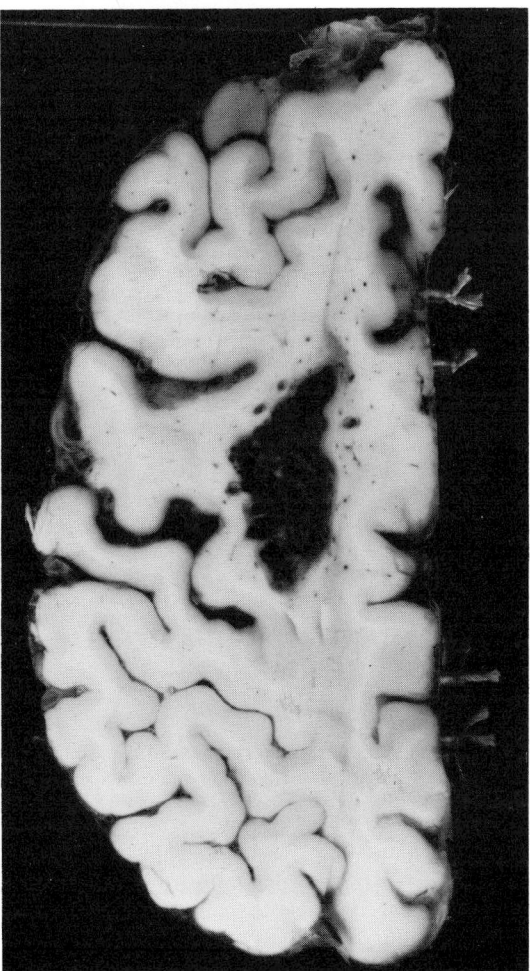

Figure 14. A horizontal section of the right cerebral hemisphere from the same case as shown in Figure 12. The arteriovenous malformation extended like an inverted pyramid from a broad base on the cerebral cortex to a small tip abutting against the lateral ventricle.

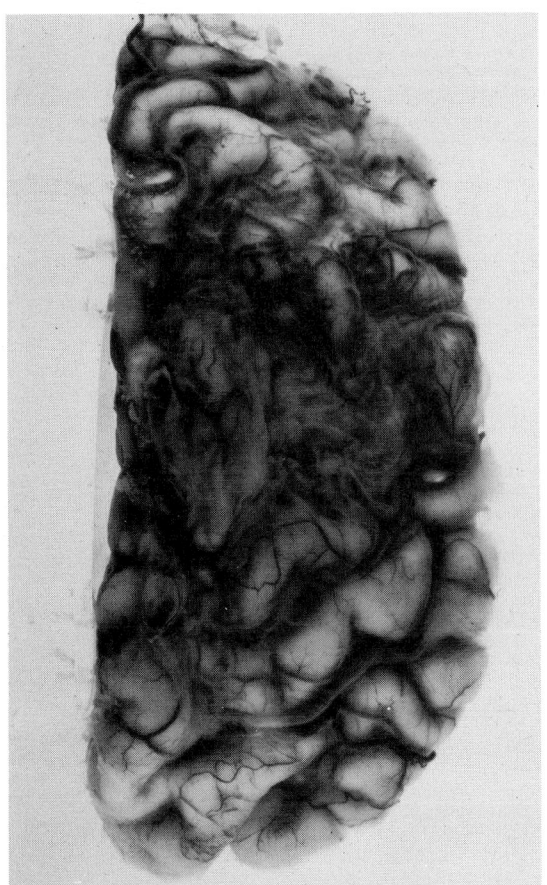

Figure 13. Superior aspect of the right cerebral hemisphere, showing a large arteriovenous malformation that had caused headaches and seizures during life.

Besides bleeding, arteriovenous malformations may "steal" blood from the surrounding brain, and may cause a significant increase in cardiac output. Likewise, patients with large arteriovenous malformations may have a variety of symptoms and signs aside from those directly related to bleeding, such as headaches, cranial bruits, convulsive seizures, mental deterioration, or a hemispheric neurologic deficit. Therefore, in contrast to intracranial aneurysms, arteriovenous malformations may frequently be diagnosed by angiography before they bleed. On the other hand, arteriovenous malformations tend to bleed earlier in life than aneurysms, with the peak incidence in persons between 15 and 20 years.

Surgical treatment by occlusion of the ipsilateral carotid arteries or of the arterial branches directly feeding the arteriovenous malformation does not have lasting value since collateral feeders quickly enlarge and the malformation persists. Repeated embolization of these malformations with plastic spheres of graded sizes or with other materials introduced via the internal carotid artery in the neck to promote intravascular thrombosis has proved to be a satisfactory alternative in some cases. But adequate control in many instances requires surgical excision of the entire malformation if its location and size will permit such a procedure. It may also be necessary to perform a craniotomy to evacuate an intracerebral hematoma even if the malformation cannot be resected.

The symptoms of untreated arteriovenous malformations tend to increase with time, and recurrent episodes of bleeding are common. The prognosis of lesions treated surgically depends on the size and location of the malformation, and the extent of cerebral destruction from intracerebral hemorrhage, direct surgical trauma, and cerebral infarction due to arterial interruption. As a general rule, about 60 per cent of patients from whom it is possible to excise an arteriovenous malformation will be free of symptoms or have only minimal symptoms, and another 20 per cent will be partly disabled but still able to work.

SPONTANEOUS INTRASPINAL HEMORRHAGE

Angiomatous Malformations[2, 3, 12]

The various types of angiomatous malformation encountered intracranially are also encountered within the spinal canal, but it is the location of the lesion in respect to the cord rather than the pathologic type that usually determines the clinical syndrome that results. A lesion that is partially or totally intramedullary will usually cause thrombotic infarction of or hemorrhage into the adjacent spinal cord (hematomyelia), with a resultant myelopathy, whereas a lesion that is primarily extramedullary but intradural will often cause subarachnoid hemorrhage or will compress the adjacent cord by its bulk. Typically, in both types patients will experience a progressive loss of spinal cord function, punctuated by sudden and often painful increases in their neurologic deficits with each episode of hemorrhage.

Myelography will often reveal the abnormal vessels as serpentine defects in the oil column. Often they may also be studied in better detail by selective arteriography, frequently via transfemoral catheterization of the intercostal artery or arteries that feed the malformation.[2, 3]

Despite the relative ease with which these lesions may be diagnosed, the results of treatment have been quite disappointing. Even with careful removal of the accessible malformations by means of microneurosurgical techniques, the damage that has already been done to the cord remains, and the surgical interruption of feeding arteries may cause further ischemia and infarction of the cord adjacent to the malformation.

Neoplasms

Neoplasms of various sorts account for a significant percentage of the cases of spontaneous spinal subarachnoid hemorrhage, so they must be considered in the differential diagnosis of these cases along with angiomatous malformations.

Spinal Epidural Hemorrhage

Patients suffering from a spinal epidural hemorrhage typically experience severe back pain at the level of the hemorrhage, associated with a rapidly progressive paraparesis or quadriparesis. The bleeding usually originates from some point in the extensive epidural venous plexus within the spinal canal, and it may be initiated by minor trauma, such as stretching or sneezing. Also, a number of these patients are receiving anticoagulant medication at the time of onset of their hemorrhage.

It is extremely important that diagnosis be made early, by history, physical examination, and myelography, so the clot can be evacuated surgically as soon as possible, With early diagnosis and operation, it may be possible to completely restore or significantly improve neurologic function. This is even more important in view of the fact that few of these patients ever have another such hemorrhage.

SELECTED REFERENCES

Krayenbühl, H., Maspes, P. E., and Sweet, W. H.: Progress in Neurological Surgery, Volume 3. Chicago, Year Book Medical Publishers, 1969.
  In this book are 12 comprehensive papers by various experts dealing with virtually all aspects of the treatment of spontaneous intracranial hemorrhages due to aneurysms, arteriovenous malformations, microangiomas, and hypertension.

Sahs, A. L., Perret, G. E., Locksley, H. B., and Nishioka, H.: Intracranial Aneurysms and Subarachnoid Hemorrhage. A Cooperative Study. Philadelphia, J. B. Lippincott Company, 1969.
  This 296-page volume constitutes a detailed analysis of 6368 cases of intracranial aneurysms and subarachnoid hemorrhage that were contributed to a cooperative study from 18 medical centers in the United States and one in England between 1958 and 1965. It represents the largest and best-analyzed series of such cases.

Vinkin, P. J., and Bruyn, G. W.: Handbook of Clinical Neurology, Volumes 11 and 12, Vascular Diseases of the Nervous System. Amsterdam, North-Holland Publishing Co., 1972.
  These two volumes contain 47 chapters (1415 pages) by world authorities and include exhaustive reviews of various aspects of spontaneous intracranial and intraspinal hemorrhage.

REFERENCES

1. Barrows, L. J., Hunter, F. T., and Banker, B. Q.: The nature and significance of pigments in the cerebrospinal fluid. Brain, 78:59, 1955.
2. Djindjian, R., Houdard, R., and Hurth, M.: Les angiomes de la moelle. Paris, Sandoz Editions, 1969.
3. Doppman, J. L., DiChiro, G., and Ommaya, A. K.: Selected Arteriography of the Spinal Cord. St. Louis, Warren H. Green, 1969.
4. Drake, C. G.: Ligation of the vertebral (unilateral or bilateral) or basilar artery in the treatment of large intracranial aneurysms. J. Neurosurg., 43:255, 1975.
5. Fisher, C. M.: Cerebral miliary aneurysms in hypertension. Am. J. Pathol., 66:313, 1972.
6. Fisher, C. M.: Clinical syndromes in cerebral thrombosis, hypertensive hemorrhage, and ruptured saccular aneurysm. Clin. Neurosurg., 22:117, 1975.
7. Forster, D. M. C., Steiner, L., and Håkanson, S.: Arteriovenous malformations of the brain. A long-term clinical study. J. Neurosurg., 37:562, 1972.
8. Krayenbühl, H., Maspes, P. E., and Sweet, W. H.: Progress in Neurological Surgery, Volume 3. Chicago, Year Book Medical Publishers, 1969.
9. Luessenhop, A. J., and Presper, J. H.: Surgical embolization of cerebral arteriovenous malformations through internal carotid and vertebral arteries. Long-term results. J. Neurosurg., 42:443, 1975.

10. Millikan, C. H.: Cerebral vasospasm and ruptured intracranial aneurysm. Arch. Neurol., *32*:433, 1975.
11. Nibbelink, D. W.: Cooperative aneurysm study: Antihypertensive and antifibrinolytic therapy following subarachnoid hemorrhage from ruptured intracranial aneurysm. *In* Whisnant, J. P., and Sandok, B. A. (Eds.): Cerebral vascular diseases. Ninth Conference. New York, Grune & Stratton, 1975, pp. 155–165.
12. Odom, G. L.: Vascular lesions of the spinal cord: Malformations, spinal subarachnoid and extradural hemorrhage. Clin. Neurosurg., *8*:196, 1962.
13. Odom, G. L.: Ophthalmic involvement in neurological vascular lesions. *In* Smith, J. L. (Ed.): Neuro-Ophthalmology. Springfield, Ill., Charles C Thomas, Publisher, 1964, pp. 1–96.
14. Paillas, J. E., and Alliez, B.: Surgical treatment of spontaneous intracerebral hemorrhage. J. Neurosurg., *39*:145, 1973.
15. Pool, J. L., and Potts, D. G.: Aneurysms and Arteriovenous Anomalies of the Brain. New York, Hoeber Medical Division, Harper & Row, 1965.
16. Sahs, A. L., Perret, G. E., Locksley, H. B., and Nishioka, H.: Intracranial Aneurysms and Subarachnoid Hemorrhage. A Cooperative Study. Philadelphia, J. B. Lippincott Company, 1969.
17. Scott, W. R., New, P. F. J., Davis, K. R., and Schnur, J. A.: Computerized axial tomography of intracerebral and intraventricular hemorrhage. Radiology, *112*:73, 1974.
18. Vinken, P. J., and Bruyn, G. W.: Handbook of Clinical Neurology, Volumes 11 and 12, Vascular Diseases of the Nervous System. Amsterdam, North-Holland Publishing Co., 1972.
19. Wilkins, R. H.: Hypothalamic dysfunction and intracranial arterial spasm. Surg. Neurol., *4*:472, 1975.
20. Yasargil, M. G., and Fox, J. L.: The microsurgical approach to intracranial aneurysms. Surg. Neurol., *3*:7, 1975.

V

CRANIOCEREBRAL INJURIES

Guy L. Odom, M.D.

Accidental injury has become the fourth leading cause of death in the United States with the increase in the number of motor vehicles, and the leading cause in the age group of 1 to 44 years. Approximately 50,000 deaths a year result from automobile accidents in this country. It is estimated that injuries to the head occur in 72 per cent of persons involved in automobile accidents and 1 of every 10 such injuries is dangerous or fatal.

Classification of Craniocerebral Injuries

Scalp
    Laceration
    Subgaleal hematoma
Skull
    Fracture, simple vs. compound
        Linear
        Depressed
Cerebrum
    Concussion
    Contusion
    Laceration
Hemorrhage
    Extradural
    Subdural
    Subarachnoid
    Intracerebral
Penetrating wounds

Although this classification may be helpful, most patients have a combination of these injuries, not a single one. In severe accidents, Braunstein reports that 44 per cent of the patients with head injuries sustain injuries to other parts of the body.

Initial Examination

It is frequently difficult to make a definite diagnosis or to evaluate a patient completely from a neurologic standpoint immediately after an injury. In this complex situation one must determine whether the patient is in *shock,* whether *multiple injuries* have occurred, whether there is *evidence of increasing intracranial pressure,* and whether there is *evidence of spinal cord involvement.*

The Question of Shock and Airway

The presence of vascular *shock* and the adequacy of the *airway* are the two most important clinical determinations to be made when the patient is first examined, and these two problems are given priority over all other aspects of the examination and immediate therapy. The presence of shock usually indicates that the patient has sustained multiple injuries and the examiner's attention should be directed to other organs of the body, even though the patient may be unconscious.

A severe head injury alone seldom results in shock unless there has been extensive scalp laceration with profuse bleeding that has been unattended.

The most common causes of shock associated with head injuries are rupture of an abdominal organ, intrathoracic bleeding, and fracture of the femur or pelvis. The treatment of shock demands priority over everything else, *unless* it is obvious that the patient has an *extradural hematoma.* It is essential that the patient *not be moved* for x-rays or other procedures until the usual methods are carried out to combat shock. No attempt is made to repair scalp lacerations during the initial phase of observation. The wound should be covered with a sterile dressing and a tight elastic bandage applied. If large arterial bleeders are present, the vessels may be clamped or ligated, and repair or further examination of the wound is deferred until the patient's condition has stabilized.

The maintenance of an adequate airway is as essential as treating shock. The air passage may become obstructed by blood, mucus, and vomitus. This may be avoided by the use of suction and positioning with someone in constant attendance. In extensive facio-maxillary injuries or in the unconscious patient with respiratory difficulty, tracheotomy may be a lifesaving procedure.

Associated Spinal Injuries

The early recognition of a spinal injury is of extreme importance in order to prevent further damage to the spinal cord. This is seldom a problem in the conscious patient, but it may be difficult to determine in the unconscious person. In the comatose patient, the absence of deep reflexes in the lower extremities, diaphragmatic respirations, and the failure of painful stimulation to produce reflex movement in the lower portion of the body while it does so over the arms or shoulders indicates involvement of the spinal cord.

Observation and Treatment

At the time of the initial clinical evaluation, if the patient has a closed head injury, it may be necessary to observe the patient for a period of time to determine whether the problem will require surgical or nonsurgical treatment. This decision may depend upon whether signs of increasing intracranial pressure due to intracranial hematomas or cerebral edema develop. The parameters to be monitored include level of consciousness, blood pressure, pulse, respiration, pupils, eye movements, motor responses to command or pain, and electrolytes.

If personnel and facilities are not available for surgery, the patient should be immediately transferred, if not in shock, to a neurosurgical center.

One of the first changes to ocur with rising intracranial pressure may be a *decrease in level of consciousness*. The patient becomes restless, confused, and lethargic. If intracranial pressure continues to rise, the patient becomes stuporous and finally comatose.

Blood pressure, pulse, and respiration should be recorded every 15 minutes for 1 to 2 hours, then every 30 minutes, and finally every hour depending on the individual case. *Rising blood pressure and slowing of pulse rate* and *irregular respirations* are indications of acute increased intracranial pressure.

The pupils should be checked each time the vital signs are recorded. Unilateral dilation of the pupil followed by fixation to light is indicative of third nerve compression from herniation of the medial aspect of the temporal lobe over the edge of the tentorium.[9, 19] Bilateral constriction and fixation of pupils suggest pontine involvement and poor prognosis. The spinociliary reflex is useful in determining brain stem involvement. A normal reflex results in ipsilateral pupillary dilatation in response to pinching of the skin of the neck and is lost in progressive brain stem dysfunction.

Rising intracranial pressure may produce *changes in motor function* such as increasing hemiparesis, increasing spasticity on one or both sides with increased muscle tone, increased deep tendon reflexes, ankle clonus, and Babinski sign. The development of decorticate posturing (lower extremities extended and rigid

with upper extremities flexed at the elbows) and decerebrate posturing (upper and lower extremities extended and rigid) is indicative of progressive midbrain involvement.[8]

In recent years various methods have been devised for continuous measurement of intracranial pressure. By these methods early elevation in intracranial pressure can be recognized and appropriate treatment undertaken before irreversible pathological changes occur. Tindall et al.[17] recommends that when pressure remains above 30 mm. Hg hyperventilation be employed by assisted or controlled ventilation, and that mannitol be administered intravenously in a dosage of 1 to 2 gm. per kg. over 30 to 60 minutes. He also uses glucosteroids but states that their effectiveness in head injury has not been conclusively proven.

Electrolytes should be checked every 2 to 3 days. Electrolyte imbalance, which has been found to occur following cerebral injury, may produce confusion, drowsiness, coma, and convulsions.[13] This syndrome may be difficult to differentiate from expanding intracranial lesions.

Scalp Laceration

A scalp wound, whether single or multiple, may involve the underlying skull and should always be considered a potentially serious problem. The scalp should be shaved widely about the laceration and thoroughly cleansed. The wound is then palpated with a sterile glove in an attempt to determine whether there is involvement of the underlying skull. The scalp edges are debrided and closed in layers without tension. When there is a scalp defect that cannot be closed primarily, a local pedicle scalp flap may be needed to close the defect and cover the underlying exposed bone or dura.[10] If this is done, it is necessary to outline the flap to maintain maximal blood supply and venous drainage. If the secondary defect cannot be closed without tension, a skin graft is used.

Linear Skull Fracture

Linear skull fractures seldom present a problem unless they extend into air spaces (otorrhea and rhinorrhea), cross middle meningeal channels, become widely separated (tear of underlying dura), or are compounded. In the latter instance, the fracture line is thoroughly inspected for trapped particles of hair or other foreign material between the bone edges of the fracture line. With a blow to the head it is not unusual for the edges of the linear fracture to spring open several millimeters and immediately close, retaining foreign debris in the fracture line. When this occurs, it is necessary to debride the bone edges by placing a trephine opening adjacent to the fracture line and removing a narrow strip of bone from both sides of the fracture with rongeurs.

One of the most serious complications of linear skull fractures is cerebrospinal fluid rhinorrhea. Fractures involving the cribriform plate or the posterior wall of the frontal sinus are the most frequent causes of this complication, which opens a pathway for infection into the subarachnoid space. If there is not an associated compound depressed fracture, the patient can be followed for 7 to 10 days to determine if the drainage will stop. During this period of time, the head of the bed is elevated, antibiotics are given, and the patient is advised not to blow his nose. If the leak does not cease spontaneously, the dural tear is closed by exploring the anterior fossa by means of a bilateral frontal craniotomy.[10]

Cerebrospinal fluid otorrhea is a leak of subarachnoid fluid from the external auditory meatus and is caused by fractures extending into the petrous ridge. These patients are treated conservatively and seldom require surgery to close the dural tear.

In cases of linear fractures with separation of the bone edges, there may be laceration of the underlying dura with herniation of cerebral tissue. This complication occurs more frequently in children and may result in a leptomeningeal cyst that may progressively increase in size.[15, 16]

Depressed Fracture

In simple depressed fractures there are two instances when the fracture may be treated conservatively: first, if the inner table is depressed several millimeters and there is no associated focal neurologic deficit; and, second, if the depressed fragment overlies the sagittal or transverse sinus. In the latter situation, the underlying venous sinus may have been lacerated by the sharp edge of the depressed bone and elevation of the fragment may necessitate ligation of the sinus to control hemorrhage.

Simple depressed or simple comminuted depressed fractures are treated by outlining a suitable scalp flap that will extend several centimeters beyond the margins of the involved bone. After the scalp has been reflected from the depressed fragments, the periosteum is incised and separated between the fragments and the intact skull. A burr hole is then placed in the skull adjacent to the depression with a piecemeal elevation of the fragments. Care must be taken to separate the dura from the inner surface of each individual fragment. If the dura is torn, there may be contusion, laceration, or hemorrhage into the underlying cortex. If the dura is intact but bluish in color it should be opened and underlying hemorrhage or contused cortex removed. After careful hemostasis, the dura is closed and bone fragments replaced.

The seriousness of the compound depressed fracture depends upon associated laceration of the underlying dura and cortex or subdural or intracerebral hemorrhage. These wounds are frequently contaminated by foreign material and must be cleansed thoroughly and debrided. The comminuted depressed bone fragments are removed and occasionally edges of the intact skull must be debrided with rongeurs. If the dura is discolored it should be opened to be certain that there is not an associated subdural hematoma or contusion or hemorrhage in the underlying cortex. The devitalized brain is removed and the dura is closed. If the edges of the dura cannot be approximated, a small fascial graft is inserted. The scalp is closed with through-and-through steel sutures. Drains should not be used.

Carrington, Taren, and Kahn[3] report that in compound comminuted depressed fractures in children, the bone fragments may be replaced without danger of infection after they are thoroughly cleansed. In 76 cases treated by means of this technique, infection occurred in only two cases and in these there was no spread of infection intracranially.

Extradural Hemorrhage

Extradural hemorrhage most commonly occurs from a tear of the middle meningeal artery and accompanying veins secondary to a linear fracture in the temporal bone, and initially is seldom associated with cerebral involvement (Fig. 15).

The typical history of an extradural hemorrhage is that of a minor head injury with a short period of unconsciousness.[7] There is then an interval during which the patient is alert and has no neurologic involvement. In a short time, however, progressive severe headache, nausea, and vomiting may develop. These symptoms are followed by impairment in state of consciousness, which at first may be very gradual and later abruptly change to coma. During the period of lethargy, there may be decrease in voluntary movements on one side of the body. As the intracranial pressure increases, the blood pressure becomes elevated, with slowing of the pulse rate. The accumulation of blood displaces the medial aspect of the temporal lobe over the edge of the tentorium, with compression of the oculomotor nerve which produces dilatation of the pupil.[8, 16] Bilateral rigidity and extension of the extremities may occur. The hematoma must be evacuated at this time without additional diagnostic studies. If surgery is delayed, further herniation of the hippocampal gyrus occurs with compression of the posterior cerebral artery at the edge of the

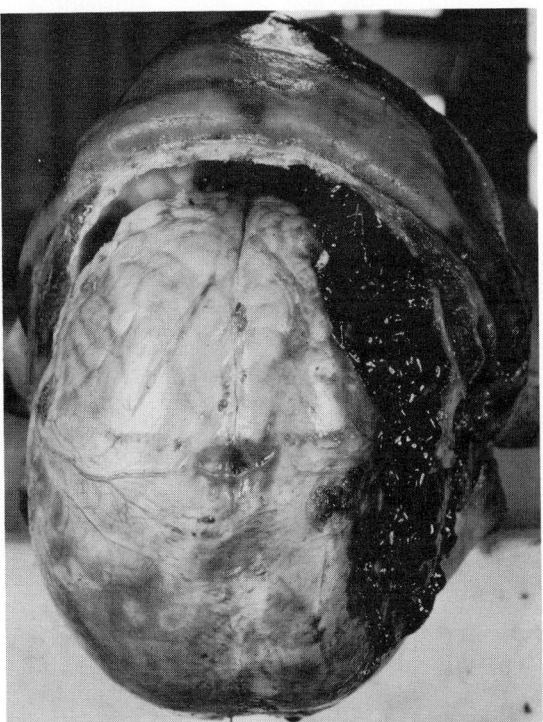

Figure 15. Autopsy specimen revealing an extradural hematoma on the right.

tentorium and infarction of the occipital lobe. This further increases intracranial pressure and results in midbrain hemorrhage and death.

If an extradural hemorrhage is suspected, a trephine hole should be placed in the temporal bone immediately, instead of awaiting further developments. The evacuation of an extradural hemorrhage is carried out by means of a subtemporal craniectomy. Endotracheal anesthesia is used to provide an adequate airway. The entire side of the head is prepared and draped. An incision is made in the temporal region, 2 to 3 cm. anterior to the ear with the lower end of the incision extending down to the zygomatic arch. A trephine opening is placed in the bone and rapidly enlarged with rongeurs. The clot is removed by suction and if the site of bleeding is not obvious, the middle meningeal artery should be followed down into the middle fossa and the foramen spinosum packed with a small piece of cotton and bone wax. If a third nerve palsy was present before operation, the dura should be opened and the middle fossa explored for a hippocampal herniation. If a molded herniation is encountered, it should be removed by suction or the edge of the tentorium should be sectioned. During the closure the dura is sutured to the periosteum to prevent reaccumulation of blood in the epidural space and displacement of the dura and brain.

Subdural Hematoma

Subddural hematomas are divided into acute, subacute, and chronic types. This division is a rather arbitrary one depending upon the time between injury and surgical intervention. Acute subdural hematomas are considered to be those that deteriorate and require surgery during the first 24 hours, subacute those requiring surgery 2 to 14 days after the injury, and chronic those requiring surgery after 14 days.

The symptoms of an acute subdural hematoma occur immediately after the injury and are difficult to differentiate from those of an extradural hematoma. The patient with acute subdural hematoma usually sustains a severe head injury with contusion of the cerebrum as well as bleeding into the subdural space. The type of operation indicated depends upon the consistency of the clot. If the clot is liquid, it can be evacuated by multiple trephinations and a small temporal craniectomy. A temporoparietal skull flap is required if a solid clot is encountered. The wound should be drained. Acute subdural hematomas may occur bilaterally; therefore, if such a lesion is encountered on one side, an exploratory trephination should be done on the opposite side as well. The operative mortality of acute subdural hematomas during the first 24 hours is 82 per cent.[1]

Chronic Subdural Hematoma. The injury responsible for a chronic subdural hematoma may be rather trivial and in a number of cases may not be recalled as part of the history. Headache is the most common complaint and may be progressive from the time of the accident. Progressive focal neurologic signs and lethargy may occur, with papilledema and pupillary inequality; however, it is not infrequent for patients to be free of headache and focal neurologic signs.[2] To complicate the diagnostic problem, cerebrospinal fluid

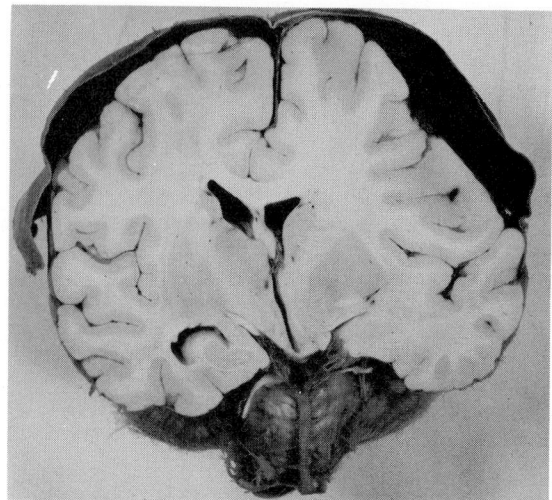

Figure 16. Autopsy specimen revealing bilateral subdural hematomas.

pressure may be normal in spite of the presence of a large chronic subdural hematoma.

X-rays of the skull may or may not reveal a fracture. Poppen reported fractures in only 8 of 119 patients.[14] The pineal gland may be displaced away from the side of a unilateral lesion, but may remain in the midline in bilateral subdural hematomas (Fig. 16). Poppen reported displacement of the pineal gland in 40 of 119 patients,[14] and Brock in 22 of 114 cases.[1]

The brain scan is helpful in screening patients for intracranial mass lesions and may reveal subdural hematomas that were unsuspected from a clinical

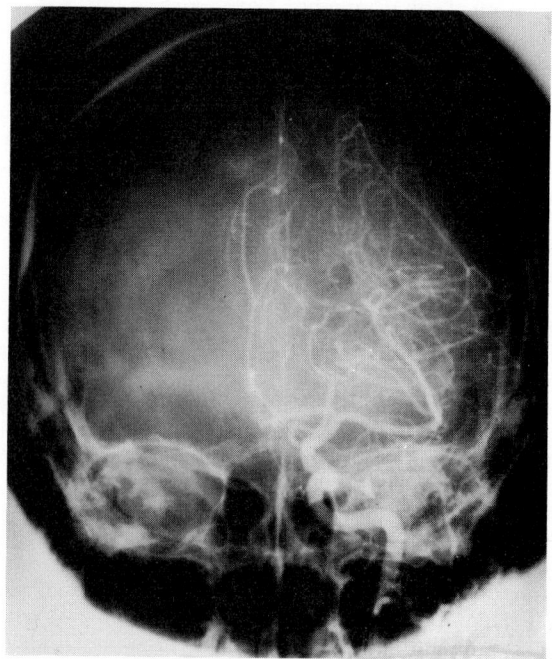

Figure 17. Carotid arteriogram revealing a chronic subdural hematoma on the left.

standpoint. Approximately 80 per cent of patients with chronic subdural hematoma have a positive brain scan.[4, 20] Contusion of the scalp and subgaleal hematoma may be confused with subdural hematoma on brain scans.

Pneumoencephalography or arteriography[18] may be necessary to establish the diagnosis of a chronic subdural hematoma. Arteriography is usually the procedure of choice, since it does not change intracranial dynamics. The arteriographic pattern of chronic subdural hematoma (Fig. 17) is very typical, with the convexity of the displaced vessels toward the midline and displacement of the anterior cerebral artery toward the opposite side. If there is inward displacement of cortical vessels and no shift of the anterior cerebral artery, a bilateral subdural hematoma should be suspected and looked for by angiography or burr holes.

The chronic subdural hematoma can usually be evacuated by a small subtemporal craniectomy with frontal and parietal trephination. The temporal incision should be placed as part of the anterior limb of a temporoparietal skull. This is done in case there is solid clot that cannot be removed by through-and-through irrigation or in case postoperative recurrence of the hematoma necessitates a flap as a second procedure. The outer membrane is removed in the exposed area and the inner membrane is incised in a stellate fashion after it is gently separated from the arachnoid. The dura is left open beneath the temporal muscle to permit the escape of fluid from the subdural space.

SELECTED REFERENCES

Browder, J.: A résumé of the principal diagnostic features of subdural hematoma. Bull. N. Y. Acad. Med., *19*:168, 1943.
This is an excellent review of the symptoms and signs in 289 cases of subdural hematoma.

Jefferson, G.: Tentorial pressure cone. Arch. Neurol. Psychiatr., *40*: 857, 1938.
This article contains a very good review of the literature and an excellent discussion of the pathophysiology of the tentorial pressure cone.

Kahn, E. A., Crosby, E. C., Schneider, R. C., and Taren, J. A.: Correlative Neurosurgery. Springfield, Ill., Charles C Thomas, Publisher, 1969.
This text contains an excellent chapter devoted to closure of various types of scalp defects with pedicle flaps and grafts.

Langfitt, T. W.: Clinical methods for monitoring intracranial pressure and measuring cerebral blood flow. Clin. Neurosurg., 22:302, 1975.
An excellent review of the different methods that have been advocated for measuring continuous intracranial pressure.

Tindall, G. T., Patton, J. M., Dunion, J. J., and O'Brien, M. S.: Monitoring of patients with head injuries. Clin. Neurosurg., 22:332, 1975.
An excellent discussion of the parameters to be monitored in individual head injuries.

REFERENCES

1. Brock, S.: Injuries of the Brain and Spinal Cord and Their Coverings. New York, Springer Publishing Company, 1960.
2. Browder, J.: A résumé of the principal diagnostic features of subdural hematoma. Bull. N. Y. Acad. Med., *19*:168, 1943.
3. Carrington, K. W., Tarne, J. A., and Kahn, E. A.: Primary repair of compound skull fractures in children. Surg. Gynecol. Obstet., *110*:203, 1960.
4. Cowan, R. J., Maynard, C. S., and Laster, K. R.: Technetium-99m pertechnetate brain scans in the detection of subdural hematomas: A study of the age of the lesion as related to the development of a positive scan. J. Neurosurg., *32*:30, 1970.
5. Echlin, F.: Traumatic subdural hematoma—acute, subacute and chronic; analysis of 70 operated cases. J. Neurosurg., *6*:294, 1949.
6. Echlin, R. A., Sordilo, S. V. R., and Garvey, T. Q., Jr.: Acute, subacute and chronic subdural hematoma. J.A.M.A., *16*:1345, 1956.
7. Gurdjian, E. A., and Webster, J. E.: Extradural hemorrhage. Int. Abstr. Surg., *75*:206, 1942.
8. Jefferson, G.: Bilateral rigidity in middle meningeal hemorrhage Br. Med. J., *2*:683, 1921.
9. Jefferson, G.: Tentorial pressure cone. Arch. Neurol. Psychiatr., *40*:857, 1938.
10. Kahn, E. A., Crosby, E. C., Schneider, R. C., and Taren, J. A.: Correlative Neurosurgery. Springfield, Ill., Charles C Thomas, Publisher, 1969.
11. Langfitt, T. W.: Clinical methods for monitoring intracranial pressure and measuring cerebral blood flow. Clin. Neurosurg., 22:302, 1975.
12. McLaurin, R. L., and Intor, F. T.: Acute subdural hematoma. Review of ninety cases. J. Neurosurg., *18*:61, 1961.
13. McLaurin, R. L., King, L. R., Elam, E. B., and Budde, R. B.: Metabolic response to craniocerebral trauma. Surg. Gynecol. Obstet., *110*:282, 1960.
14. Poppen, J. L.: Chronic subdural hematomas. Geriatrics, *10*:49, 1955.
15. Schwartz, C. W.: Leptomeningeal cysts from a roentgenological viewpoint. Am. J. Roentgenol., *46*:160, 1941.
16. Taveras, J. M., and Ransohoff, J.: Leptomeningeal cysts of brain following trauma. J. Neurosurg., *10*:233, 1953.
17. Tindall, G. T., Patton, J. M., Dunion, J. J., and O'Brien, M. S.: Monitoring of patients with head injuries. Clin. Neurosurg., 22:332, 1975.
18. Webster, J. E., Dawson, R., and Gurdjian, E. S.: The diagnosis of traumatic intracranial hemorrhage by angiography. J. Neurosurg., *8*:368, 1951.
19. Woodhall, B., Devine, J. W., Jr., and Hart, D.: Hemolateral dilation of pupil, hemolateral paresis and bilateral muscular rigidity, in diagnosis of extradural hemorrhage. Surg. Gynecol. Obstet., *72*:391, 1941.
20. Zingesser, L. H.: Scanning in diseases of the subdural space. Sem. Nucl. Med., *1*:41, 1971.

VI _____

INTRACRANIAL INFECTIONS

Robert H. Wilkins, M.D.

The number of patients with infections amenable to neurosurgical treatment is relatively small, but because of the wide variety of infectious agents and the different pathologic lesions they can incite, this area remains a challenge for the neurosurgeon.

Cranial Osteomyelitis, Epidural Abscess, Subdural Empyema[3, 4, 5, 8]

A cranial bone may be the site of hematogenous spread of a bacterial infection from another area of the body, but more often it becomes involved by adjacent spread from an infected paranasal sinus, by a penetrating wound, or by an operative infection involving a craniotomy flap. Pott's puffy tumor is such a frontal osteomyelitis, with marked overlying soft tissue swelling, that is secondary to frontal sinusitis.

Treatment is centered around the surgical removal of the infected bone, with simultaneous treatment of any coexisting sinusitis. Appropriate systemic antibiotics are administered, and an adequate margin of normal bone is removed with the specimen to minimize the risk of recurrent infection. A cranioplasty may be performed later for cosmetic and protective reasons, but at least a year should be allowed to pass, during which there is no evidence of inflammation in the area, before the plate is inserted. Otherwise, this large foreign body will serve as a focus for a further inflammatory response.

An epidural infection is usually a well-confined bacterial abscess associated with one or more of the previously mentioned infections, and it is drained at the same time the coexisting osteomyelitis or sinusitis is treated. A subdural infection, on the other hand, is usually an empyema rather than an abscess, since the developing infection easily dissects open the subdural space to cover the surface of an entire cerebral hemisphere. Subdural empyema may begin by the extension through the dura mater from without, or through the arachnoid from within; or it may result from the operative infection of a subdural hematoma. In any event, a subdural empyema is usually treated by immediate evacuation through multiple trephine openings or craniotomy in order to avert an almost certain fatality. Drains are usually left in the subdural space, to be removed days later, after all drainage has ceased.

Meningitis[1, 5, 6]

Bacterial meningitis as such is not a surgical disease, and all but the most resistant or unusual forms will usually respond to systemic antibiotics. But if recurrent bouts of meningitis occur, the neurosurgeon may become involved in the search for and treatment of cerebrospinal fluid rhinorrhea, a midline cranial or spinal dermal sinus tract, or some other portal of entry for organisms into the central nervous system.

Also, in a certain number of patients recovering from meningitis, effusions will develop in the subdural spaces over the cerebral hemispheres, or hydrocephalus due to the obstruction of subarachnoid pathways concerned with the normal absorption of cerebrospinal fluid will occur. Subdural effusions ordinarily occur in infants, and frequently may be cured by repeated aspiration with needle and syringe through the coronal suture. Occasionally large unilateral or bilateral craniotomies are necessary for evacuation of the effusions and removal of coexisting subdural membranes that are formed by the same inflammatory process, and rarely the subdural fluid must be shunted into other areas of the body, such as the heart or peritoneal cavity.

Encephalitis, Cerebritis, Brain Abscess[3–5, 7]

The neurosurgeon may be fooled into exploring and resecting an area of severe viral encephalitis, thinking it is a malignant glioma. Herpes simplex, for example, may cause a necrotic and cystic mass in the temporal lobe that closely resembles a brain tumor. However, even if the correct diagnosis is suspected preoperatively, biopsy of the lesion may be of value for verification. Furthermore, resection of such a lesion, or some type of decompressive operation, may also be necessary if steroids and other medical measures are inadequate to control the severe elevations of intracranial pressure that frequently accompany encephalitis.

The term cerebritis is usually reserved to describe the focal area of cerebral inflammation that immediately precedes the development of a bacterial brain abscess. Such areas of cerebritis may arise from:

1. Natural extension of an infection through the meninges. In this way, mastoiditis may lead to an abscess in the ipsilateral temporal lobe or cerebellar hemisphere, or frontal sinusitis may produce a frontal lobe abscess.

2. Hematogenous spread from some other site, especially either from the lungs, pleura, or heart, or from other areas of the body via congenital heart defects that permit the paradoxical embolism of infected material. Brain abscesses that originate in this manner are distributed among the various areas of the brain in proportion to the vascular supply, so a large number occur in the territory of the middle cerebral arteries.

3. Artificial inoculation through the meninges, as by a compound depressed skull fracture.

Typically, the patient with a brain abscess uncomplicated by meningitis has no systemic signs of infection, such as fever, tachycardia, or leukocytosis. The abscess presents clinically, and by skull x-rays, electroencephalography, brain scan, computerized axial tomography, cerebral angiography, and pneumoventriculography, as an intracranial mass that must be differentiated from a neoplasm, hematoma, or some other type of space-consuming lesion (Fig. 18). Bacteriologically, these abscesses contain one or more of a variety of organisms. Anaerobic or microaerophilic bacteria can be discovered frequently if appropriate techniques are employed, but even so, a large percentage of brain abscesses are found to be sterile.

The neurosurgeon ordinarily prefers to delay operating on a brain abscess until its wall has become dense enough to withstand surgical manipulation without rupturing. For this reason he often waits for about 2 weeks, while the patient receives intravenous antibiotics, before attempting a total excision of the abscess (Fig. 19). However, because of the degree of inflammation and reactive cerebral edema, the surgeon may be forced into operating earlier to prevent cerebral herniation and death. Under these circumstances, excision of the necrotic and poorly defined area of cerebritis may not be technically feasible; aspiration and drainage may be preferred. Aspiration and drainage may also be the treatment of choice of a well-encapsulated abscess if it is located in a vital area of the brain that might be irreparably damaged by an attempt at total excision of the abscess. Under these circumstances, colloidal barium sulfate may be injected into the abscess cavity after its aspiration so that its size may be followed radiographically.

No matter which operative technique is used, there is a high incidence of seizures among survivors of abscesses of the cerebral hemispheres, which justifies the prophylactic administration of anticonvulsants in most of these patients.

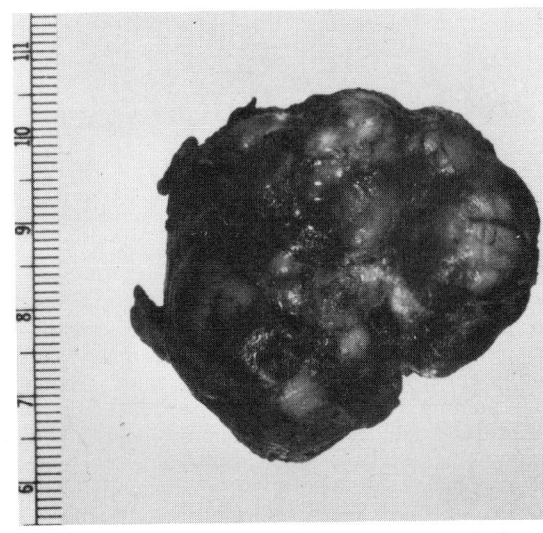

Figure 19. Operative specimen of a totally excised brain abscess.

Other Types of Intracranial Infections[2, 5]

Tuberculosis, sarcoidosis, and infections with various fungi sometimes cause a basal meningitis that obstructs the outflow of cerebrospinal fluid from the fourth ventricle. The resultant hydrocephalus may require a shunt. If an intracerebral or intracerebellar tuberculoma or fungal granuloma is formed, it may require excision like any other brain tumor, provided that the patient also receives appropriate drug therapy to combat his systemic illness.

The parasitic infections, especially echinococcosis and cysticerosis, present a problem to neurosurgeons in some countries, but are too seldom seen in the United States to justify further discussion here.

SELECTED REFERENCE

Ojemann, R. G., (Ed.): Clinical Neurosurgery, Volume 14. Baltimore, Williams & Wilkins Company, 1967.
This excellent volume contains 18 papers by a variety of distinguished authors covering all aspects of intracranial and intraspinal infections. It constitutes a review of the entire field, complete with numerous references.

REFERENCES

1. Dodge, P. R., and Swartz, M. N.: Bacterial meningitis—a review of selected aspects. II. Special neurologic problems, postmeningitic complications and clinicopathological correlations. N. Engl. J. Med., 272:954, 1003, 1965.
2. Fetter, B. F., Klintworth, G. K., and Hendry, W. S.: Mycoses of the Central Nervous System. Baltimore, Williams & Wilkins Company, 1967.
3. Gurdjian, E. S.: Cranial and Intracranial Suppuration. Springfield, Ill., Charles C Thomas, Publisher, 1969.
4. LeBeau, J., Creissard, P., Harispe, L., and Redondo, A.: Surgical treatment of brain abscess and subdural empyema. J. Neurosurg., 38:198, 1973.
5. Ojemann, R. G. (Ed.): Clinical Neurosurgery, Volume 14. Baltimore, Williams & Wilkins Company, 1967.
6. Swartz, M. N., and Dodge, P. R.: Bacterial meningitis—a review of selected aspects. I. General clinical features, special problems and unusual meningeal reactions mimicking bacterial meningitis. N. Engl. J. Med., 272:725, 779, 842, 898, 1965.
7. Victor, M., and Banker, B. Q.: Brain abscess. Med. Clin. North Am., 47:1355, 1963.
8. Wright, R. L.: Postoperative Craniotomy Infections. Springfield, Ill., Charles C Thomas, Publisher, 1966.

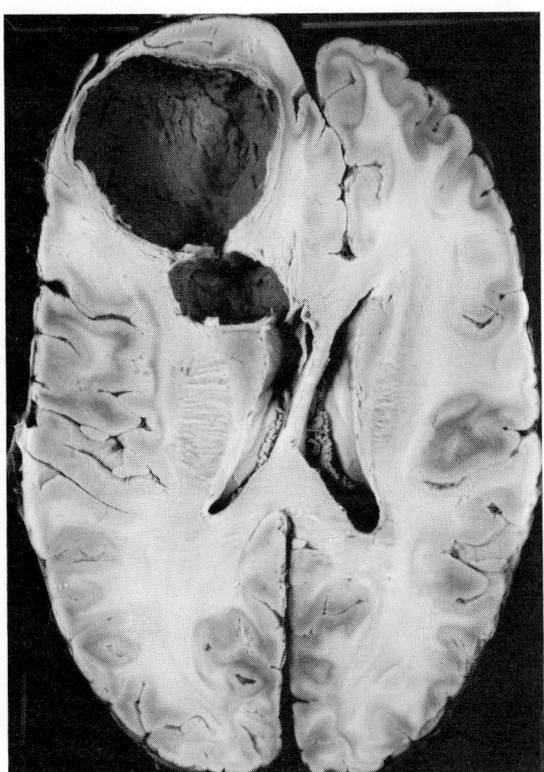

Figure 18. Brain abscess, left frontal lobe. A "daughter" abscess, posterior to the main lesion, had ruptured into the left lateral ventricle as the terminal event in this case.

VII

SPINAL TUMORS

M. Stephen Mahaley, Jr., M.D.

Spinal tumors can be conveniently divided into three major categories based upon location: extradural, intradural-extramedullary, and intramedullary. The most common extradural tumors are the malignant metastatic carcinomas, most frequently from the lung in males and from the breast in females. Intradural-extramedullary tumors include benign meningiomas and nerve sheath tumors. Intramedullary neoplasms are usually gliomas: ependymomas or astrocytomas. All of these lesions occur with about equal frequency in males and females except meningiomas, which are more common in females. As regards metastatic carcinoma, the upper dorsal region seems to be the level of highest frequency. Not included in this discussion are certain congenital lesions, such as angiomas, dermoids, lipomas, and syrinx, or infectious processes such as tuberculoma, abscess, and gumma.

Symptoms and Signs

Pain, fairly constant but worse at times on reclining, is a common early symptom because of the frequency of nerve root involvement and traction placed upon meningeal and vascular structures. The site of spine pain may locate the lesion itself, and the radicular component may identify the spinal root(s) involved. As a root is compressed or destroyed by tumor growth, the appropriate neurologic deficit of numbness, weakness, and reflex change may become apparent. When spinal cord compression or destruction occurs, particularly in the cervical or lumbar segments, a lower motor neuron deficit may be observed at the level of the lesion. More significantly, though, a myelopathy will be evident in terms of weakness and numbness distal to the lesion, with hesitancy or incontinence. On examination, a motor and sensory level may be evident with bladder signs of autonomic nervous system dysfunction. An absolute and total neurologic deficit of this type is certainly a late consequence of spinal tumors, and the prognosis for significant recovery of neurologic function when such a deficit has been present for more than a short while is very poor. For this reason, it is imperative that spinal tumors be accurately diagnosed early and that therapy be begun before a complete neurologic deficit develops.

Diagnosis

Plain spine films may reveal changes indicative of neoplasia. Metastatic tumors frequently cause erosion of the vertebral body or pedicles or both, with collapse or compression fracture of the body in some instances. With intradural tumors, the entire spinal canal over several segments may be widened. The routine chest film may reveal an unsuspected primary neoplasm, or such may be found by physical examination of the

breast, lymph nodes, or prostate gland. When an obvious bony change corresponding to the clinical spinal level of disease is not seen, lumbar puncture and myelography become essential. When the Queckenstedt test reveals a block, only 1 to 2 ml. of Pantopaque will be needed to outline the lower level of the lesion. Cerebrospinal fluid removed should be examined for protein content and the presence of inflammatory or neoplastic cells. Characteristic myelographic defects are seen in the anteroposterior view in Figure 20, helping to differentiate the extradural, intradural-extramedullary, and intramedullary lesions. The skin of the back lateral to the midline should be marked at the level of the lesion under fluoroscopic control dur-

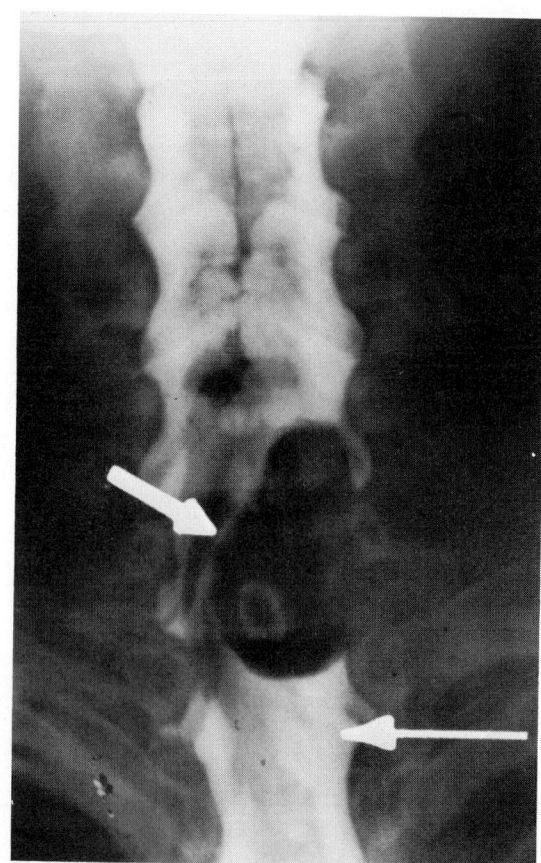

Figure 20. Myelogram showing an intradural-extramedullary meningioma at the seventh cervical segment. The thin arrow shows a broad dye column on that side of the spinal canal with the halftone shadow of the cord displaced toward the opposite side. The broad (upper) arrow shows the medial border of the tumor mass itself.

ing myelography for subsequent localization of the skin incision at surgery.

Treatment

The most common extradural neoplasm is metastatic carcinoma. When this is fairly obvious by virtue of a known primary lesion and appropriate radiographic spine changes produced by the lesions, a decision has to be made as to whether surgery would likely accomplish any useful purpose. If there is no neurologic deficit but adequate evidence of bony infiltration, then one may elect to treat with radiation therapy or chemotherapy. When there is a complete neurologic deficit that has been present for more than a few days and there is evidence of a primary carcinoma elsewhere, then it is often decided that surgical decompression would not likely restore neurologic function or otherwise aid the patient. However, when there is any doubt as to the metastatic origin of the tumor or when the neurologic deficit is only partial or recent, then surgical biopsy and decompression may yield two important results: diagnosis is certain and decompression may permit improvement of the neurologic status at least for a time or until adjunctive therapy can be instituted.[2] When the need for tissue for diagnosis is not essential and when neurological deficit is mild, the use of steroids may afford improvement, and their use should be considered while making plans for surgery or in instances where radiotherapy instead of surgery seems advisable.[1]

As regards intradural-extramedullary tumors, surgery is essential. A profound neurologic deficit from a benign meningioma compressing the spinal cord may show amazing improvement after tumor removal, which is usually curative as well. The same is true with nerve sheath tumors. Intramedullary tumors require surgery for diagnosis and may be totally resected (ependymomas) or may be only partially resectable (astrocytomas) owing to poor demarcation of neoplasm from surrounding cord tissue. When total resection is impossible or doubt is present regarding any remaining tumor, then postoperative radiation therapy is considered.

Rehabilitative therapy plays an important role in the subsequent management of many of these cases. Great care must often be given to the problem areas such as bladder care and prevention of pressure sores when a neurologic deficit is present. Physical and occupational therapy will assist in the functional recovery of the patient, and occasionally psychiatric assistance is required.

REFERENCES

1. Clarke, P. R. R., and Saunders, M.: Steroid-induced remission in spinal canal reticulum cell sarcoma. J. Neurosurg., 42:346, 1975.
2. Vieth, R. G., and Odom, G. L.: Extradural spinal metastases and their neurosurgical treatment. J. Neurosurg., 23:501, 1965.

VIII

RUPTURE OF LUMBAR INTERVERTEBRAL DISCS

Barnes Woodhall, M.D.

Low back pain and sciatica may well be the price that the human animal has paid for his unique ability among animals to stand on his own feet and walk without falling down.

Both Bradford and Spurling[1] and Hanreats[3] in their respective monographs have described the early and modern history of these health problems and this unique ability of the human animal has been pointed out by La Barre.[4] Sporadic reports over some decades suggested the true relationship between disc rupture and sciatica, but these were either confused or overlooked by the established feeling that these small protrusions from the disc were true tumors called "chondroma." In 1934, Mixter and Barr resolved this issue with a convincing demonstration that a protruding portion of a degenerated intervertebral disc was the common cause for sciatica.[6] Within six years, some 49 fresh reports confirming this paper were available. One later report in monograph form is highly readable.[8]

The cause of ruptured disc has been variously attributed to trauma, to an inherited connective tissue defect, and to aging. As to the factor of aging, Hanreats charts the incidence of lumbar disc protrusions at its peak about the third decade and suggests that certainly the common dehydration of aging is not a precipitating factor. From these data, he writes that this looks very much like a predisposition and he describes a number of families with such a predisposition. Any experienced neurosurgeon might describe similar familial trends. Connective tissue is the product of the metabolism of cells derived from primitive mesenchyme, in large part from fibroblasts. In terms of biochemistry, mixtures of polymeric materials derived from this cell are characteristic of cartilage, tendons, intervertebral discs, arteries, the corium of the skin, and various fluids and secretions. A slow but growing understanding exists concerning the relationship between chemical components and biological functions in this field. One simple mucopolysaccharide is known, hyaluronic acid. Its molecular weight is grossly reduced in rheumatoid arthritis and restored to normal values with cortisone. In ruptured discs, as compared to age-controlled normal discs, the concentration of hyaluronic acid is markedly reduced.[5] The total polysaccharide content is reduced from 30 per cent of the dry weight in normal human samples to 5 per cent of the dry weight in herniated samples. The chondroitin sulfate moiety of the polysaccharide fraction is reduced to a larger extent than is the keratosulfate. The collagen content of the herniated samples rises to 60 per cent of the dry weight from a normal value of 30 per cent. Ultracentrifuge patterns of herniated chondroitin sulfate show increased polydispersity; the kerato-sulfate fraction appears similar to the normal. A small but detectable amount of chondroitin B was isolated from herniated samples.[2]

These changes are qualitatively similar to those seen as a result of aging. Are these changes then the result of premature aging secondary to repetitive or acute trauma, to weight-bearing in the erect human form, or to predisposition? From these and related biochemical studies, the direct injection of chymopapain into the ruptured disc under radiographic techniques has been advocated by highly reputable orthopedic surgeons. The procedure is potentially dangerous and should be considered as a continuing experimental enterprise at this time.

As noted above, the most common cause of low back pain with radicular involvement is a ruptured disc at either the fourth or fifth lumbar interspace (Fig. 21). In the classic syndrome, intermittent attacks of low back pain are usually associated with pain radiating down the posterior aspect of the thigh and calf. The pain is aggravated by coughing and sneezing. Numbness may involve the foot and lower leg, and motor weakness or reflex and sensory changes may occur. Other findings can be classified as mechanical. These consist of scoliosis, paravertebral muscle spasm, limitation of forward bending, limitation of straight leg raising, positive Lasegue's sign, sciatic tenderness, and positive popliteal compression tests. These may occur with a protrusion at either the fourth or fifth in-

terspace and are never helpful in localizing the involved root. Neurologic findings such as reflex changes or motor weakness may be indicative of the level of the involved nerve root.

Scoliosis, paravertebral muscle spasm, and flattening of the lumbar curve are protective mechanisms that splint the back to prevent further compression of the tense nerve root. Limitation of straight leg raising, positive Lasegue's sign, and positive popliteal compression tests result from stretching the already tense spinal nerve over the protruded disc.

The neurologic signs result from compression of the spinal nerve and consequent changes within the nerve. A ruptured disc at the fifth lumbar interspace with involvement of the first sacral nerve root may weaken the gastrocnemius and soleus muscles (resulting in weakness of plantar flexion), which is best tested by requesting the patient to walk or stand on tiptoe; the ankle jerk may be decreased or absent and numbness and decreased sensation to pinprick may involve the lateral aspect of the leg and the fourth and fifth toes.

Involvement of the fifth lumbar nerve root at the fourth lumbar interspace produces weakness of the anterior tibial, peroneal, and extensor hallucis longus (with weakened dorsiflexion of foot and big toe). Weakness of the extensor hallucis longus may be detected when dorsiflexion of the foot and toes is attempted. The big toe on the involved side is not flexed as much as that of the uninvolved side. The knee jerk may be decreased, and numbness and decreased sensation to pinprick may involve the anterolateral aspect of the leg, the dorsum of the foot, and the big toe (Fig. 22).

Although some 90 per cent or more of ruptured discs appear at the fourth and fifth lumbar interspaces, a few may occur at the third or second interspaces. Multiple protrusions may occur, and massive protrusions may give the clinical picture of cauda equina paraplegia with bilateral leg pain, marked motor weakness, saddle anesthesia, and urinary retention. In terms of differential diagnosis, metastatic carcinoma of the spine, spinal cord tumors, carcinoma of the cervix and rectum, spondylolisthesis, various gradations of lumbar spondylosis, infections, and Marie-Strumpell arthritis all may simulate the clinical picture of a ruptured disc.

Unless the clinical history and neurologic-mechanical findings are classic for a single space ruptured disc, myelography with Pantopaque is required. Shapiro has devoted a small monograph to this diagnostic tool. Progress, from the use of spinal air by Dandy to the serendipity of Sicard and Forestier's finding of Lipiodal to newer media, forms a tidbit of neurosurgical history.[9] A number of short-term, personalized records of results of intervertebral disc surgery make rather pleasant reading. In one such unpublished study of 1000 cases, there were but 84 instances of operative failures (recurrent sciatica) with 54 recurrences at the same interspace, 9 disc ruptures at another interspace, scar fixation of the nerve root in five cases, intractable sciatica, cause not established but requiring spinothalamic cordotomy in 2 cases, and 14 clinical recurrences treated conservatively.

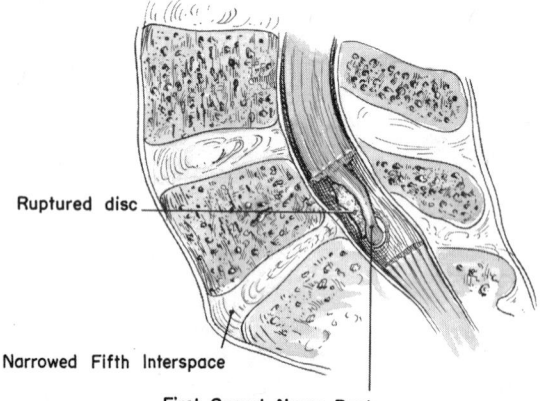

Ruptured disc

Narrowed Fifth Interspace

First Sacral Nerve Root

Figure 21. Diagram of cross section of lumbosacral spine illustrating a fragment of disc tissue rupturing through the posterior longitudinal ligament and compressing the first sacral nerve—a simple variant of this syndrome.

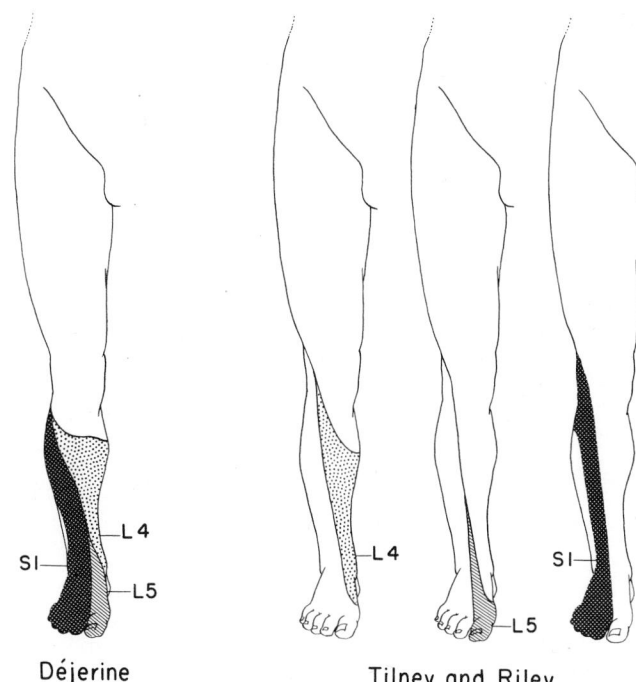

Figure 22. Commonly accepted variations in the sensory pattern of disc protrusions at the third, fourth, and fifth lumbar interspaces, involving lumbar roots 4 and 5 and sacral 1.

Déjerine

Tilney and Riley

A significant contribution to the life history of 1123 patients with evidence of a ruptured intervertebral disc treated by operation or by conservative measures may be found in a 20-year follow-up study by the Veterans Administration.[7] In spite of the modifying influences of Army Service, changing administrative decisions, and definitive therapy by many physicians, the findings can be accepted by knowledgeable persons. The value of this monograph is enhanced by a selective bibliography over the years 1945 to 1970.

An equally comprehensive review of this subject may be found, with a comprehensive appendix and bibliography, from Scandinavian sources.[10]

SELECTED REFERENCES

Bradford, F. K., and Spurling, R. G.: The Intervertebral Disc with Special Reference to Rupture of the Annulus Fibrosis with Herniation of the Nucleus Pulposus. Springfield, Ill., Charles C Thomas, Publisher, 1944.
This is a small monograph of personal experience by surgeons who, quite early after the report by Mixter and Barr, contributed strongly to the understanding of the disc syndrome. The early brief chapters on embryology, anatomy, physiology, and pathology serve as an introduction to the clinical studies. Case reports and 258 references up to 1941 embellish this very readable production.

Hanreats, P. R. M. J.: The Degenerative Back and Its Differential Diagnosis. Amsterdam, Elsevier Publishing Company, 1959.
This book qualified as a treatise on the subject. With the exception of some deficiencies in modern biochemistry, it is a thoughtful, very well documented study that points directly to one conclusion, "the syndromes often thought to point to the existence of hernia nucleus pulposus were certainly not, we found, pathognomonic for this affliction." This is a meticulous enterprise and, in part at least, the reader needs some experience to aid the process of full digestion.

Semmes, R. E.: Ruptures of the Lumbar Intervertebral Disc. Springfield, Ill., Charles C Thomas, Publisher, 1964.
This is a brief description of the author's experience in the surgical treatment of some 6000 patients with this syndrome. Dr. Semmes is a highly respected neurosurgeon, interested always and in many ways with the careers of younger neurosurgeons. This is a personal primer, and the operative illustrations are superb.

REFERENCES

1. Bradford, F. K., and Spurling, R. G.: The Intervertebral Disc with Special Reference to Rupture of the Annulus Fibrosis With Herniation of the Nucleus Pulposus. Springfield, Ill., Charles C Thomas, Publisher, 1944, p. 158.
2. Davison, E. A., and Woodhall, B.: Biochemical alterations in herniated intervertebral discs. J. Biol. Chem., 234:2951–2954, 1959.
3. Hanreats, P. R. M. J.: The Degenerative Back and Its Differential Diagnosis. Amsterdam, Elsevier Publishing Company, 1959, p. 690.
4. La Barre, W.: The Human Animal. Chicago, The University of Chicago Press, 1968, p. 386.
5. McClure, C., Holland, G. C., and Woodhall, B.: A method for the quantitative determination of hyaluronic acid in the human intervertebral disc. Science, 119:189, 1954.
6. Mixter, W. J., and Barr, J. S.: Rupture of the intervertebral disc with involvement of the spinal canal. N. Engl. J. Med., 211:210–215, 1934.
7. Nashold, B. S., Jr., and Hubrec, Z. (Ed.): A Twenty Year Follow-up. Saint Louis, The C. V. Mosby Company, 1971.
8. Semmes, R. E.: Ruptures of the Lumbar Intervertebral Disc. Springfield, Ill., Charles C Thomas, Publisher, 1964, p. 80.
9. Shapiro, R.: Myelography. Chicago, Year Book Medical Publishers, Inc., 1962.
10. Spangfort, E. V.: The lumbar disc herniation: A computer aided analysis of 2,504 operations. Acta Orthop. Scand., (Suppl.), 142:1–95, 1972.

IX

CERVICAL DISC LESIONS

Guy L. Odom, M.D.

For a clear understanding of the problem of cervical disc lesions, they must be divided into several categories: (1) the lateral soft disc protrusions, (2) the foraminal spur (hard disc), (3) the midline soft disc, and (4) the midline hard disc (cervical spondylosis or osteoarthritic bony proliferation). The symptoms, surgery, and results of therapy cannot be grouped together.

UNILATERAL SOFT DISC PROTRUSIONS

This syndrome was first described by Semmes and Murphey[19] in 1943 and since then has become recognized as the leading cause of neck and radicular arm pain. Although numerous reports have appeared in the literature, very little has been added to their original description.

The most common cervical disc lesion is the lateral soft disc protrusion. In large series,[13, 15, 18] approximately 80 per cent of the lesions are soft lateral discs, with lateral hard discs and midline hard and soft discs making up the balance. The majority of these lesions (90 per cent) are located at either the fifth or sixth cervical interspace,[6, 13] are aggravated by movement (wryneck), and are followed by subscapular, anterior chest (precordial), and radicular arm pain. A characteristic complaint is that the pain is aggravated by hyperextension of the neck.[6, 13, 15, 16, 19, 20] The anterior chest pain on the left may be confused with angina pectoris; in fact, two of the first four cases reported by Semmes and Murphey[19] were treated for angina before the correct diagnosis was established.

Ruptured Intervertebral Disc at the Fifth Cervical Interspace, with Compression of the Sixth Cervical Nerve Root. The pain, paresthesias, or numbness may extend into the thumb. The biceps reflex may be decreased or absent, and there may be weakness of the biceps muscle. The area of sensory impairment will vary, but may correspond to the distribution of the pain or paresthesias, with involvement of the thumb or the thumb and the second digit.

Ruptured Inervertebral Disc at the Sixth Cervical Interspace, with Compression of the Seventh Cervical Nerve Root. The pain and paresthesias may extend into the second and third digits, the triceps reflex may be decreased or absent, and the triceps muscle may reveal decrease in tone and marked weakness.

Ruptured Intervertebral Disc at the Fourth Cervical Interspace, with Compression of the Fifth Cervical Nerve Root. The pain or paresthesia seldom extends into the digits, and is usually located over the region of the deltoid. Reflex changes are rare, but the biceps reflex may be decreased. The muscle most commonly involved is the deltoid and at times there may be profound weakness of this muscle.

Ruptured Intervertebral Disc at the Seventh Cervical Interspace, with Compression of the Eighth Cervical Nerve Root. The pain or paresthesia may extend into the fourth and fifth digits, the deep reflexes of the extremity are not involved, and muscle weakness is usually restricted to the intrinsic muscles of the hand.

Roentgenograms

X-rays of the cervical spine should include anterior-posterior, lateral, and oblique views. The films are never diagnostic but may reveal reversal of the cervical curvature, narrowing of the intervertebral space, and foraminal spurs. Odom and associates[15] found that abnormal changes in the x-rays coincided in only 30 per cent of the cases with myelographic defects due to soft disc protrusions.

Pantopaque myelography has proved a reliable diagnostic procedure as to localization of the protrusion or spur.[18] The myelographic defect may vary from a small filling defect of the nerve root to a large cut involving the dural sac (Fig. 23).

Discography

Cervical discography has been reported as a helpful diagnostic procedure by Cloward,[3] Robinson et al.,[17] and Dohn.[7] The procedure is performed by injecting 0.2 to 0.3 ml. of a water-soluble contrast medium into the nucleus pulposus of one or more intervertebral discs. If the contrast medium remains within it the disc is normal, but if it extrudes the disc is ruptured or degenerated. We have never considered this procedure to be a helpful diagnostic aid.

Treatment

A period of conservative therapy should be tried for all patients unless they have marked motor weakness. The patient is placed in halter traction and receives physical therapy and sedation. We have not been impressed by the number of patients in whom conservative therapy has succeeded if the diagnosis has been confirmed by myelography. It is strongly recommended that all patients treated conservatively be checked periodically for motor weakness.

Indications for operation include failure to respond to conservative therapy and development of motor weakness.

Surgery

POSTERIOR APPROACH. Operation is performed with the patient in the sitting position with the neck flexed. Endotracheal anesthesia is used and the patient is hyperventilated moderately to avoid the negative phase of respiration because of the potential hazard of air emboli when patients are operated upon in the sitting position. A skin incision is made from the third cervical vertebra to the tip of the spinous process of the seventh cervical vertebra. The muscles are sepa-

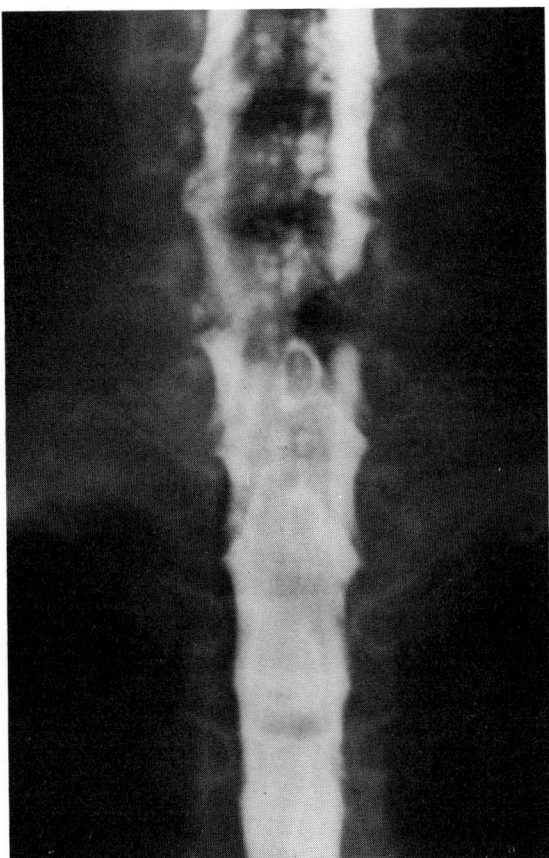

Figure 23. Pantopaque cervical myelogram with filling defect due to a unilateral ruptured intervertebral disc between sixth and seventh cervical vertebrae on the right.

rated subperiosteally from the spinous processes, the lamina, and facets. When exposing the sixth interspace, the laminae of the fifth, sixth, and seventh cervical vertebrae should be exposed in order to obtain an adequate lateral exposure. The medial portion of the inferior facet is then removed by rongeurs. The high-speed air drill is used to remove an additional portion of the inferior facet and the medial portion of the superior facet of the corresponding vertebra (Fig. 24A). Gauze packing should be avoided in the wound when the high-speed air drill is used and the ligamentum flavum should be left intact during this part of the procedure. A technique should be developed to leave a thin rim of bone over the nerve root, which is then removed with a curet (Fig. 24C). It is always wise to shift from the ordinary burr to the diamondhead burr when the removal is close to the nerve root. After the nerve root is exposed, the ligamentum flavum is removed by sharp dissection from between the corresponding lamina. As the ligamentum flavum is elevated, the underlying extradural veins are carefully separated from the ligamentum flavum and small cottonoid patties are placed in the extradural space above and below the nerve root in order to compress the veins. A small portion of the lateral lower portion of the upper lamina and the upper lateral portion of the

lower lamina is removed with rongeurs. The removal should be sufficient to obtain an adequate exposure above and below the dural sleeve of the nerve root. The anterior portion of the spinal canal is then palpated with a blunt dissector and the nerve root is retracted upward or downward to determine whether there is a posterior lateral protrusion of the disc. It must be stressed that the dura should never be retracted during the procedure if damage to the spinal cord is to be avoided. When a protrusion is encountered, an incision is made in the thinned-out annulus over the dome of the protrusion and this will permit soft disc to bulge immediately through the incision. Pressure is then placed on the adjacent part of the annulus with the blunt dissector and additional disc material is milked through the opening (Fig. 24D). Care should be taken to carry the inspection well out into the foramina. All free fragments of disc material are removed but no attempt is made to curet the interspace as is done in the lumbar area. The wound is closed in anatomic layers. The patient is permitted out of bed on the first postoperative day and is usually out of the hospital on the seventh or eighth postoperative day.

FORAMINAL SPUR. A similar approach is used for the foraminal spur syndrome, but a more extensive facetectomy is performed, exposing the nerve root farther out into the intervertebral foramen. If the spur is large and the root is very tight, the diamond burr is used to drill a hole just below the nerve root in the superior lateral margin of the vertebra and above the nerve root in the inferior lateral margin of the vertebra above. With a small curet it is then possible to break off the thin spur without traumatizing the nerve root.

ANTERIOR APPROACH WITH FUSION. Those interested in the anterior approach for the removal of cervical intervertebral disc and fusion are referred to the procedures described by Cloward,[3] Robinson et al.,[17] and Kempe.[12]

ANTERIOR APPROACH WITHOUT FUSION. A variation in the anterior approach to lateral soft disc protrusions and spondylosis has been reported by Hirsch et al.,[10] Boldrey,[1] Susen,[22] Murphey and Gado,[14] and Hankinson and Wilson.[9] They simplify the procedure by removing only part of the disc and not doing a fusion. Their results compare favorably with those obtained by fusion with unilateral soft disc protrusion and multiple level discectomies for spondylosis.

UNILATERAL FORAMINAL SPURS (HARD DISC)

The clinical syndrome produced by the foraminal spur is identical to that produced by soft disc protrusion and usually cannot be differentiated until the lesion is exposed at surgery. Semmes and Murphey[19, 20] believe that the radicular pain due to disc lesions is produced by soft protrusion and that radicular arm pain is not associated with foraminal spurs (hard disc). The postoperative results are not as good as with soft disc protrusions. Haft and Shenkin[8] report excellent or good results in 83 per cent of patients and Odom et al.[15] in 76 per cent.

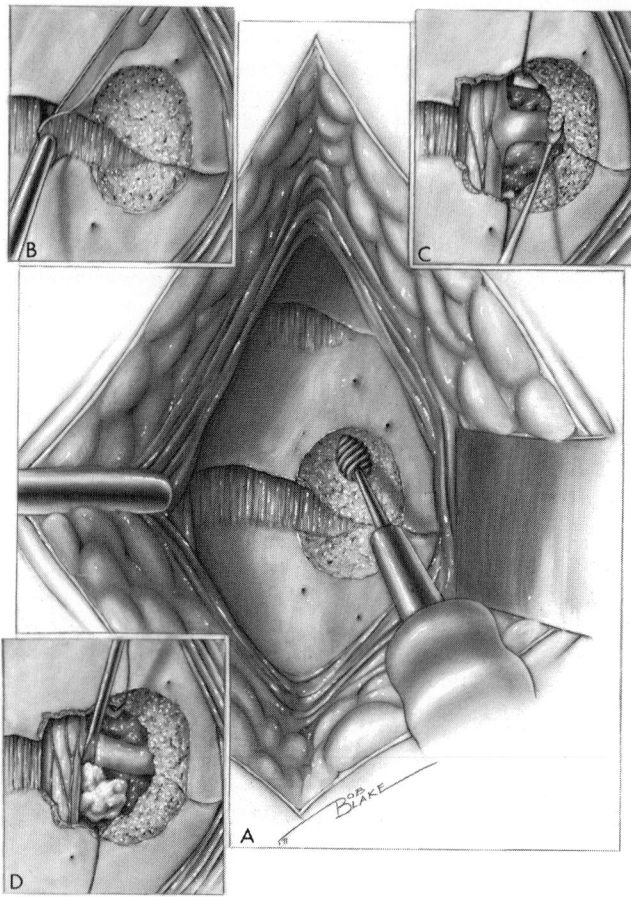

Figure 24. *A*, Unilateral exposure of laminae of C6 and C7 on the right with beginning removal of facets. *B*, Removal of ligamentum flavum. *C*, Exposure of nerve root with removal of small portion of laminae of C6 and C7. Additional bone over nerve root removed with curet. *D*, Disc material forced out from beneath nerve root and dura.

CERVICAL MYELOPATHY SECONDARY TO CERVICAL SPONDYLOSIS

Brain et al.[2] must be given credit for clarifying the syndrome of cervical myelopathy associated with cervical spondylosis. They stressed the fact that cervical cord and nerve root involvement due to degenerative disc disease was not uncommon in the older age group and that the neurologic symptoms were due to cord compression by the bony ridge or interference with blood supply to the cord. Holt and Yates[11] studied 120 cervical spines removed at autopsy from elderly patients and found some degree of degeneration of the intervertebral disc in 110 cases, and in 46 of these it was severe. The degeneration is most common in the midcervical area.

The symptoms may vary from patient to patient owing to the fact that the ridging or degenerative changes may occur at one or multiple levels in the cervical area. Brain et al.[2] reported single lesions in 18 cases and multiple lesions in 20. The onset may be with weakness or paresthesias in the upper or lower extremities and occasionally radicular upper extremity pain. The deep reflexes are hyperactive, with a decrease in the biceps or triceps reflex if the sixth or seventh cervical nerve root is involved by a foraminal spur.

The syndrome may be confused with amyotrophic lateral sclerosis, neoplasm, and syringomyelia.

X-rays of the cervical spine are helpful, but more than 50 per cent of the patients in this age group may have degenerative changes in the cervical discs that are of no clinical significance.

Pantopaque myelography is essential to determine whether the diameter of the spinal canal is compromised by a bony ridge associated with a degenerative disc (Fig. 25). The degree of cord involvement is associated with the variation in the diameter of the cervical canal. The diameter of the canal may also be impinged upon posteriorly by the ligamentum flavum with extension of the neck. For this reason, precautions must be taken to avoid hyperextension of the neck during myelography.

Surgery

The surgery of cervical myelopathy secondary to cervical spondylosis has been the subject of much debate during the past decade concerning posterior laminectomy vs. anterior discectomy and fusion. In cases with a single ridge the procedure of choice seems to be an anterior approach, with removal of bony ridge and interbody fusion, whereas if there are multiple levels, a posterior laminectomy with dural graft is the

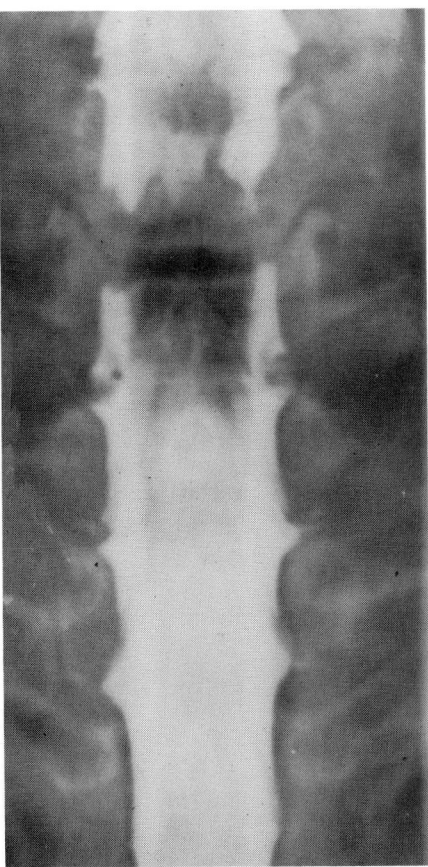

Figure 25. Pantopaque cervical myelogram with transverse defect secondary to cervical spondylosis.

The authors report a review of 52 anterior cervical discectomies without fusion in 13 cases of acute cervical disc herniations and 38 cases of degenerative cervical disc disease or cervical spondylosis. They discuss the indications, techniques, and results.

Scoville, W. B.: Types of cervical disk lesions and their surgical approaches. J.A.M.A., *196*:479, 1966.
The author presents a review of 741 consecutive operable cervical disc lesions, of which 607 (82 per cent) were soft discs and 95 (13 per cent) were hard lateral discs, a total of 95 per cent being unilateral disc lesions. He is a strong advocate of the posterior approach for removal of unilateral disc lesions.

REFERENCES

1. Boldrey, E. B.: Anterior cervical decompression (without fusion). Presented at the American Academy of Neurological Surgery, Key Biscayne, Florida, 1964.
2. Brain, W. R., Northfield, D., and Wilkinson, M.: The neurological manifestations of cervical spondylosis. Brain, *75*:187, 1952.
3. Cloward, R. B.: The anterior approach for removal of ruptured cervical disks. J. Neurosurg., *15*:602, 1958.
4. Connolly, E. S., Seymour, R. J., and Adams, J. E.: Clinical evaluation of anterior cervical fusion for degenerative cervical disc disease. J. Neurosurg., *23*:431, 1965.
5. Crandall, P. H., and Batzdorf, U.: Cervical spondylotic myelopathy. J. Neurosurg., *25*:57, 1966.
6. Davis, C. H., Odom, G. L., and Woodhall, B.: Survey of ruptured intervertebral discs in the cervical region. N. Carolina Med. J., *14*:61, 1953.
7. Dohn, D. F.: Anterior interbody fusion for treatment of cervical disk conditions. J.A.M.A., *197*:897, 1966.
8. Haft, H., and Shenkin, H. A.: Surgical end results of cervical ridge and disk problems. J.A.M.A., *186*:312, 1963.
9. Hankinson, H. L., and Wilson, C. B.: Use of the operating microscope in anterior cervical discectomy without fusion. J. Neurosurg., *43*:452, 1975.
10. Hirsch, C.: Cervical disc rupture: Diagnosis and therapy. Acta Orthop. Scand., *30*:172, 1960.
11. Holt, S., and Yates, P. O.: Cervical spondylosis and nerve root lesions. Incidence at routine necropsy. J. Bone Joint Surg., *48B*:407, 1966.
12. Kempe, L. G.: Operative Neurosurgery. Volume 2, Posterior Fossa, Spinal Cord and Peripheral Nerve Disease. New York, Springer-Verlag, 1971.
13. Murphey, F.: Fourth Annual R. Eustace Semmes Lecture, Southern Neurosurgical Society Meeting, January 23, 1971.
14. Murphey, M. G., and Gado, M.: Anterior cervical discectomy without interbody bone graft. J. Neurosurg., *37*:71, 1972.
15. Odom, G. L., Finney, W. H. M., and Woodhall, B.: Cervical disk lesions. J.A.M.A., *166*:24, 1958.
16. Peet, M. M., and Echols, D. H.: Herniation of the nucleus pulposus. Arch. Neurol. Psychiatr., *32*:924, 1934.
17. Robinson, R. A., Walker, A. E., Ferlic, D. C., and Wiecking, D. K.: The results of anterior interbody fusion of the cervical spine. J. Bone Joint Surg., *44A*:1569, 1962.
18. Scoville, W. B.: Types of cervical disk lesions and their surgical approaches. J.A.M.A., *196*:479, 1966.
19. Semmes, R. E., and Murphey, F.: The syndrome of unilateral rupture of the sixth cervical intervertebral disk with compression of the seventh cervical nerve root. A report of four cases with symptoms simulating coronary disease. J.A.M.A., *121*:1209, 1943.
20. Semmes, R. E., and Murphey, F.: Ruptured intervertebral disks: Cervical, thoracic and lumbar, lateral and central. Surg. Clin. North Am., *34*:1095, 1954.
21. Stoops, W. L., and King, R. B.: Chronic myelopathy associated with cervical spondylosis. Its response to laminectomy and foramenotomy. J.A.M.A., *192*:281, 1965.
22. Susen, A. F.: Simple anterior cervical discectomy without fusion. Presented at the American Academy of Neurological Surgery, San Francisco, California, 1966.

operation of choice. The laminectomy should extend two vertebral levels above and below the most caudal and rostral ridge. In multiple ridges, it is usually necessary to remove five or six laminae.

SELECTED REFERENCES

Brain, W. R., Northfield, D., and Wilkinson, M.: The neurological manifestations of cervical spondylosis. Brain, *75*:187, 1952.
These authors must be given credit for clarifying the problem of cervical myelopathy associated with cervical spondylosis. The article contains an excellent review of the literature prior to 1952, and a superb discussion of symptomatology, pathology, and surgical results.

Cloward, R. B.: The anterior approach for removal of ruptured cervical disks. J. Neurosurg., *15*:602, 1958.
This author is responsible for popularizing the anterior approach to cervical discs. His operative technique for the removal of cervical intervertebral discs by an anterior approach, followed by vertebral body fusion, is given in detail.

Hankinson, H. L., and Wilson, C. B.: Use of the operating microscope in anterior cervical discectomy without fusion. J. Neurosurg., *43*:452, 1975.

X

PERIPHERAL NERVE INJURIES

Barnes Woodhall, M.D.

The modern historical era of peripheral nerve surgery began with Weir Mitchell's book recounting his experiences in the Civil War, published in 1872.[5] This volume also contains a number of earlier accounts, including Paré's record of lance wounds of peripheral nerves. It is fair to say that wars and their wounds account for the majority of laboratory and clinical studies in this special field of surgery.

The basic problem in peripheral nerve repair can be stated quite simply. The surgeon must understand and then adjust the conflict between two forces, one, the continuing and virtually irresistible drive of axonal regeneration, and two, an equally significant barrier at the point of injury, derived from both mesenchymal tissue efforts at local repair and degeneration of all components of the distal nerve segment, distal receptor organs, and distal muscle, skin, and bone tissues.

An appreciation of the finer details of nerve structure is essential when one proposes to suture a divided nerve segment. The term *epineurium* designates the thin but relatively tough sheath of connective tissue that surrounds the aggregated fascicles of a nerve. This is the structure that the surgeon attempts to suture, by one means or another, to restore the continu-

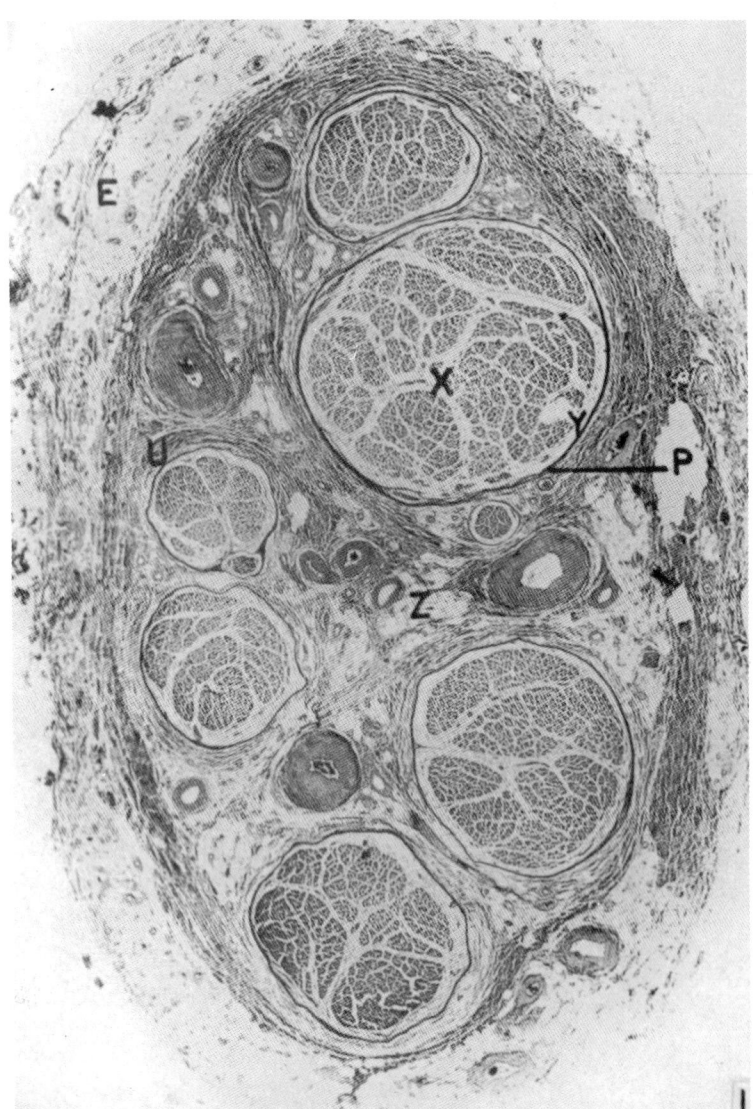

Figure 26. *1,* There is some vascular pathologic change and intrafascicular edema in this cross section of a common peroneal nerve. E represents the epineurium and P the perineurium. U shows thicker sheaths blending with interfascicular tissue and the perineurium. ×22.5.

Illustration continued on opposite page

ity of nerve segments. It fuses with the interfascicular connective tissue that binds the nerve fascicles together and carries the larger blood vessels and the vasa nervorum. The interfascicular tissue may contain various amounts of fat. Longitudinally oriented blood vessels are present beneath and on the epineurium and traverse the interfascicular space. They may represent a large vessel such as the arteria concomitans of the median nerve, and nerves are also fed by irregularly spaced segmental vessels such as the common to the ulnar nerve in the region of the medial epicondyle. The surgeon makes use of their longitudinal orientation to prevent rotation of nerve segments preparatory to suture. Hemorrhage from these vessels poses a technical problem as well.

Each fascicle is surrounded by a thin sheath of laminated connective tissue, the *perineurium.* The internal architecture of the fascicular pattern of a nerve is highly variable, being influenced by the site in any nerve trunk at which it may be examined, by the merging of sensory and motor axons, and by the migration of an emerging nerve branch. The surgical significance of fascicular pattern has been overemphasized, since the usual longitudinal extent of an injury plus the removal of damaged nerve ends will make improbable the suture of true mirror images.

Within each fascicle are numbers of myelinated and amyelinated nerve fibers, the latter often occurring in clusters, which vary in size and number depending upon their function and the cross-area of the individual nerve. The *axon,* protected by its myelin sheath and its component parts, is derived from a centrally placed neuron. Its axoplasm is fluid, viscous, and granular; it moves centrifugally with a force that cannot be denied and represents, as a mass, the structure that the surgeon hopes by his efforts to link up with a motor endplate or a sensory end organ. This task, from the point of view of the microanatomist, appears to be virtually an impossible one (Figs. 26 and 27).

The student of peripheral injury must understand as

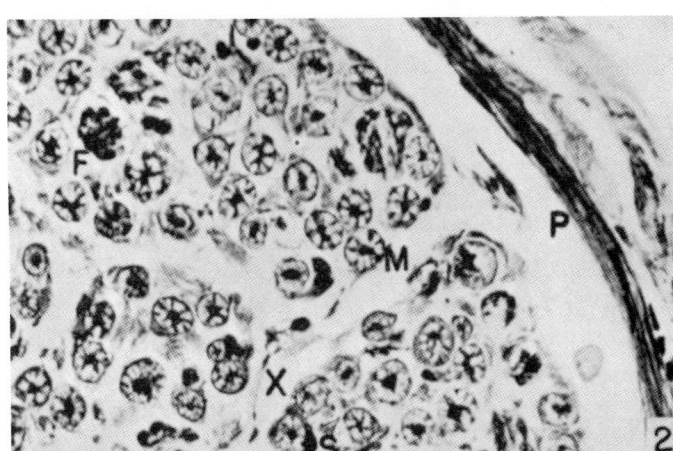

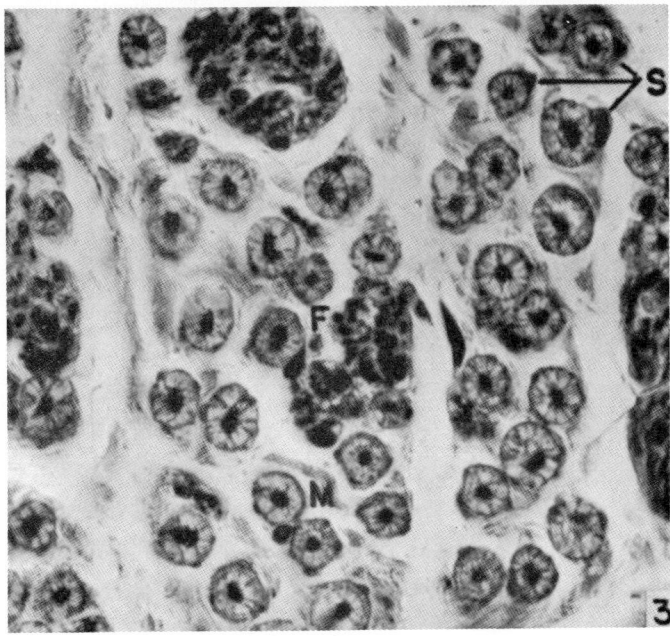

Figure 26 *Continued. 2* and *3,* Cross section at ×600 *(2)* and ×1000 *(3),* with myelinated fibers (M) and clusters of amyelinated fibers (F). In a few places Schwann cells are seen around the myelinated fibers. (From Lyons, W. R., and Woodhall, B.: Atlas of Peripheral Nerve Injuries. Philadelphia, W. B. Saunders Company, 1949.)

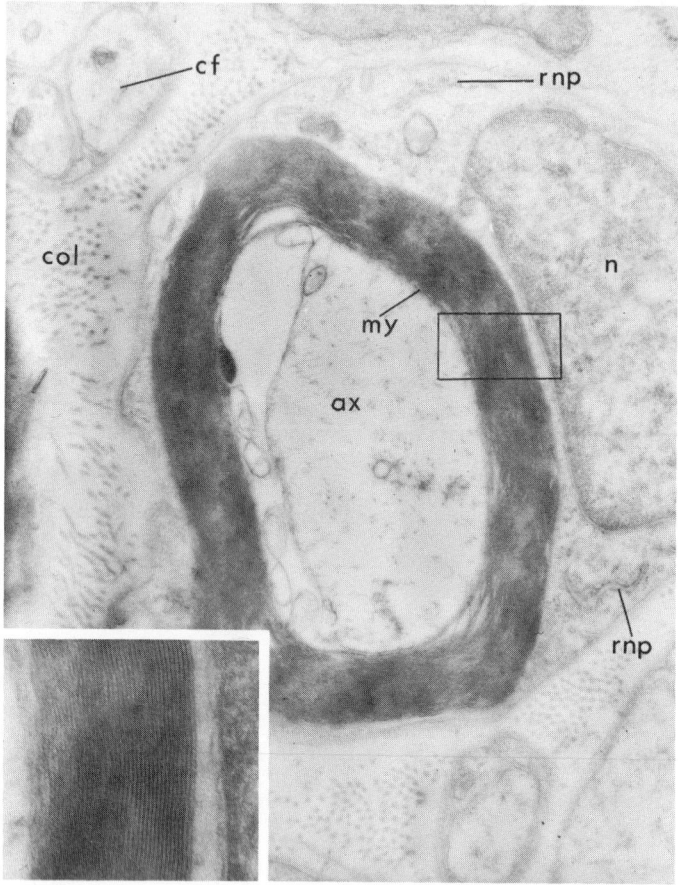

Figure 27. Electron micrograph of cross section of normal rat sciatic nerve. Note the rnp particles, the axon (ax), the myelin (my), the C fiber (cf), the collagen (col), and the Schwann cell nucleus (n). ×32,000. The inset illustrates the concentric and periodic myelin sheath. ×88,000. (From Boone, S. C., and Woodhall, B.: J. Surg. Res., 4:413, 1964.)

well the metabolic response to injury and regeneration as this occurs at three levels: (1) the anterior horn cell of the spinal cord and the dorsal nerve root ganglion cell, (2) the proximal nerve stump, and (3) the distal nerve segment and associated end organs.[2] A knowledge of the gross anatomy of the peripheral nervous system and of the characteristic clinical signs of injury to major peripheral nerves is another primary prerequisite to peripheral nerve repair. This may be obtained from specialized monographs devoted to the subject.[3, 7, 8] Beyond these points, the student enthralled by pathologic processes may care to peruse a reference volume on normal and pathologic anatomy.[4]

The Acute Pathology of Peripheral Nerve Injury

When the intact human nerve is transected at the operating room table by a surgical cutting instrument, the nerve ends retract some 4 per cent of their normal length between points of fixation. The thin epineurium is intact about its severed circumference, the proximal fascicles pout for a distance of perhaps 1 mm. beyond the epineurium, and there is hemorrhage from divided vessels at the point of severance. In the majority of accidental nerve injuries, the application of force is vastly different from that implied in surgical division by a cutting instrument. The application of force through the media of kitchen knives, clasp knives,

broken glassware, pottery, water faucets, beer bottles, window and automobile glass, steel fragments, broken bones, and civilian-type gunshot wounds implies the additional factor of stretch, with resulting damage over a considerable portion of the affected nerve segments.

When such accidental nerve injuries are visualized at emergency operation, much more complicated injuries may be seen, which may be placed in four broad categories: (1) complete nerve division, (2) partial nerve division, (3) a contused or swollen nerve segment in continuity, and (4) a relatively normal-appearing nerve. In complete nerve division, the epineurium is frayed and may be split longitudinally in either proximal or distal nerve segment. Hemorrhage occurs from the divided nerve ends and within the nerve substance as well, at varying distances from the point of severance. In partial nerve division, intact fascicles may herniate through lateral epineural lacerations. Intact fascicles become edematous at the point of maximal force. The divided fascicles retract within the intact cuff of epineurium. The extent of neuronal damage is difficult to assess, both in partial nerve division and in those cases in which the epineurium is quite intact and the nerve trunk is swollen and hemorrhagic. At a time period of 3 weeks to 1 month after injury, the extent of the injury to a peripheral nerve becomes much more apparent, largely as a result of peripheral nerve regenerative and healing processes.

The acute peripheral nerve wound may in addition be associated with fracture, vascular injury, tendon injury, and loss of skin. Neither the surgeon nor the patient may be fully prepared for the disciplined effort of meticulous nerve repair. This is the time for recognition of the extent of the injury, control of hemorrhage, closure of the wound to insure normal healing, appropriate splinting, and support of denervated muscles. In essence, it is the first step in preparation for an elective procedure at a time period 3 to 4 weeks after injury. Three alternatives to this procedure are indicated. The first has to do with preservation of the extremity in cases of major vascular injury. In such instances, vessel repair is mandatory as a primary procedure. The second alternative is found in rare cases of traumatic limb amputation in which replantation of the limb or finger seems feasible. The third alternative to deferred nerve suture is found in accidental section of nerves in the operating room or in simple, clean wounds involving small nerves such as the digital nerve.

Favorable Prerequisites for Deferred Nerve Repair

1. The patient, his wound, and the surgeon are well prepared for definitive nerve repair. The patient has been evaluated in terms of fitness for local or general anesthesia. The raw, primary wound has healed without infection. The surgeon has now available a reasonably accurate diagnosis supported by electromyography, and he has escaped the errors of misidentification common to primary nerve repair.

2. As Ducker has pointed out, the spinal cord neuron has re-established its metabolic function and is prepared to support, after 2 weeks, the multiple sprouting of axons in the proximal stump. By the same time token, the neurolemmal tubules of the distal segment are free of debris and open for the downgrowth of new fibers (Fig. 28).

3. After 3 weeks, repair and regenerative processes have clearly defined the proximal neuroma and the distal glioma in completely severed nerves (Fig. 29). In so-called neuromas in continuity, intraneural injury can be identified by palpation as nodules and such injuries are in prime condition for proximal and distal electrostimulation. If the primary wound exploration has not disclosed complete nerve division, local anesthesia is preferable for deferred exploration so that sensory stimuli can be evaluated by the patient.

4. Suture line tension must be avoided, and the clean, well-healed primary wound at 3 weeks post injury allows free access to the techniques of overcoming nerve defects after resection of pathologic proximal and distal nerve ends. These include free mobilization of nerve segments, transposition, and limb posturing.

In substance then, at 3 weeks after the primary injury, the surgeon and his patient both stand on a very firm foundation. The surgeon can assume the stance of a radical exploration with real hopes of understanding the exact extent of injury to peripheral nerve and other structures. At the same time, lacking evidence of complete nerve division, the surgeon can assume a

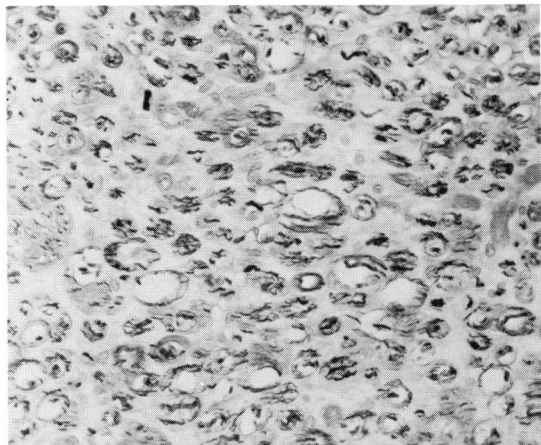
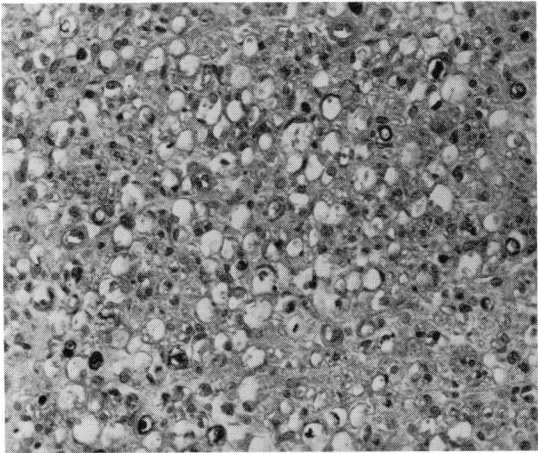

Figure 28. *Top,* Proximal cross section following resection of proximal neuroma 4 weeks post injury. Note open tubules and regrowth of axons. *Bottom,* Distal cross section from same case. Note open tubules free of debris with minimal connective tissue change. (From Woodhall, B.: Surg. Clin. North Am., *31:*1369, 1951.)

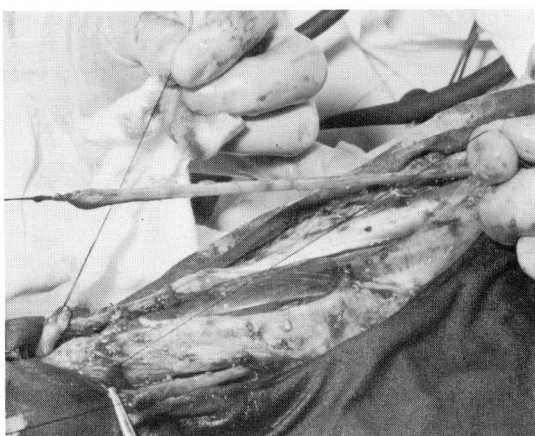

Figure 29. Deferred median nerve operation at 4 weeks for complete nerve division. Note proximal neuroma at right and distal glioma at left, with wide exposure for mobilization of nerve segments. (From Woodhall, B.: Surg. Clin. North Am., *31:*1369, 1951.)

conservative operative approach, close the wound, and further monitor the degree and usefulness of spontaneous regeneration.

The third time period commonly used in peripheral nerve repair is 3 months after injury, or so-called late repair, when degenerative changes in the distal nerve segment and in all tissues of the denervated extremity will progressively prejudice the quality of peripheral regeneration. Without firm objective evidence of spontaneous regeneration, this wait-and-see policy is to be condemned. The long-term results of peripheral repair conducted at various time intervals after injury and other data related to nerve regeneration under the influence of various types of trauma may be found in Sunderland's book[8] and in a Veterans Administration study published some years after the end of World War II.[11]

The Technique of Repair

The additional armamentarium for nerve repair is not formidable. It includes a nerve stimulator delivering short faradic stimuli of variable intensity, fine forceps for handling delicate epineurium, sharp No. 11 scalpels for nerve segment section, both 0.003 inch tantalum swedged sutures and No. 5 swedged ophthalmic silk sutures, and perhaps gelatin sponge for curbing hemorrhage and surrounding the region of the nerve suture. More recently Ducker and his associates under the stimulation of their own experiments and studies during the Vietnam war have advocated the use of Silastic cuffs to cover the suture line.[1]

It is advisable to cleanse the entire extremity in any acceptable technique. Drape it in such a manner that all muscle movements and joint positions may be observed or passively attained. The use of a tourniquet rests with the experience or customs of the operating surgeon.

The skin incision is planned to encompass and then resect the original injury scar, and to include any potential longitudinal extension that may be necessary for mobilization purposes. It is marked in a series of gentle curves and placed transversely across joint creases. The nerve segment may lie quite superficially at the point of injury, and dissection is more safely commenced to expose the proximal and distal nerve segments. As the proximal nerve segment is identified and followed toward the point of injury, in a region where motor branches arise, the proximal nerve segment should be stimulated to ascertain the presence of intact nerve branches that may arise just proximal to the lesion and may be embedded in scar tissue. Proximal nerve stimulation may also elicit a peripheral response through the point of injury, strongly suggesting the occurrence of a neuroma in continuity. A normal distal nerve segment is then identified and dissected toward the point of injury.

When the anatomically complete or practically complete nerve division of lacerating wounds is found, the potential nerve defect should be measured that might exist after resection of the pathologic nerve ends and then the surgeon must survey the possibilities of overcoming this defect by the methods at his disposal. In almost every instance, this will require extensive mobilization of distal and proximal nerve segments.

This must be done with careful effort to preserve both the blood supply and the integrity of branches. In order, the second choice for making up nerve defect has to do with posturing the extremity, flexing of the hand on the wrist, flexing of the elbow, or flexing of the foreleg on the thigh. The third choice of making up nerve defect has to do with transposition of the nerve segment, and this is virtually always indicated with lesions of the ulnar nerve in the region of the elbow and with median nerve injuries in the region of the heads of the pronator teres. Actual transplantation of the nerve segments medially may be necessary with extensive nerve defects in the radial nerve at the midarm level, and removal of the head of the fibula may be indicated in extensive defects of the peroneal nerve in the upper foreleg. Critical resection lengths have been established for the major peripheral nerves beyond which nerve suture rarely shows regeneration. Fortunately such defects are rarely obtained in civilian-type injuries.

It is well to mark the position in the extremity of the respective nerve segments by single epineural sutures of fine silk placed at corresponding points of the nerve circumference. This prevents undue rotation of the mobilized and resected nerve ends at the time of suture. Various ingenious nerve clamps have been devised for sectioning of nerve segments, but a clean deliberate cut with a sharp No. 11 scalpel is equally satisfactory. The proximal section may be made at the base of the proximal neuroma and should be reviewed if any residual neuroma is present. The distal section should always err on the side of generosity. If necessary, at this time the proposed suture line bed may be revised.

A number of epineural sutures should be used just sufficient to provide accurate apposition of the epineurium without undue buckling of the nerve segments. Stay sutures are inadvisable except under conditions of unusual tension. The use of the operating microscope will facilitate both the recognition of nerve fiber damage and repair procedures.

Immobilization of the suture point in a light plaster cast for 3 to 4 weeks, with control of postured joints, promotes wound healing and may prevent suture line disruption. Such disruption may occur without obvious cause and may be detected by x-ray visualization of the suture line, if tantalum wire or marking sutures have been used. The actual technique of this end point, the suture, is of far less import than the principles of treatment outlined earlier in this report. With the mobilization of the extremity, the continuing protection against the development of deformities, intermittent use of electrical diagnostic measures, and the use of orthopedic transplants to correct muscle function are some parts of the approach to postoperative care. These can be found in major treatises.

Although this account has to do primarily with incised or compound nerve injuries, mention should be made of the involvement of major nerve trunks by traction, by concomitant bone injury, by compression, and by certain complications of vascular injury. All four represent acute conditions with unique pathologic sequelae and should receive the benefit of specific therapy.

Traction or stretch injuries, particularly of the brachial plexus and of the peroneal nerve, occur in the former instance with vehicular accidents and in the latter with forced adduction of the thigh on the lower leg. In all forms of traction palsy, force is directed along the longitudinal extent of the nerve segment with disruption of all constituents of the nerve segment. Intraneural hemorrhage and mesenchymal repair lead to collagenization of a nerve trunk over many centimeters of its length and make resection and repair rarely possible. In the common brachial plexus palsy, myelography of the cervical segment of the spinal cord may demonstrate actual avulsion of nerve roots. If no evidence of regeneration is present after 24 months in brachial plexus palsy, amputation of the upper extremity is often indicated. The peroneal type of traction palsy is best treated with a drop-foot brace and similar rehabilitation measures.

Simple bone fracture with peripheral nerve injury is a common combined injury, and the most common example is fracture of the humerus with radial nerve paralysis. Seddon has estimated that the chances are 5 to 1 in this combined injury that the radial nerve component will represent axonal degeneration without significant disruption of the supporting tissues of the nerve trunk.[6] Regeneration will therefore follow the customary course of axonal growth, roughly 1 mm. a day. In the usual spiral fracture of the humerus, reinnervation of the most proximal muscle, the brachioradialis, should occur therefore within 4 to 5 months after injury. In this particular nerve, with its relatively rough motor function and great capacity for regeneration, it is safe to observe such a combined injury for this period of time. In instances of peripheral nerve injury, the distance from the assumed point of nerve injury to the motor nerve entrance of the next muscle in line of innervation should be estimated. If function cannot be detected clinically or by electrodiagnostic data at the assumed time for reinnervation, exploration is mandatory.

An evaluation of sensory recovery is peculiarly important in the disabling median nerve injury that may accompany anterior displacement of the distal fragment of the humerus in supracondylar fractures of that bone. A similar situation is found at the wrist, where anterior displacement of either of the forearm bones may compromise the rather close confines of the medial nerve at this point. Dislocation of the hip and shoulder may stretch or compress major nerve trunks. Spontaneous recovery is the rule. Fracture of the ramus of pubis may lacerate the sciatic nerve, and if paralysis of this nerve is associated with radiating pain upon pressure over the area of injury, exploration is indicated. Fracture of the clavicle may be followed by brachial plexus palsy if excessive callus forms during healing. Rather common syndromes designated as the carpal tunnel syndrome, tardy ulnar palsy, and the thoracic outlet syndrome are well-documented instances of chronic compression syndromes of nerve tissue. The details of their recognition and treatment are available in major treatises. The student should be aware of another common syndrome of accessory nerve division following simple surgical procedures such as lymph node biopsy in the posterior cervical triangle.

This is accompanied by disabling and often unrecognized paralysis of the trapezius muscle.[10] In virtually all peripheral nerve injuries, the surgeon is confronted with some form of accompanying pain, and the strange and eclectic history of the treatment of pain deserves special and concentrated attention.[9]

Summary

An effort has been made from a number of biologic points of view to suggest that the repair of peripheral nerve injury secondary to the usual lacerating wounds of civilian life is not a surgical emergency. On the other hand, this documented biologic evidence suggests that primary emergency nerve suture is followed by a high incidence of failure of functional nerve regeneration. A sequence of primary wound débridement and closure, followed by early deferred nerve repair as an elective procedure, has been proposed as the best answer to the majority of these common problems. One of the most respected modern peripheral nerve surgeons, Mr. H. J. Seddon, has stated the premise in clear terms: if he himself were to suffer a peripheral nerve wound, he would suggest that his surgeon defer definitive surgery until he (the patient), the surgeon, and the wound were all in fit shape for such an important matter.

SELECTED REFERENCES

Ducker, T. B., Kempe, L. G., and Hayes, G. J.: The metabolic background for peripheral nerve surgery. J. Neurosurg., *30*:270, 1969.
This is a superb summary of neuronal metabolism and metabolic responses in the proximal and distal nerve segments that accompany peripheral nerve injury. Such metabolic alterations are related to the time of surgical repair and are derived from personal investigations and from pertinent literature (73 references).

Haymaker, W., and Woodhall, B.: Peripheral Nerve Injuries. Principles of Diagnosis, 2nd ed. Philadelphia, W. B. Saunders Company, 1953.
This is a relatively simple and highly usable treatise, derived from experience with war injuries, but from its basic design valuable as an approach to the understanding and treatment of civilian-type injuries. It is a primer on the nature of a peripheral nerve injury, its diagnosis, and its surgical anatomy.

Lyons, W. R., and Woodhall, B.: Atlas of Peripheral Nerve Injuries. Philadelphia, W. B. Saunders Company, 1949.
This is another basic neuropathologic reference volume concerned with definitions, normal peripheral nerve anatomy, and the pathologic changes in complete nerve division, neuromas in continuity, nerve sutures, and nerve grafts. Gross and light microscopic photographs are used to illustrate the material.

Seddon, H. J. (Ed.): Peripheral Nerve Injuries. London, The Nerve Injuries Committee of the Medical Research Council, Her Majesty's Stationery Office, 1954.
Another superb, inclusive, and readable record of British wartime experience in this field, an experience readily transferred to civilian-type injuries. The chapter on nerve grafting and the histopathology of nerve grafts represents a good introduction to that subject.

Sunderland, S.: Nerves and Nerve Injuries. Baltimore, Williams & Wilkins Company, 1968.
This is a monumental enterprise, the result of activities in the laboratory and the clinic spread over the years 1940 to 1957. It is clearly a reference book, but an adequate table of contents and a superb index allow the student ready access to any particular problem. Part VIII under the heading of "individual nerves" is uniquely valuable to the student for the understanding of both open and closed nerve injuries. There are countless references, but the volume is fundamentally the work of a man of considerable scholarship.

White, J. C., and Sweet, W. H.: Pain and the Neurosurgeon. A Forty-Year Experience. Springfield, Ill., Charles C Thomas, Publisher, 1969.

A virtual repository of total knowledge and a 40-year personal experience of the senior author in the neurosurgical methods of relieving pain. The first 48 pages are concerned with pain following peripheral nerve injuries, but the student at least should continue with those pages concerned with "pain following amputation" and "other varieties of peripheral neuralgia."

Woodhall, B., and Beede, G. W.: Peripheral Nerve Regeneration. A Follow-Up Study of 3656 World War II Injuries. Washington, D. C., Veterans Administration Monograph, U.S. Government Printing Office, 1956.
This is one of several monographs published by the Veterans Administration after World War II. As its Introduction states, "This monograph is not a textbook of peripheral nerve surgery.... From the data presented in the body of the monograph, certain surgical conclusions have been reached or, when necessary, restated so the informed surgeon can treat a new peripheral nerve injury with a firm concept of the result he will attain under the diverse and many factors that influence such an injury." It is not easy reading, but neither is regeneration an easy subject.

REFERENCES

1. Ducker, T. B., and Hayes, G. J.: Experimental improvements in the use of silastic cuff for peripheral nerve repair. J. Neurosurg., 28:582, 1968.

2. Ducker, T. B., Kempe, L. G., and Hayes, G. J.: The metabolic background for peripheral nerve surgery. J. Neurosurg., 30:270, 1969.

3. Haymaker, W., and Woodhall, B.: Peripheral Nerve Injuries. Principles of Diagnosis, 2nd ed. Philadelphia, W. B. Saunders Company, 1953.

4. Lyons, W. R., and Woodhall, B.: Atlas of Peripheral Nerve Injuries. Philadelphia, W. B. Saunders Company, 1949.

5. Mitchell, S. W.: Injuries of Nerves and Their Consequences. Philadelphia, J. B. Lippincott Company, 1872.

6. Seddon, H. J.: Nerve lesions complicating certain closed bone injuries. J.A.M.A., 135:691, 1947.

7. Seddon, H. J. (Ed.): Peripheral Nerve Injuries. London, The Nerve Injuries Committee of the Medical Research Council. Her Majesty's Stationery Office, 1954.

8. Sunderland, S.: Nerves and Nerve Injuries. Baltimore, Williams & Wilkins Company, 1968.

9. White, J. C., and Sweet, W. H.: Pain and the Neurosurgeon. A Forty-Year Experience. Springfield, Ill., Charles C Thomas, Publisher, 1969.

10. Woodhall, B.: Operative injury to the accessory nerve in the posterior cervical triangle. Arch. Surg., 74:122, 1957.

11. Woodhall, B., and Beede, G. W.: Peripheral Nerve Regeneration. A Follow-Up Study of 3656 World War II Injuries. Washington, D. C., Veterans Administration Monograph, U.S. Government Printing Office, 1956.

XI

CONGENITAL ABNORMALITIES

M. Stephen Mahaley, Jr., M.D.

Congenital aneurysms and arteriovenous malformations have been discussed elsewhere as vascular lesions. Many of the remaining congenital abnormalities represent midline cranial or spinal problems, and it has been postulated that they stem from a common basic embryonic defect, a permeability abnormality in the rhombic roof of the fourth ventricle.[8]

Hydrocephalus

The production, movement, and reabsorption of cerebrospinal fluid is now recognized as an extremely complex interaction between bulk flow, active transport, and facilitated diffusion. It is subject to a variety of physiologic and pathologic influences.[5, 13]

Two types of congenital hydrocephalus are recognized: communicating and noncommunicating, referring to whether or not the ventricular fluid communicates with the subarachnoid space. The noncommunicating variety may take the form of a stenosis or occlusion of the aqueduct of Sylvius or an impermeable rhombic roof. A child with hydrocephalus evident at birth classically has enlargement of the head, a wide and tense fontanelle, prominent venous channels in the scalp, and downward displacement of the globes within the orbits ("setting-sun" appearance). The head circumference should be carefully measured and the child examined for other congenital abnormalities, since multiple lesions are not uncommon. Transillumination of the head in a totally dark room should be attempted, since this finding in patients with anencephaly or extreme loss of cortex indicates a grave prognosis and usually interdicts surgery. X-rays of the skull are often helpful as regards the relative proportions of the various cranial fossae and the general configuration of the cranium. A transcoronal ventriculogram permits estimation of the thickness of the cortical mantle and may illustrate the actual site of obstruction of cerebrospinal fluid flow (Fig. 30). Arnold-Chiari malformations[4] and Dandy-Walker syndromes[2] probably represent variations on this same theme, the differences relating to specific mechanical displacements of structures in the posterior fossa.[8]

Surgical correction generally takes the form of a shunt procedure, the ventriculoatrial shunt being most commonly used at this time.[11] The decision to perform this procedure has to take into account the severity of the hydrocephalus, the presence or absence of other more serious congenital anomalies, and the general medical condition of the patient. The decision is often as difficult to make as it is to set down hard and fast rules for making it. The shunt, once performed, is subject to complications. Obstruction of the ventricular or atrial end of the shunt or infection of the shunt mechanism can necessitate removal or revision. Elective revisions have been recommended as the child grows and bony lengthening displaces the cardiac catheter,[11] and considerable work has been done regarding the management of the infected shunt.[7, 14] The majority of these children are shunt-dependent

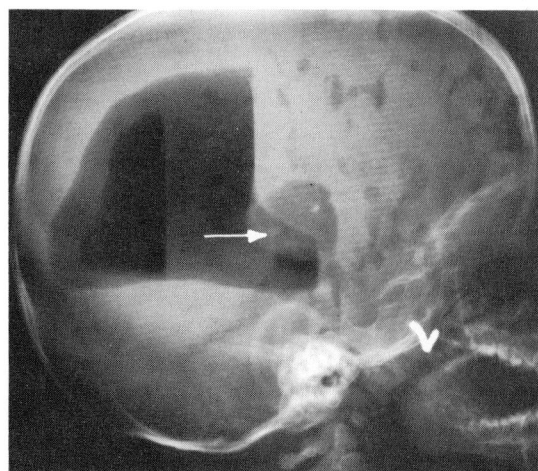

Figure 30. Ventriculogram, showing hydrocephalus secondary to aqueductal occlusion (arrow). Air (dark areas) is seen to fill part of the enlarged lateral and third ventricles, with the dilated proximal part of the aqueduct attached at the floor of the third ventricle.

after surgery, although clinical trials are now attempting to develop shunt independence, as part of the neurosurgical treatment.[6]

Meningomyelocele and Encephalocele

These lesions represent congenital midline defects with absence of bony covering (spina bifida or cranium bifidum), protrusion of a meningeal sac through this opening (meningocele), and oftentimes a herniation of nervous tissue into the sac (myelocele and encephalocele). If the meningeal sac is extremely thin over the surface, leakage of cerebrospinal fluid may be present at birth or develop shortly thereafter, permitting bacterial contamination and meningitis. Occasionally the meningeal sac is deficient in the midline, thus exposing the underlying nervous tissue, with free flow of cerebrospinal fluid (rachischisis); this condition is most often accompanied by the severest of neurologic deficits and represents the most difficult to manage neurosurgically.

Each child should be examined carefully to ascertain the extent of neurologic involvement at and below the level of the lesion; leg movements, response to pain, and anal sphincter tone are commonly impaired. The meningeal sac (Fig. 31) should be transilluminated to see if nervous tissue can be outlined. Other congenital anomalies should be sought, especially hydrocephalus.

The decision regarding surgical closure of these defects is often a difficult one because of (1) the small size of the patient, (2) the severity of the neurologic deficit often present, and (3) the associated congenital anomalies that may exist. If the patient with a meningocele is known to be hydrocephalic, then the hydrocephalus problem should be treated first and the meningocele later. If the midline defect is severe and leaking spinal fluid, with absence of neurologic function below the level of the lesion, the case may be considered hopeless, although there are those who would disagree and would insist on early surgical correction of almost all such defects.[3, 9, 15] If the midline defect is covered by healthy skin, then there may be no need for early surgery, the advantages to delay being severalfold: a chance to observe the patient longer for any evidence of hydrocephalus, time for the patient to outgrow the newborn period prior to being subjected to a surgical procedure, and the opportunity to carefully evaluate neurologic function as the child gets older. When a meningocele shows areas of extremely thin epidermis or when a small leak of cerebrospinal fluid is seen or suspected, surgical closure is advised at an early date, unless the seriousness of the neurologic deficit weighs against attempted repair. The primary aims of surgical repair are: (1) protection of underlying nervous tissue, (2) prevention of meningitis, (3) improvement of the mechanical inconvenience and cosmetic unpleasantness of a midline defect and mass, and (4) in a broad sense, improvement of the quality of existence of the patient.

Encephaloceles are usually located in the occiput, subfrontal (nasal), or forehead areas. The indications and aims of surgical repair are similar to those of meningoceles.[12] Nasal encephaloceles may mimic nasal polyps and should be suspected when such lesions are seen in children.

Syringomyelia and Hydromyelia

These congenital abnormalities refer to the presence of a pocket of fluid trapped within the cord substance

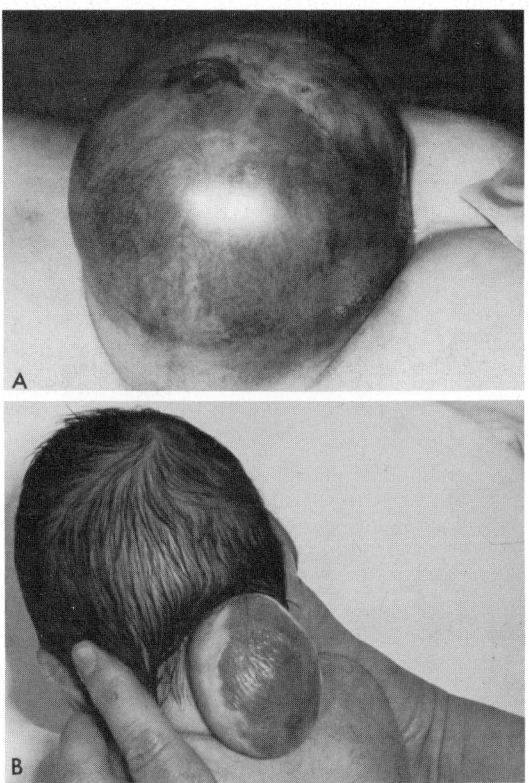

Figure 31. *A,* Lumbosacral meningocele, with buttocks to the right. *B,* Craniocervical meningocele.

(syringomyelia) or central canal (hydromyelia) more or less isolated from normal pathways of spinal fluid flow. These lesions may also stem from basically a permeability problem at the level of the rhombic roof during embryonic development.[8] However, the typical symptoms of a suspended sensory deficit to pain and temperature, a lower motor neuron dysfunction at the level of the lesion, and distal long tract signs may not appear until later in life, apparently as a result of gradual enlargement of the fluid pocket during life. The lesion is most commonly seen in the lower cervical and upper dorsal spinal areas but may extend the entire length of the spinal cord and occasionally into the brain stem.

Diagnosis may be aided by evidence of widening of the spinal canal on plain spine films and by myelographic evidence of an intrinsic mass lesion of the cord. Treatment involves creation of a communication between the fluid cavity and the subarachnoid space and, in cases of hydromyelia in which a communication exists with the fourth ventricle, plugging of the cervical canal opening at the obex.

Craniosynostosis

Premature closure of fusion of one or more of the cranial sutures results in a form of craniosynostosis.[17] The cranium will appear short in the anterior-posterior direction when the coronal suture alone is fused (brachycephaly) or narrow in the lateral dimension with sagittal suture closure (scaphocephaly). These single suture premature closures are largely cosmetic problems. Premature fusion of several or all (oxycephaly) cranial sutures can result in brain damage and visual loss as development occurs within an unnaturally rigid enclosure. The problem of oxycephaly must be distinguished at birth from that of microcephaly, in which the primary defect is one of congenitally poor brain development with secondary small head. X-rays of the skull are helpful, since microcephaly will usually show overlapping, unfused sutures at birth while oxycephaly will show fused sutures and often a thinning of the calvarium due to increased intracranial pressure. It is usually advisable to correct a craniosynostosis problem surgically as soon after birth as possible. The earlier prematurely fused sutures are opened, the better the chance for a more normal shape to the head and lesser the likelihood of impairment to the underlying developing brain.[16]

Dermal Sinus and Dermoid

These congenital defects result from persistence of somatic ectoderm in the vicinity of the midline mesodermal elements (muscle and bone) or the neuroectoderm (brain, spinal cord, or cauda equina).[1] The dermal sinus consists of a cutaneous opening which is usually quite small, located in the sacral (Fig. 32) or suboccipital areas, and connecting to the deeper midline structures by virtue of a sinus tract. The lining of this sinus contains dermal elements (sweat glands, hair follicles, and sebaceous glands) along its length and periodically extrudes debris via the surface orifice. This tract may terminate as a cul-de-sac inside the spinal canal and is then referred to as a dermoid, or a dermoid may exist in the spinal canal without ap-

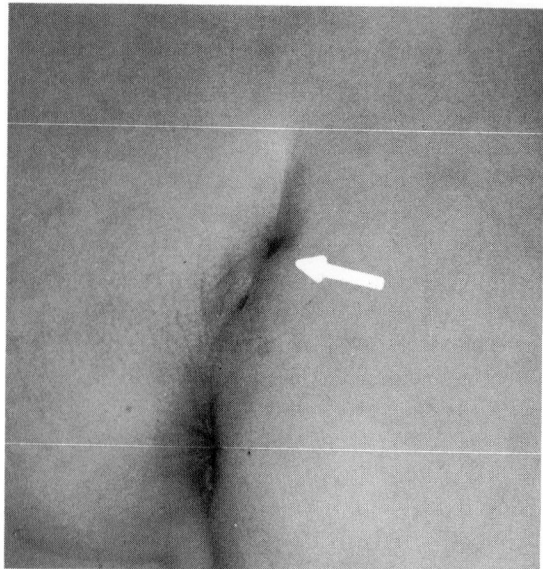

Figure 32. Dermal sinus. The characteristic cutaneous opening of a dermal sinus (arrow) is seen in the midline above the sacral area and just cephalad to the anal opening.

parent connection with the surface skin. A sinus tract or dermoid extending into the spinal canal may rupture and create meningitis. Indeed, a child with recurrent unexplained bouts of meningitis due to Staphylococcus or *Escherichia coli* should be examined carefully for the possible presence of a dermal sinus. An intraspinal dermoid may present with signs and symptoms of an intraspinal tumor. Careful examination of the midline skin may reveal the sinus opening or an overlying skin angioma or tuft of hair. X-rays of the spine or skull may reveal a bony opening through which a sinus tract passes. It is generally advised that any such midline tracts be explored and excised, with the exploration carried into the spinal canal when necessary to resect an extradural or intradural dermoid.

Diastematomyelia

Another of the congenital midline spinal defects consists of the presence of a spicule of bone arising perpendicularly from the dorsal surface of a vertebral body, usually in the lower thoracic spine, and often extending superiorly to the overlying laminal arch. This bony spicule effectively divides the spinal canal, cord, and surrounding meninges and acts as a source of traction on these structures as the child grows, resulting in leg weakness, numbness, and incontinence. A plain spine anterior-posterior x-ray may reveal the bony spicule, and a myelogram usually demonstrates division of the subarachnoid space by the bone. Surgical resection of the spicule can usually be accomplished without difficulty, often with improvement in the neurologic symptoms.

Congenital Scalp Defects

Agenesis of areas of the scalp are rare, usually located in the midline, and associated with skin defects elsewhere as well.[10] The entire thickness of scalp may be absent, or there may be a partial loss of skin. In order to prevent infection, protect the underlying tissues, and improve appearance, these lesions are usually treated with excision of the margins and closure primarily or with a full-thickness graft.

SELECTED REFERENCES

Matson, D. D.: Neurosurgery of Infancy and Childhood, 2nd ed. Springfield, Ill., Charles C Thomas, Publisher, 1969.
  This text is a "must" for all interested in diagnosis and treatment of childhood neurosurgical disturbances. It is the most complete and comprehensive text of its kind.

Gardner, W. J.: The Dysraphic States. Amsterdam, Excerpta Medica, 1973.
  The popular "rhombic roof" theory for the origin of various congenital anomalies of the CNS is evident throughout this complete review of the topic.

REFERENCES

1. Bailey, I. C.: Dermoid tumors of the spinal canal. J. Neurosurg., 33:676, 1970.
2. Benda, C. E.: Dandy-Walker syndrome or so-called atresia of foramen megendie. J. Neuropath. Exp. Neurol., 13:14, 1954.
3. Bunch, W. H., Casa, A. S., Bensman, A. S., and Long, D. M.: Modern Management of Myelomeningocoele. St. Louis, Warren H. Green, 1972.
4. Chiari, H.: Uber Veranderungen des Kleinhirns infolge von Hydrocephalie des Grosshirns. Dtsch. Med. Wochenschr., 17:1171, 1891.
5. Davson, H.: Physiology of the Cerebrospinal Fluid. London, J. & A. Churchill, 1967.
6. Epstein, F., Hockwald, G., and Ransohoff, J.: A volume control system for the treatment of hydrocephalus: Laboratory and clinical experience. J. Neurosurg., 38:282, 1973.
7. Fokes, E. C., Jr.; Occult infections of ventriculo-atrial shunts. J. Neurosurg., 33:517, 1970.
8. Gardner, W. J.: The Dysraphic States. Amsterdam, Excerpta Medica, 1973.
9. Heimburger, R. F.: Early repair of myelomeningocele (spina bifida cystica). J. Neurosurg., 37:594, 1972.
10. Kasnik, E. J., and Sayers, M. P.: Congenital scalp defects: Aplasia cutis congenita. J. Neurosurg., 42:32, 1975.
11. Matson, D. D.: Neurosurgery of Infancy and Childhood, 2nd ed. Springfield, Ill., Charles C Thomas, Publisher, 1969.
12. Mealey, J., Jr., Ozenitis, A. J., and Hockey, A. A.: The prognosis of encephaloceles. J. Neurosurg., 33:209, 1970.
13. Milhorat, T. H.: Hydrocephalus and the Cerebrospinal Fluid. Baltimore, Williams & Wilkins Company, 1972.
14. Perrin, J. C. S., and McLaurin, R. L.: Infected ventriculoatrial shunts. A method of treatment. J. Neurosurg., 27:21, 1967.
15. Sharrard, W. J. W., Zachary, R. B., Lorber, J., and Bruce, A. M.: A controlled trial of immediate and delayed closure of spina bifida cystica. Arch. Dis. Child., 38:18, 1963.
16. Shillito, J., Jr., and Matson, D. D.: Craniosynostosis: A review of 519 surgical patients. Pediatrics, 41:829, 1968.
17. Taveras, J. M., and Wood, E. H.: Diagnostic Neuroradiology. Baltimore, Williams & Wilkins Company, 1964.

XII

NEUROSURGICAL RELIEF OF PAIN

Blaine S. Nashold, Jr., M.D., and
Harry Friedman, M.D.

Not everyone has a soul of fire, and, in actual human life, even in the case of the great mystics, the struggle against pain exacts a high price.

  — Lerche

Pain is not a simple sensory event but a complex neural and psychological phenomenon that involves the entire nervous system. Humans differ remarkably in their individual reactions to pain and suffering, and when severe pain is unrelieved, a state of suffering may intervene that threatens the very existence of the person. Our understanding of the anatomy and physiology of pain perception in man has evolved slowly simply because pain is a private matter and direct observations in man have their limitations. Someone has said that in order to relieve pain totally the nervous system must be destroyed, and yet we know that section of the dorsal roots and spinal cordotomy are time-honored neurosurgical operations that can relieve pain.

Although the free nerve endings of the C fibers are considered the primary receptors that signal pain, recent physiologic evidence indicates that these free nerve endings also function as receptors for other kinds of sensation. At the peripheral end, fine cutaneous afferent activity appears to be a necessary condition for the sensation of pain. Although the functional localization of pain is important, recent physiologic work emphasizes spatial and temporal mechanisms that are involved in the coding of sensory experience within the central nervous system.

The success of spinal cordotomy in relieving pain is related to the anatomic organization of pain and thermal fibers in the lateral spinothalamic tract. Edinger delineated the spinothalamic tract in 1889, but its function was not known until 1905 when Spiller noted the loss of pain and temperature in a patient with a discrete tuberculoma in the anterior quadrant of the spinal cord.[1, 7] Martin, in 1912, at the urging of Spiller, carried out the first thoracic cordotomy.[8] Although the lateral spinothalamic tract is of considerable importance in the transmission of painful and thermal sensations, recent anatomic evidence indicates that additional pathways are available for the transmission of

pain. The lateral spinothalamic tract is a phylogenetically recent pathway with its input directly into
the sensory thalamus. Pain transmission over the
spinothalamic route has a rapid transit time to the
thalamus where higher levels of integration occur
through the thalamocortical connections. A definite
topographic scheme of the body's sensory image exists
within the cord and the thalamus, the input from the
facial region being medial to that from the body, and
from the leg regions, lateral. Pain resulting from electrical stimulation of the spinothalamic pathways is
usually experienced by the patient as a sharp, well-
demarcated sensation referred to a localized region of
the body.

In contrast to this, the diffuse pain pathways appear
to have multiple routes through the spinal cord with
distribution to the midbrain, thalamus, and hypothalamus; these spinoreticular pathways are phylogenetically older than the newer lateral spinothalamic
tracts and have been designated the paleothalamic
system. They may be crossed or uncrossed tracts,
which are composed of short chains of neurons that
make several synaptic connections at successive rostral levels in the central nervous system. Pain transmitted via these routes appears to be slower in transit
to higher levels and the sensation experienced by alert
patients during stimulation is ill-defined and unpleasant, being diffusely localized to the regions in the central parts of the body, including the head, chest, or abdomen.

Pain can be thought of as either a primary or secondary symptom. In most cases it is a secondary symptom
usually originating from some underlying pathologic
change, correction of which will relieve the pain. However, when the pathologic state cannot be eradicated,
as may be the case in metastatic malignant disease,
the pain may be relieved by a specific neurosurgical
operation.

Pain as a primary symptom results from physiologic
or pathologic involvement of the pain pathways within
the central nervous system. A painful dysesthesia occurring after surgical cordotomy, tractotomy, or thalamotomy is an example of primary pain syndrome.
Other examples include the pain of the thalamic syndrome or painful phantom limb. Central pain syndromes often occur after trauma, vascular occlusion,
tumor, degenerative disease in the central nervous
system (multiple sclerosis), or infections (herpes zoster). The patient describes this kind of pain as intense, burning, crushing, or tearing, and it can be
aggravated by the slightest sensory stimulation. An
emotional upset will intensify the patient's pain, as
can psychiatric disturbances. These patients often
become drug addicts and undergo permanent personality changes. Numerous theories have been proposed to
explain central pain as the presence of hyperirritable
neurons at the site of injury in the diffuse pain tracts,
the diversion of noxious impulses from the spinothalamic tract into the paleothalamic system, or the release
of the thalamus from cortical inhibition.

Neurosurgical treatment of central pain has not
been completely successful, although tractotomy and
thalamotomy have been used in a limited number of
patients.

NEUROSURGICAL OPERATIONS FOR PAIN

The neurosurgeon must consider certain facts before
recommending an operation to relieve pain. The
neurosurgical operation must not be done as a last
resort or in desperation. Most failures to relieve pain
are due to delay in surgical treatment. The neurosurgeon should be consulted early, before the occurrence of drug addiction or suffering. Long-established
pain leads to a state of suffering that is to be avoided.
Ideally the benefit from the operation should last for
the lifetime of the patient.

Neurosurgical operations for the relief of pain can
be divided into four types: (1) anatomic interruption
pathways subserving pain or the destruction of sensory integration regions in the central nervous system
(rhizotomy, cordotomy, tractotomy, thalamotomy,
cingulotomy); (2) sympathectomy for the relief of causalgia and sympathetic dystrophy; (3) pituitary ablation to relieve pain from metastatic tumors under hormonal influence; (4) electroanalgesia to relieve pain,
by stimulation of peripheral nerves or the dorsal column of the spinal cord.

The simplest operation for pain relief is a section,
avulsion, or alcohol injection of a peripheral nerve. It
has the advantage of relieving pain originating from a
small localized area. In trigeminal neuralgia, injection
or avulsion of one of the peripheral branches of the
fifth nerve may give several years of relief. When the
pain recurs or involves larger areas of the face, the
gasserian ganglion may be sectioned or lightly traumatized by rubbing, adding additional long periods of
relief. One disadvantage of sectioning a peripheral
nerve is the return of the pain with its regeneration.
The sensory loss from a dorsal rhizotomy involves a
larger area, but at least three to four of the nerve
roots must be sectioned to produce an analgesic zone
equal to one dermatome. Dorsal rhizotomy may be
useful in relieving pain originating from the neck,
shoulder, thorax, or abdominal wall, but it is usually
unsuitable if the pain involves the arm or leg, since total loss of sensation in these regions often reduces the
usefulness of the limb.

Spinal cordotomy still remains the most useful
operation for the relief of widespread pain in the torso
and extremities (Fig. 33). It is especially helpful when
the pain orginates from thoracic or abdominal regions.
The surgical section is performed opposite the site of
the pain in the anterolateral quadrant of spinal cord
at least six cord segments above the origin of the pain,
to allow for some degree of postoperative regression of
the sensory level. The analgesia resulting from a cordotomy covers the opposite half of the body with the
level beginning several segments below the cord section. For the most complete relief of pain, the entire
lateral spinothalamic tract must be sectioned, since an
incomplete cut, for example, may result in the sparing
of sensation in one region or another with the persistence of the pain. An open surgical cordotomy has a
mortality of 10 per cent and the cord section can be
done at two different spinal levels, usually cervical
(C1–C3) and thoracic (T1–T2), and in the case of the
cervical operation the analgesic level reaches up to the
clavicle, involving the arm to varying degrees but

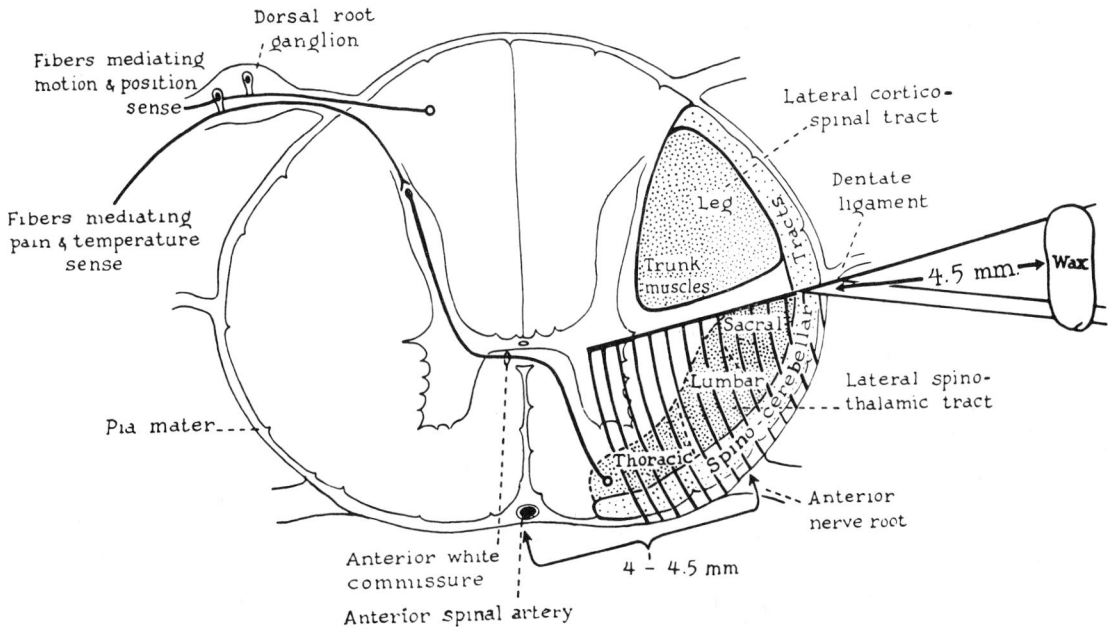

Figure 33. Cross-sectional drawing of thoracic cord showing extent of incision in anterolateral cordotomy. (From Kahn, E. A., Bassett, R. C. Schneider, R. C., and Crosly, E. C.: Correlative Neurosurgery. 1955. Courtesy of Charles C Thomas, Publisher, Springfield, Ill.)

with the densest analgesia over regions of thorax, abdomen, and leg. A thoracic cordotomy produces contralateral analgesia beginning in the lower thorax (Fig. 34). A well-executed unilateral lumbar cordotomy should result in good pain relief in 85 per cent of cases, whereas with a high cervical cordotomy relief occurs 50 per cent of the time. After unilateral cordotomy as a rule complications are few, with normal bladder, bowel, and sexual function. Postoperative

complications such as an ipsilateral hemiparesis or monoparesis can occur if the surgical incision involves the nearby corticospinal tract. A bilateral cordotomy performed either in the cervical or thoracic cord has higher overall operative risks and the postoperative deficits are greater; most of these operations should be restricted to patients with widespread carcinoma whose life expectancy is limited. Bilateral cordotomy at either level seriously interferes with the bladder, bowel, and sexual function.

Percutaneous cervical cordotomy, introduced by Mullan in 1963, has proved useful in patients who could not withstand the operative rigors of an open cordotomy.[3] The percutaneous cordotomy is done with local anesthesia, with roentgenographic control of a coagulating needle which is guided into the anterolateral quadrant of the spinal cord between the first and second cervical vertebrae (Fig. 35). The direction and depth of the needle are controlled by roentgenograms, and electrical stimulation can be used to test the location of the needle tip within the cord tissue. The lateral spinothalamic tract can be coagulated unilaterally or bilaterally by means of a high-frequency electrical current. Such operations can be done quickly by experienced surgeons with a minimum of surgical trauma. It is, however, a blind operation, so the surgeon must exercise great care not to misplace the lesion and cause additional neurologic deficits. One risk of the percutaneous technique is that the high bilateral cervical cord lesions may interfere with breathing and after surgery patients have died in their sleep of respiratory failure. A percutaneous cordotomy is best suited for a poor-risk patient with a short life expectancy. Long-term chronic pain is best not treated by the percutaneous technique because of the occur-

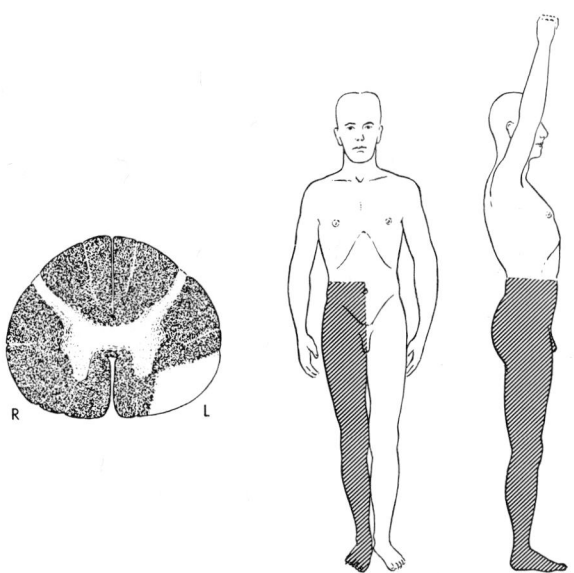

Figure 34. Extent of analgesia after thoracic cordotomy. Area of cord involved is shown in section on the left.

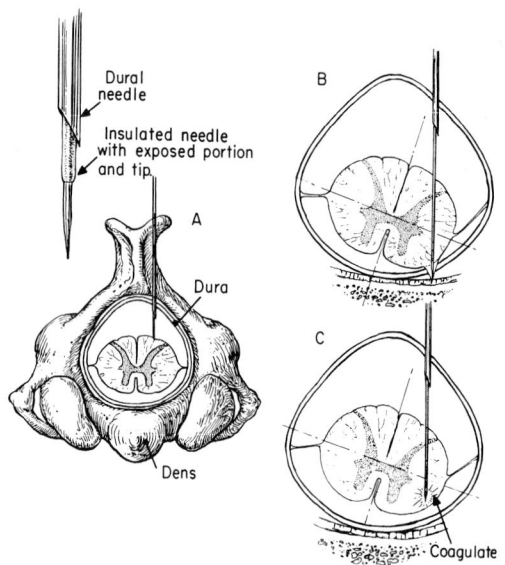

Figure 35. Percutaneous cordotomy using posterior approach; anterior and lateral introductions of needle also are possible.

rence of late failures and the risk of recurrence of the original pain or even more serious risk of a postoperative painful dysesthesia.

Pain involving overlapping areas of the head, neck, or arm can be difficult to control by a single surgical operation owing to the overlapping of the cranial and cervical nerves in the head and neck. Stereotactic operations at midbrain or thalamic levels have relieved these widespread cranial and cervical pains. A stereotactic medullary tractotomy can be performed to selectively interrupt pain involving the individual divisions of the trigeminal nerve. The first open surgical section of the spinothalamic tracts in the midbrain was performed by Walker in 1942, producing an analgesia of the opposite half of the body.[9] However, the open medullary or mesencephalic tractotomies were associated with a high mortality (7 per cent) and morbidity, with one serious drawback being the risk of a postoperative dysesthesia. Since 1947, using the human stereotactic instrument, Spiegel and Wycis and others have coagulated the mesencephalic pain tracts by introducing a small probe into the mesencephalon via a frontal burr hole (Fig. 36).[6] The mortality rate has been reduced to 1 per cent, with good relief of pain, and although postoperative dysesthesias still occur, they are less frequent. Postoperatively there is usually loss of upward gaze and occasional diplopia that may complicate recovery.

Stereotactic lesions in the thalamus or the cingulum have been successfully employed to relieve widespread pain causing suffering. A unilateral thalamic lesion (centrum medium or parafascicular nucleus or both) is often sufficient for relief of the pain of extensive carcinoma. The relief is thought to be due to interruption of sensory integration at higher levels in the central nervous system. A thalamic lesion does not alter the threshold for pain, and no analgesia occurs despite the

relief of the patient's pain. An added risk of the thalamic operation may be an interference with memory or speech mechanism and in some patients the relief of the pain is short-lived.

When suffering is the most prominent clinical feature in a patient with intractable pain, it can best be relieved by a medial dorsal thalamic or cingulate gyrus lesion interrupting the cingulum. The beneficial effect of the thalamic lesion is thought to be due to the interruption of the thalamofrontal connections, while a cingulate lesion exerts its effect by interfering with some circuits in the limbic system. Frontal leukotomy can no longer be recommended as an operation for the relief of pain.

Painful Phantom Limb

The loss of an arm, leg, or breast or the penis will result in a phantom sensation. The neural organization of one's conscious awareness of his own body scheme requires a period of learning when the sensory patterns of the body schema are organized within the sensory cortex. A person with congenital absence of a limb has no phantom sensation. After an amputation, the phantom image seems fixed in the person's awareness. The patient's awareness of the traumatic circumstances surrounding the loss of his limb appears to

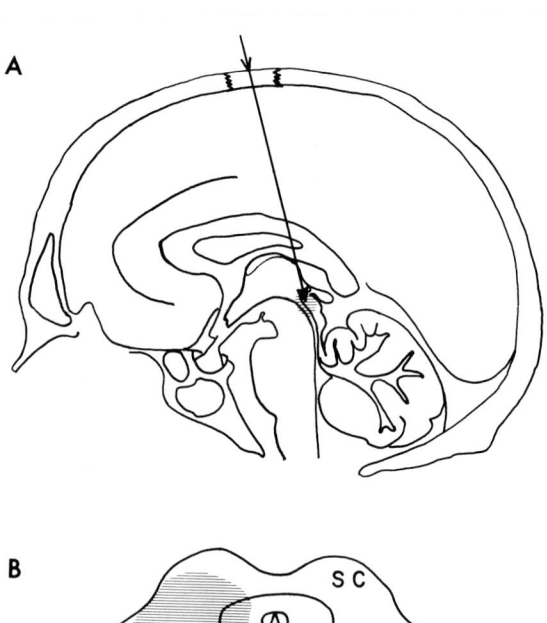

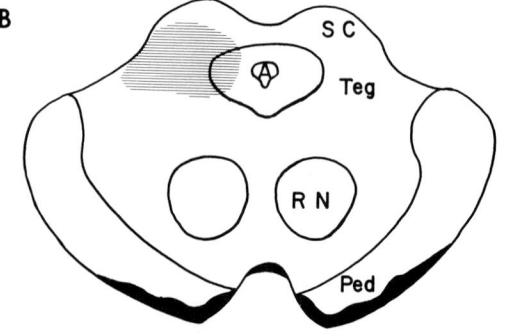

Figure 36. A, Sagittal section of brain shows target tract to midbrain. B, Cross section of mesencephalon at superior colliculus. Area of therapeutic lesion shown on the right.

exert some influence on whether or not he may experience the phantom sensation. Normally the phantom sensation will fade away by retracting into the end of the stump, but the patient is often aware of its posture and may even be able to move the missing fingers or toes. Before an amputation a wise surgeon forewarns his patient about the possible postoperative occurrence of the phantom sensation.

When the phantom sensation is accompanied by pain, surgical treatment may be necessary. The presence of pain intensifies and prolongs the phantom sensation and when the pain is relieved the phantom fades. A painful phantom often follows a traumatic avulsion of the brachial plexus that tears the nerve roots from their attachment to the spinal cord. The arm becomes insensitive and flaccid and the pain is described as burning, tearing, or crushing, and its intensity seems to heighten the patient's awareness of his phantom limb. Injury to the substantia gelatinosa in the spinal cord at the point where the dorsal roots are avulsed may be the site from which the pain originates. A high cervical cordotomy, stereotactic mesencephalic tractotomy, or thalamotomy has relieved the pain, while resection of the arm or leg area of the parietal sensory cortex relieves neither the pain nor the phantom. Amputation of the painful arm after brachial avulsion is of no value in relieving the pain.

Surgical Sympathectomy for Relief of Causalgia and Sympathetic Dystrophy

Causalgia is a syndrome characterized by severe "burning pain" and autonomic dysfunction that occurs after partial injury to large nerve trunks. The first detailed clinical description appeared in 1864 when Mitchell, Morehouse, and Keen examined Civil War veterans with gunshot wounds of the arm or leg that had injured major nerve trunks.[2] The etiology of this disorder is unknown but the symptoms are more likely to occur after injuries to large peripheral nerves such as the brachial plexus, or the median or sciatic nerve. Usually the nerve lesion is incomplete, with only a partial sensory loss in the involved painful limb. The physiologic basis for the pain and its association with autonomic dysfunction is not understood, but some have postulated that the burning dysesthesia results from short-circuiting of C fiber impulses or the shunting of efferent sympathetic impulses via the injured somatic nerve, which in turn activates the pain fibers. If the disorder persists for too long a time without relief, drug addiction and psychoneurosis may complicate the surgical treatment. The burning pain of causalgia (hyperpathia) usually involves the hand or foot, with the skin of the extremity becoming smooth and glossy in appearance along with loss of the hair. The vasomotor disturbances appear with sweating and coldness involving the limb. The patient becomes irritable, fearful, and protective of his injured limb, and as time passes without relief of his pain, he withdraws from social contacts and avoids bright lights and loud noises, and the slightest emotional problem will aggravate his pain. He may find temporary relief by bathing his painful limb in tepid running water. The symptoms are dramatically relieved by a block of the sympathetic nerves to the involved limb, and a cure results after surgical sympathectomy.

The second group of painful disorders associated with pain and autonomic dysfunction is sympathetic dystrophy, which occurs after trauma of a less specific degree to extremities or joints. The pain is not usually burning as in causalgia but vasomotor disturbances can occur, with vasospastic phenomena, cyanosis, sudomotor dysfunction, and trophic skin changes in the involved limb. Diagnostic sympathetic nerve block often relieves the symptoms and surgical sympathectomy may be curative. Psychoneurosis is not uncommon in these patients, and their disorder is oftentimes complicated by personal problems associated with litigation or compensation claims. Ill-advised surgery may tend to magnify the entire symptom complex.

Relief of Pain by Pituitary Ablation

Bone pain caused by metastases from breast or prostatic tumor will dramatically subside after ablation of the pituitary gland. The relief of pain is probably related to a reduction or loss of the effects of pituitary growth hormone, which has a direct stimulating effect on these tumors. As the pain subsides, the tumor nodules also diminish in size and the lesions in the bone seen on the roentgenogram often resolve with recalcification. Pituitary ablation should be considered only after oophorectomy in women, or following the removal of the gonads in males. Hypophysectomy exerts its best effect in premenopausal women and the most satisfactory results are noted if the pituitary gland is completely ablated to produce a significant drop in the levels of the growth hormone. Complete surgical removal of the pituitary can be accomplished through a subfrontal craniotomy, but recently stereotactic ablations have been carried out by introducing lesion probes into the sella turcica (Fig. 37). The overall operative risks are less following the stereotactic operation and the gland can be destroyed by either freezing, heat coagulation, or implanting radioactive yttrium. Postoperatively these patients must be maintained on hormone replacement, often combined with Pitressin if diabetes insipidus appears. Pituitary ablation can be followed by many pain-free months during which time the patient's overall condition improves and life becomes bearable.

Relief of Pain by Electroanalgesia

In 1967, Wall and Sweet found that during stimulation of a peripheral nerve, pain sensation was reduced over the distribution area of the stimulated nerve.[11] They proposed that the electrical activation of A fibers of the peripheral nerve in some way interfered with the perception of the painful stimulus, probably at the spinal cord level. Wall had already shown, in animals, that when the activity of the larger A fibers in peripheral nerves was increased by electrical stimulus there occurred a concomitant inhibition of the smaller pain fiber activity within the spinal cord.[10] Later, Shealy et al. noted that stimulation of the dorsal column of the cat, which is made up entirely of the large A fibers, reduced the animal's reaction to noxious stimuli.[5] The

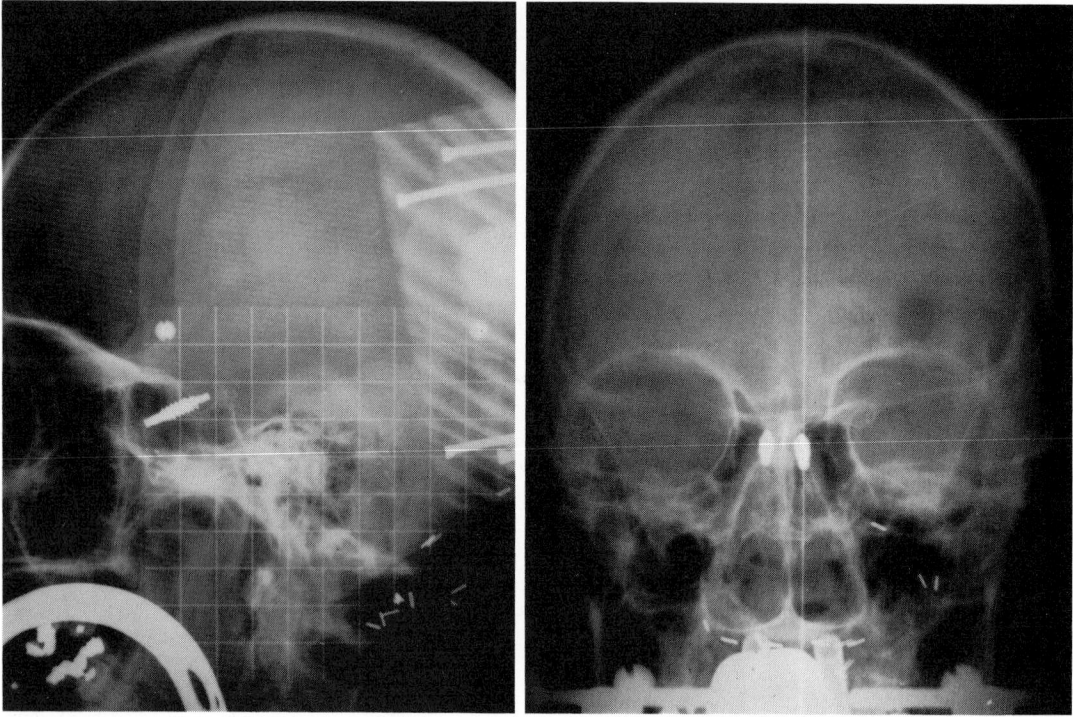

Figure 37. Skull x-rays of female patient with intractable pain from metastatic breast cancer. Yttrium pellets introduced transsphenoidally for pituitary ablation.

term "electroanalgesia" was coined, although the neurophysiologic mechanism responsible for the pain relief was not known. Sweet originally employed the electrical stimulation technique to successfully relieve pain originating from an injured peripheral nerve. A pair of platinum electrodes is placed in contact with the nerve trunk above the level of the injury and a minature RF receiver, which is attached to the stimulating platinum electrodes, is buried beneath the skin. The patient carries out self-activation of the painful nerves by an electrical signal transmitted through the skin of the RF receiver by a small portable RF generator. The patient can vary either the frequency or strength of the stimulating current in order to find a level of stimulation that relieves his pain. Later, in 1970, Shealy and Mortimer reported on the implantation of stimulating electrodes to activate the dorsal columns of the spinal cord in patients with pain from widespread carcinoma.[4] The device was inserted through a laminectomy at either the cervical or thoracic level but always above the segmental level of the body from which the pain originates. Self-activation of the dorsal columns by the patient resulted in his experiencing a paresthesia over the painful region with reduction of the pain. The technique, although still new as a mode of treatment, seems promising, and its greatest potential is based on the concept that the nervous system is not physically disrupted but the "on-going" neural activity related to pain perception is in some way altered by the introduction of an extrinsic electrical impulse, thereby preserving the physical integrity of the central nervous system.

SELECTED REFERENCES

Cassinari, V., and Pagni, A. C.: Central Pain: A Neurosurgical Survey. Cambridge, Mass., Harvard University Press, 1969.
    A concise monograph of the physiologic and clinical aspects of central pain.

Knighton, R. S., and Dumke, P. R.: Pain. Boston, Little, Brown and Company, 1966.
    International symposium on new concepts of pain, stressing both clinical and research aspects.

Spiller, W. G.: The occasional clinical resemblance between caries of the vertebral and lumbothoracic syringomyelia, and the location within the spinal cord of the fibres for the sensations of pain and temperature. Univ. Penn. Med. Bull., *18*:147, 1905.
    Classic paper on the functional role of the lateral spinothalamic tracts by a founder of American neurology.

Sternbach, R. A.: Pain: A Psychophysiological Analysis. New York, Academic Press, 1968.
    An overview of pain and suffering from the psychiatric and psychologic point of view.

White, J. C., and Sweet, W. H.: Pain and the Neurosurgeon. A Forty-Year Experience. Springfield, Ill., Charles C Thomas, Publisher, 1969.
    A 40-year experience of the neurosurgical treatment with detailed clinical data combined with anatomic and physiologic correlations.

REFERENCES

1. Edinger, L.: Vergleichend-enturick-lungsgeschichtliche und anatomische Studien und Bereiche des Central-nervensystems: II. Uber die Fortsetzung der hintern Ruckenmarks wurseln Zum Gehirn. Anat. Anz., *4*:121, 1889.
2. Mitchell, S. W., Morehouse, G. R., and Keen, W. W.: Gunshot wounds and Other Injuries of Nerves. Philadelphia, J. B. Lippincott Company, 1864, p. 164.
3. Mullan, S., Harper, P. R., Hekmatpanah, J., Torres, H., and Dobbin, G.: Percutaneous interruption of spinal pain tracts by means of a strontium[90] needle. J. Neurosurg., *0*:931, 1963.

4. Shealy, C. N., Mortimer, J. T., and Hagsfors, N.: Dorsal column electroanalgesia. J. Neurosurg., *32*:560, 1970.
5. Shealy, C. N., Mortimer, J. T., and Reswick, J. B.: Electrical inhibition of pain by stimulation of the dorsal columns. Anesth. Analg., *46*:489, 1967.
6. Spiegel, E. A., Wycis, H. T., Marks, M., and Lee, A. J.: Stereotactic apparatus for operation on the human brain. Science, *106*:349, 1947.
7. Spiller, W. G.: The occasional clinical resemblance between caries of the vertebral and lumbothoracic syringomeylia, and the location within the spinal cord of the fibres for the senations of pain and temperature. Univ. Penn. Med. Bull., *18*:147, 1905.
8. Spiller, W. G., and Martin, E.: The treatment of persistent pain of organic origin in the lower part of the body by division of the anterolateral column of the spinal cord. J.A.M.A., *58*:1489, 1912.
9. Walker, A. E.: Relief of pain by mesencephalic tractotomy. Arch. Neurol., *48*:865, 1942.
10. Wall, P. D.: Control of impulses at the first central synapse in cutaneous pathways. *In* Eccles, J. C., and Schade, J. P. (Eds.): Physiology of Spinal Neurons. Progress in Brain Research, Volume 12. New York, Elsevier, 1964.
11. Wall, P. D., and Sweet, W. H.: Temporary abolition of pain in man. Science, *155*:108, 1967.

XIII

NEUROSURGICAL TREATMENT OF EPILEPSY

Blaine S. Nashold, Jr., M.D.

Epilepsy can be defined as a paroxysmal, excessive, neuronal discharge within the brain orginating from either cortical or subcortical regions. Although the brain is the site of the dysfunction, there occurs a sudden disruption of function of the body or mind and the symptoms produced by the epileptic seizure are a reflection of the part of the brain involved.

The epileptic neuron exhibits an instability of its cellular membrane and the abnormal neuronal discharge is due to excessive depolarization with possible fluctuation in activity associated with repolarizing and hyperpolarizing mechanisms. Although these intrinsic neuronal mechanisms are of prime importance, extrinsic factors affect the irritable neurons, such as excessive afferent bombardment from distant regions of the brain, or systemic metabolic changes may alter the local chemical milieu of the hyperirritable neurons.

Epilepsy is a serious social and medical problem, and it is estimated that 1 in 200 persons suffers from seizures, although an accurate figure on the exact numbers of persons who have an attack at some time in their lives is unknown. The incidence of epilepsy is increasing; this increase is largely due to the survival of persons who would have died of brain injuries or other cerebral abnormalities acquired in early life. This has been brought about by the use of antibiotics and the improvements in medical care that have saved many children who might have died of meningitis, brain abscess, encephalitis, severe head injury, or brain tumor. It should be noted that seizures may result from any pathologic process that is capable of affecting the structure and function of the brain; therefore, the causes of seizures are numerous, and include congenital anomalies, disorders occurring during intrauterine life, birth injuries, infections, trauma, vascular anomalies, metabolic and nutritional disturbances, tumors, degenerative diseases, and specific genetic disorders. In man, surgical treatment is usually reserved for those patients who exhibit intractable focal epilepsy originating from either trauma, infection, or vascular anomalies. Traumatic epilepsy can be severe and persistent, regardless of the kind of injury or the length of the interval between injury and the onset of seizures. Trauma is a common source of epilepsy, and the insult to the brain may occur either at birth or later in life. It has been estimated that the overall incidence of post-traumatic epilepsy in the American veteran of World War II is 28 per cent, whereas it is 11 per cent in men who sustained a closed head injury associated with varying degrees of concussion. In a group of 1000 civilians who sustained an uncomplicated blunt head injury, the overall incidence of epilepsy was 1 per cent; however, the incidence increased to 50 per cent if the dura and brain were penetrated.

Clinical Classification of Epilepsy

Various clinical classifications of seizures have been proposed; the most recent, by the International League Against Epilepsy, divides seizures into three types:

1. *Partial seizures* beginning locally, usually without loss of consciousness. The clinical types in this group include the focal motor and jacksonian seizures with somatosensory or autonomic symptoms or both, partial seizures with affective or cognitive symptoms, psychosensory illustrations, and hallucinations, and the electroencephalographic abnormality is usually focal.

2. *Generalized or major seizures* beginning bilaterally symmetrically or without local onset. The clinical types include absences and myoclonic, atonic, and akinetic seizures, and the electroencephalographic abnormality is either a 3 per second spike wave or polyspikes and wave discharges.

3. *Unilateral seizures, clonic, tonic,* without impaired consciousness, with focal spikes and waves or focal slow waves recorded in the electroencephalogram.

The modern foundations for the surgical treatment of epilepsy were laid at the end of the nineteenth century by two Englishmen, John Hughlings Jackson and Victor Horsley. It was Jackson who formulated the concept that epileptic seizures originate from hyperirritable neurons in the central nervous system, and he also showed that the pattern of the clinical seizure depends upon its anatomic location in the brain, and stressed the importance of carefully recording in the clinical history the sequence of events during the epileptic seizure. In 1886, at the urging of Jackson, Victor Horsley performed the first subpial cortical resection of the "hinder end of the superior frontal sulcus" in a 22-year-old Scotsman who had suffered from focal seizures caused by a depressed skull fracture sustained as a child.[2]

Later, Foerster showed the value of systematic electrical stimulation of the cerebral cortex in patients with post-traumatic focal epileptic seizures and he successfully performed surgical excision of the cortical scar in these patients with significant relief of their post-traumatic epilepsy.[1] It was Penfield and Jasper who introduced the careful clinical analysis of seizure disorders combined with extensive cortical stimulation and simultaneous electroencephalographic recordings performed prior to the surgical excision of the epileptic focus.[4] Krynauw, in 1950, performed the first cerebral hemispherectomy for intractable seizures due to infantile hemiplegia.[3] At the present time, stereotactically implanted cortical and subcortical electrodes are being used to evaluate the electrographic abnormalities of subcortical epilepsy prior to the placement of a sterotactic lesion.

It has been estimated that about 5 per cent of epileptics may be considered as candidates for surgical treatment. Psychomotor seizures orginating from a unilateral temporal focus can be relieved by surgical excision of the anterior temporal lobe in about 75 per cent of patients. It is important that every epileptic patient be given an adequate trial (2 to 3 years) of anticonvulsant medication directed by a neurologist before the final decision to operate is made.

Clinical Evaluation of Seizures for Surgery

A detailed historical account of the patient's seizure pattern is the first important step in the clinical analysis. The reports of the seizure pattern as observed by the patient's family or the medical staff often add important clues that will aid in the cerebral localization of the epileptic focus. The kind of aura experienced by the patient must be determined, along with the physical and psychologic factors that influence the duration of the attacks and the occurrence of postictal phenomena. The nature of the aura gives an important clue as to the possible location of the irritable epileptic focus in the brain. For example, olfactory and epigastric sensations, dreamy states, fear, and automatisms point to involvement of the mesial temporal lobe, while more complex sensory or motor behavior may suggest involvement of the brain stem. Visual and auditory hallucinations or illusions may originate from temporoparietal association cortices, while complex motor behavior may point to involvement of the supplementary motor cortex in the frontal lobe. It is also important to discover which extrinsic factors seem to precipitate or modify a patient's seizure; examples of such factors are the effects of bright lights, noises, or cutaneous stimuli that may activate reflex sensory seizures. The psychologic changes occurring before, during, or after a seizure often give important clues as to the location and severity of the brain involvement. Seizures may be influenced by normal metabolic changes such as hypoglycemia or the hormonal alteration in women associated with their menstrual periods.

Clinical tests should include roentgenography of the skull, electroencephalography, brain scanning, carotid Amytal test, and psychological testing. The plain roentgenogram of the skull of an epileptic may reveal an old depressed skull fracture, or in the case of a patient with temporal lobe epilepsy or infantile hemiplegia the cranial vault may be deformed or smaller on the side of the damaged hemisphere. The pneumoencephalogram may reveal a porencephalic cyst, enlarged ventricles, or focal dilation of the temporal horn, indicating the area of the brain lesion, and in addition angiography can give valuable information as to the extent of vascular anomalies.

The most important single clinical test for the evaluation of epilepsy is electroencephalography. Multiple scalp electroencephalograms are necessary prior to surgery, plus specialized electroencephalographic recordings such as those using nasopharyngeal electrodes in the patient with temporal lobe seizures. The recording electrodes can be placed directly on the surface of the cortex or implanted stereotactically in the deeper regions of the brain (Fig. 38). The electroencephalographic recordings from these electrodes give valuable information on the degree and extent of epileptic involvement in the deeper brain regions that may not be evident from routine scalp electroencephalogram (Fig. 39). Drugs, sleep, or photic or direct electrical stimulation may be necessary to activate the electroencephalographic focus. Prior to the surgical excision direct electrocortical recordings can be made on the surface of the exposed cerebral cortex to aid in the delineation of the size and shape of the epileptic focus (Fig. 40). Confirmation of the location of the epileptic focus must depend not only on the information from the clinical history but also on the corroborating findings from the radiologic and electroencephalographic evaluation.

The indications for consideration of surgical resection of an epileptic focus are as follows:

1. The attacks should be numerous and resistant to treatment.

2. The attacks should constitute a significant family and social handicap.

3. The epilepsy should have been present for at least 2 years.

4. Careful clinical evaluation should give reasonable evidence of an objective abnormality of the brain as judged by one or all of the following: skull roentgenogram, pneumoencephalogram, angiogram, or electroencephalogram.

5. Repeated electroencephalograms must show the persistence of the focus and its fixed location and this location in the brain should be confirmed by radio-

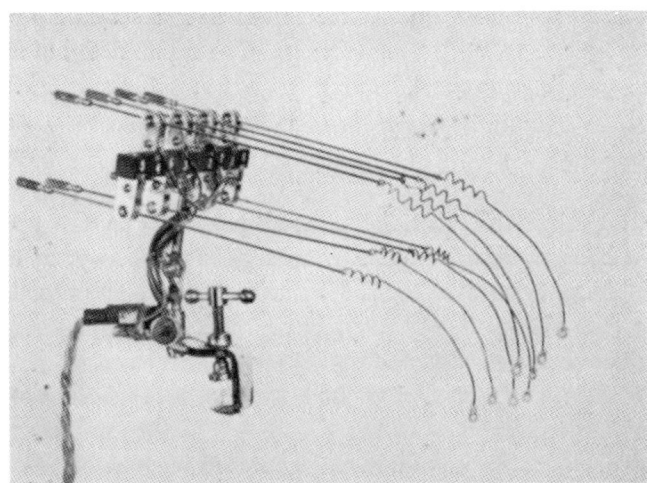

Figure 38. Electrodes used by Penfield for direct electrocorticogram on exposed brain. (From Penfield, W., and Jasper, H.: Epilepsy and the Functional Anatomy of the Human Brain. Boston, Little, Brown & Company, 1954.)

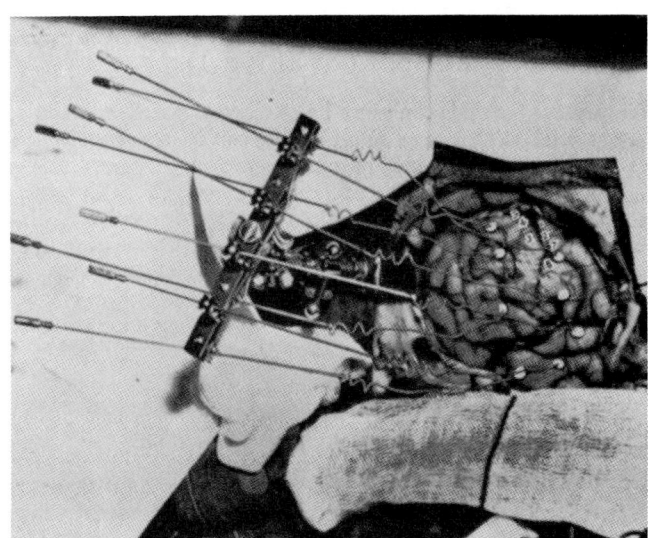

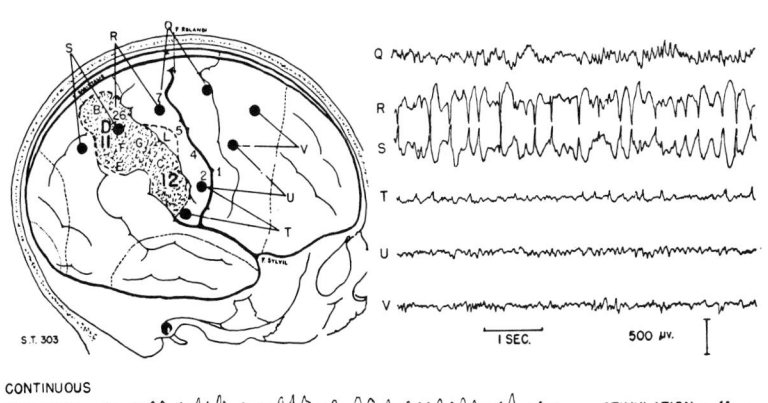

Figure 39. Focal cortical seizures. Note afterdischarge following stimulation within the area of high-voltage rhythmic spikes. The onset of the patient's attack was reproduced at points 11 and 12. (From Penfield, W., and Jasper, H.: Epilepsy and the Functional Anatomy of the Human Brain. Boston, Little, Brown & Company, 1954.)

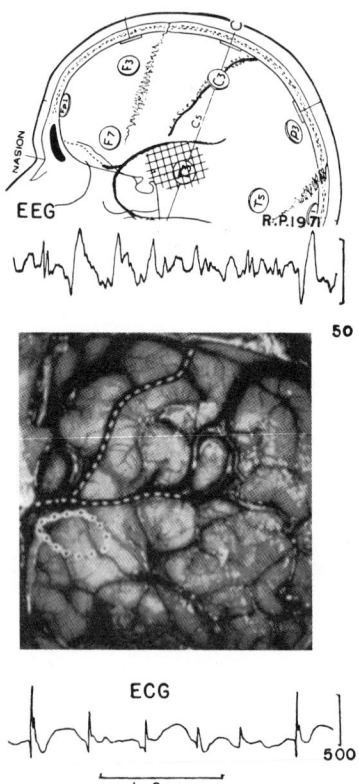

Figure 40. Spike focus, first temporal convolution. Localization of spike focus on border of tumor. Upper picture shows electroencephalographic abnormality recorded from scalp. The lower picture shows exposed temporal lobe with the spikes recorded from area outlined in black dots. (From Penfield, W., and Jasper, H.: Epilepsy and the Functional Anatomy of the Human Brain. Boston, Little, Brown & Company, 1954.)

graphic or angiographic studies and the clinical history.

6. One must deal with a mature brain, which means waiting a longer time before operating for epilepsy in young children or adolescents; however, temporal lobe epilepsy occurring in adolescents may be an exception to this rule, since relief occurs in about 75 per cent of these patients regardless of their age.

7. The presence of psychiatric disturbance warrants serious consideration for surgery.

Surgical Treatment of Temporal Lobe or Psychomotor Epilepsy

The surgical treatment of unilateral temporal lobe epilepsy has been highly successful with relief in about 75 per cent of the patients. This means that in most patients anticonvulsants can be stopped 1 year after temporal lobectomy. Brain injury sustained either at birth or postnatally may be a source for temporal lobe epilepsy, since it is thought to produce sclerosis of the mesial temporal structures. The cause of this pathologic sclerosis, however, may be unknown in certain patients and the brain tissue removed at surgery may reveal microscopic arteriovenous anoma-

lies or hamartomas. It is well known that the higher rates of cure after surgery for epilepsy occur in those patients in whom a definitive pathologic lesion can be demonstrated in the excised brain tissue.

The epileptic phenomena reported by patients during temporal lobe seizures include auditory illusions, hallucinations, feeling of fear, visual illusions, amnesia, déjà vu phenomena, and olfactory sensations. During or after the seizure the patient may exhibit aggressive behavior, automatism, memory changes, or simple alterations in awareness.

Two kinds of temporal lobe seizures have been recognized. Uncinate seizures originate from the region of amygdaloid nucleus in the mesial part of the temporal lobe. The person experiences olfactory hallucinations and somatic sensations such as strange feelings in the head, chest, or neck along with a visceral aura with rising or falling epigastric sensation. There may be unilateral or bilateral tonic motor effects during and especially after the seizure, and the patient remains confused, exhibiting automatic and irrelevant behavior in the period of postictal amnesia. Lateral temporal cortex seizures originate from the lateral temporal cortex and are more complex in their behavioral expression, with auditory phenomena, changes in physical or perceptual events, fear, illusion, déjà vu, and postictal behavioral disorders (Fig. 40). Electrical stimulation of the abnormal epileptic cortex in the region of the temporal lobe focus at the time of operation or with depth electrodes may set off the patient's seizure pattern, and greatly aid in its location.

Infantile Hemiplegia with Intractable Epilepsy

Intractable epilepsy due to infantile hemiplegia can be successfully relieved by surgical excision of the diseased cerebral hemisphere plus the basal ganglia. The hemiplegia may be caused by an acute cerebral insult occurring at or just after birth, and whether or not birth trauma, vascular occlusion, or vital infection may be primarily responsible for the development of this type of epilepsy is not known. In some patients the brain injury probably results from an acute occlusion of the middle cerebral artery. The pathologic consequence of this massive cerebral insult is the development of widespread cerebral scarring followed by intractable epilepsy. The epileptic attacks often involve the hemiplegic side, but generalized seizures also can occur and are very resistant to medical therapy. These children, when they are examined, exhibit hemiatrophy of the body opposite the injured hemisphere. The cranial cavity on the side of the cerebral insult is often smaller and skull roentgenogram may show an elevation of the bones of the sphenoid or petrous pyramid, while the pneumoencephalogram reveals a dilated or deformed ventricular system. Angiography often demonstrates a threadlike atrophic middle cerebral artery, which carries a minimum of blood to the injured cerebral hemisphere, and its blood supply often comes via collateral circulation from either the anterior or posterior cerebral arteries. An insult to the left cerebral hemisphere does not usually affect speech development if it occurs before the patient is 5 years of age, and resection of the damaged left hemisphere causes no speech defect. These children often show some degree of mental retardation, which may improve after surgery as a result of removal of the adverse influence on brain function of the epilepsy combined with anticonvulsant drugs. In addition to these physical signs, the electroencephalographic observations are of importance in the diagnostic evaluation. The electroencephalographic abnormalities originate from widespread epileptic foci in the damaged hemisphere. They are often greater in the central regions of the brain, but isolated epileptic activity may occur in other lobes of the brain as well as in the opposite cerebral hemisphere. The occurrence of bilateral electroencephalographic abnormalities does not contraindicate surgery, since the epilepsy in the uninvolved hemisphere often subsides after removal of the damaged brain tissue.

At surgery the diseased cerebral hemisphere and the basal ganglia are removed and pathologic examination of the brain tissue reveals intense scarring in the cortex and white matter, with intense astrocytosis and obliteration of the cerebral blood vessels. Children tolerate the operation well, but occasionally defective absorption of cerebrospinal fluid may follow the hemispherectomy, requiring correction by a ventricular shunt. After surgical excision of the hemisphere, little motor or sensory defect is superimposed on the hemiplegic side and the reduction of seizures is usually immediate, with improvement of the electroencephalographic pattern from the remaining brain. Anticonvulsant medication can often be reduced; this improves the child's alertness and his I.Q. No brain is better than bad (epileptic) brain, and so every effort should be made to relieve the seizures in these children.

Stereotactic Treatment of Epilepsy

Spiegel and Wycis were the first to use stereotactic methods to treat epilepsy; they noted improvement of myoclonic seizures in a few persons following coagulation of the basal ganglia.[5]

The childhood epilepsies often originate from the subcortical regions of the brain. The most common disorders are centrencephalic epilepsy (petit mal), myoclonic jerking, and reflex sensory signs. Patients in this group are among the most resistant to treatment. Stereotactic techniques using implanted electrodes in the thalamus, brain stem, and basal ganglia are now being used to investigate these disorders in an effort to devise surgical treatments. Temporal lobe seizures associated with emotional instability or hyperactive aggressive behavior have been relieved by

stereotactic lesions in the amygdaloid region. There occurs a normalization of the patient's behavior even though his seizure pattern may not be significantly altered. At times better control of the attacks can be achieved with lesser amounts of anticonvulsants. Reduction in the number of major motor seizures (grand mal) have followed stereotactic lesions in the Forel-H field and thalamic lesions, which are believed to block the conduction pathways of the epileptic spread to deeper regions of the brain stem responsible for the major clonic and tonic seizure with loss of consciousness. These newer stereotactic approaches to the surgical treatment of epilepsy still have limited clinical application, but they have increased our understanding of the distribution of epileptic activity in the subcortical regions of the brain.

SELECTED REFERENCES

Krynauw, R. A.: Infantile hemiplegia treated by removal of one cerebral hemisphere. J. Neurol. Neurosurg. Psychiatr., *13*:243, 1950.
The first neurosurgical report of hemispherectomy for relief of intractable seizures.

Penfield, W., and Jasper, H.: Epilepsy and the Functional Anatomy of the Human Brain. Boston, Little, Brown and Company, 1954.
A detailed analysis of seizure disorders using extensive electroencephalographic evaluation and direct electrical stimulation of the brain at the time of excision of the epileptic focus. The modern foundation of the neurosurgical treatment of seizures is based on these observations.

Speigel, E. A., and Wycis, H. T.: Stereoencephalotomy. Part 2: Clinical and Physiological Application. New York, Grune and Stratton, 1962.
The first detailed analysis of seizure disorders and their treatment using stereotactic technique.

Taylor, J. (Ed.): Selected Writings of John Hughlings Jackson. Volumes 1 and 2. New York, Basic Books, 1958.
A collection of Jackson's papers on epilepsy and epileptiform convulsions in volume one, and his observations on the evaluation and dissolution of the nervous system in volume two. Jackson's concepts of the functioning of the central nervous system are still the basis for modern neurologic thought.

REFERENCES

1. Foerster, O.: Zur operativen Behandlung der Epilepsie. Dtsch. Z. Nervenheilkd., *89*:137, 1926.
2. Horsley, V.: Brain surgery. Br. Med. J., *2*:670, 1886.
3. Krynauw, R. A.: Infantile hemiplegia treated by removal of one cerebral hemisphere. J. Neurol. Neurosurg. Psychiatr., *13*:243, 1950.
4. Penfield, W., and Jasper, H.: Epilepsy and the Functional Anatomy of the Human Brain. Boston, Little, Brown and Company, 1954.
5. Spiegel, E. A., and Wycis, H. T.: Stereoencephalotomy. Part 2: Clinical and Physiological Application. New York, Grune and Stratton, 1962.

XIV

STEREOTACTIC NEUROSURGERY

Blaine S. Nashold, Jr., M.D.

Clarke and Horsley in 1906, seeking a method of producing localized lesions in the cerebellar nuclei of animals with minimal damage to the cerebellar cortex, devised the first animal stereotactic instrument.[4, 5] Since then the stereotactic technique has been used extensively in neurophysiologic and neuroanatomic laboratories, and much of our knowledge of brain function has been based on data gathered by this technique; one of the greatest advantages of stereotactic neurosurgery has been the use of small exploring probes that can be safely introduced into the thalamus, midbrain, or cerebellum.[10]

In 1947, Spiegel and Wycis applied the stereotactic technique to man and so began the exploration of these deeper regions of the brain in patients suffering from epilepsy, involuntary movement disorders, and psychiatric disturbances.[18] A breakthrough occurred in Parkinson's disease with relief of tremor and rigidity following lesions of the globus pallidus and, later, thalamic lesions.[3] Cooper has carried out extensive thalamic surgery for the therapeutic relief of parkinsonian tremor, intention tremor, and other involuntary movements, and low mortality and good clinical results.[19] The overall mortality of stereotactic operations is less than 2 per cent and the morbidity averages 2 per cent. The serious complications include hemiplegia, aphasia, hyperkinesis, ocular dysfunction, convulsive seizures, altered mentation, and hypothalamic dysfunction.

The basic principle in the use of stereotactic surgery is that of localizing a point in space and defining its position with respect to or relative to some suitable frame of reference. The precise location of the point can be defined numerically or graphically. Most stereotactic frames use a right-angled reference system after the cartesian coordinate system of the French mathematician and philosopher Descartes. The cartesian system is convenient to use, and it is relatively easy to construct a physical system on these principles that allows the surgeon to locate the tip of the probe or electrode at a particular point in space, defined by its three coordinates. Furthermore, the position of the tip can easily be changed by any desired amount in any one of the three mutually perpendicular directions.

Stereotactic Surgical Technique

The neurosurgical techniques necessary for stereotactic operations require the use of a precision stereotactic instrument that can direct probes into various subcortical regions through a small burr hole in the skull (Fig. 41). The intracerebral target is determined from the coordinates of a special stereotactic atlas of the human brain with sections in the coronal, sagittal, and horizontal planes (Fig. 42). At the time of operation localization of the intracerebral target is made

from outline of the ventricular system on an x-ray film. Specific internal landmarks in the brain are used, such as the anterior and posterior commissure, which can be visualized. Then the position of the brain target can be determined from the measurements on the x-ray film and these coordinates can be translated to the stereotactic frame to direct the introduction of the brain probe.

The normal anatomic variations of the human brain, often altered by central nervous system diseases, may cause a certain degree of imprecision in exact target localization; however, these variations can be minimized by using electrical stimulation or electroencephalographic recordings of the brain tissue in or near the target area. The cerebral target can therefore be identified by its anatomic, physiologic, and electrical characteristics, and, for example, activation or suppression of parkinsonian tremor following electrical stimulation or cooling of the thalamus can be a useful technique to localize the position of therapeutic lesion in the thalamus that will relieve the tremor.

Electrographic recordings from the thalamic and midbrain nuclei have not been as helpful in the precise nuclear localization as expected; however, evoked electrical responses produced by the stimulation of a peripheral nerve have been employed for localization in the sensory regions of the central nervous system. The implantation of depth electrodes adds to the understanding of distribution and characteristics of the epileptic activity originating from these deeper cerebral regions, but as yet no definitive method of treatment has evolved for relief of epilepsy of subcortical origin.

The ideal technique for producing a therapeutic lesion in the central nervous system of man has as yet not been perfected, however. At present three methods are employed: use of the mechanical leukotome, thermal coagulation, and freezing coagulation. Each of these techniques has certain advantages and disadvantages that must be considered by the stereotactic surgeon, but currently coagulation by heat and by cold are the most popular methods and the clinical results from the two seem about equal. The current era of brain exploration and mapping compares with the earliest efforts of Horsley, Foerster, and Penfield, who pioneered the exploration of the cortical mantle in man.

Complications of Stereotactic Surgery

The immediate operative complications of stereotactic surgery include acute subdural hygroma, subdural hematoma, and intraventricular hemorrhage, which are due to tapping the lateral ventricles or passage of the probe through the brain. Late complications are related to the effects produced by the lesion and may

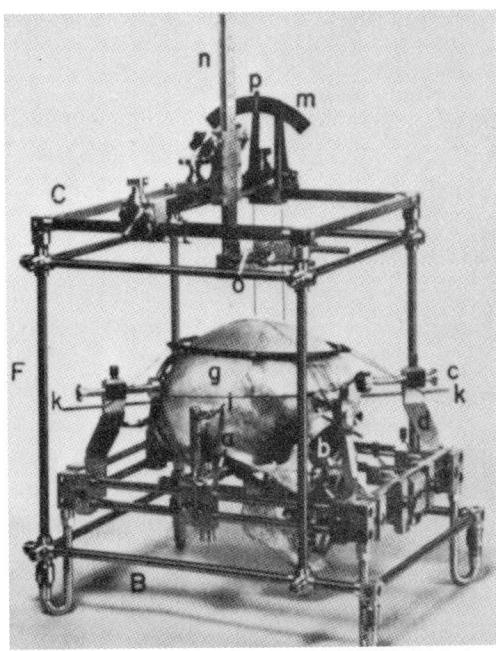

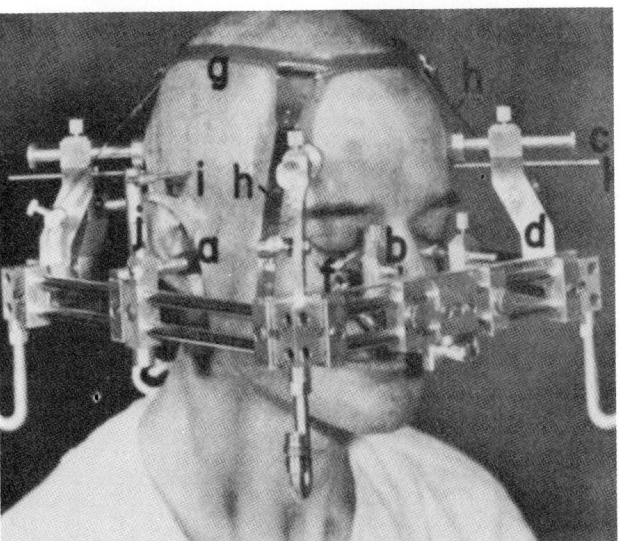

Figure 41. Human stereotactic instrument devised by Spiegel and Wycis. Upper picture shows complete stereotactic instrument and electrode carrier. Lower picture shows baseplate attached to patient's head, electrode carrier applied later after placement of burr hole in skull. (From Spiegel, E. A., et al.: Science, *106*:349, 1947.)

include hemiparesis or speech defects of varying degrees (2 per cent), hyperkinetic movements due to misplaced lesions (2.5 per cent), convulsive seizures (rare), and change in mentation (transient).[14]

Disorders Treated with Stereotactic Surgery

Treatment has been carried out in persons with a variety of involuntary movement disorders due to extrapyramidal disease, for relief of painful syndromes,

for palliation of epilepsy and mental disturbances, for injection of radioactive material into brain tumors, for thrombosis of intracranial aneurysms, and for the recovery of foreign bodies from the depths of the brain.[12, 20, 21]

To date, patients with parkinsonism represent the largest group treated by stereotactic surgery. The etiology of parkinsonism is unknown and the nature of the pathophysiology is still obscure, although recent evidence points to a biochemical disturbance of catecholamine metabolism in the basal ganglia or subthalamic region. In some parkinsonian patients the dopamine content in the basal ganglia may be reduced and replacement with L-dopa administered orally has dramatically relieved the akinesia and rigidity. Tremor, when it is a major disabling symptom, can best be relieved by a therapeutic lesion in the ventrobasal complex of the thalamus with periods of relief from tremor lasting as long as 8 to 10 years in about 70 per cent of the patients.

Athetosis, chorea, dystonia, spasmodic torticollis, and ballismus are also serious disabling involuntary movements that are under active study and treatment by the neurosurgeon using stereotactic techniques.[6] These hyperkinetic disorders are usually nonprogressive. Their pathophysiology remains obscure, and current efforts at drug therapy have been disappointing. Chorea, ballismus, and dystonia can be successfully reduced by stereotactic lesions localized to the ventrolateral thalamus and the adjacent subthalamic region. Athetosis and spasmodic torticollis have not been successfully relieved by stereotactic thalamic lesions. Recently therapeutic lesions involving the dentate nucleus of the cerebellum have been reported to reduce athetoid movements, but these operations are still in a stage of experimental development.[9, 15]

Mental Disorders. Spiegel and Wycis, interested in improving the surgical techniques of frontal leukotomy, developed the first human stereotactic instrument for making lesions in the medial dorsal thal-

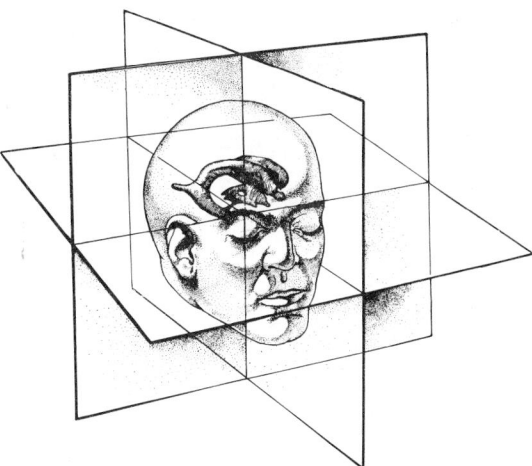

Figure 42. Intersecting planes used to determine intracranial target area during stereotactic surgery. (From Todd-Wells Manual of Stereotactic Procedures.)

amus of psychotic and psychoneurotic patients.[17] They noted long-lasting relief in the patients with anxiety and depression who had previously failed to respond to psychotherapy, drug, or shock treatments alone or in combination. Localized stereotactic lesions made in the mesial temporal lobe in epileptic patients with severe behavioral disorders have resulted in an amelioration of the behavior disorder but have not always altered the epilepsy. Severely hyperkinetic children have been relieved by bilateral amygdaloid lesions without alteration in their intelligence or general ability to function.[13] Recently patients with violent and aggressive behavior have shown improvement after a stereotactic lesion was made in the posteromedial hypothalamus.[16] Bilateral lesions of the cingulate gyrus of the frontal lobes have successfully relieved certain patients with affective disorders, severe psychosis, and intractable pain.[2, 8] Greater use of these techniques to treat and investigate mental disorders can be expected in the future.

Brain Tumor. The stereotactic techniques have had limited use in exploring brain tumors either by tapping deep-lying cystic tumors for the recovery of brain biopsies or for introduction of radioactive materials into cystic lesions. Stereotactic transfrontal or transsphenoidal hypophysectomies to destroy the anterior pituitary gland will satisfactorily relieve pain due to metastatic cancer from the breast or prostate. The symptoms of acromegaly can be arrested by stereotactic ablation of the pituitary gland.[21]

Other Uses of Stereotaxy. Although the method is new, certain intracranial aneurysms or arteriovenous anomalies may be treated by stereotactic surgery. A special probe is introduced through a burr hole to the site of the vascular anomaly. Obliteration of the aneurysmal sac may be done with heat or with an ingenious technique that employs a magnetic probe placed on the dome of the aneurysm.[1, 11] A suspension of iron particles is then injected into the sac of the aneurysms; the iron particles are held in the aneurysm by the magnet, resulting in coagulation and obliteration of the sac. The method may prove useful in those lesions inaccessible to direct surgical attack or could be used in poor-risk surgical patients to tide them over the critical period of time during the first 2 weeks after rupture of the aneurysm when rebleeding may occur and is often fatal.

Stereotactic neurosurgical techniques are new and still in early stages of development. New applications in the treatment of neurologic disorders can be expected in the future, along with the enriching of our knowledge of the function of the human subcortex, a hope expressed by Clarke and Horsley five decades ago.[4]

SELECTED REFERENCES

Alksne, J. R., Fingerhut, A. G., and Rand, R. W.: Magnetically controlled metallic thrombosis of intracranial aneurysms. Surgery, 60:212, 1966.
The use of stereotactic method employing magnetic thrombosis of intracranial aneurysms.

Clarke, R. H., and Horsley, V.: On a method of investigating the deep ganglia and tracts of the central nervous system. Br. Med. J., 2:1799, 1906.

The first report in 1906 of the development and design of the stereotactic instrument for lobotomy.

Narabayashi, H., Nugao, T., Saito, Y., Yoshida, M., and Nagahata, M.: Stereotaxic amygdalotomy for behavioral disorders. Arch. Neurol.,9:1, 1963.
The modification of abnormal human behavior by specific stereotactic lesions in the amygdaloid nucleus of the temporal lobe.

Spiegel, E. A., and Wycis, H. T.: Stereoencephalotomy. Part II: Clinical and Physiological Applications. New York, Grune and Stratton, 1962.
The first detailed clinical use of stereoencephalotomy in the treatment of involuntary movements, pain, mental disorders, and epilepsy.

Spiegel, E. A., Wycis, H. T., Marks, M., and Lee, A. J.: Stereotactic apparatus for operation on the human brain. Science, 106:349, 1947.
The first report in 1947 of the development of a human stereotactic instrument.

REFERENCES

1. Alksne, J. R., Fingerhut, A. G., and Rand, R. W.: Magnetically controlled metallic thrombosis of intracranial aneurysms. Surgery, 60:212, 1966.
2. Ballantine, H. T., Jr., Cassidy, W. L., Flanagan, N. W., and Marino, R., Jr.: Stereotactic anterior cingulotomy for neuropsychiatric illness and intractable pain. J. Neurosurg., 26:488, 1967.
3. Bertrand, C., and Martinez, N.: Experimental and clinical surgery in dyskinetic disease. Confin. Neurol., 22:375, 1962.
4. Clarke, R. H.: Atlas of Photographs of the Frontal Sections of the Cranium and Brain of the Rhesus Monkey, Baltimore, The Johns Hopkins Hospital Reports, Special Volume, 1920.
5. Clarke, R. H., and Horsley, V.: On a method of investigating the deep ganglia and tracts of the central nervous system. Br. Med. J., 2:1799, 1906.
6. Cooper, I. S.: Relief of juvenile involuntary movement disorders by chemopallidectomy. J.A.M.A., 164:1297, 1957.
7. Cooper, I. S.: Clinical and physiologic implications of thalamic surgery for dystonia and torticollis. Bull. N.Y. Acad. Med., 41:870, 1965.
8. Foltz, E. L., and White, L. E.: Pain relief by frontal cingulotomy. J. Neurosurg., 19:89, 1962.
9. Heimburger, R. F.: Dentatectomy in the treatment of dyskinetic disorders. Confin. Neurol., 29:101, 1967.
10. Horsley, V., and Clarke, R. H.: The structure and functions of the cerebellum examined by a new method. Brain, 31:45, 1908.
11. Mullan, S., Raimondi, A. J., Dobben, G., Vailati, G., and Hekmatpanah, J.: Electrically induced thrombosis in intracranial aneurysms. J. Neurosurg., 22:539, 1965.
12. Mullan, S., Vailati, G., Karasick, J., and Malis, M.: Thalamic lesions for control of epilepsy. Arch. Neurol., 16:277, 1967.
13. Narabayashi, H., Nugao, T., Saito, Y., Yoshida, M., and Nagahata, M.: Stereotaxic amygdalotomy for behavioral disorders. Arch. Neurol., 9:1, 1963.
14. Nashold, B. S., Jr.: Operative complications due to stereotactic surgery. Confin. Neurol., 30:325, 1968.
15. Nashold, B. S., Jr., and Slaughter, D. G.: Stimulation and lesions of the deeper regions in the cerebellum of man. J. Neurosurg., 31:172–186, 1969.
16. Sano, K., Yoshioka, M., Ogashiwa, M., Ishijima, B., and Ohyl, C.: Posteromedial hypothalamotomy in the treatment of aggressive behavior. Confin. Neurol., 27:164, 1965.
17. Spiegel, E. A., and Wycis, H. T.: Stereoencephalotomy. Part II: Clinical and Physiological Applications. New York, Grune and Stratton, 1962.
18. Spiegel, E. A., Wycis, H. T., Marks, M., and Lee, A. J.: Stereotactic apparatus for operation on the human brain. Science, 106:349, 1947.
19. Stellar, S., and Cooper, I. S.: Mortality and morbidity in cryothalamectomy for parkinsonism. J. Neurosurg., 28:459, 1968.
20. Sugita, K., Sato, O., Takaoka, Y., Mutsuga, N., and Tsugane, R.: Successful removal of intracranial air-gun bullet with stereotaxic apparatus. J. Neurosurg., 30:177, 1969.
21. Wycis, H. T., Baird, H. W., III, and Spiegel, E. A.: Long range results following pallidotomy and pallidoamygdalotomy in certain types of convulsive disorders. Confin. Neurol., 27:114, 1966.
22. Zervas, N. T.: Technique of radiofrequency hypophysectomy. Confin. Neurol., 26:143, 1965.

44

DISORDERS OF THE MUSCULOSKELETAL SYSTEM

I ——————————————————————————————

FRACTURES AND DISLOCATIONS: GENERAL PRINCIPLES

John M. Harrelson, M.D.

The treatment of fractures and dislocations requires a knowledge of the anatomy, physiology, and biomechanics of the musculoskeletal system. While a fracture represents a disruption in the continuity of a bone, it also represents a major soft tissue injury. The fracture surgeon must be aware of the soft tissue structures adjacent to a fracture site and be alert for neurologic and vascular components of the injury. Since many fractures occur in a setting of violent trauma, full evaluation of each patient is necessary, and the surgeon must be prepared to deal with major injuries in other tissue systems.

Mechanism and Classification of Fractures

When sufficient force is applied to a bone, fracture results. When a single fracture line is produced, it is referred to as a *simple* fracture. When multiple fracture lines and bone fragments exist, the fracture is said to be *comminuted*. When penetrating injury has produced a fracture or when fracture fragments have protruded through the skin, an *open* fracture exists. When no such wound is present, the fracture is classified as *closed*. The distinction is important, since open fractures are likely to be contaminated with pyogenic bacteria. The treatment and prognosis of open fractures are significantly different from those of closed fractures.

The force necessary to produce a fracture may be transmitted to the skeleton in a variety of ways. The direction and rate of application of the force govern to some extent the pattern of the fracture and the associated soft tissue injury. When a bending moment is applied to bone, a simple transverse or oblique fracture line usually results. When a direct blow or crushing force is applied to bone, a comminuted open frac-

ture often results. There is usually severe soft tissue injury as well. When torque or twisting force is applied to bone, a spiral or oblique fracture results. When compression force is applied along the longitudinal axis of a bone, an impacted fracture may result. This type of fracture usually occurs at the junction between the metaphysis and diaphysis, where the cortex becomes thin. The diaphyseal portion of the bone is usually impacted into the metaphyseal fragment. Traction force applied to a bone may also produce fracture. Vigorous or violent muscle contraction may produce avulsion of portions of bone where major tendons attach.

Fractures in children deserve special consideration. The periosteum is extremely tough in children, and their bones are much more resilient and less brittle than those of adults. Bending moments applied to the bone of a child may result in a "greenstick" fracture in which there is distraction of the cortex on the convex side and compression of bone on the concave side. There will be angulation at the fracture site but no other displacement. Fractures may occur through the physeal plates and result in future growth disturbance. The parents should accordingly be cautioned. When fracture occurs entirely within the physeal plate and there is no displacement of the epiphysis relative to the metaphysis, anatomic reduction produces good results with no disturbance in growth. When the fracture line extends part way through the physeal plate and then through either the adjacent metaphysis or epiphysis, accurate anatomic reduction is mandatory in order to avoid future growth disturbance. When compression forces have produced a fracture across the physeal plate, growth disturbance is a likely result. More subtle trauma may also produce fractures. In the elderly patient with osteoporosis or in the patient with a metabolic bone-wasting disease, the activities of daily living may be sufficient to produce fracture in diseased bone. Such injuries are referred to as *pathologic* fractures. The most common cause of the pathologic fracture is metastatic carcinoma, in which fracture occurs through a deposit of tumor that has eroded and weakened bone. Fracture may occur in healthy bone with the repetitive application of minor trauma. Such fractures are called fatigue or stress fractures and may be seen in the metatarsals after a long hike or in the tibia or femur in individuals who are vigorously training for athletic activities.

Acute Complications

When a fracture occurs, there is bleeding from the broken bone ends and from the adjacent soft tissues involved in the injury. A rapidly enlarging hematoma envelops the fracture site. Since most fractures occur as a result of significant force, the bone ends are frequently displaced. This displacement is increased by the pull of those muscles that cross the fracture site and may further increase the extent of soft tissue injury.

The initial evaluation of the fracture patient requires a careful neurologic and vascular examination. The proximity of major nerves to bone makes them vulnerable to injury from adjacent fracture fragments. Direct arterial injury may also occur as a result of penetration by a sharp bone fragment. More often, vascular insufficiency of a fractured limb is the result of swelling from the fracture hematoma with compression of adjacent vessels. When bleeding occurs within a closed compartment, muscle ischemia progressing to eventual muscle necrosis may develop. This situation exists with bleeding into the anterior compartment of the leg or into the volar compartment of the forearm. The surgeon must be aware of these syndromes and be prepared to do a decompressive fasciotomy.

Adjacent organ injury occurs with certain fractures. Fractures of the rib cage may rupture the lung, produce lacerations of the liver, or penetrate the spleen. Fractures of the pelvis, particularly those in which there is disruption of the symphysis pubis, may produce rupture of the bladder. Spinal fracture introduces the risk of injury to the spinal cord. Bleeding from spinal fractures into the retroperitoneal space may produce a temporary paralytic ileus. With fractures of the femur or pelvis or with multiple fractures, the hemorrhage at the fracture sites may be sufficient to produce hypovolemic shock.

In a small number of fractures, the syndrome of fat embolization occurs. This respiratory complication of multiple fractures is most frequently seen in those patients who have been in hypovolemic shock. The clinical signs develop within the first 12 to 72 hours following injury. Tachypnea and dyspnea are the first signs of decreasing pulmonary function caused by fat embolism. Small punctate petechiae develop over the chest and abdomen. The patient shows confusion and delirium progressing to coma without associated localizing neurologic signs. These mental changes are the direct result of decreasing arterial oxygen tension. The chest x-ray in patients with fat embolism shows a diffuse patchy infiltrate throughout both lung fields.

The urine shows free fat particles and the serum lipase may be elevated. Early recognition of a developing fat embolization syndrome is essential. The symptoms may be sudden in onset and the patient may deteriorate rapidly, with fatal results. The earliest clinical signs of a developing syndrome are rising pulse and respiratory rates. A falling arterial Po_2 is a more sensitive indicator of impending problems. It has been our custom to draw daily arterial blood gases for the first five days after injury in patients with major skeletal trauma. When the syndrome of fat embolization is recognized, administration of corticosteroid hormones is of benefit. Large doses are continued for three to five days and then abruptly stopped. Oxygen is administered by tent, intubation, or tracheostomy as necessary. A volume respirator may be necessary in severe cases.

Principles of Fracture Treatment

Reduction. Fractures are displaced as a result of either etiologic trauma or the pull of muscles crossing the fracture site or both. In order to reduce a displaced fracture, the patient must first be relieved of his pain by either local anesthetic injection or systemic analgesics. It is then necessary to overcome the spasm of those muscles bridging the fracture site, allowing restoration of length of the fractured member and correction of angulation and rotation. The reduction of a fracture may be accomplished in several ways.

Manipulative reduction can be accomplished by the examiner in fractures of the distal portion of the extremities, where one can manually overcome the pull of those muscles bridging the fracture site. When the fracture is more proximal (humerus, femur), the muscle spasm is too great for manipulative reduction. In this situation it is necessary to apply steady, prolonged *traction*. For femoral fractures, this is accomplished by inserting a transverse pin through the proximal tibia or distal femur and placing the patient in bed with continuous pull on the pin. The muscle spasm is gradually overcome, length is restored, and alignment is achieved. It is sometimes acceptable to use skin traction by applying strips of felt to the extremity with adhesive and attaching them to the appropriate amount of weight. Some fractures are not appropriately treated by either manipulative reduction or traction. Such fractures may require surgery and *open reduction*. When open reduction is required, it is usually accompanied by some form of internal fixation of the fracture. Fractures that are inherently stable and in acceptable alignment require no reduction.

The goal of reduction is restoration of length of the extremity, correction of angulation and rotation, and apposition of the bone ends. Once reduction has been accomplished, fracture healing requires that the bone be immobilized.

Some fractures require excision of a portion of bone rather than reduction and immobilization. Comminuted fractures of the patella are appropriately treated by excision of the patella and repair of the patellar tendon rather than by attempts at reduction. Fractures of the radial head with severe comminution of the articular surface are best treated by excision of the radial head and replacement with a prosthesis. In both of these situations, excision is performed to avoid a painful irregular articular surface. Prosthetic replacement is also required in fractures of the neck of the femur in elderly patients. In this situation the articular surface is not comminuted. Rather, healing is prolonged in these fractures and the circulation to the femoral head is disrupted. Overall rehabilitation of the elderly patient is significantly shortened by removing the femoral head and replacing it with a prosthetic component.

Immobilization

Immobilization of fractures may be accomplished in a variety of ways. Impacted fractures with inherent stability may require only a sling or soft dressing for comfort. Fractures requiring operative reduction also require internal fixation. Fractures about the hip are treated in this way because of their inherent instability when treated by other methods and because of the morbidity associated with prolonged bed rest or cast immobilization. Most fractures of the extremities can be appropriately treated by plaster immobilization. While the many advantages of plaster are well recognized, it should be borne in mind that improperly applied plaster may create more injury than it treats. The surgeon should be familiar with proper plaster technique. The cast should be appropriately padded and smooth on its inner surface and should not be constricting.

Since a bone participates in joint motion at both ends, it is necessary to immobilize the joint above and below the fracture site. Thus, forearm fractures require long-arm plaster immobilizing both the wrist and the elbow. Plaster maintains the reduction that has been achieved, provides rigid immobility, and relieves pain. A well-reduced, rigidly immobilized fracture should not require a significant amount of analgesic. Swelling occurs at a fracture site and, since a plaster cast is rigid, increasing pressure within the cast will be heralded by increasing pain in the extremity and progressive numbness and diminished circulation of the digits. All fracture patients are cautioned to watch for these signs and should be examined the following day for assessment of the cast and the neurovascular status.

Skeletal traction is used not only to achieve reduction of fractures but to maintain relative immobilization of the fracture. The injured part is placed at rest either on an appropriate splint or on the bed while traction is being applied. Traction is continued until the fracture is stable enough to allow cast or brace immobilization.

Open Fractures

An open fracture should be treated as an *emergency*. Surgical débridement of the wound is required. Since open fractures are usually the result of more violent trauma, other major injuries may be present. When the patient has been fully evaluated and his condition is stable, débridement is performed in the operating room as a formal surgical procedure. All devitalized tissue is removed, with special attention given to devitalized muscle. Macerated skin edges are debrided and the wound thoroughly irrigated with saline containing antibiotics. Bone ends, which may have embedded dirt, paint or other material, are debrided by

sels, and tendons. Repair of nerves and tendons in an open fracture wound is rarely indicated. Vessels require repair if the circulation to the extremity is in jeopardy. When débridement is completed, a decision must be made about stabilization of the fracture. Internal fixation devices are not desirable in a contaminated wound. The use of skeletal traction with a transverse pin placed at some distance from the fracture is acceptable. Cast immobilization with a window overlying the wound is also suitable. The *wound* should be dressed open. Even in minor open fractures, we find little to recommend the practice of immediate closure. The morbidity from delayed closure at five to seven days following débridement is minimal compared to the consequences of infection. Intravenous antibiotics are administered during the first several days following injury. The wound should be cultured at the time of delayed closure. Where extensive skin loss has occurred, split thickness grafting or pedicle flap grafting may be required.

Fracture Healing

When a fracture occurs, a hematoma rapidly develops about the bone ends. As pressure from the hematoma increases, interstitial edema develops in the adjacent soft tissues and there is some degree of venous congestion. Leukocytes invade the hematoma, producing a sterile traumatic inflammatory reaction. Primitive mesenchymal cells within the periosteum and the medullary canal on either side of the fracture line differentiate into primitive osteoblasts and begin to proliferate. These changes are appreciated microscopically at 48 to 72 hours. By this time there is also the development of early granulation tissue about the periphery of the hematoma. This granulation tissue contains other primitive cells from adjacent fascial planes, which also differentiate into osteoblasts.

This proliferation of osteogenic cells and the early primitive bone that they produce constitute the "fracture callus." If the fracture fragments are in apposition and rigidly immobilized, bone growth progresses until the two fracture fragments are united by a network of primitive new bone. As this bone matures, constant remodeling occurs and the trabeculae become oriented to the long axis of the bone.

If there is motion at the fracture site, the primitive mesenchymal cells may differentiate into chondroblasts. If the motion is not excessive or if the fracture site is subsequently rigidly immobilized, this cartilaginous tissue calcifies and is gradually replaced by new bone by the process of endochondral ossification. When distraction of the fracture fragments is present or when muscle is interposed between the fracture fragments, dense fibrous tissue develops between the fracture ends. Again, if rigid immobilization is achieved this fibrous tissue may ultimately be replaced by bone. If in the latter two situations rigid immobilization is not achieved, nonunion results. When motion is persistent at the fracture site the differentiation of cartilage progresses. A cleft develops between the layers of cartilage covering each fracture fragment, and cells at the periphery of this cleft differentiate into synovial cells, producing a *pseudarthrosis*. If distraction at the fracture site is allowed to persist, a dense fibrous scar develops between the bone ends, producing a *fibrous nonunion.* Compression of a fracture enhances fracture healing. This principle is used in treatment. Fractures of the tibial shaft may be treated in a walking cast, allowing the patient to bear weight across the fracture site. The compression principle may be used with internal fixation devices. Plates have been designed that allow rigid internal fixation of long bone fractures, with compression exerted at the fracture site. Fracture healing is also affected by the available blood supply to bone involved. In general, cancellous bone at the metaphyseal ends of long bones has a richer blood supply than the diaphysis. Fractures in these areas heal more rapidly than shaft fractures. Long bones with more overlying muscle have a greater blood supply. The shaft of the femur, enveloped by muscle, has a better blood supply than the distal tibia, which is subcutaneous in one third of its circumference. Fractures of the tibial shaft traditionally are slower to heal.

Late Complications

The soft tissue injury that accompanies a fracture results in scarring of the adjacent muscles, ligaments, and tendons and produces limitation of motion of the joints adjacent to the fracture. Fractures occurring close to a joint produce more limitation of motion than fractures of the midshaft. Once the fracture has healed, rehabilitation of the extremity involves rehabilitation of the soft tissues. Physical therapy in the form of active and passive exercises may be necessary. Tendons may become adherent to the underlying bone, and subsequent surgical release may be necessary. Because of the muscle atrophy that has resulted from inactivity, stasis edema is usually present after fracture and gradually diminishes as muscle tone and strength return.

Nonunion of a fracture, either as a pseudarthrosis or a fibrous nonunion, may develop for the reasons mentioned. When an established nonunion is present, operative intervention is usually indicated. Surgical removal of the fibrocartilage or scar tissue that has formed at the fracture site and apposition of fresh bone ends is necessary. It is desirable to bone graft the nonunion at the time of surgery. Bone is obtained either from the patient (autogenous) or from a donor (homologous). The bone graft serves as a mineral lattice for new bone formation and becomes incorporated in the fracture callus. It is gradually replaced by osteoclastic resorption and subsequent new bone deposition, a process known as "creeping substitution."

When a fracture heals with unacceptable angulation or rotation, a *malunion* has occurred, The disability from malunion may be cosmetic or functional or both. The functional disability from malunion may be immediately apparent (rotary malalignment of a forearm fracture, which limits pronation and supination) or may not develop for some time (valgus malalignment of a distal tibial fracture producing subsequent degenerative arthritis of the ankle). Malunion requires surgical intervention for correction. Osteotomy is performed either at the old fracture site or at a more appropriate level and the angular or rotary deformity is corrected. In almost all fractures, some degree of shortening occurs. In the upper extremities, shortening is seldom noticeable and is rarely a functional disability. In the lower extremities, if shortening exceeds one half inch, a shoe lift may be required. In children, fracture often results in stimulation of the physeal growth plates throughout the involved extremity, and overgrowth of that extremity may occur. In some fractures there is loss of circulation to the involved bone with subsequent avascular necrosis. This situation occurs in fractures of the femoral neck in the elderly patient, in fracture dislocations of the talus in any age group, and in fractures through the waist of the carpal navicular bone. Avascular necrosis usually results in collapse of the articular surface of the involved bone and the development of subsequent degenerative arthritis.

Fractures that involve articular surfaces may eventually result in traumatic arthritis. Even with accurate anatomic reduction, the process of healing may produce irregularities on the cartilaginous surface with ingrowth of fibrous tissue and/or fracture callus. Once the congruity of the joint has been lost, gradual deterioration usually occurs. The rate at which degenerative arthritis develops depends on the degree of incongruity, the age of the patient, and the amount of injury to the articular surface at the time of fracture.

II ————

FRACTURES OF THE SPINE

James R. Urbaniak, M.D.

A diagnosis of fracture of the spine ("broken neck" or "broken back") is a terrifying matter to a patient and his family. It frequently signifies that a major disaster has occurred and implies that the patient may be crippled or paralyzed for life. Fractures of the vertebral column are common, but less than 10 per cent of spine fractures are associated with neurologic deficit. More than 90 per cent of spine fractures involve only the skeletal structure, and if proper treatment is instituted, the prognosis is excellent. All patients who complain of pain or tenderness in the neck or back after an injury must be suspected of having a fracture of the spine until proven otherwise. The attending physician should determine the neurologic involvement in the initial assessment, as the early neurologic status greatly influences both the course of treatment and the prognosis.

Trauma subjects the vertebral column to one of five types of violent forces: flexion, flexion and rotation, extension, vertical compression, and direct shearing. If these forces produce motion greater than the physiologic range of the spine, a fracture or dislocation will occur. The spinal cord usually terminates between L1 and L2, and in the cervical and thoracic spinal canal it occupies about 50 per cent of the available space. In the lumbar area the cauda equina is the only neural element in the canal and therefore has much free space in the spinal canal. The anatomic relationship of the vertebral supporting structures, the neural elements, and the type of forces (flexion, compression, etc.) determine the amount of displacement, stability, and neurologic involvement in spinal injuries. The specific injuries and treatment will be discussed individually.

THE CERVICAL SPINE

When a patient complains of pain in the neck after an injury, a fracture or dislocation of the cervical spine should be suspected. A careful history concerning the *method* of the injury is important. If the patient complains of neck pain or tenderness, a complete neurologic examination is followed by cervical spine roentgenograms. The radiographs should include anteroposterior, right and left oblique, lateral, and open-mouth odontoid views. If these are negative, then gentle lateral flexion-extension views of the cervical spine should be obtained to exclude an unstable cervical spine. The physical examination is the most important aspect of the evaluation. If the patient has pain, tenderness, or decreased motion of the neck, or neurologic symptoms or signs, the cervical spine must be immobilized until a complete set of roentgenograms is obtained.

Fractures of the Atlas—Jefferson's Fracture

In 1920, Sir Geoffrey Jefferson described the mechanism of the fracture of the first cervical vertebra. The injury occurs from an axial load on the top of the head. The resultant of the forces is exerted laterally on the ring of C1, and the arches fracture at the thinnest and weakest points (Fig. 1A). Usually the spinal cord is not damaged, as the canal of the atlas is normally large and with the fracture, the fragments spread outward to increase the neural canal. The fracture can usually be diagnosed on the lateral cervical spine roentgenograms, but special films such as the submental vertex view better delineate the injury.

If the neurologic examination is normal, the fracture may be managed conservatively with head halter traction in bed for a few days to allow the acute edema

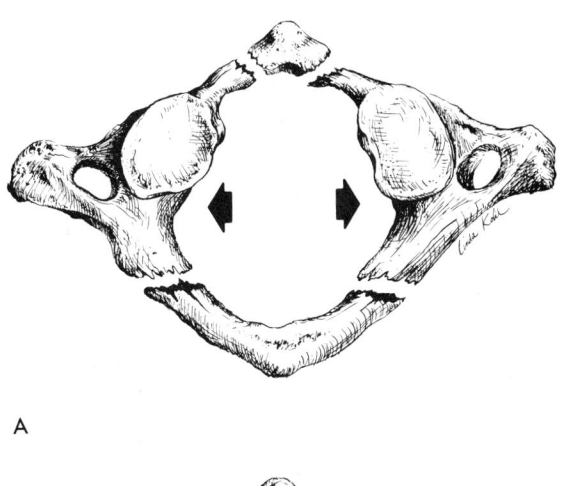

A

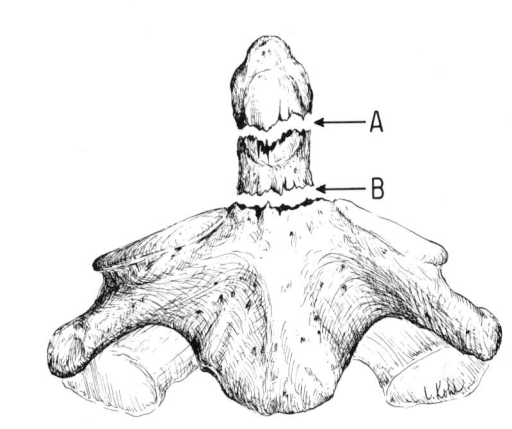

B

Figure 1. *A,* Jefferson fracture. Fracture of the arches of C1 secondary to an axial load. The resultant of the forces, indicated by the arrows, produces the fracture at the thinnest areas of the arch. *B,* A fracture of the odontoid may occur at the waist (A) or at the base (B). The fracture at the base is more stable and usually heals with immobilization. A fracture in the waist of the odontoid is less stable and may require surgical fusion for stabilization.

and pain to subside. A four-poster brace (Duke design) (Fig. 2A) or a cervical collar for six to eight weeks is adequate treatment. If instability on the flexion-extension views or neurologic symptoms or signs occur, then skeletal traction with skull tongs or a halo should be used for two to three weeks; then either a four-poster brace with a head band or preferably a halo cast for three months after injury is indicated (Fig. 2B).

Fractures of the Odontoid

An understanding of the anatomic relationships of the first two cervical vertebrae is essential for a discussion of their injuries. Rotation of the atlas about the odontoid process of the axis accounts for about half of the rotary movement of the head. The dens is held adjacent to the anterior arch of C1 by the transverse ligaments and the alar ligaments. It is important to remember that the dens, spinal cord, and empty space each occupy one third of the spinal canal at the level of the arch of the atlas (the "rule of thirds"). On a lat-

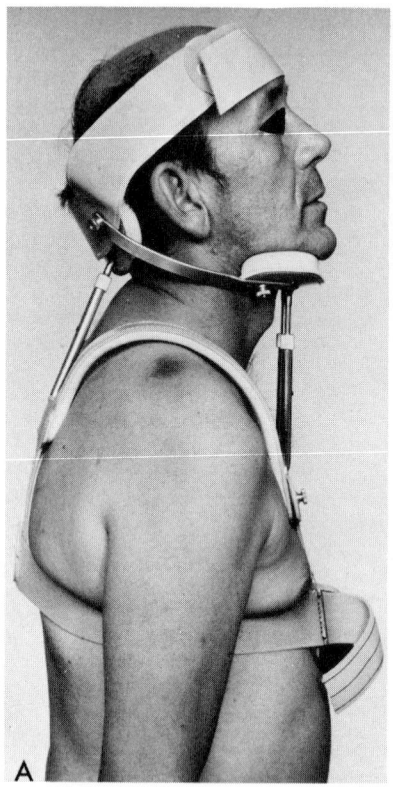
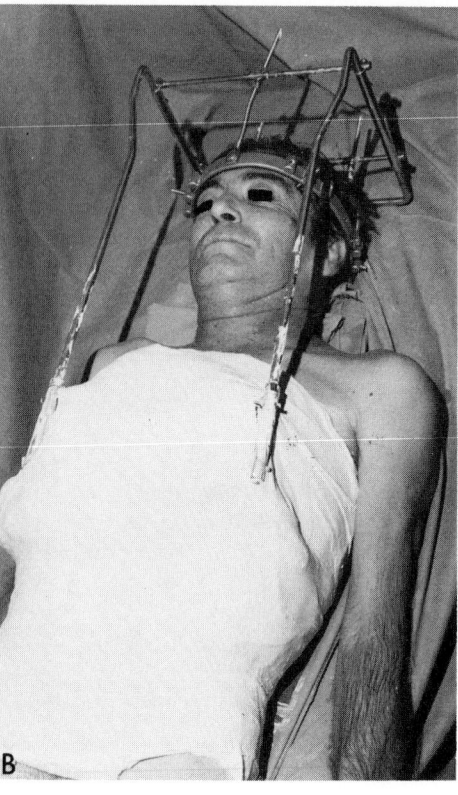

Figure 2. *A*, A four-poster brace (Duke design). The uprights with the chin piece and occiput pad limit flexion and extension of the cervical spine, and the addition of the head band restricts rotation at C1–C2. Ear lobe must be opposite shoulder tip. *B*, Halo cast. The halo, which has four screws inserted in the outer table of the skull, provides for rigid fixation of the cervical spine. The halo may be used for cervical traction in the recumbent position or attached to a cast. The patient may be ambulatory in the halo cast.

eral roentgenogram centered at C2, the predental space is 3 mm. or less in the adult. A predental space of 5mm. indicates rupture of the transverse ligaments, and a predental space of 12 mm. means that all ligaments have been ruptured.

Transverse or alar ligament ruptures are uncommon unless there are predisposing factors such as rheumatoid arthritis, posterior pharyngitis, or ankylosing spondylitis. If such a rupture occurs and the odontoid is intact, cervical myelopathy is a frequent and grim complication.

Fractures of the odontoid (dens) however, occur relatively frequently and represent about 10 per cent of cervical spine fractures. Odontoid fractures, as well as transverse ligament injuries, occur from falls or blows on the head, auto accidents, and sports such as gymnastics. Fractures of the odontoid may occur at two anatomic areas—the base or the waist of the odontoid (Fig. 1*B*).

The diagnosis is often delayed because of the difficulty of visualizing the area on routine films. If the injured patient complains of neck or occipital pain or headaches, or has torticollis, the odontoid area should be examined thoroughly. Lateral views centered at the C2 vertebra and open-mouth views of the odontoid usually allow adequate visualization of the odontoid region. However, tomograms of lateral flexion-extension views and anteroposterior lateral bending views are often helpful.

Immediately or *early* myelopathy occurs in less than one fourth of the patients with fractured odontoids.

However, *delayed* myelopathy may occur in as many as three fourths of patients in whom union or adequate reduction has not been achieved. Fractures through the base of the dens involve primarily cancellous bone of the body of the axis. These fractures are more stable and usually unite during three months of immobilization in a four-poster brace with head band or a Minerva jacket (Figs. 2*A* and 3).

Fractures through the waist of the dens are the most common. Their management is more difficult than the basilar fracture. These fractures should be reduced in extension over a double mattress, with traction (usually head halter is sufficient). After swelling subsides, the patient is maintained in a reduced position with a four-poster brace and head band, a plaster cast, or a halo cast. Although union will usually occur in three to four months if satisfactory reduction and mobilization are achieved, the nonunion rates may be as high as 40 per cent. Operative arthrodesis and wiring of C1 to C2 through a posterior approach are indicated if union is not achieved at three to six months.

Fracture of the Pedicle of the Axis (Hangman's Fracture)

A fracture through the pedicles of C2 usually occurs from a severe extension injury of the neck, such as an auto accident or fall. This injury has been labeled the hangman's fracture because autopsy studies have demonstrated that a long drop with a rope about the neck with the knot in the submental position will

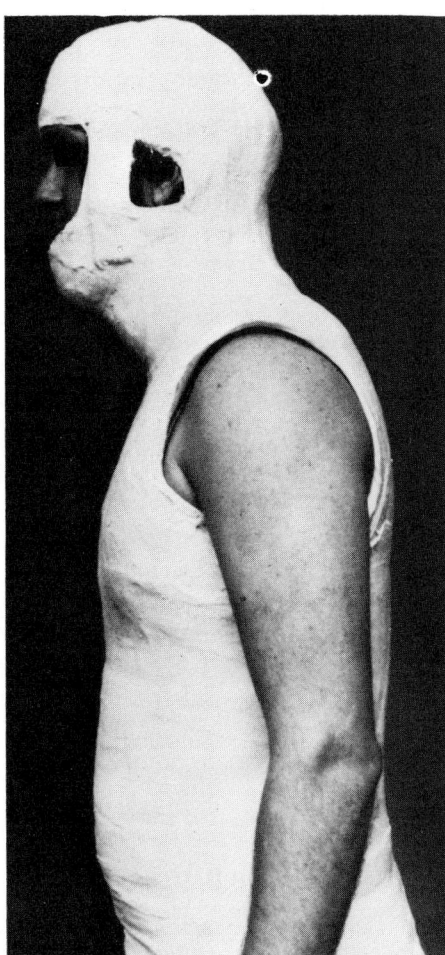

Figure 3. A Minerva plaster jacket provides good stability for unstable fractures of the upper cervical spine. The halo plaster cast generally gives more stability and comfort.

however, they must be interpreted with caution, as a spinal block may be secondary to edema rather than interference from a bone fragment or ruptured disc.

Fractures of the cervical spine may be stable or unstable and may or may not involve the spinal cord or nerve roots. Fractures and dislocations of the cervical spine result from forces of flexion, extension, lateral bending, rotation, and axial loads, or various combinations of these forces. An understanding of the mechanism of injury and accurate diagnosis of the type of fracture or dislocation enables the physician to determine both the stability and the neurologic status and to establish a method of treatment.

Compression Fractures of the Cervical Vertebral Bodies

Compression fracture of a cervical vertebral body secondary to flexion forces may range from very mild to very severe injury. If there is no comminution of the body, no tearing of the posterior longitudinal ligament, and no dislocation of the facets, then the fracture is stable. Rarely are there any associated neurologic lesions with these injuries, and the head and neck are adequately stabilized for comfort with minimal bracing such as a soft or hard cervical collar.

In contrast, the comminuted ("bursting" or "tear drop") fracture is usually a disastrous injury with a high incidence of severe and permanent spinal cord damage. This injury is frequently caused by hyperflexion of the neck, as in a diving accident. The fragments of the vertebral body are pushed posteriorly and cause a sudden impact on the spinal cord. This fracture is very unstable and requires skeletal traction for attempted reduction and stabilization. Traction may be necessary for three to four months. This fracture may also be managed by anterior resection of the fragmented vertebral body and disc material, and interbody fusion with a bone graft.

Dislocations of the Cervical Spine

Dislocations of the cervical spine most commonly occur at the interspaces between C3 and C7. The injury is caused by a flexion-rotation force, with dislocation of the facet and disc and tearing of the posterior longitudinal ligaments (Fig. 4). One or both facets may be jumped and locked. Associated fractures of the facets or other posterior elements may occur with the dislocation. These injuries may be associated with a variable degree of neurologic loss, ranging from none to complete quadriplegia. As a rule, the neurologic injury is less severe than with the "bursting" or "tear drop" compression type of fracture. A lateral roentgenogram demonstrates the forward dislocation of the vertebral body and the jumped and locked facets. An anteroposterior projection in which there is rotation of the spinous process from the midline suggests a jumped and locked facet. Oblique roentgenograms and pillar views (projected at 45 degrees to delineate the facet joints and lateral masses) are valuable for accurate interpretation of the fracture-dislocation.

Fractures and dislocations of the cervical spine are managed in a similar manner to fractures and dislocations in other parts of the skeleton; the fragments must be realigned and the dislocation reduced. If there

produce this fracture. Usually C2 anteriorly subluxes on C3 because the disc bond between these two vertebral bodies is broken.

Cord compression is rare because the neural canal is enlarged with forward displacement of the body of C2. The posterior elements remain behind. Non-union is rare; the fracture can be managed by a four-poster brace or Minerva plaster cast for three months. Operative fusion is rarely indicated.

Fractures and Dislocations of C3 to C7 Vertebrae

Fractures and dislocations of the *lower cervical spine* are common. The majority are caused by vehicular accidents, others by diving into shallow water, falls, and sports injuries. After neurologic assessment of the patient who has a suspected cervical spine injury, precise roentgenograms are obtained. If C7 is not visualized, the patient's shoulders should be pulled caudalward and pressure applied to the feet in a cephalad direction for clear views of the lower cervical spine. Spinal fluid manometrics, including the Queckenstedt test, and myelography frequently give useful information;

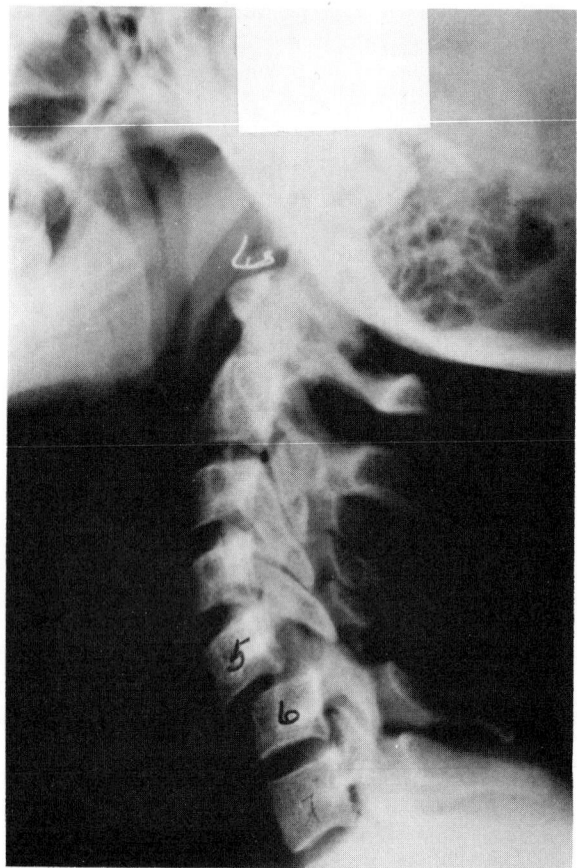

Figure 4. A dislocation of the cervical spine. This injury may or may not produce cord or nerve root damage. Reduction is usually achieved by relaxation and skull traction with tongs. Surgery is sometimes necessary to achieve reduction and stabilization.

is neurologic involvement, the reduction is more urgent. Most dislocations can be reduced by traction and manipulation; only a few require operative reduction.

After the diagnosis and neurologic status have been ascertained, skeletal traction is applied. Many dislocations will reduce easily when traction is applied. Beginning with 15 pounds of traction, the weight is increased gradually over a two-hour period with the patient awake and cooperating. Serial roentgenograms are obtained with each five-pound increment of weight. The weight is increased up to 35 or 40 pounds. If reduction is not achieved with this amount of weight and muscle relaxation, then a bony block or soft tissue interposition may exist. Increasing the weight will not result in a physiologic reduction and may be detrimental to the disc bonds and neural tissues. If the reduction cannot be achieved with 40 pounds of traction, then gentle manipulation after complete muscle relaxation under general anesthesia is the next step. If this maneuver is not successful, then operative reduction and wire fixation and fusion with a bone graft are performed.

If closed reduction is achieved, as usually occurs, the patient may be maintained in skeletal traction for seven to 10 days and then placed in a four-poster brace with head band, a halo brace, or a Minerva plaster cast.

In general, the easier the reduction, the more unstable the fracture or dislocation. Serial lateral roentgenograms are valuable in determining the projected stability of the cervical spine. If calcification is seen in the anterior longitudinal ligament by six weeks, then spontaneous interbody fusion is usually assured. At three months, lateral flexion-extension radiographs out of the brace or cast are obtained, and if stability is apparent, the treatment is discontinued. If instability is present, then posterior or anterior cervical fusion is performed. Laminectomy for fracture-dislocation is seldom indicated. The major indications for laminectomy are (1) progressive worsening of the neurologic status when the posterior elements are comminuted, (2) bony spicules in the spinal canal, and (3) late nerve root pain.

Fractures of the Posterior Elements

Lateral bending or compression forces may result in fractures of a unilateral facet or pedicle. Avulsion fractures of the spinous processes are caused by sudden severe muscle contraction (clay shoveler's fracture) or a direct blow. The fractures are stable and there is not neurologic loss. They may be managed by muscle relaxants, analgesics, and a soft collar until the patient is comfortable.

THE THORACOLUMBAR SPINE

It is important to recognize the relationship of the neural elements to the thoracolumbar skeletal structures when evaluating and treating injuries in this location. The spinal cord usually terminates at the lower margin of the L1 vertebra (Fig. 5). Caudal to L1 the spinal canal contains only spinal roots, the cauda equina. Whereas the spinal cord occupies nearly half the spinal canal in the thoracic area, the neural canal has considerable free space below L1. Therefore, fractures or dislocations in the lumbar area require considerably more displacement to produce neurologic damage than fractures in the thoracic spine. A bursting fracture in the cervical or thoracic area may result in catastrophic neurologic loss, whereas a similar fracture in the lumbar area may produce no neurologic deficit. Because of the anatomic structure of the terminal cord and roots (Fig. 5), spinal injuries cephalad to T10 involve only the cord, from T10 to L1 both the cord and roots, and caudal to L1 only the roots. Individual spinal roots may be injured as they exit through the intervertebral foramina by skeletal disruption. Because the sympathetic ganglia are located anterolateral to the vertebral bodies, fractures of the vertebral bodies or transverse processes frequently result in paralytic ileus.

Diagnosis

The history of the mechanism of the injury is helpful in the evaluation of the patient with a suspected thoracolumbar injury. Usually, there is a clear episode

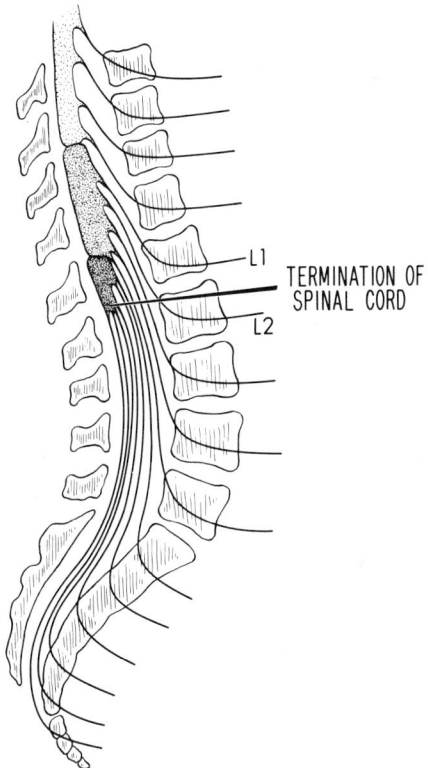

Figure 5. The spinal cord terminates at the L1 vertebra. The cauda equina, composed of spinal roots, is caudal to L1. These relationships are important in the diagnosis and treatment of fracture-dislocations of the dorsolumbar spine.

of sudden violence followed immediately by severe back ache and muscle spasm. In the osteoporotic patient, a rather minimal incident, such as bending to lift an object or a missed step, may result in a compression fracture of the dorsal spine. However, most thoracolumbar fractures follow such violent forces as falls from high places, automobile collisions, diving injuries or the fall of a heavy object onto the back.

Careful documentation of the onset of partial or complete loss of motor or sensory function of the lower extremities is essential for purposes of management and prognosis. If a spinal injury is suspected, the patient should be initially examined in the position in which he is first seen. A brief neurologic examination to determine the motor and sensory status of the lower extremities should first be performed. The clothing should be removed to allow detailed inspection of the spine. If the patient is in the supine position, the examiner's hand may be gently positioned to palpate each spinous process for tenderness. The patient may then be gently rolled to the lateral position for inspection for swelling, abrasions, ecchymosis, or distortions such as spasm, a "step-off," or gibbus.

A complete neurologic evaluation is essential in all individuals with suspected spine injuries. This should be performed prior to the roentgenographic studies. The intercostal and abdominal muscles should be examined as well as motor, sensory, and reflex testing of

the extremities. The anal sphincter tone and bulbocavernous reflexes must be included in the evaluation. In the sensory testing, particular attention should be given to the perianal region, as many cord levels are represented in this small cutaneous area.

Complete loss of motor and sensory function, *including perianal sensation,* during the first 24 hours after injury indicates complete cord injury. The bulbocavernous reflex usually recovers within the first 24 hours. Recovery of this reflex in the presence of complete anesthesia and paralysis is definite evidence that the patient will not recover functional motor power of the lower extremities.

Anteroposterior and lateral roentgenographic views generally demonstrate the fractures or dislocations in the thoracolumbar area. However, right and left oblique projections are usually helpful in the lumbar area and frequently laminograms are necessary to delineate accurately the type of injury. As in the cervical spine, the indications for myelography in the patient with an acutely injured spine continue to be controversial. A complete myelographic block may occur from edema. Also, a complete block may be present in the absence of neurologic deficit and vice versa. Accurate interpretation of the physical findings and skeletal damage on roentgenographic studies usually provides sufficient information to determine the type of lesion and the locus of the neurologic injury. However, myelography is indicated when there is no apparent fracture or dislocation and neurologic loss is present, or when the skeletal findings on roentgenograms do not correlate with the neurologic findings. Pretreatment myelography allows the surgeon to determine if a block is relieved after reduction, provided that the contrast is left in the subarachnoid space.

CLASSIFICATION AND MANAGEMENT

In violent accidents the spine may be subjected to one of the following forces: pure flexion, flexion and rotation, flexion and distraction, vertical compression, extension, lateral bending, or shearing. When these traumatic forces exceed the physiologic limits of the spine, then fractures or dislocations peculiar to the particular forces usually result. Although most authors attempt to categorize spine fractures and dislocation as stable or unstable, based on the mechanism of the injury, such a cataloging is not always distinct.

A spine fracture or dislocation is considered stable if the fragments are not likely to move and cause neural damage during the healing phase. Conversely, if movement and neural damage is likely, then the injured spine is labeled unstable. The instability may be acute or chronic, depending on whether displacement is threatening immediately or a progressing deformity occurs during the extended healing process. Although classification into stable and unstable spine fractures and dislocations is not absolute, this scheme is practical from a management standpoint if the physician is cognizant that each injury must be individualized. The goal is to maintain or achieve a painless functional back, which to a great degree means maintenance or restoration of spinal stability.

STABLE INJURIES

Flexion

Pure flexion injuries are the most common of all thoracolumbar skeletal failures. Compression anteriorly and distraction of the posterior ligaments, which do not pull apart, results in the wedge compression-fracture of the vertebral body (Fig. 6A). These fractures most commonly occur at the thoracolumbar junction.

The flexion injuries are acutely stable, and neurologic loss is uncommon. Progressive angulation may occur during the healing phase, although neurologic changes rarely accompany the deformity.

These fractures may be very painful, especially at the level of the injury. Paralytic ileus secondary to hemorrhage about the sympathetic ganglion or reflex pain referral is common. The patient should be admitted to the hospital and placed at bed rest on a firm mattress. Analgesics, central nervous system depressants, and muscle relaxants are administered. Since there is an increased incidence of thromboembolic disease in patients with thoracolumbar fractures, anticoagulation therapy is indicated. The patient should be encouraged to move about in bed and may become ambulatory as soon as he is comfortable (three to five days). If the compression wedging is greater than 50 per cent of the body height, then either a three-point brace or a plaster jacket to attempt to hold the spine in hyperextension is used. This bracing is utilized for three to four months to prevent progressive angular deformity. This, however, is almost impossible without

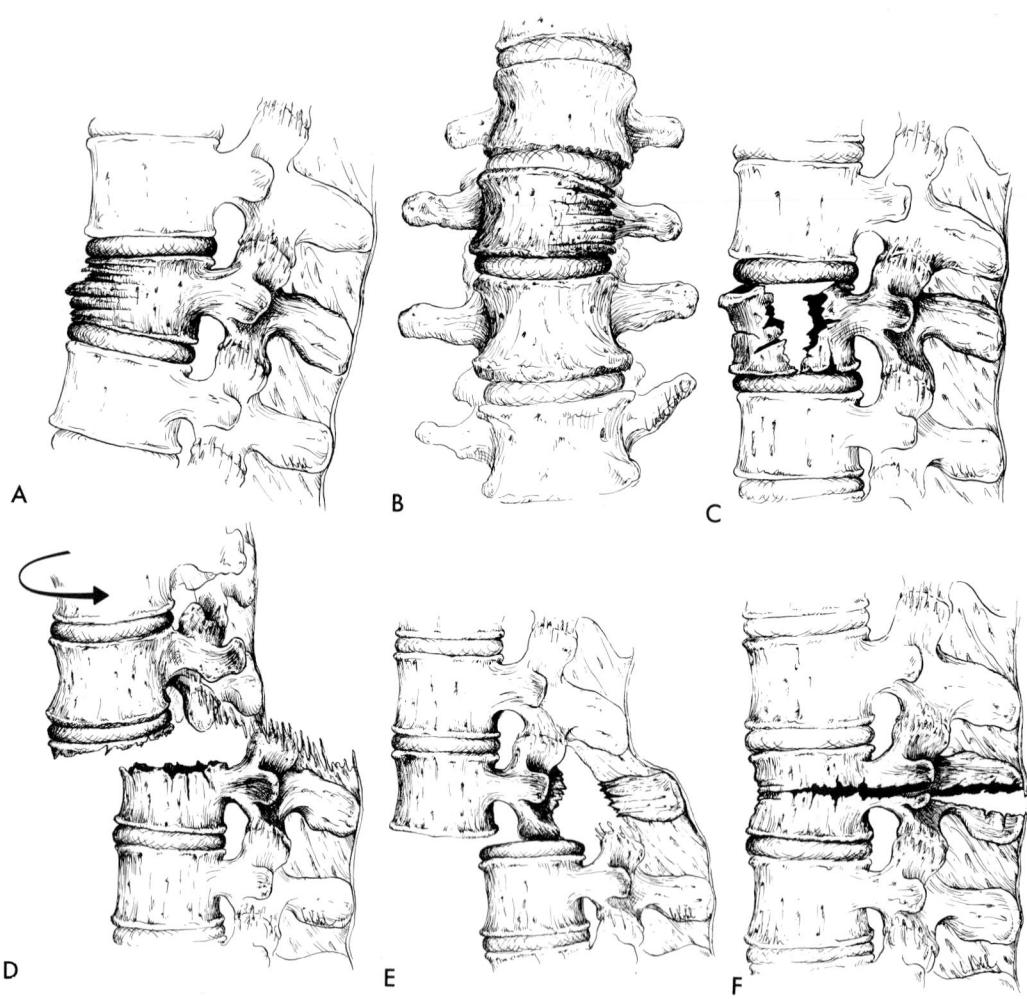

Figure 6. *A,* A wedge compression fracture of the dorsolumbar spine. The posterior elements and ligaments remain intact. This fracture is stable, and neurologic loss is uncommon. *B,* A lateral wedge compression fracture of the vertebral body is a stable fracture and usually without neurologic loss. *C,* The "burst" fracture of the lumbar vertebral body. These fractures are usually stable, but neurologic loss may result from posterior displacement of the fragments into the spinal cord or roots. *D,* The unstable flexion-rotation injury of the dorsolumbar spine. Neurologic loss is common with this injury and reduction and stabilization by surgery are usually indicated. *E,* The anteroposterior "shear" fracture of the lumbar spine. This fracture is generally stable above T10, but unstable below this level. *F,* A "Chance fracture" is a horizontal splitting of the neural arch and vertebral body. It is secondary to a flexion-distraction force and may or may not be stable.

operative stability. If the compression is less than 50 per cent, then a dorsolumbar corset is frequently helpful in decreasing discomfort, although it offers less immobilization. It is not uncommon for patients to have prolonged complaints even though the fractures are stable and heal.

Extension

Although extension fractures commonly occur in the cervical spine, they are rare in the thoracolumbar area. An avulsion fracture of the anterior region of the vertebral body may occur, but the posterior ligaments remain intact. These fractures are stable, and neurologic deficit is rare. Treatment for comfort is all that is required, as these injuries are relatively benign.

Lateral Bending

Lateral bending forces may produce a lateral wedge fracture of the vertebral body (Fig. 6B). These fractures are uncommon, stable, and usually without neurologic damage. The initial symptoms are treated similar to wedge compression fractures, and a corset for comfort is all that is necessary.

Vertical Compression

Compression fractures secondary to axial forces are of two types: intervertebral disc protrusion into the vertebral end-plate, and the "burst" injury. These fractures most often occur in the lumbar area.

In the young patient with a healthy intervertebral disc, a violent vertical force will result in protrusion of the nucleus through the end-plate into the softer cancellous bone of the vertebral body. The traumatic Schmorl's node is visualized on the lateral roentgenograms. These fractures are stable, and no neural deficit occurs. The patient is treated with a few days of bed rest, analgesics, and a corset for a few weeks. Chronic pain persists occasionally.

The "burst" fracture is caused by a severe compressive force of the magnitude sufficient to produce a vertical fracture that joins the damaged superior and inferior end-plates of a vertebral body. Outward displacement of the fragments is characteristic, but the spinous processes are not separated (Fig. 6C). Although this fracture is quite stable, neurologic loss may occur because of the posterior encroachment of the fragments into the spinal canal. If no neurologic deficit is present, these fractures are treated with bed rest until the acute pain subsides. A plaster or plastic jacket to hold the spine in extension for three to four months is recommended. Spontaneous fusion usually occurs, but deformity persists.

If there is neurologic involvement, usually from fragments impinging on the cauda equina, then the surgeon must decide whether decompression is indicated. Posterior decompression, which is seldom helpful or indicated, may lead to undesirable instability and therefore should be accompanied by operative fusion. Posterior stabilization with the Harrington device has been helpful. Anterior decompression by resection of all or parts of the fragmented vertebral body shows promise of being the procedure of choice in this situation. Replacement of the resected body with autografts to obtain intervertebral body fusion and

spinal stability is necessary if anterior decompression is performed.

UNSTABLE INJURIES OF THE THORACOLUMBAR SPINE

Rotation-Flexion Injuries

The combination of rotation and flexion is the most common mechanism producing fracture-dislocation of the thoracolumbar spine. The injuries are recognized on roentgenograms by a fracture through the vertebral body (or intervertebral disc disruption) and fractures and rotation of the posterior structures of the vertebra (Fig. 6D). These injuries are extremely unstable. In fact, they are so unstable that spontaneous reduction may occur by positioning the patient. However, since these are the most unstable of all spine injuries, care must be taken in handling the patient. Therefore, when this injury is suspected, the roentgenograms must be accurately evaluated to determine the integrity of both the anterior and posterior supporting structures. These fracture-dislocations most often occur in the transitional area of T10 to L1 and are associated with a high incidence of neurologic loss.

The most important principle in the management of these injuries with or without neural deficit is to achieve and maintain reduction. Operative reduction and internal fixation are the most reliable means to achieve stability. Most authorities now agree that laminectomy is contraindicated even though neurologic loss is present. This procedure only produces more instability and permits inadequate removal of the offending bony elements anterior to the spinal canal. The neural elements can best be decompressed by reduction of the displaced vertebral elements. A limited laminectomy or removal of a pedicle to explore the neural canal anteriorly may be indicated in selected patients, for example, if an associated ruptured disc is suspected. After reduction of the spine, fixation may be achieved by various metallic devices such as Harrington rods, Weiss springs, or Meurig-Williams plates. If internal fixation is used, the patient remains at bed rest for two to six weeks and then is walked in a plaster jacket, corset, or three-point brace for three to four months or until there is radiographic evidence of spinal fusion.

Shear Fractures

After severe trauma, a vertebra may be displaced in a lateral or anteroposterior direction (Fig. 6E). The pedicles or articular processes are usually fractured in the process. If this injury occurs in the thoracic region above T10, it is stable, but complete paraplegia usually occurs. When shearing occurs in the lumbar region, it is usually very unstable and there is often neurologic sparing because of the relatively large free space of the neural canal at this level. The unstable shear fractures are managed in the same way as rotation-flexion injuries.

Flexion-Distraction Injuries

The "chance fracture" is a fracture in the lumbar spine in which there is horizontal splitting of the vertebral bodies and the neural arch through the pedicles

(Fig. 6*E*). Flexion-distraction forces such as occur in a seat belt injury best describe the pathomechanics. In the past, this fracture has been considered a stable fracture, but recent evidence discloses that in some instances this fracture may be unstable. Therefore, stabilization with the Harrington rod may be indicated in the management of this injury.

SELECTED REFERENCES

Fielding, J. W.: Atlanto-axial rotary subluxation. J. Bone Joint Surg., *51A*:1672, 1969.
  A lucid description of C1-C2 subluxation.

Holdsworth, F. W.: Fractures, dislocations and fracture-dislocations of the spine. J. Bone Joint Surg., *45B*:6, 1963.
Holdsworth, F. W.: Fractures, dislocations and fracture-dislocations of the spine. J. Bone Joint Surg., *52A*:1534, 1970.
  These two articles contain classic descriptions of spinal fractures and their management.

Lewis, J., and McKibbin, B.: The treatment of unstable fracture-dislocations of the thoraco-lumbar spine accompanied by paraplegia. J. Bone Joint Surg., *56B*:391, 1974.
  A method of surgical management of spine injures.

Nickel, V. L., Perry, J., Garrett, A., and Hepenstall, M.: The halo. J. Bone Joint Surg., *50A*:1400, 1968.
  A good description of the Halo apparatus.

Rockwood, C., and Green, D.: Fractures. Vol. 2., Chap. 12. Philadelphia, J. B. Lippincott, 1975.
  The chapters on cervical and lumbar spine injuries are thorough and well illustrated.

Whitesides, T. E., Kelly, R. P., and Howland, S. C.: The treatment of lumbosacral fracture-dislocations. J. Bone Joint Surg., *52A*:1267, 1970.
  A surgical approach to spine fracture-dislocations.

REFERENCES

1. AAOS Course on the Cervical Spine. New York, 1974.
2. Bailey, R. W.: The Cervical Spine. Philadelphia, Lea & Febiger, 1974, p. 263.
3. Blockey, N. J., and Purser, D. W.: Fractures of the odontoid process of the axis. J. Bone Joint Surg., *38B*:794, 1956.
4. Burke, D. C.: Hyperextension injuries of the spine. J. Bone Joint Surg., *53B*:3, 1971.
5. Chance, C. Q.: Note on a type of flexion fracture of the spine. Br. J. Radiol., *21*:452–453, 1948.
6. Chesire, D. J. E.: The stability of cervical spine following the conservative treatment of fractures and fracture-dislocations. Paraplegia, 7:193–203, 1969.
7. Commission on Spine Injuries. Denver, Colorado. J. Bone Joint Surg., *52A*:1273, 1970.
8. Garber, J. N.: Fracture and dislocations of the cervical spine. AAOS Symposium on the Spine. St. Louis, The C. V. Mosby Co. 1967, pp. 18–53.
9. Guttman, L.: Spinal Cord Injuries, Comprehensive Management and Research. Oxford, Blackwell Scientific Publications, Ltd., 1973, p. 694.
10. Jefferson, G.: Fracture of the atlas vertebra: Report of four cases and review of those previously recorded. Br. J. Surg., 7:407, 1920.
11. Katznelson, A. N.: Stabilization of the spine in traumatic paraplegia using Harrington rods. Paraplegia, 7:33–37, 1969.
12. Kaufer, H., and Hayes, J. T.: Lumbar fracture-dislocations. J. Bone Joint Surg., *48A*:712, 1966.
13. McCraw, R. W., and Ruschi, R. M.: Atlanto-axial arthrodesis. J. Bone Joint Surg., *55B*:482, 1973.
14. Rennie, W., and Mitchell, N.: Flexion distraction fractures of the thoracolumbar spine. J. Bone Joint Surg., *55A*:386–390, 1973.
15. Roaf, R.: A study of the mechanics of spinal injuries. J. Bone Joint Surg., *42B*:810–823, 1960.
16. Roberts, J. B., and Curtiss, P. H.: Stability of the thoracic and lumbar spine in traumatic paraplegia following fracture or fracture-dislocations. J. Bone Joint Surg., *52A*:1115, 1970.
17. Schneider, R. C., Livingston, K. E., Cowe, A. J. E., and Hamilton, G.: Hangman's fracture. J. Neurosurg., *22*:141, 1965.
18. Smith, W. S., and Kaufer, H.: Patterns and mechanisms of lumbar injuries associated with lap seat belts. J. Bone Joint Surg., *51A*:239, 1969.
19. Stryker, W. S.: Simple compression fractures of the dorsolumbar spine. J. Bone Joint Surg., *49A*:204, 1967.
20. Taylor, A. R.: The mechanism of injury to the spinal cord in the neck without damage to the vertebral column. J. Bone Joint Surg., *33B*:543, 1951.
21. Taylor, A. R., and Blackwood, W.: Paraplegia in hyperextension in cervical injuries with normal radiographic appearances. J. Bone Joint Surg., *30B*:245, 1948.
22. Thompson, H.: The "halo" traction apparatus. J. Bone Joint Surg., *44B*:655, 1962.
23. Weitzman, G.: Treatment of stable thoraco-lumbar spine compression fractures. Clin. Orthop., 76:16–122, 1971.

III

FRACTURES AND DISLOCATIONS OF THE SHOULDER, ARM, AND FOREARM

Donald S. Bright, M.D.

The size of the glenoarticular surfaces is about one third the size of the articular surface of the humeral head. The humeral head is in 30 degrees of retroversion. Stability of the shoulder is maintained by a thick capsule—"the shoulder cuff" and the overlying muscles. Superiorly the ligaments and the acromion stabilize the joint. The humerus abducts 90 degrees on the scapula and the scapula abducts 60 degrees on the thorax. *Neurovascular structures* in the extremity lie in the axilla and may be injured as a result of trauma.

FRACTURES OF THE SCAPULA AND HEAD OF HUMERUS

Mechanism of Injury. The majority of fractures are caused by a fall on an outstretched arm. If the force is in the direction of the humerus, an impacted fracture results. Additional torque may cause fracture of the greater or lesser tuberosity or the shaft. Direct blows in vehicular injuries or as a result of a seizure cause the most severe fractures and fracture-dislocations.

Clinical Findings. Patients present with tenderness, swelling, pain, and limited motion.

Several classifications of shoulder injuries are available, but that of Neer[27-29] is acceptable. Classification is based on the segments of the shoulder (humeral head, greater tuberosity, lesser tuberosity, and humeral shaft). Neer classifies fractures into one-, two-, or three-part fractures, depending on how many of the segments are displaced from each other. Nondisplaced fractures are classified as one-part fractures even though fracture lines may exist between any number of these segments.

In order to assess any fracture, a complete roentgen series is necessary. This consists of an anteroposterior view of the shoulder and an axillary or true lateral view. This is often unobtainable because of pain. A trauma series[34] consists of two roentgenograms taken at right angles to each other while the arm is at the side. One x-ray is perpendicular and the other parallel to the plane of the scapula. A transthoracic projection or a stereoprojection may help.

Treatment. Impacted fractures or those without significant displacement are treated by partial immobilization, with the arm at the side in a padded sling, and a limited chest wrap. Within seven to 10 days, passive and then active motion of the shoulder is started. This motion consists of circumduction exercises with the forearm in the sling. Active exercise should be continued until maximum range of motion is obtained. This may take several months.

The most common two-part fracture involves either the greater or lesser tuberosity or the humeral shaft. If the greater tuberosity is displaced more than 1 cm., interference with abduction and external rotation should occur. If significant angulation of the displacement of the shaft is present, closed reduction is attempted. Open reduction is rarely necessary.

Fractures with three major parts displaced usually have to be treated by operative reduction and internal fixation if closed reduction fails to give satisfactory alignment. Wires, screws, and intramedullary rods are necessary to maintain apposition of the fragments, but none of these methods is sufficient to allow recovery of a full range of motion. Moderate limitation of motion therefore occurs.

Fractures with four-part displacement produce significant injury to the articular surface of the humeral head with disruption of the blood supply. Early prosthetic replacement of the humeral head is usually indicated if the glenoid is intact and the patient's health will permit the procedure.

The most common fracture-dislocation is an anterior shoulder dislocation with a fracture of the greater tuberosity. After reduction, the greater tuberosity usually is in a satisfactory position. Fracture dislocations that include three-part fractures will require open reduction and internal fixation or prosthetic replacement of the humeral head.

The most common type of articular fracture is caused by the pressure of the anterior or posterior glenoid rim on the humeral head when dislocation occurs.

ANTERIOR DISLOCATIONS

Mechanism of Injury. The common mechanism is forced abduction and external rotation, levering the head against the anterior inferior capsule and rupturing the capsule at its glenoid attachment. After dislocation the pressure of the glenoid rim on the posterior articular surface causes a compression injury that is permanent. Depending on the applied forces during trauma, the head may lie anteriorly, inferiorly, or medially (Fig. 1). These acute injuries most often occur in young active individuals. A few patients can voluntarily dislocate their shoulders. Rarely, congenital imbalance does result in dislocation.

Clinical Findings. The arm is held immobile at the side, and the acromion is prominent with a defect below this. The patient cannot actively move his hand across his chest. The most common neurovascular involvement is the axillary nerve, which supplies the deltoid muscle and sensation to the lateral aspect of the arm. In severe injuries, more than one segment of the brachial plexus is damaged.

Treatment. Reduction is accomplished with sedation, regional or general anesthesia, and traction on the arm after surrounding muscles are relaxed enough to allow the head to relocate. Straight longitudinal or anterior traction accompanied by lateral pressure on the humeral head is effective. Another way to slowly reduce the dislocation is to tie 20 pounds to the wrist and place the patient in the prone position with the arm suspended for 10 minutes. After reduction is obtained, the extremity is placed in a sling and the arm is held in internal rotation for three weeks. Protected range of motion exercises are initiated. Abduction and external rotation should be avoided for three months. Recurrence is a common complication in the younger individual[35] and less common in the older.

RECURRENT ANTERIOR DISLOCATIONS

The incidence of recurrent anterior dislocations varies from 30 to 60 per cent in active individuals. After two or three recurrences, operative repair is usually desirable. Good results have been reported with many procedures. The Bankart operation repairs the torn capsule and labrum.[2, 3] The Putti-Platt procedure[32] excises the labrum and replaces it with the subscapularis tendon. The subscapularis muscle insertion is transferred laterally in the Magnuson-Stack procedure[22, 23] after the capsule is repaired. The Bristow procedure transfers the coracoid process with muscles attached to the anterior rim of the glenoid.[16, 21] In elderly or debilitated individuals, unrecognized long-standing dislocations do occur.

Partial dislocations or subluxations have been more frequently recognized.[7] Active individuals have the feeling of instability accompanied by pain. A shoulder arthrogram demonstrates the ballooning or tear of the capsule. An anterior repair is usually necessary.

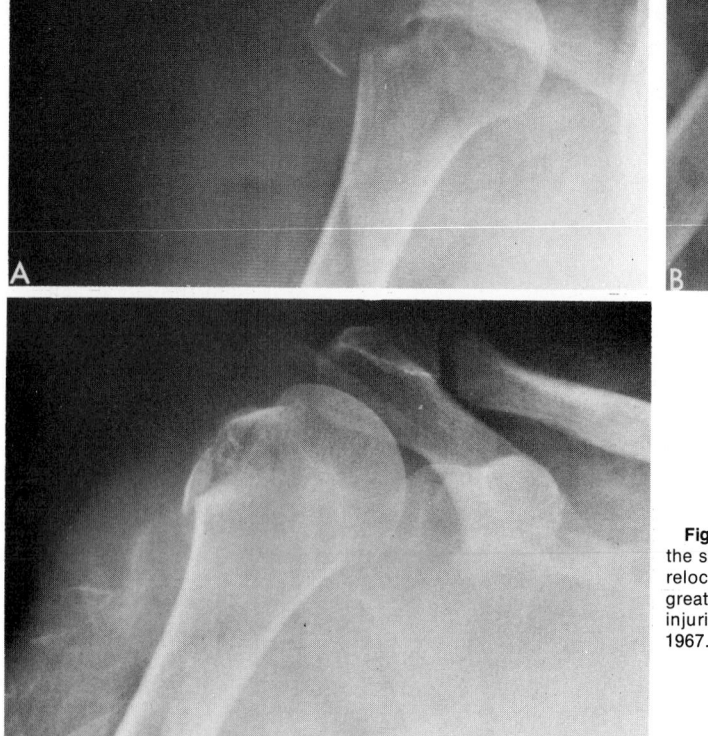

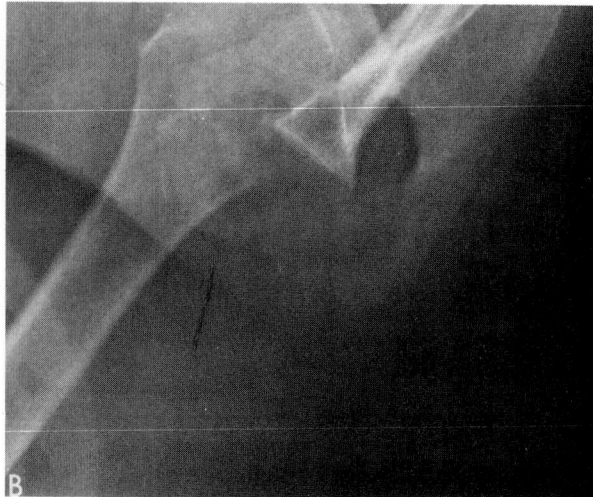

Figure 1. AP and axillary lateral of subcoracoid dislocation of the shoulder with associated fracture of the greater tuberosity. After relocation using traction, there is satisfactory apposition of the greater tuberosity. (From Allman, F. L., Jr.: Fractures and ligamentous injuries of the clavicle and its articulation. J. Bone Joint Surg., *49*:1, 1967.)

INFERIOR DISLOCATIONS

This injury is produced by straight abduction of the shoulder with the humeral head levered directly inferiorly.

POSTERIOR DISLOCATIONS

These are rare injuries and usually occur from seizures, a direct anterior force, or habitual dislocations. An unrecognized dislocation may be misdiagnosed as a "frozen shoulder." The average time from occurrence to diagnosis in one series was eight months.[17] The patient holds the arm in the adducted and internally rotated position. Roentgenographic interpretation is difficult. Routine anteroposterior projection may be misinterpreted as normal. Axillary lateral views are difficult to obtain because of pain. Roentgenogram in the plane of the scapula[34] will demonstrate this dislocation. The capsule is torn pos-

teriorly and the glenoid creates a depression in the anterior surface of the humerus. This may be quite large, leading to an unstable shoulder. Traction may reduce this injury. The arm is immobilized in external rotation and abduction. In dislocations recognized late, an open reduction capsular repair and bone block may be necessary.

ROTATOR CUFF INJURIES

The rotator cuff (supraspinatus, infraspinatus, and teres minor) stabilizes the shoulder in the glenoid and gives strength through abduction and rotation. Injuries occur in active individuals by full abduction and external rotation. In middle-age or older individuals, injuries can occur spontaneously or by repeated activity.

Patients present with pain in the shoulder, tenderness beneath the acromion, and decreased strength in the abducted and externally rotated positions.

Roentgenograms are usually normal, but may show calcifications or a small avulsion fracture of the greater tuberosity. An arthrogram will demonstrate dye leaking from the joint capsule in the area of the rotator cuff in the acute injury.

The majority of patients can be treated with analgesics and range of motion exercises. Repair is indicated in severe acute or chronic injuries and in active individuals; rarely is operation necessary in older patients. In late tears the humerus may ride through the defect in the torn tendon with impingement of the greater tuberosity on the acromion. This may result in painful limited shoulder motion and require repair of the rotator cuff tendon as well as resection of one third of the acromion.

FRACTURES AND DISLOCATIONS OF THE CLAVICLE

Anatomy. The clavicle is S shaped, and is the only bony connection between the thorax and upper extremity. Proximally it is fixed to the thorax by the strong sternoclavicular joint and the costoclavicular ligaments. Distally the clavicle broadens out and is fixed to the scapula by the acromioclavicular and coracoclavicular ligaments. A fibrocartilaginous meniscus lies between the distal clavicle and the acromion. Horizontal stability is maintained by the acromioclavicular ligaments and vertical stability by the coracoclavicular ligaments. Deep to the scapula is the subclavian artery and the brachial plexus. When the clavicle is fractured the weight of the arm tends to carry the scapula downward and the pull of the pectoralis brings the shoulder forward, thereby shortening the clavicle.

Mechanism of Injury. Direct lateral trauma produces either a fracture of the middle third of the clavicle or a sternoclavicular disruption proximally. Direct blows usually produce fractures in the proximal two thirds. A fracture may occur as the result of a fall on the shoulder. The shoulder is depressed and the clavicle abuts against the first rib. As the shoulder continues its downward motion, either the clavicle fractures at its distal third or an acromioclavicular separation occurs. Smaller forces produce stretching of the ligaments, and greater forces can tear the acromioclavicular and coracoclavicular ligaments.

In fractures of the distal third, if the coracoclavicular ligaments are intact, the fragments are held in good apposition. If the ligaments are present on the proximal fragment only, the distal fragment will ride upward.

Clavicular fractures may occur as the infant passes through the birth canal. Lateral pressure on both shoulders produces fractures of the midportion of the clavicle. These heal readily.

Clinical Findings. Infants and children cry and will not move the affected extremity. There is painful crepitation of the clavicle, and the roentgenogram is confirmatory. In older patients the deformity is obvious. Acromioclavicular injuries present with tenderness over the joint, and the clavicle tenting the skin in complete separations. Diagnosis of sternoclavicular dislocations is more difficult. Local pain is present with motion of the arm, or there may be venous congestion, decreased circulation of the involved extremity, or tracheal injuries, depending on whether the clavicle is anterior or posterior.

The diagnosis of sternoclavicular dislocation is difficult to make radiographically. Hobbs[18] and Rockwood and Green[34] have described two different ways to better delineate the dislocations. Fractures of the shaft of the clavicle are seen on the standard projections, and injuries to the acromioclavicular joint are usually obvious. If subluxation is suspected, then an anteroposterior view of both shoulders that includes the clavicles with the patient standing and holding 10-pound weights in each hand will accentuate the deformity.

Treatment. Sprains and posterior subluxation of the sternoclavicular joint can be treated with figure-of-eight dressings holding the shoulder back. Dislocations are treated in a similar manner with additional pressure over the joint. Posterior dislocations generally need to be reduced under general anesthesia. The clavicle is pulled forward with the use of a towel clip through the sterilized skin.

Fractures of the shaft of the clavicle in children can be treated with a comfortable figure-of-eight soft dressing. Union is rapid, and remodeling takes place with growth. In older individuals a lump results where the bones override and callus forms. Improved reduction can be obtained by pulling the shoulder backward with a figure-of-eight dressing. Functional recovery is good, but a lump usually remains. Fractures of the distal third with gross displacement can be treated in a similar manner, although occasionally pin fixation is helpful.[30, 31] Sprains of the acromioclavicular joint without significant displacement can be treated with a protective sling. Moderate subluxation of the joint with a few millimeters of displacement can be treated with a protective sling or strapping. This involves a strap passing around the elbow and over the clavicle. That puts an upward force on the arm and a downward force on the clavicle. This must be kept in place for three or more weeks.[41, 42]

Complete acromioclavicular dislocations can be treated with either the above-mentioned strap for six weeks or a variation of it utilizing plaster. The closed method is sufficient in most individuals.[1, 42] Even if reduction is not accomplished, the patients often achieve good function of the extremity. If impingement of the distal clavicle occurs, then later resection of a segment can relieve these symptoms. Reduction and repair of the acromioclavicular ligament[5, 36] are done occasionally. Reconstruction of the coracoclavicular ligaments[6, 19] may be helpful.

Complications. The most frequent complication of clavicular fractures is the malunion of the fracture with a visible lump. More serious complications involve sternoclavicular dislocations with lacerations of the vena cava,[43] pressure on the trachea,[33] and brachial plexus compression.[24] Acromioclavicular joint injuries produce impingement of the clavicle to the acromion when the arm is abducted. Post-traumatic arthritis does occur.

Nonunion of the clavicle is rare, but does occur. Open reduction, plate or intramedullary rod fixation, and bone grafting are usually successful in adults.

FRACTURES OF THE SCAPULA

The body of the scapula is flat and held securely against the ribs by the surrounding muscles. It is fixed firmly to the clavicle and articulates with the humerus. Fractures of the body and spine are usually caused by direct trauma. There is often associated rib, shoulder, or vertebral injuries. The patient usually holds the arm to the side, and any motion, especially abduction, is painful.

Treatment. Treatment is by a protective sling and initiation of early motion. Because of the stabilizing effect of surrounding muscles and good blood supply, healing is usually rapid, with moderate functional loss.

Fractures of the glenoid may occur with direct trauma to the shoulder causing a compression type fracture. In anterior and posterior dislocations, either the anterior or posterior rim may be avulsed by the capsule. Fractures of the neck of the scapula are caused by a lateral blow and are usually impacted fractures. Fractures of the neck and glenoid, unless severely displaced, can usually be treated by protective splinting and early institution of motion. Since the shoulder is a non–weight-bearing joint, disruptions in the congruity of the articulation produce less long-term disability than the same injury in a larger, weight-bearing joint.

The coracoid process can be either avulsed by coracoclavicular ligaments, fractured by an anterior shoulder dislocation, or avulsed by a pull of the attached muscles. There is local pain and tenderness to palpation. The majority of these fractures do well without any specific treatment. If there is a wide separation of fragments in a young person, then a reduction should be performed.[29]

FRACTURES OF THE SHAFT OF THE HUMERUS

Anatomy. The humeral shaft is cylindrical proximally and broadens distally. The major neurovascular structures are located medially except for the radial nerve, which courses laterally. The muscles of the arm and gravity act on midshaft fractures to produce shortening and varus angulation. In fractures below the insertion of the deltoid muscle, the proximal fragment is abducted by the deltoid, while the biceps, triceps, and coracobrachialis adduct and shorten the distal fragment. In fractures above the insertion of the deltoid and below the insertion of the pectoralis major, the distal fragment is drawn into abduction by the deltoid while the proximal fragment is adducted by the pectoralis major.

In fractures above the insertion of the pectoralis major, the distal fragment is held in alignment while the proximal fragment is abducted by the rotator cuff and internally rotated by the subscapularis.

Mechanism of Injury. The majority of these fractures are caused by direct trauma or a fall on the arm. Bending movements cause transverse fractures, while torsional forces cause spiral fractures.

Clinical and X-ray Findings. Pain, tenderness, and instability of the arm are obvious. Radial nerve involvement is relatively common and should be suspected in all cases.

Treatment. Open fractures are treated as emergencies with immediate débridement. Injuries to the vascular structures, either directly or indirectly, should likewise be treated as emergencies with appropriate arteriograms, internal injury exploration, and repair or grafting of the artery. Nerve trauma is usually treated by reduction of the fracture and not by immediate operation.

After emergency treatment has been administered, then the principles of treatment to be considered are the method of initial immobilization and alignment of the fragment. After stability has occurred in five to seven weeks, shoulder and elbow motion should be initiated.

Undisplaced Fractures. These can be treated by padding the axilla, placing the arm in, and wrapping the arm to the chest. Early protective motion is started in two to three weeks, and healing occurs in about 10 weeks. The arm only may be splinted, leaving the elbow free to move.

Displaced Fractures. Several methods have been utilized for the treatment of these fractures. The hanging cast[10, 11, 37] is useful. A light-weight cast is applied extending from the level of the fracture to the hand. A sling is placed under the involved axilla and over the opposite trapezius through a loop or rope fixed to the forearm cast.

The alignment of the fragments can be controlled by the length of the sling and the position of the hoop on the forearm cast, either dorsal or volar. This will change the rotation and angulation at the fracture site in three planes. During the first three weeks of treatment the patient is kept in an upright or semisitting position because the weight of the arm and the cast provides traction and aligns the fracture. Periodic x-rays are necessary, and early shoulder motion is initiated. Pendulum exercises with the cuff still attached maintain shoulder motion. Finger and hand exercises are encouraged.

A coaptation splint[8, 13, 15] consists of a single 10- to 15-thickness splint applied from the axilla, around the elbow, and over the deltoid with light padding and nonelastic wrapping. This holds the fragments in alignment, and a sling is used for comfort. This has the advantage of allowing earlier elbow, wrist, and hand motion and often gives the patient more comfort initially than the hanging cast. Adjustment and alignment are more difficult.

Patients who have associated injuries or who are bedridden for other reasons can be treated by traction through an olecranon pin or by skin traction. Traction aligns the fragments, but care must be taken to prevent overpull of one fragment or pressure on the radial nerve or injury to the ulnar nerve from the pin.

In fractures associated with vascular injury, rapid internal fixation of the fragments is done prior to repair of the vessels, if the time interval from injury to repair is not greater than four hours.

In established nonunions or in fractures with soft

tissue interposition, open reduction and fixation with metallic devices is necessary.

The humerus is the common site of pathologic fractures caused by metastatic tumors, and these may be treated by local radiation and/or chemotherapy, and the fracture may heal. More commonly, however, there is a large defect in the bone with gross instability of the humerus. The patient is often uncomfortable, and open fixation is done followed by appropriate treatment of the tumor. Healing is delayed longer in these patients. If extensive bone loss is present, then methylmethacrylate supplements the metallic fixation.

Prognosis. Closed, nondisplaced, and minimally displaced fractures heal in six to 10 weeks and allow functional use of the arm for light activities. In severely displaced or comminuted fractures associated with neurovascular injuries, the prognosis is guarded. Associated fractures of the elbow or shoulder worsen the prognosis.

Complications. The radial nerve may be injured in open fractures or fractures at the junction of the middle and distal thirds of the humerus. At this point the nerve is in close proximity to the humerus. In the majority of instances, the injury is a result of stretching or bruising, and function will return within several weeks to six months. It is safe to wait for at least three months to determine if regeneration will occur.[38, 40] The electromyogram will demonstrate early regeneration. In open fractures involving the radial nerve or in fractures with soft tissue interposition, exploration of the radial nerve is indicated. Delayed suture is acceptable, but the decision depends on the lesion.

Established nonunion is more common in transverse than in oblique fractures. Fixation with a plate or intramedullary rod and bone grafting is indicated.[9, 12, 20, 26]

FRACTURES ABOUT THE ELBOW

Fractures about the elbow are common. In the younger age group, epiphyseal injuries occur frequently after a fall. In the older patient, fractures are often open and caused by motor vehicles. At any age, fractures about the elbow are difficult to treat.

The discussion will include fractures of the distal humerus (supracondylar, transcondylar, and intracondylar fractures), fractures of the humeral condyles and epicondyles, dislocations of the elbow, fractures of the olecranon, and fractures of the radial head.

Anatomy of the Elbow. The elbow joint consists of three articulations within one synovial capsule. The ulnar-humeral joint provides stability and allows flexion and extension. Pronation and supination occur between the radius and capitellum and the distal radial-ulnar joint. The medial and lateral collateral ligaments give stability to the joint. The brachial artery and median nerve pass volar to the joint and are subject to injury in severe fractures or dislocations. The ulnar nerve coursing behind the medial epicondyle is subject to early or late compression.

External landmarks of the distal humerus are the medial and lateral epicondyles, which serve as muscle attachments for the flexors and extensors of the wrist and hand. The articular surface of the humerus, made up of the trochlea and capitulum, are angled anteriorly 30 to 40 degrees with the shaft of the humerus. The trochlea has a central groove that is directed laterally in extension, and this determines the carrying angle (normal, 15 degrees).

The radial head is palpable on the lateral side of the elbow. The neck is stabilized by the annular ligament and just distal to this is the bicipital tuberosity to which the biceps tendon attaches.

SUPRACONDYLAR, TRANSCONDYLAR, AND INTRACONDYLAR FRACTURES

Mechanism of Injury. Supracondylar fractures occur as a result of a fall on the outstretched hand or flexed elbow. The majority have volar angulation of the fracture and dorsal displacement of the distal fragment. These fractures are usually proximal to the widest portion of the distal humerus and are extrasynovial. Serious complications result from direct trauma to the neurovascular structures.

Transcondylar fractures are interarticular and involve the capitellum and trochlea. The intracondylar T or Y fractures are caused by severe trauma in the elderly. Associated soft tissue injury and comminution of one fragment are noted frequently. The ulna is wedged between the condyles, and the muscle attachments of the epicondyles cause persistent displacement.

Clinical Findings. Pain and swelling are present. Neurovascular complications are suspected with these fractures. Close observation is essential, and prompt aggressive treatment is necessary if vascular insufficiency occurs.

Treatment. Undisplaced fractures are treated by immobilization for two or three weeks, after which motion is initiated gradually. Displaced fractures are reduced with traction and held by plaster molding over the displaced fragment. The carrying angle and volar angulation of the condyles should be re-established. With a severely displaced fracture or with concomitant soft tissue injury, Dunlop's modified side arm traction or an olecranon traction pin should be used to align the fragments and protect the neurovascular structures. In displaced intercondylar fractures, open reduction and anatomic alignment are usually necessary.

Complications. The most serious complication is Volkmann's ischemia with subsequent contracture. Some loss of motion is usual and loss of the carrying angle may occur in supracondylar or transcondylar fractures. Most severe interarticular fractures produce pain and marked limitation of motion.

FRACTURES OF THE CONDYLES, EPICONDYLES, AND ARTICULAR FRACTURES

Mechanism of Injury. These fractures are caused by varus, valgus, and compression forces on the elbow.

Clinical Findings. Condylar fractures produce instability and loss of motion. Epicondylar fractures produce instability. Articular fractures decrease motion.

Treatment. Fractures involving the articular surface must be reduced anatomically. Epicondylar fractures may be treated closed unless the fragment is interarticular.

EPIPHYSEAL INJURIES

Either the medial or lateral epiphysis can separate in children. Treatment usually consists of closed reduction and a sort of immobilization. Injury to the epiphyseal plate may result in growth disturbance and angular deformity either medially or laterally.

DISLOCATIONS OF THE ELBOW

Posterior dislocation is caused by a fall on the outstretched arm, resulting in dislocation of the radius and ulna. Neurovascular structures are not affected, although arterial injury occurs occasionally. Anterior dislocations are caused by a blow on the flexed elbow. Dislocation of the radial head can occur as an isolated injury anteriorly or posteriorly. Dislocation of the ulna alone occurs rarely. Associated fractures of the coronoid process, medial epicondyle, or radial head do occur when dislocation occurs.

Clinical Findings. Elbow motion is limited. There is deformity, and the neurovascular structures are usually intact. Median nerve injury occurs occasionally.

Treatment. Gentle pull on the olecranon followed by flexion usually relocates the dislocation. After reduction, the elbow should be carried out through a reasonable range of motion to test stability. If the dislocation is stable, immobilization for one to two weeks is recommended. Protective splinting is done for an additional two weeks.

Complications. In simple dislocations, a functional range of motion usually results. Myositis ossificans, however, can produce mild or severe limitations in elbows of a small percentage of patients. Neurovascular complications occur occasionally.

FRACTURES OF THE OLECRANON

These usually result from a direct blow or fall on the flexed elbow. On examination the area is painful, and the patient is unable to extend his elbow against gravity.

Undisplaced fractures are treated by splinting at 60 degrees of flexion. Displaced fractures must be opened, aligned, and stabilized with either wires or an intramedullary screw. Avulsion fractures or fractures involving a small piece of the olecranon can be excised and triceps surae attached to ulna. The entire proximal fragment can be excised in the elderly patient and the triceps repaired.

Prognosis depends on an anatomic reduction of the fracture, early active motion, and rigid internal fixation. The nonunion rate is low with good fixation.

FRACTURES OF THE RADIAL HEAD

These fractures usually occur by indirect trauma from a fall on the outstretched hand. The radial head is compressed against the capitellum with a fracture of a portion of the head, or the radial neck is fractured.

In children, the "nurse maids elbow" is caused when the radial head is pulled distally through part of the annular ligament by forcible traction and pronation. Reduction is accomplished by supination of the forearm and is accompanied by an audible or palpable click.

Clinical Findings. Diagnosis is made by noting direct tenderness over the radial head with limited motion in supination and pronation.

Treatment. Nondisplaced fractures are treated with early motion. Fractures involving less than 30 to 50 per cent of the head are treated by splinting until swelling resolves; then motion is initiated.

In fractures involving more than 50 per cent of the radial head, the entire head may be excised early, or later if symptoms persist. In severely comminuted fractures, early excision of the head is advisable. A silicone prosthesis may be a useful substitute. Complications after excision of the radial head include limited pronation and supination and subluxation of the distal radial-ulnar joint.

FRACTURES OF THE DISTAL FOREARM

Anatomy. The distal radius articulates with the scaphoid and lunate and participates in the radioulnar joint, allowing pronation and supination of the forearm. The distal ulna is covered by a fibrocartilaginous articular disc. The distal radius angulates 15 to 30 degrees ulnarly and has a 10-degree volar tilt. The epiphyseal plates of the radius and ulna are particularly susceptible to injury in children.

Mechanism of Injury. Fractures are produced when the patient falls forward or backward. The carpal bones may be driven into the articular surface of the radius with an anterior or posterior lip fractured.

Pathology. A *Colles fracture*[14] is a transverse fracture of the distal radius with dorsal and radial displacement. In the Smith fracture[39] the distal fragment is displaced volarly. Barton[4] described a fracture dislocation of the distal articular lip either anteriorly or posteriorly.

Clinical Findings. Examination shows swelling, limited motion, median nerve compression, and edema of the hand. In displaced fractures there is deformity as well as crepitation.

X-ray Findings. These clarify the location and determine involvement of articular surfaces, degree of displacement, and change in the normal volar and ulnar angulation. Epiphyseal injuries in children often involve a section of the metaphysis or a longitudinal fracture of the epiphysis.

Treatment.   Undisplaced fractures may be treated by three to four weeks of immobilization. Early finger motion is encouraged. Displaced fractures or epiphyseal injuries should be reduced under regional anesthesia, avoiding repeated forceful manipulation. The Colles fracture is reduced by first disimpacting the fracture, then placing traction on the hand and forcibly applying pressure to the dorsum of the distal fragment with volar pressure over the distal fragment. The wrist is immobilized in 10 degrees of flexion and 20 degrees ulnar deviation (Fig. 2). Epiphyseal injuries are reduced in a similar manner; however, redisplacement of the fragments is common, since the epiphyseal plate is smooth.

A *Smith fracture* is reduced by the reverse maneuver. Displaced fractures should be splinted to include the elbow, elevated for 48 hours, and early finger mo-

tion encouraged. Immobilization is carried out for four to six weeks. Open cross pin fixation is rarely necessary.

A *Barton fracture* is reduced by angulating the hand toward the fragment, relaxing the capsule, and pressing the fragment into place. If a large fragment is involved, internal fixation may be necessary.

Prognosis and Complications.   Undisplaced or minimally displaced fractures and epiphyseal injuries usually result in satisfactory function. Articular fractures and fractures in the elderly have a more guarded prognosis. There may be persistent angulation, but more importantly the loss of wrist motion and finger flexion may result because of swelling of the hand.

Other complications include median nerve dysfunction, sympathetic dystrophy, rupture of the extensor pollicis longus as it passes across the fracture frag-

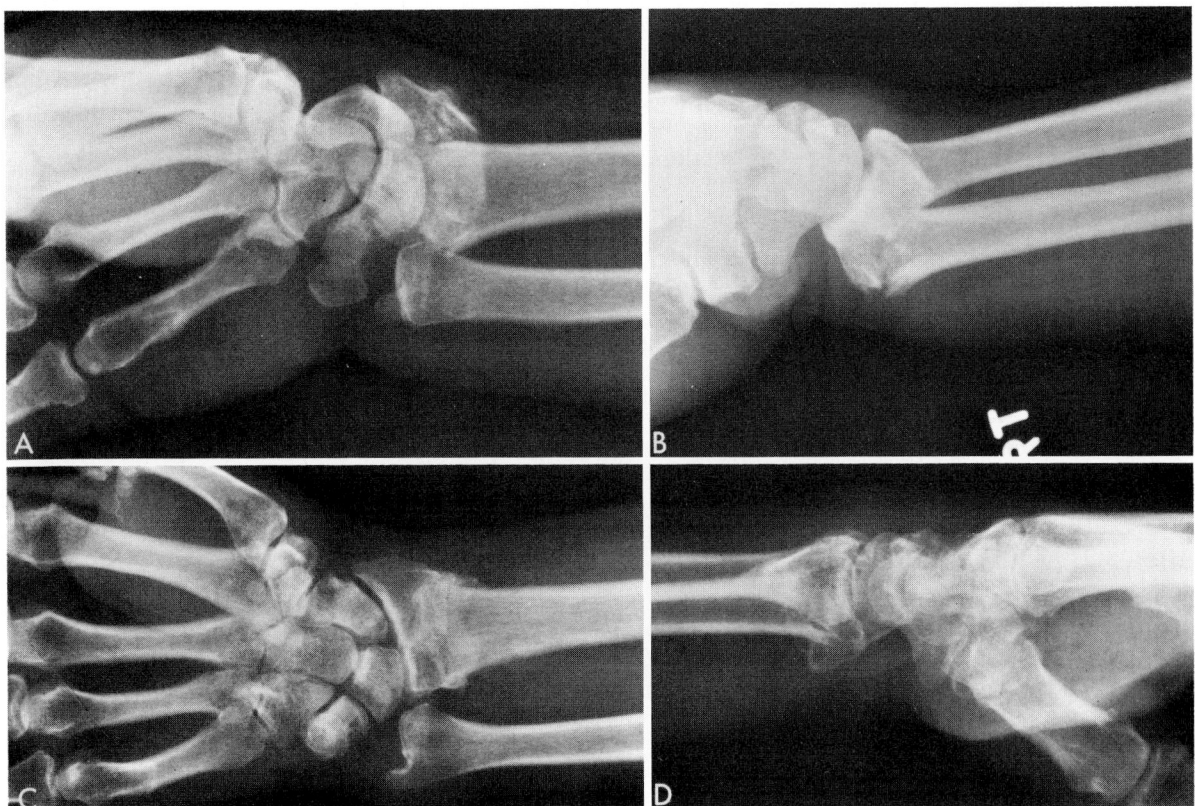

Figure 2.   *A* and *B,* Fracture of the distal radius with dorsal displacement, shortening, loss of the normal volar and radial tilt of the wrist in a 66-year-old white female. *C* and *D,* Two months post reduction and immobilization in a dorsal plaster splint. Satisfactory restoration of radial length with the articular surface at neutral. Apposition was on maintaining full finger motion.

ments, shoulder stiffness, and malunion. Nonunion is rare. Children should be observed for at least one year to assure that the epiphysis is growing normally.

FRACTURES OF THE SHAFT OF THE RADIUS AND ULNA

The radius and ulna articulate with each other proximally and distally. Proximally the radial head rotates within the radial notch of the ulna. A fracture of either bone causes the unfractured bone to articulate abnormally. The radius is connected with the ulna by a tough fibrous interosseous membrane, which acts as a hinge for the radius to rotate around the ulna and for muscle origins. The maintenance of the interosseous space is necessary for the normal articulation of the radius and ulna.

Mechanism of Injury. Direct blows or penetrating injuries can cause fracture to either or both bones. A fall on the outstretched arm causes direct rotational stresses. Both bones may be fractured. Also, a fracture of the ulna can occur with dislocation of the radial head (Monteggia's fracture). Similarly, the shaft of the radius may be fractured at the proximal one third with dislocation of the distal ulna (Galeazzi's fracture). Fractures alter the biomechanics of the forearm in several ways: (1) a change in the normal interosseous membrane space limits rotation; (2) the proximal and distal radioulnar joints may disrupt; (3) neurovascular injuries may occur; (4) muscle pull can be changed, i.e., radial fractures proximal to the insertion of the pronator teres result in supination of the proximal radial fragment, and fractures distal to the insertion of the pronator teres produce a balanced muscle pull (Fig. 3).

X-ray Findings. X-rays should delineate the location and type of fracture, rotational deformities, and the condition of the joint above and below.

Clinical Findings. Pain, instability, and deformity are present and a careful evaluation of the neurovascular status must be made, since arterial and venous circulation may be compromised, causing Volkmann's ischemic contracture. This presents early with pain on passive extension of the fingers, followed by an inability to fully flex and extend the digits. Progressive necrosis of the forearm muscles in varying degrees may occur.

Treatment. The most important initial aspect of treatment of forearm fractures is to prevent neurovascular compromise. Special attention is given to avoid arterial insufficiency, to recognize impending Volkmann's contracture, and to excise open fractures. Arterial insufficiency should be treated by arterial repair, whereas Volkmann's ischemia should be treated by decompression and improvement of arterial and venous blood flow. Open fractures should be debrided, irrigated, and left open. Appropriate anesthesia is essential.

Criteria for acceptable reduction of forearm fractures are more rigid than for other extremity fractures. The normal interosseous space must be maintained, since this is necessary for maximum pronation

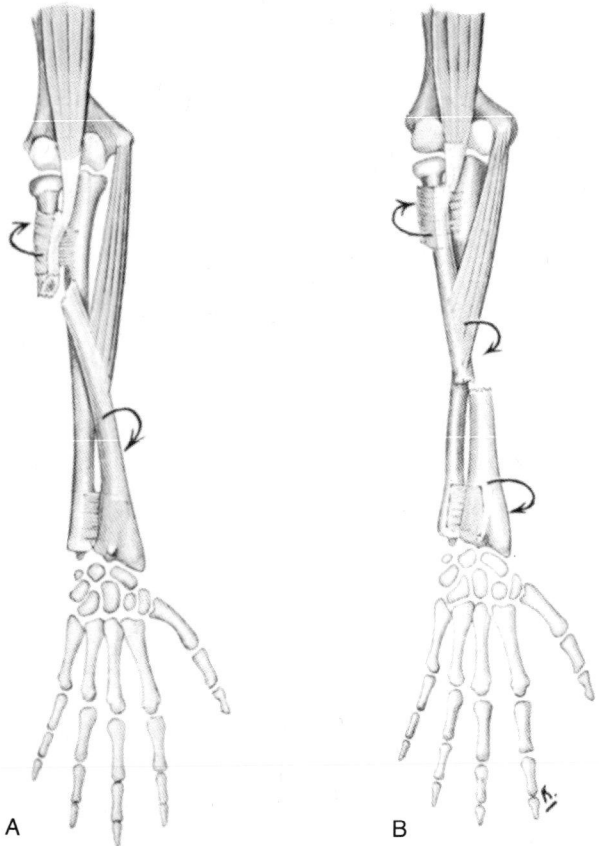

A   B

Figure 3. *A,* Fractures of the upper shaft of the radius. The proximal fragment is supinated and the lower fragment pronated. *B,* Fractures of the middle or lower shaft of the radius. The proximal fragment is in the mid position and the lower fragment is pronated. (From Watson & Jones: Fractures and Joint Injuries, 4th ed. Vol. II, Edinburgh, E. & S. Livingston, 1955.)

and supination. Closed treatment is satisfactory for fractures of one or both bones in children, undisplaced fractures of both bones, and fractures of the distal ulna and the proximal radius. Further growth of the child will usually correct angulation and overriding, but not rotational deformities.

Reduction is obtained by traction, molding of plaster over the fracture, and immobilization of the arm in a long arm cast for 10 to 12 weeks.

Fractures of the radius proximal to the insertion of the pronator teres are immobilized in supination. Most other fractures are immobilized in the mid position. The position of rotation is determined clinically and radiographically.

Open reduction should be considered for (1) both bones in adults; (2) the shaft of the ulna with dislocation of the radial head in adults; (3) the distal third of the radius with dislocation of the distal ulna; (4) a single bone fracture of the proximal ulna or the distal third of the radius with significant displacement; and (5) segmental fractures. Open reduction is considered in these instances because better alignment can be maintained and earlier motion initiated.

Important principles in the open treatment of fractures include rigid fixation with either a plate or an intramedullary rod, stripping the periosteum, and maintaining the interosseous space. Many authors prefer to add a bone graft at the fracture site.

In Monteggia's or Galeazzi's fractures, not only must the fracture be rigidly fixed, but the dislocated proximal radius and distal ulna must be relocated.

Complications. The most serious complication of forearm fractures is neurovascular compromise. Constant evaluation of the neurovascular status is necessary to prevent this.

Nonunion occurs 5 to 10 per cent of the time with closed treatment, and more frequently with open treatment. Malunion is more common with closed reduction and can prevent full rotation of the forearm. Rotational complications are common, and complete pronation and supination are not achieved in severe fractures. Rotation should be assessed systematically. Osteomyelitis occurs with open fractures or open reduction. Once established, rigid fixation should be maintained until the fracture is united. Other complications include elbow stiffness, finger stiffness, and reflex sympathetic dystrophy.

SELECTED REFERENCES

Bankart, A. S. B.: The pathology and treatment of recurrent dislocation of the shoulder joint. Br. J. Surg., 26:23–29, 1939.
A classic description of recurrent dislocation of the shoulder.

Blazina, M. E., and Satzman, J. S.: Recurrent anterior subluxation of the shoulder in athletics—a distinct entity. J. Bone Joint Surg., 51A:1037–1038, 1969.
In this paper, subtle injuries of the shoulder are emphasized.

Caldwell, J. A.: Treatment of fractures in the Cincinnati General Hospital. Ann. Surg., 97:161, 1933.
This paper considerably altered the treatment of the fractured humerus.

Helfet, A. J.: Coracoid transplantation for recurring dislocation of the shoulder. J. Bone Joint Surg., 40B:198–202, 1958.
In this paper, a description of the Bristow operation is presented.

Neer, C. S., II: Articular replacement for the humeral head. J. Bone Joint Surg., 37A:215–228, 1955.
A description of the early use of shoulder prostheses.

Neer, C. S., II: Displaced proximal humeral fractures. Part II, Treatment of three-part and four-part displacement. J. Bone Joint Surg., 52A:1090–1103, 1970.
In this paper, a classification of fractures of the shoulder is presented.

Osmond-Clarke, H.: Habitual dislocation of the shoulder. The Putti-Platt operation. J. Bone Joint Surg., 30B:19–25, 1948.
This is a classic paper concerning habitual dislocation of the shoulder.

REFERENCES

1. Allman, F. L., Jr.: Fractures and ligamentous injuries of the clavicle and its articulation. J. Bone Joint Surg., 49A:774–784, 1967.
2. Bankart, A. S. B.: Dislocation of the shoulder-joints: In Robert Jones' Birthday Volume. A Collection of Surgical Essays. London, Oxford University Press, 1928.
3. Bankart, A. S. B.: The pathology and treatment of recurrent dislocation of the shoulder joint. Br. J. Surg., 26:23–29, 1939.
4. Barton, J. R.: Views and treatment of an important injury to the wrist. Med. Examiner, 1:365, 1838.
5. Bateman, J. E.: Athletic injuries about the shoulder in throwing and body-contact sports. Clin. Orthop., 23:75–83, 1962.
6. Bearden, J. M., Hughston, J. C., and Whatley, G. S.: Acromioclavicular dislocation: Method of treatment. J. Sports Med., 1:5–17, 1973.
7. Blazina, M. E., and Satzman, J. S.: Recurrent anterior subluxation of the shoulder in athletics—a distinct entity. J. Bone Joint Surg., 51A:1037–1038, 1969.
8. Bohler, L.: The Treatment of Fractures. Supplementary volume. New York, Grune & Stratton, 1966.
9. Boyd, H. B., Lipinski, S. W., and Wiley, J. H.: Observation on nonunion of the shaft of the long bones with a statistical analysis of 842 patients. J. Bone Joint Surg., 43:159, 1961.
10. Caldwell, J. A.: Treatment of fractures in the Cincinnati General Hospital. Ann. Surg., 97:161, 1933.
11. Caldwell, J. A.: Treatment of fractures of the shaft of the humerus by hanging cast. Surg. Gynecol. Obstet., 70:421, 1940.
12. Campbell, W. C.: Ununited fractures of the shaft of the humerus. Ann. Surg., 105:135, 1937.
13. Charnley, J.: The Closed Treatment of Common Fractures. Baltimore, Williams & Wilkins, 1961.
14. Colles, A.: On the fractures of the carpal extremity of the radius. Edinburgh Med. Surg. J., 10:182–186, 1814.
15. DePalma, A. F.: The Management of Fractures and Dislocations, 2nd ed. Philadelphia, W. B. Saunders Company, 1970.
16. Helfet, A. J.: Coracoid transplantation for recurring dislocation of the shoulder. J. Bone Joint Surg., 40B:198–202, 1958.
17. Hill, N. A., and McLaughlin, H. L.: Locked posterior dislocation simulating a "frozen shoulder." J. Trauma, 3:225–234, 1963.
18. Hobbs, D. W.: Sternoclavicular joint: A new axial radiographic view. Radiology, 90:801–802, 1968.
19. Kennedy, J. C., and Cameron, H.: Complete dislocation of the acromioclavicular joint. J. Bone Joint Surg., 36B:202–208, 1954.
20. Kuntscher, G.: Intramedullary surgical technique and its place in orthopedic surgery: My present concept. J. Bone Joint Surg., 47A:809, 1965.
21. May, V. R., Jr.: A modified Bristow operation for anterior recurrent dislocation of the shoulder. J. Bone Joint Surg., 52A:1010–1016, 1970.
22. Magnuson, P. B.: Treatment of recurrent dislocation of the shoulder. Surg. Clin. North Am., 25:14–20, 1945.
23. Magnuson, P. B., and Stack, J. K.: Bilateral habitual dislocation of the shoulders in twins, a familial tendency. J.A.M.A., 144:2103, 1940.
24. McKenzie, J. M. M.: Retrosternal dislocation of the clavicle. A report of two cases. J. Bone Joint Surg., 45B:138–141, 1963.
25. Moseley, H. F.: Athletic injuries to the shoulder region. Am. J. Surg., 98:401–422, 1959.
26. Muller, M. E.: Treatment of nonunions by compression. Clin. Orthop., 43:83, 1965.
27. Neer, C. S., II: Articular replacement for the humeral head. J. Bone Joint Surg., 37A:215–228, 1955.
28. Neer, C. S., II: Degenerative lesions of the proximal humeral articular surface. Clin. Orthop., 20:116–124, 1961.
29. Neer, C. S., II: Displaced proximal humeral fractures. Part II, Treatment of three-part and four-part displacement. J. Bone Joint Surg., 52A:1090–1103, 1970.
30. Neer, C. S., II: Fractures of the distal clavicle with detachment of the coracoclavicular ligaments in adults. J. Trauma, 3:99–110, 1963.
31. Neer, C. S., II: Fractures of the distal third of the clavicle. Clin. Orthop., 58:43–50, 1968.
32. Osmond-Clarke, H.: Habitual dislocation of the shoulder. The Putti-Platt operation. J. Bone Joint Surg., 30B:19–25, 1948.
33. Paterson, D. C.: Retrosternal dislocation of the clavicle. J. Bone Joint Surg., 43B:90–92, 1961.
34. Rockwood, C. A., and Green, D. P.: Fractures. Philadelphia, J. B. Lippincott, 1975.
35. Rowe, C. R.: Prognosis in dislocations of the shoulder. Clin. Orthop., 82:84–86, 1972.
36. Rowe, C. R.: Symposium on surgical lesions of the shoulder. Acute and recurrent dislocation of the shoulder. J. Bone Joint Surg., 44A:977–1012, 1962.
37. Scientific Research Committee, Pennsylvania Orthopedic Society. Fresh midshaft fractures of the humerus in adults. Penn. Med. J., 62:848, 1959.
38. Seddon, H. J.: Nerve lesions complicating certain closed bone injuries. J.A.M.A., 135:691, 1947.
39. Smith, R. W.: A treatise on fractures in the vicinity of joints and on certain forms of accidental and congenital dislocations. Dublin, Hodges & Smith, 1854.

40. Stewart, M. J.: Fractures of the humeral shaft. *In* Adams, J. P. (Ed.): Current Practice in Orthopedic Surgery. St. Louis, The C. V. Mosby Co., 1964.
41. Urist, M. R.: Complete dislocation of the acromioclavicular joint. J. Bone Joint Surg., 45A:1750–1753, 1963.
42. Urist, M. R.: Complete dislocation of the acromioclavicular joint. The nature of the traumatic lesion and effective methods of treatment with an analysis of 41 cases. J. Bone Joint Surg., 28:813–837, 1946.
43. Worman, L. W., and Leagus, C.: Intrathoracic injury following retrosternal dislocation of the clavicle. J. Trauma, 7:416–423, 1967.

IV

FRACTURES OF THE CARPAL BONES

J. Leonard Goldner, M.D.

Because *carpal scaphoid fractures* are the most frequent injury to the wrist joint, the major emphasis of this section will be on injuries involving the carpal scaphoid.

Wrist Motion. Movement of the wrist joint occurs at the radiocarpal and intercarpal joints. Volar flexion takes place between the radius and the proximal carpal row and allows placement of the hand in numerous positions. Interference with the articular surfaces of the distal end of the radius and the proximal carpal row impedes both flexion and extension.

Elevation of the hand through motion at the wrist joint occurs primarily at the intercarpal joints between the capitate and the lunate (Fig. 1*B*). Limitations between those articulations decrease the full potential of hand action for complex maneuvers. The scaphoid participates in the activities of both carpal rows.

Scaphoid movement observed by image intensification demonstrates the upward motion of the scaphoid on dorsiflexion and the effect that a fall on the outstretched hand has on the distal segment of the scaphoid. The scaphoid articulates with the trapezium and the lunate and is covered partially by the radius. On the lateral roentgenogram of the wrist the distal part of the scaphoid is directed toward the volar aspect of the wrist at the point where it articulates with the trapezium. Thus, the scaphoid makes a stepoff from the proximal carpal row to the distal carpal row (see Fig. 6*B*).

Radial and ulnar deviation (Fig. 2) results in movement of the scaphoid both into and away from the distal radius and demonstrates the effect of different positions on the intact scaphoid and on the fractured scaphoid. Not only does a fall on the outstretched hand result in dorsiflexion, but also a position of either radial or ulnar deviation and a torque movement are part of the force that results in a fracture. Experimentally, as much as 3000 pounds per square inch may be necessary to fracture the scaphoid.

Surface Anatomy. Certain critical points that must be examined after known trauma to the hand are demonstrated in

Figure 1*A*. The dot at the base of the thumb coincides with the snuff box and the distal end of the scaphoid. The next dot is over the styloid process of the radius and the dorsum of the scaphoid. The dot in line with the third and fourth digits

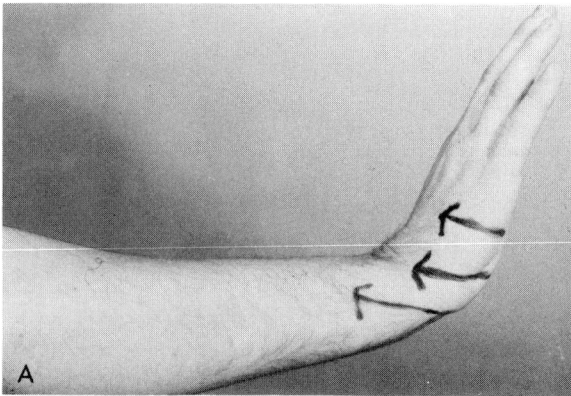

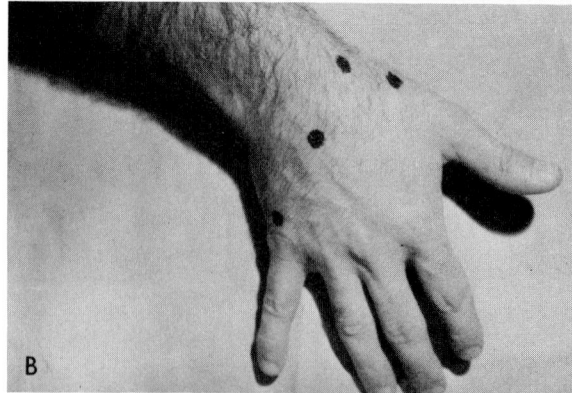

Figure 1. *A,* Position of the hand and forearm usually associated with "fall on the outstretched hand." Arrows represent lines of force that might occur. *B,* The dots correspond with common areas of fracture of the hand, the base of the thumb, the proximal carpal row, and the base of the metacarpal.

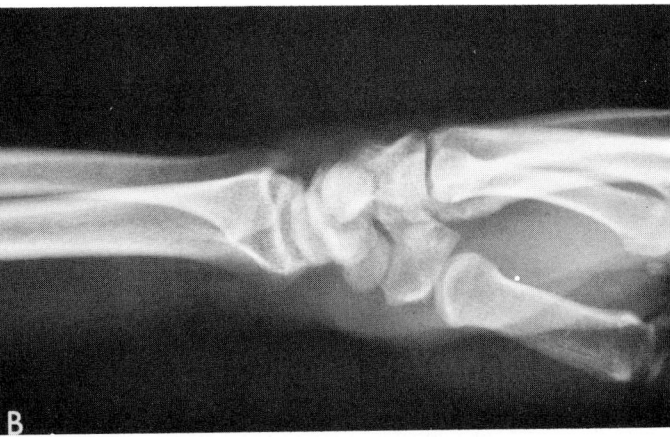

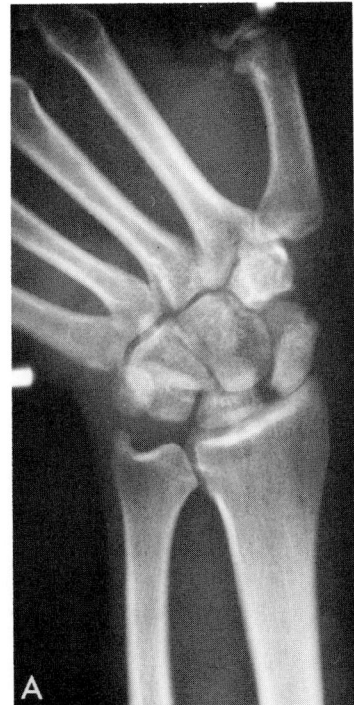

Figure 2. *A*, Space between the lunate and the carpal scaphoid indicative of rotary subluxation of the carpal scaphoid. Instability between scaphoid and lunate. *B*, Incongruity of the lunate and the scaphoid. Internal fixation and reconstruction of ligaments required.

is over the lunate, and the marking over the fifth metacarpal is the point where a fracture of the metacarpal neck occurs. Figure 1*B* shows the outstretched hand with the possible lines of force that occur depending on how the individual breaks the fall. The lowest line of force may result in Colles' fracture, whereas the upper may cause a metacarpal fracture. The central force would be involved in a carpal injury.

Differential Diagnosis of Carpal Scaphoid Injuries

1. *Rotary subluxation of the scaphoid* occurs as a result of a tear of the ligament between the scaphoid and the lunate (Fig. 2). Once this ligament is avulsed or ruptured, the relationship between the lunate and the scaphoid is distorted. The scaphoid can then move in a superior and interior direction without maintaining its usual relationship to the lunate. The space between the two carpal bones enlarges, and this is the pathognomonic sign on the roentgenogram. The patient complains of a popping and clicking in the wrist joint associated with pain and limited motion. The condition is not easily diagnosed unless suspected.

2. *Rupture of the flexor carpi radialis tendon* results from a fall on the outstretched hand and separation of the insertion of the flexor carpi radialis at a point where it is attached under the thenar muscles. A chip of bone may separate with the tendon, or, in patients over 35 years old, the tendon itself may rupture partially or completely. This tendon is also one affected by aging of collagen, and localized partial ruptures may occur with minimal trauma. Pain is at the point that coincides with the scaphoid on the volar surface of the wrist.

3. A *fracture of the styloid process* of the radius may result from a fall on the outstretched hand or a direct blow (Fig. 3*A*). This area coincides with the body of the scaphoid. Compression of the styloid process may cause pain at approximately the same location as does compression of the scaphoid.

4. A *trapezium fracture* such as occurs with a direct fist blow or a fall on the radial, deviated, closed hand may also be confused with the fractured scaphoid. Usually the swelling and pain are closer to the thumb than is the fractured scaphoid, and the mechanism of injury is slightly different.

5. *Extensor carpi radialis longus avulsion* from the first metacarpal occurs as a result of a forceful injury in ulnar deviation, a direct blow, or a downward stroke such as hitting the ground with a golf club. The area of localized tenderness is almost directly over the anatomic snuff box and is similar to that present when the carpal scaphoid is fractured. However, the roentgenogram will not show a fracture, and the volar aspect of the wrist will not be painful.

6. An *extensor carpi radialis brevis tendon avulsion* may occur as a result of forceful volar flexion of the wrist. Palpation at this point results in pain at the base of the third metacarpal, which is slightly distal to the point where the scaphoid would be tender if fractured.

7. *Osteochondral fracture of the distal radius* as a result of an injury simulates the fractured scaphoid. The mechanism of injury, the radiologic findings, and pain primarily on the dorsal and radial aspects of the wrist will aid in differentiating this injury from the carpal scaphoid fracture.

8. *Lunate dislocation or fracture* causes pain on the dorsum of the wrist more to the center of the wrist area and less on the radial side. Wrist motion is

limited, and the roentgenogram will show distortion of the proximal carpal row.

Special Clinical Problem Related to Carpal Scaphoid Injury

The alterations that occur with a trans-scaphoid perilunar dislocation are shown in Figure 3. The irregularity of the scaphoid is evident, and the space between the scaphoid and the lunate is obvious. The carpal area is distorted. Roentgen projections from the volar and dorsal surfaces provide different but essential visualization. The lateral, oblique, and anteroposterior views demonstrate the fractured scaphoid and the great distortion between the capitate and the lunate.

This injury is best treated by manipulation and internal fixation, either by open or closed reduction using percutaneous fixation in order to avoid a prolonged excessive position of flexion and to maintain good apposition between the scaphoid fragments, as well as assuring anatomic positioning of the lunate. The incision or exposure will extend from the dorsal aspect of the radius around the radial aspect to the volar side.

Anatomic Physiology of the Carpal Scaphoid

Blood Supply. The carpal scaphoid specimen from a cadaver cleaned of its soft tissue attachments will show many perforations that represent entrance and exit points of blood vessels. These points of perforation are directly related to the survival or death of bone fragments after trauma. Figure 4

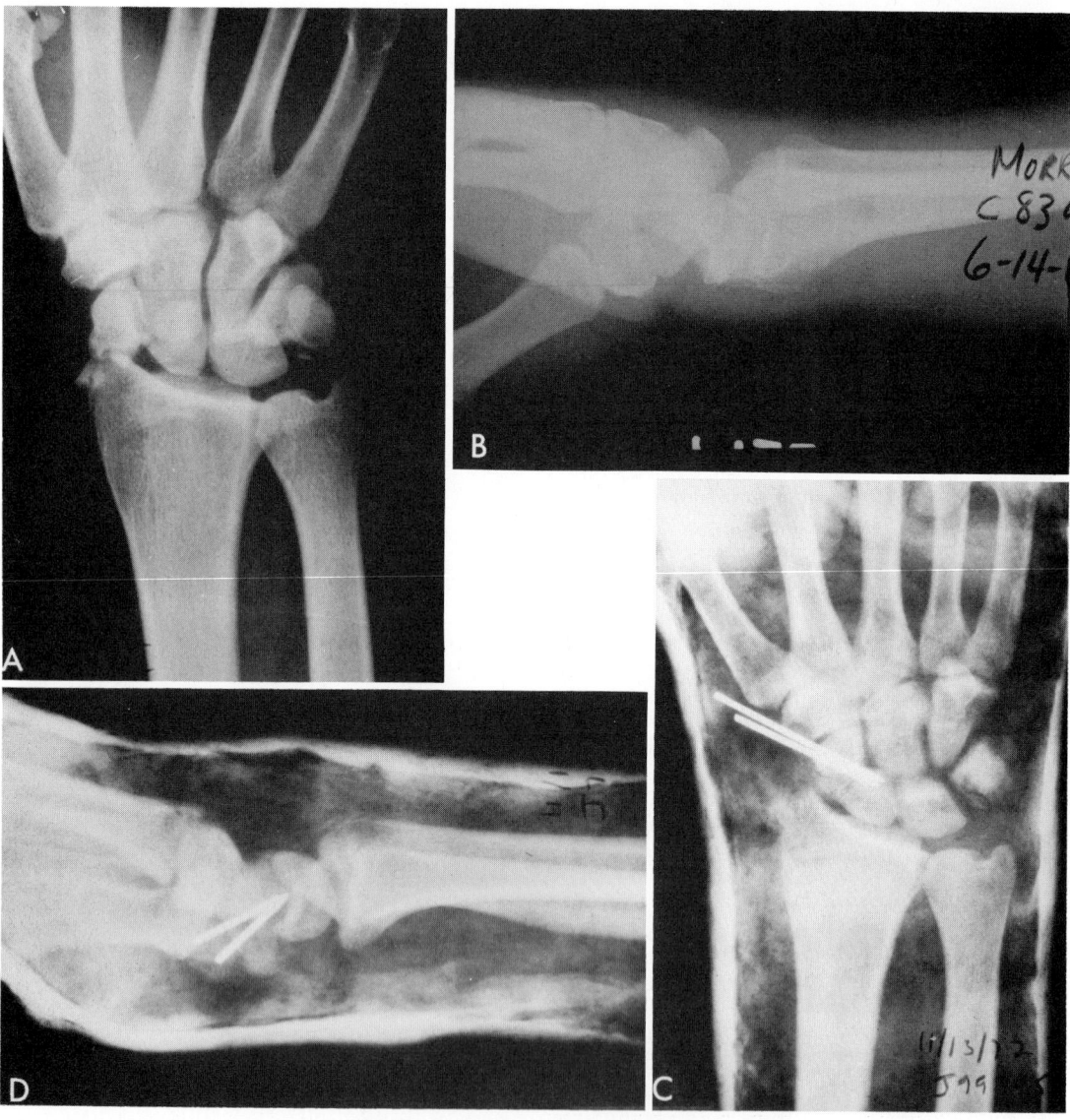

Figure 3. *A*, Fracture of the carpal scaphoid with disruption of the adjacent carpal bones, compatible with trans-scaphoid perilunate dislocation. *B*, Traction and rotation improved position, but the scaphoid fragments are only moderately apposed. *C*, Two weeks later the position was still incomplete and open operation was done for fixation of the carpal scaphoid fragments in order to maintain contact of the fragments and close apposition to the lunate. *D*, Lateral view showing the scaphoid fragments in anatomic position. Fixation is by smooth pins which can be removed easily. Satisfactory union occurred.

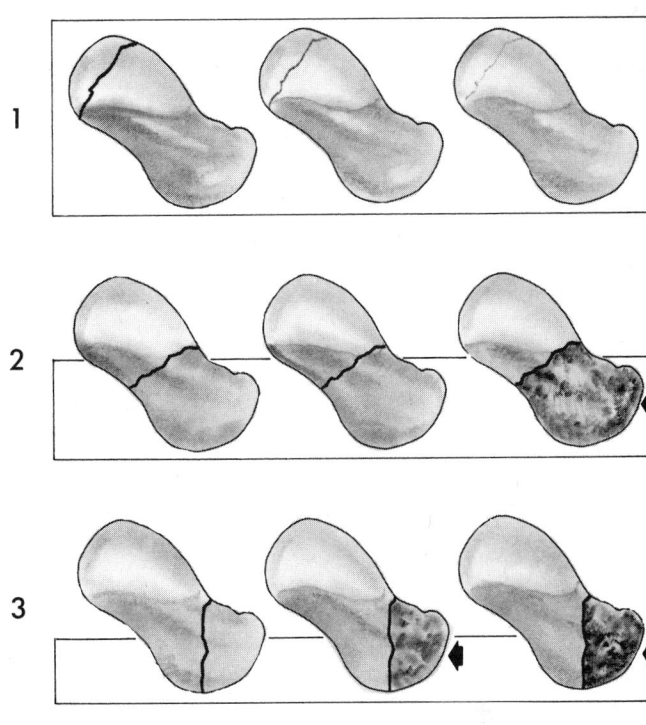

Figure 4. Diagrammatic representation of blood supply of the carpal scaphoid, which affects both healing and the development of avascular necrosis.

shows 9 different patterns of blood supply and demonstrates certain specimens with most of the blood vessels distally, others with a few vessels proximally. This pattern of blood vessel distribution indicates that the proximal segment is most likely to undergo avascular necrosis after trauma. Figure 3A is the prereduction roentgenogram of the transscaphoid perilunar dislocation. Note the large gap in the scaphoid and the location of the fracture. The proximal fragment is likely to undergo temporary avascular necrosis until the fragment is revascularized by "creeping substitution."

Clinical Assessment of the Painful Wrist

Pain. Radial and ulnar deviation will result in pain on the radial side of the wrist. Stress must be applied in certain instances if the fracture is occult. Forced dorsiflexion causes most pain. Individuals required to do pushups will do them with the closed fist and a straight wrist rather than by dorsiflexing the wrist. Pressure in the snuff box causes pain, but this maneuver must be differentiated from pressure over the radial artery, which also is painful. Pain can be reproduced by having the patient put extreme pressure on the fingertips with the wrist in the dorsiflexed position. Percussion of the second metacarpal head directed toward the radius may produce pain. Rotation of the hand against resistance frequently causes pain on the radial aspect of the wrist. The patient is asked to supinate and the examiner attempts to pronate against resistance, and vice versa. *Palpation of pain points* on the volar, radial, and dorsal aspects of the wrist will elicit pain reaction at one or all of these locations.

Roentgen Projections. Specific orders must be given to the technician in order to obtain proper roentgen projections. These should include anteroposterior views with the wrist in both ulnar and radial deviation, pronated oblique and supinated oblique views, and a lateral view in dorsiflexion and volar flexion. Occasionally, a posteroanterior view is helpful if there is a question of rotary subluxation of the carpal scaphoid.

SPECIAL ROENTGENOGRAPHIC TECHNIQUES. Roentgen projection at the time of the original injury may not demonstrate the fracture because of impaction and absence of absorption. At 10 to 14 days after injury, however, decrease in bone density at the fracture site and physiologic absorption do occur and a repeat roentgenogram at this time may demonstrate the fracture. If the clinical findings are positive and strongly suggestive, but the routine roentgenogram does not show a fracture, then special views and techniques include (a) magnification roentgenogram, which may bring out interruption of trabeculae and an occult fracture, (b) tomography, which may show a fracture at a level deeper than the surface projection allows, (c) repeat stress roentgenogram after injection of the wrist joint with a local anesthetic, and (d) a videotaped visualization of the wrist after injection with the local anesthetic. The importance of detecting the fracture is related to the length of time and the kind of immobilization that must be done. There are numerous instances of "sprained wrists" treated by a simple soft dressing that results in nonunion of the carpal scaphoid which, if treated for 8 to 10 weeks in an appropriate plaster cast, would have united and eliminated the impairment that occurs as a result of a nonunion of the scaphoid.

Treatment

One must be cautious about accepting the diagnosis of a "sprained wrist." If the mechanism of injury is in keeping with that which might usually cause a fractured carpal scaphoid, the wrist should be treated with the plaster splint or plaster cast for 10 days. The roentgenogram should be repeated, the wrist should be maneuvered and manipulated, and if a fracture is seen, then a permanent plastic or plaster cast is applied. The usual length of time of immobilization is three to four months, although as long as 10 months may be needed in certain instances (Fig. 5).

Occasionally, a special type of plastic splint can be applied in order to allow an athlete to continue playing competitive sports. A segment of the thumb may be left out of the cast in order to allow a student or an executive to write (Fig. 6A and B). Treatment must be pragmatic as well as physiologic.

Immobilization and Fixation. The hand and wrist are placed in a position that corresponds with the location and kind of injury that has occurred. If the injury resulted from a dorsiflexed hand, then volar flexion is a logical position for replacement of the fragments. If ulnar deviation was part of the mechanism of injury,

then radial deviation should allow impaction of the fragments (Fig. 6A and B).

In certain fractures there is impingement of the radial styloid on a fracture of the carpal scaphoid. In ulnar deviation the fragments are spread, in radial deviation a moderate compression is allowed, and the radius covers the scaphoid. Radial deviation and 10 degrees of flexion will provide good compression, provided that the styloid does not spread the fragments. Figure 6A shows an extremity in a cast below the elbow with the base of the thumb included. If the individual must have the thumb for writing, part of the plaster can be removed and only the metacarpal immobilized. My experience is that the cast should be changed about every 10 to 14 days for the first six weeks. After that a water resistant, porous cast can be applied that can be immersed in water without losing its strength. Figures 6C and D shows plastic tape and "light cast," both used successfully in athletes.

Fixation of the fragments should be done early. The position will depend on the mechanism of injury, but radial deviation in 10 degrees of flexion will usually provide compression or apposition of the fragments.

The cast should be molded carefully, extend proximally over the muscles of the forearm, and follow the

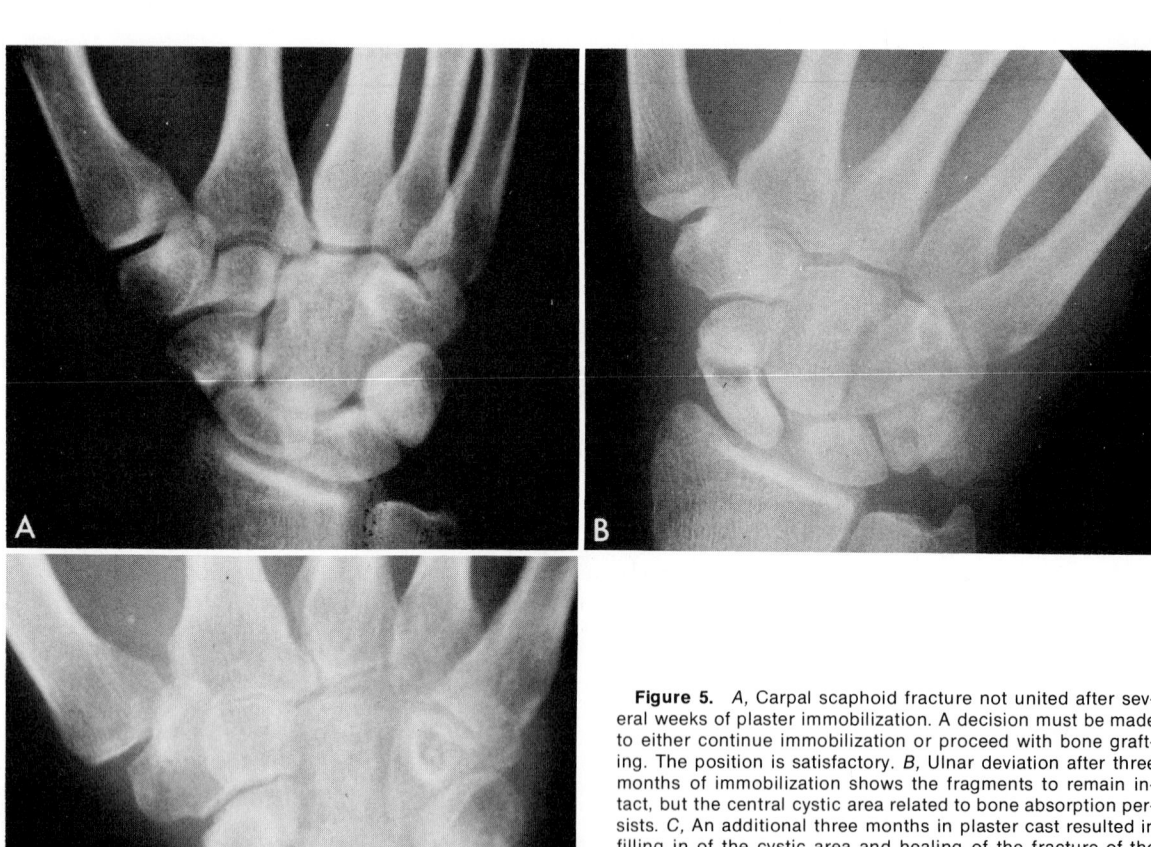

Figure 5. A, Carpal scaphoid fracture not united after several weeks of plaster immobilization. A decision must be made to either continue immobilization or proceed with bone grafting. The position is satisfactory. B, Ulnar deviation after three months of immobilization shows the fragments to remain intact, but the central cystic area related to bone absorption persists. C, An additional three months in plaster cast resulted in filling in of the cystic area and healing of the fracture of the carpal scaphoid with complete motion resulting without pain.

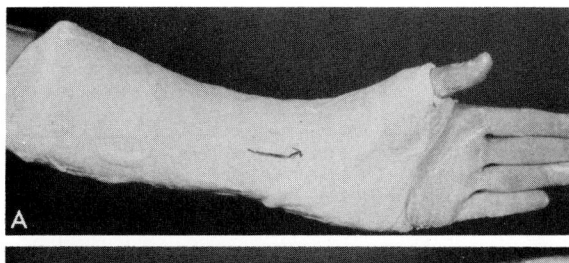

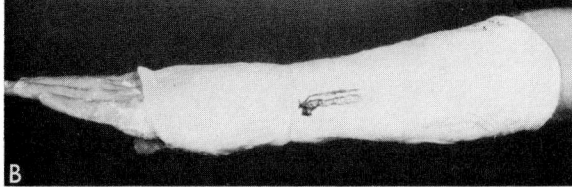

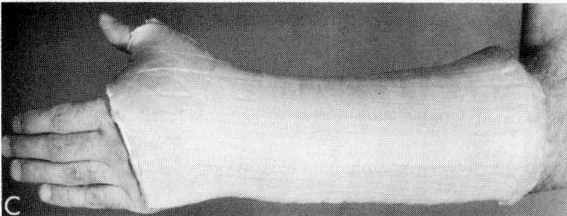

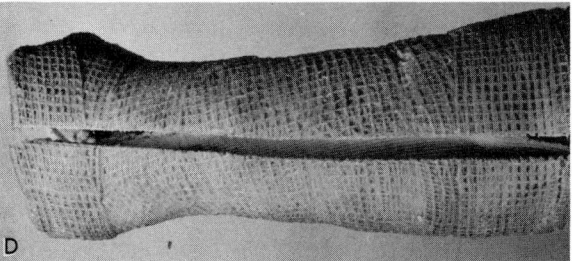

Figure 6. *A,* Well fitting short arm cast is sufficient to immobilize the carpal scaphoid fragments. The contour of the forearm is used for molding of the plaster, thereby eliminating the need for cast above the elbow. *B,* In many instances, radial deviation and volar flexion give the best contact. The thumb metacarpal is included, but the distal joint is free so that the individual can handle a pen or do certain other activities related to work or education. *C,* Synthetic "Lightcast." This is water repellent and durable. The patient can use this for several weeks or months in ways that are more convenient and more comfortable than the standard plaster cast. "Lightcast" is usually used in the secondary stages of healing. *D,* Plastic tape over a carpal scaphoid soft wrapping is safe for temporary use during an athletic activity. This kind of wrapping is allowed by game officials whereas plaster or metal, even though padded, are not permissible.

contour of the forearm (Fig. 6*A* and *B*). The cast should not be circular but should be contoured and quadrilateral. Minimal padding should be used throughout so that when edema subsides, fixation will be adequate. The styloid process of the ulna and the radial styloid should be carefully covered with a small piece of felt to avoid cast pressure on the skin. The cast should be molded into the palm and the fingers free at the metacarpophalangeal joints and distally.

Postreduction roentgenograms are taken if warranted by the condition of the fragments prior to application of the cast. If the gap is wide, then an x-ray should be taken to be certain that the gap is closed.

Special Complex Problems Affecting the Carpal Scaphoid

Figure 3*A* shows disruption of the scaphoid through the waist and distortion of the carpus at the intercarpal joints. After closed manipulation, the position of the scaphoid was relatively anatomic, but a small segment of bone that arose from either the scaphoid or the styloid of the radius was still visible. Figure 3*C* shows that the relationship between the proximal and distal carpal row has been re-established, and the lateral view shows satisfactory position. Percutaneous pin fixation was done primarily to stabilize the scaphoid and incidentally to provide at least soft tissue fixation between the proximal and distal rows of the carpus.

Delayed Healing

The cause of delayed union or nonunion is usually delayed diagnosis. A "sprained wrist" is not an acceptable diagnosis until fracture of the carpal scaphoid is completely ruled out.

In other situations, when the diagnosis is made but the reduction is incomplete, inadequate apposition of the fragments may result in nonunion. With certain complex injuries, such as trans-scaphoid perilunar dislocation, percutaneous fixation with pins may provide complete stabilization whereas no fixation or only one pin may result in instability.

Pathology Associated with Nonunion or Malunion

Osteonecrosis may occur at the fracture site owing to a great force associated with the injury, or multiple small fractures may occur and affect the quality of bone healing.

Avascular necrosis results from inadequate blood supply and depends on the anatomic makeup of the scaphoid and the location of the fracture in relationship to the major arterial vessels (Fig. 4*A*).

Traumatic arthrosis results from cartilage damage at the time of the original injury, incongruity of cartilaginous surface secondary to malposition or malunion, or hypermobility from nonunion.

Excision of one or both fragments of an ununited scaphoid may result in satisfactory wrist function and motion for a year or two, but the long-term follow-up has generally been unsatisfactory because of radial deviation and traumatic arthrosis.

Reconstructive Procedures for Nonunion of the Carpal Scaphoid

The author has reviewed a five-year group of scaphoid nonunions treated by autogenous iliac bone grafting to the carpal scaphoid through a volar incision. This treatment resulted in 11 of 12 nonunions healing satisfactorily.

Use of the radial styloid process for the bone graft has a greater morbidity because of involvement of the articular surfaces of the radius. Eight of 12 nonunions healed satisfactorily.

A dorsal approach for nonunion and grafting is not recommended. Four were attempted, and four failed.

Other Treatment Attempted When Bone Grafting Is Not Indicated

Proximal carpalectomy: Five patients showed satisfactory motion, reasonable strength, and relief of pain.

This is a good compromise if bone grafting or prosthetic replacement fails prior to selecting arthrodesis.

Arthrodesis of the wrist showed good strength, elimination of pain, but limitation of activities of daily living.

A metallic prosthesis was only occasionally successful. Three were put in and three have been removed.

Silicone prosthesis: Eight have been put in and five removed. The principle is good, but the prosthesis is not entirely satisfactory, and improvement in design is needed.

SELECTED REFERENCES

Barnard, L., and Stubbins, S. G.: Styloidectomy of the radius in the surgical treatment of non-union of the carpal navicular. A preliminary report. J. Bone Joint Surg., *30A*:98–102, 1948.
This report encouraged other investigators to examine the problem of nonunion of the carpal scaphoid and to examine the biomechanics of the radial carpal joint. The article focuses on the problem of non-union of the carpal scaphoid.

Campbell, R. D., Jr., Thompson, T. C., Lance, E. M., and Addler, J. B.: Indications for open reduction of lunate and perilunate dislocations of the carpal bones, J. Bone Joint Surg., *47A*:915–937, 1965.
This article emphasizes the complexity of recognizing and managing dislocations of the carpal bones. Diagnostic roentgen techniques, the interpretation of the roentgenogram, and the selection of treatment are emphasized.

Linsheid, R. L., Dobyns, J. H., Beabout, J. W., and Bryan, R. S.: Traumatic instability of the wrist: Diagnosis, classification and pathomechanics, J. Bone Joint Surg., *54A*:1612–1632, 1972.
These authors present a biomechanical background of persistent instability of the wrist after trauma. Relationship between the carpal bones and their location in the wrist joint depends on loss of stability of intercarpal ligaments and the dorsal and volar capsule.

Difficulties associated with recognition of instability and treatment are emphasized.

Russe, O.: Fracture of the carpal navicular: Diagnosis, non-operative treatment, and operative treatment. J. Bone Joint Surg., *42A*:759–768, 1960.
This author popularized a volar incision and cancellous bone grafting through this volar approach for nonunion of the carpal scaphoid. The rate of bone union was increased significantly, and the morbidity associated with the bone grafting was decreased.

Soto-Hall, R., and Haldeman, K. O.: The conservative and operative treatment of fractures of the carpal scaphoid (navicular). J. Bone Joint Surg., *23*:841–850, 1943.
These authors emphasize the problem of treatment as it relates to injuries of the carpal scaphoid. The need for operation is recognized if nonoperative treatment fails.

REFERENCES

1. Agerholm, J. C., and Lee, M. L.: The acrylic scaphoid prosthesis in the treatment of the ununited carpal scaphoid fracture. Acta Orthop. Scand., *37*:67–76, 1966.
2. Crock, H. V.: Post-traumatic erosions of articular cartilage. J. Bone Joint Surg., *46B*:530–538, 1964.
3. Goldner, J. L., Hutchinson, F., and Verhoogen, A.: Treatment of fractures of the carpal scaphoid, review of results – 20 years. Unpublished data, 1975.
4. Goldner, J. L.: Diagnosis and treatment of trauma involving the carpal scaphoid. Presentation, Academy Day, American Academy of Orthopedic Surgeons, Portland, Maine, September, 1975.
5. Hart, V. L., and Gaynor, V.: Roentgenographic study of the carpal canal. J. Bone Joint Surg., *23*:382–383, 1941.
6. Stewart, M. J.: Fractures of the carpal navicular (scaphoid): A report of 436 cases. J. Bone Joint Surg., *36A*:998–1006, 1954.
7. Swanson, A. B.: Silicone rubber implants for replacement of the carpal scaphoid and lunate bones. Orthop. Clin. North Am., *1*:299–309, 1970.

V

FRACTURES AND DISLOCATIONS OF THE HAND

J. Leonard Goldner, M.D.

Hand digits are exposed to many forces that may result in bone or joint trauma. The dexterity of the professional musician, the surgeon, the magician, and numerous other individuals depends on flexibility of joints and coordinated action of the digits. The digits are encompassed by soft tissues that provide oxygenation, nutrition, and the numerous kinds of sensation as well as the ligaments for stability and tendons for mobility that make the finger more than a senseless, stiff appendage. Avoidance of hand and finger injuries is a part of preventive medicine. Admonition to children about placing the hand near moving objects and advice to adults participating in athletics are part of this campaign to prevent soft tissue trauma, joint injuries, and fractures. Once the injury occurs, the physician must be able to diagnose the pathologic process and either provide care for the patient or direct the patient to an appropriate source so that care can be obtained.

We meet our environment with our hands and feet, and the digits are usually uncovered and are vulnerable stationary or moving objects. Sports activities, industrial machines, and excessive cold all may cause injury to the various components of the fingers and thumb. Fractures of the metacarpals and phalanges are estimated at 10 per cent of all fractures that occur. Higher estimates have been given for those working in industry.

The individual joints in each digit have an indirect effect on the total function of the digit. If the proximal interphalangeal joint has been injured and fibrosis occurs, the fingertip cannot be brought to the distal palm crease. If the distal interphalangeal joint has been affected by a ruptured extensor tendon, the distal phalanx remains in flexion and interferes with dexterity of the involved digit and the adjacent digits. The metacarpophalangeal joint, if limited by trauma, affects the degree of flexion of the adjacent digit, or, if the metacarpophalangeal joint is held in flexion, the adjacent fingers cannot be straightened completely.

Functional Anatomy of the Hand

The functional anatomy of the hand must be understood in order to diagnose and treat bone and joint injuries of the hand.

The distal transverse crease on the volar aspect of the wrist corresponds to the carpal bones. The radial artery, median nerve, and ulnar nerve are readily injured at that level.

The transverse crease in the palm corresponds to the metacarpophalangeal joints. The proximal crease of the fingers is located in the midportion of the proximal phalanx, the middle crease is opposite the proximal interphalangeal joint, and the distal crease opposite the distal joint.

The first metacarpal has an epiphysis at the proximal end, as do the proximal phalanges of the fingers. The second through fifth metacarpals have an epiphysis at the distal end.

As the fingers are flexed to make a fist, their line of action results in convergence, with the center of each nail pointing toward the carpal scaphoid. None of the fingers is flexed in a straight line, which means that immobilization should never occur with the nail in line with the corresponding metacarpal. The position of immobilization and the prevention of malrotation can best be determined by observing the position of flexion in a normal, uninjured hand. Splints and plaster and dressings should hold the digits in the position of physiologic alignment (Fig. 1).

The ulnar three fingers must be flexed together, and also extended almost in unison. The index finger requires partial flexion of the long and ring fingers when full flexion is done. Individual variations do occur but the usual pattern is that just described. The thumb can be flexed almost completely

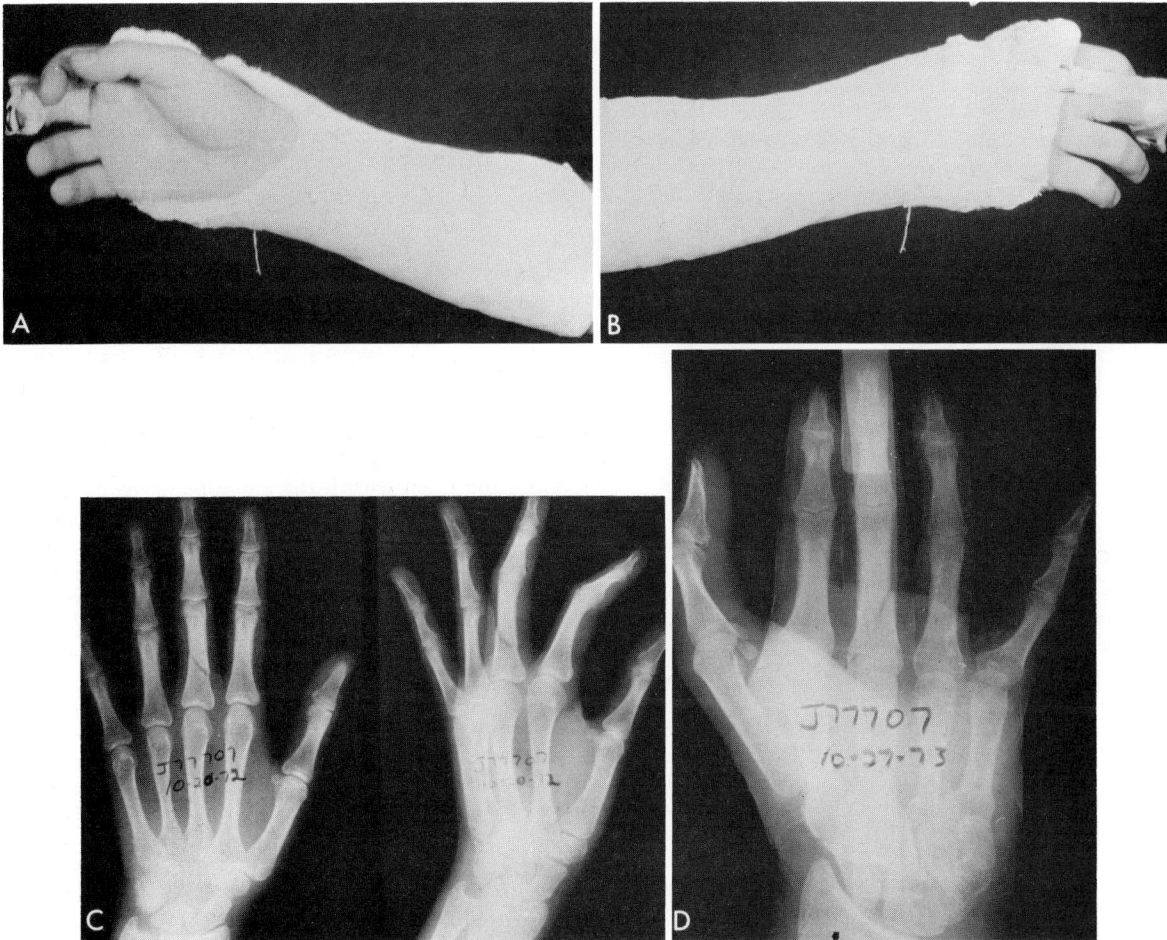

Figure 1. *A,* One method of managing phalangeal fracture. The plaster gauntlet serves as a base for the dorsal aluminum splint. The tape immobilizes the digit for a few days, and the dorsal splint blocks extension. Distal fragment of the phalanx is held in flexion, and early active motion is encouraged. *B,* Other digits are freely movable. Splint can be adjusted, and the digit visualized throughout the entire treatment. *C* and *D,* Long oblique fracture with malrotation, proximal phalanx. Pre- and post-reduction and splinting.

without simultaneous action of the adjacent fingers, although about 10 per cent of the population has connections between the flexor digitorum profundus of the index finger and the flexor pollicis longus.

The extensor aspect of the hand demonstrates the extensor communis tendons to be subcutaneous, the anatomic snuff box is evident at the base of the thumb, and the multiple skin creases over the finger joints are available so that the skin is not excessively tense when all joints are placed into the flexed position.

EXAMINATION OF THE HAND

The injured part may be examined prior to obtaining the history or after details concerning the accident have been elicited. A pattern of assessment must be established and followed meticulously, including the history, occupation, hand dominance, and accurate data concerning the injury (when, where, how, why? What is the time interval between injury and examination? What is the treatment and by whom?).

The *circulation* is tested by compressing the nail bed, observing the color of the digit, and comparing the temperature. A pale finger is usually the result of a diminished arterial blood supply. A blue finger suggests venous congestion. Elevation and depression of the extremity may provide information quickly about venous and arterial viability.

Sensation is tested by light touch, pressure, two point discrimination, and sharp point. The sensory deficit may be profound if the digital nerve is lacerated completely or may be minimal if the nerve was contused by trauma. The initial examination in a closed wound will not necessarily determine accurately whether or not the digital nerve has been lacerated. In an open fracture with sensory loss, the assumption is that the digital nerve has been lacerated or severely contused if the sensory deficit exists.

Motor function may be limited because of deformity or pain. However, an effort is made to determine active flexion and extension of the interphalangeal joints, motion at the metacarpophalangeal joint, rotation of the base of the thumb, and thumb joint voluntary control. The wrist is also tested.

Joint motion may be limited by either intra-articular or extra-articular damage or by injury to the extensor or flexor tendons, which would indirectly eliminate distal or proximal interphalangeal joint motion or both. Each joint is tested by isolating it from the adjacent joints. The patient attempts voluntarily to bend the tip of the finger, the middle joint, and the metacarpophalangeal joint. The examiner must differentiate rebound motion from voluntary motion. For example, voluntary flexion of the tip may be done and when the flexors are released the tip then rebounds to extension. This suggests that the extensors are functioning but they actually may not be. In the reverse, active extension may be possible and rebound flexion occurs, causing confusion concerning action of the flexors. The intrinsic function may be present, resulting in extension of the tips and seemingly performing as if extensor communis action were present.

The normal hand is the best model for obtaining a pattern of hand examination and the physician must refer to the wrist, thumb, and finger motion of the normal hand both in flexion and extension in order to perform a meaningful examination of the abnormal or injured hand.

The *closed* wound is examined meticulously to determine the site of disruption of bone and soft tissue. The tendon insertion should be palpated, the collateral ligaments detected, stability of the joints determined, and reasons for angulation obtained. Terminology providing description of the alignment is consistent. **Dislocation** means that the articular surfaces are not touching or congruous and that the restraining ligaments have been torn, and probably the capsule as well. **Subluxation** means a partial displacement of one part of the joint on the other but with less severe distortion than a dislocation. Soft tissue interposition may exist in either instance and prevent full reduction. The term "reduction" refers to the action required to obtain anatomic alignment.

Edema may result from hemorrhage, extravasation of joint fluid, intracellular swelling, or prominence of a segment of the articular surface or the involved bone.

Open wounds should be equated with the mechanism of injury. Was the skin avulsed by a circular ring, was the digit twisted by a turning wheel, was the palm penetrated by a sharp irregular edge, was the hand caught in a hot or cold roller? Was the ball that injured the hand large or small, and did it hit the tip of the finger or the middle of the finger? Was the thumb twisted in the loop of the ski pole or was it caught on the rope attached to the boat that was pulling the water skier out of the water?

Open wounds are examined cautiously. Both sides of the hand are inspected. Swelling on the dorsum may result from penetration on the volar surface. The examiner should wear a mask, use sterile gloves and instruments, and do minimal probing until adequate peripheral anesthesia has been obtained and the patient is in a location where definitive treatment can be completed.

Once the preliminary examination has been completed, the open wound is managed in a definitive way, preferably in the operating room area or in an operating room within the emergency room. The open fracture must be managed with major consideration for the blood supply of the part, tendon and nerve injury, and intrinsic muscle injury. By way of caution, the safest approach to the management of open wounds is adequate wound excision of all aspects of the wound and delayed or secondary closure.

A *foreign body* should be suspected in any open or penetrating injury. Many objects are not radiopaque, such as wood, clothing, most forms of glass, and certain plastics.

Experience has shown that all open wounds may be treated open, and that the importance of tissue damage is in the order of circulation, nerve, tendon, and then skin. Circulation must be restored as quickly as possible either by direct suture of digital nerves or major parts of the blood supply, or by releasing edematous soft tissue to decrease external pressure or vascular spasm. Digital nerves do not require primary repair, nor do lacerated flexor tendons. Open joints must be cleansed but can be maintained open for 24 to

48 hours without detriment to the articular surfaces. Angulation of bones should be corrected early but not at the risk of damage to adjacent soft tissues. A stable skeleton, however, decreases persistent irritation to the adjacent vascular structures and decreases the chances of infection in open wounds; however, elongation of the digit to its original length may again compromise the circulation. The concept of treating open wounds open until such time as it is safe to close them with direct suture, additional skin, or by allowing secondary healing, will eliminate many complications that occur in wounds treated both by the expert and by the less experienced.

Roentgen Examination

Multiview exposure of the hand or the digit involved is essential to accurate diagnosis. Usual views are posteroanterior, pronation and supination oblique, and direct lateral. Direct lateral exposures must be taken of the individual digits rather than of the hand as a whole. Laterals of the metacarpals and the wrist pose no problem in positioning. The addition of a 10 degree supination film for the ulnar side of the hand and a 10 degree pronation film for the radial side of the hand adds more information than the true lateral.

The *xeroradiogram* may be useful in determining the presence of nonradiopaque foreign bodies such as glass or wood. Bone detail may be determined better with this technique than with a standard roentgenographic exposure.

Magnification roentgenograms are helpful in determining occult fractures of the carpal bones or the phalanges.

Stress views taken with the joint open in a direction away from the injured ligaments will give more information about the extent of the dislocated joint than will a plain exposure.

The postreduction or posttreatment roentgenogram is usually taken through plaster, or an aluminum splint, or a dressing of some kind. A portable roentgenogram before the dressing is applied may be helpful when percutaneous pin fixation is used or when an intra-articular fracture is being manipulated prior to determining whether open reduction is needed. The few extra minutes required for taking the roentgenogram may save a second anesthesia and an additional procedure.

Anesthesia

Relief of pain associated with trauma is essential if diagnosis and treatment are to be successful. Sensory and motor examination must be completed, however, before local or regional anesthesia is given. In children, the circulation can be examined with minimal difficulty, but motor power and sensation are not determined as readily as in the adult. Accordingly, these details may not be as complete in the child as in the adult but without detriment to the patient, since primary nerve or tendon repair can always be delayed without compromising final function.

Manipulation and realignment of a phalanx requires some relaxation of the extensor and flexor tendons of the forearm. Fracture of the phalanx or an intra-articular injury in the digit can be managed by local infiltration, digital nerve block in the metacarpal area for a particular finger, and in certain instances, median or ulnar nerve block at the wrist and su-

perficial radial nerve injection at the level of the styloid process of the radius.

Several modalities of local and regional anesthesia can be used to supplement each other. Penetrating wounds can be managed by local infiltration and a peripheral nerve block; a fracture of the proximal phalanx of the index finger can be treated by local infiltration, metacarpal digital nerve block, and median block at the wrist. All of these injections can be done serially and, if followed by a waiting period of five minutes, will provide adequate anesthesia for any type of manipulation.

The use of a blood pressure cuff as a tourniquet applied after the extremity has been elevated for five minutes will also provide motor weakness in the long extensors and flexors that will decrease the likelihood of abnormal pull of these muscles on fractures of the hand after manipulation. The patient can tolerate a tourniquet for about 25 minutes with minimal discomfort. After about 15 minutes of tourniquet elevated to 300 mm. Hg in the adult and 250 mm. Hg in the child, motor weakness of the muscles supplied by median, ulnar, and radial nerves will occur, with the radial muscles weakening first, the median second, and the ulnar last.

Digital block can be accomplished by injecting anesthetic material into the webspace where there is adequate room for swelling and dorsally on either side of the metacarpal neck with the needle extending down to the palmar fascia. A circular injection should not be used, nor should epinephrine.

Intravenous anesthesia should not be used in children or adults unless the physician is prepared to leave the tourniquet elevated for about 45 minutes so that the anesthetic material can be fixed in the tissues of the forearm. Care must be taken in utilizing this procedure by having resuscitation equipment available. This technique is ideal in the operating room and for adults. Axillary block is ideal in both adults and children for multiple fractures about the hand and wrist. This can be supplemented with the use of a tourniquet and systemic analgesia for almost all kinds of injuries.

Supraclavicular brachial block should be avoided, as the incidence of pneumothorax is 20 to 25 per cent if done by individuals who are not doing the procedure regularly and consistently.

Complications associated with the use of local or regional anesthesia are rare, but they do occur and the physician must be prepared to deal with syncope, hypotension, convulsions, and anaphylactic reactions. This means that even with a local infiltration, one must have oxygen, a positive pressure bag, an airway, and intravenous medications immediately available.

Generally, open wounds should be treated in the operating room where adequate assistance, instrumentation, and equipment are available, where the traffic is limited, and where the proper protection of the patient from air-borne and other infections can take place.

OPEN WOUNDS AND IMMOBILIZATION

At the time of the initial wound excision, all tight fascial compartments must be opened, joints irrigated, and uncompromised circulation established. No effort is made to repair digital nerves or flexor tendons if the wound has been caused by high velocity missile, severe crush, human or animal bite, or high pressure. Fractures, however, should be immobilized with small fixation pins, but the joint should not be crossed with the pins. Pins should not be placed through the extensor retinaculum (Fig. 2).

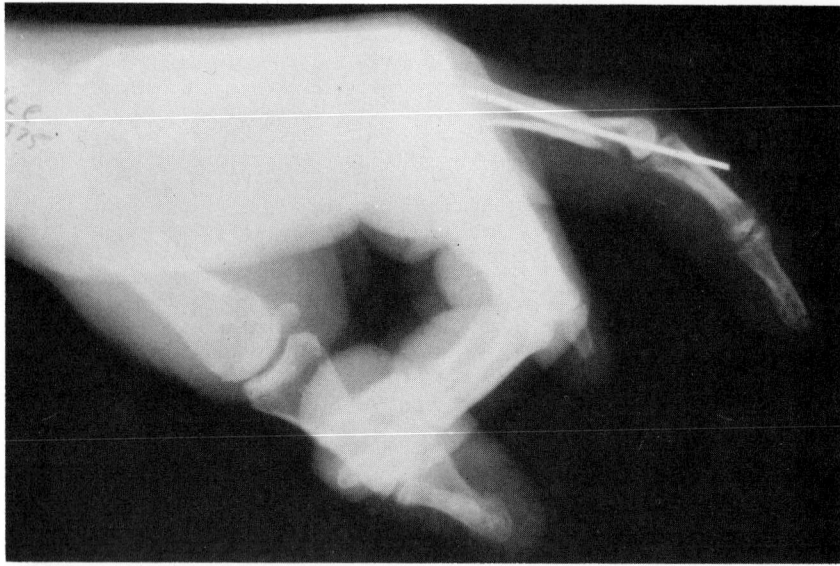

Figure 2. Pin fixation utilized to stabilize fracture of the distal phalanx. Pin was placed across the joint. Limited motion due to arthrofibrosis resulted. **This procedure is not advisable.**

DEFINITIONS OF FRACTURES AND DISLOCATIONS

The *distal phalanx* includes the pulp of the finger, the fingernail, the germinal layer, the attachment of the extensor tendon, and the flexor tendons.

The *middle phalanx* is the bone distal to the proximal phalanx. It is covered by extensor mechanism and includes the insertion on the volar surface of the flexor sublimis. It is also covered by the tendon of the flexor digitorum profundus.

The *proximal phalanx* articulates with the metacarpal head and makes up part of the proximal interphalangeal finger joint. The oblique fibers of the lateral bands and the intrinsic muscles cover it radially and ulnarward, and there are the extensor tendon on the dorsum and the flexor tendons on the volar surface. The proximal phalanx is longer than the middle and distal phalanges.

The *metacarpal* articulates with the proximal phalanx. The large articular surface provides a wide range of flexion, extension, abduction, adduction, and rotation. This joint is critical in maintaining full motion of the finger joints. The rotary as well as hinge motion at this joint makes it possible for the individual to perform dextrous actions with great ease. The piano player depends primarily on the metacarpophalangeal joints for motion. The joint is stabilized by the collateral ligaments, the dorsal capsule, and the volar capsular ligaments, and movement of the phalanges is carried out by the extensor and flexor tendons.

Rotation of the digits is dependent on coordinated action of the flexors and extensors. The fingertips as they are flexed are directed toward the radial side of the hand, all converging somewhat and not moving in a straight line.

The fourth and fifth metacarpals are mobile. The third metacarpal has a few degrees of motion, the second metacarpal is fixed, and the first metacarpal is hypermobile, when compared with the others.

The growth lines or epiphyses of the phalanges are proximal and adjacent to the joint. The growth lines of the metacarpals are distal, except for that of the first metacarpal, which is proximal.

The first ray or digit has one metacarpal and two phalanges and a complex system of coordination depending on the intrinsic muscles of the thumb as well as the extensors and flexors.

Stabilization of the thumb at the carpometacarpal joint is dependent on articulation with carpal bones, supportive ligaments that are strong but flexible, and the extensor and abductor muscle tendon units as well as the flexors.

ANATOMIC REGIONS OF FRACTURES

Distal Phalanx

Closed Fracture—Crushing Type Injury. The fingernail may be elevated by hematoma. Release the hematoma trapped in the space between nail plate and nail bed by inserting the tip of a No. 15 knife blade after the digit has been cleansed with soap and water and antiseptic. A hole is made directly in the center of the nail plate. Once the plate is perforated, the knife is twisted three or four times to enlarge the hole. An alternate method is to use the round end of an open paper clip that has been heated in a flame for sterilization.

Open Fractures. The most important aspect of the open fracture of the distal phalanx is not the bone injury but the skin and soft tissue damage. Initial treatment consists of wound excision. If the wound is contaminated, it is treated open and closed at five to seven days with a skin graft or shifting of local flaps. If the wound is clean and noncontaminated, then immediate split skin grafting or local flaps can be used to provide closure.

Damage to the germinal layer of the nail plate will result in irregular growth of the nail. The degree of damage and the area of involvement may determine whether the nail plate, the germinal layer, and the nail bed can be saved partially or completely.

Avulsion Fractures. A dorsal segment of bone is elevated when the extensor digitorum communis is involved by an acute flexion injury. The superior aspect of the articular surface may make up part of the fragment. If the fragment is small, simple extension of the distal phalanx to a neutral position and temporary flexion of the proximal interphalangeal joint will result in sufficient apposition to allow healing. An uncomplicated way of managing this injury is to use a dorsal plaster splint extending from the tip of the nail plate to the metacarpophalangeal joint with the distal joint extended 10 degrees and the proximal joint flexed about 20 degrees. This allows compression of the digit, decreases edema, and provides immediate relief of pain. After a week, the proximal interphalangeal joint can be released and a dorsal aluminum splint covering only the distal interphalangeal joint is shaped and applied with clear tape. The splint should be on constantly but can be changed every few days without losing position of the distal phalanx. This splint allows the patient to use the pulp of the finger and avoids plaster or complicated metal splints or internal fixation.

If the patient is in the age group where cooperation is not possible or if the patient's reliability is questionable, then a circular plaster splint is applied and left in place for three weeks.

A fracture fragment attached to an extensor tendon should be treated as early as possible after the injury. Alignment and function, however, can be obtained as late as two or three weeks after the injury, but each week of waiting decreases the chances of maximum recovery. If the fracture fragment is 50 per cent of the articular surface, and if the collateral ligaments have been damaged, percutaneous pin fixation may be necessary; or, occasionally, open operation is done in order to restore the fragments and provide fixation and maintain joint stability. This type of treatment is not required very often.

Avulsion of a Fragment from the Flexor Surface. This occurs when the flexor digitorum profundus is forcibly pulled off to its distal phalangeal insertion. This usually occurs with a hyperextended digit as a result of a forcible blow or fall. The diagnosis is made by the history of a fall on the outstretched hand. The findings show swelling of the digit, inability of the patient to flex the distal joint, and a palpable mass at the base of the finger or in the palm. Roentgenograms may show the fragment of bone proximally in the digit.

Treatment requires open operation in order to reattach the flexor tendon to the point from which the fragment was avulsed. This is usually done by using a polypropylene figure-of-eight suture through the distal end of the tendon and attached just proximal to the fragment. The suture is brought through the distal phalangeal area on either side of the fingernail and tied over a button. Two interrupted sutures of nonabsorbable material are also placed through the tendon and the fragment into the adjacent soft tissues. Im-

mobilization is maintained in a dorsal plaster splint including the finger, hand, wrist, and forearm for a total of three weeks, followed by protection for an additional three to six weeks.

Other Injuries of the Distal Phalanx. Trauma may result in a single chip fragment, a multiple stellate fracture, or a fracture into the distal interphalangeal joint. The extensor tendon may be attached to the fragment and displaced, or the volar capsule may be torn so that subluxation occurs. Swelling of the pulp of the digit and injury to the nail bed, the germinal layer, and the nail plate may occur. Treatment varies depending on whether the lesion is intra-articular or entirely extra-articular and on how much of the soft tissue is involved. The extra-articular lesion is treated by application of a soft compression dressing and a plaster or aluminum protective splint. This is worn for seven to 10 days and can be changed to a less bulky dressing as soon as pain subsides. If the lesion is intra-articular, special attention is given to alignment of the fragments and maintenance of position. Occasionally pin transfixion may be indicated, but usually splinting is adequate.

Interphalangeal Joint and Middle Phalanx

The proximal and distal interphalangeal joints are stabilized by the main and accessory collateral ligaments. Collateral ligament tears or avulsions result in temporary instability. In most instances realignment and splinting will allow the collateral ligament to heal without persistent instability. Fragments of bone may be attached to the collateral ligaments and detected on the roentgenogram.

The volar capsule prevents excessive hyperextension and aids in preventing malrotation. A tear of the capsule may occur either with or without the fragment attached to it.

The extrinsic muscles such as the extensor digitorum communis, the flexor digitorum profundus, and the flexor digitorum sublimis all affect the position of fragments after trauma has occurred. The force of the initial injury directs a distal or proximal fragment in one or the other direction, and the natural pull of the attached tendon either aggravates this or neutralizes it, depending on the mechanism of injury.

The intrinsic muscle attachments also affect the position of the fragments by the extensions of the lateral band mechanism across the proximal phalanx, onto the sides of the proximal interphalangeal joint, and over the dorsum of the middle phalanx and participation in the insertion of the tendon into the distal phalanx. Active muscle contraction of the lumbrical and the interossei influence the position of the fragments and deformity of the digit.

The primary force of the flexor digitorum profundus tends to result in dorsal bowing of the fragments, whereas the pull of the flexor digitorum sublimis results in volar angulation. Rotary deformities and radial and ulnar deviation may also depend on the intrinsic tendon pull as well as the force of the original injury.

A fracture through the distal end of the proximal phalanx of the thumb with volar angulation at the fracture site and dorsal displacement of the distal

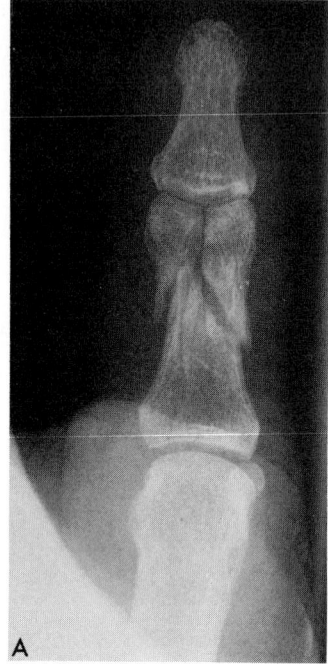

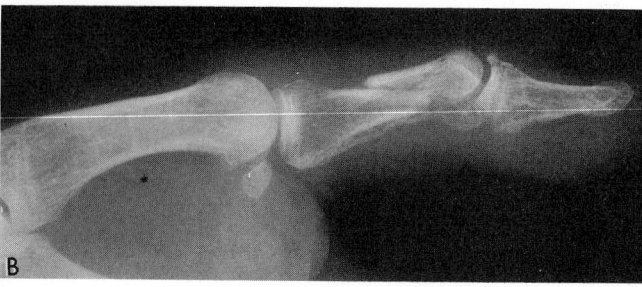

Figure 3. *A*, Fracture of proximal phalanx of the thumb with dorsal displacement of the distal fragment. An additional x-ray view is needed to determine if intra-articular injury has occurred. *B*, Fracture through the distal articular surface of the proximal phalanx. Closed manipulation and dorsal plaster splint are usually sufficient for management of this injury. Percutaneous pin fixation can be used if stability cannot be maintained.

fragment is shown in Figure 3. This is an intra-articular injury and must be reduced anatomically.

A chip fracture at the interphalangeal joint indicating collateral ligament tears is shown in Figure 4. These may be a subtle suggestion of more extensive instability, but as long as the major phalanges can be placed in anatomic alignment, a position which decreases tension and stress on the collateral ligaments, adequate healing usually occurs.

Dorsal dislocation of the middle phalanx with tearing of the volar capsule and disruption of the dorsal capsule is a serious injury that may be overlooked. The finger joint area is swollen and may be mistaken for a "sprained finger." The lateral roentgenogram demonstrates the displacement and the fragmentation. Treatment includes regional block at the metacarpal level. The patient is placed in a supine position on the table, countertraction is arranged with a loop of cloth over the lower arm, the elbow is flexed at right angles, the wrist is in dorsiflexion, and traction in slight extension is applied to the digit and held for about one minute. As the traction is exerted in the longitudinal direction, a gentle but firm compression is applied to the dorsum of the middle phalanx, and the digit is flexed. Flexion is continued until the finger is down to 70 degrees. A light plaster splint is then applied to the dorsum, and a roentgenogram is taken in the lateral as well as in the anteroposterior plane.

Proximal Phalanx

Injuries to the proximal phalanx may be divided as follows: (1) *Oblique fractures* through the shaft usually include a rotary element. The distal fragment may be displaced to the radial or ulnar aspects of the digit and the condylar segment either superiorly or inferiorly (Fig. 1). (2) An alternate type of injury is a *transverse*

fracture with resulting dorsal angulation. The fragments bow against the extensor tendon, with deformity aggravated by contraction of the flexor digitorum sublimis and profundus. The initial force is usually one that will displace the distal end of the phalanx. (3) *A fracture through the mid portion* of the proximal phalanx with volar angulation presses the long flexor tendons, and causes a resulting flexion deformity of the proximal interphalangeal joint. The acute phase with resulting pull of the involved forces aggravates the deformity. Realignment of the fragments restores full range of flexion at the proximal and distal interphalangeal joints, whereas persistent deformity may result in adherence of the flexor digitorum sublimis tendon to the periosteum and bony fragments during the course of healing and cause a fixed contracture of the proximal interphalangeal joint in the flexed position.

A shaft fracture with the angulation of the distal fragment and also the direction of the fragments at the fracture site is shown in Figure 5. Treatment depends on adequate relaxation of the extrinsic and intrinsic muscles, which can usually be managed by regional nerve block and manipulation of the distal segment of the digit while countertraction is being applied to the proximal segment of the hand with the elbow flexed, the wrist dorsiflexed, and the metacarpophalangeal joint stabilized.

For the oblique fracture, derotation is accomplished and the joints on either side of the phalanx are flexed. For dorsal angulation, the distal segment is directed upward and the proximal joint flexed. When the angulation is volar, the distal segment is manipulated downward and the interphalangeal joint remains in flexion. A dorsal plaster splint with the wrist held in full dorsiflexion, the metacarpophalangeal joints flexed to about 70 degrees, and the interphalangeal joints flexed to 80 degrees is sufficient to maintain reduction. Soft compression material is placed in the palm and the rotation is determined by judging the position of the fingernail in relationship to the palm when all joints are in full flexion. Immobilization for three weeks is usually adequate, and an interval change prior to removing the splint assures that loss of position does not occur.

Proximal dorsal compression injuries of the proximal phalanx result when the distal fragment is forced upward and the proximal fragment is stabilized by the collateral ligaments (Fig. 6). The dorsal cortex is compressed, the angle between the articular surface and the shaft may be angulated as much as 50 degrees, and the muscle balance between the extensors, the flexors, and the intrinsic tendons is distorted. Edema

on the dorsum of the digit masks the true deformity. A flexed position at the proximal interphalangeal joint occurs as a result of increased tension on the flexor digitorum sublimis. Roentgen diagnosis may be difficult, as the anterior posterior film is misleading, since minimal radial or ulnar angulation occurs. The lateral view of the phalanges may be hidden by the adjacent digits, and the oblique view may not show the true extent of the deformity. A roentgenogram should be taken with the digits in the position in which they are not overlapping completely, from both the radial and the ulnar side. Also, if the patient closes the fingers to make a fist and rotary views are made, any existing malalignment will be evident.

Treatment requires satisfactory regional block, counter and straight traction, and a strong, forcible flexion manipulation that is done with the collateral

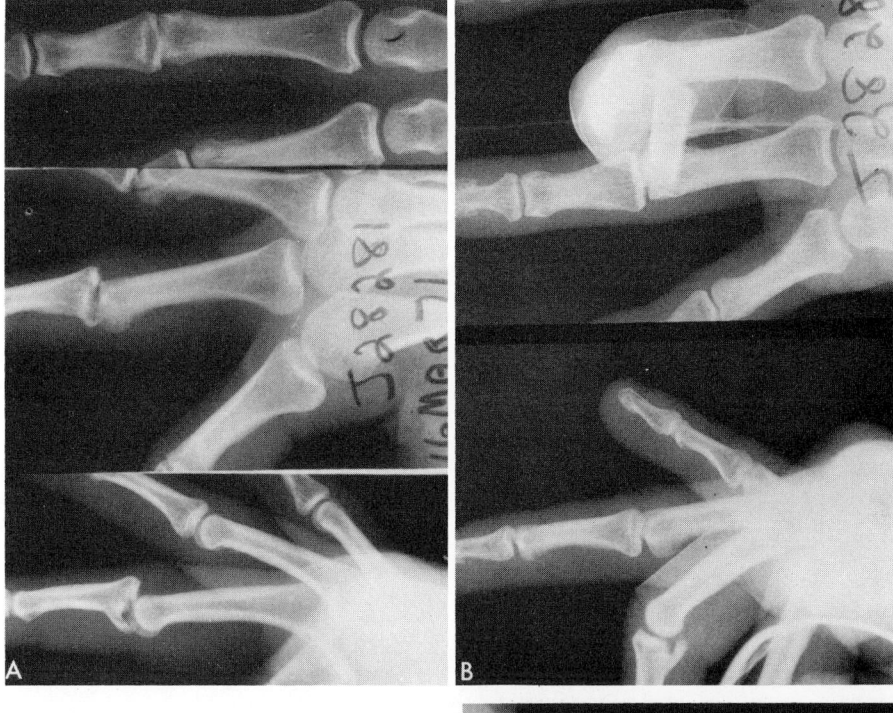

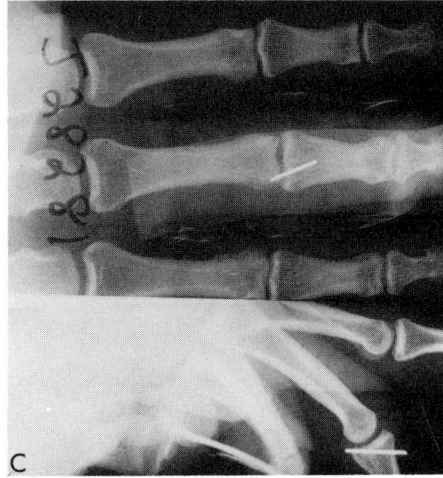

Figure 4. *A*, Proximal interphalangeal joint, dorsal fracture dislocation with involvement of articular cartilage. Multiple views give a better representation of the fragments that are displaced and the soft tissues involved. Both the dorsal capsule and the volar capsule are affected. *B*, The flexed lateral view shows where the volar capsule has been pulled off the proximal end of the proximal phalanx with a chip of bone, part of which is intra-articular. *C*, Fixation of the articular fragment with small fixation pins assures articular congruity. However, cartilage damage and cartilage necrosis must be avoided in doing this kind of operation. The pins should not penetrate the joint, as this prevents early motion.

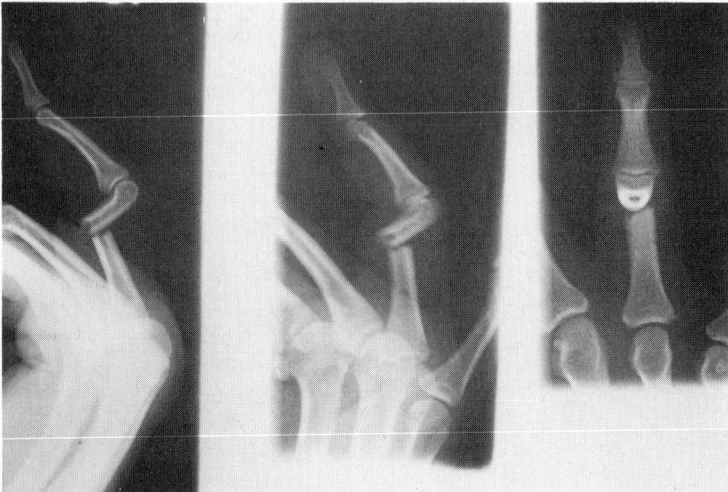

Figure 5. Fracture of proximal phalanx with dorsal angulation of the distal fragment, volar bowing at fracture site. Influence of the extensor tendon and the intrinsic muscles affects the angulation.

ligaments under tension when the metacarpophalangeal joints are flexed. The thumb of the physician should be directly under the proximal fragment as the fulcrum, and the index finger compresses downward on the distal fragment. Immobilization is maintained with the metacarpophalangeal joints and the interphalangeal joints in flexion.

A *condylar split* fracture involving the distal end of the proximal phalanx is an intra-articular fracture. Collateral ligaments are attached to each of the condyles and the intercondylar area is spread one or two millimeters. Figure 3 shows the displacement of the condyles. Dorsal or volar displacement of the condylar fragments may complicate alignment. Direct longitudinal traction tightens the collateral and the retinacular ligaments and affects the position of the condyles. Once the fragments are replaced and the middle phalanx is flexed, the position can be maintained by flexing the digit over an aluminum splint. A shorter plaster cast into which is incorporated a volar aluminum splint, is applied to the hand and the wrist and the lower forearm. The involved digit is flexed at the metacarpophalangeal joint and at the interphalangeal joint and held to the aluminum by clear tape, which is wrapped or in individual pieces not under tension and in such a way that each turn of tape overlaps the next most proximal turn. Edema is avoided by uniform application. Rotation is corrected and the nail plate is directed toward the radial aspect of the palm. Position is maintained for approximately a week and retaping is done. At that time, the joint is taken through a moderate range of motion. Immobilization is continued for about three weeks and the digit is protected for an additional two weeks, although an active range of flexion and extension is attempted several times each day. If the condyles are malrotated and adequate position cannot be obtained by manipulation, then percutaneous pinning with a fixation pin

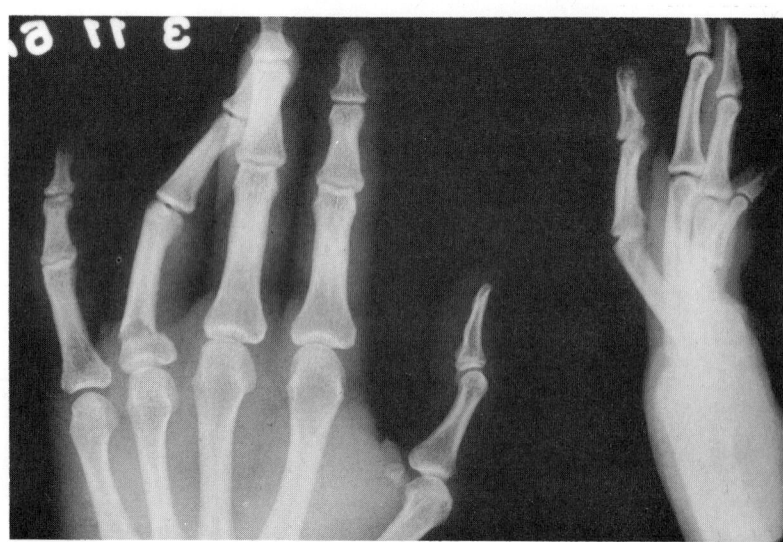

Figure 6. Fracture of the proximal phalanx with volar angulation, distal segment; affected by extensor digitorum communis and the middle phalanx flexed by intrinsic muscles. Fracture at the base of the proximal phalanx of the ring finger with malrotation, impaction, and dorsal angulation of the distal fragment.

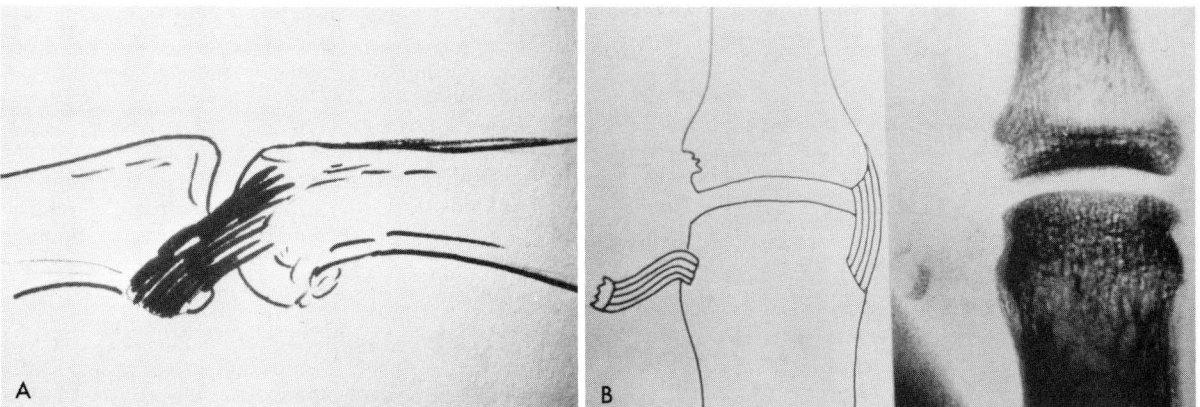

Figure 7. *A,* Accessory collateral ligaments of metacarpophalangeal joint of the thumb. Tear of this ligament may pull a bone fragment off and require open operation for fixation. *B,* Diagrammatic representation of the avulsed fragment with the collateral ligament either under or outside the retinaculum. With this much displacement, operative repair is indicated.

can be done; or open operation is carried out and the condyles are replaced and held with internal fixation. The latter procedure requires experience.

Dislocation and chip injuries at the metacarpophalangeal joint or the proximal interphalangeal joint depend on the direction of force by which the fragments are displaced. Dorsal dislocation of the proximal phalanx at the metacarpophalangeal area may result in partial tear of the capsule and displacement of the dorsal capsule and extensor mechanism (Fig. 7). Relocation is not difficult, and immobilization in the flexed position is usually sufficient. A serious articular and vascular injury may occur with dislocation of the metacarpal head and displacement of the proximal phalanx. The head protrudes through a tear in the capsule and may be entrapped by the collateral ligament or the flexor tendon or both. If the dislocation is unrecognized, then vascular insufficiency may occur. Amputation has resulted from this kind of injury as a result of inadequate early reduction or lack of recognition of the displaced fragments. One must be prepared to proceed with an open operation if replacement of the fragments is not done with relative ease and without constant manipulative forces. Figure 8A shows the position of fragments. A review of the anatomic relationship of the proximal phalanx to the metacarpal and the soft tissue structures, including the digital artery, vein, and nerve, will demonstrate the likelihood of trauma to these structures.

Chip fractures of the metacarpophalangeal joint result from a traction release of either the collateral ligament from the phalanx or the metacarpal head. Occasionally an osteochondral fracture of the metacarpal head occurs and the segment is within the joint. Chip fractures are managed by alignment and dorsal plaster fixation for about 14 days. The osteochondral fracture usually requires an open operation and complicated procedure to provide fixation of the osteochondral fracture.

Fractures through or involving the epiphysis require information about the different zones of the epiphyseal plate, including the germinal layers and the zone of

proliferating cartilage adjacent to the metaphyseal side of the epiphyseal plate. If the fracture occurs through the germinal cells, then the epiphysis will cease growing or grow in an irregular way. If the frac-

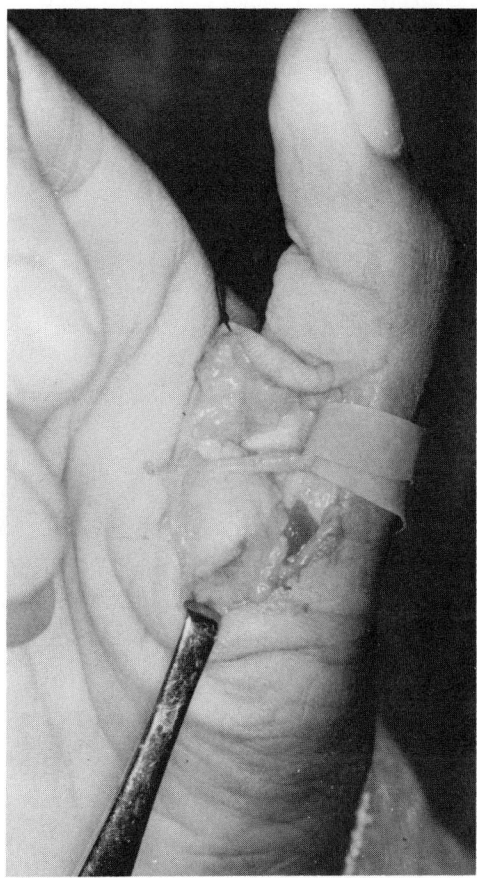

Figure 8. Dislocation of the metacarpophalangeal joint of the thumb with flexor tendon and capsule preventing relocation. Open operation necessary.

ture is through the junction of the metaphysis and the diaphysis, then growth will not be disturbed and healing will occur rapidly. The displaced fragments of the epiphysis are assessed by appropriate roentgenographic studies. Anatomic reduction should be attempted so that the cartilage fragments will heal and growth potential will not be disturbed.

The Metacarpals

These fractures can be divided as follows: (1) *Fracture of the metacarpal head* with intra-articular involvement and dorsal or volar angulation of the fragments (Fig. 9A to C). (2) *Fractures of the metacarpal neck* with dorsal or volar angulation with a rotary element (Fig. 9A and B). (3) *Transverse fractures* through the shaft of the metacarpal. (4) *Oblique fractures* through the shaft of the metacarpal (Fig. 11A to C). (5) *Dislocation* of the base of the metacarpal with emphasis on first, fourth, and fifth metacarpals. The concepts involved in managing these injuries depend on a knowledge of the anatomy and the forces involved in causing these injuries.

Fracture through the neck of the fifth metacarpal is a common injury caused by a direct blow. This is known as a "boxer's fracture," and occurs from a dorsal force applied directly to the metacarpal head. The head is displaced downward, the shaft bows dorsally, and the tip of the little finger rotates toward the radial side of the palm. Considerable soft tissue swelling

usually occurs, and the alignment of the fragments cannot be determined from external examination. Roentgenographic exam will show the angulation on the oblique and lateral views (Fig. 10).

Realignment is dependent on upward replacement of the metacarpal head and flexion of the proximal phalanx so that the collateral ligaments are under tension. The fact that the fifth metacarpal shaft is mobile decreases the reduction pressure on the metacarpal head and requires a firm manipulation of the fragments so that maintenance of reduction will occur within the fracture itself and not be the result of strongly applied external forces. If the proximal phalanx is flexed and the wrist is dorsiflexed, then a dorsal splint applied to the ring and little fingers with a small amount of soft dressing in the palm is usually sufficient. Longitudinal traction with pins, internal pin fixation, or complicated external compression splints are not advisable. The damage that results to the proximal interphalangeal joint of the finger may be more serious than the residual deformity that occurs if the fracture is not reduced anatomically.

Thumb Metacarpal Fractures. Fractures at the base of the thumb are usually caused by a fall on the hand, a twisting mechanism which involves the projected thumb, or a direct blow of the fist against a firm object. Lesions can be classified as follows (Fig. 12): (1) Intra-articular fracture through the proximal end of the metacarpal, leaving a fragment held by the inter-

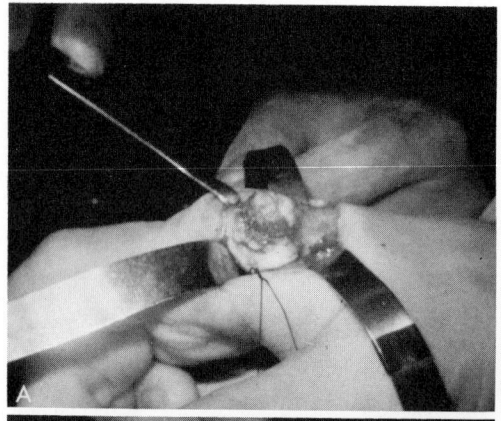
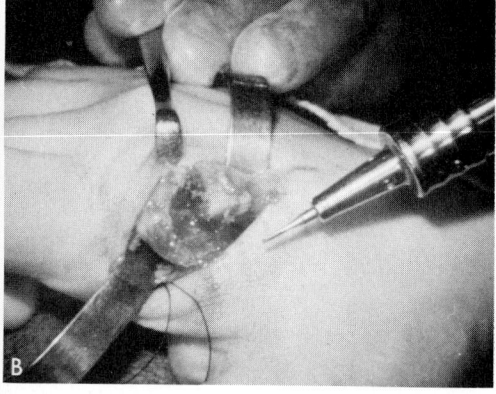
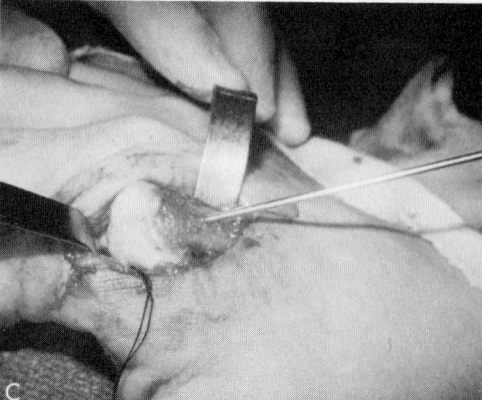

Figure 9. Open operation of severe displacement of fracture of the metacarpal head. Reattachment of collateral ligaments, dorsal capsule and pin fixation necessary. Limited motion resulted but satisfactory function occurred.

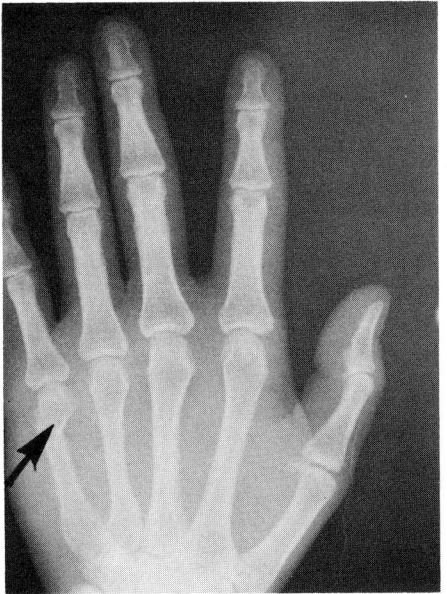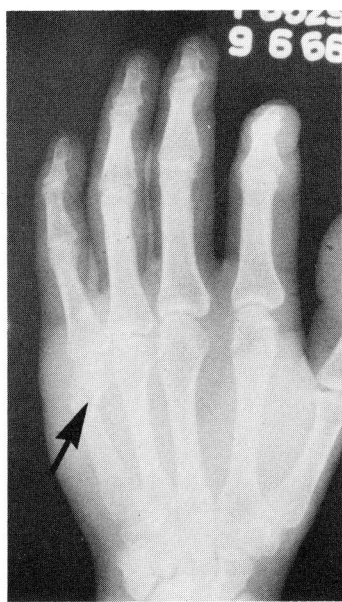

Figure 10. Fracture through neck of the fifth metacarpal with volar angulation of distal fragment and dorsal bowing at the fracture site. Re-alignment should be attempted, but minimal treatment is better than overtreatment.

metacarpal ligament, and the base of the metacarpal displaced laterally out of the joint by pull of the abductor pollicis longus (Bennett's fracture). (2) A comminuted intra-articular fracture of the proximal end of the metacarpal (Rolando's fracture). (3) Fracture through the metaphysis, not intra-articular, with angulation dorsal or volar. Other variations may occur, but these are the basic types of fractures.

The muscle pull that affects the ultimate position comes from the adductor pollicis longus acting on the

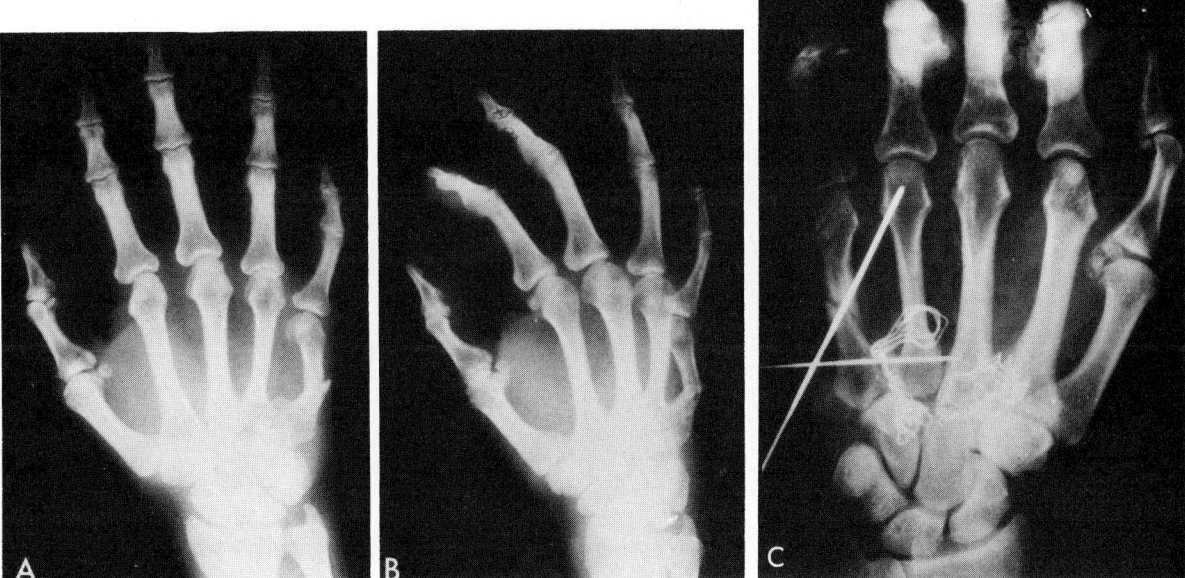

Figure 11. Shaft of the fifth metacarpal fractured with volar angulation of the distal fragment and dorsal bowing at the fracture site. Realignment requires flexion of the metacarpophalangeal joint, upward displacement of the distal segment of the distal phalanx and correction of malrotation. Closed fixation may be difficult, and pin fixation (*C*) is desirable. Bone substance had been lost by the saw causing the injury, and bone grafting, realignment, and release of the metacarpophalangeal joints had to be done at a later time to provide maximum function.

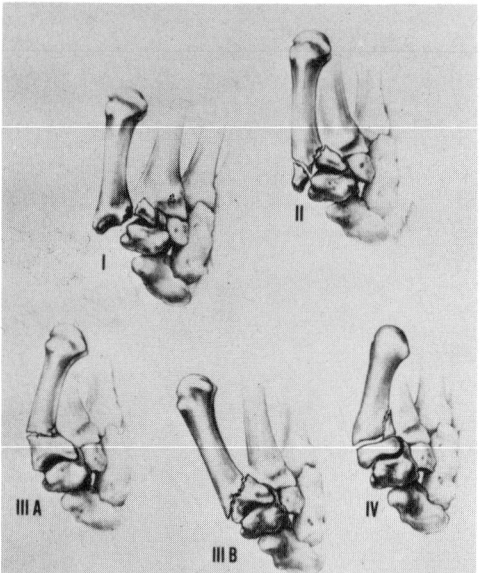

Figure 12. Diagrammatic representation of various fractures occurring at the base of the thumb: *I*, Bennett's fracture. *II*, Rolando's fracture. *IIIA, B,* and *IV,* Variations of fracture at the base of the thumb affecting metaphysis and possibly the epiphyseal plate. (From Green, D. P., and O'Brien, E. T.: South. Med. J., *65*:807, 1972.)

proximal end of the proximal phalanx, which pulls the thumb toward the palm and the metacarpal into external rotation. The strong force presented by the abductor pollicis longus displaces the base of the metacarpal away from the joint. The extensors pollicis longus and brevis act on the metacarpophalangeal joint and the metacarpal and tend to displace the head forward and the metacarpal in external rotation.

Treatment of the displaced thumb fracture will depend on the type of injury. The intra-articular frac-

ture with two segments is managed as demonstrated in Figure 13. A force must be applied to the base of the metacarpal, directing it inward. Traction occurs simultaneously, as does abduction and extension of the metacarpal head. The metacarpophalangeal joint must be held in flexion to prevent the action of the extensor pollicis longus on the distal metacarpal, and the widened web space with the thumb in the abducted extended position insures maintenance of the stabilization. Percutaneous pin fixation inserted just distal to the articular surface of the first metacarpal and directed toward the base of the second metacarpal in line with the neck of the third metacarpal should allow the first metacarpal shaft, the fragment on the inner metacarpal ligament, and the base of the second metacarpal to be held adequately to maintain the reduction. This is followed by application of a light plaster splint or cast, which maintains the position described.

The pre- and postinjury roentgenograms are shown in Figure 14. Satisfactory positioning has been obtained by manipulation. The fragments are held by the percutaneous pin. Open operation is seldom necessary. This is done only if soft tissue interposition has occurred or if a large fragment is malrotated and prevents joint congruity. The comminuted fracture at the base may be treated either by percutaneous pin fixation or by traction obtained by placing a transfixion pin through the base of the proximal phalanx or the neck of the metacarpal. Seldom do we depend on the traction mechanism, but prefer the direct plaster fixation or percutaneous pin. The fracture at the base of the thumb which does not include the joint is managed by manipulation, realignment, and plaster fixation with the thumb in wide abduction and the metacarpophalangeal joint in flexion (Fig. 13*B*).

Injuries at the *metacarpophalangeal joint* of the thumb usually include chip fractures of the ulnar collateral ligament, the fragment being avulsed from the

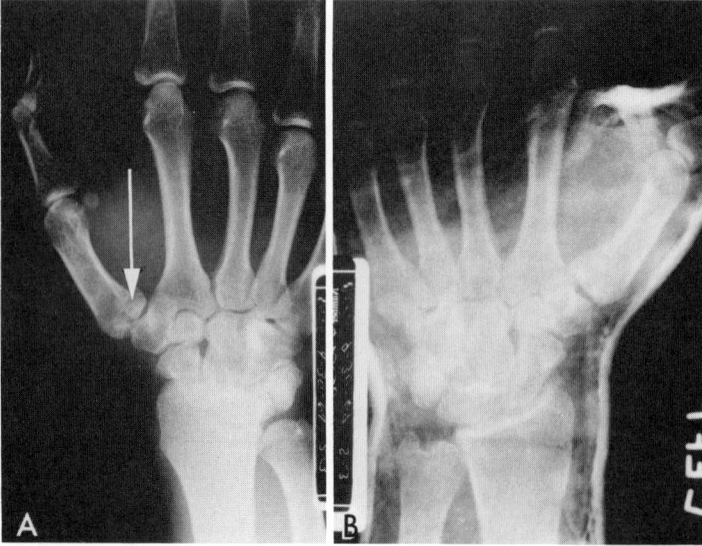
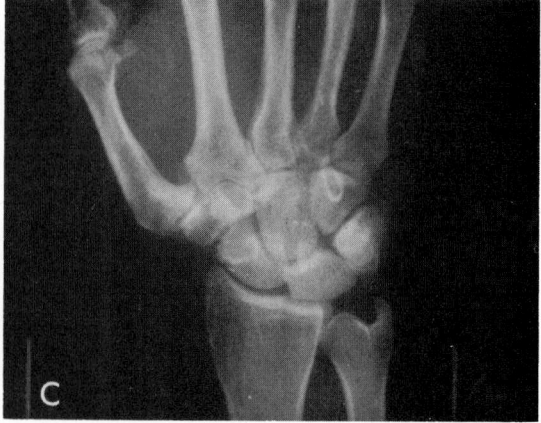

Figure 13. Fracture at the base of the thumb through medial tip of first metacarpal with dislocation. Cast has been applied, fracture realigned. *A,* Fracture; *B,* realigned with cast; and *C,* healed fracture.

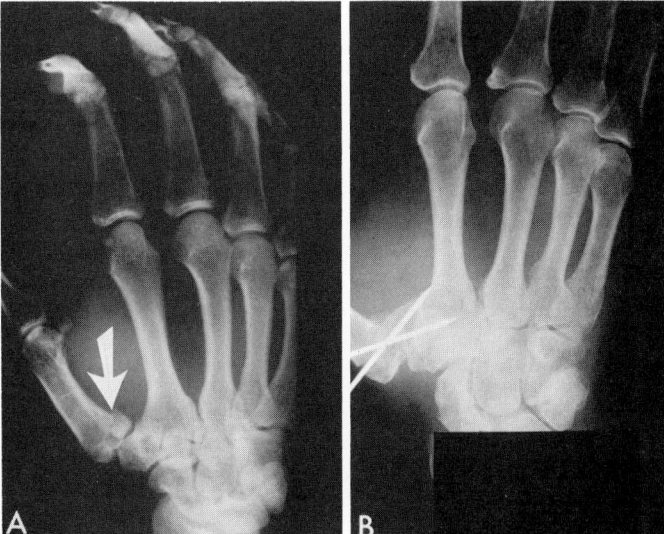

Figure 14. Fracture dislocation of the base of the thumb with two-pin fixation because of instability.

phalanx or from the metacarpal neck or in the central segment. In addition to the collateral ligament injury, the deep capsular ligaments and the dorsal capsule are usually torn, causing the phalanx to displace volarward and radially. In most instances, these injuries can be detected by clinical examination after regional block has been done and by appropriate roentgenograms showing the displacement of the phalanx under stress. The stress roentgenogram is not essential but is desirable if there is a question about the extent of the soft tissue injury. Treatment can be managed satisfactorily by application of a plaster or plastic water-repellent cast that holds the phalanx in the neutral adducted position and realigns the metacarpal and the phalanx. Protection is necessary for a minimum of four weeks and additional protection for an additional four weeks, during which time range of motion exercises can be carried out several times each day.

In certain instances, when congruity of the joint surface cannot be obtained or when the individual involved is not willing to undergo six weeks of immobilization and still not be absolutely certain that stability is present, then open operation can be recommended. There are many instances, however, in which athletes have been treated by plastic tape and splint fixation with strong immobilization. This has allowed them to continue with their athletic endeavors without the interruption of any open operation.

GENERAL PRINCIPLES OF TREATMENT

Aluminum splints can be shaped, bent, and contoured to fit the dorsal surface of the involved interphalangeal joints. A dorsal aluminum splint held on by clear tape can be used for mallet finger, for a dislocated joint, for a chip fracture, and for an oblique fracture. The splints do not have to be complicated, nor do they have to be padded excessively. The splint is usually applied without padding and can be bent to contour, but it must be narrower than the width of the finger. The splint also should be firm enough to

require bending by a lightweight pair of wire benders. If the splint can be bent readily by the physician, then it is not strong enough. Most splints should be applied to the dorsal rather than the volar surface. The ends may be bent over the tips of the fingers, depending on the type of injury that has occurred.

If a slight amount of elongation and traction of the fracture and the digit is needed, then the splint can be incorporated into a plaster gauntlet on the volar surface and the splint and the finger bent simultaneously and held in place with external tape.

Plaster splints are useful and readily available for treatment of hand fractures. The position of the wrist, metacarpophalangeal joints, and interphalangeal joints determines the success of the plaster splint treatment. The wrist must be dorsiflexed to stabilize the metacarpals and relax the extensor tendons. The metacarpophalangeal joint should be flexed at least 60 degrees in order to assure proper rotation. The interphalangeal joint should be extended or flexed, depending on the type of injury. Plaster splints can be about six thicknesses, covered by sheet cotton, and applied directly to the skin with a small amount of protective padding over the area involved. The bony prominences are padded with felt. The splint is then applied when wet, and the hand and the digit are held in the appropriate position. The splints are then wrapped on by narrow sheet cotton and then by bias-cut stockinette or more plaster. An uninvolved digit is usually included for additional protection, although this digit should not be included more than a few days. The plaster splint is changed every five to six days and the joints carried through a range of motion.

Prolonged periods of fixation of fractures of the hand are not necessary. The roentgenogram is not a good guide to the length of time that the hand should be immobilized. Twenty-one days is usually sufficient for most fractures and ligamentous injuries. Protection is followed for an additional three to four weeks, but range of motion exercises are initiated promptly.

Compression dressing is an adjunct.

SELECTED REFERENCES

Eaton, R. G.: Joint injuries of the hand. Springfield, Ill., Charles C Thomas, Publisher, 1971.
This monograph gives the author's experience in management of hand fractures. The clinical cases provide examples of how to diagnose and treat specific problems related to fractures and dislocations of the hand.

Goldner, J. L.: Trauma to the extensor mechanism at its attachment to the distal phalanx of the digits. *In* Current Practice in Orthopedic Surgery. St. Louis, The C. V. Mosby Co., 1964, pp. 143–152.
This article gives the mechanism of injury, a description of the associated deformities, and recommendations for closed treatment, as well as operative treatment in those instances when the closed treatment fails.

Riordan, D. C.: Fractures about the hand. South. Med. J., *50*:637–640, 1957.
This is a brief but clear article that provides methods of diagnosis and accepted forms of treatment for common fractures of the hand by an individual who has wide personal experience with hand fractures.

Stark, H.: Troublesome fractures and dislocations of the hand. Instructional Course Lectures, Am. Assoc. Orthop. Surg., *19*:130–149, 1970.
Common fractures of the hand are covered in this article. The author gives details concerning diagnosis and treatment. Good illustrations are included.

Wilson, J. N., and Rowland, S. A.: Fracture-dislocation of the proximal interphalangeal joint of the finger. J. Bone Joint Surg., *48A*:493–502, 1966.
The anatomy, mechanism of injury, and treatment are well described. This article provides the reader with a good background in the management of small joint fracture-dislocations of the hand.

REFERENCES

1. Coonrad, R. W., and Goldner, J. L.: A study of the pathological findings and treatment in soft tissue injury of the thumb metacarpophalangeal joint. J. Bone Joint Surg., *50A*:439–451, 1968.
2. Kaplan, E. B.: Dorsal dislocation of the metacarpophalangeal joint of the index finger. J. Bone Joint Surg., *39A*:1081–1086, 1957.
3. Kaplan, E. B.: The pathology and treatment of radial subluxation of the thumb with ulnar displacement of the head of the first metacarpal. J. Bone Joint Surg., *43A*:541–546, 1961.
4. McCue, F. C., Honner, R., Johnson, M. C., Jr., and Gieck, J. H.: Athletic injuries of the proximal and interphalangeal joint requiring surgical treatment. J. Bone Joint Surg., *52A*:937–956, 1970.
5. Neviaser, R. J., Wilson, J. N., and Lievano, A.: Rupture of the ulnar collateral ligament of the thumb (gamekeeper's thumb): Correction by dynamic repair. J. Bone Joint Surg., *52A*:1357–1364, 1971.
6. Stener, B.: Displacement of the ruptured collateral ligament of the metacarpophalangeal joint of the thumb. J. Bone Joint Surg., *44B*:869–879, 1962.

VI

FRACTURES OF THE PELVIS, FEMUR, AND KNEE

Donald E. McCollum, M.D.

Pelvic fractures are most commonly the result of pedestrian injuries. In older patients fractures of the pelvis more commonly occur from trivial injury such as a fall. Pelvic fractures are life-threatening and death occurs in as high as 20 per cent. Complications most frequently associated with pelvic fractures include hemorrhage, urologic injury, visceral injury, other skeletal injury, and head injuries.

The pelvis is a rigid ring made up of pubic rami, ischium, acetabulum, ilium, and sacrum, joined by tough fibrous tissue at the symphysis and sacroiliac joints. Disruption at one point does not produce instability; disruption at two points allows displacement, as the paravertebral muscles shorten; prolonged skeletal traction is necessary for reduction and maintenance of the fracture in a position that can produce satisfactory function.

Classification

An example of a *stable* pelvic fracture is shown in Figure 1*A*, although fractures of the pubic rami are present on both sides. The ring is broken only at one point and the fracture is stable and should be treated with bed rest only for a period of three weeks. In an unstable pelvic fracture (Fig. 1*B*), the ring is disrupted at two points. The strong paravertebral muscles attached to the rim of the pelvis tend to displace the lateral fragment upward. Disruption is shown both at the symphysis and through the sacroiliac joint in Figure 1*C*. The fracture is unstable and for satisfactory results the symphysis must be reduced. An abduction fracture, in which the pelvis is disrupted and spread at two points in the ring, is depicted in Figure 1*D*. In this type of fracture a pelvic sling is frequently helpful to close the gap in the superior and inferior pubic rami.

Minor Fractures

Minor fractures include fractures of the ilium, unilateral fractures, pubic rami, and avulsion fractures of points of muscle attachment. Fractures of the anterior superior spine occur in athletes by forcible contraction of the sartorius muscle. Treatment requires only bed rest with the hip in flexion for 10 days. The anterior inferior iliac spine is occasionally avulsed by forcible contraction of the rectus muscle, and treatment is similar. Sprinters may avulse the ischial tuberosity by

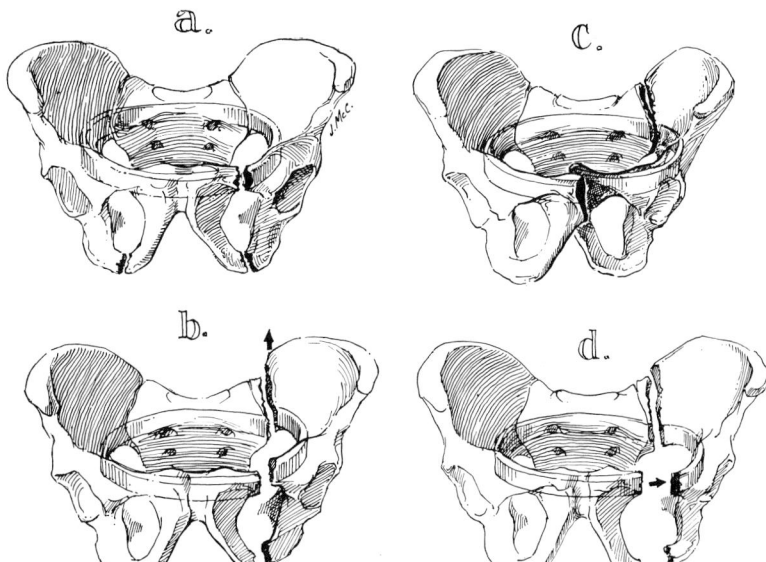

Figure 1. Classification of pelvic fractures into stable and unstable groups. *a* is a stable fracture because the ring is broken only at one point. The remaining three are unstable.

forceful contraction of the hamstrings. Bed rest or crutches allow healing to occur spontaneously. Swelling of the thigh may be massive, and pain may be severe. The displaced avulsion fracture frequently heals by fibrous union. The patient becomes asymptomatic after one to two years, but his athletic ability may be reduced.

Sacroiliac Fractures

Sacroiliac fractures in the conscious patient may be suspected when compression of the anterior superior iliac spine toward the midline produces pain in the sacroiliac region. Local tenderness over the sacroiliac joint is frequently present. Fracture of the ilium or the sacrum adjacent to the joint is more common than actual disruption of the fibrous syndesmosis. If pubic fracture is also present, the fracture is unstable, and the ilium is pulled upward by the paravertebral muscles, the upward displacement of the ilium might be overlooked by the unsuspecting examiner, but displacement of the pubis on the same side directs attention to the sacroiliac joint. Undisplaced isolated fractures are best treated with bed rest for three to four weeks. The unstable fracture must be immobilized with bed rest for 10 to 12 weeks, with longitudinal traction on the lower extremity in order to prevent upward displacement and painful nonunion in the sacroiliac joint.

Sacrum and Coccyx

Fractures of the sacrum and coccyx are treated by bed rest until the patient is comfortable, following which they may be mobilized with crutches. Frequently, after fractures of the sacrum, fibrosis may occur about the sacral nerve roots and persistent pain may be present. Persistent coccygeal pain may be the result of traumatic arthritis of the sacrococcygeal joint or more commonly is due to muscular damage to the urogenital diaphragm. Surgery is seldom indicated and frequently makes the condition worse. Treatment of chronic coccygeal pain following injury should consist of a foam rubber coccydynia pad, which relieves pressure on the coccyx, and hot sitz baths to relieve tenderness.

MAJOR FRACTURES OF PELVIS

Major fractures of the pelvis most frequently result from crush injuries occurring to the passenger within an automobile, to the pedestrian struck by an automobile, or to the patient falling from a height. These fractures are discussed apart from minor pelvic fractures because their morbidity and mortality differ greatly. Spear found this fracture to be the third most common cause of death from automobile accidents. They are frequently associated with other internal injuries to urethra, bladder, and abdominal organs. The most common complication of this fracture is that of massive hemorrhage in the retroperitoneal space, which occurs from the plexus of veins and arteries lining the inner pelvic wall.

Treatment of the *unstable pelvic fracture* varies widely. Watson Jones recommended manipulation of the fracture with the patient on his side, followed by application of a spica cast. The incidence of pelvic thrombophlebitis and pulmonary embolism is high in patients with this fracture, and casts should be avoided if possible.

Key and Conwell recommend heavy longitudinal traction and a pelvic sling, followed by manipulation if radiographic improvement does not occur. Open reduction of these fractures is difficult unless the surgeon has wide operative experience in fractures of the pelvis. Infection rates are extremely high and in some series approach 50 per cent. Because of the frequent complications, surgery is not recommended. Skeletal traction with a Steinmann pin in the distal femur, combined with the careful use of a pelvic sling, will restore most of these fractures to stability. Traction must be held for 12 weeks or until callus is apparent. The functional result in a healed unstable pelvic fracture is almost always better than the radiographic appearance.

ACETABULAR FRACTURES

Although acetabular fractures frequently occur in combination with many other pelvic fractures, they require separate treatment because the prognosis for function is worse than in other pelvic fractures. Inadequately treated fractures of the acetabulum eventually result in traumatic arthritis of the hip. Anatomic reduction is much more important, and surgical interference more often indicated.

Three major types of acetabular fractures occur. All can be caused by force transmitted in the longitudinal axis of the femur to the acetabulum. The position of the femur at the time of impact determines which type of fracture occurs. With the femur in adduction and flexion, a segment of posterior rim is avulsed, and posterior dislocation of the femoral head occurs. As the position of the femur progresses in abduction and external rotation, a central fracture with fracture line vertical (ischioacetabular) occurs. Further abduction produces a central fracture with the fracture line horizontal. Prognosis is different in each.

In rim fractures with posterior dislocation (Fig. 2), the blood supply to the femoral head is disrupted, and aseptic necrosis occurs in approximately 50 per cent of patients. This fracture should be treated as an emergency. Reduction should be prompt, with the patient under spinal anesthesia or general anesthesia and radiographic control available. The dislocation usually reduces easily. Should reduction not be done easily with gentle upward traction with the hip flexed, the femoral head may be trapped by a band of posterior capsule or by pyriformis tendon. Open reduction is then necessary, and internal fixation of the rim fragment should be done through a posterior approach.

In fractures with a vertical fracture line, the acetabular roof remains intact. Longitudinal traction may improve the position of the fragments, and the femoral head may be pulled back beneath the roof. Despite persistent displacement of the medial wall, a good functional result is usually obtained. Traction must be maintained for 12 weeks. Traumatic arthritis frequently occurs after this injury, but the patient may have many years of useful function before this complication ensues. Manipulation of the medial wall into a better position can be accomplished by very gentle manual pressure through the vagina in females or through the rectum in the male.

When the fracture line is horizontal or comminuted, as seen in Figure 3, the acetabular roof is completely disrupted. Lateral traction in addition to longitudinal traction can be accomplished best by crossed Steinmann pins in the greater trochanter. Rowe and Lowell found this combined treatment to produce the best results when held for 12 weeks, followed by crutches for three months. Although the femoral head is still

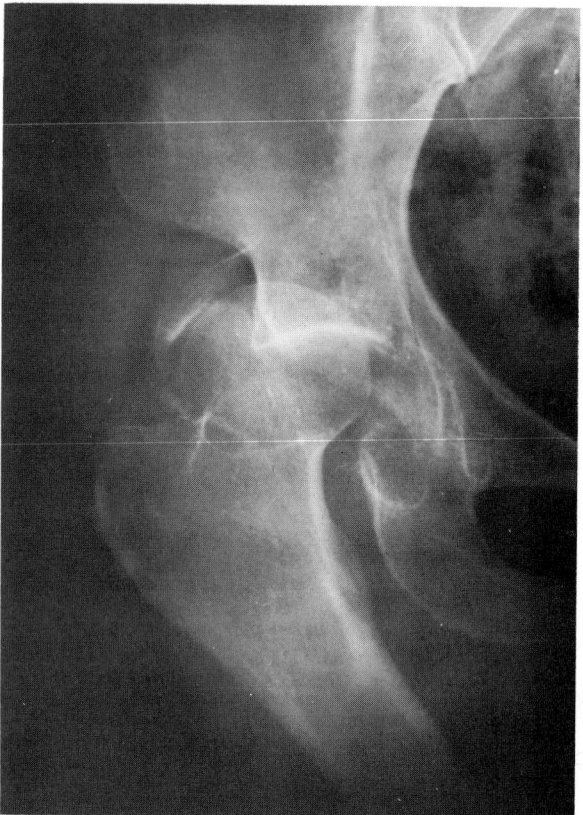

Figure 2. This rim fracture occurred from a dashboard injury. Note the fragment of posterior acetabulum above the femoral head. Reduction was unstable and the fracture was subsequently opened from a posterior approach and the posterior rim fracture fixed with staples.

displaced medially, the joint space remains good (Fig. 3). Operation is difficult, and results of open reduction are seldom better than those obtained with traction.

COMPLICATIONS OF PELVIC FRACTURES

Hemorrhage

Peltier found that the most common complication of pelvic fractures was massive hemorrhage. Bleeding may occur from laceration of hypogastric vessels by fractures extending into the sciatic notch. Shock occurs rapidly, as evidenced by decrease in vital signs, urine output, central venous pressure, and an enlarging psoas shadow. Patients must be given massive transfusions to correct shock and maintain urine output. If bleeding continues after replacement of total blood volume, arteriography should be considered. Arteriography is most helpful in fractures into the sciatic notch, ilium, or posterior ischium. If bleeding points are demonstrated, bleeding can frequently be controlled by injection of 10 ml. of autogenous blood clot into the afferent artery. If lacerations of the common iliac or external iliac artery can be demonstrated by arteriogram, they should be treated openly with ligation. Lesser arteries should be located and obliterated by closed methods.

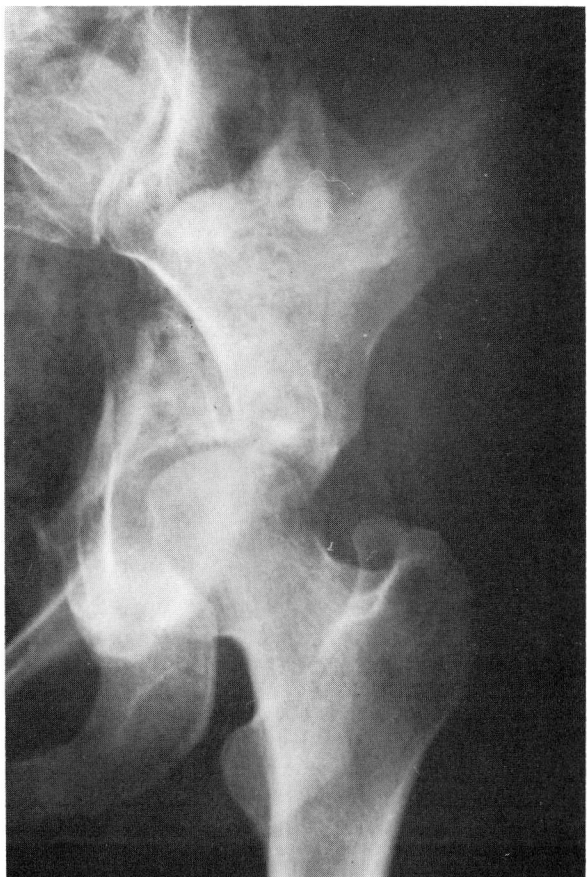

Figure 3. Comminuted central fracture dislocation of the acetabulum resulting from a lateral blow on the greater trochanter. Partial reduction was obtained immediately by gentle manipulation of the fracture fragment by vaginal manipulation and maintained by longitudinal traction. Some central fracture dislocation persists, but the fracture has filled in and the patient has essentially a normal gait with little or no pain.

Lower Urinary Tract

The bladder rests against the pubic bones and when empty is seldom injured. As the bladder extends, it may fill most of the true pelvis and rise above the symphysis, where it becomes vulnerable to either intraperitoneal or extraperitoneal rupture. Injuries to the lower urinary tract (bladder and urethra) occur in 14 per cent of all pelvic fractures and must be sought for by urethrogram, cystogram, and intravenous urogram.

If the injury is above the urogenital diaphragm, induration in the suprapubic region may be caused by perivesical hematoma. Extraperitoneal rupture of the bladder may present as a smooth rounded mass above the pubis, while intraperitoneal rupture produces no palpable mass and no induration, but produces ileus, abdominal rigidity, and rebound tenderness in the conscious patient.

If the injury occurs below the urogenital diaphragm, tenderness and swelling are usually found in the perineal area. Ecchymoses may be present in the skin of the perineum. Rectal examination must be done in all patients with pelvic fractures and may reveal hematoma, displacement of the prostate gland, or tenderness when disruption of the supramembranous urethra has occurred.

If urethrogram shows the urethra intact, a retrograde cystogram should be done with a 14 or 16 French catheter, injecting only 250 to 300 ml. of dye. The passage of a blind catheter without urethrography is condemned because it may enter and drain blood from the perivesical space simulating extraperitoneal rupture of the bladder. Rupture of both bladder and urethra are surgical emergencies requiring immediate urinary diversion and repair.

Rectum

The rectum lies directly on the sacrum, where it is well protected but may be lacerated by ischial or sacral fractures. Examination of the rectum for defects or fresh blood should be done in every pelvic fracture. The uterus, vagina, and vulva are rarely damaged, but compound fractures may extend into these structures.

Neurologic

The sciatic nerve is most frequently damaged by fractures of the pelvis extending into the ilium or the sciatic notch, by fracture of the ischium with displacement, or by posterior dislocation of the hip. The peroneal division of the sciatic nerve is more often damaged than the tibial division. It can be recognized easily by failure to contract the hamstrings and dorsiflex the foot in the conscious patient or by failure to dorsiflex the foot in withdrawal in the semiconscious patient. The obturator nerve lies in the obturator canal on the medial aspect of the acetabulum and may be damaged by central fracture dislocations of the hip. Paralysis of the obturator nerve can be recognized by inability to contract the adductor muscles and by spotty hypalgesia over the medial aspect of the thigh. The femoral nerve is seldom damaged directly by fractures of the pelvis but may be damaged by anterior dislocation of the hip. It more commonly is secondarily involved by compression from a hematoma which often occurs following fracture about the pelvis and hip.

Pulmonary

In a review of 151 patients, Spear found the most common cause of death to be post-traumatic pulmonary insufficiency. This syndrome has been referred to by other authors as "shock lung." The respiratory distress syndrome can be recognized by a significant change in blood gases, with decreasing oxygen tension and rising carbon dioxide. It is best managed by steroids and positive pressure oxygen.

Because of damage to retroperitoneal venous plexuses, pelvic thrombophlebitis and pulmonary embolism constitute a major threat to these injured patients. Body casts are almost never indicated. Low molecular weight dextran may be used cautiously as prophylaxis against thromboembolic phenomenon only after significant bleeding has ceased. Trunkey recommends low-dose heparin (2500 to 5000 units every 6 hours) after bleeding has ceased.

Although *fat embolism* occurs more frequently in fractures of long bones, it is also seen as a complication of fractures of the pelvis. Forty-eight to 72 hours after injury, the patient becomes confused, there is a sudden drop in hemoglobin which is unexplained by blood loss, arterial oxygen decreases as measured by blood gases, and small petechiae appear in the conjunctiva and over the upper chest. Chest x-ray may show hazy infiltrates throughout both lung fields. Fat globules are frequently present in the urine but are not of diagnostic help, as they are present with most major fractures. Prompt treatment by oxygen, blood replacement, and steroids in the form of prednisone 60 to 100 mg. per day is necessary to prevent permanent brain damage.

Traumatic arthritis frequently develops following acetabular fractures. Although function after treatment with prolonged traction is frequently much better than the radiologic appearance, after an undetermined number of years, the joint space begins to narrow, and the typical radiologic signs of post-traumatic arthritis develop. These are characterized by subchondral sclerosis and the development of cysts in the acetabulum and in the femoral head. Range of motion gradually diminishes as pain increases. Weight bearing becomes more difficult and constant pain eventually ensues. Such a complication in the adult is best managed by total hip replacement. This procedure is seldom indicated in younger patients and is almost never indicated as a primary procedure. However, the older patient with either rheumatoid arthritis or hypertrophic arthritis of the hip who sustains an acetabular fracture or a fracture of the head or neck of the femur may be rehabilitated faster and with less discomfort by primary total hip replacement.

FRACTURES OF THE HIP AND UPPER FEMUR

Fracture of the proximal femur is most common in elderly females but may occur at any age. Before the twentieth century, fracture of the femur was almost universally *fatal* due to pulmonary, renal, and cardiac complications. Survival was slightly better when these elderly patients were treated by Royal Whitman's method of closed reduction and cast immobilization, and a healing rate of 30 per cent was clearly unacceptable.

The most rapid progress in the treatment of this very common injury was made by Smith-Peterson in the 1930's in development of a technique of open reduction, impaction, and internal fixation with a triflanged nail. Advances have been rapid since then by addition of side plates, multiple pin fixation, and prosthetic replacement.

CLASSIFICATION

The most logical classification of hip fractures is one based upon prognosis. In any fracture, healing de-

pends not only on fixation, but more importantly on blood supply. Blood supply is marginal and more subject to damage in that portion of the femur which is intracapsular, making prognosis for these fractures much worse than for those which occur below the intertrochanteric line outside the capsule.

Intracapsular fractures include fractures of the head of the femur, impacted subcapital fractures, and displaced subcapital and neck fractures. Since there is no periosteum on the femoral neck, healing must be by endosteal callus. Fixation must be rigid and yet allow impaction as the fracture line resorbs. The femoral head receives only a small amount of its blood supply from the pelvic side of the joint through the ligamentum teres. Its major blood supply arises from the vascular ring at the base of the neck. The retinacular arteries pierce the capsule and run up the neck to enter the head in the subcapital area. These retinacular vessels may be damaged by torsion of fracture fragments or by intra-articular pressure from hematoma.

Fractures of the femoral head occur most often in posterior fracture dislocation of the hip. Either the central portion of the head is avulsed by the ligamentum teres or a quadrant of the head may be sheared off by the projecting lip of the acetabulum. This injury almost always occurs when the knee strikes the dashboard of a car. The intra-articular fragments seldom heal and continue to cause pain and result in traumatic arthritis. The treatment of choice is prompt open reduction of the hip with removal of the loose fragments and repair of the capsule. If the dislocation is stable following repair, the patient can be mobilized rapidly on crutches. However, if manipulation allows redislocation, the patient should be maintained in simple Buck's traction for a period of three weeks to allow soft tissue healing.

Impacted subcapital fractures are relatively undisplaced fractures in which the neck of the femur is telescoped into the head (Fig. 4). They may be impacted into either varus or valgus. Some authors believe that most impacted fractures are stress fractures. Large numbers of uniting trabecular fractures have been found in femoral necks of patients with senile subcapital fracture. The patient may present with minor groin pain with radiation to the knee. The initial films may not reveal the fracture line, and it frequently becomes visible only as the resorption phase of healing occurs. The elderly patient with hip pain must be treated for a fracture even though no injury is obvious by x-ray. Otherwise, the undisplaced fracture may become displaced, as shown in Figure 4, thus increasing the chances of disruption of blood supply to the femoral head.

The impacted valgus fracture is stable and may be managed conservatively by bed rest and skin traction for comfort. However, frequent x-rays must be taken in order to recognize and correct progressive displacement of the head which occurs as the resorption phase of fracture healing occurs. Many apparently stable subcapital fractures have been allowed to slip into an unstable varus position despite bed rest with traction,

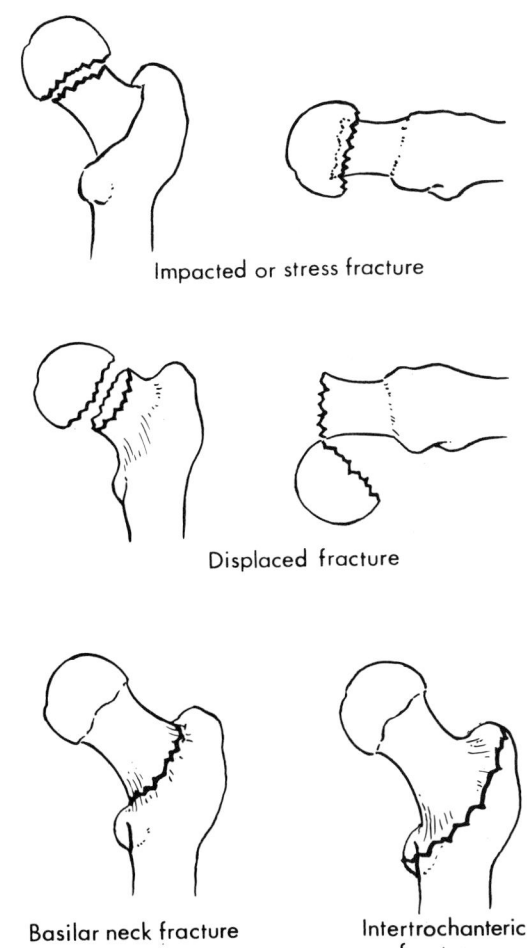

Impacted or stress fracture

Displaced fracture

Basilar neck fracture   Intertrochanteric
                                  fracture

Figure 4. Fractures of the neck of the femur. The impacted fracture above is frequently seen without trauma and may represent a stress fracture. If not treated properly, it may become displaced as shown in the middle drawing. The basilar neck and intertrochanteric fractures occur outside the vascular ring and blood supply is usually intact.

frequent. In both of these fractures, bleeding occurs within the hip joint, and the resultant intracapsular pressure rapidly exceeds the pressure in capsular vessels, resulting in thrombosis. Displacement of the fragments destroys the metaphyseal and endosteal vessels, markedly reducing blood supply to the head.

These fractures should be treated as emergencies; reduction should be accomplished under general or spinal anesthesia within 24 hours, and fixation should be rigid. The rate of avascular necrosis rises with delay, and even with immediate reduction approaches 25 per cent. When moderate displacement is present, reduction can be accomplished by gentle abduction and internal rotation. The Leadbetter maneuver described for more severe displacement is seldom necessary, and may cause additional comminution of the neck. In younger patients, if anatomic reduction cannot be obtained by manipulation, the capsule should be opened anteriorly and the fragments reduced under direct vision. Although the rate of aseptic necrosis is high, the patient may remain asymptomatic for six or seven years or more.

In young patients with good bone density, multiple pin fixation is adequate and is preferable to a triflanged nail or lag screw, which is likely to displace the fracture or destroy more endosteal blood supply. The lower pins must rest on the inferior calcar femorale; otherwise, the varus deformity will recur as the pins settle through the hollow neck seeking support, allowing the head to displace inferiorly off the calcar.

In older patients with osteoporotic bone or in fractures lower in the femoral neck, fixation between head and shaft may require a side plate, as seen in Figure 5. The unthreaded lower end of the screw allows the fracture to collapse as bone resorption occurs and the nail protrudes further into the head of the femur. The screw is inserted by means of a guide wire first, and the fracture is impacted. The nail is then driven over another guide wire parallel to the first so that it rests on the calcar. Insertion of the screw before insertion of the nail prevents distraction of the fracture site as the triflanged nail is driven into the head.

Impaction at the time of surgery, collapse at the fracture site as resorption occurs, and rigid fixation are provided by the telescoping Richards' screw and side plate. Many surgeons prefer this appliance for lower neck and stable intertrochanteric fractures. Union of the displaced subcapital or neck fracture may require six to twelve months before weight bearing can be allowed.

In the elderly or debilitated patient (Fig. 6), reduction and fixation should be done when possible, but if perfect reduction cannot be obtained, then prosthetic replacement is desirable in order to mobilize the patient more quickly. Prostheses should be used only as a last resort in younger patients, as eventually they become painful and require further surgery. A non-fenestrated prosthesis makes conversion of the painful prosthesis to a total hip replacement much easier. Prosthetic replacement is most easily accomplished through a posterior approach.

and the safest course is pinning with several pins. Multiple pins destroy less of the endosteal blood supply to the femoral head and are less likely to disimpact or displace the head than insertion of a triflanged nail. Since only the metaphyseal and endosteal blood vessels are interrupted in the undisplaced subcapital fracture, and the retinacular vessels remain intact, healing usually occurs without difficulty if adequate immobilization by either closed or open means is maintained. Aseptic necrosis of the femoral head occurs less frequently after impacted fractures, but collapse of the head with recurrence of pain may develop as late as five or six years after the injury. Nevertheless, the patient has been given several years of essentially normal function following a relatively minor procedure.

Displaced subcapital fractures and fractures of the neck of the femur are much more difficult to manage, and nonunion and avascular necrosis are much more

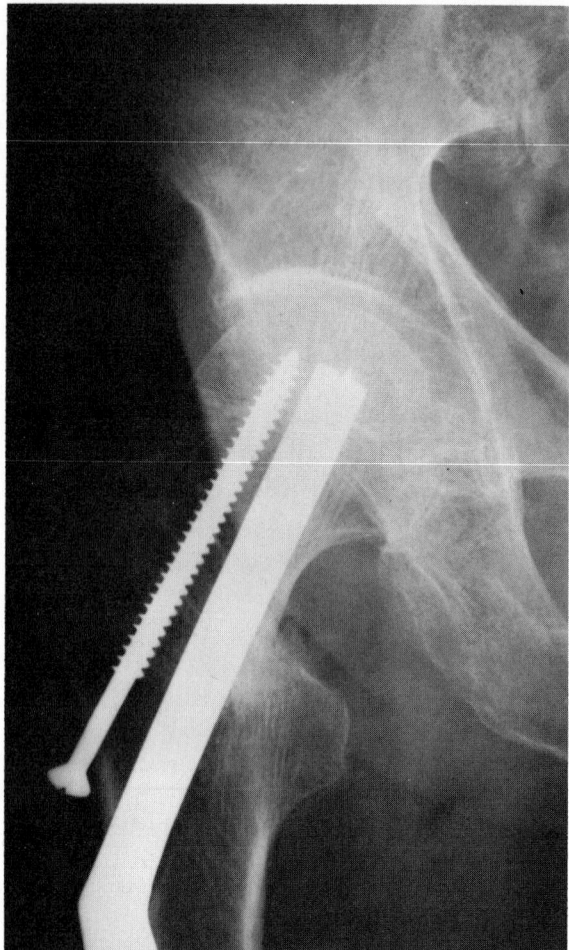

Figure 5. This basilar neck fracture occurred in an 80-year-old woman. Blood supply to the head remains intact. Owing to osteoporosis, fixation with pins is not adequate. The fracture was reduced by gentle abduction and internal rotation and was then impacted with a Venable screw. A Jewett nail with a four-hole side plate was then inserted up the neck and allowed to rest on the calcar and driven into the head. Although the patient walked the following day, union occurred uneventfully.

INTERTROCHANTERIC FRACTURES

Intertrochanteric fractures occur below the inferior attachment of the hip capsule, outside the vascular ring supplying the femoral neck and head. Blood supply is excellent, and aseptic necrosis occurs rarely. If adequate stability can be obtained, union in a functional position almost always occurs. Thus, a functional classification of intertrochanteric fractures depends upon stability rather than blood supply.

Stability in intertrochanteric fractures requires both support along the medial calcar and a lateral buttress to prevent the femoral shaft from shifting medially where it tends to be drawn by the pull of the adductors. Muscle forces about the hip result in varus deformity at the fracture site and medial displacement of the shaft. Boyd's classification into stable and un-

stable fractures is useful in determining the difficulty of fixation and prognosis (Fig. 7).

Type I fracture is a linear break along the intertrochanteric line. Reduction is easily accomplished by abduction, and the fracture is stabilized firmly with a nail plate or lag screw and plate. Healing occurs in 12 weeks or less. *Type II* fracture is comminuted. The medial calcar is difficult to stabilize, and no lateral buttress is present. If fixation is attempted as for Type I, the appliance either bends or breaks, cuts out of the head, or allows the shaft to shift medially or to collapse into varus. The *Type III* is unstable and may be combined with Type I and II. A *Type IV* fracture extends through the trochanter in at least two planes and extends into the shaft. Either a special appliance or a modified technique is necessary to restore stability.

UNSTABLE INTERTROCHANTERIC FRACTURES

The result of deforming forces in unstable intertrochanteric fractures is well illustrated in Figure 8.

Dimon and Hughston in an analysis of 302 trochanteric fractures found 140 to be unstable. They have analyzed the deforming forces present in unstable fractures and suggest that the shaft be shifted me-

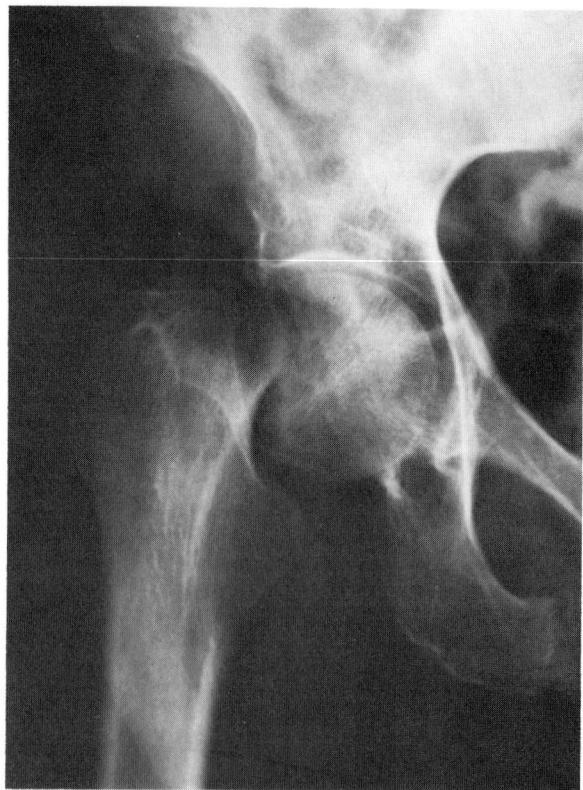

Figure 6. Reduction was not possible in this displaced subcapital fracture in this 78-year-old female. In order to mobilize the patient, the head was replaced with an A. T. Moore prosthesis. She was able to ambulate within five days with a walker.

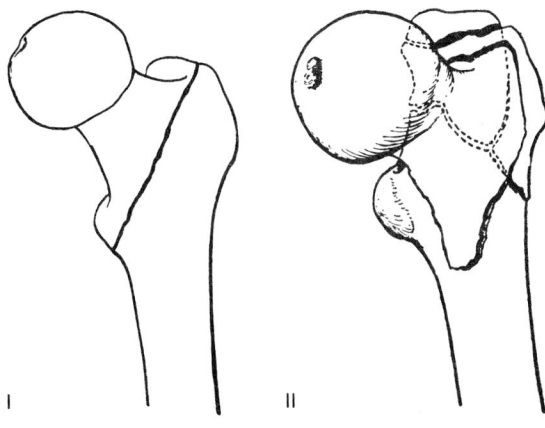

Figure 7. Boyd's classification of intertrochanteric fractures. Type I is stable and can be fixed successfully with a triflanged nail and side plate. In Types II and IV support along the medial calcar is not present and must be restored in order to keep the fracture from collapsing. In Type III, or subtrochanteric fracture, the adductors tend to pull the shaft medially allowing the head to penetrate into the acetabulum. (From Boyd, H. B., and Griffin, L. L.: Classification and treatment of trochanteric fractures. Arch. Surg., *58*:858, 1959.)

HIP FRACTURES IN CHILDREN

Intracapsular fractures in children are uncommon, but complications are common and include growth disturbance, avascular changes, nonunion, malunion, and partial ankylosis. For epiphyseal growth to continue, reduction must be anatomic and fixation secure. These goals can best be met by open reduction and internal fixation.

Transepiphyseal fractures may occur with severe trauma, or minor trauma may cause complete disruption of an epiphyseal line already weakened by chronic slipping capital femoral epiphysis (Fig. 9). Reduction should be accomplished by gentle abduction, internal rotation, and fixation by two or more parallel Knowles pins or screws.

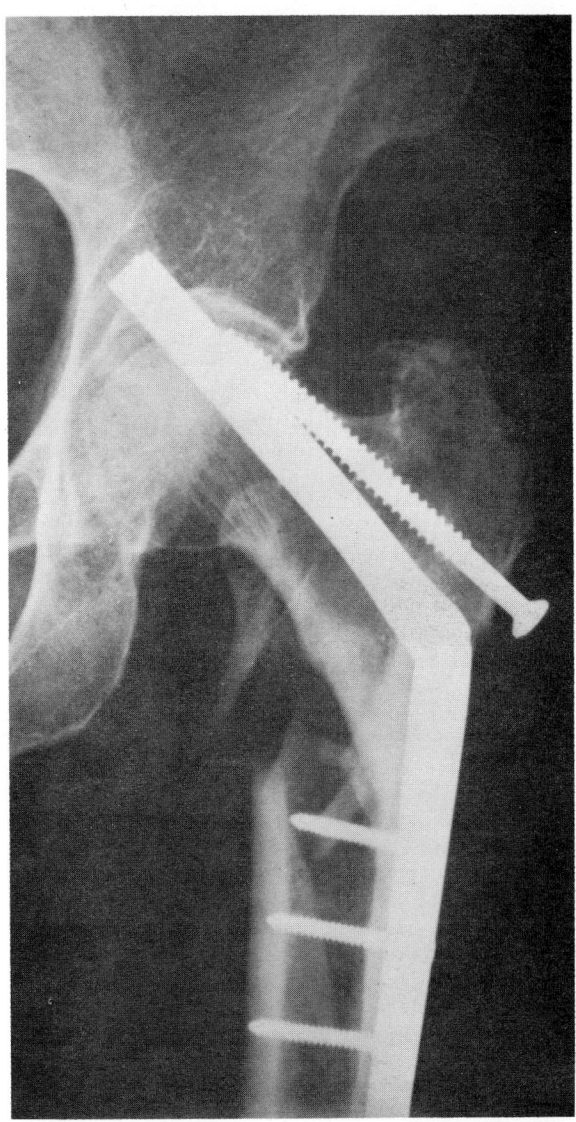

Figure 8. In the Type IV fracture, medial support is not present and ordinary means of fixation are not adequate. The proximal fragment tends to collapse into varus, and the shaft tends to shift medially, allowing the nail to penetrate into the hip joint. (From Zickle, R. E.: A new fixation device for subtrochanteric fractures of the femur. Clin. Orthop., *54*:115–123, 1957.)

dially, a short valgus nail be inserted, and bony support be restored to the medial calcar.

In reviewing a group of patients treated with displacement for unstable fractures, Roberts found that they had more limitation of hip and knee motion than those that were fixed anatomically. Zickel has created a device that stabilizes the subtrochanteric fracture in the anatomic position. The Zickel nail consists of a short intramedullary rod that is driven down the shaft of the femur across the fracture site approximately half the length of the femur. By means of a guide, a triflanged nail is then driven through a hole in the intramedullary rod and up the neck of the femur and into the head. The intramedullary rod tends to prevent medial shift of the shaft of the femur and the triflanged nail tends to prevent varus deformity of the fracture.

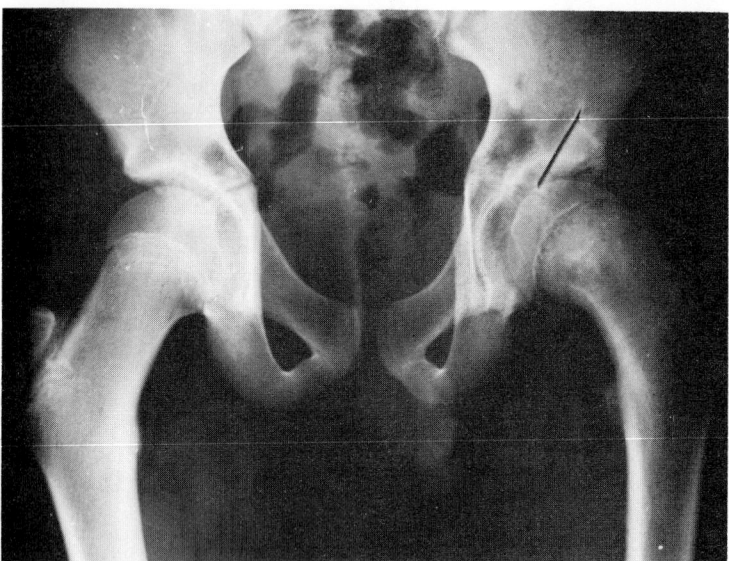

Figure 9. This child had complained of minor left hip pain for some weeks. However, while playing baseball he suddenly had acute onset of left hip pain and was unable to bear weight. Note the widening of the left proximal femoral epiphysis. There has been a sudden acute slip of the capital femoral epiphysis following trauma superimposed on a chronic slip of the capital femoral epiphysis. Reduction was obtained by gentle abduction and internal rotation and the capital femoral epiphysis was fixed with two Knowles' pins.

Fractures of the neck of the femur produce a high incidence of avascular necrosis of the head of the femur in children. Minimal motion further destroys the metaphyseal and retinacular arteries and must be prevented by anatomic reduction and internal fixation. Multiple pins are easier to insert with power tools, as the neck of the femur in a growing child is very resistant. Nails should not be used, as they are likely to distract the fracture and destroy endosteal blood vessels. Immobilization of a neck fracture by plaster in a child is nearly impossible, and nonunion frequently results.

Intertrochanteric and subtrochanteric fractures in children are best managed with traction and plaster. In fractures below the lesser trochanter, the gluteus medius abducts the proximal fragment, and it is flexed by the iliopsoas muscle. In younger children the fracture may be reduced shortly after injury and the child immobilized in a body cast with the hip flexed and abducted, placing the distal fragment in line with the proximal one. The thick periosteum in younger children prevents marked displacement, and solid union occurs in four to six weeks. Bryant's traction is seldom necessary and requires constant nursing care. The combination of elevation of the extremity, extension of the knee producing tension in the popliteal artery, and compression of the calf by skin traction may result in gangrene of the extremity.

In the older child, subtrochanteric fractures are easily managed by 90-90 traction with a femoral pin which is maintained for 10 to 14 days for stability to occur, followed by plaster immobilization for 10 to 12 weeks.

Avulsion fractures of the lesser trochanter and less commonly the greater trochanter occur mostly in athletes. Open reduction is seldom necessary despite considerable displacement. Bed rest with simple Buck's extension or Russell's traction allows pain and muscle spasm to subside in 10 to 12 days, following which the patient can be mobilized comfortably on crutches.

FRACTURES OF THE FEMUR

Fractures of the femur can be divided into four areas—subtrochanteric, midshaft or diaphyseal, supracondylar, and condylar. Each level must be managed differently because the deforming forces acting on the fragments tend to produce different deformities and require different methods of fixation. Fractures in any of these areas may be either closed or open. Most open femoral fractures not due to gunshot wounds are compounded from within, when the femoral shaft penetrates the subcutaneous tissue and skin; as the deformity is corrected, the bone ends sink within the thigh, contaminating the deeper tissues. These sometimes small and benign appearing wounds should be opened widely, and all traumatized tissue should be debrided thoroughly, irrigated copiously, and left open for secondary closure. Nothing is gained by debriding a compound wound and closing it. Necrotic tissue and hematoma provide an ideal culture medium for gas gangrene.

The patient with a fractured femur has undergone severe trauma and must be evaluated carefully. Loss of two to three units of blood within the thigh may not be apparent, and shock may ensue without warning. The hip joint and knee joint must be seen radiographically, or else an associated hip dislocation or supracondylar fracture may be missed. In fractures of the lower third of the femur, nerves and vessels lie close to the bone and can be damaged either by the initial injury or by faulty management.

In subtrochanteric fractures the proximal fragment is flexed, externally rotated, and abducted. The distal fragment is pulled medially by hamstrings and adductors, which produce overriding and shortening. Reduction is difficult in the adult, and nonunion frequently results from closed methods. Open reduction using the fracture table and radiographic control assures proper alignment and union and allows the patient to be ambulatory with crutches in seven to 10 days. Fixation with a nail and side plate affords the simplest internal fixation if there is present a buttress of bone below the nail to prevent medial migration. If no buttress is present, the double nail designed by Zickel may be necessary.

Fractures of the diaphysis or midshaft are usually stabilized by the linea aspera or by a heavy layer of periosteum in children. Reduction is usually easily obtained by traction using a pin in the tibial tubercle, with the extremity supported by a Thomas splint and a Pearson attachment. In a younger child, reduction can often be maintained by skin traction followed in seven to 10 days by application of a body cast after stability has occurred. In older children, skeletal traction may be necessary for reduction. Immobilization by traction or cast requires 16 to 20 weeks in the adult and 8 to 12 weeks in a child. The pin may be threaded or unthreaded. Placement in the tibial tubercle avoids tissue planes that communicate with the fracture, reducing the likelihood of infecting the hematoma.

One of the most significant advances in the treatment of fractures of the femoral shaft was first reported by Smith and later popularized by Mooney. This method of treatment maintains the fracture in balanced traction until swelling diminishes and tenderness subsides. At this point, with the patient still in traction, a lightly padded cast brace is applied over an elastic stump sock of Spandex. Total contact must be obtained, and a quadrilateral socket is molded to fit the proximal thigh. Polycentric hinges are applied to the knee, which is later windowed to allow knee motion. The fracture is stabilized by the hydrodynamic effect of the compressed thigh muscles, and Mooney feels that function of the muscles adjacent to the fracture stimulates healing; early knee motion preserves function. In a review of 150 fractures, he found that all healed within three and one half months, and knee motion was 80 per cent of normal on removal.

The technique is most useful in fractures of the middle and distal shaft. The transverse fracture (Fig. 10) is ideally suited for the cast brace, but if properly used, even comminuted fractures can be mobilized early, and union is rapid. For those with limited experience, the technique is easier if the cast brace is applied at five to seven weeks, after more stability is present. A fracture table can be used, and the tibial pin may be left in place for traction at night. Experienced orthopedists may be able to apply a cast brace within 24 to 48 hours following a fracture. The weight of the leg produces traction and maintains length while the patient is up and about and the leg is kept in traction while the patient remains at bed rest.

Supracondylar fractures are treated initially by traction with the knee in extension, and the cast brace applied after three to six weeks. Alignment can be corrected by wedging. The cast brace usually remains in place for eight to 10 weeks. Shortening is usually no greater than with traction alone.

OPEN REDUCTION OF SHAFT FRACTURES

Transverse or short oblique fractures of the femur between the isthmus (upper third) and the flare of the condyles are best suited for intramedullary nailing.

This technique was begun by Küntscher in 1940 using a cloverleaf nail. For the patient with no other injuries, the intramedullary nail allows the patient to ambulate with crutches within a week after surgery, and hospital stay can be as short as 10 days. Some authors feel that healing is delayed by destruction of endosteal vessels in reaming the shaft to receive the nail. Knee motion is seldom lost, and return to work is more rapid than with other methods. Comminution is a contraindication to intramedullary nailing.

SUPRACONDYLAR FEMORAL FRACTURES

Supracondylar femoral fractures may result from automobile dashboard injuries, a short fall from a

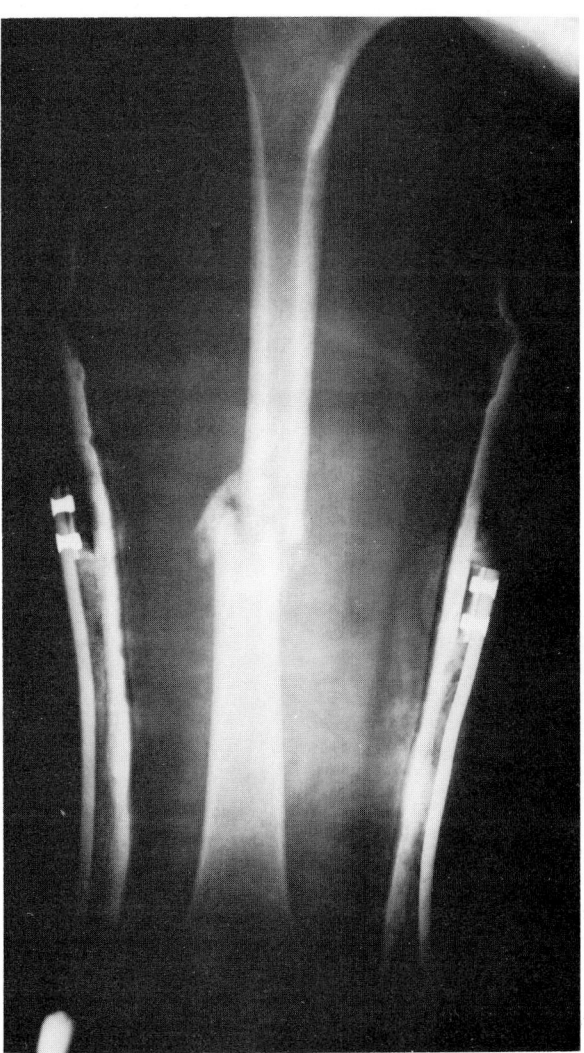

Figure 10. The transverse fracture is ideally suited for treatment by means of a cast brace. In this young man a Steinmann pin was inserted in the tibia, and he was maintained in traction for 10 days. At 10 days, a cast brace with the pin left in place was applied. Rotation was prevented by pelvic band; early knee motion was begun through the cutout stability by the polycentric hinges.

standing position, or a free fall from a height. The more comminuted fractures are usually the result of a free fall or bumper injury. Contraction of the gastrocnemius pulls the distal fragment posteriorly (Fig. 11), but uncontrolled flexion does not occur unless there is overriding of the fragments. Treatment of this fracture with traction in 90 degrees of flexion produces varus angulation of the distal fragment and allows the shaft to shift forward. The most common residual deformity is that of varus and internal rotation of the distal fragment. This alignment occurs as the distal fragment is held in neutral by traction applied through a pin in the tibia, and the proximal fragment externally rotates and angulates medially, producing a varus deformity. This deformity can be prevented by inserting the wire further posteriorly on the medial side, thus externally rotating the distal fragment.

Neer found that the best position for traction treatment of supracondylar fractures was 20 degrees flexion of the knee with a Pearson attachment beneath the distal fragment. Flexion deformity occurred only with violent injury. In the undisplaced fracture, aspiration and casting is all that is required. He found that closed treatment by this method produced union by the fifth week and results were satisfactory in 90 per cent of patients. Patients accepted stiffness of the knee better than deformity.

Closed treatment frequently results in limited motion of the knee. Open reduction allows better apposition of joint surface, and internal fixation allows faster mobilization. In a review of 110 fractures in 1967, Neer found that methods of fixation at that time were inadequate to allow early motion and recommended closed treatment with traction. In a later study with Shelton, he described a fixation device that was found superior to the inadequate blade plate. Open reduction should be considered when traction fails to produce adequate alignment, when comminution prevents early motion, in the elderly patient with arthritis, or when soft tissue interposition is present.

Through a lateral incision the articular fragments are reduced and held to each other with Steinmann pins. The condyles are then fixed with cancellous screws or Barr bolts and fixed to the shaft by means of the side plate with cortical screws (Fig. 12). The average patient should attain knee flexion of 90 degrees within three months after the fracture. When adequate reduction can be obtained with traction, cast bracing at three to four weeks will allow ambulation with crutches and early knee motion.

Supracondylar fractures in children are uncommon. A much more common injury is epiphyseal separation of the distal end of the femur, usually combined with a shaft fracture. If treated promptly these fractures are easily reduced but tend to redisplace if treated in plaster. Either percutaneous pinning with multiple smooth pins or open reduction should be considered. Survival of the epiphyseal plate is dependent upon anatomic reduction and maintenance. Premature closure of the epiphyseal plate usually occurs and may require epiphyseal arrest on the opposite side. Following asymmetric damage to the epiphyseal plate, both linear and angular deformities occur, and corrective osteotomy may be necessary.

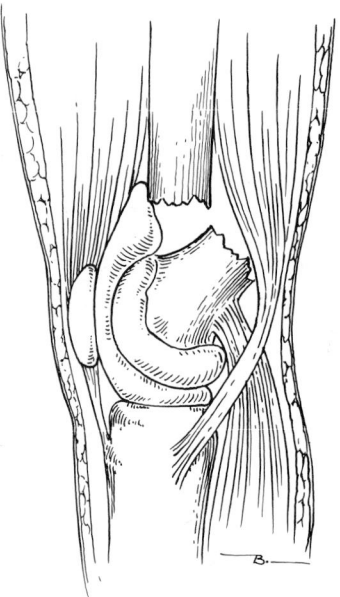

Figure 11. In supracondylar fractures associated with displacement, the distal fragment is drawn into flexion in relationship to the tibia by the pull of the gastrocnemius. This displacement occurs only with severe trauma. In the routine supracondylar fracture, 90 degrees of flexion is not necessary to reduce the fracture.

FRACTURES OF THE PATELLA

The patella is vulnerable to injury, lying in its subcutaneous position on the hard surface of the femoral condyles. Fractures occur by direct injury from the dashboard of an automobile or indirectly by contraction of the massive quadriceps muscle. Both mechanisms can occur simultaneously as the patient attempts to avoid falling by extending the knee; the patella separates, the knee collapses, and the patella strikes the ground.

Fractures due to direct injury are most often stellate, comminuted, and frequently compound. Displacement is usually minimal. Indirect fractures may occur in either the upper, middle, or lower third and may be widely separated, indicating extensive tearing of the retinaculum. If the extensor retinaculum is torn, active extension of the knee is not possible and open reduction is mandatory.

Fractures of the patella are relatively easy to diagnose because of the subcutaneous position of the fragments. Effusion is usually marked and ecchymosis is extensive. Extension may be limited by a tense effusion. If fragments are undisplaced, aspiration of hematoma and immobilization in a padded cylinder cast is sufficient treatment, and motion can be started at three to four weeks.

If the fracture fragments are separated, open reduction and repair of the retinaculum are necessary. If the two fragments are approximately equal in size, they are approximated by a heavy gauge wire inserted through two longitudinal drill holes in each fragment

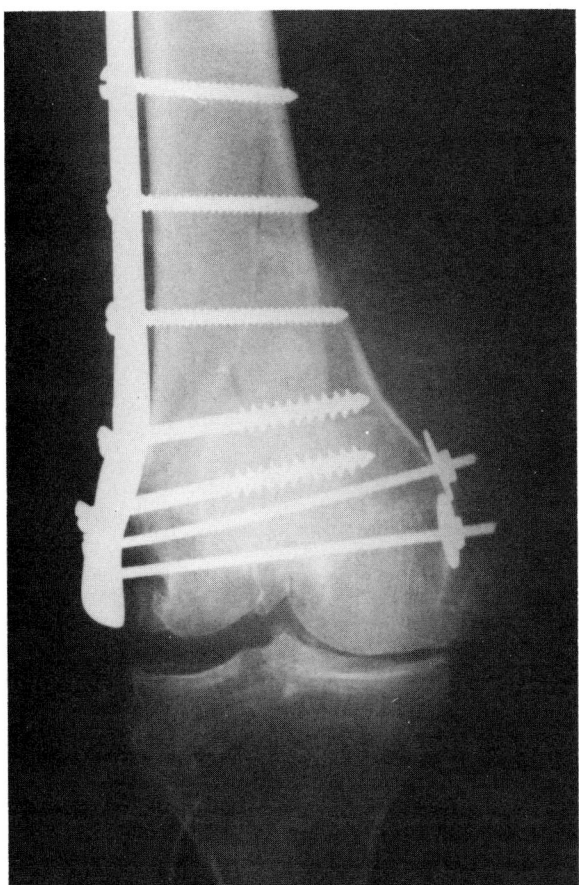

Figure 12. The comminuted supracondylar fracture in this 79-year-old female was opened, the condyles were reduced to each other and held in place with Steinmann pins, following which Barr bolts were passed across the femoral condyles; the plate was then attached to the femoral shaft with cortical screws. Motion was started at three weeks. At 12 weeks, 80 degrees of knee motion was present.

(Fig. 13). Circumferential wiring is more difficult, and accurate reduction is less certain with this method.

In comminuted or stellate fracture with displacement, total patellectomy and repair of the retinaculum produce an excellent result without the almost certain complication of chondromalacia. Immobilization must be maintained for four weeks and forceful extension limited for another four.

In fractures where the superior or inferior fragment constitutes less than one third of the patella, the smaller fragment should be excised and the remaining quadriceps or patellar tendon repaired with interrupted figure-eight nonabsorbable sutures. The knee is then immobilized in extension for four weeks in a cylinder cast. During this time full weight bearing is allowed. Activity is limited for another four weeks.

Fractures of the patella must be differentiated from a bipartite patella. When suspected, radiographs of the opposite knee may reveal the same condition. The fragments are surrounded by cortical bone with rounded margins, as opposed to the jagged, sharp margins in a peripheral fracture.

DISLOCATION OF THE KNEE

Dislocations of the knee result from violent trauma, most commonly motorcycle accidents, bumper injuries, and athletic injuries, or a fall from a height (Fig. 14). The cruciate ligament must be torn, as well as the joint capsule. Displacement of the tibia may be anterior, posterior, lateral, or medial, but anterior dislocation is most common. Although partial disruption of major ligaments must be present for dislocation to occur, most dislocations will be stable following reduction. Kennedy found both collateral ligaments to be intact at the time of delayed repair in six knees.

Most knee dislocations are easily reducible, and alignment may be normal by the time the patient arrives in the emergency room. Absence of deformity may be misleading, as severe vascular or nerve damage may be present. If the knee is still dislocated at the time of first examination, the deformity should be corrected as soon as possible by gentle longitudinal traction. The only knee deformity that does not reduce easily is the posterolateral dislocation. This injury can be recognized by the presence of a dimple over the medial joint line below the very prominent medial femoral condyle, which frequently projects through a buttonhole deformity in the medial capsule. The dimple is produced by invagination of the medial ligament into the joint. Open reduction must be done through a

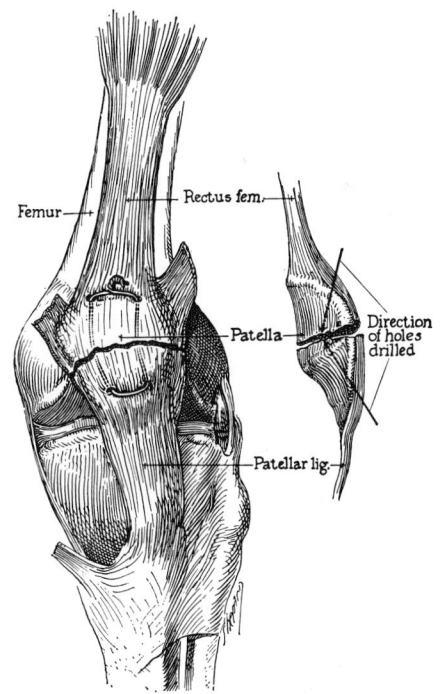

Figure 13. In the transverse fracture of the patella where the fragments are approximately equal in size, wiring of the fragments through vertical drill holes is the treatment of choice. If marked displacement is present, the retinaculum must be torn, and it must be repaired out to the extent of the medial and lateral collateral ligaments. After wiring of the patella and repair of the retinaculum, motion can be started at approximately three weeks.

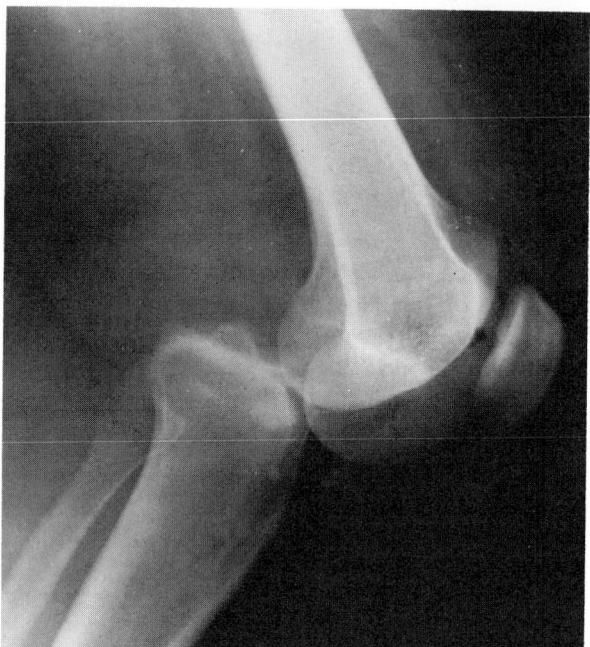

Figure 14. Lateral x-ray demonstrates a posterior dislocation of the tibia. Reduction was obtained by gentle longitudinal traction. Following five weeks in plaster, the knee was relatively stable and a good range of motion was re-established after three months.

medial incision; the rent in the capsule is enlarged and alignment restored by gentle traction.

Most dislocations of the knee will be stable after treatment with cast immobilization for six weeks. The greatest cause of morbidity from this injury is nerve and vascular damage. Goldner and Ford found peroneal palsy in half of their patients, and Shields found vascular damage in 40 per cent of 26 patients. The popliteal artery and vein are firmly fixed above and below the popliteal space, and hyperextension of the knee or anterior displacement of the tibia may either tear completely or produce enough intimal damage to cause thrombosis. Peripheral pulses must be checked carefully on first examination and followed closely for several days. If pulses are diminished or there is any question about the continuity of vessels, immediate exploration of the popliteal space should be done. Arteriography is time consuming and probably unnecessary, as vascular damage is always within a few inches of the joint line. Replacement by prosthetic artery or vein graft may be necessary.

Anterior or posterior compartment syndrome frequently follows knee dislocations and should be suspected when the patient continues to complain of severe pain in the leg following reduction. Pulses may be absent, but tissue ischemia can progress although pulses are palpable. Normal tissue pressure is zero. As tissue pressure rises, tissue perfusion decreases significantly at a level 20 mm. below diastolic pressure. When it equals diastolic pressure, tissue perfusion ceases, although distal pulses may still be present. As it approaches systolic pressure, pulses disappear.

When pain is persistent, tissue pressure should be measured by the method of Whitesides.

SELECTED REFERENCES

Boyd, H. B., and Griffin, L. L.: Classification and treatment of trochanteric fractures. Arch. Surg., *58*:858, 1949.
  This classic article analyzes 300 trochanteric fractures and was one of the first articles to differentiate between stable and unstable trochanteric fractures. The use of an additional side plate to prevent medial migration of the femur was suggested in unstable Type III fractures.

d'Aubigne, R. M.: Management of acetabular fractures in multiple trauma. J. Trauma, *8*:333, 1968.
  This study analyzes 210 patients with acetabular fractures. The author emphasizes that fractures of the acetabulum are frequently overlooked because of other injury. A classification based on prognosis of acetabular fractures is presented. Early surgery and open reduction are advocated and have been shown to produce better long-term results.

Dimon, J. H., and Hughston, J. C.: Unstable intertrochanteric fractures of the hip. J. Bone Joint Surg., *49G*:440, 1967.
  In an analysis of 302 trochanteric fractures, 140 were found to be unstable, most of them owing to comminution of the medial calcar with a large posterior fragment. A method of reduction by an osteotomy of the greater trochanter and shifting the shaft medially is described in order to prevent the late complications in unstable fractures.

Ford, G. L., and Goldner, J. L.: Dislocation of the knee joint. N.C. Med. J., *20*:463–468, 1959.
  This article, although it includes only 10 patients with dislocation of the knee, contains an excellent bibliography of the subject. Treatment by closed reduction and immobilization is advocated. The high incidence of circulatory and nerve palsy complications is emphasized.

Mooney, V., Nickel, V. L., Harvey, J. P., and Snelson, R.: Cast brace treatment for fractures of the distal part of the femur. J. Bone Joint Surg., *52A*:1563–1578, 1970.
  The technique described in this article has probably changed the management of fractures of the femur more than any other development in the past century. The techniques of applying the cast brace and of managing the patient are clearly outlined. Healing appears to be more rapid with a cast brace and physiologic function is better maintained than with either treatment with prolonged traction or open reduction and internal fixation. Mean healing time for all fractured femurs was 14.5 weeks.

Neer, C. S., Grantham, S. A., and Shelton, M.: Supracondylar fracture of the adult femur. A study of 110 cases. J. Bone Joint Surg., *49A*:591–613, 1967.
  This analysis of 110 supracondylar fractures recommended the closed treatment of this injury. The most common deformity which results from supracondylar fracture is that of internal rotation and varus deformity, which can be prevented by placing the tibial pin used for traction in a position of external rotation. Prior to this article, most authors recommended that the supracondylar fracture be treated in a position of 90 degrees of flexion, which the author in this series has shown actually aggravates the deformity by shifting the femoral shaft forward.

Reynolds, B. M., et al.: Pelvic fractures. J. Trauma, *13*:1011–1014, 1973.
  This comprehensive review of 273 fractures emphasizes the severity of pelvic fractures. The complications are clearly outlined and their management is well discussed. Open reduction of pelvic fractures with massive bleeding is discouraged. Preferably bleeding points should be localized by arteriography and hemorrhage controlled by the injection of autogenous blood clot unless major vessels are involved.

REFERENCES

Fractures of the Pelvis

1. Conolly, W. B., and Hedberg, E. A.: Observations on fractures of the pelvis. J. Trauma, *9*:104–11, 1969.
2. d'Aubigne, R. M.: Management of acetabular fractures in multiple trauma. J. Trauma, *8*:333, 1968.
3. Dunn, W., and Morris, H. D.: Fractures and dislocations of the pelvis. J. Bone Joint Surg., *50A*:1639–1648, 1968.

4. Holdsworth, F. W.: Dislocation and fracture dislocations of the pelvis. J. Bone Joint Surg., *30B*:461–466, 1948.

5. Kadish, L. J., et al.: Angiographic diagnosis and treatment of bleeding due to pelvic trauma. J. Trauma, *13*:1083–1085, 1973.

6. Key, J. A., and Conwell, H. E.: Management of Fractures, Dislocations, and Sprains. St. Louis, The C. V. Mosby Co., 1951.

7. Knight, R. A., and Smith, H.: Central fractures of the acetabulum. J. Bone Joint Surg., *40A*:1–16, 1958.

8. Malgaigne, J. F.: Treatise on Fractures. Philadelphia, J. B. Lippincott, 1859.

9. Miller, W. E.: Massive hemorrhage in fractures of the pelvis. South. Med. J., *56*:933–938, 1963.

10. Pearson, J. R., and Hargaddon, E. J.: Fractures of the pelvis involving the floor of the acetabulum. J. Bone Joint Surg., *44B*:550–561, 1962.

11. Peltier, L. F.: Complications associated with fractures of the pelvis. J. Bone Joint Surg., *47A*:1060–1069, 1965.

12. Reynolds, B. M., et al.: Pelvic fractures. J. Trauma, *13*:1011–1014, 1973.

13. Rowe, C. R., and Lowell, J. D.: Prognosis of fractures of the acetabulum. J. Bone Joint Surg., *43A*:30–59, 1961.

14. Schlonsky, J., et al.: Functional disability following avulsion fracture of the ischial epiphysis. J. Bone Joint Surg., *54*:641–644, 1972.

15. Spear, C. V., et al.: Vascular and adjacent soft tissue injuries associated with fractures of the pelvis. South. Med. J., *68*:142–144, 1975.

16. Trunkey, D. D., et al.: Management of pelvic fractures in blunt trauma injury. J. Trauma, *14*:912–923, 1974.

Fractures of the Hip

17. Albright, J. P., and Weinstein, S. L.: Treatment for fracture complications. Arch. Surg., *110*:30–36, 1975.

18. Boyd, H. B., and Griffin, L. L.: Classification and treatment of trochanteric fractures. Arch. Surg., *58*:858, 1949.

19. Boyd, R. J., Burke, J. F., and Colton, T.: A double blind clinical trial of prophylactic antibiotics in hip fractures. J. Bone Joint Surg., *55A*:1251–1258, 1973.

20. Carnesale, P. G., and Anderson, L. D.: Primary prosthetic replacement for femoral neck fractures. Arch. Surg., *110*:27–29, 1975.

21. Coventry, M. B.: The treatment of fracture dislocation of the hip by total hip arthroplasty. J. Bone Joint Surg., *56A*:1103–1127, 1974.

22. Crawford, H. B.: Conservative treatment of impacted fractures of femoral neck. J. Bone Joint Surg., *42A*:471–479, 1960.

23. Dimon, J. H., and Hughston, J. C.: Unstable intertrochanteric fractures of the hip. J. Bone Joint Surg., *49G*:440, 1967.

24. DiStefano, V. J., et al.: Stable fixation of the difficult subtrochanteric fracture. J. Trauma, *12*:1066–1070, 1972.

25. Epstein, H. C.: Posterior fracture dislocation of the hip: Long term follow up. J. Bone Joint Surg., *56A*:1103–1127, 1974.

26. Evarts, C. M., and Fail, E. J.: Prevention of thromboembolic disease after elective surgery of the hip. J. Bone Joint Surg., *53A*:1271–1280, 1971.

27. Fielding, J. W.: Subtrochanteric fractures. Clin. Orthop., *92*:86, 1973.

28. Frankel, V. H., Burstein, A. H., Brown, R. H., et al.: Biotelemetry from the upper end of the femur (abstract). J. Bone Joint Surg., *53A*:1023, 1971.

29. Freeman, M. A., et al.: The role of fatigue in the pathogenesis of senile femoral neck fractures. J. Bone Joint Surg., *56B*:698–762, 1974.

30. Jewett, E. L.: One piece angle nail for trochanteric fractures. J. Bone Joint Surg., *23*:803–810, 1941.

31. Kelly, R. P., and Yarbrough, S. H.: Post fracture dislocation of the femoral head and retained medial head fragment. J. Trauma, *11*:97–108, 1971.

32. Laros, G. S.: Current views of hip fracture. Arch. Surg., *110*:18–19, 1975.

33. Laros, G. S.: Intertrochanteric fractures. The role of complications of fixation. Arch. Surg., *110*:37–40, 1975.

34. Leadbetter, G. W.: A treatment for fracture of the neck of the femur. J. Bone Joint Surg., *15*:931–940, 1933.

35. Lunceford, E. M.: Use of the Moore self locking Vitallium prosthesis in acute fractures of the femoral neck. J. Bone Joint Surg., *47A*:832–841, 1965.

36. Mulholland, R. C., and Gunn, D. R.: Sliding screw fixation of intertrochanteric femoral fractures. J. Trauma, *12*:581–591, 1972.

37. Pankovich, A. M.: Primary internal fixation of femoral neck fractures. Arch Surg., *110*:20–25, 1975.

38. Roberts, A., et al.: A comparison of the functional results of anatomic and medial displacement valgus nailing of intertrochanteric fractures of the femur. J. Trauma, *12*:341–346, 1972.

39. Rydell, N.: Biomechanics of the hip joint. Clin. Orthop., *92*:6, 1973.

40. Sarmiento, A.: The unstable intertrochanteric fracture: Treatment with a valgus osteotomy and I beam nail plate. J. Bone Joint Surg., *52A*:1309, 1970.

41. Shelton, M. L.: Subtrochanteric fractures of the femur. Arch. Surg., *110*:41–48, 1975.

42. Smith-Peterson, M. N., Cave, E. F., and Van Gorder, W.: Intracapsular fracture of the neck of the femur. Arch. Surg., *23*:715–759, 1931.

43. Von Langenbeck, B.: Verhandl, d. deutsch. Geselloch, Chir., 1878, p. 92.

44. Welch, R. B., et al.: Total hip replacement as a salvage in traumatic lesions about the hip. Surg. Gynecol. Obstet., *140*:708–714, 1975.

45. Whitman, R.: A new method of treatment for fractures of the neck of the femur. Am. J. Surg., *36*:746, 1902.

46. Zickel, R. E.: A new fixation device for subtrochanteric fractures of the femur. Clin. Orthop., *54*:115–123, 1957.

Fractures of the Femur

47. Brown, A., et al.: Internal fixation for supracondylar fractures of the femur in the elderly patient. J. Bone Joint Surg., *53B*:420–424, 1971.

48. Carr, C. R., and Wingo, C. H.: Fractures of the femoral diaphysis. A retrospective study of the results and costs of treatment by intramedullary nailing and by traction and a spica cast. J. Bone Joint Surg., *55A*:690–700, 1973.

49. Clawson, D. K.: Closed intramedullary nailing of the femur. J. Bone Joint Surg., *53*:681–692, 1974.

50. Connoly, J. F., et al.: Femoral and tibial fractures combined with injuries to the femoral or popliteal artery. J. Bone Joint Surg., *53A*:56, 1971.

51. Dencker, H.: Is the length of hospitalization for patients with femoral shaft fracture shortened by intramedullary nailing? Acta. Orthop. Scand., *35*:67–73, 1964.

52. Fitzpatrick, C. B.: The treatment of fractures of the shaft of the femur by closed intramedullary nailing. J. Bone Joint Surg., *57B*:255, 1975.

53. Kunscher, G.: Intramedullary surgical technique and its place in orthopedic surgery. J. Bone Joint Surg., *47A*:809–818, 1965.

54. Laing, P. G.: Blood supply of the femoral shaft: Anatomical study. J. Bone Joint Surg., *35B*:462–466, 1953.

55. Mooney, V., Nickel, V. L., Harvey, J. P., and Snelson, R.: Cast brace treatment for fractures of the distal part of the femur. J. Bone Joint Surg., *52A*:1563–1578, 1970.

56. Neer, C. S., Grantham, S. A., and Shelton, M.: Supracondylar fracture of the adult femur. A study of 110 cases. J. Bone Joint Surg., *49A*:591–613, 1967.

57. Olerud, S.: Operative treatment of supracondylar–condylar fractures of the femur. J. Bone Joint Surg., *54A*:1015–1032, 1972.

58. Peltier, L. F.: A brief history of traction. J. Bone Joint Surg., *50A*:1603–1615, 1968.

59. Riggins, R. S., Garrick, J. G., and Lipscomb, P. R.: Supracondylar fractures of the femur. A survey of treatment. Clin. Orthop., *82*:32–36, 1972.

60. Schneider, H. W.: Use of the four flanged self-cutting intramedullary nail for fixation of femoral fractures. Clin. Orthop., *60*:29–39, 1968.

61. Shelton, M. L., Grantham, S. A., Neer, C. S., and Singh, R.: A new fixation device for supracondylar and low femoral shaft fractures. J. Trauma, *14*:821, 1974.

62. Stewart, M. J., Sisk, T. O., and Wallace, S. L.: Fractures of the distal third of the femur. J. Bone Joint Surg., *48A*:787–807, 1966.

63. Street, D. M.: One hundred fractures of the femur treated by means of the diamond shaped medullary nail. J. Bone Joint Surg., *33A*:659–669, 1951.

Fractures of the Knee

64. Anderson, L. D. *In* Crenshaw, A. H. (Ed.): Campbell's Operative Orthopaedics, 5th ed. St. Louis, The C. V. Mosby Co., 1971.

65. Ford, G. L., and Goldner, J. L.: Dislocation of the knee joint. North Carolina Med. J., *20*:463–468, 1959.

66. Griswold, A. S.: Fractures of the patella. Clin. Orthop., 4:44–56, 1954.
67. Kennedy, J. C.: Complete dislocation of the knee joint. J. Bone Joint Surg., 45A:889–904, 1963.
68. Magnuson, P. B.: Fractures. 2nd ed. Philadelphia, J. B. Lippincott, 1936.
69. Reckling, F. W., and Peltier, L. F.: Acute knee dislocations and their complications. J. Trauma, 9:181–191, 1969.
70. Shields, L., Mital, M., and Cave, E. F.: Complete dislocation of the knee: Experience at the Massachusetts General Hospital. J. Trauma, 9:192–215, 1969.
71. Taylor, A. R., Arden, G. P., and Rainey, M. H.: Traumatic dislocation of the knee. A report of 43 cases with special reference to conservative treatment. J. Bone Joint Surg., 54B:96–102, 1972.
72. Whitesides, T. E., et al.: A simple method for tissue pressure determination. Arch. Surg., 110:1311–1313, 1975.

VII

FRACTURES OF THE TIBIA, FIBULA, ANKLE, AND FOOT

Frank H. Bassett, III, M.D.

FRACTURES OF THE TIBIAL PLATEAU

The upper end of the tibia flares at the metaphysis to form two condyles, which articulate with the femoral condyles. The medial condyle or plateau has a biconcave articular surface, while the lateral plateau is concave in the frontal projection but convex in the sagittal plane. Between the two articular surfaces are two distinct intercondylar eminences, which articulate with the femoral condyles during flexion and extension like the flanges on the wheel of a train. In flexion, when the articular surfaces of the tibia are in contact with the diverging femoral condyles posteriorly, the intercondylar eminences do not contact the femoral condyles, and rotation of the leg is possible. When the knee extends, and the intercondylar eminence fits snugly into the converged portion of the femoral condyles, no rotation is normally possible, and the tibial plateaus are compressed firmly against the distal femur (Fig. 1).

Forced flexion of hyperextension injuries may result in avulsion *fractures of the intercondyloid eminence.* This commonly occurs in children with falls from a bicycle or skate board. Avulsion results from excessive tension on the anterior cruciate ligament, which inserts just anterior to the eminence. Partial avulsion, when the bony surface of the fragment is still in contact with the intercondyloid fossa, permits easy reduction of the eminence by extension of the knee. Displaced fragments, especially when rotated, often require open reduction and suture fixation.

When the knee joint is subjected to external stresses, a wide spectrum of damage can result depending on the amplitude and direction of the forces, as well as the relationship of the femoral and tibial condyles at the time of injury. The pathology ranges from tears of the semilunar cartilage and ligamentous injury to fractures of the tibial plateaus or femoral condyles. The cancellous condyles of the tibia, particu-larly the lateral plateau, are injured most commonly by a valgus or abduction force in a middle-aged or elderly person. Other mechanisms of injury are compression fractures resulting from falls from a height or

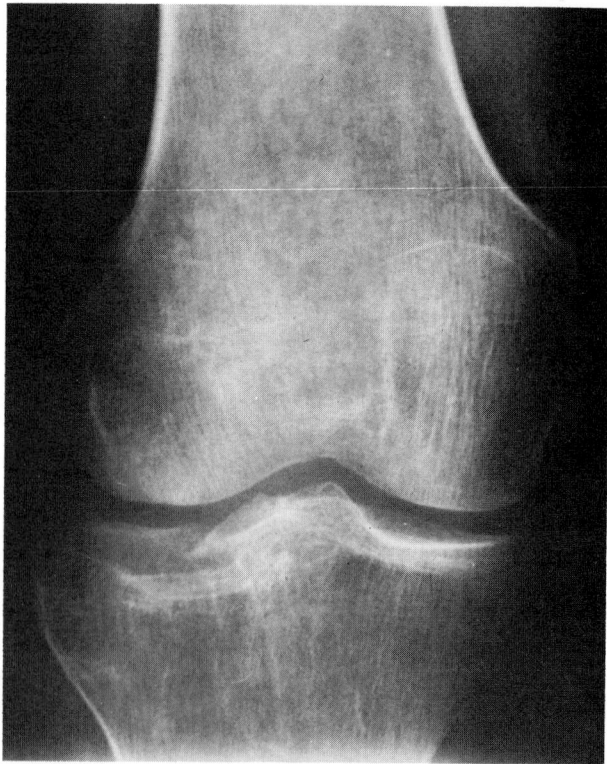

Figure 1. Roentgenogram showing central depressed fracture of the lateral tibial plateau. This was less than 5 mm. The patient was treated with active motion in bed using skin traction. The patient regained full knee motion and is free of pain.

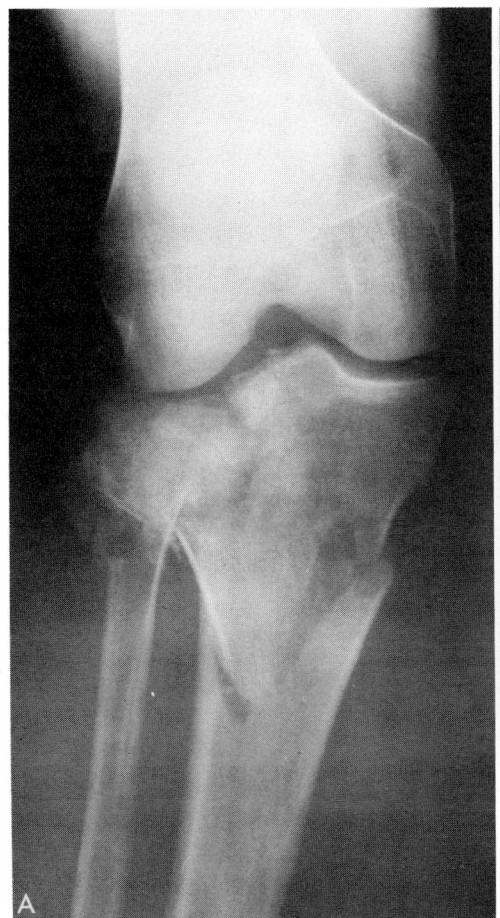
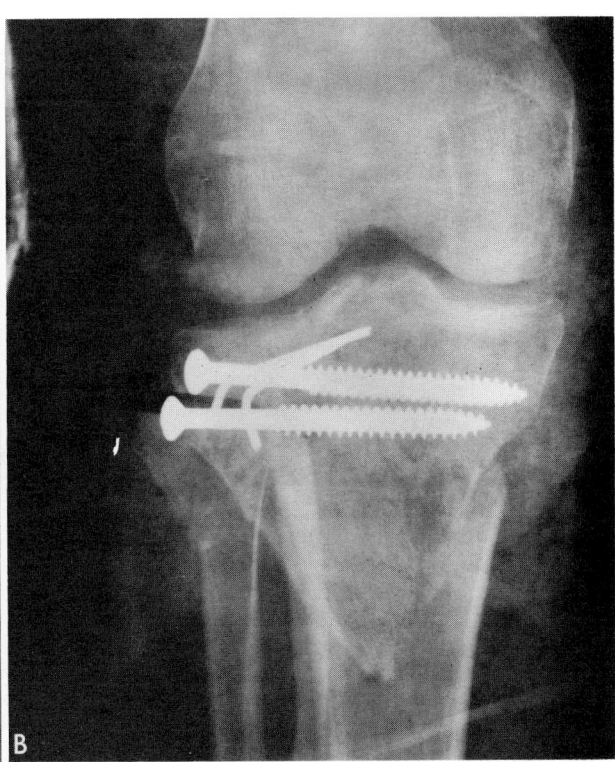

Figure 2. *A,* Severely comminuted fracture of the lateral tibial plateau extending into the tibial shaft. The medial plateau and intercondylar eminence are also separated from the tibial shaft by fracture. The knee was grossly unstable. *B,* Postoperative fixation devices to realign normal anatomy of the articular surface of the tibia.

a direct blow to the proximal tibia with the knee in flexion. The fractures include local depression of the center of the condyle, a split depression of a portion of the periphery of the plateau, and total depression of the entire condyle. A comminuted fracture involving both plateaus is one of the most serious and difficult to treat of the tibial plateau fractures.

The patient with a plateau fracture presents with localized pain over the involved plateau, and there will be swelling and local tenderness. A *genu valgus* deformity may be present if the lateral plateau has been depressed. A depressed medial plateau fracture will present with *genu varus.* These fractures often are associated with damage to the collateral and cruciate ligaments. The distal circulation, particularly the neurovascular function of the anterior compartment structures of the leg, should be evaluated. Edema and hemorrhage from a lateral plateau fracture can occlude the anterior tibial artery, and ischemic necrosis of the anterior compartment structures is a likely and common sequela. Immediate decompression by fasciotomy is indicated to prevent irreversible necrosis of the involved structures.

Roentgenograms of the knees, including both oblique views, are valuable in determining the exact location of the fractures and the extent of displacement.

One fourth of plateau fractures are undisplaced. They can usually be treated in a long leg, nonweight-bearing cast for four weeks. At that time, knee motion should be started and weight bearing progressed so that in 10 to 12 weeks full weight bearing is achieved.

Local depression fractures usually involve the posterior portion of the plateau. Collateral and cruciate ligament damage is unusual with this fracture. Closed reduction of the depressed segment by manipulation under general or spinal anesthesia often is successful. Reduction is maintained by a long leg cast, with the knee in extension, for six to eight weeks.

When a *central portion of the plateau* is depressed and is less than 5 mm., minimal instability results (Fig. 1). Early motion, done in bed with light skin traction, prevents knee stiffness, and normal knee function is expected. Meniscal injury is not common. However, when the central fragment is depressed greater than 5 mm., surgical elevation of the fragment is required. Surgical elevation of the fragments usually leaves a cavity within the plateau, and cortical bone grafts from local surrounding bone are necessary to prevent recollapse of the elevated segment.

A split depression, if greater than 5 mm. and/or associated with ligamentous injury, is an indication for open reduction. The articular surface must be restored to its normal anatomic position and the split fragment impacted against the remaining undisturbed plateau by a compression device, either a woodscrew or a cancellous compression screw. Many surgeons use a tibial bolt. When the depressed fracture involves the medial plateau, maintenance of reduction may be difficult. Weekly roentgenograms should be taken for three weeks to observe for loss of reduction. Open reduction and bolt or screw fixation often is necessary.

Comminuted plateau fractures, involving one or both plateaus, often are associated with intra-articular damage to the intercondylar eminence. Avulsion of cruciate ligaments with a fragment of bone should be restored to its normal position at the time of surgical correction of the plateaus (Fig. 2).

Regardless of the type of fracture, anatomic restoration of the articular surface is the goal of treatment. Wide exposure of the joint is indicated and should be approached inferior to or beneath the meniscus, leaving it attached to the meniscofemoral portion of the capsule. This permits better visualization of the articular surface and avoids direct damage to the meniscus. Internal fixation, using compression screws or tibial bolts, will maintain stable reduction and allow early movement of the knee joint in an effort to regain a normal range of motion. Unless severely deranged, the meniscus should not be removed. Torn capsular ligaments must be sutured anatomically.

Postoperatively, once union has occurred, knee motion should be initiated and a rigid, well-supervised rehabilitation program should be prescribed. This is especially true when ligamentous laxity persists.

FRACTURES OF THE TIBIAL SHAFT

The tibia is subcutaneous throughout its entire length. Therefore, fractures of the tibial shaft are often of the open variety. Transverse, oblique, spiral, and comminuted fractures are all common to the tibia. The stability of such fractures depends not only on the type of fracture but also on the integrity of the fibula. Oblique, spiral, and comminuted fractures are basically unstable. A thorough roentgenographic examination of the entire fibula is mandatory in such cases to look for concomitant fractures of the fibula, either above or below the site of the tibial fracture.

Open fractures of the tibia demand early, thorough irrigation and débridement of the wound. Basic principles of wound care include open treatment to permit adequate drainage, followed by wound inspection and secondary closure five to seven days after the injury. In such cases, care of the wound is equally or more important than care of the fracture itself. Following initial wound toilet, reduction of the fracture should be completed and the limb immobilized in a well-padded long leg cast. Wound inspection and closure can be done through appropriately placed windows in the cast at the proper time.

Fractures of the tibial shaft are often associated with extensive soft tissue damage, and a thorough evaluation of the neurovascular function in the extremity is mandatory on a daily basis. At the first sign of deficiency, the cast should be split to avoid excessive compression.

Reduction of open or closed tibial fractures requires general or spinal anesthesia to control muscle spasm. Correction of any angular and rotary deformity can usually be achieved manually by manipulation and traction (Fig. 3). In the case of an oblique or spiral fracture, maintenance of reduction can be a problem. If the application of a long leg cast does not maintain reduction, then percutaneous transfixion of the proximal and distal tibia with Steinmann pins may help maintain length and reduction when they are incorporated into the plaster cast (Fig. 3*D*).

Weight bearing on the involved extremity in a well-fitted walking cast is permissible as soon as soft tissue swelling and pain permit. This usually hastens the healing. Even with comminuted fractures, loss of length is usually minimal.

The indications for open reduction and internal fixation of fractures of the shaft of the tibia include extensive soft tissue injury, immobilization that cannot be maintained by external support, a patient with multiple fractures in whom care will be greatly facilitated by strong internal fixation, and some extremely unstable fractures that cannot be reduced or maintained by closed methods.

Complications of fractures of the tibial shaft include delayed union and nonunion, and these are seen most commonly in the open or infected fractures. Other well-known complications are fat embolus, deep vein thrombosis with subsequent ankle and leg swelling, and arthrofibrosis of the ankle and subtalar joints.

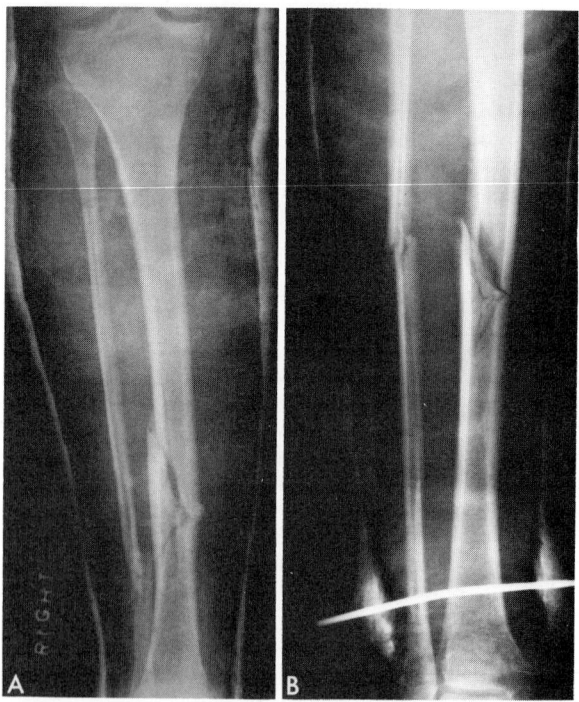

Figure 3. *A,* Comminuted fracture of the tibia and fibula reduced by closed manipulation and held in a plaster cast. Although unstable, position was held by plaster fixation alone. *B,* Unstable oblique fracture of the midshaft of the tibia. Fracture reduction could not be maintained by plaster fixation alone. A Steinmann pin was inserted above and below the fracture site and incorporated into the plaster to help maintain length for stability purposes.

FRACTURES OF THE FIBULA

Fractures of the fibular shaft usually are of little consequence. The distal one fourth to one third of the fibula is important in providing integrity to the ankle joint and therefore is of great importance in the management of fractures involving the ankle joint. However, solitary fractures of the fibula resulting from direct blows usually require little treatment other than a protective cast for just one or two weeks for comfort and the control of swelling. When spiral fractures involve the neck of the fibula, particular attention should be directed to the evaluation of peroneal nerve function because of the close proximity of the nerve to the fibula in this region.

FRACTURES AND FRACTURE-DISLOCATIONS OF THE ANKLE

The distal fibula extends approximately 1 cm. further than the medial malleolus and provides the major stabilizing support for the ankle joint. Fractures of the lateral malleolus or the distal fibula are commonly seen with rotational angular forces. The strong ligaments about the ankle and the skeletal mortice can be damaged in various combinations, depending on the direction of the stress. With abduction and external rotation forces, rupture of the deltoid ligament or an avulsion fracture of the medial malleolus presents the most minor of the injuries. With more force, the anterior tibiofibular ligament fibers are torn, which tends to open the ankle mortice anteriorly. A spiral fracture of the fibula at the level of the distal tibiofibular joint results. If abduction is the major stress, then splitting of the interosseous membrane between the tibia and the fibula occurs concomitant with fracture of the fibula above the mortice. Lateral displacement of the foot and ankle is common. Closed reduction demands regaining the entire length of the fibula by traction, internal rotation of the foot at the ankle, and application of a long leg cast with the knee flexed 20 to 30 degrees. Anatomic reduction is the goal of treatment. If reduction cannot be achieved or cannot be maintained because of the unstable nature of the fracture, then screw fixation of the medial malleolus, repair of the torn deltoid ligament, intramedullary fixation of the fibula, and repair of the torn tibiofibular ligament are indicated (Fig. 4). Occasionally a portion of the posterior aspect of the distal tibia accompanies the lateral fracture dislocation of the ankle, and the so-called "trimalleolar" fracture exists. Accurate reduction of the displaced posterior tibial fragment is indicated if it represents 20 per cent or more of the weight-bearing surface of the tibia. This so-called third malleolar fracture results from avulsion by the intact posterior tibiofibular ligament.

Union can be expected in eight weeks, following which full weight bearing and exercises to regain ankle and subtalar joint motion can be started.

Inversion injuries to the ankle usually produce tears of the lateral ligaments. Such an injury represents the so-called "ankle sprain." However, when inversion is forceful enough with the foot in the neutral or dor-siflexed position, avulsion fractures of the lateral malleolus and a shearing fracture of the medial malleolus can result. Such fractures of the medial malleolus are usually at the level of the tibial plafond and are more vertical in orientation than the avulsion fracture of the medial malleolus, which occurs below the level of the plafond and are the result of a traction force as seen in the abduction-external rotation bimalleolar fracture. With the inversion bimalleolar fracture, stability may be a problem, and if so, internal fixation may be indicated.

FRACTURES OF THE FOOT

Fractures of the hindfoot constitute serious injuries from an end result, functional standpoint. Displaced fractures of the *talus,* although rare, can produce severe, long-standing disability due to avascular necrosis of the body of the talus. Vertical fractures to the neck of the talus, the result of a dorsiflexion injury to the foot, often result in significant damage to the intraosseous blood supply to the talus. Undisplaced fractures of the talus can be simply treated by plaster immobilization for nine to 10 weeks. Nonunion is not usually a problem, and avascular necrosis is rare. However, when the fracture is displaced, accurate reduction is mandatory. Avascular necrosis is a common sequela and when the displaced fracture is associated with a posterior dislocation of the body of the talus, avascular necrosis is inevitable. Open reduction and anatomic realignment are required when closed reduction fails, which is the case in most of the displaced fractures of the talus. Union of the fracture occurs in 10 to 12 weeks. When avascular necrosis is present it becomes evident on roentgenograms by the time the fracture has healed. Prolonged plaster protection may provide some chance at revascularization. However, post-traumatic arthritis of the ankle and subtalar joint and collapse of the body of the talus are common outcomes, and arthrodesis at the ankle or triple arthrodesis may become necessary to relieve pain and minimize the long-standing disability.

Fractures of the os calcis, the result of a fall or jump from a height, are another serious fracture of the foot. This fracture often extends into the subtalar joint and leads to painful post-traumatic arthritis. When such fractures are seen before serious swelling occurs, manual manipulation of the fracture in an effort to restore the proper alignment of the calcaneous can minimize disability. Whereas open reduction and anatomic realignment of the os calcis is recommended by some, the results often lead to failure except in the hands of those with great experience in the treatment of this fracture (Fig. 5). A bulky soft dressing, immobilized in a plaster cast long enough to reduce swelling of the foot, is recommended by many who suggest that the expected post-traumatic arthritis of the subtalar joint is inevitable and that early motion and early return to function will provide as many good results as treatment by open reduction and attempts at manipulation. When pain and post-traumatic arthritis continue to be problems, triple arthrodesis is the treatment of choice (Fig. 5C).

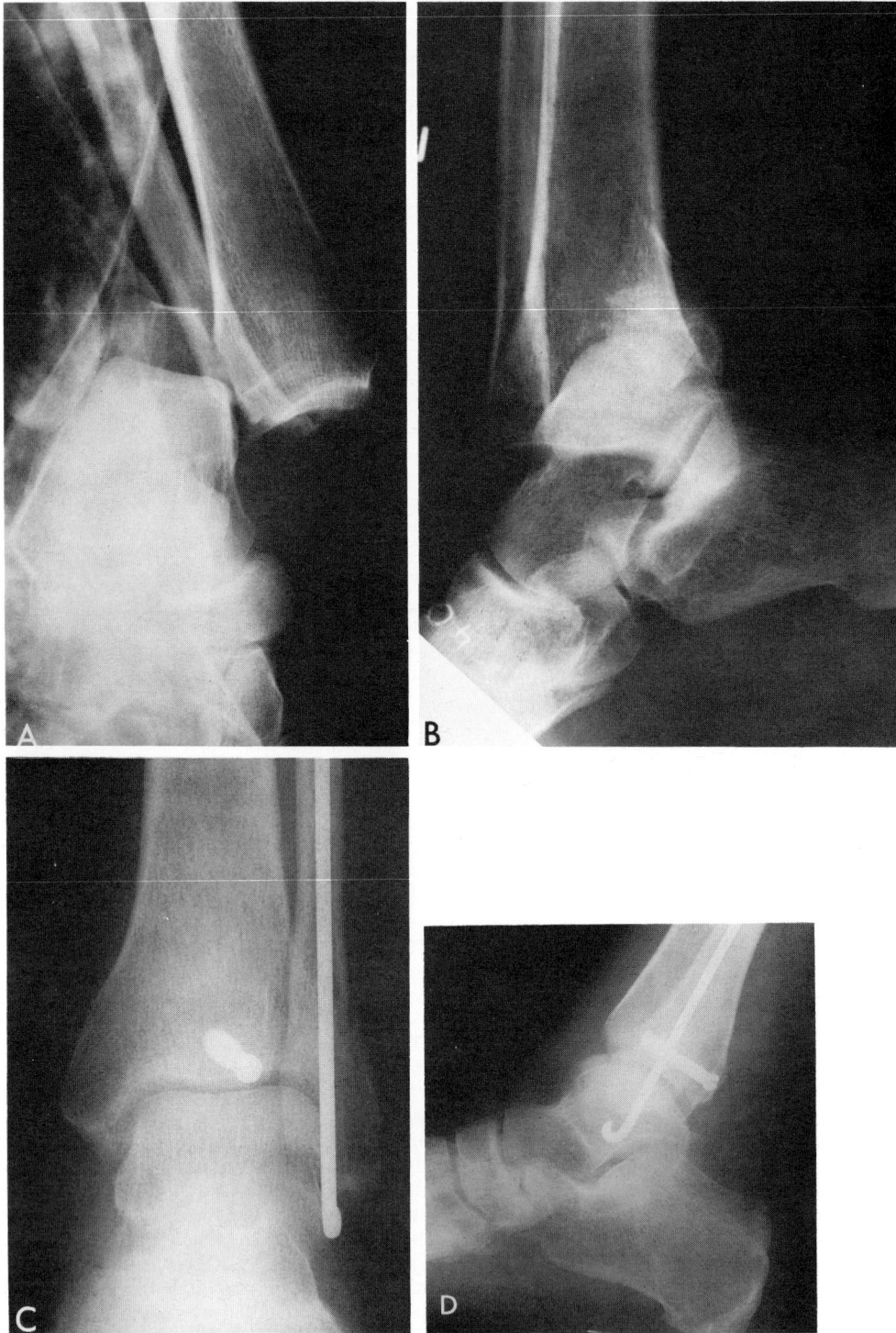

Figure 4.   *A* and *B*, Roentgenograms showing typical external rotation and abduction fracture of the ankle. The deltoid ligament was torn, the fibula was fractured obliquely just above the joint, and a large portion of the posterior tibia was avulsed, which included about 20 per cent of the weight-bearing surface. *C* and *D*, Postoperative x-rays showing screw fixation of the posterior tibial fragment and intramedullary fixation of the fibula. The deltoid ligament was repaired.

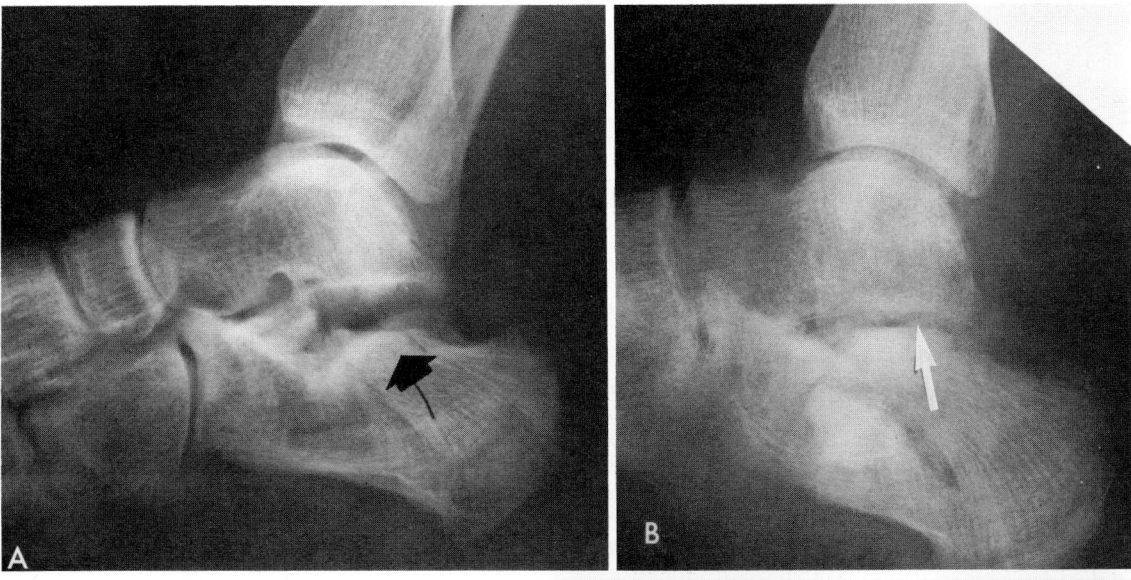

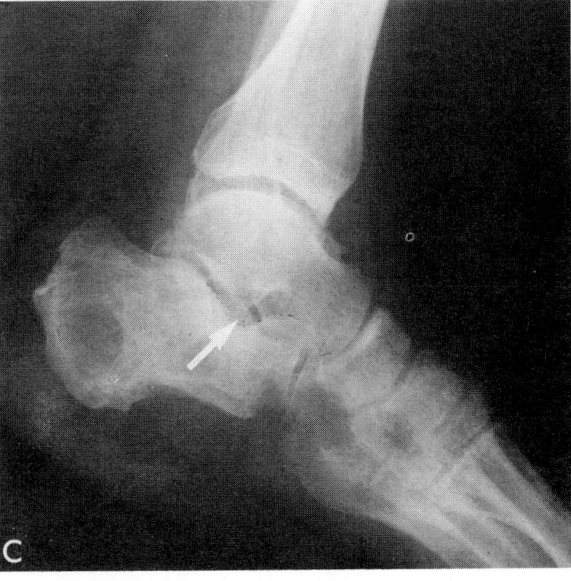

Figure 5. *A,* Severely comminuted fracture of the os calcis with depression and splitting of the posterior facet of the subtalar joint (see arrow). *B,* Postoperative film showing elevation of the posterior facet, which was held in place by a bone graft. Normal tuber angle of the os calcis was not completely achieved. *C,* Old fracture of the os calcis with persistent depression (see arrow) associated with post-traumatic arthrosis of the subtalar joint. A triple arthrodesis was necessary for the relief of pain.

Fractures through the midfoot, the navicular and cuboid bones, are rare without serious soft tissue damage from direct trauma and often are associated with other fractures or dislocations about the foot. Dislocations of the tarsal-metatarsal joints can result from direct trauma such as a crush injury from a falling object or from indirect forces centered at the tarsal-metatarsal joint level from a twisting or hyperflexion force. The spectrum of dislocations ranges from complete dislocation of all five tarsal-metatarsal joints to the dislocation of just one or two. Occasionally a divergent dislocation occurs, with the first metatarsal dislocating medially and the other metatarsals dislocating laterally. Closed reduction of the dislocation is to be attempted by traction on the forefoot. If closed reduction is not possible, then open reduction of the dislocations, followed by Kirschner wire fixation, may be necessary. Damage to the dorsalis pedis artery due to avulsion at the level where it enters the space be-

tween the first and second metatarsal bones can lead to massive swelling of the foot and subsequent compression of the posterior tibial artery, which can cause forefoot gangrene. Surgical decompression of the posterior tibial artery or ligation of the torn dorsalis pedis may become necessary to prevent this complication.

Fractures of the metatarsals can involve the necks, shafts, or bases, depending on the direction of the force and the mechanism of injury. Fractures of the neck of the metatarsals can be impacted as the result of a direct longitudinal force or can be oblique, the result of indirect twisting forces. Anatomic reduction usually is not necessary unless the metatarsal heads are displaced into the plantar surface of the foot, where future weight bearing would be painful. Fractures of the shaft of the metatarsals can be transverse, oblique, or comminuted, depending on whether the trauma is direct or indirect. Fractures of the bases of the metatarsals, even when slightly displaced, usually produce no long-term ill effects and can be treated conservatively in a padded plaster cast. Avulsion of the styloid process at the base of the fifth metatarsal is the result of an inversion force, with avulsion resulting from traction by the peroneus brevis tendon. A short leg walking cast for three to five weeks usually controls pain and permits early union.

Stress and fatigue fractures of the metatarsals are common and should be suspected in anyone who presents with pain and puffiness in a foot following excess activity to which he is unaccustomed, such as walking or jogging. Such fractures are self-limited, and treatment is aimed at creating comfort by the application of a weight-bearing cast.

Fractures of the phalanges usually do not require reduction unless badly deformed. Longitudinal traction on the toe will usually reduce the fracture, following which it can be maintained by a padded cast extended out distal to the toe for a week to 10 days. Simple strapping of the toe to one of the adjacent normal ones will then provide sufficient stability and immobilization to permit an uncomplicated union.

REFERENCES

Fractures of the Tibial Plateau

1. Hohl, M.: Tibial condylar fractures. J. Bone Joint Surg., *49A*:1455–1467, 1967.

2. Kennedy, J. C., and Bailey, W. H.: Experimental tibial-plateau fractures. J. Bone Joint Surg., *50A*:1522–1534, 1968.
3. Porter, B.: Crush fractures of the lateral tibial table. J. Bone Joint Surg., *52B*:676–687, 1970.
4. Rasmussen, P. S.: Tibial condylar fractures. J. Bone Joint Surg., *55A*:1331–1350, 1973.
5. Rockwood, C. A., and Green, D. P.: Fractures. Philadelphia, J. B. Lippincott, 1975.

Fractures of the Tibia

6. Nicoll, E. A.: Fractures of the tibial shaft. A survey of 705 cases J. Bone Joint Surg., *46B*:373–387, 1964.
7. Rockwood, C. A., and Green, D. P.: Fractures. Philadelphia, J. B. Lippincott, 1975.
8. Sakellarides, H. T., Freeman, P. A., and Grant, B. D.: Delayed union and nonunion of tibial-shaft fractures. A review of 100 cases. J. Bone Joint Surg., *46A*:557–596, 1964.
9. Sarmiento, A.: A functional below-the-knee cast for tibial fractures. J.Bone Joint Surg., *49A*:855–875, 1967.

Fractures of the Ankle

10. Lauge-Hansen, N.: Fractures of the ankle. II. Combined experimental-surgical and experimental-roentgenologic investigations. Arch. Surg., *60*:957–985, 1950.
11. Rockwood, C. A., and Green, D. P.: Fractures. Philadelphia, J. B. Lippincott, 1975.

Fractures of the Foot

12. Hawkins, L. G.: Fractures of the neck of the talus. J. Bone Joint Surg., *52A*:991–1002, 1970.
13. King, R. E.: Axial pin fixation of fractures of the os calcis (method of Essex-Lopresti). Orthop. Clin. North Am., *4*:185–188, 1973.
14. Rockwood, C. A., and Green, D. P.: Fractures. Philadelphia, J. B. Lippincott, 1975.

VIII

AMPUTATIONS AND LIMB SUBSTITUTIONS

Frank W. Clippinger, M.D.

Amputation is one of the oldest surgical procedures known to the medical arts, and we have had amputees of one kind or another with us since before the dawn of civilization. Leprosy, ergotism, and punishment are no longer major causes of amputation in the Western World, but trauma, neoplasm, and dysvascular conditions are now common enough that there are nearly a half million amputees in the United States alone. Considering this much experience, it is surprising that there is anything left to be said about level selection, surgical technique, or rehabilitation of the amputee. It is a fact, however, that practice has not kept up with existing knowledge and technology. Amputation is not a procedure known for universal excellence.

Traditionally, surgeons have taken a negative approach to amputation, being trained and oriented toward saving both "life and limb" in a literal sense. They tend to perseverate and may resort to amputation only after months of pain, debilitation, and ex-

pense, and even then, amputation has been done with apology and a psychological sense of failure. Surgeons like to forget their failures, and until recent years, amputees were relegated to a limbo of self-rehabilitation without medical support, expert knowledge, or a definite plan of action.

The surgeon's responsibility does not end when the wound is healed and the sutures have been removed. He must guide his patient through an emotionally difficult postoperative period and to do so, he must know something about prosthetic rehabilitation. The surgery must be planned with knowledge of the prosthesis to be fitted, even if the operating surgeon is not himself going to direct the rehabilitation phase of treatment.

When timed properly and with consideration to physical restoration, amputation is not destructive; it is a form of reconstruction that may be elected whenever the outlook is such that a well-fitted prosthesis

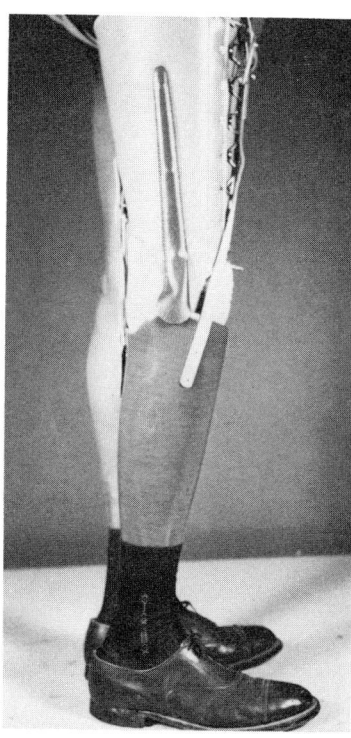

Figure 1. A so-called "conventional" below-knee prosthesis, with a carved wood socket and metal knee joints. The leather thigh lacer serves partially as a suspension mechanism and also takes some of the weight-bearing load. A posterior strap prevents hyperextension, and an anterior strap connected to a waist belt aids suspension and keeps clothing from being trapped between the stump and the socket. The ankle is articulated and foot is of wood or felt.

contracture prevention, strengthening of muscles controlling the stump, and wrapping the stump with elastic bandages in an effort to stabilize stump size by hastening the atrophy of muscles no longer used. Implementation of this program was influenced by both economic and physiologic factors. It was important, particularly in civilian practice, to fit the proper amputee at the proper time to avoid unnecessary expenditure of limited funds for prostheses that would or could not be used.

The prosthesis available at that time was ordinarily made of wood with either a carved or a molded leather socket that was attached to a leather thigh lacer (Fig. 1). Most of patient's weight was applied on the proximal portion of the stump, leaving the distal end of the stump free, movable, and subject to stretching on weight bearing. The skin changes that ensued imposed definite limitations on scar placement, stump length, and shape. While a few amputees were fitted with definitive prostheses as early as six weeks after surgery, the average time between amputation and prosthetic fitting as recently as 1960 was 7.2 months.

The single factor that has influenced the lot of the amputee most since 1950 is the use of plastic materials and reliable molding techniques, making possible a prosthetic socket that fits the stump intimately throughout its entire length (Fig. 2). Total contact fit with its advantageous distribution of pressures, sensory feedback from the stump end, and the potential use of the entire length of the stump as a lever arm and weight-bearing area has made it possible to fit al-

will provide a better result for the patient than can be obtained in a reasonable length of time with further attempts at salvage.

Modern surgical techniques for amputation were developed during the latter half of the nineteenth century as an outgrowth of medical advances such as general anesthesia and the principle of asepsis. Methods of handling bone, muscle, nerve, and skin evolved that are still appropriate today.

Prosthetic restoration and rehabilitation of the amputee proceeded in a hit-or-miss fashion until after World War II. At that time, the large number of amputees returning from the Armed Forces stimulated the United States Army and the Veterans Administration to take a hard look at the state of the art. Funds for research became available and for the first time, physicians and engineers became deeply involved in the study of the problems of the amputee. The results of these studies included new and detailed information regarding the mechanics of gait, energy expenditure, prosthetic alignment principles, recognition of the causes of gait defects, hand function, and the development of better prosthetic components and techniques. For the first time, a definite program of treatment for the amputee appeared that was directed toward preparing the amputee to wear a prosthesis. This program emphasized, over a period of weeks or months,

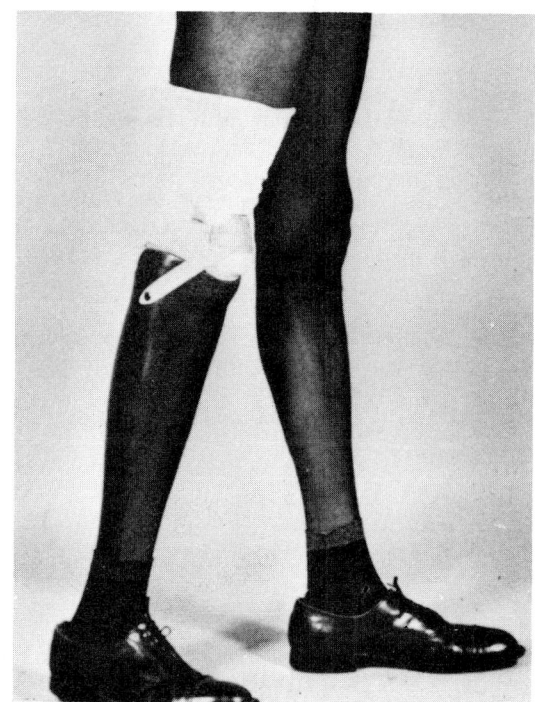

Figure 2. Patellar tendon-bearing prosthesis with a total-contact plastic socket. It is suspended by a supracondylar strap, as pictured, or by a removable wedge that clips over the medial femoral condyle. A SACH foot is usually used.

most any stump. Length is no longer an important consideration and the scar can be placed anywhere, making it possible for the surgeon to use all viable skin to the best advantage.

LEVEL SELECTION

The literature is full of advice on selection of level or "site of election" for amputation (Fig. 3). We learn that partial foot amputations other than the transmetatarsal level, long below-knee amputations, knee disarticulations, and elbow disarticulations are not advisable. These limitations are the result of extensive experience with the wood and metal prostheses, and if that is what the prosthetist is going to make, "sites of election" are sound. If, however, the available prosthetist is capable of working with plastic and can make total-contact sockets, as most prosthetists now can, the viability of skin is the only critical factor determining length of the stump. To be sure, the supramalleolar, long below-knee, and knee and elbow disarticulation levels are more difficult to fit and there are certain prosthetic disadvantages, but the longer lever and greater surface area offer some benefits to the amputee. In addition, good postamputation reconstructive surgery and better prostheses obviate many of the disadvantages of some amputations through the hindfoot.

The dysvascular patient with actual or impending gangrene may present something of a problem of judgment in selecting a level. While radioactive isotope uptake and thermography will give some information as to the status of the tissue, there are no readily available and reliable clinical tests to make this determination for us. Skin temperature, oscillometric determinations, arteriography, and the presence or absence of pulses all give information about circulation but not the information needed to determine viability of skin at a given point. Because of this, it has long been the practice of some surgeons to play it safe and amputate above the knee, particularly when femoral pulses are absent. In 1963, the ratio of above- to below-the-knee amputations in the United States was approximately 2 to 1. In some clinics, it is now 1 to 20. An above-knee amputation for vascular insufficiency is done when gangrene is impending to the knee level or in sudden catastrophic occlusion of the distal aorta or common iliac artery.

It is extremely important to save the knee when possible. The difference in disability is sufficiently great that the presence of the knee often determines whether an elderly patient can ambulate effectively in a prosthesis.

SURGICAL PRINCIPLES

For the purpose of considering surgical technique, amputations can be divided into two kinds—elective procedures where there is some freedom of fashioning skin flaps and selecting the level, and urgent procedures for trauma, fulminating infection, and gan-

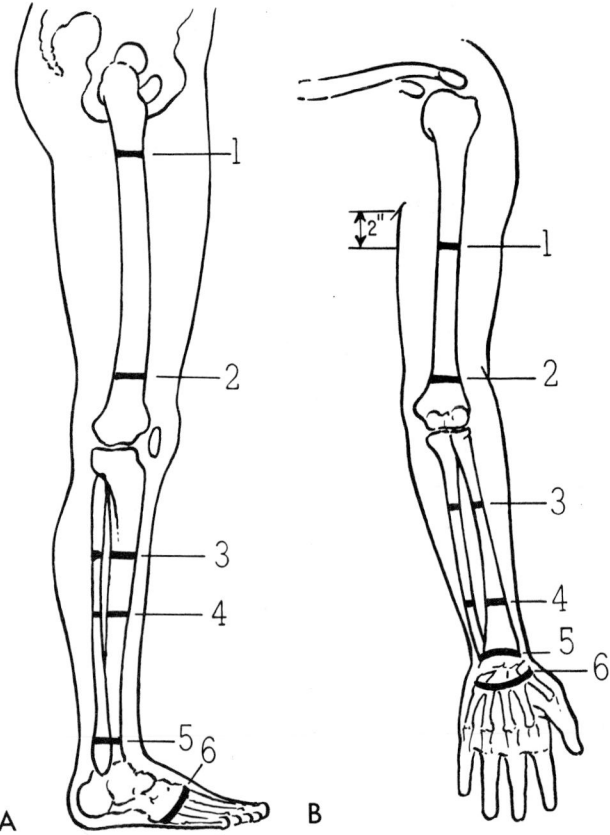

Figure 3. Traditional amputation levels. *A,* In the lower limb, amputation above 1 must be fitted with a hip disarticulation prosthesis because of the short stump. The area between 1 and 2 is fitted with the usual above-knee prosthesis with a quadrilateral socket and either pelvic band or suction suspension. Amputations between 2 and the knee joint do not have sufficient room in the prosthesis for a swing phase control knee mechanism and must be fitted with freeswinging outside joints. 3 and 4 are the conventional "sites of election" for below-knee amputations. Amputations between 4 and 5 are more difficult for the prosthetist, but offer some advantage to the amputee. Amputations below 6 require little in the way of a prosthesis; a toe filler and a steel shank in the shoe usually suffice.

B, Amputations through the upper limb above 1 require a modified socket over the shoulder, and active motion of the shoulder joint is not possible. Between 1 and 2, a conventional above-elbow prosthesis can be fitted. Between 2 and the elbow, an outside elbow joint must be used, but active humeral rotation is possible. Amputations through the forearm above 3 produce a very short forearm lever, and in some instances a geared elbow joint must be used to provide sufficient flexion of the forearm segment. Between 3 and 4, a conventional below-elbow prosthesis is used. Amputations below 4 allow some active pronation and supination. Transcarpal amputation (6) requires a prosthesis, but some hook function is provided by the stump alone.

grene, in which the viability of muscles and the areas of healthy skin are important factors.

If infection is a distinct possibility, as in wet gangrene, osteomyelitis, or severe trauma, the amputation wound, like all others in similar situations, should be left open. In years past, circumferential guillotine amputation was recommended in these instances because it could be performed very rapidly and with relative safety. The guillotine procedure has the distinct disadvantage, however, of requiring an extensive revision with significant shortening of the bone. An alternative is to fashion flaps in the usual manner but to leave the wound open with the intent to perform a delayed primary closure at the appropriate time—usually three to five days later. If this is done, the flaps should be a little longer than normally would be made because they have a tendency to swell to some extent and shorten. This may be prevented in some instances by one or two large through-and-through stay sutures from front to back, preventing retraction of the skin but leaving the wound open sufficiently for proper drainage. A rigid postoperative dressing can be used. Skin traction may be helpful in young amputees, but in the face of borderline circulatory status, this may produce a slough.

When infection is not a major hazard, a closed amputation may be planned.

The skin flaps are fashioned in a manner appropriate to the level selected, and the fascia is divided at the level of the skin incision. The underlying muscle is tapered from the level of the bone to the end of the flap. It should be remembered that a cylindrical stump is desirable if a total-contact socket is to be used, rather than the thin tapering bony stump that was felt to be advantageous in an open-end, proximally weight-bearing socket.

The periosteum is divided at the level at which the bone is to be sectioned, and periosteal tags are removed to prevent spur formation. The periosteum is not stripped from the proximal bone as was once advocated.

The bone should be divided cleanly and ragged or sharp edges removed with a rongeur or rasp.

The major blood vessels are separated and doubly ligated individually to prevent the possible formation of arteriovenous fistulae.

Major nerves are identified, pulled downward, and sharply sectioned. They are allowed to retract above the level of the cut muscle. A divided nerve attempts to regenerate, producing a terminal neuroma, and to date no techniques have been devised that prevent this from occurring. A neuroma should be expected, but it should be buried deep in soft tissue where it is not trapped in scar or irritated by the prosthesis. A large vasa communicans can be cauterized or ligated. In a dysvascular patient, this is rarely a problem.

When the surgeon is satisfied that there is no excessive bleeding, the wound may be closed by suturing the posterior deep fascia to the anterior, bringing some muscle over the end of the bone. The skin is closed with whatever suture the surgeon desires. The use of monofilament suture material such as plastic and wire has been advocated because of its reduced tendency to produce local tissue reaction. It should be remembered, however, that these materials have a tendency to cut through skin in the presence of edema, and in addition, the cut ends of the suture may be uncomfortable to the patient.

The skin margins should be handled with meticulous care, particularly in patients with impaired circulation. The use of toothed thumb forceps should be avoided. There should be little or no tension on the skin. The presence of "dog ears" is not disadvantageous. These ordinarily disappear in two or three weeks and their removal may impair irrevocably the circulation to the flaps.

Most major amputation wounds should be drained. A large hematoma can be catastrophic. Drains can be either Penrose or suction type and should be removed after 24 to 48 hours.

POSTOPERATIVE CARE

Immediate application of prosthetic devices at the time of the amputation has been advocated in recent years (Fig. 4). In selected situations, this technique has some definite benefits to the amputee. This is especially true in amputations through the upper extremity wherein a terminal device and shoulder harness can be applied at the time of the amputation and the patient started on immediate use of his extremity. This lessens the psychological impact of the loss of the extremity and starts the rehabilitative phase immediately.

Whether or not a prosthetic device is actually used, the rigid dressing developed as part of this program has very definite advantages. It has been claimed that healing of the wound is enhanced. What is more likely, however, is that edema and hematoma are controlled and the tissue is immobilized, decreasing some of the factors that complicate healing. Patients are more comfortable in this dressing and require less analgesic medication and for a shorter period of time than in bulky dressings.

A rigid dressing is applied as follows: In the upper limb, the wound is covered with a light soft dressing over which is wrapped either sheet cotton or a sterile

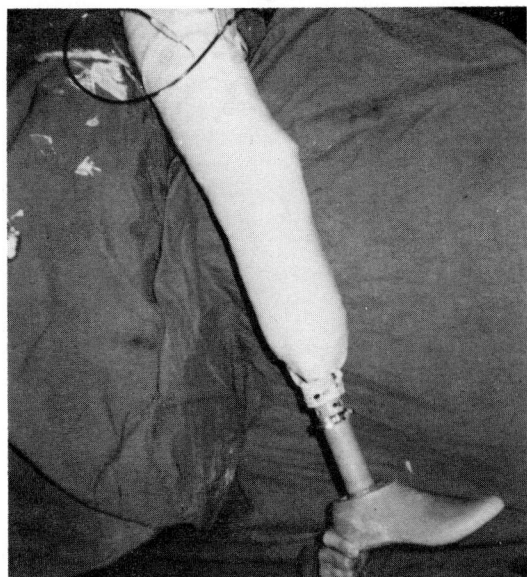

Figure 4. A long below-knee amputation with a rigid dressing and shin-foot unit applied in the operating room. Note the suction drainage tube. This is an excellent postoperative dressing, whether or not the shin-foot unit is used.

knitted stump sock. Plaster is applied snugly and molded well with even compression. Suspension is important and the plaster should be well molded around the humeral epicondyles in a below-elbow amputation and should be suspended by a shoulder harness in an above-elbow level. If the dressing slips distally in the first 48 hours after the operation, it is important to replace it immediately, as edema may occur very rapidly.

In the lower limb, the technique developed by Burgess is advised, and, in essence, is as follows: A thin dressing is applied and the distal end of the stump is covered with either 2 or 3 fluffed 4 × 4 gauze sponges or a polyurethane foam pad. A sterile knitted stump sock is pulled over the stump. Felt pads are used to enhance pressure on areas which will tolerate them, and to relieve pressure in the areas between the pads such as over the crest of the tibia and the surface of the patella. The use of elastic plaster in the deeper layers of the cast makes it easier to apply even pressures and makes the plaster conform accurately to the shape of the stump. The cast is brought well above the knee level and is molded over the femoral condyles with the knee kept in 5 to 10 degrees flexion. An auxiliary suspension is added, consisting of a strap incorporated in the cast and attached to a prefabricated waist belt.

A similar rigid dressing can be applied in above-knee amputations, although it is much more cumbersome to do so, because it has to be incorporated into a corset or extended around the pelvis as a spica to prevent the cast from loosening and shifting distally.

If desired, a pylon fitting and prosthetic foot can be applied and the patient may start on touchdown weight bearing the following day.

The drain in the wound is removed the day following surgery. The cast is left in place for seven to 10 days unless the patient is developing signs of wound complications such as fever, increasing white blood cell count, or significant pain, whereupon the cast should be removed and the wound inspected immediately. If the wound appears satisfactory at the end of a week, plans can be made for fitting a removable prosthesis. A definitive limb can be made at that time, although it should be remembered that the muscles within the stump will atrophy to some extent and a change of socket will probably be necessary within several weeks. A temporary prosthesis with a well-fitted total-contact socket and an endoskeletal pylon with adjustment capability and a SACH foot attached has some definite advantages (Fig. 5). The socket can be changed readily and the prosthesis can be aligned precisely as the patient learns to use it and develops his gait pattern. Stump socks are added as shrinkage occurs and the socket is changed as needed. The patient may return to his usual activities including employment wearing a temporary prosthesis. Because of concern of liability in what appears to be an unfinished device, some prosthetists and employers have been reluctant to allow unrestricted function. It is, however, to the patient's advantage if he can resume full activity as rapidly as possible, and this is usually within four to six weeks of his operation.

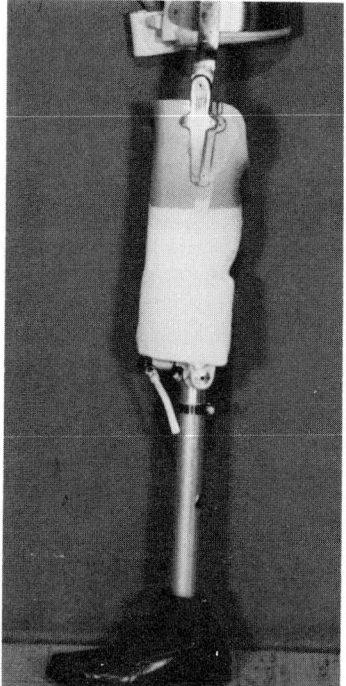

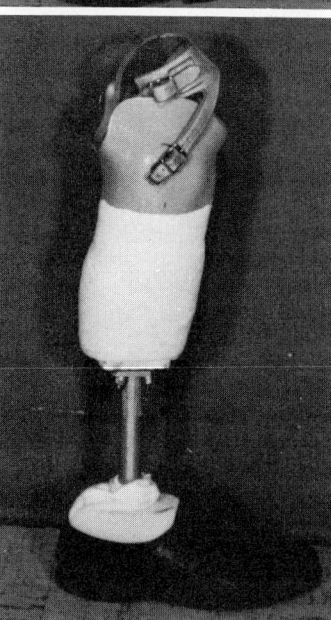

Figure 5. Removable temporary or preparatory prosthesis with total contact plastic socket. While not cosmetic, the fit and walking characteristics are identical to those of the definitive limb.

AMPUTATIONS OF THE LOWER EXTREMITY

Amputations of the lower extremity produce some physical impairment, and the degree of disability is directly related to the level of amputation. Amputations at any level below the knee will permit most normal activity including, in the teenager and the younger adults, athletics such as golf and tennis. Most occupations are available to the below-knee amputee with

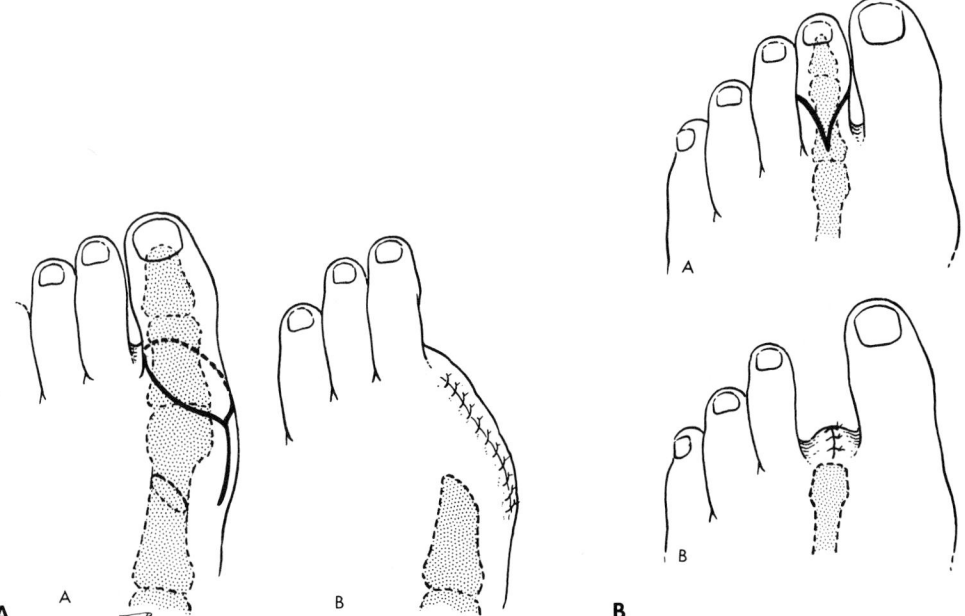

Figure 6. *A,* Amputation of the great toe usually includes the metatarsal head. A racket-shaped incision is used. *B,* Amputation of the second, third, and fourth toes utilizes lateral flaps when available, and the proximal phalanx is disarticulated. Amputation of the fifth toe is done with a technique similar to that for the great toe.

the exception of a few wherein personal safety is dependent on sensation in the foot, such as walking on scaffolds or girders or on slippery surfaces around high-speed machinery. The degree of success depends not only upon the level of amputation but upon an active rehabilitation program and precise fitting and alignment of the prosthesis.

AMPUTATIONS OF TOES AND FOREFOOT

Amputation of one or more toes (Fig. 6) has a minor effect on ambulation, consisting of a slight loss of pushoff power. The amputation is performed through a racket-shaped incision. Any part of the toe may be amputated, but a very successful level is disarticulation at the metatarsophalangeal joint. When the great toe or the little toe is amputated, however, it is often advisable to remove the metatarsal head, thus preventing a prominence with ensuing development of painful plantar callous or corn.

The prosthesis, if any, consists of foam, cotton, or lambswool in the toe of the shoe.

Transmetatarsal amputation (Fig. 7) does affect pushoff power to a significant degree. It should be remembered, however, that most elderly individuals do not normally utilize foot pushoff as part of their usual gait, but propel themselves forward with their knee and hip extensors.

A plantar flap is used to prevent a tender scar on the weight-bearing portion of the foot, and the plantar

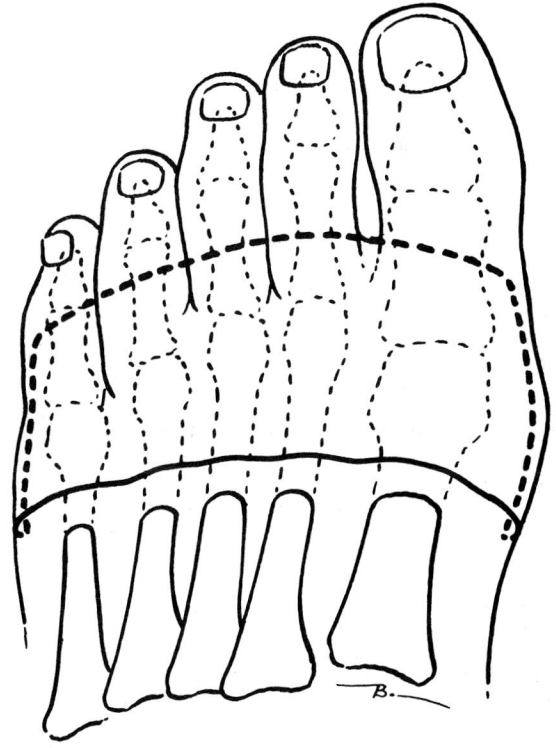

Figure 7. Transmetatarsal amputation and tarsometatarsal disarticulation. The plantar skin usually has the better circulation and the resulting dorsal scar is likely to become tender.

skin usually carries the better circulation. A steel shank in the shoe and a toe filler are all the prosthesis that is necessary.

TRANSTARSAL AMPUTATION

Amputation through the tarsus, such as Chopart's level, has not been popular in America because it can produce imbalance in the remaining muscles that often causes an equinovarus deformity of the foot with unsatisfactory weight bearing and a tender scar. This occurs because the peroneals and dorsiflexors are sectioned and the triceps surae and posterior tibial are unopposed. It is, however, a useful amputation level in young patients wherein some reconstruction is possible. Full distal weight bearing and length are maintained and a prosthesis is not mandatory for ambulation. At the time of surgery, the anterior tibial and toe extensor tendons should be inserted into the remaining bone. The Achilles tendon may be lengthened, and an ankle arthrodesis with the foot in 5 degrees dorsiflexion produces a stable weight-bearing stump. In the past, another disadvantage of this level of amputation was the type of prosthesis available, which was heavy, cumbersome, and prone to breakdown. A high shoe or boot can be used but has some cosmetic disadvantages. In recent years, the development of material such as high density polypropylene has made possible a light, durable prosthesis that can be worn inside the shoe and under the sock, decreasing most of the cosmetic problems.

SYME'S AMPUTATION

The Syme's amputation has been advocated for many years as an alternative to either long below-knee levels or amputations through the hind foot. When successful, a very durable end-bearing stump is produced that may allow full weight bearing for short distances without a prosthesis. Disadvantages of the Syme's amputation are that it requires a prosthesis as complex as that for the below-knee level and produces a bulbous stump that is not always acceptable from a cosmetic standpoint, particularly to women.

A transverse anterior incision is made at the ankle joint to the anterior portion of both malleoli. A vertical incision is then made directly downward from the anterior tip of the medial malleolus, around the bottom of the foot, and then upward to the tip of the lateral malleolus. The talus is disarticulated from the tibia, and the talus and os calcis are carefully dissected from the heel flap. The dissection must be subperiosteal to preserve the integrity of the plantar fat pad. If fat necrosis ensues, full weight bearing is limited. The tibia and fibula are divided at the level of the joint line. Removal of the malleoli and distal tibial flare has been advocated by some in an effort to decrease the unsightly bulbous end of the stump.

Postoperatively, the heel pad must be kept centered over the end of the tibia until it has had time to heal into position. Classically, this has been accomplished by the use of adhesive tape. A pin through the heel flap into the tibia has also been advocated, but this increases the chance of a tender distal scar.

The prosthesis requires both a socket and a foot and must be fitted quite accurately because the stump tends to rotate within the prosthesis. Excessive rotation produces friction, skin irritation, and the development of painful callouses over the area of the scar.

AMPUTATIONS THROUGH THE LEG

In the United States, amputations through the tibia are performed more frequently than at any other level in the lower extremity. With modern prosthetic techniques, any level of amputation between the tibial tubercle and the ankle joint can be fitted with a satisfactory prosthesis. It is more difficult, however, for the prosthetist to fit a very long or supramalleolar stump, because the socket has to incorporate any mild deformity such as tibia vara, and the prosthesis must be aligned empirically rather than dynamically with adjustable devices.

In elective situations, the technique outlined by Burgess has been successful in most cases (Fig. 8). A long posterior flap is planned with little or no anterior flap, since the posterior part of the leg in most instances carries the better blood supply.

An anterior incision is made perpendicular to the tibia and extends two thirds of the distance posteriorly on the calf, both medially and laterally. The posterior flap is cut relatively square and should be one to one and a half inches longer than the diameter of the calf at the level of the anterior incision.

The anterior and lateral compartment muscles are divided at the level of the anterior incision. The posterior muscles are beveled from the posterior aspect of the tibia to the end of the flap and are not dissected from the subcutaneous tissue. Any muscle that is at all questionable can and should be resected. While quite helpful, muscle is not a mandatory component for a functional amputation stump.

The fibula is divided with a slight lateral bevel at or one half inch proximal to the level of the tibial section. This is longer than has been recommended in the past but if a total-contact socket is to be used, a cylindrical rather than a tapering stump is desirable. The tibia is divided with an anterior bevel. A power, hand, or

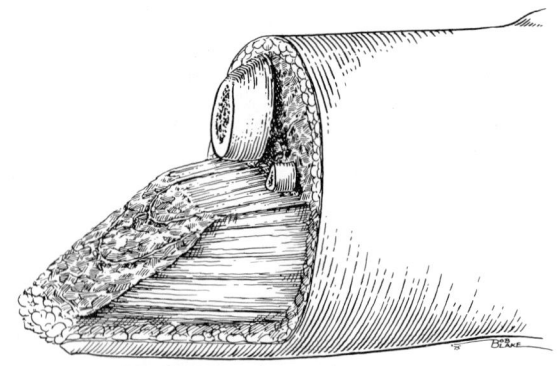

Figure 8. Below-knee amputation. A long posterior flap is used, and the posterior muscles are tapered from the posterior aspect of the bone to the end of the flap. The closure should not be tight, and "dog ears" should not be removed.

Gigli saw can be used, but if the latter is selected, great care must be taken to avoid injury to the skin.

In amputations at or about the tibial tubercle, the fibula can be resected. It has a tendency, if left in place, to angulate, as there may be insufficient interosseous membrane remaining to hold it in position. An angulated fibula makes a bulge that is difficult to fit comfortably in the socket. If the head of the fibula is removed, the lateral collateral ligament and the biceps tendon should be reattached to the tibia, and the peroneal nerve should be sectioned above the knee joint to prevent its neuroma from occurring in a position where it is vulnerable to pressure against the prosthesis.

Recently, some surgeons have advocated creation of a synostosis between the tibia and the fibula at all levels below the knee. This may have some long-term advantages, but it does prolong the rehabilitation phase significantly.

The prosthesis most commonly fitted on new amputees consists of a total contact "patellar tendon bearing" plastic socket with a so-called "SACH" foot (Fig. 2). This Solid-Ankle-Cushion-Heel foot does not incorporate an articulated ankle joint, but allows simulation of plantar flexion at heel strike by compression of a soft sponge heel component. Both the socket fit and the alignment must be precise. The socket distributes weight over the entire surface area of the stump, with a large proportion of the force applied to the area of the patellar tendon, the medial condyle of the tibia, the lateral aspect of the fibula, and the popliteal space. Some distal pressure is provided and this is indeed advantageous, as it seems to increase proprioceptive feedback. The prosthesis is worn over wool or cotton stump socks.

The prosthesis is suspended by one of several different methods. Of these, the most commonly used is a circumferential strap at the supracondylar level of the thigh, which may be attached in turn to a waist belt. Various methods of suspending the prosthesis from the femoral condyles have been developed and are useful in many cases. In fact, this method provides the most secure suspension available. It is accomplished by providing medial and lateral extensions of the socket to the supracondylar level and fitting them snugly. A removable medial socket brim or wedge insert allows the patient to don and doff his prosthesis comfortably and can be made sufficiently snug that when the prosthesis is in place, the adductor tubercle becomes a suspension point. Very short stumps can be fitted with a "PTS" socket, which is suspended by means of a removable socket liner that incorporates the wedge and, in addition, presses just above the patella, limiting full extension of the knee and providing an additional suspension point from the patella itself.

The theoretical disadvantage of a patellar tendon-bearing prosthesis has been the tendency to develop genu recurvatum because there is no mechanical stop to prevent hyperextension at the knee. This problem is solved for the most part by aligning the prosthesis with the knee in 5 to 10 degrees flexion, which, in addition to starting with the knee slightly flexed, shortens the lever arm from the ball of the foot at toe-off that produces a strong extension moment at the knee.

AMPUTATION THROUGH THE KNEE AND LOWER FEMUR

Disarticulation through the knee joint has been performed for many years but has been discouraged in the United States, principally because of prosthetic problems. The advantages of a knee disarticulation are that it provides both a long lever controlled by full musculature and a fully end-bearing stump. The disadvantages are that the stump is bulbous and hence difficult to fit with a convenient and cosmetic prosthesis, and the excessive length prohibits the use of a swing phase controlled prosthetic knee mechanism. This may not be as important as once thought, since most above-knee amputees after the first few weeks allow their knees to be free swinging and do not often adjust their friction control. The biggest disadvantage of a knee disarticulation is that it requires as much skin for coverage as the short below-knee stump and the latter provides better function.

The knee disarticulation operation is performed by fashioning a long anterior flap utilizing the skin to just below the level of the tibial tubercle, and a short posterior flap making the suture line in the popliteal space. The hamstring tendons should be sutured to the patellar tendon in the intercondylar notch of the femur, thus retaining the active action on the hip joint provided by the rectus femoris and the hamstrings. There is some advantage in leaving the patella in place, although it can be removed if necessary.

A modification of a knee disarticulation is the Gritti-Stokes amputation, which was devised originally to prevent the spread of infection into the thigh but also provides an end-bearing stump that is slightly shorter than the knee disarticulation. In this procedure, the posterior surface of the patella is removed and the patella is fused to the roughened end of the femur. The disadvantage of this procedure is that not only does it require considerable time for union to occur, but the nonunion rate is high and the patella often slips off the end of the femur, producing an irregular and tender stump that is difficult if not impossible to fit comfortably. The Gritti-Stokes amputation is not recommended except in very unusual circumstances.

AMPUTATIONS THROUGH THE THIGH

In amputations through the thigh as much femur should be retained as possible. Long stumps are more powerful than short ones, more muscle balance is maintained, and control of the prosthesis is easier for the patient. When the femur is short, the hamstrings and adductors have been significantly weakened by resection, and the stump tends to go into a flexed abducted position.

In this amputation, the anterior and posterior flaps should be of about equal length, each being made approximately two thirds the diameter of the thigh at the level of amputation. Odd-shaped flaps may be used if necessary to retain bone length.

The prosthesis for the above-knee amputee involves a total contact socket that is somewhat quadrilateral in shape to accommodate the muscle groups in the thigh and to provide an area posteriorly to fit against the ischium for weight bearing. The limb is suspended either by a waist belt that is attached to a prosthetic hip joint or by negative pressure, the so-called "suction socket." In the suction socket, no stump sock is worn and the skin of the thigh is directly against the inside of the socket. The prosthesis is donned by pulling the stump into the socket with a piece of stockinette that is pulled out through a hole distally. The hole is then plugged with a one-way valve that allows air out but not in, providing a certain amount of negative pressure in the swing phase of the gait. The advantage of this type of fitting is that the pistoning between the stump and the socket is minimized and some rotation of the hip is possible. The disadvantages are that it is necessary to maintain an extremely accurate fit and it is difficult for an elderly individual to don. Another disadvantage is that, in some instances, air will leak in while the wearer is seated, which is then expelled when he stands, with the production of antisocial noises.

The socket is attached to a knee joint that contains a mechanism to control or brake heel rise in the swing phase of gait. Many mechanical knee joints have been devised in an attempt to provide normal knee function. None of these fulfills all the requirements. In normal walking, two major events happen in the knee. During stance phase, as the heel strikes the ground, the knee flexes slightly as part of the shock absorbing mechanism, and continues to flex slightly until the foot is flat on the ground. As the heel rises and the foot plantar flexes, the knee straightens to the pushoff phase of walking. As the toes leave the ground, the knee is again flexed.

While the prosthetic knee can be extended actively to some extent by the patient's extending his hip with his foot fixed to the ground, this action is relatively weak, and stability of the knee joint must be obtained by the alignment of the prosthesis. The knee of the artificial limb cannot allow flexion during the stance phase of walking; otherwise the knee would buckle and the patient would fall. The pivot point of the knee joint is placed posterior to the weight-bearing line of the prosthesis, and the knee must remain in full extension through the entire stance phase of walking.

As the toes leave the ground, the hip and knee flex, allowing the foot to clear as the leg swings forward. Normally, the knee flexes to about 60 degrees and is checked by contraction of the quadriceps muscle. At this point, the quadriceps extends the knee gradually during the forward swing of the leg. Just before the heel strikes the ground, the hamstring muscles contract to slow knee extension to prevent it from snapping into extension. When the amputee walks, only the hip extension component of this action can occur and that only when the foot is already on the ground. A braking mechanism must be incorporated into the prosthetic knee to slow the extending leg, smoothly simulating the normal action of the hamstring muscles. There are knee joints available to provide either mechanical or hydraulic assist in controlling the swing phase and also to provide increased stability during stance. These additional features, however,

increase weight, cost, and the necessity of maintenance.

Alignment of the above-knee prosthesis is critical, and the prosthetist usually accomplishes this by the use of an adjustable device in which all components of alignment can be changed as the patient walks until a smooth, cosmetic, and economical gait is developed.

HIP DISARTICULATION AND HEMIPELVECTOMY

Hip disarticulation and transpelvic amputations are performed for malignant lesions or irreparable high thigh trauma. Fortunately, the operation is not indicated frequently, since lack of a thigh stump makes even more difficult the control of a prosthesis.

Two major types of incisions are used; both avoid scars about the ischium. The first, Pack's technique, is a racket-shaped incision with the handle of the racket centered over the anterior iliac spine and curved medially and downward about two inches below the perineum. The incision is carried across the posterior thigh to about three inches below the greater trochanter and upward to join the racket handle. The femoral artery is ligated, the leg elevated to empty it of blood, and the femoral vein then ligated. The adductors, hip rotators, rectus femoris, iliopsoas, and sartorius muscles are all sectioned at their tendinous attachments. The femoral, obturator, and sciatic nerves are pulled down and sectioned. The fascia lata is divided below the insertion of the tensor fascia lata muscle and the gluteus maximus is divided from its insertion on the linea aspera.

The hip joint is then entered along the acetabular rim. The head of the femur is dislocated and the leg completely detached. The wound is closed by approximating the gluteus maximus tendon to the adductor muscle origins. Deep fascia is sutured and the skin is closed to produce a more or less vertical anterior scar.

Another type of incision results in an anterior transverse scar. For this, the incision begins over the femoral vessels about one inch below the inguinal ligament, curves medially four inches below the pubic tubercle, and sweeps posteriorly to create a long posterior flap and then forward to the point of origin. The remaining steps in completing the disarticulation are essentially as described above.

Hemipelvectomy is performed in essentially the same fashion as the racket incision except that the dissection is done on both the outer and inner sides of the pelvis, and the pelvic bone is disarticulated either at the pubic symphysis and sacroiliac joint or through the bone adjacent to these joints. The iliac vessels and sciatic nerve are divided at the intrapelvic level and the wound is closed.

The prostheses provided for the hip disarticulation and the hemipelvectomy are similar (Fig. 9). The socket is made of plastic and encases the pelvic area. Weight bearing in the hip disarticulation is on the ischial tuberosity and in the hemipelvectomy on the contralateral ischial tuberosity, buttressed by an extension of the socket into the flank and lower rib cage on the side of the amputation. The prosthetic hip joint

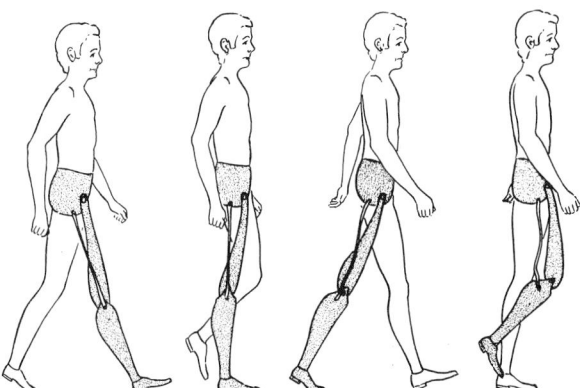

Figure 9. Walking with a prosthesis for hip disarticulation or hemipelvectomy requires control of both hip and knee joints.

is placed well anteriorly, providing flexion for the swing phase and for sitting, but providing automatic stability in stance phase, as it is always anterior to the center of gravity of the body. The patient flexes his hip by tilting his pelvis forward, the bumper on the socket contacting the thigh piece, forcing it forward into a flexed position. The remainder of the gait is essentially that of any other above-knee amputation.

All amputations at or above the knee have some innate disadvantages. The patient cannot lift the weight of his body with his prosthesis and hence must go up stairs one step at a time with his sound side. He has difficulty controlling his knee going down inclines, and because of the pendulum action of the shin-foot segment, he has considerable difficulty running.

AMPUTATIONS OF THE UPPER EXTREMITY

Amputation of the upper extremity is usually necessitated by trauma, occasionally by malignancy, and rarely by peripheral vascular disease. The psychological impact of these amputations is even greater than that of amputation of the lower extremity. The hand is not only used to manipulate the environment, but also to communicate and to express emotions. Throughout history, we have never put the upper extremity amputee in a favorable light; he has been thought of as deformed and grotesque and is usually cast as a villain.

It is most important to rehabilitate upper extremity amputees rapidly, to prove to them that they can continue to care for themselves and make a living and that life can go on in a relatively normal fashion. Immediate postsurgical fitting of a prosthetic device has definite advantages. We have not, however, been as successful in providing a replacement prosthesis for the upper as we have for the lower extremity amputee. We can supply power and motion in only a comparatively gross fashion, and cosmesis is attained at the expense of function. The most functional terminal device is still, indeed, a hook and will remain such until we can find some means of substituting for the complex action of the intrinsic muscles of the hand.

Cosmesis is important because the hand is always in public view, and some amputees are willing to sacrifice function in order to obtain the best possible cosmetic replacement. Cosmetic gloves made of polyvinyl and similar materials incorporating normal skin creases, veins on the dorsum, and even hair, have been available for years. Color matching is somewhat limited, however, not because it is difficult to reproduce skin tones, but because the normal opposite hand continually changes shade with position and season, and this cannot be reproduced.

Sensation is also an extremely important modality in hand function. Surgeons involved with hand reconstruction are aware that no matter how well joint motion and motor function are restored, unless the hand retains significant proprioception and two point discrimination, its functional potential is never realized. While there is some sensory feedback for the amputee from the prosthesis by means of pressure from the harness and the stump-socket interface, intrinsic sensation from the terminal device has not been possible. Current research efforts to provide this electrically by means of transducers in the terminal device stimulating either nerves within the stump or skin elsewhere are promising, and it is hoped that this research will lead to the development of practical sensory feedback mechanisms.

CONTROL OF UPPER EXTREMITY PROSTHESIS

Prostheses for the upper extremity consist of a hook or hand terminal device, a harness to supply force from proximal muscles, and appropriate segments between them, including a socket for the stump (Fig. 10). The socket is made of molded plastic from a cast of the stump and provides total contact with the skin. As in

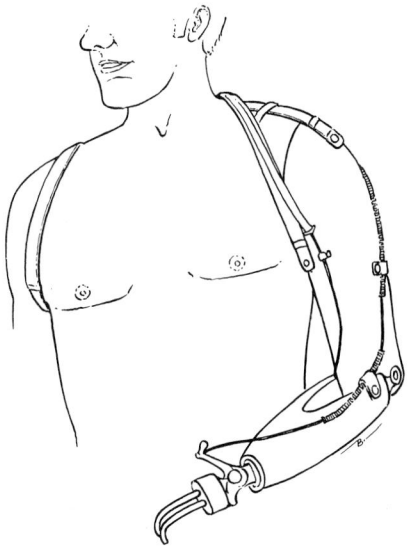

Figure 10. Prosthesis for the above-elbow amputee includes socket and arm segment, forearm, terminal device, harness, cable from harness that provides motion at the elbow and controls the terminal device, and control cable for the elbow lock.

the lower limb, the socket itself may include a means of suspension. Ordinarily, active control is provided only for the terminal device and the elbow, other joint action being either purely passive or eliminated entirely.

In the usual prosthesis, the harness, made of web strap, extends from the opposite axilla, across the back of the shoulders, to a cable that in turn activates the appropriate joints. A Bowden cable, which includes a tube-like housing through which the cable slides, in the manner of the choke cable of an automobile, has proved to be most efficient. In the above-elbow prosthesis, the housing is omitted across the elbow joint, thus allowing the elbow to be moved. With the elbow in a locked position, the cable travel is transmitted to the terminal device, activating it. Motion is initiated by the patient's either abducting his scapulae or flexing the shoulder on the prosthetic side. The elbow is locked by shrugging the shoulder, which pulls on a second cable that activates the elbow lock. Flexion and extension of the wrist are usually omitted, although there are prosthetic wrist units for special situations in which the wrist position can be present in flexed and extended positions. Pronation and supination are passive, and the desired position is set by rotating the terminal device with the opposite hand.

In recent years, other sources of force have been explored, including myoelectric control. In this system, myoelectric potentials from active voluntary contraction of muscles in the stump are picked up by electrodes in the socket, amplified, and used to switch on and off electric motors in the prosthesis. Opening and closing of the terminal device, pronation and supination, and elbow flexion and extension can be provided. Such systems are available and are useful in selected amputees. They are not at present in wide use in America, although many patients have been fitted with these devices in Europe. Myoelectric prostheses have the disadvantages of expense, increased maintenance requirements, and the loss of the sensory feedback provided by the conventional harness. The latter has been the most common cause of rejection by patients.

AMPUTATION THROUGH THE HAND AND CARPUS

When the hand is jeopardized, the surgeon must make every effort to save any useful digits that have adequate sensation and skin coverage. Two digits that will appose and have sensation will provide better function than any prosthesis, and even one digit can be opposed by a simple post prosthesis to provide prehension. If no digits are available, preservation of the carpus and part of the hand will provide some active function. This amputation ordinarily requires a long palmar flap to insure durable skin over the end of the stump. Flexion and extension of this stump are useful when a prosthesis is not worn, and pronation and supination are preserved. A prosthesis for this amputation is similar to that for higher levels, with a terminal device activated by a shoulder harness and cable.

WRIST DISARTICULATION

For many years, disarticulation of the radiocarpal joint was thought to be unfavorable because of poor stump coverage, breakdown of skin, and difficulty fitting the prosthesis. Total-contact sockets have obviated these disadvantages, although it is at the expense of some cosmesis, since the wrist area is somewhat bulky. In most cases, full or nearly full pronation and supination are preserved by this amputation. The forearm lever is strong and a short socket can be provided. About two thirds of the pronation and supination that are available in the forearm can be transmitted to the prosthesis.

AMPUTATION THROUGH THE FOREARM

In amputation through the forearm, all available length should be retained, although stumps up to the level of the radial tubercle and insertion of the biceps tendon can be fitted satisfactorily with a prosthesis. Anterior and posterior skin flaps of equal length are ordinarily made, forming a terminal scar. The socket of the prosthesis is attached to a cuff about the posterior aspect of the arm and is held in place with either a leather or a plastic strap, or in the case of short stumps, metal hinges at the elbow. In very short stumps, the socket may be suspended by the condyles of the humerus, making the arm cuff unnecessary, although this is at the expense of decreasing stability. This type of fitting, known as a Münster socket, is not appropriate for heavy activities. In all prostheses for amputation above the wrist disarticulation level, most of the pronation and supination needed are provided passively by rotating the terminal device on the socket.

SHORT BELOW-ELBOW AMPUTATION

When most of the forearm must be sacrificed, the elbow joint should be saved if possible, even if muscles are weak and its range of motion is limited. A socket fitted to the short stump may be attached to the forearm of the prosthesis by gear mechanism incorporated in the elbow hinge. This is usually a two-to-one ratio allowing two degrees of flexion of the forearm for every degree that the stump flexes. Obviously, power is lost and it may be necessary to reinforce flexion by the cable from the shoulder harness. In some cases, where there is insufficient range of motion of the elbow and insufficient power, the short below-elbow stump can still be used to activate an elbow joint lock.

ELBOW DISARTICULATION

When the forearm is disarticulated at the elbow or the amputation occurs at a higher level, a mechanical elbow joint is required to position the terminal device. The elbow joint must allow free voluntary flexion and extension activated by the shoulder harness, and it must provide locking at multiple positions for stability.

Amputation through the elbow joint produces a stump too long to fit the standard elbow joint mechanism. A special component incorporating an external lock is available, making this amputation practical.

An advantage to elbow joint disarticulation is the rotational stability provided for the socket by the flaring humeral condyles. A disadvantage is the problem of adequate skin coverage and prominent subcutaneous bony areas which can be uncomfortable within the socket. Flaps are made of equal length when skin is available but may be fashioned in any way that will allow proper coverage.

The triceps tendon may be sutured to the biceps and brachialis muscles over the joint surface. The lateral extensor muscle stump is trimmed to form a thin pad when it is drawn across the front of the joint and sutured to the medial epicondyle. The skin flaps are then closed in the usual manner.

SUPRACONDYLAR AMPUTATION

Although amputation may be done through the condyles of the humerus, the most frequent site is 2 to 2 1/2 inches above the joint line. Equal skin flaps are made. Some surgeons have advocated sectioning the triceps tendon as low as possible, and suturing it over the end of the bone to the fascia of the biceps muscle.

ABOVE-ELBOW AMPUTATION

Amputation through the shaft of the humerus to within 2 1/2 inches of the anterior axillary fold does not alter significantly prosthetic considerations. Above this level, however, the conventional above-elbow socket will not retain the stump and an extension of the socket over the anterior and posterior surfaces of the shoulder must be used. This limits effective arm and shoulder motion. As much length as possible should be preserved. The surgical technique for above-elbow amputation is similar to that for amputations lower in the arm. The triceps muscle is tapered from front to back to provide a thin musculofascial cover over the bone where this is practical.

The prosthesis for above-elbow amputations contains the usual forearm and terminal device, but most provide a mechanical elbow attached to the socket. The elbow joint provides flexion by means of a cable, with extension activated by gravity. An elbow-locking mechanism must be provided either by the shoulder elevator or by a manual locking lever. The elbow must be locked to permit the cable to act on the terminal device.

SHOULDER AND SCAPULOTHORACIC DISARTICULATION

Amputations through the shoulder or scapulothoracic joints are ordinarily performed for neoplasm, and are quite disabling.

An incision is made along the distal perimeter of the deltoid muscle from the coracoid process to the poste-rior axillary fold. A second incision connects these across the lower axilla. The neurovascular bundle is identified in the interval between the coracobrachialis and short head of the biceps and the axillary artery and vein and thoracoacromial artery are doubly ligated at this level. The median, ulnar, and musculocutaneous nerves are pulled downward, sharply sectioned, and allowed to retract. The deltoid muscle is detached from its insertion on the humerus and reflected upward with the skin flap. The coracobrachialis and short head of the biceps are divided in their attachment to the coracoid, and the pectoralis muscle is divided through its tendon of insertion in the anterior aspect of the humerus. The arm is placed in external rotation and the anterior capsule and shoulder cuff are entered with the section extending proximally to include the supraspinatus. With the arm held in internal rotation, the external rotators and teres major are divided from their attachment to the humerus. Section of the triceps muscle and the inferior capsule completes the severance of the limb. Suturing the cut ends of muscle together over the glenoid prevents a hollow from developing under the acromion.

The flap containing the deltoid muscle and overlying skin is then sutured to the skin margin in the lower axilla, completing the procedure.

There are two techniques described for scapulothoracic disarticulation or "forequarter" amputation. The anterior approach (Burger technique) starts the incision just lateral to the insertion of the sternocleidomastoid muscle on the clavicle, extends along the course of the clavicle to the acromioclavicular joint, over the acromion to the spine of the scapula, and then distally along the vertebral border of the scapula to its inferior angle. The lower portion of the incision starts at the middle third of the clavicle downward and laterally along the deltopectoral groove, crossing the axilla horizontally and joining the upper incision at the inferior angle of the scapula. The clavicle is exposed and the pectoralis major is dissected from the clavicle. The external jugular vein may be sectioned, but this is usually not necessary. The clavicle is divided with a bone cutter or Gigli saw just lateral to the insertion of the sternocleidomastoid muscle and the major portion of the clavicle may, if necessary, be removed. The pectoralis major and minor are divided at their insertions, thus exposing the neurovascular bundle. The subclavian artery and vein are doubly ligated and divided as far proximally as practical, and the brachial plexus is identified and likewise pulled down, sectioned, and allowed to retract. The latissimus dorsi and axillary fascia are divided from their humeral attachments. With the arm and scapula brought forward, the trapezius, the rhomboids, and the serratus are divided from their attachments to the scapula. If necessary, the skin flaps are trimmed to conform and the wound is closed. A drain is placed in the wound and a compression dressing is applied.

Prostheses for both shoulder and scapulothoracic disarticulations must be fitted over the upper chest, both anteriorly and posteriorly. Because of the limited sources of power and the number of joints that must be controlled, use of prostheses for these levels of amputation is quite limited. Sites from which to obtain force to activate the prosthesis include only the opposite shoulder, chest expansion, and, in the case of shoulder disarticulation, shoulder shrugging. It is for these levels that externally powered prostheses are really needed and are under development. It is hoped that these devices will be available for our patients on a routine basis in the near future.

SUMMARY

Amputation, particularly at a distal level, need not be the catastrophe that it appears to be on the surface. The major disadvantage of amputation over other ablative surgery, such as gastrectomy or pneumonectomy, is that its effect is immediately visible to the patient and produces a psychological sense of loss that can be a problem, even though this is one instance in which we have the possibility of restoring function with prosthetic replacement. The sooner rehabilitation is started, the more effective it is, and it is the uncommon amputee who cannot be restored to a relatively normal existence. A positive approach is necessary with support from everyone involved—the physician, the therapist, the prosthetist, the vocational counselor, the patient, and his family.

REFERENCES

1. Aldredge, R. H., and Thompson, T. C.: The technique of Syme amputation. Bone Joint Surg., 28:415–426, 1946.
2. Anderson, M. H., Bechtol, C. O., and Sollars, R. E.: Clinical Prosthetics for Physicians and Therapists. Springfield, Ill., Charles C Thomas, Publisher, 1959.
3. Boyd, H. B.: Anatomic disarticulation of the hip: Surg. Gynecol. Obstet., 84: 1947.
4. Burgess, E. M., Romano, R. L., and Zetti, J. H.: The management of lower extremity amputations. Veterans Adm., TR 10–6, 1969.
5. Burgess, E. M.: Sites of amputation—election according to modern practice. Clin. Ortho., 37:17, 1964.
6. Clippinger, F. W., Avery, R., and Titus, B. R.: A sensory feedback system for an upper extremity amputation prosthesis. Bull. Prosth. Res., Veterans Adm. 10–22, 1974.
7. Fields, W. S., and Leavitt, L. A.: Neural organization and its relation to prosthetics. New York, Intercontinental Med. Book Corp., 1973.
8. Flur, B., and Wilson, A. B.: Construction of patellar tendon bearing below knee prostheses. Berkeley, University of California Press, 1961.
9. Glattley, H. W.: A statistical study of 12,000 new amputees. Southern Med. J., 57:1373–1378, 1964.
10. Goldner, J. L., Clippinger, F. W., and Titus, B. R.: Use of temporary plaster or plastic pylons preparatory to fitting a permanent above knee or below knee prosthesis. Bull. Prosth. Res., Veterans Adm., 10–13, 1970.
11. Klopsteg, P. E., and Wilson, P. D.: Human limbs and their substitutes. New York, Hofner Publishing Co., 1968.
12. Littlewood, H.: Amputations at the shoulder and at the hip. Br. Med. J., 1:381–387, 1922.
13. McCullough, N. C., III, Shea, J. D., Weaver, W. D., and Sarmiento, A.: The dysvascular amputee—surgery and rehabilitation. Curr. Probl. Surg., Oct., 1971.
14. Mital, M., and Pierce, D. S.: Amputees and their prostheses. Boston, Little, Brown and Co., 1971.
15. National Academy of Sciences: Below Knee Prosthetics. Washington, D.C., 1968.
16. National Academy of Sciences: The Geriatric Amputee. Washington, D.C., 1971.
17. National Academy of Sciences: The Child With an Acquired Amputation. Washington, D.C., 1972.
18. Park, G. T., and Ehrlich, H. E.: Exarticulation of the lower extremities for malignant tumor: Hip joint disarticulation and sacroiliac disarticulation. Ann. Surg., 123:965–985, 1946; 124:1–27, 1947.
19. Pederson, H. E.: Lower extremity amputations for gangrene. Amer. Acad. Orthop. Surg., 15: 1958.
20. Radcliffe, C. W., and Foort, J.: The patellar tendon bearing below knee prosthesis. Berkeley, University of California Press, 1961.
21. Sarmiento, A., Gilmer, R. E., and Finneston, A.: A new surgical-prosthetic approach to Syme's amputation: A preliminary report. Artif. Limbs, 10:52–55, 1966.
22. Wilson, A. B.: Limb prosthetics today. Artif. Limbs, 7:1–42, 1963.

IX

INFECTIONS AND NEOPLASMS OF BONE

John M. Harrelson, M.D.

INFECTIONS OF BONE

Osteomyelitis is the general term used to denote infection of bone. While most of the organisms responsible for soft tissue infections can also produce osteomyelitis, the majority of bone infections are the result of *Staphylococcus aureus*. The location, clinical presentation, and course of osteomyelitis vary depending on the offending organism and the age of the patient. Staphylococcus and other pus-forming bacteria usually produce an acute fulminating infection of bone, or "pyogenic osteomyelitis." Tuberculosis and other nonpyogenic organisms produce a less aggressive granulomatous type of infection. It is convenient to consider these two types of osteomyelitis separately.

PYOGENIC OSTEOMYELITIS

Suppurative infection of bone occurs in one of two ways. Blood-borne bacteria from an active focus of soft tissue infection (furuncle, upper respiratory infection, urinary tract infection) may lodge in bone and establish an abscess. This mechanism is referred to as "hematogenous osteomyelitis." Bacteria may also reach bone from the external environment (penetrating wounds, open fractures, surgical incisions) and establish "exogenous osteomyelitis." The development of antibiotics has greatly reduced the incidence of both types of osteomyelitis and has significantly improved the prognosis. Prior to the antibiotic era, the mortality rate from pyogenic osteomyelitis was 20 to 30 per cent, and survivors could expect significant crippling effects of the disease. Today, death is rare and residual disability has been greatly minimized.

Hematogenous osteomyelitis is primarily a disease of childhood, occurring most frequently between the ages of 5 and 15. Males are affected three times more frequently than females. The location of osteomyelitis is dependent on several anatomic factors. In the growing child, the afferent arterial supply to bone enters through the nutrient artery and through small periosteal vessels penetrating the cortex. As these vessels reach the arteriolar level in the metaphysis at each end of the bone, they enter into numerous sinusoidal veins adjacent to the physeal plate in which flow is significantly diminished. These metaphyseal veins with sluggish blood flow provide an ideal location for the lodgement of bacteria and subsequent establishment of infection. Thus, hematogenous osteomyelitis in children is most frequently seen in the metaphyseal ends of long bones.

The adjacent epiphysis has a separate blood supply which enters through the joint capsule. The physeal plate has no traversing blood vessels and acts as a further barrier to the spread of infection from the metaphysis to the adjacent epiphysis and joint. The femur, tibia, and humerus are most frequently affected, in that order. Other tubular bones and flat bones are less commonly involved. With bony maturity, ossification of the physeal plate occurs, and the circulation of the epiphysis and metaphysis merges. The characteristic of sluggish blood flow is lost. Thus, osteomyelitis in adults is less frequent and may occur at any point within a long bone.

Hematogenous osteomyelitis most frequently involves bone with a rich blood supply. Exogenous osteomyelitis is more common in these bones with the least soft tissue covering. The distal tibia, the metacarpals, and the phalanges are most frequently the sites of open fractures or penetrating injury and subsequent infection, although any bone may be involved.

Pathologic Considerations

As the invading bacteria reach the metaphyseal veins and begin to multiply, the initial host response is an infiltration of polymorphonuclear leukocytes. This combination of bacteria and leukocytes constitutes an abscess. As a result of the bacterial multiplication and interstitial edema, pressure increases within the rigid structure of the metaphysis, producing capillary destruction, thrombosis, loss of circulation, and subsequent death of the trabecular bone within the abscess. Increasing pressure produces localized pain.

In the early stages of the disease, infarction of a portion of the metaphysis does not produce any observable radiographic change. As the process continues, granulation tissue develops about the periphery of the abscess and with it there occurs osteoclastic resorption of the living bone in this area. The isolated necrotic bone within the abscess cavity is called a *sequestrum.* About the periphery of the granulation tissue the host bone makes an effort to isolate the infectious process. New bone is deposited in this area and is called the *involucrum.*

Because of the pain and subsequent diminished activity, disuse osteoporosis develops within the affected extremity. Increased circulation to the bone as a result of the infection accelerates the development of osteoporosis. Radiographs taken at 12 to 14 days following the onset of infection reveal a central area of increased radiodensity (sequestrum) surrounded by a zone of relative radiolucency (granulation tissue), surrounded in turn by an area of increased radiodensity (involucrum). Generalized diminished radiodensity of the remainder of the long bone is the result of osteoporosis.

If the host is successful in repelling the infection at this stage, gradual obliteration of the abscess cavity with fibrous tissue occurs. This area is subsequently replaced by new bone, ultimately leaving no evidence of the infectious process. More frequently, the host is unable to contain the infection as an isolated abscess and continued growth of bacteria occurs. New areas of bone become involved as the process spreads outward toward the periosteum. Purulent material percolates through the haversian and Volkmann's canals of the cortex and reaches the subperiosteal space. With increasing pressure, pus dissects along the subperiosteal plane, stripping the periosteum from the underlying cortex. This robs the cortex of its major source of blood supply and extends the area of infarction. The subperiosteal spread of infection is limited at each end of the long bone by the adherence of the periosteum to the metaphyseal-physeal junction. The impermeability of the physeal plate prevents the spread of infection to the epiphysis. Thus, the entire shaft of the bone from one metaphysis to the other may be involved. From the inner surface of the elevated periosteum, osteoblasts begin to lay down new bone and form a periosteal involucrum (Fig. 1).

At this point, the infection may rupture through the periosteum into the adjacent soft tissues and ultimately to the skin, where it produces a draining sinus tract. Fragments of necrotic bone (sequestrum) may be extruded. If the sinus is large enough to extrude the entire sequestrum, subsequent healing may occur with obliteration of the abscess cavity by fibrous tissue. However, this situation rarely occurs. Usually the sequestrum is too large for complete extrusion and it remains as a foreign body, perpetuating the infection. Even with complete extrusion, the rigid nature of bone prevents collapse of the abscess cavity and greatly reduces the likelihood of total obliteration of the infection.

Adherence of the periosteum to the metaphysis and the impermeability of the physeal plate usually protect the adjacent joint from infection. In infants below the age of 12 months there are vessels

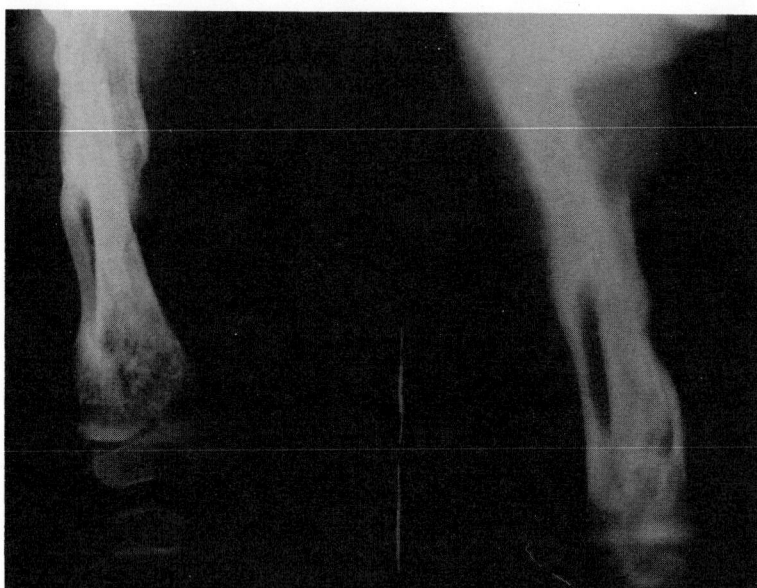

Figure 1. Notice the periosteal new bone (involucrum) which formed along the entire shaft of the femur. The central femoral cortex is necrotic and represents a sequestrum.

that traverse the physeal plate. Osteomyelitis in this age group may produce adjacent pyarthrosis. The hip joint, in any age group, is vulnerable to infection with osteomyelitis of the proximal femur because the capital femoral epiphysis lies within the joint capsule. Metaphyseal infection of the proximal femur may permeate the outer cortex and enter the joint directly (Fig. 2).

Clinical Considerations

The onset of hematogenous osteomyelitis is usually abrupt. The patient presents with high fever, generalized malaise, and pain in the involved extremity. A history of preceding infection may be obtained. Early in the course of the disease, there may be generalized swelling of the extremity without erythema. A sterile sympathetic effusion of adjacent joints may be present. Because of protective spasm of the muscles in the involved extremity, the patient will not voluntarily move the limb, a phenomenon known as "pseudoparalysis." The patient is toxic and irritable, and even the slightest manipulation of the extremity produces paroxysms of pain. Extremely gentle digital palpation along the course of the extremity will usually localize the nidus of infection.

Laboratory examination reveals a leukocytosis exceeding 15,000, mild to moderate anemia, and a markedly elevated erythrocyte sedimentation rate. In approximately 50 per cent of cases, blood cultures will be positive. In the first seven to 10 days of the disease there are no evident bony changes on x-ray, but subtle soft tissue changes can be recognized. As a result of inflammation and swelling of the extremity, the normal soft tissue shadows produced by muscle, fascial planes, and subcutaneous tissue are obliterated. This change will be seen throughout the entire course of the involved long bone. Comparison radiographs of the opposite extremity may be helpful. Within 10 to 14 days bony changes will be evident on x-ray, consisting

first of mottled lucency of the involved metaphysis followed by periosteal elevation and new bone formation.

A number of other conditions may simulate acute osteomyelitis in children. Ewing's sarcoma, acute rheumatic fever, leukemia, scurvy, acute septic arthritis, and acute juvenile rheumatoid arthritis may all mimic the clinical picture of acute osteomyelitis. Careful examination of the involved extremity is required to distinguish acute osteomyelitis from acute pyarthrosis. In osteomyelitis, tenderness is usually located over the metaphysis of the long bone, and gentle manipulation will allow motion of the adjacent joints. In contrast, acute pyarthrosis produces swelling localized at the joint level, and the patient will not tolerate any joint motion. In acute rheumatic fever and acute juvenile rheumatoid arthritis, the tenderness is similarly located over the joint, and more than one joint may be involved.

Because of the widespread use of antibiotics, the pre-existing nidus of soft tissue infection may not be identified. When antibiotic therapy has been used for a preceding soft tissue infection, the subsequent clinical course of osteomyelitis may be considerably more benign and the true diagnosis not recognized until the infection is well established. In adults, osteomyelitis characteristically presents a more benign picture. Often the infection will be limited to the metaphysis without spread to the subperiosteal space. Generalized toxicity is less and symptoms are usually localized to the site of infection.

The organism most frequently encountered in hematogenous osteomyelitis is *Staphylococcus aureus* (90 per cent). In neonates and infants Streptococcus may be the etiologic agent. These two bacteria produce the fulminating clinical picture described above. Less frequently, gram-negative organisms may produce osteomyelitis. In particular, Salmonella osteomyelitis may be seen as a complication of sickle cell anemia and will often involve the diaphysis of a long bone rather than the metaphysis. The gram-negative organisms characteristically produce a less virulent infection than gram-positive cocci.

Exogenous osteomyelitis is most frequently the result of open fracture. In that the infection results from a contamination of an existing wound, any organism may be involved. If the fracture wound has been closed, the subsequent development of infection may produce the same symptoms as seen in hematogenous osteomyelitis, though to a lesser degree. As a rule, the infection is limited to the site of injury and produces localized erythema and swelling. The continued multiplication of bacteria may cause spontaneous dehiscence of the wound with a discharge of purulent material. When the periosteum has been disrupted, as in the case of fracture, periosteal elevation is not seen as a result of infection. Rather, there is local destruction of bone at the fracture site.

Treatment

The treatment of acute hematogenous osteomyelitis begins immediately upon recognition. Once blood cultures have been obtained, antibiotics are administered intravenously without awaiting the results of culture. Since *Staphylococcus aureus* is the most frequent offending organism, penicillin in combination with methicillin is used. Blood cultures do not always reveal the etiologic agent. If there are enough localizing physical findings or confirmatory radiographic changes, the subperiosteal space may be aspirated with a large-bore needle and material obtained for gram stain and culture. Care must be taken not to contaminate an adjacent sterile joint. If no material is obtained on penetrating the periosteum, the needle may be advanced through the cortex into the metaphysis and an aspirate obtained for culture.

The maintenance of fluid and electrolyte balance and the correction of an existing anemia with whole fresh blood are also necessary. Antipyretics are required to control fever, and anticonvulsants may be necessary. Immobilization of the involved extremity is accomplished by the use of bivalved plaster. Immobilization allows the extremity to rest and reduces muscle spasm and pain. Bivalved plaster is preferred in order to allow inspection of the extremity. In most instances the administration of intravenous antibiotics produces improvement within 24 hours. If the patient's condition does not improve, surgical intervention is required.

The surgical principles in the treatment of osteomyelitis are the same as for the treatment of any soft tissue abscess and consist of incision and drainage. The surgical approach depends upon both the location and the extent of infection. When possible, the incision should be placed to allow subsequent dependent drainage. If the infection is confined to the metaphysis without periosteal elevation and if the dissection of pus within the subperiosteal space has not occurred, then a cortical window is created in the metaphysis, and the pus under pressure, together with the necrotic sequestrum, are removed. Care is taken not to damage the adjacent physeal plate. This procedure is called saucerization. Care must also be taken not to strip the periosteum widely, since this interrupts the blood supply to the underlying cortex and allows extension of the infection. The wound is packed open to allow drainage, and the extremity is immobilized in plaster.

If the infectious process involves the majority of the shaft of the bone, then closed suction irrigation may be used. A cortical window is created in the same manner as described above and two perforated polyethylene catheters are inserted into the medullary canal through separate stab wounds. The incision is then closed. One catheter is used as an inlet for irrigation fluid containing antibiotics and the other is attached to suction, allowing a closed system of continuous irrigation of the medullary canal. The catheters remain in place for five to 10 days and are removed when the infection appears to be under control.

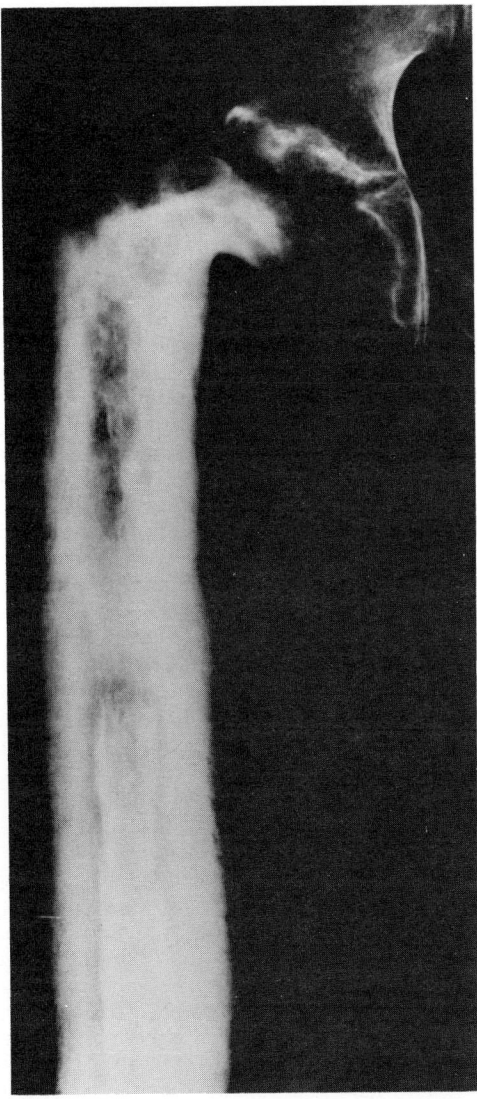

Figure 2. This child has osteomyelitis involving the entire femoral shaft. The central portion of the bone is the old femoral shaft, which is now necrotic and represents a sequestrum. Notice that the hip joint has been involved because the hip capsule extends beyond the capital femoral physeal plate.

Intravenous antibiotics are continued for a minimum of two weeks, followed by appropriate oral antibiotic therapy for an additional four weeks. Antibiotic treatment is discontinued when all clinical signs of infection are absent and the sedimentation rate returns to normal. When the acute infectious process is under control, the limb is removed from the bivalved plaster several times each day for gentle motion of adjacent joints. This prevents arthrofibrosis and maintains normal joint motion. The resumption of activity with the involved limb depends on the extent of bone destruction and the rate of healing. If a large area is involved, the return to full weight bearing and normal activity may require many months in order to avoid pathologic fracture.

The best treatment of exogenous osteomyelitis is prevention. Open, contamined fracture wounds should be debrided and packed open and closed as a delayed procedure in five days if there are no signs of infection. When a fracture wound has been closed and infection has developed, the wound must be opened widely and redebrided to allow complete drainage. Any nonviable bone at the fracture site is removed. Immobilization of the limb is mandatory. Adequate cultures are obtained and the appropriate antibiotics selected depending on bacterial sensitivity.

With the use of antibiotics, death is rarely seen in osteomyelitis. The ultimate degree of disability depends upon many factors. The location of infection, the extent of bony destruction, the involvement of adjacent joints, the virulence of the organism, and the rapidity with which treatment is started all affect the ultimate outcome. If the infection is successfully controlled by antibiotics or a combination of antibiotics and surgery, then ultimate eradication of the infection is possible. In some cases it is not possible to eliminate the infection completely. When the extent of bony involvement is great and complete sequestrectomy is not possible, draining sinus tracts may develop and indicate the beginning of chronic osteomyelitis. The infection may be quiescent for many months or years only to flare up periodically with drainage, fever, and swelling. The sinus tract becomes lined with squamous epithelium and, in long-standing cases, may undergo metaplasia and develop squamous carcinoma within the tract. Chronic cases that cannot be adequately controlled by antibiotics and local measures may require amputation of the extremity and fitting with a prosthesis to eradicate the infection and provide better function.

TUBERCULOUS OSTEOMYELITIS AND PYARTHROSIS

Like hematogenous osteomyelitis, the incidence of skeletal tuberculosis has decreased significantly in recent years. The development of effective antimicrobial agents is partly responsible. An improved standard of living that reduces overcrowding and malnutrition has also contributed to the reduction of pulmonary (human type) tuberculosis. The identification of diseased cattle and the pasteurization of milk have reduced the frequency of gastrointestinal (bovine type) tuberculosis.

Skeletal tuberculosis is the result of hematogenous seeding of tubercle bacilli from a pre-existing pulmonary or gastrointestinal focus. This organism most frequently involves the joints and adjacent bone rather than the metaphyseal area of long bones. The intervertebral discs of the lower thoracic and upper lumbar spine and the adjacent vertebrae are the most frequent sites of skeletal tuberculosis (approximately 30 per cent of all cases), the hip and knee joints being the next most frequently affected. Tuberculosis, like hematogenous osteomyelitis, is a disease of childhood. Older statistics indicate that the majority of cases occur in children between the ages of five and 15 years. However, there seems to be a decline in the number of childhood cases and an increase in the incidence of skeletal tuberculosis in adults.

Pathologic Considerations

Following hematogenous inoculation, tubercle bacilli lodge in the subchondral bone of the epiphysis, in the joint capsule, or in the synovial membrane. The initial host response is an infiltration of lymphocytes, plasma cells, and monocytes. The histologic appearance of the tuberculous lesion in bone in every way resembles that seen in visceral tuberculosis. Histiocytes (epithelioid cells) appear and may aggregate to form Langhan's giant cells. There is considerable fibroblastic proliferation. Caseous necrosis surrounded by a granulomatous inflammatory response constitutes the classic tubercle. The destruction produced by granulomatous inflammation is characteristically slow. Within the joint, destruction tends to occur first at those areas where the joint surfaces are not in constant apposition. In the knee joint this destruction occurs at the joint margins, producing a "corner defect" on x-ray. In the hip joint such lesions appear at the superior border of the femoral neck or in the inferior medial aspect of the joint away from the weight-bearing area. Erosion of articular cartilage in the weight-bearing area is a late development and accounts for the preservation of joint space seen on early x-rays. As the destruction proceeds, the joint becomes filled with caseous necrotic products and fragments of articular cartilage, material called "rice bodies" because of its appearance. In some cases, the joint or disc space infection may erupt into the adjacent soft tissues, burrow along a fascial plane, and eventually penetrate the skin, producing a chronic draining sinus tract that exudes caseous necrotic material.

Clinical Considerations

The destruction of bone and articular cartilage by tuberculous infection is a slow process, and symptoms are correspondingly insidious in their development. The patient complains of a dull ache in the area of the affected joint, often worse at night than during the day. Since the skeletal lesion is preceded by a visceral infection, the patient will often appear debilitated. A history of weight loss and easy fatigability may be obtained, as may a history of close contact with a family member with known tuberculosis.

Spinal involvement with tuberculosis produces diminished motion at the thoracolumbar level and protective paraspinal muscle spasm, which holds the back hyperextended. When the tuberculous process has escaped the confines of the disc space and adjacent vertebrae, a large paraspinal abscess may be produced. As the spine becomes weakened, collapse of the vertebral column may occur, forcing the caseous necrotic debris into the spinal canal and producing neurologic deterioration ranging from paraparesis to complete paraplegia. Prior to the development of effective antituberculous drugs, this clinical pattern of spinal tuberculosis was more common. The paraspinal abscess, which develops about a focus of tuberculous infection, may extend for some distance beneath the paraspinal muscles. It is not uncommon to see a patient with spinal tuberculosis present with a mass in the buttock or medial thigh that represents a soft tissue extension of the paraspinal abscess beneath the psoas muscle. The mass characteristically does not produce overlying erythema and is known as a "cold abscess."

The chief radiographic change in tuberculous spondylitis is narrowing of the disc space at the affected level. The outlines of the adjacent end-plates become smudgy in appearance. As the disease progresses, the interspace narrows and a kyphotic deformity develops. Destruction of the adjacent vertebral end-plates follows. If a paraspinal abscess is present, it will usually produce a soft tissue shadow on x-ray. Calcification may occasionally be seen within the abscess.

In the joints of the extremities, there is mild synovial thickening and effusion. Some increased local heat over the joint is seen, but erythema is usually lacking. Mild limitation of motion, muscle atrophy, and a limp are present. There may be enlargement of the proximal regional lymph nodes.

Laboratory examination reveals a normal to slightly elevated white count, an elevated erythrocyte sedimentation rate, and mild anemia. The tuberculin skin test is almost always positive. The patient should be questioned about previous BCG vaccination. Synovial fluid from the involved joint will be turbid, with a poor mucin clot and a lowered glucose level. The white cell count will be elevated, with an increased number of mononuclear cells. The synovial fluid sediment should be examined for acid-fast bacilli and a portion retained for culture.

Radiographs of tuberculous diarthroidal joints will show generalized osteoporosis with preservation of the joint space and distention of the joint capsule. The earliest bony changes consist of erosion of the joint margins at the point of capsular attachment to the epiphysis. Similar defects may occur within the epiphysis itself, and the infection may cross the physeal plate into the adjacent metaphysis. When the hip joint in children is involved, progressive capsular distention may interrupt the blood supply to the capital femoral epiphysis, resulting in its death and gradual disappearance (Fig. 3).

Treatment

The development of effective antituberculous drugs has radically altered the treatment of this disease. In the past, a patient's primary defense was his own immune system. If the lesion eventually showed signs of healing, arthrodesis of the joint was performed with

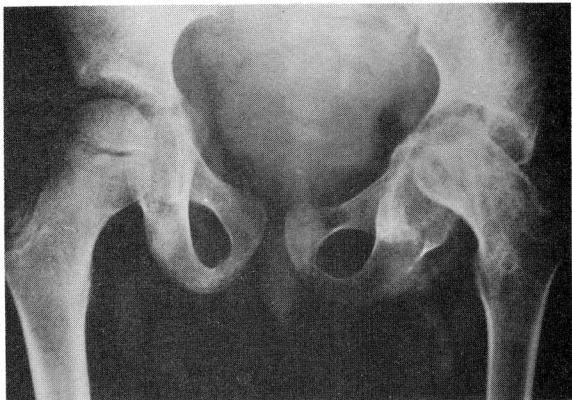

Figure 3. In this case of tuberculosis of the hip joint, the capital femoral epiphysis has been destroyed, probably owing to loss of blood supply. Notice the narrowing of the joint space and osteoporosis of the pelvis and femur on the involved side. There is very little reactive bone formation.

the joint in the functional position. Today arthrodesis is less frequently required.

The initial treatment of skeletal tuberculosis consists of appropriate antituberculous drugs (isoniazid, PAS, streptomycin, ethambutal) and protection of the involved joint. For spinal tuberculosis, the use of bedrest or plaster immobilization is recommended during the initial phase of chemotherapy. As healing occurs, gradual resumption of activity is allowed. Joints in the lower extremities are put at rest either by traction or by the use of bivalved plaster. Daily gentle range of motion exercises are performed to maintain joint function. If there is no significant evidence of healing after six to eight weeks of antituberculous therapy, then localized foci within the epiphysis may be carefully removed by curettage. Arthrodesis of the joint may still be required if there is excessive joint destruction.

ACUTE PYOGENIC ARTHRITIS

Joint infection with pyogenic organisms occurs as a result of hematogenous seeding of the joint, extension of adjacent osteomyelitis, or penetrating wounds of the joint. Hematogenous pyarthrosis is most commonly seen in children below the age of five. *Staphylococcus aureus* is the most common etiologic agent, although Streptococcus, Gonococcus, and Pneumococcus may be etiologic. The condition is almost always monarticular, although rarely several joints may be affected. The hip joint is most frequently involved.

Pathologic Considerations

The infiltration of polymorphonuclear neutrophils following inoculation of the joint is similar to that of pyogenic infection elsewhere. The initial irritation of the synovial membrane causes an increased production of synovial fluid and effusion. As neutrophils and bacteria accumulate within the joint, the intra-articular pressure rises. The combination of toxic bacterial products, lysosomal enzymes, and increased pressure produce gradual destruction of the articular cartilage. This destruction begins in the weight-bearing portion of the articular surface and progresses toward the periphery. If the full thickness of the articular cartilage is destroyed in any area, the infection may gain access to the underlying subchondral bone of the epiphysis. Rupture of the joint capsule owing to increased pressure allows access to the adjacent soft tissues. The infection may rupture through the overlying skin and form a draining sinus tract.

Clinical Considerations

The onset of pyogenic arthritis is acute, with fever, irritability, and pain. In the early stages of infection a limp may develop, which rapidly progresses to severe pain preventing ambulation. On examination there is swelling, overlying erythema, and exquisite tenderness to direct palpation or any attempt at joint motion. Even jarring the bed may produce acute pain. Pseudoparalysis is present. Careful digital palpation without moving the affected joint will aid in distinguishing metaphyseal osteomyelitis from acute pyarthrosis.

Laboratory studies show elevation of the white count and erythrocyte sedimentation rate. Aspiration of the involved joint under careful sterile conditions reveals a cloudy, turbid synovial fluid with a cell count ranging from 50,000 to 200,000 cells per cu. cm. These cells are at least 90 per cent polymorphonuclear neutrophils. The gram stain will show organisms in about 50 per cent of cases. The joint fluid should be retained for aerobic and anaerobic culture. The blood culture will frequently be positive.

In performing joint aspiration, a large-bore needle should be used. Small-bore needles may become plugged with edematous synovium or proteinaceous debris within the joint and prevent retrieval of synovial fluid. Care should be exercised to avoid damage to the underlying epiphyseal bone or articular cartilage.

Radiographs in the early stages of septic arthritis reveal no bony change. There is distention of the joint capsule due to increased pressure within the joint, and an abnormally widened joint space may be seen. In severe cases, there may be pathologic dislocation of the joint. With persistence of the infection in untreated or inadequately treated cases, destruction of the articular cartilage produces eventual narrowing of the joint space.

Treatment

Pyogenic arthritis is an emergency. Once the diagnosis has been established, intravenous antibiotics are administered without awaiting the results of culture. A broad-spectrum antibiotic is selected and may be changed depending on the results of subsequent sensitivity testing. Supportive measures include fluid and electrolyte maintenance and the use of antipyretics. The affected joint must be put at rest to prevent any further cartilage damage. Since pressure within the joint is one of the destructive mechanisms, traction is generally more appropriate than plaster immobilization.

If the initial joint aspiration reveals a serosanguin-eous fluid, the infection is in its early stages. In this situation, the joint may be irrigated with sterile saline and the patient observed during the first 24 hours of antibiotic therapy. Usually this treatment produces a marked improvement, with a fall in the temperature and diminished local symptoms. Reaspiration of the joint may be performed at intervals to confirm a reduction in the cell count. Repeat cultures are obtained on each aspiration to determine sterility. If improvement fails to occur, surgical incision and drainage of the joint are required.

If the initial joint aspiration produces thick pus, then antibiotic therapy alone is unlikely to be adequate. At this stage, there is a thick edematous synovial membrane and a considerable amount of intra-articular necrotic debris, which prevents adequate antibiotic penetration. Surgical incision and drainage should be performed. Some feel that all infections of the hip joint should be drained primarily in addition to antibiotic therapy, since aspiration of the hip joint is difficult and the circulation to the capital femoral epiphysis is threatened by the increased intra-articular pressure. Active and passive joint exercises are begun as soon as the infection is controlled in order to maintain normal joint function.

NEOPLASMS OF BONE

Primitive mesenchymal tissue gives rise to cartilage, bone, fibrous tissue, and marrow elements, the four basic tissue components of the mature skeleton. From each of these tissue types there may arise benign or malignant neoplasms. The skeleton may also be the site of neoplasms ordinarily associated with soft tissues. Hemangioma, hemangiosarcoma, lipoma, and liposarcoma may be rare primary bone tumors. Metastatic disease from soft tissue sarcomas and carcinomas frequently involves the skeleton.

Since the treatment of many skeletal neoplasms may involve radical surgery and/or the use of chemotherapy and irradiation, accurate diagnosis is essential. A complete clinical history and good biplane radiographs are the first steps in evaluating the patient with a skeletal neoplasm. When minimally symptomatic or asymptomatic lesions are clearly benign by x-ray, biopsy may not be necessary.

When biopsy of a lesion is required, several considerations should be borne in mind. Many skeletal neoplasms do not have a uniform histologic appearance. The biopsy specimen should be adequate enough to obtain representative material for histologic examination. For this reason, we advise against the use of needle biopsy technique except in lesions which are difficult to approach surgically. The placement of the biopsy incision should take into account the possibility of future radical local resection of the lesion and should allow for complete removal of the biopsy site with the specimen. If the lesion is potentially malignant, it is generally inadvisable to exsanguinate the extremity with an Esmarch bandage before inflating the pneumatic tourniquet. The pathologist should be consulted prior to the biopsy and should be present in the operating room at the time of surgery. He is thus aware of both the gross appearance of the lesion and the origin of the biopsy material relative to the radiographs. These procedures aid in making an accurate diagnosis and rendering intelligent future treatment.

Other ancillary studies are often used in the diagnosis of skeletal neoplasms. Tomography is helpful in localizing deep lesions (pelvis, spine) and may bring out radiographic detail not appreciated on plain films. Arteriography may distinguish between malignant and benign lesions and gives anatomic information about the vascularity of the lesion which is helpful if local resection is required. A bone scan may also provide information when the extent of the lesion is not fully appreciated on x-ray and when multiple lesions are present.

TUMORS OF CARTILAGINOUS ORIGIN

Osteochondroma

The osteochondroma is the most common benign neoplasm of bone. This lesion is composed of normal osseous and cartilaginous tissue and is considered by some to be a hamartoma and not a true neoplasm. Occurring with equal frequency in males and females, the osteochondroma is usually discovered during the teenage years as a result of local mechanical symptoms. The metaphyseal end of long bones is the most common site, with 50 per cent occurring in the distal femur. Any bone may be involved, including ribs, pelvis, and vertebrae.

The radiographic appearance of this lesion is that of a bony stalk arising from the metaphysis and usually pointing away from the adjacent epiphysis (Fig. 4). The end of this stalk is irregular and covered with a cartilaginous cap of varying thickness. Growth of the lesion stops when growth of the adjacent epiphysis stops. The bony stalk is in continuity with the underlying cortex of the long bone and is covered by a reflection of periosteum. The stalk may be thin with a pedunculated cartilaginous cap or broad and sessile with the cap closely adherent to the adjacent normal cortex.

Osteochondromas are probably the result of ectopic rests of epiphyseal cartilage. The junction between the cartilaginous cap and the underlying trabecular bone shows endochondral bone formation like the epiphyseal plate, although less orderly. Grossly the cartilaginous cap has the appearance of cartilaginous lesions elsewhere in the body. The surface is lobulated, pearly white, and opalescent. Overlying the osteochondroma one often finds a bursa. Inflammation of this bursa may lead to discovery of the lesion. Osteochondromas are usually solitary. Multiple osteochondromatosis is recognized as a familial disease. Grossly and histologically these lesions are in every way similar to the solitary osteochondroma.

The treatment of an osteochondroma depends upon symptoms. If a lesion is producing mechanical difficulty adjacent to a joint, excision is indicated. These lesions may be cured by excision flush with the cortex of the underlying bone with care taken to remove the periosteal envelope surrounding the bony stalk. Incomplete excision may result in recurrence.

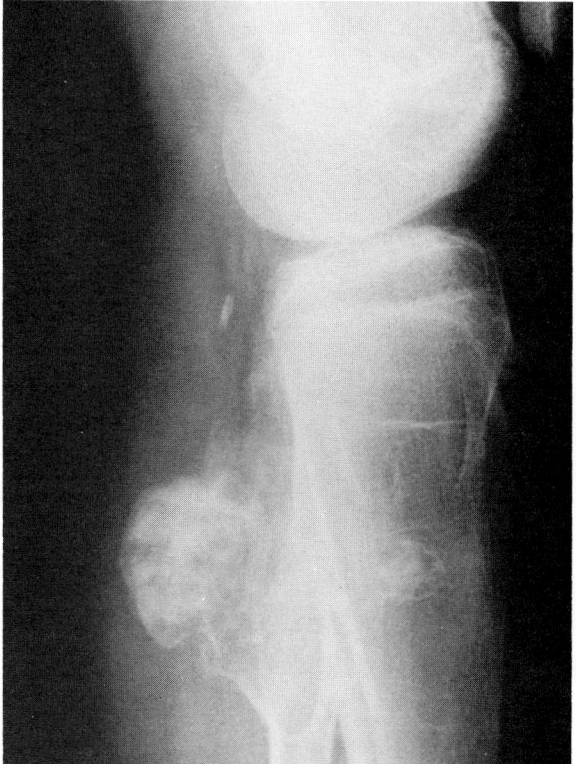

Figure 4. This child has multiple osteochondromatosis. Notice the lobulated bony stalk arising from the posterior portion of the fibula. This stalk is covered by a large cartilaginous cap not seen on x-ray.

Malignant degeneration of osteochondromas may occur rarely in solitary osteochondromas and more frequently in multiple osteochondromas. Those lesions closer to the midline of the body (scapula and pelvis) are statistically more likely to undergo malignant degeneration. Evidence of growth of an osteochondroma (solitary or multiple lesions) after epiphyseal closure of the bone involved is an indication for removal. Malignant degeneration in these lesions occurs in the cartilaginous cap and chondrosarcoma results. For this reason, careful x-ray follow-up of known osteochondromas is indicated.

Enchondroma

The enchondroma is a benign growth of hyaline cartilage within the medullary cavity of a bone. Like the osteochondroma, this lesion is considered to arise from ectopic cartilaginous rests and is considered by some to be a hamartomatous growth. Enchondromas have an equal sex distribution and most often occur in the phalanges, metacarpals, and metatarsals. They may appear in other long bones and in the pelvis, scapula, and ribs. Often they are discovered incidentally when x-rays are obtained for other reasons. When symptomatic, they present either as swelling of the bone involved with mild tenderness or as a pathologic fracture through an existing lesion.

Radiographically the enchondroma produces a lucent defect, usually in the metaphyseal region of a

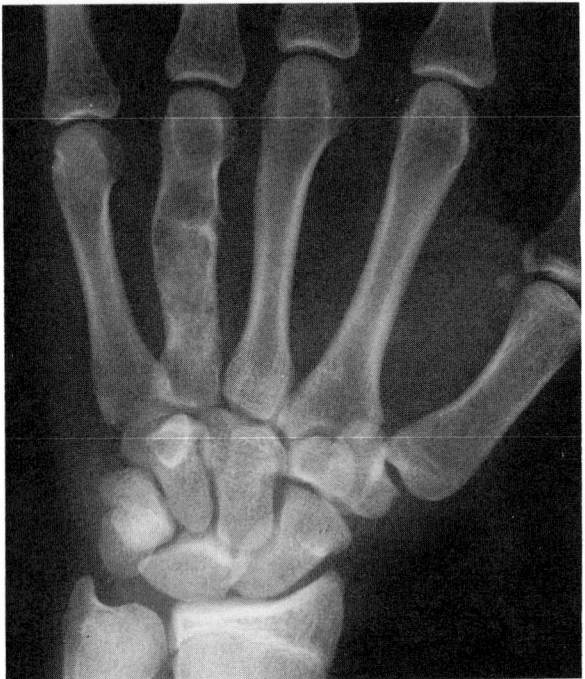

Figure 5. The lesion in the fourth metacarpal has expanded and thinned the overlying cortex. There is stippled calcification within the center of the lesion. This enchondroma was cured by curettage and bone grafting.

required. For the symptomatic benign enchondroma, curettage and bone grafting are the accepted treatments of choice. The rate of recurrence is low with adequate curettage.

Chondroblastoma

The chondroblastoma is a benign lesion of cartilaginous origin first identified as a separate entity in 1931 by Codman. Prior to that time it had been grouped with giant cell tumors of bone. The chondroblastoma occurs in the epiphyses of long bones, usually in the second decade of life. This tumor probably originates from ectopic cells of the physeal plate, which begin to proliferate sometime in the second decade. The chondroblastoma occurs more frequently in males (2:1). The symptoms are variable but usually consist of the insidious onset of aching pain, usually at night, referred to the joint adjacent to the lesion. There may be some limitation of motion, mild effusion of the joint, and synovial thickening.

The radiographic appearance of this lesion is characteristic. Eccentrically placed within the epiphysis, it has a smooth border with only a slight sclerotic margin and may have central areas of stippling that represent calcification within the substance of the tumor. There may be involvement of the physeal plate and metaphysis adjacent to the lesion (Fig. 6). Grossly these lesions are grey to grey-yellow and gritty to the

long bone. The margins of the lesion are well defined, with sclerotic reactive bone (Fig. 5). The overlying cortex may be expanded and thinned. Varying degrees of stippled calcification may appear within the lesion.

Grossly an enchondroma is blue-white and translucent. Microscopically one sees lobules of hyaline cartilage with a mild degree of cellular atypia and a slight increase in cellularity compared with normal hyaline cartilage.

The enchondroma, like the osteochondroma, has a malignant potential for degeneration into a chondrosarcoma. Since these lesions are usually asymptomatic, any clinical evidence of recent growth or pain should raise the suspicion of malignant degeneration. Radiographic evidence of erosion through the cortex by an enchondroma is a sign of malignant behavior.

Enchondromas may occur as multiple lesions in the same patient. In 1899 Ollier described the multiple metaphyseal cartilaginous lesions known now as Ollier's Disease. Multiple enchondromatosis may be associated with multiple cavernous hemangiomas, a condition first reported in 1881 by Maffucci. In multiple enchondromatosis, growth disturbance in early childhood may be one of the first manifestations of the disease. Distortion in both length growth and angular growth may be seen.

The likelihood of malignant degeneration in multiple enchondromatosis is higher than for the solitary lesion. Those lesions located centrally (pelvis, scapulae, spine) are more likely to become malignant. Regular x-ray survey in patients with multiple lesions is

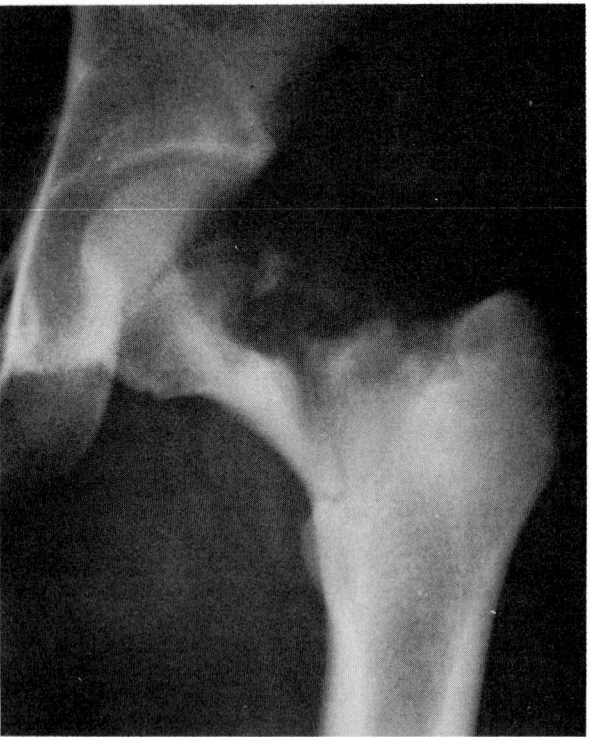

Figure 6. This rather aggressive chondroblastoma began in the epiphysis and subsequently has involved the superior femoral neck. Notice the lack of sclerotic borders to the lesion. A pathologic fracture has occurred through the femoral calcar.

touch as a result of the calcification. The articular surface of the adjacent joint may be penetrated by the tumor mass.

Histologically these lesions are highly cellular. The primary cell is usually described as polygonal in shape, with oval to round nuclei. In numerous areas of the tumor these cells produce a chondroid matrix. Multinucleated giant cells can be found throughout the lesion and are usually in the more cellular areas of the tumor. Hypercellularity often leads to a mistaken diagnosis of malignancy, particularly chondrosarcoma. Reactive bone may be found in the periphery of these tumors, leading to the mistaken diagnosis of osteosarcoma. Areas of focal calcification may be seen throughout the tumor, particularly in areas where a rich chondroid matrix has been deposited.

One of the points of controversy regarding the chondroblastoma is the occasionally aggressive local behavior that implies malignancy. Though generally considered a benign tumor, the chondroblastoma may occasionally penetrate the joint surface or the cortex of the bone involved and invade the adjacent soft tissues. There are scattered reports of pulmonary metastases from chondroblastoma.

Conservative treatment in the form of curettage and bone grafting is indicated. Care must be taken to preserve the adjacent articular cartilage. When the epiphyseal plate is involved, epiphysiodesis may be required. Incomplete removal will result in recurrence. Irradiation has not proved beneficial.

Chondromyxoid Fibroma

Like the chondroblastoma, the chondromyxoid fibroma is an uncommon benign skeletal neoplasm of cartilaginous origin. As the name implies, there are other cellular elements present. This tumor is most frequently found in the second and third decades of life, is evenly distributed between the sexes, and has a predilection for the metaphyseal ends of long bones. The distal femur and proximal tibia are the most common sites, although lesions involving the bones of the upper extremity, hands, feet, vertebrae, skull, and pelvis have been reported.

The usual presenting symptoms are dull aching pain in the area of the neoplasm or the slow development of a painful mass. Radiographically this lesion is eccentrically located within the metaphysis, usually with some expansion and thinning of the overlying cortex. A sclerotic margin surrounds the tumor. Some central sclerotic septae may produce a lobulated appearance on x-ray. Grossly the specimens are well circumscribed and present a lobulated firm outer surface which has the appearance of cartilage. Despite the myxoid element to this tumor, it lacks the gelatinous consistency expected of that tissue.

Histologically this tumor contains three basic tissue elements. The cartilaginous portion may consist of distorted hyaline cartilage similar to the enchondroma, although this tissue usually does not predominate. In certain areas the chondrocytes may resemble the benign chondroblastoma with polygonal cell borders and relative hypercellularity. Myxomatous areas within the tumor are identified by stellate cells within a pale blue background matrix. This myxomatous tissue may be highly bizarre and suggest malig-

nancy. Fibrous septae may be seen dividing the tissue into distinct lobules. Multinucleated giant cells are common. Because of the broad spectrum of histologic appearance, care must be taken not to erroneously diagnose this as a malignant lesion.

There is a risk of local recurrence following curettage, which is reported as high as 25 per cent in some series. For this reason en bloc excision is to be preferred over curettage when possible. Autogenous or homologous bone graft is used to fill the defect.

Chondrosarcoma

Malignant cartilaginous tumors may arise from preexisting benign neoplasms of bone. Malignant degeneration of a benign precursor produces a secondary chondrosarcoma. Malignant cartilaginous tumors may arise de novo in bone and are designated primary chondrosarcomas. Chondrosarcoma is the third most common primary malignant neoplasm of bone. The majority of chondrosarcomas are thought to be primary rather than secondary.

Chondrosarcoma shows a slight male predominance and occurs most frequently in the fourth, fifth, and sixth decades of life. In contrast to other malignant neoplasms of bone, which tend to occur in the peripheral skeleton, chondrosarcoma is most frequently encountered in the central flat bones (pelvis, scapula, sacrum), although any bone may be involved. Rarely are these tumors found in the small bones of the hand or foot or in the facial bones. The chondrosarcoma grows slowly and patients with tumors of the extremity usually present with a history of local pain and swelling about the lesion that may have been present for months or years. Tumors within the pelvis grow silently without symptoms for a considerable period of time unless located near sensitive structures such as the sciatic or femoral nerves. There are no specific laboratory data that aid in the diagnosis of chondrosarcoma.

Radiographically this tumor demonstrates calcification occurring within the body of the tumor outlining a lobulated pattern. Calcification may be sparse and peripherally located or may be dense enough to obliterate the surrounding bone detail. Heavily calcified lesions are more differentiated. Poorly differentiated, more aggressive lesions tend to show less calcification and, when located centrally or within the pelvis, may be difficult to diagnose radiographically. The use of arteriography is helpful in evaluating pelvic lesions, more for the anatomic information it provides about the location of the tumor relative to other structures than for any specific information about malignancy. More aggressive tumors tend to be more vascular (Fig. 7).

On gross examination, the surface of a chondrosarcoma has a lobulated, cauliflower-like appearance. Malignant behavior is typified by invasion of adjacent muscles and entrapment of muscle fibers between lobules of tumor. Outgrowths of tumor may extend for some distance along a fascial plane. When previous needle biopsy has been performed, tumor may be found growing up the needle tract to the surface of the skin. On cut section the surface is pearly white and opalescent. There may be areas of degeneration and liquefaction within the center of the tumor. Areas of calcification appear as dense, chalk-white areas on the cut surface.

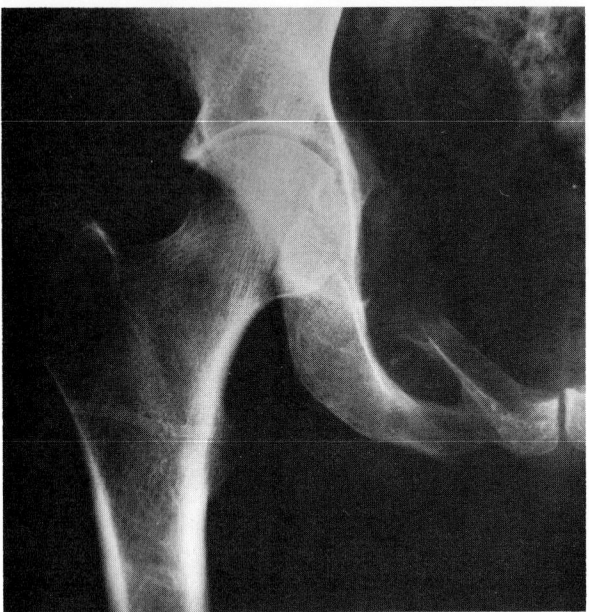

Figure 7. Chondrosarcoma. This lytic lesion has destroyed the pubic ramus from the level of the acetabulum to the mid portion of the obturator foramen. There is minor stippling within the defect. This lesion was an aggressive chondrosarcoma.

The histologic appearance of the chondrosarcoma is variable. Some lesions show well-differentiated hyaline cartilage with minimal cellular atypia, and the diagnosis of malignancy may be difficult. The radiographic appearance, the gross appearance, and the clinical behavior of the tumor must be taken into account in making the diagnosis. In lesions less well-differentiated, the usual characteristics of malignancy will appear. Variations in nuclear size and shape, hypercellularity, multiple nuclei per cartilaginous lacunae, and mitotic figures will be seen. In some areas reactive bone formation is encountered. It is important to determine whether this represents malignant bone formation or reactive bone formation, since the former implies a diagnosis of osteosarcoma with a more grave prognosis.

At the present time, total surgical excision of a chondrosarcoma is the treatment of choice. Since this tumor has a high incidence of local recurrence, meticulous technique should be employed to avoid contamination of the operative field. Curative excision may require amputation of the limb involved and should include total removal of any previous biopsy site or tract. Any biopsy of a suspected chondrosarcoma should be planned in such a way that the biopsy incision can be removed with subsequent definitive surgery.

Local recurrence of this tumor is the rule, and metastases occur late. Extension of the tumor along fascial planes and blood vessels is frequently seen. When pulmonary metastases occur they tend to be located peripherally within the lung. Because of the slow growth of this lesion, excision of pulmonary metastases may be considered in appropriate cases.

Radiation therapy has not proved effective in the control of chondrosarcoma. There are currently studies underway evaluating the effectiveness of various chemotherapeutic agents (adriamycin, methotrexate), but no definitive answers have been obtained.

TUMORS OF OSSEOUS ORIGIN

Osteoid Osteoma

This benign lesion of bone was described by Jaffe in 1935 and is considered by some to be an inflammatory lesion. Most observers feel that this is a true benign neoplasm of bone. The osteoid osteoma is a solitary, exquisitely painful lesion. Bones of the lower extremity are most frequently affected, although almost any bone may be involved. This tumor most often occurs in the first and second decades of life and is more common in males.

The most common presenting symptom is pain, which may be described as mild to intense. The pain is of a persistent nature that is neither accentuated by activity nor relieved by rest or immobilization. Often the pain will be totally relieved by the use of aspirin. In some patients the pain may be increased by the use of alcohol.

Because these lesions are small and sometimes difficult to demonstrate on x-ray, many patients will have seen several doctors and will be thought to have an emotional problem rather than true physical complaints. Also, these lesions may sometimes mimic other diseases. Osteoid osteomas of the vertebral arch may simulate intervertebral disc disease, including radiating leg pain.

The radiographic appearance of the osteoid osteoma depends on the location. When these lesions are located in cancellous bone, they present as a central radiolucent defect surrounded by a dense cloud of sclerotic bone. In lesions of long standing, the sclerosis may obscure the radiolucent center or "nidus" on routine films. Tomography may be required to identify the lesion. The osteoid osteoma may also be located in cortical bone. In this position it produces thickening of the cortex, again with a radiolucent nidus. It is this dense surrounding sclerosis that has led some to consider this lesion an inflammatory one.

Grossly the osteoid osteoma has a red, friable center surrounded by a dense margin of sclerotic bone. In older lesions the central zone may be obscured by progressive bony sclerosis and difficult to identify.

The microscopic appearance of the osteoid osteoma is characteristic. Peripherally there is dense reactive new bone formation. The central nidus is composed of a fine network of close-packed trabeculae of partially mineralized osteoid. The surfaces of these trabeculae are usually lined with benign osteoblasts. In older lesions, mineralization of the nidus may be seen and usually begins centrally. The nidus is vascular, with numerous small capillary channels. Nerve endings have been demonstrated within the nidus.

The osteoid osteoma is completely cured by en bloc excision, which allows identification of the lesion and assures complete removal. Because these lesions are small, x-ray control in the operating room may be required to assure proper localization. In some locations, en bloc excision may not be feasible and curettage is necessary. Incompletely curetted lesions may recur.

The relief of pain is immediate following excision. There is some belief that these lesions will gradually disappear with time. Because the pain has been known to persist for many years, surgery is usually indicated.

Osteoblastoma

The osteoblastoma is a benign solitary lesion of bone. This lesion occurs most frequently in the vertebral column, although almost any bone may be involved. A fairly uncommon lesion, the osteoblastoma has no apparent sex predilection. Patients in the first three decades of life are most frequently affected.

The most common presenting complaint is pain in the region of the lesion. The symptoms are comparable to those of the osteoid osteoma although generally not as severe. Relief by aspirin and exacerbation by the use of alcohol are not seen with this tumor.

Radiographically the osteoblastoma produces a central radiolucent defect with a surrounding zone of sclerotic bone. Peripheral sclerosis is not nearly as exuberant as that of the osteoid osteoma and may be lacking altogether. Whereas vertebral osteoid osteomas are found only in the neural arch of the vertebrae, the osteoblastoma is characteristically located within the vertebral body. When present in long bones, there may be widening of the transverse diameter of the bone and periosteal elevation.

Because the osteoblastoma shares certain characteristics with the osteoid osteoma, it is called by some a "giant osteoid osteoma." One of the differences between these lesions is the greater size of the osteoblastoma, which exceeds 1 cm. and may range up to 10 cm. in diameter. Grossly the cut surface of the osteoblastoma is a purplish red as a result of its vascularity. It is the microscopic appearance of the osteoblastoma that most resembles the osteoid osteoma. The central area is composed of primitive disorganized bars of osteoid surrounded by benign osteoblasts. There may be calcification occurring within some of the central zones of osteoid. The lesion is richly supplied with capillaries, and multinucleated giant cells are seen throughout.

The osteoblastoma is most appropriately treated by en bloc excision or curettage, whichever seems most appropriate to the location of the lesion.

Osteosarcoma

With the exception of multiple myeloma, the osteosarcoma is the most common malignant primary neoplasm of bone. This tumor occurs with a frequency of about 1 in 100,000, or about 2,000 cases per year in this country. Osteosarcoma usually affects those in the second decade of life (the mean age being 15 years). Occurring in the metaphyseal ends of long bone, the distal femur is the most frequent site (30 per cent), followed by the proximal tibia and proximal humerus in that order. Almost any bone may be involved.

The most common presenting symptom is pain at the site of the tumor, which has been present for one or two months. There may be local swelling and some increased heat in the area. When the tumor is near a joint, there may be limitation of motion. A small percentage of patients present with a pathologic fracture as their initial complaint.

Radiographically there are areas of new bone formation and areas of lytic destruction. Within the metaphysis of a long bone, this tumor classically produces a "sunburst" appearance, which consists of trabeculae of bone oriented at right angles to the cortical surface beneath the periosteum. These trabeculae are mixed reactive and malignant bone. Some tumors may be almost purely lytic in nature, while others may produce abundant amounts of both malignant bone and surrounding reactive bone (Fig. 8).

Histologically one sees a disorderly deposition of osteoid surrounded by malignant osteoblasts. Nuclear atypia, hyperchromatism, and bizarre mitoses are

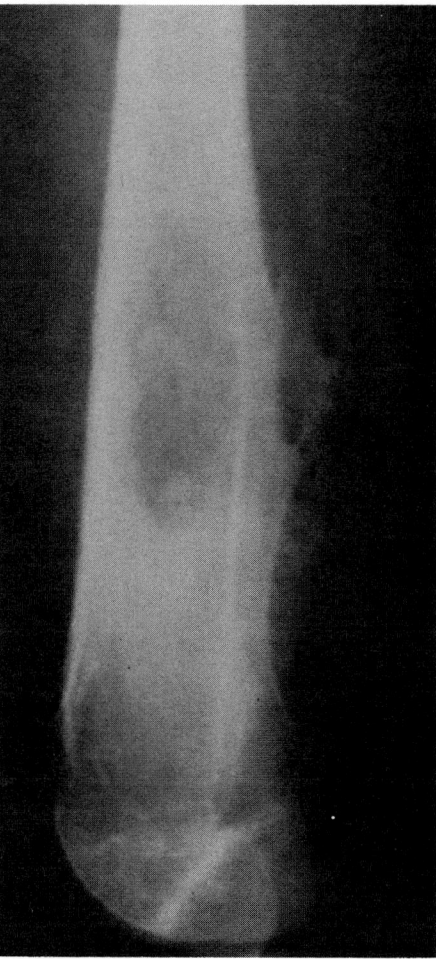

Figure 8. This lateral x-ray of the distal femur of a 14-year-old girl shows a central radiolucent defect in the femoral metaphysis, with periosteal elevation overlying the lesion. There has been erosion through the femoral cortex. Notice the "sunburst" appearance of the subperiosteal new bone along the posterior femoral cortex. This is the typical appearance of an osteosarcoma.

seen. In addition to the malignant bone production seen in an osteosarcoma, there may be areas of malignant cartilage and fibrous tissue. Despite the amount of these tissues present, if malignant bone is being produced, the lesion should be classified as an osteosarcoma in terms of its prognosis.

The treatment of osteosarcoma requires amputation of the limb at a level above the tumor. It has been recognized that osteosarcoma may produce satellite lesions within the medullary canal of the bone involved proximal to the major lesion. These "skip lesions" are usually not seen on x-ray and are discovered only on pathologic examination of the specimen. For this reason, many believe that amputation should be carried out through the joint above the bone involved. Others have followed the practice of amputation through the bone involved at a level proximal to the tumor. Although the incidence of skip lesions varies in different reports from 5 to 25 per cent, the overall survival figures for patients treated by disarticulation above the bone involved versus amputation through the bone involved do not vary significantly. The five-year survival rate of patients treated by radical amputation for osteosarcoma is approximately 20 per cent. Since the late 1950's, a number of patients have been treated by megavoltage irradiation of the lesion followed by delayed amputation three to six months later if no metastases are demonstrated. The overall five-year survival figures for this treatment also approximate 20 per cent.

The average length of time between diagnosis and the development of pulmonary metastases is six months. The average length of time between diagnosis and death from metastases is one year. Approximately 80 per cent of those patients who will die of their metastases do so within the first two years following diagnosis. Because osteosarcoma is known to invade blood vessels early in the course of development, it is now assumed that pulmonary microemboli are already present at the time the diagnosis is made. It would further appear that approximately 20 per cent of patients have some innate resistance to their tumor or that their tumor is less virulent.

In recent years adjunctive chemotherapy has been used as a means of treatment. Adriamycin and methotrexate are the two most promising agents. Used in combination with initial radical amputation, the early figures show a disease-free rate of 50 per cent or better at two years in several small series. This would indicate that the overall five-year survival may well be improved by this form of treatment. There are also studies underway at this time regarding immunotherapy as a means of adjunctive treatment. The early figures from these studies would also indicate that survival may be improved by the use of immunotherapy.

TUMORS OF FIBROUS ORIGIN

Nonossifying Fibroma

This lesion is most likely not a true neoplasm but a focal developmental defect. Occurring primarily in children and located in the metaphysis of long bones,

this lesion is also known as a benign metaphyseal cortical defect or fibrous cortical defect. These lesions are usually an incidental finding on radiographs taken for other reasons. Rarely they may be large enough to create weakness in the bone involved and lead to pathologic fracture. The nonossifying fibroma occurs with equal frequency in males and females. The lower extremities are most often involved, and there may be multiple lesions.

The nonossifying fibroma is located eccentrically in the metaphysis of a long bone lying immediately beneath the cortex, which may be somewhat thinned. There is a distinct sclerotic margin to the intramedullary portion of the lesion. The central portion is relatively radiolucent and appears to be divided by bony septae (Fig. 9).

Grossly the contents of a nonossifying fibroma are soft and yellow to brown. Histologically one sees swirls of fibrous tissue containing numerous multinucleated giant cells and lipid-filled histiocytes. In

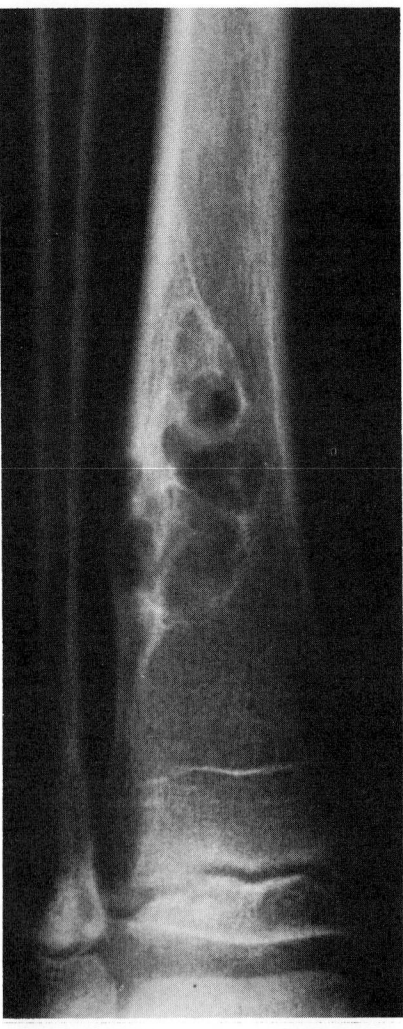

Figure 9. This eccentrically located metaphyseal lesion has smooth sclerotic borders on the medullary side and has expanded the overlying cortex. This appearance is typical of a nonossifying fibroma.

lesions of considerable age, cholesterol clefts may be seen.

The natural history of the nonossifying fibroma is one of gradual healing as the patient matures. There is no indication for surgery unless the lesion is demonstrated to be increasing in size and threatening a pathologic fracture. Curettage and bone grafting are curative.

Giant Cell Tumor

This uncommon neoplasm arises in the third and fourth decades of life and is almost invariably found in the epiphyses of long bones, with subsequent involvement of the adjacent metaphyses. This anatomic location helps distinguish it from almost all other skeletal neoplasms. The presence of a radiolucent defect in an epiphysis strongly suggests the diagnosis of giant cell tumor. Beyond this, the appearance of this lesion may vary considerably. In the slowly growing, less aggressive forms, the lesion presents as a central radiolucent defect, usually eccentrically located within the bone involved with thinning and expansion of the overlying cortex. Thin bony septae within the center of the lesion produce a loculated appearance. There is usually extension into the adjacent metaphysis. In more aggressive tumors, rapid growth of the lesion may produce a poorly demarcated edge with little sclerotic bone peripherally. There may be penetration of the overlying cortex, with extension of tumor into the adjacent soft tissues.

Grossly the tumor is red-gray in appearance with areas of soft yellow material representing lipid deposits and areas of brown stained tissue indicating local hemorrhage. There may be areas of cystic degeneration.

It is the microscopic appearance of this tumor from which the name is derived. Numerous multinucleated giant cells are found within a fibrous stroma. Focal areas of hemorrhage and collections of lipid-filled histiocytes are seen. Reactive bone formation within the lesion (which produces the septae seen on x-ray) is common and must not be mistaken for malignant bone formation, leading to the erroneous diagnosis of osteosarcoma.

The giant cell tumor may be benign or malignant. In well-selected series it is estimated that 20 to 30 per cent of these tumors will behave in a malignant fashion. Within the basic histologic definition of this lesion there may be considerable variation. Efforts have been made to grade this tumor on the basis of its fibrous stroma and on the number of giant cells present. In general, those tumors with poorly differentiated fibrous stroma have a higher likelihood of local recurrence and pulmonary metastasis than well-differentiated tumors, although the latter may occasionally show malignant behavior. Since the histologic appearance may vary from area to area within the same tumor, extensive sampling of the lesion is necessary and needle biopsy of the lesion is to be discouraged.

Curettage and bone grafting are the accepted methods of treatment of giant cell tumors. Local recurrence may be high with this method of treatment. When feasible, en bloc resection of the tumor and bone grafting are desirable. Recently, liquid nitrogen cryotherapy combined with curettage has been used in an effort to reduce local recurrence. There is no evidence that irradiation is of any therapeutic benefit. There is some evidence to suggest that irradiation may induce malignant change within these lesions. Recurrent, locally aggressive lesions may require amputation.

Fibrosarcoma

Fibrous tissue within the marrow cavity may give rise to primary fibrosarcoma of bone. This uncommon skeletal neoplasm is seen most frequently in the lower extremities (50 per cent), although almost any bone may be involved. There is a wide age distribution of this lesion, with the highest incidence in the third and fourth decades of life. Symptoms vary according to the location of the lesion and the rate of growth.

Fibrosarcoma produces a variety of patterns on x-ray, all of which basically involve destruction of bone. The lesion may be well circumscribed within the metaphysis, with thinning or penetration of the overlying cortex. If the growth is slow, there may be a thin sclerotic border. With more rapid growth the border is usually ill defined. In contrast to this "geographic" pattern of growth, this tumor may produce a picture of mottled destruction from permeative growth within the bone.

The microscopic appearance of bone is similar to that of its soft tissue counterpart. Malignant fibroblasts of varying degrees of differentiation are seen. Multinucleated giant cells are present in some tumors.

Wide local excision is the treatment of choice where feasible. If the lesion cannot be locally resected, amputation through the joint above is recommended. Radiation therapy has not proved to be of benefit. Chemotherapy of fibrosarcoma is under investigation at this time. In most series, a 30 per cent five-year survival rate can be expected with adequate treatment.

TUMORS OF MARROW CELL ORIGIN

Ewing's Sarcoma

This fortunately uncommon malignancy occurs most frequently in the first and second decades of life. It is included here as a tumor of marrow cell origin, although some believe that it arises from endothelial cells. Although almost any bone may be involved, long bones of the extremities are the most frequent site of Ewing's sarcoma.

Patients present with complaints of local pain and swelling in the region of the tumor. There may be fever, leukocytosis, and an increased erythrocyte sedimentation rate. These findings, together with the early radiographic appearance of Ewing's sarcoma, may lead to a mistaken diagnosis of osteomyelitis. In some patients the onset is less abrupt and patients may present with a large local tumor mass that has been present for many months.

The radiographic appearance of Ewing's sarcoma in the diaphysis of a long bone is one of periosteal elevation or "onion skin" appearance as a result of permeation of the cortex by tumor. In this respect the lesion may resemble osteomyelitis. In other locations the radiographic changes are less distinct. In general, this tumor produces bone destruction of varying degrees. The changes may be slight, suggesting chondrosarcoma, or may be extensive and rapid, suggesting an osteolytic osteosarcoma. Grossly the tumor may be partially necrotic, resembling purulent exudate. Areas of hemorrhage may be seen. Microscopically the tumor is composed of uniform round cells gathered in nests or cords and separated by fibrous septae. They have a hazy appearance and indistinct cytoplasmic borders. Difficulty may arise in distinguishing this tumor from metastatic neuroblastoma and reticulum cell sarcoma of bone.

Histochemical staining for glycogen may aid in the differential diagnosis. Some Ewing's sarcomas contain glycogen on PAS staining or on electron microscopic examination, whereas glycogen is absent in reticulum cell sarcoma.

The overall five-year survival rate for Ewing's sarcoma treated by amputation of the limb involved is less than 10 per cent. In recent years the use of radiation therapy to the entire bone involved combined with chemotherapy has produced longer disease-free periods and higher survival rates.

Reticulum Cell Sarcoma

In contrast to the Ewing's sarcoma, reticulum cell sarcoma is primarily a disease of adults, occurring in the later decades of life. It produces symptoms of local pain and swelling which, in contrast to the Ewing's sarcoma, may be quite slow in their development.

Radiographically this tumor produces subtle permeative destruction of bone. Arising within the medullary cavity, it may extend a considerable distance along the shaft of the long bone. Periosteal elevation may occur but is relatively uncommon. The cortex is gradually thinned and eroded and pathologic fracture may result (Fig. 10).

Histologically this tumor is composed of solid sheets of reticulum cells with varying degrees of differentiation and a background fibrous stroma. A reticulum stain may be helpful in the diagnosis and aids in the distinction of this lesion from Ewing's sarcoma.

Irradiation and chemotherapy are considered the treatment of choice and should include the entire bone involved. Amputation does not improve the survival rate, since this lesion may be multifocal.

Plasma Cell Myeloma

This malignant neoplasm of marrow cell origin is the most common primary malignant neoplasm of bone. It is most often seen in the late decades of life and more frequently in males than in females. The disease may vary from a solitary lesion to widespread skeletal involvement.

The symptoms vary from local pain and discomfort to systemic symptoms of anemia, fever, hypercalcemia, and renal failure related to the extensive skeletal involvement and the abnormal production of immunoglobulins.

This neoplasm characteristically produces lytic destruction of bone. Usually there is a "punched out" lesion with little or no accompanying sclerosis. The absence of reactive bone formation is borne out by the

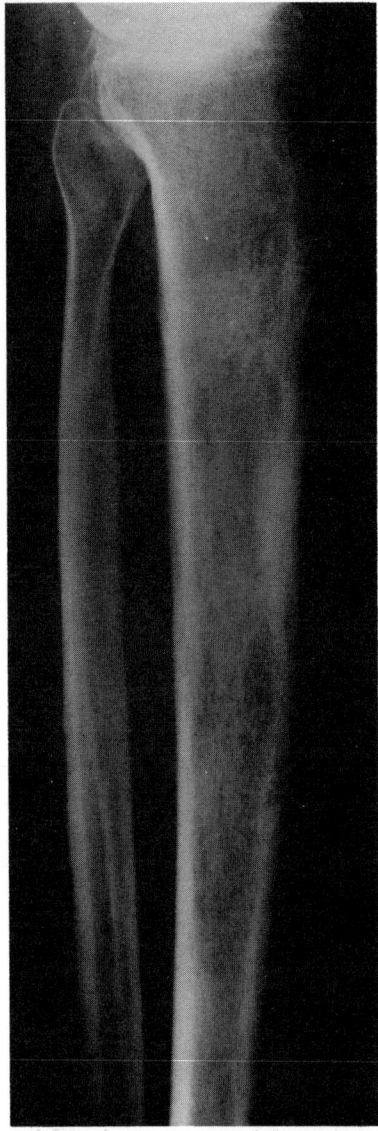

Figure 10. This lateral view of the tibia shows permeative destruction of bone throughout the upper third of the tibial shaft. There is mottled lucency both in the cortex and cancellous bone. This appearance is typical of the reticulum cell sarcoma.

observation that the lesions of myeloma are often silent on a bone scan. Pathologic fracture may be seen as an initial finding.

The diagnosis of myeloma is made by marrow aspiration and the demonstration of abnormal plasma cells. In patients with disseminated disease, Bence Jones protein may be found in the urine in approximately 50 per cent of cases. Serum electrophoresis will demonstrate an abnormal amount of globulins. Urine electrophoresis is also helpful when the diagnosis is in doubt and may show abnormal proteins in patients with a normal serum electrophorectic pattern.

Microscopically myeloma produces sheets of plasma cells. Usually these are fairly well-differentiated cells in which the eccentric nucleus and peripheral arrangement of chromatin within the nucleus can be identified. The more undifferentiated lesions may present a diagnostic problem in which the accessory laboratory data will be helpful. With the exception of biopsy for diagnosis or the treatment of pathologic fracture, the treatment of myeloma is nonsurgical. Currently, chemotherapy is the treatment of choice.

REFERENCES

1. Aegerter, E., and Kirkpatrick, J. A., Jr.: Orthopedic Diseases: Physiology, Pathology, Radiology, 4th ed. Philadelphia, W. B. Saunders Company, 1975.
2. Allen, A. R., and Stevenson, A. W.: A ten year follow-up of combined drug therapy and early fusion in bone tuberculosis. J. Bone Joint Surg., 49A:1001, 1967.
3. Barnes, R., and Catto, M.: Chondrosarcoma of bone. J. Bone Joint Surg., 48B:729, 1966.
4. Boland, A. L.: Acute hematogenous osteomyelitis. Orthop. Clin. North Am., 3:225, 1972.
5. Clowson, D. K., and Dunn, A. W.: Management of common bacterial infections of bones and joints. J. Bone Joint Surg., 49A:164, 1967.
6. Dahlin, D. C.: Bone Tumors, 2nd ed. Springfield, Ill., Charles C Thomas, Publisher, 1967.
7. Dahlin, D. C., and Coventry, M. D.: Osteogenic sarcoma. A study of 600 cases. J. Bone Joint Surg., 49A:101, 1967.
8. Dahlin, D. C., and Henderson, E. D.: Chondrosarcoma, a surgical and pathological problem. Review of 212 cases. J. Bone Joint Surg., 38A:1025, 1956.
9. Dahlin, D. C., Cupps, R. E., and Johnson, E. W.: Giant cell tumor: A study of 195 cases. Cancer, 25:1061, 1970.
10. Enneking, W. F.: Principles of musculoskeletal pathology. Gainesville, Florida, W. F. Enneking, M.D., 1970.
11. Friedman, M. A., and Carter, S. K.: The therapy of osteogenic sarcoma — current status and thoughts for the future. J. Surg. Oncol., 4:482, 1972.
12. Hustu, H. O., Pinkel, D., and Pratt, C. B.: Treatment of clinically localized Ewing's sarcoma with radiotherapy and combination chemotherapy. Cancer, 30:1522, 1972.
13. Jaffe, H. L.: Metabolic, generative, and inflammatory diseases of bones and joints. Philadelphia, Lea and Febiger, 1972.
14. Jaffe, H. L.: Tumors and Tumorous Conditions of the Bones and Joints, 2nd ed. Philadelphia, Lea and Febiger, 1961.
15. Jaffe, N.: Recent advances in the chemotherapy of metastatic osteosarcoma. Cancer, 30:1627, 1972.
16. Kelly, P. J., and Karlson, A. G.: Musculoskeletal tuberculosis. Mayo Clin. Proc., 44:73, 1969.
17. Morrey, B. F., Bianco, A. J., Jr., and Rhodes, K. H.: Septic arthritis in children. Orthop. Clin. North Am., 6:923, 1975.
18. Morrey, B. F., and Peterson, H. A.: Hematogenous pyogenic osteomyelitis in children. Orthop. Clin. North Am., 6:935, 1975.
19. Morton, D. L.: Immunological aspects of neoplasia: A rational basis for immunotherapy. Ann. Intern. Med., 74:587, 1971.
20. Pritchard, D. J.: Granulomatous infections of bones and joints. Orthop. Clin. North Am., 6:1029, 1975.
21. Rhodes, K. H.: Antibiotic management of acute osteomyelitis and septic arthritis in children. Orthop. Clin. North Am., 6:915, 1975.
22. Rosen, G., Suwansirikul, S., et al.: High-dose methotrexate with citrovorum factor rescue and adriamycin in childhood osteogenic sarcoma. Cancer, 33:1151, 1974.
23. Spjut, H. J., Dorfman, H. D., Fechner, M. D., and Akerman, L. V.: Tumors of Bone and Cartilage. Fasc. 5, 2nd ser. Washington, D.C., Armed Forces Institute of Pathology, 1971.
24. Stetson, J. W., DePone, R. J., and Southwick, W. O.: Acute septic arthritis of the hip in children. Clin. Orthop., 56:105, 1968.
25. Sweetnam, R., Knowelden, J., and Seddon, H.: Bone sarcoma — treatment by irradiation, amputation or a combination of the two. Br. Med. J., 2:363, 1971.
26. Tachdjian, M. O.: Pediatric Orthopedics. Philadelphia, W. B. Saunders Company, 1972.
27. Waldvogel, F. A., Medoff, G., and Schwartz, M. N.: Osteomyelitis: A review of clinical features, therapeutic considerations and unusual aspects. N. Engl. J. Med., 282:198, 260, 316, 1970.

X

THE HAND

J. Leonard Goldner, M.D.

The hand is an organ system requiring special study and a particular understanding of anatomy, biomechanics, and the physiology of all the modalities of sensation and fine coordination. Each part of the composite is a complete unit. From a neurologic standpoint, the opposite cerebral cortex and all the neural pathways must be intact for normal hand function. Peripheral nerve distribution is related to motor power, strength, and skin sensitivity. The pattern of innervation by each of the major peripheral nerves must be determined quickly and accurately, not only to provide early treatment but also to determine the method of late reconstruction. The physiology of nerve injury and regeneration and the technical aspects of micro- and macrosurgery, as they relate to nerve repair, must be learned in order to provide maximum anatomic realignment and functional recovery.

Management of skin deficiencies and deformities includes an understanding of free skin grafting, the use of pedicle skin flaps, and the management of local skin in order to release and prevent contractures. The place for the skin incisions, the excision of skin contractures, and the treatment of hand problems are shown in Figure 1. The flexor and extensor tendons are part of an intricate system of muscle-tendon units that function in a coordinated way. The tendons are covered by specialized epitenon and peritenon, which provide smooth gliding and rapid motion. The blood supply of the tendon is unique and, if interrupted, leads to localized fibrosis and constriction. Tendon ruptures, lacerations, and erosions are all involved in the many pathologic conditions that affect bending and straightening of the fingers (Fig. 2). Tendons can be freed of scar tissue, repaired if lacerated, temporarily replaced if they are scarred severely, elongated by lengthening, permanently replaced by autogenous

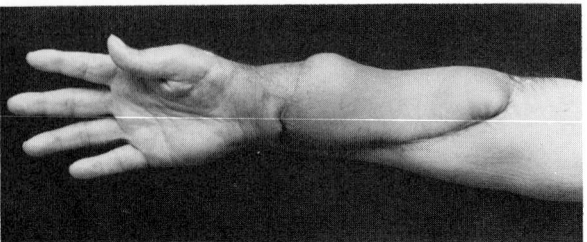

Figure 1. Severe injury involving skin, peripheral nerves, flexor tendons and the forearm bones. Initial management included meticulous wound excision, irrigation, and relief of all tension on closed compartments. The abdominal pedicle flap was then applied, and subsequently reconstructive procedures have included nerve repair and tendon transfers. The patient has a functional hand, no pain, and a good range of motion. Use of a pedicle flap is helpful in providing coverage, allowing tendons to glide under skin with good nutrition, and provides tissue through which another operation can be done without risk.

grafting, and transferred from one point of function to another when a particular deficiency occurs. The elasticity of a muscle-tendon unit, the importance of the muscle excursion, and the relationship of a muscle-tendon to the adjacent joints must be considered when early and late treatment is being planned and completed.

The joints of the wrist and hand are dependent on articular cartilage, and the biochemistry of cartilage and collagen are part of the consideration related to maintaining joint function. The various forms of arthritis or trauma that affect articular cartilage will directly and indirectly alter the range of joint motion and, in turn, decrease strength and dexterity. Damaged joints can be replaced by silicone-Dacron prostheses, and damaged tendons can be temporarily replaced by silicone-Dacron rods. The development of a medical grade silicone has provided the surgeon with

joint and tendon replacements that were not as readily available as they are now.

The vascular and lymphatic channels are essential to the nutrition of the hand, which makes the difference between viability and nonviability after trauma or excision of pathologic tissue. Open arterial channels are essential to oxygenation of tissue. Free venous outflow is also essential to the viability of skin, subcutaneous tissue, and muscle. During the past few years, development of improved microsurgical techniques, with high magnification for visualization, and the development of small instruments and miniature needles with fine suture have provided the surgeon with the proper equipment to suture vessels as small as 0.5 mm. These developments have made replantation a feasible procedure.

DIAGNOSTIC METHODS

Technical equipment and tests desirable for diagnosis and determination of the adequacy of treatment include the following:

1. *The thermogram* provides information about blood flow into the extremity. Stellate ganglion block, after the original thermography pattern has been established, will give visible evidence of increased blood flow.

2. *A Doppler ultrasound technique* will provide audible signals directly dependent on blood flow in the finger or the entire hand.

3. *Arteriography and venography* provide a visible pattern of the veins and the arteries after injection of contrast medium. Plain roentgenograms and xeroradiograms give information about foreign bodies, soft tissue changes, and details concerning osseous structure. Magnification roentgenograms are helpful in determining microinjury to the bones and joints.

4. *Development of electronic flowmeters,* based on the principle of skin contact, blood volume, and a write-out on the cathode ray oscilloscope, provides immediate information about small volumes of blood within the part. Immediate information can be obtained about the viability of a part without depending on the presence of cyanosis, paleness, or erythema and without depending on skin temperature.

5. *Electromyography and nerve conduction speed,* using the special electromyogram units and the nerve conduction unit, are a part of the routine examination in determining a diagnosis when the patient has evidence of motor impairment or sensory involvement. Speed of nerve transmission will provide information about nerve compression lesion in various parts of the extremity. Also, information about closed nerve injuries and data concerning nerve regeneration can be determined from this apparatus.

6. *Other diagnostic tests and instruments:*
   a. *Sweat testing* with tincture of iodine and starch-oil mixture determines the presence of acetylcholine and cholinesterase (Fig. 3).
   b. *Peripheral nerve blocks* provide information about anomalous innervation. Multiple nerve injections will determine anatomic variations and provide the surgeon with information con-

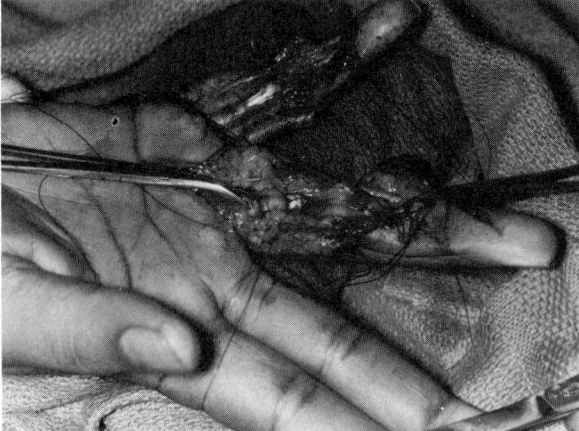

Figure 2. This child fell on a sharp object and lacerated flexor tendons and digital nerves in both the ring and little fingers. Delayed repair is being done, which included suture of a digital nerve in each digit and suture of the flexor digitorum profundus tendons within each digit after the annular ligaments had been trimmed. Satisfactory flexion power resulted.

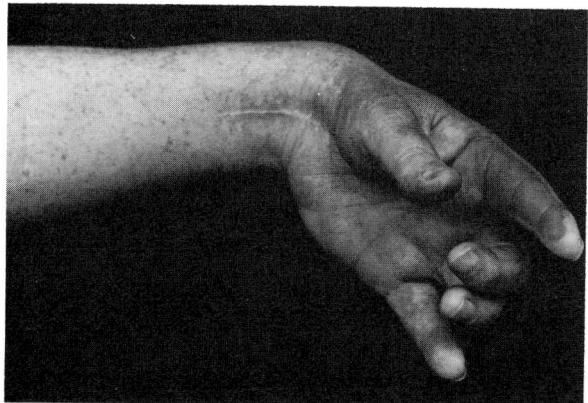

Figure 3. This hand and forearm deformity occurred when the patient was young and had an open fracture of the forearm bones, which resulted in compression of the brachial artery at the elbow. Ischemic contracture occurred, and ischemia of the median nerve resulted. Many years later, reconstructive procedures were done in order to improve the patient's ability to flex and extend the fingers and use the hand for hooking and grasping.

cerning suspected nerve lesions in spite of the absence of certain expected weakness in particular muscle groups, and sensory skin abnormalities which persist in spite of suspected nerve lesions.

c. *Hand gripper* (dynamometer) provides a baseline of strength for the uninvolved hand as compared to the hand with the lesion and also a series of readings in the same hand, dependent on nerve regeneration that occurs in time, improvement of joint function, and improvement of muscle strength.

d. *Pinch meter* provides the same kind of information concerning strength of pinch between thumb and index, and thumb and the adjacent fingers, with comparison between the uninvolved and the involved hand or fingers. The pinch meter is used at the initial examination and at regular intervals subsequently to provide a curve with a pinch designated over a specified time period (Fig. 4).

e. *Stellate ganglion block,* prior to and after flowmeter testing, will give information about blood volume and determine if certain pain patterns are relieved by stellate ganglion blocking. This gives information regarding the value of sympathectomy in the management of vascular insufficiency and pain.

f. *Transcutaneous nerve stimulator* is a relatively new apparatus, which can be placed on painful areas in the hand in order to alter the severity of unpleasant sensory output and change the quality and type of sensory input. If the transcutaneous nerve stimulator is partially helpful and if peripheral blockade of the nerve eliminates pain, then the peripheral nerve stimulator can be placed about the nerve and attached to an external power pack that provides partial or complete relief to the painful peripheral nerve, which has been mapped so that the sensory fibers can be read-

ily localized (see section on peripheral nerve stimulator).

HISTORICAL ASPECTS

Abraham Colles, Professor of Surgery at the Royal College of Surgeons in Dublin, Ireland, in his treatise, "Treatment of Fractures of the Distal End of the Radius," outlines the diagnosis and treatment of this fracture clearly. He also described a student and professor who, while dissecting a body in the anatomy laboratory, cut their fingers. Colles described an ascending infection with streaks running up the arm and shoulder, extensive abscess formation, and a high fever. The professor died, but the student lived. Colles recommended that in the future persons working in the anatomy laboratory should wash wounds with turpentine if they were cut during a dissection.

Dupuytren, as Professor of Surgery in Paris, described hyperplasia of the palmar fascia. The condition was subsequently named after him and is called *Dupuytren's contracture.* Duchenne wrote a book entitled "The Physiology of Motion," in which he showed the true action of living muscles, and was the author of "Muscles of the Forearm."

The muscular forces that act on flexion of the forearm, on pronation, and on supination are so distributed that only one muscle produces each of these movements independently of the other movements, or that only one muscle produces simultaneous flexion and supination, or flexion and pronation. Thus, the brachialis is an independent flexor; the brachial biceps is a flexor supinator; the muscle called *long supinator* (brachioradialis) is a flexor pronator, and the three muscles – the supinator, pronator teres, and pronator quadratus – are independently supinators and prona-

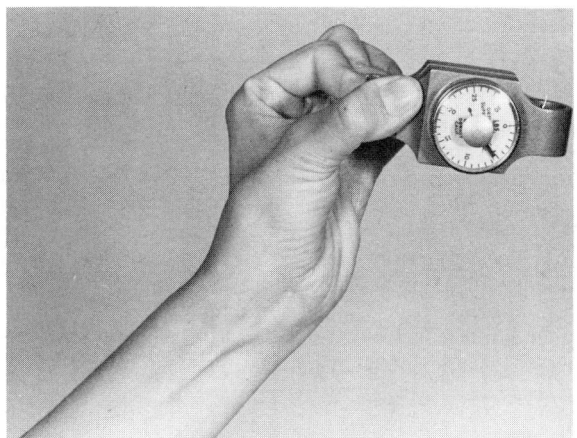

Figure 4. This patient had a laceration of the ulnar nerve in the mid-forearm secondary to an accident in the kitchen. She lost over half of her ability to grasp and pinch. The strength of pinch was five pounds per square inch as compared with a normal of twenty pounds. A delayed nerve repair was done, and subsequently multiple tendon transfers were completed in order to improve her pinch, grasp, and hook. The hand now approaches normal with partial motor and sensory regeneration after the nerve repair and reinforcement that has resulted from the tendon repair.

tors. No one will fail to recognize the usefulness of this mixed flexion-supination or pronation produced by the same muscles. These movements produced without special effort are very frequent in the activities of the upper extremity. It is also important for the skillful use of the hand that pronation and supination be made independent of flexion and extension of the forearm. Only on very strong effort do all the muscles participating in these movements contract synergistically.

S. Weir-Mitchell, a native of Philadelphia and an American neurologist working in Civil War hospitals, treated many patients with severe burning pain, usually in the arm and hands. This resulted from nerve lesions associated with gunshot wounds or fractures. He named the condition *causalgia*. During and after World War I, American surgeons received training in management of extremity trauma. Under the guidance of French surgeons, the technique of débridement (wound excision) was learned. Primary closure was avoided, and Dakin tubes of hypochlorite solution were placed into the wound. Primary closure was not performed; delayed closure was completed at a later time if spontaneous closure of the wound had not occurred.

Sterling Bunnell and Summer Koch were pioneers in the utilization of atraumatic surgical treatment in the mangement of hand injuries and in the reconstruction of hand problems. Koch advocated "forks not fingers" and emphasized the use of a face mask, gloves, and sterile instruments in managing acute injuries of the hand in the emergency room. Numerous clinical and laboratory investigators proposed new concepts that account for advances in management of acute trauma and reconstructive surgery during and since World War II. Kaplan described the surgical anatomy of the hand and forearm and has emphasized many of the anomalies that must be recognized in order to perform accurate reconstructive operations. Diagrammatic representations of live anatomic dissections have assisted many surgeons in developing operative procedures that have been used to solve special problems related to hand function. Milford, in a monograph on the extensor mechanism, delineates the anatomy of that aspect of the complicated action of the extensor and the intrinsic muscles. Numerous articles in the literature relate the function of the extensor and intrinsic mechanism to hand contractures (Goldner), as well as injury to the extensor mechanism, and contractures resulting from burns. Landsmeer emphasized the biomechanics and the anatomic arrangement of the extensor hood of the proximal interphalangeal joint. Electromyographic studies have provided the anatomic information about the functional hand.

ANATOMY AND KINESIOLOGY OF THE HAND

HAND EXAMINATION

Surface Anatomy

The surface anatomy can be studied continuously by referring to the volar and dorsal surface of the hand.

The uninvolved hand of the patient should always be examined first. The creases and wrinkles on the dorsum of the digits and the back of the hand correspond to joints. This skin elasticity allows accommodation of skin tension in both flexion and extension. Flexion of the fingers causes the loose skin to tighten and provide a full range of motion without tension or blanching. On the dorsum of the hand, the subcutaneous attachments are loose and provide space for fluid accumulation as well as swelling and for these reasons, incisions made on the dorsum of the hand separate more readily than those on the volar surface. The points of attachment of skin creases on the dorsum of the hand are important in preventing scar formation and shifting of the skin, and in addition assist in mobilizing skin after closed dorsal injuries. Attachments between the dermis and the dorsum of the extensor mechanism should be maintained if possible, and incisions should not be made at right angles to the skin creases. Large flaps undermined on the dorsum must be protected by meticulous hemostasis and external compression dressings.

The large and small veins on the dorsum of the hand should be saved whenever surgical incisions are made. The presence of these veins diminishes postoperative or posttraumatic edema. Subcutaneous nerves are readily visible after the skin is incised. These nerves *must not be damaged*. Many chronic pain syndromes result from interference with cutaneous nerves. Starting distally and reviewing the surface anatomy from distal to proximal, one sees the nail plate, the eponychium, the paronychium, the germinal layer of the nail, and the distal interphalangeal joint skin creases, all of which have an important relationship to each other. Trauma or infection in this area can be managed rationally if one knows the anatomy.

Extensor Mechanism of the Hand

Blanching of the dorsum of the proximal interphalangeal joint, which is apparent when the fingers are in full flexion, emphasizes the flexibility of the extensor mechanism and outlines the relationship of the extensor tendon to the condyles of the proximal phalanx. The extensor digitorum communis tendon is centralized over the metacarpal head and, on full flexion, the tendon shifts to both the radial and the ulnar sides and can be moved 5 to 6 mm. by rotation of the proximal phalanx (Fig. 5).

The *lateral bands* of the intrinsic tendons reinforce the joint retinaculum at the level of the proximal interphalangeal joint and, as finger flexion occurs, these lateral attachments are forced to the radial and ulnar sides; as extension occurs the lateral segments condense in the midline.

Skin over the dorsum of the web between the thumb and the index finger is flexible and pliable, and serves as a guide to the physiologic position of the thumb. The web fold at the base of the thumb should be visible, straight, and smooth if the abducted thumb is rotated and positioned properly in a dressing. If this skin fold is altered or not readily visible, then the thumb is inappropriately positioned while being immobilized in splint, brace, or cast.

The transverse creases and skin folds on the dorsum of the wrist coincide with the base of the metacarpals, the location of the carpal bones, the distal end of the ulna, the tubercle of the radius, and the origin of the extensor pollicis longus muscle. The relationship between the extensor pollicis longus and the extensor carpi radialis longus and brevis muscles is evident when the wrist is extended and the thumb is hyperextended and abducted.

Prominence of the extensor pollicis longus at the level of the metacarpal phalangeal joint of the thumb can be altered by rotation of the thumb. The thumb shifts radiad or ulnad with thumb rotation, and the flexibility of this joint on the ulnar side is evident. The indentation between the extensor pollicis longus, the extensor pollicis brevis, and the third tendon of this group—the abductor pollicis longus—is used to

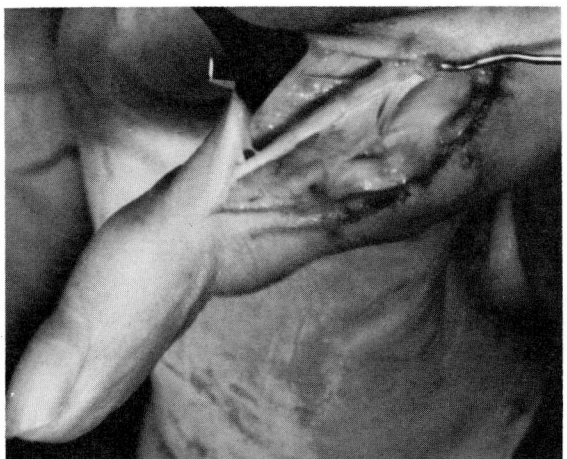

Figure 5. The extensor mechanism has been exposed through a lateral incision. There is a flexion deformity of the distal phalanx because of partial avulsion of the attachment of the common tendons. The central segment of the extensor tendon over the proximal interphalangeal joint shows the area where this tendon becomes adherent to the middle phalanx after complete partial rupture distally. This bowstringing displaces the proximal phalanx forward and causes stretching of the volar capsule and secondary tension on the flexor tendon. This aggravates the distal joint deformity (mallet finger). (Reprinted with permission of Harper and Row from Surgery of the Hand, J. L. Goldner, 1970.)

locate the carpometacarpal joint of the thumb (see Fig. 7). The annular ligament that restrains the abductor pollicis longus and the extensor pollicis brevis over the radius is directly over the radial tubercle. This area may be involved with tenosynovitis.

The appearance of intrinsic muscles of the hand is an important guide to myopathy or neuropathy. The size of the muscle mass between the first and second metacarpals is an index of the integrity of the interosseous muscles. The depth of the furrows between the metacarpals and the prominence of the abductor digiti quinti all provide information about the condition of the intrinsic muscles. In peripheral nerve injury, peripheral neuropathy, aging, or nerve root compression atrophy may result in thinning of the muscle mass and deepening of the space.

The flexibility of the metacarpals differs in that the first is most mobile and the fifth metacarpal is also movable. The two central metacarpals are stable, and the fourth provides both dorsal and volar motion as flexion and extension are completed. The strength of grip is partially dependent on both the mobility and stability of the metacarpals. The more strength utilized in gripping, the more depressed are the ulnar muscles and the metacarpals. Displacement of the distal end of the fourth and fifth metacarpals toward the volar surface must be utilized when casts and braces are being applied. A view of the metacarpal heads end-on shows them to be covered only by extensor tendon and skin and, in the flexed position, the second metacarpal is about 6 mm. more dorsal than the fifth metacarpal.

Volar Surface Anatomy. The skin on the volar surface of the hand is more firmly fixed than that on the dorsum; the skin creases are attached and movement of the skin does not affect the underlying vessels or nerves appreciably. The middle and distal skin creases coincide with the proximal and distal interphalangeal joints, whereas the proximal skin crease corresponds to the middle of the proximal phalanx and not to the metacarpal phalangeal joint. The distal palm crease coincides with the metacarpal phalangeal joints, and

at this level provides a guide for placement of plaster splints and casts. If the apparatus extends distal to the proximal skin crease, then motion at the metacarpal phalangeal joints is limited partially or completely. Any soft or rigid dressing applied to the hand with the intent of providing limited active motion should stop at the level of the distal palmar crease. This skin mark does coincide with the proximal end of the annular ligament of the flexor tendons and acts as a landmark to the digital nerves and arteries and isolation of the bands of palmar fascia. Penetrating wounds in this area frequently injure digital nerves and vessels without actual damage to the flexor tendons.

The web spaces between the digits are U-shaped rather than shaped like a V. The corner or edge of the web coincides with the proper digital nerve, which is located on the volar aspect of the digits and coincides with the radial and ulnar borders of the finger pads.

The proximal skin creases at the base of the digits coincide with the separation of the flexor digitorum sublimis tendons into two segments, and there the flexor profundus becomes subcutaneous and superficial to the sublimis.

The radial aspect of the midpalmar crease forms the distal end of the thenar crease which lies over the radial and ulnar digital nerves of the index finger, and in its central segment over the motor branch of the median nerve which supplies the thenar nerve. Under this same crease is the point where the median nerve separates into the common digital nerves that supply sensation to the median nerve of the hand. This includes all of the volar aspect of the thumb, the index and long fingers, and one half of the ring finger. The index finger receives double innervation, with the radial aspect being innervated by a superficial radial nerve as well as the median, and the ulnar aspect of the thumb receives innervation from the superficial radial nerve.

The thenar muscles include the opponens, abductor pollicis brevis, and the flexor pollicis brevis, and these are visible when the thumb is pressed against an adjacent digit. The hypothenar muscles are not readily separated into isolated muscle bellies by palpation or visualization, but if the digit is abducted and flexed, then the individual muscle units will become prominent (Fig. 4). The transverse creases on the volar aspect of the wrist are over the transverse retinacular ligament, the medial cutaneous branch of the median nerve, the median and ulnar nerves and their arteries, the condensation of the origin of the palmar fascia, and the wrist and thenar flexor tendons. The carpal bones are the junction between the forearm and the hand and provide smooth wrist joint motion in the dorsal and volar planes, as well as ulnar and radial deviation and a moderate amount of circumduction. The stabilizing ligaments of the wrist connect the radial styloid with the carpal scaphoid and the trapezium; on the ulnar styloid the ligaments connect the triquetrum, pisiform, and the triangular fibrocartilage. These ligaments also provide a scaffolding for blood supply of the carpal bones.

Carpal Motion

Volar flexion occurs mainly in the radial carpal joint and, to a lesser degree, in the intercarpal joints. Displacement of the fragments of a fractured carpal scaphoid depends on the position of motion of the hand. Dorsiflexion may elevate the radial fragment and enlarge the fracture area; ulnar deviation may separate the fragments. Volar flexion may bring the fragments together, and radial deviation may impact them even more. Dorsiflexion of the wrist occurs in the midcarpal joints primarily and, to a lesser degree, in the radial carpal joint. Radial deviation, as observed on cineradiography, is primarily in the midcarpal articulations, whereas ulnar motion is in the radial carpal joint.

At the metacarpal phalangeal joints, the proximal phalanges move toward the ulnar side of the hand as flexion occurs and is compounded of volar deviation and rotation of the phalanx on the metacarpal head. The articular surface of the metacarpal head is covered with hyalin cartilage that is thicker on the volar surface than on the dorsum. The joint is lined with a layer of synovium contiguous to, but separate from, the capsule of the joint. The capsule is attached distal to the hyalin articular surface of the proximal phalanx and proximal to the articular surface of the metacarpal head. When the capsule becomes contracted, the phalanx cannot be flexed completely. The collateral ligaments make up part of the radial and ulnar capsule and provide stabilization of the joint by preventing excessive radial or ulnar deviation, volar subluxation, or malrotation. Part of the ligament course is directly to the proximal phalanx from the metacarpal neck, and the other segment joins the volar fibrocartilage or the volar plate anterior to the metacarpal phalangeal joint. Contracture of these ligaments results in limited flexion of the phalanx. Tear or stretch of the ligament causes ulnar or radial instability. The unilateral contracture results in an appearance with malrotation of the digit, which is confused because of excessive ulnar rotation. The volar fibrocartilaginous plate is attached to the base of the proximal phalanx and to the anterior surface of the neck of the metacarpal. If this joint is maintained in extension for several months, the volar tissues become adherent to the hyalin cartilage of the metacarpal head, another factor limiting flexion of the phalanx.

Extensor Mechanism of the Digits

The intricate but practical structures of the extensor mechanism covering of the fingers provide flexibility for the extensor tendon and attachments of the extensor digitorum communis to the proximal phalanx in the form of a sling, a common unit for action of the lumbrical tendon and interosseous muscle, and a covering for the metacarpal heads sufficient to allow a boxer to traumatize this area for many years without permanent damage. The central portion of the hood includes the extensor digitorum communis on the dorsum, the dorsal capsule, and the synovium under it. The transverse fibers of the radial and ulnar retinaculum extend to the volar surface and attach to the transverse intermetacarpal ligament on each side of the joint. The retinaculum can be separated easily from the underlying collateral ligaments and capsule but less easily from the volar plate.

Traction on the extensor digitorum communis tendon elevates the proximal phalanx by a slight action on this entire phalanx. Forcible traction on the extensor communis tendon results in extension of the middle phalanx through a few degrees because of direct attachment of the extensor tendon to the proximal phalanx (Fig. 6).

Separation of the dorsal capsule from the proximal end of the proximal phalanx may result in volar subluxation of the phalanx, which, in turn, affects centralization of the extensor digitorum communis. In another instance, laceration of the extensor communis at the level of the metacarpal head will decrease the range of extension of the proximal phalanx. The effect of the lumbrical tendon on the middle phalanx of the digit is through the retinaculum at the metacarpal phalangeal joint through the oblique retinacular ligaments that make up the volar condensation of the lateral bands, which are the tendons of the intrinsic muscles. The metacarpal phalangeal joint of the thumb includes two sesamoids encapsulated in the cartilaginous plate that covers the palmar aspect of the joint. The flexor pollicis longus tendon rests between the two sesamoid bones, and the tendon is covered by a fibrous canal, the annular ligament, which is responsible for the "trigger thumb" mechanism. The flexor pollicis brevis inserts into the radial sesamoid and also into the radial tubercle of the proximal phalanx. The three thenar muscles are the abductor pollicis brevis, the flexor pollicis brevis, and the

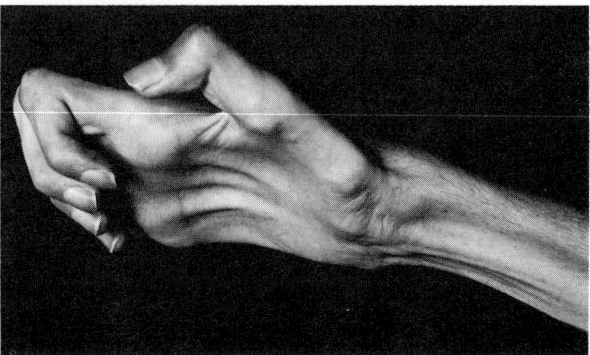

Figure 6. Muscles supplied by the median and ulnar nerves have been affected by a stretch injury of the brachial plexus. Intrinsic muscles are paralyzed; the flexor pollicis longus is contracted; the skin markings are obliterated. The flexor digitorum sublimes are prominent, and the metacarpal heads are visible. (Reprinted with permission from Harper and Row from Surgery of the Hand, J. L. Goldner, 1970.)

opponens pollicis. The muscle inserts into the radial tubercle of the proximal phalanx and the radial sesamoid and some other fibers run toward the extensor mechanism.

The extensor hood of the metacarpal phalangeal joint of the thumb functions in the same way as that of other metacarpal phalangeal joints. The extensor pollicis longus is on the ulnar side of the dorsum of the thumb, and the extensor pollicis brevis reinforces the radial side. The integrity of the ulnar or radial collateral ligaments controls deviation of the proximal phalanx.

The interphalangeal joints of the digits are hinge joints with the synovial and capsular covering on the dorsum and with extensions of the lateral band of the intrinsic tendons over the radial and ulnar aspects of the joint.

A small tubercle is present on the proximal end of the middle phalanx, and the middle band of the extensor tendon inserts into the phalanx at this point. The retinaculum of the proximal interphalangeal joint extends from the common extensor attachment on the dorsum to the volar fibrocartilage (see Fig. 5). The retinacular ligament is reinforced in the central area by oblique fibers that participate in extension of the middle phalanx. Contractures of these joints in extension depend on abnormal tension on the intrinsic lateral band tendons and on shortening of the dorsal capsule and collateral ligaments.

Thenar Muscles

The thenar eminence is made up of the abductor pollicis brevis, the opponens pollicis, and two heads of the flexor pollicis brevis. The abductor pollicis elevates the first metacarpal and assists in rotating the thumb. The tendon of the abductor pollicis brevis inserts on the radial tubercle of the proximal phalanx and is adherent to the capsule of the metacarpal phalangeal joint. Because of its attachment to the oblique retinacular expansion, this muscle assists in flexing the proximal phalanx and in extending the distal phalanx. The thenar muscles work in unison to provide elevation, rotation, and opposition of the thumb.

Hypothenar Muscles

The enlargement of the ulnar side of the hand includes the abductor digiti minimi, flexor brevis minimi, opponens digiti minimi, and the palmaris brevis. The abductor digiti minimi is usually divided into two longitudinal parts with its origins and insertions being primarily ligamentous. This muscle is inserted into the lateral tubercle of the base of the proximal phalanx of the little finger and into the expansion of the extensor tendon. It functions as a dorsal interosseous muscle. Contracture of the lateral muscles in the hand of the patient with rheumatoid arthritis results in the little finger being "pulled away" from the ring finger. The flexor brevis digiti minimi lies on the volar surface of the hypothenar area with a small separation between it and the abductor muscle of the little finger. Through this interval run the deep branches of the ulnar artery and nerve into the subtendinous part of the palm of the hand. The opponens digiti minimi is deep to the flexor brevis and inserts into the shaft of the fifth metacarpal. This muscle aids in stabilization of the ulnar grip and participates in the action of "cupping" of the palm. The opponens pollicis winds around a part of the first metacarpal. This muscle lies under the abductor brevis and acts primarily as an internal rotator and stabilizer of the first metacarpal. The flexor pollicis brevis is on the volar surface of the metacarpal and under the abductor brevis. One head of the flexor brevis originates from the volar carpal ligament and in the region of the flexor carpi radialis tendon; the other head originates from the volar surface of the trapezium and from the capitate tendon that inserts into the radiosesamoid and radial tubercle of the proximal phalanx. This muscle also attaches to an expansion into the extensor mechanism and assists in extending the distal phalanx of the thumb.

The adductor pollicis consists of two parts, one of which is transverse and the other oblique. The transverse head attaches to the volar crest of the third metacarpal; the oblique head attaches to the ligaments around the capitate, the trapezium, and the covering of the flexor carpi radialis. The heads insert separately or together into the ulnar tubercle at the base of the proximal phalanx and partially into the lateral band mechanism of the extensor tendon.

Extrinsic Muscles of the Hand and Wrist—Dynamic Considerations

All flexor tendons function simultaneously to bring the fingertips into the palm. The flexor digitorum profundi bend the tips of the fingers, and the flexor digitorum superficialis tendons bend the proximal interphalangeal joints. The tip of the thumb is flexed by the flexor pollicis longus. As the fist is formed, the extrinsic flexors and the intrinsic muscles designated as hypothenar and thenar function in a coordinated way (Fig. 7).

At the wrist, the flexor superficialis tendons are volar to the tendons of the flexor digitorum profundi. The superficialis tendons are retrieved for tendon transfer as individual tendons from the index and long fingers. The ring and little finger tendons usually lie in the same sheath but can be separated by traction. Occasionally they are united in the midpalm area. Traction on the superficialis tendons at the wrist results in flexion of the proximal interphalangeal joints of the fingers, accompanied by complete relaxation of the distal joints. The flexor digitorum profundus tendons at the wrist are covered by a synovial sheath that is thickened by aging, rheumatoid arthritis, or trauma. Enlargement of this sheath fills the carpal canal and results in compression of the median nerve. The flexor profundus tendons are connected to each other by multiple bands of tendons which result in simultaneous action of the long, ring, and little fingers. If one of these digits is held in flexion, the other two cannot be straightened completely or, if one of these digits is maintained in extension, flexion of the adjacent fingers cannot be done individually. A lesser number of bands extend from the ulnar three digits to the index finger. For this reason, the index finger functions more independently. The thumb functions most independently but, in 10 per cent of the general population, the tip of the thumb and index finger function simultaneously.

In the midpalmar area, the flexor digitorum superficialis tendons are more volar than the flexor profundus tendons. Both enter the fibrous annular ligaments and the synovial sheaths. Opposite the metacarpal phalangeal joints, the superficialis becomes more dorsal and the profundus tendon more volar. Thus, at the level of the proximal crease of the finger, the flexor profundus is a single volar tendon, and the flexor superficialis is dorsal and separated into two segments. This is the point where the flexor superficialis is retrieved for use as a tendon transfer. The annular ligament is incised, the flexor superficialis isolated from both the radial and ulnar sides, and the flexor profundus tendon retracted. At the level of the midportion of the proximal phalanx of the finger, the flexor superficialis tendon joins and forms the chiasma tendinum as a dorsal covering of the flexor digitorum profundus and moves freely on the periosteum of the middle phalanx during flexion and extension. The flexor digitorum sublimis separates distal to this, with one segment inserting into the proximal radial aspect of the middle phalanx and the other into the ulnar aspect. This tendon diminishes hyperextension of the proximal interphalangeal joint. The flexor profundus tendon is attached to the flexor digitorum superficialis by vincula, and both are contiguous and encapsulated by an annular ligament and a synovial sheath. The profundus tendon inserts into the distal phalanx after passing over the volar capsule of the distal joint.

Extrinsic Extensor of the Fingers, Thumb, and Hand

The extensor pollicis longus extends the distal phalanx of the thumb and to a lesser degree the proximal phalanx of this digit, as well as elevating and externally rotating the first metacarpal. The tendon is located toward the ulnar aspect of the metacarpal phalangeal joint and displaces toward the web spaces if pathologic conditions such as degenerative arthrosis, rheumatoid arthritis, or trauma exist. The extensor pollicis longus crosses the extensor carpi radialis

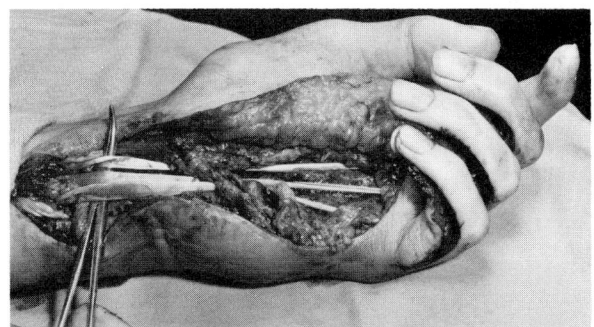

Figure 7. This patient has had a laceration of eight flexor tendons in the palm of the hand. Primary repair had been attempted by the physician who first saw the patient. Adhesions occurred, and extensive fibrosis resulted throughout the palm. A second attempt had been made at tendon grafting from the base of the palm with the flexor digitorum sublimis tendons, but these had become adherent, and the digits were non-functioning. Two years after the initial injury, one year after the second operation, the extensor tendons visible here were taken from the foot and the grafts were passed from the wrist into the fingers. Neurolysis was done at the same time. After several months of splinting, exercise bracing and resolution of fibrosis, improvement in function did occur. The current approach to this problem would utilize silicone rods to substitute for the fibrotic tendons. The initial treatment should be done by a surgeon who is experienced and well prepared for extensive operative procedures with appropriate instruments, assistants, and adequate magnification. (Reprinted with permission from Harper and Row from Surgery of the Hand, J. L. Goldner, 1970.)

longus at the wrist level just prior to where the wrist tendon inserts into the second metacarpal. The thumb extensor also crosses the extensor carpi radialis brevis just prior to where the extensor brevis inserts into the third metacarpal. The extensor pollicis longus enters a fibro-osseous canal just before the tendon enlarges to enter the muscle belly. It passes dorsal to the extensor carpi radialis longus and brevis and is subcutaneous and readily palpable throughout the entire length of the first metacarpal. Rotation of the thumb toward opposition makes the extensor pollicis longus less noticeable. External rotation of the thumb and abduction place the extensor pollicis longus in relief.

The extensor pollicis brevis lies in a common sheath with the abductor pollicis longus at the level of the styloid process of the radius. The extensor pollicis brevis passes slightly toward the ulnar side of the metacarpal phalangeal joint, makes up part of the dorsal hood, and acts primarily on the proximal phalanx. In some individuals, the extensor pollicis brevis can be removed without alteration of thumb function, but in others, removal of this tendon lessens the force of extension of the proximal phalanx and results in a flexion deformity of that joint. The extensor pollicis brevis and the abductor pollicis longus may be involved in stenosing tenosynovitis in the region of the radial styloid. The multiple segments that make up the abductor pollicis longus may be covered by separate fibro-osseous sheaths. This point is important in successful management of this syndrome.

The extensor tendons that provide elevation of the proximal phalanges at the metacarpal phalangeal joints all pass over the metacarpal heads through the dorsal hood that makes up the extensor expansion. This expansion spreads out on each side of the metacarpal phalangeal joints and aids in stabilizing the extensor tendons centrally. The expansion inserts on the deep transverse intermetacarpal ligament and into the volar fibrocartilage of the joint. The extensor mechanism over the proximal phalanx consists of heavy central slip into which course the radial and ulnar lateral bands in an oblique direction. These three units join at the midportion of the middle phalanx and pass distally, where they again divide into three bands that are interconnected. The midband continues to the middle phalanx and inserts into the posterior tubercle of this bone. It adheres to both the dorsal capsule and the proximal phalanx. The two lateral bands are attached to the central slip at the level of the proximal phalanx, but at the proximal interphalangeal joint, they follow a separate course until they enter the distal interphalangeal joint region, where they again form into a single tendon that inserts into the base of the distal phalanx. The lateral bands are dorsal with reference to the axis of the proximal and distal interphalangeal joints when the digit is in extension. The lateral bands move with flexion and extension, in that in flexion the bands are toward the volar surface whereas in extension they are toward the dorsal surface. When fixed contractures occur, these bands influence the position of the digit in relationship to either flexion or extension of the interphalangeal joints.

The thumb metacarpal joint is covered by a dorsal expansion through which run the long and short extensors. Transverse fibers fix this hood to the sides of the joint, particularly in the area of the adductor pollicis. Through this attachment, the adductor pollicis affects extension of the distal phalanx, but to a much lesser degree than occurs by the attachments of the intrinsic muscles on the radial side of the thumb. Thus, extension of the distal phalanx of the thumb is possible even if the extensor pollicis longus and brevis tendons are lacerated or paralyzed. The resistance maintained by the distal phalanx, however, is diminished considerably when compared with the force provided by an intact extensor pollicis longus. The extensor digiti minimi on the ulnar side of the extensor digitorum communis activates the proximal pha-

lanx of the little finger. These two tendons usually course on the radial side of the extensor carpi ulnaris, which is in a special tunnel on the ulnar side of the distal end of the ulna. The double tendon insertion into the little finger and index finger provides greater coordinated activity of these two digits.

Fascial Spaces of the Hand

Fluid accumulation in the hand may pass from one area to another or spread locally through potential fascial spaces. A potential space is in the subcutaneous region on the dorsum of the hand. This space extends into the dorsum of the forearm proximally and distally into the fingers and is completely separated from the extensor tendons. The latter have their own tendon sheaths and are protected from closed fascial spaces. A second space exists between the fascial sheath that separates the subcutaneous space from the tendon sheath. The third space is located between the extensor digitorum communis and the posterior interosseous fascia. All of these spaces are important anatomic features in managing crush injuries. Blood or purulent exudate may accumulate in any or all of these spaces (Fig. 8).

The *palm* has two major spaces, referred to as the thenar and midpalmar spaces. The *thenar* space is delineated on one side by the adductor pollicis in the depth of the hand, at which point this muscle is covered by the adductor fascia. On the ulnar side, the space is limited by the septum located between the third metacarpal and adhesions to the crest of the synovial bursa of the flexor tendons. The latter area is designated as the ulnar bursa. On the radial side there is union of the thenar fascia with the midpalmar fascia. On the volar surface the space is covered by the flexor tendons of the index and long fingers and their tendon sheaths and more superficially by the midpalmar fascia. Proximally, this thenar space is closed by the junction of the radial and ulnar digital synovial sheaths known as the *radial* and *ulnar bursae,* and the extensors move the wrist and the anterior interosseous fascia. Distally, the space opens toward the first and second interdigital folds.

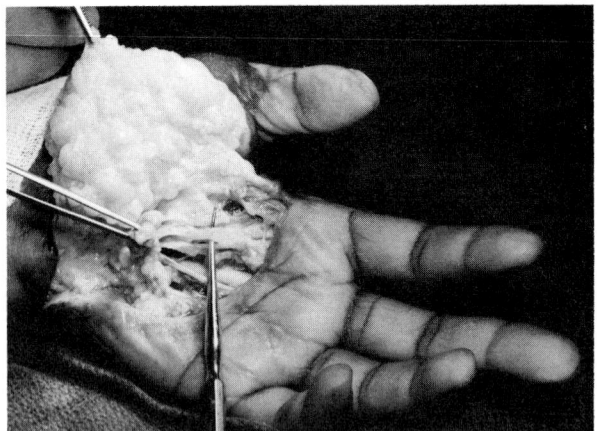

Figure 8. The palm of the hand has been exposed in order to excise contracted palmar fascia, to complete a tenolysis procedure of the flexor tendons to the fingers, and to identify the digital nerves so that they can be freed from surrounding scar tissue. These changes were secondary to a roller injury. A large primary abdominal flap had been applied to provide protection. Operating through the flap at a later time gave adequate tissue for closure without skin contracture. The fascial spaces of the hand are not clearly defined after severe trauma. (Reprinted with permission from Harper and Row from Surgery of the Hand, J. L. Goldner, 1970.)

The *midpalmar space* is on the ulnar side of the hand and in the depth of the palm. Anteriorly, the flexor tendons of the right and little fingers and their synovial sheaths and the midpalmar fascia delineate this space. Posteriorly, the potential opening is limited by the anterior interosseous fascia over the interosseous muscles of the third and fourth intermetacarpal spaces. On the ulnar side, these potential spaces are closed by the anterior interosseous fascia, the fascia covering the hypothenar muscles, and the midpalmar fascia, all of which join together to make one thick band. The midpalmar space is limited on the radial side by the connection of the distal synovial sheath designated as the ulnar bursa with the crest of the third metacarpal. Proximally, the contact of the digital synovial sheath bursae, with continuation of the anterior interosseous fascia, closes the space. The potential area of the enlargement at the wrist is made by relationship between the flexor tendons and their synovial digital sheaths and the fascia covering the pronator quadratus muscle. This is the reason that the area separates easily when a tendon transfer through the interosseous membrane is being performed. This potential sheath can be enlarged by hemorrhage, edema fluid, or purulent exudate that may arise from the hand or from a torn pronator quadratus muscle such as that which accompanies a Colles' fracture. Heavy fascial retinacular bands around the wrist are present on both the volar and dorsal sides. The volar retinaculum covers the median nerve and the flexor tendons, and the dorsal carpal ligament protects the extensor tendons. Both restrain the long tendon of the hand. The hand will function without these heavy restraining ligaments, but maximum strength, dexterity, and activity are obtained more readily if all the retinacula are intact.

The *palmar fascia* separates the deep structures of the hand from the skin. More proximally this fascia concentrates into the midpalmar fascia and is a condensation of the tissue between the thenar and hypothenar eminences. The midpalmar fascia is a firm, heavy, fibrous membrane approximately triangular in shape and connected at the thenar-hypothenar fascia coverings. The fibrous ends that extend from the midpalmar fascia course toward the index and the little fingers and are of unequal thickness. They run parallel and superficial to the flexor tendons of the fingers and form a strand of thicker fibers known as pretendinous bands. These course over the flexor surfaces of each finger, with those of the index and long fingers going into the distal part of the midpalmar fascia, running transversely from the ring to the little finger in a formation of a superficial transverse ligament. In palmar fibromatosis (Dupuytren's contracture), this tissue is fibrotic, nodular, and shortened.

BLOOD SUPPLY TO THE HAND

The radial and ulnar arteries and their numerous branches bring blood into the hand. The median artery, which is usually small, occasionally is as large as the radial or ulnar arteries and may contribute significantly to the arterial system. This artery is a branch of the palmar interosseous vessel that joins the deep palmar arch and forms a large arterial trunk. The radial artery divides into muscular branches in the forearm. At the level of the pronator quadratus muscle a branch arises that runs parallel to the border of the muscle and joins a similar branch from the ulnar artery. These branches are known as the volar-radial and volar-ulnocarpal arteries. The palmar carpal arteries form an arch with the plexus that supplies the palmar aspect of the wrist joint. A dorsal carpal arch is formed on the dorsal aspect of the wrist under the extensor tendons by a radial dorsal and ulnar dorsal branch. These form a network that supplies the dorsal metacarpal arteries. The metacarpal arteries supply the dorsum of the fingers. They communicate freely with the palmar

digital arteries from the superficial palmar arch. The latter arch is made up of the superficial branch of the radial artery that anastomoses with the end branch of the ulnar artery under the midpalmar fascia. The common digital arteries supply the individual digital vessels.

The *deep palmar arch* is located dorsal to the flexor tendons on the palmar interosseous fascia. It is formed by the end of the radial artery that perforates the space between the two heads of the first dorsal interosseous and passes into the palmar aspect of the hand where it supplies the branch to the thumb (the princeps pollicis) and to the volar index radial artery. This branch joins the deep branch of the ulnar artery that penetrates the hypothenar muscles into the retrotendinous space of the hand.

The *venous system* of the hand consists of the deep and superficial veins. The deep veins run with arteries. These veins follow the deep palmar and superficial palmar arches, the palmar and volar carpal arches, and the volar metacarpal branches, which are all outflow branches. The proper volar digital arteries do not have venae comitans. All the deep veins intercommunicate with the dorsal veins. The superficial veins are, for the most part, dorsal and consist of the dorsal digital and metacarpal veins which drain into the basilic vein on both the ulnar and radial sides.

The *lymphatic system* consists of two or three vessels that accompany the corresponding proper digital arteries and form a superficial volar system that is quite dense and a dorsal system that is less dense. The deep arteries are also accompanied by lymph channels. The ulnar collateral vessels communicate with the ulnar artery collectors, and the posterior lymphatic vessels communicate with the posterior interosseous trunk of the forearm.

WRIST FLEXOR AND EXTENSOR TENDONS

The flexor carpi radialis tendon is located just to the radial side of the median nerve and enters a special tunnel under the crest of the trapezium. The flexor carpi radialis inserts into the base of the second metacarpal. The fibrous sheath over the distal end of this tendon may become constricted secondary to trauma or arthrosis and cause pain at the base of the palm. The close relationship between the flexor carpi radialis and the median nerve occasionally accounts for irritation of the median nerve secondary to tenosynovitis of the flexor carpi radialis.

The palmaris longus partially covers the median nerve and inserts into the apex of the palmar fascia and varies in size from a thin slip of tendon to a wide, flat tendon. Occasionally the muscle belly extends to the wrist and may cause compression of the median nerve. The palmaris longus is absent in about 25 per cent of the general population, and the surgeon must pay particular attention to testing for the presence of this tendon prior to tendon grafting. Muscle testing may cause the flexor superficialis to bulge into the subcutaneous area of the wrist and simulate the palmaris longus. The palmaris longus assists in elevation and rotation of the metacarpal and, if present, supplements the action of the abductor pollicis brevis.

The flexor carpi ulnaris inserts into the pisiform bone. The tendon is covered at least 50 per cent by muscle fibers at the wrist level and extends to the volar capsule ligament, joining this structure to form a roof for the ulnar artery and nerve. The flexor carpi ulnaris tendon protects the ulnar nerve and artery at the wrist level and provides an easy point of recognition of these structures when a local nerve block is to be done. The extensor carpi ulnaris passes through a groove on the ulnar side of the distal end of the ulna and is covered by an annular ligament. Tenosynovitis may occur at this point. A synovial cyst may form in the patient with rheumatoid arthritis as the synovial sheath covering this tendon becomes irritated by constant ulnar deviation. The tendon inserts into the midportion of the fifth metacarpal, and can be used as a tendon transfer both because of its length and because it is more of an ulnar deviator than a dorsiflexor and can thus be readily spared. The extensor carpi radialis brevis is the prime dorsiflexor of the hand. This tendon inserts into the base of the third metacarpal and is in direct relationship with the extensor carpi radialis brevis, which inserts into the base of the second metacarpal. The latter tendon is primarily a radial deviator of the hand but also assists in dorsiflexion. Both tendons are dorsal to the extensor pollicis longus.

NERVE SUPPLY TO THE HAND AND WRIST

The median, radial, ulnar, and musculocutaneous nerves provide sensory and motor supply of the hand. These nerves arise from the brachial plexus, which, in turn, originates from the cervical roots. The median nerve in the hand is primarily sensory, but it also innervates the major thenar muscles. The ulnar nerve is both sensory and motor and supplies most of the small muscles of the hand. The radial nerve is primarily sensory in the hand, supplying the back of the hand and the radial aspect of the index finger and the ulnar aspect of the thumb. The wide sensory distribution of the superficial radial nerve overlaps the usual sensory contribution of the median nerve. Anatomic variations are frequently noted. On the volar side of the hand, the sensory midline passes from the tip of the ring finger through the length of the digit to the wrist. The radial side is supplied by the median nerve, and the ulnar side by the ulnar nerve. On the dorsum, the line of division consists of a longitudinal line from the center of the tip of the ring finger to the proximal interphalangeal joint of that digit. The horizontal line then passes over the dorsum of the proximal interphalangeal joints of the ring, long, and index fingers, and the area within these lines is supplied by the median nerve. The dorsum of the little finger, the ulnar half of the two distal phalanges, and the entire proximal phalanx of the long finger, as well as the dorsum of the hand on the ulnar side, are supplied by the dorsal branch of the ulnar nerve. The radial side of the proximal phalanx of the index finger and occasionally the radial aspect of the index over the middle and distal phalanges are supplied by the radial nerve. The dorsum of the thumb and the ulnar aspect of the thumb are supplied by the superficial radial nerve. The skin around the dorsum of the thumb and over the metacarpal phalangeal joint is frequently supplied by a branch of the musculocutaneous nerve.

Motor nerves of the intrinsic muscles of the hand derive from the median and ulnar nerves. Innervation of the extrinsic muscles is derived from all three nerves (median, ulnar, and radial). On the volar side of the forearm and hand, the *median* nerve supplies the flexor pollicis longus, the flexor digitorum profundus of the index and long fingers, and the flexor carpi radialis, as well as the pronator quadratus and pronator radii teres. The thenar muscles, with the exception of the deep part of the flexor pollicis brevis and the adductor muscle, are usually supplied by the median nerve. The ulnar nerve innervates the deep portion of the flexor pollicis brevis, the adductor, and the hypothenar muscles; also, all the interossei and the third and fourth lumbricals are innervated by the ulnar nerve. The flexor carpi ulnaris and the flexor digitorum profundi to the ring and little fingers are innervated by the ulnar nerve. Certain anomalies of the hand occur frequently. The entire flexor pollicis brevis may be innervated by the ulnar nerve. The abductor pollicis brevis and half of the flexor digitorum profundus of the long finger may be innervated by the ulnar nerve. Most frequent crossover innervation is where the ulnar nerve distally carries fibers to the small muscles of the hand usually supplied by the median nerve. The *radial* nerve innervates all of the extensor muscles of the hand and wrist, as well as the abductor pollicis longus and the extensor pollicis brevis. This nerve is seldom involved in anomalous innervation patterns.

DIGIT FLEXION AND EXTENSION

The extrinsic muscles originate in the forearm and their tendons extend to the fingers and thumb. They provide extension of the fingers and flexion of the digits. The small muscles within the hand make up the thenar and hypothenar groups and are located on both the volar and the dorsal aspects of the hand. These are referred to as the intrinsic muscles. All muscles perform synergistically and depend on other sets of flexors and extensors for maximum strength and range of motion. Each has a vascular and neural supply, both of which are essential to provide maximum strength. The flexor digitorum profundus originates high on the forearm and divides into four parts. A segment to the index finger divides proximally and is partially separated from the tendons directed to the ulnar three digits, which are closely interrelated within the midpalmar area. Individual flexion of the index finger is possible through about 30 degrees; at that point, the other profundus tendons begin to function. The profundus tendons activating the ulnar three digits have minimal individualization. If one digit is held in extension, limited flexion of the adjacent digits is possible; if the index finger is held in extension, the ulnar three digits can be flexed almost to the palm. This same relationship exists for the motion of extension. If the long finger is held in extension, extension of the adjacent digit at the metacarpal phalangeal joint is limited (see Fig. 3).

The *flexor digitorum sublimis* is superficial to the flexor profundus and covers the median nerve proximally in the forearm. Each flexor sublimis muscle-tendon unit is separate from the adjacent fingers, and individual action of the fingers in performing flexion is possible. Occasionally the flexor sublimis tendons of the ring and little fingers are removed for tendon transfer at the base of the ring finger, and a connecting slip between the two tendons prevents easy removal until the attachment in the palm is recognized and the two tendons are separated.

The *flexor pollicis longus* is almost completely isolated from the other finger flexor tendons, although full flexion of the thumb usually causes a few degrees of bending of the index finger, indicating partial union between these two muscles. The flexor pollicis longus may have an accessory proximal head and cause contracture of the thumb secondary to elbow injuries as the accessory head attaches to the medial epicondyle of the humerus. The muscle belly of the flexor pollicis longus may be involved in isolated anterior interosseous compression syndromes, in localized ischemic contracture, or in lacerations. If extensive wrist injuries occur, the distal end of the flexor pollicis longus may retract beneath the thenar muscles or may become attached proximally to other adjacent tendons. The action of the thumb tendon on the uninvolved side should be tested before tendon repair or tendon transfer is attempted.

The three major wrist flexor muscles stabilize the hand, assist in providing a strong grip, and aid in strong flexion of the wrist joint, as well as in providing ulnar and radial deviation of the hand. These muscles may be used for reinforcement of the flexor tendons of the fingers and thumb on both the flexor and the extensor sides. The palmaris longus is frequently absent but, when present, may insert into the fascia of the abductor pollicis brevis and provide both abduction and partial rotation of the first metacarpal, in addition to flexion of the wrist. Particular attention should be given to the insertions of the wrist flexor tendons.

INTRINSIC MUSCLES OF THE HAND

The short muscles of the hand are separated into four groups: the intrinsic, the lumbrical, the hypothenar, and the thenar muscles (Fig. 9).

Interosseous Muscles. The interossei are divided into palmar and dorsal groups, with the three palmar muscles pulling the phalanges toward the midline and assisting in flexion of the metacarpal phalangeal joints of the index, ring, and little fingers. The site of insertion of these muscles accounts for the development of ulnar deviation of the little finger if the motor branch of the ulnar nerve is injured. The four dorsal interossei insert on the radial aspect of the index finger, on both the radial and ulnar sites of the long finger, and on the ulnar aspect of the ring finger (Fig. 9). These muscles flex the proximal phalanges of these digits and spread the fingers. Occasionally, short masses of muscle originate from the carpal bones or from the base of the metacarpals on the dorsum of the hand and appear as enlargements similar to cysts or other bone or soft tissue lesions. These accessory muscle masses are similar to the muscle belly of the extensor digitorum brevis on the dorsum of the foot. Recognition of these muscle abnormalities is important in differential diagnosis. There are many variations in the insertions of the dorsal and volar interossei. In general, radial interossei tend to insert into bone with lesser insertions into the extensor hood, whereas the volar interossei usually insert into the lateral band expansion. The nerve and vascular supply of the interossei and the close relationship of the muscle bellies of these intrinsic muscles to the metacarpals account for changes in these muscles after injury of the hand in the metacarpal region or alterations of the intrinsic tendons as seen in rheumatoid arthritis. Changes in vascular or nerve supply affect the intrinsic muscles. Fibrosis of the interossei and lumbricals results in flexion of the metacarpal phalangeal joints and extension of the interphalangeal joints. Motion of the interphalangeal joints is then limited and the range of flexion and extension is diminished. Rapid finger action and the ability of the patient to spread the digits diminishes. The action of the small muscles is affected by displacement of metacarpals, by malunion of the metacarpal shaft, and by angular deviation of the phalanges.

Lumbrical Muscles. These muscles originate from the flexor digitorum profundus tendons. The area of origin varies from 3.5 to 4 cm. and extends from a level of the pisiform bone proximally. When the fingers are flexed, the lumbricals are pulled into the carpal canal and recede proximally to the distal end of the radius. Except for the first lumbrical, which is on the radial side of the metacarpal phalangeal joint of the index finger, the lumbrical muscles pass between the heads of the metacarpals. The boundaries of the muscles, as they pass from the hand to the fingers, include the transverse intermetacarpal ligament dorsally, the metacarpal phalangeal joints laterally, the superficial transverse ligament, palmar fascia, and interdigital fat volarly. The muscle is volar to the axis of flexion and extension of the metacarpal phalangeal joint. It is normally not an extensor of this joint. The lumbrical insertion is usually on the radial side to the lateral band and more dorsal than the interosseous insertion.

INFECTIONS OF THE HAND

Thumb and Finger Infections

Acute suppurative tenosynovitis, midpalmar and thenar space infections, and extensive infection of the quadralateral space of the forearm occur infrequently. However, certain special situations can occur, in the case of human bites and pyogenic infections in diabetics or other persons having major systemic disease, which demand prompt attention and the use of bacteriostatic and bactericidal drugs systemically and locally.

Involvement of one or two digits does occur frequently, and the problem is a serious one if the infection progresses without treatment. The cause and treatment of the thumb and finger infections are important so that sensation, strength, and motion of the digits can be maintained and amputation avoided. The physician should be aware of (1) mechanism of injury, (2) causative organism, (3) anatomic localization, (4) differential diagnosis, and (5) principles of treatment, which include selection of medication, methods of immobilization, techniques of incision and drainage, and choice of anesthesia.

The structures of the fingertip include (1) the nail plate, (2) the eponychium, (3) the hyponychium, (4) the nail matrix, (5) the lateral skin folds, (6) the nail root, and (7) the nail bed. On the volar surface of the thumb and fingertips are sensory pads with cutaneous ridges for fingerprints, the digital nerves with wide distribution of sensory branches, fatty tissue between the fingers, septum, and the composite insertion of the flexor tendon and its sheath into the distal phalanx, which has a thin periosteal cover. Cellulitis or abscess involving the tip of the digit requires consideration of each of these tissues alone or as a group, with the extent of involvement depending upon the degree of infection. Early treatment of a damaged cuticle (eponychium) will prevent bacterial infection which results in formation of an eponychia or paronychia.

Dorsal Infections of the Hand

Eponychia. If the cuticle is traumatized by rubbing, biting, scraping, or injury, cellulitis and subsequent

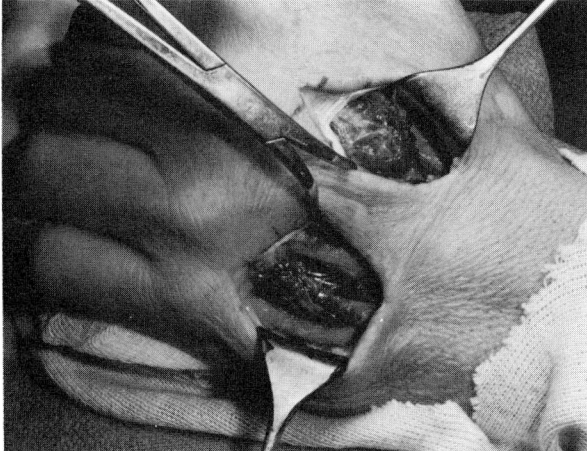

Figure 9. The dorsum of the hand contains a network of veins and lymphatics, and the dorsal fascia extends from one metacarpal to the other and covers the interossei muscles. Nerve and blood supply of the interossei are protected from injury to the dorsum of the hand. The small muscles may become fibrotic after trauma due to swelling or interference with the arterial supply. Contracture then affects the metacarpal phalangeal joints and the interphalangeal joints. The small muscles provide over a third of the strength of hand grip. (Reprinted with permission from Harper and Row from Surgery of the Hand, J. L. Goldner, 1970.)

abscess formation may result. A foreign body under the skin flap may be the initiating mechanical cause of an infection. Early treatment is accomplished by soap and water, petrolatum or lanolin, and careful cleansing of the skin edges. A break in the eponychium should be treated by using a local antibiotic ointment, a bandaid, and protective gloves for household work. If the inflamed area is covered, the individual will not constantly rub and irritate that affected part and healing will progress more rapidly. If infection progresses, a paronychia results.

Paronychia. This condition starts as a subcuticular or intracutaneous infection, with exudate developing in a localized area, which eventually spreads around under the base of the fingernail, elevating it from the nail matrix and eventually the nail bed. If a small collection of purulent material cannot be localized and expressed, complete drainage is indicated as early as possible by an incision that allows the lateral and proximal folds of the nail to be exposed. This may be done under digital block anesthesia without the use of epinephrine in the anesthetic. A pointed knife blade is inserted between the skin and the nail in order to incise the eponychium from within outward, on either side of the base of the nail. This allows the skin flap to be turned upward for adequate drainage. Wet dressings, petrolatum gauze, antibiotic ointments, and regular reopening of the drainage area will prevent the skin from adhering until infection has been controlled. If more extensive drainage is needed for a deeper abscess, the incisions are extended proximally in the skin fold, the skin edges are raised upward along with the dorsal skin over the nail bed, and the proximal end of the fingernail is excised. A small segment of nail, rather than the entire fingernail, can be removed. The infection, if chronic and severe, may be sufficient to destroy the nail matrix, the nail bed, and ultimately the phalanx. Thus, in order to avoid loss of bone and even the phalanx, treatment should be complete, aggressive, and early. Incisions adjacent to the eponychium should be avoided, as the remaining skin flaps may necrose. Also, the incisions over the extensor tendons should be avoided, since these may cause direct extension of the inflammatory process. The nail matrix should not be damaged while the fingernail is being removed. When the new nail forms it may be somewhat irregular, and several months will elapse before a smooth nail regenerates. Chronic paronychia, particularly in the female, may be due to Candida or Monilia. Local treatment by fungicidal ointments should be initiated; however, appropriate cultures should be obtained prior to extensive antibiotic therapy, if local treatment appears to be unsuccessful.

Subungual Foreign Body or Cellulitis

This condition usually begins as an infection at the tip of the digit and progresses to abscess formation, as a result of damage to the nail plate that separates it from the nail bed. Minimal hemorrhage occurs, the dermis is exposed, and continued trauma of the nail plate results in cellulitis and secondary infection caused by a material that has accumulated under the nail plate. Early treatment should consist of trimming of the fingernail as close to the nail bed as possible, soap and water cleansing, use of antibiotic ointment locally, and bandaid dressing. A foreign body, such as a lead pencil point, a sliver of wood, or a granule of plaster, may be wedged between the fingernail and the nail bed, causing discomfort, cellulitis, and local infection. If the foreign body is deep and has been unrecognized for several days, the nail should be trimmed, the finger soaked, and local ointments applied, and the foreign body will localize. Gentle pressure after a few days or a week will usually result in extrusion of the foreign body at that time. For example, a child may break the tip of a lead pencil under the nail and only a dark spot is visible. Extensive probing and attempts at immediate removal are not indicated. The nail should be trimmed, the digit kept clean and protected, and the foreign body will usually extrude within a week or ten days with general compression. Tetanus toxoid should be given if the patient has not been protected previously. Subungual lesions or paronychia-like swellings which do not respond to ordinary treatment should be suspected of being caused by fungus, foreign body, or neoplasia such as epithelioma or keratoacanthoma.

Subungual Hematoma

This condition usually results from direct trauma, and early treatment is necessary because of pain. Blood may be removed by drilling a hole into the center of the nail plate, by puncturing the nail plate with a sharp pointed knife blade, or by using the heated round end of a paper clip. The hole should be placed away from the nail matrix. Pain will be relieved but danger of infection does exist. If the hole is made with sterile technique, if the nail bed is not perforated by the knife blade or paper clip, and if wet dressings, antiseptic ointments, and immobilization are used, there is little danger of complication. The fingernail should be examined after the holes have been drilled and, if there is dirt under the nail or if the nail is long, the edge should be trimmed and the dirt and foreign body removed. This will prevent secondary infection, as well as unnecessary motion of the nail on the nail bed. The fingertip is treated just as one would trim or treat an ingrown toenail after removing the segment of the nail. If the fingernail separates from the nail bed over a wide area, as a result of either the initial crush injury or the upward elevation of the nail plate by hemorrhage, the nail, even though loose, should not be removed but should be compressed and allowed to cover the underlying tissue until fibrosis protects the nail bed and a new nail develops.

Folliculitis

Folliculitis, cellulitis, and carbuncle may occur on the dorsum of the digit as a result of trauma, direct invasion of bacteria into the hair follicles, or infection secondary to foreign body. Careful cleansing of the adjacent areas with soap and water, frequent wet dressings, removal of hairs from the center of the infected follicle with sterile forceps, and application of antibiotic ointment usually localize folliculitis. If, however, the area is squeezed with dirty fingernails, traumatized by the patient's fingertips several times a day, or not adequately cleansed, a spreading cellulitis will develop and a carbuncle with involvement of proximal lymph nodes may occur. Local incision for drainage, systemic therapy, immobilization, and wet dressings are necessary for treatment of the carbuncle.

Volar Hand Infections

Fingertip Infections. The extent of an infection on the volar aspect of the fingertip or thumb varies according to the type of injury, duration of infection, degree of bacterial invasion, and local resistance. An epidermal abscess with purulent material localized between the epidermis and the dermis, if treated early, will not spread to the deeper tissues. This lesion requires incision of the epidermis, drainage of the pus, application of wet soaks, and antibiotic ointment. If the infection extends through the dermis, the pad of the digit becomes involved. The anatomic arrangement of the fibrous septum may prevent spreading of the infection to the middle phalanx and to the tendon sheath. The attachment of the volar distal skin crease to the deep fascia is a barrier and restrains the infection to the distal phalangeal area. The superficial lesions are called epidermal abscess and subepidermal abscess. If adequate drainage is not done, then a deep infection may form within the pad of the finger. This is usually caused by *Staphylococcus aureus,* which may destroy the fat within the septa and burrow under the periosteum into bone or into the flexor tendon sheath. This results in a purulent tenosynovitis that spreads proximally and may destroy the tendon. If the infection invades the phalanx, osteomyelitis may result. If swelling and pain persist, systemic antibiotics are insufficient to abort the infection. The pain may be so severe that the patient attempts to puncture the swollen tip with a razor blade or a needle. Treatment should be done under a digital nerve block, so that a lateral incision can be used, reflecting the digital nerve and the skin flap, and draining pus from within the septa. The flexor tendon sheath should not be punctured during the incision and drainage. Petrolatum gauze is then applied and a bulky soft dressing is used, on top of which is placed a plaster splint to provide absolute immobilization of the digit. Wet dressings are then applied through the dry dressings, and additional wet dressings are placed on top. Broad-spectrum antibiotics such as tetracycline or cephalosporin can be used. The wound should be dressed daily and the flaps spread in order to prevent accumulation of pus. If treatment is initiated by one not accustomed to treating pulp space infections, the initial incision is usually inadequate and too small. However, extensive fish-mouth type incisors are unnecessary and undesirable.

If the entire finger pad is distended with pus, the digit flap may extend from one side of the fingertip to the other, with the central limb as close to the tip of the nail as possible in order to avoid damage to the sensory area. Retraction of the finger pad may occur unless the dressings are applied in such a way that the pad is maintained distally. Blood supply of the distal phalanx may determine which segment of bone is involved in fingertip infections. A paronychia may involve the proximal portion of the distal phalanx because of its relationship to the nail bed and to the

phalanx. A pulp space infection or felon may involve the distal segment of the phalanx, with minimal change in the proximal portion of the bone. This relationship of the distal phalanx to the dorsal and volar aspects of the fingertip is important and should be considered when incision and drainage are being accomplished. Osteomyelitis usually occurs late and by direct invasion. It should be avoided early with adequate treatment.

Human bites, because of the depth of trauma and mixed infection, may result in periarticular fibrosis sufficient to cause joint arthrodesis or even amputation of a digit. The complications and sequelae are usually due to a puncture wound which involves the tendon sheath or the joint surface and is followed by secondary infection involving all of the periarticular and peritendinous structures. Once the volar plate and the collateral ligaments are damaged and the flexor tendons are adherent, the chances of obtaining a functioning finger are minimal. Amputation may then be necessary. Treatment of the human bite requires special attention and careful observation. Initial treatment includes adequate wound excision, HyperTet antitoxin or a tetanus toxoid booster, whichever is indicated, antibiotic therapy, and immobilization. The wound is always left open after excision is done and, if a joint is perforated, this is opened and drained and left open. Wet dressings are used, the hand is immobilized in a compression dressing, and the wound is allowed to close spontaneously.

Hand Infections in Diabetics

The prognosis of a severe hand infection in a diabetic is less favorable than in an individual not affected with this systemic disease (Fig. 10). All minor hand infections should be treated with great caution; all major hand infections should be drained immediately. Even cellulitis should be drained if elevation and antibiotics for a period of 8 to 16 hours do not result in improvement. Any indication of tendon sheath infection, even though early, should be seriously considered for open drainage, wet dressings, and antibiotic therapy. These patients should always be hospitalized and observed frequently and carefully. Deep infections of the finger or hand frequently result in loss of flexor tendons and in partial amputation of the part involved.

Bacteriologic Factors

The extent of destruction of the finger or part of the hand depends primarily on the causative organism. The physician should be aware of the organisms and the behavior of each that are involved in hand infections. Detailed information should be placed on the request for culture to the bacteriology laboratory, so that special media or special environmental conditions can be utilized. In every instance the culture should include aerobic and anaerobic environment and the use of special media if gonococcal infection is suspected. If typical or atypical tuberculosis is suspected, the bacteriologist should be notified accordingly. Sensitivities of the organisms are essential so that appropriate medications may be selected. These organisms have certain characteristics:

1. *Staphylococcus aureus* produces necrotizing

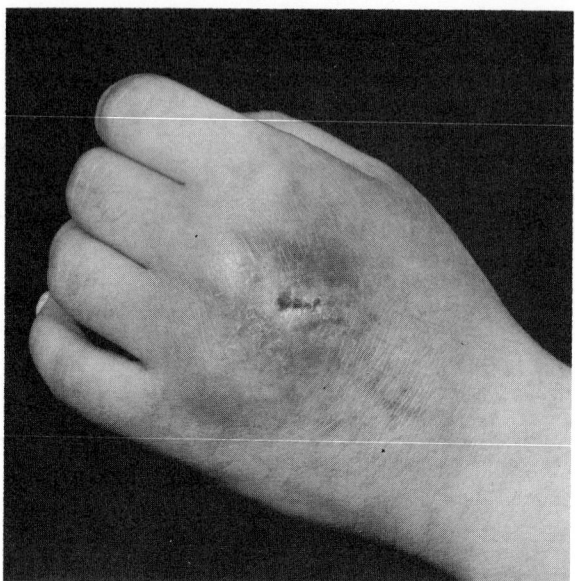

Figure 10. This patient had trauma with the resulting open fracture. The patient was a diabetic. A large subcutaneous abscess developed. The abscess extended into the intermetacarpal area and involved the interosseous muscles. Drainage had been delayed for several days. This is the residual condition of the hand after surgical incision, wet soaks, elevation and antibiotics. Contractures have occurred, and severe deformity will persist. (Reprinted with permission from Harper and Row from Surgery of the Hand, J. L. Goldner, 1970.)

toxins and has hemolytic and leukocytic properties. The coagulase-positive organisms, which destroy a serum clot, are always destructive. A high percentage of staphylococcus strains are resistant to pencillin but sensitive to synthetic penicillin or tetracycline. Certain strains, which initially are sensitive to particular medications, may eventually become resistant in the hospital environment. Certainly, early drainage is more important than it was several years ago when antibiotics were more consistently effective. The use of local applications and irrigations, such as bacitracin in a concentration of 1000 units per ml., or combination of 1 per cent neomycin solution with hydrocortisone, 21-sodium succinate (Solu-Cortef) 1 mg. per ml., is effective in giving high concentrations of drugs without producing toxic effects from the drugs.

2. *Streptococcal infections* are usually caused by group A beta-hemolytic strains; strains in groups C and G may also be responsible. These three groups produce fibrinolysin, deoxyribonuclease, hyaluronidase, and erythrogenic toxin. Nonhemolytic Streptococceae are secondary invaders and may cause a chronic infection. The patient with a streptococcal hand infection shows cellulitis, lymphangitis, lymphadenopathy, fever, and systemic toxic reaction. The organism may metastasize and, for this reason, should be treated early and vigorously with intravenous penicillin G. In general, none of the organisms in group A is resistant to penicillin G or to tetracycline. The nonhemolytic organisms, however, may be resistant.

3. *Symbiotic infection* is caused by nonhemolytic Streptococceae and hemolytic *Staphylococcus aureus,* as described by Meleny et al., has a characteristic appearance, and progresses steadily until it is brought under control. Staphylococceae may be found on routine culture, but special attention must be paid to isolating the microaerophilic Streptococceae. A necrotizing fasciitis occurs. (This kind of infection is more frequent in diabetics or individuals who have nutritional deficiency or inadequate immunogenic capabilities.) Treatment includes wide surgical excision and use of systemic antibiotics, local bacitracin, and local chemicals such as sodium hypochloride (Dakin's) solution or activated zinc peroxide. The hyperbaric chamber should also be utilized if the condition becomes widespread and cannot be controlled by local methods. Any hand infection that does not respond readily to drainage, wet dressings, and antibiotics should be suspected of being a symbiotic infection or one caused by some unusual organism. Furthermore, the bacteriologist should be made aware of the possibility of a symbiotic infection so that special techniques in isolating the organism can be utilized. Otherwise, *Staphylococcus aureus, Bacillus pyocyaneus,* Proteus, and enterococci will predominate in the culture. Symbiotic infection, of which anaerobic Streptococcus is the most prominent organism, occurs also in the human bite. The human bite may also contain pathogenic actinomyces, fusiform bacilli, and spirochetes.

4. *Erysipelothrix rhusiopathiae* (Streptothrix) produces swine erysipelas. It survives on decomposing fish, shell fish, or meat. The organism penetrates the skin through a small abrasion or wound and causes infection in fish handlers. Suppuration ordinarily does not occur, but the condition is accompanied by lymphangitis, lymphadenitis, swelling, and a tense, shiny appearance to the digit. This accounts for the term *erysipeloid.* Ordinarily, surgical excision is not indicated in treating this condition, but careful differential diagnosis must be made before operation is undertaken. Incision and biopsy may be necessary. Penicillin is the antibiotic of choice, and it should be continued for several days in order to prevent recurrence of infection.

5. *Mycobacterium tuberculosis—typical* may cause finger joint involvement as well as tenosynovitis or skin or bone lesions. Tuberculous dactylitis is usually seen in children.

6. *Mycobacterium marinum* (atypical—photochromagen) causes a chronic granuloma of the hand or a subacute inflammation, which may be difficult to recognize from chronic tenosynovitis or chronic inflammation of the fingers or hand. The organism usually enters through a break in the skin and is usually associated with either a swimming pool injury or fish handling or some form of marine exposure. The culture must be incubated at 32 degrees centigrade, rather than 37 degrees, on Löwenstein-Jensen medium. Treatment includes the use of ethambutol and rifampin.

7. *Treponema pallidum* may cause a primary lesion that could be mistaken for a paronychia. Tertiary lesions may involve tendon sheaths, bones, or joints.

8. *Pasteurella multocida* is common in the animal kingdom and is found in humans secondary to cat bite. The area involved may become painful and swollen and be accompanied by a secondary lymphadenitis and lymphangitis. Osteomyelitis may occur. The bacteriologist should be informed about the possibility of this infection, since the organism may resemble a gramnegative bacterium. All cat bites should be treated by careful local cleansing, followed by penicillin for five to seven days. The patient should receive tetanus toxoid or antitoxin (HyperTet).

9. *Pasteurella tularensis* may affect humans who are bitten by a tick or a deer fly, which introduces the organism through the skin of the hand. A papule occurs which later ulcerates and forms a granuloma.

10. *Bacillus anthracis* is an aerobic spore-forming organism found in sheep, cattle, horses, and swine. There may be a gangrenous ulcer on the hand, secondary lymphadenitis, septicemia, and further complications. Penicillin is effective against this organism.

11. *Neisseria gonorrhoeae* may produce a tenosynovitis or arthritis difficult to differentiate from the usual pyogenic infection. Smear for Diplococcus and culture on special media may aid in the diagnosis. Penicillin is used for treatment.

12. *Actinomyces bovis* enters the skin through an abrasion or break in the skin and may affect individuals working with cattle, swine, or horses. A granuloma occurs that resembles tuberculosis. Sinus formation usually results and the lesion may spread gradually to the dorsum of the digit or the hand. This infection may occur as a palmar swelling with intermittent sinus formation resistant to any kind of treatment. Culture of the material from unexplained chronic nodules should be given to the mycologist with adequate information and, if Actinomyces is present, the fungus will be recovered. Treatment includes systemic penicillin and potassium iodide.

13. *Blastomyces dermatitidis* may occur in the fingers as a pustule which becomes larger and spreads peripherally. The center heals, leaving a central scar with a spreading perimeter. If osseous lesions occur in the digits, they may be secondary to pulmonary disease. The diagnosis is made by smear and culture, and treatment is with dihydrosystilbamadine or amphotericin B. Special precautions are necessary when using these medications.

14. *Sporotrichum schenckii* is a fungus that may be introduced into the extremity through abrasions caused by thorns. An abscess develops and spreads to the regional lymphatics, resulting in multiple granulomata, which occur along the course of the lymphatics and ulcerate as the area is ruptured. Potassium iodide is the drug of choice. The medication must be used for a long period of time under careful supervision.

15. *Coccidioides immitis* may involve the hand and the ulnar and radial bursae, but its presence is a relatively rare condition. The mycologist should be informed if the patient has been traveling in a geographic area where the disease is endemic.

Gram-negative organisms, chronic infections, or hand infections in diabetic patients or those with inadequate immunity should be recognized and treated by adequate incision, excision of necrotic tissue, and identification of the organisms. If the organisms are sensitive to gentamicin, then this antibiotic should be used early and in adequate dosage.

DIFFERENTIAL DIAGNOSIS OF HAND INFECTIONS

Trauma

A traumatized fingertip with resulting swelling may resemble a digit invaded by a pyogenic bacterium. Also, secondary infection may occur following the primary traumatic injury. Persistent pain, increased swelling, and increased heat are indicative of secondary infection.

Acute Calcification of the Hand Tendons

This condition involving the interosseous tendons or fascia resembles infection because of sudden onset, swelling, increased heat, and severe pain. The patient may have elevation of temperature and even an elevated sedimentation rate. This soft tissue calcification may occur on the dorsal, medial, or lateral aspects of the digit and along the course of the lateral band mechanism. The absence of trauma, laceration, puncture wound, or malaise, and a normal white blood count tend to eliminate pyogenic infection. A slightly elevated body temperature and roentgen evidence of soft tissue calcification aid in distinguishing this condition from an acute infection. The roentgenogram may show no calcification. If additional signs of infection do not occur, even though pain persists, then incision can be avoided. Repeat roentgenogram will usually show calcification within 48 hours and local injection with triamcinolone or use of roentgen therapy may be beneficial. Acute calcification is usually found at the metacarpophalangeal joint area, the insertion of the flexor carpi radialis, the insertion of the flexor carpi ulnaris into the pisiform, and in the fingertip at the insertion of the flexor profundus or in the collateral ligament of the interphalangeal joints.

Acute Gout

Acute gout causes sudden pain, asymmetrical swelling, and limitation of joint motion. Temperature elevation frequently occurs, and the white blood count sedimentation rate may be elevated. Roentgenograms are usually negative. The deposits occur on the dorsum of the digit along the intrinsic muscle mechanism, although they may be seen within the joint and involve the synovium. Specific questions about the possibility of gout, detection of an elevated uric acid, and satisfactory response to colchicine, Benemid, and/or allopurinol aid in both diagnosis and treatment. Premature incisions should be avoided.

Acute Osteoarthritis

Acute osteoarthritis may involve the distal interphalangeal joints. The lesion is usually asymmetric and begins on the dorsal, medial, and lateral aspects of the joint. The area may be red, enlarged, and painful. Progression is usually slow, and the x-ray will show narrowing of the joint eventually. A single joint is usually involved at one time; however, several joints may be affected. Treatment is by immobilization, antiinflammatory medications, and local injection if necessary. Occasionally, resection arthroplasty or arthrodesis is indicated.

Unrecognized Trauma

Fracture of the metaphysis or diaphysis may result in swelling, limited motion, and diffuse erythema and pain even though original trauma was not recognized. White blood count is usually normal, temperature is not elevated, and pain subsides if the digit or part involved is immobilized. X-ray evidence of an incomplete fracture may aid in the diagnosis. In questionable situations, the digit should be immobilized in an aluminum splint for 24 hours. Pain will usually subside sufficiently to localize the site of the injury and soft tissue trauma and to eliminate the possibility of infection.

Foreign Body

A foreign body may simulate swelling and cause granuloma formation without signs of acute infection. Such items as wooden splinters, thorns, glass particles, needle tips, fish hooks, and human hair may cause chronic painful swellings which are accompanied by foreign body fibrosis. These lesions should be removed by careful dissection using anesthesia and tourniquet.

Glomus Tumor

This lesion involves the nail bed and causes persistent discomfort. Chronic persistent pain, absence of swelling, and a bluish discoloration under the nail together with a perforating lesion seen on x-ray of the phalanx support a diagnosis of glomus tumor. Treatment is excision of the entire flap, which includes the nail plate, nail bed, and periosteum superiorly in order to excise the circumscribed lesion on the undersurface of the flap and the bone.

Systemic Conditions

Lesions from Boek's sarcoid, pulmonary osteoarthropathy, multiple enchondromata, and metastatic neoplasms, or localized primary bone neoplasms may be differentiated by appropriate roentgenograms, by history, and by biopsy.

Clostridial Infections

Clostridii tetanus and *Clostridii welchii* may cause serious local and systemic infections. Tetanus can be avoided by use of a tetanus toxoid, HyperTet, and by adequate excision of puncture wounds or traumatic injuries.

Clostridii welchii is a gram-positive spore former that thrives in anaerobic, ischemic, and traumatized tissue. This infection may be prevented by careful wound excision, extensive wound irrigation, and avoidance of wound closure if the injury has occurred in a location where spore formers are expected. Delayed wound closure or delayed skin grafting can be done safely and without compromising tendon gliding, joint function, or recovery of maximum hand activity.

TREATMENT CONCEPTS OF HAND INFECTIONS

Certain "do's and don'ts" are important in the successful treatment of thumb and finger infections.

Do's. (1) *Do* take a careful history; examine the entire extremity carefully as well as the hand. (2) *Do* think of conditions other than infection that might account for the presenting signs and symptoms. (3) *Do* attempt to make a specific diagnosis before starting drug therapy. There is a safe waiting period. (4) *Do* wait for abscess localization before incision in most instances, although occasionally if the tendon sheath is involved, early incision may be performed without an abscess being present. Use immobilization, elevation, wet dressings, and antibiotics, both before and after incision. (5) *Do* use adequate anesthesia, either general or local nerve block, for draining an abscess. Use a tourniquet if the tendon is to be exposed or if a deep abscess in the digit or palm is suspected. (6) *Do* administer appropriate tetanus prophylaxis if there has been a laceration or puncture injury associated with the infection.

Don'ts. (1) *Do not* incise every painful, swollen digit. (2) *Do not* make incisions on the finger pads either vertically or horizontally unless the infection has already localized in this area. (3) *Do not* injure the digital nerves or the motor branch of the median or ulnar nerves when making necessary incisions for drainage. (4) *Do not* attempt to drain fingertip abscesses with a puncture type incision. (5) *Do not* close human bites or puncture wounds. (6) *Do not* close puncture wounds or lacerations when the injury has occurred to the hand in dish water, fishing water, sand, or dirt. (7) *Do not* forget to obtain adequate material for bacteriologic culture; give special instructions to the bacteriologist concerning type of injury and organisms suspected; ask for determination of organism sensitivity to particular medications.

HAND TRAUMA—ACUTE

Multiple tissue involvement requires an understanding of methods of skin replacement, recognition of vascular insufficiency (venous and arterial), understanding of nerve regeneration and repair, realization of the effect of trauma and ischemia on muscle function, and understanding of fractures and healing. A child's extremity that had been caught in a washing machine wringer is shown in Figure 11A. The rollers continued to move in spite of the presence of a large object. Note the damage to the dorsum of the thumb, the swelling of the extensor surface of the extremity, the area of skin erosion, and the discoloration of the adjacent epidermis. This wound occurred four days prior to this examination. The circulation of the hand, the sensation, the motor power were intact, no fractures occurred, and no epiphyseal injury resulted. The inner aspect of the arm where compression had occurred along the epicondylar region of the elbow is shown in Figure 11B. The radial and ulnar pulses were intact, finger flexion and extension were complete, swelling was present, but there appeared to be decreased sensation along the course of the ulnar nerve. Undoubtedly, a direct injury to the nerve had occurred.

Treatment consisted of dressings with physiologic saline, excision of the wounds with the patient under general anesthesia, and a split skin graft four days after wound excision and preparation of the underlying tissue. Meanwhile, com-

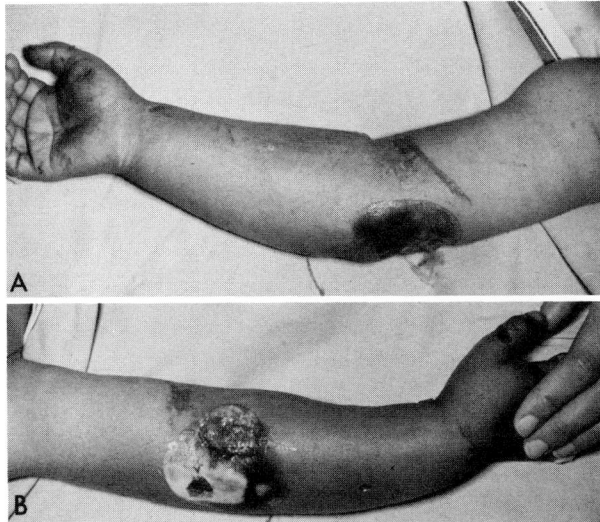

Figure 11. *A,* This child's arm was caught in a washing machine wringer. Note the diffuse edema of the forearm and the areas of skin damage around the elbow. Edema may result in ischemia of the forearm muscles. *B,* The dorsum of the forearm and arm shows skin damage in keeping with severe external compression. The points that require critical assessment are the forearm flexor and extensor muscles and the peripheral nerves.

pression dressings were used and the circulation, sensation, motor power, and tension of the anterior and posterior compartments of the forearm were monitored several times each day.

Roller injuries in children may result in insufficient blood supply to the forearm muscles or extensive venous congestion. The major goal is to prevent vascular complications involving muscle, especially infection. Hospitalization is essential for observation, and the extremity should be inspected several times each day. Aggravation of pain, pain on attempted extension of the fingers, loss of motor power, or obvious sensory diminution are all danger signs and should lead to surgical decompression of the forearm if any one of these symptoms occurs.

Compartment Decompression

Crush injuries, high pressure injections, and internal hemorrhage may lead to compartmental pressure considerably higher than the arterial blood pressure. If the compartmental pressure is too high, a tamponade effect will result. Arterial blood cannot get out of the compartment, and a relative ischemia occurs. In other instances, if the pressure is below diastolic pressure, then perfusion is not adequate and relative ischemia occurs.

Areas Requiring Incision for Decompression. (a) The digit after a grease gun, pain gun, or high pressure injection. (b) The hand and wrist level after crushing, hemorrhage, or excessive edema. This requires relief of the transverse retinacular ligament at the wrist and into the midpalmar area. (c) The skin and fascia of the forearm extending from the wrist to the midarm including lacertus fibrosis, the deep fascial compartments over the flexor carpi ulnaris, and in certain instances the edge of the flexor sublimis muscles, which compress the median nerve and the median or radial arteries.

Open Trauma to the Extensor Surface of the Hand

A hand injured by the crushing effects of a heavy weight is shown in Figure 12. The dorsal skin has been partially avulsed, the extensor tendons are exposed, the metacarpals were fractured, and osteochondral injuries occurred to the metacarpophalangeal joints. The objectives of treatment are (a) to prevent infection, particularly gas gangrene; (b) to provide stability of the skeleton and adequate skin coverage as soon as is practical; and (c) to replace or maintain damaged extensor tendons.

The initial treatment included brachial block anesthesia, application of a tourniquet to 300 mm. Hg, and wound cleansing with soap, water, and a soft brush. The wound was excised and the damaged skin trimmed; the extensor tendons were all exposed but were intact. The fractured metacarpals were recognized by direct observation and by roentgenogram. Crossed fixation pins were inserted with a motorized drill. Pins should not traverse the joints if this can be avoided. The wound was dressed open and additional necrotic tissue was excised at 48 and 72 hours. Wet dressings were begun at five days, and by ten days after the injury, the granulating bed was sufficient to accept a split skin graft from the thigh to the back of the hand. The metacarpophalangeal joints were held at 75 per cent flexion and the interphalangeal joints at 10 per cent flexion while the skin was maturing. Plaster splints were formed at three weeks and active motion was started. The extensor tendons moved through a full range of motion during the recovery phase, and the range of flexion was adequate to bring the fingertips to the palm. Metacarpal fractures healed at about eight weeks, but motion began at approximately fourteen days after the grafts were done.

These examples demonstrate a safe, proven method of management of open hand wounds. Concepts can be summarized as follows: (a) *Primary wound excision* is followed by delayed skin closure or delayed skin coverage. The period of delay may vary from five to 10 days depending on the severity of the injury. Immediate wound closure is not essential and there is a certain risk involved as it relates to development of infection and vascular insufficiency. (b) *Lacerated digital nerves* are best recognized and left unattended at the time of the acute injury. Nerve repair can be done anywhere from five days to five months after initial injury, an ideal time being from 21 to 42 days. In certain instances, delayed primary repair is performed when the wound is closed at five to seven days. The concept behind delayed nerve repair is to allow localization of the traumatic segment of the nerve, which provides more information about trimming the nerve prior to repair. (c) For *flexor tendons* lacerated at the distal palm or within the finger, and if the laceration is accompanied by crushing or multiple digit trauma, the safest approach is to avoid traumatizing the tendon by attempted repair. Skin coverage is obtained and at a later date a secondary repair is done with alternatives which include (1) use

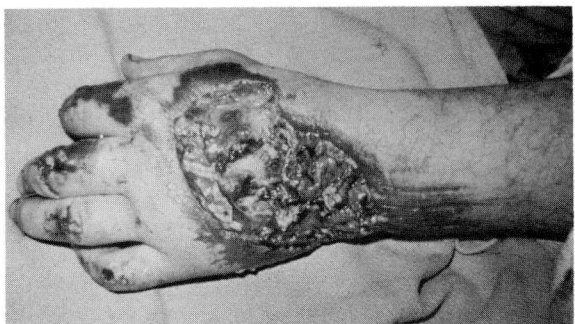

Figure 12. Both the dorsum and the volar aspects of the hand show loss of skin, fascia, extensor tendons and multi-tissue injury at all levels. Meticulous wound excision, irrigation, and coverage with a pedicle flap are essential in restoring a useful hand.

of a silicone rod followed eventually by free tendon graft, (2) delayed repair which provides an end-to-end suture of the tendon, or (3) a delayed tendon graft which utilizes either the palmaris longus, the extensor digitorum communis, or the plantaris tendon to replace the fibrotic or severed distal portion of the tendon. Primary repair of tendons does have a place in relatively young patients whose injuries have been the result of sharp lacerations not accompanied by crushing injury. (d) Fixation of fractures involving the diaphysis or the metaphysis can be done at the time of acute trauma. The wounds, however, are left open. If a crushing injury occurs with multiple fractures and the wounds are closed, then percutaneous pin fixation or manipulation with external plaster splint fixation or open reduction, depending on the type of fracture that occurred, can be accomplished (see section on hand fractures). A delay in fracture fixation for one or two days, depending on the condition of the hand, has merit if repair of the fracture requires considerable manipulation and more exposure. In general, fractures can be stabilized by either external or internal means at the time of the original wound excision.

TENDON INJURY AND REPAIR

Tendon continuity is necessary for transmission of force from the muscle belly to the hand or digits. Each muscle tendon unit has vascular supply, nerve supply, and gliding mechanism, all of which insure good nutrition and smooth activity. Disruption of a tendon causes loss of motion of the digit and diminished strength (Fig. 13). The severity of tendon injury varies according to the location of the loss of continuity, the mechanism of injury, conditions that exist at the time of the injury, the particular tendon involved, and the anatomic location of the laceration in relationship to the muscle-tendon unit. A tendon laceration directly over a joint is more serious than an injury at the musculotendinous junction. Maximal tendon function requires full thickness skin coverage, epitenon and

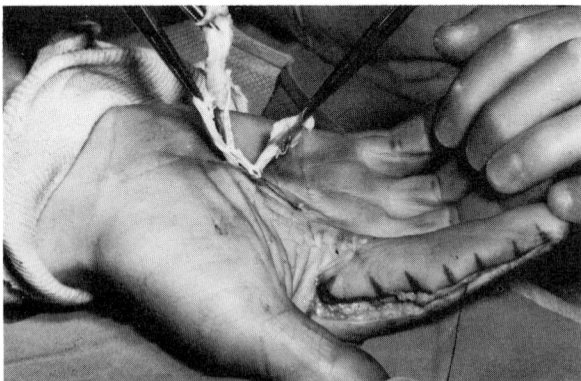

Figure 13. The flexor digitorum sublimis and profundus are firmly adherent in the palm. Both have retracted after a laceration at the base of the digit. This much fibrosis is frequently recognized in the region of the distal palm or proximal finger after an attempt at primary repair by the surgeon who only occasionally does tendon repairs. Tendon grafting was necessary in order to restore improved use of the finger. Delayed primary repair is an acceptable approach to lacerations in this region of the hand. (Reprinted with permission from Harper and Row from Surgery of the Hand, J. L. Goldner, 1970.)

teritenon to protect the tendon from surrounding adhesions, and muscle belly of adequate strength.

Healing of Tendon

The strength-duration curve shows that healing is weak at 21 days, but of sufficient strength to tolerate active contraction of the muscle. At six weeks external elastic traction can be applied if the force is not excessive. At three months, moderate stress can be applied to the flexor tendon in both flexion and extension. At eight months, full tensile strength has been recovered. The healing tendon forms a strong bond as fibroblasts realign, collagen matrices unite, blood vessels invade the area of healing, and the fibroblasts migrate from the periphery to the centrum in order to establish a bond. The peripheral covering adheres to the tendon throughout its entire length early during the period of healing. A tenoma is formed and this gradually matures. The degree of shortening or lengthening of the tendon should be within the limits of the tension-strength curve. If the tendon is shortened, too much stretch is applied to the muscle mass and maximum strength will not be obtained. A contracture will result.

Concepts Concerning Repair of Injuries Tendons

Primary repair of an injured tendon requires meticulous cleansing of the wound, gentle handling of tissue, and re-establishment of continuity with nonabsorbable, nonreactive, strong suture material. If the area of repair is within an annular ligament such as at the base of the fingers, adhesions to the annular ligament may result in diminution of gliding and contracture will result. Primary repair is acceptable if the surgeon is experienced, if the wound is exceptionally clean, and if there has been no crushing of the tendon or surrounding tissues. In almost any instance, delayed repair is safe and acceptable and can be determined as the treatment of choice if the local wound is contaminated, if the trauma is severe, if the patient's condition will not allow prolonged operation, and if the surgeon is not experienced in complicated tendon repair.

Prerequisites for Successful Tendon Repair

(1) The operative procedure is done with minimal trauma. Wound cleansing is complete and thorough, and neutral soap and saline are used when irritation is present. (2) The extremity is prepared as a bloodless field by using a pneumatic tourniquet at 280 to 300 mm. Hg. A safe, acceptable time for elevation of the tourniquet is two hours. (3) Adequate lights, experienced assistance, microsurgical instruments, strong, nonreactive, nonabsorbable suture, and magnification are essential. (4) Skin incisions should correspond to natural skin lines. (5) The surgeon should be familiar with special problems related to the anatomy of lacerated tendons so that retrieval, mobilization, and identification of the tendons can be done easily. (6) Familiarity with multitissue injuries, i.e., skin, bone, joint, nerve, and vascular, is necessary. In the presence of multiple tissue trauma, repair of tendons is best avoided.

The greater the trauma, the more active is peritendinous fibrosis and adhesions to surrounding tissue. Excessive irritation of the tendon results in extreme fibrosis. Tendon ends are held together by relaxing adjacent joints. Sutures are placed in such a way that they have a strong purchase on the involved tendon ends and penetrate the lacerated margins with accuracy and finesse, and are buried in such a way that they will not cause adhesions to surrounding tissues. Sutures are placed as a double figure of eight with two turns on either side of the tendon, and the knot is tied either proximal or distal. Several circumferential sutures of fine synthetic material are added for improved fixation.

Postoperative Care after Tendon Repair

Postoperative immobilization with plaster splints is mandatory and requires inclusion of a joint above and below the involved laceration. The position of the extremity depends on the particular tendon involved.

1. If a flexor tendon laceration occurs at the middle phalanx of the long finger, 20 degree wrist flexion, flexion of the metacarpophalangeal joint, and flexion of the interphalangeal joints of the index, long, and ring fingers should be maintained to avoid unusual pull by the adjacent tendons. A dorsal plaster splint is sufficient to provide tendon immobilization. A volar splint is contraindicated, since, if the splint slips away from the hand, the digit will be forced into extension and the tendon will be ruptured.

2. Repair of a lacerated wrist tendon requires elbow flexion and wrist flexion through about 45 degrees. The fingers may be relaxed and allowed to move.

3. Immobilization of the extensor tendons depends on the location of the injury, which joints are involved, and whether or not the tendon is part of the common extensors in the forearm.

Special problems related to laceration and repair of flexor tendons are demonstrated in the several figures designated. The legends describe in detail the problem that occurs and the method of management.

Technique of Tendon Grafting

A midlateral or midmedial incision is made for exposure of the tendon. The neurovascular structures are reflected toward the volar surface with the flap. An alternate method of exposure is zigzag incision with a 45 degree angle incision extending from the distal volar crease to the proximal crease and in turn a second oblique incision going to the radial aspects of the proximal phalanx. The neurovascular structures are isolated and a small rubber dam placed around the nerve and artery (Figs. 14A and B). The flaps are reflected, the annular ligaments identified, and the proximal and distal ligaments trimmed. The cruciate ligaments between the annular ligaments are opened so that the lacerated adherent tendons can be resected and as much of the annular ligaments as possible is saved.

Each volar capsule is identified at the metacarpophalangeal joint, as well as at the proximal interphalangeal and the distal interphalangeal joint. If the capsule has been torn or injured during the original trauma, then a delayed repair is done. The distal stump of the profundus tendon is isolated and resected so that 6-mm. segments remain attached to the distal phalanx. The lumbrical is identified and, if fibrosed, it is resected. It is not wrapped around the anastomosis site. The flexor sublimis is identified and removed at the wrist and usually used as the free tendon graft. The flexor digitorum profundus is identified in the base of the palm and cut back until good tendon is identified within the mass of the lumbrical. The proximal anastomosis is done as an end-to-end suture if the tendon graft and the flexor profundus are of the same diameter. Immobilization is done by a compression dressing from the fingertips to above the elbow, and a dorsal plaster splint from the fingertips to the mid arm in order to keep the elbow flexed, the wrist flexed at 30 degrees, the metacarpophalangeal joints flexed at 60 degrees, and the interphalangeal joints flexed at 10 degrees.

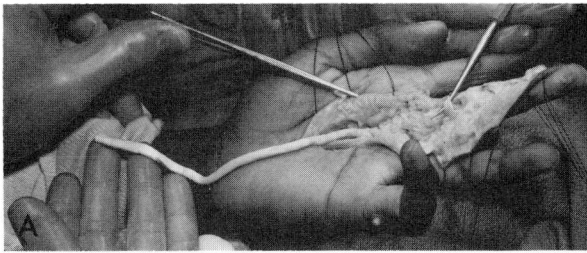
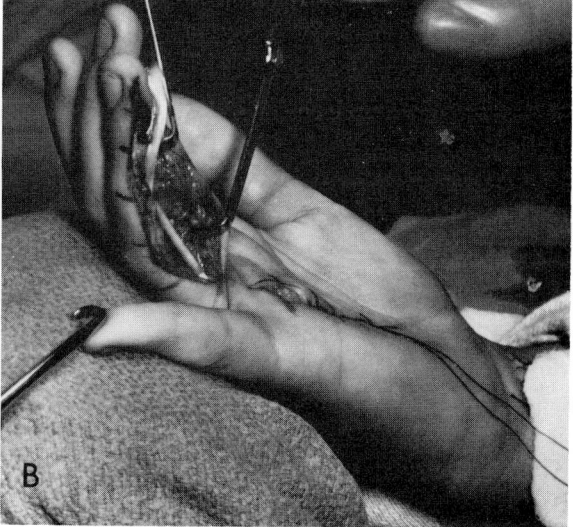

Figure 14. *A,* Free flexor tendon graft to the long finger is being completed. Original laceration was at the base of the digit, and attempted repair has failed. Three annular ligaments have been constructed. The flexor profundus proximally is being used as a motor, and the free tendon graft has been taken from the flexor digitorum sublimis. If excessive scarring is present, a silicone rod is inserted first and the flexor tendon is used later as an autogenous graft.

B, A free tendon graft is being done to salvage a finger which has been affected by laceration through the proximal finger crease for which a repair had been attempted primarily. Fibrosis occurred, and an effort at a short tendon graft had failed. The entire digit has been opened, annular ligaments have been reshaped and made more narrow. The free tendon graft extended from the fingertip to the base of the palm. A digital nerve laceration was repaired. Eventually the patient could flex the fingertip to within one centimeter of the distal palm crease and extension was almost complete. (Reprinted with permission from Harper and Row from Surgery of the Hand, J. L. Goldner, 1970.)

Complete immobilization is indicated for 21 days and partial immobilization for an additional 21 days.

Tendon Repair—Special Problems

Avulsion of the Flexor Digitorum Profundus from Insertion. The tendon retracts to the base of the digit or into the palm, depending upon the force causing the avulsion; the vinculum prevents excessive retraction. Primarily, treatment is to isolate the tendon proximally with the insertion made distally, and to reattach the tendon to the point of initial insertion. Delayed repair after 21 days may be managed in the same way. However, if the tendon has retracted in such a way that it has become adherent to itself, it cannot be used for replacement and must be excised and a free tendon graft used.

Laceration of Flexor Digitorum Profundus Distal to the Flexor Digitorum Sublimis Insertion. The proximal tendon retracts to the base of the digit or into the palm. Primary repair is possible, but usually not desirable if the wound is contaminated or if undue trauma has occurred. Delayed repair at seven to 21 days or even as long as six weeks can be done by mobilizing the tendon proximally, maintaining the annular ligaments, and suturing the tendon within the finger. Distal advancement more than 1 cm. is never advisable.

Laceration of Flexor Digitorum Profundus at the Base of the Digit. Primary repair in exceptional circumstances should be done by a surgeon who is familiar and experienced in tendon operations. Reasonable success can be expected, but in most instances delayed repair is advisable or free tendon grafting will provide a continuity without a suture line at the base of the digit. In young adults and children, free tendon grafts threaded through or around the intact flexor digitorum sublimis tendon provide sufficient restoration of strength, fingertip mobility, and dexterity to make this procedure useful and advisable. The palmaris longus or pedal extensor digitorum communis provides a satisfactory graft.

Free tendon grafts should not be used in "older" patients unless absolutely essential, as fibrosis of the digit and limitation of motion in the adjacent fingers may occur during the period of immobilization.

Laceration of Flexor Tendons in the Arm

When both flexor tendons are lacerated at the level of the metacarpophalangeal joint, flexion of the proximal interphalangeal joint and distal interphalangeal joints is not possible. Motion at the metacarpophalangeal joint can be maintained by the interossei and the lumbricals. The time and kind of repair depend on the circumstances associated with the initial injury. Primary repair is possible in certain instances, but delayed repair for 7 to 21 days is safe and acceptable. This kind of operative procedure should be done by the surgeon experienced in the anatomy of the hand and aware of the various techniques necessary to provide a satisfactory tendon junction with minimal fibrosis. In certain instances both tendons can be repaired, particularly when the suture lines do not directly coincide with each other. In other situations, the flexor profundus is repaired, and the flexor sublimis can be sacrificed. Whenever possible, however, both tendons should be sutured.

Nerve injuries associated with tendon lacerations may be repaired as primary procedures if the initial injury is clean and sharp with minimal trauma. Alternatively, a safe and reasonable way to manage the nerve is to wait 7 to 21 days and do the repair at the same time that the tendon repair is done. Flexion of the wrist provides relaxation of the tendons and mobilization of the nerve, and there is no technical difficulty in repairing tendons and nerves during the same operative procedure. There is clinical and experimental evidence to show that Surgicel wrapped around the nerve temporarily prevents adhesions between the tendon and nerve. Occasionally, when an unusual amount of fibrosis exists in a delayed repair, a thin sheet of *silicone* is placed between the tendon and the nerve or between repaired tendons in order to prevent adhesions. The silicone is removed at a later time once healing has occurred and range of motion has increased.

Lacerations of Flexor Tendons at the Base of the Palm

Tendon injuries in this area are usually associated with laceration of the median nerve. The nerve separates into sensory branches to the thumb, index, and long fingers and also into the motor segment to the thenar muscles. The transverse retinacular ligament confines the four flexor sublimis tendons, the flexor digitorum profundus tendons, and the median nerve. Tendon repair at this level requires mobilization of the nerve and tendons at the wrist, isolation of the distal segments at the mid and distal palm, and preservation of the superficial vascular arch. All profundus tendons are repaired by using nonabsorbable polyester sutures as double figures of eight and by supplementing these with fine circumferential interrupted sutures. The flexor digitorum sublimis tendons are also repaired, provided that the amount of fibrosis is not excessive and that the length of time between injury and repair has not been so long that inherent shortening of the tendons has occurred. Wrist and finger flexion will provide adequate relaxation during the healing period. Nerve and tendon repairs are done meticulously with appropriate magnification, fine suture, and careful postoperative immobilization for a minimum of three weeks. Excessive stretching of the nerve during the period of mobilization must be avoided.

CONCEPT OF DELAYED TENDON REPAIR

Flexor Pollicis Longus Tendon—Delayed Repair by Advancement, Free Graft, or Direct Suture. The patient who has had a laceration of the thumb may have other conditions that preclude primary repair of a laceration of the flexor pollicis longus. If the condition of the wound, the patient's general condition, or other factors such as nonavailability of an experienced surgeon exist, the lesion may be treated by delayed tendon repair. The choice of procedure depends on the location of the laceration. The operative management of a laceration or avulsion of the flexor pollicis longus tendon differs from that of a similar injury to one of the flexor digitorum profundus tendons, as the thumb tendon is distinctly different from the other digit flexor tendons. The thumb is the most important digit of the hand and must have maximum possible strength and stability as well as good mobility of both the carpometacarpal and the interphalangeal joints if grasp and pinch are to be normal.

Anatomical Studies. The flexor pollicis longus is an individual unit except in rare instances when the thumb flexor is partially united with the flexor profundus of the index finger. This variation at the base of the hand may complicate the operative repair.

A second difference between the flexor of the thumb and the deep finger flexors is the absence of the flexor digitorum superficialis tendon and lumbrical muscle in the thumb. The long thumb flexor moves two phalanges and passes through two annular ligaments, one being at the level of the proximal phalanx, and the other proximal to the metacarpophalangeal joint. The vinculum of the flexor pollicis longus, which attaches to the proximal part of the proximal phalanx, is more often absent than present. When absent, retraction of the proximal segment of the lacerated tendon is inevitable. The excursion of the flexor pollicis longus is 10 to 12 mm., whereas that of the profundus tendons of other digits is about 5 mm. A significant feature related to the method of repair is the large number of anatomical segments. Three to 4 cm. of the thumb flexor tendon have no muscle fibers attached to it at the wrist. This muscle-free segment proximal to the transverse retinacular ligament allows tendon lengthening of several centimeters close to the musculotendinous junction without risk of impingement of the suture line on the ligament when the thumb is in full extension and the wrist is dorsiflexed.

The thumb flexor can be exposed at any point along its course. The soft tissues overlying the palmar aspect of the tendon at the level of the metacarpal include the abductor pollicis brevis, the flexor pollicis brevis, the motor branch of the median nerve, and the origin of the common digital nerves of the thumb and of the index and long fingers from the median nerve. Exposure of the tendon in this area must be done with caution, and tendon repair in this region will depend on many factors.

Seventy-three patients with lacerated flexor tendons of the thumb were reviewed. This group showed the location of these lacerations and provided information about the common sites of injury.

Classification of Tendon Lacerations. Treatment depends upon the location of the laceration and the severity of the problem. The patients are divided into *tendon* group, *scar* group, and *joint* group. In this modified classification, injuries of the digital nerve are ignored. In the tendon group, the lacerations of the flexor pollicis longus with no scarring or joint impairment are included. The scar group includes injuries complicated by moderate to severe fibrosis around the site of laceration by demonstable soft tissue contracture. In the joint group are the injuries that have caused fibrosis and joint involvement with periarticular contracture in addition to disruption of the tendon. Associated nerve and tendon injuries in addition to those of the flexor pollicis longus were repaired at the time of delayed operation. One or both digital nerves, if lacerated, were repaired, and other finger flexors or major lacerations of the median and ulnar nerve can also be repaired. Retraction of the flexor pollicis longus occurs frequently after the proximal segment is separated from the distal segment. This tendon segment is frequently found at the wrist, and physicians unfamiliar with the anatomic characteristics of the tendon will find that efforts at primary repair result in failure.

Technique of Direct Tendon Suture. End-to-end suture is used for repairs done at the wrist proximal to the transverse retinacular ligament. After mobilization of the proximal and distal segments of the tendon, a double figure-of-eight suture of 3-0 polyester is used to provide tensile strength. Interrupted sutures of 4-0 polyester are inserted peripherally as interrupted horizontal mattress sutures to provide additional strength and to insure a smooth tendon surface at the site of repair. If the suture line enters the tunnel at the base of the palm, the portion of the tunnel traversed by the suture line is excised.

Direct end-to-end suture in the area of the distal phalanx is done after all or part of the distal annular ligament has been excised and the tendon ends freshened. A pull-out suture can be used to obtain the direct end-to-end anastomosis, and this is supplemented by horizontal mattress sutures. The suture lines are wrapped with Surgicel, as this has been shown experimentally to diminish peritendinous adhesions temporarily.

ADVANCEMENT WITH OR WITHOUT LENGTHENING

A laceration in the distal phalangeal area, not more than 1 cm. from the insertion of the flexor tendon, is managed by advancement of the proximal tendon segment, with attachment of its distal end to or under a small remnant of the remaining distal stump. The bone is roughened and a figure-of-eight 3-0 polyester suture is placed through the end of the proximal segment through the distal stump, and two limbs of the suture exit through the skin on either side of the nail plate. The suture is tied over a plastic button or a firm rubber protector. No bone hole is made. Reinforcing sutures are placed between the small remnants of the distal stump and the advanced tendon.

If advancement of more than 1 cm. is required, the tendon is lengthened at the musculotendinous junction proximal to the transverse retinacular ligament at the wrist. A Z-lengthening is performed with the free ends of the tendon sutured in a button hole fashion using synthetic suture. Reinforcement of the area of lengthening is provided by a free tendon graft obtained from the adjacent flexor carpi radialis or distal segment of the tendon removed from the thumb. The combined procedure of advancement and lengthening is less complicated than a free tendon graft, since it utilizes a tendon already in situ, a tendon that is of the same caliber as the original one, and may retain part of its original blood supply. The proper tension is relatively easy to judge.

FREE TENDON GRAFT

When a laceration occurs between the wrist and the metacarpophalangeal joint and the patient is seen immediately, the area may be operated upon and an end-to-end anastomosis done. This same method of treatment could be determined if the laceration were seen within 14 to 21 days after injury. As a rule, however, the level of metacarpophalangeal joint is arbitrarily established as the point proximal to which free tendon graft should be done.

The graft is taken from the palmaris longus, from one of the extensor digitorum communis tendons of the toes, or from the flexor digitorum superficialis of the ring finger. The anastomosis at the musculotendinous junction of the flexor pollicis longus is placed far enough proximal to the transverse retinacular ligament so that the suture line does not impinge on the ligament or at complete extension of the thumb. The graft is sutured to the proximal segment of the tendon at the wrist using a button hole technique and nonabsorbable synthetic suture. A free graft is passed along the original course of the flexor pollicis longus into the thumb, and the length of the graft is determined by certain maneuvers that can be applied to determine the length of any free tendon graft.

Postoperative Care

A dorsal plaster splint is used to immobilize the hand, forearm, and elbow for a minimum of 10 days after operation. A volar splint is avoided because if it slips distally, undue tenson may be applied to the repaired tendon. The flexed elbow tends to diminish dependency of the hand and prevent the dressing from migrating distally. The wrist is held in 30 degrees of flexion in order to relieve tension on the proximal and distal suture lines in the thumb. When the postoperative splint is removed, a shorter dorsal plaster splint is used for an additional 12 days in order to protect the thumb from forceful extension. This regimen of external immobilization is followed after lengthening at the wrist and distal advancement and after free tendon graft. After tendon advancement without lengthening, however, active motion of the digit is started in a limited way at 10 days in adults and at three weeks in children. The button is left in place for a minimum of four weeks and occasionally for five weeks if the flexion contracture of the distal joint is resistant and external splinting is necessary to improve extension. Active flexion exercises using wooden blocks of appropriate size, compressible plastic putty, hand grippers of varying resistance, firm aluminum extension splints for night use, and elastic outriggers for day use are all successful in improving range of motion. Forceful stretching and heavy work are to be avoided for at least eight weeks. Formal physical therapy is used occasionally, but in most instances, a properly planned home program is sufficient to regain maximum strength and range of motion.

Overall results depend on the initial injury, the location of the laceration, the age of the patient, and the kind of operative procedure done, as well as the classification of the laceration. Patients in the scar and the joint group do not do as well as patients in the tendon group. There is definitely no correlation between the delay in treatment and the end result in the different treatment groups.

COMPLICATIONS OF INJURIES OF THE FLEXOR TENDON OF THE THUMB

1. *Nerve involvement:* A compression syndrome involving either the main trunk of the median nerve at the wrist or the digital nerves in the thumb. This is probably the result of edema beneath the transverse retinacular ligament. Also, direct involvement of the digital nerve during the approach to the flexor tendons and placement of the graft must be considered.

2. *Separation of the tendon from the muscle belly:* The proximal portion of the lacerated tendon may be firmly adherent to the muscle belly because the tendon has coiled up on itself after retraction into the wrist. While traction is being applied during reconstruction in an effort to improve the excursion of the muscle tendon unit, the tendon may avulse at the musculotendinous junction. A tendon transfer using a flexor digitorum superficialis is usually advisable, since a free tendon graft to a fibrosed muscle belly will probably not be successful.

3. *Tendon adhesions limiting extension:* In certain instances, when more than one tendon graft has been attempted and has failed, secondary tenolysis may be required in order to improve excursion and range of motion of the thumb. Occasionally, in a delayed end-to-end suture, localized adhesions may prevent full extension of the thumb and tenolysis is necessary.

4. *Tendon bow-stringing:* This occurs at the level of the metacarpophalangeal joint after excision of the proximal annular ligament while the repair is being done, or it may be due to adhesions of the proximal annular ligament as a result of the original injury. Bow-stringing limits finger extension, reduces excursion, and causes flexion deformity of the distal interphalangeal joint. Hypersensitivity in the thumb over the bow-stringing tendon does occur.

Silicone as an Adjunct in Treatment of Tendon Repair and Tendon Fibrosis

Severe trauma, infection, or multiple tissue injuries result in a flexor or an extensor mechanism making restoration of tendon gliding and, in turn, digit function, difficult or impossible. The introduction of silicone rods, silicone sheeting, and, in the future, permanent artificial tendons represents a step forward in reconstruction of the damaged hand.

Silicone Rod Prior to Autogenous Flexor Tendon Grafting

If the gliding surface of the involved digit is fibrotic and regular, if annular ligaments need reconstruction because of damage to the major canals at the base of the finger, and if joints are limited in motion, then a free tendon graft will usually not succeed. Use of a silicone rod (3 mm., 4 mm., or 5 mm.) will provide that initial stage during which pulleys are reconstructed, joints are mobilized, and a pseudosheath forms around the silicone rod (Fig. 15). The distal end is attached by a Dacron suture to bone or the residual tendon stump, the annular ligaments are reconstructed at the anatomic points

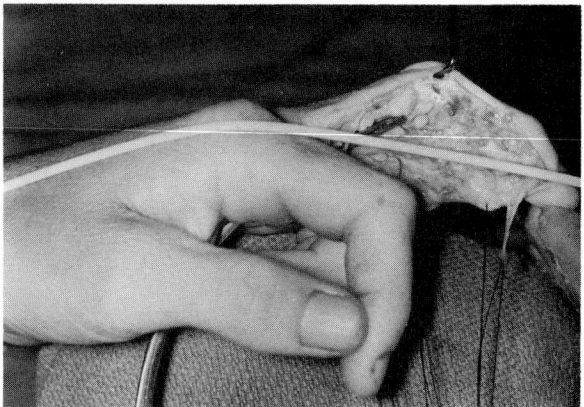

Figure 15. A flexor tendon injury resulted in severe fibrosis throughout the course of the tendon. The scarred tendon has been removed, annular ligaments reconstructed, digital nerve prepared for suture, and a silicone rod will be inserted into the digit from the tip to the wrist to act as a stimulus to pseudo-sheath formation. At a later time, the rod is removed and a biologic autogenous tendon graft is inserted.

over the middle phalanx, at the distal end of the proximal phalanx, and at the level of the metacarpophalangeal joint. Both the flexor digitorum sublimis and the flexor profundus tendons are removed back to the base of the palm and/or wrist and the silicone rod is inserted from the tip of the digit to the wrist level. The rod is not attached proximally so that passive motion will allow unimpeded gliding proximally and distally, whereas, if the rod were attached to an active muscle, several weeks or months would be necessary to provide a maximum range of motion, and in the meantime, buckling would occur when flexion was attempted because of the impedance of the muscle tendon attachment.

After a maximum range of motion has been recovered and when the neural and vascular recovery is adequate, then a free tendon graft, usually the extensor digitorum communis, is sutured to the proximal end of the silicone rod at the wrist and the distal attachment of the rod is released. Traction is applied to the rod, and the free tendon graft is threaded through the base of the palm, the mid palm, and the digit without extensive exposure. The tendon graft is attached to the flexor digitorum profundus of the involved finger or fingers proximally and is attached to the distal stump or bone with a pull-out suture. A period of immobilization is absolute for 21 days, with limited motion for an additional four weeks. An outrigger elastic traction splint, a protective night splint in either flexion or extension depending on the condition of the finger, and active exercise with the patient concentrating on each interphalangeal joint make up the postoperative exercise program.

The use of the silicone rod has provided a way of upgrading severely traumatized digits one or two classifications better than if the silicone rod had not been used. A Grade IV digit indicates damage to the skin, nerve, tendon, bone, and joint. Free tendon grafting to that digit or primary repair of tendons usually fails. The initial management is one of prevention of infection, which would indicate that delayed or secondary repair of the tissues after initial wound excision is a safe, acceptable method of treating the finger. Once skin has healed or been replaced, then the silicone rod is inserted. During this time the severity of the injury decreases as joints are mobilized, nerve regenerates, and the pseudo-sheath is being formed. A Grade IV digit may be upgraded to a Grade II digit, at which time, the autogenous free tendon graft is done with reasonable chance of success, whereas, if it had been done on a Grade IV digit, failure would have occurred.

Silicone Tendons on the Extensor Aspect of the Hand

Severe damage to the dorsum of the hand may result in avulsion of the extensor tendons, damage to the extensor hood, and inability of the patient to actively elevate the digits, including the thumb. The skeleton is stabilized by pin fixation, the joints are mobilized, a split skin graft or pedicle skin graft is used to fill soft tissue defects, and autogenous tendons or fasciae latae or silicone tendons are then used, depending on the severity and extent of the previous injury. In many instances, silicone rods are inserted from the middle of the middle phalanx to the musculotendinous junction of the extensor digitorum communis. These tendons may be left in place for several weeks, and a pseudo-sheath forms around them. Occasionally, the pseudo-sheath will act as a tendon in itself and the further addition of autogenous tendons can be delayed. In other situations, when greater strength and mobility are desired, the tendon graft is added through the pseudosheath in the same way that the free tendon graft is used on the flexor surface. Combinations of silicone rods and silicone joints are now possible. A patient who has received a severe crushing injury to the metacarpophalangeal joint of the index finger and loss of the extensor tendon can be managed in this way. Because of severe damage to the articular surfaces, because arthrodesis of that joint is not desirable, a silicone-Dacron joint is inserted to replace the damaged metacarpal head. The alternate to arthrodesis is resection, and the silicone-Dacron joint can be inserted for several years. If it fails to function mechanically, it can be resected and the remaining pseudosheath provides a reasonably stable reaction. The combined tissue replacement also requires a silicone cord to replace the extensor tendon. The silicone rod will serve as a replacement tendon for several months and eventually be replaced by an autogenous tendon graft.

Silicone sheeting of varying thickness is available as interposition material. The silicone can be anchored to tissues in a plane that allows the tendon to glide over the silicone rather than adhere to the underlying surface, producing large numbers of fibroblasts. Examples of clinical cases in which silicone has been used are: (a) Silicone sheeting placed between a flexor digitorum sublimis and profundus after repair in the palm of the hand. The silicone sheeting was left in the palm for three months, during which time tendon healing had occurred and the tendons glided on the silicone and did not adhere to each other. The silicone was then removed. (b) Silicone sheeting placed between tendons that had been adherent to bone after a fracture of a proximal phalanx in which the flexor digitorum sublimis had become adherent to bone and caused a flexion contracture of the digit. Tenolysis was done, and the silicone sheeting was placed between tendon and bone and removed four months later. A pseudosheath had formed, and the tendon was no longer adherent to bone. The contracture had been corrected.

The volar capsule at the distal interphalangeal joint, if damaged in the flexor tendon injury, may adhere to the flexor graft and cause a flexion deformity of the distal phalanx. At the time the tendon graft is inserted into the distal tendon stump, a piece of silicone sheeting is placed between the tendon and the volar capsule. During the healing phase and during the early motion, the flexor tendon graft will not adhere to the volar capsule and there is less chance for the occurrence of a flexor deformity. The silicone sheet is removed at a later time.

THE EXTENSOR AND INTRINSIC MUSCLE MECHANISM OF THE HAND

Physiologic function of the hand depends on coordination and intact intrinsic muscle mechanism and the extrinsic muscles. Injury to any part of this system results in deformity. Trauma to the central segment of the extensor tendon, to the lateral oblique tendons anywhere along their course, or to the dorsal extensor hood results in an imperfectly functioning digit. Ischemic contracture of the intrinsic muscles, fibrosis of the intrinsic tendons, thermal injury of the dorsal tissues, or contracture of the collateral ligaments results in predictable anatomic changes and specific deformities. Roller injuries or direct crushing injuries involving the extensor mechanism are examples of trauma that causes extensor intrinsic contracture.

"Claw Deformity"

Laceration of the median and ulnar nerves at the wrist results in paralysis of the interosseous, lumbrical, thenar, and hypothenar muscles. The thumb assumes the position of external rotation and adduction, opposition is absent, the concave surface of the palm becomes convex, the metacarpophalangeal joints hyperextend, and the distal joints assume a position of flexion. Flexion of the wrist from the cicatrix accentuates the overactive pull of the extensor tendons against the fibrotic flexor tendons (see Fig. 6). The characteristics of this "claw" position are skin contracture on the dorsum, shortening of the extensor tendons and dorsal fascia, adherence of the dorsal hood and capsule, and contracture of the collateral ligaments of the metacarpophalangeal joints. The dorsal interossei function as extensors of the phalanges rather than flexors because the axis of rotation is toward the dorsal surface. The volar capsule of this joint invaginates into the joint and adheres to the metacarpal head. These deformities limit active or passive flexion of the metacarpophalangeal joints. External splinting and early repair or replacement of damaged structures decrease the severity of these contractures, although the "intrinsic minus deformity" persists. A high injury to the median and ulnar nerves causes minimal clawing of the fingers as the flexors are paralyzed, and the unopposed action of the extensors results in less deformity. Once the nerves are repaired, the extrinsic flexor power returns and the distal interphalangeal joints become more flexed. Persistent intrinsic muscle paralysis maintains the "claw" position. External pressure over the proximal phalanges replaces the stabilizing effect of the intrinsic muscles and results in extension of the distal segments of the digits by increasing tension of the extensor digitorum communis and the lateral band mechanisms. Thus, even in the absence of the intrinsic muscles, the interphalangeal joints can be straightened actively. A substitute for intrinsic muscles can be obtained by one of several operations.

Capsulodesis. Plication and shortening of the volar capsule of the metacarpophalangeal joints are performed through a palmar incision and will result in sufficient contracture, providing active extension of the interphalangeal joints by producing a deformity at the metacarpophalangeal joints that prevents them from extending beyond zero degrees. This operation improves the grasp moderately by providing a better mechanical advantage for action of the flexor digitorum sublimis in the flexed position of the metacarpophalangeal joints rather than in the hyperextended position. However, the improved strength is about 75 per cent less than that provided by normal intrinsics. This operative procedure is used for patients with insensitive hands, such as those with leprosy or brachial plexus injury. It does have limited application. Capsulodesis may stretch if the individual applies excessive force to the digits.

Passive Intrinsic Transfer. This is accomplished by utilizing a tendon graft from the extensor carpi radialis longus, leaving the graft attached at the insertion of this tendon and passing the tendon from the dorsum to the volar aspects of the transverse metacarpal ligament and inserting the tendon into the radial intrinsic tendons of the proximal phalanges. This provides a flexion contracture and prevents hyperextension at the metacarpophalangeal joint. This procedure does not add strength but does improve position and provides a mechanism whereby the extensor digitorum communis can act to straighten the interphalangeal joints. Wrist flexion and wrist extension augment the effect of the extensor digitorum communis muscle and tendons on the fingers.

Active Intrinsic Transfer. This may be done in one of several ways. The advantage of the active transfer is that a strong muscle is used to provide an additional motor to flex the metacarpophalangeal joints and, in turn, to provide extension of the interphalangeal joints either by attaching the intrinsic transfer to the oblique fibers of the intrinsic muscles or by attaching the tendon into bone or the annular ligament distal to the metacarpophalangeal joint in order to provide active flexion of the metacarpophalangeal joint. The transfer depends on the secondary effects of the extensor digitorum communis to straighten the interphalangeal joints (Fig. 16).

A flexor digitorum sublimis tendon can be split into two segments back to the wrist level. One tendon is passed on the volar surface of the hand through the lumbrical canal and inserted into the oblique fibers of the index finger. The second tendon is passed subcutaneously on the dorsum under the extensor pollicis longus and into the tendon of the first dorsal interosseous. This transfer will provide almost normal strength and replace the intrinsic muscles of the index finger. A sublimis tendon from the long finger is pulled out in the palm and split into three separate tendons, after which one segment is inserted into the radial aspect of the lateral band mechanism of the long, ring, and little fingers. The tension is adjusted so that the metacarpophalangeal joint is in 45 degrees of flexion and the interphalangeal joints are at 5 degrees of flexion when the wrist is flexed 30 degrees. This transfer provides improved power in flexion of the metacarpophalangeal joints and active assistance of extension of the interphalangeal joints.

Tendon transfer to proximal phalanx as a substitute for paralyzed intrinsic muscles uses bone as an anchor rather than the oblique fibers of the lateral band mechanism. The advantage of this procedure is that there is less likelihood of an intrinsic contracture occurring after the tendon transfer. Fibrosis does occur where the hole is drilled into the bone and excessive contracture at the metacarpophalangeal joint may occur. A single tendon is implanted into a drill hole on the radial aspect of each digit.

The tendon used to replace the intrinsic muscles can be sutured directly into the annular ligament at a point distal to the metacarpophalangeal joint of the involved digit. If the annular ligament is used as the anchor point there is minimal likelihood of contracture of the intrinsic tendons. Adjustment of tension of the tendons is slightly more critical than when the tendons are inserted into the intrinsic tendons, since the axis of rotation is farther away from the point of insertion of the tendon and thus requires increased tension on the tendon in order to maintain limited extension at the metacarpophalangeal joint.

Alternative Active Transfer. When muscles on the volar aspect of the forearm are weak, such as might be the case when a high median nerve injury exists, or when extensive fibrosis has occurred in the flexor muscle mass and individual transfer cannot be spared, then the extensor carpi radialis longus can be detached from its insertion, passed through the interosseous membrane or around the radial side of the forearm, and used as a major motor for the intrinsic transfer. This tendon can be elongated by four tendon grafts from the extensor digitorum communis or from the plantaris tendon. These tendons are inserted into the oblique fibers of the lateral band mechanism on the radial aspect of the proximal phalanx of the index, long, ring, and little fingers. These tendons are passed through the carpal canal and follow the course of the lumbrical muscle and tendons. The advantage of this transfer is that the active motor is strong, it is synergistic with flexion and extension of the interphalangeal joints of the fingers, and the tendon insertion is into a point that directly affects flexion of the proximal phalanges and extension of the interphalangeal joints.

Alternate Transfer for Passive Substitute for Paralyzed Intrinsic Muscles. If sufficient motors are not available on either the volar or the dorsal surface of the forearm, then an alternative to capsulorrhaphy is a free tendon graft sutured to the volar aspect of the transverse retinaculum at the wrist with the distal end inserting into the oblique fibers of the lateral band. This transfer, in order to be successful, depends on a satisfactory range of flexion at the metacarpophalangeal joint and active dorsiflexion and volar flexion of the wrist joint.

Joint Fusions or Augmentation of Tendon Transfers. After severe median and ulnar nerve injuries or combinations of radial nerve and median or ulnar trauma, a sufficient number of strong muscles are not available for tendon transfer, and arthrodesis of interphalangeal joints or the wrist joint may be necessary in order to provide adequate stabilization and maximum function of the fingers. Osseous fusions are done after tendon procedures are completed.

Arthrodesis of the wrist is performed when insufficient dorsiflexors are present to maintain the wrist at neutral or in an elevated position.

Arthrodesis of the interphalangeal joint and shortening of all the fingers will improve pinch and grasp. Osseous fusions are done after the tendon transfers are completed.

Metacarpophalangeal joint fusion is performed in certain instances of irreparable ulnar nerve injury, occasionally in median nerve injury when an opponens substitution is planned, and for traumatic arthrosis.

Extension Contracture of the Hand Due to Direct Trauma. Avulsion, crushing, or thermal injuries involving the dorsum of the hand may result in contracture of the structures over and around the metacarpal phalangeal joints. Release of the dorsal contracture will depend on the condition of the articular surfaces of the metacarpal phalangeal joints. If the articular cartilage is intact, then release of skin, subcutaneous tissue, dorsal fascia, and extensor tendon proximal to the joint will decrease the contracture. Intra-articular excision of the collateral ligaments and release of the volar capsule will allow the proximal phalanx to be flexed to anywhere from 45 to 90 degrees, depending on the severity of the contracture. Fixation pins are passed from the proximal phalanx to the metacarpal neck to maintain a corrected position. If the skin excision was necessary and the tendons are intact, then a split skin graft is sufficient to cover the defect. If the extensor

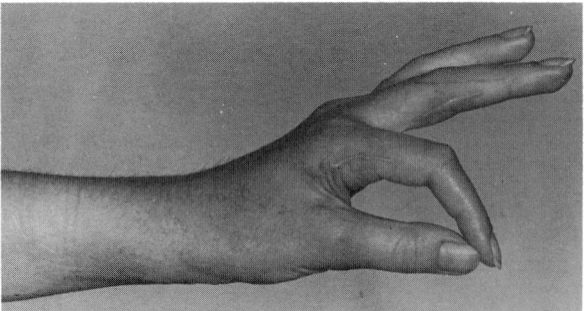

Figure 16. This patient has had multiple tendon transfers to the hand in order to improve pinch, grasph, and hook. The flexor digitorum sublimis tendons from the long and ring fingers were used to replace the interossei and had been weakened by a laceration at the wrist. Pinch approaches normal, and clawing of the fingers has been eliminated.

tendons are fibrosed or severely damaged, then a pedicle flap is necessary to protect the underlying tissue.

The order of tissue correction depends upon the condition of the joints. In most instances the flap is applied first, since maintaining the fingers in flexion is difficult while the hand is attached to the abdomen. Management of the metacarpophalangeal joint articulation includes consideration of maintenance of joint articulations and correction of contracture, replacement of extensor tendons, and replacement by adequate skin graft or pedicle flap. If the articular surfaces are damaged, then resection of the joint and replacement by silicone-Dacron joint has been successful. The fascia lata replacement of the dorsal hood is also possible, with the distal ends of the fascial strips being anchored to the extensor tendon over the proximal phalanx of each digit or by anchoring the fascia lata into the drill hole in bone. Proximally, the fascia lata is attached to the extensor digitorum communis at the musculotendinous junction. If the extensor digitorum communis muscle is fibrotic, then the adjacent extensor carpi radialis longus muscle tendon unit can be detached from its insertion, mobilized proximally, and used as an active motor of the extensor tendon grafts, whether they be extensor tendons from the feet, or fascia lata grafts.

Isolated Metacarpal Phalangeal Joint Injury. A severe injury involving the articular surfaces of the metacarpophalangeal joint accompanied by skin loss and destruction of the dorsal extensor hood may be treated by resection and replacement with a silicone-Dacron graft. An alternative is arthrodesis, but this is less desirable because of the effect of the stiff metacarpophalangeal joint on the flexion and extension of the adjacent fingers. Arthrodesis of the metacarpophalangeal joint of the index finger causes less difficulty than arthrodesis of the ulnar three digits, which are closely interrelated in the actions of flexion and extension.

The use of *silicone substitutes* provides a way of maintaining a reasonable range of motion at the metacarpophalangeal joint, and the use of a silicone rod for either the extensor tendon or the flexor tendon gives a method of reconstruction of the major components of the joint and the extrinsic tendons, thereby avoiding arthrodesis or amputation.

HAND RECONSTRUCTION AFTER THERMAL INJURIES

The severity of the original hand burn determines, in part, the magnitude of residual deformity. Other factors such as long delay in skin coverage, malposition of the digits during immobilization, and prolonged periods of immobility may result in unnecessary deformities. Positioning of each individual digit and the metacarpophalangeal joints must be considered when the initial and subsequent dressings are applied and when necrotic tissue is excised. If ligamentous and skin contractures do result, operative procedures will be necessary to alleviate the joints and contracted skin. Tissues that may be involved alone or in combination are (1) skin and superficial fascia, (2) dorsal extensor tendons, tendon sheaths, and deep fascia, (3) metacarpophalangeal joints with the extensor hood, the dorsal and volar capsule, and the collateral ligaments, (4) interphalangeal joints and the extensor tendon and dorsal hood and volar capsule, and collateral ligaments, (5) intrinsic muscles and tendons, (6) all palmar soft tissues including skin, fascia, tendons, and capsule, and (7) articular surfaces of all joints.

Burns Involving Skin and Superficial Fascia

Relatively early placement of skin grafts prevents severe contractures. If a dorsal keloid results at the metacarpophalangeal joint, extension contracture occurs. If the keloid occurs on the palmar surface, then a flexion deformity may result at the interphalangeal joints, either full flexion or full extension is impossible, and blanching of the skin at points of contracture is evident. Contractures about the thumb may limit flexion of the distal joint, abduction, rotation, and opposition. The little finger may become ulnar deviated and abducted.

Operative Technique. The tourniquet at 300 mm. Hg is used while the dissection is being done. The tourniquet is released prior to application of the skin graft so that bleeding points can be cauterized. The thickness of the skin graft varies according to the surface to be covered and the condition of the recipient site. The keloid is excised down to the subcutaneous fat and tendon sheaths, and the dorsal veins are left intact. Peripheral margins of the excised areas extend distal to involved joints and both medial and lateral to the vertical axis in order to minimize recurrent scar contracture.

If multiple joints are involved, their contracture is diminished and fixation pins are placed across the joints, avoiding articular surfaces. Metacarpophalangeal joints are fixed at 90 degrees, proximal interphalangeal joints at 90 degrees, and the distal joints at 45 degrees in order to correct extension contractures. Elongated interdigital web spaces are excised, longitudinal scars interrupted by making the incisions irregular, and diamond-shaped segments of split skin graft held in place by cotton ball compression dressings used to eliminate hematoma. Sutures are inserted through the volar surface of the hand to provide stability for the stent.

Nail bed and nail plate irregularities occur, and the heat affects the germinal cells as well. Treatment depends on the severity of the deformity. The fingernail and nail matrix may be removed, but the nail plate remains as a donor site for a split skin graft or spontaneous fibrosis. If the structures are deformed so that a nail will not regenerate, then the nail plate, nail bed germinal layer, and part of the phalanx are removed and closed when the volar flap is done.

Burns Affecting Skin, Tendons, and Ligaments

Operative procedures for correcting this deformity include skin replacement, tenolysis of the common extensor tendons, release of the dorsal hood of the metacarpophalangeal joint, and excision of the dorsal volar capsule and collateral ligaments.

Metacarpophalangeal Joint Contracture

Operative procedure includes either excision of the dorsal skin with the distal margins extending past the metacarpophalangeal joints and into the web spaces, or, if the skin is not severely contracted, vertical incisions for release of the metacarpophalangeal joints of the extensor mechanism. Tenolysis of the extensor tendons is done, the extensor hood is elevated by blunt and sharp dissection without destruction of any segment of the hood, and the dorsal and volar capsules are released. The collateral ligaments are excised. The incisions on both the radial and ulnar aspects of the joint through the extensor hood are necessary in order to excise the collateral ligaments and free the volar capsule. A fine fixation pin is inserted through the base of the phalanx and across the neck of the metacarpal, in order to avoid the articular surface of the metacarpal head. The pins are left in place for ten days, a dorsal plaster splint is substituted for the pins, and several weeks of splinting, external traction, and active and passive exercise are necessary.

Burn Causing Proximal Interphalangeal Joint Contracture

This deformity may occur in extension or in flexion. Mild extension contracture occurs when the skin is loose and abundant, when the skin is not adherent to bone, and when heat has not destroyed the extensor tendon or the lateral band mechanism. This contracture can be diminished by tendon and ligament release and lengthening. The contracture may occur when the extremity is being splinted and when the actual burn has not affected the hand but has involved the axilla, forearm, and arm. More severe contractures occur if direct damage to the joint area has occurred and when the extensor tendon has been damaged, the dorsal capsule scarred, and the collateral ligaments and intrinsic lateral band mechanisms fibrosed.

The choice of treatment of the severe contracture is between arthrodesis and arthroplasty, and the latter is usually not possible.

Flexion Contracture of the Entire Digit

This deformity, usually due to a volar scar, necessitates excision of the scar through incisions that extend from the midradial to the midulnar aspect of the digit, removing all of the fibrous skin and subcutaneous tissue. The digital nerves and arteries are isolated; the annular ligaments and attached volar capsule may require release. A fixation pin is then used to hold the joint in extension and a split skin graft is applied, which is held in place by a stent stabilized by sutures. The skin graft can be placed directly on the flexor tendon sheath and the digital nerves, as the blood supply is adequate for survival. If the contractures are old and severe, limited extension and correction are obtained at the first operation, and the second procedure is done at a later time, after nerve and vascular tissues have stretched. Recurrence of flexion contracture occurs in the growing child, and excision of fibrosis and release of deformity may be necessary every few years until the child reaches maximum growth. Volar thumb contractures and palmar fibrosis are managed by wide, deep excision, so that all tight skin lines are released and the defect is replaced by a full thickness skin graft from the groin or a split thickness skin graft from the thigh.

Burn Contractures Affecting Multiple Tissues, Including Deep Soft Tissues, Bones, and Joints

Severe burns result in destruction of skin, tendon, periarticular ligaments, and articular surfaces. Contractures after such severe tissue damage are difficult to prevent. Joint mobilization is difficult to achieve and arthrodesis, partial joint excision, or amputation may be necessary.

Severe flexion of the proximal interphalangeal joint is accompanied by excessive flexion of the distal joint, caused by over-pull of the flexor digitorum profundus and damage to the extensor mechanism. Improved position and strength may occur after arthrodesis of the proximal interphalangeal joint in 50 degrees flexion and arthrodesis of the distal interphalangeal joint in 15 degrees flexion. When interphalangeal joints are arthrodesed from flexion to extension, mortising or peg fitting of the fragment is not necessary. When multiple digits are operated upon, the joints are shaped to fit, and pin fixation is then done in a consecutive way, so that the digits can be aligned with each other.

The alignment of one or several fingers is determined by placing a gentian violet mark in the palm at a point where each fingertip should touch when flexed. The mark is then made on the fingernail and flexion is attempted. This alignment is maintained by insertion of two crossed fixation pins at each joint, either proximally or distally, depending on which is involved.

Arthrodesis of the finger joint from the extended position to the flexed position is more difficult to accomplish because of looseness of the volar capsule and the need to remove more bone. A digit that is arthrodesed must always be shortened, either from extension to flexion or flexion to extension. The ends of the phalanges are cut back, the digits are shortened moderately, and mortising is done between the proximal end of the middle phalanx, grooved volarly, and the distal end of the proximal phalanx is pegged distally. The peg is then placed into the groove in the proper position of flexion. A central fixation pin, extending from the midportion of the middle phalanx to the proximal phalanx, provides correction of rotation and lateral and medial angulation and gives a basic position before the crossed pins are inserted. Small bone chips are packed in the crevices.

The final position of the digit is determined by the occupation of the patient and by the range of motion at the metacarpophalangeal joint. If the patient handles large objects such as sacks or barrels, the digit is fixed in more extension. If smaller objects are handled, then a greater degree of flexion is used.

Metacarpal head resection may be necessary if hyperextension deformity at the metacarpophalangeal joints is old and will not correct by the usual release of skin, tenolysis, and excision of collateral ligaments. Resection of one or more of the metacarpal heads allows the phalanges to be placed in the neutral or slightly flexed position. Arthrodesis of the metacarpophalangeal joints should be avoided if possible, as this places a great handicap on the ultimate range of flexion of the digits. Even prosthetic replacement can be considered, although metacarpal head resection is usually sufficient, and the only arthroplasty possible, since the skin is frequently not healthy enough to tolerate a prosthesis. Partial or complete carpalectomy may be necessary when skin and joint contractures have been present for a long period of time. If deformity has been present for over a year, dorsal carpalectomy with removal of the carpal scaphoid, the lunate, the triangularis, the trapezium, the lesser multangular, and the capitate bone may allow the hand to be brought up to zero degrees. If additional elevation of the hand is needed, then skin and tendon lengthening on the volar wrist surface can be done. A part of a digit or even of an entire finger and metacarpal (ray) may be amputated in order to eliminate the stiff useless digit and to provide the full thickness pedicle flap with sensation, in order to cover adjacent tissue.

COMPRESSION NEUROPATHY OF THE HAND AND FOREARM

The diagnosis of compression neuropathy of the median, ulnar, and radial nerves is easily missed even though the syndrome is widely recognized. The physician may delay in arriving at a diagnosis until motor weakness or muscle atrophy occurs, or until sensory diminution is quite profound. An early diagnosis is desirable in order to provide the patient with relief of pain and complete restoration of motor power.

Each nerve may be compressed either at a low level within the hand, at the wrist, or at a high level around the forearm and the elbow.

Digital Nerve Compression in the Fingers or Thumb

Compression of the digital nerves of the thumb by a bowling ball or by harp strings results from external irritation of the digital nerve. Unless one determines the patient's vocation or avocation, the relationship between it and the numbness, tingling, and paresthesias may be overlooked.

Thumb. The edge of a bowling ball may irritate the ulnar or radial digital nerve at the thumb, depending on the position in which the ball is held and the way the ball is released. Perineural fibrosis occurs. The nodule in the digital nerve is painful to pressure and the skin distal to the nerve becomes hypesthetic. *Treatment:* Initially, bowling should be stopped. After several weeks the irritation should diminish. A ball with a larger thumb hole, as well as change of grip, should prevent the condition from recurring. Operative procedure is usually not indicated.

Harp Player's Thumb. Certain musicians' strumming thumbs sting, with the thumb irritating the digital nerve either radially or ulnarly. Pain and hyper- or hyposensitivity results. The individual with a lesion must rest the thumb and change the way that the strings are moved. *Treatment:* Operative procedure is not indicated, but change in the method of activity is.

Finger Compression. Finger compression of the digital nerve at the base of the finger, either by a nodule associated with palmar fibromatosis or compression of the nerve by fascial bands in the distal palm, can usually be determined by a detailed history and careful examination. *Treatment:* Relief of the compression.

Nerve Compression by Alterations of the Finger Joints

Individuals with osteoarthritic nodules at the distal or proximal joints may have both temperature change with cool weather, indicating compression of the digital artery, and paresthesias or hypesthesia associated with compression or tethering of the nerve due to exostosis. The neural symptoms usually regress spontaneously once the nerve becomes acclimated to the change in the joint architecture.

Compression of the Median Nerve Within the Hand

Patients with compression of the median nerve distal to the transverse crease at the wrist show compression under the distal third of the ligament, in the palm where direct trauma may have occurred, or directly under the transverse retinacular ligament at the base of the palm, or at the wrist just proximal to the beginning of the transverse retinacular ligament. Occasionally compression is found in the region of the motor branch of the median nerve where a fascial ring is present that protects the nerve as it enters the thumb muscles.

Compression of the Median Nerve at the Wrist (Carpal Tunnel Syndrome)

Compression of the median nerve in the carpal tunnel, frequently recognized in recent years, was described in 1913 by Marie and Foix. Other published reports occasionally indicate existence of compression of the median nerve at the wrist. At operation, compression of the nerve by the transverse retinacular ligament causes flattening of the nerve and obliteration of the vascular supply and enlargement of the nerve proximal to the ligament. The nerve may be slightly narrowed at the point of compression, with no other major findings. Occasionally, the ligament may be tight, but definite compression is not noted. Electromyography can be done to determine polyphasic action potentials, and nerve conduction studies will also assist in determining the presence of slow conduction.

Other Causes of Median Nerve Compression at the Wrist and in the Hand

(1) Repeated minor trauma. (2) Synovial sheath hypertrophy of the flexor digitorum profundus or flexor pollicis longus tendons. (3) Trauma usually forgotten by the patient. (4) Mass on the volar aspect of the wrist such as ganglion, aberrant calcification, hypertrophic fat pad, or vascular dysfunction may result in burning and paresthesias, as well as weakness. (5) Elongated muscle belly of the palmaris longus filling the carpal canal. (6) Distal extension of the flexor digitorum sublimis muscle bellies under the transverse retinacular ligament. (7) New growth such as neurofibroma, neurolemmoma, or lipohemangioma. (8) Displacement of the carpus or disruption of the distal radius due to fracture or dislocation may result in immediate or delayed nerve compression against the nerve. (9) Digit amputation resulting in adherence of digital nerves distally or in the palm, associated with cutting of the nerves or tenosynovitis, may cause tethering of the median nerve proximally and paresthesias.

Treatment

Neurolysis performed by release of the transverse retinacular ligament at the wrist, from a point proximal to the ligament to the midpalmar extension, is usually sufficient to eliminate the compression, provide regeneration of motor fibers, and result in complete recovery of sensory diminution.

Neurolysis and tenosynovectomy are necessary in rheumatoid arthritis when the thickened proliferating synovium may be edematous and space filling to such an extent that release of the transverse retinacular ligament alone may be insufficient to decompress the nerve entirely. The hypertrophied proliferative synovium around the flexor digitorum profundi tendons should be excised after releasing the transverse retinacular ligament. This decrease in volume of the tissues within the carpal canal usually precludes recurrence of median nerve compression.

Neurolysis including splitting of the epineurium and limited fascicular release: Prolonged localized compression of the median nerve at the wrist as a result of positioning of the wrist in acute flexion may result in the firm compressive band secondary to external force on the median nerve. This usually occurs under the thickened portion of the transverse retinacular ligament and may leave a sulcus on the volar aspect of the nerve on either side of which is palpable, firm neuroma in continuity. The lesion may be a flattened segment of a centimeter in length under the thickened portion of the transverse ligament, or, if the compression is proximal to the transverse retinacular ligament, there is a flattening under the uppermost proximal portion of the ligament and the firm neuroma proximal to the ligament itself.

If the lesion is toward the palm, the compression can be due to external force by the distal end of the transverse ligament and the neuroma in continuity is located distal to the edge of the most distal limit of the ligament.

Neurolysis of the median nerve and excision of a prominence caused by malunion of the distal end of the radius after Colles fracture, or unreduced dislocation of the lunate causing compression, or a perilunar fracture-dislocation with an unreduced segment of the carpal bone causing pressure.

Repeat neurolysis, due to recurrent fibrosis or incomplete neurolysis, requires careful isolation of the median nerve and the motor branch as it enters the intrinsic muscles of the thumb. The epineurium is split longitudinally under magnification so that the fascicles are clearly seen and the thickened or adherent epineurium is elevated proximally and distally. If interfascicular adhesions are abundant, then the fascicles are carefully separated with the fine, sharp instrument under magnification in such a way that the fascicles are not damaged.

The indications for this kind of decompression, in my opinion, are (1) complete motor and sensory loss due to total interruption of conduction; (2) complete sensory interruption with association of pain and very little evidence of regeneration after several months of observation; (3) complete or partial motor loss associated with partial sensory diminution; and (4) persistent pain and paresthesias in spite of satisfactory motor strength and only moderate sensory impairment.

Compression of the Median Nerve by the Pronator Radii Teres

As the nerve passes under the *pronator radii teres,* the space for its accommodation is limited. Hypesthesia and paresthesias occur in tennis players who have been practicing or participating several hours a day. Hypertrophy of the pronator muscle may result in compression over a 3 to 4 cm. distance. Treatment usually consists of limiting the length of time that the individual is allowed to play and eliminating efforts at building forearm muscles by weight lifting or hand grasping. Rarely is release of the insertion of the pronator muscle or the origin of the pronator muscle necessary.

Compression of the median nerve at the elbow by the lacertus fibrosis does occur in muscular individuals who are participating in repetitive exercise. Treatment of the median nerve compression is accomplished by releasing the lacertus fibrosis under local anesthesia. The median nerve is isolated and the patient is asked to open and close the hand in order to observe the diminished pressure of the underlying muscle mass on the median nerve as it is forced against the lacertus.

Compression of the median nerve by the proximal edge of the origin of the flexor digitorum sublimis does occur if ischemia contracture is present or if repetitive activities occur, or if the forearm muscles are affected by scleroderma or a similar collagen condition. Splitting of the proximal end is sufficient to relieve the pressure. Compression of the median nerve by a *supracondyloid* process on the medial aspect of the humerus or by the accessory origins of the pronator radii teres does occur occasionally and, if recognized by palpation and by roentgenogram, can be relieved by simple excision of the fibrous band or the osteochondral exostosis.

Compression Neuropathy—Median Nerve

Compression of the anterior interosseous nerve, a motor branch of the median nerve, occurs in the proximal one third of the forearm. This nerve supplies the flexor pollicis longus and the flexor digitorum profundus to the index finger. The nerve may be affected by direct trauma or by repetitive motions that result in fibrous bands or hypertrophy of the deep muscles, with primary interruption of motor conduction to the involved muscles. Treatment may require neurolysis if internal conditions have caused the lesions or may consist of merely waiting for regeneration if external trauma has caused the temporary denervation.

Compression Neuropathy—Ulnar Nerve Compression Within the Hand

A. *Hook of the hamate:* The sensory branches of the ulnar nerve supply the volar aspect of the little finger and half or all of the volar surface of the ring finger. As the sensory component of the ulnar nerve is split off from the motor branches just distal to the pisiform bone, nerves to the fingers follow a course to the ulnar aspect of the hook of the hamate. Degenerative arthritis or trauma may result in irritation or tethering of the sensory nerves at this point and result in intermittent paresthesias or hypesthesia of the sensory area usually supplied by the ulnar nerve. Occasionally, the sensory nerve splits into two segments proximal to the hook of the hamate with one branch coursing to the radial and the others to the ulnar side around the hook of the hamate. Tethering or compression may occur at this point also.

B. *The sensory branch of the ulnar nerve* is within a canal encased by firm, fibrous tissue on its radial side (Guyon's), and the nerve may be compressed or constricted at this point. This is the most common site of compression of the nerve in the hand and it may be due to external trauma such as repetitive blows from a stapler or using the hand to strike the edge of a knife, or the patient's complaint of sensory impairment may have some other personal or occupational characteristic that accounts for the irritation of the nerve.

C. *Thrombosis of the ulnar artery* can result in enlargement of the artery secondary to inflammatory response, or organization of the thrombus produces a firm object within the canal that may cause compression of the contiguous nerve.

D. *Proximally the edge of the canal* may compress the nerve just at the point where the common nerve separates into motor and sensory. This may occur in individuals who have gained a large amount of weight rapidly, or in those who have connective tissue fibrosis resulting in compression of the nerve by the edge of the fibrous canal.

E. *Compression of the ulnar nerve:* The pressure of a

wristwatch band or movement of the flexor carpi ulnaris due to repetitive activity such as twisting the handle of a motorcycle, or compression and position of the wrist and hand while riding a bicycle may result in ulnar nerve compression.

Treatment of Ulnar Compression Lesions in the Hand

The essential aspect of treatment depends on a correct diagnosis. The detailed and careful history usually requires the physician to ask searching and revealing questions about the patient's daily activities. The carpenter may use the heel of his hand to compress small objects while he is working; the physician may have a tight elastic wristwatch band around the wrist that has resulted in a neuroma in continuity. The patient may sleep with the head supported by hands, palms against each other, and the base of the palm where the ulnar nerve is located is compressed. A secretary striking an office stapler many times each day or a man who has been cutting off fish heads for years by striking the back or a large knife with the heel of the right hand may have developed an ulnar neuropathy secondary to the recurrent blows. Once the diagnosis is made, the action causing the compression should be discontinued. Usually the nerve requires exploration to be certain that there is no neoplasm involved and that the compressing mechanism is eliminated. Occasionally, hypertrophic or accessory muscles may affect the nerve or encroach on the canal. The thrombosed artery should be resected.

Ulnar Compression at the Elbow

The ulnar nerve may be compressed at the *intermuscular septum* located just proximal to the medial condyle of the humerus. This fibrous ridge must be incised so that its firm edge will not compress the nerve as elbow flexion is completed. This is usually done at the time the ulnar nerve is transferred in the patient who has symptomatic motor and sensory changes.

Ulnar nerve compression *within the ulnar groove* of the humerus: A hypermobile nerve located on the medial aspect of the humerus may be compressed by the external restraining annular ligament that holds the nerve within the groove or by excessive motion of the nerve as the forearm is flexed. As flexion is completed, the loose nerve slides forward and is compressed by both the annular ligaments and the epicondyle.

The flexor carpi ulnaris muscle has a firm, fibrous sheath encasing it at the level of the proximal ulna. The ulnar nerve penetrates this muscle and is surrounded by the fibrous fascial covering of the flexor muscle. If the nerve is affected by anterior displacement or by any of the factors that might lead to fixation associated with position of the arm, the edge of the fascia causes compression of the nerve distally and enlargement of the nerve proximally.

Treatment of Ulnar Nerve Compression at the Elbow

Once the diagnosis is made by a careful history, the localized point of sensitivity of the nerve at the elbow is determined and confirmed by nerve conduction studies and electromyography. The nerve can then be relocated in such a way that external or internal compression does not persist. The usual method of treatment is to isolate the ulnar nerve through a medial posterior incision at the elbow. The sensory branch to the joint is sacrificed, and the distal motor branches into the flexor carpi ulnaris are identified and inspected so that the nerve can be moved anteriorly. The annular ligament and the interosseous fibrous ridge are incised. A thick subcutaneous layer of tissue is left on the skin and three nonabsorbable sutures are placed through the subcutaneous tissue and into the fascia over the forearm flexor muscles. Sutures are placed in such a way that the surgeon's little finger can be inserted both proximally and distally adjacent to the nerve without difficulty. This assures adequate room for the nerve at these points. Cutaneous nerves are spared. A posterior splint is applied for seven to 10 days so that the subcutaneous tissue undergoes primary healing and makes recurrent compression of the nerve unlikely.

Alternative ways of managing the nerve are: (a) Excision of the medial condyle of the humerus to allow the nerve to remain in its usual position. This may be satisfactory, but the nerve may continue to be affected by its posterior position. (b) The nerve may be placed under the muscle mass of the forearm flexors. This is done in management of early ulnar neuropathy in the patient with leprosy. Occasionally, however, the nerve becomes compressed by the large muscle mass and has to be released. This procedure is performed in the patient with leprosy in order to keep the nerve warm, since the mycobacteria do not survive in a warm environment.

Compression Neuropathy of Radial Nerve

Compression lesions of the radial nerve occur infrequently. From an anatomic standpoint, however, the nerve is vulnerable at the *junction of the upper and middle thirds of the arm* where it passes in the musculospiral groove. The nerve can be compressed by displacement of the humerus or by external compression such as the "Saturday night palsy." A compression lesion may result if the relaxed extremity is resting over a firm object against the nerve which is close to the humerus. The same kind of compression can occur if one "falls asleep" on the extremity when the arm is resting on a firm object. Compression of the radial nerve at the distal third of the humerus results from injury to the humerus at the point where the nerve courses from posterior to anterior over the interosseous membrane. This compression lesion is usually from without in, or due to a fracture of the humerus compressing the radial nerve.

Posterior interosseous nerve compression occurs where the radial nerve courses around the neck of the radius and enters the supinator. Repetitive actions may cause hypertrophy of the supinator muscle and compress the nerve, or a constant rotary effect of the radius against a nerve moving in a small canal may result in flattening and limited conduction. Treatment of the posterior interosseous nerve compression syndrome requires decompression of the nerve after the history, the physical findings, and the electrical studies have confirmed the diagnosis. The nerve is decompressed and the flattened area recognized. Epineural splitting may be necessary, and incision of the supinator muscle is usually required. Results after treatment depend on the duration of the compression and the severity of the nerve injury. In many instances, the lesion is unrecognized for years and operative treatment is not helpful. In others, if the compression is not severe and the nerve is released relatively early and the repetitive physical activities are not resumed, then improvement does occur. Tendon transfers may be used to supplement the nerve decompression if improvement does not follow after several months of observation.

Compression of the Sensory Component of the Radial Nerve

Hypesthesia or hyperesthesia on the dorsum of the thumb and index finger may be related to compression of the cutaneous branch of the radial nerve where this nerve is compressed between the sheath of the brachioradialis and the shaft of the radius, or where the nerve is affected by enlargement of the abductor pollicis longus at the wrist when this tendon is associated with tenosynovitis. Trauma about the wrist joint or the base of the thumb may also affect the sensory conduction of the radial nerve and cause primary compression. The syndrome is diagnosed by detecting a sensory deficit or an area of hyperesthesia in the course of the cutaneous branch. Release of the nerve from the fibrous canal where the nerve emerges from under the tendon of the brachioradialis will eliminate the aspect of the problem. If the nerve is compressed distally, either by adhesions to the annular ligament or by a watch band, a bracelet, or intermittent trauma, the lesion can usually be improved by elimination of the external compressing force.

Peripheral Nerve Repair: Primary Versus Secondary

The decision to repair a nerve at the time of primary injury or to wait for delayed repair is not absolute, nor an all-or-none decision. There are factors in favor of each procedure, and whichever is chosen does not necessarily jeopardize the end result. However, if all factors concerned are not taken into consideration and the decision is based only on a primary or secondary action, then the end result may be jeopardized. If one wishes to determine evidence, enough nerves have been sutured by enough individuals with scientific background to arrive at an opinion on a statistical basis. However, the measurement of excellent, good, fair, or poor end results has not been standardized, and investigators who have attempted to present data concerning primary versus delayed or secondary repair have not always followed the same standards. The decision to perform a peripheral nerve repair either primarily (within a few hours after injury), delayed (within five to ten days after injury), or secondarily (any time after three weeks) depends on the mechanism of injury, the physiology of nerve repair, the surgeon's experience, and the magnitude of the multiple tissue injury.

Diagnostic studies that indicate whether a nerve has been completely or partially severed depend on as-

sessment of the autonomic nerves, including sweat glands, fingerprints, and peripheral circulation. Also, sensory end plates are tested by heat, cold, touch, sharp and dull pressure, and two-point discrimination. Muscle testing is done to determine the presence of intrinsic muscles of the hand and the extrinsic extensors and flexors. The percussion test (Tinel's sign) is used to determine hypersensitivity at a point of injury and to follow evidence of regeneration, tapping from distal to proximal toward the point of injury. Electromyography three weeks after injury will give information about the existence of action potentials, denervation, and alteration of the conduction time.

Preparation of the nerve for suturing should include: (a) Adequate mobilization both proximally and distally, without fear of damaging blood supply. (b) Preparation to transfer median nerve anteriorly in the forearm and ulnar nerve anterior to the epicondyle. (c) Release of transverse retinacular ligament at the wrist to eliminate postoperative compression and likelihood of median and ulnar compression during regeneration. (d) The nerve is stabilized, held firmly on a wooden spatula, and cut quickly and firmly at right angles with a fresh razor blade. (e) The peripheral vessels and the alignment of the fascicles are determined with appropriate magnification (three to four power gives satisfactory alignment for identifying fascicles and for matching the ends). (f) Spring-loaded needle holders and small jeweler type forceps are used to handle the epineurium and the fascicles. (g) Taper cut needles with 6-0 polyester suture are used for alignment and stabilization of the nerve, placing the first suture at zero degrees, the next at 60 degrees, and a third at 120 degrees. Gentle tension is placed on the suture. A Keith needle is used to align the fascicles and prevent them from bulging. Interrupted 8–0 sutures are then placed between the major tension guide sutures and watertight repair is done. Tension on the sutures must be sufficient to close the epineurium but not to wrinkle or disalign the fascicles.

Wound care in closing includes wrapping of Surgicel or Gelfoam around the nerve repair to protect it from rapid adhesions of surrounding tissue. This is similar to a plasma clot. The wound is drained if necessary. The fascia is not closed, nor is the subcutaneous tissue, and the skin is closed with interrupted sutures. The wrist is flexed 10 to 15 degrees, the elbow to 90 degrees, both to relieve tension on the nerve and to prevent dependency. A dorsal plaster splint is applied, but *no* splint is applied to the concave side, since slippage may result in increased tension on the nerve. At 10 days the entire dressing is removed, the joints are eased somewhat, and a new dorsal splint is applied for an additional 14 days. At that time, flexion of the joint is initiated, but extension is allowed only to the point of resistance by the skin. Protection is continued for a minimum of six weeks. Gradual extension is resumed without stretching until full mobilization has occurred.

Digital Nerve Lacerations

Digital nerves are pure sensory nerves. There is a wide margin of safety in performing delayed repair of a digital nerve. A digital nerve is best repaired when the surrounding tissue is in satisfactory condition, when adequate magnification and materials are available, and when other aspects of the finger inury have been assessed and can be treated, either simultaneously or in another stage. Repair of digital nerves, anywhere from three weeks to six months after injury, will result in satisfactory regeneration of the nerve and recovery of reasonable action of the sensory receptors. Ideally, five to seven days is physiologically correct, and anatomically this is a time when the epineurium has condensed somewhat. Since the digital nerve is entirely sensory, there is less need for geographic alignment. Evidence shows that the digital nerve repaired even a year after laceration can result in improvement in sensory reception in the area supplied by that nerve.

Anomalous Innervation

About 25 per cent of the general population appears to have some elements of anomalous motor and/or sensory innervation in the hand. This is determined by electrical stimulation at motor points in the forearm and hand and observation of the resulting digit motion. The major clinical detection has been done by utilizing peripheral nerve block, both at the high levels and low levels, in a patient who has had a known nerve laceration. The most *common motor crossover* (Martin-Gruber anomaly) is illustrated by median nerve muscles of the hand being innervated by the ulnar nerve. This means that if the median nerve is lacerated at the wrist, the motor fibers from the median nerve proximal to them have already shunted into the ulnar nerve and are carried by the ulnar nerve into the hand and into the intrinsic muscles, such as the abductor pollicis brevis and the flexor pollicis brevis. These anomalous innervations then provide the hand with active muscles that ordinarily would have been lost with this kind of nerve injury.

The same applies for sensory variations, in that lacerations of a nerve in the palm may result in loss of only part of the sensation of the index finger, since a large surface of the index finger may obtain sensory supply from the radial nerve. Also, for example, the ring finger may obtain all of its sensation from the ulnar nerve.

The factors of anomalous innervation, both sensory and motor, must be considered in determining the result of a peripheral nerve repair. If sensory and motor nerve blocks are not done, if electrical studies are not obtained, then the sensory and motor recovery thought to be related to the nerve itself may be misleading. Experience has shown that any peripheral nerve injury can be managed by delayed repair or secondary repair without compromising the end result, provided that the delay is within an arbitrary three-month period. Primary repairs may be possible, but the comparative results, when all controllable factors are considered, indicate that delayed repair is comparable physiologically and legally and, in certain instances, is the treatment of choice. The difference in success of one or the other is not all or none in ideal circumstances. Primary repair, if done inadequately and in a situation where this repair is not advisable, may give an end result that is less desirable than a delayed repair.

TENDON TRANSFERS FOR IRREPARABLE PERIPHERAL NERVE INJURIES

Concepts Concerning Tendon Transfers

Motor deficits in the hand may result from such conditions as poliomyelitis affecting the anterior horn cells, trauma to the cervical nerve roots or peripheral nerves, neoplasia causing destruction of a peripheral nerve, and familial diseases that cause nerve atrophy. All of these conditions are amenable in varying degrees to treatment by tendon transfer. Restoration of strength to a single muscle or group of muscles depends on the physiologic behavior of a normal nerve-muscle unit. Prerequisites for a successful restoration of finger and hand motion depend on a balance between flexors and extensors, a painless range of motion at all joints, and preservation of automatic function of grasp and release. There are certain muscles on the flexor and extensor surfaces of a forearm that can be detached distally and transferred in order to provide motion of a part that performs an action opposite to that usually done by the muscle. For example, the extensor carpi radialis longus can be transferred from its dorsal attachment to the volar aspect of the forearm and can function as a substitute for the flexor digitorum profundus muscles or as a primary motor muscle for opposition of the thumb. It can also act as a wrist flexor if the other flexors have been used for transfer elsewhere. Each muscle unit must be considered in terms of the relationship between the length of the muscle and the tension it produces, the excursion of the muscle in its original position as compared with its new position, and the adaptation of a muscle to function in a new position while performing a different action. This peripatetic activity of muscle-tendon units allows the surgeon to restore function even when certain muscles are irreparable.

Analysis of Hand and Forearm Deformity

The plan of treatment is outlined after all data have been collected. Several different operative procedures may be available for any one muscle deficit. The goal of treatment should be directed toward providing maximum strength of grasp and pinch, maximum stability and endurance, minimal contracture or tenodesis effect if active motors are available for transfer, and maintenance of adjacent joint function whenever possible. The muscle-tendon units should not be expected to provide strength and function to any greater extent than that demonstrated by the muscle to be transferred in its physiologic position. Tendon transfer should be done in the presence of a mobile wrist. This allows maximum or ideal tension to develop when the wrist is flexed or extended, rather than requiring maximum tension on the involved digit over a stable wrist. A wrist arthrodesis is best done as a last step rather than the first in the reconstructive procedure.

Muscle Testing

The surgeon who is planning to do a tendon transfer must be aware of both the weakness and the strength of the remaining muscles of the upper extremity. Accurate testing of a muscle to be transferred is essential. In most instances, a muscle loses part of its original strength during the process of the transfer. The muscle to be tested prior to transfer is placed in a position of maximum function and the patient is then asked to contract the muscle and hold the part against resistance. Substitution patterns must be recognized, as the pure action of any muscle seldom occurs.

Other Assessments

Sensory examination of all kinds, determination of range of joint motion, detection of contractures, appraisal of the adequacy of skin coverage, and the condition of the arterial and venous circulation are all part of the preliminary procedures.

TREATMENT FOR SPECIFIC PERIPHERAL NERVE INJURIES

The peripheral nerves that innervate the upper extremity will be considered both alone and in combination with other nerves, beginning distally and progressing proximally. The assumption is made that only the peripheral nerves are involved and that other systems and tissues are physiologic.

Low Median Nerve Lesions – Tendon Transfers

Opposition is attempted but cannot be done because of atrophy of the opponens and abductor pollicis brevis. The patient's ability to oppose is weak, and the flexor pollicis longus provides almost all of the available strength in flexion. Prerequisites for tendon transfers include (a) a strong flexor pollicis longus, (b) a strong extensor pollicis longus, (c) a wide web space without contracture, (d) a stable metacarpal phalangeal joint, (e) a stable pulley in the region of the pisiform bone, and (f) a strong motor for transfer.

Procedure. The flexor digitorum sublimis in the ring finger is detached at the base of the digit and isolated at the wrist. The tendon is passed under the flexor carpi ulnaris as a pulley and subcutaneously to the proximal phalanx of the thumb. The distal end is anchored into the proximal phalanx and the lateral band of the extensor mechanism. This provides opposition, improves pinch, and insures better utilization of extensor and flexor muscles. Details concerning the technique for isolating and anchoring the tendons have been described in detail.

High Median Nerve Lesion – Tendon Transfer

The opponens pollicis and abductor pollicis brevis are reinforced by a tendon transfer even if the median nerve lesion is proximal to the innervation of the flexor digitorum sublimis. The innervated flexor digitorum sublimis of the ring finger is isolated at the wrist, and the distal 3 cm. of the flexor carpi ulnaris tendon is detached and extended into and sutured to the extensor carpi ulnaris tendon, thereby forming an indirect dynamic pulley. The paralyzed flexor digitorum sublimis is then passed through this pulley and into the proximal phalanx of the thumb, just as one would accomplish a routine opponens transfer. The proximal end of the flexor carpi ulnaris is used as an active motor by suturing it into the musculotendinous junction of the flexor digitorum sublimis.

Accessory Transfers in High Median Nerve Lesion. The flexor pollicis longus is reinforced by the brachioradialis in order to maintain thumb strength in flexion. The flexor digitorum profundi of the index and long fingers are reinforced by transfer of the extensor carpi radialis longus. The opponens pollicis and abductor pollicis are reinforced by the paralyzed flexor digitorum sublimis around the distal end of the flexor carpi ulnaris–extensor carpi ulnaris used as a motor. Accessory procedures include either arthrodesis of the metacarpal phalangeal joint or the distal interphalangeal joint of the thumb, depending on stability.

Low Ulnar Nerve Injury – Tendon Transfers for Irreparable Lesions

A lesion of the ulnar nerve at or near the wrist or base of the palm will result in paralysis of the hypothenar muscles, all the interosseous muscles, one half of the flexor pollicis longus brevis, the palmaris brevis, and the adductor pollicis. Clawing of the ulnar two digits occurs and, to a lesser degree, the long finger cannot be completely extended.

The operative procedures to be considered are: (a) Adductor pollicis substitution by flexor digitorum sublimis of the long finger passed through the interosseous membrane, under and over the extensor carpi ulnaris as a distal pulley, below the extensor digitorum communis, and into the adductor insertion, anchoring the tendon into bone. (b) Interosseous and lumbrical muscles of the ring and little fingers, substituted by the flexor digitorum sublimis of the ring finger. (c) First dorsal interosseous muscle substituted by extensor carpi radialis longus and a free tendon graft; or a split flexor sublimis of the ring finger with one half to the first lumbrical and one half to the first dorsal interosseous. If adductor pollicis transfer is not possible because of lack of motors, then arthrodesis of the metacarpal phalangeal joint of the hypermobile thumb will provide reasonable stability and moderate improvement in strength.

High Ulnar Lesions – Tendon Transfers

The ulnar innervated intrinsic muscles of the hand, the flexor carpi ulnaris, and the flexor digitorum profundus units to the ring and little fingers and part of the long finger, if paralyzed, weaken the hand noticeably and limit all activities requiring pinch and grasp. A list of possible tendon transfers that would improve grasp and pinch include: (a) Flexor digitorum profundus reinforced by extensor carpi radialis longus to long, ring, and little fingers. (b) Adductor pollicis reinforced by flexor digitorum sublimis through the interosseous membrane and under pulley of the extensor carpi ulnaris, with insertion into proximal phalanx of the thumb. (c) First dorsal interosseous reinforced by flexor digitorum sublimis of the ring finger with one half into the lumbrical and one half dorsal cutaneous. (d) Intrinsic muscles of ring and little fingers reinforced by little finger sublimis to radial intrinsic muscles of the little finger and tenodesis of the right finger to transverse retinacular ligament of the wrist (passive tenodesis). (e) Index finger strengthening by transfer of flexor digitorum sublimis of index finger to oblique fibers of lateral band at the same digit.

Combined High Median and Ulnar Lesions — Tendon Transfers

Digit flexors are restored by transferring the extensor carpi radialis longus to the flexor digitorum profundus tendons. The flexor pollicis longus is reinforced by the brachioradialis and, in certain instances, the distal joint of the thumb is arthrodesed. The metacarpal phalangeal joint of the thumb is arthrodesed if this joint is unstable. Opposition and abduction of the thumb are secured by transfer of the flexor digitorum sublimis, around the flexor carpi ulnaris, which if denervated can be formed into a pulley by use of extensor carpi ulnaris as an active motor to the flexor digitorum sublimis. The first dorsal interosseous is reinforced by either the extensor indicis proprius or the extensor pollicis brevis, and the metacarpal phalangeal joint of the thumb is arthrodesed.

The techniques for each of these tendon transfers are described in detail by the author in another publication.

Low Radial Nerve Lesions — Tendon Transfers

The extensor pollicis longus, the abductor pollicis longus, and the extensor pollicis brevis action are replaced by transferring the extensor carpi radialis longus from the base of the second metacarpal to the rerouted extensor pollicis longus. This one muscle will replace all three muscles if proper tension and direction are obtained. The extensor digitorum communis, which is paralyzed, is reinforced by transferring the flexor carpi ulnaris around the ulnar border of the wrist or through the interosseous membrane through the pronator quadratus to the extensor digitorum communis tendons, after the dorsal retinacular ligament has been incised. The extensor carpi ulnaris is reinforced with a flexor digitorum sublimis of the ring finger to restore full ulnar deviation and to replace the paralyzed extensor carpi ulnaris after the flexor carpi ulnaris has been moved for tendon transfer. Other muscles that might be used for transfer are the brachioradialis, which is still functioning in a low radial nerve lesion, or the flexor digitorum sublimis of the long and ring fingers. The pronator radii teres and the flexor carpi radialis are both available for transfer, depending upon the patient's hand dominance and requirements for strength.

High Radial Nerve Lesions — Tendon Transfers

The extensor carpi radialis longus brevis is reinforced by the pronator radii teres at the musculotendinous junction of the extensor muscle that is paralyzed. Also, the flexor digitorum sublimis of the ring finger is isolated at the wrist, detached, and transferred through the interosseous membrane to the extensor carpi radialis brevis insertion. The extensor pollicis longus is redirected toward the line of abductor pollicis longus and reinforced by using the flexor digitorum sublimis of the long finger, either through the interosseous membrane or directly around the radial border. The extensor digitorum communis is reinforced by the flexor carpi ulnaris, detached from its insertion, and passed either through the interosseous space or around the ulnar border. These transfers provide adequate strength, grasp and pinch, and control of the hand and the fingers as well as the thumb in performing actions of extension.

HAND-TENDON TRANSFERS IN RHEUMATOID ARTHRITIS: CONCEPTS CONCERNING PATHOLOGY OF TENDONS AND JOINTS AFFECTED BY RHEUMATOID ARTHRITIS

Operative procedures for repair of tendon separations or muscle weakness are not as reliable in rheumatoid arthritis as they are in instances in which trauma has caused the tendon rupture. The differentiation of a hand problem in a patient who has rheumatoid arthritis rather than some other, nonprogressive condition is important in determining a method of treatment. For example, a patient with rapidly progressive rheumatoid disease or lupus erythematosis will not be helped by tenosynovectomy, nor will multiple direct tendon repairs be successful. Soft tissue procedures should be done only when the patient's condition is reasonably well stabilized. A remission may occur after several months or several years. A surgeon should be prepared to undertake tendon transfers or joint replacements with less effort devoted to re-establishing continuity of a ruptured tendon or prolonging function of the joint by synovectomy alone.

Special Considerations

The silicone rod is an adjunct to the management of ruptured flexor tendons in rheumatoid disease. The rod may be used as the first step in tendon grafting when tendon transfers are not practical at the first operation. A digit affected by rheumatoid arthritis may show disruption of the entire flexor mechanism of the finger. Synovectomy, construction of pulleys, and placement of the surgical rod constitute the initial procedure. Subsequently, a tendon graft can be used to replace the rod.

Joint arthrodesis is another form of treatment used in lieu of tendon repair. Deformity at the level of the metacarpophalangeal joint of the thumb may occur secondary to rupture of the extensor pollicis brevis and displacement of the dorsal hood. Joint arthrodesis rather than direct repair of the tendon improves strength and maintains function, whereas efforts at reconstruction of a joint, if the articular surface is severely damaged, will be unsuccessful. Displacement of the extensor hood at the level of the metacarpophalangeal joint or rupture of the common extensor at the wrist level may require joint replacement and tendon transfer, since re-establishing finger extension depends on joint mobility, elimination of intrinsic contracture, and utilization of a good muscle-tendon unit as a substitute for the ruptured tendons. Effort devoted to the repair of tendons or immobilization of joints in the presence of persistent deformity will be wasted. Repair of proximal interphalangeal joint deformities, such as hyperextension of a finger or dorsal rupture causing a flexion deformity, will not be successful with the usual kind of stabilizing reconstruc-

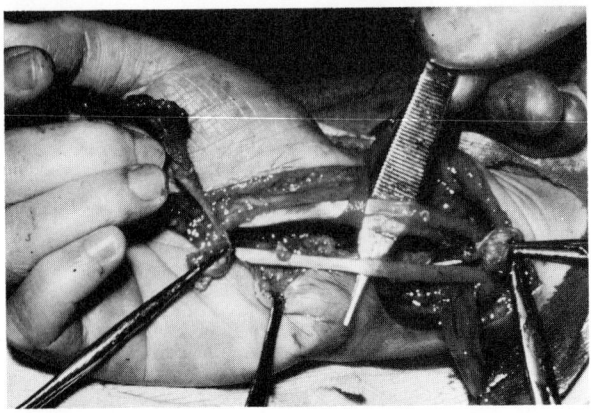

Figure 17. These flexor tendons are surrounded by a diffuse thickening of the synovial sheaths. Synovectomy is helpful in maintaining the integrity of flexor tendons and preventing erosion and destruction. The synovial material is removed from the mid-palm to the lower forearm and a pseudo-sheath re-forms within several weeks. An early active exercise program is essential in order to prevent peripheral adhesions of one tendon to another. (From Goldner, J. L.: Tendon transfers in rheumatoid arthritis. Orthop. Clin. North Am., 5:2, 1974.)

tion about this joint. Tenotomy and joint replacement or tenotomy alone followed by extensor tendon reinforcement may be successful, whereas treatment directed to isolated repair of the extensor mechanism or tightening of the volar capsule and release of the intrinsic lateral bands alone may not be successful.

Compression neuropathies in rheumatoid disease may be accompanied by a florid tenosynovitis at the wrist or at the elbow, and rupture of the flexor tendons in the carpal canal does occur (Fig. 17). When release of the volar transverse retinacular ligament is done in a patient with rheumatoid arthritis, a flexor synovectomy of proliferating synovium may diminish the chances of tendon rupture in the future. The dorsal retinacular ligament stabilizing the extensor digitorum communis tendon at the wrist level and the proliferating synovium in this area with erosion of the distal ulna lead to rupture of the extensor digitorum communis of the two ulnar digits. On the radial side of the hand, the extensor pollicis longus may rupture at the level of the musculocutaneous junction, and the extensor carpi radialis longus and brevis occasionally separate near their insertion into the carpal bones. Tendon ruptures around the wrist may be either delayed or eliminated if synovectomy is performed, if irregular osseous structures are removed, and if ligamentous compression is diminished.

Pathologic Process in Rheumatoid Arthritis

This aspect of the disease needs to be re-emphasized. Synovitis, the destructive action of lyosome enzymes, and the invasion of connective tissue by granulation tissue with collagen destruction lead to tendon attrition at the critical points. Treatment in the rheumatoid patient is directed toward producing remission. Anti-inflammatory medication may reduce proliferation of synovial tissue that erodes tendon and cartilage, and destruction may be halted or limited. Synovectomy may protect the finger joints and the partial remission obtained may indirectly protect the adjacent tendons, but even this concept is not completely established (Fig. 17).

The different patterns of rheumatoid disease affect the end result after operation. The patient involved in a single episode may have a remission and no recurrence for several years. Tendon reconstruction will be relatively successful. The patient who has had two or three recurrences followed by short remissions offers a more difficult challenge in medical management and surgical prognosis. Stenosing tenosynovitis, for example, is an isolated lesion in a patient who has had a single episode of rheumatoid arthritis and does not present a major problem. However, the patient who has never gone into remission and in whom multiple digits are involved with stenosing tenosynovitis represents a problem that requires every effort to obtain a remission and as much local treatment as possible in order to diminish pain and avoid progressive deformity. Splinting, local injections of anti-inflammatory medications, and occasionally surgical release are necessary. Excessive release of the annular ligaments in the palm, however, may result in deviation of the flexor tendons, bow-stringing of tendons, and aggravation of ulnar deviation of the digits. The concept of treatment of the whole patient must not be forgotten.

In the patient with systemic disease who develops tendon rupture, the usual periods of tendon immobilization may not apply. End-to-end union of tendons should not be attempted, but interweaving or button hole junctures should be used for strength and dependability. Special attention should be given to suture material because the point where the knot is made is the weakest. The use of nonabsorbable suture is advised. Restoration of the maximal strength of a repaired tendon or at the juncture of a transferred tendon may take four months before adequate stress can be applied and months more before development of maximal strength. Twenty-one days have been utilized as a minimal time for tendon union, but 35 days is a safer figure to bear in mind. Mobilization can begin at three weeks, but without forceful stretching or undue stress. Tendons repaired on the flexor surface can be moved in three weeks but should be protected for several weeks longer and any flexion deformity stretched slowly. Elastic traction is safe and helpful. Extensor tendons should be protected for at least six weeks and occasionally even for 12 weeks. Tensile strength is low early in the course of healing and gradually increases with time. Successful management of the rheumatoid patient with tendon ruptures depends on the awareness of the systemic disease patterns, understanding of the pathologic process that caused the rupture, a plan to provide a tendon substitute by transfer if possible, utilization of a safe technique that provides strong junctures held by nonabsorbable suture, a plan for postoperative management that provides early motion but protects healing tendons, and persistent efforts at maintaining the patient in total remission if possible.

CONGENITAL DEFECTS

Congenital defects occurring in the upper extremities are classified and related to either a systemic problem or a limb bud deficiency. Our goal is to obtain a hand or upper extremity that has maximum function and resembles the normal as closely as possible.

Etiology

Malformations of the hand and upper extremity are classified as *endogenous* (a deficiency of germ plasm which may be hereditary) or *exogenous,* which are secondary to an intrauterine alteration. Historical information may assist in establishing the cause of the malformation, but frequently the history alone is insufficient. Certain conditions are known to be hereditary, however, and advice given to the parents about a future child can be positive with regard to the frequency of occurrence and the chance of a deformity occurring in another child.

Syndactyly, symphalangism, and supernumerary digits are examples of hereditary deformities. Penetrance varies and for this reason a generation may be skipped.

Certain teratogenic agents are recognized as affecting the developing fetus. Thalidomide affects the upper extremities, and certain anomalies of the upper limb occur in the period of gestation as follows: absence of the limb in the third or fourth week, absence of hand at the fifth and sixth weeks; digital absence in the seventh week, and digital stunting in the eighth week (Ingalls, T. H., in Barskey, A. J.).

Classification

Classification may be derived from the morphologic patterns of the anomalies and grouped into several entities according to the parts that have been affected by specific embryologic failures. The six groups used for this classification are:

   I. Failure of differentiation
  II. Arrest of development
 III. Focal defects
 IV. Duplication
  V. Overgrowth
 VI. General conditions

A large number of subgroups are present, and the reader is referred to the work of Swanson, Barksy, and Entin for details.

Treatment of Congenital Anomalies

Failure of Differentiation of Parts. Forearm—synostosis of radius and ulna. These patients show a fixed deformity usually in pronation. A moderate flexion deformity occurs and progresses as the child gets older. Rotation of the forearm is not possible, but the extremity is rotated at the shoulder joint. In most instances when the fixation is stabilized at neutral between pronation and supination, nothing is required in the way of treatment. However, if excessive pronation occurs, the child has difficulty in lifting a flat object, and treatment is in the form of a rotary osteotomy of the radius and the ulna, distally in the metaphysis. The fragments are fixed with two fixation pins in a position of 20 degrees supination. This is a compromise between excessive pronation and excessive supination. Other variations occur such as dislocation of the radius and radial or ulnar deviation of the wrist associated with alterations of the length of the radius or the ulna.

Hand—Carpals. Coalition of carpal bones or absence of a part of the carpus may cause limitation of wrist motion but no major deficiency.

Metacarpals. Short metacarpals may be associated with pseudohyperparathyroidism. Metacarpal deformities are occasionally related to systemic conditions with abnormalities of the mucopolysaccharide. Metacarpals may be unsegmented, giving rise to finger deformities. Two metacarpal heads may be present, articulating with a thick phalanx, and one segment may require removal.

Digital Anomalies

Syndactyly. Uncomplicated syndactyly consists of skin joining the digits but no bone or cartilage junction. The deformity is frequently bilateral and most commonly is between the long and ring fingers. There is a familial kind of syndactyly which is dominant and repetitive. Operative treatment can be performed after six months of age. There is no urgency involved, but frequently the family desires to have the deformity corrected as soon as this is safe. The base of the digits where the web is formed as the separation is being done ultimately should be square or U-shaped and not V-shaped. A triangle of skin is formed at the base and the central portion excised, or a flap of skin is elevated and folded from volar to dorsal. A curved incision on the dorsum prevents contracture and allows isolation of the neurovascular structures from the dorsum prior to incision of the volar aspect. A full thickness skin graft from the groin is a safe way of filling the defect if a large amount of loose skin is not available locally. In most instances a skin graft is needed and is desirable. The graft is taken as a full thickness fat-free piece of skin with the donor site being closed by subcutaneous and nonabsorbable sutures and a pull-out prolene suture in the dermis. The donor skin is applied after the tourniquet is released and is sutured in place with 4-0 chromic catgut so that the child does not have to be disturbed to remove the sutures. A bolus of cotton balls is tied over the graft and saturated with Zephiran and glycerine solution. Special attention is given to the flap area at the base so that the donor skin and all recipient areas are compressed and no dead space exists. A long arm plaster cast is used to immobilize the part and is left in place for seven days. The bolus is then removed, warm water soaks are started, and a protector splint is used for an additional two weeks. There is little danger of joint stiffness in young patients.

Complex Syndactyly

The fingernails or nail beds are united and the distal phalanx is usually common to both fingers. Existence of bone union requires separation as early as is feasible, and delay is not recommended beyond one year.

Contractures

A thumb web contracture is the most common contracture within the hand, although contractures of the proximal interphalangeal joint of the other fingers occur reasonably frequently. The flexor digitorum sublimis is contracted as well as the skin and the overlying fascia.

Ganglia. A ganglion is the most common enlargement of the hand. In young individuals the lesions are probably developmental abnormalities. Trauma may aggravate the prior existence and call attention to the lesion. Aging is associated with lesions arising from the joint lining, which penetrate the capsule and communicate with the joint by a pedicle.

Confirmation of the anatomic relationship has been done by injecting contrast media into the joint. The contrast passes through the pedicle into the lesion. Conversely, if contrast is injected into a ganglion, the pressure differential and the valve effect usually prevent the contrast from entering the joint. Prior to excision of a ganglion, 0.1 ml. of methylene blue is injected into the lesion. This becomes fixed by the lining cells and allows the surgeon to locate the pedicle easily and excise it, the capsule, and the local synovium, thereby preventing recurrence. The most common site of a ganglion is the dorsum of the hand. The lesion arises from the scaphoid-lunate articulation or the scaphoid-trapezium joint. On the volar aspect of the wrist, the lesion frequently arises from the trapezium-metacarpal or trapezium-scaphoid joint. Patients with early or late rheumatoid arthritis may show a synovial cyst that resembles a ganglion. The mechanism of formation is somewhat the same, except that the inflammatory process is more extensive and the lesions are more diffuse, with a wider base.

Treatment of dorsal or volar wrist ganglia requires meticulous excision. A tourniquet should be used, placing the tourniquet in the upper arm at 280 mm. Hg; local or regional block is satisfactory. The procedure should be performed in a well-equipped operating room, with adequate assistance, and can be done on an outpatient basis. The skin incision follows the skin creases; the superficial veins and the cutaneous nerves are retracted, particularly the branches of the superficial radial nerve. The extensor pollicis longus is identified and isolated with a tape. The extensor carpi radialis longus is identified and retracted. The ganglion, if previously injected with methylene blue, will appear as a deep colored dome. Dissection is done slowly and carefully, remaining outside the lesion and following the peripheral borders down to the pedicle. When the pedicle is identified, the capsule and joint lining are excised, attempting to maintain the pedicle within the base of the lesion. Once the ganglion is removed, the articular surface of the involved bone will be evident. The remaining defect is left open. This fills in with fibrous tissue and, prior to that, incompleteness of healing allows synovial fluid to exit and not accumulate. The tourniquet is released, bleeding points are coagulated, sutures are placed in the skin only, and a compression dressing is applied. Early motion is encouraged so that the capsule will not adhere to the underlying osseous surface.

Other Sites of Ganglia Formation

Volar Aspect of the Annular Ligament. Just distal to the metacarpophalangeal joint, this lesion is moderately painful, firm to compression, and frequently unnoticed for many months. It does not move as the finger flexes or extends. The lesion can usually be punctured by a No. 18 needle after

Xylocaine has been injected. If the patient is told to compress the lesion several times each day, eventually it may regress spontaneously. Rarely does the lesion have to be excised.

A ganglion involving the flexor carpi radialis tendon at its insertion or the trapezium scaphoid joint on the flexor surface can be treated by observation, aspiration, and only occasionally by excision. If there is a question about the diagnosis, the lesion can be aspirated and the mucoid material obtained in the syringe will establish the diagnosis.

Mucous Cysts. A mucous-filled enlargement may occur on the dorsal aspect of the distal interphalangeal joint of the digit. These are usually eccentric on either side of the extensor tendon. The cyst may be hard, may occasionally break with compression, and occasionally becomes ulcerated. The roentgenogram usually shows an osteophyte or narrowing of the joint. The cyst arises from the joint, acts as a synovial cyst, and does contain mucoid material. A small early lesion may be managed by incision and cauterization with silver nitrate. A larger or recurrent lesion should be managed by excision of the skin, the cyst, curettage of the underlying osteophyte, and placement of either a local flap or a split skin graft.

Giant Cell Tumor (Fibroxanthoma) Tendon Sheath. These lesions may be noted in individuals who have hypercholesterolemia. The lesion is usually adjacent to a flexor tendon or a joint. The lesions may be fixed and immobile and cause compression of the adjacent cortex evident on x-ray. There is evidence that giant cell tumor is the end phase of a localized xanthoma. Histologically, the lesion may be grossly yellow if the predominant cell is a lipid-containing histiocyte. The lesion will be yellow and gray if there are fewer histiocytes and more fibrocytes and giant cells. The totally gray, firm lesion is a mature giant cell tumor with fibrocytes and foreign body giant cells. Once the diagnosis is established, if the lesion is in a critical position, such as involving the joint capsule, total excision is not necessarily desirable. Total excision in a patient with a tendency to joint fibrosis may cause a finger contracture with greater deformity than if the diagnosis is made, partial excision is done, and the condition is observed. It is usually a slow growing lesion, and total extirpation is not essential.

Glomus Tumor. These lesions may be located in any region of the body, but the most frequent site of occurrence is a digit. The lesion is usually located in the subungual tissue. It arises from a glomus body, which physiologically aids in heat regulation of the vasomotor system. The lesion is usually minute and well localized, varying in size from a few millimeters to a centimeter. No visible evidence of the lesion may be evident early, but a point of exquisite tenderness can be isolated. Grossly, the lesion is purplish or deep red. The lesion may be best removed by a lateral incision on the digit, elevating the entire nail plate and nail bed, and isolating the lesion as it compresses bone.

Tumors of the Hand Bones. Tumors or neoplasms of the hand skeleton are relatively rare. The lesions are usually benign, although primary malignant tumors as well as metastatic lesions do occur. The clinical findings, in addition to roentgenography, will usually provide a tentative diagnosis and establish a course of treatment. Ultimately, a biopsy is essential in confirming or establishing the diagnosis.

Enchondroma. These lesions may be solitary or multiple and comprise 90 per cent of the tumors arising in the bones of the hand. These lesions are never malignant in the young patient, and only rarely do they show sarcomatous changes in the elderly. Many of the solitary enchondromata are discovered initially because of pathologic fracture. A patient complaining of vague aching in the hand, fatigue in one or two digits, or soreness on compression may have a lesion when the x-ray is taken. Occurrence of the lesion appears to have a racial variation in that it seldom occurs in the black but occurs more frequently in the white, and the author has seen many patients in Japan with enchondromata.

Solitary enchondromata usually occur in the proximal phalanx, although they may occur in the middle phalanx or a metacarpal. Seldom, if ever, have they been noted in the carpal bones. Roentgenographic findings include an ovoid, lytic lesion which is expansile, with the appearance of few bubbles. It is usually eccentric, thins the cortex, and shows a thin sclerotic margin in the one area of the lesion. There may be stippling in the center and a few spots of calcification. The differential diagnosis includes epidermoid inclusion cyst or a solitary cyst. Multiple enchondromas are not difficult to determine. If a fracture accounts for recognition, the lesion should be splinted for a few weeks until early healing occurs. The enchondroma can then be excised and bone grafting used to fill the defect. Excision should be as complete as is possible without disrupting all of the cortex that maintains length. One entire cortex should be excised so that pockets and crevices do not persist. The entire crater is curetted meticulously and then irrigated. Cancellous bone chips from the bone bank are then packed firmly into the lesion. The bone graft eventually amalgamates and recurrence is rare.

Osteochondroma. These lesions are usually solitary and occur second in frequency to the enchondroma. They are noted by a prominence which is not painful, and the prominence is usually near the metaphyseal segment of the bone. Exception to this is the solitary lesion of the distal phalanx. These lesions of the hand may be pedunculated or sessile and, although they are usually benign, a malignant change is occasionally noted. Films show the mass projecting from the cortical outline. Those with a stalk are more readily detected, whereas those that are flat are less apparent. The lesion is managed by meticulous excision. The periosteum is not elevated, and the lesion is excised *in toto*. If the distal phalanx is involved, the nail bed and plate are elevated and the plate is allowed to remain as protection for the underlying soft tissues. If multiple lesions exist, only those that are symptomatic should be removed.

Solitary Bone Cyst. This lesion contains fibrous connective tissue and small amounts of brown or yellow fluid. The lesion may be eccentric, with enlargement of the cortex. These cysts usually occur in the distal half of the metacarpal or a proximal portion of the proximal phalanx. The lesion may be discovered by a pathologic fracture or by incidental x-ray. The epiphysis of the second through the fifth metacarpal is distal, and the cyst begins in the area directly adjacent to the epiphyseal plate. The cyst may fill the medullary canal and expand the cortex, and the cortex may become very thin and eccentric. There may be a smooth sclerotic margin and there may be some loculation. The lesion can usually be recognized on the roentgenogram. Excision of the thinning cortex, removal of the lining, and packing with bank bones are usually sufficient to eliminate the lesion. Fluid is usually present and is removed.

Osteoid Osteoma. This lesion occurs rarely in the hand and is usually accompanied by a long history of aching pain noted more at night than during the day. Aspirin usually decreases the pain. It is recognized by the clinical history, as well as soft tissue swelling and sclerosis of one segment of a phalanx, with the sclerotic area being the central nidus. A ring of lesser density surrounds the nidus. The lesion may occur in the tubular bones of the hand and in the carpal bones. The proximal phalanx is the site of most frequent occurrence, the metacarpal is next, and the carpal bones last. Of these, the scaphoid is the bone in which the lesion occurs most frequently.

X-rays are helpful not only in localizing the osteoid os-

teoma, but also in detecting the exact site of the lesion in relationship to the medullary canal and the cortex. The nidus appears in the cortical part of bone and around this is the area of radial lucency. Tomography will be helpful in locating the lesion exactly, since treatment consists of excision and the nidus must be excised in order to obtain a cure.

TECHNIQUE RELATED TO EXCISION OF BONE LESIONS OF THE HAND. If the terminal phalanx is replaced by an enchondroma or an epidermoid inclusion cyst, the cortex and the pathologic material can be excised and iliac bone used to replace the phalanx. The cartilaginous articular surface is intact, and the expanding nail plate and nail bed will decrease in size after the lesion is removed. Amputation should be avoided if possible. The same holds for the glomus tumor if it involves much of the phalanx. A malignant lesion involving the distal phalanx is best managed by amputation of the part.

Aneurysmal Bone Cyst. This is a vascular lesion that results in absorption of bone and expansion of the cortex. The diagnosis is based upon a swelling in an area that has been uncomfortable for several months. Trauma may have been noted, but the exact cause of the aneurysmal cyst has not been determined. The affected bone may enlarge rapidly and require operation for biopsy and excision. The roentgenogram shows the cortex to be expanded and a lacy pattern of ossification exists throughout the late lesion. The entire circumference of the involved bone is usually affected. The differential diagnosis includes a giant cell tumor of bone, which contains more cellular material but which may bleed sufficiently to resemble an aneurysmal bone cyst. Treatment of a giant cell tumor of the hand requires more extensive excision than an aneurysmal bone cyst, although the latter may recur and progress and require deletion of a digit or a segment of the hand. A hemangioma of the bones of the hand will show more destruction of bone and more adjacent soft tissue involvement. The malignant hemangioma progresses more rapidly and shows more vascularity on arteriography.

TREATMENT OF ANEURYSMAL BONE CYST. The lesion should be diagnosed by a quick section, and biopsy excision should be attempted at the primary operation. Clinical appearance is suggestive of lesions that should be managed by local excision rather than simple curettage and, for this reason, the operative procedure must be well planned. A certain amount of soft tissue sacrifice, such as intrinsic muscles, must be expected. If the patient is seen after biopsy has been obtained and the lesion continues to progress, then the second operative procedure may require resection of an entire metacarpal or phalanx, or extensive bone and soft tissue resection, followed by bone grafting. The operative procedure should be done under tourniquet control. Resection of most or all of the lesion is necessary in order to control bleeding. Low dose radiation therapy is indicated if incomplete resection has been done because of existence of adjacent critical structures such as major nerve branches or a large vascular arch.

Giant Cell Tumor of Bones of the Hand. This lesion does occur in the phalanges and the metacarpals of the hand but has not been noted in the carpal bones. The confusion between giant cell tumor of the hand and aneurysmal bone cyst continues, with the latter diagnosis being most frequent, and the tissue from the aneurysmal bone cyst does resemble that seen in small biopsy from giant cell tumor. Treatment necessitates excision of the lesion followed by bone grafting. A sufficient amount of cortex may be left, and the articular surfaces may persist so that loss of the joint may be avoided. The use of tightly packed iliac cancellous bone and adequate peripheral cortical bone may be sufficient to maintain substance of the phalanx of the metacarpal and assist in avoiding recurrence of the lesion.

Malignant Lesions of Bones of the Hand

Metastatic Lesions of the Hand. Soft tissue malignancies in the distant parts of the body may metastasize to the hand, and bone tumors may also metastasize to bones of the hand. Chondrosarcoma of bone has been reported as metastasizing to the hand, probably from pulmonary tissues through the arterial tree.

Metastatic tumors to the hand may occur from tumors of the lung and the breast. Metastatic tumors of the hand usually present as the initial lesion recognized in a patient who has a primary carcinoma of the lung. Recognition of the hand lesion by the roentgen appearance and pain leads to diagnosis of the pulmonary lesion. Treatment usually consists of ray deletion or excision of the part in order to decrease pain, swelling, and hemorrhage. Metastatic tumors from the breast respond to radiation therapy and chemotherapy. The lesion is diagnosed either by aspiration or direct biopsy. Metastatic lesions from the gastrointestinal tract to the hand occur occasionally, as do lesions from malignancies of the thyroid, kidney, prostate, and uterus.

PRIMARY MALIGNANT TUMORS OF THE HAND

Malignant Hemangioma

This lesion may either begin in soft tissue and invade bone or begin in bone and invade soft tissue. Satellite lesions may occur in adjacent soft tissue. Cortical destruction occurs, pain is severe, and the lesion is locally invasive. Spread is by regional lymph nodes and by venous metastases.

Treatment necessitates complete excision of the lesion either by deletion of a portion of the hand or amputation at a point where skin coverage can be obtained without vascular lesions within the skin flap. Radiation therapy is used only if partial hand amputation is done. Biopsy of regional nodes is helpful in determining whether lymph node dissection should be done, radiotherapy used, and chemotherapy considered.

Chondrosarcoma

This lesion develops from a tumor that was originally an enchondroma or a sessile osteochondroma. Transformation from a benign to a malignant lesion is rare but should be suspected if the lesion is growing rapidly in elderly individuals.

Once the biopsy confirms the alteration of the lesion to one that is malignant, then local resection, partial hand amputation, or complete hand amputation is selected as the method of management, depending on the size of the lesion, the location of the lesion, and whether or not the lesion can be resected completely.

Osteogenic Sarcoma

This primary malignant bone tumor may occur in the phalanges or in the metacarpals. Diagnosis is made by existence of a suspected lesion because of pain, swelling, and local tenderness. The x-ray appearance is suggestive of a neoplastic change, and the biopsy will confirm the diagnosis. Considerations as to the origin of the lesion must include the following: (a) prolonged exposure to radiation for many years, (b) metastatic lesion from a known primary osteosarcoma, and (c) alteration of a previously existing lesion in the hand such as Paget's disease. Treatment requires local resection of the part involved.

Arteriovenous Fistulas

These lesions are believed to arise from the failure in differentiation of the common embryonic anlage into true artery and vein, and the short circuiting of blood as a result of persistent communication between the vessels. The pathologic process may be limited to the finger, to several fingers, or to part of an extremity, and the lesion may become prominent as the patient ages. Chronic ulceration of the digit owing to trauma may bring the lesion to one's attention. The size of the fistula will determine whether the bruit or thrill is detected. Differential diagnosis includes consideration of: (a) A capillary hemangioma involving muscle. This is a lesion with dilation of both veins and arteries, which may involve intrinsic muscles of the hand. (b) Venous angioma which may be a dilation primarily on the venous side of the circulatory tree. Phleboliths, small areas of calcification, and moderate erosion of bone may occur because of external compression. (c) Traumatic false aneurysm may result in persistent bleeding, slight enlargement of soft tissue over the deficit in the artery, and the presence of a bruit intermittently.

Diagnosis of the arteriovenous fistula is confirmed and visualized by arteriography. Flowmeter studies such as the Doppler instrument or the electronic flowmeter can provide additional information about the location of the multiple vessels and detect flow through both arterial and venous channels. The arteries leading to the fistula will be dilated, and the arteries distal to the fistula will show inadequate filling. There will be pooling of the arteriographic contrast in the region of the fistula. The characteristic appearance of the arteriogram, showing distal veins filling early even though proximal arteries are not yet completely filled, demonstrates the anatomical characteristic of the arteriovenous fistula.

The success of treatment depends upon the size of the lesion, the length of time it has been present, and the multiplicity of the communications. One way of treating the lesions successfully is to isolate the major vessels just proximal to the beginning of the arteriovenous fistula, and to excise the connecting veins and arteries on one side of the digit from proximal to distal. An interval of several weeks is allowed and the vessels on the opposite side are resected. There is usually sufficient arterial blood flow and venous outflow from the skin, tendons, and metacarpals and phalanges to allow maintenance of arterial inflow and venous outflow so that ischemic necrosis will not occur. After local resection, pain and cold intolerance may be a problem. Stellate ganglion blocks, sympathetic blocking agents, and occasionally sympathectomy are necessary.

Lymph Vessel Lesions of the Hand

Simple Lymphangioma. This lesion is usually congenital and noted at birth. The enlargement is somewhat spongy, relatively small, and well circumscribed. Histologically the lesion is one of anastomosis of spaces and vessels of small and medium caliber with thin cellular septal strains and an endothelial lining of the spaces that is flat or cuboidal. The lesion is excised at the time that the diagnosis is being established.

Cavernous lymphangioma. These lesions are congenital, grow slowly, and are composed of dilated lymphatic sinuses filled with lymph and occasionally blood. The lesion on the hand may be extensive and difficult to excise, and require numerous stages of excision and skin grafting. Constricting bands at the base of the digits aggravate swelling of the fingers, and part of the treatment is excision of the constricting bands and re-establishment of subcutaneous flow of fluid. After the constricting bands have been excised, future treatment depends upon the degree and extent of persistent swelling.

SELECTED REFERENCES

Barsky, A. J.: Congenital Anomalies of the Hand and Surgical Treatment. Springfield, Charles C Thomas, Publisher, 1958.
This monograph describes the frequent and infrequent congenital deformities of the hand that are amenable to some type of reconstructive operation. The classification is helpful in assimilating the information and in understanding the reasons for the kind of treatment recommended. The author's descriptions are related to both cosmetic improvement and function.

Boyes, J. H.: Flexor-tendon grafts in the fingers and thumb. An evaluation of end results, J. Bone Joint Surg., *32A*:489–499, 531, 1950.
End results are based on the kind of finger treated initially. The operative procedure selected is important and the expectations are reasonably well standardized if biological approach to the problem of tendon laceration is followed. In an ideal situation, the flexor tendon graft will be successful in about 90 per cent of the cases.

Burkhalter, W. E., Butler, B., Metz, W., and Omer, G.: Experiences with delayed primary closure of war wounds in the hand in Vietnam, J. Bone Joint Surg., *50A*:945–954, 1968.
These authors review the concept of delayed closure of wounds and apply it to the severely traumatized hand. They have shown that delayed closure of five to seven days, or even longer, is compatible with excellent restoration of function with minimal morbidity. The importance of accepting the concept of delayed closure is not difficult when one reviews the clinical cases and the statistics presented.

Eyler, D. L., and Markee, J. E.: The anatomy and function of the intrinsic musculature of the fingers. J. Bone Joint Surg., *36A*:1–9, 18–20, 1954.
A detailed description of the anatomic arrangements of the interossei and lumbricales as it relates to function of the specific muscles and their action on the major joints of the fingers.

Goldner, J. L.: Surgery of the Hand. Practice of Surgery, Chapter 5, pp. 1–81.
Many clinical problems are discussed in this material, which is arranged in a problem-oriented way: the legends, the entire case history in many instances.

Hunter, J. M., and Salisbury, R. E.: Flexor tendon reconstruction in severely damaged hands. J. Bone Joint Surg., *53A*:829–858, 1971.
These authors emphasize the concept of silicone interposition rod in managing severely damaged hands. They were able to upgrade a digit with severe scar to one with greater range of motion than prior to reconstruction with limitation of scar formation. This concept is one of the great advances in hand surgery.

Kaplan, E. B.: Functional and Surgical Anatomy of the Hand, 2nd ed. Philadelphia, J. B. Lippincott, 1965.
The descriptions of the anatomic dissections are correlated with clinical syndromes. The importance of the anatomic arrangement of structures of the hand are evident as one reads the clear details related to the normal anatomy.

Littler, J. W.: The severed flexor tendon. Surg. Clin. North Am., *39*:435–447, 1959.
This author's wide experience with flexor tendon grafting will provide one with a background of clinical selection of patients, and the techniques should be followed if a successful range of motion is to be obtained in the finger.

Verdan, C. E.: Primary repair of flexor tendons. J. Bone Joint Surg., *42A*:647–657, 1960.
Lacerations of the flexor tendons were managed by primary repair by this author. He is meticulous, with excellent technique. Primary repair of tendons can be successful if the selection of patients and the experience of the operating surgeon are of high caliber.

Wrenn, R. N., Goldner, J. L., and Markee, J. L.: An experimental study of the effect of cortisone on the healing process and tensile strength of tendons. J. Bone Joint Surg., *36A*:588–601, 1954.
This experimental study confirms the physiologic process of tendon healing and shows that systemic injections of cortisone acetate prevented peripheral adhesions from occurring but also delayed the development of tensile strength. Once the corticosteroid was discontinued, rapid massive fibroblastic response occurred. If active motion persisted, fewer adhesions resulted with the corticosteroid than without. However, the systemic effects of corticosteroid did not justify prolonged use of this drug in eliminating adhesions tempo-rarily. Local use of Gelfoam, without steroid, resulted in a smaller number of adhesions and a greater tensile strength. This article embodies the concepts of a collagen-blocking agent or a local interposition membrane which is absorbable as two methods that will require further investigation in order to prevent tendon adhesions after trauma.

REFERENCES

1. Goldner, J. L., and Irwin, C. E.: An analysis of paralytic thumb deformities. J. Bone Joint Surg., *32A*:627–39, 1950.
2. Goldner, J. L.: Deformities of the hand incidental to pathological changes of the extensor and intrinsic muscle mechanisms. J. Bone Joint Surg., *35A*:115, 1953.
3. Goldner, J. L.: Function of the Hand Following Peripheral Nerve Injuries. American Academy of Orthopaedic Surgeons, Instructional Course Lecture, Volume X, Ann Arbor, Michigan, 1953.
4. Bell, G. E., Jr., and Goldner, J. L.: Compression neuropathy of the median nerve. South. Med. J., *49*:966–972, 1956.
5. Kelley, J. M., and Goldner, J. L.: Radial nerve injuries. South. Med. J., *51*:873–883, 1958.
6. Goldner, J. L., and Clippinger, F. W.: Excision of the greater multangular bone as an adjunct to mobilization of the thumb. J. Bone Joint Surg., *41A*:609, 1959.
7. Goldner, J. L.: Reconstructive surgery of the hand following thermal injuries. Clin. Orthop., *13*:98–113, 1959.
8. Goldner, J. L.: Thumb and finger infections. Am. Surg., *28*:12–25, 1962.
9. Goldner, J. L., and Urbaniak, R.: The clinical experience of silicone-dacron metacarpal phalangeal and interphalangeal joint prostheses. J. Biomed. Mater. Res. Symposium, *4*:137–163, 1973.
10. Goldner, J. L.: Trauma to the extensor mechanism and its attachment to the distal phalanx of the digits. Curr. Prac. Orthop. Surg., *1*:143–151, 1963.
11. Goldner, J. L.: Tendon transfers for irreparable peripheral nerve injuries of the upper extremity. Orthop. Clin. North Am., *5*:343–375, 1974.
12. Groves, R. J., and Goldner, J. L.: Restoration of strong opposition after median nerve or brachial plexus paralysis. J. Bone Joint Surg., *57A*:112–115, 1975.
13. Eguro, H., and Goldner, J. L.: Bilateral thrombosis of the ulnar arteries in the hand. Plast. Reconstruct. Surg., *52*:573, 1973.
14. Urbaniak, J. R., and Goldner, J. L.: Laceration of the flexor pollicis longus tendon: Delayed repair by advancement, free graft, or suture. J. Bone Joint Surg., *55A*:1123–1148, 1973.
15. Clippinger, F. W., Goldner, J. L., and Roberts, J.: Use of electromyography in determining treatment and prognosis of peripheral nerve injuries. J. Bone Joint Surg., 1962.
16. Goldner, J. L.: Biological principles of repair and regeneration of nerve and tendon. South. Med. J., *64*:121–122, 1971.
17. Goldner, J. L.: The injured hand: A panel by correspondence. Arch. Surg., *103*: 1971.
18. Goldner, J. L.: Transfers in rheumatoid arthritis. Symposium on tendon transfers in the upper extremity. Orthop. Clin. North Am., *5*:425–444, 1974.
19. Urbaniak, J. R., Bright, D. S., Gill, L. H., and Goldner, J. L.: Vascularization and the gliding mechanism of free flexor-tendon grafts inserted by the silicone rod method. J. Bone Joint Surg., *56A*: 1974.
20. Seddon, H. J.: Electrical Phenomena in Sural Disorders of Peripheral Nerves. Baltimore, Williams and Wilkins, 1972, pp. 577–677.
21. Önne, L.: Recovery of sensibility and pseudomotor activity in the hand after nerve suture. Acta Chir. Scand. (Suppl. 30), 1962.
22. Moberg, E.: Objective methods for determining the functional value of sensibility in the hand. J. Bone Joint Surg., *40B*:454, 1948.
23. Bunnell, S.: Surgery of the Hand, 3rd ed. Philadelphia, J. B. Lippincott, 1956.

Rheumatoid Arthritis

24. Bunnell, S.: Surgery of the rheumatoid hand. J. Bone Joint Surg., *37A*:759, 1955.

25. Clayton, M. L.: Surgical treatment at the wrist in rheumatoid arthritis. J. Bone Joint Surg., *47*:741, 1965.
26. Goldner, J. L.: Surgery of the hand. *In* Practice of Surgery. Hagerstown, Maryland, Harper and Row Publishers, Inc., Chapter 5, pp. 1–22.
27. Kestler, O. C.: Reconstruction of the deformed arthritic hand. Ann. Surg., *131*:218, 1950.

Hand Bone Tumors

28. Jaffe, H. L.: Tumors and tumor conditions of the bone and joints. Philadelphia, Lea & Febiger, 1958.

29. Coley, D. L.: Neoplasms of bone. 2nd ed. New York, Hoeber, 1960.
30. Curtis, E. M.: Congenital arterial venous fistulae of the hand. J. Bone Joint Surg., *35A*:917–928, 1953.
31. Harkins, G. A., and Sabiston, D. C., Jr.: Lymphangioma in infancy and childhood. Surgery, *17*:811, 1960.
32. Pack, G. T., and Ariel, I. M.: Tumors of the Soft Somatic Tissues. 2nd ed. New York, Hoeber, 1964.
33. Stout, A. P.: Hemangiopericytoma: A study of 25 new cases. Cancer, *2*:1027, 1949.
34. Stout, A. P.: Tumors of the soft tissues. Armed Forces Institute of Pathology, Atlas of Tumor Pathology. Washington, D.C., 1953.

45

REPLANTATION OF THE EXTREMITIES

G. Rainey Williams, M.D., and J. Michael Kelly, M.D.

The first successful replantation of an amputated human extremity was performed in 1962. Experience with such procedures has rapidly increased. Techniques have improved, allowing successful replantation even at the digital level. Its newness and the importance of proper patient selection justify considering limb replantation as an entity.

HISTORICAL ASPECTS

Man's long-standing interest in restoration or replacement of severed human parts is amply demonstrated in legend, illustrations,[20] and reports[8] of crude surgical maneuvers. Modern surgical investigation directly related to replantation began in 1887 when Halsted divided and repaired all structures of the hind limb of dogs except the femoral artery and vein.[10] These experiments were stimulated by Dr. Halsted's interest in postmastectomy edema and were not reported until 1922. In 1903, Hopfner described experiments in which dogs' limbs were amputated and replanted using a nonsuture method of vascular anastomosis, with maintenance of viability up to 11 days in one animal.[13] Shortly thereafter, Carrel and Guthrie were also able to replant an extremity in a dog with short-term survival.[5] In 1908, Carrel described a dog leg homograft that survived for 22 days.[4] Very few experimental attempts at replantation were recorded between 1908 and the report of Lapchinsky[18] in 1960. Subsequently, several investigators have described experimental replantation and have added a substantial amount of information regarding the technique and physiologic effects of extremity replantation.[6, 7, 24, 32, 33]

In 1944, a protocol for replantation of amputated human extremities was formulated and published.[9] In 1962, a 12-year-old boy presented at the Massachusetts General Hospital shortly after sustaining a traumatic amputation of the right arm below the shoulder. Dr. Ronald Malt, then a resident in surgery, made the decision to attempt replantation, summoned a number of surgical colleagues, and promptly performed the first successful limb replantation. The efforts of a number of laboratory workers and particularly the careful, objective report of successful limb replantation in two patients by Malt and McKhann[21] stimulated worldwide interest in replantation.

The first successful replantation at a digital level was performed by Komatsu and Tamai on July 7, 1965.[17] The laboratory development of techniques and instrumentation for microvascular surgery has stimulated increasing interest and experience in digital replantation.

CLINICAL EXPERIENCE WITH REPLANTATION

Replantation experience, including all levels of amputation, numbers several hundred patients. Operations have been carried out in many geographic areas and it is of interest that the largest single institutional series are from China[30] and Australia.[25] It is likely that the total number of replantation procedures performed is considerably greater than that reported. Variations in the completeness and timing of scientific reporting allow only general conclusions to be drawn from the recorded clinical experience.

Age

Replantation has been reported in patients from 20 months[27] to nearly 60 years[14] of age. It is quite clear that the best functional results have been obtained in younger patients. The long period of rehabilitation and the decreasing likelihood of good functional recovery with increasing age suggest that replantation should be attempted only in the most ideal situation in patients over 45 years of age.

Level of Amputation

Replantation of the upper extremity has been performed at virtually every level. Perhaps because of the size of the blood vessels involved, initial success has been somewhat more likely in the higher amputations. The ultimate functional recovery is considerably better with more distal wounds, probably because nerve regeneration is more complete after distal injuries.

Etiology of Amputation

Attempts at replantation have followed traumatic amputation due to a wide variety of wounding agents, including automobile accidents, industrial machines, clothes dryers, and assorted sharp instruments (machetes, meat cleavers). Experience indicates clearly that sharp, incised wounds are more favorable for both initial and long-range successful replantation. In general, avulsion wounds have resulted in less complete neural regeneration, and replantation after such wounds should be attempted only under special circumstances. Wounds that would be considered too dirty for primary closure or in which the time interval dictates against primary closure should certainly not be considered acceptable for attempted replantation.

Results

The success rate in achieving extremity viability is approximately 75 per cent for major upper extremity replantations and just over 50 per cent for digital replantations. Because it seems likely that the most successful cases have been reported, these may be optimistic figures. Early failure has usually been described as due to circulatory inadequacy or infection. Late failure has virtually always been due to faulty innervation.

With current techniques, the end result after extremity replantation is never perfect. For practical purposes, the end result is dependent upon the extent of nerve regeneration. Experience with extremity replantation confirms the long accepted observation that peripheral nerve regeneration is more complete (1) in young persons, (2) in sharply incised wounds, and (3) in more distal wounds. The collected replant material does not permit correlation of either technique or timing of nerve repair with the ultimate degree of regeneration. Many surgeons now feel that primary repair of nerve trunks by epineural or interfascicular suture is highly desirable when possible. Early secondary

repair has been successfully performed in many instances. It is also not possible to define accurately functional success in extremity replantation. In general, the procedure is considered successful if the patient and the evaluating physician feel that the extremity function is preferable to that of currently available prostheses (Fig. 1). Using this criterion, the outcome of replantation operations has been termed successful in a high percentage of patients reported.

Incomplete Traumatic Amputation

It is obvious that the incompletely severed extremity offers virtually the same surgical challenge as complete amputation. Reviews of replantation have customarily not included cases of incomplete amputation because the presence of a viable tissue pedicle introduces so many variables into the assessment of results that even general conclusions become impossible. It is recognized, however, that one of the principal benefits of the recent interest in extremity replantation is a trend to more careful assessment of the badly injured extremity and the consequent salvage of extremities that might formerly have been amputated.

Bilateral Replantation

A single instance of bilateral upper extremity replantation is known.[34] The patient was a 12-year-old boy who sustained bilateral complete amputation of the upper extremities above the midhumeral level. Replantation was completed, but circulatory failure necessitated amputation of one arm and infection necessitated amputation of the other below the elbow, improving the outlook for prosthetic function. This experience suggests that bilateral replantation is technically feasible and is of interest in that no cardiovascular systemic effects were observed.

Summary

Experience with upper extremity replantation is encouraging. Better understanding of the basic processes

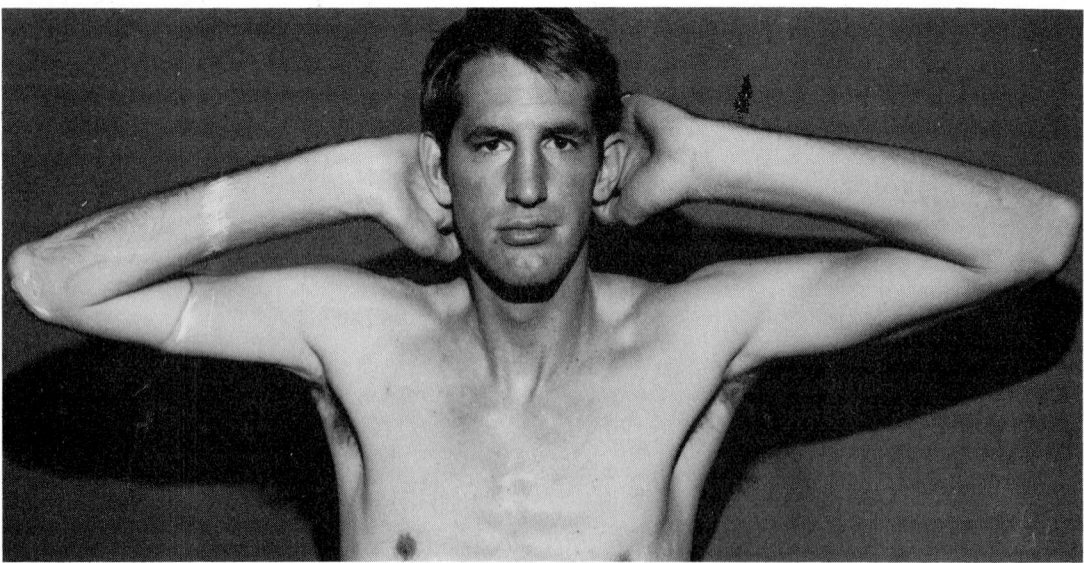

Figure 1.   Photograph of a patient 14 months after replantation of a severed right arm. (From Williams, G. R.: Monogr. Surg. Sci., *3*:53, 1966.)

involved and particularly of peripheral nerve regeneration should lead to improved results.

BASIC CONSIDERATIONS IN REPLANTATION

Extremity replantation involves many basic considerations. Most obvious is the necessity for detailed anatomic knowledge. Even more than with many other operations, surgical restoration of an amputated extremity requires knowledge of wound healing, the factors that influence healing, and the time required for the healing process. Currently, inadequate understanding of the healing process of peripheral nerves is the greatest single cause of imperfect results after replantation. The observation that infection is a major cause of early failure after limb replantation emphasizes the need for knowledge of surgical microbiology and for understanding the methods of minimizing, detecting, and treating bacterial infection. A basic problem shared with other vascular procedures but uniquely severe in replantation is the phenomenon of ischemia and restoration of blood flow. Several important questions regarding ischemia and restoration of flow may be posed. What is the maximal period of ischemia that will allow restoration of function by re-establishing circulation? What factors modify the period of permissible ischemia and, particularly, how can this period be prolonged? What problems are associated with restoration of blood flow and how can these be minimized or prevented?

Ischemia

When blood flow to an extremity is completely interrupted (as in traumatic amputation), the available oxygen is quickly exhausted and anaerobic metabolism begins. Ultimately, an irreversible state is reached when restoration of blood flow will no longer result in recovery. The length of time between the onset of ischemia and the state of irreversibility varies widely from one tissue to another. Skeletal muscle is the tissue in an extremity that is most sensitive to ischemia, followed by skin, fat, nerves, and bone. In experimental preparations, the ability of skeletal muscle to contract after electrical stimulation diminishes after 2 hours of ischemia and is totally lost after 4 hours.[11] Few gross or microscopic changes can be detected in ischemic muscle until 4 to 6 hours after ischemia is produced, although depletion of glycogen and ATP has been described.[28] Most studies of the maximal period of tolerance for ischemia have involved re-establishing flow after varying periods of ischemia in a variety of experimental preparations and studying the morphologic, physiologic, or biochemical changes that occur.[12, 19] When flow is restored in experimental preparations, necrosis of some skeletal muscle cells follows an ischemic period of about 2 hours duration, and necrosis is very extensive after an ischemic period of 8 hours.[31] There is some species variation in the resistance of muscle to ischemia and presumably this is true of other tissues. In the rat, the permissible period of skin ischemia is about 8 hours.[36] It is generally stated that fat, nerve, and bone are more resistant to ischemia, but precise experimental definition is lacking.

Basic studies of the effect of ischemia on skeletal muscle and skin, briefly cited in the preceding paragraph, suggest that an extremity replanted with adequate restoration of circulation after 6 to 8 hours should survive with good recovery of skeletal muscle contractility. This has been confirmed by limb replantation experiments in dogs.[33]

For obvious reasons, extension of the tolerable period of limb ischemia is desirable in clinical replantation. The oldest and perhaps most widely used agent to accomplish this is hypothermia. Presumably, hypothermia slows the metabolic processes that lead to an irreversible state. The optimal degree of hypothermia and the exact period of protection that might be offered by hypothermia are not precisely defined. Lapchinsky has reported survival of a replanted, cooled dog leg after 25 hours.[18] It seems significant that cooling during the period of ischemia has been shown to minimize some of the events, particularly edema, that follow restoration of circulation.[7]

Clearing the vasculature of the amputated extremity by perfusion should theoretically prevent the intravascular coagulation of blood and might remove some of the metabolic products of anaerobic metabolism. Such clearing has been shown to be useful in prolonging the life of experimental animals after replantation.[7] The efficacy of several perfusates in clearing the microcirculation has been studied and the most effective was found to be saline with heparin.[22] Prolonged perfusion using nonoxygenated solutions has no rationale.

Restoration of Circulation

When blood flow is re-established to an ischemic limb, femoral arterial flow rapidly rises to a level exceeding the preamputation flow in the experimental animal.[35] In addition, there is a marked increase in bleeding from the distal muscle ends and a visible reddening of the skin, which has been described as reactive hyperemia. An increase in limb weight occurs rapidly for approximately 2 hours and then increases very slowly for about a week, at which time the edema begins to subside.[7]

Studies of the microcirculation of both skin and muscle show that after ischemia of more than a few minutes' duration the restoration of flow in major vessels is not followed by uniform flow in the microcirculation.[36] Rather, the return of flow is patchy, with some areas filling well and others not at all. The role of lymphatic interruption in the formation of edema is not clear, but there is some evidence that lymph channel reconstruction in the experimental animal reduces the extent of edema.[18]

The principal recognized systemic effect of restoration of blood flow to a replanted extremity is the frequent development of shock. The appearance of shock after replantation is not consistent, but it has been described both clinically[23] and experimentally.[18] This shock has been extensively investigated and at least three explanations for its appearance have been suggested. Most evidence suggests that the shock is due to blood and fluid loss into the replanted extremity.[7, 24] Fluid loss into a traumatized extremity was carefully studied by Blalock in classic studies that showed that traumatic shock was not due to a tissue-elaborated toxin.[1] The same conclusion with regard to tourniquet shock[37] and replantation shock[7, 35] was reached after experiments by others. Since shock is not universally encountered after experimental replantation, it seems probable that the original condition of the animal, the blood loss during the amputation, the amount of fluid administration during the procedure, types of anesthesia, and perhaps other factors have served to confuse the experimental results. The concept that a vasodepressor toxic substance is elaborated in ischemic tissue and causes shock on restoration of circulation has had proponents since the work of Cannon.[3] The question is not whether such a substance might be elaborated after prolonged ischemia[29] but whether the effect is clinically significant under the conditions in which replantation might be attempted. Recent experiments again indicate that it is unlikely that a tissue toxin of significance is elaborated during periods of ischemia of up to 8 hours.[35] Mehl has suggested that shock in the postreplant period is due to fall in pH, and improved survival using an amine buffer in his experiments was impressive.[23] Certainly this work demonstrates the importance of control of pH, whether it is the primary cause of shock or secondary to it.

TECHNICAL CONSIDERATIONS

The Decision to Attempt Replantation

Replantation should be considered in every instance of upper extremity traumatic amputation. Since the functional result of replantation is imperfect at best and since the procedure entails definite risk to the patient, a number of factors should be carefully considered before a decision is made to proceed with the replant operation. The operation is more strongly indicated in young than old persons, both because of the significance of extremity loss and because the reported results of functional recovery in younger patients have been more favorable. The wound should be one that is acceptable for primary repair. Wounds that are badly contaminated and grossly avulsed should probably be excluded from consideration. The presence of significant associated injury should be carefully ascertained and probably constitutes a contraindication to replantation. The time interval between wounding and anticipated restoration of circulation should be less than 10 hours, although this is not an absolute figure. If the extremity has been promptly cooled and the circulation can be cleared during the first 8 hours, the time interval may be up to 20 hours. Finally, the impact of replantation, the expectation of multiple operations, and the necessity for at least 2 years of rehabilitative therapy should be considered in each patient.

Lower extremity replantation is indicated only in exceptional circumstances, such as loss or threatened loss of the other leg. The principal reason for this is that the function of the lower leg is relatively well accomplished by available prostheses. Also of importance is the fact that a shortened, anesthetic lower extremity is a constant and significant handicap during the period between replantation and very unpredictable nerve regeneration. It is obvious that improved methods of managing peripheral nerve injury will alter the indications for attempting to replant lower extremities.

The Replantation "Team"

All aspects of replantation are integral to other more common surgical procedures, yet experience indicates that preliminary review of the subject by all personnel to be involved will avoid recurring problems and improve the likelihood of success. Laboratory experience with the procedure is strongly recommended.

General, vascular, and orthopedic surgical skills are necessary for major replantation, and microsurgical skills are required for digital replantations. At least two, and as many as four or five, surgeons should compose the replantation team.

The anesthesiologist should be sensitive to the likelihood of hypovolemia. He should anticipate rapid, sizable blood loss when the extremity circulation is re-established. The problem of replantation shock and acidosis should be recognized and prevented or promptly treated by administration of blood, fluid, and bicarbonate.

Specialized facilities are required in the postoperative period, and the availability of physiotherapy and a spectrum of rehabilitative services is highly desirable.

Steps in Replantation

Control of bleeding from the amputation wound and careful assessment of the general condition of the patient and of the extremity are preliminary to making a decision to attempt replantation. Preoperative x-ray examination of the extremity and the wound is usually indicated. In avulsion injuries, x-ray examination of the cervical spine is indicated to rule out evidence of nerve root avulsion. If such evidence is present, myelography should be performed prior to attempting what might be a hopeless replantation. The extremity should be cooled by immersion in a sterile iced solution. When operating room conditions are available, the vasculature of the extremity should be cleared with balanced salt solution to which heparin and an antibiotic have been added. An intravenous infusion set is adequate, and the perfusion is discontinued when venous drainage becomes clear. Occasionally, extraction of thrombus material by means of a balloon catheter may be necessary. Both the extremity and the amputation wound are carefully prepared for replantation. In addition to mechanically cleaning the skin surrounding the wounds, extensive irrigation of the wounds with large volumes of sterile saline is important. Bone stabilization and fixation are initial steps in replantation (Fig. 2). It is essential to shorten the bone at all levels of amputation to allow approximation of other structures. The type of bone fixation depends upon the degree of comminution of the fracture and the anatomic level. A variety of intramedullary devices and plates have been used successfully, and evidence does not strongly favor one method over another. When bone fixation is complete, reconstruc-

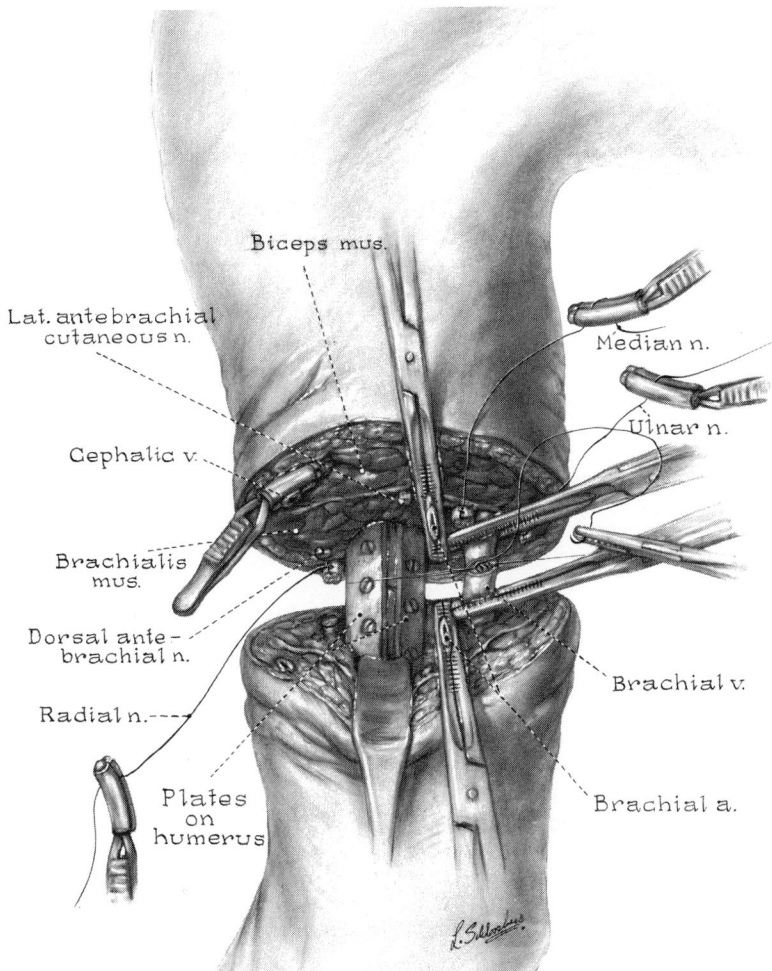

Figure 2. An illustration of the steps in upper extremity replantation. Bone fixation by plates is visible, the venous anastomosis is being performed, arterial anastomosis will follow, and nerves have been identified for approximation.

Biceps mus.

Lat. antebrachial cutaneous n.

Median n.

Cephalic v.

Ulnar n.

Brachialis mus.

Dorsal antebrachial n.

Radial n.

Brachial v.

Plates on humerus

Brachial a.

tion of the veins is begun. This is perhaps the most critical technical step in the replantation procedure. As many large veins as possible should be identified and careful anastomoses performed. Gentle dilation of the vein ends and placement of traction stay sutures allow construction of accurate, maximal-size, end-to-end anastomoses. Very fine synthetic suture is placed with continuous or interrupted technique. Following completion of at least two, and perferably several, venous anastomoses, the arterial anastomosis is performed. In amputations distal to the bifurcation of the brachial artery, both the radial and ulnar arteries should be repaired. Vein grafts from the saphenous system can be used to bridge gaps in either arteries or veins. On release of vascular clamps, hemorrhage from the distal muscle ends should be anticipated. This is apt to be massive, and transfusions will usually be necessary at this time. Establishing hemostasis will involve time, pressure, and patient ligation of multiple bleeding points. At this point, débridement of the amputation wound should be completed, as non-vascularized tissue can be accurately identified for the first time. Thorough débridement is important in preventing infection, and its value cannot be overemphasized.

Management of the divided peripheral nerves is controversial. Early opinions were generally that secondary definitive nerve suture should be performed.[32] Experience with exceedingly difficult secondary operations in dense scar and the hazard of vascular damage have convinced many surgeons that primary nerve suture should be performed when possible. Very careful interfascicular suture using magnification gives the best chance for a useful regeneration. Repair of the muscles is then performed by means of interrupted sutures in the muscle fascia. Subcutaneous tissue and skin closure is routine. Drainage of the wound is indicated in many instances. If adequate skin coverage is unavailable, grafting may be necessary, and tendon, bone, nerve, and vessels must be covered by flap tissue. Following the completion of the procedure, the arm should be elevated and protected by padded splinting in a position of function.

Postoperative Management

Postoperative care of the replanted extremity involves efforts to maintain circulation, protect the extremity against injury, and preserve functional capacity until nerve regeneration occurs. Anticoagulant therapy, fasciotomy, and methods of minimizing edema should be considered in the early postoperative period. The failure of heparin to improve results in experimental replantation and the complications often associated with effective levels of heparin have led to the recommendation that it not be used routinely after replantation proximal to the hand. Heparin and/or dextran are generally used after digital replantation. Fasciotomy may be critical in maintaining adequate circulation and should be performed freely but probably not routinely. Edema is controlled principally by elevation, gently and carefully applied elastic compression, and careful attention to serum protein level. The formation of edema is rapid in the first few hours after replantation, and care to avoid constricting dressings in this period is important.

The anesthetic arm is protected by padding, frequent position changes, and skin care. Physiotherapy should be employed very early in the postoperative period to preserve range of motion and joint function in the extremity. Muscle stimulation is added when healing of the wounds is well established. The cooperation, advice, and assistance of a physiotherapy unit is invaluable in the management of these patients and probably essential in obtaining a satisfactory functional result.

The risk of infection is minimized by appropriate selection of patients, careful and complete débridement, good surgical technique, and early, adequate antibiotic therapy. Antibiotic administration is begun prior to the replantation operation, and high intravenous doses of broad-spectrum antibiotics are continued for several days. Prophylaxis against tetanus should not be forgotten. Life-threatening infection is an indication for amputation.

Hypovolemia and its attendant cardiovascular and renal problems is the principal threat to the patient in the early postoperative period. Blood replacement prior to and during the replantation procedure should be as complete as possible, and further blood and fluid administration may be required as fluid is sequestered in the extremity in the postoperative period. Careful attention to blood pH, serum electrolytes, and urine output should allow prompt correction of abnormalities before major damage occurs.

The postoperative replantation patient requires far more than the usual psychological support from the managing team. The attempt to save an extremity will involve a long rehabilitation period, several subsequent operations, and a lengthy period of doubt about the extent of functional recovery. The managing physician and the many ancillary personnel involved in such procedures must realize the importance of establishing good rapport and maintaining support during this long period of treatment.

Most patients will require one or more secondary procedures for nerve repair or grafting, and many will require subsequent orthopedic reconstructive procedures. These are not unique to replantation. Wound infection is not as destructive to nerve repair as it is to the healing of bone or tendon.

During the long period of convalescence following extremity replantation, frequent review of the course, problems, and outlook by all participating personnel is important. The best interests of the patient are served by appropriate timing of subsequent procedures, recognition of problems, and prompt recognition of failure if it should occur. The difficult decision to amputate a replanted extremity is often made more easily and promptly by a multidiscipline review of the patient's progress.

REPLANTATION OF DIGITS

The replacement of any amputated part distal to the distal wrist crease, whether it be single or multiple digits or amputation through the metacarpal bones, is considered to be digital replantation. The development of microsurgical techniques for repair of vascular and neural injuries and clinical success in digital replantation, first achieved by Komatsu and Tamai in July, 1965,[17] created a surge of interest in digital replantation that is still increasing in momentum. Currently, success rates of 40 to 70 per cent are being reported in series of digital replantation procedures.[16, 25, 26, 30]

Indications for Replantation

The selection of patients for digital replantation takes into account the same factors mentioned for more proximal replantation. Specifically, replantation is indicated with multiple injuries or single amputation of a thumb or index finger. A single, complete, or incomplete amputation in any of the three ulnar digits should be replanted only if there are extenuating circumstances.

Operative Techniques

The steps in digital replantation are similar to those in major extremity amputation. Skeletal fixation is achieved initially, followed by repair of the extensor mechanism and dorsal veins, with an attempt made to repair at least two dorsal veins and the dorsal skin. Following repair of the above structures, the volar surface of the finger or thumb is approached, with digital arterial repair being accomplished initially. Finally, the neural anastomoses are followed by the flexor profundis tendon suture and volar skin closure. The neural and vascular anastomoses are carried out using an operating room microscope and employing well-documented microsurgical instruments and technique.[2, 15] All digits to be replanted should be shortened in bony length in order to allow vascular anastomoses without tension. Failure of digital replantation has most often been associated with inordinate tension on the venous anastomosis with subsequent thrombosis.

Postoperative Management

Of extreme importance following this precise technical accomplishment is diligent postoperative care. Observations should be made at half-hourly intervals of the color and capillary return of the replanted digit. With any suspicion of a venous or arterial thrombosis, the individual is returned to the operating room for operative evaluation of the anastomotic site and reanastomosis. The digit will exemplify a reactive hyperemia in like manner to the extremity of a major replant. In digital replantation, in contrast to major extremity replantation, anticoagulants are used in the form of heparin for a period of approximately one week to ten days in conjunction with aspirin and dipyridamole. Immobilization of the extremity is continued for a period of four weeks, at which time active and passive motion exercises are undertaken as one would in general digital rehabilitation following traumatic injury to the osteotendonous structures.

Discussion

The primary aim in replantation surgery is to obtain extremity survival. Of equal importance, satisfactory function must be achieved. The major limiting factor to satisfactory function seems to be tendon motion. Subsequent reconstructive procedures will restore satisfactory tendon motion in a significant percentage of replanted digits. Satisfactory survival and function after digital replantation is dependent on the availability of microsurgery. The general principles of hand reconstructive surgery must be followed.

SELECTED REFERENCES

Malt, R. A., and McKhann, C. F.: Replantation of severed arms. J.A.M.A., *189*:716, 1964.
  This is the original description of the first successful human replantation experience, which, more than any other factor, stimulated interest in the possibility of extremity salvage by replantation.

Nabseth, D. C., Mayer, R. F., and Deterling, R. A., Jr.: Experimental basis of limb replantation. Adv. Surg., *2*:35, 1966.
  This is an extensive review of the pertinent literature concerning the experimental basis for limb replantation, including the authors' investigative experience.

O'Brien, B.McC.: Replantation surgery. Clin. Plast. Surg., *1*(3):405, 1974.
  An excellent review of the subject of both major and digital replantation by an authority.

REFERENCES

1. Blalock, A.: Experimental shock; cause of low blood pressure produced by muscle injury. Arch. Surg., *20*:959, 1930.
2. Buncke, H. J., Jr., and Schulz, W. P.: The suture repair of one-millimeter vessels. *In* Donaghy, R. M. P., and Yasargil, M. S. (Eds.): Microvascular Surgery. St. Louis, The C. V. Mosby Co., 1967.
3. Cannon, W. B.: Traumatic Shock. New York, D. Appleton and Co., 1923.
4. Carrel, A.: Results of the transplantation of blood vessels, organs, and limbs. J.A.M.A., *51*:1662, 1908.
5. Carrel, A., and Guthrie, C. C.: Complete amputation of the thigh, with replantation. Am. J. Med. Sci., *131*:297, 1906.
6. Eiken, O., Nabseth, D. C., Mayer, R. F., and Deterling, R. A., Jr.: Limb replantation. I. The technique and immediate results. Arch. Surg., *88*:48, 1964.
7. Eiken, O., Nabseth, D. C., Mayer, R. F., and Deterling, R. A., Jr.: Limb replantation. II. The pathophysiological effects. Arch. Surg., *88*:54, 1964.
8. Gibson, T.: Early free grafting: The restitution of parts completely separated from the body. Br. J. Plast. Surg., *18*:1, 1965.
9. Hall, R. H.: Whole upper extremity transplant for human beings: General plans of procedure and operative technic. Ann. Surg., *120*:12, 1944.
10. Halsted, W. S., Reichert, F. L., and Reid, M. R.: Replantation of entire limbs without suture of vessels. Trans. Am. Surg. Assoc., *40*:160, 1922.
11. Harman, J. W.: Histological study of skeletal muscle in acute ischemia. Am. J. Pathol., *23*:551, 1947.
12. Harman, J. W., and Gwinn, R. P.: Recovery of skeletal muscle fibers from acute ischemia as determined by histologic and chemical methods. Am. J. Pathol., *25*:741, 1949.
13. Hopfner, E.: Uber Gefassnaht, Gefasstransplantation und Reimplantation von amputierten Extremitaten. Arch. Klin. Chir., *70*:417, 1903.
14. Inoue, T., Toyoshima, Y., Fukusumi, H., Uemichi, A., Inui, K., Harada, S., Hirohashi, K., Kotani, T., and Shiraha, Y.: Replantation of severed limbs. J. Cardiovasc. Surg., *8*:31, 1967.
15. Jacobson, J. H.: Microsurgery. Curr. Probl. Surg., *3*:56, 1971.
16. Kleinert, H. E., and Kasdan, M. L.: Anastomosis of digital vessels. J. Ky. Med. Assoc., *63*:106, 1965.
17. Komatsu, S., and Tamai, S.: Successful replantation of a completely cut-off thumb. Plast. Reconstr. Surg., *42*:374, 1968.
18. Lapchinsky, A. G.: Recent results of experimental transplantation of preserved limbs and kidneys and possible use of this technique in clinical practice. Ann. N.Y. Acad. Sci., *87*:539, 1960.
19. LePage, G. A.: Biological energy transformation during shock as shown by tissue analyses. Am. J. Physiol., *146*:267, 1946.
20. Malt, R. A.: Clinical aspects of restoring limbs. Adv. Surg., *2*:19, 1966.
21. Malt, R. A., and McKhann, C. F.: Replantation of severed arms. J.A.M.A., *189*:716, 1964.
22. Mehl, R. L., Paul, H. A., and Shorey, W. D.: Patency of microcirculation in the traumatically amputated limb—a comparison of common perfusates. J. Trauma, *4*:495, 1964.
23. Mehl, R. L., Paul, H. A., Shorey, W. D., Schneewind, J., and Beattie, E. J., Jr.: Treatment of "toxemia" after extremity replantation. Arch. Surg., *89*:871, 1964.
24. Nabseth, D. C., Mayer, R. F., and Deterling, R. A., Jr.: Experimental basis of limb replantation. Adv. Surg., *2*:35, 1966.
25. O'Brien, B. McC.: Replantation surgery. Clin. Plast. Surg., *1*(3):405, 1974.
26. O'Brien, B. McC., and Miller, G. D. H.: Digital reattachment and revascularization. J. Bone Joint Surg., *55A*:714, 1973.
27. Rosenkrantz, J. G., Sullivan, R. C., Welch, K., Miles, J. S., Sadler, K. M., and Paton, B. C.: Replantation of an infant's arm. N. Engl. J. Med., *276*:609, 1967.
28. Scully, R. E., Shannon, J. M., and Dickerson, G. R.: Factors involved in recovery from experimental skeletal muscle ischemia produced in dogs. I. Histologic and histochemical pattern of ischemic muscle. Am. J. Pathol., *39*:721, 1961.
29. Selby, D. M., Haddy, F. J., and Campbell, G. S.: Vasodilator material in ischemic tissues. Surg. Forum, *15*:232, 1964.
30. Sixth People's Hospital, Shanghai: Severed Limb Replantation Research Institute: The understanding and progress of replantation of severed limbs and digits. Chin. Med. J., *1*:3, 1973.
31. Strock, P. E., and Majno, G.: Vascular responses to experimental tourniquet ischemia. Surg. Gynecol. Obstet., *129*:309, 1969.
32. Williams, G. R.: Replantation of amputated extremities. Monogr. Surg. Sci., *3*:53, 1966.
33. Williams, G. R., Carter, D. R., Frank, G. R., and Price, W. E.: Replantation of amputated extremities. Ann. Surg., *163*:788, 1966.
34. Williams, G. R., Frank, G. R., and Barkett, V. M.: Unpublished data.
35. Williams, G. R., Stamatis, J. J., and Garrett, D. H.: Response to reestablished circulation in the ischemic extremity. Surg. Forum, *22*:174, 1971.
36. Willms-Kretschmer, K., and Majno, G.: Ischemia of the skin. Am. J. Pathol., *54*:327, 1969.
37. Wilson, H., and Roome, N. W.: Effects of constriction and release of an extremity: Experimental study of tourniquet. Arch. Surg., *32*:334, 1936.

46

SURGICAL DISORDERS OF THE SKIN

Kenneth L. Pickrell, M.D.

In the average adult, the skin has a superficial area of 10,000 to 18,000 sq. cm.; it accounts for about 15 per cent of the total body weight. Its thickness varies from 1.5 to 5 mm., depending upon the location, age, sex, race, and state of nutrition. It is thinnest on the eyelids, penis, and labia minora, and thickest on the palms, soles, shoulders, and back. Infants and the very old have the thinnest skin. Sweat glands are abundant almost everywhere except the glans penis and labia minora. Sebaceous glands are profuse on the face, neck, and back; they are absent on the palms and soles. Sexual differences are involved in the distribution of hair, mainly on the face, neck, chest, and pubis.

The skin as an organ is vulnerable to a wide variety of diseases and conditions. Aging is accompanied by loss of elasticity and wrinkling. Degenerative changes result from excessive exposure to the sun and radioactive elements (see Fig. 4). Reactions to chemicals and drugs are common.

MICROBIOLOGY OF THE SKIN

Resident bacteria are found chiefly in the stratum corneum (keratin layer) and the openings of the pilo-sebaceous apparatus. Gram-positive cocci of several types are found essentially everywhere. A number of diphtheroids are widely distributed, especially in moist areas; gram-positive rods are found in moist areas also. *Pityrosporon ovale* is classified as a resident fungus.[13] The number of resident bacteria is said to remain relatively constant unless altered by antibiotics or temperature. Those with oily skin have larger numbers of organisms, and more organisms are present in hot, humid weather. Despite the superficial position of the resident bacteria, it is virtually impossible to sterilize the skin. Body odor is influenced by the bacterial flora. Resident gram-positive bacteria act on the eccrine (sweat) and apocrine (scent) secretions to produce the characteristic odor of the axilla. The use of deodorants that contain aluminum salts reduces the number of gram-positive organisms, thereby reducing or eliminating the odor. The normal pH of the skin, 4 to 6, retards the growth of many skin orga-

nisms; streptococci are more affected than staphylococci. The pH of the skin is largely the result of lactic acid from sweat and amino acid residues from keratinization.[23] Intact skin presents a formidable defense against entry by pathogenic organisms, but traumatized skin (burns, penetrating wounds, crush injuries, and so forth) presents a favorable site and environment for their growth.

SKIN PERMEABILITY

One of the major functions of the skin is to provide a barrier: from inside out and outside in. A very effective barrier is provided against loss of electrolytes, proteins, carbohydrates, lipids, and significant amounts of water from the internal environment. *Percutaneous absorption* is the passage of substances from the outside of the skin through the epidermis and dermis into the circulation. Well-absorbed substances are lipid-soluble substances, phenolic and arsenical compounds, hormones, gases, vitamins (A, D, K), insecticides, and so forth. Absorption through the palms and soles is poor because of the thick keratin layer. Skin absorption can be increased by increasing the temperature and moisture.

REGULATION OF BODY TEMPERATURE

Sweating is a major function of the skin because of its role in regulation of body temperature by evaporative cooling. Each liter of sweat is capable of removing 540 calories of heat from the body.[13] The most important stimuli for sweating are heat, muscular exercise, and a neuroendocrine reaction (fright, cold sweat). Thermoreceptors in the skin are stimulated by an increase in temperature (summertime). Similarly, thermoreceptors in muscle are stimulated by increased temperature of blood from working muscles. The heat center in the hypothalmus induces sweating when the temperature of blood circulating through it is elevated. *Emotional sweating* affects primarily the glands of the face, neck, palms, and axilla. *Reflex sweating* after eating spicy or hot foods affects primarily the face. Sweat glands are innervated by sympathetic nerves of both cholinergic and adrenergic type.[13]

Sweat is hypotonic with a pH range of 3.8 to 6.5 and a specific gravity of 1.001 to 1.006. It contains little or no protein, fat, acetone, or alkaline phosphatase. There are significant amounts of sodium, chloride, calcium, and iodide.[13] In *congenital ectodermal dysplasia* sweat glands are sparse and show lack or absence of function. Affected persons do not sweat adequately and hence they cannot cool their bodies in a hot environment.

Sweating from the skin must not be confused with the *circulation of fluid in the skin,* for in the latter there are three structures with membrane function: (1) dermal capillaries and lymphatics, which are concerned with escape and reabsorption of fluid and metabolites; (2) the basal membrane, which is permeable to water and most electrolytes; and (3) the barrier layer of keratin (stratum corneum), which is essentially impermeable to electrolytes but allows some passage of water and permits free passage of carbon dioxide.

HISTOLOGY OF THE SKIN

Epidermis

The epidermis is an avascular cellular structure that varies in thickness from 0.06 mm. on the eyelids to 0.8 mm. on the palms and soles. The border between the epidermis and the dermis is irregular because numerous cone-shaped dermal papillae reach or push upward and indent the inner surface of the epidermis. The ridges of epidermis separating the papillae appear in histologic sections as pegs and therefore are referred to as *rete pegs,* although the term *rete ridges* might be preferable (Figs. 1 and 2). If one could separate or peel off the epidermis from the dermis, it would look like the inside of an egg carton.

Layers of Epidermis. The epidermis is divided into four layers of cells: (1) the basal layer, (2) prickle layer or stratum malpighii, (3) granular layer or stratum granulosum, and (4) the horny layer of keratin or stratum corneum (Fig. 2). An additional layer, the stratum lucidum, is present between the granular and the horny layers, but it is conspicuous only in the epidermis of the palms and soles. The cells in the various layers represent different stages in the gradual evolution and maturation of the basal cells into cornified cells and do not actually represent different types of cells.

BASAL LAYER. The basal layer divides the epidermis from the dermis; two types of cells are present: basal cells and melanocytes. The basal cells are columnar in shape with their long axis vertical. These cells are active metabolically and mitotically and are the source of keratinocytes. It is from this layer that basal cell cancer develops. Basal cells frequently contain melanin, especially in dark-skinned persons; the pigment is transferred to them from the melanocytes. Mitotic figures may be present, denoting regeneration. In

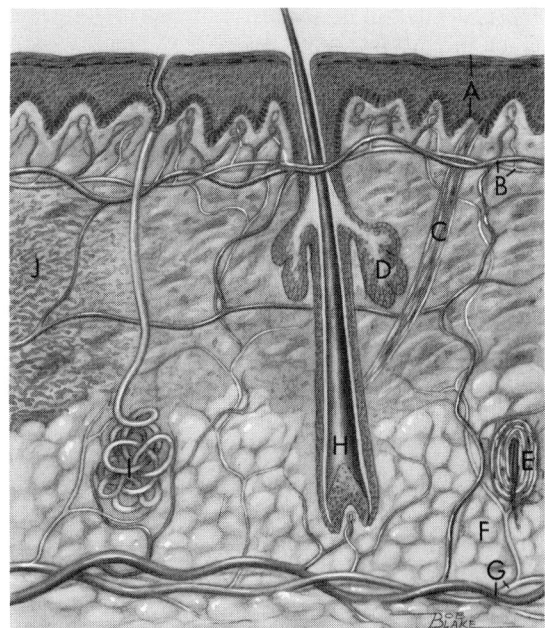

Figure 1. Drawing of normal skin: A, epidermis; B, capillaries; C, arrectores pilorum muscle; D, sebaceous gland; E, pacinian corpuscle; F, adipose tissue; G, blood vessels and lymphatics; H, hair; I, eccrine sweat gland; J, collagen, which gives substance to the skin.

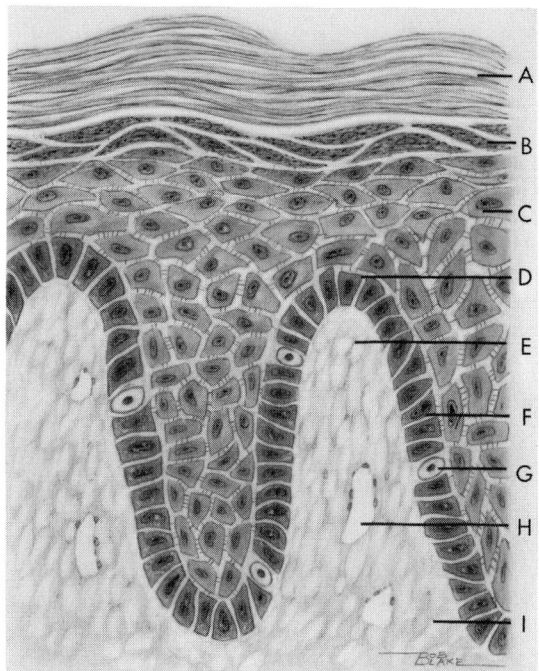

Figure 2. Drawing of normal epidermis from dorsum of hand, high magnification. Four layers are recognized: A, stratum corneum or keratin or horny layer; B, stratum granulosum or granular layer; C, stratum malpighii or prickle layer (note the presence of intercellular bridges); D, basal layer, which divides the epidermis from the dermis (an additional layer, stratum lucidum, not shown, is present between the granular and keratin layers, but it is conspicuous only in the epidermis of the palms and soles); E, papillae of dermis; F, mitotic figures, which can be seen in basal and prickle layers; G, melanocytes, clear cells, scattered in the basal layer; H, capillaries; I, collagen and elastic tissue.

the normal epidermis, the cells of the prickle layer show more mitoses than cells of the basal layer. *Melanocytes* are of neural origin and are wedged in between the basal cells.

PRICKLE LAYER. The prickle layer (stratum malpighii) is located immediately above the basal layer. The cells are larger and more spherical and are connected by prickles or intercellular bridges, which are formed by opposing protrusions of the cell membrane of neighboring cells. These prickles or intercellular bridges hold them together but do not represent avenues of passage of material from one cell to another. Between the cells, however, is a potential space, which in life appears to contain intercellular fluid and makes possible the exchange of nutrients and waste. As the cells pass upward, they become more egg-shaped with their long axis parallel with the skin surface. This is the layer from which squamous cancer arises.

GRANULAR LAYER. The granular layer (stratum granulosum) comes next and it is three to four cells thick. The cells are flattened with their long axis parallel to the surface. The cytoplasm contains basophilic granules called *keratohyalin* and the nucleus is undergoing degeneration. In areas of imperfect keratinization, *parakeratosis,* the granular layer is absent. The granular layer is normally absent from mucous membrane, in the lips, mouth, and vagina. The mucous membrane in the mouth normally possesses no granular cells and no horny cells. Here the epithelial cells in their migration from the basal layer to the surface first become vacuolated, and then shrink and desquamate.

STRATUM LUCIDUM. The stratum lucidum comes next; however, it is well developed only on the palms and soles.

HORNY, KERATIN LAYER. The horny layer (stratum corneum) is the outermost layer and is composed of anuclear dead cells, keratin, surface lipids, and dirt. This layer is responsible for the "bathtub ring." The cells of the horny layer normally desquamate in an orderly fashion; desquamation and cell production are geared so that one controls the other. The stratum corneum remains at approximately the same thickness unless the balance is disturbed.

Under normal conditions, it takes approximately 26 to 28 days for an epithelial cell to migrate from the basal layer to the surface. Mitoses occur mainly in the basal and prickle layers. The *mitotic index,* the number of dividing cells per 1000 cells, varies from 2 to 8 or higher, depending upon the number of desquamated cells, since the thickness of the epidermis remains quite constant. Mitotic activity is greatest during rest and sleep; it is reduced during activity, in a cool environment, and during stress and starvation. Methotrexate and other anticancer drugs depress division of cells not only in the skin but in other organs also.

Epidermal Appendages. Hair and nails are keratinizing appendages; the other appendages are glandular—the eccrine, apocrine, and sebaceous glands.

Eccrine (sweat) glands are present everywhere in the skin, being most numerous on the palms and soles and decreasing in concentration from the head and neck to the extremities. The secretory cells are large, cylindrical cells that contain glycogen, which disappears on sweating (Fig. 2).

Apocrine (scent) glands are located chiefly in the axilla, groins, labia, scrotum, and pararectal areas. They are tubular glands that are located in the deep derma; the duct usually opens into a hair follicle above the sebaceous gland. Since the ducts do not open directly onto the surface, and since the secretory part of the gland is approximately 10 times larger than the secretory coil of eccrine glands, infections are extremely resistant to local antibiotics and emollients (see hidradenitis, Fig. 28).

Sebaceous glands are present everywhere except in the palms and soles. Their greatest concentration is on the head and face. Sebaceous glands are composed of several lobules. They are alveolar, holocrine glands; that is, they have no lumen and their secretion is formed by decomposition of their cells. They usually empty into the upper part of the hair follicle. Cyst formations are common; cancer forming in sebaceous cysts is rare; the author has never seen a case in 35 years. Sebaceous cysts are most common in adolescence and early adult life (Fig. 3). Cysts in the lower forehead, root of the nose, and brow areas must be dif-

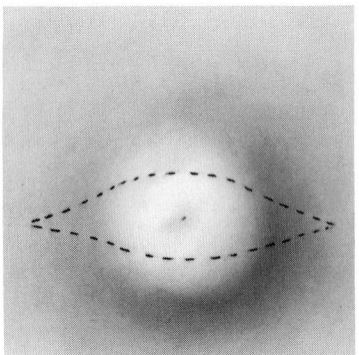 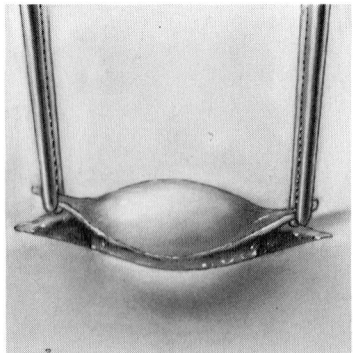 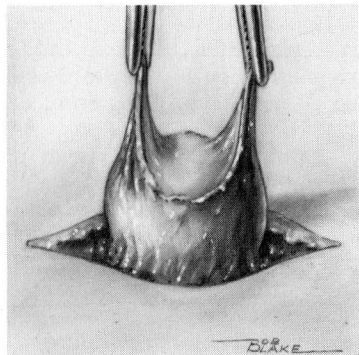

Figure 3. Method of excision of sebaceous cyst. Sebaceous cysts are intimately fused with the skin, and in the very center the obstructed orifice and duct can be seen. Since the skin is usually very thin because of underlying pressure, one should use rather wide elliptical incisions, the ends of which then serve as handles to remove the cyst without rupture.

ferentiated from dermoid cysts, which may have an intracranial extension, and encephaloceles (see Fig. 27).

Dermis (Cutis, Corium)

The dermis constitutes the bulk of the skin; it is thickest on the nape of the neck (where sebaceous cysts and carbuncles are common), back, palms, and soles. It is intimately related to the epidermis, which it supports and nourishes and into which the epidermal appendages grow.

The dermis is composed of three types of fibers: collagen, elastic, and reticulum; it also contains blood vessels, lymphatics, nerves, cells, and ground substances (see Fig. 2).

Collagen forms about 95 per cent of the connective tissue of the dermis. The bundles and fibers are held together by amorphous ground substance. It is generally accepted that collagen is formed extracellularly by the action of fibroblasts. Collagen bundles are only slightly extensible, but since they are wavy, they permit some stretching of the skin. A few fibroblasts are interspersed between the collagen bundles (see keloids, Fig. 6).

Elastic fibers entwine among the collagen bundles. Elastic fibers are wavy and therefore only small portions are seen in histologic sections. Selective tissue stains must be used, such as Verhoeff's stain. There is progressive loss of elastic fibers in actinic (solar) keratoses (see Fig. 4).

Reticulum fibers are not visible with routine stains but stain with silver, as Foot's stain. They probably represent immature or young collagen fibers (precollagen), and are the first fibers to form during wound healing. They are replaced gradually or transformed into true collagen.[18] Large numbers of reticulum fibers are present in mesodermal tumors, such as histiocytomas, sarcomas, and lymphomas.

Dermal blood vessels consist of capillaries, arterioles, and venules arranged in numerous anastomoses and arcades, abnormalities of which result in hemangiomas (see Figs. 20 to 22). There is prompt vascular response in infections (heat, redness), shock, and trauma (vasodilatation in burns and vasoconstriction in lacerations and injuries due to cold and so forth).

A special vascular structure, *the glomus,* occurs most abundantly in pads and nail beds of the fingers and toes. The glomus is concerned with temperature regulation and represents a special short-circuit device connecting an arteriole with a venule. The glomus cells are in intimate association with a rich network of nonmyelinated nerve fibers.[10]

Lymphatic vessels begin as fluid spaces between the cells of the epidermis, which then circulate between the collagen bundles as loops in the papillae, leading down through the dermis into the subcutaneous tissues and lymph channels. The response of the lymphatics to trauma and infection (lymphangitis) is prompt and marked. Distant dissemination of cancer is most often due to invasion of the lymphatics, less often vascular or hematogenous invasion.

Muscles of the skin are mainly involuntary or smooth muscles. The arrectores pilorum when they contract produce "gooseflesh." The tunica dartos of the scrotum and the muscle fibers in the nipple and areola contract markedly when exposed to cold. The facial muscles of expression and the platysma muscles of the skin of the neck are striated or voluntary muscles.

PATHOLOGIC PROCESSES OF THE EPIDERMIS

Localized hyperplastic lesions of the skin are of importance to the surgeon because they may be mistaken for cancer or melanoma. Certain terms are common in skin pathology and need to be defined. *Acanthosis* is a hyperplastic thickening of the prickle cell layer, the rete malpighii, and is a frequent finding in neurodermatitis and psoriasis. *Hyperkeratosis* is thickening of the stratum corneum, the keratin layer, as seen in senile keratoses and warts. It is associated with increased thickening of the granular layer. *Parakeratosis* signifies imperfect keratinization with retention of nuclei in the horny layer, a common finding in psoriasis and in inflammatory dermatoses. *Dyskeratosis* applies to changes in the epidermis suggestive of developing malignancy, including loss of cell polarity and increase in the number of mitoses, changes that are summed up in two descriptive words: atypicality and jumbling, the latter referring to the loss of normal, orderly cell arrangement. *Pseudoepitheliomatous hyperplasia* is a wild, but benign, overgrowth of the prickle cell layer which is seen frequently in infectious granulomas.

HYPERPLASIA

Seborrheic Keratosis

This hyperplasia is a benign basal cell papilloma. The lesions are frequently multiple and occur on the forehead, cheek, nape of the neck, and upper back, usually in persons over 50 years of age. The lesions are raised, soft, and greasy, and sometimes wartlike. They may be markedly pigmented and look like a scorched lima bean stuck on the surface. The lesions show little tendency to malignant change. They may be removed by excision, dermabrasion, or currettage in the clinic or office (see Fig. 15).

Solar (Actinic, Senile) Keratosis

This lesion, in the beginning, is small and firm, and occurs frequently on the face, posterior neck, and hands in older persons with little skin pigment (redheads and blonds, persons with blue eyes) who have been exposed excessively to the sun (farmers, ranchers, commercial fishermen, and "sun worshipers"). The condition is a premalignant one, with a strong tendency to develop into squamous cancer (Fig. 4). Surgical excision and pathologic examination are recommended so that an accurate diagnosis can be made.

Leukoplakia

This lesion of mucous membranes (lips, mouth, vagina) is analogous to the senile keratosis of the

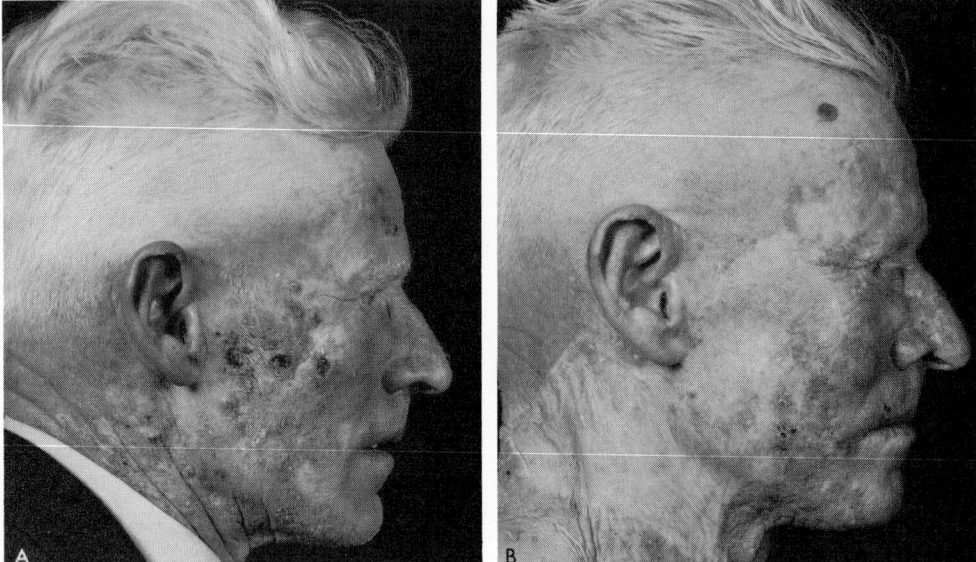

Figure 4. *A,* A 45-year-old commercial fisherman with extensive actinic changes in the skin frequently referred to as *farmer's* or *sailor's disease.* There were many hyperkeratoses and early squamous cell cancers in his thin, dry skin after prolonged exposure to the sun and wind. *B,* The forehead, lateral cheeks, and neck were resurfaced with heavy split grafts. Postoperative photograph taken 3 years later shows beginning changes occurring on the nose and maxillary rim of the graft. (See Fig. 19, xeroderma pigmentosa.)

skin. As the name, white patch, implies, it takes the form of white patches of thickened mucous membrane (Fig. 5). It is often associated with chronic irritation, either physical (sharp, jagged teeth) or chemical (snuff, smoking, alcohol). Intraoral lesions are frequently multiple and are decidedly premalignant, of the squamous cell type. The irritating factors should be stopped and if prompt regression does not occur, the lesions should be excised, and skin grafted if necessary to close the mucous membrane defect without tension.

Verruca Vulgaris (Verruca Juvenilis)

The common wart is the result of invasion of the epithelial cells by a specific virus. Warts occur in childhood through adolescence and early adult life and affect chiefly the fingers and hands. The warts occur in crops because of autoinoculation. Although the condition may be painful and troublesome owing to cracks, fissures, and bleeding, and psychologic trauma may be severe, the condition is self-limited and the lesions will eventually disappear without any residual scar-

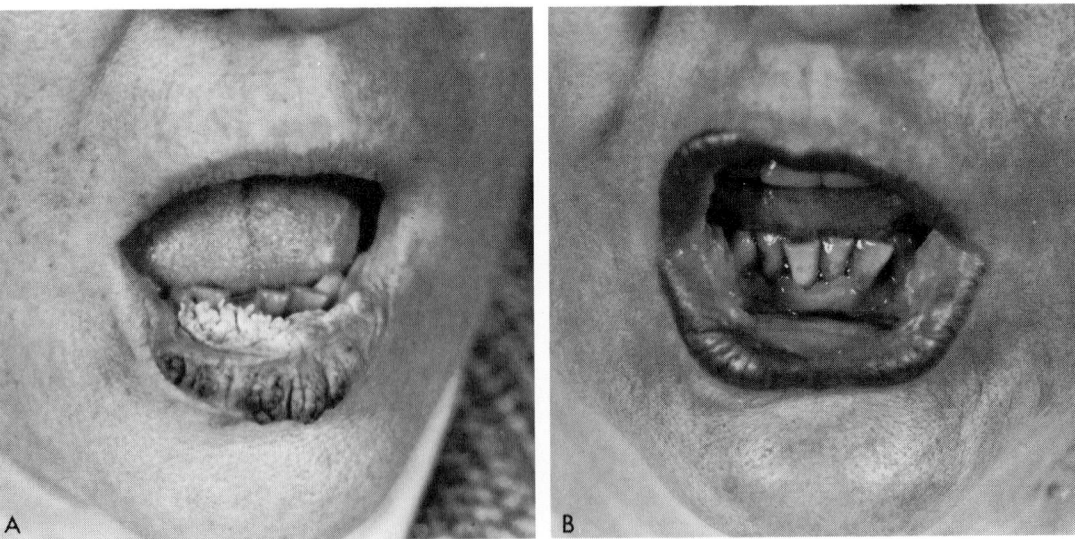

Figure 5. *A,* A 54-year-old woman, an excessive cigarette smoker of many years, with extensive leukoplakia and squamous papillomas of the cutaneous and buccal surfaces of the lip. The lesions were excised widely and grafted. *B,* Postoperative photograph taken 1 year later. (See also Fig. 13.)

ring. Excision is of doubtful value. Dermatologic assistance by electrodesiccation or freezing with liquid nitrogen may be helpful.

Verruca Plantaris (Plantar Wart)

Verruca plantaris is the most troublesome of all warts. Located on the sole of the foot, over the metatarsal heads or the os calcis, the wart is usually covered by a thickened, cornified epithelium. Compression by the pressure of the weight of the body in standing is very painful. Corrective shoes and orthopedic appliances may be helpful. If the condition persists, excision and either the use of a split-thickness graft or the rotation of a contiguous flap may be necessary. Plantar wart must not be confused with a corn or callus, both of which are due to pressure and friction. In the corn or *clavus*, keratinization is developed as a dense localized plug (see Fig. 17).

BENIGN TUMORS OF FIBROUS TISSUE

Keloid

Keloid, from the Greek root *chele* (crab's claw), is a dense fibrous tumor of the skin that occurs after injury. That the fibrous tissue represents an overgrowth is evident from the fact that a keloid extends not only above the surface of the skin but also laterally to involve areas that were not affected by the original injury. This characteristic is the chief finding in the clinical differentiation of keloids from hypertrophic scars. The color of a keloid may vary from red (when it may still be in an active phase) to pink (when its activity is subsiding) to white (when it is mature or quiescent). Telangiectatic vessels usually traverse the surface. Pruritus may be profound and very difficult to control.

Etiology. There is a strong individual predisposition and a family tendency in some instances. Black and other dark-skinned persons are particularly vulnerable. Some areas of the body are more susceptible than others: sternum, deltoid region, lateral cheeks, ears, and neck. Thermal burns of the face and neck and grease burns of the hands will frequently result in keloids (Fig. 6).

Treatment. Since the lesion may recur following excision, and possibly in greater extent, it must be looked upon as a locally recurrent, yet benign, tumor. If the keloids are young, less than 3 months, and are still in an active phase, benefit may be obtained from radiation.[6] In 3 to 6 months the lesions become organized; the cells mature and are less radiosensitive. Intralesional injection of steroids may reduce itching and result in some softening; however, our results have been far from impressive.

If the keloid is small, as in those which follow piercing of the ear lobe, it may be excised, but should receive two radiation treatments of 200 R, one treatment the day of excision and a similar treatment when the sutures are removed, usually around the sixth day. The results are excellent for small keloids when this regimen is followed.[6] In dark-skinned patients, who are the ones most frequently affected, two irradiation treatments of 300 R each may be necessary.

When the keloids are large and involve important functional areas, such as the face, neck, hands, and forearms, surgical excision and split-thickness grafting then become procedures of necessity (Fig. 6). Wide excision, beyond the keloid into normal skin, and grafting will frequently give a pleasing result. The split-thickness graft should be taken from the thigh or buttock, not the abdomen, and it should be thin, 0.010 to 0.012 (dermatome setting), to lessen the possibility of a keloid developing in the donor area. In a true keloid, former, "prophylactic" irradiation, in small doses, may be given over the donor area in 3 to 4 weeks. The effect of radiation is to produce rapid maturation of the fibroblasts with diminution of the vascularity of the fibrous tissue. It should be reserved only for use as an early postoperative measure. However, a word of caution: in certain persons, despite meticulous attention to lines of elasticity of the skin and to techniques of excision and suture, development of hypertrophied scars or keloids may follow even minimal trauma. Consult Peacock and Van Winkle's excellent volume on *Surgery and Biology of Wound Repair.*[18]

Fibroma

A pure fibroma is rare. Nearly all tumors known as fibromas are qualified in some way by such terms as dermatofibroma (which is not just a fibroma of the skin), neurofibroma (which is more than a fibroma of nerve), fibroadenoma, and so forth.

Two types are described: The hard fibroma, *fibroma durum*, occurs primarily on the face and extremities as an elevation of the skin. The soft fibroma, *fibroma molle*, is a soft, pedunculated tumor of connective tissue that differs from a papilloma of the skin in that the bulk of the tumor is its subepithelial portion. Neither fibroma molle nor fibroma durum is regarded as a premalignant lesion though the point of origin of fibrosarcoma of the skin and subcutaneous tissues is a matter of speculation. Either one may occur in conjunction with von Recklinghausen's disease, or neurofibromatosis. The distinction between a soft fibroma and a well-differentiated fibrosarcoma may be difficult for the pathologist, unless he knows the clinical history.

Pachydermatocele is a type of pendant fibroma of the skin and subcutaneous tissue that occurs in association with von Recklinghausen's disease. The lesions are present from birth but may increase markedly in size. Their tissue weight may cause distortion of regional soft tissues, and underlying bones may be enlarged because of their vascularity. The term "pachydermatocele" comes from the thick, corrugated appearance not unlike that of the skin of an elephant (Figs. 7 and 8). Surgical excision, in stages if the tumor is large, is advised. The tumor may be extremely vascular because of loose areolar tissue and abundant large vascular sinuses. These sinuses have no contractility, as do normal blood vessels, and control of hemorrhage may be difficult.

Lipoma

Lipomas are among the commonest and the most benign of tumors. They usually occur singly, but may be multiple. The tumor consists of normal fat, arranged

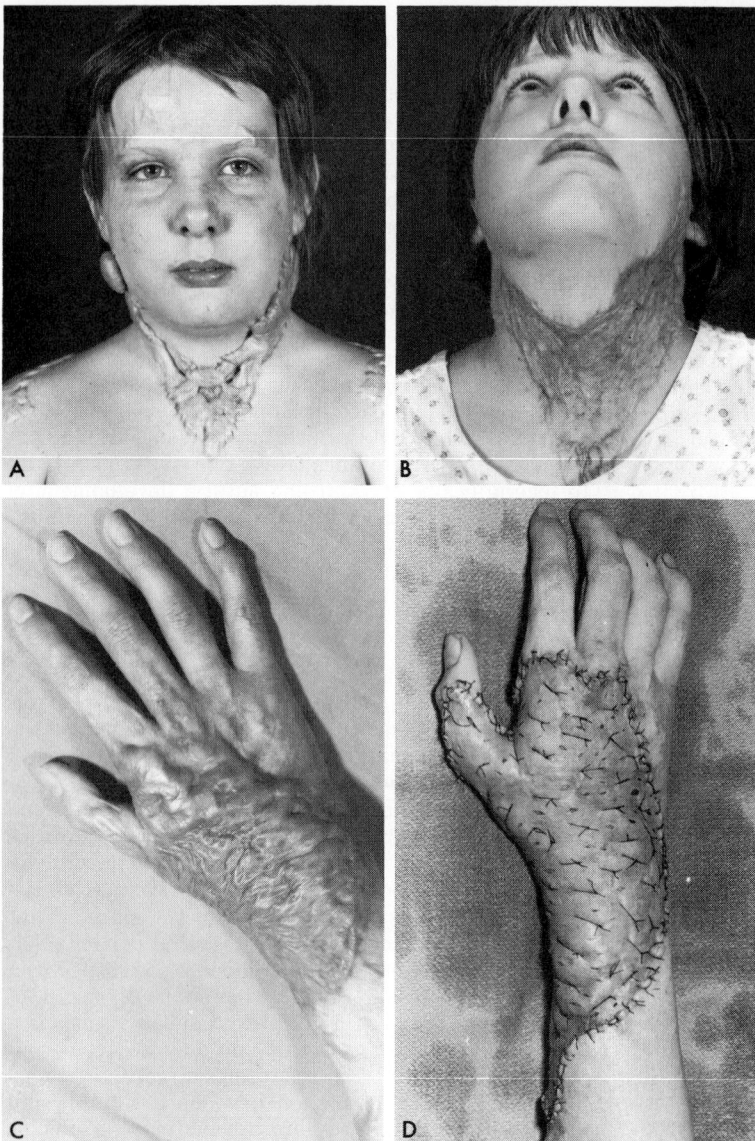

Figure 6. *A*, An 11-year-old girl with extensive keloids of the neck resulting from flame burns 2 years previously. The keloids had extended above and beyond the original areas of injury. Since it was impossible for her to extend her head, the keloids were excised and skin from the buttock was grafted. *B*, Postoperative photograph 1 year later shows some wrinkling of the graft but no recurrence of the keloid. *C*, Extensive keloids of the hand of a 27-year-old woman resulting from flaming paraffin-plastic burns 1 year previously. *D*, The entire keloid was excised and skin, 0.015 inch thickness, was grafted from the buttock.

in lobules and separated by fibrous septa and enclosed in a very delicate capsule. Although often of small size the tumor may grow tremendously, but still remains benign. It forms a soft, painless mass that moves readily over the fascia. The overlying skin is frequently dimpled owing to fibrous bands passing from it down between the lobules. The fat of which the tumor is composed is not affected by purposeful reduction or the general wasting of disease. Surgical excision is recommended if the lipoma is large; small ones are only a nuisance. Complete extirpation cannot be guaranteed because of the very thin capsule, since the boundary between the lipoma and the surrounding normal adipose tissue may be indistinct and deceptive.

Xanthoma

Xanthoma is the name applied to a group of conditions rather than to a single type of tumor. Three types are recognized: *Xanthelasma* is characterized by a small, yellow patch in the medial aspects of both upper and lower eyelids. It usually occurs in persons over middle age and frequently in those with abnormal cholesterol or fat metabolism. Therefore, xanthelasma of the eyelids is not a tumor, but rather a cutaneous manifestation of an abnormal cholesterol-lipid metabolism. The lesions are readily amenable to surgical excision; however, they may recur because of the underlying faulty metabolic process. On pathologic examination, there is a deposit in the tissues of a finely divided lipoid substance, cholesterol ester. *Xanthoma multiplex* is a condition in which groups of yellow nodules are scattered over the trunk and extremities, occurring most often in young people, and usually associated with a disturbance of cholesterol metabolism, hypercholesterolemia, or lipemia. It may be associated with diabetes mellitus and biliary ob-

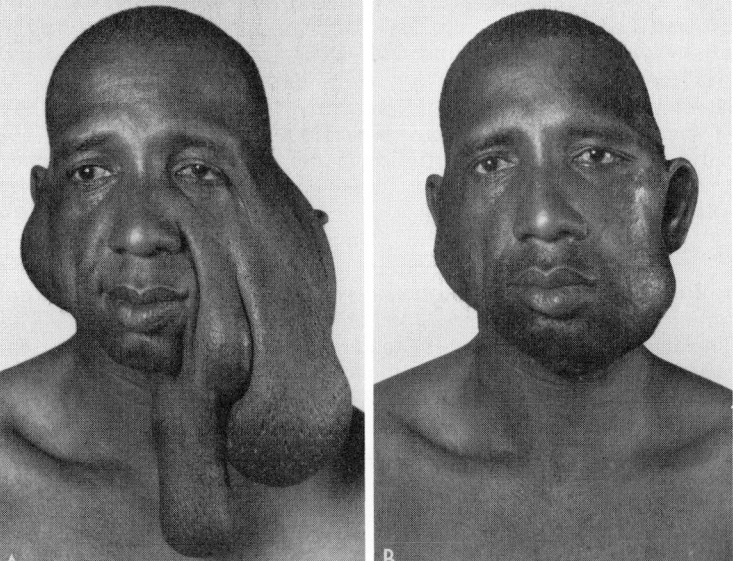

Figure 7. *A*, Pachydermatocele in a 38-year-old man, which had grown to its present size in 10 years. He also had many peripheral nodules that had not grown. These tumors are soft but not compressible. They are extremely vascular but no bruit is heard. The tumor was excised in one operation. *B*, Postoperative photograph taken 1 year later.

struction. The nodules are not true tumors. *Heterogeneous xanthomatous masses* are fibromas of the tendon sheaths of the hand and forearm. They may be associated with trauma or infection. All of the lesions have a characteristic bright yellow color which gives the condition its name. Most authorities hold that the color is due to the presence of the cholesterol ester.[2, 12] As stated, xanthomas are probably not true tumors in the strict sense of the term: they may represent more of a granuloma than a neoplasm. Xanthomatous

changes, however, may be encountered in giant cell tumors of bone and other connective tissue tumors.

Gardner's Syndrome

Gardner's syndrome is usually an inherited disorder characterized by fibrous skin tumors, cystic skin lesions, osteomatosis, dental abnormalities, and polyposis of the colon. Fibromas and cystic lesions, usually epidermal inclusion cysts, appear in childhood. They are usually multiple, though variable in number, and

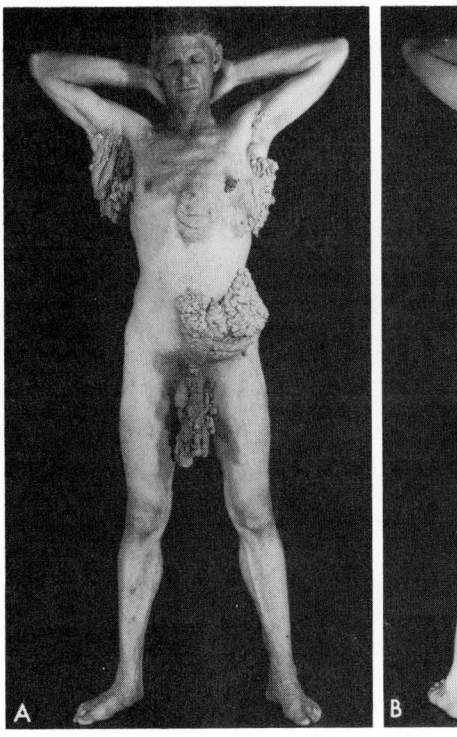
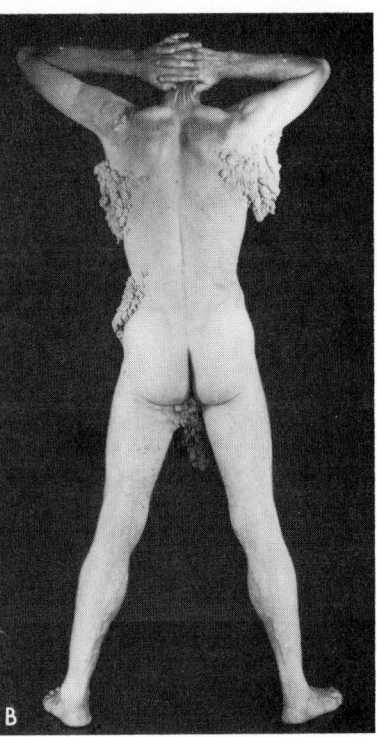

Figure 8. Diffuse neurofibromatosis of von Recklinghausen's disease. The cutaneous tumors of this 45-year-old man ranged from small nodules to large hanging masses which were excised and grafted in stages.

most numerous on the face, scalp, and trunk. Benign osteomas tend to develop, especially in the membranous bones of the face and skull. Dental abnormalities consist of supernumerary teeth, missing teeth, odontomas, and dentigerous cysts with abnormalities of the maxilla and mandible. Multiple adenomatous polyps may appear later in the colon and rectum, and may become malignant (Fig. 9).[16] (See also Chapter 35-VII.)

Rhinophyma

Rhinophyma, from the Greek *rhis* (nose) and *phyma* (growth), is a disease process rather than a neoplasm. The disease is also known as pseudoelephantiasis nostrum, acne hypertrophica, cystadenofibroma, whiskey-rum nose, and many other names. This slowly growing tumor involves only the lower half of the nose and usually spares the skin of the maxillary regions (Fig. 10). Rhinophyma starts as a hypertrophy of the sebaceous glands and subcutaneous tissue. Large lobulated masses of soft tissue develop in which are located large dilated pores. Telangiectatic vessels may course over the humpy surface, giving the nose a red appearance; hence the name whiskey-rum nose. However, the condition is entirely unrelated to alcohol; in fact, in an analysis of approximately 70 personal patients, there was not a single excessive drinker in the group.[15] Sebum may accumulate between the hypertrophied lobules and produce a foul odor; but the main complaint of the patient is the unsightliness of the nose. The condition itself is benign, but cases of basal and squamous cell epitheliomas developing in the area of involvement have been cited. Rhinophyma occurs primarily in men.

Treatment. Some investigators feel that acne rosacea may be a precursor of rhinophyma; if so, early der-

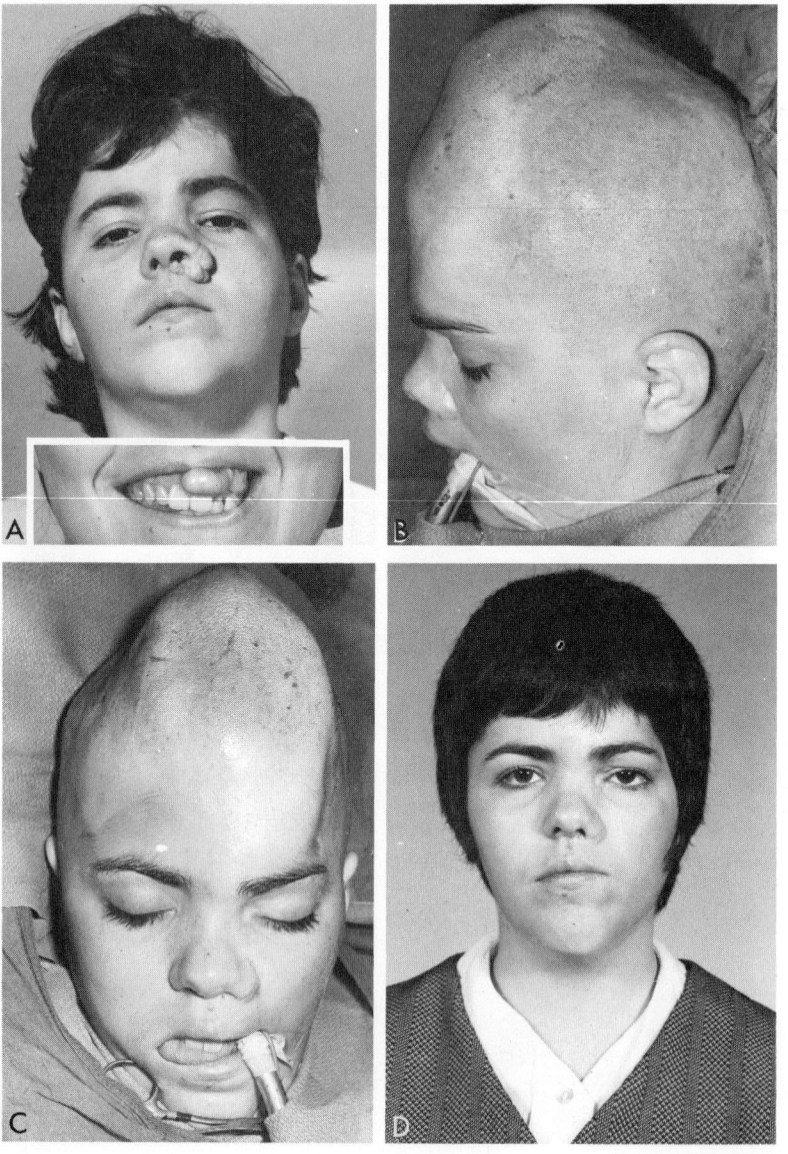

Figure 9. *A*, An 11-year-old girl with early lesions of Gardner's syndrome: fibromas of the alar wing and nasal vestibule and osteofibromas of the alveolus (insert). The lesions were excised. *B* and *C*, At 15 years, there was marked oxycephaly due to a large osteoma or exostosis projecting from the skull, which involved both the frontal and parietal bones. The osteoma was removed through a midline incision. It was 7 cm. thick. *D*, Two years postoperative photograph, at 17 years, shows normal craniofacial features.[14]

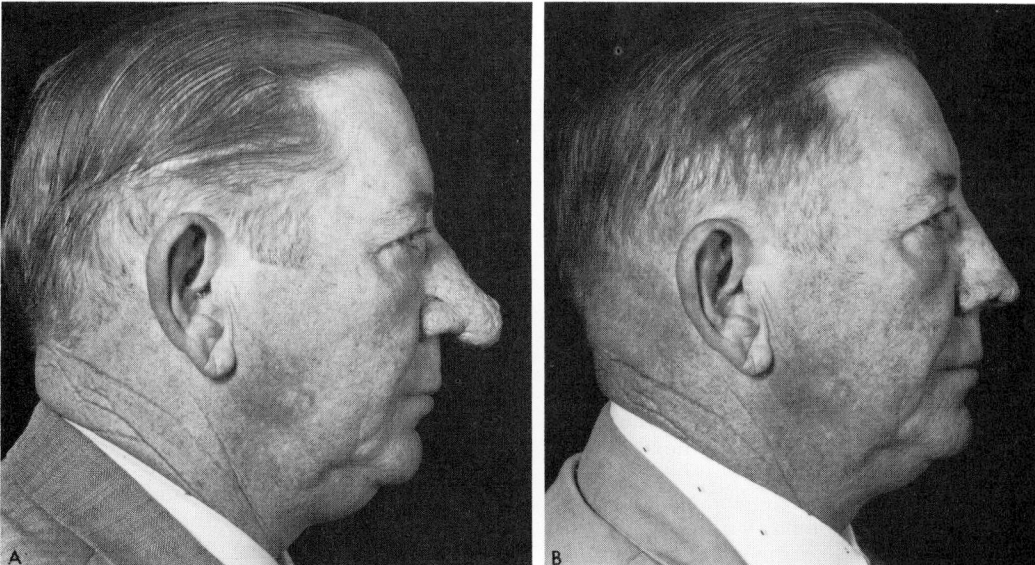

Figure 10. *A,* A 60-year-old engineer whose nose began to enlarge about 10 years prior to admission. The nose was shaved down and sculptured in one operation under local anesthesia. *B,* Postoperative photograph taken 1 year later.

matologic treatment may be beneficial. But once the rhinophyma is fully developed, no treatment other than surgery is of value. The simplest technique, which is very effective, is to shave down the hypertrophied tissues to a normal nose level with a No. 10 or 15 scalpel or an ordinary safety razor blade. The procedure may be performed under local infiltration or block anesthesia. Bleeding points are electrocoagulated. Nitrofurazone (Furacin) dressings are changed daily. Re-epithelialization will take place promptly and the transition between the "new nose" and the adjacent skin becomes almost undetectable (Fig. 10).

Pseudoxanthoma Elasticum

Pseudoxanthoma elasticum is a congenital disorder of the elastic fibers or an "elastotic degeneration of collagen." The skin, eyes, and vascular system are affected. The skin lesions consist of yellow papules and plaques, which are arranged in a crepelike pattern parallel to the folds of skin which may hang in drape-like folds on the neck, axilla, and groin (Fig. 11). In the eyes, angioid streaks of the fundi are found, with progressive impairment of the vision. The cutaneous lesions and the angioid streaks constitute the *Grönblad-Strandberg syndrome.* Cardiovascular manifestations include decrease or absence of peripheral pulse, intermittent claudication, angina, and cardiac decompensation. Rupture of vessels may lead to gastric hemorrhage or bleeding into the subarachnoid space. Pathologic changes in the skin are diagnostic: in the middle and deep dermis there is considerable accumulation of swollen, fragmented, and irregularly

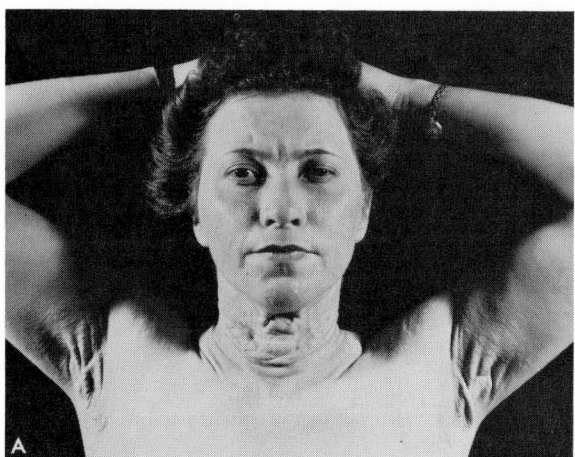
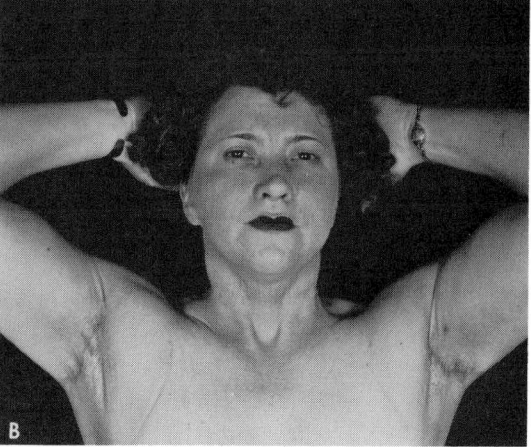

Figure 11. *A,* Characteristic appearance of pseudoxanthoma elasticum with pendulous reduplication of the flexural folds of the neck and axilla due to loss of elastic tissue. When the skin was stretched, the exaggerated folds remained unchanged for a considerable time. The color and texture of the skin were similar to those of a chamois. The deformity was corrected by excision of the redundant tissues after extensive undermining. *B,* Postoperative photograph taken 3 years later.

clumped fibers staining as do elastic fibers. The collagen fibers are normal. The angioid streaks probably represent degeneration of elastic fibers of Bruch's membrane in the retina.[9] There is no effective therapy. Plastic surgical removal of the excessive folds of skin has been helpful from the psychologic and cosmetic standpoints.

MALIGNANT TUMORS OF FIBROUS TISSUE

Fibrosarcoma

Fibrosarcoma may be the prototype of *sarcoma*, which is a malignant tumor of mesenchymal origin. It is the most frequent of the malignant tumors of soft tissues. Fibrosarcomas and sarcomas of the skin and soft tissues are considered as actually one neoplasm, since those arising in the soft tissues below the skin often invade it.[2, 25]

The tumor may occur at any age, and may grow in a slow, persistent fashion for some years, without causing the patient concern. The common sites are the trunk and lower extremities. The gross appearance may be dangerously deceptive, for a desmoplastic reaction in the surrounding tissue may cause the formation of a false capsule, from which the tumor may be shelled out. However, this statement should not be interpreted as a degree of benignity of the tumor, for it is highly malignant. *Microscopically* the tumor is composed of spindle-shaped fibroblasts separated by varying amounts of collagen; the cells and fibers tend to run in bundles which either curve gently and interlace or bind almost at right angles.

The tumor spreads principally by invasion; therefore, there is the ever-present danger of recurrence due to incomplete removal of the primary lesion. Involvement of the lymph nodes is rare. In the poorly differentiated forms, distant metastasis may occur by hematogenous invasion. Fibrosarcomas of the skin are almost all well differentiated, with superficial rather than deep spread. Nodularity in the operative incision may be the first clue to recurrence, and a more radical extirpation is indicated immediately.

There are many other types of sarcoma that originate in and attack literally every body system and organ: bone, tendon sheaths, nerve, brain, breast, pleura, retroperitoneum, uterus, and so forth.

Liposarcoma

Liposarcoma is the second most common malignant tumor arising in the subcutaneous tissues. The most common sites are the lower extremity: leg and buttock. Like the benign lipoma, the tumor may reach tremendous size. The lipoma, however, never develops into a liposarcoma. On cut surface, liposarcoma is soft and may be mucoid. Like the fibrosarcoma, it is dangerous because of its tendency to infiltrate and invade locally, rather than to metastasize.

Myxosarcoma

Myxosarcoma is a cutaneous and subcutaneous malignant disease characterized by multiple semicystic lesions that have a bluish color and occur most frequently on the extremities. The diagnosis presumes the acceptance of primary myxoma as a true tumor, in contrast to the theories that explain myxoma as a development by mucoid change of fibromas and neurofibromas.[2, 12] The tumor is characterized as low in degree of malignancy. *Microscopically* it is differentiated from fibrosarcoma by the formation of mucin-containing matrices in which the spindle-shaped cells of sarcoma are found. The lesions are best treated by wide excision; local recurrence may occur; metastases are rare.[13]

Angiosarcoma

Angiosarcoma (malignant hemangioma, hemangioendothelioma, hemangiopericytoma) is a malignant tumor of angioblastic origin, occurring in any region of the body. The tumors are soft in consistency and blue in color owing to the presence of large vascular sinuses, rupture of which may cause external hemorrhage. Angiosarcomas may grow very rapidly and are highly malignant. Surgical excision may be unsatisfactory because of the large size and mass of vascular tumor. Radiation therapy may be a necessary and valuable adjunctive treatment. If the lesion involves an extremity, amputation may become a procedure of necessity.

Rhabdomyosarcoma

Since these tumors extend directly to the skin, they are considered here, briefly, with tumors of the skin. They may occur in any body area. They may be confused with liposarcoma and fibrosarcoma. The author has seen two cases in which the tumor involved the lips. The tumor develops within or is attached to striated muscle. Since the tumor is resistant to radiation, wide surgical excision is the treatment of choice. Spread takes place through both the blood and lymph systems.

Leiomyosarcoma

Leiomyosarcomas occur on any part of the surface by direct extension to the skin from the underlying tissue. Some pathologists feel that these tumors arise in the smooth muscles of blood vessels or from the arrectores pilorum. Occasionally they behave as benign tumors; however, they usually resemble fibrosarcomas in their clinical manifestations and course.

Kaposi's Sarcoma

Kaposi's sarcoma is a malignant tumor of the skin that usually starts on the hands or feet as multiple nodules that are reddish to purple in the early stages. There is considerable controversy regarding its pathogenesis; the neurovascular system, the reticuloendothelial system, and the lymphatic system have all been indicated as the primary focus. On microscopic examination, one sees vascularity, pigmentation, elastic fibers, round cell infiltration, and the spindle cells of sarcoma.[9] Kaposi's sarcoma is looked upon as a slowly developing vascular and connective tissue tumor of the skin and subcutaneous tissues, which metastasizes via the lymphatics.

Dermatofibrosarcoma Protuberans

Dermatofibrosarcoma protuberans is a fibrous tissue tumor of the skin and subcutaneous tissues that is of low-grade malignancy. The tumor starts as a firm cutaneous or subcutaneous nodule covered with normal epidermis. It may occur on the scalp, torso, and extremities. On microscopic examination, the picture is that of a fibroma, rich in fibroblasts, which progresses to the characteristic appearance of fibrosarcoma. Wide surgical excision is the treatment of choice; the tumor is radioresistant. Local recurrences may be anticipated unless the primary excision is radical (Fig. 12)

Lymphangiosarcoma

Lymphangiosarcoma is a rare tumor that may occur in lymphedematous extremities or the scalp. The tumor may develop in the lymphedematous arm after radical mastectomy for cancer. The tumor appears as an ecchymotic area with induration and overlying vesiculation. Nodularity develops and the local appearance of the tumor is quite similar to that of Kaposi's sarcoma. The tumor is highly malignant; either radical excision of the area or amputation of the extremity is necessary to effect a cure.

Neurosarcoma

Neurosarcoma (neurofibrosarcoma, neurogenic sarcoma, malignant neurolemmoma) represents malignant degeneration of neurofibroma or of neurolemmoma. The tumor invades the skin from the underlying tissues. The author has recently seen two young patients with large neck masses that were diagnosed as malignant plexiform neurofibromas, and it

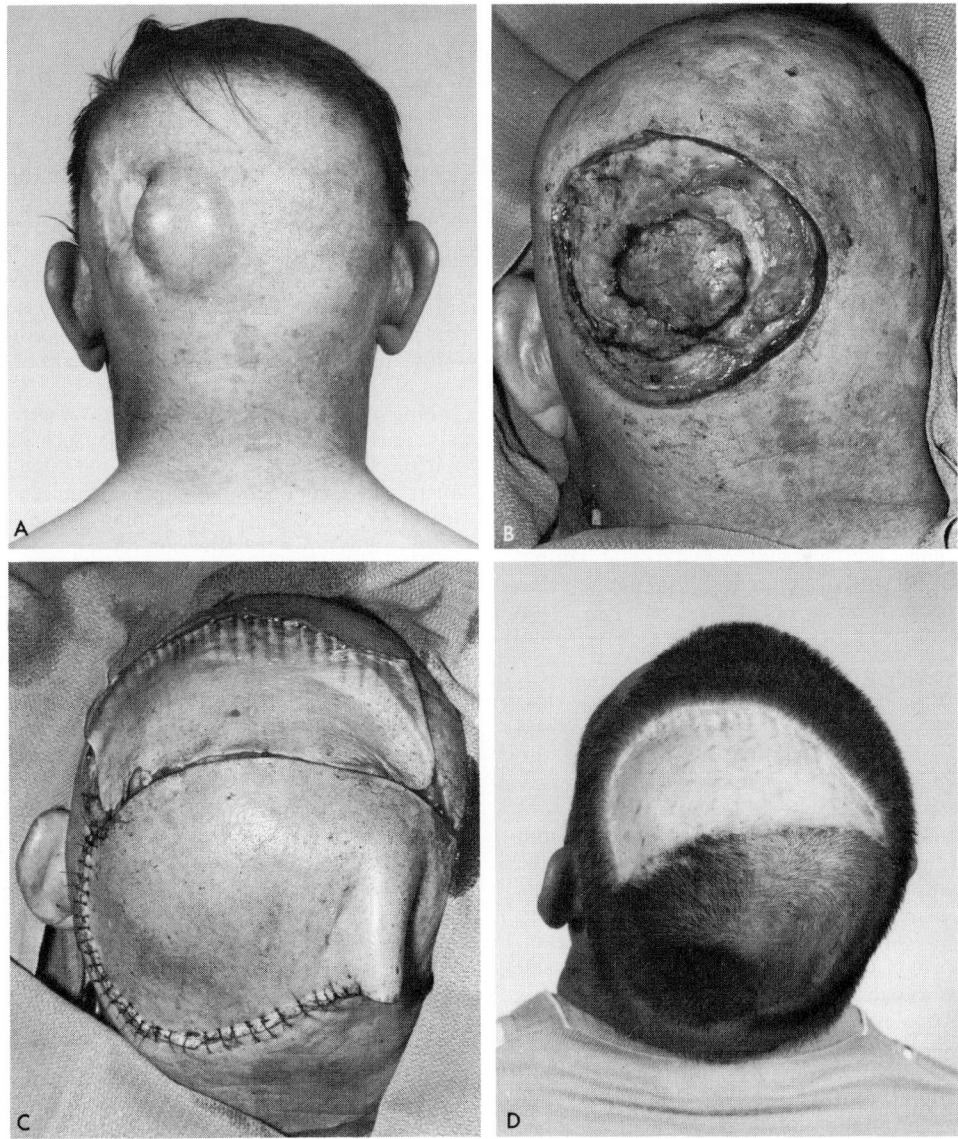

Figure 12. *A,* A 40-year-old man with a recurrent dermatofibrosarcoma protuberans of the occipital area, which had been removed 2 years previously at another hospital. Since the tumor had invaded the skull, a craniectomy was performed. *B,* The large operative defect and dura were covered with a direct transfer scalp flap; a split graft from the buttock was applied to the flap donor area. *C,* Three weeks later the "dog ear" or pedicle was divided and tailored to complete the reconstruction *(D).*

was thought that they represented malignant transformation of von Recklinghausen's disease, since there were other stigmata of the disease present. The tumor grows rapidly by local invasion. Radiation therapy may be helpful.

Von Recklinghausen's Disease

Von Recklinghausen's disease (neurofibromatosis) is characterized by brown macules (café au lait spots) and soft pedunculated and sessile cutaneous neurofibromas (see Figs. 7 and 8). The tumor represents a diffuse proliferation of peripheral nerve elements; according to Anderson, "the tumors of this group may contain nerves with sheaths, nerves without sheaths, sheaths without nerves (containing Schwann cells) and about all this there are masses of fibrous tissue."[2] The lesions may be single and localized (but are not encapsulated), but much more often they are multiple. When numerous, they constitute the classic neurofibromatosis of von Recklinghausen. There may be literally hundreds of neurofibromas growing from cutaneous nerves; there may also be involvement of the spinal and intercostal nerves with dumbell-like extensions into the chest. The deeper growths are prone to malignant change. In the common cutaneous form, soft nodules in the skin are distributed widely over the body. When proliferation occurs inside the nerve sheaths, rendering the nerve thick, tortuous, and ropelike, the condition is known as *plexiform neuroma;* it occurs frequently in the neck, involving the cervical nodes. Peculiar soft overgrowths of connective tissue may occur, causing the skin to hang in great folds, perhaps with enlargement of an extremity—a condition known as *elephantiasis neuromatosis.*

On microscopic examination, the characteristic tissue has a tangled structure; the tissue does not show palisading or whorls. Superimposed upon this reticular mass is a varying amount of tissue of the Schwann type showing palisades and whorls. With special stains, nerve fibrils can be seen passing through the mass; this never occurs in neurolemmoma.[9]

CANCER OF THE SKIN

Cancer of the skin occurs primarily on exposed areas; because of its accessibility, especially on the face, it offers an unparalleled opportunity for early diagnosis and treatment. When a lesion attracts attention early and is readily accessible to observation and treatment, its nature and course are more likely to be understood than those of tumors arising in deeply situated organs. From the viewpoint of early recognition, skin cancers are in particularly favorable position. However, in spite of the intensive educational crusade against cancer during the past decade, one is still confronted with a relatively large group of patients with active lesions who, in many instances, have been "followed and treated" for long periods.

Too much emphasis cannot be placed on the importance of early biopsy and complete eradication of the cancer. Inadequate therapy, whether with surgery or irradiation, only results in residual and recurrent cancer, which may require an extensive or a destruc-

tion operation for cure. Furthermore, oft-repeated procedures may actually accelerate the growth of the tumor. This has been stressed by cancer surgeons and radiation therapists. I share and repeat the statements of my mentors, principally Dr. Robert Ivy, Dr. Jerome Webster, Dr. Hayes Martin, and the late Drs. John Staige Davis, Ferris Smith, and Vilray Blair: It is not so much the lack of treatment or the selection of the type of treatment that has handicapped the recurrent cancer patient, but the lack of conviction and the use of temporizing methods or puttering treatment that have lowered the quality of our results. Further, every extensive cancer did not become so overnight, but it began as a small, seemingly insignificant lesion, which continued to increase progressively in size. Cutaneous cancer accounts for 50 to 60 per cent of all types of malignant lesions seen by the family physician. This section is presented for the student and young physician and not the specialist. It is hoped some of the following guides will be of help.

Predisposing Factors. Skin cancers tend to develop more frequently in blond persons, and those with thin, dry skin. They occur rarely in the yellow races of the Orient and the olive-skinned Italians, Spanish, and South Americans, and almost never in the black race. However, those persons (predominantly men) with "Scotch-type" skin (blond hair and beard, blue eyes, thin skin) who, because of their outdoor occupations or habits (farmers, ranchers, commercial fishermen, sailors, and "sun worshipers"), are exposed for long periods to intense sun and wind frequently do incur skin cancers; however, the precursor is usually an area of hyperkeratosis (see Fig. 4).

General Statements about Skin Cancer. Squamous cell cancer may develop in areas of postradiation dermatitis. Ulcerations occurring in old burn scars are favorite sites for the development of squamous cell cancer. While skin cancers may occur at any age, there is a definite predilection for men over 50 years of age. Basal cell cancers of the face are much more common than squamous cell cancers, accounting for more than three fourths of all cases in some reports.[2, 19, 23]

All cancers arising on the mucous membrane surface of the lip are squamous cell (see Fig. 13). Numerically, most epitheliomas of the skin of the face are basal cell, at least in their beginning, but some of these may change later to squamous cell. However, there is an exception—those lesions which develop in hyperkeratoses on the skin of men who have had a lifetime exposure to sun and wind are squamous cell from the beginning. On the face of an individual, one lesion may develop into a basal cell cancer, while a neighboring lesion may be a squamous cell cancer. Squamous cell cancers metastasize. Basal cell cancers do not metastasize, but they should be regarded as elusive and invasive and are highly malignant locally (see Fig. 14).

Pathologic Considerations. The characteristic histologic feature of the malignant cell is its power of unlimited multiplication, in contrast to the orderly migration and maturation of epithelial cells as outlined previously. Structurally, these cells are anaplastic and may tend to revert to embryonal form (undifferentiated). Generally speaking, the more they differ from

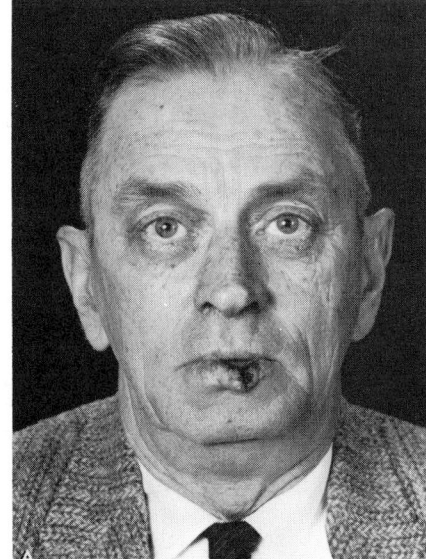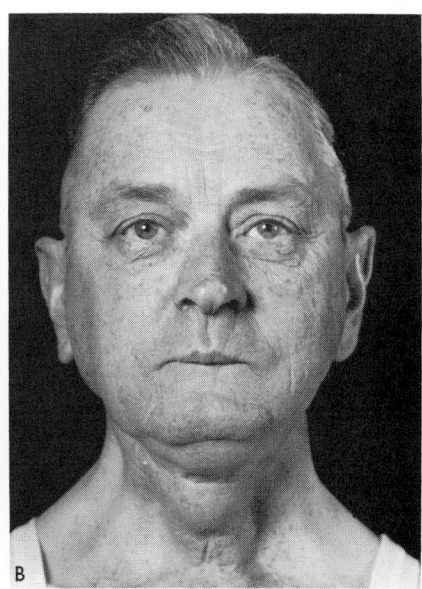

Figure 13. *A,* A 55-year-old man with a squamous cell cancer of the lip of 1 year's duration. The greater part of the lower lip was removed and reconstructed with cheek advancement flaps. A two-stage bilateral neck dissection was performed to remove metastatic nodes. *B,* Postoperative photograph taken 10 years later.

the normal cell and structure, the nearer they approach the embryonal type, the more malignant is the lesion. When the variation is slight, the degree of malignancy may be low; when the variation is marked, the degree of malignancy may be high. On this basis of differentiation of cells, that is, their ability to resemble and mimic the cells from which they originated, Broder grouped cancers into four grades.[2, 7, 19] Grade I is least malignant, since less than 25 per cent of the cells are undifferentiated (75 per cent or more are normal). Grade IV cancers are the most malignant, because most of the cells are undifferentiated and only 25 per cent or less resemble the parent

cell. In between are Grades II and III, Grade II being less malignant and Grade III more malignant. It should be emphasized, however, that this is a microscopic-pathologic classification of cell differentiation and that virulence and evident activity of growth are by no means synonymous, either clinically or by Broder's grading system.

Squamous Cell Cancer

This tumor, commonly known as epidermoid carcinoma, occurs wherever squamous or transitional epithelium is found. In this chapter we are concerned with squamous cell cancer of the skin, but it may develop in

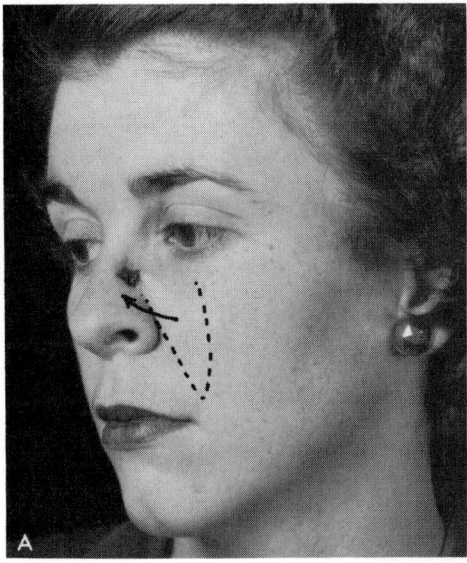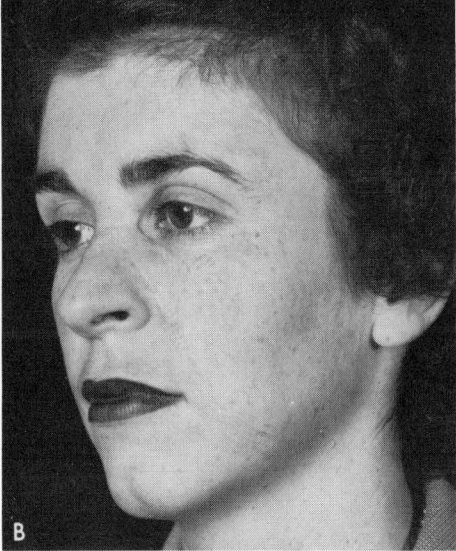

Figure 14. *A,* A 25-year-old woman with a burrowing basal cell cancer of the side of the nose of 1 year's duration. At operation, the cancer was found to extend into the interior of the nose and to involve the maxillary process. The operative defect was reconstructed with an interpolated flap from the nasolabial crease, as shown. The flap was subsequently trimmed and tailored. *B,* Postoperative photograph taken 5 years later.

mucous membranes lined by stratified squamous epithelium, such as the tongue, mouth, and esophagus. A favorite site is the junction of skin and mucous membrane, such as on the lip, nostrils, eyelid, penis, and vulva.

Squamous cell cancer develops frequently in areas of previous skin change: from solar keratoses or hyperkeratoses, old burn scars (Marjolin's ulcer), an ulcer of long standing, or radiation dermatitis. The difference between an early squamous cell cancer and a keratosis may not be apparent clinically and therefore the lesion should be biopsied or excised or both.

Typical squamous cell cancers, such as occur on the lower lip, may be preceded by an area of leukoplakia or what was thought to be a "fever blister." The transformation from a benign lesion to a squamous cancer may be detected as a slight thickening or a small nodule. Ulceration occurs and is frequently followed by the development of a crusty overgrowth (Fig. 13) in a bulky or papillomatous, cauliflower-like growth which, at the same time, may burrow into the deeper tissues. Pain is not prominent until late in the disease. Squamous cancers are quite malignant from the beginning and may metastasize quite early to the

regional lymph nodes. This is particularly true of squamous cancers arising in the mucous membranes of the mouth, tongue, parotid, and pharynx; in fact, a metastatic mass in the neck may be the "prime mover" to get the patient to his physician. If the lesion in question is large and the clinical diagnosis is in doubt, a small portion may be removed, usually without local anesthesia, for histologic study. If it is small, the entire lesion may be removed by excisional biopsy under local anesthesia.

Pathology. Squamous cell cancers invade the dermis early as solid columns of epithelial cells. The cells show varying degrees of atypia including variation in size, shape, and depth of staining, numerous mitoses, and so forth. Abnormal keratinization is manifested by whorls of keratin or horny pearls near the surface. As the cancer invades the dermis, the squamous cells may be arranged in a concentric manner, as "cell nests" or "epithelial pearls," which, although highly characteristic of squamous cell cancer, may be absent in rapidly growing tumors and in the esophagus, where cornification does not normally occur. A well-known feature to pathologists is an infiltration of the dermis by chronic inflammatory cells,

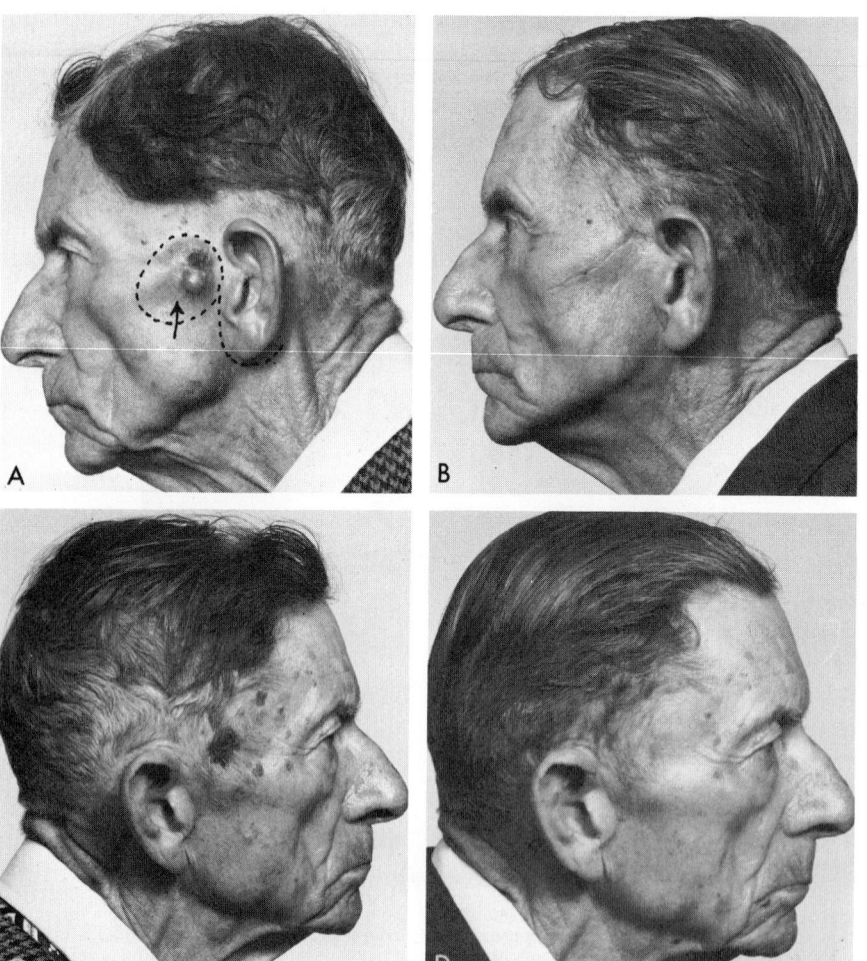

Figure 15. *A,* A 68-year-old man with a squamous cell cancer of the left zygomatic area and, *C,* multiple benign seborrheic keratoses of the right temple. *B,* The cancer was excised widely and then cheek and neck skin were advanced superiorly, in face lift fashion, to close the operative defect. The seborrheic keratoses were surgically abraded (sanded). Re-epithelization should occur in two to three weeks, as shown in *D.*

particularly plasma cells, just deep to the neoplastic epithelium.[9]

Treatment. All lesions should be biopsied. It is essential that an accurate pathologic diagnosis be established. It is imperative that the tumor be removed or destroyed completely. Many dermatologists treat small lesions by electrodesiccation. I personally feel that squamous cell cancers are best treated by wide excision. Even rather extensive lesions may be removed with local or block anesthesia supplemented by intravenous diazepam (Valium). Before any treatment is undertaken, an x-ray of the chest and a careful examination of the regional lymph nodes of the neck should be made.

Basal Cell Cancers

Basal cell cancers should be regarded as elusive, treacherous, and highly, locally malignant, even though they do not metastasize to distant parts (Fig. 14). These lesions are deceptive: they appear and behave like benign lesions in their early stages, but unless removed widely, they will recur and destroy everything in their path of invasion.

Basal cell cancers arise most frequently in the midportion of the face, the so-called seborrheic areas. They develop at an earlier age than squamous cell cancers. The lesions may arise in otherwise normal skin, de novo, and without a prodromal keratosis as frequently occurs in squamous cell cancer. Early lesions rarely show rapid growth; in fact they appear to be quite indolent. There is no pain or discomfort and hence it not infrequently happens that patients defer seeking advice until the disease is well advanced.

The appearance of an early lesion is quite characteristic (Fig. 14): it may resemble an intracutaneous button, in that there is a firm, slightly elevated edge which may surround the lesion partially or completely. The edge may be pearly or gray-blue in color and may have a scalloped appearance. In early lesions, the ulceration in the center is shallow. The lesion is somewhat indurated, and so it looks and feels like a button. However, striking variations in the clinical picture may be encountered. While slow growth and progression is the general rule, any rapid change should be acted upon promptly, for it may be indicative of change from a basal cell lesion to a basosquamous or a pure squamous cell cancer.

I refer to the primary lesion, described in the previous paragraph, as a *button-type basal cell cancer.* However, there are two other types which should be borne in mind. The *field-fire basal cell cancer* is usually a large, flat lesion with an active edge surrounding a central scarred area. It may be serpiginous and the peripheral manner of spread has been compared to that of a fire in a field. The edges are active and spreading, whereas the central area may seem, often falsely, to have burned itself out. This field-fire type of cancer may actually be due to the coalescence and spread of several multicentric lesions.

The third type of basal cell cancer is the highly invasive *rodent ulcer.* This is the most difficult lesion to eradicate and, therefore, one of the most dangerous. The surface lesion may appear quite innocuous; however, there is usually extensive invasion in and beneath the skin—hence the designation *submarine or iceberg type of progression and spread.* What is actually seen on the surface may bear little resemblance to what is found beneath it. Favorite and dangerous sites for the development of basal cell cancers are the nose and along the lower eyelid and inner canthus (Fig. 14). In these special locations basal cell cancers seem to have a definite predilection for burrowing deeply, and unless they are removed early and completely, they may cause widespread destruction or even death.

Pathology. The microscopic appearance consists of solid masses of darkly stained cells that extend downward from the basal layer into the dermis and subcutaneous tissues. The columns extend down to a uniform level; their ends have an expanded club-shaped appearance—a geographic arrangement of bays, capes, and promontories. The peripheral nuclei maintain a palisade arrangement.[9]

Treatment. It is advisable to perform a biopsy to verify the clinical impression. Small lesions may be treated by excisional biopsy. Irradiation is quite effective in the treatment of early lesions, but much less effective when the lesions are advanced. We believe that wide surgical excision is the treatment of choice. If the surgeon receives pathologic clearance that all margins are free of tumor, on the basis of frozen section studies, primary repair may be undertaken immediately. When in doubt, one should wait for final pathologic clearance before reconstructing the defect. This is doubly important if a free graft or a flap is to be used, and is especially true with basal cell cancers around the orbit.

The physician who treats cancer is, in reality, treating a patient with cancer. Cancers are malignant and a life is at stake. Each far-advanced cancer was at one time a small, perhaps seemingly insignificant lesion. Our aim should be to educate the public so that they will seek advice early. Then the remainder is up to us and is our responsibility. The final result depends on how early the patient seeks advice and the adequacy of the treatment administered. Our aim should be to eradicate the lesion completely and, at the same time, to leave a minimum of disturbance of function and disfigurement.

MELANOMA*

Melanomas are the most malignant and the most treacherous of all the cancers that develop in the skin. The lesion may be described as an area of pigmentation, present for a few months or several years, that suddenly has changed in character. These changes are usually subtle and may consist of increase in size and depth of color; onset of seepage of clear serum or frank bleeding; nodule or tumor formation; ulceration and formation of satellite pigmented macules (ink spots) (see Figs. 16 and 17). The appearance of satellite lesions around the primary site is an ominous sign that the melanoma is growing, and biopsy, with study of permanent sections, not frozen sections, should be

---

*See also Chapter 23-II.

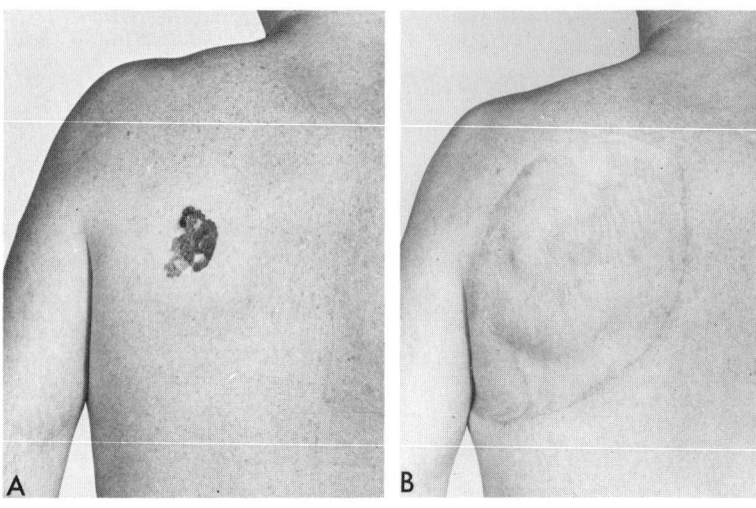

Figure 16. *A,* This 48-year-old man knew that he had a pigmented lesion of the left scapular region for at least five years. While boating his wife noted increase in size and pigmentation; these are characteristic and ominous signs of melanoma. *B,* Radical excision of the entire area and into the axilla was performed with immediate application of split thickness skin grafts cut from the left buttock and thigh. The patient was immunized with BCG and his own killed melanoma cells grown in tissue culture.[24] Postoperative photograph taken two years later.

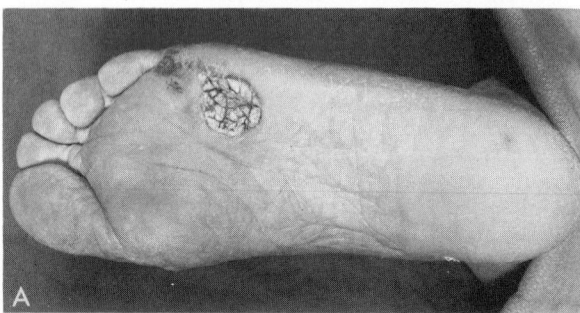

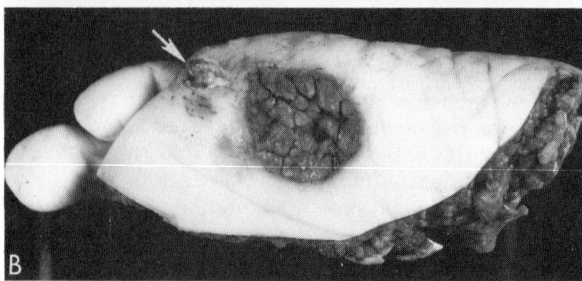

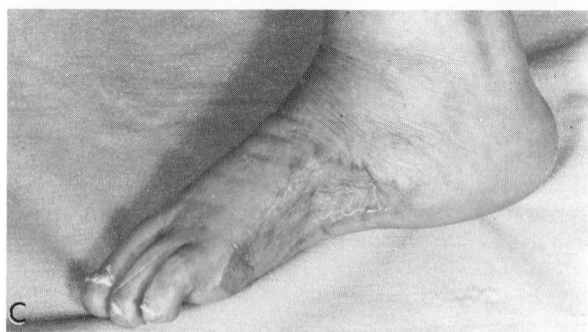

Figure 17. *A,* A 60-year-old woman with a melanoma developing near the base of the little toe, adjacent to a plantar wart that had been present for several years. *B,* A biopsy (arrow) confirmed the diagnosis and a ray amputation was performed that included the fourth and fifth metatarsals. A split thickness graft was applied to the raw area after one week when a granulation tissue base had developed. The patient was immunized with BCG and killed melanoma cells. She remains well and has a good functioning-walking foot three years later, as shown in *C.*

performed immediately. Metastases occur early through the lymphatics, and enlarged regional lymph nodes may be the initial sign noticed by the patient. Later, metastases occur through the bloodstream and become widespread.

Treatment. Wide excision and grafting is the first treatment and this should be performed immediately, followed by exploration and dissection of the regional lymph nodes if there is any enlargement. Regional perfusion of the extremities with alkylating agents was popularized by Creech and Kremintz.[8]

However, the long-term results have been disappointing. Recently, Seigler and associates[24] have reported excellent results with the use of BCG vaccine, and with the patient's killed melanoma cells as an immunologic adjuvant in the total body defense against the melanoma.

MISCELLANEOUS SKIN LESIONS

Intraepithelial cancer or carcinoma-in-situ is seen frequently on the skin. The layers of the epidermis show evidence of dyskeratosis—cellular "unrest" and malignant transformation, with acanthosis, loss of polarity, and increased mitosis. There is no invasion of the dermis and the neoplastic change is confined to the epidermis.

Pseudoepitheliomatous hyperplasia is, in essence, the reverse of carcinoma-in-situ. It is a benign proliferation of the epidermis, the result of chronic irritation. Elongated pegs of epithelium, seemingly frustrated in their attempt to cover the surface, grow downward.

In *Bowen's disease* the picture is one of modified carcinoma-in-situ, the anaplasia being less marked. It is a relatively inactive form of cutaneous malignant disease. The lesion is usually solitary and may be mistaken for a solar keratosis or an early basal cell epithelioma. Excisional biopsy is recommended.

Keratoacanthoma resembles squamous cell cancer both clinically and histologically, although it is a benign lesion (Fig. 18). An important characteristic is

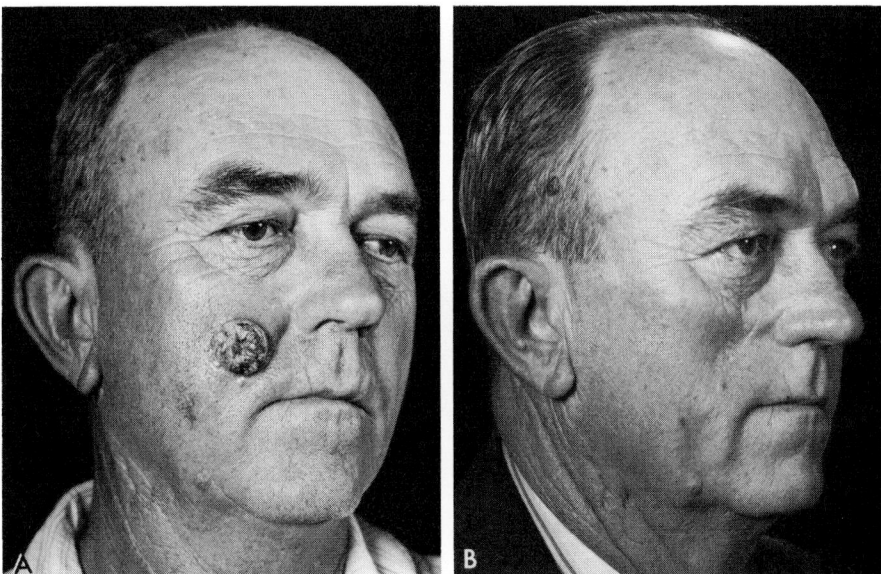

Figure 18. *A,* A 52-year-old man with a characteristic keratoacanthoma: the lesion grew to its present size in 2 months; it was round, elevated, dome-shaped, cherry red, and friable. Since the lesion is benign, radical excision is not necessary. *B,* Postoperative photograph taken 1 year later.

the fact that the tumor, which is usually single, may grow with extreme rapidity, to 2 cm. or more in a month. It is a round, elevated, dome-shaped lesion that is cherry red and friable. There is no discomfort. Some investigators feel that the causative agent may be a virus. The major differentiation is between it and squamous cell cancer. Its rapid growth and its mushroom-like appearance should not be relied upon implicitly; therefore, biopsy is necessary. Surgical removal is recommended, although radical excision is not necessary.

Adenoacanthoma or *pseudoglandular squamous cell carcinoma* has a predilection for the skin of the face and ears. The surface has a verrucous appearance; the lumina are filled with desquamated cells—this may be seen both clinically and on histologic study. The lesions are confined to the surface and have little tendency to metastasize. Surgical excision is recommended.

Cylindroma or *adenoid cystic carcinoma* is a circumscribed but poorly encapsulated infiltrating tumor, taking origin in the subcutaneous tissues, most commonly from the ducts of the parotid (Stenson's) and submaxillary (Wharton's) glands. The growth is slow but relentless and invasion and metastasis may occur. Histologic examination is characteristic: there are anastomosing cords of small dark cells that are arranged around tubules in a "Swiss cheese" pattern.

Xeroderma pigmentosum is a rare disease of children who show extremely abnormal sensitivity to sunlight. The condition begins in early life with hyperpigmentation of the exposed parts which then deepens; atrophy and tightening of the skin is followed by ectropion of the eyelids and lips. Both squamous and basal cell cancers develop and metastasis may occur. We have resurfaced the entire face of a boy, shown in Figure 19, with split- and full-thickness grafts.[26] However, the condition recurred in the grafted areas

within 5 years, even though protective measures were taken: sun screen ointments, wide-brim hats, long sleeves, gloves, and so forth. The prognosis is poor; few patients survive their adolescence. Radiation therapy is contraindicated since the skin is already damaged severely. The basic vulnerability is inherited in a recessive pattern. The two sexes are equally susceptible. Clinically this condition in childhood resembles severe radiodermatitis in the adult.

Calcifying epithelioma of Malherbe is usually a solitary, well-circumscribed, indurated tumor firmly attached to the skin but freely movable over the deep tissues. It occurs most frequently on the face and upper extremities, and in the author's experience, children show a definite predilection. Microscopically the lesion consists of fragments of what have been termed "mummified basal epithelium" with varying amounts of calcium. Anderson[2] feels that it is probably not a true neoplasm, but a mummified epidermal cyst.

Hemangiomas (Vascular Nevi)

Nevus is a general term to designate pigmented neoplasm of vascular and epidermal origin. In infants and children, nevi make up the largest group of benign tumors.

The *hemangioma* or *vascular nevus* has its origin in the angioblastic layer of embryonic mesoderm. It is a tumor of independently growing vascular channels. Small hemangiomas have little connection with the surrounding vascular tree; large and extensive tumors have "feeder" vessels that may be tremendous. Hemangiomas are classified pathologically into two groups: capillary and cavernous (Figs. 20 to 22).

Capillary hemangiomas are very common in infancy and childhood and are of two varieties. The *strawberry hemangioma* (hemangioma simplex) is composed of masses of capillaries lined with embryonic endothelium. The *congenital port-wine stain* is lined with adult-

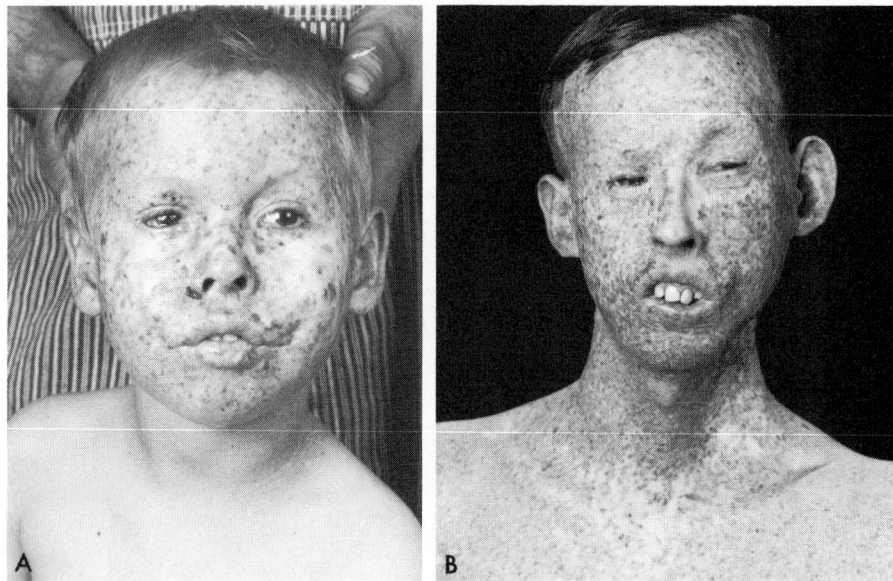

Figure 19.   *A,* A 4-year-old boy with advanced changes in the skin of the face and neck characteristic of xeroderma pigmentosa. Many cancers, both basal and squamous cell, were present. In stages, the entire skin of the face—forehead, eyelids, nose, lips, and cheeks—was removed and resurfaced with split- and full-thickness grafts; however, the same condition recurred in the grafts in spite of protective meassures: limited exposure, wide-brim hat, sun screen lotions, and so forth. *B,* Postoperative photograph taken 10 years later, patient 17 years of age. (From Woolf, R., et al.: Plast. Reconstr. Surg., *24:*214, 1959.)

type endothelium. The strawberry hemangioma looks somewhat like a strawberry that has been cut in half and placed on the skin, cut side down. They are usually bright red, raised above the surface, and quite circumscribed. Their growth may be very rapid—from the size of a pea to several centimeters in 4 to 6 weeks. Port-wine stains are present at birth, may vary in coloration from pink to purple, and are usually flat and not raised,

except slightly, above the surrounding skin surface. Pressure will cause blanching; however, the color will return immediately when the pressure is released. They do not grow or increase in size in themselves, although their dimension increases with the normal growth and development of the part. They frequently follow roughly the distribution of the trigeminal nerve of the face, along the frontal, maxillary, and mandibu-

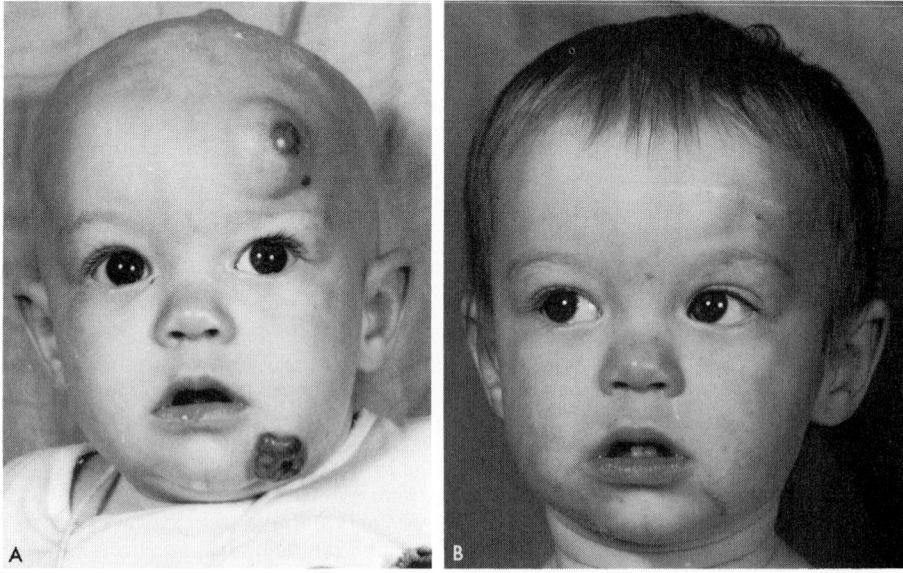

Figure 20.   *A,* A 4-month-old child with rapidly growing hemangiomas of the chin and forehead. She also had large vascular nevi on the elbow and back. All were excised. The hemangioma on the chin was of the capillary variety; that on the forehead was of cavernous origin; those on the elbow and back were juvenile hemangioendotheliomas. While the classification of hemangiomas is a pathologic one, it may be difficult to ascribe an exact diagnosis from the clinical appearance. *B,* Postoperative photograph taken 6 months later.

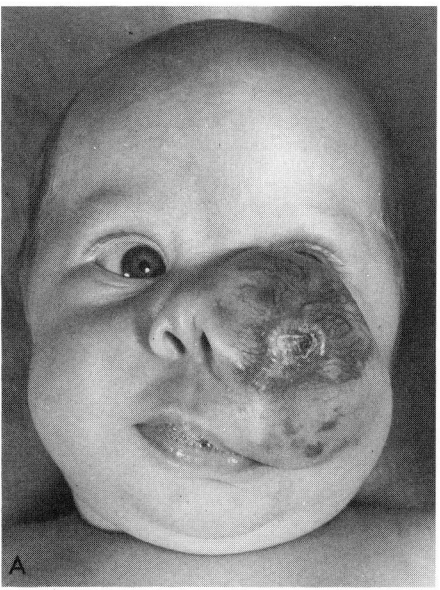
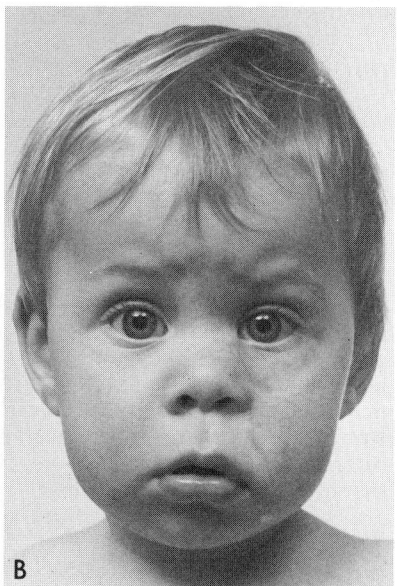

Figure 21. *A,* A two-month-old baby with a terribly deforming, rapidly growing hemangioma, which began from a tiny red spot in the maxillary region at one month. Prednisone therapy was not effective. Because of unrelenting progression of the tumor, it was totally excised in a single operation at three months. Pathologic studies disclosed the tumor to be a hemangioendothelioma: a hemangioma with malignant-like potential and characteristics. *B,* Postoperative photograph at two years, following two revision procedures on the nose and lips.

lar branches; however, they have nothing to do with the nerve. Generally port-wine stains do not cross the midline of the face. Hemangiomas are not painful until ulceration occurs (see Fig. 22).

Cavernous hemangiomas are soft, bluish, compressible tumor masses which on pathologic examination are composed of large, thin-walled venous sinuses. They may reach tremendous size gradually over a period of months. Because of their thin epithelial covering, ulceration or bleeding may occur. Frank hemorrhage may be difficult to control because of the lack of supporting stroma to permit the normal vascular re-

traction and clotting mechanism to work effectively. Cavernous hemangiomas rarely undergo complete regression.

Treatment. Many small hemangiomas in infants will regress and disappear; pediatricians will verify and confirm this statement. The regression is due to fibrosis, possibly initiated by trauma. These are frequently referred to as sclerosing hemangiomas. In them, the capillaries become partially or completely obliterated. The surgeon usually does not see these. However, a large number of hemangiomas will grow with extreme rapidity and can be quite alarming

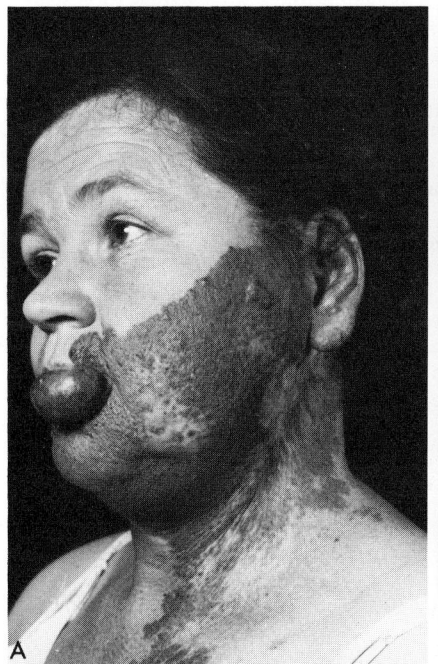
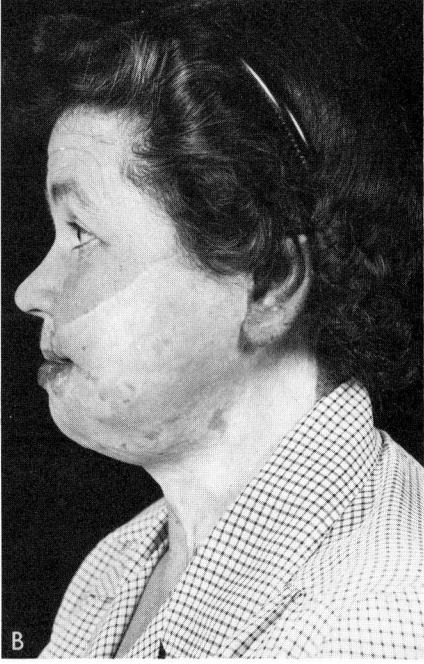

Figure 22. *A,* A 55-year-old woman with an extensive deep purple colored port-wine stain of the cheek and neck, and a large cavernous hemangioma of the lower lip. The entire hemangioma of the face, lip, and neck was excised in a single sitting. Delayed split thickness skin grafts, approximately 15/1000 inch in thickness and cut from the thigh, were applied one week after excision. *B,* The result about one year later. The patient is not wearing cosmetics.

because of their location in rather critical areas: eyelids, nose, lips, cheeks, neck, hands, and vulva. For a physician to give assurance to already anxious parents that the hemangioma will regress or disappear may invite medicolegal trouble, for their course is extremely variable. We believe that early excision is the treatment of choice. This avoids the possibility of uncontrollable growth and the resulting deformity, and also the fear and apprehension of the parents. A fine surgical scar is far to be preferred to a rapidly growing, ulcerated hemangioma whose future course remains in doubt (Fig. 20). Zarem and Edgerton[28] and Brown et al.[4] have reported quite marked regression of rapidly growing hemangiomas in early infancy using prednisone for 4 to 6 weeks.

Although radiation has been used in the treatment of hemangiomas, there are distinct disadvantages and contraindications that must be kept in mind. Radiation should not be given over the penis, testicles, vulva, or ovaries, or over epiphyseal growth centers, especially of the fingers, toes, jaws, and tooth buds because of the danger of interference with these growth centers. The ocular lens is very susceptible to radiation; therapy over hair-bearing areas will produce permanent alopecia, and unless the normal skin is shielded and protected, radiation dermatitis may result as a late complication.

The port-wine stain may be cosmetically one of the most deforming of all vascular nevi when it involves the face. There is no uniformly successful method of treatment. Excision and resurfacing with skin grafts may be desirable when the stain is deep red or purple; however, grafts from another part of the body to the face will not have the same color and texture, and the seam or edge where the grafts join the normal skin may be quite visible even when cosmetics are used. Tattooing with insoluble dyes has been quite successful in some instances when the discoloration is not marked. The recent improvements and better methods have been reported by Thompson.[26] Dermabrasion and electrodesiccation have been disappointing in our experience. Port-wine stains are totally radioresistant, since the endothelial lining is of adult variety. The use of Cover-Mark is recommended in women; men do not like to use cosmetic agents (see Fig. 22).

While hemangiomas are considered benign lesions, on rare occasions malignant change may occur. *Three malignant entities have been described:* metastasizing hemangioma, hemangiopericytoma, and hemangioendothelioma. *Hemangioendotheliomas* in children increase in size with great rapidity, and because of this fulminating rate of growth, closely resemble a true malignant tumor. *Hemangiopericytomas and metastasizing hemangiomas* are uncommon in children, and when they do occur, the tumor is more orderly in arrangement and metastasizes later than its adult counterpart (see Fig. 21).

Pigmented Nevi (Moles)

The common mole and its variants constitute the second broad category of cutaneous tumors of congenital origin. They are among the most common tumors of childhood and adult life. The exact origin of the pigmented nevus is still argued: Masson's neurogenic theory and Allen's epidermal theory are the two most widely accepted concepts. Masson feels that the nevus cell is derived basically from the tactile end organs of nervous tissue within the dermal and basal layers of the epidermis. Allen's epidermal theory suggests that the nevus arises from the basal layers of the skin by a process of "abtrophung" or dropping off of cells containing the enzyme melanogenase from the basal layer. The argument is of academic-pathologic interest only and it does not influence the treatment.[2, 20, 21]

The classification of pigmented nevi is a pathologic one; it should be emphasized that the clinical appearance of nevi is deceiving and unreliable. In general, they fall into five major groups: (1) intradermal nevus, (2) junctional nevus, (3) compound nevus, (4) blue nevus, and (5) juvenile melanoma. All are present during childhood, but many, particularly the junctional nevi, do not become apparent until puberty.

Intradermal nevus, the common mole, may assume a wide variety of sizes, shapes, and colors. It occurs anywhere except on the palms, soles, and genitalia. On histologic section it is composed of masses or cords of nevus cells which contain varying amounts of pigment. As the term implies, the intradermal nevus is located beneath the basal cell layer in the dermis. It does not possess malignant potential.

The *junctional nevus* may occur anywhere, particularly on the hands, feet, and genitalia. They may not become apparent until puberty, when they may appear quite suddenly and in multiples. The junctional nevus varies in size, shape, and degree of pigmentation. Clinically it is not always possible to distinguish a junctional nevus from an intradermal nevus or common mole, except by its location. Histologically, it is composed of irregular masses of cells within the epidermis, in or above the basal cell layer, which have lost some degree of cohesion. This loss of cohesion is manifest by the formation of "clear cells" either within the epidermis or in the prolongations of the epidermis.[9] Although the lesion is benign, the presence of junctional activity may be the forerunner of malignant change. Some girls and women regard a mole of the face as a beauty spot. Any change in size or coloration demands immediate removal.

The *compound nevus* is generally manifest in infancy as a large pigmented lesion which may occupy the face (Figs. 23 and 24), extremity, or trunk. In the latter location, it is frequently referred to as a bathing trunk nevus, for the greater part of the trunk may be involved. Microscopically, it is an intradermal lesion with superimposed areas of junctional change. While it is considered a benign lesion, the author has had two children as patients in whom there was rapid and devastating malignant change resulting in death.

The *blue nevus* is an uncommon tumor similar to the mongolian spot of childhood. It occurs about the face, the dorsum of the hands, the feet, and the buttocks. Pathologically, the cells are spindle-shaped. Unlike the mongolian spot, the blue nevus does not fade or disappear. While the blue nevus is a benign lesion, malignant change may occur.

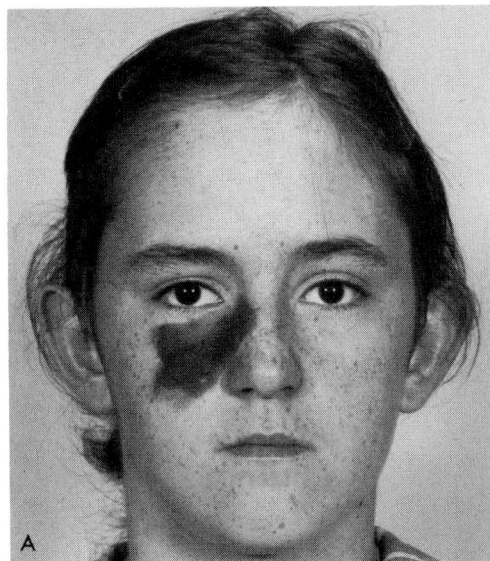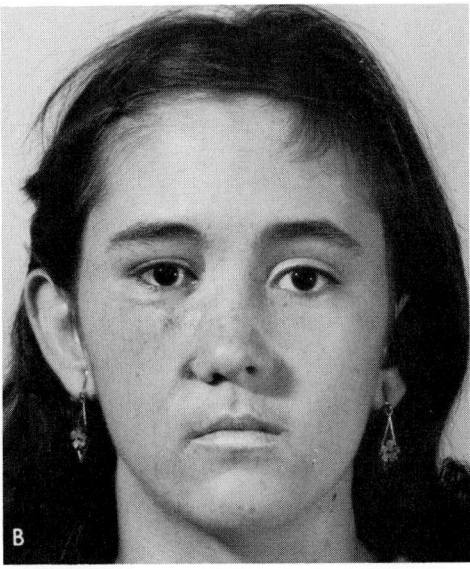

Figure 23. *A*, A 13-year-old girl with a benign compound nevus of the right side of the nose and maxillary region. In three stages, the nevus was excised and the cheek was advanced superiorly. *B*, Postoperative photograph taken 3 years later.

Juvenile melanoma occurs only in the prepubertal child; it varies markedly in size, shape, and color. On microscopic examination it is identical with malignant melanoma; however, the clinical course does not correspond with the histologic picture, for it is considered by Pack[17] and other authorities to be a benign lesion.

Treatment. Surgical excision is the treatment of choice of pigmented nevi. Pathologic evidence of the benign nature of the lesion and the adequacy of removal is proof positive of clinical safety. Malignancy cannot occur in a mole that has been completely excised. The crux of the problem, however, lies in the decision as to which nevi should be removed. The author feels that any pigmented lesion occurring in an area of chronic stress and irritation such as the shave area of the face and neck and the belt or bra line and those occurring on the palms, soles, and genitalia all should be removed, for the best treatment of melanoma is the prophylactic removal of its precursor. In addition, any pigmented lesion that has changed in size or character, with increased pigmentation, satellite lesions, or other changes, should be removed immediately under block or local anesthesia, with the anesthetic injected at some distance from the lesion. Procrastination may be fatal.

Lymphangioma

Lymphangiomas are true tumors of lymph vessels, analogous in some ways to hemangiomas, which are tumors of blood vessels. They are much less common than hemangiomas. They are usually present at birth and constitute a proliferation of lymph vessels to form a wormlike mass. Lymphangiomas are common on the face and neck (Figs. 25 and 26) and also in the tongue where they are the cause of macroglossia.

Lymphangiomas are of three clinical types: simple or capillary, cavernous, and cystic. Capillary lymphangiomas occur superficially and present a shiny, wartlike surface which may be reddish purple in color. Pressure on the excrescences may yield a serous fluid. The skin of the face and mucous membranes of the lip and tongue are favorite sites.

Cavernous lymphangiomas, like cavernous hemangiomas, are more deeply situated and consist of a loose framework of connective tissue in which are numerous single or multiple communicating lymphatic cysts. These tumors are found most frequently in the neck and axilla.

Cystic hygromas may represent a late stage of the cavernous type. Some authorities feel that cystic hygromas are at the outset cavernous lymphangiomas that have become dilated with lymph because of either a change in drainage or an alteration in the function of their endothelial lining. These are cystic tumors which may reach tremendous size, involving the lower face, with extension into the neck on one or both sides, and downward beneath the clavicle into the pectoral region and axilla. Since they occur frequently in the newborn in the face and neck (Fig. 26) an immediate tracheostomy may be necessary to prevent suffocation.

Etiology. It is generally agreed that lymphangiomas develop from embryonic sequestrations of lymph buds which continue to grow and increase progressively in size and, as shown, may reach tremendous proportions.

Treatment. If the lymphangioma involves the face and neck, a tracheostomy may be a life-saving procedure. Since cystic hygromas are frequently multiloculated with cysts that may vary tremendously in size, aspiration with a Luer syringe and a lumbar puncture needle of large bore may result in "tapping" or decompressing some of the larger cysts, as a temporary measure. Surgical excision is recommended. When the

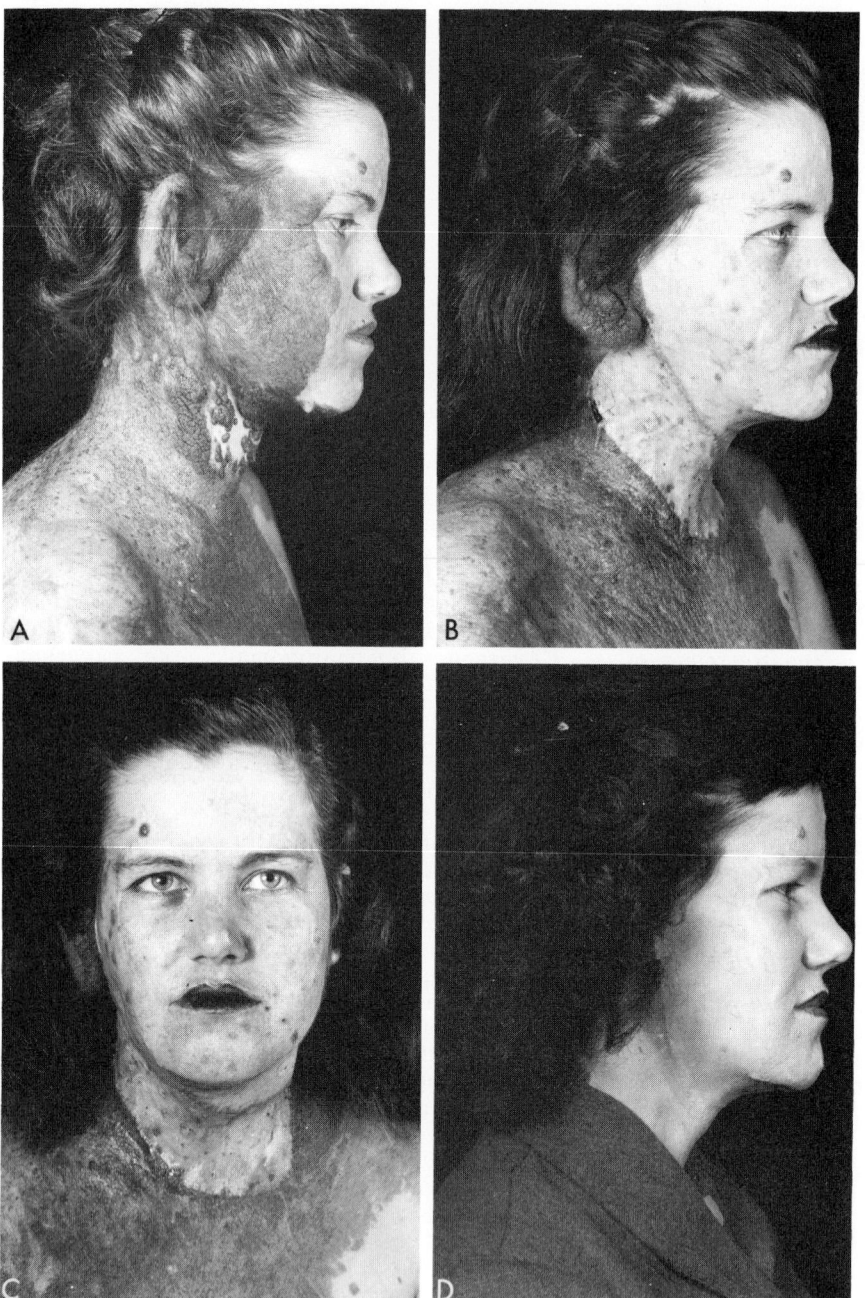

Figure 24. *A,* A 20-year-old girl with a large hairy compound nevus of the face, neck, and chest. *B* and *C,* In two operations, the nevus was excised first from the cheek and the area grafted with a split thickness skin graft from the buttock. Two weeks later, a similar procedure was performed on the neck. A third operation was performed at three months when the nevus was excised from the upper chest and grafted. *D,* Postoperative result at one year. Split thickness grafts will take cosmetic agents quite well. Although men will wear hair pieces, they will not use cosmetic agents.

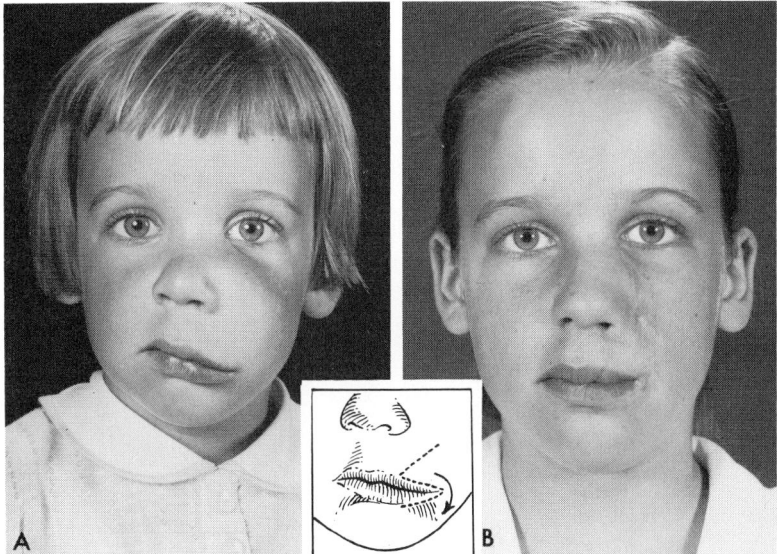

Figure 25. *A,* A 4-year-old girl with a diffuse, noncystic lymphangioma of the maxillary region, cheeks, and lips, producing severe asymmetry and macrostomia. The tumor was first removed through incisions in the nasofacial and nasolabial creases. The lips were then repositioned with interpolated flaps, using the Z-plasty principle, as shown in the inset. *B,* Postoperative photograph taken at 10 years.

tumor mass is well localized, operation is a procedure of choice, as to time. When the mass is large, diffuse, and infiltrating, operation becomes a procedure of necessity. If remnants are left behind, the condition will recur. Cystic hygromas are not radiosensitive.

Cysts

Sebaceous cysts (epidermal inclusion cyst, wen) are cutaneous swellings that develop as the result of blocking of the anatomically constricted necks of the sebaceous glands by sebum. They are lined by flattened epidermal cells. The scalp, face, neck, and retroauricular areas are favorite locations. Surgical excision is the treatment of choice (see Fig. 3). To prevent recurrence, the entire cyst must be removed without rupture. Redness over the cyst area is evidence of infection and is a contraindication to excision. Infected areas should be treated by incision and drainage, with definitive excision at a later time. Multiple cysts in the retroauricular area require the removal of a large ellipse of cyst-bearing skin.

Milia (whiteheads) are minute, multiple, white cutaneous cysts that occur commonly on the forehead, nose, and cheeks. They develop from mechanical blocking of the outlet of sebaceous glands. They may occur in skin grafts, especially if the remnants of the original skin are present, and also after dermabrasion procedures for acne and postacne scarring. They respond nicely to incision with a No. 11 scalpel or needle.

Dermoid cysts are congenital lesions located near embryonic lines of fusion. Those of the face are regarded as cysts originating from faulty fusion of the embryonic facial processes. They occur commonly on the forehead, base of the nose, and brow areas (Fig. 27), on the scalp, especially the occiput, over the abdomen and back, in the median raphe of the scrotum and perineum, and in the ovaries. The cysts are usually soft and elastic; they do not exhibit adherence

to the skin as sebaceous cysts do. The tumors contain various epidermal structures including hair and sebaceous material. They are lined by stratified squamous epithelium and are benign. Surgical excision is recommended on an inpatient basis under general anesthesia, even for the small cysts of the brow area. On occasion, the presenting cutaneous cyst is but the outer manifestation of an hourglass dermoid cyst with intracranial extension.

Mucous retention cysts occur primarily on the buccal surface of the lower lip as a soft, fluctuant mass. The overlying mucous membrane is normal unless the cyst has been bitten or traumatized. Surgical excision under local or block anesthesia is recommended. A sticky mucoid fluid occupies the cyst.

Synovial cyst is a degenerative cyst of the finger occurring most frequently over the distal interphalangeal joint and adjacent nail bed. The cysts appear suddenly as dome-shaped painless swellings and contain a clear to yellow viscid fluid. They arise from the joint capsule or tendon sheath. Fluid re-collects after drainage; therefore, excision under block anesthesia is recommended. A small skin graft is usually necessary since the tissues cannot be reapproximated.

Ganglia are small, round, tense, subcutaneous swellings occurring most commonly over the wrist but also over the tendon sheaths of the hands and feet. They progress slowly and are mildly painful. They may result from trauma, either accidental or occupational. They contain a glycerin-jelly–like fluid. Microscopically the wall of the ganglion is composed of collagenous tissue and may or may not be lined with synovial cells. Surgical excision with block anesthesia and tourniquet, using a transverse incision, is recommended. At operation ganglia are found to be adherent to the synovium or to a tendon sheath and frequently extend down in between the wrist bones. The complete excision of a ganglion requires an operative assistant to retract the margins of the wound, tendons,

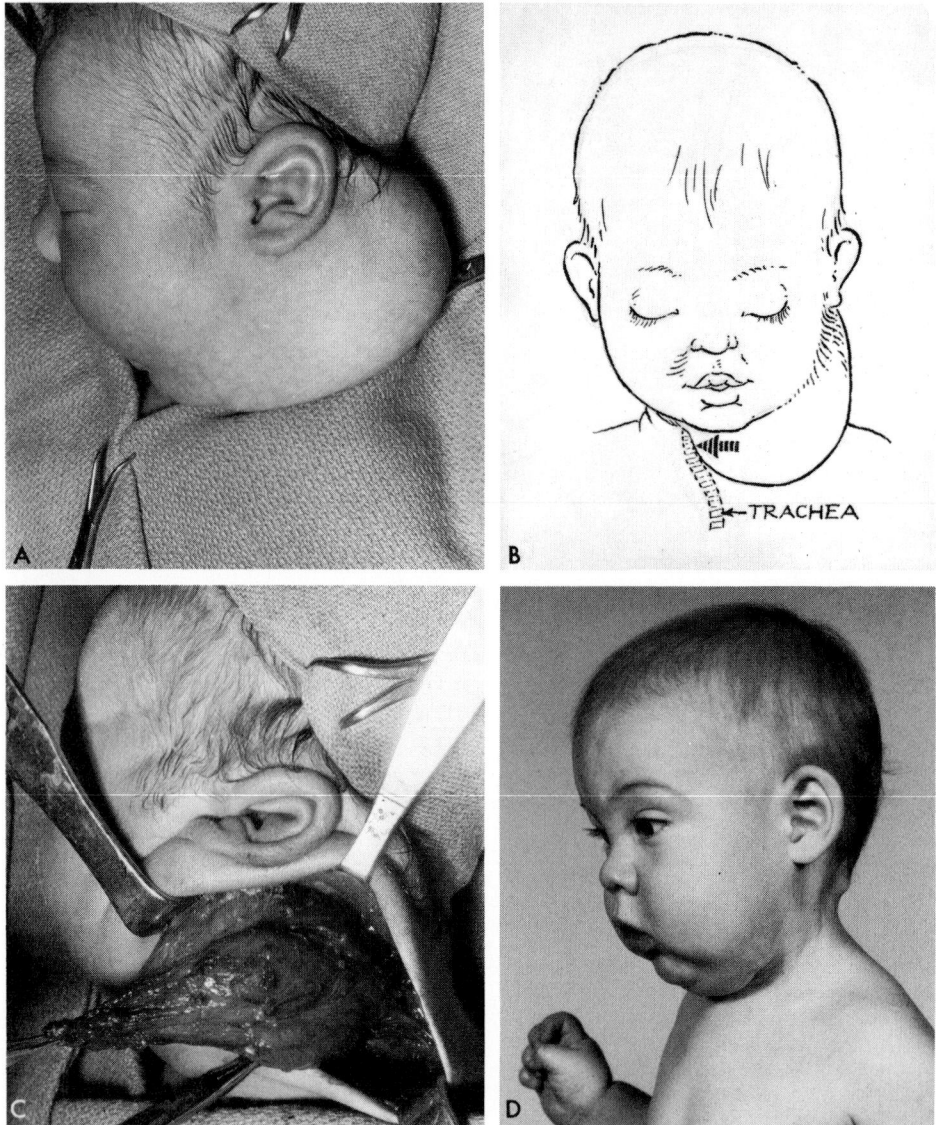

Figure 26. *A*, A 3-day-old infant with a large cystic lymphangioma (hygroma) of the neck producing tracheal deviation, compression, and obstruction, as shown in *B. C*, The tremendous lymphangiomatous mass extended beneath the sternum and to the right side of the neck. *D*, Postoperative photograph taken at 9 months shows no residual tumor.

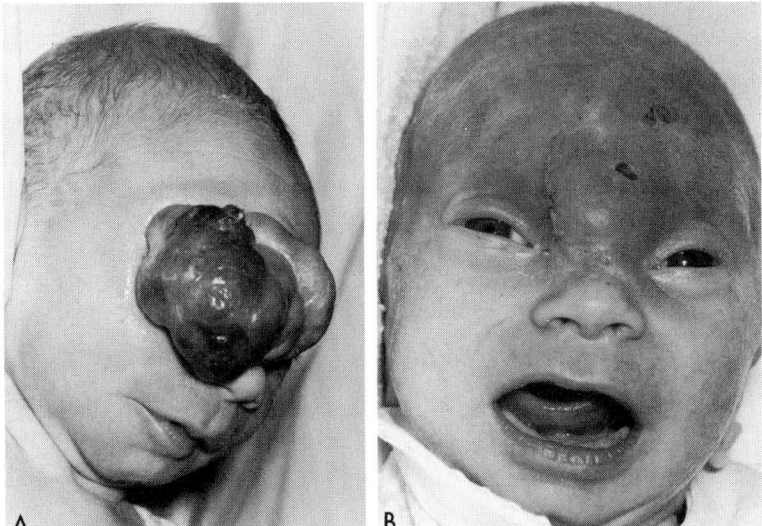

Figure 27. *A,* A 10-day-old baby with a large dermoid cyst of the interbrow area. The main mass was removed without difficulty; a periosteal flap from the frontal bone was used as a seal over the dura and to encourage bone regeneration. *B,* Postoperative photograph taken 2 weeks later.

and deep structures; the dissection can be a difficult one. The entire cyst must be removed as protection against recurrence.

Hidradenitis (apocrinitis) is a chronic, cicatrizing, suppurative process involving the apocrine (scent) glands. A better term is apocrinitis, since hidradenitis refers more generally to an inflammation of the sweat glands. The disease is most common in the second and third decades and is three times more common in women than in men. The axilla (Fig. 28) is affected much more frequently than the groin and perineum. Many conditions have been incriminated as contributing to the development of the disease: hyperhydrosis (excessive sweating), poor hygiene, the use of chemical depilatories and deodorants, trauma from shaving, and so forth. Locally, duct obstruction by keratin plug-

ging, followed by rupture of the apocrine glands into the dermis and subcutaneous tissue, coupled with superimposed infection, is the mechanism of development of this progressive, chronic process. Because of the anatomic arrangement of the duct orifice, which opens into a hair follicle above the sebaceous gland, infections are extremely resistant to emollients and local antibiotics. Pain is severe; disability in bilateral cases may be marked.[3]

In cases that are refractory to medical management, wide excision becomes a procedure of necessity. If the operative defect cannot be closed primarily (use catgut subcutaneously because of infection), one may use an advancement flap or free graft. The axilla thereafter will be dry, since the eccrine (sweat) glands have been removed also (Fig. 28).

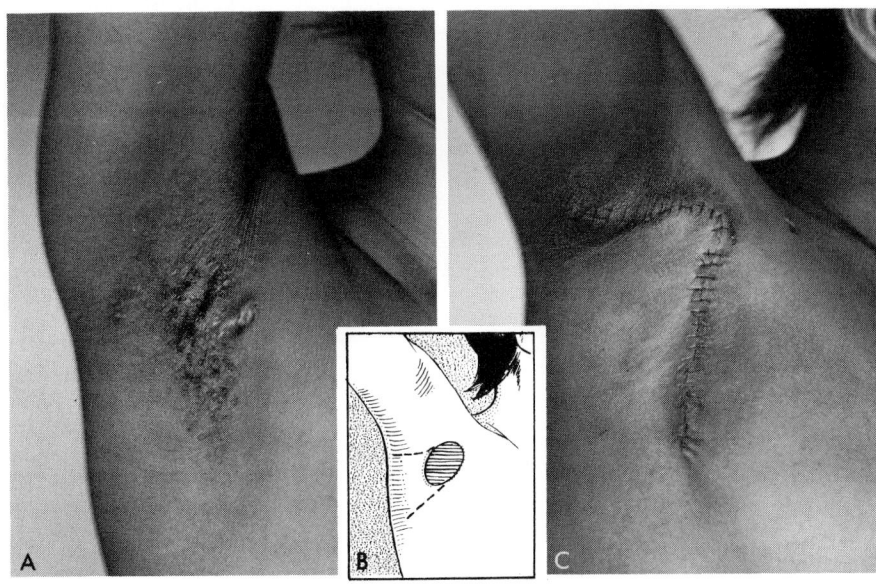

Figure 28. *A,* Characteristic appearance of hidradenitis suppurativa of the axilla with multiple draining sinuses. The use of local antibiotics and emollients is of limited value because of the deep-seated infection. *B,* Operative defect following excision of all of the axillary sweat glands and outline of posterolaterally based advancement flap. *C,* Result 7 days after primary closure.

SELECTED REFERENCES

Burian, F.: Plastic Surgery Atlas. New York, Macmillan Company, 1968.
A splendid three-volume atlas written by the late Professor Burian, Chairman of the Institute of Plastic Surgery, Prague.

Conley, F.: Cancer of the Head and Neck. Washington, D. C., Butterworth, 1967.
A collection of papers presented at the International Workshop on Cancer, New York City, May 10–14, 1965.

Converse, J. M. (Ed.): Reconstructive Plastic Surgery, 2nd ed. Philadelphia, W. B. Saunders Company, 1977.
An exhaustive five-volume work covering the entire field of reconstructive plastic surgery.

Domonkos, A.: Andrew's Diseases of the Skin. Philadelphia, W. B. Saunders Company, 1971.
An outstanding and profusely illustrated dermatology text.

Gaisford, J. C.: Symposium on Cancer of the Head and Neck. St. Louis, The C. V. Mosby Company, 1969.
A splendid collection of papers on head and neck cancer by more than 50 authors.

Grabb, W. C., and Smith, J. W.: Plastic Surgery, A Concise Guide to Clinical Practice. Boston, Little, Brown and Co., 1968.
A concise but exhaustive guide for both the student and surgeon in practice.

MacComb, W. S., and Fletcher, G. H.: Cancer of the Head and Neck. Baltimore, Williams & Wilkins Company, 1967.
An excellent volume written by an outstanding head and neck cancer surgeon and an outstanding radiologist.

Martin, H.: Surgery of Head and Neck Tumors. New York, Paul B. Hoeber, Inc., 1957.
A profusely illustrated atlas on head and neck cancer by a world authority from Memorial Hospital, New York.

May, H.: Plastic and Reconstructive Surgery, 3rd ed. Philadelphia, F. A. Davis Company, 1971.
A magnificent volume on general reconstructive plastic surgery.

McGregor, I.: Fundamental Techniques of Plastic Surgery, 4th ed. Baltimore, Williams & Wilkins Company, 1968.
A primer on plastic surgery principles and techniques recommended especially for students and house officers.

Pack, G. T., and Ariel, I. M.: Treatment of Cancer and Allied Diseases. Volume III. 2nd ed. New York, Hoeber Medical Division, Harper and Row, 1962.
A fine book on all types of neoplastic disease; concise and to the point

Paletta, F. X.: Pediatric Plastic Surgery. St. Louis, The C. V. Mosby Company, 1967.
An excellent little book. Pediatric patients are not just small people, for their treatment demands knowledge that is applicable directly to them.

Stark, R. B.: Plastic Surgery. New York, Harper and Row, 1962.
An excellent volume dealing with the general principles of excisional and reparative surgery.

Thompson, D. E., Frost, H. M., Hendrick, J. W., and Horn, R. C.: Soft tissue sarcomas involving the extremities. Southern Med. J., 64:33, 1971.
An excellent review of the literature and the authors' experiences providing an up-to-date categorization of sarcomas and histologic criteria.

Ward, G. E., and Hendrick, J. W.: Diagnosis and Treatment of Tumors of the Head and Neck. Baltimore, Williams & Wilkins Company, 1950.
Among the first of the books to be devoted exclusively to cancer of the head and neck; a classic.

REFERENCES

1. Allen, A. C.: A reorientation on the histogenesis and clinical significance of cutaneous nevi and melanomas. Cancer, 2:28, 1949.
2. Anderson, W.: Boyd's Pathology for the Surgeon, 8th ed. Philadelphia, W. B. Saunders Company, 1967.
3. Armstrong, D., and Pickrell, K. L.: Axillary hidradenitis suppurativa. Plast. Reconstr. Surg., 36:200, 1965.
4. Brown, S. H., Neerhout, R. C., and Fonkalsrud, E. W.: Prednisone therapy in the management of large hemangiomas in infants and children. Surgery, 71:168, 1972.
5. Callaway, J. L. (Chairman and Professor of Dermatology, Duke University Medical Center): Personal communication.
6. Cavanaugh, P. (Director, Radiation Therapy, Duke University Medical Center): Personal communication.
7. Conway, H.: Tumors of the Skin. Springfield, Ill., Charles C Thomas, Publisher, 1956.
8. Creech, O., Jr., and Krementz, E. T.: Regional perfusion in melanoma of limbs. J.A.M.A., 188:855, 1964.
9. Fetter, B. (Professor of Pathology, Duke University Medical Center): Personal communication.
10. Freier, D. T., and Lindenauer, S. M.: Subcutaneous glomus tumor. Am. J. Surg., 120:359, 1970.
11. King, G. D., and Salzman, F. A.: Keloid scars. Surg. Clin. North Am., 50:595, 1970.
12. Lever, W. F.: Histopathology of the Skin. Philadelphia, J. B. Lippincott Company, 1961.
13. Lewis, G. M., and Wheeler, C. E.: Practical Dermatology, 3rd ed. Philadelphia, W. B. Saunders Company, 1967.
14. Masson, P.: Pigmented nevi; nerve tumors. Les naevi pigmentaires, tumeurs nerveuses. Ann. Anat. Pathol., 3:417, 1926.
15. Matton, G., and Pickrell, K. L.: The surgical treatment of rhinophyma; an analysis of 57 cases. Plast. Reconstr. Surg., 30:403, 1962.
16. Neale, H. W., Pickrell, K. L., and Quinn, G. W.: Extra-abdominal manifestations of Gardner's syndrome. Plast. Reconstr. Surg., 56:92, 1975.
17. Pack, G. T.: Prepubertal melanoma of the skin. Surg. Gynecol. Obstet., 86:374, 1948.
18. Peacock, E. E., Jr., and Van Winkle, W., Jr.: Surgery and Biology of Wound Repair, 2nd ed. Philadelphia, W. B. Saunders Company, 1977.
19. Pickrell, K. L., and Georgiade, N. G.: Surgical treatment of early carcinoma of the face. Postgrad. Med., 27:406, 1960.
20. Pickrell, K. L., and Georgiade, N. G.: Plastic surgery conditions in infancy and childhood. Postgrad. Med., 27:704, 1960.
21. Pickrell, K. L., and Masters, F. W.: Tumors of the head and neck in infancy, childhood and adolescence. Plast. Reconstr. Surg., 12:10, 1953.
22. Pickrell, K. L., Kelley, J. W., and Marzoni, F. A.: The surgical treatment of pseudoxanthoma elasticum. Plast. Reconstr. Surg., 3:700, 1948.
23. Pillsbury, D. M., Shelley, W. B., and Kligman, A. M.: Dermatology. Philadelphia, W. B. Saunders Company, 1957.
24. Seigler, H. F., Shingleton, W. W., and Pickrell, K. L.: Intralesional BCG, intravenous immune lymphocytes, and immunization with neuraminidase-treated tumor cells to manage melanoma. Plast. Reconstr. Surg., 55:294, 1975.
25. Thompson, D. E., Frost, H. M., Hendrick, J. W., and Horn, R. C.: Soft tissue sarcomas involving the extremities. Southern Med. J., 64:33, 1971.
26. Thompson, H. D., Douglas, L., and Monroe, I.: Surgical tattooing: An experimental study (Part II). Plast. Reconstr. Surg., 39:291, 1967; also 37:536, 1966.
27. Woolf, R., Kepes, J., Georgiade, N., and Pickrell, K.: Xeroderma pigmentosa. Plast. Reconstr. Surg., 24:214, 1959.
28. Zarem, H. A., and Edgerton, M. T.: Induced resolution of cavernous hemangiomas following prednisone therapy. Plast. Reconstr. Surg., 39:76, 1967.

47

GYNECOLOGY: UTERUS, OVARIES, AND VAGINA

Charles B. Hammond, M.D.

INTRODUCTION AND HISTORY OF GYNECOLOGY

Gynecology is that branch of medicine which deals with diseases of the female genital tract. In practice, however, it includes some aspects of internal medicine, obstetrics, and endocrinology, as well as multiple other areas of interest that are common to any surgical specialty.

The art and practice of gynecology dates to the ancient Egyptians, the time of the Old Testament, and the early Greeks, when most thoughts and practices of gynecology were vested in superstition and based on empiricism derived from observation. Rules concerning menstruation and sexual conduct are recorded in Lev. 15:19–32. Soranus, Hippocrates, and Galen taught about diseases of the uterus and observed mental attitudes and traits in women that they related to the uterus and its humors. The visible events of female physiology were so steeped in folklore and myth that it was not until the emergence of scientific medicine in the Middle Ages that gynecology actually profited from objective observation of the human body. Gynecology advanced as medical science as a whole prospered, but at perhaps a slower pace because of the persistence of the fantasies surrounding human reproduction, many of which remain in the twentieth century.

Modern gynecologic surgery dates from 1809, when Ephraim McDowell of Kentucky performed the first ovariotomy for a large ovarian cyst. The operation was a success and laid the foundation for abdominal and pelvic surgery. Many others provided significant discoveries: In 1817, Langenbeck reported the first vaginal hysterectomy. In 1842, Long and, in 1846, Morton introduced ether anesthesia. In 1849, Mattauer and, in 1852, Sims described successful closure of vesicovaginal fistula, a common complication of obstructed labor in that time. In 1860, Hodge described the vaginal pessary for support of the prolapsed uterus. In 1861, Pasteur noted living organisms lead to fermentation and tissue destruction. In 1867, Lister conceived and published his principles of antisepsis. In 1878, Freund performed the first successful abdominal hysterectomy for cancer of the uterus. In 1884, Tait reported excellent success with abdominal operation for ruptured ectopic pregnancy. In 1895, Röntgen discovered x-rays. In 1898, the Curies discovered radium; Kelly described the operative cure of bladder and urethral prolapse and published a two-volume text of operative gynecology.

The twentieth century began with Wertheim describing a radical operation for cancer of the cervix and Landsteiner discovering the major human blood groups. Other contributions include: In 1903, Cleaves treated the first patient with cancer of the cervix with radium. In 1908, Hitschmann and Alder demonstrated the cyclic physiologic changes of endometrium. In 1921, Sampson described pelvic endometriosis and published his theory of "retrograde menstruation." In 1923, Allen and Doisy isolated estrogen. In 1928, Aschheim and Zondek discovered human chorionic gonadotropin. In 1929, Allen and Corner isolated progesterone. In 1935, Stein and Leventhal described the polycystic ovary syndrome. In 1936, Hamblen first induced human ovulation with gonadotropins of nonhuman primates; Colebrook and Kenny first used antibiotics (sulfanilamides) to treat human puerperal infections. In 1941, Papanicolaou and Traut published the classic monograph on vaginal cytology for cancer screening. In 1949, Barr discovered the sex chromatin body; Li, Simpson, and Evans isolated human follicle-stimulating hormone. In 1951, Brunschwig reported exenterative pelvic surgery for advanced or recurrent cervical cancer. In 1956, Li, Hertz, and Spencer first cured metastatic choriocarcinoma with chemotherapy; Tjio and Levan identified the normal human karyotype as 46 chromosomes. In 1958, Gemzell reported successful ovulatory induction with human gonadotropins; Pincus introduced oral contraceptives.[17, 19]

The accomplishments of these men, plus many others, have enabled gynecology to become a broadly based discipline. While this chapter is not intended to be a complete treatise on the diagnosis and management of gynecologic disorders, it is hoped it will provide a summation of the current and accepted knowledge of the specialty. Ideally, it will stimulate the reader to more in-depth study regarding specific problems.

EMBRYOLOGY AND ANATOMY

A knowledge of embryology is necessary for proper understanding of gynecology, particularly as it relates to such problems as congenital malformations, hermaphroditism, endocrine interrelationships, and generative neoplasms. The external genitals develop from the genital tubercle, a group of cells found at the caudal end of the body (Fig. 1). The urogenital sinus develops from part of the ventral entodermal cloaca. The lower portion of the vagina originates from the genital tubercle and provides an invading epithelium which covers the external genitalia, the vagina, and the vaginal part of the cervix. Externally, the clitoris forms first, then the labia minora, and finally labia majora. The hymen forms from the unfolding of the urogenital sinus. As the urogenital sinus unfolds it joins the müllerian tubercle developing cephalad as the upper vagina. At this stage the urethra acquires a separate orifice.

The urogenital ridge is formed on each side of the posterior body cavity. From these primordial cells develop the ovaries, the wolffian ducts and bodies, and the müllerian ducts. The müllerian ducts develop into the tubes, uterus, cervix, and upper vagina. To form these latter three structures the müllerian ducts must fuse in the midline, and aplasia of one duct or failure of fusion may result in several congenital malformations. The ovaries develop from coelomic epithelium covering the surfaces of the wolffian bodies. This epithelium forms early into a sex gland anlage and at this stage histologic sexual differentiation is not evident. When ovarian development occurs, primordial follicles appear and remain inactive until gonadotropic stimulation begins at puberty. The wolffian ducts are the forerunner of the male reproductive system and undergo regressive changes in the female which cause them to become vestigial. Remnants of the wolffian ducts persist in the normal female as ductal structures which may become manifest clinically as Gartner's duct cysts, usually seen in the vagina, parovarian cysts, and as hydatid of Morgagni.[5]

The External Genitalia (Fig. 2)

The female external genitals, or vulva, include the mons veneris, which is a fat pad over the pubic symphysis into which the labia majora blend. It is covered with skin which contains sweat glands and hair follicles. The labia majora are the most lateral structures of the external genitalia and do not acquire full growth until puberty. After menopause, atrophy may occur. These structures are covered with skin which contains sweat glands, hair follicles, and sebaceous and sudoriferous glands beneath the squamous epithelium. The underlying tissue is adipose and the round ligaments insert into the upper ends of the labia majora. The labia minora are medial to the majora and are covered with skin containing sweat glands but no hair follicles. The labia minora extend from the clitoris anteriorly and continue to the perineum. Anteriorly they pass over the top of the clitoris to form the prepuce and join below the clitoris to form the frenulum. Growth and configuration of the labia minora are influenced by estrogen. The clitoris is composed of two roots which traverse the pubic rami to unite beneath the symphysis in the clitoridal body and terminate in the upper portion of the glans, which is exposed. The covering of the glans is modified cutaneous tissue. The clitoris contains two corpora cavernosa and is erectile.

The urethral meatus is situated below the clitoris and above the vaginal orifice. Lateral to this meatus open Skene's ducts, which lead from paraurethral glands. Bartholin glands are

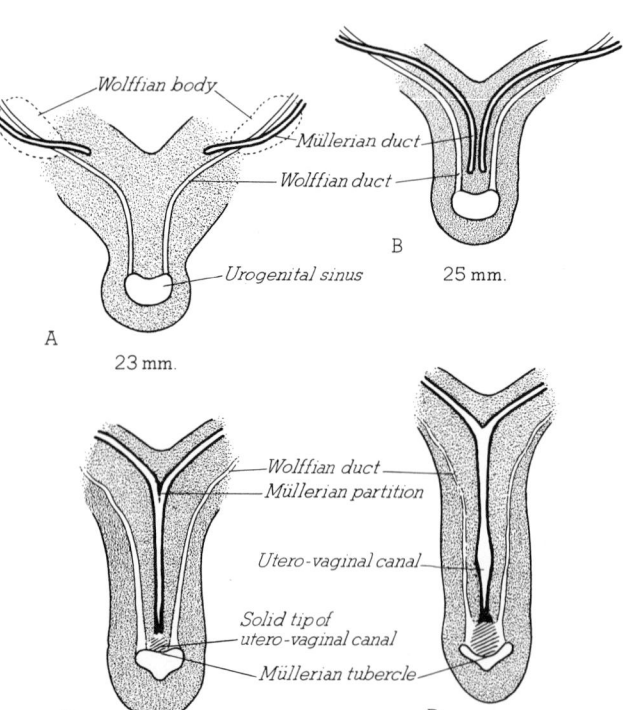

Figure 1. Relationships of müllerian and wolffian ducts during early genital development. (After Koff, A. K.: Contributions to Embryology. Washington, D.C., Carnegie Institute of Washington, 24:61, 1933.)

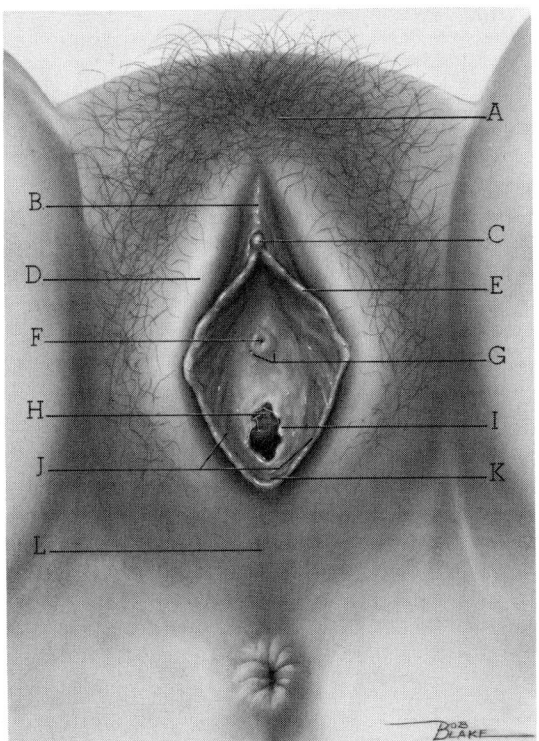

Figure 2. The external genitalia. A, Mons pubis. B, Prepuce. C, Clitoris. D, Labia majora. E, Labia minora. F, Urethral meatus. G, Skene's ducts. H, Vagina. I, Hymen. J, Bartholin glands. K, Posterior fourchette. L, Perineal body.

fascia of the levator ani and coccygeus muscles. The deep transverse perineal muscle is covered on both sides by fascia and the three structures constitute the urogenital diaphragm. The urethra and vagina perforate this diaphragm which stretches as a wall across the space between the ischiopubic rami. The deep layer rests between the deep transverse perineal muscle and the pubococcygeal portions of the levator ani sling.

The perineal muscles divide into deep and superficial portions, sphincter urethrae, and bulbocavernosus and ischiocavernosus muscles. The superficial transverse perineal muscles arise from the ischial tuberosity on either side and insert into the central perineal tendon. They blend with the anal sphincter muscle and with fibers from the bulbocavernosus muscles. The bulbocavernosus muscles surround the vaginal orifice and have a sphincteric contractile effect arising anteriorly from the clitoris and inserting posteriorly into the perineal body. The ischiocavernosus muscles arise from the medial borders of the ischial rami and clitoris, and course posteriorly and laterally to insert into the ischial tuberosity. The sphincter muscle of the urethra is attached to the periurethral structures and fans laterally on either side to attach to the pubic rami. The deep transverse perineal muscle lies below the superficial muscle and attaches in the midline of the perineal body.

The Internal Genitalia (Fig. 4)

The Vagina. The vagina is a muscular tube lined with stratified squamous epithelium that is histologically similar to the mucosa of the cervix and vulva. It does not contain

located at four and eight o'clock at the vulvovaginal orifice, and are compound racemose glands that connect to the surface by a single tubule lined by transitional epithelium. The gland acini are lined by a single layer of cuboidal epithelium. In its normal state the gland usually cannot be seen or palpated. The hymen divides the external and internal genitalia and may be a fibrous structure. The aperture varies greatly in size and shape and may be imperforate.

The Muscles and Fascia of the Perineum (Fig. 3)

The superficial fascia of the perineum consists of outer and deep layers, both continuous with the layers of the anterior abdominal wall; the outer layer is called Cruveilhier's fascia and is continuous with Camper's fascia of the anterior abdominal wall; the deep layer of the superficial perineal fascia is called Colles' fascia and is continuous with Scarpa's fascia of the abdomen. The outer layer of superficial fascia forms the greater part of the labium majus and is continuous with the superficial fascia of the thigh. The deep layer of superficial fascia, Colles' fascia, is a strong membrane adding support to the urogenital structures. This fascia is firmly attached laterally to the medial surface of the thigh, being continuous with the fascia which covers the saphenous vein opening. It becomes attached to the deep fascia along the posterior border of the superficial transverse perineal muscle and blends on either side into the median raphe of the perineum.

The deep perineal fascia consists of obturator fascia, infra-anal fascia, and fascia of the bulbocavernosus, ischiocavernosus, and transverse perineal muscles. The obturator fascia forms the lateral wall of the ischiorectal fossa, and meets the infra-anal fascia deep in the fossa. The infra-anal fascia is the

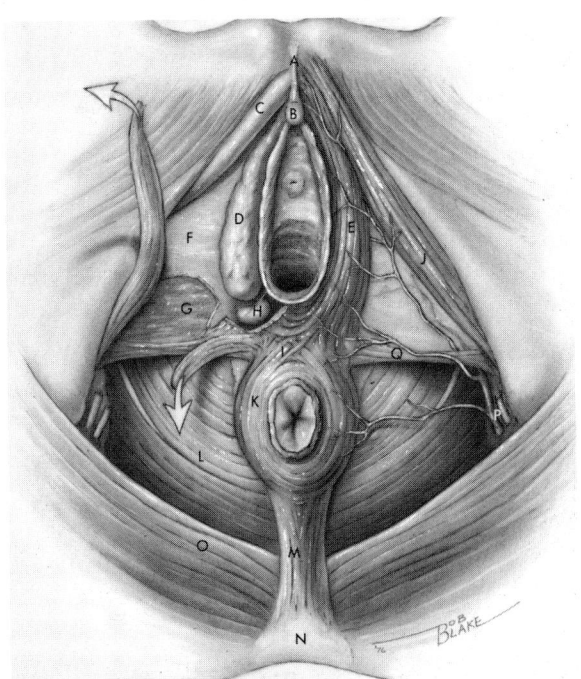

Figure 3. The muscles and fascia of the perineum. A, Suspensory ligament of clitoris. B, Clitoris. C, Crus of clitoris. D, Vestibular bulb. E, Bulbocavernosus muscle. F, Inferior fascia of urogenital diaphragm. G, Deep transverse perineal muscle. H, Bartholin's gland. I, Perineal body. J, Ischiocavernosus muscle. K, External anal sphincter. L, Levator ani muscle. M, Anococcygeal body. N, Coccyx. O, Gluteus maximus muscle. P, Pudendal artery and vein. Q, Superficial transverse perineal muscle.

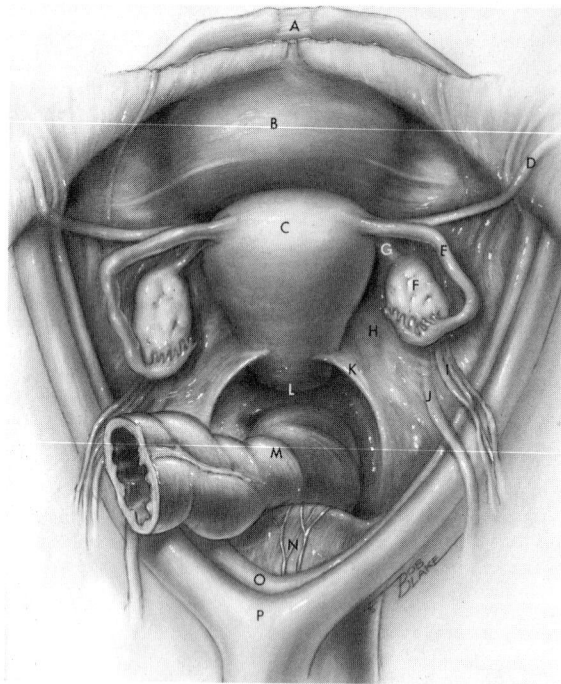

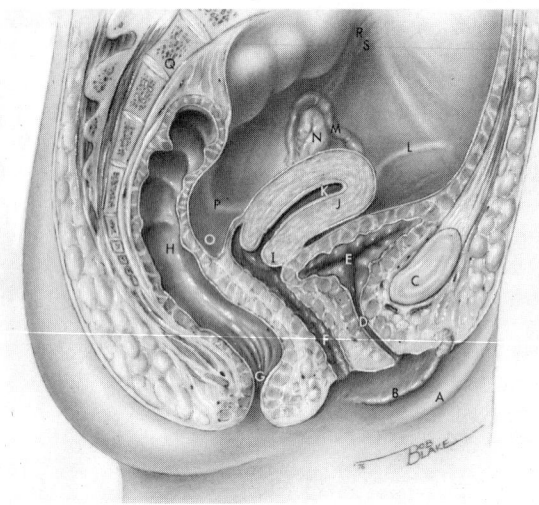

Figure 4. The internal genitalia. *Front view:* A, Symphysis pubis. B, Bladder. C, Corpus uteri. D, Round ligament. E, Fallopian tube. F, Ovary. G, Utero-ovarian ligament. H, Broad ligament. I, Ovarian artery and vein. J, Ureter. K, Uterosacral ligament. L, Cul-de-sac. M, Rectum. N, Middle sacral artery and vein. O, Vena cava. P, Aorta. *Side view:* A, Labium majus. B, Labium minus. C, Symphysis pubis. D, Urethra. E, Bladder. F, Vagina. G, Anus. H, Rectum. I, Cervix uteri. J, Corpus uteri. K, Endometrial cavity. L, Round ligament. M, Fallopian tube. N, Ovary. O, Cul-de-sac. P, Uterosacral ligament. Q, Sacrum. R, Ureter. S, Ovarian artery and vein.

The vaginal axis is toward the sacral promontory and the cervix is suspended at the upper end, surrounded by the anterior, posterior, and lateral fornices. The upper two thirds of the vagina is supported by the paravaginal fascia and the paracervical tissues, the lower one third by the perineal body.

The Cervix. The inferior portion of the uterus, the cervix, is a fibromuscular organ covered with stratified squamous epithelium. The portio vaginalis of the cervix arises in the vaginal fornices and ends at the external cervical os at the entrance of the endocervical canal. This squamocolumnar junction is the most common site of origin of squamous cell carcinoma. The endocervical canal is lined by columnar epithelium, and racemose glands, lined with similar epithelium, are in the fibromuscular stroma. Such glands, if obstructed, may form nabothian cysts on the cervical surface. The nulliparous cervical os is round, but parturition changes this to a horizontally flattened orifice. The cervix is the most common site of genital malignancy in women.

The Uterus. The uterus is a hollow, fibromuscular-walled organ between the bladder and rectum and consists of cervix and fundus. The organ is pear-shaped, and in nonpregnant women measures approximately 8 cm. in length and weighs 30 to 100 gm. The fallopian tubes and the cervical canal communicate with the uterine cavity which is lined by the endometrium. The endometrium proliferates in response to estrogen and becomes secretory with progesterone, and bleeds as it sloughs when hormonal support is withdrawn or inadequate. The uterine fundus is covered by peritoneum except in its lower anterior portion, where the bladder is contiguous with the lower uterine segment and the peritoneum is reflected, and laterally where the folds of the broad ligament are attached. The uterus is supported by condensations of endopelvic fascia and fibromuscular tissue laterally at the base of the broad ligaments, the cardinal ligaments, and the uterosacral ligaments. The round ligaments arise from the cornual areas, pass through the external inguinal ring, and insert in the upper labia majora. The broad ligaments support laterally and the uterovesical fold anteriorly. None of these last three provide major uterine support.

The Oviducts. The fallopian tubes arise from the superior portion of the lateral borders of the uterus, superior to the attachment of the round ligaments, and are patent. The distal ends, the fimbriae, open into the abdominal cavity and the proximal ends into the uterine cavity. The tubes are lined by a single layer of low columnar epithelium, some ciliated, arranged in a branching or "frond" pattern. This structure is divided into interstitial, isthmic, ampullar, and fimbriated portions. The wall is thin, with two muscular layers and an outer layer of peritoneum within the upper borders of the broad ligament.

The Ovaries. The normal ovary is a white, almond-shaped structure measuring 2 by 3 by 3 cm., and is located on the posterior surface of the broad ligament and inferior to the fallopian tube. The nerves, lymphatics, and blood vessels enter the ovary at the point of attachment to the broad ligament, the hilus. Lateral support of the ovary is the infundibulopelvic ligament, which extends to the pelvic sidewall and medial support is to the uterus by the utero-ovarian ligament. The ovary has a cortex and medulla. Germinal epithelium, a single layer of cuboidal cells, covers condensed fibrous tissue called the tunica albuginea. Follicles originate within the ovarian cortex and are composed of the basic embryonic complement; no new follicles are formed after birth. The medullary portion of the ovary is occupied by blood vessels, lymphatics, nerves, and connective tissue and contains remnants of wolffian body precursors. The ovary is an endocrine and a generative organ. Parafollicular granulosa cells produce estrogen and, after ovulation and corpus luteum formation, progestins. Androgens are produced by stromal cells, particularly in the hilus.

glands or hair follicles but individual cells produce mucus. The superficial layer is not keratinized. During menstrual life the vagina has transverse folds called rugae. After menopause the vaginal walls become thin and atrophic, reflecting the lack of estrogen as seen in the childhood years. The adult vagina measures 12 to 13 cm. in depth, and in nulliparous women there is coaptation of the anterior and posterior walls.

The Urinary System. The kidneys and ureters arise from the metanephros and a diverticulum from the wolffian duct in both sexes. The ureters vary from 28 to 34 cm. in length, the right about 1 to 2 cm. shorter than the left. The ureter is not of uniform caliber. The abdominal part of the the ureter lies behind the peritoneum on the medial part of the psoas muscle and is crossed obliquely by the ovarian vessels. It enters the pelvis by crossing either the termination of the common, or the commencement of the external, iliac vessels. The pelvic ureter runs at first downward on the lateral wall of the pelvis, then medially and forward toward the lateral aspect of the cervix about 1.5 cm. from the exterior of the cervix. In this course it is accompanied by the uterine artery. The uterine artery then crosses over the ureter and ascends between the leaves of the broad ligament to enter the uterus laterally. Blood supply of the ureter arises from branches of the renal, ovarian, hypogastric, and inferior vesical arteries.

In the female, the uterus, cervix and upper vagina are behind the bladder and it is separated from the uterus by the vesicouterine fold. Below this peritoneal fold the bladder is connected to the cervix and upper vagina by areolar tissue. The bladder is stabilized by ligamentous attachments at its inferior portion or base, near the exit of the urethra, and at the vertex. The remainder is free to move. The basal attachment is to the internal investing layer of deep fascia on the pubic bone by strong fibrous bands. The arterial supply of the bladder is the superior, middle, and inferior vesical arteries, derived from the anterior hypogastric artery, the obturator and inferior gluteal arteries, and the uterine and vaginal arteries.

The female urethra is a narrow membranous canal about 4 cm. long extending from the internal to the external urethral orifice. It is placed behind the symphysis, embedded in the anterior vaginal wall, and its direction is obliquely downward and forward. The resting diameter is about 6 mm. The urethra perforates the fasciae of the urogenital diaphragm where it acquires longitudinal folds. Many small paraurethral glands open into the urethra.

The Rectosigmoid Colon

The sigmoid colon forms a loop that averages 40 cm. in length and normally lies in the pelvis. It begins vertically from the left side of the pelvis as the continuation of the descending colon, passes transversely across the front of the sacrum to the right side of the pelvis, curves on itself and turns toward the left to reach the midline at the level of S3, where it bends inferiorly and terminates in the rectum. The colon is completely surrounded by the peritoneum and forms a mesentery which diminishes in length from the center. The sigmoid loop is fixed at its junctions with the two other parts of the colon, and the central portion has considerable mobility. The rectum is continuous with the sigmoid colon. From its origin at the third sacral vertebra, the rectum passes downward, lying in the sacrococcygeal curve, and extends in front of, and below, the tip of the coccyx. It then turns posteriorly into the anal canal. The rectum is approximately 12 cm. long and is dilated near its distal end to form the rectal ampulla. The peritoneum is applied to the upper two thirds of the rectum, covering it at first anteriorly and laterally, but more inferiorly covering its anterior surface only. The distal 5 cm. is devoid of peritoneal covering. The arterial supply of the rectum is derived from the superior hemorrhoidal branch of the inferior mesenteric artery. The anal canal is supplied by the middle hemorrhoidal branch of the hypogastric artery, the superior hemorrhoidal branch of the inferior mesenteric artery, and the inferior hemorrhoidal branch of the internal pudendal artery.

The Blood Vessels of the Pelvis (Fig. 5)

The ovarian arteries arise from the front of the aorta just below the renal arteries. The left ovarian vein empties into

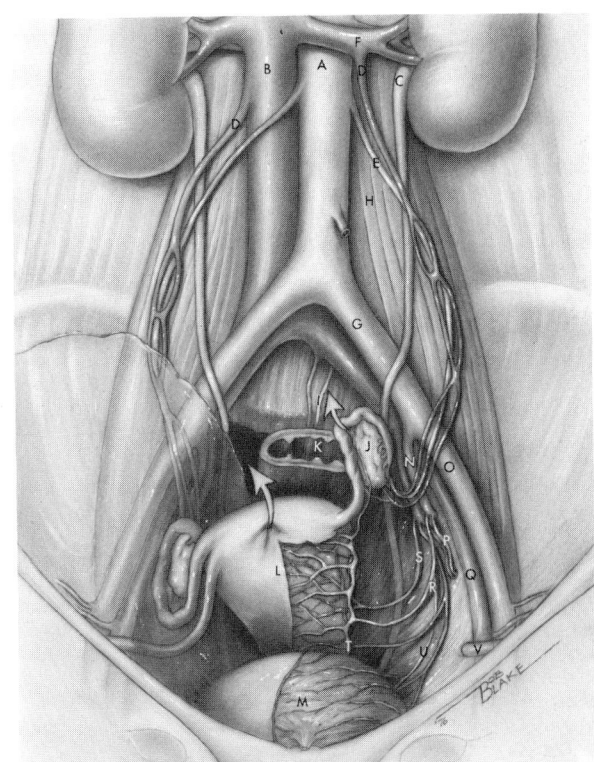

Figure 5. Blood supply of the pelvis. A, Aorta. B, Inferior vena cava. C, Ureter. D, Ovarian vein. E, Ovarian artery. F, Renal vein. G, Common iliac artery. H, Psoas muscle. I, Middle sacral artery. J, Ovary. K, Rectum. L, Corpus uteri. M, Bladder. N, Internal iliac (hypogastric) artery, anterior branch. O, External iliac artery. P, Obturator artery. Q, External iliac vein. R, Uterine artery. S, Uterine vein. T, Vaginal artery. U, Superior vesicle artery. V, Inferior epigastric artery.

the left renal vein; the right ovarian vein empties into the vena cava just inferior to the renal vein. The ovarian vessels follow a downward course and pass between the layers of the infundibulopelvic ligament and the broad ligament to reach the ovary. Small branches divide to supply the ureter and fallopian tube. The main branches unite with the uterine vessels on the side of the uterus and small branches supply the round ligaments.

The iliac vessels originate as the common iliac arteries from the aorta at the L4 vertebral level and slightly to the left of midline. Each is about 5 cm. long, and just below the S1 level divides into the internal iliac (hypogastric) artery and the external iliac artery. The common iliac veins closely follow the arteries and join inferiorly and to the right of the aorta to form the vena cava. The external iliac vessels lie on the lateral walls of the pelvis above the psoas muscles, behind the peritoneum, to pass beneath the inguinal ligaments through the femoral canal to become the femoral artery and vein. The inferior epigastric vessels arise from the external iliacs immediately superior to the ligament. The hypogastric (internal iliac) vessels pass inferiorly and posteriorly along the border of the great sciatic notch. The hypogastric vessels are 3 to 4 cm. in length before they divide into anterior and posterior branches. The anterior branch provides the main blood supply to the bladder and forms the middle hemorrhoidal, obturator, internal pudendal, inferior gluteal, uterine, and vaginal arteries. The uterine artery arises from the anterior branch of the hypogastric artery and passes medially on the levator ani muscle toward the junction of the cervix and the uterus. At the level of the internal os the vessels turn superiorly and follow a tortuous route between the leaves of the broad ligament to join the ovarian arteries. An inferior branch of the uterine artery turns inferiorly on either side to form the cervical arteries. The vaginal artery arises from the hypogastric artery below the level of the uterine artery and sends branches to the vagina, bladder, and rectum. The internal pudendal artery is the most caudal extension of the hypogastric artery and supplies the external genital organs. This vessel emerges from the pelvis between the piriformis and coccygeus muscles, crosses the ischial spine, and passes through the lesser sciatic foramen to enter the perineum. The artery traverses the lateral wall of the ischiorectal fossa and supplies the erectile tissue of the vulva.

The Lymphatics of the Pelvis (Fig. 6)

The lymphatics of the pelvis parallel the vascular channels. The external iliac nodes are interposed in the drainage pattern of the deep inguinal nodes, the fundus of the bladder and the uterus, cervix, and upper vagina. The external iliac and hypogastric drainage occurs via the common iliac nodes. The hypogastric nodes surround the hypogastric vessels and receive drainage from the cervix, uterine fundus, upper vagina, bladder, urethra, and lower ureter. The obturator nodes reside in the obturator fossa, lateral to and surrounding the obturator nerve, and receive channels from the cervix, uterus, and part of the buttocks. The sacral nodes receive

branches from the cervix and uterus and reside in the sacral concavity. The rectal lymphatics course posteriorly to the sacral nodes also. The vulva drainage takes place via subcutaneous ascending lymphatics to the superficial and deep inguinal nodes and femoral nodes which also receive the lymphatics from the lower portions of the vagina and urethra. The lower extremity lymphatics lead to the femoral and inguinal nodes. Cross drainage in this region may occur via Cloquet's node (femoral canal) to deep nodes of the pelvis.

The Nerve Supply of the Pelvis

The sacral plexus arises from the fourth and fifth lumbar and the first four sacral cord segments. The pudendal nerve originates from the second, third, and fourth sacral segments. The plexus rests in the hollow of the pelvis over the piriformis muscle. The branches of the plexus contain fibers of sympathetic and parasympathetic nerve trunks. The parasympathetic fibers are efferent preganglionic to pelvic viscera, and afferent from the pelvic organs. The sympathetic fibers arise from the hypogastric sympathetic plexus. The levator ani, coccygeus, and sphincter ani muscles receive branches from the pudendal plexus. The pudendal nerve leaves the pelvis through the greater sciatic foramen, crosses the ischial spine, and re-enters the pelvis via the lesser sciatic foramen. It accompanies the pudendal vessels and sends branches to the sphincter ani muscle and sensory fibers to the labia majora, while another branch supplies the perineal muscles. The dorsal nerve of the clitoris also arises from the pudendal nerve.

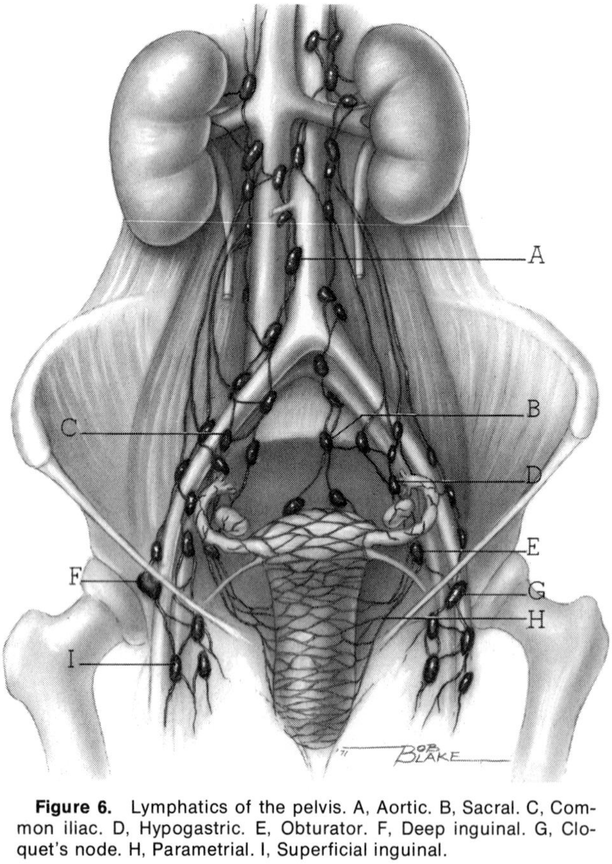

PHYSIOLOGY AND ENDOCRINOLOGY

The interactions of physiologic and endocrinologic mechanisms cannot be separated in any adequate summary of the function of the female genital system. Numerous workers have identified the interrelationships between the central nervous system, hypothalamus, pituitary, ovary, and other endocrine systems. Dependence of the pelvic structures, breasts, skin, other organs, and many metabolic processes on estrogen and progesterone has been demonstrated.[5, 6, 12, 13, 15]

Hypothalamus, Pituitary, and Gonadotropins

The hypothalamus (Fig. 7) serves as the primary control center for reproductive endocrine systems. This system is essentially dormant until late childhood when activation begins and certain hypothalamic cells become capable of releasing short-chain peptides to the anterior pituitary via the hypophyseal portal system. In experimental animals, and probably also in man, these humoral agents, or releasing factors, cause the anterior pituitary to produce and release follicle-stimulating hormone (FSH) and luteinizing hormone (LH). Physiologic, pathologic, and even psychologic problems can alter these interrelationships.

The pituitary gonadotropins, FSH and LH, are necessary for normal ovarian function and, via the hypothalamus, are in turn regulated through feedback mechanisms from ovarian estrogen and progesterone (Fig. 8). FSH arises from the basophilic cells of the anterior pituitary, is transmitted through the blood, and stimulates maturation of the ovarian follicle and parafollicular cells to produce estrogen. FSH, which can occasionally be found in small amounts in the urine of young girls, increases in amount just prior to puberty,

Figure 6. Lymphatics of the pelvis. A, Aortic. B, Sacral. C, Common iliac. D, Hypogastric. E, Obturator. F, Deep inguinal. G, Cloquet's node. H, Parametrial. I, Superficial inguinal.

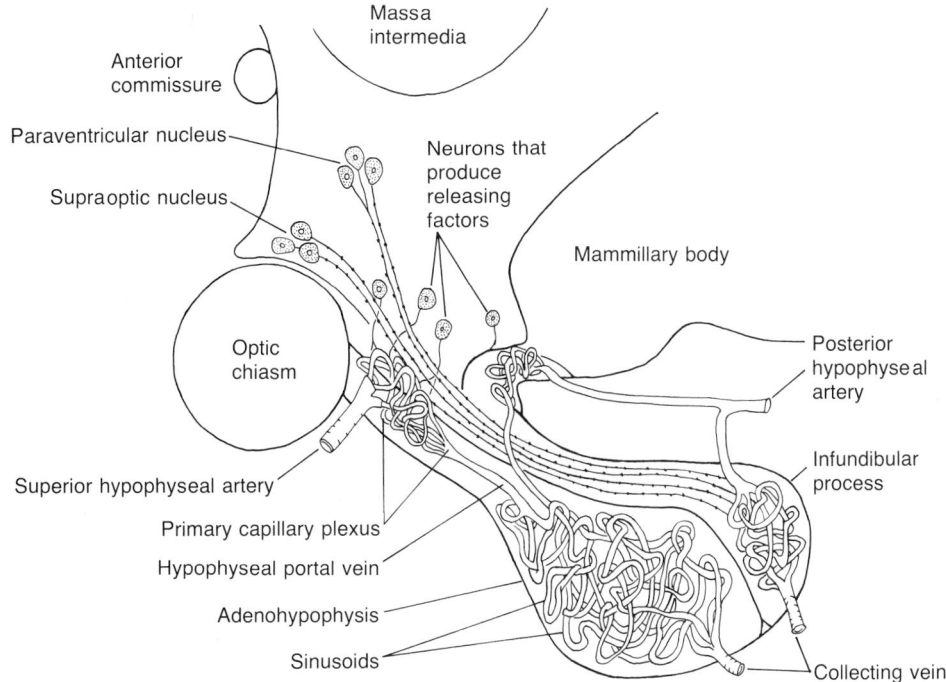

Figure 7. Neural and vascular connections from the hypothalamus to the pituitary. (Redrawn from Radford, H. M.: Proc. Aust. Soc. Anim. Prod., *6*:19, 1966.)

and is found in large amounts in the urine of mature women. After the ovarian failure of menopause, there is a sharp rise in urinary and plasma FSH as the hypothalamus attempts to correct resultant hypoestrogenism. In ovulating women FSH is elevated during the follicular phase of the cycle, then rises sharply at midcycle during ovulation. FSH levels are relatively low during the luteal phase of the cycle. Luteinizing hormone (LH) complements FSH secretion and the two provide a synergistic effect on ovarian function.

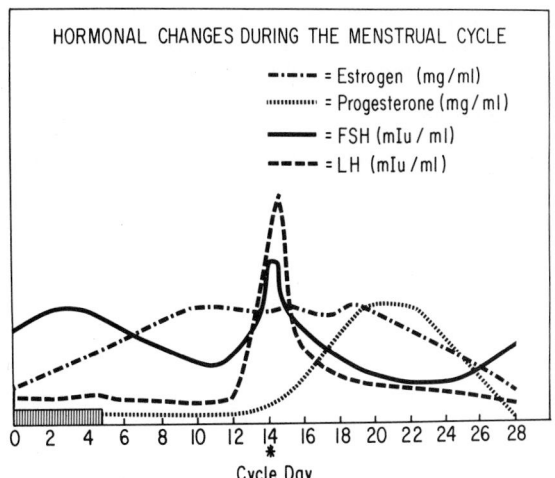

Figure 8. Hormonal changes during the menstrual cycle. Menses, days 0–5; ovulation, day 14.

LH levels are relatively low during the follicular and luteal phases of the menstrual cycle but rise sharply for a 72-hour span surrounding ovulation. Luteinizing hormone, acting on the FSH-stimulated follicle, can cause ovulation. LH also stimulates the interstitial cells of the ovary and may be an integral part of corpus luteum maintenance. Excessive amounts of sex steroid hormones, estrogen, progesterone, or androgens, will inhibit hypothalamic-pituitary secretion.

Ovarian Function (Fig. 9)

During infancy and childhood the ovary is dormant, owing to low gonadotropin production, but is capable of being stimulated if these hormones are present. The beginning of puberty and the age of menarche vary considerably between individuals, but the usual age for the first menstrual period is from 12 to 15 years. The age of menarche may vary normally from the tenth to eighteenth year. The early menstrual periods are usually irregular and anovulatory. Later, regular ovulatory cycles usually ensue. At puberty there is a spurt in somatic growth, probably due to growth hormone production by the pituitary and the growth effect of increased ovarian estrogen on bone. Later in adolescence higher levels of estrogen result in epiphyseal closure.

Before puberty the primordial follicles develop in the deeper portions of the ovary, and after puberty the maturing follicle migrates to the surface of the ovary. After achieving full maturation, the graafian follicle ruptures and the ovum is extruded into the peritoneal cavity, usually around the fourteenth day of the cycle. With rupture of the follicle, the corpus luteum is

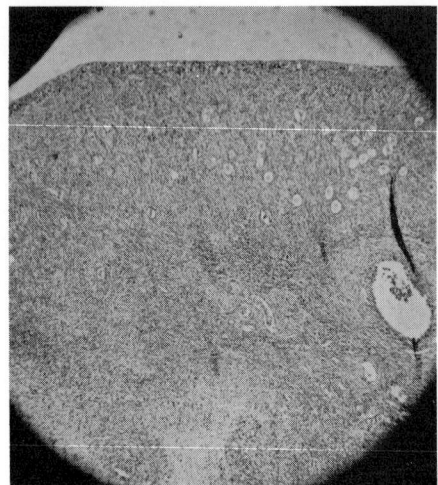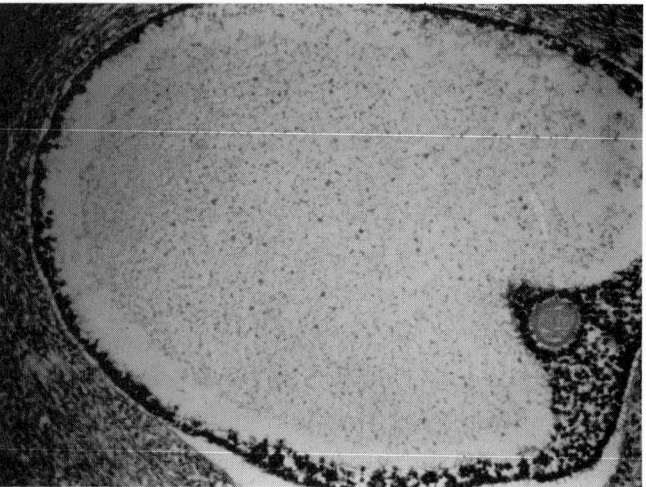

Figure 9. Human ovary with multiple primordial follicles (left) and a higher-power view of a maturing follicle (right).

formed. It persists for 14 days in a normal cycle. Should pregnancy occur, the corpus luteum will persist for approximately 12 weeks before beginning regression. After ovulation the corpus luteum shows hypertrophy and vascularization of the theca lutein cells. The granulosa cells about the follicle become enlarged and polyhedral and are transformed into lutein cells. Progesterone, produced in small amounts just prior to ovulation, is now produced in large amounts. About 4 days before menses the corpus luteum regresses and loses the ability to produce progesterone unless human chorionic gonadotropin from pregnancy sustains corpus luteum function.

Menopause occurs with waning of ovarian function, usually between 45 and 53 years of age. With intrinsic failure of the ovary, there is atresia of the follicles and failure of estrogen production, which is at first sharp but later becomes more gradual, with a minimal amount of estrogen production extending for several additional years. With decline of estrogen the breasts atrophy, the pelvic structures become smaller, and the vaginal mucosa becomes thin and smooth.

Estrogen

Many studies have demonstrated that oophorectomy performed on the immature female is followed by persistent infantile characteristics of genital tissues. If the gonads are removed from a mature female animal, the uterus and breasts atrophy. The human ovary produces primarily estrone, 17β-estradiol, the most potent naturally occurring estrogen, and estriol. These estrogens are produced primarily in the theca interna cells. Preadolescent girls and women beyond the menopause secrete little estrogen. The adult, cycling woman produces 10 to 55 μg. of the various estrogens each day, with a low level during menses which increases steadily until ovulation. After ovulation there is a slight decline, then significant levels persist until 2 to 3 days prior to menses. The placenta and adrenal glands also produce estrogens.

The estrogens are lipids with the same phenanthrene nucleus as the other steroids, from which they are distinguished by a phenolic ring A (Fig. 10). In addition to natural estrogens, chemicals with estrogenic activity have been synthesized. These include diethylstilbestrol, hexestrol, dienestrol, and, most recently, a group of 17 α-ethinyl steroids. The various estrogens are rapidly metabolized by the liver and are conjugated with glucuronic and sulfuric acid. These conjugated compounds are excreted 60 per cent in urine and 40 per cent in bile and feces and by other routes.

The principle physiologic function of estrogen is stimulation of endometrial growth, myometrium, other tissues of müllerian origin, the vulva, and the breast. Estrogen is responsible for uterine and tubal contractility and is the feminizing hormone that at puberty brings about the secondary sex characteristics: mammary growth, primarily of ductal tissue, and the adult female fat pad distribution. A variety of metabolic processes are also influenced by estrogen, notably plasma protein production, bone matrix stabilization, and lipid metabolism.

Progesterone

Progesterone is the other steroid hormone produced by the ovary (Fig. 10). The corpus luteum begins to secrete this hormone just before ovulation and throughout the luteal phase of the cycle. The placenta and adrenal glands also produce progesterone. It is synthesized in the body from cholesterol via pregnenolone and is converted by the ovary to estrogens and small amounts of testosterone. The production rate of progesterone from the ovary and adrenal glands of a normal adult female is approximately 3 mg. per 24 hours during the follicular phase of the cycle and 22 mg. per 24 hours during the luteal phase. Progesterone is readily synthesized for both oral and parenteral use. Natural progesterone is deactivated by gastric secretions. Synthetic progestins are abundantly

OH

ESTRADIOL

ESTRONE

ESTRIOL

PROGESTERONE

PREGNANEDIOL

Figure 10. Structural formulas of three prominent natural estrogens, and progesterone and its main urinary metabolite, pregnanediol.

available and are useful for treating menstrual disorders and endometriosis and for inhibition of ovulation.

Progesterone is essential for the maintenance of pregnancy; initially it is produced by the corpus luteum and later by the placenta. It has not been of major use as a drug for quieting uterine activity or labor. There is some evidence that progesterone reduces tubal activity. Progesterone is responsible for the acinar and lobular development in the breast and for characteristic changes seen in cervical mucus and in cervical and vaginal cytology. Progesterone is thermogenic and basal body temperatures are 0.2 to 0.8° F. higher in the latter half of the ovulatory cycle.

Genital Structures

The female genitalia are responsive to estrogen. In the child these structures are immature and thin and begin to maturate only with pubescence and the onset of ovarian function. The vulva is thin and not prominent. The vaginal epithelium, which is quite thick at birth because of maternal gestational hormones, rapidly regresses to a thin membrane and pH is neutral. With puberty the vagina thickens, glycogen storage increases, and pH becomes more acid. The cycling woman's vagina normally contains diphtheroids and Döderlein's bacilli, which aid normal vaginal secretion and acidity. After menopause, the vagina again becomes thin and loses the normal rugal pattern, and pH slowly rises. Exfoliated vaginal cells may be stained and microscopically examined for histologic changes that occur with the varying hormonal patterns (Fig. 11).

The cervix of the child is disproportionately larger than the fundus, but after puberty this ratio is reversed. As in the vagina, the cervical epithelium undergoes cyclic changes during the menstrual cycle, but these are less than those seen in the endometrium. The racemose glands of the endocervix are dormant in children but initiate secretion of mucus after puberty. Under the dominance of estrogen the cervical mucus increases, is thin and watery, and forms a "fern" pattern when dried (Fig. 11). When progesterone is present cervical mucus is opaque, thick, and tenacious and does not "fern." After menopause cervical mucous production declines as estrogen production declines.

The myometrium of the adult woman normally undergoes spontaneous rhythmic contractions. The uteri of castrates lose this rhythmicity. Hypertrophy of myometrium occurs when higher levels of estrogen are

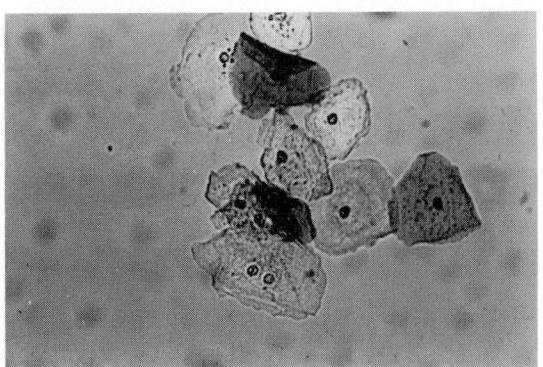

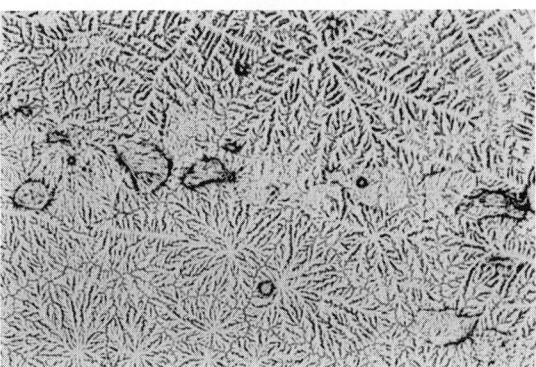

Figure 11. Estrogen effect on exfoliated vaginal cells (left) and cervical mucus (right) with the characteristic "fern" pattern.

present, and uterine atrophy occurs after menopause. The endometrium reflects generally the levels of estrogen and progesterone. Estrogen causes proliferation of the endometrium and its vascular channels. Progesterone transforms proliferative into secretory endometrium with glandular and stromal features that promote possible implantation. Endometrial biopsy is a simple office procedure that may allow precise interpretation of ovarian hormonal production (Fig. 12).

The fallopian tube epithelium also reflects ovarian hormonal changes through cyclic modification, maturation, and regression changes. The tubal musculature possesses an intrinsic peristaltic action believed to aid tubal transport. The action of cilia of certain tubal cells may also be involved in transport. Estrogen appears to influence these activities.

CYTOGENETICS

During the past 15 years observations on the chromosomal etiology of gonadal defects have led to a much better understanding of these problems.[9, 16] In 1938 Turner described seven young girls in whom short stature, sexual infantilism, webbing of the neck, and cubitus valgus were prominent clinical features. These patients were found to have high levels of pituitary gonadotropins, suggesting inadequate ovarian responsiveness, and at laparatomy were found to have either no ovarian tissue or rudimentary streaks of tissue where ovaries should have been. The terms "ovarian agenesis" and "gonadal dysgenesis" were introduced to signify a chromosomally caused gonadal defect.

In 1949 Barr and Bertram demonstrated a characteristic chromatin mass present as a satellite structure on the nuclear membrane of a significant percentage of cells from normal females, but not present on cells of males. This "Barr body" has since been shown

to be the condensed chromatin of the second X chromosome of the normal female complement of XX and its detection can aid in the evaluation of "chromosomal sex." Examination of blood smears from females shows that a percentage of polymorphonuclear leukocytes have "drumstick" projections not seen often in males. In 1956 Tijo and Levan accurately identified the normal human chromosomal karyotype as 46, 22 pairs of autosomes and two sex chromosomes. The normal female sex chromosomal complement is XX; that of the male is XY (Fig. 13).

With these discoveries more fundamental studies of chromosomal aberrations as causes of gonadal defects became possible. Recent studies have shown that sex chromosomal aberrations such as Turner's syndrome, Klinefelter's syndrome, and XXX and XXXY patterns are caused by nondisjunction. Other gonadal defects may occur as a result of mosaicism, chromosomal translocation, isochromosome formation, and deletion during the course of meiosis or mitosis. Problems of pseudohermaphroditism in certain patients suggest mutation of sex chromosomes to yield paradoxical function (testicular feminizing syndrome).

It seems clear that chromosomal surveys should be done in a larger group of patients, particularly those with primary amenorrhea in whom abnormal chromosomal constitutions can be expected in up to 40 per cent.

THE GYNECOLOGIC HISTORY AND EXAMINATION

An adequate history remains a prerequisite for intelligent diagnosis and treatment. All elements of a general medical history are essential to adequate evaluation of pelvic complaints. The gynecologic history should include:

Present illness: A chronological story of the patient's prob-

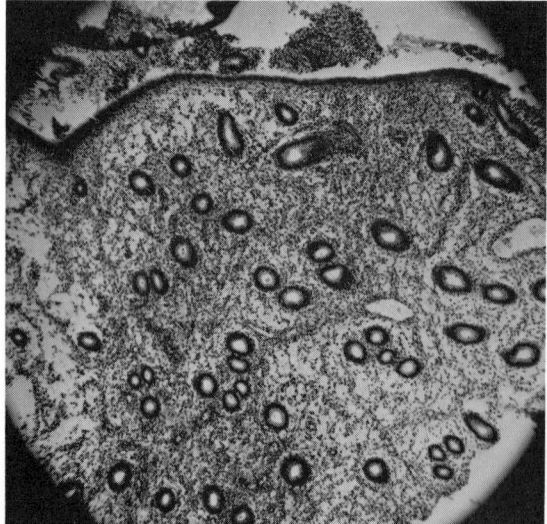
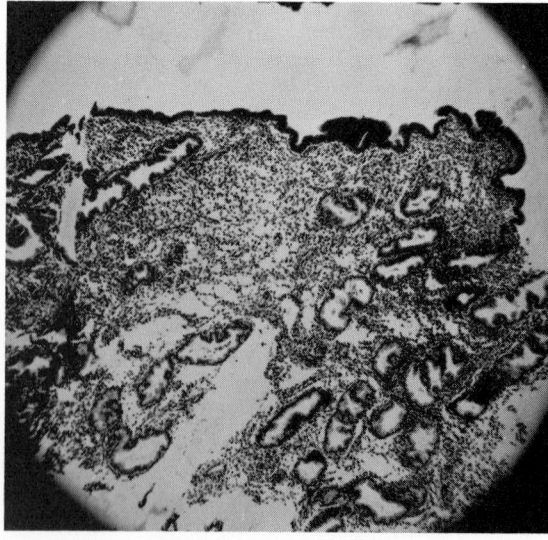

Figure 12. Endometrial biopsies demonstrating the proliferative pattern of estrogen dominance (left), and the secretory effects of progesterone after ovulation (right).

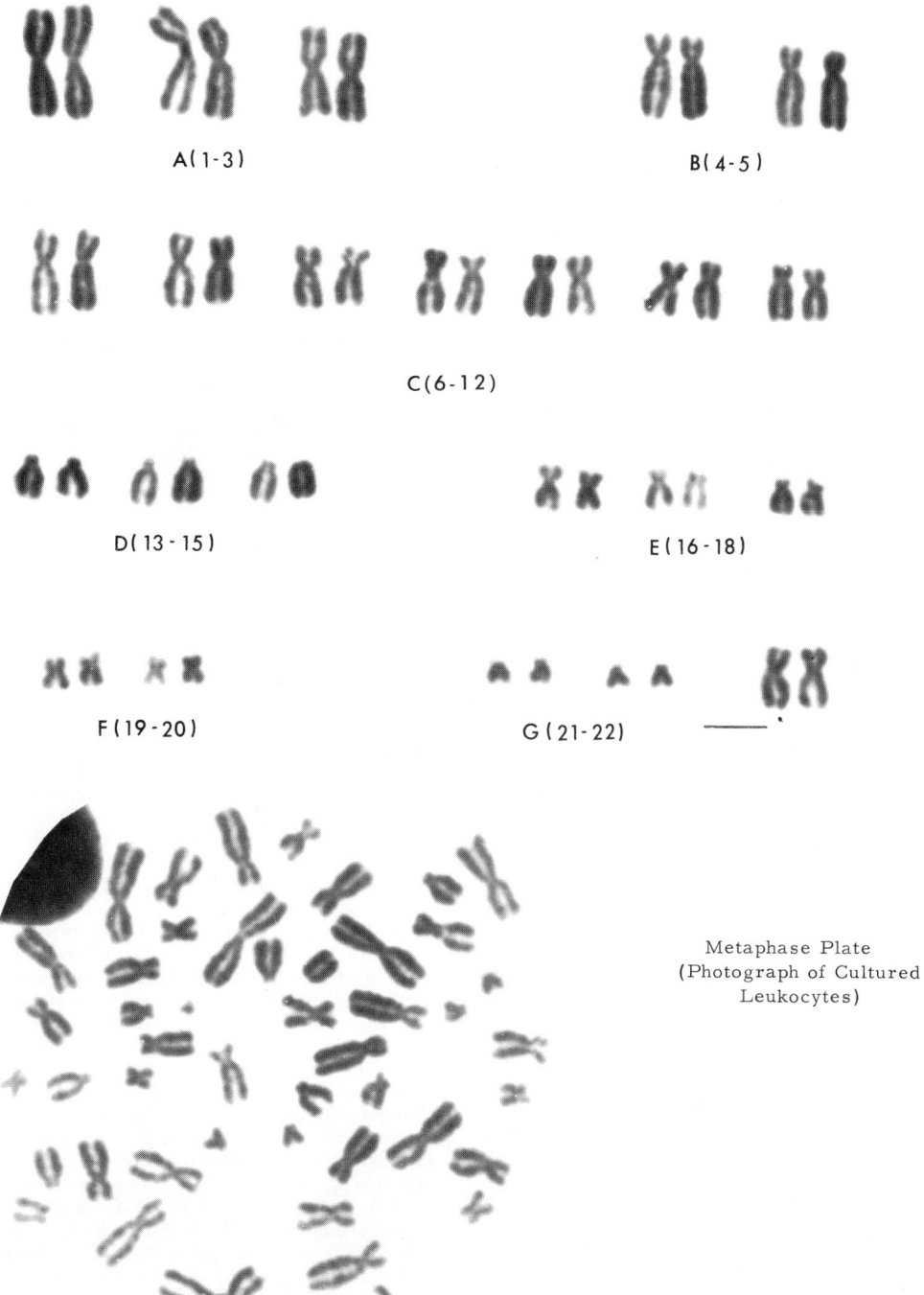

Figure 13. Metaphase plate of the normal female karyotype with XX sex chromosome pattern. (Courtesy of Dr. A. C. Christakos.)

lem, relating symptoms, signs, dates, effects of other organ function, and prior investigation or therapy.

Menstrual pattern: Age at onset of menses; frequency, duration, and amount of flow; menstrual irregularities; date of the first day of the two most recent episodes of menstrual bleeding; history of pain with menses and its location, character, and duration, any vaginal bleeding between periods or after contact as douching or coitus; and any other major physiologic or pathologic changes associated with menses.

Vaginal discharge: Amount, type, color, relation to menses, itching, and previous vaginal infections and therapy.

Obstetric history: Each pregnancy should be listed chronologically with comments about duration, complications, delivery, and the puerperium.

Marital history: The dates of marriages, contraceptive techniques and duration of use, frequency of coitus, and dyspareunia.

Other factors: Sensations of pressure, incontinence, urinary symptoms, bowel complaints, pelvic or abdominal surgery including findings and complications, and a thorough general and endocrine systems review.

The normal woman dislikes a pelvic examination and presents herself for examination with reservation. Gentleness, privacy, and dignity are necessary, and a female chaperone should always be present for assistance, patient reassurance, and protection from possible legal embarrassment. Each step in the pelvic examination should be explained briefly to the patient to gain her confidence and cooperation. The pelvic examination is done with the woman in the lithotomy position with the legs placed in stirrups. Before being placed on the table, the patient should empty her bladder. The chaperone aids in positioning of the patient and drapes her.

The first part of the pelvic examination consists of inspection of the external genitalia for evidence of infection, neoplasia, hypertrophy, atrophy, or trauma. Specific note is made about skin texture, hair patterns, clitoridal size, Skene's ducts, and Bartholin glands. The groins should be examined. The speculum examination is next and a variety of instruments of different sizes and shapes are available. There is no substitute for adequate equipment and lighting. The instrument should be approximately body temperature and lubricated slightly. The vaginal wall and cervix should be inspected for size, shape, and evidence of atrophy, infection, trauma, bleeding, or neoplasia. Specimens can be obtained for cancer cytologic study, hormonal interpretation, and bacteriologic examination. The vagina should be inspected again during withdrawal of the speculum, particularly the anterior and posterior surfaces which may have been covered initially by the blades of the speculum. The patient then performs the Valsalva maneuver while the support of the bladder, rectum, and uterus is visualized and note is made of any stress incontinence.

The examiner then proceeds to the bimanual part of the examination, introducing the first two fingers of one hand into the vagina and palpating above the symphysis with the other hand (Fig. 14). The physician attempts to determine the consistency, size, shape, and mobility of the uterus. After the uterus is palpated, the adnexal regions are felt. Next, it is important to palpate the parametrial and paracervical areas. Finally, a combined rectovaginal examination should be done. In children and virgins, a rectal examination may be all that is possible because of the intact hymen. A child's small speculum or Kelly cystoscope may aid visualization and appropriate smears should be obtained.

LABORATORY AND CLINICAL TESTS

Cytologic Studies

Approximately 20 per cent of cases of cancer in women arise in the genital tract. The most useful techniques for the early detection of genital malignant diseases are the pelvic examination and Papanicolaou studies. It should be routine to utilize these techniques for all new patients and at yearly intervals at least thereafter. Not only can early malignancy be detected but also premalignant changes may frequently be discovered. Malignant and preinvasive lesions arising from the genital organs exfoliate tumor cells which may traverse the intermediate structures and collect in the vaginal pool and on the surface of the cervix. Malignant cells from the vagina and the cervix will be present in 90 per cent of patients with these lesions. If the tumor is of the vulva, it may be missed unless the external genitals are carefully exam-

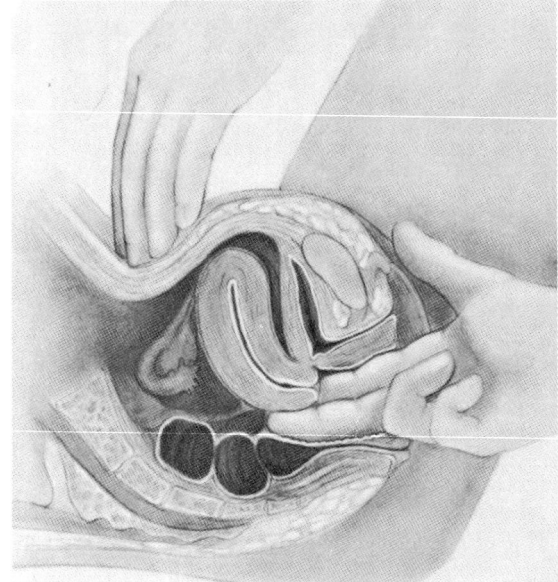

Figure 14. Bimanual pelvic examination. The examiner inserts two fingers into the vagina and places the other hand on the lower abdomen. The structures of the pelvis are then outlined between the two hands. (From Nelson, J. H., Jr.: Atlas of Radical Pelvic Surgery. New York, Appleton-Century-Crofts, 1969.)

ined and direct scrapings obtained from suspicious areas. For endometrial or uterine smears best results are achieved by passing a fine probe, sound, or small brush into the uterine cavity and obtaining direct smears. Malignant tumors of the tubes or ovaries rarely exfoliate cells that can be collected on routine pelvic examination.

Exfoliated cells are collected by aspiration or gently scraping and evenly spread onto glass slides, then immediately fixed in an equal solution of ether and 95 per cent alcohol. Deeper scraping may yield basal cells of different cytologic patterns which may confuse the unwary cytologist. Delay in fixation may allow drying and cytologic alteration. After fixation and Papanicolaou staining, slides should be studied microscopically by an experienced cytologist for cytologic changes compatible with malignancy.

Papanicolaou cervical cytology offers a high degree of accuracy, but can be no better than the material collected. If gross infection or blood and mucus are present, care must be exercised to provide sufficient material for study. Such cytologic studies should be used in the detection of premalignant disease or hidden or occult malignant disease, and for follow-up of patients after treatment of malignant disease. *Cytologic studies should never be used as an indication for surgical or irradiative therapy;* rather, they should lead the examiner to diagnostic surgical studies to provide adequate tissue for histopathologic diagnosis.

Fresh vaginal smears also may be of aid in evaluating the hormonal status of the patient. Such vaginal smears are made by obtaining a drop of material from the vaginal pool. For hormonal studies the material is evenly spread on a slide, then stained (Papanicolaou, eosin Y, or Shorr's) and microscopically examined for biologic changes that occur with estrogen or progesterone (see Fig. 11). Such hormonal values are reported as the maturation or cornification index. Vaginal material obtained for study of the etiology of vaginal infection is mixed with saline, placed on a slide, and microscopically examined for the presence of *Trichomonas vagin-*

alis or *Candida albican* (Fig. 15). Cultures are required for positive identification of vulvovaginal fungi.

Cervical Studies

While Papanicolaou cytology is the major tool in the screening for premalignant cervical or vaginal neoplasia, other techniques also may be of use. Gross visualization of the cervix is mandatory and any suspicious areas should be biopsied, usually without anesthesia. The cervix may be painted with an iodine solution, such as Schiller's stain, with which normal cells rich in glycogen stain darkly, whereas neoplastic cells do not take the stain. This technique, as well as colposcopy or colpomicroscopy (microscopic visualization of the cervix in situ), can serve to direct biopsies for histologic diagnosis. If abnormal Papanicolaou smears have been reported, use must be made of either multiple biopsies or cold-knife conization of the cervix, which removes the exocervix, including the squamocolumnar junction, and the endocervical canal (Fig. 16). The important fact is not to miss the diagnosis of invasive carcinoma. Presumption of a benign or premalignant diagnosis on the basis of cytology alone may result in a patient with occult invasive carcinoma receiving inadequate therapy.

The colposcope (Hinselman, 1924) and the colpomicroscope (Antoine, 1954) have recently become most valuable tools in the evaluation of suspected neoplastic genital lesions. Magnification, coupled with various staining techniques, allows an accurate *in vivo* analysis of genital neoplasia and enables the examiner to direct biopsies to suspicious lesions which might not be noted during a nonmagnified evaluation. Other cervical studies include investigation of cervical mucus for various hormonal changes such as spinn-barkeit and ferning (see Fig. 11) produced by estrogen or progesterone.

Cervical smears and cultures are quite important for the diagnosis of gonorrhea, but all too often negative results are obtained because of faulty technique. To properly obtain cervical cultures a vaginal speculum is inserted and the cervix is wiped clean with cotton swabs. Through compressive force of the blades of the speculum on the anterior and posterior cervix, the mucus of the endocervical glands is "milked" into the endocervical canal. A sterile culture swab is introduced into the endocervical canal, with care not to contaminate the swab with other vaginal secretions. One such swab is spread on a slide, dried, stained with Gram's stain, and examined under high microscopic power for the classic gram-negative intracellular diplococci. Another swab is immediately plated onto Thayer-Martin medium, and then incubated in carbon dioxide for culture identification. One should never inform a patient that she unequivocally has gonorrhea on the basis of a smear, although therapy can be initiated. Diagnosis of this disease without culture identification may be fraught with legal hazard.

Endometrial Studies

The endometrial biopsy is used to study hormonal effects, fertility, and ovulatory factors and, on occasion, to aid in the diagnosis of malignancy. The procedure is done without anesthesia and discomfort is minimal. By the insertion of a fine curet several samples of endometrium can be obtained for histopathologic examination. Endocrine changes are reflected quite adequately through such endometrial biopsy techniques and, by timing the biopsy to the latter half of the menstrual cycle, the presence of progesterone and ovulation can be detected. For conditions of abnormal bleeding or abnormal genital cytology the endometrial biopsy or fluid washing (irrigation of the uterine cavity) may provide tissue adequate for diagnosis. If the diagnosis is negative, however, an indicated dilation and curettage should seldom be replaced by endometrial biopsy, since the tissue sampled by curettage is considerably greater and diagnosis more accurate.

Pregnancy Tests

Pregnancy may be detected by a variety of tests that detect the presence of human chorionic gonadotropin (HCG). Most biologic tests have been replaced by immunologic tests which give a positive result with a urinary level of 0.5 to 1.0 IU per milliliter, concentrations that are usually achieved 2 weeks after the first missed menstrual period. False-positive pregnancy tests can occur. As HCG and pituitary luteinizing hormone (LH) cross-react, these tests are intentionally set at higher levels to reduce false-positive results from the hypergonadotropinuria of normally timed or premature menopause. To adequately measure normal pituitary gonadotropins, 0.005 IU per milliliter or less, sensitive biologic assays on urinary concentrates or the new, highly sensitive radioimmunoassay must be employed.

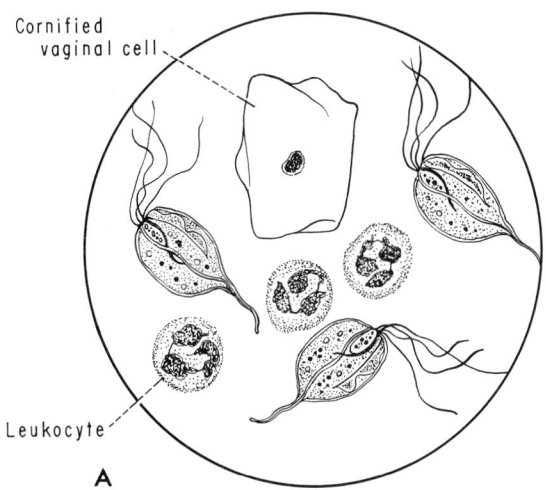

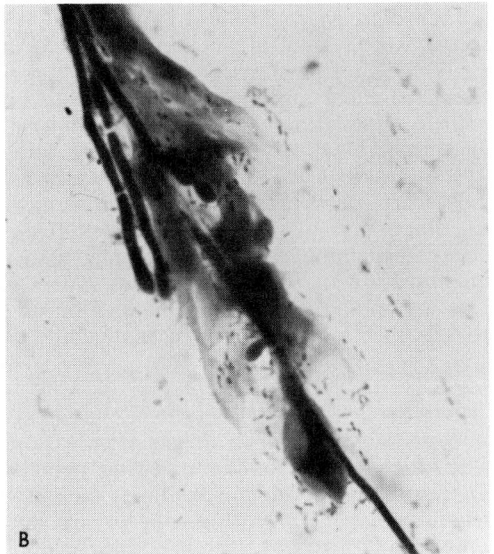

Figure 15. Preparations of vaginal secretions showing: *A*, trichomonads, about one-half the size of a cornified vaginal cell but larger than leukocytes, and *B*, the fiber-like mycelia of *Candida albicans*. (From Gynecology: Principles and Practice by Robert W. Kistner. Copyright © 1964, Year Book Medical Publishers. Used by permission.)

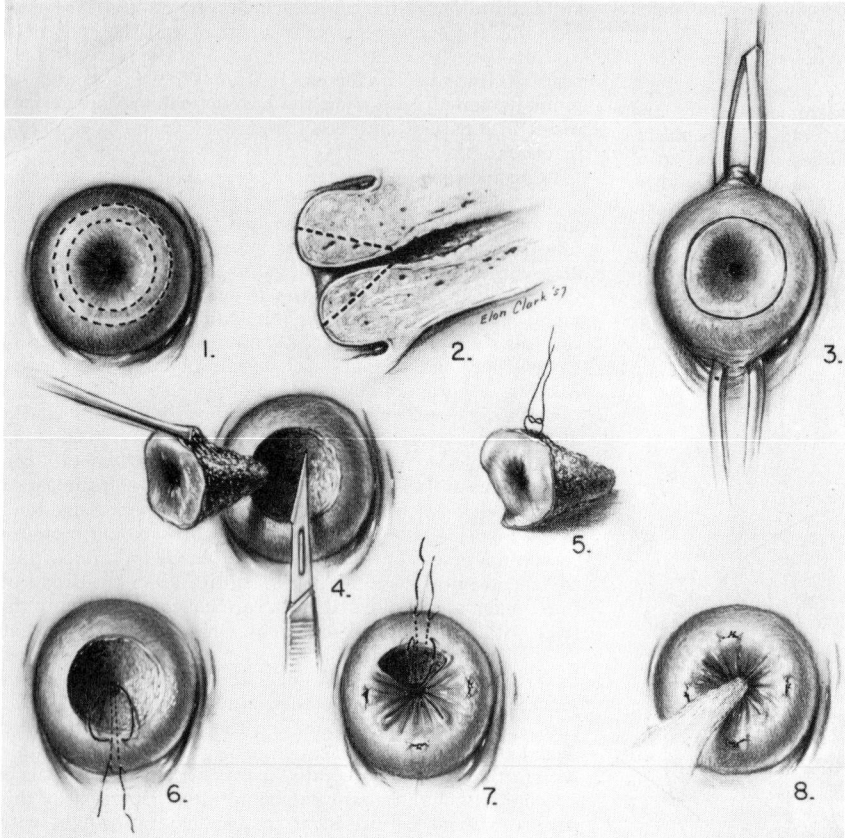

Figure 16. Technique of cold-knife conization of the cervix. (From Parker, R. T.: Obstet. Gynecol. Survey, *24*:691, 1969.)

Other Studies

Several other diagnostic tests should be mentioned. Hysterosalpingography is a technique by which a cannula attached to the cervix allows the uterine cavity and fallopian tubes to be filled with a radiopaque dye.[6] By appropriate x-ray techniques the endometrial cavity and tubes can be outlined quite adequately. Laparoscopy and culdoscopy are techniques by which the pelvic viscera can be directly visualized by a transperitoneal route and with a minimum of morbidity.

CONGENITAL ANOMALIES

Imperforate Hymen

An imperforate hymen may lead to retention of mucus or blood, causing hematocolpos, hematometrium, hematosalpinx, and even hemoperitoneum. Such defects are rarely recognized until after puberty and the onset of menses, and may present as primary amenorrhea, pelvic pain, or a palpable abdominal-pelvic mass. Diagnosis is based on careful examination of the external genitals, which reveals a bulging hymen without communication with the vagina, and a fluctuant pelvic mass that lies anterior to the rectum. With adequate surgical drainage the distended structures will promptly return to normal.

A transverse vaginal septum is rare but may present in similar fashion to that of imperforate hymen. A vertical vaginal septum occurs with failure of müllerian fusion. In both cases the septum can be partial or complete. Therapy, if necessary at all, is surgical excision.

Defects of Müllerian Fusion (Fig. 17)

Other defects in müllerian fusion can present a spectrum of congenital anomalies. As one tube and half of the uterine fundus, cervix, and upper vagina arise from each müllerian duct, improper fusion can result in duplication of part or all of the system. One abnormality is uterus didelphys with two vaginas, cervices, and uteri, each with a separate tube and ovary. Such patients can present with pelvic pain due to obstruction of outflow of blood from one uterine horn, as an intra-abdominal crisis if pregnancy occurs in a rudimentary uterine horn that cannot expand properly, or as an undiagnosed pelvic mass. Therapy, if indicated, is surgical excision or reconstruction.

Dysgenesis

There are a variety of defects of the female genital tract due to hypoplasia or aplasia of its various components. Such defects may occur either primarily or as secondary underdevelopment due to lack of estrogen. Congenital absence of both ovaries is rare, but absence of one tube or ovary at birth is not unusual. There are cases of complete absence of the vagina, usually associated with absence of the uterus, and congenital absence of the uterus despite a normal vagina. In these patients the testicular feminizing syndrome should be suspected, in which the gonad is testicular, yet secondary sexual characteristics are feminine. Most of these patients present with primary amenorrhea and are infertile. Jacobs has shown that 40 per cent of patients with primary amenorrhea have demonstrable chromosomal abnormalities or sex inversions of some type. Buccal smears and karyotypic studies are therefore important. In patients with vaginal agenesis a normally functional vagina can be surgically created by dissection or progressive dilation of the potential space between bladder and rectum. Skin grafting may be required. Such reconstruction should be delayed until just prior to marriage as repetitive dilation is mandatory to retain patency. If the primary defect is due to ovarian abnormalities, replacement of estrogen provides a growth stimulus to the genital structures. In patients with testicular feminization the intra-abdominal gonad should be removed in late adolescence because of the high rates of malignancy during the third and fourth decades of life.

Hermaphroditism

True hermaphroditism, a medical rarity, exists when male and female gonadal tissue is present in the same person. Most hermaphrodites are pseudohermaphrodites, or persons who possess the genitalia of one sex and gonads of the opposite sex. Chromosomal studies are of use in evaluating such patients and the reader is referred to excellent review articles of Miller and Simpson.[9, 16] A male pseudohermaphrodite has testes with the genitalia of a female. An example is the testicular feminization syndrome. A female pseudohermaphrodite has ovaries but the external genitals resemble those of a male. Such persons usually have a combination of anatomic maldevelopment and congenital adrenal hyperplasia. In these patients excess androgen from the hyperfunctioning fetal adrenal cortex results in persistence of the urogenital sinus and marked hypertrophy of the clitoris. The vagina, cervix, uterus, tubes, and ovaries are present but hypoplastic and nonfunctional. Patients with these abnormalities usually present with problems in sexual identification or with primary genital failure at puberty with amenorrhea or male hypogonadism. Therapy is fraught with problems, as the patient's personality, age, and psyche must be carefully weighed in

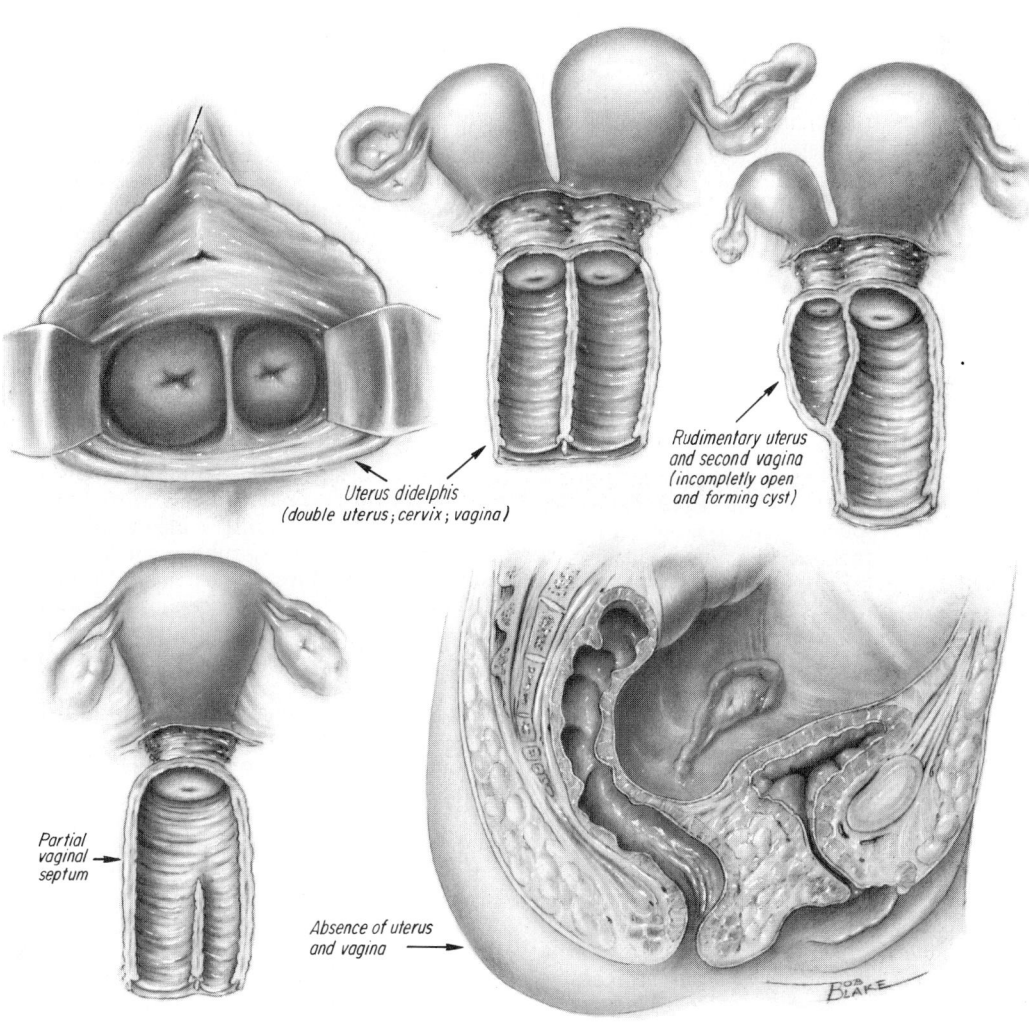

Uterus didelphis
(double uterus; cervix; vagina)

Rudimentary uterus
and second vagina
(incompletly open
and forming cyst)

Partial
vaginal
septum

Absence of uterus
and vagina

Figure 17. Abnormalities of genital formation.

relation to anatomy. In some cases it may be best to assist and encourage the patient to continue to live as previously identified, even if gonadal biopsy shows her to be of the opposite sex. In other patients it may be appropriate to reverse the previous sexual identification by surgery and hormone administration.

During the evaluation of patients with congenital anomalies of the female genital system, one should always evaluate the urinary system. Associated urinary anomalies are quite common, occurring in as many as 50 per cent of such patients.

Wolffian Duct Persistence

Other congenital anomalies of the female genital system consist of those derived from remnants of the mesonephric duct or the wolffian duct and body, which normally regress during female genital development. The most common of these is the parovarian cyst which arises from the upper wolffian duct and may grow as large as 20 cm. There are no symptoms specific to a parovarian cyst to differentiate it from an ovarian cyst. The treatment is surgical excision with preservation of the tube and ovary. A similar cyst, the hydatid of Morgagni, may also develop near the distal end of the fallopian tube. Significant enlargement of these cysts is rare, and only under unusual circumstances is their removal mandatory. Similarly, the wolffian system may give rise to Gartner's duct cysts. As the lower portion of the wolffian duct courses along the lateral vaginal wall, remnants persist and may later form this tubular cystic tumor mass. Only if dyspareunia develops because of excessive size is surgical excision indicated. Finally, remnants of the mesonephric system may remain in the cervix, broad ligament, and ovarian hilus and develop into bizarre varieties of malignant neoplasms. These include clear cell tumors, adenocarcinomas, and mixed tumors.

THE VULVA

The gynecologist faces an exceptional variety of problems in the area of the external genitals. Trauma, allergy, inflammatory conditions, infections, degenerative changes, and neoplasia give rise to disorders ranging from minor annoyances to major hazards to life.

The vulva is rich in pigment, which increases in pregnancy. Vitiligo of the vulvar skin is no different from the same lesion in other locations, nor does it require treatment. Vitiligo should not be confused with leukoplakia, in which the skin is whitish, but thickened and leathery. Various skin eruptions involving the body as a whole may affect the vulva and appear as do other lesions elsewhere on the body. Varicose veins of the vulva often are found in association with varicosities of the lower extremities, and pregnancy may cause further hypertrophy. Therapy consists of lower extremity and vulvar support and ligation or injection in the nonpregnant state. A severe direct blow to the vulva may be complicated by subcutaneous hematoma formation. Such a hematoma may dissect widely beneath the fascia of the vulva and it is usually necessary to carry out surgical evacuation. It

is frequently difficult to isolate bleeding points and packing is often required. Vulvar lacerations should be cleansed and sutured as lacerations elsewhere on the body.

Glandular Lesions

The vulvar glands are subject to a variety of disorders. Skenitis usually occurs as a consequence of gonococcal infection. In the acute phase an exudate may be expressed from ductal orifices and the patient often has dysuria and other symptoms of urethral irritation. In chronic infections secondary organisms are usually present and on occasion these glands may become abscessed and require surgical drainage. Antibiotic therapy is indicated for both acute and chronic infections. Infections and cysts of Bartholin glands are common. A Bartholin abscess should be treated with heat until fluctuant, and then sharply incised on the mucocutaneous junction between the vagina and vulva. After drainage the margins of the incison are marsupialized with interrupted sutures of fine chromic catgut. Bartholin abscesses may occur from gonococcal infection but more commonly other organisms are involved. Antibiotic therapy is indicated in cases of significant cellulitis or systemic symptoms, but drainage remains the treatment of choice. Bartholin cysts may be marsupialized or excised, but the latter procedure is usually associated with significant blood loss. Small asymptomatic Bartholin cysts usually require no treatment unless biopsy is necessary to exclude malignancy. The vulva is also a common site of sebaceous cysts. These may be removed if they become greatly enlarged or secondarily infected. Rarely, one may find vulvar apocrine tumors, hidradenomas, as raised, red, sessile masses less than 5 cm. in diameter. These are treated by wide local excision.

Vulvitis

Vulvar irritation occurs from a variety of causes, allergic, infectious, degenerative, or neoplastic. Pruritus accompanied by vaginal infection or vulvar skin change suggests allergy as the underlying cause. Usually the sensitivity is due to undergarments made of synthetic fibers or washed with harsh detergents. Other contact irritants can include soaps, vaginal lubricants or sprays, rubber condoms, and spermicidal foams or jellies. Other causes of vulvar irritation include pediculosis pubis or mechanical irritation from obesity, clothing, or menstrual pads. Intestinal parasites may remain on the vulva and cause irritation. Systemic diseases as Hodgkin's disease, diabetes mellitus, leukemia, congestive heart failure, and anemia may cause vulvar irritation. Inadequate nutrition, poor hygiene, and vitamin deficiencies also have been associated with vulvar irritation. The basic principles of management of a patient with vulvitis are to search thoroughly for a diagnosis, treat any specific infectious disease, investigate possible allergies, and then keep the area clean and dry and avoid trauma from scratching, harsh soaps, drugs, ointments, or rubbing with a towel.

The most common cause of vulvar irritation is an infectious vulvovaginitis caused by either *Candida albicans* or *Trichomonas vaginalis* or both. The vulva appears swollen and red and may be excoriated and secondarily infected. Mycotic vulvovaginitis is a common problem among diabetics, oral contraceptive users, and persons receiving systemic antibiotics. Diagnosis is based on fresh-preparation identification of yeast or Trichomonas (see Fig. 15). Therapy is discussed in the section dealing with vaginitis. For both types of infection immediate relief is obtained by additional use of topical creams containing hydrocortisone, or nystatin (Mycostatin), as well as the general instructions for nonspecific vulvitis.

Follicular vulvitis may occur and penicillin treatment and local therapy are recommended. Another cause of infectious vulvitis is herpes progenitalis infection with painful vesicular eruptions. Treatment is supportive. Finally, condylomata acuminata, or venereal warts, occur as a presumed infectious vulvitis of viral origin but also are associated with any irritating vaginal discharge. These benign epithelial neoplasms may be few or many, even to covering the entire perineum and extending onto the vagina or cervix (Fig. 18). Therapy is topical use of podophyllin or 5-flourouracil. Cautery is used for the more extensive forms of the disease but requires an anesthetic.

Recently, there has been a near epidemic of sexually transmitted vulvovaginitis caused by *Herpes progenitalis* (*H. simplex*, Type II). This infection is characterized by vesicular eruptions which are extremely painful and often are secondarily infected when the patient is seen. Current therapy includes warm baths in water containing potassium permanganate, drying, and systemic analgesics. The use of various dyes and ultraviolet light have now fallen out of use. The duration of this infection is usually limited to 1 to 2 weeks, but it may recur.

Other venereal diseases may present as vulvar lesions. These include the primary chancre of syphilis or the moist, grayish patches (condylomata lata) of secondary syphilis. After dark-field examination for diagnosis, therapy consists of penicillin or its substitute. Granuloma inguinale is a rare infectious disease of the vulva caused by the Donovan bacillus. A scraping of the serpiginous lesion may reveal the intracellular Donovan body. Streptomycin, chloramphenicol (Chloromycetin), and tetracyclines are most useful agents for this disease. Lymphogranuloma venereum is a disease of viral origin, associated frequently with inguinal adenitis, multiple draining sinuses, and rectal stricture. The diagnosis is made by the Frei skin test. Chloromycetin and tetracycline are useful, as are the sulfonamides. Chancroid is caused by the gram-negative Ducrey's bacillus. It appears as a small papule 2 to 4 days after exposure, and afterward becomes an indurated and punched-out lesion with soft edges and a purulent surface. Inguinal adenitis, often suppurative, is a frequent occurrence. Chancroid is treated with sulfonamides, although other broad-spectrum antibiotics may be useful.

Degenerative Diseases of the Vulva

There are three degenerative diseases of the vulva, all occurring most frequently after menopause. All result in itching, pain, dyspareunia, and frequent secondary infection. These diseases are more commonly seen after vulvar irradiation or premature menopause. The incidence of vulvar carcinoma is increased with these lesions and biopsy should be employed when necessary to rule out neoplasia. Papanicolaou cytology of scrapings is of aid.

Kraurosis vulvae is a disease in which the vulva appears shrunken and dried. Leukoplakia, another degenerative vulvar disease, presents initially as a hypertrophic lesion and later as an atrophic problem. The skin is whitened and leathery. Lichen sclerosus et atrophicus may be difficult to differentiate from either kraurosis or leukoplakia. This is a slowly changing, chronic, localized lesion but, unlike the other two problems, tends to involve the skin of the thighs. In all three lesions an intense pruritus frequently occurs and excoriation with secondary infection is often noted. Approximately 50 per cent of vulvar carcinomas are found in areas of these degenerative lesions, and both cytologic smears and biopsy should be frequently used. Treatment of these three lesions is symptomatic with relief of pruritus a primary goal. Topical and systemic estrogens may offer some aid. Local excision is frequently necessary and with more extensive lesions simple vulvectomy may be required.

Carcinoma-in-situ of the Vulva

Bowen originally described a preinvasive cancer of the skin of the vulva and others have noted a high incidence of this disease associated with previous venereal disease. Carcinoma-in-situ of the vulva may appear in a woman who has leukoplakia, kraurosis vulvae, or lichen sclerosus et atrophicus, with or without pruritus. The diagnosis should be made only after adequate histologic study shows the criteria of intra-

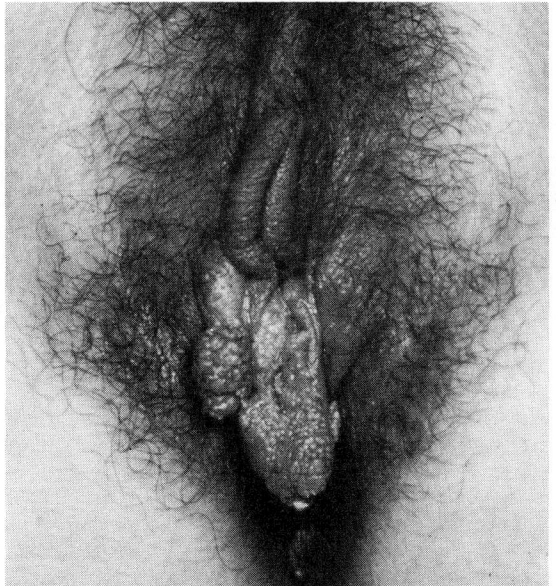

Figure 18. Condylomata acuminata. These growths may appear anywhere on the vulva. They may be either broad and confluent or papillary. (Courtesy of Mr. C. P. Jones.)

epithelial changes characteristic of epidermoid carcinoma, but without invasion. Treatment should be simple vulvectomy in most instances. In patients with carcinoma-in-situ of the vulva, up to 35 per cent may have a second genital malignant lesion. In approximately 15 per cent of patients with either intraepithelial or invasive carcinoma of the vulva carcinoma of the vagina or cervix later develops. Thus, patients with carcinoma-in-situ of the vulva should be carefully followed.

Carcinoma of the Vulva (Fig. 19)

Vulvar cancers compose about 3.5 per cent of all genital cancers, and the peak incidence occurs in the seventh decade of life. Way reports that among patients with vulvar cancer 20 per cent were between 20 and 50 years old, 26 per cent were in the sixth decade, and 40 per cent were in the 61 to 70 year age range.[20] In approximately half of the patients the cancer develops in areas of pre-existing leukoplakia, kraurosis vulvae, or lichen sclerosus et atrophicus, and others report a high incidence of syphilis and other vulvar venereal diseases among these patients. Most patients with vulvar carcinoma complain of a mass on the vulva or perineum, ulceration or vulvar irritation, or pruritus. Bleeding and pain may be additional findings. Any firm tumor or ulceration must be biopsied and the biopsy should include the primary lesion and some adjacent normal tissue. There is an average patient delay of 20 months from discovery of some vulvar abnormality.

Carcinoma of the vulva is usually squamous (95 per cent) but adenocarcinoma, melanocarcinoma, basal cell carcinoma, and Paget's disease are reported. Squamous cancer may arise anywhere on the vulva, but lesions of the labia majora or labia minora are most frequent. Most squamous cancers of the vulva are rather well differentiated. Adenocarcinoma of the vulva usually arises from Bartholin glands, but may develop from paraurethral glands or embryonic cell nests. Melanocarcinoma is an infrequently found vulvar cancer, as is Paget's disease, a slowly spreading ulcerative eczematoid lesion of the vulvar skin, which is thought to be an adenocarcinoma of the apocrine sweat glands of that region. Basal cell carcinoma of the vulva is most frequently seen on the labium majus but may appear on other structures. Microscopically, basal cell carcinoma shows extensive proliferation of the cells of the basal layer of the epidermis, which invade the dermis beneath and usually present as a crater-like ulcer. Unlike other varieties of vulvar cancer, basal cell carcinoma usually does not metastasize but grows deeply into underlying or adjacent tissues. Some basal cell cancers have squamous cell carcinoma elements.

Vulvar cancer tends to spread by local extension and lymphatic metastasis. The frequency and sites of metastasis are dependent upon the size, location, and differentiation of the vulvar lesion. Of those in whom the primary lesion is less than 1.5 cm. in diameter, approximately 12 per cent have positive lymph nodes. However, if the vulvar lesion measures 1.5 to 3.0 cm. in diameter, the incidence of lymph node metastasis is 45 per cent. Way found lymph node metastasis in 62 per cent of cases of anaplastic cancer, but if the primary tumor was well differentiated the incidence of lymphatic metastasis was only 35 per cent. The primary lymphatic drainage of the vulva is via superficial inguinal lymph nodes of that side. From there, the lymphatics drain via Cloquet's node to the external iliac nodes and up the aortic chain. Contralateral vulvar drainage may occur, however, even from well-lateralized lesions. The upper vulvar areas, principally around the clitoris, may drain directly to Cloquet's node, which then may be involved with tumor while the superficial inguinal nodes are negative. Vulvar lesions in the perineal, Bartholin, or posterior fourchette areas may involve the rectovaginal septum, rectum, or vagina and may metastasize via the deep pelvic nodes. Way has demonstrated the difficulty of detecting inguinal node metastases by palpation, as many enlarged nodes will not contain metastases, while nodes normal to palpation may have tumor cells when microscopically examined.[20] In general, however, if the primary vulvar lesion is small and the superficial inguinal lymphatics and Cloquet's node are negative, it is unlikely that the deeper nodes will be involved. Metastasis may also occur to the skin of the thigh, pubis, groin, and to the bladder, urethra, upper vagina, or retrovaginal septum. Blood-borne metastases are unusual.

The treatment of vulvar cancer is surgical. Radiotherapy has been of little use for primary or recurrent disease, and is contraindicated because of the risk of intense vulvar necrosis. Basal cell carcinoma and Paget's disease of the vulva should be treated with wide and deep local excision of the tumor and, if it is large, hemivulvectomy should be done. Removal of regional lymph nodes is not indicated. The prognosis is generally excellent, but these patients should be followed closely for local recurrence. *Such operations*

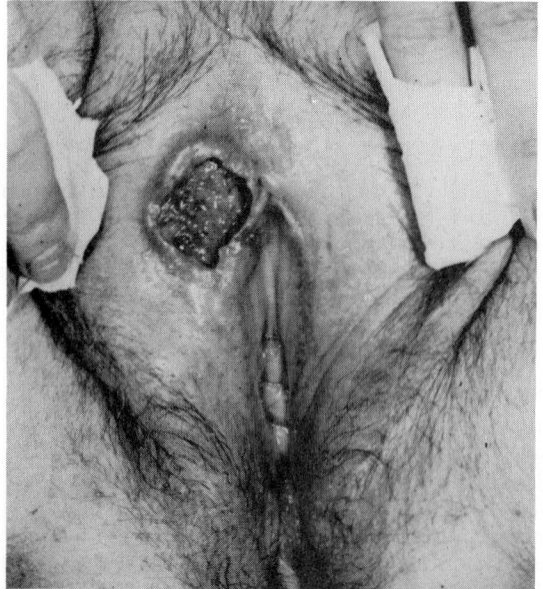

Figure 19.   Carcinoma of the vulva. (Courtesy of Mr. C. P. Jones.)

as local excision, hemivulvectomy, and simple vulvectomy have proved to be inadequate therapy for the other forms of vulvar cancer. Most authors have outlined appropriate therapy as including at least a block dissection of the vulva, in continuity, removing the skin, subcutaneous tissues, and lymphatic tissues of the groins, vulva, and perineum as one specimen. Controversy exists as to whether all patients should also have a retroperitoneal node dissection to include removal of the femoral, iliac, and obturator nodes. These procedures are usually done as a one-stage operation, but may be divided, with the deep node dissection performed later. Utilizing the radical vulvectomy and node dissections, one can expect a 5-year cure rate of over 80 per cent in patients without positive nodes, and a 5-year survival of 47 per cent of patients with positive inguinal nodes. Overall, the 5-year cure rate after surgical therapy of cancer of the vulva is approximately 60 per cent. If the vulvar lesion involves the vagina, rectum, or urethra, then pelvic exenteration may be the operation of choice. Recurrence of surgically treated vulvar cancer may occur at the skin margins of the primary operation or in the skin of the groin. Distant metastases may also develop. Therapy of recurrent vulvar cancer with local excision or chemotherapy may provide palliation.

THE VAGINA

The stratified squamous epithelium of the vagina is histologically similar to epithelium of the cervix and the skin of the vulva, and responds by proliferation to estrogen. The vagina of the child and that of the postmenopausal woman are similar in that the epithelial layer is quite thin, is easily traumatized, and is subject to a variety of infections. The normal adult vagina contains diphtheroids, Döderlein's bacilli, and anaerobic streptococci. This flora converts glycogen of vaginal cells to lactic acid, which maintains the vagina with an acid pH and enhances normal secretions.

Vaginitis

Vaginal inflammation can occur from protozoan, fungal, bacterial, or viral infection and also from deficiencies of estrogen. *Trichomonas vaginalis* is a common protozoan organism causing pruritus, tenderness, and dyspareunia. Trichomonas vaginitis is characterized by a foamy, greenish yellow vaginal exudate; the vaginal walls are erythematous and tender. The diagnosis of this infection is made by high-power microscopic examination of fresh preparations of the vaginal discharge and identification of the flagellated, motile organisms which are the size of leukocytes (see Fig. 15). There is uncertainty about the epidemiology of trichomonas vaginitis, but it is seen most commonly among sexually active women. The male sexual partner may harbor these organisms without symptoms and promptly reinfect the woman who has been treated successfully. This infection is also frequently seen in chronically ill and debilitated women and in women with other pelvic infections. Current therapy consists of oral metronidazole (Flagyl) for both sexual partners.

Candida albicans is probably the most frequent and bothersome cause of vaginitis. The wide use of antibiotics and oral contraceptives predisposes to this fungal infection, as does diabetes mellitus. Symptoms are vaginal discharge, vulvar and vaginal irritation, and itching. Inspection reveals a "curdy" white vaginal exudate, intense vaginal erythema, and a white watery discharge. Diagnosis is made from fresh preparations of vaginal discharge which microscopically reveal the mycelia as threadlike fibers or budding forms (see Fig. 15). Cultures on Sabouraud's medium may be necessary to identify the etiology of low-grade vaginitis. Therapy consists of the intravaginal application of Mycostatin suppositories each night for 2 weeks, including during the menses if it occurs. There is a tendency for vaginal moniliasis to recur and in these patients one should consider evaluation for diabetes mellitus. If such a patient is taking oral contraceptives, their use may have to be temporarily terminated until the infection is controlled.

Vaginal irritation can occur in the patient with insufficient estrogen to maintain normal vaginal thickness. Infection of this thin, atrophic, easily traumatized vagina is nonspecific and caused by a variety of usually nonpathogenic bacteria. Treatment is replacement of systemic or topical estrogen. *Haemophilus vaginalis* can also cause severe vaginitis. Treatment with sulfonamides or tetracyclines is usually successful after smear or culture diagnosis is made. Herpes simplex virus may result in an intense, painful vaginitis that is associated with a granular surface and vesicular eruptions. The diagnosis is made clinically and by serial serum antibody determinations. Therapy is supportive but, fortunately, the disease usually terminates within 2 to 3 weeks. Gonorrhea is an occasional cause of vaginitis in the child. The diagnosis is made by smear and culture and therapy with penicillin is recommended. Children with vaginitis should be examined for intestinal parasites and intravaginal foreign bodies. Rarely do these last three causes of childhood vaginitis produce similar problems in the adult.

Dysplasia and Intraepithelial Carcinoma of the Vagina

Dysplasia of the vaginal epithelium may be the source of abnormal genital smears even if the cervix is normal or absent. Treatment consists of excision or cryosurgery to remove abnormal epithelium. Intraepithelial carcinoma may also develop, most commonly in patients treated previously for other lower genital tract cancers. These lesions may occur at the apex of the vagina in patients after hysterectomy or may be multifocal in areas remote from the vaginal apex. As in dysplasia, intraepithelial carcinoma of the vagina causes no specific symptoms. Diagnosis is suspected from genital cytology and confirmed by biopsy. Therapy can be by irradiation or surgery, either partial or total colpectomy. These lesions justify the close follow-up suggested for patients, even adequately treated, who have had other lower genital tract cancers. Results of therapy are excellent.

Carcinoma of the Vagina

Primary carcinoma of the vagina is a rare lesion, and most are epidermoid in variety. Postcontact bleeding is the usual presenting complaint. Many patients with invasive vaginal carcinoma have previously had other preinvasive or invasive epidermoid lesions of the lower genital system. Primary vaginal cancer may occur in any location, but prognosis is considerably more grave if the lesion is situated anteriorly. The current classification of primary vaginal cancer (International Federation of Gynecology and Obstetrics) includes: Stage I, limited to the vaginal mucosa; Stage II, subvaginal tissue involved, but not to the pelvic wall; Stage III, tumor extended to the pelvic wall or to the symphysis, but not fixed to the symphysis; Stage IV, tumor fixed to symphysis, outside the pelvis, or proved by biopsy to involve the bladder or rectum. Treatment may be by irradiation or surgery. Rutledge's most recent review of radiation therapy of primary vaginal carcinoma describes the type of treatment varying according to the location of the vaginal lesion. In general, it consists of 3000 to 5000 rads of external irradiation followed by 5000 to 3000 rads of intravaginal radium by sources specifically designed to deliver the radiation to the primary lesion. He reports survivors as follows: Stage I, 16 of 22 patients; Stage II, 19 of 25 patients; Stage III, 3 of 14 patients; Stage IV, 3 of 16 patients. Complications of therapy are relatively low, but include radiation cystitis and proctitis. Individualization of therapy was recommended.[14] Exenterative surgery may be used as primary therapy or therapy for recurrence. Results of primary surgical therapy are not as good as those achieved with irradiation, and the operative and postoperative morbidity and mortality are significant.

The vagina may also be the site of other histologic types of cancer, including melanocarcinoma, sarcoma, and mesonephric adenocarcinoma. Melanomas of this organ have an extremely poor prognosis, regardless of therapy utilized. Only 3 of 30 patients reported in the literature have survived 5 years or longer. Surgery should be radical, usually exenterative, and should include removal of the regional lymph nodes. Sarcoma of the vagina, the so-called "sarcoma botryoides," is most frequently seen in children and the prognosis is grave. Irradiation is ineffective and radical surgery is only of limited success. These tumors are thought to be of mixed mesodermal origin. Primarily vaginal adenocarcinoma, while rarely seen in the past, is more common now in women who were exposed to diethylstilbestrol in utero. These tumors usually become symptomatic shortly after puberty. Older women may occasionally have similar lesions from mesonephric remnants or paraurethral glands. Treatment is usually exenerative or irradiational.

DEFECTS OF PELVIC SUPPORT

The major support of the uterus and vagina is provided by the cardinal ligaments, condensations of endopelvic fascia at the bases of the broad ligaments. The round, broad, and uterosacral ligaments are more important in maintaining uterine position than in providing support. Support from the vaginal side of the bladder and rectum is provided by the pubocervical fascia, which is not true fascia but condensed connective tissue in the vesicovaginal and rectovaginal septum. The distal vagina is also supported by the perineal body. Overdistention of these supporting structures, usually by childbirth, may give rise to a variety of defects in pelvic support. Frequently, these defects cause few symptoms until atrophy after menopause results in further weakness. Such defects include cystocele, urethrocele, rectocele, enterocele, and uterine descensus (Fig. 20).

Cystocele and Urethrocele; Stress Urinary Incontinence

A cystocele is a herniation of the anterior vaginal wall with secondary relaxation, descent, and protrusion of the bladder floor into the vaginal introitus. Cystocele is usually accompanied by urethrocele, and not infrequently by some degree of uterine descensus or rectocele. The classic symptoms of cystocele are vaginal protrusion and recurrent cystitis which occurs because of incomplete bladder emptying. A large cystocele may be relatively asymptomatic. Surgical repair is indicated not for the size of the cystocele, but rather for its symptoms. A common problem asso-

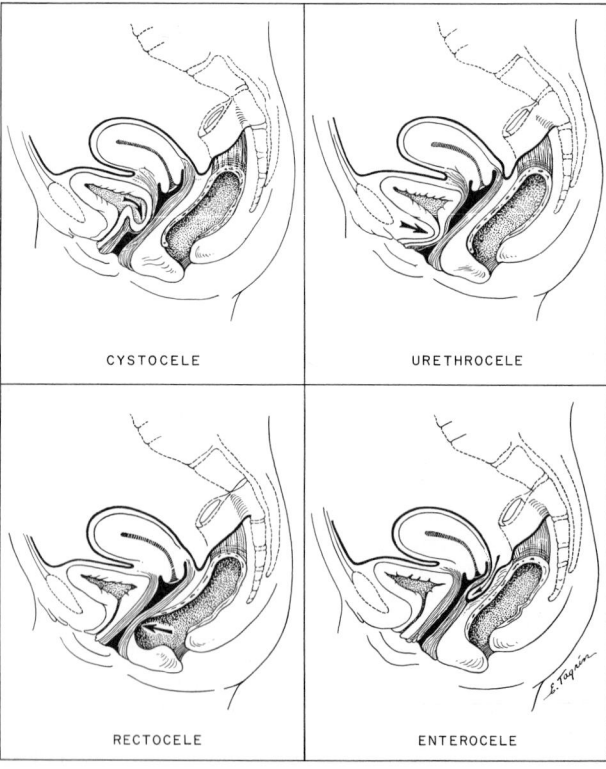

Figure 20. Diagrammatic representation of the four most common types of pelvic floor relaxation: cystocele, urethrocele, rectocele, and enterocele. Arrows depict sites of maximal protrusion. (From Gynecology: Principles and Practice by Robert W. Kistner. Copyright © 1964. Year Book Medical Publishers. Used by permission.)

ciated with cystocele is urethrocele and together they may produce flattening of the vesical neck, predisposing to stress urinary incontinence. Stress incontinence can be identified by observation of bladder support during Valsalva maneuver. If pressure and elevation lateral to the urethrovesical junction inhibits the incontinence (Marshall test), good results can be expected from surgical repair. Such supporting surgery should be postponed until childbearing has been completed, for delivery after repair will usually be accompanied by return of the defect. The primary surgical repair is usually anterior colporrhaphy, frequently performed with vaginal hysterectomy. This operation includes separating the overlying vaginal mucosa from the bladder and urethra, followed by plication of the pubocervical fascia beneath these organs before reclosure of the vaginal mucosa. Elevation and narrowing of the urethrovesical neck are the keys to success of the procedure. Anterior colporrhaphy will provide successful repair in approximately 85 per cent of patients with stress urinary incontinence. Such procedures as the retropubic Marshall-Marchetti-Krantz cystourethropexy or suburethral sling techniques may offer good results for the remaining patients.

Rectocele

Rectocele is protrusion of the rectal wall toward the vaginal canal. In this condition, the paravaginal tissue which is normally interposed between the vagina and rectum becomes attenuated and lacerated during delivery. Symptoms of rectocele are vaginal protrusion and sacculation of the rectal wall when fecal material is propelled into the anal canal. Defecation may require digital pressure to the posterior vaginal wall to force the feces from the sacculation back into the ampulla. Such problems may be reduced by posterior colpoperineorrhaphy by which the rectovaginal fascia is rebuilt and the pubococcygeus and lower levator ani muscles are joined. Most patients with rectocele also have some associated cystocele or uterine descensus. Thus, vaginal hysterectomy and anterior colporrhaphy must be combined with the posterior repair for best results. In addition, combined repairs may be mutually supporting, as the posterior repair may provide extra support for cystourethrocele. Nonoperative treatment is usually unsuccessful.

Enterocele

Pelvic enterocele is a herniation of the peritoneum of the cul-de-sac with invagination of the sac into the rectovaginal septum. A sliding hernia may develop in this space, usually created by labor, delivery, or vaginal hysterectomy. An enterocele of considerable size may exist without symptoms, but most will provoke pelvic pressure, pain, and posterior vaginal protrusion. Enterocele may be difficult to separate from rectocele, but combined rectovaginal examination, or examination with the patient in the standing position, will usually clarify the problem. Enterocele may be surgically repaired by vaginal or abdominal approaches, but the gynecologist usually utilizes the former to allow repair of other associated defects. From either approach, surgical repair of enterocele consists of plication of the uterosacral ligaments and

obliteration of the cul-de-sac. If there is accompanying rectocele it should be repaired.

Prolapse of the Uterus

Uterine prolapse, or procidentia and descensus uteri, occurs when the uterus and its adjoining structures herniate through the vaginal canal. Prolapse is described as first, second, and third degree in severity, the latter being protrusion of the entire uterus from the vagina, with the entire vagina inverted as a consequence. While congenital weakness of the supporting tissues may rarely cause uterine prolapse, the most frequent cause is childbirth. The symptoms of uterine prolapse are protrusion of the cervix or uterus through the introitus. Prolapse frequently is associated with cystocele or rectocele and these defects may cause presenting symptoms. Other symptoms include backache, significant pelvic pressure, and ulceration or bleeding of the prolapsed structures. Uterine prolapse cannot be cured by nonoperative means, but can be supported by a pessary in most patients if surgery is not feasible. Uterine prolapse is best approached vaginally for surgical repair since abdominal procedures are usually inadequate. Successful procedures include vaginal hysterectomy and repair of the pelvic diaphragm, procedures that preserve the uterus while resupporting these structures, and total colpocleisis if coital function is never again anticipated.

BENIGN DISEASES OF THE CERVIX

The portio vaginalis of the normal cervix is covered with squamous epithelium that is similar to that of the vagina. In the nulliparous woman the external cervical os is a centrally located, small, round opening connecting with the endocervical canal. After childbearing, the external os is longitudinally flattened. Mucus-secreting columar epithelium lines the endocervical canal and its junction with the squamous epithelium of the cervical portio is the squamocolumnar zone.

Cervicitis

Cervical infection, in one form or another, is one of the most frequently encountered gynecologic lesions. Acute cervicitis is rarely seen except in gonorrhea, in patients with acute vaginitis from *Trichomonas vaginalis* or *Candida albicans,* in patients with puerperal endometritis, or in patients with retained intravaginal foreign bodies. The cervix is erythematous and edematous, and leukocytic infiltration is prominent. Pain and tenderness are rarely prominent symptoms, but a purulent discharge is frequently seen. Diagnosis is made by appropriate smears and cultures (see Laboratory Tests) and therapy with topical or systemic antibiotics usually is curative.

In chronic cervicitis the cervical mucus is mucopurulent and profuse. The histologic changes seen in chronic cervicitis are variable and are present to some extent in nearly all women. Cellular changes such as metaplasia, epidermization, and hyperplasia of the basal cells are frequently seen. Often seen are erosions or eversions of the cervix. An erosion is a true ulcer of the cervix, while the eversion is formed by columnar epithelium of the endocervical canal proliferating downward, forming a lowered squamocolumnar line. Orifices of the cervical mucus-secreting glands may become obstructed to form nabothian cysts. A mucopurulent discharge may be the only symptom of chronic cervicitis, although postcontact bleeding, infertility, and, rarely, pain may occur. Diagnosis is based on cytology and biopsy, but one must remember that while cervical cytologic studies are very effective in the discovery of early cervical cancer with an intact surface epithelium, they are much less reliable when an erosion is present. Colposcopy, colpomicroscopy, and iodine staining may be of aid in localizing areas for biopsy. Any suspicious or eroded area should be biopsied before treatment. Therapy of chronic cervicitis is usually by electrodesiccation, by ultrarefrigeration (cryosurgery), or with silver nitrate. Cautery should include the involved exocervix and endocervical canal, and rarely requires an anesthetic. These methods destroy the infection of the columnar area and allow the squamous epithelium to grow over the area. Repeated cautery, surgical conization, and, on occasion, even hysterectomy (if childbearing is ended) may be necessary for severe chronic cervicitis.

Cervical Polyps

Polyps may arise from the endocervix and are rarely malignant. The usual symptom is postcontact bleeding. They appear as single or multiple, cherry red growths protruding from the external cervical os. Such polyps may be removed by biopsy or dilation and currettage, with cauterization of the pedicle. One must not overlook uterine or other cervical causes of abnormal bleeding which may be the symptom of other, more severe, pelvic disease. Another polypoid hyperplastic lesion, atypical endocervical hyperplasia, may develop in oral contraceptive users. The gross appearance is that of a polyp and histologically it may resemble adenocarcinoma. This is not a malignant lesion, however, and will regress with discontinuation of use of the contraceptive pills.

CANCER OF THE CERVIX

Invasive carcinoma of the cervix is the most common pelvic malignant disease and accounts for 15 per cent of cancers of women. At birth there is a probability that 2.3 per cent of our female population will eventually have cervical cancer; and it is currently estimated that 10,000 women die in this country each year from these neoplasms. It is encouraging that, during the past 15 years, primarily through early detection, the death rate from cervical cancer has declined from 21.8 to 11.5 per 100,000 population. Invasive carcinoma of the cervix should be a preventable disease, as regular examinations and frequent use of today's diagnostic techniques should enable detection of nearly all patients with preinvasive cervical carcinoma, a totally curable disease.

The average age of occurrence of carcinoma of the cervix is 48 years, with the majority of patients be-

tween 35 and 55 years of age. However, many authors have reported cervical cancer in women as young as the teens and as old as the eighth decade. Much has been written about the etiology of cervical carcinoma. Epidemiologic studies show peak instances of this disease among women of low socioeconomic status, among those who begin coitus and childbearing at an early age, and among women with multiple sexual partners. Heredity seems to play a small role. The theory of a viral relationship has been advanced, suggesting that a virus transmitted through intercourse is responsible for cervical cancer.[2, 3]

Cervical Dysplasia

Dysplastic changes may be seen in epithelium exfoliated or biopsied from the cervix. While this is not a diagnosis of malignancy, patients with cervical dysplasia should be followed with cytologic studies every 4 to 6 months, for it has been found that carcinoma-insitu of the cervix will develop in a significant percentage of these patients over the subsequent several years. Dysplasia may resemble carcinoma-in-situ of the cervix, but the abnormal cells do not extend through the full thickness of epithelium. Cervical biopsy should be frequently employed as well as the colpomicroscopic and iodine staining techniques. Recent studies suggest the lesions, and many patients with limited dysplasia do quite well without treatment.

Preinvasive or Carcinoma-in-situ of the Cervix

Bowen in 1912 described a preinvasive malignant lesion of the skin and in the same year Schottlander, Rubin, and Schiller described preinvasive carcinoma of the cervix. During the next 30 years this interesting lesion was only noted, but ultimately it was described as a precursor to invasive carcinoma of the cervix. It remained for Papanicolaou and Traut, in 1941, to develop the cytologic evaluation of exfoliated cells that suggests the need for biopsy and adequate tissue study. Histopathologically, carcinoma-in-situ consists of cellular changes in the squamous epithelium of the cervix that are compatible with cancer, but evidence of invasion in the underlying stroma is absent. Glandular epithelial replacement by neoplastic cells may be mistaken for invasion and it is important that this differentiation be made. Other benign conditions that may confuse diagnosis are atypical basilar hyperplasia and the metaplasia and hyperplasia of glandular elements frequently seen in pregnancy. The peak incidence of carcinoma-in-situ is approximately 35 to 40 years of age. *There are no gross lesions or symptoms of carcinoma-in-situ of the cervix.* The use of Papanicolaou cytology screening and adequate biopsy techniques are discussed in the Laboratory Tests section of this chapter. The diagnosis of carcinoma-in-situ is made by histologic review of biopsy specimens (Fig. 21).

The treatment of carcinoma-in-situ of the cervix is abdominal or vaginal hysterectomy with excision of 2 to 3 cm. of upper vagina. The tubes and ovaries are usually left in place in younger women. Radical hysterectomy and pelvic lymph node dissection is not in-

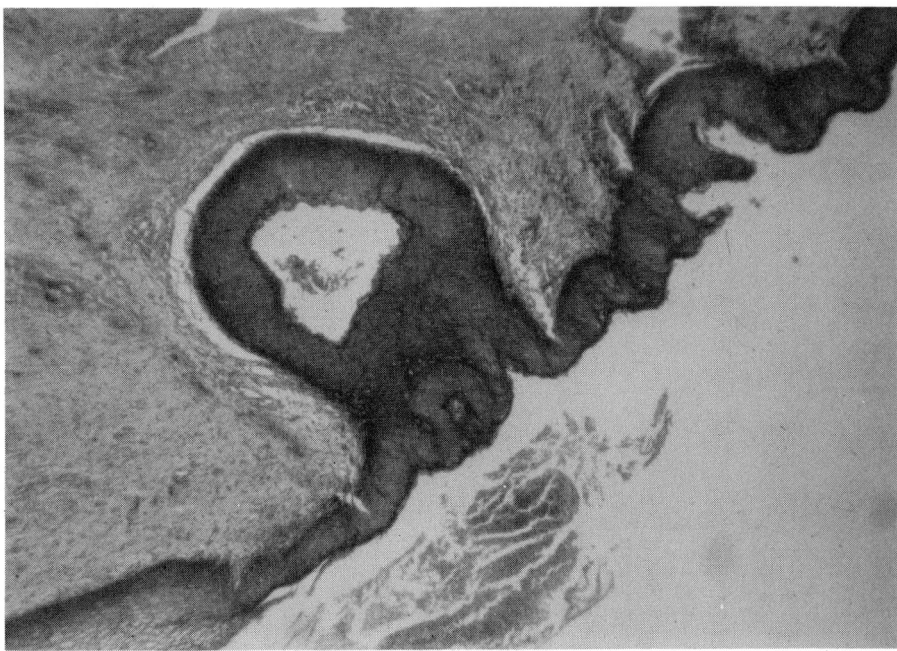

Figure 21. Carcinoma-in-situ of the cervix. Note sharp demarcation between normal and malignant epithelium (lower border) and the glandular epithelial involvement. (Courtesy of Dr. D. E. D. Jones.)

dicated for this lesion. Results of therapy are uniformly good and 5-year survival approaches 100 per cent.[10] Radiation therapy may be indicated for carcinoma-in-situ, but it usually results in ablation of ovarian function and may cause the same side effects as radiation therapy for invasive carcinoma.[8] As carcinoma-in-situ is a disease of younger women the question of allowing continued reproduction prior to hysterectomy has been raised. If the patient has normal smears after conization and desires to have more children, we have allowed her to do so and deliver vaginally. Hysterectomy is recommended after childbearing is ended, even if cytologic findings are benign. If the smears remain positive after conization, hysterectomy is suggested at that time. If abnormal smears are detected during pregnancy, cervical conization is used for diagnosis, or quadrant biopsy in later pregnancy and when there is no obvious lesion present. If carcinoma-in-situ is detected the pregnancy is allowed to continue with vaginal delivery. If invasive carcinoma is present, adequate therapy is begun immediately.[10]

Microinvasive Cancer of the Cervix

There has been considerable debate as to both the diagnosis and treatment of microinvasive carcinoma of the cervix, a condition in which carcinoma-in-situ exists and there is less than 5 mm. of invasion present. Data showing lack of nodal metastasis have led to treatment of patients as if the lesions were only carcinoma-in-situ. Results of this treatment in microinvasive cancer of the cervix are equally as good as those of full radical surgery or irradiation, and morbidity has been much less.

Carcinoma of the Cervix

Approximately 95 per cent of cervical cancers are squamous, the remaining 5 per cent usually being adenocarcinoma. Most often the adenocarcinoma arises from the mucus-secreting epithelium of the cervix, but rarely adenocarcinoma may arise in mesonephric duct remnants. Squamous cell, or epidermoid, carinoma of the cervix usually arises at the squamocolumnar junction. Varying degrees of microscopic differentiation are found. A halo of carcinoma-in-situ is frequently found around the invasive cancer or on the vagina.

There are no symptoms of early carcinoma of the cervix; the first symptoms of bleeding, usually postcontact, or a blood discharge, do not begin until ulceration is present. More advanced cervical cancers cause symptoms referable to invasion of adjacent organs (bladder, rectum, ureter) or to distant metastasis. Pain is a sign of advanced cervical cancer.

Although cytologic findings and clinical appearance may strongly suggest carcinoma of the cervix, the diagnosis can be made only by histopathologic study. In the presence of an obvious exophytic lesion, as is found in more than 80 per cent of patients with even early cervical cancer, tissue may be easily obtained by punch biopsy. If the lesion is endophytic, or if the punch biopsy shows carcinoma-in-situ, or less, conization may be mandatory to fully evaluate abnormal cytologic studies. Broken and ulcerated epithelium and proliferating tissue that bleeds easily upon touch are most valuable clinical signs, particularly when such lesions involve the squamocolumnar junction. Colposcopy and staining techniques may aid direction of biopsies.

If treatment of cervical cancer is adequate, the single most important factor in prognosis is the extent of disease when therapy is begun. For this reason each patient should have a careful pelvic examination, cystoscopy, proctoscopy, intravenous pyelography, and x-rays of the chest and bones so that the extent of the disease may be established. Staging of cervical cancer is arrived at by entirely clinical evaluation and is made before treatment is initiated (Fig. 22). Such staging should not be changed at any later time. We currently utilize the classification for clinical staging of cervical carcinoma provided in 1966 by the Cancer Committee of the International Federation of Gynecology and Obstetrics:

Stage 0
    Carcinoma-in-situ (preinvasive or intraepithelial).
Stage I
    Carcinoma confined entirely to the cervix (IA, early stromal invasion; IB, all other Stage I lesions).
Stage II
    Carcinoma extends beyond the cervix but has not reached either the pelvic sidewall or the lower third of the vagina. (IIA, no parametrial involvement; IIB, parametrial involvement is present).

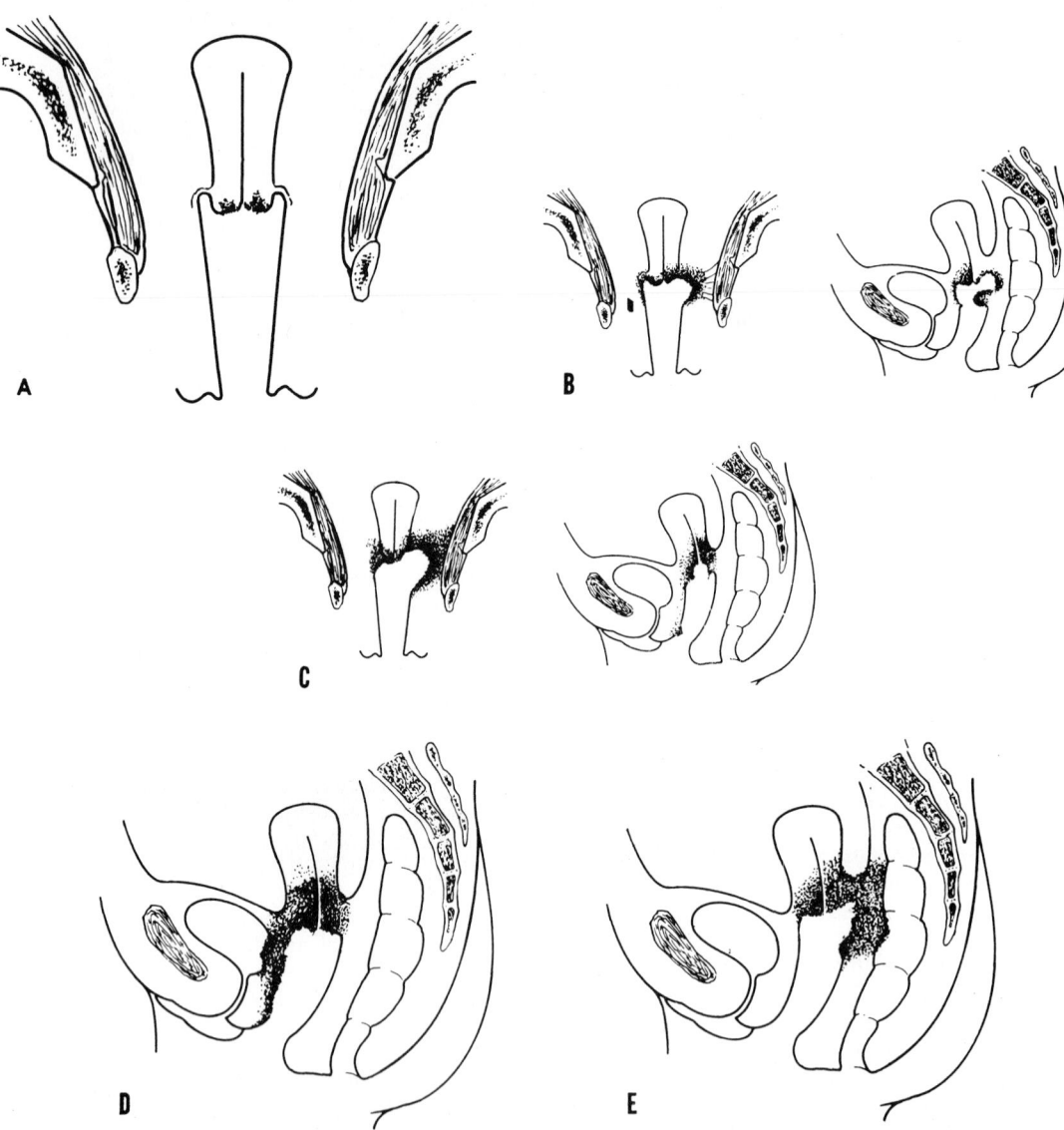

Figure 22. Stages of carcinoma of the cervix. *A*, Stage I, the cancer is confined to the cervix. *B*, Stage II, the cancer is confined to the parametrium on one or both sides, and is not fixed to either pelvic wall. Or the cancer involves the upper one-third of the vagina. *C*, Stage III, the cancer has spread to one or both pelvic walls, or has invaded the lower one-third of the vagina. *D*, and *E*, Stage IV, the cancer involves the bladder or the rectum, or it has spread beyond the pelvis. (From Taylor, E. S.: Essentials of Gynecology, 4th ed. Philadelphia, Lea & Febiger, 1969.)

Stage III

Carcinoma has reached the pelvic sidewall or the lower third of the vagina.

Stage IV

Carcinoma involves the bladder, rectum, distant nodes, or distant areas.

While clinical staging is done before therapy, it is useful to understand the significance of such staging on disease spread. The most common method of tumor spread, and the most frequent cause of patient death, is direct extension of cervical cancer to involve the vagina, uterus, parametrium, pelvic sidewall, ureter, bladder, and rectum. More than 50 per cent of patients who die with cervical cancer die of ureteral obstruction and uremia. Fistula formation from ureter, bladder, and rectum is not infrequently seen, and bleeding may be a serious complication. Carcinoma of the cervix also has a propensity for lymphatic metastasis. Lymphatic drainage of the cervix is via the hypogastric and obturator lymph chains to the iliac and then aortic nodal systems. Vertebral lymphatic metastases may also occur. Morton and others have shown positive lymph node metastases in the following percentages of clinically staged cases of cervical carcinoma: Stage I, 16.5; Stage II, 31.9; Stage III, 46.7; and Stage IV, 80.8.[3] In addition to the clinical staging, the size of the primary cervical lesion has also been shown to influence the frequency with which lymph node metastases are found: less than 1 cm., rare metastases; 1 to 3 cm., 17 per cent with metastases; greater than 3 cm., 52 per cent with lymph node metastases. These latter two factors of lymphatic node metastasis are variable and of little use in the therapy of a given patient. Other studies have shown that lymphatic spread beyond the pelvic nodal chains is present in more than 40 per cent of patients who die of cervical cancer. Autopsy data demonstrate distant metastases in many patients dying of carcinoma of the cervix and nearly every organ may be involved. Most common sites of distant metastases include: liver, 16 per cent; lung, 14 per cent; vertebrae, 9 per cent; and other bony metastases, 9 per cent.

Treatment of Cervical Cancer. Carcinoma of the cervix can be effectively treated by surgery or irradiation, *but treatment does not include simple hysterectomy or nonindividualized radiotherapy.* No other major lesion requires more critical selection of techniques and methods of therapy. The present operation for cancer of the cervix (Stages I and IIA) is an extended hysterectomy (Wertheim) which removes the parametrial tissues, the upper third of the vagina, and perhaps the adnexa, and a pelvic node dissection which removes the iliac, hypogastric, ureteral, obturator, and lower aortic lymph nodes. The radical operation for cancer of the cervix has two primary disadvantages: first, there is a 7 to 8 per cent incidence of ureteral or bladder fistula; and second, few surgeons are qualified to undertake the operation and perform it satisfactorily. Certain patients with Stage IV carcinoma, those with only rectal or bladder involvement, may be candidates for primary surgical therapy by pelvic exenteration. The results of primary surgical treatment for cervical cancer are perhaps best demonstrated by Brunschwig's data from 703 patients managed by the choice of operations just noted.[1] That study showed 5-year survivals of: Stage I, 78.8 per cent; Stage II, 53.0 per cent; Stage III, 31.3 per cent; Stage IV, 19.7 per cent. The numbers of patients with Stages III and IV disease were small. The operative mortality was 2.3 per cent and a high rate of postoperative urinary fistulas was reported. Most gynecologists now reserve the primary surgical treatment of carcinoma of the cervix for those patients with smaller Stage I or early Stage II lesions.

Most clinics favor primary radiation treatment of cancer of the cervix. The purpose of therapy is to deliver to the lesion and to areas of possible pelvic spread sufficient radiation to destroy the cancer and still not cause irreparable damage to surrounding tissues. Most therapists employ a combination of external supervoltage therapy, such as from cobalt-60 units, and intravaginal, contracervical, and intracervical irradiation with radium. In our clinic external cobalt-60 radiotherapy is initially delivered to a dosage of 4000 to 6000 rads to the entire pelvis, over a 4 to 6-week course. This is followed by one or two radium applications to deliver 4000 to 6000 rads to the primary cervical lesion. In Stages I and II disease we tend to deliver the higher dose by radium; in Stages III and IV disease the higher dose is usually administered by external cobalt-60. Total dosage administered by the two routes approximates 10,000 rads. As in surgery, the prognosis with primary radiation therapy for carcinoma of the cervix varies with the clinical stage present at the time therapy is begun. The usually accepted figures for 5-year survival with this type of treatment are: Stage I, 86.4 per cent; Stage II, 60.0 per cent; Stage III, 26.3 per cent; Stage IV, 8.8 per cent.[3, 8]

As with surgery, there are complications of radiation therapy for cervical cancer. These problems include radiation sickness, leukopenia, pelvic infection, proctitis, cystitis, small bowel injuries, vaginal stenosis, menopausal symptoms, radiation necrosis of vagina and cervix, skin reaction, and fistulas. Many of these problems may develop only at long intervals after therapy and management is based on conservatism, exclusion of extant carcinoma, and surgical repair when indicated. Estrogen replacement may alleviate many of the symptoms and does not appear to influence the likelihood of recurrence of carcinoma.

Regardless of the type of therapy utilized, patients with carcinoma of the cervix must be followed frequently and regularly. We speak hopefully of 5-year "cures," but there are significant numbers of patients in whom recurrent disease will develop 10 or 20 years later or who later have other malignant lesions of the genital tract. Follow-up should include frequent cytologic study and appropriate biopsy. Secondary treatment for therapeutic failures, with surgery or further irradiation, have provided limited success. Chemotherapy has been of palliative aid only.

BENIGN UTERINE DISEASE

Various benign uterine diseases occur, including leiomyoma uteri, adenomyosis, endometrial hyperplasia, and polyps. Abnormal bleeding, uterine enlargement, and pain are the usual symptoms associated with these diseases, but the primary difficulty is to achieve an accurate diagnosis.

Leiomyoma Uteri

Uterine leiomyomas, also called myomas, fibromyomas, or fibroids, are the most common cause of benign uterine enlargement and are seen in 20 per cent of women. The incidence is higher in the Negro race. Leiomyomas originate from the smooth muscle cells of the myometrium and vary in size from microscopic to large enough to fill the entire abdomen. Such tumors may be single but are more often multiple. On cut section these solid tumors have a white, glistening appearance with a characteristic whorl pattern. There is no true capsule but compressed peripheral fibers form a pseudocapsule. Microscopically, smooth muscle cells are arranged in interlacing muscle bundles, interspaced with varying amounts of connective tissue and hyaline material. Such tumors may be submucous, intramural, subserous, pedunculated, parasitic, cervical, or interligamentous (Fig. 23).

The symptoms of leiomyoma vary according to location; some may produce severe complaints, others none at all. The three most common symptoms are abnormal bleeding, pain, and uterine enlargement. Abnormal bleeding, usually cyclic but profuse and prolonged, is most frequently due to submucous tumors which distort the overlying endometrium and interfere with normal hemostatic mechanisms. Occasionally a submucous or cervical myoma may be extruded and also cause abnormal bleeding. Abnormal bleeding is the most common indication for hysterectomy for leiomyoma, but caution must be taken to exclude other causes, as a malignant lesion may coexist with myoma. Often a curettage may be mandatory to make this differentiation. Rapid enlargement is another symptom of concern in patients with leiomyoma, as 1 to 2 per cent of such tumors may undergo sarcomatous

change or degeneration of other nonmalignant varieties. Estrogen, including the synthetic estrogens of oral contraceptives, may cause enlargement of myomas. Myomas tend to regress after menopause and any enlargement of these tumors demands prompt removal of the uterus. Slow enlargement of leiomyomas during the menstrual years frequently occurs with a minimum of symptoms. Surgical removal is not mandatory for slow growth or moderate size unless other symptoms occur. Pelvic pressure, frequency of urination, and sciatic or hip pain from pressure on pelvic nerves can be symptoms of uterine leiomyoma. Tenderness in a myoma is usually caused by degeneration or by impairment of the blood supply. Cystic changes and calcification can follow degeneration. Significant pain or tenderness usually warrants hysterectomy. Infertility is not infrequently seen in patients with myomas, nor is abortion, but in the former it is not known whether the infertility or the myoma is primary. The increased rate of abortion is attributed to poor uterine distensibility and compression. While uterine myomas are usually recognized without difficulty in the operating room, their preoperative diagnosis may be quite difficult especially if the myoma involves primarily one of the adnexa.

The treatment of leiomyoma demands individualization for each patient. Some tumors require no treatment if small and asymptomatic and semiannual examination only is warranted. If a young patient who desires further childbearing has symptomatic leiomyomas, then multiple myomectomy is a useful surgical procedure. In larger or more symptomatic myomas in a woman who has completed her reproduction, hysterectomy is the treatment of choice.

Adenomyosis

Invasion of the myometrium by endometrium, adenomyosis, is a frequent cause of uterine enlargement and pain. Grossly the uterus is enlarged, fibrotic, and

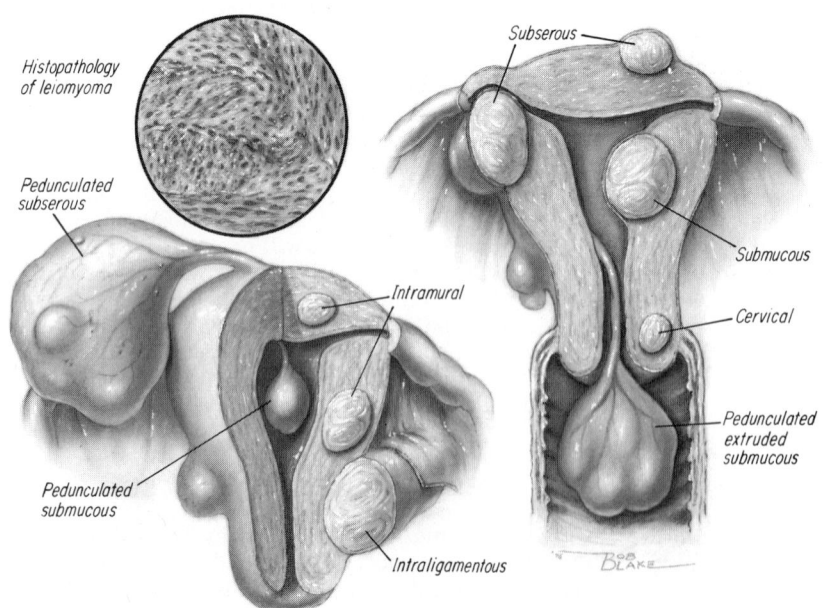

Histopathology of leiomyoma

Pedunculated subserous

Subserous

Intramural

Submucous

Cervical

Pedunculated submucous

Intraligamentous

Pedunculated extruded submucous

Figure 23. Leiomyoma uteri.

thickened and on cut section the areas of endometrial growth and loculated menstruation may be quite apparent.

The classic symptoms and signs of adenomyosis are acquired dysmenorrhea occurring in the 35 to 40-year age group, menstrual irregularities with cyclic, prolonged, and profuse flow, and an enlarged, tender uterus. Treatment is hysterectomy, although hormonal suppression (pseudopregnancy regimen with estrogen and progesterone) may provide relief without removal of the uterus.

Endometrial Hyperplasia and Polyps

Hyperplasia of the endometrium, causing abnormal uterine bleeding, is a common problem of women. Women near menopause, or less frequently in early adolescence, are most frequently affected. The basic problem is anovulation and failure of corpus luteum formation without production of progesterone. Continued stimulation of the endometrium by estrogen brings about proliferation, overgrowth, and cystic hyperplasia of the endometrium. Areas of the thickened endometrium may form polyps. Cycles become irregular with intervals of amenorrhea associated with other intervals of intermenstrual spotting or bleeding. Pelvic examination is usually nonrevealing and curettage produces copious amounts of endometrial scrapings. Microscopic examination shows hyperplasia of the epithelium and stroma. The cells lining the glands are nonsecretory and the stroma often contains cells with frequent mitotic figures. Cystic changes of the glands may be present.

Curettage is useful in diagnosis and for treatment, as it removes the hypertrophied endometrium and leaves a fresh surface for endometrial regeneration. Because of the frequency of recurrence of hyperplasia, the administration of cyclic progesterone will aid in prevention of recurrence and promote cyclic menses. If endometrial hyperplasia recurs, it may proceed to atypical or adenomatous hyperplasia, and then to carcinoma-in-situ, which may lead to endometrial cancer. Recurrent abnormal bleeding requires repeated curettage for diagnosis and proper therapy.

Adenomatous hyperplasia is diagnosed when there is marked proliferation, with the glands being closely packed and the stroma quite dense and hyperplastic. This adenomatous pattern closely resembles adenocarcinoma and is felt to be a precancerous lesion. Diagnosis of this lesion is by currettage. While cyclic progesterone will be of aid for most patients, hysterectomy is probably the treatment of choice for the older patient who has completed her reproduction.

MALIGNANT DISEASES OF THE UTERUS

Adenocarcinoma of the Endometrium

Adenocarcinoma of the endometrium, the second most prevalent gynecologic cancer, is seen most commonly among postmenopausal women. The peak incidence occurs in the 50- to 70-year age group, but one must suspect the condition as early as the third decade if there is bleeding irregularity. Postmenopausal bleeding is the cardinal symptom of endometrial cancer and must be considered as due to malignancy until proved otherwise. Prolonged, profuse, or irregular bleeding may occur in the premenstrual woman. Papanicolaou cytologic study may yield negative results, as the exfoliated cells may not reach the vaginal pool. Cervical stenosis with secondary hematometrium or pyometrium is frequently present and can be identified by passage of an endocervical probe. Fractional curettage is the diagnostic method of choice and only in this fashion can the diagnosis be established as well as the degree of cervical involvement, an important factor influencing therapy. Histologically, adenocarcinoma of the endometrium has wide variations in differentiation and in stromal invasion by the glandular epithelial cells, and, finally, there is a highly undifferentiated type in which neither glandular nor stromal elements can be identified.

The etiology of endometrial cancer is unknown. There does appear to be a relationship to prolonged estrogenic stimulation, as in patients with estrogen-producing ovarian tumors. Newer studies also suggest a higher incidence of endometrial adenocarcinoma in women given high-dose estrogen replacement therapy for menopausal symptoms. Such studies require further documentation. Other frequently associated findings in patients with endometrial adenocarcinoma are obesity, diabetes, hypertension, and low parity.

Endometrial cancer is usually a polypoid lesion growing into the endometrial cavity, and only late in the disease does myocardial or cervical involvement occur (Fig. 24). Uterine size is usually normal to slightly increased in women with early cancer of the endometrium. Uterine enlargement and irregularity occur in advanced disease or disease associated with hematometrium or leiomyoma. In addition to direct extension to adjacent structures, adenocarcinoma of the endometrium may spread through the extensive lymphatic anastomosis at the upper uterus between the tube and ovary. Thus, the tubes and ovaries are frequent sites of early metastases. Besides this direct lymphatic extension of endometrial cancer, these tumors may spread by regional and distant lymph node metastasis to the pelvic and aortic nodal chains. The incidence of such lymph node metastasis is rare when only the uterine fundus is involved (2 per cent) but frequent if the primary lesion is near the cervical junction (50 per cent). Hematogenous dissemination may also occur, and the most frequent sites are the peritoneal surfaces, lungs, liver, and skin. Local recurrence in the apex of the vagina, vaginal walls, and perineum occurs in 10 per cent of patients who have been treated for endometrial cancer.

The usual clinical staging of endometrial cancer includes: Stage 0, preinvasive or carcinoma-in-situ of the endometrium; Stage I, the growth is confined to the uterine body; Stage II, the carcinoma involves the corpus and the cervix; Stage III, the tumor extends outside the uterus but not outside the true pelvis; Stage IV, the carcinoma has extended outside the true pelvis or has involved the mucosa of the rectum or bladder.[3] The location of the primary neoplasm in the uterus, the degree of anaplasia of the cells, and the gross size of the uterus influence the prognosis of the patient and the effectiveness of treatment.

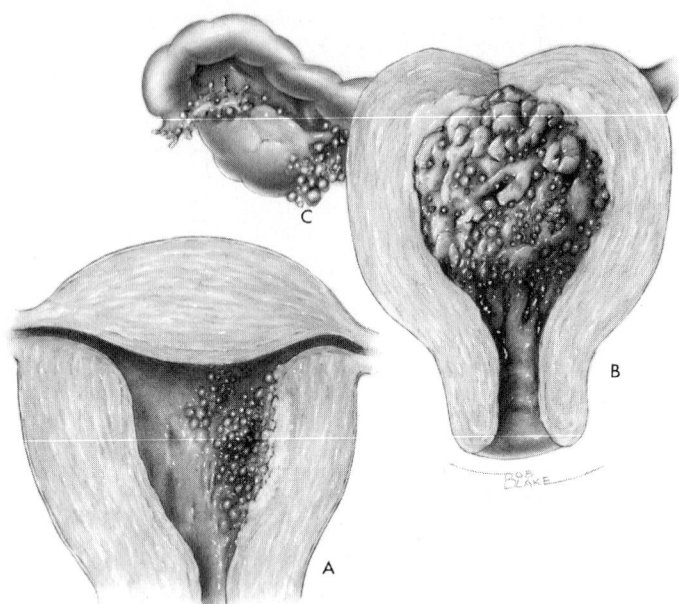

Figure 24. Carcinoma of the endometrium. *A*, Stage I. *B*, Stage III, myometrial invasion plus. *C*, Ovarian extension or metastases.

The treatment of adenocarcinoma of the endometrium is primarily surgical. Many clinics supplement the surgical treatment with preoperative intrauterine radium application or preliminary deep x-ray or cobalt-60 therapy to the pelvis. There is considerable disagreement as to whether preoperative radiotherapy enhances survival rates, but it does seem clear that such treatment will reduce vaginal recurrence after appropriate surgical therapy. Nolan has shown that in Stage I disease in which the uterus is small, preoperative radiotherapy does not improve survival, but in other Stage I lesions the survival may be increased by a factor of 10 per cent.[3] If the cervix is involved by endometrial carcinoma, or Stage II disease, preoperative treatment with irradiation followed by radical Wertheim hysterectomy with pelvic lymphadenectomy may be indicated. The survival rate for patients with cancer spread beyond the uterus is poor, regardless of whether surgery, irradiation, or a combination of the two methods is used. Approximately 30 per cent of patients with recurrent or metastatic adenocarcinoma of the endometrium will benefit from large doses of parenteral progesterone (Delalutin or Depo-Provera), usually those with tumors that are well differentiated histologically. Other forms of chemotherapy have been of little aid. External pelvic radiotherapy or transvaginal irradiation and intravaginal radium may provide palliation for locally recurrent adenocarcinoma of the endometrium.

The prognosis for adenocarcinoma of the endometrium is generally good, but results of larger series are frequently difficult to compare owing to differences in tumor size, differentiation, stage, and type of treatment. Of those patients selected for surgery because of an operable lesion, with and without preoperative irradiation, approximately 60 per cent will survive 5 years.[3, 8]

Sarcoma of the Uterus

Sarcomas may arise from the endometrium, myometrium, cervix, a leiomyoma, or uterine blood vessels. These diseases are most frequently seen in the fifth decade and a rare sarcoma of the cervix, sarcoma botryoides, is seen in infants. The incidence of corpus sarcoma is much higher than that of sarcoma of the cervix. As all elements of the uterus are mesodermal in origin, and mesodermal rests may be present, mixed tumors may occur. A wide spectrum of histopathologic types can be found. Rapid uterine enlargement is a prominent sign of uterine sarcoma and abnormal bleeding may or may not be present. Pain, anemia, and weight loss are late symptoms. Pulmonary metastases frequently occur early. Surgical excision of the uterus, tubes, and ovaries is the recommended treatment for sarcoma of the uterus. The prognosis after treatment varies with the type and extent of the original tumor. The sarcomas arising in myomas generally appear to be of low malignancy and thus have a relatively good prognosis, with 45 to 50 per cent of patients with operable lesions surviving. There are very few survivors among patients with the other types of uterine sarcoma despite appropriate surgery for patients with operable lesions. Radiotherapy may offer benefit. We are currently exploring a combination approach, with extirpative surgery and combination chemotherapy with simultaneous methotrexate, actinomycin D, and chlorambucil, followed by external pelvic irradiation with cobalt-60. The initial results are encouraging but warrant further investigation.

PELVIC INFECTION

Acute Pelvic Infection

Acute pelvic infection may occur after pelvic surgery or result from other causes, but by far the most frequent etiology is gonorrhea. The initial symptoms of gonorrhea usually occur within 3 to 6 days after inoculation and consist of urethritis, skenitis, bartholinitis, cervicitis, and vaginal discharge. Tubal involvement is usually a later symptom and does not occur until after a menstrual period. At this time the gonococcus spreads rapidly from the endocervix, across the endometrium, and involves the endosalpinx. It is in the fallopian tube that the major infection and damage occurs. The tube becomes acutely inflamed and edematous, and its lumen fills with a purulent exudate. The tubular, peritubular, ovarian, and pelvic peritoneal surfaces are rapidly involved. Pelvic abscess may develop.

The signs and symptoms of acute pelvic infection are those of pelvic peritonitis with bilateral lower abdominal pain and tenderness, temperature of 38 to 39° C., and signs of peritoneal irritation with direct and rebound tenderness and muscle spasm. On pelvic examination one may be able to express pus from the paraurethral glands or cervix, exquisite tenderness is present with cervical manipulation and in the adnexal areas, and there is a thickened, doughy feeling in the tubular areas. Bilaterality of pain is an important point in differentiating acute pelvic infection from appendicitis, and the fever of the former disease is usually higher. The diagnosis of acute pelvic infection is made by cervical smear and culture (see Laboratory Tests).

Therapy is based on the degree of peritonitis and fever. If significant peritonitis is present or the temperature is greater than 38.5° C., hospitalization is indicated and intravenous antibiotic therapy recommended. Treatment in this situation consists of administration of penicillin, streptomycin, or ampicillin. This intensive treatment, plus analgesia, elevation of the head to encourage pelvic localization of pus, and parenteral fluid replacement, is continued until the acute symptoms have subsided, and then oral therapy is begun and continued on an outpatient basis for a week. Total therapy should include more than 5 million units of penicillin so as to adequately treat unrecognized syphilis which the patient may have contracted at the same time as the gonorrhea. If the presenting symptoms are not severe, one can treat the patient entirely as an outpatient. The patient should be examined twice weekly to follow her progress and exclude pelvic abscess. Surgery is not indicated for acute pelvic infection unless pelvic abscess drainage is required. If the abdomen is opened for an erroneous preoperative diagnosis but acute pelvic infection is found, no further surgery is indicated and the abdomen is closed and antibiotic therapy initiated. If significant pelvic contamination with pus is present, cul-de-sac drains are inserted.

Pelvic Abscess

This condition may follow acute pelvic infection, pelvic surgery, septicemia, puerperal endometritis, appendicitis, or peritonitis of any cause. The abscess may be localized in the cul-de-sac, or between the leaves of the broad ligament, or it may be tubo-ovarian in location. If gonorrhea is the primary etiology, the purulent exudate will usually not contain the organism, since it is short-lived in such conditions. Secondary organisms such as colon bacilli, anaerobic organisms as bacteroides, streptococci, and staphylococci may be present in large quantities. The signs and symptoms of pelvic abscess are elevation of temperature and

pulse, pelvic or lower abdominal pain, and leukocytosis. If the abscess is anteriorly placed, as in an interligamentous pelvic abscess, one may discover a tender, fluctuant mass on abdominal examination. Pelvic examination is usually quite helpful. A cul-de-sac abscess bulges into the posterior vaginal fornix and displaces the cervix anteriorly. Interligamentous abscesses may bulge into the lateral fornix and displace the cervix to one side. Treatment of pelvic abscess consists of surgical drainage. Posterior colpotomy is performed to drain a pelvic abscess localized in the cul-de-sac, and loculations are digitally opened, and large drains are left indwelling. Antibiotics should be used after surgery. Other pelvic abscesses may be drained vaginally, but may require anterior extraperitoneal drainage or abdominal exploration for removal of involved structures and drainage. If a pelvic abscess ruptures intra-abdominally, there is significant morbidity and mortality from disseminated infection. In that event the uterus, tubes, and ovaries should be removed and adequate drainage and antibiotic coverage instituted.

Chronic Pelvic Infection

Included among chronic pelvic infections are chronic salpingo-oophoritis, pyosalpinx, hydrosalpinx, and tubercular salpingitis. Chronic salpingo-oophoritis is one of the major complications of gonorrhea. The patient may have few complaints. Since the endosalpinx was intensely involved in the acute infection the tube may be agglutinized. Pyosalpinx is one of the chronic destructive lesions of gonorrhea in which the tube is dilated, closed, and filled with pus. Hydrosalpinx results from pyosalpinx in which the purulent material is replaced by a serous fluid. Chronic oophoritis may develop after ovarian surface involvement, and often the tube and ovary are involved in a single inflammatory process. The classic pattern of chronic pelvic infection is one of quiescent intervals interspaced with flares of more acute inflammation. After the initial infection, usually gonococcal, anaerobic organisms invade and involve these tissues. Tuberculous salpingitis is now a fairly rare problem in this country, and the process usually involves the endometrium and adjacent structures as well. The dense adhesions of pelvic viscera to bowel and omentum are outstanding features of this disease, and these structures may be covered with a caseous exudate.

Chronic pelvic infection may be treated medically or surgically. The important elements of medical therapy are rest, heat, and antibiotic therapy. Sedation and analgesia will usually be required. Penicillin, ampicillin, clindamycin, and tetracycline are the oral antibiotics utilized. Those patients who have recurrent pain or abnormal uterine bleeding from reduced ovarian function caused by chronic pelvic infection are often difficult to relieve of symptoms. This disease is a common gynecologic complaint and surgical therapy is often required. The only cure for chronic, recurrent pelvic infection is surgical removal of the uterus, tubes, and ovaries. Surgery should always be delayed, if possible, until maximal medical control has been obtained. Estrogen replacement is indicated for the younger woman if both ovaries are removed.

BENIGN DISEASES OF THE OVARY

Benign ovarian tumors may be solid or cystic and may represent a "functional" process or neoplasia. While these growths are usually small, they may persist or become massively enlarged. The judgment as to the necessity of surgical removal should be based on size, duration of symptoms, the interval of persistence of the smaller lesions, and the age of the patient. Most classifications of such benign tumors include ovarian cysts, non-neoplastic and neoplastic, and solid ovarian tumors.

Many authors report that more than 90 per cent of ovarian growths discovered in women less than 30 years old are benign. In the 30- to 50-year age group, 80 per cent are benign. After 50 years of age approximately half of such ovarian growths are malignant. Others, excluding the frequently seen follicle and corpus luteum cysts, report the likelihood of the various benign ovarian growths as: endometrial cysts, 33 per cent; simple cysts, 26 per cent; serous and mucinous cystadenomas, 19 per cent; dermoids, 15.2 per cent; others, 2 per cent.[3] The most frequent sign of benign ovarian growths is slow abdominal enlargement. Other symptoms are pain and tenderness from torsion of the pedicle and interference with the blood supply. Less than 10 per cent of such growths are associated with aberrations in the menstrual cycle. Amenorrhea or irregular bleeding may accompany follicle or corpus luteum cysts, polycystic ovaries, or endometrial cysts. Unless quite large, most benign ovarian tumors rarely cause pressure on adjacent pelvic structures. Most commonly, such ovarian growths are asymptomatic and discovered on routine pelvic examination.

The benign, non-neoplastic ovarian cysts are usually of "functional" origin. The follicle cyst represents failure of a developing follicle to rupture or regress and rarely exceeds 8 cm. in diameter. Corpus luteum cysts occur from hemorrhage into the corpus luteum, and these blood-filled cysts have the yellow granular color of the normal corpus luteum while the follicle cyst is filled with clear fluid. Both usually regress over a 4- to 8-week period. The theca lutein cyst and the luteoma of pregnancy are also functional cysts resulting from the high levels of circulating chorionic gonadotropin of normal pregnancy and trophoblastic disease. They regress after pregnancy is terminated. Germinal inclusion cysts occur in the cortex of the ovary and represent inward growth of the germinal epithelium which has undergone cystic change. These cysts are thought to be the origin of the neoplastic serous cystadenoma. Polycystic ovaries are enlarged with multiple small follicular cysts and leuteinization of the stroma, and have a thickened capsule. The etiology is unknown but may relate to tonic elevation of luteinizing hormone.

The benign neoplastic ovarian cysts are most frequently the endometrial cyst or "chocolate" cyst of pelvic endometriosis (Fig. 25) or the simple cyst. These may achieve large size, especially the latter. Serous and mucinous cystadenomas arise from neoplastic changes in germinal epithelium and often reach considerable size. These cystic tumors are multilocular,

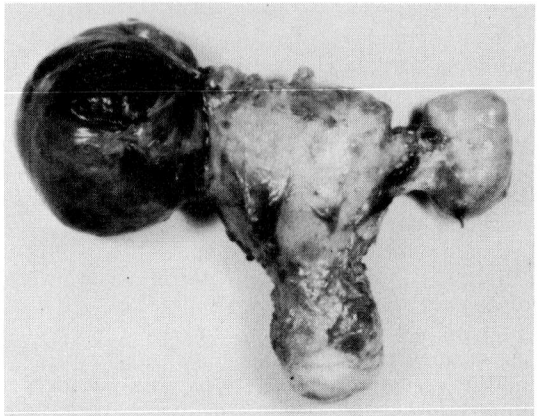

Figure 25. "Chocolate" cyst, endometrioma of the ovary with attached hysterectomy specimen.

have smooth capsules, and usually replace the entire ovary. Histologic examination reveals an adenomatous pattern or tall columnar cells producing mucin, respectively. The benign teratoma, or dermoid cyst, is a common ovarian tumor, benign in more than 99 per cent of patients. The gross appearance is that of a smooth-coated, gray tumor which usually replaces the ovary. Microscopically, ectodermal and mesodermal structures are found with hair, teeth, bone, and cartilage present. Approximately 25 per cent of dermoids are bilateral and, thus, if one ovary is involved, the other should be opened and inspected.

The solid benign ovarian tumors include the Brenner tumor, which is thought to arise from Walthard inclusion rests in the cortex of the ovary. This tumor grossly resembles the ovarian fibroma, another benign solid tumor. Ovarian fibromas are occasionally the cause of Meigs' syndrome with concomitant sympathetic hydrothorax and ascites. Other solid ovarian tumors include the rare androgen-producing Leydig cell tumor, or hilus cell tumor, and the neuroma, angioma, papilloma, and fibroadenoma. The most important decision facing the surgeon who finds a solid ovarian tumor is to differentiate benign from malignant.

The treatment of benign ovarian growths is primarily surgical removal with conservation of all normal ovarian tissue possible. The functional cysts, follicle and corpus luteum, should regress in a relatively short interval and do not require surgery unless rupture and hemorrhage have occurred. These will not infrequently be found during surgery for other reasons and do not require treatment. The majority of the other benign cystic and solid ovarian tumors will usually replace or destroy any remaining ovarian tissue in the involved gonad, and oophorectomy, preserving the tube, is often indicated. Endometrial or "chocolate" cysts are an exception, and after all involved ovarian tissue is resected one attempts to leave even a small amount of normal ovarian tissue for future fertility. In any event, bilateral oophorectomy is rarely indicated in the young woman unless one is *sure* malignancy is present. If there is any doubt, the abdomen should be closed even if reoperation is needed at a later date. In general, we have felt that if an un-diagnosed ovarian mass is larger than 6 cm., or if it persists without diminution in size for longer than 3 months, exploration should be done. Acute torsion or significant hemorrhage may require immediate surgery.

OVARIAN CANCER

The incidence of cancer of the ovary varies considerably in different reports because of the wide range of criteria accepted for making this diagnosis. Among the adenomatous tumors there is a broad group of borderline cases. Most series report that ovarian cancer accounts for 4 to 6 per cent of all cases of malignant disease in the female. Most investigators report incidences of histologic types as serous cystadenocarcinoma, 60 per cent; pseudomucinous carcinoma, 15 per cent; solid undifferentiated adenocarcinoma, 10 per cent; granulosa cell carcinoma, 6 per cent; dysgerminoma, 2 per cent; and other rare types (arrhenoblastoma, teratoma, mesonephroma), 7 per cent. The ratio of benign ovarian tumors to malignant ovarian tumors is 4 to 1, until the peak incidence of ovarian cancer at 40 to 60 years of age, when the ratio is 1 to 1.[3]

The International Federation of Gynecology and Obstetrics has adopted the following clinical classification, based on clinical studies and surgical exploration, for staging primary carcinoma of the ovary.[8]

Stage I
    Growth limited to the ovaries.
Stage II
    Growth involves one or both ovaries with extension of the cancer to other areas within the pelvis.
Stage III
    Growth involves one or both ovaries with widespread intraperitoneal metastasis to the abdomen.
Stage IV
    Growth involves one or both ovaries with distant metastasis outside the peritoneal cavity.

Several factors need to be stressed in regard to ovarian cancer. First, the delay in diagnosis is reprehensible: 50 per cent of ovarian cancers are neglected by the patient and 25 per cent by the physician who does not examine the patient in more than 60 per cent of cases. Second, 30 to 50 per cent of ovarian cancers are inoperable at the time of diagnosis and in only 20 per cent can the tumor be entirely removed surgically. Third, only 11 per cent of patients have suspicious or positive Papanicolaou cystologic findings. Fourth, as expected, the survival is greater the earlier the stage of the disease at the time of diagnosis. As the overall survival of ovarian cancer has improved only slightly in the past 20 years, we must strive for earlier diagnosis.[3, 11]

Ovarian cancer occurs more frequently in Caucasians, and the mean age at diagnosis is 51 years. Fifty-eight per cent of patients are postmenopausal. Childbearing may have some effect in reducing the likelihood of ovarian cancer. It is suggested that a family history of cancer, exposure to pelvic irradiation, and previously existing benign ovarian tumors may increase the likelihood of development of cancer of the ovary.[3, 11]

Signs and Symptoms

The signs and symptoms of ovarian cancer may be only those of an enlarging tumor in the pelvis. Parker reported 56 per cent of his patients complained of pain and 46 per cent of abdominal swelling. He also reported 31 per cent had experienced at least a 10-pound weight change, usually loss, and 22 per cent had either abnormal or postmenopausal bleeding.[11] There may be ascites with unilateral or bilateral hydrothorax. Anemia is frequently seen in advanced disease. Pelvic examination may reveal firm nodular implants of metastatic tumor in the cul-de-sac and pelvic viscera. As noted, there are often no early symptoms of ovarian cancer. Every woman should have an annual pelvic examination before age 40 and more frequently thereafter. The diagnosis is made histopathologically and the differential diagnosis between benign and malignant ovarian tumors cannot be made until operation. The gross examination of the tumor at surgery is usually helpful, as papillary growths on the surface of a cystic or semicystic tumor, or papillations on the inside of the tumor, are suggestive of malignancy (Fig. 26). Solid ovarian tumors that are lobulated or have hemorrhagic areas in the capsule are usually malignant. Peritoneal cell washings should be obtained with any suggestive ovarian tumor.

Treatment

The reader is referred to the many excellent reviews on the various types of therapy for ovarian cancer.[3, 7, 8, 11] Results of all therapy, however, remain poor and various proponents report limited success with a variety of therapeutic regimens. There is general agreement that total abdominal hysterectomy, bilateral salpingo-oophorectomy, and possibly omentectomy should be carried out, even if some tumor is left behind. As the 5-year survival for Stage I ovarian cancer is only 60 per cent, and only 20 per cent of patients explored have disease as limited as Stage I, most investigators feel supplemental therapy is mandatory for all patients with ovarian cancer. Radiotherapy and chemotherapy have both been used with moderate palliative success. Total pelvic and abdominal irradiation, intraperitoneal radioisotopes, alkylating agents, and combination chemotherapy are of significant palliative aid in nearly half of patients so treated.[7, 8, 11]

MALIGNANT TROPHOBLASTIC DISEASE

Malignant gestational trophoblastic diseases are relatively rare cancers of women but are of major importance. Even if metastases are present, essentially all patients with these tumors can be cured. It is tragic for a woman to have an erroneous diagnosis of "anaplastic metastatic cancer" made and the diagnosis of trophoblastic malignancy overlooked. As these tumors frequently present with the symptoms of metastases, it is useful for any physician who treats women of reproductive ages to be aware of the patterns of these diseases.

Malignant trophoblastic disease may follow any type of pregnancy, including abortion or term live

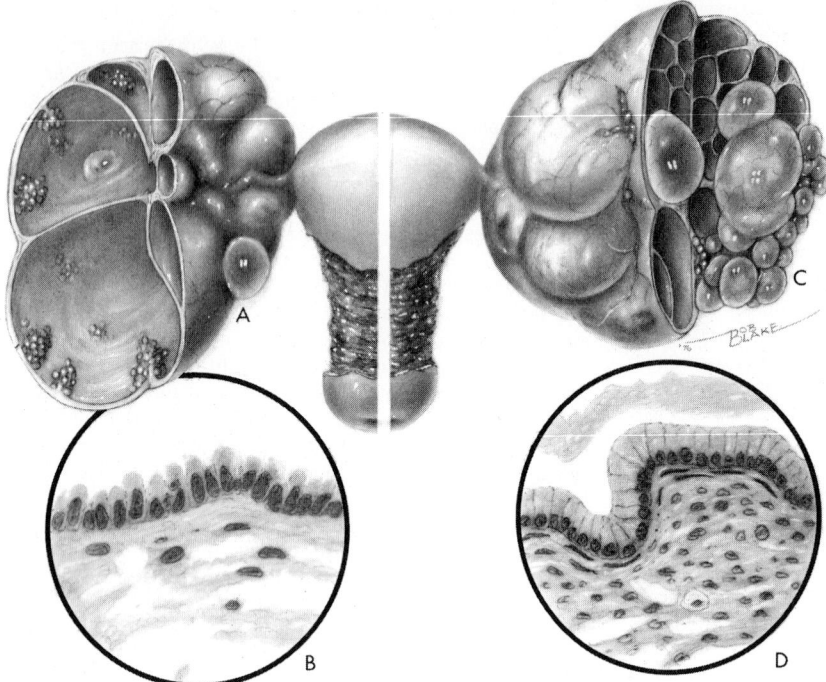

Figure 26. Ovarian carcinoma. *A,* Cystic, papillary. *B,* Microscopic view of *A. C,* Pseudomuconius. *D,* Microscopic view of *C.*

birth, although more than half the tumors occur after hydatidiform mole. Tissue diagnoses include invasive mole (chorioadenoma destruens), choriocarcinoma, and anaplastic trophoblastic tissue. Irregular uterine bleeding is a common presenting sign, but patients present with amenorrhea, uterine rupture, or the sequelae of distant metastasis to lung, vagina, brain, bowel, kidney, and elsewhere. The anaplastic pattern of the placental trophoblasts, with or without preservation of the pattern of the villus, may be seen histologically. Fortunately, all of these tumors produce a hormone identical to human chorionic gonadotropin (HCG) which can be measured in higher levels by pregnancy tests (positive in 75 per cent of these patients) or by sensitive biologic or radioimmunologic techniques. The finding of a suspicious metastatic lesion, with or without pelvic symptoms, should lead to HCG testing. If the HCG level is elevated and normal pregnancy can be excluded, one should strongly suspect malignant trophoblastic disease.

Considerable assistance for physicians treating patients with suspected malignant trophoblastic disease can be obtained from any of the several trophoblastic disease centers in this country. Treatment consists of intensive chemotherapy with methotrexate or actinomycin D, given alone or in combination with surgery or irradiation. With appropriate and intensive therapy essentially all patients with these diseases can be cured, even when metastases are present.[4]

AMENORRHEA

Amenorrhea is defined as the absence of menses at the time a woman should be menstruating and may be classified as primary or secondary. Most investigators feel a patient should be without menses for at least 6 months before the diagnosis of amenorrhea is made. Amenorrhea occurs physiologically in pregnancy and lactation. Menstruation is based on the interaction of the central nervous system, hypothalamus, pituitary, ovary, uterus, and other glands and their hormones (see Physiology and Endocrinology).

Primary amenorrhea, in which the patient has never had menses, may occasionally be due to abnormalities of central nervous system or pituitary gland, but much more commonly occurs from gonadal, adrenal, or uterine defects. Most girls will begin menses by 18 years of age, and failure of menstruation by this age warrants careful examination, chromosomal testing, hormonal assays, and, on occasion, visualization of the gonad. Gonadotropin assays will frequently provide the appropriate direction for further study, as these levels are increased in cases of ovarian failure or abnormal function and are usually reduced with central nervous system or pituitary gland diseases. Congenital absence of the uterus always, and endometrial disease frequently, result in amenorrhea while gonadotropins are normal.

Secondary amenorrhea, or cessation of menses, may be due to a variety of problems. Space-occupying lesions of the central nervous system, hypothalamus, or pituitary result in absence or low levels of gonadotropins and amenorrhea. Pituitary tumors or infarction can also yield similar results. Skull films, visual field examinations, appropriate contrast studies, and hormonal studies may aid in making these diagnoses. However, one must always remember the symptom of amenorrhea may precede the diagnosis of such lesions by a span of years and prolonged follow-up is mandatory. Psychiatric illnesses may interfere with gonadotropin release and result in amenorrhea. Ovarian problems as polycystic ovaries and premature ovarian failure may cause secondary amenorrhea and in these patients gonadotropins will be normal and elevated, respectively. Acquired failure of endometrial responsiveness may also cause secondary amenorrhea, as can significant dysfunction of the thyroid or adrenal glands. Treatment is based on the appropriate diagnosis.

ECTOPIC PREGNANCY

An ectopic pregnancy is one in which the ovum implants and develops outside the normal location, the uterine cavity. Ninety-five per cent of ectopic pregnancies are tubal, with the greatest percentage of these occurring in the dilated ampulla, that portion of the distal tube immediately proximal to the fimbriated end. Less common sites of ectopic pregnancy are abdominal, ovarian, and interligamentary (Fig. 27). Abdominal ectopic pregnancy usually occurs after tubal abortion with secondary reimplantation elsewhere in the abdominal cavity. The incidence of all types of ectopic pregnancy is approximately 1:150 births.

Despite the fact that the ovum is implanted outside the uterine cavity, the uterine endometrium is converted into a decidua similar to that of normal pregnancy. The size and consistency of the uterus also changes in ectopic pregnancy. The cervix and body of the uterus soften and the corpus may enlarge to a size compatible with a 6- to 8-week intrauterine pregnancy. All of these changes are due to the production of placental hormones from the ectopic embryo. As ectopic placental function declines, as usually occurs in tubal pregnancy, the hormonal support declines and irregular uterine bleeding begins. The decidua is usually discharged in fragments, but may on occasion be expelled intact as a decidual cast.

The duration and eventual outcome of tubal ectopic pregnancy are determined primarily by the area of tube involved. If the ovum implants in the relatively large ampullary region of the tube, the pregnancy will usually continue longer than one in the narrow isthmus. Local bleeding from trophoblastic invasion continues and increases, and blood dissects the ovular sac from the tubal wall. With complete separation, the ovular sac is usually extruded from the end of the tube and, unless a major vessel is involved, bleeding terminates. More often, however, the process is prolonged and repeated bleeding episodes yield a pelvic hematoma. In other areas of the tube, the tubal wall is less distensible and the lumen is narrower and tubal rupture is inevitable as the trophoblasts invade and blood collects. Ectopic pregnancies in the narrow isthmic segment usually rupture in 6 to 8 weeks, while those in the interstitial portion, where the tube traverses the uterine wall, continue for 14 to 16 weeks before rupture. Rupture is usually into the peritoneal cavity and is accompanied by sudden and significant bleeding. Tubal pregnancies may regress spontaneously with either the ovum dying at an early age or being extruded from the tubal ostium without significant bleeding.

The classic symptoms of ectopic pregnancy are a history of infertility or pelvic disease, light vaginal bleeding beginning within 2 to 4 weeks after the first missed period, and sharp and fleeting lower abdominal pain. Eventually the patient experiences sudden severe abdominal pain and shock as the tube ruptures. On examination one usually notes the signs of early pregnancy such as cyanosis and softening of the cervix and uterine enlargement. The most important pelvic finding prior to tubal rupture is a unilateral tender mass. In patients with pelvic hematoma the cul-de-sac may be "doughy" and distended. Signs of peritoneal irradiation may be present. Fever is a rare finding, but progressive anemia is frequently observed. Pregnancy tests are positive in about one half of patients with unruptured tubal pregnancy, the discrepancy being due to low levels of chorionic gonadotropin produced by the functional restricted placenta.

The diagnosis of an unruptured tubal pregnancy is not difficult to make when classic symptoms are present but, unfortunately, the symptoms are frequently atypical and the pelvic findings misleading. A high index of suspicion is one's most valuable adjunct. Culdocentesis, or large-gauge needle perforation of the cul-de-sac, may reveal considerable old dark blood and strongly suggest pelvic hematoma. Laparoscopy or culdoscopy may allow visualization of the ectopic embryo. Posterior colpotomy, or vaginal incision into the cul-de-sac, not only allows accurate diagnosis, but the skillful operator can remove the embryo in approximately 50 per cent of tubal pregnancies through this incision. Although it is usually possible to diagnose tubal pregnancy with reasonable accuracy, problems such as uterine abortion, salpingitis, appendicitis, or ruptured corpus luteum or follicular cysts may produce signs and symptoms causing confusion in diagnosis. In uterine abortion the period of amenorrhea is usually longer, the amount of vaginal bleeding is greater, and pain is less severe, more midline, and cramping in nature. No adnexal mass or tenderness is present. Salpingitis and appendicitis usually present with signs of infection and there has been no amenor-

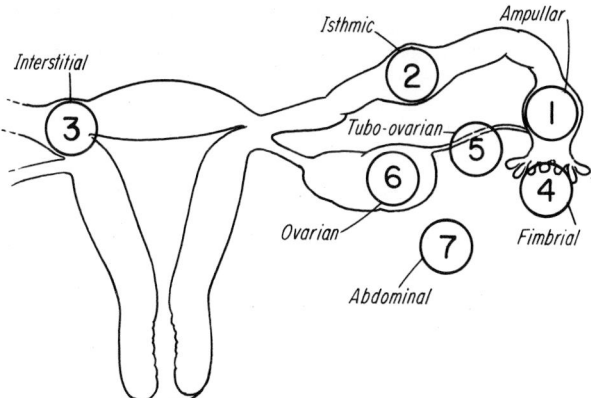

Figure 27. Ectopic pregnancy. Diagram shows the various implantation sites numbered in order of decreasing frequency of occurrence.

rhea or irregular bleeding. Ruptured cysts, particularly those of the corpus luteum, usually are not associated with prolonged amenorrhea. Follicular cysts tend to rupture at midcycle. In both varieties an occasional patient may require surgical exploration for control of hemorrhage.

The treatment of ectopic pregnancy consists of surgical removal of the involved tube and replacement of blood loss. Prompt blood replacement and surgical intervention are mandatory, but the patient's condition should be stabilized prior to surgery if at all possible. General anesthesia should be used. Abdominal pregnancy is treated by removal of the fetus and ligation of the umbilical cord near its insertion into the placenta. Owing to the intense vascularity of the placenta, it is usually best to leave it in situ. Prognosis with prompt management is good and mortality from ectopic pregnancy has been reduced to 1 to 2 per cent. Recurrence of ectopic pregnancy in the remaining tube occurs in about 10 per cent of patients.

SELECTED REFERENCES

The following books were utilized heavily in the preparation of this chapter, and a number of the illustrations were drawn from them. For detailed and factual information about gynecology, the reader is recommended to them all:

Brewer, J. I.: Textbook of Gynecology, 4th ed. Baltimore, Williams & Wilkins Company, 1967.

Kistner, R. W.: Gynecology, Principles and Practice. Chicago, Year Book Medical Publishers, 1964.

Nelson, J. H.: Atlas of Radical Pelvic Surgery, New York, Appleton-Century-Crofts, 1969.

Novak, E., Jones, G. S., and Jones, H.: Textbook of Gynecology, 8th ed. Baltimore, Williams & Wilkins Company, 1970.

Parsons, L., and Ulfelder, H.: An Atlas of Pelvic Operations, 2nd ed. Philadelphia, W. B. Saunders Company, 1968.

Reid, D. E., Ryan, K. J., and Benirschke, K.: Principles and Management of Human Reproduction. Philadelphia, W. B. Saunders Company, 1972.

Taylor, E. S.: Essentials of Gynecology, 4th ed. Philadelphia, Lea & Febiger, 1969.

REFERENCES

1. Brunschwig, A.: The surgical treatment of cancer of the cervix. Am. J. Roentgenol., *102*:147, 1968.
   Dr. Brunschwig and the group at Memorial Hospital in New York became leading proponents for the radical surgical treatment of gynecologic malignant disease. This group popularized exenterative surgery and proved it a useful operation. Techniques, results, and complications are reviewed.

2. Fluhmann, C. F.: The Cervix Uteri and Its Diseases. Philadelphia, W. B. Saunders Company, 1961.
   Diseases of the cervix, including cervical cancer, are reviewed in detail in this book. The illustrations and material are excellent. Any student of gynecologic disease should utilize this valuable test.

3. Gusberg, S. B., and Flick, H. E. (Eds.): Corscaden's Gynecologic Cancer, 4th ed. Baltimore, Williams and Wilkins Co., 1970.
   This text, now in its fourth edition, is one of the standards about gynecologic malignancy. Cancers of the vulva, vagina, cervix, uterus, tube, and ovary are discussed in detail. Etiology, epidemiology, natural history, diagnosis, and therapy are well reviewed. The bibliography is excellent.

4. Hammond, C. B., and Parker, R. T.: The diagnosis and treatment of trophoblastic malignancy. Obstet. Gynecol.. *35*:132, 1970.
   The authors review the history of trophoblastic malignancy,

including the work of Hertz's group at the National Institutes of Health who popularized chemotherapeutic treatment. The article reviews the experience at Duke University in more than 100 patients with these cancers, approximately half with metastases. More than 93 per cent of patients were cured. Methods of chemotherapy and the roles of surgery, combination chemotherapy, and arterial chemotherapy are discussed.*

5. Huffman, J. W.: The Gynecology of Childhood and Adolescence. Philadelphia, W. B. Saunders Company, 1968.
   This textbook has been long needed by gynecologists and other physicians who care for pelvic problems of the young girl. The chapters dealing with embryology, endocrinology, oncology, and functional disorders are exceptionally strong.

6. Israel, S. L.: Diagnosis and Treatment of Menstrual Disorders and Sterility, 5th ed. New York, Hoeber Medical Division, Harper & Row, 1967.
   As the title suggests, this book deals primarily with sterility and its multiple causes. Menstrual dysfunction is also quite adequately reviewed. The reader is referred to it for further details regarding these problems.

7. Julian, C. G., and Woodruff, J. D.: The role of chemotherapy in the treatment of primary ovarian malignancy. Obstet. Gynecol. Survey, *24*:1307, 1969.
   In 1969, this excellent journal began a monthly, detailed review article and this paper is from that series. The detail, clarity, and bibliography are excellent. It summarizes the current knowledge and therapy for chemotherapy of ovarian cancer, a tumor particularly responsive to this form of treatment.

8. M. D. Anderson Hospital and Tumor Institute: Cancer of the Uterus and Ovary. 11th Annual Clinical Conference. Chicago, Year Book Medical Publishers, 1969.
   This institution is well known for its contributions to gynecologic oncology. The details about treatment and follow-up of results for cancers of the cervix, uterus, and ovary are quite good, particularly the sections on radiotherapy and chemotherapy.

9. Miller, O. J.: The sex chromosome anomalies. Am. J. Obstet. Gynecol., part 2, *90*:1078, 1964.
   This article is one of the first detailed summaries of chromosomal aberrations that can result in gonadal and extragonadal defects. The article is commended for its clarity and completeness.

10. Parker, R. T.: The clinical problems of early cervical neoplasia. Obstet. Gynecol. Surgery, part 2, *24*:691, 1969.
    This article presents the problems, findings, therapy and results in more than 1000 patients with early cervical neoplasia. The entire issue of the journal is devoted to various problems with these diseases and the reader will profit from its detailed study.

11. Parker, R. T., Parker, C. H., and Wilbanks, G. D.: Cancer of the ovary. Am. J. Obstet. Gynecol., *108*:878, 1970.
    Ovarian cancer remains a diagnostic and therapeutic problem of major proportion. This article reviews the past 20 years experience with these diseases at Duke University. The influence of histopathologic diagnosis, clinical staging, positive cell washings and ascites is discussed. The effects of surgery, radiotherapy, and chemotherapy are reviewed.

12. Richardson, G. S.: Ovarian Physiology. Boston, Little, Brown and Company, 1967.
    This monograph discusses in considerable detail what is currently known about ovarian physiology and is suggested for better basic understanding of this subject and its influence on gynecologic disease.

13. Rutledge, F. N.: Cancer of the vagina. Am. J. Obstet. Gynecol., *97*:635, 1967.
    Primary vaginal carcinoma remains a poorly responsive malignant lesion, regardless of the therapy chosen. This article reviews the experience of the M. D. Anderson Hospital with radiotherapy for this tumor, and the results are the best reported.

14. Sherman, R.: Human Ovulation Induction. Springfield, Ill., Charles C Thomas, Publisher, 1969.
    Anovulation and amenorrhea are perplexing problems for both diagnosis and therapy, particularly if fertility is desired. With the advent of newer drugs capable of allowing ovulation induc-

tion, this timely text reviews the problems, studies, findings, and treatment schedules that offer the best chance of success.

15. Simpson, J. L., and Christakos, A. C.: Hereditary factors in obstetrics and gynecology. Obstet. Gynecol. Survey, *24*:580, 1969.
    This excellent review article summarizes the more current chromosomal aberrations that can result in gonadal and extragonadal defects. The bibliography is most adequate.

16. Speert, H.: Obstetric and Gynecologic Milestones. New York, Macmillan Company, 1958.
    This book, subtitled "Essays in Eponymy," explores the discoveries and men who have contributed to this specialty. It is recommended to all practitioners of this area of medicine and to any student of medical history.

17 Speroff, L., Glass, R. H., and Kase, N. G.: Clinical Gynecologic Endocrinology and Infertility. Baltimore, Williams and Wilkins Co., 1973.
    This is a superb book of factual details regarding gynecologic endocrinology. It is current and easily read. While not encylopedic, this book provides a formulation of clinical diagnosis and management founded on physiologic principles.

18. . Taylor, E. S.: Essentials of Gynecology, 4th ed. Philadelphis, Lea & Febiger, 1969.
    This general textbook of gynecology was particularly useful to the author. The organization, graphic material, and detail of presentation are excellent.

19. Way, S.: Carcinoma of the vulva. Am. J. Obstet. Gynecol., *79*:692, 1960.
    The names of Taussig, Bassett, Twombly, Collins, and others all come to mind during any discussion of vulvar cancer. Dr. Way must certainly be included among those who have made major contributions to our knowledge of these diseases and their surgical treatment. This article summarizes his experience.

20. Williams, R. H. (ed.): Textbook of Endocrinology. 5th ed. Philadelphia, W. B. Saunders, Company, 1974.
    This classic textbook on human endocrinology contains considerable detail about human reproductive endocrinology. Concise and detailed information is presented about the physiology and biochemistry of this system.

48

THE URINARY SYSTEM

John T. Grayhack, M.D.

The production, transport, storage, and discharge of liquid waste by the human body are accomplished by an integrated system which includes functions varying from delicately controlled, highly complex cellular mechanisms to those of a rather gross muscular conduit. The kidneys, ureters, bladder, and urethra are located extraperitoneally in the abdomen and pelvis (Fig. 1). The embryologic development of the upper urinary tract is complex. The adult renal parenchyma, the metanephros, arises from the mesoderm of the nephrotome after sequential lysis of the pronephros and the mesonephros. Fusion of the ureter,

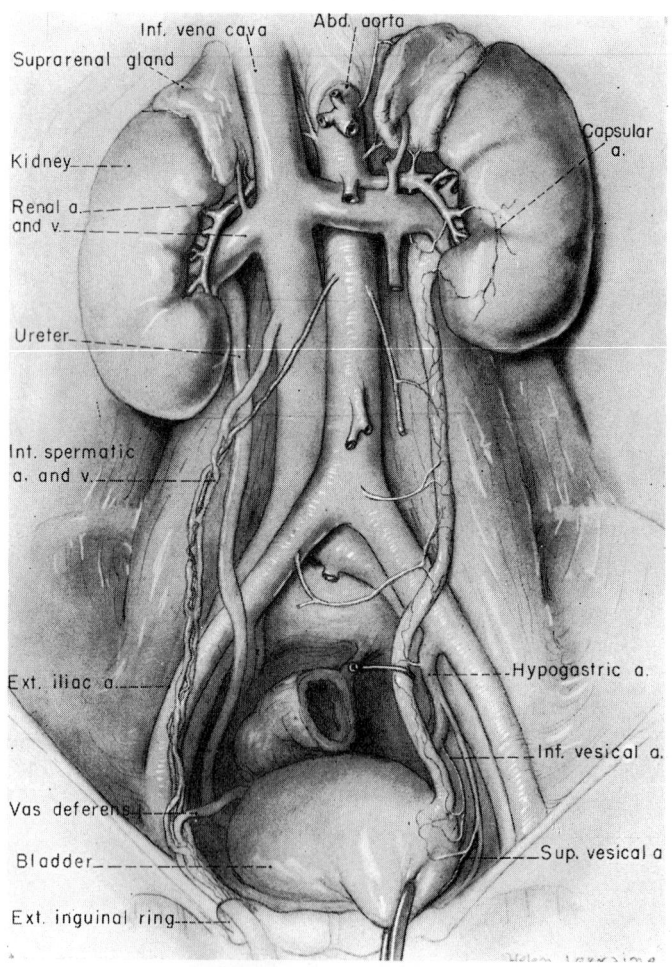

Figure 1. Gross anatomic relationships of the organs composing the urinary tract.

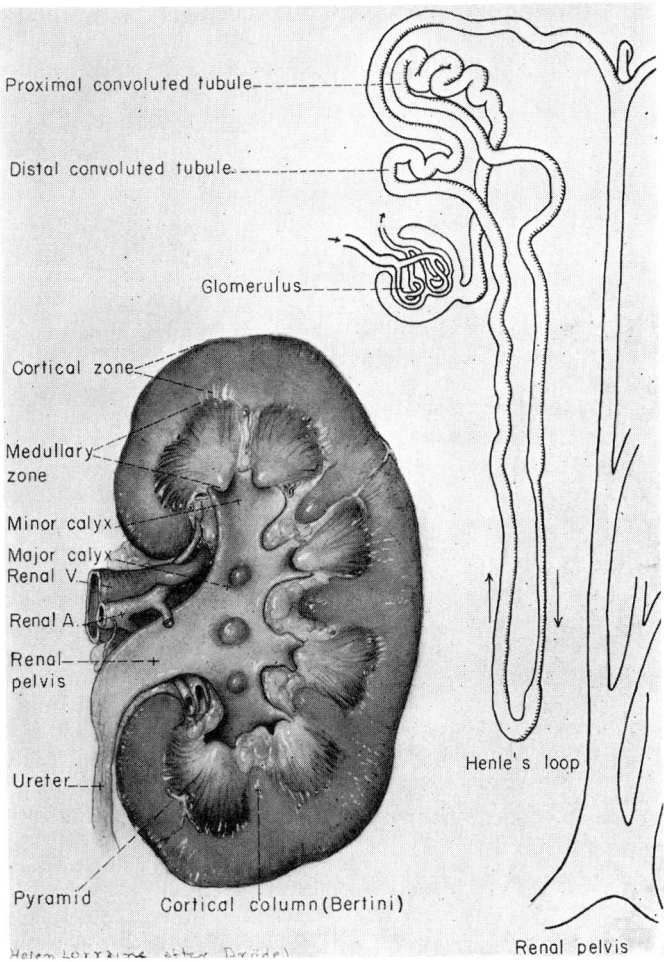

Proximal convoluted tubule

Distal convoluted tubule

Glomerulus

Cortical zone

Medullary zone

Minor calyx

Major calyx

Renal V.

Renal A.

Renal pelvis

Ureter

Pyramid   Cortical column (Bertini)

Henle's loop

Renal pelvis

Figure 2. Cross section of kidney showing gross anatomic relationships. *Inset,* Diagrammatic representation of the nephron shown joining a collecting duct. (From Dodson, A. I. *In* Campbell, M. F. (Ed.): Urology. Philadelphia, W. B. Saunders Company, 1954.)

which arises from the wolffian duct, with the mesoderm of the nephrogenic cord is necessary for the normal development of collecting tubules and functioning nephrons. As the kidney matures, it migrates upward from the region of the fourth to the first lumbar vertebra and rotates so that the original dorsal border becomes the convex lateral border. The superior pole of the left kidney may lie as high as T10 or as low as L2. X-ray measurements indicate a length of 12.6 ± 0.8 cm. by a width of 5.9 ± 0.4 cm. in females and a length of 13.2 ± 0.8 cm. by a width of 6.3 ± 0.5 cm. in males. The right kidney is slightly lower than the left and slightly smaller. The arterial blood supply is derived from the aorta; the venous blood flow enters the vena cava.

The kidney is divided into the peripherally situated cortex, which contains the glomeruli and portions of the tubules, and the centrally located medulla, composed primarily of portions of the tubules and the collecting ducts (Fig. 2). The initial step in urine formation is the physical process of filtration accomplished in the glomerulus of the nephron. The glomerular filtrate is modified in the tubules by

reabsorption of solute and water as well as secretory activity. The urine is delivered from the papilla through the collecting ducts into the minor calyx. The urine that enters the calyx is normally excreted essentially unmodified. The calyces, pelvis, ureter, and bladder are lined by transitional epithelium. Transport of urine is accomplished with development of pressures exceeding 35 cm. H_2O by a coordinated contraction of the smooth muscle surrounding the epithelium. The volume of urine retained in the pelvis is small. Once urine enters the ureter peristaltic activity results in its prompt delivery to the bladder. Unlike the pelvis and the ureter, the bladder, which derives its arterial blood supply from branches of the hypogastric artery, is a reservoir with the capacity for storage of urine for hours. Periodic integrated contraction of this smooth muscle reservoir results in normal micturition with minimal postvoiding residual urine. The mechanism of normal voiding and its neurogenic control are discussed briefly in the section on neurogenic bladder.

Historically, operative procedures for removal of bladder calculi were undoubtedly carried out by the ancients. In the middle ages, itinerant lithotomists who retained the secrets of their art for their family carried out this procedure. However, the development of urology as a recognized, respected surgical specialty depended primarily on the introduction of specialized roentgenographic and endoscopic diagnostic techniques. Specialized therapeutic procedures were conceived and improved once diagnoses could be established with regularity. Similarly, proper treatment today demands accurate diagnosis. This in turn requires a painstaking history, a complete physical examination, a careful examination of the urine with employment of special tests as indicated, and utilization of appropriate x-ray, isotope, and endoscopic studies. All are essential to establish a diagnosis.

A patient may have a life-threatening disease of the genitourinary tract with few if any symptoms. However, the following symptoms are suggestive of urinary tract disease.[18, 45]

Nocturia, awakening at night to void, is unnecessary for the normal person. Nocturia may be caused by lower urinary tract disease, such as bladder neck obstruction, neurogenic dysfunction, infection, and calculus; metabolic disorder, such as diabetes mellitus or diabetes insipidus; congestive heart failure; renal failure; and habitual excessive fluid or drug intake.

Frequency: The normal person voids three to five times a day. Increased frequency may be due to organic or psychogenic causes. Diurnal frequency in the absence of nocturia suggests a functional disorder.

Polyuria means larger than normal total urine volume and is characteristic of metabolic disorders, renal disease, and excessive fluid intake.

Oliguria is utilized to describe diminished urine volume; usually 400 ml. is considered the minimal obligatory urine output.

Anuria is complete suppression of urine formation.

Urgency is a precipitious desire to void, making control difficult or impossible.

Dysuria means pain or discomfort on urination. When it is severe, it is called strangury. Bladder spasm or tenesmus often follows voiding in the presence of an irritated or infected bladder.

Hesitancy denotes undue delay and difficulty in initiating voiding.

Intermittency is the term used to describe the interrupted urinary stream thought to be due to detrusor fatigue in the presence of bladder neck obstruction. Usually there is an associated decrease in size and force of the urinary stream.

Incontinence is involuntary loss of urine. It is further characterized as true when caused by abnormalities such as sphincter injury or fistula; as paradoxical or overflow when resulting from urinary leakage from an overdistended bladder; as stress when associated with coughing or straining, or as urgency when it is preceded by a desire to void as may occur with neurogenic dysfunction or inflammatory lesions.

Pyuria is used to denote the presence of pus in the urine. It is due to inflammation and may be associated with an undesirable odor.

Crystalluria due to precipitated urinary solutes is similar in gross appearance to pyuria.

Hematuria may be gross or microscopic, painless or painful. Hemoglobinuria, beeturia, red bladder dyes, and the brick-dust color of uric acid crystals may be confused grossly with hematuria. Hematuria may be further characterized by its relationship to the act of micturition. Initial hematuria is noted only at the beginning of urination and usually is secondary to pathologic change distal to the neck of the bladder. Terminal hematuria is noted at the end of urination and is secondary to pathologic change in the region of the trigone, bladder neck, and posterior urethra such as a calculus, bladder neoplasm, or prostatitis. When blood is passed throughout urination, the descriptive term total is utilized. The common causes for hematuria vary with age and sex (Table 1). Although there are more than 100 causes for hematuria, consideration of tumor of the bladder, tumor of the kidney, stone, tuberculosis, acute hemorrhagic cystitis, trauma, and blood dyscrasia as causes of gross hematuria in the adult is a useful diagnostic framework. Benign prostatic hypertrophy is probably the commonest cause of bleeding in males over the age of 55. Blood dyscrasias have assumed greater importance with the increased use of anticoagulants.

Lithuria is used to describe the passage of urinary calculi.

Pneumaturia, passing gas in the urine, may be due to an enterovesical fistula, gas-forming organisms, or urologic instrumentation.

Pain from a renal lesion may vary from a dull, aching flank discomfort to a severe, sharp flank pain radiating into the lower abdomen or the gluteal region. The pain may be episodic or persistent. Often, it is associated with anorexia, nausea, and vomiting. No relationship is evident to the intake of food or to movement. Occasionally, as in the presence of ureteral reflux, the pain may be precipitated by voiding, or as

TABLE 1.   Common Causes of Hematuria in Various Age Groups Listed in Order of Frequency

Male and Female				Male			Female		
1–5	5–10	11–30	31–40	41–50	51–60	31–40	41–50	51–60
Inf. Gl. Neph.	Gl. Neph. Inf.	Inf. Cal. Bl. Neo.	Inf. Bl. Neo. Cal.	Bl. Neo. Cal. Inf.	Bl. Neo. B.P.H. Cal. Inf.	Inf. Cal. Bl. Neo.	Inf. Cal. Bl. Neo.	Bl. Neo. Inf. Cal.

Inf.—Inflammatory lesion; Gl. Neph.—glomerulonephritis; Cal.—calculus; Bl. Neo.—bladder neoplasm; B.P.H.—benign prostatic hypertrophy.

in the occasional rare instance in which renal ptosis is obstructing, by the assumption of an erect position. In general, renal pain is as likely to awaken a patient as to occur during waking hours. Usually, with severe discomfort the patient tends to move about restlessly and to indicate the site of discomfort by grasping the flank between his thumb and forefingers. Renal disease may be responsible for bizarre abdominal complaints.

Pain from ureteral colic often causes flank discomfort associated with severe abdominal discomfort, nausea, and vomiting. As the site of the calculus or clot responsible for the discomfort progresses inferiorly, the pain tends to radiate into the lower abdomen, the genitalia, and occasionally the thigh. If a calculus lodges at the ureterovesical junction it may also cause associated frequency, urgency, and dysuria.

Pain from bladder disease is often dull and aching and confined to the suprapubic area. It may, as in the case of an acute infection, be severe and associated primarily with voiding or a desire to void. Discomfort of the glans penis, particularly at the end of voiding, often results from a lesion in the region of the neck of the bladder.

All patients with urologic complaints deserve a complete physical examination, including a neurologic evaluation. Inspection of the abdomen in the presence of a distended bladder may disclose a lower midline mass tending to flatten rather than accentuate the lower abdominal crease. Neither the distended bladder nor the hydronephrotic kidney is easy to delineate on palpation. Palpation of the kidney should usually be initiated with the patient supine and with one examining hand on the flank and the other hand anteriorly on the abdomen. Utilization of both the lateral margin and tips of the fingers of the anterior examining hand is an aid in the examination. Observation of the changes in position of a palpable mass with respiration and change to a lateral or erect position of the patient is of value in identifying the mass, as in recognition of a landmark such as the renal hilum. In a child, a hydronephrotic kidney can occasionally be seen by transillumination. Sudden pressure in the costovertebral angle may elicit pain in the diseased kidney; this does not require delivery of a blow to the flank. On many occasions the site of maximal abdominal tenderness is best localized by examination with a single finger or by having the patient cough or strain and identify the site of discomfort. Pressure over a full bladder often precipitates a desire to void. Percussion will often assist in recognition and delineation of an enlarged kidney or a distended bladder.

Accurate diagnosis is usually dependent on judicious utilization of the many laboratory studies now available. This in turn requires an understanding of the tests and their limitations.

Urinalysis[31] should be preceded by cleansing of the genitalia, particularly in the female. In the male a two- or three-glass urine specimen assists in localizing the abnormality found in the urinary sediment. The first glass should contain the initial 30 to 60 ml. and the third glass, if employed, the final 30 ml. of voided urine. In the female, midstream urine should be utilized; if properly collected, the sample is likely to reflect the findings in the urinary tract, particularly if negative. Under some circumstances, catheterization is required in the female to obtain a representative specimen. Assessment of findings on urinalysis and urine culture is discussed in the section on infection.

Evaluation of total and often individual renal function is of importance in patients with suspected or proved disease of the urinary tract.[21, 34] Clinically, evaluation of total renal function is achieved by measurement of the degree of retention in the blood of endogenous wastes such as *urea* or *creatinine* and excretion of these substances or of exogenous chemicals such as *inulin, para-aminohippurate,* or *phenolsulfonphthalein.* The blood urea nitrogen is a less accurate indicator of renal function than the serum creatinine level. Although both substances are excreted primarily by glomerular filtration, the amount of the former available for excretion is variable. For example, excessive protein breakdown following hemorrhage may result in a marked increase in total urea production. Creatinine is produced in essentially constant amounts. The blood urea level often seems more indicative of the clinical status of the patient, although urea itself is a nontoxic substance. In clinical practice, the creatinine clearance test is popular. It is a satisfactory measure of glomerular filtration rate and may be performed in most hospital laboratories. Inulin clearance, an extremely accurate measure of glomerular filtration, is utilized as an investigative tool. Para-aminohippurate is secreted by the proximal tubule and is a measure of renal plasma flow. All these excretory tests are dependent on total urine collection for accuracy and may yield inaccurate results in patients with significant residual urine unless this is corrected. A variety of tests that utilize infusion of radioactive substances such as ^{125}I or ^{131}I diatrozoate, ^{57}Co or ^{58}Co cyanocobalamin (vitamin B$_{12}$), or labeled chelates of ethylenediaminotetraacetic (EDTA) and diethylenetriaminopentaacetic acid (DTPA) have been employed to evaluate total renal function successfully. Despite the obvious advantages in avoiding the need for total urine collection, these tests have usually been reserved for clinical investigation rather than clinical practice. Knowledge of the concentrating ability of the kidney is of value in assessing renal functional status and in studying patients with possible diabetes insipidus. Individual renal function may be assessed crudely by cytoscopic observation of concentration of a chromogen such as indigo carmine excreted by each ureter or more accurately by the insertion of ureteral cathers bilaterally and collection of individual urine for clearance studies—split function studies.

In addition, the *radioisotope renogram* may be utilized to indicate the functional status of the individual kidney in a qualitative fashion (Fig. 3). This test is carried out by placing a scintillation counter over each renal area and measuring the accumulation of radioactivity following the intravenous injection of an organic iodide labeled with isotopic iodine, either ^{131}I or ^{125}I. Computerized analysis has permitted quantitation of individual renal function with radioactive scanning techniques.[36]

Development of special instruments, useful in both

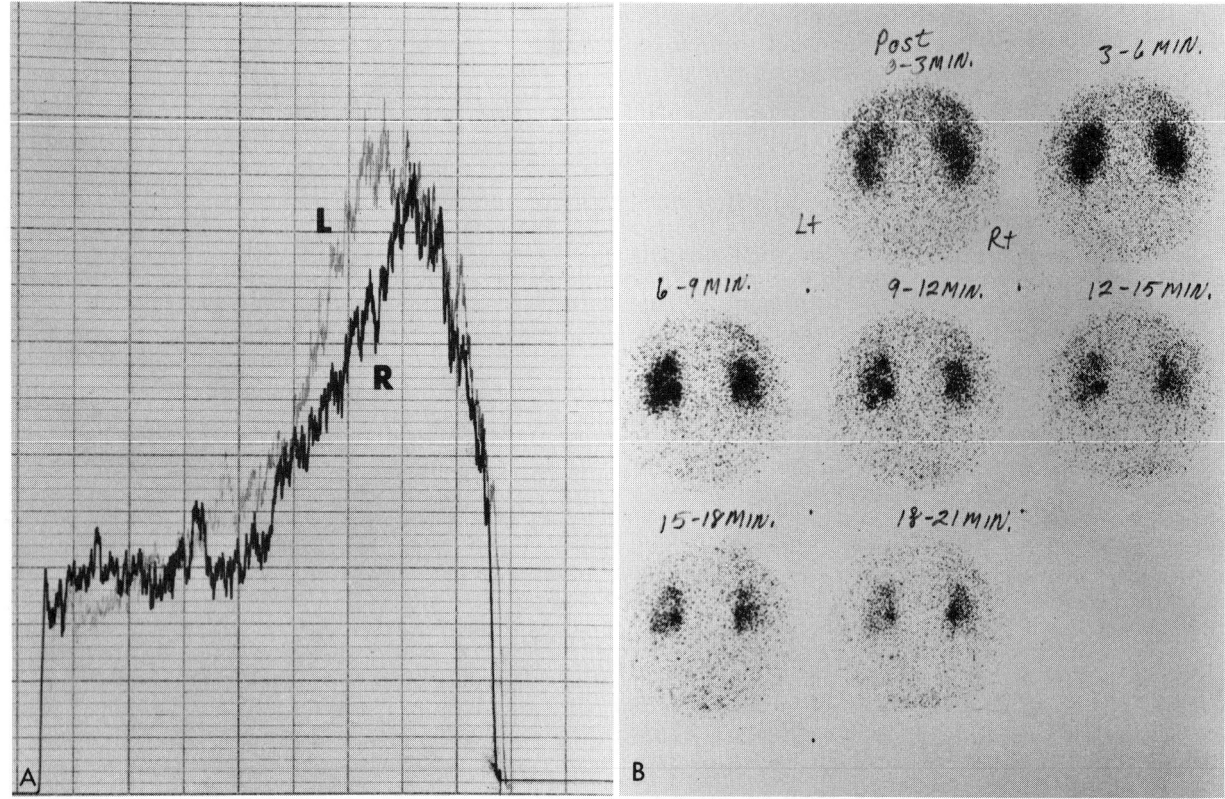

Figure 3. Radioactive renogram (*A*) is a graph of the accumulated radioactivity in the renal area following intravenous injection of labeled (^{131}I or ^{125}I) organic iodide. The initial phase represents the vascular spike. This is followed by an accumulation of radioactivity dependent on renal function and finally by a decrease in radioactivity dependent on excretion. In this renogram, a small, minimally obstructing stone causes a slight delay in excretion on the left. A simultaneously obtained renal scan (*B*) adds anatomical information and aids in interpretation of the study.

diagnosis and treatment, has greatly benefited the patient with genitourinary disorders. *Catheters* of varying construction have been utilized since ancient times. They are employed to bypass and relieve obstruction, to measure residual urine, to introduce and remove solutions or other substances, or to collect specimens. These hollow tubes come in varying sizes and are made of a variety of materials (Fig. 4). Properly utilized for a reasonable indication, they can provide important information and may be lifesaving; employed indiscriminately in an unskilled fashion, they can cause serious complications.

Cystometry (Fig. 5), a method of assessing the pressure response of the bladder to distention, may be performed by infusing fluid through a urethral or suprapubic catheter and recording the pressure response. Bladder capacity and voiding pressure may be noted. This method is of value in evaluating neurogenic dysfunction, especially when drugs modifying the response of the autonomic nervous system are utilized in conjunction with the test.

A *bougie* (Fig. 6) is an acorn-tipped instrument usually utilized for calibration of the urethra.

Sounds are metal instruments of various shapes primarily employed to dilate the urethra. A *filiform* is a thin threaded guide used to bypass a difficult stric-

ture or tortuous area of the urethra and act as a guide for larger, less flexible sounds or catheters.

Direct visualization of the bladder and urethra has been achieved by development of an excellent group of endoscopic instruments. In general, the *cystoscope* combines a hollow tube or sheath with a light source and a lens system. Employment of water as an irrigating fluid distends the portion of the lower urinary tract being studied and permits visualization. Proper combinations of instruments permit complete inspection of the lower urinary tract. In addition the instruments may be utilized to pass other diagnostic aids such as ureteral catheters and may be employed for a number of therapeutic purposes such as ureteral stone extraction and fulguration of bleeding areas or bladder neoplasms.

The *resectoscope* is an endoscopic instrument that permits excision of prostatic and bladder tissue through the urethra. The tissue is excised with a movable wire loop by employing a high-frequency current; bleeding is controlled by fulguration.

Diagnostic ultrasound is the most readily available and least costly of a growing number of noninvasive imaging devices that rely on physical phenomena. The technique depends on conversion of electric signals into acoustic beams by a transducer and detection of

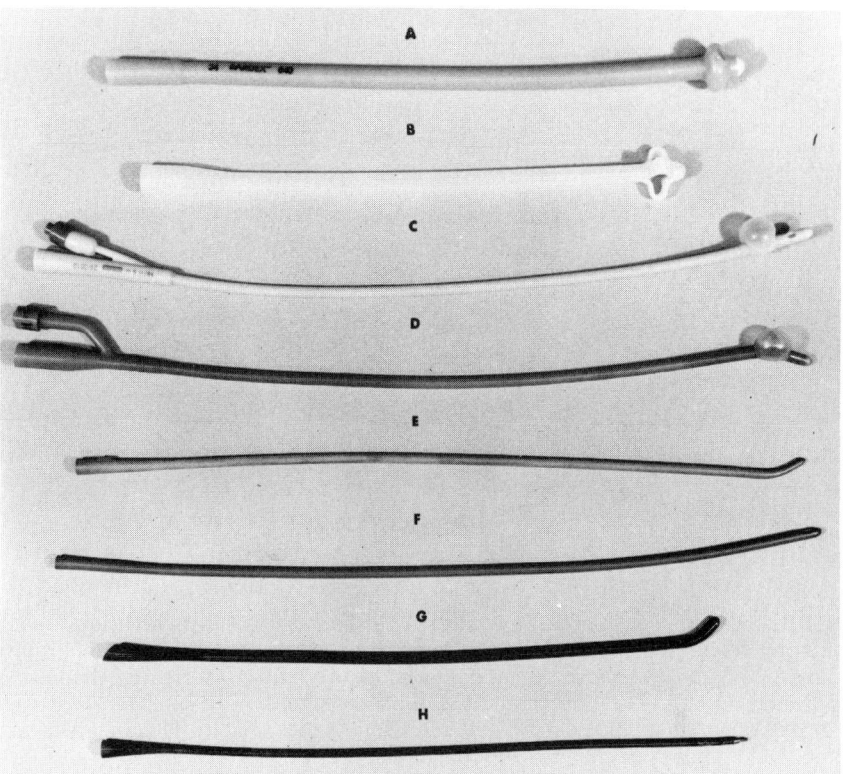

Figure 4. Types of catheters: *A*, de Pezzar latex catheter; *B*, Malecot Silastic catheter; *C*, Foley Silastic catheter; *D*, Coudé tip Foley latex catheter; *E*. Red rubber coudé tip catheter; *F*, Red rubber Robinson catheter; *G*, Woven silk coudé catheter; *H*, Woven silk Phillip's following catheter.

reflected or echo beams by the same transducer. Useful information is obtained by connecting the reflected pulse to an electronic signal that can be recognized. Commonly the information is generated to permit display on an oscilloscope screen in the form of echo amplitude versus depth (A mode) or as two dimensional images (B mode). The B mode scan or one of its modifications provides the most diagnostic information in urology (Fig. 7). Ultrasound studies are useful in identifying the size and position of the kidney, the gross configuration of the renal collecting system, the presence and ultrasonic characteristics of renal masses, the relationship of the kidney to the other abdominal organs and mass lesions, and the configura-

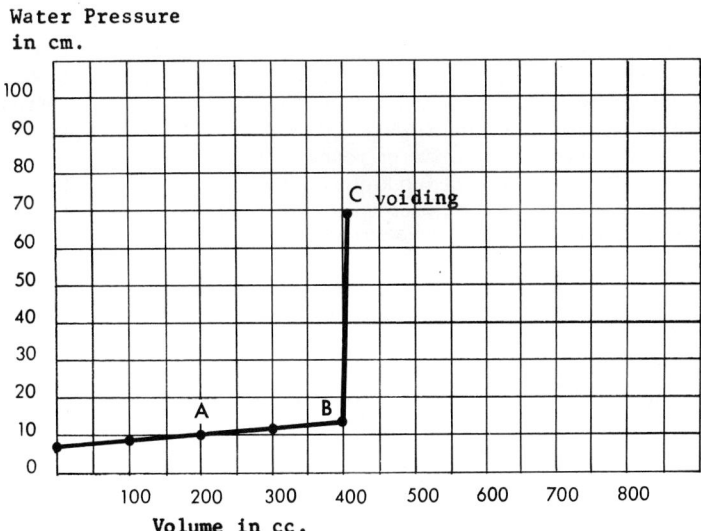

Figure 5. Normal cystometrogram. Pressure response is recorded to gradual or intermittent filling of the bladder. First desire to void (A) is usually at 150 to 250 ml. Sensation of discomfort (B) precedes voiding. Voiding pressure is usually 40 cm. H_2O or more. Residual urine determination and testing of sensation of bladder to heat and cold are carried out as part of the test. The initial pressures may be set at 0 or utilized as a zero point as in this drawing.

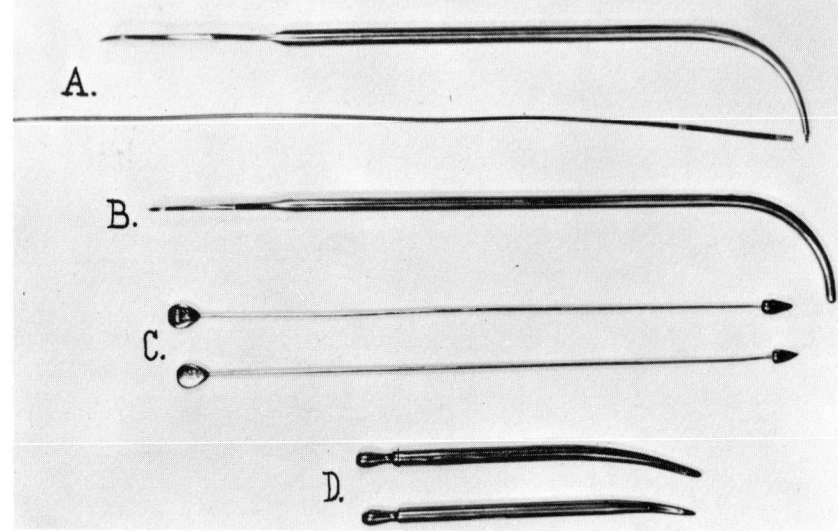

Figure 6. Urethral instruments. *A*, Filiform and LeForte (following) urethral sounds. *B*, Van Buren urethral sound. *C*, Otis bougie à boule. *D*, Walther female dilator-catheter. Many other specialized instruments exist for diagnostic and therapeutic manipulation of the urethra.

tion of the bladder and its contents. Ultrasound is proving useful in percutaneous manipulative procedures such as cyst puncture and insertion of renal drainage tubing. The role that ultrasound or computerized x-ray imaging devices will play in diagnosis and management of diseases of the urinary tract is likely to be an expanding one.

Roentgenographic study of the urinary tract has been a great asset in increasing accurate diagnosis of genitourinary disorders.[14] A scout film of the abdomen taken with a soft tissue technique (KUB — kidneys, ureter, bladder) may demonstrate normal structure — e.g., the size, shape, and position of the kidney, the psoas shadow, and the bony structures of the pelvis and lumbar spine (Fig. 8). In addition, significant abnormalities such as soft tissue masses or radiopacities representing possible calculi may be seen. Visualization of the various portions of the urinary tract by employing contrast media has added to the value of x-ray as a diagnostic tool. These studies should always be preceded by a plain film to permit accurate interpretation.

The *intravenous pyelogram* (Fig. 9) is a technique for achieving visualization of the urinary tract that employs the intravenous injection of an organic iodide and is dependent on renal function. The contrast medium is excreted primarily by glomerular filtration and concentrated because of reabsorption of water. The collecting system of the kidney is visualized as an opacity because of the absorbed x-rays. Visualization can usually be improved by increasing water reabsorption as occurs in a dehydrated patient. Administration of large amounts of contrast medium increases the amount filtered and may achieve visualization even in patients with some degree of impaired renal function.

The *nephrotomogram* (Fig. 10) is an x-ray study that combines the prolonged injection of large amounts of an organic iodide contrast medium with tomography. The contrast medium is concentrated homogeneously by functioning renal tissue. Nonfunctioning vascular tissue such as a neoplasm shows irregular pooling of the medium; avascular tissue such as a cyst lacks

opacification. Use of a body-sectioning x-ray technique such as tomography aids visualization by reducing interfering shadows overlying an organ.

Aortography (Fig. 11) is an x-ray technique utilized to visualize the renal arteries. It is dependent on delivery of a sizable concentrated bolus of contrast medium to the renal arterial system and is independent of function. The contrast medium is commonly introduced through a needle placed in the lumbar aorta from the back or through a catheter threaded into the lumbar aorta from the femoral artery. The retrograde catheter technique is favored by most and has the advantage of allowing selective catheterization of individual renal arteries (Fig. 11).

X-ray studies utilizing intravascular injection of contrast media introduce the risk of various allergic reactions, including anaphylactic shock. Damage to the arterial system or the kidney may also occur after intra-arterial injection. The possibility of these infrequent complications must be recognized.

A *radioactive renal scintiscan* (Figs. 2 and 12) may be carried out by injecting radioisotope-labeled compounds such as chlormerodrin ^{197}Hg or ^{99m}Tc-diethylenetriaminopentaacetic acid which are concentrated throughout the functioning renal tissue. Areas composed of nonfunctioning tissue, such as cyst or tumor, fail to concentrate the isotope. The routine renal scan provides information similar to that obtained with a nephrotomogram. Modifications of the method employing computerized analysis permit assessment of individual renal function.[36]

Combinations of instrumentation and instillation of contrast media have the advantage of permitting complete visualization of the portion of the urinary tract being studied without relying on function. They are disadvantageous in that instrumentation must be possible and that it introduces risk, although minimal, of infection, bleeding, or perforation.

The *retrograde pyelogram* (Fig. 13) is accomplished by the instillation of contrast media through a small catheter inserted in the ureter or wedged into the ureteral orifice.

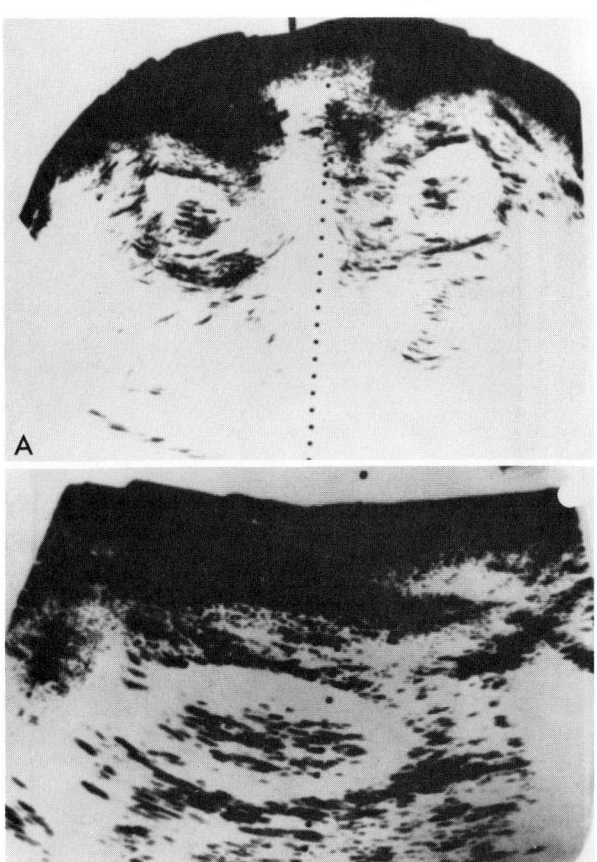

Figure 7. Ultrasound study of the kidney. Transverse ultrasonic B-mode study of the kidneys (*A*) demonstrating the echo patterns caused by the renal parenchyma and the renal calyces and pelvis; longitudinal ultrasonic B mode study of the right kidney (*B*).

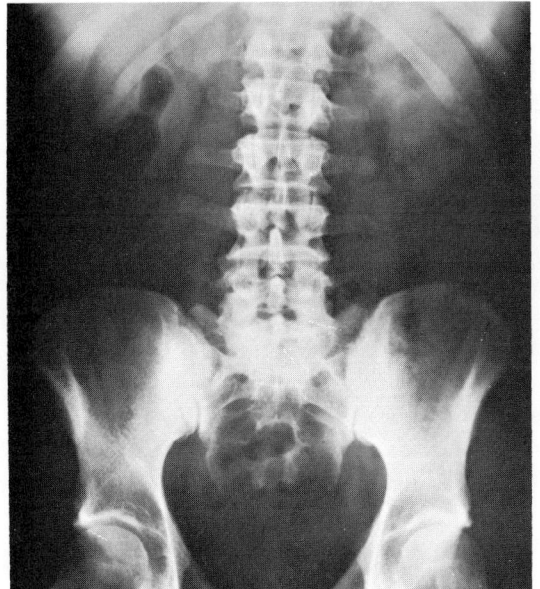

Figure 8. KUB. The renal and psoas shadows are visible as well as the bony structures. An estimate of renal size as well as evaluation of renal shape and position is possible. Small radiodensities in the left side of the pelvis represent phleboliths.

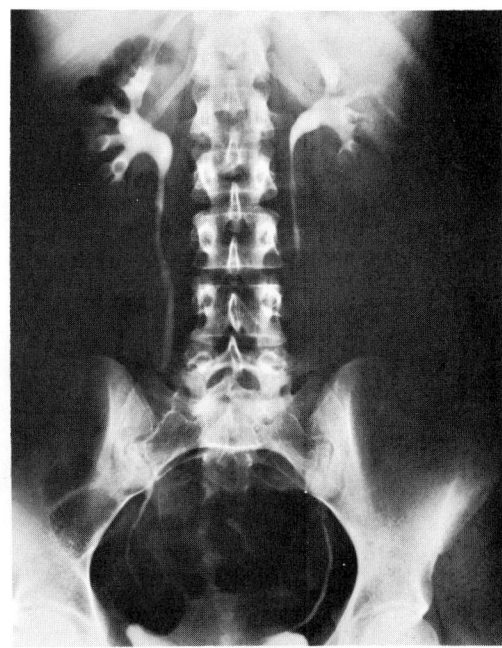

Figure 9. Intravenous pyelogram. Excellent visualization of the renal collecting system is achieved bilaterally. The distal collecting tubules are faintly visualized near the tip of the papilla, causing a fanlike effect within some of the minor calyces. The calyces do not lie in one plane, so that they may be seen in an "end-on" view at times. The patchy visualization of the ureter is the result of normal peristaltic activity.

The *retrograde cystogram* (Fig. 14) is made by gravity instillation of contrast media through a catheter into the bladder. This study has considerable value in demonstrating ureteral reflux and in delineating abnormalities such as bladder diverticula and urinary extravasation. X-rays taken as the patient voids the contrast medium may disclose ureteral reflux, or bladder neck or urethral disease.

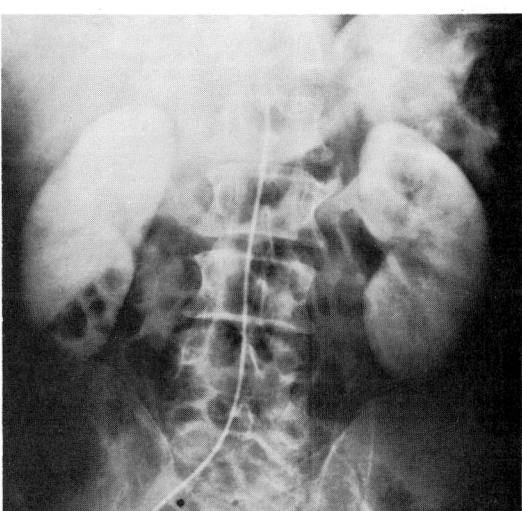

Figure 10. Nephrogram. Opacification of the renal parenchyma resulting from functional accumulation of contrast medium by kidney. Tomogram technique is unnecessary in this postaortogram study because of absence of interfering shadows.

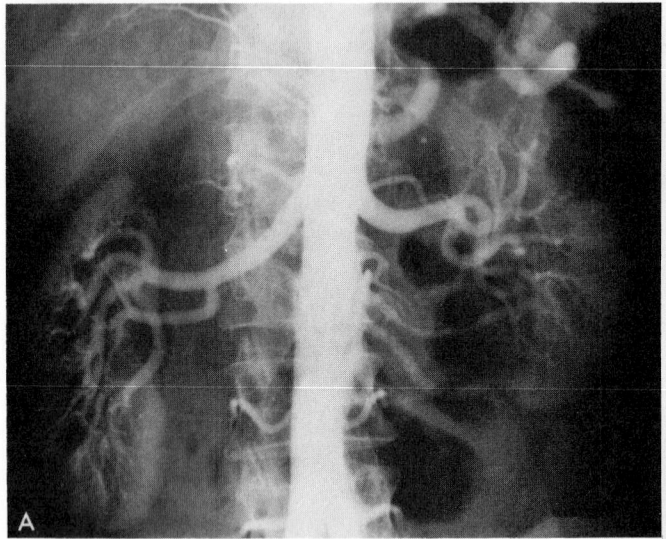
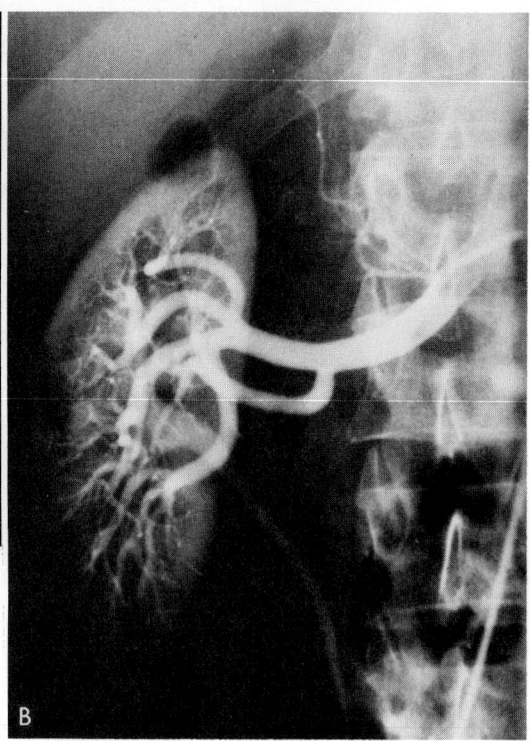

Figure 11. A, Abdominal angiogram performed by injection of contrast media through a catheter inserted percutaneously into the femoral artery and guided into the abdominal aorta, B, Selective renal arteriogram by the retrograde technique.

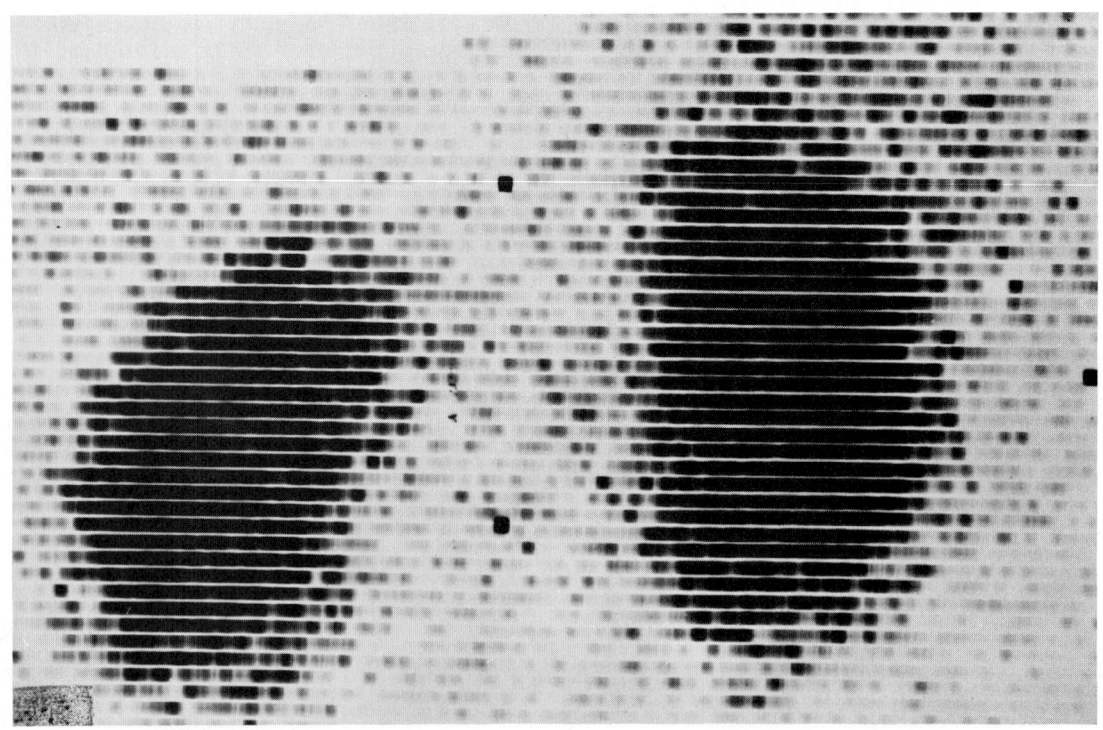

Figure 12. Mercury-203 renal scan. Functioning renal tissue concentrates the radioisotope.

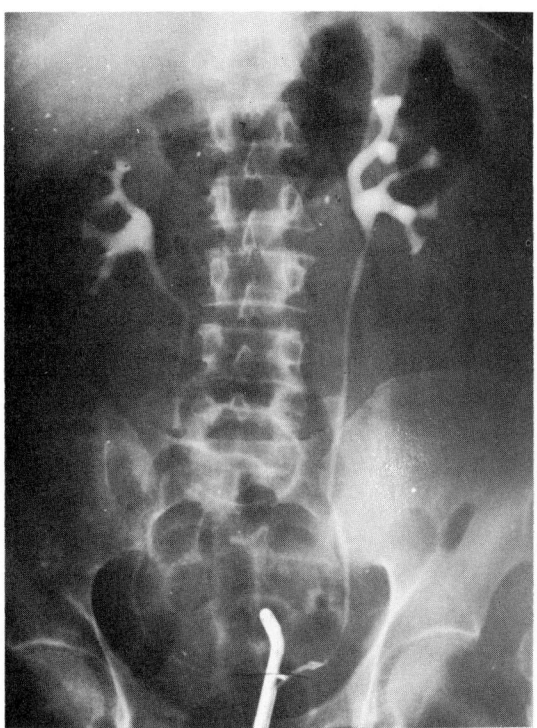

Figure 13. Retrograde pyeloureterogram obtained by instillation of an organic iodide through an acorn-tip ureteral catheter.

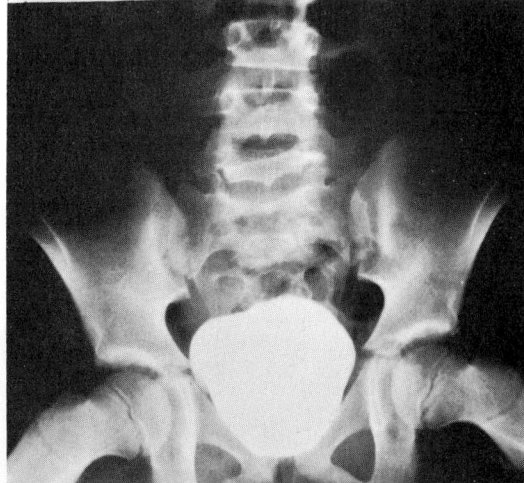

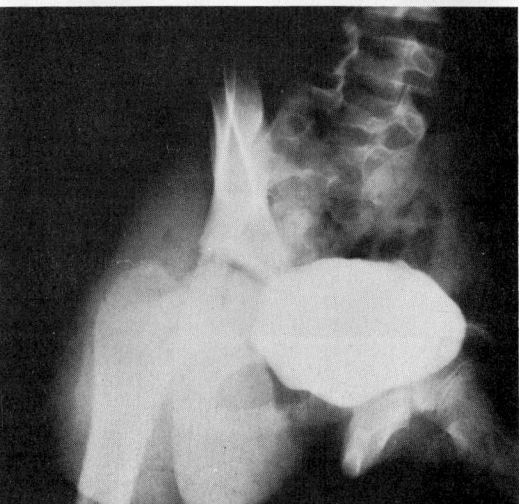

Figure 14. Retrograde cystogram. Anteroposterior and oblique views of bladder filled with opaque medium instilled in a retrograde manner. Note that the bladder wall is smooth, filling defects are absent, and the contour is nearly symmetric.

A *retrograde urethrogram* (Fig. 15) accomplished by instilling a thick contrast medium in the urethra may also be of assistance in demonstrating urethral lesions such as strictures and diverticula.

CALCULOUS DISEASE OF THE URINARY TRACT[7, 8, 50, 51]

Calculous disease of the urinary tract has been the object of diagnostic and therapeutic effort since ancient times. A urinary calculus is usually composed of a crystalline component and an organic matrix. Table 2 lists the common crystalline compositions of calculi received from patients and the frequency with which they are found. The organic matrix is a mixture of mucoprotein and mucopolysaccharide. The factors initiating calculus formation are controversial. However, a typical calculus can be made to form artificially without an organic matrix. On the other hand, so-called matrix calculi with crystalloids present in minute traces form clinically. Currently, the crystalloid component is thought to be critical under ordinary circumstances.

Areas of high incidence of stone formation are recognized throughout the world. The etiologic factors in this phenomenon are unknown. In general, stone formation is facilitated by factors that increase solute concentration in the urine, alter urinary pH, and provide a nidus for precipitation. Recognized abnormalities contributing to stone formation are stasis; infection with alteration in pH and nidus formation; im-

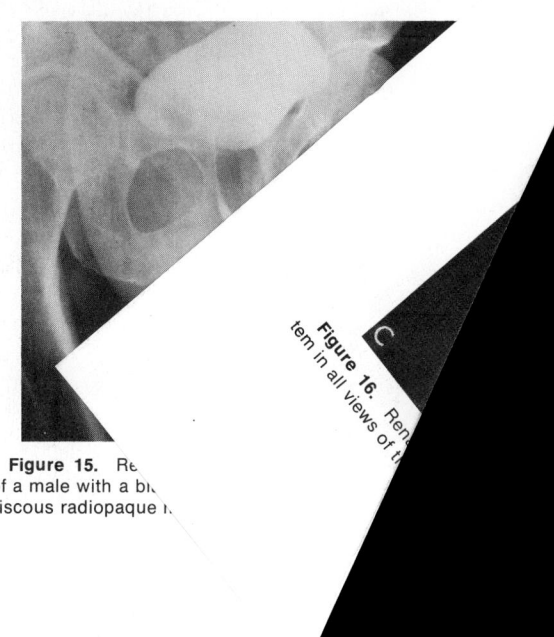

Figure 15. Re
of a male with a bl
viscous radiopaque i.

Figure 16. Ren
tem in all views of t

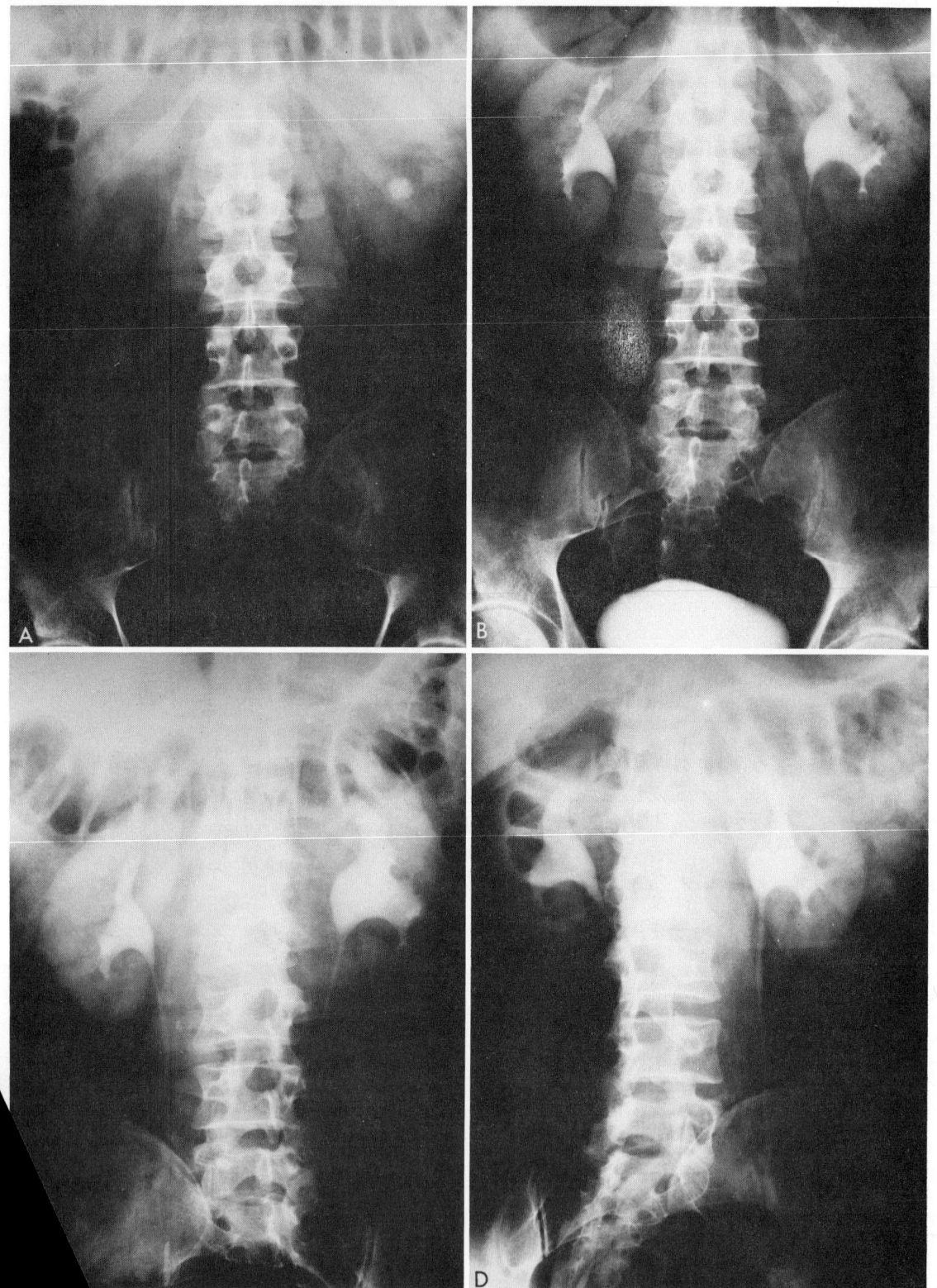

al calculus. Radiopacity in left renal area on KUB: the opacity maintains a constant relationship to the renal collecting sys-
e intravenous pyelogram, supporting the diagnosis of renal calculus.

mobilization impairing transport of urine and altering calcium metabolism; dehydration; metabolic disorders, e.g., hyperparathyroidism, hyperuricemia, cystinuria, and oxalosis; hypercalciuria secondary to neoplasm or sarcoidosis, or occurring without apparent cause; vitamin D intoxication; prolonged ingestion of excessive quantities of milk and absorbable alkali, the so-called milk-alkali syndrome; acquired or iatrogenic gastrointestinal malabsorptive disorders; abdominal renal function altering urine composition, e.g., renal tubular acidosis or Fanconi syndrome; and a foreign body, e.g., catheter.

The patient with urinary tract calculi may present with any one or a combination of symptom complexes: pain, severity, and site being dependent on the site and effect of the calculus; systemic or local symptoms of infection including fever, chills, frequency, dysuria, urgency, and pain; hematuria; anuria, if complete obstruction of the only functioning or both kidneys develops; or uremia characterized by nausea, vomiting, diarrhea, mental confusion, somnolence, muscular irritability, and weight loss.

Physical findings in the presence of an uncomplicated urinary calculus are minimal. There may be slight abdominal or costovertebral angle tenderness and muscle spasm with guarding over the site of a ureteral calculus. If infection or obstruction is present, characteristic physical findings may be evident.

Urinalysis usually discloses the presence of erythrocytes but not always. Leukocytes may be present with or without associated bacteria. The pH of the urine may assist in reasonable speculation regarding the composition of the calculus once its presence is established. Calcium oxalate, uric acid, and cystine calculi usually are found in acid urine. Crystals such as the hexagonal crystal of cystine may be present. Determination of calcium or cystine excretion and culture of the urine may aid in evaluation of cause or complications of calculous disease.

The diagnosis depends primarily on indirect methods of evaluating the urinary tract, namely, roentgenography. The plain film of the abdomen usually discloses a radiopacity due to the calculus (Fig. 16), provided that the size and composition of the stone permit sufficient absorption of the x-rays to cause this, and that surrounding or overlying structures permit its recognition. The radiopaque stones are primarily those containing a heavy metal, such as calcium or magnesium; cystine calculi are radiopaque presumably because of their sulfur content. Uric acid calculi are radiolucent and therefore not seen on a plain film. Not all radiopacities seen on x-ray of the abdomen are urinary calculi. It is necessary to establish a constant relationship of the opacity to the urinary tract to justify the presumptive diagnosis of urinary calculus. To achieve this, visualization of the urinary tract by intravenous or retrograde pyelography is necessary. Radiolucent calculi cause a filling defect on pyelography (Fig. 17). Calculi may be diagnosed by other indirect methods such as the clank resulting when a urethral sound strikes a bladder stone or the scratch resulting on a waxed ureteral catheter when it bypasses a ureteral calculus, but these methods are primarily of historical interest. On the other hand, direct visualization of bladder calculi by cystoscopy is commonly employed and is extremely useful. Extension of endoscopic techniques for visualization of calculi in other areas is being investigated.

The therapy of urinary calculi may consist mainly of observation to prevent serious complications from occurring. Medical therapy utilizing such rational measures as forcing fluid and alteration of urinary pH in uric acid and cystine calculi may be initiated. Drugs such as allopurinol in patients with uric acid calculi and penicillamine in patients with cystine calculi may be given to reduce production or excretion of components of the calculus. Chemotherapeutic and antibiotic agents are useful in the prevention and treatment of urinary infection. Surgical procedures may be urgently necessary to correct the complication result-

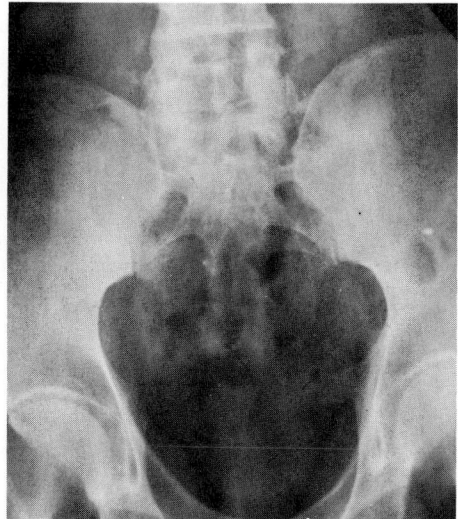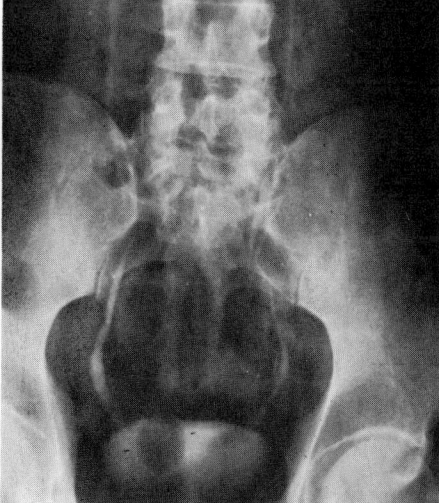

Figure 17.   Radiolucent bladder calculus not evident on scout film (KUB) but appearing as a filling defect in the cystogram of the intravenous pyelogram.

TABLE 2. Composition of Urinary Calculi*

Urinary pH usually acid; urine usually sterile:	
Calcium oxalate, CaC_2O_4	33%
Calcium oxalate + apatite	34%
Uric acid, $C_5H_4N_4O_3$	6%
Cystine, $(-SCH_2CH(NH_2)-COOH)_2$	3%
Urinary pH usually alkaline; urine usually infected:	
Apatite	3%
Carbonate, $Ca_{10}(PO_4\ CO_3OH)_6(OH_2)$	
Hydroxyl, $Ca_{10}(PO_4)_6(OH)_2$	
Magnesium ammonium phosphate, $MgNH_4PO_4$	19%
Pure (0.3%) + Mixed (18.5%)	
Calcium hydrogen phosphate, $CaHPO_4$	2%

*Data from Prien, E. I., and Prien, E. I., Jr.: Am. J. Med., 45:654, 1968; hydrated state of crystals is ignored in formula presented.

ing from the presence of urinary calculus. Surgical removal of calculi may be accomplished by various techniques, both endoscopic and open. Obstruction, infection, and recurrent or persistent pain are the usual indications for surgical intervention.

Between 10 and 20 per cent of patients with urinary calculi develop so-called "malignant stone disease," a life-threatening process.

URINARY TRACT INFECTION[1, 17, 26, 28, 35, 45, 47, 48]

Bacteriuria may be defined as significant presence of pathogenic bacteria in the urine. Bacteriuria is usually thought to be indicative of a urinary tract infection. However, if an infection in the urinary tract is defined as a tissue reaction resulting from the presence of a foreign organism, bacteriuria and urinary tract infection need not always be synonymous.

In any consideration of urinary tract infection, the resistance of the normal urinary tract to infection must be emphasized. Consequently, persistence or recurrence of urinary tract infection must be assumed to be associated with a local or systemic abnormality. Systemic abnormalities such as malnutrition, diseases causing severe liver dysfunction, or diabetes mellitus may contribute significantly to the development and persistence of infection. The local factors usually considered are urinary stasis and the presence of a calculus, essentially a foreign body (Fig. 18). Urinary stasis may result from obstruction, neuromuscular dysfunction, or a congenital or acquired abnormality such as ureteral reflux. The presence of any foreign body such as an indwelling catheter or a calculus acts as a nidus for continued infection and makes eradica-

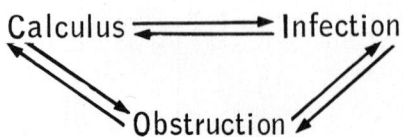

Figure 18. Diagram depicting interrelationship of obstruction, stone formation, and urinary tract infection.

tion of infection extremely difficult, if not impossible. Trauma is a third local factor which is employed experimentally to permit development of infection and which has probable clinical significance in the urinary tract infections developing after instrumentation and in the common occurrence of so-called "honeymoon cystitis."

Bacteria do not enter the urinary tract by normal filtration. The routes by which they do enter the urinary tract are *hematogenous,* as in the coccal infections of the kidney; *ascending,* as in the presumed entrance of bacteria into the bladder via the female urethra or into the kidney from the bladder; *direct extension,* as in the bladder infection at times associated with a diverticulitis of the colon; and *lymphatic.* The organisms infecting the urinary tract are commonly gram-negative bacilli. However, infections of the urinary and adjacent genital organs may be caused by parasites such as Echinococcus, primarily in the kidney, and *Schistosoma haematobium* and *mansoni,* primarily in the bladder; by protozoa, such as Trichomonas, primarily in the prostate and the female urethra, and by *Entamoeba histolytica;* by yeast, usually occurring in debilitated patients treated repeatedly with antibiotics; by the tubercle bacillus, and by other specific organisms such as the Gonococcus which causes an anterior urethritis in the male. The common bacterial organisms causing urinary tract infection are *Escherichia coli, Pseudomonas aeruginosa, Aerobacter aerogenes, Proteus vulgaris,* Staphylococcus, Streptococcus, *Alcaligenes faecalis,* and Paracolon organisms. Among these, Proteus is recognized for its ability to split urea with liberation of ammonia. The resulting alkalinization may be important, not only in stone formation, but also in permitting persistence of infection. Subcellular forms of bacteria such as protoplasts may play a role in the persistence of urinary tract infections.

The patient presenting with an acute urinary tract infection has symptoms related to the site and severity of the infection. Acute pyelonephritis is usually associated with flank pain, chills, fever, and often nausea and vomiting. Acute cystitis is associated with frequency, dysuria, urgency, suprapubic pain, and hematuria. The patient with a chronic urinary tract infection may experience the symptoms associated with acute urinary tract infection chronically or periodically or may be virtually asymptomatic until renal failure develops.

The physical findings in urinary tract infection vary with the site and severity of the infection. Marked flank tenderness and muscle spasm are characteristic of acute pyelonephritis. The patient with chronic pyelonephritis may have only equivocal flank tenderness or no abnormal physical findings. Occasionally, a physical finding makes a diagnosis highly probable, as in the beading of the vas or the scrotal fistula seen with tuberculosis of the vas deferens and epididymis.

Examination of the urine is the most important tool employed in establishing a diagnosis of urinary tract infection. Gross inspection of the urine may yield valuable clues. As an example, the first portion of the voided urine of the patient with prostatitis usually contains shreds.

The number of white blood cells that must be present on microscopic examination of the urine to cause suspicion of a urinary tract infection is not clearly established. If the uncentrifuged urine is employed, 10 white cells per 20 high-power field must be regarded with suspicion. If a 10 ml. random midstream urine sample is centrifuged at 2500 rpm for 5 minutes, one or two white blood cells per high-power field requires further evaluation. One or more red blood cells per high-power field must be regarded as abnormal. White cell casts in the urinary sediment are a significant abnormality and are indicative of renal infection, past or present, until this presumption has been disproved. Visualization of bacteria on a wet smear or on Gram stain of the urine is an excellent indicator of bacteriuria. Occasionally, as in the gonococcal infections, the stained smear remains an important method of establishing a diagnosis.

A persistently alkaline urinary pH or the finding of abnormal amounts of protein may be the result of urinary tract infection, although other causes warrant equal consideration.

The urine culture is the definitive laboratory test for establishing the presence of bacteria in the urine and the diagnosis of urinary tract infection. Identification of the bacteria is of value in directing therapy and sensitivity testing is of even greater assistance. Normal urine is sterile. The sterility is maintained in the bladder but because the urethra frequently contains a few bacteria, the urine collected after passage through the urethra often contains bacteria. Passage of a catheter through the urethra also occasionally yields a contaminated urine and is not entirely free of risk. The problem, then, is to obtain a urine sample that satisfactorily reflects the status of the bladder urine and to obtain this with a minimum of risk. Urine may be obtained by voiding, catheterization, or suprapubic aspiration. A voided urine sample should be obtained after satisfactory cleansing of the genitalia by utilizing a two- or three-glass collection technique for urine to be examined microscopically and by employing a midstream specimen for culture. The voided urine reflects the bacteriologic status of the urinary tract more accurately in the male than in the female. In either sex it has a great significance if it is sterile and free of abnormality on examination of the sediment. In an attempt to assess the significance of finding bacteria in the urine, quantitative techniques have been employed to count numbers of bacteria present. Because urine is an excellent culture medium and because the bladder is a reservoir usually emptying at 3- to 4-hour intervals, one can predict that bacteria present in the bladder will multiply and be present in great numbers in the urine. Observations have confirmed this postulation. Further, on studying urine samples obtained by both catheter and voided techniques there seem to be two groups, one with little or no bacterial growth, and a second with more than 100,000 colonies per milliliter. The finding of a colony count exceeding 100,000 organisms per milliliter is employed clinically to increase the probability to over 90 per cent that bacteria found in the urine are representative of the state of the bladder urine. However, with a voided urine, particularly in the female, this may represent contamination or mishandling of the specimen. Furthermore, a urinary tract infection may be present with a colony count of less than 1000 colonies per milliliter. Routine use of the catheter increases the reliability of the urine sample, particularly in the female. However, catheterization of a patient with a sterile urinary tract may introduce a urinary tract infection. Therefore, as much reliable information as possible should be obtained from the voided specimen. Catheterization is a valuable tool and should be employed when indicated. Separate microscopic and culture studies of urine obtained by voiding or catheterization from various portions of the urinary tract may assist in identification of the sites of infection.

Biopsy may yield isolated evidence of infection of a genitourinary organ in rare instances. The x-ray studies of the upper urinary tract may be characteristic of a urinary tract infection such as tuberculosis and occasionally chronic pyelonephritis. The presence of characteristic anatomic changes makes a diagnosis highly probable even in the absence of bacteriologic confirmation on examination of the urine.

Although infection of any portion of the urinary tract constitutes a risk to other organs and both ascending and descending infection occur, isolated infection of an organ such as the bladder or prostate does occur and is relatively common. Although the possible effect on renal function is of primary concern, not all or even the majority of urinary tract infections are pyelonephritis. In addition to local effects of a urinary tract infection, the systemic effects of a chronic infection, such as weight loss, weakness, and easy fatigability, may be evident. Furthermore, the bacteria in the urinary tract are a potential cause of bacteremia, septicemia, and occasionally bacteremic shock.

Once the diagnosis of infection is established, the fact that a single urinary tract infection in the male, or a recurrent infection in the female, is likely to be related to an underlying systemic or local cause must be emphasized. Stasis, stone, diabetes, and other abnormalities must be sought by repeated examination.

Treatment should be directed at elimination or control of the underlying causes for the infection, elimination of the bacterial agent by employment of antibiotic or chemotherapeutic agents indicated by culture, and re-examination at intervals following treatment to be certain that the infection has been eliminated.

OBSTRUCTION OF THE URINARY TRACT [9, 17-19, 38, 41]

Obstruction to the free egress of urine in response to normal contracture of the musculature of any portion of the urinary tract results in a series of events that may eventually result in destruction of the portions of the urinary tract above the obstructive site. The sequence of events following an obstruction may usually be divided into the following stages:

Trauma. The site of the obstruction and the urinary tract above it may show hemorrhagic areas. The urine above the site may increase in both volume and hemoglobin content.

Muscular Hypertrophy. Muscular hypertrophy is presumably related to development of increased pressure required to overcome obstruction. The portion of the urinary tract just above the obstruction shows these changes first. In the urinary bladder, the hypertrophied muscle associated with a distal obstruction is evident on gross inspection as prominent ridges called trabeculae.

Dilatation and Destruction. Dilatation resulting in anatomic changes such as hydroureter, hydronephrosis, and caliectasis, which are recognized as a consequence of obstruction, may be marked. With progression there is usually replacement of functioning muscle or nephrons by fibrous tissue.

Etiology

The causes of an obstructive lesion in the urinary tract may be *congenital* or *acquired, intrinsic* or *extrinsic* (Fig. 19). The obstruction may be partial or com-

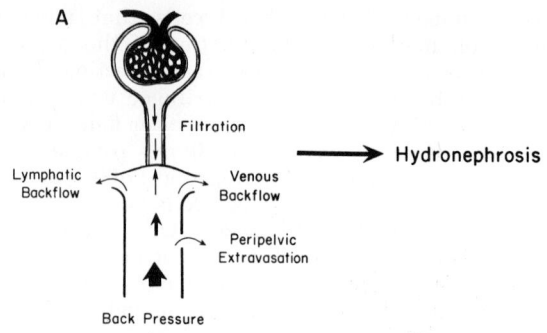

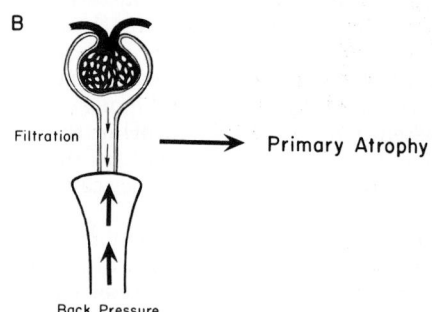

Figure 20. *A* represents the mechanism by which hydronephrosis is thought to develop; if reabsorption failed, as shown in *B*, it is postulated that a small contracted kidney would result from primary atrophy.

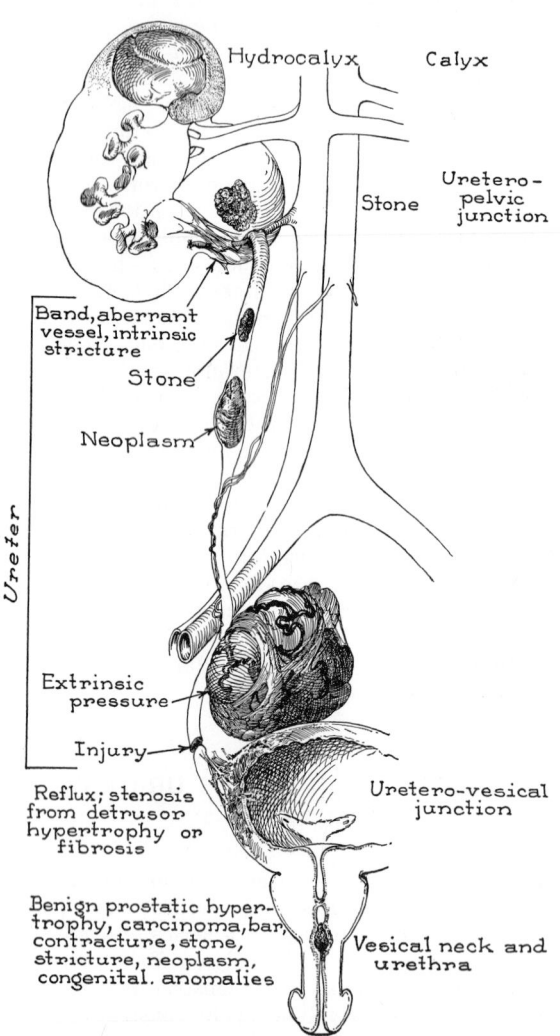

Figure 19. Causes of urinary tract obstruction (From Hinman, F., Jr. *In* Campbell, M. F., and Harrison, J. H. (Eds.): Urology, 3rd ed. Philadelphia, W. B. Saunders Company, 1970.)

plete. The effects of an obstructive lesion depend on the site, degree, and duration of the obstruction. Any obstructive lesion below the site of the ureteral orifices is likely to affect the functional status of both kidneys and to subject them both to any complications that may occur.

With regard to the development of hydronephrosis, the kidney is unique in that even after total obstruction urine formation continues (Fig. 20). After the development of an obstructive lesion, the intraluminal pressure above the site of obstruction rises rapidly. One would suspect that as this pressure reached filtration pressure glomerular filtration would cease and tubular secretion would be minimal. However, active reabsorption of urine occurs by pyelovenous, pyelolymphatic, tubulovenous, and tubulolymphatic routes and by peripelvic extravasation. This permits continued urine formation by filtration. Although there is an immediate increase in renal blood flow with an acute obstruction, this rapidly diminishes to levels well below normal. The resulting anoxia adds to the tissue destruction resulting from the back-pressure. This sequence of events, continued secretion of urine with gradual destruction of tissue, probably accounts for the dilatation of the kidney usually found as the result of ureteral obstruction. Otherwise, primary atrophy would be expected. Experimentally, respiration of cortical tissue falls markedly within 48 hours after obstruction, but the respiration of medullary tissue is unaltered. Anaerobic glycolytic ability of the cortical tissue increases markedly in the same period after occlusion.

Clinical Symptoms

The patient with urinary tract obstruction may present with one of the following symptom complexes: obvious symptoms related to obstruction, as in the patient with bladder neck obstruction presenting with hesitancy, intermittency, decrease in size and force of the urinary stream, frequency, and nocturia; symptoms related to the primary pathologic disturbance causing the obstruction, as in the patient presenting with hematuria from stone or bladder tumor; symptoms related to the presence of an abdominal mass, such as the epigastric distress that may accompany a hydronephrosis, and symptoms resulting from the complication of the obstruction, as in the patient presenting with nausea, vomiting, diarrhea, muscular irritability, mental confusion, and somnolence as the result of renal failure, or in the patient presenting with chills, fever, and flank pain as the result of infection of an obstructed kidney.

The significant physical findings in a patient with obstruction may be those associated with the lesion causing the obstruction, such as the enlarged prostate causing bladder neck obstruction. They may be due to the enlarged, distended organ, such as the palpable midline abdominal mass associated with dullness on percussion characteristic of a distended bladder. They may be the result of the development of a complication of an obstruction, such as the flank tenderness and muscle spasm associated with infection of the obstructed kidney.

Unfortunately, there are no findings characteristic of obstruction on urinalysis or blood chemistry studies. The findings on urinalysis may be due to the primary pathologic disorder, such as red blood cells seen with a calculus, or to a complication such as bacteria or pyuria seen with a urinary tract infection. Similarly, findings of elevated serum creatinine, blood urea nitrogen, serum phosphorus, and serum potassium associated with decreased serum calcium, characteristic of renal failure, raise the question of the presence of an obstructive lesion but do not assist in establishing this diagnosis.

The diagnosis of an obstruction in the urinary tract is dependent on one of the following: demonstration of abnormal retention of urine by recovery by catheter, by visualization of dilatation and delayed drainage by intravenous pyelography, or by showing abnormal retention of contrast medium instilled in a retrograde fashion; demonstration of the obstructing lesion by cystoscopic visualization of the obstructing prostatic tissue or x-ray visualization of the calculus, or demonstration by cystoscopy or cystogram of secondary disorders usually due to obstruction such as trabeculation and diverticulum of the bladder.

Treatment is directed toward relieving the obstruction (Fig. 21). This is often easily accomplished by as simple a maneuver as passage of a catheter. The effects of even long-standing obstruction including renal failure are potentially reversible with this relief. Whereas provision for unobstructed drainage of the urinary

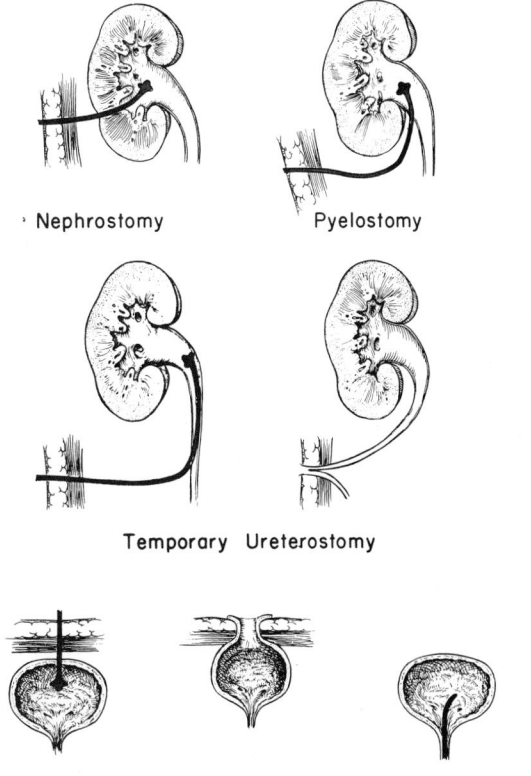

Figure 21. Representative methods of achieving temporary diversion of urine at various sites in the urinary tract.

tract is essential, correction of the cause of obstruction is frequently elective.

DISEASES OF THE KIDNEY AND URETER

ANOMALIES OF THE KIDNEY[2, 3, 11, 53]

Anomalous development of the upper urinary tract can be life-threatening in the patient with renal hypoplasia or polycystic renal disease, or may predispose to acquired disease, as in partial ureteral duplication. Urogenital malformations account for 35 to 40 per cent of all congenital abnormalities and are frequently one of multiple abnormalities. In some patients, an association of particular defects exists, such as aneurysm of cerebral vessels with polycystic kidney and nerve deafness with congenital renal parenchymal failure. Anomalies of the genital organs and kidney frequently coexist. The complex embryologic development of the kidney with serial maturation of the pronephros, mesonephros, and metanephros, the independent development of the collecting system prior to joining the renal parenchyma, and the ascent and rotation from a pelvic to a flank position provide multiple opportunities for maldevelopment of the upper urinary tract. The renal anomalies are usually classified as anomalies of number, including bilateral agenesis, unilateral agenesis, and supernumerary kidney; anomalies of position, including simple ectopia such as pelvic kidney, crossed ectopia with or without fusion, and nephroptosis or movable kidney; anomalies of form, including horeshoe, disk, L-shaped, lump, hourglass, lobulated, and round kidney; anomalies of rotation; anomalies of volume and structure, such as hypoplasia, congenital hypertrophy, solitary cyst, multicystic disease, parapelvic cyst, sponge kidney, and polycystic disease; and anomalies of the renal pelvis, including duplication or so-called double kidney, and congenital hydronephrosis.

All these lesions have clinical importance. Knowledge that a patient without an abdominal scar may have been born with only one kidney can be critical even if the incidence of this abnormality is one in 1200. Recognition that a palpable mass may be a functioning renal mass can prevent serious errors in diagnosis and treatment. The relative frequency of urogenital abnormalities requires consideration of this possibility in patients with abdominal complaints or physical findings of an obscure nature. These lesions may become manifest at any age. Employment of modern diagnostic techniques should permit uniformly accurate assessment of the anatomic status of the upper urinary tract.

CYSTIC DISEASE[1, 2, 12, 17, 25, 46]

Solitary cysts of the kidney are probably the most common renal mass recognized clinically. They are thought to result from a malunion or obstruction of the tubules when the etiology is congenital, and from tubular obstruction associated with localized vascular insufficiency when the lesion is acquired. Solitary renal cysts are bluish, thin-walled, smooth masses characteristically containing a clear serous fluid with small quantities of albumin, chlorides, globulin, urea, cholesterol, epithelial cells, and leukocytes. They are rarely seen before adulthood and are most common in the fourth, fifth, and sixth decades. Renal cysts are often asymptomatic. They may be associated with slight flank discomfort, mild gastrointestinal complaints, or infrequently with hematuria. Even less commonly, the cyst may be associated with excessive production of erythropoietin and consequent polycythemia. Infection of the cyst is a possibility. Demonstration of a thin-walled avascular mass on nephrotomography and arteriography makes a diagnosis of solitary cyst highly probable, but not certain. Aspiration of the cyst and instillation of contrast medium increases the probability of accurate nonoperative diagnosis. Definite diagnosis is dependent on observation of the characteristic gross and histologic appearance in the absence of neoplasm. The treatment of solitary renal cyst is partial excision of the cyst wall with oversewing of the remaining edge. If nonoperative differentiation of solitary cyst and renal neoplasm were certain, many would not require operative therapy.

Peripelvic cyst is essentially a simple serous cyst located in the hilum of the kidney. It characteristically exerts lateral pressure on the collecting system and shows no evidence of renal parenchymal distortion on aortography or nephrotomography.

Medullary sponge kidney is a term applied to describe a dilatation of the distal collecting tubules of the kidney. This anatomic deformity probably results from either a developmental defect or an acquired abnormality. The characteristic dilated tubules seen at the renal papilla on intravenous pyelography suggest the diagnosis. Tuberculosis lesions of the kidney may mimic the changes seen in medullary sponge kidney. Rarely the lesion may be localized to one segment of the kidney and partial resection may be employed because of complications such as persistent infection or calculous disease.

Medullary cystic disease of the kidney is an infrequent lesion often associated with renal failure and salt losing. At present this disease has no surgical significance.

Multicystic renal disease usually presents as an abdominal mass in infancy. Older patients may complain of dull abdominal pain. The lesion consists of multiple thin-walled cysts resembling a bunch of grapes. There is no associated renal parenchyma. The ureter is characteristically rudimentary and not connected with the cystic mass. Unfortunately, an abnormality of the opposite kidney may be associated with this lesion.

Congenital polycystic disease is an inherited renal abnormality. The adult variety is probably transmitted as a mendelian dominant, the infant variety as a recessive. The disease must be considered bilateral. Pathologically, Oasthanondh and Potter have described four types of polycystic disease: Type I, due to hyperplasia of interstitial portions of the collecting tubules; Type II, due to inhibition of ampullary activity resulting in marked reduction of the number of generations of tubules derived from the ureteral bud; Type III, consisting of multiple developmental renal defects; and Type IV, due to urethral obstruction. In polycystic disease the kidneys are usually several times larger than normal and studded with cysts of varying sizes. Cysts of the liver and pancreas and aneurysms of the circle of Willis are recognized as associated lesions infrequently.

Clinically, the disease becomes manifest either in infancy or in early adulthood. Some patients with polycystic disease have a normal life expectancy. The symptoms calling attention to polycystic disease are pain, hematuria, abdominal mass, and the symptoms of renal failure or hypertension. The physical examination characteristically discloses palpable, irregular enlarged renal masses bilaterally. Hypertension is common. Urinalysis characteristically shows proteinuria; pyuria and hematuria may be present. Evidence of renal failure may become apparent on testing as the disease progresses. The diagnosis is made from the history, the physical findings, and the demonstration on intravenous or retrograde pyelography of bilateral renal enlargement with flattening of the minor calyces, elongation of the infundibula, and other evidences of multiple space-occupying lesions (Fig. 22). Progressive renal failure is the rule in recognized disease in the adult.

Hematuria, infection, obstruction, and calculous dis-

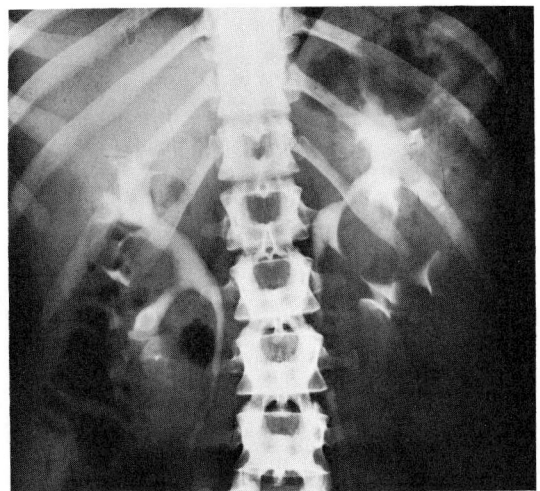

Figure 22. Intravenous pyelogram demonstrating typical configuration of polycystic renal disease. Note enlarged renal shadow, flat minor calyces, and deformity and elongation of infundibulum.

ease occasionally require surgical intervention in these patients. All attempts to preserve renal function permanently have been unsuccessful to date. The disease presents a continuing challenge because many of the patients have satisfactory renal function when first seen. At present, they constitute a group for whom renal transplantation is often ultimately advised.

CONGENITAL OBSTRUCTION OF THE UPPER URINARY TRACT[2, 18, 19]

Although obstruction at the ureterovesical junction and other sites may have a congenital basis, congenital obstruction of the upper urinary tract occurs most frequently at the ureteropelvic junction. Obstruction at the ureteropelvic junction may be due to an aberrant renal vessel, adhesions, intrinsic stenosis, and perhaps a functional abnormality of this segment, either alone or in combination. The lesions may be bilateral. The patient with a congenital ureteropelvic junction obstruction usually presents with intermittent flank pain, often associated with nausea and vomiting, hematuria, or evidence of a urinary tract infection. In children, an abdominal mass is commonly palpable. The lesion may not become symptomatic until early adulthood or late in life. The diagnosis is usually established by x-ray studies demonstrating the dilatation of the pelvis or calyces characteristic of a hydronephrotic kidney and the site of obstruction at the ureteropelvic junction (Fig. 23). Functional impairment may be sufficiently great to prevent visualization by intravenous pyelography.

Decisions to operate on the patient with a congenital obstruction are guided by the presence of functional impairment, complications such as infection or stone, and symptomatic complaints related to the obstruction. Whether removal of the hydronephrotic kidney or repair of the obstruction is the preferable course depends on assessment of the probable degree

of function retained in the diseased kidney, as well as the status of the opposite kidney. Of course, the age and general condition of the patient are important. A number of ingenious techniques have been devised to permit repair of a stenotic ureteropelvic junction with a high degree of success.

ANOMALIES OF THE URETER[2, 3, 11, 53]

Anomalies of the ureter and kidney are often associated. However, the ureteral anomalies are usually considered separately to facilitate presentation. The following is a commonly employed classification: anomalies of number—agenesis, duplication, triplication; anomalies of form, caliber, and structure—aplasia, congenital stricture, congenital valves, megaloureter, congenital diverticula; and anomalies of origin and termination—ectopia, ureterocele, blind ending, ureteropelvic defect, postcaval ureter.

From a clinical standpoint, the anomalies of origin and termination are of primary importance. *Ureteral ectopia* in the female may be the cause of a disturbing clinical symptom complex which requires knowledge

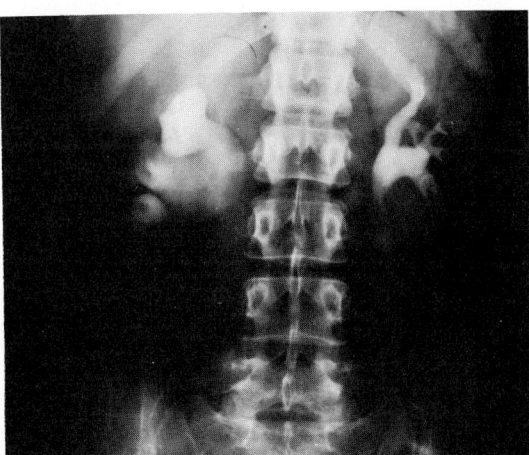

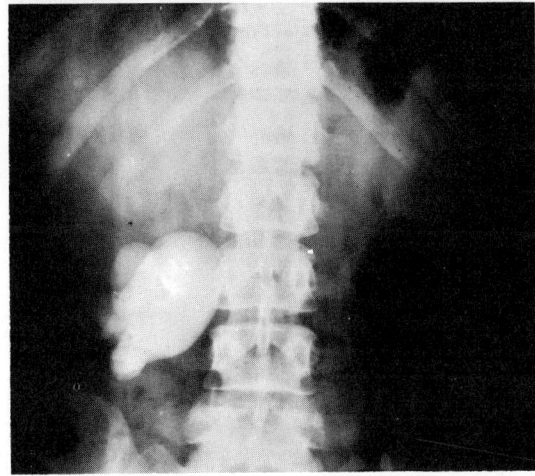

Figure 23. Intravenous pyelogram demonstrating typical deformity of hydronephrosis resulting from ureteropelvic junction obstruction. Note abrupt absence of contrast medium below this site.

of its existence to permit its recognition and treatment. The patient presents with a history of constant dribbling incontinence with intermittent normal voiding. Usually, the offending ectopic ureter is in the upper segment of a duplicated collecting system. The extravesical source of the urinary leak can be demonstrated by instilling a colored fluid into the bladder and observing the persistent loss of clear urine. The site of the extravesical orifice can often be demonstrated. Removal of the portion of the kidney supplying the aberrant ureter is the common method of treatment.

Ureterocele is a cystic dilatation of the lower end of the ureter. The ureteral orifice is narrowed. The intravesical dilatation of the ureter is covered externally by bladder mucosa and lined internally by ureteral mucosa. The lesion is of importance because it may be a cause of significant obstruction to the ipsilateral ureter and also because it may give rise to mechanical obstruction to the bladder neck with its attendant complications, particularly renal failure. The lesion can often be recognized by a characteristic cobra-head deformity of the lower ureter on intravenous pyelography. Cystoscopic examination yields the definite diagnosis.

NEOPLASMS [4, 13, 23, 40, 54, 55]

Renal neoplasms may be benign or malignant, primary or secondary. A satisfactory classification is presented in Table 3. Clinically, carcinoma of the kidney, the so-called hypernephroma, is the common (80 to 85 per cent) primary adult malignant disease. Nephroblastoma, Wilms' tumor, is the common primary renal tumor of infancy and childhood. Metastatic involvement of the kidney by lesions such as lymphosarcoma, leukemia, and carcinoma of the breast occurs with greater frequency than the clinical recognition would indicate.

Renal Cell Carcinoma

Carcinoma of the kidney occurs predominantly in persons in the 50 to 70 year age group and very infrequently in those under 30 years of age. Males are affected about twice as frequently as females. Each kidney is involved with about equal frequency. Histologically two cell types are recognized, clear and granular. In addition, a variable degree of differentiation of the tumor cells can be recognized which permits histo-

TABLE 3. Abbreviated Classification of Renal Tumors

Tumors of mature renal parenchyma—adenoma, adenocarcinoma

Tumors of immature renal parenchyma—nephroblastoma (Wilms' tumor)

Tumors of renal pelvis—transitional cell, squamous cell

Other primary renal tumors—hemangioma, hamartoma, fibroma, leiomyoma, sarcoma

Secondary renal tumors—carcinoma of breast, sarcoma

logic grading of the tumor. The ultimate prognosis is better with the more differentiated (Grade I) tumor than with the undifferentiated (Grade IV). Metastasis from renal cell carcinoma is both hematogenous to the lungs, liver, and bone in addition to the renal vein, and lymphatic to the regional lymph nodes. Although a renal cell carcinoma can be induced in the male hamster with estrogen and in the rat with dimethylnitrosamine, no etiologic relationship has been established for the human renal cell carcinoma.

The common symptoms associated with primary renal tumor are the triad of hematuria, mass, and flank pain. Any of these may be present alone. When all three are present the lesion is usually far advanced. In addition, fever is often associated with renal carcinoma and either erythrocythemia or anemia may be. The primary renal lesion is often silent and found only when systemic symptoms such as weakness, fatigue, anorexia, and weight loss signal the presence of a neoplasm.

Physical examination may reveal a flank mass which is firm and nodular. The lesion may be so sizable that it is fixed, and definite identification of its association with the kidney is impossible.

Clinical recognition of a renal mass is primarily dependent upon x-ray studies. The plain film of the abdomen may show evidence of distortion of the renal outline (Fig. 24A). Retroperitoneal carbon dioxide injection or tomograms may serve to demonstrate this more clearly. The intravenous pyelogram may reveal nonfunction, usually due to obstruction of the renal vein, or may show distortion of the collecting system compatible with the presence of a space-occupying lesion in the renal parenchyma (Fig. 24B). The nephrotomogram is of considerable assistance in further identifying the renal mass and in indicating the vascularity of the lesion (Fig. 25). The aortogram identifies the abnormal arterial and venous pattern frequently seen with a renal carcinoma (Fig. 26).

Those x-ray studies which simply indicate the presence of a mass do not establish the presence of a renal carcinoma. Any lesion that occupies space in the kidney, such as a carbuncle, a tuberculous granuloma, or a simple cyst, may cause similar distortion. Of these, the simple serous cyst is seen with five to eight times the frequency of a renal neoplasm. The renal cyst is avascular so that demonstration of blood supply to the mass on nephrotomography or aortography makes the diagnosis of renal neoplasm highly probable. Unfortunately, the demonstration of an avascular lesion does not eliminate the possibility of the presence of a tumor that has undergone necrosis, a well-recognized phenomenon. Ultrasound studies are being utilized to attempt to differentiate solid from cystic masses by demonstrating the presence or absence of internal echoes.

The presence of symptoms such as hematuria or pain increases the probability that a renal mass is a neoplasm. Histologic study of the lesion is required to establish its nature. Although needle biopsy and examination of aspirated material have been utilized for this purpose, the presumed danger of spread by these techniques has made them unpopular. At present, open exploration and biopsy, if necessary, are utilized in most instances to establish the diagnosis.

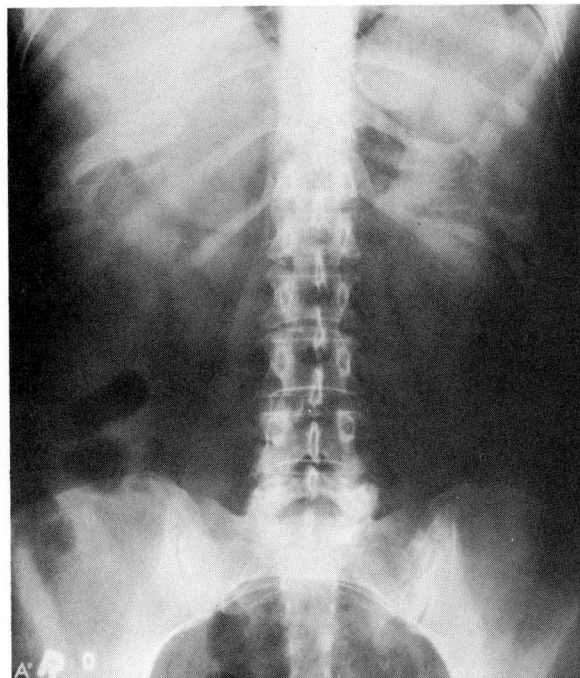

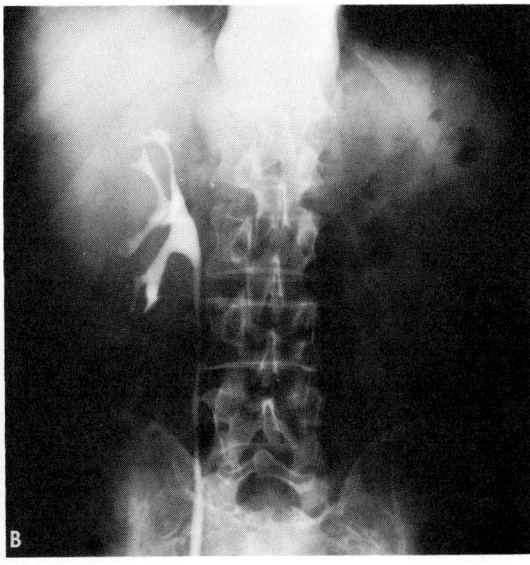

Figure 24. *A,* KUB demonstrating a mass at the lower pole of the right kidney. *B,* Retrograde pyelogram demonstrating deformity of collecting system by a mass occupying the midportion of the right kidney.

The established method of treatment for carcinoma of the kidney is excision of the kidney with its surrounding fat, Gerota's fascia, and adherent peritoneum. The regional nodes and ipsilateral adrenal gland are removed systematically by some. The desirability of occlusion of the renal vessels prior to manipulation of the renal neoplasm has been repeatedly emphasized on theoretical grounds. Prior to nephrectomy, the

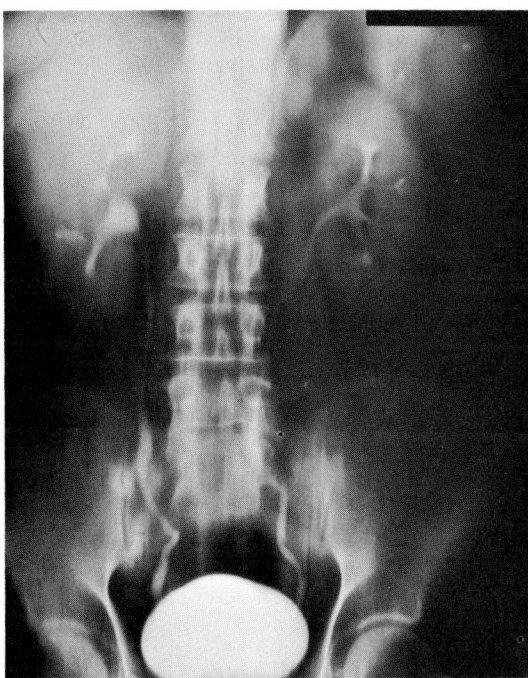

Figure 25. Nephrotomogram demonstrating an opacified mass at the upper pole of the right kidney. Opacification following injection of contrast medium indicates vascularity of a mass and is typical of a neoplasm.

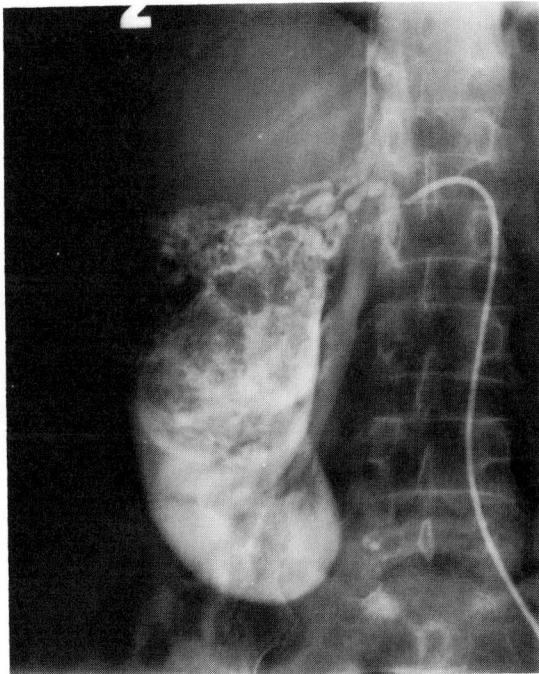

Figure 26. Aortogram demonstrating extreme vascularity with pooling of contrast medium in the right kidney typical of renal cell carcinoma. Rapid visualization of veins is characteristic of arteriovenous fistula.

presence of a contralateral kidney with life-sustaining functional ability is essential. Knowledge of the absence of demonstrable metastases at common sites is important. Biochemical evidence of liver malfunction does not necessarily indicate metastases and may reverse with the excision of the neoplasm. X-ray therapy prior to or following nephrectomy may be therapeutically useful. The chemotherapeutic agents and hormones such as progesterone must be regarded as having a limited role in the treatment of this disease.

Except for isolated experiences with highly select groups, the 5-year survival rates for patients with renal carcinoma subjected to nephrectomy have approached 50 per cent in recent communications. The 10-year rate approximates 30 per cent in these studies. Renal neoplasm is one of the tumors known to undergo spontaneous remission of metastatic lesions. This regression has occurred after nephrectomy in a few patients. The lesion is also known occasionally to follow an indolent course with metastases developing as late as 20 years after removal of the primary growth.

Carcinoma of the Renal Pelvis and Ureter

Carcinoma of the renal pelvis is most common in the fifth, sixth, and seventh decades. Males are affected four times as often as females. Each kidney is affected with equal frequency. Bilateral tumors occur in less than 5 per cent of the patients. The common pelvic neoplasm is a transitional cell one, although adenocarcinoma and squamous cell tumors occur. The prognosis with the latter lesion is uniformly bad. Transitional cell carcinoma tends to be associated with development of multiple lesions in the ureter and bladder either because of multicentric origin or because of metastatic spread or implantation. Other sites of metastases are lung, liver, bone, and lymph nodes. As with bladder tumors, the greater the degree of infiltration of the tumor, the poorer the prognosis. All tumors, even the typical papilloma, are to be regarded as potentially malignant.

Hematuria is the common symptom in a patient with a tumor of the renal pelvis. Pain may accompany the passage of a clot or tissue fragment in the ureter. Physical examination commonly reveals no abnormality. The diagnosis is suspected by the demonstration of filling defects on intravenous or retrograde pyelography (Fig. 27). In a pyelogram of good quality these defects may represent tumor, a nonopaque calculus, blood clot, or air. Urinary cytology and repeat x-ray studies carried out after passage of 2 to 3 weeks often help to differentiate these. Tissue obtained with a ureteral brush is being employed with increasing frequency to establish the diagnosis.

The treatment of choice in the presence of a normal contralateral kidney is nephroureterectomy with removal of a cuff of adjacent bladder. If a portion of the ureter remains, neoplasm develops in about 50 per cent of the patients. The 5-year survival rate after nephroureterectomy is approximately 50 per cent. Occasionally, local resection or destruction of a transitional cell neoplasm of the pelvis or ureter has apparently resulted in long-term survival without recurrence.

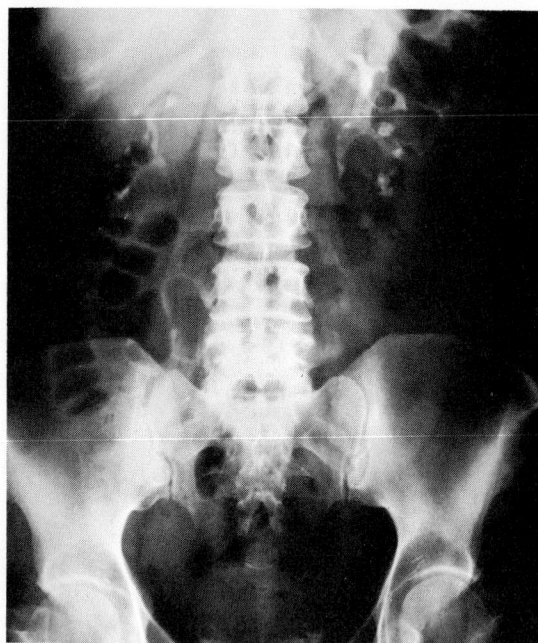

Figure 27. Intravenous pyelogram demonstrating filling defect of left renal pelvis compatible with transitional cell tumor. Similar deformity may be caused by blood clot and nonopaque calculus. Retrograde pyelogram confirmed the filling defect. Exploration revealed a transitional cell carcinoma of the renal pelvis.

Nephroblastoma of the Kidney (Wilms' Tumor)

Nephroblastoma of the kidney is a mixed tumor containing epithelial, muscular, and connective tissue elements. In a recent survey, 89 per cent were recognized before or at 6 years of age, 64 per cent being identified before 4 years of age. An occasional nephroblastoma is seen in an adult. There is no predilection for sex or side. Metastasis occurs by direct invasion of organs such as the liver, spleen, and intestine or by blood-borne spread to the lung, bone, and occasionally brain. Bilateral tumors do occur, perhaps as often as 5 per cent of the time.

An abdominal mass discovered in an infant by a parent or an examiner is the frequent presenting complaint in the presence of a Wilms' tumor. About 20 per cent of the abdominal masses noted in children arise from the genitourinary tract; about one third of these represent malignant neoplasm. Pain and vomiting are occasionally associated with a Wilms' tumor. Gross hematuria is an infrequent complaint, being present in about 15 per cent of the patients. Fever of an irregular character and degree may be present.

On physical examination, the characteristic mass noted on palpation is usually spherical, or variable consistency from soft to rubbery, and confined to the flank. The desirability of avoiding repeated palpation of the flank in the presence of Wilms' tumor has been emphasized by many surgeons. Hypertension has been noted in association with Wilms' tumor in 60 to 95 per cent of the patients.

The diagnosis is established by the studies employed to establish the presence of a renal cell carcinoma, although aortography is employed with less regularity in the child. Nonfunction on intravenous pyelography is unusual in Wilms' tumor, as is calcification of the mass seen on x-ray. The collecting system is usually distorted by the mass. Hydronephrosis is usually differentiated from Wilms' tumor by the x-ray studies. Neuroblastoma, another common retroperitoneal tumor of infancy and childhood, is more difficult to identify; these tumors show a much higher incidence of calcification. Tuberculosis, retroperitoneal lymph gland tumors, and pancreatic, splenic, and hepatic enlargement may cause confusion.

The basic treatment of Wilms' tumor is nephrectomy. The tumor is very radiosensitive; x-ray therapy is employed preoperatively infrequently and postoperatively commonly. In addition, the nephroblastoma is responsive to the administration of chemotherapeutic agents, the most widely used at present being actinomycin D and vincristine. Various combinations of surgery, x-ray therapy, and chemotherapy are currently being evaluated.

The prognosis of patients with Wilms' tumor is improving. Recently combinations of therapeutic modalities have resulted in prolonged survival of a number of patients with metastatic disease and an overall control rate approximating 80 per cent.[15] Survival for a period equal to the time required for the initial tumor to become clinically manifest (age plus gestation period) has been utilized as an indicator of control of the neoplasm by Collins. A 2-year survival period seems to be of equal value.

RENAL INFECTIONS[1, 17, 28, 32, 35, 45, 47, 48]

Renal infections are commonly divided on the basis of the infecting organism into *nonspecific,* which includes the common pathogenic organisms, and *specific,* which includes tuberculosis, actinomycosis, and echinococcosis. Routes of entry of infection include hematogenous, lymphogenous, ascending, and direct extension.

Pyelonephritis is the term applied to the common diffuse parenchymal infection of the kidney. As the name implies, both the pelvis and parenchyma are involved. The exact incidence of pyelonephritis is difficult to determine. Clinically, it is definitely recognized in less than 1 per cent of hospital admissions. Histologic evidence of chronic pyelonephritis has been reported to be present in 2.8 to 9 per cent of autopsies. The incidence of an active lesion is high at death, but the significance of this observation is questionable. In younger groups, the lesion is found predominantly in women; in the older age groups, men are more often affected. The common infecting organisms are *Escherichia coli, Pseudomonas aeruginosa, Aerobacter aerogenes, Proteus vulgaris,* Staphylococcus, Streptococcus, *Alcaligenes faecalis,* and Paracolon organisms.

The kidney with acute pyelonephritis is a swollen, tense organ with multiple subcapsular whitish areas. The mucous membrane of the pelvis and calyces may be edematous and erythematous. Microscopically, there are accumulations of leukocytes with some lymphocytes and plasma cells scattered between and within tubules but usually sparing the glomerulus.

The patient with acute pyelonephritis may first note the onset of frequency, dysuria, and urgency followed by the onset of chills, high fever, and flank pain, often associated with nausea and vomiting. At other times the chills, fever, and flank pain occur initially, often followed by frequency, urgency, and dysuria. Characteristically, the patient has a tachycardia and appears ill. Flank tenderness is often marked. When bacilluria on wet smear, stain, or culture is accompanied by symptoms of chills, high fever, flank pain, and the findings of flank tenderness, the urinary tract infection present is presumed to have affected the kidney. A moderate leukocytosis is usually present.

Treatment is administration of a chemotherapeutic or antibiotic agent selected initially on the basis of findings on smear and continued or changed on the basis of culture and sensitivity studies when they become available. General supportive measures such as the maintenance of fluid balance initially by the administration of intravenous fluids, and then by encouraging copious oral intake, and use of analgesics or antipyretic agents are essential. Urinary output and body weight should be observed. As in all patients with a bacteremia due to a urinary tract infection, bacteremic shock may develop in a few of these patients. The response to therapy of a patient with an uncomplicated pyelonephritis is usually prompt. Following the subsidence of the acute episode or during it, if it does not respond promptly, a search for local and systemic causes of the infection should be initiated. In addition to looking for evidence of obstruction and calculous disease, the possibility of ureteral reflux should be considered, especially in patients with repeated episodes of acute pyelonephritis. If urinary stasis is present, relief, at least by catheter drainage, may be required to allow control of the infection. Subsequently, correction of the primary cause of the stasis, such as removal of an obstructing stone or relief of an intrinsic ureteral stenosis or bladder neck obstruction, may be accomplished. Evidence that the pathogenic bacteria have been eradicated should be sought by culture rather than by relying upon absence of symptoms as evidence of cure of the infection.

Chronic pyelonephritis may be associated with a predisposing cause or may occur without a contributory abnormality which can be recognized with current techniques. Grossly, the kidney with chronic pyelonephritis is a pale, firm, shrunken organ with scarred, irregular surface depressions and adherent capsule. Etiology of an end-stage or contracted kidney is difficult to identify with certainty. The pelvis and calyces may be normal or thickened and fibrotic.

Microscopically, lymphocytes, plasma cells, monocytes, and neutrophils may be present. Fibrosis of the medulla and cortex with involvement of the glomeruli may be seen. The tubules may be normal or dilated with their lumen containing colloid-like casts. Varying degrees of sclerosis may occur in the arteries. Fever, chills, flank pain, frequency, dysuria, and urgency, symptoms of recurring or persistent urinary tract infection, may be present. Or, the patient may be esentially asymptomatic until nausea, vomiting, diarrhea, gastrointestinal bleeding, muscular irritability, drowsiness, weakness, and fatigue, symptoms of renal failure, develop. Urinalysis may show white cell casts, white blood cells, and protein alone or in combination.

Diagnosis is complicated by the occasional absence or intermittent presence of bacteria from the urine in patients with long-standing disease. Recognition of the infecting organisms by smear or culture is essential to establish the diagnosis of urinary tract infection. Similarly, isolation of the organism from ureteral urine supports the involvement of the upper urinary tract in the infectious process. X-ray changes of reduced renal size, irregular renal contour, calyceal blunting or clubbing, and infundibular narrowing are often sufficiently suggestive to make the diagnosis highly probable. Renal biopsy may assist in establishing the diagnosis of chronic pyelonephritis. In this type of chronic infection, search for and correction of a contributory cause such as bladder neck obstruction secondary to benign prostatic hypertrophy or neurogenic bladder dysfunction assumes great importance.

Treatment is directed to control or elimination of the bacterial infection by prolonged administration of antibiotic or chemotherapeutic agents indicated by culture. Repeated urine cultures are utilized to guide therapy. Careful, repeated evaluation of renal function is essential to permit evaluation of the effects of therapy. The importance of repeated search for underlying local or systemic cause for the infection cannot be overemphasized. Occasionally, chronic pyelonephritis may be unilateral; if the infection cannot be eliminated, nephrectomy may be necessary. Similarly, unilateral chronic pyelonephritis may occasionally be a cause of renovascular hypertension which may be alleviated by nephrectomy.

A form of renal damage in which the tip of the papilla is partially or completely destroyed occurs in association with diabetes and obstruction. The necrotic papilla often sloughs. This condition, known as *papillary necrosis,* has recently been recognized in association with other abnormalities, such as sickle cell trait and massive prolonged intake of analgesics, particularly phenacetin.[30] The sloughing papilla can obstruct and necessitate measures to relieve the obstruction. Bacterial infection may contribute to the development of papillary necrosis and lead to serious complications such as septicemia.

Urinary tract infection and pyelonephritis are recognized complications of *pregnancy.* The incidence of recognized pyelonephritis in pregnancy approximates 2 per cent. The hydroureteronephrosis which is commonly present, particularly on the right side, is an important contributory factor. These upper tract changes are thought to be due to mechanical pressure on the ureter and to some degree of ureteral hypotonia. There is an accompanying increase in vascularity and some edema of both upper and lower urinary tracts. Recent observations indicate that ureteral reflux may play a role in the etiology of pyelonephritis of pregnancy. The diagnosis is established as in the nonpregnant female. Treatment is similar to that usually employed but may include use of the knee-chest position or in unusual circumstances insertion of a ureteral catheter to reduce urinary stasis. Postpartum evaluation is essential in these patients. Evidence of persistence of infection or any deviation from expected course demands a search for etiologic factors not related to pregnancy.

Staphylococcic infections of the kidney are generally hematogenous and are usually related to a focus elsewhere in the body. The infection is primarily in the cortex of the kidney. It may subside or progress to multiple abscesses, carbuncle formation, or, if rupture into the perinephric space occurs, a perinephric abscess.

Symptoms vary considerably with the stage of the infection and the patient's status. Generally chills, high fever, lumbar or abdominal pain, and generalized malaise and weakness are present. Tenderness in the renal area and occasionally an enlarged kidney may be evident on physical examination. Leukocytosis is usually marked. The urine may show a few red and white cells on microscopic examination. Isolation of the organism is characteristically difficult. Both urine culture and smear should be utilized.

X-ray studies may show evidence of renal enlargement, obliteration of the psoas shadow, and curvature of the spine away from the infected kidney. The intravenous or retrograde pyelogram may show deformity characteristic of a space-occupying lesion or may show little deviation from normal. With perinephric involvement, either directly or indirectly, fixation of the kidney develops which prevents normal movement on respiration or the assumption of an erect position. This finding can be demonstrated by lack of blurring of the renal image on x-ray during respiratory movement. Radionuclide scanning with galium, arteriography, and ultrasound studies may add useful information.

Treatment is primarily by antibiotic therapy if the lesion is confined to the kidney. Often sensitivity studies are not available and selection of the antibiotic is empiric. If a perinephric abscess is present, or if the response to therapy is poor, suggesting a persistent renal abscess, surgical drainage is necessary. Nephrectomy is rarely required.

Perinephric abscess may develop from causes other than staphylococcic infection of the kidney. The infection of the perinephric space may be metastatic or may result from a suppurative process in adjacent organs. It may be secondary to renal infection other than a cortical abscess, such as calculous pyonephrosis. Physical, laboratory, and x-ray findings are similar to those of renal abscess, except that distortion of the renal collecting system is often absent. In general, the patients have symptoms for a prolonged period before a diagnosis is established. Perinephric abscess should be considered in any patient with prolonged sepsis of unknown etiology. Needle aspiration of the perinephric space may assist in establishing the diagnosis. Treatment is by incision and retroperitoneal drainage. If renal disease is present and severe, primary or secondary nephrectomy may be necessary.

Tuberculosis of the urinary tract is a hematogenous disease which, in the United States, usually is secondary to pulmonary tuberculosis. The primary tuberculous lesion may heal, while the renal tuberculosis progresses. The initial renal lesions are in the renal cortex in the glomeruli. The medulla is involved secondarily. Initial bilateral involvement is thought to be the rule. Bilateral or unilateral healing of the disease follows the initial hematogenous dissemination in some patients. Once the medulla is involved, the disease tends to progress and cavitation in the region of the renal papilla occurs. Renal tuberculosis is found in males more often than females. Its highest incidence is in the third decade.

The symptoms associated with renal tuberculosis are those of secondary tuberculous cystitis. Hematuria, dysuria, frequency, urgency, and nocturia draw attention to the presence of this urinary tract infection. Flank pain, usually mild but occasionally of a severe degree, may also be present. Physical examination may disclose evidence of genital tuberculosis, such as a scrotal fistula, beading of the vas deferens, or irregular nodular involvement of the prostate and seminal vesicles. The findings on urinalysis may vary from gross hematuria and pyuria to minimal microscopic hematuria and pyuria or in some instances to a normal urine. Bacteriologic studies of the urine, including smear and culture, permit accurate diagnosis. Usually three, pooled, morning urine samples, or concentrates of 24-hour urine samples, are utilized for study. Repeated bacteriologic studies are often necessary to establish the diagnosis.

Active, diffuse tuberculosis may be present without x-ray evidence. The classic changes noted on intravenous pyelogram are calcification, evidence of a renal mass, ulceration of the papilla causing a moth-eaten appearance, and stricture formation in the infundibulum. A nonfunctioning mass of putty-like calcium deposits is characteristic of the autonephrectomy seen as a result of a far-advanced tuberculous infection. Tuberculosis of the ureter secondary to renal tuberculosis may result in stricture formation or in a dilated fibrotic ureter that becomes almost "lead pipe" in character and that has a gaping "golf hole" type of orifice. Tuberculosis of the bladder is characterized by ulceration and tubercle formation.

Currently, the majority of patients with urinary tuberculosis are treated with antituberculous drug therapy. Usually, this includes streptomycin, isoniazid, and para-aminosalicylic acid. Variations in this drug regimen may be necessitated by the patient's tolerance or by the development of a drug-resistant organism. In vitro sensitivity testing aids in the selection of a variety of alternative therapeutic regimens. Nephrectomy for persistent active unilateral tuberculous infection, or because of secondary infection of a poorly functioning kidney, is occasionally necessary. Similarly, surgical correction of a ureteral structure following therapy or a procedure to enlarge the small contracted bladder which persists after treatment may be required. In general, tuberculosis of the ureter and bladder are secondary to renal tuberculosis, and even prior to institution of chemotherapy they would subside once the renal tuberculosis had been eliminated. Genital and urinary tuberculosis are commonly associated.

RENAL AND URETERAL CALCULI[8, 50, 51]

Calculi may occur in the kidney at any age but are more common in the third and fourth decades. They may be single or multiple, impacted or free. The calculi may be confined to the tubules at the tip of the papilla as in nephrocalcinosis (Fig. 28), may be a cast of the collecting system as in a staghorn calculus (Fig. 29), or may be in any of a variety of shapes. In about 15 per cent of patients the calculi are bilateral. They may result in renal destruction by causing obstruction, infection, or both.

Renal calculi may cause pain, hematuria, or symptoms of vague abdominal distress. They may be entirely asymptomatic even when large and causing serious renal damage. Characteristically, renal calculi cause severe, sharp flank pains which are often acute in onset and present intermittently. The pain may radiate into the lower abdomen or buttocks and is often associated with nausea, vomiting, and gross or microscopic hematuria. The patient usually moves about restlessly seeking relief. At other times, gross hematuria or routinely discovered microscopic hematuria may be the only indication of the presence of the calculus. Not infrequently, the symptoms or urinary findings of a urinary tract infection will prompt evaluation leading to the diagnosis.

Physical findings in patients with renal calculi may be entirely normal or may yield nonspecific evidence of renal disease, such as tenderness, muscle spasm, or a palpable mass. Tenderness and muscle spasm are usually minimal even when present. On microscopic examination of the urine sediment, hematuria is present in about 75 per cent of patients even in the absence of colic. Pyuria and bacilluria may be present. Occasionally, characteristic crystalluria is noted. Observations of the urinary pH may assist in directing attention to the composition of the calculus. The diagnosis is usually dependent on x-ray demonstration of the calculus. In the presence of a calcium-containing stone, a radiopacity maintaining a constant relationship to the kidney and its collecting system will usually be demonstrated on plain film of the abdomen and intravenous or retrograde pyelogram. If the calculus is composed of uric acid, or another nonopaque substance, its presence will be evident only as a filling defect on visualization of the urinary tract with contrast media.

Treatment of renal calculi is dependent on their size, composition, and the presence or absence of symptoms or complications such as infection or obstruction. A cause for the calculus is always sought and an attempt made to correct it. Observation utilizing analgesics for relief of acute episodes of pain, forcing fluids, and employing such measures as alkalinization and administration of allopurinol in known uric acid calculi, or alkalinization and d-penicillamine in known cystine calculi, may be indicated. If life or renal function is threatened, or if symptoms are severe with little hope of spontaneous passage of the calculus, removal by incising the renal pelvis or the renal parenchyma or both may be indicated. If the kidney is destroyed, if infection is confined to one stone-bearing kidney, or if the condition of the patient dictates, unilateral nephrectomy may be the desirable course. The recovered stone should always be analyzed to serve as a guide for future therapy.

Ureteral calculi are presumed to arise in the kidney

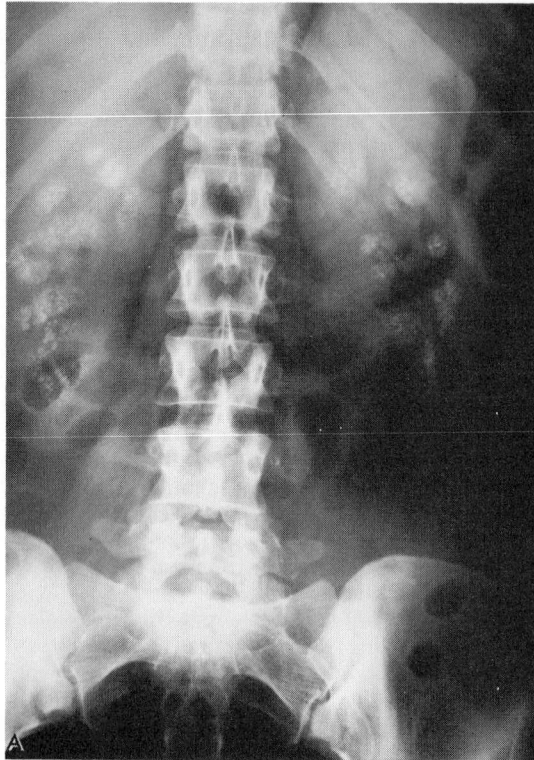
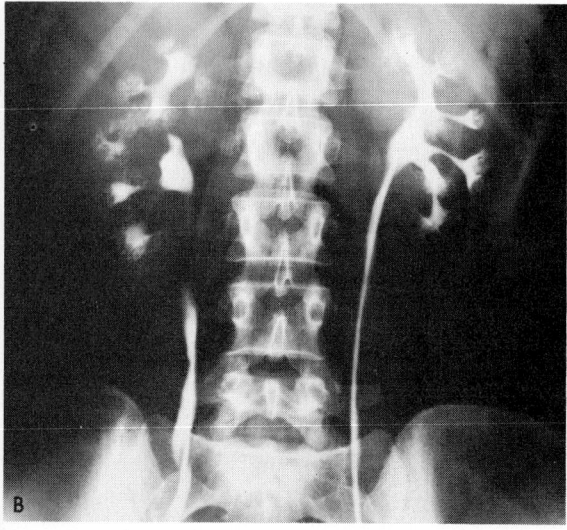

Figure 28. Nephrocalcinosis. *A*, Typical stippled calcification of kidneys, demonstrated on pyelography (*B*) to be associated with collecting ducts in the tip of the papillae.

and pass into the ureter. Their composition is essentially the same as that of renal calculi. They occur primarily in middle age and with equal frequency on each side. Men are affected about twice as frequently as women. Pain, either typical colic or indefinite or in-

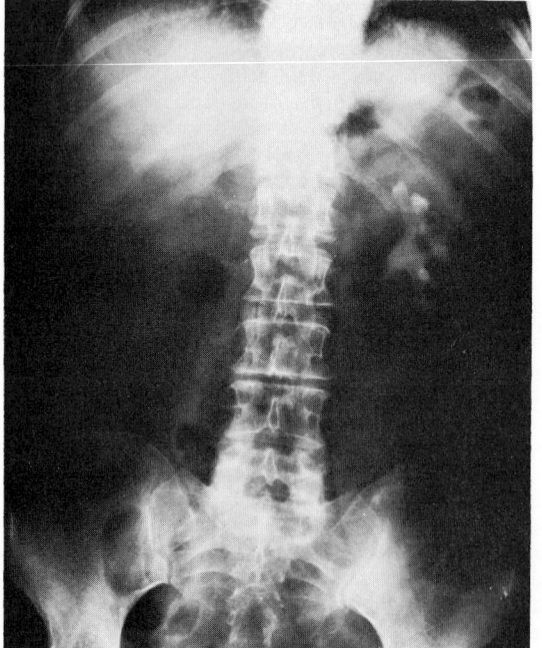

Figure 29. Staghorn calculus. Radiopaque calculus is seen to be a cast of the collecting system of the left kidney.

distinct abdominal discomfort, is present in the overwhelming majority of patients. Hematuria, symptoms of infection, or anuria may also cause the patient to seek aid. The local physical findings are usually limited to minimal localized tenderness. Flank tenderness and guarding may be noted when obstruction is present.

Urinalysis shows red blood cells in most patients with ureteral calculi. A ureteral calculus may be present in the absence of abnormality on urinalysis, but this finding should increase suspicion that a presumed diagnosis of ureteral calculus is in error. The diagnosis is established by x-ray studies. Demonstration of a constant relationship of a presumed stone to the urinary tract is essential. Most ureteral calculi pass spontaneously. They tend to impact at the ureteropelvic junction, the area over the iliac vessels, or in the lower third of the ureter, particularly in the ureterovesical area. Relief of pain of ureteral colic often requires large amounts of narcotics. Nausea and vomiting may necessitate fluid replacement. If symptoms are prolonged, they may be relieved by bypassing the calculus with a catheter. Similarly, catheter drainage of an obstructed kidney may be necessary to permit control of infection. Persistent obstruction, infection, and severe recurrent pain are the general indications for operative removal of ureteral calculi. Instrumental removal of stones is frequently accomplished with a variety of baskets and catheters; most limit the use of baskets to stones in the lower third of the ureter.

The operative approach employed for ureterolithotomy is dependent on the site of the impaction of the calculus. Every effort should be made to recover all stones and analyze them. A search for an etiologic factor, such as hyperparathyroidism, should be made routinely. Measures such as elimination of infection and obstruction and encouraging fluid intake should be undertaken to prevent recurrence.

VASCULAR DISEASE OF THE KIDNEY[17, 44, 49]

Diseases of the renal artery have been recognized with increasing frequency since aortography became a relatively safe, readily available diagnostic tool. These arterial lesions have clinical importance if they are a cause of bleeding, contribute to renal functional impairment, or cause alteration in renal blood supply sufficiently severe to stimulate excessive production of renin and consequent hypertension.

Aneurysm of the Renal Artery

Arteriosclerotic saccular aneurysm of the renal artery is commonly asymptomatic. Occasionally, rupture of the aneurysm causes massive hemorrhage or the aneurysm may be associated with hypertension. Typically, these lesions are recognized as faintly calcified ringlike shadows near the hilum of the kidney. If the lesion is small, asymptomatic, and seemingly completely surrounded by calcification, treatment is not necessary. If bleeding or hypertension secondary to the aneurysm occurs, or if the aneurysm has a significant uncalcified portion, resection of the aneurysm or nephrectomy may be desirable. Bleeding is rarely associated with a calcified aneurysm. In addition to the saccular aneurysm the renal artery may be the site of a dissecting aneurysm, poststenotic aneurysm, multiple microaneurysms, or a fusiform aneurysm. When present, they are often associated with fibrotic stenosis of the renal artery in hypertensive patients.

Arteriovenous Fistula

Arteriovenous fistula, either extrarenal or intrarenal, is also being recognized with increasing frequency. Trauma, accidental or surgical, including needle biopsy, and neoplasm are the common causes of the acquired fistula. Some are thought to be congenital in origin. Pain, hematuria, and symptoms related to hypertension and congestive failure may be presenting complaints. A localized bruit is the outstanding physical finding. The diagnosis is made by rapid visualization of the renal veins on aortography. The treatment has shifted in recent years toward a reconstructive approach rather than nephrectomy.

Occlusive Disease

Occlusive disease of the renal artery has assumed clinical importance with the recognition that it is a cause of hypertension. It has become increasingly apparent that renovascular hypertension may run almost any course. However, a renal cause should be particularly suspected in patients with hypertension of abrupt onset, in patients under 35 years of age, in patients with malignant hypertension of abrupt onset, in patients with symptoms of atherosclerosis preced-

ing the onset of hypertension, and in patients with an epigastric bruit.

Atherosclerosis is the commonest cause of occlusive lesions of the renal artery. These lesions are usually well localized and characteristically occur near the orifice of the renal artery, although other sites are affected. The second group of occlusive arterial lesions is characterized by constriction of the arterial lumen by fibrous replacement of a portion of the arterial wall. These lesions were formerly designated fibromuscular hyperplasia, but actual hyperplasia of the smooth muscle of the media is uncommon. Medial fibroplasia is the more appropriate term for the common fibrous replacement of the muscle of the media. This lesion occurs eight to nine times more frequently in women than in men. About half of the patients have bilateral lesions, which are characteristically located in the middle and distal thirds of the renal artery. The remainder of the fibrous lesions are designated intimal or subadventitial fibroplasia because of the location of the collagen. Each constitutes about 10 per cent of this group. Subadventitial fibroplasia also occurs mostly in young women and usually involves the right renal artery predominantly.

An abdominal bruit is the only physical finding suggesting the presence of renal artery stenosis. Establishing the diagnosis of a significant renal artery lesion is dependent on laboratory studies. The intravenous pyelogram may show a discrepancy in renal size of 1 cm. or more, a delay in the appearance or absence of contrast medium, or a late hyperconcentration of contrast medium on the side of the arterial lesion. The radioactive renogram is almost always abnormal on the affected side, but the nature of the abnormality may be variable. The aortogram will show evidence of an anatomic lesion of the artery which may or may not have functional significance. Differential renal function studies assist in determining this and also provide information of considerable value in formulating plans for treatment. Characteristically the urine from a kidney with a significant renal artery lesion is reduced in volume, shows a slight decrease in sodium concentration, and marked increase in the concentration of creatinine, inulin, and para-aminohippurate. Currently, determination of renin levels in the renal venous effluent of each kidney and in the systemic blood is the most reliable method for identifying a kidney responsible for hypertension. Segmental artery disease and renal infarct may also cause hypertension.

Treatment of renovascular hypertension is dependent on the general condition of the patient, the nature of the renal artery disease, and the bilateral status of the renal parenchyma. When surgical correction is indicated, reconstruction of the renal artery, bypass of an arterial lesion, partial nephrectomy, and nephrectomy all are utilized depending on these findings. Relief or marked improvement in the hypertension may be expected in about three fourths of the patients treated when properly selected.

Renal failure as a consequence of major renal artery disease has been recognized infrequently. This possibility warrants consideration in patients with renal failure of unknown etiology despite its infrequent occurrence because the possibility of reversal of the renal malfunction exists.

Renal Vein Thrombosis

Renal vein occlusion has been recognized infrequently in the past, and then almost always in infants. The infants usually present with evidence of systemic illness, hematuria, and an abdominal mass. Blood studies often show a diminished platelet count. Adults present with lumbar or abdominal pain, occasionally an enlarged kidney, and occasionally symptoms and findings compatible with the nephrotic syndrome. Cardiac failure is a frequent associated finding. As methods of visualizing the renal veins become more accurate and available, diseases of the renal vein are being recognized more frequently. In children nonoperative treatment is apparently associated with a significant incidence of renal functional recovery. In adults, medical and surgical treatment have been employed too infrequently to assess their relative merits.

Renal and Ureteral Trauma[10, 20, 42, 43]

Renal trauma may be secondary to a penetrating injury or to a blunt force. Penetrating injuries of the abdomen usually require exploration and, therefore, constitute less of a problem in diagnosis than does blunt abdominal trauma. Although renal trauma usually follows severe injury and is often associated with injury of other organs, seemingly minor falls or blows may occasionally produce severe renal injury. Aside from the direct effect of force on the kidney, injury may apparently result from the forceful whiplike movement of the kidney on its pedicle. Although spontaneous renal rupture occurs infrequently, the kidney diseased by reason of obstruction or tumor is more easily injured by trauma than is a normal kidney.

The types of renal injury are depicted in Figure 30. Depending on the type and extent of injury, the immediate complications of renal injury are those related to blood loss and urinary extravasation. Rarely, in bilateral injury or injury of a single kidney, acute renal failure may be a primary result of the renal trauma.

Hematuria is the primary finding in trauma to the urinary tract. It is often gross but may be microscopic or absent. Abdominal pain is usually present, located in the flank or upper abdomen, and variable in severity. Physical examination may disclose evidence of shock as well as local tenderness, swelling, and ecchymosis. Usually, muscle spasm is marked in the flank and upper quadrant of the abdomen. A mass is usually not palpable early in injuries other than renal pedicle injuries. An expanding mass with recurrent signs of severe blood loss is evidence of a type 3 or pedicle injury.

The diagnosis is usually made by the finding of hematuria associated with the physical findings suggesting renal trauma and evidence of renal malfunction or distortion on pyelography. In addition to providing evidence of renal abnormality, the intravenous pyelogram provides invaluable evidence of the presence of a contralateral functioning kidney. Other

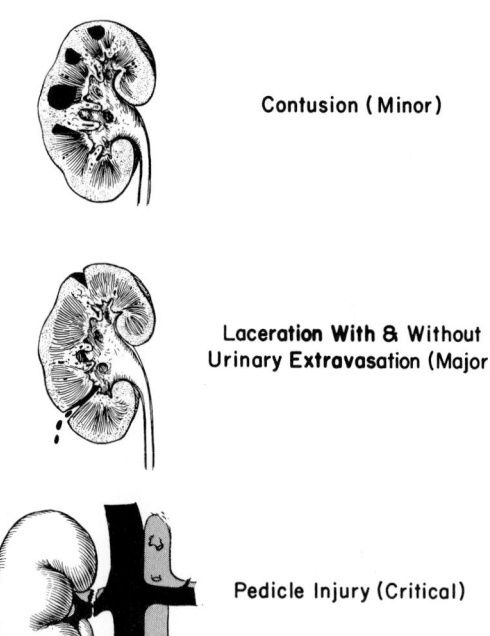

Contusion (Minor)

Laceration With & Without Urinary Extravasation (Major)

Pedicle Injury (Critical)

Figure 30. Diagram representing the various types of renal injury. Laceration with urinary extravasation usually requires drainage. Pedicle injury demands prompt control of hemorrhage.

x-ray studies such as aortography, nephrotomography, or mercury scan may be indicated to delineate the extent and nature of the trauma. The possibility that the hematuria noted may be related to lower urinary tract injury must be kept in mind and investigated, usually with a cystogram, in any questionable instance.

If a diagnosis of renal pedicle injury is suspected by the clinical course of the patient, prompt exploration and control of the hemorrhage are indicated. Even in these circumstances demonstration of a contralateral functioning kidney by intravenous pyelography is usually possible by temporary restoration of the blood pressure and a single film taken after injection of contrast medium on the way to the operating room. With the exception of pedicle injury and possibly thrombosis of major renal vessels, other renal injuries associated with blunt trauma usually do not require immediate intervention. Bed rest, analgesics for relief of pain, and observation coupled with investigation of renal status as indicated by the patient's course constitute the usual treatment. Aside from hemorrhage, the presence of urinary extravasation or development of infection may necessitate surgical intervention. If an operative procedure is performed, it may vary from simple drainage to partial or total nephrectomy. Usually, a delay of 2 to 3 days after trauma before exposure of the kidney simplifies the surgical procedure. The majority of patients with renal injury can be treated without operative intervention. Upper urinary tract extravasation is better tolerated than lower urinary tract extravasation and is not subjected to drainage by all urologists. Secondary hemorrhage from renal parenchymal injury may occur and dictates caution in allowing the patient out of bed. In many instances in patients with multiple injuries, the ideal treatment of the renal injury must be compromised.

Ureteral Injury

Ureteral injury is an uncommon complication of penetrating or blunt trauma. In penetrating trauma, symptoms from other injuries usually mask any symptoms due to ureteral involvement. In blunt trauma, evidence of urinary tract involvement is so slight that diagnosis of ureteral injury is delayed. Tenderness and muscle spasm due to urinary extravasation and development of signs of infection usually cause x-ray evaluation of the urinary tract. Intravenous or retrograde pyelography discloses the urinary extravasation and often identifies the site of injury. Drainage of extravasated urine and relief of obstruction are essential. Reconstruction of the disrupted ureter may be attempted by a number of techniques. In the past the resultant damage associated with injury and delay in recognition has made nephrectomy a frequent necessity. The ureter is subject to iatrogenic injury with much greater frequency than it is to injury from external trauma. These injuries result from both open surgical and endoscopic surgical techniques. Some of the more common types are seen in Figure 31. These may result in silent destruction of the kidney from unilateral hydronephrosis or in acute renal failure if a single ureter or both are ligated. Urinary extravasation with eventual infection and fistula between the ureter and the skin, vagina, or uterus is more common. In treating iatrogenic ureteral injuries, both relief of obstruction

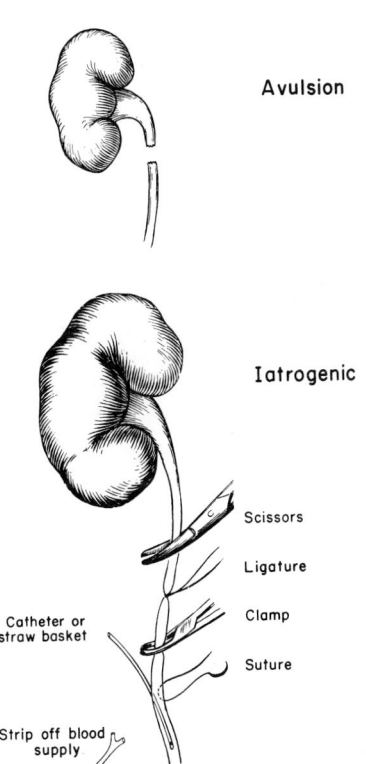

Figure 31. Diagrammatic representation of various types of ureteral injury.

Avulsion

Iatrogenic

Scissors

Ligature

Clamp

Catheter or straw basket

Suture

Strip off blood supply

and drainage of extravasated urine must be achieved promptly. Reconstruction of the defect may then be attempted as indicated by the general and local condition of the patient.

THE BLADDER

ANOMALIES[2, 3, 11, 53]

Agenesis and *duplication* of the bladder occur but are very rare. *Congenital diverticulum* is difficult to differentiate from acquired diverticulum and is recognized infrequently. The presence of muscle fibers in the diverticular wall, thought to be characteristic of congenital lesions, is probably not a valid differential feature. The symptoms of a congenital and an acquired diverticulum are similar.

Exstrophy of the bladder is an embryologic catastrophe in which there is an absence of the lower abdominal and anterior vesical walls. The posterior bladder wall is exposed. There is an accompanying epispadiac deformity of the urethra and separation of the pubes. This abnormality occurs in about 1 in 50,000 births, with males predominating 3 to 1. Muecke has produced the defect experimentally in the chicken by utilizing a plastic graft to interfere with normal cloacal membrane regression. In addition to the social inconvenience occasioned by total incontinence, upper urinary tract infection is common and often leads to death. Attempts to reconstruct the bladder are infrequently successful and diversion of the urine by placing the ureters in the large bowel, or in an isolated loop of ileum with an external orifice, is necessary (Fig. 32). Retained exstrophic epithelium has been the frequent site of adenocarcinomatous change in the past.

Urachal abnormalities vary from persistent fistula due to the failure of closure of the allantoic duct to cyst formation, persistent umbilical sinus, or a diverticulum of the dome of the bladder due to failure of fusion of a portion of the duct.

Ureteral reflux may be congenital in origin. The responsible defect is a maldevelopment of the trigone of the bladder with the trigone being large and the ureter being laterally placed with a short intramural tunnel. At times, these defects are accompanied by a thin-walled bladder with a large capacity, so-called *megacystis syndrome*.

TUMORS OF THE URINARY BLADDER[22, 33, 52]

Malignant tumors of the urinary bladder account for about 3 per cent of the deaths from cancer in the United States. Males are affected approximately 2.5 to 4 times as often as females. Epithelial tumors are rare in children but may occur at any age in adults. The peak incidence is in the sixth and seventh decades in both males and females. The overwhelming majority of bladder neoplasms are epithelial in origin. Grossly, they are commonly exophytic, protruding into the vesical lumen. They may vary from a papillary configuration with a narrow stalk and multiple frondlike

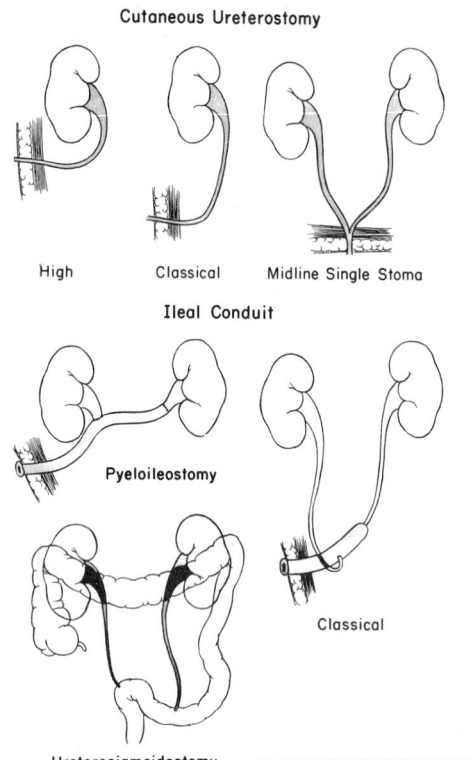

Figure 32. Methods of permanent supravesical diversion.

projections to a sessile serpiginous growth. Ulceration and encrustation with calcium salts may occur. Approximately 40 per cent of the tumors involve the trigone and an additional 45 per cent the posterior and lateral bladder walls. Multiple tumors are common, being present in approximately 25 per cent of the patients on diagnosis, and becoming evident in as many as 50 per cent of the patients with a so-called benign papilloma in a 5-year period.

Classification of the epithelial tumors of the bladder has been and is confusing. Histologically, these tumors are primarily transitional or squamous in cell type. Undifferentiated carcinoma, adenocarcinoma, and mucus-forming adenocarcinoma are also recognized. Some utilize a designation of benign papilloma for well-differentiated epithelial tumors; others prefer to utilize the term Grade I carcinoma because patients with these tumors show a tendency to reappearance of neoplasm as well as to development of a more advanced neoplasm. Grading of the tumor on the basis of cellular differentiation has clinical significance; the most differentiated tumors are designated Grade I and the undifferentiated or poorly differentiated, Grade IV. Degree of cellular differentiation varies throughout a tumor approximately 50 per cent of the time. The transitional, squamous, or undifferentiated cell type of the tumor is commonly maintained throughout.

The demonstration by Jewett and Strong that depth of infiltration of a bladder tumor is related to the presence of recognizable metastasis at autopsy was an important observation (Fig. 33). They observed no evidence of metastasis in patients with invasion confined

to the submucosa, and metastatic spread in 14 per cent of patients with invasion confined to the muscularis, and in 74 per cent of the patients with invasion of the perivesical tissue. Subsequent clinical experience has tended to confirm the potential survival without evidence of neoplasm in patients with superficially infiltrating lesions and the poor prognosis of patients with deeply infiltrating lesions.

Nonepithelial tumors of the bladder are mesenchymal in origin and may be benign such as fibroma or leiomyoma, or malignant such as sarcoma. Metastases to the bladder are unusual.

Bladder cancer is known to be associated with exposure to two chemicals, beta-naphthylamine and xenylamine. In addition, a higher incidence of bladder tumors is recognized in smokers than in nonsmokers. Bladder infestation with *Schistosoma haematobium* is also recognized as predisposing to the development of a bladder neoplasm.

Gross hematuria is the presenting complaint in about 70 per cent of the patients with bladder neoplasm. The hematuria is usually total but may be initial or terminal. Microscopic hematuria is present in an even greater proportion of patients. Symptoms of vesical irritability, such as urgency, frequency, and dysuria, constitute the other common group of complaints in patients with bladder tumors.

Physical examination is usually normal in the patient with a bladder tumor unless the lesion has spread beyond the bladder. The diagnosis of a bladder neoplasm warrants serious consideration in any patient with gross or microscopic hematuria, or recurrent episodes of vesical irritability. Presence of a filling defect on the cystogram of the intravenous pyelogram or on a retrograde cystogram should increase the suspicion of a bladder tumor. Definitive diagnosis is dependent on cystoscopic visualization of a mucosal abnormality and biopsy with confirmation of the presence of a neoplasm on histologic examination. Studies of urinary cytology may yield evidence of neoplastic change not identified by cystoscopy. In any patient with a bladder neoplasm, the kidneys and ureters should be visualized to eliminate the possibility that a transitional cell neoplasm of the upper urinary tract is seeding the bladder.

Once the diagnosis of bladder neoplasm is established, clinical staging of the neoplasm is important to permit rational therapy and prognosis. Staging is based on the pathologic observations correlating

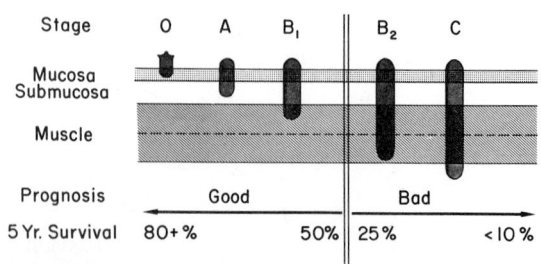

Figure 33. Staging of bladder tumors (after Jewett). Solid vertical bars indicate depth of infiltration. If lymph node or prostatic involvement is demonstrated, "D" classification is utilized by some.

tumor spread with degree of tumor invasion as confirmed and modified by clinical experience. The gross appearance of the bladder tumor assists in staging, with the more advanced lesions tending to have a broader, flatter base with evidence of fixation of the bladder wall. Similar fixation of the bladder wall may be evident on retrograde cystography. The single most important observation in staging is the depth of infiltration of the bladder tumor. To allow assessment of the infiltration, an adequate biopsy of the tumor and of the muscle at its base, as well as deep biopsy of any other suspicious area in the bladder and prostate, is essential. If biopsy indicates infiltration limited to the superficial portion of the muscle, prognosis is good. Infiltration deep in the muscle is associated with a poor prognosis. Bimanual examination under anesthesia is also of value in clinical staging. Persistent induration of any type indicates a poor prognosis, but this is particularly true if the induration extends beyond the bladder. If an infiltrating tumor is recognized, assessment of the pelvic lymph nodes by excisional biopsy or less accurately, by lymphangiography, becomes important to accurate staging; random biopsies of cystoscopically normal bladder epithelium also warrant consideration to assist in decisions regarding therapy. If histologic evidence of invasion of the prostate or involvement of the iliac lymph nodes is obtained, the prognosis for cure becomes so poor that vigorous therapeutic attempts are usually avoided in favor of palliative procedures. In general, evidence of lymphatic invasion on biopsy is a poor prognostic sign as is evidence of ureteral obstruction. Squamous carcinomas often are of a higher stage than indicated by biopsy.

Therapy of bladder tumors may be curative or palliative. The results achieved with any type of therapeutic approach seem more related to the stage of the tumor at the initiation of therapy than to the therapy itself. Untreated, the majority of the patients with carcinoma of the bladder die directly or indirectly from their disease. Renal failure from obstruction and infection is a prominent cause of death. Carcinomatosis is also common, with frequent involvement of the regional nodes, liver, lungs, and vertebrae in that order. Uncontrolled hemorrhage from the bladder tumor also contributes to mortality.

Attempts to eradicate the neoplasm employ surgery or radiation therapy. Operative procedures utilized in the treatment of bladder tumors are directed to the local destruction or excision of the neoplasm or to removal of the entire bladder. The procedures utilized in local destruction of the neoplasm include:

1. Transurethral fulguration or transurethral excision and fulguration carried out with an endoscopic instrument per urethram; this is limited by size and location of the lesion.

2. Suprapubic excision and fulguration through a cystotomy incision; the excision is followed by local destruction.

3. Segmental resection of bladder with or without ureteral reimplantation. Location and extent of the tumor have limited the utilization of partial excision of the bladder, as has the tendency for tumors to be multiple. Current techniques for ureteral reimplantation have permitted more enthusiastic employment of

this technique when adequate resection requires sacrifice of the intravesical ureter.

4. External radiation and various techniques for local application of radon packs, radon seeds, and radioactive suture materials.

5. Instillation of chemotherapeutic agents has been utilized with some success in noninvasive tumors.

6. Cystectomy is employed in the treatment of higher-stage neoplasms, multiple recurrent tumors, or failures by locally destructive techniques. It is rarely employed in the presence of metastases to iliac nodes or the prostate unless some local complication, such as bleeding, dictates the palliative removal of the bladder. Currently several groups are utilizing radiation therapy immediately before planned surgical excision. Cystectomy necessitates diversion of the urine. Utilization of an ileal conduit to divert the ureteral urine to the skin (see Fig. 32) affords the best long-term results currently. However, the surgical procedure involves moderate risk. For this reason diversion of the ureter to the skin is employed at times. Placement of the ureters into the intact large bowel is also employed. It has the advantage of providing urinary continence. The disadvantages of this technique are its frequent failure to preserve renal function and the development of hyperchloremic acidosis in some patients from the reabsorption of urine by the bowel.

Palliation of the patient with bladder neoplasm may be a very difficult problem. The local complications of hemorrhage, frequency, pain, and ureteral obstruction may necessitate utilization of the procedures employed in an attempt to eradicate the neoplasm. Locally destructive procedures or urinary diversion often provides required relief.

INFLAMMATORY LESIONS OF THE BLADDER[32, 45]

Bacterial cystitis is characterized by urinary frequency, nocturia, urgency, and dysuria. In women acute hemorrhagic cystitis is probably the commonest cause of hematuria. As in any urinary tract infection, cystitis may be secondary to upper or lower urinary tract disease or to a systemic illness and requires thorough evaluation if recurrent or persistent in the female. Males should be evaluated after a single episode. Classically, the diagnosis is based on the symptoms, the finding of a two-glass pyuria, and the identification of bacteria by smear or culture.

The symptoms of *tuberculous cystitis* are those of bacterial cystitis. Hematuria is often present. The small contracted bladder is rarely seen at present. Tuberculous cystitis is usually secondary to tuberculosis of the upper urinary tract.

Interstitial cystitis[6] is an inflammatory disease of the bladder, the etiology of which is unknown. It occurs predominantly in women. Frequency, nocturia, urgency, dysuria, and lower abdominal pain are prominent symptoms. The physical examination reveals no abnormality. The urinalysis and urine culture are normal. The diagnosis is established by the demonstration, on cystoscopy carried out under anesthesia, of an extremely small bladder capacity and evidence of ulceration and cracking of the bladder wall with hydraulic distention. Hydraulic distention of the bladder is also therapeutic, temporarily increasing bladder capacity. Other therapy has included instillation of various mild caustic solutions into the bladder. Occasionally, intractable discomfort and frequency necessitate use of a patch of bowel to increase bladder capacity and on occasion diversion of the urine has been necessary.

URETERAL REFLUX[2, 53]

Despite development of high voiding pressures by the detrusor muscle, urine does not normally reflux from the bladder into the ureters on voiding. The oblique submucosal course of the intravesical ureter combined with normal ureteral peristalsis is thought to prevent backflow of urine from the bladder into the ureter. Ureteral reflux has come to be recognized as an important abnormality of the urinary tract contributing to persistent or recurrent infection. The role of reflux in the production of renal damage in the absence of infection is equivocal. The recognized causes of ureteral reflux are congenital deformity, bladder outflow obstruction, neurogenic dysfunction, surgical alteration of the intravesical ureter, and infection. It is important to recognize that infection may be the cause as well as result of ureteral reflux. Patients with reflux commonly present with symptoms of persistent or recurrent urinary tract infection. Occasional intermittent flank pain with voiding may be present. Although reflux may be identified by cystoscopic techniques employing a chromogen or by isotope studies, the voiding cystourethrogram and the retrograde cystogram have permitted recognition of this phenomenon with ease (Fig. 34). Ureteral reflux has been recognized with greater frequency in children than in adults, and in females than in males. In some patients, reflux may subside with elimination of a contributory cause, such as infection or obstruction. In others, institution of simple techniques, such as double and triple voiding, coupled with treatment of infection, eliminates infection and prevents renal damage. When the intravesical ureter is abnormal, restoration of the normal anatomic relationship of the bladder and the tunneled intravesical ureter may be achieved by any of a number of techniques, usually employing reimplantation of the ureter. With elimination of reflux, the control of infection is usually possible.

BLADDER CALCULI[49]

In the United States, bladder calculi are a disease of the adult male. In other parts of the world, children are primarily affected. Calcium oxalate stones are the commonest type found in the bladder. They may assume a mulberry or jackstone configuration. Many patients present with symptoms of urinary tract infection. Dull or sharp pain, aggravated by movement and relieved by rest, and hematuria are the common complaints in the absence of infection. The pain may be referred to the tip of the penis. Occasionally, the patient experiences periodic retention from the ball

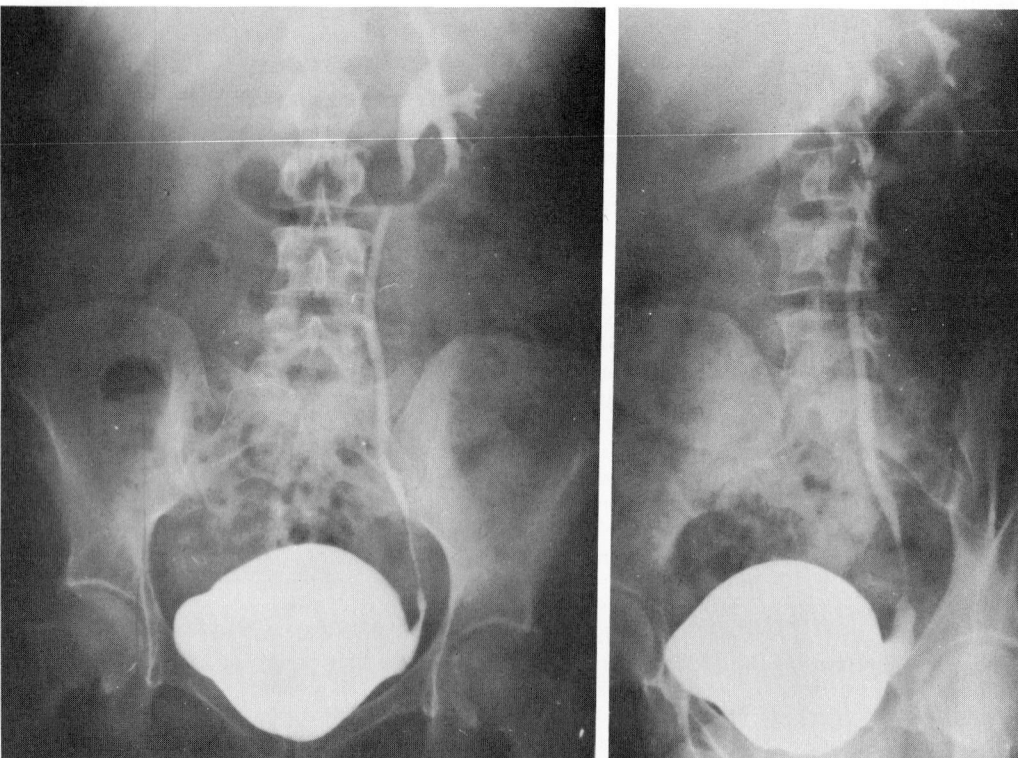

Figure 34.   Ureteral reflux on left demonstrated on cystogram study in adult female with recurrent left pyelonephritis.

valve action of the calculus or passes calculi per urethram. The physical examination rarely aids in establishing a diagnosis. The urinalysis characteristically shows red blood cells and may disclose white blood cells. Only about half of the bladder calculi are visible on x-ray, either because of their size, composition, or overlying structures. Characteristically, stones lying free in the bladder lie in the midline. Whenever bladder calculi are present in the adult, the possibility of urinary stasis either on an obstructed or a neurogenic basis becomes paramount. Other causes of calculus formation also warrant consideration. Treatment consists in removal of the stone either by endoscopic or open surgical techniques. Often, smaller calculi may be removed by irrigation through an endoscopic sheath. Fracture of the calculus may be carried out by either a blind or a visual technique to facilitate its transurethral removal. If an open surgical technique is utilized, the suprapubic route is usually employed. After removal of the calculi, prevention of recurrence is dependent on correction of the underlying cause for their development.

BLADDER DIVERTICULUM[32, 45]

A bladder diverticulum is an outpouching of the bladder wall. It may be congenital or acquired. Differentiation on the basis of etiology is often difficult; it seems probable that a congenital abnormality may play a role in the diverticula developing as the result of obstructive lesions. The majority of bladder diverticula are associated with and probably secondary to obstruction at or distal to the bladder neck. Neurogenic bladder dysfunction may also lead to their formation.

Diverticula of the bladder may be single or multiple, small or large. They form most commonly in the region of the ureteral orifices on the posterior or lateral bladder wall. The diverticular wall usually consists of bladder mucosa with few, if any, investing muscular fibers. The patient with a bladder diverticulum usually presents with symptoms of bladder neck obstruction such as hesitancy, intermittency, weak urinary stream, and nocturia. None of these symptoms suggests that the bladder neck obstruction has been complicated by the development of a diverticulum. The presence of a urinary tract infection or bladder calculus may result from the stasis of urine occasioned by a nonemptying diverticulum and cause symptoms leading to its discovery. Occasionally, an asymmetric lower abdominal mass will be evident on inspection or palpation of the abdomen of a thin patient, but the physical examination rarely aids in establishing the diagnosis.

Cystoscopic visualization of the orifice or base of the diverticulum and visualization of a smooth asymmetric outpouching of the bladder wall on retrograde cystogram are useful in establishing the diagnosis. Indirect visualization of the diverticulum by the cystogram is particularly important, because it allows an assessment of the size, the presence or absence of pathologic change on the wall, and the ability of the diverticulum to empty.

Since bladder diverticula are usually secondary to obstruction at or below the bladder neck, relief of this obstruction is essential to their treatment. If the size or configuration of the diverticulum does not permit it to empty despite relief of obstruction, or if complications of stasis such as stone or persistent infection are present, measures to ensure emptying are required. Under these circumstances the diverticulum is usually excised and the bladder wall reconstructed to eliminate the defect permitting its development. Occasionally, the presence or suspicion of a neoplasm in a diverticulum is an indication for its removal.

BLADDER TRAUMA[36, 39]

Perforation of the urinary bladder is a surgical emergency requiring prompt recognition and treatment. Spontaneous perforation is extremely rare and almost always associated with disease of the bladder, such as infection or neoplasm. Bladder rupture may result from blunt and penetrating wounds of the abdomen. A full bladder predisposes to rupture. Injuries of the bladder and urethra are associated with fractures of the pelvis with sufficient frequency to warrant consideration in patients with this type of trauma. Instrumentation and endoscopic operative procedures have assumed major importance as a cause of bladder perforation. Because a peritoneal injury may accompany the bladder injury, the extravasation may be intraperitoneal, extraperitoneal, or both. The inferior extension of the extravasated urine is usually limited by the urogenital diaphragm.

Severe abdominal pain and hematuria or inability to void are common symptoms. Tenderness, rebound tenderness, and muscular rigidity are commonly seen with perforation of the bladder. Shock is not uncommon. However, the symptoms and signs of bladder rupture may be insignificant and insidious if the possibility is not considered. Although procedures such as measuring return of instilled irrigating fluid and cystoscopy may assist in recognition of perforation of the bladder, they are often misleading. The retrograde cystogram is the most useful and reliable diagnostic tool (Fig. 35). It should always be preceded by a plain film of the abdomen because the extravasated contrast medium can be difficult to recognize in an intraperitoneal perforation.

Once the diagnosis of ruptured bladder is made or stongly suspected, treatment should be prompt because mortality increases markedly with delay. The essential therapeutic maneuver is institution of adequate suprapubic drainage. Repair of the bladder defect, although desirable, is unnecessary if adequate drainage is achieved. Repair of the peritoneal rent in patients with intraperitoneal extravasation should be carried out if possible.

NEUROGENIC BLADDER[4, 5, 6, 27, 29]

The adult urinary bladder is an integrated smooth muscle viscus that will normally act as an asymptomatic reservoir for 300 to 500 ml. of urine and will

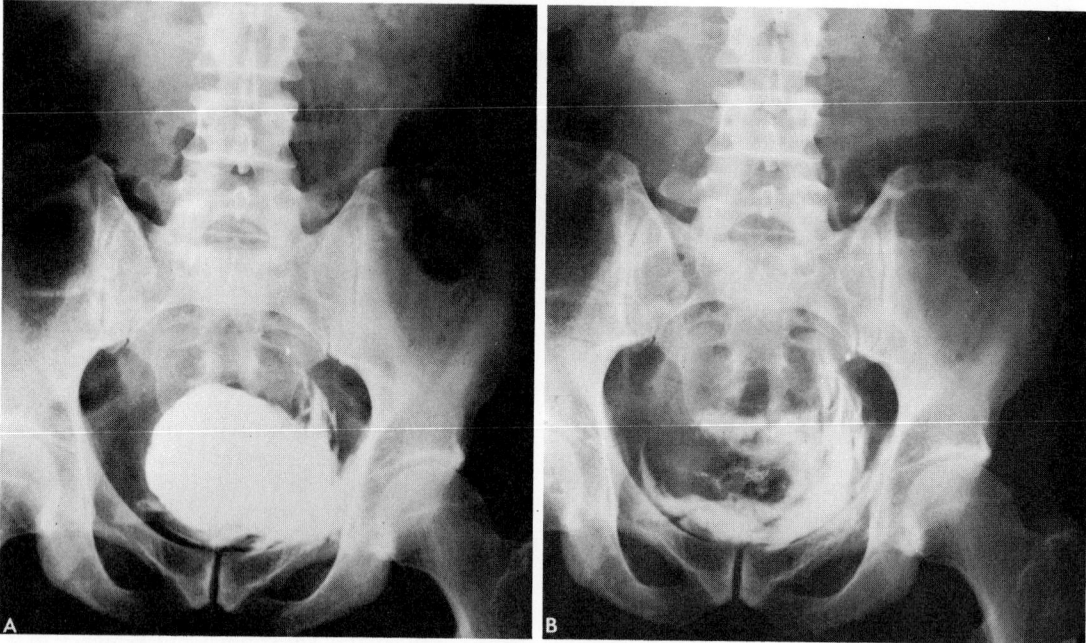

Figure 35. Retrograde cystogram demonstrating extravasation. *A*, Filling phase; *B*, postevacuation.

respond to the desire to expel this stored urine promptly with uninterrupted forceful flow. Normal function is dependent on an intact musculature and a complex control mechanism that involves both autonomic and somatic nerves.

The syncytium of smooth muscle that forms the main spherical body of the bladder, the fundus, encompasses the bladder neck as it passes into the posterior urethra. The bladder neck–urethral component of this muscular complex is assisted by a generous complement of elastic tissue in the urethra in its definite but poorly understood role in maintaining urinary continence. The striated muscle of the urogenital diaphragm and levator ani surrounding the midurethra in the female and the distal prostatic and membranous urethra in the male also play a significant role in urinary control.

The smooth muscles of the bladder and urethra receive sympathetic and parasympathetic nerve fibers (Fig. 36). The sympathetic fibers originate from T9 to L5 and course through the hypogastric nerves to the pelvic plexus. The parasympathetic fibers originate from S2 to S4 and course through the pelvic nerves to the pelvic plexus. The striated muscle of the urogenital diaphragm is innervated by the medulated fibers of the pudendal nerve, also originating from S2 to S4. All peripheral nerves contain both motor and sensory fibers. The afferent fibers carry pain, temperature, and proprioceptive sensation; the latter are related to fullness and desire to void. The important motor neurons to the smooth muscle of the bladder are parasympathetic in origin. In fact, the sympathetic innervation plays no unique role, although mounting evidence suggests that it is not without significant influence on the voiding mechanism. The reflex center for micturition is in the sacral spinal cord segments 2, 3,

and 4 (Fig. 36). Except in the untrained infant, this center is usually subject to control of the cerebral cortex.

Normally, smooth muscle is in a state of tension which is independent of central nervous system innervation. Stretching will cause a shortening of the muscle with resultant increases in tension. Even if the extrinsic nerve supply is completely divided, the bladder can store and evacuate a limited amount of urine. However, controlled accumulation of urine, as well as its timely complete evacuation, usually requires nervous control.

Initiation of *normal micturition* may be associated with a desire to void stimulated by proprioceptive impulses from bladder filling or may be volitional. With the former, release of cerebral inhibition is associated with a short latency period before detrusor contraction is initiated. The detrusor contraction shortens the urethra and increases the caliber of the urethral lumen. Relaxation of the external (striated muscle) sphincter is mediated through the pudendal nerve. The pelvic floor relaxes and sustained detrusor tone results in an uninterrupted flow of urine. Terminally, contraction of the external sphincter, bulb, and perineal musculature occurs. Attempts to void on command are associated with a longer detrusor latency period and a temporal association of pelvic floor relaxation with shortening and opening of the urethra.

Although all micturitional disturbances are manifested ultimately by detrusor dysfunction, in some, such as those related to overstretching of the bladder, direct detrusor injury may be the cause. The majority are associated with anatomic, functional, or pharmacologic interference with the primary or secondary reflex arc. The frequent combination of factors makes exact, clinically useful classification of micturitional disorders associated with neurogenic or detrusor abnormally difficult.

In assessing the individual patient with a micturitional disturbance a careful history is essential. Particular attention should be given to the following: (1) evidence of systemic disease such as diabetes or syphilis; (2) a history of utilization of drugs with recognized parasympatholytic effect such as atropine, methantheline (Banthine), or selected tranquilizers, and (3) a history suggestive or diagnostic of neurologic disease. The physical and general neurologic examination may provide evidence helpful in recognizing the possibility of and characterizing a neurogenic bladder dysfunction. Absence of rectal sphincter tone suggests a defect in the primary reflex arc. Failure of the rectal sphincter to contract with painful stimulus of the glans penis or clitoris (bulbocavernosus reflex) tends to support this supposition.

Assessment of the functional status of the upper urinary tract, by determination of endogenous serum creatinine or blood urea levels, and of the individual anatomic and crude functional status of the kidneys by use of intravenous urography is important to patient survival and care but adds little to the determination of the nature of the bladder dysfunction. A voiding cytstourethrogram may disclose a bladder diverticulum or ureteral reflux and aids in assessment of the status of the bladder neck and the urethra. Visualization of the latter assists in localizing the site of anatomic or functional obstruction. Cystoscopy and panendoscopy are useful in evaluating the bladder and urethra. Trabeculation associated with neurogenic dysfunction is variable in degree. In a bladder with deficient sensation (e.g., tabes dorsalis), trabeculation is minimal and patchy. In traumatic cord lesions, pronounced trabeculation and cellule formation may be present, depending on the degree of detrusor coordination and the duration of the abnormality. The presence of bladder lesions such as diverticula or calculi can have a marked influence on bladder function. Endoscopic procedures permit recognition of obstructing prostatic tissue and evaluation of the functional status of the external sphincter.

The most important objective observations with

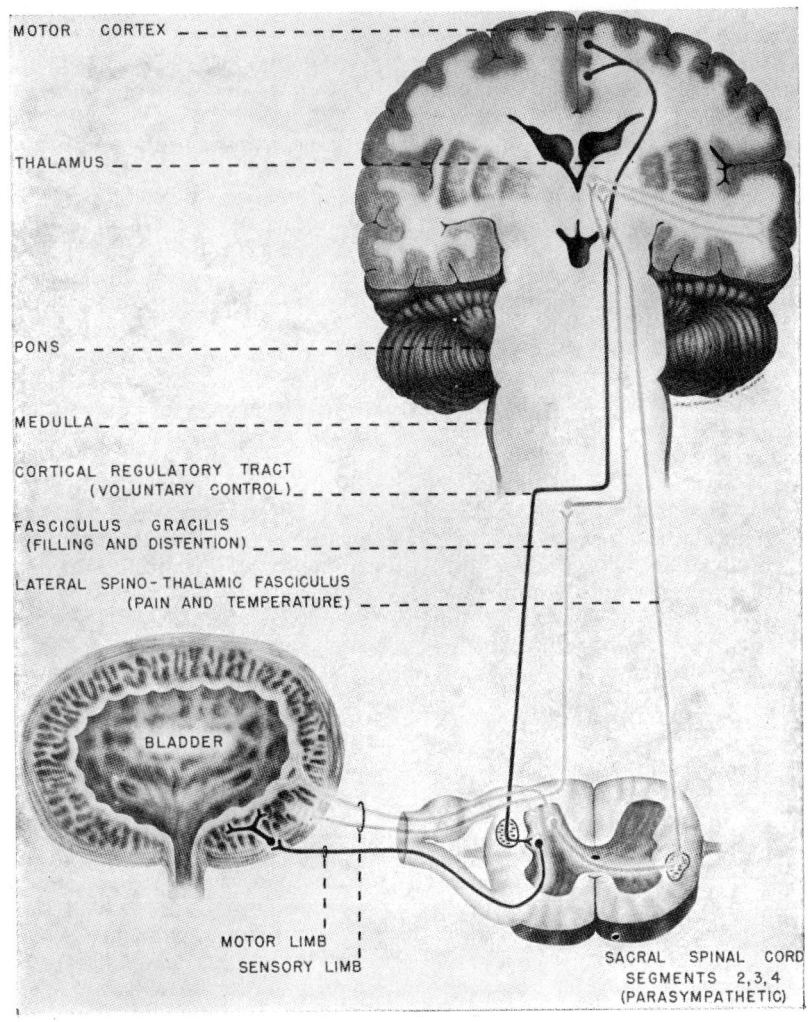

Figure 36. Diagram of major nerve pathways of importance in controlling bladder function. (From Lapides, J. *In* Campbell, M. F., and Harrison, J. H. (Eds.): Urology, 3rd ed. Philadelphia, W. B. Saunders Company, 1970.)

regard to bladder function and neurologic disease are provided by knowledge of the bladder capacity and of efficiency of voiding or achieving bladder emptying, and by observation of variation in sensation, bladder pressure, and contraction in response to filling (cystometrogram). An effort should be made to determine the amount of urine usually voided and the residual urine. Bors suggests 250 ml. rather than 300 ml. as a minimal normal capacity. He advocates considering residual urine in relation to bladder capacity (normal up to 20 per cent of capacity in upper motor neuron lesion and 10 per cent of capacity in lower motor neuron lesion) rather than as an absolute amount. After the residual urine is measured, the exteroceptive sensation of the bladder is tested by instillation of cold and hot water. If a neurologic lesion involves the upper motor neurons but not the conus or cauda equina, part or all of the sterile water is expelled promptly. Cystometry (see Fig. 5) consists of intermittent (50 ml. per minute) or continuous infusion of water at body temperature through a catheter with observation of first desire to void (150 to 250 ml.), feeling of fullness (350 to 450 ml.), and pressure response of the bladder. The intravesical pressure increases minimally until bladder capacity is reached; no spontaneous detrusor contractions are evident. On instruction to void the normal patient generates a pressure exceeding 50 cm. H_2O and often voids around the catheter. Administration of 2.5 mg. of bethanechol (Urecholine) subcutaneously increases the pressure response to filling up to 15 cm. H_2O in adults with a normal bladder and to a much greater degree in patients with a sensory- or motor-paralytic bladder. In addition to these tests sphincter resistance can be measured by determining the pressure required to overcome the sphincteric contraction. Electromyographic studies of the urinary and rectal sphincter have been utilized as investigative tools and have been informative.

Depending on degree and duration, overdistention of the bladder causes functional and probably anatomic changes in the bladder musculature and should be avoided at all times. Recognition of the undesirable effect of overdistention on bladder function is particularly important immediately after spinal cord injury. During this period (designated *spinal shock*) the bladder acts as a denervated organ and is unable to empty. Prevention of overdistention is essential and can be accomplished by intermittent urethral catheterization, indwelling urethral catheter, or suprapubic cystostomy. The method utilized will depend on the skill and availability of personnel and on the patient's condition. Every effort should be made to avoid urinary tract infection. Periodic catheter changes and sterile irrigation of the bladder to prevent stone formation are important aspects of care. Detrusor function is monitored periodically until return of voiding seems likely, at which point the catheter is removed.

A number of factors influence the type of neurogenic dysfunction resulting from a nerve lesion. The location of the nerve lesion is important. Lesions of the reflex arc (lower motor neuron) leave the detrusor more or less on its own (Fig. 37). Lesions above the sacral reflex center (upper motor neuron) affect the modification of the voiding reflex mediated through the sacral

reflex center. Incomplete, selective (sensory or motor), and combinations of upper and lower motor lesions occur clinically, making exact correlation of bladder function difficult and often unpredictable. However, a loose classification of neurogenic bladder dysfunction that usually correlates with the major aspects of the neurologic lesion is useful (Table 4).

The *uninhibited neurogenic bladder* results from decreased cerebral inhibition of bladder reflexes due to a defect in the corticoregulatory tract (Fig. 37, 1). In the normal infant, urination occurs whenever vesical or other regional stimuli reach a sufficient height to act through a lower motor neuron reflex arc. As the child grows older, bladder training allows the cerebral cortex to exercise an inhibitory effect over this simple reflex arc so that reflex emptying can be delayed. Inhibition is obtained first during the waking hours and subsequently becomes so patterned that it is present even during sleep so that enuresis ceases.

In some children, however, the cerebral inhibitory control does not become developed, perhaps as a result of deficient pathways or from psychologic defect, and the child continues to have uninhibited contractions (Fig. 38). There is then urinary frequency during the daytime and enuresis at night. The characteristics of this type of bladder are normal or increased tone and decreased capacity without residual urine.

Two types are recognized: congenital and acquired. In patients with the congenital type, administration of atropine in dosage sufficient to atropinize a child, if effective, is diagnostic of the uninhibited neurogenic bladder and, in addition, is therapeutic. Patients with the acquired type, that is, those with cerebral or high cord damage, are less susceptible to this form of treatment, although tranquilizers with parasympatholytic effects such as imipramine produce beneficial effects at times.

The *reflex (automatic) neurogenic bladder* typically results from complete transection of the cord at a level above the conus (Fig. 37, 2). It may also result from a disturbance of the suprasegmental arc that simulates transection of the cord. The result is a reflex arc running from the bladder to the sacral cord, synapsing and running back to the bladder. The bladder, then, is an organ controlled by a simple reflex. The lesions that cause this syndrome are usually injuries to the thoracic or lumbar cord that result in paraplegia. Characteristically the bulbocavernosus reflex is present and hyperactive.

The diagnosis of reflex neurogenic bladder rests upon locating the site and degree of injury and determining the type of bladder function that results. The bladder empties by reflex activity arising either from intrinsic stimuli from the bladder wall or from extrinsic stimuli that provoke mass movement. The patients have no real sensation of vesical filling, but the increasing size of the bladder as the urine accumulates produces sensations within the abdomen that they may interpret as fullness of the bladder. Urination occurs without warning as soon as the reflex arc is closed by summation of afferent stimuli.

Two major types of reflex bladders are recognized. The more usual is the spastic type; the other is the so-called normal reflex neurogenic bladder. The former is seen in patients with spasticity of the extremities. It is

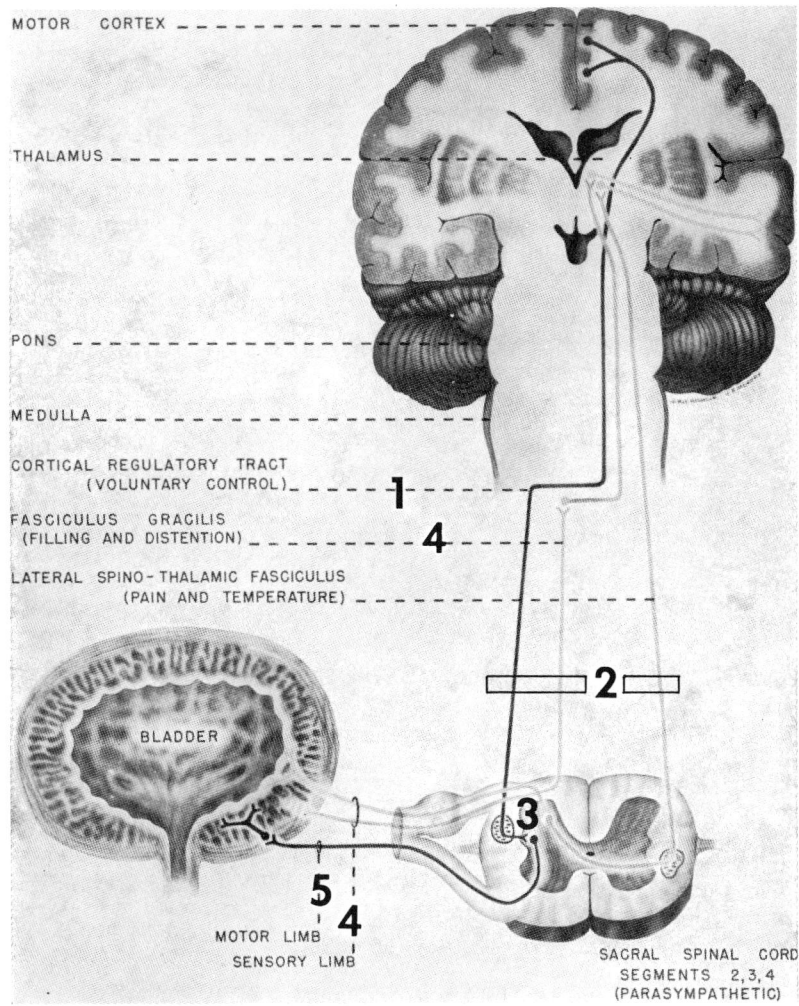

MOTOR CORTEX

THALAMUS

PONS

MEDULLA

CORTICAL REGULATORY TRACT
    (VOLUNTARY CONTROL)

FASCICULUS GRACILIS
(FILLING AND DISTENTION)

LATERAL SPINO-THALAMIC FASCICULUS
    (PAIN AND TEMPERATURE)

BLADDER

MOTOR LIMB
SENSORY LIMB

SACRAL SPINAL CORD
SEGMENTS 2,3,4
(PARASYMPATHETIC)

Figure 37. *1*, Site of typical lesion resulting in an uninhibited neurogenic bladder; lesion anywhere along the corticoregulatory tract, including an intracranial site, can be responsible. *2*, Complete transection of spinal cord above reflex center, a typical cause of a reflex (automatic) bladder. *3*, Lesions involving both limbs of the reflex arc produce an autonomous neurogenic bladder. *4*, Interruption of the sensory limb of the lower reflex arc or the long afferent tracts to the brain results in sensory paralytic bladder. *5*, Lesions of the lower motor neurons or motor fibers result in a motor paralytic bladder. (Modified from Lapides, J. *In* Campbell, M. F., and Harrison, J. H. (Eds.): Urology, 3rd ed. Philadelphia, W. B. Saunders Company, 1970.)

characterized by small capacity with more or less residual urine. The spasticity and small capacity necessitate frequent urination that is precipitant and inconvenient (Fig. 39). The goal of therapy is a so-called normal reflex neurogenic bladder. If this is obtained, bladder capacity may be as high as 300 ml. Visceral sensation of bladder filling may be enough to give the patient opportunity to reach a convenient place for voiding. Residual urine is low.

The therapeutic aim is first to remove all irritative foci, since the bladder is a purely reflex organ with sensory stimuli arising within the bladder wall itself, both from the mucosa and from the muscle as a stretch reflex. Bladder infection and calculi increase the sensory component of the reflex arc and cause increased stimuli for contraction.

A period of observation with restudy after several months is necessary to re-evaluate the effect of eliminating these sources of sensory stimuli. If spasticity

persists, blocking of the sensory nerve impulses is necessary and may be accomplished either by alcohol block or by sectioning the sacral roots. Intradural alcohol injection of the lower spinal cord blocks all long reflexes and produces an autonomous neurogenic bladder. The result is greater capacity and relative freedom from the inconvenient reflex voiding of the reflex bladder. A more direct approach is to block the sensory roots of the third, fourth, and fifth sacral nerves to cut off the sensory components arising from the irritable bladder and so interrupt the reflex arc. The bladder is then free to relax and to attain a normal capacity. In addition, the irritative stimuli arising from the posterior urethra are cut off, releasing the reflex spasm of the sphincter. Thus, sphincteric tone is more nearly normal. These procedures may assist patients with reflex bladders to regain almost normal control.

The *autonomous neurogenic bladder* results from

TABLE 4. Characteristics of Neurogenic Bladders

I. Uninhibited	II. Reflex (Automatic)	III. Autonomous	IV. Sensory (Atonic)	V. Motor
	Site of Lesion (see Fig. 37)			
Cerebral or high cord (underdeveloped central control)	A and B: Upper neuron	A and B: Lower neuron	Dorsal columns	Anterior horn cells
	Characteristics			
Voiding reflexes to filling are not suppressed	A, Spastic (imbalanced): Bladder takes part in general hypertonicity B, "Normal" (balanced): Bladder independent of control but reflex arc functions well	A, Flaccid (imbalanced): No external nervous control, but atonic B, "Normal" (balanced): No external nervous control, but bladder tone adequate for urethral resistance	Loss of sensation allowed excess filling, ending in flaccidity and atony	Sensation normal, but motor paralysis
	Disease Process			
A, Congenital: Delayed development of inhibitory pathway B, Acquired: Hemiplegia, brain tumors, multiple sclerosis	A and B: Transection of cord	A and B: Transection of conus or cauda equina	Tabes, pernicious anemia, multiple sclerosis, diabetes, syringomyelia	Poliomyelitis
	Symptoms			
Enuresis, urgency, and frequency; occasional incontinence	A: Reflex, involuntary voiding without sensation B: Same; occasional trigger zones cause voiding	A: Overflow incontinence B: Continence by periodic forceful evacuation	Painless overflow incontinence	Painful overflow incontinence
	Tone			
Normal or increased	A: Increased B: Normal or increased	A: Decreased B: Decreased	Decreased (late)	Increased (early)
	Capacity			
Decreased	A: Decreased B: Normal or increased	A: Increased B: Increased	Increased	Increased (late)
	Residual Urine			
0	A: 20–50 ml. B: 0–50 ml.	A: ±300 ml. B: 30 ml.	500 ml. +	300 ml. +
	Treatment			
Atropinization (parasympathetic block)	A: 1, Remove irritants (infection, calculi); 2, sacral neurotomy; 3, alcohol subarachnoid block B: None	A and B: 1, Presacral neurectomy; 2, pudendal block; 3, TUR; 4, Credé (5, Urecholine)	1, Preserve bladder tone; 2, evacuate with straining (3, presacral neurotomy if sphincter tight; 4, pudendal block; 5, Urecholine)	Catheter drainage expectantly
	Results			
Good in children	A: Fair if treatment prolonged. B: Good	A: Poor B: Fair	Poor	Good

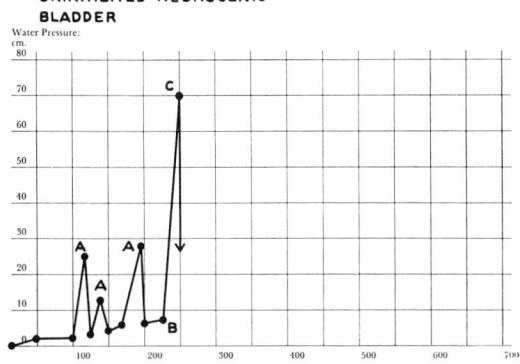

CYSTOMETROGRAM

UNINHIBITED NEUROGENIC
BLADDER

A. DESIRE TO VOID.
B. STRONG DESIRE TO VOID.
C. VOIDED AROUND CATHETER.

MANY SMALL CONTRACTIONS, NOT CONTROLLED BY
PATIENT, ENDING IN STRONGER CONTRACTION AND
VOIDING.

Figure 38.

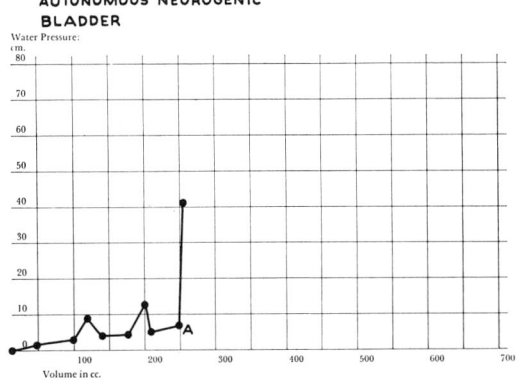

CYSTOMETROGRAM

AUTONOMOUS NEUROGENIC
BLADDER

A. STRAIN TO VOID.

NO SENSATION OF FILLING.
VOIDS BY STRAINING AND LITTLE REFLEX ACTIVITY.

Figure 40.

section of the cauda equina and conus, usually by trauma, but occasionally by inflammatory lesions and often from such congenital anomalies as meningocele with spina bifida. In contrast to a lesion across the spinal cord above the conus, a lesion through the cauda equina leaves the bladder autonomous (Fig. 37, 3; Fig. 40), possessing little or no outside reflex arc. It acts merely by the intrinsic reflex arc through the detrusor ganglia.

The bulbocavernosus reflex is usually absent, and saddle anesthesia is present. Bladder sensation is diminished and coordinated reflex stimulus to the detrusor is absent. The bladder fills against the intrinsic detrusor tone and urination is irregular and incomplete. Depending on the degree of resistance at the

vesical neck, the patient will be able to void more or less of the bladder contents by increasing abdominal pressure or by the use of manual pressure over the bladder. The capacity of the bladder may be as great as 350 ml. but the amount of residual urine is, of course, also quite high.

Treatment of these patients is directed at balancing urethral resistance against intravesical pressure. For emptying to occur, the ineffective detrusor contractions, supplemented by the pressure of the abdomen and the hand, must overcome urethral resistance. If urethral resistance is too high, retention of urine will result. On the other hand, if urethral resistance is too low, incontinence occurs.

Several measures have been proposed to decrease urethral resistance, since the strength of detrusor contraction can seldom be affected directly by therapy, even by such agents as the parasympathomimetic drugs.

Pudendal nerve block and section, either unilateral or bilateral, will cause partial paralysis of the external sphincter. Transurethral resection of the prostatic urethra, especially when definite obstructive elements are seen with the panendoscope, will quantitatively reduce urethral resistance. Often more than one resection must be done to secure a good result, since initial overenthusiasm can result in total incontinence.

The *sensory neurogenic bladder* occurs after interruption of the sensory side of the lower reflex arc or the long afferent tracts to the brain (Fig. 37, 4). Tabes dorsalis, occasionally pernicious anemia and multiple sclerosis, and syringomyelia are followed by this dysfunction. The patient does not know when his bladder is full because the afferent stimuli are cut off, so that after a time gross overdistention occurs, which results in atony. This atonic bladder devoid of motor power is the end result of the sensory defect. The bladder has a large capacity and urination occurs by overflow during straining. Incontinence often brings these patients to the physician. They are able to empty their bladders only by forceful abdominal pres-

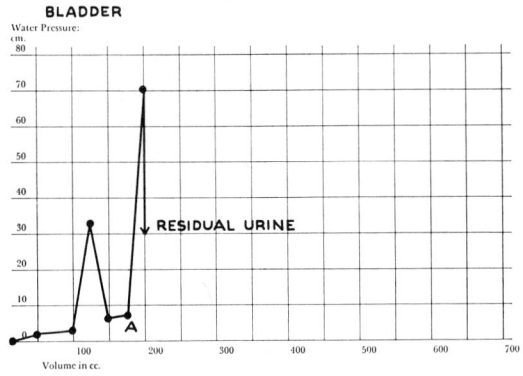

CYSTOMETROGRAM

AUTOMATIC NEUROGENIC
BLADDER

RESIDUAL URINE

A. UNABLE TO RESIST VOIDING.

REFLEX CONTRACTIONS, UNCONTROLLED, DURING
FILLING, ENDING IN FORCEFUL, INCOMPLETE EMPTYING.

Figure 39

sure and manual compression. A cystometrogram shows a low filling pressure with a very large capacity and no contractions of any sort. Cystoscopically, fine trabeculations are seen. The neck of the bladder is open and relaxed, as are the other portions of the detrusor. The external sphincter is not involved by the atony, and so its resistance is the cause of the retention of urine and overflow incontinence.

The object of treatment is primarily preventive. If the patients are seen early, before bladder tone is destroyed, they can be instructed to void at predetermined intervals, perhaps every 2 or 3 hours. Their bladders then will not become overdistended. After overdistention and atony have occurred, the object of therapy can only be to reduce the amount of residual urine and hope for return of bladder tone. The patient should be instructed to strain at each voiding and supplement the straining by manual pressure on the bladder. Bethanechol chloride (Urecholine) may be of some assistance in increasing detrusor activity. In very severe cases, a period of drainage by an indwelling catheter will occasionally reduce capacity to a more normal level and restore some tone. The fundamental disease process should be treated. Transurethral resection of the bladder neck is of little value to these patients, since the bladder neck is already widely open. Section of the pudendal nerve, either unilaterally or bilaterally, in certain cases will promote reduced urethral resistance because of partial paralysis of the normally active external sphincter and so will decrease the amount of residual urine.

The *motor neurogenic bladder* is the result of loss of the motor side of the reflex arc (Fig. 37, 5). It is seen with poliomyelitis, trauma, and tumor. Sensation is normal and so distention is painful, but overdistention occurs because the bladder is unable to contract as a result of loss of efferent stimuli to the detrusor. The cystometrogram is normal initially except for absence of detrusor contraction. Treatment consists of prompt institution of catheter drainage to avoid overdistention and atony while recovery of the nerve lesion occurs. If a partial motor lesion persists, use of bethanechol (Urecholine) may assist in restoration of function. If a complete motor lesion persists, the outlook for functional recovery is grave.

In summary, the initial treatment of the bladder with a neurogenic dysfunction should be directed to minimizing bladder damage by preventing overdistention by catheter drainage, avoiding or minimizing infection, and reducing the risk of stone formation by encouraging ambulation and high fluid intake. Subsequent to this the nature of the bladder dysfunction should be clarified by careful assessment of the neurologic state of the patient and his bladder. Return of the bladder to a stable functional state may require many months after injury. The ultimate goal of therapy is a functional state of the bladder that will insure preservation of renal function and will permit the patient to lead as normal an existence as possible while accomplishing this. A combination of preventive and active therapeutic measures is often necessary to achieve this desired goal. Active therapy may include such diverse measures as administration of drugs to control infection and modify neuromuscular response, mechanical modification of the bladder neck and external sphincter utilizing transurethral techniques, and various blocking and surgical procedures to modify the nerve supply to the bladder. Both the temporal and quantitative aspects of these measures are important to the results obtained. At times preservation of renal function or other serious complications from an unmanageable bladder require abandoning the organ and diverting the urine.

SELECTED REFERENCES

Glenn, J. F., and Boyce, W. H. (Eds.): Urologic Surgery, 2nd ed. New York, Hoeber Medical Division, Harper & Row, 1975.
  This multiauthor text presents modern concepts of indications for and complications of various surgical therapeutic endeavors as well as detailing the surgical technique. Preoperative and postoperative care is discussed.

Grayhack, J. T. (Ed.): Year Book of Urology. Chicago, Year Book Medical Publishers.
  This reference book is published yearly. It contains abstracts of significant works contributed to each of the major areas of urology during the year. References to major recent contributions in a field are available by consulting several Year Books in sequence.

Harrison, J. H., Gittes, R. F., Perlmutter, A. D., Stamey, T. A., and Walsh, P. C. (Eds.): Campbell's Urology, 4th ed. Philadelphia, W. B. Saunders Company, 1977.
  The three-volume standard reference text in urology contains 88 chapters written by recognized authorities. The detailed written text is well illustrated. An excellent list of selected references is appended to each chapter to assist the interested student.

Witten, D. M., Utz, D., and Myers, G. (Eds.): Emmett's Clinical Urography, 4th ed. Philadelphia, W. B. Saunders Company, 1977.
  This four-volume reference work describes the diagnostic techniques commonly employed in urology and illustrates the radiographic findings in various pathologic states.

REFERENCES

1. Allen, A. C.: The Kidney: Medical and Surgical Disease, 2nd ed. New York, Grune and Stratton, 1962.
2. Amar, A. D., Culp, O. S., et al.: Malformations: Encyclopedia of Urology. Berlin, Springer-Verlag, 1968.
3. Arey, L. B.: Developmental Anatomy, Rev. 7th ed. Philadelphia, W. B. Saunders Company, 1974.
4. Bennington, J. L., and Kradjian, R. M.: Renal Carcinoma. Philadelphia, W. B. Saunders Company, 1967.
5. Bors, E.: Neurogenic bladder. Urol. Survey, 7:177, 1957.
6. Bors, E., and Comarr, A. E.: Neurologic Urology. Baltimore, University Park Press, 1971.
7. Bowers, J. E., and Lattimer, J. K.: Interstitial cystitis. Surg. Gynecol. Obstet., 105:313, 1957.
8. Boyce, W. H.: Surgery of renal calculi. In Glenn, J. F., and Boyce, W. H. (Eds.): Urologic Surgery, 2nd ed. New York, Hoeber Medical Division, Harper & Row, 1975, p. 169.
9. Bricker, N. S.: Obstructive uropathy. In Strauss, M. B., and Welt, L. G. (Eds.): Diseases of the Kidney. Boston, Little, Brown and Company, 1963, p. 728.
10. Carlton, C. E., Scott, R., Jr., and Guthrie, A. G.: Initial management of ureteral injuries: Report of 78 Cases. J. Urol., 105:335, 1971.
11. Campbell, M. F.: Urology in infancy and childhood. In Campbell, M. F., and Harrison, J. H. (Eds.): Urology, 3rd ed. Philadelphia, W. B. Saunders Company, 1970, p. 1379.
12. Dalgaard, O. Z.: Bilateral polycystic disease of the kidneys. Acta Med. Scand. (Suppl.), 328, 1957.
13. Deming, C. L., and Harvard, B. M.: Tumors of the kidney. In Campbell, M. F., and Harrison, J. H. (Eds.): Urology, 3rd ed. Philadelphia, W. B. Saunders Company, 1970, p. 885.
14. Dodson, A. I.: Anatomy and surgical approach to the urogenital tract in the male. In Campbell, M. F.: Urology. Philadelphia, W. B. Saunders Company, 1954, p. 1.
15. Graham, J. B.: Renal malignancies. In Glenn, J. F., and Boyce, W. H. (Eds.): Urologic Surgery, 2nd ed. New York, Hoeber Medical Division, Harper & Row, 1975, p. 73.

16. Grayhack, J. T.: Renal Surgery. *In* Glenn, J. F. and Boyce, W. H. (Eds.): Urologic Surgery, 2nd ed. New York, Hoeber Medical Division, Harper & Row, 1975, p. 48.

17. Heptinstall, R. H.: Pathology of the Kidney, Boston, Little, Brown and Company, 1966.

18. Hinman, F.: Principles and Practice of Urology. Philadelphia, W. B. Saunders Company, 1935.

19. Hinman, F., Jr.: The pathophysiology of urinary obstruction. *In* Campbell, M. F., and Harrison, J. H. (Eds.): Urology, 3rd ed. Philadelphia, W. B. Saunders Company, 1970, p. 313.

20. Hodges, C. V., Gilbert, D. R., and Scott, W. W.: Renal trauma, J. Urol., *66*:627, 1951.

21. Holland, J. M., Grayhack, J. T., and Del Greco, F.: The kidney. *In* Preston, F. W., and Beal, J. M. (Eds.): Basic Surgical Physiology. Chicago, Year Book Medical Publishers, 1969, p. 455.

22. Jewett, H. J.: Tumors of the urinary bladder. *In* Campbell, M. F., and Harrison, J. H. (Eds.): Urology, 3rd ed. Philadelphia, W. B. Saunders Company, 1970, p. 1003.

23. King, D. R.: Diagnostic Ultrasound. St. Louis, The C. V. Mosby Company, 1974.

24. King, J. S., Jr.(Ed.): Renal neoplasia. Boston, Little, Brown and Company, 1967.

25. Kropp, K. A., Grayhack, J. T., Wendel, R. M., and Dahl, D. S.: Morbidity and mortality of renal exploration for cysts. Gynecol. Obstet., *125*:803, 1967.

26. Kunin, C. M.: Epidemiology and natural history of urinary tract infection in school children. Bull. N. Y. Acad. Med., *40*:767, 1964.

27. Kuru, M.: Nervous control of micturition. Physiol. Rev., *45*:425, 1965.

28. Lattimer, J. K.: Tuberculous infections and inflammation of the urinary tract. *In* Harrison, J. H., et al. (Eds.): Campbell's Urology, 4th ed. Philadelphia, W. B. Saunders Company, 1977.

29. Lapides, J.: Neuromuscular vesical and ureteral dysfunction. *In* Campbell, M. F., and Harrison, J. H. (Eds.): Urology, 3rd ed. Philadelphia, W. B. Saunders Company, 1970, p. 343.

30. Lindvall, N.: Renal papillary necrosis. Acta Radiol. (Suppl.), 192, 1960.

31. Lippman, R. W.: Urine and the Urinary Sediment: A Practical Manual and Atlas. Springfield, Ill., Charles C Thomas, Publisher, 1969.

32. Lowsley, O. S., and Kerwin, T. J.: Clinical Urology. Baltimore, Williams & Wilkins Company, 1944.

33. Marshall, V. F., et al.: Bladder Tumors: A Symposium. Philadelphia, J. B. Lippincott Company, 1956.

34. Merrill, J. P.: The Treatment of Renal Failure, 2nd ed. New York, Grune and Stratton, 1965.

35. O'Grady, F., and Brumfield, W. (Eds.): Urinary Tract Infections. New York, Oxford University Press, 1968.

36. Prather, G. C.: Injuries of the bladder. *In* Campbell, M. F., and Harrison, J. H. (Eds.): Urology, 3rd ed. Philadelphia, W. B. Saunders Company, 1970, p. 852.

37. Radionuclide Studies of the Genitourinary System I & II. Semin. Nucl. Med.,*4*:1, 1974.

38. Rao, N. R., and Heptinstall, R. H.: Experimental hydronephrosis: A microangiographic study. Invest. Urol., *6*:183, 1969.

39. Reynolds, C. J.: The diagnosis and a new treatment of traumatic rupture of the posterior urethra. South. Med. J., *35*:825, 1942.

40. Riches, E.: Tumors of the Kidney and Ureter. Edinburgh, E. & S. Livingston, 1964.

41. Schirmer, H. K. A., et al.: Renal metabolism with proximal or distal ureteral occlusion. Surg. Gynecol. Obstet., *123*:539, 1966.

42. Scholl, A. J., and Nation, E. F.: Injuries of the kidney. *In* Campbell, M. F., and Harrison, J. H. (Eds.): Urology, 3rd ed. Philadelphia, W. B. Saunders Company, 1970, p. 785.

43. Scott, R., Jr., Carlton, C. E., Jr., and Goldman, M.: Penetrating injuries of the kidney: An analysis of 181 patients. J. Urol., *101*:247, 1969.

44. Simon, N., Franklin, J. S., Bliefer, K. H., and Maxwell, M. H.: Clinical characteristics of renovascular hypertension. J.A.M.A., *220*:1209, 1972.

45. Smith, D. R.: General Urology, 8th ed. Los Altos, Calif., Lange Medical Publications, 1975.

46. Spence, H. M., et al.: Cystic disorders of the kidney—classification, diagnosis, treatment. J.A.M.A., *163*:1466, 1957.

47. Stamey, T. M.: Localization and treatment of urinary infections: Role of bactericidal urine levels as opposed to serum levels. Medicine, *44*:1, 1965.

48. Stamey, T.: Urinary Infections. Baltimore, Williams & Wilkins Company, 1972.

49. Stewart, B. P., Dustin, H. P., Kiser, W. S., Meaney, T. F., Straffon, R. A., and McCormack, L. J.: Correlation of angiography and natural history in evaluation of patients with renovascular hypertension. J. Urol., *104*:231, 1970.

50. Straffon, R. A., and Higgins, C. C.: Urolithiasis. *In* Campbell, M. F., and Harrison, J. H. (Eds.): Urology, 3rd ed. Philadelphia, W. B. Saunders Company, 1970, p. 681.

51. Symposium on Stones. Am. J. Med., *45*:649, 1968.

52. Wallace, D. M. (Ed.): Tumors of the Bladder. Vol. 2. Monographs of Neoplastic Disease at Various Sites. Edinburgh, E. & S. Livingston, 1959.

53. Williams, D. I.: Urology in Childhood. Berlin, Springer-Verlag, 1958.

54. Witten, D. M., Utz, D., and Myers, G. (Eds.): Clinical Urography, 4th ed. Philadelphia, W. B. Saunders Company, 1977.

55. Wolff, J. A.: Advances in the treatment of Wilms' tumor. Cancer, *35*:901–904, 1975.

49

THE MALE GENITAL SYSTEM

James F. Glenn, M.D.

HISTORICAL ASPECTS

The development of genitourinary surgery constitutes an important and provocative chapter in surgical history. Painful and disabling conditions of the genitourinary system were recognized by the ancients; early Egyptian hieroglyphics depict phimosis and bladder calculi. Anatomic interest in the lower urinary tract and the male genital system was defined in early Greece; Herophilos of Chalcedon, the Father of Anatomy, described the genital organs in 300 B.C. and is credited with naming the prostate, a term indicating that the gland guards or stands before the bladder. Lower urinary tract obstruction was recognized as a principal cause of bladder stone, and both suprapubic and perineal vesicolithotomy were practiced without benefit of anesthesia in the earliest civilizations, attended by extreme morbidity and mortality due to infection, hemorrhage, and injury of the gastrointestinal system. The lithotomists or "cutters for stones" were recognized in the Hippocratic Oath which declares, "I will not cut persons laboring under the stone, but will leave this to men who are practitioners of this work."

Early catheters were devised of straws, quills, and hollow instruments of horn, bone, and various metals. Ultimately, catheters of rubber and synthetic substances permitted comfortable instrumentation and alleviation of urinary obstruction. Diagnostic evaluation of the lower genitourinary tract evolved with cystoscopic techniques; in 1879, Nitze developed the cystoscope employing Edison's incandescent bulb. Discovery of the roentgen ray in 1895 added another modality of diagnosis, and radiographic contrast materials such as colloidal silver, introduced by von Lichtenberg in 1906, allowed further urographic evaluation of the urinary tract. Excretory urography was discovered serendipitously by Rowntree and associates in 1923,[29] and Swick, working in von Lichtenberg's laboratories in 1929 and 1930, employed a pyridine ring iodine compound, "uroselectan," for successful excretory definition of the urinary tract.

Little clinical attention was given to disorders of the prostate before 1900. Indeed, a classic text of 1858, Morland's *Diseases of the Urinary Organs,* deals exten-sively with kidney disorders, stones, inflammatory conditions of the bladder, urethral abnormalities, and other urologic difficulties, but states only that "an enlarged prostate may be mistaken for stricture." The first total prostatic enucleation was probably accomplished in St. Peter's Hospital by Sir Peter Freyer of London in the latter part of the nineteenth century. Shortly before the turn of the century, Hugh H. Young accomplished successful "operative removal of the enlarged prostate that was causing the obstruction to urination. At operation a finger was inserted through the opening into the bladder and found a large rounded mass projecting about three inches into the bladder cavity. With the assistance of a gloved finger in the rectum, it was not difficult to shell out this great mass from within the prostatic capsule, thereby removing the obstruction—my first prostatectomy."[42] Perineal prostatectomy was probably first accomplished in this country by Goodfellow. A transurethral cold "punch" operation was the forerunner of modern transurethral prostatic resection, the latter introduced by Davis and others in the early 1930s.

Modern perception of disorders of the male genitourinary system includes an advanced understanding of the physiology of the genital system, the endocrinology of sexual disorders, and the biochemistry of diseases of the prostate, seminal vesicles, and external genitalia. Recognition of the enzymatic and hormonal capabilities of the male genital system has permitted more accurate diagnosis and definitive therapy in a host of threatening conditions including carcinoma of the prostate, testicular tumors, benign prostatic hypertrophy, and male genital infections.

ANATOMY

The organs of the male genital tract include the prostate gland and seminal vesicles, the penis and its incorporated urethra, and the scrotum and scrotal contents. The male genitourinary system functions for purposes of copulation and reproduction, hormone production, and urinary excretion.

The prostate gland, seminal vesicles, and Cowper's glands

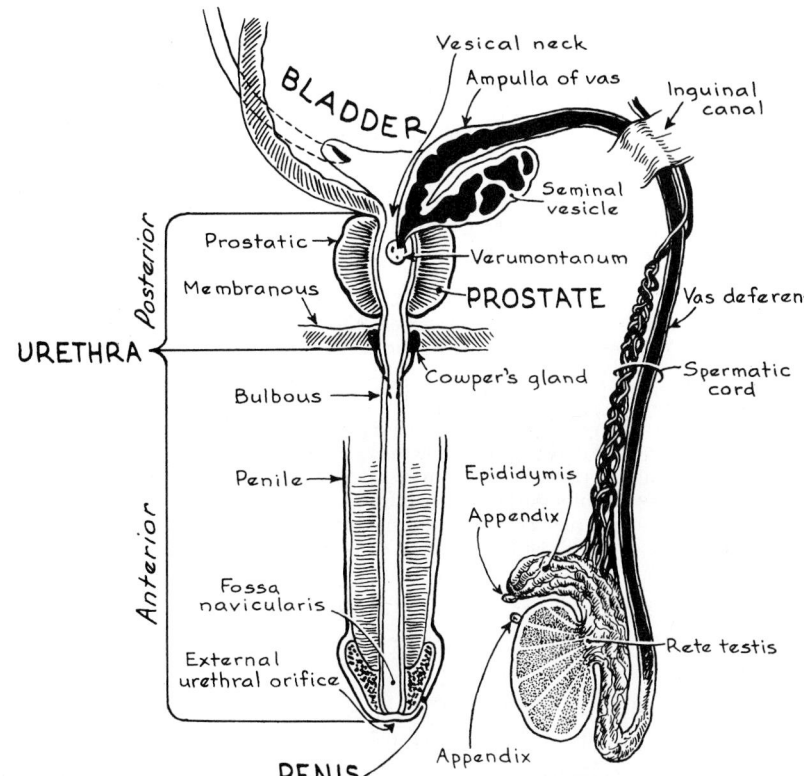

Figure 1. Schematic representation of the male genital system.

produce secretions that serve to lubricate the system and provide a vehicle for storage and passage of spermatozoa. In addition, the prostate gland is essential to normal erectile capacity of the penis. The penis, composed of two vascular erectile bodies, the corpora cavernosa, also incorporates the corpus spongiosum, which contains the male urethra. The paired testes produce both male hormones, predominantly testosterone, and spermatozoa, the former in the interstitial cells and the latter in the seminiferous tubular portions. The epididymides, lying in intimate contact with the testes, serve as the collecting system for sperm, which are transported along the efferent tract composed of the vasa deferentia and ejaculatory ducts, emptying into the posterior urethra at the verumontanum of the prostate.

Prostate Gland

The prostate is a fibromuscular glandular organ that surrounds the vesical neck and proximal portion of the male urethra. The prostate of the normal young adult male is approximately 20 gm. in weight and consists of two portions, an anterior group of glands intimately associated with the urethra and a posterior portion of more fibromuscular character. Embryologically, the gland derives from five epithelial evaginations of the posterior urethra that constitute alveolar glands emptying into the urethra.

The inferior vesical and internal pudendal arteries provide the blood supply to the prostate, entering the gland posterolaterally at the vesical neck. Venous drainage of the prostate gland is complex and diffuse, with plexuses over the anterior and lateral aspects of the gland that drain into the internal iliac veins. The nerve supply of the prostate derives from the pelvic plexus of the autonomic system. Intercommunicating lymphatics of the prostate, bladder, seminal vesicles, vasa

deferentia, and rectum provide drainage into the internal and external lymphatic systems.

Of considerable surgical importance is the difference in embryologic origin of the anterior and posterior portions of the gland. The anterior portion, consisting of periurethral glandular structures, gives rise to the hyperplasia and hypertrophy of benign enlargement and bladder outlet obstruction in older men. The posterior segment, a musculoglandular structure, is the most frequent site of origin of prostatic carcinoma.

The prostate lies immediately beneath the bladder, and in the presence of prostatic enlargement, the adenomatous hyperplastic gland is separated from the bladder only by mucosa and fibromuscular strands of the vesical neck. The gland is supported anteriorly by the puboprostatic ligament, inferiorly by the urogenital diaphragm or external urinary sphincter, and posteriorly by the rectal wall which is separated from the prostate by an obliterated pelvic reflection of peritoneum, the dual-layered Denonvilliers' fascia. In the presence of adenomatous hyperplasia and hypertrophy of the prostate, the fibromuscular outer portion of the gland is compressed and distended peripherally, constituting the surgical capsule of the prostate. A distinct cleavage plane is recognized between the adenoma and the surgical capsule in benign enlargement.

Traditionally, urinary control is attributed to the involuntary function of the internal sphincter or vesical neck and the voluntary control of the external sphincter or urogenital diaphragm. It is probable that advanced benign prostatic hypertrophy may irreparably compromise the sphincteric action of the vesical neck, and prostatic surgery may further compromise function of the internal sphincter mechanism. Diffuse, infiltrating carcinoma of the prostate may interfere with action of the vesical neck or the external sphincter.

Seminal Vesicles

The seminal vesicles are paired monotubular convoluted structures, lying beneath the base of the bladder and under the trigone. Posteriorly, they are invested by Denonvilliers' fascia, which separates them from the anterior wall of the rectum. The two seminal vesicles fuse medially with the ampullae of the vasa, forming the ejaculatory ducts that open at the verumontanum. The seminal vesicles secrete a mucoid vehicle for spermatozoa and elaborate fructose; a high free fructose level in seminal vesicle fluid is apparently necessary to maintain viability of spermatozoa. The muscular wall of the seminal vesicle is contractile, and ejaculation is accompanied by muscular contraction that expels the ejaculate through the ejaculatory ducts into the posterior urethra.

Cowper's Glands

Cowper's glands are small paired glands lying between the layers of the urogenital diaphragm at the junction of the bulbous and membranous portions of the urethra. The ducts of Cowper's glands empty into the bulbous urethra, providing an alkaline secretion that serves as a lubricant during sexual activity. Inflammatory and neoplastic diseases of Cowper's glands are extremely rare.

Penis

The penis serves the dual function of copulation and excretion of urine by the male. It consists of two parallel erectile compartments known as the corpora cavernosa, which are situated dorsolaterally, as well as the corpus spongiosum penis that invests the urethra and terminates distally in the glans penis, also an erectile body. Each corpus cavernosum and the corpus spongiosum are enveloped in fascial sheaths, and all three corpora are surrounded by the dense fibrous Buck's fascia.

The principal blood supply of the penis is through the dorsal arteries that course over the superior surface of the corpora cavernosa, lying deep to Buck's fascia. The principal blood supply is derived from the internal pudendal arteries, while venous drainage is through the dorsal veins of the penis communicating with the prostatic plexuses. Penile erection is induced by engorgement of the erectile tissue of the corpora, principally the corpora cavernosa. The exact mechanisms of erection are not fully understood, but compe-

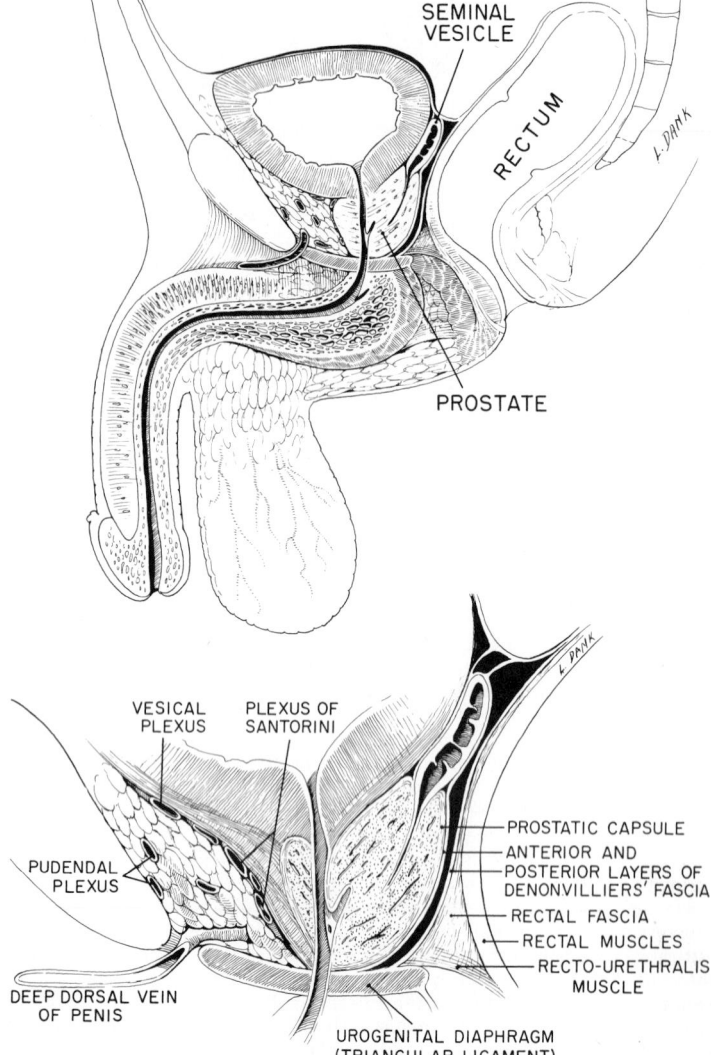

Figure 2. The anatomic relationships of the prostate gland. (From Brendler, H. *In* Glenn, J. F., and Boyce, W. H.: Urologic Surgery, 2nd ed. Hagerstown, Md., Harper & Row, 1975.)

tence of the pelvic blood supply and autonomic nervous system are essential. The corpora cavernosa take origin from the ischiopubic rami as the crura, these fusing in the perineum. Further fixation of the penis is provided by the suspensory ligament that connects the root of the penis to the pubis.

Lymphatic drainage of the penis is abundant, and that from the shaft of the penis, the corpora cavernosa, and the skin passes to the superficial and deep inguinal nodes, communicating thence to the iliac nodes. Lymphatic drainage of the glans penis parallels that of the urethra to the subinguinal, external iliac, and deep pelvic nodes, while lymphatics from the urethral mucosa drain to the hypogastric nodes. Skin of the penis differs from other skin in its paucity of sebaceous glands, its elasticity, and the extensive blood supply. These factors contribute to ready healing and permit extensive surgical reconstruction. The redundant foreskin, subject to extensive inflammatory involvement, may become constricted distally to produce phimosis, or proximal to the glans to produce paraphimosis.

Male Urethra

The male urethra consists of two major portions, the posterior urethra and the anterior urethra, each with two subdivisions. Beginning most proximally at the neck of the bladder, the posterior urethra consists of the prostatic portion and the membranous urethra. The prostatic urethra is analogous to the entire urethra of the female and is liberally invested with periurethral glands that are subject not only to enlargement, but also to acute and chronic infectious processes. The verumontanum opens in the floor of the prostatic urethra proximal to the apex of the prostate gland. The membranous urethra lacks periurethral glands, though Cowper's glands are located in the urogenital diaphragm lateral to the membranous urethra, the site of external or voluntary sphincteric action. The prostatic and membranous portions of the urethra are relatively fixed by the puboprostatic ligaments and the inherent stability of the urogenital diaphragm, while the urethra distal to the urogenital diaphragm is relatively mobile. In instances of pelvic injury including fracture, rupture or transection of the urethra is quite common at the junction of the membranous posterior urethra and the bulbous anterior urethra.

The anterior urethra includes the bulbous or perineal portion of the urethra, beginning at the urogenital diaphragm and extending to the penoscrotal junction, and the distal penile or pendulous urethra. The bulbous urethra exhibits a larger caliber than the remainder of the male urethra, and is richly invested with periurethral glands, often the site of gonococcal infection with subsequent fibrosis, cicatrix, and stricture. The penile or pendulous portion of the anterior urethra begins at the penoscrotal junction and extends distally to the external urethral meatus, just proximal to which a bulbous enlargement, the fossa navicularis, constitutes a nozzle-like effect that produces a unified urinary stream. The pendulous urethra is also invested with periurethral glands that may be the site of infection, and the narrow caliber of the pendulous urethra renders it more sensitive to irritation by a catheter.

Scrotum

The scrotal sac, consisting of two lateral compartments fused in the midline, encloses the testes, the epididymides, and the terminal portions of the spermatic cords. The dartos muscle is intimately attached to the corrugated skin of the scrotum, rich in sebaceous glands, providing for muscular contraction of the scrotal sac in response to temperature changes or sexual excitation. The principal function of the scrotum is to provide for maintenance of temperature control of the testes, since spermatogenesis is optimal at a temperature several degrees lower than that within the abdominal cavity. The alternate contraction and relaxation of the scrotum, in conjunction with similar contraction and relaxation of the cremasteric muscles of the spermatic cord, allow for maintenance of testicular temperature within a narrow and precise range. The blood supply of the scrotum arises from the femoral, internal pudendal, and inferior epigastric arteries, with venous drainage paralleling the arterial supply and emerging laterally. Lymphatic drainage of the scrotum is into the superficial and deep inguinal nodes, communicating with the femoral system. The loose character of scrotal skin permits accumulation of large quantities of lymph, extravasted urine, or blood, and in the presence of such accumulations, venous and lymphatic drainage is compromised, predisposing to gangrene or other serious infectious processes.

Testes

The testes are the essential organs of male reproduction, two in number, ovoid in form, averaging 4 to 5 cm. in length and 2.5 to 3.5 cm. in width in the normal adult male. Posteriorly, the testes are intimately attached to the epididymides and the terminal portions of the spermatic cord. The factors that control the descent of the testes from the abdominal cavity into the scrotum are probably hormonal. A poorly defined fibrous structure, the gubernaculum testis, is possibly associated with descent, which occurs during the latter phases of gestation. The peritoneum anterolateral to the testis evaginates into the scrotum and, following descent of the testicle, this processus vaginalis is obliterated, leaving around the testicle two layers of peritoneum that become the tunica albuginea, investing the testicle itself, and the tunica vaginalis, providing a cushioning sac around the testis.

Since the testis arises from the wolffian body on the genital ridge in close proximity to the kidney, it is not surprising that the blood supply of the testis arises from the aorta just beneath the renal arteries. Further blood supply follows the course of the vas deferens and may be sufficient to maintain testicular viability in instances in which the spermatic artery is divided. Venous drainage of the testis is through the multiple veins of the pampiniform plexus to the spermatic vein, which emerges from the upper end of the cord. On the right, the spermatic vein empties into the vena cava below the right renal vein, while on the left the spermatic vein empties into the main renal vein. Increased hydrostatic pressure, particularly on the left, may result in dilatation of the pampiniform venous plexus, producing varicocele. Lymphatic drainage of the testis is through the spermatic cord to the common iliac and para-aortic nodes, the latter communicating across the midline and with the mediastinal and supraclavicular chains. Testicular nerves derive from the aortic and renal plexuses, which in turn communicate with the solar plexus. Traumatic injury of the testicle may produce acute abdominal pain because of these interdigitating pathways, and intra-abdominal disease may cause referred pain in the testis.

Histologically, there are two principal portions of the testis: the seminiferous tubules, which are responsible for spermatogenesis, and the interstitial or Leydig cells, which elaborate androgenic hormones, predominantly testosterone. Because of the required relative hypothermia necessary to spermatogenesis, seminiferous tubule function may be impaired in the cryptorchid or maldescended testis, while hormonal function may be unimpaired, even in the intra-abdominal undescended testicle.

Epididymides

The epididymides are cordlike structures lying along the posterior aspect of each testis, the head of each epididymis resting upon the superior extremity of the testis and the tail attached to the inferior extremity of the testis. The medial surface of each epididymis attaches to the terminal portion of the spermatic cord through which blood, nerve, and lymphatic supply are received. A dozen or more tubular efferent ducts take origin from the rete testis, providing the system for collection of sperm. Sperm are then transmitted into the vasa deferentia, which are continuations of the ducts of the epididymides, passing up the spermatic cord and retroperitoneally to the ampullae of the seminal vesicles with which they conjoin to form the ejaculatory duct on each side. The principal blood supply of the epididymis is from the spermatic artery, which also supplies the testis, but the deferential artery, arising from the superior or inferior vesical artery, follows the course of the vas deferens and also provides some of the vascular supply of the epididymis. Venous drainage corresponds to the arterial supply, and the lymphatic drainage of the epididymis parallels that of the testis. The prime function of the epididymides is to provide a conduit for spermatozoa, but the epididymides also contribute to maturation of spermatozoa, sperm recovered from the body or tail of the epididymis exhibiting a greater degree of maturation and fertilizing capacity than those recovered from the head of the epididymis. Senescent deterioration of interstitial cells with concomitant decrease in androgen production will result in involution of epididymal epithelium.

Spermatic Cord

The spermatic cord, suspending each testicle with its attached epididymis, comprises the vas deferens, the spermatic artery, the pampiniform plexus of veins, the lymphatic drainage system of the scrotal contents, and the autonomic nerve supply to the testicle and its appendages. The cord is surrounded by fibers of the cremasteric muscle, which assist by contraction and relaxation in maintenance of optimal testicular temperature as well as providing for testicular retraction with sexual excitation or in the primitive fright reaction.

The vasa deferentia are tubular structures of 2 to 3 mm. in diameter, providing a narrow lumen for transport of spermatozoa, which are propelled by contraction of longitudinal smooth muscle fibers. Vasectomy, an operation for purposes of sterilization or prevention of retrograde infection of epididymides and testes, is accomplished by division of the vas, with or without excision of a small segment of each ductus deferens, and ligation of each divided end of the tubular structure. Successful restoration of continuity of the vasa – vasovasostomy – may be accomplished by meticulous surgical reanastomosis, a procedure that may be successful even after many years of interruption of continuity.

The pampiniform plexus is subject to venous dilatation and stasis, varicosities of this system being termed varicocele. Because of the complexity of the venous drainage in this plexus, direct surgical intervention for venous ligation is tedious; a more direct approach is to the single spermatic vein at the level of the internal inguinal ring where the pampiniform plexus becomes confluent into a single channel. Division of the venous drainage at this point is successful in preventing further stasis and will obviate the varicocele.

The processus vaginalis, the evaginated portion of the peritoneum, may not be obliterated after descent of the testis and may persist in part, producing hydrocele of the spermatic cord, or in toto, permitting partial or complete indirect inguinal hernia. In instances of incomplete or maldescent of the testis, the processus vaginalis remains patent, and orchidopexy must be accompanied by simultaneous repair of the potential or overt hernia.

PROSTATE GLAND

While all of the intricacies of the prostate gland have not yet been defined, clinical observation and basic investigation have elaborated prostatic function and provided insight into management of the various disorders that can affect this unique male organ. Normal prostatic function is apparently dependent upon androgens, principally testosterone, which is metabolized to dihydrotestosterone and androstenediol, substances of similar androgenicity. The prostate is capable of elaborating specific enzymes, principally lactic dehydrogenase and acid phosphatase. The interrelated physiologic and endocrinologic functions of the prostate are responsible for normal sexual function and provide certain clues to the etiology of benign prostatic enlargement as well as carcinoma of the prostate.

Congenital Anomalies

Complete absence of the prostate gland in an otherwise normal male has not been observed. However, failure of normal development and maturation of the prostate may be associated with the intersex states and male gonadal failure. Congenital contracture of the vesical neck at the point of juncture of prostate and bladder may cause severe urinary obstruction. Congenital valves of the prostatic urethra – mucosal folds that may be diaphragmatic or alar – occur relatively frequently and cause profound obstructive uropathy in some cases; early diagnosis and prompt treatment by endoscopic or open surgical removal of valves can prevent ultimate and inevitable renal failure. Congenital müllerian cysts predispose to obstruction and infection, presenting as midline masses beneath the gland and base of the bladder, treated by open surgical removal.

Trauma

Fracture of the bony pelvis may often result in laceration and transection of the membranous urethra just distal to the prostate, and urinary extravasation as well as bleeding may displace the prostate and bladder superiorly. Occasional penetrating wounds of the prostate due to gunshot wounds or perineal straddle injuries have been reported. The most common cause of prostatic injury is inexpert urethral instrumentation, generally in the course of urethral dilation in treatment of stricture, though injury at the time of rectal surgery is occasionally encountered. The usual concomitant of prostatic injury is damage to the external urinary sphincter, which lies in proximity to the distal portion of the gland, with fibrosis, stricture, and possible secondary sphincter damage.

Prostatic Infections

Problems of prostatic infection constitute a significant fraction of urologic practice. Infectious agents that may involve the prostate gland include the spectrum of gram-negative organisms that most frequently involve the urinary tract, gram-positive cocci, gonococci, various mycotic organisms, mycobacteria, trichomonads, and Candida species. The usual route of infection is ascending through the urethra, the potential for such exogenous infection being enhanced by stricture, diverticulum, or other abnormality of the urethra, though hematogenous and lymphatic routes of access have been incriminated, and descending infection through the urinary tract may occur, as with tuberculosis, which almost always involves first the kidney and later the organs of the lower genitourinary tract.

Acute Prostatitis

Suppurative acute prostatitis is generally a disease of younger men, but may be seen from pubescence throughout the life span. The organisms most commonly involved are the gram-negative group, principally *Escherichia coli*. Acute gonococcal prostatitis is relatively uncommon, but the involvement of the periurethral glands by gonorrhea predisposes to inflammation and stricture, which invite secondary gram-negative infection in the prostate. Stamey and others have demonstrated both bacteriostasis and a bactericidal effect of prostatic fluid, indicating that there are natural defense mechanisms inherent in the prostate gland.[36] Simple prostatic congestion may predispose to acute prostatitis. The usual symptoms of acute prostatitis include urgency and frequency of urination with severe dysuria and stranguria. There may be perineal aching and rectal discomfort, the patient sometimes complaining of a feeling of constipation. Chills and fever and even bacteremia may ensue. Edema may predispose to acute urinary retention. Examination discloses an exquisitely tender prostate that is diffusely indurated and enlarged. Urinalysis will usually reveal pyuria and often the offending organisms can be cultured. Prostatic massage should be accomplished most gently if at all, seeking to avoid bacteremia. Prostatic secretions will be filled with purulent debris, and the stained smear may reveal bacteria.

Instrumentation should be avoided in the acute phase of prostatitis unless there is associated urinary retention that demands catheterization. Vigorous antibiotic therapy with a broad-spectrum agent such as ampicillin or one of the cephalothin group should be initiated, pending culture and sensitivity studies. Bed rest, intermittent hot sitz baths, antipyretics, and restriction of sexual activity are necessary supportive measures. Antibiotic therapy should be continued for not less than 2 weeks, followed by a course of supplemental sulfonamides or chemotherapeutic agents in association with follow-up examination and prostatic massage.

Prostatic Abscess

Prior to the era of antibiotic therapy, prostatic abscesses were frequent sequelae of acute prostatitis, but are encountered less frequently today. Surgical drainage of prostatic abscess is required and may be accomplished by transurethral incision and resection, perineal incision and drainage, aspiration, or massage. Transrectal drainage of prostatic abscess is effective and is attended by surprisingly few complications, spontaneous healing of both the prostate and the rectal wall occurring in the majority of cases.

Chronic Prostatitis

Chronic inflammation of the prostate gland may ensue as sequel of acute prostatitis or may occur as a complication of prostatic enlargement and obstruction. Presenting symptoms usually consist of dull aching perineal discomfort with minimal but recurring symptoms of lower urinary tract irritation, frequency, and urgency with symptoms of fullness and irritability. Occasionally, urethral discharge occurs. Many patients may have chronic prostatitis without symptoms. Chronic prostatitis predisposes to associated urethritis, cystitis, vasitis, epididymitis, and even orchitis.

On examination, the prostate gland may be essentially normal in size and consistency, enlarged and boggy, or irregularly indurated and tender to palpation. Urinalysis may reveal red cells, white cells, and bacteria, or may be entirely within normal limits. Prostatic secretions, elicited by gentle massage accomplished by a sweeping motion of the examining finger over the lobes of the prostate from lateral to medial, followed by antegrade stripping of the prostatic urethra in the midline, contain pus cells with or without demonstrable bacteria. Normal prostatic secretions will contain 5 to 10 per cent WBC in the cellular elements of prostatic secretion, but greater numbers of pus cells and particularly leukocytes trapped in mucoid clumps confirm the diagnosis of chronic prostatitis.

The treatment of chronic prostatitis is often less than satisfactory. Antimicrobial agents may or may not be effective, and unless the symptoms are extremely severe and a positive culture can be elicited, antibiotics are usually avoided. Sulfonamides, nitrofurans, or other chemotherapeutic agents may be employed for chronic therapy along with urinary analgesics such as phenazopyridine (Azo-pyridon). Regular and periodic prostatic massage is probably the most beneficial modality of treatment, and must be accomplished over periods of several weeks or months. Hot sitz baths may offer symptomatic relief, and regular sexual intercourse will encourage normal drainage of inspissated secretions. Surgical intervention is not often indicated, but prolonged and severe chronic prostatitis may lead to fibrosis, scarring, contracture of the vesical neck, and prostatic calculi, these conditions sometimes requiring intervention by transurethral prostatic resection.

Prostatic Calculi

Calculi may occur in the glandular acini and ducts of the prostate gland, most often as the result of chronic inflammatory reaction with cellular necrosis, inspissation of debris, and deposition of calcific deposits. While prostatic calculi may be scattered through the gland, they most often occur near the periphery of the prostate, lying in a cleavage plane between the adenomatous periurethral glands and the fibromuscular capsule; the stony hard induration produced may be mistaken for prostatic carcinoma. Bacteria may be trapped in the interstices of prostatic calculi, contributing to perpetuation of prostatitis. Treatment is dictated by the clinical course: if the patient is asymptomatic and the urine is negative, no treatment is required, but associated obstructive or irritative symptoms, persistent urinary infection, or severe pain may necessitate prostatectomy, accomplished transurethrally or by open surgery.

Tuberculous Prostatitis

Tuberculosis of the prostate gland does not occur as an isolated entity. Genitourinary tuberculosis is always secondary to a primary infection, either pulmonary or gastrointestinal. Tubercle bacilli are transmitted hematogenously, usually to the kidney and thence to the ureter, bladder, prostate, and other genitourinary organs. However, it has been suggested that primary hematogenous spread to the prostate may occur. Symptoms may be totally absent or may be those of chronic obstruction and infection. Digital examination of the prostate may disclose stony hard induration, reminiscent of carcinoma or prostatic calculi. The diagnosis is established by demonstration of tubercle bacilli in the urine or prostatic biopsy with characteristic histologic findings of caseation necrosis and the other stigmata of tuberculosis. Medical management is indicated, employing various combinations of streptomycin, para-aminosalicylic acid, isoniazid, or other effective antituberculous drugs. Occasionally, total prostatectomy is indicated, but this procedure is almost universally accompanied by impotence and since the disease affects young males predominantly, surgical removal of the prostate is not the desirable modality of treatment.

Granulomatous Prostatitis

Chronic prostatitis may predispose to a severe multifocal, abacterial inflammatory process that is thought to be due to extravasation of prostatic excretions into the interstitium of the prostate gland, initiating the histiocytic granulomatous reaction. Examination of the prostate reveals irregular induration that mimics prostatic carcinoma. Symptoms of urinary urgency, frequency, and perineal pain usually bring the patient to the attention of the urologist. The palpatory findings of diffuse irregular prostatic induration generally demand prostatic biopsy—transperineal or transrectal needle biopsy or possibly open perineal biopsy—in order to establish the diagnosis and rule out the possibility of carcinoma. Prostatic massage and treatment of associated bacterial infection constitute the primary methods of treatment, but transurethral resection of the prostate may be required for alleviation of symptoms.

Miscellaneous Prostatic Infections

Other inflammatory processes in the prostate gland are encountered less frequently. Blastomycosis and actinomycosis have been reported as causes of chronic prostatitis, and treatment of these conditions may require surgical extirpation of the prostate gland. Moniliasis involving the urethra and prostate is usually alleviated by simple urinary acidification with concomitant treatment of the involved sexual partner. Trichomonas vaginalis may infest the prostate gland and produce symptoms and findings similar to those of chronic nonspecific prostatitis, the diagnosis being established by identification of trichomonads in the urine or prostatic secretions. Fortunately, a 10-day course of oral metronidazole for both sexual partners will usually eradicate Trichomonas infestation.

BENIGN PROSTATIC HYPERPLASIA

Benign prostatic overgrowth is the most common cause of bladder outlet obstruction in men over 50 years of age.[20] While exact mechanisms of prostatic hyperplasia are incompletely appreciated, it is recognized that adolescent development of the glandular acini and the fibromuscular matrix of the prostate is stimulated by gonadotropins and the androgens of the interstitial cells of the testes. After the age of 40, androgen production diminishes and glandular hypertrophy and hyperplasia of the prostate occur, progressing with advancing age. Typically, the glandular elements surrounding the prostatic urethra centrally—analogous to the periurethral glands of the female urethra—undergo spheroidal proliferation. The true acinar glands of the prostate and the fibromuscular capsule of the gland are displaced peripherally and compressed as the adenomatous hyperplasia progresses. A lobular pattern of growth is observed, the hyperplastic process involving the two lateral lobes of the gland or the median lobe, situated centrally and proximally beneath the bladder neck and trigone.

As the enlargement progresses, the prostatic urethra may become elongated and the caliber of the prostatic portion of the urethra may actually increase. However, the adenomatous process causes compression of the prostatic urethra, restricting the free flow of urine, sometimes associated with actual mechanical intrusion of a median lobe at the vesical outlet, predisposing to difficulty in initiating the urinary stream, maintaining it, and completing the act of bladder emptying. Mechanical pressure phenomena then may include upward displacement of the base of the bladder, fishhooking of the lower ureters due to trigonal displacement, hypertrophy of the bladder wall with trabeculation, cellule formation, and even diverticula of the bladder. Complete bladder outlet obstruction may result in decompensation of the detrusor muscle and total urinary retention.

The symptoms of benign prostatic hyperplasia are those of mechanical obstruction and the consequences of urinary stasis. In the early stages of prostatic enlargement, the patient complains of diminished size and force of the urinary stream, and as obstruction progresses, there is increasing frequency of urination, probably due to pressure of the enlarging gland beneath the trigone of the bladder. Nocturia is a similar index of the mechanical pressure of the enlarging prostate. It should be noted that nocturia normally occurs in older patients, both men and women, partially as a result of the inability of the kidney to concentrate urine, with resultant excretion of larger nocturnal volumes. However, nocturia more than once or twice nightly in the elderly male suggests mechanical pressure of prostatic enlargement as well as the possibility that the bladder is emptying incompletely with each voiding. Later, the patient with prostatic obstruction may note hesitancy and intermittency of the urinary stream, occasioned by intermittent fluttering

NORMAL PROSTATE

BENIGN PROSTATIC HYPERPLASIA

CARCINOMA OF PROSTATE

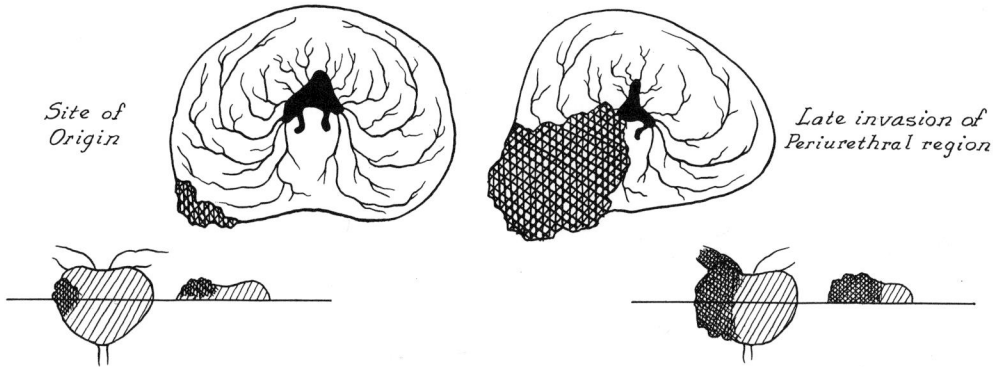

Figure 3. The normal prostate as contrasted with benign prostatic hyperplasia and prostatic carcinoma.

occlusion of the prostatic urethra by the hypertrophic lateral lobes. Terminal dribbling suggests both residual urine and pooling of urine within the prostatic urethra.[6]

Urinary bleeding may first bring the patient to the attention of the physician. Hematuria may result from prostatic enlargement with engorgement of the small mucosal vessels covering the adenomatous gland, ruptured as a consequence of straining to urinate. With progressive residual urine, infection may occur with purulent cystitis; about half of the men suffering urinary retention as a consequence of prostatic obstruction will exhibit infection. Similarly, vesical stasis of urine can predispose to the formation of bladder calculi with severe symptoms of dysuria and stranguria. Occasionally, patients may have few symptoms of bladder outlet obstruction, the syndrome of so-called "silent prostatism." Residual urines of 1000 ml. or more may produce a palpable lower abdominal mass before the patient experiences any particular symptoms, and it is not uncommon to observe bilateral hydroureteronephrosis and evidence of impending renal failure with azotemia and electrolyte imbalance.

The diagnosis of prostatic hypertrophy with bladder outlet obstruction is suggested by the history and is confirmed by careful physical and ancillary examinations. Rectal examination will reveal varying degrees of prostatic enlargement, most often symmetrical, with the prostate rubbery in consistency. As enlargement progresses, the gland protrudes posteriorly, compressing the anterior rectal wall and sometimes producing symptoms of constipation. The size of the gland may bear little relationship to the degree of symptomatic difficulty incurred by the patient, a small gland often completely obstructing the bladder outlet, whereas a large prostate three or four times normal size may produce few if any obstructive symptoms. Palpation of the distended bladder suggests incomplete emptying with significant residual urine. Cystourethroscopy will confirm the presence of prostatic enlargement and permit assessment of the degree of occlusion of the bladder neck or prostatic urethra, and the degree of bladder trabeculation and cellule or diverticulum formation.

General physical evaluation of the patient with benign prostatic enlargement is mandatory, with emphasis upon evaluation of renal function. Azotemia may occur insidiously with bladder outlet obstruction, and the usual measurements of blood urea nitrogen, serum creatinine, and creatinine clearance provide indices of renal functional capacity. The time-honored phenolsulfonphthalein (PSP) test provides a basis for evaluation of renal function as well as the degree of urinary retention; a flat curve of PSP excretion during the 2-hour interval of observation suggests severe renal functional impairment, whereas a rising curve suggests the dilutional effect of significant residual urine.

Conservative and medical measures of managing benign prostatic enlargement with bladder outlet obstruction are generally unsuccessful. Prostatic massage is of little value unless there is substantial congestion with retention of prostatic secretions. Urethral dilation is useless unless there is associated urethral stricture and should be avoided because of the danger of introducing infection. Anticholinergic drugs that induce hypotonicity of smooth muscle may effectively control symptoms of urinary frequency, but impose the risk of precipitating urinary retention. Occasionally, estrogens in small dosage may induce minimal improvement in the urinary stream, presumably through the mechanism of some prostatic shrinkage, but in general hormonal measures have been ineffective in benign prostatic hypertrophy.[28]

The decision for surgical intervention in benign prostatic enlargement is reached after evaluating a variety of factors.[32] Indications for surgery include residual urine of more than 100 ml., particularly when there is associated azotemia of any degree; persistent or recurrent urinary infection, refractory to usual therapeutic methods; gross hematuria on more than one occasion; acute urinary retention; or chronic urinary retention with overflow dribbling. To these classic indications for surgery, most urologic surgeons would add the factors of patient comfort and desire for surgery; nocturia more than two or three times nightly will interfere with rest, diurnal urinary frequency may pose a significant disability, the patient may be significantly concerned about the prospects of urinary retention, or it may be suspected that the enlarged prostate may be compromising sexual function, as it sometimes does.

There are four standard surgical procedures for removal of the obstructing enlarged portion of the prostate gland. None of these procedures constitutes total prostatectomy; all of them are designed for removal of the adenomatous hyperplastic portion of the gland, lying centrally and periurethrally. Hence, these procedures should most properly be termed prostatic

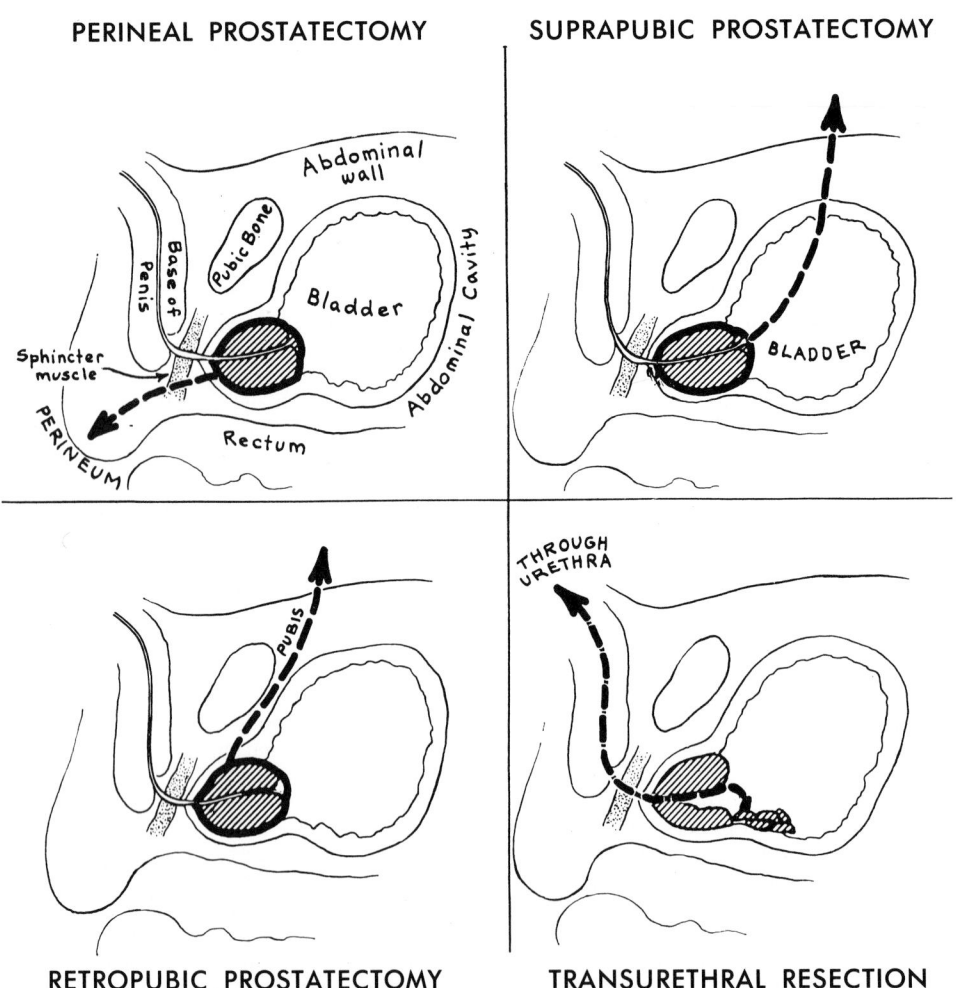

PERINEAL PROSTATECTOMY

SUPRAPUBIC PROSTATECTOMY

RETROPUBIC PROSTATECTOMY

TRANSURETHRAL RESECTION

Figure 4. The four basic surgical enucleative procedures for benign prostatic hypertrophy: perineal prostatectomy, suprapubic prostatectomy, retropubic prostatectomy, and transurethral resection of the prostate.

adenectomy rather than prostatectomy since the true prostate, compressed laterally into a fibromuscular and acinar surgical capsule, is retained after removal of the central adenomatous elements.

Suprapubic Prostatectomy

Historically, the suprapubic or transvesical method of enucleating the prostatic adenoma was the first to be generally employed. While utilized with less frequency today, this procedure still constitutes a fundamental method of surgical treatment in benign prostatic hyperplasia. A suprapubic incision, either vertical or transverse, gives access to the anterior surface of the bladder, which is then opened to give exposure of the vesical neck and the underlying prostate, a low transverse bladder incision being employed for better visualization. The mucosa surrounding the bladder neck is incised and a cleavage plane is then established between the adenomatous elements and the peripheral surgical capsule. At the apex, the prostatic adenoma is amputated from the urethra, and the enucleated adenomatous elements embrace the mucosa of the prostatic urethra. The fibromuscular surgical capsule that remains will contract to relatively normal configuration, and the inner aspect of the capsule will be epithelialized by growth of mucosa down from the trigone and bladder neck and up from the membranous urethra below, this process requiring several weeks or months. Hemostasis may be enhanced by direct fulguration and by mattress sutures, particularly at the posterolateral aspects of the vesical neck, the site of entry of the principal arterial supply. A urethral catheter is introduced and some surgeons prefer to inflate the balloon within the prostatic fossa, effecting tamponade against further bleeding. A second suprapubic mushroom catheter is usually employed as well. Surgical mortality rates of 1 to 5 per cent are generally recognized,[5] and the morbidity of suprapubic prostatectomy tends to be somewhat higher than that incurred with the other operative approaches to benign prostatic hyperplasia. However, suprapubic or transvesical prostatectomy remains a useful procedure, particularly when there is a very large median lobe or intrusion of the prostate well within the bladder cavity.

Perineal Prostatectomy

Perineal enucleation of the hyperplastic prostate was popularized at the turn of the century by Young. Perineal prostatectomy is particularly suitable to the large, low-lying prostate. The patient is placed in the extreme lithotomy position, giving access to the perineum, where a transverse incision in the shape of an inverted U is made anterior to the rectum. The rectum is separated from the posterior aspect of the prostate. The prostatic capsule is incised, and sharp and blunt dissection is employed to free the adenoma from the interior of the prostatic surgical capsule. The adenoma is amputated from the urethra distally and at the bladder neck. Hemostasis is effected with absorbable suture material at the vesical neck. A Foley catheter is inserted into the bladder through the urethra and the capsulotomy opening is closed to re-establish continuity. A rubber wick or drain is employed in the

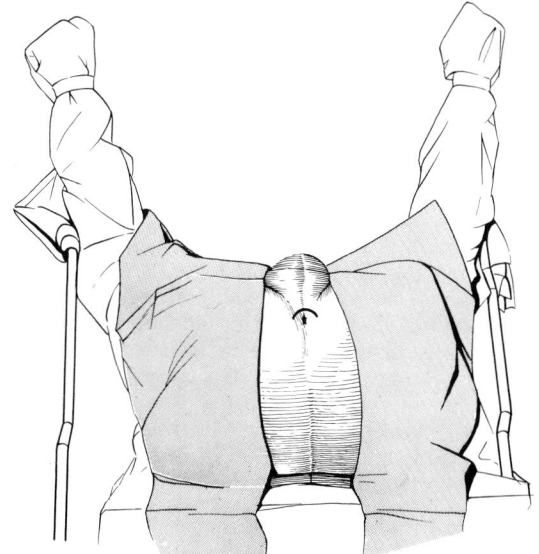

Figure 5. Position of patient and standard incision for perineal prostatectomy. (From Brendler, H. *In* Glenn, J. F., and Boyce, W. H.: Urologic Surgery, 2nd ed. Hagerstown, Md., Harper & Row, 1975.)

perineal incision. Catheter drainage is generally maintained for 7 to 10 days. The perineal procedure carries a lower mortality and morbidity than suprapubic prostatectomy,[3] but hospitalization is usually somewhat longer. The procedure offers the advantage of good control of bleeding, and it is thought that the extreme lithotomy position promotes venous return and minimizes operative vascular complications.

Transurethral Prostatic Resection

The emergence of endoscopic transurethral surgery was dependent upon the development of adequate lens systems, the incandescent bulb, and later fiberoptics, the refinement of electrical current for purposes of cutting and coagulation, and the ingenious combination of these advances into instruments satisfactory for surgical purposes. Transurethral prostatectomy has become the most commonly employed form of surgical treatment of benign prostatic hyperplasia with obstruction. Endoscopic resection of the enlarged prostate is most suitable in the smaller prostatic adenomas, those under 40 or 50 gm. in total resectable weight. It is better to resect the smaller fibrotic glands than to attempt difficult open surgical enucleative procedures.

The patient is placed in the lithotomy position and the urethra is calibrated with progressive urethral sounds. The resectoscope sheath is introduced into the bladder and the working element is positioned. Under direct vision, the wire loop is employed to cut away fragments of the obstructing adenoma. These fragments are subsequently evacuated from the urinary bladder. Constant irrigation is required, employing a nonelectrolytic isotonic irrigant of satisfactory optical properties such as commercially available solutions of glycine, urea, or mannitol-sorbitol mixtures. Saline cannot be employed, since it is an electrolyte solution that will dissipate the electrical current, and glucose cannot be utilized because of its stickiness. An isotonic solution must be employed, since fluid extravasated into the circulation may cause hemolysis with subsequent acute tubular necrosis. The electrical current passed through the wire loop may be modified as a high-frequency, high-amplitude cutting current or as a low-frequency, low-amplitude coagulating current for control of bleeding. An adequate resection is concluded when the fibers of the surgical capsule of the prostate have been visualized in all quadrants and there is no residual obstructing adenomatous tissue. Hemostasis is insured and a balloon catheter is left indwelling for 3 or 4 days. Operative mortality is minimal, usually only 0.1 to 0.5 per cent; hospitalization is generally a matter of a week or less; and morbidity and complications are minimal in patients properly selected for transurethral prostatic surgery.

Retropubic Prostatectomy

The retropubic route to prostatic enucleation was popularized by Millin[23] and is ideally suited to the rather high-lying larger gland with little if any intravesical component. The patient is operated on in the supine position and a transverse suprapubic incision is preferred. The anterior surface of the prostate is exposed and the surgical capsule is incised trans-

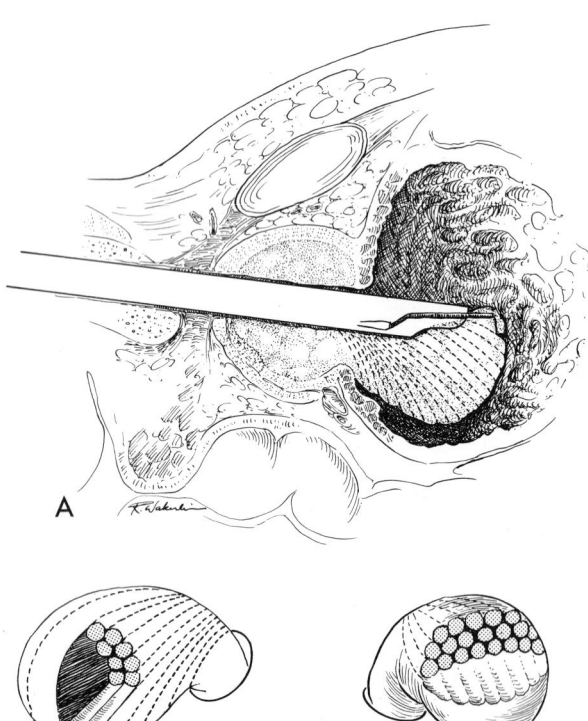

Figure 6. Transurethral resection of the prostate gland, here depicting resection of an enlarged median lobe of the prostate. (From Thompson, I. M. *In* Glenn, J. F., and Boyce, W. H.: Urologic Surgery, 2nd ed. Hagerstown, Md., Harper & Row, 1975.)

versely. Under direct vision, enucleation of the adenomatous portion of the gland is initiated by sharp dissection and completed bluntly. The adenoma is amputated from the urethra distally and from the bladder neck proximally. With a retractor in the prostatic capsulotomy, the vesical neck is visualized and hemostasis is achieved by fixation sutures of absorbable material. The prostatic fossa is fulgurated when necessary. A catheter is passed through the urethra and into the bladder and the capsulotomy is closed with absorbable suture. The procedure is modified by some surgeons who prefer to employ a vertical capsulotomy, extending the incision superiorly on the anterior surface of the bladder to gain added exposure of the bladder neck and the interior of the bladder itself. There are no contraindications to such an incision, which transects the region of the vesical neck, and exposure may be improved by this approach, particularly when there is a median lobe extending intravesically. In general, only a single urethral catheter is employed, and this is usually removed 5 to 7 days postoperatively. Problems of postoperative urinary incontinence are minimal with retropubic prostatectomy, morbidity is approximately equivalent to that of transurethral resection though hospitalization may be somewhat longer, and the operative mortality is only slightly greater than that of transurethral surgery, considerably less than that reported with suprapubic prostatic enucleation.

Long-term complications following prostatic surgery for benign adenomatous hyperplasia are relatively minimal. Since the surgical capsule is retained, sexual potency is usually unaltered, sometimes even improved, by these enucleative procedures. Urinary incontinence may occur as a permanent result of any form of prostatectomy for benign enlargement, but tends to be more prevalent after perineal prostatectomy and transurethral resection. Even here, the incidence of true and total urinary incontinence is minimal, probably no more than 1 per cent. The retained surgical capsule may afford an opportunity for regrowth of further adenomatous tissue, possibly requiring a second operative procedure. Retained adenomatous elements similarly may regrow and reobstruct. It has been estimated that 10 per cent of patients undergoing transurethral resection may have recurrent prostatic obstruction at a later date, necessitating another operative intervention, while recurrent adenomatous obstruction is seen with less frequency after the open procedures.

MEDIAN BAR OBSTRUCTION

Median bar is the term applied to the fibrous obstruction that can occur on the inferior vesical lip posteriorly, most often of congenital origin. If the fibrotic process extends entirely around the vesical neck, the condition is termed contracture of the vesical neck, which may be the result of chronic prostatitis. Not infrequently, patients may exhibit contracture of the vesical neck after previous prostatic enucleation of one sort or another, and such obstruction can demand secondary operative intervention. It should be reiterated that even the small prostate may obstruct and that diagnosis of median bar formation or contracture of the vesical neck can be established only by cystoscopic examination. Treatment of median bar or contracture of the vesical neck may be accomplished endoscopically or by open surgical revision. Endoscopic methods include transurethral resection with the electroresectoscope or with the cold-knife Thompson instrument, while some authorities—Keitzer and Turner-Warwick—recommend transurethral incision of the vesical neck with the cold knife. Severe compromise of the vesical outlet by median bar or contracture may be managed by suprapubic revision of the bladder neck, often employing the Bradford Young Y-V-plasty. Repeated instrumentation and dilation of the contracted vesical neck is ineffective and may predispose to fibrosis that aggravates the obstruction.

CARCINOMA OF THE PROSTATE

Adenocarcinoma of the prostate gland is the most common malignant disease of men over 65 years of age.[34] As a cause of death, carcinoma of the prostate is surpassed only by cancer of the stomach and colon in men. Autopsy studies by Rich have established the fact that prostatic cancer, occult or overt, is present in about 15 per cent of men over the age of 50 years.[33] It is estimated that the prevalence rate of prostatic carcinoma may be up to 20 cases per 100,000 population at the present time, and as the geriatric population increases, so must we expect an increase in prevalence of prostatic carcinoma. Squamous cell carcinoma of the prostate remains a relatively rare occurrence, and sarcoma of the prostate, still rarer, is generally seen only in the first two decades of life.

The etiology of prostatic carcinoma remains unknown. Alterations in the estrogen-androgen balance of a person have been incriminated, but clinical definition of hormonal imbalance as an etiologic factor remains to be accomplished. No definite carcinogens potentially responsible for prostatic carcinoma have been identified. Sexual activity is apparently not a factor, prostatic carcinoma having been observed in both celibate groups and those men with histories of extensive sexual activity. Infection, nonspecific or venereal, has not been incriminated as a causative factor. Metabolic alterations in the prostate may play a role; in benign prostatic hypertrophy, marked increases in the concentration of both zinc and magnesium have been observed, whereas in prostatic carcinoma there is a considerable increase in zinc concentration alone.

Prostatic carcinoma most often has its origin in the posterior capsular region of the gland, that segment of the gland which originates as the posterior element of the five embryologic components of the gland. Inves-

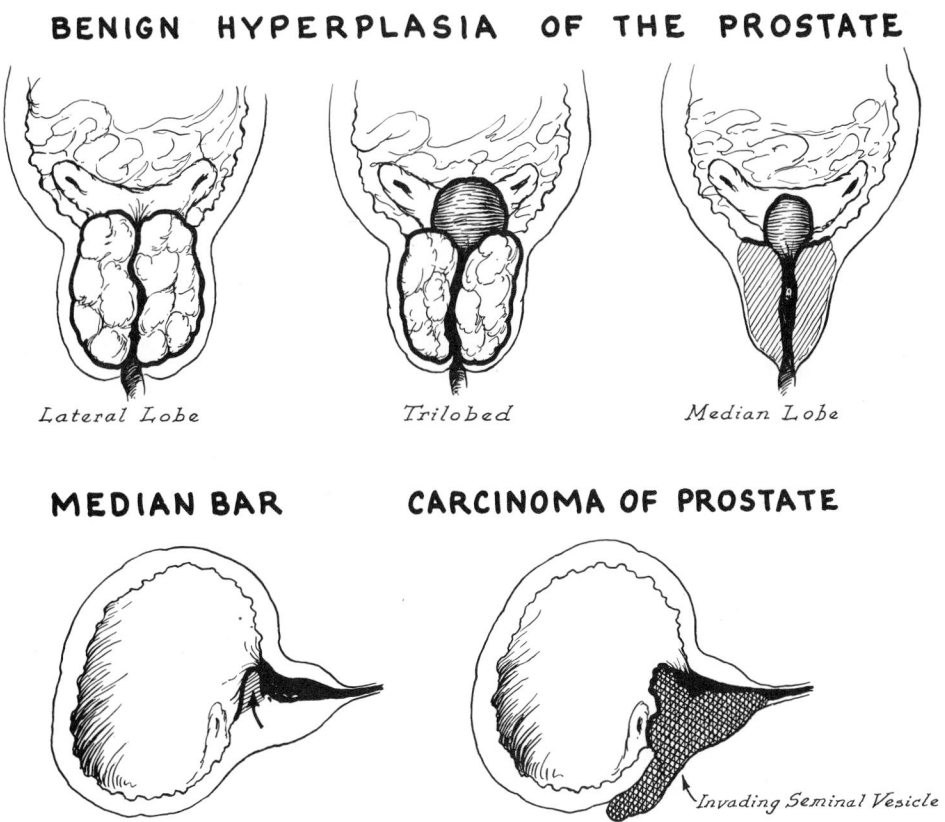

BENIGN HYPERPLASIA OF THE PROSTATE

Lateral Lobe　　*Trilobed*　　*Median Lobe*

MEDIAN BAR　　**CARCINOMA OF PROSTATE**

Invading Seminal Vesicle

Figure 7. Vesical outlet obstruction may be occasioned by benign prostatic hyperplasia, median bar formation, or prostatic carcinoma.

tigators are agreed that adenocarcinoma of the prostate does originate in glands that are metabolically and biologically active rather than in those that are atrophic, and the acinar elements in the fibromuscular surgical capsule of the peripheral prostate are frequently of an atrophic nature. There are variations in biologic behavior of prostatic cancers among those persons in whom the malignant lesion is peripheral as opposed to those who have a more centrally located paraurethral tumor, suggesting that different groups of glandular elements within the prostate may give rise to tumors of varying malignant potential.

Prostatic tissue may elaborate a variety of enzymes, including acid phosphatase and lactic dehydrogenase.[31] Nearly 40 years ago, it was recognized that phosphatases with principal activity in the acid range were produced in significant quantities in the prostate gland, and it was subsequently realized that tissue of prostatic origin, such as metastatic adenocarcinoma of the prostate, had similar capacity to elaborate acid phosphatase.[16] Measurement of serum acid phosphatase has become a standard modality in the identification of prostatic carcinoma, an elevation in the serum level signifying either advanced local disease or appreciable metastatic activity. Since acid phosphatase is richly concentrated in normal prostatic tissue as well, even prostatic examination or massage may elevate the serum level for up to 36 hours after rectal palpation.[14] Acid phosphatase is prevalent in other tissues as well, notably the erythrocyte, and tartrate fractionation of acid phosphatase is capable of differentiating that fraction of the enzyme that is of prostatic origin, though current studies would indicate that total serum acid phosphatase determination is at least as sensitive an index of prostatic carcinoma, either locally or metastatic. Normal levels of serum acid phosphatase do not rule out prostatic carcinoma, since those patients with small local lesions will not exhibit phosphatase elevations, prostatic tumors of a low order of metabolic activity may not produce such elevations, and even patients with advanced osteoblastic metastatic disease may on occasion display normal serum acid phosphatase values.

Lactic dehydrogenase (LDH) activity in human serum probably reflects glycolytic activity in all body organs and tissues. Prout and his co-workers have demonstrated alterations in the pattern of the five isozymes of LDH in patients with advanced and progressive prostatic carcinoma. It is suggested that the observed elevations of LDH isozymes IV and V in patients with advanced prostatic carcinoma reflect increased glycolytic activity within the tumor itself or in its metastatic foci. Most interesting has been the observation of reversion to normal of these elevated isozymes when adequate hormonal control measures have been initiated.[31] Serial estimation of LDH and its isozymes may thus provide an accurate laboratory method for assessment of therapeutic efficacy in the management of prostatic carcinoma.

The prostate gland is also known to be a source of fibrinolytic factors. Normal seminal fluid has significant fibrinolytic activity, possibly enhancing motility of sperm, attributed to the release of fibrinolytic activators from prostatic epithelium. Plasminogen, the

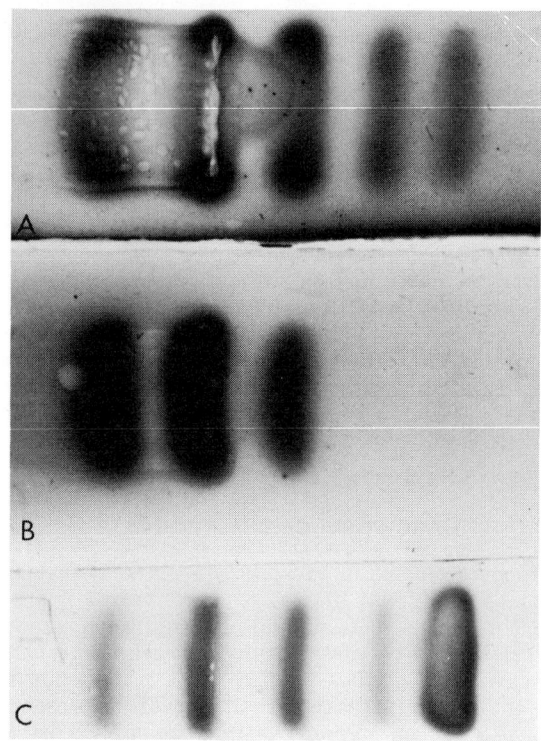

Figure 8. Alterations in the electrophoretic pattern of the enzyme lactic dehydrogenase (LDH) occur with prostatic carcinoma. *A,* From left to right, elevations of the isozymes IV and V are noted in a patient with active prostatic carcinoma. *B,* After hormonal therapy isozymes IV and V disappear. *C,* With exacerbation of prostatic carcinoma elevations of isozymes IV and V, particularly the latter, are observed. (Courtesy of Dr. George R. Prout, Jr.)

precursor of plasmin, is a fibrinolytic protease found in many tissues including the prostate. In prostatic carcinoma, increased fibrinolytic activity predisposes to spontaneous bleeding and hemorrhage, particularly after prostatic surgery. Prostatic carcinoma may predispose to increased production of plasminogen, though the source of fibrinolytic activity in the blood of patients with prostatic carcinoma has not yet been identified.

It has been estimated that prostatic cancer must be present for 2 to 5 years before it becomes clinically evident by rectal palpation. Growth rate of prostatic carcinoma seems to follow a logarithmic curve, and as the tumor increases in size, there is a concomitant increase in the ability to violate the natural tissue planes and penetrate into the periprostatic areas, predisposing to metastatic disease. On this basis, it has been suggested that only those tumors of more than 1 cc. in volume and having significant biologic potential will metastasize.

Unfortunately, early symptoms of prostatic carcinoma are generally lacking.[41] Since the majority of prostatic tumors occur in the periphery of the gland, encroachment on the urethra is a late manifestation of the disease. Irritative obstructive symptoms therefore do not signal the presence of the cancer, and it is only in advanced prostatic carcinoma that lower tract symptoms occur. Occasionally, patients may present with bone pain, usually lumbosacral, as a manifestation of metastatic disease long before local urologic symptoms occur. At the present time, there are no satisfactory screening methods for prostatic carcinoma other than routine and regular rectal examination. In the examination of 5856 men in the Cancer Detection Clinic of the University of Minnesota, 75 unsuspected carcinomas of the prostate were detected.[12]

In essence, the diagnosis of prostatic carcinoma must be based upon suspicion. Every man over the age of 50 should have mandatory rectal examination, and the finding of areas of induration and irregularity should suggest the diagnosis. Characteristically, prostatic carcinoma is stony hard in consistency and must be differentiated from focal tuberculosis, granulomatous prostatitis, and prostatic calculi. The isolated prostatic nodule should be regarded with the highest suspicion and other appropriate diagnostic maneuvers should be undertaken, including serum acid phosphatase determination, bone survey, possible marrow aspiration for tumor cells, and an appropriate form of biopsy. In advanced cases of local disease, there is usually little doubt as to the diagnosis. The prostate becomes nodular and irregular with extension of the indurated process beyond the confines of the gland, culminating in fixation of the prostate to the surrounding structures. At this stage of the disease, the patient is usually experiencing significant symptoms.

Definition of the stage of prostatic disease is aided by ancillary clinical and laboratory determinations. Bone survey may disclose metastatic lesions, classically osteoblastic in character, though poorly differentiated prostatic tumors occasionally produce osteolytic bone lesions. Bones most often involved are those of the pelvis and lower spine, though ribs, skull, and the long bones may also be involved. Even in the absence of radiographically demonstrable metastatic lesions, prostatic tumor cells may be evident in the bone marrow, and sternal or iliac aspiration may not only confirm the diagnosis but also indicate an advanced stage of prostatic carcinoma. Serum acid phosphatase determination constitutes a necessary step in diagnostic evaluation, since an elevated acid phosphatase frequently indicates metastatic activity, precluding cure by radical prostatic surgery. Intravenous urography and cystourethrography are useful radiographic techniques in evaluating degrees of lower tract obstruction due to advanced prostatic carcinoma. Cystourethroscopy is negative at early stages, but is useful in assessing the degree of bladder outlet obstruction occasioned by advanced prostate cancer.

The metastatic patterns of prostatic carcinoma are unique and interesting. Most common manifestations of metastatic disease are bony lesions in the sacrum and lumbar spine, but it is thought that earlier metastases occur in the iliac nodes, prompting some surgeons to advocate abdominal exploration as a method of assessing extent and stage of disease. Paradoxical metastases to the brain and skull with no intervening metastatic lesions in the lung or other bones may occur via Batson's plexus, the spinal venous system that communicates directly with the periprostatic veins. Pulmonary lesions may be isolated nodular metastatic defects or diffuse multiple seedlike lesions reminiscent of miliary tuberculosis. In advanced stages of the disease, metastatic adenocarcinoma of the prostate may be observed in virtually every organ including such unlikely sites as the testes, the skin of the scrotum, and the adrenal glands.

The treatment of prostatic carcinoma is, fortunately, a relatively bright page in the annals of cancer therapy. Observations by Huggins and his associates more than 30 years ago led to recognition of the androgen dependency of prostatic tumors and the corollary therapeutic response of these tumors to estrogen administration. These observations and subsequent investigations demonstrated the efficacy of hormonal management and provided the basis for the first genuinely effective chemotherapeutic approach to malignant disease. In addition, cure of prostatic carcinoma through surgery in the early stages of the disease has been practical for more than half a century. Most recently, advanced radiotherapeutic technique has provided yet another approach to control and possible cure of prostatic cancer.

Surgical Treatment

The potential for surgical cure of early carcinoma of the prostate was demonstrated shortly after the turn of the century. The efficacy of radical perineal prostatectomy has subsequently been elaborated by Jewett, Dees, and others. Clearly, radical prostatectomy, involving removal of the entire prostate and the seminal vesicles, can constitute cure only when the malignant process is confined to these tissues, with no contiguous or distant spread. It is estimated that as many as 10 per cent of patients presenting with prostatic carcinoma are in an early stage that is amenable to radical surgery. In general, the indications for radical prostatectomy include the isolated or localized prostatic malignant process, anticipated life expectancy of 10 years or more, good general condition of the patient with no significant ancillary disease, and the absence of demonstrable metastatic lesions as evaluated by radiologic survey, marrow aspiration, and normal serum acid phosphatase. Radical prostatectomy may be accomplished by the classic perineal methods of Young or Belt, and in recent years the retropubic approach to radical prostatectomy has been found successful by many. Complications of radical prostatectomy include impotence, a 2 to 5 per cent incontinence rate, and a surgical mortality of approximately 5 per cent. However, the efficacy of radical prostatectomy is apparent in various reports, Dees recording a 60 per cent 10-year survival following radical perineal prostatectomy as compared with a 22 per cent 10-year survival with palliative therapy and a 30 per cent 10-year survival with hormonal manipulation measures.[9]

Hormonal Management

While hormonal manipulation cannot afford cure of prostatic carcinoma, excellent and prolonged control can be achieved. The survey by Nesbit and Baum in 1950 documents the enhancement of survival of patients with prostatic carcinoma undergoing endocrine

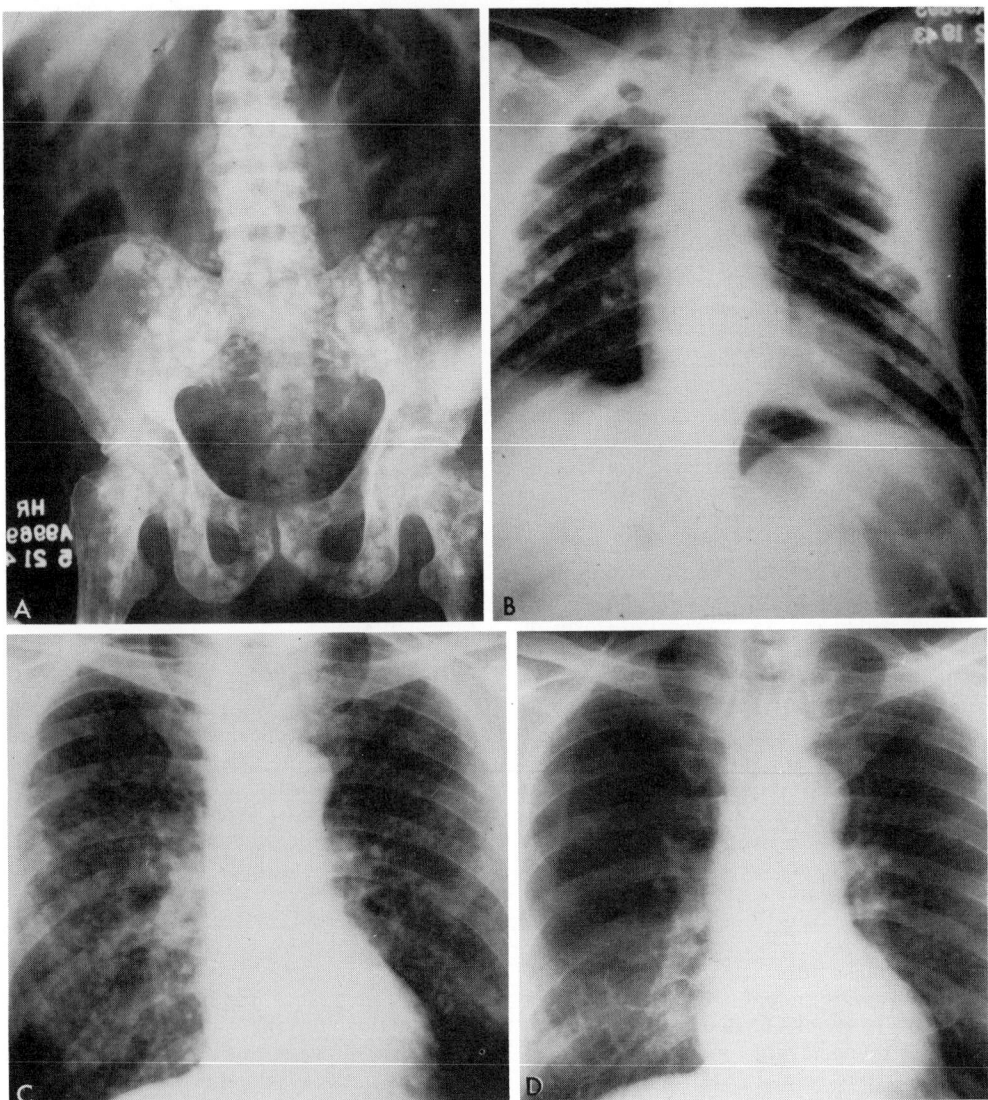

Figure 9.   Patterns of metastatic prostatic carcinoma include *(A)* multiple osteoblastic bony lesions, particularly in the pelvis and lumbar spine; *(B)* nodular pulmonary lesions and osteoblastic metastases in the ribs; and *(C)* miliary pulmonary metastases that regress *(D)* after adequate hormonal management.

therapy.[27] The oral administration of exogenous estrogens, bilateral orchiectomy, or a combination of orchiectomy and estrogens may be employed, the latter approach offering the most significant palliation and effective method of control. Alyea, reporting experience with castration and simultaneous initiation of estrogens, given as diethylstilbestrol, 0.5 to 1.0 mg. daily by mouth, observed a 30 per cent 10-year survival, irrespective of stage and grade of disease at the time of diagnosis.[1]

Since the adrenal gland is also responsible for production of a significant fraction of total-body androgens, bilateral adrenalectomy has been employed as an additional endocrinologic palliative measure in control of advanced prostatic carcinoma. Surgical or radiotherapeutic ablation of the pituitary may be similarly effective in palliation of advanced disease. The administration of exogenous cortisone or its derivatives may result in "medical adrenalectomy" with suppression of endogenous adrenal function, such therapy having the added advantages of inducing an anabolic state, producing a sense of well-being and a moderate euphoria, and diminishing the discomfort of advanced metastatic disease without the trauma of major surgery. Other measures of hormonal manipulation include the utilization of progestational agents and cyproterone acetate as additional modalities of treatment in advanced prostatic carcinoma. Recently, utilization of estrogens in dosage of 5 mg. per day and more has been subjected to some criticism on the basis of evaluation by a Veterans Administration cooperative research group; patients receiving larger doses of

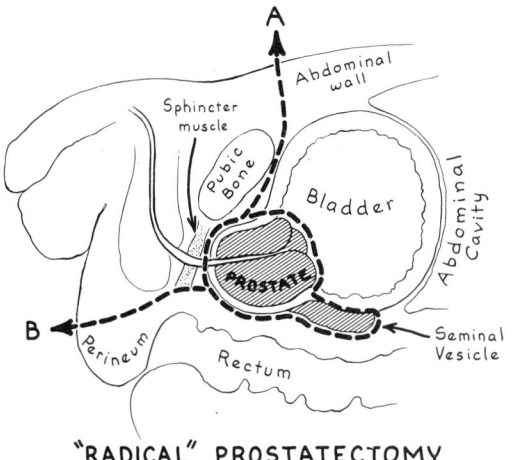

"RADICAL" PROSTATECTOMY

Figure 10. Schematic representation of radical prostatectomy, removing the prostate, seminal vesicles, and contiguous tissues by the retropubic method (A) or by radical perineal prostatectomy (B).

estrogens exhibited a substantial increase in mortality rates, predominantly from vascular complications of thrombosis involving cerebral and cardiac vessels, and it has been recommended that hormonal therapy be withheld until the disease becomes symptomatic.[39] This view, however, is not universally shared, and retrospective analyses fail to support the view that estrogen therapy increases the mortality rate for patients with prostatic carcinoma. At the present time, it is generally held that bilateral orchiectomy with simultaneous institution of estrogen therapy in modest dosage is the procedure of choice in advanced prostatic carcinoma that is beyond the realm of surgical cure. To such hormonal manipulation may be added the other modalities noted, and there is also the potential for secondary radical prostatectomy following adequate local response and regression of prostatic cancer. Finally, the implementation of hormonal measures does not preclude the utilization of radiation therapy as an adjunctive modality of treatment.[21]

Radiation Therapy

Prior to the advent of cobalt equipment and high-voltage apparatus, standard radiation therapy was effective only in the diminution of bone pain due to metastatic disease. A significant addition to the therapeutic armamentarium was the introduction of radioactive gold solution for interstitial radiation of the prostate and surrounding tissues. Flocks, reporting on 4000 cases of prostatic carcinoma, indicated a 40 per cent improvement in the 5-year survival rate among patients treated by such interstitial instillation of radioactive gold through perineal exposure of the gland.[11] Additional efforts to treat metastatic disease include the utilization of radioactive isotopes of phosphorus and strontium that are selectively absorbed by metastatic bone lesions of high metabolic activity. Most recently, carefully planned radiotherapy of prostatic carcinoma, employing external sources, has been advocated. Such radiation therapy may, of course, be employed for locally inoperable disease, as an adjuvant to hormonal therapy, and possibly as a primary therapeutic method in localized malignancy, though such utilization has yet to be demonstrated to be as effective as the radical surgical approach.[24] Complications of radiation therapy include inflammatory reaction with cystitis, urethritis, and proctitis, as well as potential stricture or slough.

SEMINAL VESICLES

The seminal vesicles, lying posterior to the bladder and uniting distally into the ejaculatory ducts that empty into the prostatic urethra, are paired tubular structures, functioning to produce mucous secretions that serve as the vehicle for sperm. The seminal vesicles are relatively inert, functioning as a reservoir for semen until ejaculation occurs, at which time muscular contraction causes the expulsion of ejaculate. Abnormalities of the seminal vesicles are relatively uncommon. Rarely, one of the seminal vesicles may be congenitally absent or exhibit cystic anomalies, usually associated with ipsilateral absence of kidney and ureter. Because of the secluded and protected location of the seminal vesicles, they are infrequently involved in trauma.

The most common clinical problems related to the seminal vesicles are those of inflammation and involvement by malignancy, due to the intimate connection of the seminal vesicles with the prostate and the base of the bladder. Chronic lower urinary tract infection may cause seminal vesiculitis, usually seen in association with chronic prostatitis, and obstruction of the ejaculatory ducts at the ampullae may predispose to abscess of the seminal vesicle. Diagnosis of such inflammatory disease is made by digital rectal examination; the dilatation and induration of the seminal vesicles can be readily appreciated, whereas the normal seminal vesicle is difficult to palpate. Massage and stripping of the seminal vesicles will produce purulent debris, confirming the diagnosis.

Primary carcinoma of the seminal vesicles is extremely rare. However, the communication of the seminal vesicles with the prostate, lying within the same fascial planes and subserved by the same lymphatic system, predisposes to early spread of prostatic cancer to the seminal vesicles. For this reason, radical prostatectomy demands the removal of the contiguous seminal vesicles. The surgical approach to the seminal vesicles may be perineal, retropubic, or transperitoneal, the method selected depending upon diagnosis; benign cysts of the seminal vesicles are best approached abdominally, whereas removal of the seminal vesicles with the prostate in cases of prostatic carcinoma is most readily accomplished by perineal exposure.

COWPER'S GLANDS

Cowper's glands are paired secretory organs lying in contiguity with the bulbomembranous urethra, draining through ducts in the floor of the bulbous urethra. They function to produce the clear mucoid secretion that serves as a lubricant to sexual function and implements ejaculation. Normally, Cowper's glands are not palpable, but occasionally infection may supervene, usually secondary to urethritis, predisposing to enlargement that is palpable on rectal examination distal to the prostate in a paraurethral position. Diagnosis of infected Cowper's glands is established by expression of pus per urethram, and treatment is usually conservative, though transurethral or perineal incision and drainage may be required. Carcinoma of Cowper's glands is extremely rare, but produces perineal pain, difficult urination, and a stony hard mass that presents rectally and perineally. Rectal fistulae may occur. Radical surgery is indicated.

PENIS

The penis serves the dual function of incorporating the male urethra and serving as the male organ of copulation. There are three erectile tissue compartments of the penis, the two corpora cavernosa situated dorsolaterally and the corpus spongiosum, which invests the urethra and terminates distally in the glans penis. The loose integument of the penis permits elasticity for erection. The mechanism of erection relates to both psychic and nervous stimuli, which produce engorgement of the corpora cavernosa and, to some extent, the corpus spongiosum. Neurophysiologic studies indicate that there is a center localized to the medial frontal lobe that is a positive locus for penile erection. Certain anterior thalamic nuclei and the mamillary bodies may be involved.

CONGENITAL ANOMALIES

It is fortunate that congenital anomalies of the penis are rare, since abnormalities of the genitalia may be the cause of severe anxiety and psychologic distress, not only to the patient but to the parents of the newborn male as well. Rare anomalies of the penis include duplication (double penis) and congenital absence of the penis in an otherwise normal male, the latter condition probably treated best by sex conversion surgery, since there are no adequate surgical methods for construction of a satisfactory erectile phallus. Microphallus may be managed successfully.

Phimosis

The normal foreskin of the penis provides a covering for the glans, the redundant portion of the foreskin being termed the prepuce. In many newborn males, the prepuce cannot be retracted satisfactorily, infection and inflammatory reaction result, and edema, fibrosis, and scarring cause constriction of the foreskin, or phimosis. In severe cases of phimosis, trapped preputial secretions predispose to balanitis (inflammation of the glans) and balanoposthitis (inflammation of both the glans and the foreskin). Obstruction to urination may occur and urinary infection can result. Further, such chronic inflammation is thought to predispose to penile malignant disease. Accordingly, prophylactic infant circumcision has been widely practiced for many years, though the universal necessity for such routine circumcision has been questioned. When phimosis leads to such complications, dorsal slit of the foreskin may be required as an emergency measure, and circumcision should be accomplished at an appropriate time. Very often, phimosis is accom-

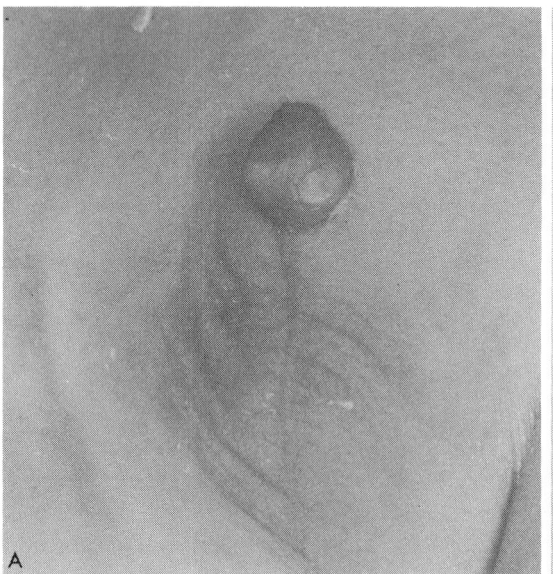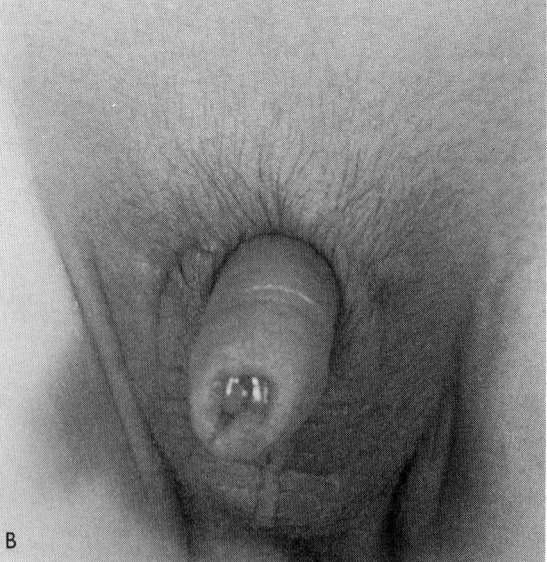

Figure 11. Congenital microphallus *(A)* is a distressing condition, but will respond to local application of testosterone preparations, response generated within 3 months as seen in *(B)*.

panied by meatal stenosis, and a urethral meatotomy may be effected at the time of circumcision. If the constricted foreskin becomes retracted and trapped proximal to the glans, severe swelling and even necrosis of the glans may ensue, a condition known as paraphimosis. Emergency surgical intervention is essential if the paraphimotic prepuce cannot be reduced manually; dorsal slit of the constricted foreskin is the procedure of choice.

Congenital Curvature

The most common congenital curvature of the penis is chordee, a fibrous constricting band along the ventral aspect of the penis that is usually associated with hypospadias, the congenital defect of the distal urethra. Epispadias, congenital absence of the upper portion of the urethra, causes dorsal deflection and curvature of the penis. In addition, abnormalities of the investing Buck's fascia may cause asymmetry of the penis with deviation.

TRAUMA

Trauma to the penis is relatively uncommon, but can cause total sexual disability. In pelvic fracture, rupture of the urethra will produce extravasation of blood and urine into the penile tissues; treatment is directed toward correction of the urethral rupture. In the erect state, the penis is subject to dislocation or even fracture, the latter condition being one of rupture of one or both of the corpora cavernosa with severe bleeding and hematoma. Immediate surgical intervention is required to repair the laceration of the investing fascia. Rupture of the veins of the penis may produce severe hemorrhage, usually best managed by catheter drainage and compression dressings. Lacerations of the penile skin and the glans are not uncommon as a consequence of masturbation, manipulation, or sexual activity, the frenulum of the penis occasionally tearing with sexual intercourse. Avulsion of the skin of the penis and of the scrotal skin may result when clothing is caught in various types of machinery, the loose integument of the genitalia being avulsed rather readily. Split-thickness skin grafts to the penile shaft take well and the cosmetic and functional results of such repair are satisfactory.

PENILE INFECTIONS

The penis is subject to infectious involvement by the various venereal diseases as well as other pathogenic bacteria and viruses. The abundant blood supply of the penile skin predisposes to excellent healing of such lesions. However, furunculosis of the penis may lead to severe cellulitis and even infection of the erectile corpora of the penis, cavernositis, most frequently due to urethritis of gonorrheal or nongonorrheal origin. Incision and drainage with appropriate antibiotic therapy constitute the treatment of choice.

Balanoposthitis

Inflammation of the glans penis and the prepuce constitutes balanoposthitis, most frequently the result of retained secretions and bacterial infection beneath the redundant prepuce, particularly when phimosis is present. Local irritative symptoms vary according to the severity of the infection, and it is thought that such chronic infections may predispose to squamous cell carcinoma of the penis. Dorsal slit of the foreskin, local measures, and antibiotics are employed initially, with circumcision the definitive method of treatment.

Condylomata Acuminata

Condyloma acuminatum is a cauliflower-like growth known as venereal wart, occurring singly or multiply on the prepuce and glans penis, and within the urethra itself. The lesions are of viral origin, usually associated with poor local hygiene, and may be transmitted from one sexual partner to another. In cases of redundant foreskin, circumcision may be beneficial in preventing recurrence. The standard method of treatment is application of 25 per cent podophyllum in benzoin on several successive occasions. Occasionally the venereal warts may achieve such size that surgical excision is necessary. Other methods of management include desiccation with dry ice, electrofulguration, and application of solutions of thio-TEPA. In advanced cases, the differential diagnosis lies between condylomata acuminata and carcinoma of the penis.

Herpes Progenitalis

Small reddened areas of the glans, prepuce, and dorsal surface of the penile shaft may become vesiculated, rupturing to leave superficial ulcerations, foci of secondary infection. This common viral infection is best managed by local cleansing and applications of bland ointments, sometimes incorporating anti-inflammatory agents.

Venereal Diseases

The principal venereal diseases to involve the penis itself are syphilis and chancroid. The primary lesion of syphilis is an ulcer or chancre, crater-like in appearance, usually occurring around the corona of the glans penis. Dark-field smear of the lesion will reveal *Treponema pallidum*. Similar chancres may be caused by sporotrichosis and tularemia, but these lesions do not usually involve the penis. The penile lesion of chancroid is a soft ulcerated area, again usually on the distal portion of the penis, later associated with inguinal buboes. Gonorrhea does not produce external penile lesions, the primary involvement being of the urethra and the paraurethral glands. Granuloma inguinale and lymphogranuloma venereum involve the inguinal lymphatics.

PENILE MALIGNANT DISEASE

Squamous cell carcinoma of the penis is the usual malignant lesion, though basal cell carcinoma and others have been described. Benign lesions such as nevi, hemangiomas, and papillomas are readily managed by local excision. Squamous cell carcinoma of the penis constitutes a more difficult challenge. It is usually seen in males of the lower socioeconomic strata, most commonly in uncircumcised men, and is a disease of filth, often the sequel of chronic balanoposthitis. Infant circumcision confers almost total immunity, though very rare cases of penile carcinoma have been reported in circumcised persons. The lesion is slow-growing and very often is obscured by the redundant foreskin. Patients tend to present with lesions in advanced stage. Persky and his associates have proposed clinical staging as follows: Stage I, limited to the glans penis or prepuce; Stage II, invasion of the corpora but without metastases; Stage III, invasive with positive regional nodes; and Stage IV, with distant metastases. Cure and survival are virtually 100 per cent in the Stage I patients, about 50 per cent in Stage II and Stage III, and nil in Stage IV.[10]

Diagnosis is established by biopsy. Treatment consists of partial or total penectomy; a proximal margin free of tumor of at least 1.5 cm. is desirable. Inguinal node dissection, with excision of both superficial and deep inguinal groups, is advocated when palpable nodes persist after amputation. Lymphadenopathy may result from the secondary infection seen in most advanced penile carcinomas. Radiation therapy in squamous cell carcinoma of the penis is relatively ineffective, but may be employed in treatment of known inguinal metastatic disease; the primary lesion should always be treated surgically. Chemotherapeutic efforts have been without avail.

SPECIAL CONDITIONS

Certain peculiar disorders of the penis or of penile function deserve special consideration, particularly since etiologic factors remain obscure in these disorders.

Peyronie's Disease

Localized plastic induration of the fibrous investments of the penile shaft was first described by the French surgeon Peyronie more than 100 years ago. Despite adequate description and an abundance of clinical observation, the etiology of the condition is unknown.[35] A firm fibrotic thickening of the fascia of the corpora cavernosa is observed, usually involving the dorsolateral aspects of the penile shaft or the intracaver-

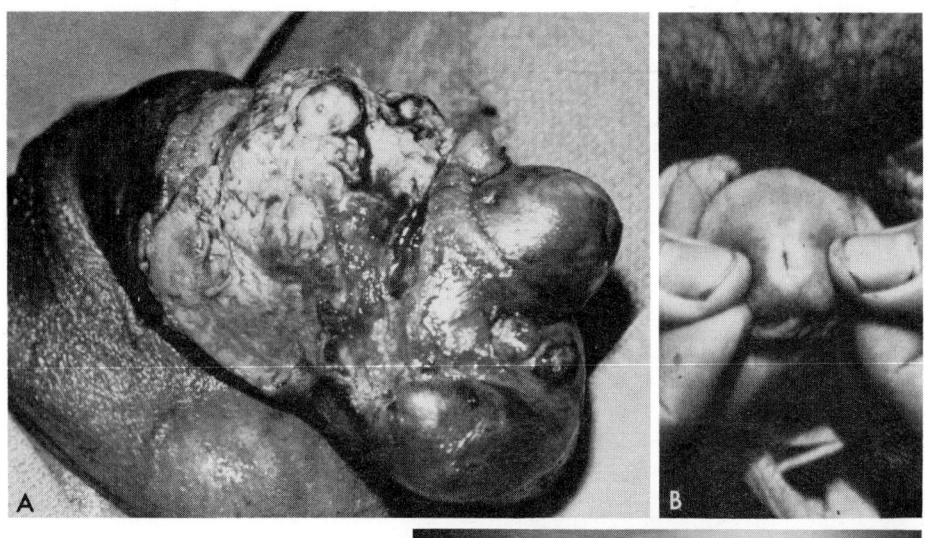

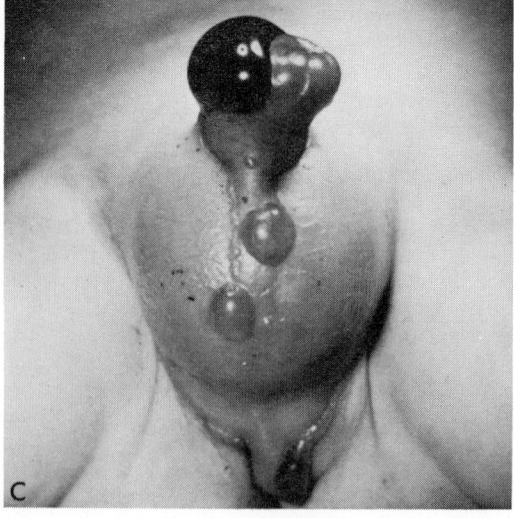

Figure 12. Penile lesions include (A) fungating squamous cell carcinoma; (B) balanitis xerotica obliterans with blanching, fibrosis, and stricture of the urethral meatus; and (C) phimosis with extravasation of urine.

nous septum between the corpora cavernosa, histologically similar to keloid or Dupuytren's contracture. The fibrous plaques themselves may be painless, but there is often compromise of erectile capability of the penis, with deviation of the penis on erection and pain as a consequence of this derangement.[4]

Patients usually note the lesion by self-examination, and they may have experienced significant deviation which interferes with intromission and coitus. Progression is slow, and spontaneous remissions are observed. Treatment is unsatisfactory; surgical excision is often unsuccessful, since recurrence of the plaquelike induration is common after excision of plaques.[17] High doses of alpha-tocopherol (vitamin E) and the oral use of potassium para-aminobenzoate (Potaba) as a fibrinolytic agent have been recommended, but successful resolution has been the exception rather than the rule. Systemic steroid therapy has not been beneficial, but local injection of high-potency corticosteroids such as dexamethasone has been reported to soften and resolve the plaques; the therapy itself—requiring weekly injections over a period of several months—is exquisitely tedious and painful. Perhaps the most effective modality of treatment at the present time is localized radiation therapy, employing 300 R in a single dose that is repeated at 3-month intervals to a total of 900 to 1200 R.

When the diagnosis of Peyronie's disease has been established, it is perhaps most important to reassure the patient that the process is not malignant. In most instances, the disease process is self-limiting with slow if any progression. Radiation therapy may alleviate any discomfort and though there may be some penile deviation with erection, sexual disability is not the rule.

Priapism

Prolonged pathologic and painful erection of the penis is termed priapism, in recognition of the Greek god of sexual excess, Priapus. Pelvic venous thrombosis predisposes to priapism, and such thrombosis is observed with metastatic malignant diseases of various sorts, leukemia, pelvic trauma, sickle cell disease or trait, trauma to the corpora, or spinal cord injury. In a majority of patients, no definite etiologic factor can be identified, and both local neural and vascular abnormalities have been incriminated as possible causes. Prompt recognition and therapy are essential, since prolonged unrelieved priapism will almost inevitably lead to subsequent permanent impotence. Immediate sedation and analgesia will sometimes alleviate priapism. Continuous spinal anesthesia has been advocated and is occasionally effective in the early hours of the condition. Classic treatment consists of insertion of large-bore needles for aspiration and detumescence, but unless pelvic venous congestion is simultaneously relieved, turbidity will recur. Thrombosis of the corpora occurs only late in the course of priapism, and accordingly venous bypass operations may be effective. The superficial saphenous vein may be employed for a corporosaphenous shunt, unilaterally or bilaterally, and a cavernospongiosum shunt may also be an effective surgical maneuver, since the corpus spongiosum is rarely obstructed in priapism.[7] A proteolytic enzyme from viper venom has been reported to cause rapid reduction in plasma fibrinogen, effective in one patient with priapism.

Impotence

While it is recognized that the aging process will diminish not only the libido but the capacity for erection as well, many men will remain potent throughout a lifetime of 90 years or more. Potency in the elderly male may be related to psychologic factors as much as to general health. Arteriosclerotic cardiovascular disease may compromise circulation to the corpora. Diabetes and other systemic disorders producing generalized neuropathies may diminish ability for erection.

Impotence may be one of the earliest signs of the Leriche syndrome, thrombotic obstruction of the iliac arteries, and the condition may be relieved by appropriate vascular surgery. Spinal cord injury may impair the capacity for erection, as may prostatic surgery, particularly perineal prostatectomy, which apparently compromises the pudendal nerves in some men undergoing such surgical treatment of benign prostatic enlargement. It should be noted that the vast majority of potent males undergoing prostatectomy remain potent postoperatively, irrespective of the surgical method employed. Radical perineal prostatectomy for malignant disease universally results in impotence. Finally, certain drugs such as the phenothiazines may impair erections and produce impotence, presumably by the adrenergic blocking effect of medication. Despite knowledge of this spectrum of potential causes of impotence, a majority of males who are otherwise healthy and who complain of an isolated problem of impotence must usually be categorized as having idiopathic or psychologic difficulties; psychiatric consultation is mandatory when the various physical causes of impotence have been eliminated.

Ejaculatory Disorders

One of the most distressing sexual disabilities of the young and middle-aged male may be premature ejaculation. Intromission may be scarcely achieved before ejaculation occurs, terminating the sexual act to the frustration of the patient and the partner. Certain organic and psychic factors can be incriminated; chronic prostatitis can increase irritability and predisposition to ejaculation, and long abstinence with attendant sexual excitation can initiate premature ejaculation. In most instances, however, the problem relates to inadequate sexual technique in the marital unit, and careful consultation and counsel may aid in overcoming premature ejaculation.

Another disorder of sexual function is retrograde ejaculation, occasionally seen as a consequence of neuromuscular disturbance of the vesical neck secondary to diabetes, spinal cord injury, and other causes of neuropathy, but most often due to surgical alteration of the vesical neck. Prostatectomy by open or endoscopic means, transurethral resection of the bladder neck, vesical outlet reconstructive procedures, and even retroperitoneal surgery with autonomic nerve damage may diminish the capacity for closure of the bladder neck, an essential ingredient of normal ejaculation, with consequent retrograde flow of ejaculate into the bladder. Once such surgical abnormality is incurred, little can be done to overcome retrograde ejaculation. In some instances, gradual narrowing of the bladder neck over a period of a year or two after prostatectomy will promote more normal ejaculation. Fortunately, retrograde ejaculation in no way diminishes sexual gratification, but it may, of course, be the cause of infertility, since sperm are deposited in the bladder rather than expelled through the urethra.

MALE URETHRA

The posterior portion of the male urethra, embryologically analogous to the female urethra, consists of the prostatic and membranous portions passing through the central portion of the prostate gland and the urogenital diaphragm or external voluntary urethral sphincter. Distal to this area, also known as the triangular ligament, lies the anterior urethra, consisting of the bulbous portion and the penile or pendulous portion. The prostatic urethra is most often involved secondarily by diseases that primarily affect the prostate gland, such as carcinoma and prostatitis. The membranous urethra within the triangular ligament that attaches to the pubic arch is a frequent site of rupture, since the prostatic and membranous urethra are relatively fixed in position with the remainder of the urethra somewhat mobile, predisposing to a shearing tear of the urethra at that point. The bulbous and penile portions of the urethra are invested with paraurethral glands that are often the site of infection, and the anterior urethra is rarely sterile in contrast to the posterior urethra, bacteria gaining entry to the distal portions of the urethra through the external meatus.

CONGENITAL ABNORMALITIES

Urethral meatal stenosis can usually be recognized by inspection and is suspected when the urinary stream is of poor caliber. Such stenosis may predispose to infection and may be a cause of enuresis. Treatment of meatal stenosis is by meatotomy. Other congenital strictures of the urethra may also be seen, often in the bulbous urethra. Open surgical repair may be favored in longer strictures, whereas lesser areas of involvement may be satisfactorily handled by internal urethrotomy and prolonged catheter drainage to provide stenting of the urethra in an open position during the phase of healing.

Urethral Valves

Congenital valves of the urethra usually cause severe obstructive uropathy with decompensation of the urinary bladder, hydroureteronephrosis, supervening infection, and consequent renal failure unless prompt and adequate treatment is instituted. Valves are mucosal or fibrous folds obstructing urethral urinary flow, usually occurring in the distal portion of the prostatic urethra at the level of the verumontanum,

taking an alar configuration and sweeping from the verumontanum to the lateral wall of the prostatic urethra or occurring as a diaphragm-like constriction of the urethra. Transurethral electroresection or destruction by fulguration is most often employed, but a retropubic transprostatic open exposure may effect surgical cure of valves. The sequelae of obstruction by urethral valves may be so severe that permanent urinary diversion is required, generally accomplished in the form of an ileal conduit, an isolated segment of ileum to which the ureters are attached at the proximal end, the distal end being brought out in the right lower quadrant as a urinary ileostomy.

Hypospadias

Varying degrees of failure of complete development of the distal urethra may be observed, termed hypospadias. The urethra may terminate just proximal to the glans (glanular hypospadias), at some point along the penile shaft (penile hypospadias), at the anterior margin of the scrotum (penoscrotal hypospadias), or in the perineum with bifid scrotum (perineal hypospadias). Associated with this defect is severe ventral curvature of the penis or chordee, which results from a fibrous band occurring in the projected course of the urethra. The embryologic defect is a failure of closure of the urethral groove. In extreme cases, particularly if there is associated bilateral testicular maldescent, the configuration of the genitalia may be so ambiguous that an intersex state results. Early and accurate diagnosis is imperative. Virtually all degrees of hypospadias demand surgical repair, for cosmetic as well as functional reasons. A classic approach is to accomplish release of chordee and penile straightening as one procedure, followed at a later date by a one- or two-stage urethroplasty. A tremendous variety of operative procedures have been advocated, and all may be

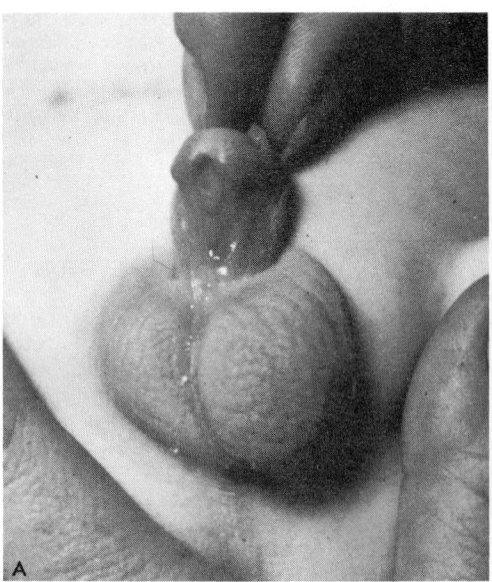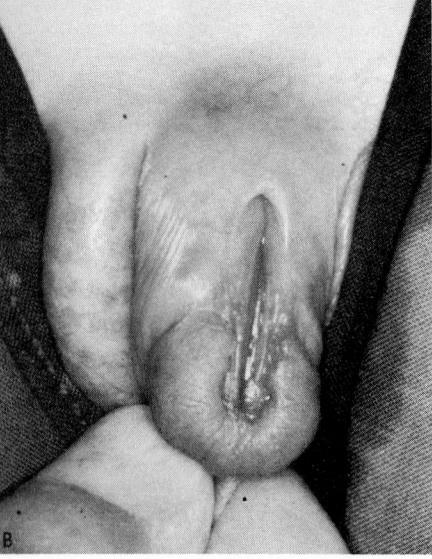

Figure 13. Urethral abnormalities include *(A)* hypospadias and *(B)* epispadias.

successful. Most recently, both Hodgson and Horton have advocated one-stage operations for release of chordee and simultaneous urethroplasty, and both of these procedures may be successful in the majority of cases. The principal difficulty encountered in surgical repair of hypospadias with associated chordee relates to achieving adequate penile straightening, imperative before urethral reconstruction is effected. The commonly employed types of urethroplasty involve construction of a skin tube from the original orifice to the coronal margin or tip of the glans. Since hypospadias and chordee are universally associated with splaying of the glans and hooded redundant dorsal foreskin, the glans can be reconstituted in conjunction with the urethroplasty, and the redundant dorsal foreskin can be mobilized and brought ventrally for covering of any defect created. The operative complications of urethroplasties of all sorts include fistula and stricture, both of which may be managed by relatively minor secondary surgical procedures.

Epispadias

Failure of development of the anterior wall of the urethra and concomitant failure of dorsal fusion of the penile corpora result in epispadias. Complete vesical exstrophy, a rare condition, is always accompanied by epispadias; epispadias alone with some degree of urinary continence is more commonly seen, perhaps as often as once in 30,000 live male births. The urethral opening may lie anywhere from the vesical neck to the glans, but if it is distal to the prostatic urethra, urinary continence and control may be satisfactory. The severe cosmetic deformity and the associated difficulty in controlling the urinary stream demand surgical correction, usually accomplished in infancy. Plastic reconstruction of the penis, closure and ventral

inversion of the urethra, and reconstruction of the bladder neck by the Young-Dees method is usually satisfactory. Unless there is complete failure of urinary control, urinary diversion is not necessary. While early repair is desirable, the child is usually better able to cooperate in achieving urinary control after the age of 3 years.

TRAUMA

Traumatic injury of the urethra most commonly occurs in association with pelvic fracture. Shearing injuries induced by external force cause rupture at the urogenital diaphragm in the region of the membranous urethra. Urinary extravasation is noted, often with extensive pelvic hemorrhage. The prostate and bladder may be displaced superiorly, well away from the distal urethra. Catheterization is impossible in such circumstances, and open surgical repair or suprapubic urinary diversion should be accomplished promptly, though primary perineal reconstruction may be most advantageous in some circumstances. The diagnosis of urethral rupture must be suspected in every instance of pelvic injury and unless the patient is able to void clear urine in a normal fashion, catheterization may be undertaken in an aseptic fashion to determine the patency and competence of the urethra. If the attempt at catheterization is unsuccessful, urethrograms may establish a diagnosis. Untreated urethral rupture, whether partial or complete, can result in urethral stricture and possible urinary incontinence. Penetrating injuries of the urethra are also observed, most commonly due to gunshot wound or stab wound. Immediate urethral reconstruction and urinary diversion by suprapubic cystotomy are advocated. Simi-

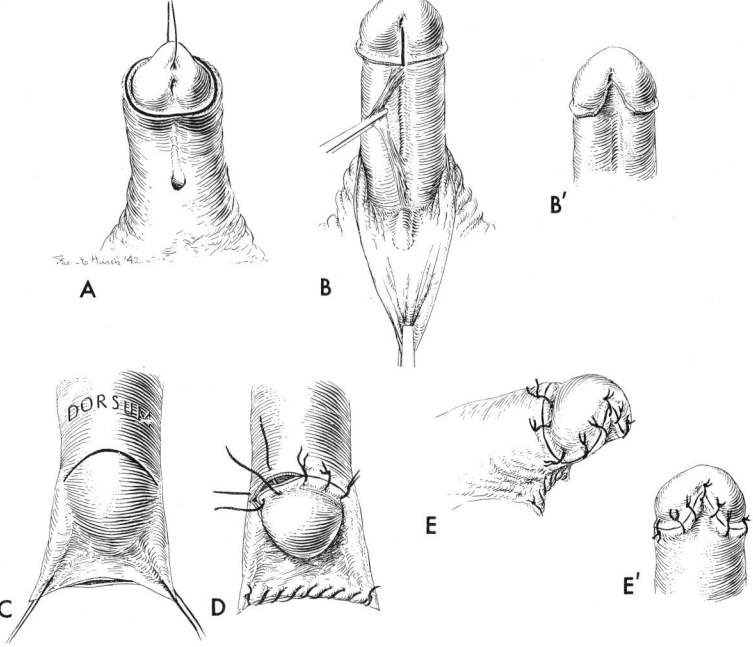

Figure 14. Nesbit technique of release of chordee, excising the fibrous band with transposition of dorsal foreskin to ventral surface of penile shaft. (From Creevy, C. D. In Glenn, J. F., and Boyce, W. H.: Urologic Surgery, 2nd ed. Hagerstown, Md., Harper & Row, 1975.)

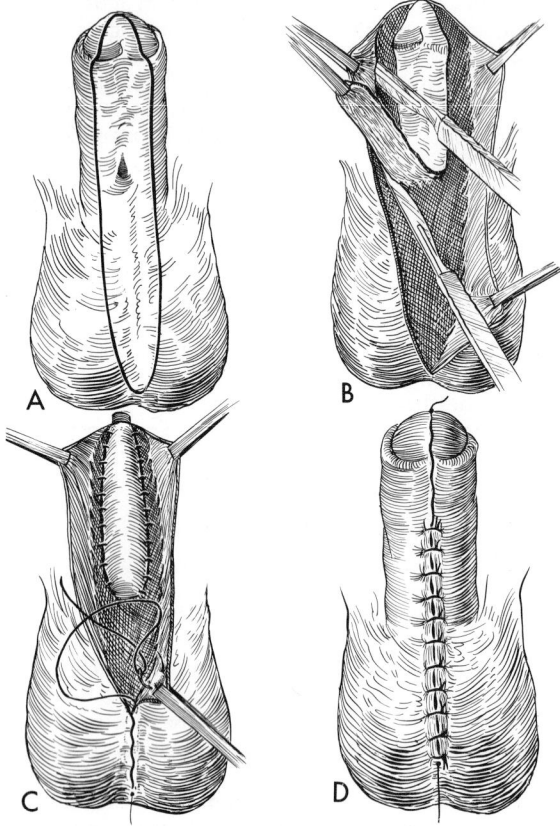

Figure 15. One technique for urethral reconstruction in hypospadias, this method the Crabtree urethroplasty, a similar procedure having been employed by Horton and Devine. (From Creevy, C. D. *In* Glenn, J. F., and Boyce, W. H.: Urologic Surgery, 2nd ed. Hagerstown, Md., Harper & Row, 1975.)

larly, straddle injuries to the perineum may cause urethral rupture, which usually demands prompt surgical intervention or prolonged catheter stenting of the urethra. Iatrogenic perforation or rupture of the urethra may occur in the course of instrumentation, cystoscopy, or urethral dilation. Pre-existing urethral strictures due to trauma or gonococcal urethritis predispose to difficult instrumentation and potential perforation of the urethra, often followed by the establishment of urethral diverticulum or false urinary passage. Periurethral abscess and attendant complications may ensue unless urethral injury of this sort is recognized. In instances of iatrogenic injury, suprapubic cystotomy for catheter drainage should be initiated along with the usual conservative supportive measures.

INFECTIONS

The urethra is subject to both gonococcal and nonspecific infections. Congenital abnormalities of the urethra such as stricture of stenosis, acquired strictures of the urethra of any cause, urethral diverticulum, or any other structural abnormality will predis-

pose to development of urethritis and will complicate management. Associated anatomic abnormalities should be treated surgically to effect maximal control of urethral infections.

Acute gonococcal urethritis results when gonococci are introduced into the urethra, finding an appropriate milieu in the relatively hypoxic recesses of the periurethral glands that invest the bulbous and penile portions of the urethra. Characteristic symptoms of gonococcal urethritis include burning on urination, frequency of urination, and a urethral discharge that is usually creamy white in character, exhibiting the typical gram-negative diplococci on the stained smear. Anaerobic culture of the urethral discharge will confirm the diagnosis. Treatment of acute gonococcal urethritis is with penicillin, ampicillin, or relatively large doses of the tetracyclines. Secondary associated gram-negative infections may demand employment of adjunctive antibiotic therapy. Untreated acute gonococcal urethritis may lead to urethral stricture through the mechanism of fibrosis and cicatrix formation, and such gonococcal strictures then dispose to the establishment of posterior urethritis and prostatitis that are refractory to usual methods of management. Gonococcal stricture may be treated by urethral dilation periodically until the stricture is relieved, or by internal urethrotomy with the Otis urethrotome or a similar instrument, with stenting of the urethra for a period of several weeks with an inlying catheter to prevent recurrence of the stenotic area.

The term nonspecific urethritis refers to those infections in which no evidence of gonorrhea can be found. Nonspecific urethritis may be due to bacterial infection or to viral infection. The typical complaint of the patient with nonspecific urethritis is of a clear viscid urethral discharge, particularly in the early morning, associated with some degree of urinary frequency and burning discomfort on urination. Prostatitis may or may not accompany the urethritis. Treatment is usually with one of the tetracyclines.

URETHRAL MALIGNANT DISEASE

Carcinoma of the male urethra is rare, only several hundred cases having been documented in the English literature.[15] Those malignant lesions occurring in the distal penile portion of the urethra are most often squamous cell carcinoma, while the more proximal tumors are transitional cell lesions. Symptoms of urethral malignant disease are hematuria, dysuria, stranguria, frequency, and ultimate urinary retention. The diagnosis is established by endoscopic visualization of the lesion and appropriate biopsy, either cystoscopically or by urethrotomy and excision under direct vision. Spread of malignancy is via lymphatics of the corpus spongiosum into the deep pelvic nodes and by venous channels. Since the diagnosis is usually established late in the course of the disease, the prognosis is poor despite radical surgical intervention. Depending upon the location of the lesion, partial urethrectomy with or without penectomy may be effective. Radiation therapy and chemotherapeutic measures are unproven as effective therapeutic modalities.

It is interesting that a high percentage of patients with carcinoma of the urethra give a history of previous venereal disease or urethral stricture.

SCROTUM

The loose skin of the scrotal sac is peculiarly adapted to house the testes, epididymides, and spermatic cords. Spermatogenesis is dependent upon critical temperature regulation and requires temperature several degrees lower than that within the abdominal cavity. Contraction of the dartos in response to cold provides added insulation for the testis, while relaxation in warm weather permits cooling to a temperature 5° to 8° lower than that within the abdomen, an optimal condition for spermatogenesis. The spermatic cords are supplied by the cremaster muscle, which contracts and relaxes in coordination with the dartos muscle.

Most common anomalies of the scrotum are associated with other developmental abnormalities such as absence of a testis or cryptorchism, in which case one compartment of the scrotum may fail to develop, a condition termed hemiabsence of the scrotum. In conjunction with complete perineal hypospadias, the scrotum may be bifid as a consequence of failure of fusion of the two compartments in the midline. Rarely, partial or complete penoscrotal transposition may be observed, all or a part of the scrotum fusing anteriorly and superior to the penis; surgical correction of penoscrotal transposition is neither complicated nor difficult and should be accomplished at an early age.

While the scrotal contents are delicate and subject to damage by even minimal trauma, the scrotum itself is not often severely injured. Blunt blows and penetrating injuries may, however, involve the scrotum, and hematomas may develop readily, since scrotal skin is rather loose and provides little hemostatic pressure effect. Partial or complete avulsion of the scrotal skin may result from injury by various types of agricultural and industrial machinery with power belt apparatus, clothing usually becoming enmeshed in the power drive with resultant tearing and avulsion of the loose skin of the genitalia. If any scrotal skin remains, the testes may be recovered. Frequently, all scrotal skin is avulsed and it is necessary to bury the testes and cords in the loose subcutaneous tissues of the inner aspect of each thigh. Penetrating and perforating injuries of the scrotum should be treated vigorously, since infection may lead to gangrene and slough.

Infections of the scrotum are usually secondary to infection of the testicles or its appendages or to urinary infection with fistula formation as seen with severe urethral stricture. Extravasation of urine may lead to extensive scrotal cellulitis and multiple fistulas through the scrotum and surrounding areas, the so-called "watering-pot perineum." The scrotum so involved is best treated by multiple incisions for drainage, with the use of many rubber wicks. Urinary diversion is mandatory, and a suprapubic cystotomy is preferable to an inlying urethral catheter. Scrotal gangrene may result from such infection, but may also be caused by mechanical, chemical, or thermal injury, and is treated by appropriate antibiotic therapy, surgical drainage, and hyperbaric oxygenation.

Localized scrotal swelling may be caused by edema associated with cardiac failure, renal disease, blood dyscrasias, ascites, or abdominal neoplasms that interfere with venous and lymphatic return from the scrotum. Similarly, large inguinal hernias may sometimes embarrass venous and lymphatic return, predisposing to edema formation. Simple edema must be differentiated from elephantiasis, classically caused by the filariae, *Wuchereria bancrofti,* and usually associated

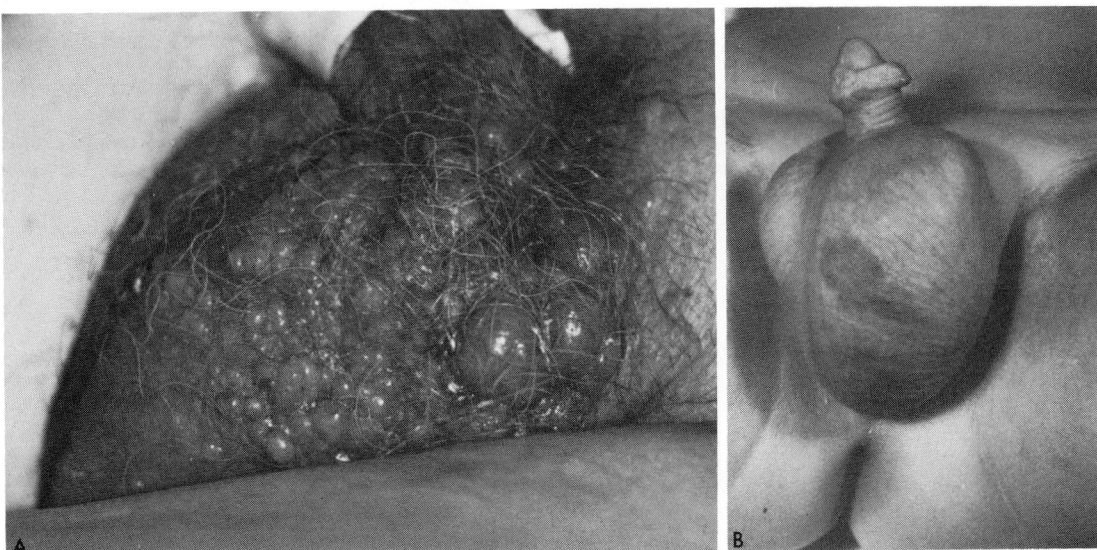

Figure 16. Unusual lesions of the scrotum include *(A)* nodular metastatic cutaneous implants of prostatic carcinoma, and *(B)* hemangioendothelioma of the scrotum.

with elephantiasis of the lower extremities. Idiopathic elephantiasis, Milroy's disease, may also involve the scrotum. Finally, inguinal node dissections or inguinal radiation therapy, employed in treatment of metastatic malignant lesions of the penis or other organs, may cause severe chronic scrotal edema. Any of these conditions of edema or elephantiasis may demand generous reduction scrotoplasty in order to effect mechanical improvement of the physical disability involved.

Tumors of the scrotum are uncommon, though benign neoplasms such as fibromas, adenomas, lipomas, and hemangiomas are occasionally seen. More commonly observed are multiple sebaceous cysts of the scrotum, sometimes demanding repeated surgical excision or incision and drainage when infection supervenes. Hemangioendothelioma of the scrotum may assume tremendous proportions and demand surgical removal. Carcinoma of the scrotal skin has been associated with prolonged exposure to chemical carcinogens and has been termed "chimney-sweeps' cancer" because of the association with that occupation; coal tar derivatives are liposoluble in the sebaceous glands of the scrotal skin. Treatment of scrotal malignant lesions requires wide local excision, sometimes associated with orchiectomy, and inguinal lymphadenectomy; radiation and chemotherapeutic agents are relatively ineffective.

TESTES

The testes, suspended in the scrotal compartments by the spermatic cords, serve a dual function, producing spermatozoa and secreting male hormones, predominantly testosterone. Impairment of spermatogenesis may occur without affecting androgen production, while the secretion of male hormones may be compromised without significant interference with spermatogenesis.[40] Most often, the two functions of the testes may be compromised simultaneously, as with severe epididymo-orchitis or the atrophy seen after hernia repair with compromise of the vascular supply of the testis. Testicular blood supply is derived from the internal spermatic arteries, which arise from the aorta below the renal arteries and course down to the internal inguinal ring and then along the spermatic cord. Venous return is accomplished through the pampiniform plexus, which merges into a single spermatic vein on either side.

CONGENITAL ANOMALIES

The most common congenital anomalies of the testes relate to anomalous location, though congenital absence of one or both testes may be observed. The testes develop within the abdominal cavity, differentiating from the primitive gonadal ridge in the early weeks of fetal life. Normally, the testis begins its migration and descent through the inguinal canal at the end of the first trimester of gestation, but various mechanical and hormonal events may impede or alter normal descent. The gubernaculum, previously thought to provide a fibroelastic cord for guidance of the testis into

the scrotal compartment, probably adds little mechanical assistance in this process. It seems most likely that the inherent functions of the testis itself are primarily responsible for the necessary ductal differentiation and descent of the normal testis.

Anorchism

The classic experiments of Jost indicate that the primitive gonad must differentiate as a testis in order to produce androgens, which are the stimulus to normal male (wolffian) ductal development. In the complete absence of testes, female (müllerian) ductal development will differentiate in feminine configuration. However, one testis may fail to develop, frequently in association with ipsilateral agenesis of kidney and ureter; monorchism is seen most often on the right and is termed the "right-sided syndrome." Rare persons are seen who exhibit no evidence of viable testicular tissue, though the external genitalia are fully differentiated in masculine configuration. In these cases, internal male ductal structures, the vasa deferentia, can be identified, usually extending to the internal inguinal ring and terminating blindly in fibrous tissue. Such persons are apparently normal males, though with a completely empty scrotum; puberty is delayed and incomplete with persistent elevation of gonadotropin levels and inadequate plasma testosterone levels. It is postulated that such persons with complete anorchism did indeed have normal testes at an early stage of gestation, but that sometime after the sixteenth week of fetal life the testes atrophied, possibly because of mechanical torsion or other interference with testicular blood supply in the course of the descent. Surgical exploration is required to establish the diagnosis, and a gratifying therapeutic response to continuing exogenous testosterone therapy will be observed: sexual maturation, cessation of growth, increased libido, and masculine redistribution of body fat and muscle mass are concomitants to treatment.

Cryptorchism

The term cryptorchism, derived from the Greek *cryptos* or hidden, should be reserved for those testes which are truly obscure, usually within the abdominal cavity and not palpable on examination. Testes lying in the course of normal descent in the inguinal canal or in ectopic locations can usually be palpated and are not truly hidden. Cryptorchid or intra-abdominal testes are observed unilaterally or bilaterally in 1 to 10 per cent of male infants. Again, the cause of cryptorchism is obscure, but a selective hormonal deficiency of the testis is suspected as a factor in such failure of descent. Occasionally, a truly cryptorchid testis will descend spontaneously at puberty or in response to parenteral chorionic gonadotropin therapy, but this is not the rule and surgical exploration with orchidopexy generally is required. The cryptorchid abdominal testis will fail in its spermatogenic function, though it may secrete adequate amounts of androgens. Spermatogenic failure is progressive, and transposition of an intra-abdominal testis to the scrotum should be accomplished before the age of 5 years to insure production of normal quantity and quality of spermatozoa. In cases of unilateral cryptorchism, the matter of surgical exploration is less critical, but in bilateral cryptorchism early surgical intervention is necessary. Exploration may be accomplished through an extraperitoneal inguinal incision, but more adequate exposure is obtained through an abdominal approach, particularly if bilateral cryptorchism exists. Cryptorchid testes are usually found retroperitoneally deep within the pelvis and in proximity to the internal inguinal ring, but may be located almost anywhere within the lower abdomen, even up in the renal fossa. It is necessary to isolate the testis with its vas and vessels, mobilizing these structures completely.[30] When the spermatic artery is short, it may be possible to bring the testis through the abdominal wall at Hesselbach's triangle, rather than through the inguinal canal, which necessitates a more devious course. Finally, since the testis may derive some blood supply from the small vessels coursing along the vas deferens, it may be feasible to divide the spermatic vessels and depend upon this collateral blood supply, permitting scrotal placement of the testis. When it is impossible to bring the testis to a palpable location within the scrotum or low in the inguinal canal, it is generally thought best to remove the testis, since there is a very high incidence of carcinoma in abdominal testes, the incidence perhaps being as much as 20 times greater than that of carcinoma in a normally descended testis. When cryptorchism is diagnosed after the age of 10 or 12 years, orchiectomy may be the preferred treatment, since such testes will rarely exhibit normal function despite adequate scrotal placement.[22]

Incomplete Descent

Incomplete descent or maldescent of the testis is the term reserved for those cases in which the testis is arrested at some point in its normal course of descent and is palpable on careful examination. The usual sites of arrest are at the internal inguinal ring, within the inguinal canal, or at the external ring. Most often, there is an associated congenital indirect inguinal hernia, since the processus vaginalis has not been obliterated at its proximal extent; there is potential for inguinal hernia, and the accumulation of normal peritoneal fluid dependently within the processus vaginalis produces communicating hydrocele. Since function of a testis in the inguinal region is less compromised than that of the abdominal cryptorchid testis, treatment may depend on other associated factors. The presence of overt hernia prompts earlier surgical correction, and bilateral maldescent constitutes cause for earlier surgical intervention. Some authorities recommend the use of chorionic gonadotropin in dosage of up to 2000 units twice weekly for 6 weeks as a stimulus to testicular descent, but in the truly arrested testis, such treatment is generally ineffective. Further, prolonged chorionic gonadotropin therapy may lead to premature pubescence and growth arrest. A brief course of chorionic gonadotropin therapy may, however, be employed in preparation before orchidopexy and herniorrhaphy, since such stimulation may improve the vascular supply and augment the potential of surgical success. Exploration is accomplished through a high inguinal incision, exposing the entire cord to the internal inguinal ring. The testis and cord are completely freed from the surrounding structures; the patent processus vaginalis is identified, opened, stripped from the cord, and excised, so that the neck of the peritoneal sac is closed; and the spermatic vessels are carefully dissected extraperitoneally in order to afford maximal cord length. The testis is then positioned in the scrotum and fixed with an external traction suture of heavy silk (Bevan technique) or attached to the fascia of the inner thigh, later to be released at a second operation (Torek procedure).

Hypermobile Testis

In many young males thought to be cryptorchid, the testis or testes are merely highly mobile, retracting into the inguinal canal in an inaccessible position owing to hyperactivity of the cremaster muscle. The simplest means of evaluation is to have the patient sit in a tub of hot water for up to 15 minutes; hypermobile testes will descend into the scrotum and will be normally palpable under such conditions. At puberty, hypermobile testes tend to situate normally within the scrotum, there is rarely any associated hernia, and surgery can be avoided.

Ectopic Testis

Occasionally, one or both testes may undergo vicarious excursion in the course of descent, coming to lodge in ectopic positions. The exact cause of such wandering ectopia is obscure, but must relate to mechanical factors. Favorite sites of testicular ectopia are symphyseal, prepubic, femoral, crural, penile, or perineal positions. Surgical correction should be accomplished for cosmetic reasons as well as to insure normal testicular function and patient comfort.

TRAUMA

Surprisingly, the testes are relatively protected against trauma despite their external position. The primitive cremasteric reflex constitutes a part of the "fight or flight" mechanism, and the testes are retracted to a protected inguinal position under extreme stress. Even in instances of avulsion of skin of the genitalia, the testes, appendages, and cords are usually undisturbed, remaining inviolate within their fascial coverings. Blunt external trauma may result in testicular hemorrhage and infarction, usually requiring surgical intervention. Penetrating wounds should be treated by surgical exploration and may be quite bizarre in character; rotary lawn mowers have been known to sweep up coat hangers, wires, and nails that impale the testes in shish-kebab fashion. Torsion of the spermatic cord may occur as a result of external trauma, compromising blood supply and threatening viability of the testis, but such torsion is usually of spontaneous variety. Surgical intervention in instances of testicular trauma should be accomplished promptly, since the risk of surgery is minimal and early surgical repair can prevent subsequent infarction, atrophy, and loss of testicular function.

INFECTIONS

Pyogenic infections of the testis are almost always secondary to spread of infection through the male ductal system, the vas deferens, and epididymis. Chronic urinary tract infection, particularly suppurative prostatitis and seminal vesiculitis, predisposes to the spread of bacteria via the vas into the epididymis and the testis. It is rare to observe pyogenic orchitis without associated epididymitis, while epididymitis may occur with virtually no involvement of the associated testis. In rare instances, systemic bacteremia may result in embolic metastatic foci of infection within the testis.

Orchitis may result from viral infection in association with mumps, usually not until after the patient has reached pubescence. Mumps orchitis produces severe local inflammatory reactions with excess accumulation of fluid within the compartment of the tunica vaginalis, the acute hydrocele of mumps. Supportive treatment is generally indicated, and aspiration of the hydrocele is usually avoided, since there is a risk of introducing bacteria and initiating a secondary infection that can result in testicular atrophy. Mechanical support to the scrotum with an adhesive bridge, bed rest, analgesics, and antipyretics constitute the first line of treatment. Smallpox, varicella, measles, influenza, and other similar infections may occasionally induce a secondary orchitis.

Tuberculous orchitis is almost always secondary to tuberculous epididymitis, the primary focus within the urinary tract generally being within the kidneys, sometimes in the prostate. Genitourinary tuberculosis of all sorts is responsive to intensive antituberculous medical management, and surgery is reserved for advanced cases of localized tuberculosis; epididymectomy, vasectomy, or epididymo-orchiectomy may be required in some cases. Syphilitic gummas may occur within the testis, and surgical removal is almost always required, since chronic draining fistulas are the rule. Fungus infections such as blastomycosis and actinomycosis of the testis are rarely observed but usually necessitate orchiectomy and continuing medical management.

The patient with an acute testicular infection is quick to appear for examination and treatment, since the condition is exquisitely painful. On physical examination, a swollen and tender testis may be observed, usually in conjunction with epididymal induration. There is increased local heat and an acute inflammatory hydrocele may be associated. Orchitis must be differentiated from testicular tumor with hemorrhage and from torsion of the spermatic cord, both conditions demanding immediate surgical intervention.

INFERTILITY

The inability of a couple to produce offspring is termed infertility or sterility. It is estimated that up to 10 per cent of marriages in this country are initially barren, approximately half of this number responding to various therapeutic measures.[2] Infertility may be attributed to the male in as many as 50 per cent of these barren marriages. Adequate evaluation of the marital unit for sterility demands assessment of the male partner and thorough evaluation of the possible factors involved. Infertility and sterility should not be confused with impotence, the latter term applied to the inability to achieve or sustain satisfactory erection for sexual intercourse.

The principal cause of male infertility is a spermatogenic defect, estimated to account for 95 per cent of cases of male infertility or sterility. Most males with such spermatogenic defects will produce sperm in some quantity, though there are usually diminished numbers of sperm and those produced are of inadequate quality, exhibiting malformations and diminished motility. Oligospermia, by definition, indicates a sperm count of less than 20 million per milliliter, and under such conditions fertility can rarely be expected. The principal causes of defective spermatogenesis include congenital inadequacy of the seminiferous tubules; testicular damage as a consequence of pyogenic infection, mumps orchitis, trauma, or infarction; Klinefelter's syndrome; hormonal defects as in hypopituitarism; and cryptorchism. Other causes of oligospermia may relate to transport of spermatozoa. Chronic prostatitis and seminal vesiculitis may result in fibrosis that impedes transport and delivery of sperm. Infection spreading into the vasa deferentia may induce fibrosis and stricture, even to the point of total occlusion of one or both vasa. Tuberculosis affecting the genitourinary system may induce similar inflammatory changes with obstruction to the conductive mechanism. Chronic suppurative prostatitis, particularly with coliform organisms, may result in impedance of sperm motility, an apparent absolute effect as demonstrated by Teague and associates. Abnormal fructose metabolism in the seminal vesicle may predispose to inadequate storage capacity and diminished numbers of spermatozoa available for fertilization.

Azoospermia, complete absence of spermatozoa in the ejaculate, may be the result of total occlusion of the sperm transport system, vasa, seminal vesicles, or ejaculatory ducts. Congenital absence of the vas and seminal vesicles may occur as an isolated anatomic defect, and congenital absence of the vasa is the rule in males with cystic fibrosis. Gonococcal epididymitis and vasitis may cause complete stenosis and azoospermia. Trauma to the vasa in the course of inguinal hernia repair or orchidopexy may result in complete obstruction. Finally, previous bilateral vasectomy, accomplished for elective sterilization or medical purposes, will quite naturally result in azoospermia.

In some instances, infertility may be due to mechanical factors with no defects in spermatogenesis or delivery of spermatozoa. Surgery of the vesical neck, particularly transurethral resection, open wedge resection, or plastic reconstruction and treatment of congenital contracture may result in an inability of the vesical neck to close with ejaculation, causing the ejaculate to be passed in retrograde fashion into the bladder rather than out through the urethra. Cystoscopic evaluation is helpful in identifying such causes of infertility.

Physical evaluation of the infertile male should include a careful and painstaking examination of the genitalia, particularly to assure that the testes are of normal size and consistency, that the epididymides and vasa are present and normal, and that there is no evidence of chronic inflammatory disease of the external genitalia. Prostatitis should be ruled out by digital examination, prostatic massage, and smear of prostatic fluid. Appropriate cultures will constitute the basis for antibiotic therapy, sometimes effective in alleviating chronic infection as a cause of infertility. Cystourethroscopic examination and radiographic studies including vasograms, accomplished by catheterization of the ejaculatory ducts or direct injection of the vasa, will help to rule out obstructive phenomena in the transport system.

Specimens of ejaculate should be examined for numbers and quality of spermatozoa. The ejaculate may be collected by masturbation technique or at the time of intercourse with a condom. The specimen should be examined within 2 to 3 hours after collection. The normal volume ranges up to 5 ml.

with an average of 3.5 ml. Fifty to 100 million spermatozoa per milliliter constitutes a normal count, and approximately 60 per cent of these spermatozoa will exhibit good motility and normal adult forms. When azoospermia exists or when there is an inadequacy of the ejaculate, testicular biopsy may be indicated, accomplished by the techniques described by Heller and Nelson. Identification of normal architecture of the seminiferous tubules and normal spermatogenesis strongly suggest the probability that obstructive or inflammatory phenomena are being overlooked, while inadequacy of the spermatogenic elements suggests congenital or hormonal deficits.[38]

In cases of mechanical obstruction such as previous vasectomy, vasovasostomy may be highly effective. Inflammatory lesions of the vasa and epididymides may be corrected by epididymovasostomy. Little can be done to stimulate spermatogenesis, though administration of thyroid preparations has been advocated and may on rare occasions improve the numbers and quality of sperm. Occasionally, chronic administration of testosterone may result in the rebound phenomenon, an increase in numbers of spermatozoa following discontinuation of testosterone. Gonadotropins are of little therapeutic value. Orchidopexy cannot be expected to improve spermatogenesis if the patient is beyond the age of 10 or 12 years. Most recently, varicocelectomy has been advocated in treatment of oligospermia. It is suggested that varicocele causes defective spermatogenesis on the basis of increased intrascrotal temperature and possible backflow of inhibiting adrenal hormones that reflux from the adrenal and renal veins down the left spermatic vein. High inguinal ligation of the left spermatic vein occasionally may result in an increased sperm count and often results in improved sperm motility, according to MacLeod, and impregnation rates as high as 44 per cent have been reported for patients undergoing such surgical treatment of varicocele when infertility is a problem.

TESTICULAR TUMORS

Neoplasms of the testis itself are almost universally malignant; only those rare fibromas of the tunica vaginalis constitute the benign tumors of the testis.[26] In contrast, extratesticular tumors within the scrotum are almost always benign, such as the adenomatoid tumors of the epididymis and cord. Because of this sharp distinction in the potential of neoplasms within the scrotum, diligent physical examination is necessary in distinguishing the site of origin of a scrotal mass. Malignant neoplasms of the testes may be of germinal or nongerminal origin, the latter tumors arising from the interstitial cells and known as interstitial cell tumors, Leydig cell tumors, or androblastomas. These are relatively rare tumors, producing excessive quantities of androgenizing hormones, which may cause virilism and precocious puberty in young males, impotence and gynecomastia in adults, and feminizing changes in the male that are analogous to those alterations observed with ovarian arrhenoblastomas in the female. Interstitial cell tumors of the testis must be differentiated from adrenal rest tumors, cells of adrenal origin being of very similar histologic character. It has been suggested that many cases of testicular tumors identified as interstitial cell neoplasms may indeed have represented unrecognized rests of hyperplastic adrenal tissue. The malignant germinal tumors of the testis arise from the totipoten-

tial cells of the seminiferous tubules and constitute a serious threat to the male population, accounting for 2 per cent of all malignant tumors, the dominant cause of death from genitourinary malignant disease in the younger adult male population. Testicular tumors are seen at all ages, but predominate in persons between the ages of 20 and 35 years. Germinal testicular tumors are categorized according to degree of cellular differentiation, which parallels malignant potential.

Seminoma

The most common of testicular malignant lesions, accounting for 35 to 50 per cent of germinal tumors, seminomas are uniform in gross and histologic appearance, characterized by slow growth and late invasion. Metastases spread via the testicular lymphatics and dominate in the iliac, aortic, and renal hilar nodes. Because of the relatively slow growth of these tumors, they may be appreciated and removed surgically prior to the development of metastases. Metastatic seminoma is responsive to radiation therapy, with 5-year survival rates in the range of 90 per cent.

Embryonal Carcinoma

Of somewhat more malignant potential, embryonal carcinoma may also be seen in the younger age group and is usually thought to be the most common testicular tumor of childhood. The histologic pattern of embryonal carcinoma is of a less differentiated form than that of seminoma, and invasion and metastases occur earlier in the course of the disease. Because of relatively rapid growth of the tumor, hemorrhage and necrosis are common. Metastases to the abdominal lymphatics and the lungs may occur as an early event.

Teratocarcinoma

Pure teratoma of the testis is relatively uncommon. Most such tumors are teratocarcinomas, embracing elements of seminoma, embryonal carcinoma, or choriocarcinoma. Tumors of the teratoma category may contain all types of tissue, and careful histologic evaluation of testicular teratocarcinoma must be accomplished, since the clinical behavior of the tumor will depend upon the most malignant element present. Prognosis of teratocarcinoma admixed with seminoma is much better than that of a teratocarcinoma with elements of embryonal or choriocarcinoma.

Choriocarcinoma

Fortunately, choriocarcinomas account for only a small number of the germinal cell tumors. The tumor is rapidly invasive, trophoblasts invading the venous system early in the course of the disease. Metastasis may be both blood-borne and via lymphatics, and has usually occurred by the time of diagnosis. Unlike choriocarcinoma in the female, which responds well to methotrexate, choriocarcinoma in the male is relatively unresponsive to chemotherapeutic measures. The prognosis is extremely poor, and the 5-year survival despite all combinations of surgical, radiation, and chemotherapeutic efforts is only about 1 per cent.

The earliest symptom of testicular tumor is a mass in the testicle, unfortunately unrecognized by most pa-

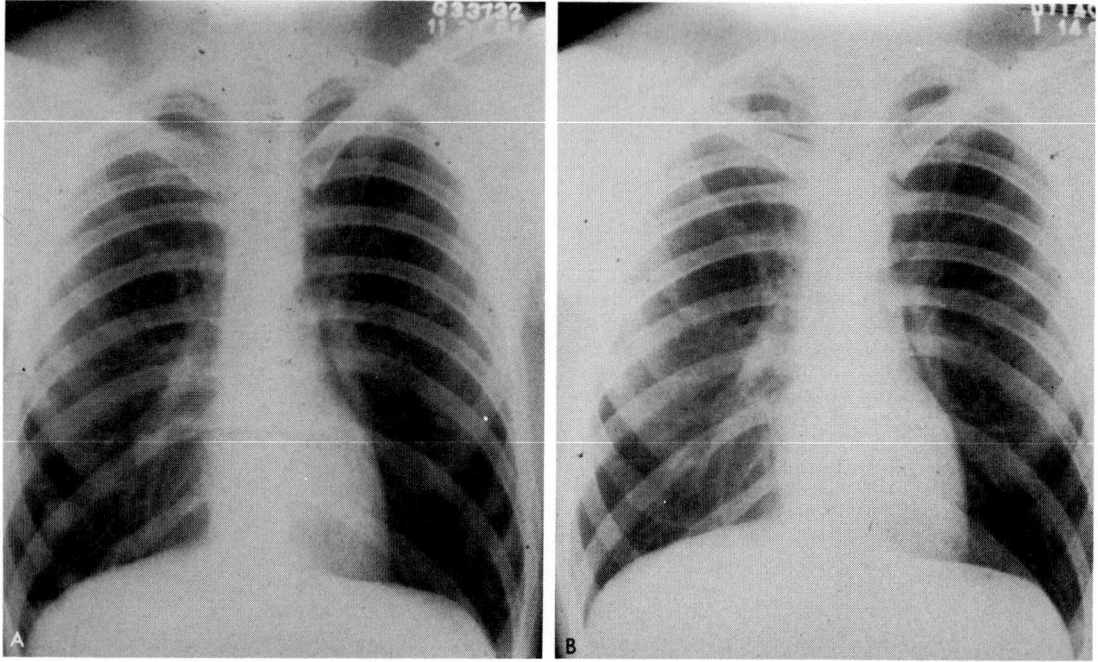

Figure 17. Metastatic testicular carcinoma, in this instance embryonal cell tumor, may manifest as pulmonary metastases *(A)* and may respond or resolve *(B)* as a consequence of intensive systemic chemotherapy. (Courtesy of Dr. John E. Dees.)

tients until there is associated pain, usually of a dull aching character. Hemorrhage within the testicle may follow minimal trauma, suggesting that traumatic injury is related to the tumor, which is probably not the case. Some of the more malignant tumors may produce hormones, measured as gonadotropins, which will induce gynecomastia. In other instances, the more malignant tumors, relatively small in the primary location, may induce an abdominal mass as an early manifestation of disease.

The successful treatment of testicular tumors demands scrupulous physical examination, a high index of suspicion, and the willingness to accomplish prompt scrotal exploration when the diagnosis is suggested. The typical testicular neoplasm is stony hard in character with a suggestion of weightiness on palpation. When the suspicion of testicular tumor is raised, extensive laboratory evaluation should be deferred and surgical exploration should be accomplished as a primary event. The approach is through a high inguinal incision, exposing the spermatic cord at its emergence from the internal inguinal ring where it is isolated. Rubber-shod clamps are applied and the testicle with its surrounding attachments can be mobilized for inspection and biopsy, and if diagnosis of testicular neoplasm is confirmed, high inguinal orchiectomy is accomplished, removing the entire cord with the involved testicle.

After orchiectomy, further diagnostic studies may be undertaken. Planograms of the chest may reveal pulmonary metastatic disease. Lymphangiograms, inferior vena cavagrams, and intravenous urograms

may give evidence of metastatic tumor. Gonadotropin levels may be assayed by 24 hour urine collection, elevations of gonadotropins being observed most commonly with choriocarcinoma, less frequently with embryonal or teratocarcinoma, and rarely if ever with pure seminoma. Bone survey may rule out skeletal metastases, a relatively uncommon event in most testicular tumors, the metastatic pattern being lymphatic and visceral.

Further treatment of testicular tumors following orchiectomy is dictated by the results of such evaluation and by the philosophy of the urologic surgeon. In most instances, it is felt that abdominal node dissection is of little value when pulmonary metastases have been demonstrated. Further, choriocarcinoma dictates against radical retroperitoneal node dissection, since its metastatic pattern is vascular in character. In other instances of testicular neoplasm, radical retroperitoneal node dissection, usually through a transabdominal approach and less commonly through bilateral thoracoabdominal exposures, is advocated as an effective modality in the control of the malignant process. Since metastatic seminoma is highly radiosensitive, many authorities question node dissection in treatment of seminoma. However, it must be pointed out that any seminoma may contain a microscopic focus of a more malignant germinal element and that metastases may reflect embryonal carcinoma, teratocarcinoma, or even choriocarcinoma that will not respond so favorably to radiation therapy. Finally, empiric radiation therapy of the abdominal and mediastinal lymphatic regions should not be condoned unless there is known metastatic disease, proven only by surgical exploration.

Because of these considerations, it is the usual practice to accomplish transabdominal radical peritoneal lymph node dissections in all instances of testicular tumor except choriocarcinoma and except when generalized metastatic disease is recognized. The efficacy of surgical node dissection has been elaborated by Staubitz and others, irrespective of ancillary radiation therapy or chemotherapy.[37] When node dissection is accomplished and there is no histologic evidence of metastatic disease, no further treatment is given. Survivals in this group of patients, irrespective of the histologic classification of the primary tumor, are extremely good. On the other hand, when positive nodes are identified or removed at surgery, radiation therapy is advisable, treating the abdomen, mediastinum, and supraclavicular areas.

When lymphatic metastases of testicular tumors respond poorly to chemotherapeutic measures, some patients with visceral metastatic disease, particularly pulmonary metastases, may respond in dramatic fashion to chemotherapeutic efforts. The most effective antitumor drugs in treating metastatic embryonal carcinoma and teratocarcinoma include actinomycin D, methotrexate, and chlorambucil, which may result in regression and 5-year cure of metastatic testicular malignant lesions. Isolated pulmonary metastases may be treated by local radiation or by surgical resection. The ultimate prognosis in testicular malignant disease, a dire condition in the young male, thus depends upon the stage of the disease at diagnosis, the histologic character of the tumor, and the vigor with which therapeutic measures are pursued. Follow-up should extend over a minimum of 5 years with regular and periodic examination, urinary chorionic gonadotropin determinations, and other modalities of evalua-

tion, in the hope of identifying recurrence of disease and initiating appropriate therapeutic measures.

EPIDIDYMIDES

The epididymides are coiled ductal structures posterolateral to the testes, with which they communicate through the rete testis, collecting spermatozoa for maturation and transport up the vasa deferentia. The upper end of the epididymis, globus major or head, accumulates sperm that are relatively immotile, sperm becoming more motile as they pass through the body and tail, globus minor, of the epididymis, which communicates with the vas. The most common abnormalities of the epididymis are inflammatory in character. Rarely, congenital absence of the epididymis and vas may be observed, though such absence is usually associated with unilateral anorchism. Occasionally, there may be a defect in fusion of the epididymis and the testis. Traumatic injuries of the epididymis are not of great clinical importance but accompany testicular injuries. Infectious epididymitis is common, particularly after puberty, but is relatively rare in the prepubescent male.

Acute nonspecific epididymitis is nongonococcal and nontuberculous, secondary to suppurative infection which usually has its origin in the prostate and seminal vesicles, spreading in retrograde fashion to the epididymis. Hematogenous and lymphatic spread of infection from a distant focus may occur but is probably quite rare. The inflammation is diffuse through the epididymis and may or may not involve the testicle concomitantly. The patient complains of severe pain and acute swelling with chills and fever and other systemic symptoms that may include headache, nausea, and vomiting. Symptoms of urinary infection such as frequency, urgency, burning dysuria, pyuria, and hema-

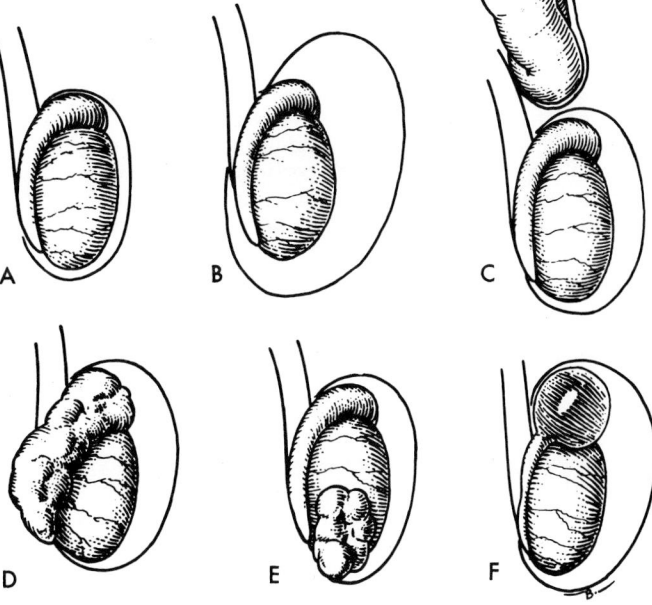

Figure 18. Common scrotal masses can be differentiated with knowledge of normal anatomy *(A)*, as compared with *(B)* hydrocele of the tunica vaginalis, *(C)* inguinal hernia penetrating the scrotal compartment, *(D)* epididymitis causing induration and enlargement of the epididymis but not the testis, *(E)* testicular tumor causing an irregular mass intrinsic to the testis, and *(F)* spermatocele or epididymal cyst arising extrinsic to the testis.

turia may be present. The epididymis and surrounding structures including the spermatic cord may be thickened by edema, swollen, and exquisitely tender to palpation. It is important to differentiate testicular swelling from epididymitis, since a mass in the testicle almost always indicates testicular tumor, and to differentiate acute epididymitis from torsion of the spermatic cord, in which the testicle generally lies high in the scrotum or even in the inguinal canal; torsion demands immediate surgical exploration, while epididymitis is treated by conservative measures. Other conditions that may confuse the diagnosis include inguinal hernia and acute hydrocele. Treatment of epididymitis consists of bed rest, elevation and support of the scrotum, application of cold packs, antipyretics, and appropriate antimicrobial agents, sometimes administered intravenously. Occasionally, suppurative epididymitis may localize into an abscess and drain spontaneously, but surgical intervention should be avoided in most instances. Acute epididymitis usually proceeds to some degree of chronic epididymitis, continuing over a period of several weeks. In past years, acute epididymitis was a common concomitant of all forms of prostatic surgery. However, utilization of routine preoperative vas ligation is extremely effective in preventing such epididymal infection, and the utilization of broad-spectrum antibiotics further diminishes the propensity for such disabling infection.

Chronic epididymitis is usually the sequel of acute epididymitis but may arise insidiously with few localizing symptoms except mass and slight tenderness. The demonstration of associated prostatic infection is an adjunct to differential diagnosis, but tumor must always be suspected when there is a relatively painless chronic enlargement of the epididymis. The most common neoplasms of the epididymis are benign and include adenomatoid tumors, leiomyomas, and cysts. Spermatocele is a diverticulum of the epididymis, containing cloudy fluid with spermatozoa, unilocular or multilocular, often confused with hydrocele since both spermatocele and hydrocele can be transilluminated. The differential diagnosis of spermatocele and hydrocele is aided by localization of the mass: hydrocele generally surrounds the testis, while spermatocele is more eccentric in location.

Other epididymal abnormalities are less common. Gonococcal epididymitis, once seen with relative frequency, is less common now, though gonorrhea continues to exist in epidemic proportion. It is probable that earlier treatment of gonorrheal urethritis diminishes the tendency to development of subsequent gonococcal prostatitis, seminal vesiculitis, vasitis, and epididymitis. Similarly, tuberculous epididymitis is rare today. Tuberculous epididymitis results in indurated asymmetric enlargement of the epididymis with nodular thickening and relatively little tenderness. Caseation necrosis may ensue, sometimes involving the scrotal wall and skin with ulceration and fistula formation. In such cases, epididymo-orchiectomy with excision of the involved portion of the scrotal wall is usually necessary. Other granulomatous reactions in the epididymis may be observed in association with syphilis or as a consequence of escape of spermatozoa with development of sperm granuloma, sometimes painful and requiring excision of the mass.

SPERMATIC CORDS AND TUNICS

The spermatic cord, composed of vas deferens, spermatic artery, venous plexus, lymphatics, autonomic nerves, and investments of cremaster muscle, terminates in the testis, which is covered by the fibrous tunics, the tunica albuginea testis, which is the capsule of the testicle, and the tunica vaginalis, which constitutes a sac partially surrounding the testis and epididymis. The entire spermatic cord is subject to inflammatory diseases, usually the result of trauma or pyogenic bacteria, termed funiculitis. The principal abnormality of the cord is torsion. Neoplasms of the spermatic cord are extremely rare, but sarcoma, usually rhabdomyosarcoma, and both invasive and metastatic malignant lesions from other structures may involve the cord. Benign tumors of the cord include adenomatoid tumor, lipoma, fibroma, and cysts, particularly hydrocele of the cord, a remnant of the processus vaginalis.

TORSION

Torsion of the spermatic cord, an axial rotation, is probably the result of an abnormally high attachment of the tunica vaginalis around the terminal cord, allowing the testicle to twist freely within the compartment, the so-called "bell clapper" deformity. When rotation of the testicle on the end of the cord exceeds 90 degrees, there may be compromise of blood supply, which causes exquisite pain and results in gangrene and subsequent atrophy of the testicle unless torsion is treated immediately. Incomplete torsion may result in partial strangulation, effects of which may be overcome if surgical intervention is accomplished within about 12 hours, whereas severe torsion with total compromise of blood supply will result in loss of the testes unless surgery is effected within about 4 hours.

Torsion is usually seen in young males and most often occurs spontaneously, even during sleep. Physical and sexual activity may predispose to torsion and aggravate it by contraction of the cremaster muscle. There is rapid onset of severe pain and swelling accompanied by nausea, vomiting, abdominal pain, and

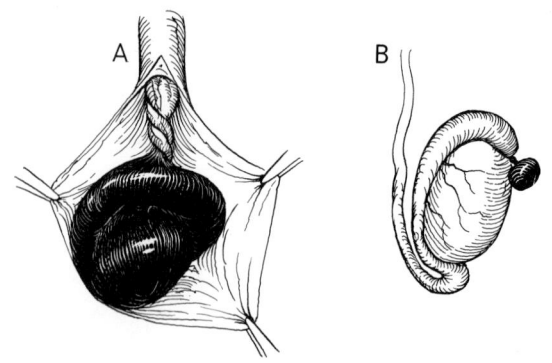

Figure 19. Torsion of the testis *(A)* is a result of twisting of the spermatic cord, usually within the tunica vaginalis; the appendix testis may also become twisted *(B)*.

even fever. On examination, the testicles seem to ride rather high in the scrotal compartment. The differential diagnosis is between torsion and epididymitis, and it should be remembered that epididymitis is almost always accompanied by evidence of prostatitis and pyuria. With torsion, the entire testicle and appendages are involved in the swelling process, while with epididymitis the prominent induration is within the epididymides and not the testes.

Torsion must always be suspected with acute onset of scrotal pain, and prompt surgical intervention is necessary.[19] In 17 of 19 patients with torsion operated upon the day of onset of symptoms, viable testes were salvaged. Any delay in surgery will diminish the prospects for salvage. When torsion is treated on one side, the contralateral scrotum should be explored; the tunica vaginalis should be opened and inverted around the testis as with hydrocele repair, and steps should be taken to surgically correct any additional defects such as deficit attachment of the epididymis to the testes.

The appendix epididymis and the appendix testis (hydatid of Morgagni) are vestigial remnants of ducts attached to the head of the epididymis and to the superior pole of the testes, respectively. These small cystic structures may become twisted, producing acute and severe pain with generalized scrotal edema. Little permanent damage or disability is incurred by torsion of these appendages, but because of diagnostic confusion, it is generally advisable to explore the scrotum when any doubt exists.

INFECTION

Infection of the spermatic cord is relatively uncommon as an isolated process, usually being an associated complication of epididymitis and prostatitis. However, isolated inflammation of the vas may occur, and the entire spermatic cord may become inflamed. Because of the rich blood supply and ample lymphatic drainage, funiculitis will generally resolve with no permanent abnormality. Vasitis may proceed to chronic inflammatory and fibrotic reaction with beading of the vas, a particularly common complication of genitourinary tuberculosis.

VAS DEFERENS

The vasa deferentia are the conduits for spermatozoa from epididymis to seminal vesicles and prostate. Thus, normal vasa are necessary to human reproduction. Since a single testis is capable of producing sufficient numbers of sperm for purposes of fertility, a single normal intact vas is all that is necessary to insure the reproductive capacity of the male. The most common anomaly of the vas is congenital absence, seen almost universally in males with cystic fibrosis. There are other isolated incidences of unilateral ductal failure with absence of the vas deferens.

While the vas is responsible for transit of spermatozoa, it may also serve as a conduit for retrograde passage of bacteria and infection of the scrotal contents, such retrograde infection being the principal cause of epididymo-orchitis. The prevalence of epididymo-orchitis in association with prostatic obstruction and prostatic surgery has prompted the employment of prophylactic vasectomy for more than 40 years. Most urologists accomplish such vasectomy in the course of prostatic surgery, though preliminary vasectomy may also be advocated as an initial step prior to surgical management of prostatic obstruction.

Vasectomy is not a new procedure, though it is gaining increased public acceptance as an elective sterilization measure at the present time. It has been estimated that up to nearly 40,000 elective vasectomies were accomplished by American urologists for purposes of voluntary sterilization in 1967, and it may be projected that even greater numbers of such procedures are being accomplished today. As an outpatient procedure under local anesthesia, a 1 cm. incision is made over each vas, or a single midline incision may be employed. The vasa are isolated, ligated, and sometimes electrocoagulated, and a small section is removed between the points of ligation. It is desirable to isolate the divided ends of the vasa in different fascial planes to prevent spontaneous recanalization. It must be remembered that spermatozoa distal to the point of ligation and stored within the seminal vesicles and prostate remain viable for several weeks. Spermatozoa disappear from the ejaculate at the rate of 50 to 70 per cent of remaining sperm with each ejaculation, and most sexually active males will have emptied all viable sperm from the reservoirs after 10 or more ejaculations. Microscopic examination of a freshly collected specimen of ejaculate should be accomplished 6 to 8 weeks after the procedure. The patient should not be pronounced surgically sterile until a negative specimen of ejaculate has been observed.

Such elective vasectomy is gaining legal as well as public acceptance. It is incumbent upon the urologic surgeon to insure that the letter of the law is met in accomplishing such sterilization operation. Conference with both the patient and spouse should be mandatory, with written request for the procedure signed by both. A waiting period should be required before the procedure is done, and it must be made clear that a follow-up examination of ejaculate is essential. It should also be explained to the couple that vasectomy must be considered a permanent sterilization measure, though there is increasing success in microsurgical reconstruction of the vasa provided an extensive segment of the vas has not been removed.

VARICOCELE

Varicocele is the term applied to dilatation and tortuosity of the veins of the pampiniform plexus, most commonly observed on the left. It has been stated that varicocele may be an indicator of left renal tumor, since the left spermatic vein system drains into the renal vein and obstruction at that point could produce dilatation of the veins of the left cord; however, varicocele is uncommonly found to be associated with renal tumor. Most varicoceles are idiopathic, though there may be a defect in the valve system of the spermatic vein, particularly on the left where the vein takes a longer course. Varicocele rarely causes symptoms, but there may be a heavy, dragging, aching sensation in the scrotal compartment. Discomfort or infertility may prompt surgical repair, accomplished by varicocelectomy, which is a tedious dissection and ligation of the multiple venous channels of the cord, or by high ligation of the spermatic vein through an incision at the level of the internal inguinal ring, giving ready access to the single vein. Following such ligation, venous collateral circulation is assumed by the deep pelvic venous system.

HYDROCELE

The tunica vaginalis, derived from the peritoneum as the processus vaginalis at the time of testicular descent, is a secretory membrane. Fluid is generated by the serous surface of the tunica vaginalis, fluid formation being enhanced by inflammation or trauma. Fluid within the tunica vaginalis is resorbed at a constant rate through the extensive venous and lymphatic systems of the spermatic cord. Hydrocele, the excessive accumulation of this serous fluid, results when there is increased production or decreased resorption, the latter condition usually being idiopathic.

Congenital hydrocele may result from failure of obliteration of the processus vaginalis, and fluid formed within the peritoneal cavity may gravitate into the tunica vaginalis. Such congenital hydroceles may fluctuate in size depending upon position of the child, and there may sometimes be an associated palpable inguinal hernia; whether a hernia exists or not, the potential for herniation is present. Occasionally, spontaneous closure of the processus vaginalis will occur during infancy and surgical intervention may not be necessary. Even in instances of complete obliteration of the processus vaginalis along the spermatic cord, there may be excessive accumulation of fluid in the tunica vaginalis in the newborn, sometimes requiring aspiration or early surgical intervention for fear of mechanical compression and compromise of testicular viability. Congenital hydrocele, particularly with associated hernia, demands surgical repair, accomplished through a high inguinal incision, giving access to the internal inguinal ring, at which point the hernia sac or processus vaginalis is ligated.

In older persons, hydrocele is frequently the result of epididymo-orchitis or trauma. If there is active pyogenic infection, the hydrocele may become infected, demanding surgical incision and drainage. Compromise of venous and lymphatic return along the cord may occur with a large inguinal hernia or as a result of herniorrhaphy with fibrosis of the inguinal canal obstructing venous and lymphatic drainage. Large intra-abdominal and pelvic masses may similarly compromise return and predispose to hydrocele. While small hydroceles may require no treatment, the swelling may assume such proportions as to cause severe discomfort and interfere with physical and sexual activity. Hydrocelectomy is accomplished by scrotal exploration with excision of redundant tunica vaginalis and retroversion of the remaining sac around the

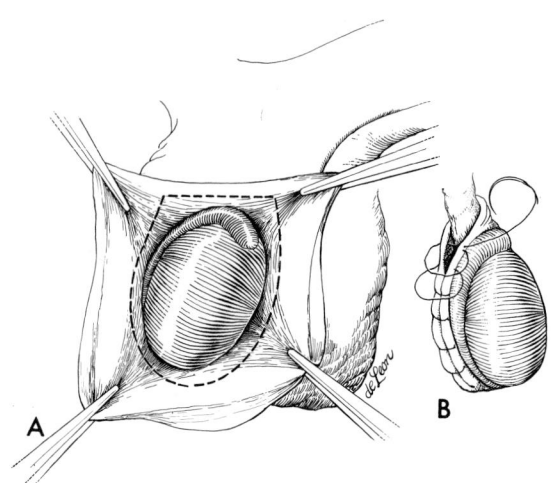

Figure 20. Repair of hydrocele involves incision of the tunica vaginalis with excision of its redundant wall *(A)* and inversion of the remaining wall *(B)* around the epididymis and terminal portion of the spermatic cord. (From Bunce, P. L. *In* Glenn, J. F., and Boyce, W. H.: Urologic Surgery, 2nd ed. Hagerstown, Md., Harper & Row, 1975.)

epididymis and terminal portion of the cord. A permanent cure may be expected by this procedure. Aspiration and injection of sclerosing materials is condemned because of the risk of infection.

INGUINAL LYMPHATICS

The superficial and inguinal lymphatic intervals constitute the principal drainage system for the external genitalia. There is interdigitation of lymphatic drainage between the superficial inguinal nodes and the deep inguinal groups, which communicate with the hypogastric and iliac nodes. Lymphatics of the penis, penile skin, and scrotum drain to the superficial inguinal group, while drainage from the urethra is to the inguinal and hypogastric nodes and that from the glans penis is to the external iliac group. Inflammatory lymphadenitis occurs with many infections of the external genitalia and is usually treated conservatively with antimicrobial agents, bed rest, and other supportive measures. Suppuration may necessitate incision and drainage. Inguinal buboes may result from chancroid, the soft chancre that usually occurs primarily on the corona of the glans penis.

Lymphogranuloma Venereum

Probably of viral origin though possibly due to L-forms, lymphogranuloma is also known as lymphopathia venereum and lymphogranuloma inguinale. Transmission of infection is by sexual intercourse, either genital or anal. Severe adenitis is sometimes associated with elephantiasis of the genitalia. Diagnosis is established by intradermal Frei test and complement fixation, though these are not positive early in the course of the disease. There may be spontaneous remission, but therapy is usually effective with sulfadiazine, tetracyclines, and chloramphenicol. Surgical excision of the involved node groups may be required, particularly if secondary infection supervenes.

Granuloma Inguinale

Granuloma inguinale is a superficial ulcerative skin lesion associated with inguinal adenitis, due to the encapsulated gram-negative Donovan body, which is transmitted by sexual contact and is related to the Friedländer and Klebsiella groups of organisms. Granuloma inguinale is seen more commonly in the south and among the Negro population. Multiple painless granulomatous lesions cause extensive scarring, which may necessitate surgical excision. Streptomycin and tetracyclines are effective in controlling the infectious process.

INTERSEX AND TRANSSEXUALISM

The intersex state is that condition in which there is ambiguity of the external genitalia or inadequate and incomplete differentiation of gonadal and ductal structures. Transsexualism, on the other hand, refers to surgical or social conversion of an individual to the opposite sex on a voluntary basis. Intersex is thus a congenital abnormality, while transsexualism may represent a psychosocial disorder.

INTERSEX STATES

The most common mode of presentation of the intersex patient is by request for sexual differentiation in the neonatal nursery. Ambiguity of the external genitalia necessitates prompt and definitive assignment of sex, reassurance of parents, and early mobilization of medical and surgical measures required to constitute the appropriate sex of the child. On occasion, the intersex patient may be seen as a rather late event, often because of microphallus, undescended testes, labial fusion, or clitoral hypertrophy noted as late as pubescence. The interested reader is referred to a number of definitive texts and monographs dealing with the various types of intersex.

True Hermaphroditism

The true hermaphrodite is the person with gonadal tissue of both sexes, manifesting as ovary and testis, ovary and ovotestis, testis and ovotestis, or two ovotestes. In such instances, relatively rare, ductal development may also be ambiguous, with male wolffian ductal structures ipsilateral to the testicular tissue and feminine müllerian ductal structures ipsilateral to the gonad with ovarian differentiation. Chromosomes are generally normal in number and buccal smear reveals XX or XY patterns. The dominant gender role, as dictated by external genital development, should be pursued and supported by medical and surgical measures. When the external genitalia exhibit severe ambiguity, it is generally best to seek a feminine role for the patient, removing male gonadal tissue and ductal structures, effecting reduction phalloplasty if necessary, and constructing a vagina when the patient reaches marriageable age if there is no vaginal canal present. As for other forms of the intersex state, satisfactory cosmetic and functional results may be achieved with the external genitalia, restoring the patient to a fully satisfactory male or female role as the conditions warrant. Endocrine abnormalities usually do not coexist, but complete removal of gonadal tissue as in instances of bilat-

eral ovotestes may demand lifelong supportive endocrine therapy in the form of appropriate estrogens or androgens.

Adrenogenitalism

The adrenogenital syndrome may occur in males or females, more commonly the latter. Congenital adrenal hyperplasia with excessive production of androgenizing steroid precursors, such as the 17-ketosteroids and pregnanetriol, results from one of several basic enzymatic defects within the gland, compromising the capability of the adrenal to synthesize cortisone and cortisol. Deficiencies of corticosteroids prompt excessive production of adrenocorticotropic hormone by the pituitary, stimulating the already hyperplastic adrenal glands to still further production of androgenizing precursors. The usual enzymatic defect is a deficiency of 11-β-hydroxylase or 21-hydroxylase. Associated hypertension may be observed, and one third or more of children so affected may exhibit a salt-losing tendency with severe vomiting and dehydration, often mistaken for the syndrome of pyloric stenosis. In the male, precocious puberty is observed as a result of the androgenizing influence: early appearance of pubic hair, growth of genitalia to adult proportions, increased muscle mass, and early epiphyseal closure leading to the terms "infant Hercules" and macrogenitosomia praecox. In the female, similar androgenizing changes occur with hypertrophy of the clitoris to the point that it simulates a penis, growth of pubic hair, fusion of the labia in the midline obscuring the urethra and the vaginal introitus behind the single perineal opening or urogenital sinus, and other stigmata including acne, hirsutism, voice changes, and the musculoskeletal changes also seen in the male. Adrenogenitalism is the most common cause of intersex, girls so affected presenting at birth with ambiguous genitalia. The diagnosis is established by demonstration of a normal female chromatin pattern (XX) and an elevation of urinary 17-ketosteroids and 17-hydroxycorticoids. Accurate assessment of urinary steroids may be accomplished in the first week of life, and appropriate definition of sex is essential during the neonatal period if subsequent emtional trauma is to be avoided. Urologic investigation of the female with adrenogenitalism should include cystourethroscopy through the urogenital sinus; introduction of the examining instrument into the vaginal introitus will permit identification of cervix, virtually certain evidence that there is a normal uterus. Once the diagnosis is established, appropriate exogenous cortisone therapy should be initiated, suppressing further pituitary activity and diminishing endogenous adrenal output of androgens. When adequate control is effected, surgical correction of the external genitalia can be accomplished; subtotal phallectomy and labioplasty will result in satisfactory cosmetic appearance of the external female genitalia. Pubic hair, seen in the older patients with adrenogenitalism, may be removed periodically with one of the liquid depilatories. Abdominal exploration is unnecessary when appropriate diagnostic measures have been accomplished, and adrenal surgery is undesirable since adequate suppression can be achieved by medical management.

The Male Intersex

Differentiation of the external genitalia to a completely masculine configuration is apparently dependent upon the fetal testes, elaborating testosterone or some other substance, sometimes referred to as müllerian-inhibiting factor. If the fetal testes fail before genital differentiation has been completed during the first trimester of gestation, ambiguous external genitalia will result. Occasionally, mechanical developmental defects may account for genital ambiguity in the male, and often such genital abnormalities are associated with massive congenital deformities of the gastrointestinal system as well. The most common ambiguity of the male external genitalia is the association of cryptorchism or incomplete testicular descent with perineal hypospadias and severe penile chordee. A male chromatin pattern (XY) can be demonstrated, and there are no associated endocrinopathies. Cystourethroscopic evaluation is helpful, since identification of a verumontanum is evidence of normal internal male ductal structures. Release of chordee and bilateral orchidopexy can be accomplished at an early age, and urethroplasty should be effected before the child reaches school age.

Maternal Virilization

In the past, it was common practice to treat abortion and habitual abortion with androgenizing drugs such as testosterone. While this mode of therapy is less frequently employed today, occasional instances of virilization of females are still observed. The administration of androgenizing agents to the mother has little or no effect on the male fetus, though there may be some precocious genital growth. In the female, the clitoris may be stimulated to considerable enlargement, assuming penile proportions. Some degree of labial fusion may also be observed, though usually the urogenital sinus is not fully formed and the urethra and vaginal introitus can be visualized. Since the influences are terminated at the end of gestation, there is no progression of the deformity. External genital reconstructive procedures are effected as with adrenogenitalism, but no continuing therapy is necessary.

Gonadal Dysgenesis

The dysgenetic testis results in varying degrees of ambiguity of the external genitalia. In males with dysplastic testes, diagnosis may not be suspected until a normal age of pubescence at which time failure of development of secondary sex characteristics points to testicular inadequacy, as with Klinefelter's syndrome. The diagnosis of gonadal dysgenesis should be approached with caution, since delayed pubescence may be a simple genetic characteristic, not indicative of any serious underlying disease process. In the male child approaching puberty with small penis and testes gonadal dysgenesis should be suspected, but the diagnosis is dependent upon testicular biopsy and should be confirmed by complete endocrine evaluation. Gonadotropins will become elevated at puberty, inducing increase in testosterone production. Measurement of urinary gonadotropins and plasma testosterone is effective in defining hypogonadal states; persistent elevation of gonadotropins with inadequate levels of testosterone supports the diagnosis of hypogonadism. Management is by medical measures.

Anorchism

The complete absence of viable testicular tissue is a rare event. Unilateral failure of testicular development, monorchism, is not uncommonly observed, and is usually unattended by any genital or developmental abnormalities. Certain males are observed, however, to lack identifiable testicular tissue, though ductal and external differentiation in normal male fashion has occurred, as indicated in the discussion of testicular anomalies.

TRANSSEXUALISM

Transsexual patients are persons who are usually normal anatomic males or females without endocrinologic abnormality.[25] For various psychosocial reasons, frequently related to events in childhood, these persons cast themselves in roles of the opposite sex and request surgical transformation. While such surgical sex conversion has been accomplished abroad and with relative discretion in the past, current public attitudes of permissiveness have allowed a more scientific ap-

proach to the problems, both psychiatric and surgical. A number of centers in this country are now actively engaged in transsexual investigation and treatment. It is much more common for males to seek conversion to female body characteristics, and such surgical conversion involves penectomy, castration, reduction scrotoplasty, and vaginoplasty as well as estrogen administration and subsequent augmentation mammoplasty by implantation of silicone prostheses. In a careful and detailed evaluation of 121 male transsexual patients followed after surgery, the result was deemed highly satisfactory in 68 per cent, and a satisfactory emotional and social readjustment in such patients is felt to be 10 times more likely than an unsatisfactory outcome. Sex conversion surgery for female transsexuals is, at present, less satisfactory. Reduction mammoplasty and complete hysterectomy are feasible, and the vaginal canal can be obliterated. Unfortunately, an erectile penis cannot be constructed, though tube skin flaps can be developed to effect a cosmetic phallus.

SELECTED REFERENCES

Creevy, C. D.: The correction of hypospadias: A review. Urol. Survey, 8:1, 1958.
The problem of hypospadias, the incompletely developed urethra, has challenged surgeons for centuries. The term hypospadias itself derives from the Greek roots meaning "under" and "to tear." This superb review, replete with lavish drawings, defines and elaborates the theory and practice of hypospadias repair. While a few of the more recent modifications of technique are not included, this survey constitutes basic information for the interested surgeon.

Federman, D. D.: Abnormal Sexual Development: The Genetic and Endocrine Approach to Differential Diagnosis. Philadelphia, W. B. Saunders Company, 1967.
The complexities of sexual differentiation and the intersex states are thoroughly presented in this compendium of current information. The normal processes of sexual differentiation are emphasized, the chromosomal and endocrinologic abnormalities associated with intersex are elaborated, and a rational approach to diagnosis and treatment of the intersex patient is presented.

Rubin, P. (Ed.): Cancer of the urogenital tract: Testicular tumors. J.A.M.A., 213:89, 1970.
This symposium, one of a series of multidisciplinary forums on malignant disease of the genitourinary system, constitutes a review and progress report relative to testicular tumors. Pathologic classification of testicular tumors, diagnostic methodology, and various aspects of treatment are emphasized with attention directed toward results of various forms of therapy. Eight authorities in the involved disciplines participate in this colloquium.

Rubin, P. (Ed.): Cancer of the urogenital tract: Prostate cancer. J.A.M.A., 210:322, 1072, 1969.
This symposium on carcinoma of the prostate is presented in two parts, one dealing with confined and localized cancer of the prostate gland and the second with advanced and metastatic prostate cancer. Ten authorities deal with incidence and detection of prostate cancer, radical surgery, hormonal manipulation, conservative therapy by transurethral resection, ancillary hormonal measures, and the role of radiation therapy, including both interstitial irradiation and definitive external radiotherapy.

REFERENCES

1. Alyea, E. P.: Early or late orchiectomy for carcinoma of the prostate? J. Urol., 53:143, 1945.
2. Amelar, R. D., and Dubin, L.: Male infertility: Current diagnosis and treatment. Urology, 1:1, 1973.
3. Bennett, A. H., and Harrison, J. H.: A comparison of operative approach for prostatectomy, 1948 and 1968. Surg. Gynecol. Obstet., 128:969, 1969.
4. Billig, R., Baker, R., Immergut, M., and Maxted, W.: Peyronie's disease. Urology, 6:409, 1975.
5. Campos Freire, J. G.: Transvesical prostatectomy with primary closure of the bladder. Urol. Int., 7:300, 1958.
6. Castro, J. E., Griffiths, H. J. L., and Shackman, R.: Significance of signs and symptoms in benign prostatic hypertrophy. Br. Med. J., 2:598, 1969.

7. Cosgrove, M. D., and LaRocque, M. A.: Shunt surgery for priapism: Review of results. Urology, 4:1, 1974.
8. Dalton, D. L., Hughes, J., and Glenn, J. F.: Foreign bodies and urinary stones. Urology, 6:1, 1975.
9. Dees, J. E.: Radical perineal prostatectomy for carcinoma. J. Urol., 104:160, 1970.
10. Fegen, P., and Persky, L.: Squamous cell carcinoma of the penis: Its treatment with special reference to radical node dissection. Arch. Surg., 99:117, 1969.
11. Flocks, R. H.: Clinical cancer of the prostate: A study of four thousand cases. J.A.M.A., 193:89, 1965.
12. Gilbertsen, V. A.: Cancer of the prostate gland: Results of early diagnosis and therapy undertaken for cure of the disease. J.A.M.A., 215:81, 1971.
13. Glenn, J. F., and Boyce, W. H.: Urologic Surgery, 2nd ed. Hagerstown, Md., Harper & Row, 1975.
14. Glenn, J. F., and Spanel, D. J.: Serum acid phosphatase and the effect of prostatic massage. J. Urol., 82:240, 1959.
15. Grabstald, H.: Tumors of the urethra in men and women. Cancer, 32:1236, 1973.
16. Gutman, A. B.: The development of the acid phosphatase test for prostatic carcinoma. Bull. N. Y. Acad. Med., 44:63, 1968.
17. Horton, C. E., and Devine, C. J., Jr.: Peyronie's disease. J. Plast. Reconstr. Surg., 52:503, 1973.
18. Johnston, J. H., and Farkas, A.: Congenital neuropathic bladder: Practicalities and possibilities of conservational management. Urology, 5:719, 1975.
19. Leape, L. L.: Torsion of the testis: Invitation to error. J.A.M.A., 200:93, 1967.
20. Lytton, B., Emory, J. M., and Harvard, B. M.: The incidence of benign prostatic obstruction. J. Urol., 99:639, 1968.
21. Marshall, V. F.: The choice of therapy for prostatic carcinoma. J. Urol., 113:285, 1975.
22. Martin, D. C., and Menck, H. R.: The undescended testis: Management after puberty. J. Urol., 114:77, 1975.
23. Millin, T.: Retropubic prostatectomy. J. Urol., 59:367, 1948.
24. Mollenkamp, J. S., Cooper, J. F., and Kagan, A. R.: Clinical experience with supervoltage radiotherapy in carcinoma of the prostate: A preliminary report. J. Urol., 113:374, 1975.
25. Montague, D. K.: Transsexualism. Urology, 2:1, 1973.
26. Mostofi, F. K.: Testicular tumors: Epidemiologic, etiologic and pathologic features. Cancer, 32:1186, 1973.
27. Nesbit, R. M., and Baum, W. C.: Endocrine control of prostatic carcinoma. J.A.M.A., 143:1317, 1950.
28. Orkin, L. A.: Efficacy of Candicin in benign prostatic hypertrophy. Urology, 4:80, 1974.
29. Osborne, E. D., Sutherland, C. G., Scholl, A. J., and Rowntree, L. G.: Roentgenography of urinary tract during excretion of sodium iodide. J.A.M.A., 80:368, 1923.
30. Prentiss, R. J., Weickgenant, C. J., Moses, J. J., and Frazier, D. B.: Undescended testis: Surgical anatomy of spermatic vessels, spermatic surgical triangles and lateral spermatic ligament. J. Urol., 83:686, 1960.
31. Prout, G. R., Jr., Macalalag, E. V., Jr., and Denis, L. J.: Alterations in patients with prostatic carcinoma after hormonal therapy. Surg. Forum, 15:486, 1964.
32. Ray, E. H., Sr.: Bladder neck obstruction due to prostatic hyperplasia: Diagnosis, treatment, and postoperative care. Am. Surg., 31:325, 1965.
33. Rich, A. R.: On frequency of occurrence of occult carcinoma of the prostate. J. Urol., 33:215, 1935.
34. Rullis, I., Shaeffer, J. A., and Lilien, O. M.: Incidence of prostatic carcinoma in the elderly. Urology, 6:295, 1975.
35. Smith, B. H.: Peyronie's disease. Am. J. Clin. Pathol., 45:670, 1966.
36. Stamey, T. A., Fair, W. R., Timothy, M. M., and Chung, H. K.: Antibacterial nature of prostatic fluid. Nature, 218:444, 1968.
37. Staubitz, W. J., Magoss, I. V., Grace, J. T., and Schenk, W. G., III: Surgical management of testis tumors. J. Urol., 101:350, 1969.
38. Stewart, B. H., and Montie, J. E.: Male infertility: Optimistic report. J. Urol., 110:216, 1973.
39. Veterans Administration Cooperative Urological Research Group: Treatment and survival of patients with cancer of the prostate. Surg. Gynecol. Obstet., 124:1011, 1967.
40. Wershub, L. P.: The Human Testis: A Clinical Treatise. Springfield, Ill., Charles C Thomas, Publisher, 1962.
41. Whitmore, W. F.: Natural history of prostatic cancer. Cancer, 32:1104, 1973.
42. Young, H. H.: Hugh Young: A Surgeon's Autobiography. New York, Harcourt, Brace and Company, 1940.

50

DISORDERS OF THE LYMPHATIC SYSTEM

Harry S. Goldsmith, M.D.

Although knowledge of arteries and veins has been documented far back into history, the lymphatic system was not described until the seventeenth century, even though Hippocrates and Aristotle had previously reported "white blood" and the existence of structures containing a clear fluid. In 1622, Gasper Asellius, Professor of Anatomy at Milan, noted ramifying cordlike structures in the canine mesentery that discharged a milky fluid when cut. Twenty-five years later, in 1647, Pecquet noted the thoracic duct, and Rudbeck, in 1653, accurately described the lymphatic system in detail. The existence of lymphatic valves, which he reported, was all but forgotten until Ryschius rediscovered them in 1721. By the end of the eighteenth century, the scientific world not only had accepted the presence of the lymphatic system, but also agreed that lymphatics absorbed various substances in their course from the periphery of the body to the thoracic duct and eventual confluence with the venous system.

COMPARATIVE ANATOMY

A true lymphatic system is found only in vertebrate animals. Lower animals with less well differentiated cardiovascular systems rely upon the venous system to perform the functions of the absent lymphatic system. Among the vertebrates, only birds and mammals possess a lymphatic system consisting of narrow, ramifying vessels endowed with valves.

The lymphatic system of all mammals parallels that of man and is characterized by a single major connection between the lymphatic and venous systems, at the jugular region. Lymph flow, which is normally centripetal and unidirectional, usually traverses at least one lymph node before draining into the thoracic duct. Afferent lymphatic channels drain from the periphery of the body to lymph nodes, and efferent vessels emerge from the nodes to form confluent main collecting channels. Groups of nodes are situated in relatively constant positions to collect lymph from a particular organ or region and, therefore, are aptly designated as regional lymph nodes. The higher the phylogenetic scale, the greater is the number of lymph nodes encountered, although the age and size of the animal also influence this number. A characteristic of mammalian lymphatics is a valve system, which is present even in small lymphatic tributaries and which insures the unidirectional flow necessary for the maintenance and regulation of normal lymph flow.

EMBRYOLOGY

Paired jugular lymph sacs are recognizable in the 6-week human embryo. These sacs enlarge and coalesce with adjacent endothelial pockets to form chains of small sacs, which are the forerunners of the major collecting lymphatics. By 9 weeks of gestation, the basic pattern of the main lymphatic channels becomes noticeable, as lymph sacs give rise to small endothelial channels, which develop into lymphatic vessels. Coincidentally, connective tissue invades and permeates the lymphatic sacs. It is by these maneuvers that the main lymphatic channels and their tributaries become delineated.

Pouchlike protuberances from the lymphatic trunks differentiate into lymph nodes, with contiguous connective tissue becoming compressed around the periphery of each node to form its capsule. Afferent lymphatic vessels develop at the periphery of the lymph node through which lymph flow enters, later exiting via the efferent lymphatic vessel on the contralateral side.

GENERAL ANATOMY

The lymphatic system is divided into three major components: (1) a network of *capillaries*, which serves to collect lymph from the various tissues and organs; (2) *collecting vessels*, which carry the lymph from the capillaries to the great veins at the root of the neck via the thoracic duct; and (3) *lymph nodes*. Other lymphoid organs, which resemble lymph nodes and are part of the reticuloendothelial or lymphoreticular system, are the tonsils, adenoids, spleen, and thymus. Lymphatic vessels that drain the small intestine are called lacteals. They are identical to other lymphatic vessels except that during the process of digestion they contain a thick, white fluid called chyle.

Lymphatic Capillaries

These small structures are necessary for maintaining fluid equilibrium within the interstitial space of the body. Lymphatic capillaries have been demonstrated in all areas of the body except for the central nervous system, cornea, inner ear, cartilage, and splenic pulp. Plexuses of these capillaries are especially extensive in the dermis and in the mucous membranes of the respiratory and digestive systems. There appears to be a direct relationship between the number of lymphatic and vascular capillaries in a particular area; i.e., the better the blood supply, the better the lymphatic drainage.

Collecting Lymphatics

Small lymphatic capillaries eventually enlarge into collecting lymphatics. These collecting lymphatics parallel blood vessels and drain through regional lymph nodes in their course toward the thoracic duct and, ultimately, the systemic circulation. As the lymphatics become confluent and extend centrally toward the thoracic duct, they normally traverse at least one, but often as many as eight to ten lymph nodes or node groups. Exceptions to this rule exist in the thyroid gland, esophagus, heart, and adrenal glands, where draining lymphatics may empty directly into the thoracic duct without passing through a lymph node.

Walls of collecting vessels possess intimal, medial, and adventitial layers, with the media containing elastic fibers and smooth muscle in proportion to the size of the lymphatic. Lymphatic vessels have their own vasa vasorum, with larger lymphatics having their own artery and vein, which in turn are surrounded by small lymphatics. The large lymphatic channels contain neural elements from the vagus nerve, lesser splanchnic nerves, and para-aortic sympathetic nerves.

Lymph Nodes

Lymph nodes, varying in size from a few millimeters to more than a centimeter, are interposed throughout the course of the collecting lymphatic channels. These lymph nodes are encapsulated and oval or bean-shaped, with an indentation along the concave surface (Fig. 1).

Lymph is brought to individual lymph nodes by afferent lymphatics which pierce the capsule's convex surface. Lymph flows into the subcapsular, cortical, and medullary sinuses within the lymph node, prior to exiting via the efferent lymphatic channel. Most commonly, there are several afferent lymphatics that carry lymph to a node, but usually only one efferent vessel.

Trabeculae, which are extensions of the capsule penetrating the nodal substance, divide the interior of the lymph node into interconnecting cavities that contain reticular tissue. The major cellular component of

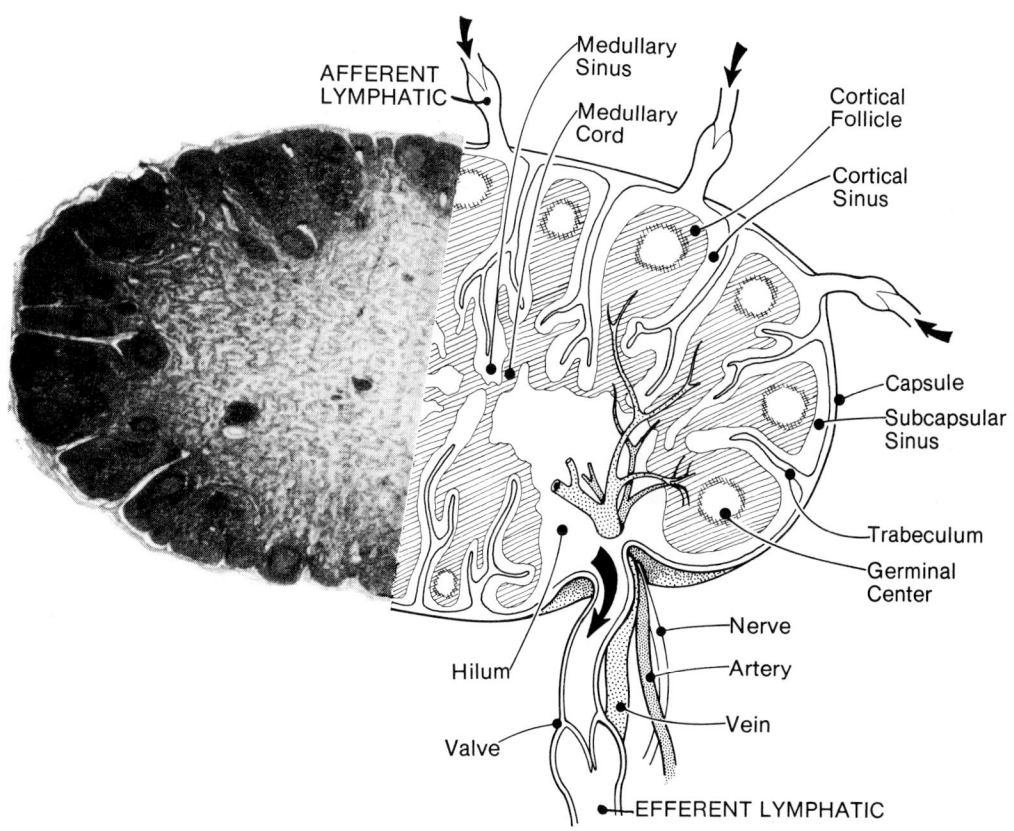

Figure 1. Anatomic and diagrammatic representation of a normal lymph node.

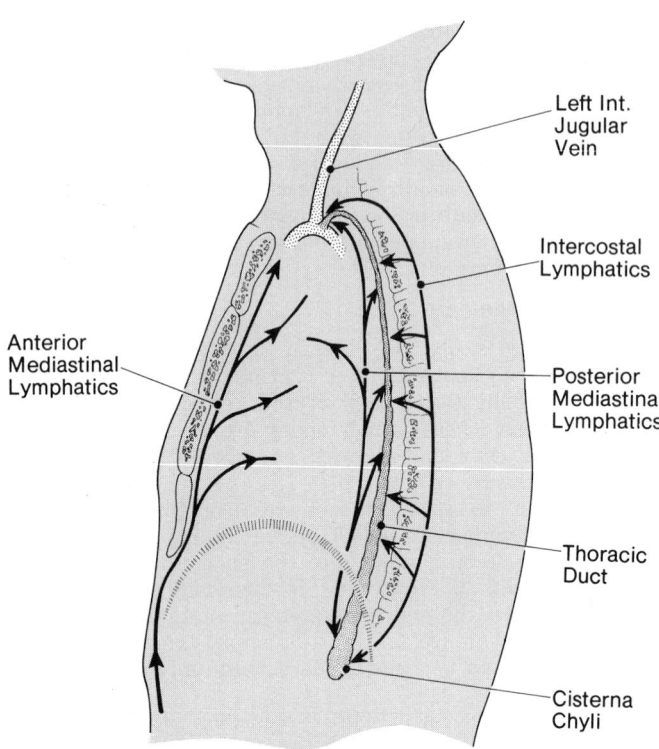

Figure 2. Supradiaphragmatic patterns of lymphatic drainage.

the lymph node is the lymphocyte, but all elements of the blood may be found in various proportions. These cells aggregate at the nodal periphery into large nodules, or follicles, making up the cortex of the node. Within the central portion of the node or medulla, lymphocytes are arranged in anastomosing cords continuous with the cortex. These medullary cords are rich in small lymphocytes, plasma cells, and macrophages. In the normal lymph node, these cells exist in equilibrium with one another, the proportion of each changing with age, diet, and hormonal milieu. At present there is no information as to how this equilibrium is controlled.

Lymph flows within the intranodal sinuses between cortical follicles and medullary cords. Within the cortical follicles, there are two distinct areas, the germinal center, which contains cells that are less densely packed and are histologically characterized by having a pale-staining and voluminous cytoplasm with abundant nuclear mitoses, and a darker-staining outer zone composed of smaller cells. The germinal center has been implicated as the site of antibody production and phagocytosis and the source of new lymphocytes.

Lymph Flow

Almost all the lymph collected throughout the body is returned to the systemic circulation by way of the thoracic duct. The thoracic duct originates as the cisterna chyli at the level of the second lumbar vertebra. The cisterna chyli receives lymph from the lower extremities, pelvic viscera and parieties, renal and suprarenal nodes, and the deep lymphatics of the abdominal wall. In addition it also receives lymph from

the stomach, intestines, pancreas, spleen, and the caudal and ventral surfaces of the liver (Figs. 2 and 3).

Immediately below the diaphragm, the cisterna chyli becomes the thoracic duct, which extends superiorly through the aortic hiatus of the diaphragm. Emptying into the caudal end of the thoracic duct are descending lymphatic trunks from intercostal and posterior mediastinal nodes. The thoracic duct ascends behind the aortic arch and left subclavian artery, rising in an arch behind the clavicle. It then crosses the subclavian and vertebral vessels, and the thyrocervical trunk, before finally emptying into the venous system at the angle of the junction of the left subclavian and internal jugular veins. The right jugular and subclavian lymphatic trunks drain into the right lymphatic duct, which in turn enters the right subclavian vein near its junction with the right internal jugular vein.

PHYSIOLOGY

The lymphatic system has two functions: (1) the uptake, transportation, and return of fluid and macromolecules from the interstitial space to the systemic circulation; and (2) protection of the host by providing a filtering system that resists infection and impedes the spread of neoplastic disease.

Ten per cent of the arterial capillary filtrate is not reabsorbed by the venous capillaries but enters the lymphatic system, to be returned to the circulation via the thoracic duct. In addition to this fluid transfer, the lymphatic system is almost totally responsible for the reabsorption of protein from the interstitial space,

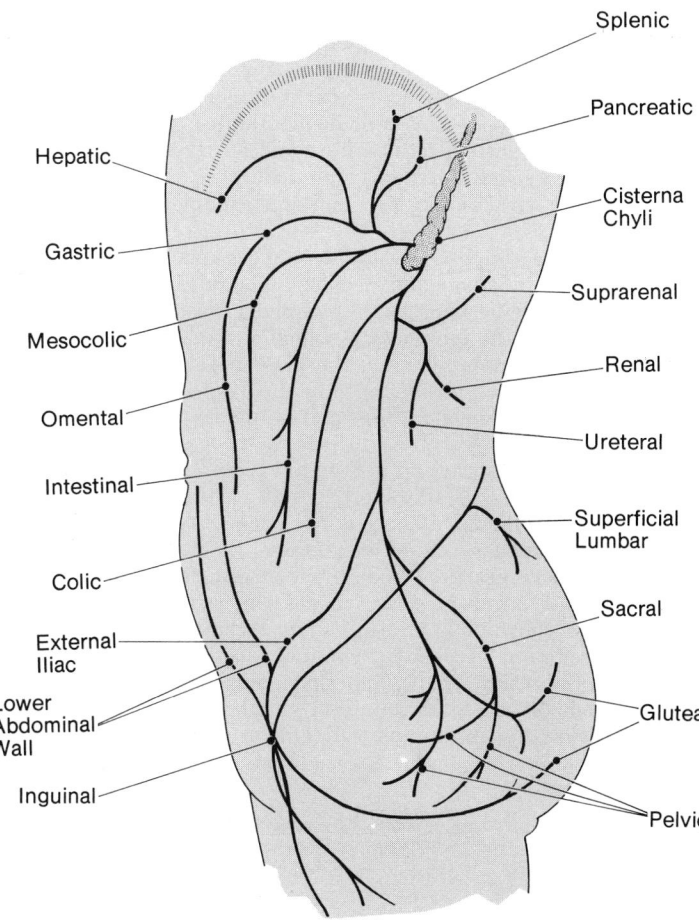

Figure 3. Subdiaphragmatic patterns of lymphatic drainage.

since only a small portion of filtered protein diffuses back into venous capillaries.

The absorption of protein-laden filtrate begins in small lymphatics, which are characterized by having openings of several micra between individual cells within the endothelial wall of the lymphatic vessel. These open intercellular junctions are superimposed upon one another, providing a valvelike action to the endothelial cells of the lymphatic wall, thus favoring the entry of fluid and large molecules into the vessel but preventing the egress of protein filtrate from these lymphatics. The spaces between individual cells become progressively smaller as the lymphatic channels enlarge, which further restricts the flow of large molecules back into the interstitial space.

Lymph is a reflection of the composition of tissue fluid in a particular area of the body. Peripheral lymph protein concentration is usually 2 gm. per 100 ml., intestinal lymph 3 to 4 gm. per 100 ml., and liver lymph protein sometimes exceeds 5 gm. per 100 ml. Thoracic duct lymph, a mixture of lymph from all areas of the body, has a protein concentration of approximately 3 to 5 gm. per 100 ml. Because the lymphatic system is also a major vehicle for fat absorption from the gastrointestinal tract, thoracic duct lymph, especially following meals, may contain a small per-

centage of fat in the form of protein-coated fat droplets called chylomicrons.

The total flow of lymph passing through the thoracic duct under basal conditions is estimated at 120 ml. per hour, so that the total amount of lymph returned daily to the bloodstream approximates the total plasma volume. Lymph return, therefore, plays an important role in the maintenance of the normal blood volume.

Normal interstitial fluid pressure is subatmospheric, approximately −7 mm. Hg. This negative interstitial pressure represents the mean pressure, with the actual pressure within the interstitial compartment varying considerably during movement of the tissues. Elevation of interstitial fluid pressure toward a more positive pressure forces fluid into the lymphatics and increases the rate of lymph flow. However, when the interstitial fluid pressure reaches atmospheric pressure, this increased pressure in the interstitial compartment compresses the adjacent lymphatics and retards lymph flow.

In addition to its function as the prime regulatory mechanism for the absorption of interstitial fluid protein and intestinal fat, lymphatic tissue is the body's major defense system. This system, which includes lymph nodes, tonsils, adenoids, spleen, and thymus, has the major responsibility for filtering bacteria, red blood cells, tumor emboli, and inanimate particles. Malignant cells or infecting organisms are removed because of the mechanical inability of tumor cells to traverse the intact lymph nodes, or by phagocytosis within the lymph nodes by reticuloendothelial cells. Viruses are apparently filtered quite inefficiently, and it has been suggested that the lymph node may serve as a center for viral replication and subsequent dissemination.

The role of the lymphatic system as a mechanism of defense against infection and neoplasia includes the production of specific immunity. Lymphoid tissue is the source of both the lymphocyte, which is necessary for cell-mediated immunity, and the plasma cell and its precursors, which are thought to be involved in the elaboration of immunoglobulins and humoral antibodies.

Malignant cells are carried to regional lymph nodes after gaining access to afferent lymphatic channels. Abundant anastomoses among lymphatics may account for the appearance of metastases in distant nodes even before proximal node involvement. If malignant cells are not destroyed after entering a lymph node, the cells continue to multiply and ultimately obstruct the efferent lymphatic channel. Continuing tumor growth within the lymph node may lead to tumor cell embolization via collateral lymphatic pathways. Occasionally, malignant cell emboli drain di-rectly into the thoracic duct or through lymphatico-venous communications into the vena cava.

The relationship between the lymphatic system and the spread of neoplastic disease was proposed by Virchow, who first noted left supraclavicular adenopathy in patients with gastrointestinal malignant disease. It was this observation that implicated the thoracic duct as the means by which cellular emboli arising from a primary tumor were deposited in distant lymph nodes.

REGIONAL LYMPH NODE ANATOMY

Head and Neck

Lymph nodes are found symmetrically on both sides of the head and neck, lying in circular and vertical chains (Fig. 4). The lymph nodes that are positioned in a circular fashion are the following: (1) *Occipital nodes*—These nodes drain the back of the scalp and are situated under the deep fascia, midway between the external occipital protuberance and the mastoid process. (2) *Posterior auricular nodes*—These nodes lie on the mastoid process under the deep fascia and drain the temporal area, the back of the pinna, and the external auditory meatus. (3) *Anterior auricular nodes*—These nodes lie in front of the tragus and drain the scalp and pinna. (4) *Parotid Nodes*—These nodes are buried under the deep fascia and lie within the substance of the parotid. The location of these

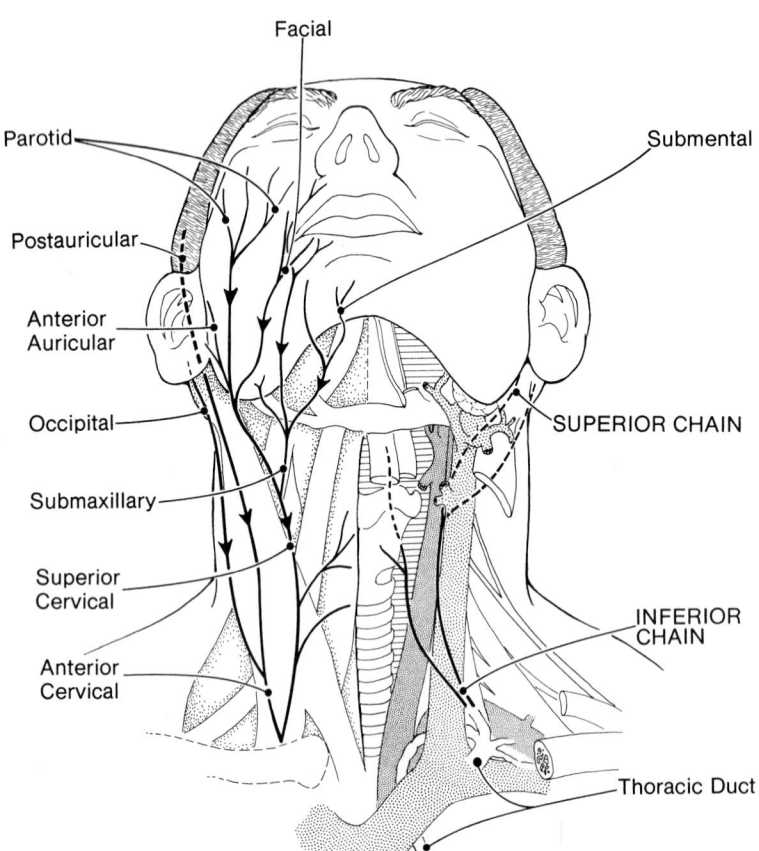

Figure 4. Lymphatics and lymph nodes of the head and neck.

nodes explains the rationale for including a superficial parotid dissection for malignant lesions of the face that have shown evidence of spread to the cervical lymph nodes. An example of this would be a melanoma of the cheek with palpable neck nodes. The parotid nodes drain the nasopharynx, external auditory canal, inner ear, and eyelids. (5) *Facial lymph nodes* – These nodes are divided into superficial and deep groups, in relation to the anterior facial and internal maxillary vessels, and drain the face, pharynx, and mucous membranes of the cheek. (6) *Submaxillary nodes* – These nodes lie within the fascia of the submaxillary gland and drain the side of the nose, cheek, angle of the mouth, upper lip, portion of the lower lip, gum, and side of the tongue. In order to be certain that these lymph nodes are removed, it is necessary to resect the submaxillary gland. (7) *Submental nodes* – These nodes lie lateral to the midline in the submental triangle. They receive drainage from the lower lip, especially on the ipsilateral side, the apex of the tongue, and the floor of the mouth. (8) *Superficial cervical lymph nodes* – These nodes lie along the external jugular vein on the sternomastoid muscle and drain the parotid area and lower portion of the external ear. (9) *Anterior cervical lymph nodes* – These nodes lie close to the midline of the neck and have a superficial and a deep group. They drain the larynx, thyroid gland, and trachea. The "Delphian" node is a member of this node group, which, when enlarged, is highly suspicious for carcinoma of the thyroid.

The vertical chains of lymph nodes in the head and neck area follow the carotid sheath from the base of the skull to the mediastinum. These nodes are extremely important clinically in the treatment of head and neck tumors, because they ultimately receive a majority of the lymphatic drainage from the head and neck. These vertical nodes are divided into superior and inferior groups by the bifurcation of the common carotid artery, at the level of the upper border of the thyroid cartilage. Several nodes of the inferior group lie between the trachea and esophagus near the recurrent laryngeal nerve and drain the thyroid gland. Efferent vessels from these nodes enter the thoracic duct on the left side, and, on the right side, enter the confluence of the subclavian vein and internal jugular vein.

The basic mechanism for the spread of cancer of the head and neck is by tumor embolization via lymphatic vessels into regional lymph nodes. If a tumor embolus cannot be destroyed within a lymph node, it may grow and overwhelm the filtering capacity of the involved lymph node. Tumors of the head and neck are known for their propensity to remain localized to the primary area and within regional lymph nodes. Eventual dissemination of the tumor occurs as a relatively late stage of the disease. These concepts, based on the recognition and importance of lymphatic drainage pathways in the head and neck, have led to the present surgical maneuvers that attempt to remove both the primary lesion and regional lymph nodes in an "en bloc" in-continuity fashion.

Breast

Knowledge of the lymphatic pathways from the breast is extremely important in understanding the natural history and rationale of proposed treatment for patients with mammary carcinoma (Fig. 5). The breast lymphatics begin around the lobules, with collecting channels following mammary ducts centripetally to the areolar area and to the subareolar lymphatic plexus. There is also a network of cutaneous lymphatics, both superficial and deep, within the skin of the breast, with unidirectional lymph flow to the axilla.

Coursing from the subareolar plexus toward the axilla are large medial and lateral collecting trunks that pass around the outer edge of the pectoralis major muscle and penetrate the axillary fascia, prior to terminating in several groups of axillary lymph nodes. In addition to these two large trunks, there are collecting lymphatics between the pectoral fascia and the breast, which perforate the pectoralis major muscles and follow the course of the thoracoacromial vessels. These lymphatics eventually drain into the nodes at the apex of the axilla. Additional lymphatic drainage pathways are present on the posterior aspect of the pectoralis major muscle, composing the transpectoral lymphatic route, and occasionally in the superior portion of the breast, forming the retropectoral lymphatic route. Between the pectoralis major and minor muscles, along the transpectoral route, lie the interpectoral or "Rotter's" nodes. From the apical, or subclavicular, nodes of the axilla, efferent lymphatic trunks emerge, run cephalad behind the clavicle, and empty into the venous system at the confluence of the internal jugular and subclavian veins.

Lymph nodes within the axilla vary in number, but meticulous pathologic clearing techniques may yield as many as 30 to 60 or more lymph nodes. The lymphatics of the breast drain into five lymph node groups within the axilla; (1) The *external mammary group*, which lies along the medial wall of the axilla and is contiguous with or within the fascia overlying the interdigitations of the serratus anterior muscle, from the sixth rib cephalad to the axillary vein. Occasionally, this group may include several paramammary nodes along the lateral edge of the pectoralis major muscle. (2) The *scapular group*, which lies along the subscapular and thoracodorsal vessels, from the lateral thoracic wall to the axillary vein. (3) The *central group*, which lies in the center of the axilla. These nodes are the largest within the axilla and are the ones most often clinically palpable. (4) The *axillary vein group*, which is found along the inferior surface of the lateral aspect of the axillary vein. (5) The *subclavicular group*, which is at the apex of the axilla and is often referred to as the apical group of nodes. These nodes are found at the point where the subclavian vein disappears behind the subclavius muscle. They are clinically important because of their proximity to the edge of the surgical field in most techniques of radical mastectomy, and because the efferent lymphatics from the other groups of axillary lymph nodes empty into this subclavicular group.

In addition to axillary lymphatic drainage pathways, the breast is drained by the internal mammary system of lymphatics and lymph nodes, which receives efferent lymphatics primarily from the central and medial portions of the breast. These lymphatics pass

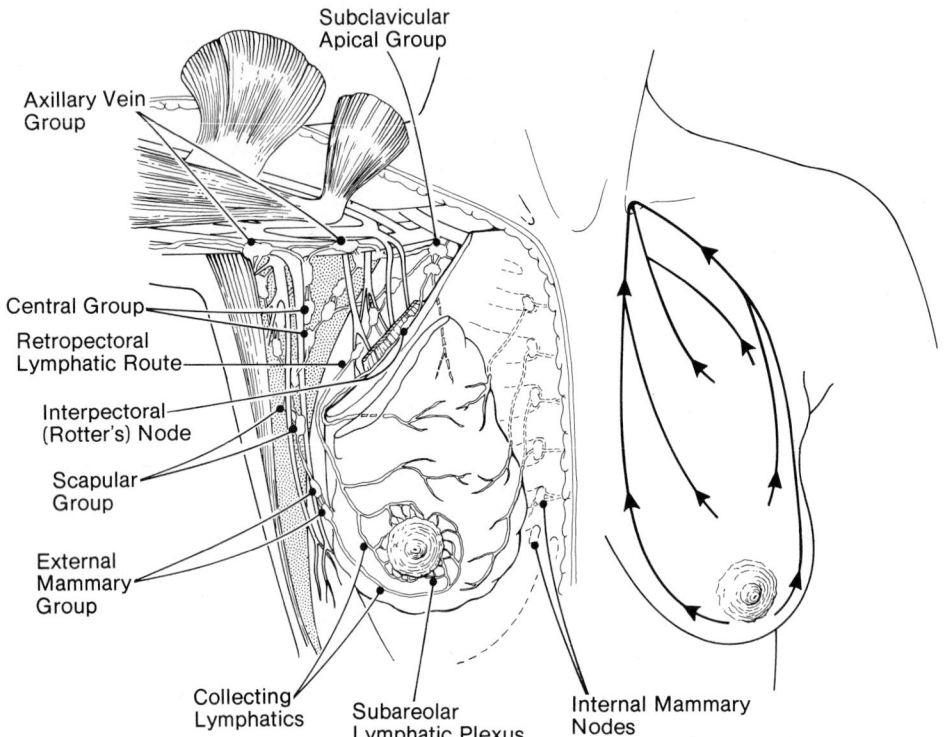

Figure 5. Lymphatic drainage of the breast.

through the pectoralis major muscle prior to emptying into the internal mammary nodes, which are situated at the edge of the sternum on the endothoracic fascia within the intercostal spaces. The internal mammary lymph nodes are small, and their efferent lymphatics drain into the thoracic duct on the left, into the lymphatic duct on the right, and, infrequently, directly into the jugular-subclavian confluence by lymphaticovenous anastomoses.

Thorax

The lymphatic vessels and nodes of the thorax may be divided into two major groups, those of the thoracic wall, or parietes, and those of the intrathoracic viscera (Fig. 6). The parietal nodes include *intercostal, diaphragmatic,* and *internal mammary* nodes. The intercostal nodes drain the posterolateral chest wall and, depending upon their location, empty into the thoracic duct or right lymphatic duct or both superiorly, or into the cisterna chyli inferiorly. Lymph nodes that lie along the diaphragm receive afferent channels from the diaphragm and from the superior surface of the liver. The internal mammary nodes have already been discussed in the preceding paragraph.

The thoracic visceral nodes consist of three groups—the anterior mediastinal, the posterior mediastinal, and the tracheobronchial nodes. The *anterior mediastinal* nodes receive afferent lymphatics from the thymus, pericardium, and internal mammary nodes. Their efferent lymphatics unite with the tracheobronchial lymphatics to form the right and left bronchomediastinal lymphatic trunks. The *posterior mediastinal* nodes receive afferent lymphatics from

the esophagus, posterior pericardium, and superior surface of the liver. Their efferent lymphatics drain into the thoracic duct, with a few channels joining the tracheobronchial nodes. The *tracheobronchial* nodes are divided into four subgroups: (1) tracheal nodes, which lie on both sides of the trachea; (2) bronchial nodes, which lie in the angle between the trachea and bronchi, and between the two major bronchi; (3) pulmonary nodes, which lie within the lung parenchyma in relation to the larger bronchioles; and (4) bronchopulmonary nodes, which lie at the hilum of each lung. Afferent lymphatics empty into all four of these groups from the lungs, bronchi, thoracic trachea, and pericardium. Their efferent trunks join with the internal mammary and anterior mediastinal lymphatics to form right and left bronchomediastinal trunks, which usually end at the jugular-subclavian confluence on the ipsilateral side, separate from the orifices of thoracic or right lymphatic ducts. Occasionally, however, they do drain directly into the thoracic duct or right lymphatic duct. Lymphatic vessels within the pulmonary parenchyma originate in superficial or deep lymphatic plexuses beneath the visceral pleura and accompany the pulmonary blood vessels before finally emptying into the tracheobronchial nodes. Connections between the superficial and deep plexuses within the lung seldom occur except at the hilum.

Esophageal lymphatic vessels form a circumferential plexus around the esophagus. These lymphatics freely anastomose with one another prior to forming confluent collecting vessels draining into the posterior mediastinal lymph nodes. The cardiac lymphatics are divided into superficial and deep plexuses, the former

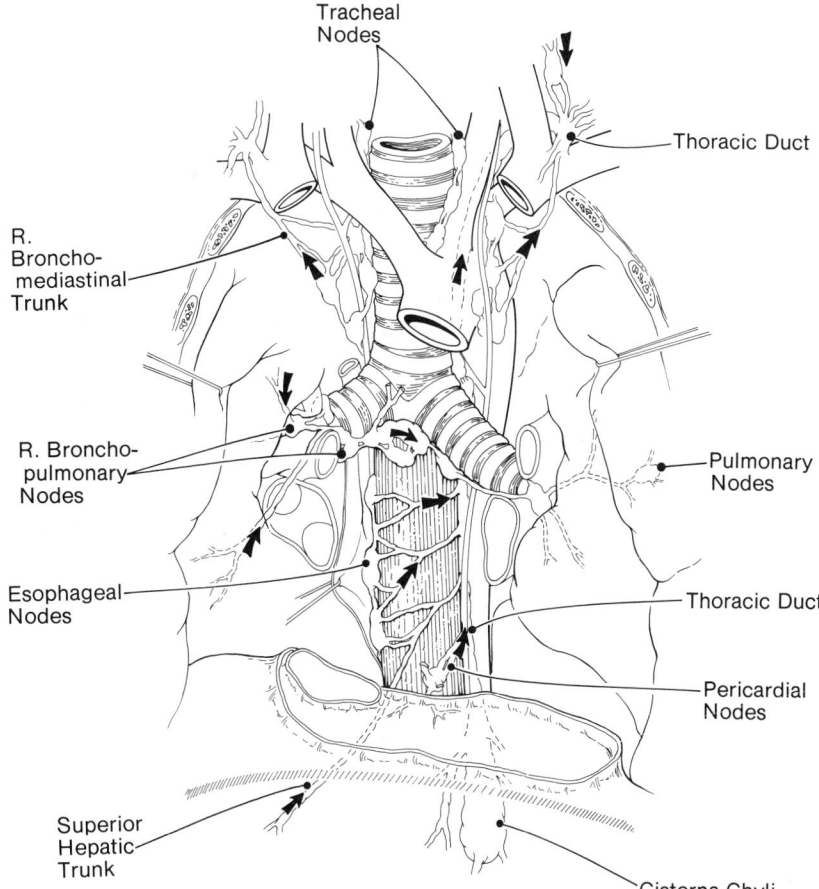

Figure 6. Lymphatic anatomy of the thorax.

being subjacent to the visceral pericardium, and the latter, beneath the endocardium. The superficial plexus receives lymph from the deep plexus prior to forming right and left collecting trunks, which then pass cephalad behind the pulmonary artery to end in the tracheobronchial lymph nodes.

Stomach and Duodenum

Gastric lymphatics are continuous with esophageal lymphatics at the proximal stomach and the duodenal lymphatics at the pylorus. There are four principal lymphatic pathways and nodal groups draining the stomach (Figs. 7 and 8). The first group is the *superior gastric* lymphatics and nodes, which receive afferent lymph from both sides of the proximal stomach before draining into the celiac para-aortic lymph nodes. The second is the *pancreaticolienal* system, which drains the lateral portion of the body and fundus of the stomach. Afferent lymphatics from these areas of the stomach accompany the short gastric and left gastroepiploic vessels before entering the pancreaticolienal lymph nodes. Efferent channels from these nodes drain into the para-aortic lymph nodes. The third set of gastric lymphatics and nodes is the *inferior gastric* group, which receives lymph from the medial half of the greater curvature of the stomach. Nodes of this group lie between the two layers of the greater omen-

tum along the distal margin of the greater curvature. Efferent lymphatics from these lymph nodes pass to the subpyloric lymph nodes and eventually empty into the para-aortic celiac nodes. The *subpyloric* system drains the pyloric area. Efferent lymphatics from these nodes drain into the hepatic and superior gastric nodes, prior to emptying into the para-aortic nodes.

Afferent lymphatics from the duodenum drain into the pancreaticoduodenal lymph nodes, which lie inferiorly and posteriorly between the head of the pancreas and the duodenum. Efferent lymphatics from these nodes run cephalad to the hepatic nodes, and caudad to the para-aortic nodes at the origin of the superior mesenteric artery.

Intestinal Lymphatics

The afferent lymphatics draining the small intestine are called lacteals and, following digestion, contain white fluid called chyle. These lacteals run between the layers of the mesentery to numerous mesenteric lymph nodes, which are arranged in groups along the course of the superior mesenteric artery. The efferent vessels from these lymph node groups drain to the para-aortic nodes.

Lymphatics of the cecal and appendiceal region are extensive, perhaps because of the abundant lymphatic tissue present with the appendiceal wall. Drainage

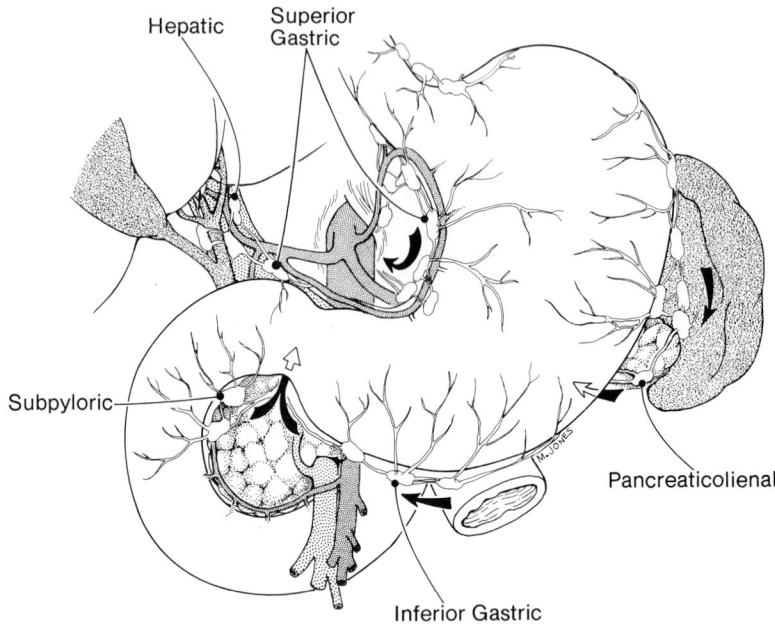

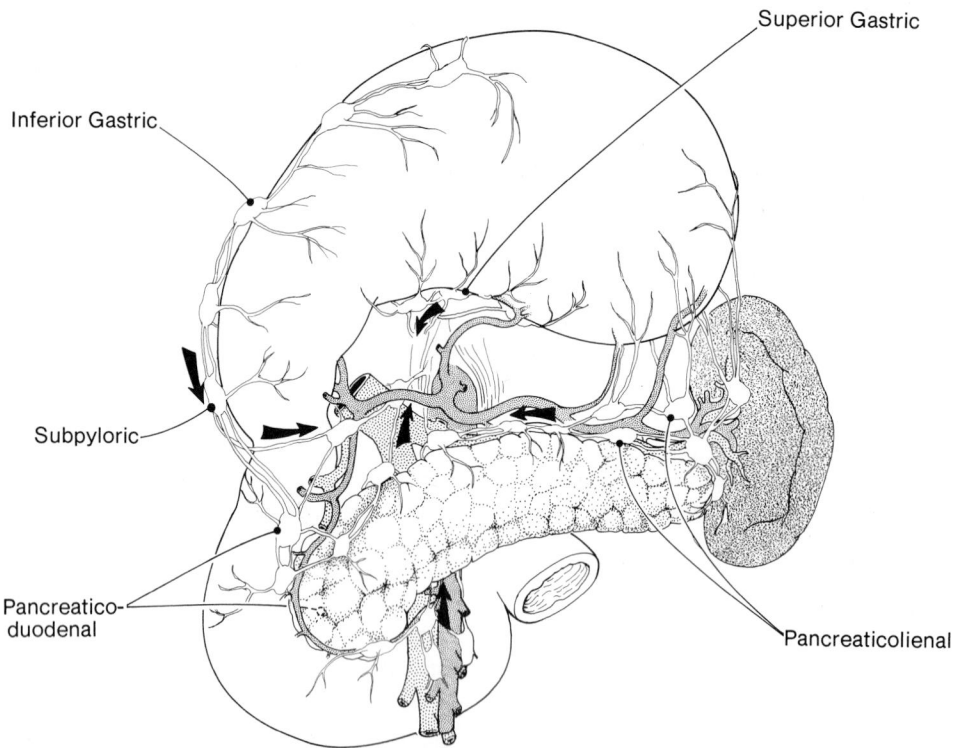

Figures 7 and 8. Lymphatic drainage and lymph nodes of the stomach and duodenum.

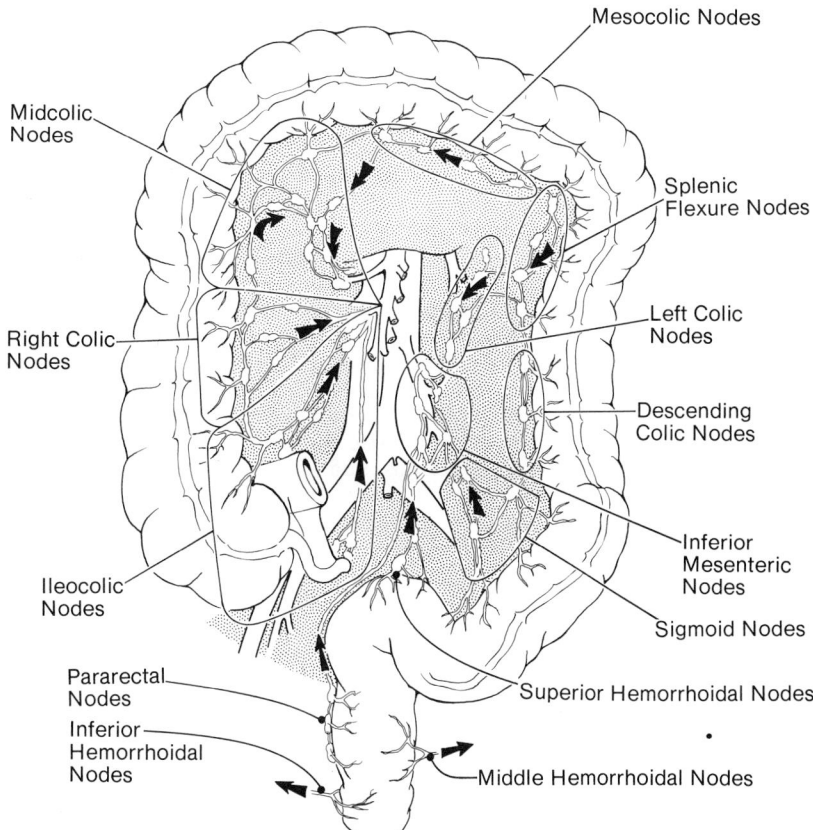

Figure 9. Lymphatic drainage and lymph nodes of the colon.

from this area ascends by way of the ileocolic lymph nodes, which are arranged along the distal ileum, the appendix, and the cecum, and which extend proximally to the trunk of the ileocolic branch of the superior mesenteric artery. These nodes drain into the para-aortic nodes (Fig. 9).

Lymphatics of the ascending and transverse colon drain to the right colic and mesocolic lymph nodes before entering the superior mesenteric nodes and ultimately the para-aortic nodes. Lymphatics of the splenic flexure, descending colon, and sigmoid colon enter a small group of lymph nodes that lie along the left colic and sigmoidal arteries and also enter another group of nodes within the sigmoid mesocolon related to the superior hemorrhoidal artery. These lymphatics eventually end in the para-aortic lymph nodes near the origin of the inferior mesenteric artery.

The rectum, anal canal, and anus drain via different pathways in spite of their close anatomic proximity. The lymphatics of the rectum traverse the pararectal nodes, which are almost contiguous with the rectum, before entering the para-aortic nodes. Lymphatics of the anal canal accompany the middle and inferior hemorrhoidal arteries and terminate in the hypogastric lymph nodes. The lymphatics of the anus accompany those of the skin of the perineum and drain primarily into the superficial inguinal lymph nodes.

Liver

Lymphatics contiguous with the falciform ligament drain both right and left lobes of the liver via two lymphatic trunks, one that accompanies the inferior vena cava through the diaphragm, and another that runs caudad and anteriorly, ending in the upper hepatic nodes which parallel the common bile duct at the porta hepatis. Lymphatics from the inferior surface of the liver drain into the porta hepatis and then to the celiac para-aortic nodes.

Deep lymphatics of the liver end in the hepatic lymph nodes, but occasionally drain cephalad in association with the hepatic veins, ending in a small group of lymph nodes at the vena cava. Lymphatics from the gallbladder and common bile duct drain to the hepatic nodes and the pancreaticoduodenal nodes. The cystic node, or "Calot's node," which lies adjacent to the common bile duct, is a member of the hepatic group of lymph nodes and is often encountered during operations for biliary inflammation and neoplasm. It should be identified when repair of the common bile duct is attempted since its relationship to the duct is almost constant.

Pancreas

Pancreatic lymphatics follow the same course as the blood vessels supplying the pancreas. These lymphatics drain into the pancreaticolienal lymph nodes, where they join other lymphatics from the spleen or empty directly into the celiac lymph nodes.

Pelvic and Retroperitoneal Lymphatics

There are both superficial and deep lymphatics in the pelvis. The former follow superficial blood vessels as they converge to the superficial inguinal lymph nodes, while the deep lymphatics parallel retroperitoneal blood vessels. The external iliac nodes drain the infraumbilical abdominal wall, the medial thigh, the external genitalia, the cervix or prostate gland, and the fundus of the bladder. The internal iliac nodes receive lymphatics from the pelvic viscera, the deeper structures of the perineum, and the buttock. The efferent lymphatics of both internal and external iliac lymph nodes are received by the common iliac nodes, which eventually drain into the para-aortic nodes.

Lumbar lymph nodes are numerous and are arranged laterally on the right and left side of the lumbar region, and centrally as the celiac, superior mesenteric, and inferior mesenteric nodes. These lumbar nodes receive efferent lymphatics from the iliac, gonadal, renal, and suprarenal lymph nodes. The efferents from the lumbar nodes either enter the cisterna chyli or connect with the lower end of the thoracic duct after piercing the diaphragm. Efferent lymphatics from the para-aortic nodes pass directly into the cisterna chyli.

The Extremities

Lymphatics of the upper extremity, both superficial and deep, follow the course of the major arm veins and pass directly to the axilla. The ulnar or basilic lymphatic vessels occasionally traverse the epitrochlear lymph nodes, and the radial, or cephalic, lymphatics occasionally drain to deltopectoral nodes. Axillary lymph nodes and lymphatics are described in the section on lymphatic drainage of the breast.

The superficial lymphatics of the leg follow the course of the greater saphenous vein medially and lesser saphenous vein laterally. Deep lymphatics of the lower extremity are not numerous, but when present, accompany the deep vascular structures. Popliteal nodes drain these deep lymphatics as well as lymphatics from the lateral aspect of the leg.

Inguinal lymph nodes are divided into superficial inguinal and subinguinal lymph nodes at the level of the confluence of the saphenous vein and the femoral vein. The superficial inguinal nodes drain the skin of the external genitalia, perineum, buttock, and the lower abdominal wall. Medial superficial lymphatics of the leg usually continue without interruption to the subinguinal group of lymph nodes, which are divided into superficial and deep systems. The deep subinguinal nodes receive the deep lymphatic trunks from the femoral vessels and from the penis or clitoris. Efferent lymphatic vessels from the inguinal lymph nodes drain above the inguinal ligament cephalad into the external iliac lymph nodes.

LYMPHANGITIS

Lymphangitis results from the introduction of bacteria into the subcutaneous tissues following an abrasion or superficial laceration of the skin. Because these cutaneous openings are the usual portals of entry, it is the superficial rather than the deep lymphatic system of the skin that is involved. The hands and feet are the most common sites for bacterial penetration and subsequent septic foci. Any organism can be the source of lymphangitis, but the most common are the beta-hemolytic streptococcus and *Staphylococcus aureus*, in that order.

Once bacteria invade and permeate the subcutaneous tissues, organisms can penetrate and progress rapidly along the lymphatic vessels. The affected lymphatics become surrounded by exudate and hyperemic areas, with the vessels gradually becoming clogged by desquamated endothelial cells, white blood cells, and coagulated lymph. The infection continues to spread along lymphatic channels until it reaches a regional lymph node. If the regional lymph node cannot contain the infection, bacteria may advance centrally to the next lymph node or may empty directly into the circulation, with resulting bacteremia or septicemia or both.

The clinical appearance of acute lymphangitis is characterized by the formation of fine, red lines, which usually spread up the arm or leg to the axillary or inguinal lymph nodes, without stopping at the epitrochlear or popliteal nodes. The erythema is the result of the inflammatory action of the invading pathogen as it progresses up the lymphatic channel. Movement of the involved extremity not only can cause discomfort but also aids in milking bacteria along the lymphatic channel. Regional lymph nodes usually become enlarged and tender within 12 to 24 hours after the first sign of infection. When there is extensive lymphatic involvement, the patient may become flushed, dehydrated, and quite ill.

Treatment of lymphangitis requires immobilization, elevation of the affected extremity, moist warm dressings, and appropriate antibiotics. Broad-spectrum antibiotics should be administered until culture and sensitivity reports are available. Surgical drainage of an area of lymphangitis is seldom required, since it is not a suppurative process. An incision into an area of inflammation can only aggravate the condition and disseminate infection. There are occasions, however, when the primary focus of infection, for example, a paronychia, should be incised, in order to afford local drainage and diminution in the number of organisms being disseminated throughout the lymphatic system.

Recovery from acute lymphangitis is usually complete, without residual lymphatic obstruction or abnormality of the lymphatic vessel. However, chronic or recurrent infection of lymphatic vessels leads to chronic lymphangitis, which may then lead to permanent damage of lymphatic structures and subsequent lymphedema.

LYMPHANGIOGRAPHY

Kinmonth, in 1955, selected the word "lymphangiography" to describe the intralymphatic injection of contrast material to visualize lymphatic vessels and the intervening lymph nodes. Earlier attempts at visualizing lymphatic vessels and nodes by injecting radiopaque material directly into a palpable lymph node had been less successful.

Technique

Following the intradermal injection of a supravital dye, such as Direct Sky Blue, a fine polyethylene catheter is secured within a stained lymphatic vessel via a surgical "cutdown." The lymphatics ordinarily used are on the dorsum of the foot for abdominal and thoracic lymphatic visualization, on the back of the hand or in the antecubital space for outlining axillary and subclavian pathways, and over the mastoid process for cervical lymphangiograms. The contrast material used for intralymphatic injection is Ethiodol, an iodine solution in an ester of poppy seed oil. This material is injected into the lymphatic at the rate of 0.1 ml. per minute, the speed of injection regulated by a constant-rate infusion pump. The maximal amount of Ethiodol used is usually 10 ml. per leg or 5 ml. per arm. Serial radiographs in several projections are taken, up to 24 hours following injection, to outline lymphatic flow, lymphatic channels, and lymph nodes.

Radiographic Appearance

Normal lymphatic vessels parallel the venous system, the major channels following the course of the greater and lesser saphenous veins in the lower extremity and the basilic vein in the upper extremity. As the dye flows toward progressively larger collecting vessels, lymph nodes are visualized as contrast material passes through them.

Lymphangiograms of the lower extremity usually show 10 to 12 lymphatic channels entering the inguinal lymph nodes. The efferent channels from the inguinal nodes are fewer in number but are of considerably larger caliber than the afferent vessels. Valves are conspicuous. Above the inguinal area, radiographs disclose iliac pathways and external, internal, and common iliac lymph nodes. Paravertebral channels carry the contrast material to the lumbar region where paravertebral or para-aortic nodes may be seen on delayed (24 hour) x-rays (Fig. 10).

The cisterna chyli and the thoracic duct are difficult to visualize radiographically. If demonstration of these structures is clinically indicated, it is necessary to massage the lower extremities and repeatedly flex and extend the hips following the injection of Ethiodol. Simultaneously, the groin and lower abdomen are massaged in order to propel contrast material in a cephalad direction. Using this technique, approximately one-fifth of subjects may demonstrate flow of dye as high as the cervical lymph nodes.

A normal lymph node on a lymphangiogram exhibits a homogenous internal architecture with a fine reticular or granular appearance. There may be a normal filling defect in the central portion at the hilum, but the contrast material is evenly distributed throughout the remainder of the node. Serial films disclose the contrast material entering the node from the peripheral afferent lymphatics, filling its central portion, and finally leaving the node via the efferent lymphatic. Customarily, nodes are more numerous

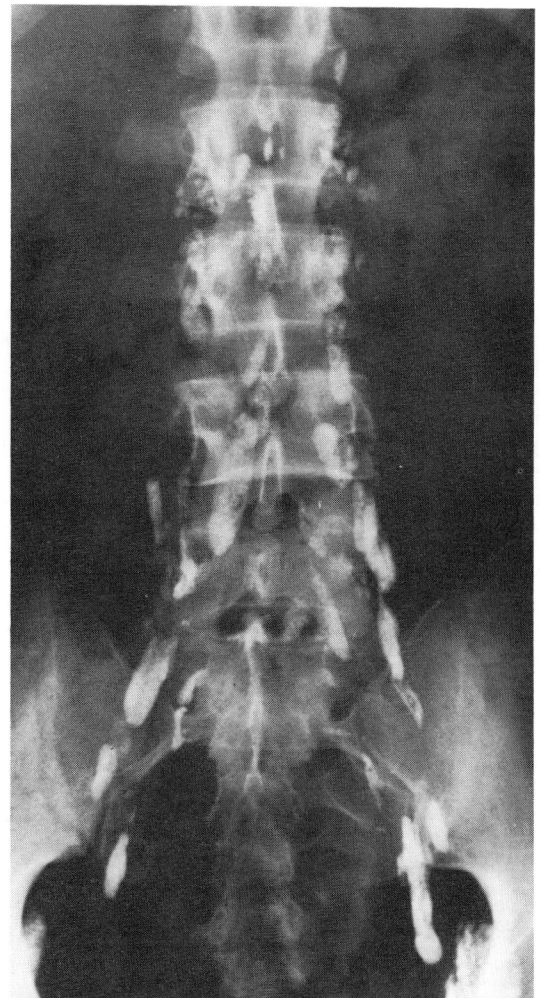

Figure 10. Abdominal radiograph obtained 24 hours after the intralymphatic injection of oily dye, showing normal lymph node arrangement and architecture. External, internal, and common iliac nodes and lumbar para-aortic nodes are well visualized.

when they are of smaller size, and conversely, they may be quite large where few in number.

Application

Initially, lymphangiography was employed primarily to differentiate among the several types of lymphedema. The uses of this technique have expanded greatly in the past decade, and include the following: (1) the study of unilateral and bilateral peripheral edema; (2) the diagnosis, prognosis, and staging of lymphomas and other lymphoproliferative diseases; (3) the evaluation of patients with chylous effusions; (4) the diagnosis of intra-abdominal, pelvic, and thoracic masses; and (5) as a guide to the surgeon in performing complete regional lymphadenectomy.

The greatest clinical experience has been gained in lymphangiography of the lower extremities, in which retroperitoneal lymphatics and nodes are visualized throughout their course. Pathologic conditions studied by this technique have included lymphatic infections and infestations, granulomatous diseases, metastastic cancer, and malignant lesions of the reticuloendothelial system, such as Hodgkin's disease and lymphosarcoma.

Complications

Occasional complications accompany lymphangiography. These are attributable either to the local effects of the surgical incision required to isolate and cannulate a peripheral lymphatic, or to a systemic reaction to the contrast material. Transient pyrexia is seen in approximately half the patients, with nausea, vomiting, headache, chills, or arthralgias reported in one fifth of patients. Wound infection has been noted in less than 10 per cent of patients undergoing lymphangiography. Complications of increasing magnitude are iodine sensitivity and anaphylaxis. Lymphangiography will cause an elevation of the serum protein-bound iodine (P.B.I.) for as long as 18 months.

The complication unique to lymphangiography is pulmonary embolization of the contrast material. The oily dye enters the pulmonary circulation via the thoracic duct, subclavian vein, and right heart, as well as by lymphaticovenous shunts below the thoracic duct. Clinical symptoms are evident in approximately 10 per cent of patients undergoing lymphangiography, and radiographic evidence of oil emboli in the lung may occur in almost half these patients (Fig. 11).

When pulmonary embolization of contrast material occurs, an alveolar-capillary block is produced in the pulmonary parenchyma. Patients in whom serial studies of pulmonary function have been done after lymphangiography show a decrease in carbon monoxide diffusion capacity of 25 per cent within 2 to 4 hours. This returns to normal over the next 2 to 3 days. Arterial Po_2 drops significantly during the first 4 hours following injection of the oily material, followed by a rapid return to normal. Measurement of vital capacity and maximal breathing capacity indicates no significant impairment of these ventilatory functions. However, the author is aware of a major hospital that routinely does not allow a general anesthetic to be administered to patients for at least one week following the performance of a lymphangiogram.

CHYLOUS EFFUSIONS

Chylothorax, chylous ascites, and chyluria are infrequently encountered clinical problems, each characterized by an effusion derived from disruption of a major lymphatic vessel. These effusions are usually rich in lipids and are milky white in color. Generally, the recognition of chylothorax or chylous ascites is made only at the time of thoracentesis or paracentesis by discovering the characteristic milky fluid instead of the serous fluid encountered with the majority of effusions. Chyluria is easily documented, since few patients ignore the passage of milky white urine.

Chylothorax

Chylothorax may follow injury to the thoracic duct, either by penetrating or closed thoracic trauma. The latter includes vertebral fracture, thoracic contusion, or indirect trauma to the thoracic duct from sudden hyperextension of the vertebral column. If there is lymphatic congestion within the mediastinum, as for instance in patients with tuberculosis, lymphoma, metastatic tumor, or filariasis, a relatively minor injury can be the precipitating factor in the disruption of the

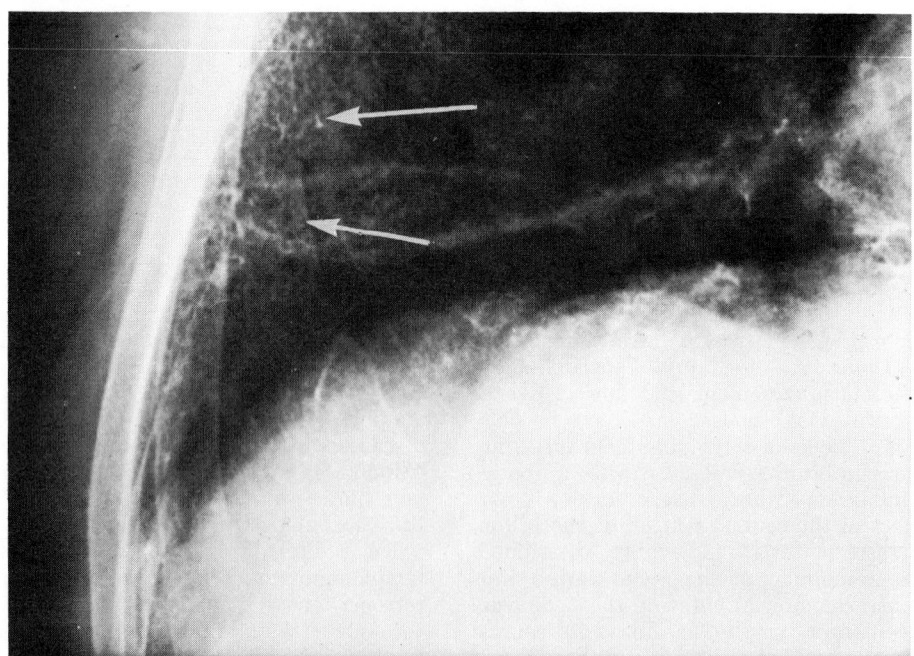

Figure 11.   PA chest radiograph showing pulmonary embolization of contrast material 24 hours after intralymphatic injection into the dorsum of the foot. The fine, reticular pattern of contrast within the pulmonary parenchyma is characteristic.

thoracic duct. When chylothorax develops secondary to malignant disease, the primary tumor is usually located in either the posterior mediastinum or the retroperitoneal region. Penetrating trauma includes direct injury to the thoracic duct by knife or gunshot, or iatrogenic injury occurring during an intrathoracic diagnostic procedure or at the time of thoracotomy.

The symptoms and signs of chylothorax are identical to those of any pleural effusion. The chylous nature of the pleural effusion is detected at the time of thoracentesis. This fluid is sterile, is usually abundant in volume, and has a high lipid content.

When a chylous pleural effusion is encountered, in the absence of an obvious cause, an extensive work-up should be undertaken, since treatment is determined by the underlying pathologic condition. This work-up may include lymph node biopsy, mediastinoscopy, and other studies to determine the presence of a lesion within the chest. Lymphangiography is the technique by which the actual site of the leak in the thoracic duct may be visualized.

Repeated thoracenteses or closed catheter drainage of the pleural cavity may be required. Frequently, these techniques control further leakage from the thoracic duct. However, thoracotomy may be necessary to ligate the thoracic duct if these maneuvers fail to control the effusion. Thoracic duct ligation may be required, even in the presence of extensive neoplastic invasion, if chylothorax is a severe problem.

Chylous Ascites

Chylous fluid is infrequently present within the peritoneal cavity at the time of birth, if an embryologic abnormality exists in the development of the lymphatic system. Usually, however, chylous ascites follows intra-abdominal lymphatic block in the area of the cisterna chyli, or less frequently, a lymphatic block within the thorax. Although chylous ascites can follow lymphatic blockage due to parasites or large inflammatory lymph nodes, the most common cause is metastatic cancer. Neoplastic invasion is reflected by dilatation of distal lymphatic vessels, lymphatic valvular insufficiency, and reversal of lymph flow. The dilated walls of distended lymphatics eventually weaken and are susceptible to rupture by minor trauma. Lymphorrhea may occur, from either the lymphatics at the site of obstruction or intestinal subserosal lymphatics. Lymphangiography in the presence of chylous ascites may demonstrate compression or distention of the lumbar collecting trunks.

In addition to the usual causes of chylous effusions, an exudative enteropathy has been described that is manifested by malabsorption, low serum calcium, increased gastrointestinal protein loss, and chylous ascites. This entity has been linked to dilatation and ectasia of the intestinal mucosal lymphatics rather than lymphatic obstruction or an abnormality of subserosal lymphatics.

Radiation therapy may prove helpful if the chylous effusion is secondary to lymph node obstruction from a radiosensitive neoplasm, such as Hodgkin's disease. Unfortunately, the treatment of chylous ascites due to invasion of lymphatic channels by metastatic tumor is rarely successful. Most often, repeated paracenteses are indicated to enhance patient comfort.

When confronted with a patient with a chylous effusion, it is always advisable to employ a fat-free diet, since a reduction in intestinal lymphatic and thoracic duct flow occurs when long-chain fatty acids are removed from the diet. If a chylous effusion rapidly recurs following aspiration, administering nothing orally may be necessary, since it has been shown that even water by mouth increases thoracic duct lymph flow. Obviously, under these conditions nutritional support must be maintained by intravenous hyperalimentation.

Chyluria

The passage of intestinal lymph in the urine, implying a communication between the urinary collecting system and the lymphatic system, is rarely encountered in the Western hemisphere. The etiology of chyluria in the overwhelming majority of cases is parasitic infestation by *Wuchereria bancrofti*, but other parasites, including Echinococcus, Ascaris, Cysticercus, and Plasmodium (malaria), have been implicated. Chyluria of nonparasitic etiology is extremely rare, but when it does occur, it usually follows trauma, or implies obstruction to the thoracic duct or cisterna chyli or both by enlarged lymph nodes, metastastic tumor, pyogenic abscess, or tuberculosis.

The pathophysiology of chyluria was described by Ackerman in 1863 and confirmed by lympangiographic studies within the past decade. Initially, partial obstruction occurs within the lymphatic vessels between the bowel and either the cisterna chyli or the thoracic duct. This obstruction leads to increased intralymphatic pressure, causing lymphangiectasis, which in turn leads to valvular incompetence and retrograde flow of chyle. Because of the fragile nature of lymphatic vessels, their close association with the renal collecting system, and lack of adequate perirenal collateral lymphatic vessels, lymphaticorenal shunts occur, resulting in chyluria.

The passage of cloudy or milky fluid in the urine may be intermittent rather than continual, since remissions of long duration can occur. The degree of chyluria is directly related to patient activity, with increased exercise causing increased lymph flow and increased chyluria. A high-fat diet also tends to increase the passage of lymph in the urine. Associated pyelonephritis occurs in a high percentage of cases of chyluria.

Lymphangiography confirms obstruction to the flow of lymph and may demonstrate not only dilated lymphatic channels with backflow toward the renal lymphatics, but even the exact site of the fistula.

The best therapy for chyluria is treatment of the pathologic process responsible for it, which, in most cases, implies the administration of antifilarial drugs. Bed rest and low-fat diet have been advocated during the course of therapy to minimize lymphatic flow.

Surgery has been advised for refractory cases of chyluria. Although controversy still exists, the surgical treatment of choice appears to be the meticulous removal of the lymphatics surrounding the renal pedicle combined with renal decapsulation. This operation has resulted in the cure of approximately 75 per cent of patients with chyluria.

TUMORS OF THE LYMPHATICS

Lymphangioma

Lymphangioma is a benign tumor of lymphatic origin encountered most frequently in young children. This tumor, commonly called cystic hygroma, is composed of soft, cystic masses which develop from lymph sacs originating from embryonic outpouchings of the venous system. Most of these lesions are found in the neck, few are located in the axilla, and the remainder are scattered throughout the body (Fig. 12). The posterior triangle of the neck is the most common single location. There is no racial or sexual predilection.

The majority of cystic hygromas appear within the first year of life, and almost 90 per cent are evident before the second year. The tumor may be large in size and, occasionally, a rapid increase in the dimensions of the mass is noted after an upper respiratory infection, probably as a result of lymphatic rupture subsequent to coughing. Another cause of sudden enlargement is hemorrhage within the lesion.

Lymphangiomas are classified into three pathologic groups: (1) *simplex*, which consists of small lymph capillaries; (2) *cavernous*, which is composed of larger lymph capillaries; and (3) *cystic*, which is the classic cystic hygroma. All three types usually coexist within the same tumor and are usually grouped together and called cystic hygroma.

Lymphangiomas contain multiple, multilocular, cystic masses, ranging in size from 0.1 to 5.0 cm. in diameter. Cysts within the larger cyst may or may not communicate. Walls are thin and delicate, and the cysts are filled with clear fluid. The endothelial lining of the cyst glistens, resembling peritoneum.

The characteristic appearance of cystic hygroma is that of a soft, cystic mass that appears fluctuant and lobulated and that is readily transilluminated. Aspiration of the cyst yields thin, watery, serous fluid, i.e.,

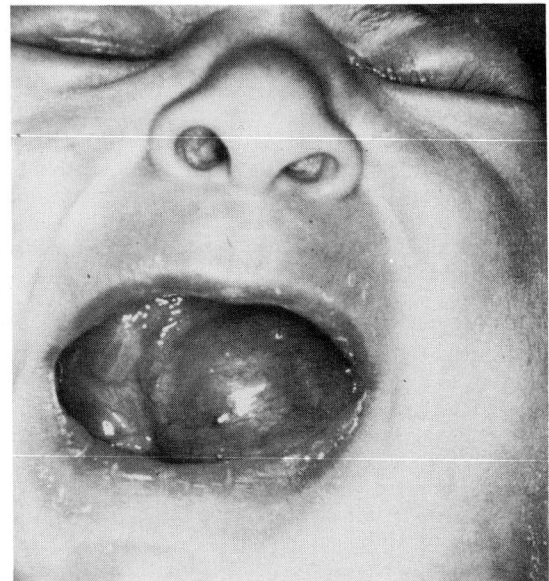

Figure 13. Lymphangioma of the floor of the mouth, necessitating urgent operation because of respiratory embarrassment.

lymph. A large cystic hygroma may cause dysphagia or dyspnea, and the rare tumor that is present in the floor of the mouth may embarrass respiration (Fig. 13). Chylothorax and chylopericardium have been infrequently reported complications. Occasional cystic hygromas extend into the mediastinum, where they may be demonstrated by chest radiography.

The only effective treatment for cystic hygroma is surgical removal. Although spontaneous regression is unlikely in large lesions, most small hygromas eventually disappear, as evidenced by the scarcity of patients in their late teens or thereafter who exhibit these lesions. Spontaneous regression occurs by irritation of the endothelial lining of the lymphatic walls, resulting in scarring and eventual obliteration, a phenomenon so frequently seen in childhood hemangiomas.

There does not appear to be any justification for early operation for this condition except in the presence of airway obstruction, repeated inflammation, or rapid enlargement. It is unnecessary and unwise to operate on an asymptomatic hygroma, exposing crucial structures in a very small neck to great surgical risk. Operation should be deferred until the patient is older, so that if surgery is still necessary, it may be performed with less chance of injury to important structures.

A cystic hygroma has no clear-cut boundaries but is simply a collection of lymphatic channels that, at their periphery, blend into the normal surrounding structures. An attempt to remove all the lymphatics, especially when they interdigitate with major nerves and vessels, may be hazardous. At operation, as much macroscopic tumor as possible should be excised, and the divided lymphatic trunks that remain should be ligated.

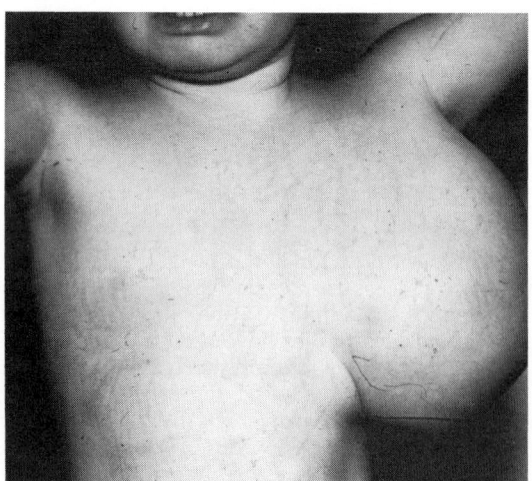

Figure 12. Lymphangioma of the axilla.

Lymphangiosarcoma

In 1948, Stewart and Treves first reported the development of lymphangiosarcoma arising in the presence of postmastectomy lymphedema of the arm. This tumor is rare, occurring in less than 0.5 per cent of patients who undergo mastectomy, and in an even smaller number of patients who have lymphedema of the lower extremity. The origin of these tumors is most likely related to lymphedema, which has been present in all reported cases. The duration of the edema is variable and has ranged from 1 to 24 years, with a mean duration of 9 years. Although most reported cases of lymphangiosarcoma have been noted in lymphedematous arms following mastectomy and radiotherapy for mammary carcinoma, this tumor has also been associated with lymphedema secondary to nonmalignant inflammatory diseases, surgical procedures, or radiation therapy alone. Despite the history of radiotherapy in a majority of patients in whom lymphangiosarcoma has developed, radiation has been considered a major cause for the development of lymphedema, rather than an apparent carcinogen per se.

Lymphangiosarcoma first appears as a blue to reddish purple discoloration or nodule in the skin. Later, small satellite nodules may form and coalesce around the original lesion (Fig. 14). The main tumor mass, as well as the satellite nodules, may ulcerate. Lymphangiosarcoma spreads by direct bloodstream invasion, resulting in visceral metastases early in the course of the disease.

Histologically, this malignant tumor shows marked lymphangiomatosis in the subcutaneous and dermal layers. Lymphatic channels are lined by endothelial cells that have foci of large, hyperchromatic, proliferating cells with bizarre, papillary, intraluminal projections. The multiple foci of abnormal cells suggest a possible multicentric origin of the tumor.

The lethal nature of lymphangiosarcoma, regardless of the treatment employed, has resulted in a pessimistic outlook. Methods of treatment have included radiation therapy, wide excision with subsequent radiotherapy, interscapulothoracic amputation with or without accompanying radiation therapy, high humeral amputation, and shoulder disarticulation, all of these with or without chemotherapy using a variety of tumoricidal agents, alone or in combination.

With these methods, only an occasional patient has survived 5 years. Half the patients are dead within 2 years of the time the appearance of the first cutaneous lesion is noted, and the mean survival time following initial definitive therapy is less than 18 months.

Because of the poor results, regardless of therapy, it is difficult to be enthusiastic about recommending any specific type of treatment. The apparent multicentricity of the disease suggests that early amputation, followed by systemic chemotherapy, might provide the best chance for survival.

LYMPHOPROLIFERATIVE DISORDERS

Malignant lymphomas or primary lymphatic neoplasms include Hodgkin's disease, lymphosarcoma, reticulum cell sarcoma, Burkitt's lymphoma, follicular lymphoma, and mycosis fungoides.

Hodgkin's disease, lymphosarcoma, and reticulum cell sarcoma account for the overwhelming majority of primary malignant lymphatic diseases and have been the subject of considerable controversy regarding classification, staging, and treatment. These neoplasms vary in clinical severity and histologic appearance, but their histologic characteristics do not necessarily correlate with their clinical course. Generally, lymphosarcoma and reticulum cell sarcoma have simple histologic patterns, with primarily a single type of proliferating cell that gradually replaces the architecture of the lymph node. Hodgkin's disease exhibits varying numbers of lymphocytes, granular cells, plasma cells, monocytes, fibroblasts, and characteristic Reed-Sternberg cells.

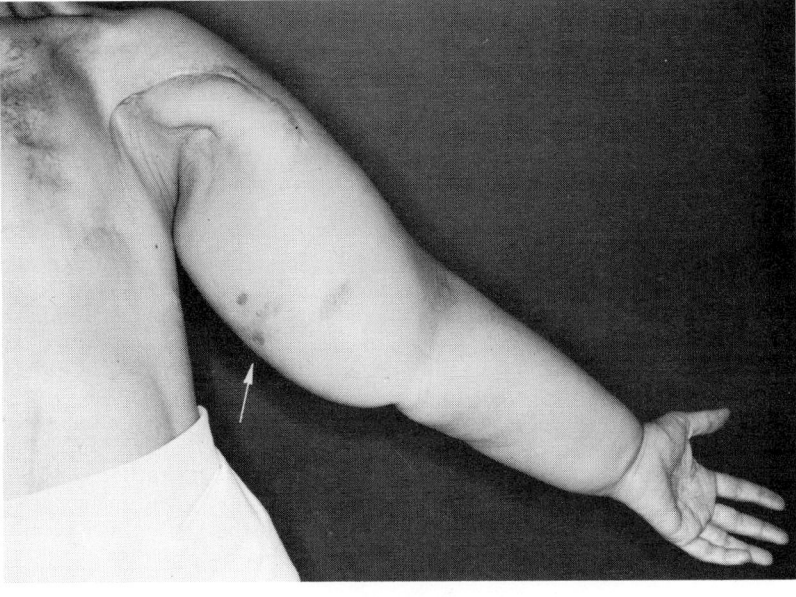

Figure 14. Fifty-one-year-old woman with 12-year history of lymphedema following radical mastectomy and radiotherapy for mammary carcinoma. Arrow denotes purple, coalescent cutaneous lesions characteristic of lymphangiosarcoma. Biopsy confirmed the diagnosis. The patient succumbed to widespread metastases less than two years later despite interscapulothoracic amputation, radiotherapy, and chemotherapy.

Hodgkin's Disease

Hodgkin's disease is a malignant process of lymph nodes that is considered unicentric in origin and is characterized by the presence of Reed-Sternberg cells with a variable proliferation of lymphocytes and histiocytes. The Reed-Sternberg cell is a large cell with abundant cytoplasm, multiple or multilobed nuclei, and prominent nucleoli.

Hodgkin's disease is clinically characterized by painless enlargement of a lymph node or group of lymph nodes, usually unilateral and frequently located in the cervical region. The disease spreads by involvement of adjacent lymph nodes so that symptoms are noted only when there is rapid enlargement of lymph nodes or when an involved lymph node impinges upon other structures. The interval between initial lymph node enlargement and progression of the disease to adjacent areas is variable, usually being much longer than that observed in lymphosarcoma or reticulum cell sarcoma.

Systemic symptoms occur early in Hodgkin's disease, fever being most prevalent. The allegedly pathognomonic Pel-Epstein fever, of alternating periods (days to weeks) of high and normal temperatures, is uncommon. If fever is an early symptom, the prognosis of the disease is allegedly poor. Lassitude, weight loss, night sweats, pruritus, and anemia with lymphopenia are additional systemic symptoms. Jaundice can occur as a result of either parenchymal liver involvement or pressure on the porta hepatis by an enlarged node, resulting in bile duct obstruction. Splenomegaly occurs in half the cases. An interesting symptom that occasionally occurs in Hodgkin's disease is pain in an involved lymph node following the ingestion of alcohol. This pain appears shortly after the alcohol is drunk and persists approximately 1 hour, the time necessary for partial oxidation of the alcohol.

Hodgkin's disease is more prevalent among Caucasians than other races, and twice as many males are affected as females. The age distribution of the disease is bimodal—a peak between 15 and 34 years of age, and a second peak over the age of 50. Extranodal Hodgkin's disease is seen infrequently, except for cutaneous manifestations that may occur in as many as one fourth of patients. These manifestations include hyperpigmentation, subcutaneous nodules, and erythematous eruptions.

In 1944, Jackson and Parker classified Hodgkins's disease into three histologic categories, Hodgkin's paragranuloma, granuloma, and sarcoma, in increasing order of aggressiveness. This classification has limited usefulness, since 80 to 90 per cent of cases fall into the granuloma category. Lukes and Butler later reclassified Hodgkin's disease into four histologic types: (1) *Lymphocyte predominance*, made up of occasional Reed-Sternberg cells and abundant lymphocytes and histocytes. This type may have a diffuse or nodular pattern, corresponds to the old paragranuloma group and has the most favorable prognosis. (2) *Nodular sclerosis*, identified by bands of doubly refractile collagen that separate the lymph node into islands of lymphoid tissue. Reed-Sternberg cells are easily visualized. (3) *Mixed cellularity*, which represents the classic Jackson-Parker granuloma. This type consists of a variety of cells including plasma cells, eosinophils, fibroblasts, and abundant Reed-Sternberg cells. (4) *Lymphocyte depletion*, characterized by few normal lymphoid cells and considerable fibrosis. Reed-Sternberg cells vary in number. In the old Jackson-Parker classification, this description corresponds to the sarcoma group and has the least favorable prognosis.

The diagnosis of Hodgkin's disease is made by histologic study of a biopsied lymph node. It is desirable to remove an entire lymph node not recently involved by inflammation, so that the pathologist has an opportunity to study nodal architecture in addition to cellular morphology.

Therapy and prognosis for patients with Hodgkin's disease are determined by accurate clinical staging. In 1966 and in 1971, an international committee proposed a classification for the clinical staging of Hodgkin's disease, which subsequently has been universally accepted. Based on the anatomic distribution of sites of involvement, this classification divides Hodgkin's disease into four distinct stages: Stage I—involvement of a single lymph node region or of a single extralymphatic organ or site. Stage II—involvement of two or more lymph node regions on the same side of the diaphragm or localized involvement of an extralymphatic organ or site and of one or more lymph node regions on the same side of the diaphragm. Stage III—involvement of lymph node regions on both sides of the diaphragm, which may also be accompanied by involvement of the spleen or by localized involvement of an extralymphatic organ or site or both. Stage IV—diffuse or disseminated involvement of one or more extralymphatic organs or tissues, with or without associated lymph node involvement.

Hodgkin's disease is further subdivided into "A" or "B" (for example, Stage IIB), describing either the absence or presence, respectively, of systemic symptoms. Fever, night sweats, and unexplained loss of 10 per cent or more of body weight in the six months preceding admission are the systemic manifestations, the presence of any of which justifies a "B" subclassification. However, weight loss of less than 10 per cent, pruritus, malaise, anemia, fatigue, leukocytosis, leukopenia, cutaneous anergy, alcohol pain, and elevated sedimentation rate are also systemic manifestations of Hodgkin's disease, but are not of sufficient significance to relegate the patient to a "B" subgroup.

To insure the accurate clinical staging of Hodgkin's disease, the following studies are desirable: (1) careful clinical history and physical examination with special attention to the presence or absence of systemic symptoms; (2) complete blood count, including differential count, hematocrit or hemoglobin, platelet count, and erythrocyte sedimentation rate; (3) chest radiographs in PA and lateral projections, plus tomograms if hilar adenopathy exists; (4) bone survey radiographs; (5) intravenous pyelogram; (6) liver function studies, including Bromsulphalein retention, alkaline phosphatase, and radioisotopic liver scan; (7) bone marrow examination, including needle biopsy of the marrow rather than simple aspiration; (8) documentation of cutaneous anergy; and (9) lymphangiography.

Until recently, hematologists and radiologists had believed that, once the tissue diagnosis of Hodgkin's disease was made, lymphangiography would confirm the clinical stage of the disease process. There is no question that lymphangiographic patterns do exist in patients with Hodgkin's disease (Fig. 15), but, despite these characteristic lymphangiographic findings, occasionally the radiographic abnormalities are indistinguishable from those encountered in pyogenic or fungal infections, other metastatic malignant diseases, or reactive hyperplasia (Figs. 16 to 18). Normally, however, the lymphangiographic findings in Hodgkin's disease occur in the following sequence. Initially, lymph nodes appear normal, but may be slightly enlarged, round, oval, or elongated, with well-demarcated peripheral sinuses. Droplets of contrast material are evenly distributed within the nodes. As Hodgkin's disease progresses, the nodes become destroyed by the malignant process, so that the resulting lymphangiogram becomes more characteristic. Lymph nodes no longer retain all the contrast material, and radiolucent filling defects become evident. Isolated neoplastic areas may produce lacuna-like filling defects that resemble moth-eaten areas of various sizes and shapes. Continued destruction of the lymph node architecture results in a coarse, foamy, cystic mottling of the lymph node pattern, caused by the contrast material being displaced to the periphery. Stasis of the entire lymph circulation may also occur. Hodgkin's

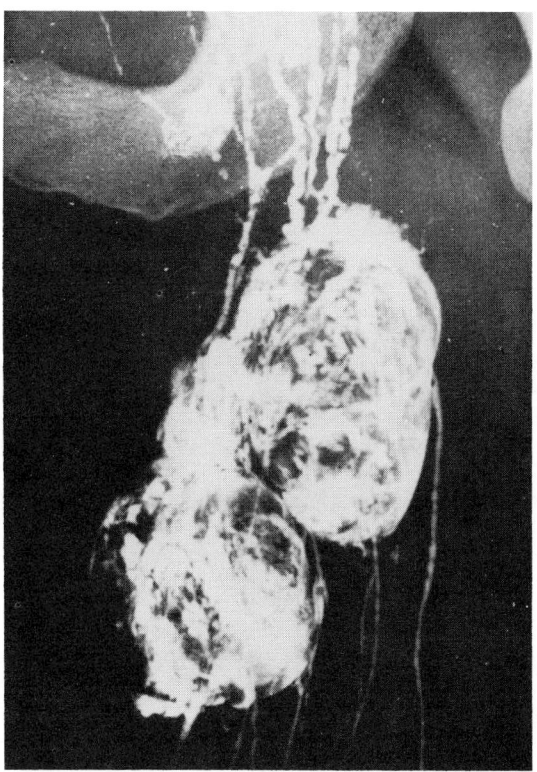

Figure 16. Enlarged inguinal lymph nodes demonstrated on 24-hour film following intralymphatic injection of oily dye, showing central and peripheral filling defects due to metastatic melanoma.

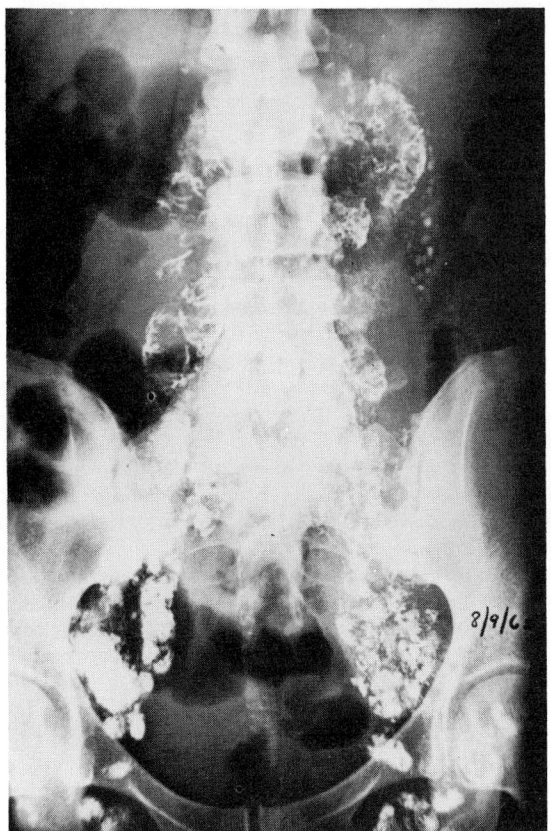

Figure 15. The lymphangiographic appearance of Hodgkin's disease involving the inguinal, iliac, and para-aortic lymph nodes. All the nodes are enlarged, with filling defects or a foamy, lacy pattern of dye distribution, or both.

disease eventually may obliterate the entire lymph node so that the contrast material is seen only in a few delicate lymphatic vessels, which skirt the involved lymph node, which is no longer itself visualized.

It should be stated that there is not complete acceptance of the value of routine lymphangiography in the clinical staging of patients with Hodgkin's disease, especially in view of the possible complications associated with the procedure. A lymphangiogram may demonstrate gross involvement of iliac and para-aortic lymph nodes but does not opacify mesenteric, celiac, or portal and splenic hilar nodes. The diagnostic reliability of the test is also open to question, since the validity rate is only 65 per cent when confirmed by a staging laparotomy.

Because staging of Hodgkin's disease has become so important in determining both therapy and prognosis, surgeons are now called upon more frequently to define the exact clinical stage of disease. Previously, the surgeon's role was merely the removal of a lymph node for histologic examination. Occasionally, laparotomy was performed in patients with hepatomegaly or abnormal liver function tests, an equivocal lymphangiogram, or splenomegaly. Other infrequent indications for laparotomy were recurrence of Hodgkin's disease after treatment, or suspicion of subsequent tumor extension following initial assessment of the disease. In those patients who underwent laparotomy, it was found that the clinical extent of disease, evaluated by lymphangiograms alone, was underestimated in almost half the patients, and in one fourth of the patients, it was necessary to restage the disease as a result of the operation.

With this retrospective evidence as a basis, several centers elected to initiate prospective studies, in which all patients with Hodgkin's disease would undergo laparotomy for clinical staging prior to initial therapy. Several significant observations have resulted. Abdominal involvement by Hodgkin's disease occurred in one fifth of the patients with normal lymphangiograms in whom no abdominal involvement was suspected. Another 20 per cent of patients with equivocal lymphangiograms, but no evidence of hepatomegaly or splenomegaly, also proved to have intra-abdominal Hodgkin's disease. Splenic involvement was difficult to ascertain before operation. Almost half of the patients with palpable or radiographically enlarged spleens failed to show splenic involvement at operation. One third of the patients with clinically normal spleens were found, at laparotomy, to have splenic involvement with Hodgkin's disease. Liver involvement rarely occurred without

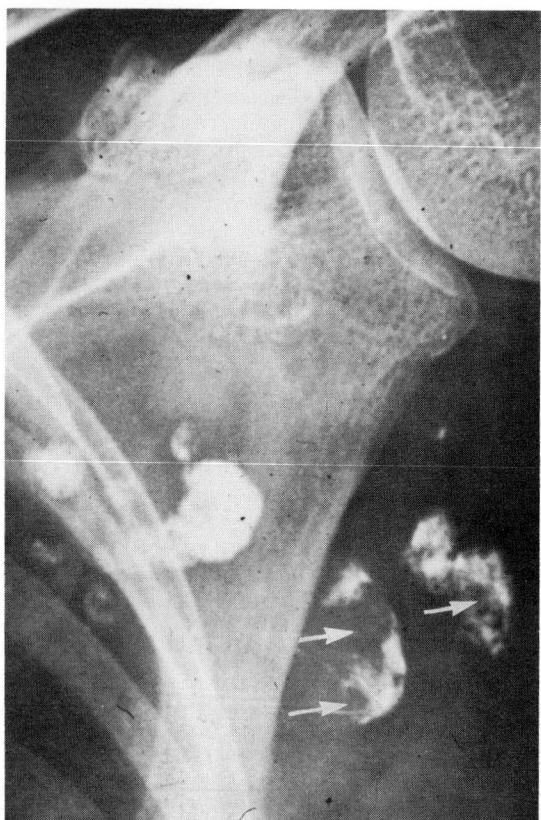

Figure 18. Lymphangiographic appearance of axillary lymph nodes enlarged and partially replaced by metastatic mammary carcinoma. Arrows indicate foci of tumor within nodes.

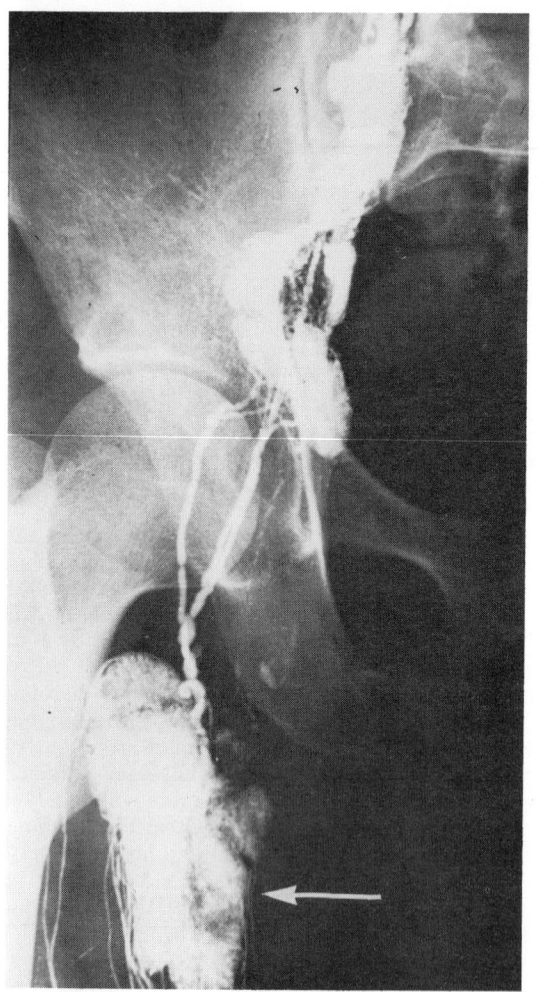

Figure 17. Enlargement of lymph nodes due to inflammation. Filling defects (arrow) caused by abscess formation within the node can be mistaken for neoplastic invasion.

concomitant splenic disease. Preoperative lymphangiographic prediction of abdominal node involvement was inconclusive, since 15 per cent of patients with negative or equivocal lymphangiograms were subsequently found to have abdominal nodal disease, and 20 per cent of patients with positive lymphangiograms did not have intra-abdominal Hodgkin's disease.

As a result of this experience with laparotomy as part of the initial work-up, surgery is at present advised for all patients with Hodgkin's disease, except those unequivocally in the Stage IV group. The maneuvers suggested at the time of surgery are as follows: (1) inspection and palpation of the abdominal viscera and retroperitoneal structures, (2) removal of all suspicious para-aortic, celiac, porta hepatis, mesenteric, splenic hilar and/or iliac nodes, (3) splenectomy, (4) liver biopsy, (5) open bone marrow biopsy from the iliac crest. In women of childbearing age, the ovaries are sutured either laterally or in the midline posteriorly to bring them out of the field of intended radiation therapy. Splenectomy is performed not only to allow its histologic examination, but also to remove a large target from the field of radiation therapy, thus decreasing possible secondary complications of left lower lobe radiation pneumonitis or radiation nephritis.

Radiation therapy is the treatment of choice for

Hodgkin's disease, and it is important that large fields be treated in continuity to avoid missing involved lymph nodes. The "mantle" field technique, as reported by Kaplan, is most commonly employed. This technique uses parallel opposing anterior and posterior fields, which are shaped to encompass all the nodes on both sides of the neck, from the mastoid tip to the supraclavicular fossa, the intraclavicular regions, both axillae, and the hilar and mediastinal nodes down to the diaphragm. Not only should the field of radiation therapy be extensive, but the dosage should be delivered with high-voltage equipment. Today's practice of using megavoltage therapy spares tissues that previously had been injured by comparable doses of low-voltage radiotherapy. Radiation burns of the skin and significant pulmonary restriction, due to radiation pneumonitis, have been minimized. In addition, severe leukopenia and thrombocytopenia have occurred less frequently since these present-day methods of radiation therapy have been employed.

Prior to the advent of clinical staging for Hodgkin's disease, prognosis was predicted by histologic classification. Clinical staging, however, has proved more accurate than histologic classification in determining the natural history of the disease, with patients in the lowest clinical stage having the best prognosis.

Present technques of high-voltage radiation therapy have not been used long enough to assess accurately long-term survival rates. Current results suggest that a majority of patients with Stages I and II disease, even in the "B" subgroup, are clinically free of disease for periods in excess of 5 years, with as many as 50 to 60 per cent of patients surviving 10 years. Improvement in prognosis has even extended to patients in Stage III who now have a relapse-free, 10-year survival rate of about 50 per cent. Patients with Stage IV disease have about a 25 per cent chance of surviving 5 years.

Patients with Stages III and IV Hodgkin's disease are frequently treated not only by radiation therapy but also with chemotherapy, using agents alone or in combination with one another. The drugs that are most often used are vincristine, nitrogen mustard, cyclophosphamide, and corticosteroids. These drugs, in addition to a variety of others, are constantly being evaluated in order to improve the efficacy of chemotherapy.

Lymphosarcoma and Reticulum Cell Sarcoma

Lymphosarcoma and reticulum cell sarcoma occur most frequently among Caucasians and involve males twice as often as females. Lymphosarcoma is two to four times more frequent than reticulum cell sarcoma. Although these tumors originate primarily within lymph nodes, 20 to 40 per cent of patients with lymphosarcoma and 30 to 60 per cent of patients with reticulum cell sarcoma have extranodal disease. Despite the usual spread of these diseases by contiguous involvement of adjacent nodes, distant metastases are frequent, and this fact has led to speculation that these neoplasms may be multifocal in origin.

Histologic sections of lymphosarcoma and reticulum cell sarcoma show a thickened capsule around matted nodes. The normal follicular pattern is lost, and there is diffuse replacement by sarcomatous cells. In lymphosarcoma, lymphocytes are present in varying degrees of maturity, whereas in reticulum cell sarcoma the cells are mainly reticulum cells. In both diseases, cells invade nodal sinuses and may extend through the node capsule into the surrounding tissues. Mitoses are frequent.

Clinically, patients with lymphosarcoma or reticulum cell sarcoma show early lymph node enlargement, which may be either unicentric or multicentric. The patient who complains of abdominal or back pain, stridor, or dyspnea may well be manifesting mediastinal or retroperitoneal nodal involvement, both of which are early symptoms in the course of these diseases. One fifth of patients with lymphosarcoma or reticulum cell sarcoma present with a systemic complaint as the first symptom of the disease.

After the initial localized symptoms occur, the disease progresses, and widespread visceral involvement is common. Effusions, both pleural and intra-abdominal, occur frequently. Hepatic parenchymal invasion or hilar node enlargement may result in jaundice. When splenomegaly occurs, it usually is late in the course of the disease. Bone lesions are demonstrated in one tenth of patients, being observed most frequently in vertebrae, femora, ribs, pelvis, and skull.

The diagnosis of lymphosarcoma or reticulum cell sarcoma is made by lymph node biopsy. Inguinal nodes should be avoided as biopsy material whenever possible, since these nodes frequently have acute and chronic inflammatory changes that add to the difficulty of accurate histologic evaluation.

Lymphosarcoma and reticulum cell sarcoma are clinically staged by means of the same criteria as are used for Hodgkin's disease. However, alternate criteria are used to allow for the frequent primary extranodal origin of both lymphosarcoma and reticulum cell sarcoma. Primary extralymphatic disease without regional lymph node enlargement is considered Stage I — for example, lymphosarcoma of the stomach, without nodal involvement. If regional node enlargement accompanies the primary extranodal disease, it is considered Stage II. When local invasion has occurred beyond the primary extralymphatic site, the disease is relegated to Stage IV even if generalized lymph node enlargement is not present.

The early stages of lymphosarcoma and reticulum cell sarcoma are usually treated with high-voltage radiation therapy. Even in the presence of advanced disease, palliative radiation therapy is indicated for such conditions as bone pain or tumor compression of a nerve.

A variety of chemotherapeutic agents are used in the treatment of advanced lymphosarcoma and reticulum cell sarcoma, the most popular being nitrogen mustard, cyclophosphamide, chlorambucil, vincristine, and corticosteroids. When effusions occur, a variety of intracavity agents may be employed, including quinacrin (Atabrine), nitrogen mustard, phosphorus-32, or ThioTEPA.

Prognosis is related to clinical stage of disease, Stages I and II demonstrating as high as 40 to 45 per cent long-term survival following therapy. Stages III and IV imply a more pessimistic outlook.

Burkitt's Lymphoma

In 1958, Burkitt described an unusual variety of lymphosarcoma among native childen in tropical Africa. He observed that this tumor accounted for almost half of all childhood malignant diseases in this part of the world. It was also noted that this tumor has a high incidence of maxillary and mandibular involvement, common association with abdominal or retroperitoneal masses, which implies ovarian or renal invasion, and infrequent involvement of the spleen or lymph nodes.

Epidemiologic data indicated that this tumor, which has since become known as Burkitt's lymphoma, occurred in areas of Africa where the temperature rarely fell below 60° F., and the rainfall was always in excess of 20 inches per year. These data suggest that Burkitt's lymphoma is infectious in origin and is transmitted by an insect vector. Another hypothesis for the etiology is that this tumor is a response to a viral infection, since two viruses have been isolated from patients with Burkitt's lymphoma, a reovirus type 3, encountered in up to 25 per cent of the patients studied, and a herpes group Epstein-Barr virus, which has been grown in tissue cultures of the lymphomatous cells.

Burkitt's lymphoma is highly sensitive to chemotherapeutic agents and, on occasion, large mandibular or maxillary lesions have rapidly disappeared following administration of systemic drugs. This disease is apparently less virulent than other malignant diseases of lymph nodes, demonstrating frequent long-term remissions.

Follicular Lymphoma

This infrequently encountered disease was initially called giant follicle lymphoblastoma because of multiple follicle-like nodules within lymphoid tissue. It was thought to have a relatively benign course but occasionally, after an indeterminate length of time, become transformed into lymphosarcoma, reticulum cell sarcoma, or Hodgkin's disease. Since all the lymphomatous diseases may histologically exhibit a follicular or a diffuse pattern at some time in their course, it is questioned whether follicular lymphoma is truly a separate entity or simply a different manifestation of the natural history of lymphoproliferative growth.

The clinical picture of follicular lymphoma occurs twice as often in men as in women, usually after the age of 40, and is characterized by extremely large lymph nodes, occasionally exceeding 5 cm. in diameter. Although systemic symptoms in this condition are rare, enlargement of liver, spleen, and retroperitoneal nodes is the rule. Diagnosis is made by lymph node biopsy, which usually shows prominent lymphoid follicles that are widely distributed throughout the node and not confined only to the cortex. The treatment of choice in follicular lymphoma is radiation therapy. If splenomegaly or hypersplenism is a problem, splenectomy or corticosteroids or both are recommended.

Mycosis Fungoides

This uncommon disease is a variant of lymphoma, in which the first manifestation is a cutaneous eruption. There are three characteristic periods defined in the natural history of this disease: (1) the premycotic period, during which the patient may complain of a nonspecific skin eruption; (2) the stage of infiltration and plaque formation, during which an intradermal infiltrate is noted; and (3) the tumor stage, wherein cellular aggregates within the skin form tumors which invade the subcutaneous tissues. Histologically, these tumors look like lymphosarcoma or reticulum cell sarcoma.

Histologic diagnosis may be made if a cutaneous lesion is biopsied in either the infiltrative or the tumor stage of the disease. However, in the premycotic period, histologically and clinically the lesions resemble psoriasis, eczema, or other benign skin eruptions.

Lymph node enlargement may occur in the infiltrative and tumor stages, but biopsy of an enlarged lymph node may not be diagnostic, because all degrees of lymphoreticular proliferation may be encountered. Lymph node morphology may remain normal despite the presence of disseminated mycosis fungoides.

Although the premycotic stage may last as long as 20 years, prognosis in mycosis fungoides is very poor. Treatment includes local therapy to the cutaneous lesions with nitrogen mustard, topical corticosteroids, or radiation therapy, alone or in combination, with or without associated systemic chemotherapy.

LYMPHEDEMA

Lymphedema of the extremities has been known since antiquity and long recognized as a consequence of lymphatic obstruction. The classification of lymphedema differentiates the primary, or idiopathic, type from secondary lymphedema, which results from the absence, obstruction, or interruption of lymphatic channels (Table 1).

Primary Lymphedema

Primary, or idiopathic, lymphedema is divided into three subgroups based upon the age at which it becomes apparent. *Lymphedema congenita* indicates lymphedema present at birth or shortly thereafter (Fig. 19). Of all patients affected by primary lymphedema, less than 10 per cent are in the congenital category. Within this group of patients with congenital lymphedema exists a unique subgroup, originally described by Milroy in 1892 as having "chronic hereditary edema." He identified 22 patients with this condition in a 97-member family representing six generations. These patients had a family history of congenital edema of the limbs. Kinmonth and his associates reported 107 patients with primary lymphedema, less than 10 per cent are in the congenital cateonly two in whom it was also hereditary. Therefore, the classic requirement that "Milroy's disease' be both hereditary and congenital makes its actual occurrence today extremely rare.

If primary lymphedema occurs between early childhood and the third decade of life, it is called *lymphedema praecox*. The largest number of patients with primary lymphedema fall into this category, with females predominating over males in the ratio of three to one.

TABLE 1. Classification of Lymphedema*

A. Primary
  1. Congenita
  2. Praecox
  3. Tarda
B. Secondary
  1. Infection and infestations
    a. Parasitic
    b. Pyogenic
    c. Fungal
  2. Mechanical, chemical, and physical trauma
    a. Abrasions or lacerations
    b. Burns
    c. Chemical irritation
    d. Radiation therapy
  3. Granulomas
    a. Lymphogranuloma venereum
    b. Syphilis
    c. Tuberculosis
    d. Sarcoid
  4. Postphlebitic
  5. Surgery
    a. Removal of lymph nodes
    b. Removal of lymph vessels
  6. Neoplastic invasion of lymph nodes
  7. Dependency edema

*Modified from Nomenclature and Criteria for Diagnosis of Diseases of the Heart and Blood Vessels. New York Heart Association, 1953.

Those patients with lymphedema occurring after the age of 30 have *lymphedema tarda*.

It is unlikely that the three classifications of primary lymphedema listed here characterize three separate pathophysiologic states. It is more likely that the natural history of the progressive lymphatic insufficiency is divisible into three different periods. If at birth there is an insufficient number of normal lymphatic channels, early lymphedema, i.e., lymphedema congenita, results. If a patient is born with lymphatics that are marginal in quality or quantity, repeated trauma throughout childhood may damage a significant number of these lymphatics, so that lymphatic drainage eventually becomes compromised. If this lymphatic inadequacy becomes evident about the time of puberty, the condition is considered lymphedema praecox. If the damage to lymphatic channels does not become manifest until later in life, the patient is placed in the lymphedema tarda group.

Prior to the advent of lymphangiography, it was assumed that primary lymphedema was most likely due to the absence of lymphatic channels. However, lymphangiography has demonstrated that lymphatic aplasia is relatively infrequent, but that hypoplasia and other lymphatic defects are responsible for the majority of cases of primary lymphedema. Kinmonth and his associates demonstrated hypoplastic lymphatics in 55 per cent of patients with primary lymphedema, but aplasia in only 14 per cent. Twenty-four per cent of patients exhibited hyperplastic, or dilated, lymphatics. An additional radiologic finding in occasional patients with primary lymphedema is reflux of contrast material from collecting lymphatic vessels to the superficial dermal plexus of lymphatics, so-called "dermal backflow" (Fig. 20).

Another small group of patients with primary lymphedema have broad, tortuous lymphatics with incompetent or absent valves, a condition designated as "lymphangiectasia." There is no familial tendency in this group, and neither sex predominates. These patients frequently have capillary angiomas over their limbs and trunks.

One third of patients with gonadal dysgenesis (Turner's syndrome) have primary lymphedema of the lower extremities at birth, caused by hypoplastic distal lymphatic vessels. This group represents a very small portion of the total number of patients with primary lymphedema.

Secondary Lymphedema

Secondary lymphedema results from the obstruction or interruption of previously normal lymphatic channels. This interference with lymph flow results in the back-up of lymph within distal lymphatic channels, which eventually becomes reflected in increased tissue fluid in the interstitial space. The distention of the in-

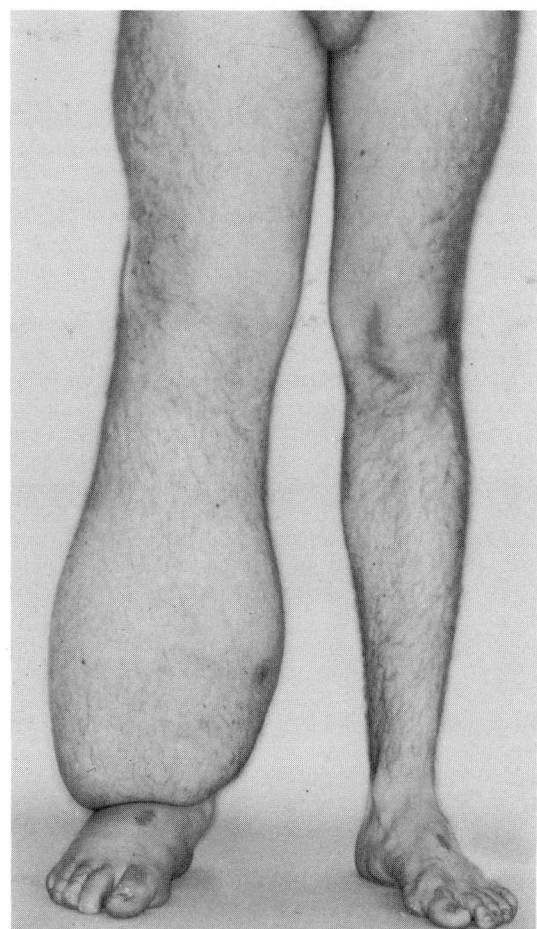

Figure 19. Congenital lymphedema. Twenty-four-year-old white male with progressive swelling of the right lower extremity noted since birth. (From Goldsmith, H. S., and De los Santos, R.: Surg. Gynecol. Obstet., *125*:607, 1967.)

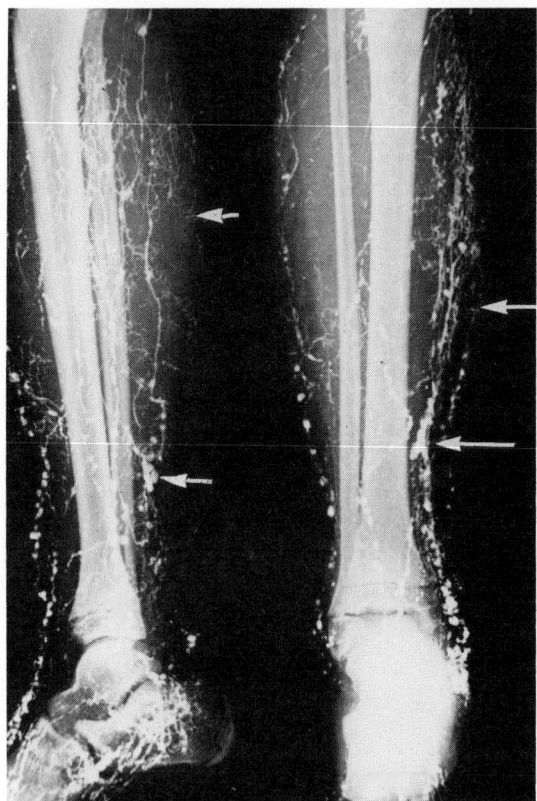

Figure 20. Lymphedema. Fourteen-year-old girl with progressive lymphedema of the right leg. Lymphangiogram demonstrates dermal backflow (upper arrows) and hypoplastic lymphatics with lymphangiectasia (lower arrows) in both lateral *(left)* and AP *(right)* projections.

toneal lymphatics, and renal pelvis. Acute symptoms result from an allergic response to the products of living and dead worms. However, microfilariae are often demonstrable in the blood without clinical symptoms.

In temperate climates, secondary lymphedema is usually due to the surgical interruption or removal of lymphatics, radiation therapy, or malignant disease. The most common surgical procedure associated with secondary lymphedema is radical mastectomy, which, in up to one quarter of patients, is followed by some degree of edema of the ipsilateral upper extremity. The temporal relationship between this operation and the onset of lymphedema is quite variable, with edema of the arm developing at any time from the early postoperative period to many years thereafter.

Radical groin dissection is another operative procedure frequently followed by edema of the ipsilateral extremity. Since any interference with *per primam* wound healing increases the likelihood of subsequent lymphedema, meticulous attention to wound care is particularly important in this operation.

Halsted first called attention to the relationship between infection and the subsequent development of lymphedema. Infection superimposed upon surgically interrupted lymphatics leads to further compromise of remaining lymphatic channels. Radiation therapy, by injuring the lymphatic endothelium, can also result in secondary lymphedema.

Malignant disease may present with secondary lymphedema as its first manifestation. Carcinoma of the cervix, with widespread pelvic involvement causing lymphedema of a lower extremity, is an example.

Treatment

Conservative measures enable the majority of patients with lymphedema to lead a relatively normal life. Recommendations for treatment include elevation of the involved extremity, prevention of infection, weight reduction, fluid and salt restriction, and local therapy using compression bandages or pulsatile air pressure devices. If fluid retention is difficult to control, diuretics may be necessary, especially in the premenstrual period.

Acute lymphangitis is particularly threatening to patients with or predisposed to the development of lymphedema. Even a minor abrasion or infection can lead to severe systemic manifestations, such as chills, high fever, and septicemia. Recurrent episodes of lymphangitis are invariably associated with progressive lymphedema, which becomes increasingly more difficult to treat effectively. Any patient with lymphedema who has had more than one bout of lymphangitis is a candidate for long-term antibiotic prophylaxis. Such therapy will render 80 per cent of patients free from further attacks of lymphangitis.

Fortunately, only a small proportion of patients with lymphedema require surgical treatment. The classic indications for surgery are the following: (1) increasing size of limb despite aggressive medical treatment, (2) significant functional impairment, (3) serious skin changes, (4) recurrent bouts of infection despite adequate attempts at prophylactic antibiotic therapy, and (5) severe emotional disturbances because of the appearance of the involved limb.

terstitial space by this increased tissue fluid puts traction on connective tissue fibers attached to lymphatic capillaries. The lymphatic valves thus become incompetent and can no longer prevent the pull of gravity from exerting its downward and peripheral effect upon the lymph column. A cycle of lymph stasis, insterstitial fluid overload, and lymphatic valve incompetence becomes established.

The most common cause of secondary lymphedema is parasitic infestation by the mosquito-borne nematode, *Wuchereria bancrofti*. The mosquitoes that carry this parasite deposit the filarial larvae subcutaneously. The larvae migrate via blood and lymphatic vessels to various sites throughout the body, where they mature into adults and produce microfilaria. The adult worms live primarily in lymphatic vessels and nodes, where repeated episodes of inflammation and infection can cause lymphatic obstruction, which in turn can result in massive lymphedema or elephantiasis.

The presumptive diagnosis of acute filariasis depends upon characteristic clinical findings in conjunction with a history of exposure to mosquitoes in an endemic area. Clinically, the patients manifest chills, fever, and malaise, which may last several weeks. Specific target areas most susceptible to inflammation are the epididymis, spermatic cord, testis, retroperi-

The large number of different operations devised to correct lymphedema are modifications of three basic procedures: (1) an attempt to stimulate the formation of new lymphatic channels, (2) the removal of large segments of lymphedematous tissue, and (3) the transfer of normal lymphatics into a lymphedematous extremity. The first of these procedures, namely the subcutaneous implantation of threads or tubes of foreign materials to stimulate lymphatic growth, has not been effective and has generally been discarded.

The second category of procedures is based on the excision of large volumes of diseased tissue, not only to improve patient appearance but in an effort to encourage anastomoses between remaining superficial lymphatics and those deep to the excised fascia. This type of operation was popularized by Kondoleon and Charles and subsequently modified by others. Unfortunately, none of these procedures has been consistently successful in alleviating the cosmetic and functional disabilities of patients with lymphedema.

New surgical techniques designed to transfer normal lymphatic channels from a healthy area into a lymphedematous limb are gaining in popularity. Thompson has suggested an operation that buries an intact dermal flap to aid in lymph drainage. This is accomplished by excising skin and subcutaneous tissue in a longitudinal plane along the edematous extremity, leaving a 1 inch wide dermal flap. This long flap is tucked into the deep tissues and sutured in place. Theoretically, the intact lymphatics within the buried flap will act as a conduit for lymphatic drainage.

Another operation advocated as a means for re-establishing centripetal lymphatic flow is the transposition of the intact omentum, with its own rich lymphatic and blood supply, into the lymphedematous extremity. It is technically possible to tailor the omentum sufficiently to allow its transfer from the peritoneal cavity into any involved limb. Connections between omental lymphatics and deep lymphatics of an affected limb have been demonstrated lymphangiographically, and the procedure has been found to be effective in approximately one third to one half of patients.

Each advocate of a particular procedure for treating lymphedema tends to be enthusiastic about the results of his favorite operation. This enthusiasm for a single procedure makes it difficult for an investigator to alternate various operations among the few patients with lymphedema he is called upon to treat. Even though the author personally continues to use omental transposition for patients with lymphedema, it is difficult at present to draw valid conclusions from available published data as to the operation of choice for the individual patient with lymphedema.

ACKNOWLEDGMENT

The author wishes to thank Dr. K. F. Lee, Professor of Radiology, Jefferson Medical College, for the lymphangiograms used in this chapter.

SELECTED REFERENCES

Glatstein, E., Guernsey, J. M., Rosenberg, S. A , and Kaplan, H. S.: The value of laparotomy and splenectomy in the staging of Hodgkin's disease. Cancer, 24:709, 1969.

This important current reference presents a study in a series of patients that forms the basis for the expanding use of exploratory laparotomy and splenectomy in "staging" patients with Hodgkin's disease. This approach is well supported by early data, but, as the authors emphasize, further investigation is needed to define and confirm its eventual clinical usefulness.

Kaplan, H. S.: Clinical evaluation and radiotherapeutic management of Hodgkin's disease and the malignant lymphomas. N. Engl. J. Med., 278:892, 1968.
This is a classic presentation on the radiotherapeutic management of Hodgkin's disease and other lymphomas.

Kaplan, H. S., and Rosenberg, S. A.: Hodgkin's disease: Current recommendations for management. Ca. 25:306, 1975.
A concise review of the various therapeutic recommendations for patients with Hodgkin's disease.

Kinmonth, J. B., Taylor, G. W., Tracy, G. D., and Marsh, J. D.: Primary lymphedema. Br. J. Surg., 45:1, 1957.
This is an excellent discussion of primary lymphedema.

O'Brien, P. H., Wallace, K., and Rambo, V. B.: Recent advances and controversies in the management of Hodgkin's disease. Surg. Gynecol. Obstet., 140:445, 1975.
A recent collective review on the problems and various treatments associated with Hodgkin's disease.

Pomerantz, M.: Lymphangiography. Surg. Clin. North Am., 49:1451, 1969.
This is a review of the various techniques and clinical indications for the use of lymphangiography together with the results.

REFERENCES

1. Aisenberg, A. C.: Hodgkin's disease—prognosis, treatment, and etiologic and immunologic considerations. N. Engl. J. Med., 270:508, 1964.
2. Alday, E. S., and Goldsmith, H. S.: Surgical technique for omental lengthening based on arterial anatomy. Surg. Gynecol. Obstet., 135:103, 1972.
3. Barrowman, J., and Roberts, K. B.: The role of the lymphatic system in the absorption of water from the intestine of the rat. Q. J. Exp. Physiol., 52:19, 1967.
4. Collette, J. M., Jantet, G., and Schoffeniels, E. (Eds.): New trends in basic lymphology. Experientia, Suppl. 14, 1966.
5. Crandall, L. A., Jr., Barker, S. B., and Graham, D. G.: A study of the lymph flow from a patient with thoracic duct fistula. Gastroenterology, 1:1040, 1943.
6. DeVita, V. T., Serpick, A. A., and Carbone, P. P.: Combination chemotherapy in the treatment of advanced Hodgkin's disease. Ann. Intern. Med., 73:881, 1970.
7. Glatstein, E., Guernsey, J. M., Rosenberg, S. A., and Kaplan, H. S.: The value of laparotomy and splenectomy in the staging of Hodgkin's disease. Cancer, 24:709, 1969.
8. Goldman, J. M.: Laparotomy for staging of Hodgkin's disease. Lancet. 1:125, 1971.
9. Goldsmith, H. S.: Lymphangiosarcoma in the lymphedematous extremity. Ca., 17:213, 1967.
10. Goldsmith, H. S.: The treatment of post-surgical lymphedema. Surg. Clin. North Am., 49:407, 1969.
11. Goldsmith, H. S., De los Santos, R., and Beattie, E. J.: Relief of chronic lymphedema by omental transposition. Ann. Surg., 166:573, 1967.
12. Goldsmith, H. S.: Long term evaluation of omental transposition for chronic lymphedema. Ann. Surg., 180:847, 1974.
13. Guyton, A. C.: Textbook of Medical Physiology, 4th ed. Philadelphia, W. B. Saunders Company, 1971, Chapter 21, The lymphatic system, interstitial fluid dynamics, and edema.
14. Hugo, H. E.: Recent advances in the treatment of lymphedema. Surg. Clin. North Am., 51:111, 1971.
15. Kadin, M. E., Glatstein, E., and Dorfman, R. F.:Clinicopathologic studies of 117 untreated patients subjected to laparotomy for the staging of Hodgkin's disease. Cancer, 27:1277, 1971.
16. Kaplan, H. S.: Clinical evaluation and radiotherapeutic management of Hodgkin's disease and the malignant lymphomas. N. Engl. J. Med., 278:892, 1968.
17. Kinmonth, J. B., Taylor, G. W., and Harper, R. K.: Lymphangiography—a technique for its use in the lower limb. Br. Med. J., 1:940, 1955.
18. Kinmonth, J. B., Taylor, G. W., Tracy, G. D., and Marsh, J. D.: Primary lymphedema. Br. J. Surg., 45:1, 1957.

19. Lewis, S. R., and Smith, J. R.: Lymphedema. *In* Converse, J. M. (Ed.) Reconstructive Plastic Surgery, 2nd ed. Philadelphia, W. B. Saunders Company, 1977.
20. Mayerson, H. S.: The physiologic importance of lymph. *In* American Physiological Society: Handbook of Physiology. Section 2, Circulation. P. Dow (Ed.). Baltimore, Williams & Wilkins Company, Volume 2, 1963.
21. Mayerson, H. S. (Ed.): Lymph and the Lymphatic System. Springfield, Ill., Charles C Thomas, Publisher, 1968.
22. Mayerson, H. S.: Three centuries of lymphatic history—an outline. Lymphology, 2:143, 1969.
23. O'Brien, P. H., Sherman, J. O., Brand, W. N., and Scarff, J. E.: Lymphangiography. Surg. Gynecol. Obstet., *126*:131, 1968.
24. Pomerantz, M.: Lymphangiography. Surg. Clin. North Am., *49*:1451, 1969.
25. Rosenberg, S. A.: Report of the committee on the staging of Hodgkin's disease. Cancer Res., *26*:Part I, 1310, 1966.
26. Rusznyak, I., Foldi, M., and Szabo, G.: Lymphatics and Lymph Circulation. New York, Pergamon Press, 1960.
27. Ruttiman, A.: Progress in Lymphology. Stuttgart, Georg Thieme Verlag, 1967.
28. Shannon, A. D., and Lascelles, A. K.: Effect of skim-milk feeding on the flow and composition of thoracic duct and intestinal lymph in young calves. Aust. J. Biol. Sci., *22*:197, 1969.
29. Thompson, N.: The surgical treatment of chronic lymphedema of the extremities. Surg. Clin. North Am., *47*:445, 1967.
30. Viamonte, M., Koehler, P. R., Witte, M., and Witte, C.: Progress in Lymphology, II. Stuttgart, Georg Thieme Verlag, 1970.
31. Yoffey, J. M., and Courtice, F. C.: Lymphatics, Lymph, and the Lymphomyeloid Complex. New York, Academic Press, 1970.

51

DISORDERS OF SYSTEMIC VEINS

John Ludbrook, M.D., F.R.A.C.S.,
and Glyn G. Jamieson, F.R.A.C.S.

FUNCTIONAL AND SURGICAL ANATOMY

The description that follows concentrates on the anatomic features of veins (particularly of the lower limbs) that are relevant either to their function or to the disorders that affect their function. The emphasis is thus somewhat different from that found in most anatomic texts.

Wall Structure

All veins that are visible to the naked eye, from venules to the venae cavae, have certain features in common. They possess *smooth muscle* in their walls, unless they are rigidly enclosed by bone or by the cranium. The more dependent a vein is in the standing posture (and thus the higher the hydrostatic blood pressure within it), the thicker is its wall in relation to the diameter of its lumen. The smooth muscle layer is thicker in the actively contractile subcutaneous veins than in the almost inert deep veins (Fig. 1). In the great veins of the trunk, the smooth muscle is arranged as a long spiral, while in the contractile subcutaneous veins of the limbs it is nearly circular in disposition. The density of *innervation* of veins by sympathetic constrictor fibers is approximately proportional to the smooth muscle content of the vein wall. Sensory endings (pain receptors, and perhaps mechanoreceptors) are present in subcutaneous veins. The *vasa vasorum* of veins, unlike those of arteries, do not communicate with the lumen.

Valves

Most veins possess valves: two frail cusps attached to a point of thickening of the vein wall (the valve ring). There is a dilatation of the vein wall immediately downstream from the valve ring (the valve sinus). There are general rules about the frequency distribution of valves, and about the direction in which they face (Fig. 2). They tend to be located immediately distal to a point of entry of a major tributary, and the orifices of the major tributaries themselves usually bear valves. In the limbs, valves usually direct blood flow from distal to proximal, and from superficial to deep. Notable exceptions are the perforating veins of the hands, feet, and forearm, in which flow is from deep to superficial. Valves occur with greater frequency distally in a limb than proximally. Valveless veins of note are venae cavae; the brachiocephalic, common iliac, renal, and hepatic veins; and the portal, mesenteric, and splenic veins.

Gross Anatomy of the Limb Veins

Each limb has three anatomically and functionally distinguishable sets of veins:

1. *Subcutaneous* (superficial). These have relatively thick, muscular walls. The major trunks run in tunnels, created by a condensation of the superficial fascia and lined by areolar tissue. Each limb has two major superficial systems of veins that intercommunicate freely with each other as well as with the deep veins. Each superficial system ends by penetrating the deep fascia to enter a major deep vein.

2. *Deep* (intermuscular, intramuscular). These have thin, scantily muscled walls. The intermuscular veins accompany named arteries, taking the form of a plexus below the level of the elbow or knee, and forming a single major vein toward the root of the limb.

3. *Perforating* (communicating) veins. These, too, are thin-

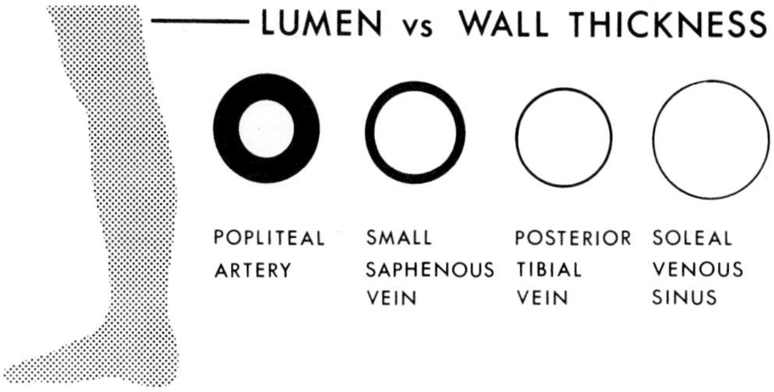

Figure 1. Relation of wall thickness to lumen diameter for an artery, subcutaneous vein, intermuscular vein, and intramuscular vein in the leg. (After Ludbrook, J.: Aspects of Venous Function in the Lower Limbs, 1966. Courtesy of Charles C Thomas, Publisher, Springfield, Ill.)

LUMEN vs WALL THICKNESS

POPLITEAL ARTERY

SMALL SAPHENOUS VEIN

POSTERIOR TIBIAL VEIN

SOLEAL VENOUS SINUS

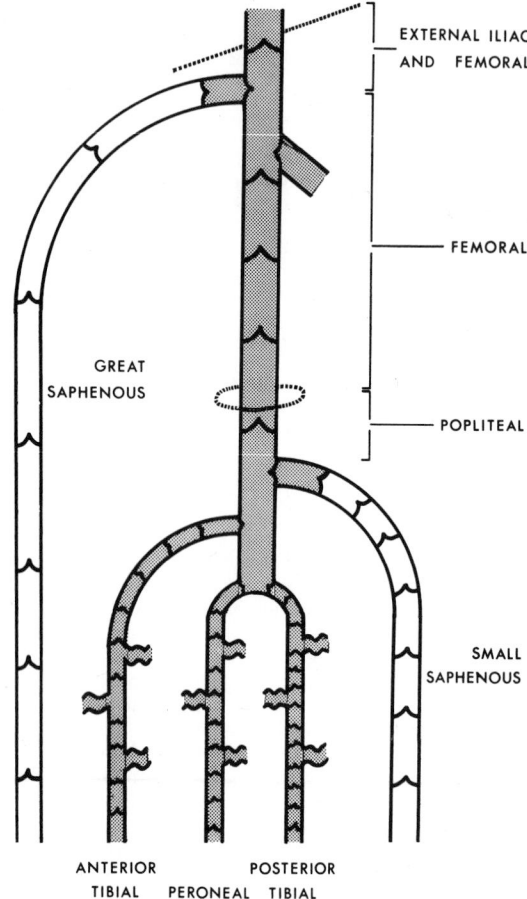

Below the knee, numerous *perforating veins* (Fig. 4) join tributaries of the great saphenous vein to the deep veins of the leg. The most important from the surgical point of view is the medial set, which joins the posterior arch complex of veins to the venae comitantes of the posterior tibial artery, and the anteromedial set running close to the periosteum of the tibia. An anterolateral set enters the anterior tibial vein. In the thigh, a perforating vein often joins the great saphenous vein (or a tributary) to the femoral vein (or its subsartorial tributary).

The *small saphenous vein* (see Fig. 3) begins at a point midway between the Achilles tendon and the posterior border of the lateral malleolus. It passes almost vertically to the middle of the popliteal fossa, accompanied by the *sural nerve* and by lymphatics. It penetrates the deep fascia at about the middle of the leg. It usually enters the deep system (the popliteal vein) in the middle of the popliteal fossa, but the precise level is variable. A posterolateral set of *perforating veins* (see Fig. 4) joins its tributaries to the peroneal vein, while less constant perforating veins enter calf muscle veins.

Figure 2. Frequency distribution of valves in the veins of the lower limb, based on averaged data from published reports. (After Ludbrook, J.: Aspects of Venous Function in the Lower Limbs. 1966. Courtesy of Charles C Thomas, Publisher, Springfield, Ill.)

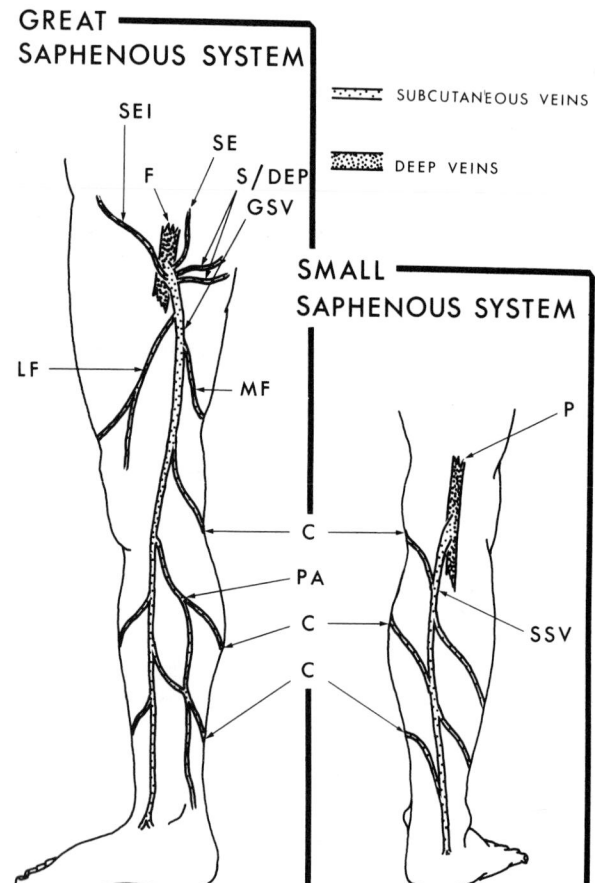

Figure 3. Diagrammatic representation of the courses and tributaries of the saphenous veins. *GSV* = great saphenous veins; *SSV* = small saphenous vein; *F* = femoral vein; *P* = popliteal vein; *SEI, SE, S/DEP, LF, MF* = superficial circumflex iliac, superficial epigastric, superficial and deep external pudendal, lateral femoral, medial femoral trubutaries; *PA* = posterior arch vein; *C* = short saphenous–great saphenous communicating veins.

walled. They pass through the deep fascia to link the superficial and deep sets of veins.

In the *lower limb,* the *great saphenous vein* (Fig. 3) begins at a point midway between the medial malleolus and the tendon of the tibialis anterior muscle, and ends by passing through an opening in the deep fascia (fossa ovalis) to enter the femoral vein at a fairly constant site 3 cm. lateral to, and 3 cm. below, the pubic tubercle. The trunk of the great saphenous vein is sometimes reduplicated (particularly in the lower thigh), and there may be a double entry into the femoral vein. In the last 5 cm. of its course the great saphenous vein receives a variable number of subcutaneous tributaries: *pudendal, epigastric, circumflex iliac,* and *medial* and *lateral femoral.*

In the leg, the great saphenous vein is closely accompanied by the *saphenous nerve.* Just below the knee it usually receives a major tributary (sometimes called the *posterior arch vein):* this collects blood from a complex of veins overlying the posteromedial aspect of the calf, and has multiple communications with the deep system. Both below and above the knee the great saphenous vein receives tributaries that run upward and medially from the *small saphenous vein.* Throughout its course the great saphenous vein is closely accompanied by *lymphatic trunks.*

PERFORATING VEINS
IN THE LOWER LIMB

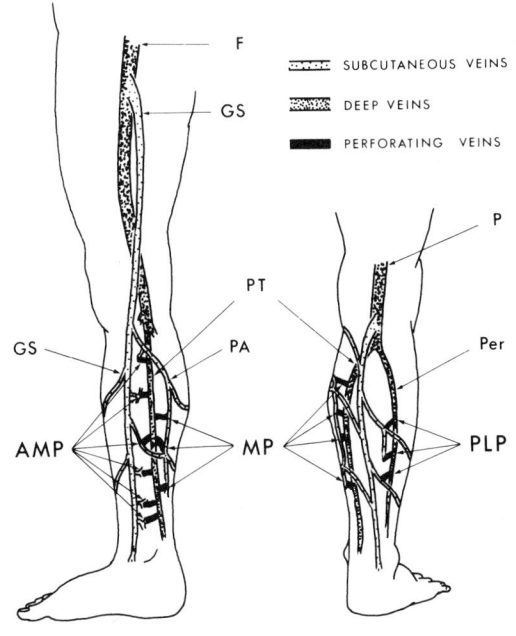

[====] SUBCUTANEOUS VEINS

[::::] DEEP VEINS

[████] PERFORATING VEINS

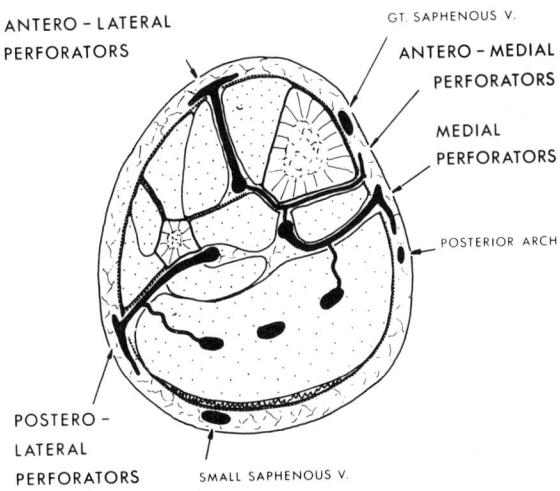

ANTERO – LATERAL
PERFORATORS

GT. SAPHENOUS V.

ANTERO – MEDIAL
PERFORATORS

MEDIAL
PERFORATORS

POSTERIOR ARCH

POSTERO –
LATERAL
PERFORATORS

SMALL SAPHENOUS V.

Figure 4. Perforating veins of the lower limb. *Top,* Medial and posterior views of the leg. *F* = femoral vein; *GS* = great saphenous vein; *PA* = posterior arch vein; *PT* = posterior tibial vein; *P* = popliteal vein; *Per* = peroneal vein; *AMP* = anteromedial perforators; *MP* = medial perforators; *PLP* = posterolateral perforators. *Bottom,* Schematic cross section at junction of middle and lower thirds of the leg.

At the root of the lower limb there are alternative routes for venous drainage from the skin, by way of the *internal pudendal vein* (scrotum, vulva), and through the *gluteal veins* (thigh below the gluteal crease): ultimately these drain into the internal iliac vein.

The *popliteal vein* is formed from the plexiform *venae comitantes* of the three main branches of the popliteal artery, and then is joined by the veins draining the gastrocnemius and soleus muscles to constitute a single (or sometimes double)

vessel behind the artery. The gastrocnemial and soleal veins are so large and tortuous that the latter have been termed *soleal venous sinuses.* At the groin the *femoral vein* lies a little behind, as well as medial to, the corresponding artery. It receives its large deep femoral tributary(ies) just below the point of entry of the great saphenous vein.

Another point of surgical import is the formation of the *inferior vena cava* by the junction of the two *common iliac veins.* The terminations of the latter are closely applied to the back of the right common iliac artery, which indents the left common iliac vein.

VENOUS FUNCTION

There are four general ways in which veins function: (1) as conduits, (2) in thermal regulation, (3) as capacity vessels, (4) and as musculovenous pumps. In individual regions or tissues of the body, variations in structure of the veins and in the nature of the tissue that surrounds them, allow one or more of these functions to be dominant.

Conduit Function

The total cross-sectional area of the veins draining a region is some two or three times greater than that of the corresponding arteries. The *resistance* to blood flow in the venous system is thus comparatively low, and postcapillary vessels contribute normally only about 10 to 15 per cent of the total resistance to cardiac output (Fig. 5). However, maximal dilatation of precapillary and capillary resistance vessels (as in violent muscle exercise) may relocate the site of maximal vascular resistance from precapillary arterioles to postcapillary venules, the latter acting as governors that prevent an uncontrolled increase in cardiac output.

The *pressure* at any point in the venous system is the sum of three components: hydraulic, hydrostatic, and transient.

Hydraulic pressure (Fig. 5) is created by the pumping action of the heart and is associated with blood flow. Under resting conditions the hydraulic pressure of blood as it enters a venous capillary is only about 15 mm. Hg and nonpulsatile, because of energy absorption by the upstream resistance vessels. In the high-flow conditions that accompany arteriolar dilatation, venous capillary pressure rises markedly and becomes pulsatile; but neither phenomenon is transmitted to macroscopic veins because the venous pathway back to the heart is wide-bore and compliant.

Hydrostatic pressure (Fig. 6) is imposed by gravity and is important because of man's upright posture. At rest, any part of the venous system that is below the level of the right atrium is exposed to a positive hydrostatic pressure equivalent to the vertical distance from the atrium. Yet the converse does not apply: at points above this phlebostatic axis, apposition of the compliant vein walls prevents a siphon effect.

Transient pressure changes originate from a number of sources. Centrally, there are pressure waves corresponding to cardiac action ("a," "c," and "v" waves), and to respiratory variations in intrathoracic pressure. In the limbs, there are pressure transients from the action of the musculovenous pumps (see later).

Thermoregulatory Function

The specialized anatomic features of cutaneous and subcutaneous veins are closely concerned with the regulation of body temperature (Fig. 7). The dermal venules, subdermal venous plexuses, and subcutaneous veins constitute an effective and important means for heat exchange with the environment (the others being the pulmonary microvasculature and sweat glands). The size of, and rate of blood flow in, the dermal venules of the hands, feet, head, and neck are in-

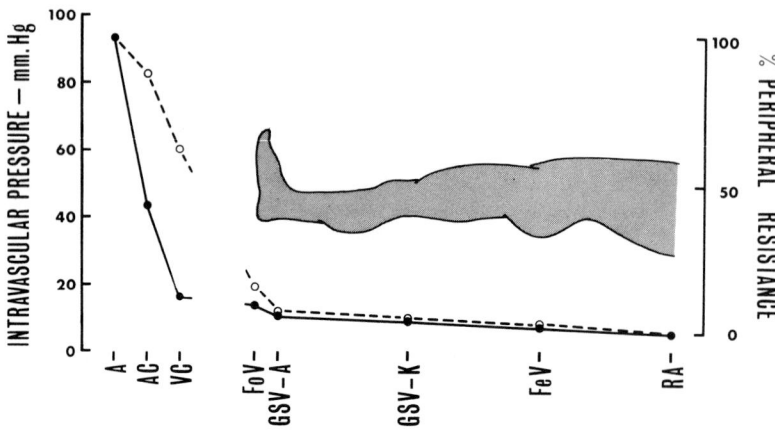

Figure 5. Hydraulic pressure gradients in the lower limb, at rest (solid line) and with maximal arteriolar dilatation (broken line). Constructed from published data. *A* = artery; *AC* = arterial capillary; *VC* = venous capillary; *FoV* = subcutaneous foot vein; *GSV-A* = great saphenous vein at ankle; *GSV-K* = great saphenous vein at knee; *FeV* = femoral vein; *RA* = right atrium. (After Ludbrook, J.: Aspects of Venous Function in the Lower Limbs. 1966. Courtesy of Charles C Thomas, Publisher, Springfield, Ill.)

versely proportional to the magnitude of the *tonic sympathetic vasoconstrictor discharge* to skin resistance vessels. The cross-sectional area of the muscular subcutaneous veins is also under *direct sympathetic control,* and there is as well a *direct temperature effect* on their smooth muscle. The juxtaposition of *deep arteries* and *veins* in the limbs constitutes a passive countercurrent heat conservation-loss mechanism, while the *disposition of venous valves in the hands and feet* ensures that all blood entering these extremities leaves by way of subcutaneous veins, and can thus exchange heat with the environment.

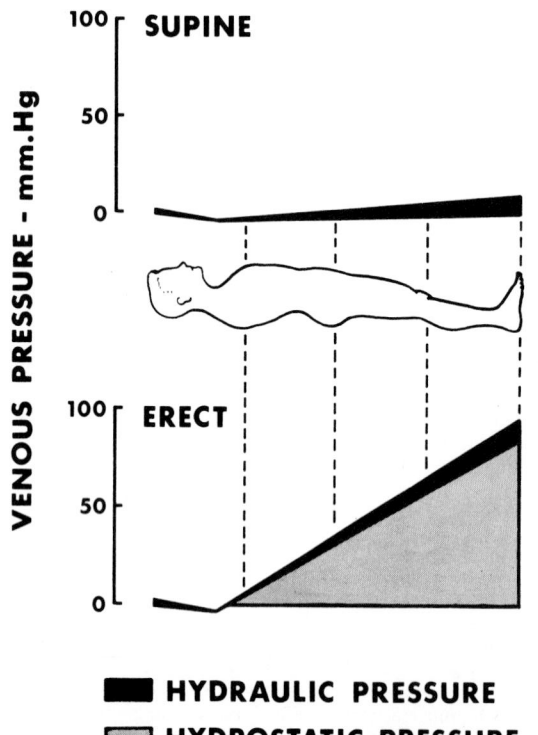

Figure 6. Schematic representation of hydraulic and hydrostatic venous pressure gradients in the supine and erect postures.

Capacity Function

It is thought that about 80 per cent of the blood volume is contained by low-pressure blood vessels: systemic veins, the right heart and pulmonary vasculature, and the left atrium. Some two-thirds of the blood volume is contained by the systemic venous system (from venules to the great veins), and most of this by deep veins.

A feature of these thin-walled, compliant, low-pressure, venous capacity vessels is that large changes in the volume of their contents induce only small pressure changes (at least over a wide, physiologic range). This is in contrast to the elastic behavior of the high-pressure arterial vessels. A consequence is that the considerable blood volume changes that may be occasioned by hemorrhage and transfusion, and the redistributions of blood occasioned by exercise, take place almost entirely within the low-pressure "compartment" of the circulation.

This pressure-volume characteristic of capacity vessels tends to assure a relatively constant filling pressure for the heart. Moreover the whole-body geometry of these vessels is such as to ensure this constancy in face of a variety of body postures, and without the need for other than fine-control active regulatory mechanisms (to which reflex control of tone in superficial veins makes a modest contribution).

Musculovenous Pumps

The valved deep veins of the limbs, and their investing muscles, constitute reciprocating pumps. The most specialized of these are in the legs, where the musculature is enclosed by a dense covering fascia (permitting the generation of high intramuscular pressures during contraction), and where the calf muscles contain large venous sinuses (which act as pump chambers). This specialization seems to be a peculiarly human charateristic, presumably associated with man's adoption of the upright posture and his ability to run.

Muscle contraction raises the pressure in the muscles of the leg by up to 250 mm. Hg. The intramuscular veins are completely emptied, and the intermuscular veins greatly compressed (Fig. 8). The valves of the perforating and deep veins direct a flush of blood up the thoroughfare deep veins, causing a modest and transient rise of pressure in the latter. During the phase of *muscular relaxation* there is a sharp pressure fall in the deep veins, then a rising slope while they refill with blood from the muscle circulation, the distal deep veins, and the subcutaneous veins (by way of perforating veins). When *rhythmic muscle contraction-relaxation* (as in walking) is continued, there is a fall of mean pressure in the superficial veins (Fig. 9) to a new steady level (from 90 to

THERMAL REGULATION

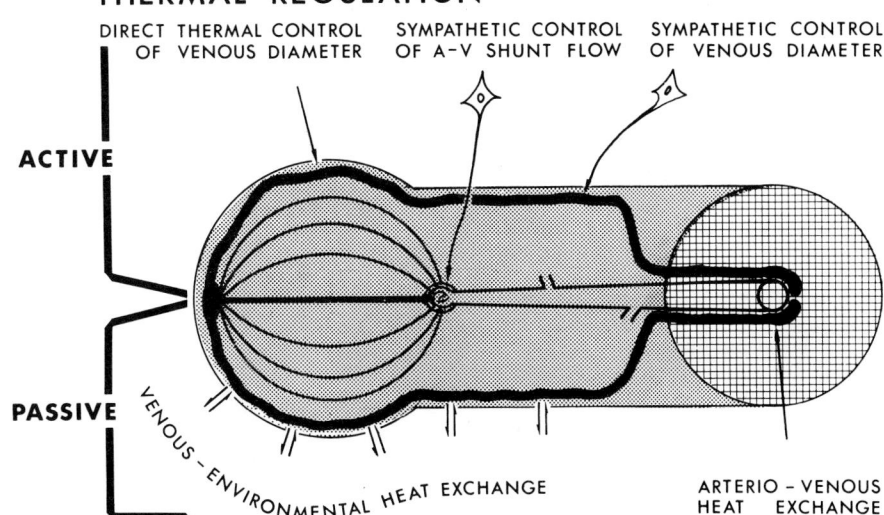

DIRECT THERMAL CONTROL OF VENOUS DIAMETER

SYMPATHETIC CONTROL OF A–V SHUNT FLOW

SYMPATHETIC CONTROL OF VENOUS DIAMETER

ACTIVE

PASSIVE

VENOUS – ENVIRONMENTAL HEAT EXCHANGE

ARTERIO – VENOUS HEAT EXCHANGE

Figure 7. Schematic representation of the ways in which thermal regulation is effected by limb veins.

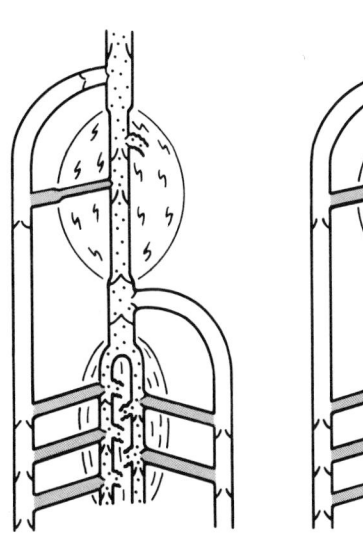
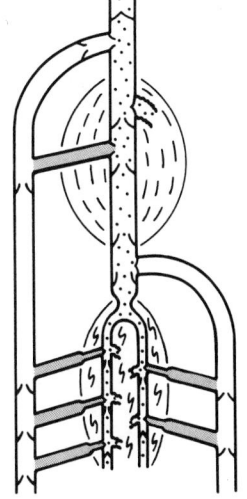

Figure 8. Schematic representation of the behavior of the lower limb veins and their valves during reciprocal thigh and calf muscle contraction-relaxation, as in walking.

☐ SUPERFICIAL

▨ COMMUNICATING   (♭) MUSCLE CONTRACTION

⬚ DEEP   (◊) MUSCLE RELAXATION

Figure 9. Diagrammatic representation of the behavior of deep and subcutaneous venous pressures in the lower third of the normal leg during intermittent calf muscle contraction, as in walking.

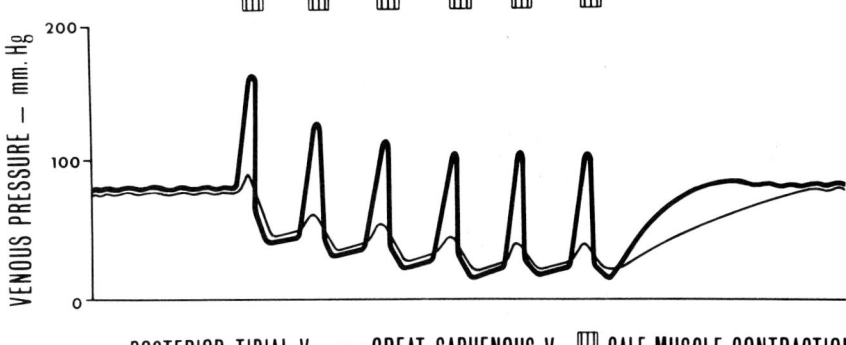

— POSTERIOR TIBIAL V.   — GREAT SAPHENOUS V.   ▥ CALF MUSCLE CONTRACTION

about 20 mm. Hg at the ankle), and also a fall in mean deep venous pressure (from 90 to about 40 mm. Hg at the ankle).

There are at least three recognizable effects of the musculovenous pumps of the leg. They constitute a genuine form of peripheral heart, or rather, *peripheral supercharger:* calf muscle blood flow can be boosted by nearly 50 per cent over that possible from cardiac action alone. The rhythmic action of the limb muscle pumps also results in a steady-state *blood volume reduction* in the lower limbs, allowing the redistribution of some 200 ml. of blood during ambulation (mainly to the pulmonary vascular bed). A third function is to minimize the accumulation of *tissue fluid* in the lower limbs, which would otherwise be considerable in the upright posture if there were a continuously maintained high subcutaneous venous pressure. Clinical manifestations of disorders of the lower limb muscle pumps occur if free outflow is obstructed (that is, there is *deep vein obstruction*), or if there is *incompetence of the valves* of the subcutaneous or perforating veins.

INVESTIGATION OF THE VENOUS SYSTEM

While enlightened physical examination remains the mainstay of diagnosis for most disorders of veins,

certain special investigations—especially phlebography—are sometimes invaluable. Nevertheless, tests on the venous system are more susceptible to observer and interpretive errors than most.

Physical Examination

Physical diagnosis of venous disorders is as much a matter of pattern recognition as of systematic clinical logic. However, special mention should be made of tests for *venous valvular incompetence* (Fig. 10) both because of their historic interest and because they sometimes allow of very accurate conclusions. Retrograde flow in the saphenous veins or their varicose tributaries may be seen as the patient stands up. This is made more evident if a proximal venous tourniquet has been applied with the patient supine and the veins empty, and then released when he is erect (*Trendelenburg test*). Segmentally placed tourniquets may identify incompetent perforating veins, by retrograde filling of the superficial veins in an isolated limb segment when the patient exercises *(Ochsner-Mahorner test)*. *Retrograde pressure waves,* or even the *thrill* of retrograde flow, can be felt by the fingers in response to

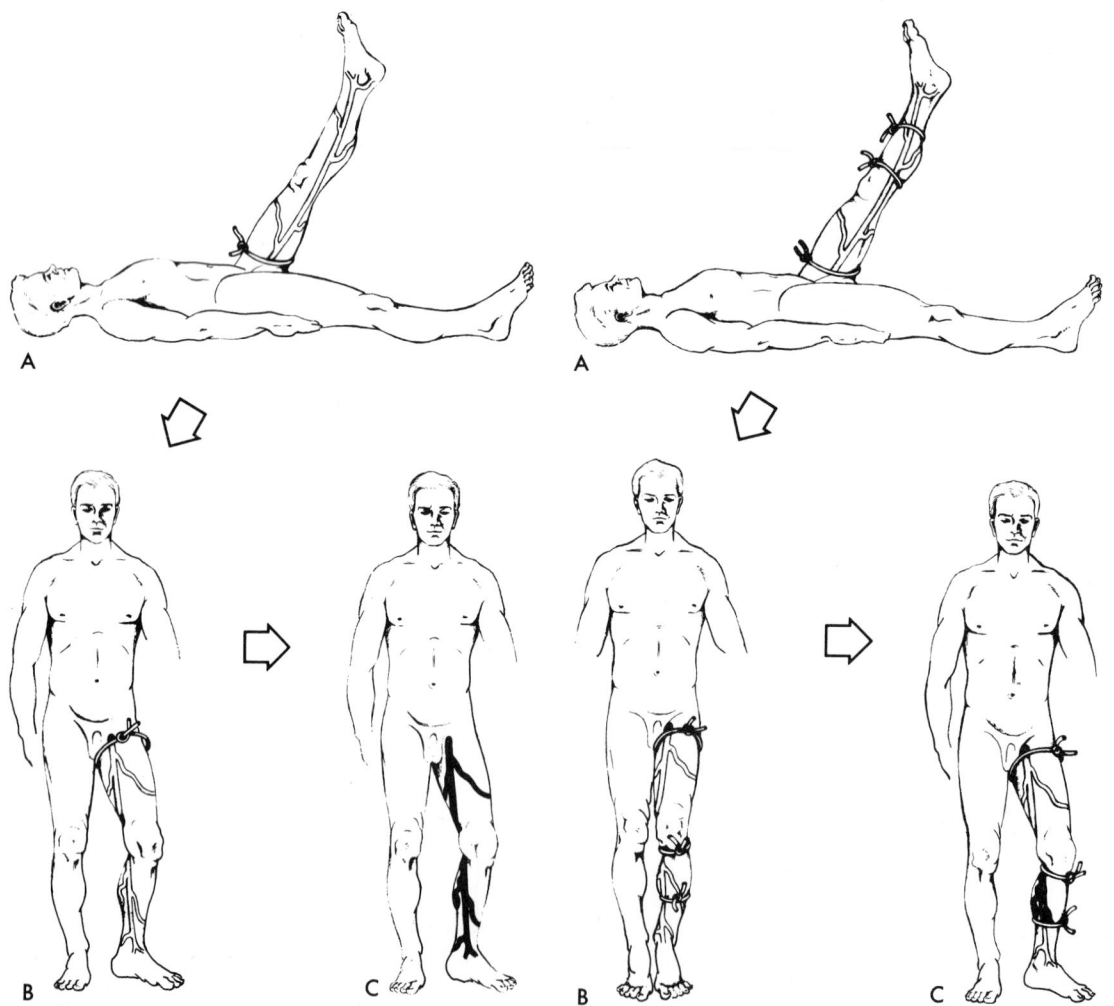

Figure 10. Tourniquet tests for venous valvular incompetence. *Left,* Trendelenburg test for great saphenous incompetence. *Right,* Ochsner-Mahorner test for perforating vein incompetence.

coughing (varicose veins, varicocele). An alternative technique is to tap the vein proximally, and sense the pressure wave by means of a distally placed finger.

Phlebography

The main uses of this technique are in detecting venous obstruction (especially by thrombus), and venous valvular incompetence (especially of perforating veins). Sources of error are streaming or layering of contrast medium; unfamiliarity with physiologic variations in profile of certain veins (e.g., iliac, subclavian); and the hasty interpretation of nonfilling as indicating thrombotic occlusion.

Techniques of upper- and lower-limb phlebography are analogous. In the case of the lower limb the usual technique is to make the radiocontrast injection into a dorsal vein of the foot, with the patient semierect, so that both superficial and deep veins fill from below up *(ascending phlebography)*. A tourniquet above the ankle may be used to encourage filling of the deep veins. Activation of the calf pump by static exercise may also help fill deep and perforating veins *(exercise phlebography)*, and by *cinephlebography* individual perforating veins with incompetent valves can be identified by the occurrence of reverse flow. When no suitable veins are available, injection of radiocontrast material into the medullary cavity of the great trochanter will regularly demonstrate the iliac veins, and into the ankle malleoli or calcaneus, the deep veins of the leg *(intraosseous phlebography)*.

To demonstrate the upper femoral vein, iliac veins, and inferior vena cava, *direct injection* into one or both femoral veins is usually necessary. The performance of a Valsalva maneuver, or rapid foot-down tilting, helps to arrest the contrast medium, and if the femoral venous valves are incompetent the contrast medium may be forced distally to outline the whole length of the femoral vein *(descending phlebography)*. Inaccessible deep veins can be demonstrated by sophisticated *orthograde* techniques or by *retrograde catheterization*.

Radionuclide Techniques

In so-called *radionuclide phlebography* technetium-99m macroaggregate injected into a distal lower-limb vein (e.g., as a preliminary to lung scanning for pulmonary embolus) can be used to produce a gamma image of proximal deep veins and to indicate obstructing thrombus. While a convenient screening method, this lacks the precision of conventional phlebography.

Local accumulation of gamma activity after remote injection of ^{131}I-labeled clotting factors or antifactors, or gamma imaging using ^{99m}Tc-labeled plasminogen activator, have been used to identify the location at which a thrombus is being formed. However, the most widely used radiopharmaceutical (and apparently the most reliable) has been ^{125}I-labeled fibrinogen, with a half-life of 60 days. Incorporation of the labeled fibrinogen into a developing thrombus is identified by means of a hand-held gamma detector and rate meter. Indices of a thrombus are the development of asymmetry in the gamma emission pattern of the two limbs, or of a rising gamma emission at one point compared with the precordial count (Fig. 11). The results of the test correlate excellently with phlebography, but it is only applicable to the lower limb below midthigh level. This test has proved invaluable in epidemiologic surveys and clinical trials of preventive measures and treatment.

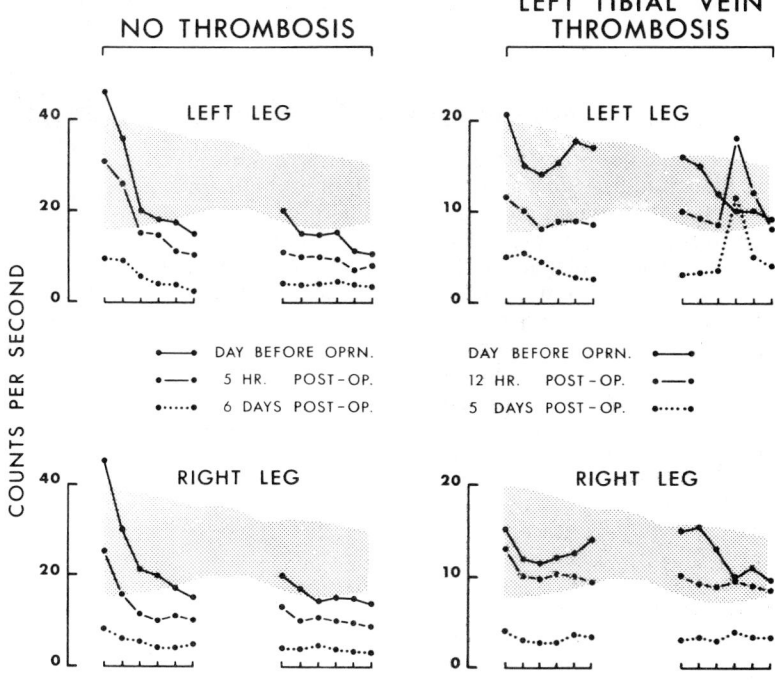

Figure 11. The ^{125}I-fibrinogen test for deep leg vein thrombosis, showing the temporal and spatial pattern of gamma emission in two patients in the perioperative period. *Left,* Normal pattern. *Right,* pattern of development of a left tibial vein thrombosis. (After Flanc, C., Kakkar, V. V., and Clarke, M. B.: Br. J. Surg., 55:742, 1968.)

Venous Pressure, Volume, and Flow

Measurements of these physiologic variables are slowly and rather hesitantly being introduced into clinical practice. Functional (in contrast to anatomic) *venous obstruction* is difficult to prove quantitatively. It can be recognized by elevation of venous pressure distal to a site of anatomic obstruction, but only when an increase in blood flow is provoked (as by exercise); and may be detectable plethysmographically by a reduction in the rate of venous emptying when the limb is elevated, or after release of a proximal venous tourniquet. Acute (thrombotic) iliofemoral venous obstruction is identifiable (though not quantifiable) by transcutaneous application over the femoral vein of a Doppler-effect ultrasonic flow probe, especially by the loss of the transient flow changes normally induced by respiration or exercise.

The presence (though not the location) of lower-leg *perforating veins* with incompetent valves can be reliably confirmed by measuring subcutaneous venous pressure near the ankle, or the corresponding volume changes in calf or foot, during ambulatory exercise. The reverse flow that occurs during calf muscle contraction in individual perforating veins with incompetent valves has been detected by the Doppler technique and by thermography.

PATHOGENESIS AND CLINICAL PATTERNS OF VENOUS DISEASE OF THE LIMBS

The possible ways in which veins and their contained blood react to disease or injury are very limited. Chief among them are thrombosis, obstruction, dilatation, and hemorrhage. Causative of these reactions are a number of more or less well understood pathogenic mechanisms. Resulting from these pathologic reactions of veins are a variety of clinical manifestations, determined mainly by the location of the affected veins.

VENOUS THROMBOSIS

The sequence of events was quite clearly described by Eberth and Schimmelbusch in 1888[8] and the main points of their description are still generally (though not universally) accepted. The process is initiated by the adherence of platelets to the endothelium and then to each other to form a platelet aggregate. On this is then deposited a fibrin mesh, which in turn induces further platelet deposition. This serial process continues until a macroscopic *white thrombus* is formed. In a vein (in contrast to an artery) the white thrombus tends to occlude the lumen, and to arrest the flow of blood in a segment between tributaries. The stagnant blood in the vein clots as if in a test tube, forming a mesh of red cells, platelets, and fibrin. This *red thrombus* exhibits other features of a test-tube clot, in that it tends to retract, and may undergo lysis.

The further behavior (Fig. 12) of a venous thrombus is the result of two competing processes. On the one hand it tends to be rapidly dissolved over a matter of

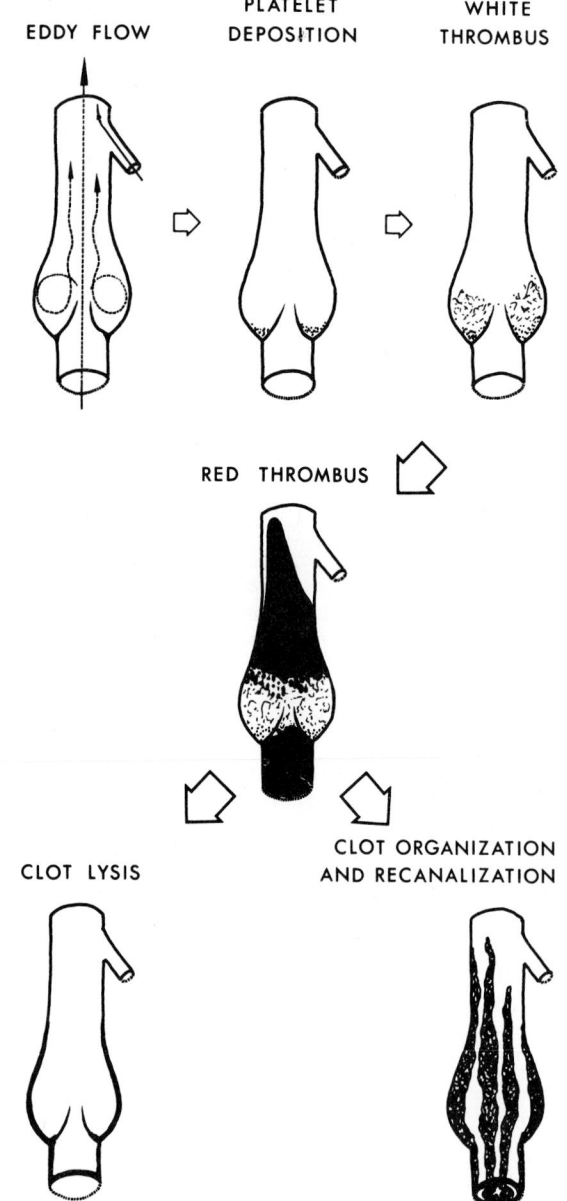

Figure 12. The pattern of evolution and resolution of a venous thrombus.

days from the action of *fibrinolysins* that are normally present in the thrombus, in the vein wall, and in the plasma. It is during this phase that large portions of a thrombus may break off and be swept as *emboli* to lodge in the pulmonary arterial tree. At the same time, a much slower process of *inflammation* in and around the wall of the vein, followed by *fibroblastic organization* of the thrombus, is going on. Provided an individual thrombus does not embolize, its fate may vary from complete dissolution, leaving the structure of the vein almost unimpaired (when the thrombus and the area of its attachment are small, and fibrinolysis is active), to its conversion into fibrous tissue (when the thrombus and its area of attachment are large, and fibrinolysis is weak). The terms *phlebothrombosis* and *thrombophlebitis* are sometimes used to describe these two patterns of pathologic (and clinical) behavior. An organized thrombus tends to become *recanalized* over a period of weeks, usually by multiple small channels. The *venous valves* are important in this whole process: first, because the initial platelet aggregate tends to occur in a valve sinus (presumably because of eddy currents), and second, because if the process of organization and recanalization has an opportunity to occur, it incorporates and then destroys the valve cusps and their function.

The etiology of venous thrombosis is complex. It is classically represented as resulting from the action of Virchow's triad: (1) reduced blood flow, (2) blood hypercoagulability, and (3) endothelial damage.[32] Over the past century opinion has swung to favor one or other of these three factors, and each still has its advocates among clinical investigators.

Subcutaneous (Superficial) Venous Thrombosis

In clinical practice a specific cause for superficial venous thrombosis can often be identified. In the case of the upper limb it is most often the result of an intravenous infusion, occasionally of bacterial cellulitis. A common association in the lower limb is with varicosity of the affected vein. Sometimes there has been a precipitating local blunt injury, and much less often infection. When recurrent thrombosis at different sites occurs *(thrombophlebitis migrans),* a systemic cause such as Buerger's disease, malignant neoplasm (especially bronchial or pancreatic), disseminated lupus erythematosus, or ulcerative colitis may be identifiable at the time or later.

Thrombosis of a subcutaneous vein is always accompanied by a vigorous inflammatory reaction. For this reason an alternative descriptive term—*superficial thrombophlebitis*—is often used. The patient almost always experiences pain, the skin over the affected vein is reddened, edematous, and hot, and there is often fever. In lean patients the thrombosed segment of vein can usually be clearly felt, but when the subcutaneous fat is thick (particularly in the lower limbs) the venous origin of the inflammatory process may be disguised. The true diagnosis may (but should not) be confused with such conditions as bacterial cellulitis, acute gout, or any one of a number of other less common inflammatory processes.

Thrombi in subcutaneous veins rarely if ever escape as emboli, even in the case of the large veins of the lower limb (because of the firm inflammatory adherence of the thrombus to the vein wall). Nevertheless, pulmonary embolism does occur in association with superficial lower limb venous thrombosis. This contradiction is explained by concomitant deep vein thrombosis, either from extension of the thrombus through perforating veins, or merely from enforced inactivity. Thus there is a good case for seeking phlebographic evidence of deep vein involvement in patients with extensive subcutaneous venous thrombosis of the lower limbs. In the absence of deep vein involvement, the treatment of superficial venous thrombosis is usually symptomatic: pain relief, local heat, possibly a heparinoid cream, compression bandaging, and continued ambulatory activity.

Deep Vein Thrombosis in the Lower Limb

The clinically important form of venous thrombosis is that which occurs in deep veins, and particularly in those of the lower limb. Such thrombi may develop at any point from the inferior vena cava downward. While reported frequency distributions of site vary according to the method of thrombus detection (autopsy, phlebography, ^{125}I-fibrinogen uptake, Doppler ultrasound), a general pattern is clear (Fig. 13). By far the majority of thrombi originate in the soleal venous sinuses of the calf, and somewhat less than half of these will propagate proximally to the axial deep veins. Less than 20 per cent originate in the iliofemoral venous segment (common and external iliac veins, common femoral vein), and a proportion of these will propagate distally. In a small minority of instances thrombi form simultaneously and independently at both locations.

Major deep vein thrombosis may occur apparently spontaneously in otherwise healthy young adults. Attempts have been made to predict venous thrombosis by means of tests of coagulation and fibrinolysis. However these have been less rewarding than certain clinical predictors: immobility from any cause, old age, obesity, the magnitude of an operative procedure or injury, myocardial infarction or heart failure, previous episodes of venous thromboembolism, varicose veins, cancer, disorders associated with thrombocytosis or blood hyperviscosity, and drugs such as estrogens.[26] The disorder is most often found in a hospital setting, and more especially in that large population of inpatients who undergo surgery or suffer from heart disease.

Following the introduction of the ^{125}I-labeled fibrinogen uptake test (see earlier), an enormous number of epidemiologic studies of deep leg vein thrombosis have been conducted. However, in any discussion of the epidemiology, the prophylaxis, or the clinical consequences of leg vein thrombosis, it is important to keep several things in mind. The ^{125}I-labeled fibrinogen test is very sensitive and reveals many calf vein thrombi which are never evident to clinical examination. As well, it fails to detect those iliofemoral thrombi that have arisen in situ, rather than by upward propagation from the calf. Are these heretofore undetected calf vein thrombi harmful to the patient? As many as half of such patients may have small pulmonary emboli, but these are detectable only by lung scanning.[3] In over 80 per cent of such patients the thrombi either lyse spontaneously or remain localized to the soleal venous sinuses. However in the remainder the thrombi propagate for a greater or lesser distance into the larger axial veins of the leg or thigh, and it is these which may become fatal pulmonary emboli or which (more commonly) may cause permanent damage to the veins. Thus in the ^{125}I-fibrinogen prospective studies it has been only these propagating thrombi that have been thought worthy of treatment; and it is only these that may produce the symptoms and signs which in more ordinary circumstances would alert the attending physician.

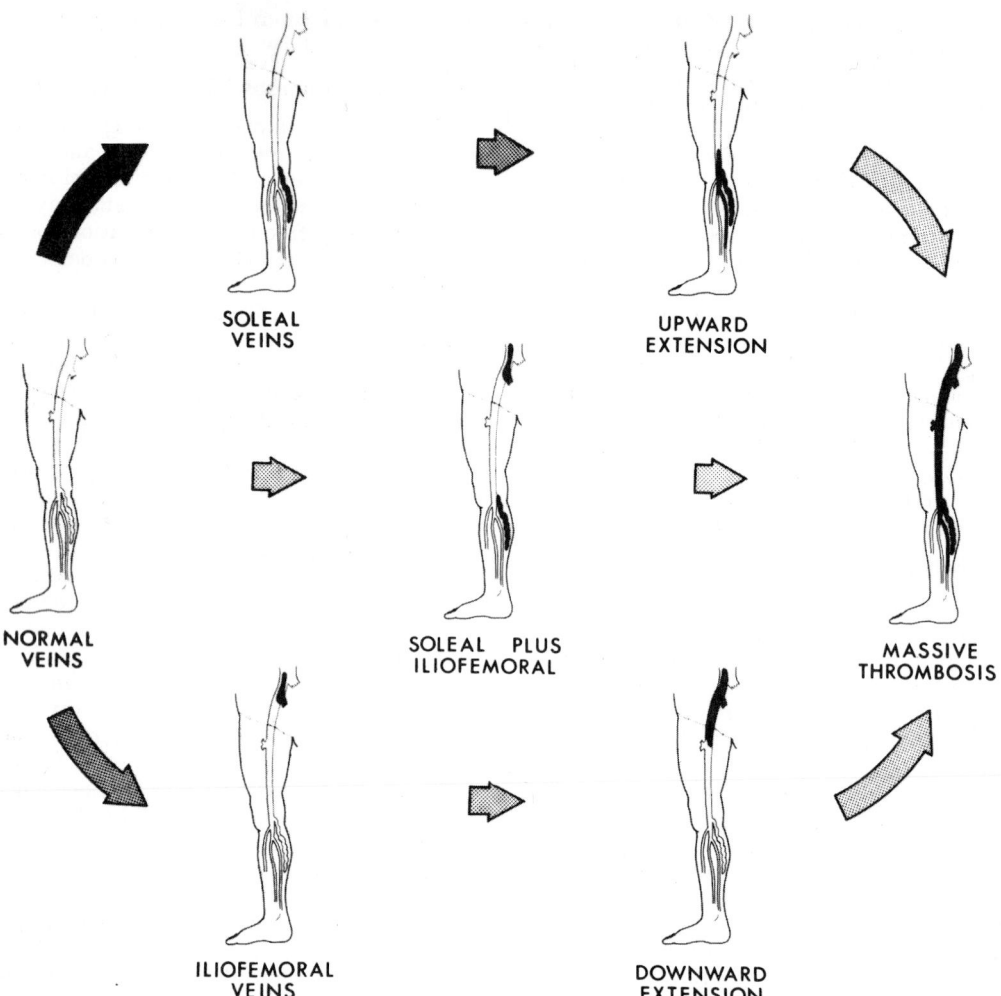

SOLEAL
VEINS

UPWARD
EXTENSION

NORMAL
VEINS

SOLEAL   PLUS
ILIOFEMORAL

MASSIVE
THROMBOSIS

ILIOFEMORAL
VEINS

DOWNWARD
EXTENSION

Figure 13.   Most commonly there is initial soleal venous sinus thrombosis, sometimes extending to axial veins, rarely as far as the iliofemoral veins. Less often thrombosis begins in the iliofemoral venous segment and may extend distally. Occasionally thrombosis commences independently at both sites.

So far as so-called postoperative deep vein thrombosis is concerned, ^{125}I-fibrinogen testing has revealed that calf vein thrombosis actually commences on the operating table in about 50 per cent of cases, and in the first few days of the postoperative period in the remainder. The attack rate in this perioperative period varies greatly, even in the same hospital, according to the type of surgical procedure. International data[12, 26] indicate the following perioperative incidences: hip operations, 37 to 74 per cent; major thoracic procedures, 26 to 65 per cent; major abdominal operations, 5 to 42 per cent; abdominal gynecologic procedures, 11 to 29 per cent; open prostatectomy, 28 to 50 per cent, and closed prostatectomy, 4 to 7 per cent. Corresponding figures after myocardial infarction are 17 to 38 per cent, and after stroke 60 per cent.

International studies[12, 26] also reveal considerable variations in perioperative attack rate within and between regions. Ranges of figures for abdominal operations are: in Britain and Europe, 23 to 42 per cent; in North America, 5 to 16 per cent; and in three widely separated tropical and subtropical areas, 12 per cent.[7, 10, 33] Reasons given for these variations include possible differences in detection technique, and ethnic, dietary, and climatic factors.[6]

The patient who develops deep vein thrombosis is not usually part of a prospective, thrombus-detection survey. It is therefore only when his thrombus is large enough to cause local symptoms (or has embolized) that he presents to his physician. The traditional symptoms of *leg (calf) vein thrombosis* are mild pain or tightness in the calf, particularly when the patient is sitting, standing, or walking. The corresponding signs are slight ankle edema, calf muscle tenderness which can be pinpointed by deep finger palpation, and pain when the foot is passively dorsiflexed (Homan's sign). It has belatedly become evident that these signs are grossly unreliable. Extensive calf vein thrombosis may (and commonly does) induce no symptoms or signs whatsoever, and conversely the traditional symptoms and signs may be due to other causes.

If it be important to establish the diagnosis beyond doubt (as is the case if prolonged and potentially hazardous therapy is contemplated, or if pulmonary embolism is suspected), phlebographic confirmation or denial of the diagnosis is essential.

In its florid form, *acute iliofemoral venous thrombosis* is easily recognizable. Sometimes there is premonitory mild soreness in the iliac fossa or groin, and a low-grade fever (even to the point of mimicking appendicitis or diverticulitis). When the main vein becomes completely occluded, the entire lower limb becomes swollen. If the patient is bedridden, this swelling may be of gradual onset and insignificant. If he is ambulant, it is common for the limb to become acutely swollen, and tightly uncomfortable, over a matter of minutes or hours. To examination, the limb is uniformly swollen up to the groin, and deeper in color than normal. Subcutaneous veins may be visibly fuller, particularly in the groin where they are acting as collaterals. To palpation, all tissue layers are edematous: not only is there pitting subcutaneous edema, but the muscle compartments are palpably turgid. Thus the limb exhibits the signs of acute venous outflow obstruction, and this has occurred either because external and internal iliac veins are both occluded, or because the main femoral vein and its deep femoral tributary are both blocked. Rarely, thrombosis of the deep system of veins may be so extensive, and so limiting to blood flow, as to threaten or cause *gangrene* of the toes, feet, or even leg (while the arterial tree remains demonstrably patent). Iliofemoral venous thrombosis should be confirmed phlebographically before drug or operative therapy is instituted. Furthermore, phlebography should be bilateral, because not infrequently a large but silent thrombus may be present in the veins of the other limb.[23]

The three common sequels to clinically evident lower limb deep vein thrombosis are pulmonary embolization (see Chapter 39), continuing obstruction to venous flow, and damage and malfunction of venous valves. *Malfunction of valves* occurs from damage caused by recanalization of a thrombus. It is clinically recognizable only when thrombosis has affected the deep and perforating veins of the leg. The manifestations are varicose veins or leg ulceration or both. *Continuing venous obstruction* is recognizable only when the thrombus occludes a major vein (iliac, femoral, popliteal) and undergoes organization rather than lysis. Edematous swelling of the limb is the chief clinical manifestation.

The aims of *prophylactic and therapeutic measures* for deep vein thrombosis are to prevent the condition itself or to prevent its sequelae, whether the latter be remote (pulmonary embolism) or confined to the affected limb (chronic venous outflow obstruction, venous valve damage and leg ulceration). Great and increasing emphasis has been placed on prophylaxis for at least three decades. The simple reason is that the incidence of the disorder in at-risk (e.g., hospital) populations is so high that the alternative approach of detect and cure is impractical. The three approaches used have been attempts to nullify one or other of the three elements of Virchow's triad. Almost all clinical trials that have used a clinical end point are of little more than historic interest, because of the low diagnostic accuracy inherent in clinical symptoms and signs. Only the demonstration of deep vein thrombosis by phlebography, or by gamma detection of ^{125}I-labeled fibrinogen, is acceptable.

It has been hard to accept *mechanical endothelial damage* as a cause for human deep vein thrombosis, and there is no evidence that prophylactic measures such as elevation of the calves from the operating table are effective.

Attempts have been made to increase the velocity of deep vein *flow*. Lower limb elevation and compression bandages probably do this, and early postoperative ambulation and leg exercises may do so. Neither approach has been shown to be effective. A more recent approach is based on evidence that venous thrombosis is commonly initiated on the operating table. Repetitive electrical stimulation and intermittent pneumatic compression of the calf muscles have been shown to lower the incidence of leg vein thrombosis. The third approach has been to alter *blood coagulability*. This can be done using full anticoagulant doses of heparin, which has to be suspended over the operative period for fear of severe bleeding; or prothrombin depressants (coumarins, inandiones), which can be continued through the operative period, provided the prothrombin time is no more than about twice normal. The efficacy of this form of prophylaxis in high-risk surgical patients, such as those undergoing hip surgery, can be regarded as established (if not generally practiced), provided it is properly carried out and precisely monitored.[4]

Low-dose subcutaneous heparin has recently been extensively studied as a prophylactic agent. In the dosage advocated (5000 I.U. subcutaneously, twice daily for 5 to 7 days, beginning just prior to operation), heparin does not affect the whole-blood clotting time. In this low dosage it forms a complex with antithrombin III (a plasma proteinase) and the complex inhibits the activation of factor Xa, a vital step in the extrinsic and intrinsic coagulation pathways. There is now unequivocal evidence that this regimen lowers the incidence of postoperative deep venous thrombosis in patients undergoing routine general surgery. However, in groups of high-risk surgical patients, such as those undergoing open prostatectomy or hip surgery, the results of low-dose heparin prophylaxis are equivocal.[4] A more important benefit of low-dose heparin may be the reduction in fatal postoperative pulmonary embolism, recently demonstrated in a very large international co-operative trial.[14]

Dextran 70 (molecular weight 70,000) was introduced as a plasma expander, but more recently it has been shown to have an antithrombotic effect. The exact mechanism of its antithrombotic action is unknown: coating of the endothelial wall and antiplatelet effects have been suggested. Nor has the optimal prophylactic regimen been established, although an intravenous dose of 500 ml. during operation and 500 ml. on the first postoperative day has been the minimum advocated. Results of trials have sometimes been conflicting, but on balance it appears that deep venous thrombosis and pulmonary embolism are significantly less frequent when dextran 70 is used in this fashion. Disadvantages are the need for an intravenous line and the possibility of circulatory overload.

Antiplatelet agents such as dipyridamole, aspirin, and hydroxychloroquine have also been assessed as prophylactic agents.[4] There is as yet unconfirmed evidence that hydroxychloroquine is effective. Reports on aspirin have been conflicting, and at present neither it nor dipyridamole can be recommended for prophylaxis. Substances which enhance fibrinolytic activity by stimulating plasminogen activator release (sulphonyl ureas, anabolic steroids) have not proved effective in surgical patients.

In summary, the only two drugs which have been accorded some degree of general acceptance in preventing deep vein thrombosis in surgical patients are dextran 70 and, more especially, low-dose heparin. Few would dispute that patients at high risk (see earlier) should be given prophylaxis, and that those at low risk (e.g., a child having a minor operation) should not. Whether patients who fall between these two extremes would benefit from prophylaxis is still unknown.

The *treatment of established deep vein thrombosis* is a separate problem from prophylaxis. Two different approaches are possible: the traditional method of using anticoagulants to prevent further thrombus formation and allowing natural lysis to occur, and the newer methods of actively promoting fibrinolysis.

The method most commonly used to prevent further thrombus formation is to administer heparin intravenously in full anticoagulant dosage for 7 to 10 days, and then replace it by the more convenient oral prothrombin-depressant agents (coumarins, inandiones). Because rethrombosis is common, there is a tendency to maintain oral anticoagulant therapy for 3 to 12 months. Defibrinogenating agents such as ancrod and reptilase (both obtained from viper venom) have been tried as potentially safer substitutes for heparin, but they have been found to be no less likely to cause bleeding complications. It should be said that there is actually no scientific evidence which proves that anticoagulation is therapeutically effective in deep venous thrombosis, but on empirical grounds most clinicians believe this therapy to be beneficial.

Fibrinolysis can be stimulated by using plasminogen activators such as streptokinase and human urokinase. There is some evidence that this form of therapy is more effective than anticoagulation, but there are some major disadvantages. It cannot be used in patients for about 10 days after an operation, as there may be serious bleeding at the operation site. Urokinase is not antigenic but is too costly for general use, while streptokinase is antigenic and can cause hypersensitivity reactions. Streptokinase has had the added disadvantage of requiring stringent laboratory control, although a simple, standardized dose schedule of streptokinase, prednisolone, and then heparin has been advocated.[1]

There were isolated reports of *surgical removal* of venous thrombi by Laewen[16] and Leriche and Geisendorf[18] before Mahorner and his colleagues[21] introduced iliofemoral venous thrombectomy in its modern form in 1957. Recent thrombi in the iliac and femoral veins

can be removed via the femoral vein at the groin, under local or general anesthesia, by means of a balloon-tipped (Fogarty) catheter.[9] Technically, and in terms of end result, the operation of venous thrombectomy is most suitably performed as soon as the condition is recognized. Unfortunately, the rather dramatic removal of large quantities of thrombus has not been matched by quality of the end result. Follow-up phlebographic studies have demonstrated rethrombosis or gross valvular damage in a very high proportion of patients,[2, 17] and comparisons of operation and drug therapy have not greatly favored operation. Nevertheless, the operation has a definite place in patients with threatened or actual venous gangrene, and possibly in the young, previously well patient in whom an iliofemoral thrombosis develops suddenly and inexplicably.

Other Forms of Venous Thrombosis

Venous thrombosis also occurs in the upper limb, the most important site being the *axillary-subclavian vein*. Thrombosis in this venous segment may occur primarily, classically in a fit young man after unaccustomed muscular exercise ("effort thrombosis").[30] The initiating factor is probably injury to the vein as it crosses the first rib. Secondary thrombosis is most commonly the result of an indwelling intravenous catheter, but can also occur after operative trauma (e.g., axillary node dissection). Pulmonary embolism from axillary-subclavian thrombosis has occasionally been reported. The venous obstruction often persists, upper limb swelling after exercise being a frequent manifestation.

Inferior vena caval thrombosis may rarely occur as a neonatal phenomenon, with swelling (and sometimes venous gangrene) in both lower limbs. In adults, the condition may also occur spontaneously, usually as an extension of bilateral iliac vein thrombosis. The commonest cause of caval thrombosis in adult life is probably *surgical caval interruption* for thromboembolism. *Renal vein thrombosis* may occur as an isolated incident, manifest as a form of nephrotic syndrome. *Hepatic vein thrombosis* may occur apparently spontaneously, in association with polycythemia vera (Budd-Chiari syndrome), or with a caval diaphragm and caval thrombosis. The main manifestations are disturbances of liver function, together with gross hepatomegaly and ascites. *Thrombosis of the portal vein* can occur in neonatal life, supposedly by extension of septic thrombophlebitis in the umbilical vein. Extensive collateral development occurs, both locally (cavernous transformation of the portal vein) and at a distance (gastroesophageal varices). Thrombosis of the portal and even splenic and superior mesenteric veins may occur in adult life in association with liver cirrhosis, and rarely as spontaneous events. Acute thrombosis of *mesenteric or omental veins* may cause an apparent or real abdominal emergency, with pain resulting from local inflammation, segmental paralysis of the gut, or even venous gangrene.

Superior vena caval or innominate vein thrombosis most often results from compression, usually by a bronchial cancer or its lymph node metastases, less often by other superior mediastinal tumors (thyroid, thymus, lymphoma). It is recognizable by swelling of the neck and face and readily visible engorgement of the subcutaneous veins of the head and neck.

Occasionally, particularly in association with septic abortion, puerperal sepsis, or tubal infection, *septic thrombi* occur in the pelvic veins. Together with signs of major venous obstruction there is high fever from septicemia, and sometimes septic pulmonary emboli occur via the iliac or ovarian veins. Septic thrombi can occur at other sites: the *cavernous sinus* from propagated facial infection, and as an iatrogenic disease from infection at the variety of sites at which *intravenous catheters* are placed.

CHRONIC VENOUS OBSTRUCTION

Whether occlusion of the lumen of a vein results in any clinical manifestation depends on the anatomic location of the affected vein and on the length of vein involved. These two factors are important in determining whether there are sufficient alternative venous pathways (collateral veins) to allow continuing venous outflow at low pressure.

Obstruction (or operative excision) of subcutaneous veins rarely results in recognizable dysfunction, because of the great number of superficial and perforating veins that can act as collaterals. Conversely, there are certain critical segments of the deep venous system in which occlusion does result in abnormalities of pressure or flow. Examples of the latter are the cavernous sinus, the subclavian vein, the superior

vena cava, the suprarenal inferior vena cava, hepatic veins, the portal vein, the right renal vein, and the iliofemoral venous segment. The consequence of venous occlusion at these critical sites is edematous swelling of the tissues in the venous watershed, dilatation of collateral veins (which may be visible if subcutaneous), and organ-specific dysfunctions such as convulsions (cavernous sinus), proteinuria (renal vein), ascites (hepatic or portal veins), and skin ulceration (lower limb veins).

The most common cause for clinically significant venous obstruction is thrombosis, whether acute (and completely occluding the lumen) or recanalized (as multiple, small, high-resistance channels).

Iliofemoral venous thrombosis that has been so extensive as to produce generalized lower limb swelling almost always results in chronic venous outflow obstruction no matter how aggressive the treatment. The manifestations of this are edematous swelling of all tissue layers of the lower limb (Fig. 14), a greater depth of color of the skin and sometimes a bluish hue, and visible and palpable subcutaneous collateral veins running from the groin onto the abdominal wall (and thence to the axilla or opposite groin). Walking or running increases the swelling and turgor, and sometimes results in a bursting, deep pain (venous claudication). Chronic venous obstruction and the edema of lymphatic obstruction are sometimes confused. A successful search for collateral veins provides a very strong index of suspicion that the limb swelling is venous in

NORMAL

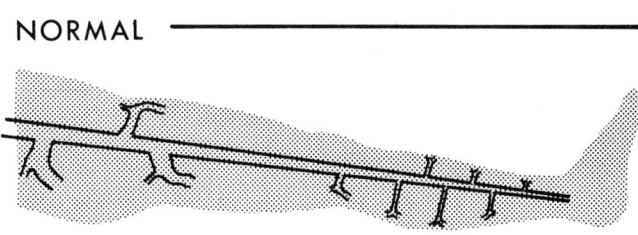

LEG VEIN THROMBOSIS

- SHORT SEGMENT
- MANY COLLATERALS
- MINIMAL EDEMA

Figure 14. The obstructive effects of leg vein thrombosis versus iliofemoral vein thrombosis.

ILIO-FEMORAL VEIN THROMBOSIS

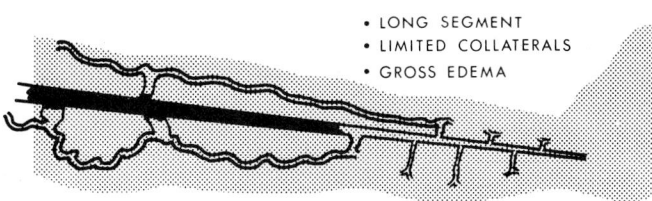

- LONG SEGMENT
- LIMITED COLLATERALS
- GROSS EDEMA

origin, though phlebography may be necessary to establish the nature and extent of the venous occlusion.

The obstruction that may result from extensive thrombotic occlusion of veins in the *lower leg* (Fig. 14) is manifest less as chronic edema (which is often mild) than as varicose subcutaneous veins and associated skin changes such as eczema, fat necrosis, or ulceration.

Uncommonly, *nonthrombotic venous obstruction* may occur. This is a misnomer, as external compression of a vein is likely to lead to secondary thrombosis. Recognition of this form of venous obstruction demands an awareness of some of the causes. In general, these are either benign lesions growing in a restricted compartment or malignant neoplasms. Among the benign lesions are aneurysms of the aorta, or iliac, femoral, or popliteal arteries; popliteal cysts, or benign neoplasms within the popliteal fossa; and rarely giant abdominopelvic tumors such as uterine fibroids, ovarian cysts, and the pregnant uterus. Among the malignant neoplasms are those of the sigmoid colon, ovary, or uterine cervix. Miscellaneous causes include retroperitoneal fibrosis and surgical misadventure.

Some success has been attained by *surgical treatment* of patients with chronic iliac or femoral vein obstruction. The most versatile technique has been to use the great saphenous vein to create a bypass.[20] An advantage of this method is that only one anastomosis is necessary, and so, it is hoped, the risk of thrombosis is reduced. It also places the valves in the direction of flow, though whether they remain competent is less certain. The technique was first used as a crossed bypass in patients with iliac vein obstruction,[27] but has also been employed as a popliteal-femoral bypass (Fig. 15). It has been reasonably successful in cases of nonthrombotic venous occlusion (neoplastic invasion, accidental or surgical damage), but much less so in post-thrombotic obstruction. Post-thrombotic stenosis, particularly of the left common iliac vein where it passes behind the right common iliac artery, has been treated by local *venoplasty* but the results have usually been disappointing. A similar technique has been used to relieve *postmastectomy swelling* of the arm when this is due to axillary vein stenosis.

The cause of superior *vena caval obstruction* (with or without thrombosis) is most often a malignant neoplasm, and radiotherapy may relieve symptoms. However, a number of ingenious resective and bypass procedures have been employed to overcome the venous engorgement of the head and neck.

Nonoperative forms of treatment — elastic stockings, massage, and diuretics — are purely palliative and no more than modestly successful.

Varicose Veins

Dilated veins commonly assume a varicose form. In most circumstances when the diameter of a vein is abnormally increased, so is its length between fixed points; that is, it becomes tortuous as well as thinwalled. The direct consequences of the dilatation are either *cosmetic* (subcutaneous varicose veins) or a greatly increased risk of *hemorrhage* (gastroeso-

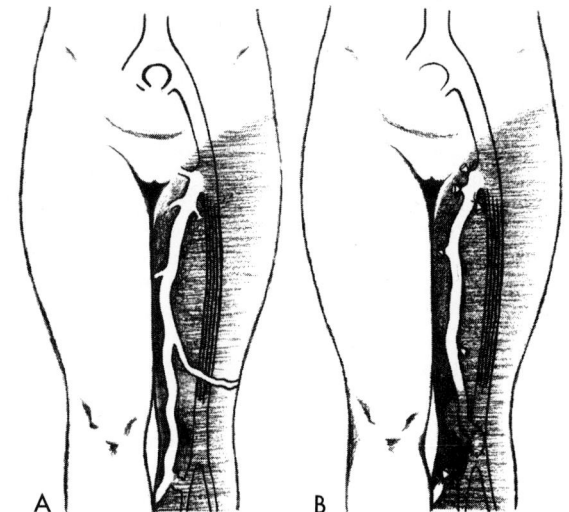

Figure 15. Popliteal-femoral saphenous bypass operation for femoral vein obstruction.

phageal varices). The cutaneous *ulceration* associated with lower limb varicose veins is a consequence of the cause of the varicose veins: malfunction of the musculovenous pumps of the leg.

Obstruction is one cause for venous dilatation — in this circumstance, of collateral veins: hence, portal vein obstruction (gastroesophageal varices), and iliofemoral or inferior vena caval obstruction (groin-abdominal wall collaterals). Rarely dilatation may result from a prolonged and great increase in systemic or regional venous pressure, due to a nearby *arteriovenous fistula* or to *tricuspid valve incompetence:* in these circumstances the dilated veins usually pulsate. However, by far the commonest causes for varicose veins of the lower limb are more or less well-defined disorders of the *musculovenous pumps*.

Primary Varicose Veins

This is a rather unsatisfactory term that is used to describe a clearly identifiable disease pattern affecting the subcutaneous veins of the lower limb. The condition is familial, though in rather a vague way: the mode of inheritance has been variously described as autosomal dominant, autosomal recessive, and sexlinked recessive. It is expressed more commonly in women than in men, and it is commoner among populations with high living standards. The underlying defect is clearly inborn, for the condition can often be recognized shortly after adolescence. It is not clear whether the primary defect is of the venous valves themselves, of the vein wall, or (more probably) of both. At all events, incompetence of subcutaneous venous valves is an invariable accompaniment. A plausible explanation, though it has not been completely proved, is that one inborn defect is absence or hypoplasia of the external iliac venous valve. Venous pressure and blood flow studies have shown that this valve is incompetent in over 95 per cent of those with primary varicose veins, and in a high proportion of young people with a family history of varicose veins (but who have not yet themselves been affected).[29] It is supposed that transient pressure rises from exertion and coughing expand the saphenofemoral junction, rendering incompetent the terminal saphenous valves. This process spreads downward in a fashion that is sequential, but that affects the tributaries of the great saphenous vein in a random manner. Thus any, or all, of its tributaries may be picked out to become varicose (Fig. 16). The small saphenous vein and its tributaries are less often affected, and then either because of incompetent subcutaneous communications between it and a varicose great saphenous vein, or because the femoral and popliteal (deep) venous valves have become incompetent (Fig. 16). Tributaries of the internal iliac vein (vulva, back of thigh) may also become varicose by a similar process (Fig. 16).

An alternative explanation that has been advanced is that the disorder is one of abnormally increased blood flow through the superficial veins, leading to dilatation in an analogous fashion to that which occurs in the case of collateral veins or an arteriovenous fistula. Two mechanisms for such an increase in blood flow have been suggested. One is that there are multiple microscopic arteriovenous shunts present in the skin. The other is that valvular incompetence in perforating veins occurs as the primary defect, causing a rerouting of deep venous blood through subcutaneous veins. On present evidence, neither of these latter explanations is as satisfactory as that of sequential valvular incompetence.

Another association with primary varicose veins has been suggested: an *aberration of endocrine function,* or an abnormal response to normal endocrine secretion. There is some evidence to support this view. The sex difference in incidence is evident before childbearing. Increase in size of varicose veins is often apparent in the first trimester of pregnancy, before vena caval obstruction by the pregnant uterus is demonstrable. A cyclic premenstrual exacerbation of varicose veins is quite common. Indeed, it is difficult to escape the conclusion that overlying the genetic basis is an endocrine effect, whether estrogenic or other, that accounts for the sex difference in incidence.

The *clinical manifestations* are chiefly cosmetic, and the demand for treatment is closely related to the sophistication of the female society, and to current fashions in clothing. The physical manifestations are not so clear-cut. Among them are aching of the legs after standing, night cramps, and swelling of the ankles. However, some care must be taken in the interpretation of these symptoms. Those in the age group that most commonly seeks medical attention for this condition (35 to 45 years) tend to notice aching legs even in the absence of varicose veins. Night cramps afflict a cross section of the otherwise normal population. In older age groups there is a variety of causes for leg pain, ranging from arterial obstruction to degenerative hip or knee joint disease. While increased tissue fluid accumulation does occur in this condition, frank pitting edema usually has some other cause. Any or all of these symptoms may be blamed by the patient (and by his unwary doctor) on visible varicose veins.

There are definite complications of primary varicose veins. They are more susceptible to thrombosis, and to laceration or blunt rupture, than normal veins. When

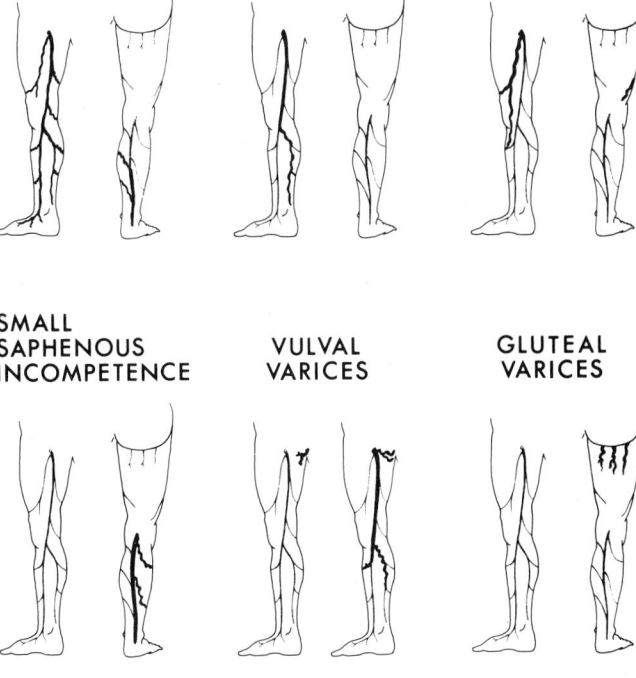

GREAT SAPHENOUS INCOMPETENCE

SMALL SAPHENOUS INCOMPETENCE **VULVAL VARICES** **GLUTEAL VARICES**

Figure 16. Patterns of primary varicose veins. *Top,* Great saphenous incompetence resulting in gross varicose veins (*left*) of great and small saphenous systems; (*center*) of the posterior arch vein; (*right*) of the lateral femoral cutaneous vein. *Bottom,* Primary small saphenous incompetence; vulval varices, from (*left*) internal pudendal incompetence of (*right*) great saphenous incompetence; gluteal varices from internal iliac incompetence.

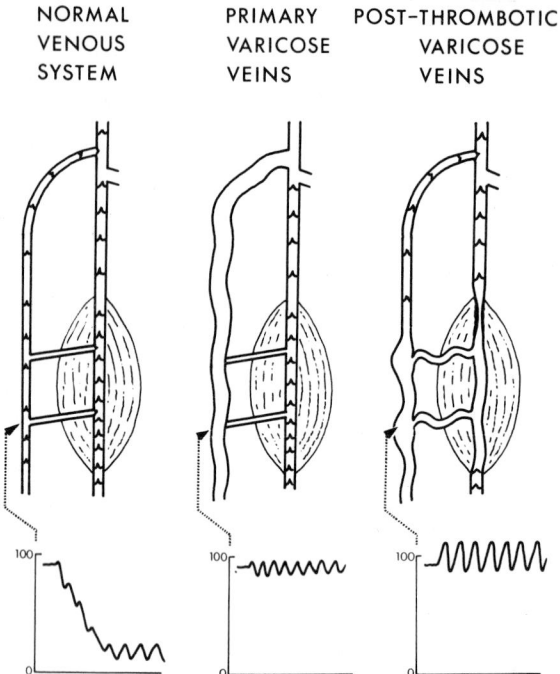

NORMAL VENOUS SYSTEM   PRIMARY VARICOSE VEINS   POST-THROMBOTIC VARICOSE VEINS

Figure 17. The causes of high subcutaneous venous pressure in association with leg ulcers. *Top,* The valvular defects. *Bottom,* The resulting ambulatory venous pressure patterns.

the varicose condition is of long standing, and especially when venous dilatation is gross, skin eczema or ulceration may occur. There is a clear association between these changes and failure of the calf muscle pump to lower subcutaneous venous pressure, just as there is clear evidence that correction of the pump defect is the major prerequisite to reversal of the skin changes. In the case of primary varicose veins, subcutaneous venous pressure fails to fall on exercise because the saphenous vein and its varicose tributaries have become wide-bore pipelines connecting the central venous pool to the skin of the leg (Fig. 17).

Gross varicose veins may have a capacity of several hundred milliliters. As a result, such patients tend to have greater postural swings of right atrial pressure, heart rate, cardiac output, and arterial pressure than normal, sometimes to the point of postural syncope.

The differentiation of primary varicose veins from the post-thrombotic variety is not always easy. Features characteristic of the former are an early age of onset (15 to 25); the ability to trace the varicose veins back to the saphenofemoral junction (and rarely the saphenopopliteal junction) by inspection, palpation, or percussion; and the ability to completely prevent reflux filling of the varicose veins by the Trendelenburg tourniquet test.

Post-thrombotic Varicose Veins

This is a useful descriptive term for the syndrome of perforating vein valve incompetence. It is presumed that prior deep vein thrombosis has resulted in a degree of deep vein obstruction, combined with damage to the valves of the deep and perforating veins. In less than half of such patients has the preceding thrombotic episode been overt, but it is now apparent that clinically unrecognized deep vein thrombosis is a rather common event in the population. In the case of perforating vein incompetence, the distending force that is exerted on the wall of the subcutaneous vein is provided by muscle contraction, which squirts jets of blood at high pressure into the superficial system (see Fig. 17): the incompetent perforating veins have become the line of least resistance for the output of the musculovenous pump. Rarely, complete *absence of deep and communicating vein valves* occurs as a congenital familial defect.

When there has been a history of florid venous thrombosis in the past, diagnosis is simple. Otherwise, the features to be described must be sought. These patients tend to be a little older than those with primary varicose veins. Post-thrombotic varicose veins are rarely as large as the primary type, and are often partly concealed by overlying eczema, subcutaneous fat necrosis, or ulceration. In theory, it should be possible to detect incompetence of the valves in affected perforating veins by means of the Ochsner-Mahorner test. In practice, because of the small size or obscurity of the varices, the result of this test is often equivocal. To complicate matters, there is often dilatation of the great saphenous vein or its tributaries, whether as a chance association, because these have acted as collateral veins round a deep venous block, or even merely from carrying the blood that is pumped in a retrograde direction from deep to superficial veins.

It has been suggested that a "flare" of intracutaneous varices over the medial malleolus is diagnostic of post-thrombotic varices, but this is not necessarily true. It has also been suggested that the dilated perforating veins can be localized by feeling the holes in the deep fascia through which they pass; but the apparent holes are more often a rim of subcutaneous fat necrosis surrounding a subcutaneous varix.

Some of the more reliable special tests to identify incompetent perforating veins have been described earlier (phlebography; venous pressure, volume and flow), but all are susceptible to observer error, and diagnosis is as accurately made on a basis of pattern recognition by an experienced clinician.

Miscellaneous Forms of Varicose Veins

When varicose veins are associated with an increase in girth (but not length) of the entire limb, care should be taken that these are not *collateral veins,* resulting from chronic deep venous obstruction (usually post-thrombotic, and usually in the iliofemoral segment).

Gross varicose veins that appear before the age of 16 to 20 years may represent one of the rarer forms of congenital anomaly. Multiple *congenital arteriovenous fistulas* often do not become evident until the growth of puberty, when a manifestation may be varicose veins of unusual distribution, which may show arterial pulsation, and over which the skin temperature is raised. A rare cause of juvenile varicose veins is congenital, often *hereditary, absence of deep vein valves.*

In adult life there are other vascular blemishes that

are usually, though by no means always, associated with primary varicose veins. Fans of *dilated intracutaneous veins* may appear in irregular patches on the lower limb. These are ugly, and are not significantly improved by the usual methods of treating varicose veins. Small (less than 1 cm.), raised, discrete, red, painful vascular anomalies are sometimes associated with varicose veins, and have been termed *angiectids*. They occur only in women, and have as their characteristic that they enlarge and become extremely painful during the premenstrual period and especially during pregnancy. They are presumed to be endocrine-determined microscopic arteriovenous fistulas. Dilated veins in the region of an *acquired arteriovenous fistula* are easily recognizable from a history of injury, increased skin temperature over the pulsating veins, and an audible local machinery murmur. The pulsating veins of gross *tricuspid valve incompetence* are widespread over the body.

Venous ("Varicose") Leg Ulcers

Apart from their association with varicose veins, these ulcers have several other distinctive features. The patient is more often obese than of normal weight for height. The ulcer is almost invariably located in the lower third of the leg—the "gaiter" area—and most often above the medial malleolus. It will invariably heal, or show signs of rapid healing, if the patient is put to bed with the affected leg elevated above heart level. The ulcer may be moderately painful when the patient is standing, but rapid and complete pain relief is to be expected from leg elevation. The appearance of the ulcer is not especially characteristic. Its size can vary from a square centimeter to the entire circumference of the lower half of the leg. While the shape is usually regular, it too is highly variable. The skin surrounding the ulcer is commonly eczematous, and almost invariably shows brown pigmentation (due both to a melanocytic reaction and to iron-containing macrophages). This skin and the edge of the ulcer are generally edematous. The wall of the ulcer can be sloping, or at the other extreme, undermined. The floor always shows pink-red granulations when the overlying slough is removed. Recurrent ulceration is associated with progressive loss of subcutaneous tissue, and a visible loss of circumference of the affected portion of the leg (indeed, a firm plaque of subcutaneous fat necrosis often precedes frank ulceration). When fat necrosis is associated with proximal swelling from chronic venous obstruction, the term "inverted bottle leg" is appropriate. The natural history of a venous ulcer is a cycle of healing and recurrence, unless cure of the underlying defect in the musculovenous pump is effected. With whichever form of varicose veins the ulcer is associated, there is the same underlying physiologic disturbance: failure of subcutaneous venous pressure to fall during ambulatory activity (see Fig. 17). Healing of the ulcer can be maintained only if this fall can be restored to near normal.

Primary varicose veins can be causative of ulceration, but only when the primary varicose veins are gross and have been evident for many years, and even then the ulceration runs rather a benign course. At

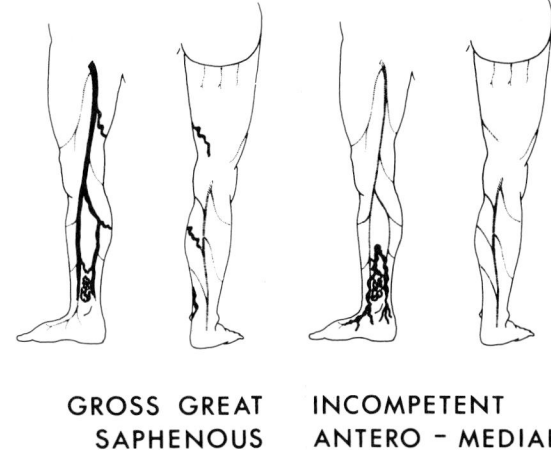

GROSS GREAT SAPHENOUS INCOMPETENCE   INCOMPETENT ANTERO - MEDIAL PERFORATORS

Figure 18. The venous pattern in venous ulceration.

least half of all venous ulcers are associated with post-thrombotic *incompetent perforating veins* (Fig. 18). Conversely, clinically recognized florid deep leg vein thrombosis is associated with a very high risk that ulceration will develop in later years. It is remarkable that in this case the varicose veins themselves are often not prominent, and indeed may sometimes be invisible beneath the base or edematous edges of the ulcer. They can nevertheless be detected when the patient is standing, by the spongy compressible quality of the tissues that lie deep to the subcutaneous scarring.

Provided the classic characteristics of venous ulcers are borne in mind, there should not be confusion with the many other forms of leg ulcer that can occur. Nevertheless, a great many patients have had actual or supposed varicose veins eradicated for nonvenous forms of ulceration, with at best no improvement, and at worst disastrous consequences. Simple *mechanical injury to the skin* of the lower third of the leg, particularly when there has been full-thickness skin loss, may be slow to heal. *Factitious ulcers* usually show surrounding scratch marks caused by the fingernails. Generalized *atopic dermatitis* is often most floridly expressed in the lower third of the legs. *Ischemic ulcers* from obliterative arterial disease are usually located on the toes or foot. However, concurrence of varicose veins and arterial disease is not uncommon, and in this circumstance an apparent venous ulcer may not heal unless arterial reconstruction is performed. A rare and bizarre ulcer is associated with the names of *Martorell*[22] and *Hines and Farber*.[11] It is an extremely painful, shallow, serpiginous, creeping ulcer, usually on the lateral side of the leg. The original descriptions associated these ulcers with arterial hypertension, but this is not a constant feature. The importance of these ulcers lies in the pain they produce, and in their tendency to recur whatever form of treatment is employed. Other unusual ulcers may be associated with *disseminated lupus erythematosus, macroglobulinemia,* and other systemic disorders that affect blood or blood vessels. *Malignant neoplastic lesions* of the skin (particularly melanoma, squamous cell cancer, and Kaposi sarcoma) may occur in the presence of varicose veins and may be mistaken for varicose ulcers. Very occasionally a *squamous cell cancer* may develop at the site of—and apparently as a result of—a very long-standing varicose ulcer.

Treatment of Varicose Veins and Venous Ulcers

There is a single rational basis for the treatment of varicose veins. It is to interrupt the valveless pathways between the subcutaneous and deep systems of veins, in order to correct the abnormality of the musculovenous pumps and in the hope that venous blood flow will be rerouted through channels with normal valves. The only controversy is as to how this should be done.

Trendelenburg[31] has the reputation for having first devised a logical operation for *primary varicose veins* in 1891, when he undertook ligation of the great saphenous vein at midthigh level. Perthes pointed out 4 years later[28] that in many of these patients the varicose veins had recurred, and suggested that the site of

ligation should be flush with the femoral vein, above the point of entry of the subterminal great saphenous tributaries. It is not clear who first systematically practiced this operation, though the credit is usually given to Homans.[13] Thus one essential component of any procedure for primary great saphenous varicose veins is division of the great saphenous vein flush with the saphenofemoral junction, and division of the tributaries that enter its last 5 to 7 cm. in order to minimize the chance of reconnection of the superficial and deep systems (Fig. 19). An entirely analogous procedure is performed at the saphenopopliteal junction if there is primary varicosity of the small saphenous vein and its tributaries (see Fig. 21).

This procedure by itself will rarely lead to a good cosmetic result, however. The pressure fall in the subcutaneous veins on exercise is restored, but while the patient is standing still the normal hydrostatic pressure still obtains in the persistently varicose subcutaneous veins. Thus a further component of treatment must be to obliterate the varicose veins themselves. This is variously done by multiple ligations through small incisions (to induce thrombosis), by excision of the varicose veins through long incisions, or by injec-

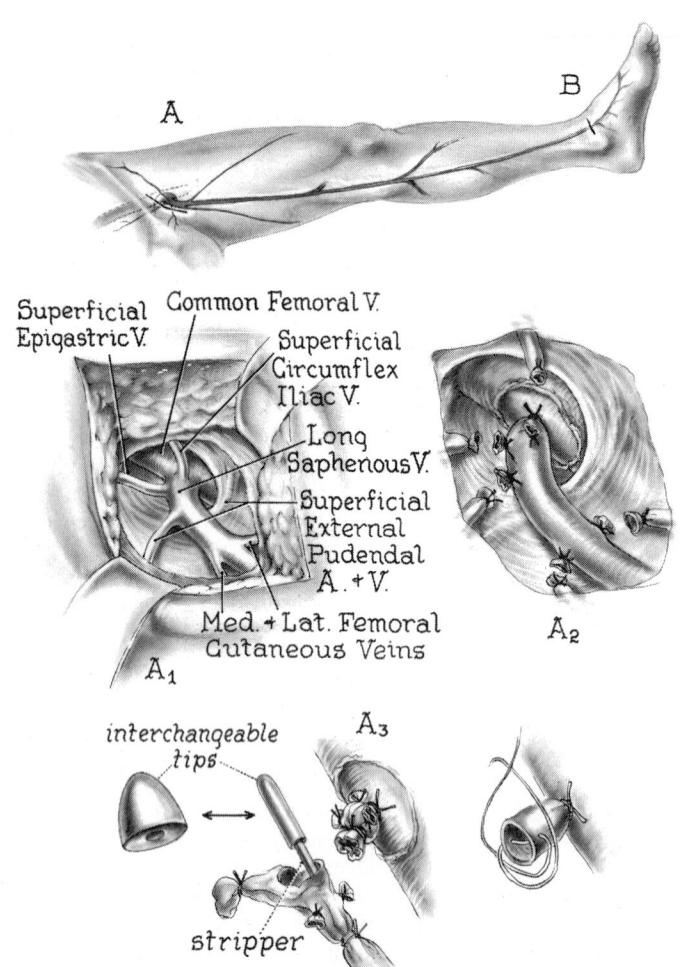

Figure 19. The procedure of flush saphenofemoral ligation. *A,* Groin incision. A_1, Exposure of the saphenofemoral junction and the terminal saphenous tributaries. A_2, Ligation and division of the tributaries. A_3, Transfixation-ligation of the great saphenous vein, and the appearance of the Myers stripper passed up from *B.* (From Venous Disease of the Lower Extremities, by A. D. McLachlin. Copyright © 1967, Year Book Medical Publishers. Used by permission.)

tion of sclerosants at a later date. The method of choice depends to some extent on the sex and age of the patient, and the perfection of cosmesis desired.

The third component of a satisfactory operation is to remove the great (or small) saphenous vein itself. This further reduces the risk of reconnection with the deep system at the groin or popliteal fossa. The technique used is to pull, or strip, out the saphenous vein from the ankle to the saphenofemoral or saphenopopliteal junction (Fig. 19 to 21). This concept was first described by Keller[15] and Mayo,[24] and perfected by Myers[25] by the use of an intraluminal braided or cabled wire leader that is passed up the lumen of the vein, and to which is attached a hemiolivary head.

Some care is necessary in the design of the appropriate operation for varicose veins of *small saphenous distribution*. Most stem from saphenofemoral incompetence, as a result of valve incompetence in the subcutaneous veins that link great and small saphenous systems (see Fig. 3). Thus the three-component operation must be applied to both systems. It is much more rarely that "primary" small saphenous incompetence occurs as an isolated event.

The surgical treatment of *post-thrombotic varicose veins* is similar in principle but different in detail. Every incompetent perforating vein must be identified and divided: the main problem is that of identification, which requires considerable experience. At physical examination the location of incompetent perforating veins can be strongly suspected from the presence of visible and palpable "blowouts" of the subcutaneous veins. Phlebography (especially cinephlebography), thermography and Doppler flowmetry (see earlier),

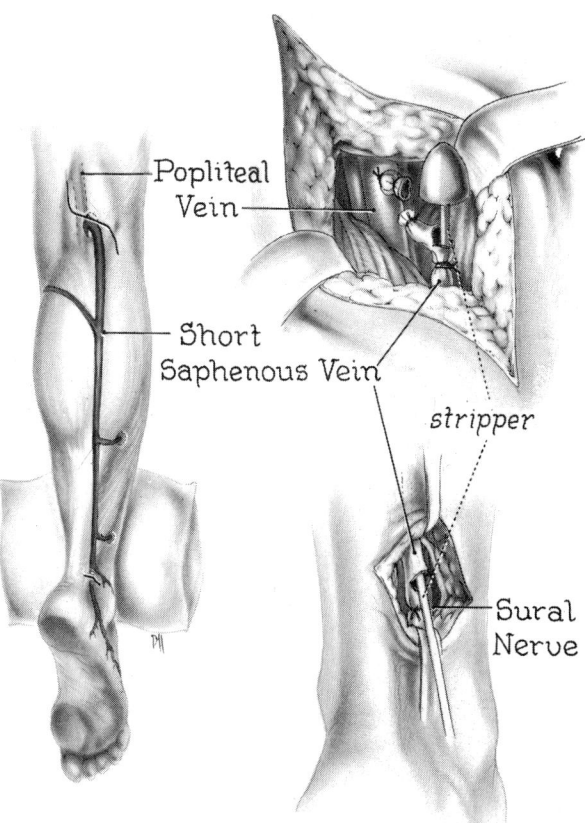

Figure 21. The procedure of flush saphenopopliteal ligation and division, and of small (short) saphenous vein stripping. (From Venous Disease of the Lower Extremities, by A. D. McLachlin. Copyright © 1967, Year Book Medical Publishers. Used by permission.)

singly or in combination, may help to enumerate and locate incompetent perforating veins.

When the skin is normal, or relatively normal, it is usual to seek the perforating veins superficial to the deep fascia, and to ligate and divide them in this plane. When there has been ulceration of the skin, and subcutaneous fat necrosis has given a wooden consistency to the tissues, it is preferable to seek them in the subfascial plane. On the medial side of the leg a vertical incision is made 2 to 3 cm. behind the subcutaneous border of the tibia, through which the medial, anteromedial, and even the posterolateral perforating veins can be located and divided (Fig. 22). Linton[19] introduced this technique in 1938 as an incision from tibial tubercle to medial malleolus, and the authors believe that this is preferable to the more limited exposure later suggested by Cockett.[5] The less-often incompetent anterolateral perforating veins can be explored through an incision over the anterior tibial compartment.

Sclerosant injection therapy is sometimes used as an alternative, or adjunct, to surgery. Ever since the technique was described in the Hippocratic writings, the popularity of this form of therapy has waxed and waned. Fegan has drawn attention to a very important prerequisite to successful sclerotherapy: if the

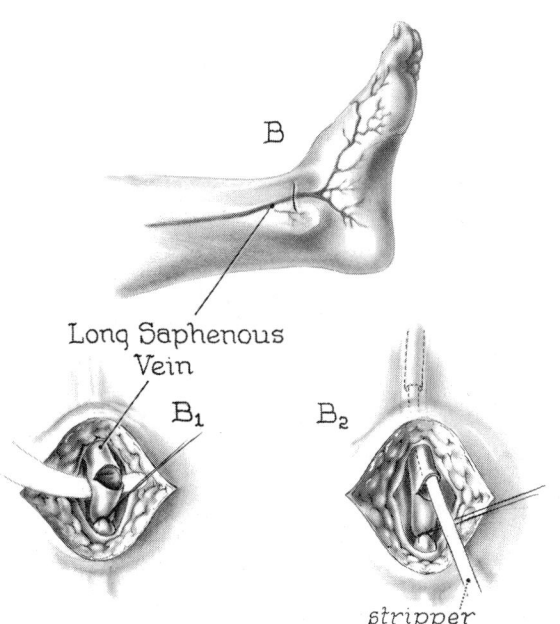

Figure 20. Introduction of the Myers stripper into the great (long) saphenous vein at the ankle. (From Venous Disease of the Lower Extremities, by A. D. McLachlin. Copyright © 1967, Year Book Medical Publishers. Used by permission.)

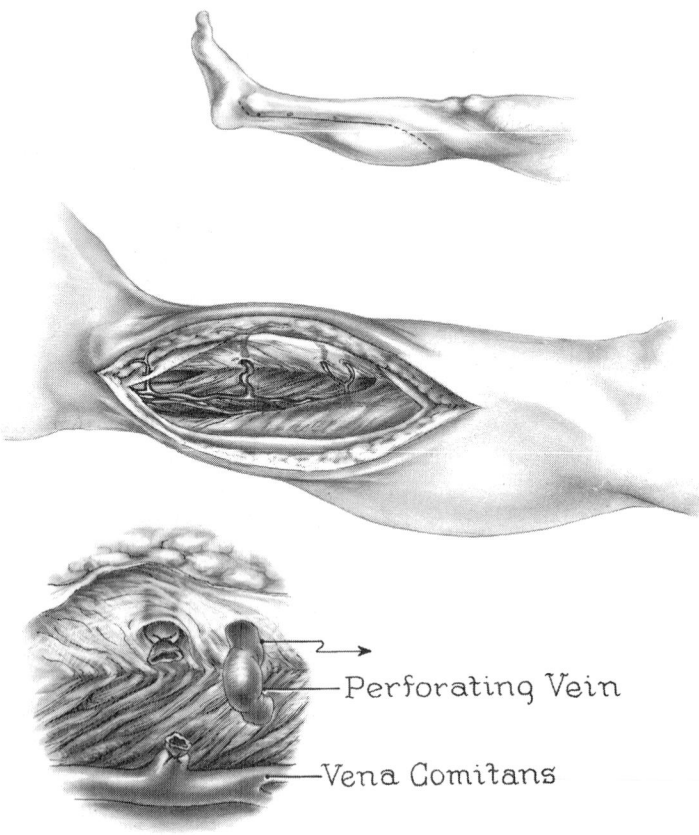

Perforating Vein

Vena Comitans

Figure 22. The Linton technique of subfascial exposure, ligation, and division of the anteromedial perforating veins of the leg. (From Venous Disease of the Lower Extremities by A. D. McLachlin. Copyright © 1967, Year Book Medical Publishers. Used by permission.)

blood is emptied out of the injected venous segment by elastic bandage compression which is continued without interruption for 6 weeks, the inflamed endothelial surfaces adhere by direct contact rather than by way of organized thrombus, and the chance of recanalization of the vein is greatly reduced. Using "continuous compression sclerotherapy" as the sole form of treatment, and 3 per cent sodium tetradecyl sulfate in benzyl alcohol as the sclerosing agent, he and others have claimed excellent results in both primary and post-thrombotic varicose veins.

Venous leg ulcers can be invariably healed by bed rest with lower limb elevation, accelerated if necessary by free split-skin grafts. Indeed, they can often be healed without hospitalization if firm bandage compression of the leg is maintained at all times when the patient is upright. The maintenance of healing depends on the extent to which the underlying venous abnormality can be corrected. This is always possible in the case of primary varicose veins, less often so in post-thrombotic varices. In the latter case, if the ulcer is a first one, if it has been present for no more than a few months, if the patient is not obese, and if only one or two perforating veins are incompetent, excellent results are obtainable by surgery. The less these conditions are met, the less the chance that anything approaching cure is possible, without the requirement that the patient wear an elastic support for the remainder of his life.

Unbiased comparison of *surgery versus sclerotherapy*

in the treatment of varicose veins presents formidable difficulties, not the least of which are how and when to assess the end result. From the evidence of attempted controlled trials, and our own and others' experiences, we offer the following conclusions. Sclerotherapy is less costly. It is the preferred initial therapy when varicose veins are small, and saphenofemoral incompetence is not evident. Surgery is the preferred initial therapy for primary varicose veins when saphenofemoral incompetence is clearly evident; and for post-thrombotic varicose veins when the skin is in good condition, and only one or two incompetent perforating veins are identifiable. Neither method does more than ameliorate the condition of the leg in which post-thrombotic damage to deep and perforating veins has been extensive, and in which there has been gross damage to skin and subcutaneous tissue.

VENOUS HEMORRHAGE

If *varicose veins* are perforated by injury, severe hemorrhage may result. The injurious agent may be chemical (gastroesophageal varices), infective (chronic venous ulceration), or mechanical (accidental, felonious, or surgical wounds). Hemorrhage is profuse either because the arterial inflow to the region finds this the line of least resistance for outflow (collateral veins), or because there is a wide pipeline to a central venous reservoir (lower limb varicose veins).

The control of hemorrhage from veins is often more difficult than of that from arteries. The wide lumen of a vein, and its often scanty musculature, mean that spasmodic constriction at the site of injury is weak and that an occluding thrombus is easily dislodged. Security from continuing or recurrent hemorrhage is achieved only by suture closure of a side defect, or by double ligation. The major practical problem is that of controlling hemorrhage until one of these definitive procedures can be performed. Some special maneuvers can be used in special circumstances. In the limbs, elevation or external counterpressure will eliminate or counteract hydrostatic pressure.

SELECTED REFERENCES

Functional and Surgical Anatomy

Hollinshead, W. H.: Anatomy for Surgeons. New York, Hoeber Medical Division, Harper & Row, 1969.
Contains a fine and current account of the gross anatomy of the venous system, especially the lower limb veins (Volume 3).

Alexander, R. S.: The peripheral venous return. In American Physiological Society: Handbook of Physiology, Section 2, Circulation. Ed. W. F. Hamilton and P. Dow. Baltimore, Williams & Wilkins Company, Vol. 2, p. 1075, 1965.
An excellent account of, and reference source for, the wall structure, valves, and nerve and blood supply of veins.

Venous Function

Ludbrook, J.: Aspects of Venous Function in the Lower Limbs. Springfield, Ill., Charles C Thomas, Publisher, 1966.
A surgically oriented account of structure and function of veins generally, but with particular reference to those of the lower limbs.

Shepherd, J. T., and Vanhoutte, P. M.: Veins and their Control. Philadelphia, W. B. Saunders Company, 1975.
An up-to-date account, with special emphasis on the physiology and pharmacology of venous smooth muscle, and the participation of veins in cardiovascular reflexes.

Investigation of the Venous System

Couch, N. P. (Ed): AMA archives symposium on diagnostic techniques in phlebothrombosis. Arch. Surg., *104*:132, 1972.
Contains informative accounts by experts of phlebography, plethysmography (standard and impedance), ^{125}I-labeled fibrinogen scanning, and use of the Doppler flowmeter, in diagnosis of deep vein thrombosis.

Ludbrook, J.: The Analysis of the Venous System. Bern, Hans Huber, 1972.
Current methods of investigating the venous system by radiology, radionuclides, pressure, volume, and flow measurements, and venous tone measurement.

Venous Thrombosis

Kakkar, V. V., and Jouhar, A. J. (Eds.): Thrombo-embolism: Diagnosis and Treatment. Edinburgh, Churchill Livingstone, 1972.
The proceedings of an international symposium which first brought together many of the people who were contributing to the knowledge explosion in this field.

Moser, K. M., and Stein, M. (Eds.): Pulmonary Thromboembolism. Chicago, Year Book Medical Publishers, 1973.
A good review of the problem, including experimental approaches, with the emphasis on the pulmonary embolic consequences of thromboembolism.

Nicolaides, A. N. (Ed.): Thromboembolism. Lancaster, Medical and Technical Publishing Company, Ltd., 1975.
An excellent and up-to-date review of deep venous thrombosis of the lower extremities, particularly concentrating on the pathogenesis, and ^{125}I-labeled fibrinogen diagnosis, of this disease complex.

Varicose Veins

Dodd, H., and Cockett, F. B.: The Pathology and Surgery of the Veins of the Lower Limb. Edinburgh, E. & S. Livingstone, 1956.

A classic account of varicose vein surgery, which is only just beginning to date (new edition in 1976).

Myers, T. T.: Results and technique of stripping operation for varicose veins. J.A.M.A., *163*:87, 1957.
A clear description of the Mayo Clinic approach to the operative treatment of primary varicose veins.

McLachlin, A. D.: Venous Disease of the Lower Extremities. Chicago, Year Book Publishers Inc., 1967.
An excellent, well illustrated, and well referenced account of the pathophysiology and operative treatment of varicose veins (and other venous disorders).

Fegan, G.: Varicose Veins: Compression Sclerotherapy. London, Heinemann Medical Books, 1967.
Details of the principles and technique of the modern injection treatment as applied to 1171 patients.

Chronic Venous Obstruction

Dale, W. A.: The swollen leg. *In* Current Problems in Surgery. Chicago, Year Book Medical Publishers, September, 1973.
An account of the clinical features and management of lower limb venous (and lymphatic) obstruction, including the use of venous bypasses (in which the author was a pioneer).

REFERENCES

1. Astedt, B., Robertson, B., and Haeger, K.: Experience with standardized streptokinase therapy of deep venous thrombosis. Surg. Gynecol. Obstet., *139*:387, 1974.
2. Barner, H. B., William, V. L., Kaiser, G. C., and Hanlon, C. R.: Thrombectomy for ilio-femoral venous thrombosis. J.A.M.A., *208*:2442, 1969.
3. Browse, N. L., Clemenson, G., and Croft, D. N.: Fibrinogen-detectable thrombosis in the legs and pulmonary embolism. Br. Med. J., *1*:603, 1974.
4. Clagett, G. P., and Salzman, E. W.: Prevention of venous thromboembolism in surgical patients. N. Engl. J. Med., *290*:93, 1974.
5. Cockett, F. B.: The pathology and treatment of venous ulcers of the leg. Br. J. Surg., *43*:260, 1955.
6. Covey, T. H., Sherman, L., and Baue, A. E.: Low-dose heparin in postoperative patients: A prospective coded study. Arch. Surg., *110*:1021, 1975.
7. Cunningham, I. G. E., and Yong, N. K.: The incidence of postoperative deep vein thrombosis in Malaysia. Br. J. Surg., *61*:482, 1974.
8. Eberth, C. J., and Schimmelbusch, C.: Die Thrombose nach Versuchen und Leichenbefunden. Stuttgart, 1888.
9. Fogarty, T. J., Cranley, J. J., Krause, R. J., Strasser, E. S., and Hafner, C. D.: Surgical management of phlegmasic cerulea dolens. Arch. Surg., *86*:256, 1963.
10. Hassan, M. A., Rahman, E. A., and Rahman, I. A.: Post-operative deep vein thrombosis in Sudanese patients. Br. Med. J., *1*:515, 1973.
11. Hines, E. A., Jr., and Farber, E. M.: Ulcer of the leg due to arteriolosclerosis and ischemia occurring in the presence of hypertensive disease (hypertensive-ischemic ulcer). Mayo Clin. Proc., *21*:337, 1946.
12. Hirsh, J., and Gallus, A. S.: ^{125}I-labeled fibrinogen scanning: Use in the diagnosis of venous thrombosis. J.A.M.A., *233*:970, 1975.
13. Homans, J.: The operative treatment of varicose veins and ulcers, based upon a classification of these lesions. Surg. Gynecol. Obstet., *22*:143, 1916.
14. Kakkar, V. V., Corrigan, T. P., and Fossard, D. P.: Prevention of fatal post-operative pulmonary embolism by low doses of heparin; an international multicentre trial. Lancet, *2*:45, 1975.
15. Keller, W. L.: A new method of extirpating the internal saphenous and similar veins in varicose conditions; a preliminary report. N.Y. Med. J., *82*:385, 1905.
16. Laewen, A.: Thrombectomy in venous thrombosis and arteriospasm. Intern. Abstr. Surg., *65*:348, 1937.
17. Lansing, A. M., and Davis, W. M.: Five-year follow-up study of ilio-femoral venous thrombectomy. Ann. Surg., *168*:620, 1968.
18. Leriche, R., and Geisendorf, W.: Resultats d'une thrombectomie precoce avec resection veineuse dans une phlebite grave des deux membres inferieurs. Presse Med., *47*:1301, 1939.
19. Linton, R. R.: The communicating veins of the lower leg and the operative technique for their ligation. Ann. Surg., *107*:582, 1938.

20. Ludbrook, J.: Postthrombotic venous obstruction in the lower limb. Arch. Surg., *106*:11, 1973.
21. Mahorner, H., Castleberry, J. W., and Coleman, W. O.: Attempts to restore function in major veins which are the site of massive thrombosis. Ann. Surg., *146*:510, 1957.
22. Martorell, F.: Las ulceras supramaleolares por arteriolitis de los grandes hipertensos. Actas Inst. Policlin., *1*:6, 1945.
23. Mavor, G. E., and Galloway, J. M. D.: Ilio-femoral venous thrombosis: Pathological considerations and surgical management. Br. J. Surg., *56*:45, 1969.
24. Mayo, C. H.: Treatment of varicose veins. Surg. Gynecol. Obstet., *2*:385, 1906.
25. Myers, T. T.: Results and technique of stripping operation for varicose veins. J.A.M.A., *163*:87, 1957.
26. Nicolaides, A. N., and Irving, D.: Clinical factors and the risk of deep venous thrombosis. *In* Nicolaides, A. N. (Ed.): Thromboembolism. Lancaster, Medical and Technical Publishing Company, Ltd., 1975, p. 193.
27. Palma, E. C., and Esperon, R.: Vein transplants and grafts in the surgical treatment of the postphlebitic syndrome. J. Cardiovasc. Surg., *6*:94, 1960.
28. Perthes, G.: Ueber die Operation der Underschenkelvaricen nach Trendelenburg, Dtsch. Med. Wochenschr., *21*:253, 1895.
29. Reagan, B., and Folse, R.: Lower limb venous dynamics in normal persons and children with varicose veins. Surg. Gynecol. Obstet., *132*:15, 1971.
30. Swinton, N. W., Jr., Edgett, J. E., Jr., and Hall, R. J.: Primary subclavian-axillary vein thrombosis. Circulation, *38*:737, 1968.
31. Trendelenburg, F.: Ueber die Underbindung der Vena saphena magna bei Unterschenkelvarican. Bruns. Beit. Klin. Chir., *7*:195, 1891.
32. Virchow, R. L. K.: Thrombose und Embolie. Frankfurt, 1856.
33. Williams, O. B., McCaffrey, J. F., and Lau, O. J.: Deep vein thrombosis in a Queensland hospital. Brit. Med. J., *1*:517, 1973.

52

PULMONARY EMBOLISM

David C. Sabiston, Jr., M.D.

Pulmonary embolism is a serious complication of a variety of medical and surgical disorders. Despite an improved understanding of this condition, its incidence continues to rise, and more than 200,000 patients are estimated to die annually of its effects in the United States and an additional 600,000 have symptomatic pulmonary embolism with recovery.[37] Although pulmonary embolism is especially apt to follow surgical procedures, most series indicate that the majority of cases are *nonsurgical,* the condition developing as a complication of a serious *medical* disorder, such as congestive heart failure, pulmonary disease, carcinomatosis, and many others. In the recent past, considerable attention has been given the fact that a high percentage of persons over the age of 40 are found to have pulmonary embolism at autopsy. Although in many the pulmonary embolus is *incidental* to death, in numerous others it either *contributes* to or is actually the principal *cause* of death.

HISTORICAL ASPECTS

It has long been recognized that thrombi may be found in the pulmonary arteries at autopsy. However, early pathologists regarded these thrombi as being *primary,* that is, arising in situ in the pulmonary arteries. In 1819 Laennec[54] described "pulmonary apoplexy," which now appears to have been pulmonary embolism. He described a typical hemorrhagic infarct and reported that "it looked like liver." In 1829 Cruveilhier[22] made the gross observation that "all arterial branches which lead to those lesions were filled with clots that branched according to the vascular tree."

Rudolf Virchow,[103] the father of modern pathology, was the first to demonstrate convincingly the *embolic* origin of the pulmonary thrombi. He noted that patients with pulmonary embolism usually had concomitant thrombosis in the systemic veins, especially in the legs or pelvis. When challenged as to whether or not such thrombi could indeed pass through the heart and into the lungs, Virchow placed pieces of muscle and rubber or thrombi recovered from patients into the veins of dogs and demonstrated their subsequent appearance in the lungs. He also emphasized age differences in the emboli and suggested that they might break off at different times and embolize in different stages of development. In addition, Virchow noted that the emboli that arrived from a distant source could be differentiated from in situ thrombi occurring *distal* to the emboli. It was his belief that the latter occurred as a result of stasis (Fig. 1). Regarding this array of contributions, William H. Welch, the American pathologist, was to state, "Between the years of 1846 and 1856 Virchow con-

structed the whole doctrine of embolism upon the basis of anatomical, experimental and clinical investigations which for completeness, accuracy and just discernment of the truth must always remain a model of scientific research in medicine."[109]

PATHOGENESIS OF VENOUS THROMBOSIS

The experimental and clinical studies that Virchow conducted on pulmonary embolism more than a century ago led to the conclusion that there were three primary factors in the pathogenesis of pulmonary embolism. These have since become known as Virchow's *triad:* (1) *stasis* or reduction of blood flow in the veins, (2) *injury* to the intimal surface predisposing to thrombosis, and (3) a state of *hypercoagulability.*

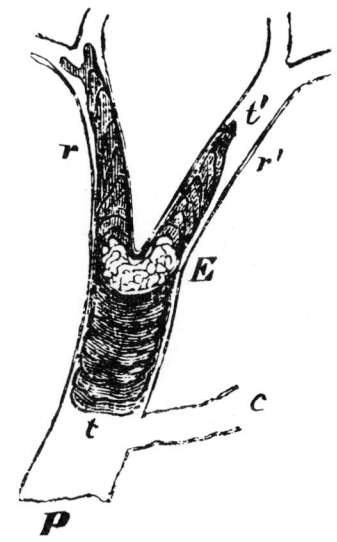

Figure 1. Illustrations taken from Virchow's original drawing depicting a pulmonary artery *(P)* occluded with an embolus *(E).* In addition, in situ thrombosis *(t)* is present which extends to the first proximal branch *(C).* A thrombus also is formed distal to the clot *(r'* and *t').* Thus, there are two types of thrombi present: (1) the thrombus that comes from a distant source and is a true *embolus;* and (2) the thrombus that forms in situ as a result of the stasis produced by the embolus. (From Virchow, R.: Die Cellularpathologie. Berlin, A. Hirschwald, 1858.)

These factors, either singly or in combination, are still thought to be of primary importance in the formation of thrombi in the systemic veins. When such thrombi become detached from the venous wall, they are swept into the circulation and pass through the heart into the lungs.

One of the more important of the factors producing thrombus formation in the systemic veins is *stasis*. It has been demonstrated that radiopaque contrast medium injected into the deep veins of the leg may take a prolonged time to clear when the patient remains in the horizontal position.[59] Moreover, Allison[8] has demonstrated that in postoperative patients radiopaque dye may remain in the calf veins up to 25 minutes after injection. Similarly, patients ill for any reason are less apt to move the extremities, and thus a situation is created that favors intravenous thrombosis.

Sites especially vulnerable to stasis and thrombosis are the sinuses of the venous valves. Here, local stasis permits the accumulation of sufficient amounts of clotting factors to initiate the primary thrombus (Fig. 2). Platelets also become adherent to the pockets created by the valves and a thrombus develops. The thrombus grows by successive deposition of aggregated platelets, leukocytes, and fibrin. From this source, propagation of the thrombus may occur upstream, or the process may spread retrograde as proximal obstruction develops (Fig. 3).

Injury is another factor favoring thrombosis. Thus, soft tissue injury either by blunt trauma or as a result of operative procedures is known to be associated with an increased incidence of venous thrombosis. *Hypercoagulability* has been defined as "the existence of an excessive amount or activity of one or more procoagulant substances, or a decrease in anticoagulant factors."[2] Thus, during pregnancy, a time when thrombosis is prevalent, the concentrations of fibrinogen, prothrombin, factor VII, Stuart factor, Christmas factor, and antihemophilic factor all are elevated,[3] and

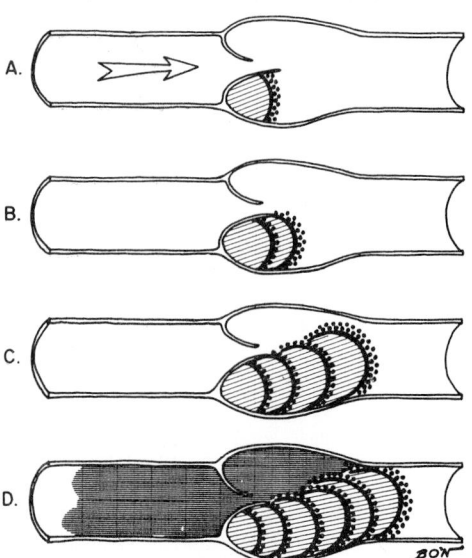

Figure 3. Diagrammatic illustration showing propagation of a deep thrombus arising in a valvar pocket with deposition of successive layers (*A*, *B*, and *C*) and retrograde extension of the thrombus after venous blockage by propagation (*D*). (From Hume, M., Sevitt, S., and Thomas, D. P.: Venous Thrombosis and Pulmonary Embolism. Cambridge, Mass., Harvard University Press, 1970.)

the risk of venous thrombosis is correspondingly increased.

PATHOLOGIC ASPECTS

During the past decade, there has been an increased awareness that pulmonary embolism (especially microscopic occlusion of the smaller vessels) is quite common. The importance of pulmonary embolism in routine autopsies is emphasized by a study demonstrating evidence of old or fresh pulmonary emboli in *64 per cent* of all persons over the age of 40.[32] Moreover, the *clinical diagnosis* of pulmonary embolism is frequently difficult to establish and its presence is often recognized for the first time at autopsy.

Although *reflex* responses are of importance in the physiologic changes following pulmonary embolism, primary emphasis should be placed upon the *mechanical* factors of arterial occlusion. This feature is well demonstrated in a classic pathologic study of 100 consecutive patients with *fatal* pulmonary embolism in which 85 had occlusion involving *one* pulmonary artery and, in addition, emboli in the *opposite* lung.[35, 36] Of the 100 patients, only 15 had emboli restricted solely to one lung, and 12 of these were more than 54 years of age and thus members of an age group with an appreciable incidence of underlying cardiac and respiratory disease. Moreover, in patients with massive pulmonary embolism in whom embolectomy is performed, it is usual to find emboli in more than one pulmonary artery.[7, 81] This evidence supports the importance of *mechanical* occlusion in the cardiodynamic sequelae of massive pulmonary embolism (Fig. 4). These data are in agreement with similar observa-

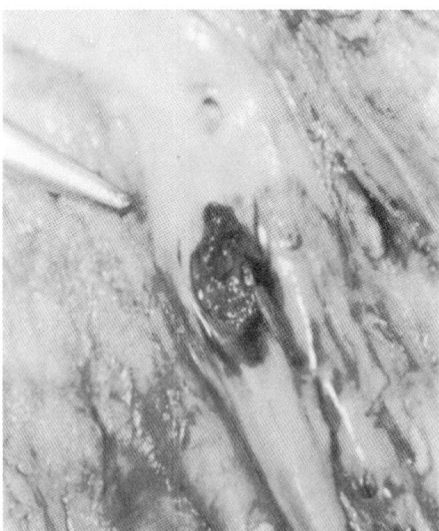

Figure 2. A primary thrombus forming in the valve pocket at the mouth of the deep femoral vein. (From Hume, M., Sevitt, S., and Thomas, D. P.: Venous Thrombosis and Pulmonary Embolism. Cambridge, Mass., Harvard University Press, 1970.)

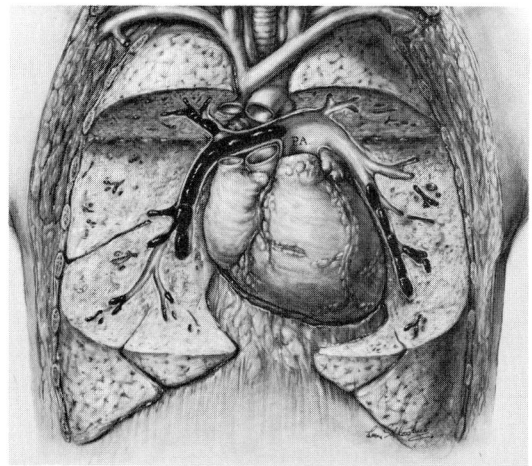

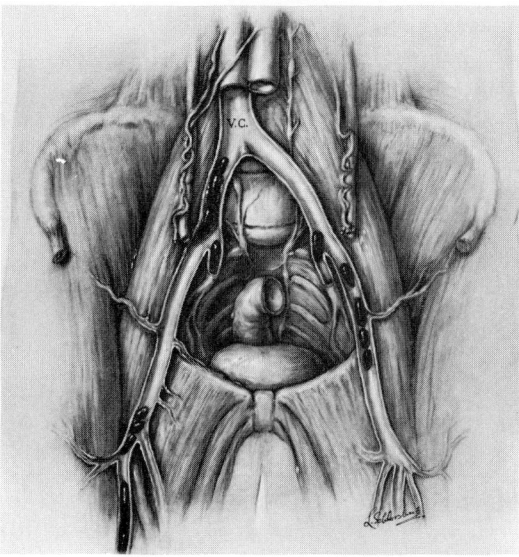

Figure 4. Illustration of the findings in a patient with massive pulmonary embolism at the time of postmortem examination. Multiple thrombi are present in the iliofemoral system. The right pulmonary artery and its branches are totally occluded by emboli. The left lower lobar pulmonary artery is also occluded. Under these circumstances, the entire output of the right ventricle must pass through the left upper lobe, which greatly increases pulmonary resistance and right ventricular work. The sudden development of this degree of pulmonary arterial occlusion produces a clinical state of severe shock, since the left ventricle receives a much diminished amount of blood to supply the systemic arterial circulation. In otherwise normal patients, 50 per cent or more of the pulmonary arterial circulation must be occluded before serious cardiovascular manifestations are produced. (From Sabiston, D. C., Jr., and Wolfe, W. G.: Ann. Surg., 168:1, 1968.)

tions upon reduction of pulmonary blood by other causes including arterial ligature, intravascular balloons, pulmonary resection, and various forms of emboli.[15, 16, 95] Following injection of experimental pulmonary emboli, reduced function of the embolized lung occurs immediately, but pulmonary function returns to near normal within several weeks.[57, 82] Similarly, marked histologic changes occur in these thrombi, with intravascular resolution and ultimate disappearance. Such resolution can be confirmed by serial pul-

monary radioactive scans, arteriography, pulmonary function studies, and gross and microscopic evaluation. The gradual dissolution can be serially demonstrated (Figs. 5 and 6).

Clinical observations also confirm the resolution of large pulmonary emboli with or without the use of anticoagulants or fibrinolysins (Fig. 7). These observations have demonstrated convincingly that the *natural history* of pulmonary embolism in most instances is one of spontaneous resolution.[31, 82, 86] This concept has become of increasing significance in a more complete understanding of the principles of diagnosis and management.

Pulmonary embolism occurs in *children* as well as in adults and in one study was found to be present in approximately 1 per cent of all children examined at autopsy, usually as a secondary manifestation of serious illness such as a respiratory infection, phlebitis, systemic infection, congenital heart disease, or rheumatic heart disease.[45] Although pulmonary embolism in children is rarely diagnosed before death, its clinical manifestations are similar to those in adults.

The emboli generally found at postmortem examination are 1.0 to 1.5 cm. in diameter, apparently having arisen in sizable veins. Their length ranges up to 50 cm. or more,[43] and they often break up after arrival in the lungs into multiple small portions with occlusion of multiple branches of the pulmonary arteries. Generally, the right pulmonary artery and its branches are more commonly involved than the left, and the *lower* lobes are preferentially involved.

The *source* of pulmonary emboli is primarily the systemic venous circulation, and the prevailing evidence indicates that the majority of emboli arise from the *iliac* and *femoral veins* (Table 1).[34, 60, 73, 78, 80, 89] While the smaller leg veins such as those of the calf may be involved, it is not as likely that such will cause serious clinical manifestations of pulmonary embolism. In other words, only thrombi produced in veins the size of the iliac or femoral vein are large enough to produce serious symptoms in most patients.

Rarely, a venous thrombus may pass through an intracardiac opening (patent foramen ovale, atrial septal defect, or ventricular septal defect) and embolize a systemic organ.[92] This is termed *paradoxical embolism* and is more apt to occur when right ventricular and right atrial hypertension are present.

In addition to the iliofemoral and pelvic veins, other possible sources of venous thrombi include the inferior vena cava, the subclavian and internal jugular veins, and the cavernous sinuses of the skull. Some have emphasized that as many as one fifth of pulmonary emboli arise from sources other than veins drained by the inferior vena cava.[39]

It is important to stress the fact that pulmonary *embolism* and *infarction* are not synonymous. Whereas pulmonary embolism is of common occurrence, pulmonary infarction is much less frequent. Pathologically, an infarct is generally a circumscribed area of local hemorrhage and demonstrates *necrosis* of the lung parenchyma. The majority of the patients with embolism do not show these features. Generally, infarcts are located peripherally in the lungs, most often in the

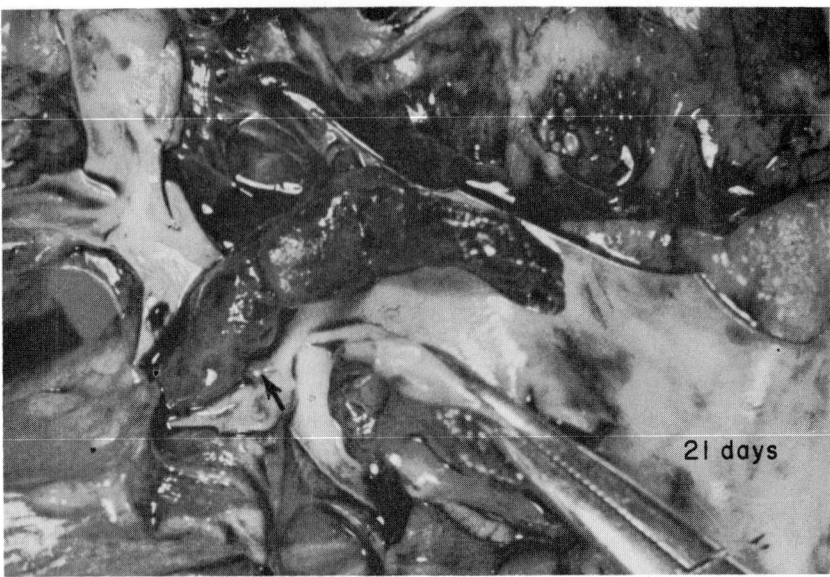

Figure 5. A large pulmonary embolus (originally produced experimentally in the inferior vena cava) is shown in the pulmonary artery 21 days after embolization. (From Sabiston, D. C., Jr., and Wolfe, W. G.: Ann. Surg., *168*:1, 1968.)

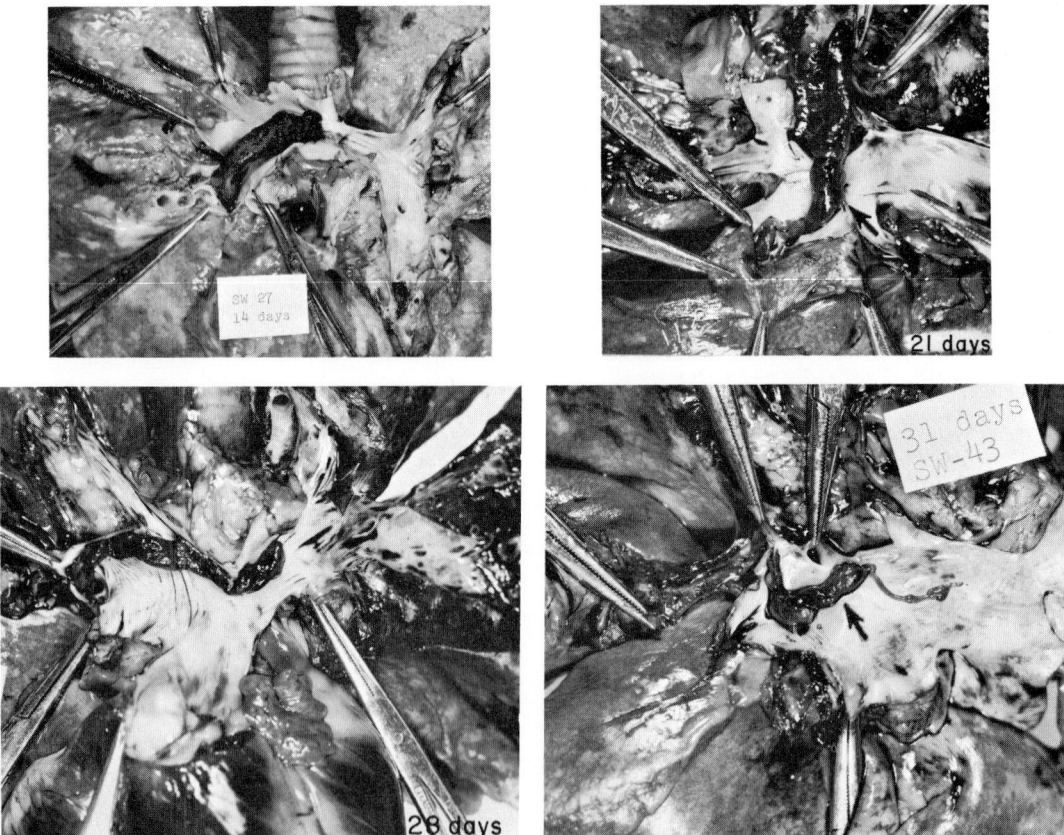

Figure 6. Progressive changes in experimental pulmonary emboli from the fourteenth to the thirty-first day. The attachments are demonstrated at the tip of the arrow at 21 days. The diameter of the embolus is definitely less by the twenty-eighth day. The embolus at 31 days demonstrates the variability in resolution in different parts of the thrombus. One end of the thrombus has been reduced to a small fragment while the remaining part is larger. (From Sabiston, D. C., Jr., and Wolfe, W. G.: Ann. Surg., *168*:1, 1968.)

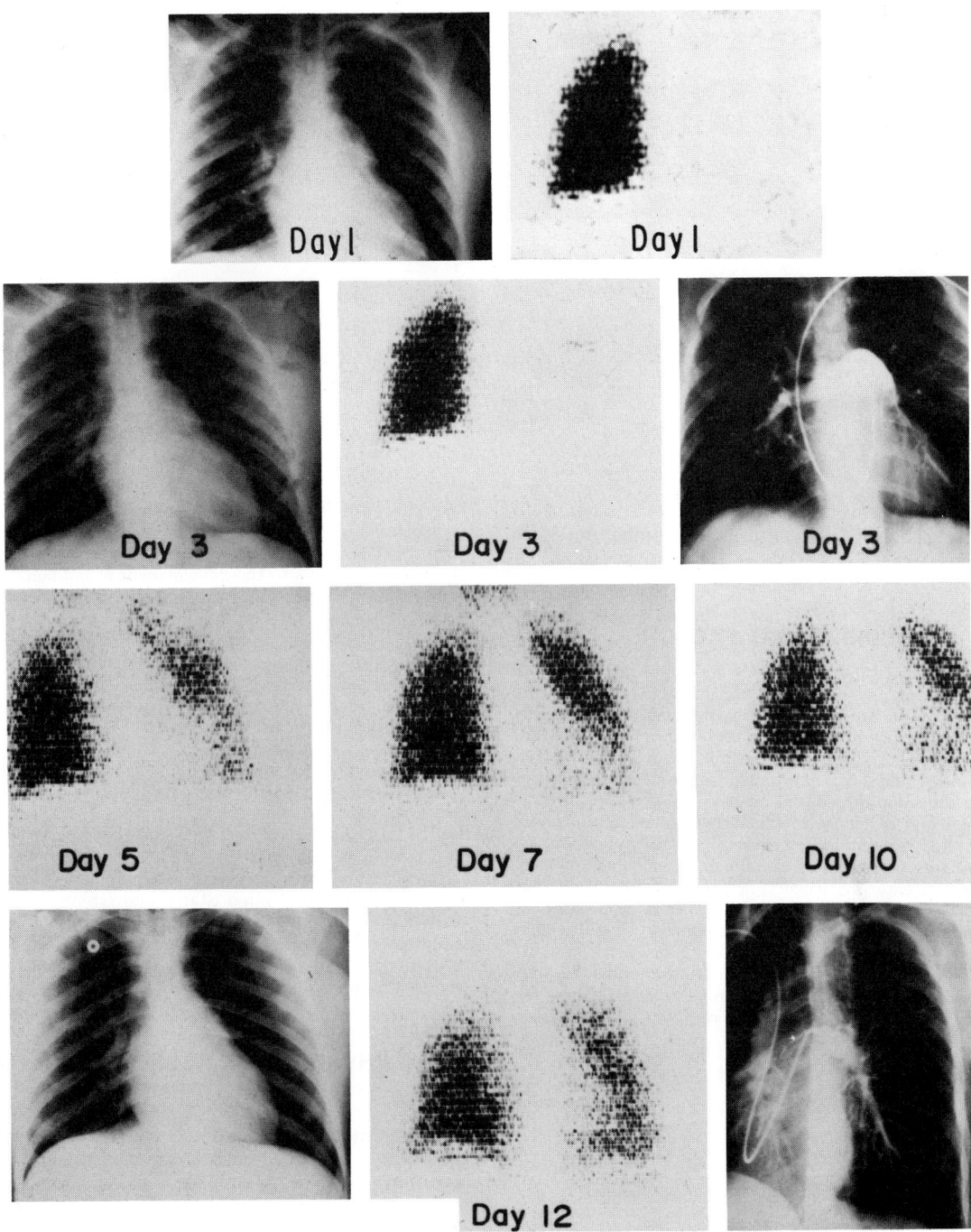

Figure 7. Serial chest films and scans following a massive pulmonary embolus to the left pulmonary artery in a 25-year-old female after a pelvic operation. On the fifth postoperative day, discomfort was noted in the left chest with dyspnea. A plain chest film taken on this day (day 1) showed diminished vascular markings (Westermark's sign). A radioactive pulmonary scan showed no evidence of pulmonary flow to the entire left lobe. Beginning on the third day after the embolus, the scan and arteriogram both show evidence of flow to the left lung. In subsequent scans and pulmonary arteriograms, resolution of the thrombus occurred with progressively increasing amounts of flow by the twelfth day.

TABLE 1.   Site of Origin of Venous Thrombi*

References	Cases with Thrombosis at Necropsy	Per Cent of Cases with Thrombi in				
		Iliac Veins	*Femoral Veins*	*Popliteal Veins*	*Soleal Veins*	*Any Deep Calf Vein*
Rosslé[80]	94	—	49	—	—	92
Neuman[73]	100	—	22	—	—	87
McLachlin and Paterson[60]	34	9	82	—	—	41
Gibbs[34]	149	—	42	—	—	65
Sevitt and Gallagher[89]	81	70		33	67	74
Roberts[78]	58	14	43	41	86	95

*From Hume, M., Sevitt, S., and Thomas, D. P.: Venous Thrombosis & Pulmonary Embolism. Cambridge, Mass., Harvard University Press, 1970.

lower lobes, and are less than 5 cm. in diameter. In one series, the proportion of infarcts to emboli was 1 to 10.[96]

PREDISPOSING FACTORS

Present evidence indicates that females are more likely to have pulmonary embolism than are males. A British study reports that in females pulmonary embolism is responsible for 110 deaths per million, as contrasted to 77 deaths per million in males.[77] There is little doubt that *age* plays an important factor and pulmonary embolism is clearly a disorder affecting the middle-aged and elderly. This relationship between age and incidence of thromboembolism is shown in Figure 8. Bed rest and lack of exercise in general are well-established antecedent causes of pulmonary embolism causing a twofold or greater incidence.[8] The presence of heart disease, especially congestive heart failure or atrial fibrillation, is particularly conducive to the development of pulmonary embolism. Following acute myocardial infarction, 34 to 37 per cent of patients have been demonstrated to have deep venous thrombosis,[58, 71] and after cerebrovascular accidents, the incidence may be as high as 60 per cent.[107] *Cancer*, particu-

larly cancer of the pancreas and prostate and carcinomatosis, is associated with a high incidence of pulmonary embolism.[20]

Surgical procedures have long been recognized as being predisposing factors to the development of pulmonary embolism. Scanning of the lower extremities after intravenous injection of radioactive fibrinogen, a simple technique which is now widely employed in the identification of thrombosis in the extremities, demonstrated deep venous thrombosis in 54 per cent of patients with hip fractures, 50 per cent of those undergoing prostatectomy, and 28 per cent of general surgical patients over the age of 40.[47]

It has long been recognized that there is a higher risk of pulmonary embolism during pregnancy and the puerperium. Pressure from the gravid uterus may act to retard venous flow from the limbs and pelvis. Infection in the postpartum patient may also give rise to septic thrombophlebitis and embolism. *Oral contraceptives* have been shown to be positively associated with the presence of pulmonary embolism in studies in both the United States and Great Britain. In a British study[61, 102] the results showed that the risk of venous thrombosis or pulmonary embolism was increased threefold in women receiving oral contraceptives and about sixfold in women who were pregnant or in the puerperium.

PHYSIOLOGIC RESPONSES TO PULMONARY EMBOLISM

The pulmonary arteries receive the total output of the right ventricle, and a characteristic and impressive feature of the pulmonary circulation is its *low* vascular resistance. This fact enables flow in the pulmonary vascular bed to be increased severalfold with minimal elevation of pulmonary arterial pressure. Despite numerous experimental and clinical studies, opinion remains divided concerning the relative importance of *reflex* versus *mechanical* effects in pulmonary embolism. The occasional finding of a small pulmonary embolus in a patient after sudden death has been cited as evidence that intraluminal occlusion of a relatively small pulmonary artery can produce death, presumably as a result of reflex mechanisms. Cur-

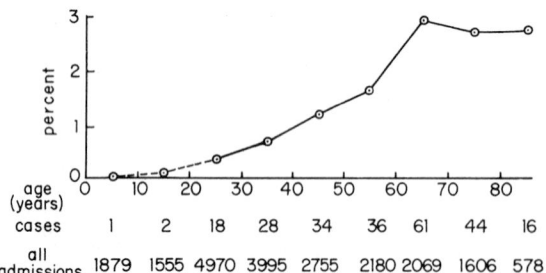

Figure 8. Graph showing the relationship of age to occurrence of thromboembolism. The ordinate represents the percentage of all hospital admissions in which a diagnosis was made clinically or at necropsy. The abscissa indicates age by decade. (From Hume, M., Sevitt, S., and Thomas, D. P.: Venous Thrombosis and Pulmonary Embolism. Cambridge, Mass., Harvard University Press, 1970.)

rently, such an explanation would rarely be accepted except under very unusual circumstances.

Experimental pulmonary embolism has been produced by many methods. The physiologic changes appear to be related to the *size* of the emboli and can be divided into those that produce *microembolism* (obstruction of terminal small arteries and arterioles) and those that produce *macroembolism* (occlusion of the larger pulmonary vessels). Considerable reduction in the diameter of the main pulmonary artery or the primary branches is required to reduce pulmonary blood flow significantly or to produce pulmonary hypertension proximal to the obstruction. It has been shown that large experimental thrombi produced in the inferior vena cava and transferred to *either* the right or left pulmonary artery 10 to 14 days later produce a minimum of cardiovascular and respiratory responses.[57] Specifically, occlusion of one pulmonary artery produces only minimal and generally insignificant changes in the central venous pressure, right ventricular pressure, pulmonary artery pressure, aortic pressure, cardiac output, total oxygen consumption, and the electrocardiogram *despite* occlusion of half the pulmonary arterial circulation. From these studies it is concluded that this type of embolism produces minimal circulatory effects that can be attributed specifically to reflex action.

Normal man usually tolerates pneumonectomy quite well. Tidal volume and oxygen consumption at rest following resection of a lung have been shown to be little changed.[16] Similarly, occlusion of one pulmonary artery by ligature or an intraluminal balloon is accompanied by few cardiodynamic changes. Patients have tolerated balloon occlusion well for periods up to 2 hours,[9] and even during exercise with similar occlusion, pulmonary arterial pressure is increased only 12 to 50 per cent while cardiac output may increase as much as threefold. Arterial occlusion of this type closely simulates the obstruction produced by large pulmonary emboli. Emphasis should be placed on the fact that such studies have been conducted in otherwise normal subjects. The presence of underlying cardiac or respiratory insufficiency is quite likely to alter this response appreciably. For example, in patients with heart disease, exercise during temporary unilateral occlusion of the right or left pulmonary artery by a balloon catheter produces a marked elevation in pulmonary arterial pressure.[95] Cardiac output does not increase significantly with exercise, and an increase in arteriovenous oxygen difference occurs. Available data suggest that resection of less than one lung is followed by only minor changes in the pulmonary arterial pressure, whereas removal of greater amounts of pulmonary tissue produces an elevation of pulmonary arterial pressure.[108]

Experimental data suggest that embolization of the lung with small particles (100 μ or less) creates *reflex* effects including tachypnea, pulmonary hypertension, and systemic hypotension that may lead to death. However, it is currently thought that microembolism of the lung is infrequently encountered as a clinical problem, although it does occur following massive blood transfusions during which platelet, leukocyte, and fibrin emboli may occlude the pulmonary microcirculation.[23] For this reason transfusion filters should be employed. Embolization with larger particles requires considerably more blockage of the pulmonary arterial system to produce significant effects. Thus, in general, the conclusion has been drawn that arterial emboli produce pulmonary hypertension by *mechanical* obstruction, while vasoconstriction is produced by arteriolar embolism and is mediated by *reflex* changes.[27] Such studies suggest that the clinical manifestations of pulmonary embolism are usually produced primarily by occlusion of the larger pulmonary arteries, a concept supported by both clinical and pathologic studies.

Cyanosis is a recognized finding in clinical pulmonary embolism, and hypoxemia is almost always present. The *cause* of reduced oxygen tension in the arterial blood has elicited considerable discussion. A number of possible etiologic factors have been advanced and include: (1) alveolar hypoventilation, (2) ventilation-perfusion abnormality, (3) decreased diffusing capacity of the lungs, (4) pulmonary edema, (5) venoarterial shunting, and (6) rapid transit of blood through the capillary bed without adequate time for oxygenation. It is apparent that a combination of these factors may be responsible, as is implied in experimental studies.[52]

Clinical evidence of *reflex bronchoconstriction* in pulmonary embolism is a subject of considerable interest.[13] Repeat pulmonary function studies after injection of intravenous heparin showed a prompt improvement in the maximal expiratory flow rate or a reduction in lung resistance.[38] Such observations are cited as further evidence of a *humoral* factor. Humoral factors mediated by platelets may be of importance in the genesis of cardiopulmonary disturbances in patients with pulmonary embolism. It is known that platelets are a concentrated source of biologically active amines. In experimental studies evidence has been obtained that 5-hydroxytryptamine (serotonin) is liberated from platelets in the process of blood coagulation and that it produces bronchoconstriction.[19]

It is well established that hypoxia elicits pulmonary vasoconstriction.[28] This response is generally considered to be a self-regulatory mechanism by which pulmonary capillary blood flow is automatically adjusted to alveolar ventilation. Such a response is classically seen in acute hypoxia as well as in the chronic hypoxia of high altitude, which has also been seen to be associated with pulmonary vasoconstriction.[12, 67] This physiologic feature should be remembered in the interpretation of the pulmonary hypertension, which is often found in association with both acute and chronic pulmonary embolism.

In summary, a combination of experimental and clinical evidence suggests that a variety of factors contribute to the changes that occur following embolism. The majority of evidence favors a primary *mechanical* basis for the physiologic changes with the belief that the blockage of the emboli themselves produces the most serious changes. It is quite clear that the *preembolic* status significantly affects the clinical manifestations, and the presence of pre-existing cardiac or respiratory insufficiency is of great importance. If the latter is present, lesser degrees of pulmonary embolism cause greater clinical responses. Evidence clearly exists for the presence of *reflex changes,* although these are in general of secondary importance. The vasoactive amines, probably arising from the emboli themselves, appear to exert a significant role.

INCIDENCE

Current statistics indicate that the incidence of pulmonary embolism is increasing, and the risk of death from pulmonary embolism following surgical procedures from a collected series is 0.11 per cent.[24] An English study over a 10-year period (1952 to 1961) showed a progressive rise in incidence,[69] and a similar rise has been observed in Germany.[62] The data for the increase in England are shown in Figure 9. Although most statistics indicate a definite increase in the incidence of thromboembolism, the causes for this increase remain unclear. Factors that are cited as being responsible include: (1) the increase in older members of the population, (2) larger numbers and greater magnitude of operative procedures, (3) increased recognition, and (4) use of hormonal agents for birth control.

DIAGNOSIS OF PULMONARY EMBOLISM

Clinical Manifestations

Pulmonary embolism is notorious for the similarity of its clinical manifestations to those of other cardiore-

TABLE 2. Clinical Manifestations in 1000 Patients with Pulmonary Embolism at the Duke University Medical Center

Symptoms	Per Cent
Dyspnea	77
Chest pain	63
Hemoptysis	26
Altered mental status	23
Dyspnea, chest pain, hemoptysis	14
Signs	**Per Cent**
Tachycardia	59
Recent fever	43
Rales	42
Tachypnea	38
Leg edema and tenderness	23
Elevated venous pressure	18
Shock	11
Accentuated P_2	11
Cyanosis	9
Pleural friction rub	8

spiratory disorders. This makes difficult the establishment of an accurate *clinical* diagnosis. The characteristic symptoms of dyspnea, chest pain, hemoptysis, and hypotension may be present in the classic example, but experience has shown that these are not sufficiently specific to permit a definite diagnosis. The following points bear emphasis: (1) many patients have underlying cardiac disease; (2) dyspnea and tachypnea are the most frequent clinical findings; (3) accentuation of the pulmonary second sound is common, whereas the more classic signs of hemoptysis, pleural friction rub, gallop rhythm, cyanosis, and chest splinting are present in only a quarter or less of patients; and (4) clinical evidence of venous thrombosis is the exception and occurs in only one third of patients.[85] The symptoms found in 1000 consecutive patients at the Duke University Medical Center are shown in Table 2.

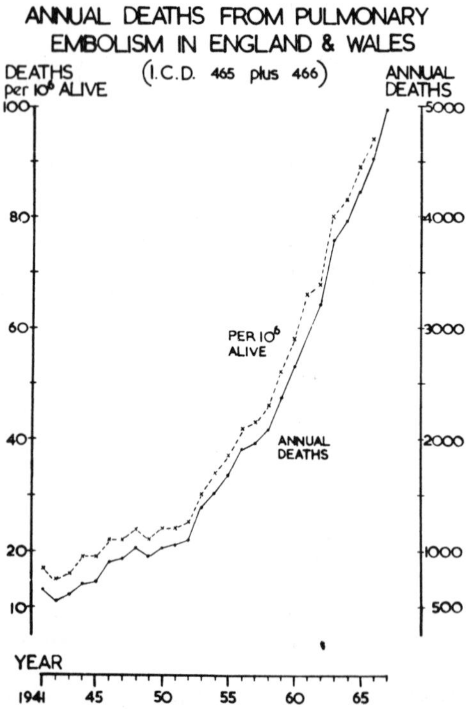

Laboratory Findings

The *plain chest* film may show diminished pulmonary vascular markings at the site of the embolus (Westermark's sign).[111] This is an inconstant and frequently equivocal sign, although it may be of aid.[99] It is apparent that the symptoms and physical signs of pulmonary embolism are frequently insufficient to establish an accurate diagnosis.

Specific serum *enzyme* changes may be helpful although are seldom conclusive. The triad of an elevated serum lactic dehydrogenase (LDH) activity, increased serum bilirubin, and a normal serum glutamic oxalacetic transaminase (SGOT) activity is often present.[105] Serum LDH is frequently elevated and the bilirubin is increased in approximately two thirds of patients. While determination of serum enzyme activity is helpful in diagnosis in patients with massive embolism and acute cardiovascular changes, the time factor is often crucial and a more rapid means of diagnosis is necessary.

The *electrocardiographic* changes have been studied

Figure 9. Graph illustrating increase in annual deaths from pulmonary embolism in England and Wales. (From Hume, M., Sevitt, S., and Thomas, D. P.: Venous Thrombosis and Pulmonary Embolism. Cambridge, Mass., Harvard University Press, 1970.)

extensively. While the electrocardiogram can be helpful, there is increasing appreciation of the fact that it cannot be depended upon for an objective diagnosis. It is probable that not more than 10 to 20 per cent of patients who subsequently are proved to have pulmonary embolism show *any* electrocardiographic changes, and of these, a still smaller number show identifiable diagnostic abnormalities.[55] Electrocardiographic alterations include disturbances of rhythm (atrial fibrillation, ectopic beats, heart block), enlargement of P waves, S-T segment depression, and T wave inversion (particularly in leads III, AV_F, V_1, V_4, and V_5). The most common abnormality is S-T segment depression, a result of myocardial ischemia from a reduced cardiac output and arterial pressure as well as increased right ventricular pressure.

Imbalance of Pulmonary Ventilation and Perfusion. The ventilatory dead space is increased in pulmonary embolism.[79] Occlusion of a major pulmonary arterial branch causes a decrease in gas exchange in the corresponding segment of the lung while alveolar ventilation continues. In a ventilated but underperfused segment of lung, the composition of the alveolar air tends to approach that of inspired air, with a low partial pressure of carbon dioxide. This air is mixed with that from the normal areas of the lung during expiration but reduces the mean alveolar carbon dioxide tension to a degree that can be detected in the expired air. Arterial carbon dioxide tension remains at a nearly normal level because of the presence of normal lung tissue. The difference between the arterial and alveolar carbon dioxide tensions therefore may be of aid in the diagnosis of pulmonary embolism.

Pulmonary Arteriography. Pulmonary arteriography is an excellent technique for demonstration of embolism. Knowledge of the normal pulmonary angiographic appearance provides a background for the evaluation of morphologic and physiologic disturbances of flow in the pulmonary vessels.[94] The arteries in the lower areas of the lung are normally larger than those in the upper portions, since they serve a larger volume of lung tissue. Major branches are readily identifiable by comparison with normal anatomic charts of the pulmonary arteries. Such vessels usually follow the branching pattern of the bronchi. Occasionally, total obstruction of the main pulmonary artery is found, usually in association with marked symptoms. In most instances, the obstruction involves lobar or segmental branches (Fig. 10). The filling defect may be sharply delineated, usually manifest as a convex shadow with a blunt end or an irregular taper. The defect should remain *constant* on several successive films in the series, and the flow may be sluggish, as shown by a small pool of contrast medium that may persist in the artery above the obstruction well into the venous phase of the angiogram. When pulmonary arteriography is performed later in the course of embolism, contrast medium may pass around the obstruction, causing delayed opacification of the artery distally. The pattern in some areas may show avascular segments that represent the result of unresolved thromboembolism.

Pulmonary Scanning. Wagner and associates[106] introduced radioisotope pulmonary scanning in 1964, and the technique has since been widely employed. The principle of the method is measurement of intravenously injected particles labeled with iodine-131, chromium-51, or technetium-99m. Macromolecules of human serum albumin (10 to 100 μ in diameter) become lodged in the pulmonary capillary bed following intravenous injection. It is thus possible to delineate the distribution of pulmonary arterial blood flow and reveal areas of decreased perfusion. It must be emphasized that lesions present on the plain chest film (such as pneumonitis, atelectasis, emphysematous bullae, or neoplasm) will uniformly demonstrate *scanning defects; therefore, these areas must be excluded from consideration.* Under these circumstances it is essential that misinterpretation be avoided by review of a simultaneous plain chest film. This technique has been found to be particularly useful in the patient with massive pulmonary embolism, especially if the plain chest film is essentially normal.

Inhalation scanning with the use of xenon-133 has been of additional aid in the interpretation of the perfusion pulmonary scan. This allows the differentiation of underperfused and underventilated areas in the lungs. It is also recognized that pulmonary embolism produces bronchoconstriction, therefore reducing the amount of air delivered to the embolized portion of the lung. Moreover, areas of the lung without pulmonary embolism may also show bronchoconstriction with reduced ventilation.

The use of *venography* is often useful in making an objective diagnosis of phlebothrombosis, particularly in the legs. It is of special significance in those patients in whom interruption of the vena cava is being considered as a therapeutic measure. The use of radioiodinated fibrinogen, although extremely sensitive in the detection of the development of new thrombi in the extremities, is less accurate in detecting thrombi in the *iliofemoral* region owing to the background of radioactivity in the urinary bladder and also to the relatively poor penetration of ^{125}I.

MANAGEMENT

Before specific therapy for pulmonary embolism is initiated, it is essential that an *objective* diagnosis be established. The two most important and reliable means of diagnosis are pulmonary *scanning* and *arteriography*. Since scanning is a simple, safe, and reliable technique, it is generally preferred. It causes the patient little inconvenience and has no appreciable risk.

ANTICOAGULANTS

Anticoagulants form the primary basis of therapy in the majority of patients. The scanning and arteriographic features of an appropriate patient for treatment with anticoagulants are shown in Figure 6. Heparin is usually employed initially, and its effect when administered intravenously is immediate. Heparin interferes with blood coagulation in at least two ways: (1) by preventing the activation of factor IX (Christmas fac-

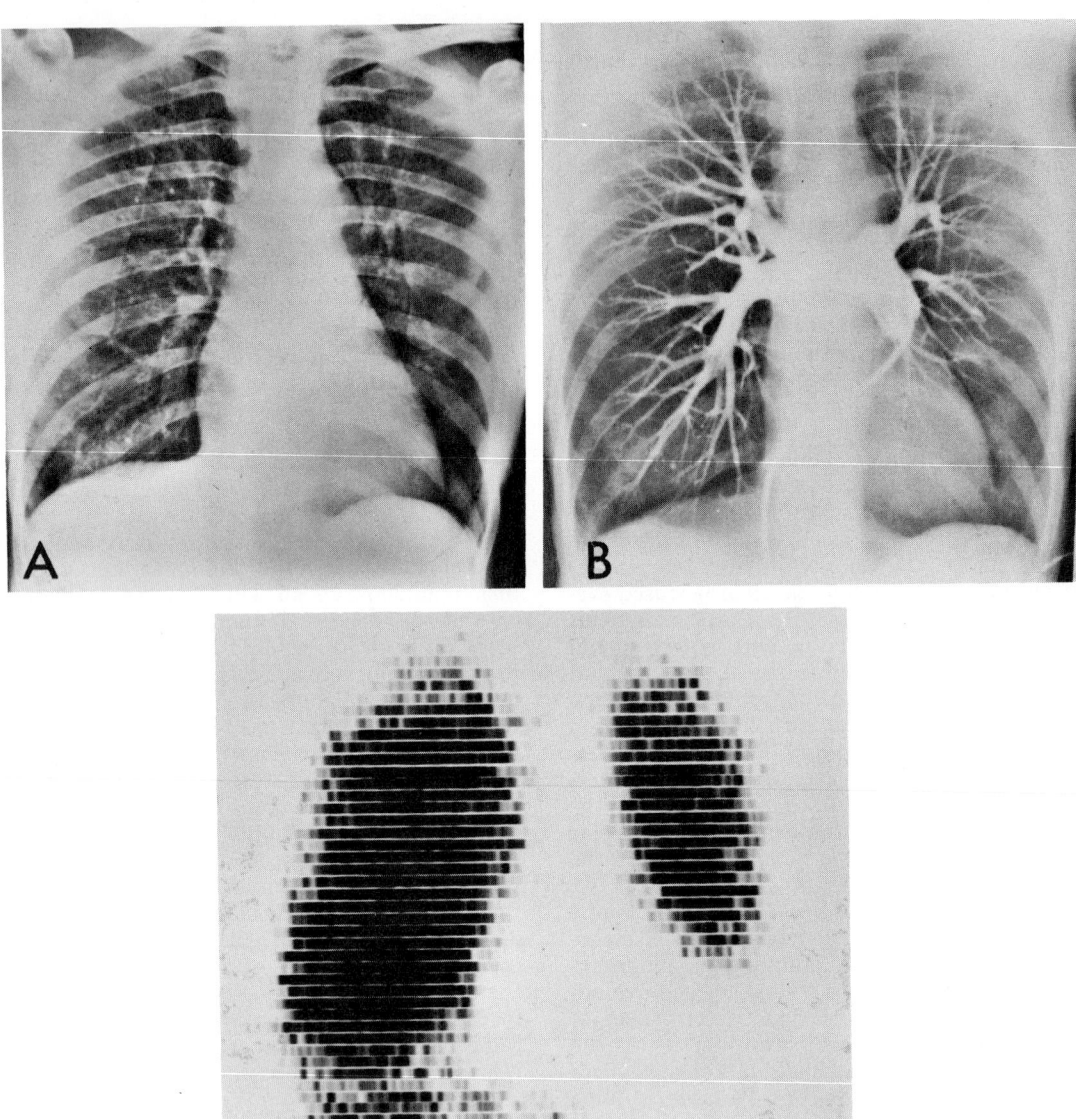

Figure 10. Films from a patient with pulmonary embolism involving the left lower lobar pulmonary artery. *A,* Slight diminution of the vascular markings to the left lower lobe is noted in comparison with those in the right lower lobe on the plain chest film (Westermark's sign). *B,* Pulmonary arteriogram illustrating occlusion of the right lower lobar pulmonary artery. *C,* Pulmonary scan showing absence of perfusion of the left lower lobe. (From Sabiston, D. C., Jr., and Wagner, H. N., Jr.: Ann. Surg., *160:*585, 1964.)

tor) by factor XI (thromboplastin antecedent) in the early coagulation sequence; and (2) by acting as a potent antithrombin in the presence of heparin co-factor. Therefore it inhibits both the *intrinsic* and *extrinsic* coagulation mechanisms. In its antithrombin effects, heparin inhibits the conversion of fibrinogen to fibrin by thrombin and in high doses prevents the action of thrombin on platelets. Heparin is largely excreted in the urine, and awareness of the renal state is important. Also, the enzyme heparinase is present in the liver, a site of some degradation.

The therapeutic level of heparin is accomplished by maintaining the clotting time twice to three times normal (20 to 35 minutes, assuming a normal clotting time of 8 to 12 minutes). The amount required varies.

In general, 15,000 units should be given intravenously as the initial dose with 5000 to 10,000 units each 4 to 6 hours thereafter to maintain the desired clotting time. At the beginning of therapy, a continuous intravenous heparin drip is the most reliable method of obtaining and controlling the extended clotting time. Later the heparin may be given subcutaneously. Heparin therapy prevents both extension of the thrombus in the venous system and the formation of distal in situ thrombi in the pulmonary arteries. Some employ quite high doses of heparin (100,000 units daily) with good results.[9, 51] The prolongation of coagulation time may be followed by either the activated partial thromboplastin time (APTT)[97] or by the Lee-White clotting time. The APTT should be maintained at approximately twice the value of the patient's preheparin activated partial thromboplastin time. If the Lee-White clotting time method is used, it should be maintained at 30 minutes or longer for effective anticoagulation.

The duration of heparin therapy is dependent upon the individual patient and the clinical course. In general, 8 to 10 days of heparin with extension of clotting time to two to three times normal is recommended, since this approximates the time necessary for the venous thrombi to become firmly adherent to the vessel wall. A continuous intravenous infusion, preferably with a small roller pump, provides a more stabilized level of anticoagulation and a reduced incidence of hemorrhage.[83] During this period, a moderate amount of thrombolysis also occurs. Customarily, oral coumarin anticoagulation is begun several days prior to the cessation of heparin therapy in order to allow the required time for adequate prolongation of the prothrombin.

Delayed postoperative hemorrhage can occur in patients receiving heparin therapy for venous thrombosis and pulmonary embolism, particularly in patients with prosthetic arterial grafts. It is thought that there is a continuous lysis and resorption of old thrombus and replacement with new thrombus at arterial prosthesis suture lines until the suture line is sealed by regeneration of new intima. Thus, patients have had serious hemorrhage as long as a month after the placement of aortic arterial grafts when maintained on heparin therapy for treatment of venous thromboembolism.[6]

The oral anticoagulant coumarin drugs have indirect and delayed action on the blood clotting mechanism. These agents act upon the liver and inhibit the production of four of the factors involved in the transformation of prothrombin to thrombin—factors XII, IX, and X and prothrombin itself. The sum of these effects has been termed "hypoprothrombinemia." The coumarin drugs are rapidly absorbed from the gastrointestinal tract and are concentrated primarily in the liver. Although short-acting, intermediate, and long-acting agents are available, one of the more commonly used is warfarin sodium. It has only a slight cumulative effect. The average loading dose on the first day is 15 to 30 mg. and on the second day 10 to 20 mg. The maximal effect is usually reached in 1½ to 2 days, and the average daily maintenance dose is usually between 5 and 10 mg. (ranges from 2 to 20 mg.). The duration of coumarin therapy is controversial, but most believe it should be continued for a minimum of 6 weeks and some advocate up to 6 months or longer. In any event, it is apparent that the local responses and subsequent course of the patient are the primary indicators. The recovery time required after maximal effect is 2 to 4 days. Administration of vitamin K counteracts the effect of the coumarin and should be employed if bleeding complications occur.

THROMBOLYTIC AGENTS

Considerable effort has been directed toward finding suitable thrombolytic agents for use in the treatment of venous thrombosis and pulmonary embolism. In the body *plasminogen* is the inactive precursor of *plasmin*, the active fibrinolytic enzyme. Under normal circumstances, plasminogen is present in the blood and tissues. Exercise, stress, and shock cause plasminogen to be activated by plasmin through a labile activator present in many tissues and especially in venous endothelium. Plasmin activity in the bloodstream is prevented by inhibitors, both by an antiactivator and by antiplasmins. Two thrombolysins, streptokinase and urokinase, have been studied extensively. Both act by transforming plasminogen to plasmin. Streptokinase is a soluble product of the metabolism of *Streptococcus pyogenes* (Lancefield Group A) and is available in a highly purified form. Since patients who have had previous streptococcal infections may be allergic to streptokinase, it can produce toxic reactions (pyrexia, dyspnea, tachycardia, and anaphylaxis). Urokinase is a strong thrombolytic agent found in human urine. In an effort to document its effects, the National Heart and Lung Institute is conducting a national cooperative study of urokinase. The initial results have demonstrated that urokinase combined with heparin therapy, as compared to heparin therapy alone, significantly accelerates the resolution of pulmonary thromboemboli at 24 hours as shown by pulmonary arteriograms, lung scans, and right-sided heart pressure measurements. *However,* no significant differences in recurrence rate of pulmonary embolism or in the two-week mortality were noted. Bleeding was a prominent complication and occurred in 45 per cent of the patients receiving urokinase as contrasted to 27 per cent of those given heparin alone. It was concluded that since the urokinase regimen did not usually achieve complete or nearly complete thrombolysis, and especially because of its hemorrhagic potential, further studies with urokinase are necessary before specific therapeutic recommendations can be made.[101] A review summarizes the present status of thrombolytic therapy.[29]

ANTI-PLATELET HYPERAGGREGABILITY AGENTS

A group of nonsteroidal anti-inflammatory drugs, including aspirin, indomethacin, and sulfinpyrazone, has been shown to inhibit the platelet release reaction, secondary ADP-induced platelet aggregation, and adherence to collagen when tested in vitro. These agents have been reported to show good antithrombotic efficacy in models, and sulfinpyrazone has been demonstrated in humans to return the increased platelet turnover to normal in thrombovascular disease.[33] In addition, pyrimidopyrimidine compounds inhibit both primary and secondary aggregation of platelets induced by ADP-epinephrine and collagen decreased platelet retention by glass-bead columns and act in part by inhibition of phosphodiesterase. Dipyridamole (Persantine) is one of these agents and has been proved to be effective in interruption of increased platelet turnover in arterial thromboembolism in man.[33] In a control study, half the patients were randomized postoperatively to receive aspirin (650 mg. twice daily) orally or, if unable to take by mouth, administered rectally by suppositories. Radioactive ^{125}I fibrinogen scans were obtained of the lower extremities of all patients. Among those receiving aspirin, 12.5 per cent developed venous thrombosis, while those in the control series without aspirin had a 20.4 per cent incidence of venous thrombosis demonstrated by the scans.[18] The use of dipyridamole in the treatment and prevention of postoperative thrombosis is less effective.[84]

PREVENTION

Much attention has been directed toward prophylaxis against thrombosis with the hope that this complication might be eliminated. However, no proven method or combination of methods currently exists for total prevention of thromboembolism. Several factors are considered of importance, including (1) physical activity, (2) elevation of the lower extremities, (3) stocking compression of the legs, and (4) prophylactic anticoagulation in selected patients.

A number of observers have recommended early ambulation and physical activity following operations or during bed rest for other illness. In a study undertaken to evaluate the role of exercise, postmortem vein dissections showed that thrombi were found in only 18 per cent of patients who had been given exercises before death, as compared with 53 per cent in controls (nonexercised and nonambulatory).[44] Other studies have been less confirmatory, including one in which the ^{125}I fibrinogen method for detection of leg vein thrombi was employed. The patients in this study group underwent an intensive regimen including vigorous leg exercises both before and after surgery, elevation of the foot of the bed, and the continuous use of elastic stockings. The correct position for maintaining the legs is shown in Figure 11. Despite such intensive efforts, the overall results fell short of those desired, with thrombosis being detected in 25 per cent of the patients on the regimen as compared with 35 per cent in controls. It is interesting that in *older* patients undergoing major surgery the incidence of thrombosis was 24 per cent compared with 61 per cent in the controls. Therefore, in the elderly this regimen appeared to have a significant prophylactic effect.

Prophylactic anticoagulation is also of proven benefit in certain patients following trauma and orthopedic disorders, including fractures of the hip.[43, 89] In 1966, the concept of "low-dose heparin" was introduced as a prophylactic measure.[90] While the dosage and duration of administration of heparin has varied among authors, the usual recommendation is an initial dose of 5000 units of heparin given two hours before operation, followed by 5000 units each 8 to 12 hours until the patient is fully ambulatory. The drug is given subcutaneously and routine coagulation tests are minimally prolonged if at all with a low risk of bleeding. It is thought that the protection offered by this regimen is in its potentiation of a naturally occurring plasmin inhibitor of activated factor X.[46]

There are now more than 20 trials of low-dose heparin administered to surgical patients postoperatively and followed with ^{125}I-fibrinogen leg scanning and/or venography for demonstration of development of venous thrombosis.[110] With only one exception, these studies have indicated a significant decrease in deep vein thrombosis in treated compared with untreated control groups.[30] Although it appears clear that the incidence of deep vein thrombosis is reduced, owing to the small number of patients in each of the trials, no definite conclusion can be reached concerning the *prevention of postoperative pulmonary embolism.* The most important studies in this field are included in a multicenter clinical trial involving over 4000 patients.[48] Despite the size of the trial group, it was not large enough to demonstrate a mortality difference between the treated and control groups. The postmortem findings revealed that large pulmonary emboli occurred in 22 of the control and in only 5 of the treated patients. There was a definite increase in postoperative bleeding in the treated group. From these data, it can be inferred, although not fully established, that the therapy provided a meaningful benefit. At present low-dose heparin is probably of most benefit in the prevention of postoperative venous thrombosis in patients over the age of 40. Moreover, there is evidence that it is of limited or inadequate value following prostatectomy,[113] after myocardial infarction,[41] and in major orthopedic procedures, particularly repair of femoral fractures and reconstructive surgery of the hip and knee. Low-dose heparin prophylaxis is also inadequate for patients with an *active thrombotic process.*[110]

SURGICAL MANAGEMENT

When anticoagulant therapy fails, several surgical procedures may be considered. It was originally thought important to interrupt the superficial femoral veins in the groin by ligature to prevent thrombi from passing into the inferior vena cava, but this procedure is rarely, if ever, indicated. An analysis of a great deal of data has shown that femoral vein ligation is less effective in preventing subsequent emboli than the use

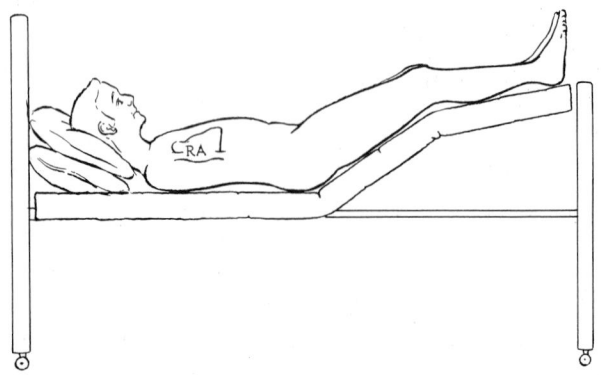

Figure 11. Correct position for lower extremities in prophylaxis of pulmonary embolism. Note the additional break at the knees. It is important that the level of the veins in the lower extremities be above the mean level of the right atrium (RA).

of anticoagulants alone. Moreover, if surgical interruption is clearly indicated, interruption of the inferior vena cava is preferred.

Venous Thrombectomy

The direct removal of venous thrombi by thrombectomy was previously recommended by a number of authors.[25, 40, 56] However, it is rarely employed today owing to the high incidence of post-thrombectomy thrombosis.[49] Moreover, massive pulmonary embolism has occurred during the course of iliofemoral thrombectomy. Most observers agree that thrombectomy is indicated in patients with *phlegmasia cerulea dolens,* since in this condition secondary *arterial spasm* is a frequent accompanying factor. Even though the venous thrombus may recur, patency of the venous lumen may persist sufficiently long to relieve the arterial spasm and permit the limb to recover. In this instance, systemic heparinization is clearly indicated in an effort to prolong the patency of the vein.

Interruption of the Inferior Vena Cava

With proper clinical indications, interruption of the inferior vena cava has been advocated by a number of authors for patients with pulmonary embolism. Some prefer total ligation[74] while others prefer the plication technique,[98] the "filter" or "screen" method,[26] or the use of plastic clips.[63, 68] Interruption of the inferior vena cava does not *completely* prevent subsequent embolism. Evidence of recurrent pulmonary embolism after ligation in as many as 20 per cent of patients has been reported.[39] Failure to ligate the ovarian vein in females is also a cause of subsequent embolism. The portion of the inferior vena cava between the ligature and the renal veins, the veins of the upper extremity and neck, the right atrium, and the right ventricle have each been shown to be the source of recurrent pulmonary emboli. Clinical evidence of this type further emphasizes the importance of considering all systemic veins as well as the right heart as potential sources of pulmonary emboli.

In summary, controversy exists at present concerning the indications for inferior vena caval interruption. One group of authors recommends the use of inferior vena caval interruption quite frequently, usually after the first attack of pulmonary embolism, irrespective of its severity. In their series, the long-term complications appeared minimal.[75] An opposing view is presented in a report of another series of cases in which the complications of inferior vena caval interruption were quite significant and the results from point of view of mortality and control of pulmonary embolism were less than desired.[76] From an analysis of recent literature, there appears to be little doubt that there has been a trend away from the use of inferior vena caval interruption. The use of the "umbrella filter," which may be passed under local anesthesia from the jugular vein and opened in the inferior vena cava just below the renal vessels, has also been advocated but not widely adopted,[64] owing to the fact that a number of these devices have migrated to the right heart and pulmonary artery.

In males, the inferior vena cava is preferably approached through a flank incision on the right side with exposure of the inferior vena cava extraperitoneally. The vena cava may then be interrupted by a direct ligature or by the placement of an appropriate clip (Fig. 12). In females, it is preferable to approach the vena cava through the transabdominal route in order to expose and ligate both ovarian veins. The duodenum is exposed by the Kocher maneuver and the vena cava interrupted just below the origin of the renal vessels.

The complications that may occur following inferior vena caval interruption as well as the mortality have been appropriately emphasized (Table 3).[11, 76] In the series at Duke, vena caval interruption by any of the techniques available has rarely been employed, and an analysis indicates that the mortality and morbidity with anticoagulant therapy is less than the operative risk of caval interruption,[93] and this view is shared by many others.[42]

In summary, an analysis of recent literature indicates that there appears to be a definite trend away from vena caval interruption in favor of anticoagulation. The use of vena caval interruption, including the

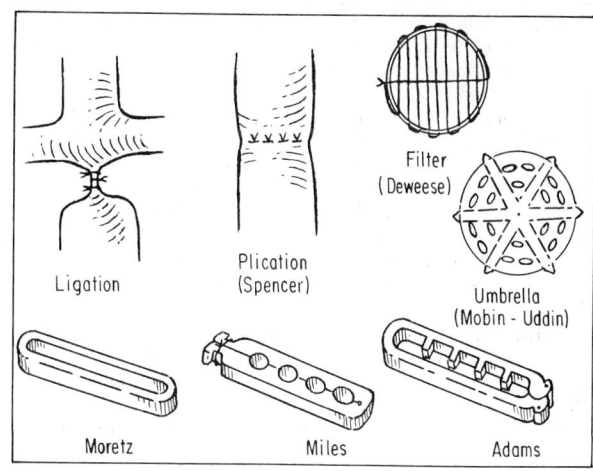

Figure 12. Diagrammatic illustration of surgical approaches for interruption of the inferior vena cava in prevention of pulmonary embolism. The umbrella and the clips shown are constructed of plastic material.

TABLE 3. Effectiveness of Inferior Vena Caval Ligation*

References	Number of Cases	Operative Mortality (per cent)	Recurrent Emboli (per cent)	Fatal Emboli (per cent)	Postphlebitic Sequelae (per cent)
Krause et al. (1963)[53]	55	5	0	0	–
Miles et al. (1964)[63]	40	15	3	0	32
Nabseth and Moran (1965)[72]	75	19	3	1	14
Bergan et al. (1966)[10]	11	9	9	0	18
Mozes et al. (1966)[70]	118	12	4	1	13
Wheeler et al. (1966)[112]	35	6	0	0	32
Amador et al. (1968)[5]	119	39	–	–	–
Moran et al. (1969)[66]	25	20	0	0	6
Ochsner et al. (1970)[75]	286	8	0	0	4
Piccone et al. (1970)[76]	72	13	36	22	33
Adams et al. (1971)[1]	38	13	8	3	43
Schowengerdt and Schreiber (1971)[88]	48	11	6	0	21
Total	922	–	–	–	–
Mean	–	14.2	6.3	2.1	–

*Adapted from Bernstein, E. F.: The place of venous interruption in the treatment of pulmonary thromboembolism. *In* Moser, K. M., and Stein, M. (Eds.): Pulmonary Thromboembolism. Copyright © 1973 by Year Book Medical Publishers, Inc., Chicago. Used by permission.

various types of filters, is largely reserved for those patients in whom heparin therapy is definitely contraindicated, in those with recurrent emboli, including those patients with cor pulmonale, and in some patients with septic pulmonary emboli, who are refractory to a combination of heparin and antibiotic therapy.

Pulmonary Embolectomy

The first pulmonary embolectomy was performed in 1908 by Friedrich Trendelenburg,[100] Professor of Surgery at the University of Leipzig. He first approached this difficult problem in the laboratory by removing a large experimental embolus from the pulmonary artery of a calf. In the original report, Trendelenburg described three patients upon whom embolectomy was performed, the longest living 37 hours and dying of hemorrhage from an internal mammary artery. In 1924, Kirschner,[51] a pupil of Trendelenburg, was the first to perform pulmonary embolectomy successfully with a long-term survivor. Despite the logical concept of Trendelenburg and the brilliant feat of Kirschner in performing it, it is generally recognized that far more patients have succumbed from embolectomy *without* extracorporeal circulation than have survived it.

In a series of 43 Trendelenburg operations performed between 1957 and 1963, there were only seven survivors, indicating again the high mortality associated with this procedure in the *absence* of cardiopulmonary bypass.[104]

In 1961, Sharp[91] was the first to use extracorporeal circulation in pulmonary embolectomy. This technique is the one generally preferred, since it permits the operation to be conducted deliberately with concomitant oxygenation of body tissues.

Indications. An increasing appreciation of the natural history of pulmonary embolism and its characteristic tendency for spontaneous lysis, a process that is clearly augmented by the administration of anticoagulants and thrombolytic agents, has brought about a reduction in the number of patients considered to be appropriate candidates for embolec-

tomy. At present, the primary indication for pulmonary embolectomy is *persistent and refractory hypotension* in a patient with massive embolism documented by either a lung scan or pulmonary arteriography. The findings from a patient in whom pulmonary embolectomy was necessary are shown in Figure 13. The immediate treatment of such patients is supportive, and many will respond to oxygen, heparinization, vasopressors, and inotropic agents. Clearly, every effort should be made to manage the patient by these means. The use of a vigorous regimen of this type has demonstrated that a number of patients previously thought to require embolectomy will respond favorably. Depending upon the severity of the clinical condition, one to several hours may be taken in an effort to restore satisfactory cardiopulmonary status. If administration of the agents described is effective in maintaining a blood pressure of 60 to 80 mm. Hg as demonstrated by a continuous intra-arterial recording, embolectomy may be deferred, particularly if renal and cerebral function is maintained.

Technique. A median sternotomy provides excellent exposure of the main pulmonary artery. The pericardium is opened and cardiopulmonary bypass is established. The main pulmonary artery is exposed and incised, and it is usually free of emboli although partially obstructing ones may be present. The emboli are removed from the right and left pulmonary arteries and their major branches. A Fogarty catheter may then be passed, with inflation of the balloon and withdrawal, to recover emboli from the smaller pulmonary arterial branches. Finally, copious irrigation with saline of the pulmonary arterial tree on both sides can be accomplished. During this portion of the procedure, general compression of both lungs with the hand forces peripheral emboli back toward the central arteries for aspiration. Following closure of the pulmonary artery, cardiopulmonary bypass is gradually discontinued, and the heart and lungs are allowed to resume their normal function. Most observers agree that after closure of the median sternotomy the inferior vena cava should be interrupted with one of the appropriate methods (ligation, plication, or clip) in order to prevent further em-

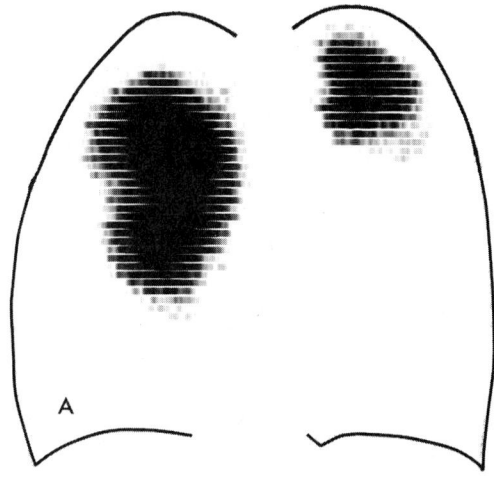

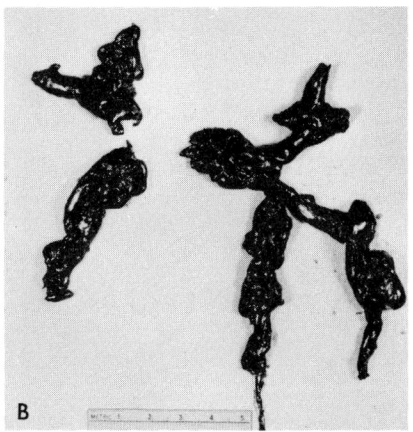

Figure 13. Illustrations from a patient with massive pulmonary embolism on the twelfth postoperative day following an orthopedic operation and accompanied by intractable shock. *A,* The pulmonary scan shows massive occlusion of the right lower and middle lobar pulmonary arteries as well as nearly all of the pulmonary arterial circulation to the left lung. *B,* Emboli removed from both pulmonary arteries at the time of embolectomy. (From Sabiston, D. C., Jr. *In* Sabiston, D. C., Jr., and Spencer, F. C. (Eds.): Gibbon's Surgery of the Chest, 3rd ed. Philadelphia, W. B. Saunders Company, 1976.)

boli. In some patients with severe cardiovascular collapse, partial cardiopulmonary bypass from the femoral vein to the femoral artery for immediate resuscitation may be necessary before the operative procedure is begun. If extracorporeal circulation is not available, an approach to either the right or left pulmonary artery can be made. In most patients with massive pulmonary embolism, one or the other pulmonary artery is primarily affected. Thus, the side with the major amount of embolus can be approached *without* the necessity for extracorporeal circulation. An anterior thoracotomy in the third interspace is quite appropriate for good exposure of the pulmonary artery. It can then be dissected to its origin, clamped, and opened for removal of the emboli while circulation and pulmonary function in the opposite lung are allowed to continue.[14, 17, 87]

Results. In a collected series of 137 patients undergoing pulmonary embolectomy, the procedure was performed with cardiopulmonary bypass in 115 patients and without it in 22.

Thrombi were found in *both* pulmonary arteries in 110 patients, whereas unilateral thrombi were found in only 20 patients. Fifty of the 115 patients operated on with bypass survived (43 per cent) although the ultimate mortality (late deaths) reduced final survival to 32 per cent. Of the 22 patients operated on without use of extracorporeal circulation, 7 had emboli in one pulmonary artery and unilateral embolectomy was performed. Each of these 7 patients survived, but only 2 of the 15 remaining patients (with bilateral emboli) survived. It is of further interest that in 7 patients the diagnosis was in error, and at the time of operation no emboli were found; all 7 patients died after operation. *These latter findings emphasize quite strongly the necessity of establishing an objective diagnosis of pulmonary embolism prior to operation, either by lung scan or by pulmonary arteriography.*[21]

Transvenous Catheter Embolectomy

In 1970, Greenfield introduced the use of transvenous catheter embolectomy. In the subsequent six years, this technique was used in 13 patients, 8 of whom were long-term survivors.[37] The catheter, with a large suction cup at the end, is passed under fluoroscopic control through the femoral vein into the pulmonary artery. The cup is positioned according to the site of the embolus as demonstrated by previous arteriography. Suction is applied with the intent that the thrombus will become firmly adherent to the cup and can be removed as the catheter is withdrawn via the femoral vein. Further experience is necessary before a full evaluation of its efficacy is established.

CHRONIC PULMONARY EMBOLISM AND COR PULMONALE

Although embolic occlusion of the pulmonary arteries is most often an acute phenomenon, recent attention has been directed toward chronic pulmonary embolism associated with cor pulmonale. This is now a well-established disorder, and despite its grave prognosis little attention has been given to its treatment.

In the recent past the diagnosis has been made with increasing frequency, and is in part a result of the more widespread use of pulmonary scanning and arteriography. The clinical manifestations of chronic pulmonary embolism are primarily dyspnea with evidence of pulmonary hypertension.

Firm indications should be present for surgical intervention. The patient clearly should have considerable dyspnea and preferably no serious additional cardiac or respiratory problems. Studies should demonstrate occlusion of the right or left main pulmonary artery and not solely occlusion of the smaller distal branches. The findings from a patient with chronic pulmonary embolism and hypertension successfully treated by embolectomy are shown in Figure 14. This patient was studied eight years later and found to have essentially normal pulmonary function, pulmonary scan, and arteriogram. At present the results obtained appear to establish a firm role for operative treatment in selected cases of chronic pulmonary embolism and hypertension.[65] This is particularly important in view of the poor prognosis of patients treated nonoperatively.

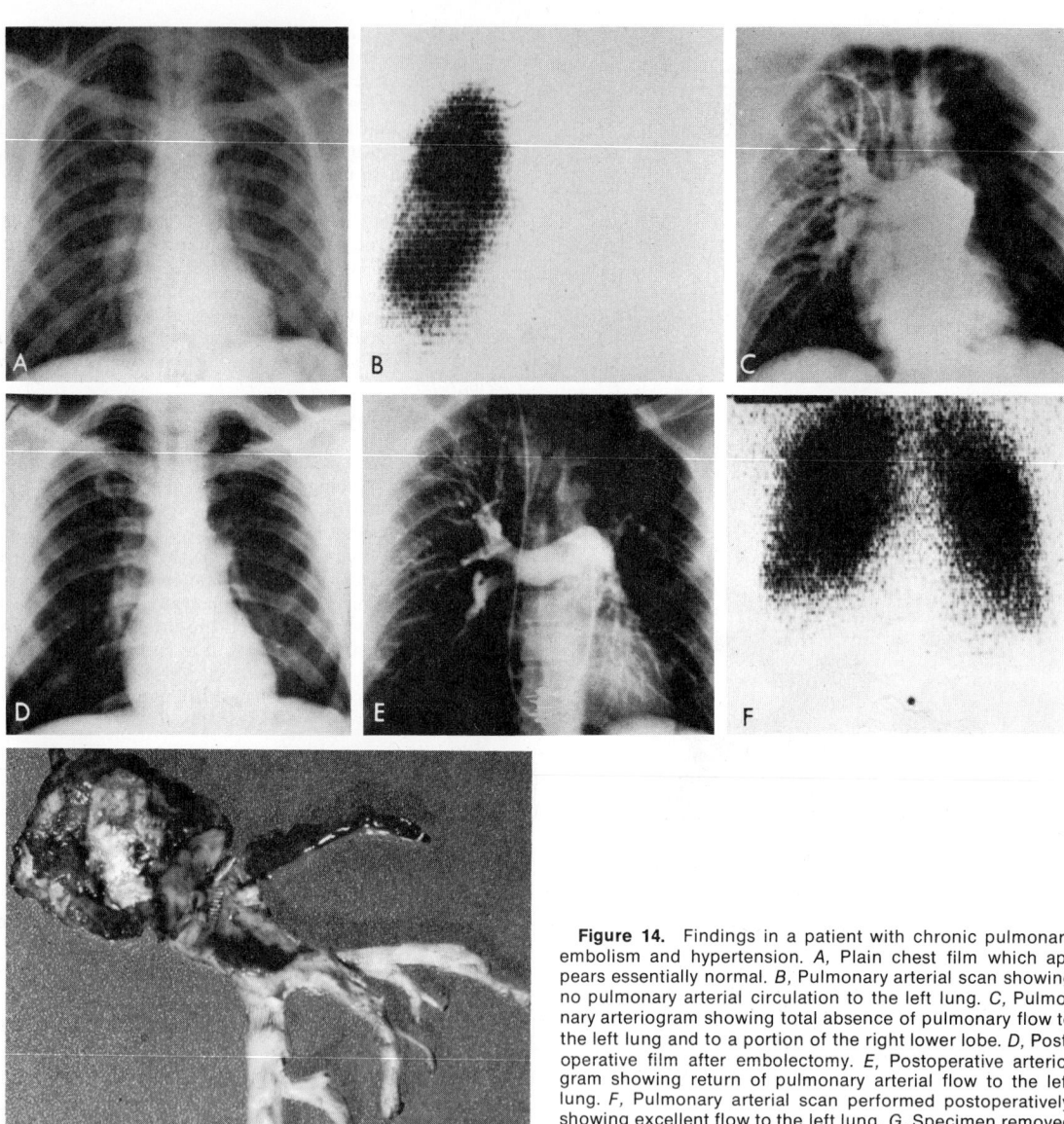

Figure 14. Findings in a patient with chronic pulmonary embolism and hypertension. *A,* Plain chest film which appears essentially normal. *B,* Pulmonary arterial scan showing no pulmonary arterial circulation to the left lung. *C,* Pulmonary arteriogram showing total absence of pulmonary flow to the left lung and to a portion of the right lower lobe. *D,* Postoperative film after embolectomy. *E,* Postoperative arteriogram showing return of pulmonary arterial flow to the left lung. *F,* Pulmonary arterial scan performed postoperatively showing excellent flow to the left lung. *G,* Specimen removed from the left pulmonary artery and its branches which microscopically was shown to be a well-organized thrombus. (From Moor, G. F., and Sabiston, D. C., Jr.: Circulation, *41*:701, 1970.)

SELECTED REFERENCES

Cross, F. S., and Mowlem, A.: A survey of the current status of pulmonary embolectomy for massive pulmonary embolism. Circulation, Supp. 1, *35*:86, 1967.
  This paper presents the data obtained from a collective survey of patients undergoing pulmonary embolectomy from a large number of centers. Emphasis is placed on the necessity for an objective diagnosis (either by scan or by arteriography). A comparison is made between the use of extracorporeal circulation and the Trendelenburg technique of pulmonary embolectomy. This represents an unusually large series for analysis.

Fishman, A. P.: Hypoxia on the pulmonary circulation. How and where it acts. Circ. Res., *38*:221, 1976.
  This is an excellent review of the effects of hypoxia on the pulmonary circulation written by an outstanding investigator. The various potential mechanisms of hypoxia and its effect are reviewed in a highly commendable manner.

Gorham, L. W.: A study of pulmonary embolism. Parts I and II. Arch. Intern. Med., *108*:8, 189, 1961.
  These companion papers emphasize the gross pathology of pulmonary embolism. Special emphasis is given the fact that in most patients with fatal embolism a substantial amount of the pulmonary

arterial bed is occluded, generally more than half. This is one of the best pathologic studies in the literature.

Greenfield, L. J.: Pulmonary embolism: Diagnosis and management. Current Problems in Surgery, Year Book Medical Publishers, Inc., April, 1976.
This is an excellent monograph, with an updated review of the entire subject. The author has had a particular interest in the use of inferior vena caval filters in the prevention and treatment of pulmonary embolism, and has also developed a transvenous catheter technique for pulmonary embolectomy.

Hume, M., Sevitt, S., and Thomas, D. P.: Venous Thrombosis & Pulmonary Embolism. Cambridge, Mass., Harvard University Press, 1970.
This monograph represents an updated source of the most recent information on the pathology, predisposing factors, mechanisms of thrombosis, and clinical features of thromboembolism. The authors are a surgeon, a pathologist, and an internist, each of whom has a particular interest in blood coagulation and thrombosis. The bibliography is extensive, and the pathophysiology of thromboembolism is described in detail. This monograph can be highly recommended.

Marshall, R., Sabiston, D. C., Jr., Allison, P. R., Bosman, A. R., and Dunnill, M. S.: Immediate and late effects of pulmonary embolism by large thrombi in dogs. Thorax, 18:1, 1963.
In this experimental study, a variety of physiologic measurements were determined following pulmonary embolism. The study emphasizes the paucity of changes that occur when only one pulmonary artery is occluded and illustrates the wide margin of pulmonary reserve.

Moor, G. F., and Sabiston, D. C., Jr.: Embolectomy for chronic pulmonary embolism and hypertension. Case report and review of the problem. Circulation, 41:701, 1970.
The use of pulmonary embolectomy for chronic pulmonary embolism and hypertension is reviewed. The diagnostic features, indications for operation, operative technique, and results are presented.

Moser, K. M., and Stein, M. (Eds.): Pulmonary Thromboembolism. Chicago, Year Book Medical Publishers, Inc., 1973.
This monograph is an excellent source of current information on all aspects of pulmonary embolism. It is composed of contributions of numerous authorities in the field as presented at a symposium on the subject.

Ochsner, A. A., Ochsner, J. L., and Sanders, H. S.: Prevention of pulmonary embolism by caval ligation. Ann. Surg., 171:923, 1970.
The authors of this paper describe an increasing utilization of inferior vena caval ligation in the treatment of pulmonary embolism. A strong position is taken concerning the necessity of ligation, and it represents what is probably the most outspoken view supporting inferior vena caval interruption.

Piccone, V. A., Jr., Vidal, E., Yarnoz, M., Glass, P., and LeVeen, H. H.: The late results of caval ligation. Surgery, 68:980, 1970.
The data in this paper emphasize the numerous and frequent complications following inferior vena caval interruption. Moreover, recurrent embolism after interruption is appreciable. These studies indicate the increasing reluctance to employ inferior vena caval interruption unless firm indications are present.

Sabiston, D. C., Jr., and Wolfe, W. G.: Experimental and clinical observations on the natural history of pulmonary embolism. Ann. Surg., 168:1, 1968.
In this paper the natural history of pulmonary emboli in the experimental animal and man is discussed. The gross and microscopic features and their changes with the passage of time are illustrated. The gradual resolution of the emboli and final disappearance in most instances are confirmed by serial scans and pulmonary arteriograms.

Sasahara, A. A.: Pulmonary angiography in the diagnosis of thromboembolic disease. N. Engl. J. Med., 270:1075, 1964.
The use of pulmonary angiography is critically appraised in this paper. The indications and diagnostic features of pulmonary angiography are well reviewed. For a detailed consideration of pulmonary arteriography, this paper is an important one.

Sevitt, S., and Gallagher, N. G.: Prevention of venous thrombosis and pulmonary embolism in injured patients: Trial of anticoagulant prophylaxis with phenindione in middle-aged and elderly patients with fractured necks of femur. Lancet, 2:981, 1959.
The studies described in this paper are classic for objective docu-

mentation of the value of prophylactic anticoagulation in high-risk patients. The authors are highly respected, and the data presented have led to a general use of prophylactic anticoagulants for special indications in a number of centers.

Wagner, H. N., Jr., Sabiston, D. C., Jr., Ilio, M., McAfee, J. G., Meyer, J. K., and Langan, J. K.: Regional pulmonary blood flow in man by radioisotope scanning. J.A.M.A., 187:601, 1964.
In this paper the original experimental and clinical studies introducing the technique of radioactive pulmonary scanning are described.

REFERENCES

1. Adams, J. T., Feingold, B. E., and DeWeese, J. A.: Comparative evaluation of ligation and partial interruption of the inferior vena cava. Arch. Surg., 172:795, 1970.
2. Alexander, B.: Blood coagulation and thrombotic disease. Circulation, 25:872, 1962.
3. Alexander, B., Meyers, L., Kenny, J., Goldstein, R., Gurewich, V., and Grinspoon, L.: Blood coagulation in pregnancy. Proconvertin and prothrombin, and the hypercoagulable state. N. Engl. J. Med., 254:358, 1956.
4. Allison, P. R.: Pulmonary embolism and thrombophlebitis. Br. J. Surg., 54:466, 1967.
5. Amador, E., Li, T. K., and Crane, C.: Ligation of inferior vena cava for thromboembolism. J.A.M.A., 206:1758, 1968.
6. Ariyan, S., and Stansel, H. C., Jr.: Further hazards of heparin therapy in vascular surgery. Arch. Surg., 111:120, 1976.
7. Baker, R. R.: Pulmonary embolism. Surgery, 54:687, 1963.
8. Barker, N. W., Nygaard, K. K., Walters, W., and Priestley, J. T.: A statistical study of post-operative venous thrombosis and pulmonary embolism: Predisposing factors. Mayo Clin., Proc., 16:1, 1941.
9. Bauer, G.: Clinical experiences of a surgeon in the use of heparin. Am. J. Cardiol., 14:29, 1964.
10. Bergan, J. J., Kinnaird, D. W., Koons, K., and Trippel, O. H.: Prevention of pulmonary embolism: Comparison of vena caval ligation, plication and filter operations in prevention of pulmonary emboli. Arch. Surg., 92:605, 1966.
11. Bernstein, E. F.: The place of venous interruption in the treatment of pulmonary thromboembolism. *In* Moser, K. M., and Stein, M. (Eds.): Pulmonary Thromboembolism. Chicago, Year Book Medical Publishers, Inc., 1973.
12. Blount, S. G., Jr., and Vogel, J. H. K.: Altitude and the pulmonary circulation. Adv. Intern. Med., 13:11, 1967.
13. Boyer, N. H., and Curry, J. J.: Bronchospasm associated with pulmonary embolism. Arch. Intern. Med., 73:403, 1944.
14. Bradley, M. N., Bennett, A. L., III, and Lyons, C.: Successful unilateral pulmonary embolectomy without cardiopulmonary bypass. N. Engl. J. Med., 271:713, 1964.
15. Brofman, B. L., Charms, B. L., Kohn, P. M., Elder, J., Newman, R., and Rizika, M.: Unilateral pulmonary artery occlusion in man. Control studies. J. Thorac. Surg., 34:206, 1957.
16. Burnett, W. E., Long, J. H., Norris, C., Rosemond, G. P., and Webster, M. R.: The effect of pneumonectomy on pulmonary function. J. Thorac. Surg., 18:569, 1949.
17. Camishion, R. C., Pierucci, L., Jr., Fishman, N. H., Fraimow, W., and Greening, R.: Pulmonary embolectomy without cardiopulmonary bypass. Am. J. Surg., 111:723, 1966.
18. Clagett, G. P., Schneider, P., Rosoff, C. B., and Salzman, E. W.: The influence of aspirin on postoperative platelet kinetics and venous thrombosis. Surgery, 77:61, 1975.
19. Comroe, J. H., Jr., Van Lingen, B., Stroud, R. C., and Roncoroni, A.: Reflex and direct cardiopulmonary effects of 5-OH-tryptamine (serotonin). Am. J. Physiol., 173:379, 1953.
20. Coon, W. W., and Coller, F. A.: Some epidemiologic considerations of thromboembolism. Surg. Gynecol. Obstet., 109:487, 1959.
21. Cross, F. S., and Mowlem, A.: A survey of the current status of pulmonary embolectomy for massive pulmonary embolism. Circulation (Suppl. 1), 35:86, 1967.
22. Cruveilhier, J.: Anatomie Pathologique de Corps Humain. Paris, J. B. Bailliere, 1829–42.
23. Dawidson, I., Barrett, J. A., Miller, E., and Litwin, M. S.: Pulmonary microembolism associated with massive transfusion: I. Physiologic effects and comparison in vivo of standard and Dacron wool (Swank) blood transfusion filters in its prevention. Ann. Surg., 181:51, 1975.

24. DeBakey, M. E.: A critical evaluation of the problem of thromboembolism. Int. Abstr. Surg., 98:1, 1954.

25. DeWeese, J. A., Jones, T. I., Lyon, J., and Dale, W. A.: Evaluation of thrombectomy in the management of iliofemoral venous thrombosis. Surgery, 47:140, 1960.

26. DeWeese, M. S., and Hunter, D. C., Jr.: A vena cava filter for the prevention of pulmonary embolism: A five-year clinical experience. Arch. Surg., 86:852, 1963.

27. Dexter, L.: Cardiovascular responses to experimental pulmonary embolism. In Sasahara, A. A., and Stein, M. (Eds.): Pulmonary Embolic Disease. New York, Grune & Stratton, 1965.

28. Fishman, A. P.: Hypoxia on the pulmonary circulation. How and where it acts. Circ. Res., 38:221, 1976.

29. Fratantoni, J. C., Ness, P., and Simon, T. L.: Thrombolytic therapy. Current status. N. Engl. J. Med., 293:1073, 1975.

30. Fratantoni, J., and Wessler, S.: Prophylactic therapy of deep vein thrombosis and pulmonary embolism. DHEW Publication No. (NIH) 75-866, 1975.

31. Fred, H. L., Axelrad, M. A., Lewis, J. M., and Alexander, J. K.: Rapid resolution of pulmonary thromboemboli in man. J.A.M.A., 196:1137, 1966.

32. Freiman, D. G.: Pathologic observations on experimental and human thromboembolism. In Sasahara, A. A., and Stein, M. (Eds.): Pulmonary Embolic Disease. New York, Grune & Stratton, 1965.

33. Genton, E., Gent, M., Hirsh, J., and Harker, L. A.: Platelet-inhibiting drugs in the prevention of clinical thrombotic disease. N. Engl. J. Med., 293:1174–1178, 1236–1246, 1296–1301, 1975.

34. Gibbs, N. M.: Venous thrombosis of the lower limbs with particular reference to bed rest. Br. J. Surg., 45:209, 1957.

35. Gorham, L. W.: A study of pulmonary embolism. Part I. Arch. Intern. Med., 108:8, 1961.

36. Gorham, L. W.: A study of pulmonary embolism. Part II. Arch. Intern. Med., 108:189, 1961.

37. Greenfield, L. J.: Pulmonary embolism: Diagnosis and management. Chicago, Year Book Medical Publishers, Inc., April, 1976.

38. Gurewich, V., Sasahara, A. A., and Stein, M.: Pulmonary embolism, bronchoconstriction and response to heparin. In Sasahara, A. A., and Stein, M. (Eds.): Pulmonary Embolic Disease. New York, Grune & Stratton, 1965.

39. Gurewich, V., Thomas, D. P., and Rabinov, K. R.: Pulmonary embolism after ligation of the inferior vena cava. N. Engl. J. Med., 274:1350, 1966.

40. Haller, J. A.: Thrombectomy for deep thrombophlebitis of the leg. N. Engl. J. Med., 267:65, 1962.

41. Handley, A. J.: Low-dose heparin after myocardial infarction. Lancet, 2:623, 1972.

42. Hirsh, J.: Venous thromboembolism: Diagnosis, treatment, prevention. Hosp. Prac., 10:53, 1975.

43. Hume, M., Sevitt, S., and Thomas, D. P.: Venous Thrombosis & Pulmonary Embolism. Cambridge, Mass., Harvard University Press, 1970.

44. Hunter, W. C., Krygier, J. J., Kennedy, J. C., and Sneeden, V. D.: Etiology and prevention of thrombosis of the deep leg veins. Surgery, 17:178, 1945.

45. Jones, R. H., and Sabiston, D. C., Jr.: Pulmonary embolism in childhood. Monogr. Surg. Sci., 3:35, 1966.

46. Kakkar, V. V., Field, E. S., Nicolaides, A. N., Flute, P. T., Wessler, S., and Yin, E. T.: Low doses of heparin in prevention of deep-vein thrombosis. Lancet, 2:669, 1971.

47. Kakkar, V.: The diagnosis of deep vein thrombosis using the ^{125}I-fibrinogen test. Arch. Surg., 104:152, 1972.

48. Kakkar, V. V., et al.: Prevention of fatal postoperative pulmonary embolism by low doses of heparin. An international multicentre trial. Lancet, 2:45, 1975.

49. Karp, R. B., and Wylie, E. J.: Recurrent thrombosis after iliofemoral venous thrombectomy. Surg. Forum, 17:147, 1966.

50. Kernohan, R. J., and Todd, C.: Heparin therapy in thromboembolic disease. Lancet, 1:621, 1966.

51. Kirschner, M.: Ein durch die Trendelenburgsche Operation geheilter Fall von Embolie der Arterien pulmonalis. Arch. Klin. Chir., 133:312, 1924.

52. Kovacs, G. S., Hill, J. D., Abert, T., Blesovsky, A., and Gerbode, F.: Pathogenesis of arterial hypoxemia in pulmonary embolism. Arch. Surg., 93:813, 1966.

53. Krause, R. J., Cranley, J. J., Hallaba, M. A. S., Strasser, E. S., and Hafner, C. D.: Caval ligation in thromboembolic disease. Arch. Surg., 87:184, 1963.

54. Laennec, R. T. H.: De l'auscultation médiate. Paris, Brossen et Chaude, 1819.

55. Littmann, D.: Observations on the electrocardiographic changes in pulmonary embolism. In Sasahara, A. A., and Stein, M. (Eds.): Pulmonary Embolic Disease. New York, Grune & Stratton, 1965.

56. Mahorner, H., Castleberry, J. W., and Coleman, W. O.: Attempts to restore function in major veins which are the site of massive thrombosis. Ann. Surg., 146:510, 1957.

57. Marshall, R., Sabiston, D. C., Allison, P. R., Bosman, A. R., and Dunnill, M. S.: Immediate and late effects of pulmonary embolism by large thrombi in dogs. Thorax, 18:1, 1963.

58. Mauer, B. J., Wray, R., and Shillingford, J. P.: Frequency of venous thrombosis after myocardial infarction. Lancet, 2:1385, 1971.

59. McLachlin, A. D., McLachlin, J. A., Jory, T. A., and Rawling, E. G.: Venous stasis in the lower extremities. Ann. Surg., 152:678, 1960.

60. McLachlin, J., and Paterson, J. C.: Some basic observations on venous thrombosis and pulmonary embolism. Surg. Gynecol. Obstet., 93:1, 1951.

61. Medical Research Council Subcommittee: Risk of thromboembolic disease in women taking oral contraceptives. Br. Med. J., 2:355, 1967.

62. Meister, H.: Ueber Thrombose und Lungenembolie. Statistische Untersuchungen an 15,130 Sektionen. Frankfurt. z. Pathol., 70:640, 1960.

63. Miles, R. M., Chappell, F., and Renner, O.: Partially occluding vena caval clip for prevention of pulmonary emboli. Am. Surg., 30:40, 1964.

64. Mobin-Uddin, K., Bolooki, H., and Jude, J. R.: A new simplified method of caval interruption for the prevention of pulmonary embolus. Circulation (Suppl. 3), 40:149, 1969.

65. Moor, G. F., and Sabiston, D. C., Jr.: Embolectomy for chronic pulmonary embolism and hypertension. Case report and review of the problem. Circulation, 41:701, 1970.

66. Moran, J. M., Kahr, P. C., and Callow, A. D.: Partial versus complete interruption for venous thromboembolism. Am. J. Surg., 117:471, 1969.

67. Moret, P., Covarrubias, E., Coudert, J., and Duchosal, F.: Cardiocirculatory adaptation to chronic hypoxia. III. Comparative study of cardiac output, pulmonary and systemic circulation between sea level and high altitude residents. Acta Cardiol. (Brux), 27:596, 1972.

68. Moretz, W. H., Rhode, C. M., and Shepherd, M. H.: Prevention of pulmonary emboli by partial occlusion of inferior vena cava. Am. Surg., 25:617, 1959.

69. Morrell, M. T., Truelove, S. C., and Barr, A.: Pulmonary embolism. Br. Med. J., 2:830, 1963.

70. Mozes, M., Bogolowsky, H., Antebi, E., Tzur, N., and Penchas, S.: Inferior vena cava ligation for pulmonary embolism: Review of 118 cases. Surgery, 60:790, 1966.

71. Murray, T. S., Lorimer, A. R., Cox, F. C., and Lawrie, T. D. V.: Leg-vein thrombosis following myocardial infarction. Lancet, 2:792, 1970.

72. Nabseth, D. C., and Moran, J. M.: Reassessment of the role of inferior vena cava ligation in venous thromboembolism. N. Engl. J. Med., 273:1250, 1965.

73. Neumann, R.: Ursprungszentren und Entwicklungsformen der Beinthrombose. Virchows Arch. Pathol. Anat., 301:708, 1938.

74. Ochsner, A.: Indications for and results of inferior vena caval ligation for thromboembolic disease. Postgrad. Med., 27:193, 1960.

75. Ochsner, A., Ochsner, J. L., and Sanders, H. S.: Prevention of pulmonary embolism by caval ligation. Ann. Surg., 171:923, 1970.

76. Piccone, V. A., Jr., Vidal, E., Yarnoz, M., Glass, P., and LeVeen, H. H.: The late results of caval ligation. Surgery, 68:980, 1970.

77. Registrar-General's Statistical Review of England and Wales, London, Her Majesty's Stationery Office, 1966.

78. Roberts, G. H.: Venous thrombosis in hospital patients: A post-mortem study. Scot. Med. J., 8:11, 1963.

79. Robin, E. D., Julian, D. G., Travis, D. M., and Crump, C. H.: A physiologic approach to diagnosis of acute pulmonary embolism. N. Engl. J. Med., 260:586, 1959.

80. Rossle, R.: Uber die Bedeutung und die Entstehung der Wadenvenenthrombosen. Virchows Arch. Pathol. Anat., 30:180, 1937.

81. Sabiston, D. C., Jr., and Wagner, H. N., Jr.: The pathophysiology of pulmonary embolism: Relationships to accurate diagnosis and choice of therapy. J. Thorac. Cardiovasc. Surg., 50:339, 1965.

82. Sabiston, D. C., Jr., and Wolfe, W. G.: Experimental and clinical observations on the natural history of pulmonary embolism. Ann. Surg., 168:1, 1968.

83. Salzman, E. W., Deykin, D., Shapiro, R. M., and Rosenberg, R.: Management of heparin therapy. Controlled prospective trial. N. Engl. J. Med., 292:1046, 1975.

84. Salzman, E. W., Harris, W. H., and DeSanctis, R. W.: Reduction in venous thromboembolism by agents affecting platelet function. N. Engl. J. Med., 284:1287, 1971.

85. Sasahara, A. A.: Clinical studies in pulmonary thromboembolism. In Sasahara, A. A., and Stein, M. (Eds.): Pulmonary Embolic Disease. New York, Grune & Stratton, 1965.

86. Sautter, R. D., Fletcher, F. W., Emanuel, D. A., Lawton, B. R., and Olsen, T. G.: Complete resolution of massive pulmonary thromboembolism. J.A.M.A., 189:948, 1964.

87. Sautter, R. D., Lawton, B. R., Magnin, G. E., and Burns, J. L.: Pulmonary embolectomy. A simplified technique. Wisconsin Med. J., 61:309, 1962.

88. Schowengerdt, C. G., and Schreiber, J. T.: Interruption of the vena cava in the treatment of pulmonary embolism. Surg. Gynecol. Obstet., 132:645, 1971.

89. Sevitt, S., and Gallagher, N. G.: Venous thrombosis and pulmonary embolism in injured patients: A trial of anticoagulant prophylaxis with phenindione in middle-aged and elderly patients with fractured neck of femur. Lancet, 2:981, 1961.

90. Sharnoff, J. G.: Results in the prophylaxis of postoperative thromboembolism. Surg. Gynecol. Obstet., 123:303, 1966.

91. Sharp, E. H.: Pulmonary embolectomy: Successful removal of a massive pulmonary embolus with the support of cardiopulmonary bypass. A Case Report. Ann. Surg., 156:1, 1962.

92. Silver, D., and Gleysteen, J. J.: Paradoxical arterial embolism. Am. Surg., 36:47, 1970.

93. Silver, D., and Sabiston, D. C., Jr.: The role of vena caval interruption in the management of pulmonary embolism. Surgery, 77:1, 1975.

94. Simon, M., and Sasahara, A. A.: Observations on the angiographic changes in pulmonary thromboembolism. In Sasahara, A. A., and Stein, M. (Eds.): Pulmonary Embolic Disease. New York, Grune & Stratton, 1965.

95. Sloan, H., Morris, J. D., Figley, M., and Lee, R.: Temporary unilateral occlusion of the pulmonary artery in the preoperative evaluation of thoracic patients. J. Thorac. Surg., 30:591, 1955.

96. Smith, G. T., Dexter, L., and Dammin, G. J.: Postmortem quantitative studies in pulmonary embolism. In Sasahara, A. A.,

and Stein, M. (Eds.): Pulmonary Embolic Disease. New York, Grune & Stratton, 1965.

97. Spector, I., and Corn, M.: Control of heparin therapy with activated partial thromboplastin times. J.A.M.A., 201:157, 1967.

98. Spencer, F. C., Jude, J., Rienhoff, W. F., III, and Stonesifer, G.: Plication of the inferior vena cava for pulmonary embolism: Long-term results in 39 cases. Ann. Surg., 161:788, 1965.

99. Torrance, D. J.: The Chest Film in Massive Pulmonary Embolism. Springfield, Ill., Charles C Thomas, Publisher, 1963.

100. Trendelenburg, F.: Ueber die operative Behandlung der Embolie der Lungenarterie. Arch. Klin. Chir., 86:686, 1908.

101. Urokinase Pulmonary Embolism Trial Study Group: Urokinase pulmonary embolism trial. Phase 1 results. A cooperative study. J.A.M.A., 214:2163, 1970.

102. Vessey, M. P., and Doll, R.: Investigation of relation between the use of oral contraceptives and thromboembolic disease. Br. Med. J., 2:199, 1968.

103. Virchow, R.: Die Cellularpathologie in ihrer Begrundung auf physiologische und pathologische Gewebelehre. Berlin, A. Hirschwald, 1858.

104. Vossschulte, K.: The surgical treatment of pulmonary embolism. J. Cardiovasc. Surg., Suppl. 197, 1965.

105. Wacker, W. E. C., and Snodgrass, P. J.: Serum LDH activity in pulmonary embolism diagnosis. J.A.M.A., 174:2142, 1960.

106. Wagner, H. N., Jr., Sabiston, D. C., Jr., Ilio, M., McAfee, J. G. Meyer, J. K., and Langan, J. K.: Regional pulmonary blood flow in man by radioisotope scanning. J.A.M.A., 187:601, 1964.

107. Warlow, C., Ogston, D., and Douglas, A. S.: Venous thrombosis following strokes. Lancet, 1:1305, 1972.

108. Weiederanders, R. E., White, S. M., and Saichek, H. B.: The effect of pulmonary resection on pulmonary artery pressures. Ann. Surg., 160:889, 1964.

109. Welch, W. H.: W. H. Welch's Papers and Addresses. Burket, W. C. (Ed.). Baltimore, Johns Hopkins Press, 1920.

110. Wessler, S.: Prevention of venous thromboembolism by low-dose heparin. A 1976 status report. Mod. Concepts Cardiovasc. Dis., 45:105, 1976.

111. Westermark, N.: On the roentgen diagnosis of lung embolism. Acta Radiol., 19:357, 1938.

112. Wheeler, C. G., Thompson, J. E., Austin, D. J., Patman, R. D., and Stockton, R. L.: Interruption of the inferior vena cava for thromboembolism: Comparison of ligation and plication. Ann. Surg., 163:199, 1966.

113. Williams, H. T.: Prevention of postoperative deep-vein thrombosis with perioperative subcutaneous heparin. Lancet, 2:950, 1971.

53

FAT EMBOLISM SYNDROME

Joseph A. Moylan, M.D.

Post-traumatic respiratory insufficiency continues to be a significant cause of death following accident. Since Zenker[23] described the anatomic findings of fat emboli in the pulmonary tissues of persons dying following injury, fat embolism has been considered one of the primary causes of post-traumatic pulmonary complication.

Ernest Von Bergmann[4] is credited with the first clinical diagnosis of the triad of findings consisting of confusion, dyspnea, and petechiae following long bone fractures. In 1879 Fenger and Salisbury[7] working at the Cook County Hospital presented the first American experience with this disease process.

Frederick Dennis[6] in his book *System of Surgery* affirmed the importance of fat emboli as a cause of collapse following injury in his "Rule of 3's." Shock causes collapse in the *first three hours* after trauma, fat emboli cause collapse *three days* after injury, and pulmonary emboli *three weeks* after accident. The initial therapeutic treatment of fat embolism using a solution of 5 per cent ethyl alcohol and 5 per cent dextrose was first described by Herrmann in 1932.[10]

Because of the protean manifestations of fat embolism, the reported incidence of occurrence has varied significantly. In studies of battlefield mortality, 10 per cent of soldiers dying during World War I had pulmonary fat embolism at autopsy, 65 per cent in World War II, and 39 per cent in the Korean war.[13, 20, 22] In a recent civilian report, Sevitt[21] reported an 80 per cent incidence of patients dying with multisystem injury. The fat embolism syndrome has increased in direct proportion to the number of automobile accidents.

PATHOPHYSIOLOGY OF FAT EMBOLISM

Two major theories have been proposed to outline the pathogenesis of the fat embolism syndrome. The first, known as the *mechanical* theory, was described by Gauss[8] in 1924 in which the fat emboli were thought to be produced by the egress of marrow fat into the blood stream at the site of injury, i.e., the fracture site. The fat emboli produce ischemic or hemorrhagic changes by temporary occlusion of the pulmonary capillary circulation. Many investigators, such as Morton and Kendall,[16] have been proponents

of this mechanism of post-traumatic respiratory failure. Arnim and Grant[1] provided experimental support to the mechanical hypothesis by demonstrating bone marrow emboli in lung capillaries after fractures of long bone in an animal model.

The other theory, the *physiochemical* hypothesis, was originally proposed by Lehmann and Moore.[12] These authors have supported the approach that neutral fats release coalase into the blood stream, forming large chylomicrons that act as emboli following trauma. The source of the neutral fats is the body fat stores or marrow cavity. These fat droplets have been reported in the 5 to 10 μ range. Continued evolution of the physiochemical theory has focused on effects of serum free fatty acids (FFA) on pulmonary function. Serum FFA are elevated in all patients following major trauma.[14] Peltier and associates[19] have clearly demonstrated the toxic effects of FFA on lung tissue. The acid substances cause disruption of the capillary alveolar membrane and alteration in lung surfactant activity, leading to edema, hemorrhage, and additional alveolar collapse. The source of the FFA may be hydrolysis of the neutral fat droplets by lipase or the mobilization of fat stores by catecholamines or both. Both the clinical course of patients developing pulmonary insufficiency following fat emboli and experimental work support the physiochemical theory. The lucid interval between the accident and the onset of the clinical syndrome of hypoxia, confusion, and petechiae, which is usually 48 hours, is thought by many authors to be the time it takes for neutral fats to be acted upon by lipase, forming FFA. Intravenous injection of unbound FFA such as oleic or arachadonic acid produce fulminant pulmonary decompensation in various animal models. Kreis and associates[11] produced lethal hypoxia, with roentgenographic and pulmonary histologic changes consistent with FES in dogs, by intravenous administration of 0.07 ml. per kg. of oleic acid. Experimentally Cahill et al.[5] demonstrated a fall in pulmonary compliance and oxygen diffusion using 0.15 ml. per kg. of oleic acid. Normally less than 1 per cent of the FFA exists in the unbound state, with albumin being the principal protein binding and transporting these poorly soluble compounds. Recent experience has demonstrated that patients developing the fat emboli syndrome have significantly lowered serum albumin levels in comparison with patients who remain asymptomatic, allowing significant portions of the elevated FFA to circulate unbound.[17] Preliminary studies with albumin administration to maintain the serum albumin level above 3.5 gm. per 100 ml. during the first 72 hours post injury show a marked reduction in the incidence of fat emboli syndrome in patients with multiple trauma. These studies contribute more evidence to the role of FFA as the etiologic agent in the pathogenesis of FES.

RECOGNITION

The fat emboli syndrome is characterized by abnormalities affecting three primary organ systems: the pulmonary, the cerebral, and the cutaneous. The patients exhibit hypoxia, confusion, and petechiae. The respiratory components begin insidiously with tachypnea, initially without distress, accompanied by tachycardia. The symptoms may progress to dyspnea and cyanosis. Cerebral signs include confusion, agitation or stupor, and coma. Petechiae are found over the upper expremities and chest, especially in the axillary areas, the conjunctiva, and the uvula.

In rare cases the syndrome is apparent in the immediate post-traumatic period; the peak occurrence, however, is 48 to 72 hours following injury (Fig. 1). This fact is helpful in the differential diagnosis of post-traumatic pulmonary insufficiency, which includes pneumohemothorax, pulmonary contusion, shock lung, and oxygen toxicity. There is no age difference and the incidence is the same in male and female, incurring the same degree of multisystem injury. However, the actual percentage of patients with fat embolism is higher in the male because of more occupational and recreational exposure in which multisystem trauma can occur, i.e., heavy industry, construction, motorcycle riding, etc.

The diagnosis is primarily a clinical one, including a history of skeletal injury, shock, respiratory distress, changes in cerebral function, and petechiae. However, there are laboratory tests that provide additional con-

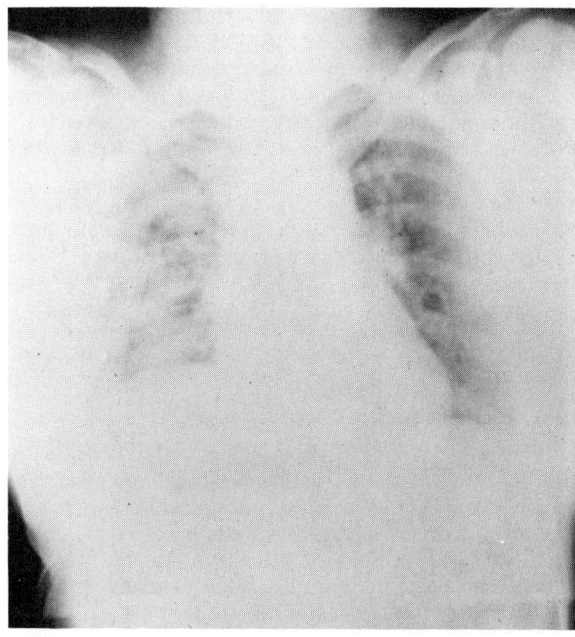

Figure 2 Diffuse fluffy infiltrate at 72 hours post injury. Patient had progressive hypoxia during the preceding 12-hour period.

firmatory data to the clinician. Chest roentgenogram demonstrates fluffy densities in both lung fields similar to pulmonary edema (Fig. 2). X-ray changes are found initially in approximately only one third of patients with this form of respiratory distress; however, in time all patients demonstrate radiologic changes. The electrocardiographic changes are nonspecific, including prominent S waves in Lead I, prominent Q waves in Lead III, varied ST changes, and right axis strain.

The value of fat globules in the urine as a diagnostic criterion is questionable,[15] since most patients have urinary fat globules following major trauma whether or not they develop fat embolism syndrome. However, the absence of fat globules in patients with respiratory distress makes the diagnosis of fat emboli as a causative factor unlikely. A similar lack of diagnostic reliability has been reported for presence of fat in the sputum.

Various hematologic changes, including thrombocytopenia, hypofibrinogenemia, and prolongation of the partial thromboplastin times have been reported in patients with fat embolism. Controlled clinical and experimental work has indicated that the clotting abnormalities are related to hypovolemic shock rather than to fat embolism. Our clinical experience shows no statistical differences in the platelet counts, fibrinogen levels, partial thromboplastin times, and prothrombin time in patients with fat embolism following multiple trauma, as compared to patients without respiratory distress who experience a similar degree of injury.[17]

Both serum lipase and tributyrinase levels have been reported in the German literature as valuable diagnostic aids for fat emboli. Investigators such as Peltier[18] and Herndon[9] have shown these enzymes to

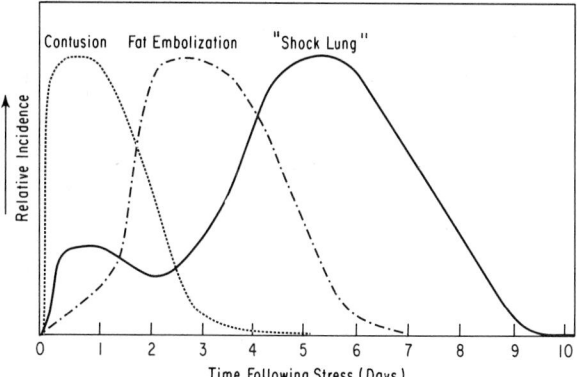

Figure 1. The peak incidence of respiratory insufficiency for fat embolism is between two and four days post injury. Pulmonary contusion is functionally significant in the first day following chest trauma and "shock lung" presents later in the course.

be elevated in many patients with fat embolism; however, the levels of lipase and tributyrinase have not correlated well with the clinical syndrome.

The most important laboratory test in the diagnosis and management of fat embolism is the arterial Po_2. An arterial Po_2 of less than 60 mm. Hg on room air is indicative of significant desaturation and the need for respiratory support. Initially, the pH may be increased and the Pco_2 slightly decreased secondary to hyperventilation in response to hypoxia. Further deterioration results in a falling Po_2, increasing Pco_2, and acidosis.

TREATMENT

Treatment of fat embolism is both prophylactic and therapeutic when the syndrome develops. Many factors have been incriminated as associated with FES, including fracture instability and shock. All fractures should be stabilized as effectively and as early as possible. The use of air splints makes fracture splinting possible at the scene of the accident.

Proper treatment of the hypovolemic shock, which occurs in patients with multiple system injuries, using rapid volume expansion with electrolyte solutions and blood, is important in minimizing post-traumatic pulmonary insufficiency. The estimation of blood loss in this patient population is difficult, especially with continued hidden blood losses in fracture sites during the first 24 to 48 hours post accident. Serial circumferential measurements of the injured limb and volume comparison with the uninjured limb, using the formula $V = \dfrac{C^2 L}{4\pi}$ (C = circumference and L = length) provides a satisfactory clinical estimation of blood loss in fracture sites. While specific value of colloid, particularly albumin, as a volume expander has been questioned during the initial resuscitation, *albumin replacement to maintain serum level above 3.5 gm. per 100 ml. during the first 72 hours post injury* has reduced the incidence of pulmonary insufficiency from fat embolism.

Historically many agents have been used in the treatment of fat emboli. Herrmann[10] first used a 5 per cent ethyl alcohol solution to treat this syndrome in 1932. Ethyl alcohol has been shown to inhibit lipase activity in vitro and in vivo; however, the efficiency of the agent in the reversing pulmonary insufficiency following fat emboli has never been demonstrated.

Heparin had been advocated for the treatment of FES because of its lipemic "clearing" capability and anticlotting property. Because of increased bleeding problems associated with the use of heparin in trauma patients and absence of demonstrated clinical value, heparin has not been extensively used.

Ashbaugh and Petty[3] reported the first use of corticosteroids in the treatment of respiratory failure with massive fat emboli. Continued patient evaluation of this agent along with experimental support has demonstrated its effectiveness in reducing the high mortality associated with FES. High doses of steroids, using Solu-Medrol (30 mg. per kg. per 24 hours in divided doses), have been recommended. The value of

the corticosteroids in reversing the toxic effects of the FFA appears to be secondary to their anti-inflammatory property. Studies show corticosteroids reduce the hypoxia secondary to experimental fat embolization.[11]

Ventilatory support using a volume ventilator via an endotracheal tube or tracheostomy has been an additional factor stabilizing and reversing pulmonary post-traumatic respiratory distress. The addition of positive end-expiratory pressure (PEEP) to the respiratory support regimen has produced an increase in the functional residual capacity and a decrease in pulmonary shunting.[2]

An organized, coordinated approach to therapy of this form of post-traumatic respiratory distress has resulted in a marked reduction of the high mortality and morbidity rates associated with this complication of major injuries.

SELECTED REFERENCES

Evarts, C. M.: The fat embolism syndrome: A review. Surg. Clin. North Am., *50*:493, 1970.

Peltier, L. F.: The diagnosis and treatment of fat embolism. J. Trauma, *11*:661, 1971.
  Both references discuss the historical background, the clinical presentation, and course of fat embolism, with one emphasizing the mechanical theory of the syndrome and the other the physiochemical. The use of laboratory evaluation and treatment modalities are discussed.

Moylan, J. A.: Diagnosis and treatment of fat embolism. Ann. Rev. Med., *28*: in press.
  A complete review including basic science and the clinical approach to the patient with fat emboli, with emphasis on prognosis and treatment.

REFERENCES

1. Arnim J., and Grant, R. E.: Observations on gross pulmonary fat embolism in man and in the rabbit. Can. J. Surg., *9*:286, 1966.
2. Ashbaugh, D. G., and Petty, T. L.: Positive end-expiratory pressure, physiology, indications and contraindications. J. Thorac. Cardiovasc. Surg., *65*:165, 1973.
3. Ashbaugh, D. G., and Petty, T. L.: The use of corticosteroids in the treatment of respiratory failure associated with massive fat embolism. Surg. Gynecol. Obstet., *123*:493, 1966.
4. Bergmann, E. B.: Ein Fall todlicher fetlenbolic. Berl. Klin. Wochenschr., *10*:385, 1873.
5. Cahill, J. M., Daly, B. F. T., and Byrne, J. J.: Ventilatory and circulatory response to oleic acid embolus. J. Trauma, *14*:73, 1974.
6. Dennis, F. S.: System of Surgery, Vol. 1. Philadelphia, Lea Brother & Co., 1895, page 533.
7. Fenger, C., and Salisbury, J. H.: Diffuse multiple capillary fat embolism in the lungs and brain is a fatal complication in common fracture: Illustrated by a case. Chicago Med. J. Examiner, *39*:587, 1879.
8. Gauss, H.: The pathology of fat embolism. Arch. Surg., *9*:593, 1924.
9. Herndon, J. H., Riseborough, E. J., and Fischer, J. E.: Fat embolism, a review of current concepts. J. Trauma, *11*:673, 1971.
10. Herrmann, L. G.: Effect of dextrose alcohol mixture upon pulmonary fat embolism. Proc. Soc. Exp. Biol. Med., *30*:588, 1932–1933.
11. Kreis, W. R., Lindenaur, S. M., and Dent, T. L.: Corticosteroids in experimental fat embolization. J. Surg. Res., *14*:238, 1973.
12. Lehman, E. P., and Moore, R. M.: Fat embolism including experimental production without trauma. Arch. Surg., *14*:621, 1927.
13. Malloy, T. B., Sullivan, E. R., Burnett, C. H., et al.: VII. The general pathology of traumatic shock. Surgery, *27*:627, 1950.
14. McNamara, J. J., Molat, M., Dunn, R., et al.: Lipid metabolism after trauma. Role in the pathogenesis of fat embolism. J. Thorac. Cardiovasc. Surg., *63*:968, 1972.
15. Morton, K. S.: Fat embolism: Incidence of urinary fat in trauma. Can. Med. Assoc. J., *74*:441, 1956.

16. Morton, K. S., and Kendall, M. J.: The failure of intravenous alcohol in the treatment of experimental pulmonary fat embolism. Can. J. Surg., *9*:286, 1966.

17. Moylan, J. A., Evenson, M. E., and Birnbaum, M.: Fat emboli syndrome. J. Trauma, *16*:339, 1976.

18. Peltier, L. F.: Fat embolism: The prophylactic value of a tourniquet. J. Bone Joint Surg., *38A*:385, 1956.

19. Peltier, L. F.: Fat embolism: The toxic properties of neutral fat and free fatty acids. Surgery, *40*:665, 1956.

20. Scully, R. E.: Fat embolism in Korean battle casualities; its incidence, clinical significance and pathologic aspects. Am. J. Pathol., *32*:379, 1956.

21. Sevitt, S.: Fat embolism. London, Butterworths, 1962.

22. Sutton, G. E.: Pulmonary fat embolism and its relation to traumatic shock. Br. Med. J., *2*:368, 1918.

23. Zenker, F. A.: Bertrage zur normalen und pathologischen. Anatomic der Lunger. Dresden, Braunsdorf, 1862.

54

DISORDERS OF THE ARTERIAL SYSTEM

I

INTRODUCTION

David C. Sabiston, Jr., M.D.

Much of the history of surgery is a record of its technical advances, and the development of surgical control of the *arterial* system represents one of the most important achievements. It is of particular significance that within the past 25 years vascular surgery has reached a state previously thought impossible. The advent of direct surgery of the arteries and the use of autografts, homografts, and arterial prostheses, together with the introduction of extracorporeal circulation, have formed the basis for these brilliant accomplishments. Moreover, there is reason to believe that these advances will continue and that much more progress lies ahead.

The beginning of *hemostasis* in wounds is recorded in ancient Chinese literature, where bandaging and use of styptics were advocated. During the era of Hippocrates, ligation of vessels was rarely practiced, and amputations were done only through the gangrenous extremity at a site where the vessels were thrombosed to assure that no significant bleeding occurred. Celsus advanced beyond the hippocratic doctrine to the point of amputation at the line of demarcation, but here again most of the vessels were thrombosed. At that time he advocated limited use of the ligature. In about A.D. 100, Archigenes was more daring and advanced the scope of amputation materially by proposing that it be performed for "gangrene, necrosis, cancer and certain callous tumors." He advocated preliminary ligation of vessels leading to the site of amputation. Antyllus made a further advance by recommending surgical treatment of aneurysms by proximal ligation of the arteries, and Galen advocated the use of Celtic linen ligatures. Despite these advances, the ligature was *rarely* used for amputations and then only as a last resort, preference being given to the actual cautery to secure hemostasis.

In 1552, Paré rediscovered the ligature and employed it instead of hot irons to control the hemorrhage in amputating the leg of an officer wounded at the siege of Danvilliers. It was this procedure that prompted Paré to state, "I dressed him and God healed him. He returned home gaily with a wooden leg saying that he had got off cheaply without being miserably burned to stop the bleeding." This operation heralded the beginning of the common use of the ligature for the control of

arterial bleeding, and Paré deserves much credit for reintroducing a forgotten principle. An excellent account of the historical facts concerning control of bleeding and the development of ligatures is found in *The History of Hemostasis* by Harvey.[11]

To William Hunter[12] is due recognition for his dissections of aneurysms and early recommendations for arterial ligature. He also was the first to recognize that an arteriovenous aneurysm represented a direct communication between artery and vein and was not a simple aneurysm. In the next century, Matas[14] first advocated endoaneurysmorrhaphy in the treatment of arterial aneurysms. Another major advance was made by Carrel and Guthrie,[4-6] with their contribution of direct suture anastomosis of arteries. It was for this and pioneering work in the transplantation of organs that Carrel was awarded the Nobel Prize in 1912. In 1906 Goyanes was the first to successfully use a venous autograft to replace a popliteal aneurysm.[10] The following year Lexer inserted a segment of saphenous vein for reconstruction of an axillary-brachial aneurysm which resulted from trauma.[13] The first successful venous autograft in the United States was by Bernheim[2] in replacement of a popliteal aneurysm. In discussing the paper, Halsted called it the "ideal operation" for this lesion. Despite these important early contributions, the use of venous autografts was rarely employed until a team of vascular surgeons working in the Mobile Army Surgical Hospitals in Korea reintroduced the technique in the management of military wounds, especially those in the lower extremities in which gangrene would have occurred requiring amputation unless the venous autografts had been employed to restore arterial continuity.[17]

In 1927, Moniz, a Portuguese neurologist, used intra-arterial injection of thorium dioxide to outline the cerebral vessels.[15] About the same time, dos Santos and associates injected a contrast medium directly into the aorta.[16] In the United States, Brooks reported the use of intra-arterial injection of sodium iodide and published beautiful arteriograms utilizing this technique in 1924.[3] An aortic abdominal aneurysm was successfully removed and replaced by an arterial homograft for the first time by Dubost in 1951.[8] Following this, thoracic aneurysms were successfully attacked by DeBakey[7] and Bahnson,[1] and these procedures were greatly augmented by the introduction by Gibbon of successful extracorporeal circulation in 1953.[9] The introduction of prosthetic arterial substitutes began in 1952, when Voorhees and Blake-more[18] first used Vinyon-N; additional study with other materials led to the present-day use of Dacron and Teflon.

SELECTED REFERENCES

Harrison, L. H., Jr.: Historical aspects in the development of venous autografts. Ann. Surg., *183*:101, 1976.
This is a very commendable and detailed description of the early use of venous autografts by Goyanes, Lexer, Bernheim, and others. These contributions are described and related to other associated scientific achievements.

Harvey, S. C.: The History of Hemostasis. New York, Paul B. Hoeber, 1929.
This excellent monograph concisely describes the history of surgical approaches to control bleeding and the development of ligatures. It is fascinating and makes excellent reading for all who desire a thorough understanding of this subject.

REFERENCES

1. Bahnson, H. T.: Definitive treatment of saccular aneurysms of the aorta with excision of sac and aortic sutures. Surg. Gynecol. Obstet., *96*:382, 1953.
2. Bernheim, B. M.: The ideal operation for aneurysm of the extremity. Report of a case. Bull. Johns Hopkins Hosp., *27*:93, 1916.
3. Brooks, B.: Intra-arterial injection of sodium iodide. J.A.M.A., *82*:1016, 1924.
4. Carrel, A.: La technique opératoire des anastomoses vasculaires et la transplantation des viscères. Lyon Med., *98*:859, 1902.
5. Carrel, A.: Suture of blood-vessels and transplantation of organs. Nobel Lecture, 1912. *In* Nobel Lectures in Physiology-Medicine. Volume 1. New York, American Elsevier Publishing Company, 1967, p. 442.
6. Carrel, A., and Guthrie, C. C.: Uniterminal and biterminal venous transplantations. Surg. Gynecol. Obstet., *2*:266, 1906.
7. DeBakey, M. E., and Cooley, D. A.: Successful resection of aneurysm of thoracic aorta and replacement by graft. J.A.M.A., *152*:673, 1953.
8. Dubost, C., Allary, M., and Oeconomos, N.: Resection of an aneurysm of the abdominal aorta: Reestablishment of the continuity by a preserved human arterial graft, with results after five months. Arch. Surg., *64*:405, 1952.
9. Gibbon, J. H., Jr.: Application of a mechanical heart and lung apparatus to cardiac surgery. Minn. Med., *37*:171, 1954.
10. Goyanes, D. J.: Substitution plastica de las arterias por las venas, ó arterioplastia venosa, aplicada, como nuevo metodo, al tratamiento de los aneurismas. El Siglo Medico, Sept. 1, 1906, p. 346; Sept. 8, 1906, p. 561.
11. Harvey, S. C.: The History of Hemostasis. New York, Paul B. Hoeber, 1929.
12. Hunter, W.: The history of an aneurysm of the aorta, with some remarks on aneurysms in general. Med. Observ. Inquir., *1*:323, 1757.
13. Lexer, E.: Die ideale Operation des arteriellen und des arteriell-venosen Aneurysma. Arch. Klin. Chir., *83*:459, 1907.
14. Matas, R.: An operation for the radical cure of aneurism based upon arteriorrhaphy. Ann. Surg., *37*:161, 1903.
15. Moniz, E.: Injections intracarotidiennes et substances injectables opaques aux rayons. X. Presse Med., *2*:969, 1927.
16. dos Santos, R., Lamas, A., and Caldas, J.: L'artériographie des membres, de l'aorte et de ses branches abdominales. Bull. Soc. Nat. Chir., *55*:587, 1929.
17. Spencer, F. C.: Deductive reasoning in the life-long continuing education of a cardiovascular surgeon. J. Cardiovasc. Surg., in press.
18. Voorhees, A. B., Jr., Jaretzki, A., II, and Blakemore, A. H.: The use of tubes constructed from Vinyon "N" cloth in bridging arterial defects. Ann. Surg., *135*:332, 1952.

II

ANATOMY

David C. Sabiston, Jr., M.D.

The function of the arterial system is delivery of blood from the heart to the tissues. For purposes of convenience, the arteries may be divided into (1) large, (2) medium-sized, and (3) small arteries. Arteries less than 100 μ in diameter are termed *arterioles*. The histologic characteristics of the arterial wall are largely dependent upon the *size* of the vessel. The *large* arteries must withstand the greatest stress and pressure and therefore contain considerable *elastic tissue* in their walls. The *medium-sized* arteries have less elastic tissue and more *smooth muscle,* and the wall of the small arteries is composed primarily of smooth muscle. At the level of the arteriole, elastic tissue is quite scant or absent. *Collagen* is present in all parts of the arterial system, with the collagen ratio becoming dominant as the arteries become smaller.

The principles of *collateral circulation* are of primary importance in all aspects of medicine, and particularly in surgery. All organs have *some* degree of collateral circulation, although the amount that occurs naturally varies greatly in the different tissues and organs and in the same organs in different subjects. For example, the subclavian artery usually can be ligated safely in the first portion, as in the performance of a subclavian-pulmonary anastomosis for congenital cyanotic heart disease (Blalock operation), since the collateral circulation around the shoulder is excellent. It is rare for ischemic symptoms to follow ligation of the subclavian at this site, and, indeed, frequently with the passage of time a pulse reappears in the radial artery as additional collateral circulation develops. Moreover, three of the four major arteries to the stomach (the left and right gastric and left and right gastric epiploic) can be ligated without significant ischemia in most subjects. With a number of other arteries the extensiveness of collaterals varies considerably from person to person, ligation producing no ill effects in some patients and ischemia in others. Finally, some arteries, such as the coronary, renal, and retinal arteries, have a very inadequate natural collateral circulation. Acute occlusion of these vessels is usually followed by serious changes of ischemia and infarction, and such arteries are referred to as "end-arteries."

The *natural* collateral circulation of a tissue or organ is important in the sequence of events following acute occlusion. In addition, the *time* involved in occlusion of an artery is of great significance. For example, with *slow* and progressive occlusion of an artery, there is ample time for collateral vessels to become *larger*. Generally, as a smaller vessel is subjected to a need for increased flow (primarily due to a pressure gradient), the vessel is apt to become *tortuous*. The latter characteristic is easily and consistently delineated arteriographically, as in chronic occlusion of the ab-

dominal aorta (Leriche syndrome). Under these circumstances, adequate arterial collaterals develop which link the branches above the occlusion with the iliac and femoral systems below. It is surprising to recognize that total occlusion of the entire abdominal aorta may produce minimal symptoms in some patients, whereas in others it results in the characteristic symptoms of intermittent claudication and impotence. Nevertheless, in the Leriche syndrome, it is rare to note gangrene until late in the disease, whereas *acute* occlusion of the abdominal aorta usually produces disastrous effects, with acute appearance of severe ischemia and gangrene of the legs if untreated.

III

PHYSIOLOGY OF THE ARTERIAL SYSTEM

Andrew S. Wechsler, M.D.

So the heart is the center of life, the sun of the Microcosm, as the sun itself might be called the heart of the world. The blood is moved, invigorated, and kept from decaying by the power and pulse of the heart. It is that intimate shrine whose function is the nourishing and warming of the whole body, the basis and source of all life. . . . The arteries are the vessels carrying blood from the heart to the body, the veins returning blood from the body to the heart, the one the way from the heart, the other toward the heart, the latter carrying imperfect blood unfit for nourishment, the former perfected, nutritious blood.

With these classic words, William Harvey delineated the conducting function of the arterial system in relation to its central propelling force, the heart. This section discusses the interrelationship between structural aspects of the arterial system and mechanics of the blood that flows through these vessels. Exploration of active and passive responses of arteries provides an initial basis for understanding disorders of blood flow.

RELATION OF BLOOD FLOW TO ANATOMIC ORGANIZATION

The anatomic conformation of the arterial system determines greatly systemic and regional effects of vascular responses. With progression from aorta to capillaries several general changes occur. These are (1) individual vessel diameters decrease with net increase in total vascular cross-sectional surface area; (2) elasticity of arterial walls decreases and muscular construction increases; (3) neural innervation becomes

maximal at the arteriolar level; (4) velocity of blood flow steadily decreases; and (5) a major pressure drop occurs across arteriolar vessels. As these changes occur, the role of arterial vasculature evolves from major systemic, hemodynamic modulation to fine regulation of flow distribution in accord with regional metabolic demand. These relationships are illustrated graphically in Figure 1.

STRUCTURAL INFLUENCES ON PRESSURE AND FLOW

Descriptors of dynamic arterial function are primarily pressure and flow, from which most other parameters can be derived. Effects of local pressure on the vascular wall are expressed by

$$T = \frac{Pr}{W}$$

where T is wall tension, P is transmural pressure, r is internal radius, and w is wall thickness. In progressing from aorta to arteriole, the ratio w/r increases. This anatomic change facilitates the major functional difference between large central arch vessels and smaller peripheral "resistance" vessels. In the great vessels, transmission of pressure from ventricular contraction generates high wall tension with resultant systolic expansion and diastolic relaxation. This is facilitated by the high content of elastic fibers and relatively low muscular organization of the great vessels.

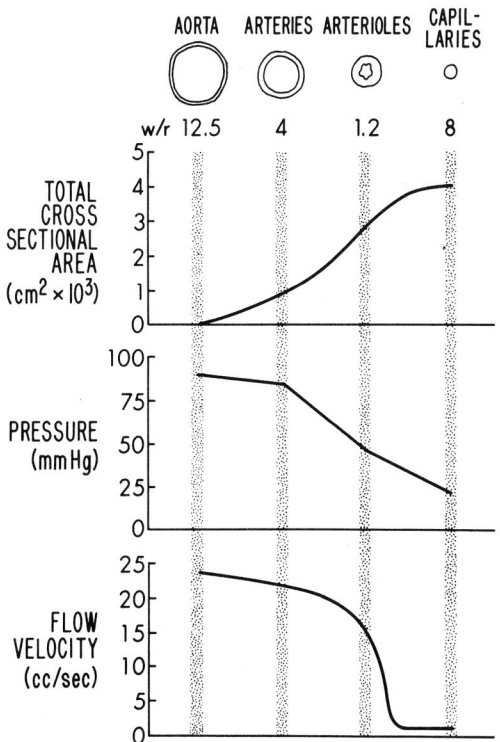

Figure 1. Profile of changes in ratio of wall thickness (w) to inner radius (r), total vascular cross-sectional area, pressure, and blood flow velocity across a systemic vascular bed from aorta to capillary vessels. The most significant changes occur at the arteriolar level.

This "windkessel" function of the great vessels modifies the pressure contour and transforms it, resulting in less pulsatile and more steady distribution of flow in the periphery. Increased stiffness in the vascular wall (generally the consequence of aging) results in more direct transmission to the periphery of cardiac events, causing increased pulse pressure independent of changes in cardiac output.

Certain definitions are required to discuss arterial physiology in vessels smaller than medium-size arteries. Terminal arteries are vessels greater than 50 microns in diameter which have an endothelium, an inner elastic lamina, and a sheath with at least two layers of well-formed vascular smooth muscle cells. The next order of vessels is arterioles, with diameters of 20 to 50 microns. These vessels are of similar construction to terminal arteries with the exception of having only one layer of vascular smooth muscle cells. They blend quickly with the metarterioles, vessels of diameters that are 10 to 15 microns. The metarterioles may have only a single layer of discontinuous smooth muscle or may be of the precapillary sphincter type, in which case they are surrounded by smooth muscle cells that, unlike terminal arteries and arterioles, do not have rich neural innervation. These precapillary sphincters are under primarily *metabolic* rather than *sympathetic neural* control and determine to a great extent which capillary beds will be perfused at any time. The capillaries are composed of a single layer of

endothelial cells, a basement membrane, and are surrounded by a reticular network of collagen fibers.

As blood flows through the arterial system, analysis of the pressure at each branch point discloses the major pressure drop to occur at the arteriolar level. The mean pressure drop associated with transition through the arteriolar bed is approximately 60 mm. Hg and is accompanied by a 60 per cent decrease in blood flow velocity. Through measurement of vascular impedance, it can be determined that the changing arterial system exhibits its greatest resistance at this level.

At the arteriolar level, the ratio of w to r increases significantly, with relatively larger amounts of muscle than elastic tissue in the vessel wall. Such a relationship makes lumen diameter at the arteriolar level very susceptible to changes in wall thickness associated with vascular muscular contraction or relaxation. With transition to the metarteriole and capillary bed, mean arterial driving pressure falls an additional 10 mm. Hg with reduction of blood flow velocity out of proportion to pressure change. Blood flow velocity, 20 to 25 cm. per second in the aorta and 5 cm. per second at the arteriolar level, decreases to 0.3 to 0.5 mm. per second in the capillaries. The reason for such a change in velocity becomes apparent when considering the systemic circulation as a series of parallel resistors. Each branch point represents addition of a resistor and, for any system, addition of a resistance in parallel always causes a net fall in total resistance. The total resistance at any point in the vascular network will be related directly to the total cross-sectional area at that juncture. By comparison, the cross-sectional area of the aorta may be estimated at 4 sq. cm., compared with the cross-sectional area of the capillary bed of 2500 to 3000 sq. cm. Thus, a small fall in pressure, a large increase in area, and diminished resistance are associated with a significant fall in blood velocity. These parameters are illustrated in Figure 1.

PRIMARY FACTORS GOVERNING FLOW IN ARTERIES

In 1839, Hagen suggested the importance of the fourth power of the radius (r^4) in determining flow through tubes. However, Poiseuille, in 1846, provided the definitive relationship between flow, radius, length, and viscosity as expressed by the formula:

$$Q = \frac{\pi \, r^4 \, (P_1 - P_2)}{8 \, L \, \eta}$$

This formula is not written exactly as in Poiseuille's equation, since contemporary symbols have been substituted for the original, but the relationships are the same. In the formula,

Q = flow
r = radius
$(P_1 - P_2)$ = the pressure difference across the length of tubing being examined
η (eta) = viscosity
L = length

The assumptions are that L is relatively great, flow is not turbulent or pulsatile, and the fluid has uniform viscosity. Errors introduced by minor deviations from these conditions are relatively small and do not alter the operational usefulness of the formula in predicting behavior of blood in the systemic vasculature. The importance of vessel radius is apparent, since flow is directly related to r^4. Since flow is equal to pressure difference divided by resistance,

$$Q = \frac{\Delta P}{R}$$

from Poiseuille's equation:

$$R = \frac{8 L \eta}{\pi r^4}$$

Expressed in this manner, resistance is *inversely* proportional to the fourth power of the radius. Within the anatomic confines of the arterial system, L remains relatively fixed and the pressure drop ($P_1 - P_2$) across most vascular beds can be determined readily.

Viscosity, however, is an important variable that is difficult to measure *in vivo*. Viscosity is an expression of "internal friction" between the lamellae of a fluid. Newton described viscosity as a "lack of slipperiness." Blood exhibits anomalous viscosity when tested in vitro because its viscosity increases with decreasing flow velocity. Its anomalous viscosity is due largely to presence of red cells in plasma. Removal of red cells and examination of the plasma demonstrates that its viscosity is constant at varying velocities, thereby behaving as a "Newtonian" fluid. In vivo, the viscosity of blood does not change with velocity as much as suggested by in vitro testing. This physiologic minimization of anomalous viscosity is due partly to axial streaming and the Fåhraeus-Lindqvist effect. Axial streaming refers to the parabolic contour of blood flow at high velocities in large tubes with axial orientation of the erythrocytes and central concentration of the erythrocyte mass in the axial stream. The greater the velocity, the greater the red cell mass is concentrated centrally and the more blood behaves as a Newtonian fluid. As blood flow occurs in small arteries (less than 200 microns in diameter), it is observed that viscosity again diminishes despite a decreased velocity. This has been attributed to separation of erythrocytes from plasma components with stacks of erythrocytes interspersed between columns of pure plasma. In this setting, blood again behaves more like a Newtonian fluid. This is the Fåhraeus-Lindqvist effect. It is extremely pronounced when considering the effect of increased viscosity associated with increased hematocrit. At the capillary level, very little effective increase in viscosity is noted, compared to the effects of increased viscosity noted in 200-micron vessels.

Viscosity increases significantly with cooling. In low-flow states with poor peripheral perfusion, effects of augmented viscosity may be great. Awareness of the effects of altered blood viscosity and regional flow and resistance become similarly important under conditions of both systemic hypothermia and chilling of an extremity.

ARTERIAL OBSTRUCTION AND TURBULENT FLOW

Flow in peripheral vessels is streamlined and laminar. As flow velocity increases, a rate is reached where flow becomes turbulent and Poiseuille's equation relating pressure change to flow becomes nonlinear. Normally, such rapid flow occurs only briefly within the heart chambers and proximal aorta during left ventricular ejection. In the presence of partial narrowing of an artery, flow is maintained if velocity of flow increases. Under such circumstances, turbulence may result as predicted from Reynold's equation:

$$Re = \frac{Vr \sigma}{\eta}$$

where Re = Reynold's number, V = mean flow velocity, r = radius, σ = density, and η = viscosity. When $Re > 1000$, turbulence develops and with increasing velocities, changes in flow become proportional to the square root of changes in driving pressure. The appearance of turbulence causes vibrations in the vessel wall, and these are audible as vascular bruits. Since turbulence is dependent upon high flow rates and pressure gradients, exercise of an extremity may precipitate turbulence by augmenting the pressure gradient across an area of stenosis. Turbulence may further impede flow to an affected extremity, since the Δ flow/Δ pressure is no longer linear.

CONTROL OF BLOOD FLOW DISTRIBUTION

In the resting state it is estimated that the muscle vascular bed receives approximately 18 per cent of the total cardiac output. During intense exercise, muscle blood flow may account for 80 per cent of the total cardiac output, with a 20-fold increase in flow. Since flow to specific regions is discussed in the appropriate chapters, for the purpose of illustration, the muscular circulatory control system will be discussed briefly to emphasize factors controlling arterial flow.

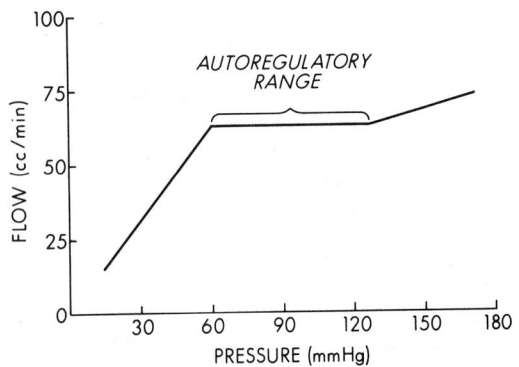

Figure 2. Schematic illustration of autoregulation. Changes in vascular radius within the "autoregulatory range" maintain constancy of blood flow despite changes in perfusion pressure. Below and above the limits of physiologic autoregulation, flow is determined passively by pressure.

Although there are certain obvious exceptions, blood supply to most major vascular beds is controlled by the process of autoregulation. Autoregulation maintains constancy of flow despite changes in pressure. Implicit in such controls is the presence of active changes in vascular tone within the perfused bed. In addition, as shown in the schematic illustration (Fig. 2), there is generally a range of pressures over which autoregulation is effective, with extremes of pressure overriding local autoregulatory responses. The relative influence of intense sympathetic stimulation in certain vascular beds may interfere with local autoregulation. Although the concept of autoregulation is easily understandable, it is difficult to quantitate. True autoregulation can be tested only in a vascular bed free from all extrinsic neural and humoral control. The vascular bed best typifying autoregulatory properties is the coronary arterial system where constancy of flow is maintained over a wide range of pressures.

Three primary theories for autoregulation of regional blood flow are commonly proposed. The first of these is the Bayliss or myogenic mechanism. Activation of vasoconstrictor smooth muscle fibers occurs whenever intraluminal pressure increases. Increased wall tension alters the resting state of the smooth muscle fibers and increases resting tone. This decreases the lumen and increases resistance, thereby reducing flow through a vessel. This concept was modified by Folkow, who suggested that increased pressure had a primary effect on precapillary sphincters. In the presence of their tonic opening and closing, flow decreases. Conversely, fall in intraluminal pressure would result in less frequent closure of precapillary sphincters, with greater flow through the regional vascular bed. In the Bayliss theory, fall in pressure results in decreased wall tension with subsequent relaxation of the constrictor fibers. Myogenic autoregulation is dependent upon effective changes in luminal diameter with small alterations in vasoconstrictor muscle fiber activity. Vessels controlling autoregulation are those with relatively large w/r ratios such as exist in vessels at the arteriolar level.

The second major hypothesis invokes metabolic autoregulation. Either the presence of a particular substrate or a metabolite causes change in vascular muscle tone. Examples of vasodilator substances are decreased pH, increased lactate, high P_{CO_2}, low P_{O_2}, and adenosine compounds. Although each of these substances has been demonstrated to produce local effects in some vascular beds, no single substance appears totally effective in all vascular beds. Other authors have suggested the importance of tissue pressure as a regulator of vascular tone. As interstitial tissue pressure rises, vasoconstrictor tone is augmented. Progressive vasoconstriction exaggerates the pressure drop at that level of the arterial system such that there is less intravascular driving pressure for transudation of fluids into the interstitial space. As interstitial pressures gradually decline, relaxation of precapillary sphincters augment flow through the capillary bed under higher driving pressures, again favoring mild transudation of fluids.

Different mechanisms of regional vascular control predominate in different portions of the arterial tree.

Thus, neurogenic influences may be extremely important in major shifts of blood flow associated with assuming the upright posture after recumbency or in acute hypovolemia. As anatomic transition to smaller vessels occurs, sympathetic innervation diminishes and autoregulatory forces predominate. Local vascular control distributes blood flow *within* most discrete vascular beds. In those zones where both vasoconstrictor fibers and strong autoregulatory forces overlap, autoregulation generally overrides sympathetic vasoconstriction. However, sympathetic activity modulates any level of basal vascular tone and influences the extent to which local autoregulation must act for a specific amount of vasodilation. Direct metabolite effects on vascular smooth muscle, generally those of vasodepression, render such muscles incapable of responding fully to neuroeffector stimulation.

Neurogenic control of blood flow distribution is mediated by sympathetic (thoracolumbar) or parasympathetic (craniosacral) components. By studying agents that block specific classes of neurotransmitters, it has been possible to identify both alpha and beta receptor responsiveness in vascular smooth muscle. Stimulation of alpha receptors by neural or humoral mechanisms results in vasoconstriction, while stimulation of beta receptors evokes vasodilation. In the presence of agents equipotent in both alpha and beta stimulation, alpha-induced constriction predominates. Treatment with specific alpha blocking agents such as phenoxybenzamine may reveal masked vasodilator effects of mixed drugs and neural stimuli. Under physiologic conditions, vasodilation in response to baroreceptor stimulation is primarily the result of sympathetic neurogenic vasoconstriction withdrawal rather than active neurogenic vasodilation. Some investigators, however, have emphasized the role of sympathetic cholinergic fibers. These fibers are unique to arterial vessels in skeletal muscle. Although contained within the sympathetic trunk, acetylcholine is released upon stimulation. Sympathetic cholinergic vasodilation is blocked completely by atropine. Demonstration of such vasodilator activity has been largely by field stimulation of large sympathetic trunks and may play a relatively minor role in normal vasomotor regulation. Worthy of mention, but also of questionable physiologic significance, is vasodilation mediated by histaminergic nerves that release histamine locally. This response is blocked by administration of antihistaminics. These, too, have not been demonstrated convincingly to play any significant role in physiologic neural vasomotor regulation. Some of these mechanisms are illustrated in Figure 3.

The relative roles of neural vasomotor regulation and autoregulation are typified by comparison of two vascular beds. Skeletal muscle, with enormous capability of altering blood flow depending upon the metabolic state of muscle, is predominantly under influence of metabolic vasomotor control. On the other hand, skin, with little metabolic function but important thermoregulatory properties, is influenced primarily by neurogenic mechanisms. In any single vascular region, neurogenic influence may shift the tonic state of the vessels toward greater or lesser constriction. On this matrix, fine metabolic control further de-

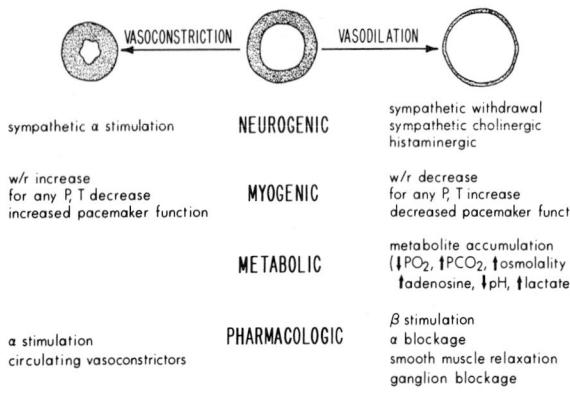

Figure 3. Primary mechanisms governing vasodilation and vaso-constriction (for details see text). No metabolite has been demonstrated to produce local vasoconstriction. Specific vasodilator metabolites are of varying effectiveness depending on the vascular region that is assayed.

termines flow distribution to smaller regions of the tissue. The two mechanisms are not generally competitive, but serve different physiologic function with some anatomic overlap.

SELECTED REFERENCES

Folkow, B., and Neil, E.: Circulation. New York, Oxford University Press, 1971.
Drs. Folkow and Neil have contributed independently a wealth of information to the scientific literature concerning control of the circulation. This text provides a superb introduction to virtually every aspect of circulatory physiology. There is in-depth discussion of regional circulations as well as some basic cardiac physiology. The text is selectively referenced and provides a good starting point for detailed reading in any area of circulation of special interest to the reader. The text stops short of overly mathematical analyses of circulatory function and yet includes enough detail to demonstrate admirably the importance of quantitation of blood flow and distribution. The sections on metabolic control of vascular function and total circulatory integration are particularly strong and reflect the major contributions of these two scientists.

Hamilton, W. F., and Dow, P.: Handbook of Physiology, Section 2: Circulation, Volume II, Chapters 24–26. Washington, D.C., American Physiological Society, 1963.
Although prepared over a decade ago, this text still serves as the primary reference source for serious students of circulatory physiology. This volume covers, among other topics, physiology of the aorta and major arteries, pulsatile blood flow in the vascular system, anatomy and physiology of the vascular wall, and resistance and capacitance phenomena in terminal vascular beds. There is also detailed discussion of regional circulations. Mathematical treatment of blood rheology is extensive, and the entire subject of physical aspects of the circulation is dealt with in depth. The text is extensively referenced, and graphic illustrations are numerous. The contributors are all accepted authorities in their respective fields. Unlike the Folkow and Neil text, considerably greater detail is present in discussing experimental methods and artifacts in studying the circulation. Recent technological advances have made some of the techniques less applicable to contemporary research, but the concepts presented are still valid.

Harvey, W.: Anatomical Studies on the Motion of the Heart and Blood. The Leake Translation, 1628. Springfield, Ill. Charles C Thomas, Publisher, 1958.

This monograph is one of the most exciting in medical literature. It is required reading for anyone who desires more than superficial knowledge of the circulation. In addition to offering Harvey's concept of the circulation, the reader is exposed to Harvey's criticism of prior circulatory concepts. The precision with which Harvey uses the power of observation to make fundamental discoveries about the circulation, and the manner in which he executed simple experiments that yielded profound results, are models for future investigators. His astuteness in postulating those aspects of the circulation which he could not see or measure are fully detailed in the text. The work is extremely readable, beautifully organized, and delightfully translated.

Mellander, S., and Johansson, B.: Control of resistance, exchange and capacitance functions in the peripheral circulation. Pharmacol. Rev., 20:117–196, 1968.
This review is one of the most frequently quoted discussions of regional vascular control. The physiologic content is very detailed without mathematical orientation. The influence of neurogenic, metabolic, and intrinsic myocyte function on flow patterns is discussed extensively, as well as effects of specific blocking agents. The role of vascular "tone" in modifying local responses is discussed, and considerable length is devoted to autoregulatory and exchange phenomena.

REFERENCES

1. Bayliss, W. M.: On the local reactions of the arterial wall to changes in internal pressure. J. Physiol., 28:220, 1902.
2. Bevegard, B. S., and Shepherd, J. T.: Regulation of the circulation during exercise in man. Physiol. Rev., 47:178, 1967.
3. Fishman, A. P., and Richards, D. W.: Circulation of the Blood: Men and Ideas. New York, Oxford University Press, 1964.
4. Folkow, B.: Description of the myogenic hypothesis. Circ. Res., 14 and 15 (Suppl. I):279, 1964.
5. Folkow, B.: Nervous control of the blood vessels. Physiol. Rev., 35:629, 1955.
6. Folkow, B.: Transmural pressure and vascular tone—some aspects of an old controversy. Arch. Int. Pharmacodyn. Ther., 139:455, 1962.
7. Glick, G., Epstein, S. E., and Wechsler, A. S.: Physiological difference between the effect of neuronally released and blood-borne norepinephrine on beta adrenergic receptors in the arterial bed of the dog. Circ. Res., 21:217, 1969.
8. Glick, G., Epstein, S. E., and Wechsler, A. S.: The role of vasoconstrictor withdrawal and histamine release in reflex vasodilatation. Am. J. Cardiol., 19:130, 1967.
9. Glick, G., Wechsler, A. S., and Epstein, S. E.: Mechanisms of Reflex vasodilatation: Assessment of the role of neural re-uptake of norepinephrine and release of histamine. J. Clin. Invest., 47:511, 1968.
10. Hamilton, W. F., and Dow, P.: Handbook of Physiology, Section 2: Circulation, Volume I. Washington, D.C., American Physiological Society, 1962.
11. Hamilton, W. F., and Dow, P.: Handbook of Physiology, Section 2: Circulation, Volume III. Washington, D.C., American Physiological Society, 1965.
12. Henry, J. P., and Meehan, J. P.: The Circulation: An Integrative Physiologic Study. Chicago, Ill., Year Book Medical Publishers, Inc., 1971.
13. Katori, M., and Berne, R. M.: Release of adenosine from anoxic hearts. Circ. Res., 19:720, 1966.
14. McDonald, D. A.: Blood Flow in Arteries, 2nd Ed. Baltimore, The Williams and Wilkins Company, 1974.
15. Mountcastle, V. B.: Medical Physiology, 13th ed. Vol. 2. St. Louis, The C. V. Mosby Co., 1974.
16. O'Rourke, M. F., et al.: Pressure wave transmission along the human aorta: Changes with age and in arterial degenerative disease. Circ. Res., 23:567, 1968.
17. Ruch, T. C., and Patton, H. D.: Physiology and Biophysics. Philadelphia, W. B. Saunders Company, 1974.
18. Whereat, A. F.: Recent advances in experimental and molecular pathology, atherosclerosis and metabolic disorder in the arterial wall. Exp. Mol. Pathol., 7:233, 1967.

IV

ARTERIAL SUBSTITUTES

William W. Krippaehne, M.D., and John M. Porter, M.D.

The perfect arterial substitute has not yet been developed. Normal arteries have often been described as the ideal vascular conduit, and autogenous arteries as the ideal arterial substitute. For long-term survival, however, these vessels leave much to be desired. Their ultimate fate is progression to atherosclerosis, which is at present the leading cause of death in the United States. Since the most frequent need for arterial replacement is in patients with degenerative arterial disease, other arterial substitutes must be used.

An *optimal* arterial substitute should (1) have persistent strength; (2) be easily, reliably, and permanently attachable to the host vessel; (3) be resistant to infection; (4) be obtainable in sterile form or easily sterilizable; (5) be available as needed and in appropriate sizes; and (6) have considerable flexibility. Moreover, such substitutes *should not* (1) leak blood on restoration of flow; (2) be subject to degeneration as encountered in other vessels; (3) incite abnormal surrounding reaction such as neoplasia; (4) incite thrombus formation within the graft; (5) occlude when flexed; or (6) damage blood constituents.

HISTORY

The dramatic advancements in arterial reconstructive surgery in the twentieth century are inextricably intertwined with the search for and development of better arterial substitutes. Many of the basic observations upon which modern vascular surgery is based were published by Alexis Carrel, often in collaboration with Charles C. Guthrie, in the first two decades of this century.

Carrel developed the modern vascular anastomotic technique based upon careful intimal approximation and the use of fine suture material.[9] He and Guthrie were the first to perform successful venous autografts in the arterial system of dogs.[12] They observed that venous autografts underwent rapid structural change, consisting primarily of a marked thickening of the connective tissue in the adventitia and media. They also noted that better results were obtained when the caliber of the vein and the artery to which it was anastomosed was similar.

The first successful arterial allograft was reported by Hoepfner in 1903.[23] Carrel performed a series of arterial allografts several years later, including detailed microscopic studies.[11] He found that fresh arterial allografts functioned well and remained microscopically normal during several months' observation. He also performed studies with viable, refrigerated allografts and nonviable, preserved allografts, work predating the development of human arterial allograft banks by almost 50 years. Carrel noted progressive arterial allograft wall thickening and hyalinization,

depending generally upon the type of preservative used and the duration of refrigeration. Nonviable grafts killed by heat, formalin, or glycerin showed rapid degeneration accompanied by a significant host fibrous reaction.[10]

Many experimental and clinical trials of various arterial replacements have been conducted following the monumental work of Carrel and Guthrie, which firmly established the feasibility of arterial substitution.[12] Numerous categories of arterial substitutes have been evaluated, including arterial autografts, allografts, and xenografts; venous autografts and allografts; textile grafts; composite or compound grafts; and solid tube grafts. Considerable evidence at present suggests that large arteries are best replaced by textile grafts, and small arteries by venous autografts of appropriate size.

ARTERIAL AUTOGRAFTS

Fresh arterial autografts are generally accepted as the ideal arterial substitute; however, they are not readily available. Technically, they are easy to handle. Their clinical function is comparable to that of a normal artery. Upon implantation the arterial wall usually retains viability of all its components. Anastomotic strength at 10 days is approximately 20 per cent, gradually rising to 70 per cent of normal artery tensile strength at 6 weeks.[15] If the arterial graft is thicker than 500 to 600 μ and revascularization of the vasa vasorum does not occur, the outer layer undergoes avascular necrosis, as has been demonstrated by Berger.[2] Geiringer,[16] Berger,[2] and others found that the inner 350 to 500 μ receives its nutrition by luminal diffusion. This process as diagrammatically depicted by Berger is shown in Figures 1 and 2. Clot surrounding the graft or suture line may delay revascularization. There is minimal or no luminal thrombus deposition if the endothelium is not damaged and if the procedure is technically correct. Varying amounts of late thrombus formation occur in rough proportion to the degree of degeneration or inflammation in or around the graft wall. A small amount appears initially at suture lines but is characteristically resorbed within 10 to 20 days. If thrombus persists, organization by capillaries and fibroblasts contributes to permanent intimal thickening and luminal narrowing. This process is similar to the fibrotic stage of human atherosclerosis.

Arterial autografts are not widely used, primarily because of the obvious problem of lack of availability. Some vascular surgeons, however, prefer to use the autogenous internal iliac artery for renal artery replacement, especially in pediatric patients, because of the reported high incidence of progressive dilatation of

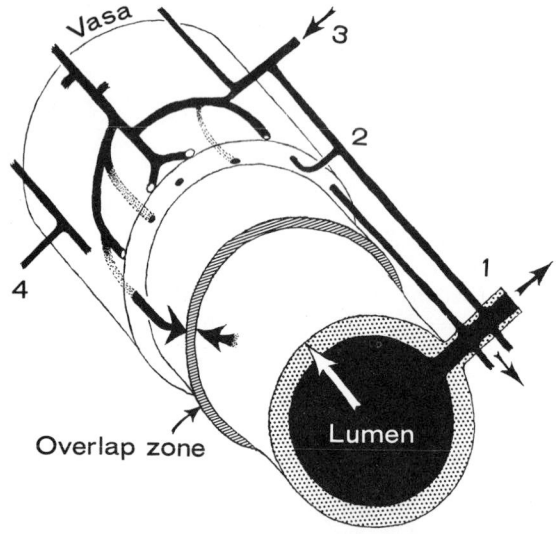

Figure 1. Diagrammatic conception of nutrition to the thoracic aortic wall. Luminal diffusion serves the inner portion of the wall. Vasa vasorum serve the outer portion. A narrower zone, the overlap zone, is served by both mechanisms. At *1*, an intercostal artery emerges. This in turn gives off branches that travel in the outer medial layer of the wall, as well as along the adventitia. At *2*, branches from the adventitial system traverse into the outer media. At *3*, connection may occur to adventitial vessels other than those derived from intercostals. At *4* is shown an adventitial vessel derived from the "nonintercostal" system. (From Berger, K., et al.: Pacif. Med. Surg., 75:367, 1967.)

length and wall thickness. In the absence of an adequate saphenous vein, good clinical results have been obtained with the use of the cephalic vein.

Five-year patency rates of saphenous vein autografts in the femoropopliteal system are in the range of 60 to 75 per cent when plotted by the life-table method. The patency rate is lower for femorotibial grafting, averaging 45 to 60 per cent. As would be predicted, the best results are usually obtained in patients with the least obstruction in the popliteal artery outflow tract. However, this is not an absolute requisite for long-term patency. Mannick has reported a patency rate of 65 per cent with autogenous vein grafts into an isolated popliteal artery without angiographic patency of the popliteal trifurcation vessels.[29]

Vein grafts in the arterial system are subject to pathologic alterations that may singly or in combination lead to graft occlusion. One of the most frequently observed changes in vein grafts is intimal proliferation, which may become sufficiently pronounced to cause luminal obstruction. The intimal thickening appears to be caused by a proliferation of smooth muscle cells associated with marked increases in collagen fibers and ground substance.[45] The cause of the intimal thickening is unknown, although simple arterial pressure has been suggested experimentally.[7] Vein grafts are also subject to atherosclerosis, fibrotic narrowing of the venous valves, fibrotic stenosis due to operative trauma, and aneurysmal dilatation. An ex-

saphenous vein autografts used in such a setting.[51] The internal mammary artery is widely used at the present time for coronary revascularization. Excellent patency rates are being reported, which is felt by many to result from a close approximation in size between the autograft and the recipient coronary artery.

VENOUS AUTOGRAFTS

Venous autografts have proved to be the best arterial substitute for small vessel replacement and are widely used at present, especially in lower extremity and coronary revascularization. The first use of a venous autograft in a patient was reported by Goyanes in 1906,[18] and followed by Lexer in 1907[28] and Bernheim in the United States in 1916.[3] The developmental story of venous autographs has been well reviewed by Harrison.[22] It was not until 1951 that the systematic application of venous autografts for the bypass of arterial obstruction in patients was reported by Kunlin.[14]

Venous autografts have a number of obvious advantages. They retain cellular viability and do not show rejection phenomena. They are more readily available than arteries, although not always in the proper size or length. Most surgeons feel that veins smaller than 4 mm. internal diameter should not be used for arterial replacement because of a high incidence of thrombosis associated with the use of such small veins. The saphenous vein is generally preferred because of its

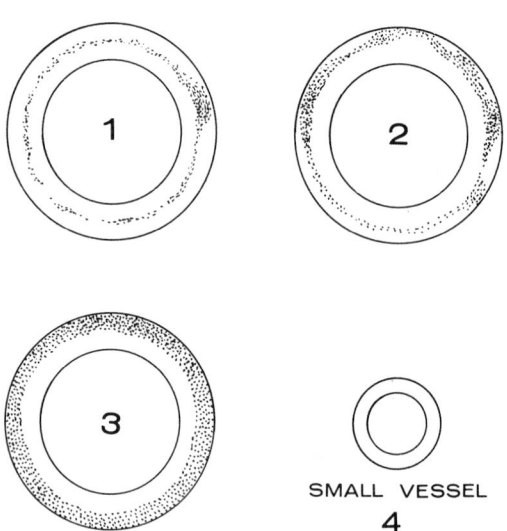

Figure 2. Diagrammatic summary of luminal diffusion and vasa vasorum zones of influence as observed in canine experiments. Necrosis is indicated by stippled areas. *1*, Results from minor trauma exemplified by aortic-aortic anastomoses, namely, freeing of the vessel ends necessary for sewing them together. This is taken to be an example of overlap zone damage. *2*, Irregular necrosis of outer wall resulting from removal of thoracic aortic segment with intercostals ligated only. *3*, Necrosis of outer wall following removal of aortic segment, plus excision of intercostal ostia. In all three instances the viable luminal diffusion zone remains of about the same order of thickness. *4*, Full wall viability of small transected and reanastomosed vessel, whose wall thickness falls within diffusion zone distance. (From Berger, K., et al.: Pacif. Med. Surg., 75:367, 1967.)

cellent review by Szilagyi and associates indicates that structural defects developed in the venous autograft in 32.7 per cent of their patients over a long period of observation.[42]

There is general agreement that vein grafts should be harvested and handled as atraumatically as possible. Vigorous hydrostatic dilatation before implantation should be avoided. Since a number of pathologic

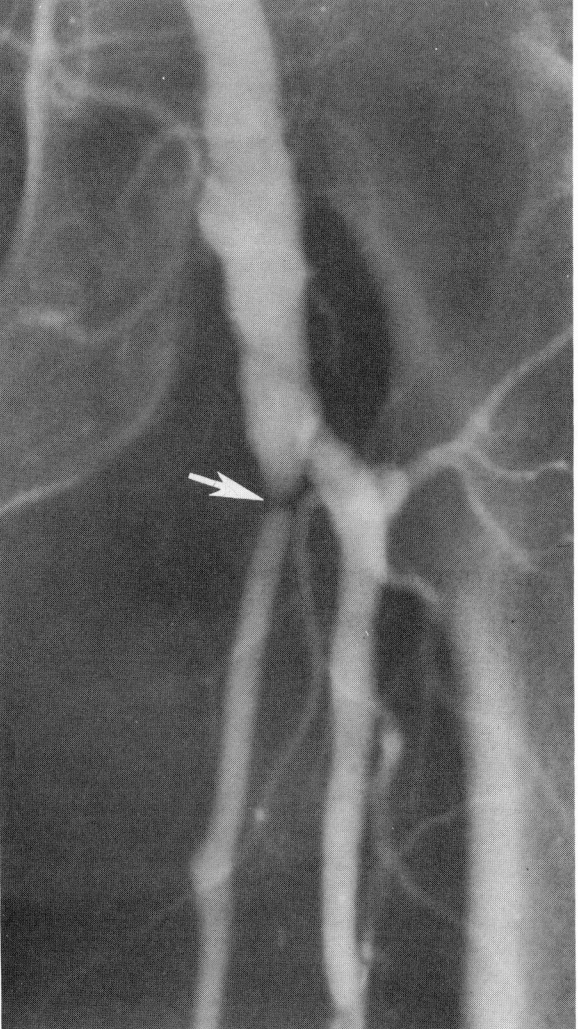

Figure 4. Routine angiogram of a femoropopliteal venous autograft one year after implantation. This close-up view of the origin of the graft from the common femoral artery shows a clinically unsuspected area of stenosis just distal to the graft origin (arrow). Elective surgical repair in this asymptomatic patient revealed a localized area of fibrous stenosis.

changes in vein grafts, which may ultimately result in occlusion, are amenable to surgical repair if discovered early, a number of authors recommend routine postoperative angiographic evaluation of the vein grafts at regular intervals. An angiogram of a well-functioning femoropopliteal venous autograft is shown in Figure 3 two years after implantation. Another graft with a clinically unsuspected proximal stenosis is shown in Figure 4.

VENOUS ALLOGRAFTS

A significant number of patients requiring arterial bypass procedures for whom an autogenous vein graft is the arterial substitute of choice do *not* possess an adequate vein because of prior vein stripping, thrombophlebitis, or venous anomalies. The use of a sa-

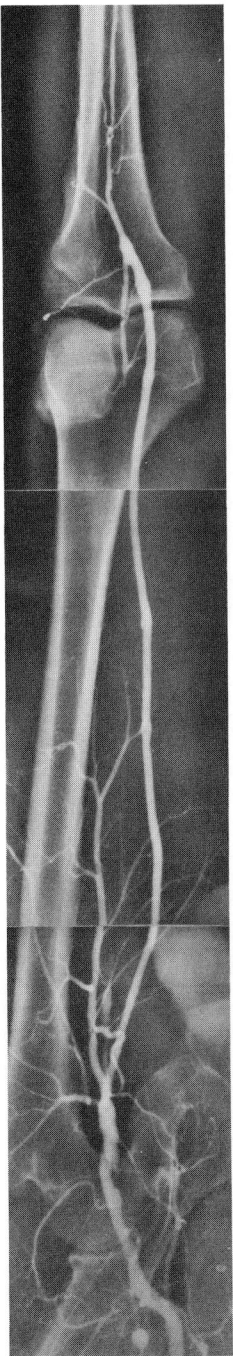

Figure 3. Angiogram of a well-functioning femoropopliteal venous autograft two years after implantation. Normal slight graft dilatation at the site of the venous valves is still present.

phenous vein allograft has been suggested for such patients.

Saphenous vein allografts were used sporadically in patients in the 1950s, but the results were poor and the procedure was generally abandoned until the early 1970s, when several reports of Tice[43, 44] and Ochsner[31] indicated encouraging results. Unfortunately, a recent report by Ochsner revealed a very high failure rate of the venous allografts after a longer period of observation.[30]

Immunologic investigations have shown that venous allografts are normally antigenic and sensitize the recipient in a predictable manner.[33] Pathologic examination has revealed significant tissue reaction, which has been most prominent at the endothelial surface of the allograft.[50] Laboratory studies suggest that immunosuppressive drugs may favorably modify host reaction to venous allografts and improve patency rates.

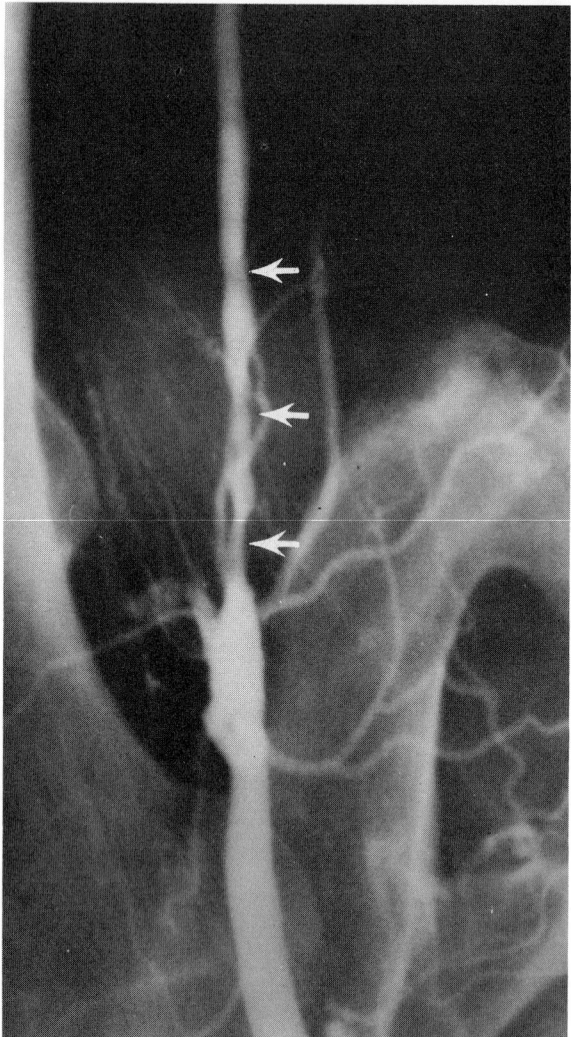

Figure 5. Angiogram of a femoropopliteal venous allograft in a patient one year after implantation. Diffuse stenosis of the proximal portion of the allograft is present (arrows). The graft subsequently thrombosed. Pathologic examination revealed diffuse fibrous thickening of all layers of the graft wall accompanied by a striking mononuclear and giant cell infiltration.

This is at present unproved in patients. Figure 5 shows an angiogram of a venous allograft within a year after implantation. Diffuse graft stenosis occurred proximally, caused by perigraft fibrosis. Weber and associates[47] have recently reported animal studies demonstrating that viable venous allografts frozen in DMSO and methylprednisolone show considerably higher patency rates upon subsequent arterial grafting than do unmodified allografts.

The use of venous allografts in patients is experimental at the present time. Their ultimate role as arterial substitutes has not yet been determined.

ARTERIAL ALLOGRAFTS

Arterial allografts were first studied experimentally by Hoepfner and Carrell, and were first used successfully in patients by Gross in 1948.[19] Early results suggested that these grafts functioned as well as autografts. Longer evaluation, however, revealed that both fresh and preserved allografts underwent progressive degenerative changes.

Allografts of the abdominal aorta, which is composed predominantly of collagen and elastin, are associated with fewer complications and longer graft function than allografts of the femoral artery, which have a much larger component of smooth muscle and elicit a much more prominent rejection reaction. All arterial allografts rapidly lose endothelium with subsequent exposure of the underlying basement membrane, collagen, and elastin. A platelet-fibrin coagulum forms on the inner surface of the graft and slowly undergoes fibrous organization, which proceeds from the suture lines at a slow rate. The central areas of allografts may never develop fibrous organization of the platelet-fibrin coagulum, and are liable to intimal ulcerations.

Allograft walls become progressively less cellular with time. After several years there is progressive thinning of the wall with loss of collagen and fragmentation of the elastic fibers. Similar degenerative changes affect both muscular and elastic arterial allografts, but occur much more rapidly with the former. Arterial allografts in patients show a high incidence of thrombosis, calcification, aneurysm formation, and rupture. Graft degeneration and clinical complications rapidly increase with time. Deterling[13] reported that 77 per cent of aortic allografts were functioning satisfactorily at 5 years, but only 38 per cent were satisfactory 10 years after implantation. Femoral artery allografts were far less satisfactory, with 36 per cent patent at 5 years and only 3 per cent patent at 10 years. Isolated reports, however, describe satisfactory clinical function of arterial allografts in certain areas. Schuster and Gross[39] report no aneurysms or occlusions in 34 patients followed an average of 5 years after short segment aortic allograft implantation for aortic coarctation. Twenty-two of the 34 grafts, however, showed calcification. Generally these grafts were placed in children and young adults, who are perhaps less likely to develop degenerative changes.

Because of the high incidence of complications, arterial allografts have been abandoned clinically in favor of more satisfactory arterial substitutes. Allografts, however, occupy an important place in the history of vascular surgery. The modern era of vascular grafting began with the successful clinical use of arterial allografts by Gross and his associates. The aortic allograft was the arterial substitute used by Oudot[32] for the first aortic bifurcation resection for Leriche's syndrome, and by Dubost et al.[14] for the first resection of an abdominal aortic aneurysm.

ARTERIAL XENOGRAFTS

Unmodified arterial xenografts produce a prominent host reaction leading to widespread damage to the layers of the xenograft wall. Their use is associated with a high incidence of thrombosis and graft disruption. Unmodified arterial xenografts are clearly not suitable for clinical use.

In recent years a modified xenograft produced from bovine carotid arteries by the technique described by Rosenberg[34] has been widely used clinically and has given satisfactory results. The graft is prepared by digestion of bovine carotid arteries by the proteolytic enzyme ficin, followed by dialdehyde starch tanning. This results in a collagenous tube essentially devoid of muscular and elastic elements. The modified graft possesses the same tensile strength as a normal artery, but is almost nonantigenic. In man the graft elicits a moderate fibroblastic reaction, but little or no inflammation. Widespread thrombus deposition on the luminal surface does not occur regularly, as it does with unmodified allografts and xenografts. The modified xenografts are lined in time by a thin layer of fibroblasts of host origin.

Modified xenografts have functioned quite satisfactorily as arterial substitutes in high-flow areas, such as iliac artery replacement. The most severe test of a graft, however, is in low-flow areas such as femoropopliteal and femorotibial bypass. In such settings these grafts have produced patency rates in the 50 to 60 per cent range for short periods of observation of under 3 years.[25, 35]

The bovine xenograft has been used to provide vascular access for hemodialysis.[4] The graft is placed subcutaneously between an extremity artery and a vein and may be punctured directly for hemodialysis.

The saphenous vein autograft remains the arterial substitute of choice in low-flow applications. The modified bovine xenograft and textile grafts yield similar results when used in such areas, but both are clearly inferior to the venous autograft.

TEXTILE GRAFTS

A milestone in the history of vascular grafting was reported in 1952 when Voorhees and his associates described the successful replacement of arteries in animals with a porous textile fabric, Vinyon-N.[46] Two years later these investigators used the same material successfully in patients.[5] This singular achievement opened the entire field of prosthetic arterial grafting and stimulated extensive laboratory and clinical research, which continues to the present.

EXPERIMENTAL STUDIES

A large number of textiles of varying composition, yarn type, and fabrication have been studied. The most detailed evaluation of prosthetic grafts was performed by Wesolowski.[48] The most important factor determining the success of prosthetic grafting in experimental animals appears to be the rate and quality of the formation of a fibrous, viable internal graft lining derived from host tissue—the so-called neointima. When a graft is first implanted, an internal layer of thrombus of variable thickness develops. Successful long-term function is associated with fibrous organization or "healing" of this initial layer of thrombus.

The most important determinant of prosthetic graft healing is the biologic porosity of the graft wall, permitting capillary and fibroblast ingrowth from perigraft tissues, with subsequent organization of the initial luminal thrombus. Totally healed grafts have a luminal surface lined by a layer of flattened cells resembling normal endothelium. It is uncertain whether these are true endothelial cells or modified fibroblasts. It is also unclear what role, if any, "fall out" healing from primitive mononuclear blood cells may play.

In the experimental animal, grafts of optimal porosity show early fibrous interstitial ingrowth and luminal healing. When the porosity is inadequate, the neointima may calcify or ulcerate, or further thrombus formation may occur.

Porosity has been described by Wesolowski as the amount of water that will pass through 1 square centimeter of graft wall under a driving pressure equivalent to 120 mm. Hg. He found that good neointima formation occurred and degenerative calcification was not seen in the animal model if the porosity was greater than 5000 ml. per min.

The body surrounds a textile graft with connective tissue, forming an outer layer called neoadventitia. The rapidly developing neoadventitia should remain stable with the neointima, which forms simultaneously but at a slower rate. The two are interconnected by collagen-vascular bundles passing through the graft interstices. Any mechanical disturbance of this process, such as the occurrence of a perigraft hematoma or seroma, may produce tearing and degeneration of the collagen-vascular bundles, which results in segmental ulceration of the neointima and new luminal thrombus formation. This inevitably results in some narrowing of the lumen. This may not be critical in vessels of large size with high flow rates, such as the aorta and iliac arteries, but it may lead to thrombotic failure when grafts are used in small arteries. If the developing neointima is over 400 to 500 μ in thickness and vascularity is not provided through graft interstices, luminal diffusion of nutrients is insufficient and late neointimal degeneration may occur.

GRAFT FABRICATION

Prosthetic grafts fabricated from a number of different materials have been evaluated clinically and experimentally. Orlon, Vinyon-N, Ivalon, Nylon, and polypropylene lose a majority of their tensile strength with time and have not given satisfactory long-term results.[21] The only materials that have functioned satisfactorily are Dacron and Teflon.

Various types of textile fabric construction have been studied. The only two that have been useful clinically are weaving and knitting. The woven graft is quite compact, with small interstices, and shows delayed intimal healing in animals. The knitted fabrication is quite porous and displays superior intimal healing, but the graft has to be preclotted before use. The knitted grafts have been more widely used clinically. Such porous grafts, however, should be used with caution in patients with platelet or coagulation defects such as may occur in advanced hepatic cirrhosis or in association with a ruptured aortic aneurysm. As the temporary plugging of small holes at the su-

ture lines and the graft interstices is primarily a function of platelet-fibrin deposition, any defect in the coagulation sytem makes the use of such grafts hazardous. A tightly woven graft is preferable under such conditions. An angiogram of an aortofemoral knitted Dacron bifurcation graft is shown in Figure 6.

Experimental studies in animals have shown that thin-walled textile grafts develop more satisfactory neointima than do thick-walled grafts. The most commonly used grafts today are fabricated from thin-walled knitted Dacron. All grafts are crimped to allow bending at flexion lines without graft occlusion. The biologic healing of grafts is significantly affected by the graft bed. Extensive clot surrounding grafts or suture lines delays or prevents capillary and fibroblast ingrowth. This may result in suture line failure, defective neointima formation, bleeding through porous grafts, pseudoaneurysm formation, or graft thrombosis. Contamination with bacteria may result in graft failure through clotting, dissolution of suture lines with hemorrhage, or continuing sepsis necessitating graft removal.

GRAFT HEALING IN MAN

Optimal criteria for graft fabrication evolved through a series of experimental studies using a variety of animals. Complete luminal healing and neointima formation occurred in all animals with the thin knitted Dacron graft, and it was assumed that similar healing occurred in man. Unfortunately, this does not appear to be the case. A recent excellent study by Sauvage and his associates documents the lack of intimal healing in prosthetic grafts in man, even after many years.[1] This obviously does not preclude long-term satisfactory graft function in high-flow applications, but it does point out the likely reason textile prostheses have been of limited success in low-flow applications. If intimal healing does not occur, the internal surface is formed of compacted fibrin, a substance that has been shown to be highly thrombogenic.[52]

The lack of complete healing of the available prostheses in man has led to a renewed search for improved prosthesis design. The most promising fabrication undergoing evaluation at present is the external velour graft.[37] The velour is composed of loops of Dacron yarn on the external surface with partial filling of the graft interstices by yarn filaments. Loose yarn appears to present a scaffolding upon which fibroblasts can migrate, leading to a more rapid and complete incorporation of the graft into the surrounding tissues, and fibrous neointimal formation. Preliminary evaluation in man has shown better healing and higher patency rates in low-flow applications than with any other prosthetic graft evaluated to date.[36] A double velour graft is also being evaluated. Figures 7A and B show the velour design in profile.

Several additional concepts in graft design are in early stages of development. One is construction of a graft composed of an expanded, highly porous form of Teflon, known as P.T.F.E. This material is composed of tiny nodules of polytetrafluoroethylene intercon-

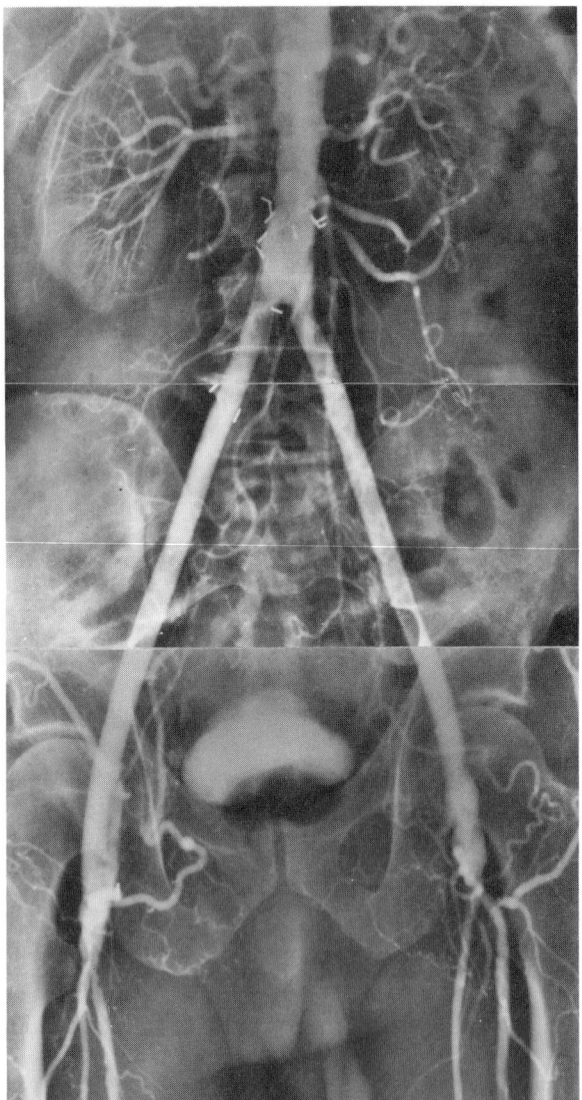

Figure 6. Angiogram of an aortofemoral knitted bifurcation Dacron graft. The graft extends from the infrarenal aorta to the common femoral arteries. The graft wall appears smooth and regular.

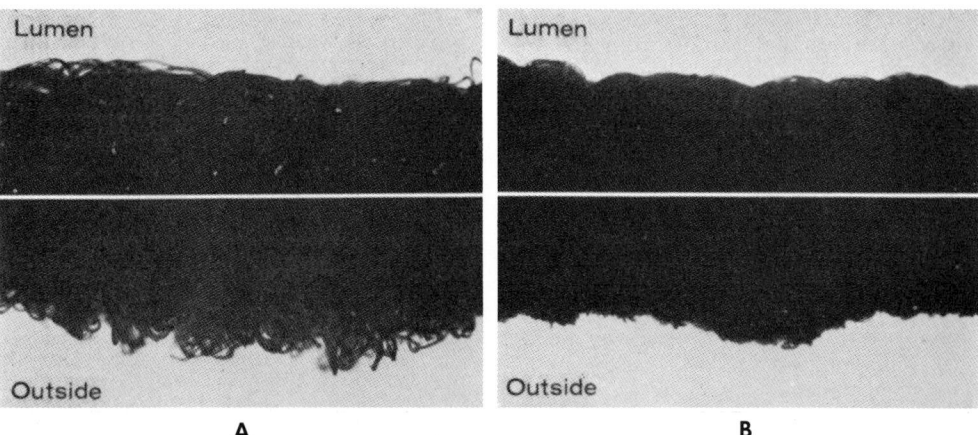

Figure 7. *A,* Photosilhouette (× 60) of surfaces of external velour graft. This graft presents some fibrillar loops to the blood, while the outside presents a great many loops that project quite markedly above the body of the yarn. The fibrillar loops are open so that fibrin, and then tissue, can surround them. *B,* Photosilhouette (× 60) of surfaces of smooth graft (Wesolowski Weavenit). The external aspect of the graft shows some projections of Dacron fibrils, but these are small and the fabric profile presented to the surrounding tissue is relatively smooth. (From Sauvage, L. R., Berger, K., Wood, S. J., Nakagawa, Y., and Mansfield, P. B.: An external velour surface for porous arterial prostheses. Surgery, *70:*940, 1971.)

nected by thin fibrils. Early reports indicate satisfactory performance as vein substitutes in several patients.[40] Experimental and clinical trials of the material as an arterial prosthesis are beginning. As yet, optimal design characteristics have not been developed.

Important studies are beginning on the application of hydrogels to synthetic polymers used in graft fabrication. These are unique compounds that are wettable, blood compatible, and appear to serve as an excellent scaffold material for the ingrowth of cells.[8]

OVERVIEW

The three types of prosthetic grafts that have been most widely used in patients are woven Dacron, knitted Dacron, and woven Teflon. All seem to function satisfactorily in high-flow applications, although the results with Dacron have generally been superior to those with Teflon.[6] None of these grafts, however, has been satisfactory for small vessel grafting. The velour concept of knitted Dacron fabrication appears to hold the most promise at present for small vessel application. Longer term evaluation will be required.

Autogenized Vascular Prostheses

An innovative and attractive concept, pioneered by Hufnagel,[24] and used clinically by Sparks,[41] is that of "autogenization" of vascular prostheses. A loose woven or knitted Dacron fabric is placed over a mandril and implanted subcutaneously or adjacent to the vessel to be bypassed. The interstices fill with collagen. Within a few weeks a compound prosthesis is formed with intimal "healing" already achieved by host fibroblasts. After removal of the mandril, the graft is anastomosed to the artery in the usual fashion. Although the initial clinical results were encouraging, longer follow-up has

revealed severe problems with this graft as currently fabricated. Hallin[20] has reported a 25 per cent incidence of aneurysm formation, and a patency rate of only 18 per cent at 29 months for grafts used in the femoropopliteal position.

Compound Grafts

The theoretical advantages of low implantation porosity in textile grafts led to the design and investigation of numerous grafts of a mixture of adsorbable-replaceable and nonadsorbable components. The most systematic studies were reported by Wesolowski.[49] Two general types of compound materials were tested — one a biologic adsorbable substance applied over stable nonadsorbable mesh, and the other an adsorbable fiber (collagen) interwoven with nonadsorbable fibers. A third category, using a very loose Dacron knit with a tanned adsorbable collagen inner liner, has also been studied.[26] The most satisfactory grafts experimentally were the mixed fiber grafts. Here biologic healing generally followed the same sequence as with textile grafts of the same biologic porosity. When the adsorbable component was replaced at a slower rate than fibrin, luminal healing was delayed. There are definable advantages to this concept: one can attain optimal biologic porosity while maintaining initial bloodtightness, and fibrinolytic or uncoagulable states do not lead to hemorrhage through the grafts. The theoretical advantages of this concept will insure further attempts toward the development of compound grafts. Adequate clinical trials have not yet been reported.

Solid-Wall Prostheses

At this writing, solid-wall prostheses are not widely accepted in clinical use. Solid-wall plastic materials of similar composition (Teflon, Dacron) to porous materials produce extensive luminal thrombus formation, usually originating at the junction of the tube with the artery. Metal tubes have been investigated. Sawyer's[38] studies in animals indicate that magnesium and aluminum conduits have remained patent for 330 days, stainless steel tubes for 30 to 40 days, and copper tubes for 1 to 7 days. Platinum tubes occlude at 1 to 2 days. Magnesium and aluminum have less tendency to precipitate blood elements electrochemically on metal surfaces. Metals high in the electromotive series lose positive ions to the solution and build up an electrical double layer with the metal being negatively charged. This process produces corrosion of metals and loss of substance.

Another method of producing a negatively charged surface on tubes has been reported by Gott.[17] Colloidal graphite is bonded to a material and treated with benzalkonium chloride and subsequently heparin. This remains firmly bonded and results in a lasting nonthrombogenic surface.

Glass tubes that activate clot formation do not remain patent. Metals and glass, being rigid, are not suitable for any location with movement. Plastic solid tubes with antithrombogenic surfaces are at present not easily, reliably, or permanently attachable to arteries. Use of solid tubes in clinical practice will depend upon further study and experimentation.

The development of prosthetic vascular substitutes has only recently begun. Under most circumstances, the best materials for large artery grafting are porous cloth prostheses because of the scarce supply of autogenous arteries. Small vessels are best replaced with autogenous veins. With further research new and better arterial substitutes will undoubtedly be developed.

SELECTED REFERENCES

Berger, K., Sauvage, L. R., Rao, A. M., and Wood, S. J.: Healing of arterial prostheses in man, its incompleteness. Ann. Surg., *175*:113, 1972.
This article reports detailed pathologic observations on arterial prostheses removed from patients. It is of pivotal importance in emphasizing the marked differences between man and the experimental animal in the healing of prosthetic arterial grafts.

Szilagyi, D. E., Elliott, J. P., Hageman, J. H., Smith, R. F., and Dal'Olmo, C. A.: Biologic fate of autogenous vein implants as arterial substitutes. Ann. Surg., *178*:232, 1973.
The authors present detailed clinical, angiographic, and pathologic follow-up information on a personal series of 377 autogenous vein bypass grafts. This excellent reference clearly documents the long-term performance of autogenous vein grafts in man.

Wesolowski, S. A., and Dennis, C.: Fundamentals of Vascular Grafting. New York, Blakiston Division, McGraw-Hill Book Company, 1963
This monograph contains a summary of most of the important historical, experimental, and clinical fundamentals of prosthetic vascular grafting.

REFERENCES

1. Berger, K., Sauvage, L. R., Rao, A. M., and Wood, S. J.: Healing of arterial prostheses in man: Its incompleteness. Ann. Surg., *175*:118, 1972.
2. Berger, K., Sauvage, L. R., Wood, S. J., and Sameh, A. A.: Endarterectomy and other surgical injuries to cardiovascular walls. Pacif. Med. Surg., *75*:367, 1967.
3. Bernheim, B. M.: The ideal operation for aneurysm of the extremity. Report of a case. Bull. Johns Hopkins Hosp., *27*:93, 1916.
4. Biggens, J. A., Remmers, A. R., Jr., Glassford, D. M., Lindley, J. D., Sarles, H. E., and Fish, J. C.: Bovine graft fistulas in patients with vascular access problems receiving hemodialysis. Surg. Gynecol. Obstet., *140*:690, 1975.
5. Blakemore, A., and Voorhees, A. B., Jr.: The use of tubes constructed of Vinyon "N" cloth in bridging arterial defects: Experimental and clinical. Ann. Surg., *140*:324, 1954.
6. Boyd, D. P., and Midell, A. I.: The use of Teflon in arterial surgery. Surg. Clin. North Am., *53*:351, 1973.
7. Brody, W. R., Kosek, J. C., and Augell, W. W.: Changes in vein grafts following auto-coronary bypass induced by pressure and ischemia. J. Thorac. Cardiovasc. Surg., *64*:847, 1972.
8. Bruck, S. D.: Biomedical applications of polymeric materials and their interactions with blood components: A critical review of current developments. Polymer, *16*:409, 1975.
9. Carrel, A.: La technique operatoire des anasomoses vasculaires et la transplantation des visceres. Lyon Med., *98*:859, 1902.
10. Carrel, A.: Latent life of arteries. J. Exp. Med., *12*:460, 1910.
11. Carrel, A.: Results of the transplantation of blood vessels, organs, and limbs. J.A.M.A., *51*:1662, 1908.
12. Carrel, A., and Guthrie, C.: Uniterminal and biterminal venous transplantations. Surg. Gynecol. Obstet., *2*:226, 1906.
13. Deterling, R. A., and Clauss, R. H.: Long-term fate of aortic arterial homografts. J. Cardiovasc. Surg., *11*:35, 1970.
14. Dubost, C., Allerg, M., and Deconomos, N.: Resection of an aneurysm of the abdominal aorta. Reestablishment of the continuity by a preserved human arterial graft, with result after five months. Arch. Surg., *64*:405, 1952.
15. Gaylis, H., Corvese, W. P., Linton, R. R., and Shaw, R. S.: The rate of healing of arterial autografts. Surgery, *45*:41, 1959.
16. Geiringer, E.: Intimal vascularization and atherosclerosis. J. Pathol. Bacteriol., *63*:201, 1951.
17. Gott, L., Whiffen, J. D., Dutton, R. C., Leininger, R. I., and Young, W. P.: *In* Sawyer, P. M. (Ed.): Biophysical Mechanisms in Vascular Homeostasis and Intravascular Thrombosis. New York, Appleton-Century-Crofts, 1965.
18. Goyanes, J.: Nuevos trabajos de cirugia vascular, substitucion plastic de las arterias por las venas o arterioplastia venosa, applicada, como nuevo metoclo, al tratamiento de las aneurismas. Siglo Med., *53*:546, 1906.
19. Gross, R. E., Hierwitt, E. S., Bill, A. H., Jr., and Pierce, E. C., II: Preliminary observations on the use of human arterial grafts in the treatment of certain cardiovascular defects. N. Engl. J. Med., *239*:578, 1948.
20. Hallin, R. W.: Complication with the mandril-grown (Sparks) Dacron arterial graft. Am. Surg., *41*:550, 1975.
21. Harrison, J. H.: Synthetic materials as vascular prostheses. Am. J. Surg., *95*:16, 1958.
22. Harrison, L. H., Jr.: Historical aspects in the development of venous autografts. Am. Surg., *183*:101, 1976.
23. Hoepfner, E.: Uber Gefassnaht, Gefasstransplantionen und replantation von amputierten Extremitaten. Arch. Klin. Chir., *70*:417, 1903.
24. Hufnagel, C. F., Gillespie, J. F., Brea, C., and Franco, W.: Introduction to the concept of "autogenization" of vascular prostheses. *In* Wesolowski, S. A., and Dennis, C. (Eds.): Fundamentals of Vascular Grafting. New York, Blakiston Division, McGraw-Hill Book Company, 1963.
25. Keshishian, J. M.: Modified bovine grafts for complex arterial problems. *In* Dale, W. A. (Ed.): Management of Arterial Occlusive Disease. Chicago, Year Book Medical Publishers, Inc., 1971, p. 185.
26. Krajicek, M., Zastava, V., and Chvapil, M.: Collagen-fabric vascular prostheses. J. Surg. Res., *4*:290, 1964.
27. Kunlin, J.: Le traitement de l'ischemie arteritique par la greffe veineuse lungue. Rev. Chir. Paris, *70*:206, 1951.
28. Lexer, E.: Die ideale operation des arteriellen und des Arteriellvenosen Aneurysma. Archiv. Klin. Chir., *83*:459, 1907.
29. Mannick, J. A., Jackson, B. T., Coffman, J. D., and Hume, D. M.: Success of bypass vein grafts in patients with isolated popliteal artery segments. Surgery, *61*:17, 1967.
30. Ochsner, J. L.: Discussion of Williams et al. Surgery, *78*:694, 1975.
31. Ochsner, J. L., DeCamp, P. T., and Leonard, G. L.: Experience with fresh venous allografts as an arterial substitute. Ann. Surg., *173*:933, 1971.
32. Oudot, J., and Beaconsfield, P.: Thrombosis of aortic bifurcation treated by resection and homograft replacement: Report of five cases. Arch. Surg., *66*:365, 1953.
33. Perloff, L. J., Reckard, C. R., Rowlands, D. T., Jr., and Barker, C.

F.: The venous homograft: An immunological question. Surgery, 72:961, 1972.

34. Rosenberg, N., Gauhran, E. R. L., Henderson, J., Lord, G. H., and Douglas, J. F.: The use of segmental arterial implants prepared by enzymatic modification of heterologous blood vessels. Surg. Forum, 6:242, 1956.

35. Rosenberg, D. M., Glass, B. A., Rosenberg, N., Lewis, M. R., and Dale, W. A.: Experience with modified bovine carotid arteries in arterial surgery. Surgery, 68:1064, 1970.

36. Sauvage, L. R., Berger, K., Mansfield, P. B., Wood, S. J., Smith, J. C., and Overton, J. B.: Future directions in the development of arterial prostheses for small and medium caliber arteries. Surg. Clin. North Am., 54:213, 1974.

37. Sauvage, L. R., Berger, K., Wood, S. J., Nakagawa, Y., and Mansfield, P. B.: An external velour surface for porous arterial prostheses. Surgery, 70:940, 1971.

38. Sawyer, P. M., Brattain, W. H., and Boddy, P. J.: In Sawyer, P. N. (Ed.): Biophysical Mechanisms in Vascular Homeostatis and Intravascular Thrombosis. New York, Appleton-Century-Crofts, 1965.

39. Schuster, S. R., and Gross, R. D.: Surgery for coarctation of the aorta. J. Thorac. Cardiovasc. Surg., 43:54, 1962.

40. Soyer, T., Lempinen, M., Cooper, P., Norton, L., and Eiseman, B.: A new venous prosthesis. Surgery, 72:864, 1972.

41. Sparks, C. H.: Die-grown reinforced arterial grafts. Ann. Surg., 171:787, 1970.

42. Szilagyi, D. E., Elliott, J. P., Hageman, J. G., Smith, R. F., and Dall'Olmo, C. A.: Biologic fate of auotgenous vein implants and arterial substitutes. Ann. Surg., 178:232, 1973.

43. Tice, D. A., and Santoni, E.: Use of saphenous vein homograft arterial reconstruction: A preliminary report. Surgery, 67:493, 1970.

44. Tice, D. A., and Zerbino, V.: Clinical experience with preserved human allografts for vascular reconstruction. Surgery, 72:260, 1972.

45. Unni, K. K., Kotke, B. A., Titus, J. L., Frye, R. L., Wallace, R. B., and Brown, A. L.: Pathologic changes in aortocoronary saphenous vein grafts. Am. J. Cardiol., 34:526, 1974.

46. Voorhees, A. B., Jr., Jaretzki, A., III, and Blakemore, A. H.: The use of tubes constructed from Vinyon "N" cloth in bridging arterial defects. Ann. Surg., 135:332, 1952.

47. Weber, T. R., Dent, T. L., Salles, C. A., Ramsburgh, S. R., Fonseca, F. P., and Lindenauer, S. M.: Cryopreservation of venous homografts. Surg. Forum, 26:291, 1975.

48. Wesolowski, S. A., and Dennis, C.: Fundamentals of Vascular Grafting. New York, Blakiston Division, McGraw-Hill Book Company, 1963.

49. Wesolowski, S. A., Fries, C. C., Domingo, R. T., Liebig, W. J., and Sawyer, P. M.: The compound prosthetic vascular graft: A pathologic survey. Surgery, 53:19, 1963.

50. Williams, G. M., ter Haar, A., Krajewski, D., Parks, L. C., and Roth, J.: Rejection and repair of endothelium in major vessel transplants. Surgery, 78:694, 1975.

51. Wylie, E. J., Perloff, D. L., and Stoney, R. J.: Autogenous tissue revascularization techniques in surgery for renovascular hypertension. Ann. Surg., 170:416, 1969.

52. Yates, S. F., Nakagawa, Y., Berger, K., and Sauvage, L. R.: Surface thrombogenicity of arterial prostheses. Surg. Gynecol. Obstet., 136:12, 1973.

V

ANEURYSMS

David C. Sabiston, Jr., M.D., and Others

An aneurysm is the dilatation of an artery full of spiritous blood.

—Fernel, 1581

An aneurysm is a localized or diffuse dilatation of an artery. Most aneurysms are designated as *true* aneurysms and contain all three layers of the arterial wall (intima, media, and adventitia). A *false* aneurysm ("pulsating hematoma") is the term applied when only the adventitia is present, as is often the situation following traumatic rupture of an artery with subsequent aneurysmal formation. It is further helpful to classify aneurysms into *saccular* and *fusiform* types. The former usually arise from a distinct portion of the wall and possess a mouth, whereas the latter involve the total circumference of the artery and represent a diffuse dilatation. Aneurysms tend to occur at certain anatomic sites, and the most common locations are shown in Figure 1.

Aneurysms may be either *congenital* or *acquired,* the latter being much more frequent than the former. Acquired aneurysms may be caused by arteriosclerosis, trauma, infection (mycotic), syphilis, or medial cystic necrosis. Although aneurysms were once untreatable, nearly all can be managed now by surgical means. Moreover, the results are usually highly satisfactory.

1. ANEURYSMS OF THE SINUS OF VALSALVA

W. Sterling Edwards, M.D., and Thomas W. Hoyt, M.D.

Aneurysms of the sinus of Valsalva take two forms, which will be discussed separately. These are (1) sinus aneurysms caused by congenital lack of attachment of the aortic media with the annulus fibrosis of the aortic valve, and (2) aneurysms of the ascending aorta, usually caused by cystic medial necrosis, which involve the aortic sinuses, the coronary orifices, and the aortic valve.

CONGENITAL ANEURYSM OF THE SINUS OF VALSALVA

A fistulous communication between the aortic sinus of Valsalva and the right side of the heart was first described by Thurman in 1840. Not until 1953, however, was the diagnosis made during life and the lesion treated surgically.[2] The surgical importance of this lesion lies in the sudden onset of symptoms and the high percentage of success of surgery.

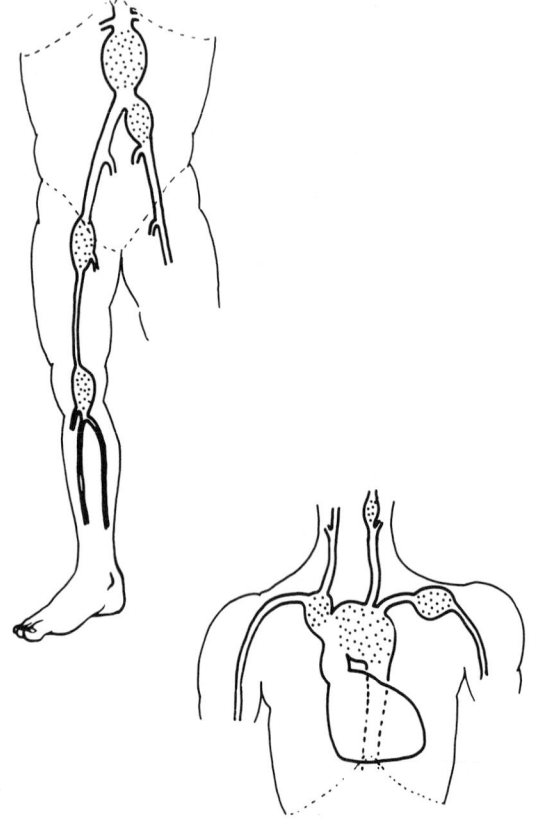

Figure 1. Common anatomic sites of arterial aneurysms. (From Ludbrook, J., and Elmslie, R. G.: An Introduction to Surgery: 100 Topics. New York Academic Press, 1971.)

Anatomical Aspects. Congenital lack of continuity between the aortic media and the annulus fibrosis of the aortic valve results in a cone-shaped bulge of tissue into one of the adjacent cardiac chambers. This lesion involves most commonly the right coronary sinus, less commonly the noncoronary sinus, and least often the left sinus.[4, 6] In the past, the etiology has been attributed to bacterial endocarditis or syphilis, but there is increasing evidence that the separation is congenital and that the infectious processes are secondary.[15] The lesions often cause no symptoms for years, until rupture occurs into a cardiac chamber, but they may be diagnosed earlier if right ventricular outflow obstruction occurs.[3] When rupture occurs, either spontaneously or as a result of superimposed bacterial endocarditis, it occurs most frequently into the right ventricle, less frequently into the right atrium, left atrium, or pericardium. Aneurysms of the left coronary sinus are relatively uncommon, and there is no reported case of rupture of this sinus. Males (80 per cent) are more frequently involved, and the average age of onset of symptoms is age forty.[1, 5, 8-11, 14]

CLINICAL AND DIAGNOSTIC FEATURES

The symptoms and signs of the sinus of Valsalva aneurysm are dependent on the intracardiac physiology. An unruptured aneurysm may be asymptomatic and without clinical signs. When the aneurysm ob-

structs the right ventricular outflow tract, a murmur similar to that of pulmonary stenosis is heard and right ventricular hypertrophy is present.[3] When rupture into a cardiac chamber occurs, clinical signs of acute aortic incompetence and/or ventricular septal defect result. There is usually a systolic-diastolic murmur, often more like that of a patent ductus than like the murmur of aortic incompetence. Left ventricular hypertrophy by x-ray and EKG and a wide pulse pressure may develop if the defect is hemodynamically significant. Right and left heart catheterization with an aortic root angiogram is necessary to define the physiology and anatomy in each case.

SURGICAL MANAGEMENT

Operation is usually not advisable for asymptomatic patients with a sinus aneurysm that has not ruptured and is not causing obstruction. In the presence of symptoms, however, surgery should be carried out promptly, since a small sinus fistula can become a large one in a relatively short time.

Operative treatment is performed with total cardiopulmonary bypass. Exposure of the fistula is obtained by opening the chamber into which the aneurysm has ruptured (Fig. 2). With the aorta clamped, the aneurysmal sac, which resembles an airfield windsock, is excised, and the congenital defect between the root of the aorta and the annulus fibrosis of the aortic valve is reapproximated with sutures. This operation can be performed with a mortality of 5 per cent or less, and long-term results are excellent. Occasionally a more complicated aneurysm, especially one involving the aortic valve, will require a combined exposure into both the cardiac chamber and the aorta.

ECTASIA OF THE ASCENDING AORTA INVOLVING THE SINUSES OF VALSALVA

All of the sinuses of Valsalva as well as the origin of the coronaries and the aortic valve may be involved in

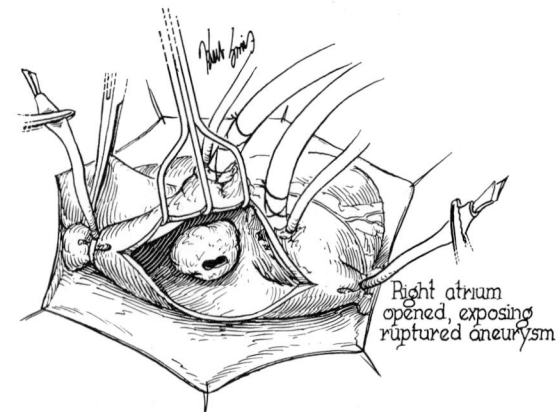

Right atrium opened, exposing ruptured aneurysm

Figure 2. Demonstration of sinus of Valsalva aneurysm with a fistula to the right atrium. A right atriotomy has been made. Following excision of the fistula, the opening into the atrium is closed directly with sutures. (From DeBakey, M. E., Dietrich, E. B., Liddicoat, J. E., Kinard, S. A., and Garrett, H. E.: J. Thorac. Cardiovasc. Surg., 54:312, 1967.)

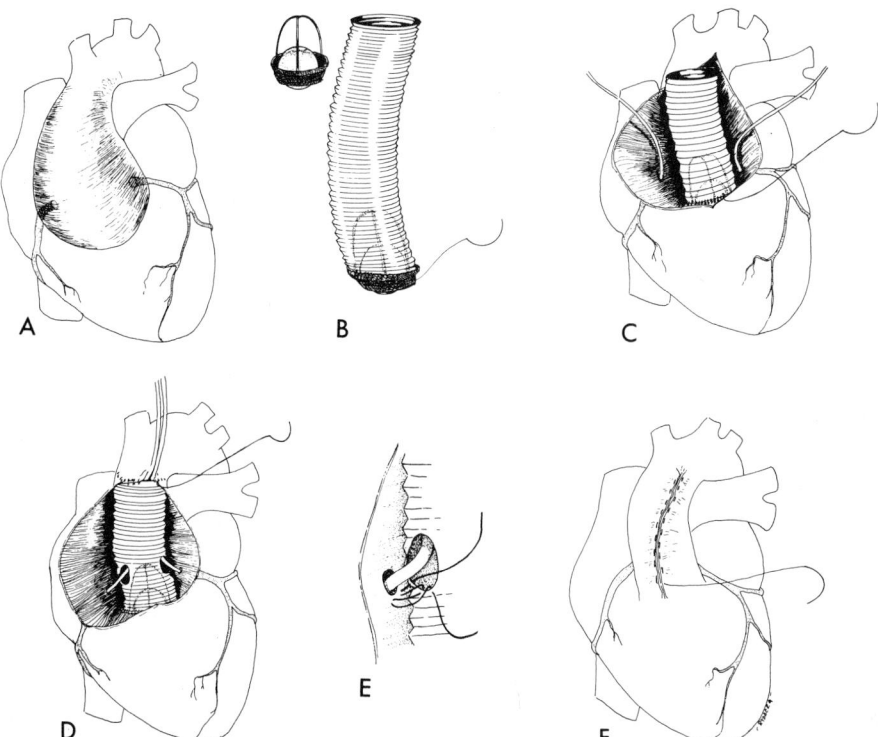

Figure 3. When ascending aortic aneurysms involve the aortic sinuses (*A*), the coronary orifices and the aortic valve, the technique demonstrated has proved safe and effective. *B*, A valve prosthesis is sutured to a woven graft. *C*, Bypass is started, the ascending aorta is opened longitudinally, and the valve is inserted in the aortic annulus with interrupted sutures. *D*, Holes are cut in the graft opposite the coronary orifices. *E*, The distal anastomosis is completed and the aneurysmal sac is closed around the graft. (From Edwards, W. S., and Kerr, A. R.: J. Thorac. Cardiovasc. Surg., *59*:837, 1970.)

a process termed "aortic ectasia" and caused primarily by a poorly understood process, "cystic medial necrosis."[4, 10] Syphilis has, in the past, caused similar pathology, but is no longer a common cause of this disease.

Pathologic Anatomy. Cystic medial necrosis can cause dissecting aneurysms as well as localized fusiform aneurysms of the ascending aorta in the absence of other stigmata of Marfan's disease. It can cause a fairly specific clinical entity, occurring predominantly in young men and involving the ascending aorta from the aortic valve to the innominate artery. There is necrosis and disappearance of muscle cells in the elastic laminae, and there may be cystic spaces filled with a mucoid material. Although these histologic findings may be found in arteries throughout the body to a lesser extent, in most cases they are strikingly limited to the ascending aorta. The fusiform dilatation may involve only the ascending aorta above the valve, but in the more advanced cases, involves the annulus of the valve, producing aortic incompetence. In this situation the coronary orifices arise from the diseased portion of the aorta, making surgical repair more difficult.

Clinical Picture. In aortic ectasia involving the sinuses of Valsalva, the major symptoms are produced by aortic valvular incompetence. Death may occur from cardiac failure or from rupture of the aorta into the pericardial sac, causing tamponade. Ascending aortic

dilatation may produce pressure symptoms on adjacent structures, particularly the superior vena cava.

Surgical Therapy. Aneurysms of the ascending thoracic aorta involving the sinuses of Valsalva require replacement of the aortic valve and the dilated aorta, including the origin of the coronaries. An effective method for performing all these requirements consists of suturing a valve prosthesis to a graft, then inserting the valve with interrupted sutures in the aortic annulus. Holes are cut in the graft where the coronary openings are attached. The aneurysmal sac is then wrapped around the graft and sutured together to minimize blood loss from this friable area. This method is safer and simpler than older methods of replacement of sinus aneurysms and effectively replaces all diseased tissue.[7]

SELECTED REFERENCES

Edwards, J. E., and Buchell, B.: The pathological anatomy of deficiencies between the aortic root and the heart, including aortic sinus aneurysms. Pathol. Anat., *12*:125, 1957.
  The most comprehensive review of the pathologic anatomy of sinus of Valsalva abnormalities by reviewing a large series of autopsy and pathology material.

Edwards, W. S., and Kerr, A. R.: A safer technique for replacement of the entire ascending aorta and aortic valve. J. Thorac. Cardiovasc. Surg., *59*:837, 1970.
  A new technique is described for replacement of the aortic valve and ascending aorta and reimplantation of the coronary arteries.

Meyer, J., Wukasch, D. C., Hallman, G. L., and Cooley, D. A.: Aneurysm and fistula of the sinus of Valsalva. Clinical considerations and surgical treatment in 45 patients. Ann. Thorac. Surg., *19*:170, 1975.
This paper reports a series of 45 patients operated upon for aneurysm and fistula of the sinus of Valsalva. The results were excellent, with a 2.2 per cent morbidity and mortality. Operative technique is discussed in detail.

REFERENCES

1. Bonfils-Roberts, E. A., DuShane, J. W., McGoon, D. C., and Danielson, G. K.: Aortic sinus fistula—surgical considerations and results of operation. Ann. Thorac. Surg., *12*:492, 1971.
2. Brown, J. W., Heath, D., and Whitaker, W.: Cardioaortic fistula: A case diagnosed in life and treated surgically. Circulation, *12*:819, 1955.
3. Bulkley, B. H., Hutchins, G. M., and Ross, R. S.: Aortic sinus of Valsalva simulating primary right-sided valvular heart disease. Circulation, *52*:696, 1975.
4. Chapman, D. W., Beazley, H. L., Peterson, P. K., Webb, J. A., and Cooley, D. A.: Annulo-aortic ectasia with cystic medial necrosis. Am. J. Cardiol., *16*:679, 1965.
5. DeBakey, M. E., Dietrich, E. B., Liddicoat, J. E., Kinard, S. A., and Garrett, H. E.: Abnormalities of the sinuses of Valsalva. J. Thorac. Cardiovasc. Surg., *54*:312, 1967.
6. Edwards, J. E., and Burchell, H. B.: The pathological anatomy of deficiencies between the aortic root and the heart, including aortic sinus aneurysms. Pathol. Anat., *12*:125, 1957.
7. Edwards, W. S., and Kerr, A. R.: A safer technique for replacement of the entire ascending aorta and aortic valve. J. Thorac. Cardiovasc. Surg., *59*:837, 1970.
8. Liddicoat, J. E., Bekassy, S. M., Rubio, P. A., Noon, G. P., and DeBakey, M. E.: Ascending aortic aneurysms: Review of 100 consecutive cases. Cardiovasc. Surg., *51* and *52* (Suppl. I):202, 1975.
9. Meyer, J., Wukasch, D. C., Hallman, G. L., and Cooley, D. A.: Aneurysm and fistula of the sinus of Valsalva. Clinical considerations and surgical treatment in 45 patients. Ann. Thorac. Surg., *19*:170, 1975.
10. Meyer, J., and Cooley, D. A.: Surgical management of patients with pathological changes involving the aortic root: Review of present techniques and proposal of a modified surgical approach. Bull. Texas Heart Inst., *2*:101, 1974.
11. Morgan, J. R., Rogers, A. K., and Fosburg, R. G.: Ruptured aneurysms of the sinus of Valsalva. Chest, *61*:640, 1972.
12. Najafi, H.: Aneurysm of cystic medionecrotic aortic root: A modified surgical approach. J. Thorac. Cardiovasc. Surg., *66*:71, 1973.
13. Oram, S., and East, T.: Rupture of aneurysm of aortic sinus of Valsalva into the right side of the heart. Br. Heart J., *17*:541, 1955.
14. Sawyers, J. L., Adams, J. E., and Scott, H. W.: Surgical treatment for aneurysms of the aortic sinuses with aorticoatrial fistula. Surgery, *41*:26, 1957.
15. Shumaker, H. B.: Aneurysms of the aortic sinuses of Valsalva due to bacterial endocarditis: Operative management. J. Thorac. Cardiovasc. Surg., *63*:896, 1972.
16. Taguchi, K., Sasaki, N., Matsuura, Y., and Uemura, R.: Surgical correction of aneurysm of the sinus of Valsalva. Am. J. Cardiol., *23*:180, 1969.

2. DISSECTING ANEURYSMS OF THE AORTA

Myron W. Wheat, Jr., M.D.

HISTORICAL ASPECTS

Dissecting aneurysms were first characterized in 1761 by Morgagni, who described the magenta-colored appearance of the involved aorta that is produced by the column of blood in the dissecting hematoma just beneath the adventitia. The first comprehensive review of dissecting aneurysms was an analysis of 300 cases by Shennan in 1934.[20] Shennan considered medial degeneration of the aorta to be the basic pathologic defect underlying aortic dissection. In 1935, the first efforts at surgical therapy were reported by Gurin, Bulmer, and Derby,[8] who attempted a localized "fenestration" operation on the right external iliac artery. The operation successfully restored the blood supply to the extremity but the patient died six days later in acute renal failure. In 1955, DeBakey, Cooley, and Creech[5] reported the first successful treatment of dissecting aneurysms and first applied the "fenestration" operation to the descending thoracic aorta for dissecting aneurysms (Fig. 4).

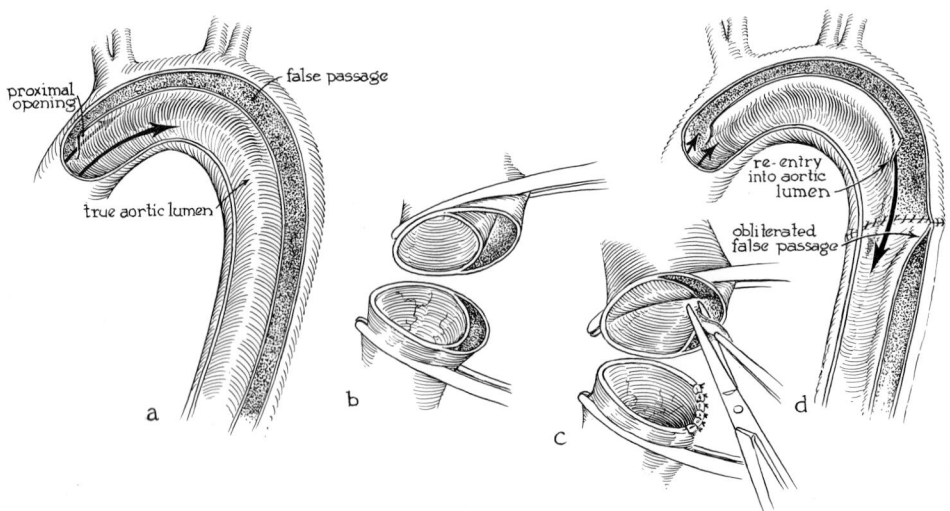

Figure 4. Drawing illustrating DeBakey, Cooley, and Creech's application of the "fenestration operation." *a*, The site of origin and extent of the dissecting process in the thoracic aorta in Case 5. *b*, The aorta has been divided. *c*, The false lumen has been obliterated distally, and proximally a segment of the inner layer is being excised to create a re-entry passage. *d*, The anastomosis is completed. (From DeBakey, M. E., et al.: Ann. Surg., *142*:586, 1955.)

INCIDENCE

Dissecting aneurysms are the most common acute catastrophe involving the aorta. They occur with a frequency of about one per 500 autopsies or about five dissecting aneurysms per million population per year, compared to ruptured abdominal aneurysms, which occur at the rate of about 3.5 per million, and ruptured thoracic aneurysms, which occur at a rate of only one per million population per year.[23]

Dissecting aneurysms occur with the greatest frequency in persons between 50 and 70 and are relatively rare in persons under the age of 40, except in those with a familial predisposition.[9] As many as 50 per cent of dissecting aneurysms seen in patients under the age of 40 may occur in pregnant women.[12] Patients with Marfan's syndrome[14] or congenital heart disease such as coarctation of the aorta or bicuspid aortic valve have an increased incidence of occurrence of dissecting aneurysms.[24]

There appears to be an increased incidence of dissecting aneurysms in the black race, and this may be related to their increased frequency of hypertension. In our own series, 60 per cent of the patients were black.[28] Eighty-seven per cent of our patients with acute dissecting aneurysm have had hypertension on admission or a history of hypertension in the past. The disease also appears to be more common in males, who account for as many as 65 per cent of the cases in some series.[28] The patient with an acute dissecting aneurysm might be typified as a black male aged 60 with known hypertension.

PATHOGENESIS

Medial degeneration of the aorta, most commonly of the cystic medial necrosis variety, is the underlying pathologic finding in most patients with dissecting aneurysms.[10] Only about two thirds of the changes are of the classic Erdheim's cystic necrosis with cystic accumulations of mucoid material, fragmented elastic lamina, and collagen fibers. In fewer than 5 per cent of cases the changes may be related to syphilis or atherosclerosis. Atherosclerotic aneurysms are rare in the ascending aorta, where about two thirds of the dissecting aneurysms originate. In the distal abdominal aorta, where atherosclerotic changes are more pronounced, and fusiform aneurysms related to atherosclerosis are common, dissecting aneurysms are rare.

The Intimal Tear

Rupture of the vasa vasorum in the outer one third of an underlying diseased media has been the major theory of origin of dissecting aneurysms of the aorta in the past.[10] The rupture of the vasa vasorum was believed to produce a hematoma in the aortic wall which was then propagated until it ruptured into the aortic lumen, admitting systolic blood and pressure to the dissecting hematoma. Although there are a few reported instances in which intramural aortic hematomas have occurred without demonstrable intimal tears, such an explanation seems unlikely in most cases of dissecting aneurysms for the following reasons:

1. The intraluminal pressure in the aorta is greater than that in the vasa vasorum 100 per cent of the time and even if a localized intramural hemorrhage should occur, a significant hematoma of the aortic media would not develop.

2. Since vasa vasorum are present only in the outer third of the aortic wall, all dissections should originate in the outer one third of the media, but they do not. Such a hypothesis does not fit with the actual findings that in most dissections there is an intimal tear and that the inner layers of the media are more frequently involved than the outer one third where the vasa vasorum are present.

3. The vasa vasorum hypothesis also does not fit with hydrodynamic data, which demonstrate that the point of greatest stress on the aortic wall is the point nearest the mainstream of the blood, i.e., the intima and inner one third of the media.[17]

4. If most or all of the dissecting aneurysms immediately involve the outer one third of the aortic wall and adventitia, many more than 3 per cent of the patients should succumb abruptly from aortic rupture after initiation of the intimal tear, whereas actually only 20 per cent die within the first 24 hours.[10]

A more likely explanation of the pathogenesis of dissecting aneurysms is as follows[27] (Fig. 5):

1. Medial degeneration of the wall of the thoracic aorta sets the stage by decreasing the cohesiveness of the layers of the aortic wall.

2. Repeated motion of the aorta related to the beating of the heart results in flexion stresses, most marked in the ascending and first portion of the descending thoracic aorta, 60 to 100 times per minute (37

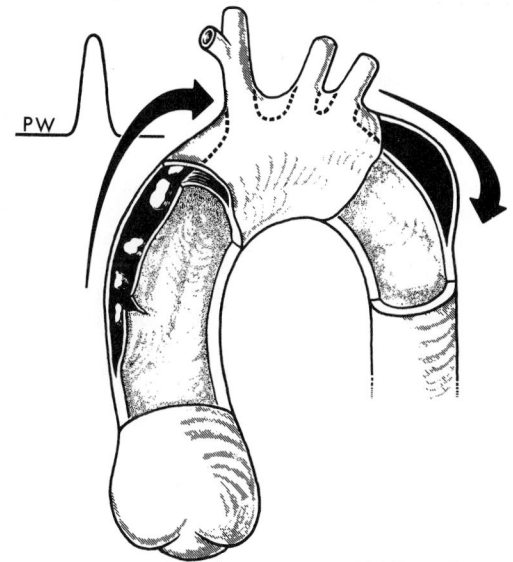

Figure 5. Diagrammatic representation of pathogenesis of dissecting aneurysms: (1) aortic wall with medial degeneration sets the stage; (2) combined forces acting on aortic wall result in intimal tear, giving aortic bloodstream direct access to weakened media; (3) resulting dissecting hematoma is propagated by pulse wave (PW) of blood produced by each myocardial contraction.

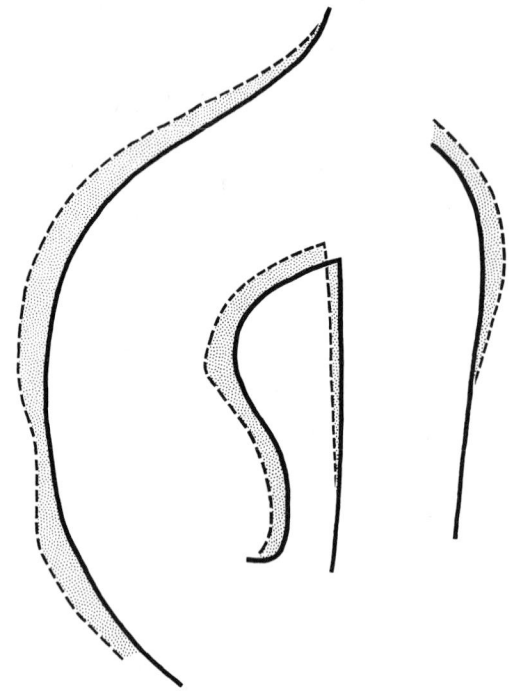

Figure 6. Superimposed tracings of aortograms, left anterior oblique projection. Solid lines with heart in systole; dotted lines, diastole. Tracings demonstrate side-to-side and "flexing" motion of ascending and first portion of descending thoracic aorta with each myocardial contraction.

million times per year). With each heartbeat, the heart, because of the rigid sternum anteriorly and the vertebral column posteriorly, moves predominantly from side to side, producing this flexing motion in the ascending aorta and in the descending aorta just distal to the left subclavian artery. The extent and frequency of this flexing action can be documented by tracing the outline of the thoracic aorta during systole and diastole in the left anterior oblique projection of aortograms and superimposing the two tracings (Fig. 6). Supportive evidence for the tendency of the aortic wall to be disrupted just distal to the left subclavian artery is also available from studies of patients suffering deceleration accidents with traumatic rupture of the aorta. Most of the disruptions occur in the area of the isthmus just distal to the left subclavian artery where mobile aorta becomes fixed descending thoracic aorta.[17]

3. Hydrodynamic forces in the bloodstream related to the pulse wave propagated by each cardiac systole act upon the wall of the aorta, most markedly in the proximal aorta.

4. A combination of the preceding three factors eventually results in an intimal tear, which leads to a hematoma dissecting into the media of the aortic wall for varying depths.

Propagation of the Dissecting Hematoma

After the intima tears and the dissecting hematoma forms, a second set of forces comes into play, those forces that propagate or extend the dissecting hematoma once it has developed. These forces include: (1)

blood viscosity; (2) pressure; (3) velocity (shearing forces); (4) turbulence; and (5) steepness of the pulse wave (dp/dt_{max}). On the basis of experimental evidence, it seems that the steepness of the pulse wave is the most important of the forces propagating the dissecting hematoma. Therefore, the forces that cause the aorta to rupture must come from the heart.[27]

The major force responsible for continuation of the dissection, the steepness of the pulse wave, involves the pulsatile nature of the blood flow in large arteries. This is known because: (1) the aorta is remarkably resistant to static pressure; (2) static pressure provides no pressure gradients as driving forces to induce shear stresses or other stresses on aortic tissue; (3) experimental models, e.g., aortas made of Tygon tubing with rubber cement intimas, dissect only when flow is pulsatile, and not when flow is nonpulsatile,[17] and experiments with dog aortas show the same relationship to pulsatile flow; and (4) in turkeys, protection from aortic rupture can be accomplished with propranolol, a beta-adrenergic blocking agent, at a dose that does not affect mean aortic pressure but does alter the quality of pulsatile blood flow.[20] Propranolol exerts its main effect directly upon the heart and decreases the steepness of the pulse wave (dp/dt_{max}).

Pressure Differentials at Sites Along the Aortic Wall

An attractive analysis of the forces that cause the progress of the dissection to continue in both a forward and a retrograde direction involves continuous pressure differentials (provided by the pulsatile nature of the blood flow) throughout the aorta. In addition to pressure differences, Womersly, in a mathematical approach to hydrodynamics, considered vessel radius (r), blood density (po), blood viscosity (n), and instantaneous blood velocities in the longitudinal (u) and in a radial (w) direction.[29] He considered the forward driving force the pressure differential along the longitudinal axis (Z) (dp/dz). From Figure 7A, if we assume that Z is finite and represents the effective distance along which, if a force were applied, dissection would occur (e.g., Z = length of the torn intima and media),

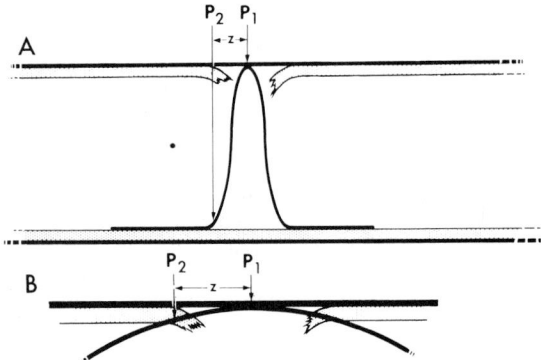

Figure 7. Steepness of pulse wave as a factor in propagating dissecting hematoma: P_1 and P_2 represent pressures on aortic wall at these two points; Z, constant and finite, equals length of torn intima and media. Driving force (ΔP) equal $P_1 - P_2$. If pressure curve is flattened, as shown in B, driving force (ΔP) will be less over distance Z than in A, where pressure curve is steep.

then the shape of the pressure pulse would determine the value ΔP ($P_1 - P_2$). In Figure 7A, the pressure profile at any time is steep, and ΔP, if Z is finite and constant, is greater than in Figure 7B, where the shape of the pressure profile is flatter. In other words, if one could flatten the pressure curve, the driving force ΔP would be less over the effective length Z. Conversely, if the pressure curve is steep (Fig. 7A), then the force driving the dissecting hematoma is increased.

Summary of Pathogenesis (see Fig. 5)

1. Medial degeneration in the wall of the thoracic aorta sets the stage by decreasing the cohesiveness of the layers of the aortic wall.

2. Repeated motion of the aorta related to the beating of the heart results in "flexion stresses" most marked in the ascending and first portion of the descending thoracic aorta.

3. Hydrodynamic forces in the bloodstream related to the pulse wave propagated by each cardiac systole act upon the wall of the aorta, most markedly in the proximal aorta.

4. A combination of the preceding three factors eventually results in an intimal tear, which leads to a hematoma dissecting into the media of the aortic wall for varying depths.

The hydrodynamic forces in the bloodstream, which are predominantly related to the steepness of the pulse wave, extend the dissecting hematoma until rupture occurs either: (1) back into the lumen of the aorta, resulting in a spontaneous cure, a rare but documented occurrence; or more likely, (2) into the pericardium or pleural cavity, leading to death in most instances within 30 days.

CLINICAL MANIFESTATIONS[10]

The patient frequently is a middle-aged black male with known hypertension who suddenly experiences excruciating pain. The pain may be described as knife-like, sharp, and often tearing or ripping in nature and is difficult or impossible to relieve with opiates. The pain most commonly is in the anterior chest or in the back between the shoulder blades. This pain does not radiate into the neck or arms as does angina pectoris.

There are frequently systolic murmurs over the heart and there may be the murmur of aortic valve insufficiency. Murmurs over the major branches of the aorta such as the carotid and subclavian arteries are secondary to partial occlusion of the vessel orifices by the dissecting hematoma (Fig. 8).

There may be a significant difference in blood pressure between the two upper extremities, further indicating the partial compression of one subclavian artery, usually the left, by the dissecting hematoma. Even though the patient may appear to be in shock, his blood pressure will usually be in the hypertensive range or he may even show marked hypertension. Occasional patients presenting in frank shock with a low blood pressure may demonstrate a rapid hypertensive response to the transfusion of only one or two units of blood.

Once the diagnosis is suspected, the patient should be placed in an intensive care unit and carefully monitored. Consultation with cardiologists should be obtained, since the most common problem in diagnosis is differentiation of acute dissecting aneurysm from acute myocardial infarction.

ROENTGENOGRAPHIC FINDINGS

Chest roentgenograms should be taken as soon after admission to the hospital as possible and will usually show widening of the mediastinum. The mediastinum will bulge to the right in dissection of the ascending aorta and show widening on the left in involvement of the descending thoracic aorta. Earlier chest roentgenograms are very helpful for comparison. The typical path of dissection of the aorta is shown in Figure 9.

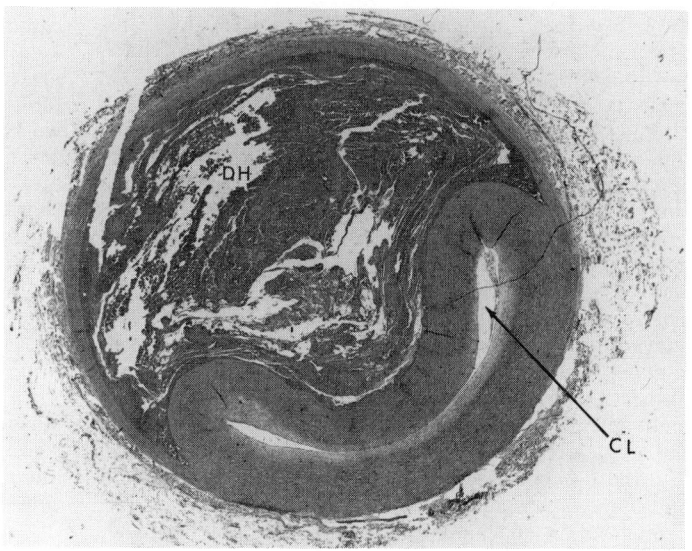

Figure 8. Low-power photomicrograph of cross section of carotid artery almost completely occluded by dissecting hematoma (*DH*). *CL* = compressed lumen.

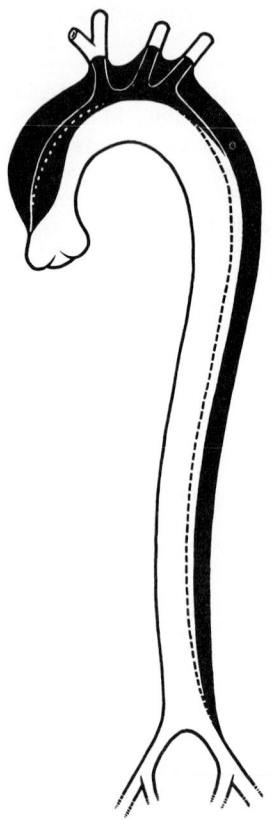

Figure 9. Diagrammatic illustration of the usual path of the dissecting hematoma (shaded area) originating from an intimal tear in the ascending aorta and re-entering in the region of the left common iliac artery.

When the dissection begins in the ascending aorta, it is usually to the right and anterior, beginning just distal to the level of the coronary artery ostia. As the hematoma advances into the arch, it is posterior and superior, and posterior and to the left in the descending thoracic aorta. If the hematoma continues into the abdominal aorta, it is most commonly posterior and to the left, with a higher incidence of dissection into the left renal artery and the left iliofemoral system than on the right side (Fig. 10).

Mediastinal widening is a highly suggestive but nondiagnostic sign of aortic dissection, since neoplastic or inflammatory processes involving the mediastinum can produce similar widening. Calcium in the wall (intima of the aorta) with obvious widening beyond the calcium of at least 4 to 5 mm. is highly suggestive but not diagnostic. The chest roentgenogram also may show a left pleural effusion, which is usually serous. The roentgenographic manifestations of dissecting aneurysm on plain films can be summarized as:[7] (1) a change in configuration of the aorta on successive films; (2) aortic wall thickening shown by displacement of intimal calcification; (3) a localized hump in the aortic arch; (4) disparity in the size of the ascending and descending aorta; and (5) mediastinal, lung, and pleural changes.

Since plain chest roentgenograms are not diagnos-

tic, aortography should be performed to either confirm the diagnosis or rule out a dissecting aneurysm. There is essentially no danger of elevating a plaque and initiating a dissection with proper technique for aortography. The aortogram manifestations of dissecting aneurysms are (Fig. 10): (1) splitting of the contrast column; (2) distortion of the contrast column; (3) alternate flow patterns; and (4) aortic valvar insufficiency.

The definitive diagnosis of dissecting aneurysms demands that the aortogram show some compression of the true aortic lumen by the dissecting hematoma.

SURGICAL TREATMENT

As previously mentioned, the first successful treatment of dissecting aneurysms of the aorta was reported by DeBakey and associates in 1955[5] and used the "fenestration" operation (see Fig. 4). The fenestration operation was an attempt to achieve, by surgical means, re-entry of the dissecting hematoma similar to the spontaneous re-entry known to occur in long-term survivors of aortic dissection. Almost 10 years later DeBakey's group reported the most successful results with surgical treatment of dissecting aneurysms in a group of 179 patients, with an overall survival rate of 79 per cent.[6] A concise classification was presented which has become the one most generally accepted (Fig. 11). This series was heavily weighted by cases of Type III aneurysm (68 per cent) in which the problems are generally less difficult and the operations are predominantly elective in patients with chronic aneurysms. Although no definition of acute was given, the mortality rate was 40 per cent for the acute variety of Type I and 19 per cent for Type III. Fifty per cent of the patients were still alive at the end of 5 years, as contrasted to Hirst's series of patients not treated surgically, of whom only 0.7 per cent were alive at 5 years.[10] DeBakey's results, truly a remarkable accomplishment, established the fact that surgery, particularly for the Type III chronic dissecting aneurysm, can be carried out with a reasonable mortality rate in experienced hands.

Today, the fenestration procedure is rarely indicated. In the ascending aorta the dissecting process is treated by (1) transection of the ascending aorta, obliteration of the false channels, and end-to-end anastomosis; (2) replacement of the ascending aorta with a woven Dacron graft; or (3) if necessary, replacement of the entire aortic root with aortic valve replacement and coronary artery implantation. In the descending thoracic aorta replacement of the aneurysm with a woven Dacron prosthesis using femoro-femoral bypass is usually the procedure of choice.[3, 19, 27, 31]

PHARMACOLOGIC TREATMENT

As a result of the high mortality rate with the surgical approach to the acute dissecting aneurysm,[11, 26] an alternate approach to the treatment of dissecting aneurysms involving intensive drug therapy was initiated in 1963.[30] Drug therapy is based on the following factors in the natural history of acute dissecting

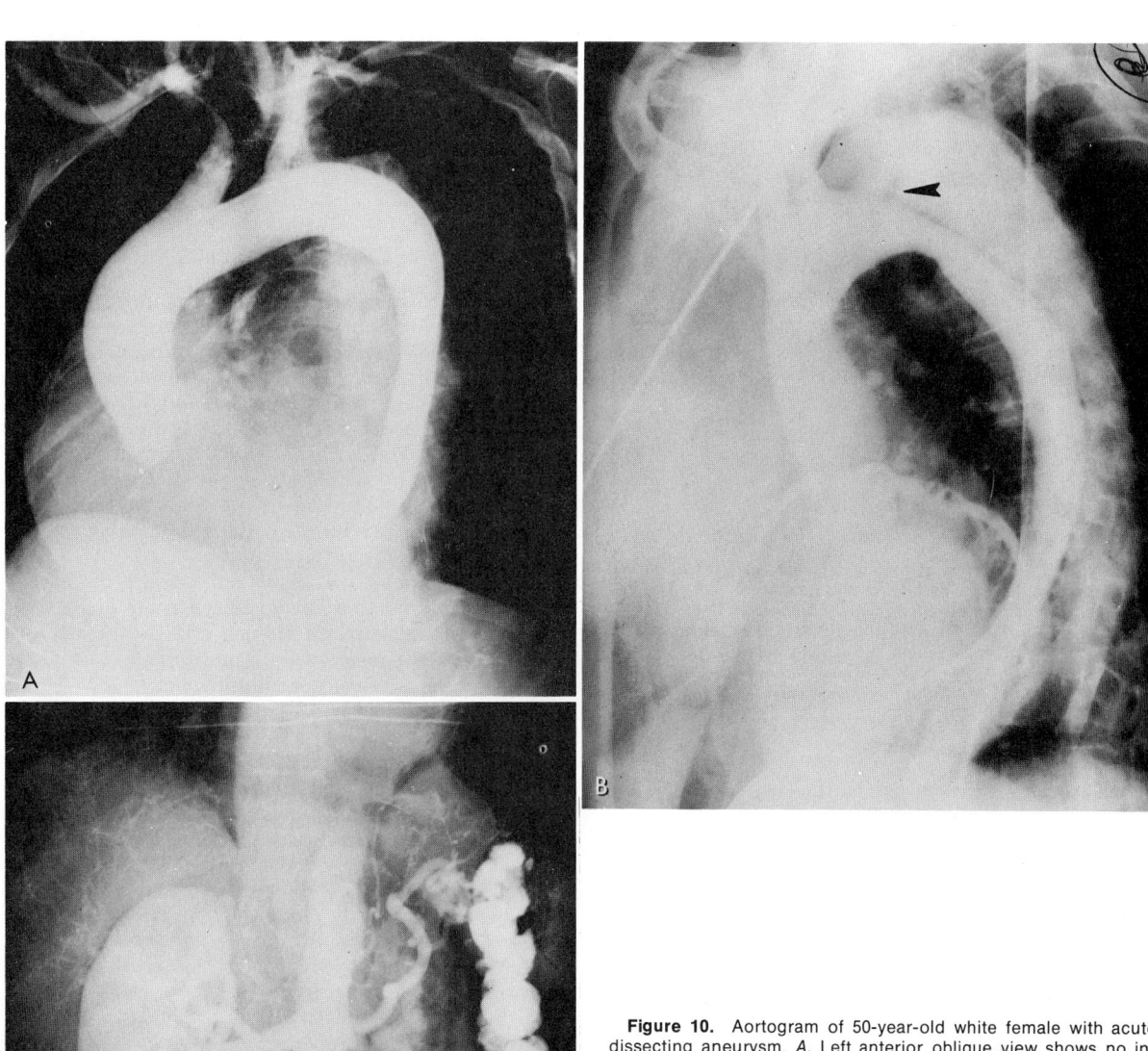

Figure 10. Aortogram of 50-year-old white female with acute dissecting aneurysm. *A,* Left anterior oblique view shows no involvement of ascending aorta or aortic valve. *B* shows site of intimal tear (arrow) with compression of descending thoracic aorta by dissecting hematoma. There is also partial visualization of the right and left coronary arteries. *C* shows continuation of false channel with re-entry into left common iliac artery. There is also compromise of the left renal artery.

aneurysms of the aorta:[10] (1) In untreated dissecting aneurysms, only 3 per cent of the patients die immediately. The mortality for untreated patients then rises rapidly to 21 per cent in 24 hours, 60 per cent in 2 weeks, and 90 per cent in 3 months. (2) The main cause of death is not the initial intimal tear but is related to extension of the dissecting hematoma with ultimate rupture and death due to hemorrhage or car-

diac tamponade or both. (3) It has been documented that acute dissecting aneurysms can occur and resolve through rechannelization or healing and present as incidental autopsy findings many years later.[2] The basic phenomenon in the progression from the intimal tear to death in the acute dissecting aneurysms is extension of the dissecting hematoma. As previously pointed out, there is considerable evidence to support

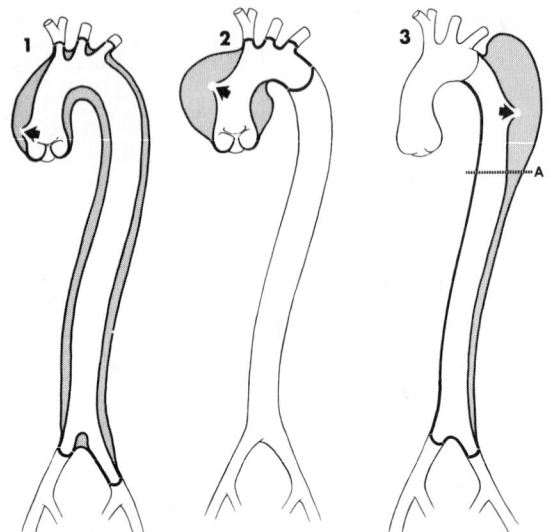

Figure 11. Classification of dissecting aneurysms of the aorta. Type I: Dissection involves ascending aorta and aortic arch and extends distally for varying distances. Type II: Dissection limited to ascending aorta. Type III: Dissection originates at or distal to left subclavian artery, extends distally for varying distances, and does not involve aorta proximal to left subclavian artery. (Modified from DeBakey, M. E., et al.: Ann. Surg., 142:586, 1955.)

period, there were seven deaths in the acute phase, with a survival rate of 86 per cent.[28] Among those patients discharged from the hospital who either died or were followed for at least a year, 84 per cent were alive at 1 year, 70 per cent at 2 years, and 62 per cent at 3 years.

CURRENT RESULTS

Since 1970, five separate groups have reported series of patients with acute dissecting aneurysms of the aorta treated both medically and surgically.[1, 3, 4, 13, 25] As shown in Table 1, prompt surgical intervention provided the best results for patients with aneurysms involving the ascending aorta: there was a mortality rate of 34 per cent with surgery, as compared to a 77 per cent mortality with drugs alone. In the descending aorta the results show a 52 per cent mortality with surgery, as compared to 23 per cent mortality with intensive drug therapy.

As indicated by these reports, dissecting aneurysms of the descending thoracic aorta continue to represent a formidable surgical challenge, and technically are, in my opinion, considerably more difficult to manage than aneurysms of the ascending aorta.

Cooley's group reports a surgical mortality of 30 per cent for aneurysms involving the descending thoracic aorta from 1964 through 1971.[19] Since 1971 in 31 patients the mortality has dropped to 3 per cent, apparently through the use of drugs to aid in the prevention of perioperative extension of the dissecting process.

Webb's group at Syracuse reports on 21 patients treated in the 1971 to 1974 period.[16] They experienced a 75 per cent mortality rate in four patients treated acutely with surgery. Resorting to a combined approach using drugs to stabilize the dissecting process, followed by definitive surgery on an elective basis, their mortality decreased dramatically to 19 per cent.

Shumacker[21] has properly re-emphasized the impor-

the thesis that the progress of the dissecting hematoma to rupture is due to pulsatile forces initiated by the heart. Therefore, drug therapy rests upon the basis of decreasing the pulsatile nature of the blood pressure to a point at which the dissecting aneurysm, instead of progressing, becomes static and heals or at least remains in a stable condition so that it can be approached operatively on an elective basis.

In our report in 1969 of the results of drug therapy involving 50 patients with acute dissecting aneurysms admitted to two different hospitals over a 5-year

TABLE 1. Summary of 185 Patients with Acute Dissecting Aneurysms Treated Medically (92) or Surgically (93)

Author	Year Reported	Ascending Aorta (100 Patients)				Descending Aorta (85 Patients)			
		Medical		Surgical		Medical		Surgical	
		Number	Survivors	Number	Survivors	Number	Survivors	Number	Survivors
Dailey[3]	1970	9	3	14	10	5	4	7	5
Attar[1]	1971	5	0	11	5	8	4	10	4
McFarland[13]	1972	6	2	–	–	10	8	–	–
Dalen[4]	1974	9	2	22	17	6	6	8*	2
Strong[25]	1974	15	3	9	5	19	15	12	7
Total		44	10	56	37	48	37	37	18
Mortality		77%		34%		23%		52%	

*Fourteen patients were initially treated with drugs, but in eight, progress of dissection was not controlled, which is an indication for surgical intervention. These eight patients are shown as surgical, since definitive surgical therapy intervened appropriately.

tance of thorough and technically high-contrast aortograms in delineating the origin and extent of the dissecting process, as well as the details of involvement of the major arterial branches. The details of involvement of major arterial branches arising from the true or false channel, or degree of obstruction, is probably even more crucial in the chronic dissecting aneurysm.

CURRENT STATUS OF SURGERY AND INTENSIVE DRUG THERAPY IN THE MANAGEMENT OF PATIENTS WITH DISSECTING ANEURYSMS OF THE AORTA[27]

Acute Dissecting Aneurysms, Symptoms Less Than 14 Days

Patients suspected of having an acute dissecting aneurysm of the aorta should be placed in an intensive care unit and monitored closely. Other cardiovascular catastrophes such as acute myocardial infarction or cerebral vascular hemorrhage must be ruled out by appropriate studies and consultations. Then:

1. Monitor electrocardiograms and blood pressure continuously, and insert a Foley catheter to follow urinary output.

2. Reduce systolic blood pressure to 100 to 120 mm. Hg (if appropriate). Use trimethaphan (Arfonad), 1 to 2 mg. per milliliter or sodium nitroprusside, 100 μg./ml.,*[15] as an intravenous drip acutely, and if necessary for 24 to 48 hours, with a flow rate to maintain the desired blood pressure (Table 2). Keep the head of the bed elevated 30 to 45 degrees to gain the orthostatic effect of the drugs.

3. Administer reserpine, 1 to 2 mg. intramuscularly every 4 to 6 hours, or propranolol, 1 mg. intramuscularly every 4 to 6 hours. (These drugs may be used in combination.)

4. Give guanethidine, 25 to 50 mg. orally twice a day.

5. Continue to monitor electrocardiogram, blood pressure, pulses, urine output, and stools for blood.

6. Take daily chest roentgenograms to check for

---

*Nitroprusside (Nipride) should be used only in the presence of sympathetic blocking agents such as reserpine, Aldomet, or propranolol to prevent reflex release of norepinephrine.

TABLE 2. Drugs Used in Management of Dissecting Aneurysm of the Aorta

Drug	Mechanism of Action	Total Effect
Reserpine	Depletes all catecholamines from all tissue stores. Neurotransmitter (norepinephrine) release diminished after nerve stimulation.	*Decreases myocardial contractility.* Sedation, depression, bradycardia (reduces cardiac output), reduces peripheral resistance, stimulates gastric secretion.
Sodium nitroprusside (Nipride)	Selectively relaxes vascular smooth muscle.	Rapid lowering of blood pressure, lowers peripheral resistance, reduces cardiac output and contractility indirectly by decreasing preload (venous return).
Trimethaphan (Arfonad)	Ganglionic blockade, direct relaxing effect on vascular smooth muscle. Histamine release.	Rapid lowering of blood pressure, lowers peripheral resistance, reduces cardiac output and contractility indirectly by decreasing preload (venous return). Produces ileus, bladder distension, and pupil dilatation.
Guanethidine (Ismelin)	Selectively depletes catecholamines from postganglionic nerve terminals, particularly in heart, gut, and blood vessels, but not in the central nervous system.	*Decreases myocardial contractility.* Postural hypotension, diarrhea, bradycardia (reduces cardiac output), decreases peripheral resistance, no C.N.S. effect.
Propranolol (Inderal)	Specifically blocks beta-adrenergic stimulation at end organ receptor (blood vessels, heart).	Bradycardia, *decreases myocardial contractility (reduces cardiac output).* Increases peripheral resistance. Mild sedation. Little hypotensive effect.
Alpha-methyldopa (Aldomet)	Metabolized to alpha-methylnorepinephrine, a weak neurotransmitter and pressor agent which replaces the more potent norepinephrine at nerve terminal. Other unknown mechanisms.	Decreases blood pressure. Sedation, little depression, reduces peripheral resistance, slight bradycardia.
Thiazides (Diuril, Hydrodiuril)	Decreased tubular reabsorption of Cl^- and Na^+; some K^+ is lost. Results in salt and/or extracellular fluid volume depletion with possibly, also, a direct cardiovascular effect.	Decrease in blood pressure.

mediastinal widening and the accumulation of pleural fluid.

The management of a typical patient is outlined in chart form in Figure 12. Usually the blood pressure response to trimethaphan or nitroprusside is rapid and can be profound if not carefully regulated. *As a rule when the blood pressure is lowered, the chest and/or back pain are dramatically relieved. The relief of pain is an important clinical guide to the effectiveness of the drug therapy in arresting the progress of the "dissecting hematoma."*

Occasional patients with acute dissection are not hypertensive. The management of these patients is similar, but trimethaphan is not used. Instead, these patients are given either reserpine or propranolol to modify the cardiac impulse.

A dose of at least 60 mg. of propranolol or 0.5 mg. of reserpine per day should be given. Aortograms should be obtained within four hours after admission or as soon as reasonably possible in order to confirm or rule out the diagnosis of acute dissecting aneurysm of the aorta. We believe it is important to visualize the aorta from the aortic valve to the abdominal aortic bifurcation in each patient (Fig. 10) initially. This study then enables the physician to know (1) the site of the intimal tear; (2) the extent of the dissecting hematoma; (3) the degree of involvement of branches of the aorta, particularly the renal arteries; and (4) the presence or absence of acute saccular aneurysms. All of these points are of paramount importance in the management of the patient. If the origin of the dissection – the intimal tear – is not clearly identified, intensive drug therapy should be continued.

If the origin of the dissection is identified, the following considerations come into play (Table 3):

In the type I dissecting aneurysm (Fig. 11) the intimal tear is in the ascending aorta. The key is involvement of the ascending aorta by the dissecting hematoma with the threat of retrograde dissection and fatal pericardial tamponade. Type I dissecting aneurysms, acute as well as chronic, can be corrected surgically (with a mortality rate of 12 to 34 per cent)[1, 3, 4, 13, 25, 27] and the threat of disaster due to retrograde dissection eliminated.

When a patient with confirmed diagnosis of acute type I dissecting aneurysm is a reasonable surgical risk, is 50 years of age or less, and has been stabilized, corrective surgery should be performed as soon as possible. Patients over the age of 50 years, generally poor surgical risks, should be continued on intensive drug therapy unless an urgent indication for surgical intervention develops (Table 3).

Patients with type III acute dissecting aneurysms are primary indications for the use of intensive drug therapy. If the patient's condition stabilizes and pain is relieved (progress of the dissecting hematoma arrested), drug therapy should be continued. After the trimethaphan or nitroprusside has been discontinued, the patient can be transferred to routine floor care and progressively ambulated while regulation of drug dosages for continued long-term care is accomplished.

Subacute and Chronic Aneurysms

Subacute aneurysms, with symptoms for more than 14 days but less than three months, and chronic dis-

TABLE 3. Dissecting Aneurysm – Treatment Indications

Drug Therapy

Initial treatment all dissecting aneurysms.
Type III aneurysm, intimal tear distal to left subclavian artery.
Community hospital lacks facilities for definitive aortography and an experienced cardiovascular surgical team.
Patient who is poor surgical risk (usually more than 50 years old).
Origin in transverse arch of aorta without extension of dissecting hematoma into ascending aorta.
Site of intimal tear not identified on aortogram.
False channel does not opacify.
Stable chronic aneurysm, duration more than 14 days.

Surgical Therapy

Types I and II aneurysms, tear in ascending aorta, or ascending aorta involved by dissecting hematoma; patient reasonable surgical risk, usually less than 50 years old.
Impending rupture of dissecting hematoma.
Progression of dissecting hematoma.
Significant aortic valve insufficiency secondary to dissecting aneurysm.
Acute saccular aneurysm.
Inability to relieve and control patient's pain.
Inability to bring arterial pressure and cardiac impulse under control within four hours.
Blood in pleural space and/or pericardium.
Compromise or occlusion of major branch of aorta.

secting aneurysms, in which the onset of symptoms occurred 3 months before, are somewhat less urgent problems. Usually the pain has subsided and the patient is in a stable condition. The diagnosis in each instance should be confirmed by aortography and the patient given appropriate doses of drugs, such as reserpine, Aldomet, guanethidine, and/or propranolol, to adequately control the cardiac impulse and the blood pressure. Surgical intervention is indicated only if there is progressive aortic valve insufficiency, compromise of a significant branch of the aorta, progressive enlargement of the aneurysm, or development of a localized saccular aneurysm (Table 3).

Follow-Up

The post-hospital management is the same for patients who have sustained an acute dissecting aneurysm and have been treated with drugs alone, or drugs plus surgery, as for those patients seen in the subacute or chronic phase. Patients should be discharged from the hospital with a systolic blood pressure no higher than 130 mm. Hg supine, and a minimal oral dosage of 0.5 mg. reserpine or 60 mg. propranolol per day. These patients should be continued on appropriate drug management for the duration of their lives because redissection is a continuing threat.

Prognosis

Patients sustaining an acute dissecting aneurysm of the thoracic aorta who are treated by drug therapy

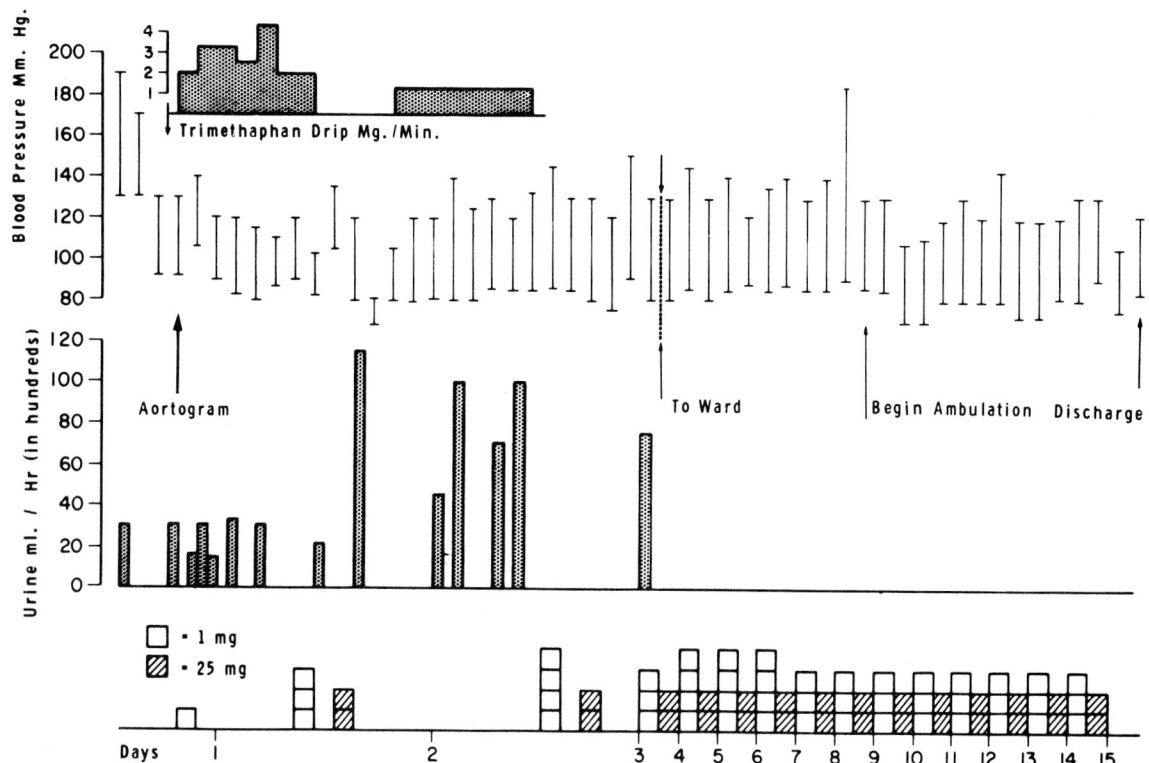

Figure 12. Graphic representation of clinical course of patient with acute dissecting aneurysm of aorta managed with intensive drug therapy. Trimethaphan drip was begun soon after admission (arrow), with prompt blood pressure response. Open squares = 1 mg. reserpine; shaded squares = 25 mg. guanethidine.

alone have an incidence of late saccular aneurysms of about 15 to 20 per cent and progressive aortic valve insufficiency of about 10 per cent.

Those patients in whom the dissecting hematoma does not opacify, who should be treated with drugs alone, do not develop saccular aneurysms and do well in general.

Patients with dissecting aneurysms involving the ascending or decending thoracic aorta who are treated surgically do well, with more than 60 per cent surviving 3 to 5 years or more.

SELECTED REFERENCES

DeBakey, M. E., Henly, W. S., Cooley, D. A., Morris, G. C., Jr., Crawford, E. S., and Beall, A. C., Jr.: Surgical management of dissecting aneurysms of the aorta. J. Thorac. Cardiovasc. Surg., *49*:130, 1969.
This report presents the largest series of dissecting aneurysms treated with surgery and also the best results with surgical therapy in this disease.

Hirst, A. E., Johns, V. J., and Kime, S. W.: Dissecting aneurysms of the aorta. A review of 505 cases. Medicine, *37*:217, 1958.
This is the most exhaustive review of the largest series of dissecting aneurysms in the literature. It should be the starting point as well as the basic source for information regarding any aspect, except therapy, of dissecting aneurysms.

Hume, D. M., and Porter, R.: Acute dissecting aortic aneurysms. Surgery, *53*:122, 1963.
This is an excellent clinical review of dissecting aneurysms, stressing the evaluation and status of treatment and, in particular, results and status of surgical treatment for acute dissecting aneurysms as of 1963.

Shumway, N. E.: Surgical therapy of dissection of the aorta. *In* Anagnostopoulos, C. E. (Ed.): Lethal Diseases of the Ascending Aorta. Baltimore, University Park Press, 1976.
In this study, a more aggressive surgical approach has been employed for acute aortic dissection. Emphasis is placed upon removal of the site of the intimal tear, obliteration of the false lumen, and restoration of aortic continuity by a prosthetic arterial graft. This surgical group believes that immediate surgical intervention is prescribed for all cases of acute aortic dissection, with the possible exception of the posterior descending group in older patients, particularly those with diffuse pulmonary disease.

Wheat, M. W., Jr., and Palmer, R. F.: Dissecting aneurysms of the aorta. Curr. Probl. Surg., July, 1971.
This monograph represents a current general review of the historical background, incidence, pathogenesis, and evaluation and current status of intensive drug therapy and surgical therapy in dissecting aneurysms of the aorta.

REFERENCES

1. Attar, S., Fardin, R., Ayella, R., and McLaughlin, J. S.: Medical vs. surgical treatment of acute dissecting aneurysms. Arch. Surg., *103*:568, 1971.
2. Conston, A. S.: Healed dissecting aneurysms. Arch. Pathol., *48*:309, 1949.
3. Daily, P. O., Trueblood, H. W., Stinson, E. B., Wuerflein, R. D., and Shumway, N. E.: Management of acute aortic dissections. Ann. Thorac. Surg., *10*:237, 1970.

4. Dalen, J. E., Alpert, J. S., Cohn, L. H., Black, H., and Collins, J. J.: Dissection of the thoracic aorta—medical or surgical therapy? Am. J. Cardiol., *34*:803, 1974.

5. DeBakey, M. E., Cooley, D. A., and Creech, O., Jr.: Surgical considerations of dissecting aneurysm of the aorta. Ann. Surg., *142*:586, 1955.

6. DeBakey, M. E., Henly, W. S., Cooley, D. A., Morris, G. C., Jr., Crawford, E. S., and Beall, A. C., Jr.: Surgical management of dissecting aneurysms of the aorta. J. Thorac. Cardiovasc. Surg., *49*:130, 1965.

7. Eyler, W. R., and Clark, M. D.: Dissecting aneurysms of the aorta. Roentgen manifestations including a comparison with other types of aneurysms. Radiology, *85*:1047, 1965.

8. Gurin, D., Bulmer, J. W., and Derby, R.: Dissecting aneurysm of the aorta; diagnosis and operative relief of acute arterial obstruction due to this cause. N.Y. J. Med., *35*:1200, 1935.

9. Hanley, W. B., and Bennett-Jones, N.: Familial dissecting aortic aneurysm, a report of three cases within two generations. Br. Heart J., *29*:852, 1967.

10. Hirst, A. E., Johns, V. J., and Kime, S. W.: Dissecting aneurysms of the aorta. A review of 505 cases. Medicine, *37*:217, 1958.

11. Hume, D. M., and Porter, R.: Acute dissecting aortic aneurysms. Surgery, *53*:122, 1963.

12. Mandel, W., Evans, E. W., and Walsford, R. L.: Dissecting aortic aneurysms during pregnancy. N. Engl. J. Med., *251*:1059, 1954.

13. McFarland, J., Willerson, J. I., Dinsmore, R. E., Austen, W. G., Buckley, M. J., Sanders, C. A., and DeSanctis, R. W.: The medical treatment of dissecting aortic aneurysms. N. Engl. J. Med., *286*:115, 1972.

14. McKusick, V. A.: Cardiovascular aspects of Marfan's syndrome; a heritable disorder of connective tissue. Circulation, *11*:321, 1955.

15. Palmer, R. F., and Lasseter, K. C.: Sodium nitroprusside. N. Engl. J. Med., *292*:294, 1975.

16. Parker, F. B., Jr., Neville, J. F., Jr., Hanson, E. L., Mohiuddin, S., and Webb, W. R.: Management of acute aortic dissection. Ann. Thorac. Surg., *19*:436, 1975.

17. Pate, J. W., Butterick, O. D., and Richardson, R. L.: Traumatic rupture of the thoracic aorta. J.A.M.A., *203*:1022, 1968.

18. Prokop, E. K., Wheat, M. W., Jr., and Palmer, R. F.: Hydrodynamic forces in dissecting aneurysms. Circ. Res., *27*:121, 1970.

19. Reul, G. J., Cooley, D. A., Hallman, G. L., Reddy, S. B., Kyger, E. R., III, and Wukasch, D. C.: Dissecting aneurysms of the descending aorta. Arch. Surg., *110*:632, 1975.

20. Shennan, T.: Dissecting aneurysms. Medical Research Council, Special Report Series 193. London, H. M. Stationery Office, 1934.

21. Shumacker, H. B., Jr., Isch, J. H., and Jolly, W. W.: Stenotic and obstructive lesions in acute dissecting thoracic aortic aneurysms. Ann. Surg., *181*:662, 1975.

22. Simpson, C. F., Kling, J. M., and Palmer, R. F.: The use of propranolol for the protection of turkeys from the development of β-aminoproprionitrile-induced aortic ruptures. Angiology, *19*:414, 1968.

23. Sorensen, H. R., and Olsen, H.: Ruptured and dissecting aneurysms of the aorta. Acta. Chir. Scand., *128*:644, 1964.

24. Strauss, R. G., and McAdams, A. J.: Dissecting aneurysm in childhood. J. Pediatr., *76*:578, 1970.

25. Strong, W. W., Moggio, R. A., and Stansel, H. C., Jr.: Acute aortic dissection—twelve-year medical and surgical experience. J. Thorac. Cardiovasc. Surg., *68*:815, 1974.

26. Warren, W. D., Beckwith, J., and Muller, W. H.: Problems in the surgical management of acute dissecting aneurysm of the aorta. Ann. Surg., *144*:530, 1956.

27. Wheat, M. W., Jr., Boruchow, I. B., and Ramsey, H. W.: Surgical treatment of aneurysms of the aortic root. Ann. Thorac. Surg., *12*:593, 1971.

28. Wheat, M. W., Jr., Harris, P. D., Malm, J. R., Kaiser, G., Bowman, F. O., Jr., and Palmer, R. F.: Acute dissecting aneurysms of the aorta. J. Thorac. Cardiovasc. Surg., *58*:344, 1969.

29. Wheat, M. W., Jr., and Palmer, R. F.: Dissecting aneurysms of the aorta. Curr. Probl. Surg., July, 1971.

30. Wheat, M. W., Jr., Palmer, R. F., Bartley, T. D., and Seelman, R. C.: Treatment of dissecting aneurysms of the aorta without surgery. J. Thorac. Cardiovasc. Surg., *50*:364, 1965.

31. Wheat, M. W., Jr.: Dissecting aneurysms of the aorta. *In* Practice of Surgery, Chapter 4 N, New York, Harper and Row, 1974.

3. TRAUMATIC ANEURYSMS OF THE AORTA

Allan M. Lansing, M.D., Ph.D.

Traumatic aneurysms of the aorta may occur as a result of penetrating or nonpenetrating trauma. Although penetrating injuries of the aorta are dramatic, steadily rising numbers of automobile accidents have increased the significance of nonpenetrating aortic trauma. The incidence of traumatic rupture of the aorta at autopsy used to be placed at 1 per cent, but more recent estimates suggest that between 10 and 15 per cent of all automobile fatalities are associated with rupture of the aorta.[11, 28]

PATHOLOGY

When blunt trauma is involved, the site of aortic injury is usually the isthmus of the thoracic aorta, that is, the region of the ligamentum arteriosum just beyond the left subclavian artery.[4, 16, 22, 28] The second most common site is just above the aortic valve, and occasionally the origin of the innominate, left carotid, or subclavian artery is involved. The much rarer injury of the abdominal aorta is briefly discussed at the end of this chapter. The pathogenesis of thoracic aortic injury was first detailed by Rindfleisch in 1893, who surmised that the aortic arch was fixed by the attachment of the great vessels, whereas the heart and the descending thoracic aorta were more mobile.[24] Thus, sudden deceleration of the body at the time of impact with differential rates of deceleration of the fixed portions of the thoracic aorta and the great vessels causes a tear involving either the intima, the intima and media, or the entire wall.[4] This tear is usually transverse, but may be ragged, stellate, or spiral. The average age of the patient is 27 years, and therefore atherosclerosis is seldom a factor in the aortic injury. Since the adventitia provides 60 per cent of the tensile strength of the thoracic aorta, survival of the patient until he is admitted to hospital usually depends upon continuity of this tissue.

Other types of injuries are much less common. Crushing injury of the thoracic aorta is extremely rare. Traumatic dissection of the thoracic aorta may also occur.[20] Multiple sites of injury of the aorta have been reported, and other associated injuries, particularly cardiac, are very common and constitute an important factor in determining the survival rate. In fact, in one large series, cardiac injuries were found in 70 per cent of the patients with traumatic injuries of the thoracic aorta.[22]

PROGNOSIS

The outcome of these injuries has been well documented in an excellent review of 275 patients by Parmley et al.[22] Surprisingly, there is no correlation between the survival rate and the extent of the disruption of the aorta, that is, partial versus complete transection. Fourteen per cent of all patients survived the initial injury and arrived in the hospital: isolated rupture of the aorta was associated with a 20 per cent initial survival rate, whereas the combination of aortic and cardiac injury resulted in only a 4 per cent initial survival rate. Thus, 80 to 90 per cent of the patients die immediately of exsanguination, while in 10 to 20 per cent, the leak is temporarily controlled by the adventitia of the aorta or the pleura.

In the patients who survive the immediate injury, delayed rupture of the aorta with massive hemorrhage is the commonest event. In Parmley's series, 66 per cent of those who survive the initial injury die within two weeks of aortic rupture, 82 per cent within three weeks, and 90 per cent within 10 weeks. In the seven patients out of 275 in this series who were still alive at the end of 10 weeks, five died of rupture within a few months and two survived operative repair. According to other reports, a few patients develop the clinical symptoms of pseudocoarctation when a flap of intima develops distal to the injury and produces partial stenosis of the aorta, with resulting hypertension in the arms and diminished blood flow to the lower part of the body.[16, 17, 19] Finally, a few patients live to develop a traumatic aneurysm, an outcome that is extremely rare, since Bennett and Cherry found only 105 cases reported up to 1967.[3] It is estimated that only 2 per cent of the immediate survivors of traumatic aortic rupture live long enough to develop an aneurysm. Even then, these lesions are rarely stable, only about 20 per cent remaining asymptomatic over five years, and nearly all developing symptoms or evidence of expansion at some time.[3] Since there is no way to predict when signs of compression of the neighboring structures, bacterial infection, rupture, or embolism will occur, repair is recommended even when the patient is asymptomatic.

DIAGNOSIS

The lethal nature of traumatic rupture of the thoracic aorta makes urgent diagnosis extremely important. Since at best only 20 per cent of the victims reach the hospital alive and over 80 per cent of these die of aortic rupture within three weeks, the clinician must be constantly aware of the possibility of this injury. The first clue is the *history of a sudden deceleration injury,* which should immediately arouse suspicion. The most important radiologic findings are *widening of the upper mediastinum* and loss of the *sharpness of the contour of the aortic knob* (Fig. 13).[9] The occurrence of both of these radiologic findings demands immediate investigation, since rupture is said to be present in 90 per cent of patients with this combination. It must be admitted that a widened mediastinum does not always indicate rupture, nor will every case of rupture present with a widened mediastinum. Further, allowance must be made for the fact that an anteroposterior supine chest film will frequently give the appearance of a widened upper mediastinum, and hence a posteroanterior chest x-ray should be performed if at all possible. The presence of

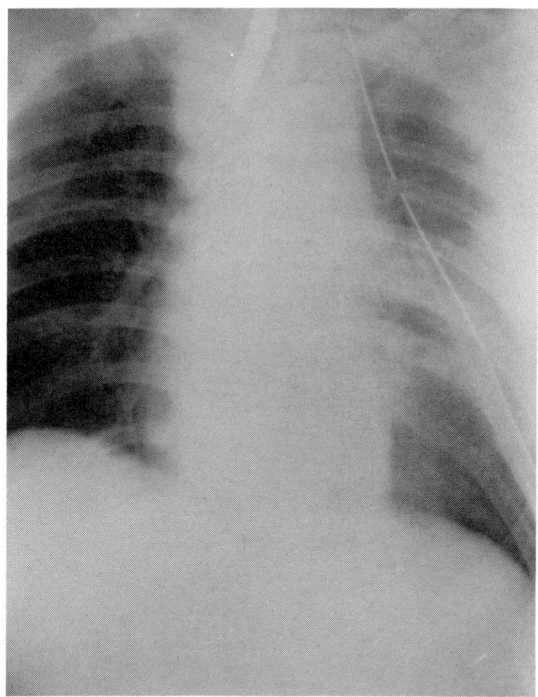

Figure 13. Chest x-ray in traumatic rupture of the aorta. Note the widened mediastinum and loss of sharpness of the aortic arch.

a left pleural effusion may also support the diagnosis, but rib fractures, pneumothorax, contusion of the lung, and other injuries do not help. Despite these limitations, if a deceleration injury has occurred, and if the mediastinum is widened with loss of contour of the aorta, the next step is an aortogram as soon as the patient's general condition and other injuries permit (Fig. 14). A high index of suspicion will lead to more frequent aortograms and a lower incidence of positive findings, but the very high mortality when the condition is missed makes this a justifiable emergency diagnostic procedure. In fact, some authorities recommend an arteriogram in all patients with sternal injuries, first rib injuries, and fractures of the clavicle that are displaced posteriorly.[7] Aortography is preferable to exploratory thoracotomy, since not only will a negative exploration in a patient who is otherwise seriously ill add significantly to his risk, but tears of the intima or media may be missed unless visualized by routine opening of the thoracic aorta.[16, 27]

In those rare patients in whom the diagnosis is missed and who survive to develop a thoracic aneurysm, the lesion is usually discovered later by an incidental chest x-ray, by the development of symptoms of compression of other neighboring structures, or by the occurrence of pain and shock when the lesion ruptures spontaneously (Fig. 15). In a few patients, the mediastinal mass appears within 24 hours of injury and is accompanied by hemothorax, increasing chest pain, and symptoms of dysphagia, tracheal or bronchial obstruction, hoarseness, and hemoptysis.

It is evident that the most important factor in successful treatment is immediate and accurate diag-

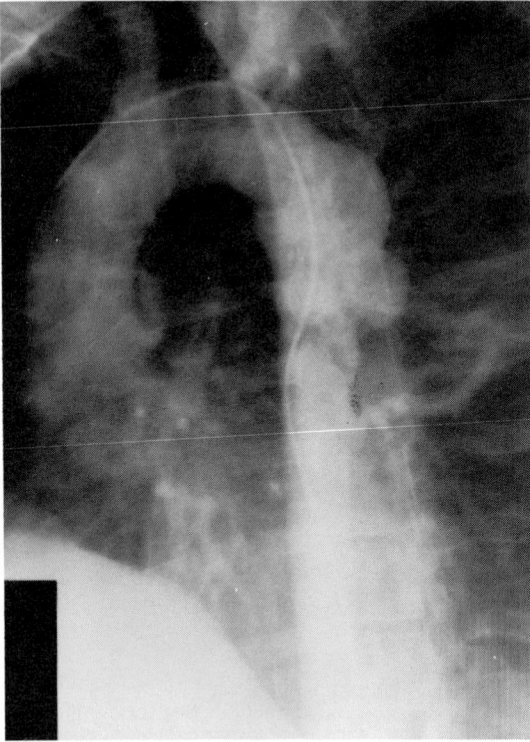

Figure 14. Aortogram in traumatic rupture of the aorta.

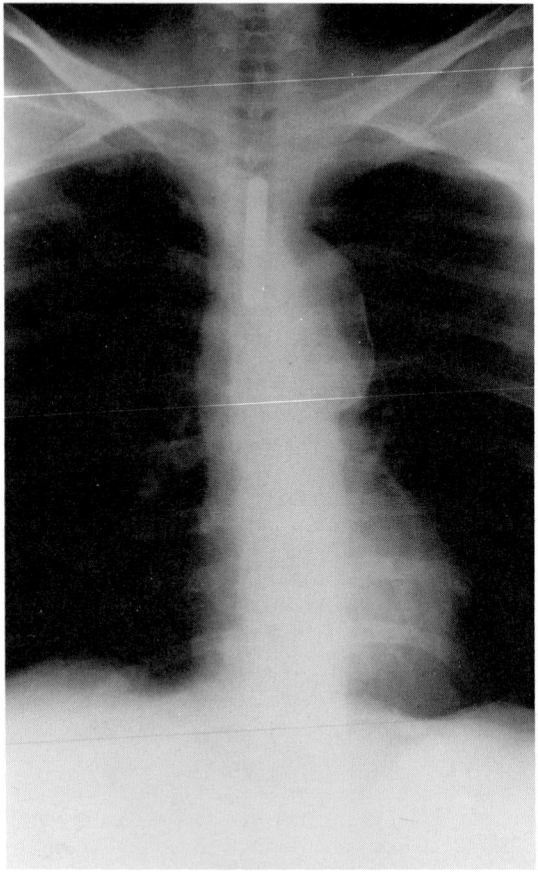

Figure 15. Chronic aneurysm following aortic trauma. Note the calcification of the wall.

nosis. In the 10 to 20 per cent of the patients who reach the hospital alive, the injury must be recognized, treated as an emergency, and urgent operative intervention undertaken. On the other hand, the rare chronic aneurysms may remain stable for many years, but should be viewed with grave suspicion and they too should be resected unless other factors contraindicate operation.

TREATMENT

Once the diagnosis is established, preparations for operation are made immediately. Resuscitation and supportive measures are instituted during this period, and other critical injuries may have to be treated first or simultaneously. If either the patient's general condition or the hospital facility is unsuitable for immediate repair, pharmacologic treatment to lower the blood pressure and reduce the pulsatile force of ventricular systole may be instituted to delay rupture of the aorta.[2] This is the same regimen that is applied in the nonoperative treatment of dissecting aneurysm, and includes the use of trimethaphan, reserpine, and guanethidine.

Since the operative treatment of these injuries will require cross-clamping of the thoracic aorta, the blood supply of the kidneys and spinal cord should be maintained during this period and back pressure on the brain and heart minimized. However, Crawford and Rubio[6] have recorded good results without any form of bypass. The first protective measure to be employed

was hypothermia, but this has been supplanted by some form of left heart bypass, as first proposed by Gerbode.[10] In this technique, a cannula is inserted into the left atrium to drain blood from the heart, and this blood is then pumped back into the femoral artery (Fig. 16). This provides perfusion of the lower part of the body during aortic cross-clamping but has the disadvantages of requiring the use of heparin, which can result in postoperative bleeding, of occasionally causing sudden rises of left atrial pressure and pulmonary edema, and of requiring a pump and the personnel to run it. An alternative procedure, femoral vein to femoral artery bypass with a pump oxygenator, avoids the risk of pulmonary congestion and disturbance of left atrial function, but still requires the use of heparin, a heart-lung machine, and technicians. These two methods are the most commonly employed today, but in complicated cases of aneurysm involving the aortic arch, total cardiopulmonary bypass and deep hypothermia followed by a period of complete circulatory arrest have been recommended so that dissection is minimized and the aortic defect can be repaired from inside the lumen of the vessel.[8]

Another technique that is available for use in all hospitals and does not require a pump or the use of heparin has been popularized by Kirsh et al.[18] and

Connors et al.[5] This consists of a temporary external shunt from the ascending aorta proximal to the lesion to the lower thoracic aorta or femoral artery beyond the lesion. The problems of bleeding from the operative area, extensive equipment, specialized personnel, and the need to use the less desirable woven grafts are thus eliminated.

After the method of bypass has been selected, the operative technique is fairly well standardized. The aortic arch is dissected within the pericardium to gain proximal control without entering the hematoma or touching the aneurysm. The aorta is encircled between the left carotid and left subclavian vessels and again distal to the lesion in its descending portion. Bypass is then established, the aorta cross-clamped, and the aneurysm or area of rupture approached directly.

In the acute cases, the tissues are usually very friable and, although direct suture repair can occasionally be accomplished, most often the lesion must be treated by resection of the damaged area and insertion of a synthetic graft.[14, 27] If the type of bypass employed requires the use of heparin, a woven graft must be used to prevent massive blood loss through the prosthesis after the clamps are removed from the aorta; otherwise, a knitted graft that will be better incorporated by the body tissues is preferable.

In the case of the chronic aneurysm, the patient's general condition is assessed to determine his life expectancy and complicating factors that might contraindicate surgical treatment. In general, however, these lesions nearly always enlarge or produce symptoms, although it may take many years for them to do so. At the time of operation, bypass using a pump or an external shunt is established, the aorta is occluded in the arch and descending portion, and the aneurysm opened (Fig. 16). Often direct suture repair can be achieved by trimming the neck of the aneurysm and approximating the aorta by sutures after the distal portion has been mobilized.[1, 15] If wide separation of the ends of the aorta prevents this, a synthetic graft is employed to restore continuity. Dissection of the tissues outside the aneurysm is kept at a minimum to decrease the chance of injury to vital structures and to lessen the degree of bleeding from the structures after the repair has been accomplished.

ABDOMINAL AORTIC INJURY

Rare cases of blunt injury of the abdominal aorta have been reported, usually associated with a longitudinal tear of the aortic wall caused by a compression injury.[22, 28] Only about 5 per cent of the traumatic injuries of the aorta involve its abdominal portion, and aneurysms are very rarely seen. Two cases of abdominal aneurysms resulting from blunt trauma and one caused by a penetrating injury have been reported.[12, 23, 25] In only one case has peripheral embolism occurred from a traumatic aneurysm of the abdominal aorta.[25] Traumatic dissection of the abdominal aorta has been reported in two cases, with

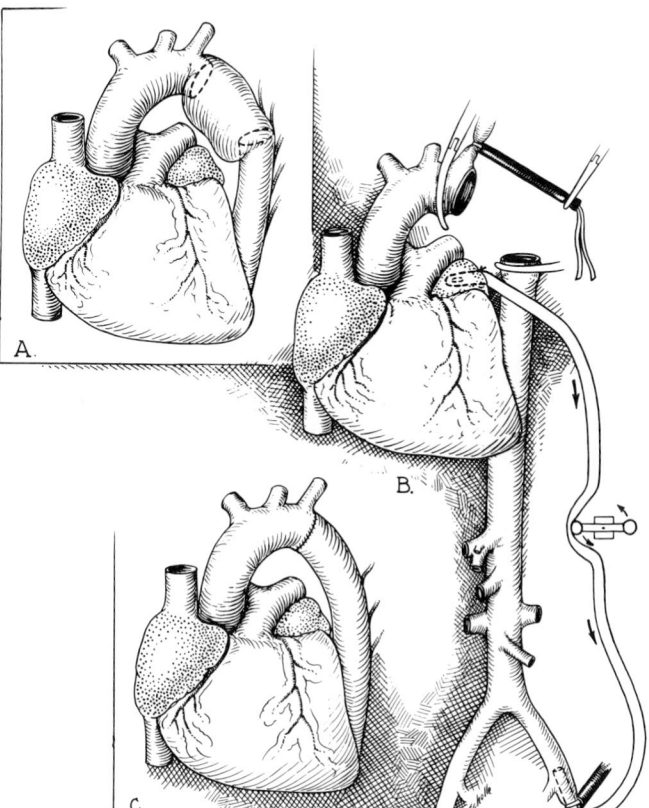

Figure 16. Technique of resection of aneurysm following aortic rupture. (From Alley, R. D., et al.: Ann. Thorac. Surg., 2:514, 1966.)

a resulting tear in the intima, formation of a flap, and occlusion and thrombosis of the terminal aorta.[13, 20]

Nonpenetrating injuries of the abdominal aorta are extremely rare, and their management is straightforward. If acute thrombosis of the aorta occurs, it must be operated upon immediately. Traumatic aneurysms of the abdominal aorta are treated by standard surgical approaches once they have been recognized. Penetrating injuries of the aorta require immediate operation even if the injury appears to have sealed off. Delay will almost universally result in a secondary fatal hemorrhage or rupture of a false aneurysm.[21]

SUMMARY

Traumatic injuries of the aorta, particularly those associated with sudden deceleration, are occurring with increasing frequency. Only 10 to 20 per cent of the patients survive to reach the hospital, and fatal secondary rupture of the aorta occurs in the majority of these within three weeks. Immediate diagnosis must be established on the basis of a history of a decelerating injury, the presence of a widened mediastinum and loss of sharpness of the aortic knob on the posteroanterior chest x-ray, and emergency aortography. Urgent operation is performed using some form of left heart bypass or an external shunt, and the lesion is usually repaired by a graft. Chronic aneurysms are rare, since most patients fail to survive this long, but when they develop, they may remain stable for several years. However, if the patient's condition permits, this lesion too should be excised and repaired by either direct suture or graft.

SELECTED REFERENCES

Bennett, D. E., and Cherry, J. K.: The natural history of traumatic aneurysms of the aorta. Surgery, 61:516, 1967.
This is an important review of the natural history of traumatic aneurysms of the aorta. The incidence of the lesion, the site, the time of death, and the prognosis in the chronic aneurysms are discussed, with excellent references to the world literature.

Connors, J. P., Ferguson, T. B., Roper, C. L., and Weldon, C. S.: The use of the TDMAC-heparin shunt in replacement of the descending aorta. Ann. Surg., 181:735, 1975.
A heparin-coated external shunt is recommended for temporary bypass to protect the spinal cord and abdominal viscera. There were two deaths in 22 elective cases, but two other patients with acute aneurysms died.

Freed, T. A., Neal, M. P., Jr., and Vinik, M.: Roentgenographic findings in extracardiac injury secondary to blunt chest automobile trauma. Am. J. Roentgenol., 104:424, 1968.
The radiologic diagnosis of traumatic injury of the aorta is well described. Emphasis is placed upon the findings in routine chest x-rays and the role of arteriography in the diagnosis.

Parmley, L. F., Mattingly, T. W., Manion, W. C., and Johnke, E. J., Jr.: Nonpenetrating traumatic injury of the aorta. Circulation, 17:1086, 1958.
This is the most complete and authoritative reference to the pathology, clinical aspects, and management of nonpenetrating injuries of the aorta. It must be read by any student of this problem.

Spencer, F. C., Guerin, P. F., Blake, H. A., and Bahnson, H. T.: A report of fifteen patients with traumatic rupture of the thoracic aorta. J. Thorac. Cardiovasc. Surg., 41:1, 1961.
This is an excellent report of an early series of 15 cases, seven acute and eight chronic. A fine review of the literature combined with a discussion of the problems makes this worthwhile reading.

REFERENCES

1. Alley, R. D., Van Mierop, L. H. S., Li, E. Y., Jagdish, K. R., Kausel, H. W., and Stranahan, A.: Traumatic aortic aneurysm. Four cases of graftless excision and anastomosis. Ann. Thorac. Surg., 2:514, 1966.
2. Aronstam, E. M., Gomez, A. C., O'Connell, T. J., Jr., and Geiger, J. P.: Recent surgical and pharmacologic experiences with acute dissection and traumatic aneurysms. J. Thorac. Cardiovasc. Surg., 59:231, 1970.
3. Bennett, D. E., and Cherry, J. K.: The natural history of traumatic aneurysms of the aorta. Surgery, 61:516, 1967.
4. Cammack, K., Rapport, R. L., Paul, J., and Baird, W. C.: Deceleration injuries of the thoracic aorta. Arch. Surg., 79:244, 1959.
5. Connors, J. P., Ferguson, T. B., Roper, C. L., and Weldon, C. S.: The use of the TDMAC-heparin shunt in replacement of the descending aorta. Ann. Surg., 181:735, 1975.
6. Crawford, E. S., and Rubio, P. A.: Reappraisal of adjuncts to avoid ischemia in the treatment of aneurysms of descending thoracic aorta. J. Thorac. Cardiovasc. Surg., 66:693, 1973.
7. DeMeules, J. E., Cramer, G., and Perry, J. F., Jr.: Rupture of aorta and great vessels due to blunt thoracic trauma. J. Thorac. Cardiovasc. Surg., 61:440, 1971.
8. Dumanian, A. V., Horksem, T. D., Santschi, D. R., Greenwald, J. H., and Frahm, C. J.: Profound hypothermia and circulatory arrest in the surgical treatment of traumatic aneurysm of the thoracic aorta. J. Thorac. Cardiovasc. Surg., 59:541, 1970.
9. Freed, T. A., Neal, M. P., Jr., and Vinik, M.: Roentgenographic findings in extracardiac injury secondary to blunt chest automobile trauma. Am. J. Roentgenol., 104:424, 1968.
10. Gerbode, F., Braimbudge, M., Osborn, J., Hood, M., and French, S.: Traumatic thoracic aneurysms: Treatment by resection and grafting with the use of an extracorporeal bypass. Surgery, 42:6, 1957.
11. Greendyke, R. M.: Traumatic rupture of aorta. J.A.M.A., 195:119, 1966.
12. Griffen, W. O., Jr., Belin, R. P., and Walder, A. I.: Traumatic aneurysm of the abdominal aorta. Surgery, 60:813, 1966.
13. Hewitt, R. L., and Grablowsky, O. M.: Acute traumatic dissecting aneurysm of the abdominal aorta. Ann. Surg., 171:160, 1970.
14. Jahnke, E. J., Jr., Fisher, G. W., and Jones, R. G.: Acute traumatic rupture of the thoracic aorta. A report of six consecutive cases of successful early repair. J. Thorac. Cardiovasc. Surg., 48:63, 1964.
15. Kahn, A. M., Joseph, W. L., and Hughes, R. K.: Traumatic aneurysms of the thoracic aorta. Excision and repair without graft. Ann. Thorac. Surg., 4:175, 1967.
16. Kaufman, J., and Storey, C. F.: Acute traumatic aneurysms of the thoracic aorta: Resection and graft replacement during cardiac massage. Am. Surg., 34:780, 1968.
17. Kinley, C. E., and Chandler, B. M.: Traumatic aneurysm of thoracic aorta: A case presenting as a coarctation. Canad. Med. Assoc. J., 96:279, 1967.
18. Kirsh, M. M., Kahn, D. R., Crane, J. D., Anastasia, L. F., Lui, A. H., Moores, W. Y., Vathayanon, S., Bookstein, J. J., and Sloan, H.: Repair of acute traumatic rupture of the aorta without extracorporeal circulation. Ann. Thorac. Surg., 10:227, 1970.
19. Malm, J. R., and Deterling, R. A., Jr.: Traumatic aneurysm of thoracic aorta. J. Thorac. Cardiovasc. Surg., 40:2, 1960.
20. Ngu, V. A., and Konstam, P. G.: Traumatic dissecting aneurysm of the abdominal aorta. Br. J. Surg., 52:981, 1965.
21. Parmley, L. F., Mattingly, T., and Manion, W. C.: Penetrating wounds of the heart and aorta. Circulation, 17:953, 1958.
22. Parmley, L. F., Mattingly, T. W., Manion, W. C., and Johnke, E. J.: Nonpenetrating traumatic injury of the aorta. Circulation, 17:1086, 1958.
23. Ricen, E., and Dickens, J., Jr.: Traumatic aneurysm of the abdominal aorta of 27 years' duration. U. S. Naval Med. Bull., 40:692, 1942.
24. Rindfleisch, E.: Zur Entshung und Heilung des Aneurysma dissecans aortae. Arch. Pathol. Anat., 13:374, 1893.
25. Smith, R., III, Perdue, G. D., Jr., Walter, L. G., Jr., and Israle, P. Z.: Post-traumatic aneurysms of the abdominal aorta with recurrent emboli to the superior mesenteric artery: A case report. Surgery, 64:736, 1968.
26. Spencer, F. C., Guerin, P. F., Blake, H. A., and Bahnson, H. T.: A report of fifteen patients with traumatic rupture of the thoracic aorta. J. Thorac. Cardiovasc. Surg., 41:1, 1961.
27. Stoney, R. J., Roe, B. B., and Redington, J.: Rupture of the

thoracic aorta due to closed-chest trauma. Arch. Surg., 89:840, 1964.

28. Strassmann, G.: Traumatic rupture of the aorta. Am. Heart J., 33:508, 1947.

4. ANEURYSMS OF THE THORACIC AORTA

Watts R. Webb, M.D., and Frederick B. Parker, Jr., M.D.

Aneurysms of the ascending, transverse, and descending thoracic aorta may be arteriosclerotic, syphilitic, degenerative (due to cystic medial necrosis), mycotic, or congenital. Arteriosclerosis is the most common cause of thoracic aneurysms, although these are still more common in the infrarenal abdominal aorta where the vasa vasorum are much less frequent.[3] Obstruction of the vasa vasorum in the tunica media leads to necrosis and aortic dilatation. Syphilitic aortitis, formerly common but now unusual owing to antisyphilitic drugs, destroys principally the medial layer (aortica elastica) of the thoracic aorta, resulting in aneurysmal dilatation of the vessel.

In 1929, Erdheim[9] described cystic medial necrosis, which is particularly prominent in patients with Marfan's syndrome. This syndrome includes other lesions such as skeletal defects, dislocation of the lens, arachnodactyly, a high and sometimes cleft palate, and sternal deformities. It may be present in a forme frust pattern with minimal stigmata. Edwards suggests that cystic medial necrosis may be a manifestation of aging. He found the postmortem incidence of cystic medial necrosis to be about 10 per cent in the first two decades of life but rose to over 60 per cent in the seventh and eighth decades in a more or less linear pattern. It is most prominent in the ascending aorta. Cystic medial necrosis allows weakening of the wall and aneurysmal dilatation, which may eventually rupture. Aortic insufficiency may result from the dilatation of the annulus, which renders the valve leaflets incapable of coapting centrally. Acute dissection of the aorta is also a significant risk in this entity. Mycotic aneurysms in this area are extremely unusual and generally represent infection of a pre-existing aneurysm. Congenital aneurysms of the thoracic aorta are generally present in the intercostal vessels in the region of a coarctation.

The pathogenesis of an aneurysm is damage to the medial elastic coat of the vessel with only the outer fibrous tissues remaining to withstand the repeated force of systolic impact. If weakening of the wall is limited in area, dilatation is localized, producing a saccular aneurysm. More diffuse weakening produces a fusiform or globular aneurysm. In addition, laminae of thrombi are deposited on the inner surfaces of the aneurysm, frequently retarding the growth of the lesion. However, these laminae are rarely organized and subsequent liquefaction necrosis often leads to further weakness, with sudden enlargement or even rupture.

Symptoms

Aneurysms of the thoracic aorta usually produce symptoms because of compression or obstruction of adjacent structures. Pain due to compression of adjacent sensory nerves is often present. The aneurysm may erode through ribs and sternum or may obstruct the innominate vein or superior vena cava, producing venous distention and edema of the neck and shoulders. Tracheal or bronchial obstruction often causes dyspnea and cough, and death by suffocation is not uncommon. Blood-streaked sputum is an ominous sign of rupture of the aneurysm into the trachea or bronchus, and death by rupture into the tracheobronchial tree, esophagus, or pleura is a common terminal event in untreated patients.

Diagnosis

In some patients, the diagnosis can be made from the history of respiratory obstruction, possibly with cough, tracheal tug, or thoracic pulsation. In most instances, the diagnosis is based on radiologic discovery of a mass contiguous with some part of the aortic shadow. Differentiation from solid mediastinal tumors may be difficult. Pulsation, for example, is misleading, as a solid tumor adjacent to the normal pulsating aorta may give the fluoroscopic appearance of expansible pulsation. Contrast visualization by direct aortography is most important and is mandatory if surgery is contemplated.

Prognosis

Prognosis of patients with thoracic aneurysms is very grave, as the average survival time is less than one year after onset of symptoms. Patients with thoracic aneurysms due to syphilis have a particularly poor prognosis. In Kampmeier's study of 188 syphilitic patients, only 18 lived longer than two years after the onset of symptoms.[10] From a total analysis of 633 patients with saccular aneurysms of the thoracic aorta, Kampmeier found that the average duration of life from the onset of symptoms was 6 to 8 months, varying somewhat with the level of involvement. Lesions of the ascending aorta and transverse arch have the poorest prognosis because of the proximity to other vital structures such as the heart, superior vena cava, and tracheobronchial tree.

Management

Excision of the aneurysm is the only effective method of surgical therapy. In previous years, injection of long lengths of fine thrombogenic wire into the aneurysm,[5] periadventitial injection of fibrogenic materials,[4] and wrapping the aneurysm with fibrogenic or reinforcing materials have all been tried without providing significant benefit. Excisional therapy of an aneurysm of the thoracic aorta was first suggested and tried unsuccessfully by Tuffier in 1902.[13] Successful and general application had to wait, however, another 50 years.[2, 7] The method of excision depends upon whether the aneurysm is fusiform or saccular. When it is saccular, tangenital excision of the aneurysm with direct closure or patch repair is adequate, but if the aneurysm is fusiform, excision and replacement are necessary.

Saccular Aneurysms

In saccular aneurysms, even when the sac is extensive, aortorrhaphy may be applied effectively so long as the neck is narrow and involves less than half the circumference of the aorta. Syphilitic aneurysms are tough and leathery and easily closed by direct suture. Others may have more friable tissue and require buttressing with synthetic felt such as Dacron or Teflon.[12] The ascending aortic lesions are easily exposed by sternal-splitting midline incisions with extension into the neck along the sternocleidomastoid muscle if necessary. Aneurysms in the distal aortic arch or thoracic aorta can be better handled by a posterolateral thoracotomy, the interspace depending on the level of the lesion.

Fusiform Aneurysms

Ascending Aorta. The technical problems in excision of fusiform aneurysms are more difficult because the entire segment of aorta must be removed and a graft inserted to bridge the defect. In the ascending aorta, this requires total bypass and some provision for myocardial protection with either local hypothermia or coronary perfusion. Since this requires full heparinization of the patient, the grafts used must be of minimal porosity (such as woven grafts) and likewise should be preclotted.

In certain patients, aortic valve insufficiency may be produced by dilatation of the aortic annulus. If the leaflets are normal, utilization of a relatively small graft with narrowing ("reefing") of the proximal annulus will allow reapproximation of the aortic leaflets and restore aortic valvular competence (Fig. 17). In other situations, aortic valve replacement may be required to correct the insufficiency. If the fusiform aneurysm extends below the coronary arteries, these arteries may have to be implanted into the graft.

Transverse Arch. Aneurysms in the arch are much more difficult to manage and carry an operative risk between 25 and 50 per cent. The major added difficulty revolves around maintenance of cerebral perfusion during the lengthy multiple anastomoses required for full arch replacement. Cerebral perfusion can be achieved by additional cannulas introduced

into the right axillary and left common carotid arteries, with flow at the rate of approximately 250 ml. per min. into each artery. Under these conditions, the brain will be safely perfused without neurologic sequelae. An additional method has been utilization of profound hypothermia at temperatures below 15°C. during the period of distal graft anastomosis and suturing to the graft a cuff of the transverse arch,[6] which includes the three major vessels (innominate, left carotid, and subclavian arteries). Utilization of this cuff reduces the number of anastomoses for the arch vessels down to one, plus the anastomoses of the graft to the transsected ascending and descending aorta (Fig. 18).

Descending Thoracic Aorta. Aneurysms of the descending thoracic aorta are similarly replaced with grafts. Perfusion of the distal aorta can be achieved by left atriofemoral artery bypass,[8] or inferior vena caval (femoral vein)–femoral artery bypass with an oxygenator, or with preheparinized shunts[11] so that general body heparinization is not required. It appears better to maintain a flow rate of 1200 to 2500 ml. per min. into the distal aortic bed with a mean renal pressure of at least 32 mm. Hg, since demonstrable renal function disappears below this level.[8]

In the thoracic aorta, the limit of safe occlusion time is determined not by damage to the heart but rather by tolerable limits of ischemia to the abdominal viscera and the spinal cord, which receive important tributaries from the lower thoracic intercostal arteries. The most important apparently is the arteria magna, which arises from a segment between the eighth thoracic and fourth lumbar vertebrae (most commonly T9 or T10). Division of this vessel may well produce paraplegia.[1] To date, no clinical method has been found for identification of this important artery. Hence, if an aneurysm in this region must be excised, one should ligate only the intercostal arteries that must be removed with the aneurysm. It may be that other factors likewise play an important role, since Crawford found no increase in paraplegia by cross-clamping the aorta without a shunt, although the occlusion time was relatively short. It appeared that reducing the aortic occlusion time, removal of minimal

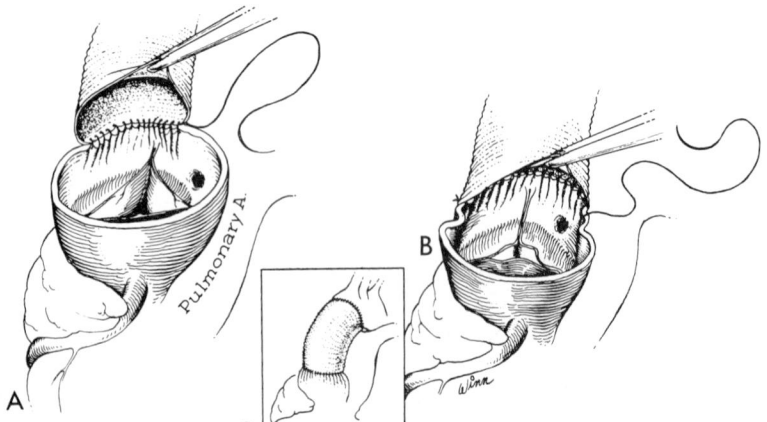

Figure 17. Diagram of surgical repair after excision of globular aneurysm of ascending aorta. *A,* Stretching of the aortic root lengthens the arc of the aortic leaflets and flattens their concave margins, which ordinarily form a semicircle. *B,* The smaller size graft is sutured to the proximal aorta with concentric reefing of the aorta. This reconstitutes the normal arc of the leaflets, allowing their coarctation and full competency. *C,* Completed repair. (From Webb, W. R., Ecker, R. R., Holland, R. H., and Sugg, W. L.: Aortic aneurysm with aortic insufficiency: Repair without prosthesis. Am. J. Cardiol., *26:*416, 1970.)

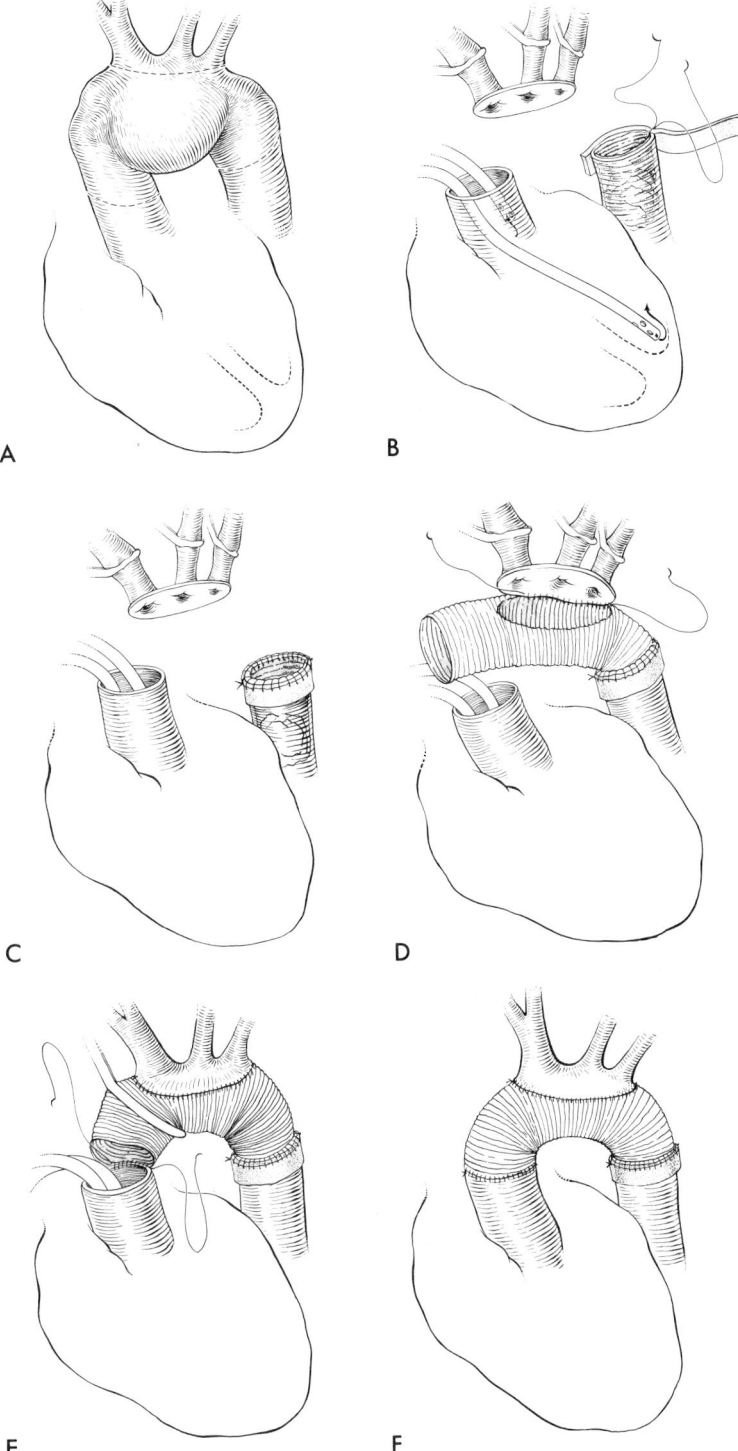

Figure 18. Operative procedure for aortic arch replacement. *A,* Lines of transection of aorta leaving cuff for great vessels. *B,* Method of left ventricular intracavitary perfusion with cold saline for myocardial protection. *C,* Inserted graft sutured from inside distal aorta with external buttressing of aorta with synthetic felt. *D,* Anastomosis of cuff of great vessels to graft. *E,* Perfusion of aortic arch and great vessels resumed during suture of graft to ascending aorta. *F,* Completed graft in place. (From Griepp, R. B., Stinson, E. B., Hollingsworth, J. F., and Buehler, D.: Prosthetic replacement of the aortic arch. J. Thorac. Cardiovasc. Surg., *70*:1051, 1975.)

segments of the aorta, and avoidance of hypotension are likewise most important. Certainly, removal of aortic segments such as in acute aneurysms from which collateral circulation to the spinal cord has not developed is more hazardous than resection of chronic aneurysms with well-developed collateral circulation.

Crawford's experience would suggest that aneurysms of the descending thoracic aorta may be safely resected under normothermic conditions without bypass, provided aortic crossclamp time is less than one hour and the blood pressure and blood volume are maintained.

Operative mortality varies with the type and location of the aneurysm and is influenced by factors such as advancing age, pre-existing heart disease, hypertension, and the acute or chronic nature of the aneurysm. Descending thoracic aneurysms of atherosclerotic origin are more likely to be found in patients with advanced age and associated heart disease and thus have an operative mortality rate of about 10 per cent. The risk falls strikingly in the younger age groups and in those who do not have complicating diseases.

SELECTED REFERENCES

Carlson, R. G., Lillihei, C. W., and Edwards, J. E.: Cystic medial necrosis of the ascending aorta in relation to age and hypertension. Am. J. Cardiol., *26*:411, 1970.

This paper analyzes the incidence of cystic medial necrosis in 250 necropsies of patients with no gross aortic abnormality. The incidence of cystic necrosis increased from 10 per cent in the first two decades to 64 per cent in the seventh and eighth decades. Subjects with hypertension always showed a higher incidence of necrosis than the control age group.

Crawford, E. S., and Rubio, P. A.: Reappraisal of adjuncts to avoid ischemia in the treatment of aneurysms of the descending thoracic aorta. J. Thorac. Cardiovasc. Surg., *66*:693, 1973.

This paper analyzes the many factors in reducing ischemic time and its effect in the treatment of aneurysms of the descending thoracic aorta.

Griepp, R. B., Stinson, E. B., Hollingsworth, J. F., and Buehler, D.: Prosthetic replacement of the aortic arch. J. Thorac. Cardiovasc. Surg., *70*:1051, 1975.

This article re-evaluates techniques for aortic arch replacement. It reports total body hypothermia with arch replacement during total circulatory arrest.

Webb, W. R., Ecker, R. R., Holland, R. H., and Sugg, W. L.: Aortic aneurysm with aortic insufficiency: Repair without prosthesis. Am. J. Cardiol., *26*:416, 1970.

This article describes the dilatation and elongation of the proximal segment of the ascending thoracic aorta with cystic medial necrosis, producing aortic insufficiency. A "reefing" technique narrows the annulus and restores competency of the valve leaflets by allowing reapproximation. Because of elongation of the aorta, some aneurysms can be resected and repaired directly without grafting.

REFERENCES

1. Adams, H. D., and von Geertruyden, H.: Neurologic complications of aortic surgery. Ann. Surg., *144*:574, 1956.
2. Bahnson, H. T.: Definitive treatment of saccular aneurysms of the aorta with excision of sac and aortic suture. Surg. Gynecol. Obstet., *96*:382, 1953.
3. Benjamin, H. B., and Becker, A. B.: Etiologic incidence of thoracic and abdominal aneurysms. Surg. Gynecol. Obstet., *125*:1307, 1967.
4. Berman, J. K., and Hull, J. E.: The treatment of aneurysms with fibroblastic agents: Experimental and clinical studies with the use of sodium dicetyl phosphate. Surg. Gynecol. Obstet., *94*:543, 1952.
5. Blakemore, A. H.: Progressive constrictive occlusion of the abdominal aorta with wiring and electrothermic coagulation. Ann. Surg., *133*:447, 1951.
6. Bloodwell, R. D., Hallman, G. L., and Cooley, D. A.: Total replacement of the aortic arch and the "subclavian steal" phenomenon. Ann. Thorac. Surg., *5*:236, 1968.
7. Cooley, D. A., and DeBakey, M. E.: Surgical considerations of intrathoracic aneurysms of the aorta and great vessels. Ann. Surg., *135*:660, 1952.
8. Cooley, D. A., DeBakey, M. E., and Morris, G. C.: Controlled extracorporeal circulation in surgical treatment of aortic aneurysm. Ann. Surg., *146*:473, 1957.
9. Erdheim, J.: Medionecrosis aortae idiopathica aptica. Virchows Arch. Pathol. Anat., *276*:187, 1930.
10. Kampmeier, R. H.: Saccular aneurysm of the thoracic aorta: A clinical study of 633 cases. Ann. Int. Soc. Surg., *17*:46, 1958.
11. Krause, A. H., Ferguson, T. B., and Weldon, C. S.: Thoracic aneurysmectomy utilizing the TDMAC-heparin shunt. Ann. Thorac. Surg., *14*:123, 1972.
12. Parker, F. B., Jr., Neville, J. F., Jr., Hanson, E. L., Mohiuddin, S., and Webb, W. R.: Management of acute aortic dissection. Ann. Thorac. Surg., *19*:436, 1975.
13. Tuffier, T.: Intervention chirurgicale directe pour un aneurysme de la crosse de l'aorte, ligature du sac. Presse Med., *1*:267, 1902.

5. ANEURYSMS OF THE CAROTID ARTERY

Jesse E. Thompson, M.D.

Aneurysms of the carotid artery in the neck are rare lesions. Reid found only 12 carotid aneurysms among 142 aneurysms in all areas treated at the Johns Hopkins Hospital through 1921.[15] Matas stated that carotid aneurysms comprised 1.6 per cent of his total aneurysm series.[18] Beall et al. listed only seven operations for carotid aneurysms among 2300 aneurysm operations during an 11-year period.[1] Raphael et al. reported only six patients with carotid aneurysms seen at the Mayo Clinic from 1936 through 1962.[14]

The majority of carotid aneurysms are due to atherosclerosis.[16] They may also be congenital[8] or result from syphilis or other infections (mycotic), trauma, fibromuscular hyperplasia, Marfan's syndrome, cystic medial necrosis, radiation therapy,[2] or follow carotid angiography or endarterectomy[7] (false aneurysms). Their usual location is the *common carotid bifurcation,* while a smaller number are located in the internal carotid and a few occur in the common carotid trunk. External carotid aneurysms are very rare. Lesions at the bifurcation are more often fusiform, while those in the internal carotid are more apt to be saccular. Carotid aneurysms are usually unilateral but may occur bilaterally.[11]

Differential diagnosis includes enlarged lymph nodes, carotid body tumors, cervical and peritonsillar abscesses,[18] branchial cleft cysts, and metastatic tumors.[21] Tortuosity and buckling of the subclavian, common carotid, and innominate arteries low in the neck, especially on the right side in hypertensive females, may simulate carotid aneurysm.[3] These latter lesions are of little prognostic significance and ordinarily require no treatment.

Carotid arteriography is the definitive maneuver for diagnosis of carotid aneurysms and proper planning of therapy (Fig. 19). It should be performed bilaterally with anteroposterior and lateral views of both cervical and intracranial vessels. It should be noted that the aneurysm may contain sufficient thrombus that the aneurysm may not appear its actual size on the arteriogram and may even show a nearly normal lumen of the vessel.

Natural History and Clinical Manifestations

An untreated carotid aneurysm is a hazardous lesion. In a study of cases recorded through 1936, Shipley, Winslow, and Walker found a 71 per cent mortality among 41 patients treated expectantly in contrast to a 28 per cent mortality in 82 patients operated

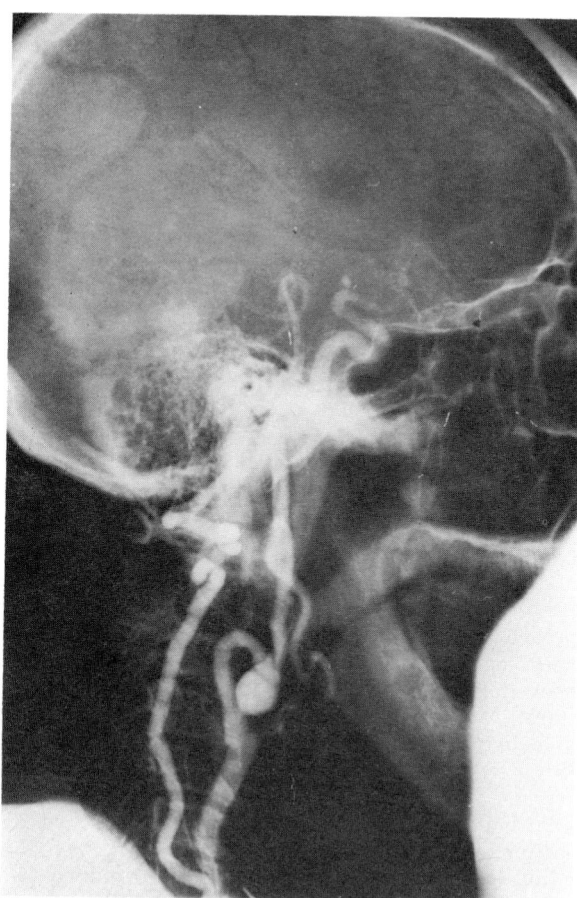

Figure 19. Lateral arteriogram showing a typical saccular aneurysm arising from the cervical internal carotid artery. (Courtesy of Dr. George Plum.)

upon.[18] The *natural history* follows four major patterns of behavior:[18] rupture with hemorrhage, cerebral embolization, thrombosis, and expansion with pressure symptoms on adjacent structures. Rupture, although rare, may result in hemorrhage from the nose, throat, or ear and produce respiratory obstruction.[16] Cerebral embolization of thrombotic material gives rise to transient ischemic attacks and frank strokes. Pressure on the vagus, glossopharyngeal, hypoglossal, and sympathetic nerves causes hoarseness, dysphagia, weakness of the tongue, and Horner's syndrome.

The most common presenting manifestation is a painful pulsating mass in the neck. Pain behind the ear and in the auditory canal is fairly frequent.[19] In addition to the symptomatology listed above, other less common presenting signs and symptoms include headache, dizziness, tinnitus, facial pain, aphasia, syncope, nausea, convulsions, pharyngeal mass, ataxia, and blurred vision.[16] A systolic bruit is usually audible over the aneurysm.

Treatment

Sir Astley Cooper was the first to ligate the carotid artery for cervical aneurysm in 1805. This patient died of sepsis, but in 1808 Cooper repeated the operation, this time successfully, and the patient lived until 1821.[4] During the 150 years following Cooper's operation, surgical therapy consisted largely of carotid ligation, with generally poor and unpredictable results.[19] Shipley et al. in 1937 reported a 28 per cent mortality associated with ligation in a collected series of 82 patients, while Matas quoted mortality of only 6.6 per cent in his personal series.[18] The incidence of cerebral complications attendant upon carotid ligation was estimated at 20 to 30 per cent.

In 1952 Dimtza first resected an atherosclerotic internal carotid aneurysm and reconstructed the artery successfully by end-to-end anastomosis.[6] In 1953 Shea et al. successfully resected a mycotic aneurysm of the common carotid and repaired the defect by end-to-end anastomosis also.[17] The English literature now records more than 70 patients who have undergone aneurysm resection with restoration of arterial continuity.[2, 9, 16]

The most common operation currently employed is resection of the aneurysm with end-to-end anastomosis, which can be done in more than half the cases, since the artery is usually tortuous and the two ends can be brought together without tension.[9, 11] If the defect is too long for primary anastomosis, repair is effected by means of a graft, either saphenous vein, autologous artery, Dacron, or bovine. Resection with lateral arteriorrhaphy is occasionally possible.[19] Endoaneurysmal reconstruction over a stent shunt has also been reported.[10]

In some cases resection with arterial reconstruction is not possible because the aneurysm extends to the base of the skull and no distal artery is available for anastomosis.[1] In these individuals carotid ligation has been the only treatment available. If the patient can tolerate ligation without neurologic symptoms, this may be done at a single stage; if not, occlusion may be accomplished gradually over several days by means of a Crutchfield[5] or Selverstone clamp.[21] Whether recently developed microneurosurgical techniques of extra-intracranial anastomosis will be applicable as definitive therapy in these difficult cases remains to be determined.[20]

False aneurysms following carotid endarterectomy present special problems in reconstruction.[7] In some cases simple patch graft repair with vein or Dacron will suffice. In others, tubular segmental reconstruction using Dacron or autologous vein or artery is necessary (Fig. 20).

Cerebral Protection

The chief hazard associated with repair of carotid aneurysms is the occurrence of neurologic deficits incident to carotid clamping. In arterial reconstructive operations when no cerebral protection has been employed, permanent neurologic deficits have occurred in 22 to 36 per cent of collected cases, and operative mortality has been 4 to 7 per cent. With the use of various methods of cerebral protection, permanent deficits have occurred in 0 to 7 per cent of patients, and mortality has been 0 to 3.4 per cent, a marked improvement over previous figures.[9, 11, 14, 16]

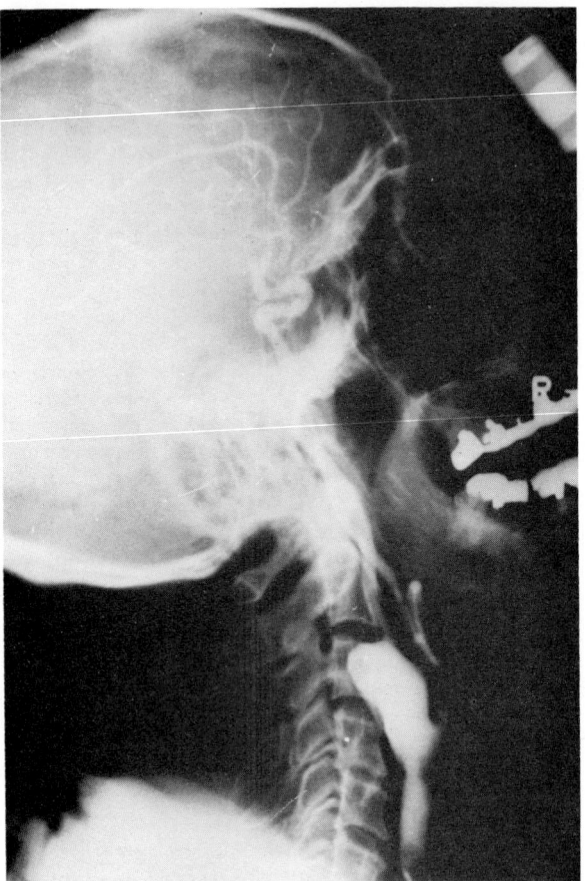

Figure 20. Right lateral arteriogram taken three years following carotid endarterectomy with Dacron patch graft using silk sutures, showing a *false aneurysm* at the site of the Dacron patch. The aneurysm was resected and replaced with an 8 mm. Dacron tube without incident, with the aid of a temporary inlying shunt.

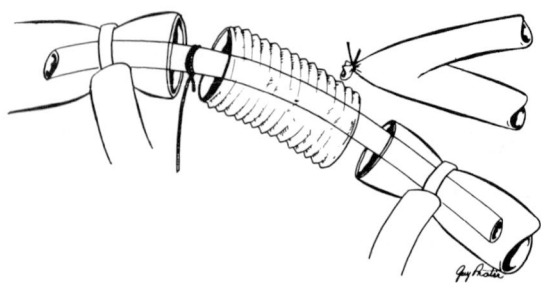

Figure 21. Technique for repair of carotid aneurysm with a tubular graft, using a temporary inlying shunt. The aneurysm has been resected, and a No. 10 French plastic shunt, previously inserted through the graft, is placed into the stumps of the common carotid and internal carotid arteries. The external carotid has been ligated. (From J. E. Thompson: "Prevention of Complications of Cerebral Arteriography and Surgery," in W. A. Dale (ed.): MANAGEMENT OF ARTERIAL OCCLUSIVE DISEASE. Copyright © 1971 by Year Book Medical Publishers, Inc., Chicago. Used by permission.)

proach 1 per cent and the incidence of permanent neurologic deficits be under 5 per cent. Results of operation in recent series have been excellent.[9, 11] Rarely, a patient with a high aneurysm and no available distal artery may require carotid ligation for life-threatening hemorrhage and suffer an obligatory stroke or death.[11]

Although not an aneurysm in the usual sense, dissection of the cervical carotid artery may occur and be clinically indistinguishable from the usual patient with cerebrovascular insufficiency. These so-called dissecting aneurysms are spontaneous and even bilateral.[12] Diagnosis is established by arteriography. Operative repair by resection or endarterectomy is the treatment of choice.

Since most carotid aneurysms are operated upon electively, one should assess the adequacy of cerebral collateral circulation prior to resection. Using regional anesthesia, one may temporarily occlude the carotid and test the patient's neurologic status.[13] More commonly, with general anesthesia one can measure the stump pressure in the occluded distal internal carotid; if this is 55 mm. Hg or higher, cerebral collateral circulation is probably adequate and one can proceed without other adjuncts. If the patient is unable to tolerate temporary clamping or has a low stump pressure, one should employ a temporary bypass shunt, which is the most reliable method for providing cerebral protection, coupled with general anesthesia.[20] Figures 21, 22, and 23 depict a technique by which this may be achieved, regardless of whether end-to-end anastomosis or graft replacement is used. Some surgeons routinely employ a shunt regardless of stump pressure levels.

With modern anesthetic techniques and appropriate cerebral protection, operative mortality should ap-

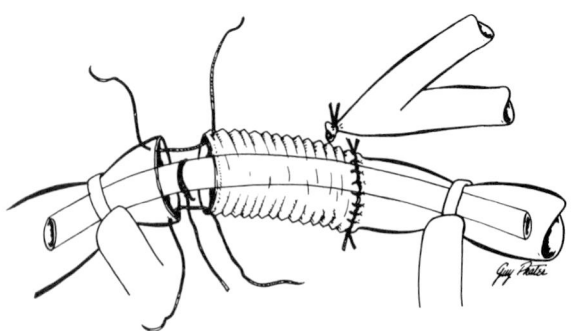

Figure 22. End-to-end anastomosis between the internal carotid and the graft is completed first. Autologous vein or artery or 8 mm. tubular Dacron prosthesis may be used together with polyester sutures. The proximal suture line between the common carotid and graft has been started. (From J. E. Thompson: "Prevention of Complications of Cerebral Arteriography and Surgery," in W. A. Dale (ed.): MANAGEMENT OF ARTERIAL OCCLUSIVE DISEASE. Copyright © 1971 by Year Book Medical Publishers, Inc., Chicago. Used by permission.)

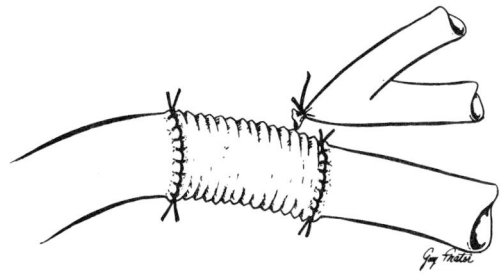

Figure 23. Anastomoses have been completed. The internal shunt is removed before the final three or four sutures are placed or tied. Interrupted sutures facilitate construction of the distal anastomosis, while either interrupted or continuous sutures may be used for the proximal suture line. The same technique of using a temporary inlying shunt for cerebral protection may be employed regardless of whether patch graft reconstruction, direct end-to-end arterial anastomosis, or tubular graft replacement is performed for restoration of arterial continuity following resection of the aneurysm. (From J. E. Thompson: Prevention of Complications of Cerebral Arteriography and Surgery," in W. A. Dale (ed.): MANAGEMENT OF ARTERIAL OCCLUSIVE DISEASE. Copyright © 1971 by Year Book Medical Publishers, Inc., Chicago. Used by permission.)

SELECTED REFERENCES

Hardin, C. A.: Surgical treatment of extracranial carotid aneurysms with excision and arterial restoration. Vasc. Surg., 7:247, 1973.
This is a detailed review of the literature with analysis of 64 cases of carotid aneurysm treated by excision and arterial restoration, with a breakdown showing the various methods of cerebral protection used during operation.

Rittenhouse, E. A., Radke, H. M., and Sumner, D. S.: Carotid artery aneurysm. Review of the literature and report of a case with rupture into the oropharynx. Arch. Surg., 105:786, 1972.
This is a concise review of the literature, with emphasis on etiology and presenting manifestations of carotid aneurysms and a listing of complications associated with surgical treatment of these lesions.

REFERENCES

1. Beall, A. C., Jr., Crawford, E. S., Cooley, D. A., and DeBakey, M. E.: Extracranial aneurysms of the carotid artery. Report of seven cases. Postgrad. Med., 32:93, 1962.
2. Bole, P. V., Hintz, G., Chander, P., Chan, Y. S., and Clauss, R. H.: Bilateral carotid aneurysms secondary to radiation therapy. Ann. Surg., 181:888, 1975.
3. Brown, G. E., and Rowntree, L.: Right-sided carotid pulsations in cases of severe hypertension. J.A.M.A., 84:1016, 1925.
4. Cooper, A.: Account of the first successful operation performed on the common carotid artery for aneurysm in the year 1808 with the postmortem examination in the year 1821. Guys Hosp. Rep., 1:53, 1836.
5. Crutchfield, W. G.: Instruments for use in the treatment of certain intracranial vascular lesions. J. Neurosurg., 16:471, 1959.
6. Dimtza, A.: Aneurysms of the carotid arteries. Angiology, 7:218, 1956.
7. Ehrenfeld, W. K., and Hays, R. J.: False aneurysm after carotid endarterectomy. Arch. Surg., 104:288, 1972.
8. Hammon, J. W., Jr., Silver, D., and Young, W. G., Jr.: Congenital aneurysm of the extracranial carotid arteries. Ann. Surg., 176:777, 1972.
9. Hardin, C. A.: Surgical treatment of extracranial carotid aneurysms with excision and arterial restoration. Vasc. Surg., 7:247, 1973.
10. Hershey, F. B.: Operation for aneurysm of the internal carotid artery high in the neck: A new and an old technique. Angiology, 25:24, 1974.
11. Kaupp, H. A., Haid, S. P., Jurayj, M. N., Bergan, J. J., and Trippel, O. H.: Aneurysms of the extracranial carotid artery. Surgery, 72:946, 1972.
12. Lloyd, J., and Bahnson, H. T.: Bilateral dissecting aneurysms of the internal carotid arteries. Am. J. Surg., 122:549, 1971.
13. Paul, R. S., Abadir, A. R., and Spencer, F. C.: Resection of an internal carotid artery aneurysm under regional anesthesia: Posterior cervical block. Ann. Surg., 168:147, 1968.
14. Raphael, H. A., Bernatz, P. E., Spittell, J. A., Jr., and Ellis, F. H., Jr.: Cervical carotid aneurysms: Treatment by excision and restoration of arterial continuity. Am. J. Surg., 105:771, 1963.
15. Reid, M. R.: Aneurysms in the Johns Hopkins Hospital. All cases treated in the surgical service from the opening of the hospital to January 1922. Arch. Surg., 12:1, 1926.
16. Rittenhouse, E. A., Radke, H. M., and Sumner, D. S.: Carotid artery aneurysm. Review of the literature and report of a case with rupture into the oropharynx. Arch. Surg., 105:786, 1972.
17. Shea, P. C., Jr., Glass, L. F., Reid, W. A., and Harland, A.: Anastomosis of common and internal carotid arteries following excision of mycotic aneurysm. Surgery, 37:829, 1955.
18. Shipley, A. M., Winslow, N., and Walker, W. W.: Aneurysm in the cervical portion of the internal carotid artery. An analytical study of the cases recorded in the literature between August 1, 1925 and July 31, 1936. Report of two new cases. Ann. Surg., 105:673, 1937.
19. Thompson, J. E., and Austin, D. J.: Surgical management of cervical carotid aneurysms. Arch. Surg., 74:80, 1957.
20. Thompson, J. E.: The development of carotid artery surgery. Arch. Surg., 107:643, 1973.
21. Webb, R. C., Jr., and Barker, W. F.: Aneurysms of the extracranial internal carotid artery. Arch. Surg., 99:501, 1969.

6. CAROTID BODY TUMORS

Jesse E. Thompson, M.D.

The carotid body is a pinkish-grey structure 3 to 4 mm. in size located within the adventitial layer on the posterior aspect of the common carotid bifurcation. Tumors of the carotid body are very uncommon and belong to the group of tumors known as chemodectomas. These are nonchromaffin paragangliomas, arising from paraganglionic tissue, probably of neural crest orgin. Normally, the cells function as chemoreceptors, sensitive to changes in Po_2, Pco_2, and pH of the blood. Similar nests of cells' are found in the glomus jugulare, middle ear, ganglion nodosum, aortic arch, innominate and pulmonary arteries, abdominal aorta, mediastinum, retroperitoneal area, and on the lung surfaces. The tumors are named according to their anatomic sites and may be multicentric, the carotid body tumors being the most common chemodectomas encountered. Although rare, some tumors apparently do produce catecholamines and the question of their relationship to multiple endocrine adenomatosis (MEA) has been raised.[4, 8, 10]

Interestingly, a high incidence of carotid body tumors has been reported from Peru among individuals living at altitudes of 6,900 to 14,000 feet, suggesting that chronic hypoxia is a stimulus for carotid body hyperplasia.[2]

Carotid body tumors are slow-growing neoplasms. Some may remain stationary for many years, while others continue to grow with progressive increase in symptoms and disability. The majority are benign but a few are malignant, as evidenced by local recurrence and spread to contiguous tissues as well as by lymphatic and hematogenous metastasis to regional nodes, lung, bones, and heart. The malignant tumors tend to occur in younger individuals under the age of 40.[6]

These tumors are usually unilateral. A very interesting characteristic is their familial incidence in some cases. When familial, the incidence of bilaterality is very high, about 25 per cent, in contrast to nonfamilial cases, where bilateral tumors occur in only 4 to 5 per cent of cases.[13]

The presenting manifestation is usually a painless mass at the common carotid bifurcation. Symptoms result from pressure on the vagus, hypoglossal, glossopharyngeal, and sympathetic nerves, and include pain in the neck or ear, carotid sinus syndrome, dysphagia, and hoarseness. Differential diagnosis includes carotid aneurysm, branchiogenic cysts, neurofibromas, and metastatic tumors.[13]

The most important recent advance in diagnosis has been arteriography. Carotid body tumors characteristically show lateral displacement of the carotid artery, separation of the internal and external divisions, and a striking vascularity (Fig. 24). Arteriography is helpful in planning operative therapy and yields important information regarding patency of carotid vessels and adequacy of cerebral collateral circulation.[11, 12]

Definitive treatment of carotid body tumors is excision. The first excision was performed by Riegner in 1880, but the patient did not survive. In 1886 Maydl removed a tumor and the patient survived but with hemiplegia and aphasia. In 1889 Albert successfully excised a tumor without ligating the carotid vessels. Scudder, in 1903, reported the first successful removal of a carotid body tumor in the United States.[10]

Over the years the major problem in treatment has been the relation of the tumor to the carotid artery, sacrifice of which has resulted in serious complications.[5] Rush, in a collective review in 1962, emphasized that when excision was accompanied by carotid ligation, operative mortality was 25 per cent and hemiplegia among survivors an additional 30 per cent. By contrast, simple excision carried an operative mortality of only 1.5 per cent and an incidence of hemiplegia of 2.9 per cent.[9]

Innovations in operative techniques have markedly improved morbidity statistics. It has been realized that the carotid artery cannot in most instances be sacrificed with impunity. The most important techni-

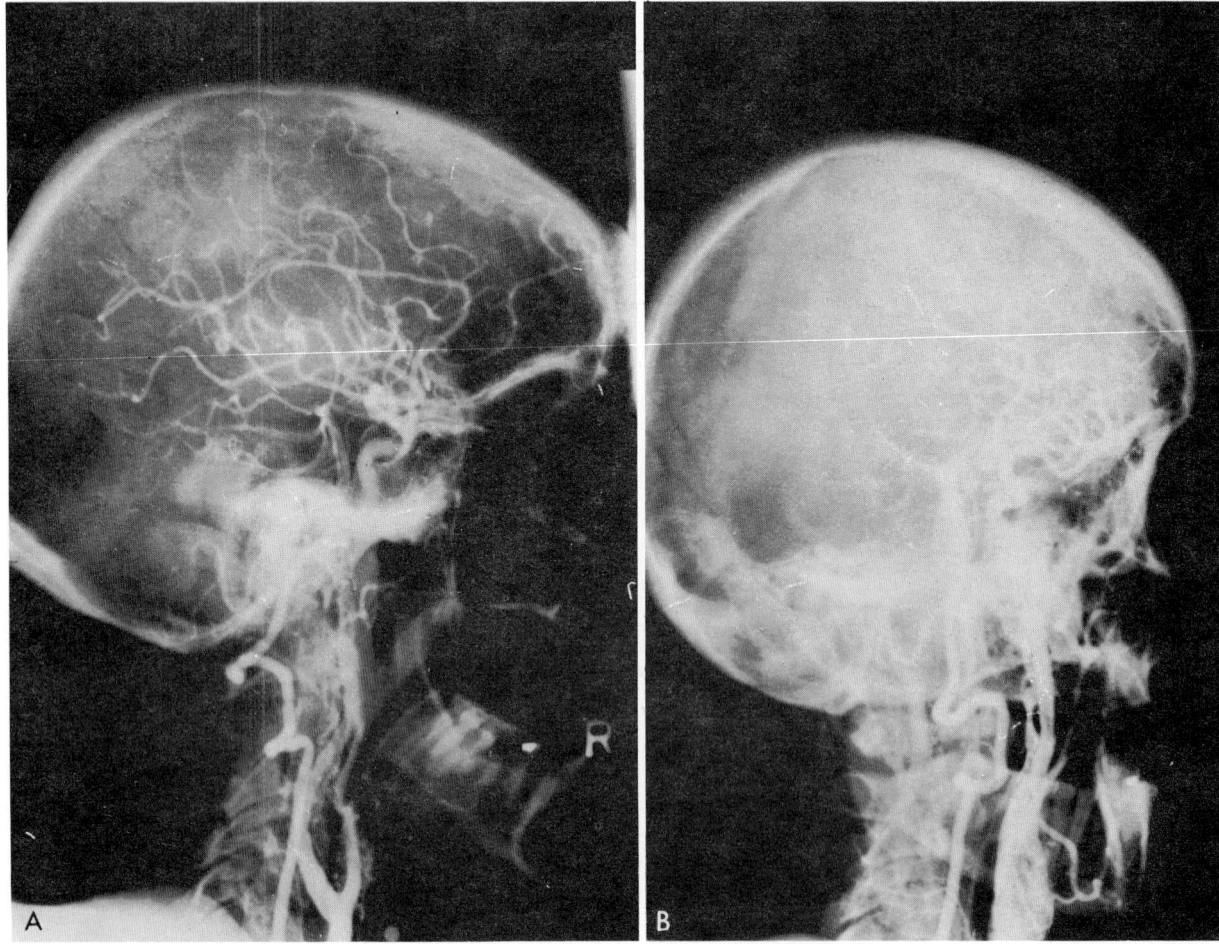

Figure 24. *A,* Lateral arteriogram of a patient with right carotid body tumor, showing the characteristic separation of the internal and external carotid arteries by the tumor at the carotid bifurcation. *B,* Later phase during arteriography of same patient, demonstrating the extreme vascularity which carotid body tumors exhibit. (Courtesy of Dr. J. H. Arndt.)

cal advance has been *subadventitial* removal of the tumors from the carotid vessels, since the media is almost never involved.[3] Meticulous dissection is carried out in the subadventitial plane. At times this requires incision into the tumor down to the media of the artery in order to enter the proper plane of dissection. With this technique the vast majority of carotid body tumors can be removed, leaving the carotid artery intact. Bilateral tumors should be removed in separate stages.

With very large, invasive, or malignant tumors the carotid artery may have to be sacrificed. If the artery is already occluded, this poses no hazard. If the artery is patent, carotid circulation may be restored by means of an artery graft, using a shunt for cerebral protection.[7, 9, 12] If no distal artery is available for anastomosis, attempts at resection should probably be abandoned.[11]

Judgment regarding therapy of carotid body tumors has swung widely over the years based on prevailing results of surgical therapy in view of the natural history of the disorder.[9] At present surgical removal is advocated for small tumors in good risk patients under the age of 50, for symptomatic lesions, and for aggressively growing and suspected malignant tumors. For the elderly asymptomatic patient, observation is generally recommended. Radiation therapy may be of value for nonresectable lesions.[10, 11]

Shamblin et al., in a collected series from the Mayo Clinic, reported a 5.7 per cent operative mortality among 90 patients with 96 carotid body tumors.[10] Several surgical series have recently been published showing no surgical mortality or serious neurologic complications.[1, 7, 11, 12] Functional results following operation are quite satisfactory.

SELECTED REFERENCES

Rush, B. F., Jr.: Current concepts in the treatment of carotid body tumors. Surgery, 52:679, 1962.
  This is a review of the subject to 1962, with emphasis on natural history of untreated tumors and the mortality and morbidity rates associated with various types of surgical therapy.

Westbrook, K. C., Guillamondegui, O. M., Medellin, H., and Jesse, R. H.: Chemodectomas of the neck. Selective management. Am. J. Surg., 124:760, 1972.
  This article clearly outlines signs and symptoms, usefulness of angiography, indications for surgical therapy, and results of treatment in the authors' large series.

Wilson, H.: Carotid body tumors. Surgery, 59:483, 1966.
  This is an extensive review pointing up morphology, physiology, diagnosis, details of surgical management, and analysis of the author's personal series of 15 cases.

REFERENCES

1. Cordell, A. R., Myers, R. T., and Hightower, F.: Carotid body tumors. Ann. Surg., 165:880, 1967.
2. Editorial: High altitude chemodectoma. Lancet, 1:1493, 1973.
3. Farrar, T., Kirklin, J. W., Judd, E. S., Jr., and Devine, K. D.: Resection of carotid-body tumors with preservation of the carotid vessels. Arch. Surg., 72:595, 1956.
4. Hewitt, R. L., Ichinose, H., Weichert, R. F., III, and Drapanas, T.: Chemodectomas. Surgery, 71:275, 1972.
5. Lahey, F. H., and Warren, K. W.: A long term appraisal of carotid body tumors with remarks on their removal. Surg. Gynecol. Obstet., 92:481, 1951.
6. Martin, C. E., Rosenfeld, L., and McSwain, B.: Carotid body tumors: A 16-year follow-up of seven malignant cases. South. Med. J., 66:1236, 1973.
7. Morris, G. C., Jr., Balas, P. E., Cooley, D. A., Crawford, E. S., and DeBakey, M. E.: Surgical treatment of benign and malignant carotid body tumors. Clinical experience with sixteen tumors in twelve patients. Am. Surg., 29:429, 1963.
8. Pollack, R. S.: Carotid body tumors—idiosyncracies. Oncology, 27:81, 1973.
9. Rush, B. F., Jr.: Current concepts in the treatment of carotid body tumors. Surgery, 52:679, 1962.
10. Shamblin, W. R., ReMine, W. H., Sheps, S. G., and Harrison, E. G., Jr.: Carotid body tumor (chemodectoma). Clinicopathologic analysis of ninety cases. Am. J. Surg., 122:732, 1971.
11. Westbrook, K. C., Guillamondegui, O. M., Medellin, H., and Jesse, R. H.: Chemodectomas of the neck. Selective management. Am. J. Surg., 124:760, 1972.
12. Wilson, H.: Carotid body tumors. Surgery, 59:483, 1966.
13. Wilson, H.: Carotid body tumors: Familial and bilateral. Ann. Surg., 171:843, 1970.

7. SUBCLAVIAN ARTERY ANEURYSMS

David C. Sabiston, Jr., M.D.

Aneurysms of the subclavian artery are most often associated with lesions producing the thoracic outlet syndrome. In this situation, the proximal subclavian artery is partially obstructed, and poststenotic dilatation and aneurysmal formation result. Thrombosis may occur, with subsequent embolization to the arterial circulation of the upper extremity. This condition is discussed further in the section on the thoracic outlet syndrome in Chapter 55.

8. VISCERAL ARTERIAL ANEURYSMS

David C. Sabiston, Jr., M.D.

Aneurysms of the visceral arteries are more common than is generally appreciated. Although in many instances these aneurysms are asymptomatic, in others they may cause catastrophic complications. The fact that these lesions are not rare is emphasized by a report in which 45 patients with splanchnic arterial aneurysms were seen in one center during a 12-year period. The most important visceral arterial aneurysms are those of the splenic, celiac, hepatic, superior mesenteric, and renal arteries. Aneurysms have also been reported of the gastroduodenal, pancreaticoduodenal, and gastroepiploic arteries. Selective arteriography of the visceral circulation has greatly aided the diagnosis of aneurysms of these arteries (Figs. 25 and 26). A number of these aneurysms have been discovered by arteriography performed for other reasons.

SPLENIC ARTERY ANEURYSMS

The most common of the visceral arterial aneurysms are those involving the *splenic artery*, representing

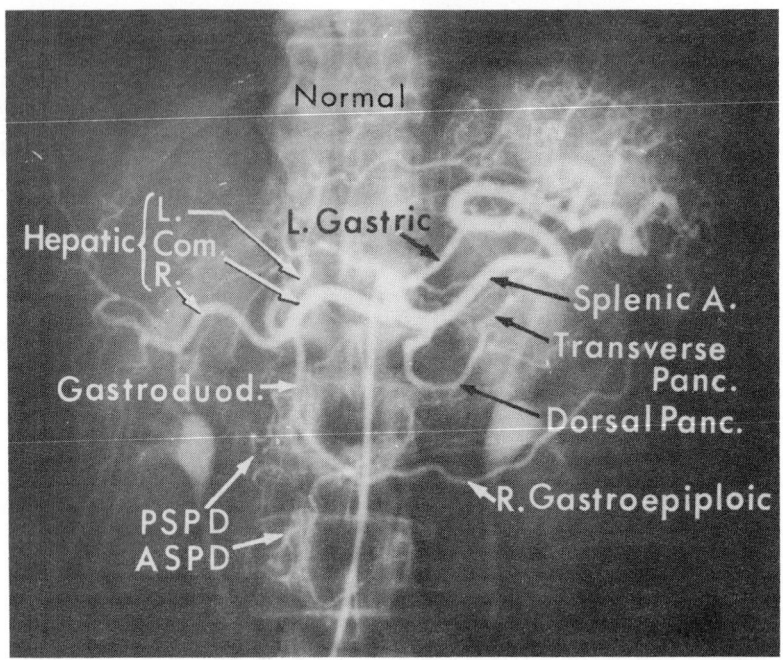

Figure 25. Selective injection of the celiac axis demonstrating normal anatomy. PSPD: posterior-superior pancreaticoduodenal artery; ASPD: anterior-superior pancreaticoduodenal artery. (Courtesy of Dr. Irwin Johnsrude.)

nearly two thirds of all such lesions. The first description of a splenic artery aneurysm was by Beaussier in 1770.[1] More than 600 aneurysms of the splenic artery have been reported.[9] These lesions are most commonly found in females, and rupture of the aneurysm during *pregnancy* is a well known complication. The most common *etiology* of these aneurysms is medial degeneration of the arterial wall. They are usually *saccular,* and the wall may contain calcium. Forty-five per cent of females with these aneurysms have had six or more pregnancies.[9] Splenic artery aneurysm may occur in association with fibromuscular hyperplasia involving the renal artery, and atherosclerosis is also a cause of these aneurysms. Congenital aneurysms are rare and are usually multiple. Mycotic lesions, usually the sequel of septic emboli in the spleen after subacute bacterial endocarditis, also occur but are rare.

The *clinical manifestations* of splenic artery aneurysms vary considerably, and many patients are asymptomatic. The most common complaint is that of vague pain in the left upper quadrant with radiation to the left subscapular region. In expanding aneurysms, the symptoms may be more prominent and become acute with rupture. The diagnosis is most often made by the discovery of a calcified lesion on abdominal roentgenograms, with objective demonstration by arteriography (Fig. 27). Physical findings are uncommon, although rarely a tender, pulsatile mass can be felt in the left upper quadrant. Generally, these lesions are small and are not palpable.

The *risk* of rupture of splenic aneurysms is difficult to determine; some reports suggest an extremely high incidence.[7] Among 40 ruptured splenic artery aneurysms recently reported, 10 resulted in death (25 per cent).[9] Operation should be recommended for most

splenic artery aneurysms, especially in pregnant patients because of the unduly high risk of rupture. The mortality of rupture during pregnancy is quite high (68 per cent in one group of 65 patients).[9] The procedure of choice is excision of the splenic artery aneurysm, usually with splenectomy.

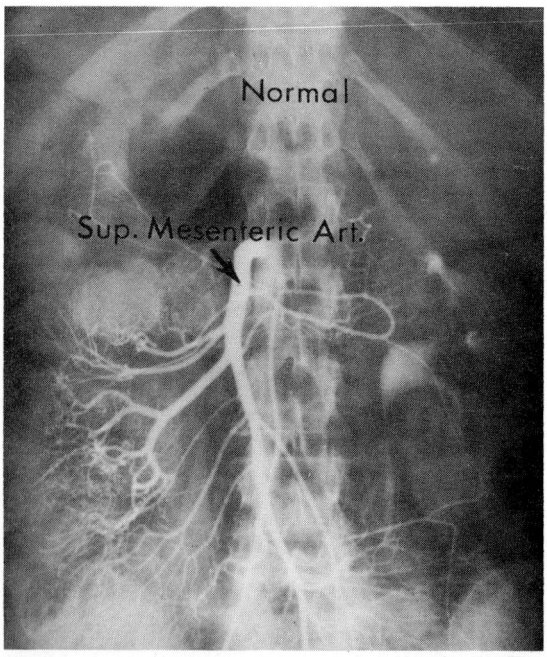

Figure 26. Selective injection of superior mesenteric artery demonstrating normal anatomy. (Courtesy of Dr. Irwin Johnsrude.)

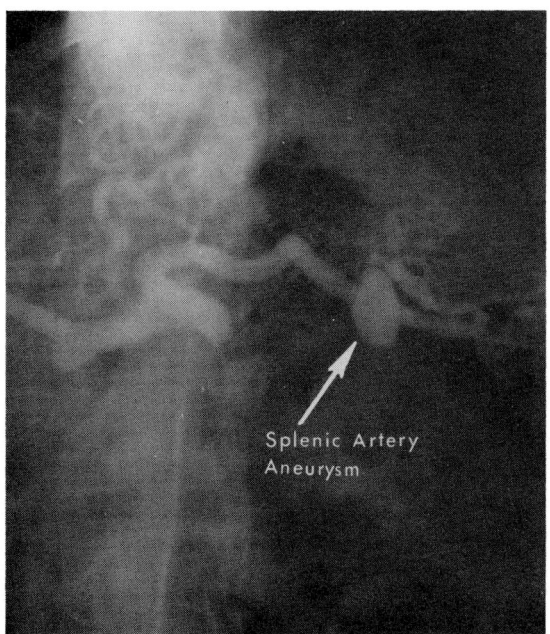

Figure 27. Splenic artery aneurysm demonstrated by selective arteriographic injection into the celiac axis. (Courtesy of Dr. Irwin Johnsrude.)

CELIAC ARTERY ANEURYSMS

Aneurysms of the celiac artery are relatively uncommon; some 50 examples can be found in the literature. Arteriosclerotic, congenital, mycotic, and traumatic types have been described. When present, the clinical manifestations are primarily those of vague abdominal discomfort. Most of the previously reported cases have been those recognized at the time of rupture. *Surgical therapy* is recommended, with excision and restoration of continuity either directly or with a graft. In a recent report, 14 patients were collected from the literature with celiac arterial aneurysms managed surgically, of whom 13 had a good result.[6]

HEPATIC ARTERY ANEURYSMS

Aneurysm of the hepatic artery was first described by Wilson in 1819,[12] and more than 200 are reported in the literature.[9] The etiology includes arteriosclerosis, infection (mycotic), trauma, and medial degeneration. Periarteritis nodosa is rarely responsible. The most prominent clinical manifestation is right upper quadrant or epigastric pain, frequently similar to that occurring in gallbladder disease. Hematemesis or melena may follow erosion into the gastrointestinal tract, as may fever and jaundice. Free rupture into the peritoneal cavity is the most serious complication of these aneurysms, and only five survivors after this complication have been reported.[9]

When the lesion is diagnosed, surgical extirpation is indicated. In a collected series of 175 patients with this disorder, only 41 were successfully treated, 37 of them in the last decade. Most aneurysms are discovered incidentally at operation, and 80 per cent are extrahepatic and can be identified during abdominal operation, whereas 20 per cent lie within the liver and are not easily palpable.[11] The procedure of choice is *excision* of the aneurysm. If the aneurysm is located proximal to the gastroduodenal artery, the lesion may be simply excised with distal ligation, since the collateral circulation through the gastroduodenal artery to the liver is excellent. If the aneurysm involves the hepatic artery *distal* to the gastroduodenal branch, preservation of arterial continuity may be necessary to prevent liver necrosis and requires aneurysmorrhaphy, direct anastomosis, or the use of a venous graft.

ANEURYSMS OF THE SUPERIOR MESENTERIC ARTERY

By 1970, 89 cases of aneurysms of the superior mesenteric artery had been reported. The majority (57 per cent) were mycotic in origin, with atherosclerosis, trauma, or medial degeneration being the cause in others. In particular, this lesion should be suspected in patients with subacute bacterial endocarditis in whom abdominal pain develops in association with an expanding, tender mass. These lesions rupture in a high percentage of patients. The first successful treatment was in 1949.[3] Since then, a total of 12 patients have been successfully managed by excision of the aneurysm.[9]

ANEURYSMS OF THE GASTRODUODENAL AND PANCREATICODUODENAL ARTERIES

Aneurysms of the gastroduodenal and pancreaticoduodenal arteries are rare, with only eight examples reported in the literature. Aneurysms of the gastric and gastroepiploic arteries are more common, with 53 patients having been reported. The majority of these lesions present with rupture, either into the peritoneal cavity or into the upper gastrointestinal tract, presenting with massive bleeding. Ligation of the aneurysm or partial gastric resection has been accomplished in approximately 30 per cent of these patients. In a recent review, 23 patients with this disorder were collected from the literature.[10]

ANEURYSMS OF THE RENAL ARTERIES

Although once considered rare, aneurysms of the renal arteries are being recognized with increasing frequency (Fig. 28). Since the first description in 1770, 345 cases had been reported by 1968.[2] These lesions constitute approximately 1 per cent of all aneurysms and occur most frequently in patients with hypertension. The lesions are located in the main renal artery or the bifurcation of the primary branches in approximately 60 per cent of cases. Approximately 15 per cent of the aneurysms are *intrarenal,* and in about a quarter there is calcification in the wall of the aneurysm. Most of the lesions are due to atherosclerosis or medial necrosis, and occurrence distal to renal artery stricture is not uncommon. *Saccular* aneurysms are the most frequent. The primary risk with these lesions is rupture. The *clinical manifestations* include the symptoms of hypertension and especially headache. Less common are symptoms of upper abdominal and flank pain. A bruit may be heard over the flank, and hematuria may be present. A palpable mass is rare (less than 10 per cent of cases). The definitive diagnosis is made by arteriography. If the renal artery is stenotic, unilateral renal ischemia can be demonstrated on the rapid-sequence pyelogram. The hypertensive mechanism is most apt to be the result of the renin-angiotensin-aldosterone mechanism, whether associated with arterial stenosis or the result of arterial emboli from the aneurysm.

The management of renal artery aneurysms includes careful preoperative demonstration of the size, type, and location of the aneurysm by arteriography. Rupture is an absolute indication for emergency operation. Those aneurysms without calcification, which represent the majority, are more prone to rupture, are associated with a high mortality, and should be managed surgically. For those aneurysms which are calcified, opinion is divided concerning their treatment, as they are less apt to rupture, although there is no doubt that they may. At present, the majority favor operation for these lesions, and in most instances it is possible to restore continuity to the renal artery and save the kidney. In one series of 72 patients, solitary aneurysms occurred in 53 and multiple lesions in 19 patients. Arteriosclerotic changes were present in nearly 30 per cent of the lesions and were considered secondary rather than primary in most instances. It was of interest that renal artery fibrodysplasia was an associated finding in 27 of the 72 patients, and 57 of the entire group

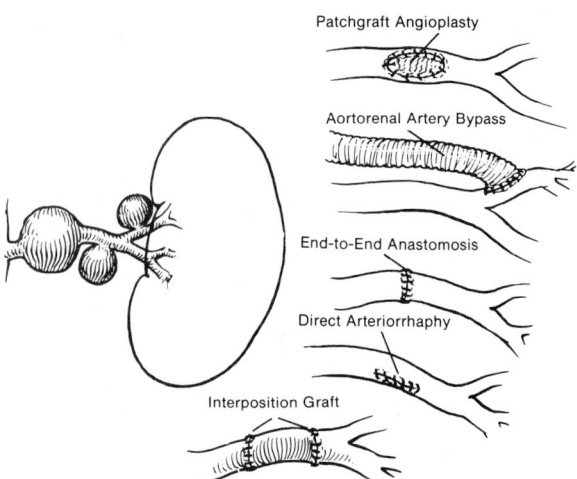

Figure 29. Surgical techniques employed in excision of renal artery aneurysms with preservation of the kidney. (From DeBakey, M. E., Lefrak, E. A., Garcia-Rinaldi, R., and Noon, G. P.: Aneurysm of the renal artery. A vascular reconstructive approach. Arch. Surg., *106*:438, 1973, with permission of authors and publisher.)

were hypertensive. Two patients in the series experienced frank aneurysmal rupture, and covert rupture occurred into the renal veins twice. Among the 72 patients, aneurysmectomy was performed on 31 occasions and nephrectomy, either partial or total, was performed 17 times. In this large series, the authors recommended operation for most lesions that are 1.5 cm. in diameter or greater. It was also emphasized that in many instances stenosis of the renal artery is present concomitantly and requires operation for associated hypertension.[8] It is also of interest that a renal artery aneurysm has been removed successfully from a solitary kidney.[5] In operative correction of these defects, emphasis is placed on vascular reconstructive approach, making every effort to avoid nephrectomy (Fig. 29).[4]

SELECTED REFERENCES

Stanley, J. C., Rhodes, E. L., Gewertz, B. L., Chang, C. Y., Walter, J. F., and Fry, W. J.: Renal artery aneurysms. Significance of macroaneurysms exclusive of dissections and fibrodysplastic mural dilations. Arch. Surg., *110*:1327, 1975.
In this review, the experience with 72 patients with renal artery aneurysms is presented. The majority of the patients were managed surgically, and the indications for operation and results are reviewed. This represents an unusually large series of patients from a single clinic.

Stanley, J. C., Thompson, N. W., and Fry, W. J.: Splanchnic artery aneurysms. Arch. Surg., *101*:689, 1970.
A very good review of splanchnic aneurysms. The natural history, diagnosis, management, and results are described.

REFERENCES

1. Beaussier, M.: Sur un aneurisme de l'artère splénique dont les parois se sont ossifiées. J. Med. Toulouse, *32*:157, 1770.
2. Cerny, J. C., Chang, C., and Fry, W. J.: Renal artery aneurysms. Arch. Surg., *96*:653, 1968.
3. DeBakey, M. E., and Cooley, D. A.: Successful resection of mycotic aneurysms of superior mesenteric artery: Case report and review of the literature. Am. Surg., *19*:202, 1953.

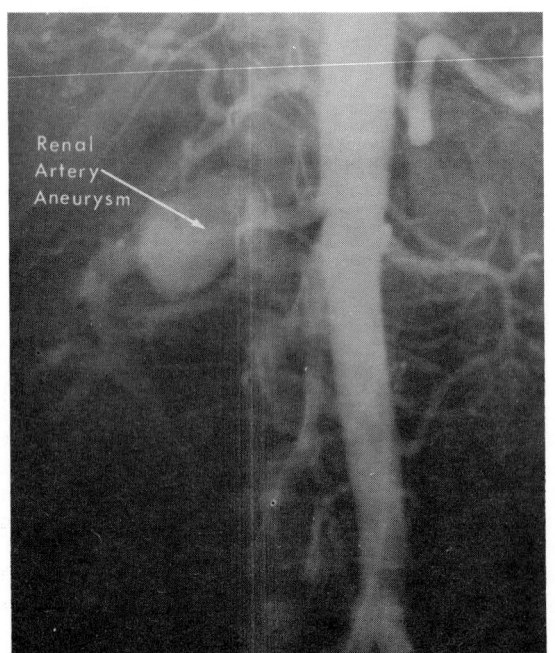

Figure 28. Aneurysm of the right renal artery. (Courtesy of Dr. Irwin Johnsrude.)

4. DeBakey, M. E., Lefrak, E. A., Garcia-Rinaldi, R., and Noon, G. P.: Aneurysm of the renal artery. A vascular approach. Arch. Surg., *106*:438, 1973.

5. Gonzales, E. T., Jr., Grimes, J. H., Seigler, H. F., and Young, W. G., Jr.: Renal artery aneurysm in a solitary kidney: Successful surgical repair. South. Med. J., *67*:368, 1974.

6. Haimovici, H., Sprayregen, S., Eckstein, P., and Veith, F. J.: Celiac artery aneurysmectomy: Case report with review of the literature. Surgery, *79*:592, 1976.

7. Owens, J. C., and Coffey, R. J.: Aneurysm of the splenic artery, including a report of six additional cases. Int. Abstr. Surg., *97*:313, 1953.

8. Stanley, J. C., Rhodes, E. L., Gewertz, B. L., Chang, C. Y., Walter, J. F., and Fry, W. J.: Renal artery aneurysms. Significance of macroaneurysms exclusive of dissections and fibrodysplastic mural dilations. Arch. Surg., *110*:1327, 1975.

9. Stanley, J. C., Thompson, N. W., and Fry, W. J.: Splanchnic artery aneurysms. Arch. Surg.,*101*:689, 1970.

10. Verta, M. J., Jr., Dean, R. H., Yao, J. S. T., Conn, J., Jr., Mehn, W. H., and Bergan, J. J.: Pancreaticoduodenal arterial aneurysms. Ann. Surg., in press.

11. Weaver, D. H., Fleming, R. J., and Barnes, W. A.: Aneurysm of the hepatic artery: The value of arteriography in surgical management. Surgery, *64*:891, 1968.

12. Wilson, J.: Lectures on the Blood, and on the Anatomy, Physiology, and Surgical Pathology of the Vascular System of the Human Body. Read before the Royal College of Surgeons, London, 1819.

9. AORTIC ABDOMINAL ANEURYSMS

David C. Sabiston, Jr., M.D.

One of the most common and most dangerous of arterial aneurysms is that encountered in the abdominal aorta. Although recognized for many years, it was not until 1951 that the first aortic abdominal aneurysm was successfully resected by Dubost in France with use of an aortic homograft.[8] Since then, thousands of aortic abdominal aneurysms have been resected, with an appreciable extension of life.

PATHOLOGIC ASPECTS

The vast majority — more than 95 per cent — of abdominal aortic aneurysms are due to atherosclerosis. Rarely, trauma, syphilis, mycotic infection, or the Marfan syndrome may be responsible. The majority of the atherosclerotic aneurysms occur in the sixth and seventh decades.

NATURAL HISTORY

The *fate* of patients with atherosclerotic aneurysms of the abdominal aorta is a subject of prime significance. Careful studies of the *natural history* of untreated abdominal aortic aneurysms have been accumulated in an effort to delineate the role of surgical treatment. In 1950, prior to the advent of surgical therapy, Estes[9] published a classic study of the natural history of abdominal aneurysms in 102 patients. In this group, 64 patients died, and in 63 per cent death was due to rupture. Only 67 per cent of these patients survived 1 year, 49 per cent survived 3 years, and 19

per cent survived to the fifth year. Similar findings were reported by Schatz[21] and Klippel (Fig. 30).[15] In another study, by Gliedman,[11] emphasis was placed upon patients with *symptomatic* aortic abdominal aneurysms. Thirty per cent of these patients were dead within 1 month after onset of symptoms, and 74 per cent had succumbed by 6 months. The death rate by the end of the first year was 80 per cent. Thus, the survival rate in this group was found to be much lower than that in a group of patients in whom aneurysms were found *incidentally* and were *asymptomatic*. Among the 49 per cent who died, only 4 per cent died from a disease that was entirely unrelated to the aneurysm or its underlying cause. Causes of death included coronary, cerebral, and renal complications of atherosclerosis (Fig. 31). Hypertension was present in 47 per cent of the patients.

CLINICAL MANIFESTATIONS

The majority of abdominal aortic aneurysms are discovered at the time of routine examination and are *asymptomatic*. In the remainder, abdominal symptoms range from vague discomfort in the epigastrium to excruciating pain. Severe pain in the flanks or back suggests leakage or actual rupture of the aneurysm and is usually accompanied by signs of blood loss.

Physical examination usually shows the presence of a pulsating mass. The smallest aneurysms are approximately 4 cm. in diameter, but the size may range upward to 20 cm. or more. The aneurysm may be tender to palpation, although this is usually not a prominent symptom. Fortunately, more than 95 per cent of abdominal aortic aneurysms arise *below* the level of the renal arteries, with the inferior mesenteric artery being the only important vessel emerging from the aneurysm. Generally, the latter is either com-

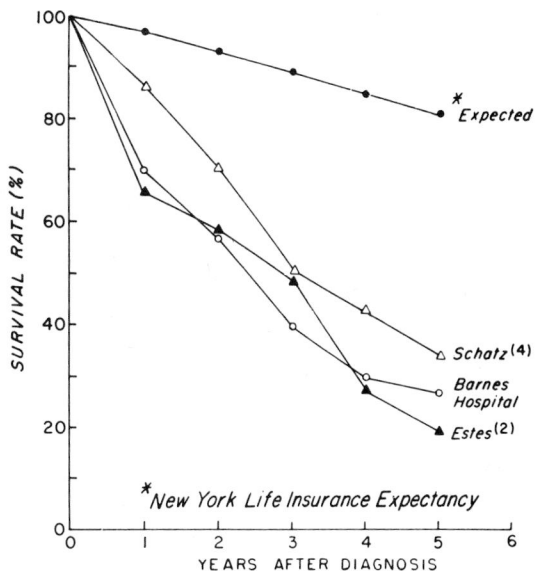

Figure 30. The natural history and survival rates among patients with *untreated* abdominal aortic aneurysms. (From Klippel, A. P., and Butcher, H. R., Jr.: Am. J. Surg., *111*:629, 1966.)

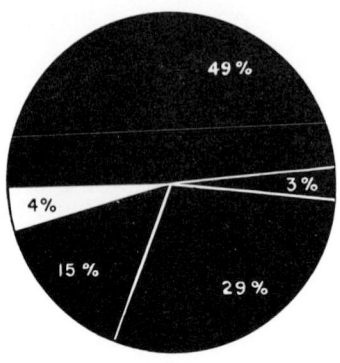

49% = Death from rupture of the abdominal aneurysm.

3% = Death from vascular rupture at another site.

29% = Death due to a disease related to cause of aneurysm.

15% = Death secondarily due to related disease (i.e., a major contributing cause of death.)

4% = DEATH DIRECTLY AND SECONDARILY DUE TO UNRELATED DISEASE.

Figure 31. Cause of death in 68 patients with an untreated abdominal aneurysm. (From Gliedman, M. L., Ayers, W. B., and Vestal, B. L.: Ann Surg., *146*:207, 1957.)

pletely occluded or severely stenotic, and this gives rise to prominent collateral circulation to the distal branches of the inferior mesenteric artery. Time should be taken to examine carefully the femoral, popliteal, dorsal pedal, and posterior tibial pulses bilaterally, particularly in reference to possible changes that may occur postoperatively.

DIAGNOSTIC STUDIES

Plain films of the abdomen frequently show calcification in the wall of the aneurysm, often best observed in the lateral view (Fig. 32). This "eggshell" appearance is essentially diagnostic. The use of lateral tomography has also been found helpful in those instances in which the calcification in the aortic aneurysmal wall is not clear on the plain abdominal films. Ultrasonography has become particularly useful in the recent past and is a very simple, noninvasive technique that not only allows an accurate diagnosis but provides information concerning the size and location of the aneurysm. Moreover, it is quite helpful in following the progress of small aneurysms in patients who are not surgical candidates owing to specific medical contraindications.[17] Arteriography is a very useful method of objective diagnosis and in addition provides much accessory information of value. With modern techniques, this procedure has become quite safe, and it is probably wise to obtain an arteriogram in most patients with a suspected or actual diagnosis of aortic abdominal aneurysm, particularly those upon whom operation is planned. Important surgical findings include suprarenal extension of the aneurysm, demonstration of stenotic lesions in the renal arteries, superior mesenteric artery or celiac axis stenosis, presence of thrombus in the aneurysm, and possibly patency of the inferior mesenteric artery.[4] Arteriography is also

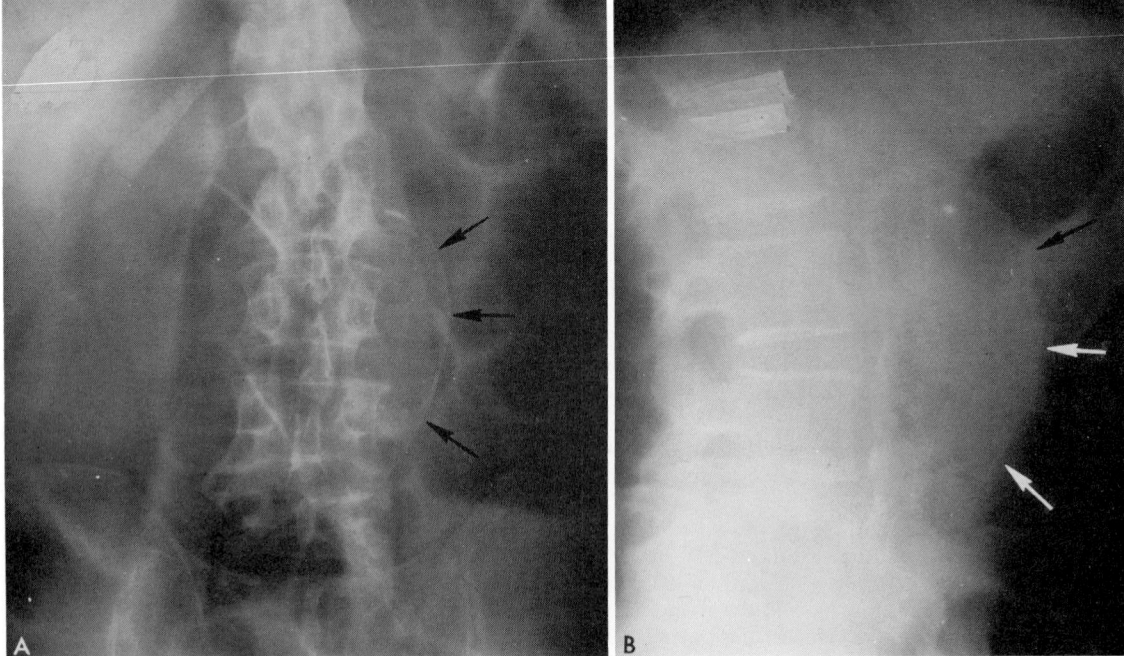

Figure 32. *A,* Plain film of abdomen of a patient with an abdominal aortic aneurysm. Note the calcium in the wall of the aneurysm outlining its border ("eggshell"). *B,* Lateral film showing calcified wall of the aneurysm.

of aid in the patient with a pulsating abdominal mass in whom neoplasm or cyst must be seriously considered in the differential diagnosis. Arteriography is *essential* for evaluation of the distal circulation in patients who have evidence of obstruction in the iliac, femoral, or popliteal arteries, since additional surgery may also be required for these lesions.

COMPLICATIONS

The complications that may be associated with untreated aortic abdominal aneurysms are largely dependent upon the size of the aneurysm. In a collective survey, patients with aneurysms less than 7 cm. in diameter had a lower mortality risk from rupture (4 to 18 per cent), whereas those with aneurysms greater than 7 cm. in diameter have a mortality rate of 72 to 83 per cent.[1] For these reasons, some believe that in *asymptomatic* aneurysms less than 7 cm. in diameter observation without operation may at times be permissible. However, should symptoms appear, resection is indicated.

Although it is clear that *rupture* is the most frequent and most serious complication of aortic abdominal aneurysms, there are additional hazards which include (1) distal embolization of the peripheral arterial system by thrombi originating in the aneurysm,[19] (2) sudden complete thrombosis,[14] (3) infection, particularly with gram-negative organisms and staphylococci,[13] (4) chronic consumption coagulopathy,[23] (5) development of an arteriovenous fistula resulting from erosion of the aortic abdominal aneurysm into the inferior vena cava,[20] and (6) aorticointestinal fistula.[18]

TREATMENT

Most abdominal aortic aneurysms should be managed by excision and restoration of arterial continuity with a prosthetic graft. Rarely, as already mentioned, small aneurysms or those in poor-risk patients may be observed if they are asymptomatic. However, the vast majority of aneurysms should be excised.

Operative Technique

Operation for excision of abdominal aortic aneurysm is best accomplished through a midline incision extending from the xiphoid process to the symphysis pubis, which provides excellent exposure. The abdominal aorta is mobilized proximally so that an arterial clamp can be placed across it for total occlusion (Fig. 33).[7] Similarly, the iliac arteries are clamped below. The inferior mesenteric artery is ligated at its origin from the aneurysm and divided. The anterior portion of the aneurysmal wall, including any thrombus present, is then removed. The posterolateral wall of the aneurysm is usually best left in place to prevent unnecessary dissection. The lumbar vessels entering the aneurysm are apt to bleed in a retrograde direction and are controlled with transfixion ligatures. A preclotted prosthetic graft of Dacron or Teflon is inserted. The graft may be either knitted or woven, the former being more apt to be infiltrated by the patient's tissues because it is more porous and the latter having the advantage that it leaks less at the time of insertion. Most prefer to perform the anastomoses with plastic sutures. Although the proximal portions of both common iliac arteries formerly were frequently resected, this is much less commonly done today. Therefore, a straight graft is usually employed, and

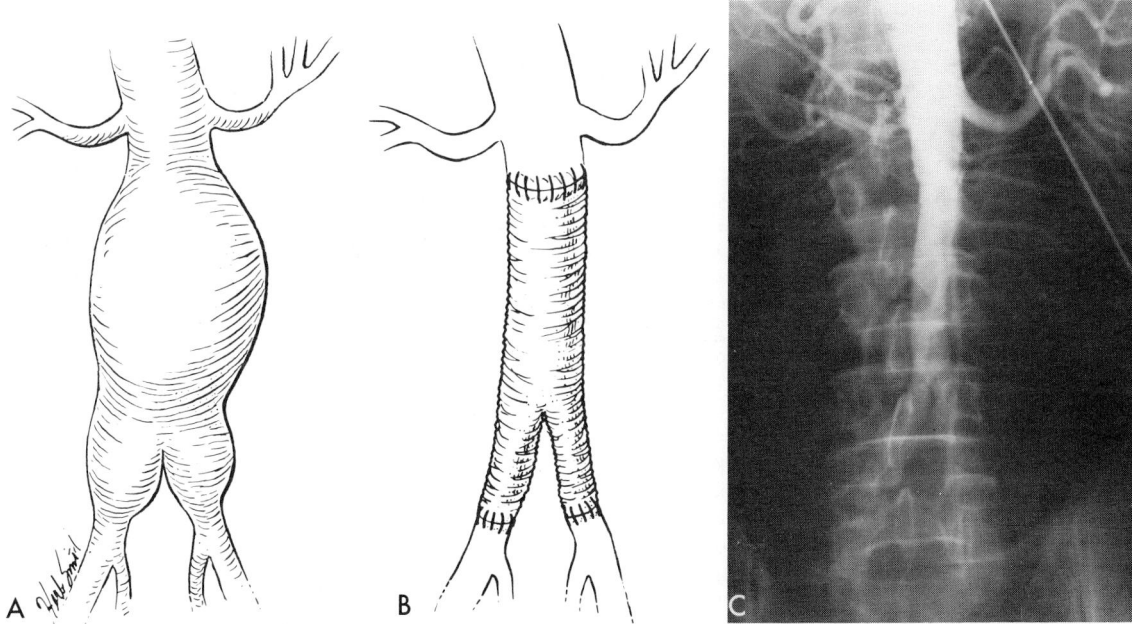

Figure 33. *A,* Characteristic type of arteriosclerotic aneurysm arising just below renal arteries and involving both common iliac arteries. *B,* Treatment by resection and replacement with bifurcation Dacron graft. *C,* Aortogram made five years after operation, showing restoration of normal circulation. In the majority of patients, it is possible to perform an end-to-end anastomosis to the distal aorta rather than to the iliacs. (From DeBakey, M. E., Crawford, E. S., Cooley, D. A., Morris, G. C., Jr., Royster, T. S., and Abbott, W. P.: Ann. Surg., *160*:622, 1964.)

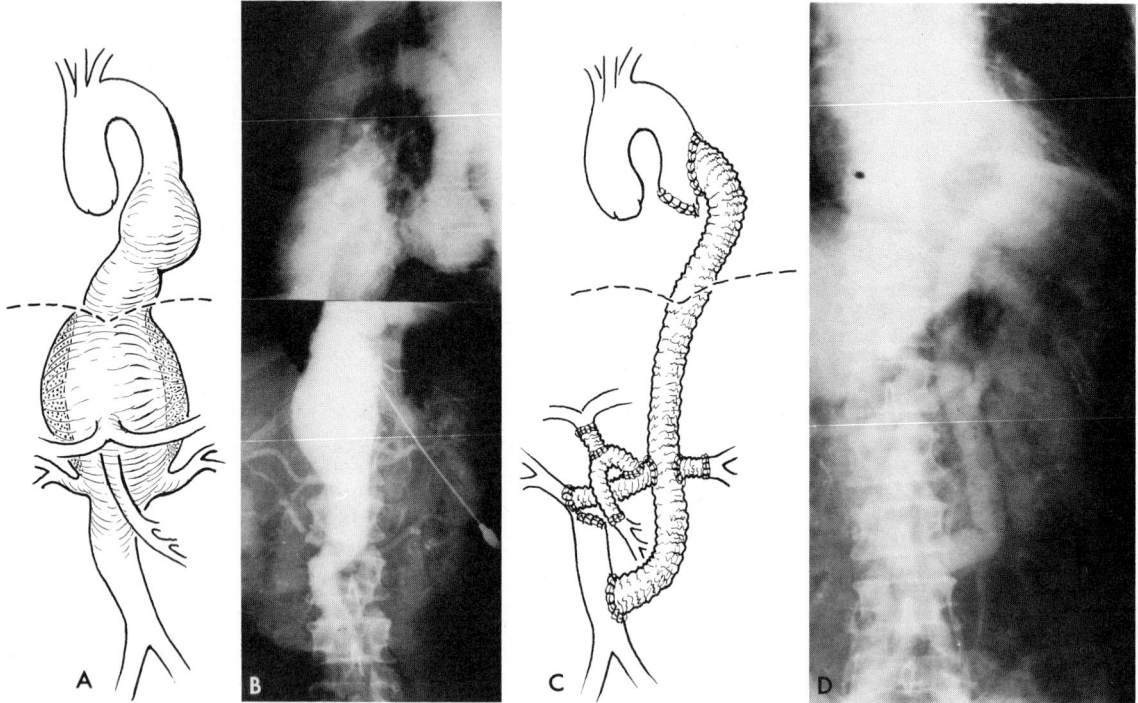

Figure 34. *A*, Drawing; and *B*, aortogram before operation, demonstrating arteriosclerotic thoracoabdominal aortic aneurysm in a 54-year-old male. *C*, Drawing illustrating method of resection and graft placement. *D*, Aortogram after operation, showing satisfactory function of graft replacements. Patient remains well five years after operation. (From DeBakey, M. E., Crawford, E. S., Garrett, H. E., Beall, A. C., Jr., and Howell, J. F.: Ann Surg., *162*:650, 1965.)

the bifurcation type is usually reserved for use when the iliac arteries are involved in an aneurysm. The results of this operation have been highly satisfactory. Prophylactic antibiotics are administered several hours preoperatively and for several days following operation.

Certain special features of the operative approach deserve emphasis. During the procedure, it is possible to dislodge thrombi from the aortic aneurysm, which may embolize distally and cause arterial obstruction. Therefore, it is important to demonstrate good back bleeding from both iliac arteries and to determine the presence of pulses in the femoral, popliteal, posterior tibial, and dorsal pedal arteries at the end of the procedure. Should discrepancy occur in postoperative pulses compared with those present preoperatively, arterial embolectomy should be considered by the Fogarty technique. Anomalies are also important and include the presence of a retroaortic left renal artery present in about 5 per cent of patients. Therefore, the left renal vein should be identified routinely in its normal anterior position, and if it is not present care must be taken to prevent injury to it when gaining proximal control of the abdominal aorta. The inferior vena cava may be transposed and found to the *left* of the aorta. In some instances, there is a duplication of the inferior vena cava, which represents a persistent left inferior vena cava. The vena cava may cross the aorta in the region of the renal vessels and constitute a circumaortic renal collar.[3] If the latter is present, division of the left inferior vena cava provides ade-

quate exposure. More than 30 patients with a horseshoe kidney associated with aortic abdominal aneurysm have been reported and present special operative problems.[2]

Rarely, aortic aneurysms are extensive and involve the lower thoracic aorta; these *thoracoabdominal aneurysms* pose difficult problems in surgical treatment. The celiac axis, superior mesenteric artery, and renal arteries may arise from the aneurysm. Therefore, surgical correction requires extensive dissection and mobilization, with tedious restoration of blood flow to each of these critical vessels. By total resection of the aneurysm and stepwise insertion of appropriate grafts, these lesions can be successfully treated (Fig. 34).[6]

In the patient presenting with a *ruptured* aortic abdominal aneurysm, an *emergency* operation should be undertaken immediately. The blood loss should be replaced rapidly, and as soon as the abdomen is entered, it is essential first to control the hemorrhage by proximal compression of the aorta. Large amounts of blood may be necessary in the resuscitation of these patients, and appropriate attention must be given to the temperature of the infused blood as well as to the administration of calcium. In those recovering from the immediate operative procedure, the effects of renal ischemia constitute the major cause of late deaths. Renal failure appearing postoperatively in these patients is usually associated with an unfavorable prognosis. However, aggressive management, including the use of early hemodialysis, often necessary for a number of weeks, may reduce the mortality and allow recovery of renal function.[5] The results in patients following ruptured aortic aneurysms have steadily improved and lower mortality figures have resulted.[22] Myocardial infarction may also occur, being precipitated by hypotension. The mortality varies between 30 and 50 per cent in operations for ruptured abdominal aortic aneurysms.[16]

POSTOPERATIVE COMPLICATIONS

Aortic abdominal aneurysmectomy is recognized to be a major operative procedure, and a number of specific postoperative complications may occur. Fortunately, the vast majority of patients recover without significant problems and are often discharged from the hospital within a week or 10 days. *Abdominal* distention, usually due to postoperative paralytic ileus, may occur and is usually self-limited. While some routinely use a nasogastric tube for several days postoperatively, this has proved to be unnecessary in at least three fourths of patients, who never require intestinal decompression postoperatively. However, if distention occurs or if a distended stomach or bowel can be demonstrated on physical examination or flat film of the abdomen, insertion of a nasogastric tube is indicated for either immediate decompression and removal or maintenance until release of the distention and return of peristalsis. Rarely, division of the inferior mesenteric artery, which is required during aneurysmectomy, may cause ischemia of the left colon, particularly the sigmoid colon. This problem should be identified prior to closure of the abdomen and if any question of viability arises, the inferior mesenteric artery should be reanastomosed to the graft. If this is not successful, the compromised colon should be exteriorized.

Bleeding from the graft retroperitoneally may occur at the suture line or through the interstices of the graft. Continuous measurement of the abdominal girth postoperatively is useful in addition to the usual measures for identification of reduced blood volume. Blood replacement may suffice if bleeding is minimal, but re-exploration should be performed if bleeding persists. Particular attention should be given the arterial circulation to the lower extremities, since emboli and thrombi may occur as a result of the operation or during the postoperative period.

Infection of the graft, especially at the suture lines, is a very serious complication, but, fortunately, is rare and occurs in less than 1 per cent in most series. Infection is particularly hazardous, since management is directed toward removal of the graft with occlusion of the terminal aorta by monofilament sutures or wire staples. Restoration of blood flow from an uninfected proximal area to the femoral vessels below, such as bilateral axillary femoral grafts, is indicated (Fig. 35).[12] Unless a procedure of this magnitude is undertaken, ultimate massive hemorrhage from the infected anastomotic site usually follows.

Rupture of the proximal suture line of the anastomosis into the duodenum or intestine also occurs and presents an equally serious complication. Occasionally, chronic bleeding occurs in such a communication, allowing time for appropriate diagnosis

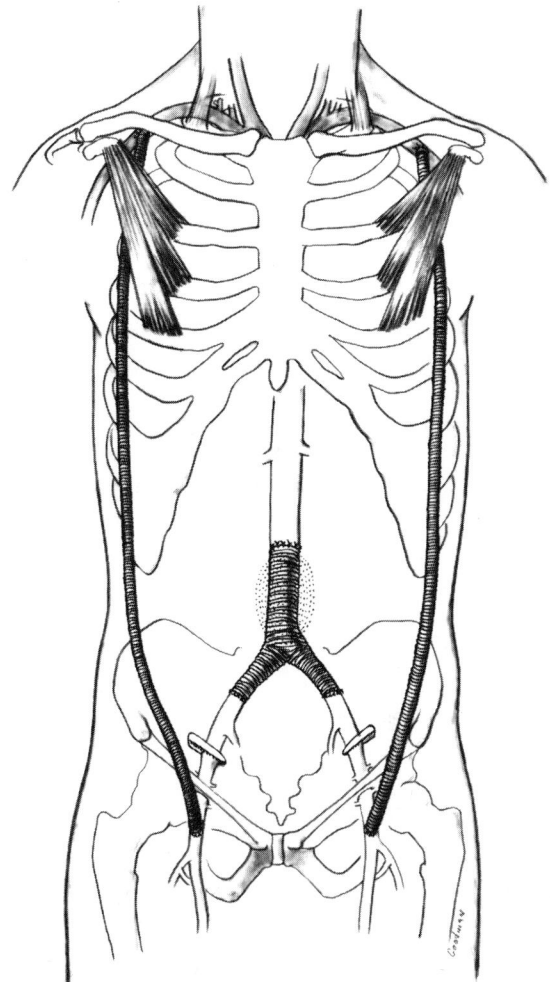

Figure 35. Diagrammatic illustration of patient with an infected aortic abdominal prosthetic graft treated with bilateral axillofemoral prosthetic grafts passed in subcutaneous tunnels on either side. The infected aortic graft was subsequently removed, with ligation of both iliac arteries and the terminal aorta. (From Hardy, J. D., and Conn, J. H. *In* Hardy, J. D. (Ed.): Critical Surgical Illness. Philadelphia, W. B. Saunders Company, 1971.)

and elective operation. In other instances, bleeding is sudden and massive, requiring emergency operation for control of the hemorrhage, closure of the duodenal or intestinal communication, and removal of the graft with appropriate reconstitution of blood flow through a noninfected area to the lower extremities.

False aneurysms also occur at the suture lines and may become manifest by *pain* or a pulsatile mass. In such instances, an appropriate diagnosis can be established by arteriography, while in other instances the first sign of such an aneurysm may be rupture.

Changes in sexual function are of considerable importance following resection of aortic abdominal aneurysms. Retrograde ejaculation has been frequently reported in as many as two thirds of patients following aneurysmectomy.[25] Loss of potency also occurs in as many as a third of patients, and these complications appear to be related to the extensiveness of the dissection at the time of operation. In the dissection, the inferior mesenteric sympathetic plexus, which lies along

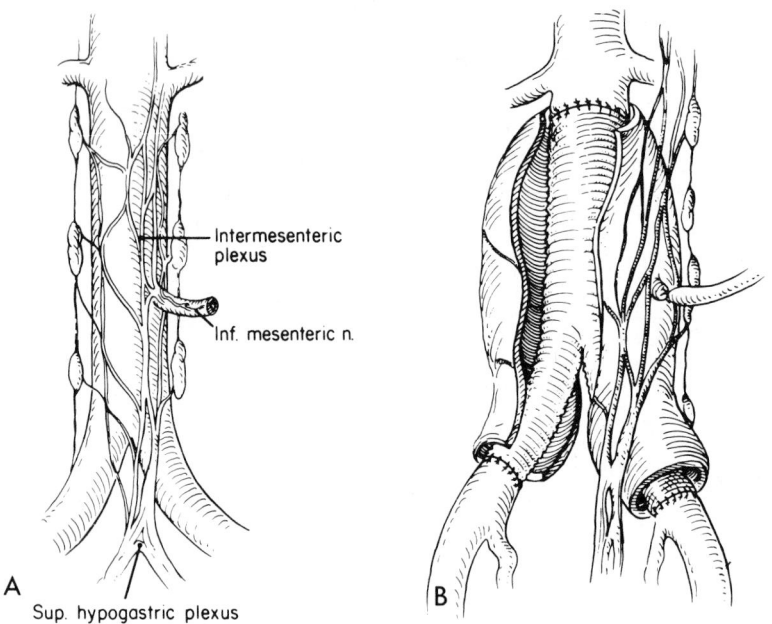

Figure 36. *A,* Normal sympathetic anatomy of distal abdominal aorta. *B,* Method of aortic aneurysmectomy preserving sympathetic plexi critical to normal sexual function. (From Weinstein, M. H., and Machleder, H. I.: Ann. Surg., *181*:787, 1975.)

the lower abdominal aorta on its left side and near the inferior mesenteric artery, should be left undisturbed (Fig. 36). If these safeguards are observed, interference with sexual function is minimized.

Spinal ischemia may follow abdominal aortic surgery.[10] Although infrequent, with less than 30 cases being reported in the literature, it appears to be somewhat more common in association with ruptured aortic abdominal aneurysms, perhaps aggravated by associated hypotension. However, rupture is not necessary and the phenomenon occurs with elective opera-

tions. The classic anterior spinal artery syndrome is characterized by paraplegia, rectal and urinary incontinence, loss of pain and temperature sensation, but with sparing of vibration and proprioceptive sense. Patients sustaining neurologic deficits in the lower extremities after abdominal aortic surgery commonly have loss of posterior column modalities.

RESULTS

Previously the mortality ranged from 5 to 18 per cent as reported in a collected review from nine medical centers in 1967,[1] but it has diminished in recent years and is now 5 per cent or lower in most centers.[24] The mortality is primarily due to associated lesions of atherosclerosis that complicate the postoperative recovery, including myocardial infarction, cerebrovascular lesions, and hypertensive cardiovascular renal disease.

The long-term results of resection of abdominal aortic aneurysms have been evaluated by DeBakey and associates, who report that 84 per cent of all patients operated on are alive at the end of 1 year, 72 per cent at 3 years, and 58 per cent at 5 years (Fig. 37).[7]

Iliac arterial aneurysms frequently occur either unilaterally or bilaterally in association with aortic abdominal aneurysms. Occasionally, an iliac aneurysm occurs as an isolated lesion. Both types should be managed by resection with prosthetic graft replacement.

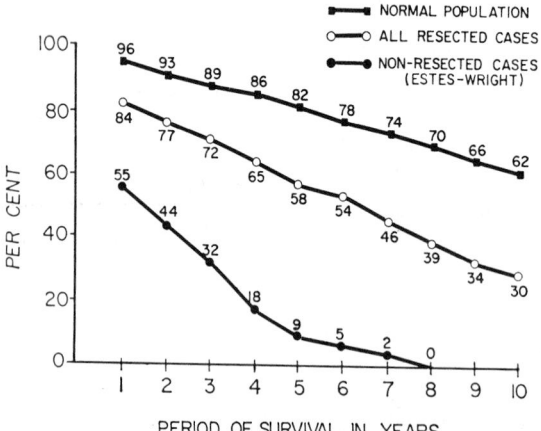

Figure 37. Life expectancy of patients with abdominal aortic aneurysm in the study of DeBakey et al., compared with that of the normal population adjusted for sex and age and with that of patients in a nonresected series by Estes and Wright and others. (From DeBakey, M. E., Crawford, E. S., Cooley, D. A., Morris, G. C., Jr., Royster, T. S., and Abbott, W. P.: Ann. Surg., *160*:622, 1964.)

SELECTED REFERENCES

Crawford, E. S.: Thoraco-abdominal and abdominal aortic aneurysms involving renal, superior mesenteric, and celiac arteries. Ann. Surg., *179*:763, 1974.

In this review, the management of 23 consecutive patients with thoracoabdominal aortic aneurysms involving the renal, superior mesenteric, and celiac arteries is presented. Emphasis is placed upon surgical technique, which depended upon the anatomic location of the aneurysm. A number of excellent illustrations are included and demonstrate the surgical procedures required. Of the 23 patients, 22 survived and did well for periods up to 13 years, indicating the feasibility of the extensive operations required in the management of these lesions.

DeBakey, M. E., Crawford, E. S., Cooley, D. A., Morris, G. C., Jr., Royster, T. S., and Abbott, W. P.: Aneurysm of abdominal aorta: Analysis of results of graft replacement therapy one to eleven years after operation. Ann. Surg., 160:622, 1964.
Long-term follow-up of the fate of patients with removal of abdominal aortic aneurysms is presented in this paper. The favorable prognosis following surgery is emphasized.

Estes, J. E., Jr.: Abdominal aortic aneurysm: A study of one hundred and two cases. Circulation, 2:258, 1950.
This is an often quoted study of the follow-up of a large group of patients with aortic abdominal aneurysms prior to the advent of surgical treatment.

Thompson, J. E., Hollier, L. H., Patman, R. D., and Persson, A. V.: Surgical management of abdominal aortic aneurysms: Factors influencing mortality and morbidity — A 20-year experience. Ann. Surg., 181:654, 1975.
The authors review a personal experience in a large group with aortic abdominal aneurysms undergoing elective resection over a 20-year period. The mortality diminished from 17 per cent during the first 7 years of the study to 5.5 per cent in the 1968–1974 period. Reasons for the diminishing mortality are presented.

REFERENCES

1. Bernstein, E. F., Fisher, J. C., and Varco, R. L.: Is excision the optimum treatment for all abdominal aortic aneurysms? Surgery, 61:83, 1967.
2. Bietz, D., and Merendino, K. A.: Abdominal aortic aneurysm and horseshoe kidney. Ann. Surg., 181:333, 1975.
3. Brener, B. J., Darling, R. C., Frederick, P. L., and Linton, R. R.: Major venous anomalies complicating abdominal aortic surgery. Arch. Surg., 108:159, 1974.
4. Brewster, D. C., Retana, A., Waltman, A. C., and Darling, R. C.: Angiography in the management of aneurysms of the abdominal aorta. Its value and safety. N. Engl. J. Med., 292:822, 1975.
5. Chawla, S. K., Najafi, H., Ing, T. S., Dye, W. S., Javid, H., Hunter, J. A., Goldin, M. D., and Serry, C.: Acute renal failure complicating ruptured abdominal aortic aneurysm. Arch. Surg., 110:521, 1975.
6. Crawford, E. S.: Thoraco-abdominal and abdominal aortic aneurysms involving renal, superior mesenteric, and celiac arteries. Ann. Surg., 179:763, 1974.
7. DeBakey, M. E., Crawford, E. S., Cooley, D. A., Morris, G. C., Jr., Royster, T. S., and Abbott, W. P.: Aneurysm of abdominal aorta: Analysis of results of graft replacement therapy one to eleven years after operation. Ann. Surg., 160:622, 1964.
8. Dubost, C., Allary, M., and Oeconomos, N.: Resection of an aneurysm of the abdominal aorta: Reestablishment of the continuity by a preserved human arterial graft, with results after five months. Arch. Surg., 64:405, 1952.
9. Estes, J. E., Jr.: Abdominal aortic aneurysm: A study of one hundred and two cases. Circulation, 2:258, 1950.
10. Ferguson, L. R. J., Bergan, J. J., Conn, J., Jr., and Yao, J. S. T.: Spinal ischemia following abdominal aortic surgery. Ann. Surg., 181:267, 1975.
11. Gliedman, M. L., Ayers, W. B., and Vestal, B. L.: Aneurysms of the abdominal aorta and its branches. A study of untreated patients. Ann. Surg., 146:207, 1957.
12. Hardy, J. D., and Conn, J. H.: Infected arterial grafts. *In* Hardy, J. D. (Ed.): Critical Surgical Illness. Philadelphia, W. B. Saunders Company, 1971.
13. Jarrett, F., Darling, R. C., Mundth, E. D., and Austen, W. G.: Experience with infected aneurysms of the abdominal aorta. Arch. Surg., 110:1281, 1975.
14. Johnson, J. M., Gaspar, M. R., Movius, H. J., and Rosental, J. J.: Sudden complete thrombosis of aortic and iliac aneurysms. Arch. Surg., 108:792, 1974.
15. Klippel, A. P., and Butcher, H. R., Jr.: The unoperated abdominal aortic aneurysm. Am. J. Surg., 111:629, 1966.

10. FEMORAL ARTERY ANEURYSMS

William J. Fry, M.D.

John Erichsen stated in his text *The Science and Art of Surgery,* published in 1877, "It occasionally, though rarely, happens that a varicose aneurysm is formed in the groin or upper part of the thigh." He further stated, "The treatment of this disease is exceedingly unsatisfactory. Of four cases in which the external iliac artery was tied, a fatal termination occurred in every instance." Bernheim, in his textbook, *Surgery of the Vascular System,* published in 1913, reported 66 cases of femoral artery aneurysm with a recovery rate of 92 per cent. He used the method advocated by Halsted of gradual occlusion of the external iliac artery in an effort to stimulate collateral circulation. Using this technique, followed by endoaneurysmorrhaphy after the method of Matas, he was able to achieve a very satisfactory cure rate, with a 6.3 per cent incidence of amputation.

The most common etiologic factor in the development of femoral artery aneurysm is atherosclerosis. With the advent of peripheral vascular reconstructive surgical techniques, an increased incidence of false aneurysms associated with aortofemoral bypass has been seen. The incidence and etiologic factors, as well as the method of management, are well outlined by Szilagyi and his associates.[6] The third most common type of femoral artery aneurysm is that associated with trauma, secondary to either penetrating or blunt injury. The common sequela of trauma in the femoral area is disruption of the femoral artery. A high incidence of false aneurysm and arteriovenous fistula formation is seen after penetrating wounds of the groin, and, although rare in the past, an increasing number of bacterial aneurysms are being observed. These are, by and large, due to bacteria resistant to the usual antibiotics. In the past, they were almost always the result of Salmonella infection. Recently, bacterial aneurysms are being seen secondary to coagulase-positive Staphylococcus infections that are resistant to most antibiotics. Aneurysmal formation anywhere in the body associated with sepsis should be suspected to have infection as the main etiologic factor. The rarest of etiologic factors in the formation of a femoral artery aneurysm is that of dissection. Arterial dissections starting in the area of the distal external iliac or in the main portion of the femoral artery are exceedingly rare. The most common sequence of events seen with dissection involving the femoral artery is a dissection originating in the aorta and continuing down into the area of the femoral artery.

The diagnosis of femoral artery aneurysm is usually self-evident on thorough physical examination. The palpation of a smooth, dilated femoral artery with expansile pulsation is, in most instances, sufficient to make the absolute diagnosis. In an occasional patient, because of obesity, scar tissue formation, or heavy musculature, some doubt may be present after careful physical examination. In such instances, the use of ultrasound scanning may be of help in delineating the size of the femoral artery.

Whenever a femoral artery aneurysm is suspected or diagnosed on physical examination, a complete arteriogram of the abdominal aorta, iliac, femoral, and tibial vessels should be obtained. We have found that 95 per cent of patients with a femoral artery aneurysm have some other associated aneurysm within their arterial tree.[3] The majority of these were associated aortoiliac artery aneurysms. Fifty-nine per cent of atherosclerotic, femoral artery aneurysms were found to be bilateral.

The natural history of atherosclerotic femoral artery aneurysms is usually one of eventual occlusion or embolization, with resulting ischemia of the lower extremity. Spontaneous rupture of an atherosclerotic femoral artery aneurysm is a rare event. Because of the musculofascial compartment surrounding the common femoral artery, exsanguination is not the usual sequence, as it is with abdominal aortic aneurysm rupture. Tamponade usually occurs with marked ischemia of the distal portion of the involved extremity. Most femoral artery aneurysms are lined with laminated thrombi. The thrombus lyses and portions are washed downstream, forming embolic occlusion in the popliteal or tibial vessels. Careful examination of the patient with a femoral artery aneurysm will usually demonstrate multiple, small, petechial hemorrhages in the distal portion of the extremity. These are secondary to microemboli from the interior of the aneurysmal sac.

Cutler and Darling classified femoral artery aneurysms, and this was further modified by Barker.[1, 2] The classification is shown in Table 4.

The techniques of reconstruction of the femoral artery after aneurysmectomy are shown in Figure 38. The preference, whenever possible, is to utilize autogenous saphenous vein. When this is not possible because of previous vein stripping or marked disparity in size, we do not hesitate to use a Dacron prosthesis. The disadvantages of using a Dacron prosthesis over a joint, with subsequent angulation, thrombus formation, and eventual occlusion are well known. We have

TABLE 4.   Types of Femoral Artery Aneurysms

Type   I   Terminating proximal to the orifice of the superficial and deep femoral arteries

Type II   Involving the superficial and deep femoral arteries

Type III   A. Femoral artery aneurysm with occlusion of the superficial femoral artery
             B. Femoral artery aneurysm with occlusion of the deep femoral artery

Type IV   Aneurysms of the deep femoral artery

Type V   Aneurysms of the superficial femoral artery

not had a problem with this in the reconstruction of femoral artery aneurysms, primarily because the prosthesis is usually very short and, therefore, not subject to the buckling seen in longer prostheses. The second drawback to the use of a prosthesis in the groin is the hazard of infection. The skin of the groin is exceedingly difficult to clean, and the chance for bacterial contamination at the time of operation is always a hazard. Meticulous cleansing of the groin, utilizing a technique of not shaving the skin until immediately prior to operation, combined with prophylactic antibiotics, has made the incidence of graft infection relatively low (1.23 per cent).[4, 5, 7] The difficulties with a cloth prosthesis in the area of the groin have led Stoney and his associates to utilize a portion of autologous iliac artery with the substitution of the prosthesis to replace this within the abdomen.[8] We have not generally subscribed to his technique, as it increases operative time, and with a relatively low incidence of graft infection, we have not felt that it was universally indicated.

The results of arterial reconstruction of the femoral artery are excellent, with a mortality rate approach-

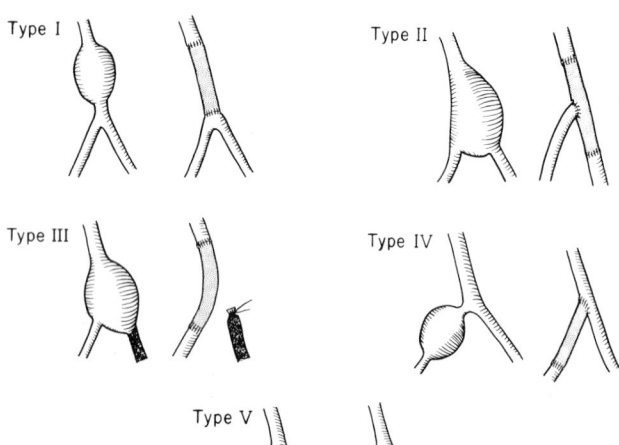

Figure 38. Methods of reconstruction of femoral artery aneurysms.

ing zero. Cutler and Darling have reported a series of 63 arteriosclerotic aneurysms treated surgically with a zero operative mortality. They, in addition, show the superiority of vein graft replacement with a 100 per cent long-term patency rate, versus a 94 per cent patency rate using a Dacron prosthesis. The numbers, however, are small enough that this is not statistically significant. We have noted similar results in a smaller series.

All patients, after repair of a femoral artery aneurysm, should be followed closely. This is particularly true in that group of patients who have a Dacron prosthesis in place. The incidence of false aneurysm formation at the suture line and secondary infection, while low, may be life- or limb-threatening if unrecognized for a long period of time. Because of the propensity of arterial aneurysms to develop at other sites, careful periodic examination is important.

SELECTED REFERENCES

Cutler, B. S., and Darling, R. C.: Surgical management of arteriosclerotic femoral aneurysms. Surgery, 74:764–773, 1973.
This is a good review of the problem of femoral artery aneurysm with the results of 45 patients treated by resectional therapy for femoral artery aneurysm.

Dent, T. L., Lindenauer, S. M., Ernst, C. B., and Fry, W. J.: Multiple arteriosclerotic arterial aneurysms. Arch. Surg., 105:338–344, 1972.
Review of the multiplicity of peripheral artery aneurysms.

REFERENCES

1. Barker, W. F.: Peripheral Arterial Disease. Philadelphia, W. B. Saunders Company, 1975.
2. Cutler, B. S., and Darling, R. C.: Surgical management of arteriosclerotic femoral aneurysms. Surgery, 74:764–773, 1973.
3. Dent, T. L., Lindenauer, S. M., Ernst, C. B., and Fry, W. J.: Multiple arteriosclerotic arterial aneurysms. Arch. Surg., 105:338–344, 1972.
4. Fry, W. J.: Vascular prosthesis infections. Surg. Clin. North Am., 52:1419–1424, 1972.
5. Fry, W. J., and Lindenauer, S. M.: Infection complicating the use of plastic arterial implants. Arch. Surg., 94:600–609, 1967.
6. Szilagyi, D. E., Smith, R. F., Elliott, J. P., Hageman, J. H., and Dall'Olmo, C. A.: Anastomotic aneurysms after vascular reconstruction: Problems of incidence, etiology and treatment. Surgery, 78:800–816, 1975.
7. Szilagyi, D. E., Smith, R. F., Elliott, J. P., and Vrandecic, M. P.: Infection in arterial reconstruction with synthetic grafts. Ann. Surg., 176:321, 1972.
8. Stoney, R. J., and Wylie, E. J.: Arterial autografts. Surgery, 67:18–25, 1970.

11. POPLITEAL ARTERY ANEURYSMS

William J. Fry, M.D.

. . . a signal instance of the living force there is in facts when they are stored in a thoughtful mind.

— Sir James Paget*

---

*Commenting on John Hunter's discovery of collateral circulation and relating it to the treatment of popliteal aneurysms.

The treatment of popliteal aneurysms has been a challenge to skilled surgeons for over 2000 years. The first recorded operation for popliteal aneurysm was by Antyllus, a Greek surgeon. in the second century A.D. He ligated the popliteal artery proximal and distal to the aneurysm and incised and packed the aneurysmal sac. John Hunter, in 1785, ligated the superficial femoral artery in a coachman with a large popliteal artery aneurysm. The leg survived and the coachman returned to his occupation, only to succumb to pneumonia four months after the operative procedure. Desault, the French surgeon, preceded Hunter in the performance of this operation seven months earlier. His operation was not based on the recognition of collateral circulation as was Hunter's. Limb salvage rates utilizing the Hunterian principle were as high as 87 per cent. Rudolph Matas advocated endoaneurysmorrhaphy for the therapy of popliteal aneurysms. He first performed this operation in 1888 and in 1920 reported a series of 154 popliteal aneurysms treated by this technique. The operative mortality was 0.6 per cent and the amputation rate was 5.2 per cent. These results represented a remarkable achievement in the days preceding arteriography, antibiotics, and adequate anesthesia.

Etiologic factors resulting in popliteal aneurysm formation are the same as those delineated in the section on femoral artery aneurysms. The majority of popliteal aneurysms seen today are secondary to atherosclerosis. The incidence of aneurysms secondary to bacterial invasion of the arterial wall is slightly higher in the popliteal area than it is in the femoral artery. As with infected femoral artery aneurysms, the Staphylococcus organism plays a very large role.

The diagnosis of a popliteal artery aneurysm is most commonly made by physical examination. The findings of an aneurysm in the popliteal space are sometimes subtle and may be missed by the inexperienced. Popliteal artery aneurysms seldom involve the distal popliteal artery and more commonly are high in the region of the knee. They may be masked by the heavy-muscled leg and without the patient properly relaxed may be very difficult to palpate. Ultrasound scanning is a readily available, noninvasive diagnostic procedure that serves as a good screening technique to make the diagnosis of popliteal aneurysm when there is some question on physical examination.

Arteriography, as with femoral artery aneurysm, is mandatory for several reasons. Popliteal aneurysms are bilateral in 47 per cent of patients. In addition to this, 78 per cent of patients with popliteal aneurysms have another aneurysm somewhere in the arterial tree. The majority, 64 per cent, are located in the abdominal aorta or iliac arteries. Popliteal artery aneurysms are notorious for being associated with distal occlusive disease. The laminated thrombus within the wall of the aneurysm forms the basis for distal embolization. The constant trauma secondary to the bending of the knee joint undoubtedly adds to fragmentation of the intraluminal thrombus. Accurate arteriography to delineate the outflow tract is always necessary prior to any operative approach in the treatment of a popliteal artery aneurysm.

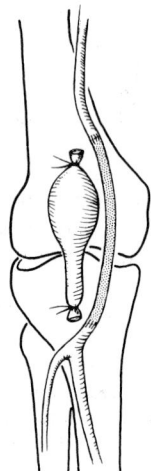

Figure 39. Preferred technique in therapy for popliteal artery aneurysm.

The most common sequela in the untreated popliteal artery aneurysm is distal arterial occlusion. Careful examination of the distal extremity in the patient with a popliteal artery aneurysm will almost always reveal areas of petechial hemorrhage secondary to small emboli. As the laminated thrombus collection progresses within the aneurysmal sac, three things may occur: (1) extensive embolization, which may occlude the outflow tract, (2) laminated thrombus, which may occlude the orifices of the popliteal trifurcation, and (3) complete thrombosis of the aneurysm. These possibilities are limb-threatening and the possibility of arterial reconstruction to maintain viability of the extremity may be slight.

Popliteal aneurysm rupture is not a common occurrence. As with the femoral artery aneurysm, the patient is not likely to exsanguinate because of the strong musculofascial compartment surrounding the popliteal artery. Rupture will usually tamponade and the resulting ischemia to the distal leg will be severe. Attempts at arterial reconstruction after rupture are difficult, and the ability to restore viability may be compromised. Large popliteal aneurysms may cause chronic or acute venous obstruction, and thrombophlebitis is not an uncommon associated finding with the acutely expanding popliteal artery aneurysm.

We have used the medial approach to the popliteal artery aneurysm. The utilization of an autogenous saphenous vein is preferred. Figure 39 illustrates the arterial reconstruction that we have routinely used in the management of popliteal aneurysms. It is impor-

tant not to attempt an excision of the popliteal artery aneurysm, as invariable damage to the popliteal vein will occur. By trapping the aneurysm as illustrated, and utilizing a proximal and distal end-to-end anastomosis, we have been able to restore blood flow with excellent long-term results.

Some prefer the posterior approach to the popliteal aneurysm. We believe that this is too extensive, and the great amount of dissection required in this approach is unnecessary. Recently, Towne and his associates have summarized their experience with popliteal artery aneurysms utilizing Dacron bypass grafts.[5] Their long-term results have been good; however, they have a patency rate of only 53 per cent at the end of seven years. While this is the only long-term follow-up of patients treated for popliteal artery aneurysms, one cannot help but question the role that a Dacron prosthesis plays in the high rate of occlusion. The utilization of the saphenous vein has allowed us an 82 per cent patency rate at four years. It is evident from Towne's report that Dacron is an adequate substitute for saphenous vein, as there was a very low amputation rate in their patients.

As for any patient having an operative procedure for aneurysmal disease, the patient who has had repair of a popliteal aneurysm should be followed indefinitely. The evidence of multiplicity of aneurysms, as well as the ever-present hazard of occlusion of either a saphenous vein or Dacron graft replacement, makes it mandatory that these patients be followed very carefully.

SELECTED REFERENCES

Edmonds, L. H., Jr., Darling, R. C., and Linton, R. R.: Surgical management of popliteal aneurysms. Circulation, 32:517–523, 1965. *An analysis of 98 popliteal aneurysms in 82 patients treated by surgery at the Massachusetts General Hospital from 1948 to 1963.*

Evans, W. E., Conley, J. E., and Bernard, V.: Popliteal aneurysms. Surgery, 70:762–767, 1971. *Excellent review of the problem.*

REFERENCES

1. Dent, T. L., Lindenauer, S. M., Ernst, C. B., and Fry, W. J.: Multiple arteriosclerotic arterial aneurysms. Arch. Surg., 105:338–344, 1972.
2. Edmonds, L. H., Jr., Darling, R. C., and Linton, R. R.: Surgical management of popliteal aneurysms. Circulation, 32:517–523, 1965.
3. Evans, W. E., Conley, J. E., and Bernhard, V.: Popliteal aneurysms. Surgery, 70:762–767, 1971.
4. Gifford, R. W., Jr., Hines, E. A., Jr., and Janes, J. M.: An analysis and follow-up study of one hundred popliteal aneurysms. Surgery, 33:284–293, 1953.
5. Towne, J. B., Thompson, J. E., Patman, R. D., and Persson, A. F.: Progression of popliteal aneurysmal disease following popliteal aneurysm resection with graft: A 20-year experience. Surgery, 80:426–432, 1976.

VI

THROMBO-OBLITERATIVE DISEASE OF THE AORTA AND ITS BRANCHES

David C. Sabiston, Jr., M.D.

Occlusive disease of the major branches of the aorta is most frequently the result of atherosclerosis. Certain arterial anatomic sites are especially susceptible to development of stenoses or total occlusion, and these are generally at the origins of vessels, where *turbulence* may be present (Fig. 1).[4] When branches of the aortic arch (innominate, carotid, subclavian) become stenotic or occluded, the symptoms produced represent ischemic disturbances due to diminution in blood flow to the cerebral circulation and to the upper extremities. In younger patients, especially women, an obliterative endarteritis, Takayasu's disease ("pulseless disease"), may produce similar symptoms.

CLINICAL MANIFESTATIONS

The subclavian artery is most commonly involved and is followed in incidence by the carotids and in-

nominate artery. The location and extent of a large number of lesions reported in one series are shown in Table 1.[1] The *symptoms* vary depending upon the nature and extent of the obstruction. Moreover, the natural development of *collateral* circulation that follows arterial occlusion and its effectiveness are of prime importance. The symptoms are primarily (1) neurologic, relating to diminished blood flow to the brain, and (2) those producing *ischemia* of the upper extremities causing claudication. The distribution of symptoms is shown in Table 2.[1] The diagnosis is confirmed by *arteriography* with use of multiple roentgenographic exposures to present the films in a series, thus demonstrating the lesion and the collateral blood supply around it.

SURGICAL MANAGEMENT

The surgical management of patients with occlusive disease is primarily accomplished by bypass grafts (Fig. 2).[1] The preoperative and postoperative obstructions as demonstrated by arteriography are shown, as well as the pressure gradient present before and after correction. The results of surgical bypass treatment are encouraging, as shown in Table 3.[1] In this series, obstruction was incomplete in 168 and complete in 244 of the arteries involved. Regardless of the extent of obstruction, the occlusive process was *segmental* in almost every instance. The surgical treatment most often is a bypass graft, but endarterectomy is at times applicable.

1. TAKAYASU'S ARTERITIS

Takayasu's disease, described by a Japanese ophthalmologist in 1908,[6] is a nonspecific arteritis affecting the thoracic and abdominal aorta and its major branches. Relatively rare in the United States, it is quite common in the Orient and usually attacks young females (85 per cent of cases). The arteritis involves all layers of the aortic wall, with proliferation of connective tissue and degeneration of the elastic fibers. Granulomatous lesions may be present with associated fusiform or saccular aneurysmal formation. Three types of this disorder are now recognized (Fig. 3).[2]

The *clinical manifestations* of Takayasu's arteritis are at first generalized and include fever, malaise, arthritis, and arthralgia. Pericardial pain, tachycardia, and vomiting may also occur. It has been suggested

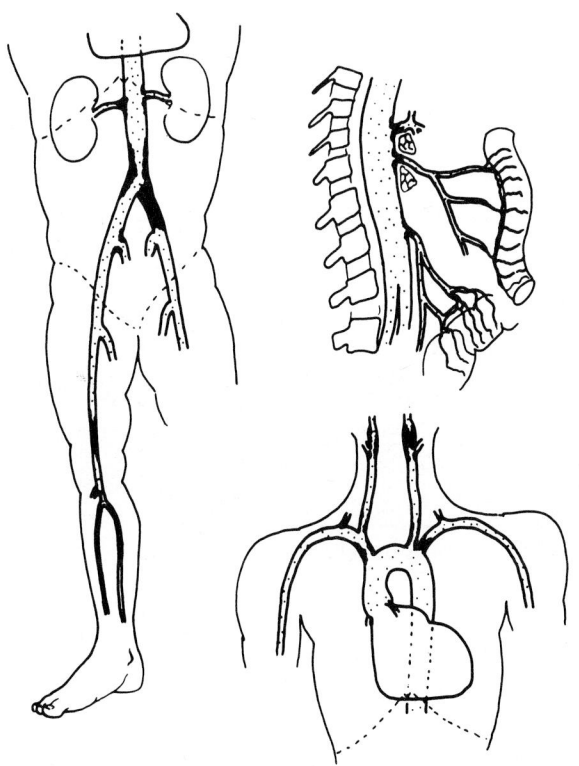

Figure 1. Anatomic sites particularly apt to become stenotic or occluded by atherosclerosis. (From Ludbrook, J., and Elmslie, R. G.: An Introduction to Surgery: 100 Topics. New York, Academic Press, 1971.)

TABLE 1.   Location and Extent of 412 Lesions in 299 Patients*

Location	Extent of Obstruction		Totals
	Incomplete	Complete	
Innominate artery	40	26	66
Right common carotid artery	5	19	24
Right subclavian artery	30	29	59
Left common carotid artery	24	37	61
Left subclavian artery	69	133	202
Total	168	244	412

*From Crawford, E. S., DeBakey, M. E., Morris, G. C., Jr., and Howell, J. F.: Surgery, 65:17, 1969.

TABLE 2.   Symptoms of Occlusion (299 Patients)*

Type of Symptom	No. of Patients	Per Cent
Neurological only	97	32
Neurological and upper extremity ischemia	124	42
Upper extremity ischemia	63	21
Systolic ear noise	3	1
No symptoms	12	4
Total	299	100

*From Crawford, E. S., DeBakey, M. E., Morris, G. C., Jr., and Howell, J. F.: Surgery. 65:17, 1969.

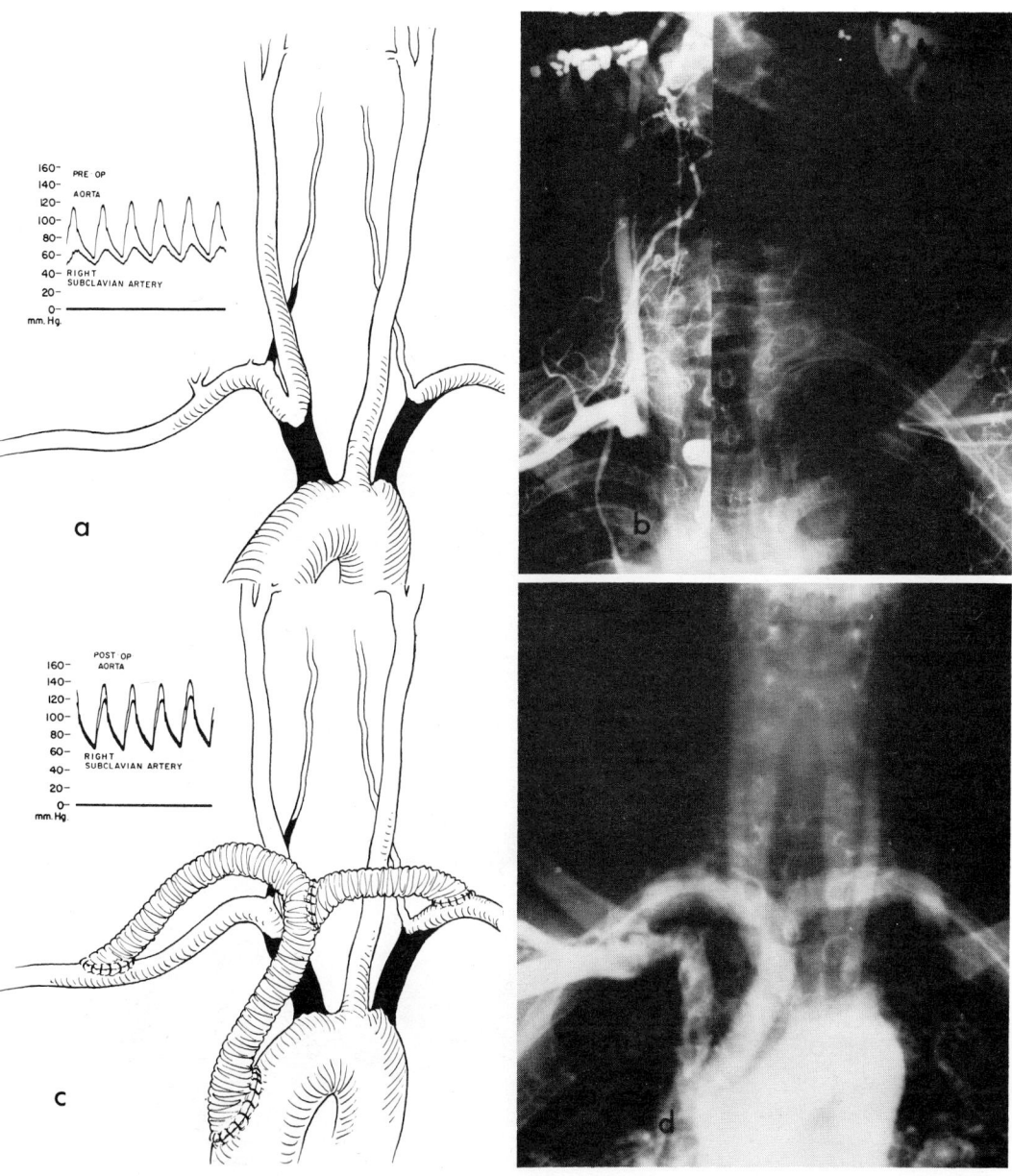

Figure 2. Patient with obstruction of innominate and left subclavian arteries, causing cerebral arterial insufficiency, and obstruction of the abdominal aorta and iliac arteries, causing both intermittent claudication and ischemic lesions of the feet. The patient was treated first at one operation by ascending aortobilateral subclavian bypass graft, and at a second operation by bilateral aortoexternal iliac artery bypass graft, relieving all symptoms. Diagram (a) and arteriogram (b) with pressure recording made before bypass show location and extent of innominate and subclavian lesions. Diagram (c) and aortogram (d) made 3 years after operation and pressure recordings made at operation after bypass show grafts in place and functioning.

Illustration continued on following page

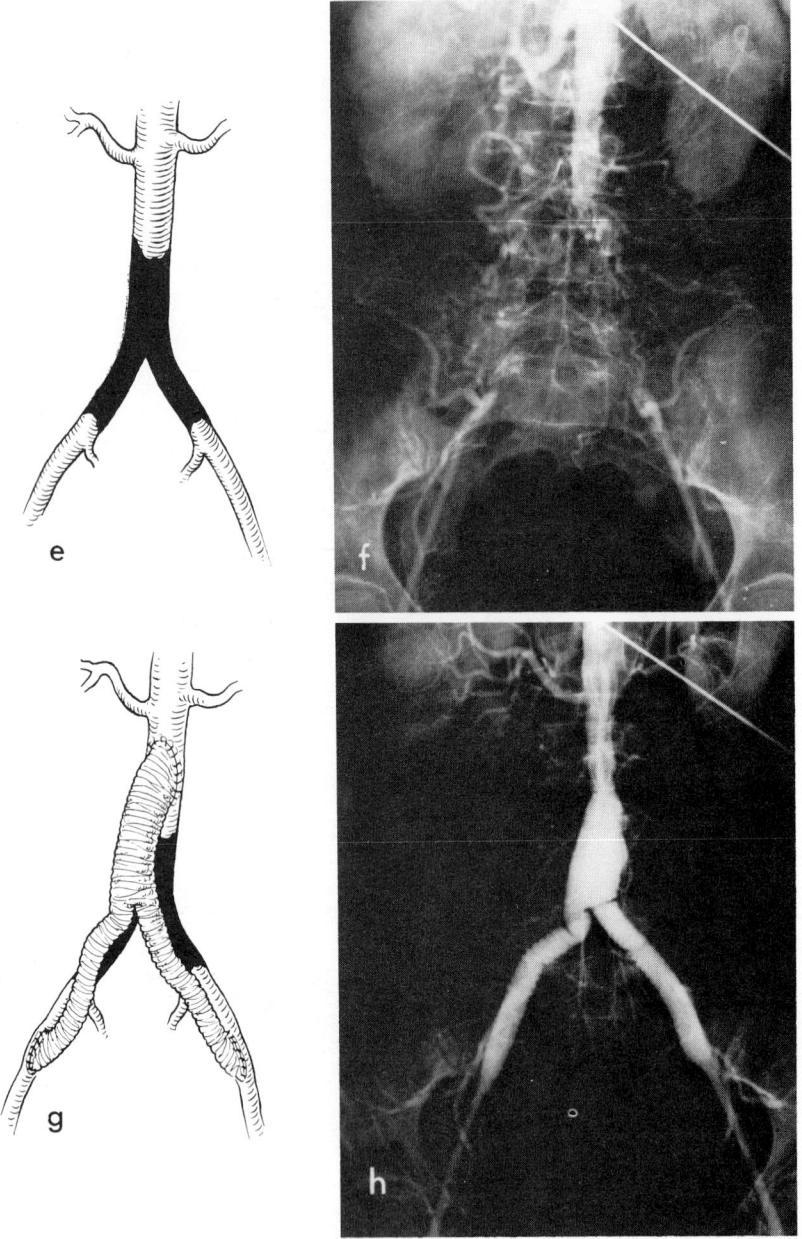

Figure 2. *Continued*
 Diagram (e) and aortogram (f) made before operation show location and extent of aortoiliac obstruction. Diagram (g) and aortogram (h) made 3 years after operation show graft in place and functioning. The patient is alive and well five years after operation. (From Crawford, E. S., DeBakey, M. E., Morris, G. C., Jr., and Howell, J. F.: Surgery, 65:17, 1969.)

TABLE 3.   Functional Results in 299 Patients with Occlusion of Great Vessels
of the Aortic Arch*

Time of Follow-up	Asymptomatic, Improved		Unimproved		Worse		Dead	
	No.	Per Cent	No.	Per Cent	No.	Per Cent	No.	Per Cent
Immediate	268	89.6	10	3.3	5	1.7	16	5.4
Late	274	91.6	3	1.0	6	2.0	43	14.4

*From Crawford, E. S., DeBakey, M. E., Morris, G. C., Jr., and Howell, J. F.: Surgery, 65:17, 1969.

that the disorder may be an autoimmune disease,[5] and steroids may be beneficial. The later manifestations are those of ischemia of both the cerebral and upper extremity circuits. Surgical treatment of Takayasu's arteritis has often proved disappointing, since the end-arterectomy site and grafts are apt to reocclude. Operation is occasionally recommended for patients with disabling symptoms.[3]

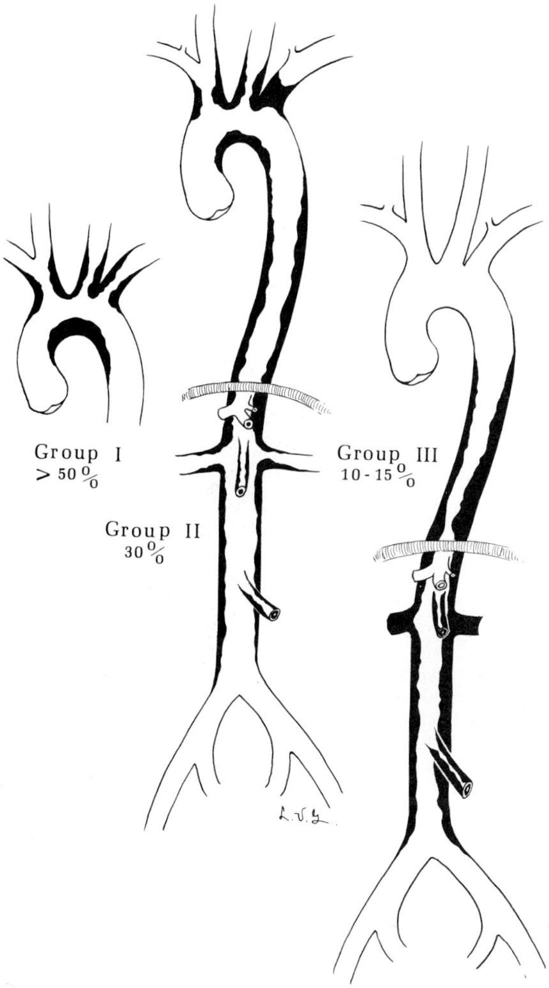

REFERENCES

1. Crawford, E. S., DeBakey, M. E., Morris, G. C., Jr., and Howell, J. F.: Surgical treatment of occlusion of the innominate, common carotid, and subclavian arteries: A 10 year experience. Surgery, 65:17, 1969.
2. Edmunds, L. H., Jr.: Trauma and occlusive disease. In Strandness, D. E., Jr. (Ed): Collateral Circulation in Clinical Surgery. Philadelphia, W. B. Saunders Company, 1969.
3. Ekeström, S., and Hansson, L. O.: Surgical treatment of "pulseless disease." Acta Chir. Scand., 128:127, 1964.
4. Ludbrook, J., and Elmslie, R. G.: An Introduction to Surgery: 100 Topics. New York, Academic Press, 1971.
5. Nakao, K., Ikeda, M., Kimata, S., Niitani, H., Miyahara, M., Ishimi, Z., Hashiba, K., Takeda, Y., Ozawa, T., Matsushita, S., and Kuramochi, M.: Takayasu's arteritis. Clinical report of eighty-four cases and immunological studies of seven cases. Circulation, 35:1141, 1967.
6. Takayasu, M.: Case of queer changes in central blood vessels of retina. Acta. Soc. Ophthal. Jap., 12:2554, 1908.

Figure 3. Clinical subdivisions of Takayasu's arteritis. The panarteritis may be localized to the aortic arch and great vessels (Group I), the distal thoracoabdominal aorta (Group III), or the entire aorta (Group II). (From Edmunds, L. H., Jr. In Strandness, D. E., Jr. (Ed.): Collateral Circulation in Clinical Surgery. Philadelphia, W. B. Saunders Company, 1969.)

Group I
> 50%

Group II
30%

Group III
10 - 15%

2.   CAROTID OCCLUSIVE DISEASE

Vallee L. Willman, M.D., and Hendrick B. Barner, M.D.

Considering the prevalence and the awesome presentation of stroke, there is little wonder that it has been described as a clinical entity since biblical times. Stroke has afflicted nine presidents of our nation and is considered to have influenced decisions of two, Woodrow Wilson and F. D. Roosevelt, during times of national emergency. The social and emotional impact of stroke on its victims and their families has been vividly described by several victims.[24, 35] In addition to causing 200,000 deaths annually in our country, stroke leaves even more people physically and emotionally crippled.[34] It is curious, then, that the importance of extracranial vascular disease as a cause of stroke has become generally recognized only in the past 20 years. Prior to 1950, the major treatises on stroke listed as etiology hemorrhage, thrombosis, and embolus, thrombosis being considered as an intracranial vascular phenomenon and embolus considered as having its origin within the heart. As recently as 1930, discussions on stroke listed hemorrhage as accounting for most instances, with intracranial thrombosis being the next most frequent cause. The failure to recognize extracranial vascular disease as a major cause of stroke is perhaps attributable to an overconcern that existed only a few years ago about the complications of cerebral arteriography, as well as the failure to examine vessels in the neck regularly in postmortem examination.

The possibility of extracranial vascular disease as a basis of stroke was suggested by Savory's report more than a hundred years ago of a woman with right hemiparesis and extracranial vascular occlusions.[32] Gowers in 1875 described a patient with left eye blindness and right hemiparesis, probably due to carotid occlusion.[21] Hunt in 1914 reported on 20 patients with hemiplegia, four of whom had diminished neck pulses.[25] Among 82 patients with evidence of cerebrovascular disease studied at autopsy, Hutchinson found that in 40 at least half of the lumen of either a carotid or vertebral artery or both was obliterated.[26] It was Fisher in two important reports (1951 and 1954) who drew attention to the relationship of disease of the carotid arteries in the neck and the several clinical patterns of cerebrovascular insufficiency.[18, 19] He described both partial and total occlusions of the carotid arteries on the basis of atherosclerosis, noting that the distal vessels were often free of disease. He suggested that operation might become a form of treatment. "It is even conceivable that some day vascular surgery will find a way to bypass the occluded portion of the artery during the period of ominous fleeting symptoms."[18] During the same year (1954), Eastcott, Pickering, and Rob reported on the resection of a stenotic area of the left carotid with relief of the recurrent signs of cerebral ischemia that had plagued the patient.[10] Reports of operative treatment of occlusion and stenosis have since appeared regularly as thousands of patients have been treated. The diagnosis and management of lesions of the extracranial vasculature are now major interests of vascular surgeons.[41]

The pathophysiology of stroke as a result of carotid artery disease has defied precise description. This is in part due to the complex and variable anatomic circulatory arrangements of the brain, the incompletely understood regulatory mechanisms of brain blood flow, the complex interrelationship of brain blood flow, the complex interrelationship of brain circulation with cardiorespiratory function, and the inability to easily assess regional brain blood flow.

The extracranial arterial blood supply of the brain is by four vessels: two internal carotids and two vertebrals. The two vertebrals join high in the neck to form the basilar. Within the cranium the two internal carotids and the basilar communicate rather freely with each other (Fig. 4). The major collateral circulation was described by Willis[39] in 1684 and is generally referred to as the "circle of Willis" (Fig. 5). Because of this arrangement, occlusion of one of the extracranial vessels is generally well compensated for by increased flow through the others. The adequacy of this collateral system, however, is limited at times by developmental or acquired variations.

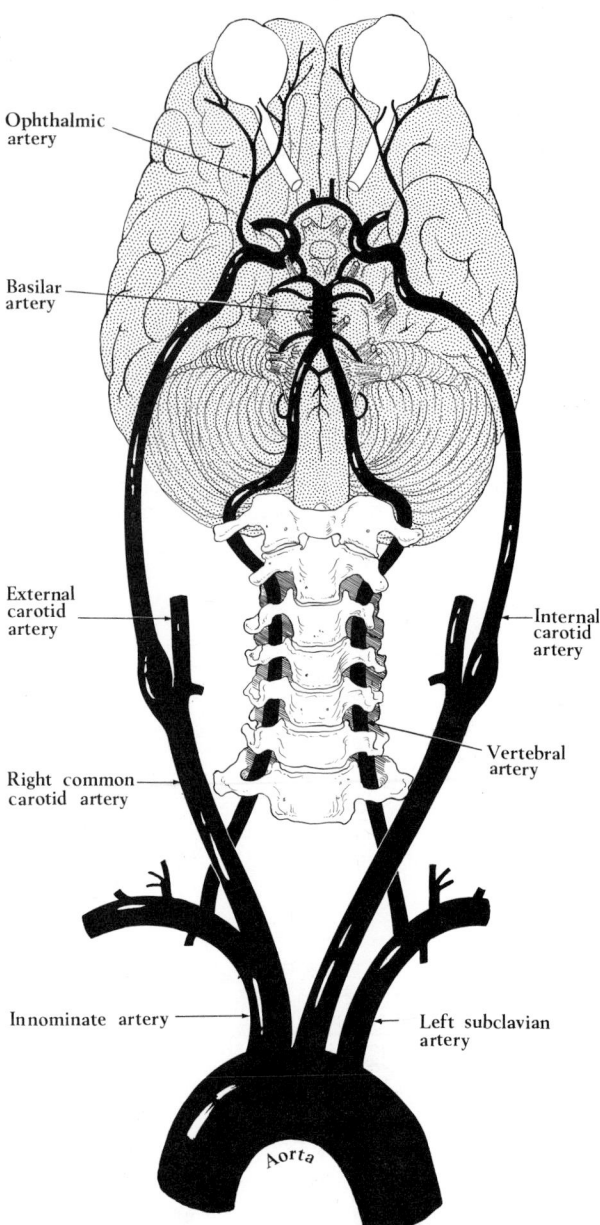

Figure 4. Diagram of major extracranial components of cerebral and ocular arterial supply. (From Wylie, E. J., and Ehrenfeld, W. K.: Extracranial Occlusive Cerebrovascular Disease. Philadelphia, W. B. Saunders Company, 1970.)

It is readily understandable that occlusive lesions in the extracranial vessels might reduce total flow to the brain below that level necessary to sustain normal brain function and thus result in stroke. It can be reasoned that lesions in the extracranial vessels progress through a stage in which brain blood flow is marginal, causing some slight aberrations in cerebral function, to the stage of occlusion, which results in clearly insufficient blood flow, with brain death and clinical stroke. Several studies have drawn a corollary between the clinical course of patients with stroke and

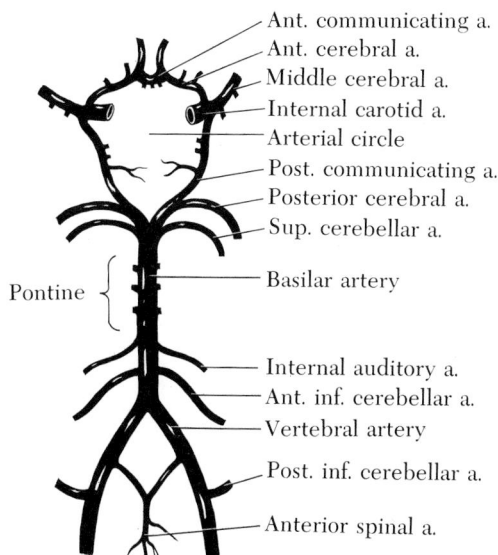

Ant. communicating a.
Ant. cerebral a.
Middle cerebral a.
Internal carotid a.
Arterial circle
Post. communicating a.
Posterior cerebral a.
Sup. cerebellar a.
Basilar artery
Pontine {
Internal auditory a.
Ant. inf. cerebellar a.
Vertebral artery
Post. inf. cerebellar a.
Anterior spinal a.

Figure 5. Diagram showing the most common configuration of the terminal branches of the vertebral and internal carotid arteries and their interconnections to form the circle of Willis. (From Wylie, E. J., and Ehrenfeld, W. K.: Extracranial Occlusive Cerebrovascular Disease. Philadelphia, W. B. Saunders Company, 1970.)

the extent of occlusive lesions in the carotids and vertebrals.[9, 17, 38] Repetitive angiographic studies have identified the natural tendency for lesions to progress.[3] In addition to continued aggregation of atheromatous material, the severity of obstruction can be enhanced by hemorrhage into the plaque itself or by thrombus formation on an ulcerated area.[40]

What is not easily explainable on the basis of decreased brain blood flow is the occurrence of brain dysfunction with only partially occlusive lesions in one carotid artery. It is well known that in most instances occlusion of one internal carotid artery is well tolerated. Why, then, should signs of cerebral ischemia occur in the presence of a partially occlusive lesion in one carotid?

Several possible explanations have been offered. One is that atherosclerosis is a generalized disease, and in most instances a process found in the internal carotid reflects the presence of multiple lesions throughout the cerebral vascular tree. Although cerebral vascular lesions are frequently multiple, they have not been found diffusely throughout the smaller vasculature of the brain. Indeed, vessels distal to a major stenosis are frequently free of disease. The occurrence of lesions in more than one of the four major extracranial vessels would logically explain variations in compensatory flow when there is flow limitation in one vessel, but it does not quite satisfy as an explanation of cerebral ischemia when lumen narrowing is no more than 50 per cent. Although a 50 per cent constriction of a carotid artery will often induce a pressure gradient across the area, experimental observations indicate that a reduction in area of approximately 90 per cent is necessary in order to reduce blood flow.[6, 13]

Transient ischemic attacks have been attributed to periods of hypotension and low cardiac output,[7, 8] yet the episodes have not been reproducible by artificially lowering blood pressure.[14, 27] Alteration in brain blood flow due to position has been proposed as a cause of transient ischemic attacks, but again the attacks have not been reproducible.

Embolization from ulcerated atherosclerotic lesions seems to offer the best explanation for transient ischemic attacks. Ulcerative lesions have been described both pathologically and radiographically.[30] (Fig. 6). Atheromatous emboli have been observed in retinal vessels[12] (Fig. 7). Fisher has observed an embolus passing through the retinal vessels of a patient who experienced repeated transient ischemic attacks, and he recognized the association of stenosis of the carotid artery on that side.[20] Platelet aggregations have been identified histologically in a patient with carotid occlusion.[28]

A characteristic of transient ischemic attacks that casts some suspicion on the embolic etiology is the tendency for the recurring clinical events to be similar, indicating that the same central nervous system area is repeatedly involved. It is of some importance that another form of repetitive central nervous system insult, that occurring with prosthetic heart valves, also has the tendency to recur in the same anatomic area and is also thought to have embolization as its basis. The flow distribution patterns of blood coursing through the carotids and over atheromatous lesions might well be so constant as to permit a high degree of selectivity for the distribution of emboli to a particular anatomic location.

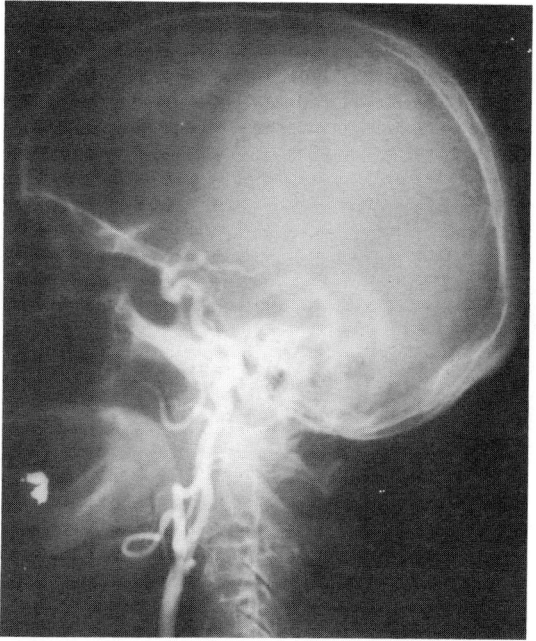

Figure 6. Left carotid arteriogram of a patient who has had transient ischemic attacks. There is an ulcerative lesion detectable near the origin of the internal carotid artery.

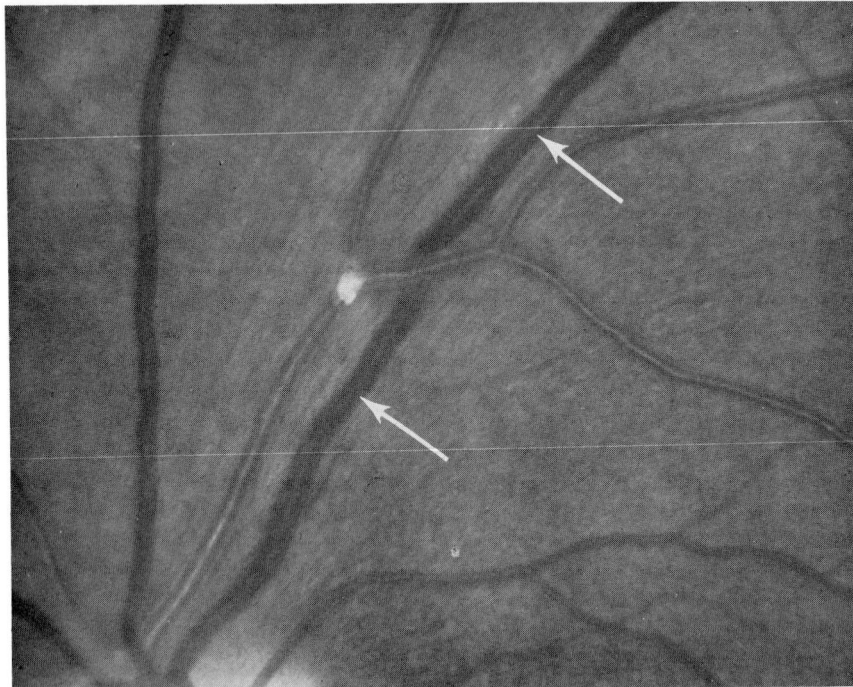

Figure 7. Atheromatous retinal embolus lodged at a bifurcation. (From Hoyt, W. F. *In* Wylie, E. J., and Ehrenfeld, W. K.: Extracranial Occlusive Cerebrovascular Disease. Philadelphia, W. B. Saunders Company, 1970.)

The usual site of internal carotid artery disease is at and just distal to its origin at the bifurcation of the common carotid. The lesions are typical of atherosclerotic lesions elsewhere in the vascular tree. At times the disease extends centrally to the base of the skull; however, it is most commonly localized to the first 3 cm. of the vessel. The carotid sinus and carotid body are located in this region of the vessel. The effect of the disease process on the function of these receptor sites has not been determined, although there is evidence that carotid baroreceptor function is strikingly modified in patients with symptoms of cerebrovascular disease.[1]

The determination of lesions of the carotid artery is made ultimately by arteriography. Thermography, ophthalmodynamometry, and pulse changes are all aids that can help make the decision for arteriography but will not provide the information necessary to decide on operation. Arteriography is indicated when there are signs and symptoms of cerebrovascular insufficiency in a patient susceptible to improvement by revascularization, or in the presence of a carotid bruit in the asymptomatic patient.

Egas Moniz is credited with introducing arteriography as a means of studying the cerebral circulation.[29] He accomplished this by direct needle puncture of the common carotid artery in the neck. This is a procedure requiring a considerable degree of care and patience and is not without complications. The inconvenience and risk are perhaps reasons why extensive use of cerebral arteriography as a diagnostic measure was slow in developing. Currently, most cerebral arteriography is performed by the introduction of a catheter into the aorta by a percutaneous technique through either the brachial or femoral artery. This allows for visualization of all four of the principal ves-

sels in the neck, a highly desirable goal in evaluating both the need for and the approach to relief of obstructive lesions (Fig. 8).

The technical details of the operative procedure for

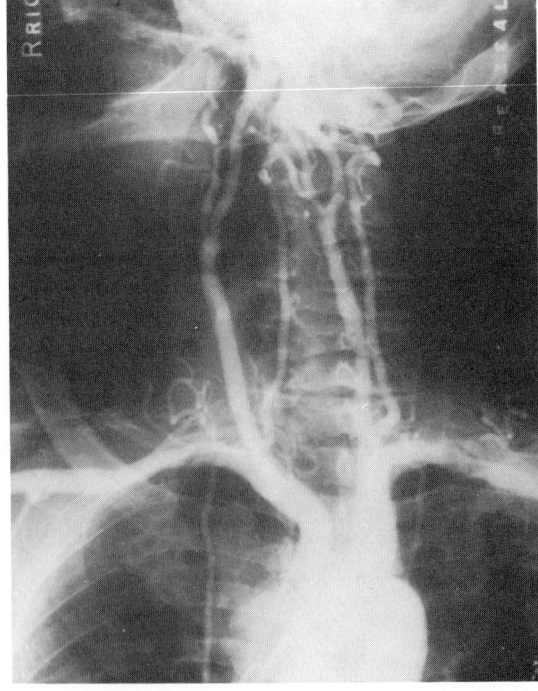

Figure 8. Contrast material injected into the aortic arch allows visualization of all four extracranial vessels supplying the brain.

carotid endarterectomy have undergone many alterations in the past decade and are not as yet standardized. Since stroke and myocardial infarction occurring during the operative period are the greatest risks, careful cardiac evaluation is important, and great attention is directed to maintaining adequate cerebral perfusion at all times. A history of angina suggesting coronary artery obstructive disease generally indicates coronary arteriography as well as carotid arteriography. The co-existence of carotid and coronary obstructive disease requires a decision as to the sequence of treatment based upon the severity of the processes and the nature of the symptoms. Preoperative medications should be administered cautiously to avoid any depression of ventilation or of cardiac output. Operation under local anesthesia was advised at one time in order to avoid the consequences of general anesthesia as well as to allow for intraoperative evaluation of the patient's motor and mental function. It has now been generally accepted that with local anesthesia there is a greater discrepancy between brain oxygen requirements and supply than with a well-conducted general anesthesia,[2, 36] and most operations are now conducted under general anesthesia with endotracheal intubation.[40] Expeditious intubation and maintenance of a high arterial Po_2 are probably the most important aspects of the anesthetic management. The proper Pco_2 maintenance remains debatable.[11, 40] Maintenance of blood pressure at or slightly above the usual preoperative level is considered important in order to maintain optimal cerebral and myocardial circulation. The maintenance of blood pressure involves the avoidance of agents that depress cardiac output or inhibit vasomotion, the meticulous replacement of blood and fluid loss, the vigorous treatment of bradycardia and other cardiac arrhythmias, and the judicious use of vasopressor agents.[40]

The patient is positioned with the head somewhat extended and turned to the side opposite the lesion. In addition to the neck, a site for obtaining a segment of vein is prepared and draped in case reconstruction of the artery requires substitution. One cannot rely on a suitable vein always being available in the neck.

The skin incision is made in the mid or upper cervical skin crease and centered on the anterior border of the sternocleidomastoid muscle. The fascia over the internal jugular vein is opened, and the common facial vein, which courses over the carotid artery, is divided. Care is taken to identify and preserve the descending branch of the hypoglossal nerve and the superior laryngeal nerve (Fig. 9). The common carotid, internal carotid, and external carotid arteries are dissected at levels not involved in the disease process and are then occluded, after the patient has been given heparin intravenously to prevent clotting in any stagnant areas. Blood pressure is measured in the internal carotid artery before and after application of occluding vascular clamps to the common carotid artery and the external carotid artery. This measurement of carotid "stump pressure" is indicative of the adequacy of collateral circulation to the brain. If it is above 50 mm. Hg, collateral circulation is adequate to support cerebral metabolism during operation and a temporary shunt is unnecessary. A lower stump pressure causes concern

for adequacy of brain perfusion during occlusion and suggests the need of a shunt during reconstruction.[23, 31] An incision is made in the anterolateral aspect of the common carotid to a point beyond the plaque. A plane between diseased intima and the media-adventitia is developed, and the obstructing lesion is removed. The artery is then carefully reconstructed; the vessel is supplemented with a vein patch if there is insufficient tissue for construction of a vessel of a size greater than that distal to the operative site (Fig. 10). Arteriograms are obtained to assess the anatomic result.

Continued surveillance of oxygenation and blood pressure is important postoperatively. The endotracheal tube is removed only when there is evidence of adequate ventilation without support. Arrhythmias and falling blood pressure are aggressively treated. Both baroreceptor and chemoreceptor function are in danger of alteration by the current operative procedures, which dissect long segments of the arteries. The loss of baroreceptor function does not seem to be of great importance, as the loss is compensated for by the several other regulatory mechanisms. Chemoreceptor function, on the other hand, although not altered by unilateral dissection, is measurably altered by bilateral carotid endarterectomy.[36] The loss of carotid chemoreceptor response in the patient with central nervous system damage, altered cardiac dynamics, and pulmonary disease could be intolerable, and the patient's survival might be dependent upon ventilatory support.

The value of operative treatment of carotid occlusions in relieving symptoms and prolonging life has not been well enough established to gain the procedure unqualified support. A remarkable attempt to evaluate carefully the role of operative treatment has been made by a large group of investigators, working in 24 different institutions, who categorized patients according to a common protocol and randomized these patients for operative treatment and nonoperative management. This effort has resulted in five reports that considerably aid in the clinical approach to the condition.[4, 5, 15, 16, 22]

Over a 5-year period (1961 to 1966), 4748 patients entered this collaborative study. Entry was on the basis of symptoms of cerebrovascular ischemia as well as, in some instances, carotid bruits in completely asymptomatic patients. The ischemic patterns were (1) transient ischemic attacks consisting of sudden onset of distinct neurologic deficit, such as paresis, dysphasia, paresthesia, or vertigo, the symptoms being transitory and clearing within a few hours; (2) steadily progressive deficit from onset that becomes a serious neurologic deficit with progression; (3) single catastrophic episode, with a severe, definitive neurologic deficit that has stabilized.

Eighty per cent of the patients had complete arteriographic study, with visualization of both the intracranial and extracranial circulation. Eighty per cent of those studied had lesions in the extracranial vasculature. This incidence is comparable to that found in recent postmortem studies. The lesions in the majority of instances were accessible to operative treatment. In nearly 70 per cent of the patients with

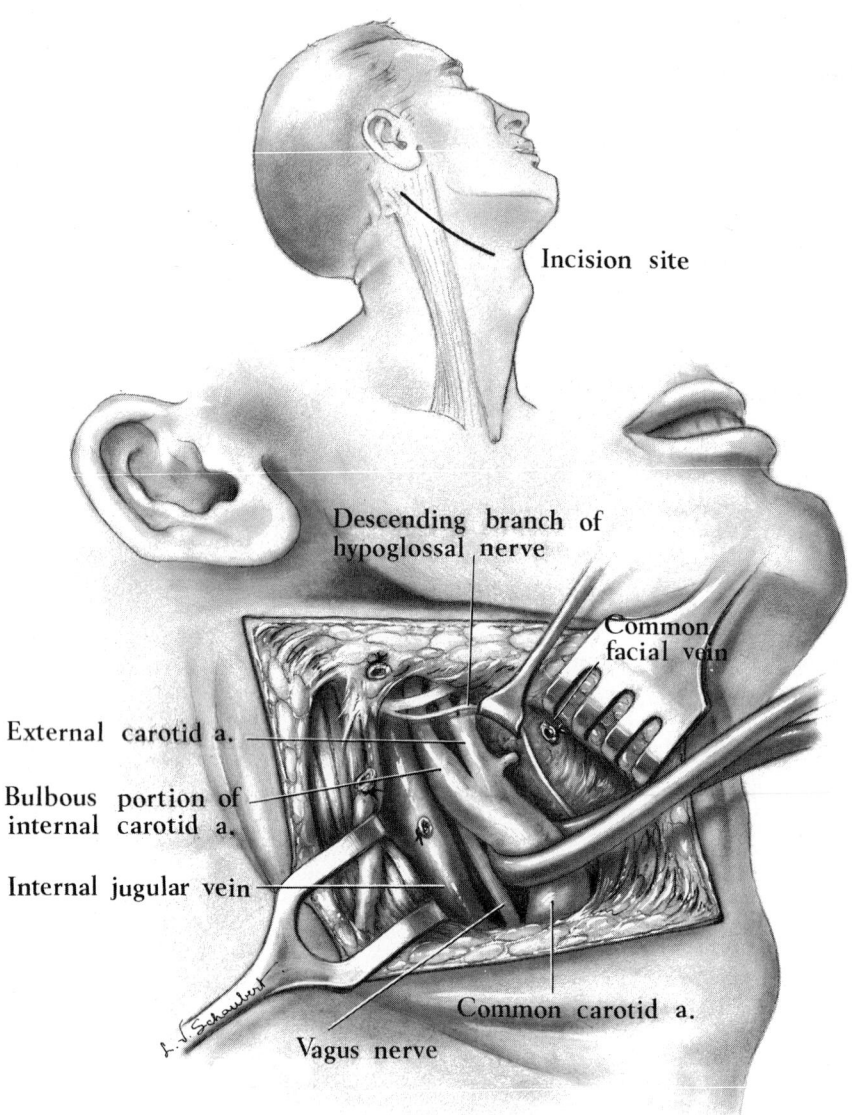

Incision site

Descending branch of
hypoglossal nerve

Common
facial vein

External carotid a.

Bulbous portion of
internal carotid a.

Internal jugular vein

Common carotid a.

Vagus nerve

Figure 9. Incision site and exposure of the carotid bifurcation area. (From Wylie, E. J., and Ehrenfeld, W. K.: Extracranial Occlusive Cerebrovascular Disease. Philadelphia, W. B. Saunders Company, 1970.)

lesions operatively accessible, the lesions were multiple. The existence of multiple lesions obviously complicates a clear relationship between lesions and the clinical pattern.

Severe complications from arteriography occurred in slightly more than 1 per cent of the patients, and clearly were related to more severe neurologic deficit. It was concluded that in patients with severe and progressive brain stem dysfunction angiographic studies should not be done until the clinical course had stabilized.

The large number of anatomic sites of obstruction and the various clinical presentations combine to make for a large number of categories coming under consideration, so that subgroups of this large group of patients are rather small, and firm conclusions are difficult to make. Data from this study suggest, however, that operation undertaken during the acute phase of a

stroke, while it is progressing, is quite hazardous, and survival is less likely than if a nonoperative course is followed. During this early period, restoration of normal arterial blood flow to an area of softened brain can result in cerebral hemorrhage.[41] In the circumstance of a stabilized single catastrophic episode, with a single carotid artery involved, operative correction offered an improved chance of survival and lessened risk of recurrent stroke. If both carotids were involved, one occluded and one stenotic, the advantage of operation was problematic. Operation is clearly of advantage in the clinical condition of ischemic attacks when one carotid artery has a partially occlusive lesion. Both survival and relief of symptoms were improved by operative correction.

Complete occlusion of an internal carotid usually results in thrombosis to the origin of the caroticotympanic arteries at the base of the skull. In this circum-

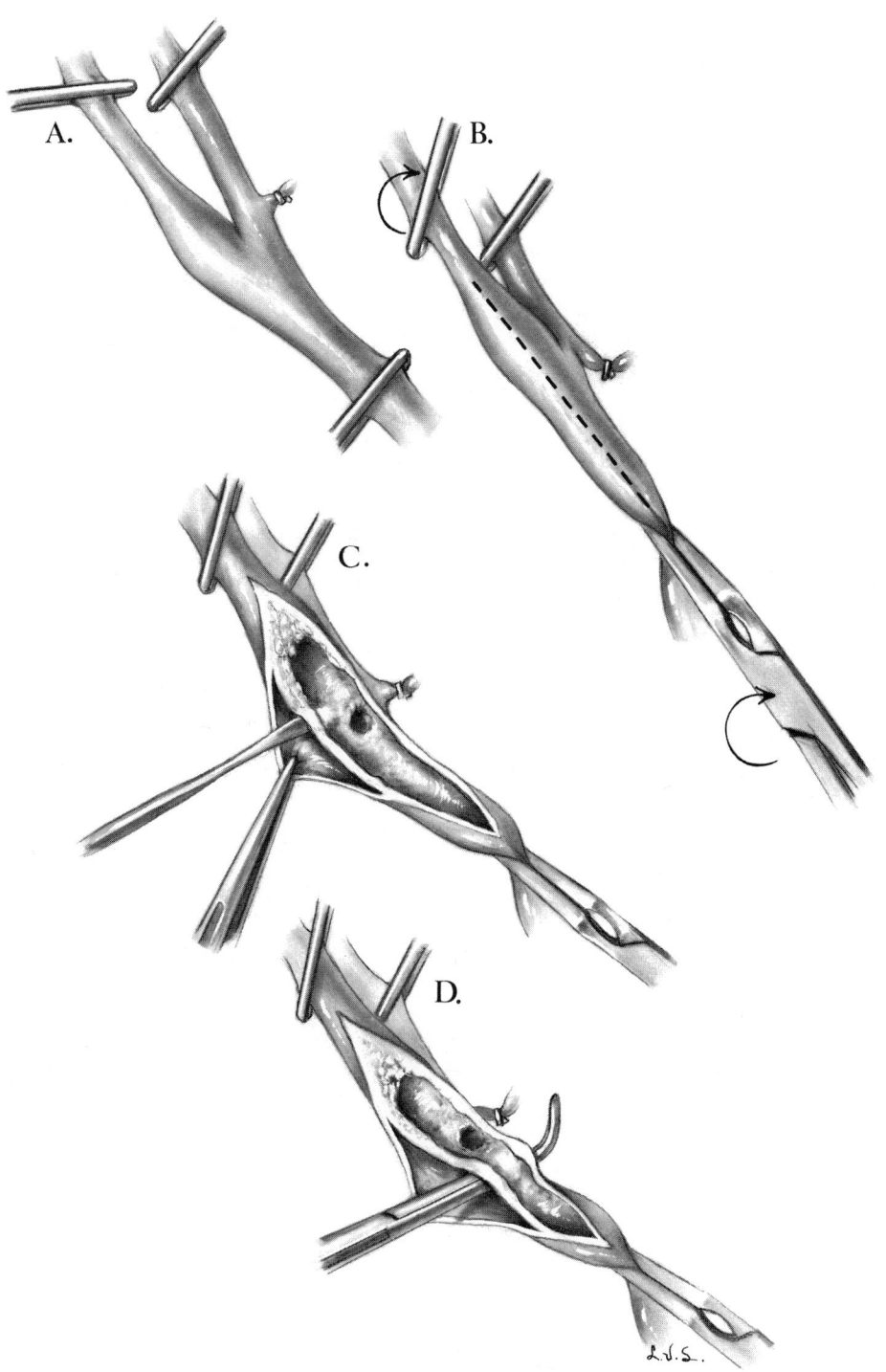

Figure 10. Technique of carotid endarterectomy. (From Wylie, E. J., and Ehrenfeld, W. K.: Extracranial Occlusive Cerebrovascular Disease. Philadelphia, W. B. Saunders Company, 1970.)

Illustration continued on following page

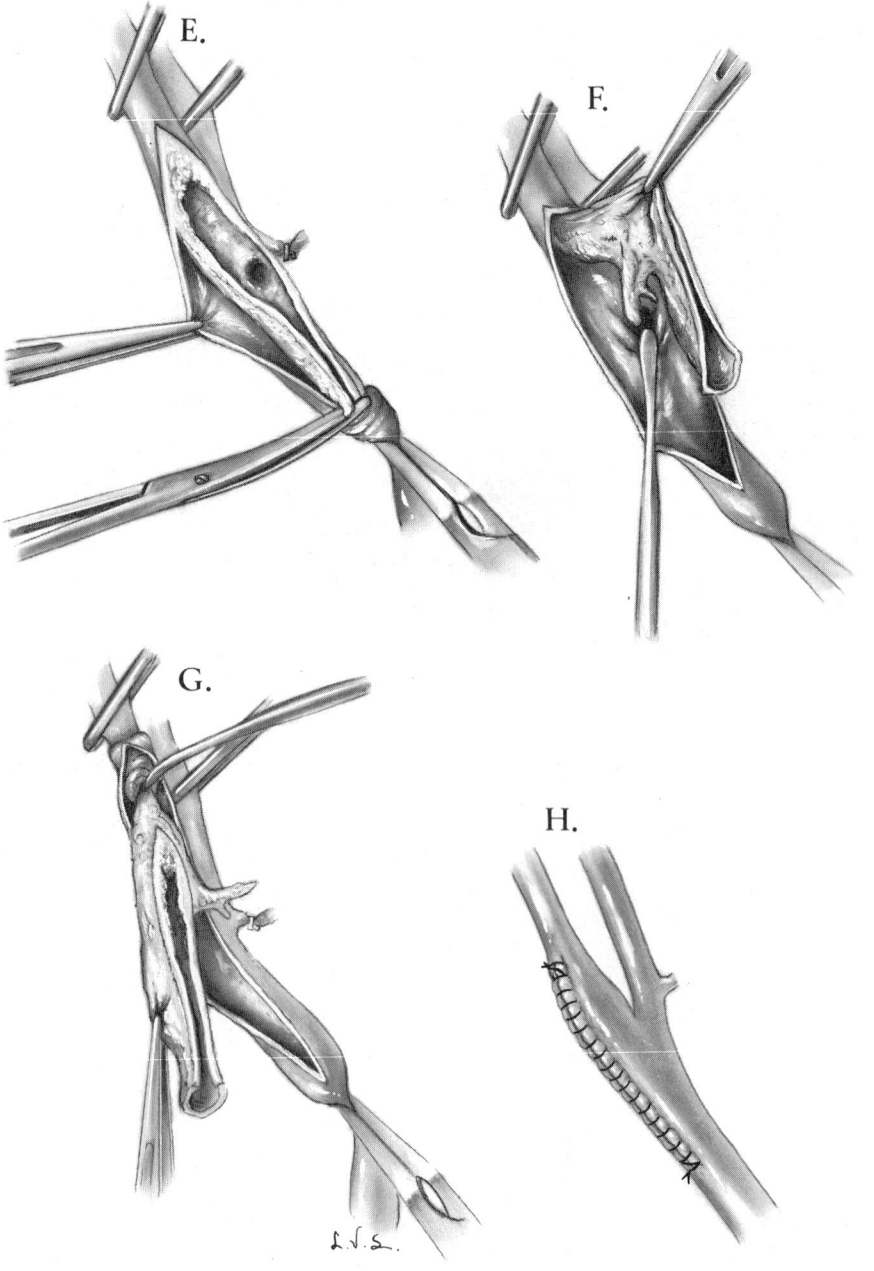

Figure 10. *Continued.*

stance, endarterectomy and thrombectomy have been infrequently successful in restoring circulation.[33] Such a lesion in conjunction with a stenotic lesion in the other carotid poses a severe threat and so far has not yielded well to treatment. The technically demanding but logical approach of bypassing such an obstruction with a vein-bypass graft from the carotid in the neck to the intracranial carotid is certain to be tried with increasing frequency.

As with many therapies, carotid endarterectomy for treatment of cerebral ischemia seems to require proper timing in the course of the disease. Unfortunately, when it is applied late in the disease, when

death of a portion of the brain has already occurred, it introduces risks equaling or outweighing the advantages. Applied early in the course of the disease, when it is prophylactic against stroke, it seems to be clearly advantageous. This is the challenge to the surgeon — to apply the procedure with such skill as to essentially avoid risk in the seemingly well patient. Current techniques certainly allow for approaching that goal. The challenge then becomes one of case finding — searching out seemingly well persons who, untreated, are unknowingly under risk of stroke. This is the most promising approach to stroke prevention in the foreseeable future.

SELECTED REFERENCES

Fields, W. S., North, R. R., Hass, W. K., Galbraith, J. G., Wylie, E. J., Ratinor, G., Burns, M. H., McDonald, M. C., and Meyer, J. S.: Joint study of extracranial arterial occlusion as a cause of stroke. I. Organization of study and survey of patient population. J.A.M.A., *203*:153, 1968.

Hass, W. K., Fields, W. S., North, R. R., Kricheff, I. I., Chase, N. E., and Bauer, R. B.: Joint study of extracranial arterial occlusion. II. Arteriography, techniques, sites, complications. J.A.M.A., *203*:159, 1968.

Bauer, R. B., Meyer, J. S., Fields, W. S., Remington, R., McDonald, M. C., and Callen, R.: Joint study of extracranial arterial occlusion. III. Progress report of controlled study of long-term survival in patients with and without operation. J.A.M.A., *208*:509, 1969.

Blaisdell, W. F., Clauss, R. H., Galbraith, J. G., Imparato, A. M., and Wylie, E. J.: Joint study of extracranial arterial occlusion. IV. A review of surgical conditions. J.A.M.A., *209*:1889, 1969.

Fields, W. S., Maslenikov, V., Meyer, J. S., Hass, W. K., Remington, R. D., and McDonald, M.: Joint study of extracranial arterial occlusion. V. Progress report of prognosis following surgery or nonsurgical treatment for transient cerebral ischemic attacks and cervical carotid artery lesion. J.A.M.A., *211*:1993, 1970.

These reports are from a study entered into cooperatively by 25 institutions in an attempt to gain a sufficient number of case studies to permit meaningful analysis of the value of treatment in a rather ill-defined entity. These are important articles not only for the extensive data and close analyses they contain, but also because this study is an excellent example of a new and important approach to the analysis of clinical information by cooperative effort.

Wylie, E. J., and Ehrenfeld, W. K.: Extracranial Occlusive Cerebrovascular Disease. Diagnosis and Management. Philadelphia, W. B. Saunders Company, 1970.

This is a complete, yet concise monograph that expertly considers all the aspects of extracranial vascular occlusion. It is particularly valuable for its elucidation of pathogenesis and discussion of diagnostic methods and selection of patients for operative treatment.

REFERENCES

1. Appenzellei, O., and Discaucts, L.: Circulatory reflexes in patients with cerebrovascular disease. N. Engl. J. Med., *271*:820, 1964.
2. Bain, J. A., Catton, D. V., Cox, J. M. R., and Spoerel, W. E.: The effect of general anesthesia on the tolerance of cerebral ischemia in rabbits. Can. Anaesth. Soc. J., *14*:64, 1967.
3. Bauer, R. B., Boulos, R. S., and Meyer, J. S.: Natural history and surgical treatment of occlusive cerebrovascular disease evaluated by serial arteriography. Am. J. Roentgenol., *104*:1, 1968.
4. Bauer, R. B., Meyer, J. S., Fields, W. S., Remington, R., McDonald, M. C., and Callen, R.: Joint study of controlled study of long-term survival in patients with and without operation. J.A.M.A., *208*:509, 1969.
5. Blaisdell, W. F., Clauss, R. H., Galbraith, J. G., Imparato, A. M., and Wylie, E. J.: Joint study of extracranial arterial occlusion. IV. A review of surgical consideration. J.A.M.A., *209*:1889, 1969.
6. Brice, J. G., Dowsett, D. F., and Lowe, R. D.: Hemodynamic effects of carotid artery stenosis. Br. Med. J., *2*:1363, 1964.
7. Corday, E., Rothenberg, S., and Werner, S. M.: Cerebral vascular insufficiency. An explanation of the transient stroke. Arch. Intern. Med., *98*:683, 1956.
8. Denny-Brown, D.: Recurrent cerebrovascular episodes. Arch. Neurol., *2*:194, 1960.
9. Drake, W. E., Jr., and Drake, M. A. L.: Clinical and angiographic correlates of cerebrovascular insufficiency. Am. J. Med., *45*:253, 1968.
10. Eastcott, H. H. G., Pickering, G. W., and Rob, C. G.: Reconstruction of internal carotid artery in patients with intermittent attacks of hemiplegia. Lancet, *2*:994, 1954.
11. Ehrenfeld, W. K., Hamilton, F. N., Larson, C. P., Jr., Hicky, R. F., and Severinhaus, J. W.: Effect of CO_2 and systemic hypertension on downstream cerebral arterial pressure during carotid endarterectomy. Surgery, *67*:87, 1970.
12. Ehrenfeld, W. K., Hoyt, W. F., and Wylie, E. J.: Embolization and transient blindness from carotid atheromata. Arch. Surg., *93*:787, 1966.
13. Eklof, B., and Schwartz, S. I.: Effects of critical stenosis of the ca-

rotid artery and compromised cephalic blood flow. Arch. Surg., *99*:695, 1969.
14. Fayekces, J. F., and Alman, R. W.: The role of hypotension in transitory focal cerebral ischemia. Am. J. Med. Sci., *248*:567, 1964.
15. Fields, W. S., Maslenikov, V., Meyer, J. S., Hass, W. K., Remington, R. D., and McDonald, M.: Joint study of extracranial arterial occlusion. V. Progress report of prognosis following surgery or nonsurgical treatment for transient cerebral ischemic attacks and cervical carotid artery lesion. J.A.M.A., *211*:1993, 1970.
16. Fields, W. S., North, R. R., Hass, W. K., Galbraith, J. G., Wylie, E. J., Ratinor, G., Burns, M. H., McDonald, M. C., and Meyer, J. S.: Joint study of extracranial arterial occlusion as a cause of stroke. I. Organization of study and survey of patient population. J.A.M.A., *203*:153, 1968.
17. Fields, W. S., Sharkey, P. C., Crawford, E. S., and Morris, G. C.: Correlation of neurologic syndromes with lesions found angiographically. Neurology, *10*:431, 1960.
18. Fisher, C. M.: Occlusion of the internal carotid artery. Arch. Neurol. Psychiatr., *65*:346, 1951.
19. Fisher, C. M.: Occlusion of the carotid artery: Further experiences. Arch. Neurol. Psychiatr., *72*:187, 1954.
20. Fisher, C. M.: Observations of the fundus oculi in transient monocular blindness. Neurology, *9*:333, 1959.
21. Gowers, W. R.: On a case of simultaneous embolism of central retinal and middle cerebral arteries. Lancet, *2*:794, 1875.
22. Hass, W. K., Fields, W. S., North, R. R., Kricheff, I. I., Chase, N. E., and Bauer, R. B.: Joint study of extracranial arterial occlusion. II. Arteriography, techniques, sites, complications. J.A.M.A., *203*:159, 1968.
23. Hays, R. J., Levinson, S. A., and Wylie, E. G.: Intraoperative measurement of carotid back pressure as a guide to operative management for carotid endarterectomy. Surgery, *72*:953, 1972.
24. Hodgins, E.: Episode: Report on an Accident Inside My Skull. New York, Atheneum, 1964.
25. Hunt, J. R.: The role of the carotid arteries in the causation of vascular lesions of the brain with remarks on certain special features of the symptomatology. Am. J. Med. Sci., *147*:704, 1914.
26. Hutchinson, E. C., and Yates, P. O.: Carito-vertebral stenosis. Lancet, *1*:2, 1957.
27. Kendall, R. E., and Marshall, J.: Role of hypotension on the genesis of transient focal cerebral ischemic attacks. Br. Med. J., *2*:344, 1963.
28. McBrien, D. F., Braddey, R. D., and Ashton, N.: The nature of retinal emboli in stenosis of the internal carotid artery. Lancet, *1*:697, 1963.
29. Moniz, E.: L'encéphalographie artérielle, son importance dans la localisation des tumeurs cérébrales. Rev. Neurol., *2*:72, 1927.
30. Moore, W. S., and Hall, A. D.: Ulcerated atheroma of the carotid artery: A cause of transient cerebral ischemia. Am. J. Surg., *114*:800, 1967.
31. Moore, W. S., and Hall, A. D.: Carotid artery back pressure. Arch. Surg., *99*:702, 1969.
32. Savory, W. S.: Case of a young woman in whom the main arteries of both upper extremities and of the neck were throughout completely obliterated. Med. Chir. Te. Land, *39*:205, 1856.
33. Thompson, J. E., Austin, D. J., and Patman, R. O.: Endarterectomy of the totally occluded carotid artery for stroke: Results in one hundred operations. Arch. Surg., *95*:791, 1967.
34. U.S. President's Commission on Heart Disease, Cancer and Stroke. Washington, D.C., U.S. Government Printing Office. Dec., 1964.
35. Van Rosen, R. E.: Comeback: The Story of My Stroke. New York, Bobbs-Merrill Company, 1962.
36. Wade, J. G., Larson, C. P., Jr., Hickey, R. F., Ehrenfeld, W. K., and Severinhaus, J. W.: Effect of carotid endarterectomy on carotid chemoreceptor and baroreceptor function in man. N. Engl. J. Med., *282*:823, 1970.
37. Wells, B. A., Keats, A. S., and Cooley, D. A.: Induced tolerance to cerebral ischemia produced by general anesthesia during temporary carotid occlusion. Surgery, *54*:216, 1963.
38. Whisnant, J. P., Martin, M. J., and Sayre, G. P.: Atherosclerotic stenoses of cervical arteries: Clinical significance. Arch. Neurol., *5*:429, 1961.
39. Willis, T.: Practice of Physick. London, S. Pordage, 1684. Part 6, p. 59.
40. Wylie, E. J., and Ehrenfeld, W. K.: Extracranial Occlusive Cere-

brovascular Disease. Diagnosis and Management. Philadelphia, W. B. Saunders Company, 1970.

41. Wylie, E. J., Hein, M. F., and Adams, J. E.: Intracranial hemorrhage following surgical revascularization for treatment of acute stroke. J. Neurosurg., *21*:212, 1964.

3. SUBCLAVIAN STEAL SYNDROME

John A. Mannick, M.D.

The *subclavian steal syndrome* occurs when there is reversal of flow in the ipsilateral vertebral artery distal to a stenosis or occlusion of the proximal subclavian or, more rarely, the innominate artery. Because of the lowering of pressure in the subclavian artery distal to the obstruction, blood flows up the vertebral artery on the unaffected side, into the basilar artery, and down the vertebral artery on the affected side to supply collateral circulation to the subclavian artery and its subsidary arterial systems (Figs. 11 and 12). Thus, blood supply is presumably "stolen" from the basilar artery and, at least theoretically, blood supply to the brain stem may be compromised.

Contorni[6] is credited with reporting the first angiographic visualization of subclavian steal in 1960; however, the potential clinical significance of this problem was not widely appreciated until the report of Reivich and his co-workers,[34] who in 1961 described two patients with clinical signs of cerebral vascular insufficiency and reversal of flow through the vertebral artery secondary to subclavian obstruction. In this report reversal of flow was demonstrated not only by angiography but by the use of the electromagnetic flowmeter at the time of surgical correction of the

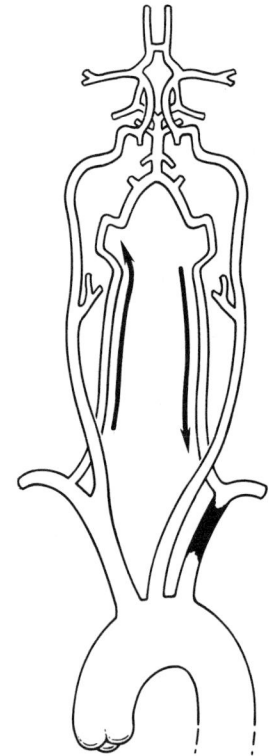

Figure 11. Diagrammatic illustration of the pattern of flow in the subclavian steal syndrome. Note the retrograde flow in the vertebral artery on the side of the lesion (after Weilbaecher).

subclavian lesion. In an editorial discussing the report of Reivich et al., C. M. Fisher introduced the term "subclavian steal syndrome." Since that time numerous reports have appeared in the literature de-

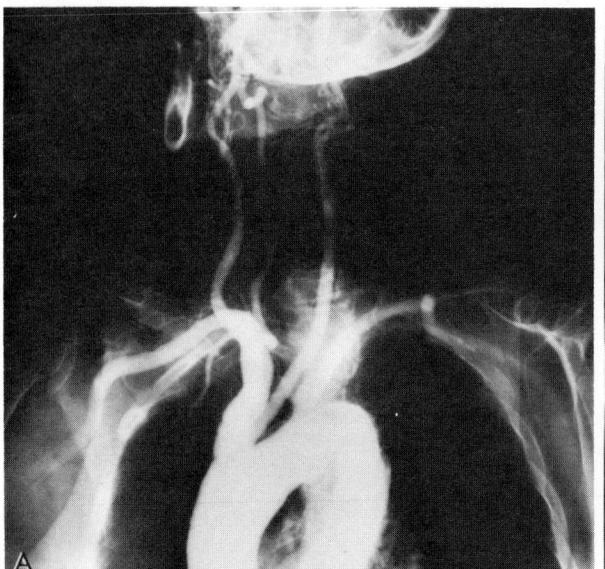
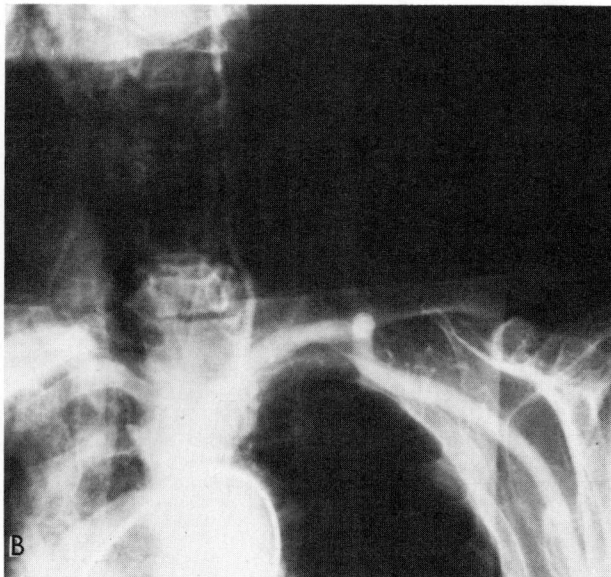

Figure 12. Early (*A*) and late (*B*) films of an angiogram of the aortic arch in a patient with the subclavian steal syndrome. In the early film a stenosis of the origin of the left subclavian artery is seen. In the late film there is retrograde flow of contrast material down the left vertebral artery filling the left subclavian artery.

scribing patients who were found to have subclavian steal by angiography.* However, there has been considerable variation in the authors' assessment of the clinical significance of the phenomenon.

Classically, the subclavian steal syndrome should be suspected in a patient who manifests symptoms of vertebral-basilar arterial insufficiency and is found on examination to have a difference in brachial systolic blood pressure of at least 30 mm. Hg between the two arms and in whom there is a *bruit* at the base of the neck or in the supraclavicular area on the affected side. The cause of the proximal subclavian obstruction is arteriosclerosis in the vast majority of instances. The left subclavian artery is involved in a greater percentage of cases (about 70 per cent) than the right.[12] The neurologic symptoms reported in patients with this syndrome include most commonly vertigo, limb paresis, and paresthesias. Bilateral (cortical) visual disturbances, ataxia, syncope, and dysarthria occur somewhat less frequently. The symptoms have been encountered initially as transient attacks of cerebral ischemia in the majority of patients. However, there have been a number of reported instances in which the symptoms progressed to complete stroke.[12, 27, 34] In patients with innominate artery stenosis, any neurologic manifestations of subclavian steal may be obscured by those caused by concomitant carotid insufficiency.

North and associates[30] in 1962 reported that symptoms of cerebral ischemia were produced by exercise of the affected arm in six of seven patients they encountered with subclavian steal. However, it is now apparent, from a review of the reported clinical experience with patients with this phenomenon, that, paradoxically, only a few have manifested neurologic symptoms in response to exercise of the involved arm, which would be expected to increase the demand for collateral blood flow.

The diagnosis of subclavian steal is made by the retrograde catheter angiography. A number of reports[11, 32, 39] have indicated that it is possible to obtain an angiographic picture falsely suggestive of subclavian steal by pressure injection of contrast material through a catheter located in the vertebral artery itself or in the subclavian artery near the vertebral origin. The force of the injection apparently alters hemodynamics so that contrast material may be forced up one vertebral artery and down the other even in the absence of any subclavian obstruction. Therefore, the angiographic diagnosis of true subclavian steal requires that the phenomenon be apparent on films obtained with the contrast medium injected into the aortic root.

An appreciation of the variable hemodynamic effects of a proximal subclavian occlusion is essential for appropriate evaluation of the significance of subclavian steal when it is encountered in an individual patient. While the retrograde flow rate in the ipsilateral vertebral artery has been shown by direct measurement to be as high as 120 ml. per minute[34] in some patients with subclavian occlusion, the simplistic assumption that the cerebral circulation is deprived of

this quantity of blood is not necessarily valid. Since flow in the major arteries is limited much more by the peripheral resistance in the arteriolar bed supplied by these vessels than by the intrinsic resistance of the major vessels themselves, it is at least theoretically possible that a normal vertebral artery, on the side opposite the subclavian lesion in a patient with the subclavian steal phenomenon, could supply adequately the posterior cerebral circulation as well as the arm on the affected side. Moreover, the basilar circulation can draw on both internal carotid arteries for collateral supply through the circle of Willis.

Conflicting experimental evidence has been reported concerning the effect of proximal subclavian occlusion on cerebral blood flow. Reivich et al.[34] and Sammartino and Toole[37] measured flow in the vertebral and carotid arteries of dogs subjected to unilateral proximal subclavian artery occlusion and observed reversal of flow in the ipsilateral vertebral artery, which increased as the affected limb was exercised. They reported that the compensatory increase in forward flow through the other major arteries supplying the brain was insufficient to make up for the flow lost through the steal phenomenon and therefore concluded that there was a net deficit in cerebral blood flow. However, Ecklof and Schwartz[10] in similar studies failed to observe a net change in cerebral blood flow with proximal subclavian artery occlusion and reversal of ipsilateral vertebral artery flow. Powers and associates[33] studied the effect in monkeys of subclavian steal on cortical blood flow measured by thermistor-tipped probes implanted in the brain substance and on auditory function in the awake state in the same animals. These workers observed, following subclavian artery ligation and the production of a subclavian steal, that there was a 10 per cent decrease in total cerebral blood flow and a 20 to 70 per cent decrease in blood flow to the brain stem. While subclavian steal failed to induce gross neurologic deficit in these experiments, there were measurable decreases in auditory discriminatory function in the awake state in these animals after production of the subclavian steal. Auditory function reverted to normal following correction of the subclavian steal. Handa and his associates,[17] who studied cerebral blood flow in monkeys with an electromagnetic flowmeter, found that subclavian artery occlusion and reversal of flow in the ipsilateral vertebral artery was accompanied by a compensatory increase in flow in the remaining three arteries supplying the brain and that there was a 6 per cent average decrease in total cerebral blood flow and no evidence of neurologic abnormality.

Early reports suggested that subclavian steal was associated with disabling neurologic symptoms in the vast majority of patients in whom it was encountered,[20, 26, 27, 30, 34] whereas increasing clinical experience led a number of observers to conclude along with Ehrenfeld and co-workers[9] that "the presence of subclavian steal is probably an asymptomatic lesion in most patients." With the realization that subclavian steal could occur, it was feared that this problem would appear in patients who had undergone the Blalock-Taussig operation for palliation of the tetralogy of Fallot, since proximal subclavian artery liga-

---

*See references 2, 4, 7–9, 14, 16, 19–23, 26–28, 30, 31, 35, 36, 38, and 40–42.

tion was an integral part of this procedure. A report by Folger and Shah[14] suggested that some patients who had undergone the Blalock-Taussig procedure had symptoms suggestive of vertebral-basilar insufficiency; however, the most prominent symptom was severe headache in these patients, a complaint not commonly observed in most other patients with the subclavian steal syndrome.[12]

Solti and associates[41] concluded that total cerebral blood flow, as measured by isotope dilution, was significantly lower in patients with the subclavian steal syndrome than in a control group of patients of roughly similar age and sex. They also reported an increase in cerebral blood flow following correction of the lesion in symptomatic patients. However, no mention was made in their report of other associated extracranial lesions of the cerebral arterial supply in the patients they studied. Mannick et al.[27] in an early report had suggested that the subclavian steal phenomenon was more likely to cause significant neurologic symptoms in patients with disease in other arteries supplying the brain.

Considerable data have resulted from the recent report of the Joint Study of Extracranial Arterial Occlusion, in which 168 patients with the subclavian steal syndrome from 24 reporting institutions were evaluated.[12] More than 80 per cent of these 168 patients had disease involving one or more of the other vessels supplying the brain. There were only 50 patients with subclavian disease only or with subclavian and vertebral artery disease. There was a 25 per cent incidence of significant complications following surgery, with an 8 per cent surgical mortality in those patients in whom the lesion was surgically corrected. It was of interest that in 34 patients treated medically or in those receiving no treatment at all, the three (9 per cent) who suffered strokes all had associated carotid disease. Of the 130 surgically treated patients, 20 had strokes at surgery or during the follow-up period (15 per cent). Of the nine asymptomatic patients in whom subclavian steal was discovered by chance in this study, none developed neurologic symptoms during the follow-up period. Patients with subclavian artery disease alone did not have strokes during the follow-up period, whether they were treated medically, surgically, or not at all.

It seems reasonable to conclude, therefore, that the subclavian steal phenomenon may frequently be a clinically asymptomatic lesion but can produce or contribute to symptoms of cerebral vascular insufficiency when it exists in conjunction with other lesions of the extracranial cerebral arterial supply, particularly carotid bifurcation lesions. Whether or not the subclavian steal phenomenon produces symptoms in a given individual is probably dependent upon (1) the size of the vertebral artery on the uninvolved side, and whether or not it is free from disease; (2) the anatomy of the circle of Willis, which may have considerable individual variation; (3) the amount of collateral circulation from other sources (particularly the costocervical and thyrocervical trunks[3, 29]) that develops to supply the arm on the affected side; and (4) the presence of other lesions in the cerebral arterial supply.

In the apparently rare instances in which the sub-clavian steal syndrome appears to be responsible for symptoms of vertebral-basilar insufficiency in the absence of other lesions in the extracranial cerebral arterial circulation, surgical correction of the lesion appears warranted and can result in amelioration of symptoms, though surgery cannot justifiably be urged for the prevention of stroke under these circumstances, since subclavian steal alone does not appear to cause stroke.[12] When the subclavian steal syndrome occurs in association with other extracranial arterial lesions, it is evident that the other significant lesions should be repaired as well. It seems likely that concomitant correction of the subclavian steal syndrome in certain of these patients should be undertaken; however, there are a number of reports of symptomatic relief of patients with subclavian steal in whom only the other arterial lesions were corrected.[9, 12]

A variety of surgical procedures[5, 7-9, 13, 15, 19, 22-24, 27, 34-36] have been recommended for correction of the subclavian steal, ranging in complexity from simple ligation of the vertebral artery on the affected side,[42] first performed by Rob in 1960,[36] to aorta-to-subclavian artery bypass graft or subclavian endarterectomy by the mediastinal or transthoracic route. The operation most frequently employed at present is the common carotid-to-subclavian artery bypass graft performed through a cervical incision. This procedure was once believed to have the potential hazard of stealing blood from the internal carotid circulation;[18] however, experimental observations[1, 25] and widespread clinical application of this operation have demonstrated that significant reduction of internal carotid flow does not occur unless there is concomitant stenosis of the proximal common carotid artery. Under such circumstances this operation is clearly not advisable. When it is normally patent, the common carotid artery apparently has the capacity in man to supply both the brain and the arm without any drop in pressure distal to the origin of the carotid-to-subclavian artery bypass graft. This procedure has the significant advantage of avoiding the impressive morbidity and mortality[7, 8, 12] associated with median sternotomy or thoracotomy in the elderly patient population in whom the subclavian steal syndrome is ordinarily encountered.

The operative approach for performing a carotid-to-subclavian artery bypass is through a transverse incision placed at the base of the neck (Fig. 13). The clavicular portion of the sternocleidomastoid muscle is divided, exposing the scalene fat pad, which is swept inferiorly to expose the phrenic nerve and the anterior scalene muscle. The phrenic nerve is carefully freed up and gently retracted medially. The scalene muscle is divided, exposing the fascia overlying the subclavian artery. The subclavian artery can then easily be freed up from the origin of the vertebral artery to or slightly beyond the lateral border of the first rib. The common carotid artery is nearby beneath the sterno-cleidomastoid muscle and is freed up from its companion structures for about two inches. Using systemic heparinization, a graft of autogenous saphenous vein or knitted Dacron is sutured end to side to the common carotid artery. An internal shunt may be employed if desired to permit carotid flow to continue while the anastomosis is performed. The distal end of

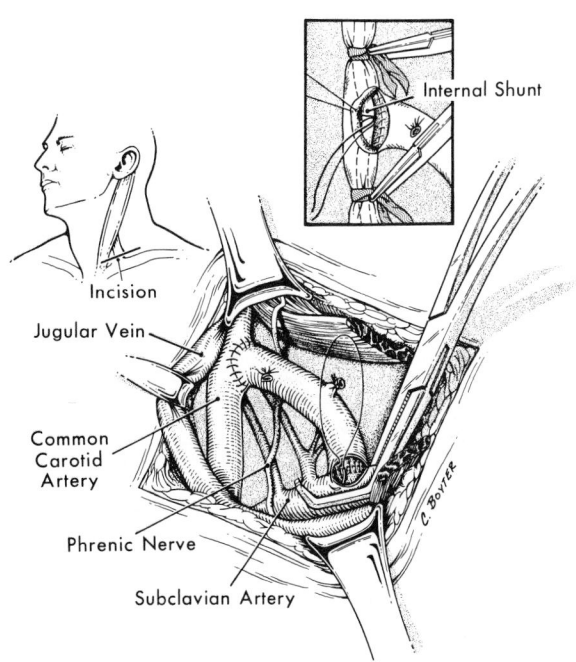

Figure 13. Diagrammatic illustration of the technique of carotid-to-subclavian bypass grafting. The incision is placed at the base of the neck. The clavicular portion of the sternocleidomastoid muscle is divided, exposing the anterior scalene muscle and phrenic nerve. The phrenic nerve is carefully spared and the anterior scalene is divided, exposing the fascia overlying the subclavian artery, which can be freed up from the vertebral origin laterally beyond the margin of the first rib. The common carotid artery is exposed through the same incision as it lies beneath the sternocleidomastoid muscle posteromedial to the jugular vein. A graft of autogenous saphenous vein is sutured end-to-side to the common carotid artery. An internal shunt (*inset*) may be used to preserve flow in the carotid artery during the time the anastomosis is performed. The shunt is removed just before completion of the suture line. The vein graft is then trimmed to size and sutured end-to-side to the subclavian artery.

the graft is then attached in similar end-to-side fashion to the exposed portion of the subclavian artery.

In order to avoid the potential hazard of operating upon the common carotid artery, several authors have recently proposed alternative methods of correction of the subclavian steal syndrome through the use of the subclavian-to-subclavian artery bypass graft[13, 15] performed through two supraclavicular incisions or the axillary-to-axillary bypass graft[24] performed through two infraclavicular incisions. Each procedure has the potential advantage of restoring normal hemodynamics in the patient with the subclavian steal syndrome without even temporarily interrupting cerebral blood supply.

The results of corrective surgery have been excellent in terms of reversal of the hemodynamic abnormalities of the subclavian steal. Relief of associated cerebral symptoms has been achieved in 75 to 80 per cent of those patients operated upon as well.[12] The operative mortality, even for carotid-to-subclavian artery bypass, is reported at approximately 5 per cent in several large series,[7, 12] a figure that is surprisingly high considering that carotid endarterectomy, a procedure of comparable magnitude performed in a similar patient population, now has an operative mortality rate in the 1 per cent range.

SELECTED REFERENCES

Diethrich, E. B., Garrett, H. E., Ameriso, J., Crawford, E. S., El-Bayar, M., and DeBakey, M. E.: Occlusive disease of the common carotid and subclavian arteries treated by carotid-subclavian bypass. Am. J. Surg., *114*:800, 1967.
In this relatively early report of carotid-subclavian bypass, the technique of the operation is well illustrated and the results in a sizable series of patients are discussed. The operation was used for occlusions of the common carotid as well as the subclavian artery. The results of grafting were excellent; however, the surgical mortal-

ity for this procedure was 4.8 per cent. The effectiveness of the operation was clearly demonstrated. Of 79 patients with symptoms of vertebral-basilar insufficiency, all but five were relieved of their symptoms without demonstrating evidence of carotid insufficiency.

Ehrenfeld, W. K., Chapman, R. D., and Wiley, E. J.: Management of occlusive lesions of the branches of the aortic arch. Am. J. Surg., *118*:236, 1969.
In this relatively early report from a group with wide experience in peripheral arterial surgery, the authors concluded that obstruction of the subclavian artery appeared to be better tolerated than obstruction of the other arteries supplying the brain and that the presence of subclavian steal was probably an asymptomatic lesion in most patients. Of 157 patients with occlusive lesions of the major branches of the aortic arch, 50 per cent were free of significant symptoms from the onset or were made so by a carotid bifurcation endarterectomy.

Fields, W. S., and Lemak, N. A.: Joint study of extracranial arterial occlusion. J.A.M.A., *222*:1139, 1972.
This is an excellent review of the fate of 168 patients with the subclavian steal syndrome treated both medically and surgically in a large number of different hospitals. The results of the study suggest that subclavian steal alone rarely if ever causes strokes and that symptomatic patients with subclavian steal are likely to have associated disease of the other extracranial arteries. There was a relatively high incidence of complications (25 per cent) and mortality (8 per cent) following surgical correction of the subclavian steal.

Powers, S. R., Jr., Roe, G. M., and Creel, W.: The relation between regional cerebral blood flow and cerebral function. Surgery, *61*:74, 1967.
In this interesting study, for the first time objective experimental evidence was presented that the subclavian steal in primates would lead to measurable neurologic deficit and a definite decrease in cerebral perfusion as measured by thermistor-tipped probes implanted in several sites in the brain. Of particular interest was a decrease in flow to the brain stem in awake animals ranging from 20 to 70 per cent of the initial control values. The animals, though grossly neurologically intact, were found to have a persistent deficit in a noise discrimination test, following production of the subclavian steal, which returned to or toward normal when the subclavian steal was corrected six months or more later.

Reivich, M., Holling, H. E., Roberts, B., and Toole, J. F.: Reversal of blood flow through the vertebral artery and its effect on cerebral circulation. N. Engl. J. Med., *265*:878, 1961.

This is the classic report describing the subclavian steal syndrome clinically and experimentally. Two patients were studied who had neurologic symptoms and reversal of flow in the left vertebral artery secondary to proximal subclavian stenosis, as demonstrated by angiography. Reversal of flow in the ipsilateral vertebral artery was demonstrated for the first time in the human at the time of surgery in one of these patients by application of an electromagnetic flow meter to the subclavian artery distal to the vertebral origin. The authors also report animal studies in which reversal of vertebral flow was demonstrated following subclavian artery occlusion. In the animal experiments they concluded that total cerebral blood flow was markedly diminished by the subclavian steal.

REFERENCES

1. Barner, H. B., Kaiser, G. C., and Willman, V. L.: Hemodynamics of carotid-subclavian bypass. Arch. Surg., *103*:248, 1971.
2. Berger, R. L., Sidd, J. J., and Ramaswamy, K.: Retrograde vertebral-artery flow produced by correction of subclavian-steal syndrome. N. Engl. J. Med., *277*:64, 1967.
3. Bosniak, M. A.: Cervical arterial pathways associated with brachiocephalic occlusive disease. Am. J. Roentgenol., *91*:1232, 1964.
4. Bryant, L. R., and Spencer, F. C.: Occlusive disease of subclavian artery. J.A.M.A., *196*:109, 1966.
5. Clark, K., and Perry, M. O.: Carotid vertebral anastomosis: An alternate technic for repair of the subclavian steal syndrome. Ann. Surg., *163*:414, 1966.
6. Contorni, L.: Il circolo collaterale vertebraovertebrale nella obliterazione dell'arterio subclavia all sua origine. Minerva Chir., *15*:268, 1960.
7. Crawford, E. S., DeBakey, M. E., Morris, G. C., Jr., and Howell, J. F.: Surgical treatment of occlusion of the innominate, common carotid, and subclavian arteries: A 10 year experience. Surgery, *65*:17, 1969.
8. Diethrich, E. B., Garrett, H. E., Ameriso, J., Crawford, E. S., El-Bayar, M., and DeBakey, M. E.: Occlusive disease of the common carotid and subclavian arteries treated by carotid-subclavian bypass. Am. J. Surg., *114*:800, 1967.
9. Ehrenfeld, W. K., Chapman, R. D., and Wylie, E. J.: Management of occlusive lesions of the branches of the aortic arch. Am. J. Surg., *118*:236, 1969.
10. Eklof, B., and Schwartz, S. I.: Effects of subclavian steal and compromised cephalic blood flow on cerebral circulation. Surgery, *68*:431, 1970.
11. Ethier, R.: Observations on retrograde vertebral artery blood flow. Am. J. Roentgenol., *91*:1245, 1964.
12. Fields, W. S., and Lemak, N. A.: Joint study of extracranial arterial occlusion. J.A.M.A., *222*:1139, 1972.
13. Finkelstein, N. M., Byer, A., and Rush, B. F., Jr.: Subclavian-subclavian bypass for the subclavian steal syndrome. Surgery, *71*:142, 1972.
14. Folger, G. M., Jr., and Shah, K. D.: Subclavian steal in patients with Blalock-Taussig anastomosis. Circulation, *31*:241, 1965.
15. Forestner, J. E., Ghosh, S. K., Bergan, J. J., and Conn, J., Jr.: Subclavian-subclavian bypass for correction of the subclavian steal syndrome. Surgery, *71*:136, 1972.
16. Gonzalez, L. L., Wiot, J. F., and Boyd, A. D.: Retrograde flow in the vertebral artery. Arch. Surg., *91*:185, 1965.
17. Handa, J., Yoshida, K., and Meyer, J. S.: Hemodynamic effects of subclavian and innominate artery ligation. Surgery, *59*:1069, 1966.
18. Harper, J. A., Golding, A. L., Mazzei, E. A., and Cannon, J. A.: An experimental hemodynamic study of the subclavian steal syndrome. Surg. Gynecol. Obstet., *124*:1212, 1967.
19. Hewitt, R. L., Weichert, R. F., III, and Drapanas, T.: Centrifugal cerebral ischemia. Arch. Surg., *101*:155, 1970.
20. Irvine, W. T., Luck, R. J., and Jacobey, J. A.: Reversed blood-flow in the vertebral arteries causing recurrent brain-stem ischaemia. Lancet, *1*:994, 1965.
21. Janeway, R., Conrad, M., and Toole, J.: Chronic reversal of vertebral artery flow. Neurology, *15*:430, 1965.
22. Javid, H., Julian, O. C., Dye, W. S., and Hunter, J. A.: Management of cerebral arterial insufficiency caused by reversal of flow. Arch. Surg., *90*:634, 1965.
23. Killen, D. A., Foster, J. H., Gobbel, W. G., Jr., Stephenson, S. E., Jr., Collins, H. A., Billings, F. T., and Scott, H. W., Jr.: The subclavian steal syndrome. J. Thorac. Cardiovasc. Surg., *51*:539, 1966.
24. LeVeen, H. H., Piccone, V. A., Jr., Diaz, C., Christoudias, G.,

25. Slade, W., and Norstrand, I.: A simplified correction of subclavian steal syndrome. Surgery, *75*:299, 1974.
25. Lord, R. S. A., and Ehrenfeld, W. K.: Carotid-subclavian bypass: A hemodynamic study. Surgery, *66*:521, 1969.
26. McDowell, H. A., Jr.: Surgical correction of vertebral steal followed by contralateral retrograde vertebral flow. Ann. Surg., *168*:154, 1968.
27. Mannick, J. A., Suter, C. G., and Hume, D. M.: The "subclavian steal" syndrome: A further documentation. J.A.M.A., *182*:254, 1962.
28. Najafi, H., Dye, W. S., Javid, H., Hunter, J. A., Ostermiller, W. E., and Julian, O. C.: Carotid bifurcation stenosis and ipsilateral subclavian steal. Arch. Surg., *99*:289, 1969.
29. Newton, T. H., and Wylie, E. J.: Collateral circulation associated with occlusion of the proximal subclavian and innominate arteries. Am. J. Roentgenol., *91*:394, 1964.
30. North, R. R., Fields, W. S., DeBakey, M. E., et al.: Brachial-basilar insufficiency syndrome. Neurology, *12*:810, 1962.
31. Piccone, V. A., Jr., Karvounis, P., and LeVeen, H. H.: The subclavian steal syndrome. Angiology, *21*:240, 1970.
32. Pineda, A., and Smith, J. L.: True and false subclavian steal syndromes. Arch. Surg., *92*:258, 1966.
33. Powers, S. R., Jr., Roe, G. M., and Creel, W.: The relation between regional cerebral blood flow and cerebral function. Surgery, *61*:74, 1967.
34. Reivich, M., Holling, H. E., Roberts, B., et al.: Reversal of blood flow through the vertebral artery and its effects on cerebral circulation. N. Engl. J. Med., *265*:878, 1961.
35. Resnicoff, S. A., DeWeese, J. A., and Rob, C. G.: Surgical treatment of the subclavian steal syndrome. Circulation, *41* and *42* (Suppl. 2):147, 1970.
36. Rob, C.: Technique of surgical therapy. *In* Millikan, C. H., Siekert, R. G., and Whisnant, J. P. (Eds.): Cerebral Vascular Diseases, Third Conference. New York, Grune & Stratton, 1961, p. 112.
37. Sammartino, W. F., and Toole, J. F.: Reversed vertebral artery flow. Arch. Neurol., *10*:590, 1964.
38. Santschi, D. R., Frahm, C. J., Pascale, L. R., and Dumanian, A. V.: The subclavian steal syndrome. J. Thorac. Cardiovasc. Surg., *51*:103, 1966.
39. Shockman, A. T.: Retrograde vertebral artery flow as an artifact of technique. Am. J. Roentgenol., *91*:1258, 1964.
40. Siekert, R. G., Millikan, C. H., and Whisnant, J. P.: Reversed blood flow in the vertebral arteries. Ann. Intern. Med., *61*:64, 1964.
41. Solti, F., Iskum, M., Papp, S., Turbók, E., and Nagy, J.: The regulation of cerebral blood circulation in subclavian steal syndrome. Circulation, *42*:1185, 1970.
42. Yum, K. Y., and Myers, R. N.: Vertebral artery ligation. Arch. Surg., *98*:199, 1969.

4. THROMBOTIC OBLITERATION OF THE ABDOMINAL AORTA AND ILIAC ARTERIES (LERICHE SYNDROME)

David C. Sabiston, Jr., M.D.

Thrombotic obliteration of the aortic bifurcation was described by Leriche in 1940.[3] In an excellent discussion of this entire subject, Leriche emphasized that the disorder is a chronic process and is associated with a specific symptom complex. Typically, the condition affects males in the 35 to 60 age group.

CLINICAL MANIFESTATIONS

The symptoms characteristic of thrombotic occlusion of the terminal aorta include (1) extreme liability to fatigue of both lower limbs, which Leriche described

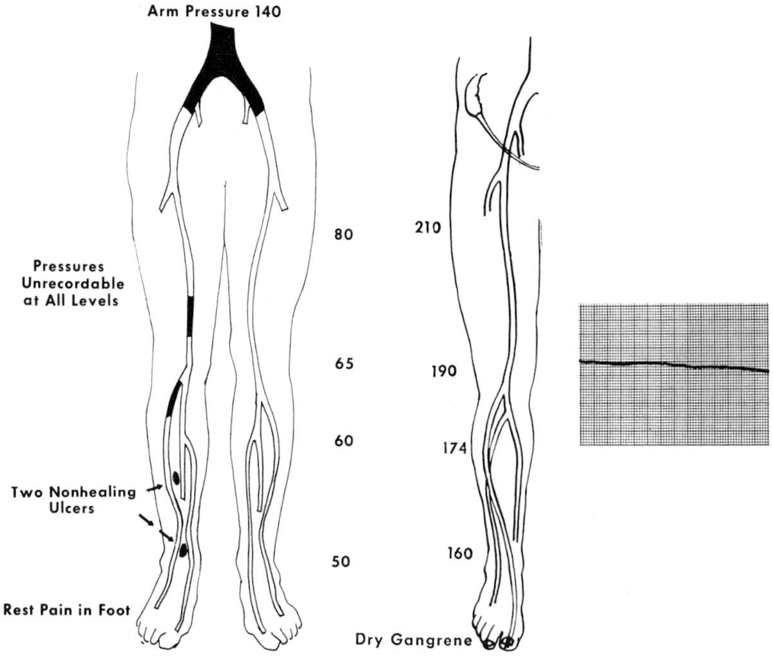

Figure 14. *A,* The extensive aortoiliac occlusion, combined with the superficial femoral artery and anterior tibial artery occlusion, reduced limb blood pressures below recordable levels. *B,* The normal ankle pressure of 160 mm. Hg and absent digit pulses placed the arterial occlusion between the ankle and digits. (From Strandness, D. E., Jr.: Collateral Circulation in Clinical Surgery. Philadelphia, W. B. Saunders Company, 1969.)

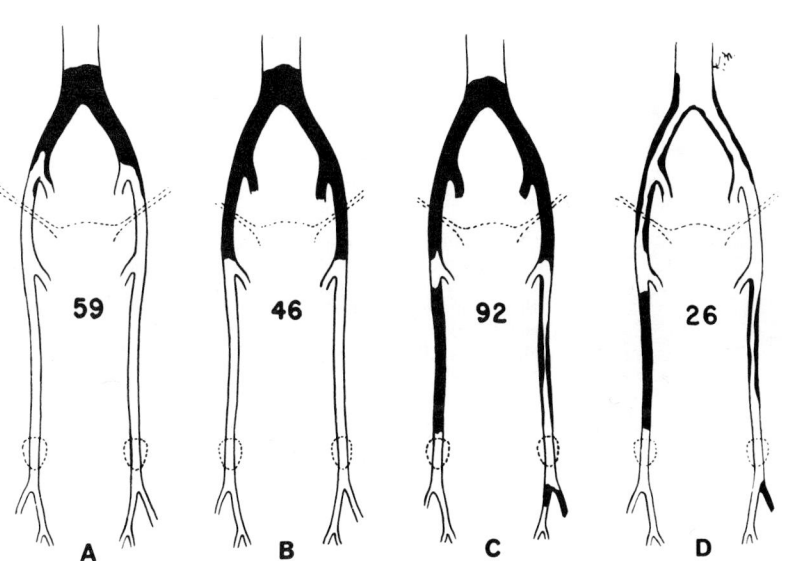

Arm Pressure 140

Pressures Unrecordable at All Levels

80

65

60

50

210

190

174

160

Two Nonhealing Ulcers

Rest Pain in Foot

Dry Gangrene

Figure 15. Schematic classification of extent of involvement in a series of patients with aortoiliofemoral arterial occlusive disease. (From Perdue, G. D., Long, W. D., and Smith, R. B., III: Trans. Southern Surg. Assoc., *82:*330, 1970.)

59   46   92   26

A   B   C   D

as a *weariness* rather than the typical intermittent claudication; (2) *symmetric atrophy* of both lower limbs without trophic changes of the skin or nails; (3) *pallor* of the legs and feet; and (4) *inability to maintain a stable erection* due to inadequate arterial flow to the penis secondary to hypogastric arterial obstruction. The physical findings include absence of pulses in the abdominal aorta and in all arteries distal to it. The physiologic changes in arterial pressure are shown in Figure 14.[8] Distal sites of segmental occlusion produce a further fall in arterial pressure, with development of ischemic ulcers.

Leriche emphasized that the disease was often well tolerated for 5 and even 10 years, but usually ended in gangrene of one or both extremities. The characteristic pathologic finding is an atherosclerotic lesion in the wall of the abdominal aorta with superimposed thrombosis. The lumen characteristically narrows gradually, and so *acute* symptoms are not apt to occur.[4]

The diagnosis is confirmed by *arteriography*, in which occlusion of the terminal abdominal aorta, and often of both common iliacs, is demonstrated (Fig. 15).[1, 6] The occlusion may involve any portion of the abdominal aorta from the renal arteries distally. The collateral circulation that develops is shown in an arteriogram in Figure 16,[2] and the anatomic collateral pathways are shown schematically in Figure 17A.[2]

It is extremely important that patients stop smoking after bypass grafts performed for the Leriche syndrome. The evidence is quite clear that thrombosis is appreciably increased by continuance of smoking.[7] The relationship showing percentage graft occlusion according to the smoking history is demonstrated in Figure 18.

SURGICAL MANAGEMENT

Although thromboendarterectomy with direct reconstitution of flow is appropriate in some patients, the majority with occlusion of the abdominal aorta are managed by bilateral bypass grafts from the aorta to the common femoral arteries (Fig. 17*B*). It may be necessary to perform a short thromboendarterectomy just distal to the renal arteries to permit a site for the proximal anastomosis. However, it is important not to disturb the aorta any more than necessary and to reduce dissection in this region to the minimum. These precautions prevent the troublesome ejaculatory complications that may otherwise result. It has been shown that thromboendarterectomy and resection of the aorta as definitive procedures for aortic thrombosis produce disturbances in ejaculation in 68 per cent of patients, whereas when bypass is chosen as the primary treatment, only 26 per cent have this difficulty.[5]

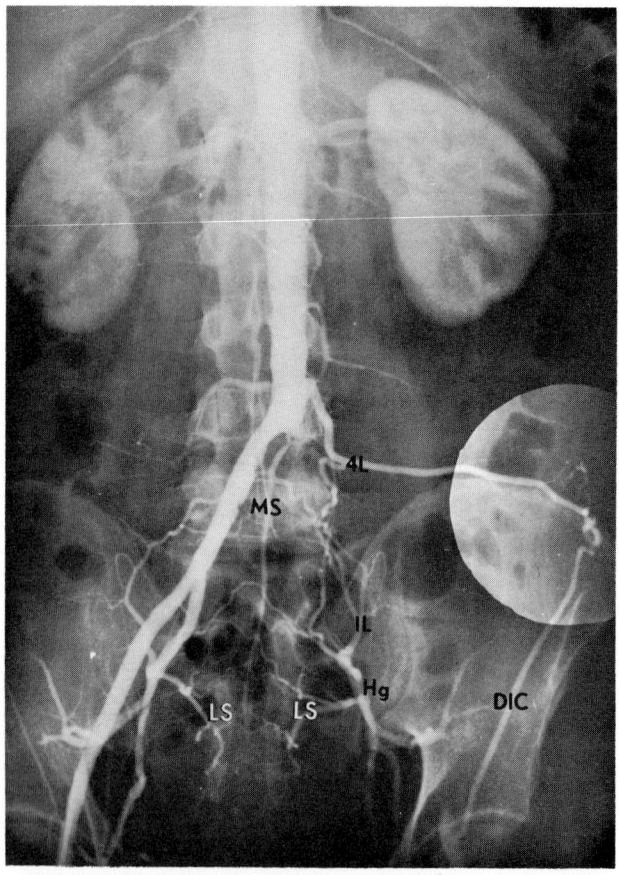

Figure 16. A 43-year-old male with left intermittent claudication. The fourth lumbar (4L) is the origin of a pathway to the femoral via the deep iliac circumflex (DIC) and to the hypogastric (Hg) via the iliolumbar (IL). The middle sacral (MS) and lateral sacral (LS) contribute to a transpelvic anastomosis to the hypogastric (Hg). (From Friedenberg, M. J., and Perez, C. A.: Am. J. Roentgenol., *94*:145, 1965.)

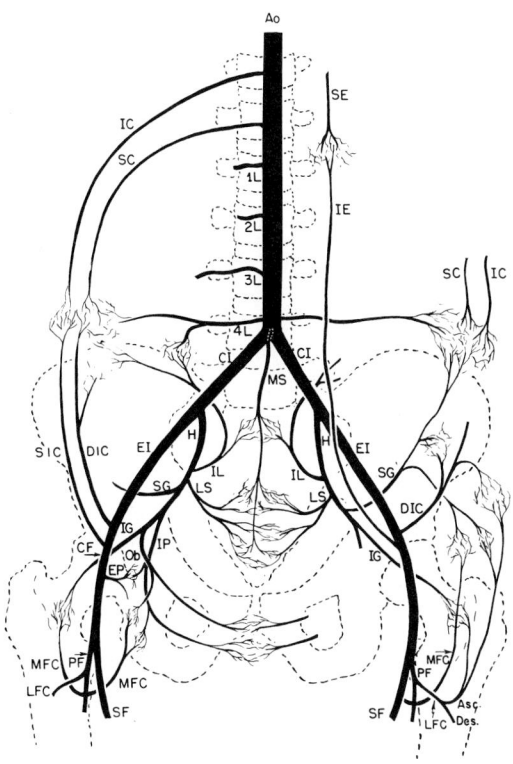

Figure 17A. Composite line drawing showing schematically the major parietal pathways of collateral circulation in aortoiliofemoral occlusive disease.

Ao	Aorta
Asc	Ascending branch
CF	Common femoral
CI	Common iliac
Des	Descending branch
DIC	Deep iliac circumflex
EI	External iliac
EP	External pudendal
H	Hypogastric
IC	Intercostal
IE	Inferior epigastric
IG	Inferior gluteal
IL	Iliolumbar
IP	Internal pudendal
L	Lumbar
LFC	Lateral femoral circumflex
LS	Lateral sacral
MFC	Medial femoral circumflex
MS	Middle sacral
Ob	Obturator
PF	Profunda femoris
SC	Subcostal
SE	Superior epigastric
SF	Superficial femoral
SG	Superior gluteal
SIC	Superficial iliac circumflex

(From Friedenberg, M. J., and Perez, C. A.: Am. J. Roentgenol., *94*:145, 1965.)

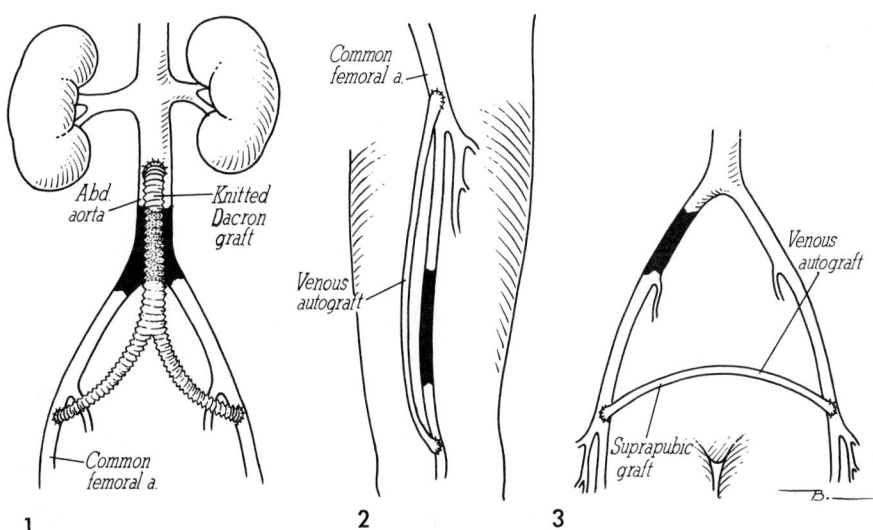

Figure 17B. Diagrammatic illustrations of various bypass grafts. *1,* For occlusion of the abdominal aorta, a bypass graft placed proximal to the occlusion can be inserted distally into each of the common femoral arteries in the groin. *2,* For occlusion of the superficial femoral artery, a venous autograft may be placed from the common femoral artery above to the femoral or popliteal artery distal to the obstruction. *3,* For unilateral iliac arterial occlusion, a suprapubic graft can be placed from one common femoral artery to the other in a subcutaneous suprapubic tunnel. Generally, under these circumstances a venous autograft is preferable to a plastic prosthesis, although the latter can be employed.

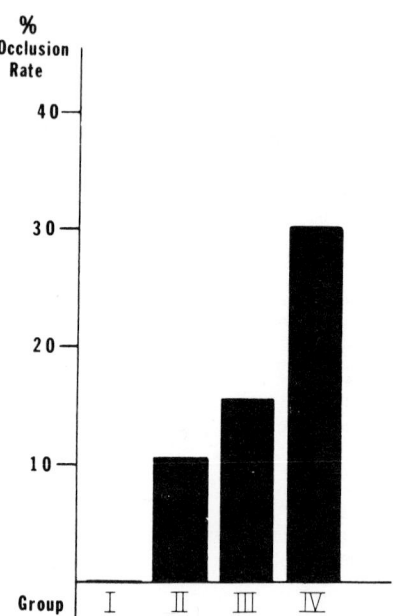

Figure 18. Occlusion rate of prosthetic grafts inserted for Leriche syndrome according to smoking history. Group I: Patients who did not smoke either before or after operation. Group II: Patients who were cigarette smokers before operation but ceased smoking postoperatively. Group III: Patients who were cigarette smokers preoperatively and who continued to smoke following operation up to one pack daily. Group IV: Patients who remained heavy smokers following operation, using more than a pack of cigarettes daily. (From Robicsek, F., Daugherty, H. K., Mullen, D. C., Masters, T. N., Narbay, D., and Sanger, P. W.: The effect of continued cigarette smoking on the patency of synthetic vascular grafts in Leriche syndrome. J. Thorac. Cardiovasc. Surg., 70:107–112, 1975.)

SELECTED REFERENCES

Foster, J. H.: Arteriography. Cornerstone of vascular surgery. Arch. Surg., 109:605, 1974.
  In this essay, the development of arteriography from its origin to the present is reviewed. Of particular significance is the fact that the author advocates more extensive use of arteriography, especially in patients with the Leriche syndrome as well as other forms of arterial obstruction.

Strandness, D. E., and Sumner, D. S.: Hemodynamics for Surgeons. New York, Grune & Stratton, 1975.
  This is an excellent and quite thorough monograph concerning the hemodynamics of the vascular system. The determinants of cardiac output and arterial and venous flow, as well as a variety of physical and physiologic aspects of the entire field are considered in detail. In addition, a number of clinical entities are used as examples to illustrate the basic physical and physiologic principles.

REFERENCES

1. Foster, J. H.: Arteriography. Cornerstone of vascular surgery. Arch. Surg., 109:605, 1974.
2. Friedenberg, M. J., and Perez, C. A.: Collateral circulation in aorto-ilio-femoral occlusive disease: As demonstrated by a unilateral percutaneous common femoral artery needle injection. Am. J. Roentgenol., 94:145, 1965.
3. Leriche, R.: De la résection du carrefour aortico-iliaque avec double sympathectomie lombaire pour thrombose arteritique de l'aorte. Le syndrome de l'oblitération termino-aortique par artérite. Presse Med., 48:601, 1940.
4. Leriche, R., and Morel, A.: The syndrome of thrombotic obliteration of the aortic bifurcation. Ann. Surg., 127:193, 1948.
5. May, A. G., DeWeese, J. A., and Rob, C. G.: Changes in sexual

function following operation on the abdominal aorta. Surgery, 65:41, 1969.
6. Perdue, G. D., Long, W. D., and Smith, R. B., III: Perspective concerning aorto-femoral arterial reconstruction. Trans. South. Surg. Assoc., 82:330, 1970.
7. Robicsek, F., Daugherty, H. K., Mullen, D. C., Masters, T. N., Narbay, D., and Sanger, P. W.: The effect of continued cigarette smoking on the patency of synthetic vascular grafts in Leriche syndrome. J. Thorac. Cardiovasc. Surg., 70:107, 1975.
8. Strandness, D. E., Jr.: Chronic arterial occlusion. *In* Strandness, D. E., Jr. (Ed.): Collateral Circulation in Clinical Surgery. Philadelphia, W. B. Saunders Company, 1969.

5. ILIAC ARTERIAL OCCLUSION

David C. Sabiston, Jr., M.D.

The iliac arteries may be individually stenosed or occluded. The symptoms are usually those of claudication of the hip and thigh associated with diminished or absent pulses in that extremity. Arteriography is diagnostic. When symptoms are unilateral, involvement of the opposite leg can often be seen on the arteriogram. Indeed, symptoms may appear in the opposite leg following operation when the patient is able to exercise sufficiently. Bypass grafts from the aorta above to the common femoral artery below are usually indicated.

6. FEMOROPOPLITEAL AND FEMOROTIBIAL BYPASS

Frederick A. Reichle, M.D.

HISTORICAL ASPECTS

The lower extremity has been the site of many of the earliest approaches in the progress of vascular surgery in the human being.[6, 39] Ligation of peripheral aneurysms was performed by the ancients, although the records of this knowledge were in large part lost during the Middle Ages. Considerable information is available on the early experimental techniques that followed the first experimental vascular anastomoses in the creation of canine portacaval shunt by Eck in 1877. Owing to considerable animal experimentation in the ensuing 20 years, Murphy first anastomosed a human artery in the distal femoral area.[30] Initial successful vein graft operations were reported in 1906 by Goyanes,[15] by Lexer[20] in 1907, and by Pringle[33] in 1913. Goyanes' and Pringle's vein grafts were performed for popliteal aneurysm and Lexer's vein replacement was performed for repair of axillary aneurysm. Weglowski[53] subsequently reported 51 vein grafts in German casualties in World War I.

The *bypass* graft was first proposed by Jeger in 1913.[17] In 1948 Kunlin[18] first performed a human bypass graft of an occluded human artery as a 16 cm. arterial replacement of the femoral artery. By 1951 he had performed 17 operations, with continued patency in seven.[19] In 1952 Voorhees et al.[50] reported that a prosthesis was capable of continued arterial function in experimental animals. More recently, distal bypasses to small vessels of the distal lower extremity have been demonstrated to be effective in limb salvage in patients with severe ischemia. Thus, the present capability of revascularization of ischemic peripheral tissues has had a relatively deliberate and prolonged experimental and clinical background, which has led to the recent extremely rapid increase in effective salvage of ischemic limbs by bypasses to any level of the distal arterial tree.

CLINICAL EVALUATION OF ARTERIAL INSUFFICIENCY OF THE LOWER EXTREMITY

Clinical History

Routine physical examination and history will correctly establish the diagnosis of arterial insufficiency of the lower extremity in the vast majority of patients. The history of claudication or rest pain is so specific that arterial insufficiency can usually be strongly suspected on the basis of the history alone. The most frequent site of claudication is the calf musculature. Calf claudication suggests occlusion of the superficial femoral artery with or without popliteal artery occlusion. Claudication may also concomitantly exist in thigh as well as buttock musculature. Claudication in the more proximal muscle groups of the lower extremity indicates occlusion or stenosis of the iliac arterial system. Patients will voluntarily relate a history of claudication that is highly specific. Claudication distance is reproducible and consistent. Prompt relief of the exercise-induced muscle pain occurs with cessation of ambulation.

Similarly, patients with rest pain usually relate a characteristic history. Rest pain is most frequently located in the most distal portion of the extremity, particularly in the toes or distal foot. With great frequency, the patient experiences onset of pain after reclining and relief of pain upon resumption of dependency of the involved lower extremity. Many patients with rest pain have associated claudication. A history typical for claudication and rest pain associated with physical findings consistent with arterial insufficiency establish the diagnosis of arterial insufficiency. Rest pain is a significantly more advanced grade of ischemia as compared to claudication alone. Operative revascularization can be highly effective in patients with gangrene or rest pain as well as in patients with claudication. Claudication is considered a relative indication for revascularization depending on the patient's age, his occupational needs for ambulation, and the extent to which claudication interferes with his daily life style.[23] Rest pain is a definite indication for arteriographic evaluation of the anatomic site of occlusion and for operative revascularization. Similarly, patients who have decreased extremity arterial perfusion and who have a history of gangrene or ischemic ulceration must undergo prompt arteriography and arterial reconstruction to prevent further tissue loss.

The differential diagnosis of lower extremity pain secondary to neuropathy as a result of pre-existing ischemia or diabetes mellitus may in some patients be difficult. The distribution of neuropathic pain may be in a sensory nerve distribution, whereas pain of ischemia most commonly is located distally in the foot, especially in the toes. Burning or shooting pain of neuropathy is different from rest pain. Rest pain is relieved or improved by extremity dependency. Neuropathic pain and rest pain may coexist. The physical examination will allow determination of the source of extremity pain in most patients.

Physical Examination

Several easily performed maneuvers as part of the physical examination will almost invariably demonstrate lack of tissue perfusion in the lower extremity and thus will corroborate the diagnosis, which can be strongly suspected on the basis of the history. Of paramount importance in the physical examination of the ischemic distal extremity is demonstration of pallor of elevation, rubor of dependency, and prolongation of the venous filling time. These tests can be done within a few minutes during routine office evaluation. These safe and easily performed observations give more clinically relevant information regarding the status of the arterial nutritional perfusion of the distal extremity than do specialized hemodynamic studies.

Although the arteriogram is of extreme importance in delineating the anatomic site of arterial occlusion and the distal runoff, the diagnosis of arterial insufficiency is established by history and physical examination. The venous filling time, if prolonged, is almost always significant. If venous filling time is normal and other signs and symptoms of arterial insufficiency are present, prolongation of venous filling time may not be significant. In the patient with venous valvular incompetency, retrograde venous filling may produce a falsely normal venous filling time in the presence of significant arterial insufficiency. Because many patients with demonstrable arterial insufficiency in the lower extremity will have associated physical findings of arterial disease in other areas, general vascular examination is important. Careful examination of the palpable amplitude of the femoral pulse is mandatory prior to distal arterial reconstruction to determine whether adequate arterial inflow from the aortoiliac system into the femoral artery is present. Auscultation over the aortoiliac areas for audible bruits and palpation for aortic dilatation must be performed. If stenosis or occlusion of the arterial inflow to the groin is suspected, preoperative arteriography must include the higher arterial tree prior to consideration of reconstruction of the femoropopliteal and femorotibial arterial system of the lower extremity. A number of specialized clinical studies are now available to assess patients hemodynamically before and after arterial reconstruction.[44]

Preoperative Arteriography

Angiographic demonstration of a patent distal vessel with an adequate arteriogram is essential in selection of patients for bypass. The site of distal anastomosis is determined primarily on the basis of the preoperative arteriogram, inasmuch as operative exploration of the distal vessel is not an adequate means of evaluating runoff, nor of selecting the site of distal anastomosis. The preoperative arteriogram must be thorough and adequate in attempting to delineate arterial runoff. The runoff of the distal patent vessel into the ramifications of the arterial tree should be demonstrated to rule out the presence of more distal stenosis or occlusion. If not bypassed, distal arterial occlusive disease may lead to early or delayed graft occlusion due to inadequate arterial run-off. In the great majority of patients, arterial run-off in a severely ischemic extremity is demonstrable on arteriogram because the viability of the extremity is of necessity maintained by collateral circulation. If no distal major vessel is visualized, the adequacy of the arteriogram must be ascertained. Demonstration of collateral vessels in the region of a nonvisualized major distal artery is considered evidence of an adequate arteriogram. In our experience, angiographically absent distal run-off precluding attempted distal bypass is uncommon. It may be necessary to film over the distal extremity for prolonged periods of time, even as long as 30 to 90 seconds, to visualize delayed filling of distal arterial run-off in tibial or peroneal arteries. If patent distal arteries are seen, limb salvage can usually be attempted by small vessel bypass (Fig. 19). Intraoperative arteriography may also be performed if the adequacy of the distal runoff is questionable on the basis of operative findings.[8, 21, 32]

Choice of Graft Material

Reversed autogenous saphenous vein is used for femoropopliteal bypass whenever adequate vein is available. If adequate ipsilateral autogenous saphenous vein is not available, contralateral saphenous vein or cephalic vein is considered. Prosthetic grafts are capable of function and limb salvage when bypasses are carried to the proximal or distal popliteal area. The rate of late occlusion is higher with prosthetics than in bypasses performed with autogenous saphenous vein.[34, 36] Prosthetic materials currently available are inadequate for use in bypassing to tibial or peroneal arteries. However, inadequacy of autogenous vein must be conclusively demonstrated prior to rejecting a given patient for bypass. At times, inadequacy of autogenous vein can be determined only after operative exploration of the vein is carried out and after operative exploration, removal, and attempted dilatation of the proposed vein graft.

RESULTS OF ARTERIAL RECONSTRUCTION IN THE SEVERELY ISCHEMIC LOWER EXTREMITY

Initial Graft Function and Initial Limb Salvage After Femoropopliteal and Femorotibial Bypass

The feasibility of limb salvage by bypasses in the ischemic lower extremity to the popliteal artery and to the tibial artery has been demonstrated.[1, 4, 5, 7, 10-14, 16, 22, 24, 26-29, 31, 47] In a recent review, initial results after femoropopliteal bypass were functional bypass and limb salvage, 182 of 224 (81.2 per cent).[36] The corresponding initial results of femorotibial bypass were functional bypass, 102 of 140 (72.8 per cent); limb salvage, 96 of 104 (68.6 per cent) (Fig. 20). Thus, the results of femorotibial and femoropopliteal bypass done primarily for gangrene, gangrenous ulceration, or rest pain indicated that bypasses to the severely ischemic distal lower extremity are capable of limb salvage in a significant percentage of individuals when bypasses are carried to the proximal or distal popliteal or to the tibial or peroneal arteries. The limb salvage capability of femorotibial grafts can be expected in view of studies in which the average flow through femorotibial grafts is in many cases equivalent to that measured in femoropopliteal grafts.

The results as described here with tibial bypass include patients in whom femoroperoneal bypass was performed as well as femorotibial bypass. In this particular group of patients, rest pain, gangrene, or ischemic ulceration was the most common indication for operation. In some patients, limiting claudication, usually occupational claudication, was considered an indication for bypass to either popliteal or tibial artery. In 224 patients undergoing femoropopliteal bypass, the indications were gangrene, 65; ischemic ulceration, 38; rest pain, 77; and claudication, 44. In 144 patients undergoing femorotibial bypasses during the same period of time at the same institution, the indications were gangrene, 54; ischemic ulceration, 28; rest pain, 47; and claudication, 11. Thus, 310 of 364 (85.1 per cent) bypasses were performed in the presence of severe ischemia (gangrene, ischemic ulceration, or rest pain). These results indicate that significant extremity salvage can be anticipated after either femoropopliteal or femorotibial bypass in the presence of severe extremity ischemia.

Long-term Results of Patients Undergoing Femoropopliteal or Femorotibial Bypass for Severe Extremity Ischemia

Late graft occlusion in patients in whom initial limb salvage is achieved is relatively low after both femoropopliteal and femorotibial bypass (Fig. 21). The long-term patency of femorotibial and femoropopliteal bypasses is listed, together with the accumulated patency rate, in Tables 4 and 5. In our total follow-up experience (1 to 11 years), delayed graft occlusion occurred in 24.6 per cent (41 of 167) of patients after femoropopliteal bypass and in 17.4 per cent (15 of 86) of patients undergoing femorotibial bypass.

After femoropopliteal bypass (autogenous vein and prosthetic) (4- to 8-year follow-up) 67.2 per cent (39 of 58) of patients are currently alive with patent bypasses or have died with patent bypasses (Fig. 22). In patients with autogenous vein bypass to the popliteal artery, 78.9 per cent (30 of 38) are currently functional or have died with limb salvage. After femorotibial bypass, 75.0 per cent (30 of 40) of patients are alive with limb salvage or have died with patent bypasses (4- to 8-year follow-up). Most patients undergoing bypasses for limb-threatening ischemia benefit substantially from revascularization to the tibial or popliteal arteries, with current limb salvage in living patients or with limb salvage until the time of death in patients dying from other causes (Fig. 22).

Mortality After Femoropopliteal or Femorotibial Bypass

In the same group of patients, mortality occurred in 7 of 224 (3.1 per cent) patients after femoropopliteal

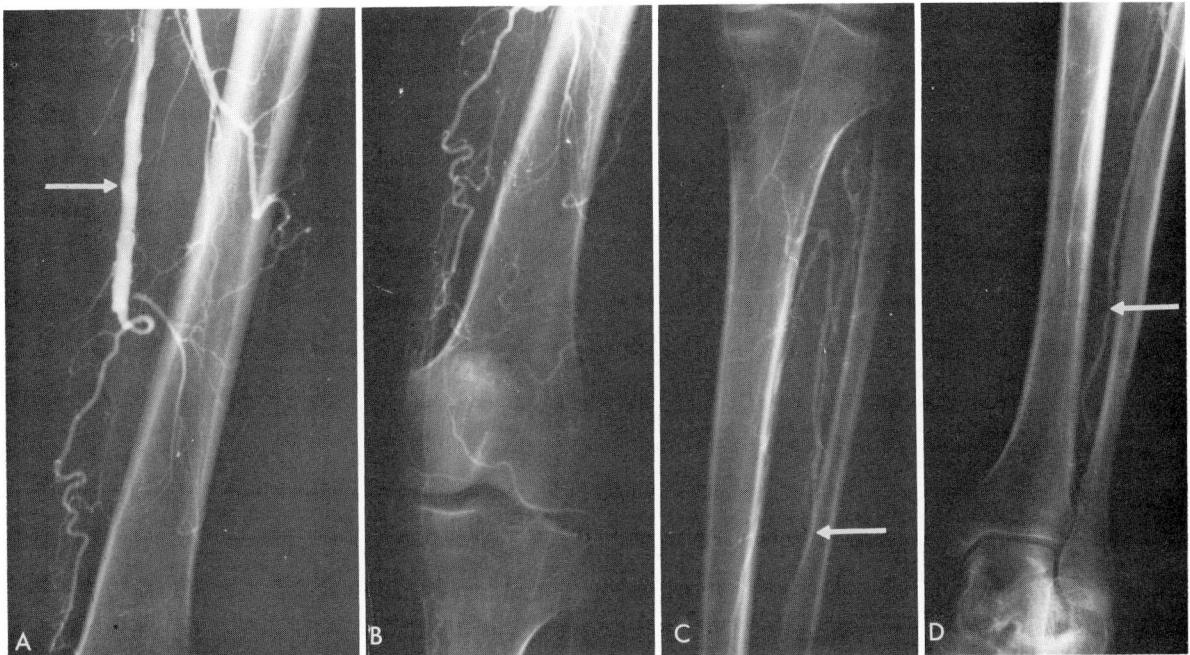

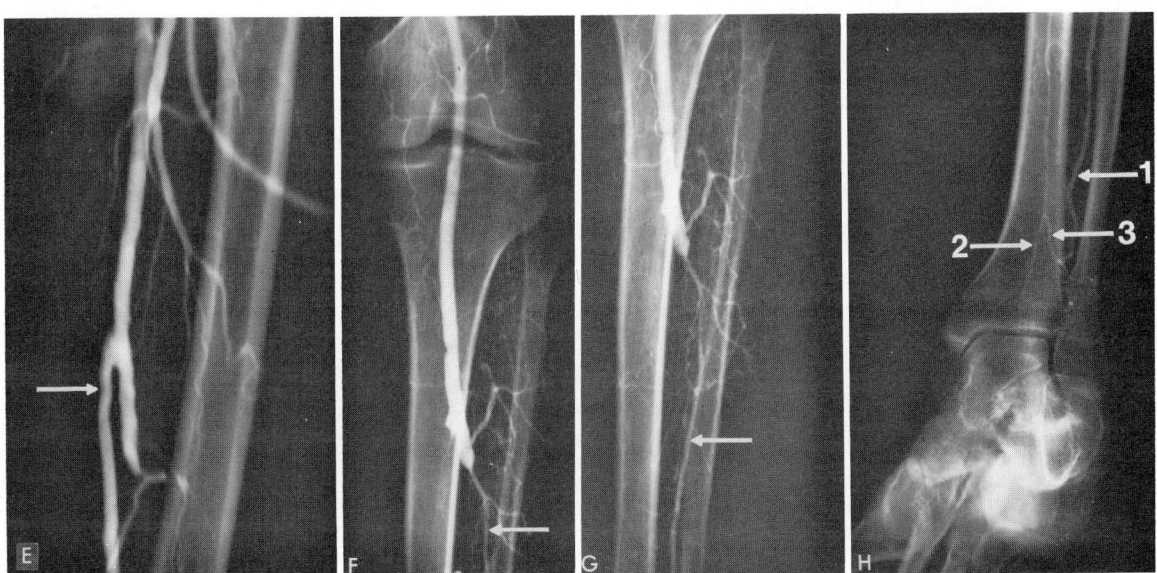

Figure 19.   *A* to *D,* Adequate preoperative arteriogram of a 58-year-old male who had rest pain of the left lower extremity. *A,* Occlusion of the midsuperficial femoral artery. *B,* Absent popliteal runoff is observed despite collaterals visualized in the region of the popliteal space, indicating adequacy of the arteriogram in this area (arrow). *C* and *D,* The peroneal artery (arrows) is visualized along its entire length to the ankle. *E* to *H,* Femoral arteriogram following femoroperoneal bypass (arrow) reversed autogenous saphenous vein anastomosed to the superficial femoral artery. *F,* Autogenous vein bypass crosses the knee joint and is anastomosed to the proximal peroneal artery. Both proximal and distal runoff into peroneal artery (arrow) is seen. *G,* Distal peroneal artery (arrow) fills. *H,* Distally the peroneal artery (1) communicates by a well-developed collateral (3) into the distal anterior tibial artery (2). This collateral is not uncommon and provides additional runoff into the foot. When the peroneal artery has collaterals visible on arteriogram, the prognosis for peroneal bypass is greatly improved. The foot developed marked heat of revascularization in the early postoperative period, and the patient gradually developed a dorsalis pedis pulse which gradually increased in amplitude in the postoperative period. (From Reichle, F. A., and Tyson, R. R.: Ann. Surg., *181*:182, 1975.)

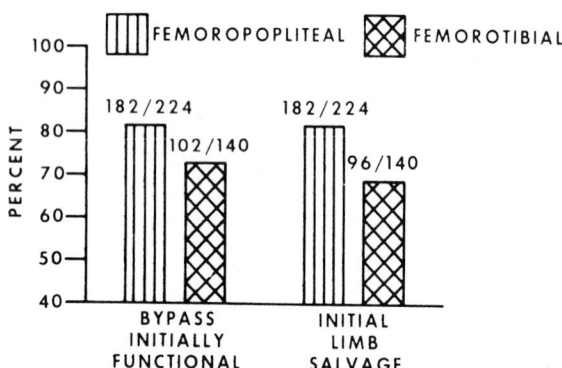

Figure 20. Incidence of bypass function and limb salvage in patients undergoing femoropopliteal or femorotibial bypass during the same period of time at the same institution. (From Reichle, F. A., and Tyson, R. R.: Ann. Surg., *182*:450, 1975.)

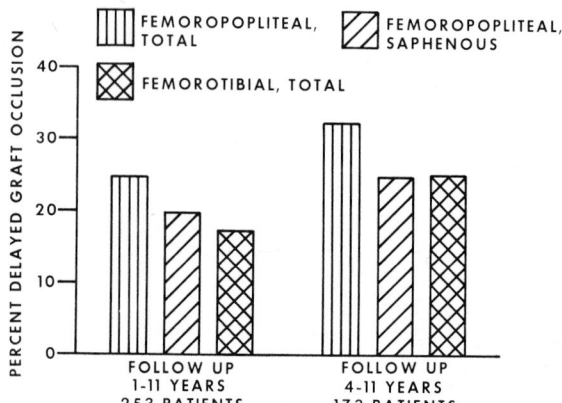

Figure 21. Incidence of delayed graft occlusion (percentage of surgically treated patients who achieve initial limb salvage and who are available for follow-up information) in patients undergoing femoropopliteal or femorotibial bypasses for severe ischemia of the lower extremity during the same period of time at the same institution. (From Reichle, F. A., and Tyson, R. R.: Ann. Surg., *182*:450, 1975.)

bypass and 4 of 140 (2.9 per cent) patients undergoing femorotibial bypass. Mortality in most of these patients was related to cardiac disease. Mortality is more common in diabetic patients. Mortality after bypass is lower than mortality generally reported for primary amputation of severely ischemic lower extremities.

Reconstruction of Femoral Profunda (Profundoplasty); Thromboendarterectomy

Alternative to femoropopliteal bypass is the possibility of reconstruction of the occluded or stenosed take-off of the profunda femoris artery in the presence of an occluded superficial femoral artery.[25] Assessment of stenosis of the profunda femoris is best done when both anteroposterior and oblique arteriograms are performed preoperatively. Superficial femoral thromboendarterectomy has the potential for prolonged patency and limb salvage in selected patients.[49] Whereas this may provide a suitable alternative to prosthetic femoropopliteal bypass, thromboendarterectomy is generally considered to be more effective in more localized

lesions and may not be feasible if heavy calcification of the media or destruction of the elastic lamina is present.

Results of Femoroperoneal Bypass

Whereas early and long-term efficacy of bypasses to anterior and posterior tibial arteries is now becoming well established, the results of bypasses to the peroneal artery are less well understood. Definite limb salvage can be achieved by peroneal artery bypass but the incidence of adequate revascularization is lower than after popliteal or tibial bypass. Therefore, in assessing the value of femoroperoneal bypass, consideration of the preoperative indications is of particular importance. In our initial observations, 35.7 per cent limb salvage (minimum of six weeks limb salvage and graft

TABLE 4. Long-Term Patency of Femoropopliteal Bypasses to Severely Ischemic Lower Extremities

Interval (in months)	Number of Bypassed Extremities at Risk	Number of Bypasses Failing	Number of Bypasses Not Observed Throughout Interval Owing to		Failure Rate In Interval (Per Cent)	Patency Rate In Interval (Per Cent)	Accumulated Patency Rate (Per Cent)
			Death	Duration of Follow-up			
0–12	224	58	16	25	28.5	71.5	71.5
13–24	125	6	16	14	5.5	94.5	67.6
25–36	89	2	7	3	2.4	97.6	65.9
37–48	67	6	2	7	9.6	90.4	59.6
49–60	52	1	4	7	2.2	97.8	58.3
61–72	40	2	5	7	5.9	94.1	54.9
73–84	26	1	3	3	4.3	95.7	52.5
85–96	19	0	1	9	0	100	52.5
97–108	9	0	2	3	0	100	52.5
109–120	4	0	0	1	0	100	52.5
121–132	3	0	0	0	0	100	52.5

TABLE 5.   Long-Term Patency of Femorotibial Bypasses to
Severely Ischemic Lower Extremities*

Interval (in months)	Number of Bypassed Extremities at Risk	Number of Bypasses Failing	Number of Bypasses Not Observed Throughout Interval Owing to		Failure Rate In Interval (Per Cent)	Patency Rate In Interval (Per Cent)	Accumulated Patency Rate (Per Cent)
			Death	Duration of Follow-up			
0–12	140	44	13	23	36.1	63.9	63.9
13–24	60	0	6	8	0	100	63.9
25–36	46	3	4	9	7.6	92.4	59.1
37–48	30	2	2	11	8.5	91.5	54.1
49–60	15	0	3	2	0	100	54.1
61–72	10	0	0	1	0	100	54.1
73–84	9	2	0	2	25.0	75	40.5
85–96	5	0	0	1	0	100	40.5
97–108	4	0	1	1	0	100	40.5
109–120	2	0	0	1	0	100	40.5
121–132	1	0	0	0	0	100	40.5

*Modified from Wheelock, F. C., and Filtzer, H. S.: Femoral Grafts in Diabetics. Arch. Surg., *99*:776, 1969.

function postoperatively) occurred in patients in whom femoroperoneal bypass was performed in lieu of primary amputation.[37] Over the same period, femorotibial bypasses produced 70.8 per cent limb salvage. Thus, a significantly lower incidence of limb salvage can be anticipated with bypasses to the peroneal artery. The observed decreased limb salvage after femoroperoneal bypass is in large part due to a relatively high incidence of graft patency without limb salvage (44.4 per cent of operated patients) following femoro-

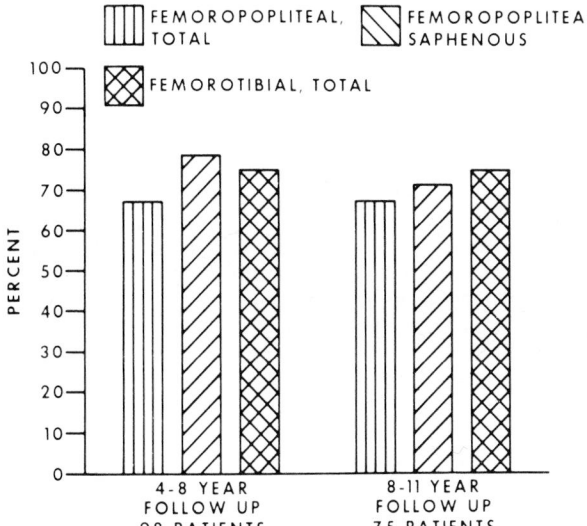

Figure 22.   Long-term follow-up of patients achieving initial limb salvage after bypass (percentage of surgically treated patients who achieved initial limb salvage and who are currently alive with limb salvage and graft function or who had limb salvage and graft function at the time of death) in patients undergoing femoropopliteal or femorotibial bypass in the same institution over the same period of time. (From Reichle, F. A., and Tyson, R. R.: Ann. Surg., *182*:454, 1975.)

peroneal bypasses. These bypasses were definitely functional in the postoperative period and at the time of subsequent distal limb amputation. The reason that bypass function without limb salvage is considerably less common after bypasses to the peroneal arteries than after bypasses to anterior or posterior arteries is presumably related to the anatomic distribution of the peroneal artery, which frequently has little distal runoff into the foot. However, in some patients extensive runoff through collaterals may contribute to continued patency of femoroperoneal bypasses. Patients in whom direct anastomosis into the arterial tree in the foot by collaterals has occurred in the course of the chronic occlusive arterial disease frequently developed heat of revascularization and loss of rest pain and healing of areas of demarcating distal gangrene and limb salvage (see Fig. 19).

Patients in the aforementioned series were operated on primarily for limb salvage, and bypasses were therefore performed in lieu of primary amputation. Preoperative indications included gangrene, gangrenous ulceration, and rest pain. In this series no patients undergoing femoroperoneal bypass had intermittent claudication as the only operative indication. As a salvage procedure, even 35 per cent limb salvage would seem satisfactory in lieu of primary amputation.

Similar to the experience with femorotibial bypasses, femoroperoneal bypasses seldom undergo late bypass occlusion after initial patency has been achieved. To date, in this series, no late bypass occlusions have occurred in any patient in whom femoroperoneal bypass resulted in patent bypass and initial limb salvage. The incidence of diabetes mellitus in patients in whom only femoroperoneal artery is patent and in whom severe ischemia is present is higher (71.4 per cent) than in patients in whom femorotibial bypass is feasible (47.7 per cent). As with femorotibial bypasses, only patients in whom an adequate autogenous saphenous vein is available as determined preoperatively or intraoperatively are candidates for bypass to the peroneal artery. Angiographic demonstration of patent distal vessels with a thorough arteriogram is essential to determine the feasibility of distal bypasses to peroneal as well as tibial arteries. Demonstration of collateral vessels in the region of a nonvisualized main distal artery is considered evidence of an inadequate arteriogram. If only the peroneal artery is visible on adequate arteriogram, bypass to the artery should be undertaken in the presence of severe ischemia if adequate autogenous vein is available. If in addition to demonstration of the peroneal artery the preoperative angiogram also demonstrates collaterals above the ankle from distal peroneal to either the anterior or posterior tibial arteries, the chance of limb salvage by successful bypass is considerably increased.

ANATOMIC AND TECHNICAL ASPECTS OF FEMOROPOPLITEAL AND FEMOROTIBIAL BYPASS

The preferred route of bypass from the femoral artery distally is generally considered to be a subsartorial tunnel in the thigh (Fig. 23).[46] The tunnel proceeds posterior to the consistently caudally directed branches of the saphenous nerve in the distal third of the thigh approximately at the level of the termination of the adductor canal. From this point distally the tunnel is best constructed along the natural course of the vessel to which the bypass will eventually be anastomosed. Accordingly, either the distal popliteal, anterior tibial, posterior tibial, or peroneal artery will be bypassed by tunnels that are directed in the same anatomic plane as the artery itself naturally follows.

The popliteal artery is exposed through a medial incision either above or below the knee (Fig. 24). The proximal popliteal space is approached by an incision carried down to the deep fascia. Opening the dense

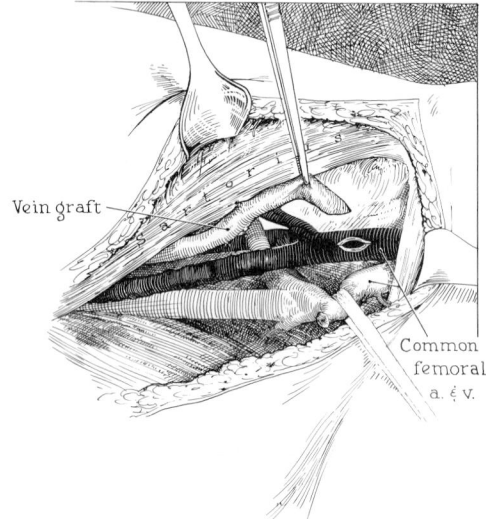

Figure 23. Operative exposure of the common femoral artery; autogenous saphenous vein graft from common femoral to popliteal artery is in its subsartorial tunnel entering the thigh and prepared for end-to-side anastomoses. (From Szilagy, D. E., Smith, R. F., and Elliott, J. P.: Arch. Surg., 89:117, 1975.)

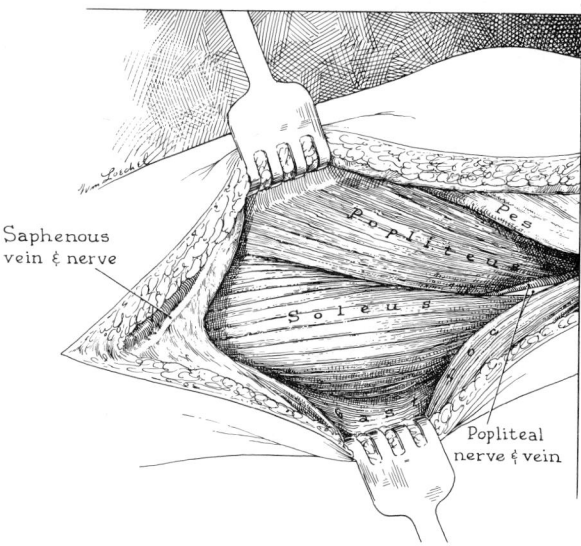

Figure 24. Approach to the distal popliteal space. The longitudinal incision is posterior to the saphenous vein and nerve. After entering the deep fascia the popliteal space is entered anterior to soleus and gastrocnemius. The popliteal neurovascular bundle is easily palpable on a posterior surface of the tibia. (From Szilagyi, D. E., Smith, R. F., and Elliott, J. P.: Arch. Surg., 89:115, 1975.)

fascia will allow direct entry into the proximal popliteal space. The artery is then readily palpable lying on the posterior surface of the distal femur. The tendons of the semitendinosus and the semimembranosus posteriorly are preserved.

The distal popliteal space is approached through an incision extending from the medial eminence of the proximal tibia and directed longitudinally and inferiorly, directly posterior to and parallel to the greater saphenous vein in this region. All incisions for popliteal or tibial arteries are carefully performed to avoid injury to the greater saphenous vein, which lies directly subcutaneously and superficial to the deep fascia. The popliteal space is then entered anterior to the medial tendon of the gastrocnemius and posterior to the tibia. The incision is carried caudally proximal to insertion of the soleus muscle on the posterior medial aspect of the tibia. Upon incision of the deep fascia, the distal popliteal space is readily entered between the popliteus muscle anteriorly and the soleus and gastrocnemius muscles posteriorly (Fig. 25). The artery is easily palpable lying on the posterior aspect of the tibia.

The proximal posterior tibial and peroneal arteries are approached by a medial incision made just posterior to the tibia and to the saphenous vein.[48] Whereas the popliteal incision was located proximal to the attachments of the soleus, in approaching the posterior tibial or peroneal artery, the tibial attachment of the soleus muscle is partially severed close to its tibial origin, and a fascial plane deep to the soleus muscle is entered. The fascial plane that is entered lies between the soleus and the flexor digitorum longus muscles. These muscles are separated to the level of the posterior tibial neurovascular bundle. The posterior tibial neurovascular bundle can be retracted anteriorly, together with the tibialis posterior muscle. Dissection

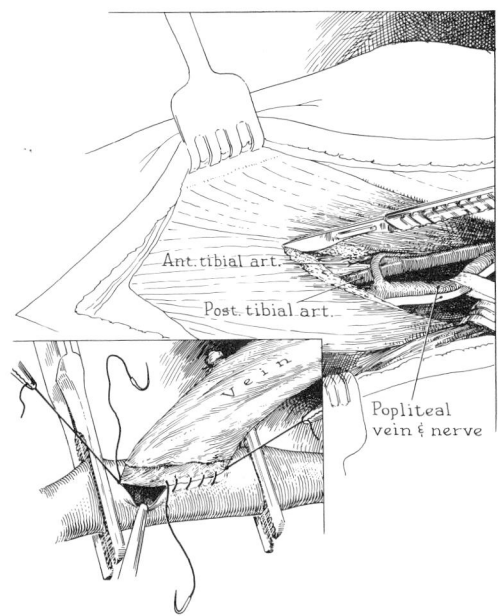

Figure 25. Exposure of the distal popliteal space and distal popliteal artery, vein and nerve. Soleus muscle can be sectioned as shown for more distal exposure of the proximal take-off of the anterior tibial artery and the origin of the tibioperoneal trunk just prior to its division into posterior tibial artery and peroneal artery. End-to-side anastomosis is preferred as shown. (From Szilagy, D. E., Smith, R. F., and Elliott, J. P.: Arch. Surg., 89:116, 1975.)

is carried into the fascial plane between the posterior surface of the tibialis posterior and the flexor hallucis longus muscles. As these muscles are separated at their fascial junction, the peroneal artery and vein will be located deep within the cleft of retracted muscles. The posterior tibial and peroneal arteries are easily located in this same plane (Fig. 26). At a varying cephalad-caudad distance, the peroneal artery may

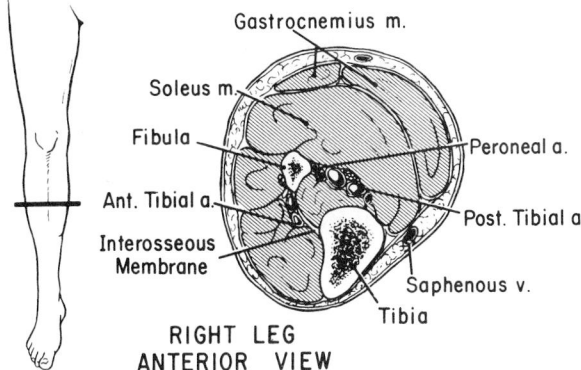

Figure 26. Cross-section of the anatomy of the leg indicating the anatomic relationships of the anterior tibial artery, peroneal artery, and posterior tibial artery. (From Dillihunt, R. C., and Ray, F.: Am. J. Surg., 127:430, 1974.)

enter the body of the flexor hallucis longus muscle. The peroneal artery usually distributes its terminal branches just proximal to the malleolar level.[37] Bypasses to the peroneal artery are performed only to the proximal half of the artery.

A tunnel for the bypass to the peroneal artery is most easily constructed in the natural plane of the peroneal artery. The easiest way technically to achieve this plane of tunneling is to enter the neurovascular bundle of the peroneal artery from inferiorly and carry the plane in a cephalad direction into the distal popliteal space. The tunnel is located between the heads of the gastrocnemius muscle and between the fibular and tibial origin of the soleus muscle. Anastomosis to the posterior tibial artery can be carried out anywhere along the length of the artery. The optimal site for arterial anastomosis is dependent in large part on the appearance of the preoperative arteriogram. Bypasses should be performed distally to known stenotic segments of artery.

The anterior tibial artery is approached by an anterolateral incision through the anterior tibial muscle. Dissection is carried down to the anterior tibial artery, which lies just anterior to the interosseous membrane at the lateral edge of the anterior tibial muscle. In the proximal leg the body of the tibialis anterior muscle is longitudinally divided. This is readily accomplished by sharp dissection through the dense fascia overlying the muscle and then by blunt longitudinal finger dissection through the longitudinally directed muscle fibers. In the more distal leg the anterior tibial artery can be approached by retracting tendons of the extensor digitorum longus and extensor hallucis longus. The tunnel for bypasses to the anterior tibial artery is constructed in the same plane as the artery in its natural course (Fig. 27). Constructing the tunnel distally from the anterior compartment proximally into the popliteal space, it is important to achieve the loose areolar plane directly down on the anterior surface of the anterior tibial neurovascular bundle. Once this plane is achieved, blunt dissection with the finger tip proximally will readily lead into the natural cleft in the interosseous membrane. After this cleft of the natural course of anterior tibial artery is entered, the distal popliteal space is then entered medially and posteriorly. If anastomosis is to be done more distally in anterior tibial or dorsalis pedis arteries, the tunnel is continued caudad beneath the substance of the tibialis anterior and beneath the tendon of extensor hallucis longus into the dorsum of the foot. In drawing the vein graft into the tunnels, it is of extreme importance that the graft not be twisted. This is of particular pertinence in the longer tunnels, where twisting can more readily occur. In this regard it is of great help to secure the vein graft to a previously placed relatively stiff plastic catheter to which the vein graft has been secured. The graft is then drawn through the tunnel without torsion (Fig. 27).

When anastomosing into more deeply placed vessels, it is of considerable importance to free a reasonably long segment of artery to which anastomosis will be performed. This will permit mobility in exposure of the vessel to be anastomosed. In the smaller vessels a low-power binocular magnifying device is of particular

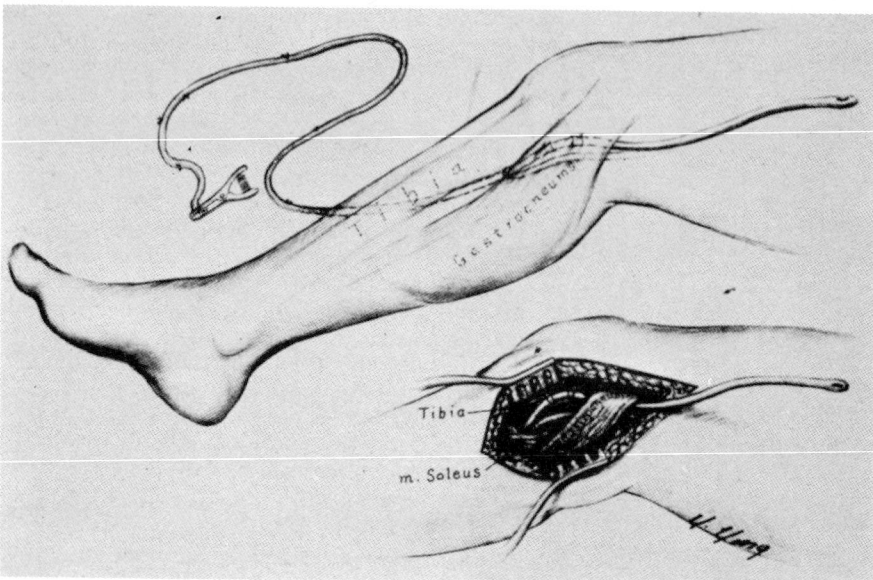

Figure 27. Technique of tunnel from popliteal space to the anterior compartment (anterior tibial artery). (From Tyson, R. R., and Reichle, F. A.: Surgery, *68*:734, 1970.)

help in constructing accurate anastomosis to distal tibial or peroneal arteries.

Regional heparinization of arteries under reconstruction is sufficient to prevent coagulation within the temporarily occluded artery. Operative systemic heparinization may alternatively be employed. Anticoagulation is not routinely administered postoperatively, inasmuch as high incidence of hematomas can be anticipated and evidence that anticoagulation prolongs function of bypasses to ischemic lower extremities is not at present available. The clinical role of other pharmacologic compounds that may minimize cellular adherence or aggregation is not clear in patients undergoing arterial reconstruction for severe ischemia of the lower extremity. This area is currently under study.

DIAGNOSIS AND MANAGEMENT OF THE DIABETIC PATIENT WITH THREATENED TISSUE LOSS OF THE LOWER EXTREMITY

Because approximately 50 per cent of patients seen with severe ischemia of the distal lower extremity have diabetes mellitus, the problem of the ischemic lower extremity in diabetic patients will be considered in more detail. Most diabetic patients with severe lower extremity ischemia have maturity onset diabetes. Inasmuch as diabetes mellitus is associated with increased cardiac, renal, and cerebral complications, the morbidity, mortality, and incidence of limb revascularization is evaluated in the diabetic patient. Early and long-term follow-up study of diabetic patients indicates that the presence of diabetes mellitus should not deter an aggressive diagnostic and therapeutic approach to revascularization of severely ischemic limbs even though limb revascularization was previously not considered feasible by bypasses distal to the knee.

The incidence of limb salvage after femoropopliteal bypass in the diabetic has been found to be quite comparable to nondiabetic patients both in our own experience and in the experience of others.[29, 38, 54] Cardiac, renal, and cerebral complications are expectedly increased in diabetic patients. Increased mortality can also be expected. Therefore, the diabetic patient with moderate ischemia (claudication alone) should be carefully evaluated from the standpoint of his general medical condition before revascularization is recommended. Limbs in diabetic patients with gangrene, gangrenous ulceration, or rest pain and severe ischemia can frequently be salvaged by distal bypass. Because patients with diabetes mellitus have an increased incidence of infections, including cellulitis and osteomyelitis, it is particularly important to differentiate ischemic from nonischemic distal extremities in diabetic patients. Therefore, diabetic patients with an ulcerating or gangrenous lesion of the lower extremity must be considered in two separate groups: (1) diabetic patients with severe ischemia and secondary gangrene and ulceration, and (2) diabetic patients without severe ischemia and with primary infection of traumatic ulcers in whom infection is in large part the cause of the threatened tissue loss. These groups will be considered separately in the following discussion of principles of treatment.

Evaluation of the Diabetic Patient with Infection and Gangrene of the Distal Lower Extremity but without Major Arterial Occlusion

Many diabetic patients with distal ulceration, gangrene, abscess, or cellulitis do not have underlying tissue ischemia. In these patients major arterial stenosis or occlusion is not a contributory factor. Frequently the amplitude of peripheral pulses is normal, bruits are not audible over the course of the major arteries, and neither history nor physical findings are suggestive of embolic or atherosclerotic occlusion of the larger arteries. In addition, the clinical observations of arterial perfusion of the extremity, including pallor on elevation, dependent rubor, and warmth of the foot are all normal. Seemingly trivial trauma (a tight shoe, a stubbed toe) is frequently the initiating event in loss of skin integrity. This may progress rapidly to a very threatening situation. The exact reasons for the vulnerability of the diabetic foot with apparently adequate vasculature is not well understood. Neuropathy is undoubtedly a factor, and structural or functional abnormalities of the microvasculature are also important etiologic factors.

Rapid clinical examination of the diabetic foot in which gangrene or ulceration is present can establish the adequacy of major artery inflow. These tests do not require the use of any specialized equipment or extensive clinical examination. All that is required is palpation of the pulses and assessment of the color and temperature of the foot and observation of the response to elevation (pallor) and dependency (rubor) of the extremity. These simple maneuvers are the best tests of adequacy of tissue perfusion. An accurate assessment of arterial tissue perfusion and the advisability of subsequent arteriography can be determined in almost all cases on the basis of this easily performed office examination. Although arteriographic examination is highly important for anatomic delineation when major vessel occlusion is expected, it does not contribute to the diagnosis or management of the patient without clinical signs of altered tissue perfusion. Therefore, this invasive study is not recommended unless the diagnosis of inadequate arterial tissue perfusion is established on the basis of clinical examination.

Evaluation of Gangrene and Ischemic Ulceration of the Lower Extremity in the Diabetic Patient with Concomitant Major Artery Occlusion

Usually the diabetic patient with a gangrenous or ulcerative lesion of the lower extremity has associated major arterial occlusion with clinical signs of diminished tissue perfusion. These patients present with gangrenous or ulcerative lesions of the distal lower extremity. In these patients, pallor on elevation of the extremity, rubor of the limb in the dependent position, a cool distal extremity, and diminished or absent distal pulses are associated with the distal gangrene or ulceration. Arteriographic delineation of the large vessel occlusion is of great importance in planning the treatment. Arteriography should be reserved for patients in whom associated ischemia is present and in whom arterial reconstruction is a definite consideration.

Therapy of Diabetic Patients with Gangrene or Ulceration but without Major Arterial Occlusion

In diabetic patients without clinical signs of altered tissue perfusion, therapy is directed at the underlying cause of the ulceration or gangrene. In these patients arterial reconstructive operations are not indicated and arteriography is generally not performed. The principles of treatment are control of infection and avoidance of the potential trauma which initiated the interruption of skin integrity. Adequate operative drainage, including, if necessary, amputation, is per-

formed. Osteomyelitic bone, if present, should be resected to establish adequate drainage.

If infection is present, particularly with systemic manifestations, antibiotic therapy is instituted. Operative drainage usually is best delayed for several hours or longer, during which the diabetic control is secured and systemic antibiotic coverage is instituted.

Treatment of Life-threatening Sepsis Caused by Infection in Ischemic Extremities

In situations that are life-threatening in the diabetic as well as the nondiabetic patient e.g., when there is clinical evidence of septicemia, at times associated with shock, emergency amputation may be required. In these patients ice packs are first applied to the distal extremity and then a proximal tourniquet is tightly secured to completely occlude arterial and venous flow. This is a temporary, atraumatic method that promptly and effectively excludes the source of sepsis from the circulation. This maneuver is performed without anesthesia or sedation. Once the patient's general condition has stabilized, operative amputation is subsequently performed, on a subsequent day, under more stable conditions.

Management of the Diabetic Patient with Distal Ulceration or Gangrene and Associated Distal Tissue Ischemia with Major Artery Occlusion and Diminished Arterial Perfusion

Therapy is directed first at control of infections, as indicated above. However, in this group of patients early anatomic delineation of the arterial occlusion by arteriography is indicated. The principal objectives of treatment are control of possible infection and prompt revascularization by arterial bypass. Arterial reconstruction with revascularization should be performed as soon as control of infection and control of the patient's diabetes have been achieved. Early revascularization is performed to stop continued progressive tissue loss. Bypasses can be very successful in the diabetic patient with gangrene or ischemic ulceration and significant limb salvage can frequently be achieved.

Bypasses in the diabetic can be performed in selected patients distally to the popliteal or to the tibial artery, depending on the preoperative arteriogram. The absence of a popliteal artery on angiogram does not preclude the possibility of salvage of the severely ischemic lower extremity. Until recently distal bypass to tibial or peroneal arteries in the diabetic was not generally recommended. However, significant limb salvage can be achieved by bypasses to tibial or peroneal arteries as well as to the popliteal artery in diabetic patients. In our initial series, eventual long-term limb salvage with a functional extremity, relief of rest pain, and healing of gangrene or a gangrenous ulceration occurred in 73.7 per cent of nondiabetic patients and in 56.1 per cent of diabetic patients.[38] Limb salvage in patients with gangrene was similar in diabetic and nondiabetic patients, whereas in patients with rest pain only, limb salvage was higher in nondiabetic than in diabetic patients. Thus, one can anticipate that primary amputation can be avoided in somewhat more than half of diabetic patients with severe ischemia of the lower extremity in whom complete chronic occlusion of the popliteal artery necessitates bypass to tibial or peroneal arteries.

The presence of severe ischemia, including gangrene or gangrenous ulceration, does not preclude the possibility of limb salvage by femoropopliteal or femorotibial bypass in diabetic patients. Concomitant management of infection is of basic importance in the diabetic patient with or without major arterial occlusion.

BIOLOGIC FATE OF ARTERIAL PROSTHETICS AND AUTOGENOUS VEIN BYPASSES

Both prosthetic materials and autogenous veins are frequently used in replacement of diseased vessels. In the femoropopliteal area autogenous vein grafts are strongly preferred to prosthetic grafts. Although the initial results with femoropopliteal bypass using currently available prosthetic tubes are similar to femoropopliteal bypass using a vein, there is a consistently higher delayed graft occlusion rate in prosthetic materials as compared to autogenous vein.[36]

The ultrastructural characteristics of Dacron bypasses have been fairly well studied by transmission electron microscopy and scanning electron microscopy with respect to eventual development of neointima and eventual development of endothelial lining.[35, 43] It is generally agreed that the cellular lining of a functioning graft in a human being is incompletely covered by a flat cell lining. Grafts removed at the time of distal arterial reconstruction have been found to be lined by collagen fibers in long-term human specimens exposed to flowing blood (Fig. 28). Despite the fact that collagen

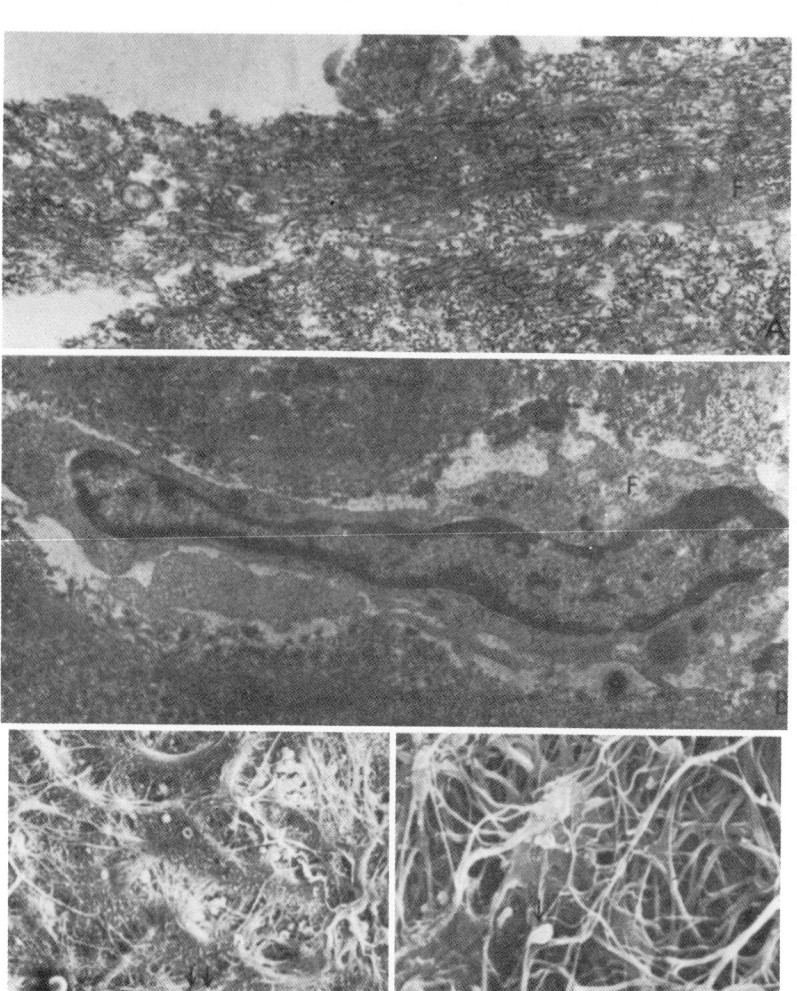

Figure 28. Intraprosthetic lining of Dacron graft from human arterial system. The graft was functional and had been functional for four years when the sample was removed at operation for purposes of distal arterial reconstruction. *A* and *B*, Transmission electron micrographs. The luminal surface appears to be composed of collagen (C). The bulk is composed of collagen and fibroblast (F). (*A*, × 9,500 and *B*, × 10,000). *C*, Scanning electron micrograph of luminal surface. This low magnification survey of the surface shows areas of closely (arrow) and loosely (double arrows) spaced fibrils. There is a limited amount of cellular infiltration in the loosely spaced area (× 240). *D*, Higher magnification of same sample. The fibers have occasional bits of material that could be platelets (arrow) (× 2,400). (From Reichle, F. A., Stewart, G. J., and Essa, N.: Surgery, 74:945, 1973.)

is a known thrombogenic material, there is no significant tendency to cellular adherence or to fibrin deposits within the arterialized surface on many of these long-term functional grafts. Thus, in the human being the eventual lining of grafts, according to current observations, is primarily a nonendothelialized lining of collagen fibrils that support graft function with little evidence of either cellular adherence or thrombogenicity in a high percentage of grafts. Numerous earlier studies done in subhuman species suggested progressive and continued endothelialization of arterialized prosthetic grafts. Despite marked similarities between routine microscopic and ultrastructural

characteristics of canine and human intraluminal deposition (neointima, pseudointima), there is a distinct difference in the extent to which these grafts endothelialize. Of the species studied with regard to prosthetic graft incorporation into the arterial system, the human grafts demonstrate the least propensity to develop an endothelial lining. Nevertheless, function of arterial prosthesis in the human being has been demonstrated for prolonged periods of time.

Autogenous saphenous vein grafts similarly are not necessarily initially covered entirely by a smooth flat cell lining (Fig. 29). However, autogenous vein grafts are generally covered by a partial endothelial lining

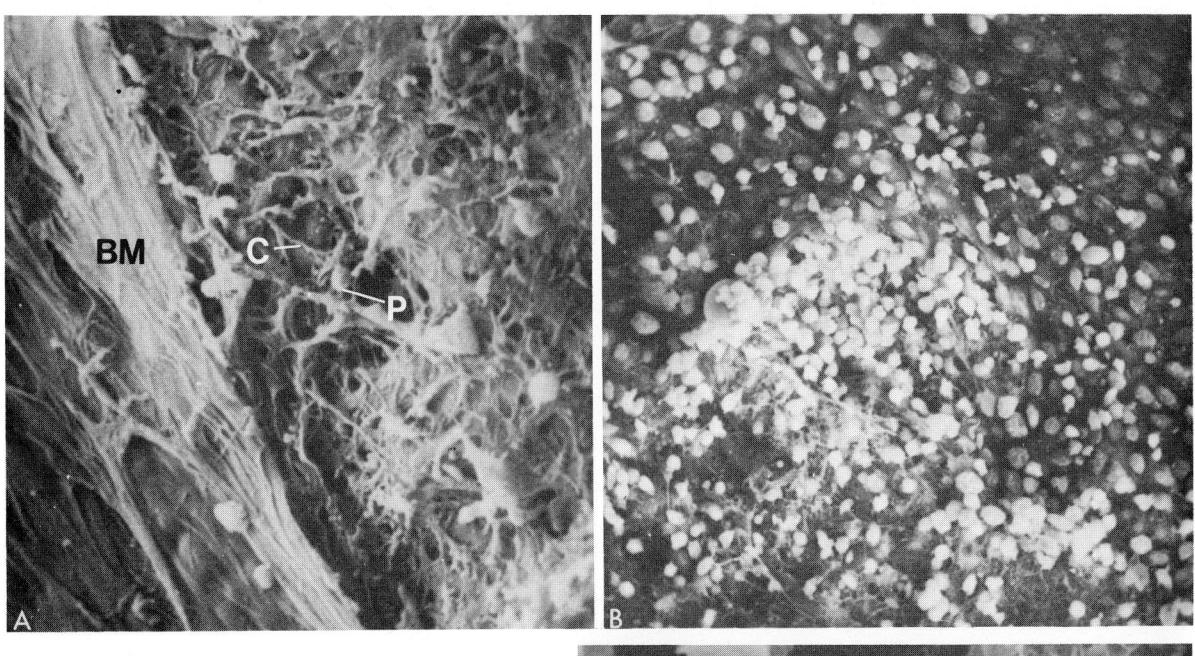

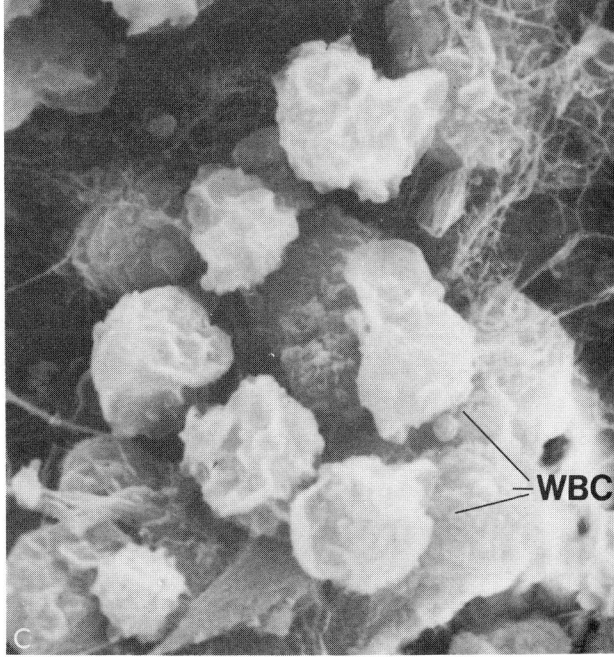

Figure 29. Seven-day functional human autogenous vein femoropopliteal bypass removed at operation at the time of distal arterial reconstruction. *A,* Scanning electron micrograph. In this area, it appears that the rather smooth, matlike basement membrane (BM) was torn, revealing the course collagen matrix (C) beneath. Surprisingly, few platelets (P) are stuck to these exposed surfaces (× 2,400). *B,* Low-power scanning electron micrograph showing an area heavily invaded by white cells. Some fibrin is associated with the white cells (× 240). *C,* Higher magnification at part of *B* showing details of the rough-surfaced white cells (WBC) and fibrin (× 2,400). (From Reichle, F. A., Stewart, G. J., and Essa, N.: Surgery, *74:*957, 1973.)

in the initial arterialization stages.[35] Despite initial incomplete endothelial lining, graft function under conditions of considerably lower blood flow without thrombosis does occur in autogenous vein bypasses as compared to the currently available prosthetic grafts. Long-term bypass function in the femoropopliteal area is superior when autogenous vein bypasses are used, in comparison to prosthetic grafts. The longevity of a prosthetic or biologic conduit depends on hemodynamic factors as well as on the fabrication and the histologic alterations within biologic graft.[2]

The most common cause of bypass failure and delayed limb loss in patients bypassed with either autogenous vein or arterial prosthetic bypass is continued, progressive arteriosclerosis obliterans of the distal arterial tree. In this process the peripheral resistance gradually increases and the flow within the bypass gradually decreases. Decreased flow then eventually leads to sudden graft thrombosis. Nevertheless, a consistent number of graft failures do occur that are attributed to primary graft failure.[3, 4, 5] Szilagyi et al. have reviewed the natural course of vein grafts.[45, 46] Although a high percentage of venous grafts are structurally sound after long-term follow-up, over 30 per cent of grafts develop structural defects related to technical mishaps or to intrinsic tissue changes, particularly subendothelial hypertrophy, layering of intimal thrombi, fibrosis of venous valves, and atherosclerosis.

Experimentally, venous grafts in the arterial system develop atherosclerosis, which includes more extensive mineralization and fibrosis than in adjacent aortic tissue.[51]

Delayed graft failure is considerably more common in the femoropopliteal area with prosthetic grafts than with autogenous saphenous vein graft. Thus, in the absence of autogenous saphenous vein the need for an improved arterial prosthesis in low-flow areas is obvious. A number of approaches in this direction are currently in progress at various centers. Evidence has been presented suggesting that improved healing of grafts can be anticipated with velour prostheses, as compared to standard woven or knitted prostheses (Fig. 30).[40, 41]

Other approaches currently under evaluation are the use of processed *human umbilical vein* graft, which is re-enforced with external loose-knit Dacron circumferentially applied over the entire graft to prevent eventual aneurysmal dilatation.[9] The healing potential and long-term function of Dacron-enforced *autogenously grown tissue tubes* is also being evaluated.[42] In this approach a previously placed mandril is removed at the time of the bypass having an autogenously grown vessel which is reinforced with Dacron mesh. Clinical and experimental investigation is currently being performed to determine the efficacy of intraoperative immersion of autogenous vein grafts

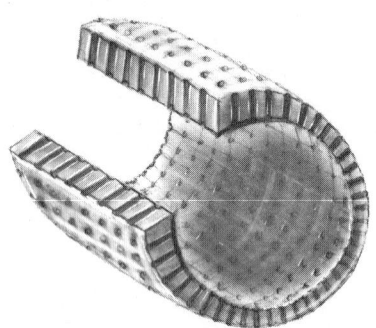

1. Both sides smooth ____

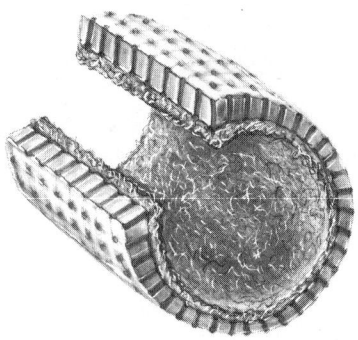

2. Internal velour _____

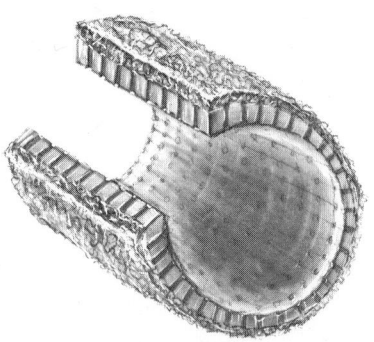

3. External velour _____

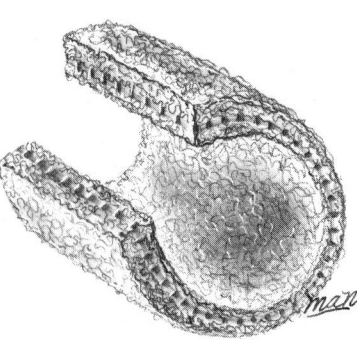

4. Double velour _____

Figure 30. Illustrations of nonvelour and velour knitted arterial prostheses. Studies, both experimental and clinical, are currently being performed to determine the practical application of the theoretically sound velour principles. (From Sauvage, L. R., Berger, K. E., Mansfield, P. B., Wood, S. J., Smith, J. C., and Overton, J. B.: Future directions in the development of arterial prostheses for small and medium caliber arteries. Surg. Clin. North Am., *54*: 213, 1974.)

in cortisone solution prior to arterial bypass.[52] These approaches to the development of an improved prosthesis are of potential importance in the femoropopliteal and femorotibial areas, inasmuch as the low-flow states encountered in the distal arterial tree predispose to graft thrombosis using currently available prostheses. At present the limb with only tibial or peroneal artery runoff and without suitable autogenous saphenous vein or cephalic vein is generally considered lost because of the lack of a suitable prosthesis for the low-flow state. The development of these and other approaches to improved arterial prostheses will be of considerable interest in the near future to determine whether improved limb salvage in patients will severely ischemic lower extremities can be achieved.

SELECTED REFERENCES

Bernhard, V. M.: Intraoperative monitoring of femorotibial bypass grafts. Surg. Clin. North Am., 54:77, 1974.
Blood flow as measured operatively through femorotibial grafts was found to be equivalent to flow measured in femoropopliteal grafts. Flow was similar in bypasses in limbs of diabetic and non-diabetic patients. These hemodynamic observations support the clinical experience which indicates that salvage of severely ischemic extremities in diabetic or nondiabetic patients can be achieved by femorotibial bypass in lieu of primary extremity amputation.

Craver, J. M., Ottinger, I. W., Darling, R. C., Austen, W. G., and Linton, R. R.: Hemorrhage and thrombosis as early complications of femoropopliteal bypass grafts: Causes, treatment and the prognostic indications. Surgery, 74:839, 1973.
The infrequent complication of early hemorrhage following bypass (technical aspects of reconstruction) and the leading cause of later hemorrhage (infection) are reviewed. Repair of early hemorrhage with preservation of the function of bypass and consideration of ligation of delayed rebleeding is recommended.

Reichle, F. A., and Tyson, R. R.: Comparison of long-term results of 364 femoropopliteal and femorotibial bypasses for revascularization of severely ischemic lower extremities. Ann. Surg., 182:449, 1975.
Successful revascularization of the severely ischemic lower extremity can be achieved by femorotibial as well as femoropopliteal bypass; the incidence of delayed graft occlusion after bypass function and salvage of the severely ischemic lower extremity is low in patients with femorotibial and femoropopliteal bypass. Bypasses to distal tibial arteries or peroneal arteries can frequently result in prolonged limb salvage in lieu of primary amputation.

Sauvage, L. R., Berger, K. E., Mansfield, P. B., Wood, S. J., Smith, J. C., and Overton, J. B.: Future directions in the development of arterial prostheses for small and medium caliber arteries. Surg. Clin. North Am., 54:213, 1974.
Newer approaches to prostheses for use in small caliber arteries are described. The concept of "velour" would theoretically provide improved healing via the trellis concept of graft construction. Other considerations in the prevention of thrombosis within bypasses in the arterial system are discussed.

Strandness, D. E., Jr.: Evaluation of the patient for vascular surgery. Surg. Clin. North Am., 54:13, 1974.
The application of specialized techniques for evaluation of success or failure of arterial reconstruction is discussed. The value of these techniques may lie in the possibility to avert failure of the reconstruction in some patients by early detection of developing problems.

Szilagyi, D. E., Elliott, J. P., Hageman, J. H., Smith, R. F., and Dall'Olmo, C. A.: Biologic fate of autogenous vein implants as arterial substitutes. Ann. Surg., 178:232, 1973.
The long-term fate of autogenous vein transplants as arterial substitutes in the femoropopliteal region indicate that autogenous saphenous vein was structurally sound and functionally unimpaired in 64 per cent of grafts 5 years postoperatively and in 44 per cent of grafts in 10 years postoperatively. Structural defects that de-

veloped in 33 per cent of grafts were due to technical mishaps or to intrinsic tissue changes (subendothelial hypertrophy, layering of intimal thrombi, fibrosis of venous valves, and atherosclerosis).

REFERENCES

1. Baird, R. J., Tutassaura, H., and Miyagishima, R. T.: Saphenous vein bypass graft to arteries of the ankle and foot. Ann. Surg., 172:1059, 1970.
2. Bernhard, V. M.: Intraoperative monitoring of femorotibial bypass grafts. Surg. Clin. North Am., 54:77, 1974.
3. Carver, J. M., Ottinger, L. W., Darling, R. C., Austen, M. G., and Linton, R. R.: Hemorrhage and thrombosis as early complications of femoropopliteal bypass grafts: Causes, treatment, and prognostic implications. Surgery, 74:839, 1973.
4. Charlesworth, D., Cave, F. D., Walker, A., and Naylor, G. P.: Femoropopliteal vein bypass: A new approach to assessing run-off. Br. J. Surg., 62:159, 1975.
5. Dale, W. A.: Grafting small arteries—Experience with 19 shunts below the knee. Arch. Surg., 86:22, 1963.
6. Dale, W. A.: Beginnings of vascular surgery. Surgery, 76:849, 1974.
7. Dale, W. A., and DeWeese, J. A.: Autogenous venous grafts for arterial repair. Surgery, 55:870, 1964.
8. Dardik, I. I., Ibrahim, I. M., Sprayregen, S., Veith, F., and Dardik, H.: Routine intraoperative angiography: An essential adjunct in vascular surgery. Arch. Surg., 110:184, 1975.
9. Dardik, I. I., and Dardik, H.: The fate of human umbilical cord vessels used as interposition arterial grafts in the baboon. Surg. Gynecol. Obstet., 140:567, 1975.
10. DeWeese, J. A., Barner, H. B., Mahoney, E. B., and Rob, C. G.: Autogenous venous bypass grafts and thromboendarterectomies for atherosclerotic lesions of the femoropopliteal arteries. Ann. Surg., 163:205, 1966.
11. Dillihunt, R. C., and Ray, M. S.: Femoral to anterior tibial artery bypass utilizing the tibial tunnel technic. Report of twelve cases. Am. J. Surg., 127:429, 1974.
12. Foster, R. P., and Yonke, B. T.: Extremity salvage: Vein bypass to the ankle and beyond. Read before the Sixth Scientific Session of the International College of Angiology. Vasc. Surg., 5:12, 1971.
13. Garrett, H. E., and DeBakey, M. E.: Distal posterior tibial artery bypass with autogenous vein graft: A report of three cases. Surgery, 60:283, 1966.
14. Garrett, H. E., Kotch, D. I., Green, M. T., Jr., Diethrich, E. B., and DeBakey, M. E.: Distal tibial artery bypass with autogenous vein grafts: An analysis of 56 cases. Surgery, 63:90, 1968.
15. Goyanes, J.: Neuvos trabajos de chirurgia vascular: Substiucoin plastica de las arterias por las venas, o arterioplastia venosa, aplicado, coma neuvo metodo, al traitamiento de los aneurismas. El Sigo. Med., 53:561, 1906.
16. Haimov, M.: The crossover femoropopliteal bypass. Surgery, 75:610, 1974.
17. Jeger, E.: Die Cirurgie der Blutgefasse und des Herzen. Berlin, A. Hirschwald, 1913.
18. Kunlin, S.: Le traitement de l'arterite obliterarte par la greffe veinoeuse. Arch. Mal. Loevr., 42:371, 1949.
19. Kunlin, J.: Treatment of arterial ischemia by long vein grafts. Rev. Chir., 70:206, 1951.
20. Lexer, E.: Die ideale Operation des Arteriellen und des arteriellvenosen Aneurysma. Arch. Klin. Chir., 83:458, 1957.
21. Liddicoat, J. E., Bekassy, S. M., and DeBakey, M. E.: Intraoperative arteriography during femoral-popliteal bypass. Arch. Surg., 110:839, 1975.
22. Linton, R. R., and Wirthlin, L. S.: Femoropopliteal composite Dacron and autogenous vein bypass grafts. Arch. Surg., 107:748, 1973.
23. Lye, C. R., Sumner, D. S., and Strandress, D. E.: The effects of femoropopliteal vein graft failure on limb function. Ann. Surg., 183:38, 1976.
24. Mannick, J. A., and Hume, D. M.: Salvage of extremities by vein graft in far advanced peripheral vascular disease. Surgery, 55:154, 1964.
25. Martin, P., Renwick, S., and Stephenson, C.: On the surgery of the profunda femoris artery. Br. J. Surg., 55:539, 1968.
26. Mavor, G. E., Krukowski, Z. H., Millar, D. G., Kasenally, A. T., and Woodruff, P. H.: The long term behaviour of autogenous vein by-pass grafts. J. Card. Surg., 16:130, 1975.

27. May, A. G., DeWeese, J. A., and Rob, C. G.: Arterialized in situ saphenous vein. Arch. Surg., 91:743, 1965.

28. McCaughan, J. J.: Successful arterial grafts to the anterior tibial, posterior tibial (below the peroneal), and peroneal arteries. Angiology, 12:91, 1961.

29. Miller, M. V.: Femoropopliteal bypass graft patency: An analysis of 156 cases. Ann. Surg., 180:35–38, 1975.

30. Murphy, J. B.: Resection of arteries and veins injured in continuing end-to-end suture. Experimental and clinical research. Med. Rec., 51:73, 1897.

31. Ortner, A. B., Berg, H. F., and Lebendiger, A.: Limb salvage through small vessel surgery. Arch. Surg., 83:102, 1961.

32. Pinkerton, J. A.: Operative arteriography: A new variation. Arch. Surg., 110:841, 1975.

33. Pringle, J. H.: Two cases of vein grafting for the maintenance of direct arterial circulation. Lancet, 1:1795, 1913.

34. Reichle, F. A., and Tyson, R. R.: Bypasses to tibial or popliteal arteries in severely ischemic lower extremities: Comparison of long-term results in 233 patients. Ann. Surg., 176:315, 1972.

35. Reichle, F. A., Stewart, G. J., and Essa, N.: A transmission and scanning electron microscopic study of luminal surfaces in Dacron and autogenous vein bypasses in man and dog. Surgery, 74:945, 1973.

36. Reichle, F. A., and Tyson, R. R.: Comparison of long-term results of 364 femoropopliteal or femorotibial bypasses for revascularization of severely ischemic lower extremities. Ann. Surg., 182:449, 1975.

37. Reichle, F. A., and Tyson, R. R.: Femoroperoneal bypass: Evaluation of potential for revascularization of the severely ischemic lower extremity. Ann. Surg., 181:182, 1975.

38. Reichle, F. A., Shuman, C. R., and Tyson, R. R.: Femorotibial bypass in the diabetic patient for salvage of the ischemic lower extremity. Am. J. Surg., 129:603, 1975.

39. Rob, C. G.: A history of arterial surgery. Arch. Surg., 105:821, 1972.

40. Sauvage, L. R., Berger, K. E., Mansfield, P. B., Wood, S. J., Smith, J. C., and Overton, J. B.: Future directions in the development of arterial prostheses for small and medium caliber arteries. Surg. Clin. North Am., 54:213, 1974.

41. Sauvage, L. R., Berger, K., Wood, S. J., Nadagawa, Y., and Mansfield, P. B.: An external velour surface for porous arterial prostheses. Surgery, 70:940, 1971.

42. Sparks, C. H.: Silicone mandril method of femoropopliteal artery bypass: Clinical experience and surgical techniques. Am. J. Surg., 124:244, 1972.

43. Stewart, G. J., Essa, N., Chang, K. H. Y., and Reichle, F. A.: A scanning and transmission electron microscope study of the luminal coating on Dacron prostheses in the canine thoracic aorta. J. Lab. Clin. Med., 85:208, 1975.

44. Strandress, D. E., Mozersky, D. J., Sumner, D. S., Baker, D. W., and Hokanson, D. E.: Noninvasive arteriography: A new approach for arterial visualization. Am. Surg., 38:494, 1972.

45. Szilagyi, D. E., Elliot, J. P., Hageman, J. G., Smith, R. F., and Dall'Olmo, C. A.: Biologic fate of autogenous vein implants as arterial substitutes: Clinical angiographic and histopathologic observations in femoro-popliteal operations for atherosclerosis. Ann. Surg., 178:232, 1973.

46. Szilagyi, D. E., Smith, R. F., and Elliott, J. P.: Venous autografts in femoropopliteal arterioplasty. Arch. Surg., 89:113, 1964.

47. Tyson, R. R., and Reichle, F. A.: Femorotibial bypass. Ann. Surg., 170:429, 1969.

48. Tyson, R. R., and Reichle, F. A.: Technique of femorotibial bypass. Surgery, 68:730, 1970.

49. Vollmar, J., Trede, M., Laubach, K., and Forrest, H.: Principles of reconstructive procedures for chronic femoropopliteal occlusions: Report on 546 operations. Ann. Surg., 168:215, 1968.

50. Voorhees, A. B., Jaretski, A., and Blakemore, A. H.: The use of tubes constructed of Vinyon N cloth in bridging arterial defects. Ann. Surg., 135:332, 1952.

51. Wagner, W. D., James, P. M., and St. Clair, R. W.: Susceptibility of autogenous venous grafts to dietary-induced atherosclerosis. Surg. Forum, 26:280, 1975.

52. Weber, T. R., Dent, T. L., Salles, C. A., Ramsburgh, S. R., Fonseca, F. P., and Lindenauer, S. M.: Cryopreservation of venous homografts. Surg. Forum, 46:291, 1975.

53. Weglowski, R.: Uber die Gefass Transplantation. Zentralbl. Chir., 52:22441, 1925.

54. Wheelock, F. C., and Filtzer, H. S.: Femoral grafts in diabetics. Arch. Surg., 99:776, 1969.

7. ARTERIAL INJURIES

Robert J. Freeark, M.D.

HISTORICAL ASPECTS

Military wounds have provided one of the major incentives to the development of arterial surgery. Ambrose Paré first used the ligature to control bleeding in warfare during the sixteenth century, replacing the brutal cautery as a means of hemostasis. Despite amputation rates as high as 50 per cent, ligation remained the principal method of treatment for arterial injuries through the time of World Wars I and II.[5]

In 1759 Hallowell[16] repaired a partially severed brachial artery by transfixing it tangentially with a pin and winding silk about it. Murphy[22] in 1897 appears to have been the first to perform successfully an end-to-end anastomosis for a traumatic arteriovenous fistula.[19] Carrel and Guthrie[2, 3] did much to advance the status of arterial repair in their animal experiments during the early 1900's, and Goyanes and later Lexer employed venous autografts for replacement of diseased arteries.[9] Pringle first successfully employed a saphenous vein graft to replace *traumatic* aneurysms in 1912.[27]

Reconstructive arterial techniques were first routinely employed during the Korean War and dramatically reduced the incidence of amputation from 50 per cent to 13 per cent. During this same conflict, the benefits of early repair of false aneurysm and arteriovenous fistula were also clearly demonstrated.[11]

Urban violence, the automobile, and iatrogenic causes are responsible for the majority of arterial injuries seen in modern surgical practice. Hand guns have replaced knives as favorite weapons of destruction and impose an ever increasing variety of injuries in nearly every region of the human anatomy. High-speed auto accidents propel both occupants and pedestrians in a manner that may tear an artery from its attached organ, stretch it beyond its limits of elasticity, or disrupt its layers as a result of direct impact or associated bony fractures. Increasing use of the arterial tree for diagnostic purposes has also been a cause of injuries. All of these injuries are, to an increasing extent, encountered in centers in which the skills and facilities are available for early recognition and repair. There remain, however, a distressing number of arterial injuries occurring in the home, on the athletic field, or at work that are unique to the physician entrusted with their care. The amputated legs of high school athletes with knee injuries and the deformed and functionless hands of children with elbow fractures are clear evidence of the need for greater awareness of these injuries.

MECHANISMS OF INJURIES

Three basic patterns of arterial injury are depicted in Figures 31 to 33. This simple classification provides a basis for understanding the pathogenesis, the clinical characteristics, and the method of diagnosis in the various types of arterial injury.

COMPLETELY SEVERED ARTERY

The completely severed artery is commonly encountered in penetrating wounds such as those inflicted by knives, missiles, or surgical instruments (Fig. 31). The severed ends characteristically constrict owing to contraction of the circular muscles and retract into the

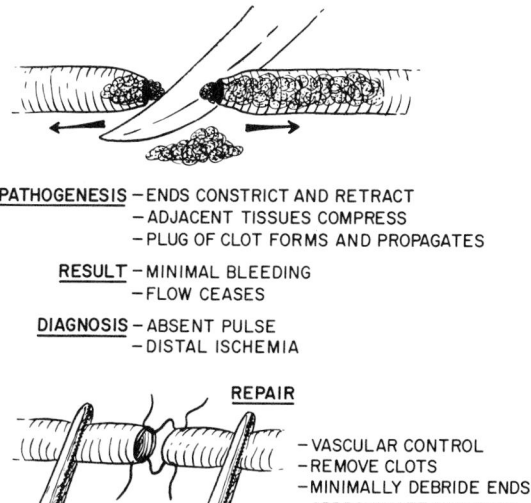

<u>PATHOGENESIS</u> –ENDS CONSTRICT AND RETRACT
              –ADJACENT TISSUES COMPRESS
              –PLUG OF CLOT FORMS AND PROPAGATES

   <u>RESULT</u> –MINIMAL BLEEDING
          –FLOW CEASES

<u>DIAGNOSIS</u> –ABSENT PULSE
           –DISTAL ISCHEMIA

<u>REPAIR</u>

–VASCULAR CONTROL
–REMOVE CLOTS
–MINIMALLY DEBRIDE ENDS
–APPROXIMATE CUT ENDS
–FINE CONTINUOUS SUTURE
 ONE LAYER, EVERTING

Figure 31. Completely severed artery.

adjacent tissue, often leaving an impressive distance between them. Bleeding usually arrests spontaneously owing to the "tourniquet" effect of the surrounding tissues and the development of a firm clot in the two ends. These clots tend to propagate proximally and especially distally, where collateral flow is sluggish. Clots in completely severed arteries seldom dislodge owing to vasoconstriction. Disruption of the entire wall and loss of blood flow in a major artery leads to the immediate disappearance of distal pulsations, which is the usual basis for the diagnosis of this type of injury.

The degree of ischemia that follows complete severance of a major artery varies with the site of interruption, the number, size, and condition of the collateral vessels, and the demands of the tissues supplied. A severed renal or carotid artery may lead to irreversible damage to the involved kidney or cerebral hemisphere in a matter of minutes, while severance of a superficial femoral artery in the upper thigh may result only in muscle pain (claudication) during later exercise. For most major extremity arteries, the skin at some point distal to the injury is pale or mottled in color and cool to the touch when compared to the uninvolved side. In addition, there may be loss of sensation, especially to cotton touch, or a feeling of numbness and tingling (paresthesias). Impairment of arterial supply to sensory nerves usually leads to a glove or bootlike loss of sensation in the involved skin, while loss of motor nerve function leads to varying degrees of paralysis. In general, because of collateral circulation, the six *P's* (pulselessness, paresthesias, paralysis, pallor, poikilothermia, and pain) are not apparent for several inches or at least one major joint below the site of arterial severance. The signs of ischemia are not always immediately apparent and may not develop until propagation of distal clot obliterates a generous collateral. Hence, the loss of distal pulses is the earliest and at times the only sign of this type of arterial injury.

Certain other exceptions to these general features of the completely severed artery are noteworthy. Certain arteries (e.g., intercostal, common iliac arteries) are surrounded by structures that either prevent their retraction into adjacent soft tissue or provide little compression of the severed ends. In patients with atherosclerosis, significant vasoconstriction does not always occur, and in patients with clotting disorders, the anticipated plug of clot may either not form or spontaneously dissolve. Under each of these circumstances, completely severed arteries may bleed excessively or recurrently.

It is also important to recognize that many important arteries do not have a distal point for palpating pulsations. The common and internal carotid, internal iliac, profunda femoris, and peroneal arteries defy evaluation by this means, and other arteries such as the renal or mesenteric vessels are not readily accessible prior to opening one of the body cavities.

PARTIALLY SEVERED ARTERY

Severance or disruption of a portion of the arterial wall is perhaps the most important arterial injury to recognize and understand (Fig. 32). This injury commonly results in serious bleeding and is the forerunner of both false aneurysm and arteriovenous fistulas. A wide variety of penetrating objects may be responsible, including knives, missiles, drill points, needles and catheters used in angiographic study and cardiovascular monitoring techniques.[32] Occasionally, partial severance occurs in association with closed injuries, usually as a result of bony fragments that lacerate a portion of the adjacent arterial wall.

The partially severed artery differs profoundly from the completely severed vessel in many important respects. Since a portion of the arterial wall remains intact, the vessel cannot retract into the surrounding tissues and enjoy the tourniquet effect that occurs with complete severance. Constriction of the circular muscle coat and retraction of the severed portions of the arterial wall cause the wound to gape, spewing forth considerable quantities of blood. If this shed blood escapes readily from the body surface or adjacent body cavity, rapid exsanguination may result. More often the overlying muscles and skin will contain the blood clot at least temporarily. This hematoma increases gradually in size and, if carefully examined, will often have a pulsatile quality and appearance, since it communicates directly with the arterial lumen. The gradual increase in size and pressure of the hematoma may force open the wound tract to the body surface or cavity and produce life-threatening hemorrhage.

The arterial lumen is seldom narrowed by partial severance, and blood that fails to exit from the defect continues to flow distally, often preventing significant ischemia. The intact portions of the arterial wall continue to transmit a pulse wave, and normal or only slightly diminished distal pulsations are usually present. In the absence of distal ischemia or pulse deficit, the partially severed artery is, therefore, difficult to diagnose by its peripheral effects and is usually detected by examination at the site of injury.

TABLE 6. Specific Arterial Injuries

Artery	Common Mechanisms of Injury	Possible Sequelae	Special Considerations
Common carotid[1, 10, 33]	Penetrating wounds of neck, blunt trauma to neck	Airway obstruction due to hematoma, cerebral ischemia, carotid jugular fistula	Treatment controversial, if neurologic deficit is present: if minor deficit—repair; if major or fixed deficit—ligation may be advisable
Internal carotid	Penetrating wounds	Cerebral ischemia	Similar to common carotid
External carotid	Penetrating wounds	None	Repair desirable— ligation well tolerated
Vertebral	Penetrating wounds	Cerebral ischemia—may bleed massively	Exposure and repair difficult; ligation usually well tolerated
Innominate[39]	Penetrating wounds of neck and chest, tracheostomy tube erosions	Cerebral and arm ischemia, innominate A-V fistulae	Need to preserve innominate vein and right carotid and vertebral artery flow
Subclavian	Fractures of clavicle and first rib, penetrating trauma, iatrogenic (needles, catheters, thoracic outlet surgery)	Intrathoracic bleeding, brachial plexus symptoms from compression, hematoma, or associated injury	Proximal occlusions may steal vertebral flow for arm
Axillary	Fractures, dislocation of humerus, penetrating wounds	Gangrene—rare	Repair desirable
Brachial	Catheter injuries, fracture and dislocation of elbow, especially in children	Gangrene—rare; ischemic symptoms—common (Volkmann's ischemic contracture)	Repair desirable
Radial	Arterial monitoring lacerations, drug abuse	Rare	Repair usually unnecessary
Ulnar	Lacerations, inadvertent injection into anomalous artery	Gangrene may follow injections of thiopental and other drugs	May ligate; heparin used for injection injuries

Table continued on opposite page

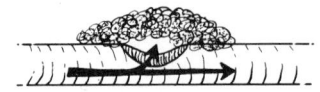

PATHOGENESIS – WOUND GAPES
           – ADJACENT TISSUES COMPRESS
           – PATCH OF CLOT

RESULT – MASSIVE BLEEDING
      – FLOW PERSISTS
      – MINIMAL ISCHEMIA

DIAGNOSIS – HISTORY OF EXCESSIVE
         OR RECURRENT BLEEDING
     – LOCAL FINDINGS
     – ANGIOGRAPHY

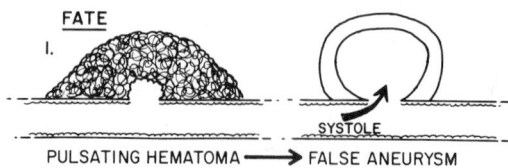

FATE
1.

PULSATING HEMATOMA ⟶ FALSE ANEURYSM
               SYSTOLE

2.

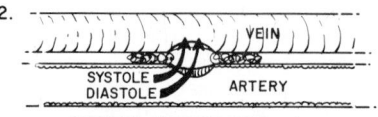

ARTERIO-VENOUS FISTULA

Figure 32. Partially severed artery.

The mass of clots may be quite large, with only a small central region in direct communication with the arterial lumen. Nevertheless, the escape of blood through the defect occurs primarily during systole, and the turbulent flow in the region is heard as a systolic bruit on auscultation or felt as a systolic "thrill" on palpation.

On occasion the initial injury that partially severs the arterial wall may simultaneously disrupt the adjacent vein. Blood escaping from the arterial defect finds the lumen of the vein a path of least resistance, and a temporary or permanent arteriovenous fistula occurs. Under these circumstances, there may be very little hematoma or evidence of bleeding in the area of the injury. Since the pressure in the venous system is far below that of even diastolic arterial pressure, there is flow through the fistulous opening during both systole and diastole leading to the development of a continuous bruit and thrill on examination. In addition, the increased flow of blood under high pressure results in a local expansion of the venous system with varicosities of the adjacent and distal veins a common accompaniment.

If the overlying hematoma effectively limits the escape of blood from the arterial defect, and the injury goes unrecognized, the course of events is highly variable. The patient may present several days after the

TABLE 6.   Specific Arterial Injuries (*Continued*)

Artery	Common Mechanisms of Injury	Possible Sequelae	Special Considerations
Thoracic aorta	Blunt (rapid deceleration), fractures of sternum, clavicle, and first and second ribs	Exsanquination; False aneurysm just distal to left subclavian	Angiography for mediastinal widening, tracheal shift, or diminished pulses
Abdominal aorta	Blunt, penetrating	Visceral or lower extremity ischemia	Repair or prosthetic graft replacement
Common and external iliac	Blunt, penetrating	Lower extremity ischemia	Repair
Internal iliac,[18, 20, 31] gluteal	Pelvic fractures	Pelvic hematoma, false aneurysms	Ligation or angiographic embolization
Renal[36]	Blunt trauma — renal pedicle injury	Hematuria, renal ischemia	Early diagnosis important; unilateral nonvisualization on IVP requires angiography
Celiac, superior and inferior mesenteric	Penetrating trauma, iatrogenic (surgery)	Variable — may cause intestinal ischemia	Repair superior mesenteric; may ligate celiac, inferior mesenteric if necessary
Common femoral	Penetrating, blunt, iatrogenic (catheters, aortic balloon pumps), anterior dislocation of femur	Leg ischemia	Repair
Superficial femoral[13, 14, 17, 26]	Fractures of femur, esp. junction of middle and lower thirds Penetrating wounds	Leg ischemia (may be minimal)	Repair
Profunda femoris[33]	Penetrating wounds, surgery (hip fractures)	Valuable collateral for later life	No distal pulse point; preserve if feasible
Popliteal[4, 10, 13, 17]	Fractures of tibial plateau, dislocation of knee, surgery of knee joint	Amputation likely without prompt and expert repair	Repair; venous repair also advisable
Anterior tibial	Fracture of tibial shaft	Anterior compartment ischemia	Repair
Posterior tibial	Dislocation of ankle, fracture of tibial shaft	Loss of artery — usually well tolerated if anterior tibial intact; posterior compartment hypertension may occur	Repair if feasible

injury with discomfort in the region of the hematoma as it expands and stretches the overlying soft tissues. The mass is often warm and tender, and the overlying skin is red. The mistaken impression that an "abscess" has developed at the site of penetration may lead to a disastrous result if incision and drainage are attempted.

In some instances the hematoma undergoes organization with fibrous tissue replacement and progressive endothelialization of its central cavity. In months to years, this process may create a very thick-walled "sac" with a smooth lining similar to that of a true aneurysm. Since the wall is composed of fibrous tissue elements not derived from the artery, it is referred to as a *false aneurysm,* and the absence of elastic fibers in the wall make its continued expansion inevitable. Since some blood continues past the fistulous opening, the distal extremity is seldom ischemic, and distal pulses are usually maintained. When large amounts of blood pass through the fistulous communication, cardiac overload may result from the efforts to supply the distal arterial bed.

The absence of ischemic changes, the preservation of distal pulses, and the potential for life-threatening hemorrhage and cardiac failure are important features of the partially severed artery.

Nonsevered Artery (Injury in Continuity)

This third category of arterial injury is commonly seen when a *blunt* force or excessive stretch is applied to the arterial wall (Fig. 33). Similar injuries may result from the passage of a high-velocity missile adjacent to the vessel or from needle or catheter wounds that penetrate the vessel without actually severing a significant portion of its outer circumference. This form of injury is characterized by a reduction or loss of flow through the artery without significant external bleeding. The findings at the site of injury are often minimal and the distal part may initially appear healthy, but signs of ischemia and loss of pulses develop over a variable period of time. This injury emphasizes the need for repeated evaluations of the arterial circulation in patients with injuries.

Gradual obliteration of the arterial lumen may result from one of several mechanisms. The intima is more susceptible to the effects of trauma and, once torn, the roughened surface may be the site of deposition of platelets, fibrin, and red cells, leading to thrombus formation. On occasion, the flow of blood may elevate the torn distal end of intima and create a false channel. The torn intima is lifted upward, becoming a flap that occludes the distal lumen. Even when both the inner and outer coats of the arterial wall remain intact, the lumen may become compromised by the accumulation of blood within the arterial wall. This "intramural hematoma" may increase in size to the extent that internal surfaces are opposed and all flow ceases.

Recognition that one or more of these changes is usually responsible for the loss of blood flow and disappearance of distal pulses in traumatized arteries has largely eliminated the concept of arterial "spasm" as a cause for arterial insufficiency. While there is little doubt that the circular muscle fibers may contract segmentally or peripherally to narrow the arterial lumen and diminish blood flow, the phenomenon is certainly a rare cause of pulse deficit and should never be invoked to explain distal ischemia or angiographic evidence of occlusion without direct inspection of the site of injury by surgical exploration.

DIAGNOSIS OF ARTERIAL INJURY

An understanding of the pathogenesis and sequelae of arterial trauma emphasizes the importance of both thoroughness and repetition in the evaluation of the arterial system in injured patients. While most arterial injuries can be diagnosed at the time of initial examination, some injuries do not become apparent until hours or even days later.

HISTORY

The mechanism of injury and the exact time and site at which it was sustained are helpful clues in the recognition of arterial injury. The magnitude of a blunt force or the length of the knife blade and its direction and depth of penetration in stab wounds are

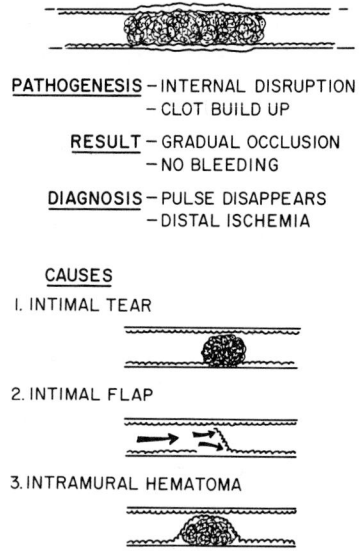

PATHOGENESIS – INTERNAL DISRUPTION
– CLOT BUILD UP

RESULT – GRADUAL OCCLUSION
– NO BLEEDING

DIAGNOSIS – PULSE DISAPPEARS
– DISTAL ISCHEMIA

CAUSES
1. INTIMAL TEAR

2. INTIMAL FLAP

3. INTRAMURAL HEMATOMA

Figure 33. Nonsevered arterial injuries.

important. The number and direction of bullets fired may be of benefit in assessing patients with missile injuries. The extent of bleeding and methods used to control or replace blood loss after injury should be ascertained from the patient or knowledgeable persons in attendance. The patient may be aware of coolness, paresthesias (numbness or tingling), loss of sensation, or severe pain in the extremity with arterial insufficiency.

EXAMINATION

The injured patient should be fully disrobed for examination of all possible sites of injury and to permit a comparison with uninjured body regions. The examination should include an assessment of the entire arterial system, including the presence and quality of all pulses in the neck, groin, and upper and lower extremities. Emphasis should be placed on the examination of the suspected area of injury and the tissues or extremity distally. The presence or suspicion of a fracture or dislocation should prompt a specific evaluation of adjacent vessels (Table 7).

The Distal Extremity

In the patient with penetrating trauma in which the area of injury may be covered by a sterile dressing, it is often wiser to begin examination of the distal extremity for pulse deficits or signs or ischemia. If a proximal tourniquet or pressure dressing has been applied, its effect must be taken into consideration during this examination.

The temperature, color, degree of venous distention, and quality of pulses should be noted and compared with those of the uninjured extremity. Loss of motor function should be evaluated by asking the patient to move digits or distal joints and to attempt to raise the

TABLE 7.   Vascular Injury Accompanying Skeletal Trauma

Bone Injury	Vascular Injury	Associated Findings
Fracture of first and second ribs	Transection of thoracic aorta	Widened mediastinum
Fracture of clavicle and first rib	Laceration and contusion of subclavian artery or vein	Diminished pulse or blood pressure in involved arm
	False aneurysm	
Dislocation of shoulder	Thrombosis of axillary artery	Diminished or absent distal pulse
Fracture of humeral shaft	Laceration of brachial artery	Diminished or absent distal pulse
Supracondylar fracture of humerus	Obstruction of brachial artery	Compartmental hypertension of forearm (Volkmann's phenomenon)
Dislocation of elbow	Disruption of brachial artery	Absent radial pulse
Fracture of ribs	Laceration of intercostal artery	Hemothorax
Fracture of pelvis	Laceration of superior gluteal artery	Massive pelvic hematoma
Anterior dislocation of hip	Femoral artery contusion	Diminished or absent distal pulse
Fracture of hip	Deep femoral artery injury during operative repair	Excessive bleeding with no pulse deficit
Fracture of femoral shaft (mid or lower third)	Occlusion and laceration of femoral artery	Distal pulsations Cold foot with loss of pulsation Cold foot with bleeding
Supracondylar fracture of femur	Laceration of popliteal artery or vein	Bleeding with diminished foot pulses
Dislocation of knee	Disruption and thrombosis of popliteal artery or vein	Diminished pulses with cold foot
Fracture of proximal tibia	Disruption and thrombosis of popliteal artery or vein	Diminished pulses with cold foot
Fracture of tibial shaft	Transection of anterior or posterior tibial artery	Diminished pulses, with cold foot; compartmental hypertension
Dislocation of ankle	Transection and thrombosis of tibial arteries	Diminished pulses

extremity. Loss of sensation to cotton touch or pin prick should be noted and its distribution plotted to determine whether it is on the basis of ischemia or associated nerve injury. In the case of nerve severance, the loss of sensation will be in a segmental or dermatomal distribution, while loss of sensation due to ischemia follows a stocking or glove type pattern.

If the examination of the distal extremity shows definite evidence of arterial injury, plans should be made for angiographic study and/or operative repair as soon as possible. It is both unwise and unnecessary to inspect the area of injury if it risks contamination or rebleeding in a patient who almost certainly requires operative repair. If, however, the distal pulses are intact, and the color, appearance, and sensation of the limb appear normal, attention should be directed to the area of injury.

The Area of Injury

If an open wound is present and particularly if there is a history of excessive bleeding, it is advisable that the examiner wear a mask and sterile gloves. When feasible, a blood pressure cuff should be applied proximal to the wound to provide an immediate tourniquet should bleeding recur. The examiner should note the relationship of the wound or missile track to major vessels and should look for evidence of excessive bleeding, either in the dressings, from the wound, or as manifested by a large hematoma. In the absence of active arterial bleeding, the examination should include palpation of the hematoma for evident pulsations and auscultation of the region for the presence of a bruit.

The circumference of the involved extremity should be measured and compared to the opposite limb at equal distances from an external landmark such as the antecubital crease or patella.

One or more of the following findings are indications of arterial injury and require immediate angiographic study or operative repair.

1. Loss or diminution of pulses distal to the site of injury.
2. Pallor, bluish mottling, or coolness in the involved extremity as compared to the opposite side.
3. Loss of sensation in a glove or stocking pattern distal to the injury.
4. History of massive external bleeding from a penetrating wound. The presence of clinical shock or the need for transfusions to stabilize such patients is almost always a reliable clue to the presence of partially severed arteries.
5. History of recurrent bleeding.
6. Large, rapidly expanding or pulsatile hematoma.
7. Presence of a systolic or continuous bruit in the region of an injury.
8. Marked venous distention of the injured extremity or part.
9. Wound or missile track adjacent to a major vessel.

DIAGNOSIS

The diagnosis of arterial injury is usually suspected on the basis of the physical examination and confirmed by arteriographic study or operative exploration. Except under special circumstances, recourse to other diagnostic techniques (oscillometry, Doppler ultrasonic flow studies, etc.) is unnecessary. Plain x-rays of the area of injury may prove helpful in demonstrating a fracture whose fragments may jeopardize an adjacent vessel (Table 7) or the presence of soft tissue swelling consistent with a large hematoma. A "negative" x-ray of the bone and soft tissues should not discourage considerations of arterial injury. This is a frequent problem in dislocations of the knee with arterial disruption, because the knee often relocates spontaneously. The radiologist's report of "no bony injury" belies the severe violence that has occurred, and the arterial injury may go unrecognized.

ANGIOGRAPHIC STUDY

Injection of a suitable contrast solution into the proximal arterial tree with exposure of multiple films at varying intervals thereafter is a safe and reliable way of confirming and localizing arterial injuries[32] (Fig. 34). While the choice of contrast material, concentration, rate of injection, site of entry, and number and projection of films will vary with the circumstances and preferences of the angiographer, the skills and equipment required should be available in any hospital that undertakes the care of injured patients. Properly performed, angiographic studies have a minimal risk of injury at the site of arterial puncture, and the currently employed contrast agents act to dilate the arterial tree, thereby improving collateral circulation to the injured or ischemic extremity.

While several authors and at least one experimental study suggest that the angiogram may be "normal" in some significant arterial injuries,[15] such is a rare occurrence, and most "false negative" angiograms are the result of attempts to interpret studies of poor quality or inadequate views of the area of injury. Experience has shown that frequent recourse to angiographic studies in patients suspected of arterial injury is the only practical and reliable way to detect or exclude these injuries.

Angiographic Findings

The angiographic findings in patients with arterial injury will vary with the type of injury sustained. Completely severed arteries and complete occlusions arising from injuries in continuity show a sudden arrest of the column of contrast material in the main artery, with passage of contrast material via collaterals to a variable extent below the site of interruption or occlusion (Fig. 35). In some patients, the collateral circulation may be sufficient to permit re-entry of dye into the more distal portions of the main artery, creating an angiographic gap at the site of injury (Fig. 36). While such collateral flow may be sufficient to prevent the development of signs of ischemia at rest, it will rarely maintain a palpable distal pulse.

Angiographic studies of partially severed arteries may show the escape of contrast material from the arterial lumen (Fig. 37). It is important to remember that the amount of contrast material outside the vessel may be relatively small in patients with a large hematoma, since the palpable mass is largely clots surrounding the arterial defect. In some patients, the resultant hematoma may actually protrude into the lumen and appear as a filling defect not unlike an arteriosclerotic plaque (Fig. 38). Any distortion of the normally smooth column of dye in the vicinity of the injury should be viewed with suspicion. In patients who develop arteriovenous fistulas, the visualization

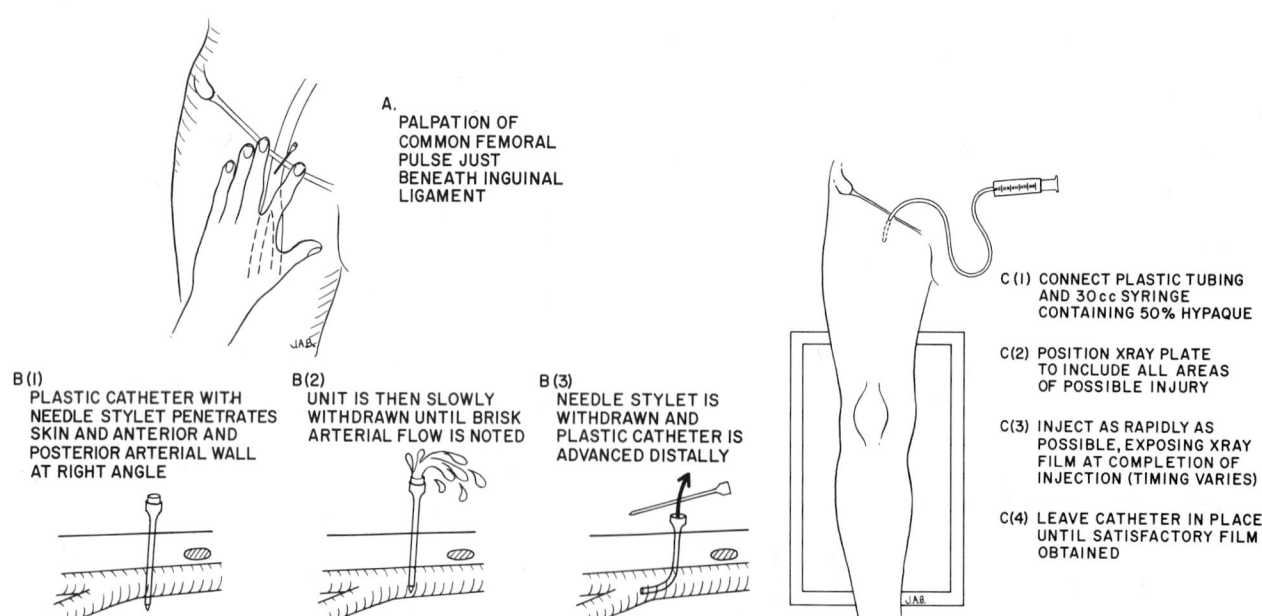

Figure 34. Technique of femoral arteriography employed in evaluation of injured lower extremity.

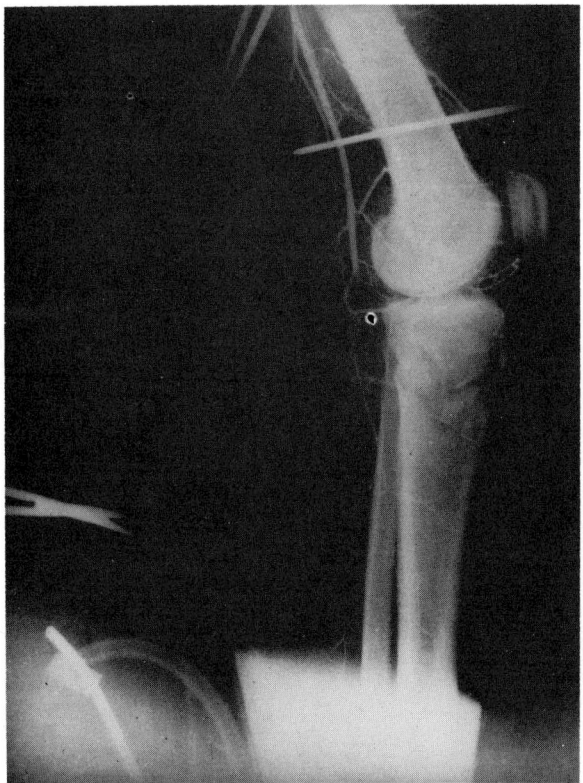

Figure 35. Arteriogram confirming complete occlusion of the popliteal artery associated with fracture of the tibial plateau. A fracture of the femur (not shown) and a pin previously placed for skeletal traction were other possible causes for the cold foot and loss of pulses in this patient.

of the adjacent venous system as well as the sac of the false aneurysm or fistulous track confirms the diagnosis (Fig. 39).

Patients with injuries in continuity are seldom subjected to angiography until a pulse deficit is noted. Under these circumstances, the angiographic picture is that of complete occlusion as described earlier. Prior to the complete loss of arterial flow, the site of injury in nonsevered arteries may be noted as an asymmetric narrowing, a filling defect, or a point at which there is a sudden change in the diameter of the arteries above and below the site of injury. Under the rare circumstances of arteriospasm leading to a pulse deficit, the artery may be symmetrically narrowed and the entire distal arterial tree appear markedly constricted. A smooth lumen is maintained, however, and complete interruption of arterial flow does not occur.

DOPPLER ULTRASONIC FLOW STUDIES

The transcutaneous Doppler ultrasound flow detection technique has proved to be a valuable addition to the management of arterial injuries.[41] An ultrasound beam of 10 megacycles per second emitted from a ceramic crystal is coupled to the skin with a gel and then passed through an underlying blood vessel. Based on the "Doppler effect," ultrasound reflected from

red cells in the blood vessel is shifted in frequency by an amount proportional to the flow velocity of the red cells. Both audible signals and waveform recordings are available for pulse examination of accessible arteries. Using the ultrasound probe as a stethoscope, systolic pressure of the forearm and ankle can be recorded by placing a sphygmomanometer cuff on the forearm or ankle, respectively. The return of flow signals in the radial or posterior tibial artery during deflation of the cuff indicates the level of systolic pressure. Since collateral flow may provide an audible signal even in the presence of arterial interruption, the adequacy of collateral flow may be assessed by measuring the systolic pressure in these arteries. A systolic pressure above 60 mm. Hg (or 50 per cent of the pressure in the contralateral, normal limb) usually indicates adequate collateral flow to maintain tissue viability. Knowledge of the status of collateral flow is helpful in determining the exact priority of arterial repair in patients with multiple injuries. In addition, the Doppler flow detection technique is of value in the determination of arterial patency when pulse examination is in doubt or when swelling or edema precludes reliable palpation of distal pulses. The technique is also useful in the detection of venous injuries and has been found to be of value in monitoring the patency of both arterial and venous reconstructions during the postoperative period.

TREATMENT

The proper application of *firm pressure* over a site of arterial bleeding is the best method for its temporary control. Attempts to find the artery or control bleeding with clamps or ligature usually dislodge clots and risk damage to adjacent structures of the arterial wall. Proximal tourniquets other than inflatable blood pressure cuffs are rarely effective and usually increase venous bleeding or aggravate arterial ischemia. Severe skeletal deformities with vascular compromise should be corrected, and the injured extremity should be splinted and kept level while the patient is transported rapidly to a well-equipped and staffed hospital. Since the success of arterial repairs is in large part determined by promptness, these injuries should receive high priority. On occasion, other life-threatening injuries may require more immediate attention (e.g., restoration of airway, control of internal bleeding, etc.), but the feasibility of simultaneous treatment of an arterial injury should be considered.

Patients with partially severed arteries who are no longer actively bleeding, or who have developed false aneurysm or arteriovenous fistula, have less urgent problems if distal pulses are preserved and no evidence of ischemia persists. Since recurrent bleeding is a constant threat, and spontaneous closure of the arterial defect is rarely observed, these patients should also be treated as soon as possible following recognition and localization of their injuries. Experience has shown that early repairs are more easily accomplished than delayed ones and minimize the hazards of bleeding and the symptoms related to the expanding hematoma.

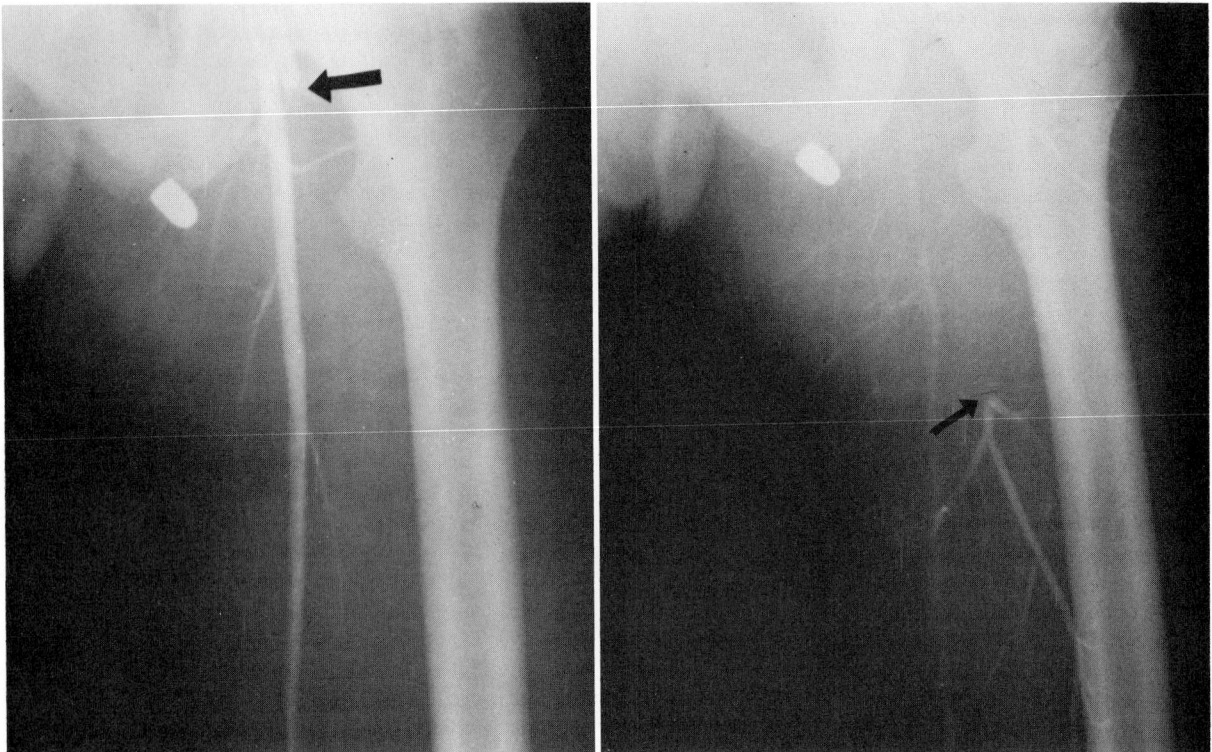

Figure 36.   Femoral arteriogram in a patient with a gunshot wound that severed the profunda femoris artery. Note that in later x-ray angiographic dye re-enters the distal artery via collaterals. The patient had excellent pedal pulses because the superficial femoral artery is intact.

OPERATIVE REPAIR

All major arterial injuries should be repaired when diagnosed, provided the tissues that they supply are viable, the general condition of the patient is satisfactory, and the risks of infection are not great. Notable exceptions include the carotid injuries in patients with a major fixed neurologic deficit and renal pedicle injuries seen after 24 hours. In injuries to the extremities, the presence of distal cutaneous gangrene or stony hard musculature makes the benefits of revascularization questionable, but successful repair may permit amputation at a lower level or preserve the viable tissues.

The operative repair should be undertaken promptly by a surgeon skilled in the techniques of vascular surgery. Repair within the first four hours after injury minimizes the extent of distal clot formation, thereby preserving collateral flow. Every hour of delay increases the effects of ischemia and diminishes the chances for a successful repair. While the techniques of operative repair vary, local considerations are outlined in Table 6 and illustrated in Figure 40. In general, the following procedure is followed.

1. Treat shock by controlling external blood loss and restoring blood volume. Assure an adequate airway and respiratory mechanism. Establish the presence and extent of all injuries and determine their priority in repair.

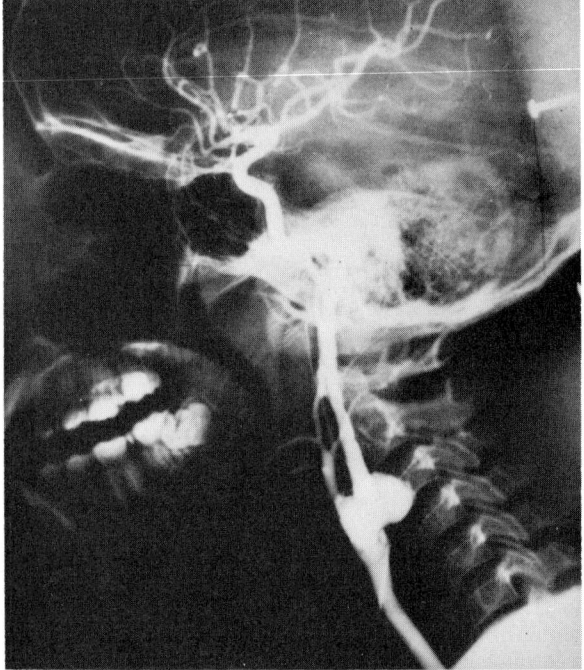

Figure 37.   Carotid arteriogram in a patient with a gunshot wound of the neck that traverses the carotid artery bifurcation. There were no abnormal neurologic findings.

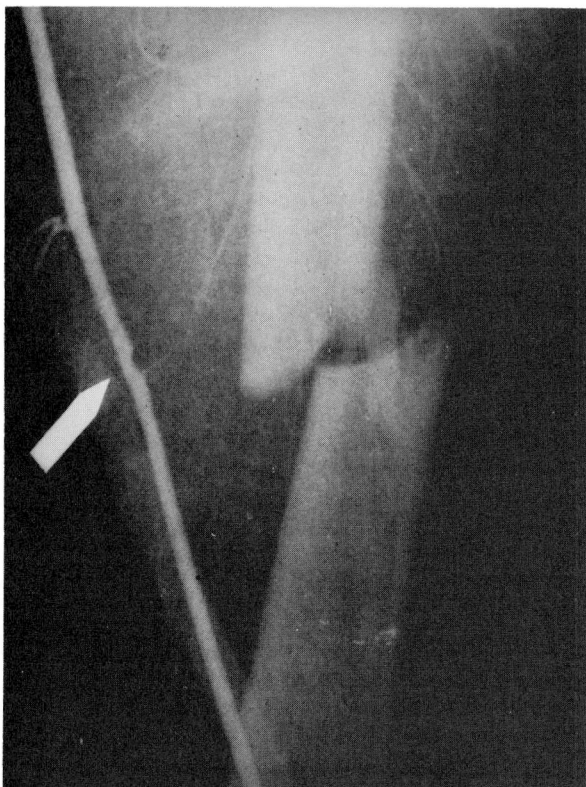

Figure 38. Femoral arteriogram in a patient with a closed fracture of the femur. Note the small filling defect at site of injury where sharp bone fragments had severed 60 per cent of the circumference of the arterial wall. Compare with Figure 37, as both are examples of angiographic evidence of partially severed arteries.

2. Initiate antibiotic and tetanus prophylaxis where indicated and arrange for assistants, equipment, arteriography, and the immediate availability of an adequate supply of type-specific and matched whole blood.

3. Prepare a wide operative field and an uninvolved lower extremity for ready access to the saphenous vein, the best and safest arterial substitute for all but the largest arteries. In an extremity injury, the entire limb and proximal torso should be prepared to assure access to all involved vessels and the operative evaluation of distal pulses by palpation or arteriography.

4. Localize the site of arterial injury by the location of the wound missile track, pulse deficits, or arteriography.

5. Incisions should be made along the pathway of the involved vessel and should utilize anatomic planes to avoid unnecessary injury to associated structures. Obtain control of the proximal pulsating artery before entering the field of injury. In the case of groin, neck, or shoulder wounds, this may necessitate entering a body cavity to assure proximal control.

6. Obtain control of the artery distal to the presumed site of injury to minimize the loss of blood from *back bleeding.*

7. Inspect or palpate the site of injury and determine the need for repair.

8. Control bleeding when present by application of vascular clamps 2 to 3 cm. proximal and distal to the site of injury. In nonsevered arteries with thrombosis and some partially severed vessels, the injured segment will usually require resection and end-to-end anastomosis.

9. Remove the proximal clot by flushing and the distal clot by milking the vessel, squeezing the distal limb, or passing a Fogarty balloon catheter (Fig. 41).[7]

10. Consider the need for and safety of systemic heparinization (5,000 to 10,000 units I.V.) and instill 20 to 30 ml. of a dilute solution of heparin (100 units per ml.) into the distal arterial tree and 5 to 10 ml. proximal to the proximal clamp.

11. Prior to anastomosis, determine the need for graft replacement by the amount of difficulty in approximating the severed ends (Fig. 34). In general, a loss of more than 2 cm. of arterial wall is required before graft replacement should be considered. Arterial anastomoses should not be performed under tension, but it is important not to interpret the retraction

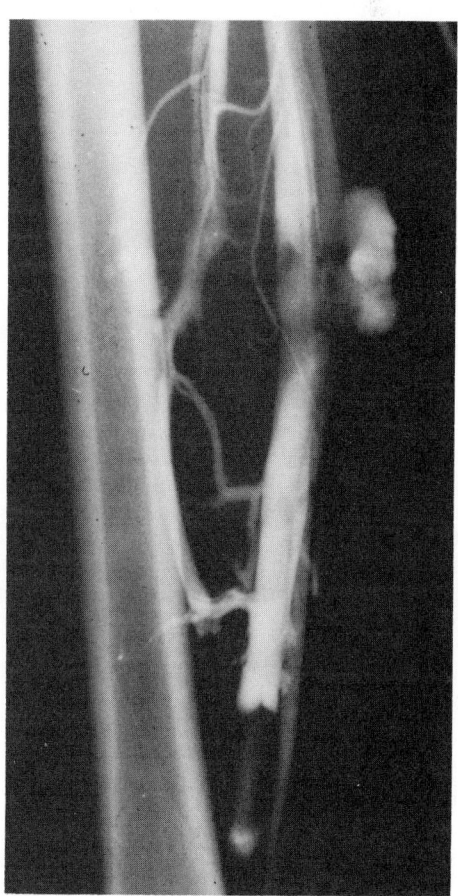

Figure 39. Femoral arteriogram in a patient with an arteriovenous fistula secondary to a gunshot wound of the thigh. Leakage of contrast material outlines the vein proximal and distal to the fistula and an associated false aneurysm at the site of injury.

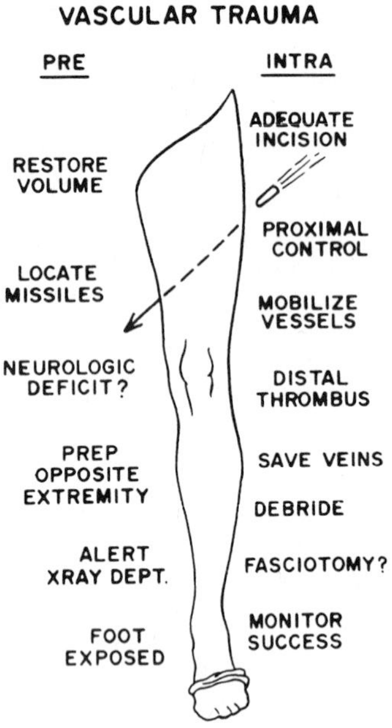

VASCULAR TRAUMA

PRE   INTRA

ADEQUATE INCISION

RESTORE VOLUME

PROXIMAL CONTROL

LOCATE MISSILES

MOBILIZE VESSELS

NEUROLOGIC DEFICIT?

DISTAL THROMBUS

PREP OPPOSITE EXTREMITY

SAVE VEINS

DEBRIDE

ALERT XRAY DEPT.

FASCIOTOMY?

FOOT EXPOSED

MONITOR SUCCESS

Figure 40. Important considerations prior to and during the operative treatment of a vascular injury to the lower extremity.

"gap" as a loss of arterial substance in making this decision.

12. Excise excess adventitia and detached or injured intima.

13. Repair using continuous fine monofilament sutures of 5-0 or 6-0 polyethylene placed approximately 2 mm. from the cut ends with "bites" 2 mm. apart. The sutures should evert the cut edge and assure a smooth internal surface at the suture line. In children an interrupted suture repair is preferred to assure circumferential growth.

14. If a graft is required, the segment of saphenous vein should be reversed in direction to assure that its valves will not obstruct flow. Prosthetic graft material is avoided if possible except for larger arteries, since it is thought to increase the risk of infection.

15. Once the repair is complete, the distal clamp is removed first and air and blood are allowed to escape through the suture line as it expands to tighten the seal. Following removal of the proximal clamp, a brief period of gentle pressure over the suture line usually provides hemostasis. Pulsation should be noted across the repair and throughout the distal vessels. The suture line should be soft and palpably free of clots or narrowing. Pulses in the distal extremity should be restored.

16. If distal pulses are not restored or the quality of arterial flow in the operative field is unsatisfactory, an operative arteriogram should be obtained to assess both the anastomosis and the status of the distal arterial tree.

17. The wound should be thoroughly debrided and explored, and other injuries identified and repaired as necessary. Drains are occasionally employed for a period of 24 to 48 hours. Every effort is made to cover the repaired artery with viable muscle and fascia in addition to closure of the skin.

18. If systemic heparinization has been employed, its effects will usually disappear over the several hours required to complete the operation, and neutralization is not required. Dressings and splints should be well padded to protect anesthetic ischemic tissues. They should be applied so as to provide for inspection of toes or fingers for capillary circulation, easy palpation of distal pulses, assessment of the musculature of the distal extremity, and ready access to the operative wound should bleeding occur. Any constriction of the limb should be avoided, and immobilization of fractures should be achieved by either skeletal traction, posterior molds, or operative fixation (see below).

POSTOPERATIVE CARE

Following surgery, every effort should be made to maintain an effective circulating blood volume with hematocrit levels above 30 per cent. Maintenance of a satisfactory perfusion pressure is confirmed by systemic blood pressure and urinary output monitoring. Systemic anticoagulation is rarely employed because of possible adverse effects upon the repair or other injuries. Agents or techniques designed to decrease platelet adhesiveness (e.g., aspirin) or blood viscosity (e.g., Dextran) or to prevent vasoconstriction (e.g., sympathectomy) are seldom the determinants of a good result.

Pulses distal to the site of arterial repair should be evaluated at hourly intervals by digital palpation or Doppler ultrasonic flow techniques. Significant

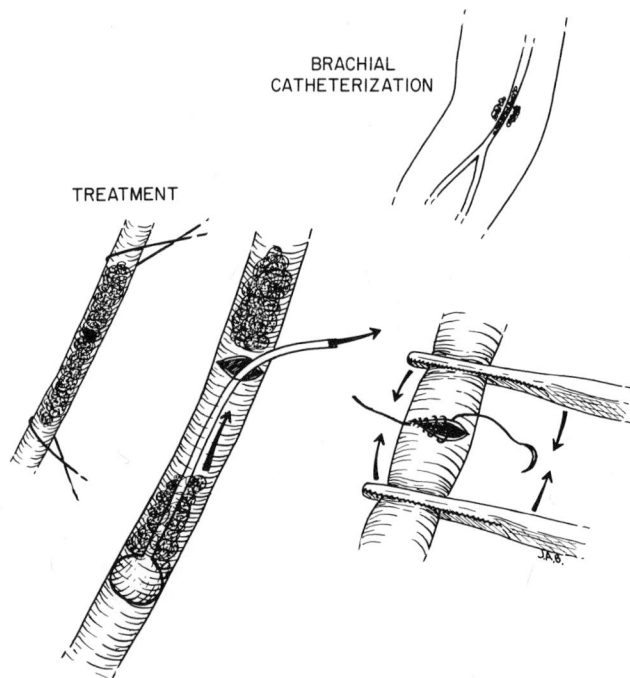

BRACHIAL CATHETERIZATION

TREATMENT

Figure 41. Steps in the operative repair of a brachial artery occlusion following catheterization for diagnostic studies.

changes in either of these findings or any increase in signs of ischemia are indications for angiographic study or re-exploration.

SPECIAL PROBLEMS

IATROGENIC ARTERIAL INJURY

Currently, a very common form of arterial injury is that which follows the insertion of a needle or catheter into an artery for purposes of angiography, collection of an arterial blood specimen, or the monitoring of arterial pressure. The large number of coronary arteriograms performed via the brachial artery at the elbow account for the relative frequency of these injuries. Thrombosis of the brachial artery with loss of the distal (radial) pulse occurs in as many as 25 per cent of these studies and appears to relate to such factors as the skill and experience of the angiographer, the size and number of catheters employed, and the duration of time the catheter is in place.[24]

While gangrene of the fingers is a rare complication, a significant number of patients experience pallor, coldness, numbness, or paresthesias in the distal extremity. Depending upon their occupation, many patients note diminished exercise tolerance in the forearm and hand.

Current practice requires prompt exploration of the site of catheterization in any patient experiencing a loss of the radial pulse following removal of the catheter (Fig. 41). In the majority, thrombosis has occurred at a site of intimal disruption, usually on the posterior portion of the wall of the brachial artery. Treatment consists of opening the thrombosed artery in a transverse direction at the site of previous arterial puncture. Direct inspection of the intimal lining with removal of attached clots or detached intima is performed proximally and distally by the passage of a small Fogarty catheter.[8] Brisk bleeding from both ends of the opened vessel is then usually observed and is readily controlled with linen tapes or vascular clamps. A meticulous transverse closure of the arteriotomy wound using fine 6-0 arterial suture is then accomplished while all tension on the severed edges of the artery is eliminated.

Additional examples of iatrogenic arterial injury include thrombosis of the radial artery following arterial blood sampling or pressure monitoring.[12] Such injuries have resulted in the loss of digits and the entire hand even when the ulnar artery was present. The subclavian and carotid arteries are occasionally injured during attempts to insert central venous catheters, perform brachial plexus or stellate ganglion anesthetic blocks, or in the course of surgical procedures to correct the thoracic outlet syndrome. Injuries to the common femoral artery and its immediate branches are also seen following catheterization of these vessels for angiographic purposes. The larger diameter of these arteries seems to protect against the development of arterial thrombosis, but intimal dissection and narrowing, recurrent bleeding, and false aneurysm are occasionally observed. Maintaining firm pressure over the site of arterial puncture for a period of at least 15 minutes following removal of the arterial catheter is the single most effective method to prevent complications following femoral angiography.

Increased awareness of the disastrous consequences of penetration into deep structures during surgery of herniated lumbar disc has largely eliminated the massive bleeding, false aneurysm, and arteriovenous fistulas of the aorta, vena cava, iliac arteries, and veins that occasionally followed these procedures.

Orthopedic procedures on the hip, knee, and shoulder area may also lead to arterial injury through accidents involving the knife, drill points, wires, screws, or plates that penetrate adjacent vessels (Fig. 42). The possibility of such injuries should be considered in any patient in whom excessive or recurrent bleeding accompanies or follows an operative procedure. Careful auscultation of the wound and judicious use of angiography will usually confirm or exclude the existence of such injuries. Severe injuries occasionally

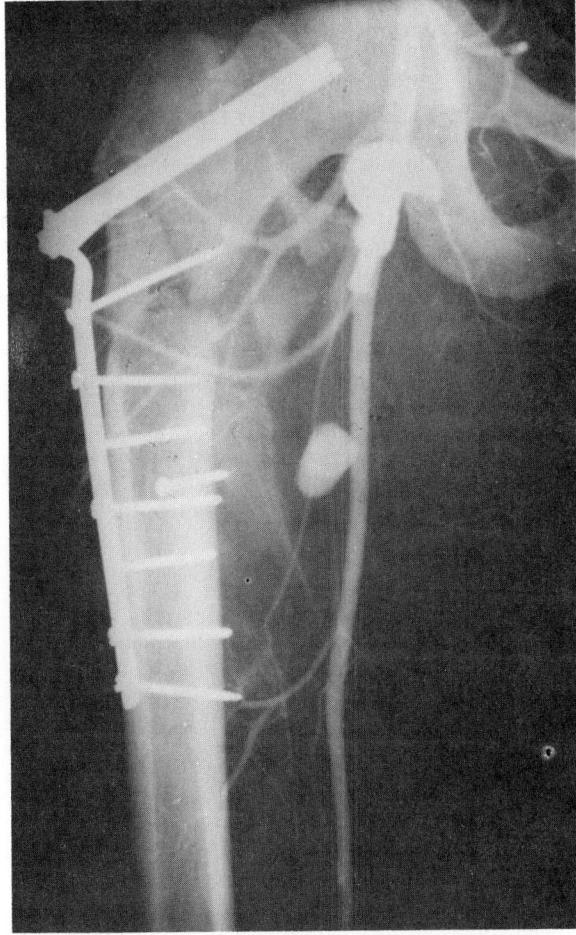

Figure 42. Femoral arteriogram in a patient with a massive swelling of the thigh following operative repair of a subtrochanteric fracture of the femur. The collection of contrast material appears to arise from the superficial femoral artery, but partial severance occurred from an orthopedic drill point involving the profunda femoris artery.

result from the accidental injection of medications into an artery during attempted venipuncture. Thiopental injections into an anomalous ulnar artery in the antecubital fossa have led to severe distal thrombosis requiring amputation of the hand.

DRUG ABUSE

An increasing number of arterial injuries in our society are a consequence of the recent surge of drug abuse. Addicts who have progressively obliterated their venous channels or inexperienced "first timers" may accidentally inject a variety of pharmacologic agents and particulate matter into arteries, with ischemia and gangrene of the distal extremity resulting. The mechanism of the ischemic changes is unclear, but true vasospasm appears unlikely.[39] Anticoagulants, rheologic agents such as Dextran, and protection of the ischemic limb are recommended methods of treatment. Exclusion of other causes of vascular injury in drug abusers is also important. In addition to local injury or infection at the site of injection, these patients may also develop compartmental syndromes from prolonged pressure over muscle groups during a period of drug-induced unconsciousness.

COMPARTMENTAL HYPERTENSION

An increase in the contents of the osseofascial compartments of the leg, thigh, and forearm may lead to a marked increase in intracompartmental tissue pressure with impairment of blood flow.[25] Arteriolar flow to the muscles of the compartment usually ceases when the tissue pressure rises to within 10 to 20 mm. of diastolic arterial pressure. Higher levels of intracompartmental pressure may ultimately lead to obliteration of flow in the major arteries that course through the compartment on their way to the distal extremity.

This sequence of events is commonly observed when muscles that have been rendered ischemic for several hours are successfully revascularized by arterial repair. Profound intra- and extracellular edema of the involved muscles creates a situation in which the strong, thick, deep fascia surrounding the extremity and overlying the compartment functions as a tourniquet that must be released if flow is to be restored.

A similar course has been described following venous occlusion, direct muscle trauma, vigorous exercise, deep burns, or hemorrhage within a closed fascial space. The forearm and calf are most frequently involved. The involved compartment becomes firm to palpation, and loss of muscle function soon becomes apparent. Loss of cutaneous sensation may result when sensory nerves that pass through the compartment are subjected to the increased pressure. Distal arterial pulsations are maintained until the more advanced stages of the condition occur. The end result of severe untreated compartmental hypertension is the loss or replacement of ischemic muscle, with fibrous tissue leading to deformity and loss of function.

Since early recognition of the syndrome permits treatment before irreversible damage has occurred, recent interest has centered on direct measurements of intracompartmental pressure by means of pressure transducers or a simple mercury manometer in line with an 18 gauge needle and plastic tubing containing air and fluid. In susceptible patients, direct or continuous measurements of the pressures in each of the muscular compartments should be made percutaneously in both extremities.[19, 38] Once the syndrome of significant compartmental hypertension is clinically or manometrically confirmed, it should be treated by an incision to release the trapped contents of the involved compartments (Fig. 43). The marked improvement in arterial flow that may follow fasciotomy of a patient with the anterior compartment syndrome is depicted in Figure 44.

The possibility of compartmental hypertension is especially great when delay in arterial repair of over six hours has led to severe muscle ischemia, or when direct trauma to muscles or impairment of venous return accompanies arterial injury. Supracondylar fractures of the humerus in children are especially prone to this complication developing in the muscles of the forearm, even in the absence of an overt arterial injury. Pain distal to the site of extremity injury is usually increased by efforts to extend the fingers. Radial pulses are usually diminished. Such a state must be

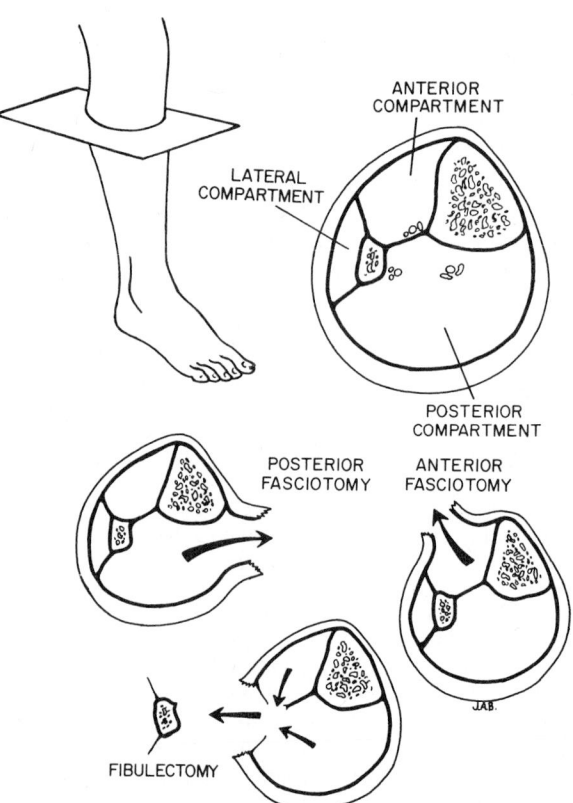

Figure 43. Diagram of the right calf, illustrating the muscular compartments and sites of incision to provide decompression when a rise in compartmental pressure occurs.

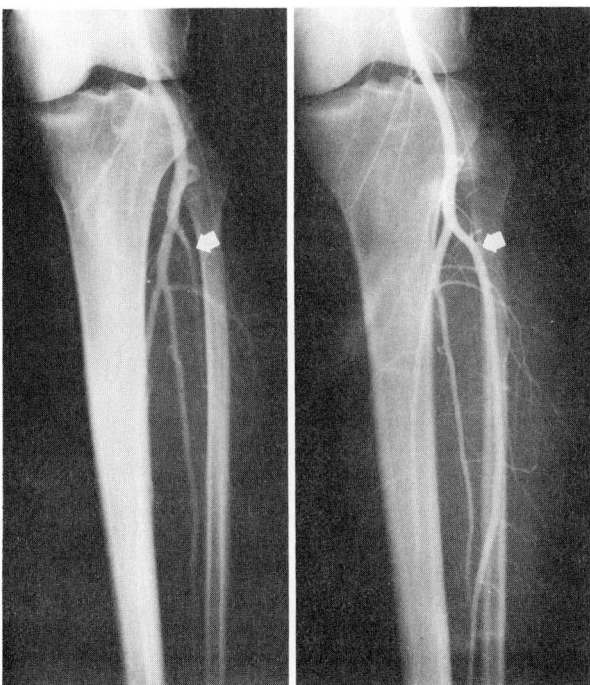

Figure 44. Pre- and postoperative femoral arteriograms in a patient with an anterior compartment syndrome secondary to femoral artery occlusion of over six hours' duration. The very small (occluded) anterior tibial artery (arrows) is much enlarged following anterior fasciotomy.

promptly investigated and usually necessitates the removal of all constricting bandages or plaster and the use of skeletal traction by means of a pin or screw in the olecranon. Failure to obtain prompt relief of symptoms by this maneuver would require exploration of the brachial artery, evacuation of the hematoma, and fasciotomy of the forearm musculature.

In the lower extremity, fractures of the shaft of the tibia may lead to severe pressure increases within either the anterior or posterior compartments of the leg. Loss of sensation may be noted in the web space at the base of the first and second digits. Careful palpation of the muscle groups in jeopardy is necessary, as well as periodic assessment of muscle function. Early measurement of tissue pressure and a high index of suspicion are essential if the tragic consequences of this condition are to be avoided.

VENOUS INJURIES

The safety of and need for repairing venous injuries has only recently been appreciated.[28, 29] Ligation of major veins impairs venous return and may jeopardize the success of arterial reconstruction by contributing to the development of compartmental hypertension. In addition, the development of chronic venous insufficiency may prove a distressing sequela. Ligation of a major vein is sometimes necessary owing to the difficulties of achieving a satisfactory repair or in the interest of reducing operative time. Under these circum-

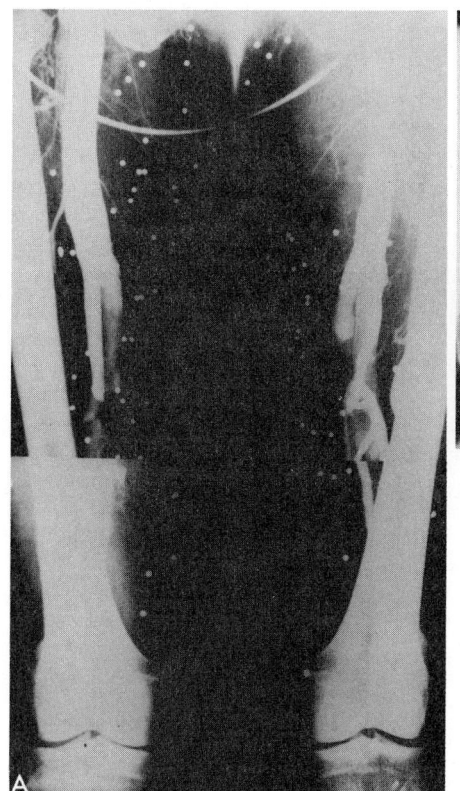

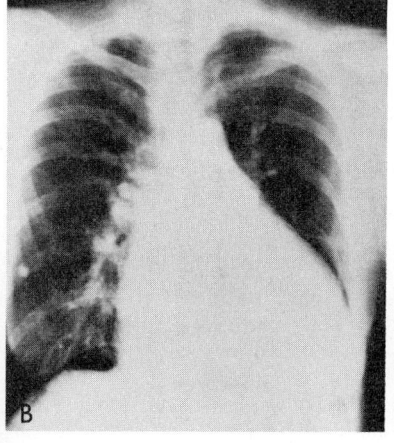

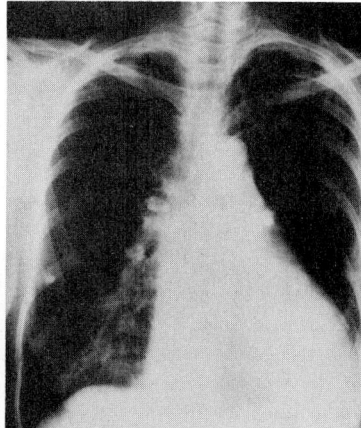

Figure 45. *A,* Bilateral femoral arteriograms in a 42-year-old female who sustained a shotgun wound to both lower extremities at age 18. *B,* The chest films are before and one month following closure of multiple bilateral femoral arteriovenous fistulas from pellets.

stances, consideration should be given to the need for performing a fasciotomy or instituting measures such as elevation, anticoagulants, and Dextran to discourage the propagation of venous thrombosis with further compromise of collateral circulation.

The repair of venous injuries is difficult and at times impossible. Thrombosis at the site of repair commonly occurs and is associated with the risk of pulmonary embolism. Nonetheless, most authorities believe that even the *temporary flow* achieved by venous reconstruction is beneficial to the total circulation and outweighs the risks involved. Reconstruction of the innominate, common femoral, and popliteal veins is especially important and should always be attempted because of the demonstrated inadequacies of collateral flow. Contrariwise, most other major extremity veins can be ligated when necessary and, with careful attention to early and late supportive measures, will be associated with satisfactory function.

FRACTURES WITH VASCULAR INJURY

The important association of arterial injuries with open or closed fractures and dislocations is outlined in Table 7.[10, 13, 14, 17, 23, 26] Recognition of the vascular injury is often obscured by the difficulties of examining the painful, swollen extremity that accompanies bony injury. More often than not, however, it is the failure to assess the status of the distal extremity or to appreciate the significance of a large hematoma, recurrent bleeding, and distal ischemia that leads to the delay in recognition of arterial injury. A distressing preoccupation with bony abnormalities seen on radiologic study is an all too common error in the care of extremity injuries and must be guarded against if tragic consequences of missed arterial injury are to be avoided.

The methods of diagnosis and principles of repair are similar to those for other arterial injuries, except for the problem of achieving stabilization of the fracture fragments adjacent to the arterial repair. The desirability of fixing the bony fragments with plates, rods, or screws prior to or immediately following arterial reconstruction must be weighed against its hazards. Not only does the orthopedic manipulation prolong the operative procedure and increase the risk of infection, especially in the case of open fractures, but, in addition, it may impair collateral circulation and jeopardize the viability of the extremity. In most extremity fractures with vascular injury, satisfactory bony reduction can be achieved by the use of external stabilization or skeletal traction without significant risk of disruption of the arterial repair. The importance of avoiding circumferential bandages or plaster casts in patients with suspected or known vascular injuries is mandatory.

In any fracture treated by closed methods, when doubt exists as to the status of the circulation or the patient complains of severe pain or loses motor function after application of a cast, the cast should be split longitudinally and all constricting elements released. If there is not prompt improvement in the patient's symptoms or findings, removal of the cast and evaluation of the tension in the muscle compartments, as well as assessment of arterial flow, is mandatory.

The prognosis in patients with vascular injury associated with fracture is clearly worsened by the presence of venous injury, delay in repair, open fracture, and the development of wound sepsis. Appropriate precautions or treatment of these factors is mandatory.

SELECTED REFERENCES

Eastcott, H. H. G.: Arterial Surgery, 2nd ed., Chapter 13. Philadelphia, J. B. Lippincott, 1973.
This is an outstanding chapter in an excellent text of vascular surgery, which reviews many fine details of diagnosis and treatment of a wide variety of arterial injuries.

Hardy, J. D., Seshadri, R., Neely, W. A., and Berry, D. W.: Aortic and other arterial injuries. Ann. Surg., *181*:640, 1975.
This is an extensive review of 360 arterial injuries encountered at one center during an 18-year period. Over 85 per cent were the result of penetrating wounds, while the majority of blunt injuries were associated with fractures and dislocations. Major veins were involved in 20 per cent. An excellent discussion regarding management of the more complicated injuries to the aortic arch, carotid, popliteal, and renal arteries is included. The principles of management and the controversies surrounding ancillary measures are well presented.

Klingensmith, W., Oles, P., and Martinez, H.: Fractures with associated blood vessel injury. Arch. Surg., *110*:849, 1965.
This is a review of 11 patients with nonpenetrating trauma. It emphasizes the seeming rarity of such injuries, but also the likelihood that they may be encountered in a private practice setting as well as the industrial clinic or urban medical center. The location, associated fracture, diagnosis, repair, and prognosis in these injuries are typical of such closed injuries and emphasize the need for early surgical intervention.

Rich, N. M., Hobson, R. W., and Collins, G. J.: Traumatic arteriovenous fistulae and false aneurysms. Surgery, 78:817, 1957.
This review of 558 injuries in the Viet Nam War provides a comprehensive but retrospective review of the diagnosis and treatment of this complication of arterial severance. It is hoped that the 7 per cent incidence will diminish as partial severance is recognized and repaired primarily.

REFERENCES

1. Bradley, E. L., III: Management of penetrating carotid injuries. J. Trauma, *13*:248–255, 1973.
2. Carrel, A.: The surgery of blood vessels. Bull. Johns Hopkins Hosp., *190*:18, 1906.
3. Carrel, A., and Guthrie, C. C.: Uni-terminal and bi-terminal venous transplantation. Surg. Gynecol. Obstet., *2*:266, 1906.
4. Conkle, D. M., Richie, R. E., Sawyers, J. L., and Scott, H. W., Jr.: Surgical treatment of popliteal artery injuries. Arch. Surg., *110*:1351, 1975.
5. DeBakey, M. E., and Simeone, F. A.: Battle injuries of the arteries in World War II. Ann. Surg., *123*:534, 1946.
6. Eastcott, H. H. G.: Arterial Surgery. Philadelphia, J. B. Lippincott, 1973.
7. Filkin, D. C., and Warren, J. V.: Arteriovenous fistulas, their effect on the circulation. J.A.M.A., *134*:1524, 1947.
8. Fogarty, T. J., et al.: A method for extraction of arterial thrombi. Surg. Gynecol. Obstet., *116*:241, 1963.
9. Goyanes, D. J.: Substitución plástica de las arterias por las venas y arterioplástica venosa, aplicada, como nuevo método, al tratmiento de cos aneurismas. Sigo Medico, Sept. 8, 1906, pp. 346, 561.
10. Hardy, J. D., Seshadri, R., Neeley, W. A., and Berry, D. W.: Aortic and other arterial injuries. Ann. Surg., *181*:640, 1975.
11. Hughes, C. W.: Arterial repair during the Korean War. Ann. Surg., *147*:555, 1958.
12. Johnson, F. E., Sumner, D. S., and Strandness, D. F., Jr.: Extremity necrosis caused by indwelling arterial catheters. Am. J. Surg., *131*:375–379, 1976.
13. Klingensmith, W., Olis, P., and Martinez, H.: Fractures associated with blood vessel injury. Am. J. Surg., *110*:849, 1965.
14. Koostra, G., Schipper, J. J., Boontje, A. H., Klasen, H. J., and Binnendijk, B.: Femoral shaft fracture with injury of the superficial femoral artery in civilian accidents. Surg. Gynecol. Obstet., *142*:339–402, 1976.

15. Lain, K. C., and Williams, G. R.: Arteriography in acute peripheral arterial injuries: An experimental study. Surg. Forum, 21:179, 1970.

16. Lambert, J. In Erichson, J. E.(Ed.): Observations on Aneurysms. London, Sydenham Society, 1844, p. 265.

17. Makin, G. S., Howard, J. M., and Green, R. L.: Arterial injuries complicating fractures or dislocation: The necessity for a more aggressive approach. Surgery, 59:203, 1966.

18. Margolies, M. M., et al.: Arteriography in the management of hemorrhage from pelvic fractures. N. Engl. J. Med., 287:317, 1972.

19. Matsen, F. A., Mayo, K. A., Sheridan, G. W., and Krugmire, R. B., Jr.: Monitoring of intramuscular pressure. Surgery, 75:702 1976.

20. Miller, W. F.: Massive hemorrhage in fractures of the pelvis. South Med. J., 56:933–938, 1963.

21. Monson, D. O., Saletta, J. D., and Freeark, R. J.: Carotid vetebral trauma. J. Trauma, 9:987–997, 1969.

22. Murphy, J. B.: Resection of arteries and veins injured in continuity—end-to-end suture. (Exp. Clin. Res.) Med. Rec., 51:73, 1897.

23. McNamara, J. J., et al.: Management of fractures with associated injury in combat casualties. J. Trauma, 13:17, 1973.

24. Nicholas, G. G., and Demuth, W. E.: Long term results of brachial thrombectomy—following cardiac catheterization. Ann. Surg., 183:436–438, 1976.

25. Patman, R. D., and Thompson, J. E.: Fasciotomy in peripheral vascular surgery: Report of 164 patients. Arch. Surg., 101:663, 1970.

26. Pradham, D. J., Jauanteguy, J. M., Wilder, R. J., and Michelson, E.: Arterial injuries of the extremities associated with fractures. Arch. Surg., 105:582, 1972.

27. Pringle, J. H.: Two cases of vein grafting for the maintenance of direct arterial circulation. Lancet, 1, 1795.

28. Rich, N. M., Hughes, C. W., and Baugh, J. H.: Management of venous injuries. Ann. Surg., 171:724, 1970.

29. Rich, N. M., Hobson, R. W., Collins, G. J., and Anderson, C. A.: The effect of acute popliteal venous interruption. Ann. Surg., 183:365–368, 1976.

30. Rich, N. M.: Vascular trauma in Viet Nam. J. Cardiovasc. Surg., 2:368, 1970.

31. Ring, E. J., Athanasoulis, S. C., Waltman, A. C., et al.: Arteriographic management of hemorrhage following pelvic fracture. Radiology, 109:65–70, 1973.

32. Saletta, J. D., and Freeark, R. J.: The partially severed artery. Arch. Surg., 96:198–205, 1968.

33. Saletta, J. D., and Freeark, R. J.: Injuries to the profunda femoris artery. J. Trauma, 12:778–785, 1972.

34. Smith, K., Ben-Menachem, Y., Duke, J. H., and Hill, G. L.: The superior gluteal: an artery at risk in blunt pelvic trauma. J. Trauma, 16:273, 1976.

35. Smith, R. F., Szilagyi, D., and Pfeifer, J.: A study of arterial trauma. Arch. Surg., 86:825, 1963.

36. Sturm, J. F., Perry, J. F., Jr., and Cass, A. S.: Renal artery and vein injury following blunt trauma. Ann. Surg., 183:696, 1975.

37. Symbas, P. N., Kourias, E., Tyras, D. H., and Hatcher, C. R. J.: Penetrating wounds of great vessels. Ann. Surg., 179:757–762, 1976.

38. Whitesides, T. E., Jr., Haney, T. C., Harada, H., Holmes, H. E., and Morimoto, K.: A simple method for tissue pressure determination. Arch. Surg., 110:1311, 1975.

39. Wright, C. B., Lamoy, R. E., and Hobson, R. W., II: Hemodynamic effects of intra-arterial injection of drugs of abuse. Surgery, 79:425, 1976.

40. Yao, S. T.: Experiences with the Doppler ultrasound flow velocity meter in peripheral vascular disease. In Modern Trends in Vascular Surgery. London, Butterworths, 1970.

8. ACUTE ARTERIAL OCCLUSION

Thomas J. Fogarty, M.D.

Reference to occlusion of the arterial circulation was first made by Harvey in 1628.[10] Labey[11] in 1911 has been credited with the first successful surgical removal of an arterial embolus. Review of the surgical literature indicates that the operative approach to acute arterial occlusion was limited by the inability of the surgeon to remove simply and effectively the embolus and distally propagated thrombus. The introduction of the balloon catheter technique[7] in 1963 simplified the technical aspects of surgery for acute arterial occlusion. Advances in the field of open-heart surgery have eliminated some of the sources of arterial emboli, and further reduced mortality by making possible correction of the cardiac disorder.

PATHOLOGY

Regardless of the source or histologic structure of an embolus, it is the location and secondary events following the impaction that determine the viability of an extremity. Following occlusion, a softer coagulum of blood forms in areas of decreased flow. Linton[13] has emphasized that this propagation of thrombus distal to the embolus is of major importance in the outcome of the disease process. Failure to recognize and to remove atraumatically the distally propagated thrombus may result in less than complete restoration of circulation and possibly in amputation. Surgeons have uniformly relied upon the presence or absence of backbleeding from the peripheral arterial bed as a guide to distal patency. Repeated clinical observations have confirmed that backbleeding is an unreliable guide to distal patency. Discontinuous thrombotic material is present in approximately one third of the cases (Fig. 46). Under these circumstances, backbleeding may be quite forceful, despite the presence of addi-

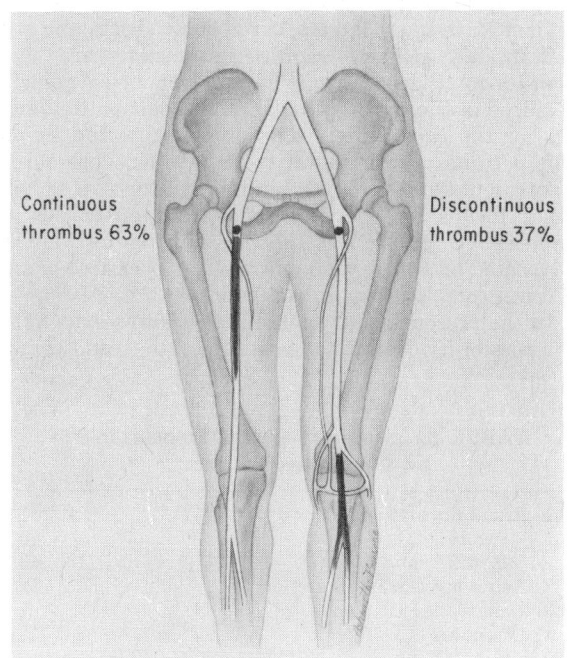

Continuous thrombus 63%   Discontinuous thrombus 37%

Figure 46. Anatomic location of distal thrombus as it relates to location of embolus.

tional distal thrombotic material. The presence of adequate collateral vessels will result in significant bleeding from the distal segment despite the fact that the more peripheral arterial bed may be totally occluded. Failure to recognize this circumstance will result in less than complete restoration of the circulation.

Arterial emboli most commonly occur in the elderly, seriously ill patient with multiple systemic diseases. Prolonged periods of surgical manipulation and general anesthesia have been considered valid deterrents to operative intervention in such patients. This has been particularly true when the clinical finding indicated that conservative measures might preserve life at the cost of limb loss or impairment of function. The balloon catheter technique is an operative procedure designed to avoid general anesthesia, reduce surgical trauma, and effectively remove all thrombotic material in a simple manner, regardless of its anatomic location.

PREOPERATIVE EVALUATION AND CARE

Patients presenting with an acute embolic occlusion should be assumed to have significant underlying heart disease. Table 8 shows the sources of arterial emboli in a series of 300 patients. The large number of patients presenting with arteriosclerotic heart disease reinforces the concept that the heart represents the site of underlying basic pathologic change.

Evaluation of cardiac function should proceed simultaneously with the examination of the peripheral vasculature. Digitalis, antiarrhythmic agents, morphine, diuretics, and heparin are drugs basic to patient care. Utilization of these agents when indicated should not delay surgical intervention.

Appropriate therapy is initiated while emergency preparation for operation is being made. The presence of congestive heart failure, cardiogenic shock, and significant arrhythmias requires intensive care unit monitoring. Placement of a central venous catheter is required in the majority of cases. In addition to allowing for the rapid administration of drugs and fluids, this permits monitoring of central venous pressures. Central placement of catheters represents a convenient means for the intravenous administration of heparin. Cannulation of the internal jugular vein as advocated by Daily[3] is simple and has been free of significant complications in our hands.

In the presence of an embolus to a lower extremity, the possibility of simultaneous emboli to mesenteric or

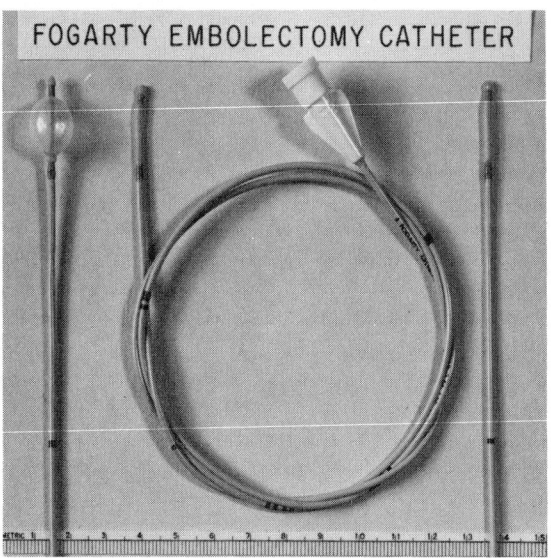

FOGARTY EMBOLECTOMY CATHETER

Figure 47. Catheter for extraction of arterial emboli.

renal arteries should always be entertained. Hematuria or abdominal complaints indicative of a possible occlusion require preoperative visualization of these vessels. Involvement of more than one extremity occurs in approximately 10 per cent of the patients and this fact should not be overlooked. Once the diagnosis of an acute arterial occlusion has been made, heparin should be given immediately and preparation for operation initiated.

INSTRUMENTATION

A balloon catheter has been developed with specific adaptations in its construction for safe, effective extraction of arterial emboli. It consists of a hollow, pliable body in graduated sizes for use in major vessels of any caliber (Fig. 47). At its proximal portion the syringe fitting provides the means for fluid exchange into a soft, distensible balloon placed at the distal tip of the instrument. The catheter is inserted into the acutely occluded vessel as far as possible. The balloon is inflated and withdrawn in the inflated position. By a mechanism of fluid displacement, the balloon maintains uniform, even contact with the vessel wall as it proceeds through areas of narrowing. This mechanism allows for removal of thrombotic material distal to stenotic areas. One surgeon manipulates both the syringe and the catheter during withdrawal. In this way it is easy to judge the amount of traction required for extraction of the occluding material as well as the quantity of fluid necessary to effect alternate inflation and deflation as the instrument proceeds through areas of arteriosclerotic narrowing or vessels of increasing or decreasing diameter.

The concept of a balloon catheter has remained basically the same since its initial introduction. There have been minor changes in the instrument itself directed at increasing its effectiveness and reducing the incidence of complications. A variety of balloon

TABLE 8. Source of Arterial Embolus in 300 Consecutive Patients

1. Atrial fibrillation	231
A.S.H.D.*	183
R.H.D.†	48
2. Acute myocardial infarction	50
3. Arteriosclerotic plaque	7
4. Unknown	12

*A.S.H.D. = arteriosclerotic heart disease.
†R.H.D. = rheumatic heart disease.

configurations and catheter materials have been evaluated. Although the utilization of double-lumen catheters and spiked balloon catheters appears attractive, significant disadvantages have been associated with their use. The utility and effectiveness of the instrument are related to its simplicity. Attempts to incorporate nonessential refinements have thus far not proved advantageous or practical.

Complications secondary to the use of the balloon catheters have been those common to all catheter techniques, and have included cases of plaque dissection, catheter tip separation, and vessel perforation. Vessel rupture can occur if the balloon portion of the instrument is overdistended in small vessels. Experience and a realization of the limitations of the instrument are the most significant factors in reducing the incidence of complications.[5]

OPERATIVE PROCEDURE

The experience with acute peripheral arterial embolization has clearly indicated that successful management of these patients is related to well-defined factors. From a technical standpoint, it must be recognized that there are varying degrees of difficulty encountered in the attempt to reestablish the peripheral circulation. Patients presenting with advanced ischemia with extensive distal propagation of the thrombus and patients presenting with significant chronic occlusive disease present the most difficult technical problems. A careful history and physical examination allow one to identify these situations.

Operative Preparation

The procedure is initiated with local anesthesia. An anesthetist should be in attendance to monitor vital signs and administer a general anesthetic if it becomes necessary. The extremity should be surgically prepared from the toes to the nipple line. A bilateral inguinal approach is utilized for aortic emboli and both extremities are prepared. An iliac embolus requires bilateral preparation. The possibility of dislodging a high iliac embolus with occlusion of the opposite extremity exists. This has not occurred in the author's experience, but the possibility is always anticipated by preparation of the opposite extremity so that the pulses may be externally palpated at the time of surgery.

An x-ray cassette should be placed under the extremities. Adequate quantities of blood should be available.

Technique

The approach to embolic occlusion regardless of the anatomic location has been through a femoral incision (Fig. 48). The common femoral artery, superficial femoral artery, and deep femoral artery are isolated and encircled with Silastic occluding pads (Fig. 48 inset). The arterial incision is made in relation to the orifice of the superficial femoral artery and deep femoral artery. A distal exploration is carried out initially and catheters should be routinely placed in the superficial and deep femoral arteries. An open deep femoral

circulation is capable of providing the margin necessary to maintain viability in many patients with advanced ischemia or in patients who had prior chronic occlusion of the superficial femoral system. Recovery of embolic material from the deep femoral artery, even in the presence of a patent common femoral artery, has been frequent in our experience. The 2F and 3F catheters are most commonly employed for exploration of the deep femoral system, while 3F and 4F catheters have been found suitable for exploration of the femoral-popliteal systems.

If there is uncertainty about adequate distal clot removal, operative arteriograms should be obtained. The presence of additional distal thrombotic material is an indication for a second incision in the medial aspect of the leg exposing the distal popliteal artery and the popliteal trifurcation (Fig. 49). Occluding Silastic pads should be placed about the distal popliteal, the anterior tibial, and the posterior tibial arteries (Fig. 49). The 2F or 3F catheter should be introduced selectively into each one of these vessels through a transverse arteriotomy. If these vessels were previously patent and uninvolved in an arteriosclerotic process, a 2F catheter should pass beyond the ankle joint. The course of the catheter can be felt by placing the hand on the distribution of the anterior and posterior tibial arteries (Fig. 49). If the progress of the catheter is impeded at the ankle joint, extension of the foot frequently permits further passage. Inability to pass the 2F catheter beyond the ankle along with the presence of angiographic evidence of obstruction beyond this point requires direct exposure of the anterior and posterior tibial arteries at the ankle. By direct manipulation of the vessel combined with gentle simultaneous probing of the catheter from the proximal end, it is possible to pass the catheter beyond the point of obstruction without the necessity of an arteriotomy. If an arteriotomy at the ankle level in either of these vessels is required, a vessel opening is made just large enough to allow for introduction of the 2F catheter. The catheter is then threaded distally, inflated, and withdrawn in the inflated condition. This maneuver frequently brings thrombotic material above the small arteriotomy. Additional attempts to extract thrombotic material should be made by the introduction of the 2F catheter into the anterior or posterior tibial vessel at the level of the popliteal arteriotomy. This maneuver avoids the necessity of enlarging the arteriotomy at the ankle level and decreases the possibility of reocclusion. Following removal of the thrombotic material, copious irrigation of the distal arterial system should be carried out with a heparinized solution.

In the presence of advanced ischemia, the simultaneous presence of major venous occlusion demands consideration. In a personal series of 300 patients, 8 per cent were found to have concomitant major venous occlusion.[8] The majority of the patients in this group had advanced ischemia with extensive distal propagation of clot on the arterial side. In this situation the vein is explored before the arterial circulation is re-established, and large venous thrombi are removed by means of venous thrombectomy catheters.[6] Prior to suture closure of the vein, the arterial circulation is re-

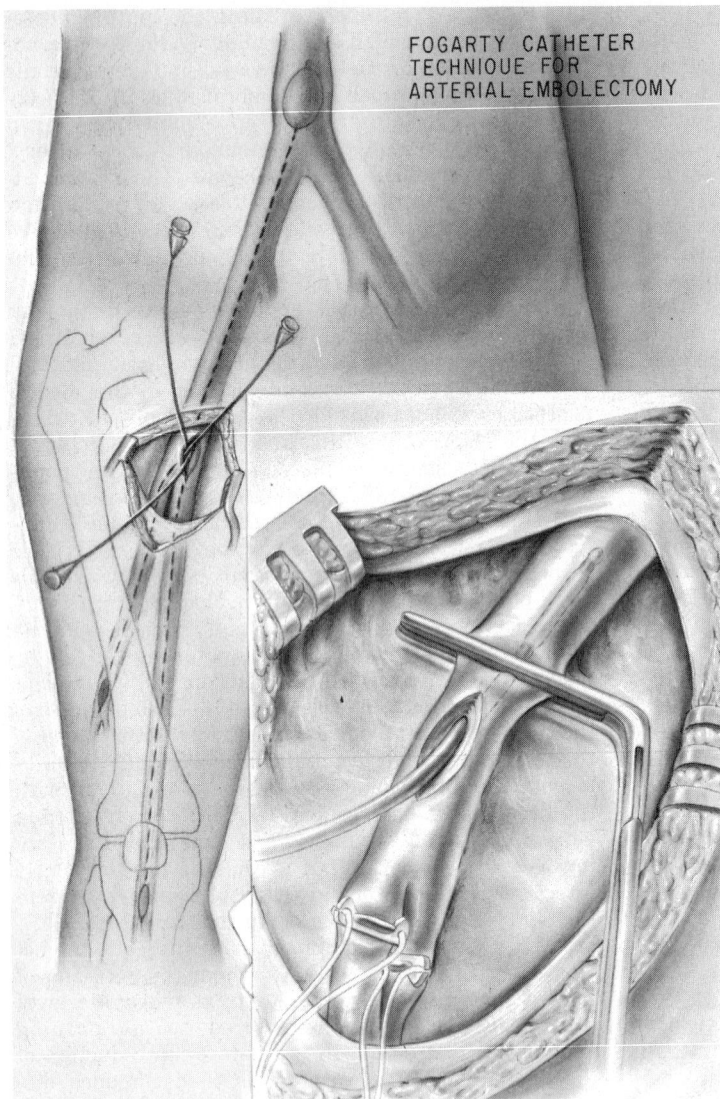

FOGARTY CATHETER
TECHNIQUE FOR
ARTERIAL EMBOLECTOMY

Figure 48. Inguinal incisions utilized for extraction of arterial embolus.

established. After removal of the arterial occlusions, the distal arterial system is irrigated with 200 to 300 ml. of a heparinized solution. The distal venous clamp is removed to allow smaller thrombi to be flushed out during this irrigation. The artery is closed first. The vein is flushed once again after re-establishment of the arterial circulation. The venotomy is closed last.

There has been reference in the literature to delaying surgical intervention in patients who present with advanced ischemia.[2] We have not employed this delayed approach, and feel that advanced ischemia secondary to acute embolic occlusion represents a surgical emergency. In these patients heparin is employed at the time of surgery and in the immediate postoperative period.

In those situations in which it is recognized that heparin should be employed in the immediate postoperative period, it has been our policy to anticipate the possible complications of hemorrhage and hematoma at incisional sites and to employ vacuum-type drainage.

Swelling of a revascularized, ischemic extremity can assume considerable proportions and requires treatment. Massive swelling that may embarrass arterial inflow is observed most frequently in those patients who present with advanced ischemia prior to surgical intervention. Capillary damage resulting in fluid exudation into ischemic tissues is a factor in this swelling. Obstruction of the venous outflow tract aggravates the problem. Failure to control immediately this edema may result in reocclusion of the arterial inflow. Fasciotomy has been required in 10 per cent of the patients who present with acute embolic occlusion. Initial decompression is carried out through small skin incisions as described by Rosato.[15] If immediate improvement is not obtained by this limited fasciotomy, the skin incisions should be extended and the deeper fascial compartments widely opened. Radical decompression requiring fibular resection is rarely necessary in patients who have an acute embolic occlusion. Patman and Thompson[14] have given an excellent review of the technique and indications for fasciotomy.

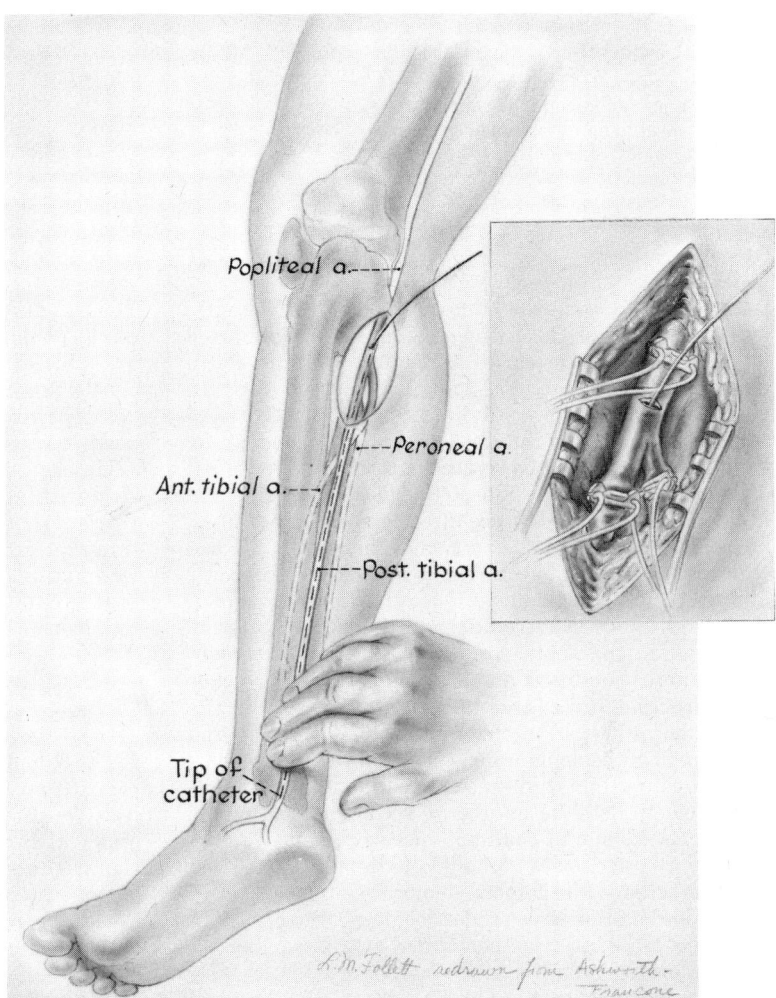

Figure 49. Exposure of popliteal trifurcation.

Immediately following restoration of arterial continuity in extremities with advanced ischemia, significant alterations in electrolytes and acid balance may occur.[4] The venous efflux of ischemic extremities following restoration of arterial continuity was studied in 10 patients (Table 9). These data clearly indicated that, following successful restoration of the circulation, there was a sudden return of very acidotic blood with a high potassium content to the heart. This metabolic effect in conjunction with pooling of blood in the revascularized extremity can result in significant hypotension. In 8 of the 10 patients studied, adverse effects were associated with clamp release, in the form of significant electrocardiographic changes or hypotension or both. The necessity of using buffering agents and antiarrhythmic agents should be anticipated at the time of clamp release. Electrolytes should be closely followed in the postoperative period. A high creatine phosphokinase level noted in the venous efflux indicates significant muscle damage.

Haimovici has described the adverse systemic effects that may occur following revascularization of the extremity presenting with advanced ischemia.[9]

EMBOLIC OCCLUSION IN THE PRESENCE OF SIGNIFICANT CHRONIC OCCLUSIVE DISEASE

A careful history and examination of the uninvolved extremity affords a reliable assessment of the peripheral circulation prior to the acute episode. The pa-

TABLE 9.   Mean Values of Biochemical Determinations on Venous Efflux of Ischemic Extremity Before and After Restoration of Flow

Ten Patients	pH	pO$_2$	pCO$_2$	K	CPK
System venous blood before embolectomy	7.38	38.2	36.4	4.3	77
Venous blood from ischemic leg before embolectomy	7.31	19.3	45.8	4.7	200
Venous blood from ischemic leg 5 minutes after restoration of flow	6.80	34.8	77.3	7.2	653.4

TABLE 10. Reconstructive Procedures Performed at the Time of Arterial Embolectomy

1. Common and deep femoral endarterectomy	14
2. Femoral-femoral crossover graft	7
3. Iliac endarterectomy	3
4. Aortofemoral endarterectomy	3
5. Aortofemoral graft	2

tient's general condition, his prior level of activity, and the extent of the pathologic change encountered at the time of operation all play an important role in determining the extent of the surgical procedure. In general, it is advisable only to attempt initially to return the circulation to its acute preocclusive state. Definitive reconstructive procedures are delayed until a more critical evaluation of the patient is possible. Major reconstructive procedures may be indicated, however, if the general condition of the patient is good when he is initially seen. Definitive procedures may be carried out, particularly if one is concerned about the viability of the extremity and the patient was active prior to the acute occlusion. Elderly patients in poor general condition are poor candidates for major reconstructive procedures. Local angioplasty of the deep femoral system in these situations is simple and quick and can be done under anesthesia. Frequently it will provide the margin necessary to maintain viability. Table 10 lists the number of reconstructive procedures carried out in conjunction with arterial embolectomy in a series of 300 patients.[8] Localized endarterectomy and femoral-femoral jump grafts are simple and can be done under local anesthesia. In 15 cases the procedure was performed at the time of initial exploration, and in 14 it was performed as a second procedure carried out during the initial hospital stay. In a total of 21 cases sympathectomy was performed; in 12 it was done in conjunction with a reconstructive procedure.

UPPER EXTREMITY EMBOLI

The management of emboli to the upper extremity is identical to that described for the lower extremity. Proximal subclavian artery emboli can be simply removed under local anesthesia by retrograde extraction. It should be borne in mind, however, that if the embolus appears to reside close to the origin of the cranial vessels, fragmentation of the embolus may occur during withdrawal, resulting in central nervous system ischemia. Thus far, this has not occurred in our experience, but the possibility should be anticipated. If there is serious doubt as to the exact location of the embolus as it relates to the orifices of the carotid and vertebral vessels, preoperative x-ray visualization should be performed.

The possible morbidity associated with upper extremity emboli should not be underestimated. Baird and Lajos noted in their study that more proximal emboli result in significantly more ischemia than the more distal brachial occlusions.[1]

RENAL, MESENTERIC, AND CAROTID ARTERY EMBOLI

The principles of management of emboli to these areas are similar to those described for management of peripheral arterial emboli. It should be borne in mind, however, that the external support provided by adjacent tissue is significantly less with vessels supplying the viscera and the brain than with the vessels of peripheral vasculature. Considerable care should be taken in introducing the catheter into these vessels. The 2F and 3F catheters are of appropriate size for distal exploration of these vessels, and the catheters are provided with a very flexible tip which significantly diminishes the possibility of perforation of the vessel. Only gentle inflation and traction should be used in removing emboli located in these areas.

Unless emboli to the internal carotid system are seen within the first few hours of onset, surgical intervention should not be considered. Hemorrhagic infarction represents a frequent and often fatal complication when attempts are made to remove emboli to the cerebral circulation, and when they are undertaken after a considerable lapse of time.

POSTOPERATIVE CARE AND MANAGEMENT

The indications for heparin in the postoperative period should be individualized for each patient. The possible presence of simultaneous venous thromboses and embolization following acute myocardial infarction represent indications for heparinization in the postoperative period.

The specific aspects of postoperative care will relate obviously to the underlying pathologic condition responsible for the embolus, the presence or absence of significant cardiac impairment, and the presence or absence of associated diseases. One's concern with the status of the peripheral vasculature should not impair the management or care of these other critical disorders. Peripheral embolization following myocardial infarction should immediately direct one's attention to the underlying cardiac lesion. Left heart catheterization and coronary artery visualization may be indicated in order to define whether or not a correctable cardiac lesion is present. The presence of significant valvular heart disease obviously deserves diagnostic investigation and surgical correction.

MORBIDITY AND MORTALITY

The aim of surgical intervention for arterial emboli is to restore the peripheral circulation to its preocclusive state. Evaluation of results is based upon restoration of pulses, relief of symptoms, and return of normal color and temperature. It is sometimes difficult to evaluate results in those patients in whom the condition of the extremity prior to the acute occlusion was unknown. Conditions such as mental confusion, concurrent illness, or death obviously preclude evaluation by exercise tolerance. Evaluation of therapy is best de-

TABLE 11. Time Interval in Relation to Advanced Ischemia

Age of Emboli	Number of Emboli	Advanced Ischemia*	Amputations
1-24 hours	193	24	3
24-48 hours	57	21	3
2-90 days	80	39	10

*Advanced ischemia = early rigor or gangrene.

TABLE 13. Associated Cardiac Procedures

Replacement of S-E ball valve:	
Aortic	2
Mitral	3
Replacement of mitral valve:	
Ruptured papillary	4
Rheumatic	12
Resection of ventricular aneurysm	5
Repair of infarct VSD	1

termined by mortality and the amputation rates. The possibility of maintaining a viable, functional extremity following acute arterial occlusion should exceed 90 per cent. The possibility of a successful procedure will obviously relate to the presence or absence of advanced ischemia. The condition of the extremity and not the duration of occlusion represents the primary determinant of operability. Reference to Table 11 indicates that even after prolonged periods of occlusion, successful surgical intervention is possible. Even in the presence of established gangrene, a lower level of amputation can often be achieved following successful embolectomy.

Failure of the initial exploration after an apparent success represents an indication for re-exploration. The most common cause for failure relates to technical factors, which on occasion can be corrected if recognized. The possibility, however, of re-embolization to the same extremity should not be overlooked. Its documented occurrence should reinforce a second-look attitude.[8]

A constant physical finding that should be cause for considerable concern after an apparently successful embolectomy is the presence of a water-hammer-type pulse. An apparently stronger than normal pulse has in our experience been associated with a high incidence of reocclusion. Under these circumstances, obstruction is present at the small artery and arteriolar level. Re-exploration should include copious distal irrigation in conjunction with venous exploration.

The mortality associated with acute arterial occlusion has in our experience been unrelated to surgical intervention. Table 12 lists the causes of death in a series of 300 consecutive patients with acute arterial occlusion. All deaths were related to cardiovascular dysfunction. Seventy-seven per cent of the patients died as a direct result of a cardiac cause. It would ap-

pear from this study and from the reviews by Levy[12] and Thompson[16] that the mortality associated with arterial embolism relates to the underlying cardiac disorder. These findings reinforce the contention that the recognition and correction of the cause for embolism should represent a very important aspect of the care of these patients. It is only through aggressive treatment of the underlying cardiac lesion that the mortality figures can be improved. With the increasing success of coronary artery surgery, patients in whom emboli develop after myocardial infarction deserve consideration for coronary visualization. The timing of such studies should relate to the general condition of the patient. Revascularization or aneurysmectomy, if indicated, should be done as soon as possible. Table 13 lists the number and kinds of associated cardiac procedures carried out in a group of 300 patients who had peripheral arterial emboli. Half of these procedures represented emergency situations and were carried out at the time of arterial embolectomy. The remaining half were semiurgent and all were carried out within one month from the time of acute occlusion.

CONCLUSION

Recognition and appropriate surgical management of the more difficult technical problems associated with acute arterial occlusion result in a decreased morbidity. The mortality associated with embolic episodes is due primarily to severe underlying cardiac disorder.

TABLE 12. Morbidity and Mortality 300 Patients, 330 Embolectomies

Limb salvage	95%
Patient survival	84%
Cause of death:	
Myocardial infarction	20
Congestive heart failure	16
Pulmonary embolus	5
Massive CVA	4
Renal failure	2

SELECTED REFERENCES

Boley, S. J., et al.: An agressive roentgenologic and surgical approach to acute mesenteric ischemia. Surg. Ann., 5:355–378, 1973.
  The article represents a review of the entire spectrum of mesenteric ischemia. A plan of diagnosis and therapy is outlined. The article emphasizes an aggressive diagnostic and therapeutic approach as the means of decreasing morbidity and mortality.

Fogarty, T. J., Daily, P. O., Shumway, N. E., and Krippaehne, W.: Experience with balloon catheter technic for arterial embolectomy. Am. J. Surg., 122:231, 1971.
  The authors report on a series of 330 embolic occlusions occurring in 300 patients. The paper emphasizes the necessity of identifying high-risk areas in terms of morbidity and mortality. An aggressive overall approach to the medical and surgical problems is presented.

Patman, R. D., and Thompson, J. E.: Fasciotomy in peripheral vascular surgery. Arch. Surg., 101:663, 1970.
  The authors review their personal experience with 164 patients who required fasciotomy. The indications for fasciotomy and the technique employed are presented. Fasciotomy, performed correctly and with proper indications, is a valuable procedure that can

result in an increased limb salvage and a decrease in morbidity. The paper is well written, and a variety of clinical situations that may require fasciotomy are detailed.

REFERENCES

1. Baird, R. J., and Lagos, T. Z.: Emboli to the arm. Ann. Surg., *160*:905, 1964.
2. Blaisdell, F. W.: Discussion of Levy, J. F., and Butcher, H. R.: Arterial emboli: An analysis of 125 patients. Surgery, *68*:973, 1970.
3. Daily, P. O., Griepp, R. B., and Shumway, N. E.: Percutaneous internal jugular vein cannulation. Arch. Surg., *101*:534, 1970.
4. Fisher, R. D., Fogarty, T. J., and Morrow, A. G.: Clinical and biochemical observations of the effect of transient femoral artery occlusion in man. Surgery, *68*:323, 1970.
5. Fogarty, T. J.: Complications of arterial embolectomy. *In* Beebe, H. G. (Ed.): Complications in Vascular Surgery. Philadelphia, J. B. Lippincott Company, 1973, pp. 95–102.
6. Fogarty, T. J.: Surgical management of acute vascular occlusion. *In* Cooper, P., and Nyhus, L. M. (Eds.): Surgery Annual. New York, Appleton-Century-Crofts, 1970, pp. 207–221.
7. Fogarty, T. J., Cranley, J. J., Krause, R. J., et al.: A method for extraction of arterial emboli and thrombi. Surg. Gynecol. Obstet., *116*:241, 1963.
8. Fogarty, T. J., Daily, P. O., Shumway, N. E., and Krippaehne, W.: Experience with balloon catheter technic for arterial embolectomy. Am. J. Surg., *122*:231, 1971.
9. Haimovici, H.: Myopathic-nephrotic-metabolic syndrome associated with massive acute arterial occlusions. J. Cardiovasc. Surg., *14*:589–600, 1973.
10. Harvey, W.: Exercitatio anatomica de motu cordis et sanguinis in animalibus (an English translation by Chauncey D. Leake). Springfield, Ill., Charles C Thomas, Publisher, 1931, p. 37.
11. Labey: cited by Mosney, M., and Dumont, N. J.: Embolie Fémorale au cours d'um rétrécissement mitral pur. Artériotomie. Guérison Bull. Acad. Med., *66*:358, 1911.
12. Levy, J. F., and Butcher, H. R.: Arterial emboli: An analysis of 125 patients. Surgery, *68*:968, 1970.
13. Linton, R. R.: Peripheral arterial embolism. A discussion of the postembolic vascular changes and their relation to the restoration of circulation in peripheral embolism. N. Engl. J. Med., *224*:189, 1941.
14. Patman, R. D., and Thompson, J. E.: Fasciotomy in peripheral vascular surgery. Arch. Surg., *101*:663, 1970.
15. Rosato, F. E., Barker, C. F., Roberts, B., and Danielson, G. K.: Subcutaneous fasciotomy. Description of a new technique and instrument. Surgery, *59*:3, 1966.
16. Thompson, J. E., Sigler, L., Raut, P. S., et al.: Arterial embolectomy: A 20-year experience with 163 cases. Surgery, *67*:212, 1970.

9. ARTERIOVENOUS FISTULA

David C. Sabiston, Jr., M.D.

There are few disorders in clinical medicine that can produce as many pathophysiologic changes as an arteriovenous fistula. This is especially true of large communications between an artery and vein that allow enormous amounts of arterial blood to pass through the fistula into the low-resistance venous bed. Many physiologic changes result from such a fistula in an attempt to compensate for the large and continuous shunt of blood from the arterial circuit.

In 1758, William Hunter recognized for the first time that an arteriovenous aneurysm was characterized by a direct communication between the artery and vein.[6] Until then, these lesions had been interpreted as simple aneurysms. Hunter designated the lesion an "aneurysm by anastomosis," with emphasis upon communication of the two vascular systems. Early surgical attempts to correct these lesions consisted primarily of *ligation* of the involved artery proximal to the fistula. Such a procedure was quite likely to be followed by gangrene of the extremity, since the blood reaching the distal extremity by arterial collaterals drained in a retrograde direction through the fistula into the venous system, thus depriving the limb of any significant arterial flow.[4] By 1886, it was emphatically recommended that the hunterian principle of ligation of the artery *proximal* to the fistula be condemned and that, instead, quadruple ligation of the artery and vein be the procedure of choice.[2] In 1875, Nicoladoni described a patient with an arteriovenous fistula in whom compression of the fistula (with cessation of flow through it) caused a decrease in the pulse rate from 96 to 64 per minute.[10] This phenomenon was described by Branham in 1890 as a "mysterious" slowing of the pulse with obliteration of an acquired femoral arteriovenous fistula.[3] Rudolph Matas called this the "Branham bradycardiac reaction," and it has since borne that name.[5]

Arteriovenous fistulas may be either *congenital* or *acquired*. Congenital fistulas in nearly every organ of the body have been described, but they are most prevalent in the extremities, where more than half of all fistulas have been reported.[15] Other common locations include the brain, lungs, neck, and kidney. Most congenital arteriovenous fistulas are accompanied by large varicose veins in and around the site of the fistula. In fact, the presence of varicose veins at unusual sites, and especially early in life, should lead one to suspect a congenital arteriovenous fistula. A pulsating mass, a continuous murmur, and signs of stasis including edema and phlebitis of the extremities are all common. Cyanosis or erythema of the skin and cutaneous hemangiomas are commonly observed. Generally, surgical excision of these lesions is indicated, and this may be difficult because of the extensive and penetrating nature of these congenital lesions. They produce manifestations similar to those of acquired fistulas.

Congenital *pulmonary* arteriovenous fistulas represent an interesting phenomenon. These lesions may be either single or multiple and are often observed for the first time on routine chest films. In addition, cyanosis, polycythemia, and clubbing of the fingers are likely to be present. These are the result of unsaturated blood flowing directly from the pulmonary artery into the pulmonary venous system without passage through the pulmonary capillary bed.[9]

Acquired arteriovenous fistulas are most frequently the result of trauma, following either incised or missile wounds. In addition, iatrogenic fistulas, especially those associated with operations on the renal pedicle and fistulas between the aorta or iliac veins and arteries secondary to intervertebral disc operations, are quite common. Rarely, erosion of an atherosclerotic aneurysm into an accompanying vein may occur, as, for example, erosion of an abdominal aortic aneurysm into the inferior vena cava.

TABLE 14.   Manifestations of Arteriovenous Fistula

		Systemic	
Pulse rate	↑	Diastolic arterial pressure	↓
Cardiac output	↑	Peripheral resistance	↓
Blood volume	↑		
Cardiac size	↑		

Local
Thrill
Continuous murmur
Increased arterial collaterals
Aneurysmal formation
Diminished pulse rate with occlusion

Physiologic changes occurring in the systemic circulation with an arteriovenous fistula are most marked in the presence of a large fistula and may be minimal to absent with a small fistula. Late manifestations of a large fistula include congestive heart failure, pulmonary edema, and death in untreated patients.

PATHOPHYSIOLOGY

The pathophysiologic changes that follow establishment of a direct communication between the arterial and venous systems are best demonstrated in the presence of a *large* fistula. Much blood flows through such a fistula, since it offers the path of least resistance. Thus, a sequence of changes occurs that is directly related to the shunt of blood from the arterial to the venous circuit. The *cardiac output* increases, the heart rate increases, and the diastolic pressure falls in the presence of *low* peripheral resistance (Table 14). Both blood and plasma volumes increase in an effort to compensate for the increased blood in the venous circuit. The heart becomes larger, primarily because of increase in size of the ventricular cavities. In the presence of large fistulas, a chronic burden is placed upon the heart that may ultimately lead to congestive heart failure. If the fistula is both *acute* and *large*, the heart may not be able to compensate adequately, with resultant pulmonary edema and death. Large experimental fistulas in animals demonstrate this feature quite strikingly.[12]

The oxygen saturation of the mixed venous blood is increased, since the shunt bypasses the capillary bed and the central venous pressure is usually increased. The *site* of the fistula in the systemic circulation is of importance, since the diameter of the vessel involved is critical. The location of the communication can be determined precisely by arteriography (Fig. 50). Much more blood will flow through a fistula of a given size in a vessel with a large diameter than in one with a smaller diameter. Thus, aortic fistulas of small size can produce more severe symptoms than larger fistulas in the femoral artery or arteries of comparable size. Occasionally, the presence of an arteriovenous fistula is responsible for the development of bacterial endocarditis, and in fact the first patient ever cured of bacterial endocarditis prior to the introduction of antibiotics was managed by surgical closure of an iliac arteriovenous fistula, after which the subacute bacterial endocarditis disappeared.[11]

LOCAL EFFECTS OF FISTULA

In addition to the systemic manifestations that arteriovenous fistulas create, there are several *local* changes of interest. An *aneurysmal dilatation* is usually present in the artery and vein at the site of the fistula. Since the arterial pressure distal to the fistula is greatly reduced (Fig. 51), an extensive collat-

Figure 50. *A,* Femoral arteriogram in a patient with a gunshot wound of the thigh and a femoral arteriovenous fistula. *B,* The site of the fistula is seen with rapid filling of the proximal femoral vein without filling distally.

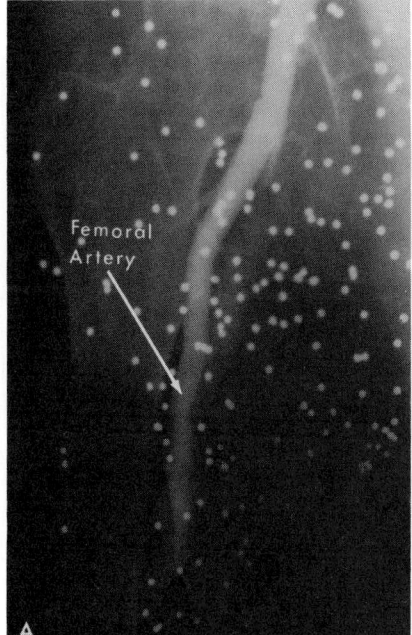
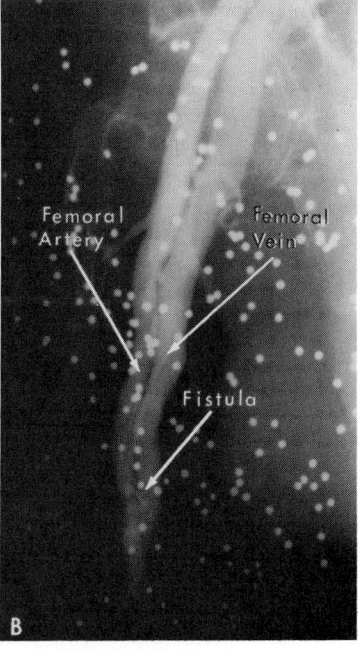

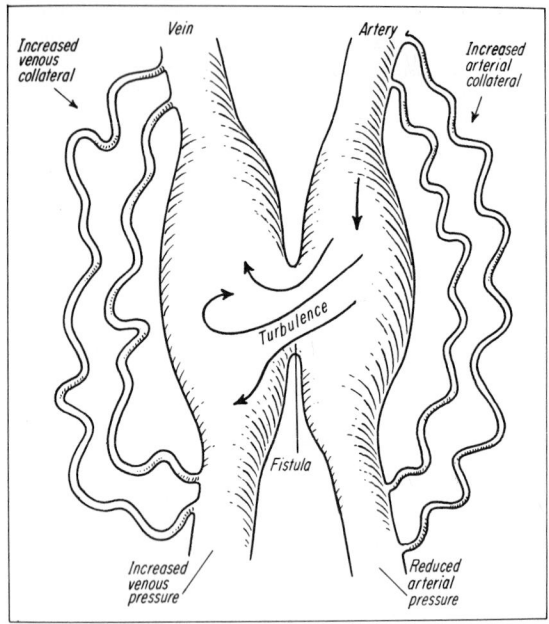

Figure 51. Diagrammatic illustration of the local changes that occur in the presence of an arteriovenous fistula. The changes shown are proportional to the *size* of the fistula. In a small fistula, these changes may be quite minimal.

Figure 52. Plethysmographic record of a 35-year-old man with a traumatic superficial femoral arteriovenous fistula. Digit pulse contours are abnormal on the left, and there is a significant depression of the ankle pressure (50 mm. Hg) distal to the fistula. (Courtesy of Dr. D. E. Strandness, Jr., Department of Surgery, University of Washington. From Strandness, D. E., Jr. (Ed.): Collateral Circulation in Clinical Surgery. Philadelphia, W. B. Saunders Company, 1969.)

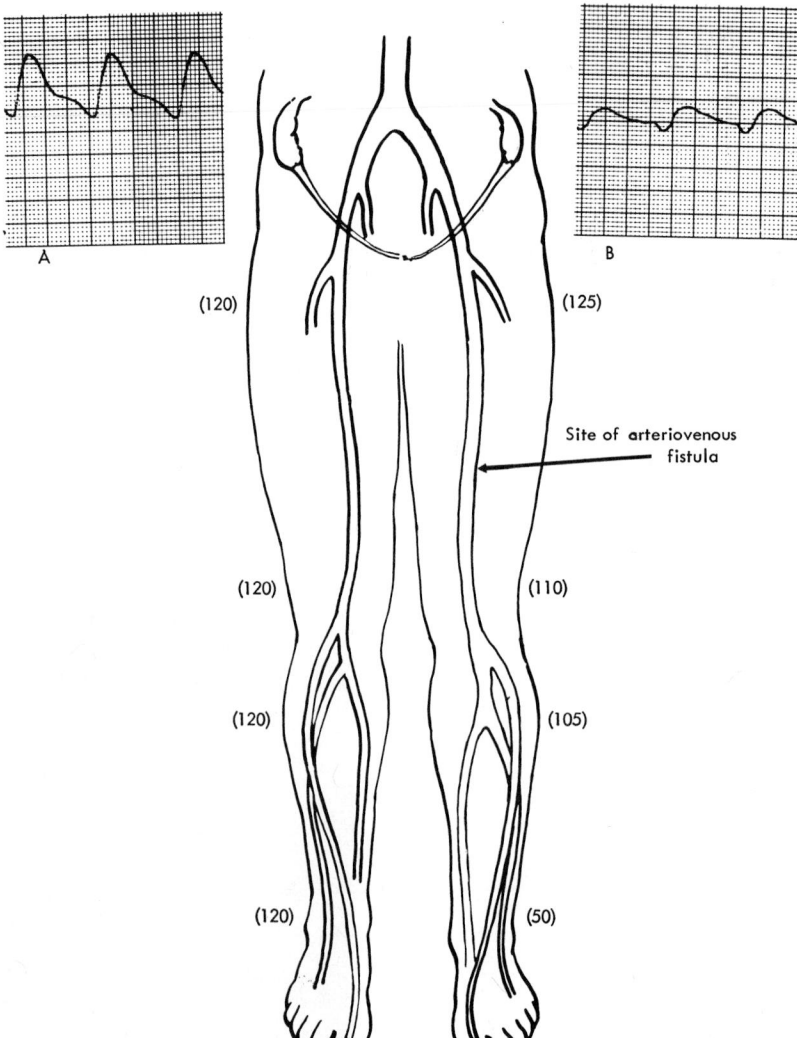

eral circulation develops from the branches of the artery arising above the fistula to those communicating below. This collateral circulation may become massive and usually results in an increase in both skin and muscle temperature. There are significant changes that occur in the *pressures* in the artery distal to the fistula and in the accompanying vein (Fig. 52).[14] When the fistula is in an extremity, the limb may have *increased length,* a fact confirmed by both experimental[8] and clinical observations.[7] There is no clear explanation for the stimulating effect of arteriovenous fistulas on bone growth, but it may be related to the fact that bone temperature is increased 1 or 2° C and to the increased blood supply.

MANAGEMENT

Since most arteriovenous fistulas are either actually or potentially symptomatic, surgical closure or excision of the lesion in the congenital type is generally recommended. Rarely, a small fistula may close spontaneously; this is recorded in 5 of 245 patients surveyed in World War II.[13] The site of the fistula can be determined by arteriography, and the surgical management of choice is usually direct repair of both the artery and the vein. If it is not possible to repair the vein satisfactorily, ligation of the vein may be necessary. Rarely, quadripolar ligation of the fistula is necessary. Thus, direct restoration of arterial continuity with closure of the fistula is the procedure of choice in the vast majority of instances. In a recent report, traumatic arteriovenous fistulas in 50 consecutive patients were corrected without a single amputation.[1]

SELECTED REFERENCES

Holman, E.: Abnormal Arteriovenous Communications. Peripheral and Intracardiac. Acquired and Congenital. Springfield, Ill., Charles C Thomas, Publisher, 1968.
  This monograph is the definitive one on the subject of arteriovenous fistula. The historical, experimental, and clinical aspects of this interesting disorder are presented in a complete and highly commendable manner.

Sumner, D. S.: Arteriovenous fistula. *In* Strandness, D. E., Jr. (Ed.): Collateral Circulation in Clinical Surgery. Philadelphia, W. B. Saunders Company, 1969.
  This section in an excellent monograph is an updated source of detailed information on all forms of arteriovenous fistulas.

REFERENCES

1. Beall, A. C., Jr., Diethrich, E. B., Morris, G. C., Jr., and DeBakey, M. E.: Surgical management of vascular trauma. Surg. Clin. North Am., 46:1001, 1966.
2. Bramann, F.: Das arteriell-venous Aneurysma. Arch. Klin. Chir., 33:1, 1886.
3. Branham, H. H.: Aneurismal varix of the femoral artery and vein following a gunshot wound. Int. J. Surg., 3:250, 1890.
4. Breschet, G.: Mémoire sur les aneurysmes. Mem. Acad. Roy. Med. (Paris), 3:101, 1833.
5. Holman, E.: Abnormal Arteriovenous Communications. Peripheral and Intracardiac. Acquired and Congenital. Springfield, Ill., Charles C Thomas, Publisher, 1968.
6. Hunter, W.: The history of an aneurysm of the aorta, with some remarks on aneurysms in general. Med. Observ. Inquir., 1:323, 1757.
7. Janes, J. M., and Jennings, W. K., Jr.: Effect of induced arteriovenous fistula on leg length: 10-year observations. Mayo Clin. Proc., 36:1, 1961.
8. Janes, J. M., and Musgrove, J. E.: Effect of arteriovenous fistula on growth of bone: An experimental study. Surg. Clin. North Am., 30:1191, 1950.
9. Moyer, J. H., Glantz, G., and Brest, A. N.: Pulmonary arteriovenous fistulas. Physiologic and clinical considerations. Am. J. Med., 32:417, 1962.
10. Nicoladoni, C.: Phlebarteriectasie der rechten oberen Extremitat. Arch. Klin. Chir., 18:252, 1875.
11. Rienhoff, W. F., Jr., and Hamman, L. D.: Subacute Streptococcus viridans septicemia cured by the excision of an arteriovenous aneurysm of the external iliac artery and vein. Ann. Surg., 102:905, 1935.
12. Sabiston, D. C., Jr., Theilen, E. O., and Gregg, D. E.: Physiologic studies in experimental high output cardiac failure produced by aortic-caval fistula. Surg. Forum, 6:233, 1956.
13. Shumacker, H. B.: Arterial aneurysms and arteriovenous fistulas. Spontaneous cures. *In* Elkin, D. C., and DeBakey, M. E. (Eds.): Surgery in World War II: Vascular Surgery. Washington, D. C., Office of the Surgeon General, Department of Army, 1955.
14. Sumner, D. S.: Arteriovenous fistula. Physiology and pathological anatomy. *In* Strandness, D. E., Jr. (Ed.): Collateral Circulation in Clinical Surgery. Philadelphia, W. B. Saunders Company, 1969.
15. Tice, D. A., Clauss, R. H., Keirle, A. M., and Reed, G. E.: Congenital arteriovenous fistulae of the extremities: Observations concerning treatment. Arch. Surg., 86:460, 1963.

10. BUERGER'S DISEASE (THROMBOANGIITIS OBLITERANS)

H. Brownell Wheeler, M.D.

In 1908, Buerger published clinical and pathologic observations on young men with severe ischemia of the extremities.[1] These patients were addicted to cigarette smoking and often had migratory superficial phlebitis. Buerger felt that his clinical and pathologic findings constituted a newly described disease for which he proposed the name "thromboangiitis obliterans." This term was selected because the acute histologic picture was highlighted by thrombosis in both arteries and veins and by a marked inflammatory reaction. The condition became more commonly referred to as "Buerger's disease," a diagnosis made frequently until recent years. However, most patients in whom this diagnosis was made suffered in actuality from arteriosclerosis. The classic syndrome described by Buerger is an uncommon, but dramatic, form of peripheral vascular disease.

CLINICAL MANIFESTATIONS

Buerger's disease occurs almost exclusively in males and begins in young adult life, usually between 20 and 35 years of age. The typical patient is a heavy smoker who began smoking at an early age. Negroes are rarely affected. Jewish men were originally reported to be particularly susceptible to the disease, but later studies failed to support this impression.[3, 7]

The diagnosis of Buerger's disease should be considered in any young male smoker with peripheral ischemia, particularly if the upper extremity is involved. The ischemic area is usually sharply demarcated, with relatively good circulation in adjacent tissues. The pain is often excruciating. Associated symptoms include migratory superficial phlebitis, cold sensitivity,

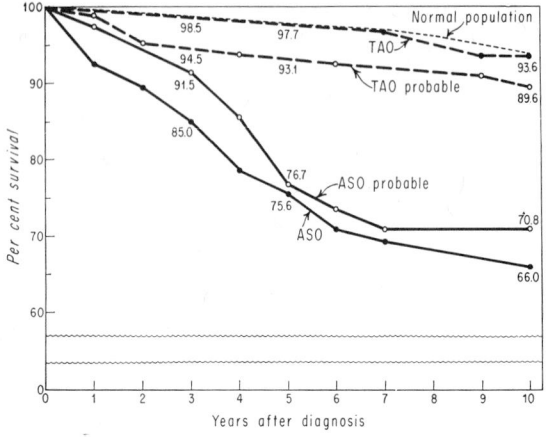

Figure 53. Widely differing 10-year survival rates in Buerger's disease (TAO) and arteriosclerosis (ASO). Confirmed cases of Buerger's disease show no significant difference from the normal population. (From McPherson, J. R., Juergens, J. L., and Gifford, R. W.: Ann. Intern. Med., 59:288, 1963.)

lize, giving a corkscrew appearance to the vessel. An unusual corrugated or rippled appearance of an artery may sometimes be seen, resembling the stem of a goose-necked lamp.[8] This finding has been attributed to severe vasospasm.

The clinical course of Buerger's disease is protracted and painful, but relatively benign. If a patient ceases smoking, prolonged remission usually occurs. However, most patients seem addicted to tobacco and continue to smoke despite all advice. They have repeated attacks and may require multiple amputations, but life-endangering complications are infrequent. Long-term life expectancy is only slightly less than that of the general population, unlike patients with comparable degrees of peripheral ischemia due to arteriosclerosis, as shown in Figure 54.[7] There is occasional involvement of visceral blood vessels, especially in the mesenteric circulation. Resection of ischemic or infarcted bowel may be required. In later life, patients with Buerger's disease often develop arteriosclerosis, perhaps more frequently and more severely than the general population.

and Raynaud's phenomenon. Exacerbations with smoking and remissions following abstinence from tobacco are particularly characteristic of Buerger's disease.

Arteriography early in the disease usually reveals segmental obliteration of arteries, especially the medium-sized arteries of the forearm and calf, with a strikingly normal appearance of the remaining vessels. The irregular plaques characteristic of arteriosclerosis are conspicuously absent. Collateral circulation in chronic cases is unusually well developed and is often described as "tree roots" or "spider legs" in appearance. Occasionally, thrombosed arteries recana-

PATHOLOGY

In the acute stage, thrombosis occurs in arteries and veins of medium to small size. Digital vessels are commonly involved, unlike arteriosclerosis.[4] Dense aggregates of polymorphonuclear leukocytes are seen within the thrombus. There is an associated panvasculitis, but the elastic lamina remains intact.[10] Unlike arteriosclerosis or periarteritis nodosa, there is no necrosis of the arterial wall. Later, microabscesses are observed, and giant cells appear within the granulation tissue. The thrombus is organized, and recanalization of the lumen may occur, as shown in Figure 54.

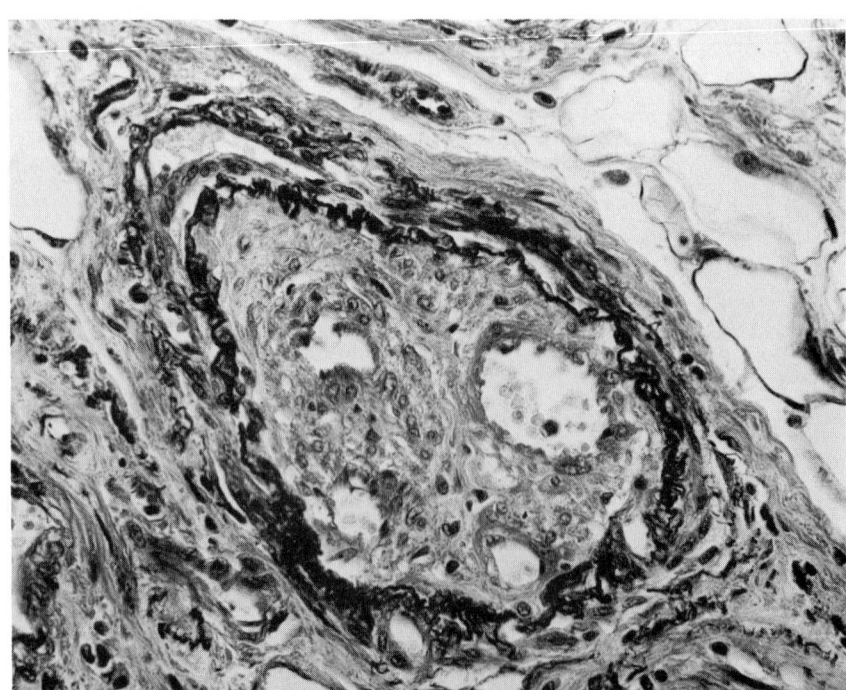

Figure 54. Chronic, well-organized arterial thrombosis in a 30-year-old man with Buerger's disease. Unlike arteriosclerosis, there is no degeneration or calcification in the vessel wall. The elastic lamina is intact, and the lumen has been partially recanalized. It would be unusual for arteriosclerosis to involve such a small artery (1 mm.). Van Giesen-Elastic Stain, × 570. (Courtesy of the Rev. Robert W. Bain, M.D., Department of Pathology, St. Vincent Hospital, Worcester, Mass.)

Older lesions show chronic inflammatory infiltrates or extensive fibrosis, which may involve peripheral nerves as well as arteries and veins. There is considerable variability in histologic findings, depending upon the state of the disease observed.[4] The most characteristic changes are seen early in the pathologic process, but the timing of amputations for ischemic gangrene usually does not permit observation of the early phases of the disease.

ETIOLOGY

A specific cause for Buerger's disease has never been demonstrated, and an interaction of multiple etiologic factors is likely. The striking association with cigarette smoking suggests a strong etiologic relationship. However, if there is a cause-and-effect relationship with smoking, it is difficult to understand why the disease occurs so rarely in women. The sex distribution suggests some role of male sex hormones. There may also be etiologic implications in the fact that patients with Buerger's disease usually come from lower socioeconomic groups. They often have a history of cold injury and of repeated fungal infections.[5] Fibrinogen levels may be elevated and a hypercoagulable state has been postulated, possibly induced through an immunologic response to fungal infection.[2] Familial predisposition has been reported, and autonomic overactivity is suggested by the association with severe peripheral vasospasm and hyperhidrosis. Any factor that causes severe peripheral vasospasm, thrombosis, or local inflammation may contribute to the development of the syndrome in a susceptible individual.

INCIDENCE

The frequency with which the diagnosis of Buerger's disease is made depends upon the criteria used to establish the diagnosis. Prior to arteriography, the diagnosis was often made clinically in any relatively young man with peripheral arterial insufficiency. The diagnosis was therefore made frequently but incorrectly. When angiographic study of patients with peripheral arterial insufficiency became routine, most patients with the diagnosis of Buerger's disease were shown to have arteriosclerosis. Based on radiographic criteria, Buerger's disease is uncommon. When the diagnosis is based solely on the histologic findings originally described by Buerger, even large teaching hospitals rarely make the diagnosis. Some investigators have even doubted the existence of Buerger's disease.[9] However, the occurrence of an infrequent, but highly characteristic clinical syndrome has never been in doubt to clinicians who have cared for such patients.[6, 7]

The best indication of the true incidence of Buerger's disease probably comes from a statistical analysis by DeBakey and Cohen of 936 World War II veterans in whom this diagnosis was made during the years 1942 to 1948.[3] Extrapolating from their data, the authors estimated the minimum incidence in the United States at seven or eight cases per 100,000 white males 20 to 44 years of age. Patients with Buerger's disease are observed much more frequently in Asia, even in populations where arteriosclerosis is rare.

MANAGEMENT

The major problem in treating patients with Buerger's disease is the management of pain, which is often excruciating. Narcotics are usually necessary, but must be used cautiously because of the frequency of drug addiction. Peripheral or sympathetic nerve blocks may provide temporary pain relief, especially when the disease is accompanied by severe vasospasm. Cervical or lumbar sympathectomy often benefits such patients. Relief of pain sometimes necessitates amputation, even if tissue necrosis has not occurred.

Every effort should be made to have the patient stop smoking, since indefinite remissions may follow abstinence from cigarettes. No specific medication has proved to be useful, although anticoagulants, low molecular weight Dextran, phenylbutazone, pyridinolcarbamate, inositol niacinate, and steroids have all been recommended. Arterial reconstruction is usually impossible because of the distal nature of the disease, but it should be considered in segmental proximal occlusions. When gangrene occurs, amputation at the lowest possible level is indicated. Unlike arteriosclerosis, it is often possible to do digital amputations with satisfactory healing.

SELECTED REFERENCES

Buerger, L.: Thromboangiitis obliterans: A study of the vascular lesions leading to presenile spontaneous gangrene. Am. J. Med. Sci., *136*:567, 1908,

The author describes his clinical observations in 30 young men with peripheral arterial insufficiency and his pathologic findings on 11 amputated legs, concluding that they constitute a new disease syndrome, which he calls "thromboangiitis obliterans." Because of the attention aroused by this article and several subsequent publications, culminating in a monograph in 1924, Buerger's own name has become attached to the syndrome.

DeBakey, M. E., and Cohen, B. M.: Buerger's Disease: A Follow-up Study of World War II Army Cases. Springfield, Ill., Charles C Thomas, Publisher, 1963.

This monograph is the largest and most detailed follow-up study of Buerger's disease, an analysis of 936 cases diagnosed in U.S. Army males in the years 1942 to 1948. It suffers from the difficulty inherent in establishing a firm diagnosis on a retrospective review of findings by many different observers. Nevertheless, it gives useful statistical information concerning incidence, prognosis, and general trends in morbidity and mortality.

McKusick, V. A. Harris, W. S., Ottesen, O. E., Goodman, E. M., Shelley, W. M., and Bloodwell, R. D.: Buerger's disease: A distinct clinical and pathologic entity. J.A.M.A., *181*:5, 1962.

This article is a convincing rebuttal to the viewpoint that Buerger's disease is merely arteriosclerosis in a younger age group. The conclusions are based on arteriographic study of all four extremities in 12 patients with Buerger's disease, as well as histopathologic study of biopsy and amputation specimens from 10 patients. No evidence of arteriosclerosis was observed in any of these patients, and angiographic and histopathologic findings consistent with Buerger's disease were documented. The authors also examined 28 additional patients and performed 24 angiograms in a Korean hospital. The findings were similar to those of American patients and are of particular interest because of the rarity of arteriosclerosis in young Korean men.

Wessler, S., Ming, S. C., Gurewich, V., and Freiman, D. G.: A critical evaluation of thromboangiitis obliterans. N. Engl. J. Med., 262:1149, 1960.

The authors fail to demonstrate the acute histologic picture described by Buerger in any of 84 patients with onset of peripheral arterial insufficiency before the age of 45. They criticize Buerger's original histologic criteria and conclude that "thromboangiitis obliterans cannot be considered an entity in either the clinical or pathologic sense." This paper was extensively quoted, and Buerger's disease was widely considered to be merely a severe form of arteriosclerosis occurring in young men.

Wessler, S.: Buerger's disease revisited. Surg. Clin. North Am., 49:703, 1969.

The senior author of a widely quoted paper doubting the existence of Buerger's disease (see above) reviews the matter in view of subsequent contradictory articles. He now accepts the definition of Buerger's syndrome as "a constellation of clinical findings." He concludes that these infrequent patients have idiopathic peripheral arterial thrombosis, possibly on the basis of systemic hypercoagulability secondary to some immunologic disorder. There is an unusually complete bibliography.

REFERENCES

1. Buerger, L.: Thromboangiitis obliterans: A study of the vascular lesions leading to presenile spontaneous gangrene. Am. J. Med. Sci., 136:567, 1908.
2. Craven, J. L., and Cotton, R. C.: Haematological differences between thromboangiitis obliterans and atherosclerosis. Br. J. Surg., 54:862, 1967.
3. DeBakey, M. E., and Cohen, B. M.: Buerger's Disease: A Follow-up Study of World War II Army Cases. Springfield, Ill., Charles C Thomas, Publishers, 1963.
4. Dible, J. H. In Cameron, R., and Wright, G. P. (Eds.) : The Pathology of Limb Ischemia. St. Louis, Warren H. Green, 1966, p. 79.
5. Hill, G. L., Moeliono, J., Tumewu, F., Brataamadja, D., and Tohardi, A.: The Buerger syndrome in Java. Br. J. Surg., 60:606, 1973.
6. McKusick, V. A., Harris, W. S., Ottesen, O. E., Goodman, E. M., Shelley, W. M., and Bloodwell, R. D.: Buerger's disease: A distinct clinical and pathologic entity. J.A.M.A., 181:5, 1962.
7. McPherson, J. R., Juergens, J. L., and Gifford, R. W., Jr.: Thromboangiitis obliterans and arteriosclerosis obliterans: Clinical and prognostic differences. Ann. Intern. Med., 59:288, 1963.
8. Schatz, I. J., Fine, G., and Eyler, W. R.: Thromboangiitis obliterans. Br. Heart. J. 28:84, 1966.
9. Wessler, S., Ming, S. C., Gurewich, V., and Freiman, D. G.: A critical evaluation of thromboangiitis obliterans. N. Engl. J. Med., 262:1149, 1960.
10. Williams, G.: Recent views on Buerger's disease. J. Clin. Pathol., 22:573–578, 1969.

11. RAYNAUD'S SYNDROME

John M. Porter, M.D.

Raynaud's syndrome defines a condition characterized by episodic attacks of constriction of the arteries and arterioles of the extremities in response to cold or emotional stimuli. These attacks are manifest clinically by intense pallor of the extremities, especially the fingers, followed by cyanosis and rubor upon warming. Recovery usually takes 15 to 30 minutes once warming is begun. Pallor occurs in almost all patients with Raynaud's syndrome and is important in establishing the diagnosis. The occurence of cyanosis and rubor is variable and may be absent in certain patients. The upper extremities are usually the more severely involved, but the feet are similarly involved in occasional patients.

HISTORY

Few topics exist in the field of vascular disease about which there has been more confusion and disagreement on terminology than Raynaud's syndrome. The syndrome was first described in 1862 by Maurice Raynaud.[14] Unfortunately, he included cases of advanced arteriosclerosis with digital gangrene despite his own statement that this syndrome was not caused by organic arterial obstruction. Some of the inconsistencies in Raynaud's publications were noted by Hutchison in 1893, who suggested that Raynaud's syndrome was not a single disease, but rather a clinical sign common to diseases of diverse etiologies.[7]

The suggestions of Hutchinson were further amplified in 1932 by Allan and Brown,[2] who proposed the separation of Raynaud's disease from Raynaud's phenomenon. These authors stated that both conditions had similar vasospastic symptoms, but that the former occurred in the absence of any underlying disease and followed a benign clinical course, whereas the latter occurred with one or more associated diseases and frequently pursued a virulent course, occasionally including digital gangrene. Critical evaluation, however, indicates that there is little justification in attempting a rigid separation of Raynaud's disease from Raynaud's phenomenon. Allan and Brown's classification was based on clinical observations alone, as detailed immunologic evaluation was unavailable at the time. Many authors have noted that certain patients develop overt connective tissue disease many years after the onset of mild Raynaud's symptoms. It appears more reasonable to refer to the condition as Raynaud's syndrome.

ASSOCIATED DISEASE

It has become clear in recent years that a large majority of patients with Raynaud's syndrome have an associated connective tissue disease, usually scleroderma.[15] Several investigators have noted that Raynaud's symptoms develop at some time in over 80 per cent of all patients with scleroderma and is the initial symptom in over 30 per cent.[4] Our own prospective evaluation of 100 patients with Raynaud's syndrome revealed an associated connective tissue disease proven or strongly suspected in 80 per cent (Table 15). Interestingly, detailed evaluations revealed some immunologic abnormality in most of the remaining patients, and some of these will likely develop overt connective tissue disease in the future.

Considerable confusion has resulted from numerous publications indicating that Raynaud's syndrome may result from a diverse group of disorders such as thoracic outlet syndrome, carpal tunnel syndrome, central nervous system disease, pneumatic hammer disease, and many others. Many of these patients indeed have long episodes of hand cyanosis, and many have severe pain. In our experience, however, they do not have

TABLE 15. Coexistent Connective Tissue Disorders in a Group of 100 Patients Evaluated for Raynaud's Symptoms

Disease or Syndrome	Number of Patients
Systemic sclerosis (scleroderma)	24
CRST syndrome*	4
Systemic lupus erythematosus	10
Probable lupus erythematosus	6
Overlap syndrome	7
Mixed connective tissue disease	6
Severe hypocomplementemia C-3	3
Morphea	2
Polymyositis	1
Glomerulonephritis	1
Erythema nodosum	1
Sjögren's syndrome	1
Suspected collagen vascular disease	15
No autoimmune disease recognized	19

*Calcinosis, Raynaud's, sclerodactyly, telangiectasia

typical episodic Raynaud's syndrome, and there is little evidence that typical Raynaud's syndrome has any causal association with this group of disorders. The vascular symptoms in many of these patients likely result from arterial occlusion secondary to trauma or embolism.

We have noted, however, as have others, that a large number of patients with Raynaud's symptoms have associated carpal tunnel syndrome. This has occurred in 15 per cent of our patients. Division of the carpal ligament has relieved the neurologic symptoms but has invariably failed to relieve the Raynaud's symptoms.

PATHOPHYSIOLOGY

The pallor in the early stage of Raynaud's attacks is caused by severe spasm of the arteries and arterioles, which results in a cessation of capillary perfusion. After some minutes the capillaries and probably the venules dilate both from hypoxia and the accumulation of metabolites. This is followed by a slight relaxation of the arteriolar spasm with the entry of a trickle of blood into the dilated capillaries, where it rapidly becomes desaturated, producing cyanosis. Rubor results from the entry of increasing amounts of blood into the dilated capillaries. The attack terminates with the entry of a normal volume of blood through the relaxed arterioles and the return of the dilated capillaries to normal.

Several indirect blood flow studies have revealed a significant reduction in digital blood flow both at room temperature and after cold exposure in patients with Raynaud's syndrome.[3, 17] This is supported by detailed angiographic studies[13] showing resting and cold-accentuated vasospasm.

The mechanism of Raynaud's attacks appears to be a further vasospastic stimulus from cold exposure or emotional distress superimposed upon chronic vasoconstriction. A controversy has raged for years as to whether the underlying abnormality is intrinsic vascular wall cold hyperreactivity or increased sympathetic nervous system activity. No conclusive evidence exists to support either theory.

Recent observations suggest a possible third mechanism. As noted, the great majority of patients with Raynaud's syndrome have numerous serum immunologic abnormalities, including a striking preponderance of antibodies to homologous nuclear constituents. Antigen-antibody immune complexes may exist in these patients and may directly or through a chemical mediator, possibly related to the complement system, produce vasoconstriction. This must occur through the sympathetic neuromuscular end-plate, since total pharmacologic blockade at this site eliminates Raynaud's symptoms.[1] The normal vasoconstrictive response to cold may be additive with underlying chronic vasoconstriction, resulting in vascular wall tension exceeding intravascular pressure, the so-called critical closing pressure.[11] Normal cold-induced vasoconstriction in low-pressure vascular beds distal to significant arteriosclerotic obstruction may also exceed the critical closing pressure, explaining the occurrence of Raynaud-like symptoms in some patients with advanced arteriosclerosis.[10]

CLINICAL DESCRIPTION

Raynaud's syndrome usually occurs in females and rarely begins after the age of 40. The symptoms are almost always bilateral. Longstanding unilateral or unidigital involvement strongly suggests localized organic arterial obstruction and not true Raynaud's syndrome. The stimulus required to produce a Raynaud's attack may be as mild as a draft from an air conditioner or hand immersion in tap water. An attack usually begins with pronounced blanching of the hands, associated with an uncomfortable sensation of numbness. Severe pain during attacks is rare. The initial pallor will usually persist as long as cold exposure continues. When the cold stimulus is withdrawn, the pallor will gradually fade and be followed by cyanosis and rubor, with a return to normal skin color in 15 to 30 minutes. Finger tip ulceration may occur in severe cases but is almost always associated with organic arterial obstruction. The arterial obstruction appears to result in many patients from the arteritis associated with connective tissue disease.

PHYSICAL EXAMINATION

The skin of the hands and fingers should be carefully inspected for any ulcerations or small hyperkeratotic areas suggesting healed ulcers. The skin should also be observed for any thinning, tightening, or telangiectasias suggestive of scleroderma. All joints should be examined for synovial thickening, effusion, or other evidence of arthritis. The status of the peripheral arterial pulses should be carefully noted. Signs of carpal tunnel syndrome should be sought with care. The physical examination is frequently completely normal in patients with Raynaud's syndrome. The diagnosis is made primarily from the history.

LABORATORY TESTS

The specific serologic tests of greatest value in detecting associated diseases include the determination of antinuclear antibody, rheumatoid factor, immunoglobulin electrophoresis, complement levels, anti-native-DNA antibody, Coombs' test, and cryoglobulins. Routine upper extremity nerve conduction velocity determinations should be performed to detect carpal tunnel syndrome. Digital temperature recovery after cold exposure and magnification hand arteriography are of value in certain patients.[13]

TREATMENT

The initial treatment of patients with Raynaud's syndrome is cold avoidance and abstinence from tobacco. In patients with mild disease no further therapy is necessary.

Regional surgical sympathectomy has been widely used for many years in the treatment of Raynaud's symptoms. Long-term results, however, have not been particularly good. While the procedure appears of lasting benefit in 40 to 60 per cent of patients with mild Raynaud's symptoms, it has been of benefit in only 20 to 30 per cent of patients with more severe symptoms.[5, 6, 8] It has been of strikingly little value in patients with Raynaud's syndrome associated with scleroderma. At present we do not use surgical sympathectomy in the treatment of Raynaud's syndrome.

The best results appear to be obtained from drugs that decrease sympathetic neuromuscular synaptic transmission. Although a wide variety of agents have been used, the best appear to be reserpine, guanethidine, and phenoxybenzamine.[3, 9, 12, 13, 16] The effect of these drugs in increasing digital blood flow has been confirmed by isotopic, thermographic, and arteriographic studies. Low drug dosages are effective, with initial dosages of 10 mg. each of guanethidine and phenoxybenzamine daily. The dosage may be incrementally increased to 40 mg. each daily if needed. Hand arteriograms on a patient with Raynaud's syndrome before and after cold exposure and before and after sympathetic blockade are shown in Figures 55 and 56.

Patients with an underlying autoimmune disease may require treatment with antiphlogistic or immunosuppressive drugs for the underlying disease. The use of such drugs alone, however, rarely results in any improvement of the Raynaud's symptoms.

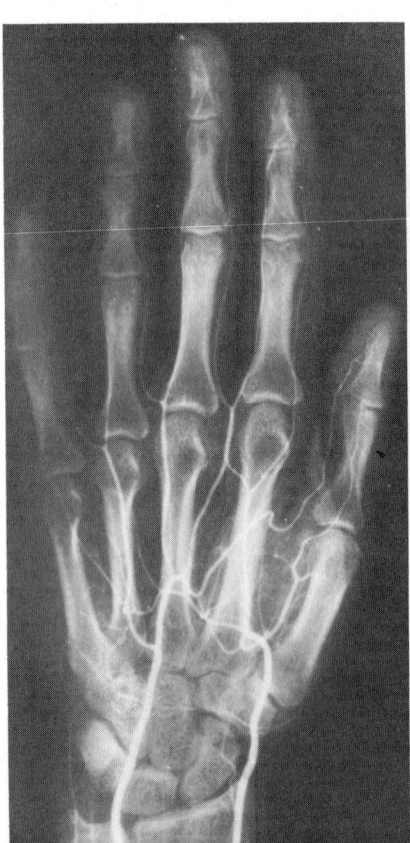 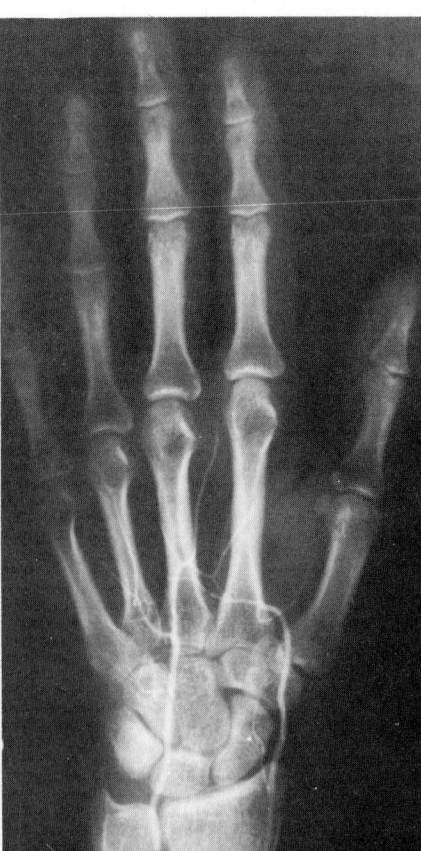

Figure 55. *Left,* Hand arteriogram in patient with Raynaud's symptoms at room temperature. Significant vasospasm is present. *Right,* Same patient after ice-water exposure for 30 seonds. A marked increase in vasospasm is present.

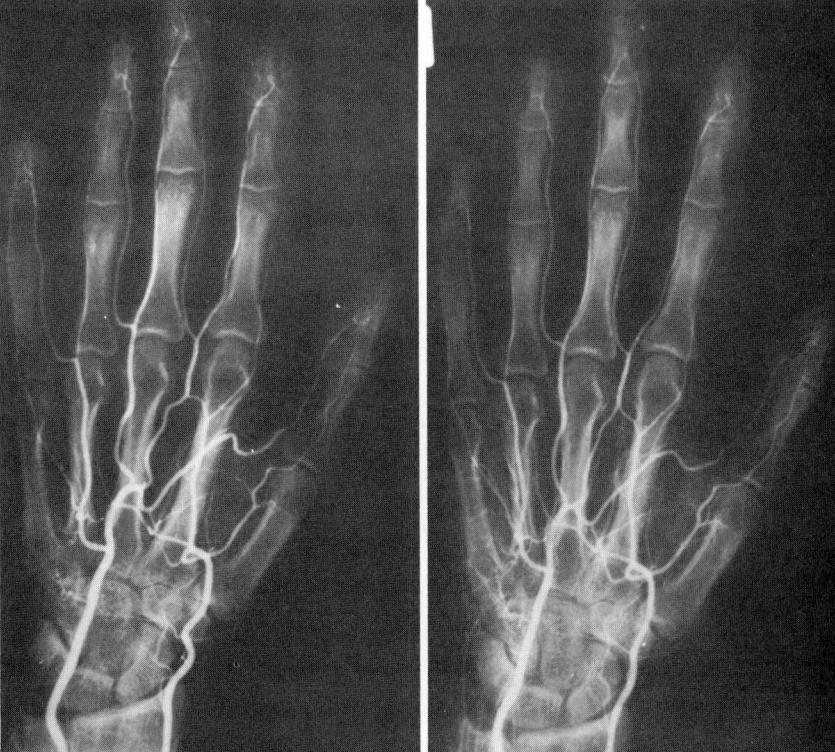

Figure 56. *Left,* Same patient as in Figure 55, 48 hours after sympathetic blockade, in this case accomplished by the intra-arterial injection of reserpine. A significant decrease in resting vasospasm is apparent. *Right,* After ice-water exposure. The vasoconstrictive response to cold is markedly diminished by sympathetic blockade.

REFERENCES

1. Abboud, F. M., Eckstein, J. W., Lawrence, M. S., and Hoak, J. C.: Preliminary observations in the use of intra-arterial reserpine in Raynaud's phenomenon. Circulation, *35*:49, 1967.
2. Allen, E. V., and Brown, G. E.: Raynaud's disease affecting men. Ann. Intern. Med., *5*:1384, 1932.
3. Coffman, J. D., and Cohen, A. S.: Total and capillary fingertip blood flow in Raynaud's phenomenon. N. Engl. J. Med., *285*:259, 1971.
4. Farmer, R. G., Gifford, R. W., Jr., and Hines, E. A., Jr.: Prognostic significance of Raynaud's phenomenon and other clinical characteristics of systemic scleroderma. Circulation, *21*:1088, 1960.
5. Gifford, R. W., Jr., Hines, E. A., Jr., and Craig, W. M. K.: Sympathectomy for Raynaud's phenomena. Circulation, *17*:5, 1958.
6. Hall, K. V., and Hillestad, L. K.: Raynaud's phenomenon treated with sympathectomy. Angiology, *11*:186, 1960.
7. Hutchinson, J.: Inherited liability to Raynaud's phenomenon, with great proneness to chilblains—gradual increase of liability to paroxysmal local asphyxia-acrosphacelus with scleroderma—cheeks affected. Arch. Surg., *4*:312, 1893.
8. Johnston, E. N. M., Symmerly, R., and Birnstingl, M.: Prognosis in Raynaud's phenomenon after sympathectomy. Br. Med. J., *1*:962, 1965.
9. Kontos, H. A., and Wasserman, A. J.: Effect of reserpine in Raynaud's phenomenon. Circulation, *39*:259, 1969.
10. Mendlowitz, M., and Naftchi, N.: The digital circulation in Raynaud's disease. Am. J. Cardiol., *4*:580, 1959.
11. Nichol, J., Girling, F., Jerrard, W., Claxton, E. B., and Burton, A. C.: Fundamental instability of the small blood vessels and critical closing pressures in vascular beds. Am. J. Physiol., *164*:330, 1951.
12. Peacock, J. H.: The treatment of primary Raynaud's disease of the upper limb. Lancet, *2*:65, 1960.
13. Porter, J. M., Snider, R. L., Bardana, E. J., Rosch, J., and Eidemiller, L. R.: The diagnosis and treatment of Raynaud's phenomenon. Surgery, *77*:11, 1975.
14. Raynaud, M.: On local asphyxia and symmetrical gangrene of the extremities. Selected Monographs. London, New Sydenham Society, 1888, p. 1.
15. Velayos, E. E., Robinson, H., Porciuncula, F. U., and Masi, A. T.: Clinical correlation analysis of 137 patients with Raynaud's phenomenon. Am. J. Med. Sci., *262*:347, 1970.
16. Willerson, J. T., and Decker, J. L.: Raynaud's disease and phenomenon, a medical approach. Am. Heart. J., *82*:572, 1971.
17. Willerson, J. T., Thompson, T. H., Hookman, P., Herdt, J., and Decker, J. L.: Reserpine in Raynaud's disease and phenomenon. Ann. Intern. Med., *72*:17, 1970.

12. CIRCULATORY PROBLEMS OF THE UPPER EXTREMITY

Donald Silver, M.D.

ARTERIAL INSUFFICIENCY

The upper extremities tolerate reductions of arterial flow much better than the lower extremities because of a smaller muscle mass and the intermittent character of the work required of them. The collateral circulation of the upper extremity is almost always sufficient to prevent distal ischemic necrosis. However, in patients with acute arterial insufficiency and insufficient collaterals, and in those whose occupation requires that they constantly use their upper extremities, ischemic symptoms and gangrene of distal parts may develop.

The arterial flow to the upper extremity may be reduced by atherosclerotic stenoses, trauma, thromboembolism, tumor, and/or compression of the subclavian-axillary arteries in the region of the thoracic outlet. Symptomatic atherosclerotic occlusions most commonly involve the innominate or subclavian arteries. The small arteries of the hand and of the fingers are next most frequently involved, and the brachial, radial, and ulnar arteries least often.

After trauma to an extremity, compression of the vessels may result from bony angulation or bone fragments, from hematomas and edema, and from direct vascular injury. The arteries may be partially or totally compressed or disrupted. If the intima is torn by the sudden stretching of an artery, blood flow may then lift the intima and produce a "flap-valve" obstruction. Penetrating wounds of the arteries may also penetrate the adjacent veins and produce arteriovenous fistulas.

Emboli are an increasing cause of arterial insufficiency, with 6 to 10 per cent of all arterial emboli lodging in the upper extremities and the majority lodging in the axillary and brachial arteries.[10] Most emboli arise in the heart, and the incidence of thromboembolic occlusion of the upper extremity parallels the increasing number of geriatric patients, with their cardiac problems. Emboli usually lodge at sites of arterial bifurcation or reduction of arterial diameters. Transbrachial and transaxillary cardiac catheterization also causes thrombotic occlusions of the respective arteries in approximately 0.5 per cent of the cases.[6]

The subclavian and/or axillary arteries may be compressed as they course through the thoracic outlet and (1) be asymptomatic; (2) cause intermittent ischemia or symptoms similar to those seen in Raynaud's disease; (3) develop poststenotic aneurysmal dilatation; and (4) when there is major compression or embolization of a mural thrombosis, cause significant ischemia of the distal portion of the extremity.

A careful history and physical examination supplemented by appropriate x-rays and angiograms should document the site and extent of the arterial occlusion and give some indication of the etiology of the insufficency.

Asymptomatic or minimally symptomatic arterial occlusions usually require no therapy. Symptomatic occlusions are treated according to the etiology, i.e., an embolus can usually be extracted using local anesthesia and an embolectomy catheter; compression in the thoracic outlet can be relieved by resecting the first rib and if necessary repairing or replacing the artery; vein grafts may be utilized to bypass chronic occlusions; and vein "patch grafts" may be utilized to enlarge short areas of stenoses.

VENOUS INSUFFICIENCY

The manifestations of venous insufficiency include edema, distention of superficial veins, tightness, aching, a reddish blue discoloration, and pain. Edema of the upper extremity from venous insufficiency is most often caused by occlusion of the axillary, subclavian, or innominate vein, or the superior vena cava. More distal venous occlusions rarely produce significant edema or chronic symptoms.

Tumors, mediastinal fibrosis, and trauma are the principal causes of thrombosis in the large central veins, although indwelling catheters for prolonged infusions are producing increasing numbers of thromboses of these veins. Thromboses of the distal upper extremity veins most often follow intravenous infusions.

The thrombosis of the axillary or subclavian vein that occurs after effort or strain[3] has been called "effort thrombosis." This thrombosis usually occurs in the dominant arm of a young or middle-aged healthy person. It usually occurs immediately after the effort, but its onset may be delayed several hours. A history of mild effort or strain with the arm abducted can be obtained in most cases. Many of the cases of effort thrombosis were probably caused by compression of the axillary vein either by the pectoralis minor tendon, by the costocoracoid ligament, or between the clavicle and first rib and, therefore, could be considered manifestations of the thoracic outlet syndrome.

An occasional patient will develop edema after effort but will not have demonstrable thrombosis of his veins. However, phlebograms usually demonstrate areas of compression of the axillary and subclavian veins in the area of the thoracic outlet. The edema, which results primarily from chronic compression and secondarily from the patient's efforts, may be effectively treated by eliminating the site of compression,[1] usually by resecting the first rib and dividing the pectoralis minor tendon.

The presence and extent of the venous thrombosis should be documented by phlebography. When there are proximal venous obstructions, the distal venous pressures, with the patient supine and the extremity at the right atrial level, will be elevated above the normal pressure of 8 to 12 cm. of saline.

Most patients with clinically significant thromboses of the veins of the upper extremity should be treated with elevation of the extremity and with heparin (provided there are no contraindications) in sufficient amounts to overcome the circulating thrombin and prolong the clotting time to three times the control value. Heparin is best given as a constant intravenous infusion, and maintained a minimum of 8 to 10 days. It is continued longer if symptoms persist. The patient is usually maintained on an oral prothrombinopenic agent for 3 to 6 months. The fibrinoloytic agents urokinase and streptokinase may also be used to accelerate the lysis of these thromboses. Although thrombectomy has been utilized to reduce the sequelae of venous thromboses,[2] most vascular surgeons utilize thrombectomy only if elevation and anticoagulation (or fibrinolytic agents) fail to restore the circulation and tissue perfusion remains altered and gangrene imminent.

CAUSALGIA

In 1872, Mitchell coined the term "causalgia"[4] to describe the burning, agonizing pain and vasomotor disturbances that occur in an occasional patient after a peripheral nerve injury. The pain of causalgia varies in intensity and is exacerbated by touching or moving a part, changes in temperature, pressure changes, or local irritants. The pain may become so agonizing that complete cessation of motion of the involved extremity ensues.

Sympathetic blockade is an excellent diagnostic and therapeutic procedure because it usually gives complete relief from pain and allows use of the previously guarded limb. The vasomotor changes also are usually completely relieved by the blockade. In a few patients, lasting relief is provided by a single sympathetic blockade. Others require repeated treatment to obtain complete relief. However, if sympathetic block gives only limited relief, operative sympathetic denervation should be performed with the expectation that complete relief of symptoms will be obtained. Active physical therapy is an important part of the postsympathectomy management.

POST-TRAUMATIC REFLEX DYSTROPHY

In some patients, causalgia-like pain develops after a trivial injury in which there is no demonstrable nerve damage. In addition to the pain, there may be edema, vasomotor disturbances, soft tissue dystrophy, and atrophy of the bone in the region of or distal to the traumatic injury. The process may follow minimal trauma, such as a sprain, or an infection, and occasionally occurs after thrombophlebitis, burns, spinal anesthesia, or herniation of nucleus pulposus. The process is called post-traumatic reflex sympathetic dystrophy, or Sudeck's atrophy because of the description of bone atrophy by Sudeck in 1900.[8]

Treatment consists of treating the local injury with supportive measures—local heat, analgesics, and so forth. Sympathetic blockade may be necessary to control the pain before physical therapy is initiated and may have to be repeated several times. Early sympathetic blockades and physical therapy are the mainstays of therapy. The majority of patients make a complete recovery with these supportive measures. However, if the supportive measures do not completely relieve the symptoms, sympathetic denervation of the involved extremity is indicated. Physical therapy is a very important adjunct during the early postoperative period.

ACROCYANOSIS

Acrocyanosis is characterized by an almost continuous painless coldness and cyanosis of the distal portions of the extremities. It is caused by constant spasm of the small arteries in response to an overactive vasomotor system. The condition should be easily differentiated from Raynaud's disease by careful history and physical examination. Treatment consists only of protection from cold in mild cases, or sympathectomy, which usually gives complete relief from symptoms, in severe cases.

ERYTHROMELALGIA

Erythromelalgia is characterized by a burning sensation in the extremities that is associated with local warmth and a reddish or cyanotic color of the skin of the affected part. It occurs most often in middle-aged men and women during times of exposure to increased heat. It may be primary or secondary, occurring in patients with hypertension, myeloproliferative disorder, diabetes, or gout. Treatment of secondary erythromelalgia should be directed toward eliminating the underlying disorder. Treatment of primary erythromelalgia is symptomatic, i.e., cooling and reducing body temperature. Sympathectomy of the involved extremity offers favorable to excellent results.[7, 9] A few patients with primary erythromelalgia have obtained symptomatic relief with methysergide maleate.[5]

SELECTED REFERENCE

Cranley, J. J.: Vascular Surgery: Peripheral Venous Diseases. Vol II. Hagerstown, Md., Harper & Row, Publishers, 1975.
This comprehensive text of peripheral venous diseases and their sequelae has an excellent section on the "Upper Extremity Obstruction Syndrome and Its Management." The section clearly distinguishes between thoracic and nonthrombotic occlusions, and outlines diagnostic and therapeutic procedures.

REFERENCES

1. Adams, J. T., DeWeese, J. A., Mahoney, E. B., and Rob, C. G.: Intermittent subclavian vein obstruction without thrombosis. Surgery, 63:147, 1968.
2. Mahorner, H., Castleberry, J. W., and Colemen, W. O.: Attempts to restore function in major veins which are the site of massive thrombosis. Ann. Sug., 146:510, 1957.
3. Matas, R.: Primary thrombosis of the axillary vein caused by strain. Am. J. Surg., 24:642, 1934.
4. Mitchell, S. E.: Injuries of Nerves and Their Consequences. Philadelphia, J. B. Lippincott Company, 1872.
5. Pepper, H.: Primary erythermalgia: Report of a patient treated with methysergide maleate. J.A.M.A., 203:162, 1968.
6. Ross, R. S.: Cooperative study on cardiac catheterization. Arterial complications. Circulation, 37(Suppl. 3):39, 1968.
7. Shumaker, H. B., Jr.: Sympathetic denervation of the extremities. Curr. Probl. Surg., July, 1965.
8. Sudeck, P.: Ueber die acute Entzundliche. Knochenatrophie. Arch. Klin. Chir., 62:147, 1900 (cited in Allen, E. V., Baker, N. W., and Hines, E. A., Jr.: Peripheral Vascular Diseases, 3rd ed. Philadelphia, W. B. Saunders Company, 1962, p. 459).
9. Telford, E. D.: Discussion on peripheral vascular lesions. Proc. R. Soc. Med., 37:621, 1944.
10. Thompson, J. E., Sigler, L., Raut, P. S., Austin, D. J., and Patman, R. D.: Arterial embolectomy: A 20-year experience with 163 cases., Surgery, 67:212, 1970.

13. VISCERAL ISCHEMIC SYNDROMES: OBSTRUCTION OF THE SUPERIOR MESENTERIC ARTERY, CELIAC AXIS, AND INFERIOR MESENTERIC ARTERY

John J. Bergan, M.D., and James S. T. Yao, M.D., Ph.D.

Syndromes of visceral artery occlusion may be acute or chronic. Obstruction of a single artery or a combination of the three main vessels supplying the abdominal contents can occur with or without symptoms, and it is now accepted that stenosis of even a single main intestinal artery might produce significant intestinal ischemia.

During the early 1900's, it was thought that chronic arterial occlusions could cause abdominal pain, but even Sir William Osler and Sir Clifford Albutt thought of abdominal angina as being a manifestation of ischemic heart disease. In 1931, Morley[28] wrote that there was no evidence that vascular pain in the abdomen ever occurred, but shortly a succinct explanation of vascular abdominal pain was given by Conner.[10] In 1936, Dunphy,[14] in a review of autopsy cases at the Peter Bent Brigham Hospital, emphasized that chronic recurrent abdominal pain might precede fatal intestinal infarction.

It was Mikkelsen[27] who suggested that corrective surgery of obstructive lesions of the mesenteric arteries might be possible, and within a year of his report Shaw and Maynard[34] published the first report of successful relief of superior mesenteric artery occlusion.

PATHOPHYSIOLOGY

The most common cause of chronic occlusion of the superior mesenteric artery, celiac axis, and inferior mesenteric artery is atherosclerosis. Other, rare occlusive lesions are curiosities and are of little clinical importance. Experimental evidence indicates that an increase in mesenteric artery blood flow occurs immediately following food ingestion. Excitation of alpha-adrenergic constrictor receptors by splanchnic nerve stimulation or adrenergic substance administration—epinephrine and norepinephrine—produces vasoconstriction. Beta receptors are present as well, and primary vasodilatation is seen when epinephrine is administered following Ilidar or ergotamine blockade.

In recent pharmacoangiography, it has been shown that epinephrine is a less potent vasoconstrictor than Pitressin, and this is explained by the fact that epinephrine stimulates both the constrictor and vasodilator receptors simultaneously.

Motor activity is the greatest influence upon mesenteric blood flow. This is important in understanding the origin of pain in intestinal ischemia. During intestinal contraction, arterial inflow decreases; during relaxation, blood flow increases. Rhythmic contractions augment flow if the muscular activity is of short duration, but strong contractions markedly decrease arterial inflow. Contractions producing intraluminal pressure of 30 mm. Hg or greater cause a decrease in blood flow, which is followed by recovery to baseline levels. Stronger contractions allow only a partial recovery.[19]

Since forceful muscular contraction is the first response of the intestine to ischemia, it may be that postprandial pain of intestinal ischemia is caused by muscular spasm initiated by intragastric food stimulation. This spasm is caused by motor activity generated in intestine supplied by arterial blood under low perfusion pressure. Decreased arterial inflow during such motor activity further stimulates the intestine to more forceful contractions. These further reduce arterial flow, and severe intestinal spasm results. This is interpreted by the patient as diffuse abdominal pain.

The most common findings in patients with chronic intestinal ischemia are postprandial pain and weight loss.[38] It is doubtful if clinically significant intestinal ischemia occurs in patients without a decrease in total body mass.

Malabsorption studies have dominated clinical investigation of chronic intestinal ischemia. These have been disappointing even in patients with severe weight loss. Among tests that have been unrewarding in study of patients with chronic intestinal ischemia are stool analyses for fat, nitrogen, and total solids; urinary excretion of administered d-xylose; serum carotene levels; vitamin B_{12} absorption; and vitamin A tolerance.[1] Of some promise is a provocative d-xylose test advocated by Fry and Kraft.[17]

Careful clinical observation of affected patients shows that, after eating, the pain intensity is sufficiently great that caloric intake is decreased and this produces weight loss. Such food habits are known as "the small meal syndrome" or "food fear." Pain-free intervals occur between meals but, as the occlusive process worsens, pain-free intervals shorten until the aching abdominal pain is almost constant.

Although conventional malabsorption tests have been disappointing, a few carefully performed balance studies such as those reported by Watt[37] have shown that malabsorption does exist in intestinal ischemia. Abnormalities of fecal fat, jejunal histology, disaccharidase activity, and bromsulphalein excretion may be demonstrated.

Other pathophysiologic manifestations of intestinal ischemia are inconstant. Patients may exhibit diarrhea or constipation.[30] Occult blood may or may not be present in the stool. The best clues to diagnosis are indirect. The patients have evidence of atherosclerotic arterial occlusive disease elsewhere. Coronary arterial occlusive disease is common. Peripheral atherosclerosis is often seen. Classically, such patients have weight loss to the point of emaciation. Thus, their abdominal pain may be thought to be due to infiltrating pancreatic carcinoma, gastric carcinoma, or chronic penetrating duodenal ulcer.

The general appearance of carcinomatosis, manifested by advanced cachexia, in a patient in whom no cancer can be demonstrated should be the best indicator that the patient may have chronic intestinal angina due to a chronic occlusion of the intestinal vessels.

Angiography is essential for definitive diagnosis of intestinal ischemia and lateral films demonstrate best the obstructive lesions at the origins of the mesenteric vessels. However, the arc of Riolan gives an important clue to presence of chronic occlusions of mesenteric arteries (Figs. 57 and 58). Atherosclerosis is the dominant lesion seen on the lateral aortogram. Since advanced plaque formation at origins of intestinal arteries is present in many patients without intestinal ischemia, careful correlation of clinical and angiographic abnormalities is necessary.

While single artery obstruction, such as isolated celiac axis stenosis, can produce all of the manifestations of intestinal angina, usually multiple lesions of celiac artery with superior mesenteric artery stenosis and/or inferior mesenteric artery occlusion co-exist.

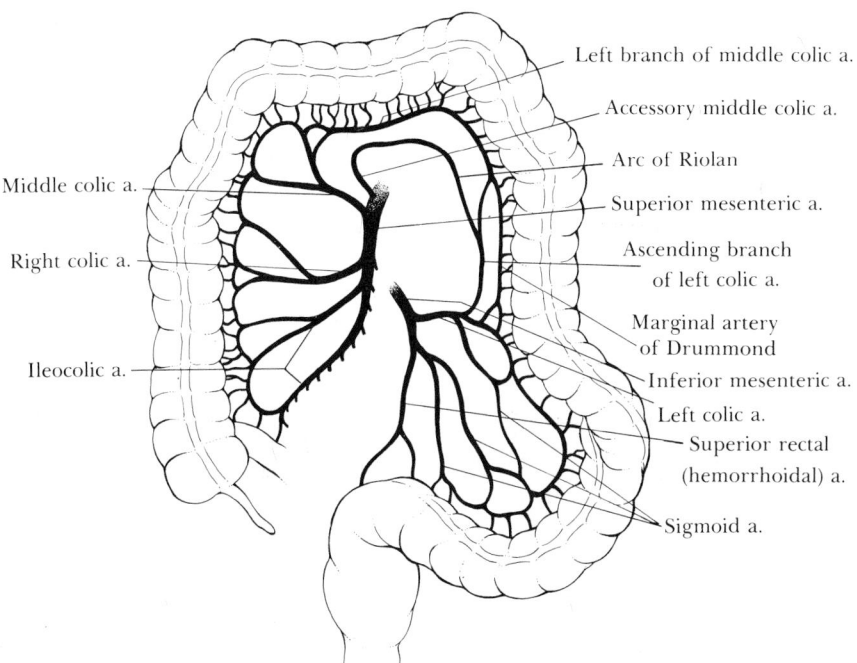

Figure 57. This diagram illustrates the normal anatomy of the superior mesenteric and inferior mesenteric arterial arborization. The arc of Riolan is indicated separate from the marginal artery of Drummond. This latter vessel may be incomplete and allow colon necrosis to occur when inferior mesenteric artery occlusion occurs. (From Ruzicka, F. F., Jr., and Rossi, P.: Radiol. Clin. North Am., *8*:1, 1970.)

INFERIOR MESENTERIC ARTERY OCCLUSION

Inferior mesenteric artery occlusion is thought to be inconsequential because this artery is frequently found to be obstructed by atherosclerosis and, on sacrifice of the artery at the time of aortic surgery, less than 1 per cent of cases exhibit colonic ischemia. Nevertheless, occasionally the inferior mesenteric artery through the arc of Riolan becomes the main source of arterial supply to the entire gut (Fig. 59). In such instances, occlusion of the inferior mesenteric artery becomes catastrophic. Rare cases of isolated colonic gangrene have been reported in which occlusion has been demonstrated only in the inferior mesenteric artery.[6]

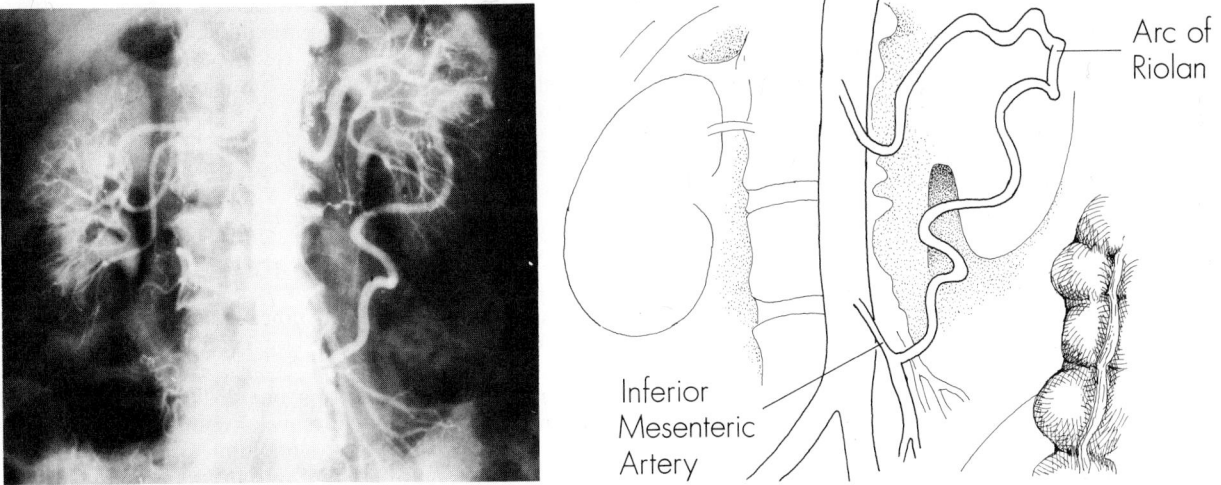

Figure 58. The arc of Riolan is an important collateral vessel to the superior mesenteric vascular bed. Its appearance on an anteroposterior abdominal angiogram is an indication of mesenteric artery occlusion.

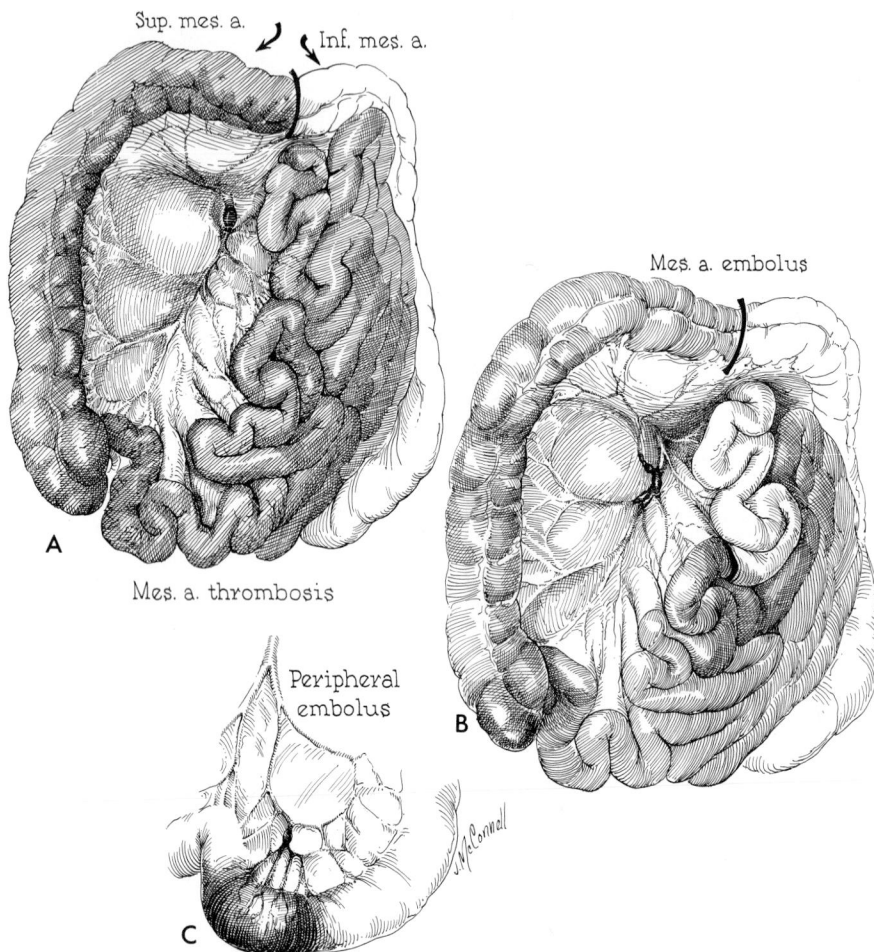

Sup. mes. a.

Inf. mes. a.

A

Mes. a. thrombosis

Mes. a. embolus

B

Peripheral embolus

C

J. McConnell

Figure 59. This diagram illustrates differences seen at operation between patients with superior mesenteric artery thrombosis and those with mesenteric artery embolization. Notice the sparing of the upper jejunal arterial supply in mesenteric embolization, and how this area is infarcted when superior mesenteric artery is occluded by atherosclerotic thrombosis. Segmental infarction of bowel may also occur when emboli lodge in peripheral mesenteric branches. (From Bergan, J. J.: Surg. Clin. North Am., *47*:109, 1967.)

SURGICAL CORRECTION

Historically, all operations advocated in treatment of peripheral arterial occlusive disease have been applied to the visceral vessels. However, thromboendarterectomy, suggested early, has been found to be needlessly complex. Bypass operations using saphenous vein or Dacron grafts have emerged as the most successful reconstructions.[23] As in coronary artery surgery, total one-stage correction of all of the lesions demonstrated on angiography is advocated now. The bypass grafts take their origin from the infrarenal lumbar aorta where the primary anastomosis can be made on the anterior surface. Grafts to the celiac axis territory are tunneled in the retropancreatic avascular plane to arrive in the lesser omental bursa. There, the distal anastomosis can be end-to-side to the common hepatic or the splenic artery. A short bypass to the superior mesenteric artery may take its origin from the lumbar aorta in the region of the inferior mesenteric artery.

In the past, single vessel reconstruction in the face of double vessel occlusions has been demonstrated to be effective.[22] Today, two or more grafts are suggested as the best way to avoid technical failure. An analysis of 246 cases giving adequate information from a total

of 357 published reports demonstrates that autologous vein bypass grafts are clearly emerging as the most favored method of correcting intestinal ischemia.[21] In these cases, early mortality of the operation was 6.5 per cent, with successful revascularization produced in 90 per cent of the patients reported. Late follow-ups of most of these cases are unavailable.

Following successful revascularization, marked weight gain is expected, but postoperative angiography is recommended, as this field of surgery is not yet settled.

CELIAC ARTERY COMPRESSION SYNDROME

Angiographic findings indicate that the celiac artery is frequently compressed by bands originating from the diaphragmatic crura. Nearly always, affected patients have no symptoms but do have an epigastric bruit. Rarely, when collateral circulation to the celiac territory is inadequate, symptoms of intestinal ischemia may be manifest. Pain occurring after meals and severe weight loss are the most reliable diagnostic symptoms.

A syndrome of celiac axis compression was first suggested in 1965.[13] This included patients generally younger than those with atherosclerosis, often female, with nonspecific intestinal complaints. A late follow-up of patients operated upon in the early days of demonstration of this syndrome indicates that many of the patients had incomplete relief of their abdominal pain and were found to have other intra-abdominal pathologic processes. While this has caused the syndrome itself to come into question,[16] it is not decided at the present time that the subject can be dismissed entirely.

SURGICAL TECHNIQUE

Surgical exposure of the celiac artery and its branches in the lesser omental bursa is relatively easy to accomplish. Following cutting of the bands surrounding the celiac axis and freeing the artery to the aortic origin, ballooning out of the vessel usually occurs. When stenosis of the origin of the vessel persists, pressures may be measured in the aorta and in the distal celiac axis, or electromagnetic flowmeter readings are taken. If flowmeter readings fail to exceed 500 ml. per min. or if an aortic/celiac pressure of 30 mm. Hg persists, direct revascularization using the bypass principle is advocated. Failure of crus cross-cutting has been salvaged by bypass grafting.

UNUSUAL CAUSES OF INTESTINAL ANGINA

Atherosclerosis and the celiac band syndrome account for nearly all causes of intestinal angina. However, specific conditions such as idiopathic aneurysm formation, allergic vasculitis, radiation arteritis, rheumatoid arteritis, systemic sclerosis, and lupus erythematosis may produce occlusive changes and physiologic intestinal ischemia.[40] Fibromuscular hyperplasia of the celiac axis and superior mesenteric artery has been reported,[32] as has mesenteric artery stenosis due to methysergide malleate.[8]

ACUTE MESENTERIC ARTERY OCCLUSION

Accurate diagnosis of the cause of acute mesenteric artery occlusion is now possible, and revascularization of ischemic gut with later resection of necrotic bowel dominates progress in treatment of intestinal infarction. This and the planned second look procedure allow greatest possibility of salvage of patients with otherwise fatal intestinal infarction.

Virtually the only treatment for intestinal infarction following Elliott's 1895 report[15] was intestinal resection. Despite nearly 100 per cent mortality, resection continues to be practiced.

The first attempted intestinal revascularization for acute occlusion was performed in 1950.[24] Surgeons were slow to attempt revascularization of the intestine in situations of acute occlusion. In the first 15 years following successful superior mesenteric embolectomy,[35] only two dozen operations were recorded. As

an increasing experience was obtained, some older teachings were shown to be wrong. For example, it was found that embolic occlusion of the superior mesenteric artery is the most frequent cause of acute mesenteric artery occlusion, and this single intestinal artery occlusion can produce bowel infarction.

A growing understanding of the pathophysiology of nonorganic intestinal ischemia emerged through the 1960's and into the 1970's. Only early diagnosis of thrombotic occlusion of the mesenteric artery remains an enigma. An understanding of treatment of mesenteric infarction has developed. It has become obvious that intestinal resection as applied to treatment of acute mesenteric infarction is followed by an unacceptable mortality: 85 to 100 per cent of cases operated upon.

PATHOPHYSIOLOGY

Following acute occlusion of the mesenteric artery, the first gross changes that occur are intense muscle contraction with accordion pleating and bluish-white rippling of the seromuscular surface.[39] Later, the bowel relaxes and the surface becomes pale with a bluish tinge. The peritoneal coverings lose their shiny appearance. Electron microscopic changes occur within ten minutes of occlusion,[7] but 30 minutes of total ischemia is required for extensive abnormalities to occur. Mitochondria are the first organelles to show damage. Fluid begins to accumulate in the infranuclear portion of the cells, and by ten minutes the cells show a washed-out appearance. Simultaneous with this is an intercellular fluid accumulation that sets the stage for epithelial slough.

Since it is the mitochondria that are responsible for ATP production through the aerobic cycle, a conversion from aerobic to anaerobic metabolism is mandatory if the cell is to survive.

After ten minutes of ischemia, changes in the rough and smooth endoplasmic reticula are seen. The smooth endoplasmic reticulum is primarily responsible for maintaining a high concentration of glucose-6-phosphatase, but it is the rough endoplasmic reticulum that is concerned with reconstituting amino acids into proteins. Lysosomal membranes remain intact, and this is indicated clinically by failure of demonstration of such enzymes in the circulating blood until bowel necrosis takes place.[36]

Ultimately, when lysosomal membranes rupture, autolytic enzymes are released that, by injuring adjacent cells, set up a vicious cycle of continuing intestinal death.[9, 18]

Much later, gross signs of hemorrhage into the mesentery are seen, and the well-known clinical features of hemorrhagic infarction are manifest. The bowel wall becomes swollen and infiltrated with blood, and the mucosa becomes necrotic. As purulent peritonitis occurs, histologically the picture is that of hemorrhagic necrosis, extensive submucosal edema, and cellular digestion from the luminal surface inward. Permeability to bacteria and fluid occurs, and a bidirectional flow of fluid develops. With this, there is a massive intraluminal loss of plasma and fluid.[33]

Successful revascularization of bowel is dependent upon knowledge that pathophysiologic changes affect the mucosa of bowel far more than seromuscular layers. In fact, the appearance of the small bowel may be deceptive. The bowel may look dead even though revascularization will allow return of viability and eventual regeneration of mucosa.[12]

Accompanying the pathophysiologic intestinal changes are profound systemic effects of acute intestinal infarction.[26] Leukocytosis above 15,000 is common. Increasing hemoglobin and hematocrit parallels hemoconcentration. Metabolic acidosis supervenes, while serum sodium, potassium, chloride, and carbon dioxide combining power remain normal. Hypoamylasemia is noted early because of the marked loss of plasma into the intestine, but later amylase levels return to normal. Late in the natural history of mesenteric infarction, the enzymes LDH, SGOT, SGPT, and CPK are all markedly elevated. The increase in LDH is thought to be due to extravasation of blood into the lumen of the bowel.[36]

SUPERIOR MESENTERIC ARTERY EMBOLIZATION

Superior mesenteric artery embolization is the most common cause of surgically treatable intestinal infarction.[3, 25] The diagnostic triad of (1) catastrophic abdominal pain in a patient with (2) a cardiac lesion that might produce embolization followed by (3) gut emptying, vomiting, and diarrhea is characteristic. To this can be added the history of a previous embolic event, which is present in more than one third of the patients, and a severe leukocytosis, present in more than two thirds of patients. Thus, a clinical diagnosis of mesenteric embolus can be made without sophisticated testing.

The cardiac lesion responsible for the embolus is atherosclerosis in two thirds of patients, and rheumatic heart disease is the next most frequent cause. Iatrogenic lesions such as cardiac valves or electrical conversion of rhythm are also important.

Diagnostic confirmation by angiography is recommended but not essential. The intra-aortic catheter is placed at the level of the first lumbar vertebra and an intra-aortic injection made. The embolus will be seen lodged near the mid-colic artery. A classic mercury meniscus sign is seen. In this location, a number of proximal collateral channels are present. These jejunal arteries occasionally allow spontaneous cure of the acute ischemia.[29] However, such return of intestinal blood flow should not be expected.

SURGICAL TREATMENT

A standard vascular exposure of the abdominal contents is utilized and the bowel is inspected. The upper portion of jejunum in the region of the ligament of Treitz is found to be normal, with pulsatile arcade vessels. Variable lengths of distal intestine are ischemic. At first, these are gray; later, they are quite dark and hemorrhagic (Fig. 59).

The mesenteric artery is palpated in the mesentery and the point of cessation of pulsations determined. A transverse incision through the peritoneum at this point allows skeletonization of the mesenteric artery and, through a transverse arteriotomy, an embolectomy with Fogarty catheter removal of propagated clot is accomplished.[2]

Following restoration of blood flow, pulsations return in marginal vessels and after an appropriate period of time, judgment is made regarding whether or not intestine should be resected. It is at this time that a decision is made for a second look procedure. If none appears necessary, the abdomen can be closed and the patient treated appropriately. It should be realized that none of the clinical signs following the first operation will assist judgment for or against a second look within the next 24 hour period.

In a review of 49 successful cases of mesenteric embolectomy, only seven have been subjected to a second look procedure and in only two of these was intestinal resection required.

Following intestinal revascularization, careful attention must be given to plasma volume and blood replacement. Plasma is lost into revascularized mesentery and gross blood into gut because of mucosal slough.

Although sudden death immediately following intestinal revascularization has been reported, recent experience has shown that cellular enzymes, histamine, free potassium ion, and gram-negative endotoxemia have not been important complications of intestinal revascularization. This is unlike observations in the experimental laboratory.[5]

ACUTE MESENTERIC ARTERY THROMBOSIS

Although postprandial pain is not a premonitory sign of intestinal infarction in patients with superior mesenteric artery embolization, it is an important finding in those patients who have mesenteric artery thrombosis. In the syndrome of thrombotic occlusion of the mesenteric artery, the acute illness develops insidiously, with a progressive, steady, sometimes collicky abdominal pain. This is pain of intestinal spasm. Half of such patients will give a history of prior intestinal ischemia manifested by weight loss, postprandial pain, and altered bowel habits. Many have manifestations of other atherosclerotic occlusions, including extremity atherosclerosis and ischemic brain and heart disease.

Following the establishment of constant abdominal pain, with or without bowel evacuation, the syndrome progresses, being characterized by systemic hypovolemia, hemoconcentration, and interstitial fluid extravasation into the splanchnic bed.[1] Later, as bowel dies, there is abdominal distention, further vomiting, and late bloody diarrhea.

As the syndrome progresses, profound leukocytosis is seen, and fever with other signs of sepsis indicates the establishment of peritonitis. At this time, a plain film of the abdomen may show dilated bowel loops, and clinically the patient appears ill out of proportion to the physical findings.

At any time bowel infarction is suspected, aortography should be performed. The intra-aortic catheter is placed at the level of the first lumbar vertebra, and anterior, posterior, and lateral films are made. If mesenteric artery thrombosis is present, a sharp cut-off of the superior mesenteric artery is seen within 1 cm. of its origin. The celiac axis may or may not be occluded and, similarly, the inferior mesenteric artery may not be visualized.

If the three vessels supplying the abdominal contents are seen to be patent, careful examination of the peripheral radicals should be done. Segmental spasm of peripheral vessels may be the only indication of a diagnosis of nonorganic intestinal infarction.

Changes in caliber of the vessels with smooth margins and symmetrical involvement indicate spasm, as opposed to the irregular margins and sharp cut-offs at bifurcations of vessels that are characteristic of atherosclerosis.

SURGICAL TREATMENT

Since pure resectional therapy for intestinal infarction results in a disastrously high mortality, attempts at revascularization are now being made. A limited degree of success has been reported.[3]

Thromboendarterectomy was used in early experience with intestinal revascularization but has been abandoned now. The operation is too time-consuming and too traumatic to the desperately ill patient with intestinal infarction. Aortomesenteric grafts are now utilized. The vessels are exposed by a standard vascular abdominal incision (Fig. 59) and the mesenteric artery dissected free of its investments in the mesentery. The infrarenal lumbar aorta is exposed and a saphenous vein graft anastomosed to the anterior surface of the aorta, led to the mesentery, and anastomosed end-to-side to the mesenteric artery itself. As much clot as possible is extracted from the mesenteric artery proximally and distally.[20]

Following revascularization, the need for intestinal resection and a second look procedure is decided upon. As in surgery for mesenteric artery embolus, the need for a second look procedure must be determined at the time of the first operation.

No attempt is made to revascularize both the superior mesenteric artery and the celiac axis, since in this emergency situation the least surgical procedure that will be effective in restoring blood supply to the gut is the one that will have the greatest success.

The attempt at revascularization is made to preserve length of small bowel and thus prevent short gut syndrome. In addition, since one of the major causes of death following resectional therapy for mesenteric infarction is intestinal fistula formation, revascularization is done to allow healing of anastomosed bowel ends.

NONORGANIC INTESTINAL INFARCTION

Nonorganic mesenteric infarction is not, strictly speaking, a surgical condition, but it must be differentiated from mesenteric infarction due to organic arterial occlusion. In nonorganic bowel infarction, a vicious cycle appears in which vasoconstriction in the mesenteric arterial bed is induced by a remote stimulus. Such a stimulus may be cardiac failure, systemic shock, or even head injury.[40] The resultant bowel ischemia allows bacterial penetration of the mucosa and subsequent sepsis and hypovolemia with decreased cardiac output causing sympathetic stimulation, which perpetuates the worsening cycle of intestinal ischemia.

Clinically, the symptoms are those of acute intestinal ischemia, with abdominal pain due to gut spasm and with gut emptying and leukocytosis. Late in the condition, melena and hematemesis are seen.

Before surgery is considered in such patients, aortography should be performed, and with the catheter placed at the level of the first lumbar vertebral body, a flush aortogram is done. In this condition, the origins and main courses of the mesenteric vessels are found to be free of occlusion.

THERAPY

Treatment of nonorganic bowel infarction should be directed at the underlying cause. The overall treatment has not been standardized; however, if nonorganic occlusion is diagnosed by aortography, the angiography catheter can be placed in the superior mesenteric artery and carefully controlled infusions of vasodilators performed. This must be done with great care under constant monitoring in the surgical intensive care unit.

The patient must be supported systemically, and frequently, massive amounts of blood, plasma, and crystalloid fluids must be given. Cardiac decompensation must be vigorously treated, and segmental resection of infarcted bowel segments may be required even if vasodilator therapy is successful.

SELECTED REFERENCES

Bergan, J. J., Dean, R. H., Conn, J., Jr., and Yao, J. S. T.: Revascularization in treatment of mesenteric infarction. Ann. Surg., *182*:430, 1975.
This study compares results of primary revascularization with primary intestinal resection in treatment of acute mesenteric artery occlusion in 48 surgical patients, pointing out the advantages of revascularization. An extensive historical resume is included.

Brown, R. A., Chiu, C.-J., Scott, H. J., and Gurd, F. N.: Ultrastructural changes in the canine ileal mucosal cell after mesenteric arterial occlusion. A sequential study. Arch. Surg., *101*:290, 1970.
The results of electron microscopic study of sequential changes in organelles of the ileal mucosa after superior mesenteric arterial occlusion is presented. Important pathophysiologic correlations are made that introduce the possibilities of an integrated study of combined biochemical and morphologic sequential changes that might occur in shock and other low flow states.

Kieny, R.: Indications and results of surgical reconstructions of arteriosclerotic intestinal arteries. Observations on 30 patients. VASA., *3*:179, 1974.
This important article emphasizes the finding of the arcade of Riolan in a normal aortogram leading to the diagnosis of chronic mesenteric arterial insufficiency. In the 30 cases described, details of surgery are presented, indicating possibilities of simultaneous reconstruction of the celiac trunk and mesenteric artery.

REFERENCES

1. Bergan, J. J.: Recognition and treatment of intestinal ischemia. Surg. Clin. North Am., 47:109, 1967.
2. Bergan, J. J.: Recognition and treatment of superior mesenteric artery embolization. Geriatrics, 24:118, 1969.
3. Bergan, J. J., Dean, R. H., Conn, J., Jr., and Yao, J. S. T.: Revascularization in treatment of mesenteric infarction. Ann. Surg., 182:430, 1975.
4. Bergan, J. J., Dry, L., Conn, J., Jr., and Trippel, O. H.: Intestinal ischemic syndromes. Ann. Surg., 169:120, 1969.
5. Bergan, J. J., Haid, S. P., and Conn, J., Jr.: Systemic effects of intestinal revascularization. Am. J. Surg., 117:235, 1969.
6. Bergan, J. J., and Selby, D. R.: Colonic infarction due to inferior mesenteric artery occlusion. Quart. Bull. Northwestern Univ. Med. Sch., 34:244, 1960.
7. Brown, R. A., Chiu, C., Scott, H. J., et al.: Ultrastructural changes in the canine mucosal cell after mesenteric arterial occlusion. Arch. Surg., 101:290, 1970.
8. Buenger, R. E., and Hunter, J. A.: Reversible mesenteric artery stenoses due to methysergide malleate. J.A.M.A., 198:558, 1966.
9. Chiu, C.-H., Scott, H. J., and Gurd, F. N.: Circulatory collapse following the restoration of blood flow to the occluded superior mesenteric artery. Surg. Forum, 21:47, 1970.
10. Conner, L. A.: Discussion of role of arterial thrombosis in visceral diseases of middle life based upon analogies drawn from coronary thrombosis. Am. J. Med. Sci., 185:13, 1933.
11. Derrick, J. R., and Logan, W. D.: Mesenteric arterial insufficiency. Surgery, 44:823, 1958.
12. Dumont, A. E., Tice, D. A., and Mulholland, J. H.: Arteriosclerotic occlusion of the superior mesenteric artery. Ann. Surg., 154:833, 1961.
13. Dunbar, J. D., Molnar, W., Beman, F. F., and Marable, S. H.: Compression of the celiac trunk and abdominal angina: Preliminary report of 15 cases. Am. J. Roentgenol., 95:731, 1965.
14. Dunphy, J. E.: Abdominal pain of vascular origin. Am. J. Med. Sci., 192:109, 1936.
15. Elliott, J. W.: Operative relief of gangrene of intestine due to occlusion of mesenteric vessels. Ann. Surg., 21:9, 1895.
16. Evans, W. E.: Long-term evaluation of the celiac band syndrome. Surgery, 76:867, 1974.
17. Fry, W. J., and Kraft, R. O.: Visceral angina. Surg. Gynecol. Obstet., 117:417, 1963.
18. Glenn, T. M., and Lefer, A. M.: Role of lysosomes in the pathogenesis of splanchnic ischemia shock in cats. Circ. Res., 27:783, 1970.
19. Grim, E.: The flow of blood in the mesenteric vessels. In Handbook of Physiology, Section II: Circulation. Vol. 2, Washington, D.C., American Physiological Society, 1963, pp. 1439–1456.
20. Gusberg, R., and Gump, F. E.: Combined surgical and nutritional management of patients with acute mesenteric vascular occlusion. Ann. Surg., 179:358, 1974.
21. Heberer, G., Dostal, G., and Hoffman, K.: Zur Erkennung und operativen Behandlung der chronischen Mesenterialarterieninsuffizienz. Dtsch. Med. Wochenschr., 97:750, 1972.
22. Jaffe, M. S.: Status of abdominal visceral circulation via superior mesenteric prosthesis. Am. J. Surg., 121:736, 1971.
23. Kieny, R.: Indications and results of surgical reconstructions of arteriosclerotic intestinal arteries. Observations on 30 patients. VSA, 3:179, 1974.
24. Klass, A. A.: Embolectomy in acute mesenteric occlusion. Ann. Surg., 134:913, 1951.
25. Liavag, I.: Acute mesenteric vascular insufficiency. A five-year material, including a case of successful superior mesenteric artery embolectomy. Acta Chir. Scand., 133:631, 1967.
26. Marston, A.: Causes of death in mesenteric arterial occlusion. I. Local and general effects of devascularization of the bowel. Ann. Surg., 158:952, 1963.
27. Mikkelsen, W. P.: Intestinal angina. Its surgical significance. Am. J. Surg., 94:262, 1957.
28. Morley, J.: Abdominal Pain. New York, William Wood & Co., 1931, p. 155.
29. Ottinger, L. W., and Austen, W. G.: A study of 136 patients with mesenteric infarction. Surg. Gynecol. Obstet., 124:251, 1967.
30. Palmer, W. L.: Clinical features of mesenteric artery insufficiency. J. Tennessee Med. Assoc., 59:152, 1966.
31. Reiner, L.: Mesenteric arterial disease. Postmortem injection studies of the mesenteric arterial circulation. Med. Sci., 12:229, 1962.
32. Ripley, H. R., and Levin, S. M.: Abdominal angina associated with fibromuscular hyperplasia of the celiac and superior mesenteric arteries. Angiology, 17:297, 1966.
33. Schennach, W., and Dorfmann, A.: Problem of acute obstruction of the mesenteric arteries. Thoraxchirurgie, 20:457, 1972.
34. Shaw, R. S., and Maynard, E. P.: Acute and chronic thrombosis of the mesenteric arteries associated with malabsorption. N. Engl. J. Med., 258:874, 1958.
35. Stewart, G. D., Sweetman, W. R., Westphal, K., and Wise, R. A.: Superior mesenteric artery embolectomy. Ann. Surg., 151:274, 1960.
36. Vyden, J. K.: The systemic effects of acute superior mesenteric vascular insufficiency. In Boley, S. J. (Ed.): Vascular Disorders of the Intestines. New York, Appleton-Century-Crofts, 1971.
37. Watt, J. K., Watson, W. C., and Haase, S.: Chronic intestinal ischemia. Br. Med. J., 3:199, 1967.
38. Wehrmacher, W. H.: Abdominal angina. Curr. Med. Dig., p. 567, Apr., 1967.
39. Welch, W. H.: Collected Papers and Addresses. Vol. I, 1920.
40. Williams, L. F., Jr.: Vascular insufficiency of the intestines. Gastroenterology, 61:757, 1971.

14. THE SURGICAL MANAGEMENT OF RENOVASCULAR HYPERTENSION

J. Caulie Gunnells, Jr., M.D. and David C. Sabiston, Jr., M.D.

The fact that obstructive lesions of the renal arteries can produce hypertension is firmly established. Moreover, surgical revascularization of an ischemic kidney is now an accepted procedure in appropriate circumstances and has produced relief of hypertension in a number of patients.

The *normal* blood pressure in the human is known to vary with age. In infants and young children, levels of 70 to 85 mm. Hg systolic with a diastolic pressure of 50 mm. Hg are within the normal range. In adolescents, a blood pressure of 100/75 is accepted as normal, whereas in the adult the upper range of normal is regarded as 140/90. Systemic arterial pressure is controlled by a number of variables, including the cardiac output, blood volume, and blood viscosity. It is thought that the most important feature determining significant and sustained renal hypertension is an elevated *peripheral resistance* as typified by the response to the *renin-angiotensin* system.

There are a number of specific causes of arterial hypertension. The forms of hypertension that are *surgically correctable* are those associated with coarctation of the aorta, pheochromocytoma, Cushing's syndrome, primary aldosteronism, and unilateral renal parenchymal disease. In addition, *renovascular* hypertension forms an increasingly important area for surgical therapy.

PHYSIOLOGIC ASPECTS

Occlusive lesions of the renal arteries are well recognized as a cause of *sustained diastolic hypertension.* The incidence of renal artery lesions and coexistent hypertension has not been established, but estimates suggest their presence in 5 to 15 per cent of the adult hypertensive population in the United States. In 1898, Tigerstedt and Bergman[14] demonstrated that an extract of kidney that they named renin was capable of producing hypertension in animals. The now-famous experiments by Goldblatt in which hypertension was produced by unilateral narrowing of a renal artery clearly documented the role of the ischemic kidney in the development of hypertension, especially when reduction in blood pressure followed removal of the involved kidney.[4] In the Goldblatt experiment, unilateral renal artery clamping resulted in *transient* hypertension, whereas sustained or persistent elevation in arterial pressure was produced either by constriction of both renal arteries or by clamp constriction of one main renal artery with removal of the contralateral kidney. In man, it has been shown that sustained arterial hypertension may result from *unilateral* renal artery obstruction. Following the Goldblatt experiments, Page and Corcoran,[9] Braun-Menendez,[1] and Helmer[6] all contributed to the early description of the renin-angiotensin system. A diminished flow of blood to the renal artery, and especially a reduction or damping of the arterial pulse pressure, is thought to represent one of the possible stimuli that elicit the renal pressor mechanism. The accepted relationships of the renin-angiotensin system are shown in Table 16.[10] The reaction of renin with its alpha globulin substrate yielding angiotensin I is ordinarily considered to be the rate-limiting response. This substance is essentially inert, but a plasmolytic converting enzyme splits off two amino acids and forms angiotensin II, an octapeptide. Angiotensin II is a powerful *vasoconstrictor*. It also evokes aldosterone secretion, and thus produces sodium retention. Angiotensin II is rapidly destroyed in the capillary circulation by tissue angiotensinases. *Renin* is the significant precursor, since the alpha globulin substrate is usually in excess, and converting enzyme is available throughout the body. Renin is apparently secreted by the kidney in response to a number of stimuli. Renin has a high molecular weight and a half-life in the bloodstream following bilateral nephrectomy of 45 minutes. Its concentration can be measured under suitable conditions of incubation by the amount of angiotensin it produces.

Much speculation has arisen concerning the physiologic role of renin.[2] Originally, its purpose was thought to be the regulation of perfusion pressure to the kidney beyond an obstructed renal artery, although more recently a broader hypothesis supports the concept that the activity of the renin-angiotensin-aldosterone axis is the primary stimulus for maintenance of body *sodium balance*.[10] This concept thoroughly explains the two classic conditions in which plasma renin activity (PRA) is increased: (1) decreased renal perfusion pressure, and (2) decreased delivery of sodium and water to the macula densa cells of the distal renal tubule. Examples of the former include renal artery stenosis, systemic hypotension, the upright posture, malignant hypertension, and afferent renal arteriolar vasoconstriction in hemorrhagic shock. Decreased sodium delivery to the distal tubules probably occurs without an obvious change in renal hemodynamics during dietary salt restriction and in certain disease states (i.e., congestive heart failure, cirrhosis of the liver, and nephrotic syndrome) accompanied by sodium retention.

The *macula densa* theory—that sodium delivery to the distal tubule is a controlling factor in renin release—is now widely accepted, although discrepancies remain. In this hypothesis, it is assumed that the macula densa cell signals the juxtaglomerular (JG) cells to release renin. It is known that patients with renovascular hypertension frequently are found to have a hyperplastic juxtaglomerular apparatus on microscopic examination.[3, 15] Angiotensin II is an extremely powerful vasoconstricting substance, with an effect approximately 10 times greater than that of norepinephrine as a pressor agent. Others have supported the *baroreceptor* hypothesis—that renin release occurs with very slight reductions in mean arterial pressure, of the order of 10 mm. Hg.[12] Thus, alteration in the arterial wall pressure is transmitted to the afferent arteriole to increase renin release in response to decreases in pressure and conversely to decrease renin release in response to increases in pressure.[18] Moreover, the ability to correct or ameliorate renovascular hypertension with the induction or injection of antirenin antibodies has added further support to a *humoral* etiology of the renovascular baroreceptor hypothesis. The sympathetic nerve theory[16, 19] encompasses the role of the autonomic nervous system in overall feedback control of renin release by the kidney. Stimulation of beta-adrenergic receptors in the renal arteriolar walls stimulates renin release, whereas blocking these receptors with drugs such as propranolol inhibits renin release.

TABLE 16.   The Renin-Angiotensin System*

α-Globulin substrate	+ Activators Renin − Inhibitors ————————→	Angiotensin I (decapeptide)
Angiotensin I	Converting enzyme ————————→	Angiotensin II (octapeptide)
Angiotensin II	————————→ Tissue peptidases	Inactive peptides

*From Romero, J. C., and Hoobler, S. W.: Am. Heart J., 80:701, 1970.

PATHOLOGIC OBSERVATIONS

The most common cause of renovascular hypertension is atherosclerosis, which is the etiologic basis in some two thirds of the patients with this disorder. The lesions are most apt to occur near the *origin* of the renal vessels from the aorta and are *segmental*, usually less than a centimeter in length (Fig. 60). Males are more commonly affected, and bilateral lesions are present in approximately a third of patients.

Fibrous and fibromuscular dysplasia is another cause of renovascular hypertension; these mural dys-

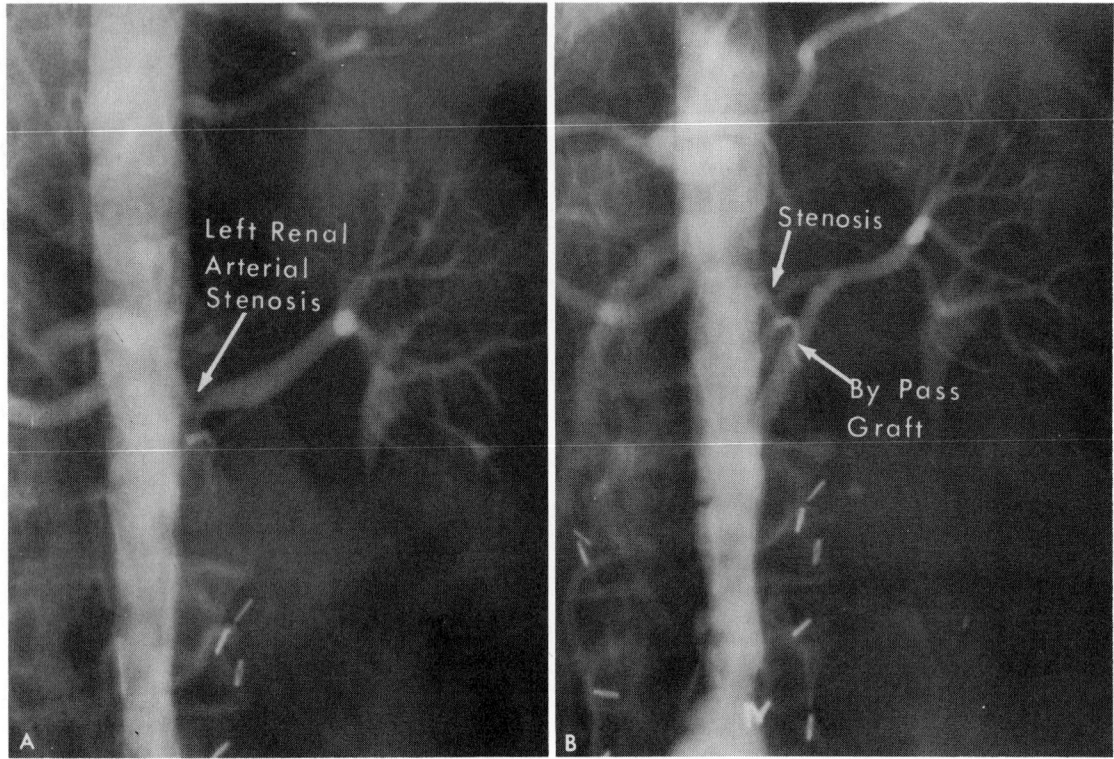

Figure 60. *A*, Arteriogram demonstrating severe stenosis of left renal artery in a patient with marked hypertension. *B*, Postoperative arteriogram after insertion of a venous autograft to bypass the stenotic lesion. The hypertension was relieved.

plasias may be classified according to the site or type of involvement (intimal, medial, adventitial). The most commonly recognized variety is termed fibromuscular medial dysplasia or hyperplasia and occurs primarily in young women. It is responsible for the disorder in approximately a fourth of patients. The microscopic lesion consists of a thickening of the media with separation and distortion of the muscle fibers by a degenerative process involving myxomatous fibrous tissue. The lesions are apt to be multiple, and the term "microaneurysms" has been used to describe their appearance, which produces a corrugated effect termed the "string of beads" phenomenon observed on arteriograms (Fig. 61).

In one series, an arteriographic diagnosis of fibromuscular medial hyperplasia of the renal arteries was made in 136 hypertensive patients.[20] In 25 of these, the lesions were minimal, and hypertension was easily controlled with medication. In 31, the lesions were bilateral, either in secondary branches of the artery or in accessory arteries, and were considered inoperable. Major lesions associated with hypertension and considered operable were found in 80 patients. The distribution of lesions determined the selection of operation, and primary nephrectomy was performed in 14 patients with unilateral disease in whom branch or accessory arteries were not amenable to arterial reconstruction. Revacularization procedures were per-

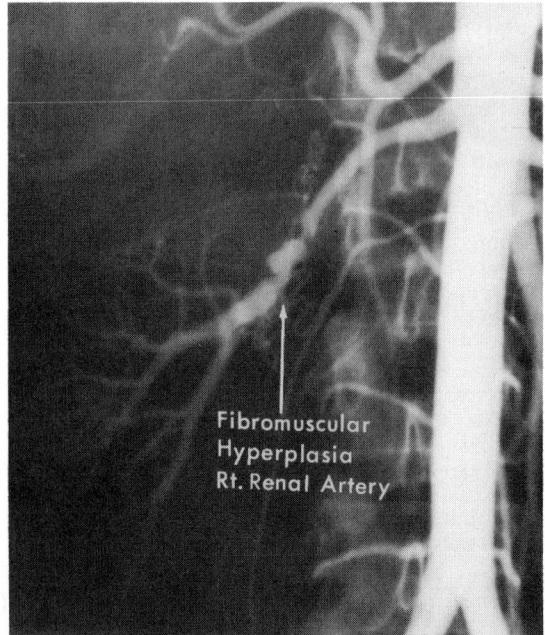

Figure 61. Arteriogram demonstrating fibromuscular hyperplasia of the right renal artery producing hypertension. Note the characteristic "scalloping."

formed in 62 patients with unilateral and 9 patients with bilateral disease of the main arteries. This disorder occurs almost exclusively in the distal three fourths of the main renal artery or its primary branches and may not be suitable for surgical correction.[7]

Other vascular lesions, including aneurysm (congenital and acquired), arteriovenous malformations, renal artery dissection, renal artery thrombosis, and emboli to the renal parenchyma, have been associated with or productive of renovascular hypertension.

CLINICAL MANIFESTATIONS

Experience has demonstrated that there are several important *clinical* diagnostic features of renovascular hypertension. These include the onset of sudden hypertension, often prior to the age of 35 or after the age of 55, with the absence of a family history and onset or worsening of the hypertension following an episode of flank pain, and the existence of malignant hypertension after the age of 55. In other words, these features would be atypical for *essential hypertension*, although it must be emphasized that a number of patients with proven renovascular hypertension exhibit none of these features.

Physical examination may reveal the most important diagnostic feature, an abdominal *bruit* located in the epigastrium or upper quadrants. This finding is present in 50 to 80 per cent of patients with *renovascular* hypertension, whereas it occurs in less than 5 per cent of those with essential hypertension. Patients with fibromuscular hyperplasia are more apt to have bruits than those with atherosclerotic lesions. Moreover, in fibromuscular disease the bruits are soft, to-and-fro, or continuous, whereas higher-pitched systolic bruits are more characteristic of atherosclerotic lesions. Patients presenting with these findings are acceptable for thorough renovascular evaluation. The appropriate studies may include angiography, split renal function studies, and renal vein renin studies. At the outset it is important to recognize that a general medical evaluation is necessary and that attention should be given to the age of the patient and duration and severity of hypertension, as well as to the presence of coexisting vascular and unrelated diseases. Emphasis must also be placed on careful assessment of overall renal function in the selection of candidates for surgery.

LABORATORY EXAMINATIONS

The initial studies of importance include a urinalysis with culture, serum creatinine determination, chest roentgenography, electrocardiography, serum potassium determination, and assessment of plasma renin activity.

ANATOMIC STUDIES

Intravenous Urography

Intravenous urography is simple, widely available, and possibly the best anatomic screening test for the presence of renovascular hypertension. It also often establishes the presence or absence of primary parenchymal renal disease. The criteria for a positive minute sequence study include the following changes in the affected or ipsilateral kidney: (1) an initial delay in the appearance time and concentration (nephrogram) of the contrast medium, followed by a paradoxical hyperconcentration of the dye in the pyelocaliceal system; and (2) a reduction in kidney length greater than 1.5 cm. A representative minute sequence urogram is shown in Figure 62. These criteria support the presence of main stem renal arterial lesions, and within these guidelines, the minute sequence intravenous urogram correlated at a level of 80 per cent with subsequent angiographic studies in detecting renal artery stenosis. The study yields a false positive result in approximately 10 per cent of patients and a false negative result in another 10 per cent of those studied. The urogram has important diagnostic limitations in detecting segmental or branch arterial lesions, bilateral renal artery disease, and bilateral parenchymal renal disease of unequal severity, and in certain congenital anomalies of the kidney.

Radioisotope Renography

The radioisotope renogram has been advocated to delineate renovascular hypertension and is characterized by three phases: (1) *vascular phase* – a rapidly ascending slope attributed to renal and extrarenal vascular radioactivity; (2) *functional phase* – a more slowly ascending second segment attributed to tubular activity and intraluminal accumulation of radioactive material; and (3) *excretory phase* – a descending slope considered to represent elimination of radioactive urine from the region of the kidney. This test has several disadvantages, including a number of false positive and false negative results, lack of a standardized technique, and necessity for specialized equipment. In addition, there are technical variables including probe placement, patient position, and state of hydration, and there is no characteristic curve that serves to differentiate renal arterial stenosis from unilateral parenchymal disease. The future role of newer techniques of noninvasive radioisotope methodology utilizing the Anger camera and rapid sequence scintillation studies may provide a wider application and greater precision of radioisotope studies in renovascular disease.

Renal Arteriography

The definitive study for the anatomic localization of a renal artery lesion is renal arteriography. This study is indicated in those patients judged to be eventual candidates for surgical therapy in whom preliminary results suggest renovascular hypertension. The percutaneous retrograde transfemoral technique[11] is quite suitable and the performance of "flush" aortography in conjunction with selective renal arterial injections of contrast media adds diagnostic precision and greater vascular detail. In addition to demonstrating the main renal arteries and potential lesions, the study provides important additional information, including the extent of post-stenotic dilatation and of

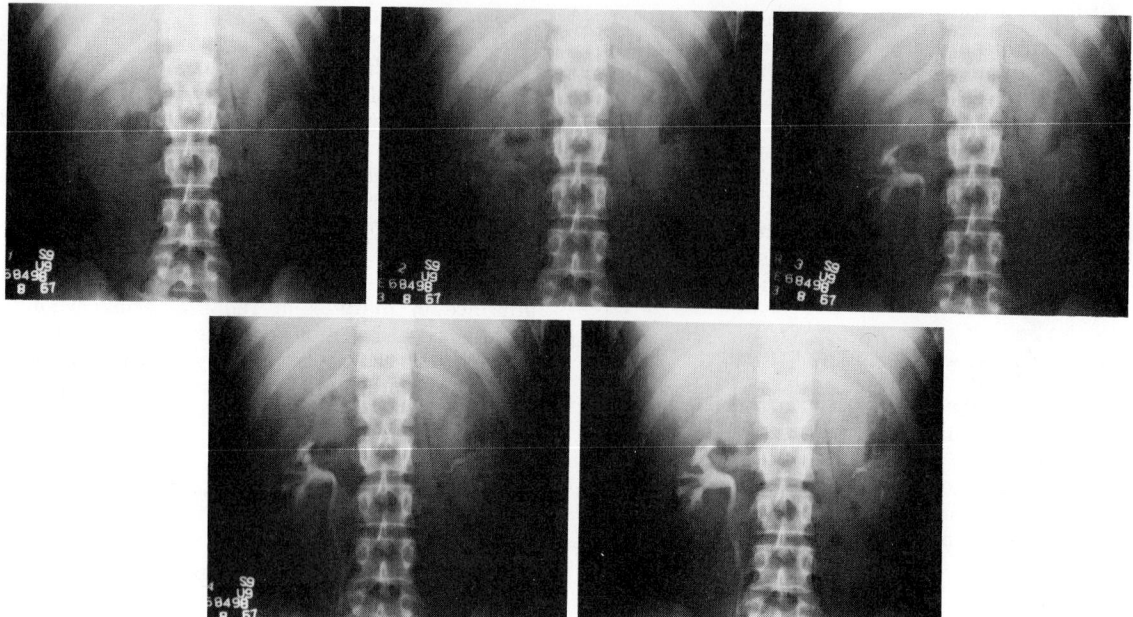

Figure 62. A positive rapid- or minute-sequence intravenous urogram. The left kidney is significantly smaller and demonstrates a delay in the appearance and concentration of the contrast medium. Paradoxical hyperconcentration is not seen in this study; delayed films not shown, only the serial one-minute films for 5 minutes.

collateral circulation, and makes possible evaluation of the extra-and intrarenal arterial anatomy. After establishing the fact that a lesion is present, it is then necessary to pursue further studies to determine whether or not the observed lesion is responsible for the hypertension.

Renal Function Studies

In addition to obtaining anatomic evidence, assessment of the function of the kidneys is of prime importance. Differential renal studies are important in estimating the functional alteration of effect of unilateral ischemia. Criteria for the physiologic or functional alteration produced by a unilateral renal arterial lesion are based firmly upon animal studies with experimentally induced renal lesions. The changes produced consist of a unilateral decrease in glomerular filtration rate, with an increased fractional reabsorption of sodium and water and increased urinary osmolality, and increased urinary concentration

of endogenous or exogenous nonreabsorbable solutes. The currently acceptable differential renal function tests (Howard, Stamey, Rapaport, and Birchall) all utilize one or more of these parameters of altered renal function as the basis of the particular study. The two most widely used techniques are those described by Howard and Stamey. The diagnostic features of these split function studies are shown in Table 17. Unfortunately, these studies require bilateral ureteral catheterization and simultaneous collection of timed urine samples from each kidney, which are analyzed for volume, sodium, urea, creatinine, and osmolality. The reliability of differential renal function studies varies considerably; however, a combined experience has reported an operative cure rate of 73 per cent for those patients with positive split function studies. At the same time, an incidence of 49 per cent surgical success is recorded in patients with *negative* studies, and therefore the overall problems related to interpretation of this test render it of somewhat limited

TABLE 17.   Criteria for Positive Split-Renal Function Studies

	Howard	Stamey
U_v (ml./min.)	50% reduction on involved side	>3:1 decreased flow from involved kidney
U_{Na+} (mEq./L.)	15% reduction from involved side	
$U_{creatinine}$ (mg.%)	Increased by 50 to 100% on involved side	
U_{PAH} (mg./100 ml.)		100% or greater concentration from involved kidney

value. In an effort to improve the diagnostic accuracy of these studies, efforts have been made to (1) assess the renal blood flow of the contralateral or normal kidney and exclude from surgery those patients who fail to exhibit a contralateral renal plasma flow of at least 200 to 250 ml. per minute in combination with a positive differential function study; and (2) combine an assessment of the degree of arteriolar nephrosclerosis (renal biopsy studies) with renal plasma flow studies. Despite these additions, the split function tests continue to be fraught with a high incidence of technical failure, postprocedural complications, unreliability in the presence of segmental and bilateral arterial lesions, and unexplained false positive and false negative results.

Plasma Renin Activity

Measurement of plasma renin activity (PRA) is of considerable help in segregating those patients in whom a humoral mechanism involving the renin-angiotensin-aldosterone system is causally related to renovascular hypertension.[2, 5, 17, 18] The value of measurement of peripheral venous plasma renin and renal vein renin activity has added greatly to the criteria for selection of patients for operative procedures. Thus far, the most experience and greatest emphasis have involved estimates of *renin* activity rather than that of angiotensin II per se. Problems in early methodology may have contributed to some of the controversy related to the diagnostic usefulness of these measurements. The bioassay of plasma renin activity, used in earlier clinical studies, has been largely replaced by radioimmunoassay techniques for the measurement of angiotensin I, which reflects and may be equated to measurements of plasma renin activity. It is worth emphasizing that clinicians must be familiar with the methodology involved and that careful assessment must be made of the conditions under which renin measurements are obtained. These conditions include body posture, sodium balance, and the presence or absence of varying pharmacologic agents, all of which may affect renin activity measurements.

The presence of an increased peripheral venous

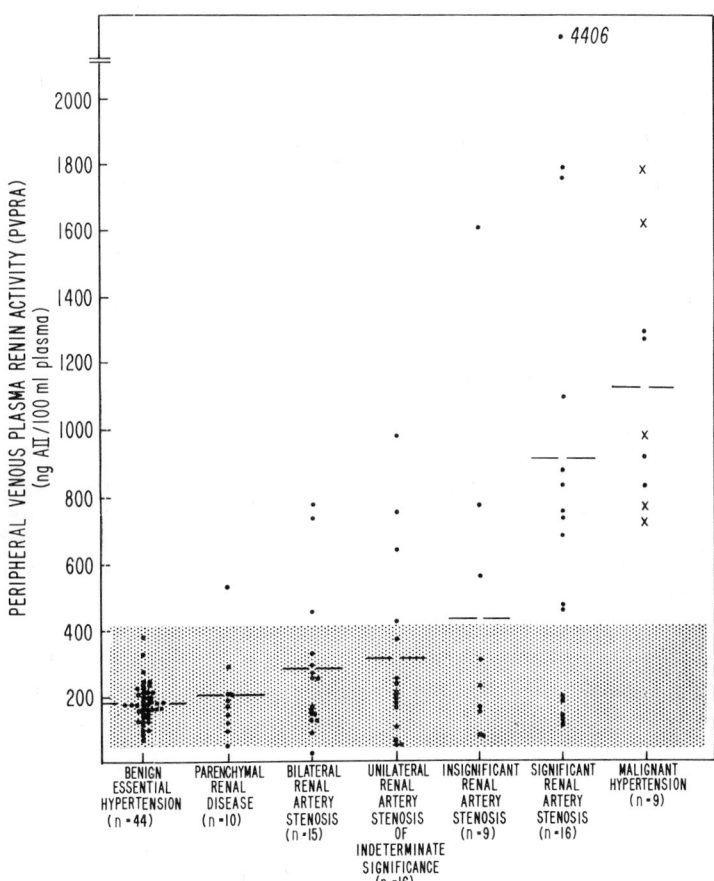

Figure 63. Peripheral venous plasma renin activity in 111 patients with a wide variety of hypertensive diseases. The four patients with malignant hypertension and parenchymal renal disease are shown in the last column on the right and identified by the closed circles (●); the remaining patients in this column (x) have occlusive renal artery lesion(s) and are also included in columns 3 to 6. (From Gunnells, J. C., Jr., McGuffin, W. L., Jr., Johnsrude, I., and Robinson, R. R.: Ann. Intern. Med., *71*:555, 1969.)

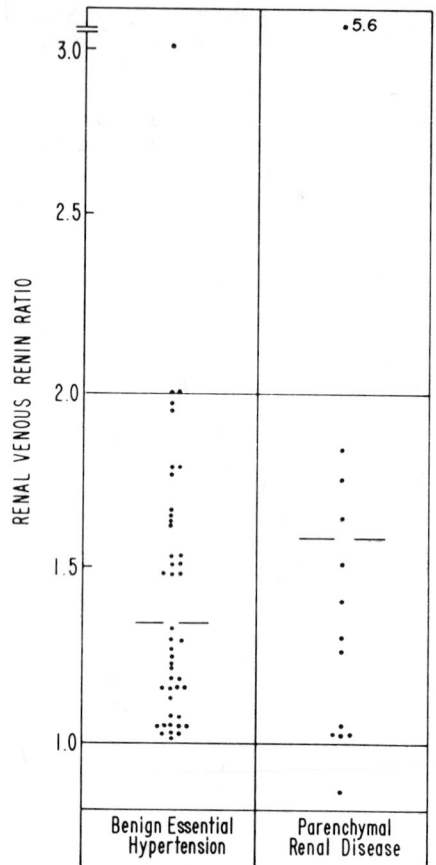

Figure 64. Renal venous renin ratios in 58 patients with normal renal arteries. (From Gunnells, J. C., Jr., McGuffin, W. L., Jr., Johnsrude, I., and Robinson, R. R.: Ann. Intern. Med., 71:555, 1969.)

measurements alone or in combination has assumed considerable importance.[5, 17] Patients with hypertension and normal renal arteries only *rarely* exhibit a renal vein renin ratio greater than 2 to 1 (Fig. 64),[5] whereas in patients with functionally significant renal artery stenosis, renal vein renin concentrations are at least 1.2 to 2 times higher in the venous blood of the involved or affected kidney than in that of the normal one. The combined use of peripheral vein plasma renin activity and renal vein renin activity measurements in determining or predicting surgical success is summarized in Table 18. Likewise, Table 19 outlines the criteria of Vaughan and Laragh[17] for predicting surgically curable renovascular hypertension utilizing both peripheral and renal vein renin sampling.

Pharmacologic Tests

The recent development of specific inhibitors of the renin angiotensin system has led to the application of new techniques in identifying patients whose hypertension may be related to overactivity of the pressor role of angiotensin II generated by the presence of renin excess.[13] Specifically, a new angiotensin II analogue (1-sarcosine-8-alanine angiotensin II; saralasin [P-113]) is a compound that competes with native angiotensin II hormone for its arteriolar receptor site. The intravenous administration of this compound to salt-restricted hypertensive patients in one reported series[13] is associated with a drop in mean diastolic blood pressure of 27 mm. Hg during the infusion in patients with either elevated peripheral venous plasma renin activity or abnormal renal vein renin ratios, whereas patients with hypertension and normal plasma renin activity exhibit no significant drop in blood pressure during such infusion. Figure 65 depicts the blood pressure fall in response to the administration of this angiotensin II analogue in a patient with renal artery stenosis and elevated plasma renin activity. Subsequent investigation has shown this type of blood pressure response under the conditions outlined above to be highly predictive of a "high renin" hypertension, as seen in functionally significant renal artery stenosis. Moreover, those patients who demonstrate a fall in blood pressure as outlined and exhibit elevated plasma renin activity with anatomic renal artery stenosis by angiography have, when submitted to surgical therapy, uniformly responded favorably to the surgery with a reduction in blood pressure. The application of this test to the identification of patients

plasma renin activity in the presence of a normal dietary sodium intake and the absence of diuretic drugs and malignant hypertension provides strong supportive evidence for functional renal arterial stenosis. An experience with measurements of peripheral venous plasma renin activity in a wide variety of clinical hypertensive diseases is shown in Figure 63.[5] Since peripheral venous renin activity measurements can be quite variable, the use of *bilateral renal vein renin*

TABLE 18. **Measurements of Renin Activity Correlated with Results of Surgical Therapy in 23 Patients**

Peripheral and Renal Venous Renin Activity	Surgical Success	Number of Patients
Patients with elevated peripheral venous PRA and greater than a twofold difference in renal venous PRA	100%	11 of 11
Patients with normal peripheral venous PRA and greater than a twofold difference in renal venous PRA	50%	4 of 8
Patients with normal peripheral venous PRA and less than a twofold difference in renal venous PRA	25%	1 of 4

**TABLE 19.   Three Criteria Obtained from Four Renin Values to Predict Curable
Renovascular Hypertension***

Samples to Collect
A. Ambulatory peripheral plasma renin and 24-hour urine sodium excretion under steady state conditions (i.e., not on day of arteriography or renal vein renin sampling).
B. Simultaneous collection of supine:
   Renal vein renin from suspect kidney (V)
   Renal vein renin from contralateral kidney (V)
   Peripheral venous or arterial renin (A)

Criteria for Predicting Cure	*Interpretation*
1. High peripheral plasma renin activity in relation to UNaV	A measure of hypersecretion of renin
2. Contralateral kidney: (V-A) = 0	An indicator of normalcy of the contralateral kidney
3. Suspect kidney: (V-A)/A = 0.48	An indicator of unilateral renin secretion
or	
(V-A)/A > 0.48	A measure of reduced renal blood flow

*From Vaughn, E. D., and Laragh, J. H.: New concepts of the renin system and of vasoconstriction-volume mechanisms. Urol. Clin. North Amer., 2:237, 1975.

for further investigation, as well as for the selection of patients to undergo corrective renovascular surgery, should add measurably to the physician's diagnostic armamentarium in the hypertensive population.

Treatment

Selection of patients for medical or surgical treatment is dependent upon the primary establishment of a strong likelihood that the hypertension is present as a *direct result* of a renal arterial lesion. In addition, one should consider the age and general health of the patient, the natural history of the disease, the feasibility of vascular repair versus nephrectomy, the comparative role of control of the hypertension with drugs, and the surgical mortality.[8] For example, elderly patients with evidence of atherosclerotic lesions elsewhere might have an operative mortality in an excessive range. Contrariwise, a young patient with a fibromuscular lesion would be an essentially ideal candidate. The majority of patients are between these two extremes, and most patients thought to have an arterial

lesion responsible for the hypertension are candidates for surgery.

The choice of surgical technique is dependent upon the nature of the occluding lesion and the individual preference of the surgeon. Segmental renal artery *resection with reanastomosis* may be feasible if the proximal and distal ends of the vessel are suitable. An anastomosis of the *splenic artery* to the distal renal artery has also been employed with good results. In properly selected patients, the stenosis can be incised and enlarged by a *vein patch angioplasty*. A saphenous vein *autograft* from the aorta to the renal artery distally with a side-to-side anatomosis at both ends is probably the most commonly used and most successful procedure. Occasionally, the renal artery can be *reimplanted* into the aorta following excision of the stenosis. Arterial *autografts* have also been employed successfully, and *endarterectomy* is the procedure of choice of several surgeons with excellent results. The closure may require a patch venous graft or the use of a prosthetic graft. *Prosthetic arterial grafts* from the aorta to the distal renal artery may also be used. *Nephrectomy* may be necessary when obstructing lesions or aneurysms are present in branch or small accessory arteries. It may also be required in patients who have failed to respond to another reconstructive procedure. The various techniques are illustrated in Figure 66.

RESULTS

Approximately 40 to 50 per cent of patients can be "cured" by surgical revascularization procedures and an additional 25 to 35 per cent "improved." The remaining 25 to 35 per cent exhibit essentially no change in their hypertension. The reported overall surgical mortality ranges between 5 and 10 per cent.

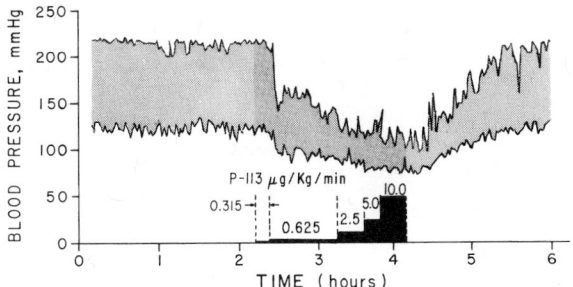

Figure 65. Automatic blood-pressure recording during Saralasin (P-113) infusion in a patient with renal arterial stenosis and high plasma renin activity. Blood pressure fell little, if at all, during P-113 infusion at 0.315 μg per kilogram per minute but fell progressively to normal levels as P-113 infusion was increased to 0.625, 2.5, 5.0, and 10.0 μg per kilogram per minute. During the first one to one and a half hours after the P-113 infusion was stopped, blood pressure returned gradually to control hypertensive levels. (From Streeten, D. H. P., Anderson, G. H., Freiberg, J. M., and Dalakos, T. G.: Use of an angiotensin II antagonist (Saralasin) in the recognition of "angiotensinogenic" hypertension. N. Engl. J. Med., 292:657, 1975.)

SELECTED REFERENCES

Hunt, J. C., Strong, C. G., and Bernatz, P. E.: Diagnosis and management of renovascular hypertension. Am. J. Cardiol., 23:434, 1969.

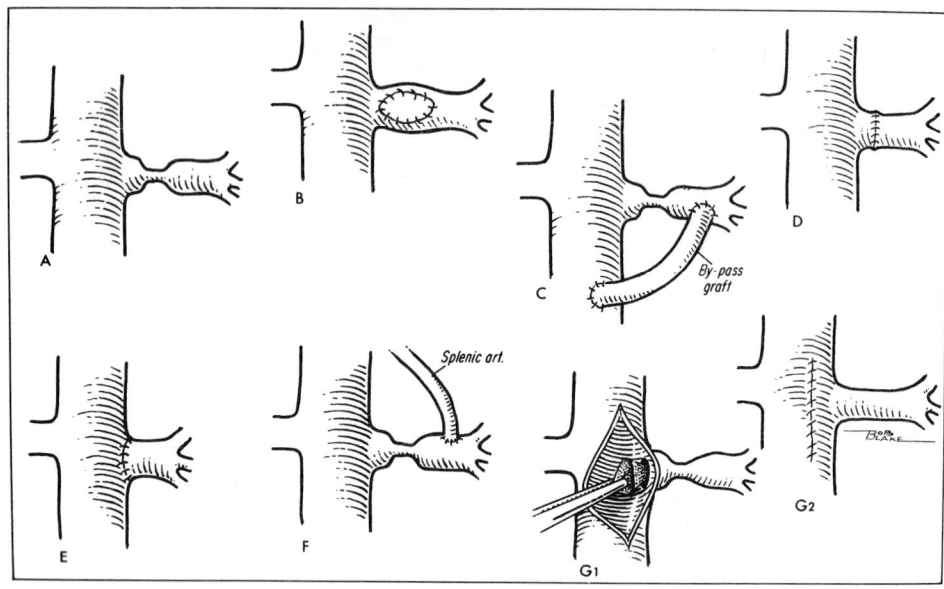

Figure 66. Diagrammatic illustration of operations designed to relieve renal arterial obstruction in renovascular hypertension. *A,* The stenosis is usually located near the origin of the renal artery. *B,* An endarterectomy performed with the use of a patch graft to prevent narrowing at the time of closure. *C,* In most patients a bypass graft from the aorta to the distal renal artery is the most satisfactory operation. The graft can be either an autogenous vein or artery or a prosthetic graft. *D,* The stenotic area is excised, with end-to-end anastomosis of the renal artery. *E,* The stenosis is excised, with reimplantation of the renal artery into the aorta. *F,* The splenic is divided and its distal end anastomosed to the side of the renal artery beyond the stenosis. G_1, The aorta is temporarily opened, with endarterectomy performed from within the aortic lumen. G_2, After endarterectomy, the aortic incision is closed.

This review considers a series of 100 patients with renovascular hypertension from the Mayo Clinic. The clinical features, laboratory data, operative procedures, and results are reviewed in detail.

Kaplan, N. M.: Clinical Hypertension. New York, Medcom Press, 1973.
An excellent book that is well organized and presents a practical approach to the overall problem of hypertension, with special reference to renovascular disease.

Kaufman, J. J. (Ed.): Management of Renovascular Hypertension. Urol. Clin. North Am., Vol. 2, No. 2, June, 1975.
This monograph contains an excellent selection of papers related to the history, pathophysiology, diagnostic evaluation, and treatment of renovascular hypertension.

Laragh, J. H.: Hypertension Manual. New York, York Medical Books, Dun-Donnelley Publishing Corporation, 1973.
This book is an extensive collection of a wide variety of papers related to the overall problem of hypertension, with a number of chapters specifically devoted to special problems of renovascular hypertension.

Wylie, E. J., Perloff, D. L., and Stoney, R. J.: Autogenous tissue revascularization technics in surgery for renovascular hypertension. Ann. Surg., *170*:416, 1969.
This summary describes the results of nephrectomy and revascularization operations for the treatment of renovascular hypertension in 190 patients. The obstructive lesions of the renal artery were caused by fibromuscular hyperplasia in 80 patients and by atherosclerosis in 110. The surgical techniques and results are discussed in detail.

REFERENCES

1. Braun-Menendez, F., Fasciolo, J. C., Leloir, L. F., Munoz, J. M., and Taquini, A. C.: Renal Hypertension. Translated by L. Dexter. Springfield, Ill., Charles C Thomas, Publisher, 1946.
2. Brunner, H. R.: Clinical implications of renin in the hypertensive patient. J.A.M.A., *233*:1091, 1975.
3. Crocker, D. W., Newton, R. A., Mahoney, E. M., and Harrison, J. H.: Hypertension due to primary renal ischemia: A correlation of juxtaglomerular cell counts with clinicopathological findings in twenty-five cases. N. Engl. J. Med., *267*:794, 1962.
4. Goldblatt, H., Lynch, J., Hanzal, R. F., and Summerville, W. W.: Studies on experimental hypertension. I. The production of persistent elevation of systolic blood pressure by means of renal ischemia. J. Exp. Med., *59*:347, 1934.
5. Gunnells, J. C., Jr., McGuffin, W. L., Jr., Johnsrude, I., and Robinson, R. R.: Peripheral and renal venous plasma renin activity in hypertension. Ann. Intern. Med., *71*:555, 1969.
6. Helmer, O. M.: Presence of renin in plasma of patients with arterial hypertension. Circulation, *25*:169, 1962.
7. Hunt, J. C., Harrison, E. G., Jr., Kincaid, O. W., Bernatz, P. E., and Davis, G. D.: Idiopathic fibrous and fibromuscular stenoses of the renal arteries associated with hypertension. Mayo Clin. Proc., *37*:181, 1962.
8. Kauffman, J. J., Maxwell, M. H., Craven, J. D., and Okun, R.: Hypertension—primary and secondary. Ann. Intern. Med., *75*:761, 1971.
9. Page, I. H., and Corcoran, A. C.: Hypertension: Review of humoral pathogenesis and clinical treatment. Adv. Intern. Med., *1*:183, 1942.
10. Romero, J. C., and Hoobler, S. W.: The renin-angiotensin system in clinical medicine. Am. Heart J., *80* 701, 1970.
11. Seldinger, S. I.: Catheter replacement of needle in percutaneous arteriography: New technique. Acta Radiol., *39*:368, 1953.
12. Skinner, S. L., McCubbin, J. W., and Page, I. H.: Control of the renin secretion. Circ. Res., *15*:64, 1964.
13. Streeten, D. H. P., Anderson, G. H., Freiberg, J. M., and Dalakos, T. G.: Use of an angiotensin II antagonist (Saralasin) in the recognition of "angiotensinogenic" hypertension. N. Engl. J. Med., *292*:657, 1975.
14. Tigerstedt, R., and Bergman, P. G.: Niere und Kreislauf. Skand. Arch. Physiol., *8*:223, 1898.
15. Tobian, L.: Relationship of juxtaglomerular apparatus to renin and angiotensin. Circulation, *25*:189, 1962.
16. Vander, A. J.: Effect of catecholamines and the renal nerves on renin secretion in anesthetized dogs. Am. J. Physiol., *209*:659, 1965.
17. Vaughan, E. D., and Laragh, J. H.: New concepts of the renin system and of vasoconstriction-volume mechanisms. Urol. Clin. North Am. *2*:237, 1975.
18. Vertes, V., and Ghose, M.: Pathophysiology of renovascular hypertension. Urol. Clin. North Am., *2*:227, 1975.
19. Winer, N., Chokski, D. S., Youn, M. S., and Freedman, A. D.: Adrenergic receptor mediation of renin secretion. J. Clin. Endocrinol., *29*:1168, 1969.
20. Wylie, E. J., Perloff, D., and Wellington, J. S.: Fibromuscular hyperplasia of the renal arteries. Ann. Surg., *156*:592, 1962.

55

DISORDERS OF THE LUNGS, PLEURA, AND CHEST WALL

I

THE DEVELOPMENT OF THORACIC SURGERY

Hiram T. Langston, M.D.

The thorax was the last of the body cavities to become a domain of surgeons because entry into it often resulted fatally. Our primary interest here concerns the steps by which the thoracic cavity was broached and the means by which security in doing so was acquired.

This is not the story of one man or one incident or even of any concise piece of research, but rather of the contributions from sundry fields of endeavor adopted by surgeons to insure that invasion of the chest for appropriate reasons could be done with ever increasing impunity.

It is clear that the first obstruction to successful intrathoracic surgery was posed by an open and uncontrolled pneumothorax. The ability to render a patient unconscious through narcosis did not alter this problem. It was obvious that the lungs had to maintain function. This problem was attacked in two basic ways. In the earlier attempts, the lung was kept inflated by application of positive pressure at the entry of the airway. In the mid 1890s, this was done by pressure chambers constructed to enclose the patient's head, or by various tubes adapted from the intubation techniques employed in laryngeal diphtheria, or by tight-fitting face masks, for example. These earlier attempts were, however, more or less isolated instances, and it seems that no clearly definable program evolved prior to early 1900.

In 1903, Sauerbruch, working with Mikulicz, developed a differential pressure chamber, reversing the approach and proposing to keep the lungs inflated by applying negative pressure to the chest. In this technique, the head remained outside the chamber at atmospheric pressure, and the thorax was enclosed within the chamber wherein subatmospheric pressure was created. Such chambers were created to house not only the patient but the entire operating team as well (Fig. 1).

In 1909, Meltzer and Auer exploited the concept of endotracheal intubation in a manner comparable to that in use today. They began with a simple tube used to insufflate the lungs and described their method as "continuous respiration without respiratory movements." Although use of endotracheal catheters and even possibly cuffed ones may date back to the experiments of Vesalius, the clinical application of the method for thoracic surgery is credited to Meltzer and Auer.

It is interesting that prior to World War II local anesthesia was frequently a favored technique of thoracic surgeons. The poor control of bronchial secretions and the ever present danger of aspiration during drainage procedures for empyema (particularly if a bronchopleural fistula existed), or of a lung abscess, dictated this technique because it insured that the patient could cough and have control over his own secretions.

Fear of the danger of deep narcosis with its obtunding effect on cough led many to combine nitrous oxide analgesia with local infiltration, particularly in operating upon tuberculosis, even while undertaking such extensive procedures as thoracoplasty. The evolution of various anesthetic agents has been of particular advantage to thoracic surgery.

The diagnostic potential of Röntgen's discovery of the x-ray in 1895 is obvious. The exciting possibilities of this discovery were so quickly recognized that attempts were being made before the end of 1896 to find practical contrast media. Although numerous investigators had studied the tracheobronchial tree of animals and patients, bronchography became an established technique only with the introduction of Lipiodol by Forestier and Sicard in 1922.

Discovery of means of inspecting remote body recesses long challenged physicians but was delayed by the problems of illumination. Visualization of the

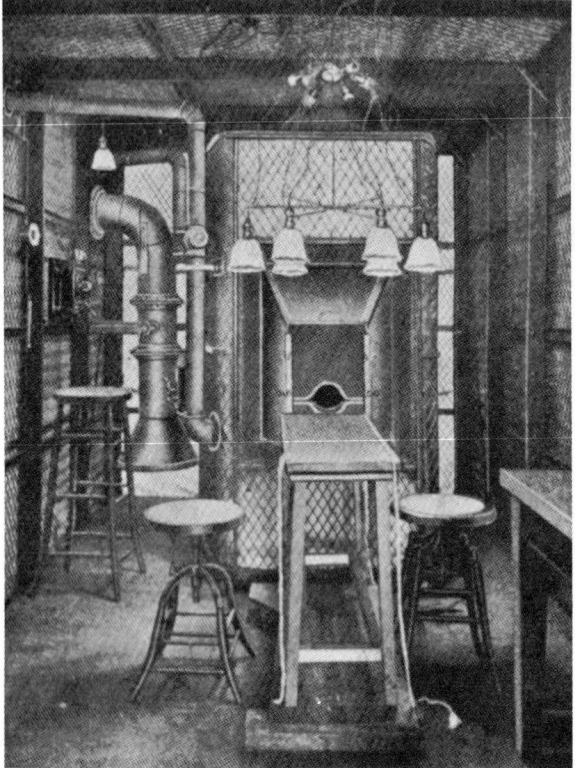

Figure 1. The Sauerbruch chamber as it was ultimately developed by Dr. H. Willy Meyer of New York City. The interior of the chamber accommodated the surgeons, the surgical table, and the patient's body below the neck. The patient's head and the anesthetist were enclosed in the smaller chamber shown at the end of the table, which provided positive pressure. This universal chamber then provided both negative and positive factors for control of surgical pneumothorax. (From Miscall, L. (Ed.): 50th Anniversary Booklet, American Association for Thoracic Surgery. New York, 1967.)

larynx under reflected light was first accomplished about 1858. It was von Mikulicz who developed esophagoscopy utilizing rigid tubes and reflected light in the early 1880s. Once direct laryngoscopic examination became feasible, inspection of the airway then followed. Killian is credited with being the "father of bronchoscopy" and demonstrated the clinical value of this technique by removing a foreign body from the bronchus in 1897.

Just at the turn of the century, Einhorn devised an esophagoscope with an auxiliary tube in the wall of the main tube that served as a light carrier to the distal end. In 1904, Chevalier Jackson combined the lighting principle of the Einhorn esophagoscope with the tube of Killian. The amazing skill acquired by the Jacksons, father and son, in the removal of foreign bodies and in the interpretation of changes induced by disease placed endoscopy apart as a highly developed field of specialization.

There is little doubt that the ability to replace blood losses by transfusion has been essential in the development of thoracic surgery and has permitted the specialty to become established. As the hazards and complications of blood transfusion, particularly the transmission of hepatitis, became more evident,

greater care in blood utilization developed. Interestingly it was in the environment of thoracic surgery that the feasibility of utilizing the patient as his own donor (autologous transfusion) was demonstrated.

To one who never treated lung abscess, bronchiectasis, or empyema before the advent of penicillin, it is difficult to describe the toxicity, the chronicity, and the fetor of patients in nontuberculous thoracic surgical wards before 1945. The tedium of postural drainage, and of serial bronchoscopies to aspirate secretions and shrink the appropriate draining bronchial orifices by topical applications, and the interminable sessions of tube and dressing changes are difficult to visualize. By eliminating the former risk of flooding the bronchial tree during operation and dispelling the dread of spreading the disease by this means, the antibiotics have truly earned their reputation as "miracle drugs." The various antibiotics, properly selected, can change the course of suppurative pneumonitis from necrosis to resolution and can reduce, if not eliminate, the sputum of the patient with bronchiectasis. The greatly enhanced curability of pneumonia has rendered empyema, bronchiectasis, and lung abscess uncommon entities in daily practice.

In tuberculosis, equally profound changes have been effected by eliminating from surgical consideration most minimal and moderately advanced lesions but preserving from death the victim of advanced disease who then becomes a candidate for surgery. The antituberculous agents have changed the surgical approach in the disease from collapse procedures to resection. By shortening drastically the period of hospitalization, these drugs have eliminated the need for many of the sanatorium beds and have permitted care of this disease in general hospitals or even on an outpatient basis. Since tuberculosis incidence and mortality figures had dropped markedly before the availability of these drugs, control of the "white plague" must be ascribed to factors other than chemotherapy (Fig. 2).

It seems strange that throughout the succession of wars no concerted opinion with respect to the management of thoracic wounds evolved. It is clear that the ancients understood the significance of a "sucking" chest wound. Advocates of prompt closure recognized the immediate physiologic benefits, but the proponents of leaving such wounds open had in mind the provision of egress for the blood and ultimately the more or less inevitable pus. Many from the latter school did use packing or other means to establish controlled forms of drainage. The apparent lack of physiologic information kept the debate alive well into World War I. It is remarkable indeed that a method of preventing unwanted entry of air into the chest while providing for egress of blood or pneumothorax air took so long to evolve as an accepted practice. The mechanical methods for providing this closed drainage were devised in the latter part of the nineteenth century. The exact credit for this contribution in terms of priority appears to be due Hewitt in 1876 in England, von Bülau in 1891 in Germany, and Subbotin in 1888 in Russia. It is likely that von Bülau applied water-seal drainage as early as 1875 and thus is generally conceded to be the originator of the method.

The treatment of purulent pleural effusions, *empyema,* has followed an evolution similar to the development of the understanding of thoracic physiology. The critical time in this area came in 1918, when the United States was mobilizing its manpower for World War I. The pandemic of "influenza" and its complications attacked the aggregates of soldiers in various army camps. This infection in recruits was often followed by streptococcic pneumonia with a high incidence of empyema. It was the current practice to provide open surgical drainage as soon as the infected effusion was recognized. In the army camps the mortality reached 30 per cent with occasional peaks in some areas of over 70 per cent.

It was undoubtedly the rather satisfactory results achieved in civilian practice with open drainage of empyema that led to a similar practice in the military hospitals. The important difference, however, seemed to be that civilian experience was obtained principally with pneumococcic infections instead of streptococcic infections. The difference in behavior between these two infections helps explain the difference in results obtained by early surgical drainage. The pneumococcus produced a heavy fibrinous exudate and the surgeon had a better chance of entering a localizing pleural abscess and much less risk of incurring a total pneumothorax at drainage. Furthermore, the pneumonic process had generally subsided before the onset of the pleural extension. Thus, pneumococcic empyemas were, in the main, postpneumonic. In contrast, the army experience involved empyema that was metapneumonic in time. Thus, when evacuation of this relatively thin pleural fluid was done by surgical drainage, an open and sucking pneumothorax often resulted, in a patient already very ill from pneumonia.

The physiologic studies performed by Graham and Bell as members of the U.S. Army Empyema Commission yielded great clarification of the pathologic physiology of pneumothorax and established the management of pleural empyema. These principles were (1) drainage, but with the careful avoidance of an open pneumothorax during the period of active pneumonia; (2) early sterilization and obliteration of the cavity; and (3) maintenance of the nutrition of the patient. Open drainage was feasible when sufficient fibrinous deposit had occurred so that an encapsulated space might reasonably be expected. This point in time was suggested by the proportion of sediment to the total amount of a pleural fluid sample aspirated and allowed to settle overnight. Thus, when a sample of pleural fluid in a container taped to the bed showed 75 to 80 per cent sediment and 20 to 25 per cent supernatant liquid, the time for drainage had probably arrived.

The principal problem in chronic pleural disease was the pleural space that persisted without being filled by the expanding lung. In very simplified terms, if the lung would not rise to meet the chest wall, the chest wall would have to be taken to meet the lung. In a rather oversimplified manner, the various steps in accomplishing this can be illustrated by the following examples of thoracoplasties. The simplest is the *Estlander* type. This consists of subperiosteal removal of appropriate lengths of ribs so that the parietal portion of the empyema cavity can collapse centrally and help obliterate the residual cavity. Over large or total empyema cavities, the procedure begins at the first or second rib and extends as far as necessary, being staged as required by the magnitude of the resection.

A further step in insuring the obliteration of the empyema cavity is typified by the *Schede* thoracoplasty. Here the full thickness of the parietal portion of the empyema space is resected—ribs, intercostal muscles, and parietal empyema wall—so as to saucerize the empyema space and allow the extracostal muscles to fall onto the visceral bed and ultimately obliterate it. This process is mutilating and slow in achieving its ultimate goal, which is, of course, final healing and cessation of drainage. The final step is to remove the visceral "peel" of the empyema in order to allow the entrapped lung to balloon out and obliterate the space. This can be combined with resection of the entire empyema sac or merely resection of the visceral coat (Fowler or Delorme) or by crosshatching the visceral peel, permitting the lung to expand through this released area to fill the chest.

During World War II, a renewal of interest in the problems of the pleura took place. During the North African campaign, it became evident to Army surgeons that blood in the pleura does in fact clot. This was contrary to the suggestion that respiratory motion tended to defibrinate blood so that intrapleural blood remained liquid, in contradistinction to extrapleural blood, which uniformly clotted. When this pleural clot became infected, the standard approach to management by drainage merely evacuated the center of the clot. The periphery of this clot remained as an organizing pleural peel.

On the conclusion that this was in fact the case, a direct attack on the problem resorted to thoracotomy and evacuation of the clot while also lifting the peel of organized fibrin from the lung surface, thereby allowing the lung to expand. The first such formal decor-

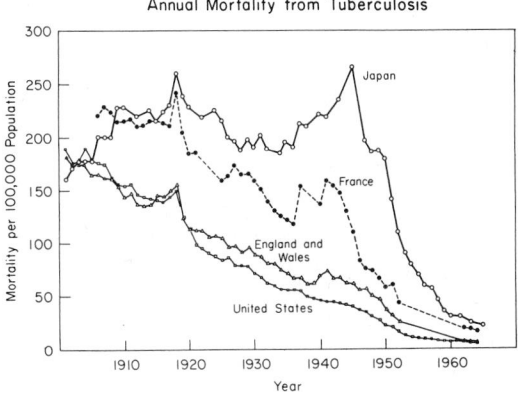

Figure 2. This graph illustrates the value of general measures in the control of tuberculosis. It is seen that the mortality rates had been steadily falling in England and Wales as well as the United States long before antituberculosis drugs became available during the mid 1940s to early 1950s. These drugs did, however, accelerate the fall in mortality rates, and this was particularly dramatic in the case of France and Japan, as depicted in this graph. The effect of a breakdown in general control measures during World War I and World War II is highlighted by the experience in the latter two countries. (From Myers, J. A.: Dis. Chest, *51*:500, 1967.)

tication was carried out by Burford in 1943. This became the established management for such an organizing hemothorax. Thoracotomy was advocated at 3 to 6 weeks after injury. At that time the "peel" was sufficiently established to permit handling with technical ease, yet had not gone on to sufficient fibrosis to make it a difficult undertaking. When infection was evident (hemothoracic empyema), an earlier thoracotomy was proper. Before this, surgeons had usually carried out a lesser procedure referred to as "turning out the clot." This limited intrapleural maneuver did in fact evacuate the clot but did not necessarily provide for prompt expansion of the lung. Suppuration was not unexpected under these circumstances because the organizing visceral peel tended to perpetuate the pleural space. Complete mobilization of the entrapped lung was carried out even in the face of infection. Although basically this was the same operation as that described by Fowler and Delorme, it was bolder and more efficacious. It was indeed a distinct conceptual contribution.

Prior to assured control of open pneumothorax, surgery for neoplasms or suppuration in the mediastinum was undertaken through an extrapleural approach, with displacement of one or both pleurae for access and maneuverability. This was a tedious technique, since disruption of the pleura changed the outlook for the procedure very decidedly. Control of surgical pneumothorax, however, permitted a free choice between an extrapleural and a transpleural approach as dictated by the exigencies of the surgical problem.

As experience accumulated with resection of lung tissue, tension pneumothorax (incident to insecure bronchial closure) and infection were common causes of death. It emerged that greater likelihood of success existed when the pleural space was obliterated by adhesions so that air leaks and the products of infection could be limited. The efficacy of this circumstance, particularly in suppuration, led to the application of various maneuvers intended to reduce the postoperative pleural space. These included performance of thoracoplasties, the paralyzing of the hemidiaphragm, and production of pleural symphysis before or after the resection.

The induction of a pneumothorax followed by talc poudrage to the healthy lobe surface under visual control through a thoracoscope and prompt (it was hoped) re-expansion of the lung represented the ultimate in a first-stage lobectomy. The chest would be entered at a later date for separation of the diseased lobe and approach to the lung root. The hilar structures were generally managed by mass ligation. The encircling ligature, rubber tubing for example, was often left in place in the anticipation that the lung would slough in 10 days to 2 weeks. The pleural space would be packed. Refinements in means of narrowing the hilum as well as securing it by sutures permitted amputation of the lobe or lung rather than sloughing. Notable was the introduction of hilar tourniquets. These were essentially cord snares used to encircle the hilum so that appropriate suturing of the hilar stump could be safely carried out after the lobe had been amputated. They were applicable to lobectomy as well as pneumonec-

tomy. In suppurative diseases, actual cautery to destroy the infected lung was also employed. This procedure was performed in stages and provided improved drainage of the area of pulmonary disease as well as extirpation of the offending portions of lung. Improved handling of the hilar structures by individual treatment of bronchus, arteries, and veins while under protection of an encircling tourniquet, and the provision of drainage for the pleura, led to improved results. From initial mortality levels of 50 and 60 per cent, Brunn could report a mortality rate of 13 per cent in a small series and Alexander a 16 per cent mortality rate in a somewhat larger group a short time after these procedures became available.

It is difficult to single out those responsible for the earliest successes with lobectomy. Amputation of some portion of lung with survival is recorded even in ancient times, and Tuffier is usually credited with the first successful resection of a tuberculous lesion by partial lobectomy in 1892. The frequency of pulmonary resection increased thereafter. For removal of an entire lung, priorities are somewhat clearer. In 1931, Nissen, working in Germany with Sauerbruch, extirpated a left lung destroyed by bronchiectasis in a staged procedure using an encircling hilar ligature of rubber, allowing the lung to slough. In 1932, Haight, working with Alexander in Ann Arbor, likewise extirpated a left lung destroyed by bronchiectasis from a young woman. The resection was staged, the hilum was encircled with rubber tubes, and the lobes were allowed to slough. This represented the first successful pneumonectomy in the Western Hemisphere.

In 1933, Graham in St. Louis removed a left lung for epidermoid carcinoma using a rubber tourniquet for control, amputating the lung, securing the hilum with suture ligatures, and then removing the tourniquet. Although there were postoperative complications, the patient, a physician, survived for 30 years. The first successful resection of a right lung is credited to Overholt in 1934.

The individual ligation technique for lobectomy had apparently been used as early as 1912 by Davies in England. This approach was repeatedly used by Churchill for lobectomies after 1938. It was Churchill and Belsey who developed *segmentectomy* for the lingular division of the left upper lobe in cases of bronchiectasis. Shortly after Graham performed his operation, Reinhoff reported pneumonectomy by individual treatment of the hilar structures. Surgical advances spurred the quest for more detailed anatomic information, and even though this did incite anatomists to respond, the practical details of bronchial and hilar anatomy were supplied originally by the surgeons themselves. The greatest utilization of segmental resection occurred in the management of pulmonary tuberculosis as popularized by Chamberlain.

Prior to the advent of antimicrobial drugs, the control of pulmonary suppuration was difficult. The medical management of bronchiectasis or lung abscess was not highly rewarding and surgical therapy was fraught with hazards. Neither approach offered great dependability or results. In the care of lung abscess, the various medical and supportive measures were applied, in the hope that the process would stabilize. If adequate drainage was not provided via the bronchial communication, external drainage was the approach of choice. After appropriate localization of the abscess and selection of the site where it contacted the chest wall and where pleural fusion was most likely, one or more ribs were resected, under local anesthesia. After it was ascertained that a pleural symphysis existed, the abscess cavity was entered, preferably by cautery, with the objective of sealing the lung parenchyma and insuring against air embolism. If symphysis was missing, gauze packing was placed and the wound closed, in the hope that this foreign body would cause symphysis to occur and be strong enough to support a drainage tract when the procedure was attempted again some 2 weeks later. Drainage from such abscesses was often prolonged, although a number of successful results were reported.

Advances in the ability to examine the esophagus by x-ray and endoscopically elicited increasing interest in this organ. The field is still developing. Prior to better control of the physiologic problems with open thoracotomy, attack on diseases in this area was primarily extrapleural and endoscopic.

The first successful resection (incidentally with long survival) of esophageal carcinoma was performed by Torek in 1913. When reporting the successful resection of a carcinoma of the esophagus with intrathoracic esophagogastrostomy 25 years later, Adams and Phemister could find only some 30 limited successes in the interim.

Efforts to reduce the ravages of *tuberculosis* began with the realization that total body rest provided the best marshaling of the defenses against the disease. This collecting of patients in one area generally provided with abundant fresh air to which was added rest and nutritious food established the sanatorium regimen. All this stimulated interest in the disease and segregated its victims, thereby reducing the contagiousness of the process. The debate that had raged over contagiousness in this disease had been solved by the work of Koch when he isolated the tubercle bacillus and demonstrated his postulates.

The observation that nature tended to immobilize and contract the chest in tuberculosis sparked the concept of achieving this as a therapeutic measure. Measures ranging from the placement of sandbags or having the patient lie on the affected side to intercostal neurectomy and scalenotomy were suggested as means of immobilizing the thoracic cage.

Introduction of air into the pleura-pneumothorax to directly rest the lung was apparently conceived by Carson about 1825, applied by Forlanini in Italy just before the turn of the century, and highly publicized by Murphy in 1898. Saugman added control to the process by introducing the manometer in 1904.

When visceroparietal adhesions prevented appropriate collapse by pneumothorax, these adhesions were divided by cautery under vision through a thoracoscope. This operation was referred to as "closed" pneumolysis and was developed by Jacobaeus in 1913. Rarely was an open approach for dividing such adhesions considered. Complications of pneumothorax were frequent and effusions of pyogenic or tuberculous etiology were common. Limitations in re-expansion were all too frequent after the requisite 4 to 6 years of collapse had transpired and were associated with a penalty in reduced pulmonary function. During the 1940s, intraperitoneal injection of air, producing *pneumoperitoneum*, was used to elevate the diaphragms and cause pulmonary collapse. Although less liable to complications, this approach was also less effective.

Phrenic nerve paralysis produced by crushing the nerve in the neck, introduced by Stuertz in 1911, enjoyed great popularity as a simple yet reversible (in 6 to 9 months) means of elevating the corresponding hemidiaphragm. Permanent paralysis by sectioning or avulsing the nerve had little usage.

The idea of resecting ribs to produce pulmonary collapse, *thoracoplasty,* probably originated with de Cerenville about 1885. The technique underwent many modifications contributed by Brauer, Friedrich, Boiffin, Gourdet, Wilms, and Sauerbruch. It finally became established as the most reliable of the collapse

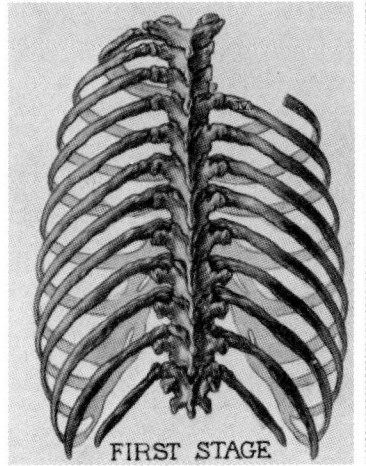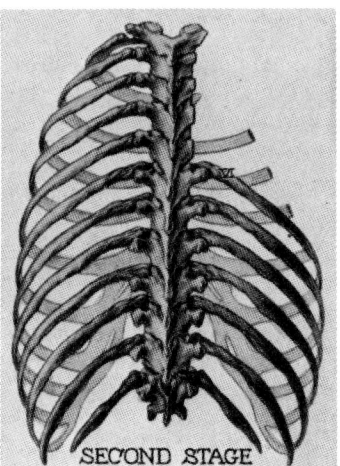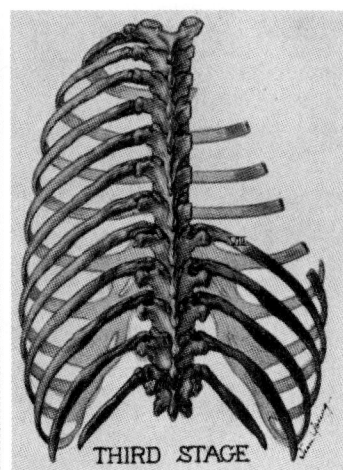

Figure 3. General schema for staged thoracoplasty as practiced by John Alexander. (From Alexander, J.: The Collapse Therapy of Pulmonary Tuberculosis. Springfield, Ill., Charles C Thomas, Publisher 1937.)

procedures. Its standard form required resection of long lengths of the upper seven ribs subperiosteally in three stages, including removal of the transverse processes of the corresponding vertebrae after the manner of Alexander and O'Brien of Detroit (Fig. 3). Further elective collapse could be provided by anterior stages if necessary. Freeing the apex of the lung in an attempt to bring an upper lobe cavity to a point for better collapse under the thoracoplasty, a procedure termed "apicolysis," was practiced by Semb of Norway in the late 1930s.

The era of chemotherapy began with the introduction of streptomycin in 1944. In 1952, isoniazid was introduced and became the keystone of chemotherapeutic regimens. Prior to this time, resection had been infrequently employed in the treatment of pulmonary tuberculosis. It was found that patients with active pulmonary tuberculosis not brought under control by chemotherapy did poorly after these earlier resections. Insistence on conversion of sputum to negative and clearing of pneumonic areas of disease to a point of radiologic stability with drug therapy greatly improved the success of resection. The lesions that remained after these points had been reached by means of chemotherapeutic control became the targets of surgical resection. The efficacy of the new and improved drug regimens (Myambutol and rifampin particularly) has now greatly changed the prognosis of this disease, and the need for surgical intervention is further reduced.

SELECTED REFERENCES

Alexander, J.: The Collapse Therapy of Pulmonary Tuberculosis. Springfield, Ill., Charles C Thomas, Publisher, 1937.
Afflicted by the very disease that led to his worldwide recognition, Alexander worked under the handicap of renal and osseous tuberculosis. This volume reflects the penchant for meticulous detail and completeness that characterized this highly disciplined man. It contains all that was of value in the management of pulmonary tuberculosis to the date of its publication in 1937. A medical counterpart, his long-time colleague, John B. Barnwell, was a contributor to the book.

Brock, R. C.: The Anatomy of the Bronchial Tree with Special Reference to the Surgery of Lung Abscess. New York, Oxford University Press, 1946.
This classic publication correlating an anatomic study of the bronchial tree with the clinical problem of lung abscess appeared at a time when antibiotics were changing surgical management in this disease from drainage to resection. It points up the relative scarcity of anatomic detail available from descriptive anatomists for the tracheobronchial tree.

Crafoord, C.: On the technique of pneumonectomy in man. Acta Chir. Scand. (Suppl. 54), 81:1, 1938.
This profusely illustrated monograph describes the experimental as well as the clinical experiences to that date. The author includes his own technique of anesthesia, thoracotomy, and management of the hilar structures.

Eloesser, L.: Milestones in chest surgery. J. Thorac. Cardiovasc. Surg., 60:157, 1970.
As invited speaker before the American Association for Thoracic Surgery in 1970, Eloesser, the oldest living member of that organization, recounted some of the milestones in thoracic surgery, to the delight of his audience.

Graham, E. A., Singer, J. J., and Ballon, H. C.: Surgical Diseases of the Chest. Philadelphia, Lea & Febiger, 1935.
This volume is a repository for the ultimate views in thoracic surgery at the time of its publication (1935). The senior author, Graham, a giant among surgeons, a legend in his own time, pushed back many frontiers in surgical physiology. In the pages of this volume, the reader will find much that is basic to the development of thoracic surgery written while history was in the making.

Hochberg, L. A.: Thoracic Surgery Before the 20th Century. New York, Vantage Press, 1960.
This interesting book of considerable size brings together the nebulous background of fable and fantasy against which the halting yet firmer steps of the early 1900s laid the foundation for successful intrathoracic surgical maneuvers.

Kent, E. M., and Blades, B.: The surgical anatomy of the pulmonary lobes. J. Thorac. Surg., 12:18, 1942.
This study by pupils of Evarts A. Graham illustrates how surgeons supplied the practical details of hilar anatomy. Even at this time, they opine that negotiating the left upper lobe hilum might be hazardous and, at times, impossible.

Langston, H. T., and Tuttle, W. M.: The pathology of chronic traumatic hemothorax. J. Thorac. Surg., 16:99, 1947.

Samson, P. C., and Burford, T. H.: Total pulmonary decortication. Its evolution and present concepts of indications and operative technique. J. Thorac. Surg., 16:127, 1947.
These two papers bring together the basic concepts evolved from the military experience of World War II concerning the fate of the blood in the pleura and what to do about it.

Lilienthal, H.: Thoracic Surgery. Philadelphia, W. B. Saunders Company, 1925.
This two-volume work is one of the comprehensive and early American texts on the subject. It represents the gleanings from a large surgical practice, described in voluminous detail, and includes many case histories that illustrate the opinions expressed. It appeared at a time when thoracic surgery was striving for stability as an emerging specialty, and clearly portrays the problems and conflicts of the era.

Meade, R. H.: A History of Thoracic Surgery. Springfield, Ill., Charles C Thomas, Publisher, 1961.
This book culminates a lifelong interest in the history of surgery and specifically that dealing with the chest. It is exhaustive in scope, accurate in detail, and factual in its content. Above and beyond this, it contains much in the way of clinical assessment that lends flavor to the drier facts of history.

Neuhof, H., and Touroff, A. S. W.: Acute putrid abscess of the lung; IV, Surgical treatment and results in eighty-six consecutive cases. J. Thorac. Surg., 9:439, 1940.
This article probably epitomizes the management of lung abscess just before the emergence of the antimicrobial era. "Medical" management was unrewarding and surgical management pre-eminent.

Nissen, R., and Wilson, R. H. L.: Pages in the History of Chest Surgery. Springfield, Ill., Charles C Thomas, Publisher, 1960.
From the pen of the surgeon who first successfully removed an entire lung from a human being, this compendium is concise, accurate, modest, and entertaining. Profusely illustrated, it is a delight to read as it unfolds the story of thoracic surgery.

Sauerbruch, F.: Die Chirurgie der Brustorgane. Berlin, J. Springer, 1920.
This publication presents the output of the dynamic and imaginative service of the man who epitomized thoracic surgery in his time. His clinic attracted worldwide visitors interested in the infant specialty. The text is profusely illustrated by artists' drawings.

Steele, J. D. (Ed.): The Surgical Management of Pulmonary Tuberculosis. Springfield, Ill., Charles C Thomas, Publisher, 1957.
This monograph, prepared by trainees of John Alexander and executed in his honor, brings together in contrast the two eras in pulmonary tuberculosis—that before and that after availability of effective chemotherapy.

II

ANATOMY

Walter G. Wolfe, M.D.

Marcello Malpighi in the seventeenth century demonstrated that the trachea terminated in dilated vesicles and not porous parenchyma. By inflating and then drying a lung, he demonstrated that membranous vesicles formed from the ends of the trachea, which terminated "in spaces and unequal vesicles." [1] These observations made it clear for the first time that air passes from the trachea in and out of the sacs in the lung and provided the anatomic basis for true conception of the respiratory process. In 1880 Christoph Theodor Aeby published a treatise that was the first work of any consequence devoted to analysis of the branching of the bronchial tree.[5] Nine years later William Ewart, a pathologist, recognizing that the human lung must be divided into yet smaller regions than lobes, described nine bronchial distributions.[5]

In 1932 Kramer and Glass,[21] to better localize lung abscess, established smaller and more accurate units within the lobes, which they named *bronchopulmonary segments*. Brock[7, 8] developed the clinical aspects of these segments and Churchill and Belsey[10] established the principle of the bronchopulmonary segments as surgical units. The importance of segmental anatomy was illustrated by Churchill and Belsey's observation that 80 per cent of patients with bronchiectasis in the left lower lobe also had involvement of the lower portion of the upper lobe. They named this segment the *lingula*. In 1943 the decisive studies of Jackson and Huber[16, 17] on the branching of the bronchopulmonary segments were reported and established the terminology accepted today.

While bronchial anatomy was of importance, development of microscopic anatomy led to the study of the lung as a physiologic unit. Malpighi described microscopic anatomy of the alveolus and used the terms "pulmonary artery" and "pulmonary vein." In 1733 Stephen Hales referred to the closed connections between artery and veins described by Malpighi as "capillary vessels."[31] The century-old question of whether alveoli of the mature lung were lined by continuous epithelium or whether the alveolar capillaries as viewed with the conventional light microscope were nakedly exposed to inspired air was resolved with electron microscopic studies of Low[25, 26] when he demonstrated a complete epithelial lining covering each alveolar surface. Electron microscopic study of the lung combined with physical and chemical studies of pulmonary tissue continues to complete and clarify the anatomy of the lung.

EMBRYOLOGY

The primordia of the principal respiratory organs appear as a medial longitudinal groove in the ventral wall of the pharynx.[1, 12] The tube is lined with endoderm from which the epithelium of the respiratory tract develops. The cephalic part of the tube becomes the larynx, followed by the trachea, and from its caudal end, two lateral outgrowths arise, i.e., the left and right lung buds. From these, the bronchi and lungs develop. The right and left lung buds are initially symmetric. Their ends, however, soon become lobulated, three lobules appearing on the right and two on the left. During the course of development, the lungs migrate caudally so that by the time of birth, the bifurcation of the trachea is opposite the fourth thoracic vertebra. As the lungs grow, they project into that part of the coelom which ultimately forms the pleural cavities.

The pulmonary arteries form from the sixth arch.[1] Each pulmonary artery is closely related to the main stem bronchus and provides an arterial partner for each new bronchial ramification. As the airway-artery pairs enter first the lobe, then the segments, and finally lobules of developing lung tissue, they assume a central location in each and project branches toward the particular subdivision of the lung. As the veins develop, they receive tributaries from the pleura and the rich vascular networks developing about the growing tips of the respiratory tree. They arch across the base of the secondary lobules toward the periphery where they turn into the planes of connective tissue that separate adjacent pulmonary lobules. Interlobular veins unite to form and serve as tributaries to intersegmental veins, which, near the pulmonary hilus, combine in most cases into the superior and inferior pulmonary veins.

ANATOMY

The respiratory system consists of the nose, nasal passages, nasopharynx, larynx, trachea, bronchi, and lungs. The respiratory tree functions proximate to the thorax and its bony and muscular components as well as to the pleura, pleural cavity, and mediastinum. The influence of pathologic changes in associated structures on the function of the respiratory system is important, and one should be familiar with these anatomic relationships and the "topographical anatomy" of the thorax[12, 37] (Fig. 1).

Chest Wall and Pleura

Beneath the skin and subcutaneous tissue, the chest wall is covered by the pectoralis muscles anteriorly, and posterolaterally the latissimus dorsi and serratus anterior muscles are encountered. In an anterior thoracotomy, the fibers of the pectoralis major may be split, exposing the intercostal muscles. However, in

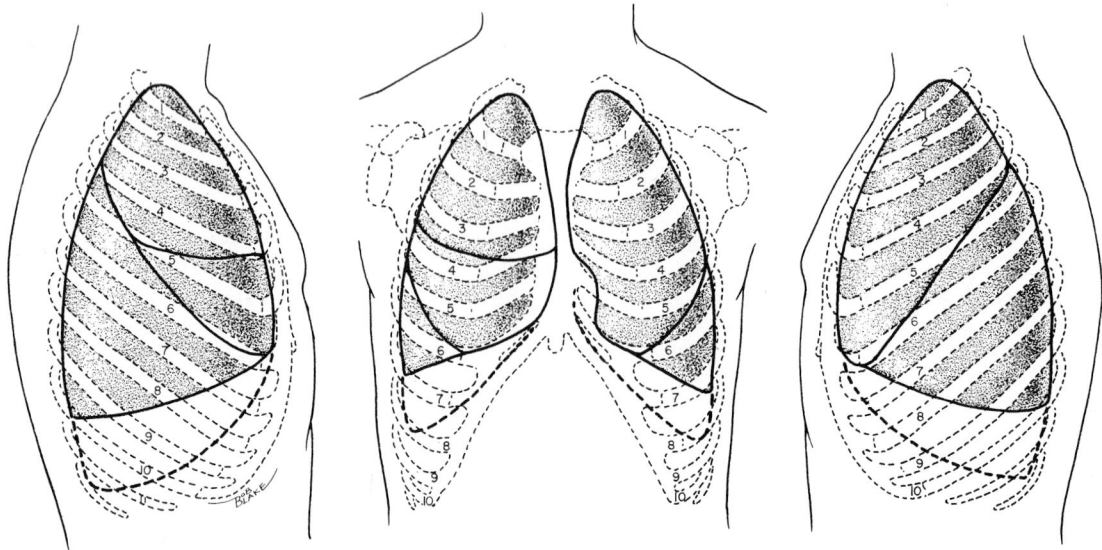

Figure 1. The relationships of the pleural reflections and the lobes of the lung to the ribs. Topographic anatomy and the relationship of the fissures of the lobes to ribs in inspiration and expiration are important in evaluation of the routine PA and lateral chest film.

the standard posterolateral thoracotomy, the latissimus dorsi is divided and then the serratus anterior divided or split. From the standpoint of chest wall mechanics and involvement of chest wall muscles, an anterior thoracotomy is usually better tolerated. However, exposure and control of thoracic structures many times is best through the posterolateral approach, which is the standard thoracotomy incision.

There are 12 pairs of ribs, seven of which are called true ribs where the cartilage articulates with the sternum and the lower five called false ribs, which are not connected directly to the sternum. The eleventh and twelfth ribs are called floating ribs, as they are not attached anteriorly. The sternum is divided into the manubrium, the body, and the xiphoid. The clavicle articulates with the sternum and the first costal cartilage. This is an important relationship, as a posterior dislocation of the clavicle can cause respiratory distress secondary to compression of the trachea by the head of the clavicle.

Muscles associated with the intercostal space are the external, internal, and transversus thoracic muscles. There are 11 intercostal spaces containing a vein, an artery, and a nerve, which course along the lower edge of each rib. All the intercostal spaces are wider in the front than posteriorly, the widest being the third.

The parietal pleura is divided into four parts, costal, cervical, diaphragmatic, and mediastinal. The costal pleura lines the ribs, cartilages, and vertebral bodies and is the thickest portion of the parietal pleura. The visceral pleura covers the lungs so firmly that it is not possible to strip it from the lung tissue under normal circumstances.

The internal mammary artery and vein rise from the first portion of the subclavian artery opposite the thyrocervical trunk and descend along the sternum to anastomose with the superior epigastric artery. The

lymphatics in the chest wall and their drainage patterns are important and will be covered in the section on carcinoma of the breast.

TRACHEA

The entrance to the trachea is guarded by the larynx. It functions to prevent aspiration and as the organ of phonation and plays an important role in production of the cough. The mucous membrane lining of the larynx is covered by ciliated epithelial cells and a few goblet cells. The epithelial surfaces in contact with food and pressure are covered by stratified squamous epithelium.[13] Except for the cricothyroid muscle, which is innervated by the external laryngeal branch of the superior laryngeal nerve, the larynx receives both motor and sensory innervation by way of the vagal accessory complex of nerve fibers. The intrinsic muscles of the larynx receive their motor innervation by way of the inferior laryngeal branch of the recurrent vagus nerve.[12]

The trachea is a fibromuscular tube 10 to 12 cm. in length and varying from 13 to 22 mm. in width, supported laterally and ventrally by approximately 20 U-shaped hyaline cartilages. The trachea originates at the level of the cricoid cartilage and descends through the superior aperture of the thorax and the superior mediastinum to its bifurcation at the level of the sternal angle (lower border of the fourth thoracic vertebra). Here it divides into the right and left primary bronchi. The spur formed at the point of bifurcation is called the carina. Half the trachea lies in the neck and the other half within the thorax.[12, 20]

The dimensions of the trachea are constantly changing with the movement of the head and neck. It is attached to a movable structure at both ends, namely,

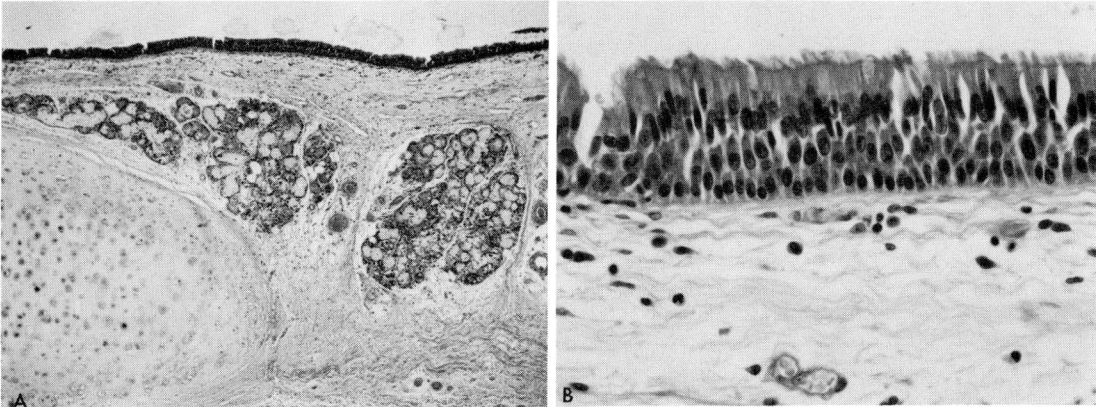

Figure 2. *A*, Photomicrograph of human trachea demonstrating the relationship between epithelium, lamina propria, submucosa, and cartilage. ×45. *B*, Pseudostratified columnar ciliated epithelium containing goblet cells resting on an elastic lamina propria. ×400.

the larynx cranially and the pericardial sac and diaphragm caudally. During forced expiration, especially when the glottis is suddenly opened as in coughing, the trachea is markedly narrowed. In young subjects the lumen may be reduced to one tenth its original size. Prior to cough, the bifurcation may ascend as much as 5 cm.[20]

The mucous membrane of the trachea rests on elastic lamina propria, beneath which is the submucosa. These layers are supported by another fibrous coat containing cartilage and smooth muscle. The dorsal membranous wall is fibromuscular. Smooth musculature elsewhere in the respiratory tree disposes in a helical arrangement about the airways; however, in the trachea it lies only in its dorsal wall. The submucosa varies in thickness with the thinnest portion on the inner surface of the cartilage and the thicker, more loosely organized portion being present on the muscular wall. In addition to blood vessels, nerves, and lymphatics, this layer contains the secretory portions of the mucous and serous glandular units. The trachea is lined with pseudostratified columnar ciliated epithelium containing goblet cells.[13] Near the basement membrane the formative cells may differentiate into new ciliated cells or goblet cells (Fig. 2).

BRONCHI

At its termination, the trachea divides into the right and left principal bronchi. The right bronchus is 12 to 16 mm. in diameter and the left 10 to 14 mm. The combined cross-sectional area exceeds that of the trachea. The right main bronchus deviates less from the axis of the trachea than does the left; this explains why foreign objects entering the trachea more often lodge in the right bronchus or one of its branches.[12, 20]

Within a primary lobe, the secondary bronchus soon divides into tertiary branches, which are remarkably constant in number and distribution. The segment of a lobe, aerated by a tertiary bronchus, is usually well delineated from adjoining segments by nearly complete planes of connective tissue. Knowledge of segmental anatomy is of great practical importance in radiology, bronchoscopy, and pulmonary surgery. Through painstaking anatomic studies of Jackson and Huber[16, 17] and others, the description of the segments of the pulmonary lobes has been completed (Fig. 3). Each segment is identified by its position in the lobe of the lung and the corresponding segmental bronchus is named for the segment it supplies (Fig. 4).

In the human lung, bronchial branches usually

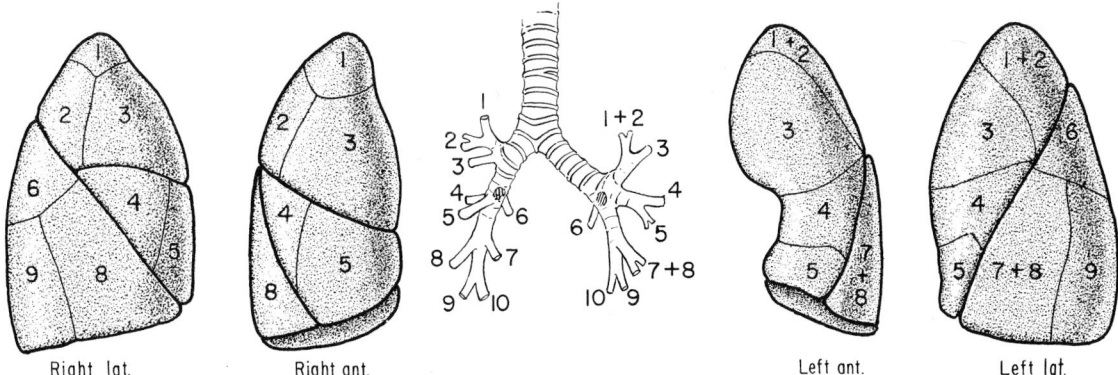

Right lat.   Right ant.   Left ant.   Left lat.

Figure 3. Segments of the pulmonary lobes. (Modified from Jackson, C. L., and Huber, J. F.: Dis. Chest, 9:319, 1943.)

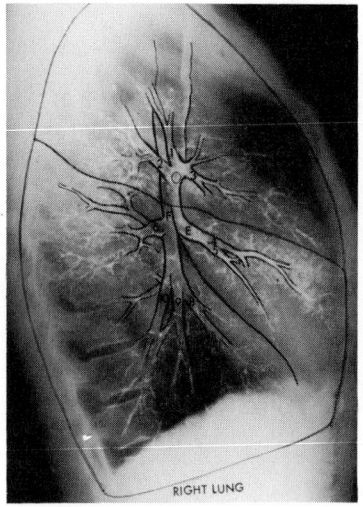
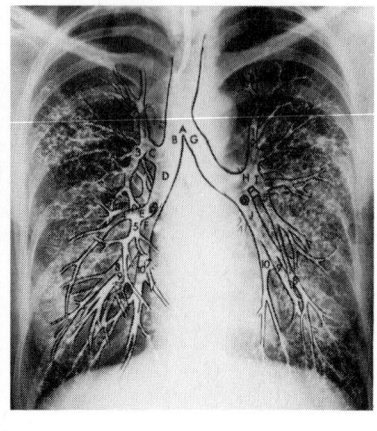
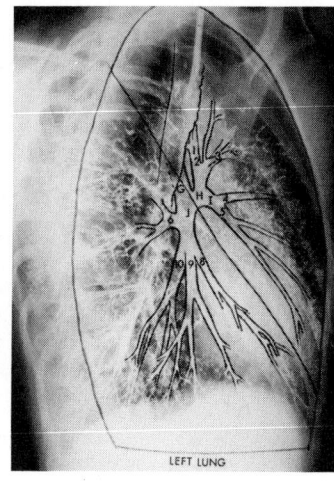

Figure 4.   Normal bronchogram. The major bronchi are indicated by the letters; segmental bronchi are numbered. Key for Figures 3 and 4:

Right

1. Apical ⎫
2. Posterior ⎬ upper lobe
3. Anterior ⎭
4. Lateral ⎫ middle lobe
5. Medial ⎭
6. Superior ⎫
7. Medial (basal) RLL ⎪
8. Anterior basal ⎬ lower lobe
9. Lateral basal ⎪
10. Posterior basal ⎭

A. Carina
B. R. main stem bronchus
C. RUL bronchus
D. Bronchus intermedius
E. RML bronchus

Left

1-2. Apical posterior ⎫
3. Anterior ⎬ upper lobe
4. Superior of lingula ⎪
5. Inferior of lingula ⎭
6. Superior ⎫
7. ⎪
8. Anterior-medial basal ⎬ lower lobe
9. Lateral basal ⎪
10. Posterior basal ⎭

F. RLL bronchus
G. L main stem bronchus
H. LUL bronchus
I. Lingula bronchus
J. LLL bronchus

arise from bifurcations, and although the resulting branches are smaller than the parent stem, their total cross-sectional area is always greater by approximately six fifths (Fig. 5). Structurally, large bronchi do not differ markedly from the trachea. Medium bronchi are distinguished by the large plates of cartilage, by the musculature, and by their relative abundance of glands (Fig. 6). The most peripheral airways containing cartilage are the terminal bronchi. The smaller bronchi have fewer glands, and are distinguished by rich venous plexuses between the muscular and cartilaginous fibrous layers. The effect of bronchial muscle contraction on venous and lymphatic channels probably plays an important role in propelling the vascular fluids toward the hilus of the lung. Also, these rich venous networks are thought to be an important factor in the warming of air en route to the pulmonary parenchyma[20] (Fig. 7).

The mucous membrane of the bronchial mucosa is made up of an epithelium, a basement membrane, and richly vascular and fibrous tunica propria. Like that of the trachea, the bronchial epithelium consists of pseudostratified ciliated and nonciliated cells, including goblet cells.[13] Peribronchial tissue consists of connective tissue that extends from the pulmonary hilus to the primary bronchioles. The peribronchium is continuous with the connective tissue investment of the ar-

terial partners of the bronchi and the connective tissue sheath of the large veins. These connections form the basis for understanding the location and spread of certain types of edema and inflammation and the paths followed by air in and about the lung in interstitial emphysema. Interestingly, the peribronchium occupies a space in which subatmospheric pressure prevails. Von Hayek[14] feels that this subatmospheric pressure plays an important role in the flow of venous blood, lymph, and alveolar fluid as well as in migration of inhaled particulate matter.

CILIATED, GOBLET, AND BRUSH CELLS

It has been demonstrated that each cilia-bearing cell has approximately 270 cilia. Each cilium originates in a basal corpuscle just beneath the cell surface and meaures approximately 0.5 μ in length and 0.14 μ in diameter. The cilium is round on cross section and contains a pair of separate central filaments and a peripheral ring of nine paired, closely branched filaments. Cilia are phylogenetically ancient structures and all cilia, whether in the plant or animal kingdom, have the same basic structure.[18, 20, 36]

Although the cilia are borne by separate cells, these many thousands of cilia beat in an organized, coordin-

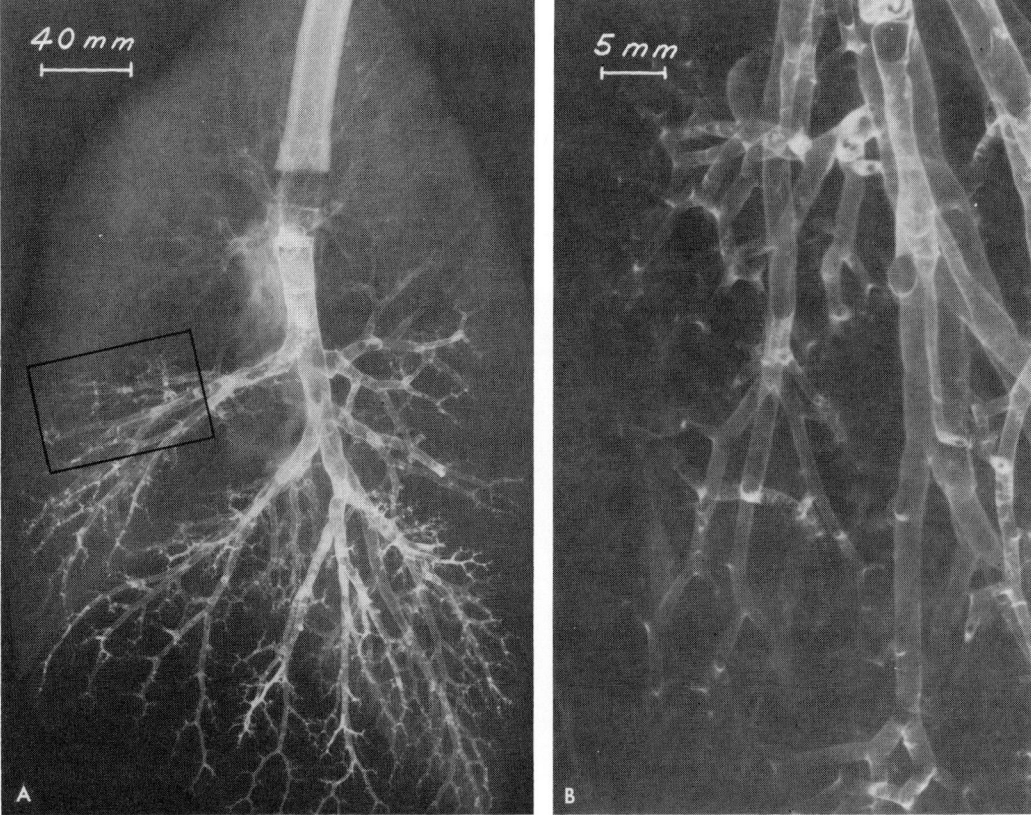

Figure 5. The airways in a postmortem human lung outlined with powdered tantalum, demonstrating in fine detail the branching of the bronchi. (From Nadel, J. A., et al.: Invest. Radiol., *3*:229, 1968.)

ated manner. Studies have shown that they beat in a whiplike fashion, the cycle of activity being divided into a rapid forward propulsive stroke and a slower recovery stroke.[18, 20, 36] This propulsion is effective in moving a superimposed carpet of mucus along with a variable number of trapped particles and cells upward toward the larynx. The rate at which particulate matter is propelled by cilia varies according to species and

that portion of the respiratory tree involved and has been recorded to be approximately 10 to 35 mm. per minute. The cilia do not beat within the viscous sheet of mucus but are bathed instead in fluid of considerably lower viscosity. The source of the fluid, factors controlling its viscosity, and rate of production are not known.[18, 27, 34] The ciliated cells disappear gradually as respiratory bronchioles are approached.

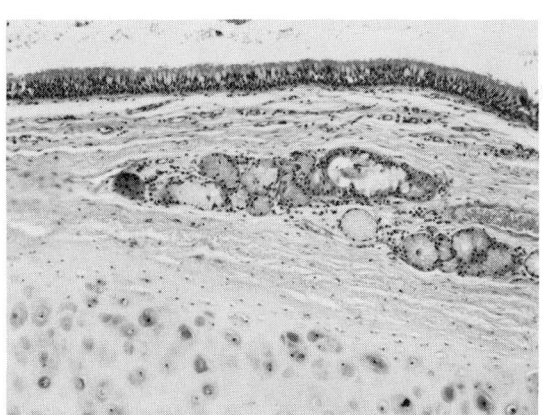

Figure 6. Section through a bronchus. The relationship of the mucosa, glands, and cartilage is essentially the same as that seen in the trachea.

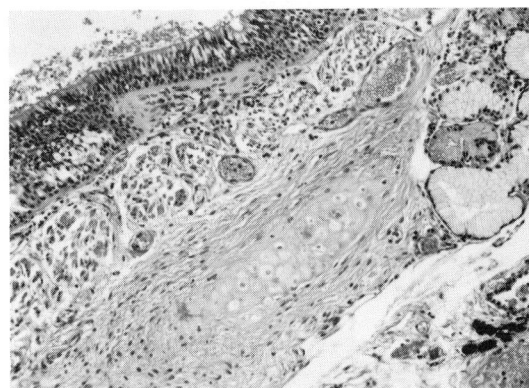

Figure 7. Section of a small bronchus. Note the prominence of the muscle layer as compared to trachea and bronchi, and the rich vascular network between the muscular and cartilaginous fibrous layer. ×100.

The nonciliated cells are the goblet and brush cells. Goblet cells occur singly and in groups between the ciliated epithelial cells. When filled with secretion, they are conspicuous by their bulging walls. In cases of chronic irritation of the tracheobronchial mucosa, there is marked increase in goblet cells at the expense of ciliated cells. It has been suggested that when mucus laden with particles of carcinogenic material has been carried to the branching point of an airway there may be a temporary stasis at that site owing to the local paucity of cilia.[20]

The brush cells are tall, standing from the basement membrane of the lumen of the airway. Electron photomicrographs demonstrate dovetailed cytoplastic processes rearing on their sides interlocking with neighboring goblet cells. This arrangement may serve to add mechanical stability to the epithelial sheet. Whether or not the brush cells are sustentacular in function or are the source of low-viscosity fluid that bathes the cilia is not known.[20, 35]

BRONCHIOLES

Bronchioles are said to have a diameter of 1 mm. or less and to be devoid of cartilage support. Of all the airways, bronchioles have the highest proportion of smooth muscle in their walls relative to the diameter of the lumen. Since small bronchi are also without connective tissue sheaths, the fibrous strands of the fibrocartilagines must extend peripherally into the mucous membrane of the bronchiole. The fibrous elements intermingle freely with the surrounding pulmonary parenchyma, exerting circumferential traction on the airway, maintaining its patency.

Bronchioles of the first order arise at the tip of the terminal bronchus and continue branching to produce three or four further divisions fully lined by cuboidal epithelium. The last to be lined is the terminal bronchiole. Estimates of the number of terminal bronchioles resulting from a single bronchus vary between 10 and 20 (Fig. 8).

A terminal bronchiole usually divides at an angle of 60 to 90 degrees into respiratory bronchioles, which in turn may give rise to further divisions. The branching of the terminal bronchiole is by no means uniform, as a single branch may be given off laterally and two or more may follow (Fig. 9). Respiratory bronchioles vary also in size (in man ranging from 1 through 3.5 mm. in length and approximately 1.5 mm. in diameter). The cuboidal epithelium stops abruptly at the entrance of the alveoli, which are lined by extremely thin squamous epithelium not revealed by conventional light microscopes. The last in a series of respiratory bronchioles usually bifurcate to produce the first in a series of alveolar ducts (Fig. 10).

ALVEOLI

The alveolar ducts terminate in one of several rotunda-like enclosures called alveolar sacs. The sacs bear a small and variable number of terminal alveoli. Like the alveolar ducts, the sacs lack proper walls and

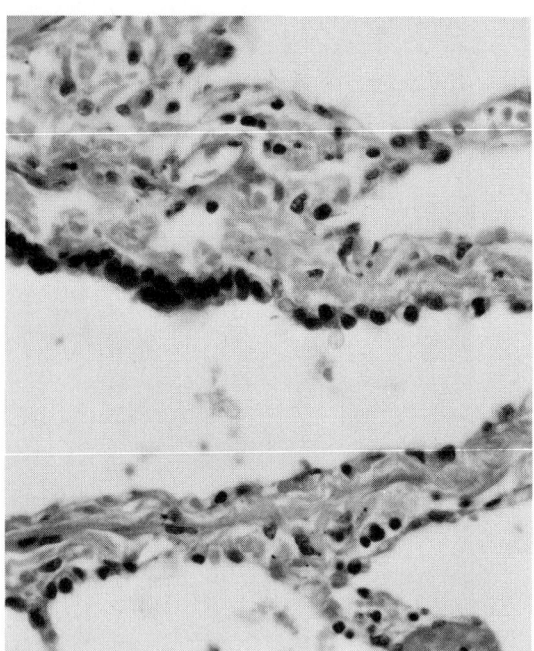

Figure 8. Section of a terminal bronchus, demonstrating the cuboidal epithelium, which grades off into a flat epithelium near the alveolar entrances. Also, a large amount of smooth muscle is evident. ×400.

open on all sides into alveoli. Each alveolus shares an entrance frame and a wall with its neighbor similar to two rooms being separated by a single wall. Because the alveoli surrounding an alveolar duct are an integral part of the pulmonary parenchyma, they are subjected to all of the stages of the respiratory cycle and to tractional forces which hold them open.

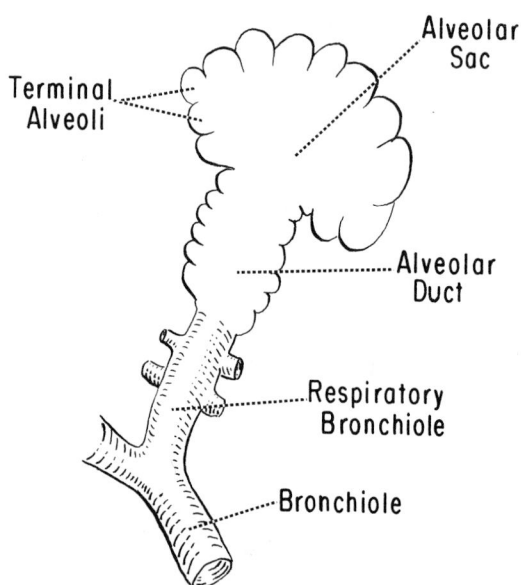

Figure 9. The relationship of the airway in the periphery of the respiratory tree. Bronchioles lead to the respiratory bronchioles, which then terminate in the alveolar duct and the alveolar sac.

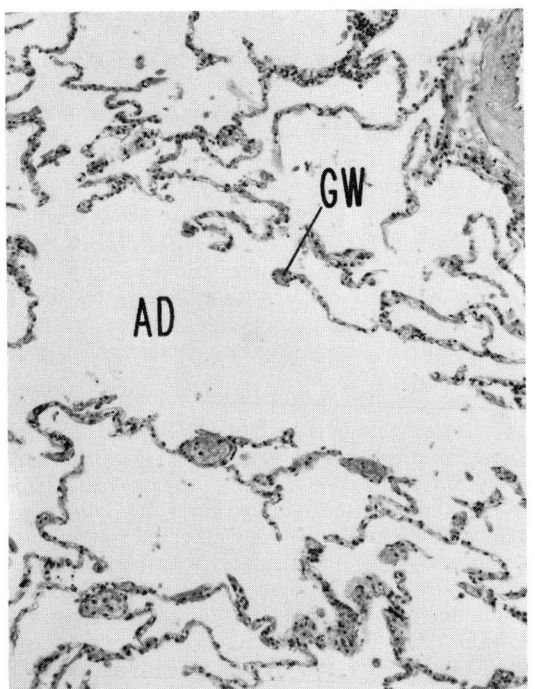

Figure 10. Section of lung demonstrating an alveolar duct (AD) with its contiguous alveoli. Note that the alveolar duct is not a structural entity in and of itself. Its walls are, in fact, alveolar septa. GW is a cross section of a collagen bundle. These bundles are important in maintaining patency of the alveolar ducts and the openings into the alveoli. They are analogous to guy wires.

Pulmonary alveoli vary considerably in shape and size with the various mammalian species, corresponding in general to body size (Fig. 11). The factors determining the dimensions in given species are not clearly understood but probably relate to a combination of factors, including the metabolic rate of the animal and the number and size of red blood cells. In man, the alveoli are approximately 160 μ in size.[20]

ALVEOLAR EPITHELIUM

The alveolar epithelial sheet rests on a basement membrane that lies on or near the basement membrane of the adjacent capillary. The structural layers composing the so-called air-blood barrier are the stratum of the alveolar epithelial cells, their basement membrane, the variable connective tissue layer, basement membrane of the capillary, and the cells of the capillary endothelium (Fig. 12).[2, 19, 25, 26, 32]

Knowledge of the structures separating the alveolar air and capillary blood is of importance. Alveolar epithelial cells are known to be sensitive to the noxious fumes and foreign particles that may be carried by the inspired air. Simple, rapid hypertrophy of the alveolar lining cell layer is possible and the cells are able to undergo metamorphosis into at least one type of alveolar phagocyte.[3, 14, 20, 29] The hypertrophy of the alveolar lining cells could provide the quantity of cells found in the pulmonary alveoli, in the alveolar cell carcinoma, and in the lung disease of sheep ("jagziekte").

There is evidence that some of the alveolar lining cells elaborate secretin products, one of importance being the surface-active fluid layer that lines pulmonary alveoli.[14, 20, 29]

ALVEOLAR CAPILLARY NETWORK

Pulmonary capillary networks are the richest in the body, so dense that openings in them are frequently smaller than the diameter of the capillaries. Since the connective tissue fibers form the principal support of the capillary networks, any disease state, such as

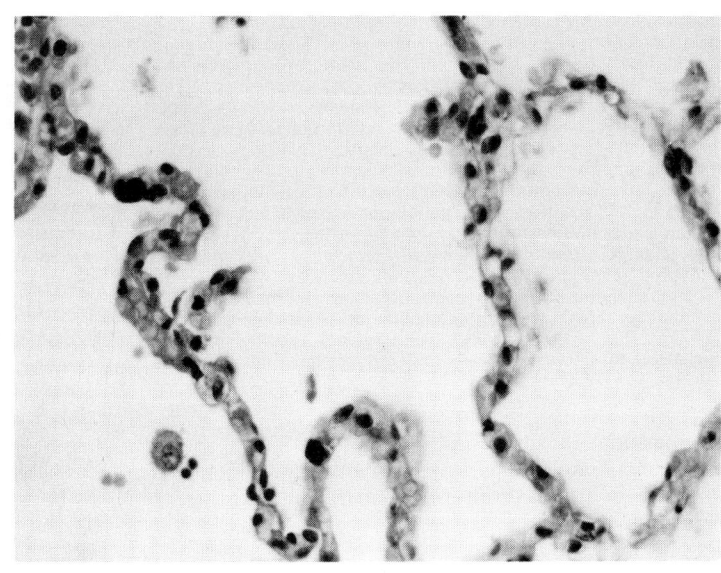

Figure 11. Section through an alveolus. Light microscopy shows the blood-air interface as a simple thin line but when it is seen by electron microscopy (Fig. 12) it is a complex structure. Endothelial and epithelial nuclei are easily seen, but the cytoplasm of these cells cannot be resolved by light microscopy. ×400.

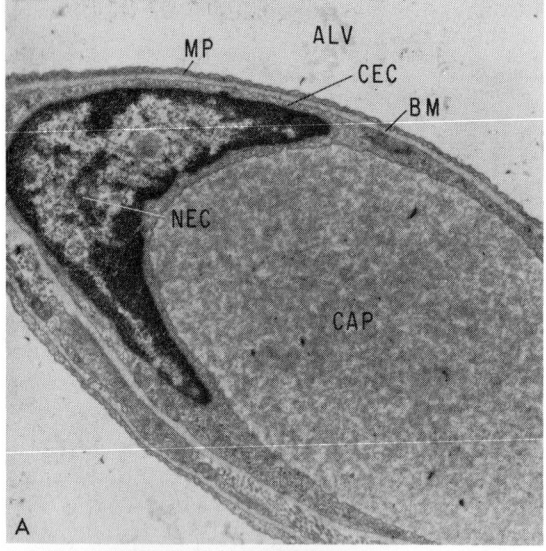

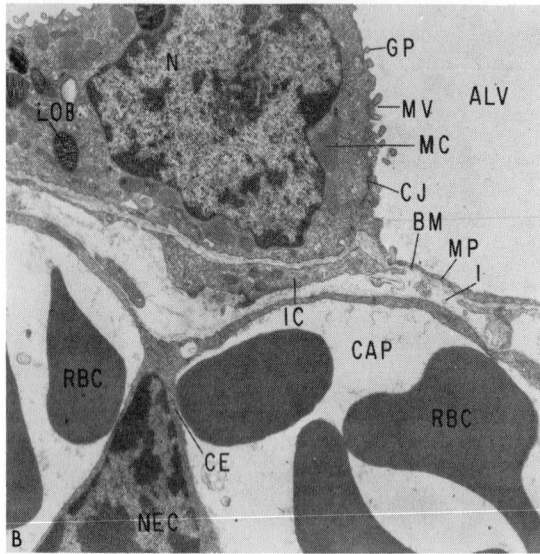

Figure 12. *A,* Electron photomicrograph of an alveolus. This demonstrates the structure of the thinnest part of the blood-air interface. Note that the blood is separated from the alveolar air only by the attenuated cytoplasm of an endothelial cell and a membranous pneumocyte joined by a basement membrane. ×6700; print magnification 13,725. *B,* Note the relationship of the granular pneumocyte to the alveolar wall. The granular pneumocyte is an integral part of the alveolar lining. This cell has been referred to as "Type II cell," "great alveolar cell," and "alveolar phagocyte." It is thought to produce surfactant; the laminated osmiophilic bodies illustrated here may be surfactant or surfactant precursors. ×6700; print magnification 13,725. N, Nucleus of granular pneumocyte; LO, laminated osmiophilic body (these cells thought to be the site of surfactant production); GP, granular pneumocyte (sometimes called the alveolar Type II or the great alveolar cell); MV, microvilli; ALV, alveolus; MC, mitochondria; CJ, cell junction; BM, basement membrane; MP, membranous pneumocyte; I, interstitium; IC, interstitial cell; CAP, capillary; RBC, red blood cell; CE, capillary endothelium; NEC, nucleus of the endothelial cell; CEC, cytoplasm of the endothelial cell.

emphysema, in which there is destruction of the alveolar wall and supporting framework would permit stretching, attenuation, and destruction of the entire capillary bed.[23]

PULMONARY AND BRONCHIAL VESSELS

The surgical anatomy of pulmonary arteries and veins, particularly their relation to each other and to other structures of the pulmonary hilus, is of obvious importance in pulmonary surgery. Knowledge of the "anatomy" of the normal pulmonary angiogram is critical so that pathologic conditions can be recognized (Fig. 13).[6, 12, 37] Pulmonary arteries and their ramifications are invested in connective tissue sleeves, permitting continuous spatial adjustments to changing positions and volumes of surrounding lung tissue. This permits marked dynamic changes in the arterial diameters while not imposing direct mechanical change on lung tissue.

Pulmonary veins do not travel the same course as their arterial partners, a feature that is in marked contrast to the systemic circulation. They course along interlobular connective tissue planes and adapt longitudinally to surrounding parenchyma but cannot withdraw from it. The direct connection of vein to adjacent lung tissue by connective tissue fibers is the anatomic device that makes their diameter largely dependent on lung volume. This arrangement provides the mechanism for promoting venous return in the special situation of the low-pressure pulmonary circuit.

Although blood from the rich pulmonary capillaries undoubtedly supplies the metabolic needs of the pulmonary parenchyma, the many servant tissues (conducting airways, pulmonary vessels, lymphoid tissue, and so forth) require their own circulation supplied by vessels derived from the systemic circulation, the bronchial arteries. These originate either directly from the aorta or indirectly via the intercostals. Bronchial arteries accompany the bronchial ramifications and eventually lose their identity along the respiratory bronchioles where the capillaries that they supply drain into the alveolar capillary network and into the pulmonary veins. There is no bronchial vein corresponding to the bronchial artery; however, there is a rich peribronchial venous network that opens at many points into the pulmonary veins. Although the bronchial veins are described, their presence in normal persons has been questioned. They may, however, appear as sizable vessels in those with diseases such as pulmonary emphysema and mitral stenosis.[11, 23]

Literature on pulmonary vascular anastomoses covers more than two centuries of anatomic studies. Weibel's studies[41] have led him to conclude that pulmonary arteries and veins are end vessels and that there is no possibility for production of the collateral circulation. He found no precapillary arteriovenous pulmonary anastomosis that might permit blood to bypass the alveolar capillary net. Extensive studies of pulmonary vasculature and its anastomotic connection have been made by von Hayek.[14] He has described arterioarterial communications between pulmonary arteries and bronchial arteries, which are distinguishable by their remarkable thickness and unusual corkscrew course in addition to the abundant longitudinal musculature. Nothing is known at present about their importance in the regulation of vascular perfusion in the lung.

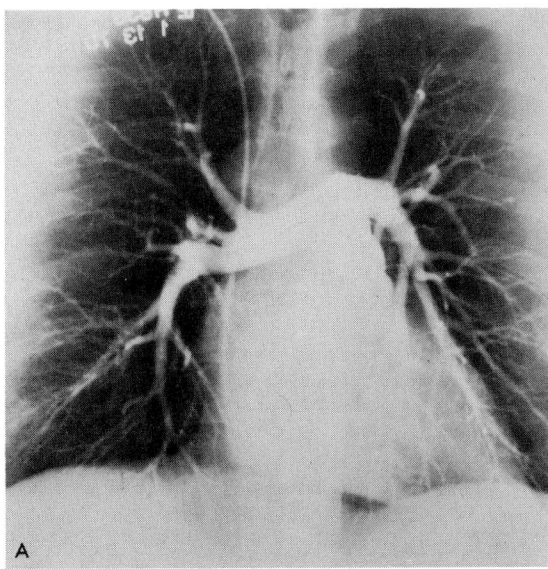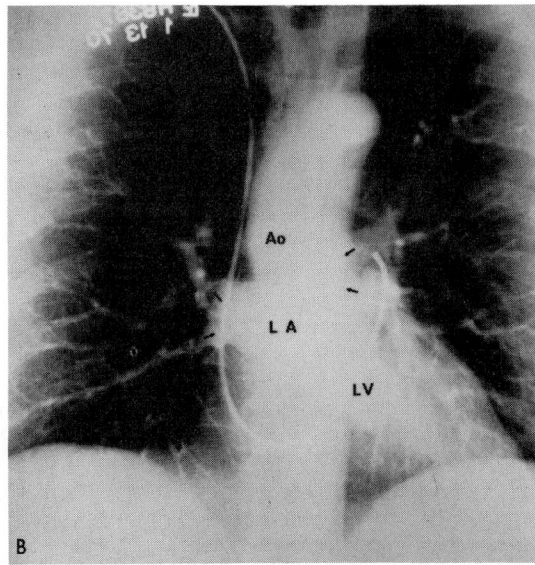

Figure 13. *A*, Normal pulmonary angiogram illustrating the branching of the pulmonary arteries in the right and left lungs to their respective lobes. *B*, Venous phase of the same arteriogram demonstrating the superior and inferior pulmonary veins entering the left atrium (arrows). AO, Aorta; LA, left atrium; LV, left ventricle.

PULMONARY LYMPHATICS

Pulmonary lymphatic vessels enter the hilar region in the second month of fetal life and continue to ramify and produce plexiform channels along the bronchi and pulmonary arteries and veins and in the subpleural connective tissue.[14, 20] According to Miller,[30] the lungs are more extensively supplied by lymphatics than the more metabolically active organs such as the liver and kidneys.

Studies of Tobin[38, 39] have demonstrated that pulmonary lymphatics do extend as far as alveoli. In most instances, the distance between the alveolus and the nearest lymphatic is extremely small. At the pulmonary hilus, the lymphatics, having gained both connective tissue and smooth muscle fibers, are relatively thick-walled and bear a histologic resemblance to the thoracic duct.

Collectively, the lymph nodes found along the lobar branches are called hilar nodes and are included in the great group of nodes about the root of the lung. The tracheobronchial nodes are usually larger on the right. On the left, one or more nodes are commonly related to the ligamentum arteriosum and thus to the recurrent branch of vagus nerve and to the vagal contributions to the anterior pulmonary plexus. Tracheal nodes form chains and are intimately related to the recurrent nerves.

NERVE SUPPLY

Histologic studies and physiologic experiments have shown both afferent and efferent fibers present in the nerves that follow the vessels and airways to the lung.[12, 20] Right and left vagus nerves send one or more bronchial branches to the smaller anterior pulmonary plexus and many others to the rich posterior pulmonary plexus dorsal to the pulmonary hilus. A great many ganglion cells are found scattered along the cer-

vical and thoracic portions of the vagus nerves. Those in the cervical vagus are thought to be sensory, whereas the thoracic vagus is considered to be motor in function. Ganglion cells often lie adjacent to bronchial mucous glands and send short fibers with nonterminal twigs to the cells of glandular epithelium.

Sympathetic nerves arise from the second to fourth thoracic sympathetic ganglia and join the vagi in formation of the pulmonary plexus. The clinical and experimental evidence points to the presence of sympathetic bronchodilator fibers having cells or origin in spinal cord levels T2 to T4.

The phrenic nerve, in addition to the usual fibers of origin in the third to fifth cervical nerves, has been found to receive various contributions from the cervical sympathetics. A number of afferent fibers from the diaphragm as well as the mediastinum also appear to ascend in the phrenic nerve.

COLLATERAL VENTILATION

In airways less than 1 mm. in diameter (bronchioles) reduction of normal traction forces in the lungs by infection, inflammation, fluid accumulation, or secretions singly or in combination may occlude the bronchial lumen. The consequences of such blockage may in some cases be offset by channels of collateral ventilation which form connections between well-aerated alveoli and those normally supplied by the occluded small airway. There are two principal mechanisms of collateral ventilation, interalveolar communications (pores of Kohn) and bronchial alveolar communications.

Alveolar pores are round to oval. Their shape and size are dictated by the delicate encirclements of elastic and other connective tissue fibers. As long as their fibrous framework is intact, the pores cannot enlarge beyond set limits. Alveolar pores may have the beneficial effect of preventing collapse of the lobules supplied by an occluded bronchiole. They may serve also as a temporary lodging place for alveolar phagocytes. Each communication may also provide pathways for the spread of fluid accumulations and for the transmission of bacteria between the communicating pulmonary lobules.[15, 29, 40]

In the past decade Lambert[22] described short, epithelial-like communications between distant bronchioles and neighboring alveoli. Such connections probably escaped discovery until recently because they are difficult or impossible to see in routine sections. They are approximately 30 μ in diameter, thus three or more times the diameter of most interalveolar pores. These communications are evidently able to remain open regardless of the degree of contraction of the bronchiolar smooth muscle. The benefit of pores may be shared only by the immediately adjacent alveoli, while the bronchiole-alveolar communications provide means of aerating hundreds of alveoli. Recently, Chen[9] has demonstrated the dynamic nature of the collateral ventilatory channels.

SELECTED REFERENCES

Boyden, E. A.: Segmental Anatomy of the Lungs, New York, McGraw-Hill Book Company, 1955.
This excellent monograph not only reviews the historical development of the segmental anatomy of the lungs, but provides the groundwork for basic concepts of functional anatomy as it can be applied surgically and to the physiology of respiration.

Hayek, H. von: The Human Lung. translated by V. E. Krahl. New York, Hafner Publishing Company, 1960.
This monograph records the sophisticated anatomy of the respiratory system. It presents some of the newest concepts and findings in the functional anatomy of the lung and is one of the outstanding contributions to this field.

Krahl, V. E.: Anatomy of the mammalian lung. *In* American Physiological Society: Handbook of Physiology. Section 3, Respiration. Vol. I. Fenn, W. O., and Rahn, H. (Eds.). Baltimore, Williams & Wilkins Company, 1964, p. 213.
This chapter on the anatomy of the mammalian lung is one of the most complete treatises on the subject. It also contains more than 200 references, many of which are the original contributions that brought knowledge of the respiratory system to its present state.

Nagaishi, C.: Functional Anatomy and Histology of the Lung. Baltimore, University Park Press, 1972.
This magnificent volume combines studies of both the gross and fine structures of the lung. It has been put together by a thoracic surgeon who clearly recognizes the importance of basic knowledge in understanding and approaching the many difficult clinical problems involving the pulmonary system.

REFERENCES

1. Arey, L. B.: Developmental Anatomy, Revised 7th ed. Philadelphia, W. B. Saunders Company, 1974.
2. Bertalanffy, F. D.: On the nomenclature of the cellular elements in respiratory tissue. Am. Rev. Resp. Dis., 91:605, 1965.
3. Bertalanffy, F. D., and Leblond, C. P.: The continuous renewal of the two types of alveolar cells in the lung of the rat. Anat. Rec., 115:515, 1953.
4. Blumenthal, B. J., and Boren, H. G.: Lung structure in three dimensions after inflation and fume fixation. Am. Rev. Tuberc., 79:764, 1959.
5. Boyden, E. A.: Segmental Anatomy of the Lungs. New York, McGraw-Hill Book Company, 1955.
6. Boyden, E. A.: The nomenclature of the bronchopulmonary segments and their blood supply. Dis. Chest, 39:1, 1961.
7. Brock, R. C.: The Anatomy of the Bronchial Tree with Special Reference to Surgery of Lung Abscess, 2nd ed. New York, Oxford University Press, 1954.
8. Brock, R. C.: The Anatomy of the Respiratory Tree. London, Oxford University Press, 1954.
9. Chen, C., Sealy, W. C., and Seaber, A. V.: The dynamic nature of

10. Churchill, E. D., and Belsey, R.: Segmental pneumonectomy in bronchiectasis. Ann. Surg., 109:481, 1939.
11. Ferguson, F. C., Kobilak, R. E., and Detrick, J. E.: Varices of bronchial veins as a source of hemoptysis in mitral stenosis. Am. Heart J., 28:445, 1944.
12. Goss, C. M. (Ed.): Gray's Anatomy of the Human Body, 28th ed. Philadelphia, Lea & Febiger, 1966.
13. Ham, A. W., and Wilson, T. S.: The Respiratory System in Histology, 4th ed. Philadelphia, J. B. Lippincott Company, 1961, p. 663.
14. Hayek, H. von: The Human Lung. Trans. V. E. Krahl. New York, Hafner Publishing Company, 1960.
15. Hesse, F. E., and Loosli, C. L.: The lining of the alveoli in mice, rats, dogs, and frogs following acute pulmonary edema produced by ANTU poisoning. Anat. Rec., 105:299, 1949.
16. Huber, J. F.: Practical correlative anatomy of the bronchial tree and lungs. J. Natl. Med. Assoc., 41:49, 1949.
17. Jackson, C. L., and Huber, J. F.: Correlated applied anatomy of the bronchial tree and lungs with a system of nomenclature. Dis. Chest, 9:319, 1943.
18. Kilburn, K. H.: A hypothesis for pulmonary clearance and its implications. Am. Rev. Resp. Dis., 98:449, 1968.
19. King, D. W. (Ed.): Ultrastructural Aspects of Disease. New York, Hoeber Medical Division, Harper & Row, 1966.
20. Krahl, V. E.: Anatomy of the mammalian lung. *In* American Physiological Society: Handbook of Physiology. Section 3, Respiration. Vol. I. Fenn, W. O., and Rahn, H. (Eds.). Baltimore, Williams & Wilkins Company, 1964, p. 213.
21. Kramer, R., and Glass, A.: Bronchoscopic localization of lung abscess. Ann. Otol., 41:1210, 1932.
22. Lambert, M. W.: Accessory bronchial alveolar channels. Anat. Rec., 127:472, 1957.
23. Liebow, A. A.: Pulmonary emphysema with special reference to vascular changes. Am. Rev. Resp. Dis., 80:67, 1959.
24. Loosli, C. G.: Intralveolar communications in normal and in pathologic mammalian lungs. Arch. Pathol., 24:743, 1937.
25. Low, F. N.: Electron microscopy of the rat lung. Anat. Rec., 113:437, 1952.
26. Low, F. N.: The pulmonary alveolar epithelium of laboratory mammals and man. Anat. Rec., 117:241, 1953.
27. Luchsinger, P. C., LaGarde, B., and Kilfeather, J. E.: Particle clearance from the human tracheobronchial tree. Am. Rev. Resp. Dis., 97:1046, 1968.
28. Macklin, C. C.: Alveolar pores and their significance in the human lung. Arch. Pathol., 21:202, 1936.
29. Macklin, C. C.: The alveoli of the mammalian lung. An anatomical study with clinical correlations. Proc. Inst. Med. Chicago, 18:78, 1950.
30. Miller, W. S.: The Lung, 2nd ed. Springfield, Ill., Charles C Thomas, Publisher, 1947.
31. Perkins, J. F.: Historical development of respiratory physiology. *In* American Physiological Society: Handbook of Physiology. Section 3, Respiration. Vol. I. Fenn, W. O. and Rahn, H. (Eds.). Baltimore, Williams & Wilkins Company, 1964, p. 62.
32. Porter, K., and Bonneville, M. A.: Fine Structure of Cells and Tissues. Philadelphia, Lea & Febiger, 1968.
33. Pratt, P. C., and Klugh, G. A.: A technique for the study of ventilatory capacity, compliance, and residual volume of excised lungs and for fixation, drying, and serial sectioning in the inflated state. Am. Rev. Resp. Dis., 83:690, 1961.
34. Quinlan, M. F., Salman, S. D., Swift, D. L., Wagner, H. N., Jr., and Proctor, D. F.: Measurement of mucociliary function in man. Am. Rev. Resp. Dis., 99:13, 1969.
35. Rhodin, J. A. G.: An Atlas of Ultrastructure. Philadelphia, W. B. Saunders Company, 1963.
36. Spock, A., Heick, H. M. C., Cress, H., and Logan, W. S.: Abnormal serum factor in patients with cystic fibrosis of the pancreas. Pediatr. Res., 1:173, 1967.
37. Thorek, P.: Anatomy in Surgery. Philadelphia, J. B. Lippincott Company, 1962.
38. Tobin, C. E.: Lymphatics of the pulmonary alveoli. Anat. Rec., 120:625, 1954.
39. Tobin, C. E.: Pulmonary lymphatics with reference to emphysema. Am. Rev. Resp. Dis., 80:50, 1959.
40. Van Allen, C. M., and Lindskog, G. E.: Collateral respiration in the lung. Role in bronchial obstruction to prevent atelectasis and to restore patency. Surg. Gynecol. Obstet., 53:16, 1931.
41. Weibel, E. R., and Gomez, D. M.: Architecture of the human lung. Science, 137:577, 1962.

collateral ventilation. J. Thorac. Cardiovasc. Surg., 59:518, 1970.

III _____

LUNG FUNCTION: PHYSIOLOGIC CONSIDERATIONS APPLICABLE TO SURGERY

Myron B. Laver, M.D.
and W. Gerald Austen, M.D.

For it is much more high and philosophical to discover
things a priori than a posteriori.

— *Robert Boyle, Sceptical Chymist, 1661*

Acute respiratory failure is a common complication in the critically ill patient, and successful prevention requires early and aggressive support of lung function. The problem is of particular concern when the operation is extensive, when the patient has been the victim of severe body trauma, or when he has a history of chronic lung disease.

Understanding of factors that control lung function will allow for early implementation of prophylactic measures, including ventilator support, and will reduce significantly the morbidity and mortality associated with abnormal blood gas exchange.

The considerations to follow will be addressed to the following aspects of lung function: (1) mechanics of gas movement; (2) distribution of ventilation; (3) distribution of blood flow; (4) blood-gas exchange; (5) diffusion of gas between upper airway and pulmonary capillary blood; and (6) respiratory failure.

MECHANICS OF GAS MOVEMENT

Ventilation is composed of three sequential phenomena: pressure change, followed by gas flow, and, finally, volume displacement. The lungs and chest wall (i.e., chest cage and diaphragm) exhibit changes in physical characteristics during the process of ventilation that can be subjected to mathematical formulations. Depending on body position, the abdominal contents may exert a highly restrictive effect on diaphragmatic motion and may in turn influence the effectiveness of pulmonary mechanics.

Action of the respiratory muscles is directed toward overcoming elastic recoil of the lung and resistance to gas flow in the major airways. Deformation of the tissues involved, or viscous resistance, is also a component of flow resistivity, but the energy required to overcome it is small, and we usually consider flow resistivity as the principal source of the work expended to achieve movement of gas.

The changes in volume, flow, and pressure characteristics for a single respiratory cycle are shown in Figure 1.

Elastic recoil (elastance) is expressed as the change of pressure produced by a step change in volume:

Elastance (cm. H_2O/ml.) =

$$\frac{\text{Pressure change (cm. } H_2O)}{\text{Volume change (ml.)}} \quad (1)$$

The reciprocal of elastance or compliance (expressed as ml./cm. H_2O) is preferred for a description of elastic property, since a change in volume is produced for which a change in pressure (P) is recorded (i.e., pressure is the independent variable). The changes in volume and pressure seen during inspiration and expiration are shown in Figure 2 (P-V curve).

Compliance of the respiratory system (i.e., volume change per unit pressure) can be calculated by noting the change in both variables (i.e., V and P) on the appropriate curves in Figure 1. At zero flow, when inspiration has been completed, the ratio between increase in lung volume and change in pressure across the lung is equal to lung compliance. Therefore:

Compliance =

$$\frac{0.5 \text{ liter}}{(8-5) \text{ cm. } H_2O} = 0.17 \text{ liter/cm. } H_2O \quad (2)$$

Figure 1 also allows calculation of resistance to flow by relating the flow-resistive pressure to the value for flow at any particular point:

$$R = \frac{P_{RES}}{\dot{V}} \quad (3)$$

where

$$R = \text{resistance (cm. } H_2O/\text{liter/sec.)}$$
$$P_{RES} = \text{flow-resistive pressure (cm. } H_2O)$$
$$\dot{V} = \text{gas flow (liter/sec.)}$$

During normal tidal ventilation, expiration is a passive process. An increased resistance to expiratory flow may be caused by a narrowing of major airways

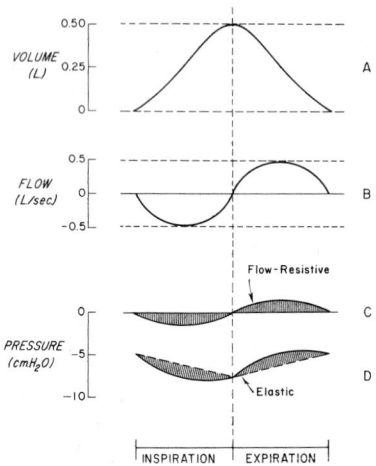

Figure 1. Changes in volume, flow, and esophageal (pleural) pressure during a complete respiratory cycle. Zero flow is recorded at three points where the flow curve crosses the x-axis. At peak inspiration, the volume displaced is approximately 0.5 liter (curve A), while the change in pressure (between points of zero flow) is from −5 to −8 cm. H_2O or 3 cm. H_2O (curve D). Thus, lung compliance equals 0.5/3 or 0.167 liter/cm. H_2O.

The dashed line on curve D was drawn between points of zero flow. The difference in pressure between dashed and solid lines on curve D, divided by the flow (curve B) recorded at the same point in the respiratory cycle, is equal to the resistance in cm. H_2O/liter/sec. Curve C is the flow-resistive curve redrawn with the ordinate equal to the pressure differences obtained from curve D. The rate of change of elastic pressure (dashed line, curve D) is constant throughout inspiration and expiration (although not strictly true, it is a permissible assumption); rate of change of flow-resistive pressure varies as flow changes (solid line, curve C). (From Mead, J., and Martin, H.: Phys. Ther., *48*:478, 1968.)

Substituting for P_{EL} in equation 4, we have:

$$W_{EL} = \frac{1}{2} \times \frac{V_T^2}{C} \qquad (6)$$

According to equation 6, a small rise in tidal volume will increase the work required to overcome elastic recoil more than a small fall in compliance. Consequently, if a patient has a low compliance, he will attempt to ventilate with smaller tidal volumes (and consequently more rapid frequencies) in order to minimize the work of breathing.

Work performed against resistance to flow (W_{RES}) is a component of the energy dissipated during respiration. This work, represented by the stippled area shown under the flow-resistive work curve in Figure 2, can be calculated by planimetry or by introducing certain simplifying assumptions. First, the rate of volume change must be obtained. Let us assume a respiratory frequency (f) and an equal distribution of time between inspiration and expiration, then duration of inspiration (sec.) = 60/2f, and the average rate of volume change will be $2V_T f$ per minute. Further details of derivation are available by reference to the original literature.[1]

Thus:

$$W_{RES} = 2R \cdot (V_T)^2 \cdot f \qquad (7)$$

where W_{RES} = flow-resistive work
R = resistance to flow
V_T = tidal volume
f = frequency

secondary to edema, spasm, excessive secretions, or external pressure, so that an otherwise passive process may be transformed into one that requires active work and greater consumption of oxygen. Thus, we may be able to eliminate the need for inspiratory work, if the patient receives controlled mechanical ventilation during or after surgery, but without influencing the need for work on expiration. To ensure proper emptying of the lung, it is best to use slow frequencies during mechanical ventilation and insist on adequate preoperative preparation whenever pre-existing lung disease may increase the possibility of retained secretions during the postoperative period.

The elastic work (W_{EL}) expended by the respiratory muscles during inspiration can be expressed as a product of the pressure generated and the volume of tidal ventilation (see Fig. 2).

$$W_{EL} = \frac{1}{2} P_{EL} \times V_T \qquad (4)$$

where V_T = tidal volume (ml.)
However, P_{EL} is related to compliance (C); therefore:

$$C = \frac{V_T}{P_{EL}} \quad or \quad P_{EL} = \frac{V_T}{C} \qquad (5)$$

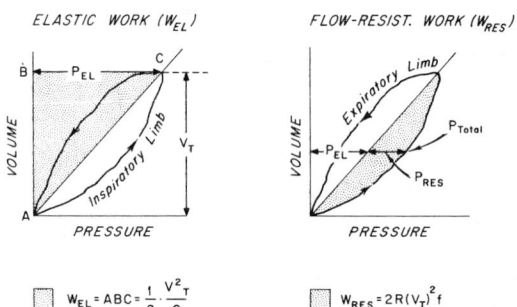

Figure 2. Calculation of the work of breathing ($W_{EL} + W_{RES}$). Work of breathing (W) is the sum of work required to overcome elastic recoil (W_{EL}) and flow resistivity (W_{RES}). The sum of the two shaded areas represents the total work of breathing. Area at left (W_{EL}) is simply the area of the triangle ABC; area at right (W_{RES}) can be obtained directly by planimetry or by applying certain mathematical assumptions. The formula in the text for W_{RES} is approximate at best and is given only to indicate relationships between work, tidal volume, and respiratory frequency. Note that work performed against elastic recoil is not frequency-dependent (f does not appear in the formula used to calculate area); on the other hand, work expended to overcome resistance to flow is frequency-dependent. Total pressure (P_{TOTAL}) developed during inspiration is the sum of elastic pressure (P_{EL}) and flow-resistive pressure (P_{RES}) as indicated in the right-hand loop. (From Mead, J., and Martin, H.: Phys. Ther., *48*:478, 1968.)

Total work is equal to the sum of $W_{EL} + W_{RES}$ (i.e., equations 6 and 7), or

$$\frac{1}{2}\frac{V^2_T}{C} + 2R\,(V_T)^2\,f \qquad (8)$$

According to equation 8, an increase in tidal volume adds considerably more work to overcome resistance to flow than an increase in respiratory frequency. This is a more complicated way of saying that the early phase of acute repiratory failure will be characterized by an attempt at compensation through an increase in respiratory frequency rather than tidal volume.

The work expended for normal breathing at rest is approximately 6 kg.-m. or 3 ml. O_2/min. or 1 to 2 per cent of body oxygen requirements (see Table 1). Oxygen consumed ($\dot{V}_{O_2}$) at rest can be estimated by measuring the change in body oxygen consumption achieved when a load (elastic or resistive) is added during the respiratory cycle. This allows us to plot the oxygen consumption for each increment of load and extrapolate the oxygen requirements under basal conditions, when no load is present.

The increase in ventilation following increasing levels of exercise leads to a disproportionate rise in oxygen consumption by the muscles of respiration. At the highest levels of exercise, the additional oxygen uptake is no longer adequate to provide the oxygen needed for the work of breathing, and the distribution of available oxygen becomes a limiting factor in performance. Failure of lung function or the inability to perform without the benefit of mechanical assistance of ventilation is generally attributed to excessive "work of breathing." Although true in principle, it implies a limitation of hemodynamic function wherein the additional oxygen consumption required by the muscles of respiration cannot be supplied by an appropriate increase in blood flow, i.e., cardiac output.

The pressure-volume relationship of the lung is significantly different during inspiration from expiration (see Figs. 2 and 3). If one removes the lung from the chest cavity and fills the lung with liquid (e.g., saline), then the pressure-volume curves obtained during inspiration and expiration are superimposed. This difference between the gas-filled and liquid-filled lung is due to the presence of surface-active material ("surfactant"), which lines the terminal airways and maintains the geometric integrity of the lung.[25, 33] The interaction between transmural pressure, surface tension, and radius of the terminal airway is defined by the Laplace expression:

$$P = \frac{2T}{R} \qquad (9)$$

where P = transmural pressure (dynes/cm.^{2})
  T = surface tension (dynes/cm.)
  R = radius (cm.)

Pressure and radius fluctuate during the normal respiratory cycle. If surface tension (T) were to remain constant throughout, then the regional differences in radii (R) would be accompanied by a greater discrepancy in regional pressure (P), and the lung would become sufficiently unstable for all high-pressure alveoli to empty into those with a low transmural pressure (see Fig. 3). This rather disadvantageous state of affairs is obviated by continuous fluctuation in regional surface tensions, and a low value is achieved at end-expiration, when terminal air units are at their lowest radius. This fluctuation in surface forces serves as a protective mechanism and provides for optimal alveolar stability at low lung volumes.

TABLE 1. Effect of Moderate and Heavy Exercise on the Oxygen Required for Breathing

Heavy exercise is accompanied by a 10-fold increase in oxygen consumption. The distribution of elastic and resistive work is reversed as compared with quiet breathing (elastic component falls from 66 to 39 per cent, and the resistive component rises from 33 to 61 per cent). A change from quiet breathing to heavy exercise, with a rise in external work performed, is associated with a fivefold rise in tidal volume but only a threefold increase in respiratory frequency. See also equation 8 in the text. Maximal voluntary ventilation is achieved by a significantly greater increase in frequency than tidal volume as compared with heavy exercise. The elastic component is smaller and the resistive component higher than during heavy exercise. An increase in minute ventilation during the postoperative period is achieved by increasing work to overcome resistance to gas flow. Thus an increase in respiratory rate is indicative of inefficient respiration and incipient respiratory failure.

Condition	External Work (kg.-m./min.)	Tidal Vol. (ml.)	Resp. Rate (breaths/min.)	Min. Vol. (L./min.)	O_2 Consumption (ml./min.)	Respiratory Work (kg.-m./min.)	(% elastic)	(% resistive)	(O_2 cost ml./min.)
Quiet breathing	0	500	15	7.5	300	0.3	66	33	3
Moderate exercise	620	1600	23	37.0	1500	5.2	57	43	52
Heavy exercise	1660	2400	48	115.0	3500	35.2	39	61	352
Maximal voluntary ventilation	0	1500	120	180	—	65.0	20	80+	—

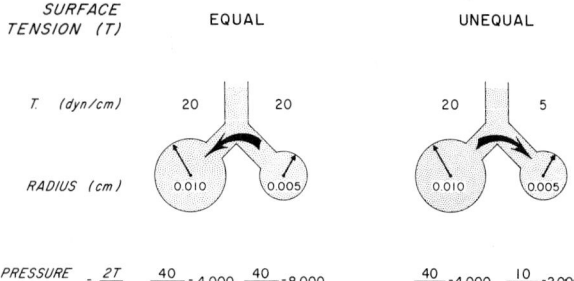

$$\frac{PRESSURE}{(dyn/cm^2)} = \frac{2T}{R}$$

Figure 3. Effect of distribution of airway diameter (R) and surface tension (T) on direction of gas flow between terminal airways. It is assumed that T remains constant during changes in volume (i.e., inspiration or expiration). At left, surface tension is equal in both alveoli; the transmural pressure for the individual gas spaces can be calculated from the Laplace expression: P = 2T/R. Since the alveolus at left is larger, its transmural pressure will be lower, and gas will flow from right to left as indicated by the arrow. If the distribution of surface tensions is unequal, then gas will flow in the reverse direction. Were this to occur in situ, then all gas spaces in the lung would empty into one alveolus and the lung would end up as a single giant balloon. Since the inhomogeneity of airway size persists in the normal lung, we must assume that changes in airway diameter (i.e., volume) are associated with continuous changes in surface tension. Thus the smallest alveoli must have the lowest surface tension in order to reaccommodate for the reduction in R. Considered in practical terms, a progressive reduction in T (as volume diminishes) serves as a protective mechanism against collapse whenever size is reduced toward a critical volume. Conversely, if surface tension is high because of pathologic changes within the lung, a large transmural pressure must be generated in order to prevent alveolar collapse. Some patients cannot achieve it in the postoperative period, and the elevated pressure can be provided only by a mechanical ventilator. (Redrawn from Nunn, J. F.: Applied Respiratory Physiology. New York, Appleton-Century-Crofts, 1969.)

several fold (0.3 to 0.9 ml. oxygen per liter of expired minute ventilation) and still keep oxygen fraction at a small level of the total oxygen consumed. If the patient with abnormal lungs requires great effort for effective alveolar ventilation, then the work of breathing may represent a significant portion of the total oxygen consumed and place an excessive load on the heart to achieve greater oxygen uptake. This problem is considered further in the section on Acute Respiratory Failure.

DISTRIBUTION OF VENTILATION

Improved respiratory care has been achieved as a direct result of better understanding of the factors controlling distribution of ventilation and perfusion and of the manner in which the lung matches these two to achieve optimal gas exchange.[3, 5, 9, 17, 20, 23, 25–27, 31, 43]

The lung is subject to gravitational forces, partly as a function of its weight and partly because of the deforming tendencies of abdominal contents applied to the diaphragm. Many of the characteristics to be described arise secondary to its mechanical inhomogeneity. The classic subdivision of lung volume shown in Figure 5 provides no information on regional variations of function (see also Figs. 6 and 7).

Gravity influences transpulmonary pressure gradient differently at the top and bottom of the lung. This is eminently obvious in the upright position when lung height may average 30 cm. in the normal adult.[12, 38]

Changes in lung structure, as in mitral stenosis or chronic obstructive lung disease, alter the compliance of the lung and the work needed to initiate gas flow. In Figure 4, normal lung mechanics are compared with the values obtained in mitral stenosis and in "emphysema." Compliance is markedly decreased in the presence of both mitral stenosis and "emphysema," while the work required to overcome resistance to gas flow is normal in association with mitral valve disease but markedly elevated in "emphysema." The expiratory limb of the pressure-volume loop in "emphysema" moves to the left of the y-axis, indicative of the work added for effective expiration. According to Table 2, both the work and oxygen cost of breathing rise significantly when respiratory frequency is elevated in the presence of mitral stenosis and chronic obstructive lung disease. However, the patient with chronic lung disease ("emphysema") is unable to achieve a significant elevation of minute ventilation, because the oxygen cost of breathing is well above normal at rest.

This inability to respond appropriately to a required rise in ventilation should alert the physician to the potential need for prophylactic ventilator support following a major operation. As noted in Table 2, a patient with normal lungs can increase the work of breathing

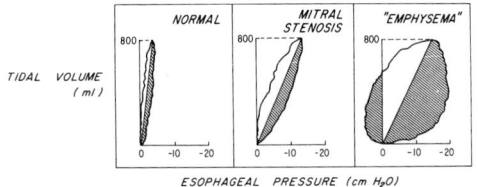

	NORMAL	MITRAL STENOSIS	"EMPHYSEMA"
LUNG COMPLIANCE (ml/cm H2O)	200	60	52
WORK AGAINST NON-ELASTIC RESISTANCE (%)	25	20	68
WORK OF BREATHING (kg m/lit. VE)	0.03	0.07	0.18

Figure 4. Mechanics of breathing in patients with mitral stenosis and chronic obstructive lung disease ("emphysema"). Slope of the diagonal line that connects the extremes of the pressure-volume loop (change in volume/change in pressure) equals lung compliance in ml./cm. H2O. A decrease in slope indicates a fall in compliance, and this is apparent in the presence of mitral stenosis or in "emphysema." Values for compliance are similar in these disorders; however, the work required to overcome resistance to flow is normal in patients with mitral valve disease but markedly increased (from 20 to 68 per cent of total work of breathing) in "emphysema." The pressure-volume loops are defined by the inspiratory limb (right of the diagonal) and an expiratory limb (left of the diagonal). During expiration, the line defining the pressure-volume relationship moves to the left of the y-axis in "emphysema," indicating the need for active work during the second half of expiration. End-expiration is at the origin. (From Turino, G. M., and Fishman, A. P.: J. Chron. Dis., 9:510, 1959.)

TABLE 2.   Work and Oxygen Cost of Breathing in Mitral Stenosis and Chronic Obstructive Lung Disease ("Emphysema") as Compared with the Normal Individual*

The increase in the oxygen cost of breathing due to a rise in minute ventilation differs little in the presence of mitral stenosis as compared with the normal person (threefold increase); however, in absolute values the rise is greater in mitral stenosis owing to elevated control values. In "emphysema," compliance decreases significantly as minute ventilation is increased, and the rise in ventilation is achieved with higher frequency and lower tidal volume than in mitral stenosis. This permits a lesser increase in the work of breathing necessary to overcome the abnormal resistance to gas flow (see equation 7). The increase in respiratory frequency requires an increase in work done against high air-flow resistance; accommodation is achieved by a reduction in tidal volume. Oxygen cost of breathing was calculated from the work of breathing on the assumption of a respiratory muscle efficiency of 5 per cent.

Diagnosis, Age, Sex	Compliance (ml./cm. H₂O)	Respiratory Rate (per min.)	Tidal Volume (ml.)	Minute Ventilation (L./min.)	Work of Breathing (kg.-m./L. of expired tidal vol.)	Oxygen Cost of Breathing (ml./L. of expired tidal vol.)
Normal	192	24	336	8.07	0.015	0.3
27, F.	195	18	876	15.8	0.030	0.6
	160	43	438	18.8	0.026	0.5
	138	63	438	27.4	0.050	0.9
Mitral stenosis	61	25	418	10.6	0.045	0.8
with severe	63	18	811	14.7	0.070	1.2
pulmonary	50	44	581	24.3	0.107	1.9
congestion	43	67	551	36.7	0.133	2.4
30, F.						
Pulmonary emphysema	54	17	576	10.0	0.17	3.0
with bronchial	36	33	380	12.7	0.19	3.4
obstruction,	18	46	349	16.1	0.23	4.1
severe						
55, M.						

*From Turino, G. M., and Fishman, A. P.: J. Chron. Dis., 9:510, 1959.

A model of lung behavior in situ is shown in Figure 6A. If a flexible spring is allowed to hang under its own weight, the upper portion is distended more than the bottom. When the spring is stretched by pull from

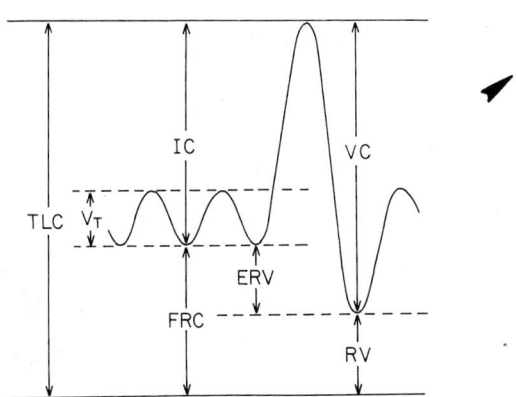

Figure 5. Subdivisions of normal lung volumes.
TLC = total lung capacity
V_T = tidal volume
IC = inspiratory capacity
FRC = functional residual capacity, i.e., lung volume at end-expiration
ERV = expiratory reserve volume
RV = residual volume, i.e., lung volume after forced expiration from FRC
VC = vital capacity, i.e., the maximal volume of gas inspired from RV
For normal values in the adult, see Table 3.

the bottom, major expansion takes place among the least distended turns. If we apply these principles to the lung, an inspiration initiated from functional residual capacity (FRC) will find apical and basal alveoli on different parts of the pressure-volume curve (Fig. 6B); for any change in transpulmonary pressure (ΔP_{base}), basal alveoli will exhibit a greater change in volume (ΔV_{base}) then alveoli at the apex (ΔV_{apex}). This difference is due to a gradient in pleural pressure, since gravity tends to keep pleural pressure in the dependent part less negative than at the apex.* The regional differences in pleural pressure are determined by: (1) height of the lung; (2) position of the diaphragm; and (3) regional characteristics of compliance. The variations found among normal lungs are small and predictable, but the volume change may be significantly different in the patient with regional pathologic change.

If one starts inspiration from residual volume, then

*At end-expiration (i.e., at functional residual capacity), the chest wall promotes lung expansion while the normal elastic recoil causes the lungs to retract. As a result, the pleural pressure is "negative" or several cm. H₂O below atmospheric pressure. When the glottis is open, the chest wall is relaxed, and pressure throughout the gas phase of the lung is atmospheric. The transpulmonary pressure (TPP) is the arithmetic difference between atmospheric and measured esophageal (or pleural) pressures.

TABLE 3. Predicted Values for Pulmonary Function Tests: Part A — Men*

1	2	3	4	5	6	7	8	9	10	11	12	13
Ht (cm)	Age (yrs)	VC	FRC	RV	TLC	$FEV_{0.75} \times 40$ (l/min)	$FEV_{1.0}$ liters	MMFR (l/sec)	$D_{Lco}SS_2$	$\dfrac{F_{Ico}-F_{EXco}}{F_{Ico}}$	$D_{Lco}SB$	ME%
155	20	3.97	2.72	1.13	5.10	136	3.6	4.3	23.8	.56	26.7	70
	30	3.65	2.72	1.30	4.95	121	3.3	3.9	21.0	.52	23.7	65
	40	3.35	2.72	1.45	4.80	106	3.0	3.5	18.2	.49	20.7	60
	50	3.04	2.72	1.61	4.65	91	2.7	3.1	15.4	.45	17.7	55
	60	2.73	2.72	1.77	4.50	76	2.4	2.7	12.6	.42	14.7	50
	70	2.42	2.72	1.91	4.35	61	2.1	2.3	9.8	.39	11.7	45
160	20	4.30	2.98	1.27	5.57	141	3.8	4.4	24.1	.55	29.0	70
	30	4.00	2.98	1.42	5.42	126	3.5	4.0	21.3	.52	26.0	65
	40	3.70	2.98	1.57	5.27	111	3.2	3.6	18.6	.48	23.0	60
	50	3.40	2.98	1.72	5.12	96	2.8	3.2	15.8	.45	20.0	55
	60	3.10	2.98	1.87	4.97	81	2.5	2.8	13.0	.41	17.0	50
	70	2.80	2.98	2.02	4.82	65	2.2	2.4	10.1	.39	14.0	45
165	20	4.62	3.23	1.42	6.04	145	3.9	4.5	24.5	.55	31.3	70
	30	4.32	3.23	1.57	5.89	130	3.7	4.1	21.7	.52	28.3	65
	40	4.02	3.23	1.72	5.74	115	3.3	3.7	18.9	.48	25.3	60
	50	3.72	3.23	1.87	5.59	100	3.0	3.3	16.1	.44	22.3	55
	60	3.42	3.23	2.02	5.44	85	2.7	2.9	13.3	.42	19.3	50
	70	3.12	3.23	2.17	5.29	70	2.4	2.5	10.6	.38	16.3	45
170	20	4.94	3.48	1.57	6.51	150	4.1	4.6	24.9	.54	33.6	70
	30	4.64	3.48	1.72	6.36	135	3.8	4.2	22.1	.50	30.6	65
	40	4.35	3.48	1.86	6.21	120	3.5	3.8	19.3	.47	27.6	60
	50	4.05	3.48	2.01	6.06	105	3.2	3.4	16.5	.43	24.6	55
	60	3.74	3.48	2.17	5.91	90	2.9	3.0	13.7	.40	21.6	50
	70	3.44	3.48	2.32	5.76	75	2.6	2.6	10.9	.37	18.6	45
175	20	5.26	3.74	1.72	6.98	155	4.3	4.7	25.2	.53	35.8	70
	30	4.96	3.74	1.87	6.83	140	4.0	4.3	22.4	.50	32.8	65
	40	4.66	3.74	2.02	6.68	124	3.7	3.9	19.6	.47	29.9	60
	50	4.36	3.74	2.17	6.53	110	3.4	3.5	16.9	.43	26.9	55
	60	4.06	3.74	2.32	6.38	94	3.1	3.1	14.1	.39	23.9	50
	70	3.76	3.74	2.47	6.23	79	2.8	2.7	11.3	.36	20.9	45
180	20	5.58	3.99	1.87	7.45	159	4.5	4.8	25.6	.52	38.1	70
	30	5.28	3.99	2.02	7.30	145	4.2	4.4	22.8	.49	35.1	65
	40	4.98	3.99	2.17	7.15	129	3.9	4.0	20.0	.46	32.1	60
	50	4.68	3.99	2.32	7.00	114	3.6	3.6	17.2	.42	29.2	55
	60	4.38	3.99	2.47	6.85	99	3.3	3.2	14.2	.39	26.2	50
	70	4.08	3.99	2.62	6.70	83	2.9	2.8	11.6	.35	23.2	45
185	20	5.90	4.25	2.02	7.92	163	4.7	4.9	25.9	.53	40.4	70
	30	5.60	4.25	2.17	7.77	148	4.3	4.5	23.2	.48	37.4	65
	40	5.30	4.25	2.32	7.62	133	4.1	4.1	20.4	.46	34.4	60
	50	5.00	4.25	2.47	7.47	118	3.7	3.7	17.6	.42	31.4	55
	60	4.70	4.25	2.62	7.32	103	3.5	3.3	14.8	.38	28.4	50
	70	4.40	4.25	2.77	7.17	88	3.1	2.9	12.0	.35	25.5	45

*From Bates, D. V., Macklem, P. T., and Christy, R. V.: Respiratory Function in Disease. 2nd ed. Philadelphia, W. B. Saunders Company, 1971.

Subdivisions of lung volume measured in seated subjects.
Ventilatory tests performed with subjects standing.
Diffusing capacity tests performed on seated subjects.

MMFR = maximal mid-expiratory flow rate
$D_{Lco}SS$ = diffusion capacity; steady-state carbon monoxide uptake with alveolar carbon monoxide measured from an end-tidal sample of gas
VC = vital capacity
FRC = functional residual capacity
RV = residual volume
TLC = total lung capacity

$FEV_{0.75}$ = forced expiratory volume at 0.75 second (the $FEV_{0.75}$ multiplied by 40 gives an approximate indication of the maximal breathing capacity in liters/min.)
$FEV_{1.0}$ = forced expiratory volume at 1.0 second
$\dfrac{F_{Ico}-F_{EXco}}{F_{Ico}}$ = fractional uptake of carbon monoxide where F_{Ico} equals the inspired and F_{EXco} equals the expired fraction of carbon monoxide
$D_{Lco}SB$ = diffusion capacity; single-breath method using helium and carbon monoxide, modified Krogh technique
ME% = closed circuit helium index; measure of FRC

Table continued on opposite page

TABLE 3. Predicted Values for Pulmonary Function Tests: Part B — Women*

1	2	3	4	5	6	7	8	9	10	11	12	13
Ht (cm)	Age (yrs)	VC	FRC	RV	TLC	$FEV_{0.75}$ $\times 40$ (l/min)	$FEV_{1.0}$ liters	MMFR (l/sec)	$D_{Lco}SS_2$	$\dfrac{F_{Ico} - F_{EXco}}{F_{Ico}}$	$D_{Lco}SB$	ME%
145	20	2.81	1.96	1.00	3.81	88	2.6	3.6	20.7	.58	19.5	70
	30	2.63	1.96	1.08	3.71	80	2.4	3.3	18.2	.55	16.9	65
	40	2.45	1.96	1.16	3.61	72	2.1	2.9	15.7	.51	14.2	60
	50	2.27	1.96	1.24	3.51	64	1.9	2.5	13.2	.48	11.7	55
	60	2.09	1.96	1.32	3.41	56	1.5	2.2	10.7	.44	9.0	50
	70	1.91	1.96	1.40	3.31	48	1.4	1.8	8.2	.41	6.4	45
150	20	3.08	2.20	1.05	4.13	92	2.7	3.7	21.1	.57	21.7	70
	30	2.89	2.20	1.14	4.03	84	2.5	3.3	18.6	.54	19.1	65
	40	2.71	2.20	1.22	3.93	76	2.2	3.0	16.0	.51	16.4	60
	50	2.53	2.20	1.30	3.83	67	2.0	2.6	13.5	.47	13.7	55
	60	2.35	2.20	1.38	3.73	60	1.6	2.3	11.0	.43	11.1	50
	70	2.17	2.20	1.46	3.63	52	1.5	1.9	8.5	.40	8.5	45
155	20	3.34	2.43	1.19	4.53	95	2.8	3.8	21.5	.56	23.9	70
	30	3.15	2.43	1.28	4.43	88	2.6	3.4	18.9	.52	21.2	65
	40	2.97	2.43	1.36	4.33	79	2.4	3.1	16.4	.49	18.5	60
	50	2.79	2.43	1.44	4.23	71	2.1	2.7	13.9	.45	15.8	55
	60	2.61	2.43	1.52	4.13	63	1.7	2.3	11.4	.42	13.1	50
	70	2.43	2.43	1.60	4.03	55	1.6	2.0	8.9	.39	10.5	45
160	20	3.60	2.67	1.32	4.92	99	2.9	3.9	21.9	.55	26.0	70
	30	3.41	2.67	1.41	4.82	91	2.7	3.5	19.4	.52	23.3	65
	40	3.22	2.67	1.50	4.72	83	2.5	3.2	16.8	.48	20.6	60
	50	3.05	2.67	1.57	4.62	75	2.2	2.8	14.3	.45	17.9	55
	60	2.87	2.67	1.65	4.52	67	1.8	2.4	11.8	.41	15.2	50
	70	2.69	2.67	1.73	4.42	59	1.7	2.1	9.2	.39	12.5	45
165	20	3.88	2.90	1.44	5.32	103	3.1	4.0	22.2	.55	28.1	70
	30	3.68	2.90	1.54	5.22	95	2.8	3.6	19.7	.52	25.4	65
	40	3.50	2.90	1.62	5.12	87	2.6	3.3	17.2	.48	22.7	60
	50	3.32	2.90	1.70	5.02	79	2.3	2.9	14.6	.44	20.0	55
	60	3.14	2.90	1.78	4.92	71	1.9	2.5	12.1	.42	17.3	50
	70	2.96	2.90	1.86	4.82	63	1.8	2.2	9.6	.38	14.6	45
170	20	4.13	3.14	1.58	1.58	107	3.2	4.1	22.6	.54	30.3	70
	30	3.94	3.14	1.67	5.61	99	2.9	3.7	20.1	.50	27.6	65
	40	3.76	3.14	1.75	5.51	90	2.7	3.3	17.5	.47	24.9	60
	50	3.58	3.14	1.83	5.41	82	2.4	3.0	15.0	.43	22.2	55
	60	3.40	3.14	1.91	5.31	74	2.0	2.6	12.5	.40	19.5	50
	70	3.22	3.14	1.99	5.21	66	1.9	2.3	9.9	.37	16.8	45
175	20	4.38	3.37	1.80	6.18	111	3.3	4.1	22.7	.53	32.3	70
	30	4.20	3.37	1.90	6.10	102	3.0	3.8	20.0	.50	29.6	65
	40	4.02	3.37	2.00	6.02	94	2.8	3.4	17.7	.47	26.9	60
	50	3.84	3.37	2.10	5.94	86	2.5	3.1	15.2	.43	24.2	55
	60	3.66	3.37	2.20	5.86	78	2.1	2.7	12.7	.38	21.5	50
	70	3.38	3.37	2.40	5.78	70	2.0	2.3	10.2	.36	18.8	45

*From Bates, D. V., Macklem, P. T., and Christy, R. V.: Respiratory Function in Disease. 2nd ed. Philadelphia, W. B. Saunders Company, 1971.
Subdivisions of lung volume measured in seated subjects.
Ventilatory tests performed with subjects standing.
Diffusing capacity tests performed on seated subjects.
For key, see Table 3, Part A.

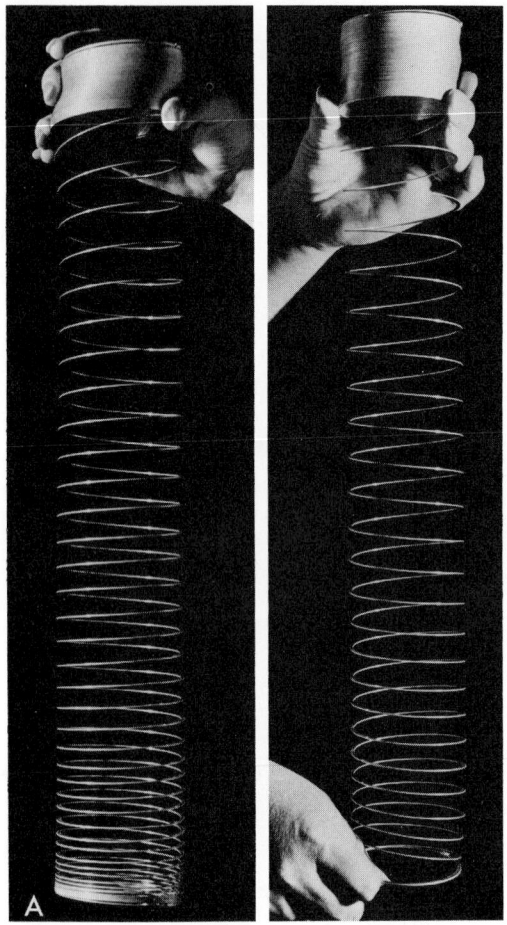

Figure 6. *A,* Model of alveolar size distribution at end-expiration and following a maximal inspiration. Behavior of the lung is qualitatively similar to a steel spring hanging under its own weight. The situation at rest (end-expiration) is shown in the left-hand panel. The top portion of the spring (equivalent to the lung apex) is stretched (alveoli are largest), while the lower segments (lung base) are barely separated (alveoli are smallest). The effect of a deep inspiration is shown in the right-hand panel where the spring is stretched by pull applied to the lower end. Note that the maximal increase in the distance between turns occurs at the bottom of the spring (i.e., basal alveoli increase in size more than alveoli at the apex).

B, Effect of inspiration from different end-expiratory volumes on regional pressure-volume changes. In the normal upright lung, pleural pressure becomes less negative (i.e., approaches atmospheric pressure) as one moves down the upright lung. Thus, the transpulmonary pressure is less at the base than apex (airway pressure equals atmospheric when the upper airway is open and there is no gas flow). The two pressure-volume curves shown in the panels at left and right characterize the changes that occur during inspiration (lung volume rises) and expiration (lung volume falls). This lack of coincidence in the pressure-volume relationship between inspiration and expiration is known as hysteresis. It is due principally to the presence of surface-active material (surfactant), which normally lines the terminal lung units. These conclusions are drawn from the finding that hysteresis disappears if the pressure-volume measurements are made in a liquid-filled lung. Differences in transpulmonary pressure between top and bottom of the lung lead to differences in terminal lung unit volume (represented by dots on the inspiratory limb of the pressure-volume [P-V] curves). An inspiration taken from FRC will cause a change in transpulmonary pressure of equal magnitude at the apex and base of the lung (i.e., $\Delta P_{apex} = \Delta P_{base}$). However, owing to different positions of the respective alveoli on the P-V curve, the alveoli at the base will expand more (ΔV_{base}) than those at the apex (ΔV_{apex}). Similarly, the slope of the curve for basal alveoli (volume/pressure = compliance) is higher than for the apical region, and so inspired air will move preferentially to the dependent part of the lung. If the lung volume is reduced, on inspiration is initiated at residual volume, then alveoli at the base will require an initial change in transpulmonary pressure before they exhibit an increase in volume. Thus, more gas moves to the apex, and the sequence of gas distribution is reversed. (Redrawn from Bates, D. V., Macklem, P. T., and Christie, R. V.: Respiratory Function in Disease, 2nd ed. Philadelphia, W. B. Saunders Company, 1971.)

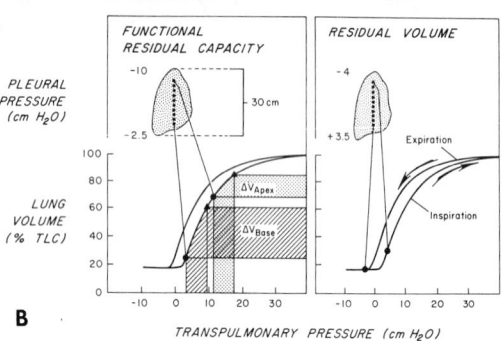

a considerable change in transpulmonary pressure will not be associated with a corresponding change in volume of basal alveoli (i.e., alveoli are on the flat portion of their pressure-volume curves), while a change in size will be evident for apical alveoli (see Fig. 6*B*). Thus, the state of lung expansion at end-expiration determines the distribution of change in volume during the ensuing tidal breath.[38] Stated a little differently, the *distribution of ventilation* (i.e., how much gas will move to where) is critically dependent on the volume history of the previous exhalation. When end-expira-

tory lung volume is normal, then the next inspirate will distribute itself preferentially to the dependent lung region, where alveoli are smaller and more compliant (they are located on the steeper portion of the pressure-volume curve). If the dependent lung is collapsed, or if its compliance is very low (e.g., Fig. 6*B*, at residual volume), then the air inspired will move preferentially to the upper lobes. The significance of such distribution to the patient with acute respiratory failure should be obvious, and its practical implications will be apparent if we consider its relationship to the

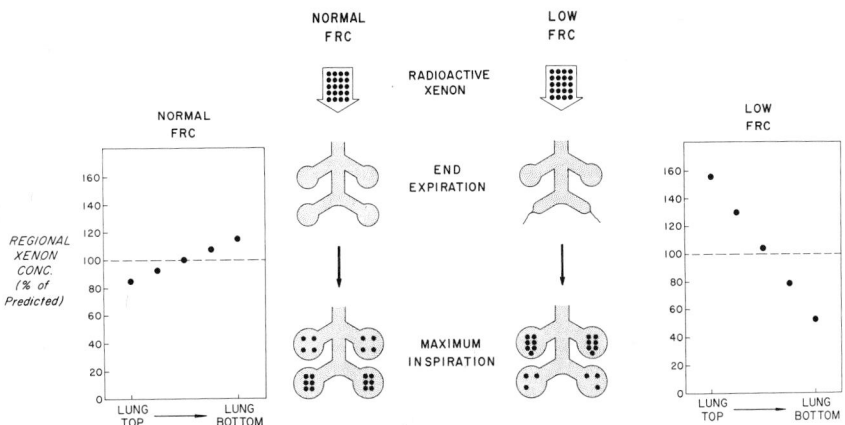

Figure 7. Effect of end-expiratory regional lung volume on distribution of an inspired breath. A bolus of radioactive xenon was injected at the beginning of inspiration, and regional radioactivity was measured with counters placed external to the chest at different lung levels. An inspiration taken from normal FRC is distributed preferentially to the dependent lung region (lung bottom). If these areas collapse on expiration, then the pattern of distribution is reversed, and the nondependent regions will receive a principal portion of the air inspired. Since perfusion of the dependent lung regions is higher than that at the apex, a marked mismatch will occur between ventilation and perfusion. Blood flowing past collapsed alveoli during the expiratory pause will not be oxygenated properly and this will contribute to the appearance of arterial hypoxemia. (From Pontoppidan, H., Laver, M. B., and Geffin, B.: Adv. Surg., 4:163, 1970. Copyright © 1970, Year Book Medical Publishers. Used by permission. Redrawn with permission from data of Milic-Emili, J., et al.: J. Appl. Physiol., 21:744, 1966.)

distribution of blood flow. Figure 7 demonstrates this phenomenon following inhalation of a radioactive gas. At normal FRC, a bolus of radioactive xenon inhaled at the beginning of inspiration moves first to the lung base. If the bases are collapsed at end-expiration, then the distribution is reversed, and most of the inspired air moves to the apex. Thus, with collapse at the lung base we face a double problem: absence of oxygenation of the blood flowing to the collapsed area during the expiratory pause, and reversal of flow during inspiration with a mismatch between normal ventilation and perfusion.

"Airway closure" can occur during normal tidal ventilation and in otherwise normal lungs. It implies cessation of continuity between upper and terminal air units and its appearance will be associated with abnormal gas exchange.[17, 21] Reference to Figure 8B will be helpful. During expiration in either the "old" or "young" normal individual, the regional concentration measured over the lung bottom diminishes abruptly. The lung volume above RV at which this occurs is known as *closing volume* (CV) and the inflection point is usually described in per cent of total lung capacity (TLC). CV is apparently reached before end-expiration in the old, normal individual (i.e., CV is above FRC) and lies at a point below the end-expiratory position in the young (i.e., CV is below FRC). When CV is below FRC, it is usually detected at 40 per cent of TLC or 20 per cent of vital capacity.

The *opening volume* is defined as the lung volume above which regional gas distribution is independent of lung volume because all airways are open and the ratios of volume to pressure change are equal throughout. This is generally assumed to take place at 65 per cent of TLC.

Age and body position are the most important determinants of CV size.[21] FRC is less in the supine than upright position, probably due to an increase in closing volume while supine. The effect of age is complex but important, particularly in view of the high incidence of respiratory complications in the elderly patient. The transpulmonary pressures active at lung base and apex as well as closing volumes in young and old adults are compared in Figure 8. The pleural pressure gradient from top to bottom of the lung is similar for the two age groups (i.e., $-10 -[-2.5] = -6.5 -[+1]$ $= -7.5$ cm. H_2O). However, pleural pressure is less negative in the older person and is reflected by a different degree of expansion of the bases and apices for the same rise in transpulmonary pressure. As shown in Figure 8B, advancing age is associated with a significant change in the distribution of ventilation. Basal alveoli, operating near the bottom of their pressure-volume curves, will change less in volume than their counterparts in the young adult, and tidal ventilation will take place near closing volume. The increased propensity for postoperative respiratory failure in aged patients may be due to less than optimal distribution of ventilation. Restriction of chest or abdominal wall motion produced by a tightly applied binder can have a significant effect on vital capacity and, more important, on functional residual capacity. This is shown in Table 4. The decrease in FRC with a reduction of chest or abdominal wall motion is due to airway closure.

The "closing volume" concept has functional rather than morphologic significance. Although the term does imply a reduction in the volume of terminal airways that participate in active gas exchange, the mode of alteration is controversial. We prefer to look upon "closing volume" as that lung volume at which the mechanical characteristics of the regional airways are altered abruptly, be this by actual collapse of terminal airways, closure of conducting airways with gas trap-

TABLE 4.   Effect of Strapping the Thoracic Cage or the Application of an Abdominal Binder on Vital Capacity and FRC*

Chest strapping caused a significant reduction in FRC, an increase of respiratory frequency, and a decrease in tidal volume, although minute volume of ventilation was not affected significantly. Following removal of the chest strap, FRC returned to normal after a deep breath. When the nitrogen concentration was monitored in expired air, the deep breath was associated with a sudden rise in N_2 concentration, suggesting that the drop in FRC was due to gas trapping.

Vital Capacity (liters)		Functional Residual Capacity (liters)
4.99	Control	3.40
2.73	Chest Restricted	2.20
6.30	Control	3.28
5.17	Abdomen Restricted	2.33

*From Caro, C. G., Butler, J., and Dubois, A. B.: J. Clin. Invest., *39*:573, 1960.

ping, or narrowing with a marked increase in resistance to gas flow. The important point to remember is not the terminology but the fact that changes in mechanical properties of the lung do occur during nor-mal ventilation, and as a consequence of advancing age, body trauma, abdominal distention, heart disease with congestive failure, and infection.[2, 4, 8, 10, 24, 28, 37]

DISTRIBUTION OF BLOOD FLOW

As with ventilation, gravitational forces and an interaction of vascular and airway pressures combine to give the lung great inhomogeneity in the distribution of blood flow.[14–16, 30] This inhomogeneity is characteristic for the normal lung and required for optimal gas exchange. An understanding of this phenomenon is enhanced if we use a model as a starting point (Fig. 9). Regardless of position (upright, supine, or lateral), the lung is subject to the effects of gravity, modified primarily, but not exclusively, by the magnitude of both pulmonary arterial and venous pressures. In the upright posture, with the upper airway open and in the absence of gas flow, alveolar pressure is the same throughout the lung. According to Figure 9, a small portion of lung near the apex is not perfused, since pulmonary artery (PA) pressure (reflected by the height of the appropriate column) does not exceed alveolar pressure. Keep in mind that we are dealing with collapsible but nondistensible blood vessels at the alveolar level (better known in physiologic terminology as Starling resistors) and that left atrial (LA) pressure is considerably lower than pulmonary artery

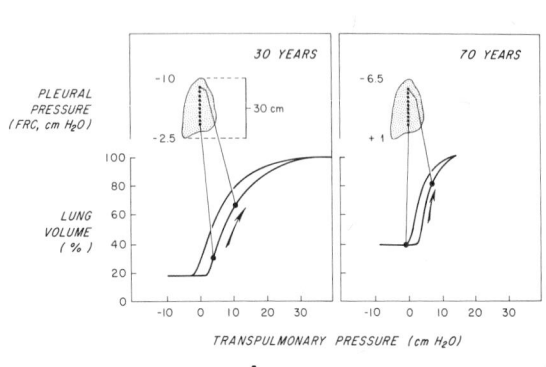

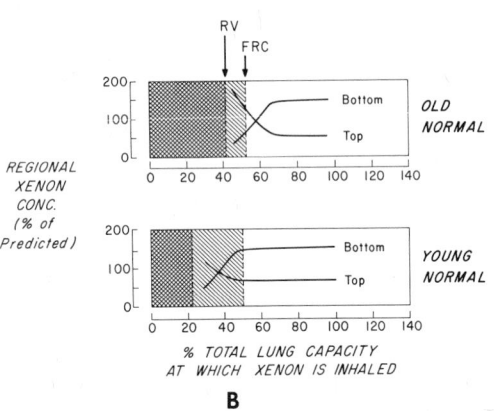

A   **B**

Figure 8.   *A*, Effect of aging on regional compliance and distribution of ventilation. Owing to a diminution of lung recoil, transpulmonary pressure (TPP) is lower in the older lung. Basal alveoli lie on a portion of the P-V curve that is near or below their closing volume. When inspiration is started, the initial change in TPP is not associated with a change in volume of basal alveoli, and gas moves preferentially to the apex. Once the critical opening pressure of basal alveoli has been overcome, their volume will increase and proceed to move around the knee of the curve on the inspiratory limb, as shown in Figure 8*B*. (Redrawn from Bates, D. V., Macklem, P. T., and Christie, R. V.: Respiratory Function in Disease, 2nd ed. Philadelphia, W. B. Saunders Company, 1971.)

B, Effect of age on closing volume. Note that the older person has a significantly higher RV than the young adult, despite little difference in FRC. If a bolus of radioactive xenon is inhaled at FRC, regional distribution of radioactivity between top and bottom of the lung will be similar in young and old persons at total lung capacity. If the regional concentration is monitored during the ensuing expiration, little regional difference will be found in the young adult at FRC. When expiration is continued below this point, a volume is reached at which the concentration of radioactive xenon at the lung decreases while the apical xenon concentration rises.

The point (per cent of TLC) at which these concentrations begin to reverse is known as the closing volume. Note that these changes occur much earlier during expiration in the old adult, implying a higher closing volume. Advancing age is associated with a greater incidence of collapse above FRC during normal tidal ventilation. It should be possible (at least in theory) to prevent such collapse by preventing complete expiration. The practical aspects of this postulate become significant when one treats acute respiratory failure by ventilation with positive end-expiratory pressure (PEEP). (From Pontoppidan, H., Laver, M. B., and Geffin, B.: Adv. Surg., *4*:163, 1970. Copyright © 1970, Year Book Medical Publishers. Used by permission. Redrawn with permission from Holland, J., et al.: J. Clin. Invest., *47*:81, 1968.)

pressure. The ventilated but nonperfused alveolus constitutes a physiologic dead space (V_D), and the area of lung where this situation prevails is defined arbitrarily as Zone I.[43] As we move from apex to lung base, pressure within the pulmonary artery will increase to overcome alveolar pressure and the collapsible tube (i.e., capillary) will open. Although the inflow portion is open, the effluent end is closed because alveolar pressure is higher than left atrial pressure. The portion of lung where this situation prevails is known as Zone II. Fluctuations in alveolar pressure during the respiratory cycle and in pulmonary artery pressure during the cardiac cycle are associated with intermittent patency of the effluent end of the capillary, and blood flow through this part of the lung is phasic in nature. *Velocity* of the liquid (cm./sec.) leaving the collapsible tube is determined by the difference between alveolar and left atrial pressures, while *acceleration* is proportional to the square root of the pressure difference across the plane of constriction (Bernoulli's principle). *Flow* (ml./sec.) across Zone II is independent of the difference between alveolar and left atrial pressures. This has been referred to as the waterfall phenomenon.*

In models similar to the one illustrated, flow through the distal portion of the collapsible tube (i.e., Zone II) is intermittent, and the tube is noted to "flutter."[32] As the effluent pressure is elevated, the collapsible tube distends, and flow depends on the difference between pulmonary artery and left atrial pressures. This is known as Zone III. Since the vessels in this zone are open at all times, resistance to flow is less

---

*The flow (ml./sec.) of water across the rim of a waterfall is independent of the height of the waterfall.

than in Zone II, but still dependent upon the diameter of the inflowing arterioles and effluent venules.

An increase in left atrial pressure will enhance fluid movement from the intravascular to the interstitial space. In fact, any body position that subjects a major portion of the lung to the pressure distribution characterized by Zone III will promote accumulation of interstitial fluid, particularly when left atrial pressure is abnormally high. This situation is illustrated in Figure 10. In the upright lung, when left ventricular failure is present, pulmonary congestion is prominent at the bases. The lateral position will compromise the dependent lung, while the supine position will jeopardize the posterior (dependent) portion of both lungs. In either case, prolonged immobilization is of little benefit for lung function, particularly in the presence of congestive heart failure. The head-down (or Trendelenburg) position carries an equal hazard. One need only consider the requirements for an abdominal hysterectomy (in which the head-down position is mandatory to facilitate exposure of the pelvic cavity) to appreciate the consequences in a patient with long-standing mitral stenosis and a high left atrial pressure. The appearance of pulmonary edema during or after operation should not come as a surprise under these circumstances.

All other factors remaining constant, a rise in pulmonary artery pressure will improve perfusion of the nondependent lung and reduce the physiologic dead space (see the next section, Blood Gas Exchange).

However, if the less well-ventilated portions of the lung are dependent, then a decrease in pulmonary artery pressure (e.g., during induced hypotension) will result in a diminution of arterial P_{O_2}. This will happen because a larger portion of total flow (i.e., cardiac output) perfuses portions of lung with diminished ventilation.

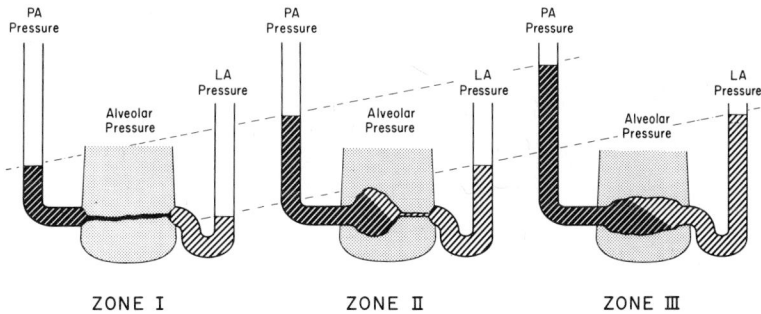

Figure 9. Effect of pulmonary artery, left atrial, and airway pressure on distribution of blood flow in the upright lung. At left, according to the model, pulmonary artery pressure is not high enough to overcome alveolar (transmural) pressure, and perfusion is nil. This is characteristic for the lung apex in the upright posture and is defined arbitrarily as Zone I.[20] Since gas movement continues during tidal ventilation while perfusion is absent, the effect is equivalent to the presence of dead space (i.e., alveolar dead space). As one moves down the lung, a level is reached where pulmonary artery pressure overcomes alveolar pressure and the inflow portion of the capillary opens. Since alveolar pressure is still higher than left atrial pressure, the effluent portion remains closed. Fluctuations in airway and vascular pressures during the breathing and cardiac cycles cause "fluttering," and blood flows intermittently. This middle portion of the lung, characterized by a pulmonary artery pressure (P_{PA}) higher than alveolar pressure (P_{ALV}), in turn higher than left atrial pressure (P_{LA}), is defined as Zone II. Zone III is the dependent part of the lung where left atrial pressure is higher than alveolar pressure and blood flows at all times. (From Laver, M. B., Hallowell, P., and Goldblatt, A.: Anesthesiology, *33*:161, 1970.)

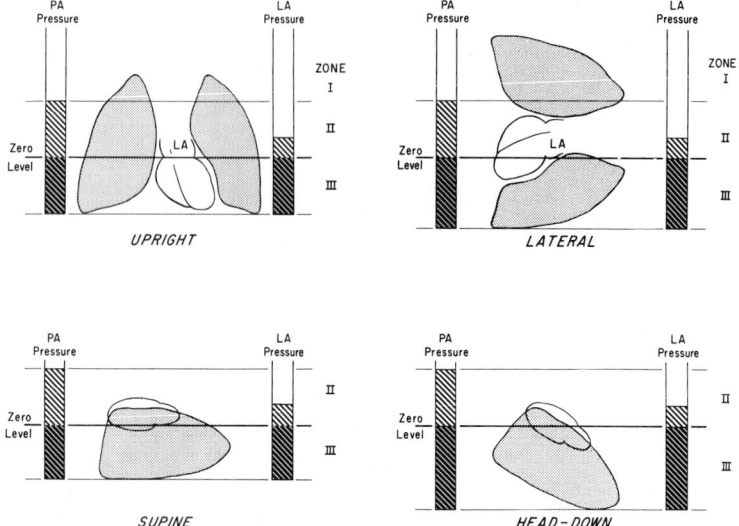

Figure 10. Effect of body position on the distribution of pulmonary perfusion. In the lateral position, all of the dependent (left) lung is Zone III. With the patient supine, the major portion of both lungs is Zone III. Pulmonary edema has a predilection for Zone III. Thus, in the lateral position, it will affect primarily the left lung; in the supine position, it will affect the posterior portion of both lungs from apex to base. The latter explains the "hypostatic pneumonia" known to appear in elderly bedridden patients. Finally, the head-down (Trendelenburg) position is the worst offender. Judging from its deleterious effects on lung function (effective left atrial pressure for the lung apex may exceed 30 cm. H₂O), there is little reason to justify its use in critically ill individuals. (From Laver, M. B., Hallowell, P., and Goldblatt, A.: Anesthesiology, *33*:161, 1970.)

It is not uncommon to find a reduction in physiologic dead space with the onset of congestive heart failure (left atrial and pulmonary artery pressures rise), only to see it return to control levels when pulmonary artery pressure returns to normal. The onset of left ventricular failure and the increase in left atrial pressure will diminish the extent of Zones I and II while increasing Zone III.

When the alveolar vessels are open continuously, blood flow will depend on the pressure gradient between pulmonary artery and left atrium. On the other hand, the rate at which water will move from the in-

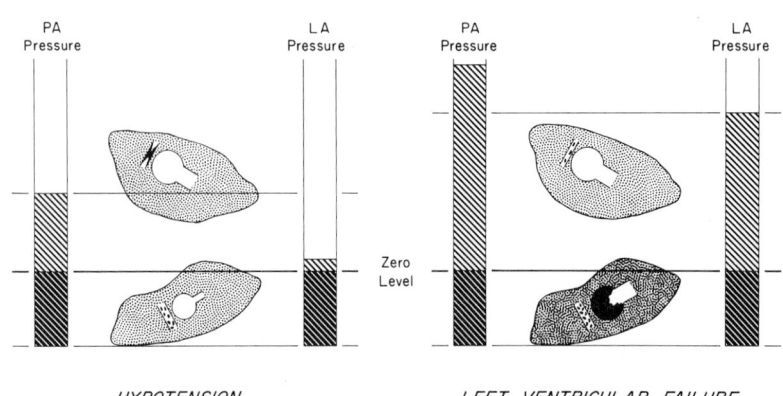

Figure 11. Effect of hypotension and left ventricular failure on the distribution of vascular pressures. The lungs were placed in the lateral position to emphasize the effect on blood gas exchange. Lowering of pulmonary artery pressure leads to cessation of blood flow in the upper (right) lung, while congestive heart failure improves perfusion of the nondependent (right) lung; however, edema formation in the dependent lung is enhanced because of the high "effective" left atrial pressure to which it is subjected. This "effective" pressure is the sum of the left atrial pressure measured at zero level (mitral anulus) plus the height of the hydrostatic column of blood below it. In the left-hand panel, the upper lung is shown to have an open, ventilated, but nonperfused alveolus. Pulmonary artery hypotension leads to an increase in physiologic dead space and a decreased efficiency of carbon dioxide removal. In the right-hand panel, the dependent lung is edematous, containing collapsed but perfused terminal airspaces. Since perfusion continues, arterial hypoxema must be present.

travascular to the extravascular space will depend on the pressure gradient between left atrium and alveolus (i.e., $P_{LA} - P_{ALV}$). A practical corollary concerns appropriate treatment of pulmonary edema. Diuresis and water restriction are important, but pulmonary edema cannot be relieved unless left atrial pressure is lowered.

Two common sources of abnormal distribution of blood flow are shown in Figure 11. Emphasis has been achieved by placing the patient in the lateral position. Hypotension associated with a fall in pulmonary artery pressure will limit perfusion of the nondependent lung, increase physiologic dead space, limit carbon dioxide removal, and reduce the efficiency of oxygenation. Thus, greater than normal ventilation (i.e., a higher tidal volume) is required to prevent arterial P_{CO_2} from rising. Left ventricular failure will improve perfusion of the nondependent lung, but the high left atrial pressure will enhance pulmonary edema in the dependent lobes. As shown in Figure 12, this can happen in a patient with congestive heart failure in whom operation requires immobilization in the right lateral decubitus position. Understanding of these principles allows derivation of some important practical points relevant to care in acute respiratory failure (see Fig. 13).

In the normal lung, ventilation and perfusion are matched, both being distributed primarily to the dependent lung. With the patient in the lateral position and the diseased lung uppermost, distribution of ventilation and perfusion are unchanged, and the degree of blood gas abnormality will be determined only by the extent of upper lung perfusion, i.e., magnitude of pulmonary artery pressure. If the collapsed lung is dependent, then its perfusion will be maximal, while ventilation will proceed preferentially to the nondependent lung (i.e., the lung with the higher compliance; see also Figure 7 for the redistribution of ventilation when inspiration is initiated in the presence of basal collapse). This mismatch will cause gross abnormalities in blood gas exchange, principally hypoxemia.

Extrinsic factors such as marked obesity may cause similar problems[13] (Fig. 14). Excessive corpulence prevents proper expansion of dependent alveoli, which, in the upright position, receive the bulk of pulmonary blood flow. Again, a mismatch between ventilation and perfusion compromises gas exchange and explains why obesity is a significant contributor to postoperative respiratory failure.

This simplistic approach to the problem of distribution of pulmonary blood flow requires further modification. Variations in blood vessel diameter are known to occur during the normal respiratory cycle. Macklin[22] noted that perfusion of the isolated lung from a reservoir containing liquids of different consistencies was associated with a contrasting response in liquid distribution during respiration. Thus, with saline as the perfusate, the liquid was pressed out of the lung during inflation; if a latex suspension was used instead, then inspiration was associated with an uptake of fluid by the lung. Based on this evidence, Macklin[22] concluded that the lung possesses a dual vasculature, which he divided into the intra-alveolar and extra-alveolar vessels, each affected differently during lung

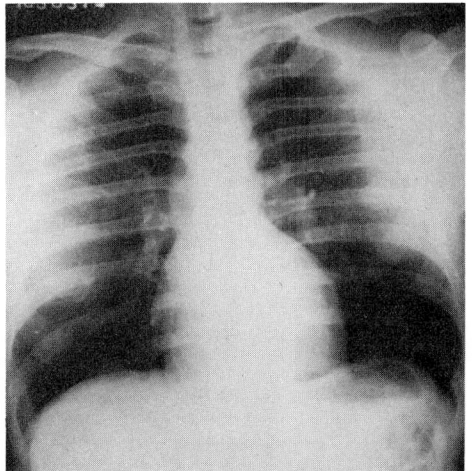

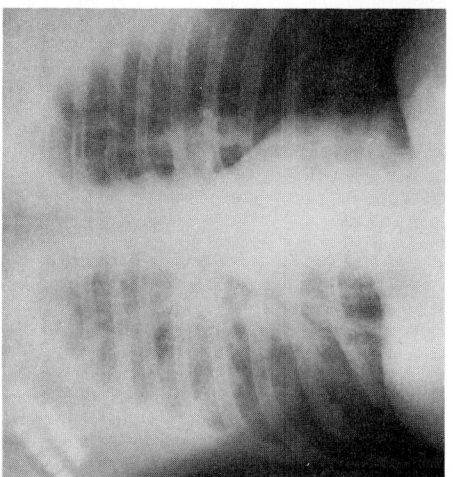

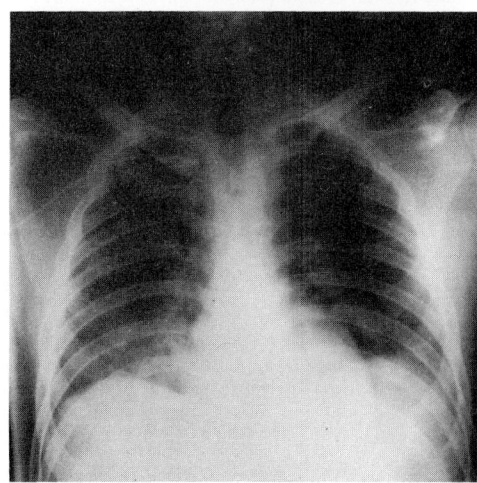

Figure 12. The practical consequence of prolonged surgery in the lateral position in a patient with congestive heart failure. The operation, left hip arthroplasty, lasted five hours. One hour postoperatively the patient developed all the clinical signs of severe pulmonary edema. The chest film at the top was taken preoperatively; the film in the center (obtained with the patient upright, taken at the time of pulmonary edema [1 hour postoperatively]), is placed on its side, similar to the position maintained by the patient during surgery. The film at the bottom was taken 48 hours later, after pulmonary edema had resolved. The most prominent congestive changes appeared in the dependent (right) lung.

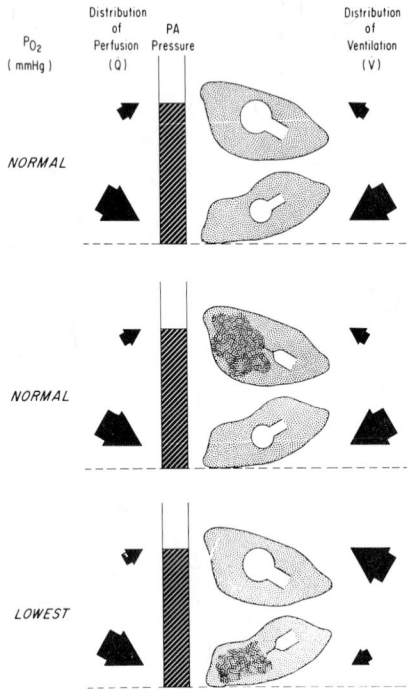

Figure 13. Effect of body position and site of airway collapse on arterial oxygenation. Distribution of perfusion undergoes only minor alteration secondary to an acute change of airway geometry. Normally, the dependent lung receives the major portion of blood flow and ventilation (*top*). If the nondependent lung contains areas of nonventilation, distribution of ventilation and perfusion remains unchanged but moderate hypoxemia will be present. The magnitude of hypoxemia will depend on the pulmonary artery pressure and the amount of blood flow ($\dot{Q}$) to nondependent lung (*center*). If the lung containing unventilated alveoli is dependent and if its compliance is low, preferential ventilation of the upper lung will occur; since distribution of perfusion remains unchanged, arterial hypoxemia will be severe (*bottom*). Arrow size reflects the relative magnitude of flow, be it $\dot{V}$ or $\dot{Q}$ (Laver and Austen, 1972).

keeps the extra-alveolar vessels maximally dilated and minimizes resistance to blood flow.

According to Figure 16, the relationship between measured pulmonary vascular resistance (PVR) and lung volume is described by an inverted bell-shaped curve with minimal PVR achieved at normal FRC.[41] An increase in lung volume above FRC (e.g., mechanical ventilation in the presence of normal lungs) will be reflected by an overwhelming effect on intra-alveolar vessels, and PVR will rise. In acute respiratory failure, when FRC may diminish to less than 50 per cent

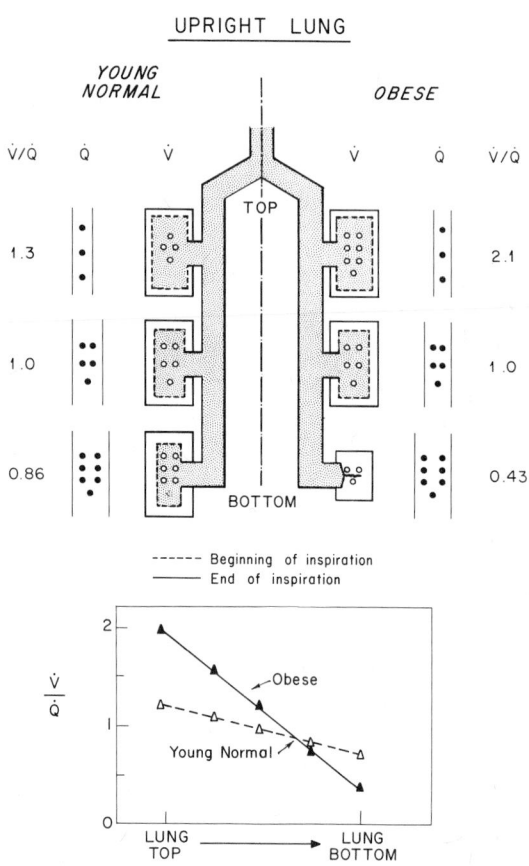

Figure 14. Distribution of ventilation and perfusion in the presence of obesity, compared with that in the normal person. A marked increase in chest and abdominal wall weight leads to underventilation of the dependent lung regions, and the distribution of ventilation in the upright lung is reversed. Circles and solid dots represent units of ventilation and perfusion, respectively. In the normal lung, *apical* $\dot{V}/\dot{Q}$ is highest, although *basal* blood flow and ventilation are greater in absolute terms. The higher apical ratio is due to the rise of perfusion as one moves from apex to base. In the obese person, progression of the $\dot{V}/\dot{Q}$ ratio from top to bottom is steeper than normal (bottom graph) because of intermittent airway closure at the base and reversed $\dot{V}$ distribution during inspiration. The obese patient comes to surgery with atelectasis built in. (From Pontoppidan, H., Laver, M. B., and Geffin, B.: Adv. Surg., 4:163, 1970. Copyright © 1970, Year Book Medical Publishers. Used by permission. Redrawn with permission from Holland, J., et al.: J. Clin. Invest., 47:81, 1968.)

expansion.* The small, intra-alveolar capillaries perfused with saline bear the brunt of the rise in airway pressure during inspiration, and flow diminishes proportionally to the increase in transmural pressure. The extra-alveolar vessels, which include arteries and veins down to vessels in alveolar septal junctions, are distended during lung expansion, and thereby their intraluminal diameter is increased (Fig. 15). The expanded airway may provide a tethering effect that

---

*Saline fills all blood vessels including the intra-alveolar capillaries. The more viscous latex suspension fills only the larger or extra-alveolar blood vessesl with lesser resistance to flow. The fact that saline is extruded during inspiration indicates the overall response of the lung with a normal FRC to a rise in mean airway pressure. If FRC is diminished by disease, then the overall response of flow to changes in airway pressure may be dictated by the behavior of the extra-alveolar vessels.

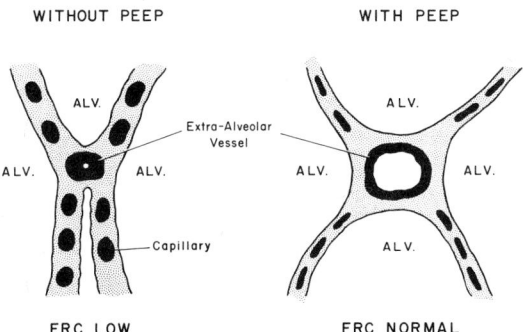

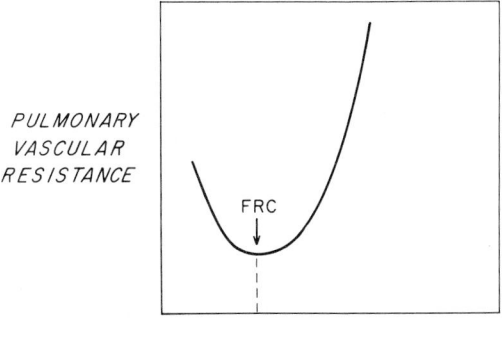

Figure 15. Effect of lung expansion on the diameter of extra-alveolar vessels. When the lung is collapsed, the supporting effect of the alveolar surface is lost, and the lumen of the extra-alveolar vessel is small. Since pressure applied to the airway (P), surface tension (T), and radius (R) are related by the Laplace equation ($P = 2T/R$), an increase in R with T remaining constant can be achieved with lesser applied pressure. A reduction in pressure at the surface results in a commensurate reduction in the interstitial pressure, and the vascular transmural pressure (VTP) gradient rises; the result is an increase in vessel diameter. If the surface tension (T) is high (often the case with respiratory failure), then the pressure applied to the airway to keep the terminal airspace open must also be high. The effective pressure transmitted to the interstitium is always a function of P and T. Two important consequences arise from these considerations: (1) Collapse or diminution in airway size leads to a narrowing of extra-alveolar (resistance) vessels and an increase in vascular resistance; flow diminishes but does not cease; therefore, airway closure is associated with hypoxemia. (2) An increase in the VTP gradient enhances the movement of water from the intravascular to the extravascular space; this implies (but does not prove) that interstitial fluid accumulation (edema) is promoted by marked distention of the lung. PEEP = mechanical ventilation with positive end-expiratory pressure. The latter is used in order to increase FRC and improve arterial oxygenation during therapy for acute respiratory failure.

Figure 16. Relationship between lung volume and pulmonary vascular resistance (PVR) in the isolated lung. Minimal resistance to blood flow is found at the normal end-expiratory position (FRC). With an increase in lung volume, pressure transmitted to the alveolar capillary has a significant effect on resistance to blood flow, which overrides the resistance-lowering effect of distending extra-alveolar vessels (shown in Fig. 15). Below FRC, collapse of terminal airways increases resistance in the extra-alveolar vessels (see Fig. 15), and overall PVR rises. (Redrawn from Thomas, L. J., Jr., Roos, A., and Griffo, Z. J.: J. Appl. Physiol., *16*:457, 1961.)

of normal, PVR is high because the tethering effect of the expanded alveolus has been lost and the extra-alveolar vessel diameter is small (see Fig. 15). Applied mechanical ventilation and the consequent increase in FRC will diminish resistance to flow, and perfusion of the lung may improve. Similarly, one may find a rise in cardiac output, when controlled ventilation is initiated in the face of respiratory failure, quite contrary to the response expected in the normal lung.

A consideration of changes in vessel diameter responsive to altered airway geometry will help us understand variations in blood flow distribution at variance with the behavior of blood flow throughout Zone III described earlier.[16] For instance (Fig. 17), if

Figure 17. Composite of factors influencing regional pulmonary blood flow in the upright lung. At the lung apex (top), the effect of pulmonary artery pressure is minimal, but mechanical factors promote maximal alveolar size and optimal diameter of extra-alveolar vessels. Blood flow is minimal. As one descends to lower portions of the lung, the influence of the pulmonary artery pressure increases but alveoli gradually diminish in size, as do the extra-alveolar vessels. As one moves down to a segment of lung below the middle, the rise in pulmonary artery pressure dominates, and flow rises to a maximum slightly above lung bottom. In the most dependent lung regions (bottom), alveolar size and extra-alveolar vessel diameter are sufficiently reduced to offset the effect of an increased pulmonary artery pressure, and blood flow is reduced. In vivo, changes in blood flow from middle to bottom of lung are less abrupt than shown in the graph at right.

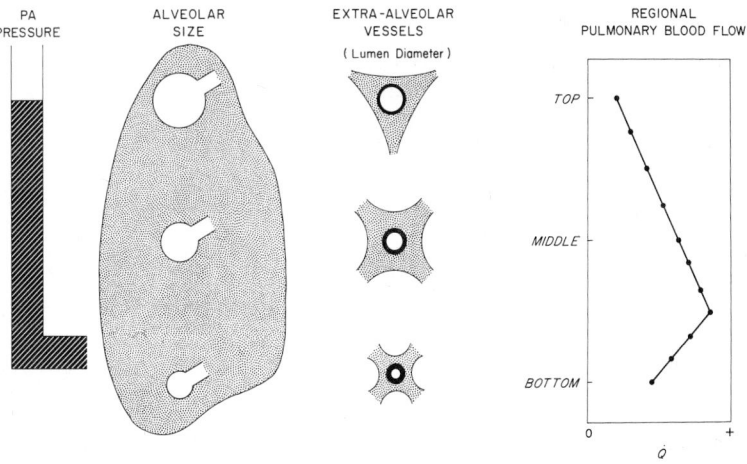

one injects minute, isotope-containing spheres into the pulmonary artery and then counts radioactivity in lung slices at different levels of the lung, one finds that blood flow to the most dependent parts decreases to a volume only slightly higher than at the apex. Thus, as one moves down the upright lung, blood flow rises as predicted by the model, until the lower third of the lung is reached. Below this point, blood flow is reduced. If we take into account the distribution of airway and vascular pressures, as well as regional differences in lung expansion with their effect on extra-alveolar vessels, we can integrate this information into a picture of how the lung behaves in situ. According to Figure 17, the volume of basal airways is smaller at end-expiration than that of their apical counterpart; as the result, basal extra-alveolar vessel diameters are reduced, vascular resistance is elevated, and blood flow is diminished. The pragmatic value of this arrangement is obvious. Blood flow past nonventilated airways is equivalent to "luxury perfusion." The lung probably does not require it for nutritive purposes; the end result is the addition of mixed venous to oxygenated blood and arterial hypoxemia. Collapse of terminal airways or a marked reduction in size influences extra-alveolar (resistance) vessels sufficiently to reduce perfusion, but unfortunately not to stop it. If the latter were the case (i.e., acute cessation of flow to nonventilated or hypoventilated areas), postoperative hypoxemia would be less of a clinical problem. Neurohumoral influences and levels of oxygenation will modify further the manner in which mechanical factors control the distribution of blood flow.[6, 7, 11, 19] Their role in the clinical setting of disturbed blood gas exchange remains to be defined.

BLOOD GAS EXCHANGE

Once the factors responsible for control of distribution of ventilation ($\dot{V}$) and perfusion ($\dot{Q}$) are defined, it is possible to consider how alterations in $\dot{V}/\dot{Q}$ will affect gas exchange, particularly oxygen uptake (i.e., arterial oxygenation) and carbon dioxide removal (i.e., arterial carbon dioxide levels).

Oxygenation

In the awake person, normal oxygen uptake and carbon dioxide elimination are maintained by an exquisite balance between ventilation ($\dot{V}$)* and perfusion ($\dot{Q}$). The normal pattern and the common deviations seen during and after surgery are presented in Figure 18. Simplification has been achieved by assuming that the lung consists of a two-alveoli system (large square boxes), each with its appropriate blood flow. Under normal conditions at rest, there is equal distribution of ventilation and perfusion to each lung. Possible sources of a deviation from normal in the arterial partial pressure of oxygen (Pa_{O_2}) are shown in part *II* of

---

*Symbols used throughout conform with established standards now in general use: See Pappenheimer, J. L.: Standardization of definitions and symbols in respiratory physiology. Fed. Proc., 9:902, 1950. (For more details, see Appendix.)

Figure 18; similarly, sources of abnormality in the arterial partial pressure of carbon dioxide (Pa_{CO_2}) are shown in part *III* of Figure 18.

Less than optimal oxygen exchange occurs as a consequence of airway collapse or marked hypoventilation (e.g., bronchial obstruction or mechanical compression of the lung), while perfusion of these airways continues. Normally, the difference between the alveolar partial pressure of oxygen ($P_{A_{O_2}}$) and arterial blood partial pressure of oxygen (Pa_{O_2}), i.e., the $P(A\text{-}aDO_2)$, is quite small. With alveolar collapse and continued perfusion, the $P(A\text{-}aDO_2)$ becomes large. The magnitude of this discrepancy in oxygenation can be analyzed readily during ventilation with 100 per cent oxygen because this maneuver simplifies calculation of $P_{A_{O_2}}$.

$$P_{A_{O_2}} = P_B - (P_{A_{CO_2}} - P_{H_2O}^T) \qquad (10)$$

where P_B = barometric pressure
$P_{H_2O}^T$ = water vapor pressure at the patient's temperature (T)
$P_{A_{CO_2}} = Pa_{CO_2}$ = arterial partial pressure of carbon dioxide (it is assumed that arterial and alveolar P_{CO_2} are equal; although this is not strictly true, the error involved is small)

Thus, the alveolar-arterial oxygen tension gradient reflects the degree of "contamination" of well-oxygenated with mixed venous blood. We say "reflects" because calculation of the right-to-left shunt must take into account the cardiac output, as we shall see.

First, keep in mind that the amount of oxygen carried in arterial blood per unit time is a product of the cardiac output ($\dot{Q}_T$ in ml./min.) and the arterial oxygen content (Ca_{O_2} in ml./100 ml.), or $\dot{Q}_T \times Ca_{O_2}$. Within the lung, blood is partitioned into: (1) flow to capillaries supplying ventilated alveoli (here the amount of oxygen picked up is the product of flow [$\dot{Q}_C$] and the oxygen content of the pulmonary end-capillary blood [$C_{C_{O_2}}$], or $\dot{Q}_C \times C_{C_{O_2}}$); and (2) blood flow past nonventilated alveoli (oxygen contributed from these areas is expressed by the product of flow ($\dot{Q}_S$) and the oxygen content of mixed venous blood ($C_{\bar{V}_{O_2}}$) or $\dot{Q}_S \times C_{\bar{V}_{O_2}}$. Thus

$$\dot{Q}_T \cdot Ca_{O_2} = (\dot{Q}_C \cdot C_{C_{O_2}}) + (\dot{Q}_S \cdot C_{\bar{V}_{O_2}}) \qquad (11)$$

Cardiac output ($\dot{Q}_T$) consists of flow to ventilated ($\dot{Q}_C$) and nonventilated ($\dot{Q}_S$) areas, or:

$$\dot{Q}_T = \dot{Q}_S + \dot{Q}_C \qquad (12)$$

Substituting for $\dot{Q}_C$ from equation 12 into equation 11 and rearranging, we obtain the "shunt equation," an expression that quantifies venous admixture:

$$\frac{\dot{Q}_S}{\dot{Q}_T} = \frac{C_{C_{O_2}} - Ca_{O_2}}{C_{C_{O_2}} - C_{\bar{V}_{O_2}}} \qquad (13)$$

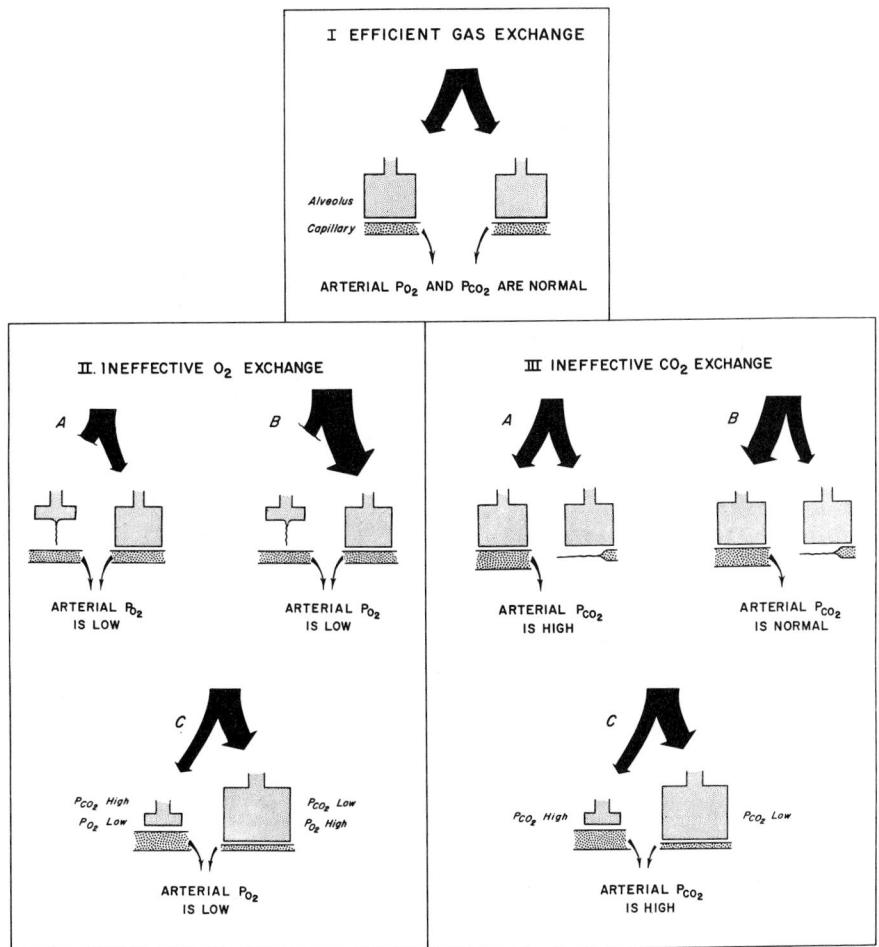

Figure 18. Effect of changes in ventilation and perfusion on arterial P_{O_2} and P_{CO_2}. Solid black arrows represent tidal volume, and differences in thickness refer to changes in magnitude of the tidal volume.

I, The normal lung is assumed to consist of two alveoli, each perfused with one-half of the cardiac output.

II, A and *B,* Acute collapse of a terminal airspace is associated with continued perfusion. The addition of mixed venous to well oxygenated blood (intrapulmonary right-to-left shunt) results in arterial hypoxemia. The extent of hypoxemia depends on the percentage of cardiac output passing nonventilated alveoli and the inspired oxygen concentration. Despite an increase in tidal volume to the ventilated-perfused airspace, oxygenation is still deficient because of the "venous admixture" effect.

II C, Marked $\dot{V}/\dot{Q}$ maldistribution (e.g., collapse of terminal airways, hypoventilation) can also result in hypoxemia. The alveolus at left receives less ventilation but most of perfusion, and the blood moving past this area is incompletely oxygenated. The reverse occurs in the alveolus at right. Since the bulk of cardiac output is underoxygenated and underventilated, arterial P_{O_2} will be low and P_{CO_2} will be high.

III A and *B,* Flow has ceased to one ventilated airspace, and this has now assumed the role of a dead space. Since it is a "variable dead space" (i.e., its effectiveness in carbon dioxide removal is dependent on the degree of ventilation and perfusion, as compared to an anatomic dead space, where gas exchange does not take place), it can be designated as an alveolar dead space. The sum of the anatomic ($V_{D_{ANAT}}$) and the alveolar ($V_{D_{ALV}}$) dead spaces is called the physiologic ($V_{D_{PHYS}}$) dead space. Changes in alveolar dead space can be produced by complete cessation of blood flow (e.g., pulmonary embolism, fall in pulmonary artery pressure due to hypotension, hemorrhage). Lesser degrees of dead space change are produced by a marked imbalance between ventilation and perfusion, as in *III C.* The arterial P_{CO_2} may be reduced to normal values if ventilation to the perfused alveolus is increased. Thus, when physiologic dead space is high, a corresponding elevation in tidal ventilation is required to maintain arterial P_{CO_2} within normal limits. (From Laver, M. B., and Austen, W. G.: *In* Sabiston, D. C., Jr., and Spencer, F. C. (Eds.): Gibbon's Surgery of the Chest, 3rd ed. Philadelphia, W. B. Saunders Company, 1976.)

The oxygen content of end-capillary blood in ventilated alveoli ($C_{C_{O_2}}$) is not accessible for direct measurement, and certain assumptions are necessary to obtain a workable expression. When 100 per cent oxygen is breathed, alveolar P_{O_2} is well above the value necessary to achieve full saturation of hemoglobin (calculable as $P_{A_{O_2}}$ in equation 10 when $P_B = 760$ mm. Hg). This facilitates calculation of pulmonary end-capillary oxygen content, as follows:

$$C_{C_{O_2}} = \underbrace{[Hb \times 1.36]}_{\substack{O_2 \text{ bound by} \\ \text{hemoglobin}}} + \underbrace{[P_{A_{O_2}} + 0.0031]}_{O_2 \text{ in solution}} \qquad (14)$$

where Hb = hemoglobin concentration in gm./100 ml.
    1.36 = ml. oxygen bound per gram of hemoglobin (one gram molecular weight of oxygen is equivalent to 22,400 ml., and four molecules of oxygen react with one gram molecular weight of hemoglobin [i.e., 66,000 gm.]. Thus, each gram of hemoglobin binds $4 \times 22,400/66,000$ or 1.36 ml. of oxygen)
    0.0031 = factor for converting partial pressure of oxygen content (ml./100 ml.) at 37°C., i.e., $\alpha \cdot 100 \cdot 1/760$, where α = Bunsen solubility coefficient for oxygen at the specified temperature

Similar conditions apply to the arterial oxygen content, whenever hemoglobin is fully saturated:

$$Ca_{O_2} = [Hb \times 1.36] + [Pa_{O_2} \times 0.0031] \qquad (15)$$

If we substitute equations 14 and 15 into equation 13, we obtain the modified shunt equation, which is considerably more useful:

$$\frac{\dot{Q}_S}{\dot{Q}_T} = \frac{0.0031 \, (P_{A_{O_2}} - Pa_{O_2})}{[Ca_{O_2} - C_{\bar{V}_{O_2}}] + 0.0031 \, [P_{A_{O_2}} - Pa_{O_2}]} \qquad (16)$$

All variables found in equation 16 are available for measurement. Samples of mixed venous blood and its oxygen content ($C_{\bar{V}_{O_2}}$) are not routinely available, but recent introduction of a technique for floating a catheter into the pulmonary artery has placed this measurement within our reach.[39]

In practice, equation 16, or the modified shunt equation, should be used only if Pa_{O_2} is above 150 mm. Hg. We have chosen this value arbitrarily on the assumption that above this value incomplete saturation of hemoglobin with oxygen introduces insignificant errors in the clinical setting. If Pa_{O_2} is below 150 mm. Hg and the patient is ventilated with 100 per cent oxygen, calculation of $\dot{Q}_S/\dot{Q}_T$ must be performed according to equations 13 and 14.

Monitoring changes in $P(A\text{-}aDO_2)$ while the patient is breathing 100 per cent oxygen is a useful maneuver for approximating the inefficiency of oxygenation, provided we remember that the changes recorded are not always indicative of a changing shunt. Examination of

equation 16 indicates that cardiac output and pulmonary right-to-left shunt are related via the Fick equation (i.e., C.O. = $\dot{V}_{O_2}/Ca_{O_2} - C_{\bar{V}_{O_2}}$). If oxygen consumption ($\dot{V}_{O_2}$) remains constant, changes in cardiac output must be reflected by simultaneous changes in $C[a\text{-}\bar{V}DO_2]$, or changes in cardiac output must be reflected by changes in $P[A\text{-}aDO_2]$, whenever $\dot{Q}_S/\dot{Q}_T$ is constant. For example, if $Pa_{O_2} = 350$ mm. Hg: (1) with a high cardiac output (i.e., $C[a\text{-}\bar{V}DO_2] = 3$ ml./100 ml. and $Pa_{CO_2} = 40$ mm. Hg, according to equations 10 and the Fick equation, $\dot{Q}_S/\dot{Q}_T = 0.25$, i.e., 25 per cent of the cardiac output perfuses nonventilated areas; and (2) with a low cardiac output (i.e., $C[a\text{-}\bar{V}DO_2] = 8$ ml./100 ml. and $Pa_{CO_2} = 40$ mm. Hg), $\dot{Q}_S/\dot{Q}_T = 0.11$, or 11 per cent of cardiac output perfuses nonventilated areas. Thus, despite a constant Pa_{O_2}, a twofold rise in cardiac output represents a proportionate rise in perfusion of nonventilated alveoli. The problem is complicated further by recent evidence that brief ventilation with 100 per cent oxygen for calculation of $\dot{Q}_S/\dot{Q}_T$ may result in increased perfusion of nonventilated lung regions and thereby increase the value of calculated shunt.[37]

Acute changes in pulmonary artery pressure (e.g. secondary to hypotension) with preferential perfusion of nonventilated, dependent lung (Fig. 11) in association with the vascular dilatation produced by high concentrations of oxygen will also alter $\dot{Q}_S/\dot{Q}_T$.[36] Conversely, pre-existent pulmonary hypertension and increased perfusion of the apices may negate the effects of increased airway pressure on ventilation of the bases, thereby eliminating the expected decrease in venous admixture.[42] Despite these complicating features certain generalizations are appropriate and useful.

A graphic presentation of equation 13 or its modified form, equation 16, is given in Figure 19. The effect that a change in alveolar P_{O_2} ($P_{A_{O_2}}$) will have on arterial P_{O_2} (Pa_{O_2}) as the intrapulmonary right-to-left shunt rises up to 50 per cent of cardiac output is shown in Figure 19A. In the face of a high $\dot{Q}_S/\dot{Q}_T$, an increase in inspired oxygen concentration to 100 per cent ($F_{I_{O_2}} = 1$ and $P_{A_{O_2}} = 680$ mm. Hg) produces a minimal rise in Pa_{O_2} above that achieved on ventilation with ambient air (i.e., $F_{I_{O_2}} = 0.21$ and $P_{A_{O_2}} = 100$ mm. Hg). This has important practical consequences. When the intrapulmonary right-to-left shunt is large and requires ventilation with a high concentration of oxygen, little will be gained by increasing the inspired oxygen concentration from 70 or 80 per cent to 100 per cent. Since prolonged ventilation with 100 per cent oxygen (24 hours or longer) is probably detrimental to the lung, and since the presence of a nonabsorbable gas (nitrogen) assists in maintaining terminal airway integrity, it is best that $F_{I_{O_2}}$ be maintained in the 0.7 to 0.8 range, although higher concentrations should be used if hypoxemia is severe.

It has been stated that in the presence of an anatomic right-to-left shunt, diagnosis of the latter can be made from the lack of change in arterial oxygenation when the patient is given 100 per cent oxygen to breathe. This is incorrect. Whether the change is large enough to be interpreted as significant depends on the

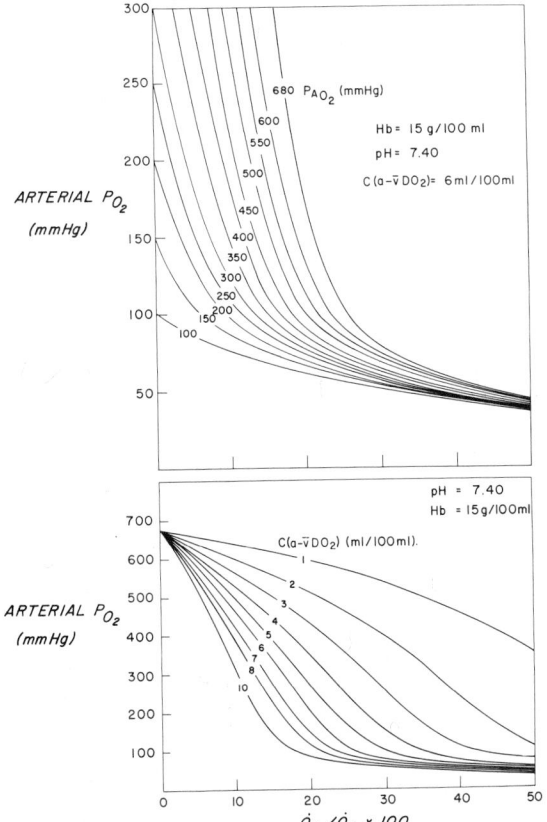

a large intrapulmonary right-to-left shunt ($\dot{Q}_S/\dot{Q}_T \times 100 = 50$) and a low cardiac output (i.e., $C[a-\overline{V}DO_2] = 10$) can be improved by an increase in cardiac output or a decrease in $C[a-\overline{V}DO_2]$. When the right-to-left shunt is large, improvement in Pa_{O_2} can be achieved only with a substantial rise in flow. However, the graph underscores the importance of cardiac output in determining the efficiency of arterial oxygenation in the critically ill patient. The same reasoning applies to changes in oxygen consumption. A rise in $\dot{V}_{O_2}$ is associated with an increase in $C[a-\overline{V}DO_2]$ and a deterioration of arterial oxygenation. The reader is encouraged to become familiar with these graphs. They provide the essence for understanding the influence of different factors on arterial oxygenation. The alinearity shown in these graphs is caused by the specific shape of the oxyhemoglobin dissociation curve[34] because Pa_{O_2} is a composite of oxygen contents taken from the linear part of the curve (ventilated and perfused airspaces, i.e., $C_{C_{O_2}}$) and its steeper, alinear portion (mixed venous blood, i.e., $C_{\overline{V}_{O_2}}$) as shown in Figure 20; Table 5 lists the factors that influence $P[A-aDO_2]$.

Carbon Dioxide

As indicated in Figure 18, part *III, A, B,* and *C,* an imbalance between ventilation and perfusion may increase the inefficiency of carbon dioxide removal. Nonperfusion of a ventilated airspace represents the same obstacle to efficient carbon dioxide removal as the addition of a mechanical dead space. To appreciate this concept, it is necessary to review the relationship between carbon dioxide output and tidal volume.

Figure 19. *Top,* Relation between arterial P_{O_2} (Pa_{O_2}) and intrapulmonary right-to-left shunt at different levels of alveolar P_{O_2} (PA_{O_2}) or arteriovenous oxygen content differences (AVO$_2$). PA_{O_2} varies according to the inspired oxygen concentration. The curves were calculated on the basis of a standard oxyhemoglobin dissociation curve (i.e., P_{O_2} at 50 per cent saturation = 26.6 mm. Hg) a pH of 7.4, and a hemoglobin concentration of 15 gm./100 ml. Note the convergence of arterial P_{O_2} values as $\dot{Q}_S/\dot{Q}_T \times 100$ rises.

Bottom, Effect of a change in the arterial minus mixed venous oxygen content (AVO$_2$) (secondary to an alteration in cardiac output or oxygen consumption) on arterial P_{O_2}. Note the marked rise in arterial P_{O_2} as AVO$_2$ falls at moderate levels of right-to-left shunt (i.e., $\dot{Q}_S/\dot{Q}_T \times 100$ range of 10 to 20 per cent). If $\dot{Q}_S/\dot{Q}_T \times 100 = 30$ per cent and AVO$_2$ = 8 ml./100 ml., arterial P_{O_2} can be raised from approximately 80 to 400 mm. Hg by a fourfold rise in cardiac output. (From "Acute Respiratory Failure in the Surgical Patient" by Pontoppidan, H., Laver, M. B., and Geffin, B. *In* Advances in Surgery, Vol. 4, by Welch, C. E. Copyright © 1970 by Year Book Medical Publishers, Inc., Chicago. Used by permission.)

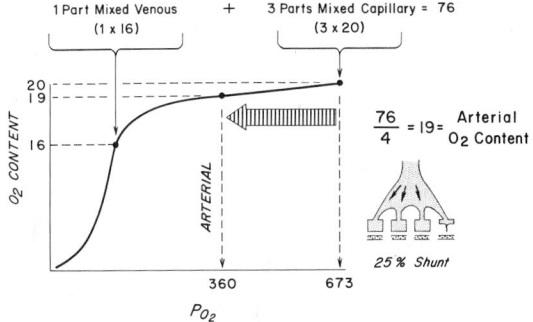

Figure 20. Effect of an intrapulmonary right-to-left shunt on arterial P_{O_2} and oxygen content during ventilation with 100 per cent oxygen. A 25 per cent right-to-left shunt is shown at right. Above full saturation of hemoglobin (i.e., P_{O_2} = 150 Torr), the relationship between oxygen content and Pa_{O_2} is expressed by a straight line (top of curve). As the mixed venous point begins to move down to the steep portion of the curve, the arterial P_{O_2} moves to the left. At this stage (Pa_{O_2} less than 100 Torr), the drop in P_{O_2} is small despite the increase in $\dot{Q}_S/\dot{Q}_T \times 100$. It is this gradual diminution in P_{O_2} that leads to convergences of the lines at high $\dot{Q}_S/\dot{Q}_T$ in Figure 15. (From Laver, M. B., and Austen, W. G. *In* Sabiston, D. C., Jr., and Spencer, F. C. (Eds.): Gibbon's Surgery of the Chest, 3rd ed. Philadelphia, W. B. Saunders Company, 1976.)

degree of right-to-left shunt. As shown in Figure 19, when $\dot{Q}_S/\dot{Q}_T \times 100$ is greater than 50 per cent of cardiac output, the resulting benefits in Pa_{O_2} are modest; when $\dot{Q}_S/\dot{Q}_T$ is less than 50 per cent, the change can be substantial.

Figure 19*B* illustrates the effect of a change in cardiac output (or oxygen consumption) on arterial P_{O_2} at different values for $\dot{Q}_S/\dot{Q}_T$. Arterial hypoxemia due to

TABLE 5. Factors that Influence the Alveolar-Arterial Oxygen Tension Difference $|P(A-aDO_2)|$*

1. Right to left shunt ($\dot{Q}_S/\dot{Q}_T \times 100$), i.e., per cent of cardiac output ($\dot{Q}_T$) flowing past nonventilated alveoli ($\dot{Q}_S$).
2. Arteriovenous oxygen content difference $C[A - \overline{V}DO_2]$).
3. Oxygen consumption ($\dot{V}_{O_2}$) through its effect on mixed venous oxygen content ($C_{\overline{V}_{O_2}}$).
4. Cardiac output ($\dot{Q}_T$)
   A. Secondary to change in $C[a - \overline{V}DO_2]$ when oxygen consumption ($\dot{V}_{O_2}$) remains constant ($\dot{Q}_T = \dot{V}_{O_2}/C(a - \overline{V}DO_2)$).
   B. Secondary to redistribution of pulmonary blood flow.
5. Inspired-oxygen concentration (uneven distribution plays a greater role when less than 100 per cent oxygen is inspired).
6. Position of the hemoglobin-oxygen dissociation curve (pH, body temperature, red cell 2,3-diphosphoglyceric acid concentration).[34]
7. Position of the arterial point (Pa_{O_2} on the oxygen-hemoglobin dissociation curve, i.e., above or below full saturation).

*The list does not include the influence of a change in distribution of ventilation or body position as discussed in the text.

Total carbon dioxide expired per breath consists of carbon dioxide removal from ventilated, perfused alveoli, represented by the volume of gas from these alveoli (V_A) times its carbon dioxide concentration ($P_{A_{CO_2}}$), or $V_A \cdot P_{A_{CO_2}}$. However, expired air is a combination from both ventilated, perfused and ventilated, nonperfused alveoli. Thus, volume of gas contributed from dead space (V_D), per breath, times its carbon dioxide concentration ($P_{D_{CO_2}}$) (i.e., $V_D \cdot P_{D_{CO_2}}$) plus $V_A \cdot P_{A_{CO2}}$ equals expired tidal volume (V_E) times the mixed expired carbon dioxide concentration ($P_{E_{CO_2}}$).*

$$V_A \cdot P_{A_{CO_2}} = V_E \cdot P_{\overline{E}_{CO_2}} + V_D \cdot P_{D_{CO_2}} \qquad (17)$$

A more practical equation is obtained with the following assumptions:

$$V_A = V_E - V_D; \ P_{D_{CO_2}} = 0; \ P_{A_{CO_2}} = Pa_{CO_2} \qquad (18)$$

The assumption that $P_{D_{CO_2}} = 0$ is not strictly true, since gas inspired into a nonperfused, ventilated alveolus is not free of carbon dioxide; however, the error introduced by the assumption is small and may be ignored.

*The quantity of carbon dioxide removed is the product of gas volume expired (V_E) and the fractional concentration of carbon dioxide in mixed expired air ($F_{E_{CO_2}}$). In the gas phase, fractional concentration and partial pressure are equivalent, but not equal ($P_{\overline{E}_{CO_2}} = F_{\overline{E}_{CO_2}} \cdot [P_B - P_{H_2O}^T]$).

Substituting the assumptions from equation 18 into equation 17, we obtain:

$$V_T \cdot P_{\overline{E}_{CO_2}} = (V_T - V_D)Pa_{CO_2} \qquad (19)$$

According to equation 19, a rise in tidal volume (V_T) is necessary to keep alveolar tidal volume ($V_D - V_T$) constant when dead space (V_D) rises. Rearranging and dividing equation 19:

$$\frac{V_D}{V_T} = \frac{Pa_{CO_2} - P_{\overline{E}_{CO_2}}}{Pa_{CO_2}} = 1 - \frac{P_{\overline{E}_{CO_2}}}{Pa_{CO_2}} \qquad (20)$$

The effects of an increase in physiologic dead space on the V_D/V_T ratio are illustrated in Figure 21. A rise in this ratio implies decreased efficiency of carbon dioxide removal and requires an increase in tidal vol-

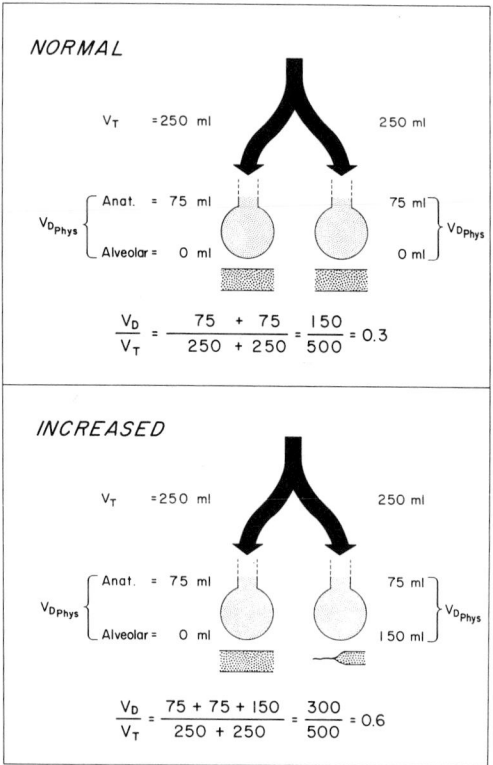

Figure 21. A schematic presentation of the influence of a rise in alveolar dead space on the V_D/V_T ratio. Physiologic dead space ($V_{D_{PHYS}}$) is the sum of anatomic ($V_{D_{ANAT}}$) and alveolar ($V_{D_{ALV}}$) dead space. $V_{D_{ANAT}}$ in the adult in milliliters is equal to body weight in pounds. Significant changes in $V_{D_{PHYS}}$ arise from changes in the ventilation-perfusion relationship. In the normal lung (top), $V_{D_{ALV}}$ is essentially zero, and the $V_{D_{PHYS}}/V_T$ ratio varies from 0.35 to 0.45. When perfusion to a major portion of the lung ceases (bottom), $V_{D_{PHYS}}$ rises and alveolar ventilation of the perfused airspace must be increased substantially if Pa_{CO_2} is to be kept within normal limits. It is not unusual to find a $V_{D_{PHYS}}/V_T$ ratio as high as 0.85 in patients with acute respiratory failure. This means that minute ventilation delivered from a ventilator must be nearly twice the estimated normal to keep P_{CO_2} at 40 Torr.

SOURCES OF MIXED ARTERIAL TO MEAN ALVEOLAR CO_2 GRADIENTS

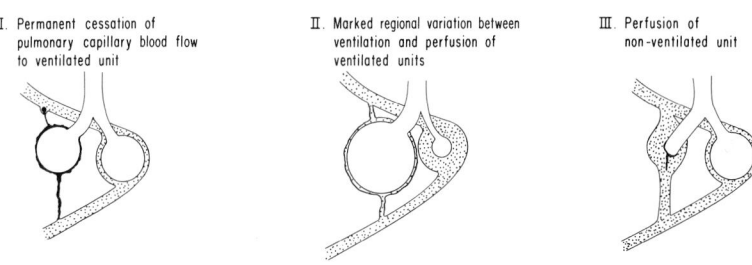

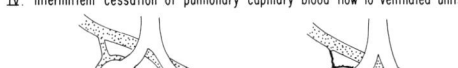

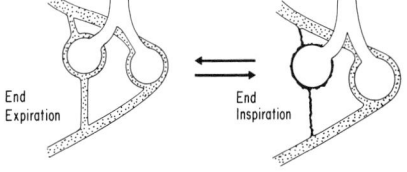

Figure 22. Potential sources of an increased physiologic dead space during and after surgery. The problem in every case is due to a marked deviation of $\dot{V}/\dot{Q}$ from normal. *I*, Permanent cessation of pulmonary capillary blood flow arises as a result of embolism or pulmonary artery hypotension. *II*, Marked regional variation between $\dot{V}/\dot{Q}$ is conspicuous in chronic obstructive lung disease and during thoracotomy. *III*, Perfusion of a nonventilated unit leads to an increase in arterial P_{CO_2} because mixed venous blood, with a high carbon dioxide content, raises the P_{CO_2} of the oxygenated and ventilated blood ("pseudo-dead space effect"). *IV*, Intermittent cessation of pulmonary capillary blood flow is common in acute respiratory failure when major portions of the lung have a low compliance, and ventilation with a high airway pressure distends excessively the high-compliance airspaces.

ume if Pa_{CO_2} is to remain constant. Changes in carbon dioxide production ($\dot{V}_{CO_2}$) can also influence Pa_{CO_2} if V_D/V_T is unaltered. A rise in $\dot{V}_{CO_2}$ (e.g., caused by a rise in temperature) will elevate Pa_{CO_2} (if ventilation is unchanged). Evaluation of arterial blood gases and lung function must take these variables into account.

Nonperfusion of ventilated alveoli is caused by pulmonary emboli, hemorrhagic hypotension, a fall in cardiac output, or a pharmacologic lowering of mean pulmonary artery pressure. Except for embolism, all these factors are associated with an increase in the size of Zone I (see Figs. 10 and 11). Carbon dioxide retention in chronic obstructive lung disease arises from a marked discrepancy between $\dot{V}$ and $\dot{Q}$. Most of the lung is hypoventilated but overperfused, while a small portion is hyperventilated but underperfused; the coalescent flow is weighted by the bulk of the hypoventilated blood, and Pa_{CO_2} remains high (Fig. 18, *III C*).

An increase in physiologic dead space secondary to or independent of a diminished cardiac output inevitably contributes to inadequate carbon dioxide removal during and after surgery, as well as in acute respiratory failure. Hypoventilation due to excessive narcotic medication or an improperly functioning ventilator is a preventable disorder and otherwise readily corrected.

Possible sources of an increased physiologic dead space are indicated in Figure 22.

We have discussed a host of variables that affect blood gas exchange in the patient subjected to surgery. However, one must not forget that age per se can also have an effect on arterial oxygenation. Table 6 lists the arterial P_{O_2} and P_{CO_2} in adults from age 30 upward. Aging is associated with a progressive fall in Pa_{O_2} but no change in Pa_{CO_2} in the absence of heart or lung disease. Although the source of the fall in P_{O_2} is not immediately obvious, it has been attributed to the higher closing volume found in the old adult.[21] Inter-

mittent airway closure lowers arterial P_{O_2} because mixed venous blood perfuses collapsed areas during the expiratory pause and passes intermittently into the arterial side without being fully oxygenated.

DIFFUSION OF GAS BETWEEN UPPER AIRWAY AND PULMONARY CAPILLARY BLOOD

Gas transport between upper and terminal airways is promoted by gas pressure gradients developed by oxygen uptake or carbon dioxide output at the alveolar-capillary boundary. The relative importance of ventilation vis-à-vis diffusion in the gas phase is illustrated by the arterial blood gas changes found in the absence of ventilatory movement. During apnea with the endotracheal tube attached to a reservoir containing oxygen, blood flowing through the lung will continue to take up oxygen, and arterial P_{O_2} will remain high. The partial pressure gradient between upper

TABLE 6. The Effect of Age on Arterial P_{O_2} and P_{CO_2} While Breathing Ambient Air at Rest*

Age Group (in Years)	No. Obs.	Pa_{O_2} (mm. Hg) Mean ± SD	Pa_{CO_2} (mm. Hg) Mean ± SD
<30 (median = 23)	38	94.2 3.31	39.0 1.8
31–40 (median = 36)	30	87.2 3.47	38.5 2.0
41–50 (median = 46)	30	83.9 4.07	39.6 2.4
51–60 (median = 55)	30	81.2 3.74	39.0 1.9
>60 (median = 71)	24	74.3 4.43	39.8 2.1

*From Sorbini, C. A., et al.: Respiration, *25*:3, 1968.

and terminal airway will be large* and will promote rapid diffusion through the gas phase. On the other hand, the P_{CO_2} gradient between alveolus and upper airway is small, and P_{CO_2} will rise in proportion to the duration of apnea.

Diffusion limitations within the lung are present from the alveolar-capillary barrier to the red cell interior and end with the reaction rate between hemoglobin and oxygen.

Two principal resistances to gas transfer exist which may be considered to be in series. The first is a composite of several layers (membrane, M) including the alveolar lining cells, basal membrane, interstitium, capillary endothelium, the plasma layer, and finally the red cell membrane. The second resistance is the reaction rate between hemoglobin and carbon monoxide, a tracer gas commonly used for quantifying diffusion properties of the lung. Using the electrical analogy for summing resistance, we have:

$$\frac{1}{R_L} = \frac{1}{K \cdot \Theta} + \frac{1}{R_M} \qquad (21)$$

where R_L = total resistance to gas transfer
  R_M = resistance of the tissue layers to gas transfer
  Θ = reaction rate between carbon monoxide and hemoglobin
  K = constant dependent on the amount of hemoglobin (i.e., red cells) in the pulmonary capillary bed

Substituting the symbol D for R in equation 23, we can write:

$$\frac{1}{D_L} = \frac{1}{V_C \Theta} + \frac{1}{D_M} \qquad (22)$$

where D_L = diffusivity of lung for the test gas (ml./min./mm. Hg)
  V_C = volume of red cells in pulmonary capillaries
  D_M = diffusivity of "membrane" component (ml./min./mm. Hg)
  Θ = reaction rate between the test gas (usually carbon monoxide) and hemoglobin (ml./min./mm. Hg)

Θ is oxygen dependent. Thus, proper assessment of D_L and D_M can be made only by defining the quantity of carbon monoxide taken up per unit time at different alveolar oxygen concentrations. Equation 21 describes a straight line (Fig. 23):

$$y = mx + b$$

*P_{O_2} in the reservoir is close to 1 atmosphere, while in mixed venous blood it is 40 to 70 mm. Hg. The gradient is sufficient to move oxygen almost as fast as it is removed by blood flow; the P_{CO_2} gradient is substantially less (mixed venous P_{CO_2} is 45 to 55 mm. Hg and upper airway P_{CO_2} near zero) and insufficient to allow for adequate removal by diffusion alone.

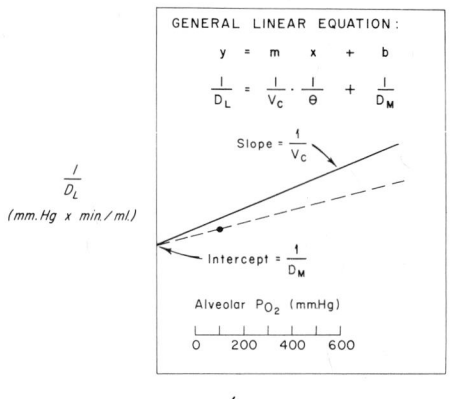

Figure 23. Effect of a change in alveolar P_{O_2} on lung (D_L) and "membrane" (D_M) diffusion capacity. The lung diffusion capacity measured with carbon monoxide ($D_{L_{CO}}$) varies according to the diffusivity of the alveolar capillary membrane ($D_{M_{CO}}$), the pulmonary capillary blood volume (V_C), and the reaction rate between hemoglobin and carbon monoxide (θ). Magnitude of the latter is dependent upon the alveolar P_{O_2}. The linear equation for diffusion shown at top can be solved for $D_{L_{CO}}$ if the measurements are carried out at different values for $P_{A_{O_2}}$. Values for θ are assumed from data obtained in vitro. If the gas transfer rate is diminished, then D_L falls and $1/D_L$ rises. The solid circle on the dashed line represents the value for D_L in a normal lung with membrane diffusivity (D_M) obtained from the y-intercept. If the pulmonary blood volume (V_C) falls, then $1/V_C$ (solid line) must rise, and a single measurement of D_L while ambient air is breathed (i.e., alveolar P_{O_2} = 100 Torr) will indicate a fall in lung diffusivity ($1/D_L$ rises) without implying a change in membrane component; i.e., the D_M intercept is constant. Comprehensive studies of diffusion have indicated that "alveolar-capillary block" is a minor contributor to hypoxemia in most disease states. (From Laver, M. B. and Austen, W. G. In Sabiston, D. C., Jr., and Spencer, F. C. (Eds.): Gibbon's Surgery of the Chest, 3rd ed. Philadelphia, W. B. Saunders Company, 1976.)

Lung diffusion capacity, expressed on the ordinate as $\frac{1}{D_L}$, is measured at different concentrations of alveolar P_{O_2} for which Θ (drawn on the abscissa) is known (Fig. 23). $\frac{1}{D_M}$ is the y-intercept, while pulmonary capillary blood volume (V_C) is equal to the reciprocal of the slope.

This type of analysis has elucidated the contribution of the "membrane" component to the abnormalities of gas exchange seen with respiratory failure. Previously, conclusions on changes of diffusivity were based on a measurement of D_L and on the assumption that D_L equals D_M without taking into account V_C or Θ. Thus, a rise of diffusivity was attributed to an "alveolar-capillary block." A single measurement of diffusivity when ambient air is breathed (e.g., $P_{A_{O_2}}$ = 100 mm. Hg) may result in an abnormally high value for D_L due to a change in pulmonary capillary blood volume (slope equals $\frac{1}{V_C}$) while D_M (the intercept) remains constant. According to recent studies,[2] the reduction of D_M is not sufficient to account for inadequate oxygenation of respiratory failure. This is even less likely to be a factor when $P_{A_{O_2}}$ is elevated during therapy.

A decrease in lung diffusivity (D_L), i.e., greater resistance to gas transfer, can be detected in the presence of pulmonary vascular congestion owing to a slight decrease in D_M and a rise in pulmonary capillary blood volume (V_C). Again, the change in D_M is not sufficiently large to justify a diagnosis of "alveolar-capillary block" as a cause of hypoxemia.

Equation 22 defines diffusivity for any gas from upper airway to the red cells. Diffusivity for oxygen can be calculated by combining the effects of (1) gas solubility on diffusivity with (2) Graham's law, which states that the ratio of diffusivity of two gases is inversely proportional to the square root of their molecular weights. Thus:

$$\frac{D_{L_{CO}}}{D_{L_{O_2}}} = \frac{\alpha CO}{\alpha O_2} \cdot \frac{\sqrt{mol.\ wt.\ O_2}}{\sqrt{mol.\ wt.\ CO}} = \frac{0.018}{0.024} \div \frac{\sqrt{32}}{\sqrt{28}} = 0.8$$

where α = Bunsen solubility for oxygen and carbon monoxide in water at $37°C$.

A clinically significant increase in D_M is seen in such disorders as pulmonary fibrosis, various "collagen" disorders, diffuse infiltration by lymphoma, and alveolar hemorrhage.

Consideration of diffusion has been exceedingly brief. However, this approach is prompted by the belief that its role in the etiology of hypoxemia is a minor one.

RESPIRATORY FAILURE

Prevention, recognition, and treatment of acute respiratory failure (ARF) in the surgical patient cannot be discussed in detail within the confines of an introductory chapter on lung function. Several recent monographs and reviews have dealt with the subject at length and will serve as appropriate references.[24, 27, 28]

Most discussions of lung function have considered gas exchange exclusively, with little attention given to its complex metabolic and hormonal functions.[18] The comments that follow are directed to clinical problems related to acute failure of adequate oxygenation.

Acute respiratory failure (ARF) is an important and frequent complication in the critically ill patient. Fashion has dictated the need for special labels proposed to help with diagnosis and, presumably, therapy. Terms such as "shock lung," "pump lung," and "adult respiratory distress syndrome" (ARDS) have found their way into the literature.[2] There is little evidence that such designations are justified. First, ARF can appear without antecedent shock and, second, it is unlikely that the pathologic physiology of abnormal gas exchange following prolonged periods of inadequate blood flow is a unique, definable entity. The term ARDS was intended to attract our attention to the similarity of ARF in the adult to that in the neonate. Unfortunately, there is nothing to suggest a common substrate for the two except profound hypoxemia.

Early ARF may exist in the absence of visible distress, and clinical experience suggests that optimal success with therapy is closely related to early, aggressive therapy intended to support both heart and lung function before the appearance of acute distress.

The causes of abnormal blood-gas exchange are many and varied. It is fair to assume that any patient who requires extensive intra-abdominal surgery, who has a history of heart or lung disease, who develops gram-negative sepsis, or who requires operation for acute trauma with massive transfusions, is at risk. Therapy is most effective if started early. Experience with mechanical ventilation has progressed sufficiently to warrant its prophylactic use whenever arterial oxygenation cannot be maintained within satisfactory limits or the hemodynamic situation is sufficiently tenuous to warrant extensive pharmacologic support. The first step to successful therapy requires an appropriate definition of ARF. In general terms, the early phase of ARF after operation is characterized by hypoxemia, decreased lung compliance, and little or no abnormality in CO_2 exchange. A set of working definitions is listed in Table 7; the common causes of ARF in the surgical patient are indicated in Table 8 and the physiologic changes shown in Figure 24.

The principal source of respiratory failure is an acute diminution of functional residual capacity (FRC), presumably secondary to a marked increase in lung fluid, either interstitial or intra-alveolar, and an increase in surface activity. The latter results in lessened stability of terminal airways, and closure or collapse ensues.

The effect of pulmonary edema on alveolar geometry is shown in Figure 25. When the duration of capillary nonperfusion is prolonged excessively (e.g., hemorrhage, pulmonary artery hypotension), loss of fluid into the extravascular space is prominent once circulation is re-established. As with pulmonary edema of cardiac origin, the excess of interstitial fluid compromises alveolar stability, fluid fills the terminal airways, and hypoxemia appears owing to continued perfusion of these nonventilated airspaces[35] (Fig. 26).

The presence of ARF implies abnormal function of both terminal air units and the pulmonary vasculature. Alterations in vascular integrity are common to gram-negative endotoxemia[8] or embolization with particulate matter secondary to massive transfusion of improperly filtered blood. Respiratory failure consequent to changes in pulmonary hemodynamic characteristics is, therefore, associated with an acute increase in right ventricular (RV) afterload, a condition poorly tolerated by the previously normal RV. Thus, proper therapy of ARF must include support of both heart and lung function. For example, the hemodynamic effects of mechanical ventilation are readily reversed by an increase in intravascular volume of red cells and plasma.[29] Although there is substantial evidence for a consistent increase in pulmonary capillary wedge or left ventricular (LV) filling pressure under these circumstances, it is less evident that this increase represents primary LV failure. Compliance characteristics of the RV are such that acute changes in after-

TABLE 7. Guidelines for Ventilatory Support in Adults with ARF

Datum	Normal Range	Indication for Tracheal Intubation and Ventilation
MECHANICS:		
Respiratory rate	12–20	>35
Vital capacity (ml./kg. of body weight*)	65–75	<15
FEV_1‡ (ml./kg. of body weight*)	50–60	<10
Inspiratory force (cm. H_2O)	75–100	<25
OXYGENATION:		
Pa_{O_2} (mm. Hg)	100–75 (air)	<70 (on mask O_2)
$P(A-aDO_2)$ (mm. Hg)**	25–65	>450
VENTILATION:		
Pa_{CO_2} (mm. Hg)	35–45	>55†
V_D/V_T	0.25–0.40	>0.60

The trend of values is of utmost importance. The numerical guidelines should obviously not be adopted to the exclusion of clinical judgment. For example, a vital capacity below 15 ml./kg. may prove sufficient provided the patient can still cough "effectively," if hypoxemia is prevented, as discussed in the text, and if hypercapnia is not progressive. However, such a patient needs frequent blood gas analyses and close observation in a well-equipped, adequately staffed recovery room or intensive care unit.
*"Ideal" weight is used if weight appears grossly abnormal.
**After 10 minutes of 100% oxygen.
†Except in patients with chronic hypercapnia.
‡First second forced expired volume.
(Reproduced with permission from Wilson, R. S., and Pontoppidan, H.: Acute respiratory failure: Diagnostic and therapeutic criteria. Crit. Care Med., 2:293–304, 1974.)

load result in increased end-diastolic volume and small changes in end-diastolic pressure. Due to limitations set by the noncompliant pericardium, an increase in end-diastolic size of one ventricle must encroach upon the size of the other. Consequently, alterations in LV filling pressure may reflect a change

TABLE 8. Common Causes of Acute Respiratory Failure in the Surgical Patient

1. Trauma (crushed chest, extensive burn, etc.)
2. Massive blood transfusion (?vascular reaction to leukocytes, platelets)
3. Embolism (e.g., fat or blood clot)
4. Sepsis (intrapulmonary or extrapulmonary)
5. Aspiration (gastric contents, drowning, etc.)
6. Abdominal distention
7. Pulmonary edema (left ventricular failure, mitral stenosis, fluid overload)
8. Prolonged loss of consciousness (head injury, drug intoxication, etc.) with inadequate lung expansion

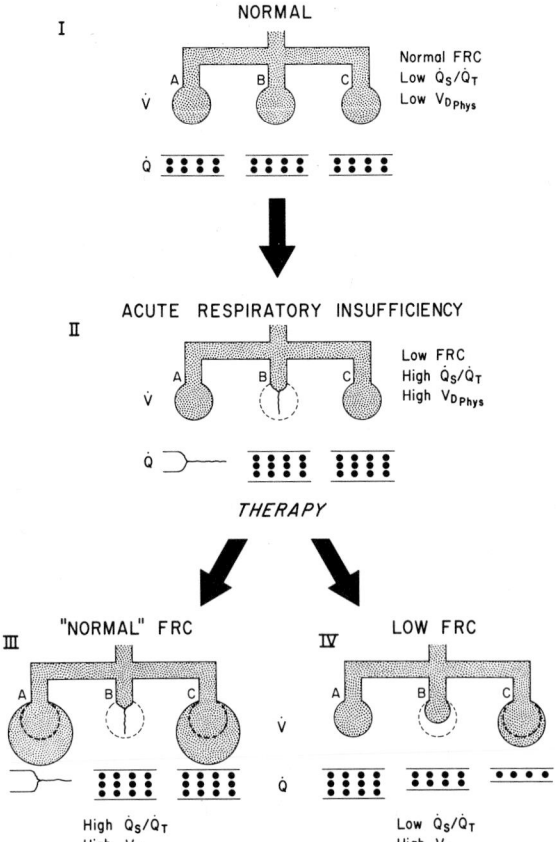

Figure 24. Common changes in lung function that accompany respiratory failure, and their response to therapy.

in ventricular compliance secondary to a modified RV end-diastolic volume. This problem has been dealt with in the animal experiment by Taylor et al.[40]

Measurement of RV volume at the bedside is not possible at this time, and interpretation of right atrial pressure (RAP) relative to atmospheric pressure is made difficult by unpredictable changes in pleural pressure when either lung compliance or intra-abdominal pressures (Fig. 27) are increased. Therefore, evaluation of hemodynamic performance in the patient with ARF is difficult and occasionally impossible without the benefit of cardiac output measurement.

The technology of extracorporeal gas exchange has progressed sufficiently to allow for extracorporeal membrane oxygenation (ECMO) support when all other measures at improved ventilation have not succeeded in alleviating the profound hypoxemia. Clinical experience with this technique is being acquired at several centers, but the data on its ultimate role in ARF remain to be established.[44]

We can summarize our brief consideration of ARF as follows:

1. In all critically ill patients arterial blood gases must be determined intermittently to ascertain the adequacy of blood gas exchange. We do not consider the timing of arterial blood gas analyses appropriate if performed only after respiratory insufficiency has set

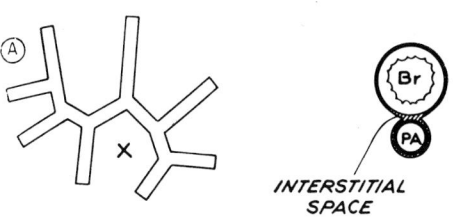

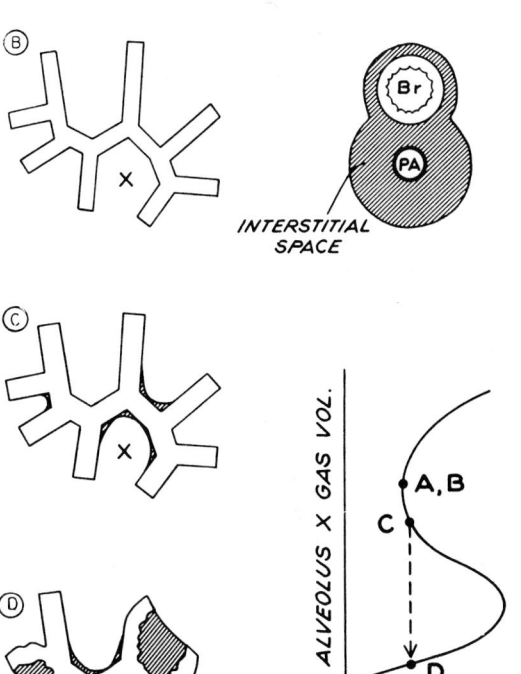

Figure 25. Effect of pulmonary edema on alveolar geometry. Edema was produced in the experimental animal by fluid overload, epinephrine infusion, or toxic damage to capillary permeability; histologic sections were obtained from lungs frozen rapidly at constant pulmonary pressure after opening the thorax. The pattern of fluid accumulation was remarkably constant regardless of the etiology of pulmonary edema. *A* and *B*, The initial accumulation of fluid was found to progress around the bronchi (Br) and pulmonary artery (PA) complex ("perivascular cuffing"), without evidence of fluid present in or immediately adjacent to alveoli. *C,* Further increase in intrapulmonary fluid volume was associated with a "thickening" of the alveolar wall, consistent with increased interstitial edema and slight decrease in alveolar diameter. *D,* Progression of interstitial edema encroaches on alveolar geometry sufficiently to cause marked instability on the volume-pressure curve. Fluid accumulates rapidly within the alveolus (intraalveolar edema) and gas exchange ceases but perfusion continues. Collapse of alveoli (i.e., apposition of alveolar walls, as noted in the unexpanded, gas-free lung of the neonate) is not evident. (From Staub, N. C., Nagano, H., and Pearce, M. B.: J. Appl. Physiol., 22:227, 1967.)

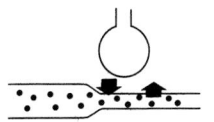

NORMAL

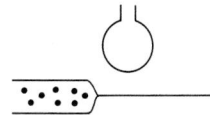

HEMORRHAGE (Hypotension)

Figure 26. Effect of an acute fall in pulmonary perfusion pressure and subsequent resuscitation on extra-alveolar distribution of fluid. Depending on the duration of arrested flow, resuscitation and re-establishment of perfusion are associated with enhanced movement of fluid into the extravascular space, ultimately sufficient to compromise alveolar integrity, as shown in Figure 25. The etiology of these changes in vascular integrity is the subject of active investigation and debate.

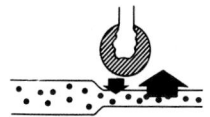

RESUSCITATION

Figure 27. Effect of intra-abdominal pressure (IAP) on right atrial pressure recorded relative to atmospheric pressure (P_{RA}^{BAR}). Right ventricular filling pressure, on right atrial transmural pressure (P_{RA}^{TM}), is equal to the difference between P_{RA}^{BAR} and pleural pressure relative to atmospheric or ($P_{RA}^{BAR} - P_{PL}^{BAR}$). An increase in intra-abdominal pressure will be transmitted to the pleural space and the right atrium, thereby causing a rise in P_{RA}^{BAR} but with no change in P_{RA}^{TM}. A patient with a distended abdomen may exhibit a high right atrial pressure (or central venous pressure) in the presence of hypovolemia and a low P_{RA}^{TM}. These problems apply also the the measurement of pulmonary capillary wedge pressures.

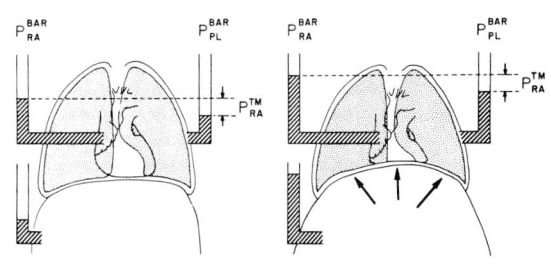

in. The recognition of incipient pulmonary failure can depend on no other tests.

2. Prophylactic ventilator therapy has proved more successful than therapy of established complications. Morbidity and mortality of this therapeutic mode, in experienced hands, has declined rapidly to a point where no patient should be denied its benefits once the need has been established.

3. Regardless of etiology, ventilator support with an adequate inspired concentration of oxygen is mandatory. Treatment of abnormal gas exchange includes appropriate support of the circulation and kidney function. Like other organs, the lung responds similarly to different stimuli, but hypoxemia is a common response to all. Pragmatism is critical if the lessons learned from basic pulmonary physiology are to find rational application in the clinical setting.

4. Acute respiratory failure occurs with frightening frequency in patients who have had no previous history of lung disease. Prevention and properly timed therapy imply recognition of the risk. Most important, and often overlooked, acute hypoxemia may be tolerated well by a patient who is otherwise chronically hypoxemic (e.g., residence of high altitude, chronic obstructive lung disease, mitral valve disease with chronic pulmonary congestion) but may be disastrous in someone whose physiologic apparatus is unprepared for the challenge.

APPENDIX: SYMBOLS FOR RESPIRATORY PHYSIOLOGY

General Variables

V	Gas volume in general. Pressure, temperature, and percentage saturation with water vapor must be stated
$\dot{V}$	Volume flow of gas per unit time
P	Gas pressure in general
F	Fractional concentration in dry gas phase
$\dot{Q}$	Volume flow of blood per unit time
C	Concentration in blood phase
f	Respiratory frequency
R	Respiratory exchange ratio in general (volume CO_2/volume O_2)
D	Diffusion capacity in general (volume per unit time per unit pressure difference)

Symbols for Gas Phase (Subscripts)

I	Inspired gas
E	Expired gas
A	Alveolar gas
T	Tidal gas
D	Dead space gas
B	Barometric

Symbols for Blood Phase (Subscripts)

b	Blood in general
a	Arterial
v	Venous
c	Capillary

Special Symbols and Abbreviations

$\overline{X}$	Dash above any symbol indicates a mean value
$\dot{X}$	Dot above any symbol indicates a time derivative
s	Subscript to denote the steady state
STPD	Standard temperature, pressure, dry (0° C., 760 mm. Hg)
BTPS	Body temperature, pressure, saturated with water
ATPD	Ambient temperature, pressure, dry
ATPS	Ambient temperature, pressure, saturated with water

Examples

V_{T_I}	= Tidal volume (inspired) (ml.)
V_D	= Dead space volume (ml.) (second subscript identifies the specific dead space, e.g., $V_{D_{ANAT}}$ = anatomic dead space; $V_{D_{ALV}}$ = alveolar dead space; $V_{D_{PHYS}}$ = physiologic dead space)
$F_{I_{O_2}}$	= Fractional concentration of oxygen in inspired gas
$\dot{V}_A$	= Alveolar ventilation (liters/min.)
$\dot{V}_{O_2}$	= Oxygen consumption (ml./min. — STPD)
$\dot{V}_{CO_2}$	= Carbon dioxide production (ml./min.-STPD)
$\dot{Q}_T$	= Cardiac output (liters/min.)
$\dot{Q}_S$	= Blood flow through pulmonary capillaries exposed to nonventilated alveoli (liters/min.)
$\dot{Q}_C$	= Blood flow through pulmonary capillaries exposed to ventilated alveoli (liters/min.)
$\dfrac{\dot{Q}_S}{\dot{Q}_T} \times 100$	= Per cent of cardiac output perfusing nonventilated areas. This is a functional definition. In normal lungs, $\dot{Q}_S/\dot{Q}_T$ measured while 100 per cent oxygen is breathed defines what is probably an anatomic intrapulmonary right-to-left shunt
$\dfrac{V_{D_{PHYS}}}{V_T} \times 100$	= Per cent of expired tidal volume distributed to physiologic dead space; $V_{D_{PHYS}}$ = sum of alveolar and anatomic dead spaces. $V_{D_{PHYS}}/V_T$ is a purely functional definition because it includes all areas that contribute to a P_{CO_2} gradient (the test gas). Thus, areas with a low $\dot{V}/\dot{Q}$ ratio are included.
$P(A-aDO_2)$	= Alveolar to arterial gradient for P_{O_2} (mm. Hg)
$P(a-ADCO_2)$	= Arterial to alveolar gradient for P_{CO_2} (mm. Hg)
$C(a-\overline{V}DO_2)$	= Arterial to mixed venous oxygen content difference (ml./ml.)
$C(\overline{V}-aDCO_2)$	= Mixed venous to arterial carbon dioxide content difference (ml./ml.)

SELECTED REFERENCES

American Physiological Society: Handbook of Physiology. Section 3, Respiration. Fenn, W. O., and Rahn, H. (Eds.). Baltimore, Williams & Wilkins Company, Vol. I, 1964; Vol. II, 1965.

These volumes are a must for the serious student of respiratory physiology. The time, effort, and expense provided to publish this superb edition will not be duplicated for years to come.

Bates, D. V., Macklem, P. T., and Christie, R. V.: Respiratory Function in Disease. An Introduction to the Integrated Study of the Lung, 2nd ed. Philadelphia, W. B. Saunders Company, 1971.
This is the standard reference for lung disease, with heavy emphasis on chronic disorders. The pioneering work performed by these authors in pulmonary physiology is reflected beautifully in their approach to the clinical problem.

Campbell, E. J. M., Agostoni, E., and Davis, J. N.: The Respiratory Muscles: Mechanics and Neural Control, 2nd ed. Philadelphia, W. B. Saunders Company, 1970.
The senior author has now expanded his original, slim monograph into a high-powered analysis of the subject. It does not read easily and requires the same care as one would accord a legal document. If one is interested in the mechanics of respiration, then this book is a must.

Caro, C. G.: Advances in Respiratory Physiology. Baltimore, Williams & Wilkins Company, 1966.
This monograph includes eight chapters, each written by an authority, on different aspects of respiratory physiology, ranging from CSF and Regulation of Respiration to Tissue Respiration. The discussion is detailed and at times complex. It is not a book for the beginner.

Fishman, A. P., and Hecht, H. H.: The Pulmonary Circulation and Interstitial Space. Chicago, The University of Chicago Press, 1969.
The proceedings of a satellite symposium on the pulmonary circulation sponsored by the 24th International Congress of Physiological Sciences consist of 27 individual papers and the ensuing discussion. The range of the contributors' interests is wide, and not all of the material is clinically relevant. The discussions and critiques of individual papers are particularly valuable.

Giuntini, C. (Ed.): Central Hemodynamics and Gas Exchange. Torino, Minerva Medica, 1971.
Proceedings of an international symposium that deals with the problem of pressure-flow relationships in the pulmonary circulation as well as regulation of pulmonary blood volume and distribution of lung water.

Scarpelli, E. M.: The Surfactant System of the Lung. Philadelphia, Lea & Febiger, 1968.
A basic, extensive, and critical review on surface active material; the chapters on pulmonary mechanics, morphology, and physiology are particularly valuable as an introduction to the subject.

West, J. B.: Ventilation/Blood Flow and Gas Exchange, 2nd ed. Philadelphia, F. A. Davis Company, 1970.
This book has been widely quoted and needs little or no introduction. Few changes characterize the second edition, but it continues with its high ratio of information per ounce book weight. One should begin here if interested to know more about lung function.

REFERENCES

This list has been biased toward an overview of lung function most relevant to the management of respiratory failure. Although many of the articles are nonclinical, patience and careful reading will make one aware of how much of what is known awaits evaluation in the critically ill patient.

1. American Physiological Society: Handbook of Physiology. Section 3, Respiration. Fenn, W. O., and Rahn, H. (Eds.). Baltimore, Williams & Wilkins Company, Vol. I, 1964; Vol. II, 1965.
2. Ashbaugh, D. G., Petty, T. L., and Bigelow, D. B.: Continuous positive-pressure breathing (CPPB) in adult respiratory distress syndrome. J. Thorac. Cardiovasc. Surg., 57:31–41, 1969.
3. Askrog, V.: Changes in (a-A) CO_2 difference and pulmonary artery pressure in anesthetized man. J. Appl. Physiol., 21:1299–1305, 1966.
4. Bates, D. V., Macklem, P. T., and Christy, R. V.: Respiratory Function in Disease. An Introduction to the Integrated Study of the Lung, 2nd ed. Philadelphia, W. B. Saunders Company, 1971.
5. Bendixen, H. H., Egbert, L. D., Hedley-Whyte, J., Laver, M. B., and Pontoppidan, H.: Respiratory Care. St. Louis, The C. V. Mosby Company, 1965.
6. Bergofsky, E. H.: Mechanisms underlying vasomotor regulation of regional pulmonary blood flow in normal and disease states. Am. J. Med., 57:378–394, 1974.
7. Berk, J. L., and Hagen, J. F.: Effect of alpha and beta adrenergic blockade on epinephrine induced pulmonary insufficiency. Ann. Surg., 183:369–376, 1976.
8. Brown, P. P., Coalson, J. J., Elkins, R. C., Hinshaw, L. B., and Greenfield, L. J.: Hemodynamic and respiratory responses of conscious swine to E. coli endotoxin. J. Trauma, 16:184–190, 1976.
9. Dolfuss, R. E., Milic-Emili, J., and Bates, D. V.: Regional ventilation of the lung studied with boluses of xenon. Resp. Physiol., 2:234, 1967.
10. Falke, K. J., Pontoppidan, H., Kumar, A., Leith, D., Geffin, B., and Laver, M. B.: Ventilation with end-expiratory pressure in acute lung disease. J. Clin. Invest., 51:2315–2323, 1972.
11. Fishman, A. P.: Hypoxia on the pulmonary circulation. Circ. Res., 38:221–231, 1976.
12. Glazier, J. B., Hughes, J. M. B., Maloney, J. E., and West, J. B.: Vertical gradient in alveolar size in lungs of dogs frozen intact. J. Appl. Physiol., 23:694, 1967.
13. Holley, H. S., Milic-Emili, J., Becklake, M. R., and Bates, D. V.: Regional distribution of pulmonary ventilation and perfusion in obesity. J. Clin. Invest., 46:475–481, 1967.
14. Howell, J. B. L., Permut, S., Proctor, D. F., and Riley, R. L.: Effect of inflation on different parts of the pulmonary vascular bed. J. Appl. Physiol. 16:71, 1961.
15. Hughes, J. M. B., Glazier, J. B., Maloney, J. E., and West, J. B.: Effect of extra-alveolar vessels on distribution of blood flow in the dog lung. J. Appl. Physiol., 25:701, 1968.
16. Hughes, J. M. B., Glazier, J. B., Maloney, J. E., and West, J. B.: Effect of lung volume on the distribution of pulmonary blood flow in man. Resp. Physiol., 4:58, 1968.
17. Hughes, J. M. B., Rosenzweig, D. Y., and Kivitz, P. B.: Site of airway closure in excised dog lungs: Histologic demonstration. J. Appl. Physiol., 29:340, 1970.
18. Junod, A. L.: Metabolism, production and release of hormones and mediators in the lung. Am. Rev. Resp. Dis., 112:93–108, 1975.
19. Laver, M. B.: Acute respiratory failure: More questions, fewer answers. Anesthesiology, 43:611–613, 1975.
20. Laver, M. B., Hallowell, P., and Goldblatt, A.: Pulmonary dysfunction secondary to heart disease. Aspects relevant to anesthesia and surgery. Anesthesiology, 33:161–192, 1970.
21. LeBlanc, P., Ruff, F., and Milic-Emili, J.: Effects of age and body position on "airway closure" in man. J. Appl. Physiol., 28:448, 1970.
22. Macklin, C. C.: Evidences of increase in the capacity of the pulmonary arteries and veins in dogs, cats and rabbits during inflation of the freshly excised lung. Rev. Can. Biol., 5:199, 1946.
23. Milic-Emili, J., Henderson, A. M., Dolovich, M. B., Trop, D., and Kaneko, K.: Regional distribution of inspired gas in the lung. J. Appl. Physiol., 21:749, 1966.
24. Moore, F. D., Lyons, J. H., Jr., Pierce, E. C., Jr., Morgan, A. P., Jr., Drinker, P. A., MacArthur, J. D., and Dammin, G. J.: Post-traumatic Pulmonary Insufficiency. Philadelphia, W. B. Saunders Company, 1969.
25. Nunn, J. F.: Applied Respiratory Physiology. New York, Appleton-Century Crofts, 1969.
26. Permutt, S., Bromberger-Barnea, B., and Bane, H. N.: Alveolar pressure, pulmonary venous pressure, and the vascular waterfall. Med. Thorac., 19:239, 1962.
27. Pontoppidan, H., Geffin, B., and Lowenstein, E.: Acute Respiratory Failure. Boston, Little, Brown and Co., 1973.
28. Pontoppidan, H., Laver, M. B., and Geffin, B.: Acute respiratory failure in the surgical patient. Adv. Surg., 4:163, 1970.
29. Qvist, J., Pontoppidan, H., Wilson, R. S., Lowenstein, E., and Laver, M. B.: Hemodynamic responses to mechanical ventilation with PEEP. The effect of hypervolemia. Anesthesiology, 42:45–55, 1975.
30. Reed, J. H., Jr., and Wood, E. H.: Effect of body position on vertical distribution of pulmonary blood flow. J. Appl. Physiol., 28:303, 1970.
31. Rehder, K., Sessler, A. D., and Marsh, H. M.: State of the art. General anesthesia and the lung. Am. Rev. Resp. Dis., 112:541–563, 1975.
32. Rodbard, S.: Flow through collapsible tubes: Augmented flow produced by resistance at the outlet. Circulation, 11:280, 1955.

33. Scarpelli, E. M.: The Surfactant System of the Lung. Philadelphia, Lea & Febiger, 1968.
34. Severinghaus, J. W.: Blood gas calculator. J. Appl. Physiol., 21:1108, 1966.
35. Staub, N. C., Nagano, H., and Pearce, M. L.: Acute pulmonary edema in dogs, especially the sequence of fluid accumulation in the lungs. J. Appl. Physiol., 22:227, 1967.
36. Steenblock, U., Mannhart, H., and Wolff, G.: Effect of hemorrhagic shock on intrapulmonary right-to-left shunt ($\dot{Q}_S/\dot{Q}_T$) and dead space (V_D/V_T). Respiration, 33:133–142, 1976.
37. Suter, P. M., Fairley, H. B., and Schlobohm, R. M.: Shunt, lung volume and perfusion during short periods of ventilation with oxygen. Anesthesiology, 43:617–627, 1975.
38. Sutherland, P. W., Katsura, T., and Milic-Emili, J.: Previous volume history of the lung and regional distribution of gas. J. Appl. Physiol., 25:566–574, 1968.
39. Swan, H. J., C., Ganz, W., Forrester, J., Marcus, H., Diamond, G., and Chonette, D.: Catheterization of the heart in man using a flow-directed balloon tipped catheter. N. Engl. J. Med., 283:447, 1970.
40. Taylor, R. R., Covell, J. W., Sonnenblick, E. H., and Ross, J., Jr.: Dependence of ventricular distensibility on filling of the opposite ventricle. Am. J. Physiol., 213:711–718, 1967.
41. Thomas, J. L., Jr., Roos, A., and Griffo, Z. J.: Relation between alveolar surface tension and pulmonary vascular resistance. J. Appl. Physiol., 16:457, 1961.
42. Trichet, B., Falke, K., Togut, A., and Laver, M. B.: The effect of pre-existing pulmonary vascular disease on the response to mechanical ventilation with PEEP following open-heart surgery. Anesthesiology, 42:56–67, 1975.
43. West, J. B.: Ventilation/Blood Flow and Gas Exchange, 2nd ed. Philadelphia, F. A. Davis Company, 1970.
44. Zapol, W., Snider, M., and Schneider, R.: Extracorporeal membrane oxygenation for acute respiratory failure. Anesthesiology, in press.

IV

BRONCHOSCOPY

Robert W. Anderson, M.D.

Since the time of its development, the bronchoscope has come to be regarded as an invaluable instrument for the diagnosis and treatment of thoracic disease. Bronchoscopy in conjunction with history and physical examination, x-rays, and laboratory examinations enables the physician, and most particularly the thoracic surgeon, to diagnose and treat conditions of a large portion of the respiratory tract with minimal discomfort and risk to the patient.

Although recent developments enable simultaneous visualization by two people during a bronchoscopic examination, clinical instruction in bronchoscopy has always been difficult by the very nature of the examination. In order to gain familiarity with the landmarks and anatomy of the tracheobronchial tree through a bronchoscope, the performance of examinations on an opened-chest cadaver is an excellent and worthwhile exercise.

HISTORICAL ASPECTS

The inspection of body orifices and cavities beyond the region of the eye was hampered initially by lack of a proper light source. In 1806, Bozzini[1] reported the use of an endoscopic instrument with a wax candle as a light source to carry out examinations of the uterus and rectum. The invention of the electric bulb by Edison in the United States began a new era in the development of endoscopy. Professor Gustav Killian[7] concluded in 1898 that it should be possible to introduce a lighted tube into the tracheobronchial tree with the use of topical cocaine anesthesia and that valuable information could be obtained from such an examination. Killian's early reports of foreign body extractions and endobronchial examinations mark him as the "Father of Bronchoscopy."

With the development of better techniques and instrumentation, bronchoscopy rapidly progressed from the art of looking into the air passages and removing foreign bodies to the science of bronchology, which is concerned with the visual examination and direct study of the anatomy, pathology, and physiology of, and also with the treatment of the diseases of, the tracheobronchial tree. The science of bronchoesophagology in America was developed by Chevalier Jackson and his associates at the Jackson Clinic in Philadelphia. For many years this group devoted themselves to the establishment and advancement of bronchoesophagology as a science, and their classic monograph on bronchoesophagology is recommended to anyone who is concerned with this field.[6]

The demonstration of the flexible bronchofiberscope by Ikeda[3] has dramatically changed the technique of examination of the tracheobronchial tree. The fiberoptic bronchoscope has obvious advantages over the rigid bronchoscope. It is easily inserted, is well tolerated by patients, and enables exploration of both segmental and subsegmental bronchi in all lobes of the lung. Probably no other diagnostic or therapeutic technique has revolutionized pulmonary surgical practice in so short a period of time. The bronchofiberscope has replaced the rigid bronchoscope in most clinics for all bronchoscopic examinations other than removal of foreign bodies or aspiration of large volumes of purulent material as in lung abscesses or massive atelectasis where the limited aspiration channel in the fiberoptic bronchoscope has proved inconvenient.

BRONCHOSCOPIC ANATOMY AND PHYSIOLOGY

The early development of bronchology was hampered by the bronchial anatomic classifications which were extremely confusing and complex. An accurate and simple nomenclature which was first outlined by Jackson and Huber[4] in 1943 now enables physicians in all fields to discuss pulmonary conditions with great accuracy. The terminology proposed by Jackson and Huber takes cognizance of the important fact that the bronchopulmonary segments are subdivisions of the lungs which function as individual units and are individually served by their own bronchus and arterial and venous blood supply. Since many disease processes are segmental in nature, it is essential that physicians diagnosing or treating chest diseases be familiar with bronchial anatomy from a radiologic, bronchographic, endoscopic, and surgical viewpoint.

An inverted schematic drawing showing the tracheobronchial tree and its bronchoscopically visible subdivisions as visualized by the endoscopist is shown in Figure 1. The trachea ends at the carina by dividing into the right and left main bronchi. The carina is an important landmark for the bronchoscopist; it should be nearly vertical and sharp if subcarinal lymphadenopathy or other distorting factors are not present (Figs. 2 and 3). The right main bronchus lies in almost the same axis as the trachea and extends for about 2 cm. before it divides into the laterally directed right upper lobe bronchus and the stem bronchus (bronchus intermedius), which is a continuation of the main bronchus. The right upper lobe bronchus commonly subdivides into three segmental branches (Fig. 4) and the bronchus intermedius divides into the anteriorly directed middle lobe bronchus and the lower lobe bronchus. The middle lobe bronchus divides into its two segmental branches while the lower lobe bronchus, after giving off the superior seg-

mental branch, then subdivides into four basilar bronchi (Fig. 5). The left main bronchus makes a greater angle with the trachea and extends about twice as far as the right main branches before dividing into the upper and lower lobe bronchi. The upper lobe bronchus subdivides into the upper division bronchus and the lingular bronchus, which then yields the superior and inferior segmental bronchi and is equivalent to the middle lobe bronchus on the right. The left lower lobe bronchus subdivides into the superior segmental bronchus and three basilar segmental bronchi.

This brief description outlines the usual pattern of the tracheobronchial tree, but anatomic variations are frequent and the presence of pathologic changes distorts normal anatomy and obscures sought-after landmarks.

The color of the bronchial mucosa, as it is visualized through a bronchoscope, depends upon the lighting source used, whether there has been trauma to the mucosa during instrumentation, and whether pathologic changes are present. A pale flesh-pink color is to be expected, but each endoscopist must become familiar with the standard of normality in his own clinic. Since many patients who undergo bronchoscopy suffer from chronic bronchitis, the distinct reddening and erythematous changes found in this disease must not be accepted as normal because of their frequent appearance. The trachea and main bronchi have a supporting framework of partially enclosing cartilaginous rings which diminish to cartilaginous plaques in the more distal secondary bronchi and finally disappear in the bronchioles. Nowhere in the bronchial tree are these rings completely encircling or rigid, and for this reason there is normal mobility of the tracheobronchial tree during respiration which includes changes in both caliber and length of the airway. The loss of this mobility suggests fixation due to some disease process.

Physiologically, the tracheobronchial tree functions as a conduit system to conduct air from the upper airway to the alveoli, where gas exchange takes place. In addition to its mechanical function of conducting air, the tracheobronchial system also acts in concert with the upper airway as a heat exchanger and humidifier to prepare the air for delivery to the alveoli. The final physiologic function of the airways is to provide a drainage and cleansing system for the lungs by means of a protective layer of mucus and retrograde ciliary sweeping action which moves particulate matter and secretions upward. The expulsive forces and peristaltic activity of the airways caused by normal inspiration and expiration are aided by forceful blasts of air during reflex-stimulated acts such as clearing of the throat or coughing.

In the normal tracheobronchial tree there are no visible secretions and their presence during a bronchoscopic examination represents an abnormality. Furthermore, the cleansing mechanisms of the airways are less efficient in protecting the alveoli against liquids than they are against particulate matter, and conditions such as bronchitis which are characterized by increased bronchial secretions result in distal airway changes as the defense mechanisms are overwhelmed.

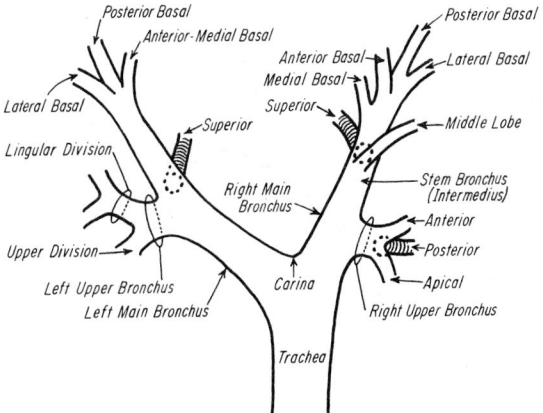

Figure 1. The inverted bronchial tree as visualized by the bronchoscopist. A rigid bronchoscope with forward-vision and right-angle telescopes allows visualization to the limits diagramed under optimal conditions. The fiberoptic bronchoscope allows visualization of the areas illustrated with relative ease.

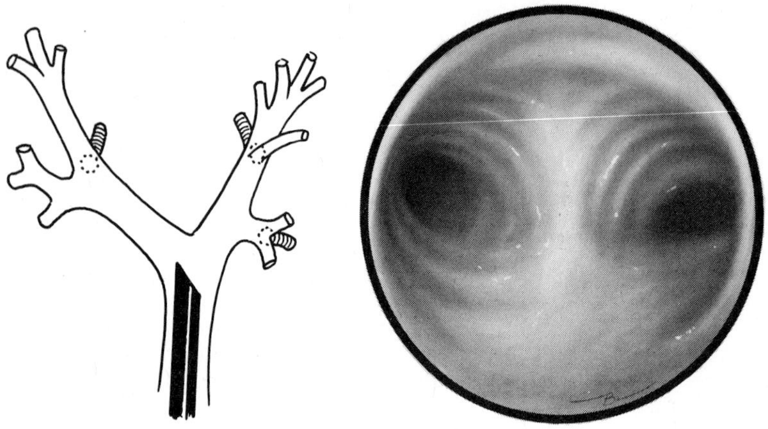

Figure 2. A normal, sharp-appearing carina during inspiration. During the expiratory phase of respiration there is some shortening and widening. Bronchial cartilage outlines are well seen and the mucosa is healthy.

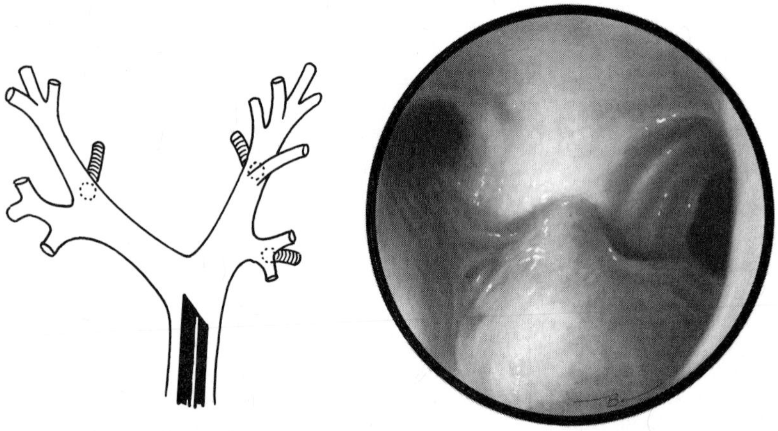

Figure 3. Widened, abnormally fixed carina caused by subcarinal lymph node metastases. The diagnosis was made by a transcarinal needle biopsy and inoperability established.

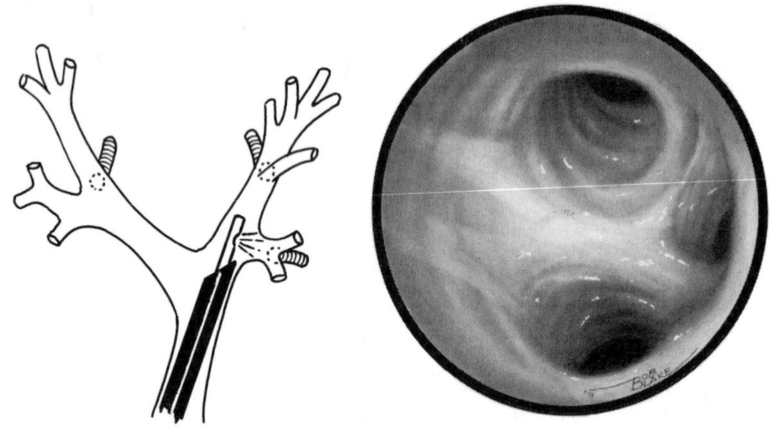

Figure 4. Normal right upper lobe bronchial orifice as visualized through the right-angle telescopic lens. The usual division into anterior, posterior, and apical branches is well seen.

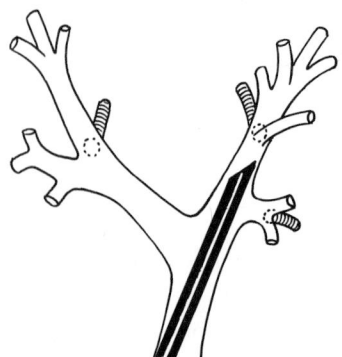

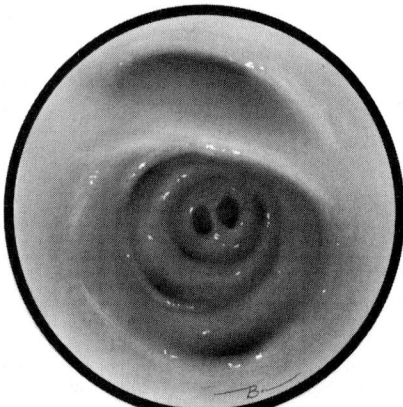

Figure 5. Termination of the right main bronchus with the middle lobe orifice seen superiorly and the superior segmented bronchus posteriorly. Distally are the basilar bronchi with the posterior basilar bronchus and its subcarina appearing in the center of the field.

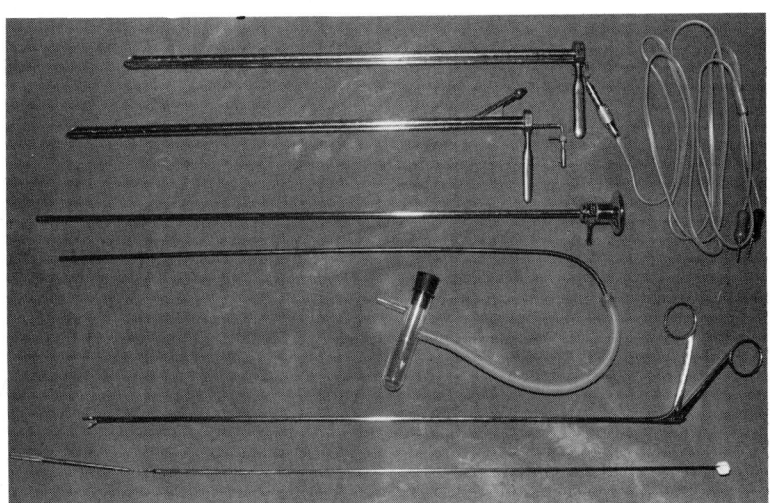

Figure 6. The standard 7 × 40 mm. broncho-scope with carrier for the light source is seen at top. Below are a side-arm ventilating bronch-oscope; right-angle Broyles telescope, which is passed through standard bronchoscope to vis-ualize upper lobes; aspirating tube; biopsy for-ceps; and sponge carrier for removal of secre-tions and cytologic smears.

INSTRUMENTATION AND TECHNIQUE

The standard rigid bronchoscope is a hollow tube with a beveled tip which has a light source at the end. These bronchoscopes are available in a variety of sizes and the 7 × 40 mm. is most commonly employed in adults (Fig. 6). Broyles developed a series of telescopes which can be inserted through the lumen of the stan-dard bronchoscope. The most useful are the forward-vision type which magnifies the lower lobe bronchi and the right-angled lens which provides a clear view of the upper lobe bronchi. The recent development of a flexible fiber bronchoscope extends the visual range of a bronchoscopic examination and has improved the diagnostic yield in more peripheral and earlier lung tumors.[9] The fiberoptic bronchoscope has an operator-controlled, flexible distal tip and can be manipulated into the far reaches of the tracheobronchial tree where cytologic specimens can be obtained under direct vis-ualization by the use of a brush (Figs. 7 and 8).

When general anesthesia is employed or the patient is in severe respiratory distress, a ventilating broncho-scope with side arm is utilized, so that insufflation of the lungs can be carried out during the course of the procedure. Ancillary equipment required for the bron-choscopic clinic includes an adjustable and reliable power source for the light employed, aspirating appa-ratus, biopsy and foreign body extraction forceps, sponge carriers, a suitable examination table, cyto-logic brushes for excoriating suspicious areas for cells, and some type of shield or spectacles to protect the op-erator's eyes during the procedure. The technique of bronchoscopy is described in magnificent detail in the works of Stradling[10] and Jackson and Jackson.[6] Only the more salient features will be discussed here.

Technique of Rigid Bronchoscopy

Although Jackson strongly advised the use of topi-cal anesthesia for all endoscopic procedures, the devel-opment of safer anesthetic drugs and muscle relaxants has made general anesthesia safe for bronchoscopic examinations. It is most important to prepare the pa-tient psychologically and pharmacologically for the procedure in order to allay his anxieties and fears. Topical anesthetics are applied to the oropharynx ei-ther by spray or swab and then dropped on the epi-glottis and cords under mirror observation. While this is being accomplished, a thorough oral examination is carried out and vocal cord motion is evaluated. Final-ly, the material is instilled into the trachea and bron-chi by dripping it through the cords or by a trans-tracheal needle puncture.

After anesthesia is complete, the patient is properly positioned in the dorsal recumbent position with the

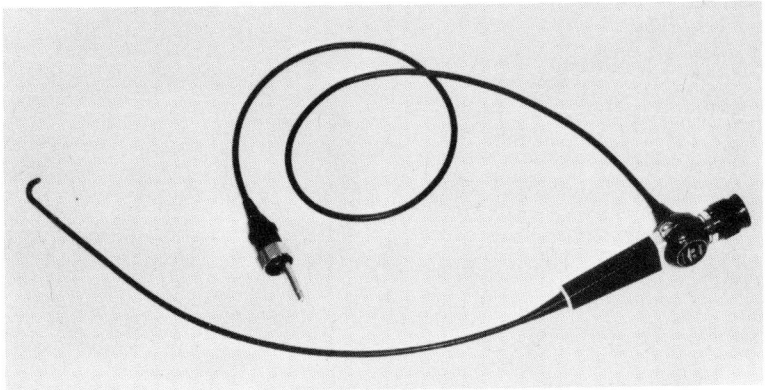

Figure 7. The flexible fiber bronchoscope, which may be introduced perorally or through a rigid bronchoscope or tracheoscope. Light is introduced from an outside power source and travels via optic fibers to the flexible distal tip, which is operator-controlled by an angle lever located near the eyepiece. Cytologic specimens are obtained from the bronchi with a brush, curet, or biopsy forceps passed through a chan-nel in the bronchofiberscope. (Courtesy of Olympus Corporation.)

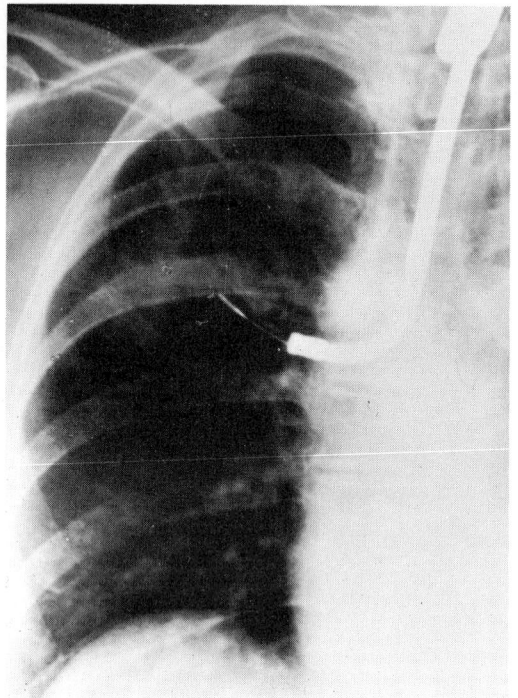

Figure 8. Bronchofiberscope passed through rigid bronchoscope into anterior segmental bronchus of right upper lobe. A cytologic brush protrudes from the tip of the instrument into the mass in the lung which appeared malignant and was cytologically confirmed to be so. (Courtesy of Olympus Corporation.)

shoulders flat, the head elevated about 5 inches, and the neck extended so that the chin points toward the ceiling (Fig. 9). While the patient's head is maintained in this position by an assistant, the bronchoscope is carefully insinuated through the cords until the trachea is identified. From this point, the examination must be methodically and gently performed and the bronchoscopist must look for details of anatomic form, mucosal coloration, nature and volume of secretions, and tracheobronchial motion. Suspicious areas should be noted during the initial examination and biopsied at the end of the procedure, since the bleeding which

occurs following biopsy makes further evaluation difficult. Aspiration must be done atraumatically and small saline lavages utilized to aid in the removal of obscuring secretions and to help liquefy purulent material so that culture specimens can be obtained.

The complications associated with bronchoscopy are usually related to adverse problems secondary to vagal stimulation, and bleeding caused by biopsy or foreign body extraction. Particular care must be exercised in biopsying areas adjacent to major vessels.

Technique of Fiberoptic Bronchoscopy

Patients should be premedicated with diazepam or meperidine and atropine 30 to 60 minutes prior to the procedure. Topical anesthesia of the nose and throat is achieved with 2 per cent lidocaine, and the fiberoptic bronchoscope is most commonly introduced transnasally. In those cases where general anesthesia is utilized, the fiberoptic bronchoscope may be passed through an endotracheal tube, through a previously inserted standard rigid bronchoscope, or through a cuffed tracheal tube to allow ventilation. Since fiberoptic bronchoscopy is so well tolerated, the use of general anesthesia is usually unnecessary.

When the fiberoptic bronchoscope has been positioned above the vocal cords, several milliliters of 2 per cent lidocaine are rapidly flushed through the cords to achieve topical anesthesia in the distal tracheobronchial tree. A successful examination is dependent on abolition of the cough reflex in the distal airways, and supplementary topical anesthesia must be instilled as required to achieve a quiet field.

The use of a soft nasopharyngeal airway as a conduit for the fiberoptic bronchoscope allows repeated passage and withdrawal of the instrument without excessive trauma to the nasal mucosa and also avoids contamination of the tip of the instrument as it passes through the nose.

Transoral passage of the fiberoptic bronchoscope has the distinct disadvantage of the patient's inadvertently damaging the fiberoptic bundles by biting the bronchofiberscope and is therefore not widely used unless transnasal passage cannot be accomplished. If the transoral route is used, a bite block should be inserted to prevent this expensive catastrophe.

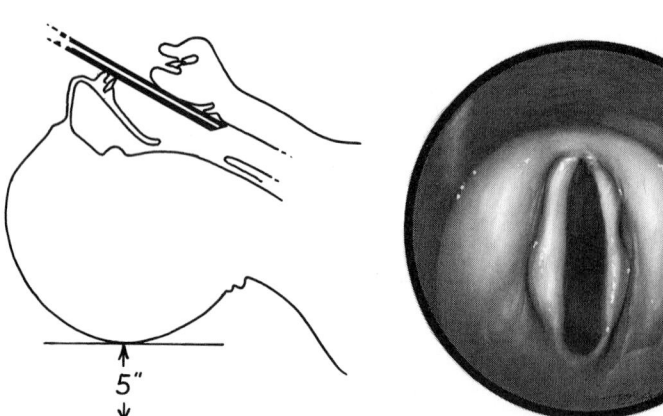

Figure 9. With the head in proper position and the bronchoscope in the midline, the epiglottis has been displaced forward by the tip of the bronchoscope and the vocal cords are well seen. The instrument can now be gently passed through the cords and into the trachea.

5"

INDICATIONS AND CONTRAINDICATIONS

Bronchoscopy is both a diagnostic and therapeutic procedure and should be performed in the presence of pulmonary disease which is undiagnosed but presents as either unexplained symptoms, signs, or radiologic findings. Diagnosed chest lesions that fail to respond to medical therapy within a short period of time may be due to underlying processes (i.e., tumor, foreign body, stenosis, and so on) and bronchoscopy is therefore indicated. Bronchoscopy is specifically indicated when there is a chronic cough, signs or symptoms of bronchial obstruction,[2] or hemoptysis; as part of any work-up for suspected lung or esophageal cancer; whenever foreign body aspiration is suspected; and in any patient for whom the inability to clear bronchial secretions is a problem. Patients being evaluated for pulmonary resection for tuberculosis or those who are found to have a positive sputum with no radiologically detectable abnormality require evaluation for endobronchial tuberculosis, and this can be accomplished only by a bronchoscopic examination.

In suppurative disease, bronchoscopy is an invaluable aid toward restoring peroral drainage.[8] Thick secretions may be removed by aspiration in pneumonia, pulmonary abscess, persistent pneumothorax, bronchiectasis, or persistent atelectasis. Specimens for culture and cytologic evaluation are obtained while a search for tumors, foreign bodies, stenotic lesions, or other etiologic factors is conducted.

The contraindications to bronchoscopy are few and the recent introduction of the flexible fiberoptic bronchoscope makes examination feasible under almost any circumstance. Disease or injury of the cervical spine which makes hyperextension impossible or the presence of an aortic arch aneurysm contraindicates rigid tube bronchoscopy, but presents no problem when a flexible fiberoptic bronchoscope is used. Status asthmaticus, massive active pulmonary hemorrhage, and severe cardiac failure or arrhythmias are relative contraindications to bronchoscopy.

At present, fiberoptic bronchoscopy appears to be the technique of choice in adult patients unless foreign body removal or endobronchial resection of a tumor is to be attempted. The complications associated with flexible bronchoscopy are minimal, but proper instruments should always be available for endotracheal intubation or insertion of a rigid bronchoscope should airway problems develop. The rigid bronchoscope is more useful for aspiration of secretions in patients who undergo endoscopy for drainage of a lung abscess or the treatment of atelectasis secondary to massive airway secretions.

TRACHEOBRONCHIAL PATHOLOGY

The pathologic changes observed in the tracheobronchial tree during a bronchoscopic examination fall into certain patterns which include inflammatory responses, bronchial distortion and displacement, new growths, and foreign bodies.

Inflammatory changes may be generalized as in bronchitis, in which the mucosa of the entire tracheobronchial tree appears reddened and hyperemic, with excessive secretions frequently noted. These secretions vary from thin mucoid material to thick purulent matter of high viscosity. The mucosa is often swollen and edematous in appearance, and normal sharp edges and contours may be obliterated by a thick enfolding carpet of swollen mucosa. Long-standing generalized bronchitis destroys the submucosal structures of the bronchial wall and the normal tone of the bronchus is lost. Areas of dilatation and puddling of secretions may occur as consequences of the loss of ciliary function and the milking action or "tussive squeeze"[5] of bronchial peristalsis during respirations. During forceful expiration, there may be complete collapse of the bronchial structures, since supporting tissue has been destroyed, and even the most vigorous expiratory efforts will fail to propel material past this obstruction.

The more common etiologic factors producing localized endobronchial inflammatory changes are pneumonia, lung abscess, bronchiectasis, foreign bodies, tuberculosis, mycotic diseases, and endobronchial tumors, particularly carcinoma. The changes noted in these conditions vary from localized mucosal erythema with purulent secretions issuing from a bronchial orifice in pneumonia or lung abscess, to granuloma formation or ulceration with scarring and stenosis in endobronchial tuberculosis or mycosis. Inert foreign bodies (e.g., metal) present for only a short time provoke only minimal local reaction, whereas long-standing irritants or vegetable matter (e.g., peanuts) may result in extensive changes with florid granulation tissue and edema. Any local inflammatory response must be explained, since a carcinoma in proximity may produce such changes, although the tumor itself may not be visible through the bronchoscope.

Hemoptysis may occur as a result of friable vascular granulation tissue in any inflammatory process or may be the result of an ulcerating or eroding tumor. Bronchial adenomas and certain other rare tumors are extremely vascular and may present as severe hemoptysis. These tumors may bleed profusely if biopsied too deeply. Bronchoscopy is often best deferred in the face of large hemorrhages, since visibility is obscured.

Defining tracheal and bronchial distortion and displacement during a bronchoscopic examination provides valuable insight as to the nature and extent of the underlying disease process. Enlarged extrabronchial lymph nodes are the usual cause of these changes, but developmental anomalies; inflammatory scarring and contraction; radiation therapy sequelae; or extrinsic pressure secondary to effusions, cysts, tumor, or diaphragmatic elevation may also cause changes. Resection of pulmonary tissue with consequent rearrangement of lobes, kyphoscoliosis, or atelectasis may also produce very confusing pictures secondary to the attendant distortion of tracheobronchial anatomy.

In the evaluation of suspected lung cancer, bronchial distortion is carefully looked for at the sites of lymph node groups which may be involved by the tumor. Widening of the carina is produced by enlarged subcarinal nodes and may confirm inoperability. Enlarged paratracheal or parabronchial nodes may cause

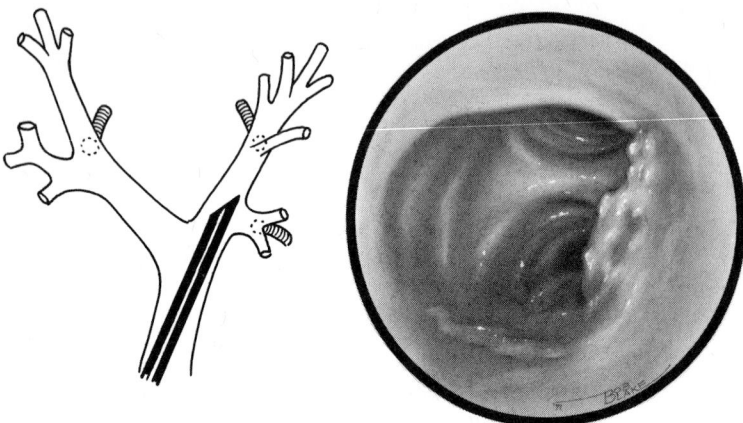

Figure 10. A squamous carcinoma protruding into the bronchus intermedius just below the take-off of the right upper lobe bronchus. A biopsy was positive and there was no evidence of inoperability. A right pneumonectomy was performed.

bronchial compression and fixation, and cautious biopsies may demonstrate invasion by tumor at these sites.

The great majority of bronchoscopically visible tumors are proved histologically to be bronchogenic carcinoma. However, the bronchoscopist's role is to define the anatomic and physiologic behavior of the tumor, since therapy is dictated by these observations as well as by the histologic identification which may result from a biopsy or cytologic study of bronchial secretions. Tumors may present as polypoid growths, as intraluminal masses which have eroded through the mucosa (Fig. 10), or as submucosal mural growths which may produce localized inflammatory changes with rigidity and partial stenosis. An unrushed and thorough examination is essential in any suspected lung tumor, and the diagnostic yield should be greater than 80 per cent if biopsies and washings for cytologic examination are judiciously performed.

PEDIATRIC BRONCHOSCOPY

A bronchoscopic examination may be performed in patients of any age, but bronchoscopy in infants should be limited to patients with suspected foreign body aspiration or evidence of bronchial obstruction. Small, delicate instruments are required, and the examination should be carried out gently and rapidly to keep laryngeal and bronchial edema at a minimum. In newborn infants and in most children below the age of 6, no anesthesia is employed for the procedure. Older children may be examined under general anesthesia or with topical anesthesia and mild sedation.

The fiberoptic bronchoscope has not proved to be useful in pediatric patients, since the smaller diameter instruments required in this age have no provision for the instillation or withdrawal of solutions, and aspirations of secretions cannot be accomplished as readily as with the rigid bronchoscope.

SELECTED REFERENCES

Holinger, P., and Andrews, A. H.: Bronchial obstruction. Signs, symptoms and diagnosis. Am. Surg., 54:193, 1941.

This article discusses the fundamental pathologic process of bronchial obstruction and the signs and symptoms it produces. The disease entities responsible for bronchial obstruction and the changes produced secondarily by obstruction are discussed in detail. The role of bronchoscopy in the diagnosis and treatment of bronchial obstruction is considered.

Ikeda, S.: Atlas of Flexible Bronchofiberoscopy. Baltimore, University Park Press, 1974.
A comprehensive monograph covering all aspects of the development and use of the fiberoptic bronchoscope. Extensive coverage of anatomy and technical aspects with a complete bibliography.

Jackson, C., and Jackson, C. L.: Bronchoesophagology. Philadelphia, W. B. Saunders Company, 1950.
In this monograph, the "Dean of American Bronchology" and his son summarize the extensive experience of the Jackson Clinic with endoscopic procedures. Recent advances in fiberoptic technology are not covered in this book, but it remains the standard work, and methodology is extensively discussed.

Stradling, P.: Diagnostic Bronchoscopy. An Introduction. London, E. & S. Livingstone, 1968.
This superb monograph provides an introduction to bronchoscopic technique and the anatomy of the tracheobronchial tree. Anyone preparing to carry out his first bronchoscopic examination will find this to be an invaluable guide. The color photographs are of the highest quality and the text is succinct and highly readable.

REFERENCES

1. Bozzini, P.: Lichtleiter, eine Erfindung zur Anschauung innerer Teile und Krankheiten nebst Abbildung. J. prakt. Heilunde, 24:107, 1806.
2. Holinger, P., and Andrews, A. H.: Bronchial obstruction. Signs, symptoms and diagnosis. Am. J. Surg., 54:193, 1941.
3. Ikeda, S.: Atlas of Flexible Bronchofiberoscopy. Baltimore, University Park Press, 1974.
4. Jackson, C. L., and Huber, J. F.: Correlated applied anatomy of the bronchial tree and lungs with a system of nomenclature. Dis. Chest, 9:319, 1943.
5. Jackson, C., and Jackson, C. L.: Peroral pulmonary drainage — natural and therapeutic, with especial reference to the "tussive squeeze." Am. J. Med. Sci., 186:849, 1933.
6. Jackson, C., and Jackson, C. L.: Bronchoesophagology. Philadelphia, W. B. Saunders Company, 1950.
7. Killian, G.: Meeting of the Society of Physicians of Freiburg, Dec. 17, 1897. Munchen. Med. Wochenshr., 45:378, 1898.
8. Peabody, J. W.: Bronchoscopic aids in medical conditions within the chest. Dis. Chest, 9:307, 1943.
9. Sackner, M. A.: Bronchofiberoscopy. Am. Rev. Resp. Dis., 111:62, 1975.
10. Stradling, P.: Diagnostic Bronchoscopy: An Introduction. London, E. & S. Livingstone, 1968.

V

DIAGNOSTIC THORACOSCOPY

James W. Mackenzie, M.D.

Thoracoscopy is the examination of the pleural cavity with an endoscope. As a *diagnostic* procedure, its main use is in patients with pleural disease in whom simpler methods have not yielded a diagnosis. It has limited application in other patients, which will be discussed later. The safety of the procedure and the highly accurate results obtained suggest that thoracoscopy should be considered before resorting to diagnostic thoracotomy in all patients with pleural disease.

Historical Aspects

Hans Jacobaeus (Professor of Medicine at the University of Stockholm, Sweden) was the originator of thoracoscopy as well as of laparoscopy about 1910.[9-11] Although he emphasized thoracoscopy as a therapeutic procedure to divide pleural adhesions during the era when induced pneumothorax was used for the control of tuberculosis, Jacobaeus also described its use as a diagnostic method. His early reports were not in English, but his 1922 report was in English and described the use of thoracoscopy as a diagnostic technique. Nevertheless, diagnostic thoracoscopy continued to be largely ignored in Great Britain and the Western Hemisphere, even though there were reports written in English which seemed to make strong cases for the selective use of diagnostic thoracoscopy.[3, 5, 6] The delay in the acceptance of diagnostic thoracoscopy was probably caused by fear of empyema and the impression that limited thoracotomy provided better inspection of the pleural cavity. Though the procedure was still used only occasionally by thoracic surgeons in the United States, the reports of Sattler in 1961, of Bergqvist and Nordenstam in 1966, and of DeCamp and his associates in 1966 and 1973 seem to have stimulated an interest in diagnostic thoracoscopy. Although these authors still seemed to favor the two-trocar system originated by Jacobaeus, their reports have emphasized the safety and diagnostic accuracy of the technique. More recently, attention has focused on the use of a fiberoptic mediastinoscope, a rigid bronchoscope, or a flexible bronchoscope as a thoracoscope.[2, 4, 7, 8, 12, 14] Miniaturized endoscopes have now been developed and they may further popularize the procedure, although at this writing their use is not clear.[1]

Anatomic and Physiologic Considerations

The procedure may be performed under either general or local anesthesia. If there is pre-existing pleural disease, complete collapse of the lung is limited by the adhesions, and respiratory distress on production of the pneumothorax is not likely. In patients without obvious pleural disease, however, the production of a large pneumothorax may cause respiratory embarrassment, particularly if there is underlying parenchymal disease. Therefore, general anesthesia with endotracheal intubation seems to be safer and more acceptable to patients. In the production of the necessary pneumothorax, air should not be insufflated into the pleural cavity, as gas emboli may be produced.

Surgeons accustomed to operating in the chest will have little difficulty recognizing the normal structures. This procedure can be performed safely in almost all patients when the amount of pneumothorax is controlled by endotracheal intubation. If there is concern regarding the respiratory status of the patient, insertion of a needle to sample arterial blood gases may be desirable. Ideal conditions for this study are provided by selective anesthesia of the dependent lung. The added complexity of this form of anesthesia and the lack of familiarity with it by most anesthesiologists limit the use of this anesthetic technique.

A hyperemic pleural reaction is highly suggestive of tuberculosis, as are the small tubercles which vary in size from 1 mm. to 4 or 5 mm. in diameter. Metastatic disease involving the pleura may be mistaken for miliary tuberculosis, but these cancerous lesions are usually larger.

Indications and Contraindications

The clearest indication for thoracoscopy is in the study of patients with pleural disease in whom simpler procedures have not provided a diagnosis. Such patients have usually undergone a study of the pleural fluid, blind needle biopsy of the pleura, and bronchoscopy. Some of these patients will have had mediastinoscopy as well.

There are other less clear-cut indications for thoracoscopy. Thoracoscopy might be considered for patients who are extremely poor risks for major thoracotomy but in whom the diagnosis of pleural-pericardial inclusion cyst (springwater cyst) seems very likely. It is possible to confirm the diagnosis by thoracoscopy. Although preoperative radiation therapy is not widely used for patients with bronchogenic carcinoma, it may be of value in treatment of patients with localized chest wall involvement. In patients in whom there is a strong suspicion of chest wall involvement but no radiologic or clinical confirmation, thoracoscopy may provide a definite answer.

Finally, peripheral lesions of the lung may be biopsied at the time of thoracoscopy. This may be a reasonable approach in patients for whom a major thoracotomy is contraindicated if other modalities have not provided histologic confirmation. Although the likelihood of spread from *percutaneous* needle biopsy of parenchymal lung lesions is extremely small, biopsy at the time of thoracoscopy would appear to provide a greater opportunity for seeding and seems inappropriate if resection is considered.

Absolute contraindications to thoracoscopy are rare. One is the lack of a free pleural space because of previous pleural disease. Thoracoscopy should certainly be avoided in acute empyema, as spread of the intrapleural infection would undoubtedly occur. In cases of trauma, thoracoscopy has been advocated to localize the site and to estimate the amount of bleeding, but such a use of thoracoscopy does not seem appropriate. Most assuredly there is not a need for thoracoscopy in all patients with the suspected or proved diagnosis of bronchogenic carcinoma.

Instrumentation and Technique

A number of authors have recommended the use of a two-trocar technique for diagnostic thoracoscopy. In this method, the pleural cavity is inspected through one site, and manipulations are accomplished by insertion of forceps through another site (Fig. 1). More recently, some authors have advocated the use of the flexible fiberoptic bronchoscope as a thoracoscope. The two-trocar system seems unduly complicated. The instruments are not readily available in most hospitals, nor is the technique familiar to most of the thoracic surgeons now practicing. The flexible bronchoscope, although more readily available, does not lend itself well to direction within the voluminous pleural cavity. For these reasons, we have preferred the technique illustrated in Figure 2.

The procedure often follows bronchoscopy and mediastinoscopy under the same anesthetic. In some patients, however, the surgeon may proceed directly to thoracoscopy. Although one may enter the pleural cavity at the time of mediastinoscopy and thereby perform thoracoscopy, access to the inferior portion of the pleural cavity is limited by this technique. It is usually better to place the patient in the true lateral position, and entry is then made into the pleural cavity at about the midaxillary line. Usually a 3-cm. incision is made at the fifth intercostal space, but adjustments are made depending upon the radiologic and clinical findings.

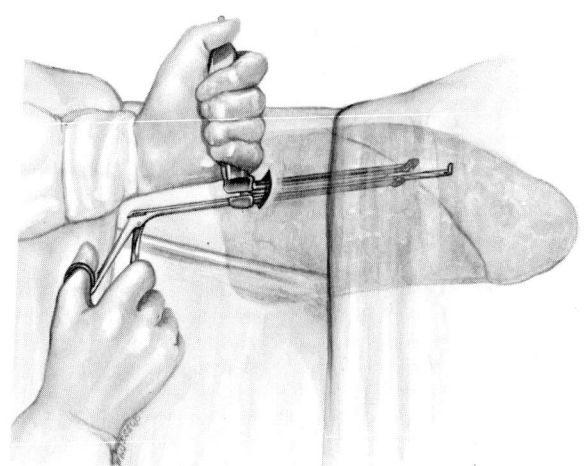

Figure 2. Use of fiberoptic mediastinoscope as thoracoscope. (From Lewis, R. J., Kunderman, P. J., Sisler, G. E., and Mackenzie, J. W.: Ann. Thorac. Surg., 21:536, 1976.)

The extracostal muscles are separated in the direction of their fibers and the intercostals are incised. All the fluid within the pleural cavity is aspirated and is sent for cytologic, bacteriologic, and biochemical studies. A finger is then inserted into the thoracic cavity to determine the extent of local adhesions, and if any are present, they are carefully broken. The fiberoptic mediastinoscope is then inserted into the pleural cavity and a careful sequential inspection is made of the surfaces of the pleural cavity. Large amounts of fibrin, if present, are sent for examination, and any obvious nodules are sampled. In the region of the superior sulcus, insertion of a rigid bronchoscope may make the procedure easier and may be supplemented by a flexible bronchoscope inserted through the rigid bronchoscope (Figs. 3 and 4). Histologic specimens are sent for frozen section as well as for bacteriologic study. If gross inspection or frozen section suggests the possibility of active tuberculosis, antituberculosis drugs are started on the day of operation. No other antibiotics are used. The pleural cavity is drained to underwater seal drainage and the chest tube is usually removed the next morning.

Although emphasis has been placed on the use of thoracoscopy as a diagnostic procedure, it may be helpful in treatment. For example, patients with spontaneous pneumothorax may continue to have significant air leak following intercostal tube insertion. If they are not candidates for major thoracotomy, thoracoscopy with divisions of adhesions may quickly seal the leak. Talc or some other escharotic agent may be instilled at this time.

Unlike bronchoscopy, the place of thoracoscopy in the treatment of patients with thoracic disease is not clear. Certainly, in patients with pleural disease of unknown etiology, thoracoscopy provides a greater degree of accuracy than blind pleural biopsy and probably provides as much information as diagnostic thoracotomy at a much smaller risk.[11, 13] Other uses of

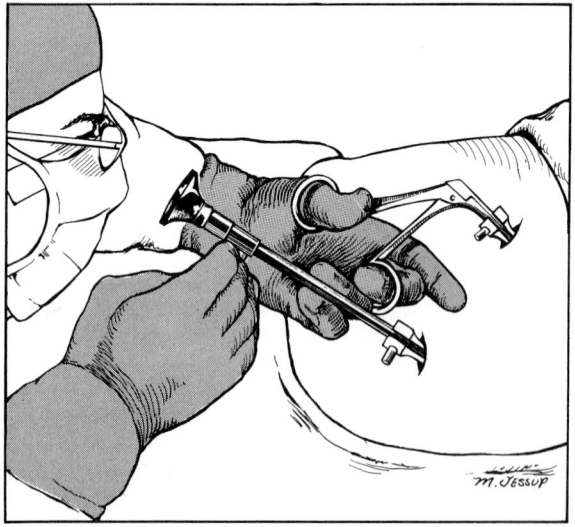

Figure 1. Two-trocar system of thoracoscopy.

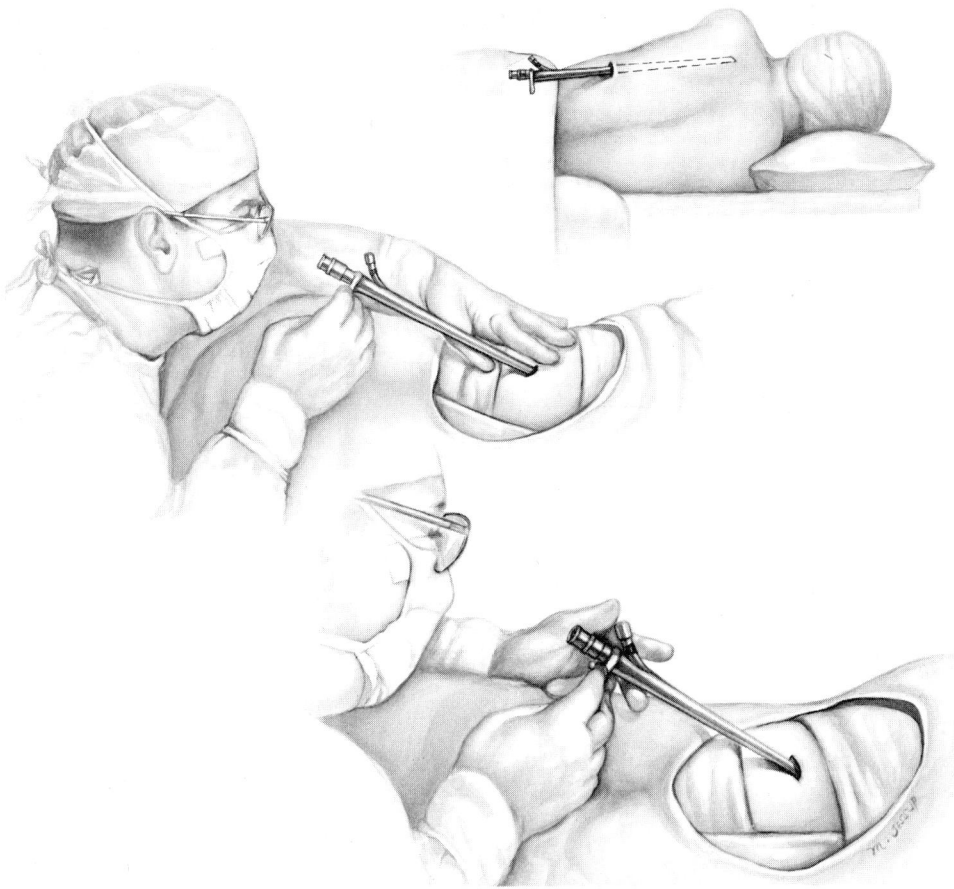

Figure 3. Use of rigid bronchoscope as thoracoscope. (From Lewis, R. J., Kunderman, P. J., Sisler, G. E., and Mackenzie, J. W.: Ann. Thorac. Surg., 21:536, 1976.)

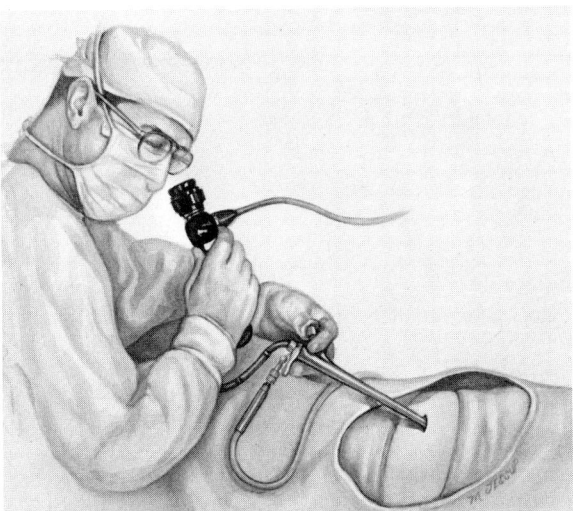

Figure 4. Insertion of flexible bronchoscope through rigid bronchoscope at thoracoscopy.

diagnostic thoracoscopy appear to be limited. The development of new equipment and apparent increased interest in this old procedure will likely lead to new indications for its use.

SELECTED REFERENCES

Bergqvist, S., and Nordenstam, H.: Thoracoscopy and pleural biopsy in the diagnosis of pleurisy. Scand. J. Resp. Dis., *47*:64, 1966.
This report of 130 patients with pleurisy is carefully done and provides comparison with other techniques for diagnosis of pleural disease. There were no deaths or significant complications. The results were far more reliable than needle biopsy and "not inferior to open thoracotomy."

DeCamp, P., Moseley, P., Scott, M., and Hatch, B., Jr.: Diagnostic thoracoscopy. Ann. Thorac. Surg., *16*:79, 1973.
This article reports a series of 126 patients who underwent thoracoscopy. The 95 per cent accuracy without any false positives was a strong stimulus for others to reconsider diagnostic thoracoscopy. Unfortunately, the two-trocar system used by the authors is not readily available nor, for that matter, is the expertise available in most hospitals. Other techniques are easier and just as rewarding.

Jacobaeus, H. C.: The practical importance of thoracoscopy in surgery of the chest. Surg. Gynecol. Obstet., *34*:289, 1922.
This article is useful mainly for its historical aspects by the developer of thoracoscopy and laparoscopy. It is primarily a discussion of the division of adhesions in patients with pneumothorax induced for the treatment of pulmonary tuberculosis. However, diagnostic thoracoscopy is also discussed, including its use in five patients with intrathoracic tumor.

Lloyd, M: Thoracoscopy and biopsy in the diagnosis of pleurisy with effusion. Q. Bull. Sea View Hosp., *14*:128, 1953.
This is apparently the first report from the United States in which the combined procedure of thoracoscopy and biopsy is advocated for the diagnosis of pleural effusion of unknown etiology. It is remarkable that this report did not stimulate greater use of diagnostic thoracoscopy in this country.

Sattler, A.: Pleural biopsy—results obtained and their practical significance. Ciba Symp., *9*:109, 1961.
Although this report does not provide much statistical information, it is distilled from what is probably the largest personal experience with thoracoscopy. These observations were instrumental in establishing rupture of subpleural blebs as the usual cause of spontaneous pneumothorax. The style of the author and the excellent illustrations make the monograph a delight to read.

REFERENCES

1. Ash, A., and Manfredi, F.: Directed biopsy using a small endoscope. N. Engl. J. Med., *291*:1398, 1974.
2. Ben-Isaac, F., and Simmons, D.: Fiberoptic pleuroscopy. Chest, *64*:388, 1973.
3. Chandler, F. G., and Morlock, M. V.: Thoracoscopy in diagnosis. Br. Med. J., *2*:982, 1938.
4. Deslauriers, J., Beaulieu, M., Dufour, C., and Michaud, P.: Mediastinopleuroscopy: A new approach to diagnosis of intrathoracic diseases. Ann. Thorac. Surg., in press.
5. Fleishman, S., Lichter, A., Buchanan, G., and Sichel, R.: Investigation of idiopathic pleural effusions by thoracoscopy. Thorax, *11*:324, 1956.
6. Geraci, C. L., and Brizzolara, L. G.: Use of the thoracoscope in the diagnosis of certain intrathoracic neoplasms. J. Thorac. Surg., *27*:266, 1954.
7. Gwin, E., Pierce, G., Boggan, M., Kerby, G., and Ruth, W.: Pleuroscopy and pleural biopsy with the flexible fiberoptic bronchoscope. Chest, *67*:5, 1975.
8. Gwin, E., Boggan, M., Pierce, G., Kerby, G., and Ruth, W.: Pleuroscopy and pleural biopsy with the bronchofiberscope. Am. Rev. Resp. Dis., *109*:690, 1974.
9. Jacobaeus, H.: Ueber die Moglichkeit die Zystoscopie bei untersuchung seroses Hohlungen anzuweden. Munch. Med. Wochenschr., *57*:2090, 1910.
10. Jacobaeus, H.: Die Thorakoskopie und ihre praktische Bedeutung. Ergeb. Ges. Med. (Berlin), *7*:112, 1925.
11. Payne, W.: Needle biopsy of the parietal pleura. Med. J. Aust., *1*:967, 1965.
12. Lewis, R. J., Kunderman, P. J., Sisler, G. E., and Mackenzie, J. W.: Direct diagnostic thoracoscopy. Ann. Thorac. Surg., *21*:536, 1976.
13. Rao, N., Jones, P., Greenberg, S., Bahar, D., Daysog, A., Jr., Schweppe, H., Jr., and Jenkins, D.: Needle biopsy of parietal pleura in 124 cases. Arch. Intern. Med., *115*:34, 1965.
14. Senno, A., Moallem, S., Quijano, E., Adeyomo, A., and Clauss, R.: Thoracoscopy with the fiberoptic bronchoscope: A simple method in diagnosing pleuropulmonary diseases. J. Thorac. Cardiovasc. Surg., *67*:606, 1974.

VI ———————————————————————

TRACHEOSTOMY AND ITS COMPLICATIONS

Hermes C. Grillo, M.D.

Tracheostomy is one of the most ancient of operations and has long been used for the emergency management of upper airway obstruction. In the past two decades, tracheostomy has been increasingly employed to control secretions in severely ill patients. More recently, tracheostomy has provided a route for ventilatory support in respiratory insufficiency. This increased use of tracheostomy has reawakened appreciation of the large number of serious complications that may follow the procedure. A new spectrum of lesions, principally associated with its use for ventilatory support, has been identified.

INDICATIONS FOR TRACHEOSTOMY

The occurrence of serious complications has caused critical reappraisal of the three classic indications for tracheostomy: (1) relief of upper airway obstruction, (2) control of secretions, and (3) ventilatory support in respiratory failure. Tracheostomy often cannot be avoided in organic upper airway obstruction, although sometimes a tube may be slipped past an obstruction transiently until definitive treatment is provided. However, the accumulation of secretions has increasingly been controlled by adequate humidification and by intensive pulmonary physiotherapy, consisting of expert instruction and assistance in cough, positional drainage, and thoracic percussion. Tracheal suctioning is used in conjunction with these measures, and occasionally transcricoid instillation of saline has been of assistance. Bronchoscopy, formerly used so frequently, is rarely necessary.

Patients with respiratory insufficiency or impending failure are usually supported by respirator with an endotracheal tube for varying lengths of time. If it appears that more than a day or so of support will be required, a nasotracheal tube is generally preferred for patients' comfort. Patients may thus be tided over a brief period of need for ventilatory support postoperatively without the need for tracheostomy. There is no firm rule about the length of time an endotracheal tube may be left in place. If it becomes clear that long-term support will be needed, a tracheostomy is usually done as an elective procedure within 5 to 7 days. Such a transfer becomes necessary because of the dangers of tube obstruction, the discomfort to the patient of a nasal or oral tube, and the considerable damage to the larynx that may result from prolonged intubation. This injury occurs especially in the posterior commissure, with damage to the arytenoid and interarytenoid area.[17]

TECHNIQUE OF TRACHEOSTOMY

Tracheostomy is only rarely an emergency procedure. The safest way to establish an emergency airway is by insertion of an endotracheal tube or, failing that, introduction of a ventilating bronchoscope. Even obstructing lesions can often be bypassed in this way or enough ventilatory force applied past an obstruction through a tube so that a patient may be maintained until a more carefully considered procedure can be done. For this reason, the simplest emergency surgical airway, an opening in the superficially located cricothyroid membrane, is rarely required.

Tracheostomy may be done under local anesthesia, with the patient supine and the neck hyperextended. An anesthetist should be in attendance to maintain a clear airway, to adjust the positioning of the endotracheal tube during the procedure, and to supply oxygen or other support as needed. The procedure should be performed in the operating room, if only to maintain the most sterile conditions and to impress the operator with the need for meticulous technique. Blind tracheotomy procedures are unnecessary and are only to be condemned because of the high incidence of complications associated with them. The speedily made vertical cutaneous incision for emergency tracheostomy has been replaced by a carefully placed horizontal incision. This avoids the late tethering scars that may follow the vertical incision. Palpation of the extended neck always reveals the position of the cri-

cothyroid membrane and the cricoid cartilage below this. The incision is placed at the level of the second tracheal cartilage and carried through the playtsma (Fig. 1). The strap muscles are separated vertically in the midline with minimal bleeding. The lower border of the cricoid cartilage is clearly defined and the incision between the strap muscles and its subjacent fascia is carried down to a point below the thyroid isthmus. The isthmus is usually divided between hemostats after careful dissection beneath it in the pretracheal plane. The thyroid tissue on either side is controlled with mattress sutures. Exact levels of the cartilaginous rings must be determined. The first cartilage must be left intact, and the opening in the trachea must be placed so that there will be no tendency for the tube subsequently to erode the first ring or the adjacent cricoid cartilage by upward pressure. The second and third cartilages (and all or part of the fourth if necessary) are incised vertically in the midline to avoid the potential danger of upward pressure by the outside of the elbow of the tube. If there is any question, it is better to incise a lower cartilage than damage a higher cartilage. Even after centuries of tracheostomy, there is little controlled work to prove the superiority of the vertical incision over the cruciate or the horizontal incision, the excision of a disc or a segment of cartilage, or the turning of a Björk or other type of flap. The tracheal opening probably enlarges to the size of the tube in most cases after some days. The important point is not to make too large an opening in the tracheal wall, whether with a flap or not, since the flap may well be destroyed or deformed. Any opening heals by cicatrization, and the larger the opening, the greater is the chance for narrowing during stomal healing. If fine retractors are used in the open trachea, even tubes with a bulky low-pressure cuff may be inserted with ease with the assistance of a little water-soluble lubricant. With such an elective procedure, hemostasis should be precise throughout.

Hypoxia and subsequent cardiac arrest, which formerly occurred during emergency tracheostomy, should not occur with this technique, since an airway has already been established. Former texts indicated the site of tracheostomy to be the suprasternal notch in the extended neck. In many, such an approach selects a midtracheal location and places the point of potential damage from cuff injury low in the trachea. The trachea is also farthest away from the cervical skin surface at this level. Further, it tends to angulate the tube more. In children and in some adults, a low incision also places the inner side of the elbow of the tube close to a high innominate artery, with greater potential for later erosive major hemorrhage.

Once the tube has been securely seated and any attached cuff is functioning satisfactorily, the endotracheal tube is withdrawn and supportive oxygenation given through a light-weight connector attached to the tube or to its inner cannula if it is a two-part tube. The skin is loosely closed with vertical mattress sutures on either side of the tracheostomy tube. The loops of the sutures on either side are passed through the flanges of the tracheostomy tube, fixing it securely in place, in addition to the usual tracheostomy tapes. Such fixation is particularly important in the first few

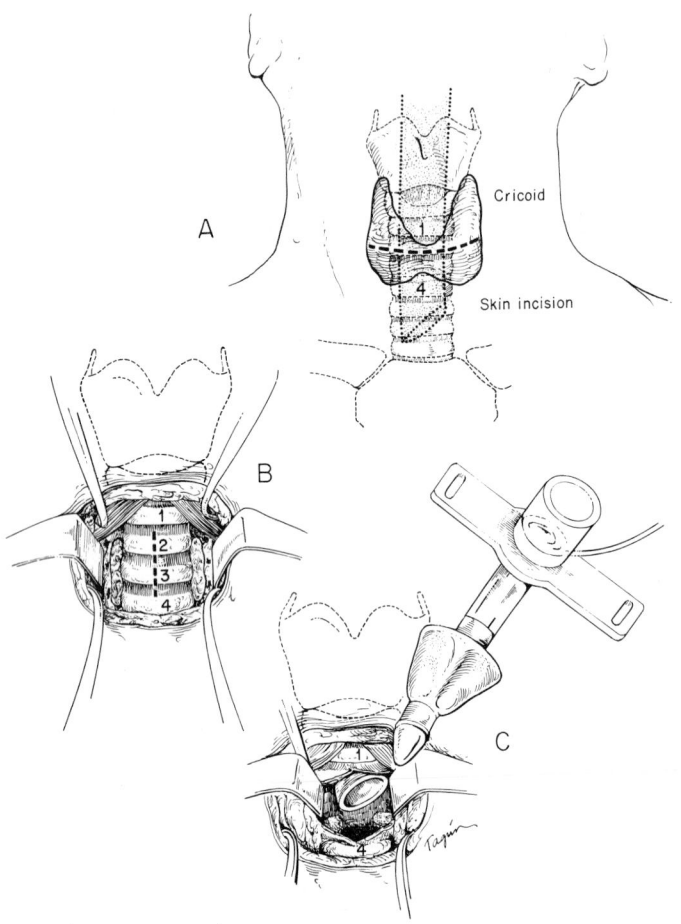

Figure 1. Technique of tracheostomy. *A,* An endotracheal airway is in place. With the patient's neck extended and centered in the midline, a short horizontal incision is made over the second or third tracheal ring after the level of the cricoid cartilage has been carefully palpated. The first and fourth tracheal cartilages are numbered. *B,* Following horizontal division of the platysma, the strap muscles are separated in the midline, the cricoid is identified, and the thyroid isthmus usually is divided and sutured to allow easy access to the second and third tracheal rings. The second and third rings are incised vertically. Occasionally an additional partial incision of the fourth ring is necessary. *C,* Smooth thyroid pole retractors are used to spread the opening in the trachea. The endotracheal tube is withdrawn to a point just above the incision. The tracheostomy tube is introduced with a small amount of water-soluble lubricant and with its large-volume cuff collapsed. The endotracheal airway is not removed until it is demonstrated that the tracheostomy tube is properly seated and permits suitable air exchange. Closure is made with simple skin sutures. The flange of the tracheostomy tube is both sutured to the skin and tied with the usual tapes around the neck. On a rare occasion when an airway cannot be established from above, an emergency incision may be necessary over the cricothyroid membrane for rapid establishment of a temporary airway.

days, especially when a vertical incision in the trachea has been used, so that displacement of the tube will not occur at a time when replacement may be difficult. Too long a tube should be avoided to prevent placement in the right main bronchus. Cuffs must be firmly fixed or cemented, if they are not an integral part of the tube, to prevent dislodgment or prolapse over the end of the tube. Suctioning during tracheostomy and immediately after its completion helps to avoid postoperative atelectasis. Prolonged suctioning, which may cause hypoxia, is avoided.

COMPLICATIONS OF TRACHEOSTOMY

Conversion of tracheostomy to a carefully performed elective procedure has largely eliminated the immediate and early complications of the procedure.[10, 14, 18] The longer-term complications of tracheostomy present largely in three ways: (1) sepsis, (2) hemorrhage, or (3) obstruction of the airway. Additional complications are tracheoesophageal fistula and persistence of the stoma. In general, the longer a tracheostomy is in place (especially with an inflated cuff), the greater is the chance that complications will occur.

Sepsis

All tracheostomies are clinically contaminated, and *Staphylococcus aureus* (often a resistant strain), *Pseudomonas aeruginosa,* and a variety of other bacteria such as *Escherichia coli* and streptococcus can be cultured. Despite this inevitability, sterile care and cleansing of the stoma and respiratory equipment must be maintained to minimize the possibility of invasive infection of the lower airway. Antibiotics are probably best reserved for use when there is evidence of tracheobronchitis, pneumonitis, or cellulitis, since their premature use will not sterilize the stoma but may merely permit other flora to establish themselves.

Hemorrhage

It has been noted that the curve of the tube may erode the innominate artery and produce late hemorrhage, especially in children, in whom the trachea is small and the artery high. Massive hemorrhage also occurs from erosion by tracheostomy cuffs or even the tip of a tube through the trachea into the innominate artery as it passes obliquely over the trachea. Bleeding from granulations or more superficial tracheal erosions is less common and usually less massive. Only immediate tamponade of a major arterial leak with an inflated cuff and prompt surgical treatment can lead to salvage. Resection of the injured artery with suture of both ends is one of the few possibilities in such a contaminated field. In the small number of cases in which this has been done successfully, neurologic problems have not yet appeared. The tracheal injury must also be handled by resection or repair.

Obstruction

Airway obstruction may occur while the tube is still in place. Cuff prolapse and its avoidance have been discussed. If a tube with an inner cannula is used, crusts may be easily cleaned. With proper humidification, obstruction of single-lumen tubes is less commonly seen. Occasionally, a valve type of crust may form at the tip of a tube so that a suction catheter may be easily passed without relieving the obstruction. If such is suspected, the only course is to change the tube. If the change is necessary early after tracheostomy, this should be done over a guiding catheter with adequate instruments and personnel available to reinsert an endotracheal tube or a bronchoscope from above in the event that the tube is not easily replaced. Occasionally, obstructive granulations also form at the tip of a tube that is still in place.

A major syndrome of postintubation airway obstruction has been recognized in the last decade[1, 7, 8, 13] (Fig. 2). It is difficult to establish absolute incidence, but it may be that as many as 15 per cent of the survivors of prolonged ventilatory therapy have had such symptoms, as well as some patients who have had no ventilatory support but simply a cuffed tracheostomy tube that was placed to prevent aspiration. *Every patient with signs of upper airway obstruction – wheezing or stridor, dyspnea on effort, episodes of obstruction from secretions – who has been previously intubated with either an endotracheal tube or a tracheostomy tube must be considered to have organic obstruction until proved otherwise.* Unfortunately, many such patients who have been discharged from the hospital are treated for asthma to the point of death or subtotal obstruction before the lesion is recognized.

Obstructive *laryngeal lesions* from prolonged endotracheal intubation may occur at vocal cord level and consist of granulation tissue or cicatrix, particularly in the posterior commissure.[10, 17] *At the stomal level,* obstruction may be due to a polypoid granuloma that forms on the healing surface of the stomal site. Narrowing and indentation at the point of cicatrization of the stoma is often seen after tracheostomy. When the stoma is large – because of overgenerous initial surgery or erosion by local infection or, most commonly, by the prying action of heavy-weight equipment that connects the tracheostomy to the ventilator – healing may produce clinically obvious obstruction. Such stomal obstruction is usually three-sided, obstructing anteriorly and laterally, since the posterior wall is intact. Occasionally, some scarring occurs posteriorly as well. A combination of granuloma and stenosis may also produce obstruction. If the tracheostomy was placed too high, erosion of the cricoid cartilage may have occurred, with loss of substance and resultant subglottic stricture, one of the most difficult lesions to correct.

At the cuff site, pressure by the sealing cuff causes varying degrees of damage.[4] Prior to the introduction of true large-volume, low-pressure cuffs, damage occurred in varying degrees in all patients in whom a cuff was inflated for more than 48 hours.[5] In the days and weeks following, erosion frequently bares numerous cartilages, leading to their fragmentation, and, eventually, total destruction (Fig. 3). Occasionally, the erosion progresses anteriorly, through the wall of the innominate artery, or posteriorly, to produce a tracheoesophageal fistula. With lesser degrees of damage, healing occurs with varying degrees of deformity and narrowing. If the tracheal wall has been deeply eroded circumferentially, a circumferential stricture results during healing (Fig. 4). This may become arrested with partial closure and produce only dyspnea on effort, or it may go on to complete closure with a fatal obstructive episode. The lengths of such strictures are extremely variable, extending from 0.5 cm. to 4 cm. Such lesions may occur with either endotracheal tubes or tracheostomy tubes, since they are due to the cuff and not to the tube itself. A far greater number have resulted from cuffs on tracheostomy tubes, since there is greater long-term exposure to them. Other factors have been implicated in the etiol-

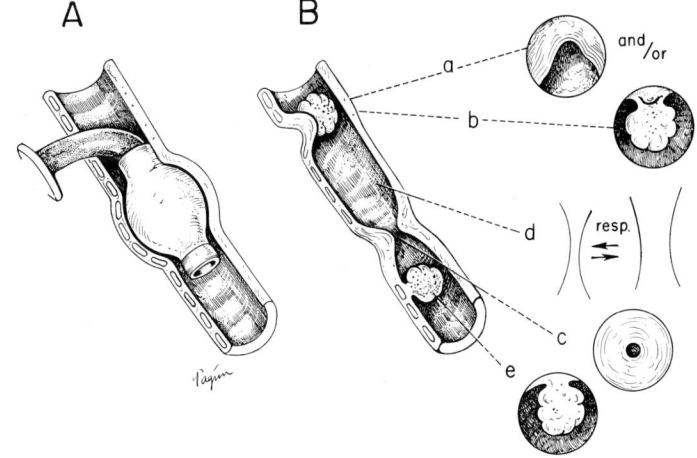

Figure 2. Obstructive lesions that may result from cuffed tracheostomy tubes. A conventional cuffed tube is in place at the left *(A)*. Sagittal and cross-sectional (bronchoscopic) views of pathologic lesions are shown at the right *(B)*. Anterolateral strictures are seen at the stoma (a) and granulomas also occur here (b). The lesions may occur concurrently. Circumferential stricture develops at the level of cuff injury (c). Between the stomal level and the cuff stricture, varying degrees of tracheal malacia may be seen; this leads to partial collapse during respiration (d). Granulomas may also occur at the level of the tip of the tube (e). (From Geffin, B., Grillo, H. C., Cooper, J. D., and Pontoppidan, H.: J.A.M.A., *216*:1984, 1971.)

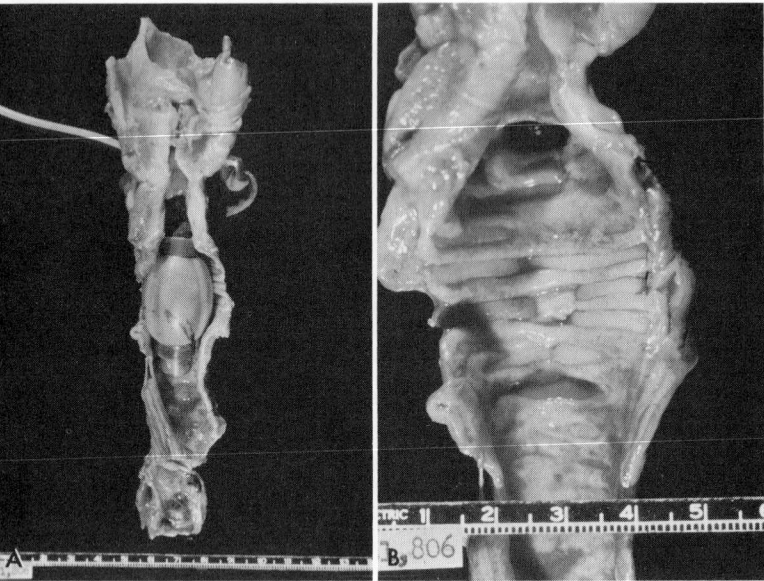

Figure 3. Tracheal injury due to a cuffed tracheostomy tube. Autopsy specimen of larynx and trachea. *A*, A metal tracheostomy tube with rubber cuff inflated had been in place for 16 days. *B*, Cartilaginous rings are exposed and fragmented at the cuff site. The tracheal wall is thinned and distended. Similar injuries occur with plastic tubes and cuffs. (From Cooper, J. D., and Grillo, H. C.: Ann. Surg., *169*:334, 1969.)

ogy of cuff strictures, including periods of hypotension, which make it easier to compress the mucosal vascular supply, bacterial infection, which is always present, and toxic products from various materials and from ethylene oxide sterilization with inadequate aeration. However, clinical, pathologic, and experimental evidence clearly demonstrates that the common denominator is pressure.[5, 6]

The tracheal cartilages *between the stoma and cuff level* are often thinned, presumably by inflammatory changes, and this segment may become malacic. With respiratory effort, the malacic segment tends to collapse, contributing to the obstructive picture. Granuloma may also form at a point of erosion by the *tip of the tracheostomy tube*. Children are more likely to show this lesion, since they are usually managed postoperatively without a cuff.

While most tracheostomies close spontaneously, a large and long *persistent stoma* will fail to close occasionally and require precise surgical repair.[16] This is apt to occur in aged or debilitated patients, in patients with metabolic disease, or in those who have been exposed to steroids.

Once a clinical diagnosis of obstruction is made, confirmation is easily obtained by simple radiologic studies (Fig. 5). Routine chest x-rays most frequently show clear lung fields. The unwary physician may treat the patient for adult-onset asthma or other vague diagnoses. Lateral neck roentgenograms will reveal tracheal deformities at the stomal level. Oblique views of the chest, which rotate the mediastinum to the side, reveal the entire trachea and demonstrate areas of narrowing at cuff level or elsewhere. A radiopaque marker taped to the skin at the site of an existing stoma or at the scar of such a stoma is helpful in pinpointing the level of a lesion. Fluoroscopy demon-

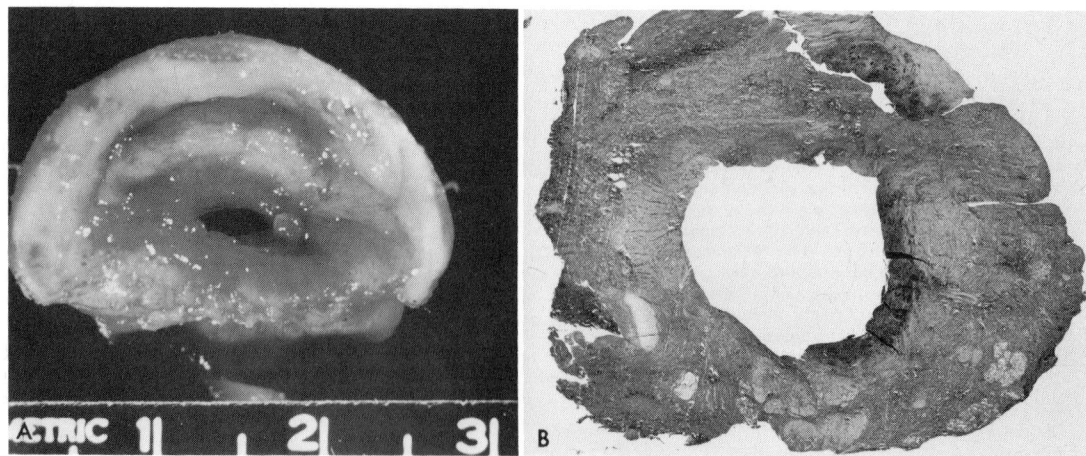

Figure 4. Tracheal stenosis from cuff damage. *A*, Gross specimen showing the typical circumferential fibrous and inflammatory lesion. *B*, Photomicrograph showing that the stricture in a severe case is composed almost entirely of scar tissue; little normal tracheal architecture identifiable. Such strictures do not respond even to prolonged dilation or splinting. (From Grillo, H. C.: J. Thorac. Cardiovasc. Surg., *57*:52, 1969.)

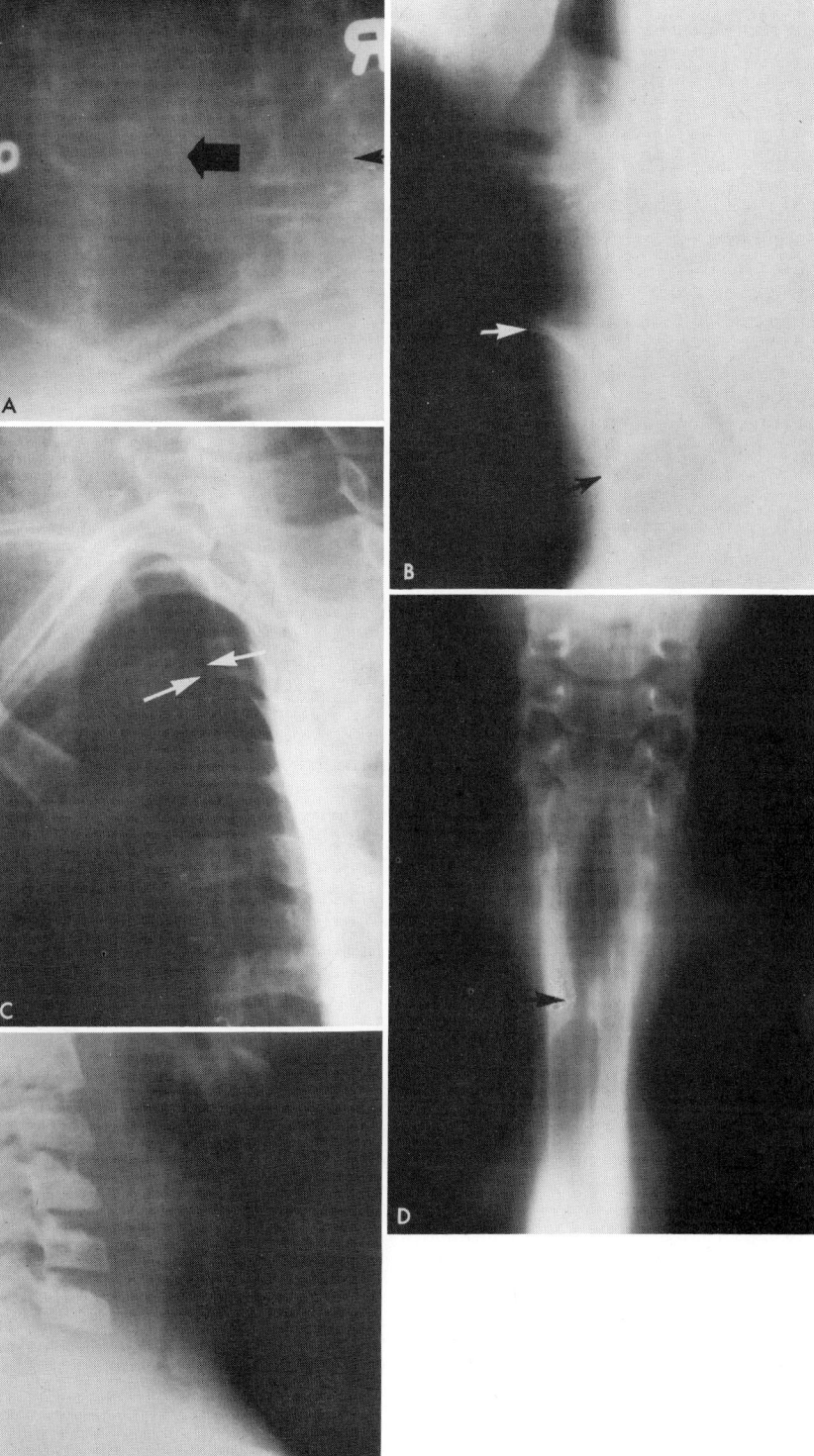

Figure 5. Roentgenograms demonstrating tracheal lesions. *A,* Granuloma at stomal site. Circular radiopaque marker is on skin at site of prior stoma. Arrow points to partially narrowed air column with large anterior granuloma visible. *B,* Stricture at tracheostomy site, shown in detail of lateral neck view. Larynx is clearly seen above. Arrows mark longitudinal limits of anterior stricture. The posterior wall of trachea is not involved. *C,* Cuff-level stenosis is demonstrated on oblique view of chest, which rotates mediastinal structures away from the trachea and shows its full length. Arrows indicate the narrowness of the airway. The lesion is circumferential. *D,* Cuff stricture shown on laminagram. The exact length of the stenosis, degree of airway narrowing, and level of stricture in relation to larynx and carina are detailed. *E,* Granuloma at level of anterior erosion by tip of tracheostomy tube, shown in lateral neck roentgenogram. In this child, a cuff had not been used.

strates the presence of malacia in the segment between the stoma and a cuff stricture. Tracheal laminagrams best define the character, the level, and the extent of a lesion, facts that are necessary to plan correction. Contrast medium produces a crisper picture but is not necessary. Insufflation of powdered tantalum avoids the possibility of obstruction that liquid media present in the tightest lesions.

Treatment. With the development of techniques of tracheal surgery that permit safe end-to-end anastomosis after resection of lengthy segments, the majority of these patients may be returned to normal function by surgical excision of the obstructing lesion and anatomic reconstruction of the upper airway.[8-10, 19] If the patient is too ill for repair or has a disease that will soon require repeated tracheostomy, conservative management is recommended. This is possible in all but those cases in which the lesion is immediately above the carina, by reinstituting a tracheostomy, dilating the stricture, and passing a fenestrated tube through it. In an occasional patient in whom the original damage was small in amount, repeated dilations or prolonged splinting with an inlying tube may produce a satisfactory airway over a long period of time. In most, however, conservative treatment will not succeed despite prolonged attempts, and a permanent tracheostomy tube is required.

One hundred forty-two patients with *tracheal stenosis* were submitted to surgical reconstruction at the Massachusetts General Hospital from 1964 through 1974. A small additional number were treated conservatively because their basic diseases did not suggest that a reconstruction would be tolerated or, more often, because they were likely to require tracheostomy again in the near future for diseases such as severe myasthenia gravis. One patient, early in the series, underwent exploration but died before resection could be done. Of the 142 surgical cases of stenosis, 137 followed intubation and 4 were post-traumatic. There were 42 postintubation lesions at the *stomal* level and 77 at the *cuff* level; eight patients had stenoses at *both* levels, and in one the lesion was of uncertain origin. Two had malacia only, six had tracheoesophageal fistulas,[12] and one had an innominate artery fistula. Fourteen of the "cuff" stenoses were in patients who had had endotracheal intubation only, one for only 48 hours. Twenty-nine of the patients incurred their strictures at the Massachusetts General Hospital and the remaining 113 were referred.

The results of aggressive surgical treatment are good. One hundred twenty-two patients had good to excellent results that were clinically satisfactory although not ideal if the patients were to stress themselves physically. Six represented failures, one predictably in completely unfavorable circumstances in which the operation was forced because of the extremely low level of the stricture. Two others exhibited factors that were not fully appreciated early in our operative experience, namely, severe accompanying tracheomalacia and destruction of the cricoid cartilage. One patient in whom there was no alternative was operated upon as a desperate measure but required ventilatory support postoperatively, which led to erosion of the suture line. There were five deaths.

Prevention. Prevention of tracheal stenosis is of key importance. Diminution in the incidence of stomal strictures was noted at the Toronto General Hospital when heavy connecting tubing was abandoned for light-weight swivel connectors.[1] A relatively low incidence of stomal strictures in a corresponding period at the Massachusetts General Hospital, where light-weight connectors were in use, confirms this observation. Obviously, the surgical stoma should not be excessively large in the first place.

Strictures have been associated with tubes of every material and with cuffs of varying types of materials. At cuff level, the principal preventive factor is elimination of pressure necrosis.[3, 6, 11, 15] The large-volume, low-pressure cuffs, which occlude the irregularly shaped tracheal lumen by conforming to the shape of the trachea rather than by expanding to distend and

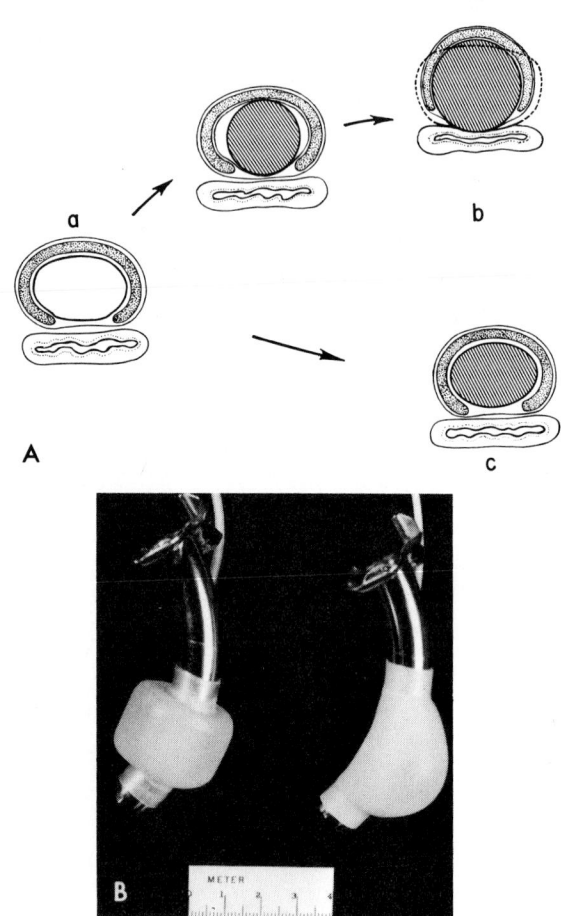

Figure 6. *A,* Diagram of the mechanism of cuff injury to the trachea and its avoidance. Above, a conventional cuff must be inflated under high pressure to effect a seal of the irregular tracheal airway. It distorts the trachea and exerts great pressure on the mucosa. Below, a cuff with large resting volume fills the irregular tracheal lumen by conforming to its shape at low intracuff pressures, below the point of elastic distention of the cuff. *B,* The experimental cuff and a Rusch cuff mounted on standard Jackson tracheostomy tubes. The new cuff (left) is shown at its resting size. It must be collapsed with gentle syringe suction for insertion. The standard cuff (right) has been inflated with 8 cc. of air. It has a high intracuff pressure, is asymmetric, and is quite rigid. (From Grillo, H. C., Cooper, J. D., Geffin, B., and Pontoppidan, H.: J. Thorac. Cardiovasc. Surg., 62:898, 1971.)

so close the airway, seem to be accomplishing this end. Such a cuff was devised initially in animal experiments and then tested clinically in patients[6, 11] (Fig. 6).

Alternative methods of safeguarding the trachea have also been proposed or used. The most promising of these methods appears to be that of intermittent inflation of the cuff with the inspiratory phase of the respiratory cycle, thereby reducing the time of exposure of the trachea to a high-pressure cuff.[2] It is entirely possible that future advances in respiratory therapy will ultimately make tracheostomy unnecessary, but this era would appear to be far off.

SELECTED REFERENCES

Andrews, M. J., and Pearson, F. G.: The incidence and pathogenesis of tracheal injury following cuffed tube tracheostomy with assisted ventilation: An analysis of a two-year prospective study. Ann. Surg., *173*:249, 1971.
This excellent study correlates the factors attendant upon respiratory therapy, the gross pathologic observations per stomam at the time of extubation, and subsequent appearance of stenosis.

Cooper, J. D., and Grillo, H. C.: The evolution of tracheal injury due to ventilatory assistance through cuffed tubes. A pathologic study. Ann. Surg., *169*:334, 1969.
The pathogenesis of tracheal injuries is traced by means of study of autopsy specimens of tracheas from patients who died while in respiratory therapy and surgically resected specimens of fully developed strictures. Pressure necrosis is identified as the major etiologic factor.

Grillo, H. C.: Congenital lesions, neoplasms, and injuries of the trachea. *In* Sabiston, D. C., Jr., and Spencer, F. C. (Eds.): Gibbon's Surgery of the Chest, 3rd ed. Philadelphia, W. B. Saunders Company, 1976.
The failure of conservative management is emphasized, and the successful application of new techniques of surgical reconstruction in the management of postintubation lesions is described in this current review of tracheal surgical problems.

Grillo, H. C.: Surgery of the trachea. Curr. Prob. Surg., July, 1970.
This brief monograph summarizes the literature on tracheal lesions and their management and presents the author's data and views on both inflammatory and neoplastic lesions of the trachea.

Lindholm, C. E.: Prolonged endotracheal intubation. Acta Anaesth. Scand., Suppl. 33, 1969.
This exhaustive study of postintubation tracheal injury emphasizes the problems created by pressure of endotracheal tubes on the posterior commissural area of the larynx. It also describe posttracheostomy injury.

REFERENCES

1. Andrews, M. J., and Pearson, F. G.: The incidence and pathogenesis of tracheal injury following cuffed tube tracheostomy with assisted ventilation: An analysis of a two-year prospective study. Ann. Surg., *173*:249, 1971.
2. Arens, J. F., Ochsner, J. L., and Gee, G.: Volume-limited intermittent cuff inflation for long-term respiratory assistance. J. Thorac. Cardiovasc. Surg., *58*:837, 1969.
3. Carroll, R., Hedden, M., and Safar, P.: Intratracheal cuffs: Performance characteristics. Anesthesiology, *31*:275, 1969.
4. Ching, N. P. H., Ayres, S. M., Spina, R. C., and Nealon, T. F., Jr.: Endotracheal damage during continuous ventilatory support. Ann. Surg., *179*:123, 1974.
5. Cooper, J. D., and Grillo, H. C.: The evolution of tracheal injury due to ventilatory assistance through cuffed tubes. A pathologic study. Ann. Surg., *169*:334, 1969.
6. Cooper, J. D., and Grillo, H. C.: Experimental production and prevention of injury due to cuffed tracheal tubes. Surg. Gynecol. Obstet., *129*:1235, 1969.
7. Geffin, B., Grillo, H. C., Cooper, J. D., and Pontoppidan, H.: Stenosis following tracheostomy for respiratory care. J.A.M.A., *216*:1984, 1971.
8. Grillo, H. C.: The management of tracheal stenosis following assisted respiration. J. Thorac. Cardiovasc. Surg., *57*:52, 1969.
9. Grillo, H. C.: Reconstruction of the trachea. Experience in 100 cases. Thorax, *28*:667, 1973.
10. Grillo, H. C.: Surgery of the trachea. Curr. Probl. Surg., July, 1970.
11. Grillo, H. C., Cooper, J. D., Geffin, B., and Pontopidan, H.: A low pressure cuff for tracheostomy tubes to minimize tracheal injury: A comparative clinical trial. J. Thorac. Cardiovasc. Surg., *62*:898, 1971.
12. Grillo, H. C., Moncure, A. C., and McEnany, M. T.: Repair of inflammatory tracheoesophageal fistula. Ann. Thorac. Surg., in press.
13. Harley, H. R. S.: Laryngotracheal obstruction complicating tracheostomy or endotracheal intubation with assisted respiration. Thorax, *24*:493, 1971.
14. Head, J. M.: Tracheostomy in the management of respiratory problems. N. Engl. J. Med., *264*:587, 1961.
15. Knowlson, G. T. G., and Bassett, H. F. M.: The pressures exerted on the trachea by endotracheal inflatable cuffs. Br. J. Anaesth., *42*:834, 1970.
16. Lawson, D. W., and Grillo, H. C.: Closure of a persistent tracheal stoma. Surg. Gynecol. Obstet., *130*:995, 1970.
17. Lindholm, C. E.: Prolonged endotracheal intubation. Acta Anaesth. Scand., Suppl. 33, 1969.
18. Mulder, D. S., and Rubush, J. L.: Complications of tracheostomy: Relationship to long term ventilatory assistance. J. Trauma, *9*:389, 1969.
19. Pearson, F. G., and Andrews, M. J.: Detection and management of tracheal stenosis following cuffed tube tracheostomy. Ann. Thorac. Surg., *12*:359, 1971.

VII ————————————

THORACIC TRAUMA

Paul A. Ebert, M.D.

Injuries of the chest occur with increased frequency, and they represent one of the most difficult and often most frustrating diagnostic complexes to the practicing physician. The thoracic cavity contains extremely vital organs, which can be injured without significant external evidence of trauma. Too often, the patient looks surprisingly well, and then suddenly shock, respiratory distress, and cardiac or respiratory arrest develop.

In patients with penetrating thoracic injuries, the potential seriousness of the condition is usually immediately appreciated by the initial examiner. On the other hand, patients suffering from blunt thoracic trauma commonly have associated injuries that occupy the physician's attention, and often the extent and potential hazard of the intrathoracic injury are not appreciated until a catastrophic event occurs. Most blunt injuries to the chest result from automobile accidents, and the majority of these patients have associated injuries. The mortality from thoracic injuries increases markedly when associated injuries are present. This may simply be a reflection of the severity of the accident, or it may be due in part to the difficulties in managing patients with multiple injuries.

It has been estimated that as many as 20 per cent of deaths from trauma result primarily from chest injuries. Surprisingly, a very small percentage of hospital deaths can be attributed to the thoracic injury. For example, only approximately 20 per cent of patients with a ruptured thoracic aorta reach the hospital alive. In injuries of the chest, the most common cause of death between the site of accident and the emergency room is respiratory insufficiency. This may be due to simple obstruction of the airway in the mouth or throat, to development of tension pneumothorax, to a sucking chest wound, or to paradoxical movement of a fractured segment of the chest wall. Many of these conditions can be treated without elaborate equipment if the initial examining physician understands the urgency required in adequate management of respiratory difficulties.

Evaluation of ventilation should be one of the physician's first concerns. This can be accomplished by simply examining the patient and estimating the force of the respirations and the amount of air inspired and expired. Obviously, if the patient has multiple secretions or blood in the nasopharynx, these should be removed to assure an adequate airway. By palpating the pulse, one can determine whether it has respiratory variation; this would suggest hemopneumothorax or pericardial tamponade. The majority of patients in shock from blood loss alone, unless they also have a severe head injury or are in intense pain, will lie quietly and will not be restless or agitated. In a patient with thoracic injuries there may be both tension pneumothorax and loss of a large amount of blood into the thoracic cavity. The major sign of respiratory insufficiency is agitation and restlessness. Of course, if the patient also has a cerebral injury, signs of restlessness and agitation may be less meaningful.

An initial precursory examination should identify any obvious open wounds of the chest. Respiratory insufficiency from a flail chest may be apparent on inspection, but frequently in a large patient the amount of subcutaneous fluid or blood will conceal the extent of paradoxical movement and make the external appearance of the skin rather smooth and concentric. The presence of crepitus or actual free movement of ribs on palpation should suggest a possible flail segment. If respiratory efforts are adequate and the chest moves symmetrically but ventilatory exchange is poor, some form of airway obstruction probably exists. The initial diagnosis of pneumothorax or hemothorax may be more difficult on physical examination than is often described. Often the involved hemithorax is diminished in volume, and there are poor respiratory excursions on the involved side. With the patient in the recumbent position, hemopneumothorax may be difficult to diagnose, since blood will lie in the posterior aspect of the thorax, while the compressed lung will be near the anterior chest wall. Breath sounds may be normal over the anterior and lateral thorax; this makes the diagnosis by physical examination alone difficult.

The neck should be examined to determine the relative position of the trachea in the suprasternal notch. In tension pneumothorax or hemothorax, the trachea may be shifted away from the involved side, and this can be a useful clinical observation. Subcutaneous emphysema and crepitance may be present in the neck about the trachea. Neck veins may be distended if there is increased intrathoracic pressure or cardiac tamponade. If percussion can be performed far enough posteriorly, a large hemothorax will be associated with a dull percussion note, whereas pneumothorax will obviously be associated with a hyperresonant sound. The aforementioned important points for evaluation of thoracic injuries should accompany a complete, thorough physical examination to evaluate other areas of the body as well. It is important to emphasize that once obvious massive hemorrhage from open arteries has been controlled by pressure, tourniquet, or vascular clamp, the chest and respiratory system demand the most attention.

It is interesting to note certain overall mortality statistics of closed chest trauma. In a review of traffic fatalities with chest injury, Kemmerer[9] found rib fractures in 39 per cent, hemothorax in 28 per cent, lung lacerations in 10 per cent, and ruptured great vessels in 10 per cent. About 40 per cent of these victims were thought to have died as a result of their thoracic injuries. It is apparent that the extent of chest injuries often is not appreciated, and institution of proper treatment is unnecessarily delayed. Perry and Galway[14] reported that 21 per cent of patients with serious chest injury reaching the hospital alive died during the first 24 hours. Associated injuries have a great influence on survival after chest trauma. Schramel[16] observed a 42 per cent mortality in patients with a significant associated injury. When a cerebral injury significant enough to cause unconsciousness for 72 hours was associated with a major thoracic injury, a survival of only 12 per cent was observed. However, in isolated thoracic injuries alone, the survival is approximately 90 per cent.

MECHANISMS OF INJURY

In the majority of incidences, it is difficult to isolate the exact mechanism of injury, since several occur simultaneously. It is important, however, to attempt to divide the mechanisms of injury so that some understanding of the etiology of internal organ damage can be appreciated. Penetrating injuries, such as bullet or knife wounds, need little explanation, since they cause injury by direct contact with the internal structure. Blunt thoracic trauma can be more complex, and the internal damage considerably more extensive than the external evidence of injury.

Direct trauma to the thoracic cage has always been a common form of injury. The victim is struck in the chest by a moving object; this may result in fractures of ribs or sternum over a localized area, but a major vascular or cardiac injury is rare. The lung may be contused by a fragment of rib driven inward, with pulmonary laceration or hemopneumothorax resulting. The majority of patients suffering direct local trauma survive, and associated injuries are uncommon. The area of the actual injury is usually clearly defined.

A *compression-type injury* of the thorax or upper abdomen may result in a specific type of damage. This is commonly seen in patients trapped in landslides, cave-ins, or building collapses. There may be direct local trauma to the thoracic cage, although in many instances no actual injury can be defined. Sustained thoracic compression causes traumatic asphyxia or cervicofacial static cyanosis. In this situation, the skin of the face, neck, and shoulders has a red to purple discoloration, and subconjunctival hemorrhages are usually present (Fig. 1). This results from blood being forced out of the thorax, with reflux cephalad through the venous system. Similar lesions can be produced experimentally by occluding the superior vena cava for approximately 10 minutes. These patients with vena caval occlusion are not asphyxiated in the usual meaning of the term, but suffer excessive oxygen removal in the capillary bed due to stasis. Compression injuries can rupture the diaphragm and contuse the lungs and the heart. In children, because of the marked pliability of the rib cage, severe thoracic

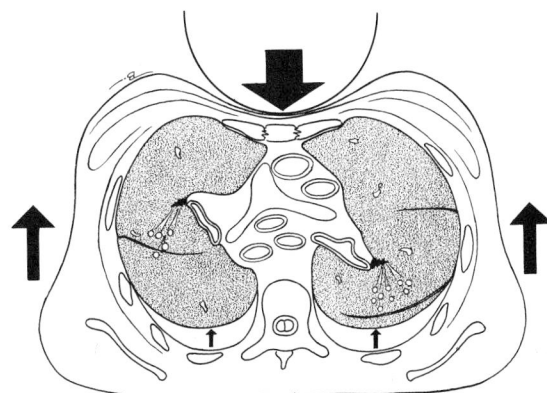

Figure 2. Diagram of a sagittal section through the thorax, demonstrating the usual point of impact over the anterior chest. The bony thorax decelerates rapidly, while the internal structures may continue to move forward. The major attachment of the lung with the least elasticity is the bronchus, and the momentum of the lung may cause this structure to tear.

compression can occur with minimal damage to the thoracic cage. Thoracic compression can result in the "crush syndrome," although it is not as common as in compression injuries of the extremities.

Deceleration-type injuries are usually classified under the broad headings of "impact" and "momentum," although most victims incur both concomitantly. Since most patients suffering blunt trauma to the chest are victims of automobile accidents, the effects of rapid deceleration are quite important. Impact injury results from direct contact of the thoracic cage with a hard object. The majority of force is dissipated against the bony thorax, with rib fractures and sternum fractures the result (Fig. 2). Contusion, laceration, and compression of soft tissues and internal organs occur. The fracture of ribs and the elasticity of the thoracic cage reduce the rate of the deceleration and lessen the likelihood of a momentum-type injury occurring to internal organs. A momentum injury results from the rapid deceleration of the body with continued movement of the internal organ. For example, the heart is attached by the great arteries and veins, but the major mass is suspended in the pericardium. Patients sustaining a major fall have impact injury, but in addition the suspended heart continues to travel and one of its attachments tears. An aortic tear in the sinus of Valsalva is common in vertical deceleration, whereas tearing of the main bronchus results when the lung continues to move after rapid deceleration in a horizontal direction.

PATHOPHYSIOLOGY

The most common thoracic injury is a simple fracture of ribs. Fracture of a rib in one place does not significantly alter the stability of the thoracic cage, but if the rib is fractured in two places, the segment between fracture sites has no stable attachment and is subject to movement related to changes in intrathoracic pressure. When several ribs are fractured in two sites, or in a single site in association with tearing of the an-

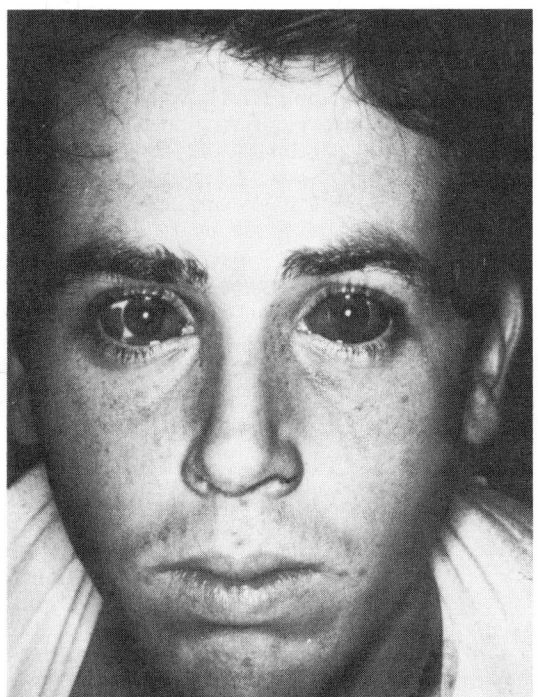

Figure 1. A young workman who was trapped in a landslide and was subjected to thoracic compression for approximately 15 minutes. Note the marked bilateral subconjunctival hemorrhage. There was red to purple discoloration and multiple petechiae over the face, neck, and shoulder areas.

terior or posterior attachments, a large segment of chest wall becomes unstable, and so-called paradoxical movement of this area occurs. The loss of structural integrity of the thoracic cage reduces the efficiency of breathing, increases the work of respiration, and limits the volume of air moved with each breath. During inspiration, the flail segment moves inward, and during expiration it moves outward. For years the inadequacy of ventilation associated with a flail chest was attributed to a pendulum-like movement of air from one hemithorax to the other in association with paradoxical movement of the chest wall. Maloney[10] showed that this "pendelluft" effect did not occur and that the paradoxical movement of the chest wall simply limited the patient's ability to create adequate negative pressure to ventilate the lungs. Respiratory insufficiency may develop from mechanical instability of the chest wall, as a result of limited ventilation due to severe pain, and from alterations in ventilation and perfusion in the lungs secondary to trauma.

Most patients suffering a combination of impact and momentum injuries are subject to some pulmonary contusion. The initial response of the lung to trauma seems to be increased fluid production with retention of that fluid. This may be in the form of edema in the walls of the alveoli or frank outpouring of fluid into the alveolar spaces with development of pulmonary edema and pneumonitis. Comroe et al.[4] emphasized that there are changes in distribution of blood flow through the traumatized lung and alterations in ventilation within these traumatized segments. Thus, a degree of ventilation-perfusion inequality develops. This simply means that the relationship of ventilation and blood flow to the alveoli may not be uniform. One area of lung may be ventilated normally, while blood flow is decreased. In another or adjacent segment, blood flow may be increased, while ventilation is normal or decreased. Certainly, in normal man, blood flow to the capillary bed is not evenly distributed; in the erect position, gravitational force acting on blood in the longitudinal vessels causes an increase in blood flow to the base of the lungs. Some changes in vascular compliance of the pulmonary arteries may also be active and tend to make flow more nonuniform. The outpouring of fluid into lung parenchyma alters ventilation-perfusion relationships. Diffusion along the capillary membranes is altered in areas of trauma, but the vast size of the pulmonary capillary bed usually permits adequate gas exchange. In some patients, the response to trauma is marked outpouring of fluid not isolated to the area of injury but involving the entire pulmonary tree. This finding has been commonly associated with severe head injury; the physiologic mechanism responsible is not well clarified, although it is thought to be related to an increase in intracranial pressure.

The physiologic shunt develops in the lung whenever blood flow through a segment of lung is greater than the ventilation to that segment. Thus, pulmonary venous blood draining the area will be incompletely oxygenated. Wilson[19] emphasized that physiologic shunting may be the earliest sign of impending respiratory failure. The ventilation-perfusion ratios are constantly changing in areas of injured lung, and the common physiologic disturbance is a reduction in oxygen content of the arterial blood. Since carbon dioxide diffusion across the alveolar membrane is approximately 20 times more efficient than oxygen transport, increased arterial carbon dioxide content is unusual. Oxygenation of the blood in capillaries is more time-consuming and is not completely accomplished in the injured lung. Increasing the oxygen content of inspired air will usually improve systemic arterial saturation. Thus, physiologic shunting can be decreased by raising the oxygen content of inspired air.

If arterial desaturation continues, some degree of tissue hypoxia occurs. The initial response is peripheral vasoconstriction, and the hypoxic tissue is thus further deprived of adequate oxygen. Patients usually become quite restless when peripheral tissue hypoxia occurs and often are quite hypertensive during this period unless associated major blood loss has occurred. There is usually an increase in the rate and depth of respiration, requiring additional work with increased oxygen consumption. Metabolic acidosis occurs, and the vicious cycle of tissue hypoxia is further amplified.

Following thoracic injury, ventilatory rate is usually increased and tidal volume is reduced. Thus, the calculated functional dead space is increased. Arterial carbon dioxide tension does not increase, although mild arterial hypoxemia has been noted when patients were breathing room air. Patients seem to be able to compensate for impaired ventilation for a period of time, but the added work of breathing to insure adequate ventilation reduces arterial oxygen content and gradually results in accumulation of carbon dioxide, with the possibility of respiratory arrest. It is important that serial measurements of blood gases be done in any patient with evidence of arterial desaturation, since patients with flail chest injuries commonly do not show signs of respiratory insufficiency for 12 to 24 hours after admission to the hospital.

Impending respiratory failure should be appreciated before the arterial carbon dioxide level is elevated. Unless there is a major defect in diffusion of gas from the alveoli to the pulmonary capillaries, arterial carbon dioxide does not become elevated until the tidal volume and dead space become nearly equal (Fig. 3). At this stage, arterial oxygen content is markedly reduced, and some type of ventilatory support is mandatory. There is only minimal reward in becoming expert in resuscitation after respiratory arrest, but great merit in recognizing and treating the early signs of respiratory insufficiency.

FRACTURE OF THE RIBS

Simple fracture of the ribs resulting from blunt trauma to the chest is probably the most common injury encountered. Simple rib fracture can be lethal if the lung is lacerated and tension pneumothorax is produced. Tearing of an intercostal artery by the bony fragment may result in hemothorax and require thoracotomy for control of hemorrhage. In blunt injuries of the chest, the finding of subcutaneous emphysema over the site of the injury almost certainly indicates that the lung was torn and air escaped from

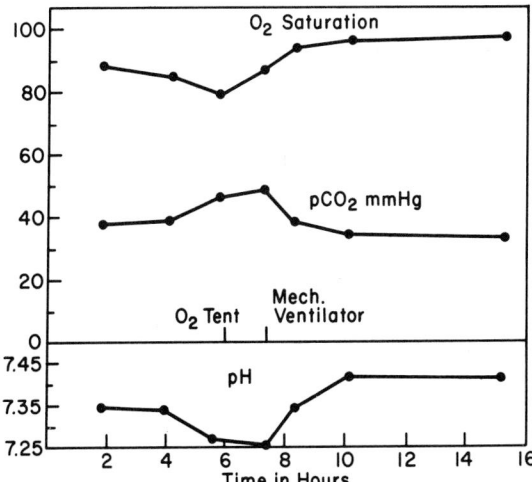

Figure 3. Measurements of blood gases in a patient with a flail chest injury. Immediately after injury, there was a decrease in the arterial oxygen saturation. Placing the patient in an oxygen tent brought only slightly improvement, and the arterial pCO_2 began to rise, suggesting further impairment in ventilation. Institution of positive-pressure ventilation with room air increased oxygen saturation, reduced the pCO_2, and raised the pH.

the lung into the pleural space and then into the soft tissues.

Most of the time simple rib fracture does not result in internal injury to the lung, and the person complains only of a sharp, knifelike pain in the rib cage. This is accentuated by breathing or movement, and the patient attempts to splint the injured side. There is a tendency to underventilate the lung on the side of injury, and the possibilities of retention of secretions and atelectasis become a major problem.

In general, strapping of the hemithorax with tape should be discouraged, since it further limits ventilatory excursion and enhances the possibility of atelectasis and pneumonitis. It is true that some relief of pain can be accomplished by strapping, but the overall benefits do not outweigh the disadvantages. Local anesthetic block of the intercostal nerves of the fractured rib and of the ribs above and below it provides considerable relief of pain. The anesthetic may last only 2 to 3 hours but often the pain is diminished because the patient breathes normally while the block is in effect. Administration of oral analgesics and expectorants is to be encouraged.

In all patients with suspected rib fractures, chest x-ray examination should be done to determine the presence or absence of pneumothorax. If a small pneumothorax is present, the physician should be alerted, as vigorous coughing and deep breathing by the patient may convert the simple pneumothorax into tension pneumothorax. If the pneumothorax is extensive, the insertion of an intercostal catheter with connection to an underwater seal is indicated. When pneumothorax alone is treated, the catheter is usually placed in the second intercostal space anteriorly. If considerable fluid or blood is present, the catheter may be inserted laterally through the sixth or seventh interspace.

TENSION PNEUMOTHORAX

A small puncture wound in the lung may produce a ball valve action in the visceral pleura and allow air to enter the pleural cavity during inspiration but prevent its escape during expiration. The lung gradually collapses and the mediastinum shifts to the opposite side (Fig. 4). The patient becomes severely dysp-

Figure 4. A, Pleurocutaneous tract and movement of the mediastinum away from the site of injury during inspiration and toward the opening during expiration. B, In a tension pneumothorax, air leaves the lung during inspiration and cannot return through the small hole during expiration. The amount trapped in the pleural space increases, and the mediastinum shifts away from the involved side.

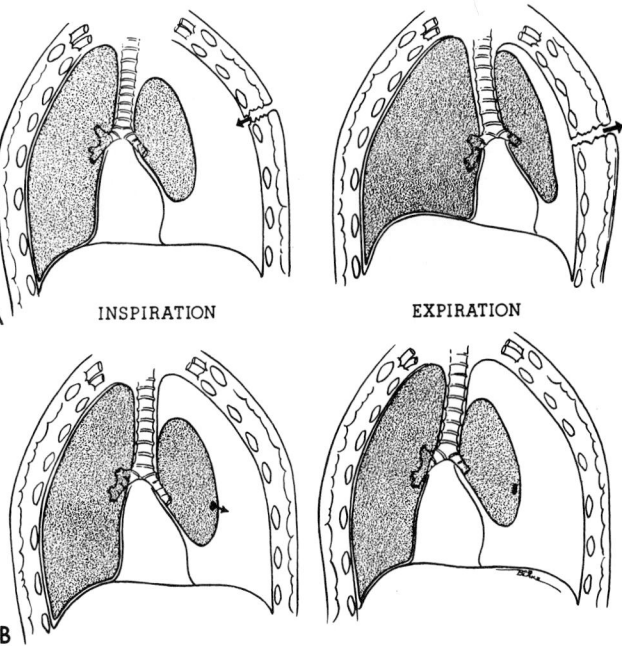

A   INSPIRATION   EXPIRATION

B

neic from compression and inability to expand the opposite lung, and respiratory arrest may ensue. The patient will usually have pain on the side of the pneumothorax, and physical examination will confirm the diagnosis. Breath sounds will be diminished and the percussion note will be hyperresonant. A needle should immediately be inserted in the chest and air aspirated. Often air will be released under pressure, and continuing decompression of the hemithorax is necessary. A chest catheter should be inserted and connected to a closed drainage system. In patients in respiratory distress with the physical findings of tension pneumothorax, needle aspiration should be performed before a chest x-ray is obtained, as this is a life-threatening emergency.

OPEN PLEUROCUTANEOUS TRACTS

A defect in the chest wall can be large enough that an open communication exists between the pleural space and the atmosphere. This is the so-called sucking-type chest wound. Often these wounds result from explosions or gunfire. The degree of respiratory distress will depend on the size of the opening. In large wounds, all air during inspiration passes through the pleurocutaneous wound rather than the trachea. This results in collapse of the lung and practically no intrapulmonary ventilation. The sound of air going through the defect is usually apparent. This rapid exchange of air through the chest wall defect results in inadequate ventilation because a positive intrathoracic pressure cannot be developed. The mediastinum shifts back and forth with each breath, and cardiac output is reduced. Immediate closure of the defect with mild external pressure will usually improve ventilation.

In most instances, an injury severe enough to cause an open thoracic wound will also injure the lung. When integrity of the chest wall is re-established by direct pressure or by a sealed dressing, the possibility of development of tension pneumothorax must be considered. In the emergency room it is best to pass a chest catheter through the wound and then restore integrity of the chest wall by applying a sealed dressing around the catheter. The catheter is attached to an underwater seal, and air leaking from the the lung will be removed. If the wound is large, a urethral catheter with a 30-ml. inflatable balloon can be inserted, the balloon inflated, and the wound sealed by gentle traction on the catheter. Surgical dressing of the defect can be accomplished, and a chest catheter can be inserted in another location to maintain expansion of the lung.

FLAIL CHEST

Fractures of four or five ribs may result in paradoxical movement of a segment of chest wall. This reduces the efficiency of breathing and limits the ability of the patient to cough effectively. Frequently the paradoxical movement of the chest wall can easily be seen, but in some cases, soft tissue swelling and hematoma obscure the magnitude of the movement. Dyspnea and cyanosis may be present when the patient reaches the hospital, and in these situations treatment is quickly instituted. Too often, the patient looks well on admission, and the extent of the flail chest injury is thought not to justify corrective measures. Spencer[17] emphasized the potential seriousness of the flail chest, which is too often not appreciated on initial examination. These patients do well for several hours, but eventually accumulations of secretions, fatigue, bronchorrhea, and decrease in pulmonary compliance render them unable to continue adequate spontaneous respiration. Hypoxia becomes more severe, and eventually retention of carbon dioxide occurs.

Many methods of immobilization of the flail segment have been tried. In emergency situations, compression of the flail segment with a soft pressure bandage or application of a sandbag will suffice until definitive treatment is available. Strapping the flail segment with tape has the disadvantage of immobilizing normal chest wall, and further limiting respiratory function. External traction has been utilized to elevate the flail segment, stabilizing it in an outward position. Towel clip traction has been quite popular; this can be effected by placing a towel clip around one of the center ribs of the flail segment and applying outward traction, especially during inspiration. Many types of soft tissue traction, suction devices, and skeletal traction have been described. Most of these are very bulky and limit mobility of the patient. Open surgical pinning or wiring of fractures of the sternum has been quite satisfactory.

The copious secretions resulting from trauma to the lung remain a major problem. Patients with signs of respiratory insufficiency secondary to flail chest injuries should be managed by means of controlled positive-pressure ventilation. Mörch et al. in 1955 showed the value of this type of treatment, emphasizing that the flail segment can be stabilized by positive-pressure breathing and the problem of hypoxia can be eliminated.[12] If the patient is in severe respiratory distress, an endotracheal tube should be placed and positive-pressure ventilation instituted immediately. A tracheostomy is performed to facilitate use of the respirator and removal of secretions. The increase of mean intrathoracic pressure has not proved harmful, even in hypovolemic patients, in whom the circulatory reflexes are assumed to be retained. Respiration may be controlled by mild hyperventilation, which produces slight alkalosis and apnea. Other physicians prefer assistance of ventilation only, but this has the disadvantage of requiring the patient to initiate inspiration and thus continually move the flail segment of the chest. Positive-pressure ventilation is necessary until the chest wall stabilizes. This may require 3 to 4 weeks; too often a patient is removed from the respirator before the chest wall is stable, and paradoxical movement resumes. Both Border[2] and Rutherford[15] suggest that positive-pressure ventilation immediately after injury should be beneficial in re-expanding atelectactic lung, reducing edema, and decreasing pulmonary hemorrhage. Experimental work has shown that a delay of 24 hours allows a post-traumatic pulmonary lesion to be established, which is much more difficult to reverse. The appearance on chest x-ray has proved to be a poor index of the extent of pulmonary dysfunction. Arterial oxygen content or the alveolar-arterial oxygen tension difference is a much more reliable index.

Long-term management of patients with crushed-chest injuries requiring positive-pressure ventilation demands expert nursing care. Absolute sterile technique must be employed during suctioning and handling of the tracheostomy tube, which should be changed at least every 48 hours. Shortly after injury, endotracheal suctioning may have to be performed frequently to remove the copious secretions. The patients are routinely given antibiotics to reduce the possibility of infection in the traumatized lung. In some instances, positive-pressure ventilation is discontinued because of the fear that a lower respiratory tract infection will develop. Ebert[6] demonstrated that pneumonitis develops in most patients with crushed-chest injuries, and positive cultures can be obtained from the trachea around the eighth to twelfth day. At this time, the general condition of the patient usually is such that proper antibiotics will control the infection (Fig. 5).

In any patient in whom positive-pressure ventilation is used, there is a risk that tension pneumothorax will develop, since the expanding lung may rub against a fragment of rib. The visceral pleura previously may have been perforated, and the fibrinous seal may be disrupted by administration of positive pressure. Thus, it is important that a routine chest x-ray be taken approximately 30 to 60 minutes after institution of positive-pressure ventilation, and the proper equipment for insertion of a chest catheter should be available.

Buford and Burbank in 1945 attributed the cause of traumatic wet lung to persistence of fluid, such as mucus, blood, or serum, in the lungs.[3] This condition lasted for several days after injury and patients were difficult to resuscitate from shock and were poor operative risks.

In patients suffering severe chest trauma, the amount of crystalloid fluid administered during the initial 48 hours after injury should be carefully calculated. The damaged capillary-alveolar membranes may leak fluid and cause increased respiratory difficulties. The lung reacts after trauma by producing an increased amount of interstitial and intra-alveolar fluid. Many patients have been made considerably worse by the injudicious use of large volumes of crystalloid fluid following trauma. In these circumstances, colloid osmotic pressure cannot hold a large volume of

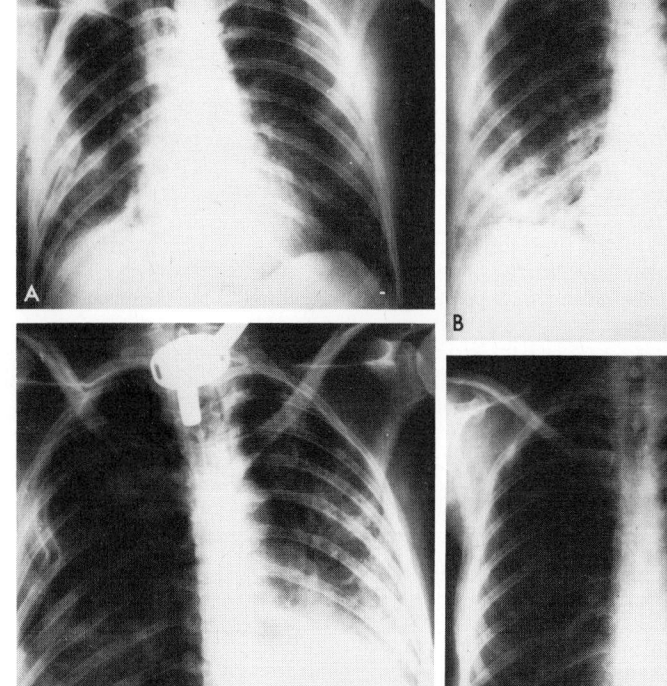

Figure 5. Sequence of x-rays following a flail chest injury. *A,* Immediate x-ray shows a chest catheter in the right thorax and a tracheostomy tube in place. The lung fields look reasonably clear. *B,* Twenty-four hours after injury, the extent of pulmonary contusion and fluid outpouring in the lung can be appreciated. *C,* Twelve days after injury, the right lung has cleared but residual pneumonitis is present on the left. *D,* Follow-up film 3 months after injury looks entirely normal.

crystalloid fluid in the vascular space, and damaged capillaries in the lung increase the amount lost into the alveoli. There is considerable variance in the individual response to injury, in that the fluid produced by the lung may be so little that it is almost unrecognized or so great that it actually drowns the patient.

Mechanical Ventilation

Whether a *volume-* or a *pressure-*regulated respirator should be used in management of flail chest injury is debated. The major advantage of the volume-regulated machine is the ability to control tidal volume and concentration of inspired oxygen. Most pressure-regulated respirators acquire their power from oxygen under pressure. If the ventilatory pressure increases, a greater concentration of oxygen is required to move the same volume of air. The problem is easily solved if compressed air is available to power the respirator.

Prolonged ventilation with high concentration of oxygen has been shown to produce changes in alveolar lining cells. These alterations are thought to be due to oxygen toxicity. Nash et al.[13] have divided these changes into two phases, an early exudative phase, with congestion, edema, hemorrhage, and fibrin, and a late proliferative phase, in which there is alveolar edema and fibroblastic proliferation with hyperplasia of the alveolar lining cells. The fundamental factors influencing oxygen toxicity are the oxygen concentration, susceptibility of the patient, and the length of exposure. In general, older patients are more susceptible than younger ones. The syndrome is progressive, and the changes are apparently irreversible. Prevention is the only known therapy, and there is no general agreement as to the length of time or concentration of oxygen required to produce alveolar changes. Prolonged ventilation with oxygen concentration no greater than 50 per cent seems to be tolerated without difficulty. However, if adequate arterial saturation cannot be accomplished with low oxygen concentrations, there is no choice but to increase the concentration of inspired oxygen. The possibility of toxic effects to the lung is realized, but the aim of treatment is maintenance until traumatized, nonfunctioning lung recovers. In all patients in whom positive-pressure ventilation is used, frequent measurements of arterial oxygen tension are necessary, and the level should be kept between 80 and 120 mm. Hg.

Prolonged use of mechanical ventilators has been incriminated as a cause of lung damage, and the term respirator lung or respirator pneumonitis has frequently appeared. Many patients who require assisted ventilation because of respiratory insufficiency have pre-existing pulmonary disease. Patients with mitral valve disease and secondary pulmonary changes often require prolonged ventilatory support after open-heart surgery. Lungs from the patients, when seen at postmortem examination, often are congested, fluid-filled, and hepar-like, and unfortunately the term respirator lung was used to describe this appearance. More often, other factors such as prolonged administration of high concentrations of oxygen, infection, prior lung disease, and postperfusion pulmonary congestion syndrome were present and were primarily responsible for the pathologic findings. These changes are uncommon in patients suffering crushed-chest injury who had normal lungs before the accident, and it is known that a properly adjusted mechanical ventilation system can function for practically unlimited periods of time if tracheal, bronchial, and pulmonary infections are prevented.

COSTOCHRONDRAL OR STERNOCHONDRAL INJURIES

A direct blow over an anterior costal cartilage may result in severe pain at the point of impact, resulting from a separation or fracture of the cartilage at either a sternal or costal junction. These injuries are extremely painful and often disabling and frustrating to the patient. Complications are rare, and the diagnosis is based on the physical findings of pain and tenderness directly over the point of the chondral junction. These cartilaginous fractures heal slowly, and the period of discomfort may be prolonged. Treatment is usually with oral analgesics.

FRACTURE OF THE STERNUM

In general, sternal fractures cause little disability except when associated with other major rib fractures. In severe flail chest injuries with associated sternal fractures, the sternum may have to be pinned or wired to provide stability of the thoracic cage. If the fracture is an isolated injury, relief of pain is only treatment necessary.

INJURIES TO TRACHEA OR MAIN BRONCHI

When blunt trauma to the chest causes a deceleration or momentum type of injury, the bronchus may be completely transected. Hemoptysis, pneumothorax, and subcutaneous emphysema usually occur, and the pneumothorax can quickly become a tension pneumothorax. Often subcutaneous emphysema of the neck appears early, and the trachea may be shifted to the opposite side (Fig. 6). Insertion of an intrathoracic tube to control the pneumothorax and air leak is important. If the patient will tolerate major surgery, direct anastomosis or bronchoplasty is recommended when the injury is recognized early. Often rupture of the bronchus is not immediately diagnosed, and it may be some time before development of pneumonitis or bronchial obstruction with distal pneumonia leads to its recognition. A ruptured bronchus heals with stenosis or occlusion. When stenosis is complete, the lung may be atelectatic and the diagnosis may remain obscure for years. If the stenosis is incomplete, air movement is partially obstructed, and coughing, due to blocking of the lumen by mucus, may occur. The likelihood of infection distal to the bronchial injury is greater when the obstructiom is incomplete. Johnson[8] emphasized that patients with severe tracheal lacera-

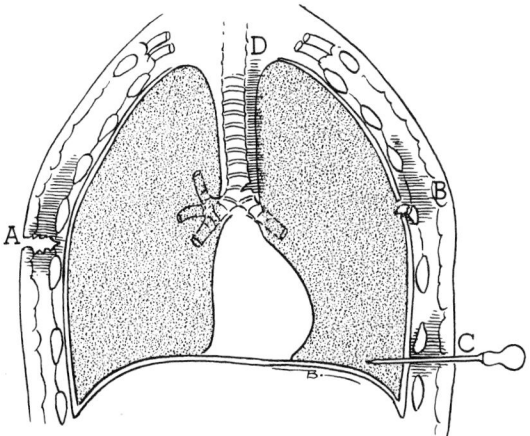

Figure 6. Possible causes of subcutaneous emphysema. *A,* Air may enter the soft tissues through external openings in the skin. *B,* A fractured rib may lacerate the parietal pleura and the lung; this results in a pneumothorax with escape of air through the parietal pleura into the subcutaneous tissue. *C,* A penetrating injury may result in subcutaneous emphysema from a combination of air entering from the outside and from a pneumothorax. *D,* A torn bronchus may cause mediastinal emphysema, which presents as subcutaneous air in the neck.

tions would be greatly improved by insertion of a tracheostomy tube. In these patients, massive air leaks usually develop, with extensive mediastinal emphysema. The tracheostomy tube lowers endotracheal pressure and decreases the amount of air escaping into the subcutaneous tissues. If the site of the laceration can be identified, it should be repaired at operation with interrupted nonabsorbable sutures (Fig. 7).

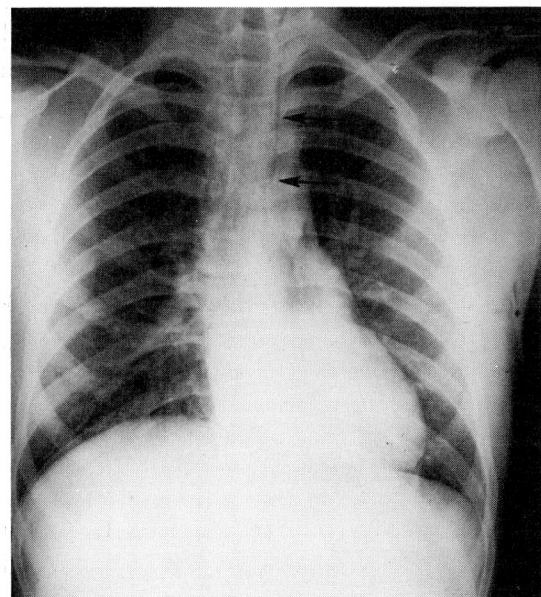

Figure 7. Chest x-ray of a patient who had been in an automobile accident with point of impact over the sternum. A small amount of subcutaneous emphysema was noted in the neck, and chest x-ray showed minimal mediastinal emphysema on the left. Bronchoscopy confirmed a tear in the left main stem bronchus, which was repaired at thoracotomy.

INJURIES TO THE HEART

Blunt trauma to the chest can cause a wide variety of cardiac injuries. Bleeding in the pericardial sac with resultant tamponade may occur. A reliable central venous pressure measurement should be obtained before aspiration of the pericardial sac is attempted. If blood reaccumulates, open thoracotomy should be considered. Contusion of the heart or actual myocardial infarction probably occurs more frequently than is appreciated. Cardiac arrhythmias are common after chest injuries and are probably related to myocardial injury. Atrial fibrillation is often seen, and the rapid ventricular response may be controlled with digitalis. If electrocardiographic evidence of myocardial injury is observed, treatment for myocardial infarction should be instituted. The late development of ventricular aneurysm has been seen after blunt thoracic injury.

Injury to the heart should be suspected particularly after a steering column injury, since the broken end of the sternum or rib may be driven into the heart, with direct rupture of the heart wall. The heart may be so severely compressed between the sternum and the vertebrae that a laceration results. Signs of cardiac failure may occur and are treated with fluid restriction, diuretics, and digitalis. If ventricular irritability is evidenced by frequent premature ventricular beats, it probably is best managed by a continuous intravenous infusion of lidocaine. Persistent tachycardia is common after chest injury, and frequent x-rays should be obtained so that signs of cardiac dilatation or frank congestive heart failure may be detected.

TRAUMATIC RUPTURE OF THE AORTA

It has been estimated that approximately 20 per cent of patients with rupture of the thoracic aorta reach the hospital alive. The majority die from exsanguination or pericardial tamponade. This subject is discussed in detail in another section.

TRAUMATIC DIAPHRAGMATIC HERNIA

The diaphragm can be injured by direct penetration or as the result of blunt abdominal or thoracic trauma. Blunt injuries to the abdomen or chest produce a marked increase in intra-abdominal or intrathoracic pressure, usually resulting in a tear in the posterior central section of the diaphragm. Occasionally, the peripheral attachments of the diaphragm may be avulsed from the chest wall. Traumatic diaphragmatic hernias occur on the left side 98 per cent of the time; the liver apparently protects the right diaphragm. The defect is usually quite large, and abdominal viscera commonly herniate into the thorax. A high degree of suspicion is necessary when the possibility of diaphragmatic hernia exists, because often only a small portion of the stomach, spleen, or liver may be present in the left chest, producing only minimal changes on routine chest x-ray. Harrington has proposed that these tears in the diaphragm occur at the time of trauma but that often actual herniation of abdominal viscera into the chest occurs much later. Dyspnea, cyanosis, and restlessness in a patient with no evidence of actual pulmonary injury should suggest that the diaphragm is incompetent.

Operative repair is indicated as soon as the general condition of the patient permits. The preferred approach has been through a left posterior lateral thoracotomy or a thoracoabdominal incision. In many of these patients, the diaphragmatic rupture is associated with multiple rib fractures or other thoracic injuries (Fig. 8). Ebert at al.[6] showed that repair of the diaphragmatic hernia should be performed in patients with flail chest, and the usual methods of managing the unstable thoracic wall should be invoked in the postoperative period. Positive-pressure ventilation will be required and will be more easily managed after visceral organs have been returned to the abdominal cavity.

In small defects of the diaphgram, the possibility of strangulation of herniated viscera must be considered. Early surgical exploration will decrease the likelihood of this complication. In some instances, the diaphragmatic hernia will not be detected for many years, and a portion of lung will be collapsed because of the space occupied by abdominal viscera. Even when operation is performed late, results should be satisfactory, because re-expansion of the collapsed lung usually results in improved ventilatory function. The defect usually can be closed by direct suture, although in some instances of long-standing hernias some type of prosthetic material or cloth may be needed to bridge the defect. The operative results are excellent, with the main difficulty being in establishing the initial diagnosis.

PENETRATING WOUNDS

Penetrating wounds of the chest are of serious concern because of the uncertainty as to whether major internal structures have been injured. One must consider the type of injury, and knowledge of the size or shape of the weapon can be extremely helpful. Unlike most abdominal wounds, which require an exploratory operation, many penetrating chest wounds do not require exploratory thoracotomy. However, a large number of these wounds are incurred in the lower left chest, and damage to the diaphragm or to intra-abdominal organs may occur, since the diaphragm lies at a much higher level than the lower limit of the rib cage. These injuries can be immediately life-threatening or, in many instances, seem highly insignificant, considering the mode of injury.

The major initial problem is that of hemopneumothorax, and most penetrating injuries of the chest require at least the insertion of an intercostal catheter connected to an underwater seal and suction. Bleeding from the lung is usually controlled by re-expansion of the lung, and thoracotomy usually is not necessary. In cardiac tamponade resulting from penetrating injuries, needle aspiration may initially provide relief but

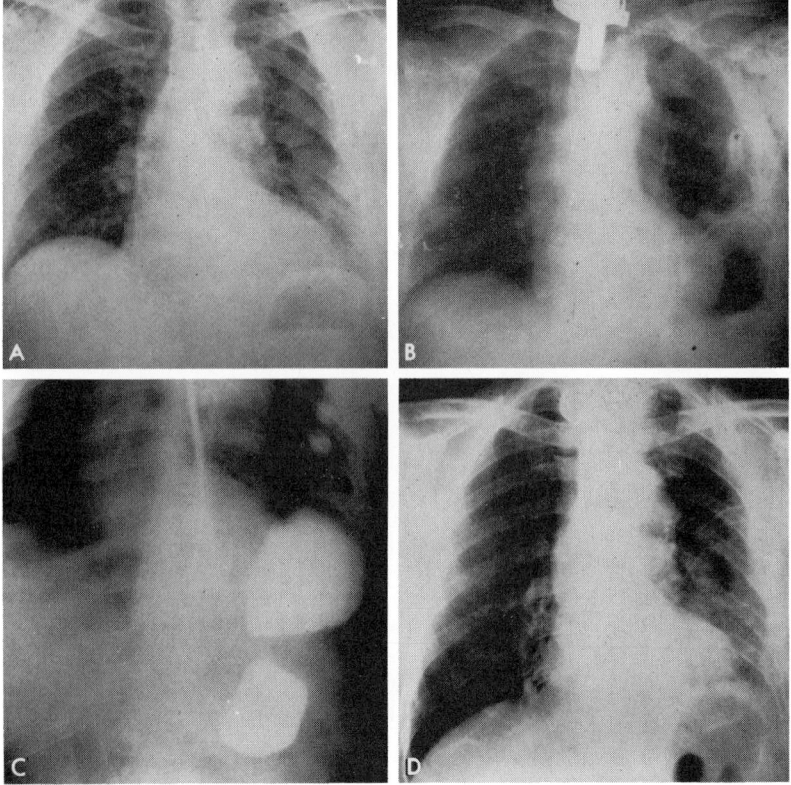

Figure 8. Sequence of chest x-rays of a patient with a left flail chest injury. *A*, The initial chest x-ray shows haziness in the left lower chest and contusion of the left lung. *B*, Two hours later, after institution of positive-pressure ventilation and tracheostomy. The suggestion of a left diaphragmatic hernia is now apparent. *C*, Radiopaque material given through the nasogastric tube confirms the presence of stomach in the left chest. *D*, Two days later, after left thoracotomy and repair of the diaphgramatic hernia.

probably should be followed by exploratory thoracotomy. Wounds of the heart should be closed by direct suture, and evacuation of blood from the pericardium may reduce the possibility of subsequent constrictive pericarditis. It should be remembered that all penetrating injuries to the chest invariably contaminate the pleural space. Blood in the thorax is partially defibrinated by movement of the lung; this facilitates evacuation by chest catheter. Antibiotics are routinely administered because of intrapleural contamination. Elimination of most of the blood in the pleural space decreases the possibility of subsequent pleuritis or empyema. Air leaks from the lung are usually controlled by maintaining adequate suction through the chest catheter.

Obviously, if blood continues to accumulate in the chest after insertion of a chest catheter, thoracotomy should be undertaken to control the hemorrhage. It is rare for significant bleeding to occur from the lung itself, but if major branches of the pulmonary artery or vein are injured, a lobectomy or even pneumonectomy may be necessary to control the hemorrhage. Intrapulmonary hematomas may develop after bullet or other penetrating injuries. These usually are asymptomatic and resolve spontaneously. Pulmonary lacerations may appear as cavitary lesions and contain a fluid level. This represents a tear in lung parenchyma, with leaking of air and fluid or blood into this space. These injuries are more common in young patients, and resolution is spontaneous, requiring an average of 6 to 10 weeks. Intrapulmonary hematomas discovered at the time of thoracotomy should be opened and the source of bleeding controlled by direct suture. The lung parenchyma is left exposed, with an intercostal catheter placed near the open area and connected to suction apparatus to maintain expansion of the lung. Development of lung abscesses in these intraparenchymal hematomas or cavities is uncommon.

SELECTED REFERENCES

Moore, F. D., Lyons, J. H., Jr., Pierce, E. C., Jr., Morgan, A. P., Jr., Drinker, P. A., MacArthur, J. D., and Dammin, G. J.: Post-Traumatic Pulmonary Insufficiency. Philadelphia, W. B. Saunders Company, 1969.
This excellent monograph considers pulmonary processes associated with trauma or other illnesses that often are responsible for respiratory insufficiency considered to be out of proportion to the primary disease. Respiratory difficulties associated with multiple fractures, sepsis, and shock are well defined. The pathophysiology of the pulmonary lesions is well illustrated, and the approach to management and prevention is emphasized. This presentation is easy to understand, and the clinical syndromes are separated by their physiologic consequences.

Nealon, T. F., Jr.: Trauma to the chest. *In* Sabiston, D. C., Jr., and Spencer, F. C. (Eds.): Gibbon's Surgery of the Chest, 3rd ed. Philadelphia, W. B. Saunders Company, 1976.
This chapter provides an excellent overview of management and evaluation of patients suffering thoracic injuries. There are good series of chest x-rays demonstrating various consequences of trauma. Many specific areas such as wounds of the heart are well covered. Certain complications of thoracic injuries such as empyema or cardiac tamponade are discussed in detail in other chapters.

REFERENCES

1. Battersby, J. S., and Kilman, J. W.: Traumatic injuries of the tracheobronchial tree. Arch. Surg., *88*:644, 1964.
2. Border, J. R., Hopkinson, B. R., and Schenk, W. G., Jr.: Mechanisms of pulmonary trauma: An experimental study. J. Trauma, *8*:47, 1968.
3. Burford, T. H., and Burbank, B.: Traumatic wet lung. J. Thorac. Surg., *14*:415, 1945.
4. Comroe, J. H., Forster, R. E., Dubois, A. B., Briscoe, W. A., and Carlsen, E.: The Lung: Clinical Physiology and Pulmonary Function Tests, 2nd ed. Chicago, Year Book Medical Publishers, 1962, Chapter 4.
5. Conn, J. H., Hardy, J. D., Fain, W. R., and Netterville, R. E.: Thoracic trauma: Analysis of 1022 cases. J. Trauma, *3*:22, 1963.
6. Ebert, P. A.: Physiologic principles in the management of the crushed-chest syndrome. Monogr. Surg. Sci., *4*:69, 1967.
7. Ebert, P. A., Gaertner, R. A., and Zuidema, G. D.: Traumatic diaphragmatic hernia. Surg. Gynecol. Obstet., *125*:59, 1967.
8. Johnson, J.: Battle wounds of the thoracic cavity. Ann. Surg., *123*:321, 1946.
9. Kemmerer, W. T., Eckert, W. G., Gathright, J. B., Reemtsma, K., and Creech, O., Jr.: Patterns of thoracic injuries in fatal traffic accidents. J. Trauma, *1*:595, 1961.
10. Maloney, J. V., Jr., Schmutzer, K. J., and Raschke, E.: Paradoxical respiration and "pendelluft." J. Thorac. Cardiovasc. Surg., *41*:291, 1961.
11. Martin, A. M., Simmons, R. L., and Heisterkamp, C. A., 3rd: Respiratory insufficiency in combat casualties. I. Pathologic changes in the lungs of patients dying of wounds. Ann. Surg., *170*:30, 1969.
12. Mörch, E. T., Avery, E. E., and Benson, D. W.: Hyperventilation in the treatment of crushing injuries of the chest. Surg. Forum, *6*:270, 1955.
13. Nash, G., Blennerhassett, J. B., and Pontoppidan, H.: Pulmonary lesions associated with oxygen therapy and artificial ventilation. N. Engl. J. Med., *276*:368, 1967.
14. Perry, J., and Galway, C. F.: Chest injury due to blunt trauma. J. Thorac. Cardiovasc. Surg., *49*:684, 1965.
15. Rutherford, R. B., and Valenta, J.: An experimental study of "traumatic wet lung." J. Trauma, *11*:146, 1971.
16. Schramel, R., Kellum, H., and Creech, O.: Analysis of factors affecting survival after chest injuries. J. Trauma, *1*:600, 1961.
17. Spencer, F. C.: Treatment of chest injuries. Curr. Probl. Surg., Jan., 1964.
18. Whitwam, J. G., and Norman, J.: Hypoxaemia after crush injury of the chest. Br. Med. J., *1*:349, 1964.
19. Wilson, R. F., Larned, P. A., Corr, J. J., Sarver, E. J., and Barrett, D. M.: Physiologic shunting in the lung in critically ill or injured patients. J. Surg. Res., *10*:571, 1970.

VIII

LUNG ABSCESS AND FUNGAL INFECTIONS

Timothy Takaro, M.D.

LUNG ABSCESS

A lung abscess is a localized area of suppuration and cavitation in the lung. This definition can encompass such diverse conditions as tuberculous, mycotic, or parasitic cavitation; bronchiectasis; infected cyst; and even pulmonary infarction with abscess formation. Cavitation of a tumor may also occur. Most of these conditions are discussed in other chapters of the text. In this section, we are concerned first with primary pyogenic lung abscesses, and second with those that occur in association with other diseases or conditions resulting in the weakening of the natural defenses of the body to infection. The former are declining in incidence, while the latter have achieved increasing prominence in recent years.[48, 77]

Pathogenesis

Edentulous patients rarely have primary lung abscesses. Primary pyogenic lung abscesses usually occur as a result of aspiration of a bit of septic debris from the oropharynx into the lung, in a patient with gingivodental disease or oral sepsis, during a period when the cough reflex is suppressed. Dental or tonsillar operations also commonly precede the development of lung abscesses. Since these episodes occur during periods of unconsciousness from alcoholism or general anesthesia, epilepsy, cerebral vascular accident, or immersion, the victim is usually in a recumbent, and often a supine, position.[83] The most direct route for the airway embolus to travel is into the right main bronchus, and the first dependent bronchus in a supine patient is that to the superior division of the right lower lobe. The posterior segment of the right upper lobe is also dependent and accessible. These two segments are therefore the most common sites of lodgment of septic emboli, and thus the commonest sites of primary lung abscesses. Esophageal disease that permits regurgitation and subsequent aspiration of esophageal contents into the lungs is another predisposing clinical setting. Rarely, an esophagobronchial fistula is the primary problem.[58]

Following the development of a severe pneumonitis in response to the embolus, liquefaction necrosis may occur. The microorganisms most commonly responsible for this chain of events are anaerobic bacteria, alpha and beta hemolytic streptococci, staphylococci, nonhemolytic streptococci, and *Escherichia coli*; other organisms are isolated less commonly.[4, 6, 30] As the liquefied necrotic material empties through the draining bronchus, a necrotic cavity containing pus and air is formed. Typically, the patient presents with a history of upper respiratory infection and is febrile and often toxic. Chest pain is not uncommon.

Hemoptysis often heralds the evacuation of the necrotic contents of the abscess cavity, and expectoration of purulent and sometimes putrid sputum will commonly follow. This may be copious or scant, and green, brown, gray, or yellow in color. The expectoration of anchovy-sauce-type sputum is suggestive of an amebic lung abscess, a rather rare condition in the United States.[82] Clubbing of the fingers can occur in as many as 20 per cent of cases.[77]

In the suppurative pneumonias of infancy due to staphylococci, clinical symptoms and signs of abscess may be overshadowed by those of toxemia, dyspnea, cyanosis, and septic shock. These may appear suddenly, or may be greatly intensified, if pyopneumothorax, due to rupture of a subpleural abscess, ensues.

The thoracic roentgenogram in lung abscess is not pathognomonic in the early stages prior to establishment of a communication between the abscess cavity and the draining bronchus. An area or areas of dense pneumonic consolidation precede the appearance of the characteristic cavitary lesion. Multiple abscesses may form multiple cavities. A distinguishing roentgenographic feature of lung abscess, the air-fluid level, is seen only on thoracic roentgenograms exposed in the upright position (or lateral decubitus, in a very sick patient). Accompanying pleural thickening, pneu-

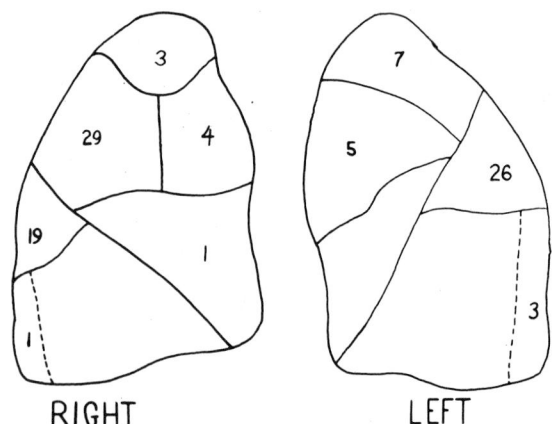

Figure 1. Diagram showing the segmental distribution in the two lungs of 98 lung abscesses due to aspiration. Note the predilection for three principal sites: the superior segment of the right lower lobe, the posterior segment of the right upper lobe, and the superior segment of the left lower lobe. (From Bernhard, W. F., Malcolm, J. A., and Wylie, R. H.: Dis. Chest, *43*:620, 1963.)

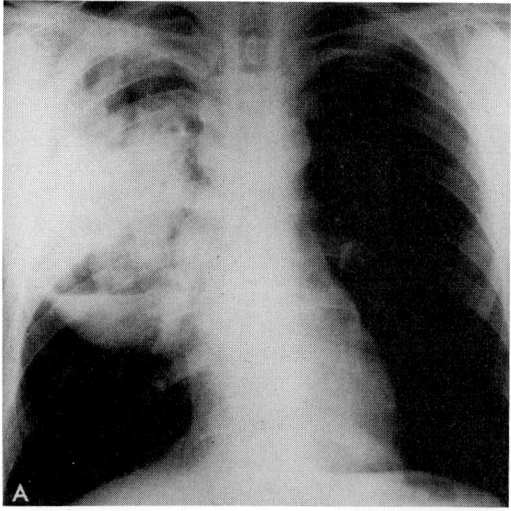

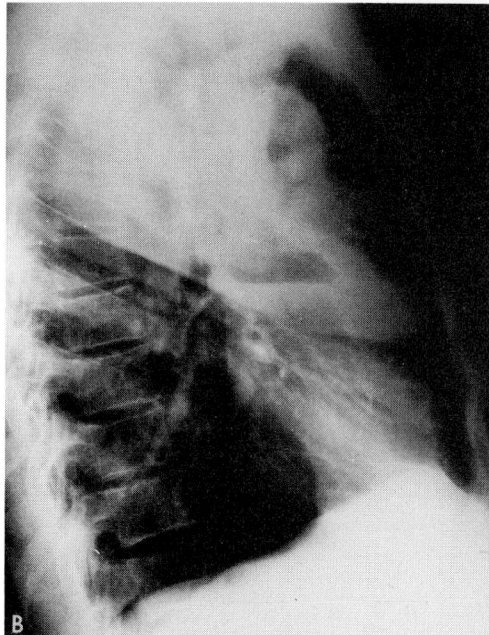

Figure 2. *A,* Posteroanterior, and *B,* right lateral, thoracic roentgenograms of a patient with a pyogenic lung abscess, from which *Klebsiella pneumoniae* and alpha streptococci were cultured. After a month of intensive antimicrobial therapy, a residual dense, thick-walled cavitary mass, 4 cm. in diameter, was resected by right upper lobectomy.

mothorax, or atelectasis may obscure or confuse this picture. Staphylococcal pneumonia of infancy, which may lead to infected pneumoceles, differs in appearance from the classic lung abscess in that the lesions are characteristically thin-walled and cystlike, and are often accompanied by pleural effusion, empyema, or pyopneumothorax. Complete or partial opacification of the hemithorax may be the presenting roentgenographic picture under these circumstances. With adequate therapy, even the most dramatic roentgenographic features may disappear completely.

Because of the availability of effective broad-spec-

trum antibiotics such as penicillin, lung abscesses can often be aborted in the stage of pneumonitis; hence, the incidence of this type of abscess has sharply declined in recent years.[77] On the other hand, much more difficult clinical problems are presented by patients, often at the extremes of age, who have serious associated diseases ranging from prematurity to incurable malignant disease, in whom therapeutic efforts have allowed survival, but without the normal defense mechanisms to enable them to combat infections successfully.[48] In such patients, lung abscess may occur as a complication of a systemic disease. Prematurity, bronchopneumonia, congenital defects requiring surgical treatment, the postoperative state itself, and the presence of other infections, blood dyscrasias, or systemic diseases are common predisposing conditions in early infancy. Systemic diseases, malignant diseases (especially of the lung and oropharynx), prolonged use of corticosteroid, immunosuppressive, or radiation therapy, and the postoperative period constitute the common conditions of the older age group in which this type of lung abscess is seen.[60] Such conditions often give rise to multiple (rather than single) abscesses, and the majority of these infections are acquired in the hospital. Bacteriologically, also, these abscesses differ somewhat from classic aspiration-type abscesses. *Staphylococcus aureus* is a common causative organism, but alpha streptococci, *Neisseria catarrhalis,* pneumococci, Pseudomonas, Proteus, *Escherichia coli,* and Klebsiella are all recognized, and occasionally, after prolonged antibiotic treatment, rather unusual bacteria are all that remain to be cultured from the sputum. There is no predilection for particular sites for these abscesses—they can occur almost anywhere, except that the right lung is more commonly involved than the left.

Treatment

The treatment of classic primary aspiration lung abscess is prolonged antimicrobial therapy.[5, 17, 30, 95] An appropriate regimen, begun even before the results of sputum cultures are known, might be penicillin G in combination with streptomycin or kanamycin; other antibiotics are used as indicated by subsequent bacteriologic studies.[5, 30] In Britain and Canada, more than in the United States, physical measures such as postural drainage and percussion are used and apparently found to be effective adjunctive measures. Bronchoscopy for diagnostic purposes, to remove a foreign body if one is present, and to provide drainage of the abscess by aspiration of the appropriate bronchus through the bronchoscope is also usually indicated. The refinement of transbronchial drainage by catheterization of the appropriate bronchus with or without fluoroscopic guidance has also been helpful.[19, 31] Surgical treatment is reserved for the complicated problems of massive hemoptysis,[49, 91] lack of response to antibiotics, and presence of a cavity that is thick-walled or of large size (6 cm. or more).[4] When a malignant lesion is suspected, or when empyema develops, surgery may also be appropriate. In most instances, resective surgery is performed—rarely is surgical drainage of lung abscesses indicated. The need for surgical resection for primary lung abscess has de-

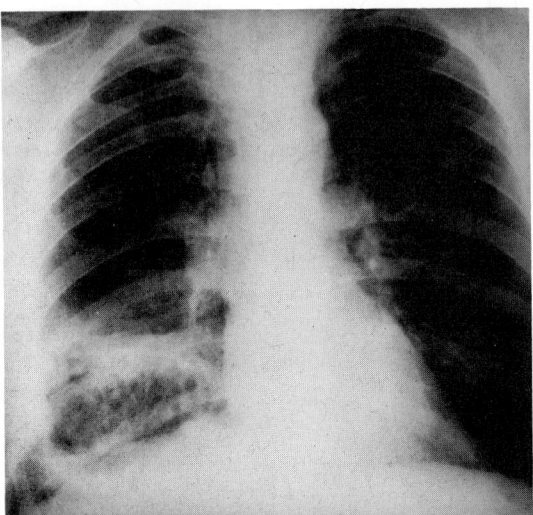

Figure 3. Thoracic roentgenogram of a patient with a huge lung abscess, right lower lobe, from which only the usually nonvirulent *Serratia marcescens* was cultured. This patient had had extensive corticosteroid therapy for severe asthma, and multiple broad-spectrum antibiotics for superimposed infection, prior to surgery. This type of abscess is currently being seen with greater frequency in similar clinical situations.

clined markedly in recent years, as the effectiveness of antibiotics has increased.[6]

The complications of lung abscesses include the occurrence of empyema, septicemia, metastatic brain abscess, and bronchogenic spread. The commonest complication is the development of chronicity.[95] A bronchiectatic, often epithelialized, residual cavity remains behind, if complete healing of the abscess has not taken place. Such a lesion is itself considered to be an indication for resection if it is symptomatic, or if infection recurs.

The mortality from primary aspiration-type lung abscess is emphatically different from that accompanying abscesses that occur as a complication of some other serious disease. The mortality from the former has declined from approximately 25 per cent, 10 to 15 years ago, to 5 per cent or less with prolonged and adequate antimicrobial therapy. On the other hand, 75 to 90 per cent of patients whose abscesses complicate some other systemic disease succumb—an appalling mortality, and a reflection of the gravity of the accompanying disease as well as of the prognostic significance of this complication.[17, 48] It is conceivable that prompt recognition and urgently applied and appropriate antibiotic therapy might in some measure alter this dismal picture.

ACTINOMYCETIC AND FUNGAL INFECTIONS OF THE LUNGS

Actinomycosis and nocardiosis have traditionally but mistakenly been classified as caused by fungal organisms. Actually the etiologic agents are bacteria belonging to the Actinomycetaceae. For convenience and common usage, they will be discussed in this section, along with fungal infections. However, the dis-

tinction is important because the treatment of infections by these two organisms differs radically from therapy for mycotic infections.

Attitudes concerning actinomycetic and fungal infections in general have changed considerably in recent years. This section emphasizes fungal infections of the *lungs,* but much of it is broadly applicable also to *systemic* infections of actinomycetic as well as mycotic origin.

Actinomycosis

Actinomycosis is caused by the anaerobic actinomycete *Actinomyces israelii,* and is characterized by abscess and sinus formation, with dense scarring. It is caused by an anaerobic or microaerophilic organism, and, therefore, special cultural techniques are required.[79]

In pathologic material, organisms with branching filaments occur in clusters or microcolonies called granules. The much larger, yellow-brown granules in draining material from abscesses or sinuses are called "sulfur granules," and again are dense clusters of organisms.[63]

Since *A. israelii* is a normal inhabitant of the oral cavity, one cannot make the diagnosis simply by recovering the organism from sputum. It must be recovered from closed tissue spaces or draining sinuses or abscesses, or shown to be invasive in histopathologic sections.

Thoracic actinomycosis is most commonly due to bronchopulmonary invasion of infectious material from the oropharynx. The infection that results may be so indolent that symptoms may be few until pleural or chest wall involvement takes place.

Empyema and chronic draining chest wall sinuses are characteristic, but insidious, nonspecific-appearing pulmonary infiltration, consolidation, or hilar mass strongly suggestive of bronchogenic carcinoma are also observed. This has been well shown by McQuarrie and others.[46, 85]

The drug of choice for actinomycosis is penicillin. Because of the dense, fibrous, avascular tissue surrounding the colonies of organisms and the concentration of organisms in dense clusters, high doses of drug must be used for long periods, and radical surgical excision should accompany antibiotic therapy, if possible. The difficulties of establishing a diagnosis in this disease also frequently result in surgical excision of the pulmonary lesions of actinomycosis, or of chest wall abscesses.[68] Empyema may require decortication or pleural drainage.[23]

Nocardiosis

Nocardiosis is usually caused by the aerobic actinomycete *Nocardia asteroides;* this organism has been isolated from the soil.[13, 65] It occurs in pathologic material in clumps or granules, made up of short or long branching filaments that are gram-positive and acid-fast. This property, as well as cultural and roentgenographic similarities, has led to confusion in the past with *Mycobacterium tuberculosis.*

Pulmonary nocardiosis may mimic pulmonary actinomycosis, tuberculosis, pneumonia, or lung abscess, both clinically and roentgenographically.[11] In the past decade, the majority of patients with nocardiosis have

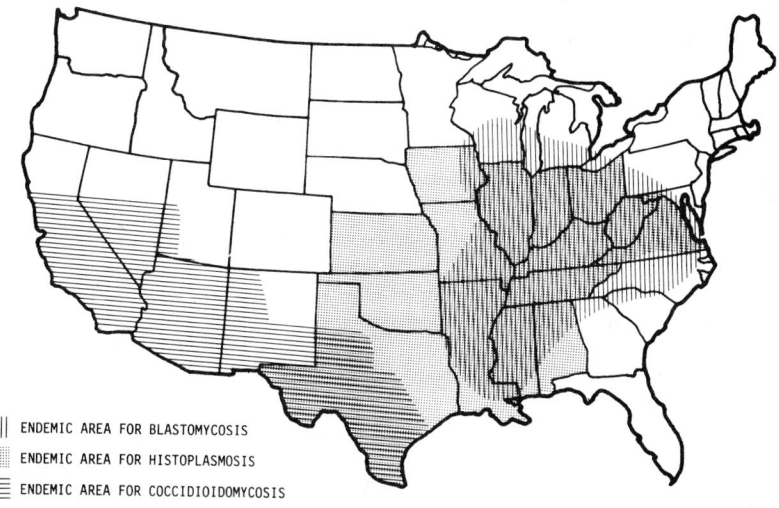

Figure 4. Map showing approximate areas in the United States recognized as endemic for North American blastomycosis, histoplasmosis, and coccidioidomycosis. (Adapted from Takaro, T. *In* Lewis' Practice of Surgery. New York, Hoeber Medical Division, Harper & Row, 1968.)

||||||| ENDEMIC AREA FOR BLASTOMYCOSIS
ENDEMIC AREA FOR HISTOPLASMOSIS
ENDEMIC AREA FOR COCCIDIOIDOMYCOSIS

had some underlying disease, such as lymphoma, leukemia, other malignant diseases, or (surprisingly) alveolar proteinosis, or have received corticosteroid therapy.[3, 22, 25] Thus, nocardiosis is more often than not an opportunistic infection, and in these situations, the prognosis is grave, even with treatment. The treatment of choice is sulfadiazine, continued on a long-term basis — a minimum of 2 months after arrest of the disease. Other drugs showing promise include minocycline and the combination of trimethoprim and sulfamethoxazole.[3, 47] On the other hand, if the disease is resectable, a cure rate of 100 per cent is reported. In many instances, the diagnosis has been made for the first time from the resected specimen.[44]

FUNGAL INFECTIONS

Formerly, blastomycosis, histoplasmosis, coccidioidomycosis, and cryptococcosis were considered to be rare, almost invariably fatal infections. Now it is recognized that benign, self-limited, and almost undetectable infections by all of these organisms are much more common. Millions of persons exhibit evidence of subclinical histoplasmosis and coccidioidomycosis, for instance, with spontaneous healing.

On the other hand, the widespread use of antimetabolites for neoplasms, of antibiotics for infections, and of steroids for a variety of conditions has given fungi such as Aspergillus, Candida, and Mucor the op-

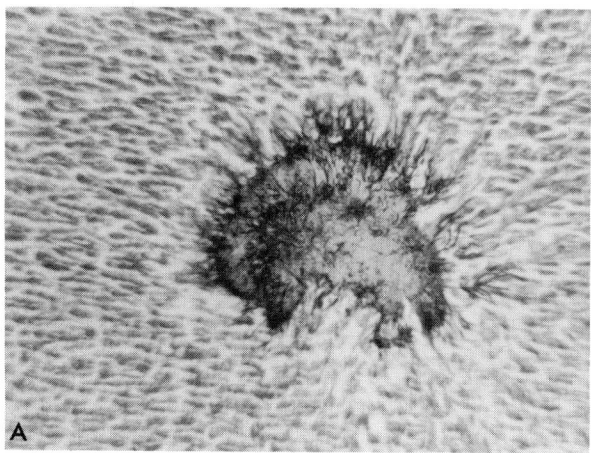

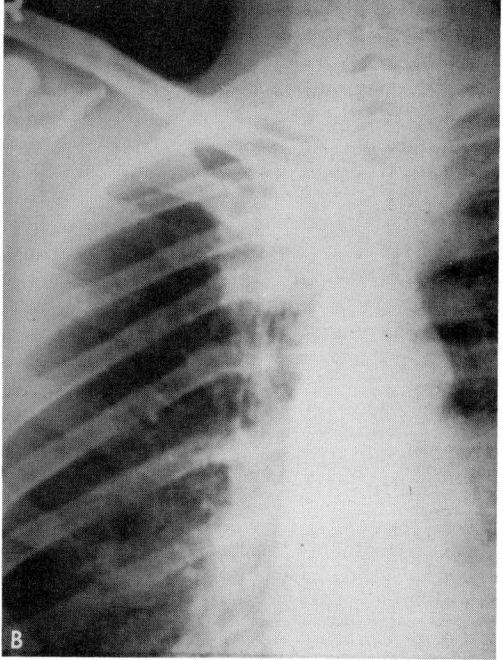

Figure 5. *A,* Actinomycotic granule showing branching filaments of a microscopic colony of *Actinomyces israelii.* Gomori stain. ×250. *B,* Thoracic roentgenogram of a patient who subsequently underwent right upper lobectomy for a suspected malignant lesion. Actinomycosis was found in the resected specimen. (From Takaro, T. *In* Lewis' Practice of Surgery. New York, Hoeber Medical Division, Harper & Row, 1968.)

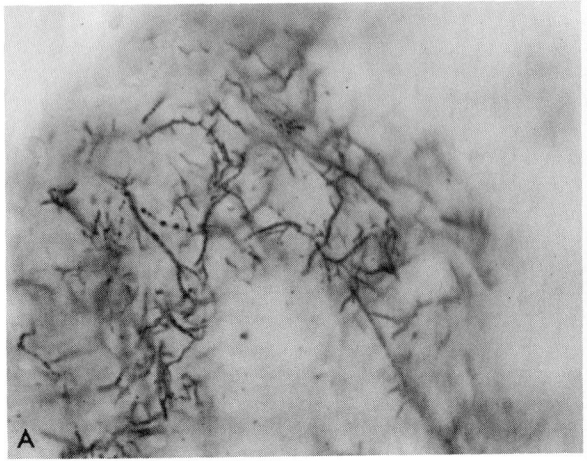

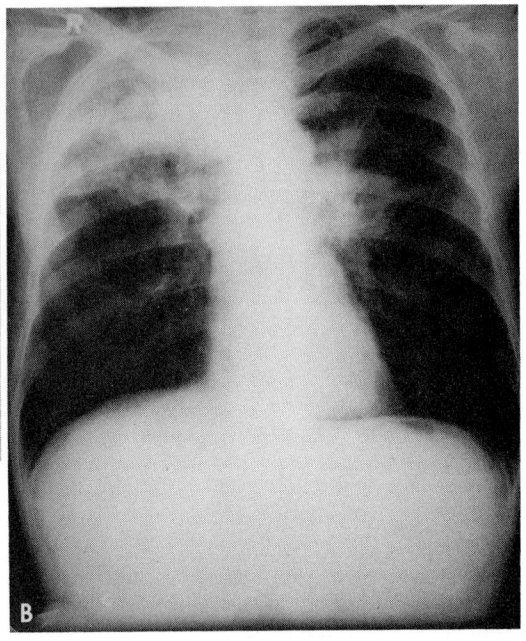

Figure 6. *A,* Organisms of *Nocardia asteroides.* Gram stain. ×1000. These organisms have been mistaken for tubercle bacilli in the past, because of acid-fast staining characteristics. *B,* Roentgenogram of thorax showing pneumonic lesion of nocardiosis. (From Takaro, T. *In* Lewis' Practice of Surgery. New York, Hoeber Medical Division, Harper & Row, 1968.)

portunity to invade the host and to cause disease. Thus, the formerly sharp line between so-called "pathogenic" and "nonpathogenic" fungi is blurred and no longer clear-cut. Both true pathogens and saprophytes *can* cause opportunistic infection—that is, invasion of the host when body defenses have been weakened or altered by drugs or disease. The surgeon must be aware of the variety of fungal infections that can beset his patient.

The surgeon is entirely dependent upon the pathologist for definitive diagnosis of these conditions, but the pathologist must rely upon the surgeon or physician to provide suspicion of fungal infection, and also to provide appropriate samples of sputum or tissue to make possible positive identification of the offending organism.[74] This is important, because serologic, immunologic, and skin tests cannot be relied upon for a definitive diagnosis,[14] and specific but rather toxic antimycotic drugs are now available for treatment (Table 1).[10]

Epidemiology

Many of the fungi causing human infection are inhabitants of the soil, and most infections are believed to be caused by direct inhalation of the organisms in contaminated dust. Thus, they are considered to be *exogenous* infections.

Three of these organisms are known to occur in the soil of specific and relatively delimited geographic areas in the United States. These are *Histoplasma capsulatum* (histoplasmosis), *Coccidioides immitis* (coccidioidomycosis), and *Blastomyces dermatitidis* (North American blastomycosis).[13] A soil reservoir is fairly well accepted for Cryptococcus, Aspergillus, and Mucor. On the other hand, candidiasis is considered an *endogenous* infection, since this yeast is part of the normal flora of human beings and animals, and is not found free in nature.

Histoplasmosis

Histoplasmosis is probably the most common of the fungal infections and occurs in the Mississippi Valley and its tributaries. The causative organism, *Histoplasma capsulatum,* is found in soil contaminated by pigeon, chicken, or bat droppings. Some 30 million persons are estimated to have been infected, judging from skin reactions to histoplasmin.[16]

The macropathology and micropathology resemble those of pulmonary tuberculosis, except for the finding of the tiny yeast cells of *H. capsulatum* in macrophages, or the capsules of nonviable organisms in the necrotic center of granulomas.

TABLE 1.   Antibiotics Effective Against Actinomycetes and Fungi*

Disease	Antibiotic
Actinomycosis	Penicillin; broad-spectrum antibiotics
Nocardiosis	Sulfadiazine; minocycline
Histoplasmosis	Amphotericin B
Coccidioidomycosis	Amphotericin B
North American blastomycosis	Amphotericin B; 2-hydroxystilbamidine
Cryptococcosis	5-fluorocytosine; amphotericin B
Aspergillosis	Amphotericin B (for invasive disease)
Candidiasis (moniliasis)	Amphotericin B; 5-fluorocytosine
Sporotrichosis	Amphotericin B; iodides
Phycomycosis (mucormycosis)	Amphotericin B; iodides
Monosporosis	None known
South American blastomycosis	Amphotericin B; sulfonamides

*Adapted from American Thoracic Society: Amer. Rev. Resp. Dis., *100*:908, 1969; Utz, J. P., Kravetz, H. M., Einstein, H. E., Campbell, G. D., and Buechner, H. A.: Chest, *60*:260, 1971; and Bennett, J. E.: N. Engl. J. Med., *290*:30 and 320, 1974.

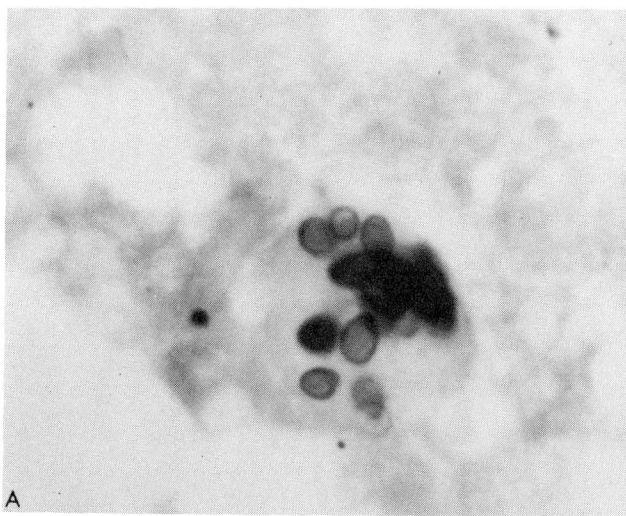
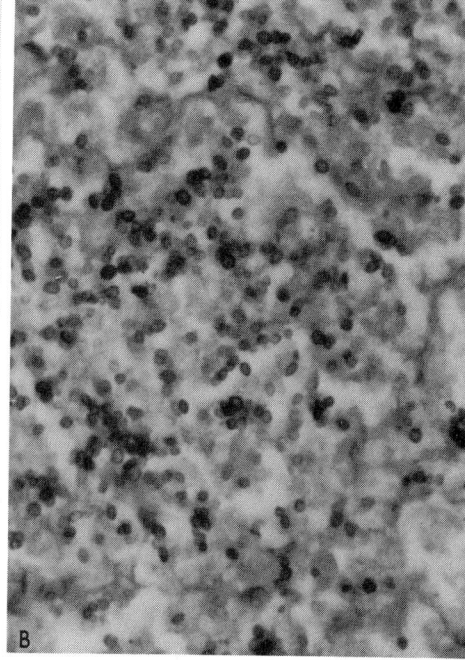

Figure 7. Forms of *Histoplasma capsulatum* found in tissues. *A*, Intracellular viable organisms. H & E stain. ×500. *B*, Nonviable capsules of *H. capsulatum* in necrotic center of a histoplasmoma. Gomori stain. ×1000. (From Takaro, T. *In* Lewis' Practice of Surgery. New York, Hoeber Medical Division, Harper & Row, 1968.)

While most cases of infection are asymptomatic, acute pulmonic infection may be accompanied by diffuse pulmonary infiltration, or scattered nodular densities, and may be characterized by an acute febrile course. By far the commonest clinical presentation of histoplasmosis is as an asymptomatic chronic granuloma, appearing on a thoracic roentgenogram as a solitary pulmonary nodule of undiagnosed etiology.

Chronic cavitary histoplasmosis resembles pulmonary tuberculosis both symptomatically and roentgenographically, although it appears to progress somewhat more slowly. In a considerable percentage of cases, pulmonary tuberculosis has been found to coexist in such patients; in many others, a mistaken diagnosis of pulmonary tuberculosis, based on roentgenographic findings, has led to hospitalization in sanatoriums. Only in the past two decades has this error begun to be recognized.[26] A wide variety of clinical manifestations of chronic histoplasmosis involving the mediastinal structures is also seen.[89]

The treatment of histoplasmosis depends upon the form of the disease that is encountered. For severe acute infections, therapy with amphotericin B, currently the only available effective drug, may be necessary. The solitary nodule may pose a problem in management. In a cooperative study of almost 1000 solitary pulmonary nodules resected in adult males, 53 per cent were found to be granulomas and 36 per cent malignant tumors.[86] Fungi, most commonly *H. capsulatum* or *Coccidioides immitis*, were isolated from the majority of these granulomas. However, since malignancy was found in such a high percentage of cases, and since the presence of calcium in a nodule does not rule out carcinoma (unless calcification is concentric, dense, or unchanged for years), exploratory thoracotomy for the undiagnosed nodule will very often be indicated, especially in adult males over forty

years of age.[41, 52, 54] On the other hand, if the diagnosis can be made by transbronchial brushing of the lesion, neither thoracotomy nor drug therapy may be necessary. Cavitary histoplasmosis, proven by culturing the organism in the sputum, should be treated primarily with amphotericin B. Pulmonary resection for chronic cavitary pulmonary histoplasmosis has often been recommended in the past,[87] but in a cooperative study involving more than 400 patients, there was no evidence that this modality, even in conjunction with amphotericin B, resulted in a greater reduction in relapses

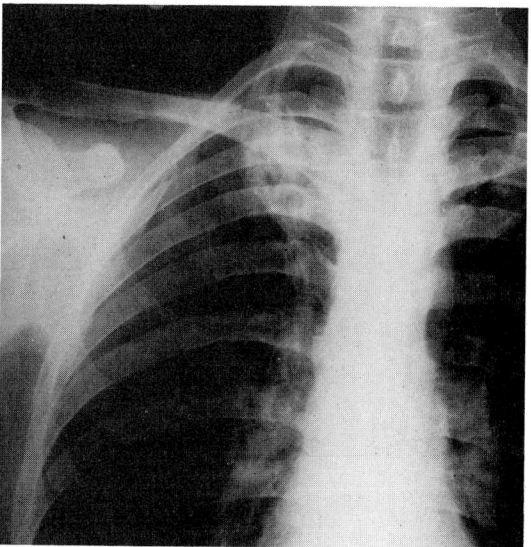

Figure 8. Thoracic roentgenogram of patient with chronic cavitary histoplasmosis who underwent upper lobectomy prior to the availability of amphotericin B. (From Takaro, T. *In* Lewis' Practice of Surgery. New York, Hoeber Medical Divison, Harper & Row, 1968.)

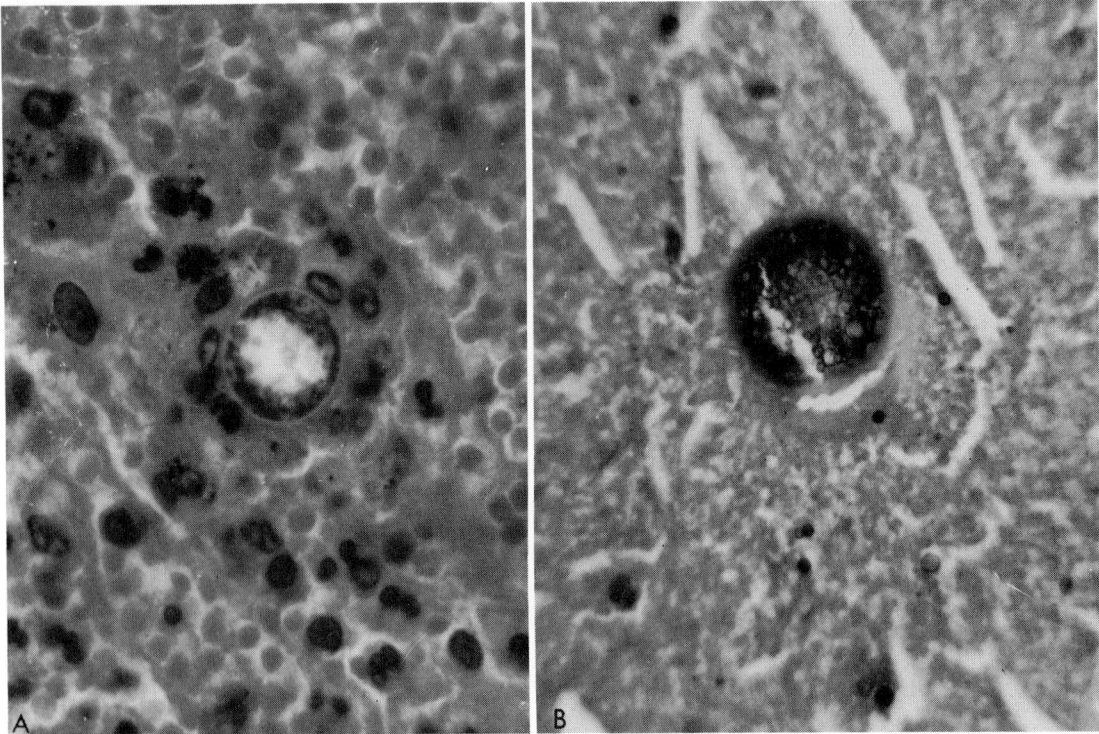

Figure 9. Spherules of *Coccidioides immitis,* packed with endospores. *A,* In a giant cell. H & E. ×500. *B,* In necrotic tissue. Gomori stain. ×250. (From Takaro, T. *In* Lewis' Practice of Surgery. New York, Hoeber Medical Division, Harper & Row, 1968.)

and deaths than did use of the drug alone.[61] On the other hand, there is general agreement that if resectional surgery is undertaken, amphotericin B should be used, until a total dosage of at least 2 gm. is reached.[1, 67, 70, 72] This can be given over a period of a month before and a month after surgery if the diagnosis is established prior to surgery. If chronic cavitary histoplasmosis is diagnosed only after surgery, treatment with 2 gm. of amphotericin B is recommended to prevent recurrence and to lower the statistically higher death rate seen in patients who have not received the drug. The treatment of mediastinal forms of histoplasmosis is variable and complicated.[89]

For disseminated forms of histoplasmosis, amphotericin B is urgently needed to prevent death.

Coccidioidomycosis

Coccidioidomycosis is caused by the dimorphic fungus *Coccidioides immitis,* which may occur in tissues in the form of large spherules packed with endospores, but also as individual small endospores (following rupture of a spherule) or as mycelial elements or hyphae (in cavities).[12, 57]

Coccidioidomycosis is also an exogenous infection occurring in the area corresponding to the zone of mesquite, found in certain well-defined regions of California, Nevada, Arizona, New Mexico, and Texas.[57] This is a region characterized by a dry, windy, dusty, hot climate. Modern irrigation has made this area a very important one from the agricultural standpoint and, therefore, also from the epidemiologic point

of view, since population growth in this zone has been rapid in the past several decades. Extensive travel through the area has helped to spread coccidioidomycosis to every part of the United States as well as to other countries. Some 10 million people in the United States are estimated to have been infected at some time in their lives with *C. immitis.*

The gross and microscopic lesions of coccidioidomycosis strongly resemble those of pulmonary tuberculosis, but with two characteristic differences. These are the occurrence of thin-walled cavities and of suppuration in coccidioidomycosis. However, thick-walled cavities, and chronic granulomas appearing as solitary nodules, as in histoplasmosis, are also common. Finally, apical or subapical infiltrates or cavities or both, indistinguishable roentgenographically from either chronic pulmonary tuberculosis or chronic pulmonary histoplasmosis, are also seen.

A history of "valley fever" while residing in an endemic area is classically obtainable, but often no clinical evidence is available of the onset of the disease. With acute cavitation, hemoptysis is the commonest symptom; with chronic infection, cough, weight loss, fever, and chest pain are the presenting complaints. Skin tests and complement fixation tests are almost always positive in active cases. The organisms can be recovered in the sputum, and also by bronchial brushing.[73]

The most effective specific therapy is amphotericin B, but many patients will require no treatment at all. The drug should be reserved for acutely ill patients and those with cavitary disease and sputum cultures positive for *C. immitis*.

While the majority of undiagnosed solitary pulmonary nodules occurring in patients in the endemic area prove to be coccidioidomas, 26 to 35 per cent are found to be malignant.[18, 69] Therefore the indications for resection of solitary pulmonary nodules in this area may be difficult to define and must be individualized, as for histoplasmosis. For cavitary lesions, the indications are clearer. They include persisting cavities 2 cm. or greater in diameter; those which are enlarging, thick-walled, or ruptured; those associated with severe or recurrent hemoptysis; those occurring in diabetic or pregnant patients; and those co-existing with pulmonary tuberculosis.[57] Drug coverage with amphotericin B is recommended by some, but it is not clear that the use of amphotericin B has resulted in significantly fewer complications of bronchopleural fistula, empyema, and recurrent cavitation.[24, 36, 52, 57, 75, 97]

North American Blastomycosis

North American blastomycosis, the third fungal infection endemic in a definable geographic area, largely east of the Mississippi River, is caused by *Blastomyces dermatitidis*, a round, thick-walled, single-budding yeast.[12, 13, 28] The disease often occurs in a cutaneous form, with chronic, indolent, usually enlarging papulopustules with thick adherent crusts and purple raised edges.[98] Biopsy in these areas may show microabscesses containing the organism. This form, with no evidence of systemic (including pulmonary) involvement, is the most favorable form of the disease. Pulmonary symptoms may be nonspecific. On the thoracic roentgenogram, cavitary, nodular, fibrotic, or disseminated lesions may be observed; bronchogenic carcinoma may be mimicked.[66, 98] Occasionally, dissemination of blastomycosis may take place following

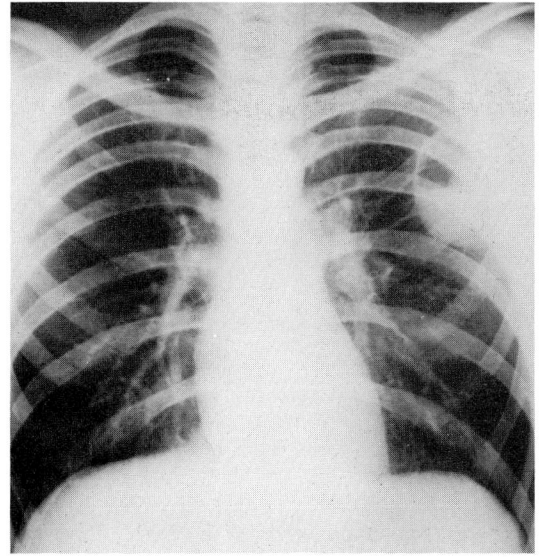

Figure 10. Cavitary lesion due to coccidioidomycosis, left lung. (From Hyde, L.: Dis. Chest (Suppl. 1), *54*:213, 1968.)

operation on an undiagnosed blastomycotic lesion. Thus, a preoperative diagnosis is of importance, in order to avoid an unnecessary operation. This may be aided by Papanicolaou smears of sputum.[88]

The two drugs considered most useful for blastomycosis are 2-hydroxystilbamidine and amphotericin B. Because of its wider margin of safety, 2-hydroxystilbamidine should be considered the drug of first choice for noncavitary disease that is not extensive, or has disseminated only to skin. For cavitary, or extensive disease, or for systemic dissemination, amphotericin B is preferable.[15] Resectional surgery is only rarely needed except for diagnosis, especially in those in whom cancer is suspected. This disease is still a serious one, with a 5-year mortality of approximately 20 per cent. The prognosis is worsened if the disease coexists with pulmonary tuberculosis.[28] Involvement of the genitourinary tract, the bones, and the nasal and oral mucosa is not uncommon.[98]

Cryptococcosis

Cryptococcosis was earlier considered to be a rare and fatal disease, often accompanied by meningitis. Now, apparently benign and indeed subclinical bronchopulmonary infections are being recognized with increasing frequency. Even the dreaded meningeal form is controllable by drug therapy.

Cryptococcus neoformans is found in nature in soil, dust, and pigeon dung. The organisms are round, budding yeast cells with thick gelatinous capsules. Opportunistic infection with Cryptococcus is frequently seen, especially in patients with lymphomas, collagen diseases, leukemias and other blood dyscrasias, diabetes, and sarcoidosis, especially after prolonged steroid or immunosuppressive drug therapy. Colonization of otherwise healthy individuals, without tissue invasion, can also occur.[32] The roentgenographic features are nonspecific and may even include pleural effusion.[72]

If cryptococci are cultured from sputum, with no demonstrable pulmonary lesion, or are isolated from lung tissue resected as an undiagnosed lesion, with no symptoms or signs of active disease (the most common way the diagnosis is made), opinions differ regarding the need for antifungal therapy.[29, 32, 62, 88] Since the mere presence of cryptococci does not necessarily denote a pathogenic process, active treatment may not be necessary if there is no evidence of central nervous system involvement and no organisms are found in spinal fluid.[29] However, now that two effective agents are available, the less toxic 5-fluorocytosine as well as amphotericin B, the proponents of treatment for proven disease have found additional support.[34, 46]

There is little controversy regarding the need for definitive treatment, if active cryptococcosis can be shown to be present by evidence of progression of a pulmonary lesion, and continued sputum positivity, or by evidence of meningeal involvement.

Aspergillosis

Aspergillosis is usually caused by *Aspergillus fumigatus*, which presents in pathologic material as a filamentous organism with coarse, septate, frag-

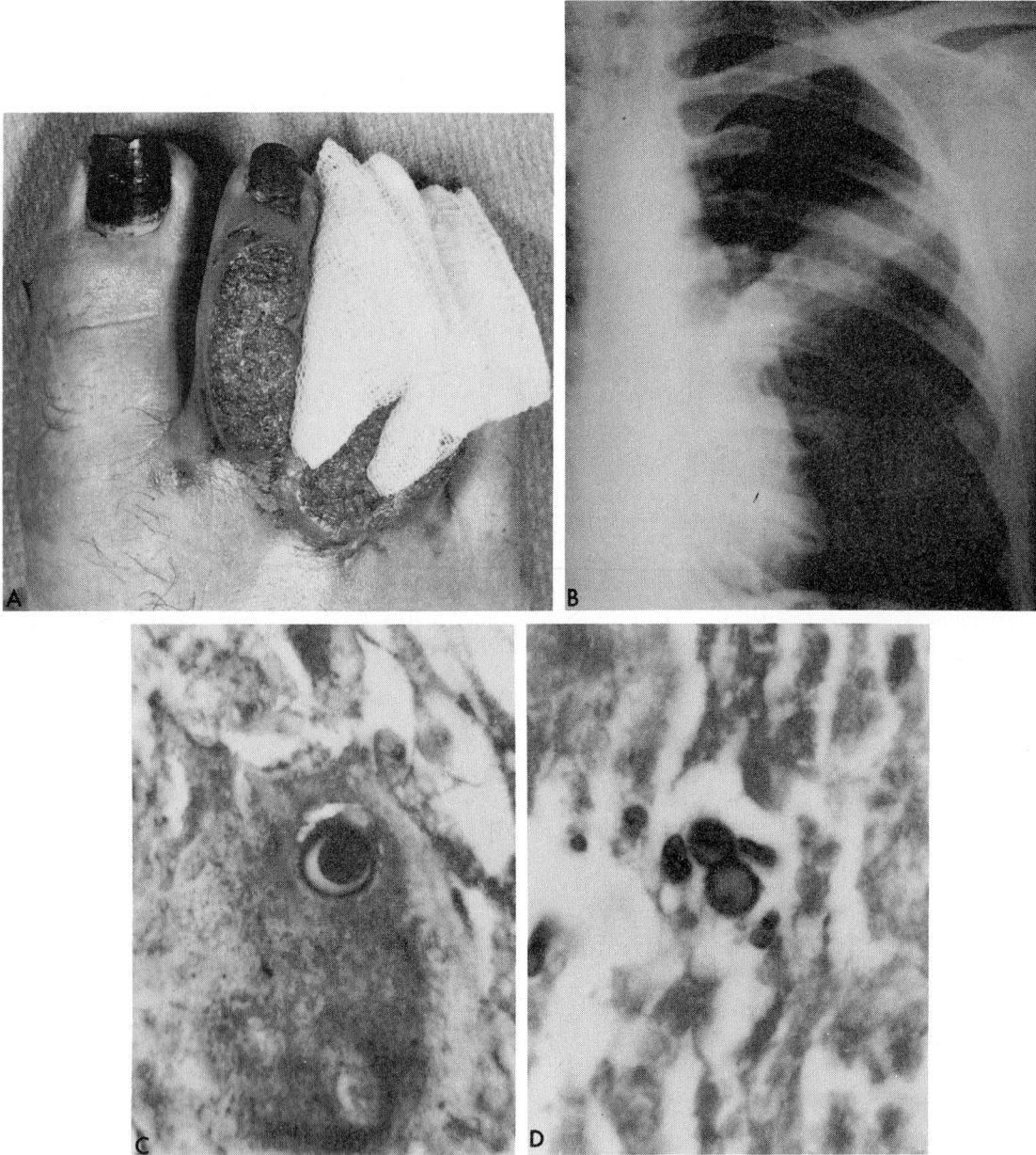

Figure 11. *A,* Skin lesions of blastomycosis on the dorsum of the toes. Biopsy of the characteristic raised edges showed multiple microabscesses containing *Blastomyces dermatitidis. B,* Blastomycotic pneumonic lesion of the lung. *C* and *D,* Organisms of *B. dermatitidis* from resected lung tissue: Thick-walled yeast form with refractile cell wall on left; single budding yeast form on right. PAS stain. ×1100. (From Takaro, T. *In* Lewis' Practice of Surgery. New York, Hoeber Medical Division, Harper & Row, 1968.)

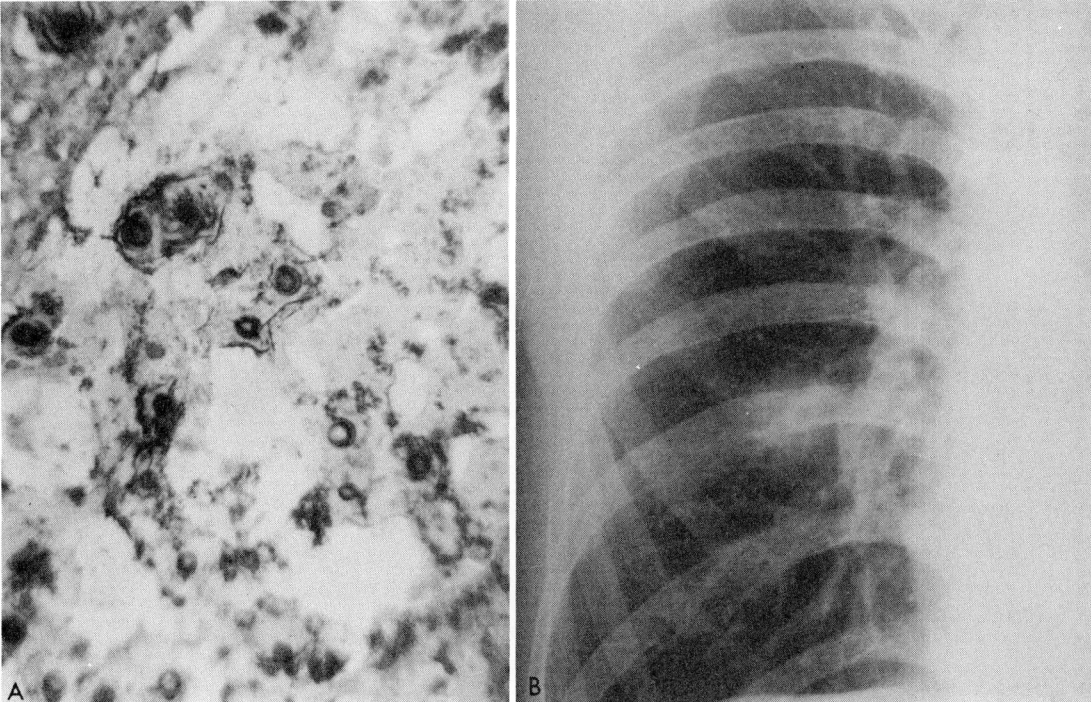

Figure 12. *A*, Organisms of *Cryptococcus neoformans* showing thick capsules. Mucicarmine. ×950. *B*, Thoracic roentgenogram showing solitary cryptococcal granuloma. This was removed by wedge resection. (From Takaro, T. *In* Lewis' Practice of Surgery. New York, Hoeber Medical Division, Harper & Row, 1968.)

mented hyphae.[13] Only rarely are characteristic vesicular spore heads identified. Of surgical interest is the tendency for this organism to invade pre-existing pulmonary cavities, there to form a rounded necrotic mass of matted hyphae, fibrin, and inflammatory cells, called an aspergilloma or fungus ball. This nondescript mass usually lies free in the cavity, and can change its location in the cavity as the patient changes his position from upright to recumbent. On the chest x-ray, a moon-shaped radiolucency adjacent to a rounded mass within a cavitary lesion is almost pathognomonic of an aspergilloma. Chronic cystic lesions of the upper lobes that remain as residua of pulmonary tuberculosis, sarcoidosis, lung cyst, or bronchiectasis commonly harbor such fungus balls; hemoptysis, occasionally severe, is the usual presenting symptom.[37]

The medical management of aspergillosis has been unsatisfactory.[33] Iodides, nystatin, hydroxystilbamidine, and amphotericin B have all been used. Surgical excision of an aspergilloma is usually curative of symptoms of hemoptysis, and should be undertaken if the patient's condition permits and pre-existing disease has not produced generalized lung damage.[20, 39] If excisional surgery is contraindicated, as it often is because of pulmonary fibrosis and respiratory insufficiency, endocavitary or endobronchial treatment with sodium iodide or amphotericin B may be helpful.[2] Aspergillus empyema is a serious complication, requiring drainage and local instillations of amphotericin B or nystatin for effective management.[42] Aspergillus endocarditis following cardiac surgery, a grave condition, is discussed under fungal endocarditis.

Fungal Endocarditis

Candidiasis is of special interest to cardiac surgeons because of the occurrence of Candida endocarditis in association with cardiac (usually valvular) lesions, over 100 cases of which are already on record.[40, 59, 80, 92] In a considerable number of patients, Candida endocarditis was diagnosed during or after prolonged and intensive antibiotic treatment for established subacute bacterial endocarditis. In another sizable group, fungal endocarditis (mostly due to Candida, but in some cases due to Aspergillus) has been reported following valve replacement.[38, 59] Heart operations offer a portal of entry through indwelling catheters, a damaged endocardial surface, and prolonged parenteral and antibiotic therapy, all of which favor the growth of this organism. The fungus is characterized by both budding yeast forms and mycelial elements.

The clinical features of Candida endocarditis are almost indistinguishable from those of bacterial endocarditis, suspicion of and treatment for which may actually aggravate the fungal infection. The finding of sterile blood cultures in the face of a clinical picture of bacterial endocarditis should dictate a search for Candida; Candida species found on blood culture must not be taken as a laboratory contaminant, but as an indication of a potentially lethal infection. Distinguishing features of Candida endocarditis are embolic episodes to major vessels, owing to the unusually large size of the mycotic valvular vegetations. In spite of potentially beneficial treatment with the combination of 5-fluorocytosine and amphotericin B, the medical cure rate is still very low and the mortality is between 80 and 90 per cent. Early surgical excision of vegetations, or when feasible of an infected prosthetic valve,

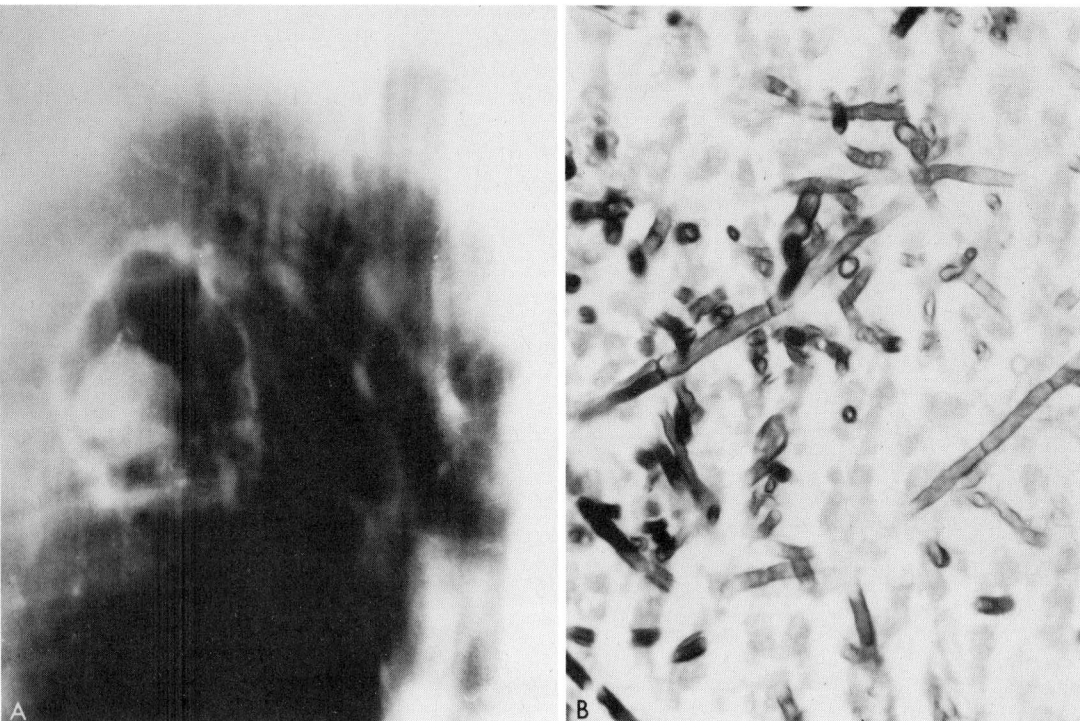

Figure 13. *A,* Laminagram showing typical aspergilloma ("fungus ball") lying free in large cavitary lesion. This ball characteristically will alter its location as the patient changes position. (From Aslam, P. A., Larkin, J., Eastridge, C. A., and Hughes, F. A., Jr.: Chest, *57:*94, 1970.) *B,* Coarse, fragmented, septate mycelia of *Aspergillus fumigatus.* (From Takaro, T. *In* Lewis' Practice of Surgery. New York, Hoeber Medical Division, Harper & Row, 1968.)

together with antifungal drug therapy, yields the best results.[40, 92] Evans poses the interesting question of the prophylactic use of antifungal agents in patients scheduled for valve replacement or organ transplantation.[21] Thus far, no cases of fungal endocarditis have been reported to occur after an aortocoronary vein bypass graft operation.[59]

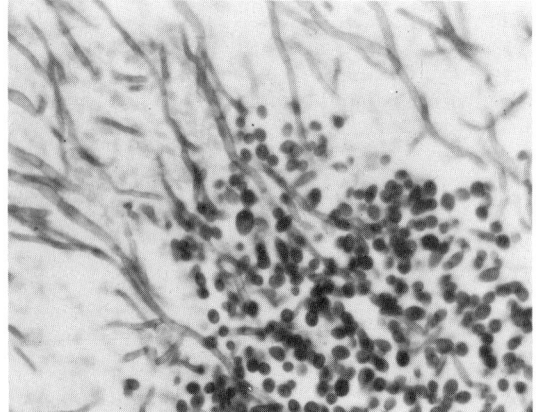

Figure 14. The organisms of *Candida albicans,* showing both mycelial and yeast forms. (From Takaro, T. *In* Lewis' Practice of Surgery. New York, Hoeber Medical Division, Harper & Row, 1968.)

Miscellaneous Fungal Infections

Sporotrichosis is caused by *Sporotrichum schenckii,* and pulmonary involvement is rare, the condition usually being encountered in its cutaneous or lymphatic manifestations. Agricultural workers and florists are especially susceptible. Localized cavitary pulmonary disease has been reported on a number of occasions recently.[8, 53, 78] Iodides are sometimes effective in lymphocutaneous sporotrichosis, and amphotericin B is sometimes effective in the pulmonary forms. However, surgical excision of localized disease appears to be the most reliable method of treating pulmonary sporotrichosis.

Phycomycosis (mucormycosis) is another rare and serious infection by any of the members of the order of fungi known as Phycomycetes.[7, 94] The organisms are characterized by broad, nonseptate hyphae, and characteristically blood vessel invasion, thrombosis, and infarction of organs are seen. Extensive necrosis of face, lungs, or brain may occur. Debilitated persons and uncontrolled diabetics seem to be especially prone to this infection. Control of the underlying disease, amphotericin B administration, and surgical excision of necrotic or infected tissue may prove to be helpful.[51, 71]

Pulmonary monosporosis is a rare mycotic infection caused by *Monosporium apiospermum.* This inhabitant of soil appears to act as a secondary invader of previously damaged lung tissue, such as a cavity, cyst, or saccule. Sometimes (but not characteristically), a

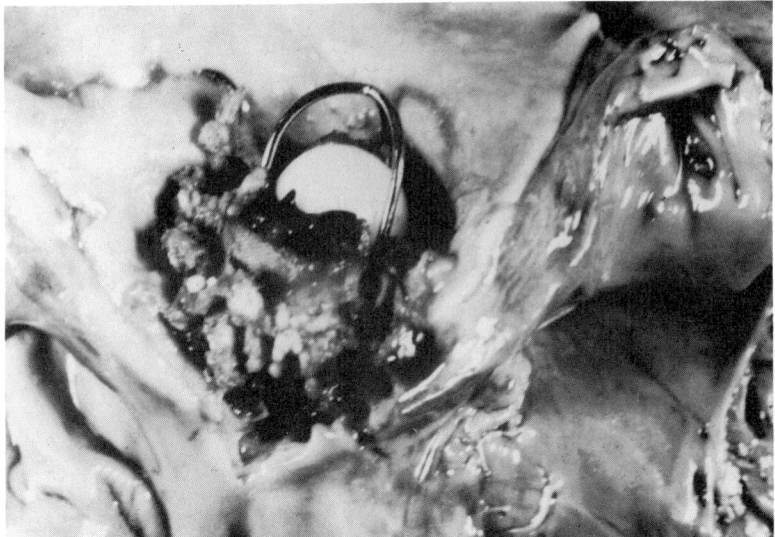

Figure 15. Fungal endocarditis due to Aspergillus species, causing aortic prosthetic dehiscence due to perivalvular tissue necrosis. More commonly, *Candida albicans* has been the etiologic agent in opportunistic fungal infections following cardiac surgery. (From Ostermiller, W. E., and Weinberg, M.: J. Thorac. Cardiovasc. Surg., *61*:670, 1970.)

fungus ball is formed. Amphotericin B has not been reported used. Localized resections have been successful in two cases.[70]

South American blastomycosis (paracoccidioidomycosis) is a chronic granulomatous infection involving the skin, mucous membrane, lymph nodes, and visceral organs, including the lungs, that is caused by *Paracoccidioides brasiliensis*, presumably a soil saprophyte. It is endemic in South America, and perhaps also in Central America, and it has now been recognized in the United States as well. The organisms resemble *Blastomyces dermatitidis* in tissues. Cavitary pulmonary disease occurs in about a third of cases. Treatment with sulfonamides is suppressive but not curative. Amphotericin B shows more promise. Surgery usually is not required.[55]

SELECTED REFERENCES

Ajello, L., Chick, E. W., and Furculow, M. L.: Histoplasmosis. Proceedings of the Second International Conference. Springfield, Ill., Charles C Thomas, Publisher, 1971.
This symposium is devoted entirely to histoplasmosis. All aspects of this disease and its etiologic agent are discussed in great detail.

American Thoracic Society: Treatment of fungal diseases. A statement by the committee on therapy. Amer. Rev. Resp. Dis., *100*:908, 1969.
This is a brief but complete statement of the current consensus regarding optimal therapy for each of the mycotic infections.

Bennett, J. E.: Chemotherapy of systemic mycoses. N. Engl. J. Med., *290*:30 and 320, 1974.
These two papers summarize the pharmacologic aspects of amphotericin-B, 5-fluorocytosine, clotrimazole, 2-hydroxystilbamidine, and iodides, i.e., the effective agents against systemic mycotic infections.

Buechner, H. A.: Management of Fungus Diseases of the Lungs. Springfield, Ill., Charles C Thomas, Publisher, 1971.
This is a clinically oriented volume emphasizing the medical management of mycotic lung infections, both common and uncommon.

Hammerman, K. J., Powell, K. E., Christianson, C. S., Huggin, P. M., Larsh, H. W., Vivas, J. R., and Tosh, F. E.: Pulmonary cryptococcosis. Amer. Rev. Resp. Dis., *108*:1116, 1973.
This paper reviews the experience of the Center for Disease Control Cooperative Mycoses Study (probably the largest series available for analysis) as well as experience reported in the literature.

Nelson, A. R.: The Surgical Treatment of Pulmonary Coccidioidomycosis. Curr. Probl. Surg., Oct., 1974.
A thorough review of epidemiologic, diagnostic, and therapeutic aspects of coccidioidomycosis from the viewpoint of a surgeon with a large experience with the disease.

Perlman, L. V., Lerner, E., and D'Esopo, N.: Clinical classification and analysis of 97 cases of lung abscess. Amer. Rev. Resp. Dis., *99*:390, 1969.
The sharp differentiation, based on clinical characteristics and on response to therapy, between primary (or simple) lung abscesses and those occurring in association with systemic disease, malignant or nonmalignant, in adults is emphasized in this review of 97 cases.

Pinkerton, J. A., Lawler, M. R., and Foster, J. H.: Pulmonary nocardiosis. Am. Surg., *37*:729, 1971.
The Vanderbilt University experience with this disease is reviewed, with emphasis on the variability of the clinical course, the diagnostic difficulties, and the management.

Schwarz, J., and Salfelder, K.: Diagnosis of surgical deep mycoses. Surg. Gynecol. Obstet., *128*:259, 1969.
This is a general exposition of the subject, with emphasis on the need for close cooperation between the surgeon and the bacteriologist for diagnostic accuracy.

Slade, P. R., Slesser, B. V., and Southgate, J.: Thoracic actinomycosis. Thorax, *28*:73, 1973.
This is an excellent and well-illustrated review, with careful documentation of the clinical aspects and management of six cases.

Takaro, T.: Lung infections and interstitial pneumonopathies. *In* Sabiston, D. C., Jr., and Spencer, F. C. (Eds.): Gibbon's Surgery of the Chest, 3rd ed. Philadelphia, W. B. Saunders Company, 1976, pp. 489–566.
This chapter presents a more detailed exposition of the subjects of lung abscess and actinomycetic and fungal infections of the lungs.

REFERENCES

1. Ahn, C., Kilman, J. W., Vasko, J., and Andrews, N. C.: Therapy of cavitary pulmonary histoplasmosis. J. Thorac. Cardiovasc. Surg., *57*:42, 1969.
2. Aslam, P. A., Larkin, J., Eastridge, C. E., and Hughes, F. A., Jr.: Endocavitary infusion through percutaneous endobronchial catheter. Chest, *57*:94, 1970.
3. Bach, M. C., Monaco, A. P., and Finland, M.: Pulmonary nocardiosis. Therapy with minocycline and with erythromycin plus ampicillin. J.A.M.A., *224*:1378, 1973.
4. Barnett, T. B., and Herring, C. L.: Lung abscess. Initial and late results of medical therapy. Arch. Intern. Med., *127*:217, 1971.
5. Bartlett, J. G., and Gorbach, S. L.: Treatment of aspiration pneu-

monia and primary lung abscess. Penicillin G vs. Clindamycin. J.A.M.A., *234*:935, 1975.

6. Bartlett, J. G., Gorbach, S. L., Tally, F. P., and Finegold, S. M.: Bacteriology and treatment of primary lung abscess. Am. Rev. Resp. Dis., *109*:510, 1974.

7. Bartrum, R. J., Jr., Watnick, M., and Herman, P. G.: Roentgenographic findings in pulmonary mucormycosis. Am. J. Roentgenol., *117*:810, 1973.

8. Baum, G. L., Donnerberg, R. L., Stewart, D., Mulligan, W. J., and Putnam, L. R.: Pulmonary sporotrichosis. N. Engl. J. Med., *280*:410, 1969.

9. Baum, G. L., Larkin, J. C., Jr., and Sutliff, W. D.: Follow-up of patients with chronic pulmonary histoplasmosis treated with amphotericin B. Chest, *58*:562, 1970.

10. Bennett, J. E.: Chemotherapy of systemic mycoses (Parts I and II). N. Engl. J. Med., *290*:30 and 320, 1974.

11. Bragg, D. G., and Janis, B.: Radiographic presentation of pulmonary opportunistic inflammatory disease. Radiol. Clin. North Am., *11*:357, 1973.

12. Buechner, H. A.: Management of Fungus Diseases of the Lungs. Springfield, Ill, Charles C Thomas, Publisher, 1971.

13. Buechner, H. A., Furcolow, M. L., Farness, O. J., Reagan, W. P., Saliba, N. A., and Abernathy, R.: Epidemiology of the pulmonary mycoses. Chest, *58*:68, 1970.

14. Buechner, H. A., Seabury, J. H., Campbell, C. C., Georg, L. K., Kaufman, L., and Kaplan, W.: The current status of serologic, immunologic and skin tests in the diagnosis of pulmonary mycoses. Report of the committee on fungus diseases and subcommittee on criteria for clinical diagnosis, American College of Chest Physicians. Chest, *63*:259, 1973.

15. Busey, J. F.: Blastomycosis. 3. A comparative study of 2-hydroxystilbamidine and amphotericin-B therapy. Am. Rev. Resp. Dis., *105*:812, 1972.

16. Carr, D., and Sutliff, W. D.: Histoplasmosis. *In* Steele, J. D. (Ed.): Treatment of Mycotic and Parasitic Diseases of the Chest. Springfield, Ill., Charles C Thomas, Publisher, 1964, pp. 31–54.

17. Chidi, C. C., and Mendelsohn, H. J.: Lung abscess. A study of the results of treatment based on 90 consecutive cases. J. Thorac. Cardiovasc. Surg., *68*:168, 1974.

18. Cohen, S. L., Gale, A. M., and Liston, H. E.: Report of a pilot study on non-calcified discrete pulmonary coin lesions in a coccidioidomycosis endemic area. Ariz. Med., *29*:40, 1972.

19. Connors, J. P., Roper, C. L., and Ferguson, T. B.: Transbronchial catheterization of pulmonary abscesses. Ann. Thorac. Surg., *19*:254, 1975.

20. Eastridge, C. E., Young, J. M., Cole, F., Gourley, R., and Pate, J. W.: Pulmonary aspergillosis. Ann. Thorac. Surg., *13*:397, 1972.

21. Evans, E. G. V.: Incidence of pathogenic yeasts among open-heart surgery patients — the value of prophylaxis. J. Thorac. Cardiovasc. Surg., *70*:466, 1975.

22. Finley, R., Kieff, E., Thomsen, S., Fennessy, J., Beem, M., Lerner, S., and Morello, J.: Bronchial brushing in the diagnosis of pulmonary disease in patients at risk for opportunistic infection. Am. Rev. Resp. Dis., *109*:379, 1974.

23. Foley, T. F., Dines, D. E., and Dolan, C. T.: Pulmonary actinomycosis. Report of 18 cases. Minn. Med., *54*:593, 1971.

24. Fosburg, R. G., Baisch, B. F., and Trummer, M. J.: Limited pulmonary resection for coccidioidomycosis. Ann. Thorac. Surg., *7*:420, 1969.

25. Frazier, A. R., Rosenow, E. C., III, and Roberts, G. D.: Nocardiosis. A review of 25 cases occurring during 24 months. Mayo Clin. Proc., *50*:657, 1975.

26. Furcolow, M. L., and Buechner, H. A.: Histoplasmosis. *In* Buechner, H. A. (Ed.): Management of Fungus Diseases of the Lung. Springfield, Ill., Charles C Thomas, Publisher, 1971.

27. Furcolow, M. L., Chick, E. W., Busey, J. F., and Menges, R. W.: Prevalence and incidence studies of human and canine blastomycosis. Am. Rev. Resp. Dis., *102*:60, 1970.

28. Furcolow, M. L., Watson, K. A., Tisdall, O. F., Julian, W. A., Saliba, N. A., and Ralows, A.: Some factors affecting survival in systemic blastomycosis. Dis. Chest (Suppl. I), *54*:285, 1968.

29. Geraci, J. E., Donoghue, F. E., Ellis, F. H., Jr., Witten, D. M., and Weed, L. A.: Focal pulmonary cryptococcosis: Evaluation of necessity of amphotericin B therapy. Mayo Clin. Proc., *40*:552, 1965.

30. Gopalakrishna, K. V., and Lerner, P. I.: Primary lung abscess. Analysis of 66 cases. Cleveland Clin. Q., *42*:3, 1975.

31. Groff, D. B., and Marquis, J.: Treatment of lung abscess by transbronchial catheter drainage. Radiology, *107*:61, 1973.

32. Hammerman, K. J., Powell, K. E., Christianson, C. S., Huggin, P. M., Larsh, H. W., Vivas, J. R., and Tosh, F. E.: Pulmonary cryptococcosis: Clinical forms and treatment. Am. Rev. Resp. Dis., *108*:1116, 1973.

33. Hammerman, K. J., Sarosi, G. A., and Tosh, F. E.: Amphotericin-B in the treatment of saprophytic forms of pulmonary aspergillosis. Am. Rev. Resp. Dis., *109*:57, 1974.

34. Hatcher, C. R., Jr., Sehdeva, J., Waters, W. C., III, Schulze, V., Logan, W. D., Symbas, P., and Abbott, O. A.: Primary pulmonary crytococcosis. J. Thorac. Cardiovasc. Surg., *61*:39, 1971.

35. Henderson, R. D., Deslaurier, J., Ritcey, E. L., Delarve, N. C., and Pearson, F. G.: Surgery in pulmonary aspergillosis. J. Thorac. Cardiovasc. Surg., *70*:1088, 1975.

36. Hyde, L.: Coccidioidal pulmonary cavitation. Dis. Chest (Suppl. I), *54*:273, 1968.

37. Israel, H. L., and Ostrow, A.: Sarcoidosis and aspergilloma. Am. J. Med., *47*:243, 1969.

38. Kammer, R. B., and Utz, J. P.: Aspergillus species endocarditis. Am. J. Med., *56*:506, 1974.

39. Karas, A., Hankins, J. R., Attar, S., Miller, J. E., and McLaughlin, J. S.: Pulmonary aspergillosis: An analysis of thirty-eight cases. Ann. Thorac. Surg., in press.

40. Kay, J. H., Bernstein, S., and Tsugi, H. K., et al.: Surgical treatment of Candida endocarditis. J.A.M.A., *203*:621, 1968.

41. Khan, T. H., Kane, E. G., and Dean, D. C.: Aspergillus endocarditis of mitral prosthesis. Am. J. Cardiol., *22*:277, 1968.

42. Krakowka, P., Rowinska, E., and Halweg, H.: Infection of the pleura by Aspergillus fumigatus. Thorax, *25*:245, 1970.

43. Kyriakos, M., and Webber, B.: Cancer of the lung in young men. J. Thorac. Cardiovasc. Surg., *67*:634, 1974.

44. Lee, B. Y., Tolete, F., and Douglass, R.: Pulmonary nocardiosis successfully treated with chemotherapy and resection. Chest, *58*:388, 1970.

45. Leffert, R. L., and Hackett, R. L.: Aspergillus aortitis following replacement of aortic valve. J. Thorac. Cardiovasc. Surg., *53*:866, 1967.

46. Lewis, J. L., and Rabinovich, S.: The wide spectrum of cryptococcal infections. Am. J. Med., *53*:315, 1972.

47. Maderazo, E. G., and Quintiliani, R.: Treatment of nocardial infection with trimethoprim and sulfamethoxazole. Am. J. Med., *57*:671, 1974.

48. Mark, P. H., and Turner, J. A. P.: Lung abscess in childhood. Thorax, *23*:216, 1968.

49. Mattox, K. L., and Guinn, G. A.: Emergency resection for massive hemoptysis. Ann. Thorac. Surg., *17*:377, 1974.

50. McQuarrie, D. G., and Hall, W. H.: Actinomycosis of the lung and chest wall. Surgery, *64*:905, 1968.

51. Medoff, G., and Kobayashi, G. S.: Pulmonary mucormycosis. N. Engl. J. Med., *286*:86, 1972.

52. Melick, D. W., and Grant, A. R.: Surgery in primary pulmonary coccidioidomycosis and in the combined diseases of coccidioidomycosis and tuberculosis. Dis. Chest (Suppl. I), *54*:278, 1968.

53. Mohr, J. A., Patterson, C. D., Eaton, B. G., Rhoades, E. R., and Nichols, N. B.: Primary pulmonary sporotrichosis. Am. Rev. Resp. Dis., *106*:260, 1972.

54. Moser, K. M.: Solitary pulmonary nodules (Editorial). J.A.M.A., *227*:1167, 1974.

55. Murray, H. W., Littman, M. L., and Roberts, R. B.: Disseminated paracoccidioidomycosis (South American blastomycosis) in the United States. Am. J. Med., *56*:209, 1974.

56. Nathan, M. H.: Management of solitary pulmonary nodules. J.A.M.A., *227*:1141, 1974.

57. Nelson, A. R.: The surgical treatment of pulmonary coccidioidomycosis. Curr. Probl. Surg., Oct., 1974, pp. 1–48.

58. Nelson, R. J., and Benfield, J. R.: Benign esophagobronchial fistula. A curable cause of adult pulmonary suppuration. Arch. Surg., *100*:685, 1970.

59. Norenberg, R. G., Sethi, G. K., Scott, S. M., and Takaro, T.: Opportunistic endocarditis following open heart surgery. Ann. Thorac. Surg., *19*:592, 1975.

60. Pappas, G., Schroter, G., Brettschneider, L., Penn, I., and Starzl, T. E.: Pulmonary surgery in immunosuppressed patients. J. Thorac. Cardiovasc. Surg., *59*:882, 1970.

61. Parker, J. D., Sarosi, G. A., Doto, I. L., Bailey, R. E., and Tosh, F. E.: Treatment of chronic pulmonary histoplasmosis. A National Communicable Disease Center Cooperative Mycoses Study. N. Engl. J. Med., *283*:225, 1970.

62. Parker, J. D., Sarosi, G. A., Doto, I. L., and Tosh, F. E.: Pulmonary aspergillosis in sanatoriums in the South Central United States. A National Communicable Disease Center Cooperative Mycoses Study. Am. Rev. Resp. Dis., 101:551, 1970.

63. Payne, W. S., Cardoza, F., and Weed, L. A.: Chronic draining sinuses of the chest wall. Surg. Clin. North Am., 53:927, 1973.

64. Perkins, W.: Pulmonary cryptococcosis: Report on the treatment of nine cases. Dis. Chest, 56:389, 1969.

65. Pinkerton, J. A., Lawler, M. R., and Foster, J. H.: Pulmonary nocardiosis. Am. Surg., 37:729, 1971.

66. Poe, R. H., Vassallo, C. L., Plessinger, V. A., and Witt, R. L.: Pulmonary blastomycosis versus carcinoma — A challenging differential. Am. J. Med. Sci., 263:145, 1972.

67. Polk, J. W.: Treatment of pulmonary histoplasmosis. Dis. Chest, 56:149, 1969.

68. Prather, J. R., Eastridge, C. E., Hughes, F. A., Jr., and McCaughan, J. J., Jr.: Actinomycosis of the thorax: Diagnosis and treatment. Ann. Thorac. Surg., 9:307, 1970.

69. Read, T. C.: Coin lesion, pulmonary, in the Southwest. (Solitary pulmonary nodules). Ariz. Med., 29:775, 1972.

70. Reddy, P. C., Christianson, C. S., Gorelick, D. F., and Larsh, H. W.: Pulmonary monosporosis: An uncommon pulmonary mycotic infection. Thorax, 24:722, 1969.

71. Reich, J., and Renzetti, A. D., Jr.: Pulmonary phycomycosis. Am. Rev. Resp. Dis., 102:959, 1970.

72. Saab, S. B., Ungaro, R., and Almond, C.: The role and results of surgery in the management of chronic pulmonary histoplasmosis. J. Thorac. Cardiovasc. Surg., 68:159, 1974.

73. Sagel, S. S.: Common fungal diseases of the lungs. I. Coccidioidomycosis. Radiol. Clin. North Am., 11:153, 1973.

74. Salyer, W. R., and Salyer, D. C.: Pleural involvement in cryptococcosis. Chest, 66:139, 1974.

75. Sarosi, G. A., Parker, J. D., Doto, I. L., and Tosh, F. E.: Chronic pulmonary coccidioidomycosis. N. Engl. J. Med., 283:325, 1970.

76. Schwartz, J., and Salfelder, K.: Diagnosis of surgical deep mycoses. Surg. Gynecol. Obstet., 128:259, 1969.

77. Schweppe, H. I., Knowles, J. H., and Kane, L.: Lung abscess: An analysis of Massachusetts General Hospital cases from 1943 through 1956. N. Engl. J. Med., 265:1039, 1961.

78. Scott, S. M., Peasley, E. D., and Crymes, T. P.: Pulmonary sporotrichosis: Report of two cases with cavitation. N. Engl. J. Med., 265:453, 1961.

79. Seabury, J. H.: Actinomycosis and nocardiosis. In Buechner, H. A. (Ed.): Management of Fungus Diseases of the Lungs. Springfield, Ill., Charles C Thomas, Publisher, 1971.

80. Seelig, M. S., Speth, C. P., Kozinn, P. J., Toni, E. F., and Taschd-jian, C. L.: Candida endocarditis after cardiac surgery. J. Thorac. Cardiovasc. Surg., 65:583, 1973.

81. Serstock, D. S., and Zinneman, H. H.: Pulmonary and articular sporotrichosis. Report of two cases. J.A.M.A., 233:1291, 1975.

82. Sethi, J. P., Gupta, M. L., and Kasliwal, R. M.: Amebic pulmonary suppuration. Dis. Chest, 51:148, 1967.

83. Shafron, R. D., and Tate, C. F., Jr.: Lung abscesses: A five year evaluation. Dis. Chest, 53:12, 1968.

84. Siegrist, H. D., and Ferrington, E.: Primary pulmonary sporotrichosis. South. Med. J., 58:728, 1965.

85. Slade, P. R., Slesser, B. V., and Southgate, J.: Thoracic actinomycosis. Thorax, 28:73, 1973.

86. Steele, J. D.: The Solitary Pulmonary Nodule. Springfield, Ill., Charles C Thomas, Publisher, 1964.

87. Sutaria, M. K., Polk, J. W., Reddy, P., and Mohanty, S. K.: Surgical aspects of pulmonary histoplasmosis. Thorax, 25:31, 1970.

88. Sutliff, W. D., and Cruthirds, T. P.: Blastomyces dermatitidis in cytologic preparations. Am. Rev. Resp. Dis., 108:149, 1973.

89. Takaro, T.: Lung infections and interstitial pneumonopathies. In Sabiston, D. C., Jr., and Spencer, F. C. (Eds.): Gibbon's Surgery of the Chest, 3rd ed. Philadelphia, W. B. Saunders Company, 1976, pp. 489–566.

90. Taylor, E. R.: Pulmonary cryptococcosis; an analysis of 15 cases from the Columbia area. Ann. Thorac. Surg., 10:309, 1970.

91. Thoms, N. W., Wilson, R. F., Puro, H. E., and Arbulu, A.: Life-threatening hemoptysis in primary lung abscess. Ann. Thorac. Surg., 14:347, 1972.

92. Turnier, E., Kay, J. H., Bernstein, S., Mendez, A. M., and Zúbiate, P.: Surgical treatment of candida endocarditis. Chest, 67:262, 1975.

93. Utley, J. R., Mills, J., and Roe, B. B.: The role of valve replacement in the treatment of fungal endocarditis. J. Thorac. Cardiovasc. Surg., 69:255, 1975.

94. Utz, J. P., and Buechner, H. A.: Mucormycosis (Phycomycosis). In Buechner, H. A. (Ed.): Management of Fungus Diseases of the Lungs. Springfield, Ill., Charles C Thomas, Publisher, 1971.

95. Weiss, W.: Delayed cavity closure in acute nonspecific primary lung abscess. Am. J. Med. Sci., 255:313, 1968.

96. Weiss, W., and Cherniack, N. S.: Acute nonspecific lung abscess. A controlled study comparing orally and parenterally administered penicillin G. Chest, 66:348, 1974.

97. Winn, W. A.: Long-term study of 300 patients with cavitary-abscess lesions of the lung of coccidiodal origin. Dis. Chest. (Suppl. 1), 54:268, 1968.

98. Witorsch, P., and Utz, J. P.: North American blastomycosis: A study of 40 patients. Medicine, 47:169, 1968.

IX

THE PLEURA AND EMPYEMA

Timothy Takaro, M.D.

THE PLEURA

The pleura is the serous membrane that invests the lungs and is reflected upon the walls of the thorax and on the diaphragm. In man, the pleura forms the lining of two complete and independent pleural sacs or potential cavities. Each extends into the neck, the retrosternal area, and the costophrenic sinuses, and also into the interlobar fissues. Familiarity with these ramifications of the pleural cavity can be extremely important, since unwitting violation of the pleural space with its special anatomic and physiologic attributes may be followed by serious consequences. Thus, the earliest experiences of surgeons with wounds penetrating into the pleural cavities, or with deliberate attempts to open them, often resulted in disaster, or near-disaster, from collapse of the lung, shift of the mediastinum, tension pneumothorax, and, later, infection.

A major surgical milestone was passed when the millimeter or two of potential space between the two layers of the pleural cavity could at last be crossed safely. This at first seemed to require that the whole operating team enter an area of negative pressure in order to operate within the thorax. Only the patient's head and neck remained outside, exposed to atmospheric pressure, when Sauerbruch's pioneering chamber was used at the turn of the century. This cumbersome arrangement was found to be unnecessary after Meltzer and Auer reported that positive-pressure insufflation of the lungs could sustain respirations, even with the chest open. The Empyema Commission's findings during World War I marked another milestone when it was understood that opening the pleural cavity to atmospheric pressure in order to drain an empyema prior to the development of adhesions limiting the extent of the infection could be catastrophic. In the years that followed World War I, intrathoracic surgery gradually evolved. Following World War II, this evolution progressed at a vastly accelerated pace, and the pleural cavities were regularly transgressed as a matter of course. These surgical developments added greatly to our knowledge of pleuropulmonary physiology and pathology.[11]

Anatomic Features

Histologically, the pleural surface consists of a uniform layer of flattened mesothelial cells without a basement membrane, beneath which are layers of areolar connective tissue containing an abundance of blood vessels, nerves, and lymphatics. The visceral pleura is thinner, remarkably elastic, and intimately attached to the underlying lung by intrapulmonary fibrous prolongations of the deeper layer of connective tissue. The parietal pleura, on the other hand, is thicker, and easily separable from the thoracic wall because of the loose layer of areolar tissue separating it from the endothoracic fascia. It is supplied by the intercostal arteries. The visceral pleura is largely supplied by the bronchial arteries. Both are relatively insensitive and pain-free, parietal pleural pain fibers probably being present mostly in the endothoracic fascia.[82]

Physiologic Characteristics

The two outstanding physiologic features of the pleural cavities are (1) the subatmospheric pressures in the normally nonexistent pleural space; and (2) the serous secreting and absorbing surface of the pleural membranes. These two characteristics seem to be interrelated. The natural elastic recoil of the lungs produces intrapleural negative pressures of −6 to −12 cm. H_2O during inspiration, and −4 to −8 cm. during expiration. Extremes of +40 cm. H_2O during the Valsalva maneuver or −40 cm. H_2O during inspiratory effort against a closed glottis are also seen.

The secreting and absorbing properties of the pleura are substantial. With special techniques, a rate of formation of 600 to 1000 ml. of fluid per day has been observed in patients, and an equal volume has been noted to be reabsorbed by the pleural lymphatics.[87] Increased capillary hydrostatic pressure, or a greater negative intrapleural pressure, tends to increase transudation into the pleural cavities. Loss of intrapleural negative pressure diminishes transudation, while increased diaphragmatic and intercostal activity increases the absorption of transudate. Particulate mat-

ter such as red blood cells can also be absorbed directly by the normal pleura.[22] All these properties may be greatly altered by disease.[9, 52]

PLEURAL EFFUSIONS

While pleural effusions are almost invariably secondary to some primary condition, they often provide the first indication of that condition. Pleural effusions are always significant. Bloody effusions are ominous, for they may signify primary or secondary pleural tumor. Therefore, attempts to make a precise diagnosis of the cause of effusion should be intelligently and persistently pursued. The finding of the classic signs of fluid — flatness, absence of tactile and vocal fremitus, diminished breath sounds, and mediastinal displacement — depends upon the size of the fluid collection and on the care with which the signs are sought.

A pleural effusion of up to half a liter may not be apparent clinically or roentgenographically in the upright position in the adult, since it ordinarily gravitates into the costophrenic sinuses and is obscured by the diaphragm. Thus, when the characteristic appearance of a "small" effusion is noted on a thoracic roentgenogram, usually considerable fluid is already present and can be obtained by a carefully performed thoracentesis. On the other hand, fluid may collect almost anywhere from the apex to the base of the pleural cavity, in one or more loculated pockets, either in contact with the parietal pleura or in an interlobar fissure. Quite uncharacteristic and often bizarre roentgenographic pictures may then result, and needle aspiration may be necessary to establish the presence of a pleural effusion and thus to differentiate it from other thoracic conditions.[16]

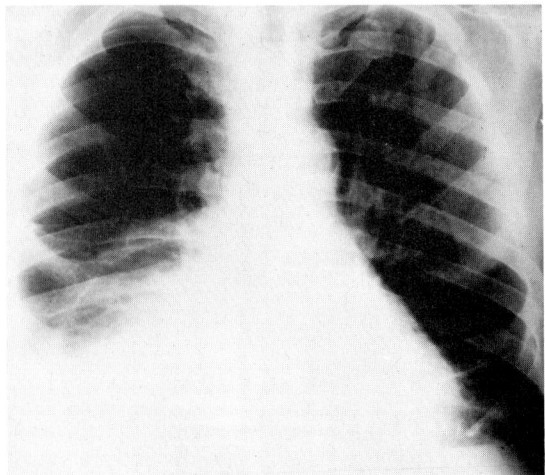

Figure 1. Pleural effusion, right base. After this thoracic roentgenogram was taken, 1300 ml. of straw-colored fluid was aspirated at thoracentesis. Surprisingly large volumes of fluid may not be apparent clinically or roentgenographically when they gravitate into the costophrenic sinuses and are partially obscured by the diaphragm. A roentgenogram obtained in the lateral decubitus position may be more revealing.

TABLE 1. Etiologic Characteristics of Pleural Effusions

	Tuberculosis	Malignancy	Congestive Failure	Pneumonia and Other Nontuberculous Infections	Rheumatoid Arthritis and Collagen Disease	Pulmonary Embolism	Fungal Infection	Trauma	Chylothorax
Clinical	Younger patient, exposure to tuberculosis, good health prior	Older patient, poor health prior to effusion	Signs and symptoms of congestive failure	Signs and symptoms of respiratory tract infection	History of joint involvement may or may not be present, subcutaneous nodules	Postoperative patient, immobilized patient, venous disease	Exposure in endemic area	History of trauma	History of trauma, known malignancy
Gross appearance	Usually serous, may be sanguineous	Often sanguineous	Serous	Serous	Turbid or yellow-green	Often sanguineous	Serous	Sanguineous	Chylous or milky
Microscopic examination	Positive for acid-fast bacilli 30 to 70 per cent of cases, cholesterol crystals	Cytology positive in 50 per cent	0	May or may not be positive for bacilli	0	0	May or may not be positive for fungi	0	Fat droplets
Cell count	5 per cent over 10,000 erythrocytes; 75 per cent over 1000 leukocytes, mainly lymphocytes	65 per cent bloody, 40 per cent over 1000 leukocytes, mainly lymphocytes	10 per cent over 10,000 erythrocytes; 10 per cent over 1000 leukocytes	Polymorphonuclears predominate	Lymphocytes predominate	Erythrocytes predominate	0	Erythrocytes	0
Culture	10 to 70 per cent pleural effusion positive; 10 to 15 per cent sputum or gastric positive	0	0	May or may not be positive	0	0	May or may not be positive	0	0
Specific gravity	75 per cent over 1.016	75 per cent over 1.016	90 per cent under 1.016 (unless pulmonary embolism)	Over 1.016	Over 1.016	Over 1.016	Over 1.016	Over 1.016	Over 1.016
Protein	90 per cent 3 g or more	90 per cent 3 g or more	75 per cent less than 3 g	3.0 g or more	3.0 g or more	3.0 g or more	3.0 g or more	3.0 g or more	Less than half plasma†
Sugar	60 per cent less than 60 mg per cent	Less than 60 mg per cent rarely	0	Occasionally less than 60 mg per cent	5–17 mg per cent; (only in rheumatoid arthritis)	0	0	0	0
Other	No mesothelial cells on cytology; will be the cause in 75 per cent of males under 25 years of age, 50 per cent of males 25 or over; tuberculin test usually positive	If hemorrhagic fluid, 65 per cent will be due to tumor; tends to continue to form after removed	Right-sided in 55 to 70 per cent	Associated with infiltrate on roentgenogram	Rapid clotting time; lupus erythematosus cell or rheumatoid factor may be present	Source of emboli may or may not be noted	Skin and serologic tests may be helpful		Fat content higher than plasma†

†From Bessone, L. N., et al.: Ann. Thorac. Surg., 12:527, 1971.

The major causes of effusions and their differentiation are outlined in Table 1. Infections (often tuberculous), tumor, and congestive failure account for at least 75 per cent of effusions in almost all types of patient populations. *Massive* effusions are due to malignancy in the majority of instances.[51] The problem of differential diagnosis often depends upon obtaining samples of either the fluid, the parietal pleura, or the lung and subjecting these to appropriate examinations.[15] This does not always solve the problem, however.

Often a specific diagnosis cannot be made from pleural fluid alone, in spite of cultures and smears for pathogenic organisms and cell blocks for tumor cells.[4]

Biopsy by needle or trephine may be expected to yield a specific diagnosis in less than half the cases in which it is attempted.[42, 69, 85] However, if the effusion is due to malignancy, a diagnosis can be established by either needle biopsy or pleural fluid cytopathology or both, in 90 per cent of cases.[75] A small open thoracotomy may be necessary to make a definitive diagnosis, since this allows the surgeon to inspect both the visceral and the parietal pleura, as well as the lung, and to select the most promising areas for biopsy. Decortication of the lung, if indicated, may also be carried out after the incision has been enlarged. The use of thoracoscopy ("pleuroscopy") with rigid endoscopes has not often been reported in recent years.[25] However, a

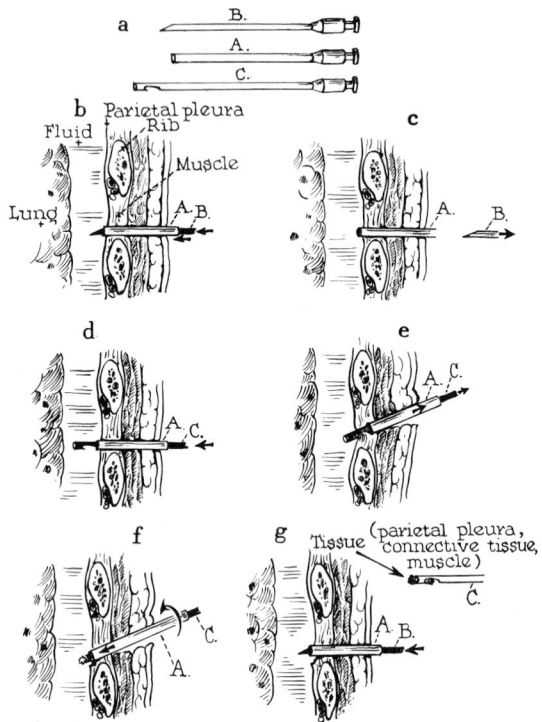

Figure 2. Diagrams illustrating a method of obtaining a pleural biopsy using the Cope needle. (From Levine, H., and Cugell, D. W.: Arch. Intern. Med., *109*:516, 1962.)

modification using the flexible fiberoptic bronchoscope has lately been advocated.[34, 78]

Pleural effusions may also occur from subdiaphragmatic or intra-abdominal processes such as subphrenic or hepatic abscesses, cirrhosis of the liver, nephritis, pancreatitis,[1, 41] or ovarian fibroma.[61] This last combination is called Meigs' syndrome. Whether passage of fluid from the peritoneal into the pleural cavities occurs through the lymphatics, or through recognized or unrecognized openings in the diaphragm, is a matter of debate.[67]

Thoracentesis is best done after careful localization of the effusion by roentgenograms in frontal, lateral, or oblique plane, or by the use of the fluoroscopic image intensifier. A syringe no larger than 20 ml., with a three-way stopcock interposed between needle and syringe, allows the most adequate control. After thorough infiltration of skin, intercostal muscle, and parietal pleura with a local anesthetic agent, the needle of appropriate caliber and length is directed just above the superior border of the lower rib of the appropriate interspace and allowed to penetrate the parietal pleura until fluid is reached, constant moderate negative pressure being applied to the syringe. When aspirating low in the costophrenic sinus, the needle tip should be directed cephalad to avoid puncturing the diaphragm. After the appropriate depth has been reached, a clamp may be placed on the needle at the level of the skin to prevent further penetration and thus to avoid injuring the lung. Removing all available fluid is usually not difficult unless a massive acute effusion is being completely evacuated. In some

instances under these circumstances, pain, discomfort, and severe coughing may be initiated. Rarely, transient unilateral pulmonary edema may occur. Thus, it may be wiser to evacuate no more than 1500 ml. of a massive effusion at the initial attempt.[93] Parietal pleurectomy is advocated for massive recurrent malignant pleural effusions, especially for those occurring in association with tumors of the lungs or breast, or of the pleura itself.[55]

"SPONTANEOUS" PNEUMOTHORAX

The accumulation of air in the pleural cavity is called "spontaneous pneumothorax" if it occurs without any apparent antecedent event. This is in contrast to iatrogenic or traumatic causes of pneumothorax, which are also fairly common. Even so-called "spontaneous" pneumothorax is almost always due to rupture of a subpleural cyst, bleb, or bulla, often in an otherwise apparently normal lung in a young (20- to 40-year-old) male cigarette smoker. Pneumothorax can occur, however, at any age, from the newborn, in whom vigorous resuscitative efforts may result in pneumothorax, to the elderly and emphysematous patient, in whom it may pose a very serious problem, especially when it occurs as a complication of ventilatory support or cardiac resuscitation.[28, 86] Rupture of a tuberculous focus as a cause is now quite uncommon. Occasionally, primary or metastatic tumor may be found in association with pneumothorax. Recurrent pneumothorax in association with menses has also been repeatedly reported.[79] Hemorrhage (hemopneumothorax) may accompany collapse of the lung due to a torn, vascular adhesion. Although this is uncommon, it may be severe enough to warrant emergency thoracotomy for control.

Symptoms depend upon the degree of collapse of the lung and on its previous condition. There may be no symptoms whatever, or severe dyspnea, hypoxemia,

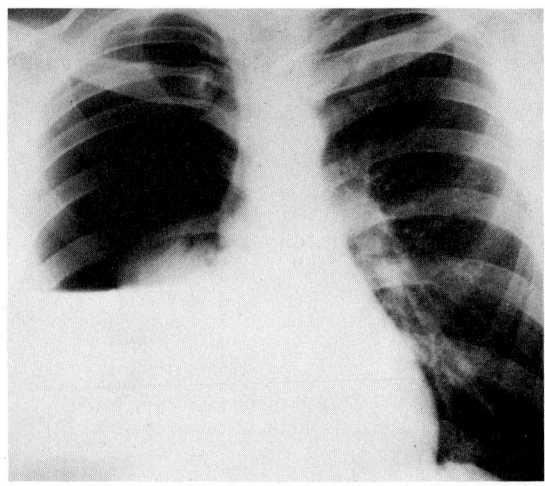

Figure 3. Thoracic roentgenogram illustrating spontaneous hemopneumothorax in a 22-year-old male. This was treated by closed tube thoracostomy and responded with prompt and complete re-expansion of the lung. The etiology was undetermined.

and even shock may be observed. Chest pain may be prominent or absent. Hyper-resonance and absent or diminished breath sounds are the characteristic physical findings.

The diagnosis is usually apparent from the roentgenogram of the chest. A film taken during expiration may help demonstrate a small pneumothorax more readily, while appropriate laminagrams of the lung may aid in the differentiation of localized pneumothorax from a large, thin-walled pulmonary cyst or pneumatocele.

Treatment depends upon a variety of factors. An initial, small (5 to 20 per cent), asymptomatic pneumothorax may safely be kept under observation. Intercostal rubber tube thoracostomy with a closed drainage system is adequate for the vast majority of patients with large pneumothoraces.[59] Prevention of recurrences is said to be favored by keeping the rubber (not plastic) tube in place for at least 4 days, to foster a sterile pleuritis. The rounded, closed-end, S-shaped needle introduced by Clagett is less traumatic and more convenient, but it lacks the desirable feature of acting as an irritant to the pleura.[28] Others have advocated the use of a small-bore polyethylene catheter inserted through a 14-gauge needle.[50] Gentle suction on either catheter or S-needle facilitates expansion of the lung. More recently, use of the Heimlich flutter-valve has been advocated.[7] This allows the patient to be ambulatory, and it can even be used on outpatients.[63] If it is unsuccessful, underwater seal drainage can be instituted for several days, or a high-volume vacuum system applied. However, if the episode is a recurrent one, or if obvious bullae or cysts are seen in the collapsed lung, open thoracotomy is advocated, with suturing, ligation, or excision of the ruptured bleb or bulla, and vigorous abrasion of especially the parietal, but also the visceral, pleura. This produces filmy adhesions and helps prevent recurrences. Excision of the parietal pleura is advocated by some observers,[12] but the consensus is against its use, as being unnecessary, more traumatic, and associated with a higher complication rate.[19, 92, 100] Subsequent thoracotomy, if it should become necessary, is rendered more difficult also. Talc poudrage, or the use of other irritants to obtain pleurodesis, is not recommended.

Appropriate antimicrobial therapy is obviously indicated if an infectious process such as tuberculosis is present.

In tension pneumothorax, or in pneumothorax developing in a patient on ventilatory support,[86] intrapleural pressures on one or both sides may rise abruptly. This is due to a valvelike mechanism that allows air to enter the pleural spaces from the lung parenchyma or airways during brief episodes of markedly elevated intrabronchial or intra-alveolar pressure, as occurs during coughing. Because of collapse of the lung and shift of the mediastinum, severe and even life-threatening respiratory distress may develop, requiring emergency needle aspiration followed by tube thoracostomy drainage. Physical findings of hyper-resonance, absent breath sounds, and mediastinal shift away from the involved side are diagnostic.

Spontaneous pneumothorax and especially tension pneumothorax in the emphysematous patient with marginal respiratory function and cor pulmonale may present a grave and sometimes insurmountable problem of management. Emergency decompression is often necessary. Monitoring of blood gases and of the electrocardiogram, assisted ventilation, tracheostomy, appropriate cardiac drugs, multiple closed thoracotomies, and open thoracotomy may all ultimately be required. To illustrate the gravity of this condition, 10 of 57 such patients in one series, and 12 of 74 in another, died of this complication, in many instances because of delayed diagnosis and treatment.[28, 86] The prognosis in the average patient with pneumothorax, however, is very good, with few recurrences if a sterile pleuritis has been successfully produced by closed tube thoracostomy.

Rarely, as with pleural effusions, rapid re-expansion of a complete pneumothorax by means of high negative pressure can be followed by ipsilateral pulmonary edema.[70] There is experimental evidence to suggest

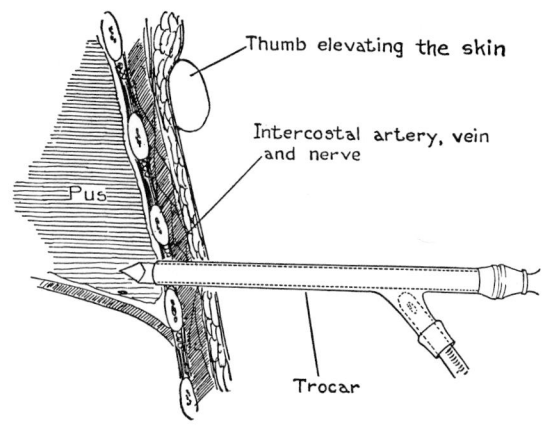

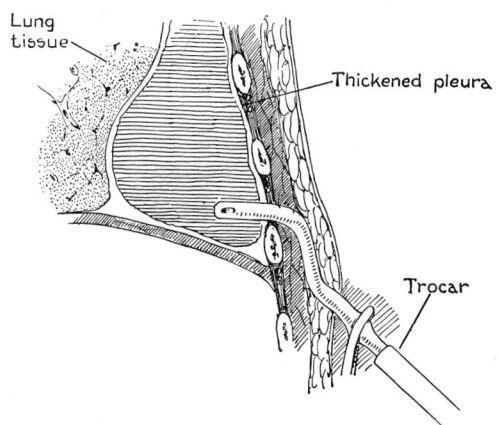

Figure 4. Diagrams illustrating a method of inserting an intercostal catheter for closed tube thoracostomy drainage. A, Step 1: Insertion of trocar into pleural space. (The patient's skin is being elevated by the surgeon's thumb to provide a flap valve for closure of the catheter tract following removal of the intercostal catheter.) B, Step 2: The intercostal catheter has been inserted through the trocar and into the pleural space. The trocar is being removed. (Note flap-valve effect produced by Step 1.) (From Cutler, E. C., Elliott, C., and Zollinger, R. M.: Atlas of Surgical Operations, 2nd ed. New York, Macmillan, 1949.)

that slower decompression, using underwater seal drainage rather than strong negative pressure, may prevent this complication.[58]

Closed pleural drainage systems should be simple, but may be more complex, depending upon the particular clinical problem.[60] Of primary importance is that the characteristics of the system used should be understood by both the responsible physician and the attending nursing staff. When little or no continuing air escape is expected, and only fluid drainage is required, simple, single-bottle, underwater-seal apparatus, or even the flutter-valve and plastic bag arrangement may be adequate.[36, 63] A two-bottle system, with a "dry trap" for the first bottle, provides a separate bottle for collection, in addition to the underwater seal, but adds to the volume of "dead space" between the pleural space and the water-seal surface. In small patients this may be of significance. When air leaks are expected, more complicated systems, involving two or three bottles, with provision for active suction, are recommended.[32, 60, 73] The first bottle may be a collecting bottle, the second a water seal, and the third a vacuum regulator with a long tube open to air, and extending under water a determinate number of centimeters to correspond with the maximal negative suction in centimeters of water required (20 to 40 cm.) Very strong suction (−40 cm. H_2O) is used occasionally, especially following segmental resections.[60] Either a wall vacuum source or a high air flow capacity, electrically driven turbine type of pump is effective. Pumps with a low air flow capacity should not be used when large air leaks, either continuous or intermittent (as during coughing), may be expected. The drainage system should function to prevent ingress of air into the pleural cavity, even when the vacuum source fails. It is equally important that the system should allow egress of large volumes of air, suddenly, whether the vacuum source is functioning or not. Time spent in understanding the physiologic and physical principles of pleural drainage systems and communicating this understanding to attending nurses will be well spent.[32, 60]

HEMOTHORAX

An accumulation of blood in the pleural cavities (hemothorax) may result from trauma to the chest wall, the lung, the mediastinal structures, or the diaphragm. It can also be found with pulmonary infarction, with pleural or pulmonary neoplasm, or following tearing of a pleural adhesion, as with spontaneous pneumothorax. It can occur as a complication of anticoagulant therapy. Hemothorax following surgery on the heart or lungs is unfortunately all too common. Partial defibrination of the blood may occur, with deposition of fibrin on the pleural surface. However, a sterile hemothorax can be completely reabsorbed, leaving little or no residue.[22] An infected hemothorax, or hemothoracic empyema, on the other hand, can lead to the development of a fibrothorax, with serious compromise of pulmonary function.[14] This is more likely to occur after war wounds and gunshot wounds, with underlying lung damage; it is less likely to occur

after a clean stab wound.[29] Hemopneumothorax is more likely to be followed by such a complication than hemothorax alone.

The management of hemothorax depends upon the rate of bleeding and the total volume bled, as well as the underlying cause. If the hemothorax is small, and bleeding has stopped, judging from clinical signs and serial roentgenograms, nothing need be done. For moderate amounts of estimated blood accumulation (500 ml. or more), a closed thoracostomy with intercostal tube drainage for complete evacuation of blood allows observation of its reaccumulation, plus re-expansion of the lung, and is preferable to needle aspiration. Continuing active bleeding, as judged from serial thoracic roentgenograms, clinical signs, or output from chest tubes, demands open thoracotomy for control of hemorrhage. It has often been observed that continuing postoperative bleeding will cease upon re-exploration and removal of blood clots, even if no active bleeding point is found.

In order to forestall the development of an imprisoning fibrothorax, and to gain re-expansion of lung compressed by blood, early decortication (within 3 weeks of the gunshot type of injury) is advocated. The fibrinous deposit will still peel off the visceral pleura readily, and pulmonary expansibility can be restored.[101] On the other hand, one should not resort to decortication precipitately, since an uncomplicated hemothorax can be completely resorbed.

CHYLOTHORAX

Chylothorax, that is, chyle in the pleural cavity, is most commonly due to trauma or tumor. The thin, fibromuscular thoracic duct that transports chyle along the length of the mediastinum from the cysterna chyli to the left subclavian vein may be ruptured anywhere along its course. Rupture above the fifth or sixth thoracic vertebra generally results in left-sided chylothorax; injury below that level often results in a right-sided collection. Because of excellent collateral pathways, the duct can be ligated with impunity.

Owing to the high fat and protein content of the milky white chyle, loss of this material into the pleural cavity can be a serious matter from the nutritional standpoint. The large volume of the effusion may also cause severe respiratory embarrassment.

Of traumatic cases, 80 per cent are the result of gunshot wounds, automobile accidents, stab wounds, and blunt trauma; and 20 per cent are iatrogenic, mostly postsurgical, usually following operations for congenital cardiovascular anomalies.[18, 33, 39] Lymphosarcomas and metastatic carcinomas account for most cases due to tumor. Aspiration or closed intercostal drainage coupled with *increased* oral fat intake is often effective, if the patient's general condition permits persistence of such therapy for 3 to 4 weeks.[8, 53, 77] If not, and if conservative measures fail to control the leakage of chyle, or if it recurs, or is voluminous (over 1.5 liters per day for an adult),[77] thoracotomy in 7 to 10 days is advocated to forestall severe nutritional depletion. The ingestion of a fatty meal or a quantity of a lipophilic dye just prior to surgery may aid in

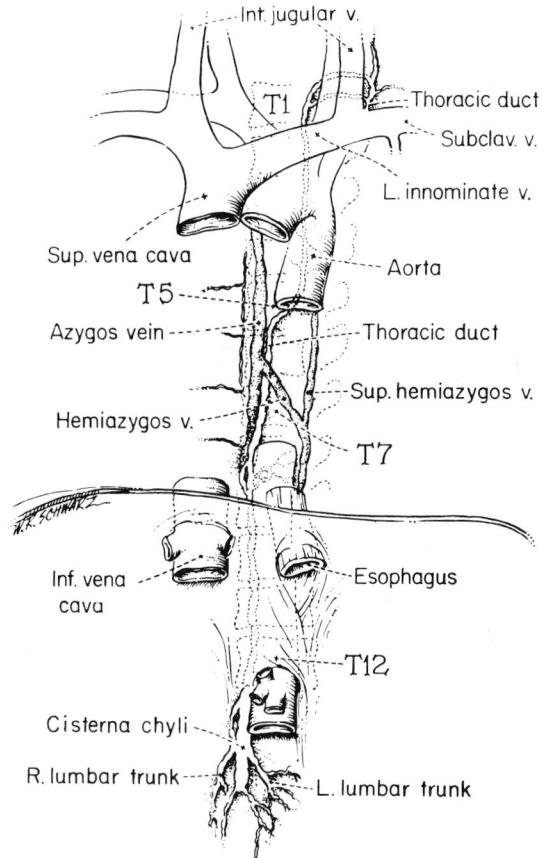

Figure 5. Diagram showing anatomic relationships of the thoracic duct. (From Williams, K. R., and Burford, T. H.: J. Trauma, 3:317, 1963.)

identifying the site of leakage.[43] Unless this leakage can be identified and controlled by suture ligation, ligation of the duct low in the mediastinum below the level of the eighth thoracic vertebra is the treatment of choice. It has been pointed out that in traumatic cases of chylothorax, surgery will usually be unnecessary, whereas in those cases due to malignant disease, it will rarely be effective.[8]

PLEURAL TUMORS

These are classified as primary and secondary. The latter are by far the more common. Primary pleural tumors are mostly mesotheliomas of which localized benign types and diffuse malignant types are recognized.[48, 66, 94] In both types, fibrous or fibrosarcomatous and epithelioid varieties are seen. Mixtures of the two histologic varieties also occur. Therefore, the pathologic classification of benign versus malignant and the differentiation from carcinoma are sometimes difficult.

Patients with localized fibrous mesotheliomas may be asymptomatic, or they may complain of symptoms of arthralgia, clubbing of the fingers, or fever.[20, 40, 89] When the solitary, often encapsulated and pedunculated, usually easily removable tumor, arising ordi-

narily from the visceral pleura, is excised, the symptoms and signs of arthralgia and pulmonary osteoarthropathy disappear, and longevity seems to be unaffected. These tumors may range in size from a few to 20 cm. or more in diameter. Rarely, they may recur.[95]

Diffuse or malignant mesotheliomas, on the other hand, cause chest pain and bloody pleural effusion containing malignant mesothelial cells.[37] These tumors are characterized by findings ranging from multiple papillary projections on both visceral and parietal pleurae to encasement of the entire lung in a thick rind of tumor, with similar findings on the parietal side. Part or all of the pleural space may be obliterated. Metastases are uncommon, except late in the disease, and are often limited to the regional lymph nodes. Extrathoracic metastases do occur, however. Death within 1 or 2 years is the rule in the majority of cases.[10]

At issue currently is the precise relationship between exposure to asbestos dust and the development of pleural hyaline plaques,[72] malignant mesotheliomas, and, even more frequently, bronchogenic carcinoma. Circumstantial evidence for a causal relation-

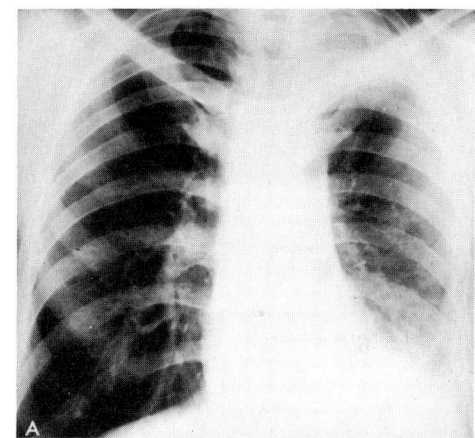

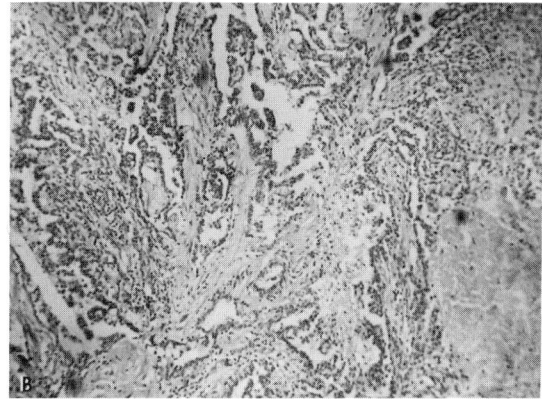

Figure 6. *A*, Thoracic roentgenogram showing marked pleural thickening around entire left lung, in an adult male. At open thoracotomy and biopsy, a pleural tumor was found that proved to be a diffuse malignant pleural mesothelioma. *B*, Reproduction of photomicrograph showing histologic pattern of pleural mesothelioma illustrated in *A*. This is only one of a variety of histologic patterns that can occur in this disease.

ship is strong and is based on experimental evidence[99] and on occupational exposure, with a high incidence of both pleural mesothelioma and bronchogenic carcinoma in asbestos workers or those exposed to asbestos.[26, 62] The identification of "asbestos bodies," the ferruginous or iron-staining foreign body capsules that coat the ultramicroscopic asbestos fibrils, in some patients with pleural mesotheliomas but also in random autopsies in 30 to 97 per cent of lungs weakens somewhat the chain of circumstantial evidence.[10, 30]

Treatment of malignant mesothelioma has been unsatisfactory. There have been no cures. A small number of 4- to 7-year survivals have been achieved by "complete" pleurectomy or pleuropneumonectomy, but the great majority of patients have succumbed within 1 or 2 years of the diagnosis, regardless of the type of treatment used. Radiation is nevertheless recommended, if excisional surgery is impossible or incomplete.[10, 48, 66]

Pleural involvement by metastatic disease is far more common than primary pleural tumor and is usually associated with implants involving the lung or with blockage of or interference with the lymphatic drainage of the visceral, parietal, diaphragmatic, or mediastinal pleura. The most common sites of primary tumor are the lung, breast, pancreas, and stomach. With direct involvement of the pleura by tumor implants, bloody fluid containing neoplastic cells can often be obtained. Various types of palliative treatment are advocated, depending upon the site of the primary tumor, the expansibility of the lung, the degree of disability from pleural effusion, and so forth. Hormonal therapy, radiation or radioisotope therapy, multiple aspirations of the chest, closed tube thoracostomy,[44] and the insufflation of talc[65] or the instillation of chemotherapeutic agents[38] have all been reported, with varying degees of palliation having been achieved.[46, 57] As noted earlier, parietal pleurectomy is sometimes helpful in controlling massive recurrent malignant pleural effusions.[55]

EMPYEMA

Pleural empyema is a collection of purulent fluid in the pleural space. It may be localized (encapsulated), or it may involve the entire pleural cavity. Empyema is classified by some authors as "acute" or "chronic," depending upon duration and pathologic reaction, but there is no sharp dividing line between the two types with respect to either time or pathologic response. A more informative but less popular differentiation between the stages of empyema might be that offered by the American Thoracic Society. *Exudative* empyema is characterized by thin fluid with low cellular content and by an underlying lung that will re-expand readily. *Fibrinopurulent* empyema is characterized by large numbers of polymorphonuclear leukocytes and by deposition of fibrin on both the visceral and parietal surfaces of the involved pleura. In this transitional phase between acute and chronic empyema, there is a progressive tendency toward loculation and delimitation of the extent of the empyema space, accompanied by beginning fixation of the lung. In *organizing* em-

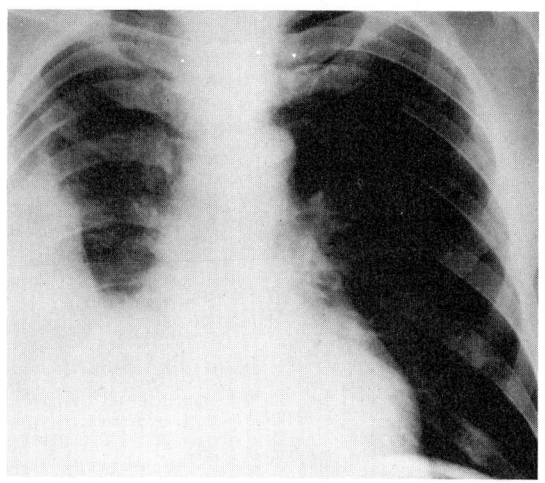

Figure 7. Roentgenogram of thoracic empyema of 2 months' duration, from which anaerobic streptococci and gram-negative bacteroides bacilli were isolated. This patient was treated by open drainage following resection of a 2-inch segment of the seventh rib. The right lung re-expanded completely and the empyema space was obliterated in approximately 2 weeks.

pyema, fibroblasts appear in the now heavier fibrin coating of the pleural membranes, and the exudate is quite thick. Over 75 to 80 per cent of the fluid consists of sediment, as is seen when the fluid is left standing. These distinctions are important, because therapy differs with each stage of the disease.

Both acute and chronic empyema in adults is relatively less common in the present era of antibiotics than it was in the past.[47, 81] In spite of the antibiotics, however, there was an impressive increase in incidence of both staphylococcal pneumonia and empyema in children during the late 1950s.[71, 88] Such recrudescences of infections can surely be expected again. Today, because of the increasing age and debility of patients with empyema who have underlying serious illness, this disease may still pose serious problems of diagnosis and management.[97]

Etiology

Acute empyema ordinarily results from a primary pathologic condition elsewhere. Most commonly, this condition is a pneumonic process in the underlying lung, such as lobar pneumonia, pneumonitis, or lung abscess.[47] This may extend to the pleura directly, by way of the lymphatics, by hematogenous spread, or by rupture of necrotic pulmonary parenchyma. The pneumonic process may itself be secondary to other conditions, such as bronchial obstruction due to bronchogenic carcinoma or a foreign body in the airway, or to bronchial infection, as seen in bronchiectasis. A ruptured emphysematous bleb with spontaneous pneumothorax may also occasionally result in empyema. Less commonly, the source of infection may be a mediastinal structure, such as the trachea or bronchi (bronchopleural fistula); the esophagus (perforation, leaking esophagogastric anastomosis),[84, 91] an abscessed lymph node; or osteomyelitis of the dorsal spine. Subphrenic or intrahepatic abscesses may spread via the rich lymphatics of the diaphragm and cause empyema. Finally, infection may be introduced into the pleural spaces from without by means of trauma, needle aspiration, or operation. Chronic empyema results from untreated or inadequately treated acute empyema. This development should be prevented if it is at all possible to do so. *Empyema necessitatis,* encapsulated empyema discharging into the subcutaneous tissues of the chest wall, is now rarely reported but still occurs.[54]

The most common bacteriologic agents responsible for empyema in the past — pneumococci and streptococci — have been displaced in importance and in frequency in recent years by *Staphylococcus aureus* and by a variety of gram-negative organisms: Pseudomonas, *Klebsiella pneumoniae, Escherichia coli, Aerobacter aerogenes,* Proteus, and Salmonella. Still more recently, a variety of anaerobic or microaerophilic bacilli have been identified with increasing frequency. These include fusobacteria, varieties of Bacteroides, and microaerophilic streptococci. Therefore, an early gram-stain of empyema fluid to provide an immediate preliminary idea of the nature of the pathogens, and special care in transporting and processing specimens to ensure isolation of oxygen-sensitive organisms, is warranted.[5] These measures will allow prompt identification of the appropriate antibiotic to use for treatment. Tuberculous empyema is now uncommon. Empyema caused by fungi is discussed in the preceding section. Amebic empyema, now quite rare, occurs usually as the result of an amebic liver abscess, with rupture into the right pleural cavity.[90]

Diagnosis

The diagnosis depends upon the detection of signs and symptoms of the underlying infectious process and of the accumulation of purulent material in the pleural cavity. This is supported and localized by the clinical examination of the patient and the roentgenographic appearance of fluid, or fluid and air, or of a pleural or interlobar opacification compatible with fluid. It is confirmed by needle aspiration with the demonstration of pus. Bacteria may not be identified if intensive antibiotic therapy has been employed previously, if the appropriate techniques for isolating oxygen-sensitive (anaerobic, or microaerophilic) organisms have not been used,[5] or if the etiologic agent is not bacterial.

Treatment

The objectives of treatment for all stages of empyema are: (1) control of the primary infection and its secondary manifestation, empyema; (2) evacuation of the purulent contents of the empyema sac and eradication of the sac, to prevent chronicity; and (3) re-expansion of the underlying lung in order to restore function. The methods used to achieve these objectives depend upon the stage of empyema being treated and the nature of the primary infection or source of contamination. These objectives are realized by the use of appropriate antibiotic therapy, based upon the bacteriologic diagnosis, and by prompt and adequate drainage. *Needle aspiration* is sometimes adequate, but only in the exudative state with thin pus. Even in this stage, insertion of an intercostal tube for *continuous closed drainage* should not be delayed if the purulent fluid cannot be completely evacuated by thoracentesis, if the fluid reaccumulates, or if infection and toxicity are difficult to control. There is an increasing trend toward the early use of closed tube drainage for all acute empyemas.[6, 47, 96, 101] For the fibrinopurulent stage, prompt use of closed tube drainage is indicated, especially if there is concern that open drainage would result in collapse of the lung. Negative pressure may have to be applied to hasten pulmonary expansion, especially in the presence of a bronchopleural fistula. The tube is often inserted through a trocar, or directly; it should be of a caliber commensurate with the type of material being evacuated and should not be permitted to become plugged. It should be placed in the most dependent part of the empyema pocket, with care being exercised to avoid perforation of the diaphgram upon insertion of the trocar. Accurate localization is greatly facilitated by the use of biplane roentgenograms of the chest or a fluoroscopic intensifier. More than one tube may be necessary. Malecot or right-angle catheters that can be inserted directly through a stab incision and pulled flush with the parietal wall of the pleural cavity are preferred by some surgeons.[76]

Open drainage accompanied by resection of a short segment of rib is used if closed tube thoracostomy is ineffective, if the pus is too thick or is loculated in multiple pockets, or if the patient's toxic condition continues.[47, 49] At this stage, the empyema is localized by adherence of those parts of visceral and parietal pleura that are not involved in the empyema. In most instances, after the pus is evacuated, the obvious locules are broken up and the empyema cavity is washed, a wide-bore tube is left in place, open to atmos-

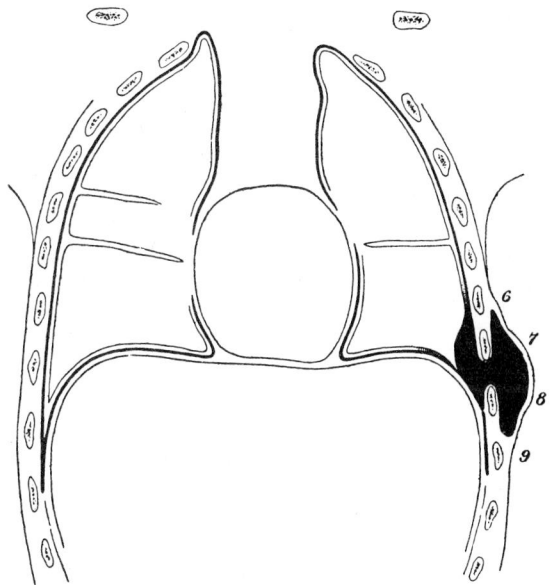

Figure 8. Diagram of empyema necessitatis showing its characteristic components: encapsulated pleural empyema, a narrow opening between the ribs through which the empyema has burrowed, and the externally presenting collection of pus in the subcutaneous tissues. (From Ashhurst, A. P. C.: Int. Clin., 4:173, 1916.)

pheric pressure. However, if it is found that the visceral pleural peel is still quite thin, and there is danger of pulmonary collapse or possible spread of empyema, the snug fit of an intercostal catheter can be duplicated by appropriate mechanical sealing of the wound around the tube and application of underwater-seal closed drainage or even negative pressure.[45, 76] Another variation, the Eloesser skin flap, originally designed for tuberculous empyema, combines some of the virtues of open and closed drainage and eliminates the need for wide-bore tubes open to air.[21, 31] With open drainage, the appropriate, most dependent site must be carefully localized roentgenographically or fluoroscopically and by repeated exploratory thoracenteses before the rib is resected. The drainage tube is removed only when the empyema sac has been eliminated, as determined by measurement of its capacity or radiographically, after introduction of contrast material.[3]

In some instances, *decortication* will achieve the goals of therapy more efficiently than open drainage. This is more likely to be true in managing infected or noninfected hemothorax, when the lung has become imprisoned by its nonelastic fibrinopurulent coat, but presumably remains expandable, and the patient is not in a toxic condition. Decortication may follow closed or open tube drainage.[13, 24, 76] Although advocated by some as primary treatment for empyema,[56] decortication is not generally advocated as primary treatment, except in unusual circumstances in which there is major pulmonary collapse and an obvious, thick visceral and parietal peel. Even here, closed drainage as a preliminary step to aid in cleansing the cavity contents and improving the patient's general condition may have a place. Infrequently, conventional *thoracoplasty* to obliterate the pleural space or Schede thoracoplasty to unroof an empyema pocket may be necessary. The use of skin flap open drainage,[76, 84] of pedicled muscle flaps as described by Maier, or of "thoracomediastinal plication" as described by Andrews[2] may be needed for complicated problems involving bronchopleural-cutaneous fistulas, if simple open drainage fails to obliterate empyema.

Treatment of empyema following pneumonectomy has changed in recent years with the observation that elimination of the empyema space is not necessary if it can be sterilized and if there is no underlying bronchopleural or esophagopleural fistula. It can be accomplished by first providing open drainage and then instilling antibiotic solutions (often neomycin alone, or in combination with other antibiotics), until the pleural cavity is sterile. The open drainage site is then closed surgically.[23, 27, 68, 83, 98]

The interesting observation has been made recently that postoperative empyema may improve the 5-year survival of patients with bronchogenic carcinoma significantly (from 18 per cent for a control group, to 50 per cent for the postoperative empyema group).[74]

Results of Treatment

The results of treatment of empyema depend upon the underlying condition, the age of the patient, and associated diseases. In Snider's series of 105 adult patients, there were 49 deaths.[81] However, in only five patients was the empyema thought to be a significant factor. In one 30-year experience involving 138 children, mortality from postpneumonic empyema remained remarkably constant (9 to 14 per cent) in spite of the fact that the time span encompassed the preantibiotic and presulfonamide periods.[6] When empyema was secondary to surgical procedures or trauma, however, the mortality rate was in the range of 60 per cent.[6, 84] On the other hand, better results in children have been reported when conservative measures could be used, including methicillin and thoracentesis alone in many cases.[17, 88] Thus some types of empyema remain a serious problem, requiring early diagnosis, accurate bacteriologic identification, and prompt and vigorous management.

SELECTED REFERENCES

American Thoracic Society: Management of nontuberculous empyema. Am. Rev. Resp. Dis., 85:935, 1962.
A statement of the Subcommittee on Surgery of the American Thoracic Society summarizing well a reasonable consensus regarding etiology, pathology, and appropriate therapy for the various phases of nontuberculous empyema.

American Thoracic Society: Therapy of pleural effusion: A statement by the Committee on Therapy. Am. Rev. Resp. Dis., 97:479, 1968.
A reasoned and detailed approach to the differential diagnosis and management of pleural effusions.

Barrett, N. R.: The pleura—with special reference to fibrothorax. Thorax, 24:515, 1970.
The Tudor Edwards Memorial Lecture, 1970; thoughts, observations, and interpretations that present a fresh insight into the structure and function of the pleura in health and in disease.

Bessone, L. N., Ferguson, J. B., and Burford, T. H.: Chylothorax. Ann. Thorac. Surg., 12:527–550, 1971.
An excellent collective review of this subject, which is complete in practically every respect and which summarizes current concepts in the management of this disease extremely well.

Eloesser, L.: Milestones in chest surgery. J. Thorac. Cardiovasc. Surg., 60:157, 1970.
A brief but fascinating recapitulation of some of the major landmarks in the development of thoracic and cardiovascular surgery, from Sauerbruch's chamber to Gibbon's pump-oxygenator.

Feingold, S. M., and Bartlett, J. G.: Anaerobic pleuropulmonary infections. Cleve. Clin. Q., 42:101–111, 1975.
One hundred such cases are presented, with bacteriologic and clinical data, emphasizing the fact that these infections are probably very commonly overlooked.

Geha, A. S.: Pleural empyema. Changing etiologic, bacteriologic, and therapeutic aspects. J. Thorac. Cardiovasc. Surg., 61:626–635, 1971.
A careful review of 85 cases, showing the evolution of this disease in the aspects indicated in the title. Reference to more recent work identifying the importance of anaerobic organisms in pleural and pulmonary infections is lacking.

Green, R. A., and Johnston, R. F.: Diseases of the pleura. In Baum, G. L. (Ed.): Textbook of Pulmonary Diseases, 2nd ed. Boston, Little, Brown and Co., 1974, pp. 941–1009.

Maier, H. C.: The pleura. In Sabiston, D. C., Jr., and Spencer, F. C. (Eds.): Gibbon's Surgery of the Chest, 3rd ed. Philadelphia, W. B. Saunders Company, 1976, pp. 370–405.
These chapters are recommended reading for a much more complete exposition of this subject, including important details of some surgical techniques.

REFERENCES

1. Anderson, W. J., Skinner, D. B., Zuidema, G. D., and Cameron, J. L.: Chronic pancreatic pleural effusions. Surg. Gynecol. Obstet., 137:827, 1973.

2. Andrews, N. C.: The surgical treatment of chronic empyema. Dis. Chest, 47:533, 1965.

3. Andrews, N. C., Ver Meulen, V. R., and Christoforidis, A. J.: Injection of contrast media in postresection pleural spaces; diagnostic, prognostic, and therapeutic value. Dis. Chest, 52:656, 1967.

4. Arrington, C. W., Hawkins, J. A., Rickert, J. H., and Hopeman, A. R.: Management of undiagnosed pleural effusions in positive tuberculin reactors. Am. Rev. Resp. Dis., 93:587, 1966.

5. Bartlett, J. G., Gorbach, S. L., Thadepalli, H., and Finegold, S. M.: Bacteriology of empyema. Lancet, 1:338, 1974.

6. Bechamps, G. J., Lynn, H. B., and Wenzl, J. E.: Empyema in children. Mayo Clin. Proc., 45:43, 1970.

7. Bernstein, A., Waqaruddin, M., and Shah, M.: Management of spontaneous pneumothorax using a Heimlich flutter valve. Thorax, 28:386, 1973.

8. Bessone, L. N., Ferguson, T. B., and Burford, T. H.: Chylothorax, Collective Review. Ann. Thorac. Surg., 12:527, 1971.

9. Black, L. F.: The pleural space and pleural fluid. Subject Review. Mayo Clin. Proc., 47:493, 1972.

10. Borow, M., Conston, A., Livornese, L., and Schalet, N.: Mesothelioma following exposure to asbestos: A review of 72 cases. Chest, 64:641, 1973.

11. Brock, L.: Evarts A. Graham: Recollections. Ann. Thorac. Surg., 9:272, 1970.

12. Brooks, J. W.: Open thoracotomy in the management of spontaneous pneumothorax. Ann. Surg., 177:798, 1973.

13. Bryant, L. R., Chicklo, J. M., Crutcher, R., Danielson, G. K., Malette, W. G., and Trinkle, J. K.: Management of thoracic empyema. J. Thorac. Cardiovasc. Surg., 55:850, 1968.

14. Burford, T. H.: Hemothorax and hemothoracic empyema. In Berry, B. (Ed.): Surgery in World War II: Thoracic Surgery. Vol. II. Washington, D.C., Office of the Surgeon General, Department of the Army, 1965, pp. 237–324.

15. Carr, D. T.: Diagnostic studies of pleural fluid. Surg. Clin. North Am., 53:801, 1973.

16. Carr, D. T., Soule, E. H., and Ellis, F. H., Jr.: Management of pleural effusions. Med. Clin. North Am., 48:961, 1964.

17. Cattaneo, S. M., and Kilman, J. W.: Surgical therapy of empyema in children. Arch. Surg., 106:564, 1973.

18. Cevese, P. G., Vecchioni, R., D'Amico, D. F., Cordiano, C., Biasiato, R., Favia, G., and Farello, G. A.: Postoperative chylothorax. Six cases in 2,500 operations, with a survey of the world literature. J. Thorac. Cardiovasc. Surg., 69:966, 1975.

19. Clagett, O. T.: The management of spontaneous pneumothorax. (Editorial) J. Thorac. Cardiovasc. Surg., 55:761, 1968.

20. Clagett, O. T., McDonald, J. R., and Schmidt, H. W.: Localized fibrous mesothelioma of pleura. J. Thorac. Surg., 24:213, 1952.

21. Cohn, L. H., and Blaisdell, F. W.: Surgical treatment of nontuberculous empyema. Arch. Surg., 100:376, 1970.

22. Condon, R. E.: Spontaneous resolution of experimental clotted hemothorax. Surg. Gynecol. Obstet., 126:505, 1968.

23. Conklin, W. S.: Post-pneumonectomy empyema. J. Thorac. Cardiovasc. Surg., 55:634, 1968.

24. Coon, J. L., and Shuck, J. M.: Failure of tube thoracostomy for post-traumatic empyema: An indication for early decortication. J. Trauma, 15:588, 1975.

25. DeCamp, P. T., Moseley, P. W., Scott, M. L., and Hatch, H. B., Jr.: Diagnostic thoracoscopy. Ann. Thorac. Surg., 16:79, 1973.

26. Demy, N. G., and Adler, H.: Asbestosis and malignancy. Am. J. Roentgenol., 100:597, 1967.

27. Dieter, R. A., Pifarré, R., Neville, W. E., Magno, M., and Jasuja, M.: Empyema treated with neomycin irrigation and closed-chest drainage. J. Thorac. Cardiovasc. Surg., 59:496, 1970.

28. Dines, D. E., Clagett, O. T., and Payne, W. S.: Spontaneous pneumothorax in emphysema. Mayo Clin. Proc., 45:481, 1970.

29. Drummond, D. S., and Craig, R. H.: Traumatic hemothorax: Complications and management. Am. Surg., 33:403, 1967.

30. Editorial: Asbestos dust—a community hazard? J.A.M.A., 209:1216, 1969.

31. Eloesser, L.: Of an operation for tuberculous empyema. Ann. Thorac. Surg., 8:355, 1969.

32. Enerson, D. M., and McIntire, J.: A comparative study of the physiology and physics of pleural drainage systems. J. Thorac. Cardiovasc. Surg., 52:40, 1966.

33. Goorwitch, J.: Traumatic chylothorax and thoracic duct ligation. Case report and review of the literature. J. Thorac. Surg., 29:467, 1955.

34. Gwin, E., Pierce, G., Boggan, M., Kerby, G., and Ruth, W.: Pleuroscopy and pleural biopsy with the flexible fiberoptic bronchoscope. Chest, 67:527, 1975.

35. Hamaker, W. R., Buchman, R. J., Cox, W. A., and Fisher, G. W.: Hemothorax: A complication of anticoagulant therapy. Ann. Thorac. Surg., 8:564, 1969.

36. Heimlich, H. J.: Valve drainage of the pleural cavity. Dis. Chest, 53:282, 1968.

37. Heller, R. M., Janower, M. L., and Wever, A. L.: Radiological manifestations of malignant pleural mesothelioma. Am. J. Roentgenol., 108:53, 1970.

38. Hickman, J. A., and Jones, M. C.: Treatment of neoplastic pleural effusions with local instillations of quinacrine (mepacrine) hydrochloride. Thorax, 25:226, 1970.

39. Higgins, C. B., and Mulder, D. G.: Chylothorax after surgery for congenital heart disease. J. Thorac. Cardiovasc. Surg., 61:411, 1971.

40. Hudspeth, A. S.: Benign localized pleural mesotheliomas presenting as arthritis. Ann. Thorac. Surg., 2:691, 1966.

41. Kaye, M. D.: Pleuropulmonary complications of pancreatitis. Thorax, 23:297, 1968.

42. Kettel, L. J., and Cugell, D. W.: Pleural biopsy. J.A.M.A., 200:317, 1967.

43. Klepser, R. G., and Berry, J. F.: Diagnosis and surgical management of chylothorax with the aid of lipophilic dyes. Dis. Chest, 25:409, 1954.

44. Lambert, C. J., Shah, M. H., Urschel, H. C., Jr., and Paulson, D. L.: Treatment of malignant pleural effusions by closed trocar tube drainage. Ann. Thorac. Surg., 3:1, 1967.

45. Langston, H. T.: Empyema thoracis. (Editorial) Ann. Thorac. Surg., 2:766, 1966.

46. Leininger, B. J., Barker, W. L., and Langston, H. T.: A simplified method for management of malignant pleural effusion. J. Thorac. Cardiovasc. Surg., 58:758, 1969.

47. LeRoux, B. T.: Empyema thoracis. Br. J. Surg., 52:89, 1965.

48. LeRoux, B. T.: Pleural tumors. Thorax, 17:111, 1962.

49. Levitsky, S., Annable, C. A., and Thomas, P. A.: Management of empyema after thoracic wounding. Observations on 25 Vietnam casualties. J. Thorac. Cardiovasc. Surg., 59:630, 1970.

50. Lindskog, G. E., and Halasz, N. A.: Spontaneous pneumothorax. A.M.A. Arch. Surg., 75:693, 1957.

51. Maher, G. G., and Berger, H. W.: Massive pleural effusion: Malignant and nonmalignant causes in 46 patients. Am. Rev. Resp. Dis., 105:458, 1972.

52. Maier, H. C.: Pulmonary and pleural lymphatics: A challenge to the thoracic explorer. J. Thorac. Cardiovasc. Surg., 52:155, 1966.

53. Maloney, J. V., Jr., and Spencer, F. C.: Nonoperative treatment of traumatic chylothorax. Surgery, 40:121, 1956.

54. Marks, M. I., and Eickhoff, T. C.: Empyema necessitatis. Am. Rev. Resp. Dis., 101:759, 1970.

55. Martini, N., Bains, M. S., and Beattie, E. J., Jr.: Indications for pleurectomy in malignant effusion. Cancer, 35:734, 1975.

56. Mayo, P., and McElvein, R. B.: Early thoracotomy for pyogenic empyema. Ann. Thorac. Surg., 2:649, 1966.

57. Meyer, P. C.: Metastatic carcinoma of the pleura. Thorax, 21:437, 1966.

58. Miller, W. C., Toon, R., Palat, H., and Lacroix, J.: Experimental pulmonary edema following re-expansion of pneumothorax. Am. Rev. Resp. Dis., 108:664, 1973.

59. Mills, M., and Baisch, B. F.: Spontaneous pneumothorax—A series of 400 cases. Ann. Thorac. Surg., 1:286, 1965.

60. Munnell, E. R., and Thomas, E. K.: Current concepts in thoracic drainage systems. Ann. Thorac. Surg., 19:261, 1975.

61. Neustadt, J. E., and Levy, R. C.: Hemorrhagic pleural effusion in Meigs' syndrome. J.A.M.A., 204:81, 1968.

62. Newhouse, M. L., and Wagner, J. C.: Validation of death certificates in asbestos workers. Br. J. Industr. Med., 26:302, 1969.

63. Pagé, A., Cossette, R., Dontigny, L., Lévy, R., Mercier, C., Pelletier, L. C., and Verdant, A.: Spontaneous pneumothorax: Outpatient management with intercostal tube drainage. Can. Med. Assoc. J., 112:707, 1975.

64. Parkes, W. R.: Asbestos-related disorders. Br. J. Dis. Chest, 67:261, 1973.

65. Pearson, F. G., and MacGregor, D. C.: Talc poudrage for malignant pleural effusion. J. Thorac. Cardiovasc. Surg., 51:732, 1966.

66. Porter, J. M., and Cheek, J. M.: Pleural mesothelioma. Review of tumor histogenesis and report of 12 cases. J. Thorac. Cardiovasc. Surg., 55:882, 1968.

67. Pratt, J. H., and Shamblin, W. R.: Spontaneous hemothorax as a direct complication of hemoperitoneum. Ann. Surg., 167:867, 1968.

68. Provan, J. L.: Management of postpneumonectomy empyema. J. Thorac. Cardiovasc. Surg., 61:107, 1971.

69. Rao, N. V., Jones, P. O., Greenberg, S. D., Bahar, D., Daysog, A. O., Jr., Schweppe, H. I., and Jenkins, D. E.: Needle biopsy of parietal pleura in 124 cases. Arch. Intern. Med., 115:34, 1965.

70. Ratliff, J. L., Chavez, C. M., Jamchuk, A., Forestner, J. E., and Conn, J. H.: Re-expansion pulmonary edema. Chest, 64:654, 1973.

71. Ravitch, M. M., and Fein, R.: Changing picture of pneumonia and empyema in infants and children: Review of the experience at the Harriet Lane Home from 1934 through 1958. J.A.M.A., 175:1039, 1961.

72. Roberts, W. C., and Ferrans, V. J.: Pure collagen plaques on the diaphragm and pleura. Chest, 61:357, 1972.

73. Roe, B. B.: Physiological principles of drainage of the pleural space. Am. J. Surg., 96:246, 1958.

74. Ruckdeschel, J. C., Codish, S. D., Stranahan, A., and McKneally, M. F.: Postoperative empyema improves survival in lung cancer. Documentation and analysis of a natural experiment. N. Engl. J. Med., 287:1013, 1972.

75. Salyer, W. R., Eggleston, J. C., and Erozan, Y. S.: Efficacy of pleural needle biopsy and pleural fluid cytopathology in the diagnosis of malignant neoplasm involving the pleura. Chest, 67:536, 1975.

76. Samson, P. C.: Empyema thoracis—essentials of present-day management. Ann. Thorac. Surg., 11:210, 1971.

77. Selle, J. G., Snyder, W. H., III, and Schreiber, J. T.: Chylothorax: Indications for surgery. Ann. Surg., 177:245, 1973.

78. Senno, A., Moallem, S., Quijano, E. R., Adeyemo, A., and Clauss, R. H.: Thoracoscopy with the fiberoptic bronchoscope. A simple method in diagnosing pleuropulmonary diseases. J. Thorac. Cardiovasc. Surg., 67:606, 1974.

79. Shearin, R. P. N., Hepper, N. G. G., and Payne, W. S.: Recurrent spontaneous pneumothorax concurrent with menses. Mayo Clin. Proc., 49:98, 1974.

80. Simon, H. B., Daggett, W. M., and DeSanctis, R. W.: Hemothorax as a complication of anticoagulant therapy in the presence of pulmonary infarction. J.A.M.A., 208:1830, 1969.

81. Snider, G., and Saleh, S. S.: Empyema of the thorax in adults. Review of 105 cases. Dis. Chest, 54:410, 1968.

82. Spencer, H.: Pathology of the Lung, Excluding Pulmonary Tuberculosis, 2nd ed. Oxford, Pergamon Press, 1968.

83. Stafford, E. G., and Clagett, O. T.: Postpneumonectomy empyema. Neomycin instillation and definitive closure. J. Thorac. Cardiovasc. Surg., 63:771, 1972.

84. Starkey, G. W. B., and Ullyot, D. J.: Pleural empyema—a grave surgical complication. Surg. Clin. North Am., 48:507, 1968.

85. Steel, S. J., and Winstanley, D. P.: Trephine biopsy of the lung and pleura. Thorax, 24:576, 1969.

86. Steier, M., Ching, N., Roberts, E. B., and Nealon, T. F., Jr.: Pneumothorax complicating continuous ventilatory support. J. Thorac. Cardiovasc. Surg., 67:17, 1974.

87. Stewart, P. B.: The rate of formation and lymphatic removal of fluid in pleural effusions. J. Clin. Invest., 42:258, 1963.

88. Stiles, Q. R., Lindesmith, G. G., Tucker, B. L., Meyer, B. W., and Jones, J. C.: Pleural empyema in children. Ann. Thorac. Surg., 10:37, 1970.

89. Stout, A. P., and Himadi, G. M.: Solitary (localized) mesothelioma of the pleura. Ann. Surg., 133:50, 1951.

90. Takaro, T., and Bond, W. M.: Pleuropulmonary, pericardial, and cerebral complications of amebiasis—a 20-year survey. Int. Abstr. Surg. (Surg. Gynecol. Obstet.), 107:209, 1958.

91. Takaro, T., Walkup, H. E., and Okano, T.: Esophagopleural fistula as a complication of thoracic surgery. J. Thorac. Cardiovasc. Surg., 40:179, 1960.

92. Thomas, P. A., and Gebauer, P. W.: Results and complications of pleurectomy for bullous emphysema and recurrent pneumothorax. J. Thorac. Cardiovasc. Surg., 39:194, 1960.

93. Trapnell, D. H., and Thurston, J. G. B.: Unilateral pulmonary edema after pleural aspiration. Lancet, 1:1367, 1970.

94. Urschel, H. C., Jr., and Paulson, D. L.: Mesotheliomas of the pleura. Ann. Thorac. Surg., 1:559, 1965.

95. Utley, J. R., Parker, J. C., Hahn, R. S., Bryant, L. R., and Mobin-Uddin, K.: Recurrent benign fibrous mesothelioma of the pleura. J. Thorac. Cardiovasc. Surg., 65:830, 1973.

96. Van de Water, J. M.: Treatment of pleural effusion complicating pneumonia. Chest, 57:259, 1970.

97. Vianna, N. J.: Nontuberculous bacterial empyema in patients with and without underlying disease. J.A.M.A., 215:69, 1971.

98. Virkkula, L., and Eerola, S.: Treatment of postpneumonectomy empyema. Scand. J. Thorac. Cardiovasc. Surg., 8:133, 1974.

99. Wagner, J. C., and Berry, G.: Mesotheliomas in rats following inoculation with asbestos. Br. J. Cancer, 23:567, 1969.

100. Young, D., Simon, J., and Pomerantz, M.: Current indications for and status of decortication for "trapped lung." Ann. Thorac. Surg., 14:631, 1972.

101. Youmans, C. R., Jr., Williams, R. D., McMinn, M. R., and Derrick, J. R.: Surgical management of spontaneous pneumothorax by bleb ligation and pleural dry sponge abrasion. Am. J. Surg., 120:644, 1970.

X

BRONCHIECTASIS

Gilbert S. Campbell, M.D.

Bronchiectasis means dilatation of bronchi. René Laennec (1781–1826) was the first to give a clear description of this condition in 1819. However, the condition had first been observed by one of his pupils, Cayol, 11 years earlier.[11]

Debate still rages as to the etiology of bronchiectasis. In 1907, Carl Beck wrote, "Bronchiectasis is, as a rule, not a disease per se, but a consequence of various affections of the lungs or bronchi."[3]

Surgeons have been aggressive leaders in the crusade against bronchiectasis, and the development of pulmonary resection was stimulated by this disease. Resection of a lung lobe diseased with bronchiectasis was attempted periodically during the nineteenth century. Because of the high mortality and morbidity, lesser procedures were undertaken, such as cautery excision with diversion of the bronchial drainage to the outside through multiple fistulas. Surgical principles underlying one-stage lobectomy were proposed by Harold Brunn in 1929. He employed intrapleural suction drainage to remove fluid and air to augment expansion of the remaining lung lobes. Rudolph Nissen performed the first successful pneumonectomy in 1931 on a 12-year-old girl with bronchiectasis. Two years later, Cameron Haight performed an identical procedure. Evarts Graham made a double advance in the third successful pneumonectomy in 1933, using a single-stage operation in a patient with bronchogenic carcinoma.[24]

Riggins stressed the morbidity in patients with advanced bronchiectasis and suppurative pneumonitis, "consisting of chronic invalidism, psychological changes varying from mild depressive states to psychopathic personalities, complete economic instability, a life alone, apart, helpless and hopeless."[27]

ETIOLOGY

Bronchial obstruction and infection beyond the bronchial obstruction are important precursors of bronchiectasis. The bronchial obstruction may result from a foreign body, plugs of tenacious mucopurulent material, tumors, and extrabronchial occlusion by lymph nodes. Mucopurulent material fills the bronchi beyond the obstruction, with subsequent infection of the bronchial wall and destruction of its muscle and elastic tissue. The diseased lung segments lose their normal cleansing power and are easy prey for further endogenous or exogenous infection. Bronchiectasis is a disease of the pulmonary parenchyma as well as of the bronchi. Pneumonitis with resultant pulmonary fibrosis may follow pertussis, measles, or other viral or bacterial infections. The theory that bronchiectasis is a result of scarring and contraction of lung tissue around bronchi was first proposed by Corrigan in 1838. He wrote, "If the fingers of the reader's hand, separated one from another, be supposed to represent a bunch of bronchial tubes, and at the intervals be supposed to be filled up with fibers undergoing a slow contraction, it is obvious that the first tendency of that contractile action will be to draw the sides of the fingers towards one another or if they were tubes to dilate them."[9]

Bronchiectasis may occur in association with situs inversus and sinusitis (Kartagener's syndrome), cystic fibrosis of the pancreas (mucoviscidosis), and agammaglobulinemia. True congenital bronchiectasis is rare. There was not a single case thought to be due to congenital malformation in a recent review of 100 cases of bronchiectasis in Alaskan native children.[17] Churchill reported that bronchiectasis in the Kartagener complex had the characteristics of acquired bronchiectasis and cited two patients with only two features of the triad (dextrocardia and absence of accessory nasal sinuses). Churchill described the moist bronchial secretion of these two patients, who were carefully treated with chemotherapy when respiratory infection occurred, in the hope that this treatment might prevent the development of bronchiectasis, which is probably acquired secondarily in Kartagener's syndrome and is not truly a congenital lung condition.[7] Culiner has suggested that congenital cystic bronchiectasis, intralobar bronchial cystic bronchiectasis, intralobar bronchial cystic disease, and the "sequestration complex" are variants of a single primary complex of bronchovascular anomalies in other-

wise normal lung parenchyma.[10] The incidence of "congenital" bronchiectasis has dropped sharply since antibiotics have become available to control acute pulmonary infections in the neonate. However, bronchiectasis is still a prominent feature of mucoviscidosis; the mucus-secreting glands of the respiratory tract as well as the pancreas produce a scanty, thick, and sticky secretion. Successful management of respiratory problems in these patients is extremely difficult.

PATHOPHYSIOLOGY

As the bronchi enter the lung, they normally become smaller as they taper and divide, and the bronchial walls become correspondingly thinner. Normal bronchi telescope during the respiratory cycle—lengthening and widening during inspiration, shortening and contracting during expiration. There is a normal peristaltic muscular contractility that tends to keep the bronchial tubes clean by moving any intrabronchial material centrally where it can be coughed free from the respiratory tract. The distinguished Toronto pathologist William Boyd has said the cough is the watchdog of the respiratory tract. Bronchiectasis damages or destroys these normal defense mechanisms.

Bronchiectasis may be classified anatomically as (1) cylindrical, (2) varicose, and (3) saccular.[26] Reid selected for study 45 cases of lobectomy with well-preserved operative specimens and technically clear preoperative bronchograms. He counted the number of bronchial subdivisions in a single bronchopulmonary segment by examining the bronchograms, operative specimens, and microscopic serial sections. With cylindrical or tubular bronchiectasis, the bronchi do not taper in their normal way but usually end squarely and abruptly. Study of the operative specimens revealed a normal number of bronchial subdivisions, many of which did not fill on bronchography because they were filled with mucopurulent secretion. With saccular bronchiectasis, the dilated bronchi are usually subpleural, and for this reason "cystic" bronchiectasis has generally been considered to involve the terminal bronchioles. However, by counting the number of generations of the bronchial tree between the hilum and the cyst, Reid redemonstrated that saccular bronchiectasis usually involves proximal divisions of the segmental bronchi (Fig. 1).

Bronchi involved with bronchiectasis undergo destruction of elastic tissue and muscular coats of the bronchial walls, with replacement by fibrous tissue. Small branch bronchi may become fibrosed and cordlike. The ciliated columnar epithelial lining may show inflammatory change plus squamous metaplasia. Mucous gland hyperplasia and excess mucus production with stagnation occur and because of the impaired cleansing function of the lung, bacteria that lodge at these sites are not properly cleared.

Liebow and his associates have demonstrated extreme enlargement of the bronchial arteries and numerous anastomoses of these vessels with the pulmonary arteries in lung segments diseased by bronchiectasis.[22] Because of these rich bronchopulmo-

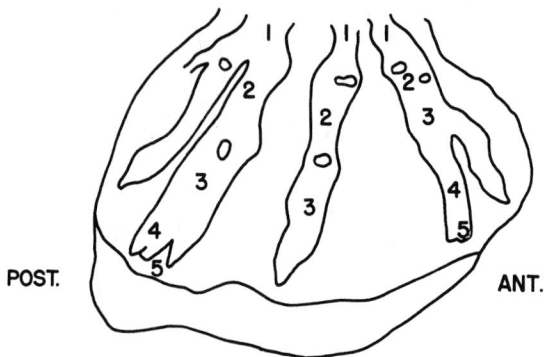

Figure 1. Diagram of lung segment with saccular bronchiectasis, showing involvement of proximal divisions of segmental bronchi. (From Reid, L. M.: Thorax, 5:233, 1950.)

tuosity of the bronchial vessels and retrograde filling of the left pulmonary artery.[1, 20]

Bronchiectasis is usually located in the basal segments of the lower lobes and is associated with involvement of the corresponding middle lobe. Ordinarily the superior segments of the lower lobes are free of disease. The lingula is diseased in 60 to 80 per cent of patients with bronchiectasis of the left basilar segments.[8] Similarly, from 45 to 60 per cent of patients with bronchiectasis of the right basilar segments will have involvement of the right middle lobe. There is approximately a 40 per cent incidence of bilateral bronchiectasis. Involvement of the upper lobes is rare but may follow scarring of old tuberculosis; the disease here is a dry type of bronchiectasis.

Blades and Dugan documented that atypical pneumonia may produce temporary dilatations of the bronchi, and repeat bronchography a few weeks later shows complete return to normal of the bronchograms. This reversible type of bronchiectasis they termed pseudobronchiectasis.[4]

Lung function tests in patients with bronchiectasis show a reduced vital capacity and forced expiratory volume at 1 second.[6] Other authors have reported reduced ventilation, depressed ventilation-perfusion ratios, and decreased perfusion in lung regions involved by bronchiectasis. They suggested that radioactive xenon studies may be helpful for patients with bilateral disease and abnormal overall lung function in whom care must be taken to preserve a maximal amount of functional tissue.[2] Uneven ventilation and air trapping may occur in bronchiectasis. Pulmonary artery perfusion of poorly ventilated segments may result in decreased peripheral arterial oxygen saturation. Macklem et al. have stressed the obstruction in the small airways in patients with bronchiectasis; the contribution of disease in small airways to hypoxia and subsequent pulmonary hypertension is real.[23]

nary anastomoses, bright red blood under systemic pressure may pour into the respiratory tree, with serious or even fatal consequences. In addition to being a troublesome source of hemoptysis, the expanded bronchial arterial supply to the diseased lung may impose an added circulatory burden on the heart, contributing to pulmonary hypertension and ultimately to the development of cor pulmonale. From the standpoint of respiratory gas exchange, the bronchial-pulmonary artery anastomoses may be beneficial, minimizing the ventilation-perfusion imbalance that would result from continued perfusion of the unventilated lung segments by pulmonary arterial blood. Advanced saccular bronchiectasis of the entire left lung may result in absence of uptake on a pulmonary scan (Fig. 2) and nonfilling of the left pulmonary artery on a pulmonary angiogram.[20] Dye injected into the descending aorta of such a patient showed marked tor-

DIAGNOSIS AND TREATMENT

Characteristically, bronchiectasis is a disease of young people—in 41 to 42 per cent onset occurs in the first decade, and in 64 to 69 per cent, before age 20.[25, 27] Since the bronchi of children are quite small, obstructive bronchitis develops readily during respiratory infections in infants and children. Some authors believe that the collateral air circulation through the pores of Kohn is not well developed in the youngster. Most cases of bronchiectasis were diagnosed as chronic bronchitis until 1922, when bronchography was introduced by Sicard and Forestier.[30] The left lung is more frequently involved in bronchiectasis than the right because (1) the right bronchus is really a continuation of the trachea and is more easily drained, (2) the left bronchus is somewhat constricted where the left pulmonary artery crosses it, and (3) the left bronchus is narrower and more easily compressed by the pulmonary artery in children.

A chronic, productive cough that persists in infants and children after an episode of measles, pertussis, or influenza may be due to secondary bronchiectasis. Septic pneumonitis and secondary bronchiectasis may

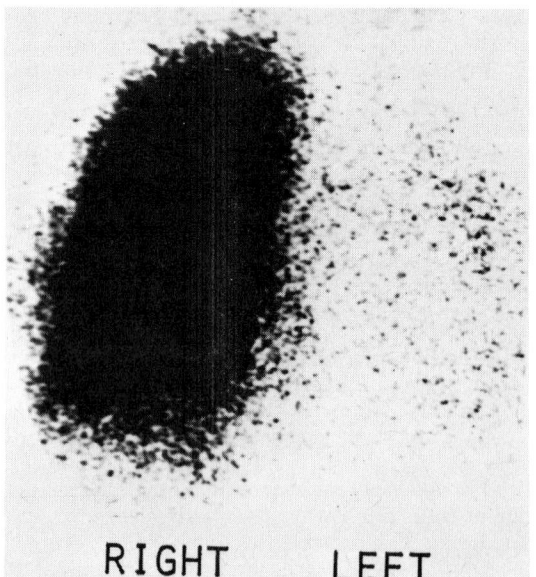

Figure 2. Lung scan from 9-year-old boy with advanced saccular bronchiectasis of left lung.

follow aspiration of foreign bodies into the bronchial tree. Cough with purulent expectoration, hemoptysis, and recurrent localized pneumonitis are important clinical manifestations of bronchiectasis. Changes in body position, especially upon arising in the morning, may produce a violent paroxysm of coughing. Coughing is stimulated by the drainage of collected pools of pus from the ectatic bronchi into the central airways. Auscultation over involved areas reveals depressed breath sounds and coarse rales. Digital clubbing is found in 25 per cent of patients.[21]

With cylindrical or tubular bronchiectasis, the x-ray film of the chest may be amazingly normal, but with saccular bronchiectasis, the diagnosis can sometimes be made on a plain chest film (Fig. 3).

Bronchoscopy is helpful in the diagnosis of bronchiectasis, enabling one to rule out foreign body, tumor, or stenosis. One can observe which bronchi are discharging pus and obtain uncontaminated material for culture.

Bronchography is the best means of demonstrating bronchiectasis (Fig. 4). When bronchography is done for preoperative evaluation, every segment of both lungs must be visualized. Preliminary postural drainage is important prior to bronchography. The presence of thick sputum not only interferes with adherence of thick viscous iodized oil to the walls of bronchi, but is often the cause of severe coughing during the bronchographic examination, giving a faulty bronchogram.

In patients with septic bronchiectasis, appropriate sputum studies and sensitivity tests lead one to the optimal antimicrobial agent. In addition to antimicrobial drugs for septic exacerbation of bronchiectasis, other forms of medical treatment are postural drainage, expectorants, cessation of smoking, and treatment of any upper respiratory problem (such as sinusitis if this exists). Local complications of

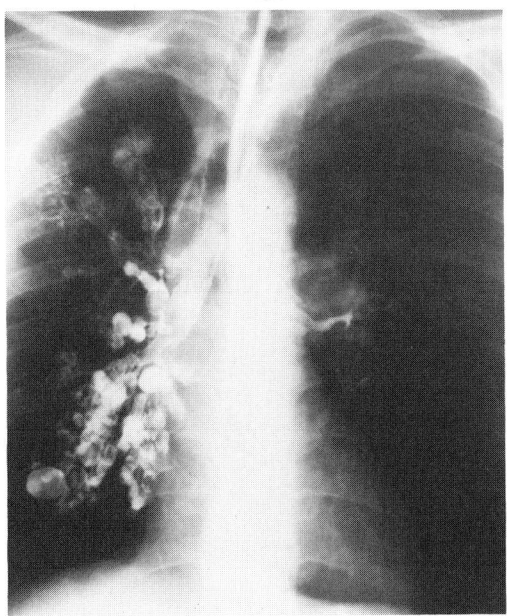

Figure 4. Bronchogram demonstrating diffuse saccular bronchiectasis of the right lung.

bronchiectasis are recurrent pneumonia, lung abscess, empyema, and pyopneumothorax. Other complications are cor pulmonale, brain abscess, and amyloid disease (rarely).

Field has made extensive follow-up studies on bronchiectasis in children.[12-16] She found that there was a trend for definite improvement in the second decade, which was maintained into the third and fourth decade. There was a sharp fall in incidence of cases of bronchiectasis between 1950 and 1960, at the time broad-spectrum antibiotics were introduced. Field recommended surgery for severe localized disease but suggested that diffuse bronchiectasis is best treated medically with postural drainage and antibiotics for exacerbations. With bilateral disease, the more involved lung should be operated upon first. Occasionally the relief of symptoms is so gratifying after an operation on one side that the remaining disease does not require resection.

Sealy, Bradham, and Young reported surgical treatment of multisegmental and localized bronchiectasis.[29] They performed pulmonary resections on 70 patients with localized disease, which they defined as bronchiectasis confined to a site distal to the bronchus of one lung, one lobe, or one segment. There were also 70 patients with generalized disease. Repeated respiratory infections were commoner in the multisegmental group. Eighty per cent of patients with localized bronchiectasis were relieved of all respiratory symptoms following surgery, whereas 36 per cent of patients with multisegmental disease were symptom-free after surgery. The right middle lobe was involved 22 times (16 per cent). During this same period, 41 patients with middle lobe syndrome[5] were operated upon, and 19 of these patients did not have true bronchiectasis.

Patients with multisegmental bronchiectasis have a tendency toward panrespiratory infections accentu-

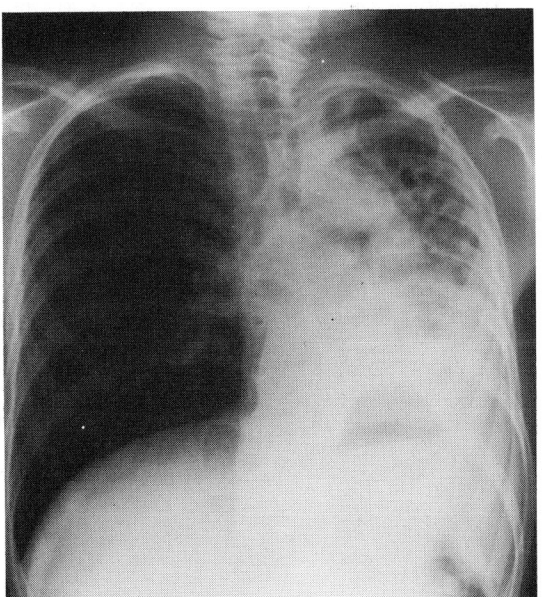

Figure 3. Chest film from same patient as in Figure 2.

ated by prolonged periods of bronchial infections, suggesting an allergic background or lowered resistance or both. The disorder tends to develop in early life, and then for an unknown reason remains stabilized once the second decade is reached. Sealy et al. were impressed by the small percentage of asthmatics in the multisegmental group. In contrast to the findings of Ginsberg et al.[18] of recurrent or new bronchiectasis, there was only one patient in the Duke series in whom new disease developed postoperatively.

Modern surgical approach to bronchiectasis is based upon the principle of conservation of pulmonary tissue. Results of surgery are far better with localized than with multisegmental disease. Patients with diffuse bronchiectasis are not good candidates for surgical treatment as a general rule.

Surgical treatment of patients with localized bronchiectasis yields excellent results with a very low morbidity and mortality. Procrastination and prolongation of nonoperative therapy in this group of patients seem imprudent. Conversely, multiple pulmonary resections in patients with diffuse bronchiectasis seem impetuous.

SELECTED REFERENCES

Field, C. E.: Bronchiectasis. Third report on a follow-up study of medical and surgical cases from childhood. Arch. Dis. Child., 44:551, 1969.
This is the third report on 54 medically treated and 111 surgically treated patients followed from childhood. The observation period averages about 21 years and spans the 1950-1960 decade when broad-spectrum antibiotics were used in patients with bronchiectasis.

Reid, L. M.: Reduction in bronchial subdivision in bronchiectasis. Thorax, 5:233, 1950.
Forty-five cases of lobectomy for bronchiectasis were selected with clear bronchograms and well-preserved resected specimens. The author notes a reduction in bronchial subdivisions in "saccular" bronchiectasis as opposed to "cylindrical" bronchiectasis.

Sealy, W. C., Bradham, R. R., and Young, W. G., Jr.: The surgical treatment of multisegmental and localized bronchiectasis. Surg. Gynecol. Obstet., 123:80, 1966.
A thoughtful study of 157 pulmonary excisional operations at Duke University emphasizing better results in patients with localized bronchiectasis as compared to multisegmental bronchiectasis.

Sanderson, J. M., Kennedy, M. C. S., Johnson, M. F., and Manley, D. C. E.: Bronchiectasis: Results of surgical and conservative management; a review of 393 cases. Thorax, 29:407, 1974.
A consecutive series of 393 cases followed for 1 to 15 years after either surgical or conservative management of bronchiectasis. The authors state that the current bias towards nonoperative management is unjustified.

REFERENCES

1. Alley, R. D., Stranahan, A., Kausel, H., Formel, P., and Van Mierop, L. H. S.: Demonstration of bronchial-pulmonary artery reverse flow in suppurative pulmonary disease. Clin. Res., 6:41, 1958.
2. Bass, H., Henderson, J. A. M., Heckscher, T., Oriol, A., and Anthonisen, N. R.: Regional structure and function in bronchiectasis. A correlative study using bronchography and [133]Xe. Am. Rev. Resp. Dis., 97:598, 1968.
3. Beck, C.: Surgical Diseases of the Chest. Philadelphia, Blakiston, 1907, p. 213.
4. Blades, B., and Dugan, D. J.: Pseudobronchiectasis. J. Thorac. Surg., 13:40, 1944.
5. Brock, R. C.: Post-tuberculous broncho-stenosis and bronchiectasis of middle lobe. Thorax, 5:5, 1950.
6. Cherniack, N. S., and Carton, R. W.: Factors associated with respiratory insufficiency in bronchiectasis. Am. J. Med., 41:562, 1966.
7. Churchill, E. D.: The segmental and lobular physiology and pathology of the lung. J. Thorac. Surg., 18:279, 1949.
8. Churchill, E. D., and Belsey, R.: Segmental pneumonectomy in bronchiectasis; the lingula segment of the left upper lobe. Ann. Surg., 109:481, 1939.
9. Corrigan, D. J.: On cirrhosis of the lung. Dublin J. Med. Sci., 13:266, 1838.
10. Culiner, M. M.: Intralobar bronchial cystic disease, the "sequestration complex" and cystic bronchiectasis. Dis. Chest, 53:462, 1968.
11. Duken, J., and Von den Steinen, R.: Das Krankheitsbild der Bronchiektasie im Kindesalter. Ergebn. Inn. Med. Kinderheilk., 34:457, 1928.
12. Field, C. E.: Bronchiectasis in childhood. Clinical survey of 160 cases. Pediatrics, 4:21, 1949.
13. Field, C. E.: Bronchiectasis in childhood; etiology and pathogenesis, including survey of 272 cases of doubtful irreversible bronchiectasis. Pediatrics, 4:231, 1949.
14. Field, C. E.: Bronchiectasis in childhood; prophylaxis, treatment and progress with follow-up study of 202 cases of established bronchiectasis. Pediatrics, 4:355, 1949.
15. Field, C. E.: Bronchiectasis. A long-term follow-up of medical and surgical cases from childhood. Arch. Dis. Child., 36:587, 1961.
16. Field, C. E.: Bronchiectasis. Third report on a follow-up study of medical and surgical cases from childhood. Arch. Dis. Child., 44:551, 1969.
17. Fleshman, J. K., Wilson, J. F., and Cohen, J. J.: Bronchiectasis in Alaska native children. Arch. Environ. Health, 17:517, 1968.
18. Ginsberg, R. L., Cooley, J. C., Olsen, A. M., and Kirklin, J. W.: An analysis of unfavorable results in the surgical treatment of bronchiectasis. J. Thorac. Surg., 30:331, 1955.
19. Graham, E. A., Singer, J. J., and Ballon, H. C.: Surgical Diseases of the Chest. Philadelphia, Lea & Febiger, 1935, pp. 575–703.
20. Hutchin, P., Terzi, R. G., and Peters, R. M.: Bronchial-pulmonary artery reverse flow. Angiographic demonstration in bronchiectasis. Ann. Thorac. Surg., 4:391, 1967.
21. Laurenzi, G. A.: A critical reappraisal of bronchiectasis. Med. Times, 98:89, 1970.
22. Liebow, A. A., Hales, M. R., and Lindskog, G. E.: Enlargement of the bronchial arteries, and their anastomoses with the pulmonary arteries in bronchiectasis. Am. J. Path., 25:211, 1949.
23. Macklem, P. T., Thurlbeck, W. M., and Fraser, R. G.: Chronic obstructive disease of small airways. Ann. Intern. Med., 74:167, 1971.
24. Nissen, R., and Wilson, R. H. L.: Pages in the History of Chest Surgery. Springfield, Ill., Charles C Thomas, Publisher, 1960, pp. 35–45.
25. Perry, K. M. A., and King, D. S.: Bronchiectasis; a study of prognosis based on a follow-up of 400 patients. Am. Rev. Tuberc., 41:531, 1940.
26. Reid, L. M.: Reduction in bronchial subdivision in bronchiectasis. Thorax, 5:233, 1950.
27. Riggins, H. M.: Bronchiectasis; morbidity and mortality of medically treated patients. Am. J. Surg., 54:50, 1941.
28. Sanderson, J. M., Kennedy, M. C. S., Johnson, M. F., and Manley, D. C. E.: Bronchiectasis: Results of surgical and conservative management; a review of 393 cases. Thorax, 29:407, 1974.
29. Sealy, W. C., Bradham, R. R., and Young, W. G., Jr.: The surgical treatment of multisegmental and localized bronchiectasis. Surg. Gynecol. Obstet., 123:80, 1966.
30. Sicard, J. A., and Forestier, J.: Méthode générale d'exploration radiologique par l'huile iodée. Bull. Soc. Med. Hop. Paris, 46:463, 1922.

XI

THE SURGICAL TREATMENT OF PULMONARY TUBERCULOSIS

W. Glenn Young, Jr., M.D., and Gordon F. Moor, M.D.

A study of the evolution of the surgical treatment of pulmonary tuberculosis is fundamental to an understanding of the entire field of current surgery of the chest. Just as the journals of the past 15 or 20 years picture the burgeoning field of cardiac surgery, the journals of the preceding 100 years or so are filled with the efforts, trials, frustrations, and successes of pioneer thoracic surgeons attempting to cope with suppurative disease of the chest, particularly tuberculosis.

Although the number of patients operated upon for tuberculosis has rapidly declined in the past few years, there are approximately 30,000 new cases of active tuberculosis being reported annually and, in addition, 3500 patients who suffer clinical relapses each year. The number of patients presented for operation remains relatively constant, and is estimated to be from 5 to 15 per cent of those admitted. Thus, the topic remains pertinent and the need exists for surgeons to understand thoroughly the vagaries of the disease and the pitfalls in its treatment.

HISTORICAL ASPECTS

The ancient Greeks recognized tuberculosis as a wasting disease and named it *phthisis,* meaning a wasting of the body, for its most conspicuous symptom. Hippocrates (470–376 B.C.) wrote the first elaborate description of the clinical disease, and apparently recognized an acute and chronic form. Hindu references to the disease were translated into Latin as consumption, from the consuming nature of the illness. The term tuberculosis was used in 1839 by Schönlein as a descriptive term for the nodule or tuber found in the lungs of patients so afflicted.

Pulmonary tuberculosis reached epidemic proportions in Europe in the eighteenth and nineteenth centuries, and one seventh of all deaths in London at the time were believed to be due to consumption. Tuberculosis was long considered to be of many varieties and origins; the unity of the disease was first recognized by Laennec (1826). The correctness of his conceptions was disputed until 1882, when Koch isolated the specific organism and reproduced the disease experimentally.

BACTERIOLOGY

Koch, in discovering the tubercle bacillus, not only identified the organism causing a disease that is still the number one infectious killer today, but also established the criteria that must be fulfilled before a particular microorganism can be accepted as the cause of a specific disease. Koch (1) found the bacillus associated constantly with the clinical disease, (2) collected it in pure culture, (3) reproduced the disease in guinea pigs and rabbits with the culture, and (4) recovered the bacillus in pure culture from the experimentally infected animals. These requirements, known as *Koch's postulates,* were introduced at a time when the infectious nature of many diseases was being recognized, and thereafter became the standard for bacteriologic research.

The avian type of bacillus was isolated in 1890 by Mafucci, and the bovine type in 1898 by Theobald Smith. The vast majority of human clinical disease is caused by the human strain *(Mycobacterium tuberculosis).*

Skin Tests

Koch, in a search for a cure for tuberculosis, turned his attention to the investigation of injection of heat-killed or chemically destroyed tubercle bacilli subcutaneously. He found that in patients with the disease this resulted in a violent systemic reaction with a high fever. The point of injection became painful and red and occasionally sloughed. Although the injection of this *old tuberculin* did not prove valuable in treatment, it did lead to a useful diagnostic skin test. Seibert and Long[14] isolated the protein fraction from the bacillus in 1937 and called it PPD (purified protein derivative). This test reagent is used most commonly in this country now.

Patients become sensitized to the protein fraction from the tubercle bacillus 2 to 4 weeks after infection with the organism. This is a delayed hypersensitivity reaction and is manifested by an area of induration 48 to 72 hours after the intradermal injection of tuberculin. Patients critically ill with tuberculosis or other disease, and especially patients with tuberculous effusions of the pleura, pericardium, meninges, or peritoneum, may fail to react to tuberculin or may react only to the stronger doses. Steroids will also decrease reactivity to the test substance.

Smear and Culture

The diagnosis of active pulmonary tuberculosis is made by identifying the tubercle bacillus in the sputum smear and is confirmed by isolating the organism in culture from sputum or gastric aspirate. A sputum specimen, preferably obtained as a fresh, early morning sample or from bronchial aspirate, is stained by the Ziehl-Neelsen method, which will identify the bacilli as brilliant red rods against a deep sky-blue background. It is sometimes necessary to examine multiple samples before a positive smear can be obtained. The human and bovine strains grow slowly, producing after 10 to 20 days small, dry, scaly colonies with corrugated surfaces. The niacin test for the human strain is based upon the findings that this bacillus is the only mycobacterium that can synthesize excess nicotinic acid.

Atypical Acid-Fast Bacilli

Atypical acid-fast bacilli are often resistant to the standard chemotherapeutic agents. Since patients infected with these organisms present a particular problem in therapy, they are often seen by the surgeon early in the course of the disease. Since 1950 there has been a rapid increase in the number of reported cases of human disease caused by the atypical mycobacteria. Before then, there were only infrequent reports in which sufficient evidence was presented to justify implication of the atypical acid-fast bacilli as the probable cause of disease. Since these organisms, unlike *M. tuberculosis* and *M. bovis,* often did not cause disease in guinea pigs, they were considered to be saprophytes and nonvirulent. Rather than there being a true increase in the incidence of atypical disease, it may be that we are today isolating and identifying the organisms more frequently.[6]

The various strains of mycobacteria differ from one another and are classified by differences in microscopic and cultural morphology, rate of growth, thermic requirements, ability to produce pigment, susceptibility to drugs, biologic activity in animal tissues, and ability to react to certain chemical and biologic tests. A wide variety of terms have been applied to the groups of acid-fast organisms that do not conform to characteristics of the classic species of *M. tuberculosis.* Runyon's classification is widely used[13] (Table 1).

It would appear from careful differential skin testing that the atypical organisms may actually be more prevalent than the human strain.[15] While thus apparently being relatively nonvirulent, they do occasionally produce human pulmonary disease, which is characteristically slowly progressive, indolent, and difficult to treat with the standard chemotherapeutic agents.

The thoracic surgeon is most likely to encounter disease caused by one of these two organisms, depending upon his geographic location.

Mycobacteria kansasii, distributed predominantly in the central United States, is responsive to drug therapy in about 80 to 90 per cent of cases, and adjunctive surgical therapy is effective in 75 to 85 per cent of the remaining cases.

M. intracellularis (Battey strain), predominant in the southeastern United States, may be found in about 8 per cent of patients with infectious sputum. This organism is notoriously resistant to drugs but fortunately pulmonary involvement is often unilateral. Good results can be expected in about 80 per cent of patients with a combination of multiple drugs and surgical therapy.

PATHOLOGY

The basic lesion in pulmonary tuberculosis follows inhalation of the tubercle bacilli and consists of a necrotizing reaction in the pneumonic process in the midlung fields and may proceed to resolution, organization and fibrosis, or caseous necrosis. The bacilli drain into the lymphatics and lodge in the hilar nodes to cause necrosis there or, in a small number of cases, may proceed to produce widespread systemic disease. The lesion in the periphery of the lung combined with hilar node involvement is called the "primary Ghon complex." This primary complex heals completely except in a few instances in which there is rapid pathologic progression. This progression may take the form of miliary tuberculosis by way of massive bloodstream infection and is often seen in early childhood, usually in the first 2 years of life.

Microscopically, the parenchymal lesion consists of a small central area of necrosis containing tubercle bacilli surrounded by a layer of epithelioid cells derived from mononuclear phagocytes. In this layer are also seen the characteristic multinuclear giant cells of the Langhans type.

Reinfection tuberculosis is almost exclusively a disease of the lungs. Chronic pulmonary tuberculosis may be the result of reactivation of an old focus in the lungs (endogenous) or may occur from reinfection (exogenous).[11, 16] It develops as a pneumonia in a segment or lobe and is usually located in the apical or posterior segment of the upper lobes or the superior segment of the lower lobes. Caseation necrosis may occur and result in liquefaction of pulmonary tissue. A cavity is formed if the necrotic process, which is surrounded by a fibrinous perifocal reaction, has involved an adjacent bronchus; this results in drainage and expectoration of the liquefield contents, which contain viable tuberculous organisms. The untreated disease process may then spread to other lobes, the contralateral lung, bronchi, the larynx, or the gastrointestinal tract.

Bronchiectatic changes occasionally accompany the destructive process of pulmonary tuberculosis, particularly in the area distal to a stenotic bronchus. This may be caused by secondary nontuberculous infection or may occur in combination with true bronchiectasis. Caseous material may rupture into the pleural space, particularly if the lesion is near the pleural surface and has not drained into a bronchus; this results in a tuberculous or mixed tuberculous and bacterial empyema. A tuberculous pleural effusion may also be hematogenous in origin. Because of the intense perifocal reaction of pulmonary tuberculosis, fibrinous

TABLE 1.   Classification of Atypical Mycobacteria (Runyon)

Group I	Photochromogens (*M. Kansasii*) (common in Southwest and upper Midwest)
Group II	Scotochromogens (frequent cause of cervical adenitis)
Group III	Nonphotochromogens (Battey-avian complex) (common in Southeast)
Group IV	Rapid growers (including *M. fortuitum*)

pleural adhesions frequently form between the visceral and parietal pleura and may obliterate the pleural space in an area adjacent to the disease process. The late stage of the disease is characterized by contraction of the lobe or lobes involved by fibrosis, with or without concomitant cavitation.

Endobronchial tuberculosis occurs as a result of infection of the bronchial mucosa by bacteria carried by liquefied necrotic material being discharged from the parenchymal lesion. The mucosa is thickened and congested and is occasionally ulcerated. Ulcerative endobronchial lesions may result in scarring and stenosis of the bronchus.

COLLAPSE THERAPY

Prior to the advent of specific chemotherapy, the most successful type of surgery directed toward pulmonary tuberculosis evolved from the idea of putting the affected part at rest, allowing the lung to "relax or collapse." Open drainage of cavitary lesions by marsupialization or tube drainage (*cavernostomy*) was employed occasionally with success, but most such direct surgical approaches were followed by unacceptable complications.

Artificial Pneumothorax

Hippocrates, using a pig's bladder and tube, introduced air into the pleural cavity to relieve the pain of pleurisy. The procedure received widespread popularity after the reporting of successful case series by Forlanini (1882, 1894) and John B. Murphy (1898).

Pneumothorax was employed in countless patients during the first 40 years of this century but often was unsuccessful in producing the desired collapse because of adhesions between the lung and chest wall, or was forcibly terminated by the appearance of pleural fluid not uncommonly infected by the acid-fast bacillus.

Extrapleural Paravertebral Thoracoplasty

The direct surgical measures to relax or compress the tuberculous lung were introduced by master surgeons of continental Europe around the turn of the century. Their fascinating story was brought to this country by classic writings of John Alexander[1, 2] and is only briefly summarized here.

Estlander first used the term *thoracoplasty* in 1879 to denote removal of ribs so as to bring the chest wall down to the lung that would not expand after drainage of empyema. De Cerenville in 1885 first applied this operation to collapse the cavity in a tuberculous lung. An internist, Ludolph Brauer, emphasized that the thoracoplasty must collapse the diseased lung in order to be as effective as pneumothorax. Friedrich, following Brauer's suggestions, performed an operation in 1907 in which he resected all of the second through the ninth ribs. He resected the periosteum, intercostal muscle, and even the nerves as well as the ribs, and four out of his first seven patients survived. Brauer then suggested that subperiosteal resection of the ribs be carried out so that they might regenerate and stabilize the chest wall. Gourdet, Wilms, Sauerbruch, and others modified the very radical operation of

Brauer and Friedrich. In addition to bringing the operation to this country, Alexander refined the "modern" operation of thoracoplasty. He carefully separated the procedure into stages and recognized the value of resection of the transverse processes in increasing the amount of collapse obtained. Alexander and Haight reported the results of paravertebral thoracoplasty from 1932 to 1934 in 119 patients. The mortality was 11 per cent, with cavity closure in 93 per cent of the survivors. In 1957, Strieder was able to report an operative mortality of 2 per cent in 99 consecutive cases.

The most important variation of the classic thoracoplasty is the so-called *plombage thoracoplasty*, a descendant of the old operation of extrapleural pneumonolysis, which was introduced by Tuffier in 1891. In this version of the procedure, an extraperiosteal pocket is developed by denuding the ribs overlying the disease area to be collapsed and filling this pocket with a "plomb" such as polyethylene spheres enclosed in a polyethylene bag.

Indications for Thoracoplasty. During the past 10 to 15 years, the standard and plombage thoracoplasties have become rarely employed operations in the surgical clinics of the country. By far the majority of patients requiring surgery are successfully treated by resection. Thoracoplasty may still be justifiably considered in certain "salvage cases" in which extensive disease, highly productive of drug-resistant orga-

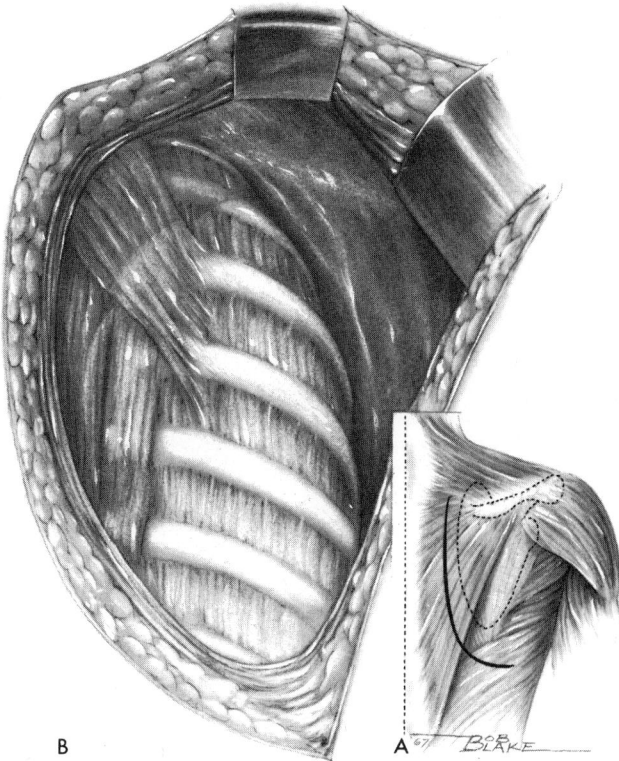

Figure 1. Technique of first-stage, standard thoracoplasty, showing incision *(A)* and exposure *(B)* following mobilization and retraction of scapula. (From Young, W. G., Jr., and Moor, G. F. *In* Sabiston, D. C., Jr., and Spencer, F. C.: Gibbon's Surgery of the Chest, 3rd ed. Philadelphia, W. B. Saunders Company, 1976.)

nisms, makes primary resection hazardous. It may also still be indicated in elderly patients as a compromise procedure.

Modified or "tailoring" thoracoplasty is used as a secondary procedure following resection when the primary operation is complicated by an infected residual space or bronchopleural fistula. In these cases, obliteration of the space can usually be accomplished in a single-stage operation without removal of the first rib or the transverse processes.

The general plan of the operation of thoracoplasty is to remove a sufficient portion of the bony chest wall to collapse the cavity-bearing portion of the lung. For the common upper lobe cavity, this usually involves removal of portions of the ribs down to the seventh or eighth (Fig. 1).

CHEMOTHERAPY

Specific chemotherapeutic agents have been introduced in the treatment of pulmonary tuberculosis during the past 25 years and have had a profound effect on the course of the disease. Case fatality and overall mortality rates have dropped faster than new case rates. The length of hospital stay for patients has been significantly shortened, and, most important for the surgeon, the drugs have allowed resectional therapy to be accomplished with an acceptable morbidity and mortality.

The plan for initial treatment is a program of chemotherapy that is so effective that bacteriostasis and conversion of sputum bacteriologic findings are achieved within 3 to 6 months, and the emergence of significant bacterial drug resistance is prevented. The treatment of patients with disease caused by drug-resistant bacilli frequently presents difficult problems. Drug sensitivity testing is helpful in selecting the most effective combination of chemotherapeutic agents.

Streptomycin (SM), isoniazid (INH), and para-aminosalicylic acid (PAS) are the major drugs used in treatment of pulmonary tuberculosis. The standard initial chemotherapy consists of a combination of INH-SM, INH-PAS, or INH-PAS-SM (triple therapy). Isoniazid is almost always included in any combination and SM-PAS is no longer recommended. Ethambutol is now frequently substituted for PAS.

Organism resistance is a serious problem and may occur early if one drug is used alone. Drug-resistant bacteria are probably present in small numbers in all infections and multiply to become the predominant organism. The objective in chemotherapy is to allow healing to occur before the drug-resistant bacteria multiply to numbers sufficient to continue the disease process. When streptomycin became available in 1944, it was found that this drug halted the progress of the disease and brought about temporary improvement of the patient's condition; this state lasted 3 to 4 months, only to be followed by progression of the disease and recurrence of organisms in the sputum. With the beginning of use of para-aminosalicylic acid in combination with streptomycin in 1946, this situation was markedly changed. Isoniazid, the third and probably most valuable of the major drugs, became available in 1952. Since then many other drugs, such as viomycin, cycloserine, pyrazinamide, ethionamide, kanamycin, and others, have been found to be moderately effective. These agents are usually held in reserve because they are more toxic, more expensive, and less effective than the basic drugs. They are particularly useful when given as an *added drug* to increase antimicrobial coverage for resectional therapy. Their primary role is in the retreatment group of patients whose organisms are resistant to some or all of three major drugs.

Isonicotinic Acid Hydrazide

Isoniazid is the most active antituberculous agent in a large family of synthetic pyridine-carboxylic acid compounds and was first synthesized in 1912. Its antituberculous activity was not recognized until 1951. The ease of administration and high efficacy were immediately demonstrated in man, but it soon became evident that the administration of isoniazid alone favored the development of bacterial resistance, just as in the case of streptomycin. In uncomplicated pulmonary tuberculosis, the average adult dose is 5 mg. per kilogram of body weight, and is usually given as 100 mg. orally three times a day. Children receive 10 to 15 mg. per kilogram of body weight for far advanced disease. The dosage may be increased to 10 to 20 mg. per kilogram in all age groups. In the high dosage ranges, pyridoxine is added in doses of at least 10 mg. for each 100 mg. of INH. Rarely, allergic manifestations or toxicity prevents its use. Toxic reactions are usually related to the nervous system. Peripheral neuritis is the most common side effect and can be prevented or treated with pyridoxine.

Para-aminosalicylic Acid

In 1941, Bernheim found that the sodium salts of benzoic and salicylic acid specifically stimulated the oxygen uptake of *Mycobacterium tuberculosis*. J. Lehman first used PAS clinically and announced his results in 1946. Para-aminosalicylic acid is a weakly tuberculostatic agent when used alone, but is very useful in delaying the emergence of resistant organisms when used in combination with other drugs, especially INH and SM. When it is used as a single drug, resistance usually develops in approximately 120 days. The chief disadvantage in the use of PAS is the frequency of side reactions. Such reactions are usually confined to the gastrointestinal tract, and include anorexia, nausea, vomiting, and diarrhea.

Streptomycin

Streptomycin was discovered by Waksman and his colleagues in 1944, and was the first chemotherapeutic agent found to be effective against *M. tuberculosis*. It was soon found that streptomycin damaged the auditory portion of the eighth cranial nerve. When it was realized that smaller doses of streptomycin were effective, and when PAS became available 2 years later, effective chemotherapy was possible with less toxicity. The dosage of streptomycin varies, depending upon the combinations of drugs selected. When it is used as one of the primary drugs, 1.0 gm. (20 mg. per kilogram) per day is usually given initially, and later the dose is decreased to 1.0 gm. twice weekly.

The following drugs are second-choice agents and are used when patients do not tolerate the major drugs, when the organisms are resistant to the major drugs, or for added coverage for resection. As previously noted, these drugs are generally more toxic and less effective than the major drugs.

Cycloserine is an antibiotic and is a fairly effective "second-line" drug used in various combinations, probably best with INH. Its primary use is in retreatment chemotherapy. The commonly accepted dosage is 0.5 gm. (10 mg. per kilogram) per day, usually given in two divided doses. Up to 20 mg. per kilogram may be given if concomitant phenytoin (Dilantin) and phenobarbital sedation is administered. In doses over 20 mg. per kilogram per day, cycloserine is toxic to the central nervous system and may cause convulsions, psychoses, dizziness, personality changes, or somnolence.

Pyrazinamide (PZA) is structurally very similar to isoniazid and may be administered orally. This drug is very effective, especially for short-term use, and is particularly suited for additional coverage for resection. Resistance develops rapidly when this drug is used alone. The recommended dosage is 3 gm. per day (40 to 50 mg. per kilogram), given orally in three divided doses. In approximately 15 per cent of the patients receiving an oral dose of 3.0 gm. per day, liver toxicity will develop, with anorexia, nausea, malaise, liver tenderness with hepatomegaly, and abnormal liver function. Two to three per cent of patients may become jaundiced. Usually these toxic manifestations will subside after the dose is decreased or administration of the drug is stopped.

Ethionamide is a good "second-line" drug for combined therapy. High concentrations of this drug are bactericidal in vitro. Some of the photochromogenic bacteria, as well as *M. tuberculosis,* are fairly sensitive to this drug. The usual adult dose is 250 mg. given twice daily with meals, and may be gradually increased to 250 mg. three or four times a day with nourishment. The most frequent untoward reaction is that of gastrointestinal intolerance, which occurs in 50 per cent or more of patients.

Ethambutol is a promising antituberculous agent, which may be used in combination with any of the other drugs. The usual adult dose is 15 to 25 mg. per kilogram per day, most often given as a single oral dose. The toxic effects usually involve the optic nerve, but fortunately this is rare and the visual disturbances are usually reversible upon cessation of administration of the drug.

Rifampin is a relatively new oral antituberculous agent developed in Italy in 1963. This drug is useful in treatment of reactivated cases or for organisms resistant to other agents. Rifampin is a very promising drug because of its effectiveness and low incidence of toxicity. The main disadvantage is that it is expensive and for that reason usually not used in the initial treatment program. It is, however, an excellent substitute for INH, ethambutol, or streptomycin when one of these "first-line" drugs is not well tolerated. Rifampin is also quite effective against *M. kansasii.* The usual adult dose is 600 mg. orally once daily, not taken with meals. The pediatric dose is 10 to 20 mg. per kg. up to 600 mg. daily.

Other drugs used in difficult retreatment problems include viomycin, capreomycin, kanamycin, thiocarlide (Isoxyl), oxytetracycline, and antithiazane.

RESECTION FOR PULMONARY TUBERCULOSIS

Historical Aspects

Although the five patients operated upon by Block (1883), Kronlein (1884), and Ruggi (1885) died following attempted partial resection of the tuberculous lung, Tuffier successfully resected the apex of the right lung of a 25-year-old man in 1891. He made an incision in the second interspace and separated the upper part of the lung in the extrapleural plane. He then passed a ligature around the lung and removed the involved area in the apex. His patient was alive 5 years later and was presented before the Surgical Conference in Paris. Subsequently, successful case reports were rare, and resection of tuberculous lung tissue was rightfully considered a dangerous mode of therapy.

Freedlander of Cleveland performed the first successful complete lobectomy for tuberculosis in 1934, and during the next several years enthusiasm was rekindled. The use of the individual ligation technique as proposed by Blades and Kent, Churchill, and others made pulmonary resection in general a safer procedure; however, in 1943 resections in tuberculous patients were still associated with a morbidity of 50 per cent or more and a mortality in the range of 25 per cent.[8] It was not until after the discovery of streptomycin and PAS and particularly after the advent of isoniazid that selective resection of tuberculous lung tissue could be performed without the fear of catastrophic spread of the infection. Segmental resection, by which maximal preservation of functioning lung tissue could be accomplished, was introduced by Churchill and Belsey in 1939.[5] In 1953, Chamberlain and his associates[4] presented a series of 300 segmental resections for pulmonary tuberculosis. Ninety-three per cent of the patients were well, and the operative mortality was 3 per cent.

Indications for Resection

The surgical approach to pulmonary tuberculosis is a valuable complement to medical therapy and when properly applied can result in a combined program that is nearly 100 per cent successful. The purpose of surgery is to remove or to assist in the healing or control of destructive residuals, which would otherwise contribute to failure of medical treatment or to reactivation of the disease process. Surgical assistance is required in a variable number of cases, depending upon selection, but the number may be as high as 20 per cent.[9] The indications for resection have become fairly well standardized:

1. An open cavity associated with positive sputum (so-called open positive) beyond 3 to 6 months after the initiation of chemotherapy. The need for surgery is

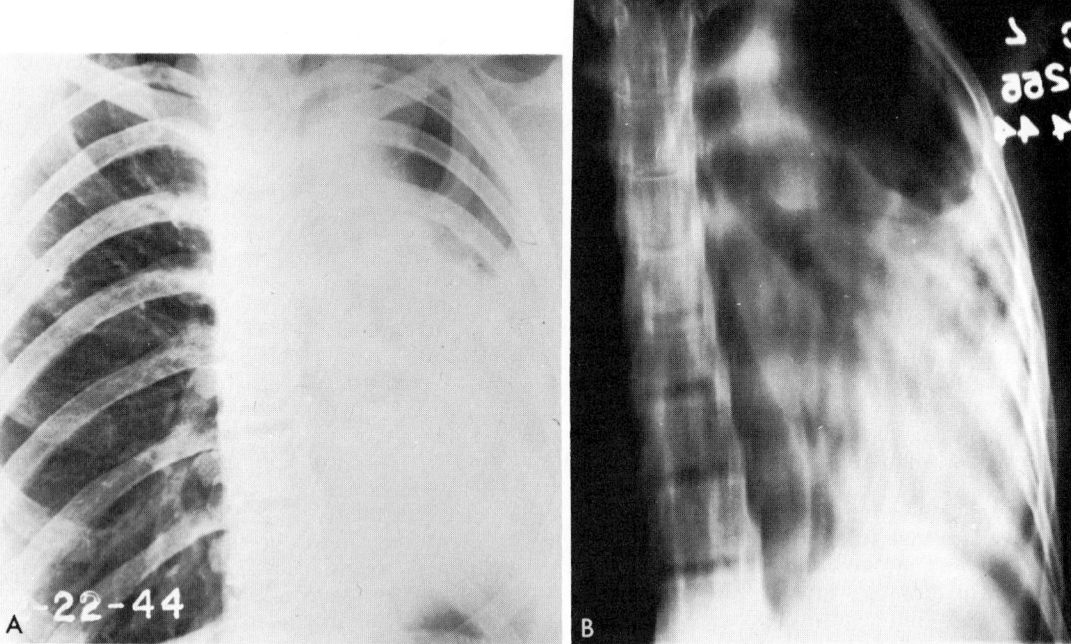

Figure 2. Plain x-ray and planigram illustrating destroyed left lung of a 33-year-old female. Candidate for pneumonectomy. (From Young, W. G., Jr., and Moor, G. F. *In* Sabiston, D. C., Jr., and Spencer, F. C.: Gibbon's Surgery of the Chest, 3rd ed. Philadelphia, W. B. Saunders Company, 1976.)

increased if the organism is resistant to one or more of the major drugs.

2. Persistent positive sputum cultures after adequate initial or retreatment programs in patients without demonstrable cavitation, but with pathologic residuals such as a destroyed lobe or lung (Fig. 2), localized bronchiectasis, bronchial stenosis with resultant atelectasis, or large residual nodular foci.

It is important that resection be performed in the first two groups before total bacterial resistance develops, and while an additional effective drug is available to increase antibacterial coverage for surgery. With increased coverage, fewer complications result.

3. Patients with negative sputum who have a residual destroyed segment, lobe, or lung; blocked cavities; tuberculomas; and significant fibrocaseous disease. In general, localized nodules larger than 2 cm. in diameter should be considered for resection (Figs. 3 and 4). Since antituberculous drugs may not penetrate dense fibrous tissue in sufficient concentration, sterilization of these lesions cannot be expected. In addition to the threat of reactivation of the tuberculous disease, the destroyed lobe may result in troublesome hemoptysis and bronchial obstruction with atelectasis and secondary infection.

4. The presence of localized infection with one of the atypical acid-fast organisms. This is an accepted indication for resection because of the organism's primary resistance to drugs and the tendency to progression or reactivation of the disease process. Therapy with INH-SM-PAS is given in spite of apparent resistance, and the decision for resection should be made early to take advantage of the organism's temporary response to chemotherapy.

5. Tuberculous bronchiectasis most commonly occurs in the upper lobes, and because of free drainage afforded the affected areas in the upright position, resection is usually not required. Bronchiectasis of the middle and lower lobes, however, is quite apt to cause subsequent difficulty because of inadequate drainage, and resection of the involved segments is often indicated (Fig. 5).

6. Recent follow-up studies of patients with cavitary disease and negative sputum (so-called open negative)

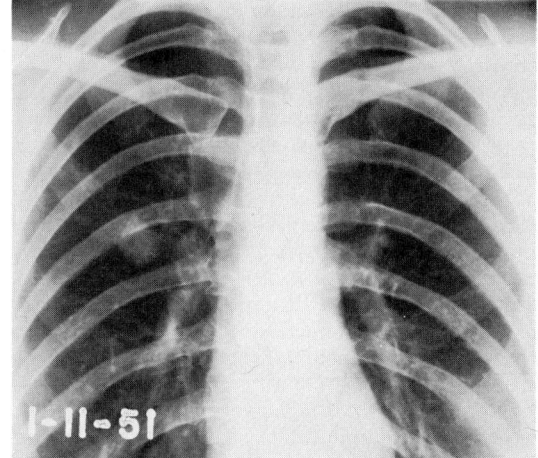

Figure 3. Solid lesion in superior segment, right lower lobe. Tuberculoma. (From Young, W. G., Jr., and Moor, G. F. *In* Sabiston, D. C., Jr., and Spencer, F. C.: Gibbon's Surgery of the Chest, 3rd ed. Philadelphia, W. B. Saunders Company, 1976.)

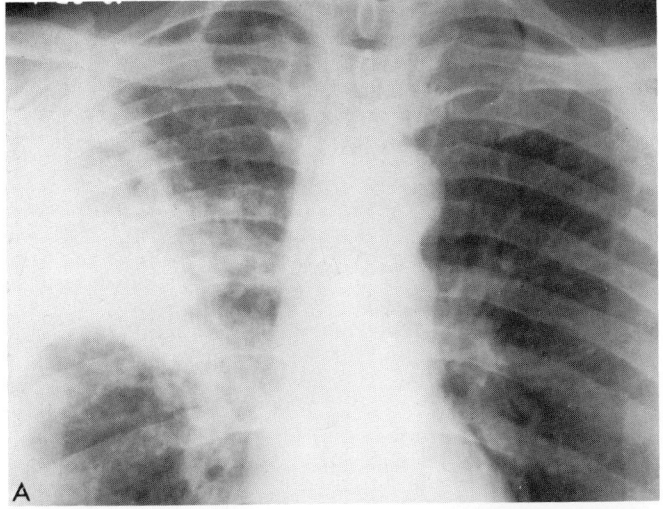

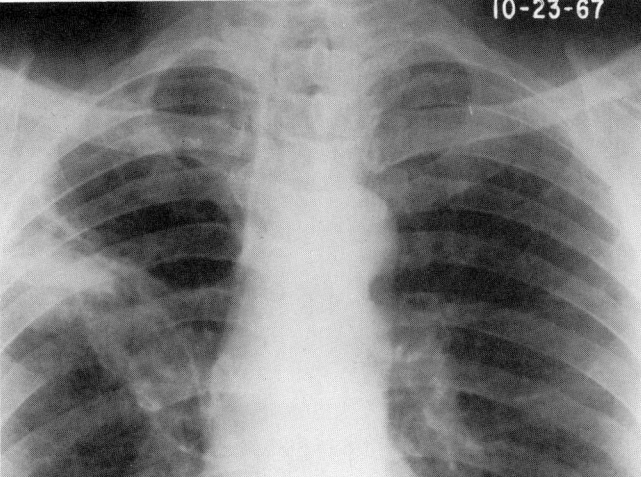

10-23-67

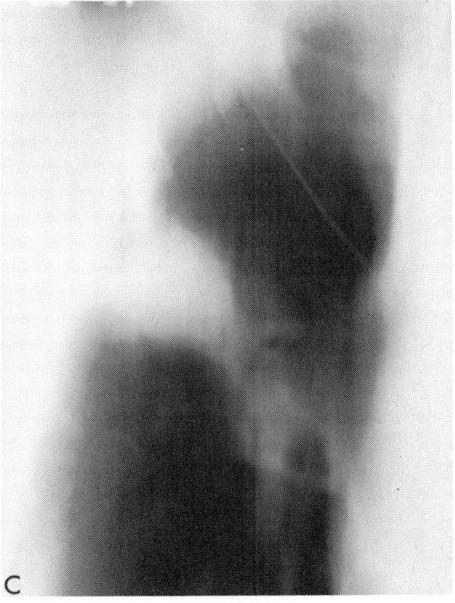

Figure 4. Forty-nine-year-old male laborer with conversion of sputum after 3 months of chemotherapy but significant residual fibrocaseous disease at 6 months. Segmental resection performed. (From Young, W. G., Jr., and Moor, G. F. *In* Sabiston, D. C., Jr., and Spencer, F. C.: Gibbon's Surgery of the Chest, 3rd ed. Philadelphia, W. B. Saunders Company, 1976.)

have shown that most of these patients do well with prolonged drug therapy. The trend in the treatment of these patients is toward the nonoperative approach. There are, however, a small number who will undergo reactivation with positive sputum and spread of their disease. Resection may be recommended in (a) patients with thick-walled cavities; (b) patients who have responded slowly, as determined by sputum conversion and by lack of radiographic improvement; (c) patients who are likely to be unreliable in taking medication or obtaining follow-up examination, such as alcoholics; and (d) those patients, men in particular, who for socioeconomic and educational reasons must perform strenuous labor for a livelihood.

7. Some tuberculous lesions will be removed because a neoplasm is suspected. In addition, concomitant tuberculosis and cancer, and the development of carcinoma in a site previously scarred by tuberculous infection, are entities that have assumed increasing importance in recent years. They require diligent observation and awareness on the part of the physician to prevent delay in the necessary resection.

8. Patients with recurrent or persistent hemoptysis,

which is often the result of an open cavity (Fig. 6), bronchiectasis, or erosion of the bronchial wall by calcified hilar lymph nodes. Emergency resection may be life-saving in a patient with massive hemoptysis.

9. Patients with pleural empyema and encapsulated unexpandable lobe or lung may need a resection as well as decortication.

Selection and Preoperative Preparation

The selection of patients for operation requires close cooperation between internist and surgeon. There is some variation of opinion regarding the timing of surgical intervention. In any event, the disease should appear stable or improving on serial x-rays. An effort should be made to convert the patient's sputum to negative before operation. This is not always possible, and undue delay carries the risk of the emergence of drug-resistant strains of bacteria. In a large number of cases, the optimal time is approximately 6 months after the institution of chemotherapy. After this period most of the reversible lesions have healed or resolved. In patients whose condition is optimal, early resectional surgery after 3 to 4 months of chemother-

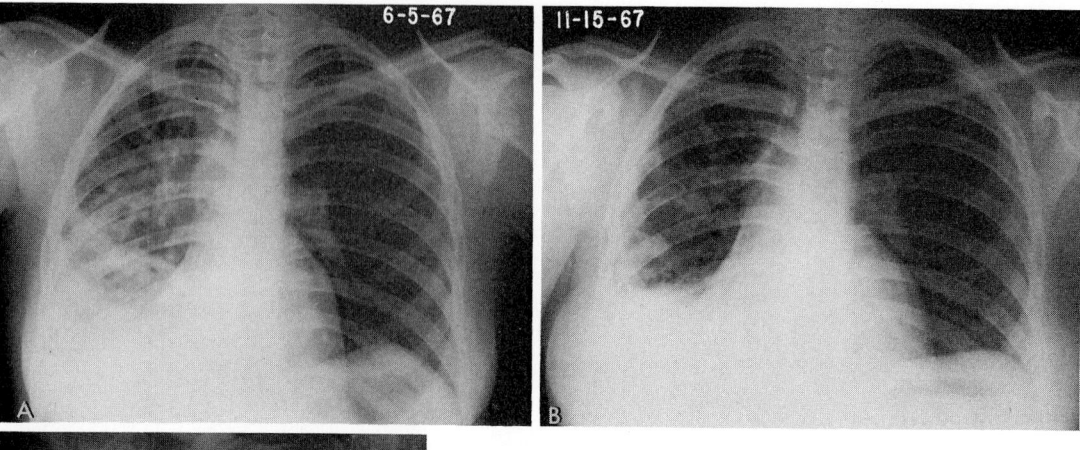

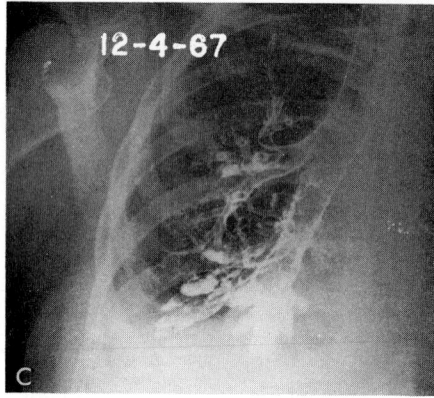

Figure 5. Lower and middle lobe tuberculosis in a 16-year-old female with resultant "bronchiectasis" despite adequate response to chemotherapy and conversion of sputum. Bilobectomy performed. (From Young, W. G., Jr., and Moor, G. F. *In* Sabiston, D. C., Jr., and Spencer, F. C.: Gibbon's Surgery of the Chest, 3rd ed. Philadelphia, W. B. Saunders Company, 1976.)

apy carries little more danger than postponement of operation and will decrease total hospital time.

Once it is seen that a patient will require surgery, a program of ambulation should be begun with improvement in general physical condition in mind. In addition to the standard preoperative evaluation, pulmonary function studies are helpful, particularly in the borderline case. Planigrams will demonstrate more clearly lesions that are to be resected. Occasionally, bronchograms are useful in demonstrating unsuspected bronchiectasis and in delineating the diseased segments. Bronchoscopy is called for in all patients to detect the unsuspected presence of bronchial stenosis, endobronchial tuberculosis, or other nontuberculous endobronchial lesions. It is wise to add a new chemotherapeutic agent to the ones already in use to protect the patient during and immediately following surgery. Pyrazinamide is an excellent drug in this context, since it is a potent although short-term drug.

The type of resection depends upon the extent of disease, as determined by preoperative x-rays, including planigrams, and palpation at the time of surgery. Wedge resection is adequate for tuberculomas and for "coin lesions" removed for diagnosis and proved by frozen section to be granulomas. Segmental resection is ideal for localized residual cavities and fibrocaseous disease. Lobectomy is perhaps the procedure of choice when the patient has active disease with positive sputum and drug-resistant bacilli. Pneumonectomy should be reserved for the patient with a destroyed

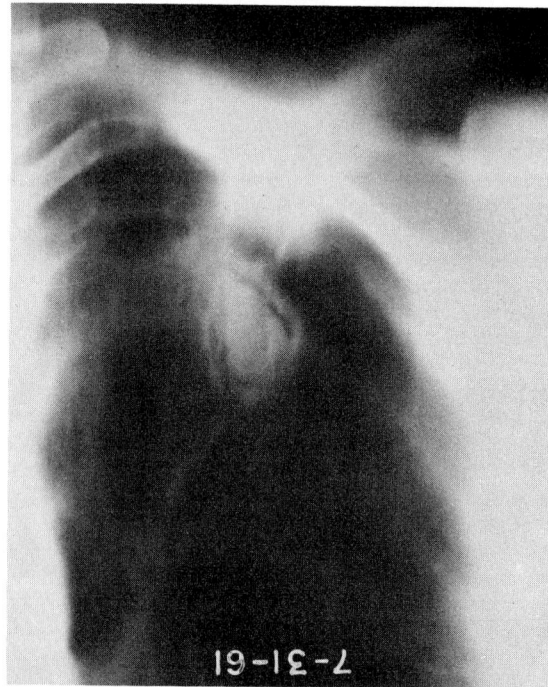

Figure 6. Residual cavitation associated with recurrent hemoptysis. The density within the cavity proved to be a "fungus ball" (aspergilloma). (From Young, W. G., Jr., and Moor, G. F. *In* Sabiston, D. C., Jr., and Spencer, F. C.: Gibbon's Surgery of the Chest, 3rd ed. Philadelphia, W. B. Saunders Company, 1976.)

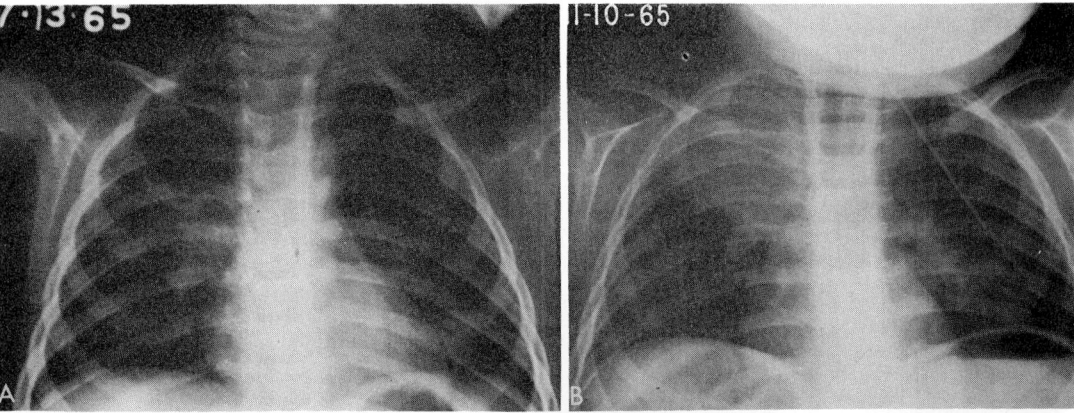

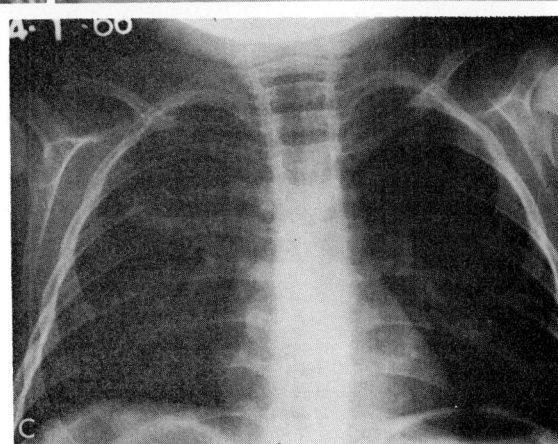

Figure 7. Pulmonary tuberculosis in a 2-year-old infant with hilar adenopathy leading to right upper lobe atelectasis. Upper lobe re-expanded and asymptomatic after prolonged chemotherapy. (From Young, W. G., Jr., and Moor, G. F. *In* Sabiston, D. C., Jr., and Spencer, F. C.: Gibbon's Surgery of the Chest, 3rd ed. Philadelphia, W. B. Saunders Company, 1976.)

lung and persistently positive sputum, recurrent hemoptysis, or secondary infection.

Resection for Childhood Tuberculosis

In the vast majority of children, standard long-term chemotherapy will cure pulmonary tuberculosis. Of almost 2000 children admitted to the Chicago Municipal Tuberculosis Sanatorium, Lees and associates[10] found that 101 (5.0 per cent) required surgery for the control of progressive primary disease or for excision of destructive residua of reinfection tuberculosis. There were two operative deaths, one late death, and no recurrence or reactivation of the disease in the 98 survivors.

The surgeon should be overly conservative, however, in advising excisional surgery for children with lobar atelectasis or obstructive emphysema accompanying the hilar adenopathy of primary tuberculosis. In the absence of secondary infection, these obstructed lobes will often return to normal as the lymph nodes regress with chemotherapy (Fig. 7), and functioning lung tissue will have been preserved.

Decortication for Pleural Tuberculosis

Although pleural effusion is still a common first sign of pulmonary tuberculosis, purulent tuberculous empyema is now rarely encountered. By the time purulent empyema becomes evident, there is usually sufficient pleural thickening and "peel" formation to produce entrapment of the underlying lung. Simple thoracentesis or even tube drainage and suction will not result in obliteration of the empyema space. For this reason, early decortication under drug coverage should be considered (Fig. 8). If complete and early re-expansion of the lung is obtained, an excellent result will ensue.

When the empyema is associated with pulmonary disease (cavitation or positive sputum or both), some form of concomitant resection will usually be required. In more complicated cases, empyema with bronchopleural fistula and secondary pyogenic infection will necessitate preliminary open drainage followed by decortication with resection (perhaps pleuropneumonectomy) and eventual thoracoplasty.

Complications of Resection

The three most important factors in the prevention of complications are (1) the correct timing of the operative procedure and early recognition of an effective chemotherapeutic program; (2) meticulous surgical technique and rapid re-expansion of remaining lung tissue; and (3) careful postoperative care.

In addition to the usual complications of thoracotomy, two major specific complications occur in tuberculous patients. These are empyema, with or without bronchopleural fistula, and bronchogenic spread of the disease. The incidence of these complications is increased when the patient has positive sputum, when

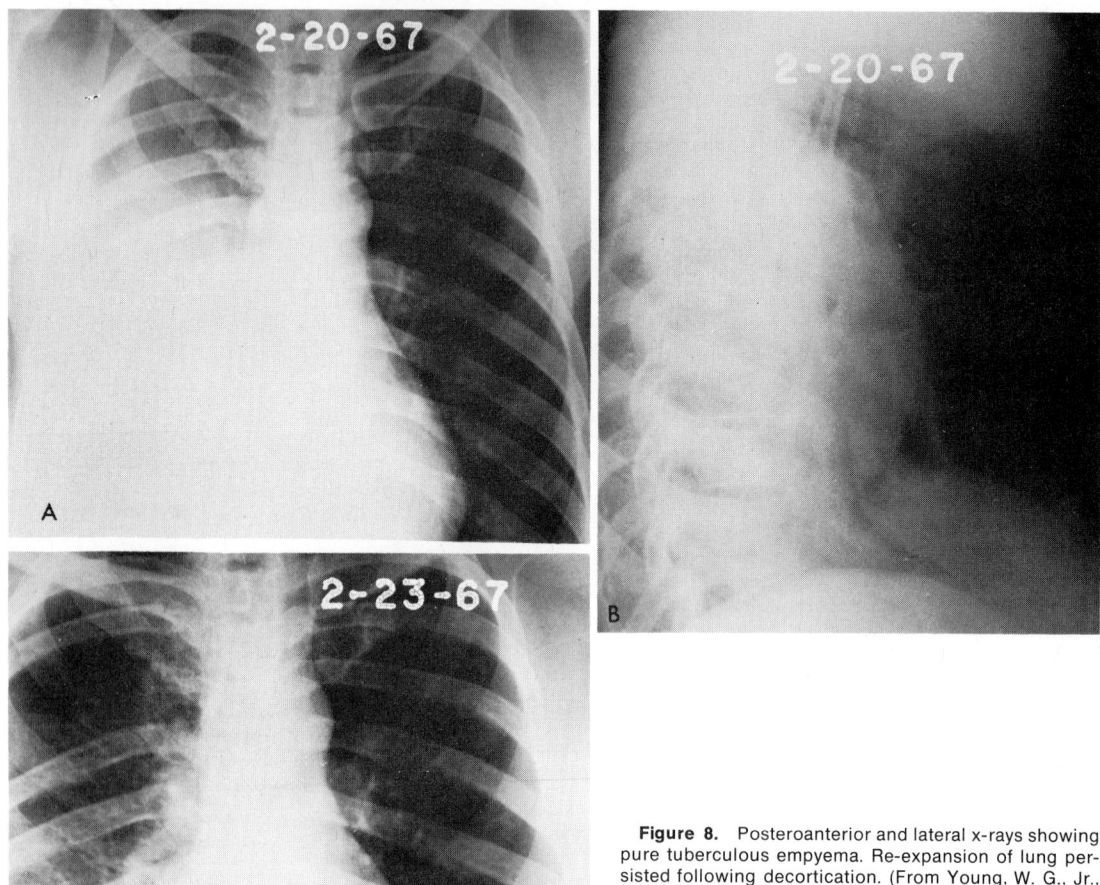

Figure 8.   Posteroanterior and lateral x-rays showing pure tuberculous empyema. Re-expansion of lung persisted following decortication. (From Young, W. G., Jr., and Moor, G. F. *In* Sabiston, D. C., Jr., and Spencer, F. C.: Gibbon's Surgery of the Chest, 3rd ed. Philadelphia, W. B. Saunders Company, 1976.)

the bacteria are drug-resistant, and when extensive resection is necessary.

Bronchopleural Fistula.   A bronchopleural fistula is said to be present if there is air or an air-fluid level in the pleural cavity. It is also present if air continues to leak via the intercostal catheter for more than 10 to 14 days and if an increasing airspace develops when the intercostal tube is clamped or removed.

The incidence of this complication has been distinctly greater in tuberculous patients than in comparable patients in whom the indication for resection was not tuberculosis. It is often the result of unsuspected or occult tuberculous disease in the bronchial stump or the result of failure of the remaining lung to fill the hemithorax. The latter is often accompanied by small alveolar air leaks. With subsequent infection of the space with tuberculous organisms, the small fistula may persist and the sputum may become positive.

It is important to differentiate between simple postresectional space problems and true bronchopleural fistulas. An asymptomatic space that demonstrates a gradual decrease in size will rarely require tube drainage and obliteration by tailoring thoracoplasty.[3] Serial x-rays will show eventual complete closure, although several months may be required. Such a benign airspace may be seen in approximately 20 per cent of cases in a series of resections. Symptomatic bronchopleural fistula will occur in 5 to 10 per cent. These cases with significant air leaks and infected pleural spaces are usually best handled by tube drainage followed by thoracoplasty to obliterate the residual space.

Spread of Tuberculosis.   This serious complication occurs in a small percentage of cases but is usually prevented by adequate added drug coverage. Spread of the disease rarely occurs if the patient's sputum is noninfectious at the time of the resection. A bronchopleural fistula, as already mentioned, may be responsible for the spread. Other factors such as techniques of anesthesia, positioning of the patient, and inefficient clearing of pulmonary secretions in the postoperative period may contribute to disease spread.

Mortality and Results

Operative mortality rates have continued to decrease during the past 15 years. In a combined study from the Veterans Administration–Armed Forces hospitals, 4126 pulmonary resections were performed between 1961 and 1966 with an overall mortality of 1.7 per cent.[12] Pneumonectomy carried a risk of 8.8 per cent (reported series vary between 2.5 and 12 per cent). The operative death rate following lobectomy was 2 per cent, segmentectomy 0.7 per cent, and subsegmental resection 0.3 per cent. It is interesting that in the Armed Forces hospitals participating in the study, 762 resections were performed with only four deaths, a mortality rate of 0.5 per cent. This would appear to represent the operative risk in a relatively young and otherwise healthy group of patients. The major fatal complications in the VA–Armed Forces study were pulmonary insufficiency or cor pulmonale and bronchopleural fistula and its sequelae.

The long-term prognosis for patients undergoing resectional therapy for pulmonary tuberculosis is excellent. A representative study, using the life-table method of analyzing results, indicates that 90 to 96 per cent of such patients will be free of disease (as determined by sputum culture and x-ray examination) at the end of a 5-year period of follow-up.[7]

SELECTED REFERENCES

Historical Aspects

Flick, L. F.: Development of Our Knowledge of Tuberculosis. Lancaster, Wickersham Printing Company, 1925.
Hochberg, L. A.: Thoracic Surgery Before the Twentieth Century. New York, Vantage Press, 1960.

Chemotherapy

Cohen, A. C.: Drug Treatment of Tuberculosis. Springfield, Ill., Charles C Thomas, Publisher, 1966.
Johnston, R. F., and Wildrick, K. H.: "State of the art" review. The impact of chemotherapy on the care of patients with tuberculosis. Am. Rev. Resp. Dis., 109:636, 1974.
Mitchell, R. S.: Control of tuberculosis. N. Engl. J. Med., 276:842, 1967.
Newman, R., Doster, B., Murray, F. J., and Ferebee, S.: Rifampin in initial treatment of pulmonary tuberculosis. A U. S. Public Health Service tuberculosis therapy trial (early results with a new drug). Am. Rev. Resp. Dis., 103:461, 1971.

Surgical Treatment

Alexander, J.: The Collapse Therapy of Pulmonary Tuberculosis. Springfield, Ill., Charles C Thomas, Publisher, 1937.
Hattler, B. G., Jr., Young, W. G., Jr., Sealy, W. C., Gentry, W. H., and Cox, C. B.: Surgical management of pulmonary tuberculosis due to atypical mycobacteria. J. Thorac. Cardiovasc. Surg., 59:366, 1970.
Neptune, W. B., Rim, S., and Bookwalter, J.: Current surgical management of pulmonary tuberculosis. J. Thorac. Cardiovasc. Surg., 60:384, 1970.
Steele, J. D.: Surgical Management of Tuberculosis. Springfield, Ill.; Charles C Thomas, Publisher, 1957.

REFERENCES

1. Alexander, J.: The Surgery of Pulmonary Tuberculosis. New York, Lea & Febiger, 1925.
2. Alexander, J.: The Collapse Therapy of Pulmonary Tuberculosis. Springfield, Ill., Charles C Thomas, Publisher, 1937.
3. Barker, W. L., Langston, H. T., and Naffah, P.: Postresectional thoracic space. Ann. Thorac. Surg., 2:299, 1966.
4. Chamberlain, J. M., Storey, C. F., Klopstock, R., and Daniels, C. F.: Segmental resection for pulmonary tuberculosis (300 cases). J. Thorac. Surg., 26:471, 1953.
5. Churchill, E. D., and Belsey, R.: Segmental pneumonectomy in bronchiectasis. Ann. Surg., 109:481, 1939.
6. Gentry, W. H.: Atypical mycobacterial infections. In Tice-Harvey Practice of Medicine. Vol. III. Hagerstown, Md., W. F. Prior Company, 1966.
7. Johnson, G., Jr., and Peters, R. M.: Pulmonary resection for tuberculosis: Life table analysis of results. Ann. Thorac. Surg., 1:634, 1965.
8. Jones, J. C.: Early experiences with resection in pulmonary tuberculosis. In Steele, J. D. (Ed.): The Surgical Management of Pulmonary Tuberculosis. Springfield, Ill., Charles C Thomas, Publisher, 1957.
9. Langston, H. T., Barker, W. L., and Pyle, M. M.: Surgery in pulmonary tuberculosis: 11-year review of indications and results. Ann. Surg., 164:567, 1966.
10. Lees, W. M., Fox, R. T., and Shields, T. W.: Pulmonary surgery for tuberculosis in children. Ann. Thorac. Surg., 4:327, 1967.
11. Medlar, E. M.: The behavior of pulmonary tuberculosis lesions; a pathologic study. Am. Rev. Tuberc., Vol. 71; part 2, 1955.
12. Mendenhall, J. T.: Report of Thoracic Surgery for Pulmonary Tuberculosis in VA–Armed Forces Study Unit Hospitals, July 1, 1965–June 30, 1966. Transactions of the 26th VA–Armed Forces Pulmonary Diseases Research Conference, Cleveland, 1967, p. 2.
13. Runyon, E. H.: Anonymous mycobacteria in pulmonary disease. Med. Clin. North Am., 43:273, 1959.
14. Seibert, F. B., and Long, E. R.: Further studies on purified protein derivative of tuberculin. Am. Rev. Tuberc., 35:281, 1937.
15. Smith, D. T., and Johnston, W. W.: Single and multiple infections with typical and atypical mycobacteria. Am. Rev. Resp. Dis., 90:899, 1964.
16. Stead, W. W.: Pathogenesis of the sporadic case of tuberculosis. N. Engl. J. Med., 277:1008, 1967.

XII ———————————————————

BENIGN TUMORS OF THE TRACHEA AND BRONCHI

Marcus L. Dillon, M.D.

Classification of benign tumors of the trachea and bronchi is fraught with several basic difficulties. First, many of these tumors have malignant neoplastic potential; second, they may be difficult to distinguish histologically from the malignant form; and third, some of the tumors are so rare that the natural history of significant numbers is unknown. In practice, the determination of whether a tumor arises from a bronchus or is malignant is frequently made after definitive removal. Peripheral lesions can seldom be differentiated radiologically from carcinoma of the lung and require removal for diagnosis. The endobronchial lesions not only may simulate carcinoma of the lung but also can be as deadly to the patient when they are associated with bronchial obstruction, distal infection, or hemorrhage. The frequency of destruction of lung tissue distal to an endobronchial lesion has led some to believe that resection of the lesion along with the distal tissue is preferable to segmental bronchial resection with anastomosis of the bronchus for benign lesions.

In the classification of tumors of the trachea and bronchi that follows, some of the tumors have considerable malignant potential, some have vascular or neurogenic origin, and some are so uncommon that the natural history is unknown, but all present clinically with features that simulate those of benign tumors of the trachea and bronchi. These lesions are listed more or less in order of frequency of occurrence.

1. Bronchial adenomas
    a. Carcinoid
    b. Salivary gland type
        1. Cylindroma (adenoid cystic)
        2. Mucoepidermoid
        3. Pleomorphic (mixed tumors)
        4. Bronchial cystadenoma (mucous gland adenoma)
2. Hamartoma
    a. Chondromatous hamartoma
    b. Congenital adenomatous malformation (diffuse hamartoma)
    c. Blastoma
3. Polyps
    a. Papillomatosis
    b. Inflammatory polyp
    c. Squamous papilloma
    d. Tumorlet
4. Vascular tumors
    a. Angiomas
        1. Hemangiomas
        2. Lymphangioma
        3. Hemangioendothelioma
    b. Pulmonary arteriovenous fistula
    c. Hemangiopericytoma
    d. Sclerosing hemangioma
    e. Pulmonary lymphangiomyomatosis (leiomyomatosis diffusa pulmonum)
5. Pseudotumors
    a. Tracheobronchopathia osteoplastica
    b. Amyloid
    c. Xanthoma
6. Granular cell myoblastoma
7. Lipomas
8. Leiomyoma
9. Fibroma
10. Chondroma
11. Neurogenic tumors
12. Myxoma
13. Plasmacytoma
14. Chemodectoma (nonchromaffin paraganglioma)
15. Clear cell tumor (sugar tumor)
16. Teratoma
17. Aberrant tissue
    a. Endometriosis
    b. Splenosis

TRACHEAL TUMORS

Benign tumors of the trachea are uncommon, but their incidence is the same as that of malignant tracheal tumors in the adult; malignant tumors of the trachea are rare in children.[8] The predominant lesions are tracheopathia osteoplastica (adult), papilloma, fibroma, hemangioma (child), and bronchial adenoma.[5] Many of the rare bronchial tumors have also been found in the trachea. Tracheal tumors have the advantage of being accessible for bronchoscopic biopsy, and, if they do not involve the tracheal wall, may be removed endoscopically. Those localized tumors which involve the tracheal wall should be removed by tracheal resection. Some of the principles of this resection are shown in Figure 1. More than 2 cm. of tracheal resection requires extended mobilization of the remaining trachea, and as much as 6.6 cm. may be removed by freeing the right hilum and inferior pulmonary ligament, transplanting the left main bronchus into the bronchus intermedius, and maintaining the head in comfortable flexion of 15 to 35 degrees;[10] additional relaxation from the larynx can be obtained

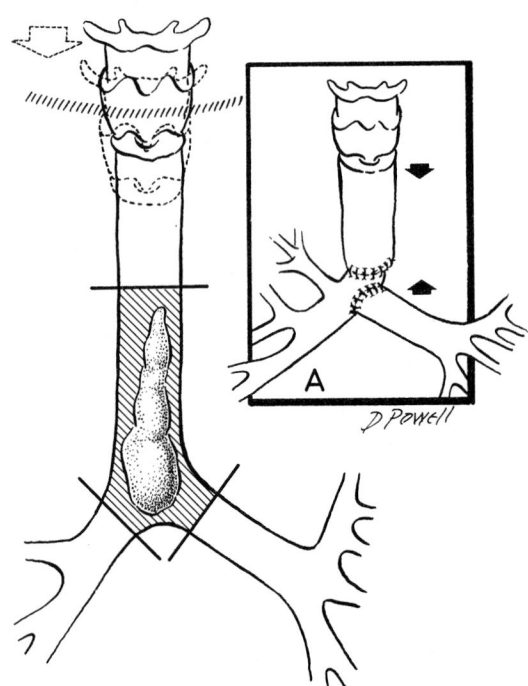

Figure 1. Diagram of a large lesion of the trachea and the extent of resection necessary for removal. Freeing of the larynx and division of the thyrohyoid and sternohyoid muscles are also represented, with displacement of the larynx inferiorly. The inset, *A*, illustrates the anastomosis of the right main bronchus, and the transposition of the left main bronchus to the bronchus intermedius.

by dividing the sternohyoid and thyrohyoid muscles transversely. Prosthetic replacement has been unsatisfactory owing to infection, disruption, and stenosis. Successful resection of all but the distal 2 cm. of the trachea has been reported; the distal tracheal stump was sutured to the back of a hole made in the sternum, which was lined by a flap of skin.

BRONCHIAL TUMORS

Clinical symptomatology of the bronchial tumors varies from none (in peripherally located lesions) to cough, dyspnea, hemoptysis, and suffocation (in proximal endobronchial lesions). The mechanisms by which the endobronchial tumors produce symptoms and changes in the lung distal to the lesion are shown

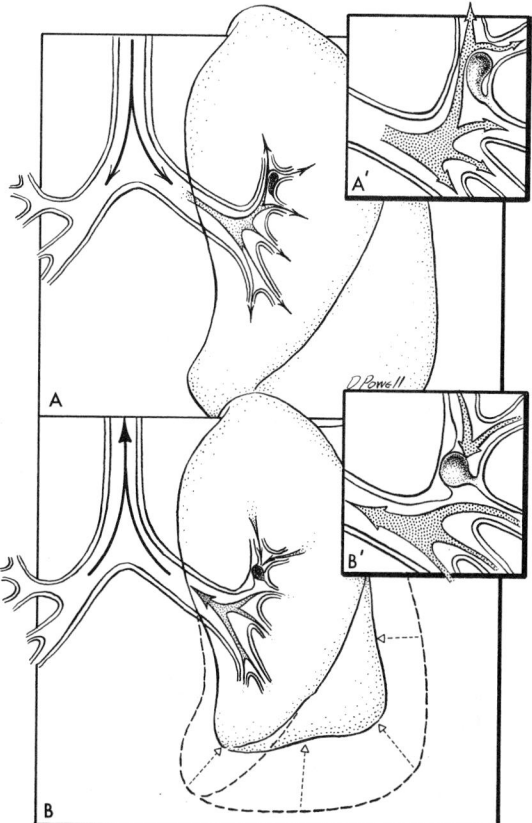

Figure 3. A, Pedunculated endobronchial tumor in the bronchus to the apical posterior and anterior segments of the left upper lobe. In the position shown, all segments are allowed to fill on inspiration. This is emphasized in A'. B, On expiration, the tumor obstructs the apical posterior and anterior segmental bronchi and prevents the segments from decreasing in size; the expiratory contraction of the left lower lobe and lingula of the upper lobe is normal. The ball valve action of the pedunculated tumor in its closed position on expiration is emphasized in B'.

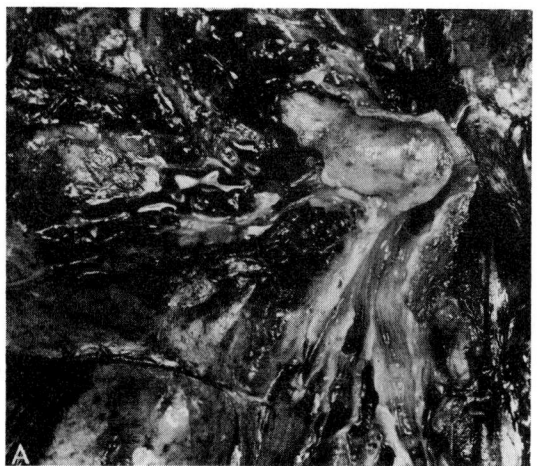

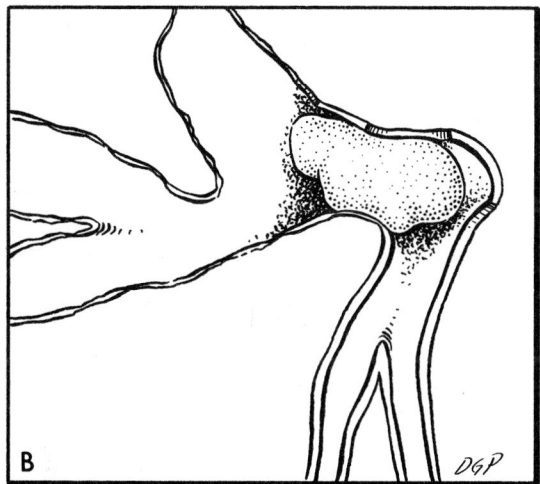

Figure 2. A, Bronchial adenoma obstructing the right upper lobe bronchus, having caused bronchiectatic changes distally in the upper lobe. The mass impinges on the lumen of the lower lobe bronchus and has not yet produced such extensive changes. This adenoma is covered by bronchial mucosa and is almost entirely endobronchial. B, Diagrammatic representation of the bronchial changes and relationships to the tumor.

in Figures 2 and 3. A partially obstructing tumor may cause localized wheezing, whereas complete obstruction of a major bronchus will cause distal atelectasis. Partial obstruction prevents adequate cleansing and contributes to recurrent distal pneumonia with necrotizing bronchitis and subsequent bronchiectasis and lung abscess. Ball valve action of a tumor will allow filling of the lung with air on inspiration and trap the air in a lobe or segment on expiration. This can be seen radiographically as lobar or segmental emphysema (Fig. 3). Involvement of the bronchial wall is frequent with the most common bronchial tumor, the bronchial adenoma. When there is bronchial wall involvement, removal of the tumor will create a defect that cannot be repaired bronchoscopically (Fig. 4). An endobronchial polypoid lesion that involves only the epithelium, as bronchial papilloma, can be removed bronchoscopically, and should be, because of the frequent recurrence in other areas (Fig. 4B).

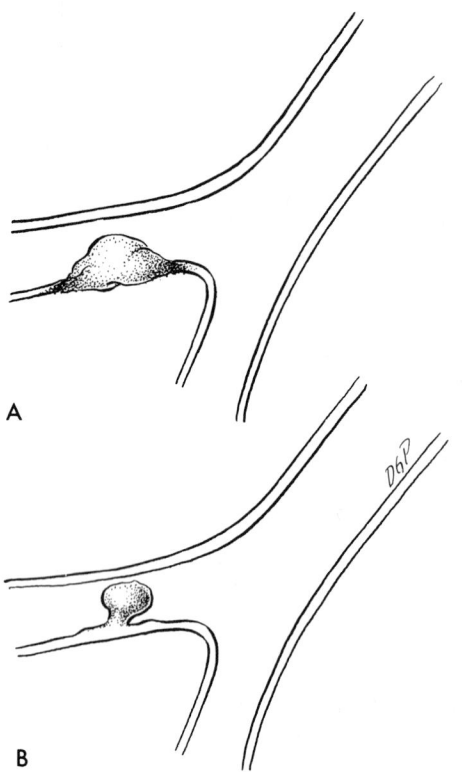

Figure 4. *A,* Involvement of the bronchial wall, common with bronchial adenomas. Complete removal of this type of tumor by endoscopy is not feasible. Pedunculated tumors not involving the wall of the bronchus, as illustrated in *B,* can at times be completely removed endoscopically.

BRONCHIAL ADENOMAS

Although Möller first described a bronchial adenoma from an autopsy in 1882, Laennec had reported a vascular bronchial polyp in 1831 that probably represented the same entity. Langston, in a critical collective review of benign endobronchial tumors, found that prior collective reviews varied greatly in tabulation, and that reclassification of tumors was common.[14] He found, after critical appraisal of the literature (prior to 1950), that it was confused, laconic, and (at times) even possibly inaccurate. It was as recently as 1965 that the first two mixed tumors of the bronchus were described by Payne, Schier, and Woolner.[23] Bronchial adenoma is the most frequently encountered benign tumor, but is rare compared to carcinoma of the lung with a 1:50 ratio. The malignant potential is reported to be 10 per cent, as determined from lymph node metastases. Approximately 80 per cent of these tumors arise from the major bronchi, and between 55 and 70 per cent are associated with distal bronchiectasis.[7] These tumors arise from the epithelium of the ducts of the bronchial mucous glands, and the carcinoid type can arise from neurosecretory cells of both the mucous glands and bronchial epithelium.[27] Payne et al. reported the incidence of the various types of bronchial adenomas to be: carcinoid, 89 per cent; cylindromatous, 8 per cent; mucoepidermoid, 2 per cent; and mixed tumors, 1 per cent.[23]

Carcinoid adenomas have the characteristic histologic appearance of carcinoid tumors in other areas.[16] Some have been found to produce ACTH and MSH, with Cushing's syndrome resulting. Calcitonin can be secreted by carcinoid adenomas as well as other nonthyroid tumors derived from cells of neural crest origin. Calcitonin overproduction by the thyroid has also been described with oat cell carcinoma of the lung, as well as calcitonin production by oat cell carcinoma. An insulin-secreting bronchial carcinoid tumor with immunoreactive insulin within the tumor has been reported. The "carcinoid syndrome," consisting of anxiety, tremulousness, temperature elevation, periorbital and facial edema, increased lacrimation and salivation, rhinorrhea, diaphoresis, explosive diarrhea, nausea and vomiting, hypotension, and oliguria, was originally attributed to the effects of serotonin produced by carcinoid tumors. As investigation continued, it was found that serotonin did not produce all of these changes, and additional factors not definitely identified, such as kinins, catecholamines, histamines, substance P, components of complement, and prostaglandins, probably contribute to producing the syndrome.[21] Carcinoid adenomas are vascular and present the real possibility of severe hemorrhage on bronchoscopic biopsy. Degeneration of the vascular component can result in calcification and ossification, which can be seen radiographically but is not a common finding. Heimburger et al. reported that two separate tumors were present in one of five patients with peripheral carcinoid adenomas at their hospital.[11] They reviewed the eleven previously reported multiple adenomas and found that they were mostly of the carcinoid type (when classified) and frequently microscopic. Spencer believes that these lesions are occasionally confused with the epithelial proliferations associated with inflammation called tumorlets and that they can be differentiated by the absence of inflammatory lesions.[27] Planned, function-preserving surgical resection produces good immediate and long-term results.[1]

Cylindromatous adenomas make up only 8 per cent of the adenomas occurring in the bronchi, but they are the most common adenomas found in the trachea. They frequently occur near the tracheal bifurcation and are vascular but seldom show necrosis or ossification. Markel and Abell (1964) described five patients with tracheal cylindroma.[20] Three were treated by partial endoscopic resection plus cobalt-60 radiation (6000 R), one had partial endoscopic resection, and one had complete endoscopic resection. Despite these inadequate resections, two of the patients were living at 8 years and 6.8 years, respectively, after operation. Three had died, one at 8 years, one at 12.5 years, and one at 13 years after treatment. Only one had distant pulmonary metastases. The authors predicted accurately that the future treatment of choice would be wide surgical excision. Cylindroma is a slow-growing, infiltrative carcinoma; however, as illustrated by this series, a 5-year survival is likely, even with less than optimal therapy, but cure cannot be expected. Cylindromas of the bronchi are best treated by resection with removal of the distal lung, which is frequently a site of infection and brochiectasis.

Mucoepidermoid adenomas usually involve the

major bronchi and frequently present as pedunculated endobronchial tumors. Reichle and Rosemond (1966)[24] reviewed the 29 reported cases and two of their own, and found no recurrences in those in whom complete resection was done. However, Welborn, Fahmy, and Gobbel (1969) reported a 28 per cent incidence of high-grade malignancy among all reported cases, with metastasis frequently by all routes.[31] Of special interest was the finding in one of their cases of an elevated urine 5-HIAA level that fell after bronchoscopic removal of the tumor. This suggests a possible relationship between tumors of mucous gland origin and those of enterochromaffin origin (carcinoid adenoma). Liebow[16] gives credit to H. F. Smetana for separating this group of adenomas and calling them "mucoepidermoid tumors" in accordance with the mucoepidermoid tumors of the salivary gland described by Stewart, Foote, and Becker.[28] A pathologic malignant counterpart was also recognized by Dr. Smetana.

Mixed tumors are so rare and so recently identified that the natural history is unknown. They have been compared to mixed tumors of the salivary gland type elsewhere in the body, in which carcinomatous transformation does occur. One patient has been reported with recurrent tumor in the stump and in nodes about the stump of the bronchus intermedius 8 years after resection. The patient was doing well 3 years after discovery of recurrence.

Mucous gland adenoma of the bronchus is a rare benign tumor that projects into the lumen and does not extend below the cartilagenous layer of the bronchial wall. It causes symptoms of hemoptysis and obstruction, and total local excision is curative.

HAMARTOMA

This term was coined by Albrecht in 1904 (from the Greek words $\alpha\mu\alpha\rho\tau\iota\alpha$ = error and $\omega\mu\alpha$ = tumor)[27] to describe tumors resulting from errors in development.

Chondromatous hamartoma characteristically presents as an asymptomatic solitary pulmonary nodule and is rarely, if ever, malignant. This is not an uncommon tumor and makes up 8 to 14 per cent of reported solitary pulmonary nodules in large series. Bateson (1965) reported that, although 80.5 per cent present as peripherally localized parenchymal tumors and 19.5 per cent present as endobronchial lesions, there is good evidence that they are similar and that the peripheral tumors arise from peripheral bronchi.[3] These tumors occur most commonly in persons between the ages of 50 to 60 years but have also been found in children. Tracheal hamartomas are rare but have been reported. Rarely has malignant change been implied. The endobronchial lesions require removal for relief of obstructive and irritating symptoms and prevention of the inevitable distal lung destruction from infection. The peripheral lesions cannot be differentiated clinically from carcinoma of the lung and require removal for diagnosis.

Diffuse hamartoma or congenital adenomatous malformation of the lung rarely presents as a clinical problem, not only because it is rare, with approximately 60 cases being reported, but also because it is usually found in premature or stillborn infants with other congenital pulmonary abnormalities. Usually a lobe or part of a lobe is involved, but it can be more extensive.[27] An adult patient with a small firm mass in the right upper lobe has been reported.

Pulmonary blastoma is a very rare tumor first described by Bernard in 1952, who believed it was benign because the patient was alive and well 15 years later. These tumors arise from embryonal lung tissue, and Spencer has found that they may ultimately metastasize by way of the bloodstream and lymphatics.[27] Only 22 cases have been reported.

POLYPS

Papillomatosis is a common laryngeal tumor of infancy and childhood. There is distal spread in approximately 2 per cent of cases, usually only to the trachea; however, bronchial and alveolar papillomatosis does rarely occur. The sex incidence is equal, and the tumor rarely occurs in adults. The incidence of recurrence has been reported to be as high as 90 per cent. The tumors tend to transplant to adjoining structures and to regress spontaneously and disappear after puberty. Local treatment of laryngeal lesions with estrogenic hormones has caused regression. Lesions have disappeared with pregnancy and reappeared after pregnancy. They have been produced experimentally in animals by mechanical and chemical irritation of the larynx and trachea. There is frequent coexistence of papillomas and warts. Papillomas have been transferred by extract to the skin of humans and the vaginal mucosa of dogs. With extracts of papillomas, Ono et al. have produced patches of growth on chorioallantoic membranes, but were unable to produce serial transplants of the growth in chick eggs.[22] Autogenous vaccine preparations from tumor tissue have prevented recurrence during the period of vaccination, with rapid reappearance between courses. Papova viruses in the crystalline lattice assembly have been found in laryngeal papilloma of a child and in the venereal warts from the mother by Boyle et al.,[4] although attempts to grow the virus in tissue culture were unsuccessful. They also demonstrated a change in a squamous papilloma after an interval of seven months to squamous cell carcinoma in an adult. Since papova viruses are DNA viruses, primarily intranuclear, and are known to be tumorigenic, the implication is one of virus-induced cancer. There is better statistical validity to the increased risk of laryngeal papillomas in children of mothers who have condyloma accuminatum. Serum complement-fixing antibodies against autologous or homologous papilloma antigens have been demonstrated in patients.[13] An interesting aspect is the finding of low serum calcium and magnesium levels in patients with laryngeal papillomas. Shilovtseva has used calcium and magnesium in treatment of rabbits with tracheal and laryngeal papillomatosis and noted a reduction in the size of papillomas.[26] In 1966, the seventh patient with bronchoalveolar papillomatosis associated with laryngeal papillomatosis was reported. Three of the seven patients have died as a consequence of their disease. Treatment of these patients may be frustrating because of the high incidence of recurrence, the frequent necessity of tracheotomy, and the need for multiple attempts at operative removal by bronchoscopy in an effort to maintain an adequate airway and prevent distal parenchymal infection over a period of many years.

Inflammatory polyps of the trachea and bronchi may be associated with laryngeal papillomatosis, chronic bronchitis, or allergic bronchitis and appear as single or multiple lesions. They are characterized by edema and inflammatory infiltration of the stalk, with squamous metaplasia of the surface. Less common is the allergic-type polyp. In the absence of squamous metaplasia, the surface is covered with ciliated columnar epithelium. In inflammatory polyps (differentiated from papillomatosis), recurrence is not common. Conservative bronchoscopic removal is the treatment of choice. Mucous polyps of the upper air passage are thought to be of this type.

Squamous papilloma is pedunculated and is usually covered with stratified squamous epithelium, often with keratinization. It occurs most commonly in the fifth to seventh decade. It is not associated with prolonged respiratory infections. Inflammatory cells are absent; however, minimal inflammation occurs if the tumor has produced obstruction with distal infection. These lesions belong to the same class of tumors as pedunculated papillomas of the skin and mucous membrane, and are localized dysplasias rather than true neoplasms. These are rare lesions.

Tumorlet is a term coined by Whitwell (1955) to describe epithelial proliferative lesions associated with chronic inflammation that resemble oat cell carcinoma morphologically but behave as benign lesions. Small peripheral carcinoids have been confused with tumorlets and are differentiated by the absence of inflammation and lung damage. Inflammatory tumorlets have been produced in rabbits by tracheal instillation of 1 per cent nitric acid. In one reported patient from whom an endobronchial tumorlet had been removed bronchoscopically, there was no evidence of recurrence at autopsy 12 years later.

VASCULAR TUMORS

Angiomas. Hemangiomatous malformation occurs in the subglottic area of the larynx and may extend into the trachea in infants. Because of the location, the consequences of these lesions can be sudden ventilatory obstruction. The lesions behave like hemangiomas of the skin in infants, with an increase in size after a month or more of life. Then, toward the later part of the first year of life, the lesions regress. The frequency of occurrence of this lesion is probably greatly underestimated, since croup is a common occurrence in infants, the engorged mass may collapse during examination and be completely missed, and, unless severe symptoms persist, examination is not done. Even at autopsy, unless they are engorged with blood they go unrecognized. Association with other vascular malformations occurs, encompassed by the term phlebarteriectasia (as telangiectases, port-wine stain, congenital arteriovenous malformations, capillary hemangiomas, and cavernous hemangiomas). Tracheotomy may be necessary to allow ventilation, along with repeated small doses of radiation to shrink the tumor. Hemangiomas may be multiple, extensive, or localized but fortunately rarely occur at the site of the usual tracheotomy.

Lymphangiomatous malformations usually present as cystic hygromas of the neck and axilla but may be associated with hemangiomas. They more frequently appear with venous hemangiomas as mixed lesions. The only case reported presenting as a solid peripheral tumor was in 1974.

Hemangioendothelioma may present histologically as part of an angiomatous malformation that contains more of the endothelial component and grossly is a more solid tumor. Hemangioendothelioma has been reported as a polypoid lesion in the trachea, treated by local excision.

Pulmonary Arteriovenous Fistula. In 1897, Churton demonstrated the lungs from a 12-year-old boy to the Leeds and West-Riding Medico-Chirurgical Society.[6] During life, the boy had a loud roaring pulmonary systolic bruit, a highly accentuated second sound, hemoptysis, epistaxis, and dropsy. Four blood-clot-filled aneurysms of the pulmonary artery in one lung and three in the other were described. The first clinical diagnosis of pulmonary arteriovenous fistula was reported in 1939, with the lesion demonstrated angiographically. The first resection was not reported until 1942, and the lesion was called a cavernous angioma. Pulsation of the whole lower lobe controlled by compression of the pulmonary artery was noted at operation. Stringer et al., in a comprehensive review, found reports of 148 patients by 1955 and emphasized that the pathologic physiology of pulmonary arteriovenous fistula is due to the shunt between pulmonary artery and vein.[30] The characteristic findings in these patients are telangiectasia, cyanosis, clubbing, exertional dyspnea, polycythemia, opacities seen in the chest x-ray, and a murmur heard over the lesion in the lung. Brain abscesses are frequent because the filtering action of the lung is bypassed. Hemoptysis is common (25 per cent) from intrabronchial rupture. The treatment is conservative surgical excision, since multiple lesions are common. The lesion is frequently found in patients with hereditary hemorrhagic telangiectasia.

Hemangiopericytoma. This is a rare lung tumor that was first described by Stout and Murray in 1942.[29] Only four tumors in the lung had been reported by 1964. The tumors are thought to originate from the pericytes (modified contractile smooth muscle cells) closely related to the capillary walls and may be benign or malignant. The diagnosis is made by removal, which also constitutes the treatment. Malignant hemangiopericytomas are somewhat radiosensitive. Of 21 cases reported through 1973, only three had metastases. Recurrences may occur years later, with the longest reported interval being 26 years.

Sclerosing Hemangioma. Sclerosing hemangiomas are unusual pulmonary tumors first described by Liebow and Hubbell in 1956.[17] They are benign tumors arising from alveolar capillary endothelial cells that do not usually involve bronchi, but do present as opacities in chest films and do cause hemoptysis as a frequent symptom. They may be multiple and may be associated with hereditary hemorrhagic telangiectasia. Localized xanthomas can be an end stage of sclerosing hemangioma.

Pulmonary lymphangioleiomyomatosis occurs almost exclusively in women from a marked proliferation of smooth muscle in the walls of the lymphatic vessels and interstitial areas of the lung. Approximately 40 cases have been reported and about 80 per cent were complicated by unilateral or bilateral chylous effusion and about 20 per cent by pneumothorax. The disease is usually progressive to death from respiratory insufficiency, with pulmonary infiltrates and honeycombing of the lungs.

PSEUDOTUMORS

Tracheobronchopathia osteoplastica is the most common benign tumor occurring in the trachea of adults. Over 20 cases have been reported.[19] It is a process of cartilagenous growth from the ecchondrosis of the tracheal rings, which ossifies and lines the tracheal submucosa with nodular projections over the rings. This can extend into the bronchi and has caused death from stenosis with distal pneumonia. Reported cases frequently represent incidental findings at autopsy or are recognized in life from routine chest films followed by bronchoscopy.

Amyloid deposits, either focal or diffuse, beneath the tracheal and bronchial mucosa occur rarely and are not associated with other amyloid lesions.[5] Amyloid also is usually an incidental autopsy finding, but it may extend into the bronchi and produce stenosis and pneumonia. Localized lesions may be removed bronchoscopically, but when there is diffuse involvement, resection is done only in those areas necessary to maintain the bronchial patency.

Xanthoma of the trachea and bronchus occurs rarely and is associated with lipoprotein disorders with fat deposits in the skin.[5] Xanthomas may arise from other pathologic processes as the end stage of sclerosing hemangioma or as maturation of a granuloma from an inflammatory process.

GRANULAR CELL MYOBLASTOMA

Granular cell myoblastoma was first described in 1926 by Abrikossoff and usually arises in the tongue, skin, or subcutaneous tissue. Forty-three have been reported of the bronchus and six have been reported of the trachea. Hormonal influence on growth has been seen in one patient, with a decrease of 50 per cent in size following delivery. They may be multiple and may occur in association with subcutaneous lesions. Local removal is adequate treatment, but because of its usual location in the large bronchi, the tumor may have caused distal pulmonary infection with destruction of the lung. Malignant forms are rare, but do occur.

LIPOMA

Lipoma of the bronchus is an uncommon benign lesion. Only 40 had been reported in the English literature by 1974; five of them had been discovered at autopsy. Bronchial lipoma was first seen bronchoscopically and successfully removed through a bronchoscope in 1927. The tumor may extend outside the bronchus and may require resection of distal lung because of bronchiectasis or pulmonary destruction from infection. Lipomas have also been reported to arise in the trachea.

LEIOMYOMA

Leiomyoma of the trachea and bronchus is a rare tumor. Of 26 cases collected by 1974 the tumor had arisen within a major bronchus in only 9. Ten tracheal leiomyomas had been reported in the English literature through 1968. One was removed by tracheal resection. Bronchoscopic removal has been used in others, but is certainly not adequate for the malignant forms. Multiple pulmonary leiomyomas have been reported in only 9 cases and must be carefully differentiated from metastatic leiomyosarcoma.

FIBROMA

Fibromas of the trachea and bronchus are rare. Leiutaud described the first tracheal fibroma in 1767, and only 37 were reported during the next 207 years. In two cases, fibroma has been reported in the trachea in children. Local excision is adequate treatment. Intrapulmonary fibromas appear in x-rays as "coin lesions" and require removal for diagnosis.

CHONDROMA

Chondroma of the bronchus is an extremely rare lesion, only seven have been reported. Four have been reported involving the trachea. It differs from a chondromatous hamartoma in that it consists of cartilage without glands or other tissue.

NEUROGENIC TUMORS

Neurogenic tumors of the lung are rare. The first bronchial neurofibroma was described in 1940, and the first excision of a solitary primary neurogenic tumor of the lung was described by Bartlett and Adams in 1946.[2] By 1951, only two benign bronchial neurogenic tumors had been reported. Schwannomatous neurofibromatous lesions have been reported to erode a bronchus. Whether the neurofibroma lesions are benign or malignant can be difficult to determine from histologic examination.

MYXOMA

Myxoma is a rare lesion described by Placitelli in 1953. In the second patient, a myxoma presented as a "coin lesion," and the patient was doing well 26 months after wedge resection. The third patient had hemoptysis and a solitary pulmonary nodule in the right lower lobe resected and reported in 1973.

PLASMACYTOMA

In 1959, Kennedy and Kneafsey reported a tracheal plasmacytoma and a right main stem bronchial plasmacytoma, which were removed locally. There was no recurrence at 4 years and at 10 months, respectively.[12] However, plasmacytoma should be considered malignant, as a variant of multiple myeloma.

CHEMODECTOMA

Chemodectomas are tumors of the chemoreceptor organs of the aorta, carotid, and jugular glomera. A glomus pulmonale has been located anatomically on the dorsal side of the main pulmonary artery. Minute, occasionally multiple glomus structures related to anastomosing pulmonary venules have been encountered in the periphery of the lung; however, their function as chemoreceptors has not been established. Of the 21 intrathoracic chemodectomas described through 1972, 10 were present in the pulmonary parenchyma. These lesions may appear benign or malignant histologically, and none has been described with abnormal physiologic function.

CLEAR CELL TUMOR

In 1963, Liebow and Castleman reported four examples of what they call benign clear cell tumors of the lung, which resemble metastases from renal carcinoma. A distinctive feature of this tumor is the immense content of glycogen, which resulted in the synonym of "sugar tumor." In a report of 12 cases in 1971, they enumerated the features which differentiate this benign tumor from metastatic renal cell carcinoma as well as from clear cell adenocarcinoma of the lung.[18]

TERATOMA

Of the 15 reported intrapulmonary teratomas, only one was endobronchial. In this patient, there was a mass in the left upper lobe surrounded by a crescent-shaped translucent area simulating a mycetoma. A left pneumonectomy was done, and the lesion was found to be an endobronchial teratoma with distal bronchiectasis.

ABERRANT TISSUE

Endometriosis of the lung was first documented by Lattes et al. in 1956 in a 34-year-old woman in whom a 1 cm. round mass developed in the right middle lobe with pregnancy.[15] She had undergone dilatation and curettage of the uterus twice in 1952, and hemoptysis

with menses had followed. On removal, the mass was found to be pulmonary endometriosis with decidual tissue. The first case of endobronchial endometriosis was reported by Rodman and Jones in 1962 in a patient with an abnormal chest film and hemoptysis during menses and a normal chest film without hemoptysis between periods.[25] This lesion was in the bronchial wall with bronchial artery supply to it.

Splenosis in the bronchus has not been reported, but Dillon et al.[9] found autotransplantation to the pleural cavity in 7 of over 75 reported cases. In their patient, who had a traumatic rupture of the spleen and diaphragm repaired 29 years previously, there was no tumor seen by chest film 22 years later. He presented with an asymptomatic mass in the left lower lung field by chest film. At thoracotomy, a 3 cm. implant was found in the parietal pleura and a 5 cm. mass imbedded in the periphery of the left lower lobe, which was removed. The mechanism of transplantation in splenosis is fragmentation of splenic tissue due to trauma, implantation at a foreign site, and development of a parasitic blood supply.

SELECTED REFERENCES

Bateson, E. M.: Relationship between intrapulmonary and endobronchial cartilage-containing tumours (so-called hamartomata). Thorax, *20*:447, 1965.
　　This article includes a rather extensive review of the literature and a detailed review of the relation of intrapulmonary and endobronchial hamartomas. It is well illustrated, and the author's argument—that they are similar lesions—is developed well.

Caldarola, V. T., Harrison, E. G., Jr., Clagett, O. T., and Schmidt, H. W.: Benign tumors and tumor-like conditions of the trachea and bronchi. Ann. Otol., *73*:1042, 1964.
　　This is a report of all benign tumors and tumor-like conditions of the trachea and bronchi encountered clinically (63 cases) at the Mayo Clinic from 1930 to 1960. It gives a thorough clinical discussion of these conditions and their frequency.

Gilbert, J. G., Mazzarella, L. A., and Feit, L. J.: Primary tracheal tumors in the infant and adult. Arch. Otolaryngol., *58*:1, 1953.
　　This is a study of one of the largest collections of primary tracheal tumors in infants and adults and has been referred to by practically all authors writing on the subject.

Grillo, H. C., Dignan, E. F., and Miura, T.: Extensive resection and reconstruction of mediastinal trachea without prosthesis or graft: An anatomical study in man. J. Thorac. Cardiovasc. Surg., *48*:741, 1964.
　　This is a study done on human cadavers to establish the maximal amount of trachea that might be removed and still permit effective reconstruction. It is pertinent and informative.

Liebow, A. A.: Tumors of the Respiratory Tract. Atlas of Tumor Pathology, Section 5, Fascicle 17. Washington, D.C., Armed Forces Institute of Pathology, 1952.
　　This fascicle has served as a study reference for 19 years. It is beautifully illustrated with both black and white and color photographs of tumors of the lower respiratory tract.

Melmon, K. L.: The endocrinologic manifestations of the carcinoid tumor. *In* Williams, R. H. (Ed.): Textbook of Endocrinology, 5th ed. Philadelphia, W. B. Saunders Company, 1974.
　　This is an excellent source giving the differences among functional carcinoid tumors in relation to their location, the biochemical substances involved, and their symptoms and treatment.

Spencer, H.: Pathology of the Lung, 2nd ed. New York, Pergamon Press, 1968.
　　This is a comprehensive reference text in the specialized study of the lung. It is especially useful as a source of both gross and microscopic pictures of all lesions of the lung except tuberculosis.

Stewart, F. W., Foote, F. W., and Becker, W. F.: Muco-epidermoid tumors of salivary glands. Ann. Surg., *122*:820, 1945.

This is an analysis of approximately 700 major and minor salivary gland tumors seen at the Memorial Hospital in New York between 1928 and 1943. The presentation of the material, utilizing color photomicrographs, is as impressive as the tabulated findings and the discussion of the various aspects of these tumors. The pathologic aspects are correlated with the clinical behavior. An understanding of the salivary-gland-type bronchial adenoma can be gained from this evaluation of salivary gland tumors.

REFERENCES

1. Baldwin, J. N., and Grimes, O. F.: Bronchial adenomas. Surg. Gynecol. Obstet., *124*:813, 1967.
2. Bartlett, J. P., and Adams, W. E.: Solitary primary neurogenic tumor of the lung. J. Thorac. Surg., *15*:251, 1946.
3. Bateson, E. M.: Relationship between intrapulmonary and endobronchial cartilage-containing tumours (so-called hamartomata). Thorax, *20*:447, 1965.
4. Boyle, W. F., Riggs, J. L., Oshiro, L. S., and Lenette, E.: Electron microscopic identification of papova virus in laryngeal papilloma. Laryngoscopy, *83*:1102, 1973.
5. Caldarola, V. T., Harrison, E. G., Jr., Clagett, O. T., and Schmidt, H. W.: Benign tumors and tumor-like conditions of the trachea and bronchi. Ann. Otol., *73*:1042, 1964.
6. Churton, T.: Multiple aneurysms of pulmonary artery. Br. Med. J., *1*:1223, 1897.
7. Condon, V. R., and Phillips, E. W.: Bronchial adenomas in children: A review of the literature and report of three cases. Am. J. Roentgenol., *88*:543, 1962.
8. Davis, C., Alexander, R. W., and DeYoung, H. D.: Splenosis: A sequel to traumatic rupture of the spleen. Arch. Surg., *86*:523, 1963.
9. Dillon, M. L., Koster, K., Coy, J., Utley, J. R., Vasquez, M., and Canlas, M.: Intrathoracic splenosis: Case report and review of the literature. South. Med. J., in press.
10. Grillo, H. C., Dignan, E. F., and Miura, T.: Extensive resection and reconstruction of mediastinal trachea without prosthesis or graft: An anatomical study in man. J. Thorac. Cardiovasc. Surg., *48*:741, 1964.
11. Heimburger, I. L., Kilman, J. W., and Battersby, J. S.: Peripheral bronchial adenomas. J. Thorac. Cardiovasc. Surg., *52*:542, 1966.
12. Kennedy, J. D., and Kneafsey, D. V.: Two cases of plasmacytoma of the lower respiratory tract. Thorax, *14*:353, 1959.
13. Klos, J., and Jezkova, Z.: A cytopathic agent in laryngeal papillomas of children. The relation of serum antibodies to the clinical course of laryngeal papillomatosis. Ann. Otol., 75:225, 1966.
14. Langston, H. T.: Benign endobronchial tumors. Surg. Gynecol. Obstet., 91:521, 1950.
15. Lattes, R., Shepard, F., Tovell, H., and Wylie, R.: A clinical and pathologic study of endometriosis of the lung. Surg. Gynecol. Obstet., 103:552, 1956.
16. Liebow, A. A.: Tumors of the Respiratory Tract. Atlas of Tumor Pathology, Section 5, Fascicle 17. Washington, D.C., Armed Forces Institute of Pathology, 1952.
17. Liebow, A. A., and Hubbell, D. S.: Sclerosing hemangioma (histiocytoma, xanthoma) of lung. Cancer, 9:53, 1956.
18. Liebow, A. A., and Castleman, B.: Benign clear cell ("sugar") tumors of the lung. Yale J. Biol. Med., 43:213, 1971.
19. Magnusson, P., and Rotemark, G.: Tracheobronchopathia osteochondroplastica. J. Laryngol. Otol., 88:159, 1974.
20. Markel, S. F., and Abell, M. R.: Adenocystic basal cell carcinoma of the trachea. J. Thorac. Cardiovasc. Surg., 48:211, 1964.
21. Melmon, K. L.: The endocrinologic manifestations of the carcinoid tumor. *In* Williams, R. H. (Ed.): Textbook of Endocrinology, 5th ed. Philadelphia, W. B. Saunders Company, 1974.
22. Ono, J., Saito, H., Igarashi, M., and Ito, M.: The etiology of papilloma of the larynx. Ann. Otol., 66:119, 1957.
23. Payne, W. S., Schier, J., and Woolner, L. B.: Mixed tumors of the bronchus (salivary gland type). J. Thorac. Cardiovasc. Surg., 49:663, 1965.
24. Reichle, F. A., and Rosemond, G. P.: Mucoepidermoid tumors of the bronchus. J. Thorac. Cardiovasc. Surg., 51:443, 1966.
25. Rodman, M. H., and Jones, C. W.: Catamenial hemoptysis due to endobronchial endometriosis. New Eng. J. Med., 266:805, 1962.
26. Shilovtseva, A. S.: The complex treatment of patients affected with papillomatosis of the larynx and trachea. Arch. Otolaryng., 89:552, 1969.
27. Spencer, H.: Pathology of the Lung, 2nd ed. New York, Pergamon Press, 1968.
28. Stewart, F. W., Foote, F. W., and Becker, W. F.: Muco-epidermoid tumors of salivary glands. Ann. Surg., 122:820, 1945.
29. Stout, A. P., and Murray, M. R.: Hemangiopericytoma, vascular tumor featuring Zimmerman's pericytes. Ann. Surg., *116*:26, 1942.
30. Stringer, C. J., Stanley, A. L., Bates, R. C., and Summers, J. E.: Pulmonary arteriovenous fistula. Am. J. Surg., 89:1054, 1955.
31. Welborn, M. B., Fahmy, A., and Gobbel, W. G.: Mucoepidermoid carcinoma of bronchus with chondroid metaplasia and elevated 5-hydroxyindoleacetic acid excretion. J. Thorac. Cardiovasc. Surg., 57:618, 1969.

XIII

BRONCHIAL ADENOMA

James W. Pate, M.D.

Episodes of frank hemoptysis, pneumonia recurring in the same area of the lung, or localized wheeze, all in an adult, strongly suggest bronchial obstruction, sometimes produced by bronchial adenoma. These are not common neoplasms, bronchogenic carcinomas being 30 to 50 times more frequent. Adenoma (ἀδέν gland and ομα tumor) implies a benign neoplasm with glandlike appearance. The term actually encompasses a group of different tumors that are not as *obviously* malignant as frank carcinoma. The group includes three clearly different neoplasms: carcinoid, cylin- droma (adenoid cystic adenoma), and mucoepidermoid adenoma. It must be recognized that there is extreme histologic and biologic variability, that most invade locally, and that some metastasize.[18] Thus, terminology is a relative and convenient convention.[7, 12] All types characteristically obstruct a bronchus and thus produce the same general pathophysiology and symptoms.[17]

A tumor that protrudes into the lumen of a bronchus partially obstructs it and therefore interferes with the smooth flow of bacterial and particulate-

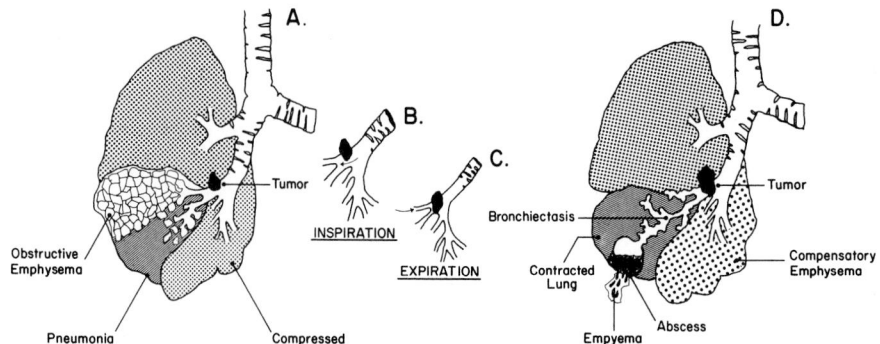

Figure 1. *A,* Bronchial adenoma with partial obstruction of bronchus; this may produce inflammatory changes and/or emphysema in distal lung. Adjacent normal lung may be compressed, adding to radiographic abnormality. *B* and *C,* On expiration, the diameter of the bronchi decreases so that a valve mechanism is common and not dependent on pedunculated or other abnormal shapes of the tumor. Therefore, obstructive emphysema is common with all forms of bronchial obstruction. *D,* Total bronchial obstruction; absorption of air results in total atelectasis, which usually results in chronic infection with bronchiectasis, pneumonitis, or abscess, which may rupture and produce empyema. With loss of volume in the obstructed area, compensatory emphysema of adjacent or, rarely, opposite lung may occur.

laden secretions from the area supplied by that bronchus. This usually leads to infection, first of the bronchus (bronchitis or bronchiectasis) and then of the parenchyma (acute, recurrent, or chronic pneumonitis). Lung abscess or empyema may follow; rarely, chronic pneumonitis simply becomes "unresolved" and leads to a fibrous mass with chronic inflammation. Partial obstruction may lead to a ball-valve effect with resultant emphysema in the involved segment (Fig. 1). The wheeze is usually more obvious on hyperventilation (as with exercise) and tends to be low-pitched, located over a large bronchus, and constant in location. Partial obstruction may persist for many years, with intermittent infections, cough, sputum production, and shortness of breath that may become severe. Total bronchial obstruction is followed by absorption of air; atelectasis replaces emphysema and results in a fibrotic, contracted lobe. Infection with either partial or total obstruction may suddenly develop into an acute tension abscess or may simply remain a chronic low-grade focus. Bronchial adenomas tend to be vascular and are frequently associated with major and repeated hemoptysis.

Radiographic examination of the chest usually reveals a smooth mass located near the hilum, but the mass may be too small to be evident.[2] Distal effects (emphysema, atelectasis, abscess, pneumonia) may predominate. Planigrams or bronchograms usually demonstrate an endobronchial mass. Bronchoscopy is almost always diagnostic and allows biopsy (which may be bloody). Except for a few patients with hormone effects, the specific type of tumor is indistinguishable on clinical grounds.

The histopathology of bronchial tumors has remained confusing and imprecise as new microscopic and behavioral characteristics are described. Sharply defined classes are artificial, since there is a *spectrum* of morphology and biologic behavior. While the two largest groups, carcinoids and cylindromas ("salivary" tumors) were described in the 1870s and 1880s, their exact origin, functions, relationships, and subgroups are not yet clear. Carcinoids appear related to oat cell

carcinoma; cylindromas are malignant; mucoepidermoid adenomas are relatives, if not parents, of mucoepidermoid carcinoma.

Carcinoids resemble cells from the neural crest which migrate to distant areas of the embryo, including the bronchi, and produce catecholamines, tryptophane derivatives, and other vasoactive compounds.[5] These cells may be the origin of bronchial carcinoids, which occur in both sexes, in most ages,[8] and with ten times the frequency of cylindromas. They are composed of small cuboid, uniform cells arranged in pseudoacini in a very vascular stroma. Variations included the "oncocytoid" type, which resembles the parathyroid oxyphilic adenoma. They are usually covered with benign bronchial epithelium, which sometimes demonstrates squamous metaplasia (leading to misdiagnosis with small biopsies). There is rarely necrosis or degeneration of stroma, although hemorrhage may be followed by calcification or even ossification. Carcinoids tend to invade, locally recur, metastasize occasionally to regional nodes, and rarely metastasize distally. They protrude in a polypoid fashion into the lumen, but, arising deep in the bronchial wall, extend into adjacent lung, where much of the tumor may be located.

These tumors are microscopically similar to intestinal carcinoids and as early as 1910 were suspected of endocrine function. Although most tumors have not been recognized to have such functions, electron microscopy has demonstrated cells of the Kulchitsky type,[3, 6] histochemistry shows elevated 5-nucleotidase and ATP activity, and there have been demonstrations of many kinins, vasoactive amines, and hormones.[14] The clinical syndromes of Cushing, "carcinoid" (gastrointestinal and/or cardiovascular), hypokalemic alkalosis, acromegaly, and hypoglycemia are reported (Toole). Similar endocrine findings occur in certain oat cell carcinomas.[16] Carcinoids may be associated with other multiple endocrine tumors or with neurofibromas, which commonly are in the same area of lung.

Biologically active agents demonstrated in these tumors have included calcitonin,[11] bradykinin, kallikrein, serotonin, histamine, growth hormone, corticotropin, parathormone, glucagon, gastrin, insulin, complement, substance P, melanotropin, antidiuretic hormone, catecholamines, and prostaglandins.

Rational therapy depends upon microscopic examination, search for metastases and other tumors, status of involved pulmonary segments (such as bronchiectasis, abscess), site, and extent of both bronchial and parenchymal involvement. Attempts at bronchoscopic removal, fulguration, and radon implantation should be reserved for the patient who cannot tolerate thoracotomy. Lobectomy or pneumonectomy may be required for total removal. Experienced pulmonary surgeons obtain good results with local bronchial resection and reconstruction in selected cases, thus preserving functioning lung tissue.[9]

Cylindromas (adenoid cystic adenomas) are of high malignant potential, sometimes referred to as adenoid cystic *carcinoma*. They are more common in the trachea[10] or large bronchi and are probably of endodermal, mucous gland origin.[16] "Cylindroma," a word coined by Billroth for orbital tumors of mixed serous and mucous cells growing in tubes, or "cylinders," is also referred to as a "salivary type" tumor. Usually, the majority of the tumor grows *outside* the bronchus. The cells are pleomorphic and dark, with frequent mitosis. They grow in a stroma of lamina propria and collagen with frequent myxomatous changes, which, with glandular mucus, give the tumor a "cartilagenous" gross appearance. These tumors metastasize more often than do carcinoids. There is a propensity for cylindromas to occur in the trachea more often then carcinoids.[15] Extensive total resection, usually lobectomy with removal of regional nodes, is indicated. Because of tracheal or main stem bronchial involvement, complicated tracheobronchial reconstruction is frequently necessary.[13] With inadequate resection, or recurrence, irradiation is indicated. The place of Cytoxan and 5-fluorouracil is not yet clear.

Mucoepidermoid tumors are variously labeled adenoomas or carcinomas. The spectrum of microscopically similar tumors includes rare, benign, polypoid mucous gland adenomas[1, 4] as well as frank epidermoid carcinomas. Behavior is similar to that of salivary gland mucoepidermoid tumors. These tumors cannot be differentiated from carcinoids and cylindromas on a clinical basis. Biopsy is necessary for diagnosis and complete resection is indicated; local removal is usually followed by recurrence or metastasis.

Rarer "adenomas" include plasmacytoma (histiocytoma), polyps (viral, papillomatous, inflammatory, and squamous polyps), and "tumorlets." *Plasmacytomas* have been reported in the trachea and bronchus, although they are usually parenchymal. Similar tumors occur more commonly in vertebrae or ribs or as part of generalized multiple myeloma. They have large, mononuclear cells with no lipid (and thus are different from xanthomas and sclerosing hemangiomas). They appear benign but infiltrate and recur and, rarely, metastasize.

Polyps (πολύσ many, πούσ foot) are pedunculated masses of mucosa, either inflammatory or neoplastic. They occur throughout the respiratory passages. Children are prone to *papillomatosis* of the larynx, which, in a few cases, involves the trachea and, less often, the bronchi. These consist of wartlike protrusions of connective tissue covered with epithelium that may be squamous or ciliated. They are usually multicentric and usually recur after removal. Papillomas are easily transplantable, frequently coincidental with cutaneous warts, and may be produced by transfer of cell-free extracts. Antibodies have been demonstrated in their hosts. Treatment is aimed at maintaining airway and bronchial toilet via bronchoscopic removal, which frequently requires multiple bronchoscopies. *Inflammatory polyps* of the bronchus are identical to the common allergic polyp of the nose or sinuses. Bronchoscopic removal is usually curative. These lesions are edematous mucosa with varying inflammatory reaction and squamous metaplasia. Similar lesions, a form of "granulation tissue," may appear about foreign bodies, particularly organic materials such as aspirated nuts or seeds, and may lead to diagnostic errors.

Squamous papillomas, analogous with cutaneous papillomas of the elderly, also occur but are of minimal clinical significance. *"Tumorlets"* are small inflammatory lesions that microscopically resemble oat cell carcinoma or carcinoids. Tumorlets, however, are associated with chronic lung disease and microscopic inflammatory reactions. An awareness of their occurrence is important in avoiding misdiagnosis.

SELECTED REFERENCES

Isawa, T., Okubo, K., Konno, K., Oshibe, M., Kidokoro, S., and Ouchi, A.: Cushing's syndrome caused by recurrent malignant bronchial carcinoid. Am. Rev. Resp. Dis., *108*:1200, 1973.
  These authors review the world's literature in regard to abnormalities of ACTH secretion and carcinoid tumors. Over 200 cases of ectopic ACTH production by tumor emphasize the location of the primary tumor in an anlagen of the foregut—lung, thymus, pancreas, and foregut. Studies of serotonin and 5HIAA are also mentioned.

Jensik, R. J., Faber, L. P., Brown, C. M., and Kittle, C. F.: Bronchoplastic and conservative resection procedures for bronchial adenomas. J. Thorac. Cardiovasc. Surg., *68*:556–65, 1974.
  The 86 per cent five-year survival of these patients obtained by use of lung-conserving operations is noteworthy as to both insight into natural history and operative techniques. A more recent editorial by the same author is found in Ann. Thorac. Surg., 19:432, 1975.

Liebow, A. A.: Tumors of respiratory tract. *In* Atlas of Tumor Pathology, Sec. 5., Fasc. 17, Washington, D.C., Armed Forces Institute of Pathology, 1952.
  This classic has excellent photographs. Although 24 years old, it offers a good starting place for study of morphology of tumors.

Spencer, H.: Pathology of the Lung, 2nd ed. New York, Pergamon Press, 1968.
  The best complete text on nontubercular pathology of the lung. As expected, it is oriented toward morphology and must be supplemented by newer chemically and clinically related material.

Toole, A. L., and Stern, H.: Carcinoid and adenoid cystic carcinoma of bronchus—collective review. Ann. Thorac. Surg., *13*:63, 1972.
  This is an excellent summary of history, morphology, histochemistry, function, and present knowledge of these tumors. Laennec's recognition in 1830, Heschl's description of adenoid cystic carcinoma in 1877, Mueller's autopsy report of 1882, and Hamprel's noting of the resemblance of bronchial and intestinal carcinoids in 1937 all lead to a detailed presentatiom of hormonal function of bronchial adenomas. Endocrinology and pharmacology are stressed.

Turnbull, A. D., Hurvos, A. G., Goodner, J. T., and Beattie, E. J., Jr.: The malignant potential of bronchial adenomas. Ann. Thorac. Surg., *14*:453, 1972.
  The observations and experience of Memorial Hospital from 1926 to 1969 are presented. The 5-year survival of slightly more than half of the patients is emphasized, although there is obvious bias in cases referred to this specialized institution.

REFERENCES

1. Allen, M. D., Jr., Marsh, W. L., Jr., and Geissinger, W. T.: Mucus gland adenoma of the bronchus. J. Thorac. Cardiovasc. Surg., 67(6):966–968, 1974.
2. Altman, R. L., Miller, W. E., Carr, D. T., Payne, W. S., and Woolner, L. B.: Radiographic appearance of bronchial carcinoid. Thorax, 23(4):433–434, 1973.
3. Bensch, K. G., Gordon, G. B., and Miller, L. R.: Studies on the bronchial counterpart of the Kulchitsky (argentaffin) cell and innervation of bronchial glands. J. Ultrastruct. Res., 12:668–686, 1965.
4. Emory, W. B., Mitchell, W. T., Jr., and Hatch, H. B., Jr.: Mucous gland adenoma of the bronchus. Am. Rev. Resp. Dis., 103(6):1407–1410, 1973.
5. Fu, Y. S., McWilliams, N. B., Stratford, T. P., and Kay, S.: Bronchial carcinoid with choroidal metastasis in an adolescent. Cancer, 33:707, 1974.
6. Gmelich, J. T., Bensch, K. G., and Liebow, A. A.: Cells of Kulchitsky type in bronchus and their relation to the origin of peripheral carcinoid tumors. Lab. Invest., 17:88–98, 1967.
7. Goodner, J. T., Berg, J. W., and Watson, W. L.: The nonbenign nature of bronchial carcinoid and cylindromas. Cancer, 14:106–119, 1963.
8. Johnson, S., Roberts, D. R., II, Oxford, B., Seidel, J. R., and Heaney, J. P.: An unusual case of bronchial adenoma in childhood. Arch. Surg., 109(6):329–331, 1974.
9. Levinsky, L., and Levy, M. J.: Tracheobronchial resection and reconstruction. A report of five cases. Isr. J. Med. Sci., 11(5):441–447, 1975.
10. Melmon, S. F., and Abell, M. R.: Adenocystic basal cell carcinoma of trachea. J. Thorac. Cardiovasc. Surg., 48:211, 1964.
11. Milhaud, G., Calmette, C., Taboulet, J., Julienne, A., and Moukhtar, M. D.: Hypersecretion of calcitonin in neoplastic conditions. Letter. Lancet, 1:462–463, 1974.
12. Payne, W. S., Schier, J., and Woolner, L. B.: Mixed tumors of the bronchus (salivary gland type). J. Thorac. Cardiovasc. Surg., 49:663, 1965.
13. Pearson, F. G., Thompson, D. W., Weissberg, D., Simpson, W. J., and Kergin, F. S.: Adenoid cystic carcinoma of the trachea. Experience with 16 patients managed by tracheal resection. Ann. Thorac. Surg., 13(1):16–29, 1974.
14. Ricci, C., Patrassi, N., Massa, R., Mineo, C., and Benedetti-Valentini, F.: Carcinoid syndrome in bronchial adenoma. Am. J. Surg., 126:671–677, 1973.
15. Roncoroni, A. J., Gene, R. J., and Fonseda, R.: Acute respiratory failure caused by a columnar cell tumor of the trachea. Resuscitation, 3(4):281–284, 1974.
16. Ryden, S. E., Silverman, E. M., and Goldman, R. T.: Adenoid cystic carcinoma of the cervix presenting as a primary bronchial neoplasm. Am. J. Obstet. Gynecol., 120:847, 1974.
17. Simpson, J. A., Smith, F., Matz, L. R., and Hodse, A. J.: Bronchial adenoma: A review of 26 cases. Aust. N. Z. J. Surg., 44(2):110–116, 1974.
18. Walker, C.: Bilateral choroidal metastases from "adenoma" of the bronchus. Br. J. Ophthalmol., 53(6):625–629, 1974.

XIV

CARCINOMA OF THE LUNG

David C. Sabiston, Jr., M.D.

During the past 50 years, primary carcinoma of the lung has increased in incidence from an obscure and rarely encountered lesion to one which is responsible for the most cancer deaths in males. This malignant tumor most often occurs in the fifth and sixth decades and currently claims the lives of one fourth of all men dying of cancer. In 1973 there were 75,933 deaths due to this disease in the United States alone, and in 1976 an estimated 93,000 new cases developed.[43] The astonishing increase in incidence during the past several decades appears to be due largely to the widespread habit of *cigarette smoking*. The most successful means of management of carcinoma of the lung is *surgical extirpation*. Although removal of a portion of the lung including lobectomy was accomplished in the 1920's, the first successful one-stage pneumonectomy for carcinoma of the lung was performed by Graham in 1933.[11] Since then, many lives have been saved by surgical management of carcinoma of the lung. In addition, irradiation has been useful in palliation, and recently the use of chemotherapy and immunotherapy has provided additional promise.

Pathogenesis

Since the sixteenth century, it has been recognized that the workers in the mines of Schneeberg, Germany, and those in nearby Joachimstal, Czechoslovakia were known to contract serious pulmonary disorders which were ultimately fatal.[7] The clinical course of a miner with this disease became quite familiar several hundred years ago and was recognized to be related to chronic exposure in the mines. The illness usually began with a chronic cough, followed by blood-streaked sputum, dyspnea, and chest pain. The miners termed this disorder *Bergkrankheit,* and they knew that this malady ultimately ended in death. The nature of the disease remained obscure until 1879 when the noted pathologist Weigert studied the condition and was the first to diagnose it as a malignant tumor. Of the 600 to 700 employed in the mines, about three quarters succumbed to carcinoma of the lung. In one study, the average estimated time of working in the mines before onset of symptoms was 17 years, and in the reported series, no patient who had been in the mines less than 13 years was found to have carcinoma. The specific etiologic agent remained unknown for a long period, since many minerals were involved, including iron, copper, silver, cobalt, arsenic, bismuth, and nickel, as well as pitchblende, which contains radium. It was estimated that during the course of 17 years a miner would have inhaled the equivalent of at least 3000 roentgens in radon gas and probably a much higher dose. The prevailing opinion today is that these pulmonary neoplasms are basically the result of radioactive particles, primarily radon, inhaled during the mining process.

Other toxic agents including chromium have also been implicated. In a recent report, an increased incidence of lung cancer eight times the normal has been described in workers exposed to chloromethyl ether. Of 14 patients who developed this lesion, 12 had oat cell carcinoma.[6]

The most important pathogenic agent in the development of carcinoma of the lung is considered to be *cigarette smoking*. In 1957, Auerbach and associates reported a painstaking and highly significant postmortem study in 117 males whose ages ranged between 22 and 88 and of whom two thirds were between the ages of 50 and 70.[1] The histories of the smoking habits in this group were carefully documented, and the entire tracheobronchial tree in each patient was studied, with more than 200 histologic sections being obtained from each. All sections were thoroughly evaluated by two or more pathologists. Of the 117 patients in the study, 34 died of bronchogenic carcinoma and *all* were smokers. Among the remaining 83 patients, all deaths were due to some condition other than pulmonary carcinoma. In this group 16 never smoked regularly or at all, 20 smoked a pack of cigarettes daily, and 47 smoked more than one pack daily. The histologic sections were studied, with four changes being evaluated: (1) basal cell hyperplasia, (2) stratification, (3) squamous metaplasia, and (4) carcinoma *in situ*. The histologic studies showed that among those who died of conditions other than lung cancer, basal cell hyperplasia, stratification, squamous metaplasia, and carcinoma *in situ* were less frequent in the group who had never smoked regularly, with a progressive increase in severity of cytologic changes in those who were moderate or heavy smokers. The same, but more extensive, changes were seen in those who died of carcinoma of the lung. These investigators concluded that the findings were fully consistent with the concept that cigarette smoking is an important factor in the causation of bronchogenic carcinoma, a position now widely held by numerous authorities. In further support of this view, another study of 6071 men aged 45 or older showed that 805 patients had bronchogenic carcinoma, *all* of whom were smokers. In a further study, the death rate for cancer of the lung per 100,000 was 3.4 in the male *nonsmoker,* 59.3 in those who smoked 10 to 20 cigarettes daily, and 217.3 in those who smoked 40 or more daily. Moreover, if a person ceases to smoke, the development of lung cancer is less likely than if smoking is continued.[14] In a study of tobacco consumption and mortality from cancer and other diseases, Dorn showed in a study of 200,000 life insurance policy-holders that regular cigarette smokers are subject to an increased risk of dying not only from lung cancer but from several other diseases as well, including cardiovascular disorders, respiratory diseases, and, to a lesser extent, other ailments.[5]

The fact that carcinoma of the lung can be produced experimentally in the dog is pathologic evidence that it is related to smoking. With a tracheostomy, dogs can be made to smoke cigarettes for prolonged periods through the tracheostomy stoma. Under these circumstances, metaplasia occurs in the tracheobronchial epithelium, later followed by a noninvasive carcinoma and finally by frank carcinoma, including metastases to lymph nodes.[13] A photomicrograph of such a lesion is shown in Figure 1. Moreover, the continuous topical application of irritants such as benzanthracene to the tracheobronchial tree also leads to the development of carcinoma.[48]

Pathologic Aspects

A variety of classifications have been advocated for primary carcinoma of the lung, and one of the most useful is (1) squamous cell (epidermoid), (2) adenocarcinoma, (3) undifferentiated or anaplastic carcinoma (including small cell, large cell, and "oat cell" carcinoma), and (4) bronchoalveolar carcinoma. Some place "giant cell" carcinoma in a separate group.[37]

Squamous Cell Carcinoma. The most common type is squamous carcinoma, with an incidence varying from 40 to 70 per cent of the total lesions. This type is characteristically associated with a history of prolonged smoking. In fact, squamous cell carcinoma of the lung is rarely seen in nonsmokers, and in one series of lung neoplasms, squamous cell lesions constituted only 1 per cent.[3] Histologically, this tumor characteristically produces keratin with the presence of intracellular bridges (Fig. 2). In the poorly differentiated forms of squamous cell carcinoma, the cytology merges imperceptibly into a pattern of anaplastic carcinoma. Most squamous cell carcinomas are centrally located in larger bronchi, and these tumors frequently metastasize to the hilar, mediastinal, and supraclavicular lymph nodes. While squamous cell carcinoma usually spreads to distant organs, it metastasizes less frequently to the brain and bone than does adenocarcinoma. Squamous tumors also have a tendency to be large, often with late discovery, and also have a propensity to undergo central cavitation due to necrosis of the tumor.

Adenocarcinoma. In most series, adenocarcinoma occurs in 5 to 15 per cent of the total group. These lesions are more apt to be in the periphery of the lung and are seen more often in females (Fig. 3). Adenocarcinoma has a tendency to metastasize to the liver, brain, bone, and adrenals in addition to lymph nodes.

Undifferentiated Carcinoma. Carcinomas with an undifferentiated cell type include those which have been previously characterized as small or round cell (Fig. 4), large cell (Fig. 5), and "oat cell" lesions (Fig. 6). In most series, this type represents 20 to 30 per cent of the total and are highly malignant lesions.

Bronchiolar Carcinoma (alveolar cell carcinoma). This lesion is now recognized as a distinct histologic as well as biologic type of primary carcinoma of the lung. While controversy still exists concerning its cellular origin, the clinical course and pathologic homogeneity are sufficient to allow it separate classification (Fig. 7). The lesion is associated with a more favorable prognosis in comparison with other types of primary lesions. In one large series, approximately two thirds of the patients seen with this disorder were *resectable* at the time of examination, with a five-year survival of 48 per cent.[30]

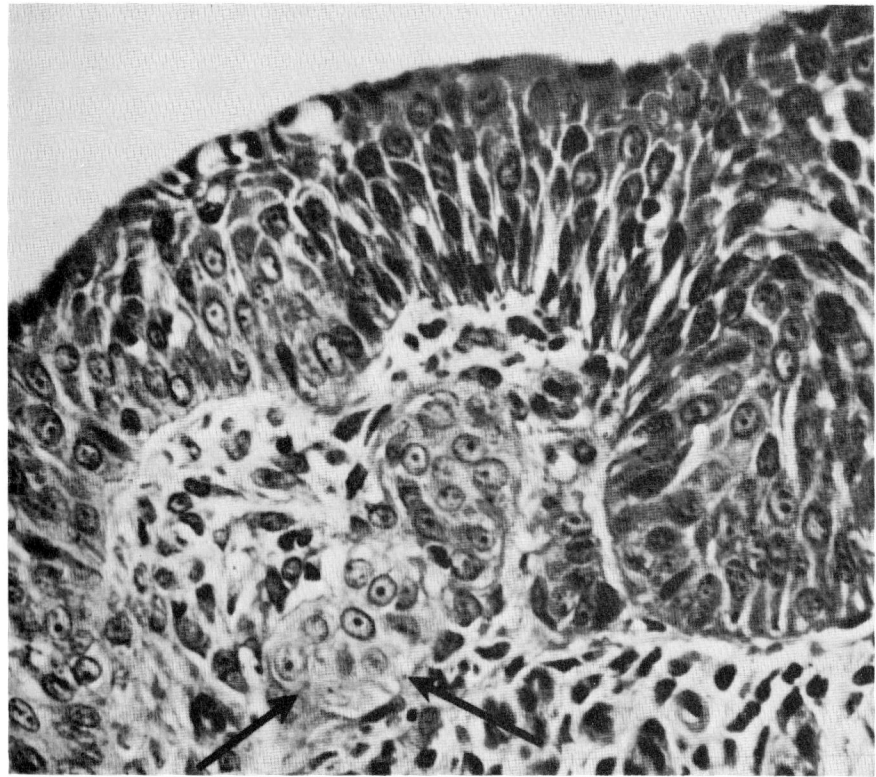

Figure 1. Invasive squamous cell carcinoma from bronchus of dog which had smoked 6210 cigarettes. The arrows indicate the area of invasion (hematoxylin-eosin ×560). (From Hammond, E. C., Auerbach, O., Kirman, D., and Garfinkel, L.: Effects of cigarette smoking on dogs. Cancer, 21:78, 1971. By permission of authors and the American Cancer Society, Inc.)

Some authors emphasize that *giant cell carcinoma,* a variant of bronchogenic adenocarcinoma, is deserving of a separate classification owing to its aggressive clinical behavior and bizarre pathologic features. Its incidence varies from 1 to 10 per cent of the total lesions.[37]

In 1938, Friedrich first described pulmonary carcinoma developing in *scars* secondary to other lung diseases.[8] A number of authors have since reported such changes occurring in the scars of tuberculosis, trauma, infarcts, pneumoconiosis, and other inflammatory lesions. Various theories have been proposed to explain the development of cancer in scars, including the fact

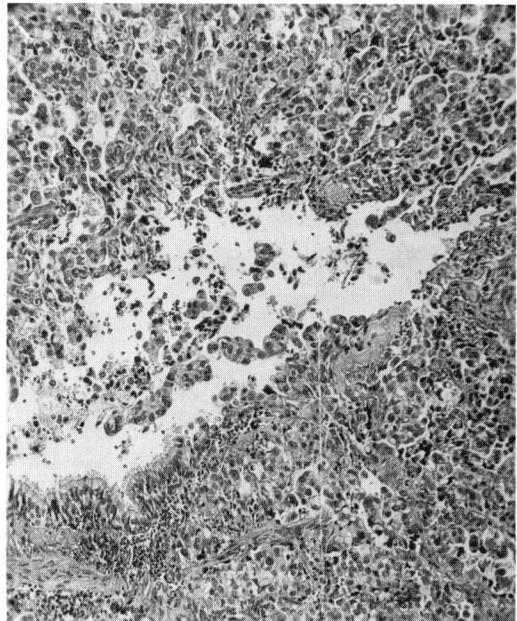

Figure 2. Photomicrograph of squamous cell carcinoma of the lung. (From Nealon, T. F., Jr., and Ching, N. P. H.: The lung, the trachea, and the pleura. *In* Nealon, T. F., Jr. (Ed.): Management of the Patient with Cancer, 2nd ed. Philadelphia, W. B. Saunders Company, 1976.)

Figure 3. Photomicrograph of adenocarcinoma of the lung. (From Nealon, T. F., Jr., and Ching, N. P. H.: The lung, the trachea, and the pleura. *In* Nealon, T. F., Jr. (Ed.): Management of the Patient with Cancer, 2nd ed. Philadelphia, W. B. Saunders Company, 1976.)

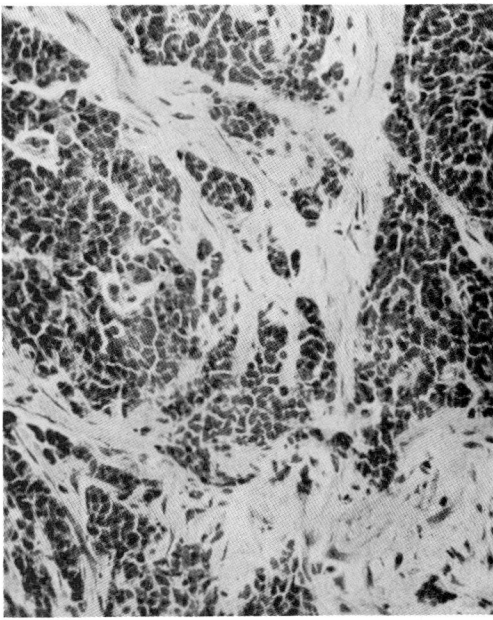

Figure 4. Photomicrograph of anaplastic small cell carcinoma of the lung. (From Nealon, T. F., Jr., and Ching, N. P. H.: The lung, the trachea, and the pleura. *In* Nealon, T. F., Jr. (Ed.): Management of the Patient with Cancer, 2nd ed. Philadelphia, W. B. Saunders Company, 1976.)

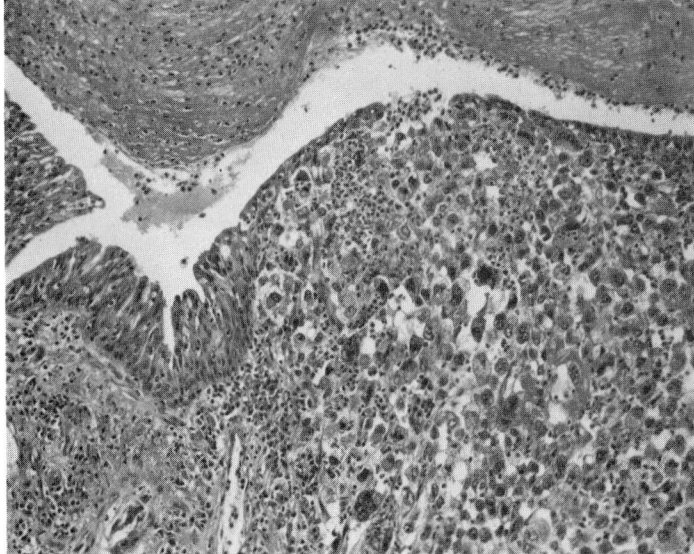

Figure 5. Photomicrograph of anaplastic large cell carcinoma. (From Nealon, T. F., Jr., and Ching, N. P. H.: The lung, the trachea, and the pleura. *In* Nealon, T. F., Jr. (Ed.): Management of the Patient with Cancer, 2nd ed. Philadelphia, W. B. Saunders Company, 1976.)

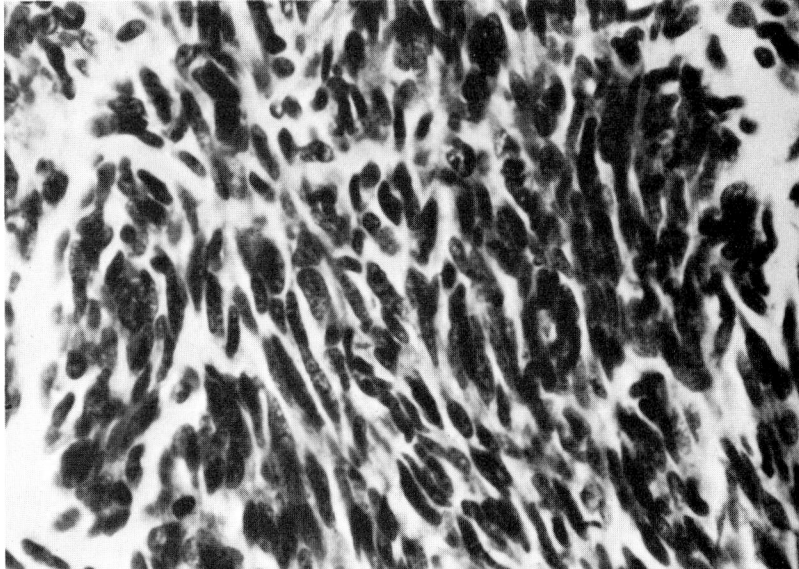

Figure 6. Photomicrograph of oat cell carcinoma.

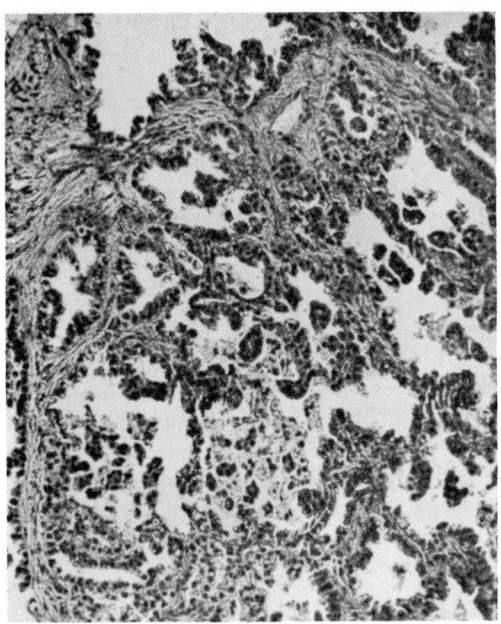

Figure 7. Photomicrograph of alveolar cell carcinoma of the lung. (From Nealon, T. F., Jr., and Ching, N. P. H.: The lung, the trachea, and the pleura. *In* Nealon, T. F., Jr. (Ed.): Management of the Patient with Cancer, 2nd ed. Philadelphia, W. B. Saunders Company, 1976.)

that blockage of the lymphatics by scar tissue causes concentration of a carcinogen-containing anthracotic pigment in the area of the lesion ultimately producing a malignant change.[47] In one report of 32 cases of cancer associated with pulmonary scars, it was shown that most are bronchoalveolar in type.[40] Despite the use of the term "scar carcinoma," there is yet no proof of this condition, since the pulmonary changes may have been due to carcinoma of the lung from the outset.

Dual primary bronchogenic carcinoma has been a subject of considerable interest and some controversy. In a recent study of 2664 patients with bronchogenic carcinoma, 34 were considered to be genuine dual primary lesions. Of these, five occurred simultaneously and 29 had a significant interval between the appearance of the two lesions.[36] Eight of the tumors were on the same side and 26 were contralateral.

Clinical Manifestations

The manifestations in patients with carcinoma of the lung range from those who are *asymptomatic* to those whose signs and symptoms are dependent upon several significant features of the disease, including (1) the anatomic location of the primary tumor, (2) the extension of the tumor into surrounding structures, (3) the presence of metastases, and (4) systemic effects due to hormonal syndromes produced by the neoplasm.[19] It is well recognized that there is clearly a symptomless phase of carcinoma of the lung. Tumors have been traced retrospectively in earlier chest films in which the lesion was present but not noted for five or more years before onset of symptoms. In one study of operable patients, a lesion was present an *average of*

three years before surgical extirpation.[38, 39] The presence of cough, hemoptysis, anorexia, and weight loss with a lesion on the chest film constitutes the most frequent clinical presentation and is highly suggestive of primary bronchogenic carcinoma (Table 1).

Cough. The commonest clinical manifestation of carcinoma of the lung is *cough,* which occurs in 75 per cent or more of patients. Most lesions which produce cough are located in major bronchi and produce irritation by neoplastic erosion of the mucosa. Sputum production often accompanies cough, and its character is dependent upon the degree of infection accompanying the lesion.

Hemoptysis. One of the most alarming symptoms to the patient is *hemoptysis,* and it is frequently the reason which prompts consultation with a physician. It is interesting that, in reported series, this symptom varies from 6 to 51 per cent, although in most series it occurs in approximately a third of patients. Occasionally, hemoptysis may be massive and constitute a surgical emergency.

Chest Pain. Approximately half the patients with carcinoma of the lung complain of chest pain when first seen by a physician. It is often described as a "heaviness," and if severe and constant pain is present, it is a poor prognostic sign, since it often signifies direct invasion of nerves and bone. Shoulder pain may be associated with an apical (Pancoast) pulmonary tumor.

Dyspnea. Some degree of shortness of breath is common in patients with carcinoma of the lung, and *wheezing* occurs in a few patients, usually the result of a large lesion producing bronchial obstruction.

Pleural Effusion. Pleural effusion may be present and if aspirated and followed by recurrence is a poor prognostic sign. Blood-stained fluid also indicates the direct involvement of the pleura with metastases. The superior vena caval syndrome occurs in about 5 per cent of patients and generally is indicative of extensive spread of the tumor to the mediastinum. Radiation therapy produces a favorable response in about half of these patients.

TABLE 1. Initial Symptoms of 2000 Patients with Bronchogenic Carcinoma*

	VA Lung Cancer Group (1969–1972)
Cough	74%
Weight loss	68%
Dyspnea	58%
Chest pain	49%
Hemoptysis	29%
Lymphadenopathy	23%
Bone pain	25%
Hepatomegaly	21%
Clubbing	20%
Superior vena cava	4%

*From Hyde, L., and Hyde, C. I.: Clinical manifestations of lung cancer. Chest, *65*:299, 1974.

Clubbing. Clubbing of the fingers is present in some 10 per cent of patients. It occurs more frequently in patients with *squamous* lesions and may disappear rapidly following removal of the tumor. Hypertrophic pulmonary osteoarthropathy has been found in 4 to 12 per cent of patients.[52] This lesion produces symmetrical proliferative subperiosteal osteitis with new bone formation and most frequently affects the distal segments of the shafts of the long bones. Chronic synovitis may cause joint pains and lead to the diagnosis of rheumatoid arthritis. It is interesting that prompt relief of this pain often immediately follows resection of the tumor. Also, vagotomy proximal to the hilum may relieve the pain of pulmonary osteoarthropathy even without resection of the primary lesion. Of interest is the fact that among 60 patients with bronchogenic carcinoma and hypertrophic pulmonary osteoarthropathy, *none* had oat cell carcinoma.[52]

Hoarseness occurs occasionally (1 to 8 per cent) and is usually the result of involvement of the recurrent laryngeal nerve with direct invasion or metastatic tumor. *Cervical lymph node* metastases occur in 15 to 20 per cent, and if scalene nodes are palpable, the likelihood that tumor is present is about 85 per cent.[10] *Dysphagia* is occasionally present (1 to 5 per cent) and usually indicates that the lesion has directly involved the esophagus. *Hepatomegaly* may be present, and at *death* approximately 35 per cent of patients have liver metastases and 25 per cent have osseous metastases. Rarely, pneumothorax occurs following penetration of the tumor through the visceral pleura.[41]

Hormonal aspects of bronchogenic carcinoma include lesions which produce clinical endocrinopathies such as adrenal hyperfunction, inappropriate diuresis, hypercalcemia, and the carcinoid syndrome. The most common hormonal manifestation is a type of Cushing's syndrome, often associated with an "oat cell" lesion. *Antidiuretic hormone* can be produced, especially from a poorly differentiated or adenocarcinoma and may produce clinical signs of mental confusion or coma with marked hyponatremia (100 to 120 mEq.). Such patients can be managed by reduction of fluid intake to less than 1000 ml. per day in order to maintain appropriate levels of serum sodium. *Parathormone* may also be secreted by bronchogenic tumors, usually squamous cell lesions, and produce symptoms of hypercalcemia, including mental confusion. Other hormonal manifestations include *hypoglycemia,* the carcinoid syndrome, and gynecomastia associated with excessive gonadotropin production.[33]

Neuromyopathies occur in patients with bronchogenic carcinoma (usually "oat cell") and may be present in as many as 15 per cent. The manifestations are divided into those of *muscular* origin consisting of a clinical picture of polymyositis and those of *neurological* origin demonstrating sensory and motor loss as well as cerebellar degenerative changes. Psychiatric manifestations may also be present.[31]

A special and well-recognized site for bronchogenic carcinoma involves the apex of the lung *(superior sulcus tumor of Pancoast).* In this position, the tumor can infiltrate the upper mediastinum and involve the cords of the brachial plexus and cervical sympathetics. Symptoms include pain in the shoulder and arm as well as in the axilla, the inner aspect of the upper arm, and in the scapular region. A Horner's syndrome may be present on that side.

Physical Findings

In many patients with carcinoma of the lung, the physical signs are esssentially absent. If bronchial obstruction is present, a wheeze may be heard in the involved area. A reduction in the intensity of breath sounds is common, and in the presence of pleural effusion signs of dullness and diminished breath sounds occur. Careful palpation of the supraclavicular, cervical, and axillary areas may reveal the presence of metastases in the lymph nodes. Evidence of weight loss, possible liver enlargement due to metastases, and painful joints may also be present.

Specific *diagnostic methods* for the definitive diagnosis of carcinoma of the lung include chest films, tomograms, sputum cytology, bronchoscopy, bronchial biopsy, bronchial brushings, and bronchial washings. Employing a combination of these, more than 75 per cent of patients can be demonstrated to have a definite histologic diagnosis of carcinoma of the lung prior to surgery.[26]

Chest Films. While carcinoma of the lung may assume a variety of roentgenographic manifestations, it most commonly presents as a mass arising in the hilar region. In other patients, a pneumonic infiltrate may be present, with or without cavitation. A pleural effusion may be present, as well as evidence of paralysis of the phrenic nerve with an elevated diaphragm on the affected side. Osteolytic lesions may be seen in the ribs or other bones as evidence of metastases. Collapse of a lobe or segment may occur with an obstructing bronchial lesion. The radiographic features of several different types of bronchogenic carcinoma are shown in Figures 8 through 16.

The perfusion *lung scan* is also useful in determining the extent of invasion of the tumor. If the scan shows a defect *larger* than the lesion itself, more than three quarters of such patients will be found to have involvement of the *regional lymph nodes,* whereas among patients in whom the scan defect is approximately *the size of the lesion,* less than a quarter will have an extension of the disease into the mediastinum.[29]

Mediastinoscopy is the direct inspection of the mediastinal structures by a small incision in the suprasternal fossa with passage of a mediastinoscope along the anterior course of the trachea. Generally, lesions arising in the proximal bronchi are more apt to be associated with the presence of mediastinal metastases. In other words, a peripheral lesion does not usually metastasize to the mediastinum *early* in the clinical course.[18] Many favor a short anterior thoracotomy in preference to mediastinoscopy, since it is simple and permits a thorough assessment of operability for hilar lesions.

Direct diagnostic *thoracoscopy* may be done, particularly in the diagnosis of effusions that do not contain malignant cells. The visceral pleura of the lung, the parietal pleura, and the diaphgram as well as pericardium can be inspected directly with a fiberoptic mediastinoscope passed through a small thoracotomy incision.[27]

Differential Diagnosis. The differential diagnosis of bronchogenic carcinoma includes pulmonary infections such as pneumonia, pulmonary abscess, tubercu-

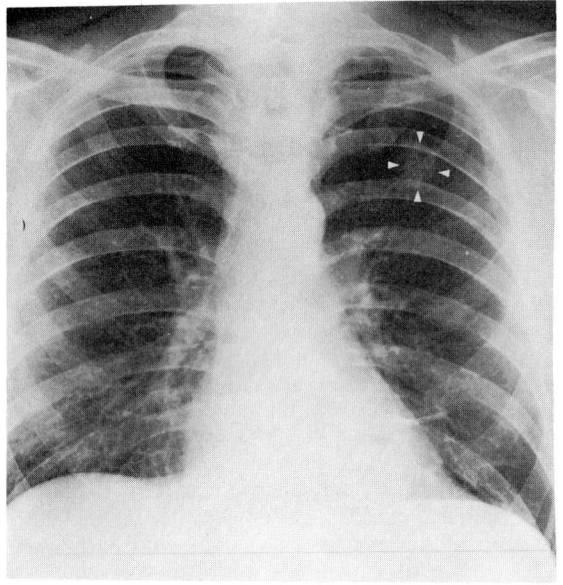

A

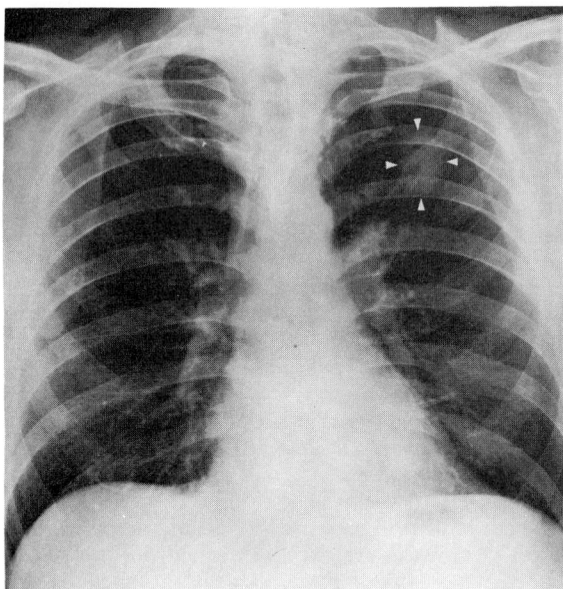

B

Figure 8. Growth of peripheral bronchogenic carcinoma: Serial films. *A,* There is a poorly defined noncalcified nodule in the left upper lobe (arrowheads). *B,* Six months later there is a marked increase in the size of the nodule (arrowheads). The diameter of the nodule is 50 per cent greater, indicating tripling of the tumor volume. Doubling of tumor volume within three months to a year suggests a malignant lesion. (From Teplick, J. G., and Haskin, M. E.: Roentgenologic Diagnosis. A Complement in Radiology to the Beeson and McDermott Textbook of Medicine, Vol. 1, 3rd ed. Philadelphia, W. B. Saunders Company, 1976.)

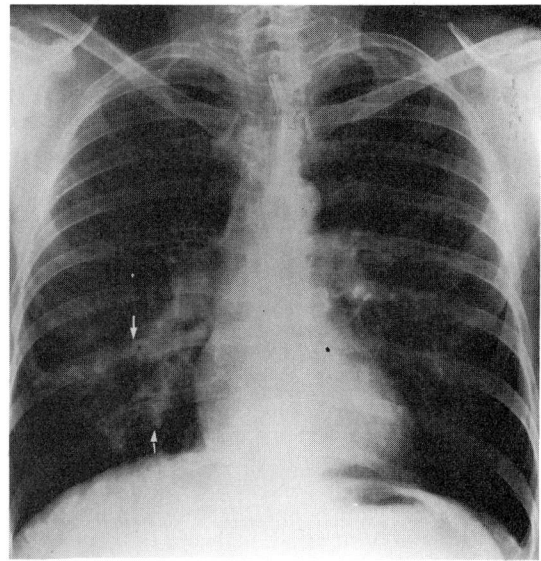

Figure 9. Bronchogenic carcinoma: Pneumonic picture. Pneumonic consolidation (arrows) with irregular borders persisted with little change over six weeks. It was a small carcinoma in the segmental bronchus. Persisting, recurring, or unresolved pneumonia, especially in a patient over 40 years of age, should be investigated. (From Teplick, J. G., and Haskin, M. E.: Roentgenologic Diagnosis. A Complement in Radiology to the Beeson and McDermott Textbook of Medicine, Vol. 1, 3rd ed. Philadelphia, W. B. Saunders Company, 1976.)

losis, histoplasmosis, and other fungal infections. Cultures for routine, anaerobic, acid-fast, and fungal organisms are quite helpful in establishing the diagnosis as well as specific sensitivity skin tests. In addition, metastatic lesions from a distant primary tumor can produce roentgenographic changes suggestive of primary bronchogenic carcinoma. Rarely, primary lymphosarcoma of the lung simulates bronchogenic carcinoma, the usual picture being a homogeneous mass that may enlarge to fill almost the entire lung field.

Surgical Management

In those patients without evidence of distant metastases or invasion of extrapulmonary structures within the chest, surgical exploration is indicated. In the majority of lesions, *lobectomy* is the treatment for most bronchogenic carcinomas. Pneumonectomy is required for complete removal of the lesions involving the left or right main bronchi or those with spread or fixation of the tumor to the hilum. For carcinomas occurring in the periphery of the lung, especially in patients with reduced pulmonary reserve or those who are high *risks* for other reasons, local ("wedge") excision can be an entirely satisfactory procedure.[45] Most surgeons favor a *posterior* thoracotomy (the so-called "standard" thoracotomy) through the fifth or sixth intercostal space for pulmonary resections, since it provides excellent exposure. However, an *anterior thoracotomy* through the third interspace is quite useful, particularly in selected patients with reduced pulmonary

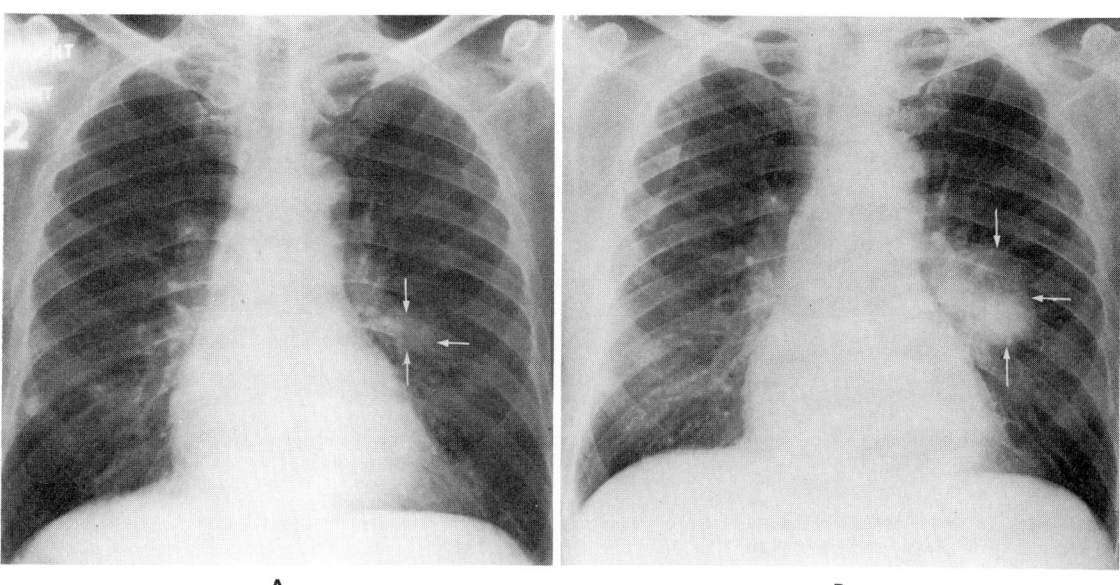

A   B

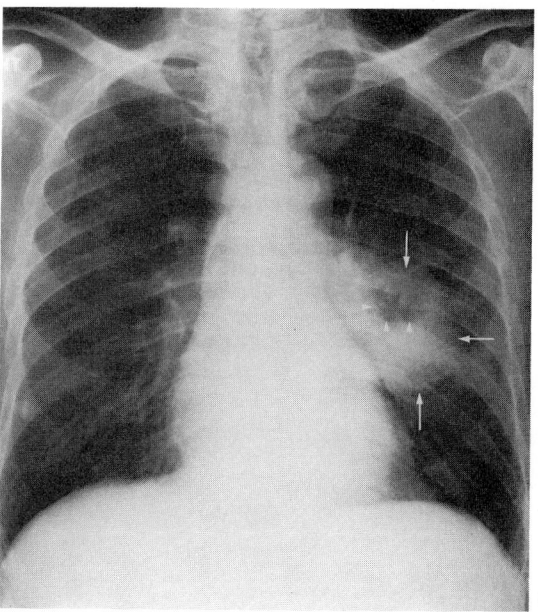

C

Figure 10. Bronchogenic carcinoma: Progressive growth and cavitation. *A,* There is a small density in the lower left hilum (arrows). The patient was asymptomatic and refused surgery. *B,* Six months later there is a marked increase in the size of the mass (arrows). The mass was lobulated but still well demarcated. *C,* Two months later the mass is even larger (arrows), and has undergone central necrosis (arrowheads). Irregularity of the cavity, with protruding nodular densities, is characteristic of a cavitating bronchogenic carcinoma. (From Teplick, J. G., and Haskin, M. E.: Roentgenologic Diagnosis. A Complement in Radiology to the Beeson and McDermott Textbook of Medicine, Vol. 1, 3rd ed. Philadelphia, W. B. Saunders Company, 1976.)

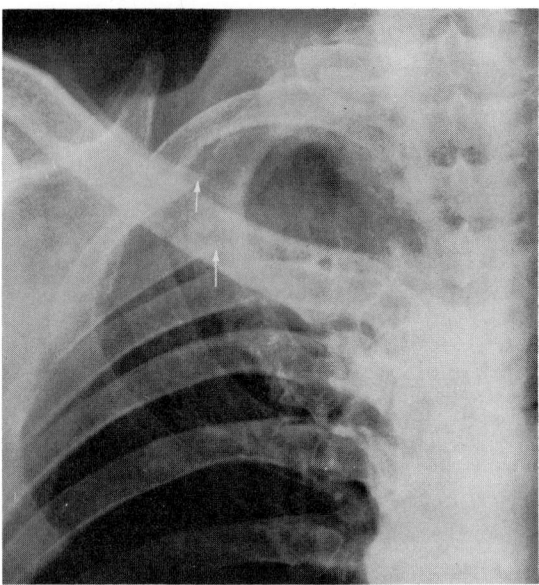

Figure 11. Superior sulcus tumor. The posterior portions of the third and fourth ribs (arrows) have been destroyed. The innocuous-appearing density in the right apex is due to an infiltrating anaplastic carcinoma that has destroyed the ribs. Tumors in the apical sulcus frequently simulate benign pleural thickenings, but rib erosion and the clinical symptoms of intractable shoulder pain and Horner's syndrome should aid in diagnosis. A superior sulcus lesion (Pancoast's tumor) may be either a squamous cell bronchogenic tumor or an anaplastic lesion. (From Teplick, J. G., and Haskin, M. E.: Roentgenologic Diagnosis. A Complement in Radiology to the Beeson and McDermott Textbook of Medicine, Vol. 1, 3rd ed. Philadelphia, W. B. Saunders Company, 1976.)

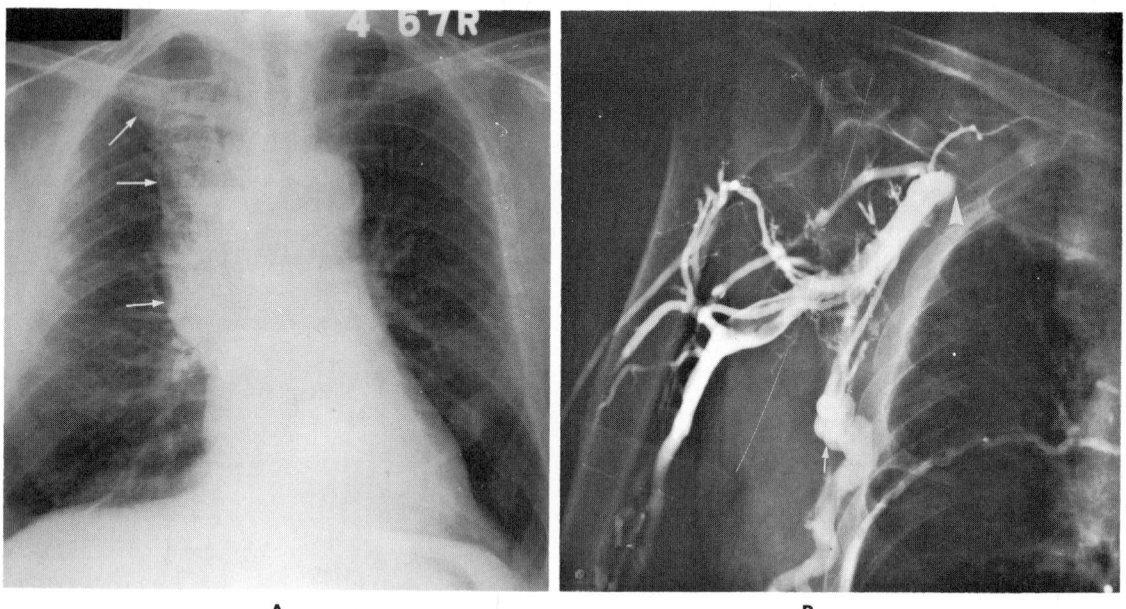

A B

Figure 12. Bronchogenic carcinoma: Superior vena caval obstruction. *A*, There is enlargement of the right hilum and widening of the mediastinum on the right (arrows) due to mediastinal extension of a bronchogenic carcinoma. There was clinical evidence of superior vena caval obstruction. *B*, Venogram reveals complete blockage of the subclavian vein (arrowhead). There are large dilated and anastomotic channels (arrow) extending between the superior vena cava and subclavian vein. In the presence of such findings, the lesion is inoperable. (From Teplick, J. G., and Haskin, M. E.: Roentgenologic Diagnosis. A Complement in Radiology to the Beeson and McDermott Textbook of Medicine, Vol. 1, 3rd ed. Philadelphia, W. B. Saunders Company, 1976. By permission of Dr. Arlyne Shockman, Veterans Administration Hospital, Philadelphia.)

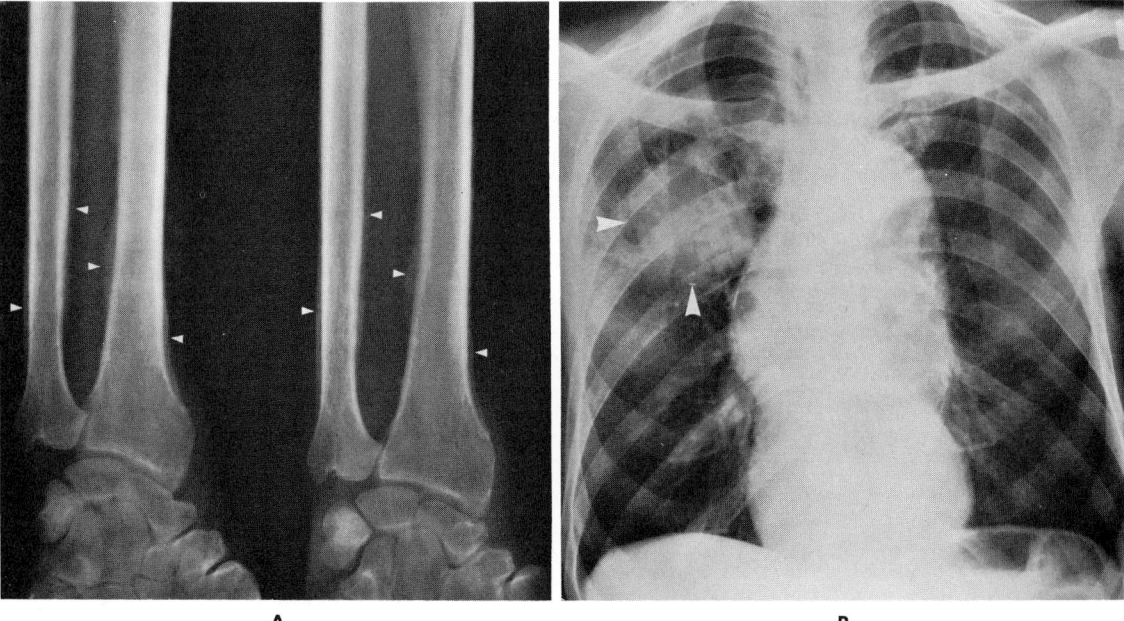

A   **B**

Figure 13. Bronchogenic carcinoma: Pulmonary osteoarthropathy. *A,* There are linear irregular areas of subperiosteal new bone formation in the distal radius and ulna (arrowheads). *B,* Large bronchogenic carcinoma is apparent in the right upper lobe (arrowheads). Following resection, periosteal reaction cleared completely. Evidence of pulmonary osteoarthropathy may occasionally be the first clue to bronchogenic carcinoma. (From Teplick, J. G., and Haskin, M. E.: Roentgenologic Diagnosis. A Complement in Radiology to the Beeson and McDermott Textbook of Medicine, Vol. 1, 3rd ed. Philadelphia, W. B. Saunders Company, 1976.)

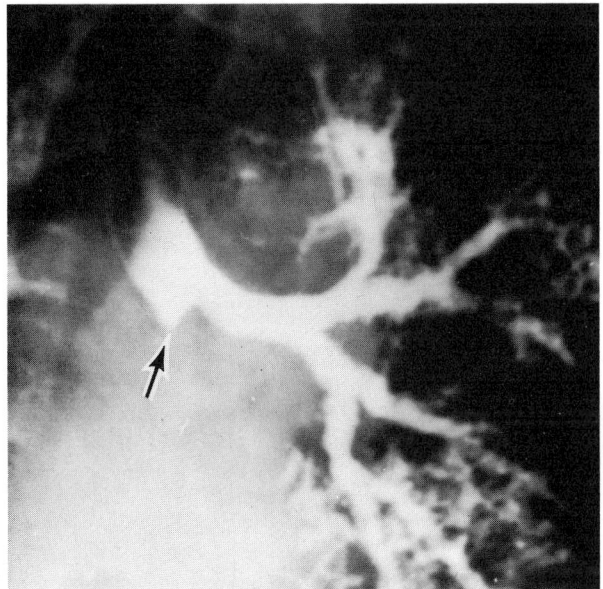

Figure 14. Bronchogenic carcinoma: Bronchogram. The dorsal branch of the left lower lobe bronchus is completely occluded (arrow) by a bronchogenic carcinoma. In a patient with a mass suspicious of bronchogenic carcinoma, bronchography will often confirm the diagnosis with evidence of narrowing or occlusion of a bronchus in the vicinity of the mass. (From Teplick, J. G., and Haskin, M. E.: Roentgenologic Diagnosis. A Complement in Radiology to the Beeson and McDermott Textbook of Medicine, Vol. 1, 3rd ed. Philadelphia, W. B. Saunders Company, 1976.)

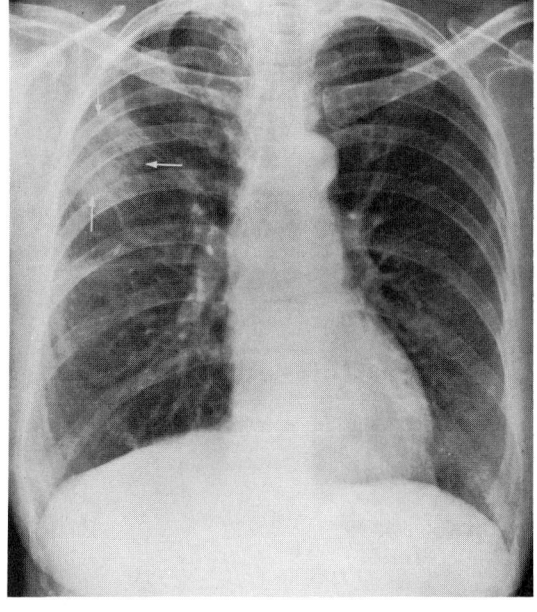

Figure 15. Alveolar cell carcinoma. Chest film in a 55-year-old woman demonstrates an ill-defined density with an indistinct lower border (arrows) in the right upper lobe. The hilar nodes are not enlarged. This picture simulated pneumonitis but proved to be an alveolar cell carcinoma. (From Teplick, J. G., and Haskin, M. E.: Roentgenologic Diagnosis. A Complement in Radiology to the Beeson and McDermott Textbook of Medicine, Vol. 1, 3rd ed. Philadelphia, W. B. Saunders Company, 1976.)

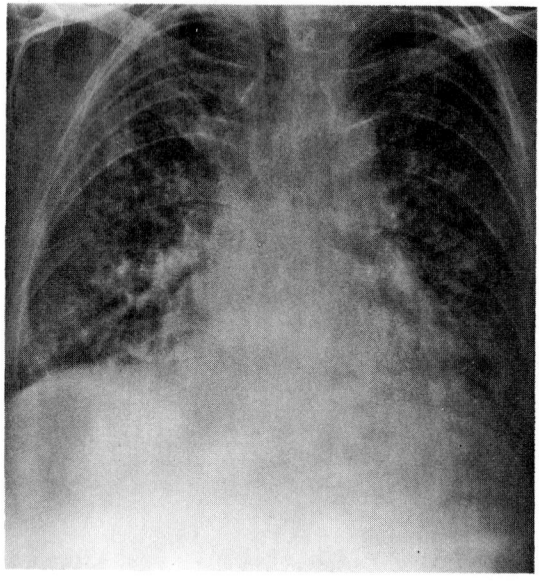

Figure 16. Diffuse alveolar cell carcinoma. There are diffuse irregular nodular infiltrates in both lung fields similar to the pattern of certain granulomatous diseases. These findings in an elderly female should suggest alveolar cell carcinoma as a possible diagnosis. (From Teplick, J. G., and Haskin, M. E.: Roentgenologic Diagnosis. A Complement in Radiology to the Beeson and McDermott Textbook of Medicine, Vol. 1, 3rd ed. Philadelphia, W. B. Saunders Company, 1976.)

reduced owing to the patient's position on the operating table; in addition, much of the lung on the side being resected is collapsed. Thus, the *anterior* thoracotomy should be borne in mind and used when appropriate.

In the technique of pulmonary resection, the use of the automatic stapling device has become an important feature and provides a more secure bronchial closure (Figs. 17, 18, and 19). With its use the postoperative complication of bronchopleural fistula is quite uncommon,[17] and experimental studies have demonstrated that bronchial healing is better with metal staples than with sutures.[42] In most resections of a lobe or a wedge excision, one or two catheters are left in the pleural cavity for drainage of blood, fluid, and possible air leak and are left in place until drainage ceases.

Evidence of Inoperability at the Time of Surgical Exploration. At the time of exploratory thoracotomy, spread of the tumor involving the parietal pleura, pericardium, heart, or other mediastinal structures is generally a sign of incurability. The presence of distant metastases to lymph nodes, liver, bones, or adrenals obviously prevents a curative resection. Similarly, the superior vena caval syndrome, paralysis of the recurrent laryngeal and phrenic nerves, and the presence of a bloody pleural effusion are contraindications. Involvement of the chest wall sometimes occurs, and most such patients are not curable. However, long-term survivors have been reported with *en bloc* resection of the tumor and chest wall, which is an acceptable means of therapy.[9, 12] Several studies have shown the importance and usefulness of the American Joint Committee's system of Staging and End Result Reporting in the long-term survival of these patients (Table 2).[49]

reserve or those who are otherwise high risks, since ventilation is much better achieved during the operation with this approach. In the *posterior* approach, the volume of thorax on the side opposite the incision is

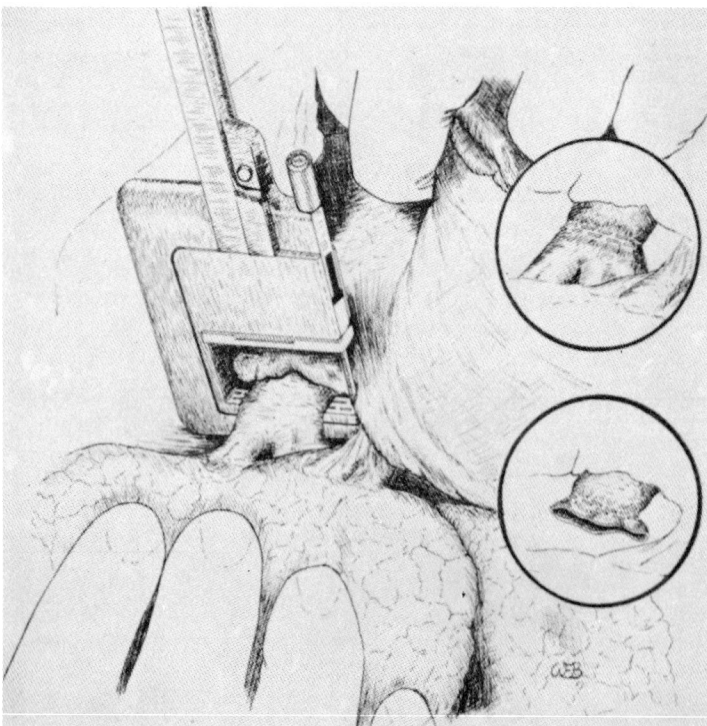

Figure 17. The main bronchus is being occluded with an automatic stapling device. (From Hood, R. M., Kirksey, T. D., Calhoon, J. H., Arnold, H. S., and Tate, R. S.: The use of automatic stapling devices in pulmonary resection. Ann. Thorac. Surg., *16*:85, 1973.)

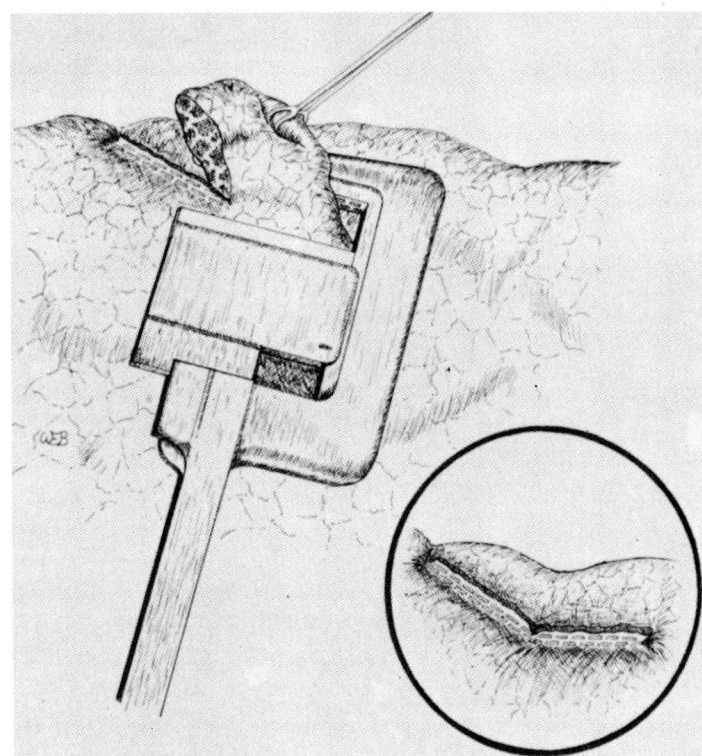

Figure 18. Stapling device for wedge resection. (From Hood, R. M., Kirksey, T. D., Calhoon, J. H., Arnold, H. S., and Tate, R. S.: The use of automatic stapling devices in pulmonary resection. Ann. Thorac. Surg., 16:85, 1973.)

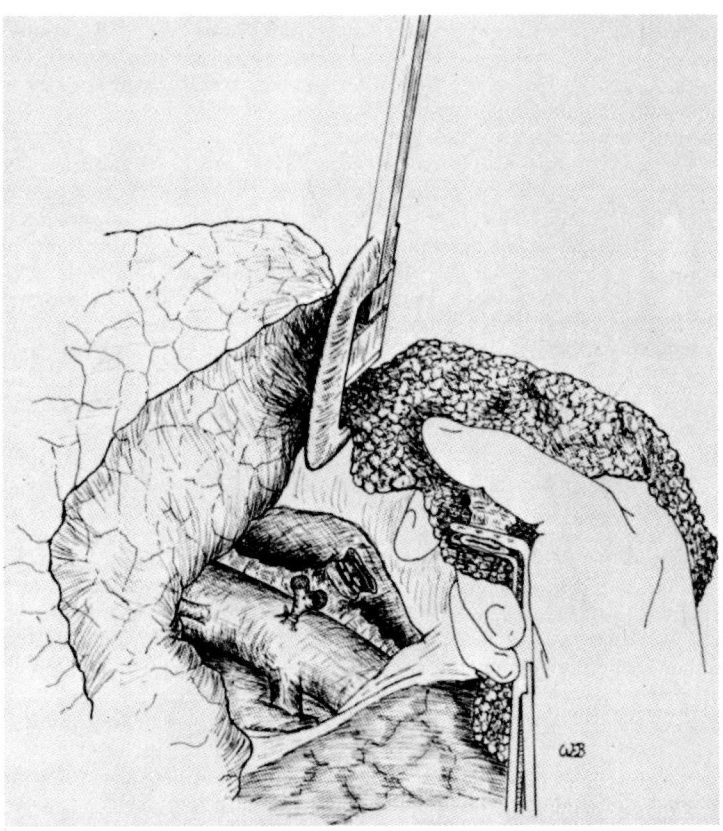

Figure 19. Use of the automatic stapling device for closure of an incomplete pulmonary fissure during lobectomy. (From Hood, R. M. Kirksey, T. D., Calhoon, J. H., Arnold, H. S., and Tate, R. S.: The use of automatic stapling devices in pulmonary resection. Ann. Thorac. Surg., 16:85, 1973.)

TABLE 2. Stage Grouping in Carcinoma of the Lung*

Occult Carcinoma	
$T_x N_0 M_0$	An occult carcinoma with bronchopulmonary secretions containing malignant cells but without other evidence of the primary tumor or evidence of metastasis to the regional lymph nodes or distant metastasis.
Invasive Carcinoma Stage I	
$T_1 N_0 M_0$	A tumor that can be classified T_1 without any metastasis or with metastasis to the lymph nodes
$T_1 N_1 M_0$	in the ipsilateral hilar region only, or a tumor that can be classified T_2 without any metastasis
$T_2 N_0 M_0$	to nodes or distant metastasis.
Stage II	
$T_2 N_1 M_0$	A tumor classified as T_2 with metastasis to the lymph nodes in the ipsilateral hilar region only.
Stage III	
T_3 with any N or M	Any tumor more extensive than T_2, or any tumor with metastasis to the lymph nodes in the
N_2 with any T or M	mediastinum or with distant metastasis.
M_1 with any T or N	

*Reprinted by permission of the American Joint Committee for Cancer Staging and End Results Reporting, Chicago, Ill.

Palliative resection may be undertaken in certain instances, especially when the tumor has produced severe bronchial obstruction or a frank abscess distal to the lesion. In other instances, severe hemoptysis provides the basis for a palliative resection to remove the primary lesion and the source of hemorrhage.

Operative Risk. Pulmonary function studies, a history of cardiac disease, and advanced age are known *risk* factors. Combinations of these are associated with a very high mortality, and in one study in patients whose maximal breathing capacity was below 59 per cent of the predicted normal, age over 69, and who had an abnormal electrocardiogram, the surgical mortality was 56 per cent.[4] The mortality of pneumonectomy is generally less than 10 per cent in most series and is frequently less than 5 per cent. Most deaths following pulmonary resection are due to cardiac complications. The mortality for lobectomy is 2 to 5 per cent.

Radiation Therapy. In most centers, megavoltage or telecobalt irradiation has been adopted, and the dosage is generally 4000 to 6000 rads given in four to six weeks when an attempt is made for cure.[44] With these dosages, minimal skin reaction and only rare spinal cord injury or radiation-induced pericarditis occur. Somewhat more frequently, esophagitis and pneumonitis are complications. For those patients with Stage I and II of the disease, who either cannot tolerate a resection due to diminished pulmonary reserve or who refuse surgery, a curative dose of irradiation should be employed. For patients with Stage III of the disease, the attempt should be limited to those in whom the tumor is confined to the involved hemithorax and can be encompassed in a 10×15 cm. portal. For those patients with Stage III disease with more extensive local spread or distant metastases, radiation should be used only in amounts sufficient to achieve palliation.

Preoperative irradiation has been advocated by some, but it is generally not employed, since randomized studies indicate that it offers little if any advantage in surgically resectable lesions. Moreover, there is no evidence that survival is lengthened in *inoperable* cases treated with radiotherapy.[50]

Occasionally, *interstitial* irradiation is employed, which may be accomplished by the placement of radioactive agents such as ^{125}I into hollow needles and inserted into the tumor mass.[15] Generally, this form of therapy is restricted to those patients in whom pulmonary resection is not possible either due to the tumor's precarious location or because of limitations imposed by the patient's marginal pulmonary reserve.

Paulson and associates have presented evidence that preoperative irradiation combined with extended radical resection in selected patients with bronchogenic carcinoma in the *superior pulmonary sulcus* yields an operability rate of 67 per cent with 34 per cent survival at 5 years and 29 per cent at 10 years.[35] This finding has not been confirmed by others.[24]

Chemotherapy has also been used in managing bronchogenic carcinoma. In a cooperative study, 2348 patients had curative resections followed by cyclophosphamide, methotrexate, mechlorethamine hydrochloride singly or in combination. The five-year survival was 24.8 per cent for the treated group and 26.2 per cent for the controls. At 10 years the figures were 13.5 per cent for the treated and 16.3 per cent for the control group.[46] On the other hand, favorable results have been reported with the use of long-term, intermittent adjuvant chemotherapy (mitomycin-C and chromomycin-A) for bronchogenic carcinoma.[22]

Immunologic Aspects of Patients with Bronchogenic Carcinoma. Depressed cellular immunity is clearly associated with a *poor* prognosis in patients with all types of malignant tumors and has led to speculation that the poor survival generally experienced with lung cancer may be related to defects in this mechanism. Immunocompetence in patients with bronchogenic carcinoma has been clearly demonstrated in both delayed cutaneous hypersensitivity skin testing[51] and *in vitro* assays of lymphocyte function.[2] Patients with depressed cellular immune mechanisms have a shorter survival and a shorter disease-free interval than those who are demonstrated to be immunocompetent. In patients sensitized to 2,4 dinitrochlorobenzene (DNCB), an antigen to which they have not been previously exposed, cancer patients with solid tumors react much less frequently (64 per cent) than do normal controls

(95 per cent). Furthermore, the cancer patient's ability to be sensitized to DNCB is associated with a *favorable* prognosis, and in nonreactive patients the prognosis is generally quite *poor*. Wells studied 75 patients with lung cancer, none of whom were receiving radiation or chemotherapy and none having had a weight loss of more than 10 per cent since onset of the disease. In evaluating delayed sensitivity, 95 per cent in each group reacted positively to at least one of the three standard microbial antigens when compared with 25 patients with benign lung disease. Conversely, cutaneous reactivity to DNCB was markedly depressed in the 75 cancer patients, particularly in those with nonresectable lesions. In a follow-up at one year, a positive correlation was found between DNCB reactivity and survival, observations which have been confirmed by others.[16] These patients also have depressed circulating levels of T-lymphocytes.[32]

Immunotherapy and chemotherapy have been employed in selected groups in order to improve long-term survival of patients with carcinoma of the lung and metastases. In one study an abstract of BCG was administered and was followed by histologic and radiographic regression in 28 per cent.[23] In another study, *Corynebacterium parvum* was given in combination with multiple drug chemotherapy in treating metastatic disease and an improved response rate occurred.[20]

Results

The poor prognosis associated with the *natural history* of bronchogenic carcinoma is demonstrated by a large study of more than 3800 patients in which those who were *untreated* had a 95 per cent mortality within one year.[34] It is usually stated that of each 100 patients with a diagnosis of carcinoma of the lung, half are found to be *inoperable* from the outset. Of the 50 per cent upon whom exploratory thoracotomy is performed, half of these (or 25 per cent of the original group) will be found to have such extensive disease that an operation for "cure" cannot be performed. Thus, the remaining 25 per cent are candidates for a *curative resection*. Of this group, 25 to 35 per cent are alive at the end of five years. However, for the series as a whole, the overall survival is only 8 to 10 per cent.

Most observers agree that the major factor which influences survival in patients with carcinoma of the lung is the extent of the tumor at the time of operation. When metastases to lymph nodes occur, the survival is significantly diminished. Generally, the *cell type* bears little relationship to survival except for the poor prognosis associated with small (oat cell) carcinoma and the improved survival which occurs with alveolar cell carcinoma.[46] In a recent study of patients undergoing what was regarded at operation as a *curative* resection, five- and 10-year survival rates were 36 per cent and 14 per cent, respectively.[25] In those patients *without* nodal metastases, the five-year survival was 49 per cent, and 31 per cent if the *hilar* nodes alone were positive. Moreover, patients with solitary peripheral lesions less than 4 cm. in diameter have a 45 per cent five-year survival after resection.[21]

SELECTED REFERENCES

Katsuki, H., Shimada, K., Koyama, A., Okita, M., Yamaguchi, Y., and Okamoto, T.: Long-term intermittent adjuvant chemotherapy for primary, resected lung cancer. J. Thorac. Cardiovasc. Surg., 70:590, 1975.
The authors used two chemotherapeutic agents to suppress local and distant recurrences in patients following resection for carcinoma of the lung. Radiotherapy was given postoperatively to patients with known residual disease. A course of long-term, intermittent chemotherapy with mitomycin-C and chromomycin-A was administered. The results were encouraging and appeared to show a difference between the treated and the untreated groups. However, caution should be taken in interpretation of these results, since it was not a randomized study.

Kirsh, M. M., Dickerman, R., Fayos, J., Lampe, I., Pellegrini, R. V., Gago, O., and Sloan, H.: The value of chest wall resection in the treatment of superior sulcus tumors of the lung. Ann. Thorac. Surg., 15::339, 1973.
These authors differ with Paulson and associates regarding the value of preoperative irradiation followed by extensive surgery in the management of superior sulcus tumors. The conclusions drawn from their data provide the reader a different point of view.

LeRoux, B. T.: Bronchial Carcinoma. Edinburgh, Scotland, E & S Livingstone, 1968.
This is an excellent text covering all aspects of bronchogenic carcinoma.

Macumber, H. H., and Calvin, J. W.: Perfusion lung scan patterns in 100 patients with bronchogenic carcinoma. J. Thorac. Cardiovasc. Surg., 72:299, 1976.
The relationship between size of the perfusion defect as seen by perfusion lung scan and size of the mass lesion as seen in the chest film was correlated with the presence of regional lymph node involvement with tumor in 100 consecutive patients with bronchogenic carcinoma. All patients underwent scanning before open thoracotomy or mediastinotomy, and each had histologic documentation of the disease. The perfusion lung scans were classified into those with (1) perfusion defect larger than the mass lesion, (2) perfusion defect of the same size as the mass lesion, or (3) no focal defect seen. Among patients with a larger perfusion defect, 84 per cent had regional lymph node involvement, whereas among patients in whom a larger defect was not present, only 23 per cent had such extension.

Paulson, D. L., and Urschel, H. C., Jr.: Superior sulcus carcinomas. *In* Sabiston, D. C., Jr., and Spencer, F. C. (Eds.): Gibbon's Surgery of the Chest, 3rd ed. Philadelphia, W. B. Saunders Company, 1976.
These authors are advocates for use of preoperative irradiation followed by radical surgery in the treatment of superior sulcus tumors. Their results are excellent but differ from those reported by Kirsh and associates.

Watson, W. L.: Lung Cancer. St. Louis, The C. V. Mosby Co., 1968.
A complete monograph which is an excellent reference source.

REFERENCES

1. Auerbach, O., Gere, J. B., Forman, J. B., Petrick, T. G., Smolin, H. J., Muehsam, G. E., Kassouny, D. Y., and Stout, A. P.: Changes in the bronchial epithelium in relation to smoking and cancer of the lung. N. Engl. J. Med., 256:97, 1957.
2. Brugarolas, A., Han, T., Takita, H., and Minowada, J.: Immunologic assays in lung cancer. N. Y. State J. Med., 1:747, 1973.
3. Cohen, S., and Hossain, S-A.: Primary carcinoma of the lung: A review of histologically proved cases. *In* Fraser, R. G., and Paré, J. A. P. (Eds.): Diagnosis of Diseases of the Chest: An Integrated Study Based on the Abnormal Roentgenogram. Philadelphia, W. B. Saunders Company, 1970.
4. Didolkar, M. S., Moore, R. H., and Takita, H.: Evaluation of the risk in pulmonary resection for bronchogenic carcinoma. Am. J. Surg., 127:700, 1974.
5. Dorn, H. F.: Tobacco consumption and mortality from cancer and other diseases. Public Health Rep., 74:581, 1959.
6. Figueroa, W. G., Raszkowski, R., and Weiss, W.: Lung cancer in chloromethyl methyl ether workers. N. Engl. J. Med., 288:1096, 1973.

7. Fried, B. M.: Tumors of the Lungs and Mediastinum. Philadelphia, Lea and Febiger, 1958.

8. Friedrich, G.: Periphere Lungenkrebse auf dem Boden pleuranaher Narben. Virchows Arch. Pathol. Anat., 304:230, 1939.

9. Geha, A. S., Bernatz, P. E., and Woolner, L. B.: Bronchogenic carcinoma involving the thoracic wall. Surgical treatment and prognostic significance. J. Thorac. Cardiovasc. Surg., 54:394, 1967.

10. Gondos, B., and Reingold, I. M.: Pathology of scalene lymph nodes. An analysis of 373 biopsies. Cancer, 18:84, 1965.

11. Graham, E. A., and Singer, J. J.: Successful removal of an entire lung for carcinoma of the bronchus. J.A.M.A., 101:1371, 1933.

12. Grillo, H. C., Greenberg, J. J., and Wilkins, E. W.: Resection of bronchogenic carcinoma involving the thoracic wall. J. Thorac. Cardiovasc. Surg., 51:417, 1966.

13. Hammond, E. C., Auerbach, O., Kirman, D., and Garfinkel, L.: Effects of cigarette smoking on dogs. CA, 21:78, 1971.

14. Hammond, E. C., and Horn, D.: Smoking and death rates—report on forty-four months of follow-up of 187,783 men. II. Death rates by cause. J.A.M.A., 166:1294, 1958.

15. Hilaris, B. S., Martini, N., Batata, M., and Beattie, E. J., Jr.: Interstitial irradiation for unresectable carcinoma of the lung. Ann. Thorac. Surg., 20:491, 1975.

16. Holmes, E. C., and Golub, S. H.: Immunologic defects in lung cancer patients. J. Thorac. Cardiovasc. Surg., 71:161, 1976.

17. Hood, R. M., Kirksey, T. D., Calhoon, J. H., Arnold, H. S., and Tate, R. S.: The use of automatic stapling devices in pulmonary resection. Ann. Thorac. Surg., 16:85, 1973.

18. Hutchinson, C. M., and Mills, N. L.: The selection of patients with bronchogenic carcinoma for mediastinoscopy. J. Thorac. Cardiovasc. Surg., 71:768, 1976.

19. Hyde, L., and Hyde, C. I.: Clinical manifestations of lung cancer. Chest, 65:299, 1974.

20. Israel, L.: Preliminary results of nonspecific immunotherapy for lung cancer. Cancer Chemother. Rep., 4:283, 1973.

21. Jackman, R. J., Good, C. A., Clagett, O. T., and Woolner, L. B.: Survival rates in peripheral bronchogenic carcinomas up to four centimeters in diameter presenting as solitary pulmonary nodules. J. Thorac. Cardiovasc. Surg., 57:1, 1969.

22. Katsuki, H., Shimada, K., Koyama, A., Okita, M., Yamaguchi, Y., and Okamoto, T.: Long-term intermittent adjuvant chemotherapy for primary, resected lung cancer. J. Thorac. Cardiovasc. Surg., 70:590, 1975.

23. Khadzhiev, S., and Kavaklieva-Kimitrova, Y. A.: Immunotherapy of lung cancer. Cancer Chemother. Rep., 4:283, 1973.

24. Kirsh, M. M., Dickerman, R., Fayos, J., Lampe, I., Pellegrini, R. V., Gago, O., and Sloan, H.: The value of chest wall resection in the treatment of superior sulcus tumors of the lung. Ann. Thorac. Surg., 15:339, 1973.

25. Kirsh, M. M., Rotman, H., Argenta, L., Bove, E., Cimmino, V., Tashian, J., Ferguson, P., and Sloan, H.: Carcinoma of the lung: Results of treatment over ten years. Ann. Thorac. Surg., 21:371, 1976.

26. Kvale, P. A., Bode, F. R., and Kini, S.: Diagnostic accuracy in lung cancer. Comparison of techniques used in association with flexible fiberoptic bronchoscopy. Chest, 69:752, 1976.

27. Lewis, R. J., Kunderman, P. J., Sisler, G. E., and Mackenzie, J. W.: Direct diagnostic thoracoscopy. Ann. Thorac. Surg., 21:536, 1976.

28. Longacre, A. M., and Shockman, A. T.: The superior vena cava syndrome and radiation therapy. Clinical response, survival, and postmortem findings. Radiology, 91:713, 1968.

29. Macumber, H. H., and Calvin, J. W.: Perfusion lung scan patterns in 100 patients with bronchogenic carcinoma. J. Thorac. Cardiovasc. Surg., 72:299, 1976.

30. McNamara, J. J., Kingsley, W. B., Paulson, D. L., Arndt, J. H., Salinas-Izaquirre, S. F., and Urschel, H. C., Jr.: Alveolar cell (bronchiolar) carcinoma of the lung. J. Thorac. Cardiovasc. Surg., 57:648, 1969.

31. Morton, D. L., Itabashi, H. H., and Grimes, O. F.: Nonmetastatic neurological complications of bronchogenic carcinoma: The carcinomatous neuromyopathies. J. Thorac. Cardiovasc. Surg., 51:14, 1966.

32. Olkowski, Z. L., McLaren, J. R., and Mansour, K. A.: Immunocompetence of patients with bronchogenic carcinoma. Ann. Thorac. Surg., 21:546, 1976.

33. Omenn, G. S., and Wilkins, E. W., Jr.: Hormone syndromes associated with bronchogenic carcinoma. Clues to histologic type. J. Thorac. Cardiovasc. Surg., 59:877, 1970.

34. Overholt, R. H., Neptune, W. B., and Ashraf, M. M.: Primary cancer of the lung. A 42-year experience. Ann. Thorac. Surg., 20:511, 1975.

35. Paulson, D. L., and Urschel, H. C., Jr.: Superior sulcus carcinomas. In Sabiston, D. C., Jr., and Spencer, F. C. (Eds.): Gibbon's Surgery of the Chest, 3rd ed. Philadelphia, W. B. Saunders Company, 1976.

36. Razzuk, M. A., Pockey, M., Urschel, H. C., Jr., and Paulson, D. L.: Dual primary bronchogenic carcinoma. Ann. Thorac. Surg., 17:425, 1974.

37. Razzuk, M. A., Urschel, H. C., Jr., Albers, J. E., Martin, J. A., and Paulson, D. L.: Pulmonary giant cell carcinoma. Ann. Thorac. Surg., 21:540, 1976.

38. Rigler, L. G.: A roentgen study of the evolution of carcinoma of the lung. J. Thorac. Surg., 34:283, 1957.

39. Rigler, L. G., O'Loughlin, B. J., and Tucker, R. C.: The duration of carcinoma of the lung. Dis. Chest, 23:50, 1953.

40. Ripstein, C. B., Spain, D. M., and Bluth, I.: Scar cancer of the lung. J. Thorac. Cardiovasc. Surg., 56:362, 1968.

41. Rose, M. E., Howard, R., Sibley, J. J., and Reilly, H. F., Jr.: Pneumothorax directly resulting from perforated bronchogenic carcinoma. Ann. Thorac. Surg., 4:160, 1967.

42. Scott, R. N., Faraci, R. P., Hough, A., and Chretien, P. B.: Bronchial stump closure techniques follow pneumonectomy: A serial comparative study. Ann. Surg., 116:205, 1976.

43. Seidman, H., Silverberg, E., and Holleb, A. I.: Cancer statistics, 1976. A comparison of white and black populations. CA, 26:2, 1976.

44. Shields, T. W.: Interstitial or external irradiation for nonresectable carcinoma of the lung. Ann. Thorac. Surg., 20:590, 1975.

45. Shields, T. W., and Higgins, G. A.: Minimal pulmonary resection in treatment of carcinoma of the lung. Arch. Surg., 108:420, 1974.

46. Shields, T. W., Robinette, C. D., and Keehn, R. J.: Bronchial carcinoma treated by adjuvant cancer chemotherapy. Arch. Surg., 109:329, 1974.

47. Spencer, H.: Pathology of the Lung. New York, The Macmillan Company, 1965.

48. Staub, E. W., Eisenstein, R., Hass, G., and Beattie, E. J., Jr.: Bronchogenic carcinoma produced experimentally in the normal dog. J. Thorac. Cardiovasc. Surg., 49:364, 1965.

49. Vincent, R. G., Takita, H., Lane, W. W., Gutierrez, A. C., and Pickren, J. W.: Surgical therapy of lung cancer. J. Thorac. Cardiovasc. Surg., 71:581, 1976.

50. Warram, J.: Preoperative irradiation of cancer of the lung: Final report of a therapeutic trial. A collaborative study. Cancer, 36:914, 1975.

51. Wells, S. A., Burdick, J. F., Joseph, W. L., Christiansen, C. L., Wolfe, W. G., and Adkins, P. C.: Delayed cutaneous hypersensitivity reactions to tumor cell antigens and to nonspecific antigens: Prognostic significance in patients with lung cancer. J. Thorac. Cardiovasc. Surg., 66:557, 1973.

52. Yacoub, M. H.: Relation between the histology of bronchial carcinoma and hypertrophic pulmomary osteoarthropathy. Thorax, 20:537, 1965.

XV

THORACIC OUTLET SYNDROME

Donald Silver, M.D.

The thoracic outlet syndrome which accounts for 0.14 per cent of patient diagnoses[19] is the preferred term for those syndromes, e.g., the cervical rib syndrome, scalenus anticus syndrome, hyperabduction syndrome, costoclavicular syndrome, pectoralis minor syndrome, and the first thoracic rib syndrome, which result from compression of the neurovascular structures to the upper extremities. The syndrome is caused by compression of the brachial plexus or subclavian-axillary artery and/or vein in the region between the thoracic outlet and the insertion of the pectoralis minor onto the coracoid process. Symptoms may arise from neural, arterial, or venous compression, or any combination thereof.

HISTORICAL ASPECTS

One of the earliest descriptions of the thoracic outlet syndrome appeared in 1860, when a Dr. Willshire reported a pulsating subclavian artery (possibly an aneurysm) that crossed a presumed cervical rib.[25] In 1861, Coote excised a cervical rib to relieve pressure on the axillary vessels and nerves.[4] Murphy in 1905[12] and Keen in 1907[10] emphasized the role of cervical ribs in the etiology of the neurovascular symptoms. In 1919, Stopford and Telford demonstrated that the brachial plexus and subclavian artery could be compressed by the thoracic rib and indicated that resection of the rib would relieve symptoms.[20]

In 1927, Adson and Coffey emphasized the role of the scalene muscles in the neurovascular compression and popularized scalenotomy as a method of therapy.[2] Various operative maneuvers were tried with varying degrees of success until 1962, when the role of the first rib, and the ligamentous and muscular attachments to it, in the pathogenesis of the thoracic outlet syndrome was reemphasized.[3, 8] Since then, the preferred form of operative therapy has been resection of the first rib with division of the pectoralis minor tendon if the symptoms are produced by hyperabduction.

ANATOMY

An understanding of the spaces of potential pressure in the thoracic outlet region is necessary for proper evaluation and treatment of this syndrome. The anterior rami of five spinal nerves, C5, C6, C7, C8, and T1 (C4 and T2 may also contribute to the brachial plexus), exit through the intervertebral foramina and form trunks that pass through the scalene triangle and then divide behind the clavicle. The divisions of the trunks reunite to form cords that surround the axillary artery as it passes behind the pectoralis minor tendon. The motor and sensory branches of the brachial plexus are usually distal to the pectoralis minor tendon.

Rami from C8 and T1 form the lowest trunk, which lies on the first rib behind the subclavian artery and is responsible for the groove in the rib (which is often attributed to the artery). The peripheral distribution of C8 and T1 provides sensory reception from the fifth finger and medial half of the fourth finger and from the medial aspect of the forearm. The motor distribution of the rami controls flexion of the wrist and fingers and innervates the intrinsic muscles of the hand.

Both subclavian arteries exit from the thorax behind the sternoclavicular joints and pass over the first rib between the scalenus medius and scalenius anticus muscles. The arteries then course laterally behind the clavicles and become the axillary arteries. The axillary arteries pass posterior to the tendons of the pectoralis minor and become the brachial arteries.

The axillary veins pass behind the costocoracoid ligaments and pectoralis minor tendons. At the edge of the first rib, each axillary vein becomes a subclavian vein which passes over the first rib *anterior* to the scalenus anticus muscle to join the jugular vein at the base of the neck before it enters the thorax as the innominate vein. Each vein courses through a narrow area consisting of the first rib and the scalenous anticus muscle posteriorly, and the costocoracoid ligament, subclavian muscle, and clavicle anteriorly.

The arteries, veins, and components of the brachial plexus may be compressed in any of several areas as they pass from the neck or the thoracic outlet into the upper extremity. The sites of compression from medial to lateral include: (1) the interscalene triangle (arteries and nerves); (2) the space between the scalenus anticus muscle and the clavicle (vein); (3) the first rib, or between the first rib and clavicle (nerves, arteries, and veins); (4) the costocoracoid fascia (nerves, arteries, and veins); (5) the pectoralis minor tendon (nerves, arteries, and veins).

Other anatomic functional causes of compression of the neurovascular structures include:

1. Cervical ribs, which occur in approximately 1 per cent of the population and are bilateral in 80 per cent of the cases. Cervical ribs compress or irritate portions of the adjacent brachial plexus and compress or elevate the subclavian artery. However, less than 10 per cent of cervical ribs produce symptoms.

2. Long transverse processes of C7, which may function as cervical ribs.

3. Abnormal first thoracic ribs. These ribs frequently fail to reach the sternum, may be attached to the sternum or to the second rib by ligaments, and may cause distortion or compression of the lowest components of the brachial plexus.

4. Postural changes during which there is downward displacement of the upper extremity and shoulder girdle. Occupations that require carrying heavy loads or working in narrow quarters so that the upper extremities are drawn forward and down are frequently associated with thoracic outlet symptoms.

5. Occupations that require hyperabduction.

6. Acquired lesions such as fractures of the first rib or clavicle with deformity or callus formation.

7. Compression by tumor in the outlet spaces.[6]

SYMPTOMS

The symptoms of the thoracic outlet syndrome vary, depending on the vessels or nerves compressed, and may be neurologic or vascular or both. Most often the symptoms are caused by neural compression.[5] The clinical manifestations rarely indicate the site of obstruction.

Neurologic symptoms consist of pain, paresthesias, and numbness, usually in the fingers and hands, in an ulnar distribution, but may occur anywhere in the upper extremity or shoulder girdle. Late neurologic defects include sensory loss, motor weakness, and atrophy.

Symptoms of arterial compression include ischemic pain, numbness, fatigue, paresthesias, coldness, and weakness in the arm or hand. These symptoms are accentuated by exercise and exposure to cold. Thromboses may occur in the compressed or poststenotic dilated areas of subclavian-axillary artery and produce distal ischemic changes. Distal embolization may also be part of the picture. The venous symptoms include pain, swelling, aching, distal edema, and cyanosis.

DIAGNOSIS

A complete history and a thorough physical examination should establish the diagnosis in most cases. The symptom complexes plus a history of trauma with fracture(s) of the clavicle or ribs or both, a history of unusual exercise or occupation, poor posture, sagging bed, and so forth, should suggest the thoracic outlet syndrome. A careful history will also indicate whether or not the symptoms are part of a generalized process such as occurs with cord tumors, multiple peripheral embolizations, osteoarthritis, and collagen or metabolic disorders.

The physical examination should be thorough, with special emphasis given to detecting the neural, arterial, and venous signs. Neural signs include sensory deficits, weakness and atrophy. Most often the sensory and motor deficits occur in the distribution of the ulnar nerve. Signs of arterial compression include weakened or absent brachial and radial pulses, a bruit in the supraclavicular or axillary space, delayed capillary blush, and occasional areas of distal gangrene. Signs of venous compression include distended veins, distal edema, and cyanosis.

The physical findings are not constant, and several examinations may be required before the thoracic

outlet syndrome is suspected. The findings may vary according to the patient's position. Except when produced by hyperabduction, compression is rarely detected when patients are examined in the supine position, but is usually readily detected when the patient is sitting or standing. There are three specific diagnostic maneuvers for the thoracic outlet syndrome.

1. Adson or scalene maneuver.[1, 2] While the physician monitors the radial pulse, the patient takes a deep breath, extends the neck, and turns the chin toward the side being examined. Disappearance or reduction of the radial pulse constitutes a positive finding. During a positive test a bruit frequently will become audible in the supraclavicular fossa, and the hand may become cool and pale. The deep breath causes elevation of the first rib, and extending and turning the neck causes narrowing of the interscalene triangle. The symptoms are caused by compression of the subclavian artery and probably the brachial plexus by the first rib and scalene muscles. If the pulse is altered before the head is turned, one should suspect the presence of a cervical rib.

2. Costoclavicular compressive maneuver.[7] While the radial pulse is monitored, the patient throws his shoulders back and downward into an exaggerated military position. Disappearance or reduction of the radial pulse with the appearance of subclavian bruit constitutes a positive finding. The results are produced by compression of the subclavian artery (or vein, or brachial plexus) between the clavicle and first rib.

3. Hyperabduction maneuver.[24] The radial pulse is monitored while the arm is passively moved into a hyperabducted position. Reduction or cessation of the radial pulse and the appearance of an axillary bruit indicate arterial compression by the pectoralis minor tendon.

Objective Examinations

Roentgenograms of the neck and chest may demonstrate cervical ribs, anomalous first ribs, prominent transverse processes, bony exostoses, calluses, abnormalities of the clavicle, and so forth. The roentgenograms also yield information about narrowing of the intervertebral foramina and tumors. Myelograms may be necessary to demonstrate a cervical disc or other causes of cervical cord compression. Arteriograms will demonstrate sites of partial or complete arterial occlusion. Arteriography should be performed with the patient's arms by his side and while he is performing the Adson, costoclavicular, and hyperabduction maneuvers. Occasionally, poststenotic dilatation or aneurysms of the subclavian artery distal to the site of compression will be demonstrated. A normal arteriogram does not eliminate neural compression as a cause of the syndrome. Phlebograms are useful to demonstrate the sites of compression of the axillary or subclavian vein. If the veins become totally or partially occluded during the hyperabduction or costoclavicular compression maneuvers, support is obtained for the diagnosis of thoracic outlet syndrome.

Plethysmography[17] has been used to document arterial compression. This technique[21] records changes in digit volume that occur with each heartbeat and can demonstrate obstruction to arterial flow. Electromyography is useful in detecting sites of compression of peripheral nerves by recording the altered response to the distal muscles to proximal electrical stimuli. Nerve conduction times between the thoracic outlet and elbow and wrist may be significantly prolonged. These conduction times return to normal range after surgical relief of the compression.[23]

MANAGEMENT

For all patients, except those with complete vascular occlusion or poststenotic aneurysm, initial management should consist of a trial of weight reduction and an exercise program directed toward improving posture, strengthening the elevators of the shoulder girdle, and avoiding hyperabduction. These measures relieve symptoms in 50[23] to 70 per cent of patients.[9, 13] Nonoperative management seems to be most successful in the obese, middle-aged female with poor posture.

Patients with major neurologic or vascular complications and those who do not respond to nonoperative management should be offered surgical intervention. A variety of only partially successful operative procedures have been devised for managing the thoracic outlet syndrome. The operative management has included excision of a cervical rib, division of the scalenous anticus muscle, resection of the clavicle, and division of the pectoralis minor tendon.[14, 18] Falconer and Li,[7] Clagett,[3] and Roos[16] have emphasized that removal of the major portion of the first rib effectively decompresses the neurovascular structures. Removal of the first rib, and of a cervical rib if it is present, has become the preferred method of treatment for the thoracic outlet syndrome.

Clagett suggested that the rib be removed through a posterior incision identical to that used for an upper thoracoplasty (Fig. 1). When the posterior approach is used, the subclavian vessels and brachial plexus are easily exposed and displaced anteriorly out of harm's way. Cervical ribs may also be easily excised through this approach, and it usually affords ample exposure for reconstructive vascular procedures that are indicated.

Roos has popularized use of a transaxillary incision for removal of the rib (Fig. 2). The author prefers this incision, which is small and is readily hidden by the arm. The vessels and nerves are lifted off the first rib when the arm is hyperabducted during surgery. Of necessity, the scalene muscles are divided during removal of the rib. The disability is minimal and the postoperative course is usually uncomplicated. Most patients may be discharged by the third or fourth postoperative day and frequently return to work in 7 to 10 days. However, reconstructive vascular procedures are more difficult through this incision, and if vascular reconstructive procedures are anticipated, the posterior approach is preferred. The posterior approach is also preferred in patients requiring reoperation for recurrent symptoms.

Resection of the first thoracic rib, and of a cervical rib if it is present, effectively removes all the potential sites of neurovascular compression that produce the thoracic outlet syndrome save one. The neurovascular structures may be compressed by the pectoralis minor tendon when positions of hyperabduction are maintained. If, because of occupation or other reasons, the patient cannot avoid these positions, division of the tendon should be undertaken and can be performed through the posterior or transaxillary incision at the time the first rib is resected.

Nelson and Jenson[15] have employed an anterior extrapleural approach for excision of the first rib, and have found this incision to be cosmetically acceptable with a minimal complication rate. However, this approach is not suitable for removing cervical ribs or anomalous first ribs.

Although the limited operations often failed to relieve the symptoms of the thoracic outlet syndrome, resection of the first rib with an occasional division of the pectoralis minor tendon offers lasting relief to over 90 per cent of the patients undergoing operation.

Recurrent symptoms requiring reoperation may oc-

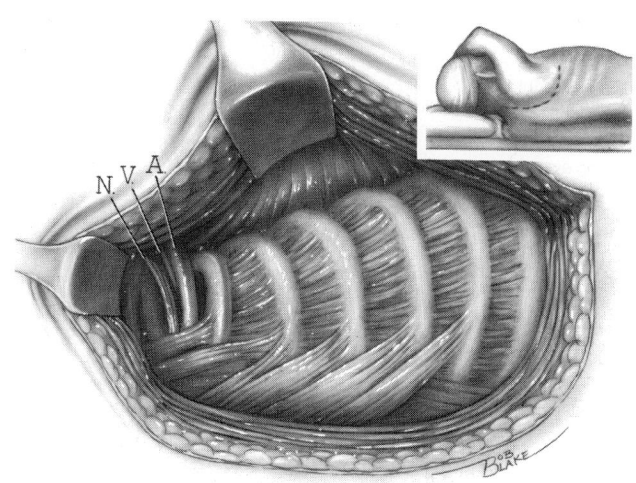

Figure 1. Posterior approach to the first thoracic rib. The surgeon is behind the patient, who is in the left lateral decubitus position. Extension of the incision cephalad along the scapula provides exposure of the first rib, scalene muscles, brachial plexus (N.), and subclavian artery (A.) and vein (V.).

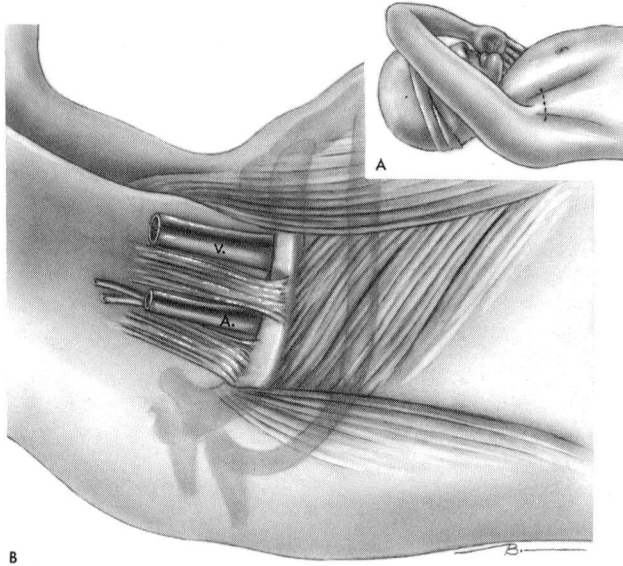

Figure 2. The transaxillary approach to the first rib provides good exposure of the first rib, scalene muscles, brachial plexus, and subclavian artery (A.) and vein (V.).

cur in 1 per cent of the patients who have had a first rib removed.[22] Many of the patients with recurrent symptoms will respond to physiotherapy and improvement of posture. However, persistent symptoms are an indication for re-resection of the first rib[22] and occasionally the second rib.

Mild poststenotic dilatation of the subclavian artery usually regresses once the compression is relieved. However, significant aneurysms of the artery should be excised and replaced with grafts, preferably vein grafts. Thrombosis of the subclavian artery should be treated by thromboendarterectomy or by replacement or bypass grafting of the involved segment. Thrombosis of the subclavian-axillary vein requires elimination of the causative factors and treatment with heparin, elevation, and an elastic sleeve until recanalization occurs. On rare occasions, a thrombectomy as suggested by Mahorner may be useful.[11]

REFERENCES

1. Adson, A. W.: Surgical treatment for symptoms produced by cervical ribs and the scalenous anticus muscle. Surg. Gynecol. Obstet., 85:687, 1947.
2. Adson, A. W., and Coffey, J. R.: Cervical rib: A method of anterior approach for relief of symptoms by division of scalenus anterior. Ann. Surg., 85:839, 1927.
3. Clagett, O. T.: Research and prosearch. Presidential Address. J. Thorac. Cardiovasc. Surg., 44:153, 1962.
4. Coote, H.: Pressure on the axillary vessels and nerve by the exostosis from a cervical rib: Interference with the circulation of the arm: Removal of the rib and exostosis: Recovery. Med. Times Gaz., 2:108, 1861; cited in Clagett.[3]
5. Dale, W. A.: Thoracic outlet syndrome. In Vascular Surgery. Baltimore, University Park Press, 1975.
6. Echo, D. A., Sickles, E. A., and Wiernik, P. H.: Thoracic outlet syndrome, supraclavicular adenopathy, Hodgkin's disease. Ann. Intern. Med., 78:608, 1973.
7. Falconer, M. A., and Li, F. W. P.: Resection of the first rib in costoclavicular compression of the brachial plexus. Lancet, 1:59, 1962.
8. Falconer, M. A., and Weddell, G.: Costoclavicular compression of the subclavian artery and vein: Relation to the scalenus anticus syndrome. Lancet, 2:539, 1943.
9. Haggart, G. E.: Value of conservative management in cervicobrachial pain. J.A.M.A., 137:508, 1948.
10. Keen, W.: The symptomatology, diagnosis, and surgical treatment of cervical ribs. Am. J. Med. Sci., 133:173, 1907.
11. Mahorner, H., Castleberry, J. W., and Coleman, W. O.: Attempts to restore function in major veins which are the site of massive thrombosis. Ann. Surg., 146:510, 1957.
12. Murphy, J. B.: A case of cervical rib with symptoms resembling subclavian aneurysm. Ann. Surg., 41:399, 1905.
13. Nelson, P. A.: Treatment of patients with cervicodorsal outlet syndrome. J.A.M.A., 163:1570, 1957.
14. Nelson, R. M., and Davis, R. W.: Thoracic outlet compression syndrome. Ann. Thorac. Surg., 8:437, 1969.
15. Nelson, R. M., and Jensen, C. B.: Anterior approach for excision of the first rib. Ann. Thorac. Surg., 9:30, 1970.
16. Roos, D. B.: Transaxillary approach for first rib resection to relieve thoracic outlet syndrome. Ann. Surg., 163:354, 1966.
17. Sanders, R. J., Monsour, J. W., and Baer, S. B.: Transaxillary first rib resection for the thoracic outlet syndrome. Arch. Surg., 97:1014, 1968.
18. Silver, D.: The thoracic outlet syndrome. In Lewis' Practice of Surgery. Vol. XI. New York, Harper & Row, 1968.
19. Silver, D.: The thoracic outlet syndrome. In Lewis' Practice of Surgery. New York, Harper & Row, 1975.
20. Stopford, J. S. B., and Telford, E. D.: Compression of the lower trunk of the brachial plexus by a first dorsal rib with a note on the surgical treatment. Br. J. Surg., 7:168, 1919.
21. Strandness, D. E., Jr., and Bell, J. W.: Peripheral vascular disease: Diagnosis and objective evaluation using a mercury strain gauge. Ann. Surg., 161(Suppl. 4): 1965.
22. Urschel, H. C., Jr., Razzuk, M. A., Albers, J. E., Wood, R. E., and Paulson, D. L.: Reoperation for recurrent thoracic outet syndrome. Ann. Thorac. Surg., 21:19, 1976.
23. Urschel, H. C., Jr., Razzuk, M. A., Wood, R. E., et al.: Objective diagnosis (ulnar nerve conduction velocity) and current therapy of the thoracic outlet syndrome. Ann. Thorac. Surg., 12:608, 1971.
24. Wright, I. S.: The neurovascular syndrome produced by hyperabduction of the arms: The immediate changes produced in 150 normal controls, and the effects on some persons of prolonged hyperabduction of the arms, as in sleeping, and in certain occupations. Am. Heart J., 29:1, 1945.
25. A mirror of the practice of medicine and surgery in the hospitals of London, clinical records, supernumerary first rib. Lancet, 2:633, 1860.

XVI

DISORDERS OF THE CHEST WALL

Mark M. Ravitch, M.D.

CONGENITAL MALFORMATIONS OF THE RIBS AND STERNUM

Deformities of the ribs and sternum are often sufficiently grotesque and obvious that one would expect them to have been recorded from ancient times. However, apart from descriptions of ectopia cordis in discussions of monsters, the congenital deformities of the type under discussion in this chapter received scant attention until the last half of the nineteenth century. The operative correction of these deformities has been largely a development of thoracic surgery since World War II. The depression deformity of the sternum, funnel chest or pectus excavatum, is by all odds the commonest. There were a few early successful operations for this, beginning with Sauerbruch's[17] in 1913 on a patient who was profoundly symptomatic and was improved. The operation for pectus excavatum was put in proper perspective by the classic paper of Ochsner and DeBakey[11] in 1939 and by the report of a series of patients presented by Lincoln Brown[4] of San Francisco in the following year. The publications of Sweet,[18] Lester,[8] and others[12] after World War II stimulated widespread interest and established the basic operative principles. The literature up to that time, and to some extent still, is replete with statements that these deformities are rare, that they are not amenable to satisfactory or lasting correction, and that in any case they cause no problems. As with most conditions, familiarity with these deformities and interest in their treatment have resulted in awareness that they occur relatively frequently. The associated physiologic, orthopedic, social, and psychologic problems are well recognized, and satisfactory operative methods for the correction of these deformities have been devised.

The sternal deformities are of three principal types: (1) depression deformities (pectus excavatum or funnel chest); (2) protrusion deformities (pectus carinatum or pigeon or chicken breast); and (3) sternal clefts (cervicothoracic ectopia cordis and thoracoabdominal ectopia cordis).

STERNAL DEFORMITIES

Depression Deformities (Pectus Excavatum, Funnel Chest, Trichterbrust, Schusterbrust)

Appearance. The deformity is marked by a sharp posterior concavity of the body of the sternum from above downward, deepest just above its junction with the xiphoid. The lower costal cartilages dip posteriorly to meet the depressed sternum so that there results a concavity from above downward and from side to side (Fig. 1). In some instances, the sternum itself is scaphoid. We recognize two principal types: (1) In the deep central deformity, in which there is a pocket that can literally hold a tennis ball or a fist, the manubrium is in proper position, and the chest on each side is well formed (Fig. 1A). This is the most striking-looking deformity, but because the remainder of the chest is properly formed, restitution to an almost normal chest wall after operation can be assured. (2) The broad, somewhat flatter deformity may go from nipple to nipple and may begin at the manubrium or may even involve a depression of the manubrium. In these patients, the chest is likely to have a narrow anteroposterior diameter on both sides lateral to the defect. The defect itself, being extremely broad, may seem not quite as impressive as the purely central defect; however, the cubic displacement of intrathoracic space is likely to be greater, and these deformities may in fact be the most significant physiologically (Fig. 1B and C). The children evidence a frequently striking paradoxical inward inspiratory motion of the sternum, a displacement of the heart invariably to the left, and frequently a forceful cardiac heave and thrust against the chest wall. In the more severe instances, with the hand placed around the left chest one can feel the imprisoned heart expanding the hemithorax with each impulse. The protuberant, potbellied abdomen is conspicuous, and as the children stand and walk the characteristic slumped shoulders, rounded back, and forward-thrust neck are noted.

Etiology. Funnel chest is a congenital deformity, most often sporadic, although familial incidence is common. We have, for instance, operated upon three children in one family whose three other siblings had varying degrees of the same deformity, operated on one father and daughter combination and seen others, and in numerous instances operated upon two siblings in a family. The deformity tends to be progressive from birth, and this, combined with the fact that it becomes more conspicuous as baby fat disappears, leads to the occasional statement that the child was perfectly normal at birth. The progression of the deformity is irregular and unpredictable. Sudden accentuation of the deformity is common during the adolescent growth spurt.

The deformity is, in general, unassociated with other congenital lesions, although it is one of the types of chest deformity that do occur in association with congenital cardiac deformities, and it is specifically associated with Marfan's disease (Ochsner and DeBakey's[11] patient had Marfan's disease). While attempts have been made to impute faulty development of the diaphragm, no developmental mechanism has been clearly demonstrated to be at fault. As reasonable as any is the suggestion that there occurs an overgrowth of costal cartilage that forces the sternum to either protrude or recede, and that under the influence of the diaphragm it is pulled posteriorly. Neither rickets nor any other disease of bone plays any part.

Physiologic Effects. Symptoms in infancy are few.

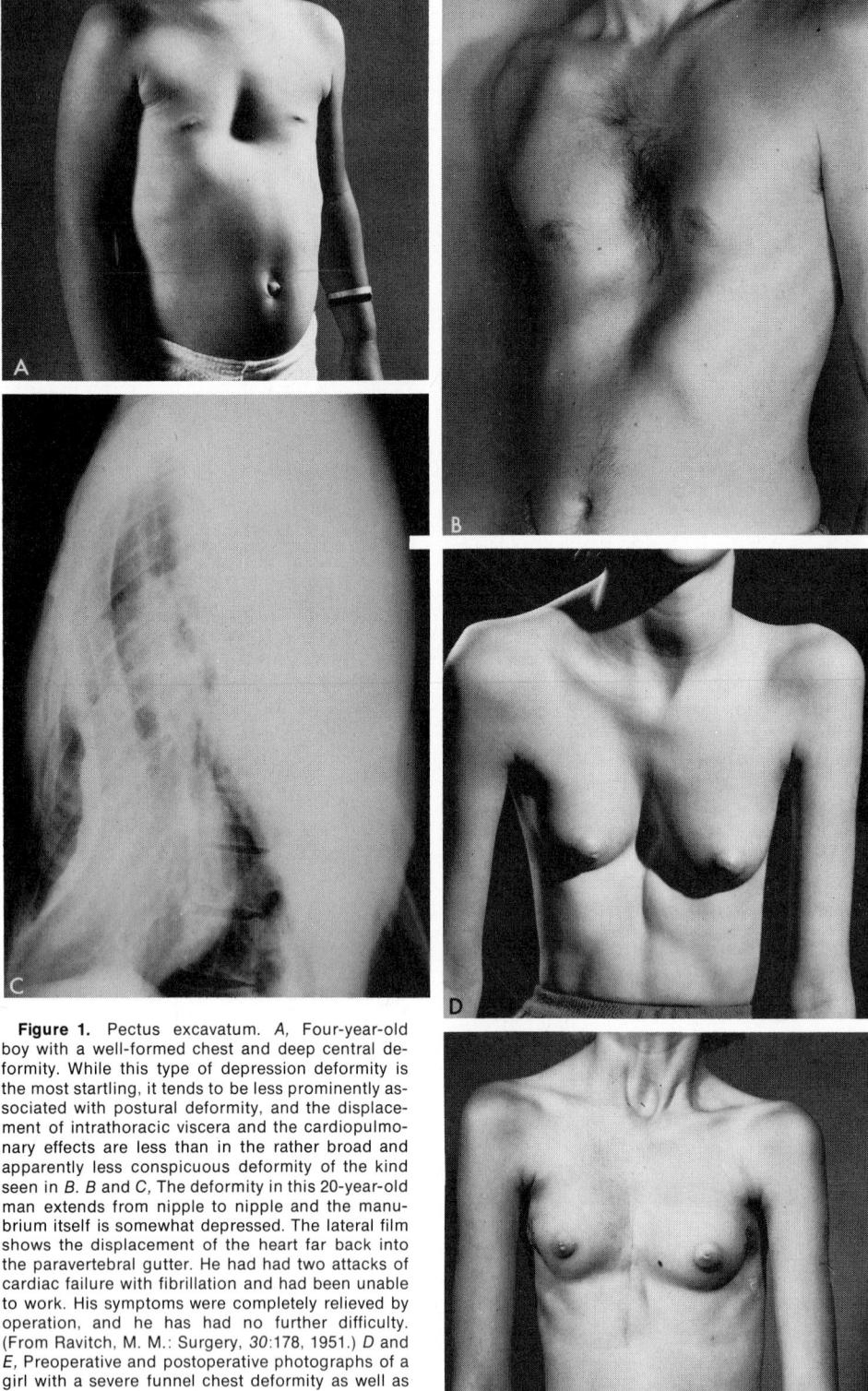

Figure 1. Pectus excavatum. *A,* Four-year-old boy with a well-formed chest and deep central deformity. While this type of depression deformity is the most startling, it tends to be less prominently associated with postural deformity, and the displacement of intrathoracic viscera and the cardiopulmonary effects are less than in the rather broad and apparently less conspicuous deformity of the kind seen in *B. B* and *C,* The deformity in this 20-year-old man extends from nipple to nipple and the manubrium itself is somewhat depressed. The lateral film shows the displacement of the heart far back into the paravertebral gutter. He had had two attacks of cardiac failure with fibrillation and had been unable to work. His symptoms were completely relieved by operation, and he has had no further difficulty. (From Ravitch, M. M.: Surgery, *30*:178, 1951.) *D* and *E,* Preoperative and postoperative photographs of a girl with a severe funnel chest deformity as well as congenital agenesis of the left lung, the combination of which produced severe limitation of exercise tolerance and unrelieved tachycardia. Note the restitution of normal thoracic contour and the inconspicuous vertical scar. The right breast is seen to be less well developed than the left, as is often the case in pectus excavatum in females.

We have seen one infant who was sufficiently difficult to feed that comment was made upon this before operation, and in whom the dysphagia was relieved after operation, and have treated a number of others in whom it was noted only after operation that the children now ate much more easily and rapidly. We and others have seen infants with severe stridor that was relieved by operative correction of the thoracic deformity. In childhood no incapacity is generally recognized, but it is frequently pointed out after operation that children who had been quiet, well behaved, "good" youngsters became energetic, tireless, and quite different in their behavior and vigor. In adolescence it is not at all uncommon to have these children described as sedentary or to have it recognized that they are somewhat less energetic than their fellows and cannot sustain activity as long. In those who undertake athletics seriously, the disability is at times obvious and the improvement after operation measurable. Physiologic evaluation of the deficit in patients with sternal depressions has been undertaken by many.[2, 5, 6, 10, 20] Cardiac murmurs are common, particularly systolic murmurs to the left of the sternum, at the base of the heart. The heart is invariably displaced to the left and rotated, as demonstrated by physical examination, plain films, angiocardiography, and electrocardiography. A fair conclusion from the extensive studies of the electrocardiographic and vectorcardiographic[19] changes would be that most of the changes seen in the records can be attributed to the displacement and rotation of the heart and to the abnormal position of the chest leads on the malformed chest. Arrhythmias of several kinds have been observed, usually intermittent and relieved by correction of the deformity. Angiocardiography shows not only the displacement of the heart but in some instances deformity of the right ventricle or atrium. Although in our experience we have cited a number of diverse and striking patients with gross physiologic defects, even to cardiac failure and atrial fibrillation[13, 20] (Fig. 1B and C), in general, physiologic measurements of cardiac and pulmonary function have not yielded the kind of documentation one would like of a significant cardiopulmonary deficit. Most studies of cardiac output and respiratory function in these patients have shown results that fall within the rather broad limits of the normal range, if often at the lower limits of the normal range. We have long thought that the fault has lain in our inability to measure the subtle decrease in function which, to cite specific examples, accounts for the boy who can hike with his scout troop on the level but falls behind on a hill, the high school boy who can "fool around" on the basketball court, but not play a game, and the college man who can volley on the tennis court, but not play a set. We have reported an 11-year-old girl with severe funnel chest and agenesis of the left lung[15] (Fig. 1D and E). She had progressively severe and disabling exertional dyspnea. A combination of two tolerable physiologic handicaps had produced an intolerable handicap. After operation she described, as a number of older patients have, a sense of freedom in inspiration, and returned to unrestricted activity; her pulmonary function tests, which had shown a restrictive respiratory defect, returned toward normal.

The literature on physiologic studies in patients with pectus excavatum is conflicting, depending to some extent upon the design of the physiologic studies. Fishman and associates[6] found no abnormalities in those respiratory functions they tested, but Weg[20] and associates, in 25 Air Force trainees with pectus excavatum and some exercise intolerance, found a decrease in the forced expiratory flow and a significant decrease in maximal voluntary ventilation. We and others have described a diastolic dip and plateau in the right ventricular pressure curve, similar to that seen in constrictive pericarditis, suggesting that the right ventricle is compressed between sternum and vertebral column, and in fact this can sometimes be seen by angiocardiography. Bevegård's[2] sophisticated studies of cardiac function yielded the information that the increase in the physical working capacity of the heart and the stroke volume were significantly less than in normal subjects in the sitting position on transition from rest to exercise, resulting in a higher pulse rate at a given oxygen uptake and explaining the lower physical working capacity. He attributes this to impaired ventricular filling. The studies from the National Institutes of Health of Beiser and others[1] confirm Bevegård's findings.

Indications for Operation. We consider operation advisable to correct an existing defect, to prevent progression of the defect with the attendant hangdog posture (and hangdog self-image) and increasing probability of physiologic disadvantage, if not necessarily disability. While the structural and physiologic effects of the deformity are the principal basis for correction of the defect, it would be a mistake to minimize the social and psychologic significance of the deformity, and considerations on these scores would of themselves warrant operation. In infants and children we advise operation for deep or progressive deformities. We have not seen significant spontaneous recession of deformities, but on the other hand are not able to predict which will progress more extensively than others. Evidence of exercise intolerance and social embarrassment are added indications in later childhood and adolescence. In general, the adults upon whom we have operated have all been severely symptomatic. The younger the child at the time of operation, the less extensive need the operation be and the more likely is an optimal result.

Technique of Operation.[14] The operation (Fig. 2), which we have evolved in the course of 30 years and some 400 operations, is based on the following considerations:

1. All of the deformed costal cartilages must be resected subperichondrially for the full extent of the deformity. The perichondrium will re-form new cartilage in the correct position.

2. The sternum must be separated from the xiphoid and from the intercostal bundles to release it for its new position.

3. A posterior sternal osteotomy above the beginning of the down curve of the deformity allows the sternum to be lifted forward in corrected position, and to be maintained there by a bone graft wedged into the osteotomy.

A great variety of other operations and techniques have been proposed, including reliance upon rigid temporary or permanent struts or upon external traction, excision and reversal of the sternum, multiple chondrotomies, and multiple sternotomies. We believe the operation described here to be the simplest and safest that will yield good results.

No mortality need be expected (the only death in our series was that of the second patient, almost 30 years ago). The operation can confidently be expected to relieve symptoms and prevent progression of the deformity. In the central deformities, the result is an essentially normal chest. In the wide deformities with a flat chest overall and sometimes with a depressed manubrium, improvement is dramatic, but parents should be forewarned that the general configuration of the chest, apart from the depressed sternum, limits the degree of restitution to a normal contour. Unsatisfactory results are likely to be due to inadequate mobilization of the sternum, insufficiently extensive resection of cartilages, or failure to devise a stable method of retaining the sternum in its new position. External traction, employed by some, is burdensome and unnecessary. In occasional adults or in very large adolescents, we employ internal Kirschner wire fixation.

Fascinatingly enough, the removal of large segments of five or six cartilages and fracture of the sternum does not cause any respiratory difficulty. We have never seen physiologic distress from the operation and have never had to use respirator support.

Protrusion Deformities of the Sternum (Pigeon Breast, Chicken Breast, Pectus Carinatum)

Clinical Manifestations. This congenital deformity, occasionally familial, and occasionally associated with congenital heart disease, shows a much wider range of variation than is seen in pectus excavatum, although we recognize two typical varieties.[21-24]

1. In the chicken breast, or classic deformity (Fig. 3), the sternum appears prominently bowed forward but is in fact chiefly made to appear so because of the parallel vertical runnels of depressed cartilage on either side. These chests function as inefficiently in the mechanics of respiration as do funnel chests, and the impingement upon the proper intrathoracic space is significant.

2. Less common is what we have termed the pouter pigeon deformity, which is characterized by a forward tilt of the manubrium followed by a posterior angulation of the gladiolus and then a reverse anterior angulation of the distal portion of the sternum, so that a sagittal section of the sternum would be Z-shaped. The sternum tends to be broad, the xiphoid to be bifid, and the sternebrae to be prematurely fused.

The grotesqueness of the various protrusion deformities in itself constitutes an adequate indication for operation, but we have been pleased to have our patients report substantially increased capacity for exercise after operation. Protrusion deformities are much less common than depression deformities and physiologic studies of patients with protrusion deformities have been few.

Treatment. The variation from patient to patient in protrusion deformities invites the exercise of a good deal of surgical ingenuity in their correction, but the general experience with the correction of protrusion deformities has been extremely satisfactory.[24] In the commoner chicken breast, or true keeled-sternum variety of pectus carinatum, we have found that, if we resect the depressed costal cartilages on either side, the lung with inspiration lifts forward the remaining perichondrium, which now, running a shorter course from the lateral limit of the rib resection to the sternum, has become redundant. If reefing sutures are taken in the perichondrium to stretch it tautly from rib to sternum, the cartilages as they regenerate provide an essentially normal thoracic contour. Ordinarily, nothing need be done to the sternum unless it is of unusual thickness or presents atypical bosses or angulations, which may be shaved away.

Sternal Clefts

Sternal clefts were in the past reported as instances of ectopia cordis. In true ectopia cordis, the infant is born with the heart partially or entirely outside the thoracic cavity, covered, if at all, only by pericardium. This generally occurs in association with a distal sternal cleft. True ectopia cordis of this kind is almost invariably associated with an internal cardiac malformation that is incompatible with life. A single infant of this kind has survived operation.[34]

The three principal types of sternal cleft are (1) superior, usually involving the manubrium and the gladiolus to the third or fourth interspace but occasionally extending almost to the xiphoid; (2) distal, involving the distal half or third of the sternum and generally part of a complex syndrome; and (3) complete sternal cleft, the rarest of all.

Superior Cervical Cleft (Cervicothoracic Ectopia Cordis). The sternum develops from paired primordia, the lateral sternal bars, which properly fuse at the ninth week. The reasons for failure of fusion in the various types of sternal cleft can only be guessed at. In the case of the superior sternal cleft, the heart is covered only by skin and pericardium. It is not actually displaced cephalad, but its prominence and the soft midline, uncovered by manubrium, make it appear to be in the neck (Fig. 4A and B). There is ample experience now to state that in the first few weeks of life there is little difficulty in freeing up or wedging out the lower ends of the two sternal bars, and bringing the sternal halves together in the midline for a complete correction of the deformity. The heart is usually normal. Without operation, as weeks and months pass, the weight of the shoulder girdle tends to hold the gap apart, and the increasing firmness of the chest wall makes approximation of the sternal halves in the midline difficult without additional procedures such as sliding chondrotomies. In still older children, even this does not avail and prosthetic reconstruction is required, with artificial materials and rib grafts, to eliminate the unsightly pulsating defect and to protect the heart and great vessels against injury. At times, a superior sternal cleft may extend almost to the xiphoid. The restitution to absolute normality of an infant with this striking deformity is accomplished with relative ease in early infancy.[27-29]

Distal Sternal Defect (Thoracoabdominal Ectopia Cordis). This is almost invariably a part of a pentalogy of

Figure 2. The operation for pectus excavatum. The pectoral muscles have been stripped to either side. The costal cartilages will be removed subperichondrially for the full extent of the deformity, in this case the third, fourth, fifth, sixth, and seventh cartilages. The sternum will be divided from the xiphoid and the intercostal bundles divided from the sternum, so that the sternum is isolated as a peninsula. The second rib will be incised obliquely from medially and in front to laterally and behind, and the sternum elevated by a posterior osteotomy in the first interspace. This will allow a chock block of rib bone to be placed in the osteotomy, wedging it open. The medial stumps of the second costal cartilages will then lie on the lateral stumps and will be sutured there. The resulting three-point fixation provides a secure fixation of the sternum in overcorrected position. In rare instances, usually in adults with very large sternums, a Kirschner wire may be placed through the sternum and across the defect, to rest on the chest wall on either side, under the pectoral muscles.

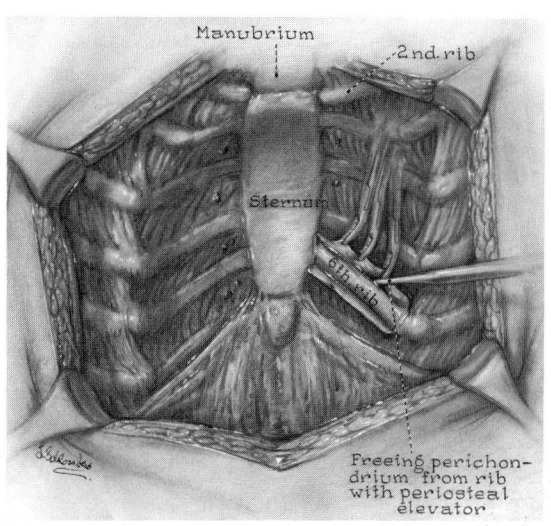

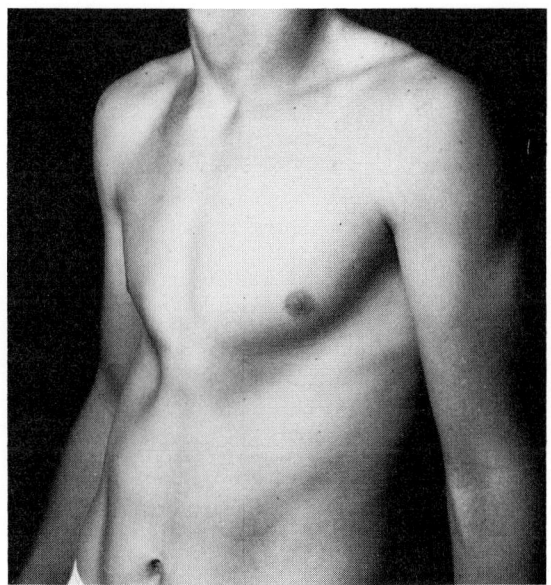

Figure 3. Pectus carinatum of chicken breast type. A 16-year-old boy referred because of a prominent sternum. In fact, it is the depression of the ribs on either side that causes the apparent prominence of the sternum. At operation, excision of four cartilages, subperichondrially, and reefing sutures in the now redundant perichondrium to provide a taut, straight course from the outer ends of the ribs to the sternum corrected the deformity very satisfactorily.

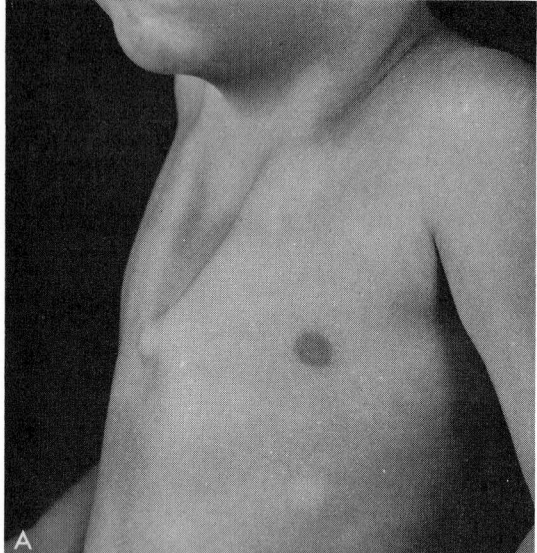

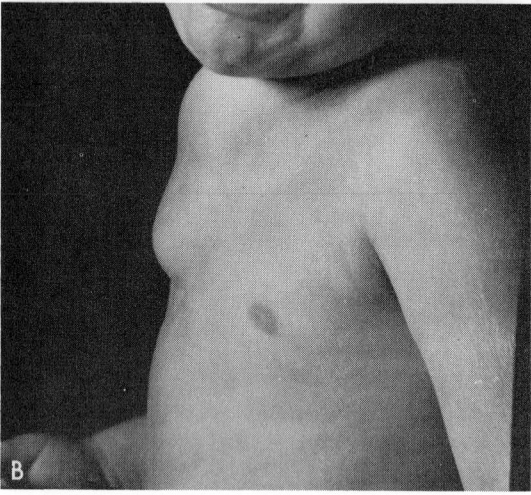

Figure 4. Cleft sternum. *A,* At rest. *B,* During forced expiration. Superior clefts of the sternum are variously V- or U-shaped. The appearance of the child as he cries explains the term "ectopia cordis," although the heart is actually not misplaced. In the newborn, defects of this kind can be corrected by direct apposition of the sternal halves. In this child, closure of the defect was made possible by sliding chondrotomies on either side. (From Sabiston, D. C., Jr.: J. Thorac. Surg., *35:*118, 1958.)

defects (Cantrell's syndrome).[26, 30, 31] (1) The distal portion of the sternum is cleft. (2) The epigastric midline is the seat of an omphalocele-like soft tissue defect or an actual omphalocele. (3) There is a ventral crescentic defect in the diaphragm. (4) The diaphragmatic pericardium is deficient as well, and the pericardium communicates with the peritoneal cavity. (5) There is an intrinsic cardiac defect, usually a ventricular septal defect, alone or as part of a complex deformity such as the tetralogy of Fallot. Occasionally there is a ventricular diverticulum.

Although the heart appears to be beating in the epigastrium, it is in fact not displaced. Operation in the first few months of life will make the midline somatic closure easiest. Closure of the diaphragm and pericardium poses no problems. The cardiac defect is treated at the time and manner determined by its nature. It has occasionally proved possible to repair the abdominal wall, the diaphragm, the chest wall, and the heart at one operation.[30, 31]

Complete Sternal Cleft. This is particularly uncommon. We have had experience with it in a single

child,[32] who had also a ventral abdominal defect, a diaphragmatic defect, and a pericardial defect but no intracardiac defect. When he was first seen at the age of 1½ years, it was no longer possible to bring the lateral sternal bars together in the midline, but a reconstruction with prosthetic material (Teflon felt) and autogenous rib grafts has resulted in a normal-appearing and normally functioning chest, now 15 years later.

RIB DEFORMITIES

A variety of bizarre deformities of the ribs occur, including missing ribs, fused ribs, and supernumerary ribs, often accompanied by other, distant, skeletal malformations as well. Each patient poses a separate problem. If there are large areas of paradoxical movement that cause respiratory embarrassment, or repeated pulmonary infections, some operative chest wall reconstruction may be considered. Most commonly, in association with these bizarre rib deformities one finds hemivertebrae, paravertebral bars of fused bone, and progressive scoliosis. It is the spinal deformity, with the possibility of progressive scoliosis, that is the serious problem and the one to which attention must usually be primarily directed, rather than to the ribs.[38, 39]

Poland's Syndrome

One anomaly of the ribs repeats itself with sufficient frequency to constitute a syndrome. This consists of absence of costal cartilages and of portions of ribs, usually the second, third, and fourth, hypoplasia or absence of nipple and breast, hypoplasia of subcutaneous fat, absence of axillary hair, absence of the costosternal portion of the pectoralis major, and absence of the pectoralis minor.[38-40] The area of absent cartilage, uncovered by muscle, and with unusually thin skin, presents a picture of conspicuous deformity, an area of striking paradoxical motion of the chest wall, and a "soft spot" that, particularly on the left side, is alarming and may actually present as a lung hernia.

The deformity is part of a spectrum of anomalies in which syndactylism, short fingers, missing phalanges, missing forearm bones, spinal anomalies, and Sprengel's deformity may also occur. The chest wall deformity may appear without the other manifestations, and the other manifestations may appear without the chest wall deformity.

Failure to correct the rib deformity may lead to progressive increase in the deformity as the cartilages above and below, unsupported and not connected to their mates, buckle and bulge.

As a substitute for the chest wall, and to provide some thickness to the tissues, we implant a sheet of prosthetic material (Teflon felt) stretched across the defect, supported by autogenous rib grafts for rigidity and some contour effect. This results in a stable chest wall, abolition of paradoxical movement, and protection of the subjacent viscera. In the absence of the pectoralis major and with deficient breast and subcutaneous tissue, the chest is still visibly asymmetric. In girls, after puberty, depending upon the degree of mammary development, prosthetic mammary augmentation may be worthwhile. The muscular absence (as after radical mastectomy) does not constitute a significant functional handicap.

ACQUIRED DEFORMITIES OF THE CHEST WALL

The physiologic cardiorespiratory embarrassment that may occur with extreme scoliosis or kyphoscoliosis is well known, and in the days when Pott's disease and grotesque hunchbacks were common, death from respiratory failure and from pulmonary hypertension with cardiac failure was well recognized. Lam[43] reported a remarkable improvement in a patient with severe "idiopathic" scoliosis in whom the progressive fatigue and dyspnea were strikingly relieved by decompression of the heart compressed by the deformed chest. We would expect that there would be patients with either scoliotic or kyphoscoliotic deformity in whom correction of a deep lateral incurvation on the concave side of the major curve might be possible, enlarging the hemithorax and permitting the lung to expand, but have never found such a patient. Block, Wexler, and McDonnell[42] demonstrated a remarkable increase in thoracic volume and pulmonary function in a 49-year-old kyphoscoliotic by the application of halo-femoral traction to stretch the patient and decrease the scoliosis. While clearly it is preferable to prevent such severe deformities and their secondary cardiopulmonary complications by appropriate orthopedic procedures early in life, it is worth bearing in mind that there may be instances in which, in addition to such measures as breathing exercises, bronchodilators, pulmonary toilet, and intermittent positive-pressure breathing that have been shown to be helpful, the basic mechanism of the disability might be attacked by procedures directed at correction of the thoracic deformity.

Fractured ribs have a remarkable capacity for springing back into shape, and deformity from this cause is uncommon. Even if double fractures of several ribs have produced a flail chest, the preferred treatment of prolonged respiratory support with a respirator maintains the segments in reasonably good position. In the rare patient in whom such segments heal in a depressed position, ultimate operative correction would be possible, although we have not ourselves seen a patient in whom this seemed advisable or justifiable.

TUMORS OF THE RIBS AND STERNUM

Tumors of the ribs and sternum are relatively uncommon. Any of the structures in the soft tissues of the chest wall may be involved in all of the histologic types of connective tissue tumors, and these may secondarily involve the ribs or sternum. A soft tissue tumor that is hard, painful, fixed to the chest wall, or growing rapidly should be considered to be malignant. Benign tumors of soft tissues (as opposed to congenital malformations such as hemangiomas and lymphangiomas) are much less common in children than in adults, and any lump in the chest wall should be viewed with suspicion.

A soft tissue tumor, or a bony tumor for that matter, must be excised with a wide margin of normal tissues on all sides, and encapsulation, real or apparent, should be neither looked for nor trusted. A soft tissue tumor involving the medial portion of the pectoralis major would therefore require resection of the chest wall to and including the pleura, whereas a tumor of similar size in the latissimus dorsi or trapezius might require only wide resection of soft tissue.

Tumors of the ribs and sternum are sufficiently uncommon that there are no large individual series, and the collected reports list scattered cases of every conceivable histologic type in all age groups. Vieta and Maier,[53] from 74 published reports on tumors of the sternum, found that the majority were malignant. Chondrosarcomas were the single commonest variety, and experience showed that pathologists had a tendency to "underdiagnose."

Chondrosarcoma was seen five to ten times more commonly arising from ribs than from sternum. The chondrosarcomas grow slowly, recur after long intervals, and ultimately cause distant metastases, or death results from inoperable local extension. Plasmacytoma of the sternum, reticulum cell sarcoma of ribs and sternum, osteogenic sarcoma, Ewing's sarcoma, and other even rarer tumors occur. Results after resection and irradiation vary for each type.

Certain valid generalizations and particularizations may be made. Malignant tumors of the ribs and sternum are more common than benign tumors, and this is true in childhood and infancy as well. Again, at all ages, metastatic tumors to the chest wall are commoner than primary tumors. The discovery of a mass fixed to the chest wall requires a systematic investigation for a possible primary tumor, the lung, thyroid, breast,and kidney being the most likely sources apart from the lymphomas. If no primary tumor can be found, operation should be undertaken as if the chest wall tumor were malignant.[44] In general, biopsy is to be avoided because (1) In the most common situation, chondrosarcoma, the histologic picture is notoriously treacherous and continues to seem benign even after the tumor has metastasized (quite the reverse of the situation with chondromas of the fingers, which look histologically malignant and are clinically benign). (2) If the skin is not attached to the tumor, it is desirable to plan the incision so that the ultimate suture line will be over intact chest wall, and this will not be possible if an incision is made directly over the tumor for biopsy. (3) Instances of seeding, even with the relatively benign chondrosarcoma, have been clearly documented.

The principles of resection of a chest wall tumor are straightforward.[45, 46, 51, 52] (1) The incision should be designed so as to fall outside the ultimate defect in the chest wall. If the skin is involved or a biopsy has been performed, a wide margin should be given the tumor from the skin on down, and the original draping planned so that appropriate flaps can be swung. (2) The chest should be entered at least one interspace away from the tumor so that a finger may be inserted to determine the extent of any visceral involvement, usually an attachment to the lung. If the lung is involved, the contiguous portion, or the involved lobe, is resected. The problem of carcinoma of the lung extending into the chest wall is discussed in the section on carcinoma of the lung. (3) For lesions involving the ribs, one uninvolved rib above and below the lesion should be resected together with all the overlying muscle externally (and the skin as indicated) and the pleura internally, and a wide margin laterally and medially should be given to the apparent area of involvement. (4) For tumors of the sternum, a similarly wide margin is required, and full thickness of the sternum must be taken together with ample lengths of costal cartilages on either side of the involved portion of the sternum. The pericardium, if adherent, should be taken with the tumor and the pleura with the attached costal cartilages.

Fortunately, very large portions of the sternum—in fact practically all of it if the upper border of the manubrium is left for attachment of the clavicles—can be removed without necessarily causing significant respiratory distress or paradoxical motion. If large areas of the costal portion of the chest wall are removed, significant paradoxical movement and respiratory embarrassment may occur. If skin has not had to be sacrificed, then for either a sternal or a costal defect we prefer a composite reconstruction, bridging the defect with autogenous rib grafts to support a tautly stretched prosthetic material such as Marlex or Teflon felt. Use of molded acrylic implants, often bonded to synthetic cloth, is increasingly reported.[49, 50] If large areas of skin have had to be sacrificed, the cutaneous defect is best compensated for by rotation of a flap. In anterior chest wall defects in females, a flap composed of a breast, the substance of which has been split from its deep side so that it may be flattened out, will cover an enormous area at a considerable distance, if need be, from the original location of the breast. The abnormality of a misplaced breast is an acceptable price to pay for this readily available and thick covering for a chest wall defect. If heavy muscle flaps (e.g., latissimus dorsi) or a large breast or both are used to cover a defect, further reconstruction of the chest wall is often unnecessary.

Chondrosarcomas may reach enormous size and still be resectable and curable. We have had the experience of finding such a tumor invading the diaphragm, a portion of which had to be resected and the diaphragm then reattached to the reconstructed chest wall. The abdominal viscera may be involved by direct extension in large but resectable and potentially curable chest wall chondrosarcomas.[47]

The presence of a parasternal ulcerating lesion in a patient who has had a radical mastectomy for carcinoma of the breast presents both a diagnostic and a therapeutic problem. The lesion may be a chronic benign ulcer in ischemic scar tissue. It may be an irradiation ulcer. It may be squamous cell carcinoma in irradiated tissue. It may be the result of chondritis following irradiation or infection. It may be persistent carcinoma or a recurrence of carcinoma from the original lesion, or it may be the result of the extension through the chest wall of a metastatic deposit originating in the internal mammary chain. Since some of the possibilities represent benign lesions and others represent curable malignant lesions, no patient with such a lesion should be abandoned without careful biopsy and consideration as to whether a chest wall resection and reconstruction should be performed. Even if one gains only 6 months or a year of life in a patient with recurrent carcinoma of the breast, a period of that duration free from pain, ulceration, and discharge would justify the excision of the tumor and chest wall reconstruction. In these patients, who have had a radical mastectomy, chest wall resection inevitably requires migration of a flap, usually the entire opposite breast.

INFECTIONS OF THE CHEST WALL

Subpectoral abscesses of remarkable size may be concealed by the pectoral muscle and breast over them. The subpectoral position of an abscess is demonstrated by the disappearance of bulge and fluctuation when the patient places his hands akimbo and tightens the pectoral muscle. The abscess may be pyogenic or tuberculous, originating from the pectoral lymph nodes, from infections of the ribs, or occasionally in communication with an empyema (empyema necessitatus). Evacuation of the abscess is performed through an incision below the pectoralis major, and appropriate therapy is directed to the underlying lesion.

Pyogenic infections of the ribs and sternum occur in association with disseminated infections. As with osteomyelitis elsewhere, the initial treatment is massive and prolonged administration of antibiotics. The thinness and softness of the cortical bone make incision and drainage of an osteomyelitic focus even less urgent than in the long bones, and the anatomic situation is such as to allow wide decortication or resection of any affected portion of the ribs or sternum. Whereas pyogenically infected rib or sternum, once adequately exposed, will generally heal, cartilage will generally not heal once the perichondrium has been breached by infection, whether resulting from an infected traumatic or operative wound or some contiguous pyogenic process. After the period of active infection and systemic reaction has been passed, the area of involved cartilage should be cleanly resected, through its full thickness, by transection of the cartilage on either side with a sharp knife, with care to avoid elevation of the perichondrium over cartilage that is to remain. The relative avascularity of cartilage renders it extremely vulnerable.

Specific Infections

Formerly, tuberculosis of the ribs, sternum, and cartilages created problems that are rarely seen in this country today. Tuberculous osteomyelitis of ribs or sternum generally perforates through the soft tissues and becomes secondarily infected. The earlier treatment of wide resection and secondary healing of the open wound has now been replaced by specific antimycobacterial therapy and expectant and limited operative treatment. A sinus or discharge a centimeter or two lateral to the sternum should be suspected of arising from the lymph nodes of the internal mammary chain; this is the route of infection that involves the costal cartilages in tuberculosis, or in the spread of cancer of the breast.

Actinomycosis of the chest wall is now similarly infrequently seen and responds to a combination of antibiotic therapy and such local operative therapy as general surgical principles dictate.

SELECTED REFERENCE

Beiser, G. D., Epstein, S. E., Stampfer, M., Goldstein, R. E., Nolan, S. P., and Levitsky, S.: Impairment of cardiac function in patients with pectus excavatum, with improvement after operative correction. N. Engl. J. Med., 287:267, 1972.

Although pectus excavatum is thought to impair cardiac performance, no consistent hemodynamic abnormalities have been identified. It was hypothesized that cardiac function might be impaired during upright exercise when the heart descends into the pectus deformity. Catheterization of the right side of the heart in six patients with pectus excavatum gave normal results, and the hemodynamic response to supine exercise was normal. In contrast, cardiac output during intense upright exercise was low in two patients, at the lower limits of normal in one, and low normal in two. The cardiac output and stroke-volume responses to mild upright exercise also differed from normal. After operative repair in three patients, cardiac output during intense upright exercise increased an average of 38 per cent, and hemodynamic responses to mild upright exercise also changed toward normal. No alterations occurred in the response to supine exercise. Thus, pectus excavatum can reduce the pumping capacity of the heart during upright exercise, and hemodynamic improvement occurs after surgical correction.

REFERENCES

Pectus Excavatum

1. Beiser, G. C., Epstein, S. E., Stampfer, M., Goldstein, R. E., Nolan, S. P., and Levitsky, S.: Impairment of cardiac function in patients with pectus excavatum, with improvement after operative correction. N. Engl. J. Med., 287:267, 1972.
2. Bevegård, S.: Postural circulatory changes after and during exercise in patients with a funnel chest, with special reference to factors affecting stroke volume. Acta Med. Scand., 171:695, 1962.
3. Brodkin, H. A.: Congenital chondrosternal depression (funnel chest): Its treatment by phrenosternolysis and chondrosternoplasty. Dis. Chest, 19:288, 1951.
4. Brown, A. L.: Pectus excavatum (funnel chest). J. Thorac. Surg., 9:164, 1939.
5. Diaz, F. V., Pelons, A. N., Valdis, F. G., Grandi, F. G. G., and Granados, A.: Pectus excavatum: Hemodynamic and electrocardiographic considerations. Am. J. Cardiol., 10:272, 1962.
6. Fishman, A. P., Turino, G. M., and Bergofsky, E. H.: Disorders of the respiration and circulation in subjects with deformities of the thorax. Mod. Conc. Cardiovasc. Dis., 27:449, 1958.
7. Howard, R.: Funnel chest, its effect on cardiac function. Arch. Dis. Child., 34:5, 1958.
8. Lester, C. W.: Tissue replacement after subperichondrial resection of costal cartilage – two case reports. Plast. Reconstr. Surg., 23:49, 1959.
9. Lyons, H. A., Zuhdi, M. N., and Kelly, J. S., Jr.: Pectus excavatum ("funnel breast"): Cause of impaired ventricular distensibility as exhibited by right ventricular pressure pattern. Am. Heart J., 50:921, 1955.
10. Mankin, H. J., Graham, J. F., and Schack, J.: Cardiopulmonary function in mild and moderate idiopathic scoliosis. J. Bone Joint Surg., 46-A:53, 1964.
11. Ochsner, A., and DeBakey, M.: Chone-Chondrosternon – Report of a case and review of the literature. J. Thorac. Surg., 8:469, 1939.
12. Ravitch, M. M.: The operative treatment of pectus excavatum. Ann. Surg., 128:429, 1949.
13. Ravitch, M. M.: Pectus excavatum and heart failure. Surgery, 30:178, 1951.
14. Ravitch, M. M.: The chest wall. In Mustard, W. T., Ravitch, M. M., Snyder, W. H., Jr., Welch, C. E., and Benson, C. D.: Pediatric Surgery, 2nd ed. Chicago, Year Book Medical Publishers, 1969.
15. Ravitch, M. M., and Matzen, R. N.: Pulmonary insufficiency in pectus excavatum associated with left pulmonary agenesis, congenital clubbed feet and ectromelia. Dis. Chest, 54:58, 1968.
16. Reusch, C. S.: Hemodynamic studies in pectus excavatum. Circulation, 24:1143, 1961.
17. Sauerbruch, D. F.: Die Chirurgie der Brustorgane, 3rd ed. Berlin, G. Springer, 1928, pp. 735–741.
18. Sweet, R. H.: Pectus excavatum. Ann. Surg., 119:922, 1964.
19. Wachtel, F., Ravitch, M. M., and Grishman, A.: The relation of pectus excavatum to heart disease. Am. Heart J., 52:121, 1956.
20. Weg, J. G., Krumholz, R. A., and Harkleroad, L. E.: Pulmonary dysfunction in pectus excavatum. Am. Rev. Resp. Dis., 96:936, 1967.

Pectus Carinatum

21. Howard, R.: Pigeon chest (protrusion deformity of the sternum). Med. J. Aust., 45:664, 1958.
22. Ravitch, M. M.: Unusual sternal deformity with cardiac symptoms. Operative correction. J. Thorac. Surg., 23:138, 1952.
23. Ravitch, M. M.: The operative correction of pectus carinatum (pigeon breast). Ann. Surg., 151:705, 1960.
24. Ravitch, M. M.: The chest wall. In Mustard, W. T., Ravitch, M. M. Snyder, W. H., Jr., Welch, C. E., and Benson, C. D.: Pediatric Surgery, 2nd ed. Chicago, Year Book Medical Publishers, 1969.

Sternal Clefts

25. Asp, K. A., and Sulamaa, M.: Ectopia cordis. Acta Chir. Scand., Suppl., *283*:52, 1961.
26. Cantrell, J. R., Haller, J. A., and Ravitch, M. M.: A syndrome of congenital defects involving the abdominal wall, sternum, diaphragm, pericardium and heart. Surg. Gynecol. Obstet., *107*:602, 1958.
27. Jewett, T. C., Jr., Hutsch, W. L., and Hug, H. R.: Congenital bifid sternum. Surgery, *52*:932, 1962.
28. Longino, L. A., and Jewett, T. C., Jr.: Congenital bifid sternum. Surgery, *38*:610, 1955.
29. Maier, H. G., and Bortone, F.: Complete failure of sternal fusion with herniation of pericardium. J. Thorac. Surg., *18*:851, 1949.
30. Mulder, D. G., Crittenden, I. H., and Adams, F. H.: Complete repair of syndrome of congenital defects involving the abdominal wall, sternum, diaphragm, pericardium and heart: Excision of left ventricular diverticulum. Ann. Surg., *151*:113, 1960.
31. Murphy, D. A., Aberdeen, E., Dobbs, R. H., and Waterston, D. J.: The surgical treatment of a syndrome consisting of thoracoabdominal wall, diaphragmatic, pericardial, and ventricular septal defects, and a left ventricular diverticulum. Ann. Thorac. Surg., *6*:528, 1969.
32. Ravitch, M. M.: Spectacular problems in surgery. Congenital absence of sternum. Surg. Gynecol. Obstet., *116*:1963.
33. Ravitch, M. M.: The chest wall. *In* Mustard, W. T., Ravitch, M. M., Snyder, W. H., Jr., Welch, C. E., and Benson, C. D.: Pediatric Surgery, 2nd ed. Chicago, Year Book Medical Publishers, 1969.
34. Saxena, N. C.: Personal communication, December, 1975.

Poland's Syndrome

35. Duhamel, B., and Glichenstein, J.: Agenesie du grand pectoral et brachysyndactyly (syndrome Poland). Chirurgie, *101*:233, 1975.

Rib Abnormalities

36. De Beneditti, M., and Chiapuzzo, A.: Malformazione Unilaterale dei Muscoli Pettorali. Arch. Ortop., *73*:408–417, 1960.
37. Epstein, L. I., and Bennett, J. W.: Syndactyly with ipsilateral chest deformity. Plast. Reconstr. Surg., *46*:236, 1970.

38. MacEwen, G. G., Conway, J. J., and Miller, W. T.: Congenital scoliosis with a unilateral bar. Radiology, *90*:711, 1968.
39. Ravitch, M. M.: Atypical deformities of the chest wall — absence and deformities of the ribs and costal cartilages. Surgery, *59*:438, 1966.
40. Sulamaa, M., and Asp, K.: Treatment of some thoracic deformities. Acta Chir. Scand., *122*:267, 1961.
41. Walker, J. C., Jr., Meijer, R., and Aranda, D.: Syndactylism with deformity of the pectoralis muscle — Poland's syndrome. J. Pediatr. Surg., *4*:569, 1969.

Acquired Deformities

42. Block, A. J. Wexler, J., and McDonnell, E. J.: Cardiopulmonary failure of the hunchback. J.A.M.A., *212*:1520, 1970.
43. Lam, C. R., and McClure, R. D.: Decompression of the heart in severe scoliosis. J. Thorac. Surg., *12*:517, 1943.

Tumors

44. Brindley, G. V., Jr.: Primary malignant tumors of the chest wall (excluding primary cutaneous neoplasms). Ann. Surg., *153*:684, 1961.
45. Dineen, J. P., and Boltax, R. S.: Problems in the management of chest wall tumor. J. Thorac. Cardiovasc. Surg., *52*:588, 1966.
46. Eijgelaar, A., and van der Haide, J. N. H.: Ergebnisse der Radikalen Brustwandresection. Thorax Chir., *20*:404, 1972.
47. Hull, D. A.: Massive chondrosarcoma of the rib with extension into the colon: Repair with tantalum mesh. Ann. Surg., *140*:886, 1954.
48. Kauffman, S. L., and Stout, A. P.: Extraskeletal osteogenic sarcomas and chondrosarcomas in children. Cancer, *16*:432, 1963.
49. Larson, R. E., Lick, L. C., and Maxeiner, S. R., Jr.: Technique for chest wall reconstruction following resection of sternal chondrosarcoma. Arch. Surg., *98*:668, 1969.
50. LeRoux, B. T.: Maintenance of chest wall stability. Thorax, *19*:397, 1964.
51. Maier, H. C.: Surgical management of large defects of the thoracic wall. Surgery, *22*:169, 1947.
52. Pickrell, K. L., Baker, H. M., and Collins, J. O.: Reconstructive surgery of the chest wall. Surg. Gynecol. Obstet., *84*:465, 1947.
53. Vieta, J. O., and Maier, H. C.: Tumors of the sternum. Int. Abstr. Surg., *114*:513, 1962.

56

THE MEDIASTINUM

H. Newland Oldham, Jr., M.D.,
and David C. Sabiston, Jr., M.D.

The mediastinum is an important subdivision of the thorax that is located between the pleural cavities. This space contains numerous organs and anatomic structures and is the site of a wide variety of primary and secondary disorders. The most important of these are infections, emphysema, and primary tumors and cysts. Other conditions such as esophageal and aortic lesions relate more appropriately to the specific organ system than to the mediastinum itself. The increasing use of chest roentgenography and the simultaneous advances in thoracic surgical techniques have emphasized the importance of accurate diagnosis and prompt surgical treatment of lesions of the mediastinum.

HISTORICAL ASPECTS

Prior to the introduction of endotracheal anesthesia, few attempts were made to operate within the mediastinum because of the hazards of collapse of the lung following entry into the pleura. The Italian surgeon Bastianelli in 1893 performed one of the earliest successful operations, removing a dermoid cyst from the anterior mediastinum after resecting the manubrium.[2] An outstanding description of early mediastinal surgery was given by Milton in 1897.[32] Working first with cadavers and later with goats, he devised a sternal splitting approach to the mediastinum that avoided entrance into either pleural cavity. Using this technique, he operated on a patient with caseating tuberculous nodes in the mediastinum, leaving the sternum and the wound open at the end of the procedure. The patient did well, and 2 days later the incision was closed without difficulty. Milton was impressed with the access afforded by this incision, and after the operation he made the prediction that a sternal splitting approach to the mediastinum might be useful for operations on valvular lesions of the heart. With the introduction of endotracheal anesthesia, which allowed the pleural cavities to be opened safely, major advances in surgery of the mediastinum rapidly followed. Although mediastinal lesions may occasionally be removed without entry into the pleura, thoracotomy with intrapleural dissection is the surgical approach most often employed. The most significant contributions leading to contemporary surgery of the mediastinum are found in the classic writings of Harrington,[21] Blalock,[4] and Heuer and Andrus.[25]

ANATOMY

The mediastinum is that portion of the thoracic cavity extending from the thoracic inlet superiorly to the diaphragms below. This space is bounded laterally by the mediastinal pleura, posteriorly by the vertebral column, and anteriorly by the sternum. Certain arbitrary divisions of the mediastinum have been made for convenience in localizing specific types of lesions. A plane extending from the lower manubrium to the fourth thoracic vertebra separates the superior from the inferior mediastinum. The inferior compartment is further subdivided by the pericardial sac into anterior, middle, and posterior compartments (Fig. 1). The superior mediastinum contains the upper trachea and esophagus, the thymus gland, and the aortic arch and its branches. Located in the anterior mediastinum are the thymus gland and adipose, lymphatic, and areolar tissues. The middle mediastinum contains the pericardium, heart, aorta, tracheal bifurcation and main bronchi, and the bronchial lymph nodes. The contents of the posterior mediastinum include the esophagus, descending aorta, and sympathetic and peripheral nerves. The various structures present in the mediastinum are shown in Figure 2. Because many lesions in the superior mediastinum extend into the anterior or posterior compartment, it has been suggested that a more practical partition would consist of only three subdivisions; anterosuperior, posterior, and middle mediastinum.

INFECTIONS OF THE MEDIASTINUM

Acute mediastinitis is a serious condition that usually produces impressive clinical manifestations. The process is found in association with a variety of disorders, including perforation of the esophagus following trauma or esophagoscopy, penetrating wounds

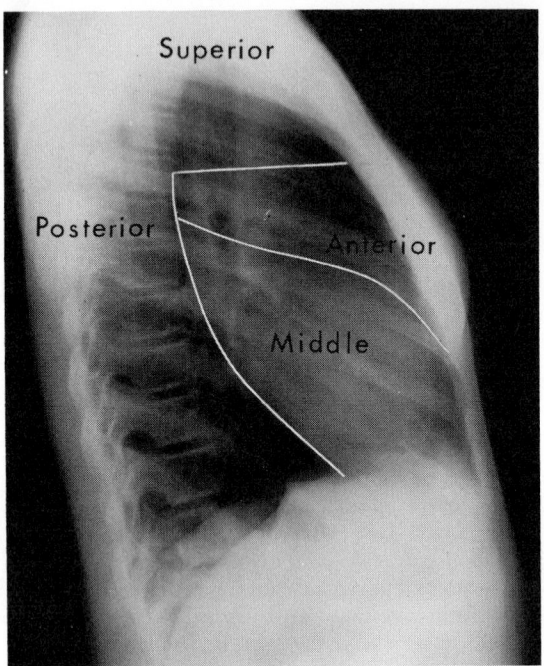

Figure 1. Anatomic subdivisions of the mediastinum superimposed on a lateral chest film.

of the thorax, esophageal leaks following surgical anastomoses, and tracheobronchial perforation. The symptoms are usually quite dramatic and are characteristically of sudden onset. High fever, tachycardia, malaise, and leukocytosis are common. Severe pain in the neck or chest is usually present. If the mediastinitis is secondary to an esophageal perforation, the pain and discomfort are most often in the neck, since the perforation is usually at the level of the cricopharyngeal muscle. Subcutaneous emphysema producing cervical swelling is nearly always found.

The treatment of the mediastinitis is directed toward the inciting cause. Antimicrobial therapy should be begun immediately as well as supportive treatment including sedation, oxygen, and careful observation. Although some patients may respond to nonoperative management alone, prompt surgical drainage is most often indicated as the safest and most certain means of controlling the infection.

Chronic mediastinitis is usually due to a granulomatous inflammatory process such as tuberculosis or one of the mycoses. Histoplasmosis commonly involves the lymph nodes of the mediastinum and has been identified as one of the agents associated with mediastinal fibrosis.[26] Antituberculosis or antifungal therapy is indicated in the presence of active infection. With progressive chronic infection, direct involvement or

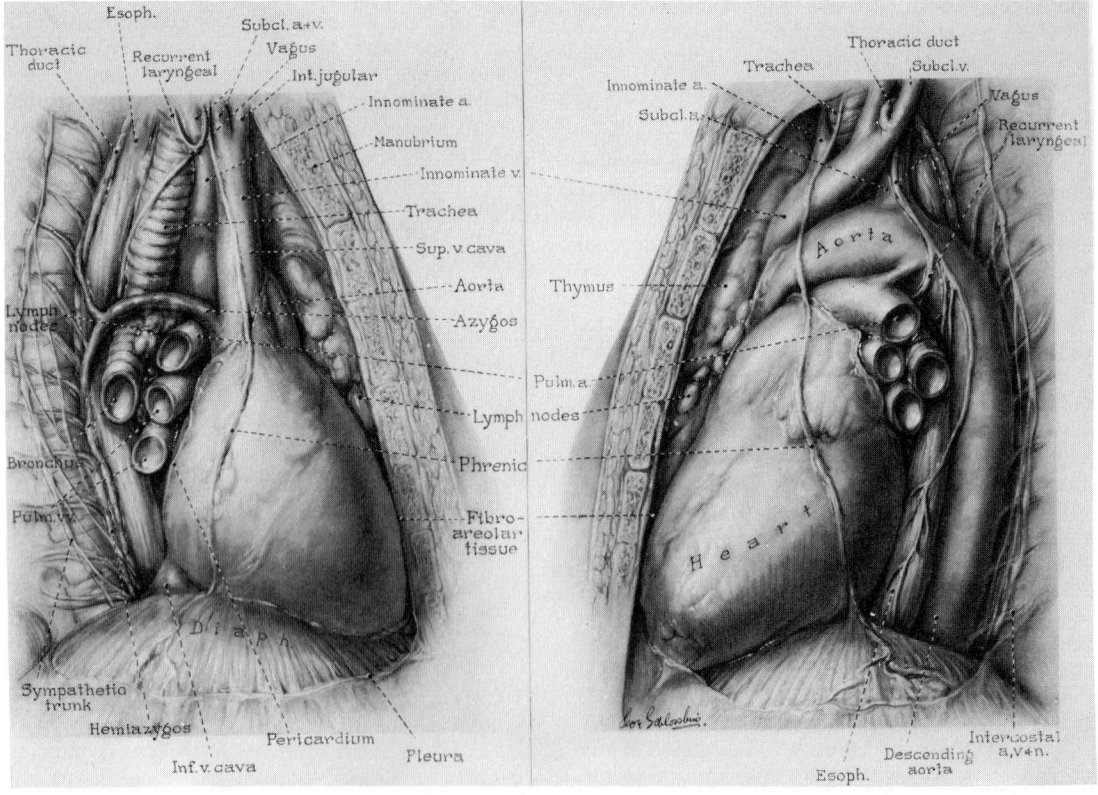

A   B

Figure 2. Anatomic structures of the mediastinum seen from the right side *(A)* and the left side *(B)*. (From Sabiston, D. C., Jr. *In* Cooke, R. E., and Levin, S. (Eds.): Biologic Basis of Pediatric Practices. New York, McGraw-Hill Book Company, 1968.)

compression of a variety of structures adjacent to the mediastinal lymph nodes may occur. This may ultimately produce obstruction of the superior vena cava, the esophagus, the trachea, or a major bronchus.

MEDIASTINAL EMPHYSEMA

The introduction of air into the mediastinum from numerous sources produces mediastinal emphysema or pneumomediastinum. The air may enter from the tracheobronchial tree, the esophagus, the neck, or the abdomen. Penetrating wounds and perforation of these structures are common causes of this condition. Blunt trauma with fracture of ribs or vertebrae is not infrequently accompanied by pneumomediastinum. Increased intrapulmonary pressure from either trauma or positive-pressure anesthesia may lead to alveolar rupture with subsequent dissection of air along the vascular structures of the lung into the hilum and then into the tissue planes of the mediastinum. In addition to these predisposing factors, "spontaneous mediastinal emphysema" is also a recognized entity.[20] In this condition mediastinal air is thought to follow interstitial emphysema of the lung, frequently occurring without specific known cause.

Mediastinal emphysema may make its clinical appearance in the deep and subcutaneous tissues of the neck and in the pleural cavity. It may also dissect into the retroperitoneal structures through the diaphragmatic hiatus. If the air within the mediastinum is under significant tension, the pressure may be sufficiently great to collapse the veins and interfere with venous return to the heart, and therefore produce clinical manifestations.

The symptoms of mediastinal emphysema include substernal pain and crepitus in the suprasternal notch and cervical region. With increasing pressure, the mediastinal air may spread to the soft tissues of the neck, chest, abdomen, and extremities. In spontaneous mediastinal emphysema, a characteristic crunching sound that is synchronous with systole is often heard over the precordium (Hamman's sign), and subcutaneous emphysema may be detectable in the cervical region. In this form of emphysema, this sign and precordial pain may be the only clinical manifestations and the disorder slowly subsides. In the more severe forms resulting from other causes, dyspnea, cyanosis, and prominence of the neck veins appear, especially if the air is under considerable tension. Rarely, circulatory failure may develop. The diagnosis is established by the clinical features as well as by roentgenography. Chest films show the presence of the air within the planes of the mediastinum dissecting also into the neck, pectoral muscles, and occasionally the extremities. The treatment of mediastinal emphysema is directed toward the inciting cause when such can be identified. The "spontaneous" form is apt to subside without producing significant sequelae. Careful observation of the patient is always indicated, so that the symptoms of increased tension and serious manifestations will be recognized promptly. Sedation and the administration of oxygen are important. Only rarely is surgical decompression necessary for the mediastinal emphysema itself, although it may be required for the underlying lesion.

MEDIASTINAL COMPRESSION SYNDROMES

Hemorrhage

Hemorrhage into the mediastinum may be due to a number of causes, but it is most commonly the result of trauma. Penetrating wounds often cause laceration of one of the major arteries or veins, and blunt trauma may be associated with transection of the aorta or other major vessels. Dissecting thoracic aneurysms are usually accompanied by significant bleeding into the mediastinum. Following cardiac surgery peformed through a sternal splitting incision, especially when cardiopulmonary bypass is used, it is not uncommon to see a large accumulation of blood within the mediastinum. Less common causes of this condition are hemorrhagic diathesis, anticoagulation therapy, uremia, infection, and bleeding from a primary tumor or cyst of the mediastinum. On rare occasions, superior mediastinal hemorrhage is seen in patients in whom no underlying cause can be established. This "spontaneous" form of bleeding sometimes follows episodes of violent coughing, and is presumably due to rupture of small mediastinal vessels during a period of markedly elevated intrathoracic pressure.[10] With progressive bleeding, mediastinal tamponade may occur, with hypotension, cyanosis, dyspnea, and venous distention, and ecchymoses extending into the neck. This syndrome is more insidious in onset than pericardial tamponade, as the mediastinum is capable of containing a large volume of blood before compression of its contents occurs. Surgical treatment may be urgently required to treat the underlying source of bleeding and to evacuate the blood causing compression.

Superior Vena Caval Obstruction

Obstruction of the superior vena cava may result from a variety of benign and malignant lesions involving the mediastinum. As the primary process that obstructs the vena cava progresses, characteristic symptoms appear. The classic features of this syndrome include increased venous pressure; edema of the head, neck, and upper extremities; dilated venous collateral channels in the chest wall; and cyanosis. The venous distention is most apparent in the recumbent position, but in most instances the veins do not collapse in the normal manner with the patient upright. The pressure in the dilated veins ranges between 20 and 50 cm. of saline. In some instances, the superior vena cava becomes occluded quite slowly and the symptoms may be insidious in onset. When the occlusion is relatively rapid, all clinical manifestations are more prominent, and edema involving the eyelids and face as well as the arms and chest may be present. Moreover, rapidly increasing venous pressure in the cerebral circulation leads to neurologic impairment.

The majority of patients with the superior vena caval syndrome have an underlying malignant tumor involving the mediastinum. The most common lesion is bronchogenic carcinoma of the right upper lobe.

Other malignant tumors including those of the thymus and thyroid may also be responsible. In less than one fourth of patients with superior vena caval obstruction, the syndrome is the result of a benign lesion. Causes of the latter include idiopathic mediastinal fibrosis, mediastinal granuloma (especially histoplasmosis), multinodular goiter, and pleural calcification.

The diagnosis of the superior vena caval syndrome is directed toward identification of the primary condition. Since more than three fourths of these patients have a malignant tumor, a histologic diagnosis is usually possible and desirable. Venous angiography will demonstrate the site of obstruction of the superior vena cava and usually shows filling of extensive collateral vessels (Fig. 3). Surgical treatment is rarely indicated in this group, since the lesions are usually inoperable. Radiation therapy produces favorable symptomatic results in many instances. Although decompression of the superior vena caval system by use of various types of grafts has been tried frequently, it has usually been unsuccessful.[47] In patients with benign lesions, the course is usually one of spontaneous regression as collateral channels develop over the chest wall. Thus, with the passage of time marked symptomatic improvement occurs, and operation is rarely indicated.

PRIMARY TUMORS AND CYSTS

A large number of histologically different tumors and cysts arise from the many anatomic structures located within the mediastinum. Since this area is also the site of numerous lymph nodes, metastases secondary to lesions in other parts of the body are also frequently found. Both benign and malignant lesions occur with considerable frequency, and a differential diagnosis is important whenever possible. Experience has shown that the majority of the primary lesions

that occur in the mediastinum can be cured by surgical means, and observation of mediastinal masses can only rarely be justified. Therefore, early diagnosis and definitive treatment are mandatory in the vast majority of patients with these disorders.

Primary lesions of the mediastinum are being recognized with increasing frequency, and in any large hospital population tumors and cysts of the mediastinum will be seen often enough to warrant a thorough understanding of their clinical characteristics. The relative incidence of the different types of mediastinal tumors and cysts in a collected series of 1000 patients is shown in Table 1. The incidence of the specific types is different in the various series, although definite tendencies for predominant lesions are apparent.[24, 29, 33, 34] Thus, neurogenic tumors are the most frequent neoplasms of the mediastinum, followed by teratodermoids and lymphomas. The incidence of various types of lesions in this collected series is quite similar to that in a report of 1064 mediastinal tumors from a single institution.[55]

Location

The division of the mediastinum into anatomic compartments as shown in Figure 1 is of value, since specific lesions characteristically arise in certain locations. The tumors and cysts most commonly occurring in each of the four compartments of the mediastinum are listed in Table 2. When a discrete mass is found in the superior mediastinum, the most likely diagnosis is thymoma or lymphoma, with tumors of the thyroid or parathyroid being less common possibilities. There are rare exceptions with each lesion, such as the occasional neurogenic tumor arising in the anterior mediastinum, or an ectopic thyroid located in the posterior mediastinum. As the tumor enlarges, it will occupy more than one compartment of the mediastinum, since there are no anatomic boundaries between them. It is not unusual to see a thymoma located in the superior mediastinum extending into

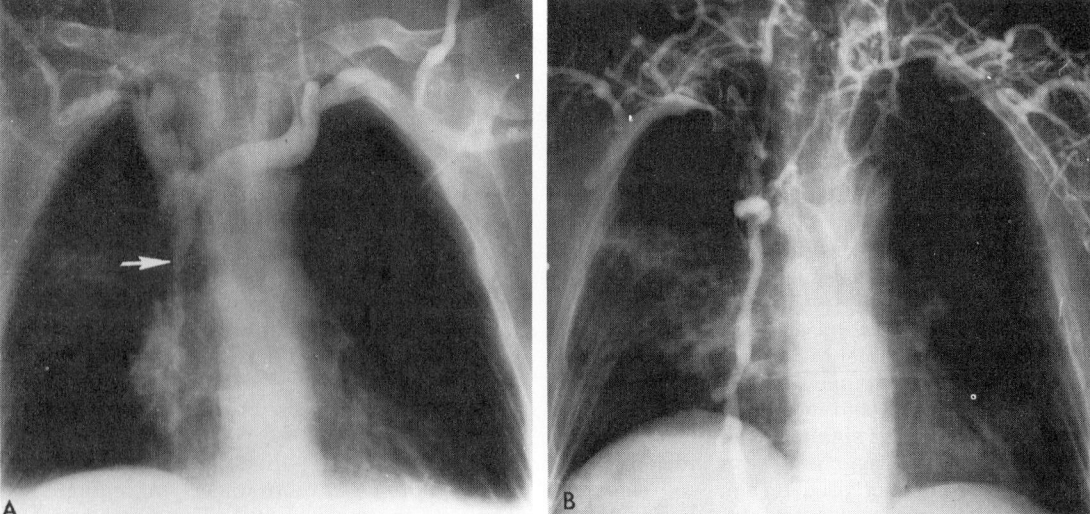

Figure 3. Venous angiogram illustrating narrowing of the superior vena cava (A). With later complete obstruction there are extensive channels bypassing the obstructed cava (B), and the azygos vein is noted as a prominent collateral pathway.

TABLE 1. Incidence of Neoplasms and Cysts of the Mediastinum
in a Collected Series of 1000 Patients*

Type of Tumor or Cyst	Herlitzka and Gale, 1958[24]	Morrison, 1958[33]	Key, 1954[29]	Harrington, 1949[21]	Oldham and Sabiston, 1967[34]	Total	Per Cent
Neurogenic tumors	35	101	10	51	43	240	24
Cysts							
Pericardial	17	13	4	7	33	74	7.4
Bronchogenic	24	23	3	10	27	87	8.7
Enteric	2	6		4	10	22	2.2
Nonspecific	4	6		8	13	31	3.1
Teratodermoids	26	36	31	40	36	169	17
Thymomas	14	47	4	8	52	125	12
Lymphomas	12	33	43		38	126	13
Other	20	26	6	30	44	126	13
Totals	154	291	101	158	296	1000	

*Excluding primary carcinoma of the mediastinum and substernal extension of cervical goiter.

the anterior mediastinum. A knowledge of the usual tumors and cysts located in each portion of the mediastinum is of help in planning the preoperative evaluation and operative procedure.

Mediastinal Tumors

Neurogenic Tumors. The most common mediastinal neoplasms in the majority of reported series are neurogenic tumors.[23, 33, 34, 45, 46] These tumors occur at any age and are most often benign, but when seen in children they have a somewhat greater tendency to be malignant. Several specific histologic types occur, including neurolemmoma, neurofibroma, neurosarcoma, ganglioneuroma, neuroblastoma, sympathicoblastoma, paraganglioma, and pheochromocytoma. Precise determination of these types may be difficult by routine microscopy, but recent descriptions of the ultrastructural morphology have helped differentiate the various tumors.[40] The typical location is in the posterior mediastinum along the paravertebral gutter, with the tumor arising from either the intercostal nerves or the sympathetic chain. There are rare reported cases of neurogenic tumors occurring in the anterior mediastinum. Most neurogenic tumors produce few symptoms, and the diagnosis is often made from an incidental chest film. Symptoms of chest pain and cough may be present and are due to pressure on adjacent structures.

Neurogenic tumors other than pheochromocytoma may exhibit hormonal activity.[19] This has been espe-

cially true of ganglioneuroma and neuroblastoma. Two syndromes have been seen: diarrhea and abdominal distention; and hypertension, flushing, and sweating. Elevated vanillylmandelic acid levels in the urine have been seen with ganglioneuroma, and the levels have returned to normal postoperatively.

Neurofibromas arise from nerve sheaths and nerve fibers of the posterior mediastinum (Fig. 4). Histologically, they are composed of a random arrangement of spindle-shaped cells lacking the uniform pattern usually seen in a neurolemmoma. Neurofibromas of the mediastinum may be seen in association with von Recklinghausen's disease, but a posterior mediastinal mass in a patient with this disease is not necessarily a neurofibroma, since meningiomas also occur with neurofibromatosis.[56] *Neurolemmomas* arise from the sheath of Schwann and microscopically show a regular pattern of elongated fusiform cells. They have been classified into several histologic types, but various theories concerning their histogenesis have produced many descriptions and names for these tumors. *Neurogenic sarcomas* (malignant schwannomas) originate by malignant degeneration from both neurolemmomas and neurofibromas. They occasionally are associated with hypoglycemia, and the blood sugar may return to normal levels after removal of the tumor. *Ganglioneuromas* originate from the sympathetic chain and contain ganglion cells and nerve fibers. These tumors occur more commonly in children than do other types of neurogenic tumors. A partially dif-

TABLE 2. Usual Location of Mediastinal Tumors and Cysts

Anterior Mediastinum	Superior Mediastinum	Posterior Mediastinum	Middle Mediastinum
Thymoma	Thymoma	Neurogenic tumor	Pericardial cyst
Teratodermoid	Lymphoma	Enteric cyst	Bronchogenic cyst
Carcinoma	Thyroid adenoma		Lymphoma
Lymphangioma	Parathyroid adenoma		
Hemangioma			
Lipoma			

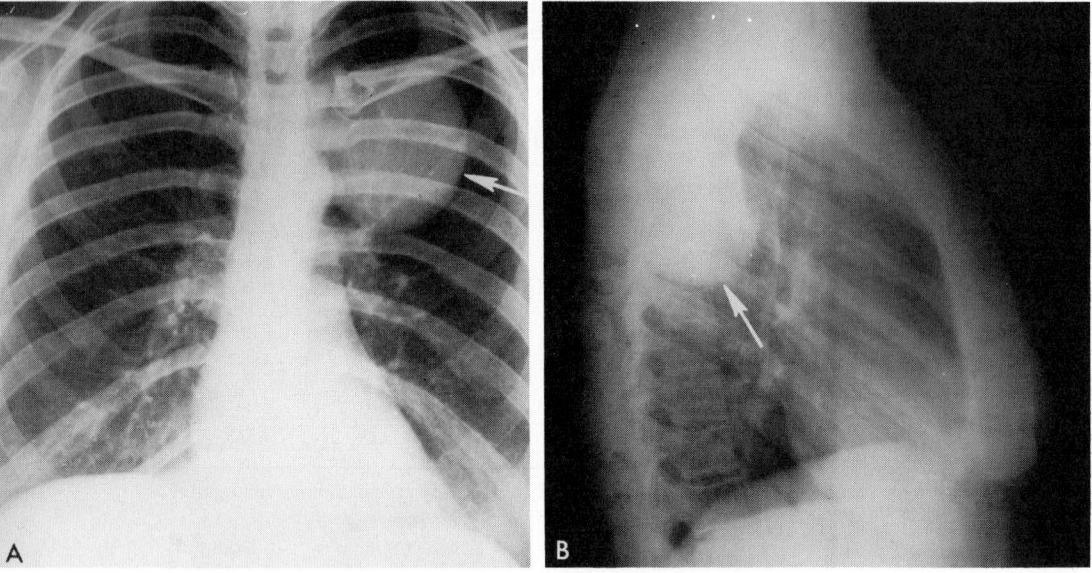

Figure 4. Chest films showing neurofibromas of the posterior mediastinum.

ferentiated type of ganglioneuroma, or ganglioneuroblastoma, may occur, and contains immature cells of the sympathetic nervous system mixed with mature ganglion cells. Ganglioneuroblastomas may behave in a benign fashion if completely excised, but they may present with widespread metastases and have the malignant potential of neuroblastomas. As many as 25 per cent of ganglioneuromas have been reported to contain immature elements with a malignant potential.

Neuroblastoma is the general term for malignant tumors of the sympathetic nervous system and includes sympathicogonioma and sympathicoblastoma. The various types are based on the histogenesis of the sympathetic nervous system. Neuroblastomas are highly invasive tumors that are most commonly seen in the retroperitoneal area in children, but also arise from any portion of the sympathetic nervous system. In spite of their very malignant nature, neuroblastomas are responsive to combinations of surgical excision, radiation, and chemotherapy. With aggressive treatment the prognosis for children with mediastinal neuroblastoma, even in the presence of metastatic disease, appears to be more favorable than for similar tumors arising in other locations.[12] Rare cases of spontaneous regression have been reported, and maturation from a malignant form to a benign form has also been documented. Immature neuroblastoma cells grown in tissue culture differentiate into mature ganglion cells.[17] Lymphocytes from children with neuroblastomas strongly inhibit the growth of neuroblastoma cells in tissue culture.[3] Histologically, neuroblastomas are composed of uniform sheets of small, round, immature cells that may form pseudorosettes.

Paragangliomas and pheochromocytomas of the mediastinum originate from derivatives of the neural crest. They arise from any portion of the chemoreceptor apparatus and are similar to tumors of the carotid body, jugular glomus, and organ of Zuckerkandl. Usually the chromaffin-positive tumors or paragangliomas are hormonally inactive, but lack of correlation between the chromaffin reaction and hormonal activity does occur. Nonchromaffin paragangliomas usually arise from the chemoreceptors and are located adjacent to the aortic arch, but they may also be found in the posterior mediastinum. Pheochromocytomas are almost always located posteriorly in the paravertebral region[9] (Fig. 5). By histologic criteria, the incidence of malignancy of paragangliomas and pheochromocytomas has been reported to be as high as 50 per cent. A more accurate index of the frequency of malignancy with these tumors is the gross appearance and presence of metastases. Based on these findings, the incidence of malignancy is probably less than 3 per cent. The hormonally active tumors present with persistent or episodic hypertension and may be diagnosed by measuring urinary catecholamine levels. Because of their location near the aorta and their extreme vascularity, these tumors may usually be visualized by means of thoracic aortography. The possibility of an associated mediastinal pheochromocytoma is an important consideration in evaluating a hypertensive patient who fails to become normotensive following resection of an abdominal pheochromocytoma.

Teratodermoid Tumors. Teratomas are tumors composed of multiple types of tissue foreign to the part in which they arise. Although the simplest form of teratoma, the dermoid cyst, appears to be different from the solid teratoma, careful microscopic examination usually reveals tissue from each germ layer rather than ectodermal tissue alone. Characteristically, mediastinal teratomas are located anteriorly, with only rare incidence in the posterior mediastinum (Fig. 6). Teratomas are usually first recognized in adult life and are rarely diagnosed in infancy. The gross appearance may vary from the smooth outline of the benign

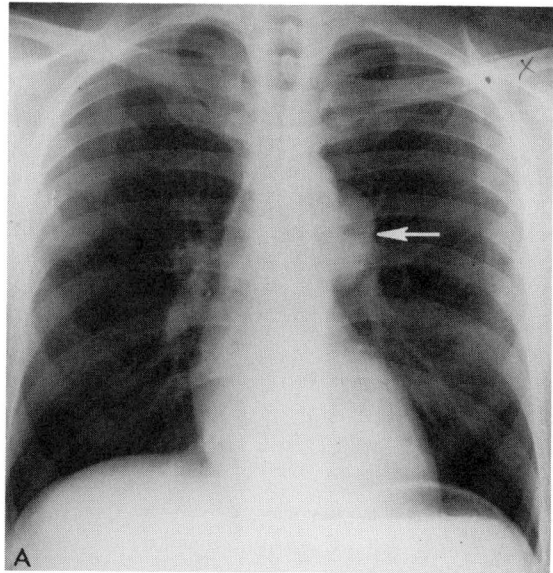
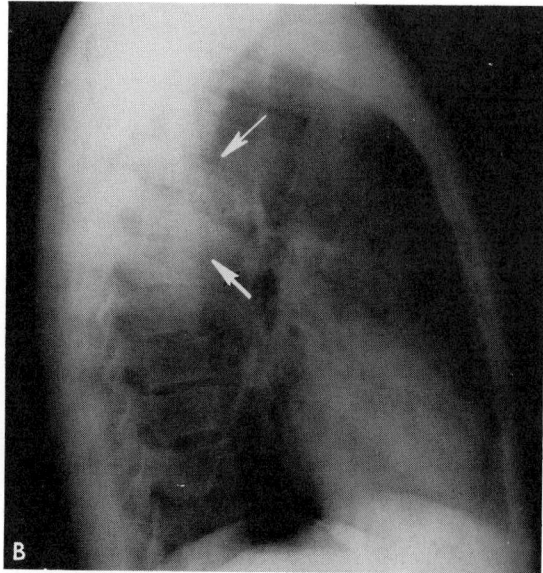

Figure 5. Chest films showing pheochromocytoma of the mediastinum that was associated with episodic hypertension.

form to a lobulated, irregular surface in the malignant type, and on sectioning they may contain hair and teeth. Microscopically, the composition ranges from predominantly ectodermal tissues in the simple cystic type to a variety of tissues of endodermal, ectodermal, and mesodermal origin in the more complex solid types. Teratomas may present as very large tumors compressing the adjacent structures, and occasionally they may rupture into the pleural space, pericardium, aorta, or vena cava. Both endocrine and exocrine secretion have been documented from components of teratomas, and the occasional finding of a surrounding

inflammatory reaction has been ascribed to the secretion of digestive enzymes.[44, 48]

Thymoma. Thymic lesions represent one of the most common types of mediastinal tumors. Rare in childhood, they usually appear in adult life. These tumors are located in the superior and anterior mediastinum and vary in their appearance on chest roentgenogram from a small, circumscribed mass to an ill-defined, lobulated density (Fig. 7).

The association of thymoma with myasthenia gravis has been recognized for many years but remains incompletely defined. The incidence of myasthenia

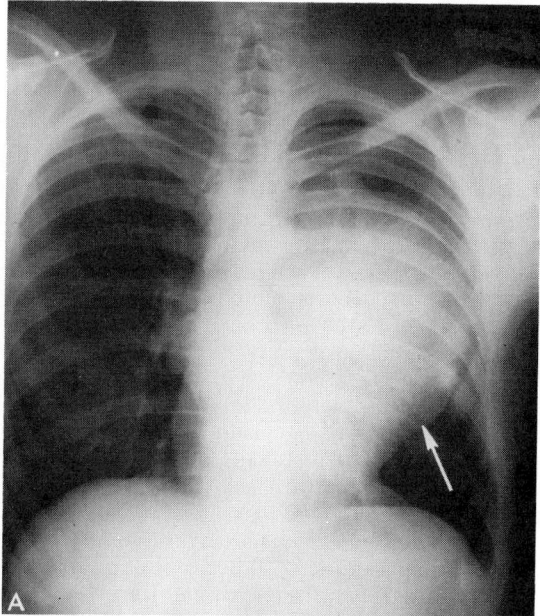
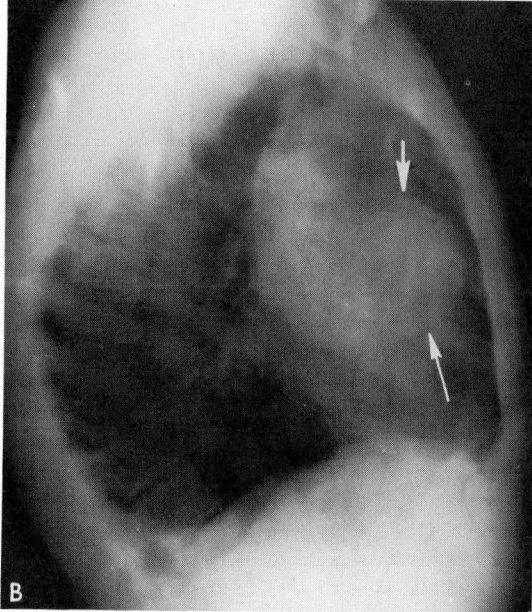

Figure 6. Chest films demonstrating teratoma of anterior mediastinum.

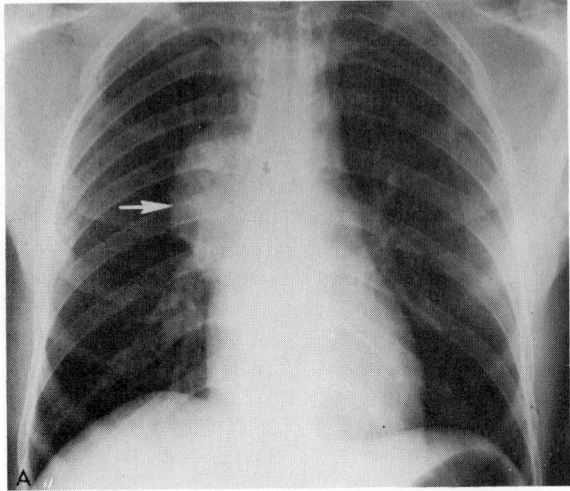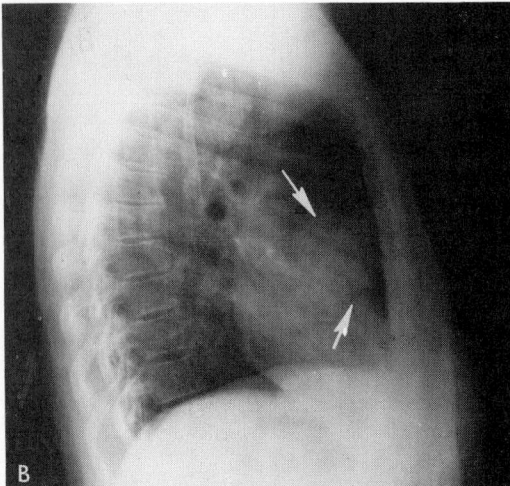

Figure 7. Thymoma of anterior mediastinum illustrated by chest films.

gravis in patients with thymoma ranges from 10 to 50 per cent, whereas the incidence of thymoma in patients with myasthenia gravis ranges from 8 to 20 per cent.[54] The beneficial effects of thymectomy for myasthenia gravis are usually greatest in female patients without a thymoma and in whom the disease has been of short duration. Patients with thymoma and myasthenia gravis in general have a much poorer prognosis than patients having a thymoma without myasthenia gravis.

One of the problems presented by tumors of the thymus is the difficulty in establishing a histologic diagnosis of malignancy. Usually, this diagnosis must be confirmed by the gross characteristics of the tumor as demonstrated by invasion into the lung, pericardium, or blood vessels. Distant metastases from malignant thymic tumors have been documented but are an unusual occurrence.

Thymomas have been associated with a wide variety of clinical conditions in addition to myasthenia gravis. There are reports of thymoma occurring with red blood cell aplasia, Cushing's syndrome, hypogammaglobulinemia, megaesophagus, and several collagen vascular disorders.[43] The exact incidence and etiology of these relationships is not well established. Carcinoid tumors may occasionally be of thymic origin, presumably arising from argentaffin cells within the thymus. No instances of carcinoid syndrome have been reported with these tumors.[27] Cysts may occur in the thymus and may be inflammatory, neoplastic, or congenital. Of these, hemorrhagic cysts within a thymoma are the most common. True congenital thymic cysts are very rare and are thought to originate from the third branchial pouch remnant and to bear no relationship to thymoma. These may occasionally be quite large and may cause symptoms due to cardiac compression.[1]

Lymphoma. The lymph nodes of the mediastinum are frequently involved with disseminated lymphoma. It is not unusual, however, for lymphoma to present primarily in the mediastinum without evidence of spread to other parts of the body. Hodgkin's disease,

lymphosarcoma, reticulum cell sarcoma, and lymphoblastoma may present as primary mediastinal tumors. These tumors are characteristically situated in the anterior mediastinum, although they may involve lymph nodes elsewhere, especially around the bronchi. By definition, all these lesions are malignant. Surgical excision is indicated in those patients in whom the lesion is localized, especially in Hodgkin's disease.[5] Radiation therapy should be employed for most patients with these conditions.

Carcinoma. Carcinoma arising within the mediastinum in the absence of any other primary source has been reported to account for 3 to 11 per cent of primary mediastinal lesions. The origin of these lesions is unclear. Since they occur most frequently in males and the most common lesion is squamous cell carcinoma, it is likely that the primary source is in the lung in many of these patients, although such an origin cannot be confirmed. It is also possible that these carcinomas may arise in previously benign cysts. The prognosis is very poor, and although radiation is usually employed, the benefits in most instances are not striking and the disease progresses rapidly.

Other Tumors. *Thyroid tumors* within the mediastinum occur quite rarely. True intrathoracic thyroid tissue or ectopic mediastinal thyroid is not to be confused with the more common mediastinal extensions of cervical goiter. Patients with mediastinal thyroid tissue are usually asymptomatic, but they may have symptoms of compression or rarely may be hyperthyroid. The diagnosis may be made with radioactive iodine scanning.[31] The vascular supply of intrathoracic goiters is usually thoracic rather than cervical, and these lesions may be visualized by thoracic angiography. The usual histologic diagnosis is thyroid adenoma. These tumors are located in the anterior mediastinum with rare exceptions.

Parathyroid adenomas occur in the anterior and superior mediastinum in 10 per cent of patients and are often embedded in thymic tissue. Rarely, an adenoma may be located in the posterior mediastinum. Most mediastinal parathyroid tumors are hormonally active, and the diagnosis is usually made after mediastinal exploration in a patient with clinical and laboratory evidence of hyperparathyroidism. Diagnostic techniques utilized in evaluating patients suspected of having a mediastinal parathyroid adenoma include the routine chest film, barium swallow, inferior thyroid artery angiography, and radioactive selenium scanning.[22, 50] Recent advances in radioimmunoassay for parathyroid hormone have been helpful, and parathyroid adenomas have been localized to the mediastinum preoperatively by selective venous catheterization combined with radioimmunoassay.[41] Although very rare, carcinoma of the parathyroid gland may occur in the mediastinum.

Mesenchymal tumors found in the mediastinum include lipomas, liposarcomas, fibrosarcomas, myxomas, tumors of muscle origin (leiomyosarcomas), and mesotheliomas.[36] All are uncommon in the mediastinum when compared to their incidence in other portions of the body. Their behavior in the mediastinum is generally no different from that in other locations. It is not unusual for soft tissue tumors to contain elements of more than one tissue type; this makes their classification difficult and accounts for the variety of descriptive names. Treatment of these tumors is surgical excision, with the malignant lesions showing little response to radiation or chemotherapy. Mesotheliomas are listed as mesenchymal tumors, although there has been some speculation concerning their exact origin. The classification as a primary tumor has even been questioned, but studies with tissue culture, histochemical techniques, and special stains have helped clarify its histogenesis.[39] It is generally thought that these tumors arise from mesothelial cells and have the potential of developing both a fibroblastic and an epithelial counterpart. They may arise from the pleura or pericardium, or may appear as a solitary mediastinal mass without an obvious attachment to a mesothelial structure. The diagnosis of benign mesothelioma must be viewed with caution, since the biologic behavior of these tumors is very unpredictable, and distant metastases may occur many years after resection of a localized lesion.[53]

Vascular and lymphatic tumors are extremely common in other parts of the body but are distinctly uncommon within the mediastinum.[37] These tumors may be seen in all age groups and are found in all portions of the mediastinum but are most characteristically located in the anterior mediastinum. The histologic types include hemangioma, hemangioendothelioma, hemangiopericytoma, lymphangioma, and lymphangiomyoma. The histologic classification depends on the morphologic structure and the relative number of endothelial cells, smooth muscle cells, and pericytes. These tumors often grow to large proportions before they are diagnosed and produce symptoms by compressing adjacent structures. Included with vascular tumors is the rare occurrence of intrathoracic extramedullary hematopoiesis. This unusual tumor is composed of hematopoietic tissue and is seen in association with spherocytic anemia and other disorders affecting the bone marrow. The mass is characteristically located in the posterior mediastinum and may be interpreted as a neurogenic tumor because of this

location. This disorder may be diagnosed by scanning after injection of radioactive gold.[38]

Seminomas are germinal tumors occurring as primary tumors of the mediastinum. In spite of the close histologic similarity between these tumors and the testicular seminomas, multiple sections of the testes have shown that the mediastinal tumors are not metastatic lesions.[28, 51] Clinically, seminomas occur in men in the third and fourth decades of life, with no diagnostic symptoms or specific radiologic findings. The rare choriocarcinomas, as opposed to seminomas, are hormonally active, causing elevation of urinary gonadotropin levels, and frequently are associated with gynecomastia. Choriocarcinomas are rapidly metastasizing, usually fatal tumors. Seminomas, however, behave like testicular seminomas, and both the primary tumors and metastatic lesions are sensitive to irradiation.

Cysts of the Mediastinum

The various cysts that arise in the mediastinum form a significant portion of the primary lesions. The cysts may originate in the pericardium, bronchi, trachea, esophagus, and thymus gland.

Bronchogenic Cysts. These cysts originate from the ventral foregut that forms the respiratory system and may occur in the mediastinum or in the lung. In the mediastinum they are usually located close to the trachea or main stem bronchi, most often immediately posterior to the carina (Fig. 8). A communication may exist with the tracheal lumen, but usually the cysts are adjacent to the trachea or connected to it by a cartilaginous tract. Histologically they are composed of ciliated respiratory epithelium, cartilage, smooth muscle, fibrous tissue, and mucous glands. Bronchogenic cysts are uncommon in infancy, but when they occur in this age group they may cause severe respiratory distress by compressing the trachea or bronchus.[15] In the older child, symptoms of cough, dyspnea, and stridor are not unusual. The roentgenogram shows a smooth density at the carinal level that may be seen to compress the esophagus on barium swallow. In the rare patient in whom the cyst communicates with the trachea, an air-fluid level may be seen within the cyst. Malignant degeneration has not been seen within a mediastinal bronchogenic cyst, but a bronchial adenoma has been found within the wall of a bronchogenic cyst.[18]

Enteric Cysts. Also called enterogenous cysts, reduplication cysts, inclusion cysts, or gastric cysts, these cysts of the mediastinum originate from the dorsal division of the foregut that develops into the gastrointestinal tract.[49] Duplications of the gut may be found at any level in the posterior mediastinum adjacent to the esophagus (Fig. 9). The cysts are smooth-walled and are composed of a muscular coat and a mucosa that may resemble that of the esophagus, stomach, or small intestine, though it is usually ciliated. They are usually attached to the wall of the esophagus but occasionally may be completely embedded within the muscularis of the esophagus. Symptoms due to pressure on the esophagus or tracheobronchial tree are common and typically occur at an early age. Since many of these cysts are lined with gastric mucosa,

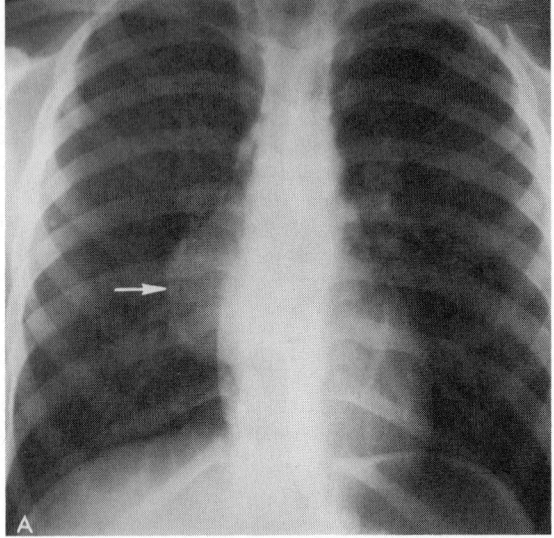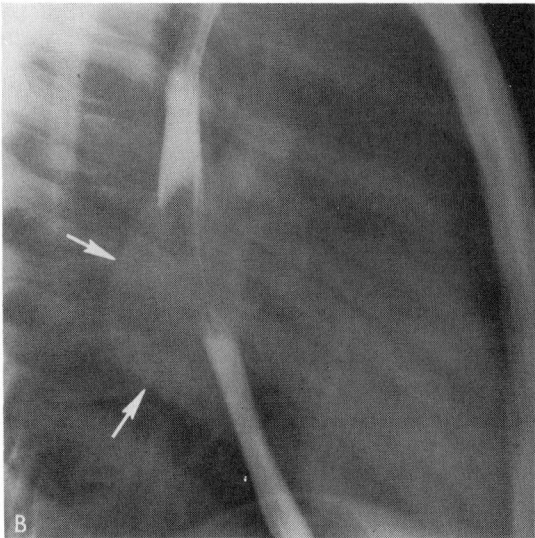

Figure 8. Chest films of bronchogenic cyst.

acid secretion with peptic ulceration, perforation, and bleeding are recognized complications.[30]

Enteric cysts are occasionally associated with vertebral anomalies, and may be attached to the meninges or spinal cord by a tract containing neural elements. This tract may be patent and may be shown by myelography to communicate with the spinal cord. Rarely, mediastinal enteric cysts may be multiple or may be associated with duplications of abdominal portions of the gastrointestinal tract, with a communication through the diaphragm between the thoracic and abdominal portions of the duplication.

Pericardial Cysts. These cysts are rather common mediastinal lesions, usually occurring at the cardiophrenic angles, especially on the right side (Fig. 10). They are thought to originate either from a fail-

ure of fusion of the primitive pericardial lacunae or from abnormal folds in the embryonic pleura.[8] The cysts either may be separate from the pericardial cavity or, more rarely, may communicate with it. The radiologic appearance of these lesions is frequently characteristic. These cysts are benign and only occasionally produce symptoms. Surgical excision is indicated, primarily for diagnosis.

Symptoms

The presenting symptoms in patients with primary tumors and cysts of the mediastinum are diverse. Although a number of lesions are found initially on routine chest films, approximately two thirds of patients have specific symptoms. The most common complaints include chest pain, cough, and dyspnea. The presence

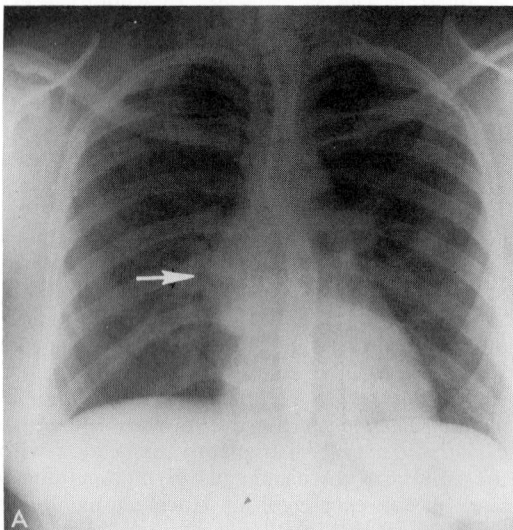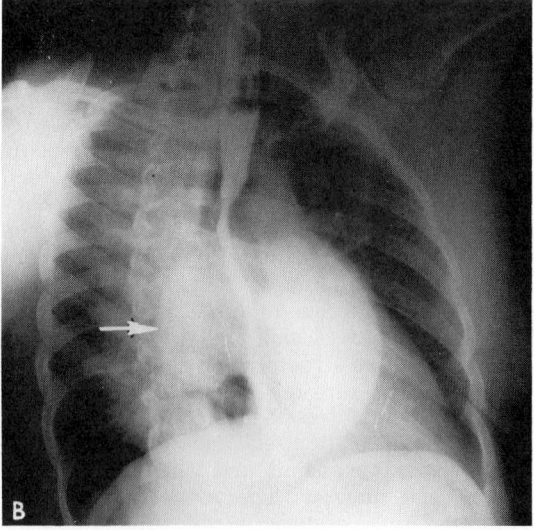

Figure 9. Chest films illustrating enteric cyst of posterior mediastinum. (From Sabiston, D. C., Jr., and Oldham, H. N., Jr. *In* Sabiston, D. C., Jr., and Spencer, F. C. (Eds.): Gibbon's Surgery of the Chest, 3rd ed. Philadelphia, W. B. Saunders Company, 1976.)

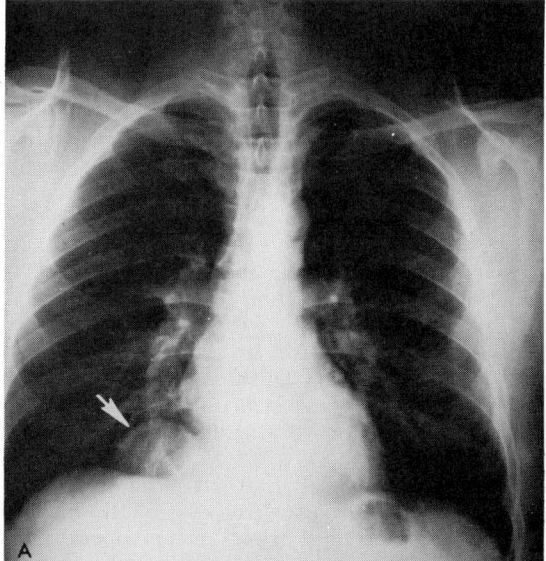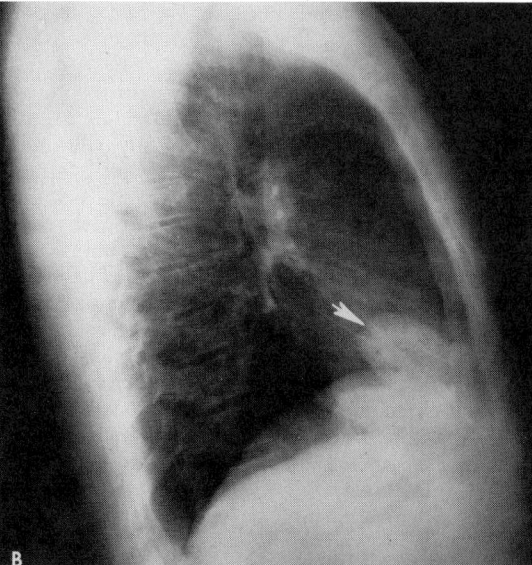

Figure 10. Chest films showing typical location of pericardial cyst in the right cardiophrenic angle. (From Sabiston, D. C., Jr., and Oldham, H. N., Jr. *In* Sabiston, D. C., Jr., and Spencer, F. C. (Eds.): Gibbon's Surgery of the Chest, 3rd ed. Philadelphia, W. B. Saunders Company, 1976.)

of symptoms in a patient with a mediastinal mass is of some significance, since such symptoms correlate with the incidence of malignancy (Table 3). The lesion is benign in 95 per cent of the patients in whom diagnosis is made from a routine chest film. In the group of patients who are symptomatic, half the lesions are benign and half are malignant.[34] The absence of symptoms is not as helpful in younger patients, as evidenced by a large series of asymptomatic young military personnel with mediastinal masses with a 60 per cent incidence of malignancy.[13]

Symptoms that suggest direct invasion of nerves, such as hoarseness, Horner's syndrome, and severe pain, are generally associated with a poor prognosis. Similarly, evidence of major vascular obstruction such as the superior vena caval syndrome is also an unfavorable sign.

It is recognized that specific syndromes are often associated with primary lesions of the mediastinum. For example, myasthenia gravis is known to occur more frequently in the presence of a thymoma. Thymomas have also been reported in association with hypogammaglobulinemia, Whipple's disease, red blood cell aplasia, and Cushing's disease. Recently several patients have been reported with mediastinal thymic

tumors and associated multiple endocrine adenomatoses.[42] Hypoglycemia is found with mesotheliomas, teratomas, and fibrosarcomas. Hypertension occurs in association with mediastinal pheochromocytomas and ganglioneuromas, and diarrhea may also be associated with these lesions. Neurofibromas accompany von Recklinghausen's disease, and vertebral anomalies are common with enteric cysts of the mediastinum. Malignant tumors of the mediastinum may produce chylothorax, and neurogenic tumors that press on the spinal cord may produce neurologic symptoms, including hemiplegia. A positive relationship between hypertrophic osteoarthropathy and neurogenic tumors has been established. Finally, many mediastinal tumors, especially those that are malignant, are associated with fever. One of the more classic types is the intermittent fever (Pel-Ebstein) characteristic of Hodgkin's disease.

Diagnosis

A careful evaluation of the history and symptoms is of much aid in localizing the mediastinal lesion and suggesting a possible diagnosis. Specific symptoms such as hoarseness and Horner's syndrome suggest pressure on the recurrent laryngeal nerve and the cervical-thoracic sympathetic chain. Back pain suggests a posterior mediastinal lesion, especially one of the neurogenic lesions arising from the intercostal nerves.

Roentgenographic studies remain the most helpful diagnostic tools. The standard chest film usually will show the anatomic location of the mass and will allow a description of its size, its relationship to adjacent structures, and its relative density, cystic or solid. Further information concerning the location and character of the mass may be obtained by fluoroscopy, barium swallow, and laminagraphy. Methods of inclined frontal laminagraphy and horizontal laminagraphy have been reported to allow a more precise

TABLE 3. **Significance of Symptoms in 164 Consecutive Patients with Mediastinal Tumor or Cyst***

	Total	Benign	Malignant
Asymptomatic†	57	54 (95%)	3 (5%)
Symptomatic	107	57 (53%)	50 (47%)

*At the Duke University Medical Center.
†Lesion found on routine chest film.

localization of mediastinal masses. Carbon dioxide pneumomediastinography has also been described for evaluation of mediastinal tumors.

The recent advances in radioisotope scanning have been applied to lesions of the mediastinum. The use of radioactive iodine for the evaluation of superior mediastinal masses is occasionally very helpful, since there have been rare instances in which the ectopic mediastinal thyroid was the only functioning thyroid tissue present. Techniques currently are being reported for the scanning of radioisotopes localized in the thymic tissue, parathyroid tissue, and heterotopic marrow.[22, 38, 52] Conceivably, these and other more refined procedures will soon allow precise diagnosis of a variety of mediastinal tumors. The use of selective venous catheterization and radioimmunoassay for parathyroid hormone is a significant advance in the preoperative localization of parathyroid adenoma in the mediastinum.[41]

Diagnostic ultrasound may be helpful in localizing mediastinal masses, and in differentiating solid from cystic lesions.[16] Needle aspiration of certain lesions demonstrated by this method to be cystic has been recommended.[14] This may have limited application to certain lesions thought to be pericardial cysts, but caution must be exercised in over-reliance on this technique, as a similar ultrasonic pattern has been described in mediastinal Hodgkin's disease.[6]

Various methods of obtaining tissue from the mediastinum have been described, including needle biopsy, needle aspiration of cystic lesions, anterior mediastinal exploration, and mediastinoscopy.[7, 11] Of these, mediastinoscopy has been the most widely used.[35] In properly selected patients, this technique will often give both a tissue diagnosis and an indication of resectability.

A wide variety of both intrathoracic and extrathoracic lesions may resemble primary mediastinal tumors and cysts. Mediastinal masses may resemble cardiovascular abnormalities, and angiocardiography may be necessary to make the proper differentiation.[35] Cardiovascular abnormalities such as aneurysms of the heart or great vessels can also resemble primary mediastinal lesions, and angiography may also be required for a proper diagnosis. Abnormalities of the vertebral column, spinal cord, or meninges may exist in the posterior mediastinum and be confused with primary mediastinal tumors. Other disease processes such as achalasia, hiatal hernia, coarctation of the aorta, mediastinitis, and many more may initially resemble tumors and cysts of the mediastinum. The experienced use of the many diagnostic tests available and the proper evaluation of the clinical presentation should in most cases lead to the proper differentiation between these abnormalities and primary tumors and cysts of the mediastinum.

Treatment

An accurate assessment of the patient's symptoms, chest film, and special diagnostic tests will lead to the proper preoperative diagnosis. The precise histologic diagnosis, however, is rarely made prior to operation. Since the incidence of malignancy is quite high, thoracotomy is usually indicated. This allows both objective diagnosis and definitive treatment. Moreover, early diagnosis and treatment are accompanied by the most favorable prognosis in those patients with malignant tumors. It is also important to emphasize that a number of benign tumors of the mediastinum may ultimately become malignant unless resection is performed. The mortality accompanying operation is quite low, and in a consecutive group of 164 patients there was no operative mortality.[34] In this series there were three postoperative deaths (1.8 per cent), and in two of the patients, who had myasthenia gravis, death followed severe respiratory complications. Of 53 patients in this series with malignant tumors, 37 required postoperative irradiation or chemotherapy for advanced lesions. Of these, 36 per cent survived 5 years or more, demonstrating the importance of obtaining an objective diagnosis and of instituting proper therapy.

It is recommended that all patients diagnosed as having a primary tumor or cyst of the mediastinum receive the benefit of expeditious preoperative evaluation followed by a thoracotomy for excision or biopsy of the lesion, with appropriate supportive chemotherapy and irradiation when indicated. The mortality and morbidity from this approach are negligible, and the relief of symptoms in patients with benign lesions and the survival rate in patients with malignant lesions are significant.

SELECTED REFERENCES

Blalock, A., Mason, M. F., Morgan, H. J., and Riven, S. S.: Myasthenia gravis and tumors of the thymic region: Report of a case in which tumor was removed. Ann. Surg., 110:544, 1939.
This classic paper describes the first successful removal of a thymic tumor associated with myasthenia gravis with subsequent symptomatic remission. The author presented 53 instances from the literature showing an association of myasthenia gravis with abnormalities of the thymus gland. This review was responsible for establishing surgical removal as the treatment for patients with myasthenia gravis and a thymic tumor.

Burkell, C. C., Cross, J. M., Kent, H. P., and Nanson, E. M.: Mass Lesions of the Mediastinum. Chicago, Year Book Medical Publishers, 1969.
This monograph presents the authors' experience in the diagnostic evaluation and treatment of patients with primary lesions of the mediastinum. Emphasis is placed on the proper use of the diagnostic tests available and on the use of radiotherapy both as an adjunct to surgery and as a palliative measure. Clinical management of patients with a mediastinal mass is illustrated by case histories of patients with each of the various disorders. This work is a concise summary of current information concerning mediastinal lesions.

Castleman, B.: Tumors of the thymus gland. In Atlas of Tumor Pathology, Section 5, Fascicle 19. Washington, D.C., Armed Forces Institute of Pathology, 1955.

Schlumberger, H. G.: Tumors of the mediastinum. In Atlas of Tumor Pathology, Section 5, Fascicle 18. Washington, D.C., Armed Forces Institute of Pathology, 1951.

Willis, R. A.: Teratomas. In Atlas of Tumor Pathology, Section 3, Fascicle 9. Washington, D.C., Armed Forces Institute of Pathology, 1951.
These three volumes of the Atlas of Tumor Pathology *from the Armed Forces Institute of Pathology are a fundamental reference for those interested in a detailed description of the gross and microscopic characteristics of mediastinal tumors. Each volume is prepared by an authority on the subject. The various histologic patterns of each type of tumor are clearly illustrated with excellent photomicrographs.*

Harrington, S. W.: Intrathoracic tumors. Arch. Surg., 19:1679, 1929.
This article presents one of the earlier series of patients with

primary tumors and cysts of the mediastinum. The excellent results obtained with surgical treatment documented the feasibility of excision of these lesions and was responsible for subsequent advances in mediastinal surgery.

Leigh, T. F., and Weens, H. S.: The Mediastinum. Springfield, Ill., Charles C Thomas, Publisher, 1959.
This monograph describes a wide variety of conditions within the mediastinum, including infections, emphysema, tumors, and cysts. A thorough description is given of the anatomy of the mediastinum, including the patterns of lymphatic drainage. The indications for and uses of the various radiographic tests available are presented. The excellent reproduction of roentgenograms adds to the value of this work.

Palva, T.: Mediastinoscopy. Chicago, Year Book Medical Publishers, 1964.
This monograph thoroughly presents the indications and techniques of mediastinoscopy as first described by Carlens. The various pathologic diagnoses obtained in this series of 295 patients demonstrate the usefulness of this procedure in a number of clinical situations. The detailed description of the anatomy of the mediastinum and the excellent color photographs of view through the mediastinoscope add to the quality of this book.

Wychulis, A. R., Payne, W. S., Clagett, O. T., and Woolner, L. B.: Surgical treatment of mediastinal tumors. A 40-year experience. J. Thorac. Cardiovasc. Surg., 62:379, 1971.
This article presents the largest series of mediastinal tumors from any single institution. The experience with 1064 patients over a 40-year period at the Mayo Clinic is concisely described, and clearly supports the methods used for diagnosis and treatment of a wide variety of mediastinal tumors.

REFERENCES

1. Alee, G., Logue, B., and Mansour, K.: Thymic cyst simulating multiple cardiovascular abnormalities and presenting with pericarditis and pericardial tamponade. Am. J. Cardiol., 31:377, 1973.
2. Bastianelli, R. Quoted by Meade, R. H.: A History of Thoracic Surgery. Springfield, Ill., Charles C Thomas, Publisher, 1961.
3. Bill, A. H.: The implications of immune reactions to neuroblastoma. Surgery, 66:415, 1969.
4. Blalock, A., Mason, M. F., Morgan, H. J., and Riven, S. S.: Myasthenia gravis and tumors of the thymic region: Report of a case in which tumor was removed. Ann. Surg., 110:544, 1939.
5. Burk, W. A., Burford, T. H., and Dorfman, R. F.: Hodgkin's disease of the mediastinum. Ann. Thorac. Surg., 3:287, 1967.
6. Cardello, F. P., McQuown, D. S., and Dollinger, M.: Ultrasound in diagnosis of parapericardial masses. J.A.M.A., 227:1124, 1974.
7. Carlens, E.: Mediastinoscopy. Dis. Chest., 36:343, 1959.
8. Drash, E. C., and Hyer, H. J.: Mesothelial mediastinal cysts. J. Thorac. Surg., 19:755, 1950.
9. Edmunds, L. H.: Mediastinal pheochromocytoma. Ann. Thorac. Surg., 2:743, 1966.
10. Epstein, A. M., and Klassen, K. P.: Spontaneous superior mediastinal hemorrhage. J. Thorac. Cardiovasc. Surg., 39:740, 1960.
11. Evans, D. S., Hall, J. H., and Harrison, G. K.: Anterior mediastinotomy. Thorax, 28:444, 1973.
12. Filler, R. M., Traggis, D. G., Jaffe, N., and Vawter, G. F.: Favorable outlook for children with mediastinal neuroblastoma. J. Pediatr. Surg., 7:136, 1972.
13. Fontenelle, L. J., Armstrong, R., Stanford, W., Lindberg, E. G., and Dooley, B. N.: The asymptomatic mediastinal mass. Arch. Surg., 102:98, 1971.
14. Friday, R. O.: Paracardial cyst: Diagnosis by ultrasound and puncture. J.A.M.A., 226:82, 1973.
15. Gerami, S., Richardson, R., Harrington, B., and Pate, J. W.: Obstructive emphysema due to mediastinal bronchogenic cysts in infancy. J. Thorac. Cardiovasc. Surg., 58:432, 1969.
16. Goldberg, B. B.: Mediastinal ultrasonography. J. Clin. Ultrasound, 1:114, 1973.
17. Goldstein, M., Burdman, J. A., and Journey, L. J.: Long term tissue culture of neuroblastomas. J. Natl. Cancer Inst., 32:165, 1964.
18. Greenfield, L. J., and Howe, J. S.: Bronchial adenoma within the wall of a bronchogenic cyst. J. Thorac. Cardiovasc. Surg., 49:398, 1965.
19. Greenfield, L. J., and Shelley, W. M.: The spectrum of neurogenic tumors of the sympathetic nervous system: Maturation and adrenergic function. J. Natl. Cancer Inst., 35:215, 1965.
20. Hamman, L.: Spontaneous mediastinal emphysema. Bull. Johns Hopkins Hosp., 64:1, 1939.
21. Harrington, S. W.: Intrathoracic tumors. Arch. Surg., 19:1679, 1929.
22. Haynie, T. P., Otte, W. K., and Wright, J. C.: Visualization of hyperfunctioning parathyroid adenoma using Se^{75} selenomethionine and the photoscanner. J. Nucl. Med., 5:710, 1964.
23. Heimburger, I. L., Battersby, J. S., and Vellios, F.: Primary neoplasms of the mediastinum. Arch. Surg., 86:978, 1963.
24. Herlitzka, A. J., and Gale, J. W.: Tumors and cysts of the mediastinum. Arch. Surg., 76:697, 1958.
25. Heuer, G. J., and Andrus, W. O.: The surgery of mediastinal tumors. Am. J. Surg., 50:146, 1940.
26. Hewlett, T. H., Steer, A., and Thomas, D. E.: Progressive fibrosing mediastinitis. Ann. Thorac. Surg., 2:345, 1966.
27. Hughes, J. P., Ancalmo, N., Leonard, G. L., and Ochsner, J. L.: Carcinoid tumour of the thymus gland: Report of a case. Thorax, 30:470, 1975.
28. Johnson, D. E., Laneri, J. P., Mountain, C. F., and Luna, M.: Extragonadal germ cell tumors. Surgery, 73:85, 1973.
29. Key, J. A.: Mediastinal tumors. Surg. Clin. North Am., 34:959, 1954.
30. Kirwan, W. O., Walbaum, P. R., and McCormack, R. J. M.: Cystic intrathoracic derivatives of the foregut and their complications. Thorax, 28:424, 1973.
31. Lindskog, B. I., and Malin, A.: Diagnostic and surgical considerations in mediastinal (intrathoracic) goiter. Dis. Chest, 47:201, 1965.
32. Milton, H.: Mediastinal surgery. Lancet, 1:872, 1897.
33. Morrison, I. M.: Tumors and cysts of the mediastinum. Thorax, 13:294, 1958.
34. Oldham, H. N., Jr., and Sabiston, D. C., Jr.: Primary tumors and cysts of the mediastinum. Monogr. Surg. Sci., 4:243, 1967.
35. Oldham, H. N., Jr., and Sabiston, D. C., Jr.: Primary tumors and cysts of the mediastinum presenting as cardiovascular abnormalities. Arch. Surg., 96:71, 1968.
36. Pachter, M. R., and Lattes, R.: Mesenchymal tumors of the mediastinum. I. Tumors of fibrous tissue, adipose tissue, smooth muscle, and striated muscle. Cancer, 16:74, 1963.
37. Pachter, M. R., and Lattes, R.: Mesenchymal tumors of the mediastinum. III. Tumors of lymphovascular origin. Cancer, 16:108, 1963.
38. Papavasiliou, C. G.: Tumors stimulating intrathoracic extramedullary hematopoiesis: Clinical and roentgenologic considerations. Am. J. Roentgenol., 93:695, 1965.
39. Porter, J. M., and Cheek, J. M.: Pleural mesothelioma: Review of tumor histogenesis and report of 12 cases. J. Thorac. Cardiovasc. Surg., 55:882, 1968.
40. Razzuk, M. A., Urschel, H., Martin, J. A., Kingsley, W. B., and Paulson, D. L.: Electron microscopical observations on mediastinal neurolemmoma, neurofibroma, and ganglioneuroma. Ann. Thorac. Surg., 15:73, 1973.
41. Reitz, R. E., Pollard, J. J., Wang, C., Fleischli, D. J., Cope, O., Murray, T. M., Deftos, L. J., and Potts, J. R.: Localization parathyroid adenomas by selective venous catheterization and radioimmunoassay. N. Engl. J. Med., 281:348, 1969.
42. Rosai, J., Higa, E., and Davie, J.: Mediastinal endocrine neoplasm in patients with multiple endocrine adenomatosis. A previously unrecognized association. Cancer, 29:1075, 1972.
43. Rubin, M., Stravo, B., and Allen, L.: Clinical disorders associated with thymic tumors. Arch. Intern. Med., 114:389, 1964.
44. Rubush, J. L., Gardner, I. R., Boyd, W. C., and Ehrenhaft, J. L.: Mediastinal tumors. Review of 186 cases. J. Thorac. Cardiovasc. Surg., 65:216, 1973.
45. Sabiston, D. C., Jr.: The digestive system: Esophagus and mediastinum. In Cooke, R. E., and Levin, S. (Eds.): Biologic Basis of Pediatric Practices. New York, McGraw-Hill Book Company, 1968.
46. Sabiston, D. C., Jr., and Scott, H. W.: Primary neoplasms and cysts of the mediastinum. Ann. Surg., 136:777, 1952.
47. Skinner, D. B., and Salzman, E. W.: The challenge of superior vena caval obstruction. J. Thorac. Cardiovasc. Surg., 49:824, 1965.
48. Sommerlad, B. C., Cleland, W. P., and Yong, N. K.: Physiological activity in mediastinal teratomata. Thorax, 30:510, 1975.

49. Spock, A., Schneider, S., and Baylin, C. J.: Mediastinal gastric cysts: A case report and review of English literature. Am. Rev. Resp. Dis., *94*:97, 1966.

50. Steiner, R. E., Fraser, R., and Aird, I.: Operative parathyroid arteriography for location of parathyroid tumor. Br. Med. J., *2*:400, 1956.

51. Sterchi, M., and Cordell, A. R.: Seminoma of the anterior mediastinum. Ann. Thorac. Surg., *19*:371, 1975.

52. Tool, J. F., and Witcofski, R.: Selenomethionine Se[75] scan for thymoma. J.A.M.A., *198*:1219, 1966.

53. Urschel, H. C., and Paulson, D. C.: Mesotheliomas of the pleura. Ann. Thorac. Surg., *1*:559, 1965.

54. Wolfe, W. G., Sealy, W. C., and Young, W. G.: Surgical management of myasthenia gravis. Ann. Thorac. Surg., *14*:645, 1972.

55. Wychulis, A. R., Payne, W. S., Clagett, O. T., and Woolner, L. B.: Surgical treatment of mediastinal tumors. A 40-year experience. J. Thorac. Cardiovasc. Surg., *62*:379, 1971.

56. YaDeau, R. E., Clagett, O. T., and Divertie, M. B.: Intrathoracic meningocele. J. Thorac. Cardiovasc. Surg., *49*:202, 1965.

57

THE PERICARDIUM

Paul A. Ebert, M.D.

HISTORICAL ASPECTS

Hippocrates in 460 B.C. described the pericardium as a smooth tunic that enveloped the heart and contained a small amount of fluid resembling urine. Lower, in the seventeenth century, described the pericardial effusion that compressed the walls of the heart and could result in death. Lancisi in 1728 elucidated the clinical and necropsy findings of constrictive pericarditis. In 1761 Morgagni recognized the danger of cardiac compression and described constrictive pericarditis of such a degree that the heart could not receive a proper quantity of blood.[20] Romero in 1819 incised the pericardium in three patients, two of whom survived.[23] Schuh and Karanaeff (1840) performed pericardicenteses for relief of massive pericardial effusion. In 1842 Chevers presented the first clear clinical picture of the development of constrictive pericarditis.[3] Kussmaul (1873) described the paradoxical pulse and rise in venous pressure on inspiration in patients with constrictive pericarditis.[15]

Resection of the pericardium was performed independently by Rehn and by Sauerbruch in 1913. Churchill in 1929 performed the first successful pericardiectomy for constrictive pericarditis in the United States. Parsons and Holman (1951, 1955)[21] and Isaacs et al. (1952)[10] reported classic experimental studies clarifying the physiologic effects of segmental compression of the heart. Many surgeons have emphasized the necessity of performing radical pericardiectomy to prevent recurrences of pericardial constriction requiring secondary operations.

FUNCTIONS OF THE PERICARDIUM

The pericardium provides a smooth serous sac that allows the heart a frictionless chamber in which to function. It is a strong fibrous material with a restraining influence against overdilatation of the heart. The pericardium may be stretched over a period of time by cardiac enlargement, but sudden changes in heart size are restricted. The pericardium may protect the heart from extension of infection from the chest, lungs, mediastinum, esophagus, and infradiaphragmatic areas.

Congenital absence of the entire pericardium is extremely rare. More commonly, small segments may be missing, and absence of small portions of the pericardial on the left side is most common. No clinical symptoms are known to result from congenital absence of the pericardium. It has been shown experimentally that without the pericardium the heart ruptures at a lower intracardiac pressure.

PERICARDIAL CYSTS

The pericardium forms from a series of disconnected lacunae, and for a brief period during developmental stages these lacunae remain as individual spaces. Occasionally, the communication with the pericardium in such lacunae persists and is called a diverticulum. If one of these lacunar cavities fails to fuse, it may remain and form a pericardial cyst or may simply atrophy. Cysts in general do not cause symptoms and are usually discovered on routine chest x-ray. The classic description of such cysts as given by radiologists is a mass lying anteriorly in the chest in either cardiophrenic sulcus. These masses may be confused with lung tumors, thymomas, and other mediastinal lesions. Cysts may become of such size that they can be incapacitating and life-threatening because of their space-occupying characteristics. (See Chapter 56, The Mediastinum.)

Pericardial diverticula are simply described as protrusions of the pericardial sac at points of weakness. These vary greatly in size, from 0.5 to 12.0 cm. They are usually more frequent on the right side and can be confused with aneurysms of the ascending aorta or with mediastinal tumors. The diverticula are rarely symptomatic, and excision is advised to establish a definitive diagnosis.

NEOPLASMS

Neoplasms arising in the pericardium are extremely rare. Such benign tumors as lipomas, lobulated fibrous polyps, and hemangiomas have been reported. Primary mesotheliomas arising from the lining endothelium have been described. Sarcomas and teratomas occasionally arise from the pericardium, and the pericardium is commonly infiltrated by primary myocardial tumors or infiltrating lung cancers.

Precordial or pleuritic pain in the left chest associated with a soft tissue mass that cannot be distinguished from the heart on chest x-ray is the usual description of acute necrosis of pericardial fat. Necrosis is thought to be due to a vascular accident with extravasation of blood and the formation of a hematoma. Hydropneumopericardium has been reported and is a rare lesion in which the clinical signs are precordial tympany and metallic splashing sounds that can be quite loud. Chest film showing air in the pericardium is conclusive. An infection may be present, and if improvement is not prompt, pericardiotomy is indicated. Air in the pericardium is also common after severe chest trauma.

PERICARDITIS

Pericarditis may occur as a primary disease process or as a secondary manifestation of a systemic disease. In its simplest form, pericarditis is an acute self-limiting inflammation most likely caused by a virus. The disease may be preceded by an upper respiratory tract infection, and symptoms vary considerably. Usually, fever is present, with the temperature around 101° F. but sometimes as high as 104 to 105° F. There is substernal or precordial pain, and a pericardial friction rub is usually heard. All degrees of severity are observed; the disease may be minimal, lasting only a few days, or symptoms may persist for weeks. Shortness of breath, shallow grunting respirations, cough, and orthopnea with a tendency to lean forward are characteristic symptoms. The pain may be sharp or dull and is usually accentuated by coughing, respiration, or activity. Commonly it is relieved by sitting up and aggravated by lying down. Leukocytosis with a predominant increase in lymphocytes is usually noted, and chest x-ray may show mild cardiac enlargement due to pericardial effusion. ST segment elevation on the electrocardiogram with absent Q waves in the presence of a pericardial friction rub is strongly suggestive of pericarditis. Pleuritis and pleural effusion may also be present.

The disease process is usually self-limiting, and complications are rare. There are isolated reports of constrictive pericarditis developing after supposedly viral pericarditis, but this is unusual. Atrial fibrillation commonly occurs, and signs of cardiac failure secondary to rhythm disturbance may be noted.

Treatment usually consists of bed rest and analgesics. Salicylates have been successful in relieving pain. If the patient does not respond to supportive treatment, steroids may be beneficial. Routine use of steroids is not encouraged, since the disease may recur when the steroids are withdrawn. Remissions are not uncommon, with pain, fever, friction rub, and even pericardial effusion frequently receding, only to recur a short time later. Heart failure is infrequent and usually can be controlled with digitalis.

Pericarditis often accompanies systemic diseases such as scleroderma, rheumatic fever, and lupus erythematosus. Sarcoidosis may involve the pericardium and heart but is rarely responsible for pericarditis. Such hypersensitivity states as serum sickness, autoimmune reactions, and various drug reactions may result in pericarditis or effusion. In cholesterol pericarditis, the pericardial fluid has a characteristic gold-paint color. The diagnosis is confirmed by pericardial aspiration and identification of cholesterol crystals. Hypothyroidism is commonly present, and pericarditis may disappear with thyroid replacement.

Acute pyogenic pericarditis may occur as a result of direct contamination of the pericardium or from septicemia or pyemia. Abscesses from below the diaphragm may rupture into the pericardial sac, or pyogenic pericarditis may result as a complication from operations on the heart, lungs, or esophagus. Severe chest pain and fever are the usual clinical signs. In the early stages, it is difficult to differentiate pyogenic pericarditis from the more common benign form. Pericardial effusion can occur more rapidly and cardiac tamponade must be expected. Tamponade may develop under these circumstances with the presence of as little as 100 ml. of fluid or pus. The electrocardiogram shows low voltage in the QRS and inverted T waves. Venous pressure is usually elevated, and a paradoxical pulse may be felt. The diagnosis is confirmed by pericardial aspiration, and repeated pericardicenteses may be necessary to evacuate accumulated fluid and pus. In most instances, resection of a costal cartilage and direct drainage of the pericardium should be performed. Very rapid forms of constrictive pericarditis have been identified, with the interval between injury and actual constriction as short as 11 weeks. Pericardial constriction occurs after cardiac surgery, but the incidence seems to be quite low.

TUBERCULOUS PERICARDITIS

Tuberculous pericarditis is thought to be secondary to tuberculosis elsewhere, with the disease spreading to the pericardial sac by direct extension from the pleura or lung, by way of lymph nodes, or through the vascular system. The onset of symptoms is usually insidious, and most often the patient is not known to have pulmonary tuberculosis.

Symptoms may be very nonspecific and include malaise, fever, sweats, pleural pain, cough, and a pericardial friction rub. In some instances, a slowly developing pericardial effusion occurs in which the fluid may be clear, straw-colored, or sanguineous. Early pericardicenteses may establish the diagnosis with the finding of acid-fast bacilli in the fluid. In many instances the skin test for tuberculosis will be negative, since a large reservoir of antibody has reacted against the massive amount of antigen in the pericardial sac. In these instances it may be several weeks after institution of treatment before an actual positive skin test will develop. Untreated patients may show progressive emaciation, toxemia, and subsequent death. The patient may die of cardiac failure, but the most common cause of death is widespread tuberculosis.

There appears to be a direct relationship between pericardial constriction and the length of time the disease is present prior to institution of treatment. Wood (1956) emphasized that pericardial constriction was a rule if treatment was delayed more than 4 months. The fibrotic process of healing, which is beneficial in pulmonary tuberculosis, is associated with a threat of pericardial contracture and constriction.

Treatment with antituberculous drugs should be started as soon as the diagnosis is established. In some cases confirmation of the diagnosis may be time-consuming; therefore, if the clinical picture is convincing, it is probably better to administer antituberculous therapy before confirmation. Single-drug therapy is ineffectual, and the combination most frequently used is isoniazid and para-aminosalicylic acid. Clinical signs of improvement usually appear within 2 to 3 weeks. Cardiomegaly, elevated venous pressure, and amount of effusion disappear more slowly. There does not seem to be any benefit in administering corticosteroids to minimize effusions and scarring.

A significant number of patients with tuberculous pericarditis will suffer the effects of pericardial constriction. As the fluid is absorbed, it becomes more viscid and more irritating to the surrounding structures. It has been postulated that the fluid then gravitates toward the diaphragmatic pericardium and that this area is subject to a longer period of irritation and thus to a greater deposition of fibrous tissue. When tuberculosis is established as a cause of effusion, drug therapy should be instituted for a period of 6 to 8 weeks. If the effusion disappears and signs of constriction occur within a short period of time, pericardiectomy is indicated. Likewise, if the effusion recurs after repeated pericardicenteses, pericardiectomy should be performed. Excellent results have been obtained when resection has been performed during the effusion stage, since the pericardium can be removed with ease. Holman and Willett[9] have emphasized that at this stage of the disease atrophy of the myocardium, fibrous infiltration, and calcification are usually not present.

Obviously it is futile to operate on febrile patients with acute toxicity and active tuberculous pericarditis. However, it is equally unwise to await a period of relative inactivity, by which time constriction and calcification have occurred. The optimal time for operation appears to be the period in the early healing phase when the patient is clinically well, aside from early signs of constriction. Constrictive pericarditis is a mechanical limitation of ventricular filling, which operative removal of the scarred pericardium will relieve. Surgical results must be evaluated in reference to the period of time during which the operation was performed. In earlier stages of thoracic surgery, the pericardium was removed only from the anterior and lateral surfaces of the heart, and recurrences were common. Shumacker and Roshe[27] have emphasized the necessity of performing a radical pericardiectomy, which includes removing the pericardium from both the anterior and posterior surfaces of the heart. When this procedure has been followed, operative results have been extremely good and recurrences uncommon.

CARDIAC TAMPONADE

Fluid or blood in the pericardial space may limit filling of the heart during diastole. This is due to the increased pressure from within the pericardium, and systolic contraction is rarely limited, whereas filling the ventricles requires a greater venous pressure. Tamponade commonly occurs after penetrating injuries to the heart in which blood escapes into the pericardial sac. The blood or fluid cannot escape through the laceration in the pericardium, and tamponade may follow. A very small amount of blood, 150 to 200 ml., may be sufficient to cause tamponade, whereas in chronic effusion the pericardium stretches over a period of time and has the capacity to contain considerably more fluid with minimal cardiac effect. In cardiac tamponade a critical point exists prior to which cardiac output is only minimally reduced. But when this critical point is reached, accumulation of a very small additional volume may reduce cardiac output, and death ensues. The treatment can be equally dramatic when removal of blood or fluid results in the quick return of blood pressure and cardiac output to near normal.

In cardiac tamponade, diastolic filling pressure rises and the amount of blood pumped per beat is reduced. Sympathetic activity increases in an attempt to maintain a normal arterial pressure, and the result is vasoconstriction. Heart rate increases and systolic ejection may become more vigorous. Venous pressure rises owing to compression of the heart during diastole, and no gradients have been demonstrated between the great veins and the right atrium during experimental cardiac tamponade. Coronary blood flow may be reduced, and myocardial failure may result from inadequate coronary perfusion.

Clinically, the patient appears to be in shock at a time when venous distention is present. Cyanosis due to marked venous stasis may be noted, and the venous pressure rather than the arterial pressure should be used as a guide to treatment, since the latter may be artificially maintained by an elevated peripheral resistance.

Treatment must not be delayed, since this is an emergency situation. Venous pressure should be obtained, and pericardial aspiration should be performed with an electrocardiogram lead attached to the needle to identify contact with the heart surface (Fig. 1). The blood or fluid can be aspirated, and a fall in venous pressure should be noted. If venous pressure rises, additional pericardicenteses should be performed. In some cases of chronic effusion, a small plastic catheter may be passed percutaneously into the pericardial sac and left in place for continual decompression. Pericardiotomy should be considered as an emergency procedure if repeated aspirations do not relieve tamponade. Pericardicenteses occasionally may result in sudden death due to laceration of a coronary artery or to ventricular fibrillation. The procedure must be considered to be serious and must be performed with care. The use of the electrocardiogram to detect contact with the heart reduces the chance of myocardial or coronary artery injury.

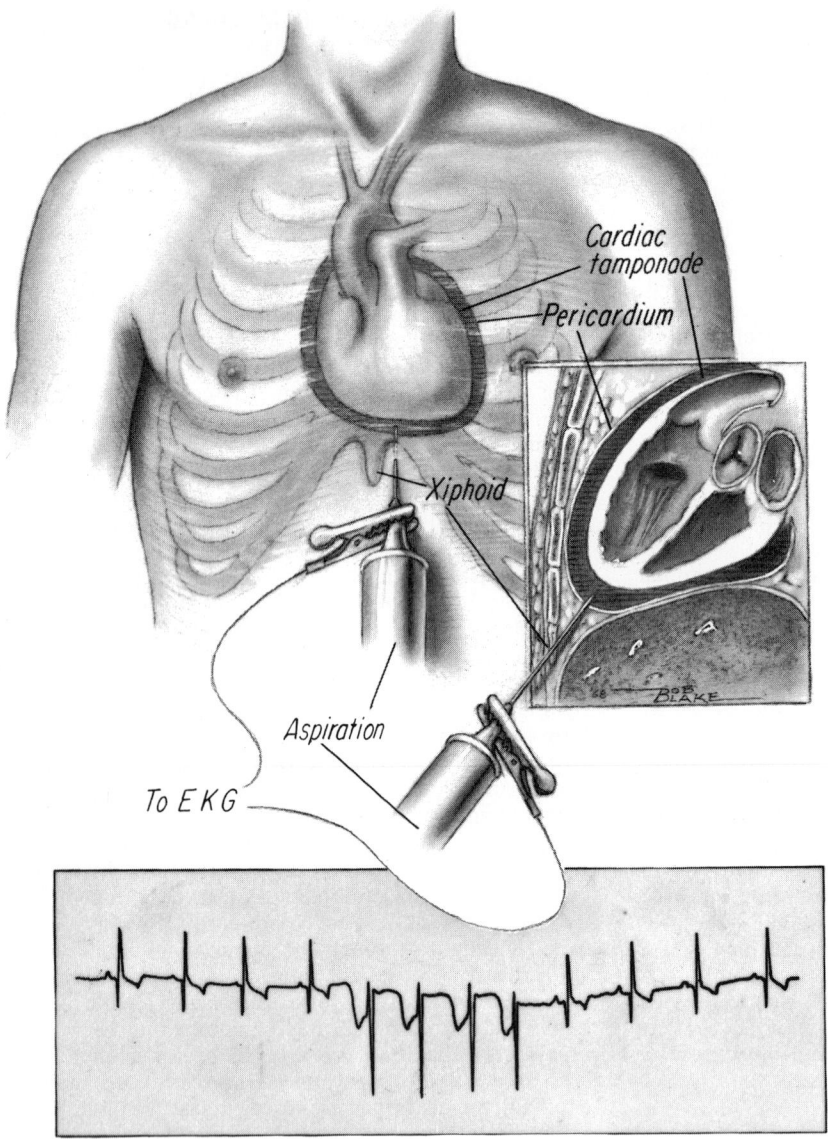

Figure 1. The technique for pericardicentesis for relief of cardiac tamponade. The needle with an electrocardiographic lead attached is introduced beneath the xiphoid. Contact with the epicardial surface of the heart produces a marked change in the electrocardiogram. The needle is withdrawn until the electrocardiogram reverts to normal. The needle may also be inserted just to the left of the sternum through the fourth intercostal space. (From Ebert, P. A. *In* Sabiston, D. C., Jr., and Spencer, F. C. (Eds.): Gibbon's Surgery of the Chest, 3rd ed. Philadelphia, W. B. Saunders Company, 1976.)

CHRONIC PERICARDIAL EFFUSION

In most cases, pericardial effusion develops over a period of time, and the heart shadow is usually markedly enlarged. The differential diagnosis is usually between pericardial effusion and marked cardiomegaly due to heart failure. In effusion, the heart sounds are usually distant, there is absence of murmurs, and shifting intensity of heart sounds is more likely to be seen. A pericardial splash or friction rub is rarely heard. Electrocardiogram usually shows low voltage, ST segment elevation, and electrical alternans of the QRS complex. In this situation the QRS complexes are regular in time but alternate in height or direction of the major deflection. ST segment elevation may be seen in acute tamponade resulting from compression of the heart and myocardial ischemia.

Numerous diagnostic techniques have been used in attempts to differentiate effusion from cardiomegaly. Echocardiography, injection of intravenous carbon dioxide, with the patient lying on his left side in order to differentiate the right atrial wall from the pericardium, and routine angiocardiography outline the heart in reference to the cardiac silhouette. Pericardicentesis is probably the most direct means of confirming the diagnosis of effusion. Repeated pericardicenteses may provide temporary relief, but surgical therapy offers the best prognosis. The creation of a window between the pericardial sac and the pleural space to drain the fluid for absorption has produced good results. Resection of the pericardium is a more definitive form of treatment (Fig. 2). Recurrences are extremely uncommon after pericardiectomy. Pericardial resection also eliminates the possibility of the development of subsequent constrictive pericarditis. Operative resection is usually fairly easy at this stage, since the pericardium is not attached to the heart. The remnant can drain into either pleural space, and excellent results have been reported.

CHRONIC CONSTRICTIVE PERICARDITIS

Constrictive pericarditis results from a chronic inflammatory process producing a fibrous thickened pericardium that surrounds the heart and limits diastolic ventricular filling. As the scar continues to shrink, further compression of the heart limits stroke volume and decreases cardiac output. In the late stages, this thickened and scarred pericardium, which becomes densely adherent to the heart, limits systolic ejection as well as restricting diastolic filling. In contrast to cardiac tamponade resulting from fluid accumulation around the heart, further elevation of venous pressure by infusion of blood or plasma results in no change in cardiac output. This reflects the severe restriction of diastolic filling imposed by the fibrous calcified pericardium.

Reduction in cardiac output means less effective perfusion to the liver, kidneys, and other tissues. Salt and water accumulation occurs; this further expands blood volume and increases venous pressure. In theory,

the function of the kidney actually worsens the condition, since increases in venous pressure and blood volume will not increase cardiac output. Diuretics are of value, since patients may undergo diuresis with the reduction of venous pressure and diastolic pressure in both the left and right heart without significant decrease in cardiac output. Lange (1956) showed that ganglionic blocking agents may reduce venous pressure without changing cardiac output.

Symptoms are usually those of heart failure, with weakness, easy fatigability, and shortness of breath. Ascites formation without peripheral edema is common. Syncopal attacks may occur with activity and are thought to be due to the inability of the heart to increase its output. Liver engorgement may cause abdominal pain.

In the late stages, the physical findings are classic; the patient's face is puffy and his abdomen is protuberant. The heart is quiet and the apex beat may or may not be felt. Sometimes a distinct diastolic shock may be palpated at the time of rapid ventricular filling. Murmurs are usually absent. Generally the liver is enlarged and ascites may be present. Peripheral edema is usually not marked. Approximately one third of the patients present with atrial fibrillation, and the

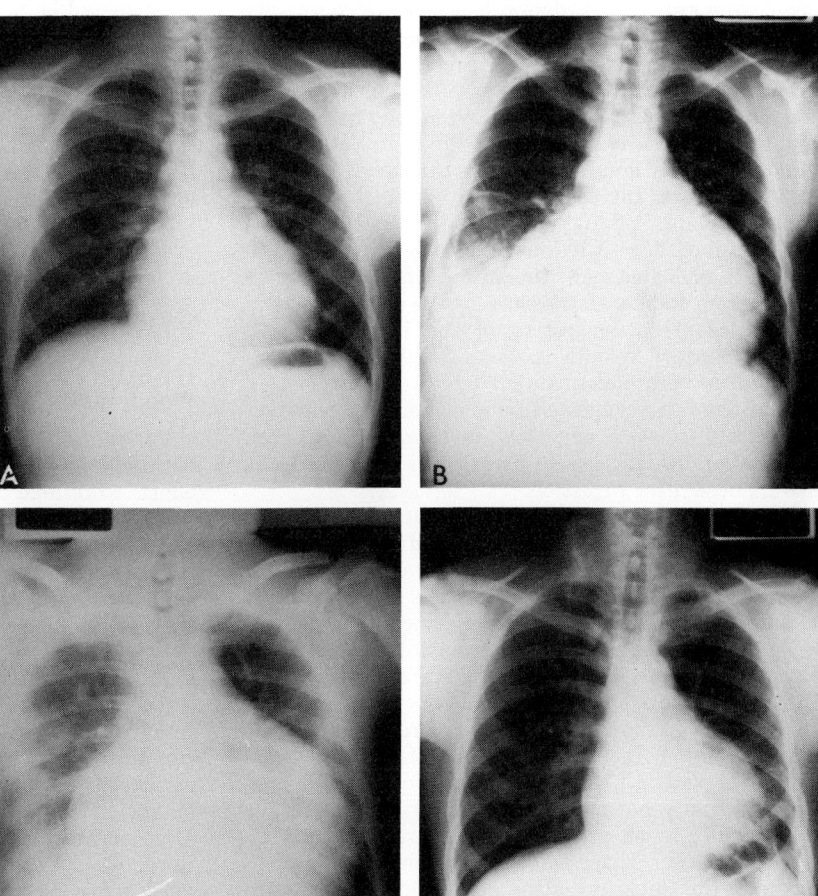

Figure 2. A sequence of chest x-rays from a patient with pericardial effusion. A, Minimal cardiac enlargement when the patient presented with malaise and night sweats. B, Two weeks later there is marked pericardial effusion. C, Repeated pericardicenteses were temporarily effective, but fluid accumulated again and the cardiac silhouette enlarged. D, Pericardiectomy was performed and 3 weeks later the chest x-ray was nearly normal.

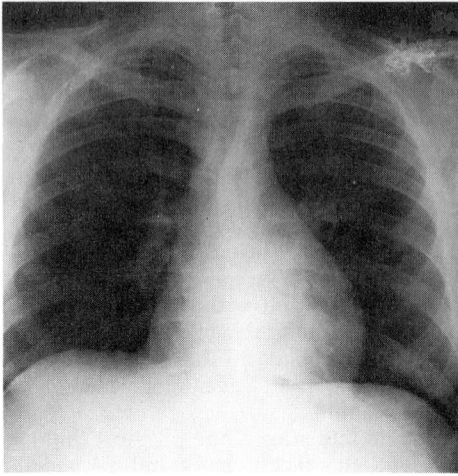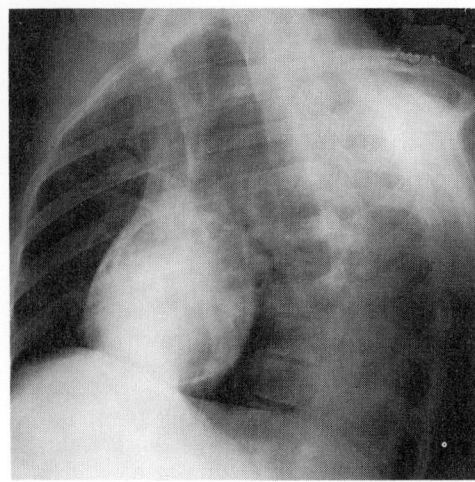

Figure 3. Posteroanterior and oblique chest x-rays from a 46-year-old male with calcific constrictive pericarditis secondary to tuberculosis. The heart size and lung markings are normal on the posteroanterior film, and calcification is not apparent. On the oblique projection, a ring of calcium almost completely encircles the heart.

peripheral pulse may be paradoxical, disappearing completely during inspiration. The arterial blood pressure is usually low, with a very narrow pulse pressure.

On chest x-ray the heart is usually normal or only moderately enlarged. Calcium deposits are commonly seen on the lateral films, and the superior vena cava may be prominent (Fig. 3). Electrocardiogram shows low voltage in the QRS complexes, and T waves are often flat and inverted. A bifid P wave may be present, with the second wave taller than the first. Serum proteins are usually low, owing to loss through the gastrointestinal tract. Increased portal pressure causes increased lymph production and increased rate of thoracic duct flow. Chylous effusions may occur in the chest and abdomen. Intestinal lymphangiectasia results from increased pressure in the capillaries and lymphatics. This congestion of the intestinal wall mucosal surface results in diminished absorption of ingested protein accompanied by an actual loss of protein from the congested lymphatics. Thoracic duct lymph will show a very low protein content, even though fluid production is increased. Fat transport is also reduced after ingestion.

The diagnosis of constrictive pericarditis is not always easy, since it can easily be confused with various forms of familial and acquired myocardiopathies. Cardiac catheterization has been the best technique in differentiating myocardial and pericardial disease. In constrictive pericarditis, the diastolic pressure in the right ventricle shows a rapid rise during early filling, with a plateau effect and a very small A wave. The systolic pulmonary artery pressure is rarely ever above 45 mm. Hg, and the right atrial pressure is always elevated. Left ventricular end-diastolic pressure is usually normal, whereas in myocardiopathies it is usually much greater, with an average as high as 15 to 18 mm. Hg. Angiocardiography is helpful in outlining the thickness of the atrial wall and the stiffness of the atrium. In a certain number of cases, the diagnosis remains uncertain and can be accurately

defined only by pericardial biopsy. This is usually performed through a small incision, with resection of the fourth or fifth costal cartilage. If the diagnosis of constrictive pericarditis is confirmed, a formal thoracotomy should be performed.

Pericardial constriction often follows suppurative forms of pericarditis, a common cause of which has been tuberculosis. Simple penetrating injuries of the heart result in hemopericardium, but this has been a rare cause of chronic pericardial constriction (Fig. 4). Blunt trauma to the chest may cause hemopericardium and precipitate scarring. In some instances the time interval between injury and pericardial constriction is considerable.

PERICARDIECTOMY

Preoperative Preparation

Patients are usually hospitalized and brought to an optimal nutritional and cardiovascular state. Vigorous efforts to relieve ascites and cardiac failure should be made by salt restriction, control of arrhythmias, adequate digitalization, and use of diuretics. Antituberculous therapy should consist of two drugs, with the possible addition of a third drug 10 days prior to operation.

Operative Technique

Adequate exposure of the heart is necessary to remove the pericardium from the anterior and posterior surfaces. A sternal splitting incision is commonly employed, although a left anterior thoracotomy with extension across the sternum into the right chest has also been advocated. The extent of pericardial resection should be determined by the operative findings; most errors have been the result of removal of an insufficient amount of the pericardium. The myocardium may be quite thinned and atrophic because of the long

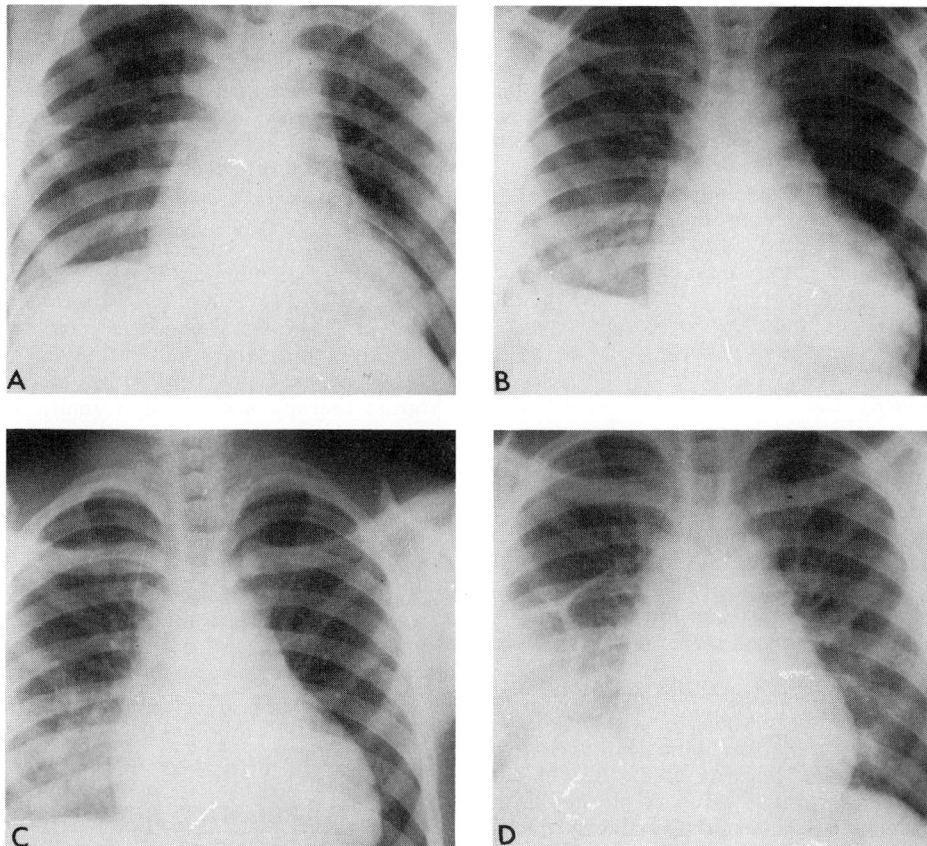

Figure 4.   Sequence of chest x-rays from an 18-year-old male stabbed in the left anterior chest with a knife. *A*, On admission the cardiac silhouette was enlarged. Blood was aspirated from the pericardial sac and the patient hospitalized 8 days. *B*, Four weeks later the cardiac silhouette was larger. There was a slight haziness in the right lower lung field and the patient remained asymptomatic. *C*, At 11 weeks symptoms of constrictive pericarditis developed, with a smaller heart but marked exercise limitation and venous stasis. *D*, Pericardiectomy was performed and the postoperative x-ray showed the heart to be smaller, with residual pleural reaction in the right chest.

period of compression by the pericardium, and care must be taken when removing the pericardium from the thin-walled right ventricle. Injury to the coronary vessels must be carefully avoided, and bleeding areas from the heart surface must be controlled by finely placed sutures. The phrenic nerves should be mobilized away from the pericardium to avoid damage to them and to allow resection of the pericardium posterior to the nerve. Small pockets of localized fluid or pus may be encountered between the epicardium and the thickened pericardium, and the epicardial lining of such pockets should be removed to lessen the chance of subsequent scarring. Oozing from the heart surface usually ceases with gentle pressure, and the pleura is opened widely on both sides. Intercostal catheters are placed in each chest for drainage.

Postoperative Care

The main concern of the postoperative period is fluid overload. Venous pressure usually falls after the constricted pericardium is removed, and intravenous fluid or blood must be administered conservatively to avoid overloading the heart or lungs. A mild cardiac stimulant may be needed if cardiac contractility decreases.

Usually a slow infusion of dilute isoproterenol will improve cardiac function. Antibiotics are usually administered for 8 to 10 days, and tuberculous chemotherapy is continued for 3 to 6 months depending upon culture reports of pericardial material. In proved cases of tuberculosis, antituberculous therapy should be continued for a minimum of 6 months, and many advise treatment for 1 year.

Salt restriction is usually necessary; however, if a profound diuresis occurs after operation, salt replacement may be indicated. Electrolytes must be closely observed, and digitalis administration usually is continued. Ambulation and exercise are gradually encouraged, since ascites and edema usually subside soon after operation.

It has been emphasized that the pericardium must be removed from the caval orifices to the right atrium to be certain of relieving ascites. In experiments in animals, Isaacs et al.[10] showed that removal of the pericardium from the right heart resulted in a decrease in central venous pressure, but the animals expired from pulmonary congestion. In other instances, removal of the pericardium from the left heart alone had no effect on venous pressure or ascites.

POSTPERICARDIOTOMY SYNDROME

Postpericardiotomy syndrome is an unusual syndrome typically characterized by fever, pericardial pain, pleural pain, pulmonary infiltrates, arthralgias, dyspnea, pericardial effusion, pleural effusion, pericardial friction rub, or any combination of these signs and symptoms. Symptoms suggesting the postpericardiotomy syndrome have been noted in 10 to 40 per cent of patients undergoing cardiac surgery, and the actual incidence may be higher, since mild cases may remain unrecognized. The sedimentation rate is elevated, and leukocytosis with an increase in lymphocytes is usually present. The electrocardiogram may show changes of pericarditis.

Cox[5] and Koucky and Milles[14] initially referred to this syndrome as polyserositis occurring after wounds of the heart. It was called postcommissurotomy syndrome because of its frequency of occurrence after mitral commissurotomy and was thought at one time to be due to reactivation of rheumatic fever. Dresdale et al.[6] observed similar symptoms after a pericardiotomy and termed the syndrome postpericardiotomy syndrome. It has been seen to occur after such minor violations of the pericardium as percutaneous left ventricular punctures.

The etiology of postpericardiotomy syndrome has received considerable speculation. It was originally thought that the syndrome represented an exacerbation of rheumatic fever, but the occurrence of the syndrome in persons without evidence of rheumatic heart disease seems to rule out this possibility. Bacterial infection was considered, but repeated cultures of pericardium or pericardial fluid in patients suffering from the syndrome did not reveal any pathogenic organism. Cohen et al.[4] noticed that there were periods of increased incidence of the syndrome with seasonal variation. This suggested the possibility of a virus infection being activated by operation and causing symptoms. Kahn and co-workers[11] in 1967 reported the isolation of parainfluenza virus from a group of patients with postpericardiotomy syndrome; this suggests that a virus infection may be responsible in some cases at least.

The possibility that the syndrome represents an autoimmune response has been suggested, the symptoms resulting from a delayed hypersensitivity reaction to damaged tissues in the pericardial cavity. The pertinent structural alterations render tissue somewhat foreign to the host, and this induces the production of autoantibody. It has been suggested that the myocardium, red blood cells, and pericardial tissue may be the organs against which the antibodies react. Van der Geld[30] detected antiheart antibodies in 21 of 29 patients with postpericardiotomy syndrome. Engle et al. (1974) noted that the antiheart antibodies could be quantitated and the serum concentration varied with the severity of clinical symptoms.

Aronstam and Cox[1] described low serum albumin associated with poor nutrition in patients with symptoms of postpericardiotomy syndrome. Reversal of negative nitrogen balance by administration of intravenous albumin resulted in clinical improvement. If collections of fluid persisted, pericardicentesis or thoracentesis was done. No evidence of the syndrome appeared in any patient showing normal blood protein levels in the postoperative period.

The syndrome is generally self-limiting and benign. The illness may last from 1 to 6 weeks, and recurrences are possible. Chronic pericardial effusion and constrictive pericarditis have not been reported to occur after postpericardiotomy syndrome. The diagnosis is based primarily on the clinical findings. Treatment is generally symptomatic, with the patient being made as comfortable as possible. Physical activity is restricted, and fever and pain are controlled by appropriate medications. Salicylates have been effective in lowering temperature and relieving pain. Stronger analgesics may be required in more severe cases. Steroid therapy may cause dramatic relief of symptoms, with temperature returning to normal. In some cases the symptoms linger and low doses of steroids are necessary for a considerable period of time. Steroid therapy is generally not recommended for the milder cases, since recurrences are common when the steroids are withdrawn.

The main complications of this syndrome are misdiagnosis resulting in failure to treat a specific infection, delay in recuperation with prolongation of hospitalization, and recurrences. Postpericardiotomy syndrome usually does not play a role in the ultimate prognosis of the patient, even though convalescence can be prolonged.

SELECTED REFERENCES

Engle, M. A., McCabe, J. C., Ebert, P. A., and Zabriskie, J.: The postpericardiotomy syndrome and antiheart antibodies. Circulation, 49:401, 1974.
This article describes the clinical course and possible etiologies of the postpericardiotomy syndrome. The immunologic significance of this rather common complication of cardiac surgery is emphasized. The findings of a heart reactive antibody that closely correlates with the clinical symptoms and the use of this as a diagnostic test in patients having persistent pain and fever after thoracotomy are demonstrated. The level of antibody is directly related to the clinical symptoms and could be used to predict recurrences.

Kirsh, M. M., McIntosh, K., Kahn, D. R., and Sloan, H.: Postpericardiotomy syndromes. Ann. Thorac. Surg., 9:158, 1970.
This review article gives an excellent résumé of the current concepts of the rather vague syndromes seen after operations on the heart. A good review of possible etiologies of the postpericardiotomy and postperfusion syndromes, such as autoimmune states, virus infection, and protein deficiencies, is presented. Treatment is outlined and the usual benign course of these syndromes emphasized.

REFERENCES

1. Aronstam, E. M., and Cox, W. A.: A new concept of the pleuropericardial syndrome. Postpericardiotomy or postcardiotomy syndrome. J. Thorac. Cardiovasc. Surg., 51:341, 1966.
2. Brawley, R. K., Vasko, J. S., and Morrow, A. G.: Cholesterol pericarditis. Am. J. Med., 41:235, 1966.
3. Chevers, N.: Observations on the disease of the orifice and valves of the aorta. Guys Hosp. Rep., 7:387, 1842.
4. Cohen, G., Dardick, I., and Greenblatt, J.: Pleurisy and pericarditis complicating myocardial infarction: The so-called post myocardial infarction syndrome. Can. Med. Assoc. J., 82:123, 1960.
5. Cox, W. M.: Wounds of the heart. Arch. Surg., 17:484, 1928.
6. Dresdale, D. T., Ropstein, C. B., Gusman, S. J., and Greene, M. A.: Postpericardiotomy syndrome in patients with rheumatic heart disease. Am. J. Med., 21:57, 1956.
7. Holman, C. W., and Steinberg, I.: The role of angiocardiography

in the surgical treatment of massive pericardial effusions. Surg. Gynecol. Obstet., *107*:639, 1958.

8. Holman, E., and Willett, F.: Treatment of active tuberculous pericarditis by pericardiectomy. J.A.M.A., *146*:1, 1951.

9. Holman, E., and Willett, F.: Results of radical pericardiectomy for constrictive pericarditis. J.A.M.A., *157*:789, 1955.

10. Isaacs, J. P., Carter, B. N., II, and Haller, J. A., Jr.: Pathologic physiology of constrictive pericarditis. Bull. Johns Hopkins Hosp., *90*:259, 1952.

11. Kahn, D. R., Ertel, P. Y., Murphy, W. H., Kirsh, M. M., Vathayanon, S., Stern, A. M., and Sloan, H.: Pathogenesis of the postpericardiotomy syndrome. J. Thorac. Cardiovasc. Surg., *54*:682, 1967.

12. Kaplan, M. H.: The concept of autoantibodies in rheumatic fever and in the postcommissurotomy state. Ann. N.Y. Acad. Sci., *86*:974, 1960.

13. Karanaeff: Paracentese des Brustkastens und des Pericardiums. Med. Ztg., *9*:251, 1840.

14. Koucky, J. D., and Milles, G.: Stab wounds of the heart. Arch. Intern. Med., *56*:281, 1935.

15. Kussmaul, A.: Ueber schwielige Mediastino-Perikarditis und den paradoxen Puls. Berlin. Klin. Wochenschr., *10*:433, 461, 1873.

16. Lower, R.: Tractatus de Corde. London, 1669. (Cited in Major, R. H.: Classic Descriptions of Disease. Springfield, Ill., Charles C Thomas, Publisher, 1932, p. 630).

17. Martin, A.: Acute non-specific pericarditis. A description of nineteen cases. Br. Med. J., *2*:279, 1966.

18. Martin, J. W., and Schenk, W. G., Jr.: Pericardial tamponade; newer dynamic concepts. Am. J. Surg., *99*:782, 1960.

19. McKusick, V. A., Kay, J. H., and Isaacs, J. P.: Constrictive pericarditis following traumatic hemopericardium. Ann. Surg., *142*:97, 1955.

20. Morgagni, G. B.: De Sedibus et Causis Morborum per Anatomen Indagatis. Venetiis, Typ. Remondiniana, 1761.

21. Parsons, H. G., and Holman, E.: Experimental segmental pericarditis. Arch. Surg., *70*:479, 1955.

22. Rehn, L.: Zur experimentellen Pathologie des Herzbeutels. Ver. Deutsch. Ges. Chir., *42*:339, 1913.

23. Romero, cited by Baizeau: Mémoire sur le ponction du péricarde au point de vue chirurgical. Gaz. Med. Chir., 1868, p. 565.

24. Roshe, J., and Shumacker, H. B., Jr.: Pericardiectomy for chronic cardiac tamponade in children. Surgery, *46*:1152, 1959.

25. Sauerbruch, F.: Die Chirurgie der Brustorgane. Vol. II. Berlin, 1925.

26. Sellors, T. H.: General observations on constrictive pericarditis with special reference to results of surgery. Minerva Cardioangiol. Europ., *4*:489, 1956.

27. Shumacker, H. B., Jr., and Roshe, J.: Pericardiectomy. J. Cardiovasc. Surg., *1*:65, 1960.

28. Soulen, R. L., Lapayowker, M. S., and Gimenz, J. L.: Echocardiography in the diagnosis of pericardial effusion. Radiology, *86*:1047, 1966.

29. Turner, A. F., Meyers, H. L., Jacobson, G., and Lo, W.: Carbon dioxide cineangiocardiography in the diagnosis of pericardial disease. Am. J. Roentgenol., *97*:342, 1966.

30. Van der Geld, H.: Anti-heart antibodies in the postpericardiotomy and the postmyocardial-infarction syndromes. Lancet, *2*:617, 1964.

31. Vieussens, R.: Traité nouveau de la structure et des causes du mouvement naturel de coeur. Toulouse, J. Guillemette, 1715.

32. White, P.: Chronic constrictive pericarditis. (Pick's disease) treated by pericardial resection. Lancet, *2*:597, 1935.

33. Wood, P.: Diagnosis of pericardial effusion by means of cardiac catheterization. Br. Heart J., *13*:574, 1951.

58

THE HEART

I

CARDIAC CATHETERIZATION

Erwin Robin, M.D., Sunilendu N. Ganguly, M.D.,
and Richard J. Bing, M.D.

HISTORICAL ASPECTS

In 1861, Chaveau and Marey performed cardiac catheterization in animals. In 1905, Fritz Bleichroeder had a ureteral catheter placed in his axillary vein from the arm and in his inferior vena cava from the thigh Forssman, in 1929, under fluoroscopic control, catheterized his right atrium from a left antecubital vein. Right heart catheterization was introduced clinically in 1941 by Cournand and Ranges and was further developed by Richards, Bing, and Dexter. Since that time, rapid advances have been made with the introduction of new methods, such as indicator dilution methods, left heart catheterization, and selective angiography.

INDICATIONS

There are no absolute contraindications to cardiac catheterization. From a clinical viewpoint, it is indicated whenever it is necessary to establish a precise and definite diagnosis. This has become increasingly important as surgical techniques have been devised for correction of more and more cardiac lesions.

PREPARATION OF THE PATIENT

The patient should be psychologically prepared. This is best accomplished by explaining the procedure and its goal, and thus gaining his confidence.

General anesthesia is neither necessary nor desirable. In adults, small amounts of a narcotic or barbiturate may be used. In children, intramuscular injection of a combination of 6.25 mg. promethezine (Phenergan), 6.25 mg. chlorpromazine (Thorazine), and 25 mg. meperidine hydrochloride (Demerol) per cubic centimeter of mixture provides good sedation. The dose varies according to the age, weight, and condition of the patient. Noncyanotic children receive 1 ml. per

20 pounds of body weight. Cyanotic children should receive a smaller dose. Newborns rarely need sedation. However, if it is needed, oral chloral hydrate may be administered in a dose of 10 to 15 mg. per pound of body weight.

The patient should fast for 3 to 6 hours prior to the study. Sedation is given 30 to 60 minutes before catheterization. Cyanotic children, because of the high viscosity of their blood, are permitted to receive fluids 2 to 3 hours prior to the procedure. As a rule, prophylactic antibiotics are not necessary.

CHOICE OF CATHETERS

Catheters are available in a variety of models and sizes (Fig. 1). Pressures are best recorded with open-end catheters. During the performance of angiocardiography, closed-end catheters are used to prevent recoil and intramural injection of contrast material.

RIGHT HEART CATHETERIZATION

Under sterile conditions and fluoroscopic control, a radiopaque catheter is inserted percutaneously or via a cutdown into a peripheral vein and passed into the right atrium, right ventricle, and pulmonary arterial vessels. In newborns, the superficial femoral or umbilical vein is used. In infants and small children, the superficial saphenous vein is usually used (Fig. 2A). In older children and adults, an antecubital vein is preferred (Fig. 2B).

Recording of Pressures

Normal values of pressures obtained during right cardiac catheterization are shown in Table 1.

Pulmonary Capillary Pressure. The pulmonary capillary pressure (also referred to as wedge pressure) resembles the left atrial pressure (Fig. 3). This is due to the fact that there are no valves between the left

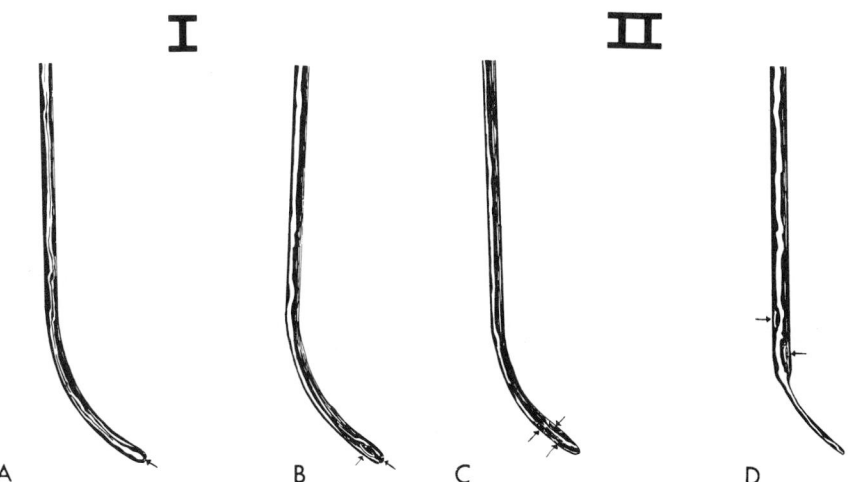

Figure 1. Catheters used during cardiac catheterization. *I*, Open-end catheter tips: A, Cournand catheter tip; B, Birdseye catheter tip with two laterally opposed eyes close to the distal tip. *II*, Closed-end catheter tips: C, NIH catheter tip with six round openings arranged in three laterally opposed pairs within 1 cm. of the tip; D, Lehman ventriculography catheter tip with four eyes arranged in two laterally opposed pairs within 4 cm. of the distal tip. (Arrows point toward openings.)

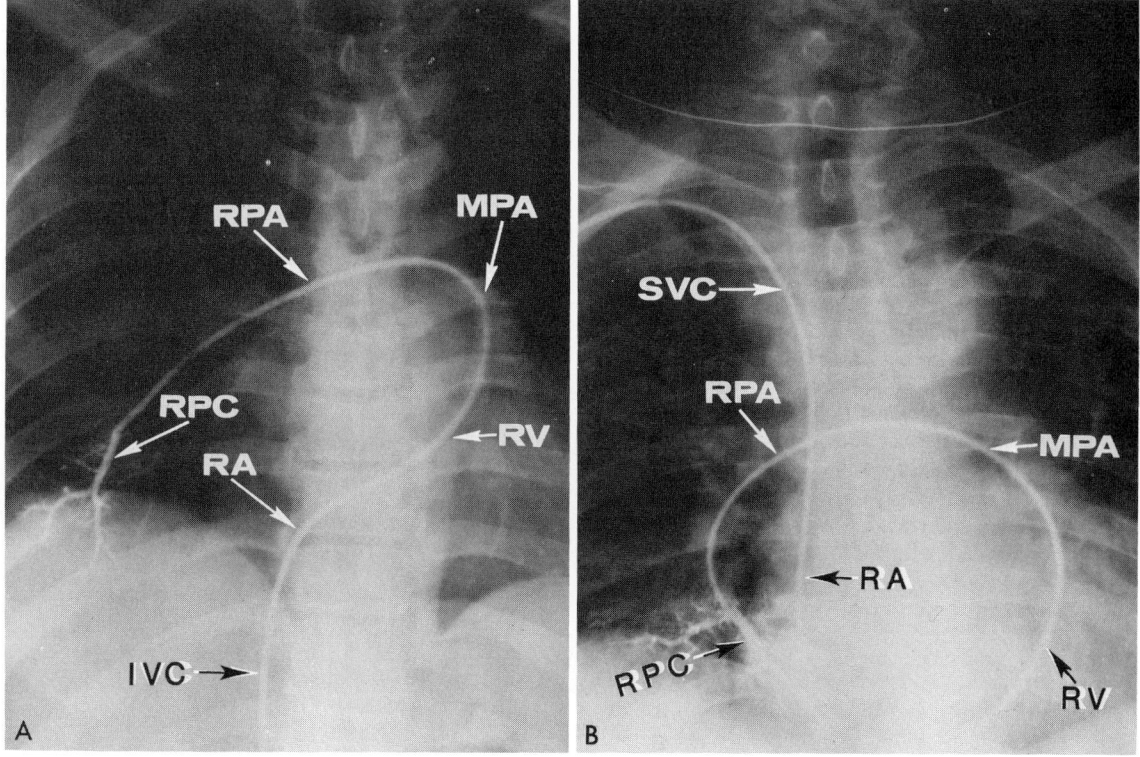

Figure 2. *A*, A catheter has been introduced into the right saphenous vein and guided through the inferior vena cava (IVC), right atrium (RA), right ventricle (RV), main pulmonary artery (MPA), and right pulmonary artery (RPA) to the right pulmonary capillary position (RPC). *B*, A catheter has been introduced into a right antecubital vein and passed through the superior vena cava (SVC), right atrium (RA), right ventricle (RV), main pulmonary artery (MPA), and right pulmonary artery (RPA) to the right pulmonary capillary position (RPC).

TABLE 1.   Normal Pressures Obtained by
Right Heart Catheterization*

| | Pressure (mm. Hg) | | |
	Systolic	Diastolic	Mean
Right atrium	5 to 7	−2 to 2	−2 to 7
Right ventricle	15 to 30	0 to 7	
Pulmonary artery	15 to 30	5 to 15	10 to 20
Pulmonary capillary			5 to 12

*Modified from Robin, E., et al. *In* Sabiston, D. C., Jr., and
Spencer, F. C. (Eds.): Gibbon's Surgery of the Chest, 3rd ed.
Philadelphia, W. B. Saunders Company, 1976.

atrium and pulmonary veins and capillaries. Incomplete wedging or wedging of the catheter tip into the wall of a tortuous pulmonary artery is a common cause of a distorted pulmonary capillary pressure tracing.

Pulmonary Artery Pressure. The pulmonary artery pressure ranges from 15 to 30 mm. Hg systolic, and 5 to 15 mm. Hg diastolic, with a mean of 10 to 20 mm. Hg.

Pulmonary hypertension is classified into hyperkinetic and obstructive types. The former type is due to a marked increase in pulmonary flow from a left-to-right shunt. During childhood and adolescence, pulmonary hypertension is more common in cases of ventricular septal defect and patent ductus arteriosus than in those of atrial septal defect.

Obstructive pulmonary hypertension may be the end result of the hyperkinetic type. In this case, the pulmonary blood flow can be normal or even decreased. Other causes are chronic pulmonary parenchymal diseases, multiple pulmonary emboli, chronic left heart failure, mitral valve disease, and pulmonary vasculitis.

Right Ventricular Pressure. A maximal systolic gradient of 10 mm. Hg between the main pulmonary artery and the right ventricle is considered normal. In pulmonic valvular stenosis, the systolic gradient between the main pulmonary trunk and the outflow tract of the right ventricle is abrupt (Fig. 4); in infundibular stenosis, on the other hand, progressive gradients are found between the main pulmonary artery, the infundibular chamber, and the right ventricle (Fig. 5).

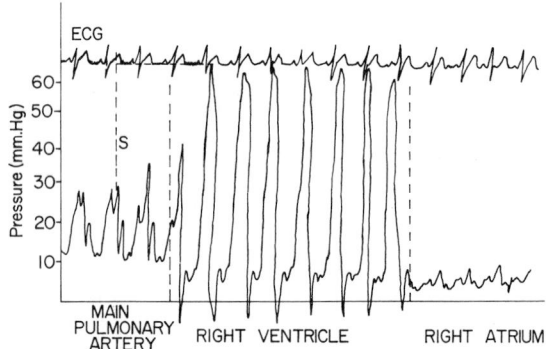

Figure 4. Pulmonic valvular stenosis: There is an abrupt systolic gradient (S) of 40 mm. Hg between the main pulmonary trunk and the outflow tract of the right ventricle at the level of the pulmonic valve. (From Robin, E., et al. *In* Sabiston, D. C., Jr., and Spencer, F. C. (Eds.): Gibbon's Surgery of the Chest, 3rd ed. Philadelphia, W. B. Saunders Company, 1976.)

In 90 per cent of cases of isolated pulmonic stenosis, the lesion is at the level of the pulmonic valve. In tetralogy of Fallot, infundibular pulmonic stenosis is present in 40 per cent, valvular stenosis in 35 per cent, and combined valvular and infundibular stenosis in 25 per cent of cases. Isolated infundibular stenosis can develop late in the course of large ventricular septal defects.

Right Atrial Pressure. The right atrial pressure curve consists of three waves, "a," "c," and "v," each of which is followed by a descent "x," "x'," and "y." The "a" wave is produced by atrial systole, the "c" wave by transmission of the right ventricular systole through the closed tricuspid valve, and the "v" wave by the inflow of blood into the right atrium during atrial diastole.

In tricuspid atresia and stenosis, in the absence of atrial fibrillation, there is a tall "a" wave; if the valve is incompetent, the "v" wave is prominent. An increase in right atrial pressure occurs in right heart failure. In constrictive pericarditis, the mean right

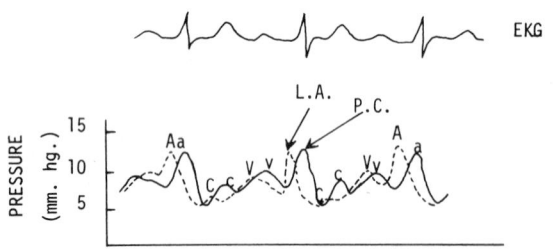

Figure 3. Simultaneous left atrial (L.A.) and pulmonary capillary (P.C.) pressures: The left atrial pressure was obtained by means of the transseptal technique. Both curves are similar in their contour and magnitude. The pulmonary capillary pressure is slightly delayed.

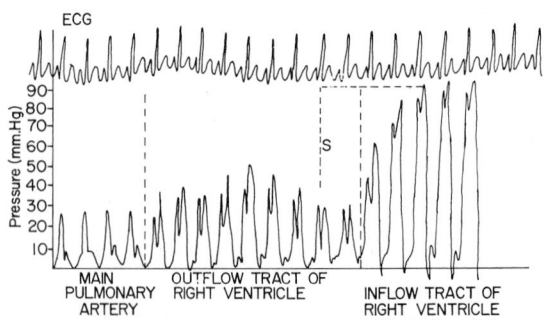

Figure 5. Pulmonic infundibular stenosis: There is a systolic gradient (S) of 40 mm. Hg between the outflow and inflow tracts of the right ventricle below the pulmonic valve. (From Robin, E., et al. *In* Sabiston, D. C., Jr., and Spencer, F. C. (Eds.): Gibbon's Surgery of the Chest, 3rd ed. Philadelphia, W. B. Saunders Company, 1976.)

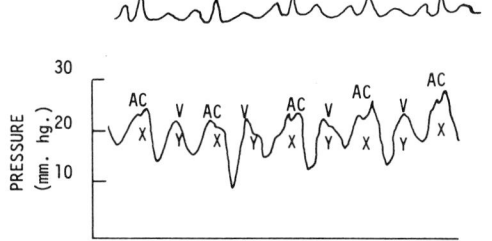

Figure 6. Right atrial pressure in a case of constrictive pericarditis: The pressure curve has an M or W shape because of the prominent and steep "x" and "y" descents.

atrial pressure is elevated, and the pressure curve assumes a distinctive pattern (Fig. 6).

Swan-Ganz Catheterization Technique

In the last two decades, hemodynamic measurements from the right heart, pulmonary circulation, and left heart have been reported in patients with acute myocardial infarction. These data have been valuable in understanding the extent of altered cardiovascular function, classifying the severity of the disease, measuring the response to treatment, and predicting the prognosis of the patient. To obviate the logistical problems of transferring ill patients to the cardiac catheterization laboratory, a flexible catheter with a small balloon at its tip was developed. Inflation of the balloon with air allows the catheter to be passed with ease from the right atrium and ventricle to the pulmonary artery. This technique can be performed at the bedside without fluoroscopy. The position of the catheter tip is verified by electrocardiographic and pressure monitoring (Fig. 7). Following recording of a pulmonary artery pressure curve, the catheter is advanced until a pulmonary wedge pressure curve is observed. The balloon is deflated and the pulmonary artery pressure curve reappears. The final position of the catheter can be checked by means of a chest roentgenogram (Fig. 8). The diastolic pressure of the pulmonary artery and the pulmonary wedge pressure can be used as indicators of left ventricular filling pressure. The catheter has been modified so that ac-

curate measurements of cardiac output by the thermo-dilution technique, monitoring of intracavity electrograms, and temporary cardiac pacing can be performed.

Sampling of Blood for Oxygen Determination and Calculation of Flow

The most commonly used method of identifying, localizing, and quantifying shunts involves the analysis of oxygen in blood drawn from the heart and the great veins and arteries. Normally, there is great variability in the oxygen in blood withdrawn from the right atrium because of laminar flow from the superior and inferior venae cavae and coronary sinus. Truly mixed venous blood is found only in the pulmonary artery.

Multiple samples of blood should be obtained in rapid succession, beginning at the pulmonary wedge position and ending at the venae cavae. At least two samples should be obtained in the right ventricle: one in the outflow tract and the other in the main cavity. In the right atrium, at least three samples should be drawn: one near the inferior vena cava, one in the middle of the atrium near the lateral wall, and the third just below the superior vena cava.

Flows are calculated according to the Fick principle (see Equations 1 and 2 at bottom of page).

If pulmonary flow is more than systemic flow, there is a left-to-right shunt. If the systemic flow is greater than the pulmonary flow, there is a right-to-left shunt.

If bidirectional shunting is present, the "effective pulmonary blood flow" must be calculated first. The "effective pulmonary blood flow" is the volume of mixed blood that, after returning to the right atrium, is aerated in the pulmonary capillaries (see Equation 3 at bottom of page).

At the level of a left-to-right shunt and downstream from it, the oxygen saturation of blood is higher than in the chamber immediately upstream. The pulmonary flow also exceeds the systemic flow. In contrast, in the right-to-left shunts the pulmonary flow is less than the systemic flow; the oxygen saturation is normal in the pulmonary veins and decreased in the peripheral arterial blood. In many cases, a bidirectional shunt is present. This results in a left-to-right shunt and a diminished oxygen saturation in the peripheral arterial blood.

Significant differences in oxygen saturation and con-

---

1. Systemic flow (S.F.) (liters/min.) $= \dfrac{O_2 \text{ consumption (ml./min.)}}{\text{Systemic A-V difference} \times 10}$ where A (vol. %) = peripheral arterial blood
V (vol. %) = mixed venous blood

2. Pulmonary flow (P.F.) (liters/min.) $= \dfrac{O_2 \text{ consumption (ml./min.)}}{\text{Pulmonary A-V difference} \times 10}$ where A (vol. %) = pulmonary vein blood
V (vol. %) = pulmonary artery blood

3. Effective pulmonary flow (E.F.) $= \dfrac{O_2 \text{ consumption (ml./min.)}}{\text{Pulmonary venous } O_2 \text{ content (vol. %)} - \text{mixed venous } O_2 \text{ content (vol. %)} \times 10}$

Then: a. left-to-right shunt = P.F. − E.F.
(liters/min.)
b. right-to-left shunt = S.F. − E.F.
(liters/min.)

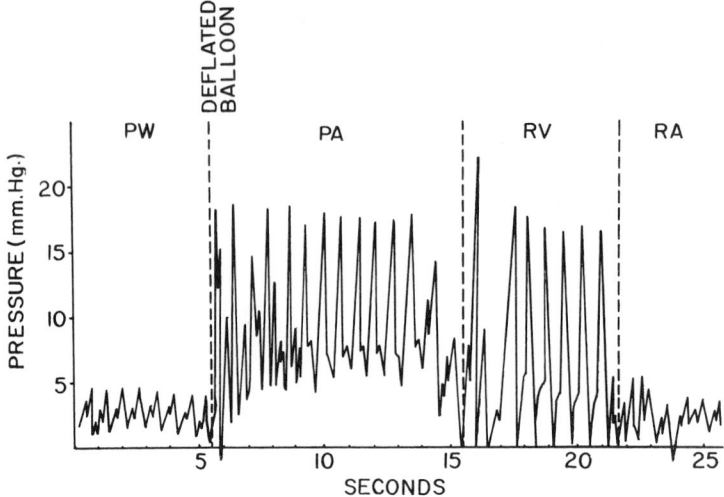

Figure 7. Pressure tracing obtained during pullback from the left pulmonary artery (PA) to the right atrium (RA) with a Swan-Ganz catheter. A left pulmonary wedge pressure curve (PW) is obtained with inflation of the balloon. With the balloon deflated a left pulmonary artery pressure curve (PA) is recorded. (From Robin, E., et al. *In* Sabiston, D. C., Jr., and Spencer, F. C. (Eds.): Gibbon's Surgery of the Chest, 3rd ed. Philadelphia, W. B. Saunders Company, 1976.)

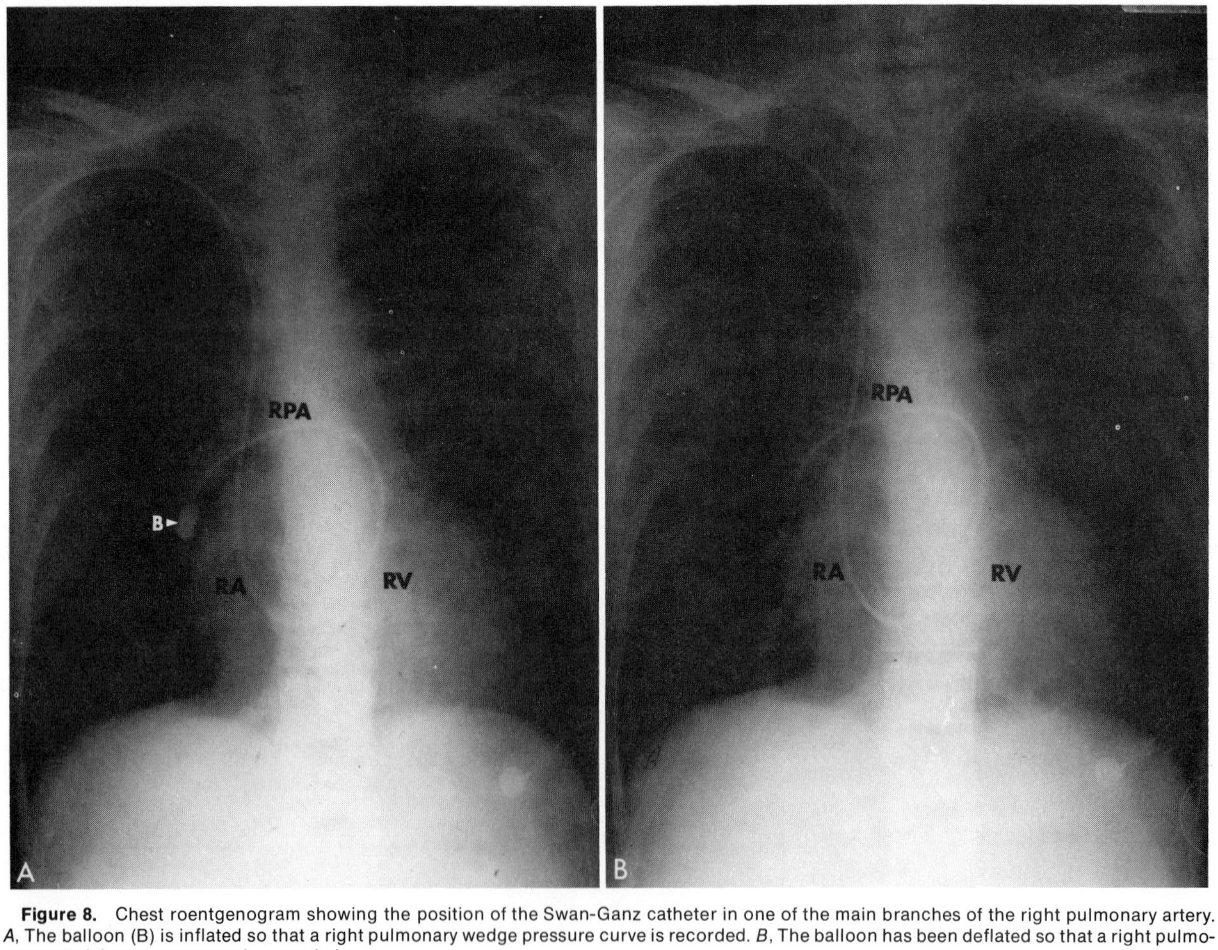

Figure 8. Chest roentgenogram showing the position of the Swan-Ganz catheter in one of the main branches of the right pulmonary artery. *A*, The balloon (B) is inflated so that a right pulmonary wedge pressure curve is recorded. *B*, The balloon has been deflated so that a right pulmonary arterial pressure curve is recorded.

TABLE 2. Significant Differences in Oxygen Saturation and Content*

	O₂ Saturation Difference (%)	O₂ Content Difference (Vol. %)	Type of Defect
SVC-RA	9.0	2.0	ASD
RA-RV	5.0	1.0	VSD
RV-PA	3.0	0.5	PDA

*Modified from Robin, E., et al. *In* Sabiston, D. C., Jr., and Spencer, F. C. (Eds.): Gibbon's Surgery of the Chest, 3rd ed. Philadelphia, W. B. Saunders Company, 1976.

tent are summarized in Table 2. Left-to-right shunts that are less than 20 per cent of the pulmonary flow are not detectable by the conventional blood oxygen saturation methods.

Oxygen Analysis

Oxygen content determination can be accomplished by the manometric method of Van Slyke and Neill or by spectrophotometry. These methods are time-consuming, and in infants multiple sampling may constitute a considerable loss of blood. By use of either transmission or reflection methods, direct analysis of blood oxygen content can be obtained rapidly by flow through cuvettes connected directly to a catheter. Oxygen tension (pO_2) may be monitored continually by means of a platinum electrode. A fiberoptic catheter incorporates instantaneous and continuous measurement of oxygen saturation without withdrawal of blood samples. The same instrument can also be used in the determination of cardiac output.

Observation of the Position of the Catheter

The position of the catheter is important in the recognition of abnormal communication between the cardiac chambers and the great vessels. If abnormal channels are encountered, serial blood samples should be drawn, and continuous pressures should be recorded.

The tip of the catheter may pass over the left side of the heart through a patent foramen ovale or atrial or ventricular septal defect. In endocardial cushion defects, either partial or complete, the position of the catheter is lower than in septum secundum defects. If the tip of the catheter is manipulated into the left ventricle, one may obtain, on withdrawal, an abrupt pressure change from the left ventricular to the right atrial form.

If an anomalous draining pulmonary vein is intubated, the shaft of the catheter will take an abnormal position in relation to the cardiac silhouette. However, distinction between an atrial septal defect and an anomalous pulmonary vein cannot be made from the position of the catheter alone.

Often the catheter may be threaded through the patent ductus arteriosus into the descending aorta. In the tetralogy of Fallot, aortic transposition, or ventricular defects in the membranous part of the septum,

the ascending aorta may be intubated directly from the right ventricle.

LEFT HEART CATHETERIZATION

The development of left heart catheterization has made it possible to assess more accurately the size and location of left-to-right shunts and to evaluate lesions of the mitral and aortic valves. Selective angiocardiography of the left heart chambers, aorta, and coronary arteries can be performed, and postoperative results can be evaluated.

The normal pressures observed during left heart catheterization are summarized in Table 3.

Pressure Relationships of the Left Heart

The diagnostic value of left heart catheterization is to a large extent based on the pressure relationships between the left atrium, the left ventricle, and the aorta (Fig. 9). The components of the normal left atrial pressure are diagnosed in Figure 10.

The "v" wave ranges normally between 5 and 15 mm. Hg, and the "a" wave between 3 and 7 mm. Hg. In auricular fibrillation, the "a" wave is absent, whereas in atrioventricular block, giant "a" waves may be present. In heart failure or valvular disease, normal pressure tracings are modified by changes in contour or height. In congestive heart failure, there is an elevation of the left ventricular end-diastolic and left atrial pressures. In mitral stenosis, there is usually an increase in the left atrial pressure and a prolongation of the "y" descent, indicating resistance to flow across the mitral valve (Fig. 11).

In mitral stenosis, the decrease in the left atrial pressure and the increase in the left ventricular pressure after the onset of its diastolic rise are such that the mitral diastolic gradient declines exponentially with respect to time. Consequently, logarithmic plotting of the gradient results in a straight line. The mitral diastolic gradient halt-time is defined as the time required for the gradient to fall to half of its initial value from the beginning of left ventricular filling (Fig. 12).

A good correlation between the mitral diastolic gradient and the severity of mitral stenosis has been found. In mild mitral stenosis the half-time is approximately 100 msec.; in moderate stenosis it is about 200

TABLE 3. Normal Pressures Recorded During Left Heart Catheterization*

	Pressures (mm. Hg)		
	Systolic	Diastolic	Mean
Left atrium			4 to 12
Left ventricle	100 to 140	4 to 12	
Aorta	100 to 140	60 to 90	70 to 90

*From Robin, E., et al. *In* Sabiston, D. C., Jr., and Spencer, F. C. (Eds.): Surgery of the Chest, 3rd ed. Philadelphia, W. B. Saunders Company, 1976.

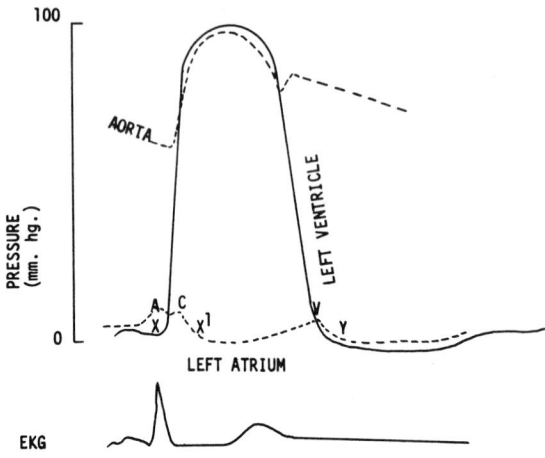

Figure 9. Pressure relationships between aorta, left ventricle, and left atrium.

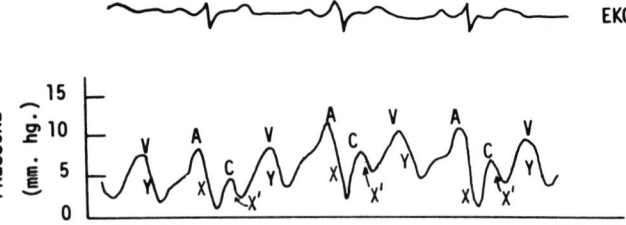

Figure 10. Normal left atrial pressure curve. The "a" wave is produced by atrial systole, the "c" wave by transmission of the rising pressure in the left ventricle through the closed mitral valve during ventricular systole, and the "v" wave by the inflow of blood into the left atrium during atrial diastole. Each wave is followed by a descent; the "v" wave is followed by the "x" descent, the "c" wave by the "x'" descent, and the "v" wave by the "y" descent. (The right atrial curve has a similar contour.)

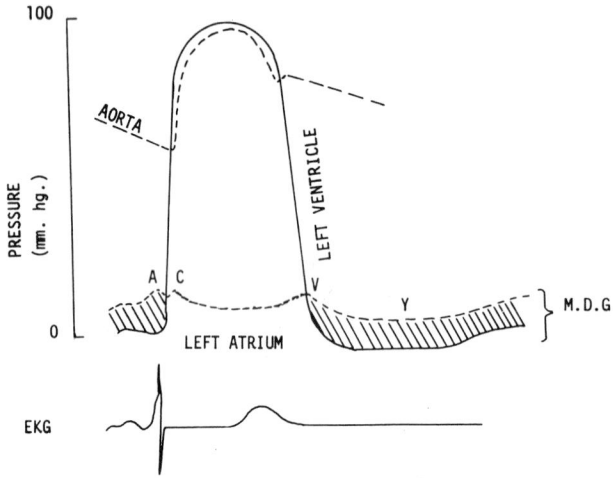

Figure 11. Mitral stenosis: There is a diastolic gradient (M.D.G.) between the left atrium and left ventricle. The "y" descent is prolonged because of the resistance to flow across the mitral valve.

Figure 12. Simultaneous left atrial (LAP) and ventricular diastolic pressures recorded in a patient with severe mitral stenosis. The diastolic pressure gradient starting at the beginning of the rise in ventricular pressure is measured at 100 msec. intervals (short vertical lines). The shaded area demonstrates the changing atrioventricular pressure gradient. LVedp = left ventricular end-diastolic pressure. (From Robin, E., et al. *In* Sabiston, D. C., Jr., and Spencer, F. C. (Eds.): Gibbon's Surgery of the Chest, 3rd ed. Philadelphia, W. B. Saunders Company, 1976.)

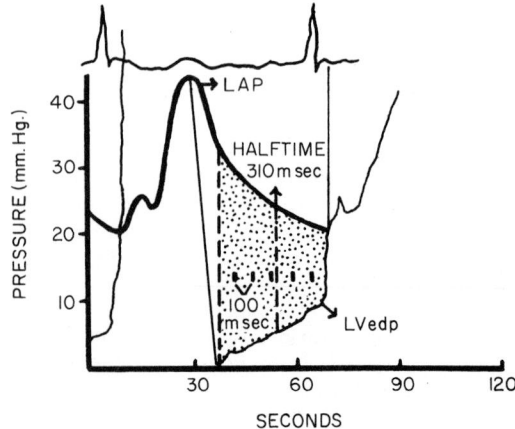

msec., and it is 300 msec. or longer in severe stenosis. Coexistent mitral regurgitation does not invalidate the results of the test. In addition, the following index has been proposed:

Mitral stenosis index =
$$\frac{\text{mitral diastolic gradient halftime (msec.)} \times 100}{\text{cardiac index (L./min./m.}^2)}$$

This index ranges from 0.4 to 0.8 in normal subjects, from 0.6 to 2.0 in patients with predominant mitral regurgitation, and from 5.7 to 10 in cases of mitral stenosis.

Although pressure contours are of value in the evaluation of patients with mitral disease, the most important criterion of the severity of mitral stenosis is the left atrioventricular diastolic pressure gradient across the mitral valve at rest and during exercise. Normally this gradient is 1 mm. or less, whereas in mitral stenosis, gradients of 5 to 30 mm. Hg at rest have been found. The gradient rises significantly with exercise. Following successful mitral commissurotomy, a marked reduction or abolition of the mitral gradient is observed.

A mitral diastolic gradient does not always indicate mitral stenosis. It may result from obstructive hypertrophy of the anterior papillary muscles, myxoma of the left atrium, anomalous myocardial hypertrophy adjacent to the mitral valve, or generalized obstructive left ventricular hypertrophy.

In mitral insufficiency, the characteristic features are a tall "v" wave (the so-called regurgitant wave) and a steep "y" descent, indicating little or no resistance to flow across the valve (Fig. 13). In combined lesions of the mitral valve, the pressure tracing reveals a combination of the findings described in mitral insufficiency and stenosis, the gradations depending on the severity of each.

The normal left ventricular pressure in man is 120 mm. Hg (100 to 140) systolic and 4 to 12 mm. Hg

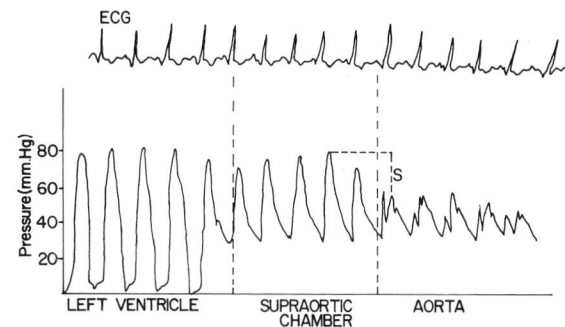

Figure 14. Supravalvular aortic stenosis: There is a systolic gradient (S) of 20 mm. Hg within the ascending aorta above the aortic valve. (From Robin, E., et al. *In* Sabiston, D. C., Jr., and Spencer, F. C. (Eds.): Gibbon's Surgery of the Chest, 3rd ed. Philadelphia, W. B. Saunders Company, 1976.)

diastolic. In infants, the systemic arterial pressure averages 60 to 70 mm. Hg. There is a difference of 10 to 15 mm. Hg between the central systolic aortic pressure and the peripheral systolic pressure, the latter being higher. Supravalvular aortic stenosis is characterized by an abrupt fall in pressure as the catheter passes the site of a narrowing above the aortic valve (Fig. 14). In congenital or acquired valvular aortic stenosis, the systolic gradient between the aorta and the left ventricle is sudden (Fig. 15). In muscular subaortic stenosis, the systolic pressure gradient shows a progressive fall between the left ventricle and the aorta similar to that described in isolated pulmonic infundibular stenosis, the site of obstruction has been localized to the left ventricular outflow tract. The ascending limb of the left ventricular pressure tracing, recorded proximally to the obstruction, generally exhibits a notch at a level that corresponds to the peak pressure distal to the obstruction (Fig. 16). Administration of digitalis, amyl nitrite, nitroglycerin, and isoproterenol or a Valsalva maneuver increases the systolic gradient (Figs. 17 and 18), whereas methoxamine and beta-adrenergic blocking agents, such as propranolol, tend to decrease the systolic gradient

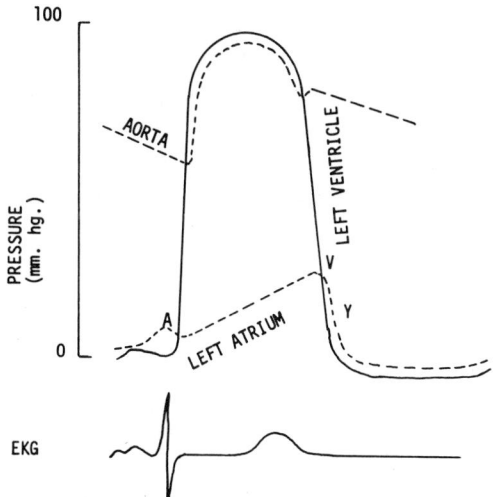

Figure 13. Mitral insufficiency: There is a prominent "v" wave and a steep "y" descent.

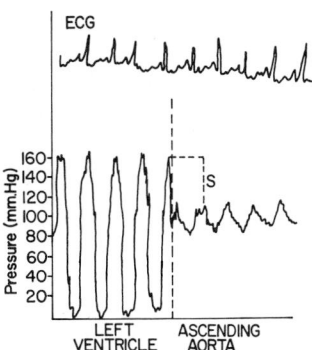

Figure 15. Aortic valvular stenosis: There is a systolic gradient (S) of 45 mm. Hg between the ascending aorta and left ventricle at the level of the aortic valve. (From Robin, E., et al. *In* Sabiston, D. C., Jr., and Spencer, F. C. (Eds.): Gibbon's Surgery of the Chest, 3rd ed. Philadelphia, W. B. Saunders Company, 1976.)

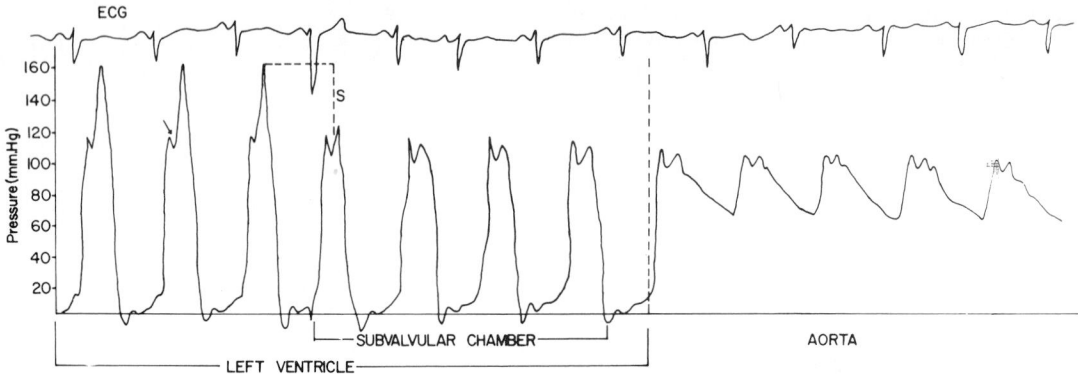

Figure 16. Subaortic hypertrophic stenosis: There is a systolic gradient (S) of 45 mm. Hg below the aortic valve within the left ventricle. The arrow denotes the notch on the ascending limb of the left ventricular pressure curve that corresponds to the peak systolic pressure distal to the obstruction. (From Robin, E., et al. *In* Sabiston, D. C., Jr., and Spencer, F. C. (Eds.): Gibbon's Surgery of the Chest, 3rd ed. Philadelphia, W. B. Saunders Company, 1976.)

(Fig. 19). There is a fall in the peripheral pulse pressure following the normal peripheral pulse pressure following the normal beat that succeeds a ventricular premature contraction (Fig. 20). In contrast, in patients with discrete supravalvular, valvular, or subvalvular stenosis, a widened pulse pressure occurs after the first normal beat following a premature ventricular contraction (Fig. 21).

In aortic insufficiency, left ventricular diastolic pressure exceeds left atrial pressure in mid-diastole and continues to rise so that the aortic and ventricular diastolic pressures are about equal at the onset of systole. The aortic pressure contour also exhibits a low diastolic pressure and a wide pulse pressure. In patients with aortic insufficiency and aortic stenosis, a combination of these signs is seen, and the brachial artery pulse pressure exhibits the so-called pulsus bisferiens.

Methods of Left Heart Catheterization

During the last 15 years, numerous methods of catheterizing the left heart have been employed clinically. These have included the transbronchial technique, the posterior percutaneous left atrial puncture technique, and the anterior left ventricular approach technique.

In recent years, these methods have been completely replaced by the transseptal left heart and retrograde aortic left heart catheterization techniques. The latter method is by far the more popular because of its relative ease and low morbidity. It can be performed percutaneously through the femoral artery or through the brachial artery via a cutdown. With either approach, the aorta, left ventricle, and coronary vascular bed can be selectively visualized. In addition, with the transbrachial route, the left atrium can be intubated from the left ventricle.

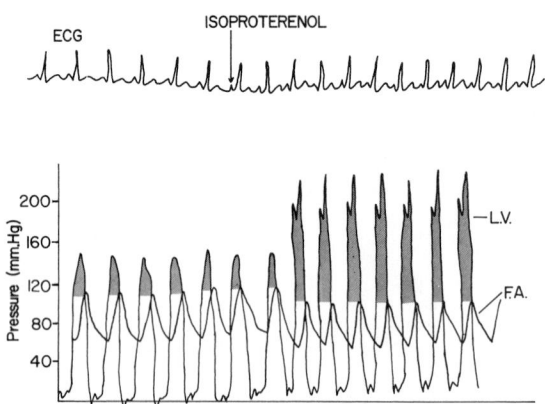

Figure 17. Effect of intravenous isoproterenol on the systolic gradient (shaded area) between left ventricle (L.V.) and femoral artery (F.A.) in subaortic hypertrophic stenosis: The baseline systolic gradient (shaded area) is about 40 mm. Hg. During infusion of isoproterenol it increases to 90 mm. Hg (shaded area). (From Robin, E., et al. *In* Sabiston, D. C., Jr., and Spencer, F. C. (Eds.): Gibbon's Surgery of the Chest, 3rd ed. Philadelphia, W. B. Saunders Company, 1976.)

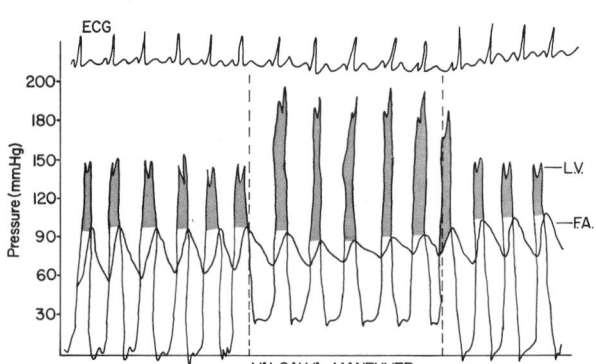

Figure 18. Effect of Valsalva maneuver on the systolic gradient (shaded area) between left ventricle (L.V.) and femoral artery (F.A.) in subaortic hypertrophic stenosis: The baseline systolic gradient (shaded area) is about 60 mm. Hg. During the maneuver it is increased to 110 mm. Hg (shaded area). (From Robin, E., et al. *In* Sabiston, D. C., Jr., and Spencer, F. C. (Eds.): Gibbon's Surgery of the Chest, 3rd ed. Philadelphia, W. B. Saunders Company, 1976.)

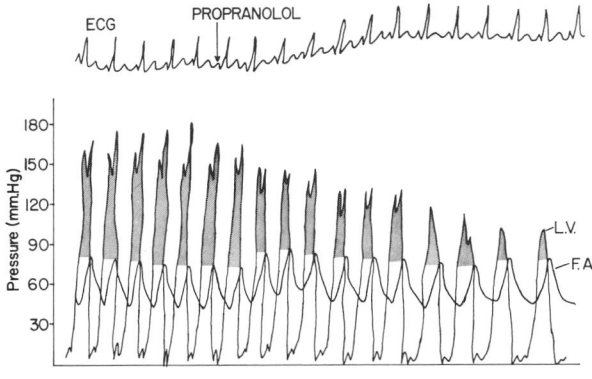

Figure 19. Effect of a beta-adrenergic blocking agent (propranolol) on the systolic gradient (shaded area) between left ventricle (L.V.) and femoral artery (F.A.) in subaortic hypertrophic stenosis: The baseline systolic gradient (shaded area) is about 80 mm. Hg. During infusion of propranolol it decreases to about 20 mm. Hg (shaded area). (From Robin, E., et al. *In* Sabiston, D. C., Jr., and Spencer, F. C. (Eds.): Gibbon's Surgery of the Chest, 3rd ed. Philadelphia, W. B. Saunders Company, 1976.)

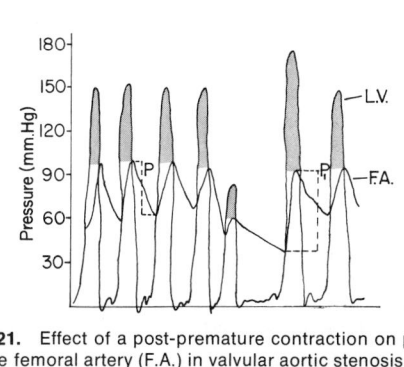

Figure 21. Effect of a post-premature contraction on pulse pressure of the femoral artery (F.A.) in valvular aortic stenosis: The baseline pulse pressure (P) of the femoral artery (F.A.) is about 35 mm. Hg. During post-premature contraction, pulse pressure (P_1) of the femoral artery (F.A.) is about 55 mm. Hg. Shaded area represents the systolic gradient between the left ventricle (L.V.) and the femoral artery (F.A.). (From Robin, E., et al. *In* Sabiston, D. C., Jr., and Spencer, F. C. (Eds.): Gibbon's Surgery of the Chest, 3rd ed. Philadelphia, W. B. Saunders Company, 1976.)

COMPLICATIONS OF CARDIAC CATHETERIZATION

Transient arrhythmias occur during every procedure. Conduction defects, knotted catheters, pyrogenic reactions, air emboli, venous or arterial spasm, thrombophlebitis, and perforation of the atria, ventricles, and coronary sinus with subsequent hemopericardium and cardiac tamponade have been reported. An increased risk is expected in cyanotic children and in patients with severe pulmonary hypertension. (See also the discussion of contrast materials under the heading Angiocardiography.)

INDICATOR DILUTION TECHNIQUES

Dye Dilution Method

The direct recording of the peripheral arterial dye dilution curve yields much information about the circulation in a relatively short time. Thus, it is possible to estimate the cardiac output and to determine the presence of shunts or valvular insufficiency. The usefulness of the technique is increased when it is employed in conjunction with right and left heart catheterization. Selective injection and selective sam-

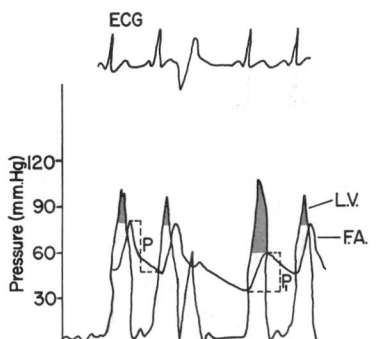

Figure 20. Effect of a post-premature contraction on pulse pressure of the femoral artery (F.A.) in subaortic hypertrophic stenosis: The baseline pulse pressure (P) in the femoral artery (F.A.) is about 35 mm. Hg. During the post-premature contraction, pulse pressure (P_1) in the femoral artery (F.A.) is about 25 mm. Hg. Shaded area represents the systolic gradient between the left ventricle (L.V.) and the femoral artery (F.A.). (From Robin, E., et al. *In* Sabiston, D. C., Jr., and Spencer, F. C. (Eds.): Gibbon's Surgery of the Chest, 3rd ed. Philadelphia, W. B. Saunders Company, 1976.)

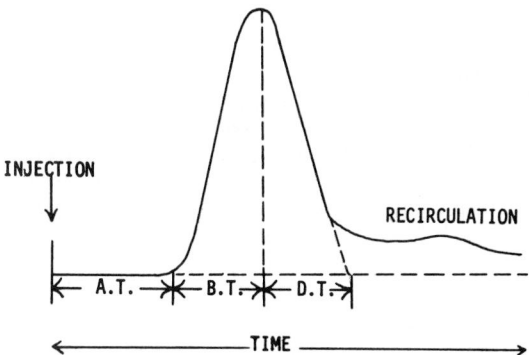

Figure 22. Diagrammatic representation of a normal indicator dilution curve: The appearance time (A.T.) represents the interval between the injection of the indicator and the appearance of the indicator at the site of sampling. The buildup time (B.T.) represents the interval between the appearance time and the time of peak indicator concentration. The disappearance time (D.T.) is represented by the downslope of the curve. To exclude any recirculating indicator, the concentration is plotted logarithmically against time (dashed segment of the downslope).

pling have made possible the localization of the sites of intracardiac and extracardiac shunts as well as the establishment of the direction of shunts. Methods for localizing incompetent valves and estimating the degree of regurgitant flow have also been described. The residual volume of the right and left ventricles can be estimated by injection of dye in the respective ventricle.

The indicator dilution techniques, helpful as they are as diagnostic aids, have definite limitations, particularly when they are used for quantitative studies. This is especially true at very low flows because of the large area under the curve and its prolonged downslope. This applies also to measurements of central volume when that volume is greatly increased. Equally important, the presence of high flow may lead to a considerable error because of the small area under the curve. At high flows, an error can be introduced because of the lag of the recording system; under these conditions, the peak of the dye concentration is often obscured. When a continuously recording densitometer is used, the flow through the sampling system must be controlled critically to avoid distortion. In the interpretation of dye dilution curves, adequate mixing of the indicator with the blood is assumed; mixing may be inadequate, however, particularly when injection and sampling sites are too close together. It is important to keep the limitations of this technique in mind when interpreting quantitative results obtained with this method.

Dye Dilution Curves. The concentration of dye in the blood is measured by recording the change in optical density of the blood by photoelectric means (decrease in the transmission of light) as the blood is drawn through a cuvette at a constant rate. Arterial sampling after rapid injection of a known amount of nondiffusible dye into the venous side of the circulation (i.e., pulmonary artery, left ventricle or atrium, or any vein) reveals a sudden appearance of the dye a few seconds after the injection. The concentration of the dye rises rapidly to a peak and then falls to a point above the baseline. A smaller, blunter peak of recirculating dye is recorded. The final dye concentration represents a state of equilibrium of dye concentration in the vascular sytem (Fig. 22).

The time course of the downstream concentration of an injected indicator is related to the flow of the volume of blood that diluted it. When the downslope of the initial appearance curve is replotted on semilogarithmic paper, it assumes a straight line. The ex-

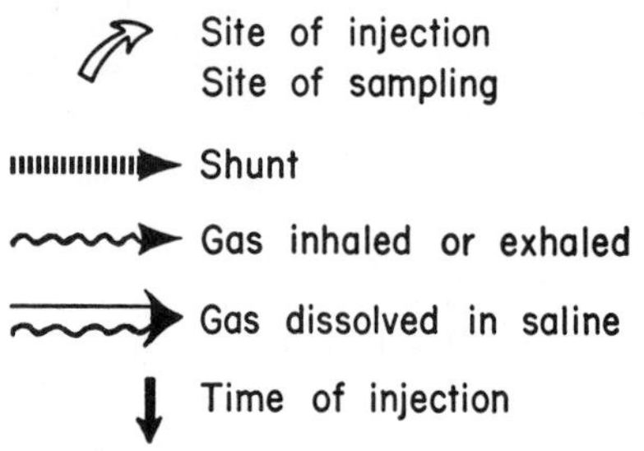

trapolation of that line to zero (or nearly zero, since the zero point is approached asymptotically) separates the area under the curve due to the first circulation of the indicator from the area due to recirculation.

The cardiac output is determined from the Stewart-Hamilton Formula:

$$F = \frac{60\ I}{CT}$$

where F = cardiac output in liters per minute, I = amount of dye injected expressed in milligrams, 60 = number of seconds per minute, C = mean concentration of dye in milligrams per liter, and T = time in seconds from the first appearance of the dye to the theoretic disappearance.

The contour of the normal dye dilution curve is modified by (1) increased central blood volume (Fig. 24b); (2) right-to-left shunts (Fig. 25); (3) left-to-right shunts (Fig. 26a); and (4) valvular insufficiency (Fig. 27).

Localization of Left-to-Right Shunts. The indicator dilution method can be utilized to locate left-to-right shunts. This is accomplished by several techniques:

1. Injection of dye in the left atrium, left ventricle, or aorta and sampling from a peripheral artery (Fig. 26b and c).

2. Injection of dye into the left atrium, left ventricle, or aorta and sampling from the right atrium, right ventricle, or pulmonary artery (Fig. 28).

3. Peripheral venous injection of dye with sampling from the right atrium or ventricle (Fig. 29).

4. Injection of dye into a branch of the main pulmonary artery and sampling from the right atrium, right ventricle, or main pulmonary artery (Fig. 30).

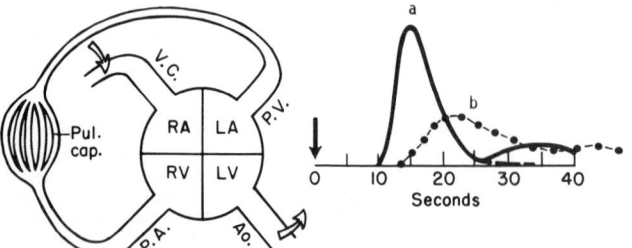

Figure 23. Symbols used in Figures 24 to 35.

(Site of injection / Site of sampling / Shunt / Gas inhaled or exhaled / Gas dissolved in saline / Time of injection)

Figure 24. The altered dye curve produced by dilution of the dye by an increased central blood volume (b). The appearance time is delayed, the peak concentration is reduced, and the disappearance time is prolonged when compared to a normal dye dilution curve (a).

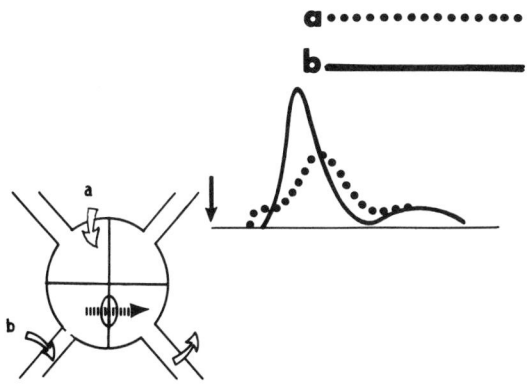

Figure 25. a, Ventricular septal defect with a right-to-left shunt. Diagrammatic representation of the dye curve showing the early appearance time of the shunted dye, which modifies the upslope of the curve. This modified upslope is produced by the portion of the dye that circulates through the abnormal pathway. b, When dye is injected downstream from the right-to-left shunt, a normal curve is produced.

Other Methods for the Diagnosis and Localization of Shunts

Included among the substances that may be used as indicators for the detection of shunts are nitrous oxide, hydrogen, sodium ascorbate, krypton-85, and iodine-131-tagged albumin. Except for ^{131}I-tagged albumin, most of these substances are not true indicators, such as tricarbocyanine (Cardio-Green), since they diffuse freely into the extracellular and often the intracellular spaces. Also, the gaseous substances are exhaled by the lung.

The Nitrous Oxide Technique. This test is based on the fact that during the first minute of inhalation of

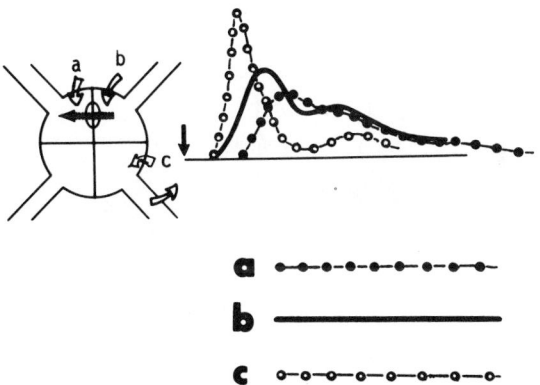

Figure 26. Atrial septal defect with a left-to-right shunt: a, The downslope of the dye curve is altered by the recirculation through the lungs of left-to-right shunted dye. The appearance time is normal and the peak concentration of the dye is decreased. b, Injected proximal to or at the site of the left-to-right shunt causes an altered downslope. The appearance time is early and the peak concentration of dye is decreased. c, Injection of dye downstream from the shunt results in a curve of normal contour with an early appearance time.

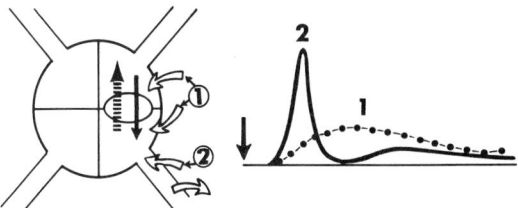

Figure 27. Mitral insufficiency: 1, Dye injected either in the left atrium or left ventricle in the presence of mitral insufficiency is diluted in increasing volumes of blood as the dye is washed back and forth through the incompetent valve. The upslope and downslope of the curve are prolonged, the appearance time is normal, and the peak concentration of dye is decreased. 2, Injection of dye at the root of the aorta results in a normal curve.

nitrous oxide, the arteriovenous difference is relatively large owing to the avid tissue uptake of the gas. The patient breathes a mixture of 50 per cent nitrous oxide with 21 per cent oxygen for a period of 30 seconds; integrated simultaneous samples are drawn from a peripheral artery and from the pulmonary artery, the right ventricle, or the right atrium. The nitrous oxide content of the blood is analyzed in a Van Slyke manometric apparatus, and an arbitrary ratio between the nitrous oxide content of the right heart blood and that of the arterial blood is determined. A value of 15 per cent or less demonstrates the absence of a shunt, while a value over 20 per cent is diagnostic of a left-to-right shunt. The tests may be repeated several times during a catheterization to permit selective sampling. The relative flow of the shunt may be quantified (Fig. 31).

The quantification, as given, also applies to the use of ^{85}Kr to be described for left-to-right shunts. The chief advantages of the nitrous oxide test are simplicity and accuracy in localizing the site of the shunt. The chief disadvantage is that the results of the tests are not immediately available to the operator because of time-consuming analysis.

The Use of Radioactive Krypton. Krypton-85 also may be used for the detection of shunts. It can be inhaled (Fig. 32) or dissolved in saline and injected into the

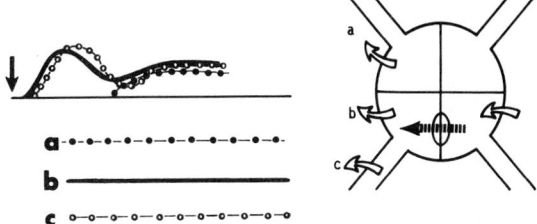

Figure 28. Ventricular septal defect with left-to-right shunt: Injection of dye into the left ventricle results in early appearance of dye in the right ventricle (b) and in the pulmonary artery (c) but not in the right atrium (a). The shunt is thus located at the ventricular level.

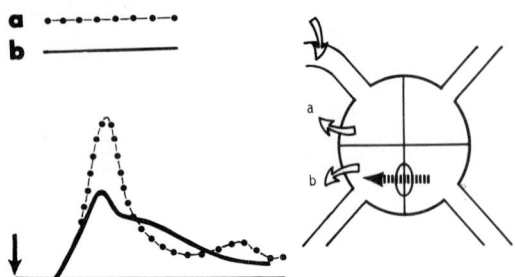

Figure 29. Ventricular septal defect with left-to-right shunt: Peripheral venous injection of dye with sample upstream from (a) or at the site of a left-to-right shunt localizes the shunt to the chamber in which an altered downslope first appears (b).

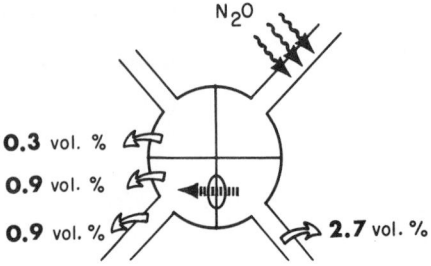

Figure 31. Ventricular septal defect with left-to-right shunt: When nitrous oxide is inhaled, there is normally a wide arteriovenous difference in the first half minute. $\frac{N_2O_{RA}}{N_2O_A} \times 100 = \frac{0.3}{2.7} = 11\%$ (less than 15%: shunt at the atrial level). However, $\frac{N_2O_{RV}}{N_2O_A} \times 100 = \frac{0.9}{2.7} \times 100 = 33\%$ (greater than 20%: left-to-right shunt at the ventricular level). The ratio of pulmonary to systemic flow =

$$\frac{100\% - 11\%}{100\% - \frac{N_2O_{RV}}{N_2O_A}} \times 100 = \frac{89}{67} = 1.33.$$

left or right circulation (Figs. 33 and 34). These tests are technically simple, and the results are immediately available. They are more sensitive in the detection of small left-to-right shunts than in the analysis of the oxygen content of blood, and they can be used in locating the site of entry of a shunt.

The Hydrogen Ion Electrode. The presence of dissolved hydrogen in the blood changes the potential difference between a platinized electrode in the blood and a silver reference electrode placed on the skin with suitable contact. The electrodes are connected directly to the D.C. input of a recording amplifier. One silver reference electrode may be used with several platinum electrodes.

For the detection of left-to-right shunts, the patient is given a breath of hydrogen, the timing of the breath being recorded from a platinum electrode at the tip of a nasal catheter. A left-to-right shunt results in an early deflection recorded by a suitably placed right heart electrode (Fig. 35). For the detection of right-to-left shunts, an arterial electrode is used. Hydrogen, dissolved in saline by being bubbled through the solution, is injected into a peripheral vein. Since the hydrogen is exhaled almost completely by the lungs during its first circulation, the appearance of a deflection on the left side of the circulation indicates a right-to-left shunt. Blood sampling is not necessary,

and multiple simultaneous recording from different sites can be obtained easily. However, hydrogen is an explosive gas; furthermore, quantification of shunts has not yet been achieved.

Sodium ascorbate also produces a potential in the presence of a platinum electrode and is used to test the electrode in situ before hydrogen is administered. Thus, sodium ascorbate is of value in the detection of shunts without blood sampling.

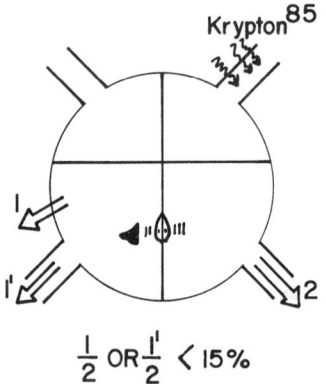

Figure 32. Localization of ventricular septal defect with left-to-right shunt with krypton-85. Inhaled [85]Kr appears rapidly in the left cardiac chambers. It diffuses freely in the interstitial and cellular compartments, and so its concentration in venous blood returning to the heart is low. Thus, in the presence of a left-to-right shunt at the ventricular level there will be an increase in the concentration of [85]Kr in the right ventricle and the pulmonary artery. As a result, the ratio of the concentration of the gas in the right heart to systemic arterial blood is increased. Normally, this ratio is less than 15 per cent. (From Robin, E., et al. *In* Sabiston, D. C., Jr., and Spencer, F. C. (Eds.): Gibbon's Surgery of the Chest, 3rd ed. Philadelphia, W. B. Saunders Company, 1976.)

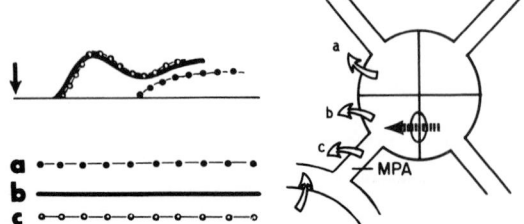

Figure 30. Ventricular septal defect with left-to-right shunt: Dye injected into a distal branch of the main pulmonary artery appears early in the right ventricle (b) and in the main pulmonary artery (c) and late in the right atrium (a).

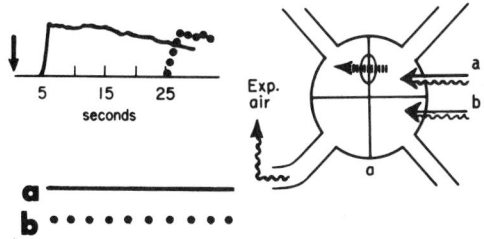

Figure 33. Atrial septal defect with left-to-right shunt: A rapid appearance time of ^{85}Kr in the expired air after a solution of the gas is injected into the left atrium indicates the presence of a left-to-right shunt at the atrial level (a). If the solution of gas is injected into the left ventricle, the appearance time will be delayed (b).

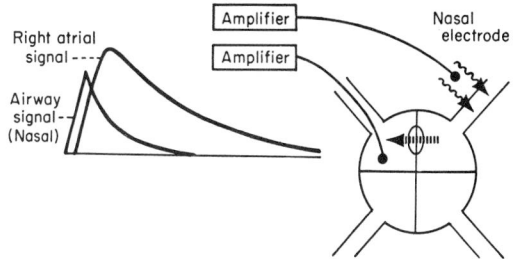

Figure 35. Atrial septal defect with a left-to-right shunt with hydrogen: The early appearance in the right atrium of a change in potential caused by inhaled hydrogen indicates the presence of an interatrial septal defect with a left-to-right shunt. The inhalation of hydrogen is timed by an electrode placed in the nose as shown in the diagram. (From Robin, E., et al. *In* Sabiston, D. C., Jr., and Spencer, F. C. (Eds.): Gibbon's Surgery of the Chest, 3rd ed. Philadelphia, W. B. Saunders Company, 1976.)

MEASUREMENTS OF CARDIAC VOLUMES

There are well-established techniques for determining cardiac volumes. When such measurements are combined with those of pressures and flows, the severity of the mechanical defects in patients with valvular and congenital heart disease and the status of left ventricular myocardial performance can be determined. With advances in cardiac surgery, these quantitative methods have become increasingly important in evaluating patients as candidates for surgery and for assessing the physiologic effects of surgery.

Cardiac output can be measured by the thermodilution technique. The indicator may be warmer or colder than circulating blood, but usually cold saline or blood is injected. The detector is a thermistor-tipped catheter. Repeated measurements may be made without withdrawal of blood. The catheter is placed beyond the aortic or pulmonic valve. A bolus of ice-cold blood or saline is injected via a second catheter into the ventricle. The thermistor temperature drops and then progressively rises as the cold solution is washed out of the ventricle. Recirculation is negligible. Cardiac output may be calculated by the Stewart-Hamilton method (Fig. 36).

The thermodilution technique yields the ventricular

end-diastolic volume for a single cardiac cycle. In vitro studies show good correlation between calculated and directly measured volumes if the pulse is less than 100 beats per min. and the end-diastolic volume is less than 300 ml.

Other indicators such as dye or isotopes may be used for the measurement of ventricular volume. The optical density associated with the washout of opaque media from the ventricle may be quantified by analysis of the cineangiocardiogram. A fiberoptic catheter system with a 95 per cent response in 0.1 second allows measurements of cardiac output and ventricular volume with indocyanine green as the indicator. The volume of one or both ventricles may be derived from washout curves obtained by precordial counting of the passage of a radioactive gamma-emitting tracer through the heart and the lungs.

Left ventricular volumes have been measured by angiocardiography. The left ventricle is treated as an ellipsoid, and its end-systolic and end-diastolic surface areas are measured on the film, with correction for magnification. Single-plane angiocardiography has also been used. Right ventricular volume is not directly determinable by radiologic techniques because of the shape of the right ventricle. By the washout methods the ejection fraction of the left ventricle is 0.3 to 0.4 and by radiologic techniques the ejection fraction is 0.5 to 0.7. Although incomplete mixing tends to cause overestimation of the ventricular end-diastolic volume, the dilution technique avoids the hemodynamic effects of opaque media and provides a rapid assessment of relative changes in right and left ventricular volumes during selected interventions. The stroke volume obtained by radiologic methods agrees well with indicator-dilution and Fick principle determinations.

The opacified left atrium is also represented as an ellipsoid so that left atrial volume can be calculated. By this method, regurgitant left atrial flow has been noted to equal or surpass effective left ventricular stroke volume.

Some of the parameters obtained from the measurements of left ventricular volumes are summarized in Table 4.

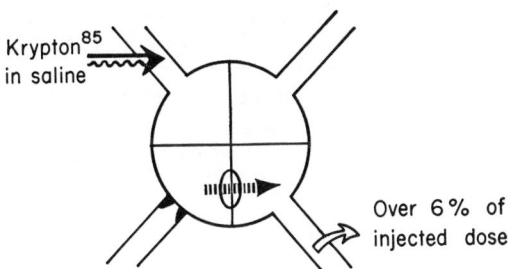

Figure 34. Ventricular septal defect with right-to-left shunt with ^{85}Kr: Since 95 per cent of the ^{85}Kr injected into the venous side of the circulation is excreted by the lungs during its first passage through the pulmonary circulation, the finding of a significant amount of radioactivity in the blood sampled from a peripheral artery indicates a right-to-left shunt. (From Robin, E., et al. *In* Sabiston, D. C., Jr., and Spencer, F. C. (Eds.): Gibbon's Surgery of the Chest, 3rd ed. Philadelphia, W. B. Saunders Company, 1976.)

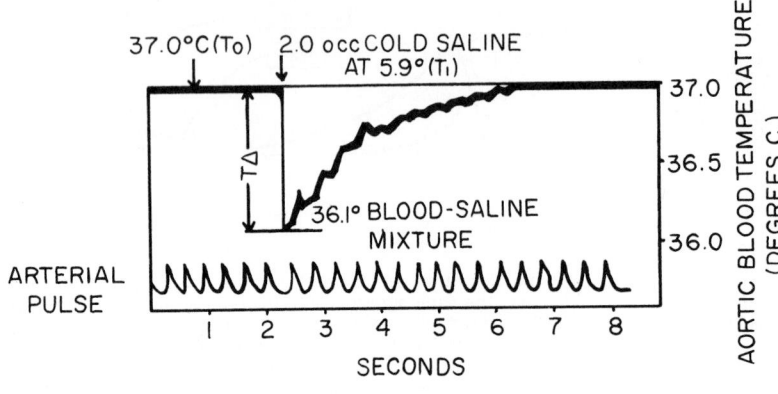

Figure 36. End-diastolic volume (EDV) of the left ventricle by thermodilution. The curve was recorded from the aorta following the injection of cold normal saline solution into the left ventricle during diastole.

$$EDV = \frac{\text{Amount of cold shared by the injectate and blood}}{\Delta T \text{ (change in the temperature of aortic blood during the first systole following injection)}}$$

$$EDV = \frac{(37.0° - 5.9°) \times 2.0 \text{ cc.}}{(37.0° - 36.1°)} = 69.0 \text{ cc.}$$

(From Robin, E., et al. *In* Sabiston, D. C., Jr., and Spencer, F. C. (Eds.): Gibbon's Surgery of the Chest, 3rd ed. Philadelphia, W. B. Saunders Company, 1976.)

INTRACARDIAC PHONOCARDIOGRAPHY

The first and second sounds are recorded throughout the heart, but the first sound reaches its maximal intensity in the ventricles and the second sound in the pulmonary artery and aorta. If a third heart sound is present, its greatest intensity is in the ventricles. The fourth heart sound is present in all patients with normal sinus rhythm: it is best recorded from the atria.

In patent ductus arteriosus, the murmur is localized to the pulmonary artery, and in pulmonic stenosis, to the pulmonary artery just downstream from the valve. In ventricular septal defect with a left-to-right shunt, the murmur is recorded in the right ventricle. In atrial septal defects, the systolic murmur is found to arise in the pulmonary artery.

Left-sided sounds and murmurs can be studied by retrograde or by transseptal left heart techniques.

The murmur of aortic stenosis originates at the level of the valve and travels distally, diminishing in intensity as the catheter is passed into the left ventricle. In aortic insufficiency, the murmur appears in the left ventricular cavity and radiates toward the apex.

The murmur of mitral stenosis is best recorded in the inflow tract of the left ventricle, and that of mitral insufficiency in the left atrium.

TABLE 4.   Values Obtained from Measurements of Left Ventricular Volumes

Parameter	Formula	Normal Values
End-diastolic volume (EDV)		70-85 ml./m.²
End-systolic volume (ESV)		25-30 ml./m.²
Stroke volume (SV)	EDV − ESV	45-55 ml./m.²
Ejection fraction (EF)	$\dfrac{EDV - ESV}{EDV}$	0.65-0.75
Stroke work (SW)	SV × Asm*	50-80 gm.-M./m.²
Function index	$\dfrac{SW}{EDV}$	1.0 gm.-M./ml.
Effective stroke volume (SVe)		45-55 ml./m.²
Regurgitant volume (Vr)	SV − SVe	0 ml.
Regurgitant fraction	$\dfrac{Vr}{SV}$	0 ml.

*Asm (mm. Hg) = mean aortic systolic pressure.

INTRACARDIAC ELECTROCARDIOGRAPHY

Intracardiac electrocardiography is the study of electrical potentials as obtained from the endocardial surface of the heart. During the performance of cardiac catheterization, a small electrode attached to the catheter serves as the exploring electrode.

Intracardiac electrocardiography has been useful for the following reasons: (1) better understanding of the genesis of the electrocardiogram; (2) precise location of the various cardiac chambers and vessels in complicated malformations; this is accomplished by the anal-

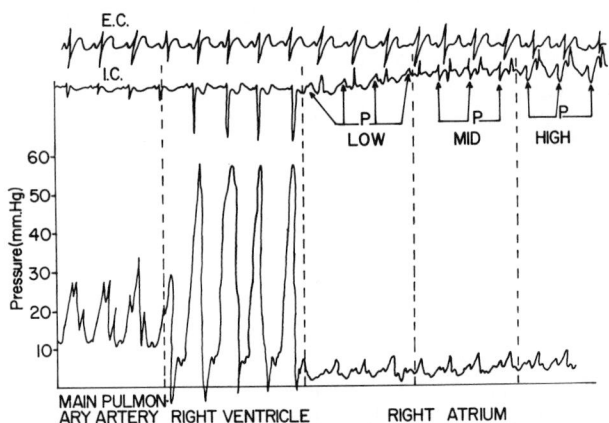

Figure 37. Intracardiac electrocardiography: Tracings from pulmonary artery to right atrium obtained from a patient with pulmonic valvular stenosis. E.C. = external electrocardiogram; I.C. = intracardiac electrocardiogram. The superior vena cava and atrial electrocardiograms consist of relatively large P waves, generally inverted in the superior vena cava and high in the right atrium, diphasic in midatrium, and positive in the lower portion of the atrium. In contrast to the large P waves, the QRS voltage within the superior vena cava and right atrium is small. The ventricular electrocardiogram demonstrates isoelectric or relatively small P waves, while the QRS complex is large. The electrocardiogram recorded from the pulmonary artery resembles the atrial electrocardiogram in that the QRS voltage is small, but differs in that the P waves are of similar magnitude to those observed within the ventricle. (From Robin, E., et al. *In* Sabiston, D. C., Jr., and Spencer, F. C. (Eds.): Gibbon's Surgery of the Chest, 3rd ed. Philadelphia, W. B. Saunders Company, 1976.)

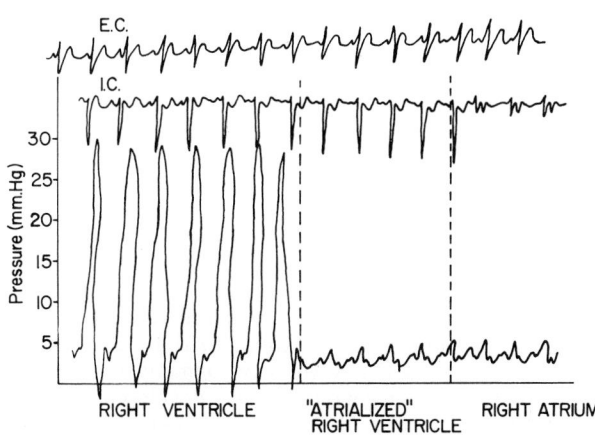

Figure 38. Intracardiac electrocardiography: Tracings obtained during pullback from right ventricle to right atrium in a patient with Ebstein's anomaly. E.C. = external electrocardiogram. There is a change from right ventricular to atrial pressure, but the intracardiac electrocardiogram (I.C.) maintains its right ventricular morphology. (From Robin, E., et al. *In* Sabiston, D. C., Jr., and Spencer, F. C. (Eds.) Gibbon's Surgery of the Chest, 3rd ed. Philadelphia, W. B. Saunders Company, 1976.)

ysis of the shape and voltage of the P waves and QRS complexes as recorded in the cardiac chambers and vessels (Fig. 37); (3) diagnosis of Ebstein's anomaly; this is accomplished by recording simultaneously intracavitary pressures and electrocardiographic patterns proximal to the tricuspid valve (Fig. 38); and (4) improved definition of atrial activity in cases of arrhythmias.

BUNDLE OF HIS ELECTROCARDIOGRAPHY

Bundle of His electrocardiography (BHE) is a useful procedure in the evaluation of arrhythmias and conduction disorders. The technique consists of passing a bipolar electrode catheter through a femoral vein or through an antecubital vein to the right atrium. The tip of the catheter lies in close proximity to the tricuspid valve. The signals from the catheter are then amplified, filtered, and recorded. Multiple surface

EKG leads should be simultaneously recorded with the BHE. The procedure is simple and safe, the morbidity being that of right heart catheterization.

The relationship of the BHE to the conduction system of the heart and to the surface EKG is shown in Figure 39.

Analysis of the BHE reveals three distinct spikes. The first spike (A) is a local bipolar electrogram recorded from the low right atrium close to the atrial septum. The second spike (H) reflects His bundle depolarization. The third spike (V) represents ventricular depolarization.

Recording of the BHE enables the breakdown of the PR interval into three components: (1) The P-A interval is an approximation of intra-atrial conduction time and is measured from the onset of the P wave on the surface EKG to the first deflection of the "A" spike on the BHE. (2) The A-H interval represents the conduction time through the A-V node. This is measured from the first high-frequency deflection of the "H"

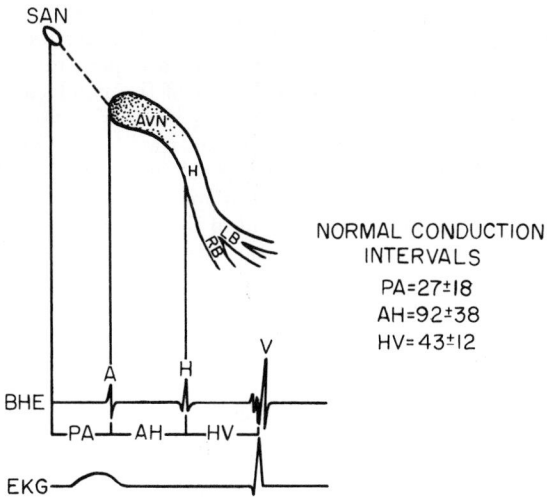

Figure 39. Diagram showing the relationship of the conduction system of the heart and the surface electrocardiogram (EKG) to the bundle of His electrogram (BHE). SAN = sinoatrial node; AVN = atrioventricular node; H= bundle of His; RB = right bundle; LB = left bundle. (Intervals from Rosen, K. M.: Catheter recording of His bundle electrograms. Mod. Concepts Cardiovasc. Dis., *42*:23, 1973.)

NORMAL CONDUCTION INTERVALS

PA=27±18
AH=92±38
HV=43±12

spike. (3) The H-V interval represents the conduction time through the His-Purkinje system and is measured from the onset of the "H" spike to the earliest appearance of ventricular activation recorded on either the BHE ("V" spike) or any of the multiple surface EKG leads. Normal conduction time values are shown in Figure 39.

Stressing the conduction system with atrial pacing may demonstrate conduction disorders not apparent during sinus rhythm. During rapid atrial pacing the normal response is an increase in A-H while H-V remains constant. At a critical paced rate, Wenckebach periods are noted proximal to the His Bundle. The increase in A-H and the development of Wenckebach periods are physiologic. The development of a block distal to the "H" spike (absent "V" spike) suggests disease in the His-Purkinje system.

In patients with first-degree atrioventricular block and narrow QRS, the conduction delay (generally atrionodal) results in a prolongation of A-H. In patients with bundle branch block, H-V may be prolonged enough to reflect itself as a first-degree atrioventricular block. In these cases, H-V prolongation reflects conduction delay in the functioning bundle branch and is a manifestation of bilateral bundle branch disease.

In patients with second- and third-degree block, three sites of block may be delineated. The block may be proximal to the His bundle, in which P waves are not followed by conducted "H" spikes. (2) The block may be in the His bundle. Two "H" spikes can be recorded, one proximal to ("H_1") and the other distal to ("H_2") the area of the block. (3) The block may be distal to the His bundle, in which P waves are conducted to the His bundle but "H" spikes are not followed by conducted QRS complexes (absent "V" spikes). This is also a form of bilateral bundle branch block.

Second-degree atrioventricular block can be divided into two types. (1) Type I block (Mobitz I, Wenckebach phenomenon) is characterized by prolongation of conduction intervals prior to the dropped beat. This occurs most commonly in the A-V node. (2) Type II block (Mobitz II) is characterized by fixed conduction intervals prior to the dropped beat. This usually reflects bilateral bundle branch disease.

In acute inferior wall myocardial infarction, complete atrioventricular block is usually proximal to the His bundle, reflecting occlusion of the right coronary artery proximal to the origin of the A-V node artery. In acute anteroseptal infarction, the block is distal to the His Bundle, reflecting septal injury and bilateral bundle branch block. In complete congenital heart block, the block is proximal to the His bundle, reflecting disruption of conduction tissue in the A-V junction.

Symptoms of dizziness, confusion, and syncope may accompany atrioventricular block at any site. However, they are more common in patients with a block distal to the His bundle. Patients with markedly prolonged H-V interval and without any manifest symptoms of block should be followed closely for the development of atrioventricular block. It should be emphasized that the decision for pacemaker implantation is based primarily on clinical symptoms.

CALCULATION OF VALVE AREAS

In order to calculate the surface area of the valves, the following general equation is used:

$$A = \frac{F}{C \times 44.5 \sqrt{P_1 - P_2}}$$

where A (cm.^{2})   = orifice area
F (ml./sec.)   = flow through orifice
44.5   = constant related to gravity acceleration
$P_1 - P_2$ (mm. Hg) = pressure gradient across the orifice
P_1 = pressure proximal to orifice
P_2 = pressure distal to orifice

Mitral Valve Area

With the foregoing formula, the mitral valve area can be calculated as follows:

$$MVA = \frac{MVF = \dfrac{CO}{DFP}}{31 \sqrt{LAm - LVmd}}$$

where MVA (cm.^{2})   = mitral valve area
MVF (ml./sec.)   = mitral valve flow
CO (ml./min.)   = cardiac output
DFP (sec./min.)   = diastolic filling time
LAm (mm. Hg)   = left atrial mean pressure
LVmd (mm. Hg) = left ventricular mean diastolic pressure (This may be assumed to be 5 mm. Hg in most cases.)

Although in the majority of cases there is a good correlation between the calculated and the actually measured surface area of the mitral valve, the following factors may introduce errors in the calculations: (1) the presence of mitral insufficiency; (2) small pressure gradients across the mitral valve; (3) left ventricular failure; and (4) changes in flow and in pressure gradients between measurements.

The average effective surface area of the normal mitral valve is about 4 to 5 cm.^{2} The surface area of the mitral valve can be narrowed down to 2.5 cm.^{2} without the presence of significant symptoms. Between 2.5 cm.^{2} and 2.0 cm.^{2}, the narrowing produces symptoms on severe exertion only. Between 2.0 cm.^{2} and 1.5 cm.^{2}, symptoms are present with moderate exertion. Below 1.5 cm.^{2}, minimal exercise may provoke severe symptoms.

Aortic Valve Area

The formula used to calculate the effective aortic valve surface area is:

$$AVA = \frac{AVF = \dfrac{CO}{SEP}}{C \times 44.5 \sqrt{LVsm - Asm}}$$

where AVA (cm.^{2})   = aortic valve area
AVF (ml./sec.)   = aortic valve flow
CO (ml./min.)   = cardiac output
SEP (sec./min.)   = systolic ejection period

$$\frac{\text{Resistance}}{(\text{dynes-sec./cm.}^5)} = \frac{\text{pressure gradient (mm. Hg)} \times 1332 \text{ dynes/cm.}^2}{\text{blood flow (cm.}^3\text{/sec.)}}$$

C   = empirical constant = 1.0
44.5   = gravity acceleration factor
LVsm (mm. Hg)   = left ventricular mean systolic pressure
Asm (mm. Hg)   = aortic mean systolic pressure

Calculations of the aortic valve surface area are not accurate in the presence of aortic insufficiency. The normal effective surface area of the aortic valve is about 3 to 4 cm.^{2} Usually the symptoms of angina and syncope do not appear until the aortic valve area measures between 0.5 and 0.7 cm.^{2}

CALCULATION OF RESISTANCE

Vascular resistance can be defined as an impedance to blood flow. This can be translated in a simplified form of Poiseuille's equation:

$$\text{Resistance (R)} = \frac{\text{pressure gradient}}{\text{flow}}$$

The result can be expressed in simple units (R). However, one can express resistance in fundamental units of force as follows (see equation at top of page).

Each unit of resistance (R) can be converted into dynes-sec./cm.^{5} by multiplying by 80.* In order to compare data obtained from infants, children, and adults resistance should be related to flow index (liters/min./m.^{2}). Thus, the formula for systemic resistance is as follows:

$$\text{SVR} = \frac{\text{Aom} - \text{RAm} \times 80}{\text{SBF}}$$

where SVR (dynes-sec./cm.^{5}) = systemic vascular resistance
Aom (mm. Hg)   = mean aortic pressure
RAm (mm. Hg)   = mean right atrial pressure
SBF (liters/min. or liters/min./m^2) = systemic blood flow

Pulmonary vascular resistance can be calculated as follows:

$$\text{PVR} = \frac{\text{PAm} - \text{LAm} \times 80}{\text{PBF}}$$

where PVR (dynes-sec./cm.^{5}) = pulmonary vascular resistance
PAm (mm. Hg)   = mean pulmonary artery pressure

LAmm (mm. Hg)   = mean left atrial pressure
PBF (liters/min. or liters/min./m.^{2}) = pulmonary blood flow

The normal values for pulmonary vascular resistance are one to three units (80 to 240 dynes-sec./cm.^{5}).

As described previously (see Pulmonary Artery Pressure. p. 2178), pulmonary hypertension can be classified in hyperkinetic and obstructive types. In the hyperkinetic type, the pulmonary artery pressure may be high in spite of a normal and fixed pulmonary arterial resistance. In contrast, in the obstructive type, the pulmonary arterial resistance is usually elevated.

MYOCARDIAL WALL TENSION AND MYOCARDIAL OXYGEN CONSUMPTION

Five determinants of myocardial oxygen consumption (MVO$_2$) have been recognized. They are (1) myocardial tension development, (2) myocardial contractility, (3) pressure-volume work and kinetic energy, (4) basal myocardial metabolism, and (5) myocardial activation. The first two factors are by far the most important ones.

The importance of myocardial wall tension in determining MVO$_2$ was first suggested by Rohde. Shortly thereafter, Evans and Matsuoka concluded from studies on the Starling heart-lung preparation that an increase in cardiac work resulting from an elevation of arterial pressure augmented MVO$_2$ to a much greater degree than a similar increment in work resulting from an increase in stroke volume. The relation of MVO$_2$ to derivatives of developed tension was also explored by using such parameters as the tension-time index (TTI) and the index of cardiac effort.

$$\text{TTI} = \text{Asm} \times \text{SEP}$$

where TTI (mm. Hg-sec./min.) = tension-time index
Asm (mm. Hg)   = mean systolic aortic pressure
SEP* (sec./min.)   = systolic ejection time

Index of cardiac effort = heart rate (beats/min.) × mean aortic pressure (mm. Hg).

Despite the good correlations between MVO$_2$ and these parameters, it was recognized that according to the law of LaPlace, the myocardial wall tension needed to produce a given ventricular pressure was increased as the volume of the ventricle enlarged.

---

*$\dfrac{1332 \text{ dynes/cm.}^2 \times 60 \text{ sec.}}{1000 \text{ cm.}^3}$

---

*SEP systolic ejection period (sec./beat) × heart rate (beats/min.).

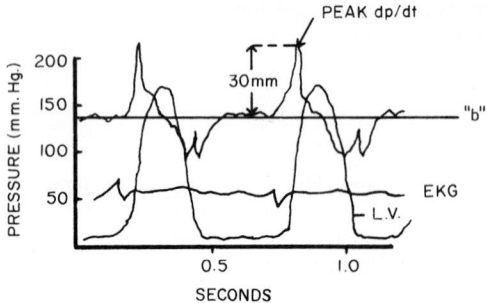

Figure 40. Peak dp/dt of left ventricular pressure. The left ventricular pressure curve (L.V.) and its dp/dt curve are recorded simultaneously. Height of the peak dp/dt curve = 30 mm. Calibration factor = 54 mm. Hg per sec. of deflection of dp/dt for the differentiator used in this case. Peak dp/dt = 30 × 54 = 1620 mm. Hg per sec. (From Robin, E., et al. In Sabiston, D. C., Jr., and Spencer, F. C. (Eds.): Gibbon's Surgery of the Chest, 3rd ed. Philadelphia, W. B. Saunders Company, 1976.)

Thus,

$$T = \frac{Pr}{2h}$$

where P = pressure
      T = intramyocardial tension
      r = radius of ventricular chamber
      h = ventricular thickness

More recent studies have confirmed that tension rather than developed pressure is the more definitive determinant of myocardial oxygen consumption.

FIRST TIME DERIVATIVE OF THE VENTRICULAR PRESSURE (dp/dt)

The first time derivative of the ventricular pressure is the rate of change of pressure with respect to time and is usually expressed as dp/dt. Its maximum value, achieved during early ventricular systole, is designated as peak dp/dt (Fig. 40).

The first requirement for an accurate measurement of the peak dp/dt is the faithful recording of the ventricular pressure through a catheter-tipped micromanometer. A conventional catheter connected to an external transducer is generally unsatisfactory unless the natural frequency response of the system equals or exceeds 30 cycles per second. The dp/dt curve is generated by coupling a differentiator to a pressure source.

Peak dp/dt of the left ventricle is greater than that of the right ventricle in normal subjects. In Gleason and Braunwald's series, left ventricular peak dp/dt ranged between 841 and 1696 mm. Hg per sec. Right ventricular peak dp/dt ranged between 223 and 296 mm. Hg per sec.

The peak dp/dt has been used in the assessment of myocardial function because of its increase following inotropic intervention and its diminution associated with depressed myocardial contractility. However, augmented preload (elevated end-diastolic volume and pressure) and afterload (increased aortic diastolic pressure) both increase peak dp/dt. Tachycardia is also associated with an increase in peak dp/dt. Thus, several parameters have been derived from dp/dt in order to eliminate the effects of the preload and afterload.

ANGIOCARDIOGRAPHY

Contrast Materials

The most commonly used preparations are sodium and methylglucamine diatrizoate (Hypaque 75 per cent or 90 per cent, Renovist 69 per cent, Renografin 60 and 76 per cent), sodium acetrizoate (Urokon 70 per cent), sodium iothalamate (Angio-Conray 80 per cent), iodopyracet (Diodrast 70 per cent), and sodium iodomethamate (Neo-Iopax 75 per cent).

Because of their hypertonicity (greater than 1500 mOsm./liter), injection of large quantities of contrast medium has been shown to cause a temporary increase in cardiac output, blood volume, and left ventricular end-diastolic and pulmonary artery pressures. In addition, an increase in heart rate and a decrease in systemic arterial pressure have been observed. In normal patients and in patients with mitral valve disease, there is a rise in left atrial pressure, the increase being more marked in the latter group.

All iodinated contrast substances are capable of producing reactions. A previous allergic history or pre-existing cerebral and renal disease should prompt careful evaluation of the indications to perform angiocardiography. Reactions are also related to the quantity, concentration, and duration of action of the material used. Because of systemic arterial vasodilation, a feeling of heat and a flushing of the skin are almost universal. Osmotic red cell agglutination can occur in cyanotic children.

Electrocardiographic changes are frequently noted. They may consist of premature atrial, nodal, and ventricular systoles. Occasionally these arrhythmias may persist for a long period of time. T waves may become flat or even inverted. The occurrence of arrhythmias may lead to temporary mitral insufficiency. A diagnosis of true mitral insufficiency is justified only if the contrast material appears in the left atrium in the absence of bradycardia or ventricular arrhythmias. The same reservations also must be made in the case of aortic insufficiency.

Selective Angiocardiography

Until 1947 peripheral intravenous angiocardiography was the most commonly used method. This technique afforded good visualization of the right heart chambers. However, a considerable degree of dilution occurred in the pulmonary vascular bed. As a result, the left cardiac chambers and aorta were ill defined.

The advantages of selective angiocardiography include (1) the injection of small quantities of less diluted radiopaque materials, (2) the injection of a radio-

TABLE 5.   Selective Angiocardiography*

I. Anomalous systemic venous return
- Persistent communication with left superior vena cava ———— Left antecubital vein
- Anomalous drainage of superior vena cava into left atrium ———— Right or left antecubital vein
- Inferior vena cava
  - Absence ———— Right or left saphenous vein
  - Anomalous return to left atrium

II. Atrial septal defect ———— Pulmonary trunk or Left atrium

III. Ventricular septal defect ———— Pulmonary trunk or Left ventricle

IV. Aorticopulmonary shunts
- Patent ductus arteriosus
- Aorticopulmonary window ———— Aorta
- Surgical shunts — Blalock / Pott's

V. Left ventricular outflow tract obstruction
- Infundibular ———— Left ventricle
- Aortic valvular stenosis ———— Left ventricle or aorta
- Aortic supravalvular

VI. Aortic anomalies
- Right – sided arch
- Vascular rings ———— Aorta
- Coarctation of aorta

VII. Coronary artery anomalies
- Coronary arterial venous fistula ———— Aorta
- Anomalous origin of coronary artery from pulmonary artery

VIII. Anomalous pulmonary venous connections
- Total anomalous pulmonary venous return
- Partial anomalous pulmonary venous return ———— Pulmonary arterial trunk
- Pulmonary arteriovenous fistula

IX. Right ventricular outflow tract obstruction
- Infundibular stenosis
- Pulmonary valvular stenosis ———— Right ventricle
- Pulmonary valvular atresia

X. Anatomy of pulmonary vascular bed
- Hypoplasia
- Dilatation
- Unilateral absence ———— Pulmonary arterial trunk or Right ventricular outflow tract
- Pulmonary branch stenosis

XI. Tetralogy of Fallot ———— Right ventricle
Double outlet right ventricle

XII. Complete transposition of great arteries Taussig–Bing anomaly ———— Right ventricle and Left ventricle

XIII. Truncus arteriosus ———— Right ventricle or Aorta

XIV. Ebstein's anomaly ———— Right atrium

XV. Tricuspid atresia ———— Right atrium and Left ventricle

*From Robin, E., et al. *In* Sabiston, D. C., Jr., and Spencer, F. C. (Eds.): Surgery of the Chest, 3rd ed. Philadelphia, W. B. Saunders Company, 1976.

paque medium in the chamber of interest so that surrounding structures do not superimpose each other, and (3) the detection of shunts by a sensitive and precise method.

Delivery of contrast material should be as rapid as possible. This is accomplished by choosing a catheter with a large lumen. Because of the possibility of recoil, the catheter should have a closed end with laterally placed holes. Injection of radiopaque material is performed either by hand or by a power injector, the latter being five times more efficient.

To study anatomic or physiologic changes, films must be taken in rapid sequence. This is made possible by rapid film changers or by image intensifiers with cine-camera attachments. Single or biplane rapid film changers can take from one to four frames per second. These machines use either precut film loaded in a cassette or roll films. This technique provides excellent anatomic details. However, the amount of radiation used is high, and the injection of contrast material cannot be monitored.

Cineangiocardiography permits recording of the passage of contrast medium by means of x-ray motion picture photography. This has been made possible by the development of amplification and intensification fluoroscopy, whereby the ordinary fluoroscopic image is converted into an electron image. The electron image is then reconverted into a light image of much increased brightness, which can be viewed by mirror optics, photographed by a cine-camera, or monitored by television. The signal can also be relayed to a video recorder for immediate replay. This method permits motion pictures from $7^{1}/_{2}$ to 60 frames per second with a 16 or 35 mm. movie camera. Thus, cardiac anatomy, as well as the direction of blood flow, can be studied while keeping the dose of radiation low.

Complications occurring during the course of angiocardiography are related to the radiopaque media and to the pressure generated by the injector. Before pressure injection, the tip of the catheter should be free in the cardiac chamber, away from the myocardial wall. The position of the catheter tip can be ascertained by the injection of small quantities of contrast material under low pressure. Myocardial extravasation of radiopaque medium occurs in about 5 per cent of cases, but the majority of cases are asymptomatic. Occasionally, perforation of the atria or ventricles occurs, resulting in cardiac tamponade. Myocardial infarction and ventricular fibrillation have also been observed. Some of the types of congenital and acquired cardiac anomalies that can be identified by the selective injection of contrast medium are summarized in Tables 4 and 5.

The indications for angiocardiography depend upon the nature of the malformation. The need for it is particularly great in complicated anomalies, since data obtained from cardiac catheterization may be misleading. Anatomic demonstration of a defect by properly obtained selective angiograms is superior or at least complementary to results obtained from catheterization.

With selective angiocardiography, the following can be accomplished: (1) assessment of the position and size of the cardiac chambers in relation to each other and to the great veins and arteries; (2) precise localization of intracardiac and extracardiac defects, including shunts; (3) assessment of the location, anatomy, and motion of the cardiac valves; (4) rough estimation of the degree of valvular insufficiency; and (5) visualization of the coronary vascular tree. Examples of selective angiocardiograms are shown in Figures 41 to 43.

Coronary Arteriography

Until the late 1950s, opacification of the coronary arteries was achieved indirectly by such methods as (1) random injection of contrast material at the root of the ascending aorta; (2) phasic injection of contrast medium at the aortic root during ventricular diastole; (3) injection of contrast material medium at the aortic root during ventricular asystole produced by acetylcholine; (4) temporary occlusion of the ascending aorta by means of a balloon catheter and injection of contrast medium above the aortic valve; and (5) differential opacification of the aortic root by means of a preformed, spiral-shaped catheter.

In 1959, Sones described a technique of *direct, selective* coronary arteriography using the transbrachial approach and a special catheter with a flexible tip (Fig. 44*A*). In 1962, Ricketts and Abrams introduced two catheters with tips formed in a way that facilitates their entrance into either the right or left coronary artery (Figs. 44*B* and *C*). Both catheters are introduced in succession in the aorta with the percutaneous transfemoral approach. In recent years the Ricketts-Abrams method has gained wide recognition following the reports of Judkins.

Indications. Coronary arteriography is indicated (1) in a patient whose symptoms, clinical course, and electrocardiographic changes are so atypical as to raise doubt regarding the diagnosis of coronary arteriosclerosis; (2) in a patient with intractable angina pectoris or heart failure in spite of adequate medical treatment and in whom coronary artery surgery is considered; (3) in the evaluation of coronary artery

TABLE 6.   Selective Angiocardiography*

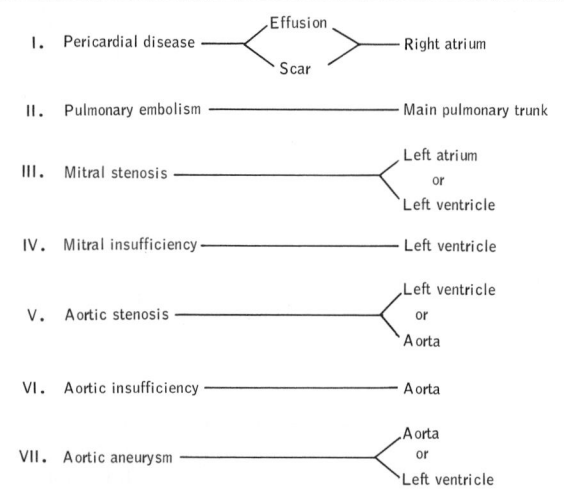

*From Robin, E., et al. *In* Sabiston, D. C., Jr., and Spencer, F. C. (Eds.): Surgery of the Chest, 3rd ed. Philadelphia, W. B. Saunders Company, 1976.

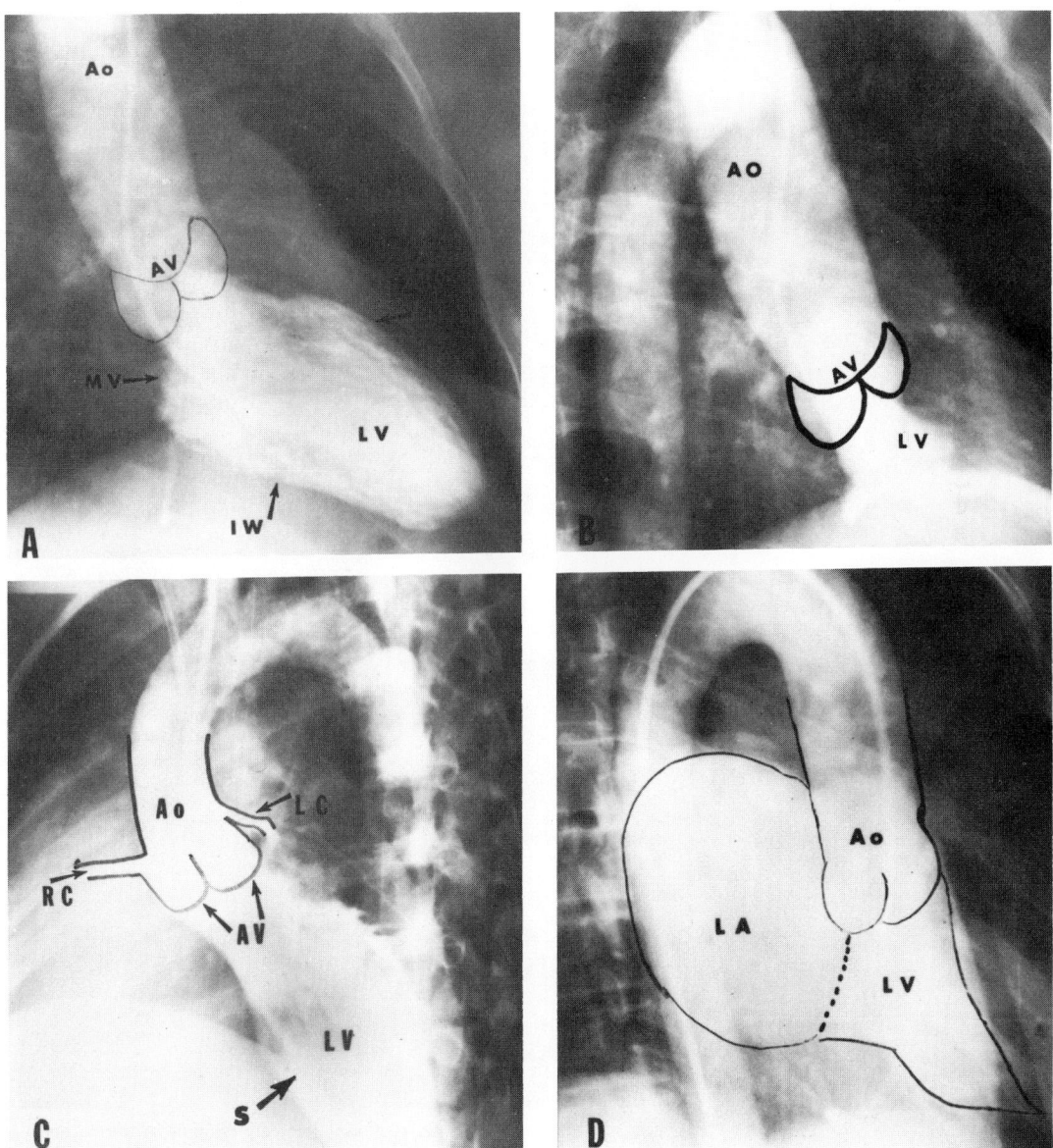

Figure 41. Left ventriculography: *A,* Normal left ventriculogram in diastole (right anterior oblique projection). *B,* Normal left ventriculogram in systole (right anterior oblique projection). *C,* Normal left ventriculogram (left anterior oblique projection). *D,* Left ventriculogram demonstrating mitral insufficiency (right anterior oblique projection). LV = left ventricle; LA = left atrium; Ao = aorta; MV = mitral valve; AV = aortic valve; IW = inferior wall; S = septum; RC = right coronary artery; LC = left coronary artery. (From Robin, E., et al. *In* Sabiston, D. C., Jr., and Spencer, F. C. (Eds.): Gibbon's Surgery of the Chest, 3rd ed. Philadelphia, W. B. Saunders Company, 1976.)

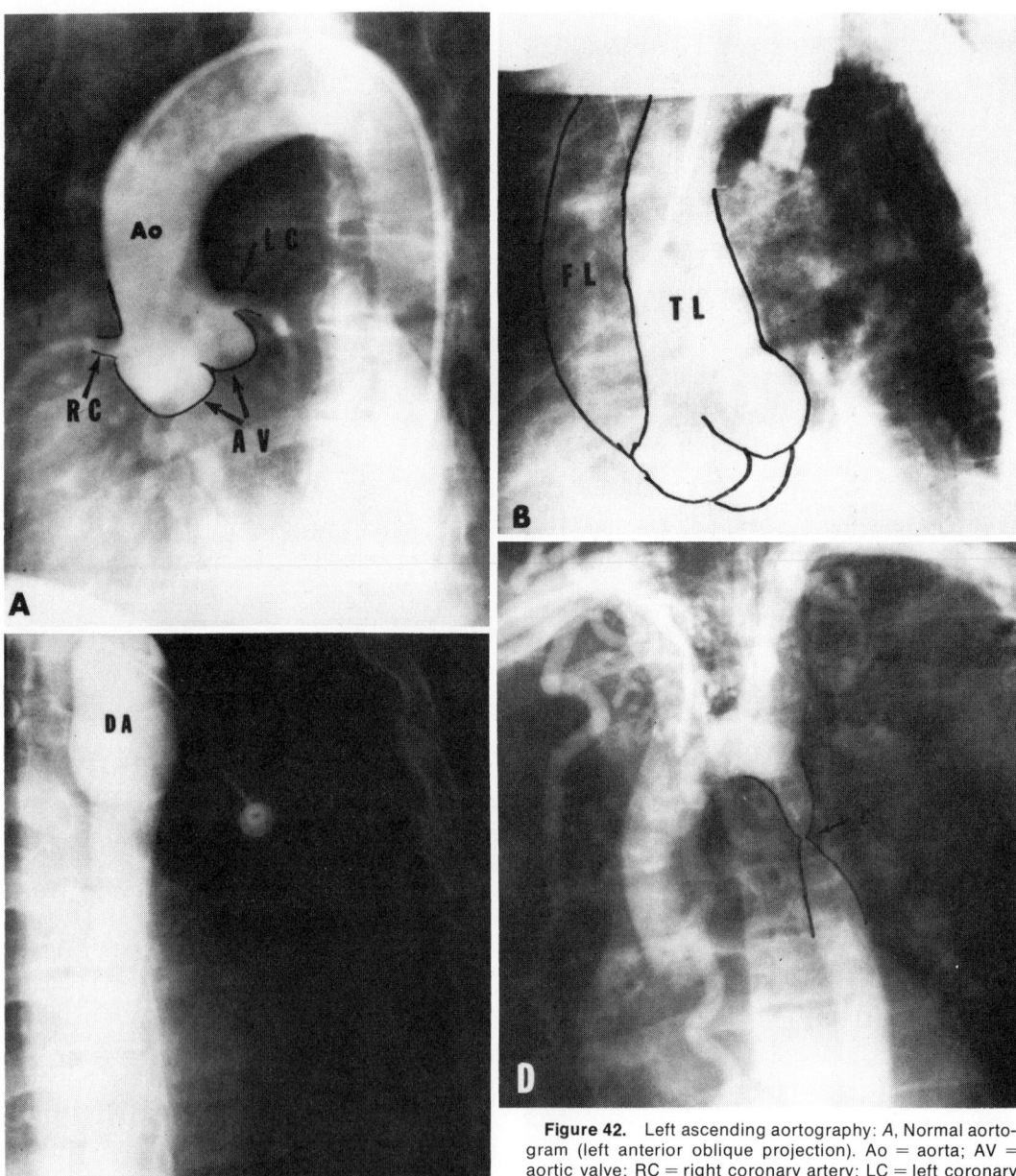

Figure 42. Left ascending aortography: *A*, Normal aortogram (left anterior oblique projection). Ao = aorta; AV = aortic valve; RC = right coronary artery; LC = left coronary artery. *B*, Dissecting aneurysm of ascending aorta. FL = false lumen; TL = true lumen. *C*, Traumatic aneurysm of the descending thoracic aorta (DA). *D*, Adult type of coarctation of the aorta. (From Robin, E., et al. *In* Sabiston, D. C., Jr., and Spencer, F. C. (Eds.): Gibbon's Surgery of the Chest, 3rd ed. Philadelphia, W. B. Saunders Company, 1976.)

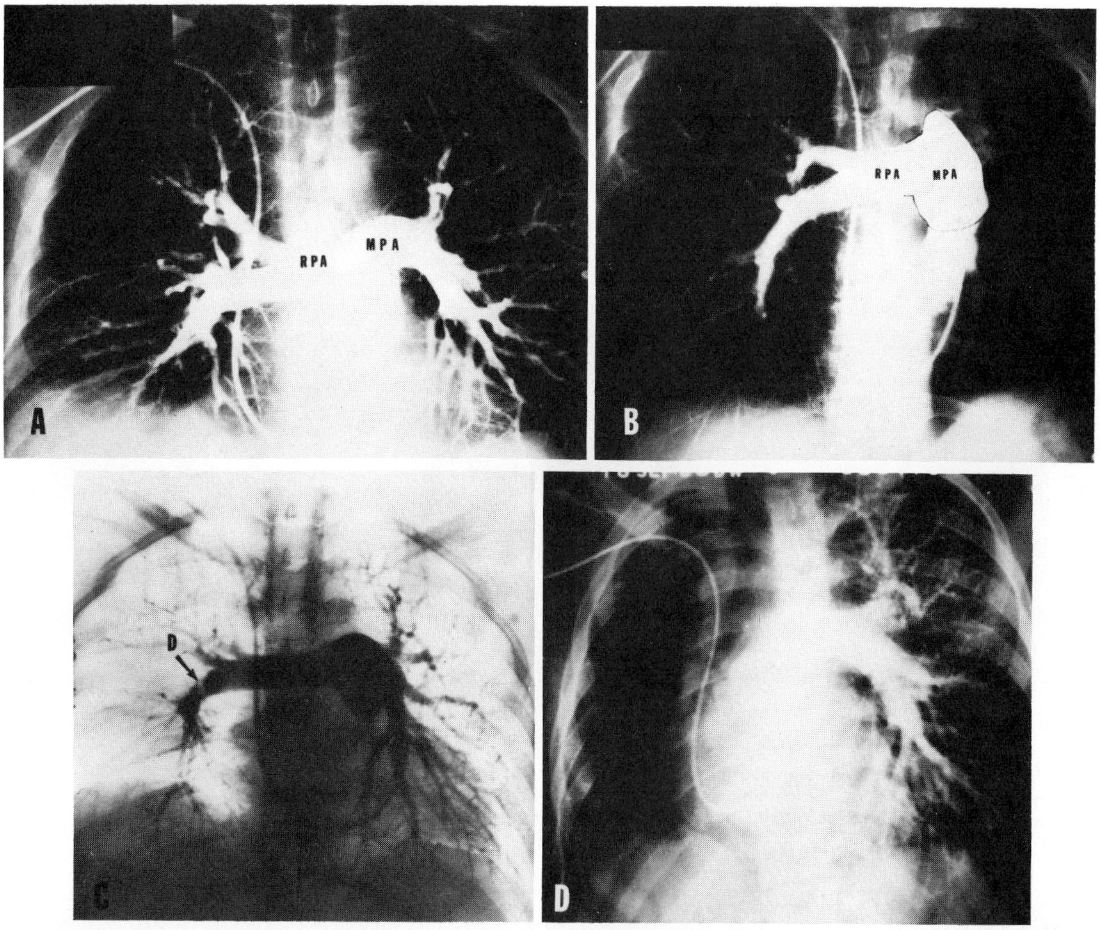

Figure 43. Pulmonary arteriography: *A,* Normal pulmonary arteriogram. *B,* Massive embolus to left pulmonary artery. *C,* Defect (D) in right pulmonary artery due to an embolus. *D,* Congenital absence of the right pulmonary artery. RPA = right pulmonary artery; LPA = left pulmonary artery. (From Robin, E., et al. *In* Sabiston, D. C., Jr., and Spencer, F. C. (Eds.): Gibbon's Surgery of the Chest, 3rd ed. Philadelphia, W. B. Saunders Company, 1976.)

and myocardial revascularization surgical procedures; and (4) in a patient with suspected congenital anomalies of his coronary arterial system.

The right and left coronary arterial patterns are shown in Figures 45 and 46.

Complications. The mortality rate attributed to coronary arteriography is less than 0.5 per cent. Ventricular fibrillation occurs in 1 to 2 per cent of patients studied. Other uncommon complications are myocardial infarction and dissection of the coronary arteries.

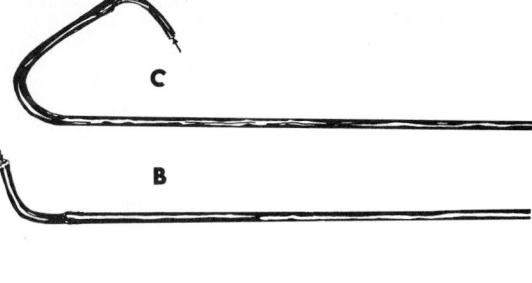

Figure 44. Catheter tips used during the performance of selective coronary angiography: *A,* Sones catheter tip; *B,* femoro-right coronary artery catheter tip; *C,* femoro-left coronary artery catheter tip. (Arrows point toward openings.)

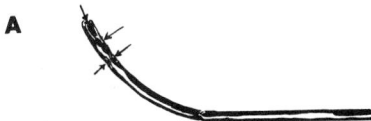

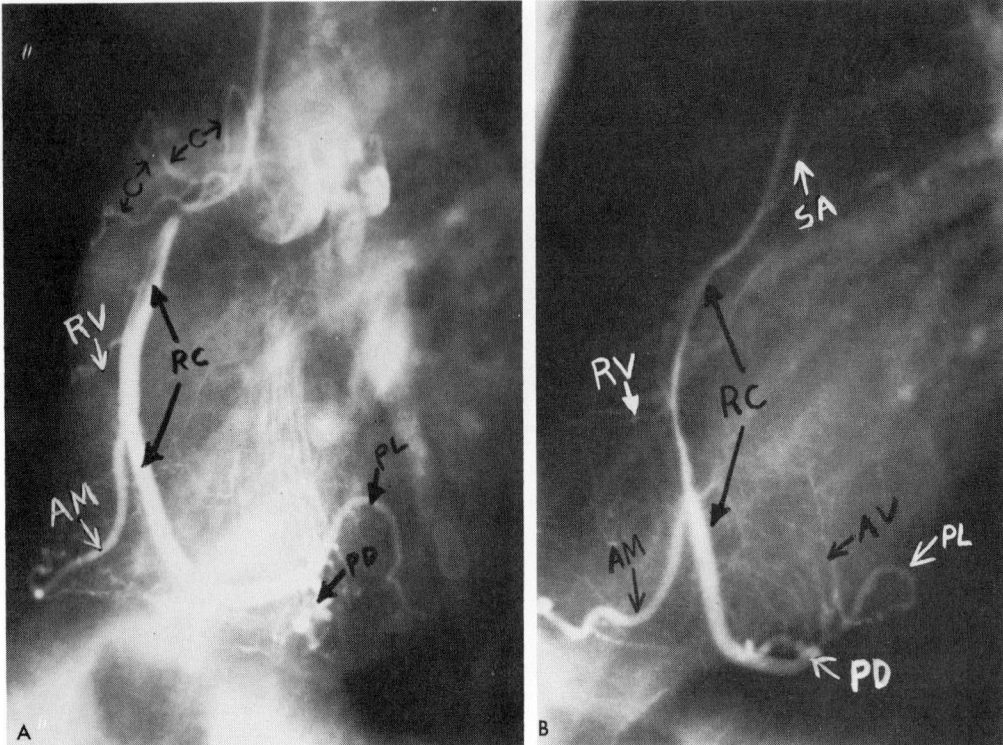

Figure 45. *A,* Selective right coronary angiogram in the left anterior oblique projection: RC = right coronary artery; C = conal branches; RV = right ventricular artery; AM = acute marginal artery; PD = posterior descending artery; PL = posterior lateral artery. *B,* Later phase in the same patient showing the sinus node (SA) and atrioventricular (AV) arteries.

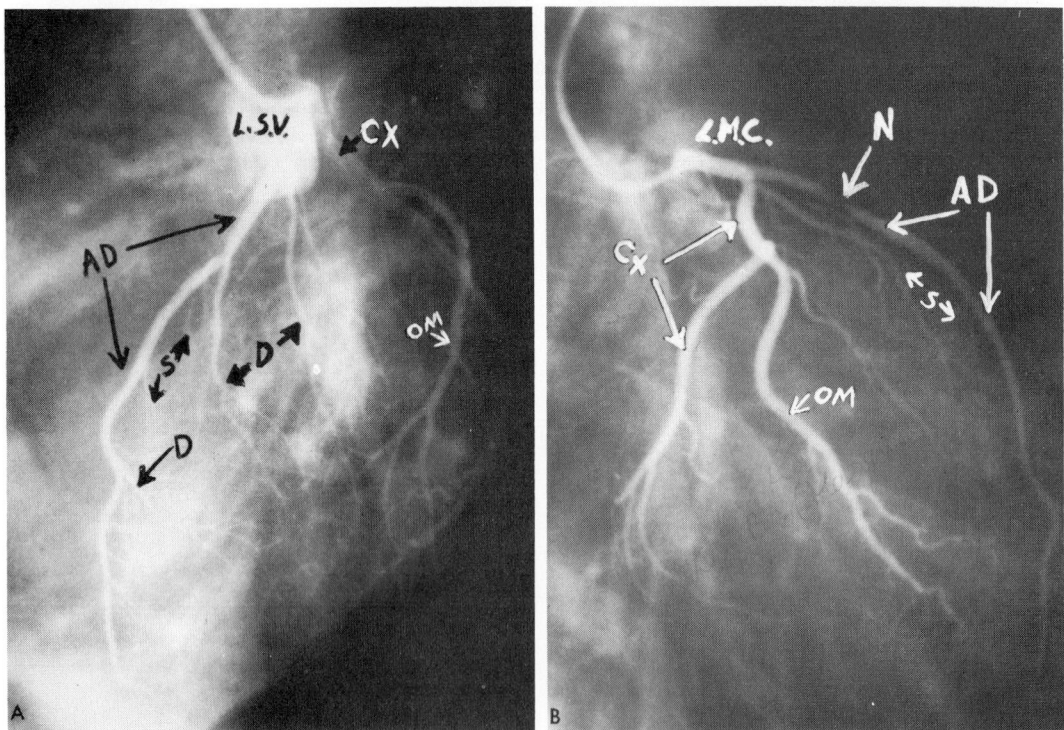

Figure 46. *A,* Selective left coronary angiogram in the left anterior oblique projection: L.S.V. = contrast material in left sinus of Valsalva; AD = anterior descending artery; CX = circumflex artery; OM = obtuse marginal artery; S = septal branches; D = diagonal branches. *B,* Selective left coronary angiogram in right anterior oblique projection: L.M.C. = left main coronary artery; N = severe narrowing involving the proximal segment of anterior descending artery (AD).

SELECTED REFERENCES

Beckmann, C. H., and Dooley, B.: Complications of left heart angiography, a study of 1,000 consecutive cases. Circulation, 41:825, 1970.
A study of 1000 consecutive left heart cineangiocardiograms is presented. Major problems were associated with the procedure in 3.1 per cent of the cases. Most cardiac complications resulted from open-end catheter angiography, especially through transseptal catheters.

Braunwald, E., Lambrew, C. T., Morrow, A. G., Pierce, G. E., Rockoff, S. D., and Ross, J., Jr.: Idiopathic hypertrophic subaortic stenosis. Circulation, Vol. 30, Suppl. IV, 1964.
This classic monograph represents the prime source of information about this most fascinating disease.

Braunwald, E., Moscovitz, H. L., Amram, S. S., Lasser, R. P., Sapin, S. O., Himmelstein, A., Ravitch, M. M., and Gordon, A. J.: The hemodynamics of the left side of the heart as studied by simultaneous left atrial, left ventricular and aortic pressure. Particular reference to mitral stenosis. Circulation, 12:69, 1955.
In six patients without mitral stenosis and in patients with mitral stenosis the hemodynamics of the left heart were studied at operation by means of simultaneous needle puncture of the left atrium, left ventricle, and aorta.

Braunwald, E., and Swan, H. J. C. (Eds.): Cooperative study on cardiac catheterization. Circulation, Vol. 37, Suppl. III, 1968.
This monograph is the latest study in the assessment of the risks of various cardiac catheterization methods in a total of 12,367 procedures carried out over a period of 2 years.

Brock, R.: The surgical treatment of pulmonary stenosis. Br. Heart J., 23:337, 1961.
This excellent presentation of the problem of congenital pulmonic stenosis is based on data obtained from 198 patients. A survey of the incidence, morbid anatomy, and clinical significance of this condition is presented. Indications and results of closed and open valvotomy are discussed.

Brockenbrough, E. C., Braunwald, E., and Ross, J., Jr.: Transseptal left heart catheterization—a review of 450 studies and description of an improved technic. Circulation, 25:15, 1962.
The technique of transseptal left heart catherization is described. This method was applied in 450 studies. The left atrium was intubated in all but two patients. The left ventricle was entered in 95 per cent of the cases. The only serious complication was accidental puncture of the aorta in three patients.

Hilder, F. J., Drake, E. H., Gale, H. H., and Ormond, R. S.: Transbrachial retrograde left heart catheterization. Evaluation of 600 consecutive cases in adults. Am. J. Cardiol., 18:52, 1966.
The transbrachial retrograde arterial approach was used in 600 consecutive adult cases. The left ventricle was intubated in 96 per cent of the cases. The failure rate of 4 per cent was due to tortuous or aberrant great arteries, tortuous aortas, calcified valves, and local arteriospasm. In 216 cases of significant aortic stenosis, the left ventricle was entered in 98 per cent of the cases.

Judkins, M. P.: Percutaneous transfemoral selective coronary arteriography. Radiol. Clin. North Am., 6:467, 1968.
The technique of coronary angiography using the percutaneous transfemoral approach and especially designed catheters is described. Results obtained in 500 patients are discussed. Reproductions of coronary angiograms are excellent.

Leonard, J. J., and Kroetz, F. W.: Lessons learned through intracardiac phonocardiography. Mod. Conc. Cardiovasc. Dis., 35:69, 1966.
A summary of the current concepts of the origin of cardiac sounds and murmurs as obtained by intracardiac phonocardiography is presented. Sounds and murmurs related to congenital anomalies such as atrial and ventricular septal defects, patent ductus arteriosus, pulmonic stenosis, and acquired defects of the mitral, aortic, and tricuspid valves are discussed.

Rosen, K. M.: Catheter recording of His bundle electrograms. Mod. Conc. Cardiovasc. Dis., 42:23, 1973.
A concise review of the physiologic basis and clinical uses of the bundle of His technique.

Ross, R. J., and Friesinger, G. C.: Anatomic and physiologic considerations in measurements of myocardial blood flow. Circulation, 32:630, 1965.
The different techniques for measuring coronary blood flow are discussed. It has not been possible to separate normal persons from patients with coronary artery disease on the basis of myocardial blood flow measurements. However, they have been useful in the study of exercise or the acute administration of drugs.

Rudolph, A. M., and Cayler, G. G.: Cardiac catheterization in infants and children. Pediatr. Clin. North Am., 5:907, 1958.
An excellent and concise report on the different cardiac catheterization techniques and their application to the evaluation of heart disease in infants and children.

Shirey, E. K., and Sones, F. M., Jr.: Retrograde transaortic and mitral valve catheterization. Physiologic and morphologic evaluation of aortic and mitral valve lesions. Am. J. Cardiol., 18:745, 1966.
The retrograde method of left atrial catheterization using the right brachial arterial approach is discussed. This technique was used in 310 patients for a total of 315 studies. The left atrium was intubated in 285 studies. In 84 per cent of cases of mitral stenosis, the left atrium was successfully catheterized. Ventricular fibrillation occurred in five cases.

Sones, F. M., Jr.: Cine coronary arteriography. *In* Hurst, J. W., and Logue, R. B. (Eds.): Heart, 2nd ed. New York, McGraw-Hill Book Company, 1970, pp. 377–385.
The technique of coronary cineangiography using the right retrograde transbrachial route is described by the man who was the first to introduce and develop the technique of direct, selective coronary arteriography. His experience with the procedure in more than 15,000 patients is discussed.

REFERENCES

1. Abrams, H. L.: Radiologic aspects of operable heart disease. III. The hazards of retrograde aortography: A survey. Radiology, 68:812, 1957.
2. Alanis, J., Gonzalez, H., and Lopez, E.: The electrical activity of the bundle of His. J. Physiol., 142:127, 1958.
3. Androuny, Z. A., Southerland, D. W., Griswold, H. E., and Ritzman, L. W.: Complications with transseptal left heart catheterization. Am. Heart J., 65:327, 1963.
4. Arcilla, R. A., Agutsson, M. M., Bicoff, J. P., Lynfeld, J., Weinberg, M., Jr., Fell, H. G., and Gasul, B. M.: Further observations on the natural history of isolated ventricular septal defect in infancy and childhood. Circulation, 28:560, 1963.
5. Arvidsson, H.: Angiocardiographic determination of left ventricular volume. Acta Radiol., 56:321, 1961.
6. Bagger, M., et al.: On methods and complications in catheterization of heart and large vessels with and without contrast injection. Am. Heart J., 54:767, 1957.
7. Bargeron, L., Clark, L. C., and Lyons, C.: Use of an electrode for continuously recording intracardiac PO_2 changes in cardiac catheterizations. Circulation, 24:881, 1961.
8. Bartle, S. H., and Sanmarco, M. D.: Measurement of left ventricle volume by biplane angiocardiography and indicator-washout techniques. A comparison in the canine heart. Cir. Res., 19:295, 1966.
9. Battro, A., and Bidoggia, H.: Endocardiac electrocardiogram obtained by heart catheterization in man. Am. Heart J., 33:604, 1947.
10. Beckmann, C. H., and Dooley, B.: Complications of left heart angiography, a study of 1,000 consecutive cases. Circulation, 41:825, 1970.
11. Bedford, D. E., and Sellors, T. H.: Atrial septal defects. *In* Modern Trends in Cardiology. London, Butterworth and Company, 1960, p. 138.
12. Bell, L. A. L., Haynes, W. F., Jr., Shimomura, S., and Dallas, D. P.: Influence of catheter tip position on pulmonary wedge pressures. Circ. Res., 10:215, 1962.
13. Beuren, A. J., and Apitz, J.: Left ventricular angiography by transseptal puncture of the left atrium. Circulation, 28:209, 1963.
14. Bing, R. J., Heimbecker, R., and Falholt, W.: An estimation of the residual volume of blood in the right ventricle of normal and diseased human hearts in vivo. Am. Heart J., 42:483, 1951.

15. Bing, R. J., Vandam, L. D., and Gray, F. D., Jr.: Physiological studies in congenital heart disease: Results of preoperative studies in patients with tetralogy of Fallot. Bull. Johns Hopkins Hosp., 80:121, 1947.

16. Bing, R. J., Vandam, L. D., and Gray, F. D., Jr.: Physiological studies in congenital heart disease: Procedures. Bull. Johns Hopkins Hosp., 80:107, 1947.

17. Björk, V. O., and Loden, H.: Left heart catheterization with selective left atrial and ventricular angiocardiography in the diagnosis of mitral and aortic valvular disease. Progr. Cardiovasc. Dis., 2:116, 1959.

18. Björk, V. O., and Loden, H.: Evaluation of mitral stenosis with selective left ventricular angiocardiography. J. Thorac. Cardiovasc. Surg., 40:17, 1960.

19. Björk, V. O., Loden, H., and Malers, E.: The evaluation of the degree of mitral insufficiency by selective left ventricular angiocardiography. Am. Heart J., 60:691, 1960.

20. Björk, V. O., Malmström, G., and Uggla, L. G.: Left auricular pressure measurements in man. Ann. Surg., 138:718, 1953.

21. Bleichroeder, F.: Intra arterielle Therapie. Berlin Klin. Wochenschr. 2:1503, 1912.

22. Bookstein, J. J., and Sigmann, J. M.: Intramural deposition of contrast agent during selective angiography. Radiology, 81:932, 1963.

23. Braunwald, E., Brockenbrough, E. C., Talbert, J. L., Folse, J. R., and Rockoff, S. D.: Selective left heart angiography by the transseptal route. Am. J. Med., 33:213, 1962.

24. Braunwald, E., Goldblatt, A., Long, R. T. L., and Morrow, A. G. The krypton inhalation test for the detection of left-to-right shunts. Br. Heart J., 24:47, 1962.

25. Braunwald, E., Lambrew, C. T., Morrow, A. G., Pierce, G. E., Rockoff, S. D., and Ross, J., Jr.: Idiopathic hypertrophic subaortic stenosis. Circulation, Vol. 30, Suppl. IV, 1964.

26. Braunwald, E., Morrow, A. G., Cornell, W. P., Augen, M. M., and Hilbish, T.: Idiopathic hypertrophic subaortic stenosis. Clinical hemodynamic and angiographic manifestations. Am. J. Med., 29:940, 1960.

27. Braunwald, E., Moscovitz, H. L., Amram, S. S., Lasser, R. P., Sapin, S. O., Himmelstein, A., Ravitch, M. M., and Gordon, A. J.: The hemodynamics of the left side of the heart as studied by simultaneous left atrial, left ventricular, and aortic pressures: Particular reference to mitral stenosis. Circulation, 12:69, 1955.

28. Braunwald, E., Pfaff, W. W., Long, R. T. L., and Morrow, A. G.: A simplified indicator-dilution technique for the localization of left-to-right circulatory shunts. An experimental and clinical study of intravenous injection and right heart sampling. Circulation, 20:875, 1959.

29. Braunwald, E., Ross, J., Jr., Gault, J. H., Mason, D. T., Mills, C., Gabe, L. T., and Epstein, S. E.: Assessment of cardiac function. Ann. Intern. Med., 70:369, 1969.

30. Braunwald, E., and Swan, H. J. C. (Eds.): Cooperative study on cardiac catheterization. Circulation, Vol. 37, Suppl. III, 1968.

31. Braunwald, E., Tanenbaum, H. L., and Morrow, A. G.: Dye-dilution curves from left heart and aorta for localization of left-to-right shunts and detection of valvular insufficiency. Proc. Soc. Exp. Biol. Med., 94:510, 1957.

32. Brock, R.: Anatomy of Congenital Pulmonic Stenosis. New York, Paul B. Hoeber, 1957.

33. Brock, R.: The surgical treatment of pulmonary stenosis. Br. Heart J., 23:337, 1961.

34. Brock, R., Milstein, B. B., and Ross, D. N.: Percutaneous left ventricular puncture in the assessment of aortic stenosis. Thorax, 11:163, 1956.

35. Brockenbrough, E. C., and Braunwald, E.: A new technique for left ventricular angiocardiography and transseptal left heart catheterization. Am. J. Cardiol., 6:1062, 1960.

36. Brockenbrough, E. C., Braunwald, E., and Morrow, A. G.: A hemodynamic technique for the detection of hypertrophic subaortic stenosis. Circulation, 23:189, 1961.

37. Brockenbrough, E. C., Braunwald, E., and Ross, J., Jr.: Transseptal left heart catheterization – a review of 450 studies and description of an improved technic. Circulation, 25:15, 1962.

38. Brown, R., Rahimtoola, S. H., Davis, G. D., and Swan, H. J. C.: The effect of angiographic contrast medium on circulatory dynamics in man. Cardiac output during angiocardiography. Circulation, 31:234, 1965.

39. Calazel, P., Gerard, R., Daley, R., Draper, A., Foster, J., and Bing, R. J.: Physiological studies in congenital heart disease. XI. A comparison of the right and left auricular, capillary and pulmonary artery pressures in nine patients with auricular septal defect. Bull. Johns Hopkins Hosp., 88:20, 1951.

40. Campbell, J. A., Klatte, E. C., and Shalkowski, R. A.: Factors influencing image quality in cineroentgenography. Am. J. Roentgen., 83:345, 1960.

41. Carleton, R. A., Bowyer, A. F., and Graettinger, J. S.: Overestimation of left ventricular volume by the indicator-dilution technique. Circ. Res., 18:248, 1966.

42. Chapman, C. B., Baker, O., Reynolds, J., and Bonte, F. J.: Use of biplane cinefluorography for measurement of ventricular volume. Circulation, 18:1105, 1958.

43. Chatterjee, K., Swan, H. J. C., Ganz, W., Gray, R., Loebel, H., Forrester, J. S., and Chonette, D.: Use of a balloon-tipped flotation electrode catheter for cardiac monitoring. Am. J. Cardiol., 36:56, 1975.

44. Chavez, T., Dorbecker, N., and Celis, A.: Direct intracardial angiocardiography; its diagnostic value. Am. Heart J., 33:560, 1947.

45. Cheng, T. O.: Myocardial infarction following transmural extravasation of contrast medium during left ventricular cineangiography. Circulation, 28:105, 1963.

46. Clark, L. C., and Bargeron, L. M., Jr.: Detection and direct recording of left-to-right shunts with the hydrogen electrode catheter. Surgery, 46:797, 1959.

47. Clark, L. C., Bargeron, L. M., Jr., Lyons, C., Bradely, M. N., and McArthur, K. T.: Detection of right-to-left shunts with an arterial potentiometric electrode. Circulation, 22:949, 1960.

48. Clark, L. C., Kaplan, S., Matthews, E. C., Edwards, F. K., and Helmworth, J. A.: Monitor and control of blood oxygen tension and pH during total body perfusions. J. Thorac. Surg., 36:488, 1958.

49. Connolly, D. C., Kirklin, J. W., and Wood, E. H.: The relationship between pulmonary artery wedge pressure and left atrial pressure in man. Circ. Res., 2:434, 1954.

50. Cope, C.: Technique for transseptal catheterization of left atrium. Preliminary report. J. Thorac. Surg., 37:482, 1959.

51. Cope, C.: Intravascular breakage of Seldinger spring guide wires. J.A.M.A., 180:1061, 1962.

52. Cournand, A., Bing, R. J., Dexter, L., and Dotter, C.: Report of the Committee on Cardiac Catheterization and Angiocardiography. Circulation, 7:769, 1953.

53. Cournand, A., Motley, H. L., Himmelstein, A., Dresdale, D., and Baldwin, J.: Recording of blood pressure from the left auricle and the pulmonary veins in human subjects with interauricular septal defect. Am. J. Physiol., 150:267, 1947.

54. Cournand, A., and Ranges, H. A.: Catheterization of the right auricle in man. Proc. Soc. Exp. Biol. Med., 46:462, 1941.

55. Cournand, A., Riley, R. L., Breed, E. S., Baldwin, E. de F., and Richards, D. W., Jr.: Measurement of cardiac output in man using the technique of catheterization of the right auricle or ventricle. J. Clin. Invest., 24:106, 1945.

56. Damato, A. N., Lau, S. H., Helfant, R., Stein, E., Patton, R. D., Scherlag, B. J., and Berkowitz, W. D.: A study of heart block in man using His bundle recordings. Circulation, 39:297, 1969.

57. Davis, F. W., Jr., and Andrus, E. C.: Mitral stenosis in facsimile. N. Engl. J. Med., 251:297, 1954.

58. Dexter, L., Haynes, F. W., Burwell, C. S., Eppinger, E. C., Siebel, R. E., and Evans, J. M.: Studies of congenital heart disease. I. Technique of venous catheterization as a diagnostic procedure. J. Clin. Invest., 26:547, 1947.

59. Dexter, L., Haynes, F. W., Burwell, C. S., Eppinger, E. C., Sogerson, R. P., and Evans, J. M.: Studies of congenital heart disease. II. The pressure and oxygen content of blood in the right auricle, right ventricle and pulmonary artery in control patients with observation on the oxygen saturation and source of pulmonary "capillary" blood. J. Clin. Invest., 26:554, 1947.

60. Dodge, H. T., Hay, R. E., and Sandler, H.: An angiocardiographic method for directly determining left ventricular stroke volume in man. Circ. Res., 11:739, 1962.

61. Dotter, C. T.: Left ventricle and systemic arterial catheterization: A simple percutaneous method using a spring guide. Am. J. Roentgenol., 6:969, 1960.

62. Dow, P.: Dimensional relationships in dye-dilution curves from humans and dogs, with an empirical formula for certain troublesome curves. J. Appl. Physiol., 7:399, 1955.

63. Dow, P.: Estimations of cardiac output and central blood volume by dye-dilution. Physiol. Rev., 36:77, 1956.

64. Duchosal, P. W., Ferrero, C., Doret, J. P., Andereggen, P., and Rilliet, B.: Les potentiels intra-cardiaques récueillis par cathétérisme chez l'homme. Cardiologia, 13:113, 1948.

65. Edwards, E. A., and Biguria, F. A.: A comparison of Skiodan and Diodrast as vasographic media: With special reference to their effect on blood pressure. N. Engl. J. Med., 211:589, 1934.

66. Enson, Y., Briscoe, W. A., Polanyi, M. L., and Cournand, A.: In vivo studies with an intravascular and intracardiac reflection oximeter. J. Appl. Physiol., 17:552, 1962.

67. Facquet, J., Lemoine, J. M., Alhomme, P., and Lefebvre, J.: La mesure de la pression auriculaire gauche par voie transbronchique. Arch. Mal. Coeur, 45:741, 1952.

68. Fegler, G.: Measurement of cardiac output in anesthetized animals by a thermodilution method. Q. J. Exper. Physiol., 39:153, 1954.

69. Feruglio, G. A.: Intracardiac phonocardiography: A valuable diagnostic technique in congenital and acquired heart disease. Am. Heart J., 58:827, 1959.

70. Fisher, D. L.: The use of pressure recordings obtained at transthoracic left heart catheterization in the diagnosis of valvular heart disease. J. Thorac. Surg., 30:379, 1955.

71. Fleming, H. A., Hancock, E. W., Milstein, B. B., and Ross, D. H.: Percutaneous left ventricular puncture with catheterization of aorta. Thorax, 13:97, 1958.

72. Fleming, P., and Gibson, R.: Percutaneous left ventricular puncture in the assessment of aortic stenosis. Thorax, 12:37, 1957.

73. Folse, R., and Braunwald, E.: Determination of fraction of left ventricular volume ejected per beat and clinical observations with a precordial dilution technique. Circulation, 25:674, 1962.

74. Forman, J., Laurens, P., and Serville, M.: Catheterization of the left cavities with micromanometry by transseptal route. Arch. Mal. Coeur, 55:601, 1962.

75. Forrester, J. S., Diamond, G., McHugh, T. J., and Swan, H. J. C.: Filling pressures in the right and left sides of the heart in acute myocardial infarctions. N. Engl. J. Med., 285:190, 1971.

76. Forrester, J. S., Ganz, W., Diamond, G., McHugh, T., Chonette, D. W., and Swan, H. J. C.: Thermodilution cardiac output determination with a single flow-directed catheter. Am. Heart J., 83:306, 1972.

77. Forssmann, W.: Die Sondierung des rechten Herzens. Klin. Wochenschr., 8:2085, 1929.

78. Fox, I. J., and Wood, E. H.: Applications of dilution curves recorded from the right side of the heart or venous circulation with the aid of a new indicator dye. Mayo Clin. Proc., 32:541, 1957.

79. Fox, S. M.: Pretracheal left heart catheterization: Difficult technique with some advantage. Circulation, 20:696, 1959.

80. Frank, M. J., and Levinson, G. E.: An index of the contractile state of the myocardium in man. J. Clin. Invest., 47:1615, 1958.

81. Freis, E. D., Rivara, G. L., and Gilmore, B. L.: Estimation of residual and end-diastolic volumes of the right ventricle of men without heart disease, using the dye-dilution method. Am. Heart J., 60:898, 1960.

82. Friedlich, A., Heimbecker, R., and Bing, R. J.: A device for continuous recording of concentration of Evans blue dye in whole blood and its application to determination of cardiac output. J. Appl. Physiol., 3:12, 1950.

83. Gasul, B. M., Dillon, R. J., Vrla, V., and Hart, G.: Ventricular septal defects. Their natural transformation in those with infundibular stenosis or with the cyanotic or non-cyanotic type of tetralogy of Fallot. J.A.M.A., 164:847, 1957.

84. Gilford, S. R., Gregg, D. E., Shadle, O. W., Ferguson, T. B., and Marzetta, L. A.: An improved cuvette densitometer for cardiac output determination by the dye-dilution method. Rev. Sci. Instrum., 24:696, 1953.

85. Gleason, W. L., and Braunwald, E.: Studies on the first derivative of the ventricular pressure pulse in man. J. Clin. Invest., 41:80, 1962.

86. Gorlin, R., and Gorlin, S. G.: Hydraulic formula for calculations of the area of the stenotic mitral valve, other cardiac valves and central circulatory shunts. Am. Heart J., 41:1, 1951.

87. Gorlin, R., Lewis, B. M., Haynes, F. W., and Dexter, L.: Studies of the circulatory dynamics at rest in mitral valvular regurgitation with and without stenosis. Am. Heart J., 43:357, 1952.

88. Graham, T. P., Jr., Covell, J. W., Sonnenblick, E. H., Ross, J., Jr., and Braunwald, E.: The control of myocardial oxygen consumption: Relative influence of contractile state and tension development. J. Clin. Invest., 47:375, 1968.

89. Greene, D. G., Carlisle, R., Grant, C., and Bunnell, I. L.: Estimation left ventricular volume by one-plane cineangiography. Circulation, 35:61, 1967.

90. Grundemann, A. M., Bosch, C., Schwantje, E. J. M., Reijns, G. A., and Verheught, A. P. M.: Retrograde catheterization of the left ventricle in aortic stenosis. Am. J. Cardiol., 6:915, 1960.

91. Hallermann, F. J., Rostelle, G. C., and Swan, H. J. E.: Comparison of left ventricular volumes by dye-dilution and angiographic methods in the dog. Am. J. Physiol., 204:446, 1963.

92. Hamilton, W. F., Moore, J. W., Kinsman, J. M., and Spurling, R. G.: Studies on the circulation. IV. Further analysis of the injection method, and of changes in hemodynamics under physiological and pathological conditions. Am. J. Physiol., 99:534, 1932.

93. Harned, H. S., Lurie, P. R., Croethers, C. H., and Whittmore, R.: Use of the whole blood oximeter during cardiac catheterization. J. Lab. Clin. Med., 40:445, 1952.

94. Hawley, R. R., Dodge, H. T., and Graham, T. P.: Left atrial volume and its changes in heart disease. Circulation, 34:989, 1966.

95. Hecht, H. H.: Potential variations of the right auricular and ventricular cavities in man. Am. Heart J., 32:39, 1946.

96. Hernandez, F. A., Rockkind, R., and Cooper, H. R.: The intracavitary electrocardiogram in the diagnosis of Ebstein's anomaly. Am. J. Cardiol., 1:181, 1958.

97. Hickam, J. B., and Frazer, R.: Spectrophotometric determination of blood oxygen. J. Biol. Chem., 180:457, 1949.

98. Hilder, F. J., Drake, E. H., Gale, H. H., and Ormond, R. S.: Transbrachial retrograde left heart catheterization. Evaluation of 600 consecutive cases in adults. Am. J. Cardiol., 18:52, 1966.

99. Holling, H. E., MacDonald, I., O'Holloran, J. A., and Venner, A.: Reliability of a spectrophotometric method of estimating blood oxygen. J. Appl. Physiol., 8:249, 1955.

100. Horger, E. L., Dotter, C. T., and Steinberg, E.: Electrocardiographic changes during angiocardiography. Am. Heart J., 41:651, 1951.

101. Hugenholtz, P. G., Gamble, W. J., Monroe, R. G., and Polanyi, M.: The use of fiberoptics in clinical cardiac catheterization. II. In vivo dye-dilution curves. Circulation, 31:344, 1965.

102. Hugenholt, P. G., Wagner, H. R., and Sandler, H.: The in vivo determination of left ventricular volume: Comparison of the fiberoptic-indicator dilution and the angiocardiographic methods. Circulation, 37:489, 1968.

103. Hunt, D., Pombo, J., Potanin, C., Russell, R. O., Jr., and Rackley, C. E.: Intravascular monitoring in acute myocardial infarction. Am. J. Cardiol., 25:104, 1970.

104. Judkins, M. P.: Percutaneous transfemoral selective coronary arteriography. Radiol. Clin. North Am., 6:467, 1968.

105. Kaltman, A. J., Herbert, W. H., Conroy, R. J., and Kossman, C. E.: Gradient in pressure across the pulmonary vascular bed during diastole. Circulation, 34:377, 1966.

106. Katz, L. H., and Feinberg, H.: The relation of cardiac efforts to myocardial oxygen consumption and coronary flow. Circ. Res., 6:656, 1968.

107. Kent, E. M., Ford, W. B., Fisher, D. L., and Childs, T. B.: The estimation of the severity of mitral regulation. Ann. Surg., 141:47, 1955.

108. Kidd, L.: The hemodynamics in ventricular septal defect in childhood. Am. Heart J., 70:732, 1965.

109. Kinsman, J. M., Moore, J. W., and Hamilton, W. F.: Studies on the circulation. I. Injection method: Physical and mathematical considerations. Am. J. Physiol., 89:322, 1929.

110. Klatte, E. C., Campbell, J. A., and Lurie, P. R.: Technical factors in selective cinecardioangiography. Radiology, 73:539, 1959.

111. Kossman, C. E., Berger, A. R., Rader, B., Brumlik, J., Briller, S.

A., and Donnolly, J. H.: Intracardiac and intravascular potentials resulting from electrical activity of the normal human heart. Circulation, 2:10, 1950.

112. Laurens, P., Bouchard, F., Brial, E.,Cornu, C., Baculard, P., and Soulié, P.: Bruits et pressions cardiovasculaires enregistrés in situ àl'aide d'un micromanomètre. Arch. Mal. Coeur, 52:121, 1959.

113. Leb, G., Derntl, F., Goldschlager, N., Cowan, C., and Bing, R. J.: Determination of effective and total coronary blood flow using Rb[84]. Am. J. Med. Sci., 257:203, 1969.

114. Lenegre, J., and Maurice, P.: De quelques résultats obtenus par la dérivation directe intracavitaire des courants électriques de l'oreillette et du ventricule droits. Arch. Mal. Coeur, 38:298, 1945.

115. Leonard, J. J., and Kreutz, F. W.: Lessons learned through intracardial phonocardiography. Mod. Conc. Cardiovasc. Dis., 35:69, 1966.

116. Levin, A. R., Spach, M. S., Anderson, P. A. W., and Capp, M. P.: Cardiac perforation following left ventricular cineangiocardiography. Circulation, 32:593, 1965.

117. Levine, H. D., Hellems, H. K., Dexter, L., and Tucker, A. S.: Studies in intracardiac electrocardiography in man. II. The potential variations in the right ventricle. Am. Heart J., 37:64, 1949.

118. Levine, H. D., Hellems, H. K., Wittenberg, M. H., and Dexter, L.: Studies in intracardiac electrocardiography in man. I. The potential variations in the right atrium. Am. Heart J., 37:46, 1949.

119. Lewis, D. H., Deitz, G. W., Wallace, J. D., and Brown, J. R., Jr.: Intracardiac phonocardiography. Progr. Cardiovasc. Dis., 2:85, 1959.

120. Lewis, D. H., Ertugrul, A. E., Deitz, G. W., Wallace, J. D., Brown, J. R., Jr., and Moghadam, A. N.: Intracardiac phonocardiography in the diagnosis of congenital heart disease. Pediatrics, 23:837, 1959.

121. Lind, J., Boesen, I. B., and Wegelius, C.: Selective angiocardiography in congenital heart disease. Progr. Cardiovasc. Dis., 2:293, 1959.

122. Litwak, R. S., Bernstein, W. H., and Samet, P.: Problems in the interpretation of left atrial, left ventricular, and mean diastolic gradients. Am. J. Cardiol., 6:1023, 1960.

123. Long, R. T. L., Braunwald, E., and Morrow, A. G.: Intracardiac injection of radioactive krypton[85]. Clinical applications of new methods for characterization of circulatory shunts. Circulation, 21:1126, 1960.

124. Lucas, R. V., Jr., Adams, P., Jr., Anderson, R. C., Meyne, N. G., Lillihei, C. W., and Varco, R. L.: The natural history of isolated ventricular septal defect. A serial physiological study. Circulation. 24:1372, 1961.

125. Luchsinger, P. C., Seipp, H. W., Jr., and Patel, D. J.: Relationship of pulmonary artery wedge pressures to left atrial pressures in man. Circ. Res., 11:315, 1962.

126. Lurie, P. R., Shumacker, H. B. Jr., Schulz, D. M., Klatte, E. C., and Grajo, M. Z.: Obstructive hypertrophy in congenital heart disease: Definition, classification, and surgical importance. Circulation, 20:732, 1959.

127. Lüthy, E., and Galletti, P. M.: In vivo evaluation of the thermodilution technique for measuring cardiac output. Helv. Physiol. Pharmacol. Acta, 24:15, 1966.

128. Mason, D. R.: Usefulness and limitations of the rate of rise of intraventricular pressure (dp/dt) in the evaluation of myocardial contractility in man. Am. J. Cardiol., 23:516, 1969.

129. Mason, D. T., and Braunwald, E.: Studies on digitalis. IX. Effects of ouabain on the nonfailing human heart. J. Clin. Invest., 42:1105, 1963.

130. Mason, D. T., Sonnenblick, E. H., Covell, J. W., Ross, J., Jr., and Braunwald, E.: Assessment of myocardial contractility in man: Relationship between the rate of pressure rise and developed pressure throughout isometric left ventricular contraction. Circulation, 36(Suppl. 2):183, 1967.

131. Mason, D. T., Sonnenblick, E. H., Ross, J., Jr., Covell, J. W., and Braunwald, E.: Time to peak dp/dt: A useful measurement for evaluating the contractile state of the human heart. Circulation. 32(Suppl. 2):145, 1965.

132. Matsuoka, Y., and Evans, C. L.: Effect of various mechanical conditions on the gaseous metabolism and efficiency of the mammalian heart. J. Physiol., 49:378, 1914.

133. McMichael, J., and Mounsey, J. P.: Complication following coronary sinus and cardiac vein catheterization in man. Br. Heart J., 13:397, 1951.

134. Meister, S. G., Banka, V. S., Chadda, K. D., and Helfant, R. H.: A balloon tipped catheter for obtaining His bundle electrograms without fluoroscopy. Circulation, 49:42, 1974.

135. Moffit, E. A., Dawson, B., and O'Neill, N. C.: Anesthesia for pediatric cardiac catheterization and angiography. Anesth. Analg., 40:483, 1961.

136. Moore, J. W., Kinsman, J. M., Hamilton, W. F., and Spurling. R. G.: Studies on the circulation. II. Cardiac output determinations; comparison of the injection method with the direct Fick procedure. Am. J. Physiol., 89:331, 1929.

137. Morrow, A. G., Braunwald, E., Haller, J. A., Jr., and Sharp, E. H.: Left heart catheterization by the transbronchial route: Technique and applications in physiologic and diagnostic investigations. Circulation, 16:1033, 1957.

138. Morrow, A G., Braunwald, E., and Ross, J., Jr.: Left heart catheterization. An appraisal of techniques and their applications in cardiovascular disease. Arch. Intern. Med., 105:645, 1960.

139. Morrow, A. G., Sanders, R. J., and Braunwald, E.: The nitrous oxide test. An improved method for the detection of left-to-right shunts. Circulation, 17:284, 1958.

140. Morrow, A. G., Sharp, E. H., and Braunwald, E.: Congenital aortic stenosis: Clinical and hemodynamic findings, surgical technique, and results of operation. Circulation, 18:1091, 1958.

141. Morrow, A. G., Waldhausen, J. A., Peters, R. L., Bloodwell, R. D., and Braunwald, E.: Supravalvular aortic stenosis, clinical hemodynamics and pathological observations. Circulation, 20:1003, 1959.

142. Moscovitz, H. L., Donoso, E., and Gelb, I. J.: The demonstration of flow murmurs by intracardiac phonocardiography. Clin. Res. Proc., 5:162, 1957.

143. Nadas, A. S., Rudolph, A. M., and Gross, R. E.: Pulmonary hypertension in congenital heart disease. Circulation, 22:1041, 1960.

144. Narula, O. S.: Recording of His bundle electrograms via the arm veins. Circulation, 46(Suppl. 2):197, 1972 (abstract).

145. Narula, O. S., and Samet, P.: Wenckebach and Mobitz II A-V block due to block within the His bundle and bundle branches. Circulation, 41:947, 1970.

146. Narula, O. S., Scherlag, B. J., Samet, P., and Javier, R. P.: Atrioventricular block: Localization and classification by His bundle recording. Am. J. Med., 50:146, 1971.

147. Nicholson, J. W., III, and Wood, E. H.: Estimation of cardiac output and blood volume by continuous recording of Evans blue time-concentration curves in man employing an oximeter. Am. J. Physiol., 163:738, 1951.

148. Nobel, F. W.: Electrical Methods of Blood-pressure Recordings. Springfield, Ill., Charles C Thomas, Publishers, 1953.

149. Nunez, V. B., and Ponsdomenech, E. R.: Heart puncture cardioangiography: Clinical and electrocardiographic results. Am. Heart J., 41:855, 1951.

150. Nutter, D. O., and Kelser, G. A.: The percutaneous intracavitary electrocardiogram in the diagnosis of arrhythmias. Ann. Intern. Med., 62:706, 1965.

151. Owen, S. G., and Wood, P.: A new method of determining the degree of absence of mitral obstruction: An analysis of the diastolic part of indirect left atrial pressure tracings. Br. Heart J., 17:41, 1955.

152. Polanyi, M. L., and Hehir, R. M.: New reflection oximeter. Rev. Instrum., 31:401, 1960.

153. Popper, R. W., Schumacher, D., and Quinn, C. H.: Cardiac tamponade due to hypertonic contrast medium in the pericardial sac following cineangiography. Circulation, 35:933, 1967.

154. Priotin, J. B., Thévenet, A., Pelissier, M., Puech, P., Latous, H., and Pourquier, J.: Cardiographie ventriculaire gauche par cathétérisme retrograde percutane fémoral. Presse Méd., 65:1948, 1957.

155. Radner, S.: Extended suprasternal puncture technique. Acta Med. Scand., 151:223, 1955.

156. Rahimtoola, S. H., Duffy, J. P., and Swan, H. J. C.: Hemodynamic changes associated with injection of angiographic contrast medium in assessment of valvular lesions. Circulation, 22:52, 1966.

157. Rapaport, E., Wong, M., Escobar, E. E., and Martinez, G.: The effect of upright posture on right ventricular volume in patients with and without heart failure. Am. Heart J., 71:146, 1966.

158. Read, J. L., Bong, E. G., and Porter, R. R.: The hazard of unrecognized catheterization of the coronary sinus. Arch. Intern. Med., 96:176, 1955.

159. Read, R. C: Cause of death in cardioangiography. J. Thorac. Cardiovasc. Surg., 38:685, 1959.

160. Reedy, T., and Chapman, C. B.: Measurement of right ventricular volume by cineangiofluorography. Am. Heart J., 66:221, 1963.

161. Reeves, T. J., Hefner, L. L., Jones, W. B., Coghlan, C., Prieto, G., and Corroll, J.: The hemodynamic determinants of the rate of change in pressure in the left ventricle during isometric contraction. Am. Heart J., 60:745, 1960.

162. Richards, D. W., Jr.: Cardiac output by catheterization technique in various clinical conditions. Fed. Proc., 4:215, 1945.

163. Ricketts, J. H., and Abrams, H. L.: Percutaneous selective coronary cinearteriography. J.A.M.A., 181:620, 1962.

164. Rodrigo, J. A.: Determination of the oxygen saturation of blood in vitro by using reflected light. Am. Heart J., 45:809, 1953.

165. Rodriguez-Alvarez, A., and Martinez de Rodriguez, G.: Studies in angiocardiography. The problems involved in the rapid, selective and safe injections of radiopaque materials. Development of a special catheter for selective angiocardiography. Am. Heart J., 53:841, 1957.

166. Rohde, E.: Über den Einfluss mechanischen Bedingungen auf die Tatigkeit und den Sauerstoffverbrauch des Warmluterherzens. Arch. Exp. Pathol. Pharmakol., 68:401, 1912.

167. Rosen, K. M., Loeb, H. S., Chuquimia, R., Sinno, M. Z., Rahimtoola, S. H., and Gunnar, R. M.: Site of heart block in acute myocardial infarction. Circulation, 42:925, 1970.

168. Rosen, K. M., Rahimtoola, S. H., Chuquimia, R., Loeb, H. S., and Gunnar, R. M.: Electrophysiological significance of first degree atrioventricular block with intraventricular conduction disturbance. Circulation, 43:491, 1971.

169. Ross, J., Jr.: Transseptal left heart catheterization: A new method of left atrial puncture. Ann. Surg., 37:482, 1959.

170. Ross, J., Jr.: Considerations regarding the technique for transseptal left heart catheterization. Circulation, 34:391, 1966.

171. Ross, J., Jr., Braunwald, E., and Morrow, A. G.: Transeptal left atrium puncture: New technique for measurement of left atrial pressure in man. Am. J. Cardiol., 3:653, 1959.

172. Ross, J., Jr., Braunwald, E., and Morrow, A. G.: Left heart catheterization by the transseptal route. A description of the technique and its applications. Circulation, 22:927, 1960.

173. Rowe, G. G., and Zarnstorff, W. C.: Ventricular fibrillation during selective angiocardiography. J.A.M.A., 192:105, 1965.

174. Rudolph, A. M., and Cayler, G. G.: Cardiac catheterization in infants and children. Pediatr. Clin. North Am., 5:907, 1958.

175. Russell, R. O., Caroll, J. F., and Hood, W. G. Jr.: Cardiac tamponade. A complication of the transseptal technique of left heart catheterization resulting in a fatality. Am. J. Cardiol., 13:558, 1964.

176. Salgado, C. R., and Galletti, P. M.: In vitro evaluation of thermodilution technique for the measurement of ventricular stroke volume and end-diastolic volume. Cardiologia, 49:65, 1966.

177. Sanders, R. J., and Morrow, A. G.: The diagnosis of circulatory shunts by the nitrous oxide test. Improvements in technique and methods for quantification of shunts. Circulation, 18:856, 1958.

178. Sanders, R. J., and Morrow, A. G.: The identification and quantification of left-to-right circulation shunts. A new diagnostic method utilizing the inhalation of a radioactive gas. Kr85. Am. J. Med., 26:508, 1959.

179. Sandler, H., and Dodge, H. T.: The use of single plane angiocardiograms for the calculation of left ventricular volume in man. Am. Heart J., 75:325, 1968.

180. Sarnoff, S. J., Braunwald, E., Welch, G. H., Jr., Case, R. B., Stainsby, W. N., and Marcuz, R.: Hemodynamic determinants of oxygen consumption of the heart with special reference to the tension-time index. Am. J. Physiol., 192:148, 1958.

181. Schafer, H., Blain, J. M., Ceballos, R., and Bing, R. J.: Essential pulmonary hypertension. A report of clinical physiologic studies in three patients with death following catheterization of the heart. Ann. Intern. Med., 44:505, 1956.

182. Scherlag, B. J., Lau, S. H., Helfant, R. H., Berkowitz, W. D., Stein, E., and Damato, A. N.: Catheter techniques for recording His bundle activity in man. Circulation, 35:13, 1969.

183. Scott, S. M., Fish, R. G., and Takaro, T.: A double needle technique for transbronchial left heart catheterization. Circulation, 22:976, 1960.

184. Scott, W. G., and Moore, S.: Rapid serialization of x-ray exposures by the radiography utilizing roll of film nine and one-half inches wide. Radiology, 53:846, 1949.

185. Scott, W. G., and Moore, S.: The development of the tautography and the advantages of automatization in cardiovascular angiography. Am. J. Roentgenol., 62:33, 1949.

186. Segal, B. L., Novack, P., and Kasparian, H.: Intracardiac phonocardiography, Am. J. Cardiol., 13:188, 1964.

187. Seldinger, S. L.: Catheter replacement of the needle in percutaneous arteriography: New technique. Acta Radiol., 39:368, 1953.

188. Shaffer, A. B., and Silber, E. N.: Factors influencing the character of the pulmonary arterial wedge pressure. Am. Heart J., 5:522, 1956.

189. Shirey, E. K., and Sones, F. M., Jr.: Retrograde transaortic and mitral valve catheterization. Physiologic and morphologic evaluation of aortic and mitral valve lesions. Am. J. Cardiol., 18:745, 1966.

190. Siegel, J. H., and Sonnenblick, E. H.: Quantification of myocardial contractility and prediction of myocardial failure. Arch. Surg., 89:1026, 1964.

191. Singleton, R. T., Dembo, D. H., and Scherlis, L.: Krypton85 in the detection of intracardiac left-to-right shunts. Circulation, 32:134, 1965.

192. Smith, C., Rowe, R. D., and Vlad, P.: Sedation of children for cardiac catheterization with an ataractic mixture. Can. Anaesth. Soc. J., 5:35, 1958.

193. Sodi Pallares, D., Vizcaino, M., Soberon, J., and Cabrera Cosio, E.: Comparative study of the intracavitary potential in man and in dog. Am. Heart J., 33:819, 1947.

194. Sones, F. M. Jr.: Cine coronary arteriography. In Hurst, J. W., and Logue, R. B.: Heart, 2nd ed. New York, McGraw-Hill Book Company, 1970, pp. 377–385.

195. Sones, F. M., Jr., and Shirey, E. K.: Cine coronary arteriography. Mod. Conc. Cardiovasc. Dis., 31:735, 1962.

196. Sonnenblick, E. H., Ross, J., Jr., and Braunwald, E.: Oxygen consumption of the heart: Newer concepts of its multifactoral determination. Am. J. Cardiol., 22:328, 1968.

197. Soulie, P., Laurens, P., Bouchard, F., Cornu, C., and Brial, E.: Enregistrement des pressions et des bruits intracardiaques à l'aide d'un micromanomètre. Bull. Soc. Med. Hop. Paris, 22:713, 1957.

198. Stern, T. N., Tacket, H. S., and Zachary, E. G.: Penetration into pericardial cavity during cardiac catheterization. Am. Heart J., 44:448, 1952.

199. Stewart, G. N.: Researches on the circulation time and on the influences which affect it. IV. The output of the heart. J. Physiol., 22:11, 1897.

200. Swan, H. J. C., Burchell, H. B., Linder, E., Birkhead, N. C., and Wood, E. H.: Symposium on diagnostic applications of indicator-dilution curves recorded from left and right sides of the heart. Part II. Mayo Clin. Proc., 33:581, 1958.

201. Swan, H. J., Ganz, W., Forrester, J., Marcus, H., Diamond, G., and Chonnett, D.: Catheterization of the heart in man with use of a flow-directed balloon-tipped catheter. N. Engl. J. Med., 283:447, 1970.

202. Van Slyke, D. D., and Neill, J. M.: Determination of gases in blood and other solutions by vacuum extraction and manometric measurement. J. Biol. Chem., 61:523, 1924.

203. Veragut, U. P., and Krayenbuhl, H. P.: Estimation and quantification of myocardial contractility in the closed-chest dog. Cardiologia 47:96, 1965.

204. Vogel, J. H. K., Tabari, K., Averill, K. H., and Blount, S. G., Jr.: A simple technique for identifying P waves in complex arrhythmias. Am. Heart J., 67:158, 1964.

205. Wagner, H. R., Gamble, W. J., Albers, W. H., and Hugenholtz, P. G.: Fiberoptic-dye dilution method for measurement of cardiac output. Circulation, 37:694, 1968.

206. Wallace, A. G., Skinner, N. S., Jr., and Mitchell, J.: Hemodynamic determinants of the maximal rate of rise of left ventricular pressure. Am. J. Physiol., 205:30, 1963.

207. Wallace, J. O., Brown, J. R., Lewis, D. H., and Deitz, G. W.: Acoustic mapping within the heart. J. Acoust. Soc. Am., 29:9, 1957.

208. Watson, H.: Electrode catheters and the diagnostic application of intracardiac electrography in small children. Circulation, 29:284, 1964.

209. Wiggers, C. J.: Dynamics of ventricular contraction under normal conditions. Circulation, 5:321, 1952.

210. Wood, E. H.: Diagnostic applications of indicator-dilution in techniques in congenital heart disease. Circ. Res., 10:531, 1962.

211. Wood, E. H., Swan, H. J. C., Fox, I. J., et al.: Symposium on diagnostic applications of indicator-dilution techniques. Mayo Clin. Proc., *32*:463, 1957.

212. Wright, J. L., Toscano-Barboza, E., and Brandenburg, R. O.: Left ventricular and aortic pressure pulses in aortic valvular disease. Mayo Clin. Proc., *31*:120, 1956.

213. Yamakawa, K., Shionoya, Y., Kitamura, K., Nagai, T., Yamomoto, T., and Ohta, S.: Intracardiac phonocardiography. Am. Heart J., *47*:424, 1954.

214. Yanof, H. M., Rosen, A. L., McDonald, N. M., and McDonald, D.

A.: Critical study of the response of manometers to forced oscillations. Phys. Med. Biol., *8*:407, 1963.

215. Zimmerman, H. A., and Hellerstein, H. K.: Cavity potentials of the human ventricles. Circulation, *3*:95, 1951.

216. Zimmerman, H. A., Scott, R. W., and Becker, N. O.: Catheterization of the left side of the heart in man. Circulation, *1*:357, 1950.

217. Zinn, W. J., Levinson, D. C., Johns, V., and Griffith, J. C.: The effect of angiocardiography on the heart as measured by electrocardiographic alterations. Circulation, *3*:658, 1951.

II

CARDIAC ARREST

Lazar J. Greenfield, M.D.

HISTORICAL PERSPECTIVE

Contemporary methods of resuscitation using expired air for ventilation can trace their origins back for thousands of years. The earliest inferences in the Bible relate the efforts of Hebrew midwives to resuscitate newborn infants during the period of Egyptian captivity in about 1300 B.C.[22] But the most specific and widely quoted reference describes the mouth-to-mouth resuscitation of the Shunemite child by Elisha in the eighth century B.C.[11] In more recent times, the manual technique of Sharpey-Schafer introduced in 1904[24] was in vogue for over 40 years, until its effectiveness was questioned by Comroe and Dripps.[5] The cycle was completed and mouth-to-mouth resuscitation restored to its rightful position of superiority based on the report of Gordon et al.[7] for the Council on Medical Physics of the American Medical Association.

Equally fascinating is the story of modern cardiac resuscitation. The identification of cardiac arrest began after the development and as a complication of general anesthesia. The first report resulted from cardiac arrest in 1848 in a young girl who was administered chloroform anesthesia in order to remove a toenail.[1] She did not recover, and the later efforts of Schiff to employ direct cardiac massage at thoracotomy were finally used successfully by Igelsrud in 1901.[23] But the problem of ventricular fibrillation seemed irreversible, even though Prevost and Batelli had demonstrated arrest of fibrillation in an animal by countershock in 1889.[17] Finally, in 1947, the studies of Carl Wiggers culminated in the successful open-chest defibrillation of a human heart by Claude Beck.[13] Later, Kouwenhoven and others developed the technique for closed-chest defibrillation and the modern era of resuscitation began. It remained for Bahnson to apply pressure to the sternum for external support of the circulation in a child, based on the observation of Knickerbocker[13] that arterial pressure was increased when the electrodes were applied to the chest wall, and then for Jude to use the technique in an adult.[12] Today these techniques are used by laymen and paramedical personnel alike and save countless lives each year.

DEFINITION AND INCIDENCE

Cardiopulmonary arrest is the unexpected cessation of effective ventilation and circulation in a person whose status may range from vigorous exertion to deep general anesthesia. The sequence of events may be initiated by unconsciousness with upper airway obstruction and asphyxiation. Even when there is a primary cardiac arrest such as from myocardial infarction or electrocution, the cause of death is always asphyxiation when circulation fails. This concept is important in the management of cardiopulmonary arrest, which must include effective oxygenation.

The frequency of cardiac arrest in the hospital is a major concern of the surgeon, and data from the Commission on Professional and Hospital Activities suggest that the frequency has increased.[18] The incidence of cardiac arrest related to anesthesia in the operating room at Duke University Hospital over a 10-year period was 1 per 1669 procedures,[26] but there is considerable variability in the statistics reported.[18] Earlier reviews suggested that approximately 500 to 600 deaths associated with anesthesia occur in the U.S. each year in University Hospitals,[2] and that figure is probably conservative considering the increasing complexity of surgery in generally older and more chronically ill patients.

PATHOGENESIS

The central nervous system is the tissue most vulnerable to interruption of circulation and oxygenation. Usually only 4 to 6 minutes of anoxia can be tolerated before the cellular damage is irreversible. After that time, the restoration of circulation may be accompanied by organ function in other areas of the body, but the loss of cerebral function represents the loss of identity and chance for recovery, and the person is legally dead.

Following cessation of circulation, the pupils begin to dilate in 30 to 45 seconds and the respiratory drive is lost after approximately 60 seconds as the medulla is depressed. The normothermic adult can tolerate only 4 minutes of this sequence in contrast to primary *respiratory* arrest when the circulation continues for several minutes. The pathophysiology of the latter situation includes many common problems:

1. *Airway obstruction* due to laryngeal spasm, mucus, or aspiration of blood, vomitus, or foreign body.

2. *Ventilatory failure* due to overdosage of paralytic drugs, myasthenia, poliomyelitis, or muscular dystrophy.

3. *Central depression* due to anesthesia, stroke, head injury, hypercapnia, or overdosage of narcotic, barbiturates, or tranquilizer drugs.

Even in the absence of primary respiratory failure, hypoxemia often contributes to the susceptibility to cardiac arrest. The clinical setting frequently involves the following:

1. *Chest trauma* producing pneumothorax, hemothorax, flail chest, or contused lung.

2. *Extensive atelectasis* in the immediate postoperative period.

3. *Pulmonary embolism* due to thrombi, fat, or air with pulmonary hypertension and hypoxemia.

4. *Reduced gas exchange* due to inhalation burn, pneumonia, congestive heart failure, septicemia, heavy metal poisoning, or multiple transfusion with particulate microembolism.

5. *Asphyxiation* due to smoke inhalation, carbon monoxide poisoning, or errors in anesthetic gas administration.

6. *Pulmonary arteriovenous shunting* due to congenital heart disease or ventilation-perfusion imbalance.

The pathogenesis of primary cardiac arrest usually is a more direct mechanical problem but may also be related to neurogenic factors. The vasovagal reflex is implicated during some procedures, and it can have a profound effect on the heart as demonstrated in tetraplegic patients whose compensatory sympathetic activity has been interrupted. In these patients simple tracheal suctioning for hypoxemia produces bradycardia and can induce cardiac arrest.[6] More commonly the causes of primary cardiac arrest include:

1. *Coronary occlusion* by thrombus, air, excessive contrast media injection, ligation, or dissection of the wall of the artery or emboli.[8]

2. *Reduced cardiac output* due to shock, arrhythmia, cardiac tamponade, myopathy, myocarditis, or direct trauma.

3. *Hyperkalemia* due to renal failure, excessive potassium administration, or rapid infusion of cold stored blood.

4. *Acidosis* due to diabetes mellitus, high intestinal fistula, starvation, hypothermia, or hypercapnia.

5. *Cardiac stimulation* by catheter, electrode, operative manipulation, electrocution, or inotropic drugs.

6. *Hypothermia* or *hyperthermia* from the environment or during extracorporeal circulation.

As a consequence of these adverse factors, the heart may cease to perform adequately in one of the following ways:

1. *Ventricular fibrillation,* which is most common following myocardial infarction and in the intensive care units where it may be anticipated by the onset of multifocal ventricular premature contractions.

2. *Mechanical asystole,* which often occurs in the operating room and is amenable to rapid treatment.

3. *Ineffective cardiac output* due to inadequate ventricular contraction often seen in association with hypoxemia or rhythm disturbances.

The mechanism of fibrillation is uncertain, but there are two major theories. One hypothesis suggests that there is a circular movement in which the cardiac action potential follows a circuitous pathway, re-entering the previously excited region after it has regained excitability. From this pathway, the impulses radiate to the remainder of the myocardium to produce the characteristic irregular, uncoordinated twitching that fails to eject blood. The second hypothesis contends that impulses are discharged at high frequency from one or more ectopic foci in the atria or ventricles. Although atrial fibrillation can revert to sinus rhythm under the influence of myocardial depressant drugs such as quinidine or procainamide, a more dramatic effect is required to defibrillate the ventricles. This conversion is accomplished by a strong electric current which places the entire myocardium in a refractory state. After depolarization, the normal S-A node should be able to resume pacing at a normal rate.

DIAGNOSIS

The recognition of ventilatory arrest is often easier than the recognition of circulatory insufficiency, since the lack of abdominal or thoracic movement and absence of breath sounds can be detected externally. Of course useless respiratory efforts will occur when there is upper airway obstruction. The diagnosis of cardiac arrest usually depends on absence of a palpable carotid or femoral pulse unless the surgeon is operating in the abdomen where the abdominal aorta is readily available. The radial pulse is not reliable for making this diagnosis. Additional support for the diagnosis is seen in the loss of normal color as skin and mucous membrane perfusion fails and loss of cerebral function is manifested by unconsciousness and dilated pupils.

Reliance upon electrocardiographic changes alone can be misleading, since electrical activity can persist long after cardiac action has become ineffective. Of more value is the immediate electrocardiographic evidence of fibrillation or premonitory arrhythmias. For this reason, the administration of general anesthesia should be accompanied by monitoring of the electrocardiogram on an oscilloscope at the least and for high-risk surgical procedures should include direct arterial pressure monitoring by an intra-arterial catheter. The latter also permits the monitoring of arterial blood gases by repetitive sampling. These measurements are important in the prevention of cardiac arrest by early treatment of the antecedent causes described previously. Vigilant monitoring by the anesthesiologist and surgeon assures that, if cardiac arrest occurs in the operating room, resuscitative measures can be instituted as rapidly as possible to increase the likelihood of effective restoration of heart action. This is certainly to be preferred to a diagnosis of cardiac arrest made by the operative evidence of lack of bleeding or dark discoloration of the blood.

Outside of the operating room, the diagnosis of cardiopulmonary arrest is made by absent arterial pulses. Even though it is known that a systolic arterial pressure of 50 mm. Hg may be present when a pulse is not palpable, a physician must act on the assumption of arrest and institute treatment without waiting for electrocardiographic confirmation or a blood pressure measurement. Delay is catastrophic in the management of cardiopulmonary arrest, and the goal of treatment is to prevent irreversible cerebral damage until more specific diagnosis and therapy can be undertaken. This is the advantage of the noninvasive external resuscitative measures to be described.

MANAGEMENT

The American Heart Association Committee on Cardiopulmonary Resuscitation (CPR) and Emergency Cardiac Care (ECC) in association with the National Academy of Sciences–National Research Council has established standards for cardiopulmonary resuscitation and emergency cardiac care.[25] These standards define a broad national program designed to provide the benefits of CPR and ECC to all segments of the population. The extension of training in basic life support to non-medical persons not only has placed greater responsibility on physicians for knowledge of the emergency medical system in their own communities, but has also increased the necessity for assurance of their own competence in CPR, since greater numbers of patients are being resuscitated and brought to the physician for further care.

BASIC LIFE SUPPORT

Following recognition of respiratory or cardiac arrest, basic life support is the emergency first-aid procedure which can maintain circulation and oxygenation until advanced life support is available. The mnemonic for basic life support is A–B–C, which refers to Airway–Breathing–Circulation. These steps must be started as rapidly as possible in the order described in the life support decision tree (Fig. 1).

The *airway* is opened by tilting the victim's head backward as far as possible using one hand on the forehead and the other behind the neck (Fig. 2). This

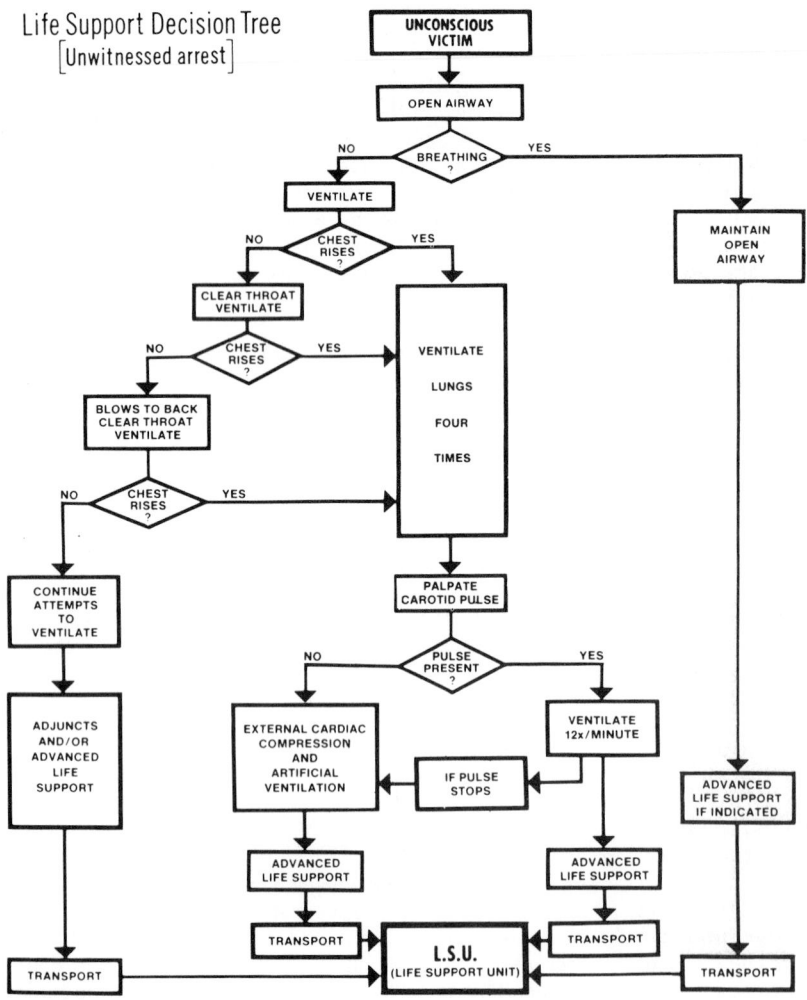

Life Support Decision Tree [Unwitnessed arrest]

Figure 1. The life support decision tree shown is the schematic management sequence for an unwitnessed cardiac arrest. (From Standards for Cardiopulmonary Resuscitation (CPR) and Emergency Cardiac Care (ECC). J.A.M.A., *227*:837, 1974.)

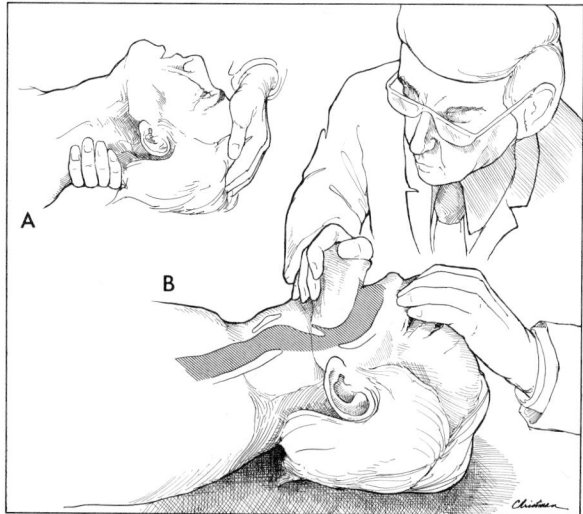

Figure 2. *A,* The initial step in resuscitation requires opening of the airway by tilting the head back and elevating the jaw if necessary to displace the tongue forward. *B,* The preparation for mouth-to-mouth resuscitation is to close the nose by compression and open the mouth. If the mouth cannot be opened, ventilation through the nose is possible if the lips are held closed.

maneuver lifts the tongue from the back of the throat, where it would otherwise obstruct the airway. Occasionally it may be necessary to displace the jaw farther forward to open the airway either by traction on the lower lip or pushing forward on the angles of the mandible.

Assuming that the patient does not begin to breathe spontaneously, artificial ventilation must be started using mouth-to-mouth or mouth-to-nose breathing. It is well established that the $F_{I_{O_2}}$ of expired air of about 0.16 is more than adequate for respiratory exchange. Although many devices have been introduced to facilitate ventilation under these circumstances, most are cumbersome and may actually increase airway resistance. In the hospital situation, an oral airway, self-inflating bag, and facemask often are available, which can improve ventilation until an endotracheal tube can be inserted.

Using either direct breathing or an anesthesia bag for ventilatory resuscitation, the inflation should be provided every 5 seconds and the victim permitted to exhale passively. The chest should be seen to expand with ventilation and air heard to escape during expiration. In infants and children, the rescuer may need to blow through both mouth and nose of the victim using smaller breaths, less backward tilting of the head, and more rapid cycles closer to every 3 seconds. Other modifications of technique are required if cervical spine injury is suspected, in which case the head should not be tilted, or in the presence of a suspected foreign body aspiration, when digital exploration of the airway is necessary.

In an unwitnessed cardiac arrest, the A–B–C sequence is initiated by four or five quick ventilations while the carotid pulse is palpated. If the pulse is absent, circulation (C) is initiated by external cardiac compression (Fig. 3). This is accomplished by compressing the lower half of the sternum approximately 2 inches, using the heels of both hands, keeping the arms straight, and maintaining a rate of 60 beats per minute. When two rescuers are present, ventilation should be performed after every fifth beat without interrupting cardiac compression, and if the rescuers are on opposite sides of the victim, they can trade places easily to avoid fatigue. When there is only one rescuer, he must perform two quick lung inflations after every 15 chest compressions, since the sternal compression does not produce adequate air exchange. Also he must increase the rate of chest compression to 80 beats per minute in order to average 60 beats per minute when the ventilation time is interposed. For infants, only two fingers are used for chest compression at rates of 80 to 100 beats per minute, and for children only one hand is applied at the level of midsternum because of the higher position of the heart in the chest.

In the event of a *witnessed* (immediately recognized) cardiac arrest or one occurring during monitoring, effective cardiac action may be restored by a blow to the sternum (precordial thump). This is delivered as a sharp blow with the ulnar side of the fist to midsternum from a distance of 8 to 12 inches, followed immediately by basic life support as outlined. It is not indicated in the presence of anoxia, as with unwitnessed

Figure 3. *A,* The correct position of the hands for cardiac compression is determined by palpation of the xiphoid with one hand and placement of the other on the sternum above that level. *B,* External cardiac compression is accomplished by depression of the sternum for a distance of 1½ to 2 inches using the heels of the hands and the weight of the rescuer at a rate of 60 beats per minute.

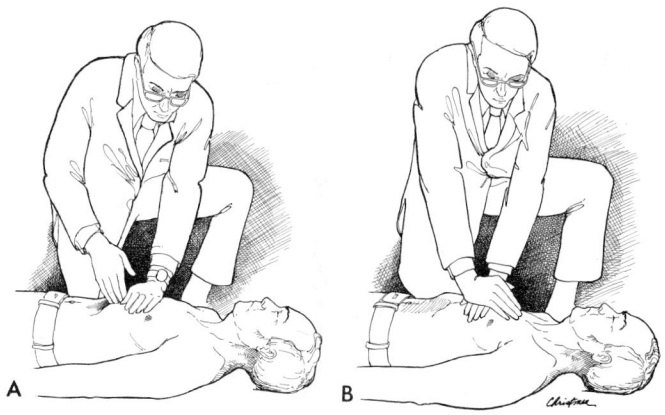

cardiac arrests, or in children. Its action is by a small electrical stimulus to a reactive heart and is most effective in asystole of short duration due to heart block.

Effective resuscitation results in a limited cardiac output of about 30 per cent of normal at best and, therefore, should be maintained without interruption of more than 5 to 10 seconds. It may take longer to intubate the patient's trachea, but the delay should not exceed 20 to 30 seconds at a time.

COMPLICATIONS OF CARDIOPULMONARY RESUSCITATION

The potential for injury to chest wall, heart, and lungs exists if CPR is applied improperly. Compression of the xiphoid, which angles downward, may cause laceration of the liver, and application of force on the parasternal region results in costochondral separation or rib fracture with its attendant complications of pneumothorax or hemothorax. Less commonly rupture of the stomach, fracture of the sternum or spleen, and fat emboli have been described.[4] These dangers can be minimized by steady, smooth compression of the sternum, keeping the fingers off the chest wall and using the heels of the hands as described.

DROWNING

Many healthy persons die annually as a result of drowning by mechanisms which relate to asphyxia in only about 10 per cent of cases.[15] Experimental studies have shown that the effects on the victim depend on the quantity and quality of fluid aspirated. During fresh water drowning, large volumes of fluid pass rapidly into the circulation, resulting in massive hemolysis and hemodilution.[28] The combination of hypoxia and hyponatremia also results in ventricular fibrillation.

The aspiration of sea water, on the other hand, which contains 3.5 per cent mixed salts, produces diffusion of salt into the circulation while fluid is drawn into the lung by osmosis, resulting in hypovolemia and hypotension.[28] Ventilation with air was noted to prevent pulmonary edema and death from near-drowning but was ineffective in preventing the ventricular fibrillation associated with fresh water drowning.[21]

Based on these studies, management should consist of:

1. Rapid mouth-to-mouth ventilation as soon as the victim is in shallow water and basic life support continued on land. Neither cardiac compression nor ventilatory support can be provided in deep water. No attempt should be made to try to evacuate water from the lungs. Ventilation with high $F_{I_{O_2}}$ should be started as soon as possible.

2. Arterial blood gas determinations should be followed closely to monitor the need for sustained positive pressure ventilation. Usually this is required for 48 to 72 hours to overcome the tendency for pulmonary arteriovenous shunting.

3. Aseptic tracheobronchial toilet should be maintained and antibiotics administered to control bacterial superinfection.

4. Examination of blood and urine for hemolysis after aspiration of fresh water often suggests the need for administration of packed red blood cells. Administration of plasma is indicated for victims of sea water aspiration. Acidosis should be corrected by administration of sodium bicarbonate, and steroids may be useful in reducing cerebral edema and the inflammatory reaction to aspiration.

ADVANCED LIFE SUPPORT

Many useful adjuncts to resuscitation are readily available in the hospital situation and can be applied while basic life support goes on uninterrupted. This would include supplemental oxygen applied by bag-valve-tube or bag-valve-mask system, oropharyngeal airway if an endotracheal tube cannot be inserted rapidly, intravenous infusion line, cardiac monitoring for dysrhythmia recognition and control, defibrillation, and definitive drug therapy to correct acidosis and restore effective cardiac rhythm and circulation. In addition, a bedboard or other firm support behind the patient's back should be used when the arrest occurs in a hospital bed. Manual or automatic chest compressors are available but are relatively awkward to use and limited to use in adults.

OPEN-CHEST CARDIAC MASSAGE

Open-chest cardiac compression may be required under certain circumstances such as following penetrating wounds of the heart or blunt chest injury when there is suspected cardiac tamponade, tension pneumothorax, or other internal thoracic injuries. In addition, it is advisable in patients with chest or spinal deformities, including severe emphysema with a barrel-chest, in which case closed-chest compression would be ineffective or dangerous. Similarly any time that closed-chest compression fails to provide effective circulation, the chest should be opened through the left fifth intercostal space and the pericardial sac opened to allow direct manual cardiac compression (Fig. 4). While the heart is rhythmically compressed with one hand, improved coronary perfusion can be obtained by compression of the ascending aorta with the other hand during diastole if the thoracotomy wound is extended and held open by a rib spreader. When the cardiac arrest occurs in the operating room during a laparotomy, the heart may be palpated and even compressed through the diaphragm. The emergency thoracotomy for direct cardiac massage allows visual assessment of the tone of the heart and presence of ventricular fibrillation, which can be corrected by direct application of electrodes for countershock. The unsterile thoracotomy is subject to infection and if the resuscitation is successful the patient should be transported to the operating room for closure of the wound under more sterile conditions which allow copious wound irrigation.

When the chest is not opened the differentiation between cardiac standstill and ventricular fibrillation

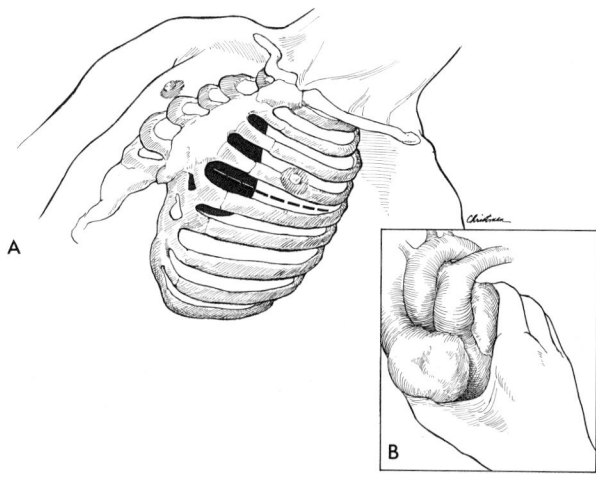

Figure 4. *A,* When open-chest cardiac compression is indicated, the incision should be made anteriorly in the fifth intercostal space as shown. The wound should be held open by a retractor if available and the pericardium opened to permit direct manual compression of the heart. *B,* Direct cardiac compression may be performed with either hand, but care must be taken to avoid excessive digital pressure on the thin-walled right ventricle, which may be perforated.

must be made by electrocardiogram. The availability of miniaturized oscilloscopes that are battery powered and packaged with a defibrillator unit has made the task of this differentiation more rapid and efficient. Generally, capacitance-discharge (DC) defibrillation is used today with the electrode pasted paddles applied to the right upper sternal border and at the apex of the heart. For an adult, the unit should be set to deliver the maximum of 400 watt-seconds. In children 60 to 100 watt-seconds should be used. After defibrillation, basic life support should be resumed immediately for sufficient reoxygenation to permit another 5-second pause to determine the cardiac rhythm.

PHARMACOLOGIC THERAPY

Effective cardiac compression provides sufficient circulation for drug action in all tissues and therefore intravenous injection usually is adequate for drug administration. An intracardiac injection not only introduces the possibility of tamponade, coronary artery injury, and pneumothorax, but it obligates cessation of cardiac compression. In the absence of a reliable intravenous route, the intracardiac injection should be made after the needle is inserted under negative pressure to insure placement in the ventricular cavity. Several drugs are essential early in the management of cardiac arrest:

1. *Sodium bicarbonate* is needed to combat metabolic acidosis and is administered in an initial dose of 1 mEq. per kg. intravenously by bolus or continuous infusion. In the presence of ventricular fibrillation, defibrillation should be performed immediately, then bicarbonate administered. If defibrillation is not successful, a second dose of bicarbonate may be ad-

ministered, but it is safer to confirm the need for the drug by arterial blood gas and pH measurement. Using the measured base deficit, the bicarbonate dose (mEq.) = $\frac{1}{2}$ base deficit $\times$ $\frac{1}{4}$ body weight (kg.). Alkalosis with secondary hyperosmolality and cerebral acidosis should be avoided, since it also adversely affects tissue oxygen unloading by hemoglobin.

2. *Epinephrine* has been one of the most effective drugs used in cardiac resuscitation[16] and the primary benefit appears to be a result of its vasoconstrictor effect, which is matched by other vasoconstrictors such as phenylephrine[20] and methoxamine.[19] The positive inotropic effects of epinephrine and other cardiotonic drugs do not improve the results of resuscitation,[9] and thus there is less need for intracardiac administration. The positive chronotropic effect of epinephrine can convert asystole to sinus rhythm or improve the rate in bradycardia. Therefore, it is indicated for all types of cardiac arrest and should be administered initially at a dose of 0.5 mg. and repeated at 5-minute intervals or as an infusion of 1 to 4 μgm. per minute.

3. *Calcium chloride* also has positive chronotropic and inotropic effects, and enhances ventricular irritability. It should be used with caution in the fully digitalized patient, in whom it may cause sinus impulse suppression. Usually it is given in increments of 5 ml. of a 10 per cent solution (0.5 gm.) at 5-minute intervals. If calcium gluconate is used, there is less ionizable calcium per unit volume and the dose should be 10 ml. of a 10 per cent solution. Neither form of the drug should be mixed with bicarbonate, which forms a precipitate.

4. *Atropine sulfate* reduces vagal tone and enhances A-V conduction, which makes it particularly useful in treatment of sinus bradycardia associated with myocardial infarction. It should be used to treat any sinus bradycardia of less than 60 beats per minute or a high degree A-V block at a bolus dose of 0.5 mg. intravenously. The dose may be repeated at 5-minute intervals until a rate above 60 beats per minute is reached or a total of 2.0 mg. has been given.

5. *Lidocaine* is a useful drug for its antiarrhythmic properties and acts to elevate the fibrillation threshold. It helps to control multifocal premature ventricular contractions, ventricular tachycardia, and the tendency for fibrillation to occur after defibrillation. It is administered intravenously in a dose of 50 to 100 mg., which can be supplemented by a continuous infusion of 1 to 3 mg. per minute. If the arrhythmia persists, procainamide (100 mg.) should be administered.

Other agents may be useful under some circumstances, such as morphine sulfate in the treatment of pain after myocardial infarction and isoproterenol for complete heart block or refractory sinus bradycardia. Propranolol also has been useful in suppression of ventricular arrhythmias, and corticosteroids may be useful in treatment of cerebral edema following cardiac arrest. Also diuretic agents, hypothermia, and controlled hyperventilation have been useful in managing the latter complication. All resuscitated patients should be placed in an intensive care facility for monitoring of electrocardiogram, urine output, blood gases, and vital signs to avoid recurrent cardiopulmonary arrest.

TERMINATION OF LIFE SUPPORT

The decision to terminate life support must be made by a physician based on the cerebral and cardiovascular status of the patient. Nonreactive pupils and lack of respiration or consciousness persisting for periods in excess of 15 to 30 minutes usually reflect cerebral death and the futility of further resuscitative effort. Similarly, absence of any cardiac electrical activity persisting after 10 minutes of resuscitation usually reflects cardiac death, although occasionally a transthoracic pacemaker lead may restore cardiac action.

In certain situations CPR is not indicated, such as in a patient with a terminal irreversible illness. Under these circumstances resuscitation is generally not wise.

RESULTS OF RESUSCITATION

As CPR became well standardized and administered by trained medical and paramedical personnel, the results of treatment improved but were still limited by the underlying disease process. In a review of 150 episodes of arrest in 137 unselected patients in a general hospital,[3] the resuscitation was successful in 35 per cent (48 of 137 patients). However, only 14 patients survived to leave the hospital. A second episode of cardiac arrest occurred in 10 of the surviving patients and 4 (40 per cent) were resuscitated successfully. A third arrest occurred in 3 patients, of whom 1 was resuscitated, but none of the patients with more than one episode of arrest were long-term survivors. In general only 12 to 20 per cent of resuscitated patients leave the hospital, but their subsequent course is encouraging. In a review of 230 patients who survived resuscitation and left the hospital, 74 per cent were alive at the end of one year and 51 per cent were alive after 3 years.[14]

The mechanism of arrest is a major determinant of survival. Initial evidence of ventricular standstill is particularly ominous and usually the likelihood of resuscitation after asystole is remote.[3] Ventricular fibrillation, on the other hand, is more encouraging, probably because it represents the earliest period of arrest as opposed to the later asystole. Approximately 30 per cent of patients in fibrillation can be resuscitated with survival.[27] However, in contrast to other major complications, younger age has an adverse effect on survival, with the best results obtained in the 40- to 49-year-old group, which showed only a 17 per cent survival rate after one month in a series of 536 patients requiring resuscitation.[29] Because of these disappointing survival rates, a more aggressive approach is warranted in those patients who have preexisting symptoms of coronary artery disease and who survive resuscitation in the community setting. In one series of 16 such patients who had hemodynamic and coronary arterial angiographic studies, 8 underwent myocardial revascularization with no operative deaths and one late death.[10] Since the first presenting symptom of coronary artery disease may well be cardiac arrest, it will probably prove worthwhile to study all unexpected cardiac arrest survivors by coronary arteriography to try to diagnose surgically treatable disease and to improve long-term survival by coronary artery bypass surgery.

SELECTED REFERENCES

Goldberg, A. H.: Current concepts: Cardiopulmonary arrest. N. Engl. J. Med., *290*:381, 1974.
This is a concise review article on the practical application of basic and advanced CPR in the hospitalized patient. It outlines management goals and methods and reviews drug therapy and dosages employed as a practical guide to resuscitation.

Kouwenhoven, W. B., and Langworthy, O. R.: Cardiopulmonary resuscitation. An account of forty-five years of research. Johns Hopkins Med. J., *132*:186, 1973.
This is a fascinating account of the history of cardiopulmonary resuscitation by a pioneer in the field whose background in electrical engineering made him uniquely suited to bridge the gap from his own discipline to medicine.

Redding, J. S.: Advances in cardiopulmonary resuscitation. Clin. Anesth., *3*:485, 1969.
From the vantage point of extensive laboratory and clinical experience, the author reviews the pathophysiology of cardiopulmonary arrest. The evaluation of adjunctive mechanical and drug therapy is outlined and the rationale for current practices presented. There is an excellent section on drowning and on the management of acute myocardial infarction.

Standards for Cardiopulmonary Resuscitation (CPR) and Emergency Cardiac Care (ECC). J.A.M.A. (Suppl.), *227*:837, 1974.
These standards represent the recommendations of the National Conference on Cardiopulmonary Resuscitation (CPR) and Emergency Cardiac Care (ECC) held in Washington, D.C., May 16 to 18, 1973, under the auspices of the American Heart Association and the National Academy of Sciences–National Research Council. The criteria of basic and advanced life-support are well reviewed and the capabilities of life-support units are detailed. A separate section on medicolegal considerations and recommendations is brief but valuable, including specific recommendations for necessary legislative action.

REFERENCES

1. Beecher, H. K.: The first anesthesia death, with some remarks suggested by it in the fields of the laboratory and the clinic in the appraisal of new anesthetic agents. Anesthesiology, *2*:433, 1941.
2. Beecher, H. K., and Todd, D. P.: A study of deaths associated with anesthesia and surgery. Ann. Surg., *140*:2, 1954.
3. Castagna, J., Wed, M. H., and Shubin, H.: Factors determining survival in patients with cardiac arrest. Chest, *65*:527, 1974.
4. Clark, D. T.: Complication following closed chest massage. J.A.M.A., *181*:337, 1962.
5. Comroe, J. G., and Dripps, R. D.: Artificial respiration. J.A.M.A., *130*:381, 1946.
6. Frankel, H. L., Mathias, C. J., and Spalding, J. M. K.: Mechanisms of reflex cardiac arrest in tetraplegic patients. Lancet, *4*:1183, 1975.
7. Gordon, A. S., Frye, C. W., Gittelson, L., Sadove, M. S., and Beattie, E. J., Jr.: Mouth-to-mouth versus manual artificial respiration for children and adults. J.A.M.A., *167*:320, 1958.
8. Greenfield, L. J., and Gaertner, R. A.: Coronary embolectomy following mitral valvotomy on cardiopulmonary bypass. Ann. Thorac. Surg., *1*:448–452, 1965.
9. Jude, J. R., Neumaster, T., and Kfoury, E.: Vasopressor-cardiotonic drugs in cardiac resuscitation. Acta Anesth.(Second Suppl.), *29*:147, 1968.
10. Kaiser, G. A., Ghahramani, A., Bolooki, H., Vargas, A., Thurer, R. J., Williams, W. H., and Myerburg, R. J.: Role of coronary artery surgery in patients surviving unexpected cardiac arrest. Surgery, *78*:749, 1975.
11. II Kings 4:32–35.
12. Kouwenhoven, W. B., Jude, J. R., and Knickerbocker, G. G.: Closed chest cardiac massage. J.A.M.A., *173*:1064, 1960.
13. Kouwenhoven, W. B., and Langworthy, O. R.: Cardiopulmonary resuscitation. An account of forty-five years of research. Johns Hopkins Med. J., *132*:186, 1973.

14. Lemire, G., and Johnson, A. L.: Is cardiac resuscitation worthwhile? A decade of experience. N. Engl. J. Med., *286*:970, 1972.
15. Moritz, A. R.: Chemical methods for determinations of death by drowning. Physiol. Rev., *24*:70, 1944.
16. Pearson, J. W., and Redding, J. S.: Epinephrine in cardiac resuscitation. Am. Heart J., *66*:210, 1963.
17. Prevost, J., and Batelli, F.: La mort par les courants électrique. J. Gen. Physiol., *1*:1085, 1899.
18. Raskind, R., Glover, M. B., and Wall, F. J.: Cardiac arrest: Part one, scope of current problem. Vasc. Surg., *6*:31, 1972.
19. Redding, J. S.: Advances in cardiopulmonary resuscitation. Clin. Anesth., *3*:485, 1969.
20. Redding, J. S., and Pearson, J. W.: Evaluation of drugs for cardiac resuscitation. Anesthesiology, *24*:203, 1963.
21. Redding, J. S., Voigt, G. C., and Safar, P.: Drowning treated with intermittent positive pressure breathing. J. Appl. Physiol., *15*:849, 1960.
22. Rosen, Z., and Davidson, J. T.: Respiratory resuscitation in ancient Hebrew sources. Anesth. Analg., *51*:502, 1972.
23. Schiff, M., and Keen, W. W. Cited in Jude, J. R.: Cardiac arrest and resuscitation. *In* Artz, C. P., and Hardy, J. D.: Management of Surgical Complications. Philadelphia, W. B. Saunders Company, 1975, pp. 108–118.
24. Schäfer, E. A.: The relative efficiency of certain methods of performing artificial respiration in man. Proc. R. Soc. Edinburgh, *25*:39–50, 1904.
25. Standards for Cardiopulmonary Resuscitation (CPR) and Emergency Cardiac Care (ECC). J.A.M.A., *227*:837, 1974.
26. Stephenson, H. E., Jr.: Cardiac arrest and resuscitation, 3rd ed. St. Louis, The C. V. Mosby Co., 1969.
27. Stiles, Q. R., Tucker, B. L., Meyer, B. W., Lindesmith, G. G., and Jones, J. C.: Cardiopulmonary arrest, evaluation of an active resuscitation program. Am. J. Surg., *122*:282, 1971.
28. Swann, H. G., and Spafford, N. R.: Body salt and water changes during fresh and sea water drowning. Texas Rep. Biol. Med., *9*:356, 1951.
29. Wildsmith, J. A., Dennyson, W. G., and Myers, K. W.: Results of resuscitation following cardiac arrest. Br. J. Anesth., *44*:716, 1972.

III

PATENT DUCTUS ARTERIOSUS, COARCTATION OF THE AORTA, AND ANOMALIES OF THE AORTIC ARCH

Henry T. Bahnson, M.D.

HISTORICAL ASPECTS

The history of these three conditions, generally included in classifications of congenital heart disease, centers on the contributions of Robert E. Gross, who in 1938 first successfully ligated a patent ductus arteriosus and thus introduced the use of surgical treatment for congenital heart disease. In 1944, Blalock and Park described experimental methods for treatment of coarctation of the aorta by anastomosis of the left subclavian artery to the distal aorta. In the following year (1945), Gross and Crafoord and Nylin independently described excision of the coarctation and primary anastomosis of the aorta, the method preferred today. Gross and his associates in 1949 used aortic homografts to replace deficiencies following excision of coarctation of the aorta, reviving a technique that had been described by Carrel and Guthrie in 1906. Gross and Ware were the first to recognize that anomalies of the aortic arch caused tracheal or esophageal obstruction that was amenable to surgical treatment and described this in 1946. In the three decades that have followed these milestones, numerous contributions have further clarified the pathophysiology and the diagnostic and therapeutic variations of these defects, and all can now be satisfactorily treated surgically.

PATENT DUCTUS ARTERIOSUS

Treatment of the patent ductus arteriosus is representative of the rapid advances made in thoracic surgery in the last 30 years. Less than three decades ago ligation of a ductus arteriosus was a "pièce de résistance" performed by a few surgeons in the country. Now, interruption is done by most thoracic surgeons, and it is considered one of the simplest operations, often performed incidentally at the time of open repair of intracardiac defects. Interruption of a ductus can be accomplished with little risk and is one of the most satisfactory and curative operations in the field of surgery of the heart and great vessels.

Pathologic Anatomy

In the majority of typical cases the only discernible abnormality is the presence of the duct joining the main, or left, pulmonary artery with the lesser curvature of the aortic arch opposite the left subclavian artery, and the channel thus conducts an aortic-pulmonary shunt of blood. The diameter may vary from several millimeters to 1 or 2 cm. It is variable in length, some of the large ducts being almost flush aortic-pulmonary connections. Aberrant positions of the ductus do occur but are rare; it is almost always on the left, even in the presence of a right aortic arch, when it joins the pulmonary artery and distal left innominate artery. The ductus, a structure present during fetal life, normally closes soon after birth. Christie (1930)[7] studied 558 infants and found that the ductus was open 2 weeks after birth in 65 per cent but that this number rapidly decreased, and only 2 per cent were open after 32 weeks and 1 per cent at 1 year. Many of these were small openings and functionally unimportant.

In most cases of patent ductus arteriosus there are no secondary changes, but in those patients with pulmonary hypertension there may be marked intimal proliferation of the medium and small pulmonary arteries, muscular hypertrophy of these vessels, and organizing or organized thrombi in the pulmonary arteries.[10] Somewhat similar pathologic findings are noted in the lungs of normal infants, but these changes regress with age and with lowering of the pulmonary arterial pressure.[12] Whether the pulmonary vascular changes are present at birth and never regress in patients with patent ductus and pulmonary hypertension, or whether they regress and then reform with the continued high pulmonary flow, has not been conclusively demonstrated. It is unlikely that this will be proved in the future, since, in view of the low operative risk, the condition will not be allowed to follow its natural course without treatment.

Clinical Manifestations

The symptoms of patients with patent ductus arteriosus vary widely from none to severe cardiac failure, the variation depending upon age, the size of the aortic-pulmonary shunt, and undetermined factors. Some children grow normally, have no shortness of breath or other limitation of activity, and lead fairly normal lives. A significant number of children are retarded in physical growth, in some instances strikingly. In many cases, particularly if the ductus is a moderately large one, the additional burden on the heart becomes apparent as the patient ages, as evidenced by loss of energy, shortness of breath, and fatigue. A typical ductus not accompanied by superimposed pulmonary hypertension or an additional cardiac defect rarely causes cardiac failure, but failure may be a problem, particularly in infants with a large ductus in whom there is pulmonary hypertension and often a high pulmonary blood flow.

Subacute bacterial endarteritis at the site of the ductus is a less frequent problem now than it was prior to the use of antibiotics. Endarteritis occurs most commonly in young adults but rather infrequently in children and is manifested by fever, weight loss, anemia, and positive blood cultures.

That the typical patent ductus arteriosus appears to be an innocuous lesion in many children may lead to the assumption that the condition is compatible with a long life and little or no disability, but such is not usually the case. Keys and Shapiro (1943) found that those who are alive at 17 years of age with a patent ductus arteriosus have a subsequent life expectancy about one-half that of the normal population. Campbell[5] has concluded, on the basis of review of his own large experience and others' reported experiences, that

by age 45, 42 per cent of patients with a patent ductus arteriosus will have died. Although his data also showed that spontaneous closure of the ductus may occur even later in life, this occurs too infrequently to justify it as a hoped-for solution to the problem.

The heart is usually normal in size or only slightly enlarged. In the presence of a large ductus it may be overactive. There may be a normal systolic blood pressure with a low diastolic level because of the run-off into the pulmonary circuit, and this may be accompanied by peripheral signs similar to those of aortic insufficiency. The murmur is a characteristic one and allows an accurate diagnosis of the condition in about 95 per cent of cases. In the typical case, it is a continuous murmur, often rumbling in systole, sometimes obscuring the pulmonary second sound, is heard most prominently in the right second to third intercostal space, and is frequently associated with a thrill. The pulmonary second sound may be accentuated. The rumbling systolic phase, the banging second sound, and the continuous murmur give the impression of machinery, the name usually applied to it. Transmission of the murmur depends largely on its intensity, the systolic phase usually being transmitted more widely than the diastolic. If the channel is small, only a systolic murmur may be heard, although the flow and turbulence are probably continuous. If the shunt of blood through the ductus is extremely large, there may be a rumbling diastolic murmur at the apex of the heart suggestive of relative mitral stenosis; there may be other murmurs due to a large blood flow through the active heart. When heart failure occurs with pulmonary hypertension, the murmur may be obscured or otherwise altered. Other variations in the murmur will be mentioned in connection with the atypical ductus.

Roentgenologic studies show the heart to be of normal size or slightly enlarged. When enlargement is significant, it is apt to be predominantly of the left atrium and left ventricle. The region of the left pulmonary artery is often full along the upper left contour of the heart. The lung fields show increased vascularity, and there may be a hilar dance, although this is not so striking in patients with a ductus as in those with a left-to-right intracardiac shunt. These changes are not specific for the patent ductus, since the picture may be similar to that of other shunts, notably a ventricular septal defect. Although it often cannot be determined by routine radiologic methods, the ascending aorta characteristically is larger in the patient with a patent ductus (by virtue of the flow through it) than in one with a ventricular septal defect. Increased pulmonary blood flow results in enlargement of the left atrium; this enlargement may be demonstrated by echocardiography, comparing dimensions of the left atrium with those of the aortic root to detect an increase in the former.[32]

A patent ductus may be an important factor in aggravation of the respiratory distress syndrome of the newborn, especially in premature infants.[21] There is a high incidence of patency of the ductus in premature infants, probably related to immaturity of the tissue in the duct which at birth begins the process of closure. Hypoxia of respiratory distress may be an added element in persistent patency, for a high level of oxygen in pulmonary artery blood enhances closure at birth. In the newborn infant with the respiratory distress syndrome, the presence of an appropriate murmur, bounding femoral pulses, unusual vascularity of the lung fields, and greater than usual right ventricular hypertrophy on the electrocardiogram should indicate the need for a diagnostic cardiac catheterization and ductal ligation if a large shunt is found. In a few cases irritation of the duct by a catheter has seemed to induce closure. The operative closure of the ductus, even in a 1 kg. infant, is well tolerated, but this is only one of many important facets in the sophisticated care of these sick infants.

Infusion of prostaglandins E₁ and E₂ has been shown to dilate the constricted ductus arteriosus, and conversely, administration of indomethacin, a potent inhibitor of prostaglandin synthetase, has resulted in constriction and closure of the patent ductus. This drug treatment of patent ductus has been most useful and efficacious in the premature newborn with respiratory distress syndrome.[15, 20]

Atypical Patent Ductus Arteriosus. When significant pulmonary hypertension exists, the patient does not present a typical picture. This may be the case in infants with an otherwise ordinary ductus. At birth the pulmonary artery pressure is elevated, but it normally falls rapidly in the first few months. Because of the reduced pressure gradient between the aorta and the pulmonary artery in neonatal life, blood does not flow continuously, and only a systolic murmur may be heard. As the child becomes older, the typical, continuous murmur appears.

On the other hand, there is a group of patients in whom moderate to severe distress is caused by a ductus and pulmonary hypertension. Dammann and Sell[10] and Ziegler[36] focused attention upon the ductus as a cause of disability and of cardiac failure in this group of infants and young children. The atypical ductus is seen most frequently in infants and young children and again in young adults, with a paucity of cases in the intermediate age. In almost all instances the ductus proves to be a large one. Infants and young children frequently are scrawny, underdeveloped, and subject to colds and infection, with dyspnea, some cardiac enlargement, and often signs of cardiac failure. The precordium is active. The murmur is usually a systolic one or one with a short diastolic element, often separated by a pause, indicating the lack of a continuous aortic-pulmonary pressure gradient. The pulmonary second sound is characteristically loud, indicative of hypertension. Radiologically the lung fields are vascular, both from increased flow and from congestive changes.

In infants and many children there is apt to be a high pulmonary blood flow with only a moderate increase in pulmonary vascular resistance. In some children and in most adults with pulmonary hypertension and an atypical ductus, there is a tendency toward lower pulmonary blood flow and high pulmonary vascular resistance. In such instances, the heart is less active and not so large. In its extreme, the atypical ductus is associated with a reverse flow, pulmonary blood entering the aorta and causing cyanosis of the toes in contrast to fingers of normal color. This late and probably irreversible stage is rarely seen in children, a fact that lends support to the concept that the pulmonary vascular changes are progressive.

Diagnosis

In 95 per cent of cases the diagnosis can be made easily and simply, largely on the basis of the charac-

teristic continuous murmur. The murmur may be simulated by a venous hum, although a hum is usually more prominent over the right upper chest, is less intense with the patient supine, and may be obliterated by compression of the jugular vein in the neck. Arteriovenous fistulas of the lung cause a similar murmur, although this type is usually high-pitched and is transmitted more widely for its intensity, and the lesion frequently can be seen in the lung field on a plain roentgenogram.

The diagnosis can be sufficiently certain and other abnormalities excluded on the basis of the murmur, roentgenogram, and electrocardiogram so that one might proceed with operation in the majority of typical cases. In others, there may still be uncertainty after use of the noninvasive diagnostic methods. Cardiac catheterization, and especially its associated cineangiocardiography, should establish the diagnosis in almost all instances with demonstration of a right-to-left shunt into the pulmonary artery and opacification of the channel or passage of a catheter through it. A more proximally located aorticopulmonary window may be hardest to differentiate, but it is relatively uncommon.

Selection of Patients for Operation

Establishment of the diagnosis in a child is sufficient indication for interruption of an uncomplicated patent ductus arteriosus. The operative risk should be little more than that of the anesthesia, and the cure is complete. Clatworthy and McDonald[8] pointed out that the operative morbidity in infants and young children is no greater than that seen in older children and advocated operation in children with symptoms when the diagnosis is established or in asymptomatic patients before the age of 5. They saw little advantage in postponing operation. Trusler et al.[33] advocate closure before age 2 years to avoid the greater psychologic trauma between ages 2 and 4. The operative risk is small; the only deaths were in infants in failure less than 6 months old. At present a new indication for ductal obliteration is in some premature infants with the respiratory distress syndrome who show signs of increased pulmonary blood flow. Interruption in some infants weighing 1 to 2 kg. has strikingly changed the course of their illness.

A difficult problem arises in treating the patient, usually an adult or older child, with pulmonary hypertension and a reverse ductus. When pulmonary hypertension is striking and in the presence of a reversed shunt, there may be such severe pulmonary vascular resistance that the patient will not tolerate the stresses of the postoperative period. Cyanosis of the toes or evidence of significant right ventricular hypertrophy as seen electrocardiographically suggests that an irreversible condition has developed. Ellis et al.[14] presented a good analysis of the problem and concluded that if the shunt is predominantly left to right but nearly balanced, operation is probably indicated but involves considerable risk. Indications are clearer for operation when the shunt is only left to right without right to left, since several studies have shown a decrease in pulmonary artery pressure and pulmonary vascular resistance after interruption of a ductus with pulmonary hypertension. The condition is more apt to be reversible in young children than in adults. When flow is predominantly right to left, there is great operative risk and little chance of benefit from the operative closure. Several studies have shown a decrease in pulmonary artery pressure and pulmonary vascular resistance after interruption of a ductus with pulmonary hypertension, but in follow-up of 68 patients after closure of a ventricular septal defect Du Shane and Kirklin[11] found that of those patients operated upon after age 2 with moderately or severely elevated pulmonary vascular resistance, over half had persistence of the high pulmonary resistance. When operated upon before age 2, over 90 per cent had a favorable result. The observations are probably applicable to patent ductus arteriosus and emphasize the need for early operation when pulmonary artery pressure and resistance are high. The condition is more apt to be reversible in young children than in adults.

In some cases, as in the tetralogy of Fallot, the ductus is a compensating structure. The ductus must not be interrupted in such cases unless the condition for which it is compensating can be corrected.

Operative Technique

Whether the ductus is surgically exposed from an anterolateral or posterolateral incision is largely a matter of personal preference. Mobilization of the aorta may be accomplished more easily through a posterolateral fourth interspace incision. However, exposure is more time-consuming and the position increases ventilatory embarrassment; we have used this approach only for the uncommon patient with a mycotic aneurysm involving the ductus or for the patient with an extremely large main pulmonary artery, which might obscure the exposure of the ductus anteriorly.

We prefer to make an incision through the third interspace, going below the breast in females (Fig. 1). The incision must extend well around laterally, with division of almost the entire intercostal muscle bundle, separating the serratus and dividing the anterior edge of the latissimus dorsi, so that one obtains good exposure well up into the axilla. In our experience this has given wide and ample exposure of the ductus, adjacent aorta, and pulmonary artery. An incision is made overlying the pulmonary artery between the phrenic and vagus nerves. If the ductus is not readily seen, it may be

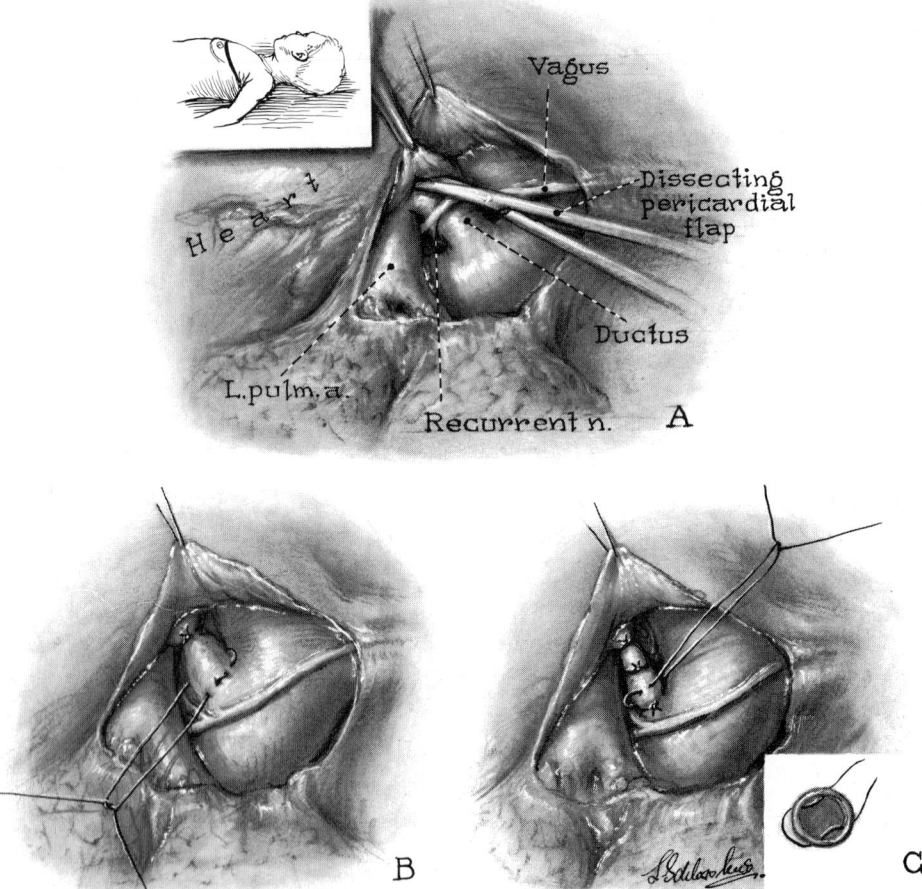

Figure 1. Operative treatment of ductus arteriosus by ligation. Incision is anterolateral in the third interspace. In females the incision circles beneath the breast. Elevation of pericardial lappet exposes the ductus. A purse-string suture, which does not enter the lumen, is placed at each end, and perforating mattress sutures are placed in between. The ductus should be obliterated over an 8 to 10 mm. distance. (From Bahnson, H. T. *In* Sabiston, D. C., Jr., and Spencer, F. C., (Eds.): Gibbon's Surgery of the Chest, 3rd ed. Philadelphia, W. B. Saunders Company, 1976.)

found by tracing the recurrent branch of the vagus nerve around the ductus and the aorta. There is usually a small lappet of pericardium extending over the ductus that should be elevated, and the ductus should be bared of its adventitia and freed of attachments.

Sharp dissection around the great vessels under direct vision is preferable to blunt, tearing dissection. The angle between the distal pulmonary artery and the ductus is particularly susceptible to injury. Attachments between the pericardium, pulmonary artery, and lesser curvature of the aortic arch should be exposed and divided. After the ductus is mobilized as much as possible and the adjacent pulmonary artery and aorta freed, a right-angle clamp may be placed around the ductus and umbilical tape passed. This clamp is probably more safely passed behind the ductus from the caudal, distal, aortic side. In order to obtain additional length slight traction may be applied on the tape and the ductus can be freed posteriorly.

There is room for personal preference also in the method of interruption of the ductus.[13] Most would agree that, theoretically, closure of any large artery can best be accomplished by division of the artery. In actual practice, however, multiple-suture ligation of the ductus with occlusion over the entire length of the ductus has given excellent results (Scott, 1950). Ligation with multiple transfixing sutures was championed by Blalock[2] (1946) at a time when division was associated with considerably greater risk than it is at present. The method is safe and satisfactory. If ligation is to be done, purse-string sutures are placed at the aortic and pulmonary ends and tied snugly, so that the flow through the ductus is nearly obliterated (Fig. 1). Two mattress sutures are then placed between these, and the ductus is obliterated over a length of 1 cm. or more.

Increased experience with the great vessels and particularly the development of finer clamps for occluding vessels have greatly reduced the risk of division of the ductus. This procedure is probably now practiced more widely than ligation. After the ductus is mobilized as much as possible, fine vascular clamps, such as the multitooth Potts ductus clamp, are placed on the aortic and pulmonary ends with sufficient room in between for division and closure (Fig. 2). When the ductus is divided, the occluding clamps must be held against the pulmonary artery and the aorta; this lessens the danger of their being pulled off and at the same time gives greater exposure for suture closure. A satisfactory method is to suture adjacent to the clamp with a mattress suture and continue back over the free edge with an over-and-over whip suture. After both openings are sutured, a sponge is held in the area for compression while the occluding vascular clamps are removed. An additional suture occasionally may be necessary to control bleeding. Suturing the lappet of pericardium across the pulmonary end of the divided ductus to tissue posterior, between the pulmonary artery and aorta, separates the two ends more completely.

If the ductus is unusually large, greater than 1.5 cm. in diameter, simple ligation is dangerous because of the possibility of the suture's tearing through the wall. Division of the ductus is advocated in such patients. When the ductus is extremely short and large, one can gain added length for closure by clamping the ductus at the pulmonary end and then cross-clamping the aorta just above and below the ductus. The ductus is then divided with sufficient cuff on the pulmonary end for closure, and the tangential opening in the aorta is closed while the aorta is collapsed. The safe occlusion time of the aorta is unknown and unpredictable,[13] but 15 minutes' occlusion is probably safe, and this should be ample to allow closure.

An alternate method of clamp application, employed routinely by several surgeons, is to use a tangential vascular clamp to occlude part of the aorta from which the ductus arises, rather than clamping the ductus itself. This is especially useful if the ductus is short.

In older adults, calcification of the ductus and adjacent aorta may make the application of clamps hazardous. In such instances a form of left heart bypass should be used, permitting occlusion of the aorta above and below the ductus.

Convalescence should be uneventful in the patient with the typical ductus. When cardiac failure, pulmonary hypertension, or endarteritis of the ductus is present, the convalescence may be correspondingly less smooth.

Results of Operation

Few operations in cardiac surgery are more satisfyingly curative than that for patent ductus arteriosus. The work of the heart is immediately lowered as the burden of the excessive shunt is removed. In 689 cases of all types at the Johns Hopkins Hospital, both typical and atypical, with and without cardiac failure, and with additional defects in a number of cases, the mor-

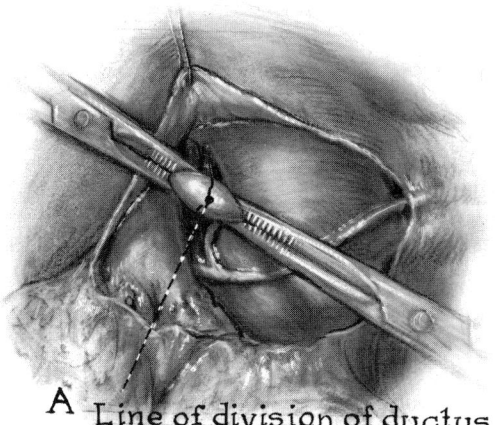
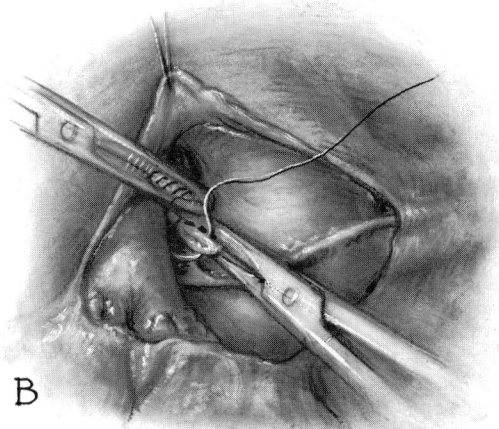

A Line of division of ductus   B

Figure 2. Treatment of ductus arteriosus by division. Anterolateral third interspace incision is used with exposure as for ligation. A thin occluding clamp is placed at each end and the ductus is divided. Pressing the clamp against the pulmonary artery or aorta after division reduces likelihood of slipping. Suture of ductus is by a continuous mattress suture adjacent to clamp, followed by whip stitch back up over the free edge. Suture of the pulmonary artery is easier when done from the patient's right side. (From Bahnson, H. T. *In* Sabiston, D. C., Jr., and Spencer, F. C. (Eds.): Gibbon's Surgery of the Chest, 3rd ed. Philadelphia, W. B. Saunders Company, 1976.)

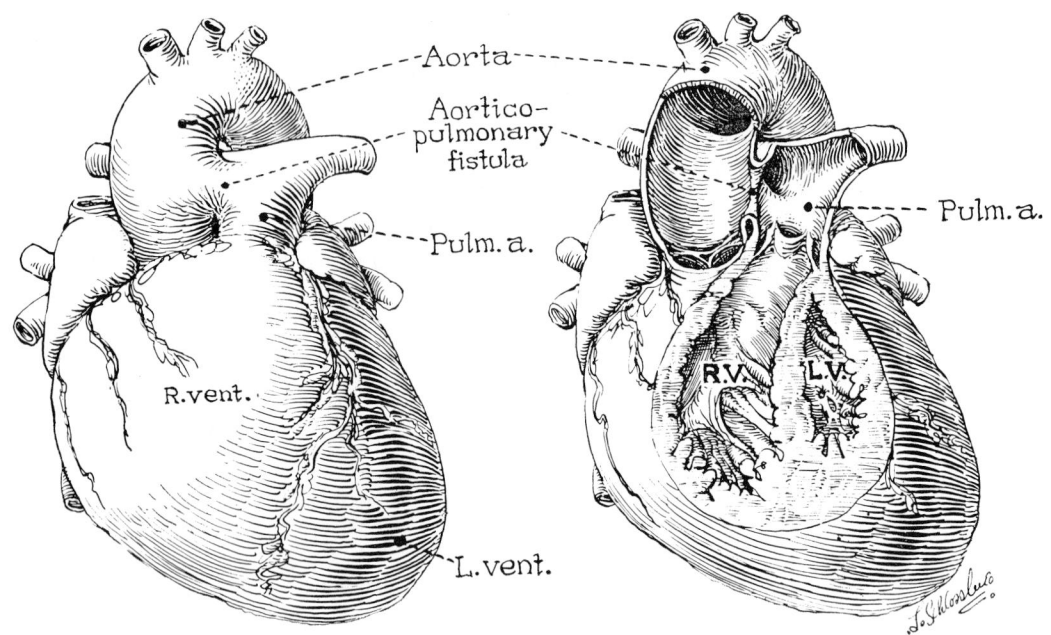

Figure 3. Aorticopulmonary window similar to that shown treated in Figure 4. Size of the fistula and its relation to the semilunar valves are variable. (From Scott, H. W., Jr., and Sabiston, D. C., Jr.: J. Thorac. Surg., 25:26, 1953.)

tality was 2.6 per cent. Gross[18] reported that in his experience in patients who had no failure or infection prior to operation the mortality was less than 0.5 per cent. In a collective review of 3986 cases, the operative mortality was 2.0 per cent with ligation and 2.1 per cent with division in children, and 4.3 and 5.2 per cent, respectively, in adults.[35]

Although patients usually are clinically entirely well after interruption of a patent ductus arteriosus, Lueker et al.[23] have demonstrated evidence of residual pulmonary vascular hyperactivity with exercise and hypoxemia. This is in keeping with other studies following operative treatment of congenital left-to-right shunt with pulmonary hypertension, showing that increased pulmonary resistance diminishes little after operation even though pressure may significantly fall with the decrease in pulmonary blood flow.

Long-term evaluation of patients who have been operated upon clearly demonstrates the value of occlusion of the ductus. In view of the low risk, prophylactic occlusion seems indicated in all children and young adults, even in the absence of symptoms. There is even greater reason for operation in most of the patients who are symptomatic. The low operative risk when balanced against the likelihood of complications and a shortened life expectancy indicates to most cardiologists and surgeons that the ductus should be interrupted in asymptomatic children and young adults. In symptomatic patients the interruption may be urgent and necessary for the control of cardiac failure.

AORTICOPULMONARY WINDOW

Aorticopulmonary window (or aorticopulmonary fenestration, fistula, or septal defect) resembles patent ductus arteriosus in its functional and clinical manifestations. In fact, differential diagnosis is difficult, and many cases have been discovered at the time of operation for patent ductus arteriosus or ventricular septal defect, the two commonly confused conditions.

Pathologic Anatomy

Between the fifth and eighth weeks of fetal life the aortic septum divides the truncus arteriosus into the aorta and the pulmonary artery. At the same time, the cardiac chambers are developing. The bulbus cordis connects the right ventricle to the pulmonary artery, and the ventricular septum separates the left ventricle and permits its attachment to the aorta. Ultimately the aortic septum from above fuses with the ventricular septum from below. Failure of development of the various septa may result in an aorticopulmonary window, a ventricular septal defect, or (if there is complete failure in development) a truncus arteriosus.

The typical fistula is anatomically located just above the aortic valve (Fig. 3) and varies in size from a few millimeters to several centimeters. Although in many instances the aorta and pulmonary artery are separate between the heart and the region of the window, in some instances the defect is located immediately adjacent to the coronary arteries and valves, and the condition may be indistinguishable externally from a truncus arteriosus in which the aortic and pulmonary valves are part of a single opening.

Clinical Manifestations

The clinical manifestations of this condition are practically indistinguishable from those of a large patent ductus. Cardiac enlargement is almost always present, along with physical underdevelopment. The murmur produced varies from a continuous to a soft systolic one, and in some instances there is no murmur at all. The murmur has been described as more superficial than that of patent ductus and may be loudest along the left sternal border in the third and fourth interspaces. As in patent ductus arteriosus with pulmonary hypertension, the pressure in the two vessels may be essentially equal, so that there is not a continuous murmur. The pulmonary second sound is usually loud, and there may be a diastolic murmur of pulmonary insufficiency. A wide pulse pressure may be noted. Increased pulmonary vascularity, often with dilatation of the main pulmonary artery, is similar to that seen roentgenologically in patent ductus arteriosus, as is the electrocardiographic evidence of left ventricular hypertrophy or both left and right hypertrophy in the presence of pulmonary hypertension.

Cardiac catheterization should demonstrate pulmonary hypertension and the left-to-right shunt into the pulmonary artery. Passage of a catheter into the aorta from the pulmonary artery close to the heart may be helpful, but the best differentiation from patent ductus, truncus arteriosus, and ventricular septal defect is by cineangiography. Even then an exact diagnosis cannot always be expected, and exploratory thoracotomy may be necessary with the realization that one may have to treat a patent ductus, truncus arteriosus, ventricular septal defect, or aorticopulmonary window.

Evaluation of the pulmonary vascular resistance is of great importance. Considerations in selection of patients for operation are similar to those given above concerning patent ductus, the operative risk being a bit greater for aorticopulmonary window.

Operative Technique

Aorticopulmonary windows have been treated by ligation, by simple clamping and division, and by division and suture during caval occlusion with hypothermia or cardiopulmonary bypass. In cases in which the defect is small or in which there is no significant pulmonary hypertension and there is sufficient room between the defect and the cardiac valves to allow mobilization, clamping and division may be used. In most cases, however, the conditions are not favorable for clamping. The vessels are large and tense with pulmonary hypertension; the right pulmonary artery seems to arise almost from the back wall of the fistula; and the vessels are easily torn during mobilization or attempted occlusion. In such instances the use of cardiopulmonary bypass converts a difficult and hazardous procedure into a relatively straightforward and easy one (Fig. 4).[9]

Results of Operation

The condition is not a common one. Pulmonary hypertension has been present in almost all instances. Decrease in heart size and relief of cardiac failure are usually impressive. In most instances the pulmonary arterial pressure falls and approaches the normal level. Whether the pulmonary vascular bed will return to normal in the majority of cases is not known, but considerations are probably similar to patent ductus. Operation should be done at as early an age as possible.

COARCTATION OF THE AORTA

Coarctation of the aorta is an important congenital cardiovascular defect that occurs in a significant number of persons. It shortens life if untreated, but it can be corrected to render the patient functionally normal.

Pathologic Anatomy

Coarctation most commonly occurs in the region of the aortic isthmus just distal to the left subclavian artery. It occurs less frequently in the aortic arch itself, and in occasional cases the constriction is in the midthoracic aorta at the level of the diaphragm or below in the region of the renal arteries.[1] In rare instances the coarctation may be multiple.

Coarctation in the aortic arch or isthmus can be helpfully classified as preductal or postductal (Fig. 5). In the preductal type, formerly called infantile because of its association with early death, the pulmonary artery communicates through a large ductus with the distal aorta, and there are usually additional major intracardiac defects, most commonly a ventricular septal defect but in a significant number of cases transposition of the great vessels, atrial septal defect, and other anomalies. The coarctation then separates the flow from the left ventricle to the head and arms and the flow from the pulmonary artery and right ventricle to the caudal half of the body through the ductus. This type of coarctation often involves the distal aortic arch along with the isthmus and tends to be more elongated or diffuse. It is generally discovered in infancy because of the striking disturbance of the circulation by the aortic obstruction in addition to the cardiac defect. Cardiac failure usually occurs, is intractable, and results in death unless correction is possible.

Interrupted aorta, or aortic atresia, is a severe form of coarctation of aorta, usually but not always associated with persistence of the ductus arteriosus. Although most cases have been found at autopsy in newborn infants, a few patients have survived to reach adulthood.

In the typical, uncomplicated, postductal type occurring in the adult, there is a localized constriction just distal to the ductus or ligamentum arteriosum. The aortic valve is bicuspid in 25 to 40 per cent of cases, but other cardiac defects are uncommon. Most patients with this type of anomaly survive to adult life. Although the typical postductal coarctation is usually localized to the region of the ligamentum arteriosum, it may involve the mouth of the left subclavian artery, may be more elongated and diffuse, or may be associated with a hypoplastic distal aortic arch.

In patients who survive beyond infancy, a number of additional features are often noted, the most striking being development of collateral circulation, as was well demonstrated by Bramwell and Jones (1941). Arteries connecting the upper and lower parts of the body, notably the internal mammary, subscapular, and lateral thoracic arteries, become dilated. These communicate with the intercostal arteries, which may be greatly dilated, thin-walled, friable, and subject to dangerous aneurysm formation. Immediately distal to

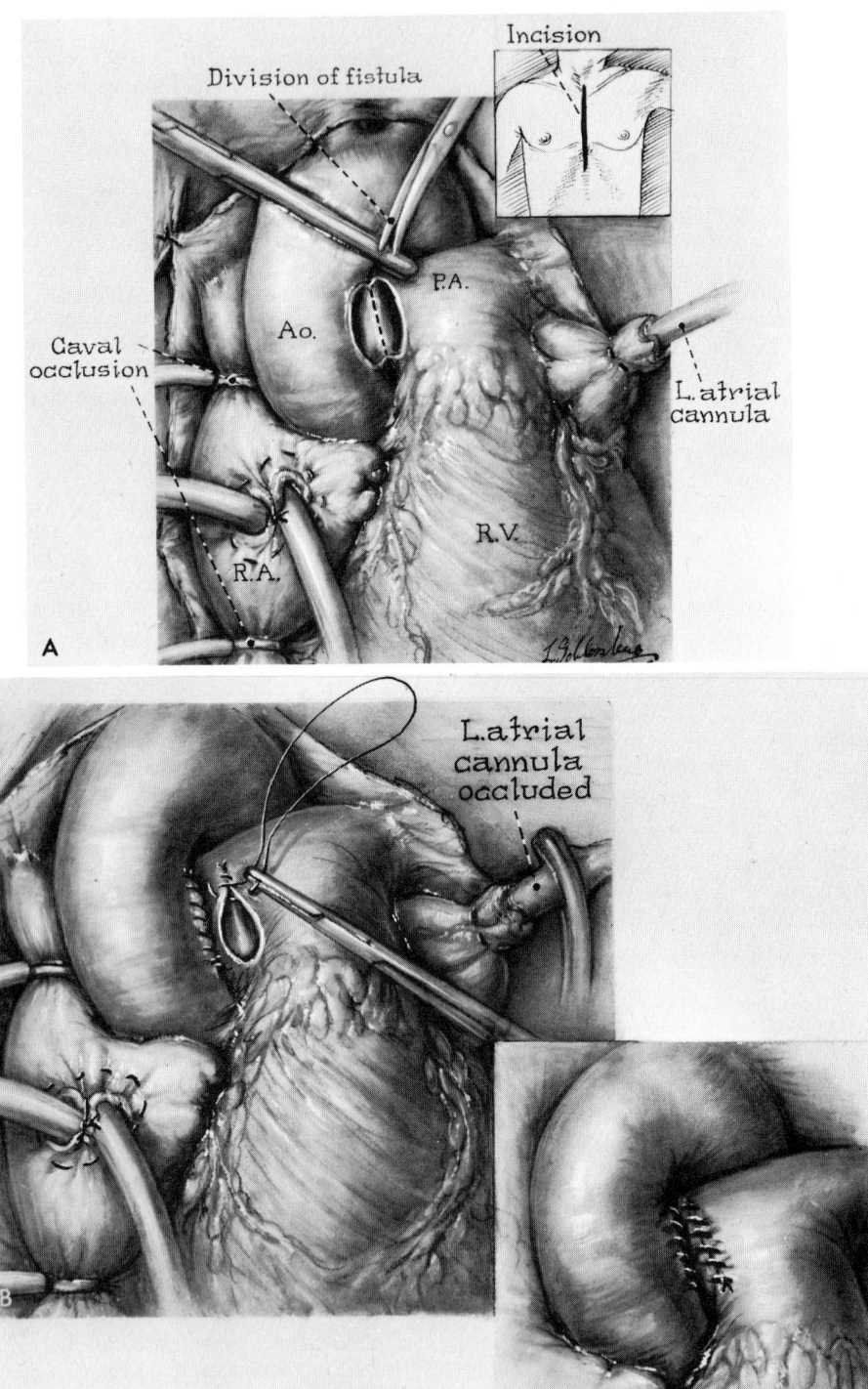

Figure 4. Closure of aorticopulmonary window during cardiopulmonary bypass. *A,* The aorta is occluded while the fistula is divided and the aortic end closed. The cannula in the left atrium through the appendage helps keep the operative area free of blood; this is clamped as closure of the aortic opening is completed and air is evacuated from the left side. *B,* The aorta is unclamped and coronary circulation is restored while the pulmonary opening is closed. (From Bahnson, H. T. *In* Sabiston, D. C., Jr., and Spencer, F. C. (Eds.): Gibbon's Surgery of the Chest, 3rd ed. Philadelphia, W. B. Saunders Company, 1976.)

POSTDUCTAL   PREDUCTAL   INTERRUPTED AORTA

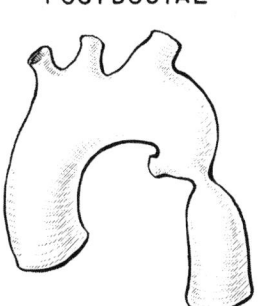 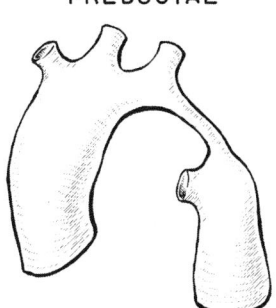 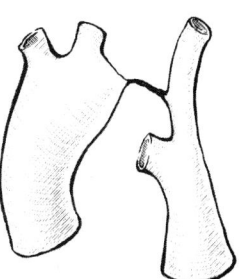

Figure 5. Sketches of representative types of coarctation.

the coarctation there is often poststenotic dilatation of the thoracic aorta, which has the appearance as much of a congenital dilation as of a functional one caused by flow through the stenotic area. There is an increased incidence of cystic medial necrosis of the ascending aorta in association with coarctation.

The etiology is unknown, although the most widely mentioned cause is in connection with the obliterative process, which causes disappearance of the aortic arches and possibly closure of the ductus arteriosus. In the unusual type of coarctation that occurs in the midthoracic aorta, there appears to be a more diffuse inflammatory process, also of unknown etiology.

Clinical Manifestations

Most children with coarctation are asymptomatic, and their condition is discovered because of a murmur or the presence of arterial hypertension discovered during a routine examination. Symptoms are more common in the adult. Headache, dyspnea, palpitation, vertigo, throbbing in the head, visual troubles, precordial pain, or symptoms of cardiac decompensation—all related to hypertension of the upper part of the body—may drive the patient to seek medical aid. General weakness is a common complaint. In a number of instances weakness and fatigue of the legs and even intermittent claudication are present, but conversely it is striking how many patients have no difficulty with the lower extremities, some even being unusually athletic before the condition is recognized.

Diagnosis is made simply and easily in almost all cases by finding a difference in arterial pulsations and blood pressure in the upper and lower extremities. A comparison of radial and femoral pulsations should be part of every complete physical examination and of course is essential in any patient with hypertension or in one who has complaints such as those just listed. Normally the pulses in the radial and the femoral arteries are synchronous, but in the presence of coarctation there is a noticeable delay in the femoral pulse. Blood pressures and pulses in both upper extremities should be compared with the same measurements in the legs, because, in rare cases, the orifice of one subclavian, usually the left, may be involved in the coarctation, giving rise to a low blood pressure in that arm. Indeed, either subclavian artery may arise below the coarctation. One case has been described in which both subclavian arteries arose from the region of the coarctation and were hypoplastic. Consequently there was no brachial hypertension. In such patients, observation of collateral circulation is most important in the diagnosis.

In addition to the pathognomonic pulse and pressure gradient, there are often pulsations in the neck and supraclavicular areas due to hypertension. A systolic murmur is often heard over the base of the heart or in the midback around the sixth or seventh dorsal vertebra. Diastolic murmurs may be heard in either place. A posterior diastolic murmur probably represents flow through the narrowed area or through the dilated intercostal arteries. Wells, Rappaport, and Sprague (1949) found posterior diastolic sounds in all 15 patients with coarctation of the aorta examined by phonocardiography. These sounds were a continuation of those noted during systole. An anterior diastolic murmur should also be carefully sought, since its presence may indicate a patent ductus arteriosus or aortic regurgitation due to a bicuspid aortic valve or dilatation of the proximal aorta.

Except in young children, enlarged collateral vessels may often be felt over the back, adjacent to the scapula, and in some cases a murmur may even be heard over these vessels. Sir Thomas Lewis in 1933 pointed out that, in the proper light, pulsations can be seen in these vessels, and he carefully mapped the circulation in this condition. The subscapular artery is often enlarged also and can be felt by compressing the subscapular tissue between the thumb and index finger. Collateral circulation should always be looked for, because the disparity of pressure and pulse characteristic of coarctation may also be caused by the Leriche syndrome and terminal aortic thrombosis.

The heart may show some increase in size, particularly of the left ventricle, but when it is unduly large, other anomalies must be considered. The upper mediastinum is often widened because of the enlarged left subclavian artery. Prominence of the left subclavian artery and the proximal and distal aorta is responsible for a characteristic notch in the upper left mediastinal shadow on the roentgenogram, giving the appearance of the number 3; the upper convexity is the proximal aorta, the notch is the coarctation, and the lower convexity is the poststenotic dilatation (Fig. 6). Notching of the ribs, as first noted by Railsbach and Dock (1929), remains one of the most characteristic radiologic features and is caused by dilatation, elongation, and tortuosity of the intercostal vessels that serve as collaterals between the subclavian arteries above and the aorta below the narrowing (Fig. 6). When present in the uncomplicated case, notching is most noticeable in the third to the seventh ribs and is bilaterally symmetric. If the distribution is more prominent in other areas or is asymmetric, one must consider an atypical coarctation or involvement of the mouth of the subclavian artery. When a subclavian artery arises from the aorta below the coarctation, notching will be present only on the contralateral side.

The electrocardiogram may vary from normal to that of a striking left ventricular hypertrophy, depending upon the severity of the coarctation and the degree of hypertension. This examination is especially important in older patients in whom changes associated with myocardial damage presage a greater operative risk.

All the signs mentioned point to an obstruction to blood flow in the aorta between the origin of the vessels to the head and arms and the origin of those to the lower extremities. In the majority of cases beyond infancy, one would be correct in assuming that the coarctation is at the junction of the arch and the descending aorta. There is an occasional patient, however, with constriction distal to the usual site. It is important to identify these cases prior to thoracotomy, since successful treatment of such a lesion often requires an aortic replacement and the area may not be readily accessible with the usual thoracotomy incision.

A satisfactory aortogram may be helpful and will demonstrate the lesion in the unusual site, but this examination is unnecessary in most instances of typical coarctation. If one is aware of the possibility of the unusual coarctation, there are several features that suggest the use of aortography. A diffuse murmur heard low in the back is unusual in the typical case

and suggests an atypical site in the back or abdomen. Notching that is most prominent in the lower ribs or the absence of notching in patients with other signs of significant aortic obstruction, such as definite hypertension or the brachial-femoral pressure gradient, is suggestive. When the coarctation is in the abdominal aorta, pulsations in the upper abdominal aorta may be palpable. If the possibility is kept in mind, one may safely reserve aortography for patients presenting any or all of the atypical signs mentioned.

Coarctation is an important cause of cardiac failure in infants, in either the preductal or the postductal site. Such children with failure are irritable and dyspneic, fail to grow and eat normally, and may have cyanosis. The baby may look quite sick, with tachypnea, tachycardia, rales over the lungs, hepatomegaly, and an overactive heart. The diagnosis may be difficult to make in sick infants, and the discrepancy in the pulses of the upper and lower extremities may not be readily apparent. Examination should be repeated until the diagnosis is clarified, although in doubtful cases aortography may be used to demonstrate the coarctation.

Prognosis

In a review of 108 infants with coarctation by Glass et al.,[16] 90 per cent of the fatalities in those under 1 year of age were due to preductal coarctation, usually in association with cardiac defects. Many infants with postductal coarctation can tolerate the failure when given nonoperative treatment and can improve, presumably as the collateral channels develop.[17] In others this is not possible and surgical relief is necessary.

Adults with typical postductal coarctation have an abbreviated life expectancy. Campbell[6] found the mean age at death to be 34 years, less than half the normal life expectancy. Reifenstein et al. (1947) reviewed a large group of patients and found that 61 per cent died in or before the fortieth year. About one-fourth of the patients lived far into adult life with no

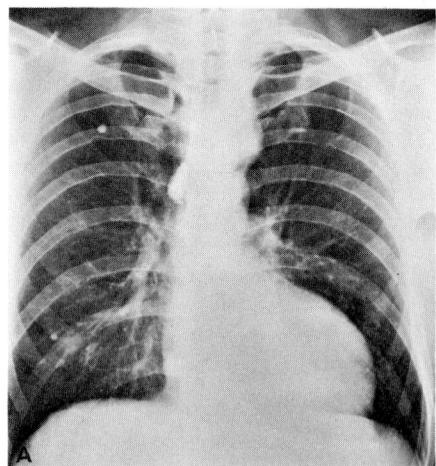
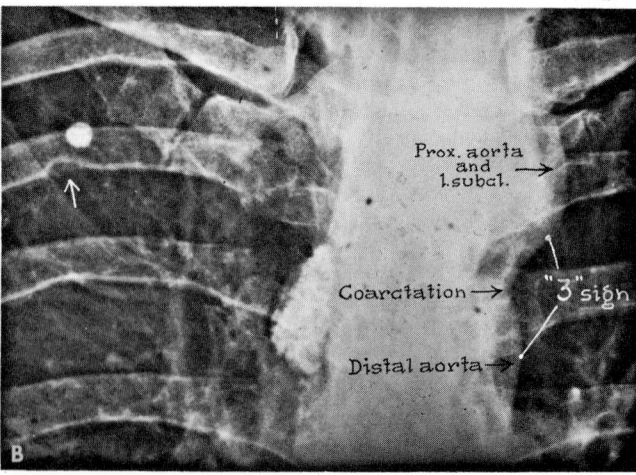

Figure 6. Roentgenologic signs, which are diagnostic but not always present in coarctation, include notching of the ribs and the "3" sign caused by the dilated proximal segment and left subclavian artery, by the constricted area, and by poststenotic dilatation. *A*, Note rounded lower left cardiac border, indicating left ventricular enlargement. *B*, Enlargement from *(A)* showing notching of rib (adjacent to calcified lesion) and "3" sign. (From Bahnson, H. T. *In* Sabiston, D. C., Jr., and Spencer, F. C. (Eds.): Gibbon's Surgery of the Chest, 3rd ed. Philadelphia, W. B. Saunders Company, 1976.)

incapacity; about one-fourth died of bacterial endocarditis or aortitis; about one-fourth died suddenly of rupture of the aorta (the aorta is susceptible to rupture both proximal and distal to the coarctation); and about one-fourth died of cardiac failure or cerebral hemorrhage resulting from the hypertensive state. It is evident that, although some subjects may live a normal life and be unhindered by coarctation, the defect is in most instances a hazardous one.

Pathologic Physiology

Physiologic studies have been concerned primarily with the cause of hypertension above coarctation of the aorta. Whether peripheral resistance of the coarctation and collateral vessels per se is sufficient cause, or whether a renal mechanism is involved, remains a controversial issue. Bing and co-workers (1948) observed no evidence of generalized increase in peripheral resistance and from their data demonstrated that the coarctation and collateral vessels alone produce sufficient increase in peripheral resistance to cause elevated pressure. On the other hand, Scott and Bahnson[29] produced coarctation experimentally in dogs, with a resultant discrepancy in femoral and carotid arterial pressures similar to that seen in clinical cases. In such animals, transplantation of a kidney to the neck and removal of the contralateral kidney caused a prompt fall in carotid pressure, although the gradient between carotid and femoral pressures remained. Perhaps there is truth in both concepts and there are some cases of coarctation of the aorta in which the resistance of the coarctation and collateral vessels alone causes hypertension and others in which there is an additional renal factor.

Selection of Patients for Operation

Almost all patients with coarctation of the aorta should be operated on at an appropriate time unless there are significant contraindications. There are degrees of coarctation, and in some patients in whom only a slight discrepancy in pressure exists between the upper and lower extremities, suggesting less total obstruction, it may be difficult to be sure that the obstruction is not more complete and that it is not simply compensated by adequate collateral circulation.

Probably the most satisfactory age for operation is between 6 and 16 years. Although technically easy in younger children, the operation is apt to be more permanently beneficial if the aorta is allowed to approach its adult size. With increasing age beyond the optimum, the operation is of greater magnitude; the aorta is more sclerotic, less elastic, and more difficult to approximate and suture, and aneurysms of the intercostal arteries are found more frequently. Hypertension also is more apt to be of a fixed nature and responds less satisfactorily to the relief of the aortic obstruction.

Operation is clearly indicated in some patients above and below the optimal age. As Gross[17] has emphasized, during the first few months of life many babies have cardiac embarrassment from uncomplicated coarctation of the aorta, but the majority of them can be supported by nonoperative means. Once compensation is gained, they often survive to later childhood without difficulty. On the other hand, there are a significant number of infants who will not survive unless surgical help can be given. In such infants the operative risk is undoubtedly high. However, Glass et al.[16] recommended that babies with symptoms in the first month of life be operated upon promptly unless they show dramatic response during a 12 hour trial of treatment with digitalis, and that babies over 1 month of age who respond to digitalis be kept on this medication until adequate compensation has taken place and operation can be performed at the optimal age.

At the other end of the age scale, some persons are unaware of coarctation of the aorta until well into adult life. Beyond the age of 30 there is some increase in the operative risk, and although statistics are not available, this almost surely rises with increased age. Of 51 patients older than 30 years treated by Dr. Blalock and his staff in their initial reported experience with coarctation, there was a 10 per cent hospital mortality as compared to a 7 per cent risk for patients in the 4 to 15 year age group. It should be emphasized, however, that there is no more specific treatment for arterial hypertension than excision of a coarctation of the aorta, and the operation should be seriously considered at any age. Successful results have been obtained in the fifth and sixth decades.

Certain conditions greatly increase the operative risk.[28] Mild to moderate aortic insufficiency may be present, caused by either rheumatic heart disease or a congenitally bicuspid valve. In a few instances the valve as well as the coarctation has been surgically treated. The risk is greater when there are significant cardiac abnormalities: mitral disease from rheumatic fever, septal defects, or myocardial damage. In almost all such cases the burden on the heart would be decreased if the hypertension due to coarctation could be relieved, but the risk may be prohibitive and operation inadvisable.

Operative Technique

Blalock and Park (1944) reported an experimental operation designed to bypass coarctation of the aorta by anastomosing the left subclavian artery to the distal aorta. This method was not attempted on a patient until Crafoord and Nylin (1945) and Gross and Hufnagel (1945) did so independently, resecting the involved area and performing end-to-end anastomosis of the divided aorta. This operation quickly became the standard one. Use of the subclavian is rarely, if ever, indicated, as sacrifice of a large number of collaterals is required.

The operation is performed with the patient in the lateral position (Fig. 7). Almost the entire length of the fifth rib is removed, as suggested by Crafoord, and the chest is entered through the bed of this rib. If the entire rib from neck to cartilage is removed, good exposure can be obtained and the removal of segments of other ribs is not necessary. In infants, incision in the fourth interspace is satisfactory. The coarctation and the arrangement of the aorta and the vessels should be inspected before the pleura is opened, because often a good view is obtained before the tissues are stained. A long incision is made in the pleura over the coarctation, the adjacent subclavian above, and the aorta below, and the pleural flaps are held back with sutures. The easier dissection is done first, namely, mobilizing the left subclavian and the adjacent aorta, the coarctation, and the ligamentum arteriosum or the

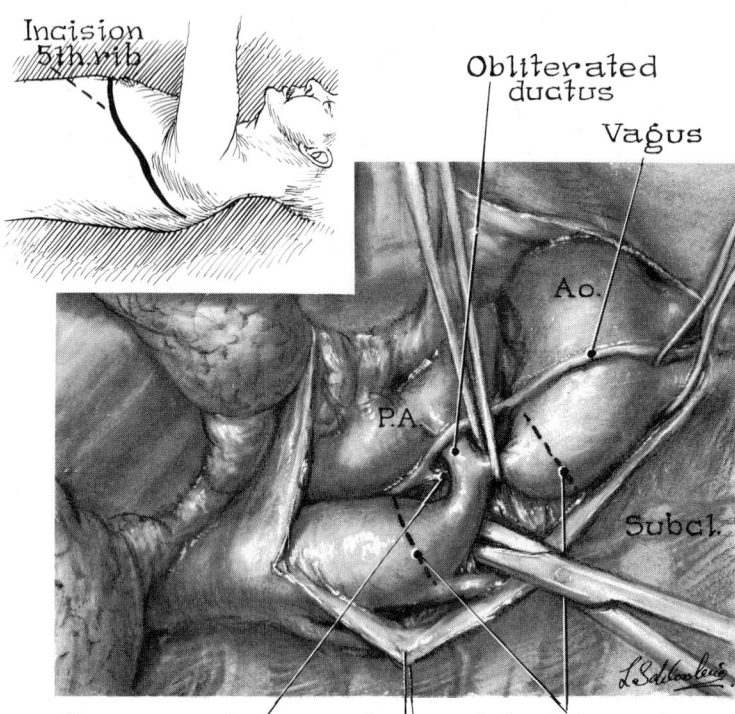

Incision
5th rib

Obliterated
ductus

Vagus

Ao.

P.A.

Subcl.

Recurrent n.　　　Lines of division of aorta

Figure 7. Operative exposure for resection of coarctation of the aorta is through the bed of the fifth rib. The entire rib is removed from neck to cartilage. The constricted segment is usually held medially by an obliterated ductus, division of which allows considerable mobility. The coarctation is held forward to facilitate dissection posteriorly. Large intercostal arteries must be carefully avoided. Division of the aorta should be through a point of normal diameter. (From Bahnson, H. T. *In* Sabiston, D. C., Jr., and Spencer, F. C. (Eds.): Gibbon's Surgery of the Chest, 3rd ed. Philadelphia, W. B. Saunders Company, 1976.)

ductus. Considerable mobility of the aorta is often obtained when the ductus or ligament is divided, so that division of this as soon as possible is helpful. If there are large intercostal arteries adjacent to the coarctation, mobilization of the aorta a short distance below may help to avoid injury to these thin-walled and sometimes troublesome collaterals.

Once this area is mobilized, the intercostals can be visualized from both sides and isolated more carefully. Great care must be exercised in dissection around the intercostal arteries, since they are friable and easily torn from the wall of the aorta. There are few places where it is easier to stay out of difficulty than to get out of difficulty than in this portion of the operation for coarctation. It is preferable to divide none of these collateral vessels, but although this is often feasible, one or two of the upper ones must usually be severed. As soon as tapes can be placed around the aorta, it can be pulled up slightly away from the vertebral column and better visualization of the posterior aspect can be obtained.

In most patients with an uncomplicated postductal coarctation, the constricted segment is short, but in some instances there is a narrow proximal aortic segment and in others a long area of marked constriction. It must be emphasized that in order to obtain relief of hypertension all of the coarctation must be removed. It is tempting to remove only a short segment and thus avoid tension in the anastomosis. If in doing this an anastomosis smaller than the diameter of the distal aortic arch is obtained, or if the ends cannot be approximated because sufficient length has been removed to relieve the constriction, some form of aortoplasty or of aortic replacement must be used.[28] Such procedures have been used in 2 to 40 per cent of cases, depending on inclination of the surgeon and the age range of his patients. Less elasticity of the aorta and greater frequency of aneurysms and atherosclerotic lesions in the adult require more frequent use of complicated reconstruction.

Various types of anastomoses may be performed. We prefer a single row of continuous 4-0 silk or synthetic sutures in adults (5-0 in young children) through all layers, the intima being everted with a mattress suture (Fig. 8). In the usual case this gives a smooth approximation of the intima of the two vessels. An overhand, noneverting suture works satisfactorily, particularly if the anastomosis is begun with eversion and efforts are made to continue the everting. In view of experimental work showing that a continuous suture may prevent growth of the anastomosis,[27] we interrupt the suture frequently on the anterior row, or, especially in children when growth is important, we use interrupted sutures for the entire anterior portion. It is often helpful to place much of the posterior row of an everting mattress suture before the vessels are closely approximated and the posterior suture line pulled up, as described by Blalock[2] (Fig. 8).

Following completion of the anastomosis, the distal clamp is removed and any necessary sutures are placed in order to obtain a tight anastomosis. The proximal clamp should be released slowly and blood given intravenously during this time. In some patients, too rapid a release of the clamp may lead to profound hypotension.

The infant with coarctation requires careful operative technique and conscientious postoperative care. Interruption of the aorta between the great vessels in the aortic arch is especially hazardous, and only a few survivors have been reported. Tyson et al.[34] advised temporary and then permanent banding of the pulmonary artery to reduce the left-to-right shunt during and after operation, and thus reduce the load on the left ventricle. Their unique success in repair of the interrupted aorta in the newborn supports this admonition.

Results of Operation

In 1601 cases collected from around the world, the average mortality was 8.6 per cent.[26] It was 6.8 per cent in patients between the ages of 4 and 15 years and significantly higher in those below age 3 or over age 30. Heart failure and pulmonary edema, often related to associated defects, and disruption of the

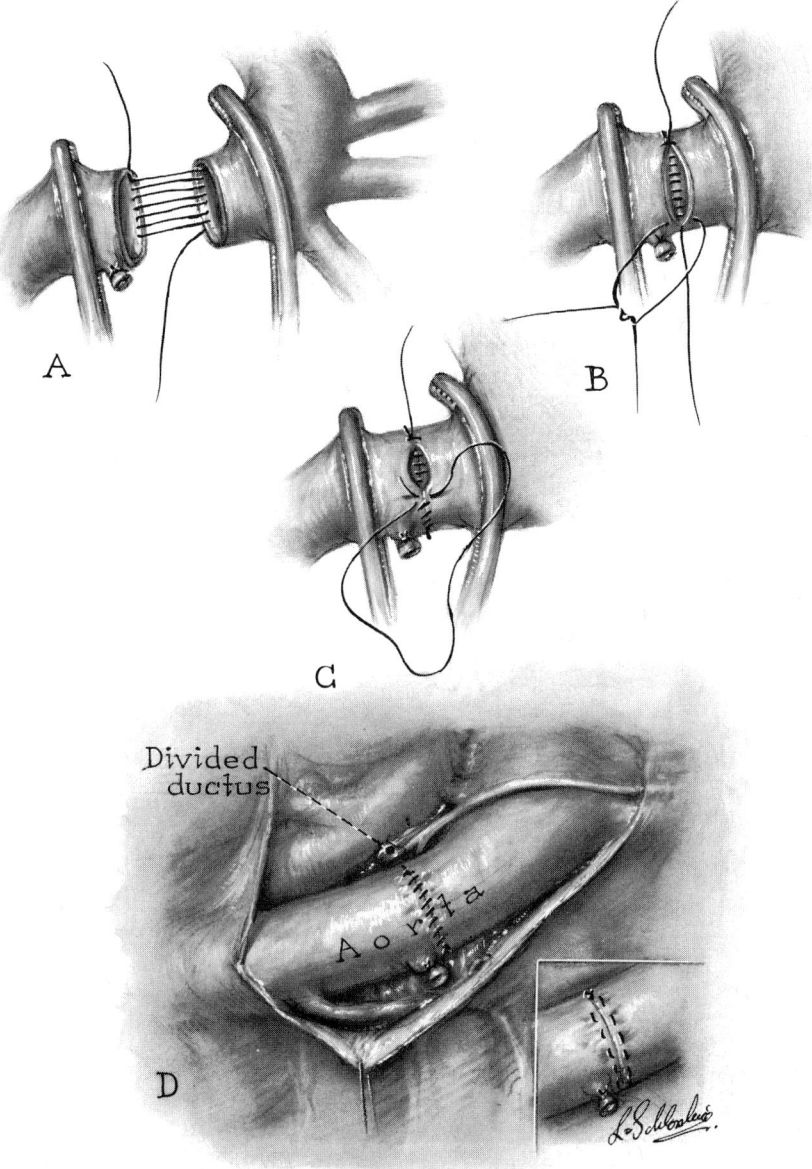

Figure 8. Anastomosis following excision of coarctation. An everting mattress suture is placed over about one-third of the posterior row before the vessels are approximated and the suture is pulled up. The anastomosis is completed with continuous over-and-over suture. Inset in *D* shows the everting mattress suture sometimes used. In children, interrupted mattress sutures are used for the entire anterior row. (From Bahnson, H. T. *In* Sabiston, D. C., Jr., and Spencer, F. C. (Eds.): Gibbon's Surgery of the Chest, 3rd ed. Philadelphia, W. B. Saunders Company, 1976.)

anastomosis, probably most often due to infection, were the most common causes of death and in conjunction with cardiac arrest or fibrillation and operative hemorrhage accounted for 72.9 per cent of the deaths.

Among the patients who survived, satisfactory relief of hypertension was obtained in 95.2 per cent, and entirely normal readings were present in 72.0 per cent. The incidence of persistent hypertension increased progressively with the age of the patient. For unknown reasons, the blood pressure does not always reach its final level immediately after operation. In the majority of patients, the pressure is normal at the time of discharge from the hospital, but it usually

remains elevated for 10 to 14 days and occasionally for several months.

One complication, which appears to be an unfortunate byproduct of the relief of hypertension, has been *necrotizing arteritis.* Although rare, this condition has occasionally been fatal. Examination shows the arteritis to be limited to the lower part of the body. Most of the clinical manifestations have been in the abdomen, causing abdominal pain and in some instances resulting in gangrene of the intestine. In about one-third of young patients operated upon with resection of the coarctation, blood pressure may rise to a higher level after operation than before—a "paradoxical hypertension." Abdominal symptoms are usually confined to this group of patients and occur in one-fourth to one-half of them (Tawes et al., 1970). Sympathicolytic drugs are indicated in such cases.[31] The cause of this complication is unknown, although it is recognized that there is increased sympathetic nerve activity following resection of coarctation (Goodall and Sealy, 1969).

A rare and distressing complication has been paraplegia or weakness of the lower part of the body after operation reported by Brewer et al.[4] to occur with an incidence of 0.41 per cent in a review of 12,532 cases. This appears to result from inadequate circulation through the anterior spinal artery, possibly resulting from interruption of important intercostal arteries or collateral vessels, emphasizing again the desirability of preserving all collaterals possible.

In the late 1960s several reports of recoarctation appeared, possibly reflecting the greater use of operation in infants earlier in the decade.[19] Restenosis has been due to insufficient resection, residual ductal or fibrous tissue, thrombosis, or failure to grow because of a constricting continuous suture.[22]

The ultimate long-term results of the treatment of coarctation are unknown. In a study of patients followed for 11 to 25 years there was a high incidence of cardiovascular disease, 78 per cent in one special group.[24] This indicates the need for early diagnosis and treatment and continued follow-up, but it is evident that surgery rests on a firm basis and has a great deal to offer most of these patients.

ANOMALIES OF THE AORTIC ARCH

Constriction by an abnormality of the aortic arch must be considered in patients, especially infants, who present evidence of tracheal or esophageal obstruction. Many anomalies of the aortic arch, of its branches, and of the great veins in the superior mediastinum are of no clinical significance, and in fact most of the reported cases were discovered incidentally. Gross and Ware in 1946, however, clearly demonstrated that embarrassing and sometimes fatal obstruction of the trachea and esophagus may arise from a double aortic arch; a right aortic arch with a ligamentum arteriosum completing a ring about the trachea; or an anomalous innominate, left common carotid, or subclavian artery.[17, 18]

Embryology

In order to understand the variations that might be encountered, it is helpful to review the embryology of the aortic arch system.[1] During the first 3 weeks of embryonic life, six aortic arches join the ventral aortic sac and the dorsal paired aortas around the interposed pharynx. The aortas caudal to the branchial arches become fused as an unpaired dorsal aorta. Figure 9A shows diagrammatically the approximate configuration of the aortic arches in the 12 mm. embryo. The embryonic subclavian artery is the seventh cervical segmental artery, which supplies the limb bud. As the heart and aortic sac move caudad and the cranial portion of the embryo elongates, the subclavian artery moves craniad on the aorta. Normally the most caudal segment of the right fourth arch

becomes obliterated as the left fourth arch takes over the majority of the cardiac output. Most of the right third arch persists as the proximal part of the carotid artery. It ultimately arises from the fourth arch, which persists as the innominate and subclavian arteries. The left fourth arch persists as the definitive aorta, and the carotid and subclavian arteries arise independently. In rare instances the left subclavian artery may ascend to the third arch, and a left innominate artery results. If the right aortic arch persists and the left arch becomes obliterated, the mirror image of the arrangement just described may occur.

If the proximal rather than the distal part of the right fourth arch becomes obliterated, the right subclavian artery arises from the unpaired aorta and courses behind the esophagus to reach the right arm. In rare instances the vessel may go between the trachea and the esophagus or anterior to the trachea. A short segment of the distal end of the right fourth arch may persist as an aortic diverticulum from which the subclavian arises. The ductus arteriosus usually connects the main or the left pulmonary artery (derived from the sixth arch) with the left aortic arch. When the proximal left fourth arch becomes obliterated, the ductus arteriosus is connected with the most distal portion of the left dorsal aorta along with the subclavian artery (Fig. 9C). If the arch becomes obliterated distal to the ductus arteriosus, this relationship is lost. When both aortic arches persist, a complete aortic ring is formed around the trachea and esophagus (Fig. 9B). In such instances the brachiocephalic vessels usually arise from the arches independently, although double aortic arches with an innominate artery have been described.

Pathologic Anatomy

A vascular ring around the trachea and esophagus may be composed of any of the several remnants of the aortic arch system. A double aortic arch results when neither of the aortic arches regresses. In such cases the ascending aorta bifurcates, one branch going to the right and behind the trachea and esophagus, and the other to the left in front of the trachea. Both limbs join behind to complete a ring around the trachea and esophagus (Fig. 10). In most instances the descending aorta is on the left side, although a right descending aorta may occur, with the aorta lying to the right of the vertebral column. Regardless of the side of the descending aorta, the smaller of the two arches is usually to the left and anterior, an important consideration in selecting the side of surgical approach.

If the left fourth aortic arch, rather than the right, disappears in the embryo, the subject is born with a right aortic arch, which ascends, passes to the right of the trachea and esophagus, and descends usually on the left, but occasionally on the right, of the vertebral column. Such an arch in itself rarely causes symptoms, although there may be some tracheal or right bronchial compression. In many such cases the ligamentum arteriosum courses from the pulmonary artery and joins the innominate artery* at its bifurcation into the carotid and subclavian. In some instances, however, the ligamentum passes from the pulmonary artery to the left of the trachea and esophagus and to the distal end of the right aortic arch, thus

---

*The innominate artery arises as the first vessel branching off the aortic arch, regardless of the side of the arch, and, hence, in this case supplies the left arm and left common carotid.

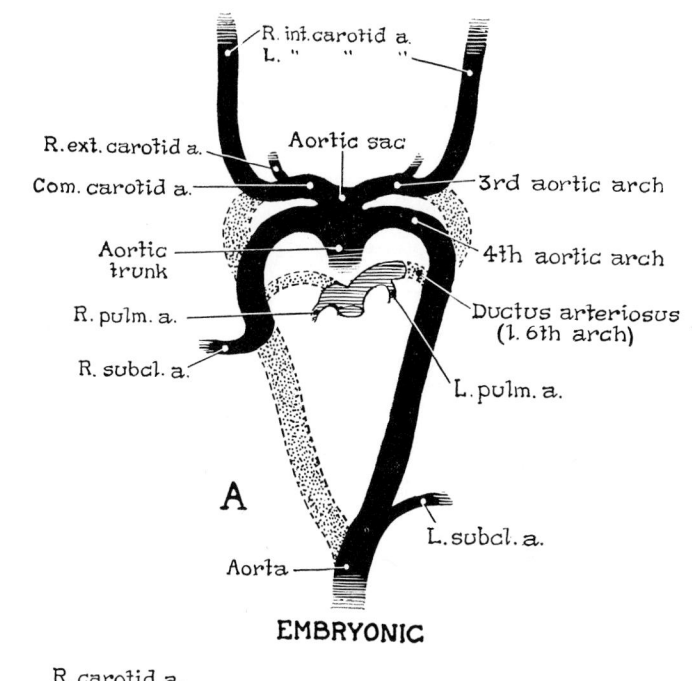

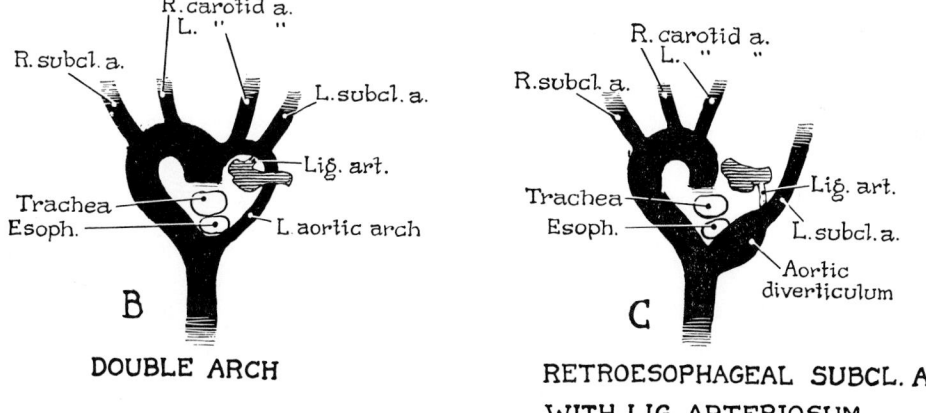

Figure 9. Development of aortic arch and anomalies. The stippled areas normally disappear. Normally only the left fourth arch persists in its entirety. Both fourth arches persist in the double aortic arch. When the right fourth arch persists and the left fourth arch disappears, the left subclavian artery is retroesophageal. A ligamentum arteriosum may join this to the pulmonary artery and complete the ring. (From Bahnson, H. T., and Blalock, A.: Ann. Surg., *131*:356, 1950.)

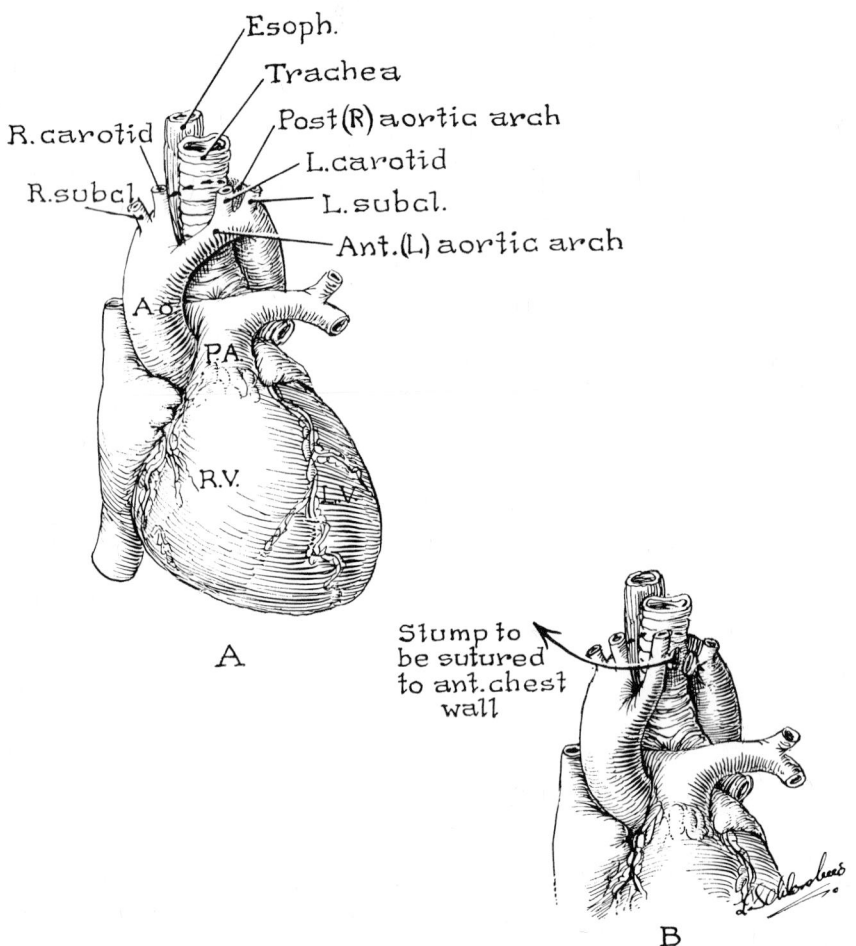

Figure 10. Double aortic arch. *A*, The larger channel is usually the posterior one and on the right. Branches of the arch arise independently. In almost all instances the descending thoracic aortic is on the left as shown. *B*, Point of division of the smaller arch is selected to preserve circulation to the branches. The left common carotid artery is then tacked to the anterior chest wall to further relieve tracheal compression. (From Bahnson, H. T. *In* Sabiston, D. C., Jr., and Spencer, F. C. (Eds.): Gibbon's Surgery of the Chest, 3rd ed. Philadelphia, W. B. Saunders Company, 1976.)

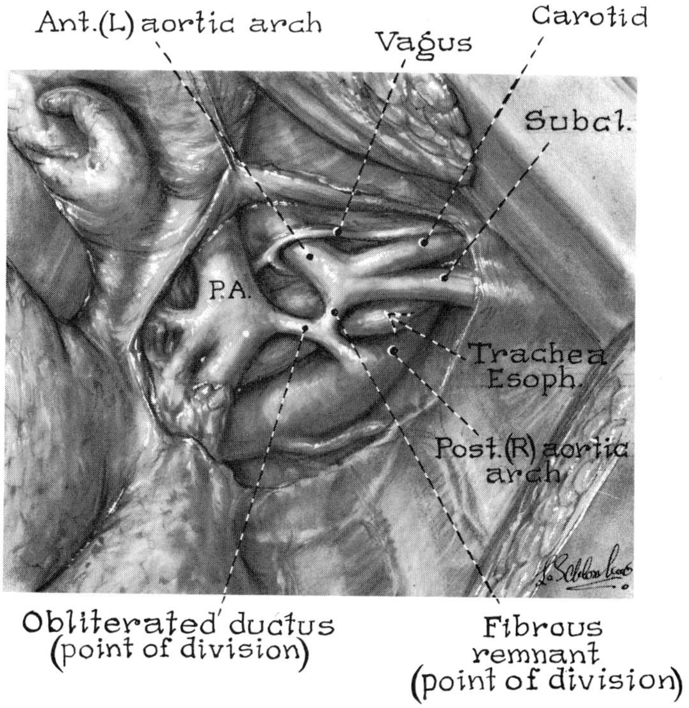

Figure 11. Operative view of tracheal ring completed by obliterated remnant of distal left arch and ligamentum arteriosum. After complete exposure of the vascular components, the proper point of division of the ligaments can easily be determined. (From Bahnson, H. T. *In* Sabiston, D. C., Jr., and Spencer, F. C. (Eds.): Gibbon's Surgery of the Chest, 3rd ed. Philadelphia, W. B. Saunders Company, 1976.)

completing a ring around the trachea and esophagus (Fig. 11). This ring may be small enough to compress and interfere with the function of the trachea and esophagus.

Of the anomalies of the branches of the aortic arch, that of the right subclavian is the most easily recognized and understood. If in the development of the aortic arch system the proximal portion of the right fourth arch disappears instead of the distal portion, the right subclavian artery will arise as the last branch of the aortic arch and course behind the esophagus (or in rare instances between the esophagus and trachea or in front of the trachea) to supply the right arm. This anomaly was clearly recognized by Bayford in 1794 and has long been known to cause "dysphagia lusoria."

Although the innominate artery normally arises to the left of the trachea, in some instances it arises farther along the arch than normal and must wind across the trachea in reaching the apex of the right chest. If the vessel is lax, no symptoms are caused, but when it is tight there may be constriction of the trachea. Similarly, if the left common carotid branches from the aortic arch farther to the right than usual, it may wind across the anterior surface of the trachea as it courses upward and to the left and may cause tracheal compression.

Of the 160 babies operated upon by Gross,[18] 40 per cent had a double arch, 25 per cent had a right arch and left ligamentum arteriosum, 12 per cent had an anomalous innominate or carotid artery, 10 per cent had an aberrant right subclavian artery, and 13 per cent had miscellaneous other anomalies.

Clinical Manifestations

Why some children with anomalies of the aortic arch remain asymptomatic and others are severely bothered is an unanswered question. Symptoms are those of tracheal obstruction, often with stridor and even a crowing type of respiration, frequent respiratory infections with secretions that cannot adequately be cleared, and a wheeze that often may be heard without a stethoscope. There may be difficulty in swallowing, and in some instances this is the complaint that brings the patient to the physician. Respiratory distress is frequently worse after eating or drinking, and aspiration pneumonia is often seen because of esophageal obstruction. The infant appears to obtain some relief by lying in a position of hyperextension, and this is frequently the preferred position. Respiratory obstruction may be exaggerated if the neck is flexed forcibly.

Symptoms may be alarming with any of the compressing anomalies, but they are usually more prominent with the double aortic arch or a right arch with a ring completed by the ligamentum arteriosum. When difficulty occurs, it is almost always evident in infancy or early childhood, many patients being under 6 months of age. Few older patients have symptoms or require treatment. The anomalous right subclavian causes difficulty principally in swallowing, there usually being little or no respiratory distress except that occasioned by dysphagia and aspiration after eating. Conversely, pressure from an aberrant innominate or carotid artery on the trachea causes predominantly respiratory symptoms.

Diagnosis

Consideration of the possibility of an aortic arch anomaly is the most important step in diagnosing the condition. Roentgenograms may show pneumonitis and in some instances the outline of the trachea and its compression. Barium swallow shows the posterior compression of the esophagus (Fig. 12), and by careful examination of the films and the direction and level of the compression, the exact anomaly can often be determined.[25] The combination of anterior tracheal compression and posterior esophageal compression justifies an almost certain diagnosis of a vascular ring. The relative sizes of the right and left arches can be determined by the size of the indentation on barium swallow. Angiocardiography may demonstrate the anomaly but is rarely necessary. A tracheogram with Lipiodol instillation may clearly identify the tracheal compression. The level and obliquity of the tracheal and esophageal compression usually allow identification of the type of vessel when obstruction is due to anomalous arteries from the aortic arch.

Operative Technique

Division of the constricting ring or displacement of an aberrant vessel has much to offer these patients in providing more room for the trachea and esophagus and in relieving their obstruction. Adequate exposure is an absolute necessity, and this usually is obtained through the left chest. The arch and the vessels arising from it, the ductus, and the fibrous tissue attached to the vascular ring must be clearly exposed. Removal of the thymus often helps.

Once adequate exposure is obtained, selection of the proper component for division is usually not difficult. In the case of the right aortic arch with a ligamentum arteriosum completing the vascular ring, simple division of the ligamentum arteriosum and mobilization of the arch should relieve the constriction. When a double arch is present, the side and position of the smaller arch must be determined. The smaller arch, usually anterior and on the left, is divided in a manner that does not interfere with circulation to the common carotid arteries. This usually means division of the arch between the left common carotid and the left subclavian arteries. The adjacent and possibly constricting fibrous tissue must be divided, and, if the divided arch and carotid in any way compress the trachea, the arch should be tacked with multiple stitches through the adventitia to the posterior surface of the sternum or chest wall in order to hold the vessel away from the trachea. Although theoretically the smaller arch can be divided at any site and circulation will continue into the branches through the distal or proximal opening, in some instances the distal end of the smaller arch is narrowed and circulation to the carotid through this opening may be curtailed.

The subclavian artery, if it is causing compression, arises as the last branch of the aortic arch; by dissecting in the posterior mediastinum, it can be mobilized behind the aorta. It can be divided with impunity, and in cases of the aberrant retroesophageal left subclavian artery, freeing of the artery from its bed and doubly ligating and dividing it is all that is required. Sufficient collateral circulation is available through the second and third portions of the subclavian artery to maintain adequate circulation to the arm. In cases of compression by an anomalous innominate or carotid artery, the continuity of the artery must be maintained. Hence, proper treatment consists of complete mobilization of the artery, division of any constricting fibrous tissue around it, and suture of the vessel away from the trachea and against the back wall of the sternum with multiple fine sutures through the adventitia.

After operation in patients in whom there has been some tracheal compression, particular care must be taken to provide an atmosphere with high humidity; there must also be close supervision of tracheobronchial secretions. Persistent tracheal obstruction may be caused by tracheomalacia or by tracheal hypoplasia resulting from tracheal pressure and narrowing present since early fetal life. Not infrequently, because of the tracheal manipulation and pre-existing obstruction, there may be respiratory obstruction and even stridor for the first few postoperative days. In rare cases this has persisted for months.[3]

Results of Treatment

Relief of the tracheal and esophageal obstruction is usually associated with dramatic clinical improvement, often evident immediately after operation. In

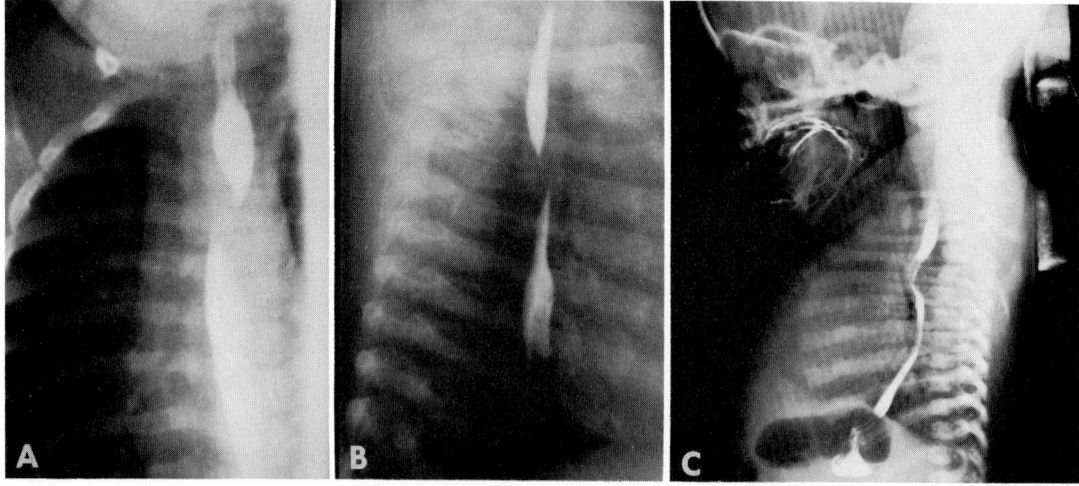

Figure 12. Roentgenograms of vascular ring. *A* and *B*, Double aortic arch. The location and direction of esophageal compression suggest a larger posterior arch coursing from above downward but with anterior compression also. *C*, Obstruction from remnant of left fourth arch and obliterated ductus as shown in Figure 11. The large posterior arch is pulled forward and compresses the trachea and esophagus. (From Bahnson, H. T. *In* Sabiston, D. C., Jr., and Spencer, F. C. (Eds.): Gibbon's Surgery of the Chest, 3rd ed. Philadelphia, W. B. Saunders Company, 1976.)

some instances there is deformity of the trachea, which may persist. No long-term follow-up of such cases is yet available, but it is likely that relief of the compression will allow the trachea to grow in a normal fashion. Persisting deformity of the tracheal cartilage is more common in patients with a double arch or a right arch with a ligamentum arteriosum.

There were 5 deaths among the 57 patients of all types treated by Gross,[17] and all 5 were among the 21 patients with double aortic arch. The age of the 57 patients ranged from 3 weeks to 12 years, the majority being under 2 years of age.

SELECTED REFERENCES

Gross, R. E.: The Surgery of Infancy and Childhood, Its Principles and Practice. Philadelphia, W. B. Saunders Company, 1953.
This is the classic text on children's surgery by the author who figured prominently in the development of surgical treatment for all the conditions discussed in this chapter.

Gross, R. E.: An Atlas of Children's Surgery. Philadelphia, W. B. Saunders Company, 1970.
This atlas is a companion piece to the textbook by the same author and shows the pathologic anatomy and operative treatment of many conditions encountered in pediatric surgery. Results of the long experience with pediatric surgery for many of the conditions are given.

Schumacker, H. B., Jr., King, H., Nahrwald, D. L., and Waldhausen, J. A.: Coarctation of the aorta. Curr. Probl. Surg., Feb. 1968.
This is a comprehensive review of the condition, including all but the most recent references.

REFERENCES

1. Bahnson, H. T.: Coarctation of the aorta and anomalies of the aortic arch. Surg. Clin. N. Amer., 32:1313, 1952.
2. Blalock, A.: The technique of creation of artificial ductus arteriosus in the treatment of pulmonic stenosis. J. Thorac. Surg., 16:244, 1947.
3. Bradham, R. R., Sealy, W. C., and Young, W. G.: Respiratory distress associated with anomalies of the aortic arch. Surg. Gynec. Obstet., 126:9, 1968.
4. Brewer, L. A., III, Fosburg, R. G., Mulder, G. A., and Verska, J. J.: Spinal cord complications following surgery for coarctation of the aorta. A study of 66 cases. J. Thorac. Cardiovasc. Surg., 64:368, 1972.
5. Campbell, M.: Natural history of patent ductus arteriosus. Brit. Heart J., 30:4, 1968.
6. Campbell, M.: Natural history of coarctation of the aorta. Brit. Heart J., 32:633, 1970.
7. Christie, A.: Normal closing time of the foramen ovale and the ductus arteriosus: Anatomical and statistical study. Amer. J. Dis. Child., 40:323, 1930.
8. Clatworthy, H. W., Jr., and McDonald, V. G., Jr.: Optimum age for surgical closure of patent ductus arteriosus. J.A.M.A., 167:444, 1958.
9. Cooley, D. A., McNamara, D. G., and Latson, J. R.: Aorticopulmonary septal defect: Diagnosis and surgical treatment. Surgery, 42:101, 1957.
10. Dammann, J. F., Jr., and Sell, C. G. R.: Patent ductus arteriosus in the absence of a continuous murmur. Circulation, 6:110, 1952.
11. Du Shane, J. W., and Kirklin, J. W.: Late results of the repair of ventricular septal defect on pulmonary vascular disease. *In* Kirklin, J. W., ed.: Advances in Cardiovascular Surgery. New York, Grune and Stratton, 1973, pp. 9–16.
12. Edwards, J. E.: Structural changes of the pulmonary vascular bed and their functional significance in congenital cardiac disease. Proc. Inst. Med. Chicago, 18:134, 1950.
13. Ekstrom, G.: The surgical treatment of patent ductus arteriosus. A clinical study of 290 cases. Acta Chir. Scand., Supp. 169, 1952.
14. Ellis, F. H., Jr., Kirklin, J. W., Callahan, J. A., and Wood, E. H.: Patent ductus with pulmonary hypertension. J. Thorac. Surg., 31:268, 1956.
15. Friedman, W. F., Hirschklan, M. J., Printz, M. P., Pitlick, P. T., and Kirkpatrick, S. E.: Pharmacologic closure of patent ductus arteriosus in the premature infant. New Eng. J. Med., 295:526, 1976.
16. Glass, I. H., Mustard, W. T., and Keith, J. D.: Coarctation of the aorta in infants. A review of twelve years' experience. Pediatrics, 26:109, 1960.
17. Gross, R. E.: The Surgery of Infancy and Childhood, Its Principles and Practice. Philadelphia, W. B. Saunders Company, 1953.
18. Gross, R. E.: An Atlas of Children's Surgery. Philadelphia, W. B. Saunders Company, 1970.
19. Hartmann, A. F., Jr., Goldring, D., Hernandez, A., Behrer, M. R., Schad, N., Ferguson, T., and Burford, T.: Recurrent coarctation of the aorta after successful repair in infancy. Amer. J. Cardiol., 25:405, 1970.
20. Heymann, M. A., Rudolph, A. M., and Silverman, N. H.: Closure of the ductus arteriosus in premature infants by inhibition of prostaglandin synthesis. N. Eng. J. Med., 295:530, 1976.
21. Horsley, B. L., Lerberg, D. B., Allen, A. C., Zuberbuhler, J. R., and Bahnson, H. T.: Respiratory distress from patent ductus arteriosus in the premature newborn. Ann. Surg., 177:806, 1973.
22. Iberra-Perez, C., Castaneda, A. R., Varco, R. L., and Lillehei, C. W.: Recoarctation of the aorta. Nineteen year clinical experience. Amer. J. Cardiol., 23:778, 1969.
23. Lueker, R. D., Vogel, J. N. K., and Blount, S. G., Jr.: Cardiovascular abnormality following surgery for left to right shunts. Observations in atrial septal defect, ventricular septal defect and patent ductus arteriosus. Circulation, 40:783, 1969.
24. Maron, B. J., Humphries, J. O., Rowe, R. D., and Mellits, E. D.: Prognosis of surgically corrected coarctation of the aorta. A 20 year postoperative appraisal. Circulation, 47:119, 1973.
25. Neuhauser, E. B. D.: The roentgen diagnosis of double aortic arch and other anomalies of the great vessels. Amer. J. Roentgen., 56:1, 1946.
26. Rumel, W. R., Bailey, C. P., Samson, P. C., Waterman, D. H., and Bing, R. J.: Surgical treatment of coarctation of aorta. Report of the Section on Cardiovascular Surgery, American College of Chest Physicians. J.A.M.A., 164:5, 1957.
27. Sauvage, L. R., and Harkins, H. N.: Growth of vascular anastomoses: An experimental study of the influence of suture type and suture method with a note on certain mechanical factors involved. Bull. Johns Hopkins Hosp., 91:276, 1952.
28. Schumacker, H. B., Jr., King, H., Nahrwald, D. L., and Waldhausen, J. A.: Coarctation of the aorta. Curr. Probl. Surg., Feb. 1968.
29. Scott, H. W., Jr., and Bahnson, H. T.: Evidence for a renal factor in the hypertension of experimental coarctation of the aorta. Surgery, 30:206, 1951.
30. Scott, H. W., Jr., and Sabiston, D. C., Jr.: Surgical treatment for congenital aorticopulmonary fistula. Experimental and clinical aspects. J. Thorac. Surg., 25:26, 1953.
31. Sealy, W. C., Harris, J. S., Young, W. G., Jr., and Callaway, H. A., Jr.: Paradoxical hypertension following resection of coarctation of the aorta. Surgery, 42:135, 1957.
32. Silverman, N. H., Lewis, A. B., Heymann, M. A., and Rudolph, A. M.: Echocardiographic assessment of ductus arteriosus shunt in premature infants. Circulation, 50:821, 1974.
33. Trusler, G. A., Arayangkoon, P., and Mustard, W. T.: Operative closure of isolated patent ductus arteriosus in the first two years of life. Canad. Med. Ass. J., 99:879, 1968.
34. Tyson, K. R., Harris, L. S., and Nghiem, Q. X.: Repair of aortic arch interruption in the neonate. Surgery, 67:1006, 1970.
35. Waterman, D. H., Samson, P. C., and Bailey, C. P.: The surgery of patent ductus arteriosus. A report of the Section on Cardiovascular Surgery. Dis. Chest, 29:102, 1956.
36. Ziegler, R. F.: The importance of patent ductus arteriosus in infants. Amer. Heart J., 43:553, 1952.

IV

ATRIAL SEPTAL DEFECTS, OSTIUM PRIMUM DEFECTS, AND ATRIOVENTRICULAR CANALS

John A. Waldhausen, M.D.,
and G. Frank O. Tyers, M.D.

HISTORICAL ASPECTS

The clinical features and pathophysiology of atrial septal defects have been studied for the past 150 years, and the first true anatomic description of septal defects was published by Rokitansky[58] in 1875. The first operation for atrial septal defect in man was reported in 1948.[49] The blind external techniques of invaginating the atrial wall into the defect[16] and of ligating the defect[49] resulted in some successful results.[2] However, incomplete closures and direction of a portion of the systemic venous return into the left atrium often followed these procedures. The blind internal technique described by Gross et al. used a rubber well sewn inside the atrial opening and allowed suturing inside the heart without direct vision.[38]

Combination of moderate hypothermia with temporary occlusion of the systemic venous return permitted accurate closure of atrial septal defects under direct vision, but even with multiple periods of venous occlusion, operating time was limited and complex defects could not be repaired.[46] In 1953 after 20 years of laboratory work, Gibbon first used mechanical cardiopulmonary bypass successfully for an operation on the human heart—closure of an atrial septal defect.[35] This is now the method of choice.

INCIDENCE

Atrial septal defect is the fifth most common congenital cardiac abnormality, occurring in one in 13,500 children under 14 years of age.[14] In the early years of cardiac surgery, atrial septal defect seemed to be the most common congenital lesion, because its relatively benign early course without treatment had permitted accumulation of a large number of patients. This also explains its low incidence, only 3 per cent, in Abbott's[1] postmortem series. It is still the most common congenital cardiac defect detected in persons over 20 years of age,[22] but in children the incidence has stabilized at approximately 7 per cent. Atrial septal defects occur three times as frequently in females as in males.

The incidence of *ostium primum* compared to that of other atrial defects can be seen in Table 1. Weidman and DuShane[73] cite a similar incidence. In contrast to ostium secundum defects, the sex distribution of ostium primum defects is equal.

At birth, persistent *common atrioventricular canal*

defects are more prevalent than ostium primum defects, but since the life span with this defect is significantly curtailed, the lesion is less common in older children and adolescents. It made up only 2 per cent of the congenital cardiac lesions in the series reported by Keith and his associates.[44] However, it represented 20 per cent of all atrial defects (Table 1). The sex incidence is equal. Down's syndrome has been reported in over 30 per cent of patients with the complete form of atrioventricular canal.[44] Minor and major associated anomalies are common.

ETIOLOGY

That atrial septal defect may result from genetic abnormalities is evidenced by its increased incidence in patients with such hereditary disorders as mongolism,[8] Turner's syndrome,[55] Ellis-van Creveld syndrome,[36] Marfan's syndrome, and the Ehler-Danlos syndrome.[74] The atrial septal defect in these disorders may be of the simple secundum variety, but more frequently single atrium (cor triloculare) or complex en-

TABLE 1. Atrial Septal Defects, Incidence of Subgroups, Hospital for Sick Children, Toronto*

Defect	Number of Cases	Per Cent of Total
Ostium secundum	307	68
Ostium primum	58	12
Atrioventricularis communis	87	20
Total	452	100
Ostium secundum	307 cases	
Isolated form		68.4
With pulmonary stenosis		10
With partial anomalous pulmonary vein drainage		7
With mitral stenosis		1
With rheumatic mitral insufficiency		0.3
With ventricular septal defect		5.0
With patent ductus		3.0
With coarctation of the aorta		0.3
Total		95

*From Keith, J. D., Rowe, R. D., and Vlad, P.: Heart Disease in Infancy and Childhood. New York, Macmillan Company, 1958.

docardial cushion defects are present. A familial incidence of atrial septal defect has been reported, and the inheritance of the defects in these cases is best explained on the basis of a dominant autosomal gene with incomplete penetrance. Prolonged A-V conduction is common among familial cases of atrial septal defect.[9] The risk to offspring of parents with atrial septal defects was 21 times greater than average,[9] but still less than 5 per cent.

Undetermined environmental influences are thought to cause the majority of atrial septal defects, however. This impression is based on the lack of association of most septal defects with known hereditary abnormalities, the high incidence of associated nongenetic abnormalities of other structures, and the lack of concordance of cardiac defects in identical twins.[71] Two environmental influences known to produce septal defects are maternal rubella infection[66] and the ingestion of thalidomide during the first trimester of pregnancy.

EMBRYOLOGY

By the fourth week of embryonic life, the venous end of the heart is composed of the sinus venosus, receiving two superior and two inferior venous channels; the primitive common atrium; and the atrioventricular canal.[24] During the fourth week, the septum primum begins to grow down from the posterior-superior aspect of the common atrium toward the endocardial cushions (Fig. 1). Its growth is temporarily arrested, and a crescentic inferior defect—ostium primum—is left just above the endocardial cushions. During the fifth and sixth weeks, growth of the septum primum resumes and the foramen primum is obliterated by union of the free edge of the septum primum with the fusing posterior and anterior endocardial cushions. The atrioventricular valves differentiate from the endocardial cushions, and the interventricular foramen is closed by proliferating tissue from the fused en-

docardial cushions and the bulbar ridges. Prior to obliteration of the foramen primum a second oval defect—the foramen secundum—is formed by cephalic degeneration of the septum primum. Later, a second septum—septum secundum—grows down from the right of the superior attachment of the septum primum between the septum primum and the left valve of the sinus venosus. It envelops the foramen secundum to form a unidirectional valve that allows passage of venous blood from the lower portion of the embryo and the placenta into the left atrium.

During the development of the interatrial septum, the sinus venosus is gradually absorbed into the atrium, and part of it eventually fuses with the posterior-superior portion of the interatrial septum. The right superior venous channel becomes the superior vena cava; the left superior venous channel becomes the coronary sinus, and the inferior venous channels become the inferior vena cava.

PATHOLOGIC ANATOMY

The morphology of interatrial defects is best understood when related to the previous section on embryology. Figure 2 shows the typical atrial septal and atrioventricular canal (endocardial cushion) defects superimposed on the normal right atrial anatomy.

Sinus Venosus and Secundum Defects

Failure of fusion of the left valve of the sinus venosus with the posterior-superior portion of the interatrial septum results in a high defect overlying the superior vena cava. This is frequently associated with absorption of a portion of the venous drainage of the right upper and middle lobes into what becomes the superior vena cava and the right atrium. As the sinus venosus defect underlies the superior caval orifice, the cava opens into both atria; there is no upper margin, and often the posterior margin is incomplete. The right upper pulmonary veins open into the superior vena cava, the middle vein opens into either atrium, and the lower pulmonary vein drains normally.[23]

Ostium secundum defects in the lower midportion of the interatrial septum result from failure of the septum secundum to close the ostium secundum. At times the defect may extend down to the inferior vena cava, leaving no atrial margin at the inferior border of the defect. If the degenerative process that produces the ostium secundum is excessive, multiple secundum defects result, or almost total lack of the interatrial septum can occur. Secundum defects are less frequently associated with venous drainage from the right lung into the right atrium, but if the defect is low, the right lower lobe may drain into what becomes the inferior vena cava. Probe patency (patent foramen ovale) of the ostium secundum occurs in approximately 30 per cent of adults[70] but is seldom of pathologic significance. There is a greater than expected incidence of mitral stenosis of rheumatic origin[65] associated with secundum defects (Lutembacher's syndrome). Other associated congenital cardiac anomalies include pulmonary stenosis, mitral regurgitation,[21, 43] and ventricular septal defects[31] (see Table 1).

Endocardial Cushion Defects

When the septum primum fails to resume its downward growth, an ostium primum defect with a crescentic upper border centered over the junction of the

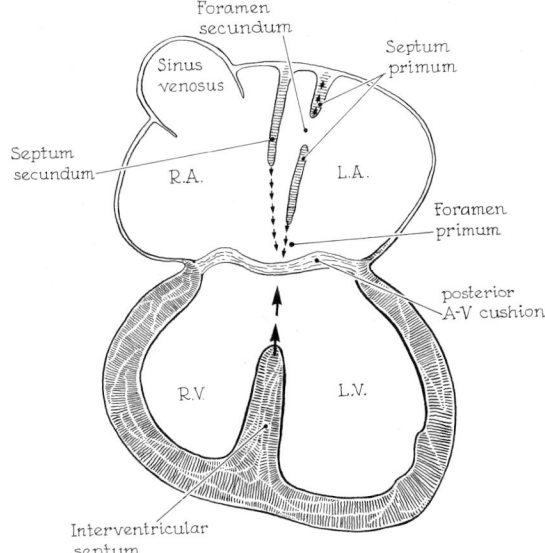

Figure 1. Embryology of the atrial septum and endocardial cushion. Arrows show direction of growth or regression of septal structures.

atrioventricular valve annuli occurs. This has also been referred to as a partial persistent common atrioventricular canal, and usually is associated with a cleft in the septal leaflets of the mitral and tricuspid valves and some abnormality of the chordae tendineae. There may be narrowing of the aortic outflow tract, resulting in the characteristic "gooseneck" deformity on cineangiocardiography[3, 10] An ostium primum defect can occur either alone, with a mitral valve cleft, or with both a mitral and tricuspid valve cleft (Fig. 3). The isolated form is uncommon (Table 2). When an ostium primum defect is associated with persistence of a high ventricular septal defect, it is known as a persistent common atrioventricular canal. Rarely the atrial portion is closed and only the valve leaflet clefts occur in association with a ventricular septal defect. An isolated mitral valve cleft or an isolated ventricular septal defect may also occur.[51] However, in the usual persistent common atrioventricular canal, the ostium primum is associated with a single atrioventricular valve with common anterior and posterior leaflets and a large interventricular septal defect, which may be almost complete.[56]

Rastelli et al.[56] observed three forms of complete atrioventricular canal.

Type I. Here the common anterior leaflet is divided into two distinct portions, one relating to the entrance into the left ventricle and one to that into the right ventricle (Fig. 4). Both portions are attached medially to the ventricular septum, while laterally they are attached to normally placed papillary muscles. The posterior leaflet is single and may or may not be attached to the septum. The membranous septum is intact.

Type II. This lesion differs from Type I in that the medial portion of each of the two distinct parts of the anterior leaflet is attached by chordae to an anomalous papillary muscle in the right ventricle (Fig. 5). The membranous portion of the septum is incompletely developed, with a defect subjacent to the aortic valve.

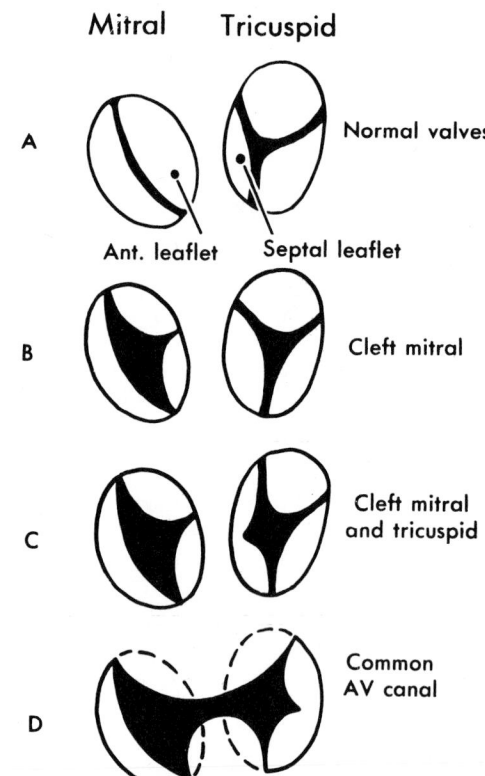

Figure 3. The mitral and tricuspid valve abnormalities seen in endocardial cushion defects. (Modified from Bedford, D. E., et al.: Lancet 1:1255, 1957.)

Type III. In this form of atrioventricular canal, the anterior leaflet is undivided and there are no attachments to the ventricular septum (Fig. 6). The membranous septum is also deficient, and an interventricular communication beneath the aortic valve results.

Type I is by far the most common (70 per cent) form of persistent atrioventricular canal if only minor associated cardiac defects are present. However, Types II

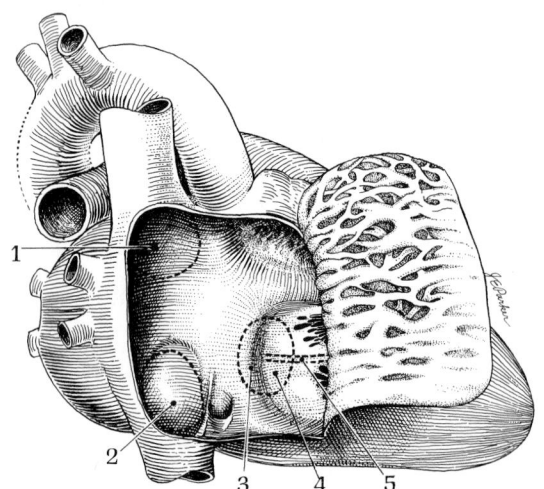

Figure 2. The different types of atrial septal defects. 1, Sinus venosus defect. 2, Ostium secundum defect. 3, Ostium primum defect. 4, Ventricular septal defect of a complete atrioventricular canal. 5, Cleft septal leaflet of mitral valve. Together, 3, 4, and 5, Complete atrioventricular canal.

TABLE 2. Incidence of Associated Abnormalities in Fifty Patients with Ostium Primum Defects of the Atrial Septum*

Type of Lesion	No. of Patients
Isolated ostium primum atrial septal defect	3+
Primum atrial septal defect with cleft mitral valve	15
Primum atrial septal defect with cleft mitral and tricuspid valves	6
Common atrium with cleft mitral valve	3
Common atrioventricular canal	23
Total	50

*From Evans, J. R., Rowe, R. D., and Keith, J. D.: Am. J. Med., 30:345, 1961.

†One patient had, in addition, a secundum atrial septal defect and pulmonary stenosis.

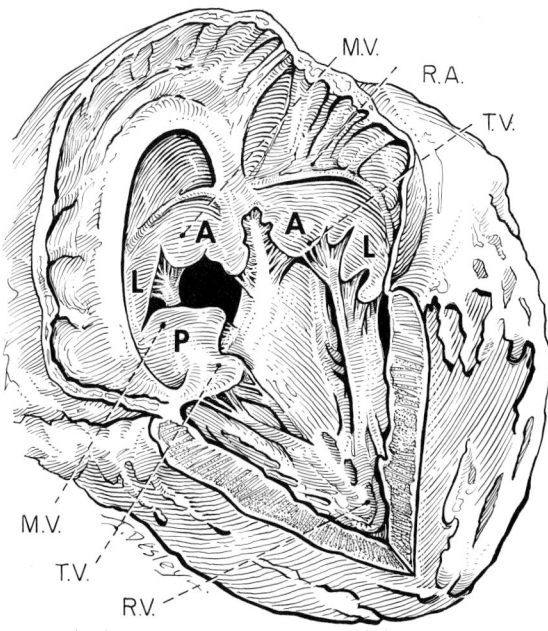

Figure 4. Most common type of complete form of atrioventricular canal as viewed from the right atrium and right ventricle. The anterior leaflet is divided into two distinct portions, both attached medially to the ventricular septum. A and P indicate common anterior and posterior leaflets of this single atrioventricular valve. L indicates a lateral leaflet. M.V. and T.V. indicate mitral and tricuspid portions of leaflets; R.A. and R.V. indicate right atrium and right ventricle. (From McGoon, D. C. *In* Cooper, P.: The Craft of Surgery. Vol. 1. 2nd ed. Boston, Little, Brown and Company, 1971.)

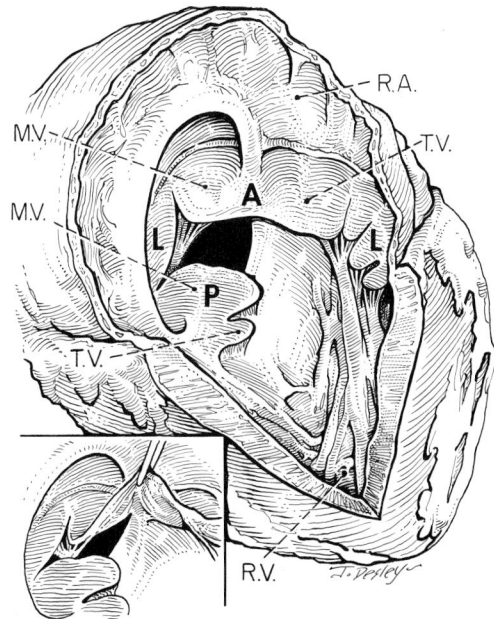

Figure 6. Complete form of common atrioventricular canal most commonly associated with other major cardiac anomalies. The undivided anterior leaflet is unattached to the ventricular septum (inset). A and P are common anterior and posterior leaflets of single, atrioventricular valve, L and L are lateral leaflets, M.V. and T.V. are mitral and tricuspid portions of common valve, and R.A. and R.V. are right atrium and right ventricle. (From McGoon, D. C. *In* Cooper, P.: The Craft of Surgery. Vol. 1. 2nd ed. Boston, Little, Brown and Company, 1971.)

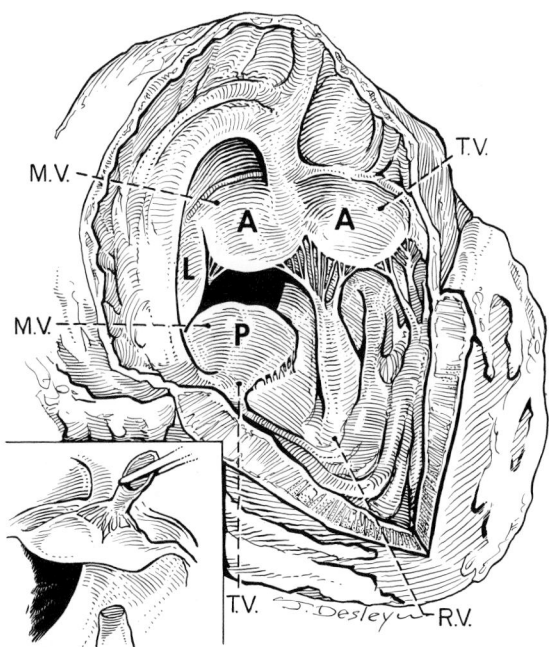

Figure 5. Complete form of atrioventricular canal in which the anterior leaflet is divided, and the medial aspect of each portion (A) is attached by chordae to a papillary muscle in the right ventricle (R.V.). P indicates common posterior leaflet, L indicates lateral leaflet, and M.V. and T.V. indicate mitral and tricuspid portions of leaflets. (From McGoon, D. C. *In* Cooper, P.: The Craft of Surgery. Vol. 1. 2nd ed. Boston, Little, Brown and Company, 1971.)

and III are most common when major cardiac malformations are associated. Posterior displacement and elongation of the bundle of His associated with this defect render the conduction system very susceptible to injury. Pulmonary vascular changes associated with pulmonary hypertension are also frequent.

Complete absence of the atrial septum, or cor triloculare, also occurs and probably results from failure of multiple embryologic processes during the development of the heart. It is usually associated with other severe congenital defects.[28]

The distribution of the various forms of endocardial cushion defects can be seen in Table 2.[31] Another lesion described in association is pulmonic stenosis, which may be valvular or combined valvular and infundibular.[59]

SECUNDUM AND SINUS VENOSUS DEFECTS OF THE ATRIUM

Physiology

In the normal heart, there is a positive pressure difference between the left and right atrium that is responsible for keeping the foramen ovale closed. This pressure gradient is reduced in small atrial septal defects but still contributes to the left-to-right shunt. Even with large defects a gradient may persist in certain patients.[30] Correlation of instantaneous pressure differences across the defect with the direction of flow, as seen by cineangiocardiography, showed the onset of flow across the defect to occur 50 to 75 milliseconds after the onset of the gradient. The major left-to-right shunt and pressure gradient occurred over an interval encompassing ventricular systole and early diastole (Fig. 7).[45] Also, there was augmentation of the left-to-right shunt during atrial contraction. In large atrial septal defects, this gradient is abolished. Direction of shunt flow then is determined to a large extent by the compliance of the right and left ventricles.[12] In infancy, the ventricles are of nearly equal thickness and compliance, but as the pressure in the pulmonary artery falls, the right ventricular muscle mass decreases, with a resultant increase in compliance. This causes more blood from the "common" atrium to enter the right ventricle and results in a gradually enlarging left-to-right shunt. As pulmonary hypertension develops later in life, hypertrophy of the right ventricle results in decreased compliance. The left-to-right shunt diminishes or even reverses and becomes a right-to-left shunt.

Even in the absence of pulmonary hypertension, some right-to-left shunting can be demonstrated in most atrial septal defects. It is due in part to streaming of blood from the inferior vena cava across the defect because of some overriding of the cava by the defect and the flap action of the eustachian valve. This small right-to-left shunt is not sufficient to cause cyanosis and usually can be detected only by dye dilution curves with injection into the inferior vena cava and sampling from the aorta or its branches.[67] However, right-to-left shunting does permit emboli from the peripheral veins and the right side of the heart to enter the systemic circulation (paradoxical embolism).[70] Pulmonary embolism (nonparadoxical embolism) is frequently associated. The paradoxical emboli usually lodge in the middle cerebral artery or one of its branches and cause stroke and occasionally brain abscess. The kidney and other viscera are less frequently involved.

Because of the proximity of the right pulmonary vein orifices to the atrial defect, there is preferential left-to-right shunting of blood from the right lung.[68] Studies of patients with atrial septal defects during exercise show that pulmonary blood flow increases in proportion to systemic blood flow in those with small left-to-right shunts. However, in patients with large shunts, pulmonary blood flow either stays the same or occasionally falls slightly,[52] which suggests that maximal output from the right ventricle has become the limiting factor.

The left-to-right shunt may be quite large and result in a pulmonary blood flow three to four times systemic blood flow ($Q_p:Q_s = 3$ to 4:1). In a series of 26 children aged 3 to 14, Levin et al.[45] found the mean left-to-right shunt to be 65 per cent (range, 59 to 74 per cent) of total pulmonary blood flow. At operation the atrial septal defects varied from 1.5 to 3 cm. in diameter. Systemic blood flow is usually normal. In spite of this large pulmonary blood flow, pulmonary hypertension is rare in children and begins to appear only in adulthood, in the second or third decade of life. Pulmonary arteries may show medial hypertrophy and intimal proliferation. The changes are rarely greater than grade 2 (Heath and Edwards classification).[42] Pulmonary diffusing capacity, as measured by $D_{L_{CO}}$, in patients with atrial septal defects is increased compared to that in normal subjects and increases in the same proportion during exercise.[5]

The large flow across the pulmonary outflow tract often results in a right ventricular pulmonary artery gradient as high as 40 mm. Hg. The pulmonary valve is normal, and after repair the flow gradient is abolished.

The physiologic changes in patients with sinus venosus defects and partial anomalous venous return are not significantly different from those in patients with ostium secundum defects.

Clinical Manifestations

Children with moderate shunts usually have few if any symptoms, and therefore the diagnosis is often made during a routine preschool physical examination. Patients with large shunts may have symptoms of fatigue, exertional dyspnea, and at times frank congestive heart failure. The structural and functional impairment that follows prolonged volume overload of the right ventricle eventually involves and leads to failure

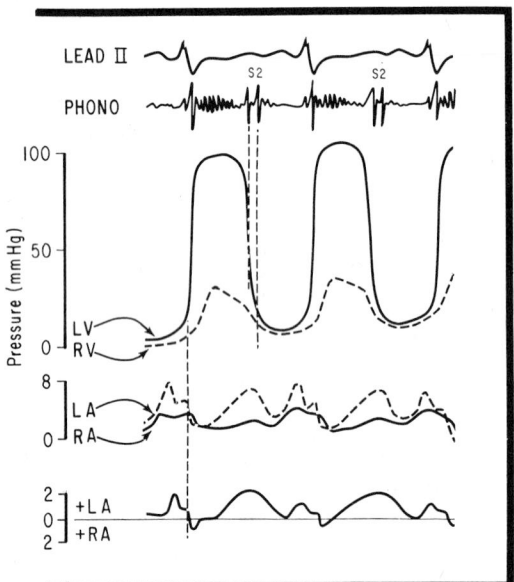

Figure 7. Intracardiac pressure dynamics in secundum atrial septum defects. The tracings were obtained with simultaneous monitoring of right and left ventricular pressures by means of Statham SF-1 pressure-tipped transducer catheters. The catheters were subsequently withdrawn to record both atrial pressures. There was no change in rate (R-R interval remained constant). All data were recorded simultaneously with the lead II electrocardiogram and the phonocardiogram in the second left interspace. A composite was made by direct overlay tracings to produce the time-aligned data as indicated.

The predominant left-to-right gradient occurred over an interval extending from midventricular systole into early diastole. The peak of the left atrial v wave was coincident with the interval of the second sound. The fluctuations in left atrial pressure can be seen to be more prominent than those of the right atrium. The transient right-to-left gradient occurred coincident with the onset of ventricular contraction. (From Levin, A. R., et al.: Circulation, *37*:476, 1968. By permission of the American Heart Association, Inc.)

of both ventricles.[32, 53] Similarly, patients with pulmonary hypertension will have exertional dyspnea and possibly cyanosis. Significant disease may, however, exist without symptoms.[73]

On physical examination, the findings are dependent upon the presence or absence of pulmonary hypertension. The typical child with a sinus venosus or secundum defect looks healthy. A right ventricular lift is palpable. The first heart sound is often accentuated, while the second is almost always split in all phases of respiration, in part as a result of delayed right ventricular emptying.[31] The second sound is often slightly increased in intensity, even in the absence of pulmonary hypertension.

Because of the increased pulmonary blood flow, there is usually a pulmonary ejection-type systolic murmur audible along the left sternal border in the second and third intercostal spaces. The large flow across the tricuspid valve results in an early diastolic murmur along the lower left sternal border.[50]

With the development of pulmonary hypertension, the pulmonary second sound increases while the systolic ejection murmur decreases and the diastolic murmur is no longer audible.

On phonocardiography the peaked jugular "v" wave exceeded the "A" wave in approximately 40 per cent of patients with atrial septal defect.[69]

Electrocardiographic Features

The electrocardiogram usually shows some variant of incomplete right bundle branch block in the first precordial lead. The mean axis of the QRS complex lies between +60 and −150 degrees, although in most patients the axis will be between +90 and +150. Prominent P waves may suggest atrial enlargement.

The vectorcardiogram shows a clockwise loop directed inferiorly and to the right in the frontal projection (Fig. 8).[31]

Radiologic Features

Slight to moderate cardiac enlargement is common (Fig. 9). Chamber analysis usually shows enlargement of the right atrium and ventricle and main pulmonary artery. Pulmonary vascular markings are increased. The left ventricle and aorta are either normal or slightly small.

Echocardiography

By measuring the size of the right ventricle and assessing motion of the interventricular septum, this study can distinguish patients with atrial septal defects from normal patients and those with patent ductus and ventricular septal defects.[25]

Cardiac Catheterization and Angiocardiography

Cardiac catheterization and oxygen measurements show a step-up in oxygen saturation in the right atrium when compared to the superior and inferior venae cavae. (Measurement of such a step-up may be inaccurate because of streaming and catheter tip location.) Partial anomalous venous return may produce similar findings, and it may be possible to differentiate it by inserting the catheter into the abnormally

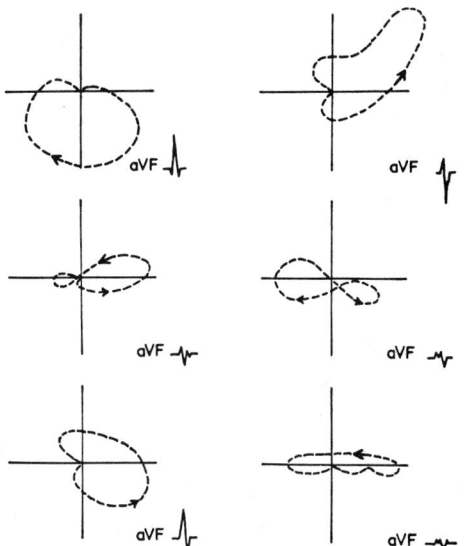

Figure 8. Frontal vector of the QRS complex computed from the electrocardiogram of six patients showing clockwise loop usually seen with secundum defects and counterclockwise loop above the horizontal plane typical of ostium primum defects. Vectors with a figure-of-eight pattern of flat loop closely applied to the horizontal axis may be seen with either secundum or primum defects. The configuration of the QRS complex in lead aVF is shown alongside the vector loop. (From Evans, J. R., et al.: Am. J. Med., 30:345, 1961.)

located orifice of the pulmonary vein. Injection of contrast medium into the left atrium during cineangiography will show the left-to-right shunt as well as the pulmonary recirculation. Injection of contrast medium into the left ventricle will help rule out an ostium primum defect with mitral incompetence. A systolic flow gradient as high as 40 mm. Hg may be detected

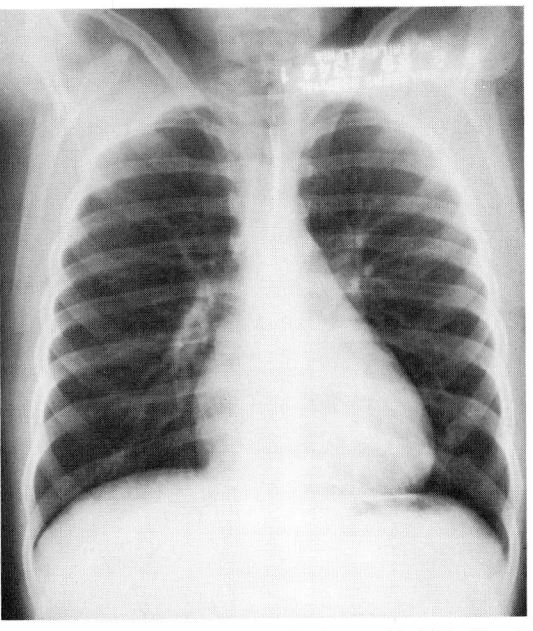

Figure 9. Chest roentgenogram of a 9-year-old child with ostium secundum defect.

across the pulmonary outflow tract. Accurate diagnosis of an atrial septal defect can usually be made from the clinical findings, the results of cardiac catheterization and cineangiocardiography, and the electrocardiogram.[26, 30]

Natural History

Prognosis is based on shunt size, but a single atrial defect is compatible with a longer life than a ventricular septal defect. Reports of patients living into the seventh and eighth decades are not uncommon. Life expectancy in two series of untreated patients was 42 and 38 years, respectively.[17]

The majority of patients have few symptoms in infancy and childhood. Nevertheless, on rare occasions congestive failure in infancy does occur in association with very large shunts and requires an aggressive therapeutic approach.[13, 40] Spontaneous closure has been reported in infancy but is a rare occurrence.

The development of pulmonary hypertension is a serious prognostic finding and usually occurs in adult life (Fig. 11). Gault et al.[34] studied 62 patients who were 40 years of age or older. Forty-five per cent were in functional class III or IV. Sixty-nine per cent had pulmonary artery hypertension, and in 28 per cent it was severe.

In other adults with moderate shunts, without significant pulmonary hypertension, symptoms develop after the onset of coronary artery disease. The decreased myocardial oxygenation and the persistent overload of the right ventricle result in congestive heart failure.[32] Cardiac arrhythmias such as atrial flutter or fibrillation are common in patients over 40 years old, although they may occur at any age.[60] A composite graphic presentation of the principal factors influencing the course of patients with atrial septal defects is shown in Figure 11.[44] Patients living at lower altitudes have less severe pulmonary hypertension than those at high elevations. The average mean pulmonary artery pressure in a group of patients under 20 years old living below 2000 ft. was 18.7 mm. Hg, whereas in a comparable group living at 4000 ft. the mean pressure was 30.4 mm. Hg.[20] Bacterial endocarditis is rare in patients with ostium secundum

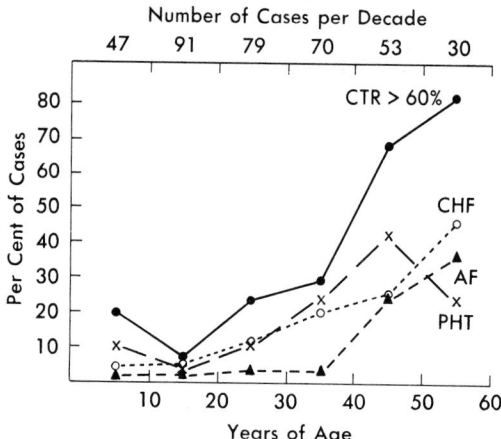

Atrial Septal Defect

Ost. secundum – 381 cases
Ost. primum – 59 cases

Figure 11. Complications in 440 patients with atrial septal defects, chiefly ostium secundum. CTR, cardiothoracic ratio; CHF, congestive heart failure; AF, atrial fibrillation; PHT, pulmonary hypertension. After the age of 40 years these complications increase significantly. (From Bedford, D. E., and Besterman, E. M. M. *In* Keith, J. D., et al.: Heart Disease in Infancy and Childhood, 2nd ed. New York, The Macmillan Company, 1967.)

defects. When it does occur, it usually involves the pulmonary valve and right ventricular outflow tract; in patients without septal defects, it is more likely to involve the tricuspid valve.[37]

Indications for Operation

Indication for operation is the presence of a shunt resulting in a pulmonary blood flow at least 1.5 times systemic flow ($Q_p:Q_s > 1.5$, where Q_p equals pulmonary flow and Q_s equals systemic flow) without severe pulmonary vascular disease ($R_p:R_s: > 0.7$, where R_p equals pulmonary vascular resistance and R_s equals systemic resistance). The optimal time for repair is between 5 and 8 years of age even if the patient is asymptomatic. Repair at any age thereafter is also indicated but is less desirable in view of such diverse factors as family responsibilities of the patient, emotional stability, pulmonary hypertension, and coronary artery disease.

Treatment

Cardiopulmonary bypass should be used in operations for closure of sinus venosus and secundum defects. This allows for precise closure as well as insertion of a patch in large defects. Furthermore, failure to recognize partial anomalous pulmonary venous drainage at the time of catheterization is of little significance, since the repair is not very difficult when cardiopulmonary bypass is used. The use of hypothermia and venous inflow occlusion has as its main virtue simplicity and the lack of need for blood to prime the extracorporeal circuit. However, the time available for intracardiac repair is limited and is insufficient for accurate repair of unforeseen complicating defects.

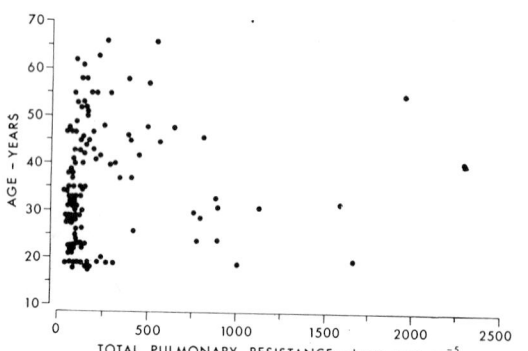

Figure 10. Relationship between patients' ages at the time of cardiac catheterization and the total pulmonary vascular resistance. (From Craig, R. J., and Selzer, A.: Circulation, 37:805, 1968. By permission of the American Heart Association, Inc.)

Normothermic cardiopulmonary bypass is usually preferred, and left ventricular drainage may be employed to avoid air embolism. Others have temporarily induced ventricular fibrillation to prevent the left ventricle from ejecting air into the systemic circulation while the right atrium is open. Through an atrial incision, the atrial septum is visualized (Fig. 12). Small defects can readily be closed with a continuous suture, but larger defects should be closed with a patch.[48] It has been shown that postoperative residual defects are common in those patients with large defects closed without a patch. Although Dacron or Teflon is quite satisfactory, we prefer to use the patient's own pericardium, since it is autogenous tissue. In the rare instances of postoperative bacterial endocarditis, bloodstream sterilization can be achieved in patients who have pericardial patches but not in those in whom synthetic material was used.[54]

Operative mortality in patients without pulmonary artery hypertension is quite low, less than 2 per cent in most series. Sellers et al.[61] reported a 1.8 per cent hospital mortality and no late deaths in 225 operations for ostium secundum defects with normal pulmonary artery pressure. Even in older patients, mortality has been quite low, and age per se should not be a contraindication to operation.[27] In patients with pulmonary artery hypertension, mortality will increase in direct proportion to the degree of hypertension, but results are still acceptable if the ratio of pulmonary vascular resistance to systemic resistance is below 0.7. Beck et al.[4] showed that in 9 of 11 patients the pulmo-

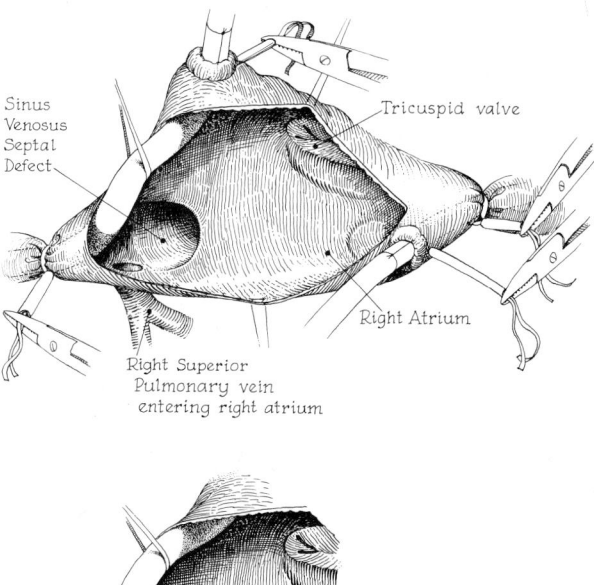

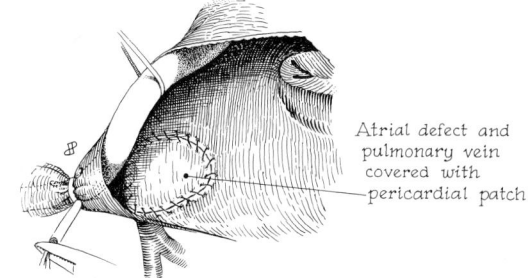

Figure 13. Repair of sinus venosus type atrial septal defect with anomalous return of right upper lobe veins.

nary vascular resistance fell from a preoperative average of 510 dynes/sec./cm.$^{-5}$ to 230 dynes/sec./cm.$^{-5}$ postoperatively. Attempts to close defects in patients in whom pulmonary vascular resistance approaches systemic resistance have been fatal or have not produced a significant fall in pulmonary artery pressure. Closure of ostium secundum defects by means of a perforated prosthesis that eventually closed completely appeared to improve survival in these very ill patients but did not alter the course of the patients' pulmonary hypertension.[14]

Repair of sinus venous defects usually requires a patch to divert the anomalous pulmonary venous drainage through the atrial septal defect into the left atrium (Fig. 13). Results are quite good and comparable to those of repair of ostium secundum defects.[19]

Thromboembolism postoperatively following closure of an atrial septal defect is well documented and occurred in 35 of 546 patients traced 2 to 15 years after closure of an uncomplicated defect. Eleven of the 35 patients succumbed to the embolism. This complication is more common in older patients and those with atrial fibrillation.[49]

OSTIUM PRIMUM DEFECT

Physiology

As in secundum defects, the left-to-right shunt is usually large and dependent upon the size of the

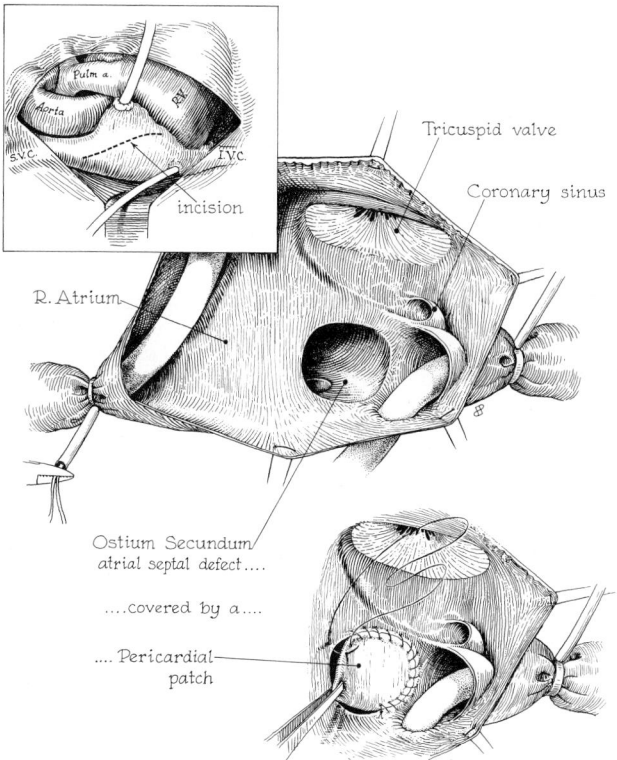

Figure 12. Repair of ostium secundum type atrial septal defect.

defect as well as upon ventricular compliance. Isolated ostium primum defects differ little physiologically from ostium secundum defects. However, a cleft mitral valve with mitral insufficiency may result in a greater left-to-right shunt. Often the regurgitant jet is ejected almost directly into the right atrium through the large septal defect. There is also volume overloading of the left ventricle. A large degree of mitral insufficiency associated with a large left-to-right shunt results in more pronounced symptoms and earlier onset of pulmonary artery hypertension than in the usual atrial septal defect.

Clinical Manifestations

The lesion is commonly discovered in infancy because of the mitral insufficiency murmur. Dyspnea and fatigue, failure to gain weight, and frequent respiratory infections are common. Congestive heart failure is not uncommon. These findings are dependent upon the degree of mitral insufficiency. The clinical features in patients with ostium primum defects without mitral regurgitation are similar to those in patients with ostium secundum defects.[31] Involvement of the tricuspid valve leads to an increased incidence and earlier onset of congestive heart failure and pulmonary hypertension.[75]

On physical examination, bulging of the left anterior chest wall and both right and left ventricular lifts are found. The pulmonary ejection murmur is more prominent than in an ostium secundum defect. The most characteristic finding is the murmur of mitral regurgitation at the apex extending out to the axilla. A mid-diastolic flow murmur across the tricuspid valve may be audible along the lower left sternal border. The second heart sound is widely split and possibly accentuated, depending upon the degree of pulmonary artery hypertension.

Electrocardiographic Features

The electrocardiogram is diagnostic and shows left axis deviation. The P waves show changes indicating atrial enlargement and the P-R interval is prolonged.[72] The vector loop shows a counterclockwise rotation to the left and superiorly in all cases (see Fig. 8).[31, 44] In most cases, the frontal plane loop lies above the isoelectric line. Delay in right ventricular activation due to volume overload is constant, while left ventricular overload is seen in those with marked mitral insufficiency.

Radiologic Features

Cardiac enlargement and increased pulmonary vascularity are more prominent than in patients with ostium secundum defects, but differentiation between the two lesions on a chest roentgenogram may be difficult (Fig. 14).

Echocardiography

Abnormalities of the mitral valve in endocardial cushion defects are well demonstrated by echo.[76]

Cardiac Catheterization and Angiocardiography

A large left-to-right shunt can be demonstrated by a step-up in the oxygen saturation from the venae cavae

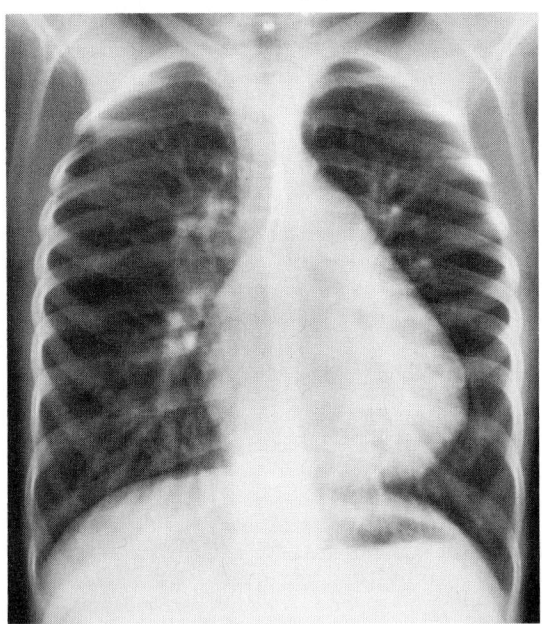

Figure 14.   Chest roentgenogram of an 11-year-old boy with an ostium primum defect with a cleft mitral valve and mitral incompetence.

to the right atrium. Often this step-up is low near the tricuspid valve, and at times, because of streaming, the increase may be detected only after entrance of the catheter through the tricuspid valve into right ventricular inflow tract; this may falsely suggest a ventricular septal defect. The left ventricular angiogram is quite diagnostic, showing the gooseneck deformity of the outflow tract as well as mitral regurgitation (Fig. 15). The gooseneck deformity is due to the abnormal mitral valve,[3] and the short nature of both the left ventricular diaphragmatic wall and the posterior aspect of the ventricular septum.[10]

Natural History

In a series of 122 patients ranging in age from 11 days to 69 years reviewed by Somerville,[63] death occurred at all ages, from 2 weeks to 56 years. The median age at death was 23 years in 18 cases collected from the literature by Fontana and Edwards.[33] The development of dysrhythmia was relatively common, occurring in 20 per cent of patients. It was a poor prognostic sign and was more common after the age of 30[31] (see Fig. 11). The arrhythmias were usually atrial fibrillation, nodal rhythm, ventricular tachycardia, or complete heart block.

Another complication is congestive heart failure, which was most common in infancy and childhood but was seen at all ages in Fontana and Edwards' series.[33] Pulmonary hypertension was more common than in ostium secundum defects, but in Somerville's review[63] only four such patients were identified and only two died of pulmonary hypertension. In the series of Ellis et al.,[29] 16 of 48 patients with ostium primum defects had significant pulmonary hypertension, although all were less than 16 years old.

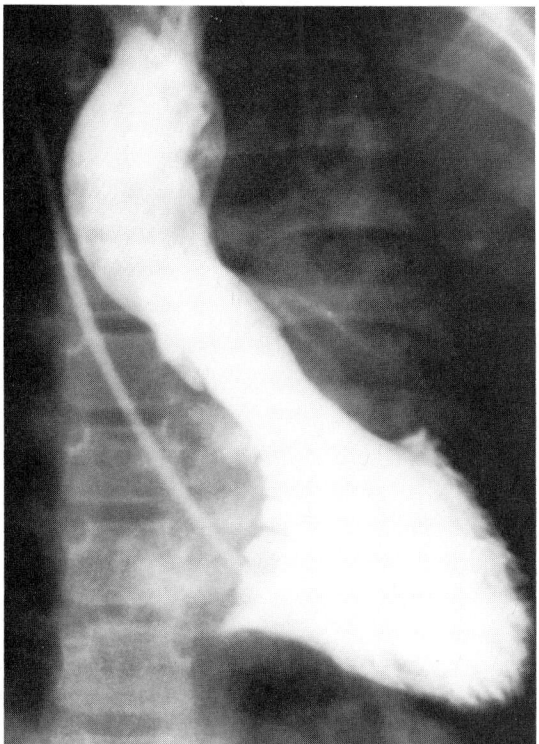

Figure 15. Frontal left ventriculogram in systole in a case of ostium primum defect. Note the elongation and narrowing of the left ventricular outflow tract. The right outline of the ventricular silhouette is scalloped and shows a deep, nonopaque indentation in the area where the two segments of the divided anterior mitral leaflet coapt. (From Moss, A. J., and Adams, F. H.: Heart Disease in Infants, Children and Adolescents. Baltimore, Williams & Wilkins Company, 1968.)

Mitral regurgitation appears to be a major determining factor in the ultimate prognosis of a patient with an ostium primum defect. Although most patients with primum defects have a shorter life expectancy, this is especially true when the lesion is associated with severe mitral regurgitation. Significant tricuspid regurgitation also worsens the prognosis.

Indications for Operation

In view of the relatively poor prognosis, virtually all patients with ostium primum defects should have repair. Shunts almost never are so small that repair is not indicated.[75] More complex is the question of mitral valve repair. Injudicious suture of a competent although cleft valve may lead to severe distortion and regurgitation or stenosis. Aortic obstruction has also been seen.[47] Clearly, all valves showing significant regurgitation during left ventricular angiography should be repaired. To omit this part of the operation can be most serious, since repair of the atrial defect destroys the "blowoff" effect through the atrial defect. It has been our practice to assess the competence of the valve carefully with cineangiography and at operation. With careful placement of sutures, valve distortion occurred in only one patient in a series of 25 ostium primum repairs. This patient had a marked

valve leaflet deficiency and ultimately required a mitral valve prosthesis.

The optimal age for repair is somewhere between 5 and 8 years, but at times earlier repair, because of cardiac failure, or later repair, because of lack of recognition, will be required.

Treatment

Defects are repaired with the patient supported by cardiopulmonary bypass. Through the right atrium, the interatrial septum is visualized and the defect inspected (Fig. 16). The characteristic low location of the defect and the lack of atrial tissue between the valve annulus and the defect make the nature of the anomaly apparent. Inspection of the septal leaflet of the mitral valve usually shows the cleft. This leaflet is carefully elevated out of the ventricle with nerve hooks. Proper anatomic approximation of the leaflet halves can then readily be accomplished with interrupted sutures.

The septal defect is closed with a patch of either pericardium or synthetic material such as Dacron. Interrupted sutures are carefully placed superficially at the inferior margin of the defect in order to avoid damage to the conduction system and complete heart block. A running suture is then used to sew the patch to the remaining atrial wall. In addition, there may be an ostium secundum defect requiring separate closure. Inspection of the tricuspid valve may also show a cleft in the septal leaflet, but repair is generally not required.

Postoperative care is not unusual save for the management of arrhythmias. Complete heart block requires the use of cardiac pacing, and pacing wires should be attached to the ventricle. However, surgically produced permanent third-degree heart block is exceedingly rare. If it is acquired, a permanent pacemaker should be implanted, since all patients with postsurgical heart block are in danger of sudden death. In some patients, preoperative heart block exists and may require permanent pacing if the ventricular rate is below 60 beats per minute.

Results have been excellent and operative mortality is quite low.[18, 29] A residual murmur of mitral insufficiency is quite common but is usually of little hemodynamic significance.

A serious complication of repair of this lesion has been the development of hemolytic anemia that is difficult to control medically. At times there is hemoglobinuria. Hemolysis results when a regurgitant jet through an incompetent, inadequately repaired mitral valve strikes the septal Teflon prosthesis, which acts like a "washboard." Repair of the valve or, at times, valve replacement may be required.[62] Replacement of the Teflon patch by pericardium may further improve the condition.

COMMON ATRIUM

This uncommon lesion represents a form of partial atrioventricular canal with absence of the entire atrial septum. The septal leaflet of the mitral valve is usually cleft, and the septal leaflet of the tricuspid

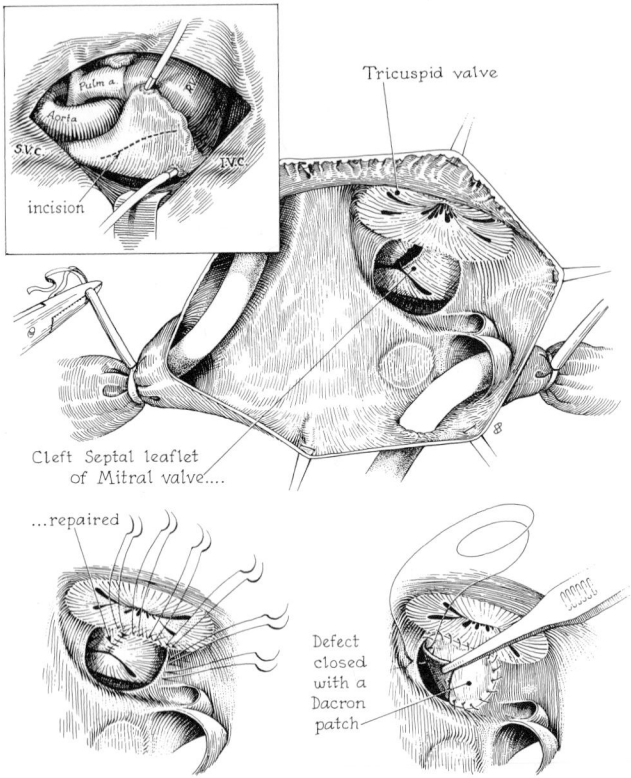

Tricuspid valve

Figure 16. Repair of an ostium primum defect with cleft mitral valve.

Cleft Septal leaflet of Mitral valve....

...repaired

Defect closed with a Dacron patch

valve may also be involved (see Table 2). Patients with this condition usually show symptoms of decreased exercise tolerance, fatigue, and dyspnea. Cyanosis may be noted on exercise. Symptoms may occur in infancy. Physical findings include a hyperactive heart, a widely split second heart sound, and a loud systolic ejection murmur at the left upper sternal border. The characteristic high-pitched holosystolic murmur due to mitral insufficiency can be heard at the apex with transmission to the axilla. The electrocardiogram is similar to that seen in patients with atrioventricular canal, while the roentgenogram shows marked cardiomegaly with increased pulmonary vascular markings owing to the large pulmonary blood flow. Cardiac catheterization shows almost complete mixing of the pulmonary and systemic venous blood, resulting in nearly equal oxygen saturation in the pulmonary artery and aortic blood. Indicator dilution curves may be of some help in demonstrating the lesion.[28] Angiocardiography shows simultaneous filling of both atria. Differentiation from total anomalous pulmonary venous return may be difficult, but many patients with this defect have an anomalous left vertical vein, and its absence lends support to a diagnosis of common atrium. Most patients require operative treatment. Contraindication to operation is primarily the severe pulmonary vascular disease, and the guidelines are similar to those for other atrial defects ($R_p:R_s$ > 0.7). The large atrial defect is closed with a Dacron prosthesis. Mitral valve repair should be performed as in the more common ostium primum defects.

PERSISTENT COMMON ATRIOVENTRICULAR CANAL

Physiology

The degree of pathophysiologic change is determined by several factors: (1) size of the ventricular septal defect; (2) degree of atrioventricular valve insufficiency; (3) degree of pulmonary hypertension; and (4) size of the atrial septal defect. Associated defects such as pulmonic stenosis or patent ductus may also significantly affect hemodynamics.

In many patients with persistent common atrioventricular canal the ventricular septal defect is large and contributes to a large left-to-right shunt. Because of the increased pulmonary blood flow and the direct pressure transmission from the left ventricle to the pulmonary artery, patients with an atrioventricular canal frequently have pulmonary hypertension. This is further aggravated by atrioventricular valve insufficiency. Indeed, right ventricular blood may eject through the incompetent common atrioventricular valve into the left atrium. This results in pressure elevation in the left atrium (in addition to the usual pressure elevation in the right atrium) and cyanosis. This cyanosis is not dependent on high pulmonary vascular resistance and therefore is not necessarily a sign of inoperability.

Clinical Manifestations

Most patients have severe symptoms early in life, and heart failure is common. Cyanosis is present in approximately 15 per cent and may be severe if there is associated pulmonary stenosis. Failure to thrive and repeated respiratory infections are common.

On physical examination, these patients are often found to be dyspneic, underdeveloped, thin infants or children with marked precordial activity and a precordial bulge. A thrill may be palpable. On auscultation the first heart sound is split and accentuated because of pulmonary hypertension. A loud holosytolic murmur from the ventricular septal defect is heard along the lower left sternal border, and is often transmitted to the back. A high-pitched murmur due to mitral insufficiency may be heard at the apex radiating into the axilla. A pulmonic ejection murmur may also be audible, as well as mid-diastolic flow murmur across the common atrioventricular valve.

Electrocardiographic Features

These are quite characteristic.[15] The mean electric axis of the QRS lies above the isoelectric line, and the vector loop in the frontal plane is directed counterclockwise. In all cases there is scalar electrocardiographic and vectorcardiographic evidence of right ventricular hypertrophy.

Radiologic Features

The heart is always enlarged (average cardiothoracic ratio, 0.62), and all four chambers are usually involved. The pulmonary artery is prominent, and the pulmonary vascular markings are increased (Fig. 17).

Echocardiography

The mitral valve abnormality can be confirmed noninvasively by echocardiography.[76]

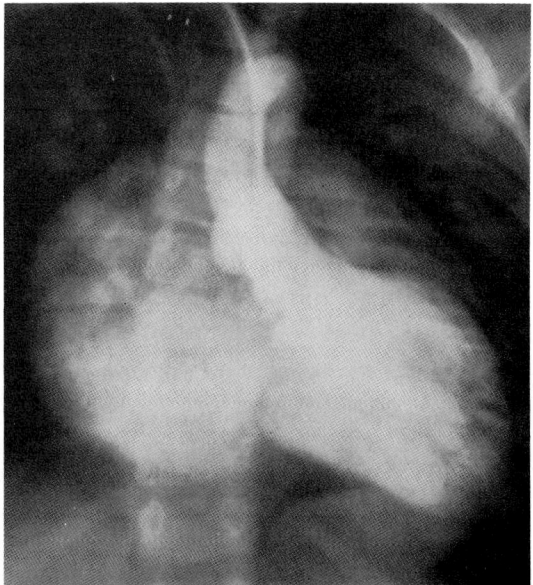

Figure 18. Frontal left ventriculogram in early systole in a case of complete atrioventricular canal with anterior common leaflet divided and attached medially to the ventricular septum. Note elongation and narrowing of the left ventricular outflow tract, with scalloping of the right border of the ventricle and a notch from which region a jet originates. (From Moss, A. J., and Adams, F. H.: Heart Disease in Infants, Children, and Adolescents. Baltimore, The Williams & Wilkins Company, 1968.)

Cardiac Catheterization and Angiocardiography

Cardiac catheterization shows an oxygen step-up in both the right atrium and the right ventricle. Pulmonary artery pressure may be quite high, while pulmonary to systemic flow ratios will usually be above 2. The majority of patients have severe pulmonary hypertension. (> 75 per cent of systolic systemic pressure $- R_p : R_s > 0.75$).

The frontal ventricular angiocardiogram demonstrates a characteristic picture. There is a long, narrow outflow tract with a scalloped right margin. A notch in the mitral valve can frequently be seen (Fig. 18). A similar left ventriculogram may be seen in patients with the partial form of persistent atrioventricular canal, as well as in those with a common atrium. If the anterior leaflet is not divided and attached to the septum, the usual picture may not be present. There may be a right-angled appearance of the right border of the left ventricle (Fig. 19). The angle's horizontal component is formed by the undivided anterior common leaflet, and the vertical side is formed by contrast medium trapped under the lateral "mitral" leaflet.

Natural History and Indications for Operation

These patients have a short life span and often die in the first or second year of life. The median age at death is 2 years, but if there are associated defects the median age is only 4 months. The cause of death in infancy is usually congestive heart failure and pneumonia. Thereafter, irreversible pulmonary vascular changes rapidly render the outlook hopeless.

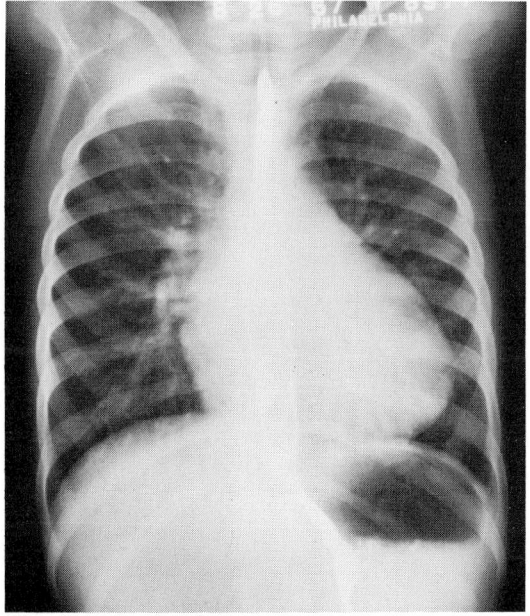

Figure 17. Preoperative chest roentgenogram of a 6-year-old girl with a complete atrioventricular canal and pulmonary hypertension in whom total correction was successful.

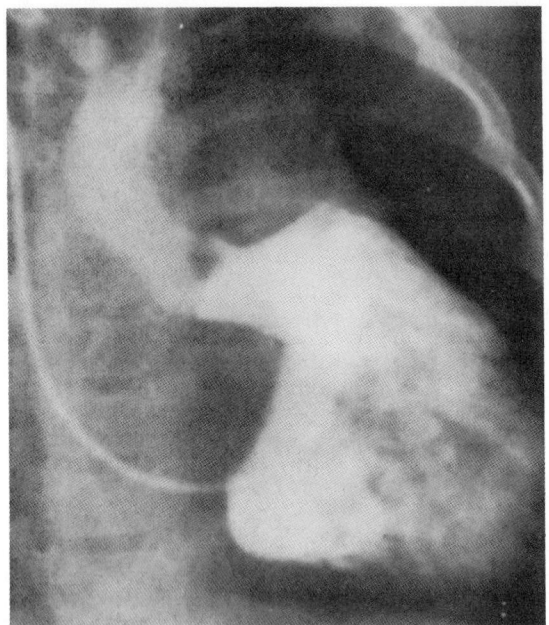

Figure 19. Frontal left ventriculogram in a case of complete atrioventricular canal with anterior common leaflet not divided and not attached to the septum. Note the right-angle appearance of the right border of the ventricle. The angle's horizontal component is formed by the undivided anterior common leaflet, and the vertical side is formed by contrast medium trapped under the lateral "mitral" leaflet. (From Moss, A. J., and Adams, F. H.: Heart Disease in Infants, Children and Adolescents. Baltimore, The Williams & Wilkins Company, 1968.)

Treatment

Initial attempts to repair this defect often failed because of lack of understanding of the complex anatomy. Persistent atrioventricular valve insufficiency and inadequate closure of ventricular septal defects were common. Surgically produced heart block was frequent, and the postoperative mortality was between 60 and 75 per cent.

With better understanding of the anatomy,[56] a new repair was developed that has proved satisfactory.[57] Since these patients often are in serious difficulty in infancy, and because of the complexity of total operative correction, palliation by pulmonary artery banding may be indicated. Somerville et al.[64] were able to provide palliation for 66 per cent of infants with a complete atrioventricular canal in whom congestive heart failure was present. Although the mortality rate is still quite high, especially when compared to that of operations for isolated ventricular septal defect in infants,[11] this operative procedure may offer the only hope for a desperately ill infant with persistent atrioventricular canal. Subsequent repair can be carried out at an age when this complex operation is feasible. The increased mortality with pulmonary artery banding in infants with persistent atrioventricular canals is related to the atrioventricular valve insufficiency and the advanced pulmonary vascular disease.

Total correction of persistent common atrioventricular canal is shown in Figures 20 and 21. Cardiopulmonary bypass is used. The right atrium is opened widely, and the details of the defect are assessed. In

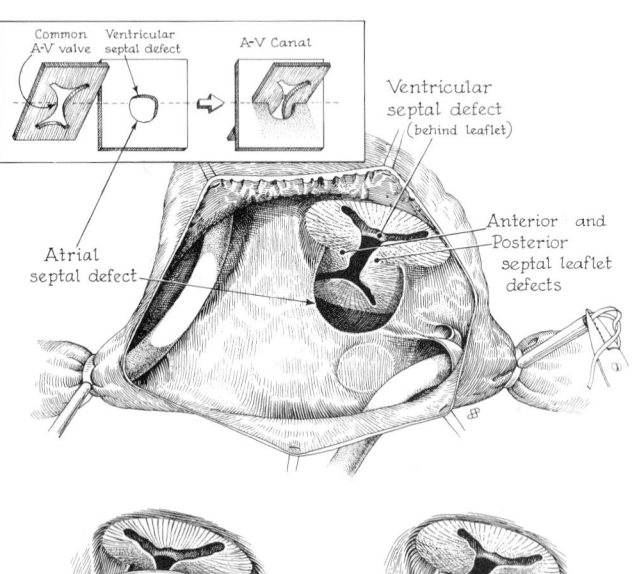

Figure 20. Repair of a complete atrioventricular canal. The anterior and posterior leaflets are divided. The mitral leaflet is repaired.

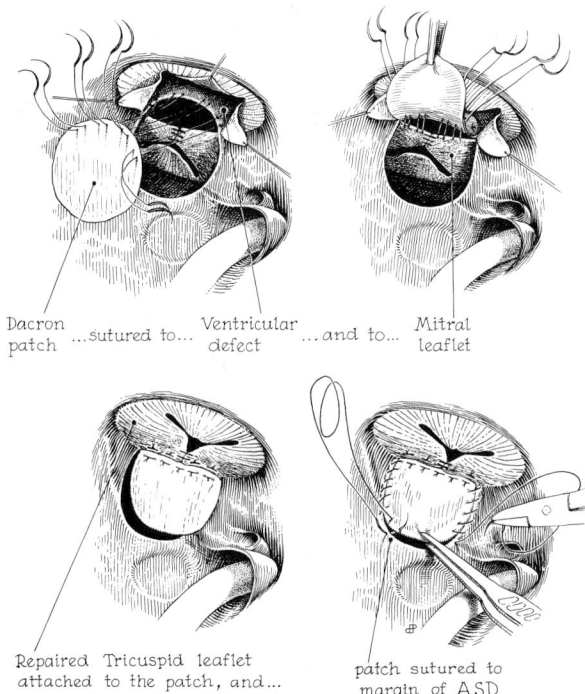

Dacron patch ...sutured to... Ventricular defect ...and to... Mitral leaflet

Repaired Tricuspid leaflet attached to the patch, and...

patch sutured to margin of ASD

Figure 21. Completion of repair of atrioventricular canal. The Dacron patch is sutured to the right of the ventricular septal defect to avoid damage to the conduction system. The valve leaflets are attached to the patch and the latter is sutured onto the atrioventricular septal defect.

the most common form, there is a common posterior leaflet with or without attachments to the ventricular septum, the anterior leaflet is subdivided and attached to the ventricular septum, and the membranous septum is closed (see Fig. 4). During correction, division of the posterior leaflet is done slightly to the right side. The "mitral" portions of the anterior and posterior leaflets are approximated with sutures, to close the "cleft" mitral valve. The defect is repaired by suturing a Dacron prosthesis to the right side of the ventricular septum. The medial portion of the mitral leaflet is then attached to the appropriate level of the patch. The cleft in the tricuspid valve is repaired and the septal leaflet attached to the right side of the patch. The patch is then sutured into the atrial portion of the defect.

In the less common form of persistent atrioventricular canal (see Fig. 6), the common anterior leaflet also will require division, but the repair is similar to that just described. In addition, the membranous ventricular septum is absent and will require closure with the patch. In the least common form of this defect (see Fig. 5), the common anterior leaflet is attached to an anomalous papillary muscle in the right ventricle, and the membranous septum is absent; repair is similar to that for the second type of persistent atrioventricular canal.

The most frequent complication of total correction is complete heart block, although this complication is much less common in recent experience.[39] This can usually be avoided, at the expense of a small residual

shunt, if the division of the leaflet is kept well to the right side of the septum and if the patch is sutured posteriorly to the divided common posterior leaflet (especially in the common form of persistent common atrioventricular canal). With this repair, the mortality has been reduced to 20 per cent. Surviving patients have done well, although most have mild to moderate mitral valve incompetence.

SELECTED REFERENCES

Cooley, D. A., and Hallman, G. L.: Surgical Treatment of Congenital Heart Disease, 2nd ed. Philadelphia, Lea & Febiger, 1975.
This monograph details the experience of a group that has managed a large number of infants and children with congenital heart disease. The book is well illustrated and adequately covers the basic operations and their results.

Gould, S. E.: Pathology of the Heart and Blood Vessels. Springfield, Ill., Charles C Thomas, Publisher, 1968.
This textbook written by a number of authors clearly details the embryology and pathologic anatomy of the various defects of the heart. It has excellent references and is of special help to the student who desires more detailed information about the morbid anatomy of the heart and great vessels.

Keith, J. D., Rowe, R. D., and Vlad, P.: Heart Disease in Infancy and Childhood, 2nd ed. New York, Macmillan Company, 1967.
This textbood of pediatric cardiology is based largely on the personal experience of the authors in one of the major pediatric centers of the world. The medical and diagnostic aspects of congenital heart disease are given particular attention.

Johnson, J., MacVaugh, H., III, and Waldhausen, J. A.: Surgery of the Chest, 4th ed. Chicago, Year Book Medical Publishers, 1970.
This monograph descibes the steps in the operative procedures of cardiothoracic surgery and is especially helpful to students and house officers who desire better understanding of the operations.

Moss, A. J., and Adams, F. H., (Ed.): Heart Disease in Infants. Baltimore, Williams & Wilkins Company, 1968.
A large number of authors contributed to this textbook of cardiology. The chapters are encyclopedic, particularly in regard to pathologic, medical, and diagnostic aspects of pediatric cardiology.

REFERENCES

1. Abbott, M. E.: Atlas of Congenital Heart Diseases. New York, American Heart Association, 1936.
2. Bailey, C. P.: Congenital interatrial connections: Clinical and surgical considerations with a description of a new surgical technique — atrioseptopexy. Ann. Int. Med., 37:888, 1952.
3. Baron, M. G.: Abnormalities of the initial valve in endocardial cushion defects. Circulation, 45:672, 1972.
4. Beck, W., Swan, H. J. C., Burchell, H. B., and Kirklin, J. W.: Pulmonary vascular resistance after repair of atrial septal defects in patients with pulmonary hypertension. Circulation, 22:938, 1960.
5. Bedell, G. N., and Adams, R. W.: Pulmonary diffusing capacity during rest and exercise. A study of normal persons and persons with atrial septal defect, pregnancy and pulmonary disease. J. Clin. Invest., 41:1908, 1962.
6. Bedford, D. E., Papp, C., and Parkinson, J.: Atrial septal defect. Br. Heart J., 3:37, 1941.
7. Bedford, D. E., Sellors, T. H., Somerville, W., Belcher, J. R., and Besterman, E. M. M.: Atrial septal defect and its surgical treatment. Lancet, 1:1255, 1957.
8. Berg, J. M., Crome, L., and France, N. E.: Congenital cardiac malformations in mongolism. Br. Heart J., 22:331, 1960.
9. Bizarro, R. O., Callahan, J. A., Feldt, R. H., Kurland, L. T., Gordon, H., and Brandenburg, R. O.: Familial atrial septal defect with prolonged atrioventricular conduction: Syndrome showing autosomal dominant patterns of inheritance. Circulation, 41:677, 1970.
10. Blieden, P. A., Randall, A., Castaneda, A. R., Lucas, R. V., Jr., and Edwards, J. E.: The "gooseneck" of the endocardial cushion defect: Anatomic basis. Chest, 65:13, 1974.
11. Boruchow, I., Waldhausen, J. A., Miller, W. W., Rashkind, W. J., and Friedman, S.: Pulmonary artery hypertension in infants

with congenital heart disease. Palliative management by pulmonary artery binding. Arch. Surg., 99:716, 1969.

12. Brannon, E. S., Weens, H. S., and Warren, J. V.: Atrial septal defect; study of hemodynamics by technique of right heart catheterization. Am. J. Med. Sci., 210:480, 1945.

13. Braudo, J. L., Nadas, A. S., Rudolph, A. M., and Neuhauser, E. B. D.: Atrial septal defects in children. Pediatrics, 14:618, 1954.

14. Braunwald, N. S., and Morrow, A. C.: The delayed closure of atrial septal defects with perforated prostheses. Surg. Gynecol. Obstet., 116:579, 1963.

15. Burchell, H. B., DuShane, J. W., and Brandenburg, R. O.: The electrocardiogram of patients with atrioventricular cushion defects (defects of the atrioventricular canal). Am. J. Cardiol., 6:575, 1960.

16. Cohn, R.: An experimental method for the closure of interauricular septal defects in dogs. Am. Heart J., 33:453, 1947.

17. Colmers, R. A.: Atrial septal defects in elderly patients: Report of three patients aged 68, 72, and 78. Am. J. Cardiol., 1:768, 1958.

18. Cooley, D. A.: Results of surgical treatment of atrial septal defects. Am. J. Cardiol., 6:605, 1960.

19. Cooley, D. A., Ellis, P. R., Jr., and Bellizzi, M. E.: Atrial septal defects of the sinus venosus type: Surgical considerations. Dis. Chest, 39:185, 1961.

20. Dalen, J. E., Bruce, R. A., and Cobb, L. A.: Interaction of chronic hypoxia of moderate altitude on pulmonary hypertension complicating defect of the atrial septum. N. Engl. J. Med., 266:272, 1962.

21. Danilowicz, D. A., Read, G. E., and Silver, W.: Ruptured mitral chordae after subacute bacterial endocarditis in a child with a secundum atrial septal defect. Johns Hopkins Med. J., 128:45, 1971.

22. Dave, K. S., Pakrashi, B. C., Woolder, G. H., and Ionescu, I.: Atrial septal defect in adults: Clinical and hemodynamic results of surgery. Am. J. Cardiol., 31:7, 1973.

23. Davia, J. E., Cheitlin, M. D., and Bedynek, J. L.: Sinus venosus atrial septal defect: Analysis of 50 cases. Am. Heart J., 85:177, 1973.

24. Davis, C. L.: Development of the human heart from its first appearance to the stage found in embryos of 20 paired somites. Contrib. Embryol., 19:245, 1927.

25. Diamond, M. A., Dillon, J. C., Haine, C. L., Chang, S., and Feigenbaum, H. Echocardiographic features of atrial septal defect Circulation, 243:129, 1971.

26. DuShane, J. W., Weidman, W. H., Brandenburg, R. O., and Kirklin, J. W.: Differentiation of interatrial communications by clinical methods: Ostium secundum, ostium primum, common atrium and total anomalous pulmonary venous connection. Circulation, 21:363, 1960.

27. Ellis, F. H., Jr., Brandenburg, R. O., and Swan, H. J. C.: Defect of the atrial septum in the elderly. Report of successful correction in five patients sixty years of age or older. N. Engl. J. Med., 262:219, 1960.

28. Ellis, F. H., Jr., Kirklin, J. W., Swan, H. J. C., DuShane, J. W., and Edwards, J. R.: Diagnosis and surgical treatment of common atrium. Surgery, 45:160, 1959.

29. Ellis, F. H., Jr., McGoon, D. C., and Kirklin, J. W.: Surgical management of persistent common atrioventricular canal. Am. J. Cardiol., 6:598, 1960.

30. El-Said, G., Ruzyllo, W., Williams, R. L., and McNamara, D. G.: Atrial pressure gradients in isolated secundum atrial septal defect and partial anomalous pulmonary venous return. Chest, 63:559, 1973.

31. Evans, J. R., Rowe, R. D., and Keith, J. D.: The clinical diagnosis of atrial septal defect in children. Am. J. Med., 30:345, 1961.

32. Flamm, M. D., Cohn, K. E., and Hancock, E. W.: Ventricular function in atrial septal defect. Am. J. Med., 48:286, 1970.

33. Fontana, R. S., and Edwards, J. E.: Congenital Cardiac Disease: A Review of 357 Cases Studied Pathologically. Philadelphia, W. B. Saunders Company, 1962.

34. Gault, J. H., Morrow, A. G., Gay, W. A., Jr., and Ross, J., Jr.: Atrial septal defect in patients over the age of forty years. Circulation, 37:261, 1968.

35. Gibbon, J. H., Jr.: Application of a mechanical heart and lung apparatus to cardiac surgery. Minn. Med., 37:171, 1954.

36. Giknis, F. L.: Single atrium and the Ellis-van Creveld syndrome. J. Pediatr., 62:558, 1963.

37. Griffiths, S. P.: Bacterial endocarditis associated with atrial septal defect of the ostium secundum type. Am. Heart J., 61:543, 1961.

38. Gross, R. E., Watkins, E., Jr., Pomeranz, A. A., and Goldsmith, E. I.: A method for surgical closure of interauricular septal defects. Surg. Gynecol. Obstet., 96:1, 1953.

39. Hardesty, R. L., Zuberbuhler, J. R., and Bahnson, H. T.: Surgical treatment of atrioventricular canal defect. Arch. Surg., 110:1391, 1975.

40. Hastreiter, A. R., Wennemark, S. R., Miller, R. A., and Paul, M. H.: Secundum atrial septal defects with congestive heart failure during infancy and early childhood. Am. Heart J., 64:467, 1962.

41. Hawe, A., Rastelli, G. C., Brandenburg, R. O., and McGoon, D. C.: Embolic complications following repair of atrial septal defects. Circulation, Suppl. 39:185, 1969.

42. Heath, D., and Edwards, J. E.: The pathology of hypertensive pulmonary vascular disease: A description of six grades of structural changes in the pulmonary arteries with special reference to congenital cardiac septal defects. Circulation, 18:533, 1958.

43. Hynes, K. M., Frye, R. L., Brandenburg, R. O., McGoon, D. C., Titus, J. L., and Giuliani, E. R.: Atrial septal defect (secundum) associated with mitral regurgitation. Am. J. Cardiol., 34:333, 1974.

44. Keith, J. D., Rowe, R. D., and Vlad, P.: Heart Disease in Infancy and Childhood. New York, Macmillan Company, 1958.

45. Levin, A. R., Spach, M. S., Boineau, J. P., Canent, R. V., Jr., Capp, M. P., and Jewett, P. H.: Atrial pressure-flow dynamics in atrial septal defects (secundum type). Circulation, 37:476, 1968.

46. Lewis, F. J., Tauffic, M., Varco, R. L., and Niazi, S.: The surgical anatomy of atrial septal defects: Experiences with repair under direct vision. Ann. Surg., 142:401, 1955.

47. Lillehei, C. W., Anderson, R. C., Ferlic, R. M., and Bonnabeau, R. C., Jr.: Persistent common atrioventricular canal. J. Thorac. Cardiovasc. Surg., 57:83, 1969.

48. Morrow, A. G., Gilbert, J. W., Baker, R. R., and Collins, N. P.: The closure of atrial septal defects utilizing general hypothermia. J. Thorac. Cardiovasc. Surg., 40:776, 1960.

49. Murray, G.: Closure of defects in cardiac septa. Ann. Surg., 128:843, 1948.

50. Nadas, A. S., and Ellison, R. C.: Phonocardiographic analysis of diastolic flow murmurs in secundum atrial septal defect and ventricular septal defect. Br. Heart J., 29:684, 1967.

51. Neufeld, H. N., Titus, J. L., DuShane, J. W., Burchell, H. B., and Edwards, J. E.: Isolated ventricular septal defect of the persistent common atrioventricular canal type. Circulation, 23:685, 1961.

52. Nielsen, J. S., and Fabricius, J.: The effect of exercise on the size of the shunt in patients with atrial septal defects. Acta Med. Scand., 183:91, 1968.

53. Phillips, S. J., Okies, J. E., Henken, D., Sunderland, C. O., and Starr, A.: Complex of secundum atrial septal defect and congestive heart failure in infants. J. Thorac. Cardiovasc. Surg., 70:696, 1975.

54. Pierce, W. S., Peckham, G. J., Johnson, J., and Waldhausen, J. A.: Gram-negative sepsis following operation for congenital heart disease: Diagnosis, management, and results. Arch. Surg., 101:698, 1970.

55. Rainier-Pope, C. R., Cunningham, R. D., Nadas, A. S., and Crigler, J. F.: Cardiovascular malformation in Turner's syndrome. Pediatrics, 33:919, 1964.

56. Rastelli, G. C., Kirklin, J. W., and Titus, J. L.: Anatomic observations on complete form of persistent common atrioventricular canal with special reference to atrioventricular valves. Proc. Mayo Clin., 41:296, 1966.

57. Rastelli, G. C., Ongley, P. A., Kirklin, J. W., and McGoon, D. C.: Surgical repair of the complete form of persistent common atrioventricular canal. J. Thorac. Cardiovasc. Surg., 55:299, 1968.

58. Rokitansky, C. F.: Die Defekte der Scheidewände des Herzens. Vienna, Bräumuller, 1875.

59. Scott, L. B., Hauck, A. J., and Nadas, A. S.: Endocardial cushion defect with pulmonic stenosis. Circulation, 25:653, 1962.

60. Sealy, W. C., Farmer, J. C., Young, W. G., Jr., and Brown, I. W.: Atrial dysrhythmia and atrial secundum defects. J. Thorac. Cardiovasc. Surg., 57:245, 1969.

61. Sellers, R. D., Ferlic, R. M., Sterns, L. P., and Lillehei, C. W.: Secundum type atrial septal defects: Early and late results of surgical repair using extracorporeal circulation in 275 patients. Surgery, 59:155, 1966.

62. Shumacker, H. B., Jr., and Herendeen, T. L.: Hemolytic anemia after repair of ostium primum septal defect and cleft mitral

valve: Surgical correction. J. Thorac. Cardiovasc. Surg., 55: 489, 1968.

63. Somerville, J.: Ostium primum defect: Factors causing deterioration in the natural history. Br. Heart J., 27:413, 1965.

64. Somerville, J., Agnew, T., Stark, J., Waterston, D. J., Aberdeen, E., Carter, R. E. B., and Waich, S.: Banding of the pulmonary artery for common atrioventricular canal. Br. Heart J., 29: 816, 1967.

65. Steinbrunn, W., Cohn, E., and Selzer, A.: Atrial septal defect associated with mitral stenosis: Lutembacher syndrome revisited. Am. J. Med., 48:295, 1970.

66. Swan, C., Tostevin, A. L., Mayo, H., and Black, G. H. B.: Further observation on congenital defects in infants following infectious diseases during pregnancy with special reference to rubella. Med. J. Aust., 1:409, 1944.

67. Swan, H. J. C., Burchell, H. B., and Wood, E. H.: The presence of venoarterial shunts in patients with interatrial communications. Circulation, 10:705, 1954.

68. Swan, H. J. C., Hetzel, R. S., Bruchell, B. H., and Wood, E. H.: Relative contribution of blood from each lung to the left-to-right shunt in atrial septal defect: Demonstration by indicator-dilution techniques. Circulation, 14:200, 1956.

69. Tavel, M. E., Bard, R. A., Franks, L. C., Feigenbaum, H., and Fisch, C.: The jugular venous pulse in atrial septal defect. Arch. Intern. Med., 121:524, 1968.

70. Thompson, T., and Evans, W.: Paradoxical embolism. Q. J. Med., 23:135, 1930.

71. Uchida, I. A., and Rowe, R. D.: Discordant heart anomalies in twins. Am. J. Hum. Genet., 9:133, 1957.

72. Waldo, A. L., Kaiser, G. A., Bowman, F. O., Jr., and Malm, J. R.: Etiology of prolongation of P-R interval in patients with endocardial cushion defect. Circulation, 48:19, 1973.

73. Weidman, W. H., and DuShane, J. W.: Defects of the atrial septum and endocardial cushion. In Moss, A. J., and Adams, F. H. (Eds.): Heart Disease in Infants, Children and Adolescents. Baltimore, Williams & Wilkins Company, 1968.

74. Wendet, V. E., Keech M. K., Read, R. C., Bistue, A. R., and Bianchi, F. A.: Cardiovascular features of Marfan's syndrome: Family studies. Circulation (Suppl. 2)32:218, 1965.

75. Weyn, A. S., Bartle, S. H., Nolan, T. B., and Dammann, J. F.: Atrial septal defect—primum type. Circulation (Suppl. 3) 32:13, 1965.

76. Williams, R. G., and Rudd, M.: Echocardiographic features of endocardial cushion defects. Circulation, 49:418, 1974.

V

DISORDERS OF PULMONARY VENOUS RETURN

Dev R. Manhas, M.D., M.S.,
and K. Alvin Merendino, M.D., Ph.D.

Abnormalities of the pulmonary veins are uncommon. These anomalies can be divided in two groups: (1) anomalous connection of the pulmonary veins, so that the pulmonary venous return enters the right instead of the left atrium; and (2) obstruction of blood flow into the left atrium due to stenosis or atresia of the pulmonary veins or cor triatriatum.[31] Abnormalities in the latter group are rare and beyond the scope of this chapter.

TOTAL ANOMALOUS PULMONARY VENOUS CONNECTION (TAPVC)

In this congenital abnormality, all pulmonary veins from both lungs fail to join the left atrium. Pulmonary venous blood instead goes to the right atrium either directly or through one of its tributaries. TAPVC constitutes about 1.6 to 2 per cent of all congenital heart anomalies.[11] In the absence of pulmonary venous obstruction, TAPVC is distributed equally in both sexes; however, there is marked male preponderance if pulmonary venous obstruction is present.[21]

HISTORICAL ASPECTS

Wilson in 1798 was the first to describe TAPVC.[7] In 1942, Brody[7] stimulated interest in this disease with an excellent review of the literature; he found 37 autopsied cases of this anomaly. Muller[29] in 1951 reported partial surgical correction by anastomosis of the end of the left atrial appendix to the side of the common pulmonary trunk. Lewis and Varco[26] in 1956 achieved the first successful open-heart correction of the cardiac type of TAPVC under direct vision using hypothermia and inflow occlusion; a few months later Burroughs and Kirklin[9] successfully employed extracorporeal circulation for repair of a similar defect. Senning[33] in 1956 performed total correction of a supracardiac TAPVC in a 21-year-old patient. Cooley and Oschner,[10] through a transatrial approach, anastomosed the posterior wall of the left atrium to the common pulmonary trunk in an infant with supracardiac TAPVC in 1957. The first successful surgical correction of infradiaphragmatic type of TAPVC was reported by Sloan and associates[34] in 1962. In 1965, Dillard et al.[12] used surface induced deep hypothermia with total circulatory arrest for total surgical correction of TAPVC in infancy. Several reviews of surgical experience have been reported in recent years.[2, 3, 6, 18-20, 30, 38, 39]

ANATOMIC AND HISTOLOGIC ASPECTS

Embryology

Primordia of the lungs develop from the foregut;[1, 14, 21] the pulmonary vascular network, formed early in the development of the lungs, initially drains into the cardinal and the umbilicovitelline system of veins. The common pulmonary vein sprouts as a small endothelial bud from the middle of the posterior aspect of the still undivided atrium. It divides into two branches, each of which further subdivides into two. Gradually, by process of differential growth, the dilated common pulmonary vein is absorbed into the enlarging left atrium up to its four subdivisions so that each subdivision becomes a pulmonary vein and opens separately into the left atrium. The pulmonary venous network in each lung establishes communication with the tributaries of the pulmonary veins and thereafter loses its connection with the cardinal and umbilicovitelline venous systems. If the common pulmonary vein persists but loses its connection with the left atrium in the early stage of embryonic life when the communication with the cardinal and the umbilicovitelline veins is still present, the latter will become the collateral channels of circulation, and various types of anomalous pulmonary venous connections will result. The most frequently used channel is the left anterior cardinal vein, which drains into the left innominate vein or the coronary sinus.[5, 8, 17]

Anatomy

The pulmonary veins may open directly into the right atrium or, more often, unite with each to form a common venous pool behind the heart.[31] This venous pool has been called by various names, such as the common pulmonary trunk and horizontal anomalous vein. From the common pulmonary trunk arises one vein, which may join the left innominate vein or any other systemic vein in the thorax or abdomen.

There is a wide spectrum of anomalous pulmonary venous connection. Blake and associates[4] reviewed 113 cases from Brook General Hospital, Walter Reed General Hospital, and the Armed Forces Institute of Pathology and reported 27 different patterns of anomalous pulmonary venous connection. Snellen and associates[36] introduced an elaborate but useful code to describe the anatomic complexes briefly and accurately. Although there are various classifications of TAPVC, one suggested by Darling et al.[11] is very popular. According to this, there are four types of TAPVC:

1. *Supracardiac type.* This is the commonest type.[5, 8] Here the central connection is to the left innominate vein via an anomalous vertical vein. Infrequently the common pulmonary trunk may drain into the superior vena cava at or below the level of the azygous vein. In this situation, the lower end of the superior vena cava is dilated, and the associated atrial septal defect is high.

The anomalous vertical vein on its way to join the left innominate vein usually passes in front of the left pulmonary artery. However, it may pass between the left main bronchus and the left pulmonary artery and be compressed between these two structures; this results in pulmonary venous obstruction.[16, 24]

2. *Cardiac type.* This is the second commonest in frequency.[5, 8] The common pulmonary trunk is connected to the coronary sinus (less often to the right atrium) through a vascular channel.

3. *Infracardiac type.* This should preferably be called the infradiaphragmatic type. A descending vein arises from the inferior portion of the common pulmonary trunk and runs downward in front of the esophagus, passes through the diaphragm at the esophageal hiatus, and joins the portal vein, ductus venosus, or rarely the inferior vena cava.[22]

4. *Mixed type.* The pulmonary veins from each lung and even from various lobes of the same lung have a different central connection in this type.

The most frequent sites of the central connection are the left innominate vein and the coronary sinus.[5, 8, 17] The incidence of various central connections is shown in Table 1.

The majority of patients with TAPVC do not have associated major cardiac defects.[5, 17] An interatrial communication is invariably present and is not considered a major cardiac defect, for it is essential to life in this condition. This communication is usually a patent foramen ovale but may be a secundum atrial septal defect. The size of the interatrial communication is one of the factors that affect the natural history of uncomplicated TAPVC;[15] patients who survive beyond the first year of life without corrective surgery have a secundum atrial septal defect.[5] Irrespective of the type of TAPVC, the heart shows some common features on gross examination. The right atrium and ventricle are usually hypertrophied and dilated; the left cardiac chambers are comparatively small but in most cases normal or only slightly hypoplastic. Microscopically, persistence of fetal pulmonary vascular pattern has been reported on histologic study of the lungs.[10]

BIOLOGIC ASPECTS

In the fetus, because the lungs are not expanded, an increased pulmonic vascular resistance exists. Con-

TABLE 1. Site of the Central Connection in Total Anomalous Pulmonary Venous Connection Unassociated with Major Cardiac Defects

Authors	Total Number of Patients	Left Innominate Vein	Coronary Sinus	Right Atrium	Superior Vena Cava	Portal Vein	Multiple Sites	Others
Burroughs and Edwards (1960)[8]	113	41	18	17	12	7	8	10
Bonham, Carter et al. (1969)[5]	58	30	16	2	3	3	2	2
Gathman and Nadas (1970)[17]	75	26	14	3	8	13	8	3
Gomes et al. (1970)[19]	59	32	10	11	5	—	1	—
Wukasch et al. (1975)[39]	125	60	18	15	15	5	9	3
Total	430	189	76	48	43	28	28	18

sequently, most of the blood from the right heart is shunted to the descending aorta via the patent ductus arteriosus. As the requirements for survival in utero require mainly an effective pump, TAPVC causes no disturbances. After birth, with the first breath the lung expands, the pulmonic vascular resistance falls, pulmonary circulation is established, and the need for a dual (pulmonic and systemic) circulation is necessary. In TAPVC, pulmonary venous blood empties into the right atrium or one of its tributaries, and a left-to-right shunt is created. In the absence of any communication between the right and left sides of the heart, the infant will die soon after birth. An interatrial communication, as already mentioned, is invariably present, and so a part of the mixture of the pulmonary and systemic venous blood goes to the left atrium, and thence to the systemic circulation. The amount of blood flow across the interatrial communication is directly related to its size.[15, 37] If the interatrial communication is large, the volume of flow to the two ventricles will depend on the pressure and distensibility of each ventricle.[8] In the absence of pulmonary artery hypertension, the right ventricle exhibits a lower pressure and greater distensibility than the left ventricle; therefore, there is more flow across the tricuspid valve than the mitral valve. As pulmonary flow is greater than systemic flow, the oxygen saturation of pulmonary venous and systemic venous blood mixture in the right atrium is very near normal and therefore cyanosis is not apparent. On the other hand, in TAPVC with marked pulmonary artery hypertension (due to pulmonary venous obstruction or increased pulmonary vascular resistance), the right ventricle becomes hypertrophied and less distensible, and the pulmonary flow is diminished. The pulmonary venous blood available for mixing is decreased, and systemic arterial oxygen saturation falls. Cyanosis is therefore encountered more often when there is marked pulmonary artery hypertension.[22]

From the foregoing it is apparent that pulmonary venous obstruction plays a significant role in the pathophysiology and the natural history of TAPVC. It is invariably present in the infradiaphragmatic type, and there are a number of reasons for this:[22] (1) the descending channel may be intrinsically narrow or may be compressed at the level of the diaphragm; (2) the hepatic vascular bed presents obstruction to a large flow; and (3) the thoracoabdominal pressure changes during respiration are yet another factor. In the supradiaphragmatic types of TAPVC, the pulmonary venous obstruction may be the result of an unusual course of the anomalous vertical vein, which passes between the left pulmonary artery and the left bronchus and is compressed at this point.[16, 24] Another site of obstruction may be a stenosis at the junction of the anomalous channel with the systemic vein. As mentioned earlier, owing to the development of pulmonary artery hypertension, cyanosis is usually present in patients with pulmonary venous obstruction, and congestive heart failure develops very early because of excessive right heart strain.[22] If compression between the left pulmonary artery and the left bronchus is the cause of obstruction, this is abetted by pulmonary artery hypertension and associated pulmonary artery

dilatation. The vicious cycle thus created has been described by Elliot and Edwards[16] as a "hemodynamic vise."

CLINICAL FEATURES

Symptoms

The signs and symptoms of TAPVC are dependent upon the presence or absence of pulmonary venous obstruction. Infants without pulmonary venous obstruction may be asymptomatic at birth.[11] The earliest problem is tachypnea, which is especially noticeable during feeding. Cyanosis may be absent or so slight that it is unnoticed by parents.[5] With the passage of time, tachypnea becomes more prominent and feeding difficulties appear. The infant suffers frequent respiratory infections and fails to thrive, and congestive heart failure usually develops by the time the baby is 6 months of age.[28] Seventy-five to eighty per cent of these infants die by the age of 1 year;[5, 8] however, an occasional patient may reach adulthood.[8, 11, 21]

The clinical picture of TAPVC with severe pulmonary venous obstruction varies markedly from that of the unobstructed form. Symptoms appear at birth or soon thereafter and include tachypnea and feeding difficulties.[22] Cyanosis is apparent at birth and cardiac decompensation appears very early. In the infradiaphragmatic type of TAPVC, cyanosis and dyspnea are aggravated by crying, straining, and so forth, owing to impediment of the flow through the anomalous channel by increased intra-abdominal pressure or the diaphragm. These infants die within a few days to a few weeks after birth.[22]

Signs

TAPVC without Pulmonary Venous Obstruction. The birth weight of these infants is usually on the low side, and most gain little weight. The infants have been described as scrawny and irritable. Tachypnea and tachycardia are invariably present. Cyanosis is usually mild and may be difficult to detect clinically.[5] It may be delayed or intermittent and appear only during exertion. Clubbing is absent initially but may be seen in older patients.

In cardiac failure, hepatomegaly is a consistent finding; distention of neck veins, peripheral edema, and pulmonary rales also may be present. Right ventricular heave can be seen in most patients. The first heart sound is distinct and loud, while the second heart sound is usually widely split and does not vary with respiration. A soft systolic murmur is heard over the pulmonic area in 75 per cent of patients;[22] a mid-diastolic flow murmur of relative tricuspid stenosis may be heard along the lower left sternal border.[25] Right ventricular failure is accompanied by a prominent third sound and a holosystolic murmur of tricuspid regurgitation.[25]

TAPVC with Pulmonary Venous Obstruction. These infants are moderately cyanotic and show signs of cardiac decompensation such as hepatomegaly, dilated neck veins, and peripheral edema. The precordium is quiet and the heart is not enlarged.[22, 23] The pulmonic component of the second heart sound is accentuated, and splitting is decreased and may be heard only in inspiration. A soft ejection systolic murmur is heard along the upper left sternal border in 50 per cent of patients.[22] A continuous murmur may be audible along the upper left sternal border in the supracardiac type.[5, 22] When heard, it usually indicates obstruction to the anomalous vertical vein,[5] although it may be occasionally heard in patients without venous obstruction.

DIAGNOSTIC STUDIES

Electrocardiogram

Right axis deviation and right ventricular hypertrophy are invariably present. The P wave is tall and peaked; this indicates right atrial enlargment. Conduction defects are uncommon.[17] The presence of a Q wave used to be considered diagnostic of TAPVC, but is not thought so now.[28]

Roentgenogram

In TAPVC without pulmonary venous obstruction, the heart is usually enlarged; this enlargement involves the right side of the heart. With a barium-filled esophagus, the left atrium is not enlarged; when the central connection is to the coronary sinus, the latter is dilated and may indent the esophagus and wrongly suggest left atrial enlargement. The pulmonary artery segment is prominent and the pulmonary vascular markings are accentuated; the aortic arch is small (Fig. 1). Classic "figure-of-eight"[35] or "snowman" configuration is seen only in TAPVC to the left innominate vein (Fig. 2).

In the presence of pulmonary venous obstruction, the heart is usually normal in size and configuration. The lung fields show a mottled, reticulated, or ground-

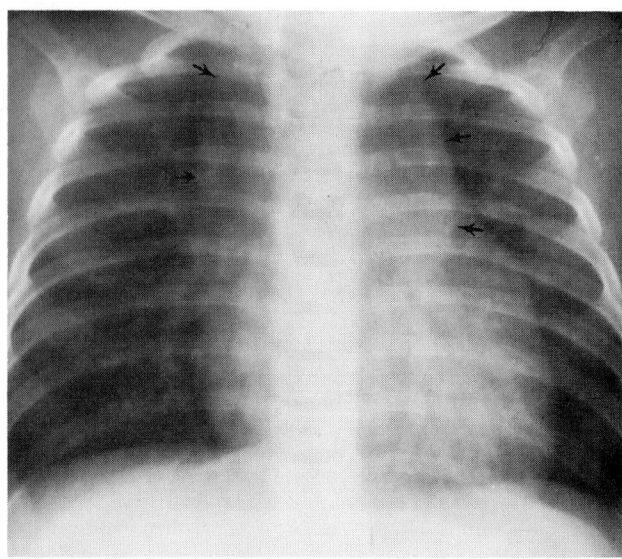

Figure 2. Roentgenogram of chest from a 5½-month-old female with TAPVC to the left innominate vein. A well-defined structure is seen both to the right and to the left of the midline which is neither thymus nor aorta. It is formed by the anomalous vertical vein, left innominate vein, and dilated superior vena cava; this imparts a "figure-of-eight" or "snowman" appearance to the cardiomediastinal silhouette.

glass appearance and prominent septal lines suggestive of pulmonary venous congestion and pulmonary edema.[22] This appearance of the lung field with a small heart is characteristic of the infradiaphragmatic type of TAPVC, although an identical appearance is seen in other types with marked pulmonary venous obstruction (Fig. 3).

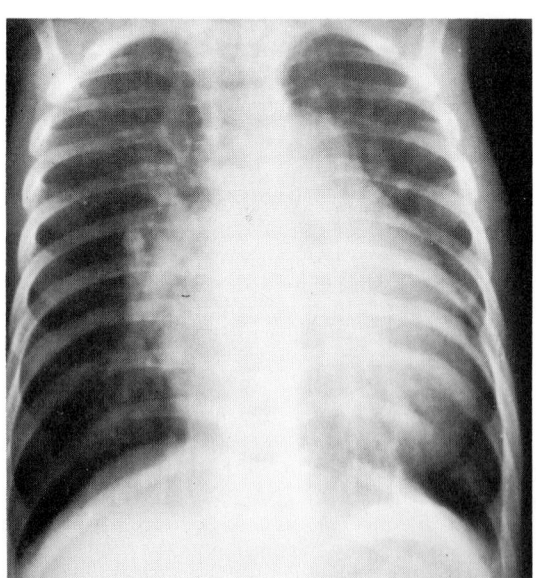

Figure 1. Chest roentgenogram of a mildly cyanotic 3-month-old male with TAPVC to the coronary sinus. Note increased pulmonary vascular markings, cardiac enlargement, and prominent main pulmonary artery.

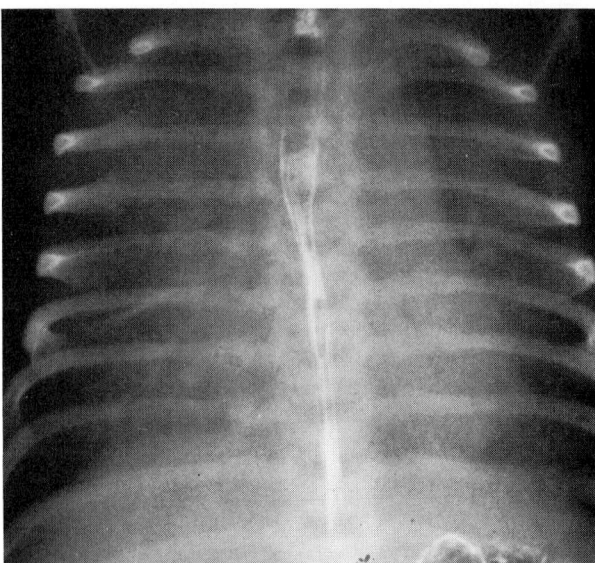

Figure 3. Roentgenogram of the chest from a cyanotic 10-day-old male with TAPVC to the portal vein. The heart size is small and the lung fields show a ground-glass appearance. (Courtesy of Dr. Stanley J. Stamm, Director of Cardiopulmonary Center, Children's Orthopedic Hospital, Seattle.)

Cardiac Catheterization

Oxygen Saturation. A step-up in oxygen saturation occurs where the pulmonary venous blood joins the systemic venous blood. When the anomalous connection is to the right atrium, oxygen step-up is seen at the right atrial level, and the oxygen saturation of blood in the four chambers of the heart, as well as in the pulmonary artery and the aorta, is equal. In the supracardiac type, the pulmonary artery blood has a higher oxygen saturation than systemic arterial blood, because the inferior vena cava blood shunts preferentially across the interatrial communication, while the superior vena cava blood streams into the right ventricle.[37] By the same token, the oxygen saturation of the pulmonary arterial blood is less than the systemic arterial blood in the infradiaphragmatic type.[17] In the presence of a large atrial septal defect, preferential flow occurs to a lesser degree.

Pressures. The right atrial pressure may be normal or higher than normal. There is a small mean gradient, in the range of 0 to 2 mm. Hg between the right and left atria.[17] The pressure in the right ventricle and pulmonary artery is usualy normal. However, in patients with pulmonary venous obstruction, the right ventricular and pulmonary artery pressure is markedly elevated and may be equal to or more than systemic pressure.[22, 23] Also, the pulmonary wedge pressure is elevated, and there is a pronounced gradient between the mean pulmonary wedge pressure and the mean right atrial pressure.[22]

Accurate measurements of pulmonary and systemic flow ratios as well as measurement of resistance are difficult in TAPVC because of difficulty in obtaining a proper mixed-venous sample.[17] In general, the estimated pulmonary blood flow is moderately increased in patients without pulmonary venous obstruction, and is nearly normal in the presence of obstruction.

Angiocardiography. Injection of contrast medium in the pulmonary artery enables one to visualize the point of entry of the anomalous pulmonary venous trunk; other associated cardiac anomalies, which are sometimes present, can also be diagnosed (Figs. 4 and 5). The mixed type of TAPVC can be better seen by selective injection of contrast medium in the right and left pulmonary artery (Fig. 6).

TREATMENT

If the defect is not corrected, 75 to 80 per cent of patients with TAPVC die within the first year of life.[8, 19] Gathman and Nadas[17] found that only 8 per cent of their patients survived up to 1 year without significant signs and symptoms. The prognosis is particularly poor in patients with pulmonary artery hypertension.[17, 19] The commonest cause of death is congestive heart failure. This natural history demands an aggressive approach in diagnosis and management.

Basically, the aims of surgical correction are: (1) to direct the pulmonary venous blood into the left atrium; (2) to interrupt the connection with the systemic veins; and (3) to repair the atrial septal defect. These aims can be achieved by total repair in one stage or by multistage procedures. Most workers recommend complete repair in one stage.[2, 3, 6, 12, 18, 19, 39]

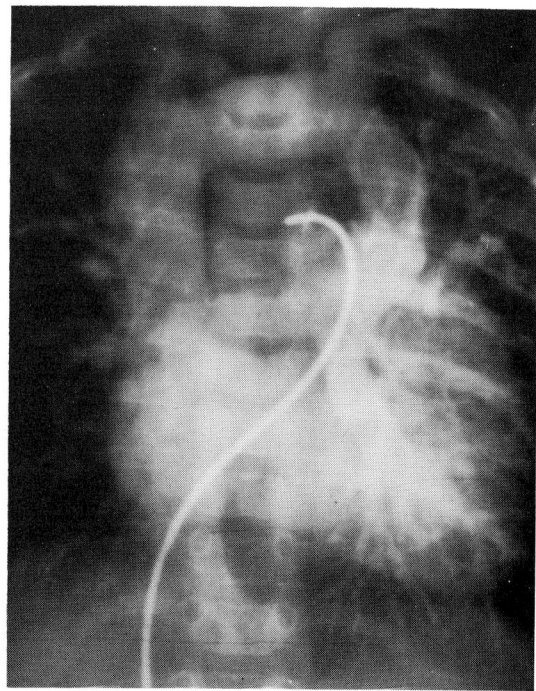

Figure 4. Angiocardiogram from a patient with TAPVC to the left innominate vein (whose chest x-ray is seen in Figure 2). The contrast material was injected through a catheter into the main pulmonary artery. The pulmonary veins from both lungs unite to form a horizontal venous confluence behind the heart, from which arises a vertical anomalous vein that joins the left innominate vein.

Total correction can be done with the aid of cardiopulmonary bypass or during deep hypothermia with total circulatory arrest.[2, 6, 12, 13] The optimal age for total correction in a relatively asymptomatic patient is 3 to 5 years; however, surgery should be considered earlier

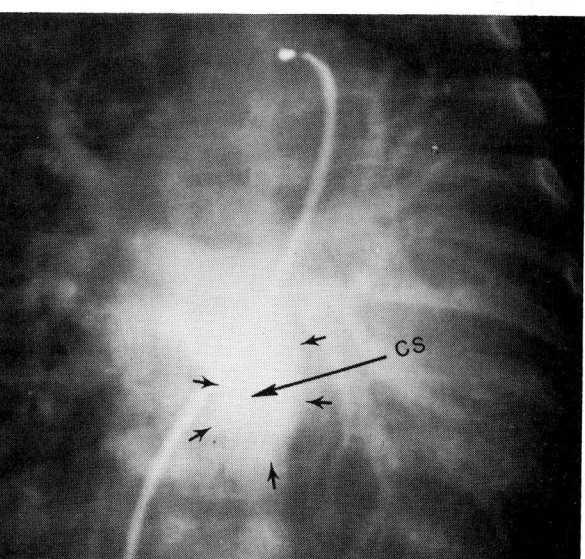

Figure 5. Angiocardiogram from a patient with TAPVC to the coronary sinus (Figure 1 shows x-ray chest of the same patient). A main pulmonary artery injection was made. The contrast material opacifies the pulmonary veins, which open into the dilated coronary sinus (CS).

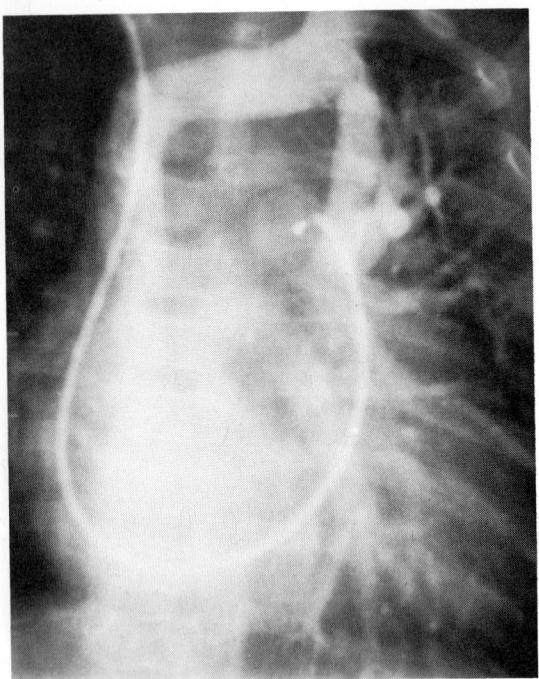

Figure 6. Angiocardiogram from a patient with mixed type of TAPVC. Selective right and left pulmonary artery injections were made. The upper lobe veins including the lingular segment drain into an anomalous vertical vein that empties into the left innominate vein. The pulmonary venous return from the right lung and left lower lobe drains into the coronary sinus.

if symptoms develop. Patients with pulmonary hypertension and pulmonary venous obstruction need total correction urgently.[17]

Supracardiac Type

Pulmonary venous blood is directed into the left atrium through a large side-to-side anastomosis between the horizontal common pulmonary venous trunk and the posterior wall of the left atrium. This can be done by rotating the apex of the heart up and performing the anastomosis posteriorly from outside, or it can be done transatrially. The most important point is the necessity of creating as large an anastomosis as possible. A small anastomosis usually produces pulmonary venous obstruction or relative obstruction aggravated by exercise. The interatrial communication is repaired, and the connection with the left innominate vein is ligated. If the anomalous connection is to the superior vena cava, a similar anastomosis is performed and the anomalous channel going to the superior vena cava is ligated (Fig. 7).

Cardiac Type

When the anomalous connection is to the coronary sinus, the foramen ovale is enlarged and the common wall between the posterior left atrium and the coronary sinus is incised or excised. Because the incision proximally frequently extends into the free pericardial sac, a continuous suture uniting the posterior atrial wall and coronary sinus for the entire length of the incision is necessary. Otherwise a serious leak posteriorly may be difficult to repair when it becomes apparent later in the procedure. This resultant defect is roofed with a Dacron patch so that all the pulmonary venous blood together with coronary sinus blood is directed into the left atrium (Fig. 8). Drainage of desaturated coronary sinus blood into the left atrium results in a right-to-left shunt without any obvious evidence of systemic desaturation or adverse effects. If the anomalous connection is to the right atrium, it can be managed in similar fashion. In repair of this type one must be careful to avoid injury to the atrioventricular node and to the conduction bundle of His, which lie below and in front of the coronary sinus opening. Likelihood of injury to the conduction bundle is less when the repair is done on a beating heart.

Infradiaphragmatic Type

Here the common pulmonary trunk is anastomosed to the posterior wall of the left atrium by an extracar-

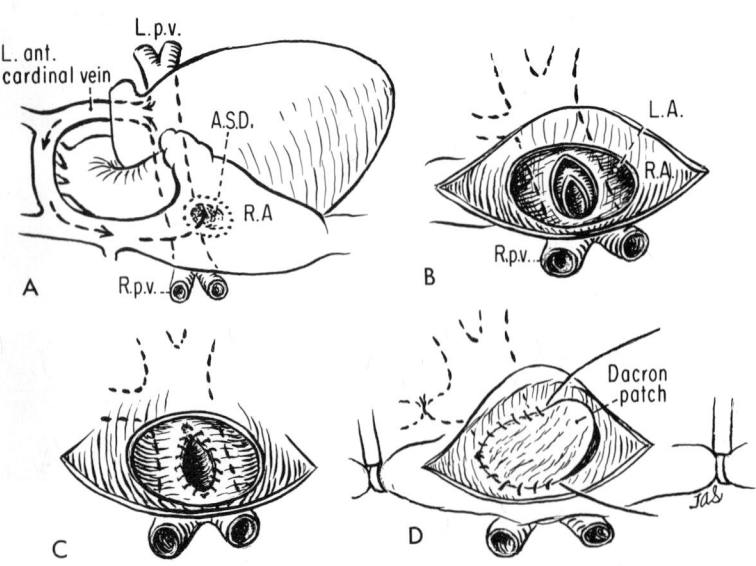

Figure 7. Operative steps for transatrial correction of the supracardiac TAPVC. *A*, Schematic representation of the anomaly. *B* and *C*, The interatrial communication is enlarged, an incision is made in posterior wall of the left atrium and anterior wall of the common pulmonary trunk, and an anastomosis is created between the two. *D*, The interatrial defect is closed with a Dacron patch and the anomalous vertical vein (left anterior cardinal vein) is ligated. R.A., right atrium; L.A., left atrium; R.p.v., right pulmonary veins; L.p.v., left pulmonary veins; A.S.D., atrial septal defect.

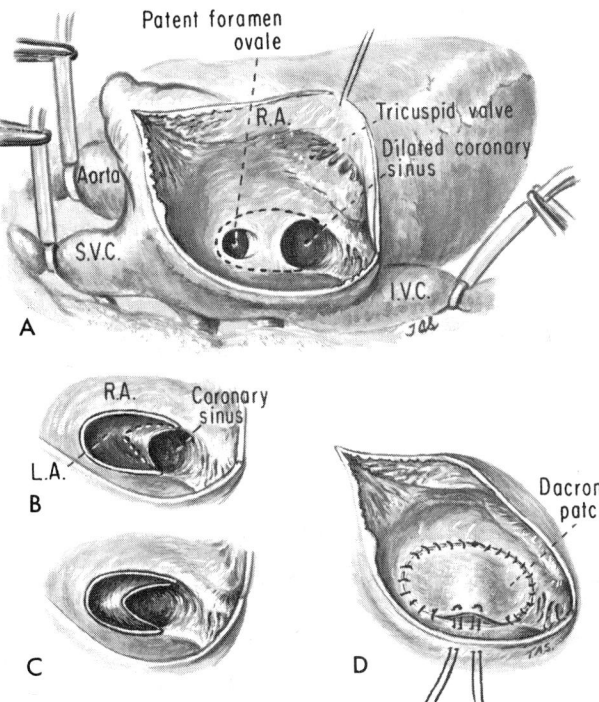

Figure 8. Operative steps for correction of TAPVC to the coronary sinus. *A* and *B*, Through a right atriotomy, the foramen ovale is enlarged and the common wall between the left atrium and the coronary sinus is excised. *C* and *D*, The resultant defect is roofed with a Dacron patch. R.A., right atrium; L.A., left atrium; S.V.C. superior vena cava; I.V.C., inferior vena cava. (From Dillard, D. H., et al.: Circulation (Suppl. 1) *35*:105, 1967. By permission of American Heart Association, Inc.)

Mixed Type

A combination of the aforementioned procedures is necessary, the choice depending on the pathologic anatomy. Because of the complicated nature of the anomaly, chances of obtaining a complete anatomic repair are not good.[39]

Multistage Correction. A large atrial septal defect allows good interchange of blood between the two atria and prolongs life in patients with TAPVC. It would appear, therefore, that creation of a large atrial septal defect should provide palliation for moribund infants. When this was done surgically, results were disappointing.[30] The technique of balloon septostomy developed by Rashkind and Miller[32] looks promising as a palliative procedure. Good results have been reported after balloon atrial septostomy in TAPVC with congestive heart failure but without pulmonary vascular obstruction.[27] It should be done at the time of initial catheterization if the interatrial communication seems small. If the patient improves after the septostomy, corrective surgery can be postponed until the child is old enough to tolerate surgical correction; if no improvement is seen following septostomy, however, immediate total correction should be considered. Mustard and associates[30] recommend leaving the anomalous channel open after anastomosis in the supracardiac type, so that it may decompress the left heart if necessary. It is ligated at a subsequent operation a few years later. Staged surgical procedures seem to have theoretical advantages; however, in actual practice the infant mortality has not been reduced, and a second operation with its inherent risk is necessary.

Acute pulmonary edema has been a common and serious postoperative complication occurring within the first 12 hours.[30, 39] Various explanations have been given for this. Some believe that the left ventricle is hypoplastic and cannot handle the circulatory load after total correction, and recommend leaving the vertical channel or the interatrial communication open to act as a safety valve for left heart decompression. The ligation of the former and closure of the latter may be done at a subsequent operation a few years later. This

diac approach in a manner similar to that used for the supracardiac type (Fig. 9). The atrial septal defect is closed and the descending anomalous vein is ligated. An end-to-side anastomosis between the descending vein and the left atrium is not recommended because of the danger of kinking and stenosis.[39]

Figure 9. Operative steps for correction of infradiaphragmatic TAPVC. *A*, Schematic representation of the anomaly. *B* and *C*, Anastomosis of the posterior wall of the left atrium with the common pulmonary trunk and ligation of the descending anomalous vein. *D*, Pattern of flow after the repair. (From Colley, D. A., et al.: J. Thorac. Cardiovasc. Surg., *51*:88, 1966.)

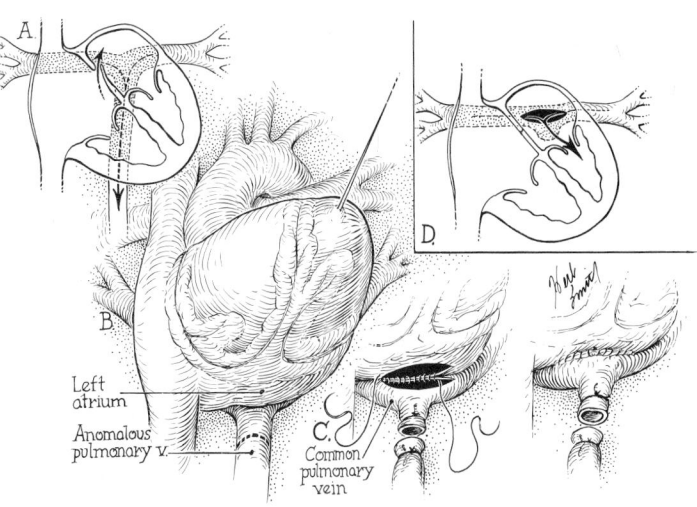

TABLE 2.   Operative Mortality According to Age in Total Anomalous Pulmonary Venous Connection

Authors	Less Than 1 Year in Age			More Than 1 Year in Age			Total		
	Number of Patients	Number of Deaths	%	Number of Patients	Number of Deaths	%	Number of Patients	Number of Deaths	%
Mustard et al. (1968)[30]	45	38	84	26	7	26	71	45	64
Gomes et al. (1970)[19]	15	7	47	44	3	7	59	10	17
Wukasch et al. (1975)[39]	63	36	57	62	9	14.5	125	45	36

explanation seems unlikely, because prior to correction in most instances of uncomplicated TAPVC the left ventricle is maintaining an adequate pressure and output. Others[25] believe that the small left atrium predisposes to pulmonary edema after total correction. However, when one realizes that the capacious pulmonary venous bed distal to the pulmonary capillaries is in a sense an extension of the left atrium, it is difficult to accept this hypothesis. Probably the most important factor is related to the size of the common vein–atrial anastomosis and the possible presence of torsion when the heart is once again distended and in circuit. Obviously, narrowing for any reason would have the same pulmonic effects as mitral stenosis. As in the patient with pure mitral stenosis, whose symptoms increase as the size of the valve orifice decreases below 1.5 sq. cm., a large anastomosis between the common vein and atrium is necessary in order to avoid an increased pulmonary venous pressure and possibly acute pulmonary edema. Another contributing factor has been proposed by Gomes et al.,[19] who think that intraoperative maneuvers that raise the pulmonary venous pressure, such as temporary occlusion of the pulmonary veins, are important factors in the production of pulmonary edema. This complication was uncommon in their experience because they avoid temporary occlusion of the pulmonary veins, and recommend opening the horizontal common vein immediately after institution of bypass occlusion of the anomalous communicating vein.

RESULTS OF TREATMENT

The results after total correction of TAPVC are summarized in Table 2. The following factors play an important role in the results after total surgical correction of TAPVC: (1) *Age*. Hospital mortality is closely related to the age of the patient. Approximately 90 per cent of patients under 6 months of age died after surgery in one series.[31] The hospital mortality was about 50 per cent in children less than 1 year of age.[19, 39] Mortality progressively decreased when surgery was undertaken after 1 year of age.[30, 39] (2) *Type of anomaly*. The cardiac type of TAPVC is comparatively easy to correct and results are comparatively better;[38] results have been poor in the mixed variety.[39] (3) *Pulmonary hypertension*. Markedly elevated pulmonary artery pressure adversely influences the natural course of this disease and increases the operative mortality. Gomes et al.[19] reported that 5 of 11 pa-

tients with pulmonary artery pressures of more than 75 mm. Hg died after total correction. Pulmonary hypertension is particularly serious in patients less than 1 year of age and carries a very high operative mortality. Pulmonary arterial hypertension almost always is secondary to pulmonary venous obstruction. (4) *Cyanosis*. Hospital mortality seems to be directly proportional to the degree of cyanosis. In patients with systemic arterial oxygen saturations of 80 to 85 per cent or less, mortality of 53 to 62 per cent has been reported.[19, 39] (5) *Size of atrial septal defect*. The presence of a large atrial septal defect appears to have a favorable influence on the course of this disease and also improves the chance of survival after total surgical correction.[30] On the other hand, when the interatrial communication was 6 mm. or less, 8 of 11 patients died after total correction in one series.[19] (6) *Deep hypothermia versus cardiopulmonary bypass*. Open heart surgery with the aid of total cardiopulmonary bypass has generally carried a high mortality when used in total correction of TAPVC in infancy. However, occasional encouraging reports have appeared in the recent literature concerning the use of conventional cardiopulmonary bypass technique.[18] At the University of Washington, deep hypothermia with total circulatory arrest has been used for correction of various congenital anomalies, including TAPVC in infancy, with gratifying results.[12, 13] Most surgeons now prefer this technique for correction of TAPVC;[2, 6] the bloodless field, the nonbeating heart, and the absence of caval cannulae greatly facilitate the performing of posteriorly placed anastomosis in the extracardiac type of TAPVC. Hypothermia and rewarming can be induced either by surface or by core using cardiopulmonary bypass.

SELECTED REFERENCES

Barratt-Boyes, B. G.: Primary definitive intracardiac operations in infants: Total anomalous pulmonary venous connection. *In* Kirklin, J. W. (Ed.): Advances in Cardiovascular Surgery. New York, Grune and Stratton, 1973, p. 127.
This excellent chapter deals with recent surgical results, techniques of surgical repair, and various factors affecting the prognosis in TAPVC.

Breckenridge, I. M., de Leval, M., Stark, J., and Waterston, D. J.: Correction of total anomalous pulmonary venous drainage in infancy. J. Thorac. Cardiovasc. Surg., 66:447, 1973.
This paper describes the results of total correction of the anomalous pulmonary venous drainage in 21 infants. Preoperative preparation, operative procedure, and postoperative care of these infants is discussed.

Delisle, G., Ando, M., Calder, A. L., Zuberbuhler, J. R., Rochenmacher, S., Alday, L. E., Mangini, O., Van Praagh, S., and Van

Praagh, R.: Total anomalous pulmonary venous connection: Report of 93 autopsied cases with emphasis on diagnostic and surgical considerations. Am. Heart J., *91*:99, 1976.

This is the largest series of total anomalous pulmonary venous connection and is admirably reviewed by a group of authors who are highly qualified to discuss both the diagnostic and surgical considerations of this often difficult congenital malformation. The illustrations are excellent, the tables are well arranged, and the overall content outstanding. It is a very thorough assessment of the entire subject.

REFERENCES

1. Auer, J.: The development of the human pulmonary vein and its major variations. Anat. Rec., *101*:581, 1948.
2. Barratt-Boyes, B. G.: Primary definitive intracardiac operations in infants: Total anomalous pulmonary venous connection. *In* Kirklin, J. W. (Ed.): Advances in Cardiovascular Surgery. New York, Grune and Stratton, 1973.
3. Behrendt, D. M., Aberdeen, E., Waterston, D. J., and Bonham-Carter, R. E.: Total anomalous pulmonary venous drainage in infants. Clinical and hemodynamic findings, method and results of operation in 37 cases. Circulation, *46*:347, 1972.
4. Blake, H. A., Hall, R. J., and Mannion, W. C.: Anomalous pulmonary venous return. Circulation, *32*:406, 1965.
5. Bonham-Carter, R. E., Caprils, M., and Noe, Y.: Total anomalous pulmonary venous drainage. A clinical and anatomical study of 75 children. Br. Heart J., *31*:45, 1969.
6. Breckenridge, I. M., de Leval, M., Stark, J., and Waterston, D. J.: Correction of total anomalous pulmonary venous drainage in infancy. J. Thorac. Cardiovasc. Surg., *66*:447, 1973.
7. Brody, H.: Drainage of the pulmonary vein into the right side of the heart. Arch. Pathol., *33*:221, 1942.
8. Burroughs, J. T., and Edwards, J. E.: Total anomalous pulmonary venous connection. Am. Heart J., *59*:913, 1960.
9. Burroughs, J. T., and Kirklin, J. W.: Complete surgical correction of total anomalous pulmonary venous connection. Report of three cases. Mayo Clin. Proc., *131*:182, 1956.
10. Cooley, D. A., and Ochsner, A., Jr.: Correction of total anomalous pulmonary venous drainage. Surgery, *42*:1014, 1957.
11. Darling, R. C., Rothney, W. B., and Craig, J. M.: Total pulmonary venous drainage into the right side of the heart: Report of 17 autopsied cases not associated with other major cardiovascular anomalies. Lab. Invest., *6*:44, 1957.
12. Dillard, D. H., Mohri, H., Hessel, E. A., Anderson, H. N., Nelson, R. J., Crawford, E. W., Morgan, B. C., Winterscheid, L. C., and Merendino, K. A.: Correction of total anomalous pulmonary venous drainage in infancy utilizing deep hypothermia with total circulatory arrest. Circulation 35 (Suppl. 1):105, 1967.
13. Dillard, D. H., Mohri, H., and Merendino, K. A.: Correction of heart disease in infancy utilizing deep hypothermia and total circulatory arrest. J. Thorac. Cardiovasc. Surg., *61*:69, 1971.
14. Edwards, J. E.: Pathologic and developmental considerations in anomalous pulmonary venous connection. Mayo Clin. Proc., *28*:441, 1953.
15. El-Said, G., Mullins, C. E., and McNamara, D. G.: Management of total anomalous pulmonary venous drainage. Circulation, *55*:1240, 1972.
16. Elliot, L. P., and Edwards, J. E.: The problems of pulmonary venous obstruction in total anomalous pulmonary venous connection to the left innominate vein. Circulation, *25*:913, 1962.
17. Gathman, G. E., and Nadas, A. S.: Total anomalous pulmonary venous correction. Circulation, *42*:143, 1970.
18. Gersony, W. M., Bowman, F. O., Jr., Steeg, C. N., Hayes, C. J., Jesse, M. J., and Malm, J. R.: Management of total anomalous pulmonary venous drainage in early infancy. Circulation, *43 and 44* (Suppl. 1):19, 1971.
19. Gomes, M. M. R., Feldt, R. H., McGoon, D. C., and Danielson, G. K.: Total anomalous pulmonary venous connection: Surgical consideration and results of operation. J. Thorac. Cardiovasc. Surg., *60*:116, 1970.
20. Gomes, M. M. R., Feldt, R. H., McGoon, D. C., and Danielson, G. K.: Long term results following correction of total anomalous pulmonary venous connection. J. Thorac. Cardiovasc. Surg., *61*:253, 1971.
21. Gott, V. L., Lester, R. G., Lillehei, C. W., and Varco, R. L.: Total anomalous pulmonary return: An analysis of thirty cases. Circulation, *13*:543, 1956.
22. Hastreiter, A. R., Paul, M. H., Malthan, M. E., and Miller, R. A.: Total anomalous pulmonary venous connection with severe pulmonary venous obstruction. A clinical entity. Circulation, *25*:916, 1962.
23. Hauck, A. J., Rudolph, A. M., and Nadas, A. S.: Pulmonary venous obstruction in infants with anomalous pulmonary venous drainage (abstract). Am. J. Dis. Child., *100*:744, 1960.
24. Kaufman, S. L., Ores, C. N., and Andersen, D. H.: Two cases of total anomalous pulmonary venous return of the supracardiac type with stenosis simulating infradiaphragmatic drainage. Circulation, *25*:376, 1962.
25. Keither, J. D., Rowe, R. D., Vald, P., and O'Hanley, J. H.: Complete anomalous pulmonary venous drainage. Am. J. Med., *16*:23, 1954.
26. Lewis, F. J., Varco, R. L., Taufic, M., and Niazi, S.: Direct vision repair of triatrial heart and total anomalous pulmonary venous drainage. Surg. Gynecol. Obstet., *102*:713, 1956.
27. Miller, W. W., Rashkind, W. J., Miller, R. A., Hastreiter, A. R., Green, E. W., Golinko, R. J., and Young, D.: Total anomalous pulmonary venous return: Effective palliation of critically ill infants by balloon atrial septostomy (abstract). Circulation, *36* (Suppl. 2):189, 1967.
28. Moss, A. J., and Adams, F. H.: Heart Disease in Infants, Children and Adolescents. Baltimore, Williams & Wilkins Company, 1968, p. 672.
29. Muller, W. H., Jr.: The surgical treatment of transposition of the pulmonary veins. Am. Surg., *134*:683, 1951.
30. Mustard, W. T., Keon, W. J., and Trusler, G. A.: II. Transposition of the lesser veins (total anomalous pulmonary venous drainage). Progr. Cardiovasc. Dis., *11*:145, 1968.
31. Nakib, A., Muller, J. H., Kanjub, V. I., and Edwards, J. E.: Anomalies of the pulmonary veins. Am. J. Cardiol., *20*:77, 1967.
32. Rashkind, W. J., and Miller, W. W.: Creation of an atrial septal defect without thoracotomy: A palliative approach to complete transposition of the great arteries. J.A.M.A., *196*:991, 1966.
33. Senning, A.: Complete correction of total anomalous pulmonary venous return. Ann. Surg., *148*:99, 1958.
34. Sloan, H. J., Mackenzie, J., Morris, J. D., Stern, A., and Sigmann, J.: Open-heart surgery in infancy. J. Thorac. Cardiovasc. Surg., *44*:459, 1962.
35. Snellen, H. A., and Albers, F. H.: The clinical diagnosis of anomalous pulmonary venous drainage. Circulation, *6*:801, 1952.
36. Snellen, H. A., Van Ingen, H. C., and Hoefsmit, E. C. M.: Patterns of anomalous pulmonary venous drainage. Circulation, *38*:45, 1968.
37. Swan, J. J. C., Toscano-Barboza, E., and Wood, E. H.: Hemodynamic findings in total anomalous pulmonary venous drainage. Mayo Clin. Proc., *31*:177, 1956.
38. Vetto, R. R., Dillard, D. H., Jones, T. W., Winterscheid, L. C., and Merendino, K. A.: The surgical therapy of extracardiac anomalous pulmonary drainage. Circulation, *23*:907, 1961.
39. Wukasch, D. C., Deutsch, M., Reul, G. J., Hallman, G. L., and Cooley, D. A.: Total anomalous pulmonary venous return: Review of 125 patients treated surgically. Ann. Thorac. Surg., *19*:622, 1975.

VI

VENTRICULAR SEPTAL DEFECTS

Nicholas T. Kouchoukos, M.D.,
and John W. Kirklin, M.D.

Isolated ventricular septal defect is the most common congenital cardiac lesion, accounting for 30 to 40 per cent of all congenital heart disease at birth.[9] The clinical signs of ventricular septal defect and the underlying pathological condition were described by Roger in 1879. By 1950, the development of cardiac catheterization techniques allowed precise delineation of the hemodynamic alterations produced by such defects. Surgical management of ventricular septal defect was first performed by Muller and Dammann,[24] who banded the pulmonary artery to reduce pressure in the pulmonary vascular system and the likelihood of development of irreversible pulmonary hypertension. The first successful repair of a ventricular septal defect was performed in 1954 by Lillehei et al.[20] using controlled cross-circulation. Development of pump-oxygenators and improvement in surgical techniques[15, 21] increased the safety with which closure of such defects could be performed. Increasing knowledge of the life history of patients with ventricular septal defects,[9] further improvements in operative techniques, and knowledge of the results of operation in various subgroups of patients have resulted in the present patient management programs for this anomaly.

ANATOMY

Ventricular septal defects, exclusive of those occurring in association with transposition of the great arteries, corrected transposition, tetralogy of Fallot, or the complete form of common atrioventricular canal, can be divided into four general anatomic types (Fig. 1).[3, 16] The largest number are the so-called *high ventricular septal defects.* Viewed from the left ventricle, they are located immediately under the aortic valve, and they most commonly lie beneath the commissure between the noncoronary and right coronary cusps (Fig. 2). Viewed from the right ventricle, these defects appear to be in the region of the membranous septum. Often, however, they are slightly ventral, or anterior, to it. They are located in the inflow portion of the right ventricle, beneath the crista supraventricularis (infracristal) and in the portion of the septum adjacent to the junction of the septal and anterior leaflets of the tricuspid valve.

Some defects, when viewed from the left ventricle, are "high" defects but lie beneath the central portion of the right coronary cusp and that part of the right cusp adjacent to the commissure between it and the left coronary cusp. Viewed from the right ventricle, they are seen to be *supracristal ventricular septal defects.* They are located in the outflow portion, or infundibulum, of the right ventricle and lie immediately beneath the pulmonary valve (Fig. 3).

A third group of defects is located beneath the septal leaflet of the tricuspid valve, further removed from the aortic valve. There is no muscular tissue between these defects and the tricuspid valve. They are often triangular in shape and

are termed *defects of the atrioventricular canal type* because of their similarity to the defects observed in the complete form of common atrioventricular canal.

Muscular ventricular septal defects are located in the inflow portion of the right ventricle, in areas other than those described previously (Fig. 4). They may be multiple and can occur with the other types of defects as well.

The location of the bundle of His must be known when surgical repair is undertaken, in order to avoid producing heart block. In high ventricular septal defects, the bundle of His is located along the posterior and inferior margins of the defect (Fig. 5). The relations of the bundle of His to the margins of defects of the atrioventricular canal type are not so constant, but presumably the bundle is located along the edge of the ventricular component of the defect from its midportion to that extremity of the ventricular septal edge of the defect near the coronary sinus. The bundle of His is generally not in danger of being damaged when supracristal or muscular defects are closed.

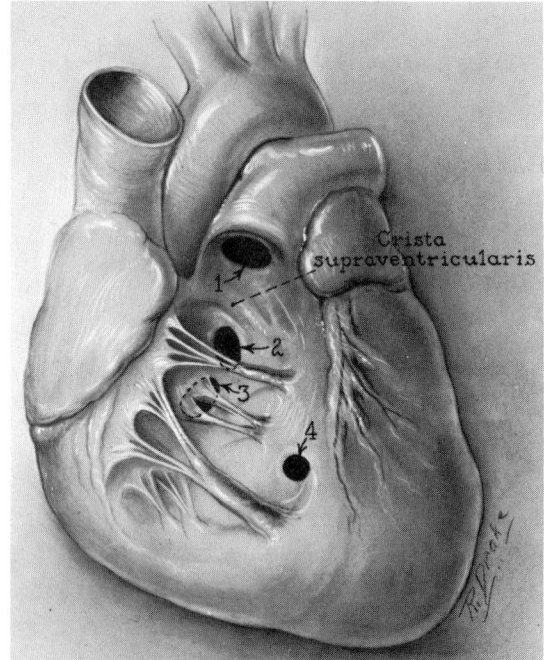

Figure 1. Schematic representation of the common locations of isolated ventricular septal defects: (1) the supracristal defect, located immediately under the pulmonary valve, but from the right ventricular aspect still under the aortic valve; (2) the most common type, the typical high defect that from the left ventricular aspect is also under the aortic valve; (3) the atrioventricular canal type of ventricular septal defect; and (4) one of the common locations of defects of the muscular portion of the septum. (From Kirklin, J. W., Harshbarger, H. G., Donald, D. E., and Edwards, J. E.: J. Thorac. Surg., *33*:45, 1957.)

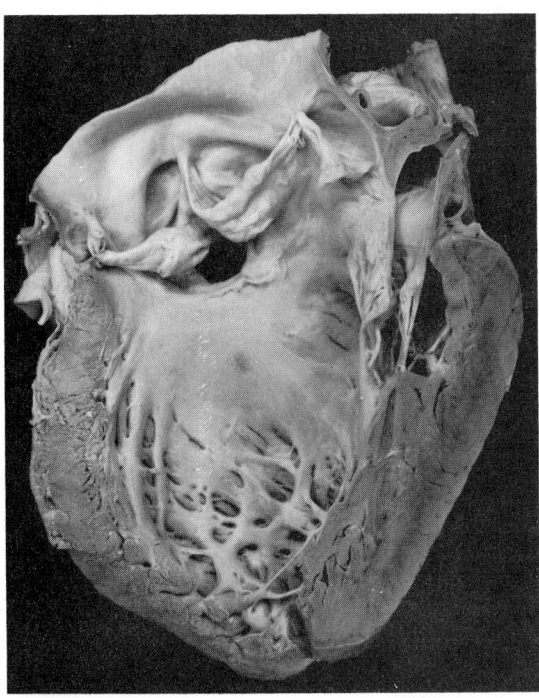

Figure 2. A high ventricular septal defect viewed from the left ventricular side. Note that it is immediately under the commissure between the right and noncoronary cusps of the aortic valve. (From Kirklin, J. W., Harshbarger, H. G., Donald, D. E., and Edwards, J. E.: J. Thorac. Surg., *33*:45, 1957.)

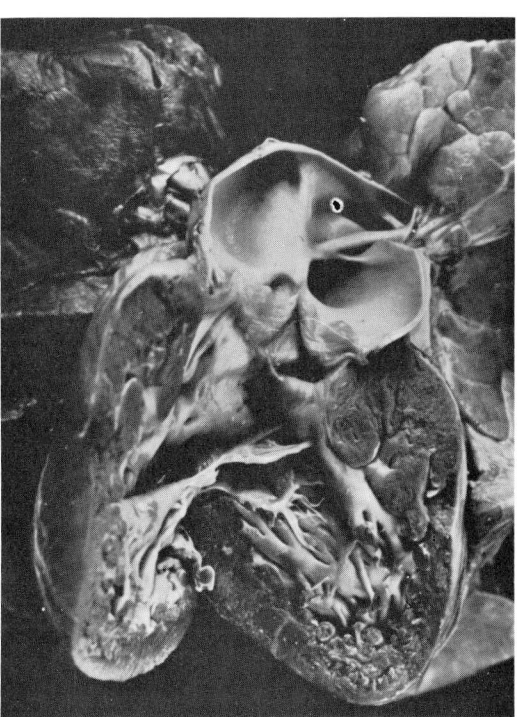

Figure 3. Supracristal ventricular septal defect viewed from the right ventricular side. Note that it is immediately beneath the pulmonary valve. (From Becu, L. M., Fontana, R. S., DuShane, J. W., Kirklin, J. W., Burchell, H. B., and Edwards, J. E.: Circulation, *14*:349, 1956. By permission of the American Heart Association, Inc.)

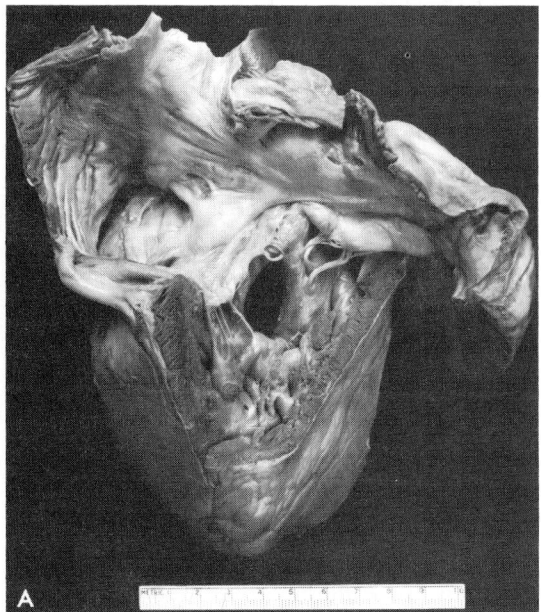

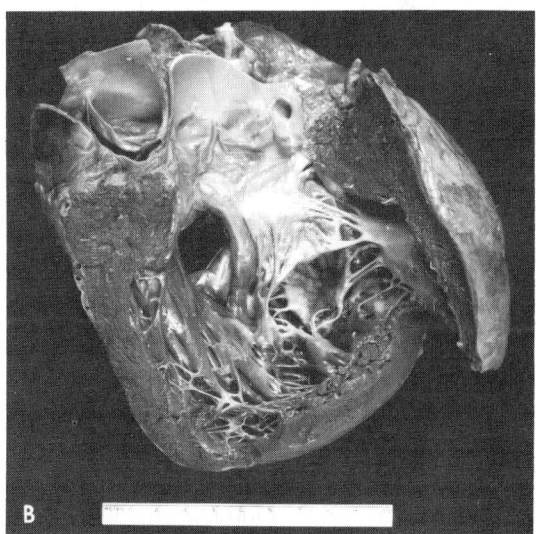

Figure 4. Muscular ventricular septal defects. *A*, The defect is near the tricuspid valve but is completely surrounded by ventricular septal muscle. *B*, This muscular ventricular septal defect, viewed from the left ventricular side, is low in the muscular septum. (From Kirklin, J. W., Harshbarger, H. G., Donald, D. E., and Edwards, J. E.: J. Thorac. Surg., *33*:45, 1957.)

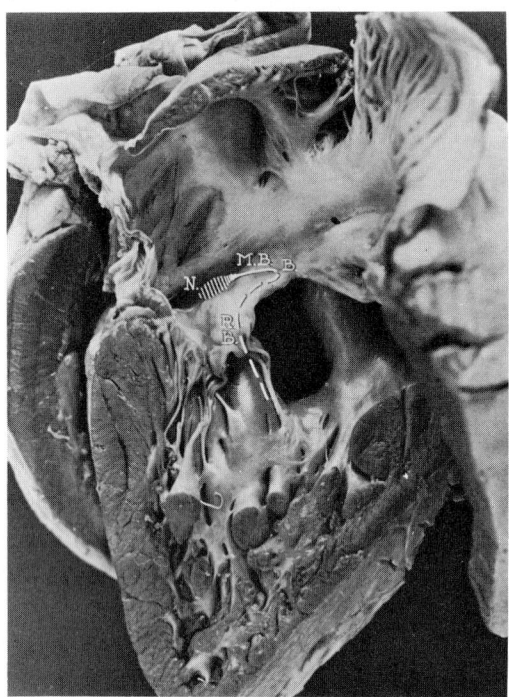

Figure 5. In this specimen, the right ventricle and right atrium have been opened. The pulmonary valve and pulmonary artery are superior and to the right. The relations of the bundle of His (M.B.B.) are illustrated. The bundle lies not in the tricuspid valve tissue but in that part of the septum immediately beneath it. One cannot be certain that the main bundle has become the right bundle (R.B.) until one reaches the level of the papillary muscle of the conus. Stitches must not be placed in these areas when repairing the defect. (From Kirklin, J. W., Karp, R., B., and Bargeron, L. M., Jr.: Surgical treatment of ventricular septal defect. *In* Sabiston, D. C., Jr., and Spencer, F. C. (Eds.): Surgery of the Chest, 3rd ed. Philadelphia, W. B. Saunders Company, 1976.)

ASSOCIATED LESIONS

In some patients with supracristal ventricular defects, aortic valvular incompetence develops, presumably as a result of progressive prolapse of the right aortic cusp through the defect.[25, 33] Abnormalities in the development of the aortic root may also contribute to the development of aortic incompetence. Peak pressure gradients between the inflow portion of the right ventricle and the outflow portion or the pulmonary artery are present in approximately one half of the patients with ventricular septal defects and aortic valve incompetence as a result of associated displacement and hypertrophy of the crista supraventricularis and its bands.[13] The prolapsed aortic leaflet may contribute to the obstruction.[29]

Occasionally patients with ventricular septal defects have associated mild or moderate degrees of infundibular pulmonary stenosis. Less commonly, there is associated valvular pulmonary stenosis. These lesions should be recognized and treated appropriately when repair of ventricular septal defect is carried out. These lesions differ morphologically from the tetralogy of Fallot, which is discussed elsewhere in this text.

Other lesions that occur with ventricular septal defect include patent ductus ateriosus, atrial septal defect, coarctation of the aorta, congenital mitral stenosis or insufficiency, and persistent left superior vena cava. These lesions are of importance when decisions are made regarding therapy and the conduct of the operation.

PATHOPHYSIOLOGY

Hemodynamics

The direction and magnitude of the shunt in patients with ventricular septal defect depend upon the size of the defect and the differences in pressure between the ventricles during systole and diastole. When the ventricular septal defect is small, it offers resistance to flow and only a relatively large pressure difference between the two ventricles, such as occurs during mid and late systole, results in significant flow across the defect. Since under these circumstances pressure is higher in the left than in the right ventricle, the shunt is left-to-right. When the defect is large, it offers little resistance to flow, and small pressure differences between the right and left ventricle then result in shunting.[12, 19] During mid and late systole, when most of the shunting occurs, the pressure differences between the two ventricles and the resultant shunting are related primarily to the relative resistance to ejection offered by the systemic and pulmonary vasculature. In diastole and early systole, a number of other factors appear to influence the magnitude and direction of the gradients and the resultant shunting, including the relative compliances of the ventricles, their diastolic pressures, and the presence of asynchronous contraction.[19] The size of the ventricular septal defect may vary during various phases of the cardiac cycle and may also influence the degree of shunting.

When a left-to-right shunt is present, pulmonary blood flow is increased relative to normal and to systemic blood flow. Flow through the left atrium and mitral valve orifice is similarly increased and thus greater work (pressure × flow) is performed by both the left and the right ventricles. Both ventricles enlarge when this work load is significantly increased by a large left-to-right shunt. The pressure and size of the left atrium increase to a degree corresponding to the magnitude of increase in pulmonary blood flow. In patients with severe pulmonary hypertension, severe elevation of pulmonary vascular resistance, and bidirectional shunting, pulmonary, left atrial, and mitral valve flow are about normal, and the left ventricle and atrium are consequently not enlarged. The right ventricle is hypertrophied.

Effects on the Pulmonary Vasculature

Patients with small ventricular septal defects (area < 1 cm.² per square meter body surface area) generally have normal right ventricular and pulmonary arterial pressures, slightly elevated pulmonary blood flow relative to systemic flow, and no pulmonary vascular disease as evidenced histologically or by the measurement of pulmonary vascular resistance (Table 1).

The hemodynamic state in patients with large ventricular septal defects is determined largely by the pulmonary vascular resistance, which in these patients may be mildly, moderately, or severely elevated because of varying degrees of hypertensive pulmonary vascular disease. The pulmonary vascular disease develops as a result of the large ventricular septal

TABLE 1. A Way of Categorizing Patients with Ventricular Septal Defects*

| Size of Defect | Pulmonary Arterial Hypertension | | Pulmonary Blood Flow | | Pulmonary Vascular Disease | | Resistance Units |
	Degree	P_P/P_S†	Magnitude of Increase	Q_P/Q_S‡	Severity	R_P/R_S§	
Small	None	<0.25	Mild	<1.4	None	<0.25	<5
	None	<0.25	Moderate	1.4–1.8	None	<0.25	<5
Large	Mild	0.25–0.45	Large	>1.8	Mild	<0.25	5–7
	Moderate	0.45–0.75	Large	>1.8	Mild	<0.25	5–7
	Severe	>0.75	Large	>1.8	Mild	0.25–0.45	5–7
			Moderate	1.4–1.8	Moderate	0.45–0.75	8–10
			Small	<1.4	Severe	>0.75	>10

*Modified from Kirklin, J. W., Karp, R. B., and Bargeron, L. M., Jr. *In* Sabiston, D. C., Jr., and Spencer, F. C. (Eds.): Gibbon's Surgery of the Chest, 3rd ed. Philadelphia, W. B. Saunders Company, 1976.

†P_P/P_S refers to the ratio between peak pressure in the pulmonary artery and that in a systemic artery (ratio between mean pressures is more commonly used, and is similar).

‡Q_P/Q_S refers to ratio between pulmonary and systemic blood flow.

§R_P/R_S refers to ratio between pulmonary and systemic vascular resistance.

defect. The pulmonary vascular resistance is expressed numerically in resistance units, normalized as to body surface area (BSA):

$$\frac{\text{Mean pulmonary artery pressure} - \text{Mean left atrial pressure}}{\text{Cardiac output/BSA}}$$

The absolute value for pulmonary vascular resistance is important, but so also is the relation between pulmonary and systemic vascular resistance, although the variability of the latter in a given patient dictates the use of caution in interpreting this ratio. Some patients with large ventricular septal defects have a low pulmonary/systemic resistance ratio (less than 0.45) and a large pulmonary blood flow relative to systemic flow. This has been termed the hyperdynamic type of pulmonary hypertension. When the pulmonary/systemic resistance ratio is between 0.45 and 0.75, indicating significant pulmonary vascular disease (see later discussion), pulmonary blood flow is only moderately elevated relative to systemic flow. When the resistance ratio is greater than 0.75, the flow across the defect is bidirectional or right-to-left and the pulmonary blood flow is similar to or less than systemic blood flow.

In normal persons, a fourfold increase in pulmonary blood flow, as occurs with exercise, can be accommodated without an increase in pulmonary artery pressure; this indicates an actual decrease in pulmonary vascular resistance under these circumstances. In patients with ventricular septal defects and moderate or severe pulmonary vascular disease, the pulmonary vasculature usually loses the ability to accommodate increases in pulmonary blood flow, caused by physiologic stresses such as exercise, by a decline in pulmonary vascular resistance. In this case, closure of the ventricular septal defect is hazardous, since pulmonary, and thus systemic, blood flow cannot increase during exercise. With the defect open, systemic blood

flow and oxygen consumption can increase, albeit by the mechanism of increased right-to-left shunting.

The elevations of pulmonary vascular resistance in patients with ventricular septal defects are associated with anatomic changes in the small arteries of the lungs.[7, 8, 34] The changes result from a decrease in the ratio between the diameter of the lumen and the total diameter of the small muscular pulmonary arteries and arterioles. In patients with moderately elevated pulmonary vascular resistance, the increase in vessel wall thickness is primarily due to increased thickness of the muscle of the media and to intimal fibrosis with actual occlusion of some of the vessels. In patients with severe elevation of pulmonary vascular resistance, the intimal proliferation is more pronounced, with widespread occlusion of the muscular pulmonary arteries and arterioles and plexiform dilatation of many of the remaining vessels.[7]

NATURAL HISTORY

Many patients with ventricular septal defects have small defects and few or no symptoms, since the left-to-right shunt is small and pulmonary hypertension and vascular disease do not develop. It is estimated that only 10 to 20 per cent of patients have large defects and incur serious difficulties.[10]

Infants born with large ventricular septal defects have moderate elevation of pulmonary vascular resistance, owing to persistence of the medial thickening of the small pulmonary arteries present in the normal fetus. As the pulmonary vessels mature in the first few weeks of life, pulmonary resistance declines, the magnitude of the left-to-right shunt across the defect increases, and symptoms develop. Such infants may die of severe congestive heart failure during this period.[23] If they survive and the hemodynamic state stabilizes, the small systemic blood flow and breathlessness, which entails a large caloric expenditure and interferes with eating, can result in growth failure. If operation is not performed, death can occur during this period, usually from congestive failure or pneumonia, and usually in the first year of life.[10]

In a small number of infants with large ventricular septal defects who survive the neonatal period, severe pulmonary vascular disease and a significant increase in pulmonary vascular resistance begin to develop by the age of 6 to 12 months. If operation is not performed and this condition progresses over the ensuing months or years until it becomes severe, these patients can no longer be considered candidates for operation because of the severity of the pulmonary vascular changes. When the shunting becomes dominantly right-to-left across the defect as a result of the hypertensive pulmonary vascular disease, the patients become cyanotic and can be considered to have Eisenmenger's complex. Operation is then contraindicated.

Another group of infants with large defects have only mild elevation in pulmonary vascular resistance in the first few years of life, although significant pulmonary hypertension and a large pulmonary blood flow are present. These children are usually of small stature and have significantly impaired exercise tolerance. If the defect is still open or unrepaired by the time the patient is about 10 years old, the pulmonary vascular disease usually begins to progress, and at the age of 15 to 20 years these patients have Eisenmenger's complex with severe elevation of the pulmonary vascular resistance, and predominant right-to-left shunting occurs across the defect. Occasionally, severe pulmonary vascular disease does not develop, and heart failure may occur in the second or third decade of life. Those patients with Eisenmenger's complex become polycythemic and eventually succumb to the complications of hypoxia and polycythemia, usually at the age of 25 to 30 years.

In some infants, the ventricular septal defect becomes smaller in size relative to the size of the heart as time passes. Pulmonary blood flow decreases because of the resistance to flow offered by the smaller defect, and pulmonary artery pressure also decreases. Although a left-to-right shunt is still present, severe pulmonary vascular disease does not develop. The growth and development of these children is quite normal. In a few of these patients bacterial endocarditis develops.[27]

Spontaneous complete closure of ventricular septal defects has been estimated to occur in 25 to 50 per cent of patients during childhood.[10] Even large defects may close in this way. Closure most commonly occurs before the age of 3 years and only occasionally after the early teen years. The mechanism of closure is usually related to ingrowth of fibrous tissue from the margins of the defect or adherence of the septal leaflet of the tricuspid valve to the margins of the defect.[10]

DIAGNOSIS

History

Infants with large ventricular septal defects do not usually have symptoms until they reach the age of 6 weeks to 3 months. At this time the pulmonary vascular resistance has fallen from the elevated levels present at birth, and this results in maximal left-to-right shunting of blood across the defect and a marked increase in pulmonary blood flow. Tachypnea, growth failure, pneumonia, and severe cardiac failure may then develop.

Many patients with ventricular septal defects are asymptomatic. Generally these are patients whose defects are small in size. Children with moderate-sized or large septal defects may demonstrate growth failure and have limitations in exercise tolerance. The growth failure is related to the size of the defect and the magnitude of the left-to-right shunt.

Patients with markedly elevated pulmonary vascular resistance and predominant right-to-left shunting across the septal defect (Eisenmenger's complex) are cyanosed, polycythemic, and severely limited in their activities.

Examination

The infant with a large ventricular septal defect and increased pulmonary blood flow characteristically presents with tachypnea and marked subcostal retraction. Severe growth failure and a lack of subcutaneous tissue are often evident. The complexion may be waxen, and evidence of profuse sweating, such as damp or matted hair, may be noted. The jugular venous pulses are prominent even when the infant is held erect. On palpation, there is often a precordial bulge, and the heart is overactive with a rapid rate. A thrill is present in the third to fifth left intercostal spaces. A loud systolic murmur is also present in this same area. The second sound at the base is usually loud and may be split. The liver and spleen are usually enlarged, and the peripheral pulses are weak.

In older children with large ventricular septal defects, a protruding sternum or pigeon breast deformity is frequently present. Presumably this results from the enlarged right ventricle pushing the sternum anteriorly during the period of growth. The heart is hyperactive, there is a right ventricular lift, and the left ventricle is enlarged. A systolic thrill is often present over the left precordium. The characteristic murmur is harsh and pansystolic and is heard best in the left fourth interspace along the sternal border. If pulmonary blood flow is large, there may be a superimposed midsystolic ejection murmur in the area of the pulmonary valve.[18] A mid-diastolic murmur is present at the apex and indicates a large flow across the mitral valve. The first sound at the base is normal. The second sound is characterized by an abnormally wide split in expiration, and the splitting is accentuated in inspiration.[18]

Patients with small defects and small left-to-right shunts have only a systolic murmur. The heart is not hyperactive, and there is no enlargement of the left ventricle or right ventricular lift. In patients with large defects and high pulmonary vascular resistance resulting in only small net left-to-right shunts or in bidirectional shunts of equal magnitude, the systolic murmur is soft and short or may be absent. There is no apical diastolic rumble and the second sound is markedly accentuated. There is no left ventricular enlargement and a right ventricular lift is prominent. When the patient is cyanotic, pulmonary vascular disease is severe and the shunt is dominantly right-to-left.

Chest Roentgenograms

As already emphasized, this and all other parts of the clinical and hemodynamic state are determined by the size of the defect and the degree of pulmonary vascular resistance.

In patients with small ventricular septal defects and small left-to-right shunts, chest roentgenograms are usually normal. Patients with large ventricular septal defects, mild elevation of pulmonary vascular resistance, and large left-to-right shunts have large pulmonary arteries, both centrally and peripherally, and therefore a large pulmonary blood flow (Fig. 6). The right ventricle and the left ventricle are enlarged, as is the left atrium. When marked enlargement of the left atrium is present in a patient suspected of having a ventricular septal defect, the presence of coexisting mitral valvular regurgitation should be considered.

In patients with large ventricular septal defects and severe elevation of the pulmonary vascular resistance, the chest roentgenogram is quite different (Fig. 7). The central pulmonary arteries appear normal in size or are enlarged, but the peripheral pulmonary arteries appear normal; this suggests a normal or decreased pulmonary blood flow. The right ventricle appears somewhat enlarged, but there is no evidence of significant left atrial or left ventricular enlargement. Aside from the enlarged central pulmonary arteries, the cardiac silhouette may appear normal.

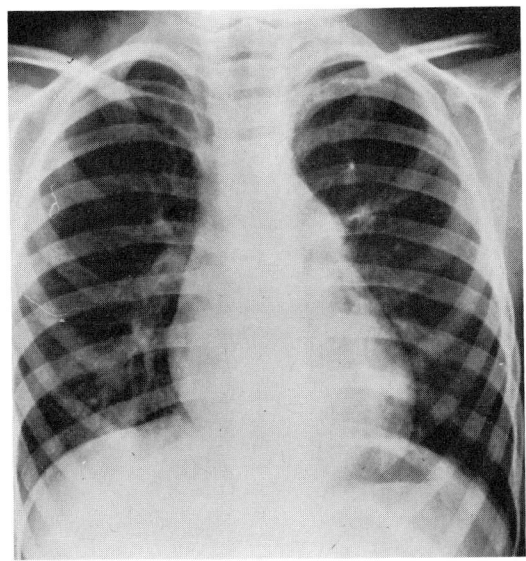

Figure 7. This chest roentgenogram is in contrast to that shown in Figure 6. The heart is not enlarged overall. The main pulmonary artery is enlarged; there is no evidence of increased pulmonary blood flow. This patient has a large ventricular septal defect, pulmonary hypertension, severe elevation of pulmonary vascular resistance, and pulmonary blood flow that is less than systemic blood flow. The condition is inoperable. (From DuShane, J. W., and Kirklin, J. W.: Circulation, 21:13, 1960. By permission of the American Heart Association, Inc.)

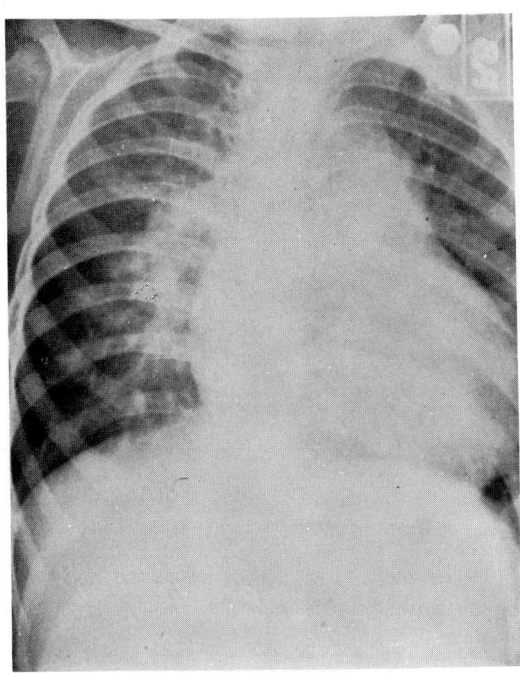

Figure 6. Chest roentgenogram of a child with a large ventricular septal defect, large pulmonary blood flow, and pulmonary hypertension, but only mild elevation of pulmonary vascular resistance. This is reflected in the evidence of left and right ventricular enlargement, enlargement of the main pulmonary artery, and marked increase in pulmonary blood flow. (From Kirklin, J. W., Karp, R. B., and Bargeron, L. M., Jr. In Sabiston, D. C., Jr., and Spencer, F. C., (Eds.): Surgery of the Chest, 3rd ed. Philadelphia, W. B. Saunders Company, 1976.)

Electrocardiogram

The electrocardiographic findings, in the absence of a conduction defect, are likewise determined by the size of the defect and the pulmonary vascular resistance.

In patients with small ventricular septal defects, the electrocardiogram may be normal. When the defect and shunt are slightly larger (Q_p/Q_s > about 1.8), the increase in left ventricular work from the large left ventricular stroke volume is evidenced by increased R wave voltage and tall peaked T waves from the left precordial leads. When the shunt is still larger, a pattern of mild right ventricular overload may be present as suggested by an RSR' pattern in the V_1 lead.

If the ventricular septal defect is large, and the left-to-right shunt is large (Q_p/Q_s > 2), but the pulmonary vascular resistance is significantly less than the systemic vascular resistance (R_p/R_s < 0.75), there is evidence of increased work of both ventricles. The R wave from the right precordial leads is tall, and when the right ventricular peak pressure is similar to the left ventricular peak pressure, it is notched on the upstroke. The left precordial leads in this situation have the pattern of left ventricular overload previously described, although there may be a deeper S wave.

When the ventricular septal defect is large and the pulmonary vascular resistance is equal to or greater than the systemic resistance, right axis deviation is usually present in the limb leads. The right precordial leads show the typical large, usually notched R waves of right ventricular hypertrophy while the left precordial leads no longer show left ventricular overload.

The Q wave usually disappears in the left precordial leads, the R wave voltage is below normal, and a deep S wave appears.

In many patients with ventricular septal defect and large pulmonary blood flow, evidence of left atrial hypertrophy is seen in the broadened and even notched P waves present primarily in the left precordial leads.

The electrocardiogram then supplements the physical findings and chest roentgenogram. Taken together, they usually provide a useful categorization of patients as to the size of the ventricular septal defect, the size of the shunt, and the magnitude of the pulmonary vascular resistance.

Cardiac Catheterization

Cardiac catheterization is indicated in all patients in whom the history, physical, and laboratory findings suggest the presence of a ventricular septal defect, except those in whom the hemodynamic derangements are minimal. The study is performed not only for confirmation of the diagnosis, but to measure pulmonary and systemic pressures and flows and to calculate resistance in the two circuits. Catheterization is also indicated when the clinical findings are atypical or when the presence of associated cardiac defects is suspected.

Angiocardiography

Injection of radiopaque contrast material into the left ventricle at the time of catheterization is essential in any patient in whom operation is contemplated. This is particularly true for infants, where information regarding the location and number of defects is of value in planning the technical details of the operation. Angiocardiographic studies are also indicated in those patients suspected of having associated defects such as aortic valvular incompetence or pulmonary infundibular or valvular stenosis.

Indications for Operation

The decision to recommend operation for an individual patient is based on knowledge of the natural history of similar untreated patients and of the results of surgical correction. Important considerations in the natural history include the presence of congestive failure or growth failure, the likelihood of development of severe pulmonary vascular disease, and the possibility of spontaneous closure. The results of surgery depend upon the initial risk of operation, its effect on pulmonary vascular disease, and the incidence of complications such as heart block or incomplete repair.

At any age, the presence of pulmonary vascular disease so severe that the pulmonary/systemic resistance ratio is greater than 0.90 is considered a contraindication to operation. If the pulmonary/systemic resistance ratio is between 0.75 and 0.90, operation is generally advised but with full knowledge of a possible unsatisfactory long-term result.[4] The presence of severe pulmonary hypertension is not a contraindication to operation if the resistance ratio is less than 0.75. Operation is usually not truly curative in older patients with established pulmonary vascular disease, however.

Prompt intracardiac repair is indicated in infants with large defects, large shunts, and pulmonary hypertension who present with left ventricular failure, recurrent pulmonary infections, severe growth failure or evidence of increasing pulmonary vascular disease. We believe that pulmonary arterial banding no longer has a place in the management of such patients.

All other patients with large ventricular septal defects should have elective repair before the age of two years. When patients with large defects are first seen after the age of two years, prompt repair is advisable unless the contraindications to repair noted above (pulmonary vascular disease) are present.

If the defect is small or moderate in size, the possibility of spontaneous closure and the general well-being of the patient support the decision to defer operation. If such defects remain patent in patients who reach the age of 10 to 12 years, the likelihood of spontaneous closure is small, and surgical repair is usually recommended.

When aortic valvular incompetence begins to develop in a child with a ventricular septal defect, closure of the defect should be undertaken to prevent further prolapse of the aortic cusps and progression of the aortic incompetence. When coexisting pulmonary infundibular or valvular stenosis is present, the ventricular septal defect is generally large and if the stenosis is severe, right-to-left shunting may be present. In these situations operation is advisable. Mild or moderate mitral incompetence in association with ventricular septal defect is not a contraindication to repair of the defect.

SURGICAL TREATMENT

Intracardiac Repair

A midline sternal splitting incision is used, and the pericardium is opened vertically to the level of the left innominate vein. Careful exploration of the pericardial cavity is performed to determine the presence of a patent ductus arteriosus, a left superior vena cava, and any anomalous pulmonary venous connections. The sizes of the various cardiac chambers are estimated, and the peak systolic pressures in the right and left ventricles and in the pulmonary artery are measured. In general, the atrial approach is preferred. The ventricular approach is utilized if the defect is of the supracristal type or if there is coexisting pulmonary valvular or infundibular stenosis. Right or left ventriculotomy may be required for some patients with multiple muscular defects.

Cardiopulmonary bypass is established using two venous cannulas, one in each vena cava, and a cannula in the ascending aorta for arterial return from the pump-oxygenator. Moderate (28°C) or profound (24 to 28°C) total body hypothermia is induced with the perfusate. A venting catheter is passed into the left atrium and the right superior pulmonary vein and is secured with a purse-string suture and a tourniquet. Tapes previously placed around the superior and inferior venae cavae are then secured tightly around the cannulas. Repair of the defect is carried out while the aorta is clamped intermittently for 10 to 15 minute intervals, releasing the clamp for three-minute intervals with the perfusate temperature at 28°C to allow perfusion of the coronary arteries. Alternatively, the myocardium can be cooled by taking the perfusate temperature initially to 12°C over several minutes and clamping the aorta for one period of 30 to 40 minutes. With either technique, if intracardiac return of blood is interfering with exposure, perfusion flow rates may be reduced to low levels or total circulatory arrest induced for brief periods.

If the atrial approach is to be used, the right atrium is opened obliquely between the caval cannulas. If an atrial septal defect or a probe-patent foramen ovale is present, this is closed by direct suture. The ventricular septal defect is then exposed by retracting the leaflets of the tricuspid valve (Fig. 8). It is not necessary to incise or disconnect the leaflets. The relations of the defect to the tricuspid valve, to the area of the ventricular septum occupied by the bundle of His, and to the aortic and pulmonary valve cusps are carefully noted. If all edges of the defect cannot be clearly visualized, it is preferable to abandon the atrial approach and to repair the defect through a right ventriculotomy.

Small defects are generally closed by direct suture and large defects are repaired with a patch of Dacron or Teflon cloth. When a patch is to be used, the first stitch is placed between the patch and the edge of the defect at the position most distant from the surgeon (Fig. 9). The edge of the patch is sutured to the anterior rim of the ventricular septal defect with a continuous suture. The posterior half of the patch is then sutured to the inferior and posterior edges of the ventricular septal defect. It is in this area that the bundle of His is located. The stitches in the ventricular septum are therefore placed 3 to 4 mm. away from the edge of the defect to avoid injury to the conduction system. As the suture line is continued posteriorly, the

region of the tricuspid annulus is approached. In this area a transition stitch is placed between the septum, the base of the septal leaflet of the tricuspid valve, and the patch. Closure of the defect is then completed by suturing the patch to the base of the septal leaflet of the tricuspid valve and extending this suture line superiorly (to the surgeon's left) until the previously placed sutures on the anterior border of the defect are reached.

When the defect is approached through the right ventricle, a transverse ventriculotomy is made in the location shown in Figure 10A. Repair of a high septal defect is similar to that just described except that the first stitch is placed through the posterior portion of the inferior margin of the defect, the base of the septal leaflet of the tricuspid valve, and then through the patch. The repair is carried anteriorly along the inferior border of the defect, the patch being sutured to the ventricular septum and the bites placed 3 to 4 mm. away from the edge of the defect (Fig. 10B). The repair is completed posteriorly by suturing the edge of the patch to the base of the septal leaflet of the tricuspid valve. Stitches are then placed between the patch and the superior margin of the defect with care to avoid injury to the aortic cusp, which lies beneath.

When the defect is of the supracristal type and lies immediately beneath the pulmonary valve, it is generally oval or triangular in shape and can be closed by direct suture. There is little danger of damage to the tricuspid valve or the bundle of His in this area. Care must be taken, however, to avoid injury to the aortic and pulmonary valve cusps.

Defects of the atrioventricular canal type, located beneath the septal leaflet of the tricuspid valve, are triangular in shape and must usually be closed with a patch. The patch is sewn into place with continuous sutures that secure it to the base of septal leaflet of the tricuspid valve along one side and to the margins of the ventricular septal defect along the other two sides. When the patch is sutured to the posterior margin, the stitches should be placed well away from the edge of the defect to avoid injury to the conduction system.

Defects in the muscular portion of the septum can usually be closed by direct suture. If these defects lie far anteriorly, it is best to place the sutures from outside the right ventricle, grasping the edges of the defect and bringing the stitch again outside the heart to be tied on the surface over bolsters of Teflon felt.

If pulmonary infundibular or valvular stenosis exists with the ventricular septal defect, valvotomy and resection of the infundibular muscle are performed prior to repair of the defect. If aortic incompetence exists in association with a ventricular septal defect, the severity of the incompetence should be assessed as accurately as possible preoperatively. If the incompetence is mild, only closure of the septal defect is indicated. If the aortic incompetence is moderate or severe, plication of the aortic leaflets should be performed through an aortotomy before closure of the septal defect.[30] This allows evaluation of the valvuloplasty through the ventricular septal defect after removal of the aortic clamp. If significant incompetence persists,

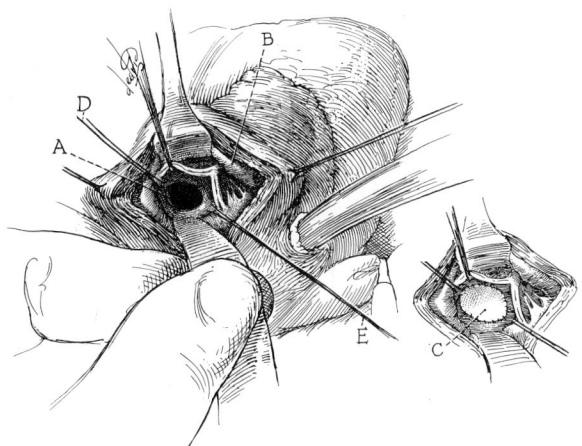

Figure 8. Repair of ventricular septal defect using the transatrial approach. *A,* Portion of aortic valve seen through defect. *B,* Anterior leaflet of tricuspid valve. *C,* Dacron velour patch in place with continuous suture. *D* and *E,* Traction sutures. (From Subramanian, S.: Primary definitive intracardiac operations in infants: Ventricular septal defects. *In* Kirklin, J. W. (Ed.): Advances in Cardiovascular Surgery. New York, Grune and Stratton, 1973, p. 145. By permission.)

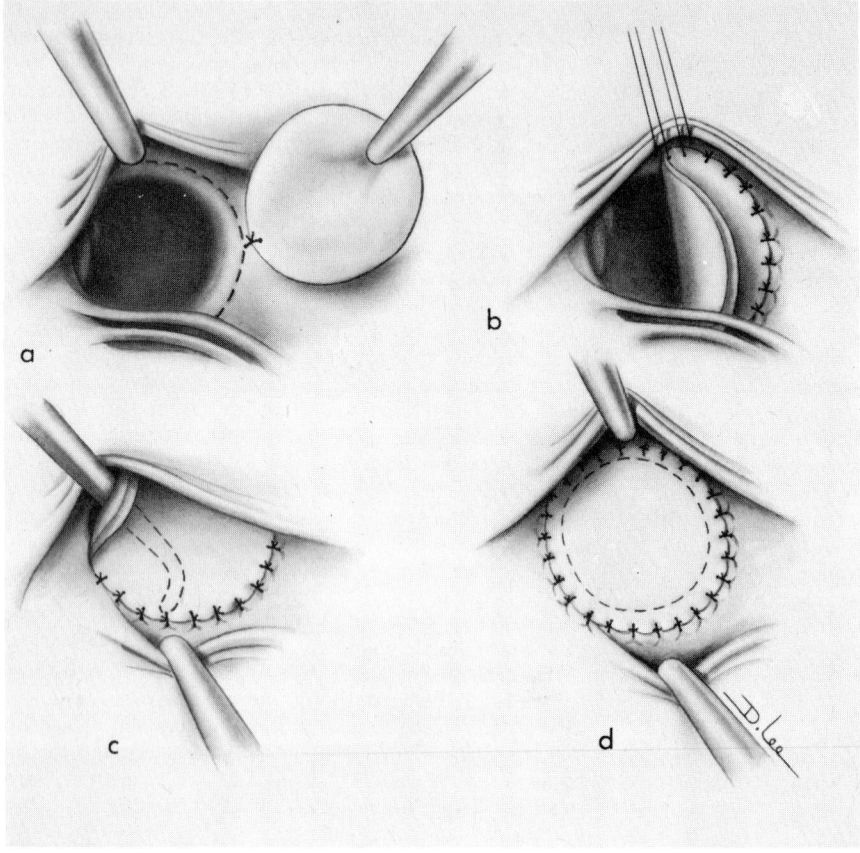

Figure 9. Steps in the repair of a large ventricular septal defect through the right atrium. The leaflets and chordae are retracted to provide visualization. In actual practice a continuous suture is used. Before the suture line is completed, a fine probe is used to detect any residual apertures, and any found are closed with additional sutures. (From Cartmill, T. B., DuShane, J. W., McGoon, D. C., and Kirklin, J. W.: J. Thorac. Cardiovasc. Surg., *52*:486, 1966.)

replacement of the aortic valve is indicated (See Section XVI).

Intracardiac repair of ventricular septal defects in infants under one year of age presents special problems because of the small size of the structures and because of the tendency to postoperative pulmonary complications. More or less standard perfusion techniques have been used with satisfaction by some surgeons in this special situation,[28] but more recently a combination of surface cooling, total circulatory arrest during the repair, and rewarming with cardiopulmonary bypass has been popularized for intracardiac surgery in infants.[2] At present, we employ the basic technique described above unless the heart is so small

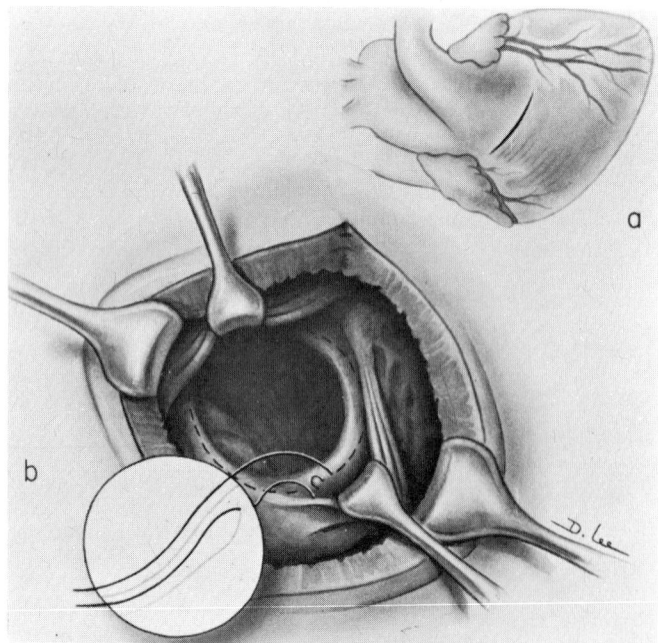

Figure 10. In infants, the right ventricular approach is usually employed for high defects; the transverse right ventriculotomy incision is illustrated (*a*). In *b*, the first stitch for the repair has been placed. This stitch is carried anteriorly along the dotted line and then to the left and anteriorly along the dotted line to the other side to complete the repair. (From Cartmill, T. B., DuShane, J. W., McGoon, D. C., and Kirklin, J. W.: J. Thorac. Cardiovasc. Surg., *52*:486, 1966.)

(usually in infants less than three months of age) that insertion of the left atrial vent is not possible. Then, without surface cooling, we induce profound hypothermia with the perfusate using one or two venous cannulas and perform the repair during total circulatory arrest.

Pulmonary Arterial Banding

We have not utilized the technique of banding of the pulmonary artery for some time. It is still used by some groups for managing infants with isolated ventricular septal defects and severe heart failure and for infants with multiple cardiac anomalies.[11, 31]

A left anterolateral thoracotomy incision in the third intercostal space is employed. The pericardium overlying the pulmonary artery is incised longitudinally, and a plane is developed between the pulmonary artery and the aorta. A band of synthetic cloth (Dacron or Teflon) is passed through the aperture behind the pulmonary artery. The band should not be too wide, to prevent excessive fibrosis.[5] The ends of the band are then placed in a right-angle clamp anteriorly and traction is placed on the band to produce the desired amount of constriction of the pulmonary artery. In such infants an indwelling arterial needle is helpful. As the band is tightened, the arterial blood pressure rises; but when the band is too tight, bradycardia and cardiac dilation occur. In addition, a fall in peripheral arterial oxygen saturation occurs as a result of the production of some right-to-left shunting as the pulmonary artery is constricted. Ideally, a pulmonary artery systolic pressure of 30 to 50 mm. Hg distal to the band with an adequate systemic pressure is optimal. Once the desired level of constriction of the artery has been achieved by the right-angle clamp, the clamp is released slightly and horizontal mattress sutures are placed through the edges of the band to secure it at the desired level. The edges of the pericardium are then approximated and the thoracotomy incision is closed in the usual fashion. One small tube is left in the pleural cavity for drainage.

POSTOPERATIVE CARE

Although the outcome of operation for closure of the ventricular septal defect is determined largely by events in the operating room and by proper preoperative selection of patients, the postoperative care is also of importance, particularly in infants.

Optimal cardiac performance is obtained by avoiding excessive injury to the myocardium during operation and by maintaining adequate ventricular enddiastolic pressure and blood volume early after operation. Fine polyvinyl catheters placed in the left and right atria are used to monitor atrial pressures for the first 24 hours after operation. If the cardiac output is greater than about 3.0 liters per minute per square meter (by measurement or clinical estimate), the left atrial pressure should be kept low (6 to 10 mm. Hg). If the cardiac output is less, maintenance of left atrial pressure at 12 to 14 mm. Hg by infusion of blood will often improve cardiac output by increasing preload (the stretch of the sarcomeres at end-diastole). Arterial pressure should also be monitored closely, particularly in infants. If mean arterial pressure and peripheral resistance are elevated above the normal levels for age, and cardiac index is low ($<$ 2.2 to 2.4 L./min./m.²), reduction of arterial pressure with vasodilating agents such as trimethaphan camsylate (Arfonad) or sodium nitroprusside (Nipride) will increase cardiac output despite a fall in left ventricular filling pressure.[1, 17] Following pressure reduction with nitroprusside, further increase in cardiac output in infants can be achieved by infusion of blood to elevate left ventricular filling pressure to levels present before infusion of the vasodilator.[1] If cardiac output remains low after these maneuvers, and cardiac tamponade is not present, use of isoproterenol or epinephrine is indicated to improve myocardial contractility. A rapidly acting digitalis preparation (Digoxin) may also be used and can be administered intravenously or intramuscularly.

Ventilation is assisted early after operation with a positive-pressure ventilator and an endotracheal tube. In most patients, this can be discontinued within a few hours after operation. If the cardiac output is low or pulmonary dysfunction is present, ventilatory assistance via an endotracheal or nasotracheal tube is continued for 24 to 36 hours. Infants require particular care of the respiratory subsystem in the early postoperative period.

Urine flow is usually adequate after operation, particularly when some degree of hemodilution of the perfusate has been employed. In those unusual situations in which cardiac output is low and oliguria is present, use of a potent diuretic such as furosemide (Lasix) is indicated.

Excessive postoperative bleeding following surgical treatment of ventricular septal defect is quite unusual. When drainage from the chest tubes in the early postoperative period is excessive, reoperation is indicated. Generally, no specific bleeding point is found, but the evacuation of clotted blood is advantageous. With very small children and infants, reoperation would be indicated after smaller amounts of chest drainage.

RESULTS OF SURGICAL TREATMENT

Hospital Mortality

Hospital mortality rates and complications are directly related to the preoperative condition of the patient (Table 2) and to the conduct of the operative procedure. At the present time, the risk for repair of small or moderate-sized ventricular septal defects and of large ventricular septal defects with mild pulmonary vascular disease is approximately 1 per cent. Properly selected patients with moderate or severe pulmonary vascular disease can be operated upon with a risk of less than 10 per cent.

In the past, operative mortality has been high following complete repair of ventricular septal defects in infants. Recent experiences suggest that this risk is approximately 10 to 15 per cent.[2, 32] Operative mortality rates in older infants have been low for some years, being approximately 5 per cent in children between six months and two years of age.[14, 22]

TABLE 2.   Hospital Mortality after Repair of Ventricular Septal Defect in Patients More Than 6 Months of Age*

Category	Patients	Hospital Deaths	
		No.	%
P_p/P_s <0.45	108	0	0
P_p/P_s 0.45–0.75	40	0	0
P_p/P_s > 0.75			
R_p/R_s < 0.45	50	3	6
R_p/R_s 0.45–0.75	39	2	5
R_p/R_s > 0.75	6	1	17
P_p < 40 mm. Hg.	13	0	0
P_{rv}/P_{lv} > 0.75	—	–	–
Totals	256	6	2

*1962 through 1965. From Cartmill, T. B., DuShane, J. W., McGoon, D. C., and Kirklin, J. W.: J. Thorac. Cardiovasc. Surg., 52:486, 1966.

Heart Block

Although permanent heart block occurred in a large percentage of patients after repair of ventricular septal defect in the early years when the operation was performed, this complication is quite unusual at present. In one group of 256 patients in whom closure of ventricular septal defects was performed between 1962 and 1965, permanent heart block did not occur in a single instance.[4] If heart block should occur at the time of operation, temporary ventricular pacing wires should be placed and connected to an external pacing unit. Permanent epicardial pacing electrodes can also be implanted and, if heart block persists in the postoperative period, a permanent pacing unit can be connected to these electrodes.

Incomplete Repair

With standardization of the operative technique, and with the use of synthetic patch material to close moderate-sized or large ventricular septal defects, the incidence of persistent or recurrent shunts approximates 10 per cent or less.[4]

Resolution of Pulmonary Vascular Disease

The late results of the surgical treatment of ventricular septal defects in patients with abnormally elevated pulmonary vascular resistance are dependent not only upon the closure of the ventricular septal defect but also upon the behavior of the pulmonary vasculature.[4, 22]

Patients with mild elevation of pulmonary vascular resistance (pulmonary to systemic resistance ratios of less than 0.45) have for the most part shown a decline or no increase in the pulmonary vascular resistance after operation. About one third of the patients over 2 years of age at the time of operation with moderate pulmonary vascular disease (pulmonary to systemic resistance ratios between 0.45 and 0.75) have no change in pulmonary vascular resistance 2 to 5 years after operation. Unfortunately, about one third of patients with moderate elevation of pulmonary vascular resistance preoperatively have a progressive increase in pulmonary vascular resistance late in the postopera-

tive period. These patients and approximately two thirds of those patients with severe pulmonary vascular disease preoperatively (pulmonary to systemic resistance ratios of greater than 0.75) do not have a satisfactory long-term prognosis because of the severity of the pulmonary hypertension at rest and the pulmonary vascular disease. With exercise, such patients have a restriction of cardiac output because of the obstructive pulmonary vascular disease. If these patients could be identified with certainty preoperatively, it would be preferable to avoid operating on them.

Progression of pulmonary vascular disease is uncommon when the ventricular septal defect is repaired before the age of 2 years.[6] This is the major reason for advising closure of ventricular septal defects in infants less than 2 years of age when there is increasing pulmonary vascular resistance.

Overall Results

The overall results of the surgical treatment of patients with ventricular septal defects in the various categories outlined previously are indicated in Figure 11. The results are excellent in most patients with small or moderate-sized ventricular septal defects and in patients with ventricular septal defects and pulmonary stenosis. Satisfactory results have also been obtained in patients with ventricular septal defects and aortic valve incompetence in whom the aortic valve is repaired or replaced.[26, 30] Nearly all patients with large ventricular septal defects and mild elevation of pulmonary vascular resistance have an excellent prognosis. Patients with large ventricular septal defects and moderate elevation of pulmonary vascular resistance may have an excellent long-term prognosis, but more severe pulmonary vascular disease develops in about one third of those over 2 years of age at the time

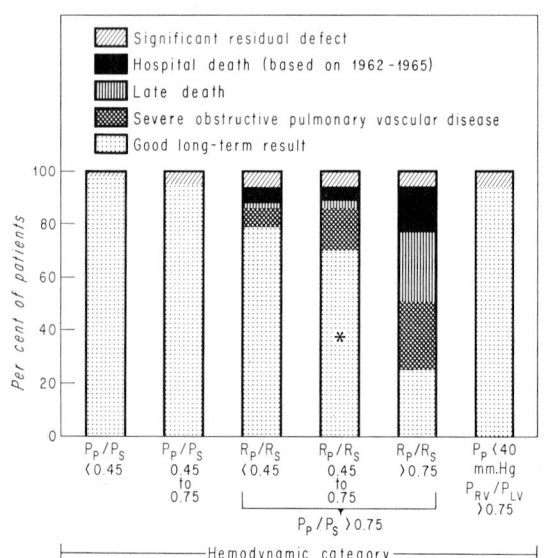

Figure 11.   Composite results of repair of ventricular septal defect in patients more than 6 months of age. (From Cartmill, T. B., DuShane, J. W., McGoon, D. C., and Kirklin, J. W.: J. Thorac. Cardiovasc. Surg., 52:486, 1966.)

of operation. Those patients who preoperatively have severe elevation of pulmonary vascular resistance have a high incidence of unsatisfactory results.

The results appear to be particularly favorable when the ventricular septal defect is repaired during the first 2 years of life.[6]

SELECTED REFERENCES

Becu, L. M., Fontana, R. S., DuShane, J. W., Kirklin, J. W. Burchell, H. B., and Edwards, J. E.: Anatomic and pathologic studies in ventricular septal defect. Circulation, *14*:349, 1956.

This paper analyzes in detail the anatomic features of ventricular septal defects in 50 hearts examined at autopsy. The precise anatomic relationships of the various types of septal defects to adjacent structures are outlined, and the defects are divided into two major groups according to their location, either in the inflow or the outflow portion of the right ventricle. In addition, the coexisting congenital anomalies of the cardiovascular system are tabulated. Although a subsequent classification (see text) has proved more useful from the surgical standpoint, the relationships of the various types of septal defects to the surrounding structures described in this paper are important to surgeons in particular.

Cartmill, T. B., DuShane, J. W., McGoon, D. C., and Kirklin, J. W.: Results of repair of ventricular septal defect. J. Thorac. Cardiovas. Surg., *52*:486, 1966.

This is a review of 447 patients having complete repair of ventricular septal defect during a 5-year period (1960 to 1965) at one institution. The patients are categorized according to the severity of the preoperative pulmonary hypertension and the pulmonary vascular resistance as compared to the systemic vascular resistance. In addition, particular emphasis is placed on the changes in pulmonary vascular resistance that occur as a result of surgical closure of the defects. The studies indicate that in some patients with only mild increase in pulmonary vascular resistance preoperatively, severe obstructive pulmonary vascular disease developed after operation. In 20 per cent of the patients with moderate elevations in pulmonary to systemic resistance, increased pulmonary vascular disease developed after operation. With these findings as the basis, specific indications for operative intervention in patients with ventricular septal defects are outlined.

DuShane, J. W., and Kirklin, J. W.: Late results of the repair of ventricular septal defect on pulmonary vascular disease. *In* Kirklin, J. W., (Ed.): Advances in Cardiovascular Surgery. New York, Grune and Stratton, 1973, p. 9.

This paper analyzes the long-term course of 68 patients with large ventricular septal defects and severe pulmonary hypertension evaluated five or more years after operation with repeat cardiac catheterization, emphasizing the effects of operation on the pulmonary vasculature. Over 90 per cent of patients less than two years of age had normal or only mildly elevated pulmonary vascular resistance late postoperatively, even when pulmonary resistance was severely elevated preoperatively. Over 50 per cent of the older patients with moderate or severely elevated pulmonary resistance preoperatively had moderate or severely elevated resistance late postoperatively and potentially unsatisfactory long-term results. On the basis of these findings, the authors advise closure of large ventricular septal defects before the age of two years.

Hoffman, J. I. E., and Rudolph, A. M.: The natural history of isolated ventricular septal defect with special reference to selection of patients for surgery. Advances Pediatr., *17*:57, 1970.

This excellent article contains an enormous amount of information regarding the natural history of patients with isolated ventricular septal defect. It deals extensively with the problems related to the severity of the disease, the frequency and the time course of spontaneous closure of ventricular septal defects, the incidence and importance of pulmonary vascular disease, and the changes in pulmonary vascular resistance that occur after surgical closure. In addition, a program is outlined for the management of patients with ventricular septal defect, particularly infants, and the indications for operative intervention are given.

Levin, A. R., Spach, M. S., Canent, R. V., Jr., Boineau, J. P., Capp, M. P., Jain, V., and Barr, R. C.: Intracardiac pressure-flow dynamics in isolated ventricular septal defects. Circulation, *35*:430, 1967.

This study characterizes the nature of intracardiac shunting in 50 children between the ages of 3 and 15 years with isolated ven-

tricular septal defects. Intraventricular pressure measurements and biplane cineangiocardiography were utilized to study the timing and the direction of flow across the defects during the cardiac cycle. Patients with moderately elevated right ventricular pressures demonstrated left-to-right shunting across the defect throughout the cardiac cycle. When pressure in the right ventricle approximated that in the left, left-to-right shunting occurred across the defect into the left ventricle during isovolumic relaxation. All patients showed a predominant left-to-right pressure gradient and shunt across the defect into the right ventricle during diastole and increase of the left-to-right pressure gradient with resultant increase of the shunt into the right ventricle during isovolumic contraction immediately before the aortic valve opened. During ventricular ejection and isovolumic relaxation, the pressure-flow relationships are affected significantly by the size of the defect and the ratio of the pulmonary to systemic vascular resistance.

Wagenvoort, C. A., Neufeld, H. N., DuShane, J. W., and Edwards, J. E.: The pulmonary arterial tree in ventricular septal defect. A quantitative study of anatomic features in fetuses, infants and children. Circulation, *23*:740, 1961.

This paper is an anatomic study of the pulmonary arterial tree of 50 fetuses, infants, and children with uncomplicated ventricular septal defect. A detailed analysis of the pulmonary arterial medial thickness and the index of medial surface area (the ratio of medial tissue to pulmonary parenchyma) was carried out. During the fetal and newborn period, both the thickness and the index of surface area of the media were generally within normal limits. The subjects between 1 and 5 weeks of age had a medial thickness and an index of medial surface area that were lower than the average values at the time of birth. In this regard, the pulmonary arterial tree in cases of ventricular septal defect was similar to that from normal newborn infants. Soon after this period, however, and particularly from 8 weeks of age on, the subjects with ventricular septal defects showed a pronounced rise both in the medial thickness and in the index of medial surface area, indicating the presence of considerable medial hypertrophy. These findings correlate closely with the development of pulmonary hypertension and with the clinical findings in patients with ventricular septal defects.

REFERENCES

1. Appelbaum, A., Blackstone, E. H., Kouchoukos, N. T., and Kirklin, J. W.: Afterload reduction and cardiac output in infants early after intracardiac surgery. Am. J. Cardiol., in press.

2. Barratt-Boyes, B. G.: Complete correction of cardiovascular malformations in the first two years of life using profound hypothermia. *In* Barratt-Boyes, B. G., Neutze, J. M., and Harris, E. A. (Eds.): Heart Disease in Infancy: Diagnosis and Surgical Treatment. Proceedings of the Second International Symposium on Surgical Heart Disease. London, Churchill Livingstone, 1973, p. 25.

3. Becu, L. M., Fontana, R. S., DuShane, J. W., Kirklin, J. W., Burchell, H. B., and Edwards, J. E.: Anatomic and pathologic studies in ventricular septal defect. Circulation, *14*:349, 1956.

4. Cartmill, T. B., DuShane, J. W., McGoon, D. C., and Kirklin, J. W.: Results of repair of ventricular septal defect. J. Thorac. Cardiovasc. Surg., *52*:486, 1966.

5. Dobell, A. R. C., Murphy, D. A., Poirier, N. L., and Gibbons, J. E.: The pulmonary artery after debanding. J. Thorac. Cardiovasc. Surg., *65*:32, 1973.

6. DuShane, J. W., and Kirklin, J. W.: Late results of the repair of ventricular septal defect on pulmonary vascular disease. *In* Kirklin, J. W. (Ed.): Advances in Cardiovascular Surgery. New York, Grune and Stratton, 1973, p. 9.

7. Heath, D., and Edwards, J. E.: The pathology of hypertensive pulmonary vascular disease. A description of six grades of structural changes in the pulmonary arteries with special reference to congenital cardiac septal defects. Circulation, *18*:533, 1958.

8. Heath, D., Helmholz, H. F., Jr., Burchell, H. B., DuShane, J. W., and Edwards, J. E.: Graded pulmonary vascular changes and hemodynamic findings in cases of atrial and ventricular septal defect and patent ductus arteriosus. Circulation, *18*:1155, 1958.

9. Hoffman, J. I. E.: Natural history of congenital heart disease: Problems in its assessment with special reference to ventricular septal defect. Circulation, *37*:97, 1968.

10. Hoffman, J. I. E., and Rudolph, A. M.: The natural history of isolated ventricular septal defect with special reference to

selection of patients for surgery. Advances Pediatr., *17*:57, 1970.

11. Hunt, C. E., Formanek, G., Levine, M. A., Castenada, A., and Moller, J. A.: Banding of the pulmonary artery. Results in 111 children. Circulation, *43*:395, 1971.

12. Jarmakani, M. M., Edwards, S. B., Spach, M. S., Canent, R. V., Jr., Capp, M. P., Hagan, M. J., Barr, R. C., and Jain, V.: Left ventricular pressure-volume characteristics in congenital heart disease. Circulation, *37*:879, 1968.

13. Keck, E. W. O., Ongley, P. A., Kincaid, O. W., and Swan, H. J. C.: Ventricular septal defect with aortic insufficiency. A clinical and hemodynamic study of 18 proved cases. Circulation, *27*:203, 1963.

14. Kirklin, J. W., and DuShane, J. W.: Repair of ventricular septal defect in infancy. Pediatrics, *27*:961, 1961.

15. Kirklin, J. W., DuShane, J. W., Patrick, R. T., Donald, D. E., Hetzel, P. S., Harshbarger, H. G., and Wood, E. H.: Intracardiac surgery with the aid of a mechanical pump-oxygenator system (Gibbon type): Report of eight cases. Mayo Clin. Proc., *30*:201, 1955.

16. Kirklin, J. W., Harshbarger, H. G., Donald, D. E., and Edwards, J. E.: Surgical correction of ventricular septal defect: Anatomic and technical considerations. J. Thorac. Surg., *33*:45, 1957.

17. Kouchoukos, N. T., Sheppard, L. C., and Kirklin, J. W.: Effect of alterations in arterial pressure on cardiac performance early after open intracardiac operation. J. Thorac. Cardiovasc. Surg., *64*:563, 1972.

18. Leatham, A., and Segal, B.: Auscultatory and phonocardiographic signs of ventricular septal defect with left to right shunt. Circulation, *25*:318, 1962.

19. Levin, A. R., Spach, M. S., Canent, R. V., Jr., Boineau, J. P., Capp, M. P., Jain, V., and Barr, R. C.: Intracardiac pressure-flow dynamics in isolated ventricular septal defects. Circulation, *35*:430, 1967.

20. Lillehei, C. W., Cohen, M., Warden, H. E., Ziegler, N., and Varco, R. L.: The results of direct vision closure of ventricular septal defects in eight patients by means of controlled cross circulation. Surg. Gynecol. Obstet., *101*:446, 1955.

21. Lillehei, C. W., DeWall, R. A., Read, R. C., Warden, H. E., and Varco, R. L.: Direct vision intracardiac surgery in man using a simple disposable artificial oxygenator. Dis. Chest, *29*:1, 1956.

22. Lillehei, C. W., Levy, M. J., Adams, P., and Anderson, R. C.: High-pressure ventricular septal defects. J.A.M.A., *188*:949, 1964.

23. Morgan, B. C., Griffiths, S. P., and Blumenthal, S.: Ventricular septal defect. I. Congestive heart failure in infancy. Pediatrics, *25*:54, 1960.

24. Muller, W. H., Jr., and Dammann, J. F. Jr.: The treatment of certain congenital malformations of the heart by the creation of pulmonic stenosis to reduce pulmonary hypertension and excessive pulmonary flow. A preliminary report. Surg. Gynecol. Obstet., *95*:213, 1952.

25. Nadas, A. S., Thilenius, O. G., La Farge, C. G., and Hauck, A. J.: Ventricular septal defect with aortic regurgitation. Medical and pathologic aspects. Circulation, *29*:862, 1964.

26. Sanfelippo, P. M., DuShane, J. W., McGoon, D. C., and Danielson, G. K.: Ventricular septal defect and aortic insufficiency: Surgical considerations and results of operation. Ann. Thorac. Surg., *17*:213, 1974.

27. Shah, P., Singh, W. S. A., Rose, V., and Keith, J.: Incidence of bacterial endocarditis in ventricular septal defects. Circulation, *34*:127, 1966.

28. Sigmann, J. M., Stern, A. M., and Sloan, H. E.: Early surgical correction of large ventricular septal defects. Pediatrics, *39*:1, 1967.

29. Somerville, J., Brandao, A., and Ross, D. N.: Aortic regurgitation with ventricular septal defect. Surgical management and clinical features. Circulation, *41*:317, 1970.

30. Spencer, F. C., Doyle, E. F., Danilowicz, D. A., Bahnson, H. T., and Weldon, C. S.: Long-term evaluation of aortic valvuloplasty for aortic insufficiency and ventricular septal defect. J. Thorac. Cardiovasc. Surg., *65*:15, 1973.

31. Stark, J., Aberdeen, E., Waterston, D. J., Bonham-Carter, R. E., and Tynan, M.: Pulmonary artery constriction (banding): A report of 146 cases. Surgery, *65*:808, 1969.

32. Subramanian, S.: Primary definitive intracardiac operations in infants: Ventricular septal defects. *In* Kirklin, J. W. (Ed.): Advances in Cardiovascular Surgery. New York, Grune and Stratton, 1973, p. 141.

33. Van Praagh, R., McNamara, J. J., and Gross, R. E.: Anatomic types of ventricular septal defect with aortic insufficiency. Circulation (Suppl. 2) *36*:256, 1967.

34. Wagenvoort, C. A., Neufeld, H. N., DuShane, J. W., and Edwards, J. E.: The pulmonary arterial tree in ventricular septal defect. A quantitative study of anatomic features in fetuses, infants and children. Circulation, *23*:740, 1961.

VII

THE TETRALOGY OF FALLOT

David C. Sabiston, Jr., M.D.

The tetralogy of Fallot is one of the most frequent of the serious congenital cardiac malformations commonly accompanied by cyanosis. Of further significance is the fact that it was among the first of the congenital heart lesions to yield to a highly successful palliative operation. A landmark in cardiac surgery was established in 1944 by Blalock and Taussig when the first successful systemic-pulmonary artery anastomosis was performed. Since then a corrective procedure employing extracorporeal circulation has been developed, and the surgical treatment of tetralogy of Fallot is now one of the most satisfactory in cardiac surgery.

HISTORICAL ASPECTS

There are a number of early descriptions of the tetralogy of Fallot, including those of Stensen (1672),[55] Sandifort (1777),[52] John Hunter (1783),[33] William Hunter (1784),[34] Farre (1814),[21] Gintrac (1824),[25] Hope (1839),[32] and Peacock (1866).[45] However, the most notable contribution was that of Étienne-Louis Arthur Fallot of Marseille, who in 1888 clearly described the clinical and pathological aspects. In these communications, Fallot referred to previously reported cases but emphasized the clinical manifestations of the malformation *during life*. His original communications appeared under the title "Contribution à l'anatomie pathologique de la maladie bleue (cyanose cardiaque)."[20] In translation, the following is Fallot's own description of the now famous *tetralogy*:

"This malformation consists of a true anatomopathological type represented by the following tetralogy: (1) stenosis of the pulmonary artery; (2) interventricular communication; (3) deviation of the origin of the aorta to the right; (4) hypertrophy, almost always concentric, of the right ventricle. Failure of obliteration of the foramen ovale may occasionally be added in a wholly accessory manner."

In his descriptions, Fallot reported 55 cases of congenital heart disease of which most were of the tetralogy type. It is remarkable that such a large number of cases could have been reported by a single author at that time.

In 1944, Blalock operated upon a severely ill infant with tetralogy of Fallot and established a subclavian-pulmonary anastomosis.[6] The child greatly benefited from the procedure, and this operation heralded the onset of a wide variety of additional cardiac procedures that were to follow. The first open correction of the tetralogy of Fallot was performed by Scott (1954), employing arrested circulation with hypothermia;[53] following the advent of extracorporeal circulation, the scope of intercardiac surgery advanced greatly. Open correction using cardiopulmonary bypass was first performed by Lillehei in 1955.[38] Although the mortality was originally quite high, it has progressively diminished.

ANATOMY

In the original description, Fallot emphasized *four* primary anatomic points, including pulmonary stenosis, ventricular septal defect, dextroposition of the aorta, hypertrophy of the right ventricle. However, it is now recognized by most that the two most *important* features of the tetralogy of Fallot are (1) the right ventricular outflow tract obstruction, which is nearly always infundibular in location, but valvar stenosis may also be present in some 20 per cent of patients, and (2) the ventricular septal defect. The overriding of the aorta is related to the location of the ventricular septal defect, and the right ventricular hypertrophy is a secondary phenomenon due to the outflow tract obstruction of the right ventricle. Emphasis should be placed upon the fact that there is a wide variation in the spectrum of the severity of the anatomic malformations in the tetralogy of Fallot.[35] The wide differences in the severity of these components have led some to urge discontinuance of the term "tetralogy of Fallot." However, from the view of both diagnosis and surgical management, the term continues to have sufficient usefulness to justify its retention. In general, a working definition of the tetralogy includes the basic principle that it is a congenital cardiac malformation with a ventricular septal defect, the size of which approximates the aortic orifice, and with pulmonary stenosis of such a degree that approximately equal pressures result in both ventricles. In addition, there are varying degrees of dextroposition (or overriding) of the aorta. Moreover, the degree and nature of the infundibular pulmonary stenosis may be quite variable. Several types of infundibular chambers have been described, depending mostly upon the size of the chamber.[9, 10] Thus, the infundibular chamber may be quite small when the outflow tract obstruction is near the pulmonary valve. At the opposite extreme, the muscular obstruction in the outflow tract may be quite proximally situated, resulting in a large infundibular chamber sometimes called a "third ventricle." Moreover, *stenosis* of the pulmonary valve is common, occurring in as many as one third of patients with tetralogy of Fallot in addition to infundibular stenosis. Occasionally, the stenosis is confined solely to the pulmonary valve without the presence of infundibular obstruction.

It becomes apparent that from the physiologic point of view the majority of patients with tetralogy of Fallot exhibit a high resistance to right ventricular emptying owing to pulmonary stenosis. Therefore, the predominant shunt is from right-to-left, with flow across the ventricular defect into the aorta. This produces cyanosis and results in elevation of the hematocrit. In those instances in which the pulmonary stenosis is less severe, bidirectional shunting may occur. In some patients, the infundibular stenosis is minimal, and the predominant shunt is left-to-right, producing what is termed clinically "the pink tetralogy." Although such patients may not appear cyanotic, they may have slight oxygen desaturation in the systemic arterial blood.

Occasionally, no communication exists between the right ventricle and the pulmonary artery. In these patients, the outflow tract of the right ventricle or the pulmonary valve is *atretic.* The pulmonary valve ring and main pulmonary artery are often quite small, although the left and right branches may be of significant size. Such infants exhibit severe symptoms and usually require operation early in life. It has also been recognized that some patients with a previous systemic-pulmonary anastomosis may experience a progression of the outflow tract obstruction in the right ventricle. Thus, the infundibular stenosis or valvar stenosis may become more severe and can become total, representing an *acquired* lesion. Under these circumstances, life is maintained solely by a previous systemic-pulmonary shunt with additional help from collateral bronchial arterial circulation.[51]

DIAGNOSIS

Clinical Manifestations

Experience has shown that the clinical manifestations of the tetralogy of Fallot vary with the severity of the anatomic malformation. Infants with pulmonary atresia manifest distress shortly after birth and usually succumb unless operation is performed. Cyanosis is common, especially with crying. In most children, cyanosis is *not* present *at birth,* probably because of a persistent ductus arteriosus. As the child grows older, dyspnea on exertion usually follows, and a characteristic position *(squatting)* is assumed by the great majority of these patients to relieve fatigue. This position has diagnostic significance and is highly characteristic of the tetralogy of Fallot. It usually produces an increase in systemic arterial oxygen saturation.

Some patients with pulmonary atresia may present desperate problems in infancy. At the opposite end of the spectrum, rare instances of longevity with a reasonably normal life have been reported. One interesting example is that of an American composer, Gilbert, who lived to the age of 60 with tetralogy of Fallot and who led a relatively productive life without surgery.[59] Such a history is obviously rare. Statistics show that the natural history for the entire group of patients with tetralogy of Fallot indicates that half reach the age of 7, one fifth reach age 14, and not more than one tenth survive to age 21 in the absence of operative intervention.[11]

Physical Examination

Cyanosis of the lips and nail beds is usually apparent, and the patient may appear to be smaller than expected for his age. The fingers and toes usually show clubbing (hypertrophic pulmonary osteoarthropathy). On palpation of the chest, a thrill is usually present anteriorly. A harsh systolic murmur is audible over the pulmonary area and along the left sternal border. Absence of a murmur in a patient suspected of having the tetralogy is suggestive of pulmonary atresia.

Roentgenograms

The chest film in the tetralogy of Fallot usually shows diminished vascularity in the lungs and absence of prominence of the pulmonary artery. In the early stages, the chest film may be normal. The shadow of the great vessels in the superior mediastinum is narrow, owing to the diminished caliber of the pulmonary artery. If cyanosis and dyspnea are quite prominent, the pulmonary vascular markings are usually markedly diminished. Later, the classic boot-shaped heart (*coeur en sabot*) may develop and is recognized as a hallmark of the tetralogy of Fallot (Fig. 1). Diminution or absence of pulsations in the pulmonary arteries can be demonstrated by fluoroscopy. Right ventricular enlargement is present and is best demonstrated in the left anterior oblique position. The barium swallow provides evidence of the side on which the aortic arch descends. This is of considerable importance, since approximately one fourth of the patients with tetralogy of Fallot have a *right* aortic arch. In fact, the presence of a right aortic arch with cyanosis is strong evidence that the malformation is indeed tetralogy of Fallot.

Blood Studies

An elevation in the hemoglobin, hematocrit, and erythrocyte count is usually present. The magnitude of hemoconcentration is generally proportional to the cyanosis. Hematocrit values may vary from normal to as high as 90 per cent, the majority being between 50 and 70 per cent. The erythrocyte count varies between normal and a high of 12,000,000. Similarly, the oxygen saturation in the systemic arterial blood is variable, usually between 65 and 70 per cent. However, in severe forms of the malformation, the arterial oxygen

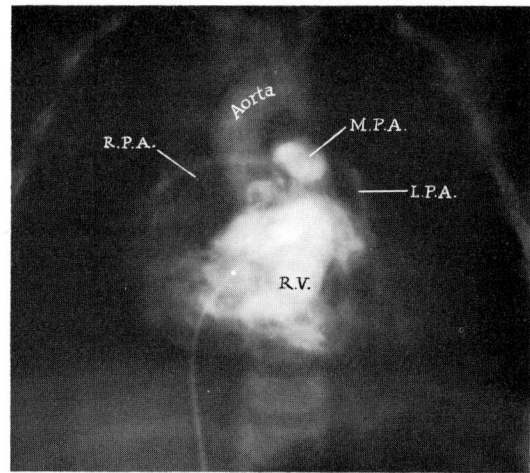

Figure 2. Angiocardiogram of infant with tetralogy of Fallot in whom pulmonary arteries are very small. An ascending aorta–right pulmonary artery anastomosis (Waterston) was performed because of serious symptoms. The infant greatly benefited from the procedure. (From Sabiston, D. C., Jr. *In* Sabiston, D. C., Jr., and Spencer, F. C. (Eds.): Gibbon's Surgery of the Chest, 3rd ed. Philadelphia, W. B. Saunders Company, 1976.)

saturation during exercise may fall as low as 25 per cent. It has been recognized that a bleeding tendency is present in many patients with the tetralogy of Fallot, especially those in whom cyanosis is intense. In the various studies that have been performed on these patients, the usual finding is a diminution in a variety of the factors responsible for blood coagulation, but none of the factors are reduced to critical levels. The platelet count and total blood fibrinogen are frequently slightly diminished, and clot retraction is sometimes poor and associated with prolonged prothrombin and coagulation times. Despite the defects in the clotting mechanism in some patients, the changes are usually insufficient to explain the hemorrhagic tendency noted at the time of operation.[30, 46]

Electrocardiogram

The electrocardiogram usually shows right ventricular hypertrophy. This is usually apparent in the standard leads and is most consistently found in the unipolar leads. The more commonly encountered findings include tall and peaked T waves, reversal of the RS ratio, and a normal PR interval and QRS duration. It is to be emphasized that if right ventricular hypertrophy is absent, the diagnosis of tetralogy of Fallot should be seriously doubted.

Angiocardiograms

The angiocardiogram is of great importance in establishing the diagnosis. Moreover, it demonstrates objectively the magnitude of pulmonary stenosis and the size of the pulmonary arteries (Fig. 2). The ventricular septal defect and overriding of the aorta are also shown (Fig. 3). An atrial septal defect may also be present. Occasionally, only one pulmonary artery is present, and in nearly all patients with a single artery, it is the left one that is absent.

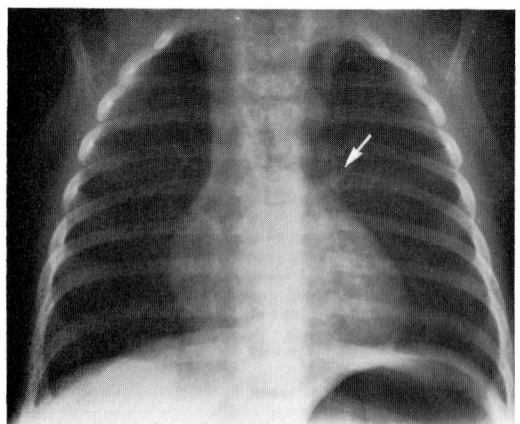

Figure 1. Chest film of infant with tetralogy of Fallot. Note diminished vascular markings in the lungs and reduced prominence of the pulmonary artery shadow. (From Sabiston, D. C., Jr. *In* Sabiston, D. C., Jr., and Spencer, F. C. (Eds.): Gibbon's Surgery of the Chest, 3rd ed. Philadelphia, W. B. Saunders Company, 1976.)

from isolated valvar pulmonary stenosis, in which the pressure in the right ventricle may be considerably greater than that in the left ventricle. Tracings also establish the level of right ventricular outflow tract obstruction and the presence of valvar stenosis.

INDICATIONS FOR OPERATION

Nearly all patients with tetralogy of Fallot should be considered candidates for surgical correction. When feasible, it is preferable to perform a corrective procedure before school age, generally at 3 to 5 years.[15] However, severe symptoms may become manifest much earlier, including the first several days of life, and an operative procedure must be performed as a life-saving measure. Most surgeons prefer to perform corrective procedures using extracorporeal circulation and hypothermia at any age.[44, 54] Others, however, prefer a systemic to pulmonary anastomosis, generally the Blalock-Taussig type, as a preliminary procedure.[12, 43, 60] Those who prefer open correction at any time emphasize that it prevents the necessity for a

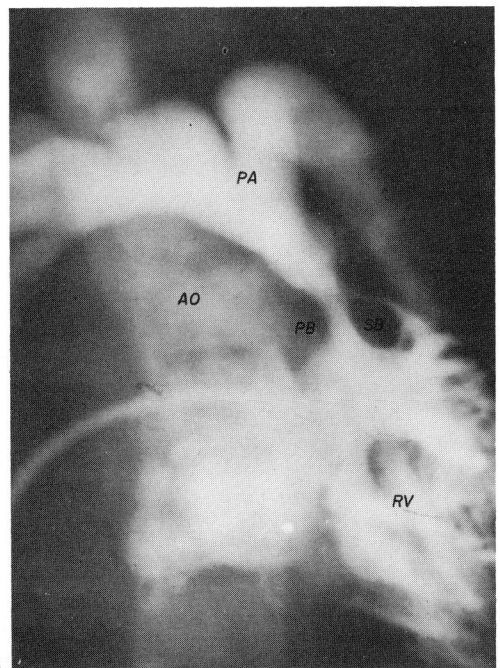

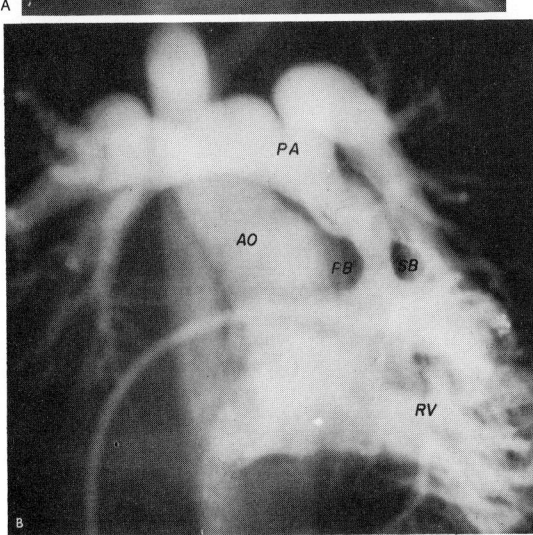

Figure 3. Obstruction in the region of the infundibulum. *A*, Frame made in systole. *B*, Frame made in diastole. The negative shadows of the hypertrophied parietal (PB) and septal (SB) bands are particularly well demonstrated. The pulmonary valve appears domed, and at operation was bicuspid, but not stenotic. The aorta (AO) is opacified by this right ventricular injection and its diameter is three times that of the pulmonary artery. The underdevelopment of the infundibulum of the right ventricle, a basic characteristic of the tetralogy of Fallot, is apparent in this angiocardiogram. RV = right ventricle; PA = pulmonary artery. (From Kirklin, J. W., and Karp, R. B.: The Tetralogy of Fallot from a Surgical Viewpoint. Philadelphia, W. B. Saunders Company, 1970.)

Cardiac Catheterization

Much valuable information is provided by cardiac catheterization (Fig. 4). The presence of equal pressures in both ventricles distinguishes the condition

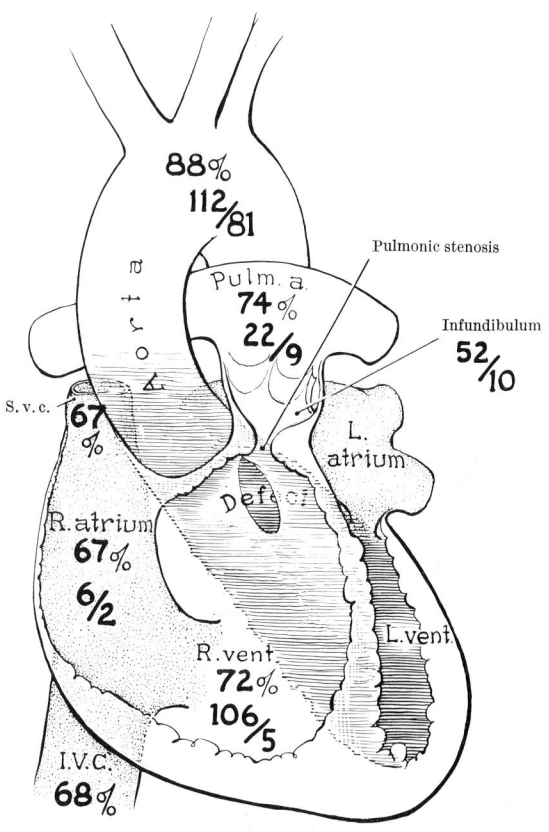

Figure 4. Diagram of results obtained at cardiac catheterization in patient with tetralogy of Fallot. This patient has a relatively high arterial oxygen saturation and represents one of the less severe anatomic types. Values for oxygen are expressed as percentage saturation. The pressures are given in millimeters of mercury. (From Sabiston, D. C., Jr., and Blalock, A. *In* Derra, E. (Ed.): Encyclopedia of Thoracic Surgery. Heidelberg, Springer-Verlag, 1959.)

second operation and that the current results are sufficiently good to support this judgment. Those who prefer an initial shunt in infancy emphasize that the overall mortality is lower than if the mortality of the later corrective operation is included. In addition, these observers are concerned about whether or not the small heart in infancy will remain corrected as growth continues, feeling perhaps that outflow tract obstruction of the right ventricle may occur. Although controversy continues concerning the preferential operation in *infancy,* as is well documented in the literature, nevertheless the majority tend to prefer open correction as the procedure of choice in most instances.[4]

SURGICAL TECHNIQUES

The most versatile of the *shunt* operations is a systemic-pulmonary anastomosis.[5, 6] Formerly performed frequently, today this procedure has its maximal usefulness in the severely ill infant in whom operation must be performed at any early age. It is becoming unusual to employ this procedure after the age of one year. The result of the procedure is to produce an increase in blood flow to the lungs. In earlier years, an alternate technique was sometimes employed, anastomosis between the left pulmonary artery and the descending aorta (Potts operation).[48] This procedure is rarely used today, since the anastomosis usually enlarges with the passage of time and produces an excessive shunt, with pulmonary hypertension and often aneurysmal formation at the site of the anastomosis.[49, 56] Moreover, a Potts anastomosis is more difficult to close at the time of subsequent correction. Another alternate technique is that of an ascending aorta to right pulmonary anastomosis (Waterston),[58] but this procedure has become less popular owing in large part to the fact that kinking and stenosis may ensue at the anastomotic site and make difficult subsequent open correction.[24]

For a *subclavian-pulmonary anastomosis (Blalock-Taussig),* the incision is generally made on the side opposite that on which the aorta descends (Fig. 5). In the majority of patients, the incision is made on the right side, since the aorta most often descends on the left. When the aorta descends on the right (20 to 25 per cent), the incision is made on the left. Ideally the subclavian branch of the innominate artery is used for the anastomosis because the angle produced at its origin from its parent vessel is better than that formed when the subclavian artery is used, as shown in Figure 6.[50] The latter arises directly from the aorta and is apt to kink at its origin when deflected inferiorly for anastomosis to the pulmonary

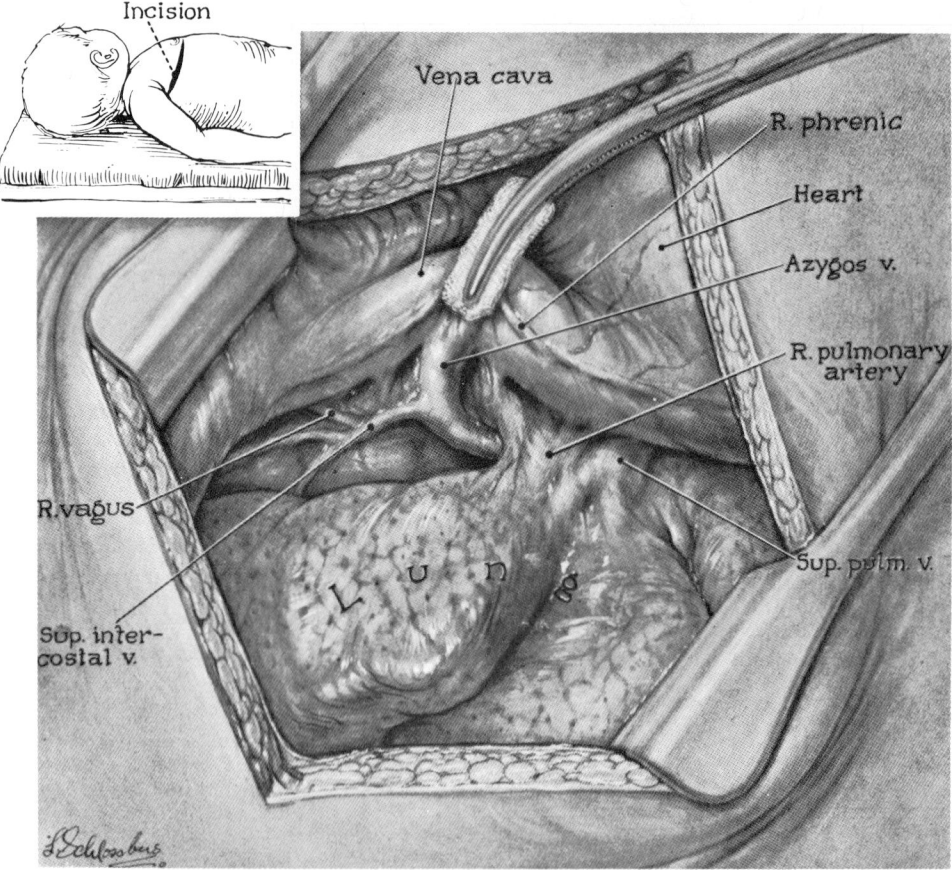

Figure 5. Initial dissection and exposure of the pulmonary artery for construction of a right subclavian–pulmonary artery anastomosis. The inset at the top shows the position of the patient on the operating table. The entry into the pleural cavity is through the second intercostal space. (From Blalock, A.: Surg. Gynecol. Obstet., *87:*385, 1948.)

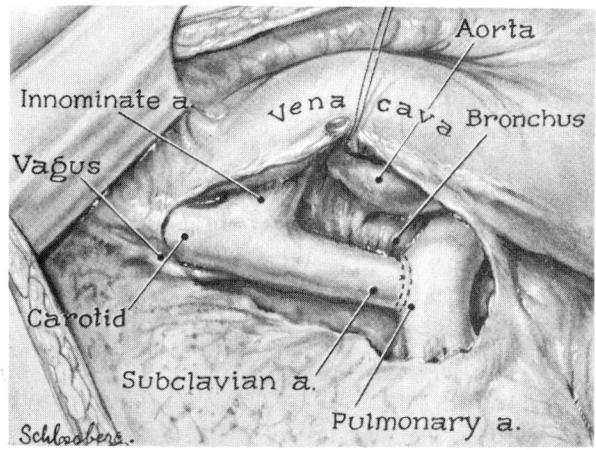

Figure 6. Completed anastomosis. Note that the subclavian artery at its origin from the innominate artery is circular. When the anastomosis is performed between the subclavian branch of the aorta and the pulmonary artery, there is usually a kink (oval shape) of the left subclavian artery at its origin; this diminishes the blood flow through the anastomosis. (From Blalock, A.: Surg. Gynecol. Obstet., 87:385, 1948.)

artery. Experimental studies have shown that approximately three fourths of the blood passing through a subclavian-pulmonary shunt is directed to the lung on the side of the anastomosis.[23]

Much attention must be paid to detail in performing the Blalock shunt, especially in the construction of the anastomosis itself. Every effort must be made to prevent constriction of the anastomosis; meticulous technique is essential (Fig. 7). Whereas the posterior row of sutures may be continuous, it is important to construct the anterior row with interrupted sutures. Use of the subclavian branch of the innominate is more difficult in patients over the age of 12, and generally the subclavian branch of the aorta is preferable.

Vascular anomalies are encountered frequently with the tetralogy of Fallot. For example, a right aortic arch is quite common, and a single pulmonary artery is occasionally seen. A retroesophageal subclavian artery occurs in approximately 5 per cent of patients and may involve either the right or left vessel. A persistent left superior vena cava occurs with about the same incidence.[42] It is quite *rare* for the retroesophageal subclavian vessels to cause dysphagia. In fact, it is usually not necessary to alter the retroesophageal relationship of the vessel in order to perform a proper anastomosis. Peripheral pulmonary arterial stenosis of the main artery or of branches has also been described.[27] In a number of patients in whom return of symptoms indicates inadequate blood flow because

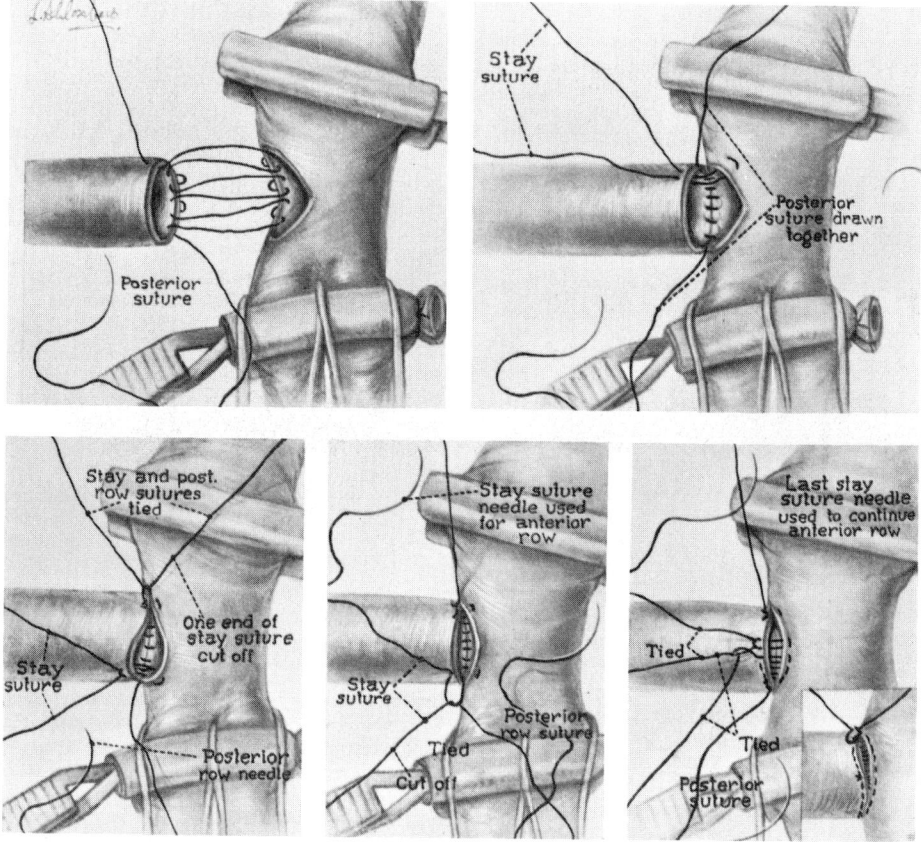

Figure 7. Technique of anastomosis of the end of the subclavian artery to the side of the pulmonary artery. The suture is an everting and continuous one for the posterior row; 5-0 or 6-0 silk is used. The anterior row is constructed by interrupted mattress sutures. The space separating each "bite" in the vessel is approximately 1 mm. (From Blalock, A.: Surg. Gynecol. Obstet., 87:385, 1948.)

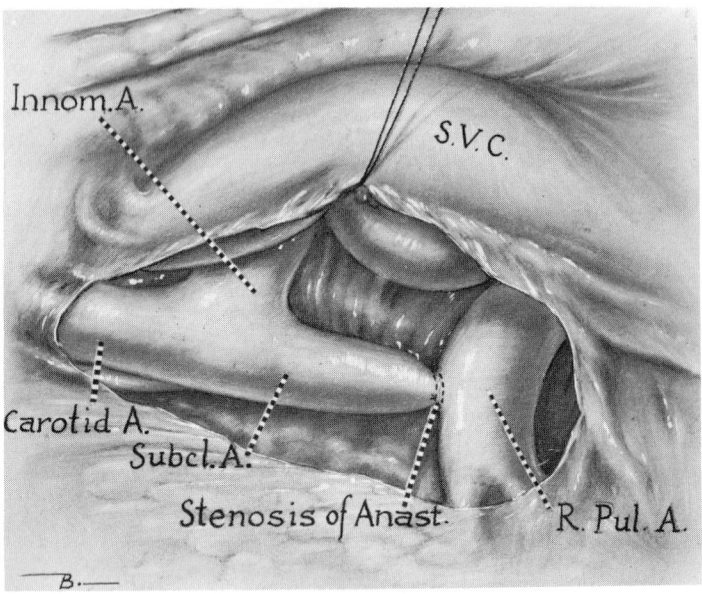

Figure 8. Illustration of late stenosis of subclavian-pulmonary artery anastomosis. This is the usual site at which the constriction occurs, and diminished systemic-pulmonary blood flow results. This situation is frequently encountered at the time of open correction when the subclavian-pulmonary anastomosis is dissected in preparation for ligation of the subclavian artery. (From Sabiston, D. C., Jr. *In* Sabiston, D. C., Jr., and Spencer, F. C. (Eds.): Gibbon's Surgery of the Chest, 3rd ed. Philadelphia, W. B. Saunders Company, 1976.)

of stenosis of the anastomosis (Fig. 8) or because of occlusion, a second subclavian-pulmonary anastomosis may be performed with benefit.[28] However, in most instances open correction is indicated if a second operation is performed.

The *ascending aorta–pulmonary anastomosis* was originally described by Waterston and has since been emphasized by several others.[14, 16] The procedure is performed through a right anterior thoracotomy entering the pleural cavity through the third intercostal space, with exposure of the as-

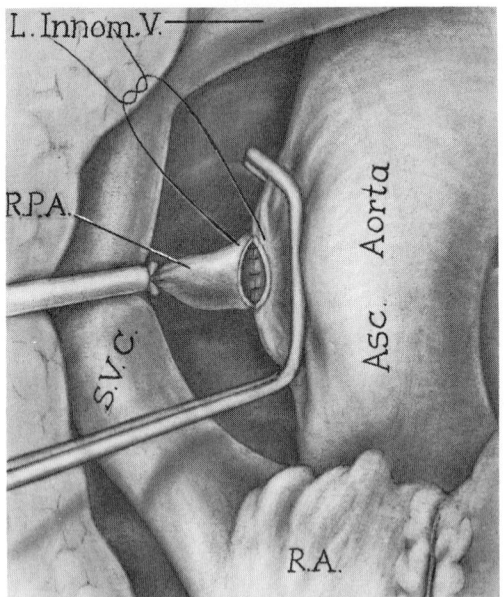

Figure 9. Ascending aorta to right pulmonary artery anastomosis (Waterston). The anastomosis has a diameter of 4 to 5 mm., and care is taken to prevent its being larger. The clamp only partially occludes the aorta, whereas it totally occludes the right pulmonary artery. Particular attention should be paid to rotating the aorta so that the communication constructed between the aorta and the right pulmonary artery is *posterior;* otherwise, kinking of the anastomosis will occur. (From Sabiston, D. C., Jr. *In* Sabiston, D. C., Jr., and Spencer, F. C. (Eds.): Gibbon's Surgery of the Chest, 3rd ed. Philadelphia, W. B. Saunders Company, 1976.)

cending aorta. The right pulmonary artery is then dissected, and a vascular clamp is placed so that one blade is beneath the pulmonary artery and the other anterior to the ascending aorta. Thus, it is possible to occlude both the right pulmonary artery and a portion of the ascending aorta with the same clamp (Fig. 9). An incision is then made in the anterior wall of the right pulmonary artery and a similar one on the lateral slightly posterior aspect of the ascending aorta. An anastomosis approximately 4 to 5 mm. in diameter is then made between the ascending aorta and the right pulmonary artery. It has proved quite satisfactory and is the preferred procedure when systemic-pulmonary anastomosis is needed within the first several months of life. This procedure has the distinct advantage of being easily corrected at the time of open correction.

Rarely, *anastomosis of the superior vena cava to the right pulmonary artery (Glenn operation)* has been advocated in the treatment of tetralogy of Fallot.[3, 26] In this procedure, the systemic venous blood from the superior vena cava passes directly into the pulmonary circulation, thus bypassing the right heart. Although the procedure has produced good results with respect to symptoms in some, more difficulty is experienced in the subsequent total correction. It is rarely employed in the treatment of the tetralogy of Fallot. A method for subsequent correction of the ventricular septal defect and relief of the right ventricular outflow obstruction following a superior vena cava to right pulmonary artery anastomosis has been described.[13]

Open Correction

Open correction is the ideal operation for the tetralogy of Fallot and is accomplished with extracorporeal circulation. Through a median sternotomy, the pericardium is opened. Major branches of the right coronary artery may pass across the outflow tract to supply the left ventricle; occasionally, the anterior descending coronary artery arises from the right coronary artery and should be avoided. Among 94 patients with tetralogy of Fallot who underwent visualization of the coronary arteries, the anterior descending coronary arose from the right coronary in 4 per cent and a single left coronary artery was present in 1 per cent. Of additional interest is that in 195 postmortem specimens of tetralogy, evidence of coronary anomalies was 5 per cent.[22] A careful estimate is made

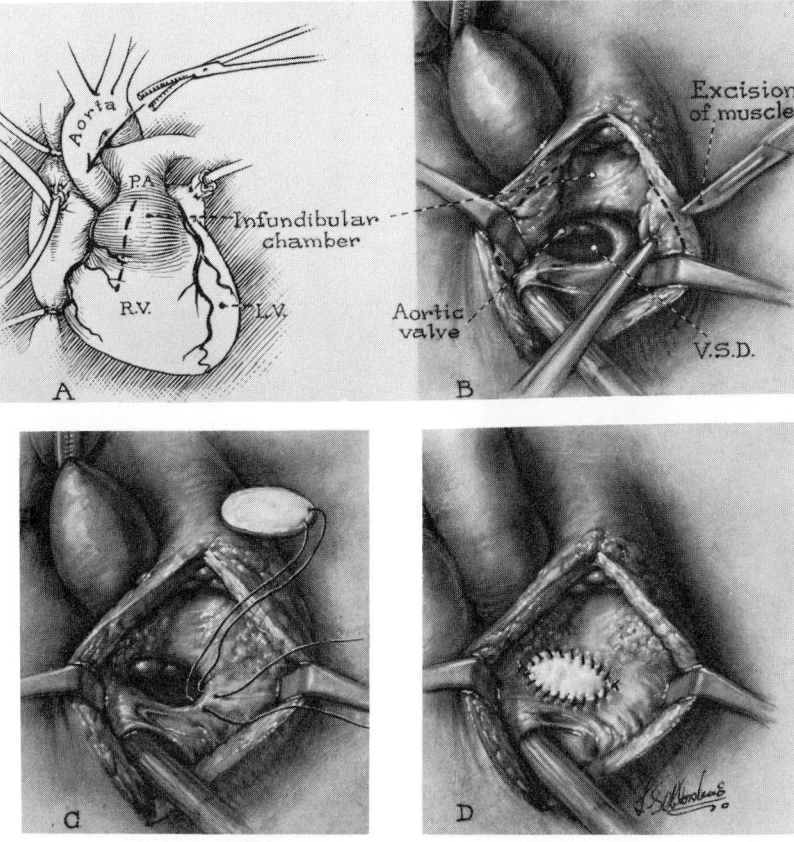

Figure 10. Steps in the total correction of the tetralogy of Fallot. *A*, Note infundibular chamber and normal distribution of coronary vessels. The superior and inferior venae cavae are separately cannulated. The left atrium is decompressed by a catheter in the left atrial appendage. *B*, Marked infundibular stenosis is present in the outflow tract of the right ventricle. The pulmonary valve is normal. The interventricular defect is of the standard type. Through the defect, the cusps of the aortic valve are easily visualized. The aorta is temporarily occluded to prevent reflux of blood that would obscure the operative field in the region of the ventricular septal defect. *C*, The placement of the initial suture in the ventricular septal defect border. Intermittent aortic occlusion is employed. *D*, Completion of placement of ventricular prosthesis. (From Sabiston, D. C., Jr. *In* Sabiston, D. C., Jr., and Spencer, F. C. (Eds.): Gibbon's Surgery of the Chest, 3rd ed. Philadelphia, W. B. Saunders Company, 1976.)

of the size of the main pulmonary artery as well as of the possible presence of valvar stenosis. The inferior and superior vena cavae are dissected, in preparation for insertion of venous cannulas into the right atrium. The left heart is vented through a catheter passed either through the right superior pulmonary vein, through the left atrial appendage, or through the left ventricular apex. A transverse or longitudinal ventriculotomy is then made in the outflow tract of the right ventricle (Fig. 10A). In a recent publication, the repair of the ventricular septal defect and infundibular stenosis was advocated through an atriotomy.[17] If valvar pulmonary stenosis is present, it is relieved by commissural incisions. The infundibular stenosis is carefully resected, with removal of all obstructing muscle (Fig. 10B). The ventricular septal defect is then identified. It is usually large and requires a plastic prosthesis for closure (Fig. 10C and D). Extreme care is devoted to the placement of the sutures, and it is important that the electrocardiogram and the atrial and ventricular contractions be monitored while these sutures are being placed. Should a pattern of heart block occur, the suture should be removed and reinserted. Intermittent occlusion of the ascending aorta is helpful when retraction and exposure of the defect produce aortic insufficiency and obscure the field. Air emboli in the coronary circulation must be pre-

vented on reopening of the aorta by the passage of a clamp to render the aortic valve completely insufficient as the aortic clamp is released. Following closure of the interventricular septal defect, the right ventricle may be closed primarily or may require a patch. When feasible, primary closure is desirable; but if primary closure produces excessive obstruction, right ventricular hypertension and a low cardiac output syndrome will ensue. If the pulmonary artery or the valvar annulus is small, it may be necessary to extend the patch across the valve ring to the proximal portion of the pulmonary artery (Fig. 11). This produces pulmonary insufficiency, but it may be unavoidable and is apt to cause few problems. Residual right ventricular pulmonary artery gradients above 50 mm. Hg can be tolerated, although if this level is to be exceeded judicious assessment of the situation is required. After the procedure has been completed and cardiopulmonary bypass discontinued, a dye dilution curve should be obtained to be certain that there is not any residual shunt present. If the dye curve shows a shunt, the heart should be reopened and the defect found and appropriately closed. The operation for correction is more difficult for patients with a previous left pulmonary artery–descending aorta anastomosis (Potts). The technique described by Kirklin is a very satisfactory one (Fig. 12).[36]

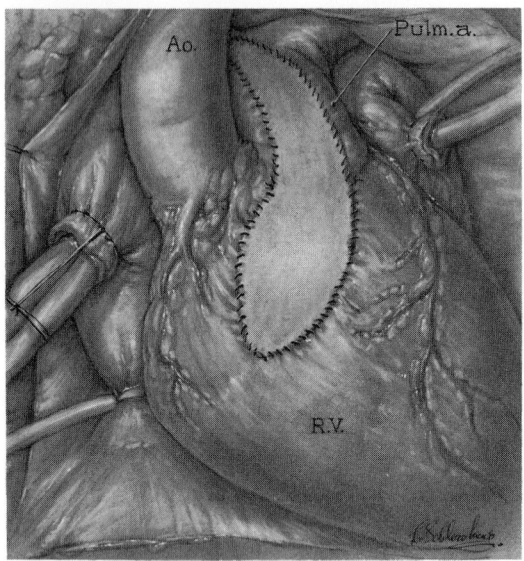

Figure 11. In this patient with atresia of the pulmonary valve ring a large plastic prosthesis was required from the bifurcation of the pulmonary artery in order to decompress the right ventricle adequately. (From Sabiston, D. C., Jr. *In* Sabiston, D. C., Jr., and Spencer, F. C., (Eds.): Gibbon's Surgery of the Chest, 3rd ed. Philadelphia, W. B. Saunders Company, 1976.)

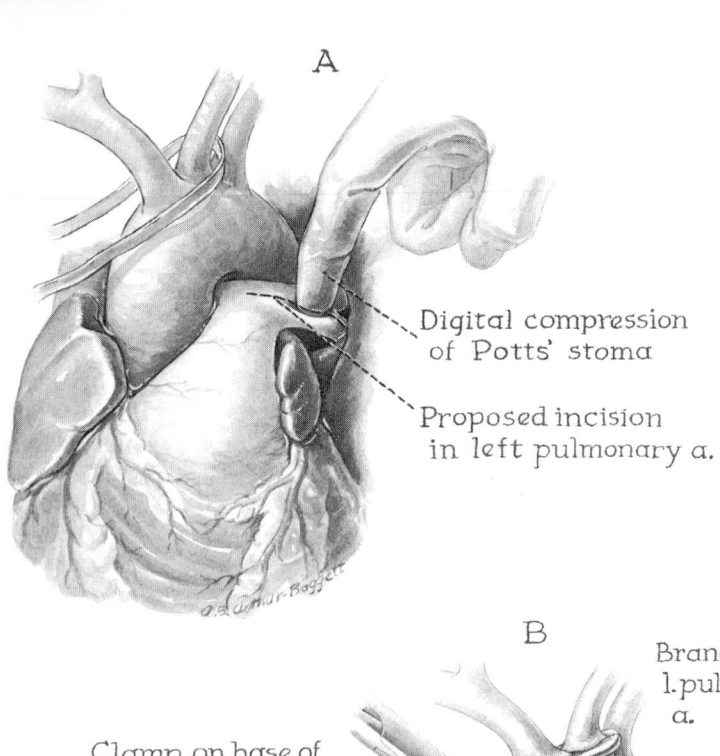

Figure 12. For closure of a Potts anastomosis, the head vessels are clamped at their origin, circulatory arrest is established, and the stoma is visualized through an incision in the left pulmonary artery. (From Kirklin, J. W., and Karp, R. B.: The Tetralogy of Fallot from a Surgical Viewpoint. Philadelphia, W. B. Saunders Company, 1970.)

RESULTS

The tetralogy of Fallot is now being corrected frequently and with an ever diminishing mortality. The results with open correction during the recent past have been impressive. The mortality in most series is now between 3 and 10 per cent.[2, 37, 40] In the majority of patients, the clinical and physiologic status is greatly improved, and good to excellent results have been reported in up to 90 per cent.[40] Some of the rarer and more severe anatomic malformations respond less well, but even these lesions are now yielding to surgery with improved results.[1, 29, 57] Following open correction, the chest film usually shows slight enlargement of the heart, and murmurs of pulmonary insufficiency may be present. In early experience with the technique of open correction, left-to-right shunts through a ventricular septal defect or reopening of the defect occurred with some frequency, but these are now uncommon.

POSTOPERATIVE MANAGEMENT

Following operation, a number of variables must be followed carefully. Adequate *pulmonary function* is maintained by the use of an endotracheal tube, generally for the first 24 hours. This permits the maintenance of relatively normal values for the arterial Po_2, Pco_2, and pH. Whenever possible, the percentage of oxygen in the inspired air is maintained between 40 and 50 per cent, with attempts made not to exceed 60 per cent to prevent oxygen toxicity. Maintenance of an adequate *cardiac output* is also of crucial importance. It is appropriate to obtain dye dilution determinations of cardiac output when indicated. In general, the cardiac output can be increased by increasing the ventricular end-diastolic pressure, as accomplished by administration of blood or fluids. The atrial pressure can be raised should this be necessary. However, if evidence of *low* cardiac output persists, a search should be conducted for other primary causes. *Cardiac tamponade* is a recognized cause of the low output syndrome and may be present. If tamponade is not present, efforts should be made to improve the contractility of the cardiac muscle; this can be accomplished by the use of digitalis if the situation is not acute, and with inotropic agents such as isoproterenol if the clinical manifestations are more serious. The use of dopamine is often quite helpful in maintaining adequate arterial pressure. Maintenance of *renal* function is also of critical importance. The urethral catheter is left in place with a desired output of at least 20 ml. per hour. It is generally necessary to limit fluid intake, especially during the first 24 hours following operation. This is due to the tendency to development of fluid retention of patients after repair of tetralogy of Fallot. On the first day, approximately 500 ml. of water per square meter of body surface should be administered. After the second postoperative day, the patient is allowed fluids by mouth but is placed on a low sodium diet (500 mg. daily). Following this, fluid intake may be regulated in accordance with total body weight, which should be obtained on accurate and reliable scales. Furosemide (Lasix) is quite helpful in controlling retained fluid and should be used as indicated. To prevent infection, especially when prosthetic materials have been used, antibiotics are given routinely. Arrhythmias, especially atrioventricular dissociation, can be a serious postoperative complication. Temporary pacemaker wires are generally inserted into the mycoardium and allowed to remain for several days in the event that such are needed. If a dissociation pattern occurs in the postoperative period, pacing may be easily instituted. If atrial fibrillation develops, rapid digitalization is indicated. In the presence of *ventricular ectopic* beats, potassium chloride is employed (3 to 5 mEq. per 10 per cent solution).

PULMONARY STENOSIS WITH INTACT VENTRICULAR SEPTUM

Pulmonary valvar stenosis with intact ventricular septum is one of the most favorable congenital cardiac lesions from the point of view of treatment. The symptoms are generally less pronounced than with the tetralogy of Fallot, although there are numerous examples of infants with extremely severe pulmonary stenosis that produces congestive heart failure. Some infants require immediate valvotomy as an *emergency* procedure, but in the majority of patients symptoms develop more slowly. In approximately three fourths of this group, the foramen ovale is patent, and with development of increased pressure in the right atrium, blood is shunted to the left atrium and cyanosis is produced. Clubbing of the fingers may appear later. Characteristically, the pulmonary valvar commissures are fused into a dome-shaped structure with a small central lumen. A *jet* of blood that is forced through the

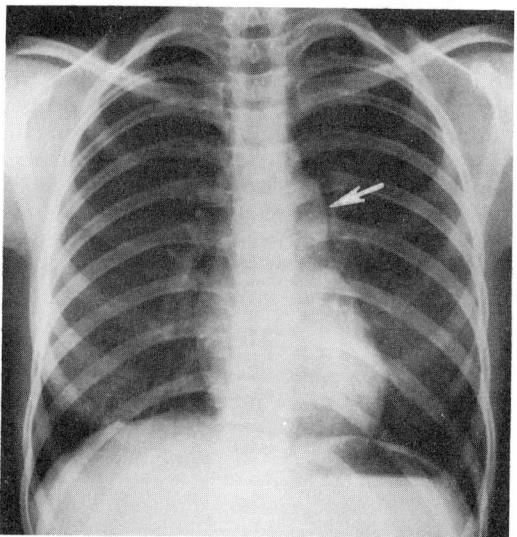

Figure 13. Chest film of patient with isolated valvar pulmonary stenosis, demonstrating typical appearance of dilatation of the pulmonary artery. (From Sabiston, D. C., Jr. *In* Sabiston, D. C., Jr., and Spencer, F. C. (Eds): Gibbon's Surgery of the Chest, 3rd ed. Philadelphia, W. B. Saunders Company, 1976.)

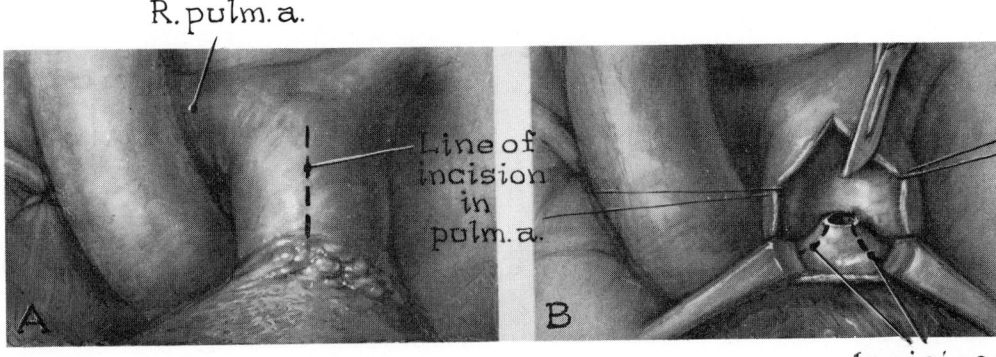

R. pulm. a.

Line of incision in pulm. a.

A   **B**

Incisions

Figure 14. Illustration of open correction of pulmonary valvar stenosis employing extracorporeal circulation. An incision is made in the main pulmonary artery, exposing the dome-shaped pulmonary valve. Radial incisions are made in each of the fused commissures, with complete opening of the valve. (From Sabiston, D. C., Jr. In Sabiston, D. C., Jr., and Spencer, F. C. (Eds.): Surgery of the Chest, 3rd ed. Philadelphia, W. B. Saunders Company, 1976.)

aperture under great pressure from the right ventricle into the pulmonary artery creates eddy currents and a prominent thrill. Poststenotic dilatation of the main pulmonary artery ensues. In rare instances, *infundibular* stenosis may be associated with valvar stenosis and an intact ventricular septum. Moreover, frank atrial septal defects are also encountered, the latter combination being termed the *trilogy of Fallot.* The clinical findings are dependent upon the severity of the valvar pulmonary stenosis and the patency of the foramen ovale.[19] Dyspnea on exertion is the most common complaint, and cyanosis is usually present in those patients with a patent foramen ovale or an atrial septal defect. A harsh systolic murmur and thrill are present over the pulmonary area; the thrill can be palpated in the suprasternal notch. The pulmonary second sound is characteristically weak or absent. The chest film is often typical, demonstrating prominence of the pulmonary artery due to poststenotic dilatation (Fig. 13). The angiocardiogram is also helpful in demonstrating the classic dome-shaped pulmonary valve with small aperture and poststenotic dilatation, or an atrial septal defect and infundibular stenosis combined with valvar stenosis. Cardiac catheterization demonstrates a gradient between the right ventricle and the pulmonary artery *without* evidence of a shunt at the ventricular level. In severe forms, the pressure gradient between the pulmonary artery and the right ventricle may exceed 200 mm. Hg.

Treatment

The original treatment of valvar pulmonary stenosis was introduced by Brock[8] and consisted of transventricular valvotomy. A valvulotome was passed through the wall of the right ventricle into the pulmonary artery to open the stenotic valve. Later, an improved valvulotome was designed for transventricular use.[47] For a number of years this approach was used with moderate success and was associated with both clinical and hemodynamic improvement.[31] Nevertheless, closed valvotomy has definite disadvantages,[39] and it is now agreed that open repair of the valvar stenosis

under direct vision produces the best results.[7] The use of extracorporeal circulation permits simultaneous correction of coexisting atrial septal defects and of infundibular stenosis when present.[41] Thus, the open approach to the correction of pulmonary valvar stenosis is most often indicated (Fig. 14).

Open correction of pulmonary valvar stenosis yields excellent results, and recurrence of the condition is rare. Moreover, the compensatory infundibular hypertrophy that frequently accompanies the valvar stenosis usually regresses with time. Although the gradient between the right ventricle and the pulmonary artery may not be totally abolished immediately after operation, regression of the secondary hypertrophy of the right ventricular outflow tract occurs and repeat catheterization later shows a marked reduction in the gradient.[18]

In addition to valvar pulmonary stenosis, *isolated infundibular stenosis* of the right ventricle may also occur as a congenital anomaly. The symptoms are quite similar to those of valvar stenosis, although the murmur may be located somewhat lower in the precordium. The angiocardiogram demonstrates the lesion with precision, and cardiac catheterization demonstrates two gradients: (1) between the pulmonary artery and the infundibulum, and (2) between the infundibulum and the right ventricle. Management of these cases is resection of the infundibular stenosis in the open heart employing extracorporeal circulation. The results are excellent.

SELECTED REFERENCES

Blalock, A., and Taussig, H. B.: Surgical treatment of malformations of the heart in which there is pulmonary stenosis or pulmonary atresia. J.A.M.A., *128:*189, 1945.
  In this paper, Dr. Blalock's first three operations for creation of a systemic-pulmonary artery anastomosis are reported. The first patient, a 15-month-old infant with severe cyanosis, had a history of multiple episodes of loss of consciousness. An anastomosis of the left subclavian artery to the left pulmonary artery was made, and the clinical improvement was striking. Two additional patients with successful results are also described. It is of interest that Dr. Blalock refers to earlier experimental work in which subclavian-pulmonary anastomoses were performed in the dog in an effort to

produce pulmonary hypertension. Although these experiments did not succeed in producing an elevated pulmonary arterial pressure, the operation was subsequently used for an entirely different purpose. This procedure was the first of many additional cardiac surgical advances.

Chopra, P. S., Levy, J. M., Dacumos, G. C., Jr., Berkoff, H. A., Loring, L. L., and Kahn, D. R.: The Blalock-Taussig operation – the procedure of choice in the hypoxic infant with tetralogy of Fallot. Ann. Thorac. Surg., 22:235, 1976.
These authors advocate systemic pulmonary anastomosis (Blalock) as the ideal procedure in the infant. It is their belief that a better long-term result is obtained using a preliminary shunt followed by open correction than by performing the definitive procedure with extracorporeal circulation as the initial operation.

Kirklin, J. W., and Karp, R. B.: Tetralogy of Fallot from a Surgical Viewpoint. Philadelphia, W. B. Saunders Company, 1970.
This is a superb monograph with excellent presentations of the anatomy, natural history, hemodynamics, clinical features, and diagnosis of tetralogy of Fallot. The techniques of palliative and open corrective surgery are superbly described and illustrated. A detailed account of the results is provided and ranks among the best in the world literature. This monograph is highly recommended for a complete analysis of the entire subject.

Lillehei, C. W., Cohen, M., Warden, H. E., Read, R. C., Aust, J. B., DeWall, R. A., and Varco, R.: Vision intracardiac surgical correction of the tetralogy of Fallot, pentalogy of Fallot, and pulmonary atresia defects. Ann. Surg., 142:418, 1955.
In this paper the original descriptions for surgical correction of the tetralogy of Fallot are provided. The paper is a classic one in the development of surgical techniques for complete correction of this malformation.

Sabiston, D. C., Jr.: Role of the Blalock-Taussig operation in the hypoxic infant with tetralogy of Fallot. Editorial. Ann. Thorac. Surg., 22:303, 1976.
In this editorial, the use of an initial systemic to pulmonary shunt procedure is contrasted with total correction of the tetralogy of Fallot in infancy. The reasoning advanced by the advocates of each of these methods is discussed in detail.

Sabiston, D. C., Jr., Cornell, W. P., Criley, J. M., Neill, C. A., Ross, R. S., and Bahnson, H. T.: The diagnosis and surgical correction of total obstruction of the right ventricle. J. Thorac. Cardiovasc. Surg., 48:577, 1964.
In this paper, the most severe of the forms of tetralogy of Fallot, those with complete obliteration of the outflow tract of the right ventricle and its communication with the pulmonary artery, are described together with the details of operative correction and results. It is interesting that in these patients who have no communication between the right ventricle and pulmonary artery and, following correction, have total pulmonary insufficiency, the subsequent course is generally surprisingly good. In other words, pulmonary valvar insufficiency can be well tolerated.

Sade, R. M., Williams, R. G., and Castaneda, A. R.: Corrective surgery for congenital cardiovascular defects in early infancy. Am. Heart J., 90:656, 1975.
In this review, the authors advocate early correction of tetralogy of Fallot irrespective of the age of the patient, including newborn infants. The results are quite good, and optimism is expressed about the long term results when the children become older.

Taussig, H. B.: Tetralogy of Fallot. In Congenital Malformations of the Heart, 2nd ed. Cambridge, Harvard University Press, 1960.
This chapter in an outstanding text of pediatric cardiology is an excellent resource for the descriptions of the clinical manifestations, physical findings, laboratory studies, and ultimate results in patients with the tetralogy of Fallot. Its author has probably examined and followed more patients with this condition than anyone else in the world.

REFERENCES

1. Allison, P. R., Gunning, A. J., Hamill, J., and Mody, S. M.: Fallot's tetralogy. A postoperative study. Circulation, 28:525, 1963.
2. Bahnson, H. T.: Discussion of Malm, J. R., Blumenthal, S., Bowman, F. O., Jr., Ellis, K., Jameson, A. G., Jesse, M. J., and Yeoh, C. B.: Factors that modify hemodynamic results in total correction of tetralogy of Fallot. J. Thorac. Cardiovasc. Surg., 52:502, 1966.
3. Bakulev, A. N., and Kolesnikov, S. A.: Anastomosis of the superior vena cava and pulmonary artery in the surgical treatment of certain congenital defects of the heart. J. Thorac. Surg., 37:693, 1959.
4. Barratt-Boyes, B. G., Simpson, M., and Neutze, J. M.: Intracardiac surgery in neonates and infants using deep hypothermia with surface cooling and limited cardiopulmonary bypass. Circulation, Suppl. 1, 43:1, 1971.
5. Blalock, A.: Surgical procedures employed and anatomical variations encountered in the treatment of congenital pulmonic stenosis. Surg. Gynec. Obstet., 87:385, 1948.
6. Blalock, A., and Taussig, H. B.: The surgical treatment of malformation of the heart in which there is pulmonary stenosis or pulmonary atresia. J.A.M.A., 128:189, 1945.
7. Blount, S. G., Jr., McCord, M. C., Mueller, H., and Swan, H.: Isolated valvular pulmonic stenosis; clinical and physiologic response to open valvuloplasty. Circulation, 10:161, 1954.
8. Brock, R. C.: Pulmonary valvulotomy for the relief of congenital pulmonary stenosis; report of 3 cases. Br. Med. J., 1:1121, 1948.
9. Brock, R. C.: Congenital pulmonary stenosis. Am. J. Med., 12:706, 1952.
10. Brock, R. C., and Campbell, M.: Infundibular resection for pulmonic stenosis. Br. Heart J., 12:403, 1950.
11. Campbell, M., and Deuchar, D. C.: Results of the Blalock-Taussig operation in 200 cases of morbus caeruleus. Br. Med. J., 1:349, 1953.
12. Chopra, P. S., Levy, J. M., Dacumos, G. C., Jr., Berkoff, H. A., Loring, L. L., and Kahn, D. R.: The Blalock-Taussig operation – the procedure of choice in the hypoxic infant with tetralogy of Fallot. Ann. Thorac. Surg., 22:235, 1976.
13. Claxton, C. P., Jr., and Sabiston, D. C., Jr.: Correction of tetralogy of Fallot following superior vena cava to pulmonary artery shunt. J. Thorac. Cardiovasc. Surg., 57:475, 1969.
14. Cooley, D. A., and Hallman, G. L.: Intrapericardial aortic-right pulmonary arterial anastomosis. Surg. Gynecol. Obstet., 122:1084, 1966.
15. Dobell, A. R. C., Charrette, E. P., and Chughtai, M. S.: Correction of tetralogy in the young child. J. Thorac. Cardiovasc. Surg., 55:70, 1968.
16. Edwards, W. S., Mohtashemi, M., and Holdefer, W. F., Jr.: Ascending aorta to right pulmonary artery shunt for infants with tetralogy of Fallot. Surgery, 59:316, 1966.
17. Edmunds, L. H., Jr., Saxena, N. C., Friedman, S., Rashkind, W. J., and Dodd, P. F.: Transatrial resection of the obstructed right ventricular infundibulum. Circulation, 54:117, 1976.
18. Engle, M. A., Holswade, G. R., Goldberg, H. P., Lukas, D. S., and Glenn, F.: Regression after open valvotomy of infundibular stenosis accompanying severe valvular pulmonic stenosis. Circulation, 17:862, 1958.
19. Engle, M. A., and Taussig, H. B.: Valvular pulmonic stenosis with intact ventricular septum and patent foramen ovale: Report of illustrative cases and analysis of clinical syndrome. Circulation, 2:481, 1950.
20. Fallot, E. A. L.: Contribution à l'anatomie pathologique de la maladie bleue (cyanose cardiaque). Marseille Med., 25:77, 138, 207, 270, 341, 403, 1888.
21. Farre, J. R.: Pathological Researches. Essay I. On Malformation of the Human Heart. London, 1814.
22. Fellows, K. E., Freed, M. D., Keane, J. F., Van Praagh, R., Bernhard, W. F., and Castaneda, A. C.: Results of routine preoperative coronary angiography in tetralogy of Fallot. Circulation, 51:561, 1975.
23. Fort, L., III, Morrow, A. G., Pierce, G. E., Saigusa, M., and McLaughlin, J. S.: The distribution of pulmonary blood flow after subclavian-pulmonary anastomosis: An experimental study. J. Thorac. Cardiovasc. Surg., 50:671, 1965.
24. Gay, W. A., Jr., and Ebert, P. A.: Aorta-to-right pulmonary artery anastomosis causing obstruction of the right pulmonary artery. Ann. Thorac. Surg., 16:402, 1973.
25. Gintrac, E.: Observations et recherches sur la cyanose, ou maladie bleue. Paris, J. Pinard, 1824.
26. Glenn, W. W. L., and Patino, J. F.: Circulatory bypass of the right heart. I. Preliminary observation on direct delivery of vena caval blood into pulmonary arterial circulation. Azygos vein-pulmonary artery shunt. Yale J. Biol. Med., 27:147, 1954.
27. Gregoratos, G., Jones, R. C., and Jahnke, E. J., Jr.: Unilateral peripheral pulmonic stenosis complicating tetralogy of Fallot. J. Thorac. Cardiovasc. Surg., 50:202, 1965.
28. Haller, J. A., Jr.: Second shunting operations for pulmonary

stenosis with cyanosis following failure of original systemic-pulmonary anastomoses. Surgery, 44:919, 1958.

29. Hallidie-Smith, K. A., Dulake, M., Wong, M., Oakley, C. M., and Goodwin, J. F.: Ventricular structure and function after radical correction of the tetralogy of Fallot. Br. Heart J., 29:533, 1967.

30. Hartmann, R. C.: A hemorrhagic disorder occurring in patients with cyanotic congenital heart disease. Bull. Johns Hopkins Hosp., 91:49, 1952.

31. Himmelstein, A., Jameson, A. G., Fishman, A. P., and Humphreys, G. H., II: Closed transventricular valvulotomy for pulmonic stenosis. Surgery, 42:121, 1957.

32. Hope, J.: A Treatise on Disease of the Heart and Great Vessels and on the Affections which may be Mistaken for Them. London, J. & A. Churchill, 1839.

33. Hunter, J.: Medical Observations and Inquiries by a Society of Physicians of London. London, 1757–1784.

34. Hunter, W.: Three cases of malformation of the heart. Case II. Medical Observations and Inquiries by a Society of Physicians in London, 6:291, 1784.

35. Johns, T. N. P., Williams, G. R., and Blalock, A.: The anatomy of pulmonary stenosis and atresia with comments on surgical therapy. Surgery, 33:161, 1953.

36. Kirklin, J. W., and Karp, R. B.: The Tetralogy of Fallot from a Surgical Viewpoint. Philadelphia, W. B. Saunders Company, 1970.

37. Kirklin, J. W., Wallace, R. B., McGoon, D. C., and DuShane, J. W.: Early and late results after intracardiac repair of tetralogy of Fallot. Trans. Am. Surg. Assoc., 83:258, 1965.

38. Lillehei, C. W., Cohen, M., Warden, H. E., Read, R. C., Aust, J. B., DeWall, R. A., and Varco, R. L.: Vision intracardiac surgical correction of the tetralogy of Fallot, pentalogy of Fallot, and pulmonary atresia defects. Ann. Surg., 142:418, 1955.

39. Lillehei, C. W., Winchell, P., Adams, P., Baronofsky, I., Adams, F., and Varco, R. L.: Pulmonary valvular stenosis with intact ventricular septum. Am. J. Med., 5:756, 1956.

40. Malm, J. R., Blumenthal, S., Bowman, F. O., Jr., Ellis, K., Jameson, A. G., Jesse, M. J., and Yeoh, C. B.: Factors that modify hemodynamic results in total correction of tetralogy of Fallot. J. Thorac. Cardiovasc. Surg., 52:502, 1966.

41. McGoon, D. C., and Kirklin, J. W.: Pulmonic stenosis with intact ventricular septum. Treatment utilizing extracorporeal circulation. Circulation, 17:180, 1958.

42. Nagao, G. I., Daoud, G. I., McAdams, A. J., Schwartz, D. C., and Kaplan, S.: Cardiovascular anomalies associated with tetralogy of Fallot. Am. J. Cardiol., 20:206, 1967.

43. Neches, W. H., Naifeh, J. G., Park, S. C., Lenox, C. C., Zuberbuhler, J. R., Siewers, R. D., Pontius, R. G., and Bahnson, H. T.: Systemic-pulmonary artery anastomoses in infancy. J. Thorac. Cardiovasc. Surg., 70:921, 1975.

44. Pacifico, A. D., Bargeron, L. M., Jr., and Kirklin, J. W.: Primary

total correction of tetralogy of Fallot in children less than four years of age. Circulation, 48:1085, 1973.

45. Peacock, T. B.: Malformations of the Human Heart. London, J. & A. Churchill, 1866.

46. Porter, J. M., and Silver, D.: Alterations in fibrinolysis and coagulation associated with cardiopulmonary bypass. J. Thorac. Cardiovasc. Surg., 56:869, 1968.

47. Potts, W. J., Gibson, S., Riker, W. L., and Leninger, C. R.: Congenital pulmonary stenosis with intact ventricular septum. J.A.M.A., 144:8, 1950.

48. Potts, W. J., Smith, S., and Gibson, S.: Anastomosis of the aorta to a pulmonary artery for certain types of congenital heart disease. J.A.M.A., 132:629, 1946.

49. Ross, R. S., Taussig, H. B., and Evans, M. H.: Late hemodynamic complications of anastomotic surgery for treatment of the tetralogy of Fallot. Circulation, 18:553, 1958.

50. Sabiston, D. C., Jr., and Blalock, A.: The tetralogy of Fallot, tricuspid atresia, transposition of the great vessels and associated disorders. In Encyclopedia of Thoracic Surgery. Heidelberg, Springer-Verlag, 1959, Vol. 2, p. 697.

51. Sabiston, D. C., Jr., Cornell, W. P., Criley, J. M., Neill, C. A., Ross, R. S., and Bahnson, H. T.: The diagnosis and surgical correction of total obstruction of the right ventricle: An acquired condition developing after systemic artery–pulmonary artery anastomosis for tetralogy of Fallot. J. Thorac. Surg., 48:577, 1964.

52. Sandifort, E.: Observations Anatomico-Pathologicae. Ludg. Bat P.v.d. Eyk et D. Vygh, 1777, Chapter 1, Figure 1.

53. Scott, H. W., Collins, H. A., and Foster, J. H.: Hypothermia as an adjuvant in cardiovascular surgery. Experimental and clinical observations. Am. Surg., 20:799, 1954.

54. Starr, A., Bonchek, L. I., and Sunderland, C. O.: Total correction of tetralogy of Fallot in infancy. J. Thorac. Cardiovasc. Surg., 65:45, 1973.

55. Stensen, Hiels (Nicholaus Steno): In Thomas Bartholin, Acta Medica et Philosophica Hafnienca, 1671/72, Vol. I, p. 302. Reprinted in Nicolae Stenosis: Opera Philosophica. Copenhagen, Vilhelm Maar, 1910, Vol. 2, pp. 49–53.

56. Stephens, H. B.: Aneurysm of the pulmonary artery following a Potts' shunt operation. J. Thorac. Cardiovasc. Surg., 53:642, 1967.

57. Theye, R. A., and Kirklin, J. W.: Physiologic studies early after repair of tetralogy of Fallot. Circulation, 28:42, 1963.

58. Waterston, D. J.: Treatment of Fallot's tetralogy in children under 1 year of age. Rozhl. Chir., 41:181, 1962.

59. White, P. D., and Sprague, H. B.: The tetralogy of Fallot. Report of a case in a noted musician who lived to his sixtieth year. J.A.M.A., 92:787, 1929.

60. Wood, W. C., McCue, C. M., and Lower, R. R.: Blalock-Taussig shunts in the infant. Ann. Thorac. Surg., 16:454, 1973.

VIII

DOUBLE OUTLET RIGHT VENTRICLE (DORV)

Robert K. Brawley, M.D.

Double outlet right ventricle, or origin of both great vessels from the right ventricle, is an uncommon defect but is potentially correctable. Numerous anatomic variations exist, but the essential characteristics of the defect are a morphologic right ventricle from which both the aorta and pulmonary artery originate and a ventricular septal defect that provides the only outlet from the left ventricle. In most patients with this defect there is absence of the normal fibrous continuity between the anterior leaflet of the mitral valve and the aortic or pulmonary valves. The aortic valve is also often higher than normal and located at about the same level as the pulmonary valve. Usually the aorta lies to the right of the pulmonary artery but can be to the left or directly anterior to the pulmonary artery. Pulmonary stenosis is frequently present, and subaortic stenosis has also been encountered.[13, 15] The ventricular septal defect is variable and can be situated above or below the crista supraventricularis or may be of the atrioventricular canal type.[16, 20, 24] A variety of associated congenital cardiovascular anomalies have also been found in these patients.[4, 10, 23]

The current understanding of the pathology and clinical features of double outlet right ventricle is based upon a number of studies.[4, 9, 10, 16, 18, 19, 25, 27] Children with this anomaly may present with clinical features suggesting tetralogy of Fallot or ventricular septal defect with bi-directional shunting depending primarily upon whether or not pulmonary stenosis is present. Although certain clinical, hemodynamic, and electrocardiographic findings may suggest double outlet right ventricle, these are not specific and accurate anatomic diagnosis requires angiographic study.[4, 9, 17, 20] Since surgical techniques now exist for the correction of many of the less common types of congenital heart disease, including at least some forms of double outlet right ventricle, precise anatomic definition of the specific anomaly is necessary. The diagnosis of double outlet right ventricle requires angiocardiographic demonstration that (1) the aorta and pulmonary artery take origin from the same ventricle that has the anatomic features of the right ventricle, and (2) fibrous continuity between the morphologic mitral valve and either the aortic or pulmonic semilunar valve is absent.[4] The diagnosis does not require that both semilunar valves be at the same horizontal level, since approximately one fourth of the patients with this condition will have the aortic and pulmonary valves located at different levels.

While the anomaly had previously been described by pathologists and recognized clinically, Witham[27] is probably responsible for stimulating increased interest in the condition and providing the term "double outlet right ventricle" with a publication in 1957 describing four patients with this malformation. In 1961 Neufeld and associates[18, 19] described 14 patients with the abnormality, which they designated origin of both great vessels from the right ventricle, and emphasized clinical differences depending upon the presence or absence of pulmonic stenosis. Also in 1961, McGoon[14] reported a successful operation in a patient with double outlet right ventricle and thereby established that some forms of the defect were amenable to intracardiac repair.

Since this malformation includes a variety of specific anatomic forms, an understanding of several terms is necessary in the description of this anomaly. When used to designate the cardiac ventricles, the terms *right* and *left* apply to the morphologic rather than the positional or functional characteristics of the ventricular chamber being described. The right ventricle possesses coarse interior trabeculations, a tricuspid atrioventricular valve, and a crista supraventricularis with its septal and parietal muscular bands. The left ventricle possesses a relatively smooth interior and a bicuspid atrioventricular valve. The term *situs solitus* designates the normal anatomic position of the viscera of the thorax and abdomen wherein the

right lung is trilobed, the left lung is bilobed, the spleen and stomach lie to the left of the midline, and the major part of the liver is situated to the right of the midline. *Situs inversus* of the viscera designates a condition in which the organs of the thorax and abdomen are opposite to their normal positions. The position or situs of the atria is the same as that of the abdominal viscera. The viscera and atria can be in situs solitus and the ventricles in situs inversus (ventricular inversion) or the viscera and atria can be in situs inversus and the ventricles in situs solitus. *Levocardia* refers to the usual position of the heart within the thorax with the apex of the heart pointing to the left. *Dextrocardia* designates the cardiac position when the apex of the heart points to the right. In double outlet right ventricle, the great arteries are said to be normally related if the aorta is to the right of the pulmonary artery and abnormally related if the aorta is to the left or anterior to the pulmonary artery. Right ventricular infundibulum or conus is the term applied to the outflow portion of the right ventricle that lies immediately below the pulmonic valve. The crista supraventricularis is the structure that forms the posterior portion or the floor of the right ventricular infundibulum and has parietal and septal limbs that constitute the lateral borders of the infundibulum. The parietal band of the crista supraventricularis normally separates the tricuspid valve from the outflow portion of the right ventricle.

Double outlet right ventricle has been classified in several different ways.[7, 10, 16, 18, 20, 21, 27] A very helpful classification[21] emphasizes the relationship of the ventricular septal defect and the great arteries, since this relationship is an important determinant of the technique for surgical repair (Table 1). Based upon the position of the great arteries and the ventricular septal defect and excluding the existence of ventricular inversion and pulmonary stenosis, there are four possible types of double outlet right ventricle (Fig. 1). In patients with normally related great arteries (aorta on the right), the ventricular septal defect will be predominantly subaortic if it is posteriorly located (Fig. 1A). This is the situation in the classic form of double outlet right ventricle. If the great vessels are normally related, the ventricular septal defect is subpulmonic if

TABLE 1.　Classification of Double Outlet Right Ventricle*

I. Situs solitus of atria and ventricles
　A. Normally related great arteries (aorta to right)
　　1) Subaortic (posterior) VSD
　　2) Subpulmonic (anterior) VSD
　B. Abnormally related great arteries (aorta to left or anterior)
　　1) Subpulmonic (posterior) VSD
　　2) Subaortic (anterior) VSD
II. Situs solitus of atria, situs inversus of ventricles
　A. Normally related great arteries
　B. Abnormally related great arteries

*Modified after Patrick, D. L., and McGoon, D. C.: An operation for double-outlet right ventricle with transposition of the great arteries. J. Cardiovasc. Surg., 9:537, 1968.

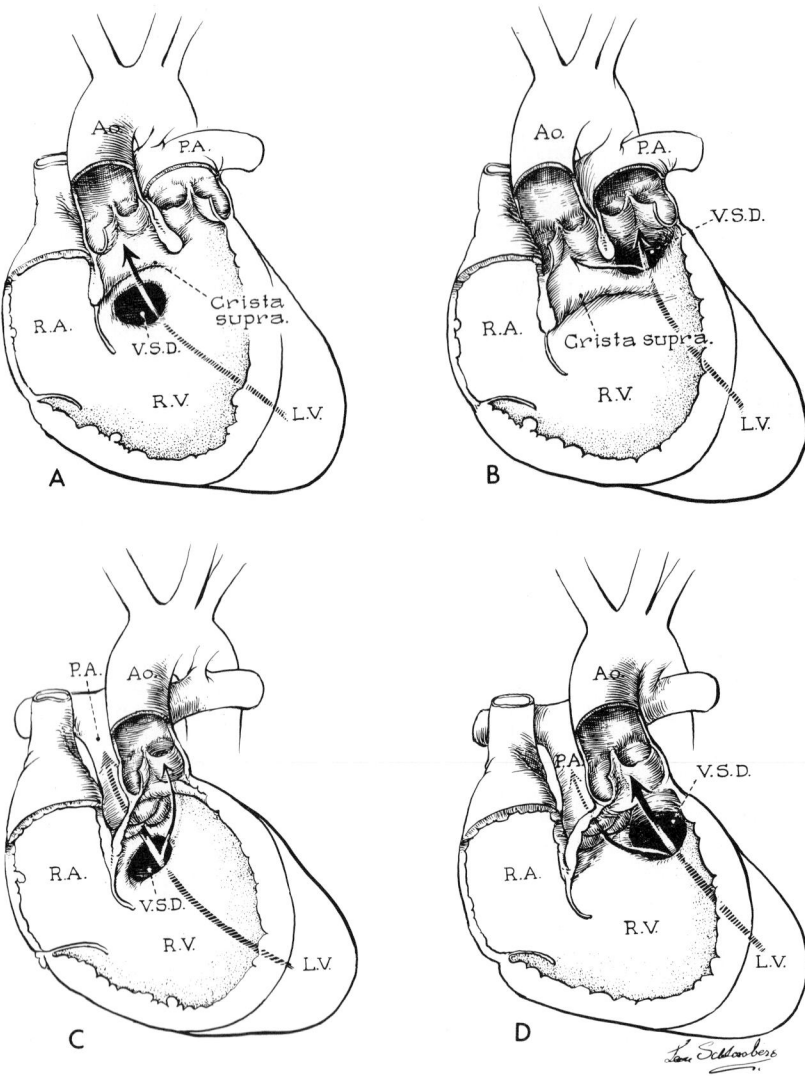

Figure 1. Diagrammatic representation of four different types of double outlet right ventricle based upon the interrelationship of the great arteries and the position of the ventricular septal defect (V.S.D.). *A,* Double outlet right ventricle with normally related great arteries and a posterior or subaortic V.S.D. *B,* Double outlet right ventricle with normally related great arteries and an anterior or subpulmonic V.S.D. *C,* Double outlet right ventricle with abnormally related great arteries and a posterior V.S.D. which, in this situation, is subpulmonic. *D,* Double outlet right ventricle with abnormally related great arteries and an anterior or subaortic V.S.D. (R.A. = Right atrium. R.V. = Right ventricle. L.V. = Left ventricle. Ao. = Aorta. P.A. = Pulmonary artery.)

it is anteriorly located (Fig. 1*B*). Usually the ventricular defect is supracristal in this anatomical combination, which is similar to that in the original Taussig-Bing heart.[21] If the great arteries are abnormally related (aorta on the left or anterior), the relationship is reversed and posterior ventricular septal defects are predominantly subpulmonic and anterior septal defects are subaortic (Figs. 1*C* and *D*). The relationship of the great arteries to the ventricular septal defect can also influence the presence and severity of desaturation of systemic arterial blood (Fig. 1).[20] When the septal defect is subaortic, the most direct pathway for ejected oxygenated left ventricular blood is through the defect and into the aorta. Desaturated blood ejected from the right ventricle is directed into the pulmonary artery. Thus, there may be little or no mixing of ventricular blood and, therefore, no peripheral desaturation unless pulmonary stenosis or increased pulmonary vascular resistance also exists. The patient with double outlet right ventricle may be severely cyanotic even in the absence of pulmonary stenosis or

elevated pulmonary vascular resistance when the ventricular septal defect is subpulmonic.

With the atria and ventricles in situs solitus, the great arteries normally related, and the ventricular septal defect subaortic, it is usually possible to construct an intraventricular tunnel that will close the interventricular communication and direct blood from the left ventricle to the aorta (Figs. 2, 3, and 4).[2, 3, 6, 7, 11, 13, 14, 22] Repair would differ in patients with situs solitus of the atria and ventricles, normally related great vessels, and a ventricular septal defect that is anterior or subpulmonic in position. In this situation, repair might be accomplished by constructing an intraventricular tunnel that would close the interventricular communication and divert blood from the left ventricle to the pulmonary artery, creating a hemodynamic situation similar to complete transposition of the great arteries. An intra-atrial baffle (Mustard procedure) would then be constructed to divert systemic venous return to the left ventricle and pulmonary venous return to the right ventricle, thereby

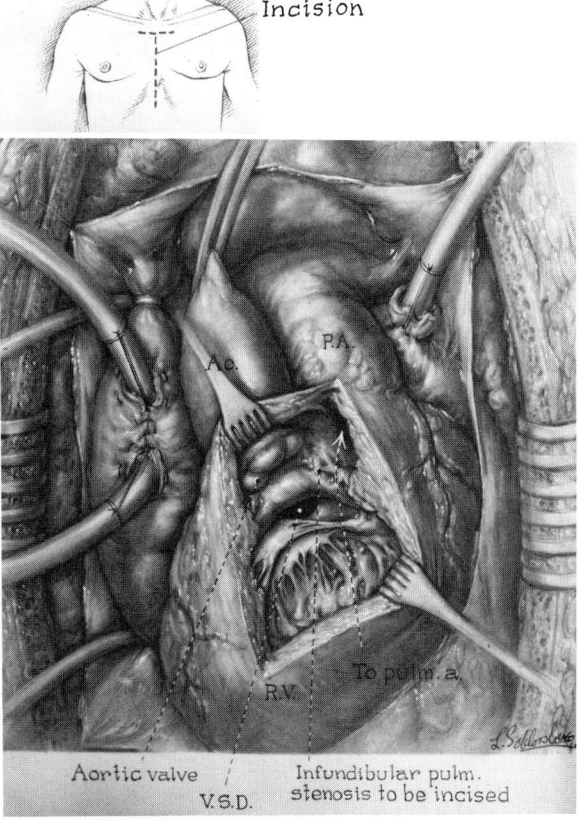

Figure 2. Drawing showing an early stage in the intracardiac repair of a patient with double outlet right ventricle. The great arteries are normally related, the ventricular septal defect (V.S.D.) is subaortic, and there is associated infundibular pulmonary stenosis and dextrocardia. (Ao. = Aorta. P.A. = Pulmonary artery. R.V. = Right ventricle.) (By permission of H. T. Bahnson.)

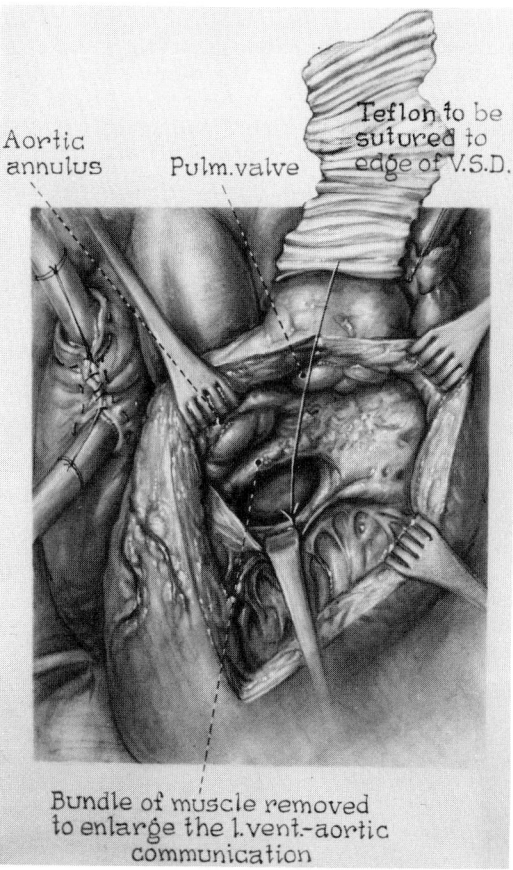

Figure 3. Drawing showing another stage in the intracardiac repair of a patient with double outlet right ventricle. Here the infundibular pulmonary stenosis has been excised and muscle has been removed from the superior rim of the ventricular septal defect (V.S.D.) in order to enlarge the outlet of the left ventricle and prevent subaortic stenosis. (By permission of H. T. Bahnson.)

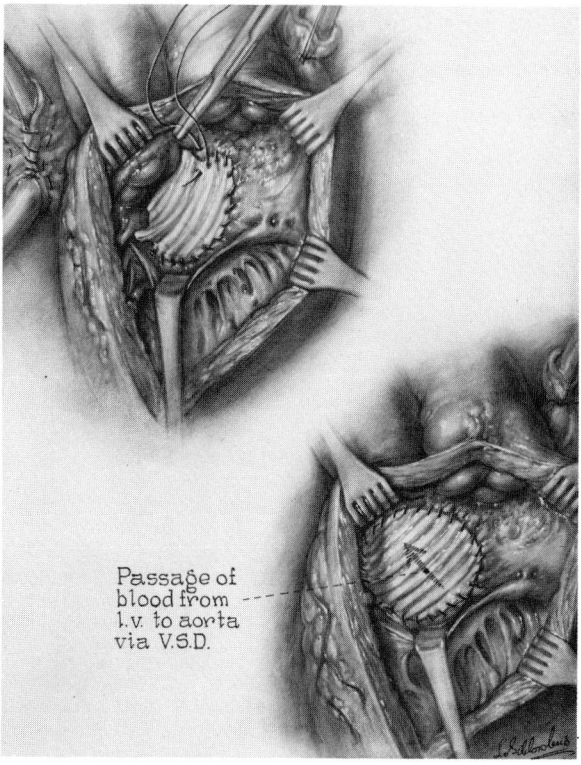

Figure 4. Drawing showing one of the final stages in the intracardiac repair of a patient with double outlet right ventricle. The Teflon patch has been placed so as to close the ventricular septal defect (V.S.D.) and direct blood from the left ventricle (L.V.) to the aorta. (By permission of H. T. Bahnson.)

restoring a normal circulation. Successful repair has been reported in patients with double outlet right ventricle, situs solitus of the atria and ventricles, and abnormally related or transposed great vessels.[1,5,12,21,25] In some of these patients with a subpulmonic ventricular septal defect, it is possible to construct an intraventricular conduit that closes the ventricular septal defect and diverts blood from the left ventricle to the aorta.[21] In other patients with double outlet right ventricle of this type, it will be preferable to construct a tunnel that closes the subpulmonic ventricular septal defect and diverts blood from the left ventricle into the pulmonary artery, thus creating a condition similar to complete transposition of the great arteries. Venous return can then be transposed by means of a Mustard procedure.[5] In patients with double outlet right ventricle, situs solitus of the atria and ventricles, abnormally related great vessels, and a subaortic ventricular septal defect, closure of the ventricular septal defect with a prosthetic patch that diverts blood from the left ventricle into the transposed aorta has been relatively easy because of the subaortic position of the ventricular septal defect (Fig. 5).[1,12,25] Surgical repair in patients with double outlet right ventricle,

situs solitus of the viscera and atria, situs inversus of the ventricles, and abnormally related great vessels has also been reported.[8] All such patients have had associated dextrocardia and pulmonic stenosis.

Pulmonary stenosis, when it exists with any of the various forms of double outlet right ventricle, must be relieved by employing one or a combination of the following: pulmonary valvotomy, infundibular resection, enlargement of the subpulmonary infundibulum with pericardium or prosthetic material, or insertion of a valve-containing tubular prosthesis between the pulmonary artery and the ventricle receiving systemic venous blood.[7]

From the foregoing discussion it follows that biplane angiocardiography is necessary to confirm the diagnosis of double outlet right ventricle and define precisely the anatomy in a patient whose clinical features are compatible with double outlet right ventricle. Particular attention should be given the position of the atria and ventricles, the relationship of the great arteries to one another and to the ventricular septal defect, the anatomy of the atrioventricular valves, and the possible existence and type of pulmonary stenosis. In the absence of pulmonary stenosis, recommendation

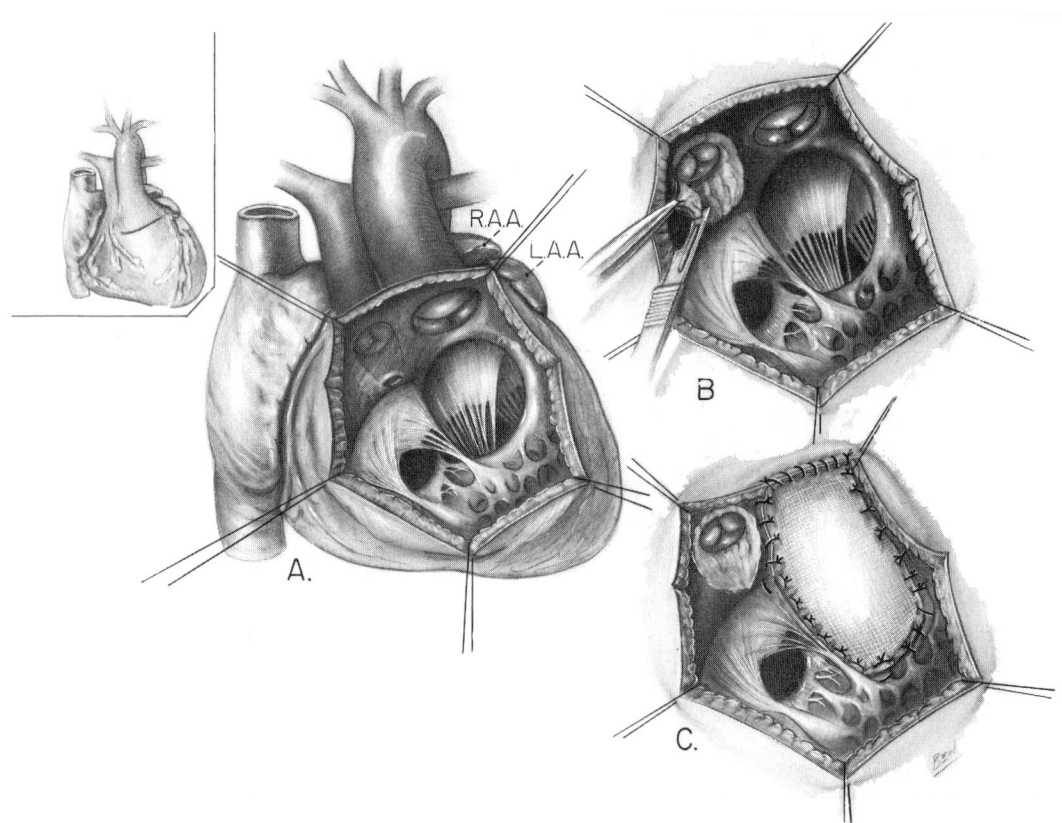

Figure 5. Drawing showing stages in the intracardiac repair of a patient with double outlet right ventricle, abnormally related great arteries, subaortic (anterior) ventricular septal defect, and associated subvalvular pulmonary stenosis and juxtaposition of the atrial appendages to the left of the midline. *A*, Intracardiac anatomy as viewed through a cutaway of the anterior wall of the right ventricle. *B*, Excision of muscle producing subvalvular pulmonary stenosis. *C*, The ventricular septal defect has been closed with a Teflon patch that diverts blood from the left ventricle into the transposed aorta. (From Danielson, G. K., Ritter, D. G., Coleman, H. N., III, and DuShane, J. W.: Successful repair of double-outlet right ventricle with transposition of the great arteries (aorta anterior and to the left), pulmonary stenosis, and subaortic ventricular septal defect. J. Thorac. Cardiovasc. Surg., *63*:741, 1972.)

for repair must be based upon calculated pulmonary vascular resistance, since operative mortality is increased when pulmonary hypertension is present.[3] The optimum time for intracardiac repair of double outlet right ventricle is approximately 5 years of age.[2, 7] If a prosthetic conduit containing a valve is to be used in the reconstruction, operation is preferably delayed until a conduit of adult size can be employed. Rapidly increasing pulmonary hypertension or severe cyanosis may necessitate surgical intervention in patients less than 5 years of age, and the decision to employ intracardiac repair or a palliative procedure such as a systemic pulmonary artery shunt or pulmonary artery banding will depend upon the specific anatomy of the double outlet right ventricle and the reconstructive procedure required in an individual patient.

SELECTED REFERENCES

Hallerman, F. J., Kincaid, O. W., Ritter, D. G., Ongley, P. A., and Titus, J. L.: Angiocardiographic and anatomic findings in origin of both great arteries from the right ventricle. Am. J. Roentgenol., *109*:51, 1970

This is an excellent article which discusses and illustrates the anatomy and angiographic manifestations of various forms of double outlet right ventricle. It is particularly helpful for the student, since it clearly defines a number of specific terms used in the description of various congenital cardiac anomalies, including double outlet right ventricle. It will also be helpful to those who are more experienced with cardiovascular disease because of the numerous pictures of angiograms that demonstrate anatomic features necessary for the diagnosis of double outlet right ventricle and several of the anatomic variations that can be present in this anomaly.

Kirklin, J. W., Kouchoukos, N. T., Bargeron, L. M., Jr., and Barcia, A: Double-outlet right ventricle (origin of both great arteries from right ventricle) with abnormally interrelated great arteries: Anatomic, diagnostic, and surgical considerations. *In* Kidd, B. S. L., and Keith, J. D. (Eds.): The Natural History and Progress in Treatment of Congenital Heart Defects. Springfield, Ill., Charles C Thomas, Publisher, 1971.

These authors have had extensive experience with the operative management of double outlet right ventricle, which they review concisely. Of particular interest is the section devoted to preoperative evaluation and planning of the operation and another section entitled "Surgical Strategy." The chapter also discusses operative repair of patients with double outlet right ventricle complicated by ventricular inversion and illustrates the technique for repair of these very complicated congenital heart defects.

Neufeld, H. N., Lucas, R. V., Jr., Lester, R. G., Adams, P., Jr., Anderson, R. C., and Edwards, J. E.: Origin of both great vessels from the right ventricle without pulmonary stenosis. Br. Heart J., *24*:393, 1962.

In this article the authors present clinical, hemodynamic, roentgenographic, and anatomic features in patients with double outlet right ventricle without pulmonary stenosis. They put forth a classification based upon the anatomical position of the ventricular septal defect. Of particular interest is their discussion of the pathways for blood flow in patients with the different types of double outlet right ventricle. They suggest that the position of the ventricular septal defect and its relationship to the great arteries can be important in determining whether or not cyanosis exists. Despite the existence of a large ventricular septal defect, complete mixing of ventricular blood may not occur because of a streaming of blood during ventricular ejection, which tends to direct blood from one ventricle into the pulmonary artery and blood from the other ventricle into the aorta.

Witham, A. C.: Double outlet right ventricle: A partial transposition complex. Am. Heart J., *53*:928, 1957.

This article is of special importance historically, since it is one of the earliest reports which stimulated clinical interest in patients with double outlet right ventricle. Four cases of double outlet right ventricle are described and divided into two groups, depending upon the presence or absence of pulmonary stenosis. One group is labeled the "Eisenmenger" type, since the clinical picture in these

patients was one of a slowly developing cyanosis due to a progressive increase in pulmonary vascular resistance and pulmonary hypertension. The second group is called the "Fallot" type, since these patients had clinical characteristics similar to patients with tetralogy of Fallot due to various degrees of pulmonary stenosis.

REFERENCES

1. Danielson, G. K., Ritter, D. G., Coleman, H. N., III, and DuShane, J. W.: Successful repair of double-outlet right ventricle with transposition of the great arteries (aorta anterior and to the left), pulmonary stenosis, and subaortic ventricular septal defect. J. Thorac. Cardiovasc. Surg., *63*:741, 1972.
2. Gomes, M. M. R., Weidman, W. H., McGoon, D. C., and Danielson, G. K.: Double-outlet right ventricle with pulmonic stenosis: Surgical considerations and results of operation. Circulation, *43*:889, 1971.
3. Gomes, M. M. R., Weidman, W. H., McGoon, D. C., and Danielson, G. K.: Double-outlet right ventricle without pulmonic stenosis: Surgical considerations and results of operation. Circulation, *43* and *44* (Suppl. I):31, 1971.
4. Hallerman, F. J., Kincaid, O. W., Ritter, D. G., Ongley, P. A., and Titus, J. L.: Angiocardiographic and anatomic findings in origin of both great arteries from the right ventricle. Am. J. Roentgenol., *109*:51, 1970.
5. Hightower, B. M., Barcia, A., Bargeron, L. M., Jr., and Kirklin, J. W.: Double-outlet right ventricle with transposed great arteries and subpulmonary ventricular septal defect. Circulation, *39* and *40* (Suppl. I):207, 1969.
6. Kirklin, J. W., Harp, R. A., and McGoon, D. C.: Surgical treatment of origin of both vessels from right ventricle, including cases of pulmonary stenosis. J. Thorac. Cardiovasc. Surg., *48*:1026, 1964.
7. Kirklin, J. W., Kouchoukos, N. T., Bargeron, L. M., Jr., and Barcia, A: Double-outlet right ventricle (origin of both great arteries from right ventricle) with abnormally interrelated great arteries: Anatomic, diagnostic, and surgical considerations. *In* Kidd, B. S. L., and Keith, J. D. (Eds.): The Natural History and Progress in Treatment of Congenital Heart Defects. Springfield, Ill., Charles C Thomas, Publisher, 1971.
8. Kiser, J. C., Ongley, P. A., Kirklin, J. W., Clarkson, P. M., and McGoon, D. C.: Surgical treatment of dextrocardia with inversion of ventricles and double-outlet right ventricle. J. Thorac. Cardiovasc. Surg., *55*:6, 1968.
9. Krongrad, E., Ritter, D. G., Weidman, W. H., and DuShane, J. W.: Hemodynamic and anatomic correlation of electrocardiogram in double-outlet right ventricle. Circulation, *46*:995, 1972.
10. Lev, M., Bharati, S., Meng, C. C. L., Liberthson, R. R., Paul, M. H., and Idriss, F.: A concept of double-outlet right ventricle. J. Thorac. Cardiovasc. Surg., *64*:271, 1972.
11. Levy, M. J., DeWall, R., Elliott, L. P., and Cuello, L.: Origin of both great arteries from the right ventricle and pulmonary stenosis: Apropos case successfully corrected. Dis. Chest, *42*:372, 1962.
12. Lincoln, C.: Total correction of d-loop double-outlet right ventricle with bilateral conus, α-transposition, and pulmonic stenosis. J. Thorac. Cardiovasc. Surg., *64*:435, 1972.
13. Mason, D. T., Morrow, A. G., Elkins, R. C., and Friedman, W. F.: Origin of both great vessels from the right ventricle associated with severe obstruction to left ventricular outflow. Am. J. Cardiol., *24*:118, 1969.
14. McGoon, D. C.: Origin of both great vessels from the right ventricle. Surg. Clin. North Am., *41*:1113, 1961.
15. Megarity, A. L., Chambers, R. G., Calder, A. L., Van Praagh, S., and Van Praagh, R.: Double-outlet right ventricle with left ventricular-right atrial communication: Fibrous obstruction of left ventricular outlet by membranous septum and tricuspid leaflet tissue. Am. Heart J., *84*:242, 1972.
16. Mehrizi, A.: The origin of both great vessels from the right ventricle: I. With pulmonic stenosis. II. Without pulmonic stenosis. Johns Hopkins Med. J., *117*:75, 1965.
17. Mirowski, M., Mehrizi, A., and Taussig, H. B.: The electrocardiogram in patients with both great vessels arising from the right ventricle combined with pulmonary stenosis: An analysis of 22 cases with special reference to the differential diagnosis from the tetralogy of Fallot. Circulation, *28*:1116, 1963.
18. Neufeld, H. N., DuShane, J. W., and Edwards, J. E.: Origin of both great vessels from the right ventricle—II. With pulmonary stenosis. Circulation, *23*:603, 1961.

19. Neufeld, H. N., DuShane, J. W., Wood, E. H., Kirklin, J. W., and Edwards, J. E.: Origin of both great vessels from the right ventricle – I. Without pulmonary stenosis. Circulation, 23:399, 1961.

20. Neufeld, H. N., Lucas, R. V., Jr., Lester, R. G., Adams, P., Jr., Anderson, R. C., and Edwards, J. E.: Origin of both great vessels from the right ventricle without pulmonary stenosis. Br. Heart J., 24:393, 1962.

21. Patrick, D. L., and McGoon, D. C.: An operation for double-outlet right ventricle with transposition of the great arteries. J. Cardiovasc. Surg., 9:537, 1968.

22. Redo, S. F., Engle, M. A., Holswade, G. R., and Goldberg, H. P.: Operative correction of ventricular septal defect with origin of both great vessels from the right ventricle. J. Thorac. Cardiovasc. Surg., 45:526, 1963.

23. Roberts, W. C., Eggleston, J. C., and Humphries, J. O.: Complex congenital cardiac malformation: Corrected transposition, origin of both great vessels from the anatomic right ventricle, common ventricle, and dextroversion. Johns Hopkins Med. J., 120:155, 1967.

24. Sridaromont, S., Feldt, R. H., Ritter, D. G., Davis, G. D., McGoon, D. C., and Edwards, J. E.: Double-outlet right ventricle associated with persistent common atrioventricular canal. Circulation, 52:933, 1975.

25. Van Praagh, R., Perez-Trevino, C., Reynolds, J. L., Moes, C. A. F., Keith, J. D., Roy, D. L., Belcourt, C., Weinberg, P. M., and Parisi, L. F.: Double outlet right ventricle (S,D,L) with subaortic ventricular septal defect and pulmonary stenosis: Report of six cases. Am. J. Cardiol., 35:42, 1975.

26. Venables, A. W., and Campbell, P. E.: Double outlet right ventricle: A review of 16 cases with 10 necropsy specimens. Br. Heart J., 28:461, 1966.

27. Witham, A. C.: Double outlet right ventricle: A partial transposition complex. Am. Heart J., 53:928, 1957.

IX

TRICUSPID ATRESIA

Harvey W. Bender, Jr., M.D.

Tricuspid atresia consists of atresia of the right atrioventricular (tricuspid) valve, varying degrees of hypoplasia of the right ventricle and infundibulum, and a defect in the atrial septum. In addition to the above abnormalities, the great arteries may be transposed, there may be a ventricular septal defect, and there may or may not be stenosis of the pulmonary outflow tract.

Tricuspid atresia accounts for 1 to 5 per cent of all congenital heart defects. The embryologic events that are altered to produce this complex are unknown. Two alternative explanations are offered.[3] The first explanation is that a differential growth rate occurs between the ventricle and bulbus cordis, with subsequent failure of adequate development of the right ventricle; tricuspid atresia is thus a secondary event. The second possible etiologic mechanism is that the atrioventricular orifice fails to migrate from its initial position overlying the future left ventricle.

Various classifications for the spectrum of abnormalities found in tricuspid atresia are currently being used. An anatomic-pathologic classification proposed by Tandon and Edwards[4] is based primarily on the relationships of the great arteries to the ventricles and secondarily on the presence or absence of obstruction to pulmonary blood flow. A clinical anatomic classification has been proposed by Rudolph.[3] Each of Rudolph's three classes has a characteristic clinical presentation. In Group I, tricuspid atresia with intact ventricular septum and hypoplastic right ventricle, infants present with hypoxemia and acidemia. Pulmonary blood flow is dependent on the presence of a patent ductus arteriosus. All systemic and pulmonary venous returns mix in the atria. The degree of cyanosis in these infants depends primarily on the size and patency of the ductus arteriosus and the ratio of systemic to pulmonary vascular resistance. In Group II, tricuspid atresia with ventricular septal defect and normally related great arteries, cyanosis occurs during the first few days of life and is then accompanied by left ventricular failure and pulmonary edema as pulmonary vascular resistance falls. Congestive heart failure develops in this group of infants within the first two to three weeks of life. In Group III, tricuspid atresia with ventricular septal defect and transposed great arteries, the infant may present with only mild cyanosis. However, the hypoplastic right (or systemic) ventricle will be unable to sustain an adequate cardiac output if there is no stenosis of the pulmonary outflow tract.

All treatment for infants with tricuspid atresia has been considered palliative. In the cyanotic infant augmentation of pulmonary blood flow is required. This is accomplished by one of three types of shunts – aortopulmonary artery shunts, subclavian to pulmonary artery shunts, or superior vena cava to pulmonary artery shunts. Few infants in Rudolph's Group I survive the first six months without treatment; in addition, operative mortality rates of 23 to 44 per cent in this group of infants have been reported. On the other hand, after the age of six months, palliative operations have a lower operative mortality (7.4 per cent), and the long-term results have been good, with 50 per cent survival reported at 15 years of age.[6]

The various types of systemic-pulmonary shunts are associated with their certain complications and results. A Potts descending aorta to left pulmonary artery shunt offers the most certain increase in pulmonary blood flow, but the anastomosis tends to grow with the child, thereby increasing the amount of pulmonary blood flow and increasing the likelihood of developing elevated pulmonary vascular resistance. The Waterston ascending aorta to right pulmonary artery shunt gives good palliation and appears to grow with the child but does not enlarge to the degree that the Potts shunt enlarges. The Blalock-Taussig subclavian artery to pulmonary artery shunt has not been used often in the very young infant but is excellent palliation for the older infant (> 6 months) or as a second palliative procedure. The Glenn operation (superior vena cava to pulmonary artery shunt) has demonstrated satisfactory relief of hypoxemia for five to seven years, but the patient may require a second shunting procedure.[2]

In those infants in Rudolph's Group II and Group III

with increased pulmonary blood flow, medical management with digitalis and diuretics should be undertaken. If this treatment regimen fails, banding of the pulmonary artery may be necessary. In all groups, a large interatrial communication is necessary. If a large ASD is not present, a balloon atrial septostomy or Blalock-Hanlon atrial septectomy is required.

In 1971 Fontan and Baudet[1] reported a new procedure to correct patients with tricuspid atresia. In this procedure, all systemic venous return is diverted through a valve-containing conduit to the lungs, and closure of the interatrial communication allows only arterialized pulmonary venous blood to return to the left atrium (Fig. 1). To prevent right atrial blood refluxing into the inferior vena cava during atrial systole, an aortic valve homograft was placed at the junction of inferior vena cava and right atrium. Obviously this procedure is only possible when the pulmonary vascular resistance is low.

This procedure as described by Fontan[1] and modified by others[5] has been performed on a relatively small number of patients. The early results have been encouraging, although the long-term effect of elevated systemic venous pressure is not known. The surgeon must bear in mind that this too is a palliative procedure and will have to be compared with the long-term results obtained with systemic-pulmonary artery shunts.

SELECTED REFERENCES

Fontan, F., and Baudet, E.: Surgical repair of tricuspid atresia. Thorax, 26:240–248, 1971.
This is the first published report of attempts to correct tricuspid atresia; two of three patients survived. The details of the operation and indications for its applicability to older children who have received shunts are discussed.

Rudolph, A. M.: Congenital diseases of the heart. Chicago, Year Book Medical Publishers, 1974, pp. 424–461.
This monograph is a personal approach to understanding the physiology and clinical presentation of a variety of congenital cardiac defects. The natural history of tricuspid atresia, progressive changes in the hemodynamics of the circulatory system, and types of operative and nonoperative treatment are clearly discussed.

Walker, D. R., Sbokos, C. G., and Lennox, S. C.: Correction of tricuspid atresia. Br. Heart J., 37:282–286, 1975.
All reports of the Fontan operation to correct tricuspid atresia are reviewed in this paper. In addition, the authors present two patients of their own. The criteria for patient selection, long-term complications of arrhythmias, homograft failure, and hepatic dysfunction are also discussed. A description of the operative procedure is included.

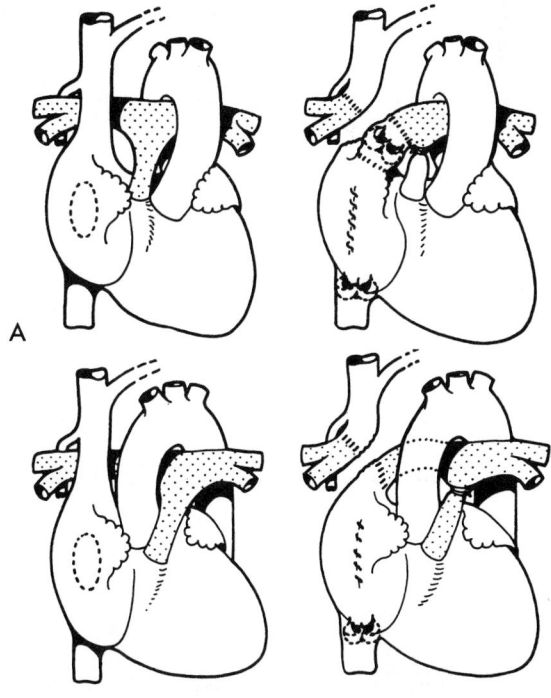

A

B

Figure 1. *A,* Fontan's operation consists of the construction of an end-to-side superior vena cava–to–right pulmonary artery anastomosis and an anastomosis between the right atrial appendage and the proximal stump of the right pulmonary artery, with interposition of a segment of aortic allograft with intact valve. The patient is then placed on cardiopulmonary bypass, the right atrium is opened, the interatrial communication closed, and a pulmonary valve allograft inserted into the inferior vena cava. The main pulmonary artery is ligated and bypass is discontinued. The last step of the procedure is division of the superior vena cava below the pulmonary anastomosis and suture closure of the two ends. *B,* In one patient, the same procedure was performed, but no allograft was used at the atrium–to–pulmonary artery anastomosis. (From Sade, R. M., and Castaneda, A. R. *In* Sabiston, D. C., Jr., and Spencer, F. C. (Eds.): Gibbon's Surgery of the Chest, 3rd ed. Philadelphia, W. B. Saunders Company, 1976. Reproduced with permission from Fontan and Baudet, 1971.)

REFERENCES

1. Fontan, F., and Baudet, E.: Surgical repair of tricuspid atresia. Thorax, 26:240–248, 1971.
2. Mathur, M., and Glenn, W. W. L.: Long-term evaluation of cava-pulmonary artery anastomosis. Surgery, 53:899–916, 1973.
3. Rudolph, A. M.: Congenital Diseases of the Heart. Chicago, Year Book Medical Publishers, 1974, pp. 424–461.
4. Tandon, R., and Edwards, J. E.: Tricuspid atresia: A re-evaluation and classification. J. Thorac. Cardiovasc. Surg., 47:531–542, 1974.
5. Walker, D. R., Sbokos, C. G., and Lennox, S. C.: Correction of tricuspid atresia. Br. Heart J., 37:282–286, 1975.
6. Williams, W. G., Rubis, L, Trusler, G. A., and Mustard, W. T.: Palliation of tricuspid atresia. Arch. Surg., 110:1383, 1975.

X _____

TRUNCUS ARTERIOSUS

Robert B. Wallace, M.D.

HISTORICAL ASPECTS

Persistent truncus arteriosus is a fascinating congenital cardiac malformation comprising between 1 and 4 per cent of congenital cardiac defects in autopsy series. The condition is characterized by a single arterial vessel arising from the heart, receiving blood from both ventricles, and supplying blood to the aorta, lungs, and coronary arteries. The pathologic anatomy was first described by Taruffi in 1875.[18] In 1949, Collett and Edwards[4] classified the defect according to anatomic types, which is the basis for the surgical classification used today. In 1965 Van Praagh and Van Praagh[19] classified truncus arteriosus and termed it "common aorticopulmonary trunk." Although their classification more clearly defines the condition in relation to its embryology, it is not a practical surgical classification.

In 1968, McGoon et al.[11] reported the first successful repair of truncus arteriosus. They employed a technique, based on the experimental work of Rastelli and co-workers,[15] in which a conduit consisting of a homograft of the ascending aorta and aortic valve was used to construct a pulmonary artery. Subsequently, Bowman et al.[3] suggested that a Dacron graft containing a porcine valve be used as the preferred conduit. Minor modifications of this technique have resulted in the current definitive treatment for truncus arteriosus.

ANATOMY AND CLASSIFICATION

Truncus arteriosus is due to a lack of partitioning of the embryonic conus during the first few weeks of fetal development and is almost always associated with a ventricular septal defect. Collett and Edwards[4] classified truncus arteriosus into four types, based on the origin of the pulmonary arteries (Fig. 1). In *type I,* a single arterial trunk gives rise to the aorta and main pulmonary artery. In *type II,* the right and left pulmonary arteries arise immediately adjacent to one another from the dorsal wall of the truncus. In *type III,* the right and left pulmonary arteries arise from either side of the truncus, and in *type IV,* the proximal pulmonary arteries are absent and pulmonary blood flow is by way of bronchial arteries. Types I and II comprised 76 per cent of Collett and Edwards' series, and type III, 13 per cent. Currently, types II and III are grouped together. Type IV, in which there are no pulmonary artery trunks, more appropriately should be considered a severe form of tetralogy of Fallot with absence of the pulmonary trunks. Thus, for practical purposes, all cases of truncus arteriosus may be classified as either type I or II of the Collett and Edwards' classification.

A ventricular septal defect immediately beneath the truncal valve has been present in all patients with truncus arteriosus except the two reported by Van Praagh and Van Praagh[19] (Fig. 2). The truncus most commonly overrides the ventricular septum or arises entirely from the right ventricle and only rarely arises to the left of the plane of the septum. Collett and Edwards[4] reported a 25 per cent incidence of common ventricle, although this was not present in any of Van Praagh and Van Praagh's series and in only one of the 180 specimens studied by Bharati et al.[1]

The truncal valve has from two to six cusps, although most valves have three cusps. Four cusps have been noted in about 25 per cent of valves and two cusps in about 5 per cent. Mair et al.[9] noted some truncal valve incompetence in 25 of 70 patients studied; however, the incompetence was considered severe in only four. The aortic arch is to the right in about 20 per cent of patients with truncus arteriosus, and an interruption of the aortic arch occurs in 10 to 15 per cent.

The left or right pulmonary artery was absent in 2 per cent of Van Praagh and Van Praagh's series and in 4.5 per cent of Bharati and associates' series; however, Mair et al.[9] noted absence of one of the pulmonary arteries in 16 per cent of their clinical series. Other defects of surgical significance occurring with truncus arteriosus include patent ductus arteriosus in 15 to 30 per cent, persistent left superior vena cava in 10 to 15 per cent, and an atrial septal defect in 20 per cent.

The pathologic changes that may occur in the pul-

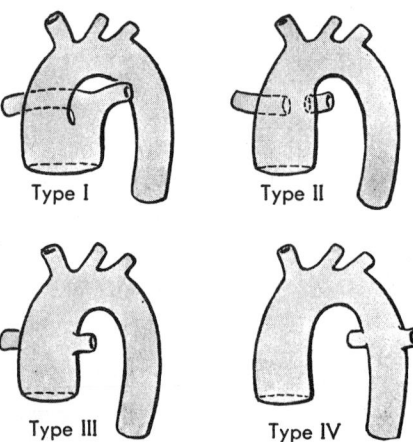

Figure 1. Anatomic types of truncus arteriosus, Collett and Edwards' classification. (From Keith, J. D., Rowe, R. D., and Vlad, P.: Heart Disease in Infancy and Childhood. New York, Macmillan Company, 1958, p. 521. By permission.)

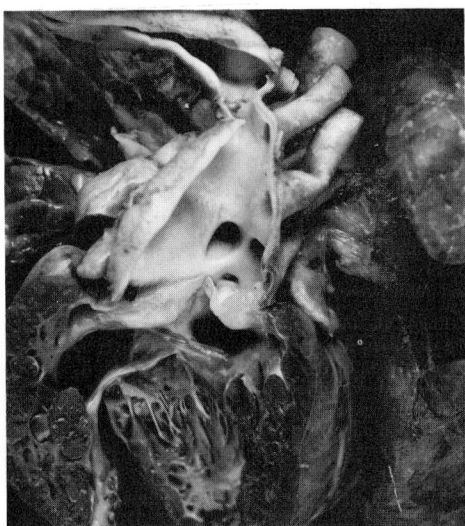

Figure 2. Pathologic specimen of type II truncus arteriosus. Right and left pulmonary arteries arise from left dorsal aspect of truncus. High ventricular septal defect is seen immediately below truncal valve. (From Wallace, R. B.: Truncus arteriosus. *In* Sabiston, D. C., Jr., and Spencer, F. C. (Eds.): Gibbon's Surgery of the Chest, 3rd ed. Philadelphia, W. B. Saunders Company, 1976.)

monary vasculature are similar to those of other conditions in which a high-pressure, left-to-right shunt produces pulmonary vascular obstructive disease, as described by Heath and Edwards.[7]

HEMODYNAMICS

All of the blood from both the left and right ventricles is ejected into the truncus arteriosus. The systemic and pulmonary venous blood mixes, and the degree of arterial oxygen unsaturation is dependent on the amount of pulmonary blood flow. Pulmonary blood flow may be limited by stenosis of the pulmonary arteries, but this is uncommon. In most instances, pulmonary blood flow (and thus arterial oxygen saturation) is determined by the resistance to flow in the pulmonary vascular bed. As with isolated ventricular septal defect, the pulmonary vascular bed in truncus arteriosus is exposed to high flow at systemic pressure—conditions that may lead to progressive changes of pulmonary vascular obstructive disease. Mair et al.[9] noted a high correlation between pulmonary vascular resistance and arterial oxygen saturation in truncus arteriosus. In their series, patients with two pulmonary arteries and no pulmonary stenosis who had an arterial oxygen saturation less than 85 per cent usually had a pronounced increase in pulmonary vascular resistance and advanced pulmonary vascular obstructive disease.

PROGNOSIS

Most patients with persistent truncus arteriosus die in early infancy from congestive heart failure. Only

three patients in Van Praagh and Van Praagh's autopsy series of 57 cases lived beyond six months of age. In Keith and associates'[8] review of 89 patients, 22 per cent survived beyond six months of age and 10 survived to the second or third decade. The causes of death for those who survived the first two years of life were generally related to pulmonary vascular obstructive disease and decreased pulmonary blood flow.

SYMPTOMS AND DIAGNOSIS

The symptoms associated with truncus arteriosus are related primarily to the amount of pulmonary blood flow. During the first few weeks of life, when pulmonary vascular resistance is normally increased, symptoms are usually absent, unless there is associated significant truncal valve incompetence.[5] With maturation of the fetal pulmonary vascular bed associated with a decrease in pulmonary vascular resistance and an increase in pulmonary blood flow, symptoms of congestive heart failure may develop. These include dyspnea, excessive perspiration, and failure to thrive. Cyanosis is not usually apparent because the arterial oxygen saturation is generally greater than 85 per cent. With the progressive development of pulmonary vascular obstructive disease and the associated decrease in pulmonary blood flow, cyanosis becomes more evident. The condition then resembles tetralogy of Fallot or ventricular septal defect with severe pulmonary vascular obstructive disease.

Physical examination usually reveals a systolic thrill and murmur over the left third and fourth intercostal spaces parasternally. The apical impulse is prominent, and there are signs of cardiomegaly. The second heart sound is single and accentuated. When truncal valve incompetence is present, a diastolic murmur follows the second heart sound.

Chest roentgenography shows cardiomegaly with biventricular enlargement (Fig. 3). The aortic arch is to the right in 20 per cent of patients, and the left pulmonary artery may be elevated from the normal position. The peripheral pulmonary vasculature is increased unless there is advanced pulmonary vascular obstructive disease. The electrocardiogram is nonspecific and usually indicates biventricular hypertrophy.

Right and left heart catheterization and angiocardiographic studies are indicated in all patients suspected of having truncus arteriosus in order to establish the diagnosis, define the anatomy, and determine the pulmonary vascular resistance. Ventricular pressures are equal, and in the absence of pulmonary artery stenosis, there are equal pressures in the ventricles, truncus, and pulmonary arteries. Oxygen saturation studies indicate bidirectional shunting at the ventricular level, the predominant shunt being left to right. Pulmonary flow and resistance should be determined by measurement of pressures and oxygen saturations in both pulmonary arteries. In patients without left or right pulmonary artery, calculations of pulmonary blood flow are complicated by bronchial flow, and thus the amount of this flow must be considered in the calculations.

Angiocardiographic studies for defining the anat-

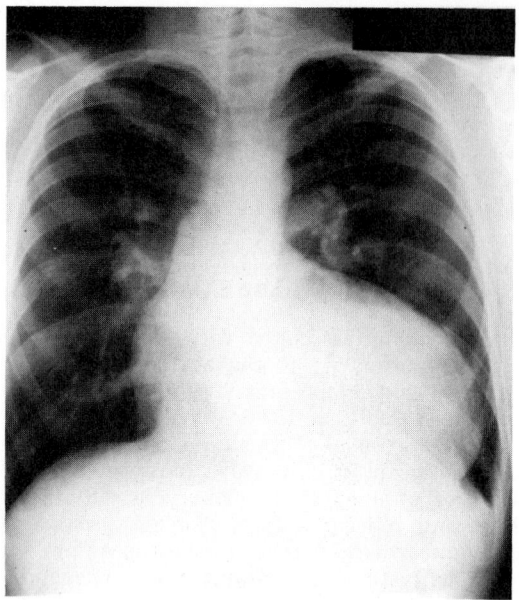

Figure 3. Chest roentgenogram of patient with truncus arteriosus showing cardiomegaly, increased pulmonary vasculature, and elevation of left pulmonary artery relative to right. (From Hallermann, F. J., Kincaid, O. W., Tsakiris, A. G., Ritter, D. G., and Titus, J. L.: Persistent truncus arteriosus: A radiographic and angiocardiographic study. Am. J. Roentgenol., *107*:827, 1969. By permission of Charles C Thomas, Publisher.)

omy require the injection of large amounts of contrast medium.[6] Injection into the right ventricle shows the ventricle to be enlarged and hypertrophied (Fig. 4). The contrast medium outlines the ventricular septal

defect beneath the truncal valve and traverses the defect, filling the left ventricle. Both ventricles eject into a single arterial trunk. Adequate visualization of the pulmonary arteries usually requires an injection into the truncus and also allows assessment of the truncal valve.

TREATMENT AND RESULTS

Medical

Medical therapy is directed at the treatment of congestive heart failure, the prevention of bacterial endocarditis, and in patients with pulmonary vascular obstructive disease, the complications of right-to-left shunts and the associated polycythemia. The high mortality rate in infants with truncus arteriosus attests to the ineffectiveness of medical management in most patients.

Pulmonary Artery Banding

Banding of the pulmonary artery was proposed by Muller and Dammann[12] to decrease pulmonary artery pressure and flow in an attempt to control congestive heart failure and to limit the progression of pulmonary vascular obstructive disease in patients with large left-to-right shunts. This procedure has been used in truncus arteriosus, as reported by Smith et al.,[16] Oldham et al.,[13] and Stark et al.[17] Although the mortality has been high in the reported series, a number of patients have been sucessfully palliated, and this has enabled them to undergo complete repair at a later age.

The procedure is best performed through a median sternotomy so that both the left and right pulmonary

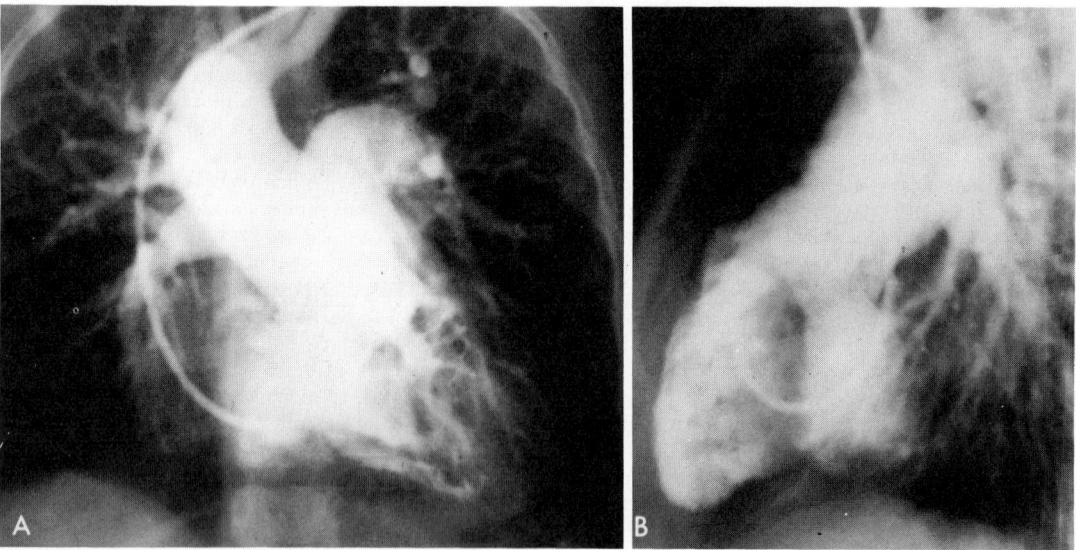

Figure 4. Angiocardiograms. Anteroposterior view (*A*) and left lateral view (*B*) after injection of contrast material into right ventricle. Both ventricles are enlarged; ventricular septal defect is present immediately beneath truncus. Right ventricular infundibulum is absent, and pulmonary arteries arise from truncus. (From Hallermann, F. J., Kincaid, O. W., Tsakiris, A. G., Ritter, D. G., and Titus, J. L.: Persistent truncus arteriosus: A radiographic and angiocardiographic study. Am. J. Roentgenol., *107*:827, 1969. By permission of Charles C Thomas, Publisher.)

arteries might be banded. The band must be fixed to prevent distal migration. If, in type I truncus, the band is placed on the main pulmonary artery, the band should be fixed proximal to the bifurcation in order to prevent disproportionate constriction of the left and right pulmonary arteries.

Systemic-Pulmonary Shunts

Billig et al.[2] have reported good palliation after a systemic-pulmonary shunting procedure. The only indication for a shunt procedure probably is when there is proximal pulmonary artery stenosis producing symptoms of inadequate pulmonary blood flow.

Complete Repair

Technique. The operation is performed through a median sternotomy incision utilizing total cardiopulmonary bypass, moderate hypothermia, and intermittent aortic cross-clamping. Cannulation is through the external iliac or femoral artery. The left ventricle is vented through an apical stab wound (Figs. 5 and 6).

The pulmonary arteries usually can be excised from the truncus as a single segment, even in type II truncus. The incision in the right ventricle is made high in the ventricle in the planned direction of the conduit. The aortic cross-clamp is temporarily released after air has been removed from the aortic root, and the competency of the valve is checked. If incompetence is severe, valve replacement must be considered. A patch is used to close the ventricular septal defect. An appropriate-sized Dacron conduit containing a porcine aortic valve is cut to proper length and is used to

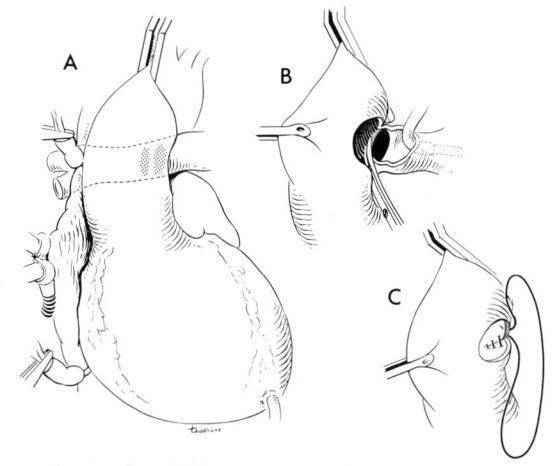

Figure 5. Surgical repair. *A,* Cardiopulmonary bypass, left ventricle vented at apex, aorta cross-clamped. *B,* Origin of pulmonary arteries excised from truncus. *C,* Closure of defect in truncus. (From Wallace, R. B., Rastelli, G. C., Ongley, P. A., Titus, J. L., and McGoon, D. C.: Complete repair of truncus arteriosus defects. J. Thorac. Cardiovasc. Surg., 57:95, 1969. By permission of C. V. Mosby Company.)

establish continuity between the right ventricle and the pulmonary arteries. The course of the conduit should be such that kinking is avoided and the closed sternum does not compress the conduit.

In patients in whom a previous pulmonary artery

Figure 6. Surgical repair (continued). *A,* Incision made high in right ventricle. *B,* Ventricular septal defect closed with Teflon patch. *C,* Dacron graft with porcine valve sutured to pulmonary arteries. *D,* Proximal end of graft anastomosed to right ventricle. (LPA, left pulmonary artery; RPA, right pulmonary artery; VSD, ventricular septal defect; RV, right ventricle.) (From Wallace, R. B.: Truncus arteriosus. *In* Sabiston, D. C., Jr., and Spencer, F. C. (Eds.): Gibbon's Surgery of the Chest, 3rd ed. Philadelphia, W. B. Saunders Company, 1976.)

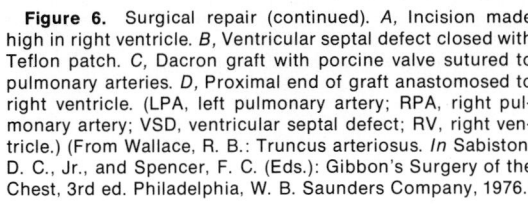
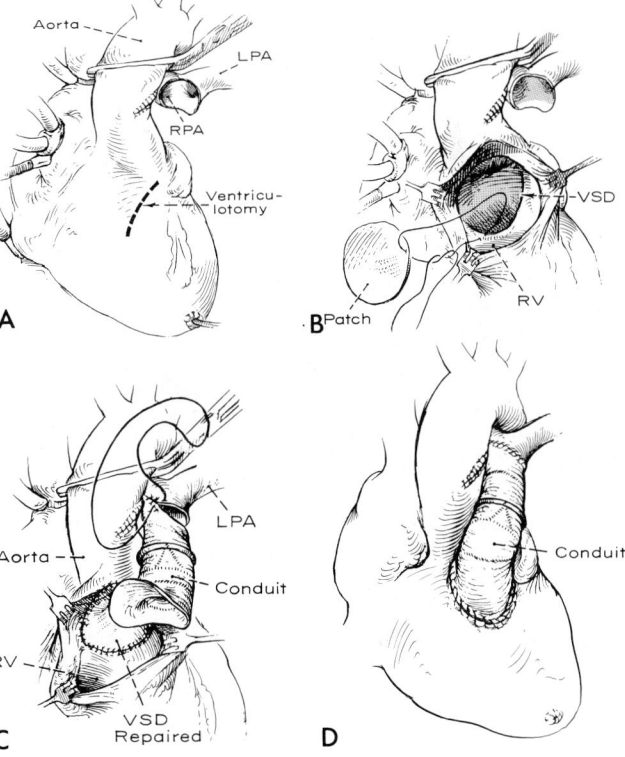

banding has been performed, the pulmonary arteries usually need to be incised to a point distal to the area of banding in order to relieve the stenosis produced by the band.[14] The distal end of the conduit is then tailored to produce an angioplastic enlargement of the pulmonary arteries (Fig. 7).

Results. In a series of 92 patients who underwent complete repair of types I and II truncus arteriosus at the Mayo Clinic from September, 1967, to February, 1975, the operative mortality was 23 per cent.[10] This series included six patients who required truncal valve replacement, two of whom died, and three patients who had an interrupted aortic arch, one of whom died.

The patient's age and the degree of pulmonary vascular resistance were important factors in the operative mortality. Five of six patients who were less than two years old did not survive. Of 13 patients in whom the pulmonary vascular resistance was less than 5 units m², none died, whereas 11 of the 28 patients (39 per cent) in whom the pulmonary vascular resistance was greater than 8 units m² died. Previous banding of the pulmonary arteries (which was done in 25 patients) did not affect operative mortality. There were four early deaths, for an operative mortality of 16 per cent.

During the latter part of the series there was a significant reduction in operative mortality. From September, 1967, to November, 1972, during which time an aortic homograft was used as the conduit, the operative mortality in 59 cases was 34 per cent. From November, 1972, to February, 1975, 33 patients had repair using a Dacron graft–porcine valve conduit, and the operative mortality was 9 per cent. Undoubtedly several factors other than the type of conduit contributed to this reduction in mortality rate.

Late follow-up on the 63 survivors (obtained through April, 1975) varied from 4 to 92 months after repair, with a median follow-up of 36 months. There were six late deaths, and these occurred 2 to 38 months after surgery. All but two of the surviving patients are considered to have good to excellent clinical results.

Calcification has occurred in all of the aortic homograft conduits. Although at follow-up only one patient had required reoperation for replacement of the conduit, other homograft conduits probably will require replacement because of stenosis.

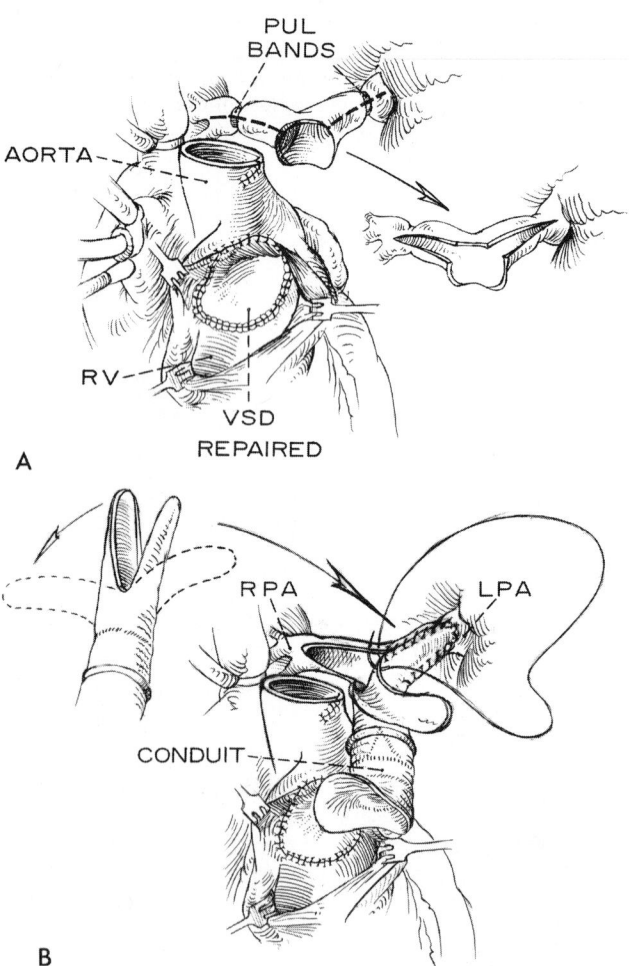

Figure 7. Complete repair with previous pulmonary artery banding. *A,* Pulmonary arteries are incised through areas of banding. *B,* Distal end of conduit tailored to enlarge the pulmonary arteries. *C,* Completed repair. (RV, right ventricle; VSD, ventricular septal defect; RPA, right pulmonary artery; LPA, left pulmonary artery.) (From Parker, R. K., McGoon, D. C., Danielson, G. K., and Wallace, R. B.: Repair of truncus arteriosus in patients with prior banding of the pulmonary artery. Surgery, *78:*761, 1975. By permission of C. V. Mosby Company.)

INDICATIONS FOR OPERATIONS

The definitive treatment of truncus arteriosus is complete repair. Although results of operation are satisfactory in patients more than two years old, the operative mortality has been high in patients less than this age. Palliative banding of the pulmonary artery likewise has had a high mortality. At the present time, the best surgical treatment for infants with truncus arteriosus is not clearly defined. Surgery should be deferred in patients about two years old in whom the symptoms of congestive heart failure can be managed medically and in whom there is no evidence of progressive pulmonary vascular obstructive disease. In infants who cannot be managed medically, the choice is between pulmonary artery banding and complete repair, both procedures being associated with a high mortality in the infant group. It is hoped that the mortality of complete repair in infancy can be reduced and thus make it the procedure of choice.

Operability in cases of pulmonary vascular obstructive disease depends on severity. In patients with both left and right pulmonary arteries, the upper limit of pulmonary vascular resistance for operability is 12 units m²; when the left or right pulmonary artery is absent, the upper limit of pulmonary vascular resistance for operability is 20 units m².

SELECTED REFERENCES

Collett, R. W., and Edwards, J. E.: Persistent truncus arteriosus: A classification according to anatomic types. Surg. Clin. North Am., Aug., 1949, p. 1245.

The anatomy, embryology, and criteria for diagnosis of truncus arteriosus based on 80 cases from the literature and the authors' material were reviewed. The embryologic discussion emphasized the development of the septal system that divides the ventricles, the conus arteriosus, and the truncus arteriosus to form two separate circulations. Two absolute criteria for the pathologic diagnosis of persistent truncus arteriosus were established: (1) that there be only one main arterial trunk leaving the base of the heart and no remnant of an atretic pulmonary trunk or aorta, and (2) that this single arterial trunk supply branches to the coronary, pulmonary, and systemic circulations. An anatomic classification of truncus arteriosus was presented in which four types were identified, the classification being based on the embryologic development of the pulmonary arteries from the sixth aortic arch. In type IV of this classification, the pulmonary blood flow is derived from bronchial arteries, and this type more appropriately should be classified as a severe form of tetralogy of Fallot with absence of the main pulmonary artery.

Hallermann, F. J., Kincaid, O. W., Tsakiris, A. G., Ritter, D. G., and Titus, J. L.: Persistent truncus arteriosus: A radiographic and angiocardiographic study. Am. J. Roentgenol., *107*:827, 1969.

The plain roentgenograms of the thorax and angiocardiograms of 30 patients with truncus arteriosus were reviewed. In all patients, the chest roentgenogram showed cardiac enlargement and signs of biventricular enlargement. A right aortic arch was present in 10 patients, and the left pulmonary artery was elevated, as compared with the right, in 19. The peripheral pulmonary vasculature was increased in 27 of the 30 patients. The authors stressed the importance of using large amounts of contrast medium (1.5 to 2.0 ml. per kg. body weight) in performing angiocardiography in order to define the anatomy accurately. Injection into the right ventricle revealed an enlarged and hypertrophied ventricle in all patients. In the anterior portion of the septum immediately beneath the truncal valve, the right ventricular infundibulum was absent and a large ventricular septal defect was present. Injection of contrast material into the truncus of 21 patients revealed some truncal valve incompetence in 14. Differentiation of types I and II defects, as well as the determination of the number of cusps in the truncal valve, was difficult.

Mair, D. D., Ritter, D. G., Davis, G. D., Wallace, R. B., Danielson, G. K., and McGoon, D. C.: Selection of patients with truncus arteriosus for surgical correction: Anatomic and hemodynamic considerations. Circulation, *49*:144, 1974.

A series of 70 patients with Collett and Edwards' types I and II truncus arteriosus underwent cardiac catheterization at the Mayo Clinic; 40 subsequently underwent surgical correction. Interruption of the aortic arch was present in four patients, three of whom underwent operation. Of the 70 patients, 25 had some truncal valve incompetence; however, the incompetence was severe in only four. In the series of 70 patients, 23 of 59 (39 per cent) with two pulmonary arteries were inoperable because of pulmonary vascular obstructive disease, and 8 of 11 (73 per cent) with a single pulmonary artery were inoperable for the same reason. Among the 40 patients who had surgery, a definite relationship was noted between operative mortality and the calculated pulmonary vascular resistance. For patients with calculated pulmonary resistances of less than 8.0 units m², the operative mortality was 18 per cent, whereas for those with resistances greater than 12 units m², the operative mortality was 100 per cent. There was a good correlation between calculated pulmonary vascular resistance and degree of pulmonary vascular obstructive disease. There also was a relationship between arterial oxygen saturation and pulmonary vascular resistance: in the absence of pulmonary stenosis, patients with arterial oxygen saturation greater than 85 per cent had pulmonary resistances less than 12 units m² whereas those with arterial saturation less than 85 per cent had pulmonary resistances greater than 12 units m². This review suggested that patients with two pulmonary arteries and a pulmonary resistance greater than 12 units m² are inoperable. A different criterion for operability must be used for patients with a single pulmonary artery.

McGoon, D. C., Wallace, R. B., and Danielson, G. K.: The Rastelli operation: Its indications and results. J. Thorac. Cardiovasc. Surg., *65*:65, 1973.

Fifty-five patients with truncus arteriosus underwent operation at the Mayo Clinic between September, 1967, and March, 1972. The overall operative mortality rate was 29 per cent. Certain factors related to death were identified. Three of the 4 patients who were less than 2 years old died, whereas only 6 of 32 patients who were between 5 and 12 years old died. The mortality rate for patients whose ratio of pulmonary resistance to systemic resistance was less than 0.6 was 19 per cent, whereas for those with a ratio greater than 0.7, the operative mortality was 75 per cent. The follow-up on patients who survived surgery (although survival was relatively short) showed favorable surgical results. The authors concluded that, when possible, definite repair of truncus arteriosus should be deferred until the child is about 5 years old, recognizing that many patients will require definite repair before this age, albeit at a higher risk with current techniques.

Parker, R. K., McGoon, D. C., Danielson, G. K., Wallace, R. B., and Mair, D. D.: Repair of truncus arteriosus in patients with prior banding of the pulmonary artery. Surgery, *78*:761, 1975.

The results of complete repair of truncus arteriosus in patients who had undergone previous banding of the pulmonary arteries were reviewed. The operative technique was described. The data indicated that previous banding of the pulmonary arteries does not increase the operative mortality at the time of complete repair. The authors recognized that the preferred surgical treatment for infants with truncus arteriosus and congestive heart failure has not been established, but they suggested that successful banding of the pulmonary arteries does not jeopardize subsequent complete repair.

REFERENCES

1. Bharati, S., McAllister, H. A., Jr., Rosenquist, G. C., Miller, R. A., Tatooles, C. J., and Lev, M.: The surgical anatomy of truncus arteriosus communis. J. Thorac. Cardiovasc. Surg., *67*:501, 1974.
2. Billig, D. M., Kreidberg, M. B., Chernoff, H. L., and Khan, M. A. A.: Systemic to pulmonary anastomosis in truncus arteriosus with reduced pulmonary blood flow. Am. J. Cardiol., *30*:288, 1972.
3. Bowman, F. O., Jr., Hancock, W. D., and Malm, J. R.: A valve-containing Dacron prosthesis: Its use in restoring pulmonary artery–right ventricular continuity. Arch. Surg., *107*:724, 1973.
4. Collett, R. W., and Edwards, J. E.: Persistent truncus arteriosus:

A classification according to anatomic types. Surg. Clin. North Am., Aug., 1949, p. 1245.

5. Gelband, H., Van Meter, S., and Gersony, W. M.: Truncal valve abnormalities in infants with persistent truncus arteriosus: A clinicopathologic study. Circulation, 45:397, 1972.

6. Hallermann, F. J., Kincaid, O. W., Tsakiris, A. G., Ritter, D. G., and Titus, J. L.: Persistent truncus arteriosus: A radiographic and angiocardiographic study. Am. J. Roentgenol., 107:827, 1969.

7. Heath, D., and Edwards, J. E.: The pathology of hypertensive pulmonary vascular disease: A description of six grades of structural changes in the pulmonary arteries with special reference to congenital cardiac septal defects. Circulation, 18:533, 1958.

8. Keith, J. D., Rowe, R. D., and Vlad, P.: Heart Disease in Infancy and Childhood. New York, Macmillan Company, 1958, p. 521.

9. Mair, D. D., Ritter, D. G., Davis, G. D., Wallace, R. B., Danielson, G. K., and McGoon, D. C.: Selection of patients with truncus arteriosus for surgical correction: Anatomic and hemodynamic considerations. Circulation, 49:144, 1974.

10. Marcelletti, C., McGoon, D. C., Danielson, G. K., Wallace, R. B., and Mair, D. D.: Early and late results of surgical repair of truncus arteriosus (abstract). Circulation, 52(Suppl. 2):101, 1975.

11. McGoon, D. C., Rastelli, G. C., and Ongley, P. A.: An operation for the correction of truncus arteriosus. J.A.M.A., 205:69, 1968.

12. Muller, W. H., Jr., and Dammann, J. F., Jr.: The treatment of certain congenital malformations of the heart by the creation of pulmonic stenosis to reduce pulmonary hypertension and excessive pulmonary blood flow: A preliminary report. Surg. Gynecol. Obstet., 95:213, 1952.

13. Oldham, H. N., Jr., Kakos, G. S., Jarmakani, M. M., and Sabiston, D. C., Jr.: Pulmonary artery banding in infants with complex congenital heart defects. Ann. Thorac. Surg., 13:342, 1972.

14. Parker, R. K., McGoon, D. C., Danielson, G. K., Wallace, R. B., and Mair, D. D.: Repair of truncus arteriosus in patients with prior banding of the pulmonary artery. Surgery, 78:761, 1975.

15. Rastelli, G. C., Titus, J. L., and McGoon, D. C.: Homograft of ascending aorta and aortic valve as a right ventricular outflow: An experimental approach to the repair of truncus arteriosus. Arch. Surg., 95:698, 1967.

16. Smith, G. W., Thompson, W. M., Jr., Dammann, J. F., Jr., and Muller, W. H., Jr.: Use of the pulmonary artery banding procedure in treating type II truncus arteriosus. Circulation, 29(Suppl. 1):108, 1964.

17. Stark, J., Aberdeen, E., Waterston, D. J., Bonham-Carter, R. E., and Tynan, M.: Pulmonary artery constriction (banding): A report of 146 cases. Surgery, 65:808, 1969.

18. Taruffi, C.: Sulle malattie congenite e sulle anomalie del cuore. Mem. Soc. Med. Chir. Bologna, 8:215, 1875.

19. Van Praagh, R., and Van Praagh, S.: The anatomy of common aorticopulmonary trunk (truncus arteriosus communis) and its embryologic implications: A study of 57 necropsy cases. Am. J. Cardiol., 16:406, 1965.

XI

TRANSPOSITION OF THE GREAT ARTERIES

Paul A. Ebert, M.D.

HISTORICAL ASPECTS

Anatomic observation of transposition of the great arteries was reported as early as 1672 by Steno, and by Morgani in 1761 and Bailey in 1779. Even in these early reports, variations in the anatomic configurations of the transposition malformation were described. Von Rokitansky[46] (1875) reported analysis of the pathogenesis of transposition and attempted to classify the various types. The clinical recognition of this anomaly during life was emphasized by Fanconi[12] in 1932. Taussig[41] in 1938 described not only the clinical manifestations of this anomaly during life but also the pathologic anatomy and hemodynamic manifestations of the disorder.

The era of surgery for transportation of the great arteries began in 1950 when Blalock and Hanlon[6] reported an ingenious method of creating an atrial septal defect to increase mixing between the two circulations. Although the mortality with this operation was extremely high in the early years of its use, the marked improvement observed in the survivors created considerable enthusiasm. In 1952, Mustard[32] attempted to reverse the transposed great arteries directly, and in the same year Bailey[4] also reversed the aorta and pulmonary artery, but neither patient survived. In 1952, Lillehei and Varco[28] transferred the right pulmonary veins to the right atrium and the inferior vena cava to the left atrium to partially correct the circulation. In 1954, Glenn and Patino[15] anastomosed the right pulmonary artery to the superior vena cava in patients with transposition of the great arteries and pulmonary stenosis. Baffes[3] in 1956 successfully transferred the right pulmonary veins to the right atrium and grafted the right inferior vena cava to the left atrium. Kay and Cross[23] (1955) and Merendino[30] (1957) attempted intra-atrial diversionary procedures to redirect venous flow into the respective ventricles. In 1959, Senning reported success in transposing the atria in a young boy. Barnard[5] in 1961 excised the atrial septum and inserted a plastic prosthesis around the orifices of the pulmonary veins, connecting the other end to the orifice of the systemic or right ventricle. Considerable enthusiasm for the management of transposition of the great vessels followed Mustard's[31] report in 1964 of an operation in which he excised the entire atrial septum and positioned a pericardial baffle in the atrium to redirect all the caval blood to the pulmonary ventricle and allow the oxygenated blood returning by pulmonary veins to enter the systemic ventricle. This procedure has received universal acceptance and has produced excellent results.

ANATOMIC ASPECTS

Transposition of the great arteries accounts for approximately 9 per cent of cases of cyanotic congenital heart disease. This lesion represents approximately 15 per cent of congenital cardiac anomalies seen at autopsy in infants less than 1 month of age. Transposition is the leading cause of death due to congenital heart lesions in the first months of life. There is a definite male preponderance, the ratio being between 2:3 and 3:1.

Complete transposition of the great arteries essentially means that the aorta and pulmonary artery are misplaced across the ventricular septum. The aorta usually arises anteriorly from trabeculated right ventricle that receives desaturated venous blood from the right atrium (Fig. 1). The pulmonary artery most commonly lies posterior to and to the left of the aorta and receives oxygenated blood from a smooth-walled left ventricle. There are many possible combinations of great artery and chamber arrangements in transposition of the great arteries, depending on rotation of the heart and the side-to-side relationships of the ventricles. Paul[34] reported that complete transposition occurred as a relatively isolated anomaly 65 per cent of the time, with only simple associated lesions such as atrial septal defect, ventricular septal defect, patent ductus arteriosus, or these in combination. When transposition occurred with situs inversus (3 per cent of cases) or asplenia (6 per cent), associated complex intracardiac anomalies also were noted.

In the normal heart, the aortic valve is inferior to and in direct continuity with the mitral valve, while in transposition it lies superior, atop the subaortic conus. Many theories of morphogenesis have been proposed, but the differential conal growth hypothesis[17] has been favored. It is postulated that in the normal heart, the subaortic segment of the conus does not grow and that dominant growth of the left-sided subpulmonary conus forces the pulmonary valve anteriorly and superiorly to the left, whereas in ordinary forms of transposition growth of the subaortic part of the conus pushes the aorta anteriorly and disrupts aortic-mitral valve continuity. Failure of the subpulmonary portion of the conus to develop maintains posterior location of the pulmonary artery and pulmonary-mitral valve continuity.

Development of the conus determines truncal rotation, and the relationship of the great arteries proximally at the semilunar valves is similar to that at the arch. There is no twist in the great arteries simply because the aorta is anterior. In less common types of transposition, development of both right and left parts of the conus thrusts both the aortic and pulmonary valves forward. If growth of the two segments is approximately equal, the valves will lie side by side at about the same height. Bilateral conus development is more common in transposition associated with malposition of the heart.

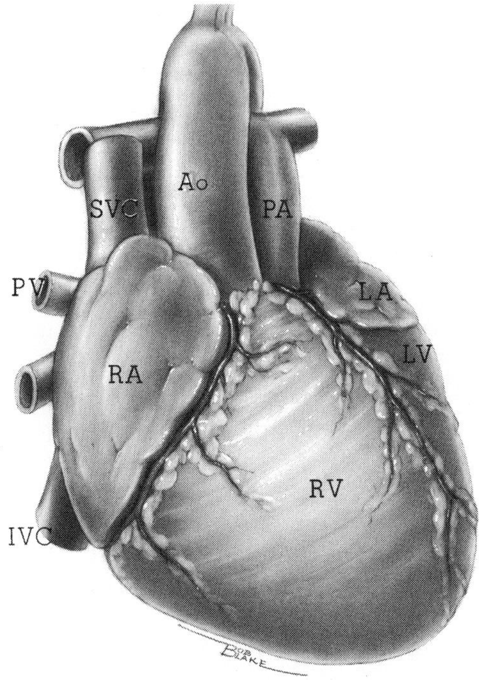

PATHOPHYSIOLOGY

The basic physiologic abnormality in complete transposition of the great arteries is that venous blood is pumped directly into the aorta while oxygenated blood is returned to the pulmonary artery. Thus, there are two separate circulations in parallel instead of in series. Oxygenated pulmonary venous blood enters the circulation only by way of intracirculatory shunts (Fig. 2). Thus, the greater the number of simple associated anomalies such as atrial septal defect, ventricular septal defect, and patent ductus arteriosus, the greater the opportunity for intracirculatory mixing of venous and oxygenated blood. Infants with these associated lesions are usually less cyanotic. When intracirculatory shunting is limited, the infant is extremely cyanotic because of recirculation of the systemic venous blood. Pulmonary flow is usually excessive, and often the pulmonary artery pressure is elevated. Heart work is increased, and the myocardium must sustain this load with marginal coronary oxygenation.

The degree of intracirculatory shunting that occurs appears to be related to simple pressure gradients present at the site of the communication. Most infants with transposition have an increased pulmonary blood flow and pulmonary venous return. As the left atrium enlarges, the foramen ovale is stretched, and this results in oxygenated blood being shunted into the right atrium and systemic circulation. A systemic-to-pulmonary shunt exists through the bronchial vessels

Figure 1. External view of the usual form of transposition of the great arteries. The aorta arises anteriorly from the right ventricle, and there is minimal if any rotation to the great vessels. The pulmonary valve lies almost directly posterior to the aortic valve. The left and right ventricles have a nearly normal relationship.

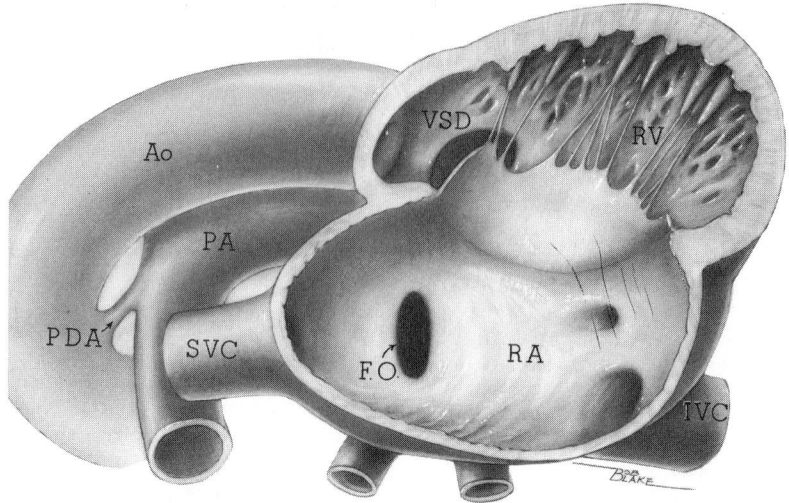

Figure 2. The common anomalies associated with transposition of the great arteries are patent ductus arteriosus (PDA), ventricular septal defect (VSD), and patent foramen ovale (FO). These intracirculatory communications facilitate mixing of arterial and venous blood between the parallel circulations. The size and number of these associated anomalies determine the degree of cyanosis.

and also through a ventricular septal defect or patent ductus arteriosus if either is present. Bidirectional shunting can usually be demonstrated across the atrial septum, but the amount of systemic blood entering the pulmonary circuit is usually related to the size of the atrial septal defect.

The pulmonary vascular resistance is usually normal or only mildly elevated in infants with transposition of the great arteries with or without an associated ventricular septal defect. Ferencz[13] observed advanced histologic changes in the lungs of children over 2 years of age, and intimal fibrosis was noted as early as 1 month of life. These changes seem to be present in most children with transposition and suggest that this malformation may be associated with a more advanced and malignant form of pulmonary vascular disease than ventricular septal defect with normal relationship of the great arteries. Whether the advanced changes are related to perfusion of the pulmonary arterial tree with oxygenated blood in association with systemic desaturation is not clear. Severe pulmonary vascular changes are present in most older children with transposition of the great arteries with associated moderate to large ventricular septal defects. Hemodynamic measurements do not completely agree with the histologic findings in children with intact ventricular septum or small ventricular septal defects, however, since the majority do not have physiologic evidence of increased pulmonary vascular resistance. It has been postulated that systemic hypoxia stimulates sympathetic activity, with a resultant increase in tone of pulmonary arterioles. Thus, after complete correction, a decrease in pulmonary vascular resistance might be anticipated in many cases.

CLINICAL FEATURES

Cyanosis and congestive heart failure are the common findings in infants with complete transposition of the great arteries. The cyanosis is usually observed by 1 week of age and is more pronounced when the ventricular septum is intact. When cyanosis appears later, there is usually significant intracirculatory shunting through a large ventricular septal defect or patent ductus arteriosus. Differential cyanosis, with the upper extremities more blue than the lower part of the body, indicates a large patent ductus and increased pulmonary vascular resistance, with pulmonary-to-systemic shunting through the ductus. Clubbing of the digits is rare before 6 months of age but may progress rapidly in the older infant. Squatting, which is so characteristic of children with tetralogy of Fallot, is rarely seen with transposition.

Birth weight is usually normal or above normal. Growth and physical development are always retarded. Anoxic spells are usually characterized by prolonged, labored breathing with increased cyanosis. The infant usually remains conscious and rarely has convulsions. These spells are due to hypoxemia from inadequate intracirculatory shunting, and metabolic acidosis results. Congestive heart failure is a common clinical finding, with dyspnea, cardiac enlargement, hepatomegaly, pulmonary rales, and occasionally peripheral edema. Symptoms of heart failure are present within the first week of life in about 10 per cent of patients but more commonly appear at about 1 month. Seventy-five per cent of these infants will have a systolic murmur even though the ventricular septum is intact. The second heart sound is single and loud because of the close proximity of the aorta to the chest wall. An apical diastolic gallop is commonly heard, and a mild diastolic apical murmur may be noted in those with an associated ventricular septal defect. The degree of pulmonary vascular obstruction cannot be assessed by auscultation, since the second sound is usually loud and single. Pulmonary valvular or subvalvular stenosis is characteristically associated with a long crescendo-decrescendo systolic murmur along the left sternal border transmitted to the right clavicular area.

The common electrocardiographic findings are right atrial hypertrophy, right or combined ventricular hypertrophy, and right axis deviation. In early infancy the electrocardiogram may appear normal for age since the newborn characteristically has right ventricular hypertrophy. These findings vary, depending on age, presence or absence of ventricular septal defect, presence or absence of pulmonary vascular resistance. Right axis deviation is usually associated with an intact ventricular septum, whereas in approximately 40 per cent of patients with a moderate-sized ventricular septal defect the axis will be normal.

The routine chest x-ray is frequently diagnostic. The important factors are progressive cardiomegaly in early infancy, an oval or egg-shaped cardiac configuration, a narrow superior mediastinum, and increased pulmonary vascular markings (Fig. 3). Characteristically, the heart is normal in size during the first 1 or 2 weeks of life, but then cardiac enlargement is observed in almost all infants with transposition of the great arteries and increased pulmonary blood flow. The pulmonary markings are prominent, and even pulmonary stenosis, unless unusually severe, does not significantly reduce the prominence of the pulmonary vasculature.

MANAGEMENT

Since most infants with transposition of the great arteries are cyanotic within the first week of life and the mortality is so high within the first 2 months, the majority usually are brought for treatment at a very early age. Cardiac catheterization should be undertaken to substantiate the diagnosis and confirm the position of intracardiac chambers. In most cases, the left atrial pressure will be greater than the right atrial pressure, and the pressure in the posterior or left ventricle will depend on the presence or absence of ventricular septal defect or pulmonary valvular or subvalvular stenosis as well as the state of the peripheral pulmonary vasculature. Catheterization must be performed in an expedient manner, as any stress in these severely ill infants increases metabolic requirements and the marked degree of cyanosis quickly results in systemic acidosis with marked reduction in arterial pH.

Once the diagnosis is confirmed in the newborn period, a balloon septostomy, performed as described by Rashkind and Miller in 1966,[35] is indicated in most of these infants. A balloon-tipped catheter is placed in a systemic vein and advanced into the right atrium and through the foramen ovale into the left atrium. The balloon is inflated with 1 to 3 ml. of contrast material so it can be visualized on the image intensifier, and then it is pulled vigorously across the atrial septum to enlarge or tear the foramen ovale (Fig. 4). This increases mixing of venous and oxygenated blood at the atrial level and has proved to be an excellent means of palliation in the very small infant. The balloon septostomy procedure can be repeated at subsequent dates if cyanosis becomes unmanageable, but results are less good as it becomes more difficult to tear or enlarge the rapidly thickening atrial septum. The more severely cyanotic infants are usually those with an intact ventricular septum and are therefore the best candidates for subsequent total correction.

Palliative Operations

Since the advent of the balloon septostomy, the necessity of performing palliative operative procedures during the first month of life has been reduced. Approximately 70 per cent of infants with transposition of the great arteries and intact ventricular septum if left untreated will not survive the first month of life. The value of performing an intra-atrial baffle correction or atrial septectomy at this young age is undecided. Both may be considered palliative, since a baffle placed in such a small heart may require modification with growth. The intra-atrial baffle has the ad-

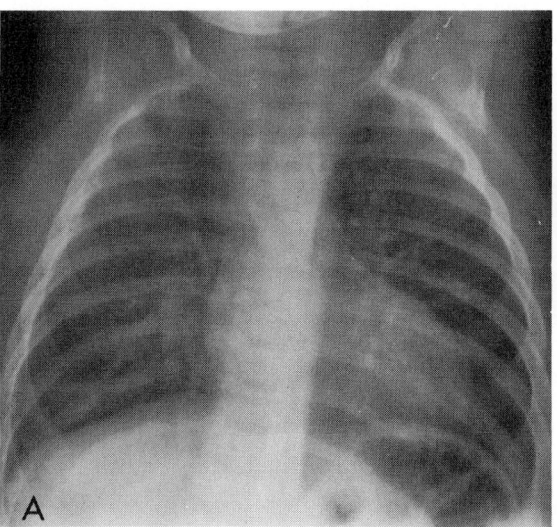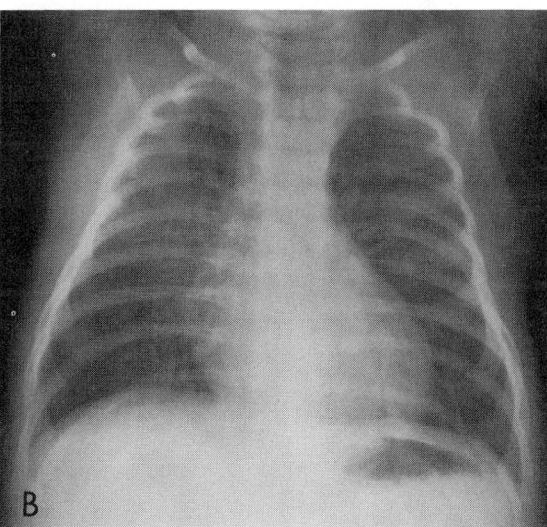

Figure 3. *A,* Typical chest x-ray of a 2-month-old infant with transposition of the great arteries showing hyperemic lung fields, narrow heart base, and the globular-shaped cardiac silhouette. *B,* Chest x-ray 3 weeks later, after creation of an atrial septal defect by the Blalock-Hanlon technique. Heart size is smaller and the lung fields are less plethoric.

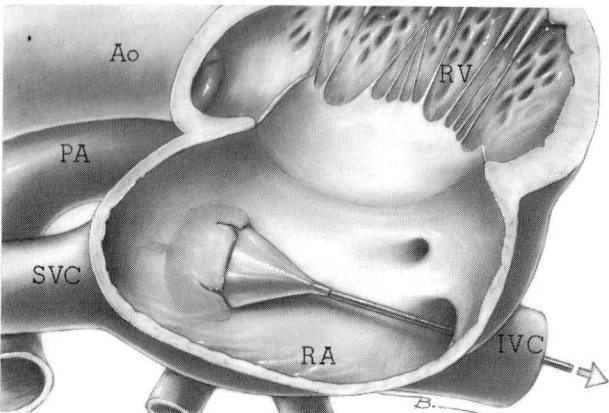

Figure 4. The size of the interatrial communication is enlarged by passing a balloon-tipped catheter through the foramen ovale, inflating the balloon, and forcefully pulling it back into the right atrium. The atrial septum is torn and the patent foramen enlarged, this facilitates increased mixing of arterial and venous blood.

vantage of separating the circulations and reducing systemic embolization and infection. If both procedures can be accomplished with similar mortality, the baffle probably has the advantage.

If an atrial septectomy is considered, the technique of Blalock and Hanlon is generally used: the right pulmonary veins and a segment of right atrium are incorporated in a partial occluding clamp so that a segment of the atrial septum included within this clamp can be excised (Fig. 5). The creation of an atrial septal defect under direct vision by inflow occlusion as recommended by Trusler in 1964 has generally carried a higher mortality than the closed procedure.

Ventricular Septal Defect

The presence of a small ventricular septal defect and only moderate elevation of pressure in the left ventricle should not cause major concern, since irreversible pulmonary vascular disease is not likely to develop. Infants with large ventricular septal defects and systemic pressure in the left ventricle present one of the most difficult problems. These infants generally are not severely cyanotic, but irreversible vascular

changes in the lungs develop at an early age if some type of protection is not afforded. Banding of the pulmonary artery is a very delicate procedure in transposition of the great arteries. If the band is too tight, pulmonary flow is reduced too much and systemic hypoxia and metabolic acidosis ensue. On the other hand, if the band is too loose, flow to the lungs will not be significantly impeded and respiratory failure or pulmonary vascular changes will occur. If a patent ductus is present, it should be closed at the time of banding. In most instances, banding alone should not be considered but should be accompanied by some type of palliative procedure to improve mixing at the atrial level. This can be either open creation of an atrial septal defect, closed creation by the Blalock-Hanlon technique, or transposition of the atrial septum as recommended by Edwards and Bargeron in 1965[10] (Fig. 6). In general, if pulmonary flow is to be reduced by banding of the pulmonary artery to protect the pulmonary vasculature, improved mixing must be provided at the atrial level to prevent cyanosis from being too severe. It is *imperative* that a high pulmonary artery pressure not be allowed to persist beyond the first months of life, as irreversible pulmonary vascular changes are likely to develop.

Left Ventricular Outflow Obstruction

This group of infants has proved to pose most perplexing problems as regards subsequent total correction. Palliative procedures probably should be designed so that subsequent total correction can be accomplished if the outflow obstruction can be relieved successfully or if a conduit can be used to bypass the obstructed valve. Since the pressure in the pulmonary artery is quite low because of the outflow obstruction, anastomosis of the superior vena cava to the right pulmonary artery has been an attractive solution but this anastomosis can only be accomplished in older children and has become less attractive as better corrective procedures have been developed. Subsequent total correction is not precluded by this procedure, but late studies of children in whom superior vena cava to right pulmonary artery shunts have been created have shown a progressive decrease in the amount of blood going to the right lung. If total correction is at-

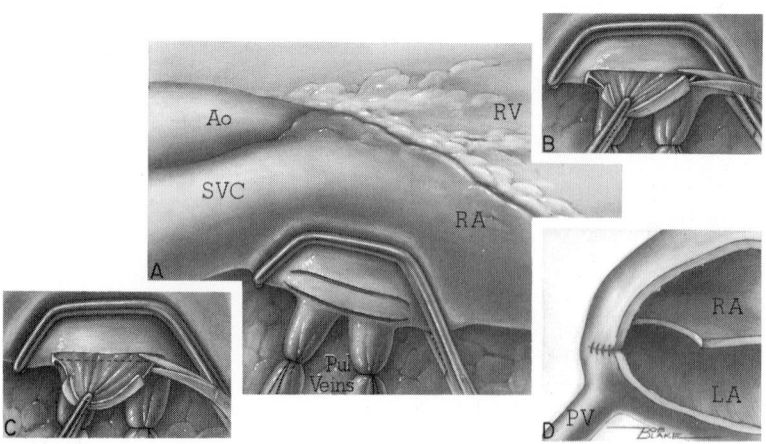

Figure 5. Creation of an atrial septal defect by the Blalock-Hanlon technique. *A,* The partial occluding clamp is placed to incorporate the interatrial groove on the right side of the atrium. The pulmonary veins are occluded, and parallel incisions are made in the right and left atria. The septum is grasped (*B*) and cut on each end. The clamp is partially released so that more septum can be pulled outward (*C*) and then excised. *D,* The two edges are sutured together; this leaves a large interatrial communication.

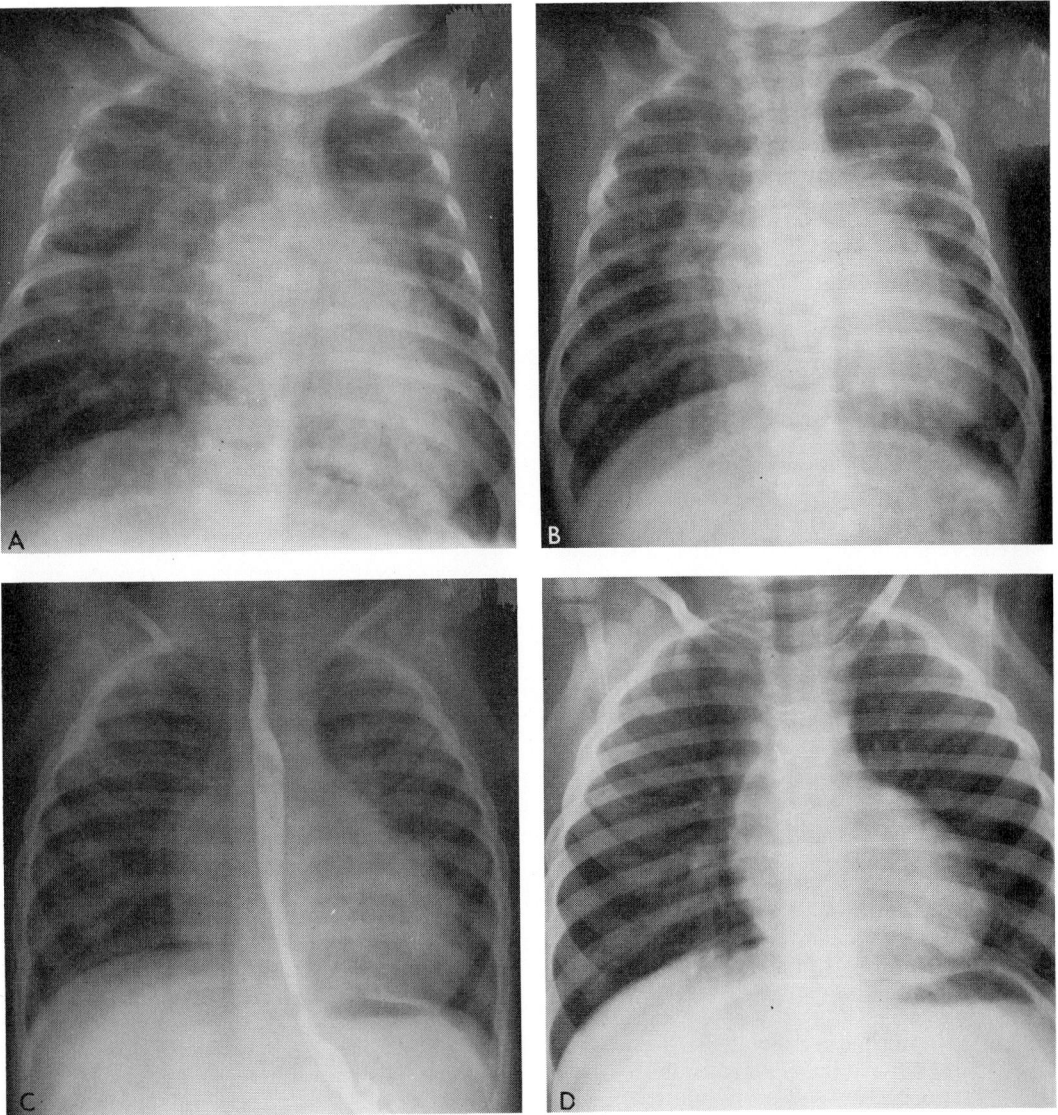

Figure 6. Sequence of chest x-rays showing: *A,* Age 3 weeks: Infant with transposition of the great arteries and a large ventricular septal defect in marked congestive heart failure. *B,* Age 5 weeks: Ten days after banding of the pulmonary artery the lung fields are less congested and heart failure is controlled. *C,* Age 3 months: Two weeks after creation of an atrial septal defect the lungs are even less congested and the heart size is smaller. *D,* Age 2½ years: Chest x-ray 6 months after removal of the pulmonary band, closure of the ventricular septal defect, and placement of an intra-atrial baffle for total correction. Heart size is reduced and lung markings are normal.

tempted, the superior vena cava to right pulmonary artery anastomosis is usually left intact, and the inferior vena cava return is diverted to the posterior atrium. In most instances, pulmonary flow is reduced and must be increased in order to relieve cyanosis. Because of the anatomic relationship of the main pulmonary artery to the aorta, it is difficult to create a satisfactory Waterston-type shunt between the right pulmonary artery and the ascending aorta. In the infant, the best solution is probably a systemic-to-pulmonary shunt between the descending aorta and left pulmonary artery or a direct anastomosis between the main pulmonary artery and ascending aorta. These should be accompanied by either balloon septostomy or creation of an atrial septal defect as a subsequent

simultaneous or separate procedure. If the child is above 1 year of age, a subclavian artery to pulmonary artery anastomosis can be accomplished. Fortunately, infants with outflow obstruction represent only a small minority of patients with transposition of the great arteries, and this type of palliation is seldom required.

Reduced Pulmonary Flow

A small percentage of infants with transposition of the great arteries have diminished pulmonary markings, and usually an intact ventricular septum, and fail to thrive after creation of an atrial septal defect either by balloon septostomy or by operation. Whether in these infants there is some difference in compliance between the right and left ventricles that causes filling of the pulmonary ventricle to be inadequate to propel blood into the lungs has not been determined. However, this group has not done well with atrial septectomy, since the atrial pressures are so similar that minimal shunting occurs. A direct open repair as described by Dillard[8] using profound surface hypothermia with circulatory arrest or Clark and Barrett-Boyes[7] using surface hypothermia, circulatory arrest, and rewarming with a pump-oxygenator system is indicated. Improvement in the technique of profound hypothermia and circulatory arrest has made the operative mortality in the infant acceptable. The technique commonly employed is surface cooling to 27 or 28° C, then opening of the chest and cooling to 15° C using the pump-oxygenator. Total circulatory arrest of 30 minutes can be safely accomplished. If longer operative time is required, perfusion for 5 minutes will allow a longer safe period. After corrective surgery the infant is rewarmed using the pump-oxygenator. The technique is commonly used up to 6 months of age and sporadically employed in older children.

Total Correction

Correction of complete transposition of the great arteries by repositioning the transposed arteries over their appropriate ventricles has been clinically successful but associated with a high mortality. A major difficulty with this technique is that if the repositioning were accomplished above the orifice of the coronary arteries, coronary flow would come from the pulmonary artery and the heart would receive desaturated blood. Jatene[29] has corrected transpositions in infants by dividing both the aorta and the pulmonary artery with removal of a "button" of aorta around the origin of the coronary arteries for repositioning and anastomosis of the coronaries into the pulmonary artery. A portion of each pulmonary artery stump is closed in order to make its diameter conform to that of the aorta. The proximal portion of the pulmonary artery is then sutured to the distal portion of the aorta and the distal part of the artery to the proximal segment of the aorta. If the coronary arteries are replanted, the question of growth of the circular suture line is unanswered and late coronary ostial obstruction may occur.

Diversion of the venous inflow at the atrial level has appeared more appealing, and Senning in 1959[39] created two large interatrial channels for crossing the systemic and pulmonary venous circulations. This was accomplished by incising, realigning, and suturing interatrial septal tissue and the right atrial free wall in order to create these separate channels. This procedure was difficult to perform, and in the small infant it was practically impossible to obtain channels of adequate size. Mustard[33] in 1964 described an operation for total correction of transposition of the great arteries, based on principles proposed by Albert,[2] that provides an intra-atrial baffle, made of pericardial tissue, to direct the systemic venous return to the posterior ventricle and allow the pulmonary venous return to enter the systemic ventricle. Surgical success with this operation has been reported to be in the range of 80 to 90 per cent, and at present this technique certainly represents the best approach to total correction.[22]

If successful palliation has been provided in early infancy by balloon septostomy or a palliative operation, or both, elective total correction is usually undertaken when the child is between 18 and 36 months of age. It may be advisable to lower this elective age to 8 to 14 months in order to reduce the possibility of cerebral thrombosis or emboli, which are common in children with transposition. Although excision of a portion of the atrial septum and interatrial groove by the Blalock-Hanlon technique allows the two atria to enlarge in a spherical form and thus facilitates total correction, the operation described by Mustard has been performed with satisfactory results in children who have had only balloon septostomy.

The operative approach is through a median sternotomy incision. A large piece of anterior pericardium is excised, the pericardium is cleaned of as much scar or fibrous tissue and fat as possible, and the venae cavae are mobilized for about 1 to 2 cm. into the pericardial orifices to facilitate cannulation. A purse-string suture is placed on the right lateral side of the atriocaval junction, and care is taken in placement of the superior vena cava catheter to avoid injury in the area of the sinus node. Total cardiopulmonary bypass is established, and the heart is electrically fibrillated to reduce the possibility of air emboli when the systemic atrium is opened (Fig. 7). The right atrium may be opened in either a longitudinal or transverse fashion. The ventricular septal defect, if present, is repaired by retraction of the leaflets of the tricuspid valve. If adequate exposure cannot be accomplished with retraction, a small, high ventriculotomy will facilitate exposure. The ventricular septal defects usually have a muscular rim owing to development of the subaortic conus. The defects are usully located just below the posterior aspect of the aortic conus, and the conduction bundle passes along the superior aspect of the lower rim of the defect. Good exposure can be accomplished and closure is rarely a significant problem. In most instances, a patch should be used for closure of the ventricular septal defect.

The atrial septum is then completely excised; care must be taken to excise completely the interatrial groove in the cephalad area between the superior vena cava and the top of the ventricular septum. The incision may extend outside the heart and require suturing of the endocardial surfaces. If the rim of the atrial septum is not completely removed between the medial junction of the superior cava and the superior border of the ventricular septum, this ridge may be too close to the pericardial baffle and obstruct flow from the superior cava. In some cases, it may be necessary to extend this incision superiorly along the medial side of the atriocaval junction and enlarge the area with a patch. A small rim is left attached to the top of the muscular ventricular septum between the tricuspid and mitral valves. This minimizes the possibility of damaging the conduction bundles when the baffle is sutured in place. The coronary sinus is generally left alone and the suture line positioned between the sinus and the tricuspid valve. The baffle is tailored so that the center portion is somewhat narrower than the

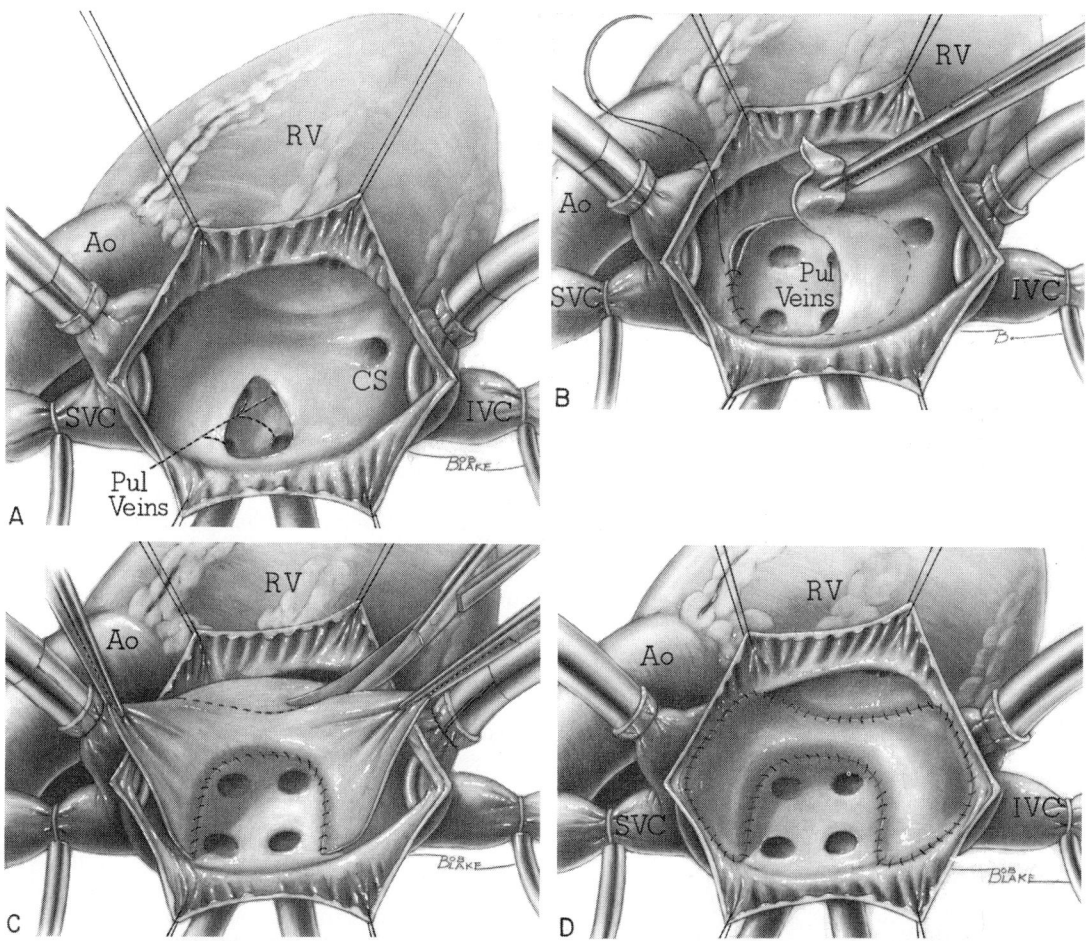

Figure 7. Total correction of transposition of the great arteries by intra-atrial diversion. *A,* The right atrium is opened, so that the atrial septum, coronary sinus, and atrial septal defect are exposed. *B,* The atrial septum is excised. If the excision extends outside the heart in the interatrial groove, it is repaired by direct suture. *C,* The pericardial or prosthetic patch is fashioned around the pulmonary veins and trimmed to fit the atrium. *D,* To complete repair, the baffle is sutured around the caval orifices and to the remnant of tissue across the top of the ventricular septum. Caval blood is now diverted posteriorly into the left ventricle, while pulmonary venous blood enters the right ventricle and then the aorta.

ends, and the center section is sutured to a position between the left pulmonary veins. The baffle is then sutured around the lateral orifice of the left pulmonary veins, and this suture line must be fairly close to the veins in order to allow adequate systemic venous return into the posterior ventricle. The suture line continues to the right across the floor of the left atrium onto the right lateral wall. The baffle is left loose to form a smooth surface as it becomes stiffer with time and will form a more natural confluence. The baffle extends over the orifices of the vena cava so that the venous catheters enter into the venous atrium. If a previous Blalock-Hanlon procedure has been performed and the interatrial septum has been removed on the right side, it is unusual to have to enlarge the systemic atrium (Fig. 8). If only a balloon septostomy has been performed, a pericardial patch is necessary to enlarge the left atrium by incorporating it in the closure of the atrium. The heart is allowed to fill with blood and care is taken to eliminate all air from the systemic ventricle. As closure of the atriotomy is accomplished and the heart is filled with blood, electrical fibrillation is discontinued and spontaneous defibrillation usually occurs. Usually, the superior vena caval catheter is removed before cardiopulmonary bypass is terminated.

One of the major complications of this operation has been associated tachycardia from an atrial origin or the creation of nodal rhythm. It seems reasonable that when such large portions of the atrium have been excised and several incisions have been made in the walls of the atrium, conduction from the sinus node to the atrioventricular node may be impaired or the scarring process about sutures may be responsible for ectopic atrial activity. The incidence of atrial flutter or supraventricular tachycardia has been high in the postoperative period, and both can be difficult to control. Definite care should be taken to preserve the sinus node, and positioning of the intra-atrial baffle in regard to the coronary sinus has been of concern. If the baffle is placed too near the atrioventricular node, it is possible that the atrioventricular node may be injured directly by suture, by scarring and fibrosis, or by ischemia produced by interruption of coronary vascular supply to the node. Thus, the suture line passing from the septal remnant between the atrioventricular orifices to the area of the coronary sinus should lie near the tricuspid valve; very delicate bites of tissue should be taken in this area. An alternative has been to eliminate the incision into the coronary sinus and extend the anterior suture line below the coronary sinus; this permits the coronary sinus to drain into the pulmonary atrium and assumes that the small right-to-left shunt will be of no significance. At present, the answer to the problem of how to avoid atrial rhythm disturbance has not been clearly defined.

The presence of pulmonary stenosis has been a most difficult problem to manage in the child with transposition of the great arteries. In most cases, this is a subvalvular stenosis that incorporates a portion of the mitral valve into the stenotic fibrotic band. Because of the posterior location of the pulmonary outflow tract and the presence of a major coronary vessel overlying the tract, it has not been possible to patch the outflow tract, as is commonly done in repair of tetralogy of Fallot. Excision or cutting of the fibromuscular components with a rongeur through a pulmonary arteriotomy has been satisfactory in some children, but complete relief of the stenosis may not be possible. If the child can be maintained to an older age, approximately 8 years, the procedure described by Rastelli[36] can be utilized. This technique is applicable in the presence of pulmonary stenosis and a large ventricular septal defect (Fig. 9). The pulmonary artery is simply divided and the end exiting from the heart sutured closed. A ventriculotomy is then performed between the aortic outflow and the ventricular septum, and an interventricular patch is positioned to divert the posterior ventricle efflux through the ventricular septal defect and out through the aorta. An aortic homograft is then placed over the ventriculotomy and connected to the pulmonary artery to carry the systemic venous blood into the lungs. If a palliative atrial septal defect has previously been created, it is closed through a separate atriotomy.

If the pulmonary stenosis is mild, then direct surgical relief through the pulmonary artery should be adequate. It must be remembered that there usually is direct continuity between the pulmonary annulus and mitral annulus in the standard form of transposition, and good visualization must be accomplished to avoid damage to the mitral valve. The ventricular septal defect is closed in the usual fashion through the tricuspid valve and a routine intra-atrial baffle procedure is performed. Although this problem affects a very small percentage of infants with transposition of the great arteries, it certainly is the most challenging and difficult aspect of the anomaly to correct.

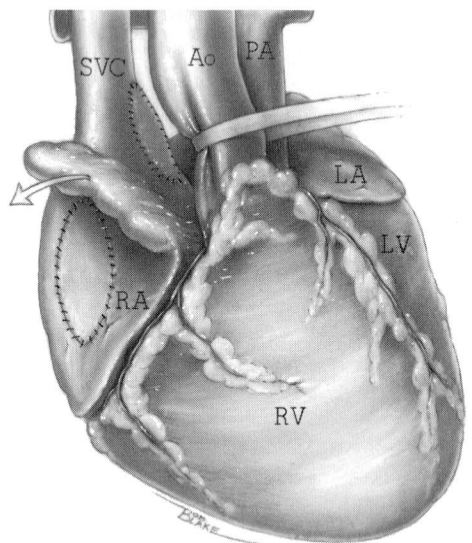

Figure 8. The atrium may require enlargement at two sites during complete correction. The right atrium may require an external patch over the lateral wall to enlarge the size of the chamber receiving blood from the pulmonary veins. In some cases, when the pulmonary veins arise more superiorly than usual, an external patch along the medial aspect of the superior caval-atrial junction is necessary to prevent obstruction of flow from the superior cava into the posterior atrium.

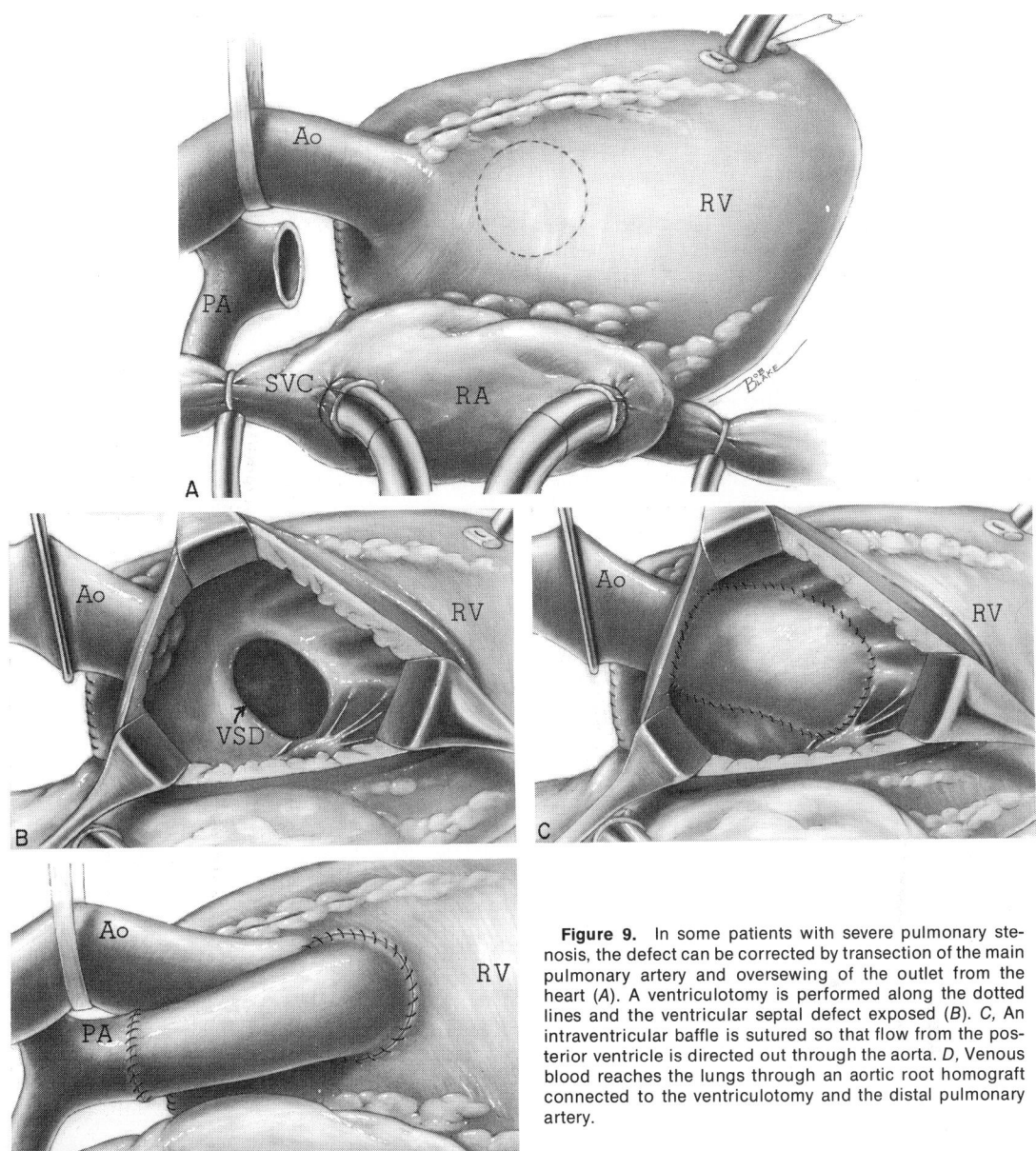

Figure 9. In some patients with severe pulmonary stenosis, the defect can be corrected by transection of the main pulmonary artery and oversewing of the outlet from the heart (*A*). A ventriculotomy is performed along the dotted lines and the ventricular septal defect exposed (*B*). *C*, An intraventricular baffle is sutured so that flow from the posterior ventricle is directed out through the aorta. *D*, Venous blood reaches the lungs through an aortic root homograft connected to the ventriculotomy and the distal pulmonary artery.

OPERATIVE COMPLICATIONS

In any operative procedure when the systemic atrium and ventricles are open, air embolus must be prevented. Fibrillation of the heart during intracardiac repair and until the entire vascular system is refilled with blood has been a useful technique. The caval tapes should be released prior to defibrillation so that the surgeon can check for any leaks around the baffle and also detect any hemorrhage in areas where sutures may have torn the atrial wall during placement of the baffle. Blood will then pass through the lungs and any air trapped in the pulmonary veins should exit through the systemic atrium. Immediately

before defibrillation, a small catheter is placed through the tricuspid valve to ensure that the ventricle is free of air.

The mediastinum must be drained well, because after correction of transposition the heart seems especially sensitive to any space-occupying lesions in the mediastinum. We have seen marked impairment of cardiac output caused by postoperative hemorrhage in the thymus. Clarke and Barratt-Boyes[7] described two cases in which postoperative pulmonary edema was relieved by reoperation and removal of a clot positioned between the right pericardium and the right atrial wall. This extreme sensitivity of these children to mild postoperative mediastinal clot may be related to the anterior position of the systemic atrium and to its somewhat small size after the intra-atrial baffle procedure. The slightest compression of the right anterior atrial wall may impair filling of the systemic ventricle and result in low cardiac output and elevated pulmonary venous pressure. Partial obstruction of the superior vena cava by the baffle may occur, since the pulmonary veins are located in the more superior aspect of the atrium, much nearer the superior vena cava orifice than the inferior vena cava orifice. Usually, partial obstruction of the superior cava will not be of clinical significance, as venous collaterals easily divert the return to the lower part of the body and into the inferior vena cava. Redundancy of the baffle may partially obstruct the mitral orifice, or if the venous pressure is too high the baffle may bulge into the systemic atrium and cause pulmonary edema.

Rhythm disturbance following total correction of transposition of the great arteries has been quite common. Nodal rhythm will be present in a large percentage of these children in the postoperative period, and often a small amount of isoproterenol will be required to increase heart rate. Adjustment to a nodal rate of 80 to 90 per minute usually occurs after the first 4 to 5 days, but the use of a cardiotonic agent is most helpful during this time. Complete heart block is not common but certainly carries the same grave prognosis as when it occurs after surgical repair of other congenital heart defects. Atrial flutter with a rapid ventricular response has been a complication in the later postoperative period, and this can be extremely difficult to control with medications. In these children, it has proved difficult to block the atrioventricular node with digitalis, and antiarrhythmic agents such as quinidine have not been especially helpful in controlling the atrial disturbance. We have seen foci of atrial activity in the left atrium and in the coronary sinus as the source of atrial tachycardia or flutter. In one patient, propranolol proved effective in controlling these episodes. In most cases, these episodes are intermittent, usually self-terminating, and, in many instances, accentuated by sympathetic activity, as when the child is excited or frightened. These disturbances in rhythm have been less common in children with nodal rhythm in the postoperative period as compared to those with some type of conducted rhythm of atrial origin whether it be from the sinus node or other areas of the atrium.

Some degree of cardiac failure may be present in the immediate postoperative period and is usually manifested as mild pulmonary congestion and occasional accumulation of fluid in the pleural cavity. Since most of these children have a strong left ventricle, it is probably not advisable to elevate venous pressure above 8 to 10 cm. H_2O. A high venous pressure can cause bulging of the baffle into the right atrium and impede pulmonary venous return by diminishing the size of the atrium. This, of course, increases pulmonary congestion and compounds the problem if the pressure in the pulmonary artery is low and the left ventricle responds to a rise in central venous pressure. Tracheostomy has usually not been necessary, but the majority of children have required the use of an endotracheal tube and positive-pressure ventilation for 24

to 72 hours. Obviously, if the pulmonary vascular resistance is elevated or mild pulmonary stenosis remains, it may be necessary to increase venous pressure to improve the function of the left ventricle and elevate cardiac output. The hourly urine output has proved to be the best index of cardiac output, and we commonly use minute amounts of isoproterenol to improve cardiac function whenever urine output decreases, even though other measurements and clinical signs remain unchanged. Mild congestive heart failure may persist for several weeks or months but responds to proper medication, such as digitalis and diuretics, and appears to be self-limiting.

RESULTS OF OPERATION

In transposition of the great arteries with intact atrial septum, total correction has been most gratifying, with operative survival between 80 and 90 per cent (Fig. 10). The presence of a small associated ventricular septal defect without evidence of pulmonary hypertension has also been associated with a high success rate. The majority of these children have been between the ages of 18 and 36 months at the time of correction, although more reports of total repair in infancy are being presented. The clinical responses have been excellent, with normal oxygen saturation and relatively unlimited activity. The pulmonary markings on chest x-ray decrease over 6 to 12 months, and progressive pulmonary hypertension has not been observed. Cardiac catheterization performed 1 to 3 years after operation has not demonstrated tricuspid insufficiency to be a major early complication, although the ability of the tricuspid valve to remain competent at systemic pressures continues to be a major unanswered question and ultimate success will depend greatly on this factor.

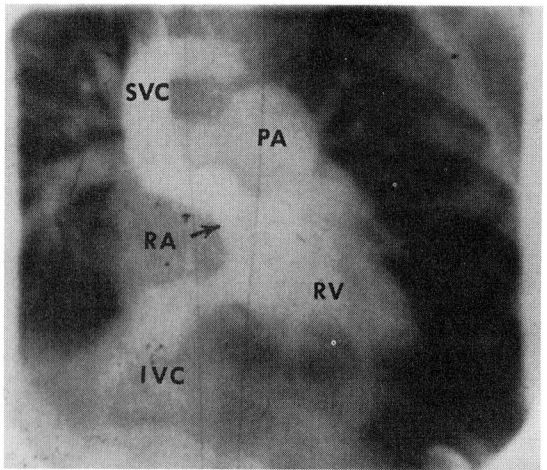

Figure 10. Postoperative cineangiocardiogram following total correction using an intra-atrial baffle. The arrow points to the baffle. Note that the blood flow from the venae cavae is directed posterior and to the left. The pulmonary venous return enters the right atrium, which is of adequate size.

SELECTED REFERENCES

Aberdeen, E., and Carr, I.: Modern Trends in Cardiac Surgery. New York, Appleton-Century-Crofts, 1968.
This monograph gives an excellent appraisal of the results of surgical treatment for transposition of the great vessels. It represents a review of the pertinent literature and presents a very large personal experience of the authors. The postoperative management and complications associated with total correction of transposition of the great vessels are well outlined.

Blalock, A., and Hanlon, C. R.: The surgical treatment of complete transposition of the aorta and pulmonary artery. Surg. Gynec. Obstet., *90*:1, 1950.
This original article opened the era of surgical treatment of transposition of the great vessels. The illustrations and text emphasize to the student the necessity of complete understanding of the anatomic relationships necessary for the planning of a successful palliative procedure. The clinical histories relate the difficulties encountered in the preoperative and postoperative management of these severely ill infants.

Mustard, W. T., Keith, J. D., Trusler, G. A., Fowler, R., and Kidd, L.: The surgical management of transposition of the great vessels. J. Thorac. Cardiovasc. Surg., *48*:953, 1964.
This excellent work describes the intra-atrial baffle procedure for total correction of transposition of the great vessels. The important details of the operative procedure are well defined, and many subtle points are emphasized to allow a better understanding of the complexity of this procedure. This paper was responsible for a complete change in thinking regarding the outlook for children with transposition of the great vessels.

Paul, M. H.: Transposition of the great arteries. In: Moss, A. J., and Adams, F. H.: Heart Disease in Infants, Children, and Adolescents. Baltimore, Williams & Wilkins Company, 1968.
This chapter clearly outlines the anatomic and embryologic development of transposition of the great vessels. Descriptions of the various types and possible positions of the great arteries and ventricles are presented. The basic pathophysiology of the circulatory anomaly is fully explained.

REFERENCES

1. Aberdeen, E., and Carr, I.: Modern Trends in Cardiac Surgery. New York, Appleton-Century-Crofts, 1968.
2. Albert, H. M.: Surgical correction of transposition of the great vessels. Surg. Forum, *5*:74, 1955.
3. Baffes, T. G.: A new method for surgical correction of transposition of the aorta and pulmonary artery. Surg. Gynecol. Obstet., *102*:227, 1956.
4. Bailey, C. P.: Surgery of the Heart. Philadelphia, Lea & Febiger, 1955.
5. Barnard, C. N., Schrire, V., and Beck, W.: Complete transposition of the great vessels: A successful complete correction. J. Thorac. Cardiovasc. Surg., *43*:768, 1962.
6. Blalock, A., and Hanlon, C. R.: The surgical treatment of complete transposition of the aorta and pulmonary artery. Surg. Gynecol. Obstet., *90*:1, 1950.
7. Clarke, C. P., and Barratt-Boyes, B. G.: The cause and treatment of pulmonary edema after the Mustard operation for correction of complete transposition of the great vessels. J. Thorac. Cardiovasc. Surg., *54*:9, 1967.
8. Dillard, D. T., Mohri, H., Merendino, K. A., Morgan, B. C., Baum, D., and Crawford, E. W.: Total surgical correction of transposition of the great arteries in children less than six months of age. Surg. Gynecol. Obstet., *129*:1258, 1969.
9. Ebert, P. A., Gay, W. A., Jr., and Engle, M. A.: Corection of transposition of the great arteries: Relationship of the coronary sinus and postoperative arrhythmias. Ann. Surg., *180*:433, 1974.
10. Edwards, W. S., and Bargeron, L. M., Jr.: More effective palliation of transposition of the great vessels. J. Thorac. Cardiovasc. Surg., *49*:790, 1965.
11. Elliott, L. P., Anderson, R. C., Tuna, N., Adams, P., Jr., and Neufeld, H. N.: Complete transposition of the great vessels. I. An anatomic study of sixty cases. Circulation, *27*:1105, 1963.
12. Fanconi, G.: Die Transposition der grossen Gefusse (das charakteristische Rontgenbild). Arch. Kinderheilk., *95*:202, 1932.
13. Ferencz, C.: Transposition of the great vessels. Pathophysiologic considerations based upon a study of the lungs. Circulation, *33*:232,1966.
14. Ferguson, D. J., Adams, P., and Watson, D.: Pulmonary arteriosclerosis in transposition of the great vessels. Am. J. Dis. Child., *99*:653, 1960.
15. Glenn, W. W. L., and Patino, J. F.: Circulatory bypass of the right heart. I. Preliminary observations on the direct delivery of vena caval blood into the pulmonary arterial circulation. Azygos vein-pulmonary artery shunt. Yale J. Biol. Med., *27*:147, 1954.
16. Glotzer, P., Young, D., and Bloomberg, A.: Sequential banding of the creation of atrial septal defect for transposition of the great vessels. J. Thorac. Cardiovasc. Surg., *46*:104, 1963.
17. Grant, R. P.: The morphogenesis of transposition of the great vessels. Circulation, *26*:819, 1962.
18. Hallman, G. L., and Cooley, D. A.: Complete transposition of great vessels: Results of surgical treatment. Arch. Surg., *89*:891, 1964.
19. Hanlon, C. R., and Blalock, A.: Complete transposition of the aorta and the pulmonary artery. Experimental observations on venous shunts as corrective procedures. Ann. Surg., *127*:385, 1948.
20. Harris, J. S., and Farber, S.: Transposition of the great cardiac vessels with special reference to the phylogenetic theory of Spitzer. Arch. Pathol., *28*:427, 1939.
21. Hightower, B. M., Weidman, W. H., and Kirklin, J. W.: Open intracardiac repair for complete transposition of the great arteries. Circulation (Suppl. 1), *33*:19, 1966.
22. Indeglia, R. A., Moller, J. H., Lucas, R. V., Jr., and Castaneda, A. R.: Treatment of transposition of the great vessels with an intra-atrial baffle (Mustard procedure). Arch. Surg., *101*:797, 1970.
23. Kay, E. B., and Cross, F. S.: Transposition of the great vessels corrected by means of atrial transposition. Surgery, *41*:938, 1957.
24. Keith, J. D., Neill, C. A., Vlad, P., Rowe, R. D., and Chute, A. L.: Transposition of the great vessels. Circulation, *7*:830, 1953.
25. Kirklin, J. W., Devlon, R. A., and Weidman, W. H.: Open intracardiac repair of transposition of great vessels: 11 cases. Surgery, *50*:58, 1961.
26. Lev, M., and Saphir, O.: A theory of transposition of the arterial trunks based on the phylogenetic and ontogenetic developments of the heart. Arch. Pathol., *39*:172, 1945.
27. Liebman, J., Cullum, L., and Belloc, N. R.: Natural history of transposition of the great arteries. Circulation, *40*:237, 1969.
28. Lillehei, C. W., and Varco, R. L.: Certain physiologic, pathologic, and surgical features of complete transposition of the vessels. Surgery, *34*:376, 1953.
29. Medical News. J.A.M.A., *234*:1102, 1975.
30. Merendino, K. A., Jesseph, J. E., and Herron, P. W.: Interatrial venous transposition, a one stage intracardiac operation for the conversion of complete transposition of the aorta and pulmonary artery to corrected transposition: Theory and clinical experience. Surgery, *42*:898, 1957.
31. Mustard, W. T.: Successful two-stage correction of transposition of the great vessels. Surgery, *55*:469, 1964.
32. Mustard, W. T., Chute, A. L., Keith, J. D., Sirek, A., Rowe, R. D., and Vlad, P.: A surgical approach to transposition of the great vessels with extracorporeal circuit. Surgery, *36*:39, 1954.
33. Mustard, W. T., Keith, J. D., Trusler, G. A., Fowler, R., and Kidd, L.: The surgical management of transposition of the great vessels. J. Thorac. Cardiovasc. Surg., *48*:953, 1964.
34. Paul, M. H.: Transposition of the great arteries. *In* Moss, A. J., and Adams, F. H.: Heart Disease in Infants, Children and Adolescents. Baltimore, Williams & Wilkins Company, 1968, p. 527.
35. Rashkind, W. J., and Miller, W. W.: Transposition of the great arteries: Results of palliation by balloon atrioseptotomy in 31 patients. Circulation, *38*:453, 1968.
36. Rastelli, G. C., Wallace, R. B., and Ongley, P. A.: Complete repair of transposition of the great arteries with pulmonary stenosis. A review and report of a case corrected by using a new surgical technique. Circulation, *39*:83, 1969.
37. Reed, W. A., Lauer, R. M., and Diehl, A. M.: Staged correction of total transposition of the great vessels. Circulation (Suppl. 1), *33*:13, 1966.
38. Rowlatt, U. F.: Coronary artery distribution in a complete transposition. J.A.M.A., *179*:269, 1962.

39. Senning, A.: Surgical correction of transposition of the great vessels. Surgery, 45:966, 1959.
40. Shaher, R. M., and Kidd, L.: The hemodynamics of complete transposition of the great vessels before and after the creation of an atrial septal defect. Circulation (Suppl. 1). 33:3, 1966.
41. Taussig, H. B.: Complete transposition of the great vessels. Am. Heart J., 16:728, 1938.
42. Taussig, H. B.: Congenital Malformations of the Heart, 2nd ed. Cambridge, Mass., Harvard University Press, 1960.
43. Trusler, G. A., Mustard, W. T., and Fowler, R. S.: Role of surgery in the treatment of transposition of the great vessels. Can. Med. Assoc. J., 91:1096, 1964.

44. Van Mierop, L. H. S., and Wiglesworth, F. W.: Pathogenesis of transposition complexes. III. True transposition of the great vessels. Am. J. Cardiol., 12:233, 1963.
45. Van Praagh, R., and Vlad, P.: Transposition of the great arteries. In Keith, D., Rowe, R. D., and Vlad, P. (Eds.): Heart Disease in Infancy and Childhood, 2nd ed. New York, Macmillan Company, 1967.
46. Von Rokitansky, C.: Die Defekte der Scheidewände der Herzens. Vienna, Bräumuller, 1875.
47. Waldhausen, J. A., Pierce, W. S., Rashkind, W. J., et al.: Total correction of transposition of the great arteries following balloon atrioseptotomy. Circulation (Suppl. 2) 41:123, 1970.

XII

CONGENITAL AORTIC STENOSIS

H. Newland Oldham, Jr., M.D.

Congenital aortic stenosis is produced by a group of malformations that cause obstruction to the flow of blood from the left ventricle into the central aorta. This obstruction may be located at, above, or below the level of the aortic valve. These lesions are not uncommon and account for 5 to 10 per cent of all congenital heart defects.[26] Current information indicates that an abnormality of the aortic valve, although not always hemodynamically significant, is the single most common congenital cardiac defect encountered.[39] It is also now recognized that there is evidence of a pre-existing congenital valvular deformity in at least one half of adult patients with isolated aortic valve lesions.[38]

There are no known etiologic or genetic factors associated with either valvular or discrete subvalvular aortic stenosis, although supravalvular stenosis may occur with derangements in vitamin D metabolism and infantile hypercalcemia. Both the aortic lesions and the associated craniofacial abnormalities seen with this type of stenosis may be induced experimentally by administration of large doses of vitamin D.[12] A genetic factor is present in patients with hypertrophic muscular subaortic stenosis, since this lesion occurs in a familial form in about one third of patients.[18]

HISTORICAL ASPECTS

Early descriptions of aortic valve disease such as that given by Riverius in 1646 primarily concerned calcific aortic stenosis in the adult.[37] In 1844 Paget described the tendency of congenitally bicuspid aortic valves to cause obstruction, and in 1886 Osler reported the occurrence of endocarditis with bicuspid aortic valves.[33, 34] The association of arrhythmias and sudden death with aortic stenosis was recognized by Cowper in 1705 in a young adult, and Thursfield in 1913 called attention to sudden death in a child with subaortic stenosis.[11, 44] Tuffier in 1913 successfully dilated a calcific aortic valve, but no further advances were made until 1950 when Bailey successfully performed a closed dilation of the aortic valve.[1, 46] In 1955 Swan and Lewis independently performed valvulotomies using hypothermia.[24, 43] With the development of extracorporeal circulation, techniques for accurate relief of various forms of congenital aortic stenosis were successfully introduced.

PATHOLOGIC ANATOMY

The four types of obstruction that occur between the left ventricle and the aorta are valvular, discrete subvalvular, supravalvular, and hypertrophic muscular subaortic stenosis (Fig. 1). The stenosis is usually limited to one of these four types, but combinations of lesions may occur together in the same patient.[42] Between 20 and 25 per cent of these patients have other associated cardiovascular defects, most commonly coarctation of the aorta, patent ductus arteriosus, ventricular septal defect, or pulmonary stenosis.

The type of obstruction in more than half the patients is isolated valvular aortic stenosis. The basic malformation is a thickening of the valve leaflets associated with varying degrees of fusion of the commissure. The annulus is usually not affected, although occasionally it is hypoplastic. The valve may be tricuspid, with partial fusion of each commissure producing a central stenotic orifice. Fusion of the commissure between the right and the left coronary cusps, producing a bicuspid valve with an eccentric narrowed opening, occurs in 60 to 80 per cent of patients with valvular stenosis.[9, 27] Less common types encountered are valves with four cusps or valves with only a single supporting commissure that functions as a monocusp.[30, 40] Histologically, the valves demonstrate fi-

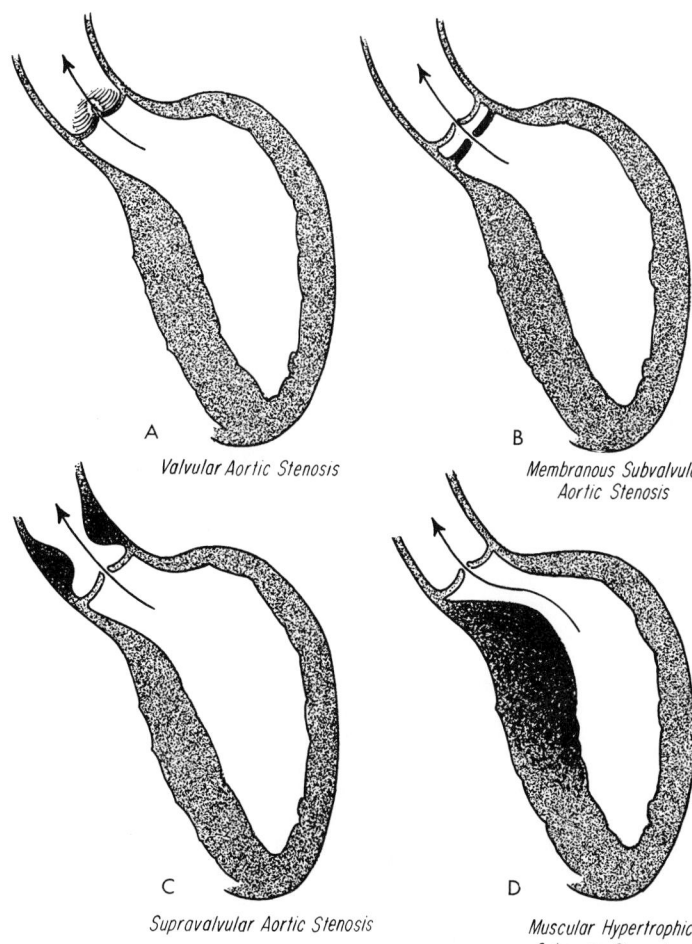

A — *Valvular Aortic Stenosis*

B — *Membranous Subvalvular Aortic Stenosis*

C — *Supravalvular Aortic Stenosis*

D — *Muscular Hypertrophic Subaortic Stenosis*

Figure 1. Diagrammatic representation of the types of congenital obstruction between the left ventricle and central aorta.

brosis and a persistence of embryonic connective tissue.[41] Infants with critical stenosis may have fibrosis of the myocardium, necrosis of the papillary muscles, and fibroelastosis.[29, 41] Calcification of a deformed aortic valve is quite common in patients over age 30 but is extremely rare during childhood.

Discrete subaortic stenosis is the second most common type of obstruction encountered and consists of a thin ring of fibrous tissue located 10 to 15 mm. below the aortic valve. This may form a concentric diaphragm with a central stenotic opening, but often the membrane is more prominent over the anterior portion of the left ventricular outflow tract and fuses at each end with the aortic leaflet of the mitral valve. The aortic valve in this situation is not stenotic, but the leaflets may be thickened, in which case mild aortic insufficiency is produced. This thickening may be due to the turbulence produced by blood ejected through the stenotic subvalvular membrane and may cause the valve to be more susceptible to bacterial endocarditis.[31]

Supravalvular aortic stenosis occurs in several anatomic forms, ranging from localized narrowing just above the valve commissures to diffuse hypoplasia of the aortic annulus and ascending aorta.[10, 36] The outer diameter of the aorta is usually normal, but may be reduced at the site of localized obstruction. The obstructing ridge is composed of fibrous tissue and elastic fibers extending from the tunica media, and it may cover the sinuses of Valsalva and produce obstruction of the coronary artery ostia. Supravalvular aortic stenosis is commonly associated with peripheral pulmonary stenosis, abnormalities of the aortic valve leaflets, coronary artery abnormalities, and craniofacial deformities.[12, 36, 48]

Muscular subaortic stenosis is a diffuse abnormality of the cardiac muscle with a broad area of hypertrophied tissue located several centimeters below the aortic valve. This type of obstruction may occur as a secondary phenomenon with other forms of aortic stenosis, or it may be a primary disorder with no other associated malformations. Microscopically, the tissue is composed of muscle fibers arranged in whorl-like masses. Electron microscopic studies demonstrate both intracellular and cell-to-cell abnormalities that are more prevalent in the region of the ventricular septum.[18]

PHYSIOLOGY

The basic hemodynamic alteration produced by obstruction of left ventricular outflow is an increase in left ventricular pressure. All four types of aortic stenosis result in a pressure gradient between the left ventricle and the aorta during the systolic ejection period. The degree of stenosis determines the pressure gradient at any given flow rate, but as cardiac output increases, the pressure gradient increases in proportion to the square of the flow rate.[16] Normal flow can be maintained through an abnormal valve at the expense of a sustained elevation of left ventricular pressure. With exercise, a doubling of cardiac output produces a fourfold increase in ventricular pressure if the systolic ejection period remains constant. Both the increase in ventricular wall tension and the increased duration of tension due to increased systolic ejection time are associated with an increase in myocardial oxygen consumption. The ventricle adapts to this prolonged pressure overload by an increase in muscle mass and a subsequent decrease in left ventricular cavity size.[17] The increased systolic ejection period results in a decrease in the length of diastole and therefore reduces coronary perfusion. Increased myocardial energy requirements coupled with a relative decrease in coronary flow ultimately result in left ventricular failure or ischemia. The development of subendocardial ischemia may be critically related to heart rate, and tachycardia may produce electrocardiograpic evidence of left ventricular strain.[23] With left ventricular failure there is a reduction in cardiac output and an increase in left ventricular end-diastolic, left atrial, and pulmonary artery pressures.

The resting cardiac output and stroke volume are usually within normal limits in children with congenital aortic stenosis. If the resting pressure gradient between the left ventricle and the aorta is less than 50 mm. Hg, or if the calculated aortic orifice size is greater than 0.7 sq. cm. per square meter of body surface area, the heart usually responds to the demands of exertion without failing. In the majority of patients with a greater degree of stenosis, manifested by a higher pressure gradient and a smaller effective valve area, cardiac output cannot be elevated by means of exercise.

The two most important sequelae of severe obstruction to left ventricular ejection are clearly increased stress on the myocardium and inability of the left ventricle to increase forward flow in response to exertion. These limitations explain the frequent occurrence of left ventricular strain, angina, and exertional syncope in children with congenital aortic stenosis.

These considerations are particularly applicable to congenital valvular, supravalvular, and discrete subaortic stenosis, all of which have a fixed area of obstruction. Hypertrophic muscular subaortic stenosis differs in that the severity of the obstruction varies, depending on the contractile state of the myocardium and left ventricular end-systolic volume. In this condition the pressure gradient is increased by infusion of inotropic drugs such as isoproterenol, by decreasing blood volume, and by the Valsalva maneuver. The obstruction is reduced by maneuvers such as increasing blood volume, general anesthesia, and administration of propranolol, an adrenergic blocking agent. A clear understanding of the effects of these influences on myocardial contraction and ventricular volume has helped to explain the different gradients measured by catheterization during varying physiologic states.[4, 32, 47]

CLINICAL FEATURES

Congenital aortic stenosis is three to four times more common in males than in females. The clinical presentation is essentially identical for each type of obstruction and the distinguishing factor is the capacity of the left ventricle to compensate for its pressure overload both at rest and during exercise. Even in the presence of significant stenosis, most patients are asymptomatic during early childhood and show normal growth and development. During later childhood, symptoms of exertional dyspnea and fatigue are common. It should be emphasized, however, that it is not unusual for children with critical stenosis to remain entirely free of symptoms, whereas others with minimal obstruction may have prominent symptoms. When the cardiac output is insufficient to meet the demands of the systemic or coronary circulation, symptoms of exertional syncope, angina, and congestive heart failure occur. These findings usually indicate a severe degree of stenosis. Approximately 10 per cent of patients with valvular aortic stenosis, however, will develop severe congestive heart failure early in life. Left ventricular failure occurring in infancy is particularly ominous and is usually fatal if untreated.[22, 35]

Physical examination demonstrates a characteristic harsh systolic murmur, most prominent over the second right interspace and usually associated with a thrill. A diastolic murmur of mild aortic insufficiency is heard in one fourth of patients with congenital aortic stenosis and is more common with discrete subvalvular stenosis. Phonocardiography characterizes the systolic murmur as the ejection type, beginning shortly after the first heart sound and ending just before the second heart sound. The second heart sound may be paradoxically split as a result of the increased duration of systolic ejection. On percussion, the heart is not found to be enlarged, but a prominent left ventricular lift is often present. The carotid pulse has a palpable slow upstroke, except with hypertrophic muscular subaortic stenosis, in which the upstroke is normal or rapid. The remainder of the physical examination is not remarkable, with the exception of the findings associated with supravalvular aortic stenosis. In this disorder a characteristic facies is frequently present, and the systolic blood pressure in the right arm is often higher than that in the left.[10, 36, 48]

The chest roentgenogram demonstrates little overall cardiomegaly, but 70 to 80 per cent of patients have evidence of left ventricular enlargement.[27] Unfortunately, the degree of enlargement does not correlate well with the severity of the stenosis, and severe obstruction may be present in children with a normal chest film. Post-stenotic dilatation of the ascending aorta is present in approximately one half of patients with moderate to severe stenosis and occurs more commonly with valvular stenosis than with the other forms of obstruction (Fig. 2). Active pulsation of the ascending aorta is seen with fluoroscopy. Calcification is rarely present in children, but its presence in a young adult is evidence that the obstruction is valvular.

The electrocardiogram has been extensively used to judge the degree of obstruction in congenital aortic stenosis. It is now realized that the electrocardiographic findings do not always correlate well with the magnitude of the pressure gradient. Stenosis that is severe enough to cause sudden death has been documented in children without any electrocardiographic abnormalities, although this is rare. In most patients with a pressure gradient of greater than 50 mm. Hg, changes of left ventricular hypertrophy and left ventricular strain are present. There is a much better correlation between these findings and the degree of stenosis in patients under 10 years of age.[5] The vectorcardiogram at times may demonstrate evidence of severe aortic stenosis despite a normal electrocardiogram.[14] Because of the difficulties in relating electro-

cardiographic findings to the presence of left ventricular overload in any individual patient, caution should be exercised in the use of these results in determining patient management.

Recent advances in diagnostic ultrasound have been helpful in evaluating the various types of aortic stenosis. Characteristic echocardiographic patterns have been described for valvular, subvalvular, supravalvular, and hypertrophic subaortic stenosis.[3, 19, 20] This noninvasive method permits localization of the site of left ventricular outflow obstruction, characterization of left ventricular performances, and in some instances estimation of the magnitude of the obstructing gradient.[19] At the present time echocardiography has not replaced the need for cardiac catheterization, but is of help in choosing the proper time for catheterization, and in following the results of surgical treatment.[4] Further refinements in these techniques may, however, eliminate the need for serial invasive evaluation of these patients.

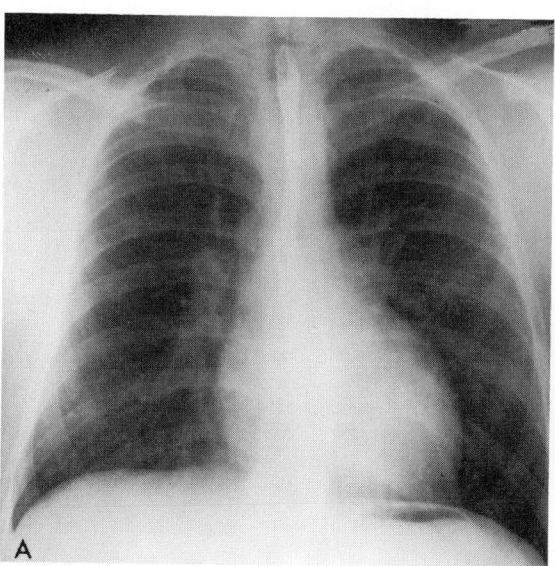

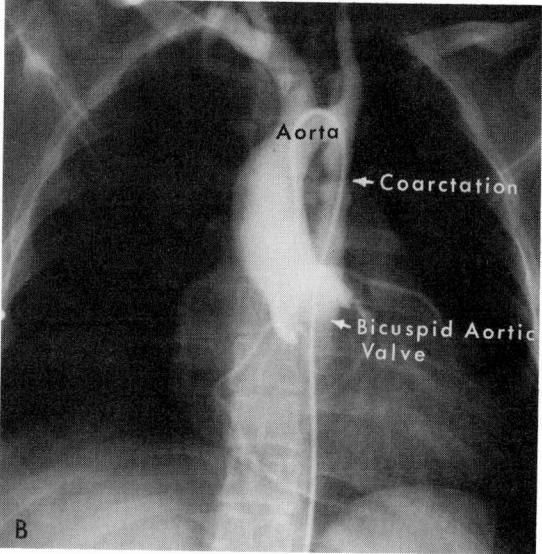

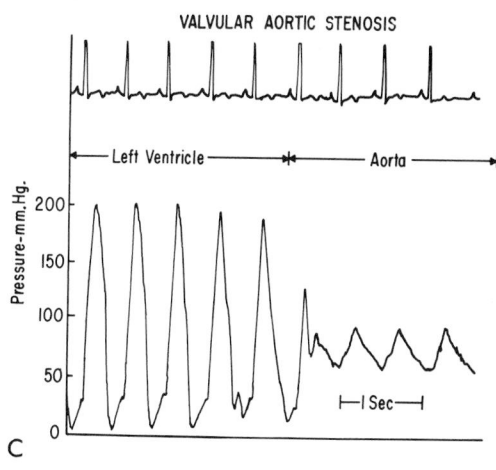

Figure 2. Valvular aortic stenosis. *A*, Chest film demonstrating slight prominence of the left ventricle. *B*, Aortogram showing a bicuspid aortic valve, post-stenotic dilatation of the ascending aorta, and associated coarctation of the descending thoracic aorta. *C*, Pressure tracing during withdrawal of a catheter from the left ventricle into the aorta, localizing the change in pressure to the level of the aortic valve.

CARDIAC CATHETERIZATION

Congenital aortic stenosis may be diagnosed accurately on the basis of clinical findings, the chest roentgenogram, the electrocardiogram, and the echocardiogram. In order to confirm the type and the degree of stenosis, and to eliminate the possibility of other associated defects, catheterization is essential. Combined right and left heart catheterization and selective angiocardiography are necessary to obtain this information. Catheterization of the right side of the heart will demonstrate any other lesions, such as a ventricular septal defect or pulmonary stenosis, that may be present, and it will also determine the presence or absence of pulmonary hypertension. Left heart catheterization is performed by either the transseptal or retrograde arterial approach. From the measurements of cardiac output and of the systolic pressure gradient between the left ventricle and the central aorta, it is possible to calculate the functional orifice area of the stenosis.[16] Selective left ventricular angiocardiography permits visualization of the level of obstruction and also allows assessment of left ventricular cavity size, ventricular wall thickness, and competency of the mitral valve (Figs. 2 to 5). If hypertrophic muscular subaortic stenosis is suspected, measurement of the pressure gradient is indicated during infusion of drugs that change peripheral vascular resistance or the inotropic state of the myocardium.[6, 32]

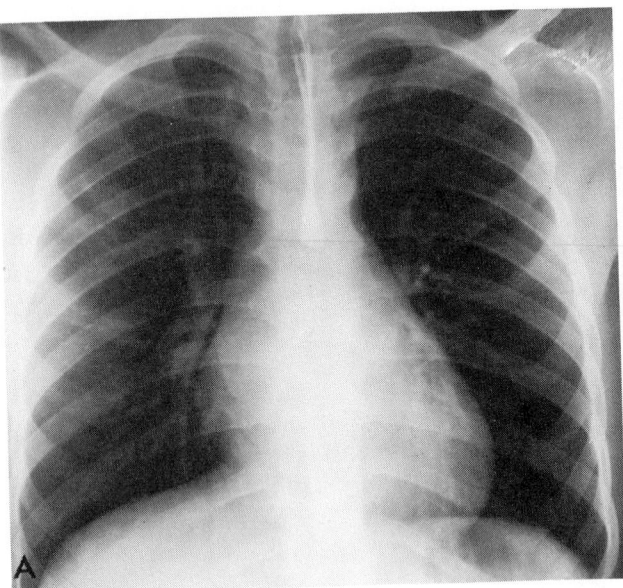

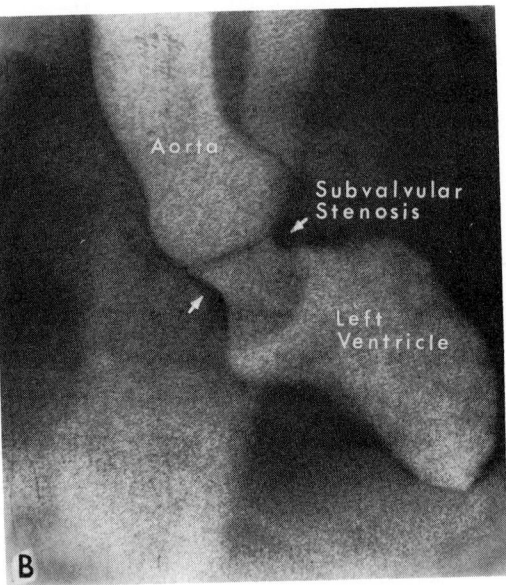

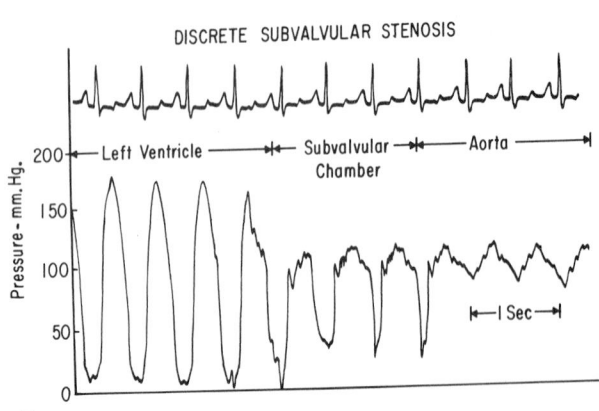

Figure 3. Discrete subvalvular aortic stenosis. *A*, Chest film. *B*, Cineangiogram during left ventricular injection, demonstrating a subvalvular membrane. *C*, Pullback pressure tracing showing systemic systolic pressure in the subvalvular chamber.

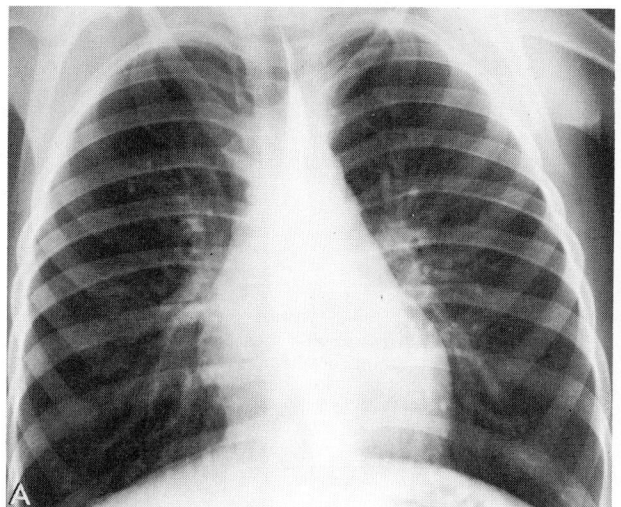

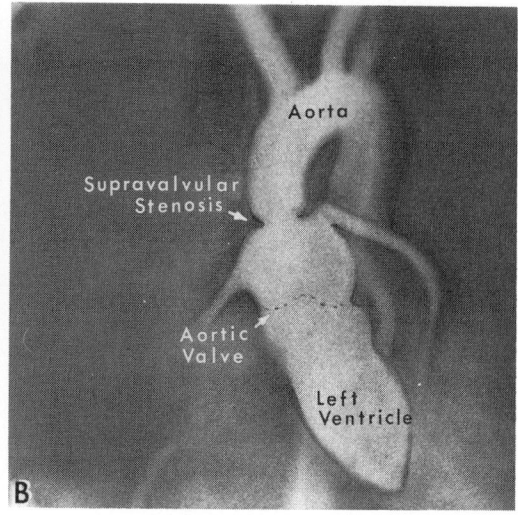

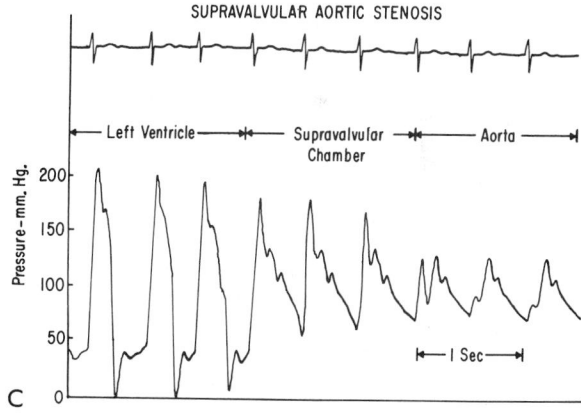

Figure 4. Supravalvular aortic stenosis. *A*, Chest film. *B*, Cineangiogram illustrating an obstructing ridge just above the origin of the coronary arteries. *C*, Pressure recording demonstrating a supravalvular zone of elevated pressure.

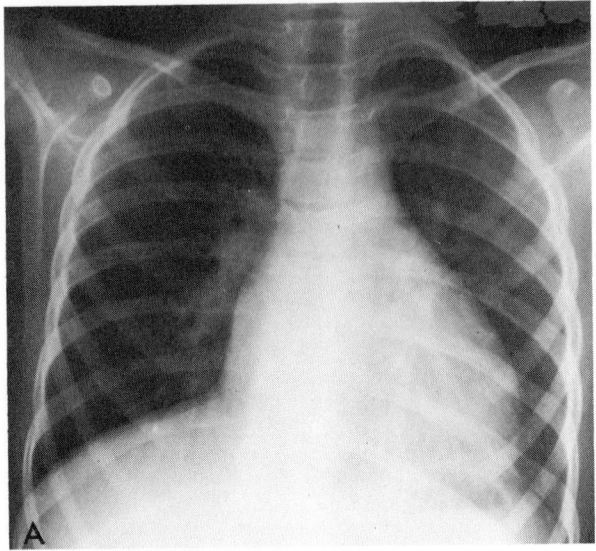

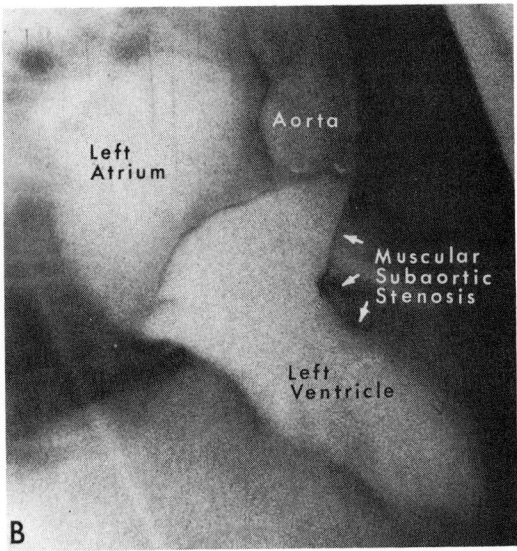

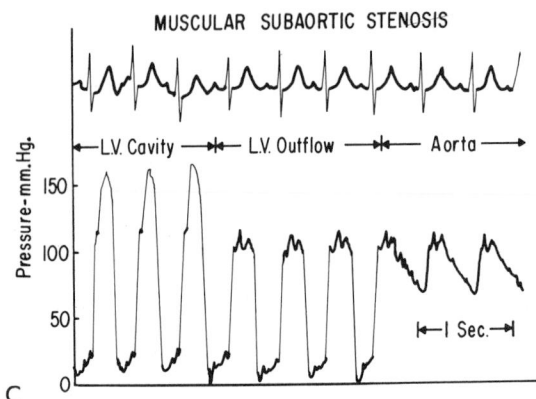

Figure 5. Hypertrophic muscular subaortic stenosis. *A,* Chest film showing considerable enlargement of the left ventricle. *B,* Left ventricle cineangiogram illustrating a broad area of muscular obstruction. The left atrium is opacified as a result of associated mitral insufficiency. *C,* Pressure tracing showing an area of systemic pressure within the left ventricular outflow tract.

NATURAL HISTORY AND OPERATIVE INDICATIONS

Careful studies of the natural history of patients with congenital aortic stenosis have been limited by the development of surgical treatment of this condition. The finding of congenitally deformed valves in most adults with isolated calcific aortic stenosis indicates the progressive nature of the obstruction over a prolonged period of time.[38] The clinical course is quite variable, with a normal life expectancy in some patients and overt cardiac decompensation or sudden death in others. Severe aortic stenosis occurring in infancy is accompanied by a high incidence of associated malformations and often causes cardiac failure and death.[7] Older children who become symptomatic usually have a moderate to severe degree of stenosis. Evaluation of initially asymptomatic children by serial cardiac catheterization showed that severe obstruction developed in more than half over a period of several years. The majority of these patients who acquired significant gradients showed no progression of symptoms or electrocardiographic findings suggest-

ing severe obstruction.[13, 28] It is therefore recommended that children with mild aortic stenosis undergo repeat cardiac catheterization after several years to identify those developing significant obstruction.[8] Sudden death is reported to occur in 1 to 19 per cent of children with aortic stenosis.[7, 15] This phenomenon, probably related to arrhythmias, is seen in most patients only after development of serious symptoms and electrocardiographic changes of left ventricular strain. It should be emphasized, however, that patients with none of these abnormal signs or symptoms have experienced sudden death.[21]

Operative treatment is recommended in a child with severe obstruction, indicated by a systolic pressure gradient greater than 50 mm. Hg or by a calculated area of stenosis less than 0.5 sq. cm. per square meter of body surface area. It is advisable, if possible, to delay operation until the child is older, because surgical exposure and techniques are easier when the structures are larger. Since as many as one fourth of infants with severe obstruction die during the first year of life, operative treatment may be indicated at this early age in spite of the increased operative risk.[7, 22]

SURGICAL TREATMENT AND RESULTS

Operative procedures are currently available for correction or palliation of all forms of left ventricular outflow obstruction. The general approach of the various types is the same, but specific methods for relief of the stenosis are quite different. Except during infancy, all operations are performed with cardiopulmonary bypass, which allows ample time and exposure for complete assessment of the defect and utilization of precise surgical techniques. The heart is exposed through a median sternotomy. Venous drainage is provided by a catheter inserted into the right atrium, and arterial inflow is directed into the femoral artery or the ascending aorta. The left ventricle is cannulated through its apex or the right superior pulmonary vein to produce a bloodless field. After the ascending aorta is clamped, a vertical aortotomy is made into the noncoronary sinus of Valsalva. Protection against myocardial ischemia is achieved by mild hypothermia, and individual perfusion of the coronary arteries may be used if extended operative time is necessary. At this point, careful evaluation of the anatomy is undertaken, with the realization that additional sites of obstruction may be present. Only after the exact nature of the lesion is established can specific methods for its correction be employed.

Valvular stenosis is corrected by incision of the fused commissures. If the valve is tricuspid, each of the three commissures is divided to within 1 mm. of the aortic annulus. With the more common bicuspid valve, the two lines of fusion are carefully separated (Fig. 6). The incomplete commissure in the left half of the bicuspid valve representing the fusion point of the right and left coronary cusps should not be incised, since this destroys the support of that portion of the valve and produces significant aortic regurgitation. It is advisable to perform a limited valvulotomy, and leave a residual gradient, rather than to abolish the gradient completely at the expense of aortic insuffi-

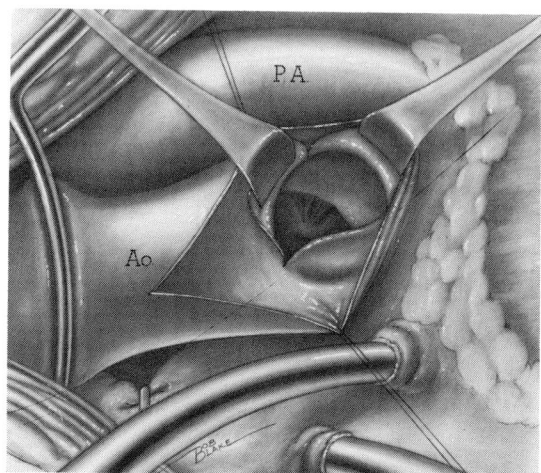

Figure 7. Discrete subvalvular aortic stenosis. The aortic valve leaflets are retracted to expose the subvalvular membrane. Partial excision of this membrane eliminates the obstruction.

cieny. In the rare circumstance when a unicusp valve is encountered, extreme care must be exercised, since it may be impossible to enlarge the valve orifice safely. Occasionally fibrosis and thickening of the valve cusps cause functional stenosis after a commissurotomy has been performed. In these rare instances it may be necessary to replace the valve with a prosthesis in order to eliminate the obstruction.[49]

The management of critical valvular stenosis in infancy may be approached in a similar manner using cardiopulmonary bypass, although the use of a brief period of inflow occlusion has produced quite favorable results.[22] Success has also been reported in infants using a closed transventricular approach to dilate the valve.[45]

Exposure of discrete subvalvular stenosis is obtained by retracting the aortic valve leaflets (Fig. 7). The fibrous membrane is partially removed in the safe portion of its circumference beneath each side of the commissure between the right and left leaflets. Extensive removal of the membrane in other areas can produce damage to the underlying structures and result in mitral insufficiency, ventricular septal defect, or third-degree heart block. The aortic valve leaflets are often thickened and may cause mild aortic insufficiency, but no attempt should be made to correct hemodynamically insignificant regurgitation.

When supravalvular stenosis is caused by diffuse hypoplasia of the ascending aorta, surgical procedures such as endarterectomy or enlarging the aorta by a long prosthetic patch may occasionally be successful, but in general the results of these maneuvers have not been satisfactory. The localized type of supravalvular stenosis is much more amenable to surgical correction. The deformed area is usually just above the commissures, so total excision of the tissue as a form of treatment is not possible. Partial excision of the intraluminal ridge is indicated if there is obstruction of the coronary ostia. Effective relief of the obstruction is achieved by suturing a patch of plastic material to

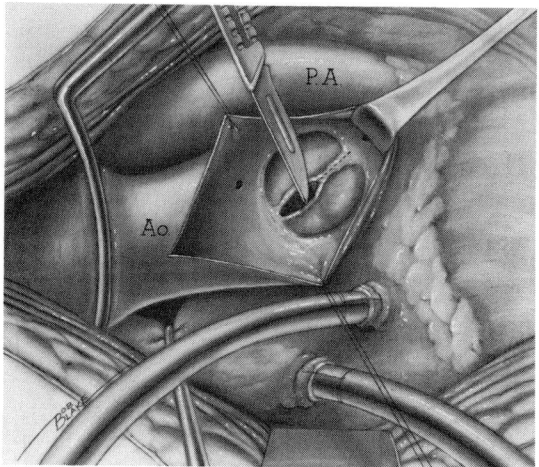

Figure 6. Valvular aortic stenosis. A longitudinal incision is made in the ascending aorta to expose the bicuspid aortic valve. The valve is incised along the line of fusion of the commissures to relieve the stenosis.

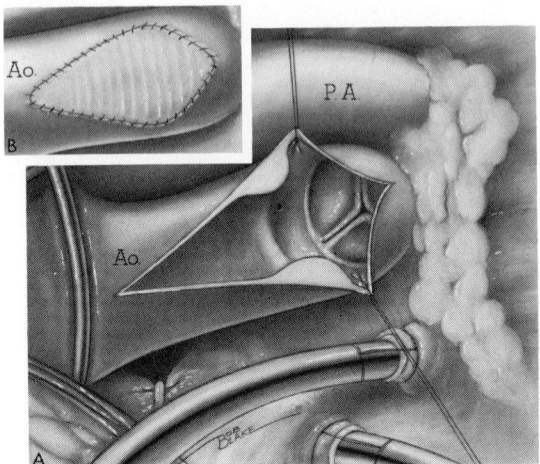

Figure 8. Supravalvular aortic stenosis. *A,* The aortotomy is performed through the ridge of obstructing tissue located just above the coronary ostia. *B,* A patch of plastic material is inserted into the aortic incision to enlarge the narrowed segment.

each side of a generous aortotomy and extending it through the constricting segment (Fig. 8).

Muscular subaortic stenosis is now recognized as a diffuse disorder of the left ventricular musculature. Pharmacologic alteration of the process by adrenergic blocking agents is occasionally helpful; however, in those patients with severe gradients, relief of the obstruction by surgical means is preferable. Numerous approaches for resection of a portion of the muscle mass have been advocated, but the transaortic route has been successfully used in most instances.[32] After the aortic valve leaflets have been retracted, the diffuse area of hypertrophy is defined by palpation through the valve. Parallel incisions are made into the muscle and a strip of tissue is excised between these cuts for a considerable distance into the ventricle (Fig.

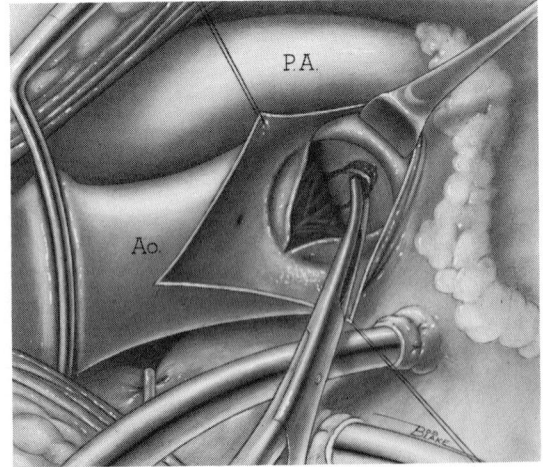

Figure 9. Hypertrophic muscular subaortic stenosis. After retraction of the aortic valve leaflets, a portion of the hypertrophied tissue is removed with a rongeur to widen the left ventricular outflow tract.

9). The incision must be properly placed to avoid perforation of the septum or injury to the conduction system.

At the conclusion of the operative procedure for the various types of aortic stenosis, simultaneous pressures should be recorded from the left ventricle and the ascending aorta to measure any residual gradient. Simultaneous determination of cardiac output by the indicator dilution method is of help in interpreting the significance of the measured gradient. It is preferable to accept a gradient of 30 mm. Hg or less rather than extend the opening and risk the production of aortic insufficiency or damage to adjacent structures. There is good correlation between the gradient recorded at the end of the procedure and measurements obtained during postoperative catheterization. In some patients with adequate correction of valvular stenosis, a gradient remains because of secondary muscular hypertrophy, but this usually resolves during the postoperative period.

The risks of surgical correction of all types of aortic stenosis are small, and the postoperative results are generally good. The long-term results following relief of supravalvular, muscular subaortic, and discrete subaortic stenosis justify an aggressive surgical approach to these disorders.[2, 25, 32, 36] The ultimate outcome following operation for congenital valvular stenosis is not as clearly established. At the present time it is not known whether opening a deformed valve during childhood will prevent the progression of subsequent stenosis and calcification during adult life. It is probable that a second operative procedure will be necessary in some of these patients, and insertion of a prosthetic valve may be required. Until these questions are answered, it seems wise to limit operative treatment for congenital valvular aortic stenosis to those patients with a significant pressure gradient or clinical findings of left ventricular compromise.

SELECTED REFERENCES

Bernhard, W. F., Keane, J. F., Fellows, K. E., Litwin, S. B., and Gross, R. E.: Progress and problems in the surgical management of congenital aortic stenosis. J. Thorac. Cardiovasc. Surg., 66:404, 1973.
This series of 188 patients with various forms of congenital aortic stenosis is the largest currently available for review. The authors stress the low operative mortality and the generally favorable results. It is apparent that some patients will require reoperation because of residual pressure gradients or progressive aortic insufficiency.

Braunwald, E., Goldblatt, A., Aygen, M. M., Rockoff, S. D., and Morrow, A. G.: Congenital aortic stenosis. I. Clinical and hemodynamic findings in 100 patients. Circulation, 27:426, 1963.

Morrow, A. G., Goldblatt, A., and Braunwald, E.: Congenital aortic stenosis. II. Surgical treatment and results of operation. Circulation, 27:450, 1963.
These companion papers represent excellent examples of the critical use of hemodynamic measurements in evaluating both the preoperative severity of congenital aortic stenosis and the results of operative intervention. A thorough analysis of the clinical findings, electrocardiographic patterns, and cardiac catheterization data from 100 children is presented. The surgical procedures used in 44 of these patients are clearly described and illustrated. Complete postoperative cardiac catheterization studies were performed in 33 patients, and the findings document the effectiveness of the methods of treatment utilized.

Friedman, W. F., Modlinger, J., and Morgan, J. R.: Serial hemodynamic observation in asymptomatic children with valvar aortic stenosis. Circulation, 43:91, 1971.

This evaluation of initially asymptomatic children by serial cardiac catheterizations demonstrated that severe obstruction developed in more than half over an average follow-up period of 6.8 years. In the majority of these patients, symptoms, electrocardiograms, and chest roentgenograms did not correlate well with the development of a significant transvalvular pressure gradient. The authors conclude that serial hemodynamic studies should be a routine part of the evaluation of asymptomatic children with aortic stenosis in order to determine properly the advisability of surgical treatment.

Morrow, A. G., Reitz, B. A., Epstein, S. E., Henry, W. L., Conkle, D. M., Itscoitz, S. B., and Redwood, D. R.: Operative treatment in hypertrophic subaortic stenosis. Circulation, 52:88, 1975.
The authors review their extensive experience over a 15-year period with the operative treatment of 83 patients with hypertrophic subaortic stenosis. Postoperative catheterization results in 52 patients clearly demonstrate successful relief of obstruction for periods up to 14 years.

Rastelli, G. C., McGoon, D. C., Ongley, P. A., Mankin, H. T., and Kirklin, J. W.: Surgical treatment of supravalvular aortic stenosis. J. Thorac. Cardiovasc. Surg., 51:873, 1966.
Surgical experience with 16 patients with congenital supravalvular aortic stenosis is presented in this article, and the literature on this unusual lesion is reviewed. The various types of supravalvular obstruction are described, and the surgical procedures recommended are clearly presented.

Roberts, W. C.: The congenitally bicuspid aortic valve. Am. J. Cardiol., 26:72, 1970.
The author gives a detailed analysis of the postmortem examination of 105 adult patients with isolated aortic valve stenosis. Sixtyseven of these patients were found to have congenitally deformed valves, and in 54 the valve was bicuspid. This paper establishes the bicuspid aortic valve as the most common congenital malformation of the heart, and supports the concept that these valves progressively stenose and finally produce the adult form of calcific aortic stenosis. This is an excellent presentation of the pathologic anatomy and the ultimate fate of the congenitally bicuspid aortic valve.

REFERENCES

1. Bailey, C. P., Glover, R. P., O'Neill, T. J. E., and Redondo-Ramirez, H. P.: Surgical relief of aortic stenosis. J. Thorac. Surg., 20:516, 1950.
2. Bernhard, W. F., Keane, J. F., Fellows, K. E., Litwin, S. B., and Gross, R. E.: Progress and problems in the surgical management of congenital aortic stenosis. J. Thorac. Cardiovasc. Surg., 66:404, 1973.
3. Bolen, J. L., Popp, R. L., and French, J. W.: Echocardiographic features of supravalvular aortic stenosis. Circulation, 52:817, 1975.
4. Bolton, M. R., Jr., King, J. F., Polumbo, R. A., Mason, D., Pugh, D. M., Reis, R. L., and Dunn, M. I.: The effects of operation on the echocardiographic features of idiopathic hypertrophic subaortic stenosis. Circulation, 50:897, 1974.
5. Braunwald, E., Goldblatt, A., Aygen, M. M., Rockoff, S. D., and Morrow, A. G.: Congenital aortic stenosis. I. Clinical and hemodynamic findings in 100 patients. Circulation, 27:426, 1963.
6. Braunwald, E., Oldham, H. N., Jr., Ross, J., Jr., Linhart, J. W., Mason, D. T., and Fort, L., III: The circulatory response of patients with idiopathic hypertrophic subaortic stenosis to nitroglycerin and to the Valsalva maneuver. Circulation, 29:422, 1964.
7. Campbell, M.: The natural history of congenital aortic stenosis. Br. Heart J., 30:514, 1968.
8. Cohen, L. S., Friedman, W. F., and Braunwald, E.: Natural history of mild congenital aortic stenosis elucidated by serial hemodynamic studies. Am. J. Cardiol., 30:1, 1972.
9. Conkle, D. M., Jones, M., and Morrow, A. G.: Treatment of congenital aortic stenosis. Arch. Surg., 107:649, 1973.
10. Cornell, W. P., Elkins, R. C., Criley, J. M., and Sabiston, D. C., Jr.: Supravalvular aortic stenosis. J. Thorac. Cardiovasc. Surg., 51:484, 1966.
11. Cowper, W.: Of ossification or petrifactions in the coats of arteries, particularly in the valves of the great artery. Trans. Phil. Tr. R. Soc. London, 5:215, 1703–1712.
12. Friedman, W. F., and Mills, L. F.: The relationship between vitamin D and the craniofacial and dental anomalies of the supravalvular aortic stenosis syndrome. Pediatrics, 43:12, 1969.
13. Friedman, W. F., Modlinger, J., and Morgan, J. R.: Serial hemodynamic observations in asymptomatic children with valvar aortic stenosis. Circulation, 43:91, 1971.
14. Gamboa, R., Hugenholtz, P. G., and Nadas, A. S.: Comparison of electrocardiograms and vectorcardiograms in congenital aortic stenosis. Br. Heart J., 27:344, 1965.
15. Glew, R. H., Varghese, P. J., Krovetz, L. J., Dorst, J. P., and Rowe, R. D.: Sudden death in congenital aortic stenosis: A review of eight cases with an evaluation of premonitory clinical features. Am. Heart J., 78:615, 1969.
16. Gorlin, R., and Gorlin, S. G.: Hydraulic formula for calculation of area of stenotic mitral valve, other cardiac valves, and central circulatory shunts. Am. Heart J., 41:1, 1951.
17. Graham, T. P., Jr., Lewis, B. W., Jarmakani, M. M., Canent, R. V., and Capp, M. P.: Left heart volume and mass quantification in children with left ventricular pressure overload. Circulation, 41:203, 1970.
18. Henry, W. L., Clark, C. E., Glancy, D. L., and Epstein, S. E.: Echocardiographic measurement of the left ventricular outflow gradient in idiopathic hypertrophic subaortic stenosis. N. Engl. J. Med., 288:989, 1973.
19. Henry, W. L., Clark, C. E., and Epstein, S. E.: Asymmetric septal hypertrophy (ASH): The unifying link in the IHSS disease spectrum. Circulation, 47:827, 1973.
20. Johnson, M. L., Warren, S. G., Waugh, R. A., Kisslo, J. A., Sabison, D. C., and Lester, R. G.: Echocardiography of the aortic valve in non-rheumatic left ventricular outflow tract lesions. Radiology, 112:677, 1974.
21. Jones, R. C., Walker, W. J., Jahnke, E. J., and Winn, D. F.: Congenital aortic stenosis: Correlation of clinical severity with hemodynamic and surgical findings in 43 cases. Ann. Intern. Med., 58:486, 1963.
22. Keane, J. F., Bernhard, W. F., and Nadas, A. S.: Aortic stenosis surgery in infancy. Circulation, 52:1138, 1975.
23. Lewis, A. B., Heymann, M. A., Stanger, P., Hoffman, J. I. E., and Rudolph, A. M.: Evaluation of subendocardial ischemia in valvar aortic stenosis in children. Circulation, 49:978, 1974.
24. Lewis, F. J.: Aortic valvulotomy under direct vision during hypothermia. J. Thorac. Surg., 32:481, 1956.
25. Lillehei, C. W., Bonnabeau, R. C., Jr., and Sellers, R. D.: Subaortic stenosis: Diagnostic criteria, surgical approach, and late follow-up in 25 patients. J. Thorac. Cardiovasc. Surg., 55:94, 1968.
26. Mitchell, S. C., Korones, S. B., and Berendes, H. W.: Congenital heart disease in 56,109 births. Circulation, 43:323, 1971.
27. McGoon, D. C., Geha, A. S., Scofield, E. L., and DuShane, J. W.: Surgical treatment of congenital aortic stenosis. Dis. Chest, 55:388, 1969.
28. Mody, M. R., and Mody, G. T.: Serial hemodynamic observations in congenital valvular and subvalvular aortic stenosis. Am. Heart J., 89:137, 1975.
29. Moller, J. H., Nakib, A., and Edwards, J. E.: Infarction of papillary muscles and mitral insufficiency associated with congenital aortic stenosis. Circulation, 34:87, 1966.
30. Moller, J. H. Nakib, A., Eliot, R. S., and Edwards, J. E.: Symptomatic congenital aortic stenosis in the first year of life. J. Pediatr., 69:728, 1966.
31. Morrow, A. G., Fort, L., III, Roberts, W. C., and Braunwald, E.: Discrete subaortic stenosis complicated by aortic valvular regurgitation: Clinical, hemodynamic, and pathologic studies and the results of operative treatment. Circulation, 31:163, 1965.
32. Morrow, A. G., Reitz, B. A., Epstein, S. E., Henry, W. L., Conkle, D. M., Itscoitz, S. B., and Redwood, D. R.: Operative treatment in hypertrophic subaortic stenosis. Circulation, 52:88, 1975.
33. Osler, W.: The bicuspid condition of the aortic valves. Trans. Assoc. Am. Physicians, 2:185, 1886.
34. Paget, J.: On obstructions of the branches of the pulmonary artery. Med. Chir. Trans., 27:162, 1844.
35. Peckham, G. B., Keith, J. D., and Evans, J. R.: Congenital aortic stenosis: Some observations on the natural history and the clinical assessment. Can. Med. Assoc. J., 91:639, 1964.
36. Rastelli, G. C., McGoon, D. C., Ongley, P. A., Mankin, H. T., and Kirklin, J. W.: Surgical treatment of supravalvular aortic stenosis: Report of 16 cases and review of literature. J. Thorac. Cardiovasc. Surg., 51:873, 1966.
37. Riverius, L.: Observations medical et curatives insignes, quebus accesserunt observations an Alles communicatae. London, M. Flesher, 1646.

38. Roberts, W. C.: The structure of the aortic valve in clinically isolated aortic stenosis. Circulation, *42*:91, 1970.

39. Roberts, W. C.: The congenitally bicuspid aortic valve: A study of 85 autopsy cases. Am. J. Cardiol., *26*:72, 1970.

40. Robicsek, F., Sanger, P. W., Daugherty, H. K., and Montgomery, C. C.: Congenital quadricuspid aortic valve with displacement of the left coronary orifice. Am. J. Cardiol., *23*:288, 1969.

41. Serck-Hanssen, A.: Congenital valvular aortic stenosis: Histologic changes in the valves and myocardium in 3 cases. Acta Pathol. Microbiol. Scand., *72*:465, 1968.

42. Shumacker, H. B., and Nahrwold, D. L.: Associated subvalvular and supravalvular aortic stenosis with aortic valve anomaly. Ann. Thorac. Surg., *9*:356, 1970.

43. Swan, H., Wilkenson, R. H., and Blount, S. G., Jr.: Visual repair of congenital aortic stenosis during hypothermia. J. Thorac. Surg., *35*:139, 1958.

44. Thursfield, H., and Scott, H. W.: Sub-aortic stenosis. Br. J. Child. Dis., *10*:104, 1913.

45. Trinkle, J. K., Norton, J. B., Richardson, J. D., Grover, F. L., and Noonan, J. A.: Closed aortic valvotomy and simultaneous correction of associated anomalies in infants. J. Thorac. Cardiovasc. Surg., *69*:758, 1975.

46. Tuffier, T.: Etat actuel de la chirurgie intrathoracique. Trans. Int. Cong. Med., London, 1914.

47. Whalen, R. E., Cohen, A. I., Sumner, R. G., and McIntosh, H. D.: Demonstration of the dynamic nature of idiopathic hypertrophic subaortic stenosis. Am. J. Cardiol., *11*:8, 1963.

48. Williams, J. C. P., Barratt-Boyes, B. G., and Lowe, J. D.: Supravalvular aortic stenosis. Circulation, *24*:1311, 1961.

49. Wittig, J., McConnell, D., Buckberg, G., and Mulder, D.: Aortic valve replacement in the young child. Ann. Thorac. Surg., *19*:40, 1975.

XIII

THE CORONARY CIRCULATION

David C. Sabiston, Jr., M.D.

A variety of distinct pathologic disorders may reduce blood flow to the myocardium and produce a serious threat to life. By far the most common cause of myocardial ischemia is coronary *atherosclerosis,* and this disorder is the greatest single cause of death among Americans today. Although the symptoms of *angina pectoris* have been known since Heberden's classic description in 1768,[52] and *acute myocardial infarction* has been recognized since the report by Herrick in 1912,[53] only in recent years has the *epidemic* nature of coronary disease been appreciated. The presence of extensive coronary atherosclerosis in otherwise healthy young males was emphasized in World War II by the incidence of fatal myocardial infarction occurring in soldiers. It was also shown in *routine* autopsies on young military casualties in the Korean conflict that 77 per cent had *gross* evidence of coronary atherosclerosis and 10 per cent showed *advanced* disease, with 70 per cent or greater occlusion of one or more major coronary arteries.[35] In a community study, coronary atherosclerosis (from 25 per cent to complete occlusion of one or more major arteries) was present in three fourths of the entire population.[98] These figures indicate the extreme prevalence of the disorder, but unfortunately its presence is usually not made manifest until serious symptoms appear.

Advances made in coronary arteriography and evaluation of ventricular function have been of great significance in the objective diagnosis of coronary occlusion and myocardial ischemia. The direct approach to myocardial revascularization by anastomosis of venous autografts from the aorta to the coronary arteries has assumed a primary position in the field of cardiovascular surgery and is currently the most frequent heart operation.

ANATOMY OF THE CORONARY ARTERIES

The right and left coronary arteries are the first branches of the aorta and arise from the sinuses of Valsalva. The right coronary artery passes deep in the right atrial ventricular groove and proceeds over the anterior surface of the heart. At the superior end of the acute margin of the heart on the right, the vessel turns posteriorly toward the crux of the heart and usually terminates as the *posterior descending* coronary artery as it passes forward on the diaphragmatic surface of the heart in the posterior interventricular groove. The right coronary artery initially branches into a number of small vessels, which anastomose on the anterior ventricle in the pulmonary conus region with corresponding branches from the left coronary artery (the arterial circle of Vieussens). It next supplies multiple ventricular branches and the sinus node artery (the latter *may* arise from the left circumflex artery). Along the acute right border of the heart, the right *marginal* artery takes origin. The right coronary artery terminates in the posterior descending artery and by an extension to the crux, and branches into an atrial ventricular nodal artery and several terminal left ventricular branches supplying the posterior surface of the left ventricle. A diagrammatic illustration of the right coronary artery and its branches is shown in Figure 1.[110]

The *left* coronary is usually about 1 cm. in length and gives rise to the *anterior descending* and *circumflex* arteries, but careful analysis has shown that an *early bifurcation* of the left main coronary artery is very common and is of importance when the left coronary artery is being perfused directly through its ostium by an indwelling cannula during open-heart surgery.[43] The anterior descending gives branches to the arterial circle of Vieussens, and several *diagonal* branches to the left ventricular surface, and as it proceeds inferiorly, gives origin to a number of anterior penetrating branches to the interventricular septum. This artery terminates at the apex of the heart, usually anastomosing with the *posterior descending* artery. The anterior descending coronary artery supplies (1) the anterior left margin of the right

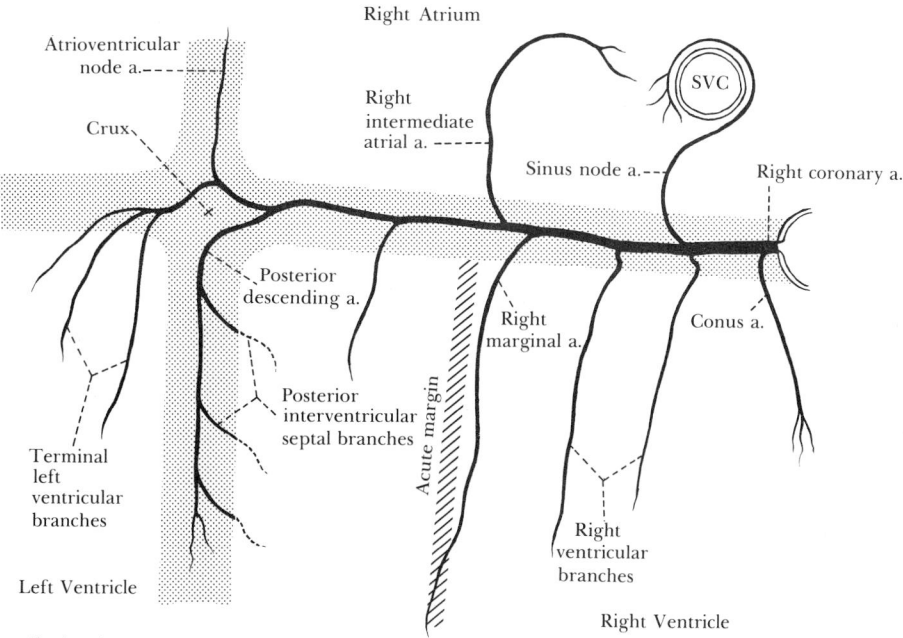

Figure 1. A schematic drawing of the right coronary artery, showing its usual branches and the common point of termination between the crux and obtuse margin of the heart. (From Winterscheid, L. C.: In Strandness, D. E., Jr. (Ed.): Collateral Circulation in Clinical Surgery. Philadelphia, W. B. Saunders Company, 1969.)

ventricle, (2) the free wall of the left ventricle, (3) the apex of the heart, and (4) the principal blood supply of the interventricular septum.

The left *circumflex* artery lies in the atrioventricular groove on the left and proceeds inferiorly and posteriorly to pass around the obtuse margin of the heart, terminating in the left marginal artery or communicating via the crux with the posterior descending coronary artery. The first branch of the circumflex artery is usually the auricular anastomotic artery (Kugel's artery). A diagrammatic illustration of the left coronary artery and its anterior descending and circumflex branches is shown in Figure 2.[110]

A *single* coronary artery occurs as an anatomic variation and has been described in more than 150 patients. The presence of a single coronary artery without other cardiac defects (59 per cent) is usually an innocuous finding. However, in some patients without other anomalies sudden death or cardiomyopathy in young adulthood or childhood occurs. This anomaly is also of interest in the perfusion of coronary arteries at the time of open-heart surgery.[95]

The *venous drainage* of the heart is via *superficial* and deep circuits. The superficial veins conduct most of the venous blood and accompany the respective coronary arteries and empty either into the *coronary sinus* (which drains into the right atrium) or into the anterior cardiac veins, the latter emptying individually into the right atrium. The deep veins communicate with both the atrial and ventricular cavities via thebesian and sinusoidal channels.

CORONARY COLLATERAL CIRCULATION

The coronary collateral circulation has been studied extensively both in the experimental animal and in the human. It is well recognized that the human heart has few *natural* collaterals of sufficient diameter to immediately deliver a significant quantity of blood in the event of a major coronary occlusion. It is for this

reason that sudden occlusion of an otherwise normal coronary artery is such a hazardous event. It has been recognized for many years that there are a number of collaterals the size of 200 microns or less present in most hearts, but these channels require enlargement over a period of time and in the presence of favorable pressure differentials in order to become functionally significant. In the experimental animal, a slowly occluding obstructing device (ameroid constrictor) can be placed on a major coronary artery and totally occlude the vessel over a period of weeks. Under these circumstances, the pressure and flow through the involved coronary artery are *slowly* reduced, during which time the natural collaterals slowly enlarge. Thus, in the experimental animal, the distal pressure following slow occlusion may progressively rise to essentially that of the preocclusion value. However, in the human the data have not shown thus far such an effective collateral circulation.

In normal humans undergoing cardiac operations for conditions other than coronary atherosclerosis, the retrograde flow from the left main coronary artery averaged 2.4 ml. per minute and from the right coronary artery 1.7 ml. per minute with respective peripheral coronary pressures of 15 and 16 mm. Hg.[45]

It is now recognized that stenotic lesions of 90 to 95 per cent or greater are required to produce *significant* collateral vessels in man. Under these circumstances, at the time of operation back pressure and back flow can be determined. The mean back pressure for totally occluded arteries varies from 30 to 40 mm. Hg, and for those arteries with less than a 90 per cent stenosis the average is only 18 to 20 mm. Hg.[78, 106]

Human studies have demonstrated that the coronary collateral circulation can appear and regress rap-

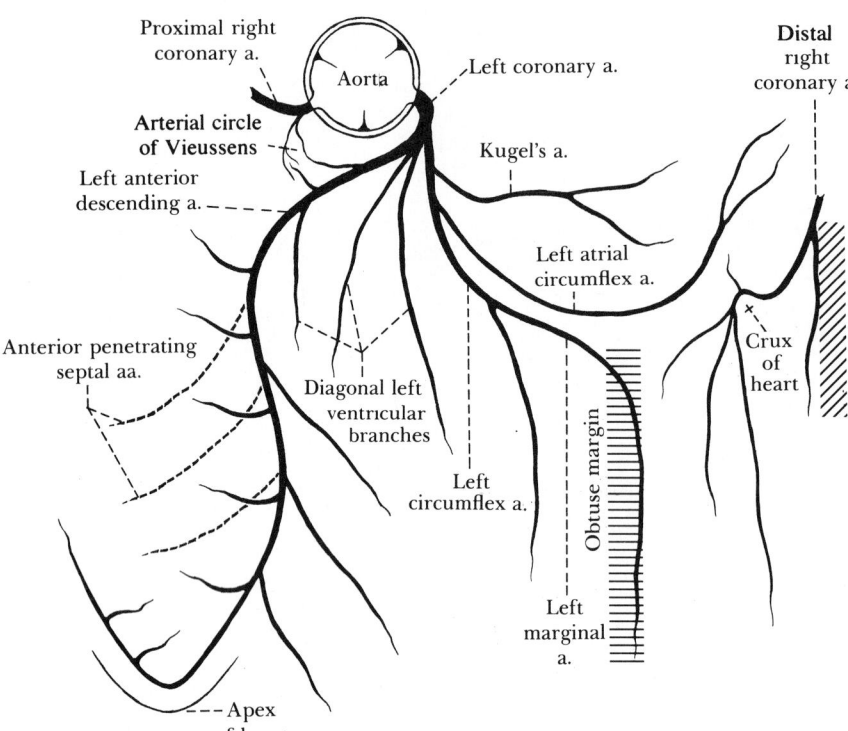

Figure 2. The left coronary artery with its anterior descending and circumflex branches. (From Winterscheid, L. C. *In* Strandness, D. E., Jr. (Ed.): Collateral Circulation in Clinical Surgery. Philadelphia, W. B. Saunders Company, 1969.)

idly according to myocardial nutritional needs and pressure gradients as may occur with the insertion of a vein bypass graft or by its subsequent occlusion. These data have been found at the time of repeat arteriography and comparison with previous films.[19]

Finally, it should be remembered that myocardial infarction may occur with minimal or even absent coronary narrowing. This has been reported to occur in as many as 7 per cent of patients with fatal myocardial infarction.[34] Coronary arterial *spasm* may account for this (Prinzmetal's *variant or atypical angina*).[55]

PHYSIOLOGIC DETERMINANTS OF CORONARY BLOOD FLOW

The average coronary blood flow in the human adult has been calculated to be 80 ml. per 100 gm. per minute (range, 66 to 93 ml. per 100 gm. per minute).[85]

Compared with other organs, the oxygen extraction is quite high (Fig. 3),[46] and the average coronary arteriovenous oxygen difference is approximately 11 ml. per 100 ml. of blood (range, 10.3 to 12.5).[85] The coronary venous Po_2 is in the range of 20 mm. Hg. These data emphasize the high oxygen *utilization* of the myocardium, which is approximately 10 ml. per 100 gm. of cardiac muscle per minute. The arterial pressure is an important determinant of flow, and generally follows an essentially linear relationship in physiologic ranges; that is, the higher the arterial pressure, the greater the coronary blood flow. It is somewhat paradoxical that during *ventricular systole* coronary blood flow decreases because of the increased resistance as the cardiac muscle contracts. Conversely, an augmentation of coronary flow occurs during *diastole* as the ventricles relax and resistance diminishes. *Thus, the heart is the only organ in the body that consistently has a greater arterial blood flow in diastole than in systole.*

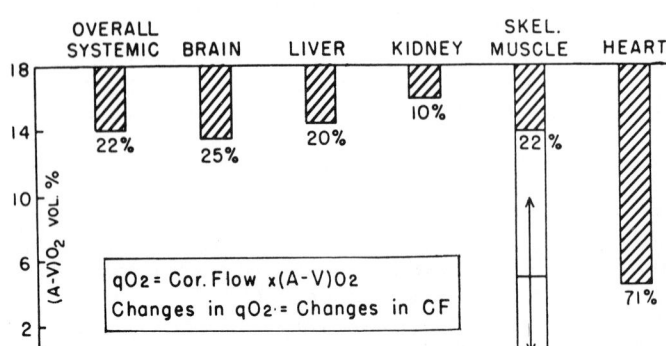

Figure 3. Systemic and regional arteriovenous oxygen extraction. qO_2 = oxygen consumption per minute. Exercising skeletal muscle extracts an increasing but varying amount of oxygen during effort (arrow). Oxygen extraction by cardiac muscle remains relatively constant and exceeds that of other organs. (From Gorlin, R.: Br. Heart J., Suppl., *33*:9, 1971.)

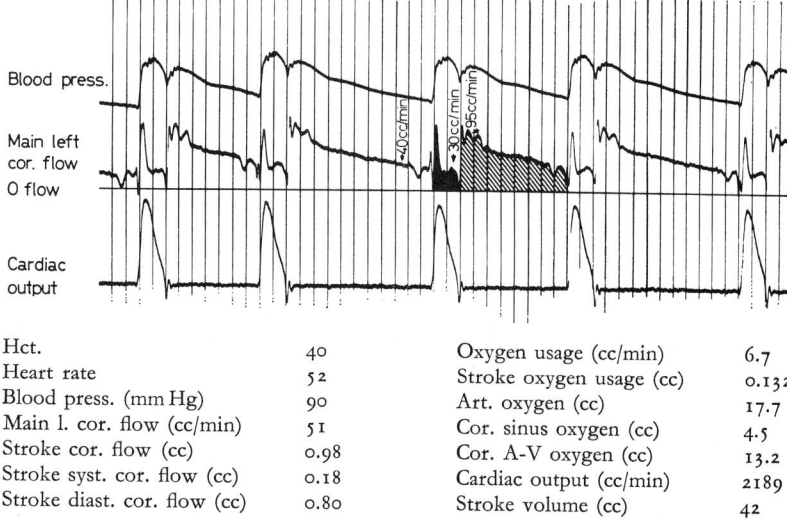

Figure 4. Data illustrating phasic aortic pressure and phasic flow in the left main coronary artery and ascending aorta obtained by means of a chronically implanted strain gauge and electromagnetic flowmeter in a dog at rest. (From Gregg, D. E. *In* Marchetti, G., and Taccardi, B. (Eds.): Coronary Circulation and Energetics of the Myocardium. Basel, S. Karger, 1967.)

Hct.	40	Oxygen usage (cc/min)	6.7
Heart rate	52	Stroke oxygen usage (cc)	0.132
Blood press. (mm Hg)	90	Art. oxygen (cc)	17.7
Main l. cor. flow (cc/min)	51	Cor. sinus oxygen (cc)	4.5
Stroke cor. flow (cc)	0.98	Cor. A-V oxygen (cc)	13.2
Stroke syst. cor. flow (cc)	0.18	Cardiac output (cc/min)	2189
Stroke diast. cor. flow (cc)	0.80	Stroke volume (cc)	42

A sequential moment-to-moment flow through the coronary circulation is illustrated in Figure 4.[48]

The most powerful *vasodilator* of the coronary circulation is hypoxemia. As the oxygen content of arterial blood is reduced, impressive increases in coronary blood flow occur without an increase in perfusion pressure, a phenomenon termed *reactive hyperemia*. A composite diagram illustrating the factors regulating coronary blood flow is shown in Figure 5.[46]

MYOCARDIAL METABOLISM

The primary problem in myocardial ischemia is the reduction in oxygen available for myocardial metabolism. Normally, the heart extracts approximately 75 per cent of the oxygen present in the arterial blood, leaving little additional to be removed during stressful situations. The added oxygen required for the heart during exercise or emotional stress is normally provided by an appropriate *increase* in coronary flow. This is made difficult if not impossible in the presence of significant arterial obstruction. The basic substrates utilized in myocardial metabolism are glucose, fatty acids, and lactate. In the presence of adequate oxygen, glucose is converted to pyruvate with production of ATP (adenosine triphosphate) in the Krebs cycle. Lactate is also converted to pyruvate. Oxidative phosphorylation of pyruvate is greatly slowed with reduction or absence of oxygen, and the lactate-pyruvate reaction may be reversed, with production of lactate in the heart. *Anaerobic* metabolism is inefficient in the heart, and although glucose is degraded, much less energy is provided. The clinical manifestations of significant myocardial hypoxemia include (1) anginal pain; (2) cardiac arrhythmias (ventricular premature systoles, ventricular tachycardia, and ventricular fibrillation) and electrocardiographic abnormalities (inversion of T waves and ST segment depression, especially with exercise); and (3) signs of cardiac failure.

PATHOLOGIC ASPECTS

Coronary atherosclerosis is a progressive disease, the earliest microscopic changes of which have been described in the newborn infant.[72] The infantile lesions consist of rupture, degeneration, and regeneration of the internal elastic membrane, together with deposits of mucopolysaccharide and proliferation of endothelial cells and fibroblasts.[72] At this early stage, it

FACTORS REGULATING CORONARY FLOW

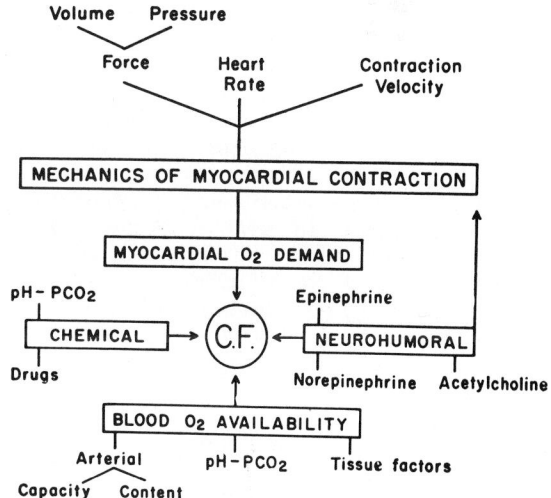

Figure 5. Factors regulating coronary flow (C.F.). These factors can be subdivided into those affecting myocardial oxygen requirements (above), those affecting oxygen availability per unit flow (below), and those acting directly on the arteriole. Neurohumoral factors can affect coronary flow not only through primary vasomotion but also through altered oxygen demand. Likewise, pH can affect both arteriolar resistance and oxygen availability. (From Gorlin, R.: Br. Heart J., Suppl., *33*:9, 1971.)

TABLE 1. Frequency of Obstructive Lesions in the Coronary Arteries Due to Atherosclerosis as Found in a Series of 300 Consecutive Patients With Coronary Atherosclerosis*

Coronary Artery	No. of Cases	—
Right	165	28.4
Left main	26	4.5
Left anterior descending	251	43.4
Left circumflex	134	23.7
Totals	576	100.0

*From Berger, R. L., and Stary, H. C.: N. Engl. J. Med., 285:248, 1971.

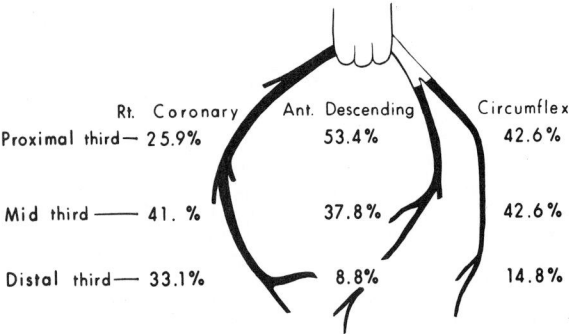

Figure 6. Localization of the stenotic lesion in the three major coronary trunks. Each coronary artery is divided into three equal segments and the percentage of the total number of lesions in each third is noted. In the anterior descending circumflex arteries, the obstructions tend to be in the proximal half, whereas the primary involvement is in the distal half of the right coronary artery. (From Berger, R. L., and Stary, H. C.: New Engl. J. Med., 285:248, 1971.)

is obvious that such lesions are quite minimal and are solely microscopic. However, *gross* lesions subsequently appear within a few years in the form of small yellow deposits of lipoid material visible beneath the intima. These lesions are present in half the hearts examined at autopsy during the second decade of life.[111] Careful pathologic studies have been done by a number of observers to assess the incidence and degree of atherosclerosis in *each* of the major coronary arteries. Nearly all of the studies have shown that the anterior descending coronary artery is the most frequently involved, followed in incidence by the right coronary, the left circumflex, the left main, and, least frequently of all, the right posterior descending coronary artery (Table 1).[3, 11, 15, 107]

It has also been noted that the more severe changes occur in the *proximal third* or *half* of the coronary arteries. In a thorough study of some 400 hearts, Schlesinger and Zoll[94] concluded that most occlusions were less than 5 mm. in length and that the majority were in the proximal third of the vessel. In a recent review of atherosclerotic lesions in 300 hearts studied primarily for an assessment of *operability* by direct bypass graft, a definite anatomic pattern was identified.[11] The usual pattern is one of *multifocal* lesions characteristically involving more than one major trunk in the same heart. The stenoses tend to be short but are contiguous with other areas of less severe coronary atherosclerosis. In general, lesions in the branches of the left coronary artery are usually proximal and originate at the bifurcation of the anterior descending and circumflex branches. However, there are appreciable numbers of distal lesions in these vessels. In the right coronary artery, the disease is more diffuse and involves primarily the proximal and middle portions of the artery. In this study, it was noted that 88 per cent of hearts with coronary atherosclerosis were anatomically suitable for a graft distal to the obstructing lesion. Further analysis indicated that bypass in *all* obstructed coronary arteries was achievable in 62 per cent of hearts, whereas of those with multiple lesions, only 27 per cent were suitable for surgical repair of *each* of the involved vessels.[11] The site of obstruction for each of the three major coronary vessels in this study is shown in Figure 6.[11]

CLINICAL MANIFESTATIONS OF ISCHEMIC HEART DISEASE

The symptoms associated with significant coronary atherosclerosis are those produced by a reduction in coronary blood flow. While coronary atherosclerosis is clearly the most common cause of myocardial ischemia, angina pectoris may also be associated with other lesions that cause a reduced coronary flow and enter the differential diagnosis. These include aortic stenosis, aortic insufficiency, syphilitic coronary ostial stenosis, hypertension, other forms of arteritis, embolism, and congenital malformations of the coronary arteries (Fig. 7).[14]

The *clinical syndrome* of angina pectoris was first described by Heberden in 1768. His original account is worth citing, since most believe that it has never been improved upon:

There is a disorder of the breast marked with strong and peculiar symptoms, considerable for the kind of danger belonging to it, and not extremely rare, which deserves to be mentioned more at length. The seat of it, and sense of strangling, and anxiety with which it is attended, may make it not improperly be called angina pectoris.

They who are afflicted with it, are seized while they are walking, (more especially if it be up hill, and soon after eating), with a painful and most disagreeable sensation in the breast, which seems as if it would extinguish life, if it were to increase or continue; but the moment they stand still, all this uneasiness vanishes.

In all other respects, the patients are, at the beginning of this disorder, perfectly well, and in particular have no shortness of breath from which it is totally different. The pain is sometimes situated in the upper part, sometimes in the middle, sometimes at the bottom of the os sterni, and often more inclined to the left than to the right side. It likewise very frequently extends from the breast to the middle of the left arm. The pulse is, at least sometimes, not disturbed by this pain, as I have had opportunities of observing by feeling the pulse during the paroxysm. Males are most liable to that disease, especially such as have passed their fiftieth year.

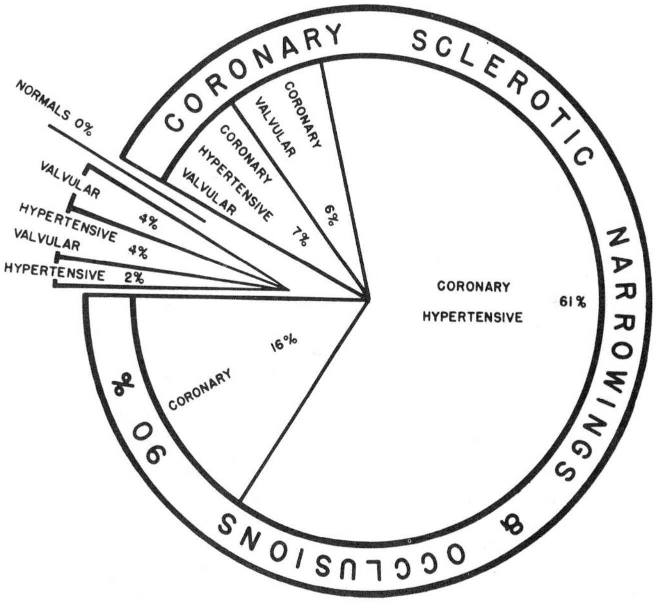

Figure 7. The etiologic basis of angina pectoris based on studies in 177 patients. (From Blumgart, H. L., Pitt, B., Zoll, P. M., and Freiman, D. G. *In* James, T. N., and Keyes, J. W. (Eds.): The Etiology of Myocardial Infarction, Boston, Little, Brown and Co., 1963.)

After it has continued a year or more, it will not cease so instantaneously upon standing still; and it will come on not only when the persons are walking, but when they are lying down, especially if they lie on their left side, and oblige them to rise up out of their beds. In some inveterate cases it has been brought on by the motion of a horse, or a carriage, and even by swallowing, coughing, going to stool, or speaking, or any disturbance of the mind. . . .

The termination of the angina pectoris is remarkable. For, if no accidents intervene, but the disease go on to its height, the patients all suddenly fall down, and perish almost immediately. Of which indeed their frequent faintness, and sensations as if all the powers of life were failing, afford no obscure intimation.

The discomfort is generally substernal in location and is described by the patient as "a pressure, choking sensation or tightness which is quite discomforting." A variety of factors, primarily exercise and emotional stress, can initiate the symptoms. Occasionally angina occurs at rest and in the recumbent position and is termed *angina decubitus*. The pain frequently radiates down the left arm and into the left neck and occasionally to the right arm.

The physical examination is frequently not remarkable in the patient with angina pectoris. Occasionally the fourth heart sound can be heard on auscultation; it has been interpreted as an increase in the amplitude of presystolic enlargement of the left ventricle.

The plain chest film is normal in the majority of patients, although cardiac enlargement may be present in those with more serious disease, especially those with heart failure. Left ventricular aneurysms of varying size may also be present. The electrocardiogram can be of substantial aid in the diagnosis of angina pectoris, although in at least half the patients it is within normal limits. Myocardial ischemia may be evidenced by the presence of inverted T waves, and especially ST segment and T wave changes, which occur during the course of an anginal episode. ST segment depression is an especially reliable sign and, if

not present at rest, may be elicited by an exercise stress test. Nevertheless, the diagnostic usefulness of exercise electrocardiography is limited, since false negative responses are frequent in patients with clinically suspected coronary disease and false positive responses are frequent in asymptomatic patients.[16]

SEVERE STENOSIS OF THE LEFT MAIN CORONARY ARTERY

Among patients with significant stenosis (70 per cent or more) of the left main coronary artery, the prognosis is poor and sudden death occurs frequently. Generally, these lesions occur in a somewhat older patient population with a more classic history of angina pectoris than coronary patients at large and with frequent calcification being seen in the area of the left coronary artery. Moreover, the EKG findings after exercise are apt to be more strongly positive with most patients in this group, showing 2 mm. or more ST depression during exercise testing. Ventricular contraction is apt to be abnormal in 60 to 86 per cent of the patients.[62, 64] This condition requires operative relief, usually on an *urgent* basis.[25, 69]

UNSTABLE (PREINFARCTION) ANGINA

It has been recognized for many years that sudden worsening of the pain pattern in a patient with angina pectoris often has ominous significance. The term *unstable angina* signifies the recent onset of angina or change in the clinical manifestations, a condition which is interposed between stable angina and frank myocardial infarction. The important clues include abrupt decrease in the tolerance for physical activity in a patient with previously stable angina, increased frequency, severity, and duration of an anginal attack, radiation of pain to sites previously not involved, such as the back, jaw, or both arms, and additional new features including diaphoresis, nausea, arrhythmia, or decreased relief of pain by nitroglycerin in amounts which were previously effective. EKG changes such as elevation or depression of ST segments or transient abnormalities of the T waves are often observed during attacks. It is essential, however, that there be no cardiac enzyme abnormalities nor any specific electrocardiographic changes indicative of myocardial necrosis.

Among the group of patients, 15 to 43 per cent have died and acute myocardial infarction developed in up to 50 per cent.[9, 74] Therefore, in view of the high risk, these patients are deserving of either intensive medical management or immediate surgical revascularization. Opinion is divided between those who prefer medical management or believe that surgical management is not imperative,[93] and those who present data showing better results following surgical management.[67, 68] A summary of the present status of therapy indicates that either medical or surgical therapy is acceptable. However, it has been shown that surgery can be performed in these patients with an acceptable mortality and with a stronger likelihood that the

anginal pain will be completely relieved in the future.[67]

CORONARY ARTERIOGRAPHY

Coronary arteriograms are essential for the *objective* diagnosis of angina pectoris caused by coronary atherosclerosis. The *selective* technique with placement of a tapered catheter *directly* into the coronary artery has been widely employed.[81] Since selective coronary arteriography was first performed by Sones in 1958, the procedure has become well established and is generally associated with few complications. However, thrombolic sequelae do occur,[18] with a mortality of 0.1 to 0.3 per cent in better series.[96] Another complication of coronary arteriography is acute *coronary occlusion.* This has been described and may require emergency bypass grafting due to life-threatening myocardial infarction.[50] Also, if *coronary calcification* as detected by fluroscopy is present, 97 per cent of such patients have been shown by arteriography to have significant coronary artery disease (greater than 70 per cent stenosis).[7] A diagram of the arteriographic pattern is shown in Figure 8.[81] An example of the normal anat-

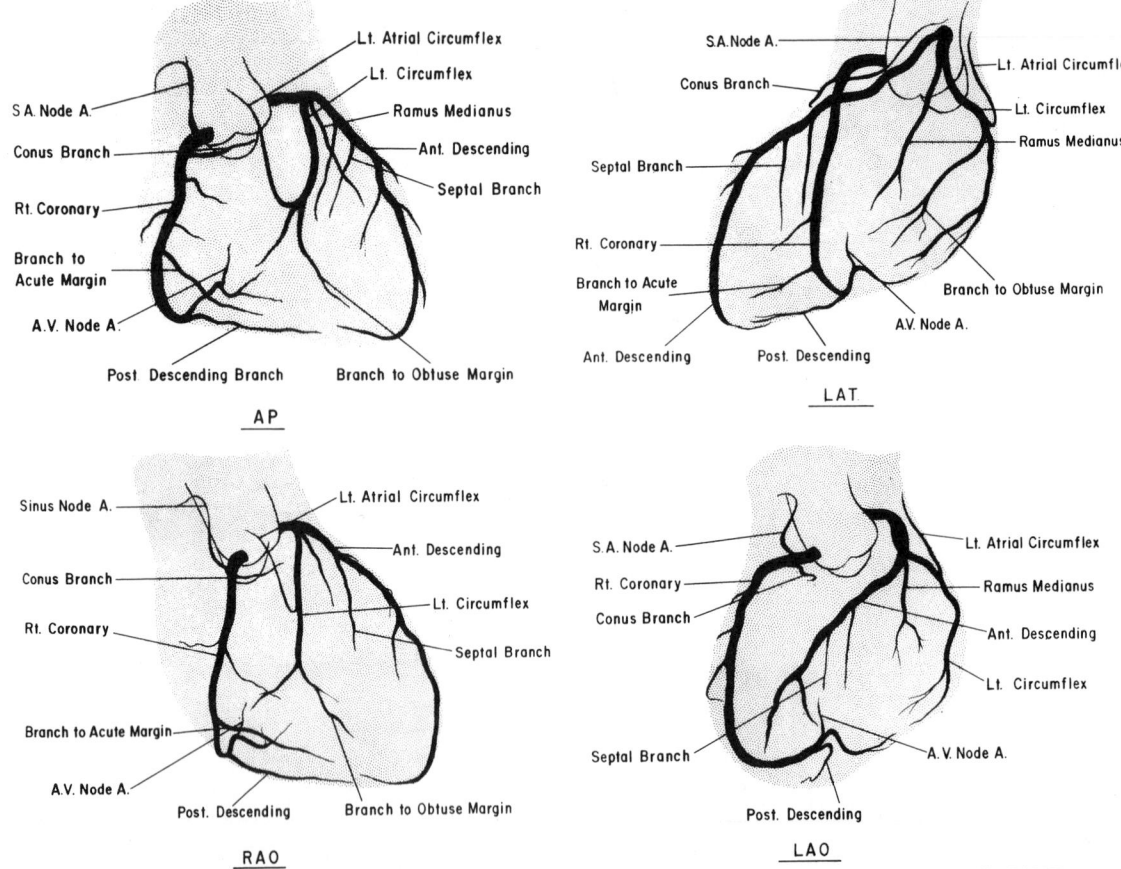

Figure 8. Anatomic representation of the coronary arteries. These vessels are represented as they would be seen on the angiogram. No attempt to convey the third dimension has been made. Careful study of the changes in position of the various branches with rotation of the heart is essential to intelligent interpretation of arteriograms. The combination of the left anterior oblique (LAO), lateral (LAT), and right anterior oblique (RAO) positions usually demonstrates all branches in profile. (From Abrams, H. L., and Adams, D. F.: New Engl. J. Med., *281*:1276, 1969.)

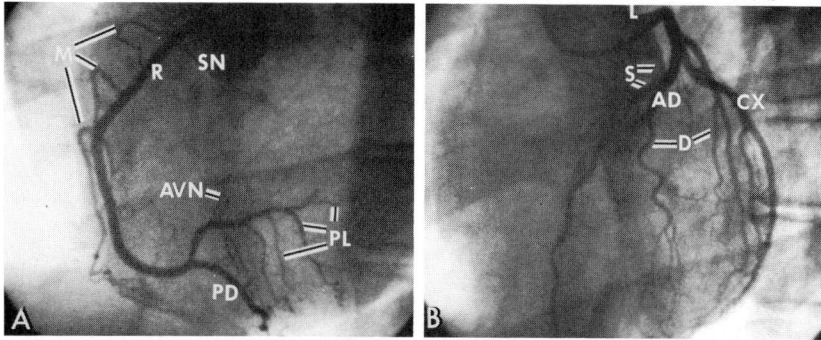

Figure 9. *A,* Right coronary arteriogram, left anterior oblique position. The right main trunk (R) supplies a series of marginal branches (M) to the right ventricle, as well as an atrial branch from which the artery to the sinus node arises (SN). After its major bifurcation and the origin of the posterior descending (PD) branch, the right coronary artery continues across the crux of the heart, giving rise to a branch to the atrioventricular node (AVN) and branches to the posterolateral aspect of the left ventricle (PL). *B,* Left coronary arteriogram, left anterior oblique projection. The main trunk of the left coronary artery (L) divides into its major anterior descending (AD) and circumflex (CX) divisions. The anterior descending division provides one or more branches to the interventricular septum (S), and a series of diagonal (D) branches to the anterolateral aspect of the left ventricle. The circumflex division contributes a series of branches distributed to the anterolateral, lateral, and posterolateral areas of the left ventricle. (From Sheldon, W. C.: Surg. Clin. North Am., *51*:1015, 1971.)

omy of the right and left coronary arteries is shown in Figure 9.[96] Obstructions are well demonstrated, together with the collateral vessels (Fig. 10).[96] For all patients being considered for surgery, coronary arteriography is essential.

Coronary arteriography is also useful in that it provides major predictive information. For example, in patients with normal or slightly to moderately abnormal coronary arteriograms, serial arteriography performed later has shown progression of the disease in the majority of patients who have *moderate* narrowing but progression or development of narrowing only occasionally in patients with *normal* to *mild* lesions.[21]

MEDICAL MANAGEMENT

The medical management of coronary atherosclerosis and angina pectoris is both general and specific. If hypertension is present, it should be controlled, and smoking should be avoided, since the vasoconstrictive effects of nicotine and its influence upon the coronary circulation are well established.[54] It has also been demonstrated that cessation of smoking in patients with myocardial infarction tends to prevent reinfarction.[108] The presence of abnormal lipoproteins in the blood should be determined (Fredrickson types) and treated appropriately. Often it is necessary to ad-

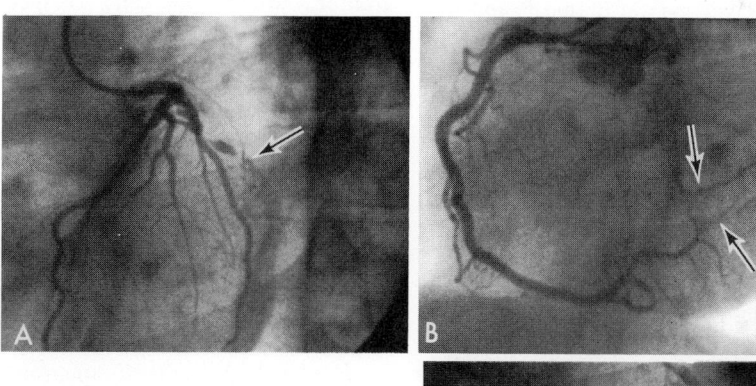

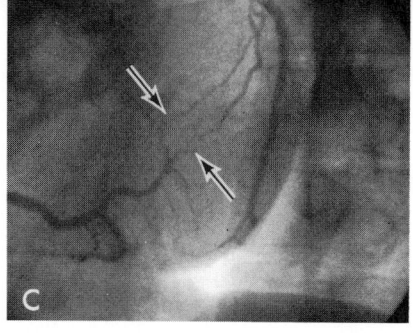

Figure 10. *A,* Left coronary arteriogram, left anterior oblique (LAO) position, demonstrating total obstruction of the proximal left circumflex coronary artery (arrow). *B* and *C,* Right coronary arteriogram demonstrating retrograde perfusion of the obstructed left circumflex branches via intercoronary collateral anastomoses with distal right coronary branches (arrows). (From Sheldon, W. C.: Surg. Clin. North Am., *51*:1015, 1971.)

just the patient's life style to reduce the likelihood of anginal attacks, especially if associated with myocardial irritability.

When making a choice between medical and surgical therapy, the *natural history* of angina pectoris should be recalled. In a number of studies, the overall annual death rate in patients with angina pectoris varies from 4 to 8 per cent or more. In a study in which groupings of patients were made according to the severity of the lesions, it was found that in patients with *one vessel* involvement the annual risk rate varied between 0.7 and 4 per cent, in *two vessel* disease the rate was 6.3 to 15.4 per cent, and in *three vessel* disease between 10 and 20 per cent.[83]

Drug Therapy

The primary basis of medical therapy is the use of agents found to be successful in controlling the pain of angina pectoris. The majority of patients obtain relief with sublingual nitroglycerin (0.4 to 0.6 mg.), and results are usually quite prompt. Many patients anticipate attacks of pain, especially with exercise or emotional stress, and can prevent them by prophylactic use of nitroglycerin. Several long-acting coronary vasodilators are available but produce variable results. The use of beta-adrenergic blocking agents such as *propranolol* is frequently effective. The pharmacologic effects of propranolol are a reduction in cardiac output, lowering of the pulse rate, and decrease in the force of ventricular contraction. Since it reduces the work load, it may produce substantial relief when administered regularly. Although much has been written concerning the use of anticoagulants in the treatment of angina pectoris and coronary atherosclerosis, there is little definitive evidence to support their use. Exercise has been advocated to aid in the development of coronary collateral circulation, and its beneficial effect has been shown both in the experimental animal[33] and in man.[66]

SURGICAL MANAGEMENT

For many years surgeons have held a prominent interest in myocardial revascularization. However, most of the procedures previously advocated have yielded in the recent past to the use of direct grafts from the aorta to the coronary arteries distal to the obstruction. This procedure has been supported widely by both cardiologists and surgeons, and the initial results are encouraging. Nevertheless, a cautious attitude remains appropriate until long-term assessment of this procedure is available. A number of distinct questions await answers that only appropriate observation will provide.

Historical Aspects

A surgical approach for relief of angina pectoris was first suggested in 1899 by a professor of physiology in Paris, François-Franck.[44] He believed that section of the cervical sympathetics might interrupt the pain fibers to the heart and ameliorate the symptoms. This procedure was first employed in 1916 by Jonnesco[59] and produced symptomatic relief in the patient. The subsequent recognition that angina pectoris was usually accompanied by a reduction in arterial blood supply to the heart led to the development of a number of surgical procedures designed to improve coronary blood flow.

Epicardial abrasion was advocated by Beck[10] in 1935 to stimulate the development of intramyocardial arterial collaterals. A number of tissues have been applied directly to the surface of the heart (omentum, pectoral muscle, pericardial fat pad, the spleen, and so forth) to promote the ingrowth of new arterial vessels to anastomose with the coronary circulation.[101] A procedure used in a large number of patients was that devised by Vineberg[102] in 1946 of *internal mammary artery implantation* into a tunnel in the left ventricle. From the implant a system of arterial communications with the intramyocardial vessels developed. Such arterial implants were demonstrated to remain patent, although the amount of blood flow that passed through them remained quite controversial. In 1957 Bailey[6] introduced coronary *endarterectomy,* a technique that was substantially modified by Longmire the following year.[65] This technique was applied primarily to proximally located lesions and was suitable for only a small number of patients, generally less than 10 per cent of the total.

In 1962, a direct aortocoronary bypass graft employing a saphenous vein was performed.[87] However, this patient later succumbed due to a cerebrovascular accident. Several years later came the notable contributions of Johnson[58] and of Favaloro[37] and their associates which led to an extensive reappraisal of the surgical approach to ischemic myocardial heart disease. It has been clearly demonstrated by these workers and others that coronary arteries as small as 1 mm. in diameter may be joined by a suture anastomosis, with prolonged patency demonstrated by subsequent coronary arteriography.

Indications for Operation

The primary indication for a surgical approach in patients with angina pectoris is for relief of severe and unresponsive anginal pain. In addition, clear indications include in appropriate circumstances refractory arrhythmias, left main coronary lesions with occlusion greater than 70 per cent irrespective of symptoms, preinfarction angina, and patients in congestive heart failure with ventricular aneurysms.

Most surgeons agree that in 80 to 90 per cent of patients with occlusive coronary artery disease the anatomy is appropriate for direct aortic-coronary grafts, provided the necessary indications for the procedure are also present. The majority of patients are likely to have more than one occlusion, and an appreciable number have three or more significant obstructing lesions, each potentially correctable by a graft. It is essential that the lesions be demonstrated accurately by coronary arteriography prior to operation. Moreover, in most instances at least 75 per cent occlusion of one or more vessels will be apparent in patients with angina pectoris. In some, especially those with evidence of congestive heart failure, a *dyskinetic* area is apt to be found in the left ventricle, with poor or paradoxical contraction. In a more severe form, these areas are actually *aneurysms* of the ventricular wall that bulge during systolic contraction. These aneurysms may contain thrombus, which may potentially embolize the systemic arteries. The dyskinetic areas may be suitable for plication or excision, depending upon their characteristics. Emergency aortocoronary bypass has been used in patients with impending or extending myocardial infarction with good results.[56] Patients with acute myocardial infarction and "power failure" (intractable shock) have also been treated successfully by direct grafts, with or without aneurysm resection.[76]

Cardiac catheterization studies have been quite helpful in documenting objective evidence of left ventricular function. In general, cardiomegaly, low ejection fractions from the left ventricle (especially below 25 per cent), increased left ventricular volume, and wide coronary arteriovenous differences (greater than 6 vol. per cent) all are associated with increased morbidity and mortality. To a lesser extent, an elevated end-diastolic pressure in the left ventricle may increase risk. However, the presence of any one of these variables does not necessarily preclude a successful surgical result. In addition, preoperative assessment and evaluation of dyskinesia, aneurysms, associated valvar disease, and diffuse myocardial damage with poor function are required in consideration of the advisability and extent of the operation planned.

Surgical Procedures

The vast majority of patients with obstructive disease of the coronary circulation who are candidates for surgery are treated with grafts of autogenous veins anastomosed between the aorta and the coronary arteries. The saphenous vein is usually chosen, and the vessel is reversed so that blood may flow in the direction of the valves. The procedure is conducted with extracorporeal circulation, although the aortic anastomosis can usually be accomplished without the use of bypass, since the aorta is relatively still and this anastomosis can be easily accomplished (Fig. 11). For the coronary artery anastomosis, bypass is instituted with cannulation of the left ventricle for continuous decompression. The body temperature is often lowered to 30° C. and the anastomosis is performed in a quiet and nonbeating heart. Meticulous attention to surgical detail is mandatory, and the anastomosis is accomplished with very fine sutures (7–0) (Figs. 12 and 13).[38] Some advocate the use of interrupted sutures, whereas others employ a continuous suture. It is essential that the anastomosis be performed distal to the obstruction and preferably in a site in which there is little involvement of the wall with atherosclerotic change. The use of magnifying glasses has been found helpful.[97] After reconstruction, electromagnetic flowmeter determinations of volume of blood flow have shown average flows for right coronary grafts of 60 ml. per minute (range, 28 to 150 ml.); of the anterior descending, 80 ml. per minute (range, 20 to 160 ml.); and of the circumflex, 75 ml. per minute (range, 60 to 90 ml.).[73] In high risk patients, an intra-aortic balloon may be inserted for counterpulsation just prior to initiation of the operation. Use of intra-aortic balloon assistance has also been found to be quite useful in those patients whom it is difficult to wean from cardiopulmonary bypass after revascularization. In such pa-

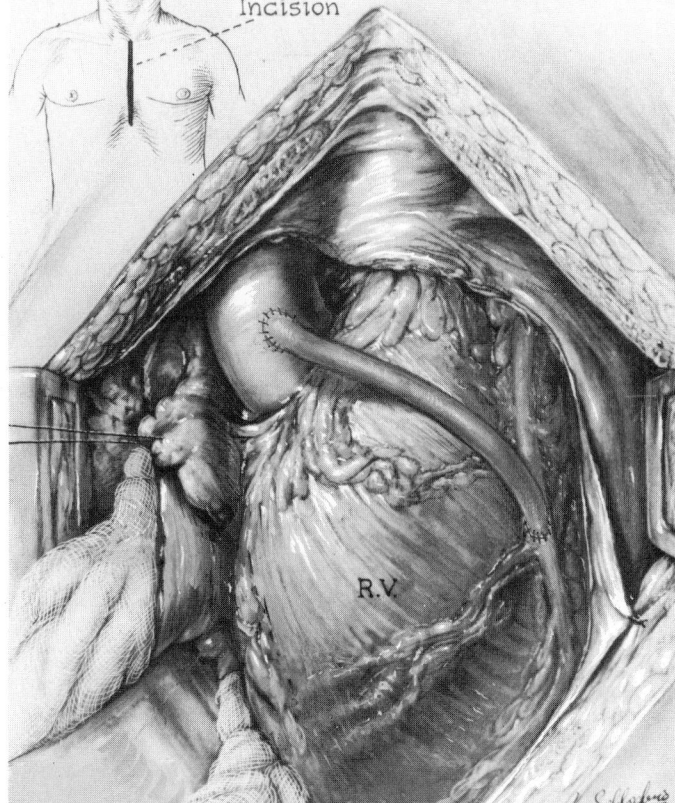

Figure 11. Illustration of anastomosis of saphenous vein autograft from side of ascending aorta to side of left anterior descending coronary artery distal to an obstruction in the anterior descending coronary artery.

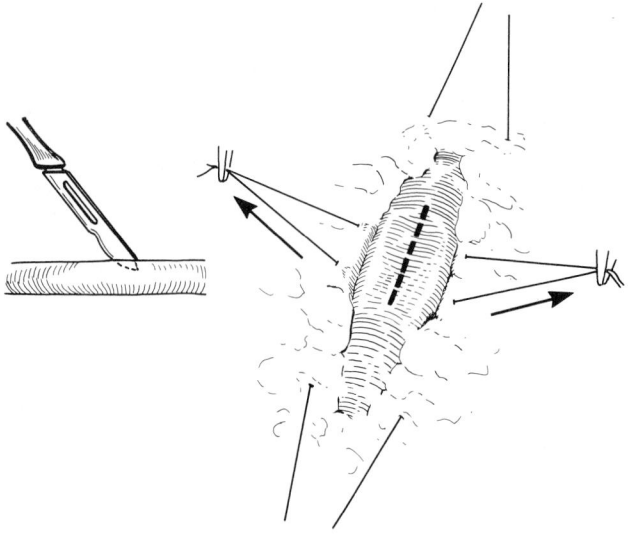

Figure 12. Dissection of the coronary artery is avoided in the left coronary artery and its divisions, except when the anastomosis is performed on the main circumflex coronary artery. A No. 15 bistoury blade is utilized to open the artery layer by layer from outside. (From Favaloro, R. G.: Surg. Clin. North Am., *51:* 1035, 1971.)

tients, its use has clearly led to increased survival[60, 105] and may be used for prolonged periods, up to several weeks if necessary.

Areas of dyskinesia or aneurysm formation may require direct correction. Occasionally mitral insufficiency results from infarction of the papillary muscles and if severe may require replacement with a prosthetic valve. A direct anastomosis of the internal mammary artery to the coronary artery has also been recommended in preference to using a venous autograft.[47]

Postoperative Management

The postoperative management of patients following revascularization procedures is of prime importance. The endotracheal tube is generally left in place for the first day, to permit adequate ventilation by a respirator. It should remain in place until satisfactory ventilation can be assured, as shown by blood gas measure-

ments of P_{O_2} and P_{CO_2}. The cardiac output is maintained by attention to the central venous pressure, which is kept as high as 150 to 200 mm. of saline (10 to 15 mm. Hg) if necessary. The use of isoproterenol and dopamine may be indicated to improve the *low output syndrome.* Similarly, various arrhythmias may develop and require the use of digitalis, procainamide, xylocaine, potassium, or electrical cardioversion. Perioperative myocardial infarction following aortocoronary bypass grafting generally occurs in 5 to 15 per cent or more of patients and in some series has been higher.[75] It is most frequent in patients with severe and extensive coronary lesions. It is of interest that this type of myocardial infarction is not usually associated with the usual clinical picture, and often there are no symptoms.

Results

The surgical mortality following aortocoronary bypass has been reported to vary between 1 and 12 per cent, depending largely upon the severity of disease.[75] It has been convincingly demonstrated that if a series is composed of *good* risk patients the mortality will be low, generally 2 to 4 per cent. Contrariwise, if a significant number of high risk patients are included, the mortality will be correspondingly higher. In a computerized study, it has been shown that in patients with one or two vessel coronary disease without involvement of the left main coronary artery the operative mortality was 1 per cent, whereas in patients with three vessel disease it was 6 per cent.[26] Thus, the differences in mortality between series, and indeed in the same series over a period of time, can be demonstrated to be directly related to the *severity* of the patient's disease. Risk factors include left main coronary stenosis, congestive heart failure, a low ejection fraction, and multivessel involvement. Others have also demonstrated that the operative risk and subjective response are related basically to the degree of ventricular function loss prior to surgery, as demonstrated by objective multivariable analysis and computer evaluation.[23]

The results in most series demonstrate an excellent

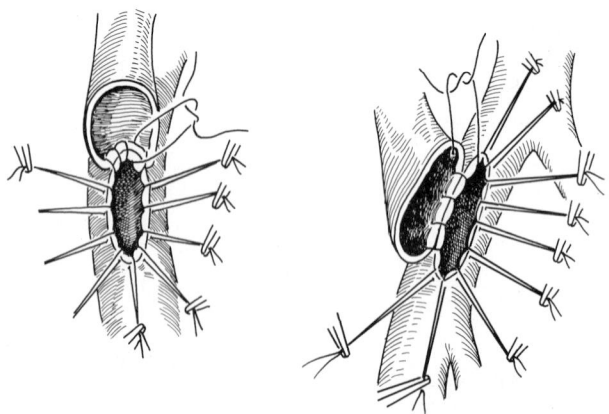

Figure 13. The anastomosis starts at the proximal end of the arteriotomy (*left*) except for the proximal segment of the anterior descending and circumflex coronary arteries. To avoid kinking of the graft, the anastomosis should start in the middle of the medial side of the arteriotomy (*right*). (From Favaloro, R. G.: Surg. Clin. North Am., *51:*1035, 1971.)

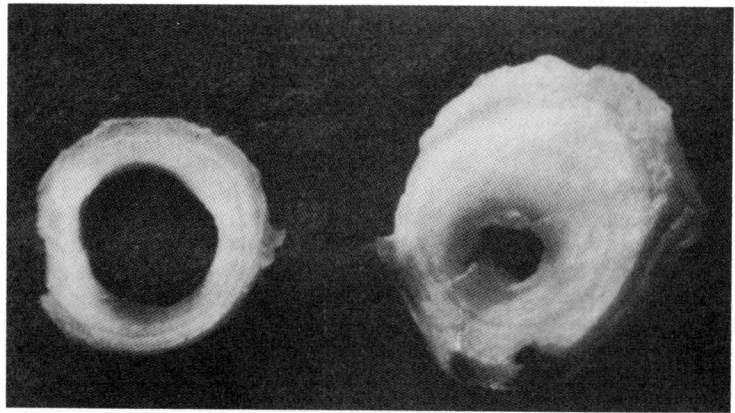

Figure 14. Segments of the vein graft showing marked narrowing of the lumen in the first portion of the graft (*right*) in comparison to the "normal" lumen-wall ratio of the distal segment of the vein graft (*left*). (From Grondin, C. M., Meere, C., Castonguay, Y., Lepage, G., and Grondin, P.: Circulation, *43*:698, 1971. By permission of the American Heart Association, Inc.)

symptomatic response, and in approximately 65 per cent, relief is complete, with no further symptoms. Distinct improvement occurs in an additional 25 per cent.[86] However, it is clear that changes in the grafts and in the coronary arteries themselves occur after revascularization. It has been demonstrated that the original stenosis present in the coronary artery may progress to complete occlusion after a bypass graft is placed distally.[4] In addition, progressive and late obstruction of the aortocoronary venous bypass graft has been demonstrated. The early patency rate during the first year after operation approximates 90 per cent in the grafts, although with the passage of time an *intimal fibrosis* may occur in the vein graft and cause obstruction (Figs. 14 and 15).[49, 103] In some instances, thrombi have also been noted. A distinctive *fibrous endarteritis* that occludes the grafts has been described in detail.[104] In one series of 100 patients, rearteriography after revascularization one to four years postoperatively showed a 55 per cent incidence of progression of the lesions *proximal* to the graft and only 7 per cent *distal* to the graft. In this series, 14 per cent of those vessels which were not grafted showed progression of the disease.[70]

Despite the encouraging results currently reported, an objective attitude is essential relative to the late results of these procedures. A critique of direct surgery of the coronary circulation for atherosclerotic obstruction would include (1) the ultimate patency rates of the grafts, (2) the development of atherosclerosis in the venous grafts, (3) aneurysmal dilatation, fibrosis, or thrombosis of the graft, (4) progression of the previously existing coronary artery disease, (5) effect of the venous graft on prevention of subsequent myocardial infarction, and (6) the extension of the life span in those patients undergoing operation as compared to survival without operation.

Reoperation after unsuccessful coronary surgery can be performed, but the technical problems are often appreciable. In a group of 21 patients undergoing reoperation, 33 per cent obtained complete relief of angina, 29 per cent some relief, and in 38 per cent there was no change. Of interest is the fact that four of the seven patients who were free of angina had perioperative myocardial infarction at the time of the second operation. The conclusion drawn is that in these patients, reoperation does not provide the same rate of anginal relief as does the first procedure.[109]

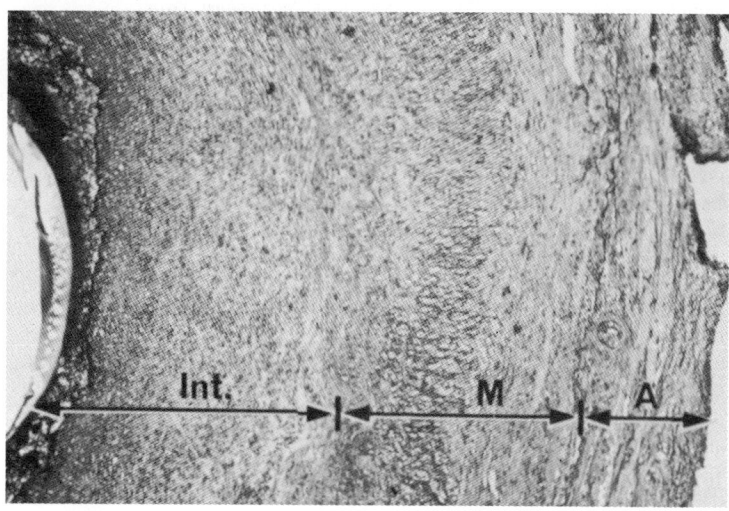

Figure 15. Histologic section of the vein graft in the area of stenosis, showing marked fibrosis of all layers, but predominantly of the intimal layer (Int.). M = media; A = adventitia. Hematoxylin and eosin, × 65. (From Grondin, C. M., Meere, C., Castonguay, Y., Lepage, G., and Grondin, P.: Circulation, *43*:698, 1971. By permission of the American Heart Association, Inc.)

VENTRICULAR SEPTAL DEFECT FOLLOWING MYOCARDIAL INFARCTION

Data obtained from postmortem studies indicate that 8 to 10 per cent of fatal cases of myocardial infarction are due to *rupture* of the heart.[79] In addition, infarction of the interventricular septum with subsequent formation of a ventricular septal defect causes death in 1 to 2 per cent of cases of acute myocardial infarction. The usual interval between the acute infarct and septal rupture is 4 to 12 days; this correlates well with histologic findings of maximal cardiac muscle degeneration. Once rupture has occurred, the prognosis is poor, as demonstrated in one series of 157 patients, of whom 24 per cent died on the first day after rupture, 65 per cent had died by the end of two weeks, and 81 per cent by two months. Only 7 per cent survived for a year after the development of a ventricular septal defect.[80]

This condition develops classically in a patient with myocardial infarction in whom shock or congestive heart failure appears. A loud, holosystolic murmur is usually heard over the apex, and two thirds of the patients demonstrate a palpable thrill. The differential diagnosis includes papillary muscle dysfunction, rupture of a papillary muscle with acute mitral insufficiency, rupture of chordae tendineae, mitral insufficiency due to left ventricular failure, and a pericardial friction rub secondary to myocardial infarction. Although clinical findings may be highly suggestive, the definitive diagnosis is made by catheterization. The data demonstrate a left-to-right shunt at the ventricular level.

Since the natural history of the disease is dismal, surgical correction is indicated in nearly all patients. Whenever possible, it is preferable to allow the infarct to heal, with operation deferred for six to eight weeks. However, the condition of the patient may not permit delay, and early or even emergency operation may be a necessity. Since currently available figures indicate that some three fourths of untreated patients will not survive for two months, it is recommended that surgery be considered before six weeks in any patient who no longer responds to vigorous medical management.

The first correction of a postinfarction ventricular defect was by Cooley in 1957.[27] These defects are usually in the apical septum and are most often associated with occlusion of the anterior descending coronary artery and with a ventricular aneurysm. *Multiple* defects are present in approximately one third of patients. The operation is performed with the use of extracorporeal circulation. An incision is made in the area of infarction in the left ventricle or through the aneurysm. If the infarct has healed (usually six or more weeks after onset), a fibrous rim may be present. If operation is done earlier, before complete healing, it may be necessary to remove a portion of the necrotic edges of the defect and to insert a plastic prosthesis for closure. The sutures may also be passed through the lower and apical portion of the normal right ventricle to buttress the VSD closure and provide additional strength. Approximately two thirds of reported patients have survived the operative procedure.

OTHER COMPLICATIONS OF ACUTE MYOCARDIAL INFARCTION REQUIRING SURGICAL MANAGEMENT

In addition to the development of ventricular aneurysms and perforation of the interventricular septum, acute myocardial infarction may produce other specific complications that require surgical management. These include *heart block, peripheral arterial emboli, rupture of a papillary muscle, pulmonary embolism, and rupture of the ventricle.* Successful management of cardiac rupture has been reported.[40] The other complications listed are discussed in appropriate sections.

CONGENITAL LESIONS OF THE CORONARY CIRCULATION

It has long been recognized that a number of congenital malformations occur in the coronary circulation.[77] The most important of these include congenital origin of the left coronary artery from the pulmonary artery, origin of the right coronary artery from the pulmonary artery, coronary arteriovenous fistulas, and coronary arterial aneurysms.

CONGENITAL ORIGIN OF THE LEFT CORONARY FROM THE PULMONARY ARTERY

The first description of origin of the left coronary from the pulmonary artery was by Abrikossoff in 1911.[2] The original report described a five-month-old infant dying with congestive heart failure and an aneurysm of the left ventricle. Photomicrographs of the ventricle showed infarction, including areas of calcification.

The prognosis of the vast majority of patients with origin of the left coronary artery from the pulmonary artery is quite poor. Keith estimates that some 95 per cent of infants born with this malformation will die within the first year of life unless surgical therapy is undertaken.[61]

Although poorly understood for many years, the pathophysiology of this malformation is now relatively straightforward. Numerous studies on postmortem specimens clearly reveal the presence of many collaterals connecting the right and left coronary arteries. In fact, when dye is injected into the right coronary artery, branches of the left coronary artery fill easily and in significant amounts.[24] It was also observed that, at the time of operation, occlusion of the left coronary at its origin caused an increase in pressure within the artery.[89, 91] Of additional significance is the fact that blood withdrawn from the left coronary artery at operation shows it to be fully saturated with oxygen. This is clear evidence that the origin of this blood is from a systemic arterial source rather than from the pulmonary artery, since the saturation in the latter is about 75 per cent. Of parallel interest is the malformation in which the *right* coronary artery arises from the pulmonary artery. In 1886, St. John

Brooks described two patients with this condition.[20] At that time, he suggested that flow in the *right* coronary artery might actually be retrograde into the pulmonary artery. It is of importance that it was discovered accidentally in the anatomic dissection laboratory.

Although most patients with this malformation demonstrate symptoms in infancy (95 per cent or more), some survive to adult life with few if any symptoms. For example, Abbott in 1927 reported a 64-year-old patient with this lesion,[1] and in another collected review,[51] 28 adults were reported with this condition.

Clinical Manifestations. The infant usually appears normal at birth, since the pulmonary arterial pressure at this age is elevated and allows perfusion of the left coronary artery from the pulmonary artery. Nevertheless, symptoms may be present at birth, especially if there are *associated* cardiac malformations. Symptoms are most apt to occur during the first several months of life as left ventricular ischemia becomes more pronounced. Once symptoms appear, the course is usually one of progressive deterioration. Unless surgery is undertaken, congestive heart failure with death is likely to follow.

Symptoms. *Tachypnea* and *dyspnea* are the two most characteristic symptoms of this condition. Coughing, wheezing, and cyanosis usually follow. One of the interesting findings that may be present may be described as the "angina of feeding," in which the infant shows evidence of pain during and immediately after feeding. As the congestive heart failure progresses, dyspnea, cyanosis, and pallor become apparent.

Physical Examination. The characteristic features include a rapid respiratory rate, tachycardia, and marked cardiac enlargement. Early in the course of the illness murmurs may not be present, since this anomaly is one of the few cardiac conditions in infancy in which congestive failure may be present without a murmur. However, with the passage of time, relative mitral insufficiency occurs as a result of left ventricular dilatation.[22] Moreover, it has been shown that infarction can involve the papillary muscles and also be a cause of mitral regurgitation as well as of dilatation of the mitral ring. The liver is characteristically enlarged, and the spleen is palpable in a smaller number of patients. Occasionally, the presenting symptoms are those of cardiovascular collapse and *shock,* similar to acute coronary occlusion in an adult manifesting marked tachycardia, hypotension, and peripheral vasomotor collapse.

Chest Roentgenography. The chest film shows enlargement of the heart, especially involving the left ventricle. Aneurysmal dilatation may be present as a result of marked thinning of the left ventricular wall. In many instances the left border of the heart extends to the lateral rib margin. Moreover, the force of ventricular contraction is much reduced and the pulsations are diminished. As a result of left ventricular failure, the pulmonary vascular markings are usually exaggerated.

Electrocardiography. The first description of myocardial ischemia in the electrocardiogram of an infant with this condition was by Bland and associates in 1933.[13] Generally, it is possible to make a relatively confident diagnosis on this basis. Tachycardia is nearly always present. The T waves are characteristically inverted in the standard leads and the ST segment in lead I may be slightly raised. The T waves in the precordial leads, especially V5 and V6, are usually inverted, and deep Q waves are frequently present. The body surface potential distribution has also been helpful in diagnosis and in providing evidence of improved coronary blood flow following surgery.[41]

Angiocardiography. The most striking feature on the angiocardiogram is the enlargement of the left atrium. The wall of the left ventricle may be quite thin, especially on its anterolateral aspect near the apex. A true ventricular aneurysm with paradoxical pulsations may be present, and mitral insufficiency is relatively common. Contrast medium passing into the aorta demonstrates a single right coronary, although selective aortography is more reliable for certain demonstration of this feature.

Aortography. When contrast medium is injected into the proximal aorta, it enters the right coronary artery as it originates from the aorta and passes through dilated collaterals which communicate with the left coronary artery. The dye can then be followed into the left circumflex and anterior descending coronaries, where it converges to enter the left main coronary artery. This finding is very impressive and conclusive, and one can see large amounts of radiopaque contrast medium flowing freely into the pulmonary artery. Thus, retrograde flow of blood in the left coronary artery can be convincingly demonstrated in such a study, and this examination establishes an objective diagnosis (Fig. 16).[90]

Cardiac Catheterization. The right ventricular and pulmonary artery pressures may be elevated. Moreover, it is usually possible to demonstrate a left-to-right shunt at the pulmonary artery level by dye injection. While the oxygen saturation may at times show a significant increase from the right ventricle to the pulmonary artery, this is not always present even when it can be demonstrated that the left coronary arises from the pulmonary artery.

The ejection fraction in patients with anomalous origin of the left coronary artery has been determined in eight preoperative patients, in whom it varied between 0.13 and 0.72. It is noteworthy that among those who died the ejection fraction was less than 0.36, whereas in the survivors the figure was more than 0.55.[71]

Pathology. The left ventricle is characteristically greatly dilated and the wall thin. The left coronary artery is *larger* than normal and numerous collateral vessels are apparent connecting the right and left coronary arteries. These are usually quite tortuous and thin-walled. The right coronary artery arises in its normal position and is also enlarged. Its branches tend to be more tortuous than usual as they communicate with the various collateral vessels. With time, and especially in adults, the right coronary artery may become quite large and increasingly tortuous. Similarly, the left coronary artery may also become quite enlarged, up to 10 mm. or more in diameter at its origin. The left coronary artery arises from the left or

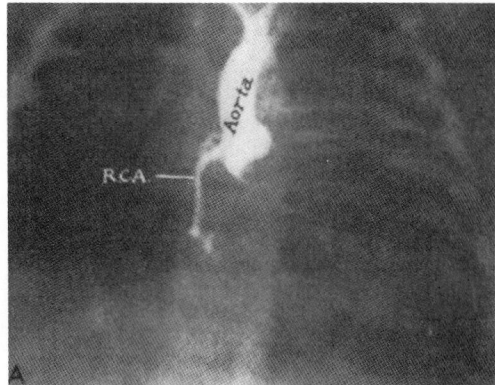

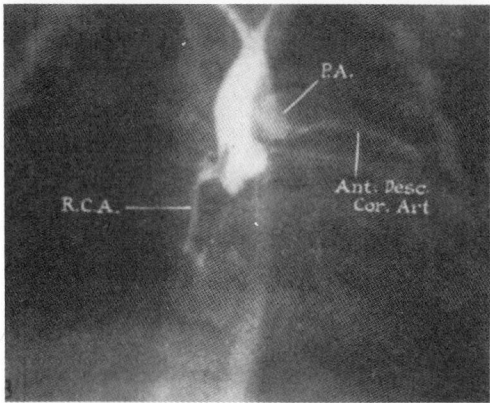

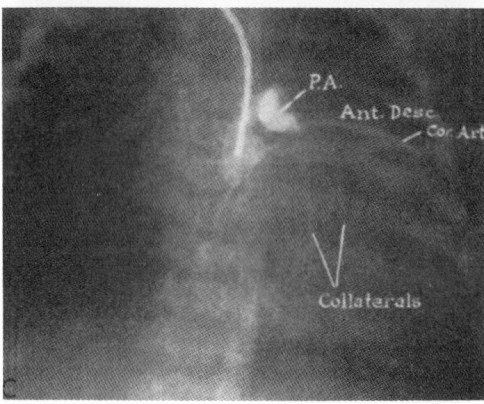

Figure 16. Several cine frames taken from a series illustrating coronary arterial filling during aortography. *A,* Filling of the right coronary as it arises normally from the aorta. Note that its size is somewhat greater than normal. *B,* Filling of the branches of the left coronary artery through collaterals from the right coronary artery. *C,* Filling of the pulmonary artery by retrograde flow from the left coronary artery. (From Sabiston, D. C., Jr., and Orme, S. K.: Cardiovasc. Surg., *9*:543, 1968.)

posterior cusp of the pulmonary artery. The branches and course of the anterior descending and circumflex branches are usually otherwise normal. On section, the left ventricle may be markedly thin and in areas is totally replaced by scar tissue (Fig. 17). Varying amounts of subendocardial fibroelastosis may be present. Calcification is often present in the fibrotic portion of the left ventricle. Infarction of the ventricle and ventricular septum may lead to infarction of the

papillary muscle producing mitral insufficiency. If the left ventricle is dilated, the mitral ring may be sufficiently enlarged to produce relative *mitral insufficiency,* preventing normal coaptation of the valve leaflets.

SURGICAL MANAGEMENT

Once symptoms appear, the prognosis without surgical treatment is very poor. Since it has been demonstrated that blood flow in the left coronary artery is reversed or *retrograde* (blood flows from the normal right coronary artery through numerous dilated collateral vessels into the left coronary), an arteriovenous fistula is created which deprives the left ventricular myocardium of a supply of blood that is badly needed. This phenomenon has been demonstrated by selective arteriography in which the contrast medium can be followed from the right into the left coronary artery with ultimate drainage in the main pulmonary artery. Moreover, at the time of operation, blood aspirated from the left coronary artery and its branches is fully saturated with oxygen, indicating that it has a systemic arterial source. In addition, occlusion of the vessel at its origin causes a marked rise in the pressure within the left coronary artery. If the blood flow were actually from the pulmonary artery, a fall in the pressure would be expected. These ob-

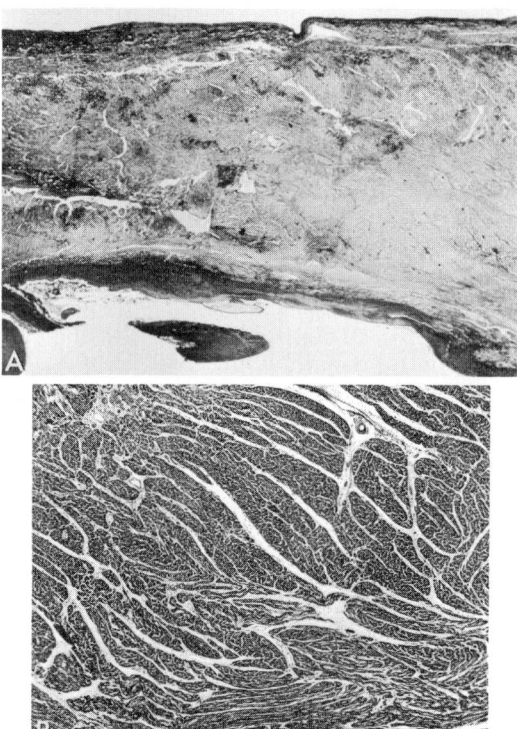

Figure 17. *A,* Histologic section of full thickness of left ventricle. Note that the left ventricular wall is almost totally replaced with scar tissue. The section represents the full thickness of the ventricle and is magnified 12 times, illustrating the extreme thinness of the left ventricle. *B,* Histologic section of right ventricular myocardium in the same patient showing normal cardiac muscle. (Published by Edizioni Minerva Medica, Turin, Italy, 1968, Nov.-Dec.)

servations led to the conclusion that *ligation* of the coronary artery at its origin would represent a logical procedure in the surgical treatment of this condition.

The ideal operation in patients with this disorder is the anastomosis of the left coronary artery to a systemic arterial source. This has been accomplished in older children and adults, and in a few infants. The technical problems of direct anastomosis of a vessel of this size in the first year of life are considerable. Moreover, ligation of the vessel at its origin has proved quite effective in this group. For example, in our own series, the last 10 infants have been managed by ligation, and eight are now alive and well. Thus, in the infant there appears to be a relatively consistent view that ligation of the vessel at its origin is the surgical procedure of choice.[5]

The appropriate form of treatment for those children who survive beyond the age of a year is more controversial. Such patients have been successfully treated by ligation of the left coronary artery,[8, 84, 88] and others have been treated by the anastomosis of the left coronary artery to the aorta by means of a venous autograft or a prosthetic graft.[28] While the direct anastomosis by means of a vein graft represents the most ideal form of therapy, the ultimate *fate* and long term patency of such grafts remain to be demonstrated. Thus, it is possible that thrombosis of the graft could result in retrograde spread of the thrombus to the left coronary arterial system. However, if the long-term patency of the left coronary following grafts can be shown, this method will clearly represent the procedure of choice, provided the mortality is within acceptable limits.

Of interest is the fact that occasionally an infant may be symptomatic early in life and then experience a remission, probably due to development of adequate coronary collaterals.[57] An infant with a left ventricular aneurysm in congestive heart failure has been reported, with resection of the aneurysm and ligation of the abnormal left coronary artery at its origin.[100] A combination procedure, resection of a left ventricular aneurysm and introduction of a saphenous vein graft from the aorta to the anterior descending coronary artery, has also been reported in a young child with anomalous origin of the left coronary artery from the pulmonary artery.[42] Direct anastomosis of the left subclavian artery to the left coronary artery has also been shown to produce good results.[82]

ANOMALOUS ORIGIN OF THE RIGHT CORONARY FROM THE PULMONARY ARTERY

In a recent report, 16 patients with anomalous origin of the right coronary artery from the pulmonary artery were reviewed. There are few if any characteristic features which permit a clinical diagnosis. It will be recalled that St. John Brooks originally described this condition in two cadavers in his anatomic dissection laboratory. Both were adults and there was no evidence that either had heart disease.

In this condition, the symptoms are rare and the patient is usually asymptomatic. In the 16 cases recorded in the literature, the abnormal artery was discovered in 11 individuals whose ages ranged from 17 to 90 years. The malformation was thought to have been associated with the death of the patient in only two instances. One of these was a 17-year-old female who died suddenly, and autopsy showed complete occlusion of the left coronary artery by a thrombus and evidence of left ventricular infarction. The other occurred in a 42-year-old patient who was asymptomatic. Three additional patients have been reported in whom the anomaly occurred in association with other congenital malformations.

Rarely, both coronary arteries may arise from the pulmonary artery, and five such infants have been reported. The survival time ranged from nine hours to five months.[99] There is also an interesting report of a child who lived to the age of seven with *total coronary arterial circulation* from the pulmonary artery.[39] This prolonged survival was due to an interventricular septal defect with pulmonary hypertension and congenital mitral stenosis. Thus, the pressure in the pulmonary artery was sufficient to force blood into the myocardial capillary bed, and under these circumstances, the child lived an amazingly long time.

CORONARY ARTERY FISTULAS

In 1865 Krause described the first patient with a coronary arteriovenous fistula.[63] Since then more than 200 examples of this lesion have been reported in the literature. It is quite likely that more patients with this disorder will be discovered in the future as a result of the widespread use of cardiac catheterization and arteriography in the investigation of patients with cardiac murmurs.

The size of the direct arteriovenous communication usually becomes larger with time. In order of incidence, the *right* coronary artery is the most frequently involved and the communication most often enters into the right ventricle, followed in incidence by drainage into the right atrium and pulmonary artery. Fistulas involving the *left* coronary artery are less common but may enter the right ventricle, right atrium, or coronary sinus. Rarely, coronary fistulas may enter the vena cava.

This lesion represents essentially a left-to-right shunt with the potential of producing an increased cardiac output and ultimately congestive heart failure. In addition, mural thrombi may form in the fistula, especially if saccular or fusiform aneurysmal dilatation is present, and lead to distal embolization. Bacterial endocarditis, anemia, and glomerulonephritis have also been reported.[92]

A number of conditions may be associated with findings similar to a coronary arteriovenous fistula and include aortic pulmonary window, sinus of Valsalva fistulas, ventricular septal defect with aortic insufficiency, pulmonary arteriovenous fistula, and fistulas of the systemic vessels, such as the subclavian and internal mammary arteries connecting with appropriate veins in the chest wall.

The most important clinical manifestation is the presence of a continuous mumur overlying the site of the fistula. The mumur may closely resemble that of a patent ductus arteriosus and, in fact, the first patient upon whom closure was ever performed was operated

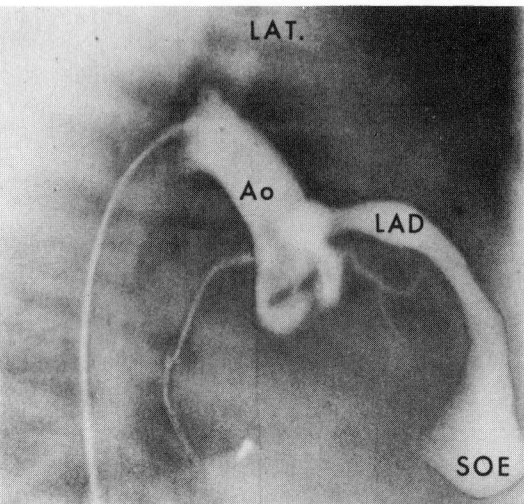
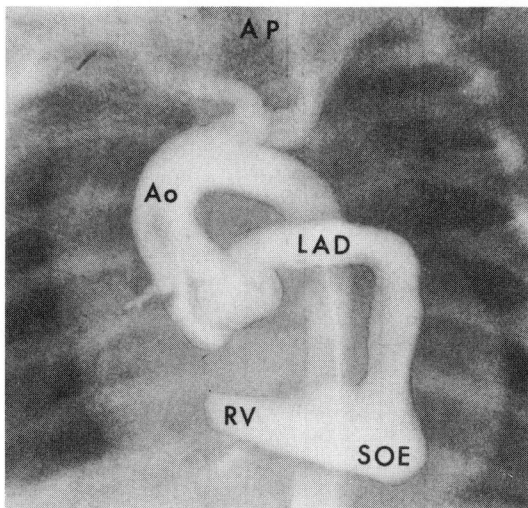

Figure 18.   Ascending aortogram of left coronary artery—right ventricular fistula showing lateral and anteroposterior views. Ao, Aorta; LAD, left anterior descending coronary artery; SOE, site of entry of fistula into the right ventricle; RV, incompletely opacified right ventricle. (From Daniel, T. M., Graham, T. P., and Sabiston, D. C., Jr.: Coronary artery—right ventricular fistula with congestive heart failure: Surgical correction in the neonatal period. Surgery, 67:985, 1970.)

upon by Bjork and Crafoord[12] in 1947 with a preoperative diagnosis of a patent ductus arteriosus. Since a ductus was not found, the pericardium was opened and revealed a fistula between an anomalous coronary artery and the pulmonary artery, which was closed. Most patients with coronary arteriovenous fistulas are *asymptomatic*, and symptoms result when complications occur. Thus, if the fistula becomes quite large and the shunt of blood from the left to the right heart is appreciable, the heart may enlarge and congestive heart failure may ultimately result. Bacterial endocarditis is a potential complication in such patients.[30]

Finally, the diagnosis is established by arteriography and cardiac catheterization. The site and magnitude of the lesion can be identified and appropriate therapy undertaken.

Although there is some controversy concerning the management of asymptomatic fistulas, most now believe that the fistulas should be closed when the diagnosis is confirmed, thereby preventing the complications that may occur. Moreover, surgical management is highly satisfactory and the mortality is negligible in these lesions. In most instances, closure is accomplished without the use of cardiopulmonary bypass, although extracorporeal circulation should be available if needed in order to eradicate the communication. Large fistulas, even in infants, can produce congestive heart failure (Figs. 18 and 19).

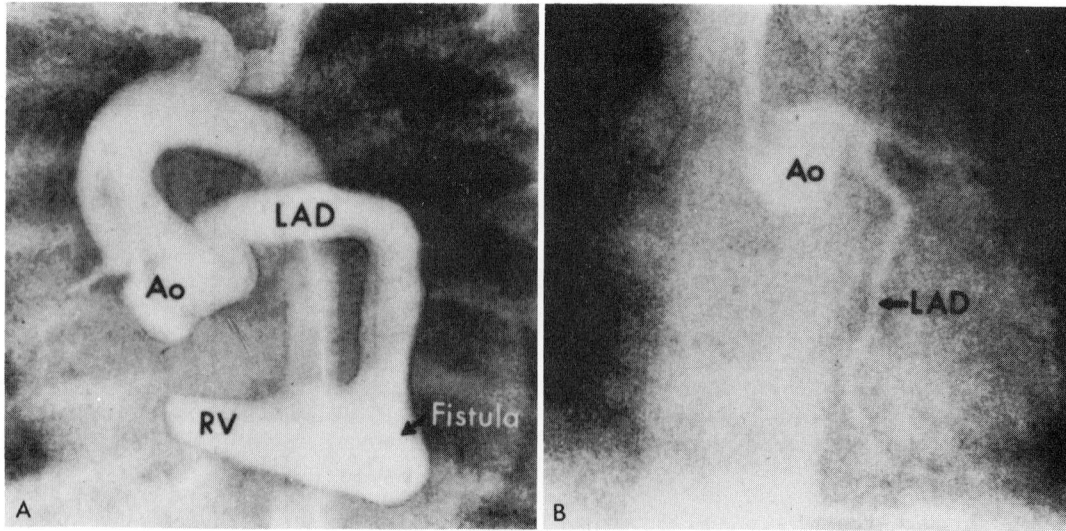

Figure 19.   *A*, Preoperative and, *B*, postoperative aortogram of patient shown in Figure 18.

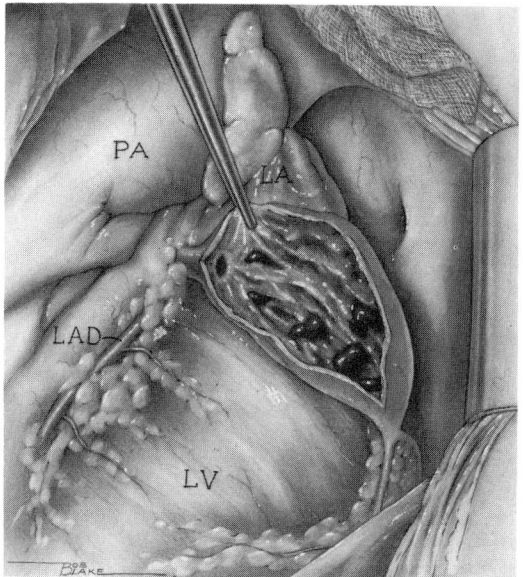

Figure 20. The numerous small fresh clots of blood are shown adherent to the rough irregular surface of the aneurysm. The proximal opening into the aneurysm was a discrete, mildly dilated vessel of good quality and normal appearing intima. The distal branches were of normal size. PA = Pulmonary artery. LAD = Left anterior descending coronary artery. LV = Left ventricle. (From Ebert, P. A., Peter, R. H., Gunnells, J. C., and Sabiston, D. C., Jr.: Resecting and grafting of coronary artery aneurysm. Circulation, *43*:593, 1971, by permission of the American Heart Association, Inc.)

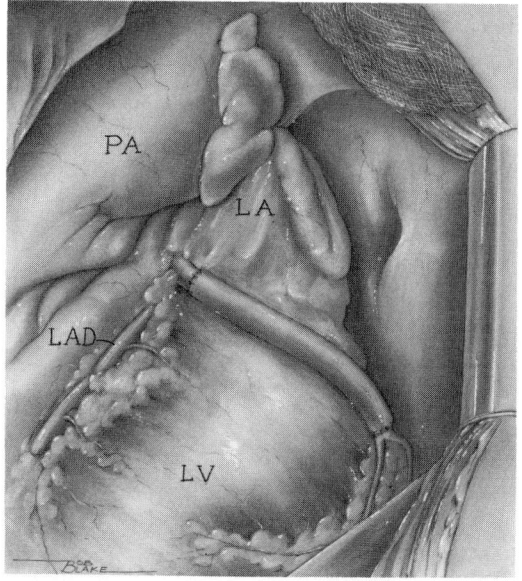

Figure 21. The entire aneurysm was excised and a segment of saphenous vein autograft interposed. There was only minimal discrepancy in the size of the autograft and the ends of the circumflex coronary artery. A continuous running suture of 7-0 Tevdek was used to complete the anastomosis. (From Ebert, P. A., Peter, R. H., Gunnells, J. C., and Sabiston, D. C., Jr.: Resecting and grafting of coronary artery aneurysm. Circulation, *43*:593, 1971, by permission of the American Heart Association, Inc.)

CONGENITAL ANEURYSMS OF THE CORONARY ARTERIES

The first congenital aneurysm of the coronary artery was reported by Bougon in 1812.[17] These lesions have been reported from infancy[29] to adult life. Congenital aneurysms of coronary arteries are rare and constitute about 15 per cent of 89 patients with these lesions.[31] Other causes of aneurysms of the coronary arteries include atherosclerosis, mycotic aneurysms, syphilis, and rheumatic types.

Most patients with this lesion are asymptomatic until specific complications occur. Patients are prone to produce thrombi, which subsequently embolize to cause myocardial ischemia and which may also rupture. Intramural coronary aneurysm has also been reported and has produced reversed flow during systole owing to bulging of the thin-walled chamber into the left ventricular cavity. The narrow neck of the aneurysm was successfully closed at operation. An example of a congenital coronary arterial aneurysm involving the left circumflex vessel is shown in Figure 20. In this patient, a mural thrombus occurred in the aneurysm, which embolized and produced acute myocardial infarction. The aneurysm was resected with insertion of a saphenous vein autograft as shown in Figure 21.[32]

If symptomatic, most agree that the aneurysm should now be removed with either primary closure if possible or substitution with a vein graft. It is especially important to remove the lesion if there is evidence that emboli from it are causing distal coronary arterial occlusion and myocardial ischemia.

In the recent past, additional aneurysms of the coronary arteries have been discovered as a result of the large number of arteriograms done for acquired myocardial ischemia. In one study, 1.5 per cent of patients so studied were found to have coronary artery aneurysms. The lesions were often multiple and were associated with extensive coronary atherosclerosis in 10 of the 11. Of 15 patients operated upon, there were 13 survivors.[36]

SELECTED REFERENCES

Abrikossoff, A.: Aneurysma des linken Herzventrikels mit abnormer Abgangsstelle der linken Koronararterie von der Pulmonalis bei einem funfmonatlichen Kinde. Virchows Arch. Pathol. Anat. Physiol. Med., *203*:413, 1911.
This is the first description of anomalous origin of the left coronary artery from the pulmonary artery. Both the gross and microscopic illustrations are excellent. The author describes in detail the clinical manifestations and postmortem findings.

Askenazi, J., and Nadas, A. S.: Anomalous left coronary artery originating from the pulmonary artery. Report on 15 cases. Circulation, *51*:976, 1975.
This is a summary of 15 infants and children with origin of the left coronary artery from the pulmonary artery managed both medically and surgically. The authors favor medical management in early life if surgical treatment can be delayed.

Baroldi, G., and Scomazzoni, G.: Coronary Circulation in the Normal and the Pathologic Heart. Washington, D.C., Office of the Surgeon General, Department of the Army, 1967.
This monograph is an exhaustive study of numerous specimens of the normal heart and those with atherosclerotic occlusive disease. It

is the most detailed of the studies of the anatomy and pathology of coronary atherosclerosis and is a classic.

Cohen, M. V., Cohn, P. F., Herman, M. V., and Gorlin, R.: Diagnosis and prognosis of main left coronary obstruction. Circulation, *45* and *46*(Suppl. 1):57, 1972.
In this presentation, the authors compare medical versus surgical management in a group of patients at one institution with severe stenosis of the left main coronary artery. They conclude that surgical management is far superior and that operation should be performed on an urgent basis to reduce complications to a minimum.

Daniel, T. M., Graham, T. P., and Sabiston, D. C., Jr.: Coronary artery–right ventricular fistula with congestive heart failure: Surgical correction in the neonatal period. Surgery, *67*:985, 1970.
Nearly 200 cases of coronary arteriovenous. fistula are reviewed. The incidence of congestive heart failure was 14 per cent. Approximately half of all patients with isolated arteriovenous fistulas were symptomatic. The age of onset of dyspnea, congestive heart failure, bacterial endocarditis, and angina pectoris is reviewed.

Falsetti, H. L., and Carroll, R. J.: Coronary artery aneurysm. A review of the literature with a report of 11 new cases. Chest, *69*:5, 1976.
In this paper, previously reported cases of coronary artery aneurysm are reviewed, together with 11 new cases reported by the authors. The etiology, pathology, and results of surgery are discussed.

Favaloro, R. G., Effler, D. B., Groves, L. K., Sheldon, W. C., Shirey, E. K., and Sones, F. M., Jr.: Severe segmental obstruction of the left main coronary artery and its divisions: Surgical treatment by the saphenous vein graft technique. J. Thorac. Cardiovasc. Surg., *60*:469, 1970.
In this paper, pioneers in the establishment of aortic-coronary bypass surgery describe their experience; their series constitutes the largest group of patients managed surgically. The indications, operative technique, and results are emphasized.

Gorlin, R.: Regulation of coronary blood flow. Br. Heart J., Vol. 33, Suppl. 9, 1971.
This paper describes the various factors that regulate coronary blood flow. It is concise and well presented.

Higgins, C. B., Wexler, L., Silverman, J. F., and Schroeder, J. S.: Clinical and arteriographic features of Prinzmetal's variant angina: Documentation of etiologic factors. Am. J. Cardiol., *37*:831, 1976.
In the recent past, much attention has been directed to the paradox of normal coronary arteriograms in patients with electrocardiographic abnormalities indicative of myocardial ischemia. The observation has been made that chest pain, S-T segment elevation, and spasm of coronary arteries demonstrated at arteriography may be the responsible mechanism for variant (Prinzmetal's) angina in some patients. In the study reported by these authors, it is concluded that coronary arterial spasm is the responsible pathogenetic mechanism of myocardial ischemia in some patients with Prinzmetal's angina and that this mechanism may be suspected from the clinical characteristics that these patients exhibit.

James, T. N.: Anatomy of the Coronary Arteries. New York, Paul B. Hoeber, 1961.
This monograph is the definitive source describing the anatomy of the coronary circulation. The work is superbly documented with numerous dissections and injections of specimens, which are carefully reproduced. This monograph is highly recommended.

Johnson, W. D., Flemma, R. J., Lepley, D., Jr., and Ellison, E. H.: Extended treatment of severe coronary artery disease: A total surgical approach. Ann. Surg., *170*:460, 1969.
This paper represents the early experience of the group who deserve primary credit for the introduction of the aortic-venous bypass graft for myocardial revascularization.

Marchetti, G., and Taccardi, B. (Eds.): Coronary Circulation and Energetics of the Myocardium. Basel, S. Karger, 1967.
This monograph records the presentations made at an International Symposium on the Coronary Circulation and Myocardial Energetics. World leaders in this field participated, and these papers form the best single source of physiology and metabolism of the coronary circulation currently available. The illustrations are excellent.

Peter, R. H.: Coronary arteriography. *In* Sabiston, D. C., Jr., and

Spencer, F. C. (Eds.): Gibbon's Surgery of the Chest, 3rd ed. Philadelphia, W. B. Saunders Company, 1976.
This is an excellent reference source for all aspects of coronary arteriography by an experienced cardiologist in the field. The illustrations and reproductions of cine arteriograms are outstanding.

Sabiston, D. C., Jr.: The coronary circulation. The William F. Rienhoff, Jr., Lecture. Johns Hopkins Med. J., *134*:314, 1974.
This is a review of the anatomy, physiology, and pathologic aspects of the coronary circulation. The data presented are based upon experimental and clinical findings in the normal and pathologic coronary circulation. The use of a saphenous vein bypass graft from the aorta directly to the coronary artery performed in 1962 is described in this paper.

Sabiston, D. C., Jr., and Orme, S. K.: Congenital origin of the left coronary artery from the pulmonary artery. J. Cardiovasc. Surg., *9*:543, 1968.
The authors describe 23 patients, ranging in age from 1 day to 31 years, with this disorder. The natural history, clinical findings, laboratory data, and ultimate course are presented.

Vlodaver, Z., and Edwards, J. E.: Pathologic changes in aortic-coronary arterial saphenous vein grafts. Circulation, *44*:719, 1971.
This is an excellent pathologic study of segments of saphenous vein used as grafts between the aorta and coronary artery. The earliest lesions were noted at one month and consisted primarily of intimal fibrotic proliferative lesions and organized thrombi. It is thought that the intimal fibrous proliferative lesion is primarily a response to arterial pressure within the segment of vein.

Vlodaver, Z., Amplatz, K., Burchell, H., and Edwards, J. E.: Coronary Heart Disease. Clinical Angiographic and Pathologic Profiles. New York, Springer-Verlag, 1976.
This is a superb monograph with excellent illustrations and narrative correlating coronary arteriograms with pathological lesions. It is an excellent reference source written by acknowledged authorities in the field and of much aid in understanding the importance of the clinical findings at the time of coronary arteriography with the pathologic lesions present in the vessels.

REFERENCES

1. Abbott, M. E.: Congenital cardiac disease. *In* Osler, W. (Ed.): Modern Medicine, 3rd ed. Philadelphia, Lea & Febiger, 1927.
2. Abrikossoff, A.: Aneurysma des linken Herzventrikels mit abnormer Abgangsstelle der linken Koronararterie von der Pulmonalis bei einem funfmonatlichen Kinde. Virchows Arch. Pathol. Anat. Physiol. Med., *203*:413, 1911.
3. Ackerman, R. F., Dry, T. J., and Edwards, J. E.: Relationship of various factors to the degree of coronary atherosclerosis in women. Circulation, *1*:345, 1950.
4. Aldridge, H. E., and Trimble, A. S.: Progression of proximal coronary artery lesions to total occlusion after aorta-coronary saphenous vein bypass grafting. J. Thorac. Cardiovasc. Surg., *62*:7, 1971.
5. Askenazi, J., and Nadas, A. S.: Anomalous left coronary artery originating from the pulmonary artery. Report on 15 cases. Circulation, *51*:976, 1975.
6. Bailey, C. P., May, A., and Lemmon, W. M.: Survival after coronary endarterectomy in man. J.A.M.A., *164*:641, 1957.
7. Bartel, A. G., Chen, J. T., Peter, R. H., Behar, V. S., Kong, Y., and Lester, R. G.: The significance of coronary calcification detected by fluoroscopy. Circulation, *49*:1247, 1974.
8. Baue, A. E., Baum, S., Blakemore, W. S., and Zinsser, H. F.: A later stage of anomalous coronary circulation with origin of the left coronary artery from the pulmonary artery. Circulation, *36*:878, 1967.
9. Beamish, R. E., and Stassie, U. M.: Impending myocardial infarction—recognition and management. Circulation, *21*:1107, 1960.
10. Beck, C. S.: The development of a new blood supply to the heart by operation. Ann. Surg., *102*:801, 1935.
11. Berger, R. L., and Stary, J. C.: Anatomic assessment of operability by the saphenous-vein bypass operation in coronary-artery disease. N. Engl. J. Med., *285*:248, 1971.
12. Bjork, G., and Crafoord, G.: Arteriovenous aneurysm on the pulmonary artery simulating patent ductus arteriosus Botalli. Thorax, *2*:65, 1947.

13. Bland, E. F., White, P. D., and Garland, J.: Congenital anomalies of coronary arteries: Report of an unusual case associated with cardiac hypertrophy. Am. Heart J., 8:787, 1933.

14. Blumgart, H. L., Pitt, B., Zoll, P. M., and Freiman, D. G.: Anatomic factors influencing the locations of coronary occlusions and development of collateral coronary circulation (Henry Ford Hospital International Symposium). In James, T. N., and Keyes, J. W. (Eds.): The Etiology of Myocardial Infarction. Boston, Little, Brown and Company, 1963.

15. Blumgart, H. L., Schlesinger, M. J., and Davis, D.: Studies on the relation of clinical manifestations of angina pectoris, coronary thrombosis and myocardial infarction to the pathologic findings with particular reference to significance of collateral circulation. Am. Heart J., 19:1, 1940.

16. Borer, J. S., Brensike, J. F., Redwood, D. R., Itscoitz, S. B., Passamani, E. R., Stone, N. J., Richardson, J. M., Levy, R. I., and Epstein, S. E.: Limitations of the electrocardiographic response to exercise in predicting coronary-artery disease. N. Engl. J. Med., 293:367, 1975.

17. Bougon: Bibl. Med., 37:183, 1912. Cited by Packard, M., and Wechsler, H. F.: Aneurysm of the coronary arteries. Arch. Intern. Med., 43:1, 1929.

18. Bourassa, M. G., and Noble, J.: Complication rate of coronary arteriography. A review of 5250 cases studied by a percutaneous femoral technique. Circulation, 53:106, 1976.

19. Bourassa, M. G., Solignac, A., Goulet, C., and Lesperance, J.: Regression and appearance of coronary collaterals in humans during life. Circulation, 49 and 50 (Suppl. 2):127, 1974.

20. Brooks, H. St. J.: Two cases of an abnormal coronary artery of the heart arising from the pulmonary artery. J. Anat. Physiol., 20:26, 1886.

21. Bruschke, A. V. G., Proudfit, W. L., and Sones, F. M., Jr.: Clinical course of patients with normal, and slightly or moderately abnormal coronary arteriograms. A follow-up study on 500 patients. Circulation, 47:936, 1973.

22. Burchell, H. B., and Brown, A. L., Jr.: Anomalous origin of coronary artery from pulmonary artery masquerading as mitral insufficiency. Am. Heart J., 63:388, 1962.

23. Carey, J. S., and Cukingham, R. A.: Subjective multivariable analysis by computer for evaluation of coronary artery bypass. Arch. Surg., 111:769, 1976.

24. Case, R. B., Morrow, A. G., Stainsby, W., and Nestor, J. O.: Anomalous origin of the left coronary artery: The physiologic defect and suggested surgical treatment. Circulation, 17:1062, 1958.

25. Cohen, M. V., Cohn, P. F., Herman, M. V., and Gorlin, R.: Diagnosis and prognosis of main left coronary obstruction. Circulation, 45 and 46 (Suppl. 1):57, 1972.

26. Conley, M. J., Wechsler, A. S., Anderson, R. W., Oldham, H. N., Jr., Sabiston, D. C., Jr., and Rosati, R. A.: The relationship of patient selection to prognosis following aortocoronary bypass. Circulation, 55:158, 1977.

27. Cooley, D. A., Belmonte, B. A., Zeis, L. B., and Schnur, S.: Surgical repair of ruptured interventricular septum following acute myocardial infarction. Surgery, 41:930, 1957.

28. Cooley, D. A., Hallman, G. L., and Bloodwell, R. D.: Definitive surgical treatment of anomalous origin of left coronary artery from pulmonary artery: Indications and results. J. Thorac. Cardiovasc. Surg., 52:798, 1966.

29. Crocker, D. W., Sobin, S., and Thomas, W. C.: Aneurysms of the coronary arteries. Report of three cases in infants and review of the literature. Am. J. Pathol., 33:819, 1957.

30. Daniel, T. M., Graham, T. P., and Sabiston, D. C., Jr.: Coronary artery–right ventricular fistula with congestive heart failure. Surgical correction in the neonatal period. Surgery, 67:985, 1970.

31. Daoud, A. S., Pankin, D., Tulgan, H., and Florentin, R. A.: Aneurysms of the coronary artery. Am. J. Cardiol., 11:228, 1963.

32. Ebert, P. A., Peter, R. H., Gunnells, J. C., and Sabiston, D. C., Jr.: Resecting and grafting of coronary artery aneurysm. Circulation, 43:593, 1971.

33. Eckstein, R. W.: Effect of exercise and coronary artery narrowing on coronary collateral circulation. Cir. Res., 5:230, 1957.

34. Eliot, R. S., Baroldi, G., and Leone, A.: Necropsy studies in myocardial infarction with minimal or no coronary luminal reduction due to atherosclerosis. Circulation, 49:1127, 1974.

35. Enos, W. F., Holmes, R. H., and Beyer, J.: Coronary disease among United States soldiers killed in action in Korea. Preliminary report. J.A.M.A., 152:1090, 1953.

36. Falsetti, H. L., and Carroll, R. J.: Coronary artery aneurysm. A review of the literature with a report of 11 new cases. Chest, 69:5, 1976.

37. Favaloro, R. G.: Direct myocardial revascularization. Surg. Clin. North Am., 51:1035, 1971.

38. Favaloro, R. G., Effler, D. B., and Groves, L. K.: Severe segmental obstruction of the left main coronary artery and its divisions: Surgical treatment by the saphenous vein graft technic. J. Thorac. Cardiovasc. Surg., 60:469, 1970.

39. Feldt, R. H., Ongley, P. A., and Titus, J. L.: Total coronary arterial circulation from pulmonary artery with survival to age seven: Report of case. Mayo Clin. Proc., 40:539, 1965.

40. FitzGibbon, G. M., Hooper, G. D., and Heggtveit, H. A.: Successful surgical treatment of post-infarction external cardiac rupture. J. Thorac. Cardiovasc. Surg., 63:622, 1972.

41. Flaherty, J. T., Spach, M. S., Boineau, J. P., Canent, R. V., Jr., Barr, R. C., and Sabiston, D. C., Jr.: Cardiac potentials on body surface of infants with anomalous left coronary artery (myocardial infarction). Circulation, 36:345, 1967.

42. Flemma, R. J., Marx, L., Litwin, S. B., and Gallen, W.: Left ventricular aneurysmectomy in infancy: Treatment of anomalous left coronary artery. Ann. Thorac. Surg., 19:457, 1975.

43. Fox, C., Davies, M. J., and Webb-Peploe, M. M.: Length of left main coronary artery. Br. Heart J., 35:796, 1973.

44. Francois-Franck, C. A.: Signification physiologique de la resection du sympathique dans la maladie de Basedow, l'epilepsie, l'idiotie et le glaucome. Bull. Acad. Natl. Med., 41:565, 1899. Cited by White, J. C.: Cardiac pain—anatomic pathways and physiologic mechanisms. Circulation, 16:644, 1957.

45. Goldstein, R. E., Michaelis, L. L., Morrow, A. G., and Epstein, S. E.: Coronary collateral function in patients without occlusive coronary artery disease. Circulation, 51:118, 1975.

46. Gorlin, R.: Regulation of coronary blood flow. Br. Heart J., 33(Suppl.):9, 1971.

47. Green, G. E., Stertzer, S. H., Gordon, R. B., and Tice, D. A.: Anastomosis of the internal mammary artery to the distal left anterior descending coronary artery. Circulation, 41(Suppl. 2):79, 1970.

48. Gregg, D. E.: The coronary circulation in the unanesthetized dog. In Marchetti, G., and Taccardi, B. (Eds.): Coronary Circulation and Energetics of the Myocardium. Basel, S. Karger, 1967.

49. Grondin, C. M., Meere, C., Castonguay, Y., Lepage, G., and Grondin, P.: Progressive and late obstruction of an aortocoronary venous bypass graft. Circulation, 43:698, 1971.

50. Guss, S. B., Zir, L. M., Garrison, H. B., Daggett, W. M., Block, P. C., and Dinsmore, R. E.: Coronary occlusion during coronary angiography. Circulation, 52:1063, 1975.

51. Harthorne, J. W., Scannell, J. G., and Dinsmore, R. E.: Anomalous origin of the left coronary artery. Remediable cause of sudden death in adults. N. Engl. J. Med., 275:660, 1966.

52. Herberden, W.: Commentaries on the History and Cure of Diseases. Boston, Wells and Lilly, 1818, p. 292.

53. Herrick, J. B.: Clinical features of sudden obstruction of the coronary arteries. J.A.M.A., 59:2015, 1912.

54. Heyden, S.: Risk Factors of Ischemic Heart Disease. Boehringer Mannheim GmbH, Mannheim, Germany, 1975.

55. Higgins, C. B., Wexler, L., Silverman, J. F., and Schroeder, J. S.: Clinical and arteriographic features of Prinzmetal's variant angina: Documentation of etiologic factors. Am. J. Cardiol., 37:831, 1976.

56. Hill, J. D., Kerth, W. J., Kelly, J. J., Selzer, A., Armstrong, W., Popper, R. W., Langston, M., and Cohn, K. E.: Emergency aortocoronary bypass for impending or extending myocardial infarction. Circulation, 43(Suppl. 1):105, 1971.

57. Ihenacho, H. N. C., Singh, S. P., Astley, R., and Parsons, C. G.: Case report. Anomalous left coronary artery. Report of an unusual case with spontaneous remission of symptoms. Br. Heart. J., 35:562, 1973.

58. Johnson, W. D., Flemma, R. J., Lepley, D., Jr., and Ellison, E. H.: Extended treatment of severe coronary artery disease: A total surgical approach. Ann. Surg., 170:460, 1969.

59. Jonnesco, T.: Angine de poitrine guerie par la resection du sympathique cervico-thoracique. Bull. Acad. Med., 84:93, 1920.

60. Kaiser, G. C., Marco, J. D., Barner, H. B., Codd, J. E., Laks, H., and Willman, V. L.: Intraaortic balloon assistance. Ann. Thorac. Surg., 21:487, 1976.

61. Keith, J. D.: The anomalous origin of the left coronary artery from the pulmonary artery. Br. Heart J., 21:149, 1959.

62. Khaja, F-U., Sharma, S. D., Easley, R. M., Jr., Heinle, R. A., and Goldstein, S.: Left main coronary artery lesions. Risks

of catheterization; exercise testing and surgery. Circulation, *49* and *50* (Suppl. 2):136, 1974.

63. Krause, W.: Z. Rat. Med., *24,* 1865.

64. Lavine, P., Kimbiris, D., Segal, B. L., and Linhart, J. W.: Left main coronary artery disease. Clinical, arteriographic and hemodynamic appraisal. Am. J. Cardiol., *30:*791, 1972.

65. Longmire, W. P., Jr., Cannon, J. A., and Kattus, A. A.: Direct-vision coronary endarterectomy for angina pectoris. N. Engl. J. Med., *259:*993, 1958.

66. Mann, G. V., Garrett, H. L., Farhi, A., Murray, H., and Billings, F. T.: Exercise to prevent coronary heart disease. Am. J. Med., 46:12, 1969.

67. Mathur, V. S., and Guinn, G. A.: Prospective randomized study of coronary bypass surgery in stable angina. The first 100 patients. Circulation, *51* (Suppl. 1):133, 1975.

68. Matloff, J. M., Sustaita, H., Chatterjee, K., Chaux, A., Marcus, H. S., and Swan, H. J. C.: The rationale for surgery in preinfarction angina. J. Thorac. Cardiovasc. Surg., *69:*73, 1975.

69. McConahay, D. R., Killen, D. A., McCallister, B. D., Arnold, M., Reed, W. A., Crockett, J. E., and Bell, H. H.: Coronary artery bypass surgery for left main coronary artery disease. Am. J. Cardiol., 37:885, 1976.

70. McLaughlin, P. R., Berman, N. D., Morton, B. C., McLoughlin, M. J., Aldridge, H. E., Adelman, A. G., Goldman, B. S., Trimble, A. S., and Morch, J. E.: Saphenous vein bypass grafting. Changes in native circulation and collaterals. Circulation, *51* and *52* (Suppl. 1):66, 1975.

71. Menke, J. A., Shaher, R. M., and Wolff, G. S.: Ejection fraction in anomalous origin of the left coronary artery from the pulmonary artery. Am. Heart J., *84:*325, 1972.

72. Moon, H. D.: Coronary arteries in infants and juveniles. Circulation, *16:*263, 1957.

73. Morris, G. C., Jr., Howell, J. F., Crawford, E. S., Reul, G. J., Chapman, D. W., Beazley, H. L., Winters, W. L., and Peterson, P. K.: The distal coronary bypass. Ann. Surg., *172:*652, 1970.

74. Mounsey, P.: Prodromal symptoms in myocardial infarction. Br. Heart J., *13:*215, 1951.

75. Mundth, E. D., and Austen, W. G.: Surgical measures for coronary heart disease. N. Engl. J. Med., *293:*13, 75, 124, 1975.

76. Mundth, E. D., Buckley, M. J., Leinbach, R. C., DeSanctis, R. W., Sanders, C. A., Kantrowitz, A., and Austen, W. G.: Myocardial revascularization for the treatment of cardiogenic shock complicating acute myocardial infarction. Surgery, 70:78, 1971.

77. Ogden, J. A.: Congenital anomalies of the coronary arteries. Am. J. Cardiol., *25:*474, 1970.

78. Oldham, H. N., Jr., Rembert, J. C., Greenfield, J. C., Wechsler, A. S., and Sabiston, D. C., Jr.: Intraoperative relationships of aortocoronary bypass graft blood flow, peripheral coronary artery pressure, and reactive hyperemia. Pathogenetic Mechanisms of Angina Pectoris. Therapeutic Implications. Satellite Workshop of the VII European Congress of Cardiology, Pisa, Italy, June, 1976. New York, Grune and Stratton, in press.

79. Oldham, H. N., Scott, S. M., Dart, C. H., Fish, R. G., Claxton, C. P., Dillon, M. L., and Sabiston, D. C., Jr.: Surgical correction of ventricular septal defect following acute myocardial infarction. Ann. Thorac. Surg., 7:193, 1969.

80. Oyamadi, A., and Queen, F. V.: Spontaneous rupture of the interventricular septum following acute myocardial infarction with some clinicopathological observations on survival in 5 cases. Presented at Pan Pacific Pathology Congress, Tripler U.S. Army Hospital, 1961.

81. Peter, R. H.: Coronary arteriography. *In* Sabiston, D. C., Jr., and Spencer, F. C. (Eds.): Gibbons's Surgery of the Chest, 3rd ed. Philadelphia, W. B. Saunders Company, 1976.

82. Pinsky, W. W., Fagan, L. R., Kraeger, R. R., Mudd, J. F. G., and Willman, V. L.: Anomalous left coronary artery. J. Thorac. Cardiovasc. Surg., *65:*810, 1973.

83. Reeves, T. J., Oberman, A., Jones, W. B., and Sheffield, L. T.: Natural history of angina pectoris. Am. J. Cardiol., *33:*423, 1974.

84. Roche, A. H. G.: Anomalous origin of the left coronary artery from the pulmonary artery in the adult. Am. J. Cardiol., *20:*561, 1967.

85. Rowe, G. G., Castillo, C. A., Maxwell, G. M., and Crumpton, C. W.: Comparison of systemic and coronary hemodynamics in the normal human male and female. Circ. Res., 7:728, 1959.

86. Sabiston, D. C., Jr.: Direct revascularization procedure in the management of myocardial ischemia. Circulation, *43:*175, 1971.

87. Sabiston, D. C., Jr.: The coronary circulation. The William F. Reinhoff, Jr., Lecture. Johns Hopkins Med. J., *134:*314, 1974.

88. Sabiston, D. C., Jr., Floyd, W. L., and McIntosh, H. D.: Anomalous origin of the left coronary artery from the pulmonary artery in adults. Arch. Surg., *97:*963, 1968.

89. Sabiston, D. C., Jr., Neill, C. A., and Taussig, H. B.: The direction of blood flow in anomalous left coronary artery arising from the pulmonary artery. Circulation, *22:*591, 1960.

90. Sabiston, D. C., Jr., and Orme, S. K.: Congenital origin of the left coronary artery from the pulmonary artery. J. Cardiovasc. Surg., *9:*543, 1968.

91. Sabiston, D. C., Jr., Pelargonio, S., and Taussig, H. B.: Myocardial infarction in infancy. J. Thorac. Cardiovasc. Surg., *40:*321, 1960.

92. Sabiston, D. C., Jr., Ross, R. S., Criley, J. M., Gaertner, R. A., Neill, C. A., and Taussig, H. B.: Surgical management of congenital lesions of the coronary circulation. Ann. Surg., *157:*908, 1963.

93. Scheidt, S., Wolk, M., and Killip, T.: Unstable angina pectoris. Natural history, hemodynamics, uncertainties of treatment and the ethics of clinical study. Am. J. Med., *60:*409, 1976.

94. Schlesinger, M. J., and Zoll, P. M.: Incidence and localization of coronary artery occlusions. Arch. Pathol., *32:*178, 1941.

95. Sharbaugh, A. H., and White, R. S.: Single coronary artery. Analysis of the anatomic variation, clinical importance and report of five cases. J.A.M.A., *230:*243, 1974.

96. Sheldon, W. C.: Cine coronary arteriography. Surg. Clin. North Am., *51:*1015, 1971.

97. Spencer, F. C.: Bypass grafting for occlusive disease of the coronary arteries. Maryland Med. J., *20:*2, 1971.

98. Spiekerman, R. E., Brandenburg, J. T., Achor, R. W. P., and Edwards, J. E.: The spectrum of coronary artery disease in a community of 30,000. A clinico-pathologic study. Circulation, *25:*57, 1962.

99. Tedeschi, C. G., and Helpern, M. M.: Heterotopic origin of both coronary arteries from the pulmonary artery. Review of literature and report of a case not complicated by associated defects. Pediatrics, *14:*53, 1954.

100. Turina, M., Real, F., Meier, W., and Senning, A.: Left ventricular aneurysmectomy in a 4-month-old infant. Alternative method of treatment of anomalous left coronary artery. J. Thorac. Cardiovasc. Surg., *67:*915, 1974.

101. Vansant, J. H., and Muller, W. H., Jr.: Surgical procedures to revascularize the heart: Review of the literature. Am. J. Surg., *100:*572, 1960.

102. Vineberg, A. M.: Development of an anastomosis between the coronary vessels and a transplanted internal mammary artery. Can. Med. Assoc. J., *55:*117, 1946.

103. Vlodaver, Z., and Edwards, J. E.: Pathologic changes in aortic-coronary arterial saphenous vein grafts. Circulation, *44:*719, 1971.

104. Vlodaver, Z., and Edwards, J. E.: Pathology of coronary atherosclerosis. *In* Sabiston, D. C., Jr., and Spencer, F. C. (Eds.): Gibbon's Surgery of the Chest, 3rd ed. Philadelphia, W. B. Saunders Company, 1976.

105. Webb, W. R.: Intraaortic balloon pumping. Ann. Thorac. Surg., *21:*571, 1976.

106. Webb, W. R., Parker, F. B., Jr., and Neville, J. F., Jr.: Retrograde pressures and flows in coronary arterial disease. Ann. Thorac. Surg., *15:*256, 1973.

107. White, N. K., Edwards, J. E., and Dry, T. J.: The relationship of the degree of coronary atherosclerosis with age in men. Circulation, *1:*645, 1950.

108. Wilhelmsson, C., Vedin, J. A., Elmfeldt, D., Tibblin, G., and Wilhelmsen, L.: Smoking and myocardial infarction. Lancet, *1:*415, 1975.

109. Winkle, R. A., Alderman, E. L., Shumway, N. E., and Harrison, D. C.: Results of reoperation for unsuccessful coronary artery bypass surgery. Circulation, *51* and *52* (Suppl. 1):61, 1975.

110. Winterscheid, L. C.: Collateral circulation of the heart. *In* Strandness, D. E., Jr. (Ed.): Collateral Circulation in Clinical Surgery. Philadelphia, W. B. Saunders Company, 1969.

111. Wolkoff, K.: Ueber die Atherosklerose der Koronararterien des Herzens. Beitr. Pathol., *82:*55, 1929.

XIV

PATHOLOGIC CHANGES OCCURRING IN VENOUS AUTOGRAFTS

James C. A. Fuchs, M.D.

Autologous saphenous vein is the most widely used graft material for the bypass of small caliber arteries. Although it was first used in 1906,[33] it is only since the 1950s that it has achieved widespread acceptance. Cumulative studies of grafts in the peripheral arterial position[14, 19] provide data concerning long-term patency and offer performance standards by which any other arterial substitute should be judged.

Since venous autografts have produced good results in peripheral arteries, they have been widely used to bypass obstruction in coronary and renal arteries.[22, 59] Follow-up studies of grafts to these organs have been quite thorough, with frequent postoperative evaluation of patency by arteriography. In addition, special histologic examinations have been performed when obtained at the time of re-exploration or at autopsy.[68] In consecutive series of patients,[12, 16, 32] such studies provided data about the incidence of a variety of distinctive histologic changes which occur.[35, 59, 68, 69]

Recently methods of investigation similar to the studies of coronary grafts have been applied to veins used in the bypass of peripheral arteries in humans.[66] Additional sporadic clinical reports[7, 8, 45, 54, 61] of pathologic changes in peripheral bypass, as well as the more extensive animal experiments,[17, 26, 36, 44, 49, 51, 52, 54, 71–74] support the fact that such changes occur in vein grafts whether in the peripheral or in the central position. Data from both human and experimental work have been combined in the following analysis in order to establish the characteristics of normal vein, the alterations brought about in preparing a vein for a graft, the changes seen postoperatively, and the features that may lead to the development of these changes.

NORMAL VEINS

To understand the distinctive changes that occur postoperatively in vein grafts, an appreciation of the normal characteristics of veins is essential. Traditional light microscopy shows the anatomy of the three layers in the venous wall (Fig. 1). (1) The *intima* consists of a thin endothelial layer on the luminal surface of the vessel. When seen in cross section, this mononuclear layer is thrown into folds along the inner surfaces of the vessel. Owing to poor staining characteristics, only the nuclei are seen distinctively with light microscopy. In fortuitous sections, in which the endothelial surface is cut tangentially, the orderly distribution of the nuclei of the endothelial cells can be appreciated (Fig. 2). (2) In the *media* are smooth muscle cells arranged in an inner longitudinal and an outer circumferential direction and interlaced with collagen and elastic fibrils. The elastic fibrils appear to

be oriented predominantly in a longitudinal direction. (3) The outer *adventitia* is frequently thicker than the media and is formed by a loose, collagenous network interspersed with vasa vasorum. Longitudinal or spirally arranged smooth muscle cells may appear in this layer. The collagen fibers blend with the surrounding adipose tissue in the case of superficial, subcutaneous veins.

More recently, transmission and scanning electron microscopic studies have provided useful information about the fine structure of veins.[48, 53, 62] These methods have been particularly valuable in defining the anatomy of the endothelial layer. Transmission electron microscopy shows the monolayer of endothelium to consist of cells with a large central nucleus and a thin cytoplasm (Fig. 3). The latter contains the usual ultrastructural organelles as well as a large number of

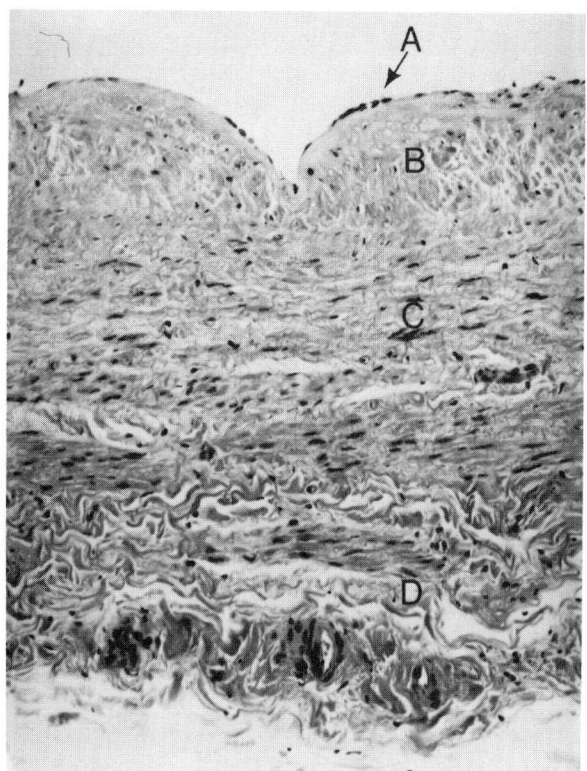

Figure 1. Normal saphenous vein (× 170, cross section with hematoxylin and eosin stain). The endothelium is seen as a monolayer of nuclei (A). Medial smooth muscle cells are arranged in an inner longitudinal (B) and an outer circular (C) fashion and are surrounded by the loose stroma of adventitia (D).

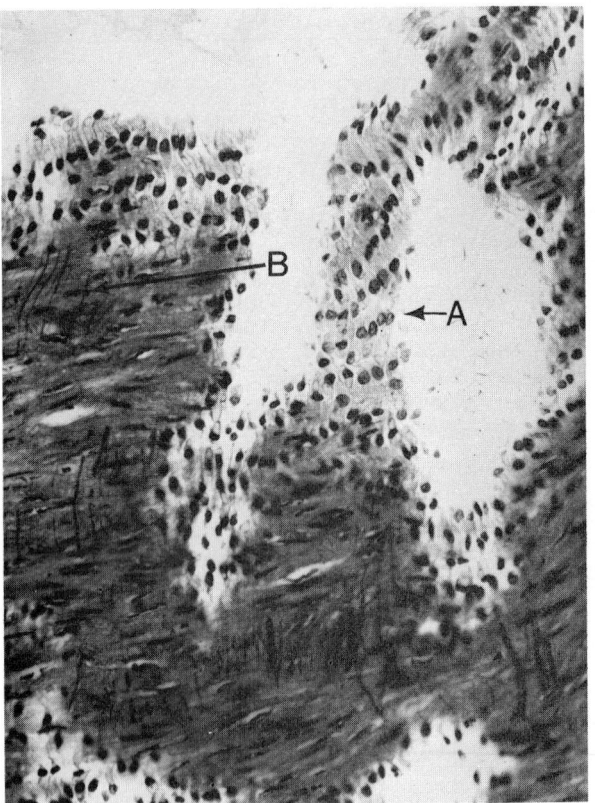

Figure 2. Canine jugular vein (× 250, longitudinal section with elastic tissue stain). The fortuitous tangential section shows the structural arrangement of the sheet of endothelium (A). The longitudinal elastic fibers can be appreciated in the media (B).

plasmalemmal vesicles, many of which are open at the cell surfaces. In addition, microvilli can be seen on the luminal border of the endothelium.

Although the technique of scanning microscopy is limited to this endothelial layer, it is invaluable in providing a three-dimensional impression of the surface (Fig. 4). One can readily appreciate the polygonal cells with their bulging nuclei and prominent intercellular ridges. Magnified views of the endothelial surface also support the presence of microvilli (Fig. 5). Electron microscopy of deeper layers of the venous wall is restricted to transmission technique. Smooth muscle cells have contractile fibers and prominent subsurface vesicles, as well as the normal ultrastructural organelles (Fig. 6). The predominent cell types in the adventitia are fibroblasts surrounded by strands of collagen.

Apart from such histologic evaluation, veins have been examined in terms of their physical[70] and biochemical properties.[28, 40, 44] Pressure-strain studies performed to determine elastic properties of veins have shown these vessels to have a highly compliant phase over physiologic ranges of venous pressure and a relatively noncompliant phase in the range of arterial pressures. Such a response is different from arteries which maintain compliance over all physiologic pressure ranges.[70]

The initial biochemical studies of venous tissue involved histochemical assay.[44] Normal vein has been found to have high degrees of lactic dehydrogenase activity and smaller amounts of other oxidative enzymes. Hydrolytic enzyme activity has also been detected in the forms of adenosine triphosphatase and esterases. Information is also available on the metabol-

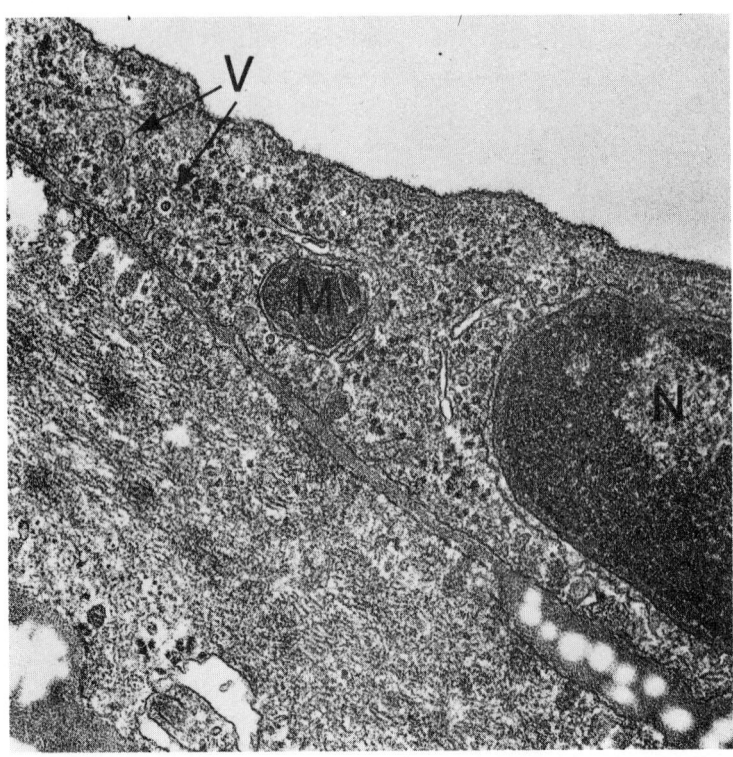

Figure 3. Canine jugular vein (× 15,000). Transmission electron micrographic view of an endothelial cell showing nucleus (N), mitochondrion (M), and vesicles (V).

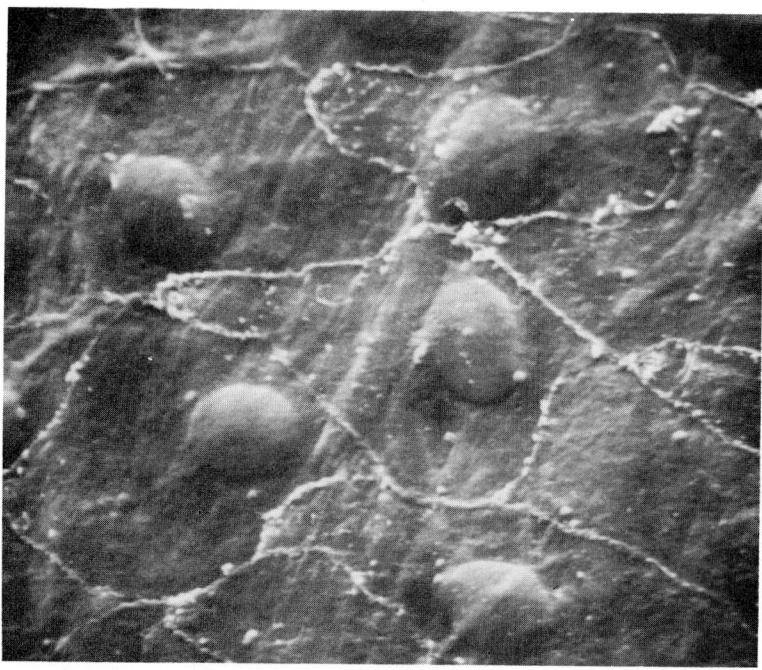

Figure 4. Canine jugular vein ($\times$ 2500). Scanning electron micrograph of the endothelial surface demonstrating polygonal cells with flat nuclei and prominent intercellular ridges.

ic activity[40] and tissue content of lipids in normal veins.[28]

AUTOLOGOUS VEIN PREPARED FOR IMPLANTATION

Under usual circumstances, a vein chosen to form a bypass must undergo preparation before it is placed into the arterial circuit, including dissection from its bed, ligation of its branches, flushing of the lumen, and distention to overcome spasm and to identify

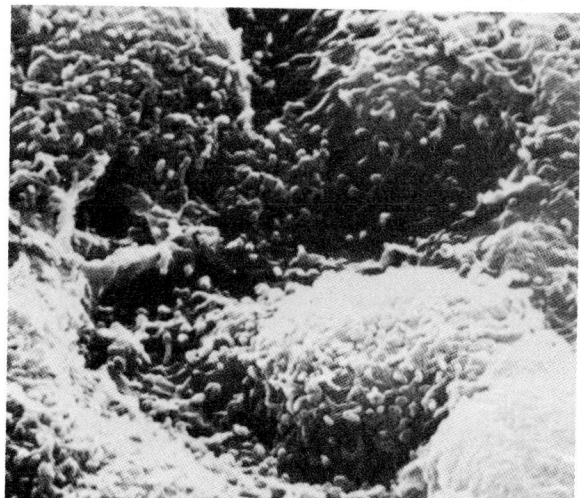

Figure 5. Canine cephalic vein ($\times$ 5355). Scanning electron micrograph showing the luminal surface to be covered with numerous microvilli (From Ramos, J. R., et al.: Ann. Surg., *183*:225, 1976.)

leaks. It may then be placed aside for a variable period of time before insertion.

The potential for these procedures to produce trauma in the vein is recognized. Histologic examination with light microscopy has demonstrated extensive sloughing of the fragile endothelium.[74] More recent scanning electron microscopic studies have shown further damage by demonstrating the adhesion and subintimal migration of polymorphonuclear cells,[64] crater formation in the endothelial cytoplasm (Fig. 7),[48, 63] and fracture and separation of the endothelial cells (Fig. 8).[48, 53] Swelling of the smooth muscle cells in the flattened medial layer has been described,[47] with accumulation of fluid and disruption of cellular membranes. In the adventitial layer, fracture of the bundles of collagen and thrombosis of the vasa vasorum can occur.[53]

Another approach to the changes induced by graft preparation involves analysis of the stress-strain relationship in normal and in prepared venous tissue.[1] Such physical investigations have demonstrated significant alterations of the stiffness or of the distensibility of the vein, depending on the preparation technique used. These physical and anatomic changes have been ascribed to a variety of types of injury. Direct physical trauma occurs with dissection of the vein, but this can be minimal if careful technique is used.[48] Unavoidable, however, is the chemotactic response of intraluminal leukocytes, which adhere to the endothelial surface and invade the subendothelial region whether surgical intervention is near or distant to the dissected vein.[62, 64] Considerable distention pressure (500 to 600 mm. Hg) can be generated with the dilatation that is often performed to overcome spasm and to detect leaks in the vein.[1, 53] The ischemic conditions that exist in the walls of vessels deprived of both intraluminal blood and vasa vasorum are sufficient to result in cellular injury.[11, 24, 48] Such alterations are

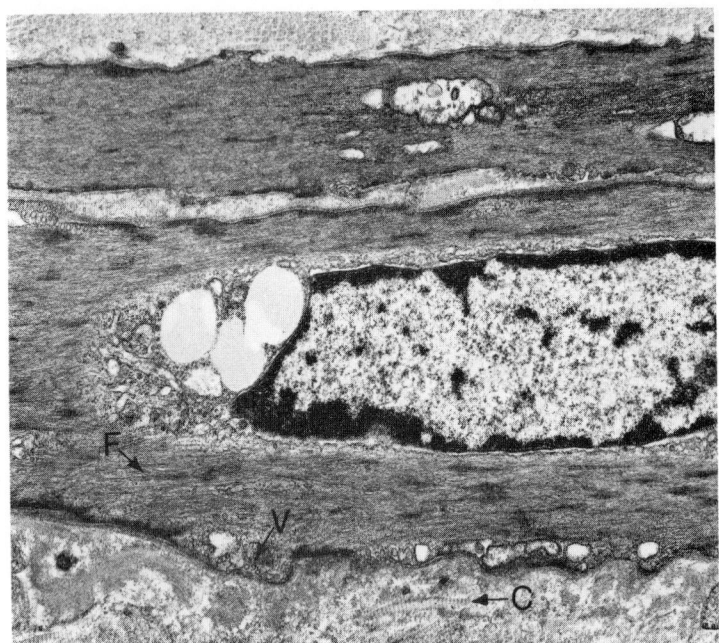

Figure 6. Canine jugular vein (× 15,000). Transmission electron micrograph of a medial smooth muscle cell showing contractile fibers (F), subsurface collection of vesicles (V), and surrounding matrix of collagen (C) and elastin.

enhanced by the nonphysiologic pH of many unbuffered crystalloid solutions used either to dilate or to maintain the veins between the time of removal and insertion.[1] All of these changes can be exaggerated by the metabolic stress of prolonged hypoxia at room temperature.

The value of listing such a variety of noxious stimuli lies in the fact that most can be minimized or eliminated. With careful dissection, maintenance of luminal blood flow, low pressure distention, and storage in cold buffered solutions, the degree of injury is small and can be reversed.[48, 65]

CHANGES IN VEINS AFTER GRAFTING

The specific pathologic changes seen in these grafts are usually related to the length of time the vein has been implanted. An *acute* phase first occurs in which changes develop in response to the new environment of high pressure and rapid flow. The intima shows areas of endothelial desquamation, and leukocytes and fibrin can be found on the denuded surface of the underlying basement membrane.[44, 53, 54] In the media are found areas of edema, focal hemorrhage, and smooth muscle cell necrosis.[7, 49] The fragmented ad-

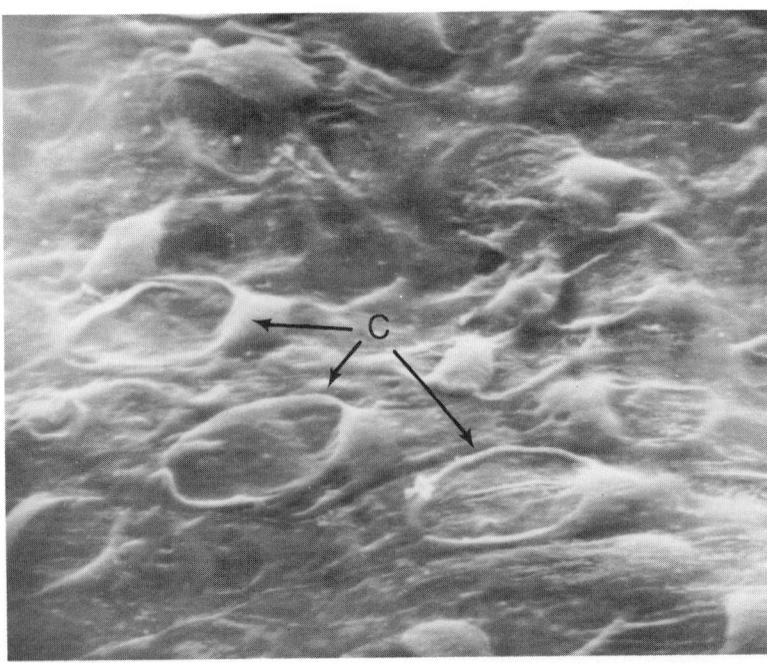

Figure 7. Canine jugular vein (× 2500). Scanning electron micrograph of a vein that has been dissected from its bed and deprived of intraluminal blood flow for two hours. Note the presence of crater-like defects (C).

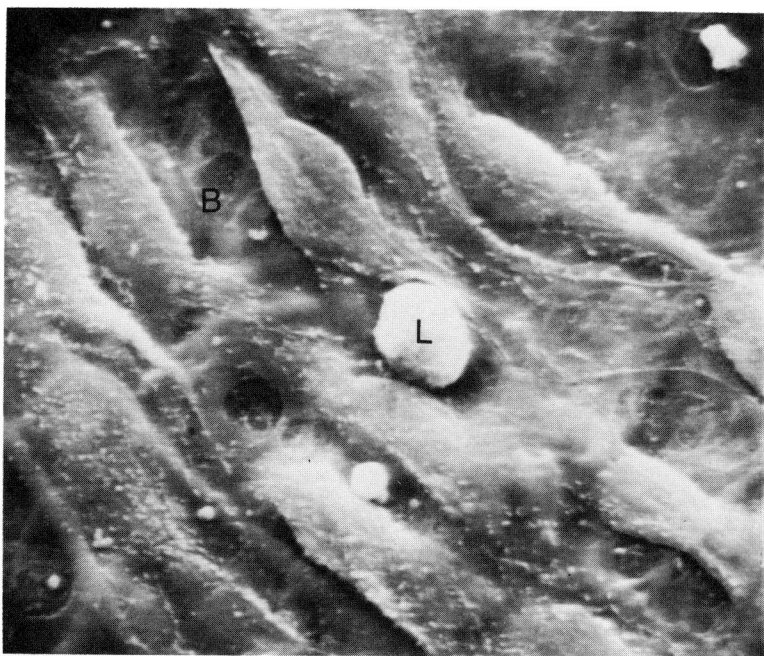

Figure 8. Canine jugular vein (× 3500). Scanning electron micrograph of vein prepared by distention of the lumen with saline. The endothelial cells have separated, exposing underlying collagen and basement membrane (B) with an adherent leukocyte (L).

ventitia remains separated from surrounding structures (Fig. 9).

Early endothelial regeneration is common and will completely line the internal luminal surface within six weeks.[54] During this period the medial layer undergoes a fibrous transformation, with collagen deposition and diminution in the number of smooth muscle cells,[53] and the surrounding adventitia becomes incorporated by a periadventitial connective layer (Fig. 10). These acute changes appear to be manifestations of the injury sustained during graft insertion and are accompanied by elevated levels of glucose-6-phosphate dehydrogenase that characterize the process of inflammation and repair.[44]

Most of this information has been provided by experimental preparations that can be excised at precise time intervals and studied extensively. The pathologic material available from the human use of this graft material usually depends on the occurrence of graft failure with subsequent loss of limb or life. When this functional failure occurs during the acute stage, it is often due to *thrombosis*. This process accounts for most instances of failure occurring within the first month after graft insertion.[68] Contributing features that possibly lead to thrombosis are volume of flow through the graft,[31, 42] the state of coagulability of the blood and blood particles,[60] the outflow available to the graft,[66, 67] and technical errors at the time of graft insertion.[12] Even if the graft is not completely occluded, foci of thrombus are often seen in the region behind the open venous valve (Fig. 11).[46] The exact incidence of thrombosis is not precisely known, but with aortocoronary bypass grafts it has been reported in unfavorable situations to be as high as 42 per cent.[42] However, the early *patency* rate in usual series with this procedure or with renal artery bypass is 90 per cent or more, suggesting that early thrombosis occurs in a relatively small number of such patients.[12, 16] In the peripheral position the immediate failure rate is higher, between 20 and 35 per cent,[19, 66] and is usually dependent on the flow through the graft as determined by the amount of disease in the distal vascular bed.

Evaluation of venous grafts in place for one to two months demonstrates a variety of well-developed pathologic changes. A characteristic *intimal hypertrophy* is well recognized both in full vein grafts and in onlay grafts.[13, 56, 61] Such changes have been termed

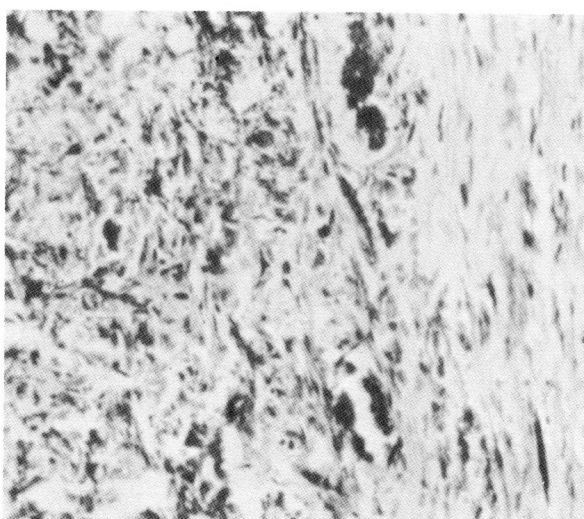

Figure 9. Canine cephalic vein (× 100). Masson trichrome stain of vein graft in place for one week. Medial smooth muscle edema, necrosis, and focal hemorrhages are prominent. (From Ramos, J. R., et al.: Ann. Surg., *183*:213, 1976.)

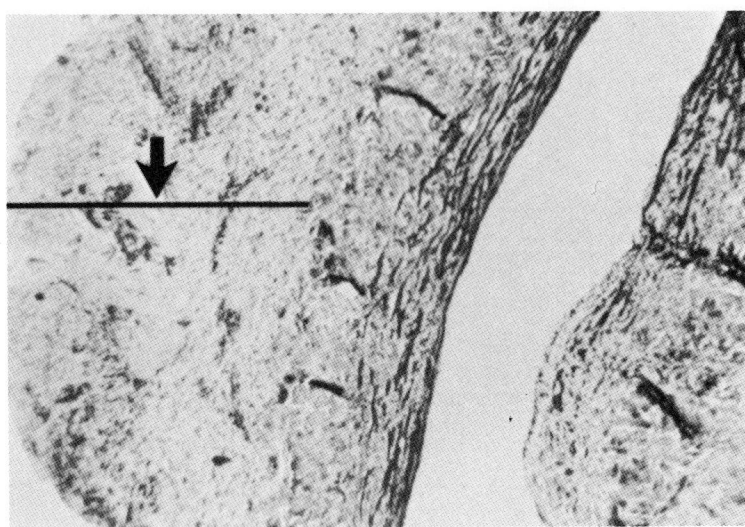

Figure 10. Canine cephalic vein (× 40). Masson trichrome stain of a graft in the arterial circuit for 15 days. Note the ingrowth of perivascular tissue adherent to the adventitia of the graft (arrow). (From Ramos, J. R., et al.: Ann. Surg., *183*:223, 1976.)

"arterialization" and are thought to follow exposure to a high intraluminal pressure. These findings have been especially noted in aortocoronary grafts.[43, 69] Thorough histologic examination of almost all grafts inserted for more than a month reveals some evidence of this process (Fig. 12), and it may proceed to a graft occlusion (Fig. 13). The fibrous nature of this prolifer-

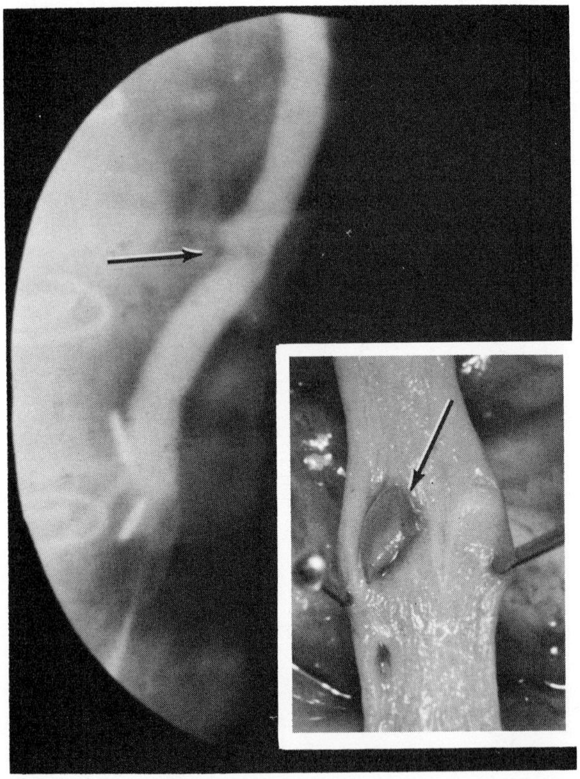

Figure 11. Angiogram and postmortem view of an aortocoronary saphenous vein graft showing thrombus beneath the cusp of a vein valve. (From Mills, N. L., and Ochsner, J. L.: J. Thorac. Cardiovasc. Surg., *71*:878, 1976.)

ative process was noted and led to the designation *intimal fibrous proliferation*.[69] With the aid of transmission electron microscopy, both fibroblasts and smooth muscle cells have been identified.[39] thus making the general term, *intimal hyperplasia,* a more accurate description. The luminal surface of this thickened layer becomes lined with endothelial cells, although these cells may be altered by the irregular underlying surface of hyperplastic tissue (Fig. 14).

The pathogenesis of this complex phenomenon is not fully understood. Implicated in the development of such a response has been exposure of the graft to arterial pressure,[10] hydraulic and shear stress factors,[9, 38] the level of serum lipids,[2] and the release of proliferative factors from the blood or the blood particles adherent to the luminal surface.[23] These changes are not limited to venous tissue, as they have been described in implanted and endarterectomized arteries.[34, 37] Intimal hyperplasia thus appears to be a basic blood vessel response regularly encountered after many procedures in vascular surgery. Such an intimal hyperplastic reaction is a common initial event in the arteries of animals with experimentally induced atherosclerosis. That these changes may lead to this disease in "arterialized" vein is borne out by the occurrence of mature *atherosclerosis* in vein grafts (Fig. 15). Fully developed atherosclerotic plaques have been recognized in long-term human grafts in the peripheral circuit[8, 20, 21, 39] and in the aortocoronary position.[5] The earliest these lesions have been seen is six months post implantation, with an occurrence rate by angiographic identification as high as 7 per cent.[66]

There is ample experimental evidence that grafted venous tissue under conditions of induced hyperlipidemia will develop atherosclerotic lesions.[26, 51, 58, 72] In fact, venous tissue has demonstrated an avidity for the uptake of serum lipids surpassing that of arterial tissue in the same species.[28, 58] Whether such serum factors are directly related to the development of graft atherosclerosis in humans is unclear, but the manipulation of these factors through diet or drug therapy provides a means of postoperative treatment that is applicable to many patients.[3, 6]

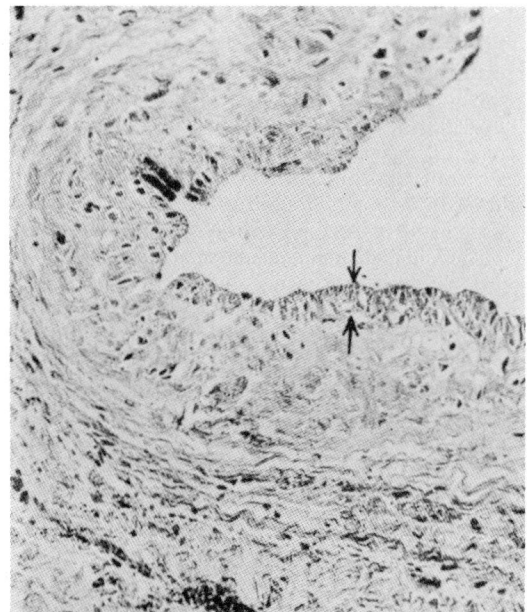

Figure 12. Aortocoronary saphenous vein graft (× 50, hematoxylin and eosin). This graft has been in place for one month and shows a minimal amount of intimal hyperplasia (arrows). (From Vlodaver, Z., and Edwards, J. E.: Circulation *44*:721, 1971. By permission of the American Heart Association, Inc.)

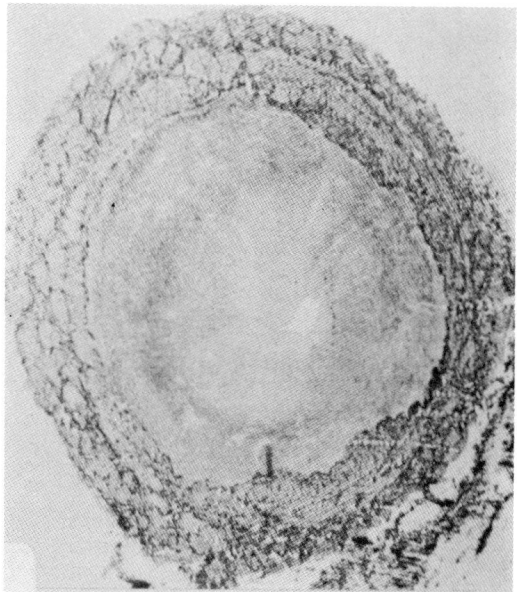

Figure 13. Aortocoronary saphenous vein graft (× 14, elastic tissue stain). After nine months this graft shows severe obstruction of the lumen with intimal hyperplasia. (From Vlodaver, Z., and Edwards, J. E.: Circulation, *44*:723, 1971. By permission of the American Heart Association, Inc.)

Histologic changes in chronic grafts are not limited to the intimal layer. In the media, the smooth muscle layer becomes variably replaced by collagen and fibroblasts, while the ingrowth of scar tissue into the adventitia brings about similar changes in the outer layer of the graft. The net result of such changes is an alteration of the elastic properties of the graft. The graft vessel rapidly becomes a rigid tube of low compliance, and its physical properties change little during the remaining life of the bypass.[41, 70]

The fibrous incorporation of the graft may become excessive at certain isolated points, producing *graft stenosis*. In large and consecutive series of both central and peripheral grafts, the incidence of this phenomenon is found to be about 7 per cent (Fig. 16).[59, 66] The origin of this process is thought to be either due to

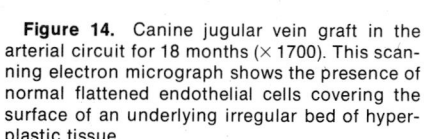

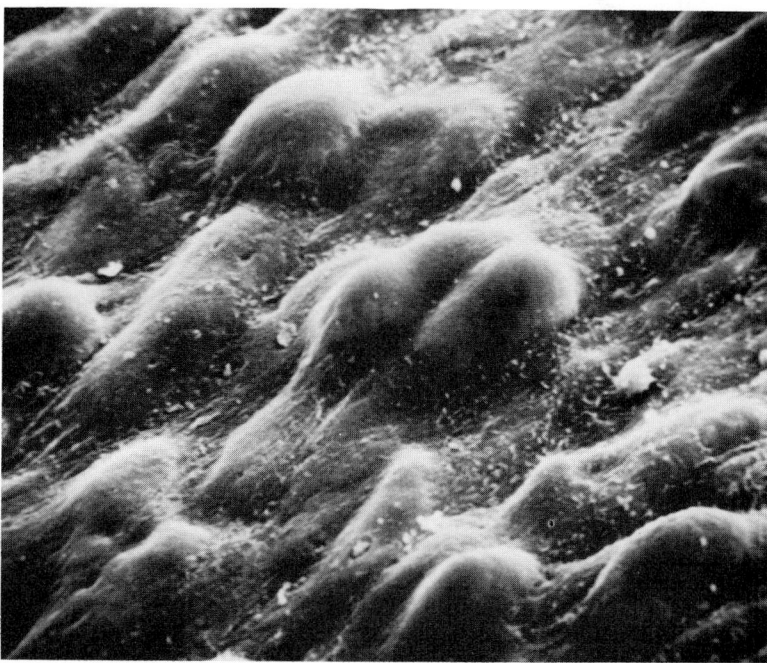

Figure 14. Canine jugular vein graft in the arterial circuit for 18 months (× 1700). This scanning electron micrograph shows the presence of normal flattened endothelial cells covering the surface of an underlying irregular bed of hyperplastic tissue.

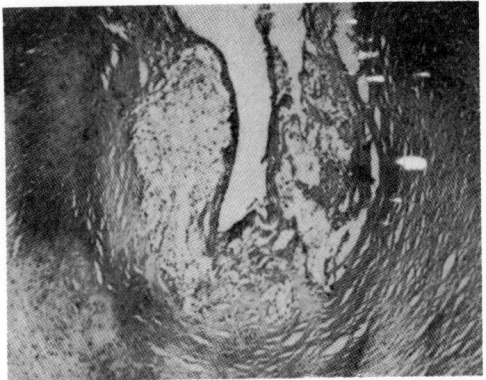

Figure 15. Vein graft (× 50, hematoxylin and eosin). After 29 months in the arterial circuit, this graft demonstrates lipid deposition in a fibrotic and hyperplastic intima, suggestive of mature atherosclerosis. (From Kern, W. H., Dermer, G. B., and Lindesmith, G. G.: Am. Heart J., *84*:773, 1972.)

trauma from clamping the graft or secondary to constriction from a suture of a branch of the graft. In both situations, the resulting scarring in the adventitia produces a narrowing of the graft that results in significant stenosis and reduction of flow.

When *fibrosis* of the *venous valve cusps* occurs, a thickened web is formed which extends into the lumen of a graft, producing severe obstruction to blood flow.[20] The incidence of stenosis due to fibrotic valves (Fig. 16) is as high as 6 per cent in the peripheral vascular location but has not been so frequently reported in the shorter, central organ grafts.[66]

Dilatation or expansion of autogenous venous grafts has often been described in the renal artery position (Fig. 17).[16, 25, 59] Repeated arteriograms have shown that almost half of the patients with this procedure have a nonprogressive, uniform enlargement of the graft averaging a 20 per cent increase in transverse diameter. It is not certain whether this dilatation is related to the higher flow which these grafts sustain or to the expanding influence of the arterial pressure in the acute postoperative period. That this change occurs early is probably due to the chronic alterations of intimal hypertrophy and adventitial collagenization that later render the graft unexpandable. In any event, these features are not applicable to grafts in the femoropopliteal position, where such uniform dilatation has not been described.

Local dilatation to the point of *aneurysm* formation has been seen in all sites of graft insertion (Fig. 16).[15,

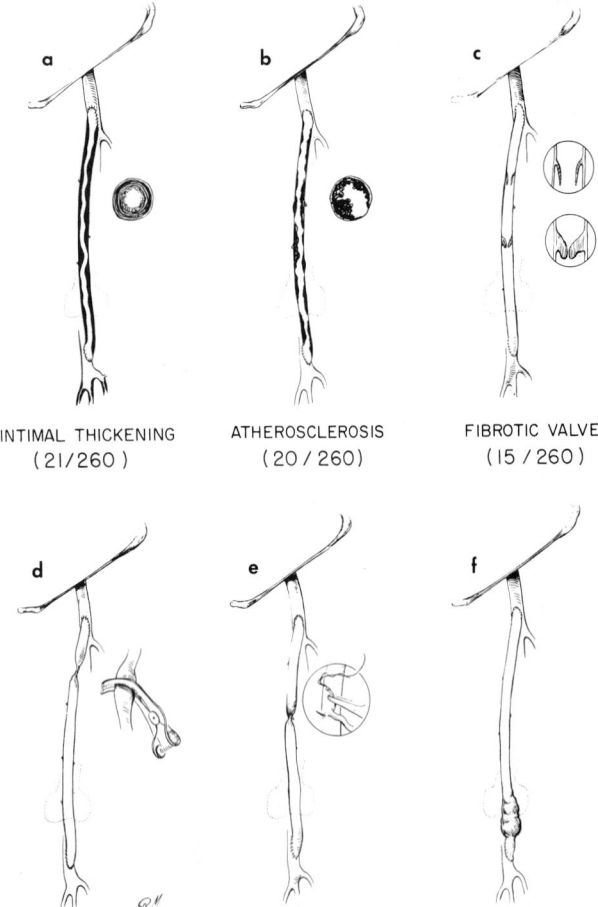

INTIMAL THICKENING
(21/260)

ATHEROSCLEROSIS
(20 / 260)

FIBROTIC VALVE
(15 / 260)

FIBROTIC STENOSIS
(11 / 260)

SUTURE STENOSIS
(8 / 260)

ANEURYSMAL DILATATION
(10 / 260)

Figure 16. Schematic representations of the pathologic changes and their incidence as demonstrated angiographically in a series of 260 patients with femoral popliteal grafts. (From Szilagy, D. E., et al.: Ann. Surg., *178*:237, 1973.)

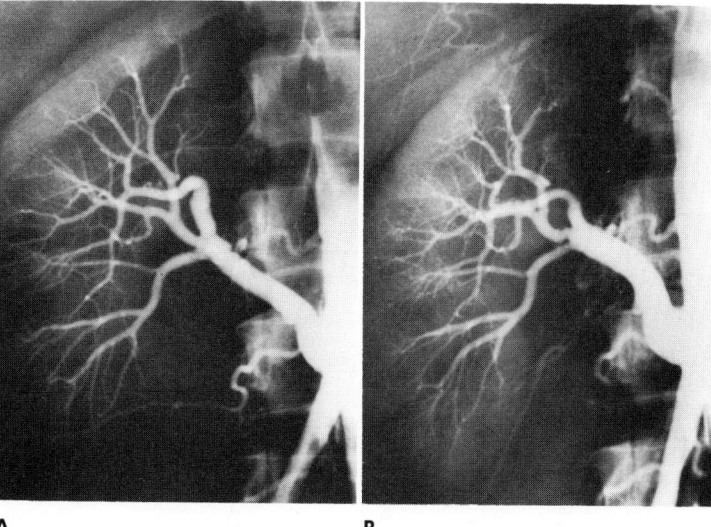

Figure 17. Expansive dilatation changes seen in an aortorenal graft seven days (*A*) and 12 months (*B*) postoperatively. (From Stanley, J. C., Ernst, C. B., and Fry, W. J.: Surgery, *74*:939, 1973.)

A   B

[18, 55, 59, 60] Although this can be associated with atherosclerosis,[15, 18] it is frequently found not to differ histologically from the nonaneurysmal portion of patent vein grafts. Although autologous venous tissue usually remains viable, spontaneous *necrosis* has been detected in a patent, functioning peripheral graft.[27] This occurs in the absence of infection and may be related to intrinsic abnormalities of the structure of the vein selected to perform the bypass.

PREVENTION

Despite the variety of the pathologic conditions that may occur, autologous vein still remains an effective arterial substitute. The value of examining the incidence of such changes lies in the possibility of eliminating features that may lead to structural alterations. Minimization of dissection injury is clearly important. The techniques of graft insertion involve meticulous application of vascular surgical principles. The length of the graft,[30] its angle of insertion,[9, 38] its configuration in the graft bed,[17, 29] and careful construction of anastomotic suture lines[67] are each of vital significance. Whether one should leave intact venous valves within the graft remains controversial.[4, 46] If occlusion of the graft becomes necessary, only the most atraumatic clamps should be used, to reduce the incidence of postoperative change. Sutures of branches must be performed to avoid compromise of the lumen.

The choice of peripheral outflow circuits is critical to the blood flow and patency of the graft.[31, 42] Early thrombosis is best prevented by adequate flow through a properly inserted graft, although platelet function and clotting factors may play a contributing role. The use of agents to suppress platelet adhesiveness and prolong platelet survival may achieve more widespread indications and acceptance.[60] Perigraft stenting has been suggested to prevent dilatation in postoperative bypasses,[50, 57] but this expansion occurs only in the renal artery bypass situation and does not appear to be sufficiently progressive to warrant intervention.

The control of atherosclerosis remains controversial. Although there is evidence to suggest that the failure of grafts may be related to hyperlipidemia,[2] it has not been shown that control of serum values will alter this situation. Nonetheless, the majority of patients requiring these procedures have abnormalities that predispose to atherosclerosis,[3, 6] and it appears reasonable to treat these factors with the appropriate diet or drugs.

The most common and least understood change, intimal hyperplasia, may result from many possible features of graft harvesting and insertion. It appears to be an inevitable feature of the adaptation of venous tissue to the arterial environment. However, this process can be minimized, and the resulting venous graft should continue as a satisfactory, functioning conduit for arterial flow in most patients.

One of the principal values of appreciation of the changes that occur in vein grafts is that many such pathologic alterations are amenable to surgical correction. This is particularly true when the lesions are localized to a short segment of the graft. Since the incidence of such changes can be as high as 30 per cent in large series, it is apparent that careful follow-up, including regular arteriography when indicated, will allow salvage of additional grafts.

SELECTED REFERENCES

Campeau, L., Crochet, D., Lesperance, J., Bourassa, M. G., and Grondin, C. M.: Postoperative changes in aortocoronary saphenous vein grafts revisited. Angiographic studies at two weeks and at one year in two series of consecutive patients. Circulation, *52*:369, 1975.

This study describes the changes occurring in aortocoronary bypass grafts as demonstrated by follow-up angiography in two large series of patients. Significant differences in patency figures after one year were found, and possible explanations by improved surgical techniques are offered.

Dean, R. H., Wilson, J. P., Burko, H., and Foster, J. H.: Saphenous vein aortorenal bypass grafts: Serial arteriographic study. Ann. Surg., *180*:469, 1974.

Serial angiography is described in 75 patients following aortorenal bypass. This valuable study evaluates the postoperative changes found with their incidence and subsequent progression in a smaller series of long-term studies.

Ramos, J. R., Mansfield, P. B., Wechezak, A., and Sauvage, L. R.: Histologic fate and endothelial changes of distended and nondistended vein grafts. Ann. Surg., 183:205, 1976.

Numerous illustrations are presented in this comprehensive study of changes in canine vein grafts. Scanning and light microscopy are employed to evaluate the timed histologic alterations seen in prepared and grafted veins. Information is given concerning the role of distention and perfusion on the subsequent changes in grafts.

Szilagyi, D. E., Elliott, J. P., Hageman, J. H., Smith, R. F., and Dall'Ollmo, C. A.: Biologic fate of autogenous vein implants as arterial substitutes: Clinical, angiographic and histopathologic observations in femoro-popliteal operations for atherosclerosis. Ann. Surg., 78:232, 1973.

A comprehensive presentation of serial angiographic studies of saphenous vein bypass grafts in the leg is offered in this outstanding study. It reveals the type and incidence of pathologic changes that can be expected.

REFERENCES

1. Abbott, W. M., Wieland, S., and Austen, W. G.: Structural changes during preparation of autogenous venous grafts. Surgery, 76:1031, 1974.
2. Allard, C., Goulet, C., Grondin, C. M., Lesperance, J., and Bourassa, M. G.: Patency of aortocoronary vein grafts and serum triglycerides, three year follow-up study. Am. J. Cardiol., 33:679, 1974.
3. Allard, C., Ruscito, O., and Goulet, C.: Preoperative serum lipid profile in surgically treated patients with coronary arteriosclerosis. Surg. Gynecol. Obstet., 133:807, 1971.
4. Baba, H., Djordjevic, M., Kiso, I., Hamada, O., Moskowitz, M. S., von Recum, A., and Kantrowitz, A.: Hemodynamic effects of venous valves in aortocoronary bypass grafts. J. Thorac. Cardiovasc. Surg., 71:774, 1976.
5. Barboriak, J. J., Pintaj, K., and Korns, M. E.: Atherosclerosis in aortocoronary vein grafts. Lancet, 2:621, 1974.
6. Barboriak, J. J., Rimm, A., Tristani, F. E., Walker, J. R., and Lepley, D. Jr.: Risk factors in patients undergoing aortocoronary bypass surgery. J. Thorac. Cardiovasc. Surg., 64:92, 1972.
7. Barboriak, J. J., Van Horn, D. L., Pintar, K., Batayias, G. E., and Korns, M. E.: Scanning electron microscope study of human veins and aorta-coronary artery vein grafts. J. Thorac. Cardiovasc. Surg., 71:673, 1976.
8. Beebe, H. G., Clark, W. F., and DeWeese, J. A.: Atherosclerotic change occurring in an autogenous venous arterial graft. Arch. Surg., 101:85, 1970.
9. Bond, M. G., Hostetler, J. R., Karayannacos, P. E., Geer, J. C., and Vasko, J. S.: Intimal changes in arteriovenous bypass grafts. Effects of varying the angle of implantation at the proximal anastomosis and of producing stenosis in the distal runoff artery. J. Thorac. Cardiovasc. Surg., 71:907, 1976.
10. Brody, W. R., Kosek, J. C., and Angell, W. W.: Changes in vein grafts following aorto-coronary bypass induced by pressure and ischemia. J. Thorac. Cardiovasc. Surg., 64:847, 1972.
11. Brody, W. R., Angell, W. W., and Kosek, J. C.: Histologic fate of the venous coronary artery bypass in dogs. Am. J. Pathol., 66:111, 1972.
12. Campeau, L., Crochet, D., Lesperance, J., Bourassa, M. G., and Grondin, C. M.: Postoperative changes in aortocoronary saphenous vein grafts revisited. Angiographic studies at two weeks and at one year in two series of consecutive patients. Circulation, 52:369, 1975.
13. Chatterjee, K. N., Warren, R., and Gore, I.: The long term functional and histologic fate of arteriotomy patches of autogenous arterial and venous tissue—observations on "arterialization." J. Surg. Res., 4:106, 1964.
14. Cutler, B. S., Thompson, J. E., Kleinsasser, L. J., and Hempel, G. K.: Autologous saphenous vein femoropopliteal bypass: Analysis of 298 cases. Surgery, 79:325, 1976.
15. Davidson, E. D., and DePalma, R. G.: Atherosclerotic aneurysm occurring in an autogenous vein graft. Am. J. Surg., 124:112, 1972.
16. Dean, R. H., Wilson, J. P., Burko, H., and Foster, J. H.: Saphenous vein aortorenal bypass grafts: Serial arteriographic study. Ann. Surg., 180:469, 1974.
17. Dedomenico, M., Sameh, A. A., Berger, K., Wood, S. J., and Sauvage, L. R.: Experimental coronary artery surgery: Long-term follow-up, bypass venous autografts, longitudinal arteriotomies, and end-to-end anastomoses. J. Thorac. Cardiovasc. Surg., 56:617, 1968.
18. De La Rocha, A. G., Peixoto, R. S., and Baird, R. J.: Atherosclerosis and aneurysm formation in a saphenous vein-graft. Br. J. Surg., 60:72, 1973.
19. DeWeese, J. A., and Rob, C. G.: Autogenous venous bypass grafts five years later. Ann. Surg., 174:346, 1971.
20. Downs, A. R.: Repair of late vein graft occlusions. Arch. Surg., 103:639, 1971.
21. Ejrup, B., Hiertonn, T., and Moberg, A.: Atheromatous changes in autogenous venous grafts. Acta Chir. Scand., 121:211, 1961.
22. Favaloro, R. G.: Saphenous vein graft in the surgical treatment of coronary artery disease. Operative technique. J. Thorac. Cardiovasc. Surg., 58:178, 1969.
23. Fishman, J. A., Ryan, G. B., and Karnovsky, M. B.: Endothelial regeneration in the rat carotid artery and the significance of endothelial denudation in the pathogenesis of myointimal thickening. Lab. Invest., 32:339, 1975.
24. Fonkalsrud, E. W., Sanchez, M., Zerubavel, R., Lasaletta, L., Smeesters, C., and Mahoney, A.: Arterial endothelial changes after ischemia and perfusion. Surg. Gynecol. Obstet., 142:715, 1976.
25. Foster, J. H., Dean, R. H., Pinkerton, J. A., and Rhamy, R. K.: Ten years experience with the surgical management of renovascular hypertension. Ann. Surg., 177:755, 1973.
26. Friedman, M.: Spontaneous atherosclerosis and experimental thromboatherosclerosis. Effect of arterial and venous environments. Arch. Pathol., 76:115, 1963.
27. Friedman, S. A., Cerruti, M. M., and Amadeo, B.: Spontaneous necrosis of a functioning saphenous vein graft. Surgery, 66:1022, 1969.
28. Fuchs, J. C. A., Hagen, P.-O., Oldham, H. N., Jr., and Sabiston, D. C., Jr.: Lipid composition in venous arterial bypass grafts. Surg. Forum, 23:139, 1972.
29. Gordon, A., Williams, J., and Buxton, B.: Changes in flow and pressure due to rotation of a saphenous vein segment. Cardiovasc. Res., 9:538, 1975.
30. Gordon, A., Williams, J., and Buxton, B.: Optimal length of a saphenous vein segment when used as an arterial substitute. Cardiovasc. Res., 9:541, 1975.
31. Grondin, C. M., Lepage, G., Castonguay, Y. R., Meere, C., and Grondin, P.: Aortocoronary bypass graft: Initial blood flow through the graft, and early postoperative patency. Circulation, 44:815, 1971.
32. Grondin, C. M., Lesperance, J., Bourassa, M. G., Pasternac, A., Campeau, L., and Grondin, P.: Serial angiographic evaluation in 60 consecutive patients with aorto-coronary artery vein grafts 2 weeks, 1 year, and 3 years after operation. J. Thorac. Cardiovasc. Surg., 67:1, 1974.
33. Harrison, L. H., Jr.: Historical aspects in the development of venous autografts. Ann. Surg., 183:101, 1975.
34. Imparato, A. M., Bracco, A., Kim, G. E., and Zeff, R.: Intimal and neointimal fibrous proliferation causing failure of arterial reconstructions. Surgery, 72:1007, 1972.
35. Johnson, W. E., Auer, J. E., and Tector, A. J.: Late changes in coronary vein grafts. Am. J. Cardiol., 26:640, 1970.
36. Jones, M., Conkle, D. M., Ferrans, V. J., Roberts, W. C., Levine, F. H., Melvin, D. B., and Stinson, E. B.: Lesions observed in arterial autogenous vein grafts. Circulation, 47 and 48(Suppl. 3):198, 1973.
37. Kabemba, J. M. and Hammond, G. L.: The fate of internal mammary arteries implanted in the normal heart with subsequent development of ischemia. Curr. Top. Surg. Res., 3:29, 1971.
38. Kennedy, J. H., Wieting, D. W., Hwang, N. H. C., Anderson, M. S., Bayardo, R. J., Howell, J. F., and DeBakey, M. E.: Hydraulic and morphologic study of fibrous intimal hyperplasia in autogenous saphenous vein bypass grafts. J. Thorac. Cardiovasc. Surg., 67:805, 1974.
39. Kern, W. H., Dermer, G. B., and Lindesmith, G. G.: The intimal proliferation in aortic-coronary saphenous vein grafts. Am. Heart J., 84:771, 1972.
40. Larson, R. M., Hagen, P.-O., and Fuchs, J. C. A.: Lipid biosynthesis in arteries, veins, and venous grafts. Circulation, 50(Suppl. 3):139, 1974.
41. Lye, C. R., Sumner, D. S., Hokanson, D. E., and Strandness, D. E., Jr.: The transcutaneous measurement of the elastic properties of the human saphenous vein femoropopliteal bypass graft. Surg. Gynecol. Obstet., 141:891, 1975.
42. Marco, J. D., Barner, H. B., Kaiser, G. C., Codd, J. E., Mudd, J.

G., and Willman, V.: Operative flow measurements and coronary bypass graft patency. J. Thorac. Cardiovasc. Surg., 71:545, 1976.

43. Marti, M. C., Bouchardy, B., and Cox, J. N.: Aorto-coronary by-pass with autogenous saphenous vein grafts: Histopathological aspects. Virchows Arch. Pathol. Anat., 352:255, 1971.

44. McCabe, M., and Cunningham, G. J.: A histological and histochemical examination of autogenous vein grafts. Br. J. Surg., 54:147, 1967.

45. McNamara, J. J., Darling, R. C., and Linton, R. R.: Segmental stenosis of saphenous-vein autografts, preventable cause of late occlusion in arterial reconstruction. N. Engl. J. Med., 277:290, 1967.

46. Mills, N. L., and Ochsner, J. L.: Valvulotomy of valves in the saphenous vein graft before coronary artery bypass. J. Thorac. Cardiovasc. Surg., 71:878, 1976.

47. Mitchener, J. S., Fuchs, J. C. A., Hagen, P.-O., and Ratliff, N. B.: Histology of prepared and grafted vein studied by differential interference contrast microscopy (DIC). Circulation, 51(Suppl. 2):219, 1975.

48. Mitchener, J. S., Ratliff, N. B., and Fuchs, J. C.: Scanning Electron Microscopy (SEM) of the Endothelium of Canine Vein Segments Prepared for Surgery. In Bailey, G. W. (Ed.): 33rd Ann. Proc. Electron Microscopy Soc. Amer., Las Vegas, Nevada, 1975, p. 524.

49. Nunn, D. B., Chun, B., Whelan, T. J., and Martins, A. N.: Autogenous veins as arterial substitutes: A study of their histologic fate with special attention to endothelium. Ann. Surg., 160:14, 1964.

50. Parsonnet, V., Lari, A. A., and Shah, I. H.: New stent for support of veins in arterial grafts. Arch. Surg., 87:180, 1963.

51. Penn, I., Schenk, E., Robb, C., DeWeese, J., and Schwartz, S. I.: Evaluation of the development of athero-arteriosclerosis in autogenous venous grafts inserted into the peripheral arterial system. Circulation, 31 and 32(Suppl. 1):192, 1965.

52. Ramirez, A., and Stallworth, J. M.: Long-term behavior of vein grafts as replacements for arterial segments within the peritoneal cavity. Surgery, 69:832, 1971.

53. Ramos, J. R., Mansfield, P. B., Wechezak, A., and Sauvage, L. R.: Histologic fate and endothelial changes of distended and nondistended vein grafts. Ann. Surg., 183:205, 1976.

54. Reichle, F. A., Stewart, G. J., and Essa, N.: A transmission and scanning electron microscopic study of luminal surfaces in Dacron and autogenous vein bypasses in man and dog. Surgery, 74:945, 1973.

55. Riahi, M., Vasu, C. M., Tomatis, L. A., Schlosser, R. J., and Zimmerman, G.: Aneurysm of saphenous vein bypass graft to coronary artery. J. Thorac. Cardiovasc. Surg., 70:358, 1975.

56. Rossi, N. P., Koepke, J. A., and Spencer, F. C.: Histologic changes in long-term autologous arterial patch grafts in coronary arteries. Surgery, 57:335, 1963.

57. Sako, Y.: Prevention of dilatation in autogenous venous and pericardial grafts in the thoracic aorta. An experimental study. Surgery, 30:148, 1951.

58. Scott, H. W., Jr., Morgan, C. V., Bolasny, B. L., Lanier, V. C.,

Younger, R. K., and Butts, W.: Experimental atherosclerosis in autogenous venous grafts. Arch. Surg., 101:677, 1970.

59. Stanley, J. C., Ernst, C. B., and Fry, W. J.: Fate of 100 aortorenal vein grafts: Characteristics of late graft expansion, aneurysmal dilatation and stenosis. Surgery, 74:931, 1973.

60. Steele, P., Battock, D., Pappas, G., and Genton, E.: Correlation of platelet survival time with occlusion of saphenous vein aortocoronary bypass graft. Circulation, 53:685, 1976.

61. Stein, A. A., Rosenblum, I., and Leather, R.: Intimal sclerosis in human veins. Arch. Pathol., 81:548, 1966.

62. Stewart, G. J., Ritchie, W. G. M., and Lynch, P. R.: A scanning and transmission electron microscopic study of canine jugular veins. Proc. of the Workshop on Scanning Electron Microscopy in Pathology, 1973, p. 473.

63. Stewart, G. J.: The role of the vessel wall in deep venous thrombosis. In Nicolaides, A. N. (Ed.): Thromboembolism Etiology, Advances in Prevention and Management. Baltimore, University Park Press, 1975, p. 101.

64. Stewart, G. J., Ritchie, W. G. M., and Lynch, P. R.: Venous endothelial damage produced by massive sticking and emigration of leukocytes. Am. J. Pathol., 74:507, 1974.

65. Storm, F. K., Gierson, E. D., Sparks, F. C., and Barker, W. F.: Autogenous vein bypass grafts: Biological effects of mechanical dilatation and adventitial stripping in dogs. Surgery, 77:261, 1975.

66. Szilagyi, D. E., Elliott, J. P., Hageman, J. H., Smith, R. F., and Dall'Olmo, C. A.: Biologic fate of autogenous vein implants as arterial substitutes: Clinical, angiographic and histopathologic observations in femoro-popliteal operations for atherosclerosis. Ann. Surg., 78:232, 1973.

67. Urschel, H. C., Razzuk, M. A., Wood, R. E., and Paulson, D. L.: Factors influencing patency of aortocoronary artery saphenous vein grafts. Surgery, 72:1048, 1972.

68. Vlodaver, Z., and Edwards, J. E.: Pathologic analysis in fatal cases following saphenous vein coronary arterial bypass. Chest, 64:555, 1973.

69. Vlodaver, Z., and Edwards, J. E.: Pathologic changes in aortic-coronary arterial saphenous vein grafts. Circulation, 44:719, 1971.

70. Wesly, R. L. R., Vaishnav, R. N., Fuchs, J. C. A., Patel, D. J., and Greenfield, J. C., Jr.: Static linear and nonlinear elastic properties of normal and arterialized venous tissue. Circ. Res., 37:509, 1975.

71. Wimberly, J. E., Symbas, P. N., and Foster, J. H.: Portal vein grafts: Microscopic study after a seven year follow-up. Surgery, 64:761, 1968.

72. Wyatt, A. P., and Gonzales, I. E.: Atheromatous lesions in arterialized vein grafts. An experimental study. Br. J. Surg., 56:194, 1969.

73. Wyatt, A. P.: Experimental atheroma in autogenous vein-grafts. Br. J. Surg., 55:860, 1968.

74. Wyatt, A. P., and Taylor, G. W.: Vein grafts: Changes in the endothelium of autogenous free vein grafts used as arterial replacements. Br. J. Surg., 53:943, 1966.

XV _____

VENTRICULAR ANEURYSM

William A. Gay, Jr., M.D.

The vast majority of ventricular aneurysms are due to acute transmural myocardial infarction with its resultant muscle necrosis and scar formation. Rarely, aneurysms may result from trauma or congenital cardiac defects.[8, 9, 21] The typical ventricular aneurysm may be described as a "thinned-out transmural scar that has completely lost its trabecular pattern . . . always clearly delineated from the surrounding muscle."[14] Although the gross pathology of ventricular aneurysms was accurately described in the eighteenth century,[12] it was more than 150 years later before the relationship of this entity with coronary occlusive disease was appreciated,[19] and it remained for Tennant and Wiggers[20] first to demonstrate the deleterious effects of acute coronary occlusion upon regional myocardial contraction in 1935.

CLINICAL MANIFESTATIONS

It is estimated that 12 to 15 per cent of recognized myocardial infarctions will result in the formation of a ventricular aneurysm.[1, 18] Until the recent advances in the treatment of patients with acute myocardial infarction, many of these patients would not have survived the early postinfarction period. The typical patient who develops a ventricular aneurysm has a stormy postinfarction course, usually marked by overt or borderline congestive heart failure or recurring arrhythmias. In the absence of other hemodynamic factors, such as mitral insufficiency or chronic myocardial fibrosis, the occurrence of congestive failure following myocardial infarction usually indicates that a large portion (20 per cent or more)[13] of the left ventricle has been involved and aneurysm formation is not unlikely. Although some patients who have aneurysms of the left ventricle may not develop symptoms for several years after infarction,[6] this course of events now seems to represent the exception rather than the rule. The most common symptom in patients with ventricular aneurysm is congestive failure (dyspnea) with palpitations and angina frequently associated and peripheral emboli occurring rarely (Table 1). Many patients will have more than one symptom: for example, dyspnea and angina with minimal effort or angina combined with palpitations. It is in these patients that suspicion should be aroused and further evaluation pursued.

While the presence of a ventricular aneurysm may be suspected from the history of left ventricular failure and/or recurrent arrhythmias following myocardial infarction, substantiation of the diagnosis requires further evaluation. An abnormal cardiac impulse is usually detectable at the apex of the heart and a ventricular gallop may often be audible. The aneurysm itself produces no cardiac murmurs, but the presence of coexisting valvular dysfunction (most commonly, mitral regurgitation) often results in characteristic findings. Although the persistence of elevated ST segments following acute myocardial infarction is very suggestive of a developing ventricular aneurysm, this finding has not proved reliable enough to be diagnostic.[4, 10, 11] Chest roentgenograms most often reveal

TABLE 2. Arteries Involved in 80 Patients with Ventricular Aneurysms

Artery	Number	Per Cent
LAD	80	100
Right	25	31
Circumflex	7	9
Diffuse	19	24

enlargement of the left ventricle. The area of enlargement may be localized more specifically by selected oblique views. Cardiac fluoroscopy may reveal systolic expansion (paradox) in the area of the aneurysm. Recent demonstration of local left ventricular dimension characteristics using the echocardiogram[7] has indicated that this noninvasive technique will unquestionably be of considerable value in screening patients with suspected ventricular aneurysms. The diagnosis of left ventricular aneurysm is substantiated by left ventriculography, preferably performed in both the AP and lateral planes. With this procedure the aneurysm may be localized, an accurate estimate of its extent made, the existence of significant valvular malfunction confirmed and, often, the presence of thrombus in the aneurysm sac noted. Although the ventricular end-diastolic pressure (LVEDP) is measured and the ejection fraction may be calculated, the functional status of the remaining left ventricular muscle is best evaluated by observing its movement on the cineventriculogram. Selective coronary arteriography is always performed in conjunction with left ventriculography. The arteriograms are most often done in the left anterior oblique and right anterior oblique projections. In eighty patients with proven ventricular aneurysms (Table 2), the left anterior descending artery was found occluded in all. In 29 of these patients there was no other significant coronary obstruction; however, 25 had occlusions of their right coronary artery, 7 had obstructive circumflex disease, and in 19 the coronary tree was diffusely involved. Not infrequently an unsuspected ventricular aneurysm is discovered in the course of coronary arteriography and ventriculography in the patient with angina. While aneurysms located on the posterior and inferior walls of the left ventricle do occur[14] and may be surgically approached, the majority of ventricular aneurysms are located in the apical and anterior portion of the heart.

TREATMENT

The treatment of left ventricular aneurysm is aneurysmectomy combined with correction of any significant valvular abnormalities and bypass of major coronary obstructive lesions. Operation is indicated in patients whose aneurysms cause symptoms. Similarly, patients whose aneurysms were discovered during the course of coronary arteriography in consideration for coronary bypass surgery should have aneurysmectomy at the time of their bypass operation. Whereas the 3-year mortality following uncomplicated myocardial in-

TABLE 1. Symptoms in 80 Patients with Ventricular Aneurysms

Symptom	Number	Per Cent
Failure	61	75
Arrhythmia	36	45
Angina	32	40
Emboli	1	1

farction is about 15 to 20 per cent, this figure is 70 to 75 per cent in patients with aneurysms[16, 18] and rises to nearly 90 per cent in 5 years. Elective surgery for ventricular aneurysms should not be undertaken earlier than two months from the time of infarction.

In 1931, Sauerbruch accidentally entered an aneurysm of the right ventricle during the course of exploring a patient thought to have a mediastinal tumor. He was able to suture the neck of the aneurysm and resect the sac successfully.[17] The etiology of that aneurysm is not known. Beck, in 1944, used a fascia lata stent to reinforce the left ventricular wall of a patient with ventricular aneurysm diagnosed preoperatively.[3] In 1954, Bailey successfully resected a ventricular aneurysm by placing a vascular clamp about its neck, excising the aneurysm, and suturing the neck closed.[2] The use of cardiopulmonary bypass in the surgery of ventricular aneurysm was applied by Cooley in 1958,[5] and this has been the technique utilized since that time. The concept of simultaneous coronary revascularization and aneurysmectomy did not become popular until the era of direct coronary surgery began in about 1968.[8]

Operation for left ventricular aneurysm is performed through a midline sternotomy incision. In the patient with a very large aneurysm or unstable hemodynamics, exposure of a femoral artery, administration of heparin, and cannulation of the artery may be wise prior to opening of the pericardium in order that cardiopulmonary bypass might be commenced rapidly should this be necessary. Additionally, the saphenous vein should be removed if coronary bypass grafting is planned as a part of the procedure. A single large venous cannula in the right atrium usually provides sufficient venous return to the oxygenator, but should grafting of the circumflex artery or one of its branches be planned, cannulation of both cavae is desirable. The left side of the heart is decompressed by a venting catheter (18 to 24 Fr.) placed into the left atrium or ventricle via the right superior pulmonary vein or the superior aspect of the left atrium between the aorta and superior vena cava. Extreme care is taken not to advance the venting catheter into the aneurysm so as not to dislodge any of the clot which is usually present. It is helpful to induce ventricular fibrillation or cardiac arrest prior to incising the aneurysm.

The steps in excising the aneurysm are depicted in Figure 1. The area occupied by the aneurysm is usually obvious by its grayish color when compared to the surrounding myocardium. When the heart is not beating and the ventricle is empty, the walls of the aneurysm may even collapse. The left anterior descending coronary artery is usually totally occluded, and the distal portion of this vessel courses along the right edge of the aneurysm sac. This vessel is only rarely suitable for bypass grafting. The aneurysm is opened in a soft, thin spot near its center, all thrombus carefully removed, and the aneurysm sac trimmed back to leave a thin rim of scar tissue (5 to 10 mm.). Clamping of the aorta is usually not necessary during this portion of the operation unless aortic regurgitation is present. Prior to closure of the left ventricle, other necessary procedures such as valve replacement or coronary bypass are performed as needed. Mitral

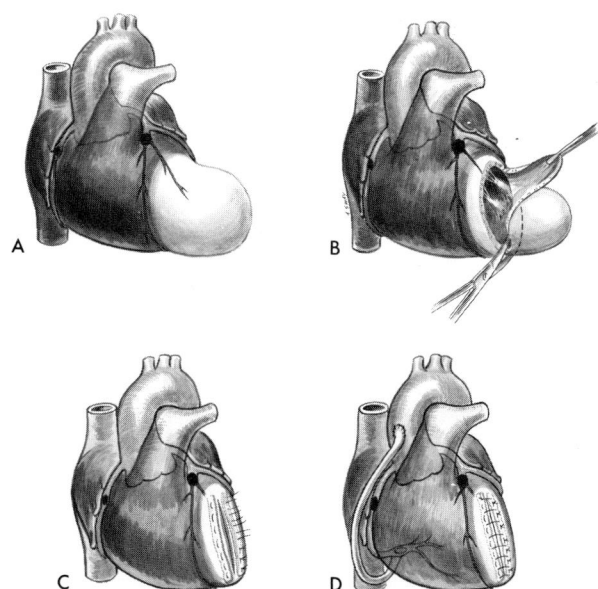

Figure 1. *A,* An apical-anterior ventricular aneurysm that has resulted from occlusion of the left anterior descending coronary artery. There is also significant occlusive disease of the right coronary artery. *B,* The aneurysm is opened and resected, leaving a 5 to 10 mm. rim of scar tissue. *C,* The ventricle is closed using sutures over Teflon pledgets and (*D*), the right coronary artery is bypassed using autologous saphenous vein.

valve replacement done through a ventricular aneurysm gives the cardiac surgeon a rare opportunity to view the mitral mechanism in its entirety. In the event that the scar from the ventricular wall extends down along the apical portion of the interventricular septum, a large patch of Teflon felt should be sutured to the left ventricular side of lower septum in hopes that this would minimize the septal paradox. The author recommends placement of the distal anastomosis of any coronary bypass grafts prior to closure of the left ventricle, largely because of the technical ease with which this can be done, even in relatively inaccessible areas, with the ventricle open. Then the ventriculotomy is closed by placing interrupted horizontal mattress sutures of 0-gauge Dacron through strips of Teflon felt placed on either side of the incision. These sutures are tied and the suture line is reinforced by a continuous simple suture of 2-0 Dacron. All air is evacuated from the ventricle, the heart defibrillated, the vent removed, proximal coronary graft anastomoses done, and bypass discontinued. During cardiopulmonary bypass, the body temperature is usually lowered to 30° C.

The operative mortality for elective excision of left ventricular aneurysm is quite low, even when combined with other cardiac procedures. Most centers report an operative mortality of less than 5 per cent for these procedures,[14] and, more importantly, it has been found that nearly 80 per cent of those patients operated upon are alive four years later. This is a complete reversal of the figures obtained prior to the availability of effective operative therapy. It is, therefore, recommended that all patients with symptomatic ventricular aneurysms have aneurysmectomy.

COMPLEX VENTRICULAR ANEURYSMS

From the clinical picture presented in the preceding paragraphs, it may be concluded that the patient with the symptomatic postinfarction aneurysm of the left ventricle who has aneurysmectomy and bypass surgery two months or more after his infarct has a better than 95 per cent chance of surviving one year and about an 80 per cent chance of surviving four years. The most important factor in these very satisfactory statistics is the two-month period between infarct and surgery. There are some patients, however, who require operation at an earlier time because of hemodynamic deterioration producing refractory heart failure or even severe cardiogenic shock. In a few of these patients the amount of left ventricular myocardium involved in the infarction is sufficient to result in an inadequate cardiac output, while in others complications such as ruptured papillary muscle or ventricular septal defect may have occurred. In these critically ill patients the only hope of survival rests upon the finding of some surgically correctable hemodynamic disturbance. The plan of choice is temporary cardiac assistance with a device such as the intra-aortic balloon pump and performance of ventriculography and arteriography then, if possible, to surgically repair the lesion.[15] If, however, there is no discrete area of ventricular dyskinesia, no ventricular septal defect, or no mitral regurgitation, or if the shock state has been prolonged so as to result in prolonged anuria, or if there is failure of the ventricle to respond, even minimally, to stimulants, operation is probably not indicated.

Because of the severity of the illness in these patients and the adverse circumstances under which many of them undergo operation, the mortality is much higher than in those having elective aneurysmectomy. If, however, hemodynamic improvement can result from operation, many of these individuals who would otherwise not have survived may go on to full recovery.

SELECTED REFERENCES

Kitamura, S., Kay, J. H., Krohn, B. G., Magidson, O., and Dunne, E. F.: Geometric and functional abnormalities of the left ventricle with a chronic, localized noncontractile area. Am. J. Cardiol., 31:701, 1973.

A concise, well-written, and easily understood overview of the pathologic physiology of ventricular aneurysms. Not only is the pathology of ventricular function explained, but the distribution of pathologic changes in the major coronary arteries is reviewed also. This article may serve the student as an introduction to the subject and the experienced clinician as an updated review.

Mundth, E. D., Buckley, M. J., Daggett, W. M., Sanders, C. A., and Austen, W. G.: Surgery for complications of acute myocardial infarction. Circulation, 45:1279, 1972.

This article, along with its companion article which follows in the same journal, may serve as a reference for the surgical treatment of the complications of acute myocardial infarction. In general, it deals with those conditions occurring in the early postinfarction period which often result in cardiogenic shock and its attendant high mortality. The companion article considers the circulatory assist devices that may be used as adjuncts to definitive surgery in the management of those conditions.

REFERENCES

1. Abrams, D. L., Edelist, A., Luria, M. H., and Miller, A. S.: Ventricular aneurysm. A reappraisal based on a study of sixty-five consecutive autopsied cases. Circulation, 27:164, 1963.
2. Bailey, C. P., Bolton, H. E., and Nichols, H.: Ventriculoplasty for cardiac aneurysm. J. Thorac. Cardiovasc. Surg., 35:37, 1958.
3. Beck, C. S.: Operation for aneurysm of the heart. Ann. Surg., 120:34, 1944.
4. Cokkinos, D. V., Hallman, G. L., Cooley, D. A., Zamalloa, O., and Leachman, R. D.: Left ventricular aneurysm: Analysis of electrocardiographic features and postresection changes. Am. Heart J., 82:149, 1971.
5. Cooley, D. A., Colling, H. A., Morris, C. G., and Chapman, D. W.: Ventricular aneurysm after myocardial infarction: Surgical excision with use of temporary cardiopulmonary bypass. J.A.M.A., 167:557, 1958.
6. Davis, R. W., and Ebert, P. A.: Ventricular aneurysm: A clinical-pathological correlation. Am. J. Cardiol., 29:1, 1972.
7. Dillon, J., Feigenbaum, H., Weymarr, A., Peskoe, S., and Chang, S.: Echocardiography in the evaluation of patients for aneurysmectomy. (Abstract) Circulation, 52(Suppl.II):135, 1975.
8. Favaloro, R. G., Effler, D. B., Groves, L. K., Westcott, R. N., Saurez, E., and Lozada, J.: Ventricular aneurysm—clinical experience. Ann. Thorac. Surg., 6:227, 1968.
9. Flemma, R. J., Marx, L., Litwin, S. B., and Gallen, W. J.: Left ventricular aneurysmectomy in a child. Ann. Thorac. Surg., 19:457, 1975.
10. Gorlin, R., Klein, M. D., and Sullivan, J. M.: Prospective correlative study of ventricular aneurysm. Mechanistic concept and clinical recognition. Am. J. Med., 42:512, 1967.
11. Groden, B. M., and James, W. B.: Significance of persistent R-ST elevation after acute myocardial infarction. Br. Heart J., 31:34, 1969.
12. Hunter, J.: An account of the dissection of morbid bodys. London, Library of the Royal College of Surgeons, 32:30, 1757.
13. Klein, M. D., Herman, M. V., and Gorlin, R.: A hemodynamic study of left ventricular aneurysm. Circulation, 35:614, 1967.
14. Loop, F. D., Effler, D. B., Navia, J. A., Sheldon, W. C., and Groves, L. K.: Aneurysms of the left ventricle: Survival and results of ten year experience. Ann. Surg., 178:399, 1973.
15. Mundth, E. D., Buckley, M. J., Daggett, W. M., Sanders, C. A., and Austen, W. G.: Surgery for complications of acute myocardial infarction. Circulation, 45:1279, 1972.
16. Nagle, R. E., and Williams, D. O.: Natural history of ventricular aneurysm without surgical treatment. Br. Heart J., 36:1037, 1974.
17. Sauerbruch, F.: Erfolgreiche operative beseitigung cines aneurysm a der rechten herzkammer. Arch. Klin. Chir., 167:586, 1931.
18. Schlichter, J., Hellerstein, H. K., and Katz, L. N.: Aneurysm of the heart; a correlative study of one hundred and two proved cases. Medicine, 33:43, 1954.
19. Sternberg, M.: Das chronische partielle herzaneurysma. Vienna and Leipsig, Franz Deutlicke, 1914.
20. Tennant, R., and Wiggers, C. J.: Effect of coronary occlusion on myocardial contraction. Am. J. Physiol., 112:351, 1935.
21. Turnia, M., Real, F., Meier, W., and Senning, Å.: Left ventricular aneurysmectomy in a four month old infant: Alternative method of treatment of anomalous left coronary artery. J. Thorac. Cardiovasc. Surg., 67:915, 1974.

XVI

ACQUIRED DISORDERS OF THE AORTIC VALVE

William H. Muller, Jr., M.D.,
and Stanton P. Nolan, M.D.

ANATOMY AND FUNCTION OF THE AORTIC VALVE

The normal aortic valve is tricuspid, and each leaflet forms a truncated parabola. The uppermost attachment of the commissures defines the distal limits of the sinuses of Valsalva, with the coronary arteries usually arising in the upper third. Pulse duplicator studies of valvular motion indicate a rapid retraction of all three cusps at the beginning of ejection to form a triangular orifice. A slow, wavelike motion of the free edge and billowing of the base of each cusp are caused by eddy currents within the sinuses of Valsalva. Occlusion of the coronary ostia by the leaflets is thus prevented, and a position is maintained that allows slight reversal of flow to result in immediate closure without regurgitation.[13] Only 20 per cent of total coronary blood flow occurs during systole.[7] Therefore, diastolic coronary blood flow is enhanced by the aortic pressure and decreased intramural pressure of the ventricles and retarded by increased right atrial and intraventricular pressures. Left ventricular ejection occurs when left ventricular pressure exceeds aortic pressure. The forward pressure gradient ceases during the first half of systole, and thereafter forward flow is maintained by a mass-acceleration effect. Closure of the normal aortic valve is accomplished by reversal of the flow rather than by reversal of the pressure gradient.[10]

PATHOLOGY AND ETIOLOGY

Rheumatic Fever

This process begins as myocarditis invading the aortic valve through the valvular ring. In the acute stage, there is edema, inflammation, formation of granulation tissue, and scarring, often resulting in thickened, scarred, contracted leaflets with rolled edges. The valvular ring frequently dilates because of destruction of its fibrous tissue. In addition, the tissues are more susceptible to degenerative alterations and may undergo atheromatous changes and calcium deposition (Fig. 1). Dilatation of the annulus may produce insufficiency with shortening or stiffening of the cusps, or stenosis may occur as a result of fusion of the commissures and agglutination of the leaflet borders.

Syphilis

Syphilitic valvular disease, now seldom seen in the United States, begins in the aorta around the vasa vasorum. Initially, there is perivascular cellular infiltration that compromises the nutrient vessels, producing destruction of the muscular and elastic layers of the tunica media as well as associated elevation and roughening of the intima. Valvular dysfunction occurs when the process affects the aortic root, producing dilatation of the valvular ring and widening of the commissures. The cusps are rarely involved except for secondary stretching and patulence, and consequently pure aortic insufficiency most commonly results. A recent review of 258 autopsy reports of aortic regurgitation[1] indicated that syphilis now accounts for less than 5 per cent of the cases. Since the coronary ostia are involved, and coronary insufficiency occurs in most of these patients, it is possible that sudden death occurs and that this accounts for the relatively few patients referred for surgical consideration.

Bacterial Endocarditis

Subacute bacterial endocarditis is characterized by the deposition of bacterial vegetations and thrombus formation on the valvular leaflets. These lesions induce inflammation and scarring or may progress to erosion and valvular perforation. The process usually occurs on a congenitally deformed valve or one damaged by rheumatic valvulitis. Either *insufficiency* or *stenosis* may result, the former being by far the more frequent lesion. Autopsy studies indicate that the inflammatory process subsides slowly over a period of several months following sterilization of the bloodstream.

Traumatic Aortic Insufficiency

Traumatic rupture of the aortic valve is rare; it most frequently occurs in a previously diseased valve and usually follows extreme muscular exertion. Blunt trauma to the chest may also cause rupture of a diseased valve, and if it is severe enough it may affect similarly a normal valve. A linear tear through a single cusp or avulsion of a commissure from the aortic wall is generally found.

Marfan's Syndrome

Marfan's syndrome is a heritable, generalized, systemic disease of connective tissue. Aortic insufficiency results when cystic medial necrosis of the aorta produces dilatation of the aortic ring and aneurysm formation. Sudden insufficiency often develops when spontaneous intimal rupture and retrograde dissection releases the commissural attachments of the valve, so that it partially invaginates into the left ventricle during diastole.[9]

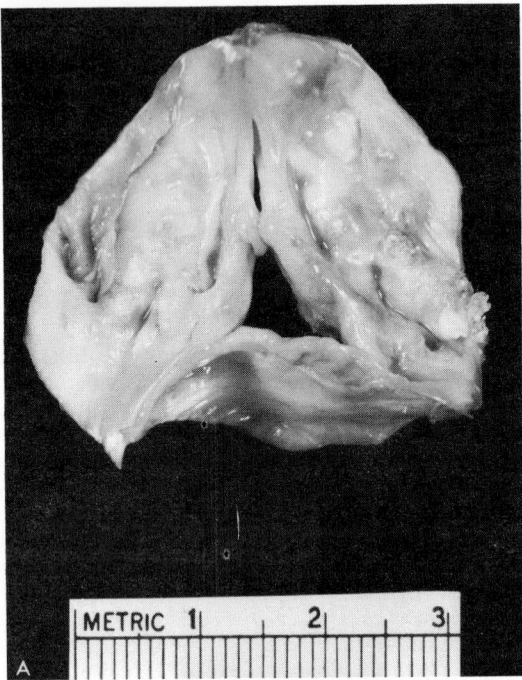

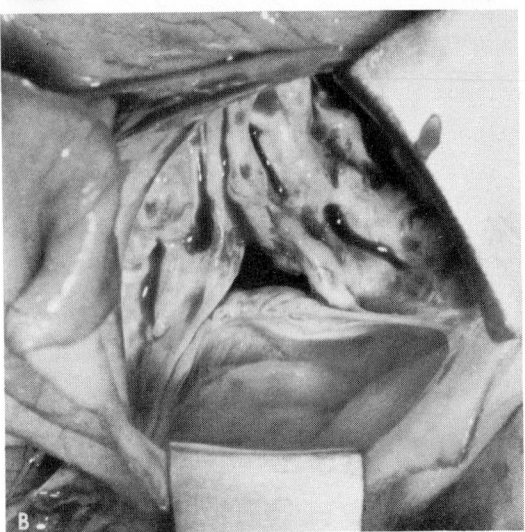

Figure 1. *A*, Photograph of the excised valve, showing dense calcification of two leaflets. *B*, Operative view of a calcified stenotic aortic valve.

Congenital Valvular Disease

Acquired disease of the aortic valve may result from a congenital deformity. Although a congenitally deformed valve may remain asymptomatic for many years, it is more susceptible to bacterial endocarditis, rheumatic fever, or, particularly, calcification and may become stenotic or insufficient. Of 59 patients between the ages of 15 and 65 years who died of valvular aortic stenosis, Roberts[14] found that only 50 per cent had signs of previous rheumatic fever and that the remaining cases of aortic stenosis were due to congenital deformities.

PATHOLOGIC PHYSIOLOGY

Aortic Insufficiency

The hemodynamic changes in aortic insufficiency result from the reflux of a significant amount of blood into the left ventricle during diastole. What constitutes a "significant" volume of reflux in the human is difficult to define. Measurements performed in the operating room prior to valvular replacement and studies from the animal laboratory indicate that greater than 50 per cent of the left ventricular ejection must regurgitate into the left ventricle before symptoms of heart failure are produced.[7]

When significant aortic insufficiency alone is present, the pulse pressure is always increased, and there is an exaggeration of the normal elevation of peripheral over central systolic pressure. Mean systemic pressure generally remains in a normal range owing to a proportional increase in systolic pressure. There is much controversy concerning the left ventricular end-diastolic pressure in this disease. However, it probably remains normal until the onset of either cardiac failure or myocardial fibrosis.

Cardiac compensation is achieved by hypertrophy and dilatation of the left ventricle. Thus, addition of the volume of reflux to the normal left atrial inflow produces an increase in the initial intraventricular tension and results in a more forceful and rapid ejection. Additional compensation is achieved by the decrease in aortic diastolic pressure, which allows an abridgment of the isometric contraction phase and prolongation of the systolic ejection time. Experimentally, it has been shown that the normal phasic pattern of coronary arterial flow persists in aortic insufficiency, and that the major portion of coronary perfusion occurs during diastole.[10] Although there may be an increase in the absolute coronary flow in aortic insufficiency, in some patients relative coronary insufficiency will develop because of cardiac hypertrophy secondary to increased myocardial oxygen consumption and a shorter diastolic coronary perfusion time.

Symptoms are rare in uncomplicated compensated aortic insufficiency. Occasionally, patients complain of nocturnal angina pectoris;[6] however, it is difficult to delineate the role played by the valvular disease from that of underlying coronary artery disease. Cardiac compensation may last for years, and the first indications of the progression of the disease are signs and symptoms of left ventricular failure.

Aortic Stenosis

The systolic pressure gradient across the aortic valve is increased by left ventricular outflow obstruction. Experimental studies indicate that diminution of the cross-sectional area of the valve orifice to one fourth its normal size must occur before a significant decrease in resting cardiac output or increase in pressure gradient is evident.

Systemic blood pressure is usually normal, although the pulse pressure is often decreased and the peripheral pulses diminished. Left ventricular aortic systolic gradients may range as high as 150 mm. Hg (Fig. 2). The resting cardiac output is normal unless failure is present; however, cardiac output does not increase

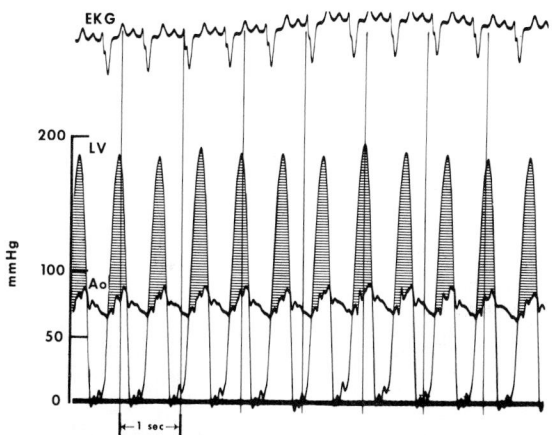

Figure 2. Simultaneous recording of the electrocardiogram (EKG), left ventricular pressure (LV), and aortic pressure (Ao) obtained at cardiac catheterization in a patient with aortic stenosis. The shaded areas indicate the pressure gradient across the aortic valve. The LV-Ao peak systolic pressure gradient is 95 mm. Hg.

with exercise in the presence of severe stenosis. Left ventricular hypertrophy and increased left ventricular diastolic volume act as compensatory mechanisms to maintain cardiac output. Prolongation of the isometric contraction phase, as well as the systolic ejection time, allows a longer period for emptying of the ventricle and compensation for the lower flow rate. These mechanisms allow maintenance of an adequate cardiac output but interfere with myocardial perfusion because the proportion of the cardiac cycle devoted to isometric contraction and systolic ejection is markedly lengthened, and the period of elevated intramural tension is increased. Thus, the duration of diastolic coronary perfusion is decreased. Coronary insufficiency in the absence of primary coronary artery disease may ensue, causing electrocardiographic changes consistent with myocardial ischemia and the symptoms of angina pectoris. However, because aortic stenosis commonly occurs in patients over the age of 40 years, the possibility of associated primary coronary artery disease must be considered. The frequent occurrence of sudden death in aortic stenosis is probably due to sudden ventricular arrhythmias secondary to inadequate coronary blood flow.

CRITERIA FOR SURGERY

The selection of patients for aortic valvular surgery is often difficult. Ideally, all patients with aortic valvular disease should undergo operation prior to the onset of *irreversible* myocardial changes. Unfortunately, there is no certain method of recognizing this state; thus, the surgeon is left with the decision to operate upon relatively asymptomatic patients whose prognosis with medical management may be good, or upon those with myocardial damage whose mortality will be higher and in whom the results will be less than satisfactory.

In general, surgery is contraindicated in anyone with active rheumatic heart disease. In those with bacterial endocarditis, surgery should be postponed, if possible, for approximately 3 months after blood cultures are negative. If one is forced to operate earlier, adequate antibiotics must be given with full knowledge that the results will not be as good. The degree of pulmonary fibrosis or emphysema, or both, if present, must be carefully determined before the decision to operate is made. Primary coronary artery disease must be recognized by preoperative coronary arteriography. If there is significant arterial narrowing, concomitant aortocoronary artery bypass should be considered.

Aortic Insufficiency

The lack of a method for quantitating the degree of aortic insufficiency results in the selection of operative candidates primarily on the basis of clinical progression of signs and symptoms. The development of angina or congestive failure indicates subsequent progressive deterioration. Cineangiocardiography may be of help in estimating the degree of insufficiency but is of limited practical aid in selecting candidates for operation. Cardiac catheterization may be helpful in patients with an elevated left ventricular end-diastolic pressure prior to the recognition of overt heart failure and may provide additional evidence of dysfunction of other cardiac valves.

Any patient with advanced aortic insufficiency should be considered a candidate for surgery. Usually, there is a history of congestive heart failure, progressive electrocardiographic changes, and radiographic evidence of progressive cardiomegaly (Fig. 3).

Aortic Stenosis

Aortic stenosis often produces no symptoms for 10 to 30 years. Once symptoms develop, however, the patient's condition is precarious, and the average life expectancy is 2 years.[12] Therefore, patients with symptomatic aortic stenosis should undergo cardiac catheterization. If electrocardiographic signs of coronary insufficiency are present, or if the history suggests such a condition, coronary angiography should be performed simultaneously in order to evaluate the coronary circulation, so that the coronary lesions may be treated at the time of operation. In the symptomatic patient, the demonstration of a systolic gradient across the valve of more than 50 mm. Hg is sufficient to justify operative intervention. Serial x-ray evidence of rapid cardiac enlargement is an ominous sign and an urgent indication for operation.

OPERATIVE TREATMENT

Operations on the aortic valve are performed through a median sternotomy. Cardiopulmonary bypass is achieved by cannulating the right atrium or the superior and inferior venae cavae and the ascending aorta or femoral artery. The aorta is occluded proximally, and the valve is exposed through a transverse or curved aortotomy. Exposure is facilitated by sump suction through the apex of the left ventricle.

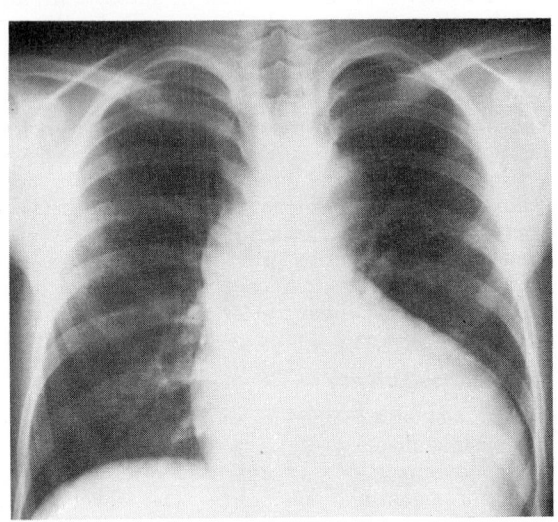
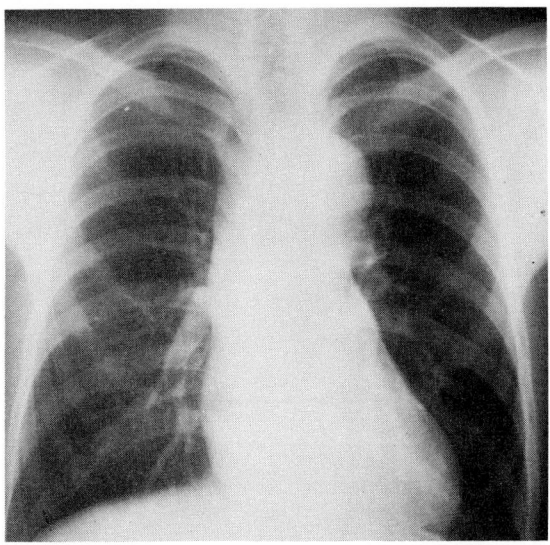

A   B

Figure 3. Roentgenograms of a patient with aortic insufficiency, demonstrating changes in cardiac size. *A*, Immediate preoperative view, poorly controlled congestive heart failure for 6 months. *B*, Six months after aortic valvular replacement, patient asymptomatic.

Coronary artery perfusion with a cannula in each coronary orifice is preferred by some surgeons. However, recent technical developments suggest that local hypothermia may also provide adequate myocardial protection.[16]

Occasionally, valvular function can be restored in the young patient by excising small amounts of calcium from the leaflets and incising the commissures to the annulus. However, in the majority of adults with acquired aortic valve disease, the entire valve must be excised and replaced.

Although many devices have been employed for aortic valve replacement, none is ideal. The most widely used are prosthetic valves, which are usually composed of a metal frame exposed or covered with cloth and containing a moving obturator. The obturator may be a sphere, disc, toroid, or hinged flap fabricated from plastic or metal[3] (Fig. 4). Tissue valves of various types have been employed for many years. In the past, these have consisted of human valves obtained at autopsy and prepared by a variety of methods, and of tissue leaflets prepared from fascia lata and dura mater.

The majority of these valves have undergone deterioration over a period of several years, and these devices are rarely used today. The most promising valve at present is the porcine xenograft.[19] These valves are harvested from pigs and fixed at diastolic pressure in a stabilized glutaraldehyde preparation. These devices have been under clinical investigation for four years and deterioration has been rare. The major advantage is the relative freedom from thromboembolic complications.

Prosthetic valves, especially if relatively small, may result in a moderate left ventricular–aortic pressure gradient. The majority carry some risk of thromboembolism, although many of the prostheses have been modified or redesigned in an effort to prevent this complication. Most surgeons advocate postoperative anticoagulants indefinitely. Xenograft valves rarely cause thrombosis or embolism; however, their long-term fate at present is unknown. Although the durability of these valves has been excellent up to four years, it should be remembered that all of the earlier tissue valves eventually demonstrate deterioration.

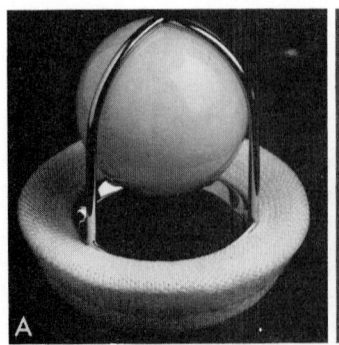
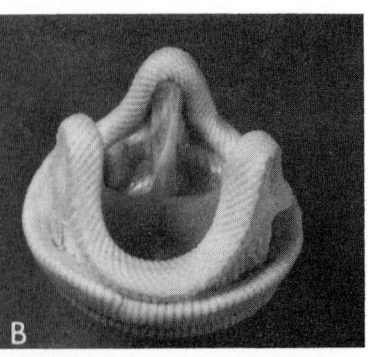

Figure 4. *A*, Starr-Edwards aortic ball-valve prosthesis with silicone rubber poppet and metal cage. (Courtesy of Edwards Laboratories.) *B*, Hancock porcine xenograft processed in stabilized glutaraldehyde and mounted in a flexible stent. (Courtesy of Hancock Laboratories.)

RESULTS OF SURGERY OF THE AORTIC VALVE

The results of aortic valvular surgery must be evaluated from several points of view: (1) the prognosis of patients with untreated aortic valvular disease; (2) the risk of operation; (3) the risk of complications secondary to the device used for valvular replacement; (4) the percentage of patients alive several years after operation; and (5) the percentage of patients living and functionally improved.

Barnhorst et al.[2] have reported results over a 9-year period in 1027 patients undergoing insertion of an aortic ball valve prosthesis. Six per cent of their patients died in the first 30 days. For those patients who survived the early postoperative period, the late mortality rate was 27 per cent at the end of 9 years. There was a correlation between the early deaths and the preoperative New York Heart Association classification. Only 4 per cent of the patients in Class II died during the perioperative period, while 15 per cent of those in functional Class IV died. Emboli occurred in 22 per cent of the patients surviving 5 years or longer; however, the embolization rate was reduced with adequate anticoagulation.

Stabilized glutaraldehyde-prepared porcine xenografts were placed in 89 patients and followed up to 45 months by Zuhdi.[19] There were no early deaths and none of the valves failed during the period of follow-up. Furthermore, there were no thromboembolic complications during this period.

IDIOPATHIC HYPERTROPHIC SUBAORTIC STENOSIS (IHSS)

Gross Pathology

IHSS is a syndrome consisting of eccentric hypertrophy of the left ventricle and particularly the outflow tract, producing severe subvalvular stenosis. Patients dying of this disease have large hearts in which the thickened left ventricular muscle encroaches on the ventricular cavity, thus narrowing the volume. There are two general types: by far the most common is asymmetric hypertrophy involving the outflow portion of the ventricular myocardium, usually including the ventricular septum; the second is a more or less symmetric diffuse hypertrophy of the entire ventricle and ventricular septum. There is often enlargement of the papillary muscles and trabeculae carneae, thickening and opacity of the endocardium, particularly in the outflow tract, and thickening of the anterior mitral leaflet. In some hearts, the texture of the hypertrophied muscle is coarser than that of adjacent, more normal-appearing muscle.

Histopathology

The histopathologic appearance varies. There is a generalized increase in the amount of interstitial connective tissue. The muscle bundles are separated by this tissue and assume a bizarre arrangement. In some instances there are endothelial-lined channels between the muscle bundles opening into the ventricular cavities. Electron microscopic examination indicates not only thickening of the fibers but shortening as well. There is an increase in the size and number of nerve fibrils, elastic tissue, and mitochondria. Pearse[13] noted that hypertrophied myofibrils were being replaced by mitochondria, and so myofibril bands were shortened. The similarity between these fibers and normal sinoatrial nodal cells and atrial muscle suggested to him that IHSS might be the result of displacement of atrial muscle or abnormal proliferation of cardiac sympathetic nerves.

Clinical and Accessory Clinical Findings

Males are affected twice as frequently as females. In 64 patients reported by Braunwald and Morrow,[3] the ages ranged from 6 to 56 years of age. All patients had systolic murmurs, and 48 of them had complaints that were believed to be related to their disease. A heart murmur was most often the first clinical manifestation of disease. Dyspnea, angina, and dizzy spells were the most common symptoms, and syncope occurred not infrequently. The heart was usually enlarged, and a systolic thrill, best felt over the lower precordium on the left, was present in about half the patients. A systolic murmur along the lower left sternal border or at the apex was present in nearly all instances. Electrocardiographic abnormalities were present in virtually all patients. Roentgenologic examination showed an increased cardiothoracic ratio in more than 50 per cent. Angiocardiography demonstrated a smaller than normal left ventricular cavity during diastole and one that appeared to be almost entirely obliterated during systole. The left ventricular wall was generally much thicker than normal and often thicker than that found in patients with valvular or membranous subvalvular aortic stenosis. The ventricular septum is often much thicker than the left ventricular wall, and the relationships of the septum and ventricular wall, as well as the decreased diastolic rate of closure of the mitral valve, may be demonstrated by echocardiography[17] (Fig. 5).

Hemodynamics

Hemodynamically, pullback pressures measured by cardiac catheterization show a marked systolic gradient from the apex to the infundibulum and no systolic gradient from the infundibulum to the aorta in many instances (Fig. 6). However, the most prominent feature is the variability of the obstruction. The pressure gradient may vary tremendously during a single study, at times increasing severalfold, diminishing significantly, disappearing entirely, or appearing when none was present initially. This is explained by the fact that the obstruction is produced by the myocardial contractions and is subject to the same regulatory influences that control the contractile state of the entire myocardium. A number of factors can be introduced to influence the degree of stenosis and are based primarily upon whether or not the ventricular volume is diminished or increased. Those factors

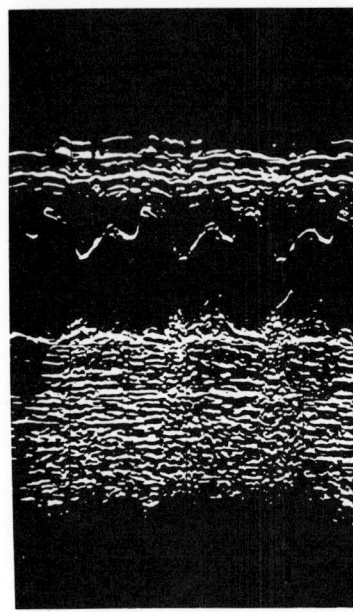

SEPTUM

MITRAL
VALVE

VENT. WALL

LUNG

Figure 5. Echocardiogram showing a large septum to ventricular wall ratio, as well as the diastolic apposition of the anterior leaflet against the ventricular septum and the decreased diastolic closure rate of the mitral valve.

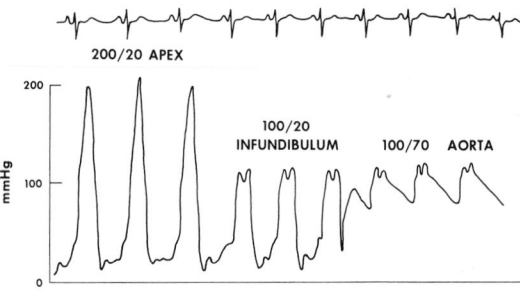

Figure 6. Pull-back pressures measured in the apex, infundibulum, and ascending aorta show a gradient from the apex to the infundibular area of the left ventricle, but no gradient across the aortic valve in IHSS.

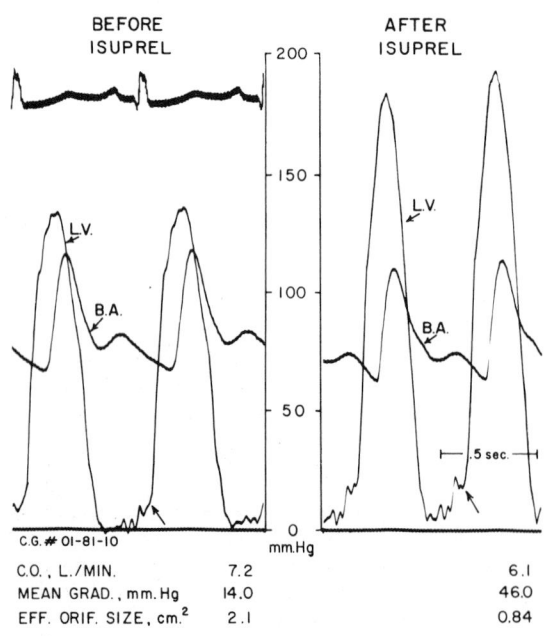

	BEFORE ISUPREL	AFTER ISUPREL
C.G. # 01-81-10		
C.O., L./MIN.	7.2	6.1
MEAN GRAD., mm.Hg	14.0	46.0
EFF. ORIF. SIZE, cm.^{2}	2.1	0.84

Figure 7. Simultaneous left ventricular (LV) and brachial artery (BA) pressure recordings from a patient with IHSS made before and after the intravenous infusion of isoproterenol. The inotropic effect of this pharmacologic agent caused the pressure gradient to increase from 14 to 46 mm. Hg, while the effective aortic orifice area decreased from 2.1 to 0.8 cm.^{2}

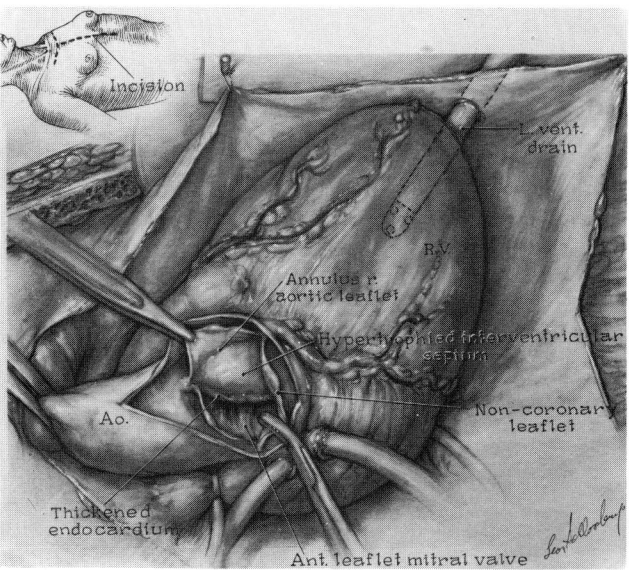

Figure 8. General operative exposure for the treatment of hypertrophic subaortic stenosis. An incision is made in the ascending aorta and extended down into the noncoronary sinus of Valsalva. The normal aortic valve is retracted, and bulging hypertrophic muscle in the interventricular septum can be seen beneath the base of the right coronary leaflet. Opposite is the anterior leaflet of the mitral valve, which is often thickened and opaque.

which reduce ventricular volume will increase the obstruction and include a decreased venous return produced by bleeding or by maneuvers to increase the intrapleural pressure, certain drugs with a positive inotropic effect on the myocardium (Fig. 7), and decreased afterloading. Conversely, those factors which increase ventricular volume reduce or alleviate the obstruction. These include an increased venous return, a negative inotropic effect on the myocardium, an increased afterload, and operations to relieve the obstruction.

Operative Treatment and Results

A number of operations have been devised to treat this disease and are directed primarily toward relieving the outflow obstruction. The most effective and frequently employed operation is that devised by Morrow (Figs. 8 and 9), which consists of approaching the hypertrophied myocardium through an aortotomy and making two parallel incisions longitudinally through the muscle mass in the outflow tract[7] (Fig. 10). These incisions are then increased in depth by digital pres-

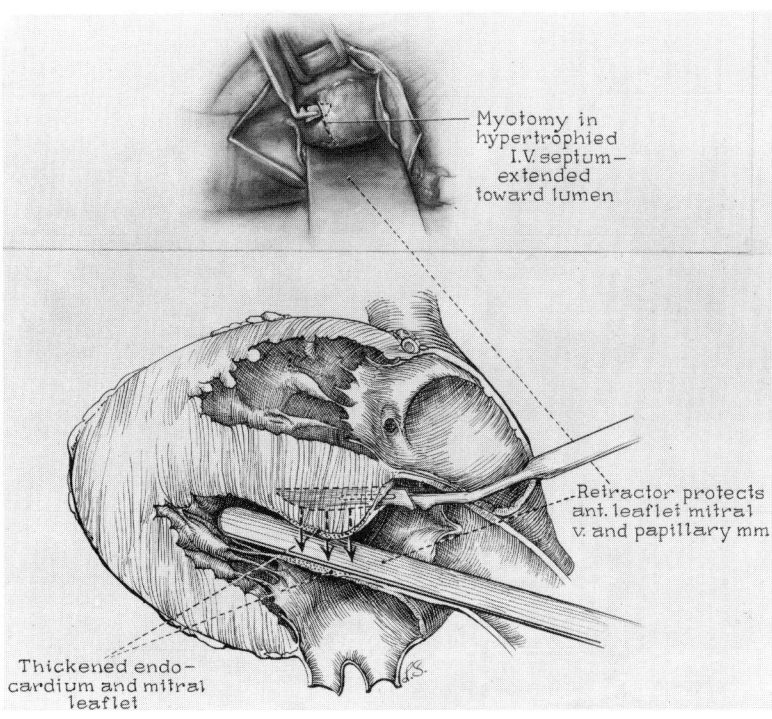

Figure 9. A flat ribbon retractor is passed through the aortic annulus to the apex of the heart, displacing and protecting the anterior mitral leaflet and papillary muscles behind it. The tip of a No. 10 knife, attached to an angled handle, is passed into the septum just below the base of the right coronary leaflet at a point 2 or 3 mm. to the right of the commissure between the left and the right coronary leaflets. The blade is inserted through the septum toward the apex for a distance of about 4 cm. and is then withdrawn as its cutting edge incises the septum with a sawing motion directed toward the ventricular lumen and the retractor.

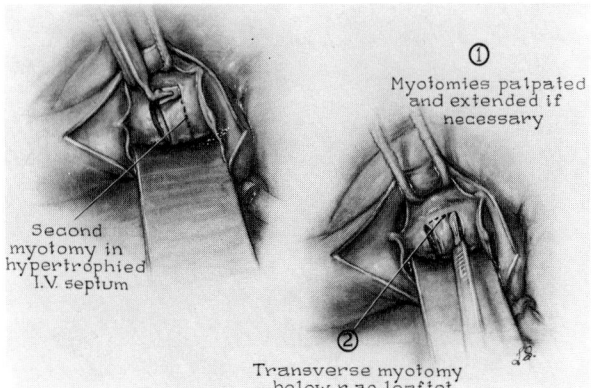

Figure 10. A second myotomy is made parallel to, and about 1 cm. clockwise from, the initial one. Both incisions are then palpated and deepened by digital pressure if necessary. At the most prominent part of the septum, the incision should be about 1.5 cm. in length. A transverse incision is then made at the base of the right coronary leaflet connecting proximal portions of the two myotomies.

sure, and the mass of tissue between them is excised with a special rectangular knife. At times, a rongeur passed through an apical incision may be necessary to reach the more distal part of the muscle mass (Figs. 11 and 12). Cooley has advocated mitral valvular replacement alone; however, it appears that this method of treatment should be reserved for specially selected cases.

The operative mortality is approximately 10 per cent. Symptomatic as well as hemodynamic results are excellent. There is no peak gradient at rest when the operation is properly executed. Maneuvers to decrease left ventricular volume and thereby increase outflow obstruction are effective only to a minimal degree in some patients. The end-diastolic pressure is reduced, and associated mitral insufficiency, when present before operation, is usually corrected.

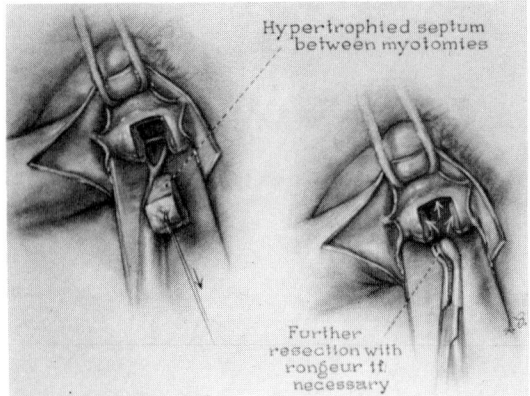

Figure 11. Traction is made on the suture, and a special rectangular knife is pushed toward the apex, freeing the muscle bar from the septum. The bar of muscle can usually be excised intact, but if it breaks or fragments, the resection is completed with the special angled rongeur.

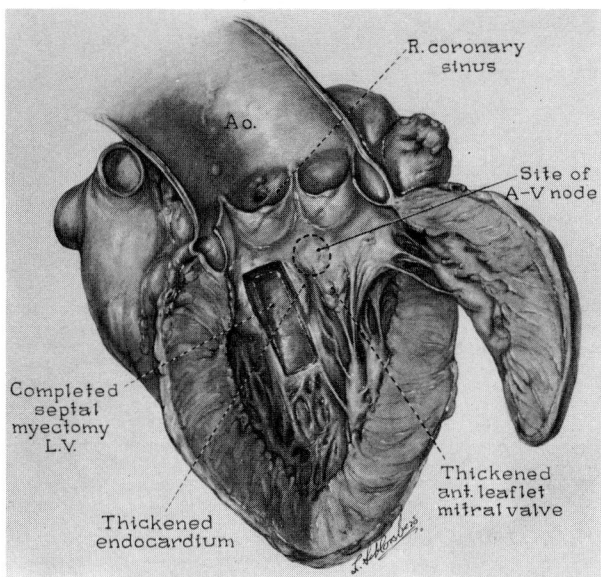

Figure 12. The appearance of the resected area of the septum and its relation to the aortic valve leaflets are shown. Also illustrated is the area of the conduction tissue which must be avoided.

SELECTED REFERENCES

Barnhorst, D. A., Oxman, H. A., Connolly, D. C., Pluth, J. R., Danielson, G. K., Wallace, R. B., and McGoon, D. C.: Isolated replacement of the aortic valve with a Starr-Edwards prosthesis: A 9-year review. J. Thorac. Cardiovasc. Surg., 70:113, 1975.
This report of 1027 operations for replacement of the aortic valve with an aortic ball valve prosthesis includes an evaluation of the effects of several factors on early and late results.

Morrow, A. G., Reitz, B. A., Epstein, S. E., Henry, W. L., Conkle, D. M., Itscoitz, S. B., and Redwood, D. R.: Operative treatment in hypertrophic subaortic stenosis: Techniques, and the results of pre and postoperative assessments in 83 patients. Circulation, 52:88, 1975.
The results are reported of the operative treatment of 83 patients with idiopathic hypertrophic subaortic stenosis. Detailed preoperative and long-term postoperative hemodynamic data are presented and the long-term results of this operation, in patients followed up to 14 years, are given.

Zimmerman, J.: The functional and surgical anatomy of the aortic valve. Fourth Asian-Pacific Congress of Cardiology, 5:862, 1969.
An excellent description and graphic representation of the dynamic behavior of the normal aortic valve is presented. The surgical implications of the normal anatomy as it relates to operative technique and prosthetic valve design are discussed.

Zuhdi, N., Hawley, W., Voehl, V., Hancock, W., Carey, J., and Greer, A.: Porcine aortic valves as replacements for human heart valves. Ann. Thorac. Surg., 17:479, 1974.
A review is presented of 89 patients undergoing xenograft aortic valve replacement and followed up to 45 months postoperatively. The results and complications associated with xenograft valves are evaluated and discussed.

REFERENCES

1. Barondess, J. A., and Sande, M.: Some changing aspects of aortic regurgitation. Arch. Intern. Med., 124:600, 1969.
2. Barnhorst, D. A., Oxman, H. A., Connolly, D. C., Pluth, J. R., Danielson, G. K., Wallace, R. B., and McGoon, D. C.: Isolated replacement of the aortic valve with a Starr-Edwards prosthesis: A 9-year review. J. Thorac. Cardiovasc. Surg., 70:113, 1975.

3. Braunwald, E., Lambrew, C. T., Rockoff, S. D., Ross, J., Jr., and Morrow, A. G.: Idiopathic hypertrophic subaortic stenosis. Circulation, 30(Suppl. 4):3, 1964.

4. Brewer, L. A., III (Ed.): Prosthetic Heart Valves. Springfield, Ill., Charles C Thomas, Publisher, 1969.

5. Cooley, D. A., Leachman, R. D., and Wukasch, D. C.: Diffuse muscular subaortic stenosis: Surgical treatment. Am. J. Cardiol., 31:1, 1973.

6. Ionescu, M. Z., Ross, D. N., Deac, R. C., and Woller, G. H.: Heart valve replacement with autologous fascia lata. J. Thorac. Cardiovasc. Surg., 60:331, 1970.

7. Levinson, G. E., Frank, M., and Schwartz, C. J.: The effect of rest and physical effort on the left ventricular burden in mitral and aortic regurgitation. Am. Heart J., 80:791, 1970.

8. Morrow, A. G., Reitz, B. A., Epstein, S. E., Henry, W. L., Conkle, D. M., Itscoitz, S. B., and Redwood, D. R.: Operative treatment in hypertrophic subaortic stenosis: Techniques, and the results of pre and postoperative assessments in 83 patients. Circulation, 52:88, 1975.

9. Morrow, A. G., Brawley, R. K., and Braunwald, E.: Effects of aortic regurgitation on left ventricular performance: Direct determinations of aortic blood flow before and after valve replacement. Circulation, 31(Suppl. 1):80, 1965.

10. Muller, W. H., Jr., Dammann, J. F., Jr., and Warren, W. D.: Surgical correction of cardiovascular deformities in Marfan's syndrome. Ann. Surg., 152:506, 1960.

11. Nolan, S. P., and Muller, W. H., Jr.: Instantaneous coronary artery blood flow in aortic insufficiency. Surg. Forum, 14:251, 1963.

12. Nolan, S. P., and Muller, W. H., Jr.: The aortic valve. Ann. Rev. Med., 16:33, 1965.

13. Pearse, A. G. E.: The histochemistry and electron microscopy of obstructive cardiomyopathy. In Ciba Foundation Symposium on Cardiomyopathies. Boston, Little, Brown and Company, 1965.

14. Roberts, W. C.: Valvular, subvalvular, and supravalvular aortic stenosis: Morphologic features. Cardiovasc. Clin., 5:97, 1973.

15. Ross, J., Jr., and Braunwald, E.: Aortic stenosis. Circulation, 38(Suppl. 5):61, 1968.

16. Sapsford, R. N., Blackstone, E. H., Kirklin, J. W., Karp, R. B., Kouchoukos, N. T., Pacifico, A. D., Roe, C. R., and Bradley, E. L.: Coronary perfusion versus cold ischemic arrest during aortic valve surgery. Circulation, 49:1190, 1974.

17. Tajik, A. J., and Giuliani, E. R.: Echocardiographic observations in idiopathic hypertrophic subaortic stenosis. Mayo Clin. Proc., 49:89, 1974.

18. Zimmerman, J.: The functional and surgical anatomy of the aortic valve. Fourth Asian-Pacific Congress of Cardiology, 5:862, 1969.

19. Zuhdi, N., Hawley, W., Voehl, V., Hancock, W., Carey, J., and Greer, A.: Porcine aortic valves as replacements for human heart valves. Ann. Thorac. Surg., 17:479, 1974.

XVII

ACQUIRED MITRAL AND TRICUSPID VALVULAR DISEASE

W. Gerald Austen, M.D., and Adolph M. Hutter, Jr., M.D.

Mitral and tricuspid valvular diseases are most often acquired disorders, and are usually the result of rheumatic fever. Within the past 30 years the prognosis for these lesions has changed as a result of remarkable advances in diagnostic techniques and cardiac surgery.

HISTORICAL ASPECTS

Surgical correction of *mitral stenosis* was first suggested in 1902 by Brunton[32] and first attempted in 1923 by Cutler and Levine.[43] The result was unsatisfactory because partial resection of the stenosed valve resulted in severe mitral regurgitation. In 1925, Souttar[174] performed a digital commissurotomy in one patient, but no significant progress was made over the next two decades. During this period, the technique of cardiac catheterization was developed, and it added immensely to the understanding of valvular heart disease. Forssmann, a urologist, presented the first radiographic evidence of right atrial catheterization in man in an operation he performed on himself in 1929.[59] In 1941 Cournand and Ranges[42] established right cardiac catheterization as a useful tool. In the late 1940s, Harken et al.,[76] Bailey,[9] and Brock,[30] working independently, successfully accomplished closed digital commissurotomy for mitral stenosis, and thus made this procedure a practical reality. The addition of techniques employing various knives or *transatrial* valvulotomes did not produce significant improvements in results. However, the subsequent development of the Tubbs *transventricular* dilator in 1959 allowed a considerably more effective commissurotomy.

Effective surgical treatment of *mitral regurgitation* had to await development of cardiopulmonary bypass techniques, beginning in the early 1950s.[66] Various forms of open annuloplasty were subsequently employed, with variable results. The introduction of the rigid-ring, ball-valve prosthesis by Starr and Edwards in 1961[178] provided a consistently successful surgical procedure for patients with mitral valvular heart disease (both regurgitation and stenosis), even in the presence of extensive valvular damage. Both the success and the complications of the early models have been taken into account in the subsequent modifications[22, 82, 83, 177, 181] and improvements of the Starr-Edwards prosthesis, and a number of other types of prostheses have been designed and clinically tested.[14, 19, 53, 85, 98, 112, 147, 194] Allograft, xenograft, and autologous tissue valves have also been employed.[13, 33, 91, 92, 155]

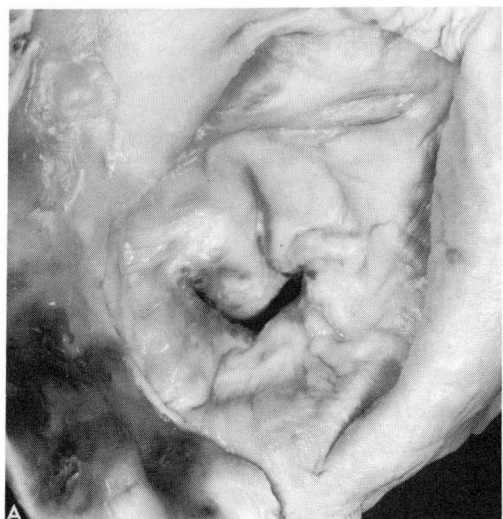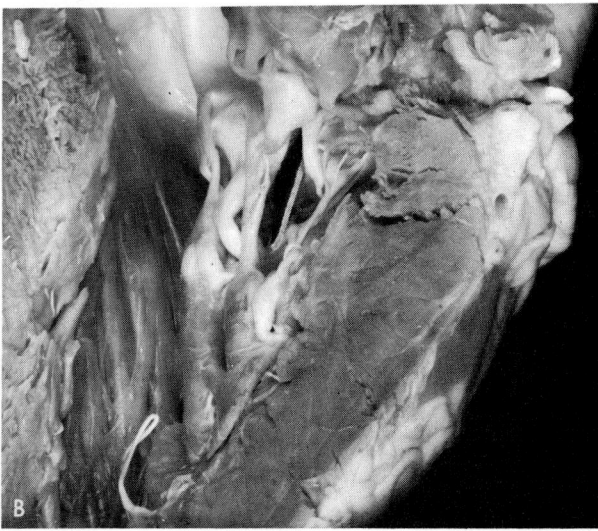

Figure 1.   Typical pathologic changes in mitral stenosis: *A,* Mitral valve viewed from atrial side. Leaflets are thickened and adherent. *B,* Left ventricular view. Thickened, fused, and retracted chordae tendineae are seen. The leaflet-chordal complex forms funnel-shaped structure with narrowed apex in left ventricle. (From Eliot, R. S., and Edwards, J. E. *In* Hurst, J. W., and Logue, R. B.: The Heart, 2nd ed. Copyright 1970, McGraw-Hill Book Company. Used with permission of McGraw-Hill Book Company.)

It has now become apparent that a significant number of patients have severe *tricuspid valvular disease* that can seriously affect the operative result following mitral or aortic valve surgery.[10, 128, 180, 188] Open valvulotomy has been shown to be helpful in patients with acquired tricuspid stenosis,[164] and annuloplasty may occasionally be of value in patients with tricuspid regurgitation. Frequently, however, valve replacement is necessary in patients with severe acquired or functional tricuspid disease.[180]

MITRAL STENOSIS

ETIOLOGY AND PATHOLOGY

Mitral stenosis is far more frequent in women than in men, the ratio being 2 or 3 to 1. Although a definite history of rheumatic fever is evident in only approximately half of patients with mitral stenosis, pathologic evidence reveals that rheumatic heart disease is the usual cause.[87] A history of Sydenham's chorea is particularly significant; rheumatic heart disease (usually mitral stenosis) will develop in up to 30 per cent of these patients, without apparent initial carditis, over the subsequent 30 years.[5] *Congenital* mitral stenosis is rare.

A number of pathologic changes contribute to narrowing of the mitral orifice secondary to rheumatic inflammation. The process is progressive, with pathologic changes occurring over a number of years after the initial attack of rheumatic carditis. The ingrowth of fibrous tissue results in a thickened, rigid leaflet. Concurrently, retraction develops, and fusion of the leaflets at the commissures produces narrowing of the orifice. Concomitantly, the chordae tendineae may become thickened, retracted, and fused, pulling the valve down into the left ventricle. In some cases, later

calcification adds to the rigidity of the valve. These combined processes result in a rigid, narrowed, funnel-shaped orifice with the apex projecting into the left ventricle (Fig. 1). The inflammatory process usually involves the myocardium and pericardium, and direct myocardial injury may occasionally produce clinical manifestations. The extent of pathologic changes is an important determinant in the choice of surgical therapy. Pliable, nonregurgitant leaflets that are stenotic primarily because of fusion respond well to commissurotomy. On the other hand, extensive fibrosis and retraction of the leaflets, heavy calcification, shortening of the chordae tendineae with fusion of the leaflets to the underlying papillary muscles, or significant regurgitation requires mitral valve replacement for restoration of good valvular function. *Restenosis* after mitral valvulotomy is common, but in properly selected patients, it usually does not occur for at least 5 to 10 years. Factors that predispose to early restenosis following commissurotomy are calcification of the valve leaflets and shortening of chordae, both of which tend to leave the leaflets immobile, favoring refusion and further stiffening of the leaflets.

PHYSIOLOGY

The cross-sectional area of a normal mitral valve measures 4 to 6 sq. cm. Gorlin and Gorlin[71] have devised a formula that includes the relationship of valve area, blood flow, and the pressure gradient across the valve and that allows a reliable approximation of the area of a nonregurgitant valve from data obtained at cardiac catheterization. As mentioned previously, it is probable that the mitral valve becomes progressively more narrowed over subsequent years after the initial attack of rheumatic carditis. Recurrent attacks of rheumatic fever hasten the process – hence the value of penicillin prophylaxis. Symptoms may appear early, but more often their appearance is delayed 20 to 30 years or more. Significant narrowing of the mitral valve is required before symptoms appear. When the valve area is 2.1 to 2.5 sq. cm., symptoms usually occur only with extreme exertion.[111] Moderate exertion may produce symptoms when the valve area is 1.6 to 2.0 sq. cm. When the valve area approaches 1.0 sq. cm., even normal activity may produce symptoms. The term "critical stenosis" is often applied to a mitral valve area this small, since the left atrial pressure and hence the pulmonary capillary wedge pressure are usually about 25 to 30 mm. Hg at rest, i.e., about the level of oncotic pressure.[71, 111] Consequently, with this degree of stenosis, the heart is unable to increase forward flow by elevations of the pressure gradient across the mitral valve without precipitating early pulmonary edema.[72, 111] The limitation of forward flow by the narrowed valve may also result in a low cardiac output. A valve area of approximately 0.4 sq. cm. is the minimal orifice size compatible with life.

The constant elevation of pulmonary capillary wedge pressure results in vasoconstriction[95, 111] and, later, structural changes in the pulmonary arterioles resulting in pulmonary artery hypertension.[70, 86, 95, 167, 190, 192] In a sense, pulmonary hypertension "protects" the pulmonary capillaries from sudden increases in right ventricular output and consequently lessens the occurrence of pulmonary congestion.[49, 111, 190] The price paid is right ventricular hypertrophy and eventual failure with secondary or "functional" tricuspid regurgitation.[111, 192] The pulmonary arterioles may become a second area of obstruction to flow, further contributing to low cardiac output.[111] Fortunately, even severe pulmonary artery hypertension in time usually recedes after effective mitral valve surgery.[26] The length of time required appears to be related to the relative contributions of *vasoconstriction* and *structural changes* to the pulmonary hypertension. On occasion, the pulmonary hypertension secondary to structural changes will take a number of months to decrease and may never return to normal.

The chronic left atrial hypertension produces left atrial enlargement and structural changes in the left atrial wall that eventually result in *atrial fibrillation*.[167] The onset of atrial fibrillation frequently precipitates pulmonary congestion because the rapid rate shortens diastolic filling time with resultant increase in left atrial pressure. Rate control by digitalis may yield dramatic results. The loss of the "atrial kick" may also be important in decreasing cardiac efficiency. The combination of atrial fibrillation and mitral stenosis results in stasis of blood in the left atrium, a condition that greatly increases the risk of left atrial clot and subsequent systemic embolization.[44, 167, 193]

CLINICAL FEATURES

The patient is often a woman in her thirties who complains of dyspnea on exertion, fatigue, or palpitations. These symptoms may be precipitated by pregnancy or atrial fibrillation. The early course is usually dominated by manifestations of pulmonary congestion – dyspnea, orthopnea, paroxysmal nocturnal dyspnea, and a nocturnal cough.[111, 167, 192] The last three symptoms result from an increased return of fluids to the lungs from dependent portions of the body in the supine position. Mild bronchitis and coughing may result in hemoptysis from engorged pulmonary veins. On occasion, massive hemoptysis can be quite frightening.[117] The fear-induced tachycardia with its attendant rise in left atrial pressure only complicates the situation. Occasionally, death can result from this complication. As pulmonary artery hypertension develops, the patient notes fewer congestive symptoms and may believe she is "better." Left-sided failure is then replaced by right-sided failure, with peripheral edema and an elevated jugular venous pressure. An engorged liver may be manifested by pain in the right upper abdominal quadrant,[184] splanchnic congestion, nausea, diarrhea, or protein-losing enteropathy. Although most patients describe a course initiated by left-sided failure followed later by symptoms of right-sided failure, about 15 per cent are seen with the features of pulmonary arteriolar hypertension alone. These patients have right heart failure with no history of pulmonary congestion, a relatively small left atrium, and often normal sinus rhythm. It may be that their pulmonary arterioles "hyper-react" with considerable constriction causing pulmonary artery hypertension early, which in turn protects the patient from left-sided symptoms and keeps the left atrium small and physiologically intact. Occasionally, hoarseness may develop from encroachment of a dilated left pulmonary artery on the left recurrent nerve (Ortner's syndrome).[57] Encroachment of the enlarged left atrium on the esophagus may give rise to dysphagia. At any time throughout this progression, the symptoms of a "low output state" may be dominant. Easy fatigability and weakness are the major early clues, and weight loss is a later sign. The physician is frequently amazed at the advanced state of incapacity a patient can reach without realizing it, because of the gradual adjustments in daily activities she has made to accommodate her disability. Precise questioning regarding the necessity of resting after minimal housework or similar activity often reveals considerable limitation of activity.

On *physical examination*, the patient may appear relatively normal. Patients with advanced disease may be thin and frail owing to long-standing low cardiac output. Ruddiness of the cheeks with mild cyanosis of the lips, fingers, and toes may be present, and is probably the result of peripheral oxygen desaturation in the low output state. There may be basilar rales, or the lungs may be clear, even in severe stenosis. The heart size is usually normal. Careful assessment of the cardiac impulse yields much information. In pure mitral stenosis, the left ventricular impulse is often normal. A sustained or diffuse impulse suggests additional aortic valve disease or mitral regurgitation. A palpable pulmonic closure sound and right ventricular lift over the parasternal area indicate pulmonary hypertension and right ventricular hypertrophy. Right-sided failure is manifested by distended neck

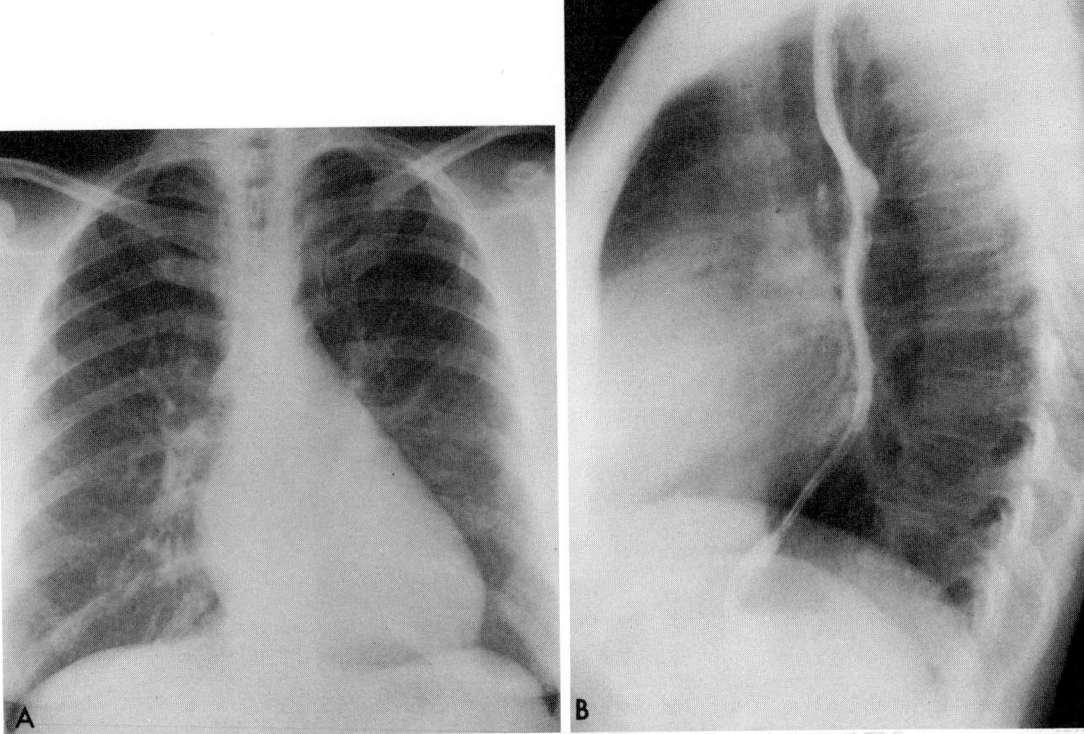

Figure 2. Typical posteroanterior and lateral roentgenograms in mitral stenosis: *A,* On posteroanterior view, left atrial enlargement is evidenced by double contour on right, elevated left mainstem bronchus, and straightening of mid left heart border. Distention of upper lobe pulmonary veins results from pulmonary venous hypertension, and dilatation of central pulmonary artery reflects pulmonary artery hypertension. *B,* On lateral view, enlarged left atrium displaced barium-filled esophagus. Left ventricle is not enlarged, but right ventricle is, and this is best seen as filling of the retrosternal space on lateral view. (Courtesy of Dr. Robert E. Dinsmore.)

veins, an enlarged liver, and peripheral edema. Predominant systolic venous waves and a pulsatile liver indicate tricuspid regurgitation, usually secondary to pulmonary hypertension and right ventricular dilatation.

The primary *auscultatory* features are a loud first heart sound, an opening snap, and a low-pitched diastolic rumbling murmur heard at the apex.[107, 192] The pulmonic closure sound is accentuated if pulmonary hypertension is present. The diastolic rumble is best heard at the apex with the patient in the left lateral decubitus position. It is often well localized and may be inaudible even an inch away. In some patients, a murmur may be heard only after exercise; in others, it may be loud enough to produce a palpable thrill. The loudness of the murmur, however, does not correlate well with the severity of the stenosis.[69] Indeed, with pulmonary artery hypertension and considerable right ventricular enlargement, the left ventricular apex may be displaced posteriorly, making the murmur inaudible (so-called silent mitral stenosis).

The earliest *radiologic* finding in mitral stenosis is left atrial enlargement. This is first evidenced by posterior displacement of the middle third of the barium-filled esophagus on the lateral view (Fig. 2).[3] In the posteroanterior view, the esophagus may be displaced

to the right. A larger atrium may elevate the main stem bronchus and may appear as an increased density extending to the right side within the cardiac shadow (double density). The overall cardiac size is often normal. Enlargement of the pulmonary artery and left atrial appendage characteristically obliterates the normal concavity in the upper and middle left heart border, producing a straightened or convex border. Right ventricular enlargement is revealed by anterior encroachment on the retrosternal space in the lateral view. Calcification of the mitral valve is rare in patients under 30 years of age.[114] When mild, it may be detected only by fluoroscopy with image amplification. Heavier calcification may be visualized on an overpenetrated film. Calcification of the left atrial wall may also be seen, and indicates a higher incidence of mural thrombi and potential technical difficulties at operation.[78] The lung fields initially reveal only distention of the upper pulmonary veins, a reflection of pulmonary venous hypertension.[106] Later, distended pulmonary lymphatics are seen as horizontal linear densities termed "Kerley's B lines,"[172] best visualized just above the costophrenic angle on the right side. Pulmonary congestion or even frank pulmonary edema may be present.

The classic *electrocardiographic* pattern demonstrates left atrial enlargement with right ventricular hypertrophy. The former is reflected by a broad, double-humped P wave in lead II (P mitrale) or by a broad, deep, negative deflection in the terminal part of the P wave in lead V_1.[126] The most sensitive indication of right ventricular hypertrophy is right axis deviation. With more severe pulmonary hypertension and right ventricular hypertrophy, a high R/S ratio in V_1 and a clockwise rotation may appear. Any evidence of left ventricular hypertrophy should prompt a search for concomitant disease, such as aortic valve disease or mitral regurgitation. Atrial fibrillation is frequently seen, and is often marked by relatively coarse fibrillation waves.[145] Unfortunately, the electrocardiogram is not a reliable guide to the severity of mitral stenosis, and may occasionally be completely normal even in cases of relatively severe mitral stenosis complicated by moderate pulmonary hypertension.[170, 192]

The echocardiogram is particularly helpful in mitral stenosis.[52, 56, 109, 131] Normally, the anterior and posterior leaflets of the mitral valve move in opposite directions during diastole on the echocardiogram, and the E to F slope of the anterior leaflet is greater than 35 mm. per second.[56] In mitral stenosis, the E to F slope is reduced, the magnitude of reduction correlating with the severity of stenosis. In addition, the posterior leaflet moves in the same direction as the anterior leaflet[52, 56, 109] (Fig. 3). The latter observation is important, since the E to F slope can be reduced in patients

with poor left ventricular filling without mitral stenosis, but in these, the posterior leaflet retains an essentially normal motion, i.e., opposite that of the anterior leaflet.[52, 56] The echocardiogram is also helpful in assessing the mobility of the mitral leaflets and the degree of calcification.[131]

In most patients with pure mitral stenosis, the diagnosis and estimation of severity can be made from clinical findings. When quantitation is needed in unclear cases, most of the pertinent information can be obtained by right heart *catheterization*. Pulmonary capillary wedge pressure (which closely reflects the left atrial pressure), the pulmonary artery pressure, and the cardiac output can be measured. The stress of exercise is often helpful in detecting significant disease either by precipitating a markedly abnormal rise in a near-normal resting "wedge" pressure or by revealing an inability to elevate the cardiac output appropriately. Prominent V waves in the wedge pressure may indicate significant mitral regurgitation. A proper evaluation of aortic valve disease, mitral regurgitation, or left ventricular function requires left heart catheterization, usually by retrograde passage of a catheter across the aortic valve. A significant proportion (15 to 30 per cent) of patients with pure mitral stenosis are found to have left ventricular dysfunction in the absence of aortic valve disease or coronary artery disease.[81] This abnormality, which may be due to old rheumatic myocarditis, can be detected by careful left heart catheterization, coronary arteriography, and left ventricular angiography. Left heart catheterization also allows precise measurement of the diastolic gradient across the mitral valve (Fig. 4), which, combined with the cardiac index and the length of diastole, permits calculation of the valve area by the formula of Gorlin and Gorlin.[71] The pulmonary capillary wedge pressure may be substituted for the left atrial pressure if a left atrial pressure is not obtained. The mean diastolic gradient in significant mitral stenosis is usually 10 mm. Hg or more, depending on the cardiac output. A smaller gradient may be significant with low cardiac output. Left ventricular angiography is the best way to quantitate mitral regurgitation (the height of the V wave in the left atrium or on the pulmonary capillary wedge trace may also be helpful), and an aortic root angiogram provides the best quantification of aortic regurgitation. Coronary arteriography is generally indicated if angina is present, if the patient is in an older age group, or if there is left ventricular dysfunction not explained by aortic valve disease or mitral regurgitation. The amount of valvular calcification is noted on fluoroscopy. Significant mitral regurgitation or heavy calcification indicates that mitral valve replacement is probably necessary rather than a commissurotomy. The assessment of aortic and tricuspid valvular disease may be important in planning surgical correction. If any hint of aortic or tricuspid valvular disease is present on clinical evaluation, catheterization may be indicated because the determination of relative severity of the different valvular lesions may be difficult on clinical grounds alone when multiple valves are diseased. If circumstances preclude catheterization, the state of the aortic and tricuspid valves should be carefully assessed at operation.

Normal Mitral Valve

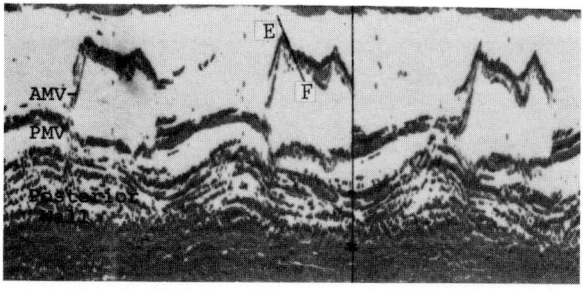

Mitral Stenosis

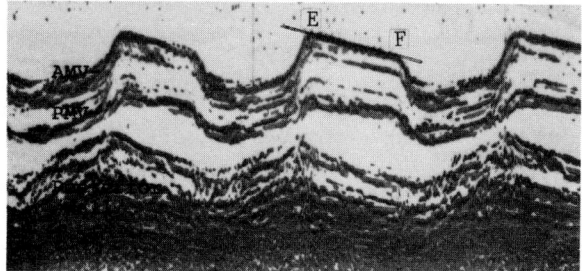

Figure 3. Echocardiograms of anterior and posterior leaflets in patient with normal mitral valve (above) and in patient with mitral stenosis (below). In mitral stenosis, the E-to-F slope is reduced and the posterior leaflet moves in same direction as the anterior leaflet. (Courtesy of Gordon S. Myers, M.D.)

R.M.

LEFT VENTRICLE   PULMONARY CAPILLARY
/0-5   30/12   MEAN = 17

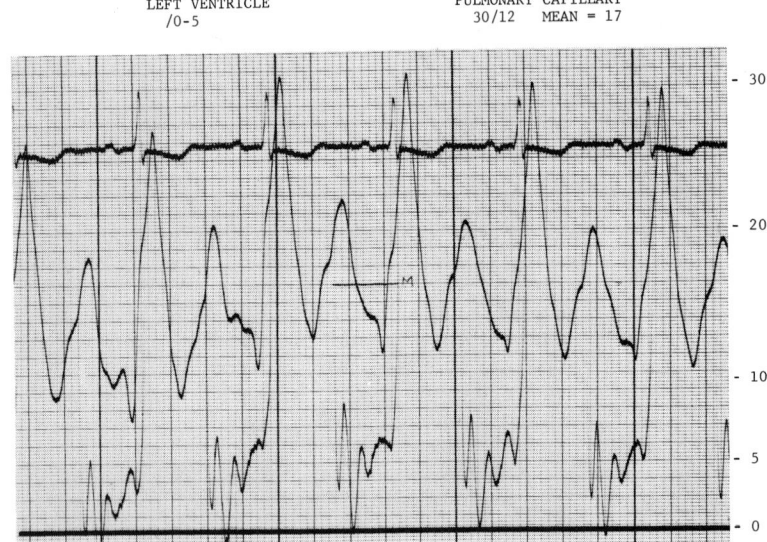

Figure 4. Typical cardiac catheterization findings in mitral stenosis: Simultaneous pulmonary capillary wedge and left ventricular pressure tracings. There is a delay in inscription of wedge pressure that represents transmission time from left atrium to right heart catheter tip. The A wave on wedge tracing is predominant, rising to 30 mm. Hg. A mean diastolic gradient of about 12 mm. Hg is present across mitral valve. (Courtesy of Dr. Charles A. Sanders.)

INDICATIONS FOR OPERATION

In general, mitral valve surgery is indicated for any patient with significant limitation from the disease despite an appropriate medical regimen; the definition of significant limitation depends on the patient and on the circumstances related to his condition. For example, a physician would decide on operation earlier for a patient without mitral regurgitation or calcification in whom a commissurotomy appeared feasible. On the other hand, in patients with a clear-cut need for mitral valve replacement, a greater degree of disability (Class III*) would usually be required to justify operation. It is important to emphasize, however, that the risk of operation is considerably greater if symptoms are allowed to progress to a far-advanced stage, and surgical treatment should be advised before this occurs. One factor that may prompt operation even in a mildly symptomatic patient is evidence of pulmonary vascular disease with increased pulmonary arteriolar resistance. Fortunately, excellent results may be achieved even when considerable pulmonary hypertension and markedly elevated pulmonary arteriolar resistance are present, although the risk of operation is greater than for patients without pulmonary hypertension. No patient should be refused operation because of the severity of pulmonary hypertension or congestive heart failure, since the prognosis for such patients with medical therapy alone is poor.

---

*New York Heart Association Functional Classification:
Class I—No symptoms on ordinary physical activity.
Class II—Symptoms on ordinary physical activity.
Class III—Symptoms on less than ordinary physical activity.
Class IV—Symptoms on any physical activity and possibly at rest.

SURGICAL THERAPY

Open Valvuloplasty and Closed Valvulotomy

Considerable discussion has taken place regarding the open versus the closed approach in the treatment of mitral stenosis.[64, 132, 135, 141] Some groups prefer open techniques for all patients, while others believe that certain patients can be treated best with a closed procedure. *Open* mitral valvuloplasty is usually accomplished through a median sternotomy or right anterolateral thoracotomy. After institution of cardiopulmonary bypass, the left atrium is incised, any thrombus is removed, and the valve is inspected. If it is primarily stenotic and if calcification is not severe enough to affect leaflet flexibility, the commissures are opened under direct vision, usually with a scalpel. Any subvalvular chordal fusion should be released if possible; this is usually accomplished by dilation with a finger or incision with a scalpel or both.

Advantages of open valvuloplasty include fewer thrombotic and calcific embolic sequelae, avoidance of hemorrhage from left atrial tears, and on occasion, more complete commissurotomy. Complications include the usual risks associated with open-heart surgery, particularly the difficulties occasionally encountered with cannulation and clotting. Care must be taken to avoid peripheral arterial embolization of valvular debris or air trapped in the left side of the heart. After cardiopulmonary bypass has been discontinued at completion of the procedure, the surgeon should insert his finger into the left atrium via a purse-string suture to estimate the operative result in the functioning heart. If possible, when the patient's cardiac output is satisfactory, left atrial and left ventricular pressures should also be measured to determine whether there is a significant diastolic gradient across the mitral valve or large V waves in the left atrium, suggesting significant mitral regurgitation. If valvular function is still inadequate, mitral valve replacement should be undertaken.

In patients with predominant mitral stenosis and moderate to no valvular calcification as determined by fluoroscopic study, we prefer a *closed* commissurotomy performed through a left posterolateral thoracotomy with removal of the fifth rib to provide adequate exposure for a closed or an open operation. Incision in the fourth or fifth interspace can also be employed, with transection of a rib if necessary, and some surgeons favor anterolateral thoracotomy in the fourth interspace. The left groin is positioned so that the femoral vessels can be cannulated if necessary. Operation should be performed in an operating room equipped for open-heart procedures with the pump-oxygenator assembled and ready for use ("pump standby") and sufficient blood available for cardiopulmonary bypass. To detect thrombus, the left atrium is inspected visually for lack of motion and the left atrial appendage is palpated. If thrombus is present, the closed operation should be converted to an open procedure; the clot can then be safely removed under direct vision, followed by valvulotomy.

If there is no evidence of atrial thrombus, a purse-string suture is placed in the atrial appendage, the appendage is incised, and a small amount of blood is permitted to flow from the incision to remove the rare, unsuspected, small thrombus. The surgeon then inserts his finger through the incision into the atrium, after which the purse-string suture may require tightening to prevent further loss of blood. The atrium should be examined digitally for thrombus and calcification, and the state of the mitral valve should then be assessed, considering the amount of regurgitation and calcification, the extent of subvalvular fusion, and the likelihood of dislodgment of calcium particles during a closed valvulotomy. An occasional group still employs temporary bilateral carotid arterial occlusion during initial insertion of the surgeon's finger into the left atrium and at valvulotomy to lessen the risk of cerebral emboli; we have not found this technique of significant value.

If thrombotic or calcific emboli from the valve or atrial wall appear to be a possibility, the operation should be converted to an open procedure. However, if it appears that a satisfactory closed valvulotomy can be carried out, i.e., when prodominant mitral stenosis exists with minimal to no valvular calcification, this is the procedure of choice. Some surgeons apply digital pressure to open the fused commissures gradually, but many groups, including our own, prefer use of the transventricular dilator[8, 65, 115] as the primary procedure (Fig. 5). After a purse-string suture is placed in a relatively avascular area at the tip of the left ventricle, an incision is made in the epicardium and a tunnel is created in the left ventricular muscle by a clamp or scissors. The closed dilator is inserted and guided through the mitral valve. To lessen the risk of mitral regurgitation, it is essential that the dilator not be enmeshed in the chordae tendineae and that it be opened only when its tip is in the left atrium. Therefore, the dilator should be positioned to traverse the subvalvular area easily, and the surgeon's finger should palpate the tip of the dilator in the left atrium. It seems reasonable that the blades of the dilator should be opened against the valve leaflets,[8] but this is probably not crucial. The dilator should initially be opened only 3.0 to 3.5 cm. and then gradually expanded. Dilation with the finger may also be helpful in addition to the mechanical dilator. No matter what technique is employed, the surgeon, with his finger in the left atrium, should intermittently assess the degree of relief of stenosis and the amount of mitral regurgitation. In addition, subvalvular stenosis should be relieved by finger fracture if possible; if necessary, this may have to be done as an open procedure with blade incision. At the end of the procedure when cardiac output is satisfactory, left atrial and left ventricular pressures should be measured if possible.

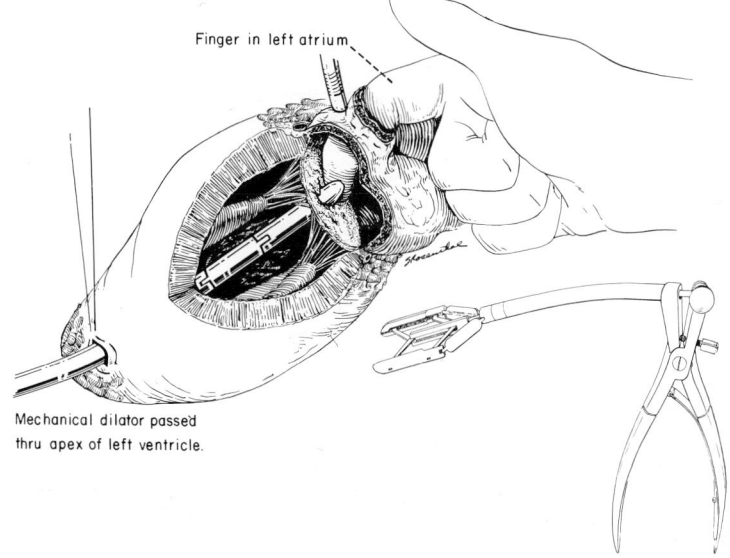

Figure 5. Use of transventricular mitral dilator for mitral stenosis: Dilator, with blades closed, is inserted through purse-string suture in tip of left ventricle and passed through mitral valve. Blades are then opened (inset) to accomplish valvulotomy.

Finger in left atrium

Mechanical dilator passed thru apex of left ventricle.

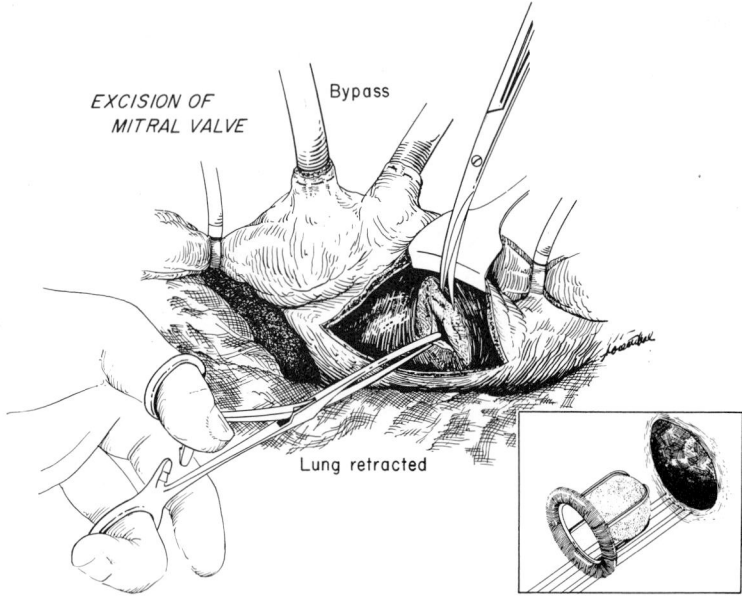

EXCISION OF MITRAL VALVE

Bypass

Lung retracted

Figure 6. Mitral valve replacement: Deformed mitral valve is excised, and (inset) Starr-Edwards prosthetic valve is inserted by means of multiple sutures to mitral annulus.

Minimal mitral regurgitation and low gradients of 3 or 4 mm. Hg across the mitral valve are acceptable.

The advantages of a closed approach over open operation are (1) it is simpler, (2) the operating time is shorter, (3) less blood is required, and (4) valvular function can be assessed in the working heart during operation. Complications associated with closed mitral valvulotomy include systemic emboli, significant mitral regurgitation, inadequate relief of stenosis, and hemorrhage from a tear in the left atrial wall secondary to insertion of the surgeon's finger.

If adequate mitral valve function cannot be achieved by a closed technique, cardiopulmonary bypass should be instituted and an open valvuloplasty or valve replacement should be performed. Arterial cannulation for cardiopulmonary bypass with a left thoracotomy can be accomplished using the femoral artery or the thoracic aorta via a purse-string suture. Venous return can sometimes be accomplished with femoral venous cannulation alone. As an alternative, a venous cannula can be inserted into the right ventricle either directly or via the pulmonary artery, with or without femoral venous cannulation.

Mitral Valve Replacement

If open mitral valvuloplasty or mitral valve replacement is planned preoperatively, a median sternotomy or right anterolateral thoracotomy is usually employed. Arterial cannulation can be accomplished using the femoral artery or via a purse-string suture in the ascending aorta. Although femoral arterial cannulation requires an additional incision, it has the advantage that the cannula is not in the main operative field, and if femoral venous cannulation is also employed, early partial cardiopulmonary bypass is readily available to extremely ill patients. However, particularly in patients with peripheral vascular disease, there is a significant incidence of arterial dissection from the trauma of the catheter tip and the retro-

grade arterial perfusion. Most groups, including our own, employ ascending aortic cannulation in most situations. Venous cannulation is usually accomplished by insertion of catheters via the right atrium into the superior and inferior venae cavae. Perfusion flow depends on the temperature of the patient, which is usually lowered to approximately 32° C.; at this temperature, a flow rate of 50 to 60 ml. per kg. is satisfactory. If the aorta is to be occluded for a significant length of time while the mitral valve is replaced, we usually lower the heart temperature further to protect the myocardium. The left atrium, which is better visualized if the right atrium is mobilized and the intra-atrial groove is exposed, is usually incised parallel to the intra-atrial groove (Fig. 6); the mitral valve is then exposed by retraction. Occasionally, because of a small atrium and consequent poor visualization, the valve may be exposed transseptally by incising both atria and the intra-atrial septum.

As mentioned previously, one of the major risks of open mitral procedures is air embolism. Many surgeons cross-clamp the aorta temporarily during valve replacement to avoid ejection of air by the left ventricle. This also eliminates the possibility of blood in the operative field resulting from aortic regurgitation, but on the other hand, it prevents coronary arterial perfusion. Because of the anoxic effects on the heart, we frequently do not cross-clamp the aorta unless there is significant aortic regurgitation. If the aorta is not cross-clamped, it is important to render the mitral valve regurgitant as soon as it is visualized; this can be accomplished by inserting a clamp or catheter through the valve. At the end of the procedure, before left ventricular ejection is allowed, the left ventricle should be aspirated with a needle and syringe. A needle should also be inserted into the upper aspect of the ascending aorta to allow air removal.

Valve replacement is usually performed if there is

significant mitral regurgitation or if the valve is so stiff and calcified that long-term relief of obstruction cannot otherwise be satisfactorily achieved. The diseased valve can be brought into better view if it is pulled toward the surgeon with a hook or clamp (Fig. 6). The valve is incised circumferentially on the inner margins of the annulus; the incision must be made well to the inside because of the proximity of the atrioventricular node and the circumflex coronary artery. In addition, overly generous removal, particularly posteriorly, can result in a tear in the left ventricular wall at the annular level with resultant hemorrhage.[119] While there has been some disagreement as to whether the papillary muscles and the attached chordae tendineae should be left intact,[113] most surgeons remove all chordae and transect the papillary muscles near the left ventricular wall. Detached chordae must be removed because they can become enmeshed in the prosthetic valve and cause dysfunction.

Suture technique in valve replacement is extremely important. Most surgeons employ multiple interrupted sutures, either figure-of-eight or mattress. If the annular tissue is soft, buttresses of Teflon felt may be helpful. Paravalvular leakage that usually results from circumferential tearing of the patient's tissue or from cutting through of the tissue by the sutures is an important complication.[1, 191] The resultant regurgitant flow, particularly in association with prosthetic valves such as the Starr-Edwards models, may lead to significant traumatic hemolysis. With proper technique, paravalvular leaks should be rare.

A variety of valve replacements are now available, of which the Starr-Edwards prosthesis has been the most commonly employed and the most extensively evaluated by clinical follow-up.[12, 22, 29, 101] If the left ventricular cavity is large enough, a Starr-Edwards prosthesis can be employed. It is important, however, not to use a prosthesis that is too large, because if the cage impinges on the left ventricular endocardium, ventricular irritability will result. The ball and cage can also obstruct left ventricular outflow. If the left ventricle is very small, it is preferable to employ a low-profile prosthesis or tissue valve. Ball variance (for example, swelling and surface irregularities) in Starr-Edwards mitral models with Silastic occluders has been uncommon, in contrast to the high incidence in early aortic models. In the earliest Starr-Edwards mitral valve, Model 6000, a considerable amount of metal was exposed on the undersurface (Fig. 7A), and embolization rates ranged between 20 and 40 per cent over a few years of follow-up.[1] The Model 6120 Starr-Edwards valve (Fig. 7B) has a cloth sewing ring composed of Teflon and polypropylene that is extended over the seat of the valve to decrease the amount of exposed metal. Within a matter of months, tissue covers the cloth; this has resulted in considerable decrease in the incidence of thromboembolism.[177] Valvular gradients have not usually been significant, although gradients of a few millimeters of mercury are common. With Model 6300, the first Starr-Edwards valve in which both ring and struts were completely covered, significant valvular gradients occurred because of valve design and tissue ingrowth; with Model 6310, gradients were not a problem, but cloth wear on the struts and valvular thrombosis caused difficulties.

In current use, the Model 6320 is completely covered with Teflon/polypropylene cloth except for small metallic studs to prevent the hollow stellite ball from hitting the cloth on the ring (Fig. 7C). It has been excellent in reducing emboli in patients receiving anticoagulants;[22] however, cloth wear has occurred both on the ring and on the struts. The most recent Starr-Edwards mitral valve, Model 6400 (Fig. 7D), is a

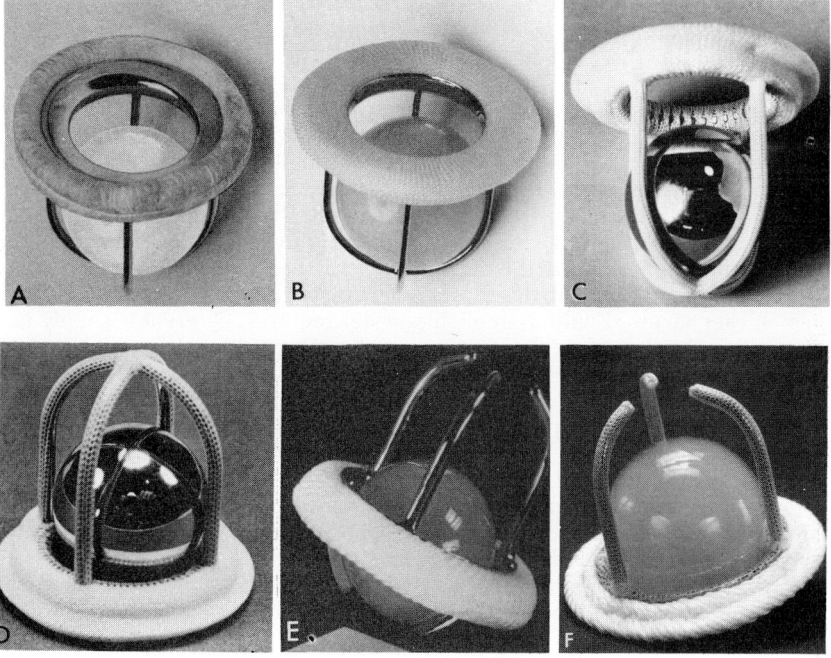

Figure 7. Caged-ball valves: *A*, Early Starr-Edwards valve (Model 6000) with Silastic ball and stellite cage; base has large area of exposed metal. This prosthesis was removed at postmortem examination; sewing ring is abnormally roughened and darkened. *B*, Starr-Edwards valve introduced in 1966 (Model 6120) with Silastic ball, stellite cage, and extended Teflon cloth sewing ring. *C*, Newer Starr-Edwards valve (Model 6320) with hollow stellite ball and stellite cage that is covered with porous Teflon/polypropylene fabric except for metallic studs projecting through orifice cloth. *D*, Most recent Starr-Edwards valve (Model 6400), the composite track prosthesis, with hollow stellite ball, stellite cage, and porous knit polypropylene covering. Orifice has exposed metallic studs, and each strut has exposed metallic track. *E*, Smeloff-Cutter valve with Silastic ball and titanium cage. Note descent of ball below sewing ring, resulting in minimal regurgitation. *F*, Braunwald-Cutter valve with Silastic ball and totally cloth-covered titanium cage. Inflow ring is covered with ultrathin polypropylene mesh, and struts as shown are covered with Dacron.

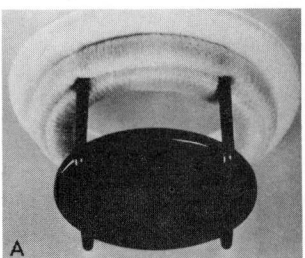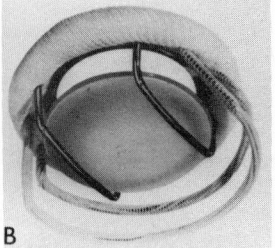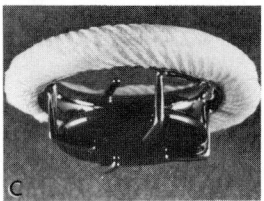

Figure 8. Caged-disc valves: *A*, Beall valve with disc and struts coated with pyrolytic carbon and Dacron velour covering the base. *B*, Kay-Shiley valve with stellite cage and Silastic disc; sewing ring may be either Teflon or Dacron cloth. This model has muscle guard designed to prevent contact between ventricular wall and disc. *C*, Cooley-Cutter valve with titanium cage, disc coated with pyrolytic carbon, and Teflon cloth sewing ring.

composite track valve in which porous knit polypropylene covers the stellite struts except for an exposed track intended to eliminate contact of the stellite ball with the cloth. In comparison with Model 6320, there seems to be an increased incidence of thromboemboli with Model 6400; this increase has not yet proved to be statistically significant. Cloth wear has not been apparent thus far.

Two other caged-ball mitral prostheses are the Smeloff-Cutter and Braunwald-Cutter valves. In the Smeloff-Cutter valve (Fig. 7E), the occluder passes through the sewing ring into the atrium; this design allows use of a smaller prosthetic ball providing a larger orifice during diastole. Although it was hoped that the Smeloff-Cutter valve would afford superior hemodynamic performance and a low rate of thromboembolism, long-term results have not confirmed this.[143] The Braunwald-Cutter mitral valve (Fig. 7F), a totally cloth-covered prosthesis with a Silastic occluder, thus far appears to be a satisfactory valve substitute;[147] although its aortic counterpart is currently unavailable because of serious difficulties with ball variance, the mitral model thus far has been free of this complication.

Some surgeons have employed low-profile, caged-disc types of prostheses rather than caged-ball valves, since the former occupy less space and require less force to move the occluder. Notable examples include the Beall, Kay-Shiley, and Cooley-Cutter valves (Fig. 8). The Beall valve has undergone several design changes because of problems with wear. In the Model 105, pyrolytic carbon superseded Teflon as the disc and strut covering; however, lethal strut fractures[68] have led to development of the most recent prosthesis, Model 106, which still utilizes pyrolytic carbon but has thicker struts. Evaluation of this model requires longer follow-up. Acceptably low rates of thromboembolism have been reported both with the Beall valve[15] and with the Cooley-Cutter valve,[194] while this complication appears to be significant with the Kay-Shiley prosthesis.[189]

The Björk-Shiley and Lillehei-Kaster valves (Fig. 9) represent another type of valvular prosthesis, the eccentric-monocusp valve. Rather than popping back and forth like the occluders in caged-ball and caged-disc valves, the occluders in these valves tilt or pivot to present only a thin cross section to blood flow when the valve is open. While this enhances hemodynamic characteristics by allowing nearly central flow,[20, 176, 187] stagnation of blood and eddy currents can occur below pivoting points where thrombi can cause complete malfunction, and in fact, this has proved to be a problem with both the Björk-Shiley[194] and Lillehei-Kaster valves.[175] When a valve of this type is used, anticoagulant treatment seems a necessity. Strut fracture has also been a problem in a recent Björk-Shiley model, but one that we believe has been overcome.

Of the various tissue valves, aortic allografts[129] have had the longest clinical trial in the mitral position.[80] Stented allografts have been used more commonly than unstented allografts, and the technique for their insertion is the same as for a prosthetic valve. The advantages of allografts include freedom from thromboembolic complications, relatively normal hemodynamic characteristics with central flow and low gradients, a very low incidence of hemolysis, and absence of abnormal valve sounds. However, healthy valves are difficult to procure in quantity, and implanted allografts have frequently been associated with a relatively high incidence of regurgitation and late failure. This has been at least partly due to harsh methods of sterilization and preservation utilizing ethylene oxide or irradiation with freeze-drying or frozen storage, for example.[104, 120, 140] Short-term cool storage of fresh valves in balanced salt solutions or tissue-nutrient media with physiologic doses of antibiotics is the most recent method of choice, but even with this more conservative technique, problems have resulted.[182]

Because of the limited quantity of allografts, valves from other species have gained popularity.[138, 139] Xenografts appear to be a logical alternative, since a greater supply is available, they can be removed from young, healthy animals immediately after death, and all required sizes are obtainable by choosing among different species. The commonest source of xenografts is the pig. Initially, finding the proper method of sterilization and preservation was also a problem with xenografts, and early preparations such as organomercurial salt solutions and formalin solutions were seen to be unsatisfactory.[37] In 1968, Carpentier et al.[38] introduced glutaraldehyde as a cross-linking factor to preserve the integrity of collagen molecules in the porcine valve, and today, this type of preservation ap-

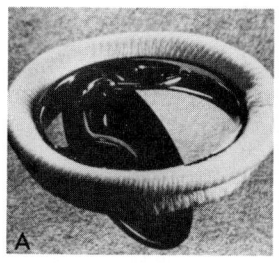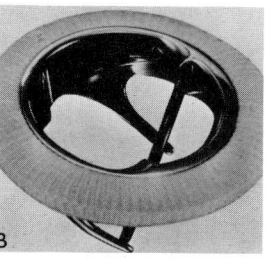

Figure 9. Eccentric monocusp valves: *A,* Björk-Shiley valve with stellite housing, disc coated with pyrolytic carbon, and Teflon cloth sewing ring. *B,* Lillehei-Kaster valve with titanium housing, disc coated with pyrolytic carbon, and Dacron sewing ring.

pears to hold great promise. The Hancock glutaralde-hyde-preserved porcine xenograft on a flexible stent (Fig. 10) is the valve of this type that has been used most extensively, and clinical results thus far have been very satisfactory in both mitral and tricuspid positions,[94, 124] as well as in the aortic position. Rates of thromboemboli with or without anticoagulants have been low, hemodynamic performance has been good, and failure of the xenograft has not yet appeared to be a significant problem. A few instances of thrombotic occlusion of this valve have been reported,[84, 94] however, and it is still too early to know what the long-term results will be.

Various types of autologous tissue have been studied for either partial or total replacement of cardiac valves, including venous tissue,[130] pericardium,[54] peritoneum,[55] and rectus sheath,[6] as well as the pulmonary valve.[116] Xenogeneic pericardium and allogeneic fascia lata have also been utilized,[90] but the autologous three-leaflet fascia lata valve[171] has received the most extensive clinical trial among the tissue-constructed valves. Unfortunately, results in both mitral and tricuspid positions have been sufficiently disappointing to cause most investigators to discontinue use of this valve for mitral and tricuspid valve replacements.[45, 156, 173] Thickened, shrunken leaflets leading to regurgitation are a common finding, and are believed to result at least partly from the pattern of blood flow through the mitral and tricuspid orifices.[122]

Our preference in mitral valve replacement continues to be the Starr-Edwards Model 6120 caged-ball valve. We certainly recognize that other mitral valve substitutes may be equally satisfactory and that sufficient study and follow-up may show them to be superior. We are particularly pleased with the Hancock

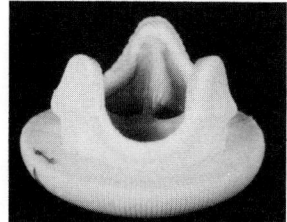

Figure 10. Hancock aortic porcine xenograft for atrioventricular valve replacement. Flexible polypropylene stent is covered with knitted Dacron.

xenograft, and we are also pleased with the Björk-Shiley eccentric-monocusp valve. We look with interest to the long-term results with the Starr-Edwards Model 6400 composite track valve and a number of other valves that we have also mentioned.

EARLY POSTOPERATIVE DIFFICULTIES

The primary postoperative difficulties that occur early after mitral valve surgery, in addition to complications already mentioned, are similar to the complications after other major cardiac procedures, and include low cardiac output or cardiac failure, cardiac arrhythmias, hemorrhage, respiratory failure, renal failure, the postpericardiotomy and postperfusion syndromes, valvular infections, peripheral emboli, and psychologic problems.

Low cardiac output and *cardiac failure* are moderately common after mitral valve procedures. Although they usually occur associated with long-standing mitral valve disease with significant pulmonary hypertension, they may occasionally result from unsatisfactory valvular repair or intraoperative myocardial damage. Cardiac failure is usually right ventricular in mitral stenosis, but occasionally may be left ventricular. In mitral regurgitation, cardiac failure is more often left ventricular, but can be right ventricular or both. Proper management of the low cardiac output syndrome or cardiac failure requires determination of the cause. Central venous pressure and left atrial pressure measurements are extremely important. Central venous pressure of 15 mm. Hg or higher[118] may be required to support cardiac output, and similar or higher pressures may be required in the left atrium.[58] If the patient is hypovolemic, infusion of blood or other colloid may reverse the low output state. Care must be taken to avoid overinfusion, as reflected by pulmonary congestion and more sensitively by lowered arterial Po_2 resulting from increased pulmonary arteriovenous shunting. Since acidosis, hypocalcemia, hyperkalemia, hypokalemia, and severe hyponatremia may have an adverse effect on myocardial function and require therapy, frequent determinations of electrolyte and blood-gas levels are essential. Digitalis glycosides should be administered carefully to avoid digitalis toxicity, especially if hypokalemia is present. In patients with volume overload or congestion, potent diuretics such as furosemide or ethacrynic acid are helpful. The low-output state frequently requires use of inotropic agents such as isoproterenol, epinephrine, or dopamine or a combination of two or three. When the ventricular rate is relatively slow, augmentation of heart rate by atrial pacing or by ventricular pacing in patients with atrial fibrillation or atrioventricular block may greatly improve cardiac output. Atrioventricular sequential pacing is sometimes effective in preserving the contribution of the atrial kick. In patients with low cardiac output and high peripheral resistance, peripheral vasodilating agents such as nitroprusside or phenoxybenzamine hydrochloride may be useful in decreasing left ventricular work and increasing forward blood flow.[50] With vasodilation, volume must be replaced simultaneously to maintain adequate cardiac filling pressures and cardiac output. Partial circulatory support may be of value in some patients with refractory but potentially reversible low cardiac output.[163]

Virtually any *cardiac arrhythmia* may occur after mitral valve surgery with a frequency much higher than that associated with standard general surgical procedures; furthermore, such an arrhythmia may have more serious consequences because it occurs in a heart unable to perform at normal efficiency. Thus, constant electrocardiographic monitoring during operation and in the first few days afterward is essential. In patients without atrial fibrillation, both temporary atrial and ventricular pacing wires are inserted, while in patients with atrial fibrillation, only ventricular pacing wires are employed. The atrial wires may be utilized as sensing electrodes in diagnosing complicated arrhythmias.[47] In addition to heart rate augmentation for improved cardiac output, atrial or ventricular pacing may be effectively employed for rate-overdrive suppression of ventricular arrhythmias, allowing reduced dependence on antiarrhythmic agents;[16] ventricular pacing is vital in patients with heart block.

Ventricular premature beats require rate-overdrive suppression or antiarrhythmic agents, especially if more than five or six occur per minute. Early after operation, intravenous lidocaine is probably the safest drug to administer for ventricular irritability. Although intramuscular procainamide is effective, it depresses the myocardium when administered in high doses.[77, 102] Phenytoin* is also effective, especially if ventricular irritability is due to digitalis toxicity;[18, 96] propranolol may also be employed in this situation. Long-term suppressive therapy may be achieved with quinidine, procainamide, phenytoin, or combinations of these drugs. Accelerated junctional ("nodal") rhythms, which occur frequently after mitral valve surgery, probably reflect transient inflammation of the atrioventricular junctional tissue adjacent to the mitral annulus. This type of rhythm is difficult to suppress pharmacologically, but it is usually benign, requiring no specific therapy and almost always disappearing with time. If the loss of atrial kick adversely affects cardiac performance in junctional tachycardia, overdrive atrial pacing at a rate slightly faster than the junctional rate can restore normally timed atrial contractions.

Atrial premature beats are frequent and do not themselves require suppression; however, they often presage atrial fibrillation, and their appearance might prompt the physician to begin administration of quinidine or digitalis in an attempt to stabilize the atrium and to prevent atrial fibrillation. Atrial flutter may cause considerable difficulty because of a rapid ventricular rate that is difficult to control with digitalis. Digitalization may convert the rhythm to atrial fibrillation or occasionally to normal sinus rhythm. In patients with atrial flutter, intravenous administration of propranolol can be effective both for rate control and for conversion to normal sinus rhythm. Because rate control in this situation is difficult to achieve with

---

*New official name of diphenylhydantoin as of July 1, 1975.

drugs, electrical cardioversion is usually performed early, either by rapid atrial pacing to "capture" the atrium or by external countershock. Atrial fibrillation is common preoperatively, and cardioversion with countershock during operation is unlikely to be successful for a prolonged period. In general, we perform cardioversion six weeks to three months after operation, usually in patients in whom atrial fibrillation has only recently begun, and the incidence of long-term maintenance of normal sinus rhythm after cardioversion in this group is high.[169] In many patients with normal sinus rhythm preoperatively, atrial fibrillation occurs during the first week or so after operation; treatment should usually be directed at control of the ventricular rate by administration of digitalis compounds. Although spontaneous reversion to normal sinus rhythm occurs frequently, rapid atrial fibrillation with significant hemodynamic depression may occasionally require early electrical cardioversion. To decrease the incidence of serious arrhythmias, proper electrolyte balance, particularly avoidance of hypokalemia and hyperkalemia, is essential. Digitalis compounds must be administered carefully to avoid toxicity.

Postoperative *hemorrhage* is much less common now than a few years ago, and is almost exclusively associated with open procedures. Of the many alterations in the hemostatic mechanism that may occur after cardiopulmonary bypass, the two most important are the effect due to circulating heparin and thrombocytopenia.[160] Protamine sulfate, 1 to 3 mg. intravenously for each milligram of heparin, is usually employed to reverse the heparin effect. Administration should be slow in order to avoid significant hypotension; on occasion, vasopressors may be required. Excessive amounts of protamine sulfate have a mild anticoagulant effect. The partial thromboplastin time serves to indicate the adequacy of neutralization of heparin; if it is still prolonged after the standard amount of protamine sulfate is administered, it is helpful to perform a protamine titration test to determine the degree of heparin neutralization. Although no treatment is usually required for platelet deficiency after cardiopulmonary bypass, platelet-rich fresh blood or platelet concentrates may occasionally be needed.

Other less common problems in hemostasis include intravascular coagulation, fibrinolysis, and difficulties related to hepatic disease.[63] Certainly the most important measure that the cardiac surgeon can take is to obtain adequate mechanical hemostasis. It is essential to monitor chest tube drainage carefully after operation, to obtain chest x-ray films periodically, and to observe the patient carefully for signs suggesting cardiac tamponade. If no coagulation defect can be determined and hemorrhage continues for more than 4 to 6 hours at high rates (150 to 200 ml. per hour), exploratory operation should be performed.

Respiratory failure is a major complication of mitral valve surgery. Before operation, all patients should be taught respiratory exercises and should be instructed regarding their use in the postoperative period. Elective ventilatory support should be employed immediately after operation to ensure adequate oxygenation. The length of respiratory support depends on the procedure performed and on the state of the lungs. Support can be discontinued a few hours after operation in the awake patient who has undergone closed mitral valvulotomy for mitral stenosis without significant pulmonary hypertension or other pulmonary problems; in patients with the same pulmonary status who have undergone mitral valve replacement, it can usually be withdrawn the day after operation. However, patients with severe, long-standing mitral valve disease with significant pulmonary hypertension are likely to require respiratory support for at least two days and sometimes longer. Measurements of arterial blood-gas levels are very helpful in determining when the respirator can be discontinued.[17] Use of a prestretched nasotracheal tube allows longer respiratory support in the occasional patient who requires it. If support is needed for more than five to seven days, however, tracheostomy should usually be performed.

Renal failure may occur after mitral valve surgery;[73] it is usually associated with operative or postoperative hypotension with secondary acute tubular necrosis.[195] Although oliguria is the usual manifestation, hemoglobinuria from prolonged cardiopulmonary bypass or renal arterial embolus from left atrial clot or mitral valvular debris may occasionally occur. Acute tubular necrosis must be differentiated from prerenal azotemia and oliguria secondary to hypovolemia or poor cardiac function. Adequate blood volume should be achieved, and the most effective cardiac action should be maintained. Occasionally, severe vasoconstriction may be present secondary to administration of catecholamines at operation and to hypothermia with resultant decreased renal perfusion. Maintenance of a normal or slightly elevated body temperature plus administration of small amounts of a vasodilator such as nitroprusside may improve urinary output. Isoproterenol, which combines a cardiac stimulatory effect with peripheral vasodilation, may be particularly helpful. If blood volume is adequate and levels of hydration and vasomotor tone are satisfactory, administration of diuretics such as furosemide or mannitol is reasonable. If the patient does have renal failure, he must be appropriately treated with fluid restriction and careful monitoring of electrolyte levels. Hyperkalemia should be managed with ion-exchange resin enemas (Kayexalate) and, if necessary, intravenous administration of glucose, insulin, and sodium bicarbonate. Peritoneal dialysis or hemodialysis may be required.[137]

A frequent complication of mitral valve surgery, occurring in perhaps a third of patients, is the *postpericardiotomy syndrome*,[60, 62] which usually consists of abrupt development of fever, pericarditis, pleurisy, and pleural effusion. The white blood cell count may be normal or elevated; rarely, a few atypical lymphocytes may be seen. This syndrome usually develops two to four weeks after cardiac surgery, but may occasionally occur as early as one week or as late as three months after operation. The cause is unknown, but an autoimmune phenomenon is suspected. After other causes of fever are excluded, treatment should consist of administration of salicylates, indomethacin, or corticosteroids in severe refractory cases, and it should usually continue for a week or more. Relapses may occur.

The less common *postperfusion syndrome*[61] consists of fever, malaise, splenomegaly, and a low white blood cell count with a high level of atypical lymphocytes in a patient who has undergone cardiopulmonary bypass and transfusions. Additional findings may include a maculopapular rash, hepatomegaly, lymphadenopathy, and hemolysis. Cytomegalic inclusion virus has been implicated in some cases.[105] Treatment is similar to that of the postpericardiotomy syndrome.

Valvular infection after mitral valve surgery is an uncommon but serious complication, particularly after replacement of the valve.[2] To minimize its occurrence, most surgeons administer high doses of antibiotics[133] directed against gram-positive organisms (primarily staphylococci), such as sodium methicillin (Staphcillin) or oxacillin. To ensure an adequate level in the blood at operation, antibiotic administration should be started preoperatively, and it is usually continued for three to five days postoperatively. If an intracardiac infection develops, aggressive antibiotic therapy is necessary. The patient should be treated for approximately six weeks with high doses of the appropriate antibiotic as determined by sensitivity studies, and then should be carefully observed to determine whether the infection has been eradicated. In patients who have undergone mitral valve replacement, infection is very difficult to eliminate by antibiotics alone. Commonly, the infection causes disruption of sutures and consequent mitral regurgitation. If antibiotics fail to eradicate the infection or if regurgitation becomes significant, the valve and any adjacent infected tissue must be removed and a new mitral valve inserted.[21]

Peripheral *arterial emboli* have already been mentioned as a significant complication associated with mitral valve surgery. Peripheral pulses should be carefully checked after operation, and signs and symptoms of cerebral, mesenteric, and renal emboli should be sought. Operative intervention for mesenteric, renal, or peripheral emboli may be necessary. In patients with mitral prostheses, sodium warfarin therapy is usually begun two or three days after operation and is continued indefinitely,[1] with the prothrombin time maintained at approximately twice normal. The incidence of emboli appears to be lessened significantly with sodium warfarin; other agents that affect platelet adhesiveness, such as dipyridamole and aspirin, may be valuable in preventing emboli as well.[185] When tissue valves are employed, anticoagulants are usually administered for approximately three to four months and then discontinued.

Psychologic problems occur commonly after mitral valve surgery, most often in patients who are very ill and who require prolonged intensive care. Patients may experience depression, agitation, disorientation, delusions, or hallucinations; treatment usually consists of mild sedation, gentle reassurance, and removal of the patient from the intensive care setting as soon as possible. These psychologic problems are transitory and are almost always resolved in a short time.

GENERAL POSTOPERATIVE CONSIDERATIONS

Because of the tendency to retain salt and water after operation, most patients are limited to 500 mg. of

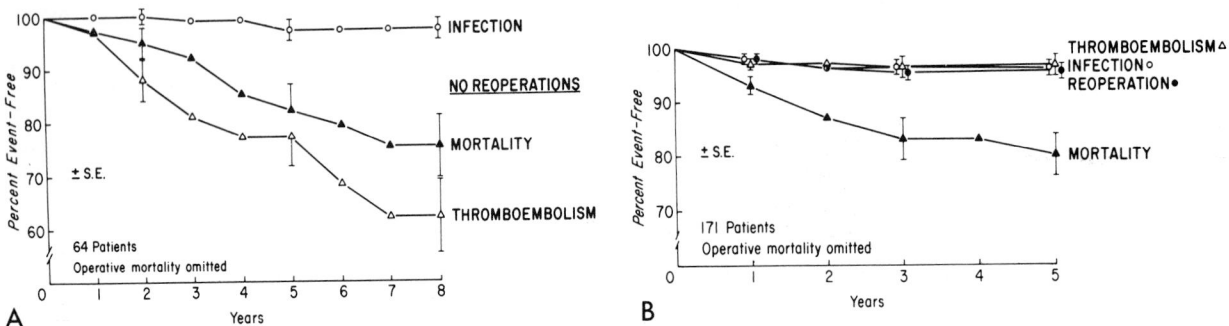

Figure 11. *A,* Mitral valve replacement with Starr-Edwards Model 6120 (noncloth-covered). Actuarial analysis of individual event-free curves in patients who survived operation and received sodium warfarin. Vertical bars denote standard errors. *B,* Mitral valve replacement with Starr-Edwards Model 6310 or 6320 (cloth-covered, composite seat). Actuarial analysis as in *A.* (From Bonchek, L. I., and Starr, A.: Am. J. Cardiol., 35:843, 1975.)

sodium and 1500 ml. of fluid per day for a few days, after which this intake is progressively increased. Following mitral valve surgery, patients are usually discharged on a low sodium diet, but many patients can manage a regular diet within a few months. Digitalis glycosides and diuretics are usually required in the early postoperative period, but by the time the patient is ready for discharge, they may have been discontinued. The amount of activity advised depends on the degree of cardiac impairment. Patients are usually permitted to dangle their feet on the second postoperative day, and are allowed out of bed on the second or third postoperative day; activity is gradually increased to full ambulation around the ward before discharge. Normal activity may be possible two or three months after valvulotomy, but may take longer after valve replacement. Patients with mild hemolytic anemia, particularly those with prosthetic mitral valves, should receive an iron supplement and folic acid until the anemia is corrected.

Patients who have undergone mitral valvulotomy or valve replacement should receive prophylactic antibiotic therapy to avoid bacteremia and valvular infection. In addition, they should receive antibiotics in association with any other operations or dental procedures and in the presence of any severe infection. Young patients with rheumatic heart disease should also receive daily antibiotic prophylaxis for rheumatic fever; penicillin is the drug of choice in the nonallergic patient.

OPERATIVE RESULTS

The operative risk of mitral surgery depends primarily on the severity of the patient's disease. In appropriately selected patients, the mortality associated with closed mitral valvulotomy should not exceed 1 or 2 per cent.[99] With open valvuloplasty in comparable patients, the results are similar. Usually, however, patients undergoing open valvuloplasty have more complicated problems, and the operative mortality is a little higher. Symptomatic improvement after closed mitral valvulotomy or open mitral valvuloplasty is

excellent; however, in 20 to 50 per cent of these patients, hemodynamically significant mitral disease *recurs* in 5 to 10 years.[99]

While rates in some early series were higher, current operative mortalities for mitral valve replacement are usually between 5 and 10 per cent,[28, 143, 147, 181, 194] and lower figures have been reported by some groups using the Hancock xenograft.[41, 84, 183] In general, the improved early survival rates are due to increase in operative and postoperative expertise and advances in technique rather than to changes in valvular design. Deaths are related to the severity of the mitral disease and to secondary myocardial and pulmonary effects, with low cardiac output, congestive heart failure, and arrhythmias being the most common causes of early fatalities.

Among the factors bearing on long-term results, both cardiopulmonary status and the type of prosthesis used are important (Fig. 11). Today, because of increased technical skill and improved mechanical valves, many surgeons are advocating operative intervention for mitral valve disease earlier than previously.[22, 157] While mitral valve replacement has classically been reserved for severely disabled patients in whom medical treatment is of little or no benefit,[127] more patients with moderate disability are now being operated on in the belief that, in carefully selected patients in this category, the risk of late morbidity and mortality related to the prosthesis is now less than if the patient did not receive surgical treatment. The death rate in the first five years after operation with the newer, improved prostheses should be approximately 2 per cent per year. Functional and hemodynamic results in most patients with newer valves are satisfactory, and rates of valve-related complications such as paravalvular leaks, infective endocarditis, and hemolytic anemia are acceptably low. Although systemic embolism continues to be a problem with prostheses and long-term anticoagulation is still a necessity, the incidence of this complication is impressively low with the newer caged-ball and caged-disc valves.[15, 147, 181, 194] With the Hancock xenograft, the incidence of thromboemboli even without anticoagulation has been almost nonexistent.[183] We remain concerned, however, about the durability of all the recent valves, both mechanical and tissue, and about the formation of valvular thrombus, especially on the eccentric-monocusp prostheses.

MITRAL REGURGITATION

ETIOLOGY AND PATHOLOGY

In contrast to the etiology of mitral stenosis, that of mitral regurgitation is varied. The most common cause of mitral regurgitation requiring operation is rheumatic valvulitis. Rupture of the chordae tendineae is also common.[152] Other less frequent etiologic factors in mitral regurgitation requiring operation include papillary muscle dysfunction or rupture, the floppy valve syndrome, and bacterial endocarditis. Females are more commonly affected by rheumatic mitral regurgitation than males, although the ratio is not as high as that in mitral stenosis. Papillary muscle dysfunction, on the other hand, occurs more frequently in men because of the higher incidence of coronary artery disease in males.

In rheumatic mitral regurgitation, the pathologic process is similar to that in mitral stenosis, but the end result favors regurgitation, probably because of a preponderance of contraction of the leaflets and chordae tendineae. Immobility of the leaflets, particularly if they are calcified, contributes to the retention of the valve in an "open" position. Why the rheumatic process produces mitral regurgitation in one patient and mitral stenosis in another is not known. As might be expected, a variable component of mitral obstruction often accompanies regurgitation in rheumatic heart disease.

Perhaps the most common cause of mitral regurgitation is papillary muscle dysfunction,[31, 34, 79, 110, 134, 146, 161] but only a minority of these patients require mitral valve surgery. Three types of papillary muscle dysfunction may be considered:[161] (1) The first is due to alteration of spatial relationships between the papillary muscles and mitral leaflets, which causes loss of their normal parallel alignment. Abnormalities of this relationship may result from left ventricular dilatation from any cause[110] and may also be an important factor in the mitral regurgitation seen with idiopathic hypertrophic subaortic stenosis.[51] (2) Intrinsic papillary muscle dysfunction due to ischemia or infarction from coronary artery disease is the most common cause of papillary muscle dysfunction.[34, 40, 46, 161] The *posteromedial* papillary muscle is most prone to abnormalities in this situation,[40, 46, 79, 161] for its major nutrient vessel, the descending branch of the dominant coronary artery, has little collateral support.[93] In contrast, the blood supply to the anterolateral papillary muscle is rich in collaterals. (3) Actual rupture of the papillary muscle occurs uncommonly, but when it does, it is usually in the setting of myocardial infarction.[46, 161, 166] Again, the posteromedial muscle appears more susceptible.[46, 166]

Rupture of the chordae tendineae may cause mitral regurgitation to a degree that is either acute and severe or insidious and chronic, depending on the number of chordae ruptured.[165, 168] Although the most common cause in the preantibiotic era was bacterial endocarditis, it is now apparent that some cases occur as a complication of rheumatic valvulitis. An increasing number of cases appear to occur as isolated spontaneous ruptures without evident pre-existing lesions;[162, 168] pathologic examination has revealed areas of lysis of elastin and collagen in these chordae.[39] Isolated spontaneous chordal rupture tends to occur in middle-aged or elderly men and usually involves the posterior leaflet.[11]

The "click-murmur" syndrome due to prolapse of one or both leaflets of the mitral valve has come to be recognized as a common cause of mitral regurgitation.[11, 75, 89, 148] Hemodynamically severe regurgitation, however, is unusual, and most symptoms are related to associated atrial and ventricular arrhythmias. This syndrome tends to run in families and may be associated with soft tissue abnormalities, such as Marfan's syndrome, and thoracic skeletal abnormalities, such as pectus excavatum, scoliosis, or straight back syndrome.[23, 159] On pathologic examination, the leaflets and chordae are thin and redundant and may show myxomatous degeneration. Other causes of mitral regurgitation include trauma,[125] active bacterial endocarditis, and massive calcification of the mitral annulus.[103]

PHYSIOLOGY

In mitral regurgitation, a variable amount of left ventricular output is directed back to the left atrium; this causes a systolic rise in left atrial pressure represented as a V wave on a left atrial or pulmonary capillary wedge pressure tracing. The extra blood is then returned as an added volume load to the left ventricle in diastole. Fortunately, the heart is capable of adapting to even large increments in volume work without great reduction in systemic blood flow. The stroke volume can be doubled without significant change in oxygen consumption, probably because the extra work is performed at low pressure.[25] This adaptive ability most likely accounts for the fact that some patients may do quite well for long periods despite severe mitral regurgitation. The volume of mitral regurgitation tends to rise in proportion to the increasing cardiac output with exercise, and it also reduces rapidly with a decline in cardiac output during rest.[108]

The physiologic and hence clinical consequences of mitral regurgitation are different in the acute and chronic forms. In acute regurgitation, the left atrium is usually small, and the rhythm is normal sinus. Thus, the high-pressure jet from the vigorous left ventricle is immediately transmitted back to the pulmonary veins. A huge V wave results, and is often associated with significant pulmonary artery hypertension (Fig. 12).[150, 162] Since left ventricular function is often quite good, exercise increases cardiac output and hence mitral regurgitation, with resultant precipitous rises in left atrial pressure. Consequently, these patients have progressive exertional dyspnea marked by frequent episodes of pulmonary edema in the presence of a good forward output. At the other ex-

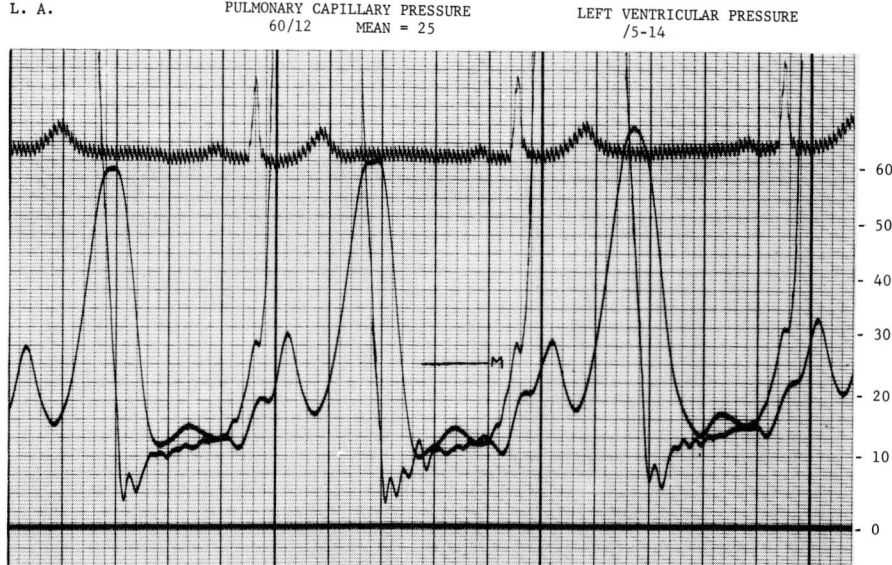

L. A.   PULMONARY CAPILLARY PRESSURE   LEFT VENTRICULAR PRESSURE
                                     60/12   MEAN = 25   /5-14

Figure 12. Typical cardiac catheterization findings in acute mitral regurgitation: Simultaneous pulmonary capillary wedge and left ventricular pressure tracings. There is normal sinus rhythm. Mean wedge pressure is elevated to 25 mm. Hg. Large V wave rises to over 60 mm. Hg without end-diastolic gradient across mitral valve. (From Sanders, C. A., Scannell, J. G., Harthorne, J. W., and Austen, W. G.: Circulation, *31*:506, 1965. By permission of the American Heart Association, Inc.)

treme, chronic mitral regurgitation is usually associated with a large left atrium that is often fibrillating. The combination of a dilated, more compliant atrium and often a poorly functioning left ventricle results in a low fixed cardiac output, small left atrial V waves, and lower pulmonary capillary pressure. In such patients, easy fatigability and weakness predominate, and acute episodes of pulmonary edema occur less frequently.

An increase in pulmonary arteriolar resistance occurs more slowly and less frequently than in mitral stenosis, probably because the left atrial pressure is elevated only intermittently, i.e., only during systole. Furthermore, owing to the absence of stasis in the left atrium, the incidence of left atrial clot is much lower than in mitral stenosis.

CLINICAL FEATURES

The major symptoms in patients with mitral regurgitation are usually dyspnea on exertion, easy fatigability, and sometimes palpitations. Pulmonary hypertension and right ventricular failure are relatively infrequent until late in the course of the disease. In acute mitral regurgitation, pulmonary congestion dominates the picture. The sudden worsening of a patient's chronic course, especially with the appearance of marked pulmonary congestion, should alert the physician to the possibility of bacterial endocarditis or ruptured chordae tendineae.

The key *physical* finding is an apical systolic murmur, which is holosystolic. This occurs with fixed regurgitation, as in rheumatic heart lesions, ruptured papillary muscle, or ruptured chordae tendineae. The murmur of papillary muscle dysfunction may be vari-

able in timing during systole.[40] The murmur of a prolapsed mitral leaflet (floppy valve syndrome) is usually late systolic and is often accompanied by a midsystolic click[11, 75] or, occasionally, an early systolic click.[89] The murmur in all types of mitral regurgitation is usually best heard at the apex and extends toward the axilla. With posterior leaflet chordal rupture, extension to the left sternal border is likely. The first heart sound is frequently difficult to hear because it merges with the onset of the murmur. The second heart sound may be widely split owing to shortening of left ventricular systole. An opening snap may be heard in 10 per cent of patients with severe rheumatic mitral regurgitation and, when present, indicates a movable and pliable anterior mitral leaflet.[136] In diastole, a loud and palpable S3 gallop represents the rapid filling of the left ventricle with the large volume of blood from the left atrium. A short filling rumble may follow the gallop. In acute mitral regurgitation with normal sinus rhythm, the small left atrium generates a loud S4 gallop. In all types of mitral regurgitation, the left ventricular impulse is abnormally wide, hyperdynamic, and of normal duration. In chronic mitral regurgitation with left ventricular enlargement, the impulse is displaced downward and to the left. Occasionally, systolic expansion of the enlarged left atrium can displace the heart anteriorly, causing a late systolic parasternal impulse. This gives a rocking sensation to the precordium on palpation and may be mistaken for the impulse of right ventricular hypertrophy.[121]

The *chest x-ray film* in patients with chronic mitral regurgitation reveals an enlarged left atrium (Fig. 13), which sometimes reaches gigantic proportions, and usually left ventricular dilatation. In spite of considerable cardiomegaly, the pulmonary vasculature may be unremarkable. Significant calcification of the mitral valve is unusual in pure mitral regurgitation. Acute mitral regurgitation in the absence of pre-existing heart disease presents a distinctive radiologic appearance of a relatively small heart with a disproportionate amount of pulmonary vascular congestion. Left atrial size is normal or only moderately increased (Fig. 14).[162]

The *electrocardiogram* is of only modest help. Left ventricular hypertrophy and left atrial enlargement with normal sinus rhythm may be seen. Atrial fibrillation is frequent in long-standing cases. Right ventricular hypertrophy may appear in later stages of the disease.

The *echocardiogram* is not so helpful in mitral regurgitation as it is in mitral stenosis, and has little quantitative value in terms of severity of the regurgitation.[56] However, it can be quite useful in diagnosing two specific causes of mitral regurgitation: mitral valve prolapse[35, 48, 56, 149] and ruptured chordae tendineae.[35, 56, 186] In each, the echocardiographic picture may be specific enough to indicate the diagnosis with reasonable certainty.

Frequently, accurate quantitation of the severity of mitral regurgitation and the functional impairment of the patient can be made clinically, without *catheterization*. However, mitral regurgitation can best be quantitated by left ventricular angiography via a catheter passed retrogradely across the aortic valve (Fig. 15). This study also provides important information about left ventricular size and the adequacy of left ventricular contraction. Left atrial or pulmonary capillary wedge pressure tracings may reveal an elevated mean pressure with tall V waves (see Fig. 12). A high left ventricular end-diastolic pressure may indicate left ventricular failure. In more severe cases, the cardiac index may be low at rest and unable to rise appropriately with exercise. Pulmonary hypertension may be present. The preoperative assessment, when indicated, of concomitant aortic or tricuspid valve disease or of significant coronary artery disease by catheterization is as important in patients with mitral regurgitation as it is in those with mitral stenosis.

INDICATIONS FOR OPERATION

Since patients with significant mitral regurgitation can function well for years with medical management and since mitral valve replacement with its attendant risks and complications is usually required for surgical correction, operation is usually reserved for patients in Classes III and IV despite appropriate medical treatment, although we are now more often considering patients in Class II. As in mitral stenosis, operation should not be delayed until the patient reaches Class IV if earlier operation is possible, because of the considerable increase in the risk of a surgical procedure in Class IV patients. Nevertheless, dramatic clinical

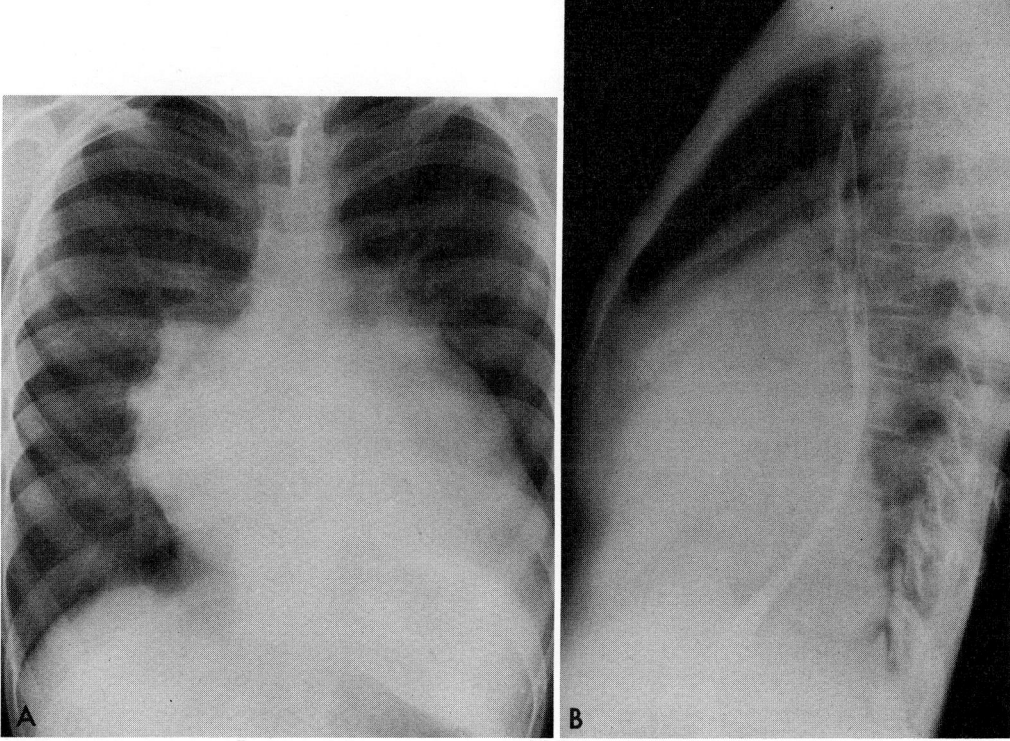

Figure 13. Typical posteroanterior and lateral roentgenograms in chronic mitral regurgitation: Chronicity of mitral regurgitation is suggested by very large left atrium. In addition, there is left ventricular enlargement. (Courtesy of Dr. Robert E. Dinsmore.)

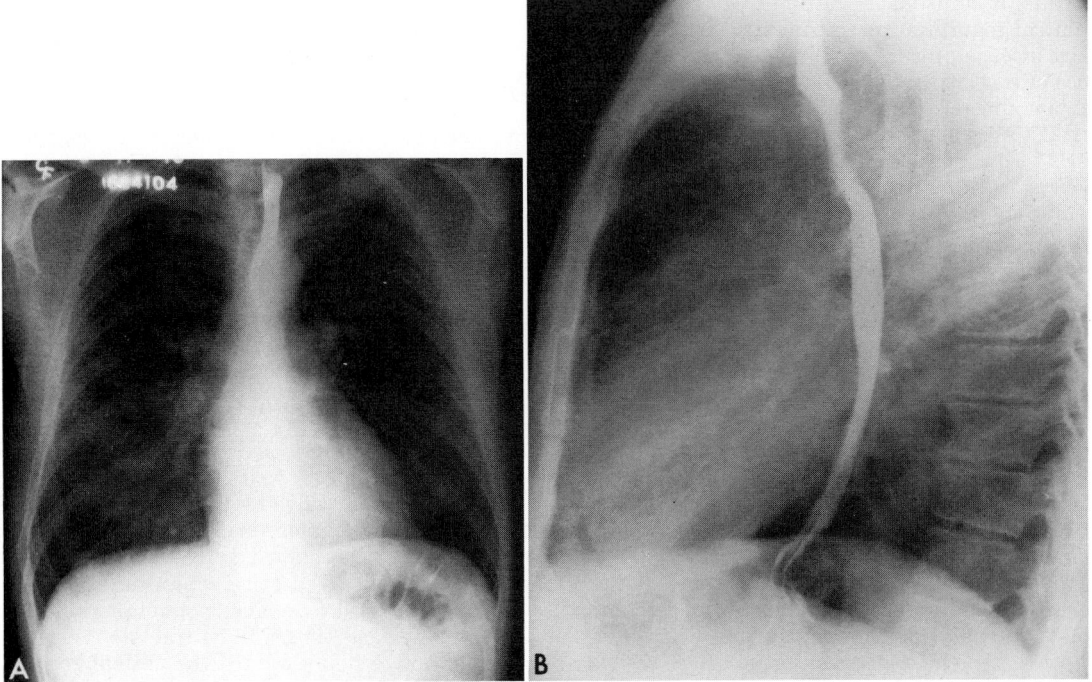

Figure 14.   Typical posteroanterior and lateral roentgenograms in acute mitral regurgitation: Combination of relatively small left atrium and marked pulmonary congestion in patient with loud apical holosystolic murmur suggests acute mitral regurgitation. In this patient, ruptured chordae tendineae with severe mitral regurgitation were found. (Courtesy of Dr. Robert E. Dinsmore.)

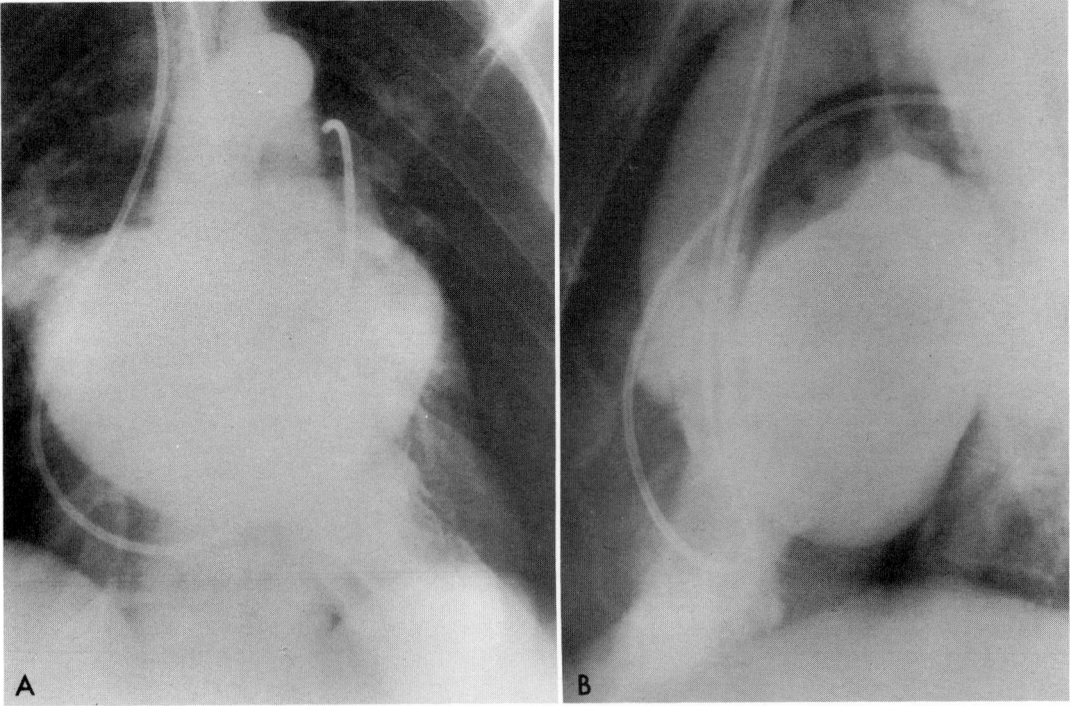

Figure 15.   Biplane left ventricular angiogram of patient with mitral regurgitation: Note dense opacification of left atrium by contrast medium injected into left ventricle through catheter passed retrogradely across aortic valve. Right heart catheter is also present with tip in pulmonary artery.

improvement can be accomplished even in Class IV patients by operation.

SURGICAL THERAPY

Operative repair of mitral regurgitation requires open-heart techniques and cardiopulmonary bypass. The usual approach is through a median sternotomy or right anterolateral thoracotomy. If significant mitral regurgitation is created or unexpectedly found during closed mitral valvulotomy, cardiopulmonary bypass can be instituted through a left lateral thoracotomy.

Mitral Valve Replacement

The standard procedure for the treatment of mitral regurgitation under most circumstances is mitral valve replacement, and many surgeons perform *only* this procedure. The technical considerations, types of valve substitutes, and operative and postoperative problems are identical to those in mitral valve replacement for mitral stenosis, and have already been discussed. We currently employ the Starr-Edwards caged-ball Model 6120 or the Hancock xenograft; in patients with mitral regurgitation, the left ventricle is usually large enough that problems such as left ventricular endocardial irritation or obstruction of outflow by the valve replacement are unlikely if the proper-sized valve is selected.

Mitral Annuloplasty

In a small percentage of patients with relatively mobile leaflets and a dilated valvular annulus, mitral annuloplasty with cardiopulmonary bypass may be considered for the treatment of mitral regurgitation. Any commissural fusion is incised, and mattress sutures are placed in the mitral annulus to narrow it; located at one or both commissures, they are usually buttressed with Teflon felt. While this technique relieves the mitral regurgitation, it does decrease the size of the mitral orifice; an orifice of approximately 3 sq. cm. should be maintained if possible. At the completion of the procedure, with cardiopulmonary bypass discontinued, the function of the mitral valve and the degree of mitral regurgitation or stenosis should be assessed by insertion of the surgeon's finger into the left atrium and also by simultaneous measurement of left atrial and left ventricular pressures. If adequate valvular function has not been achieved, mitral valve replacement should be carried out.

Mitral Valvuloplasty

Several types of valvuloplasty in addition to annuloplasty have been suggested in the treatment of mitral regurgitation. Most have now been discarded in favor of valve replacement. When the regurgitation is due to loss of leaflet substance (particularly the mural leaflet), the leaflet area can be extended and increased by insertion of pericardium or prosthetic material; this may be carried out in association with an annuloplasty as well.

When ruptured chordae tendineae are the cause of the mitral regurgitation, plication of the flail leaflet

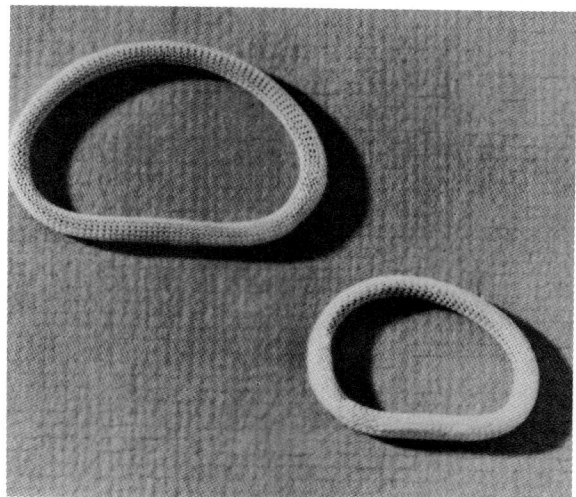

Figure 16. Carpentier valvuloplasty rings: *left*, mitral ring; *right*, tricuspid ring. These devices are stainless steel covered with jersey.

may be possible[97, 123] if the number of ruptured chordae is not too great and if their location is appropriate. Mitral annuloplasty may also be necessary. Again, the function of the mitral valve must be checked after bypass is discontinued, and if it is inadequate, valve replacement should be carried out.

Carpentier et al.[36] have introduced a technique of open valvuloplasty in which a stainless steel ring covered with jersey (Fig. 16) is sutured to the natural mitral annulus. This procedure, which entails repositioning of leaflets, remodeling of leaflets and commissures, and correction of annular dilation by staged plications, appears very promising, particularly in the correction of mitral and tricuspid valves with predominant regurgitation.

EARLY POSTOPERATIVE DIFFICULTIES AND GENERAL POSTOPERATIVE CONSIDERATIONS

The postoperative difficulties and general postoperative considerations associated with the operative treatment of mitral regurgitation are similar to those for the open operative treatment of mitral stenosis, and have already been discussed. Early valvular disruption and inadequate valvular function are additional concerns in patients who have undergone annuloplasty or other types of valvuloplasty.

OPERATIVE RESULTS

The operative results of mitral valve replacement for mitral regurgitation are similar to those for mitral stenosis. The operative mortality, ranging between 5 and 10 per cent, depends in large part on the severity and duration of the mitral regurgitation and on the secondary myocardial and pulmonary effects. Symptomatic improvement has been very satisfactory, similar to that in patients with mitral stenosis, and the five-year mortality should be approximately 2 per cent per year.

Significant late recurrence of valvular dysfunction has been associated with annuloplasty and other types of valvuloplasty. Repeated stenosis or regurgitation occurs in significant numbers of patients in whom leaflet extension procedures have been performed, and regurgitation may occur after plication for ruptured chordae tendineae. In one well-conducted series of annuloplasties, significant mitral regurgitation developed in approximately 10 per cent of patients.[151] It is hoped that these problems will not occur with long-term follow-up of patients with the Carpentier ring.

TRICUSPID VALVULAR DISEASE

ETIOLOGY AND PATHOLOGY

Tricuspid stenosis is most commonly due to rheumatic heart disease. It occurs as a clinically significant lesion in 3 to 5 per cent of rheumatic patients.[7, 100] Women are affected four to five times more frequently than men, a female preponderance exceeding that of mitral stenosis. Patients are usually between 25 and 40 years of age. Rheumatic tricuspid stenosis is essentially always associated with rheumatic mitral valve disease, generally with severe mitral stenosis.[67, 164] The pathologic changes seen in the tricuspid valve are quite similar to those found in the mitral valve in rheumatic stenosis. Leaflets are thickened, fused, and rigid; chordae tendineae are shortened and fused. Obstructing vegetations of bacterial endocarditis occasionally cause tricuspid stenosis. The endocardial thickenings seen with carcinoid may result in either tricuspid stenosis or tricuspid regurgitation.[153]

In contrast, *tricuspid regurgitation* is much more likely to be functional. Normal tricuspid leaflets are barely large enough to effect valve closure. Muscular contraction of the tricuspid ring in systole is thus an important adjunct in complete closure of the valve. Consequently, right ventricular dilatation, from any cause, may easily result in displacement of papillary muscles and dilatation of the tricuspid ring, leading to regurgitation. Organic tricuspid regurgitation may result from rheumatic retraction of the leaflets or chordae tendineae, bacterial endocarditis, carcinoid,[153] or trauma.[142]

PHYSIOLOGY

The hemodynamic effects of both tricuspid stenosis and tricuspid regurgitation result in an increased systemic venous pressure and a reduced right ventricular output. The former is manifested by right atrial enlargement, distended neck veins, hepatic engorgement, and peripheral edema. In rheumatic heart disease, the low output of the right ventricle may have the effect of "protecting" the patient from paroxysms of pulmonary congestion by preventing abrupt increases in blood flow into the pulmonary circulation. The tricuspid lesions may also significantly contribute to the systemic manifestations of low cardiac output,

i.e., easy fatigability, weight loss, and hypotension. Thus, the recognition, quantitation, and appropriate correction of tricuspid valvular disease is important in the attainment of satisfactory hemodynamic results from operation for other valvular lesions.

CLINICAL FEATURES

The clinical manifestations are determined by the coexisting mitral or aortic valvular disease. Organic tricuspid disease should be suspected, however, in a female with severe disease of the mitral or aortic valve who is seen with long-standing venous stasis and who yet has been relatively spared from frequent pulmonary symptoms such as orthopnea and paroxysmal nocturnal dyspnea.[158] Gastrointestinal symptoms including anorexia, nausea, eructations, vomiting, and pain in the right upper abdominal quadrant result from splanchnic congestion and hepatic engorgement. Cardiac cachexia may be present.

The *physical findings* are frequently missed unless specifically searched for. Of great importance is the examination of the neck veins. In normal sinus rhythm, tricuspid stenosis may cause prominent presystolic A waves in the jugular venous pulse. They are more significant if seen in the absence of manifestations of pulmonary hypertension and right ventricular hypertrophy, which also can result in large A waves. The V wave occurring around the end of systole is not as prominent as the A wave, but the Y descent following it may be slow; this indicates obstruction to right atrial emptying. In addition to peripheral edema, elevated systemic venous pressure leads to hepatomegaly and may eventually result in cardiac cirrhosis with secondary ascites and splenomegaly. A protein-losing enteropathy with low albumin and globulin levels as well as a decreased number of circulating lymphocytes may be seen.[184] On auscultation, a diastolic murmur, often higher-pitched than the rumble of mitral stenosis,[24] may be heard at the left lower sternal border. Sometimes only a presystolic murmur is heard.[144] Augmentation by inspiration (Carvallo's sign) is an important feature, but sometimes is not present.[144] An opening snap may be heard, but it may not be easily distinguished from that of mitral stenosis.[144] In the presence of atrial fibrillation, the diagnosis of tricuspid stenosis may be very difficult owing to loss of the A wave and changes in the murmur.[164]

In tricuspid regurgitation, a large systolic wave merging with a tall V wave in the jugular venous pulse is a key feature. A rapid collapsing venous pulse (sharp Y descent) following the systolic wave argues against concomitant tricuspid stenosis, especially if the collapse is followed by a brisk rebound.[144] The systolic expansion may move the ear lobe and cause the liver to pulsate. The murmur of tricuspid regurgitation is a high-pitched, usually holosystolic murmur heard at the left lower sternal border and is often increased by inspiration. The intensity of the murmur is probably better correlated with right ventricular pressure than with the amount of regurgitation.[88] Presumably, the high pressure causes a higher velocity of flow and hence a more prominent murmur. In contrast, the murmur in severe tricuspid regurgitation with a normal right ventricular pressure, as might occur with a traumatic cause, is often very soft or may be absent.[142]

The major clue to tricuspid valvular disease on the *chest x-ray film* is enlargement of the right atrium (Fig. 17). With significant right atrial enlargement, the right lower cardiac contour bulges to the right, and its convexity is increased in the frontal view. In the right anterior oblique projection, there is a local prominence posteriorly just above the diaphragm. The superior vena cava may be widened and may be seen to pulsate on fluoroscopy.

On the *electrocardiogram*, right atrial enlargement, characterized by tall peaked P waves in leads II, III, aVF, and VI, is the best clue to tricuspid valvular disease. Usually, however, the electrocardiographic pattern is determined by the associated mitral or aortic valvular disease.

Cardiac catheterization is indicated in all patients suspected of having tricuspid valvular disease who are about to have other valvular surgery. Clinical assessment alone is often inaccurate. In one series,[179] significant tricuspid valvular disease was unsuspected preoperatively in one third of the patients who subsequently had an operative procedure on the tricuspid valve. Atrial fibrillation makes the clinical diagnosis of tricuspid stenosis even more difficult, as exemplified by a series in which the diagnosis was not made in 80 per cent of such patients until catheterization.[164] At catheterization, the relatively low right-sided pressures permit quite a low gradient across the tricuspid valve, even with moderately severe stenosis. Thus, the double-lumen catheter, which allows simultaneous right atrial and right ventricular pressure tracings, is necessary[164] (Fig. 18); pullback tracings are not adequate. Right ventricular angiography to detect tricuspid regurgitation may yield many false-positive studies but very few false-negative ones.[179] A prominent right atrial V wave may indicate tricuspid regurgitation. A normal or only slightly elevated pulmonary artery pressure is helpful in differentiating organic from functional tricuspid regurgitation, for the latter is unlikely if the pulmonary artery pressure is not significantly elevated.

INDICATIONS FOR OPERATION

The decision to correct significant tricuspid regurgitation is best made after correction of the left-sided lesions at operation. Most surgeons agree that operation on the tricuspid valve can be lifesaving in a patient with severe tricuspid regurgitation who is unable to maintain adequate circulation without the pump-oxygenator. On the other hand, how often functional tricuspid regurgitation of moderately severe degree requires correction is debated.[27, 179] For patients with infective endocarditis of the tricuspid valve, Arbulu et al.[4] have been examining the long-term merits of tricuspid valvulectomy without prosthetic replacement; because of the possibility of subsequent right heart failure, they may recommend insertion of a tricuspid prosthesis late after the infection has been cured by excision, but recognize the danger of this in patients who tend to have recurrent infection, such as drug addicts.[154]

In patients with quite significant tricuspid stenosis, correction at operation for associated mitral or aortic valvular disease seems reasonable.

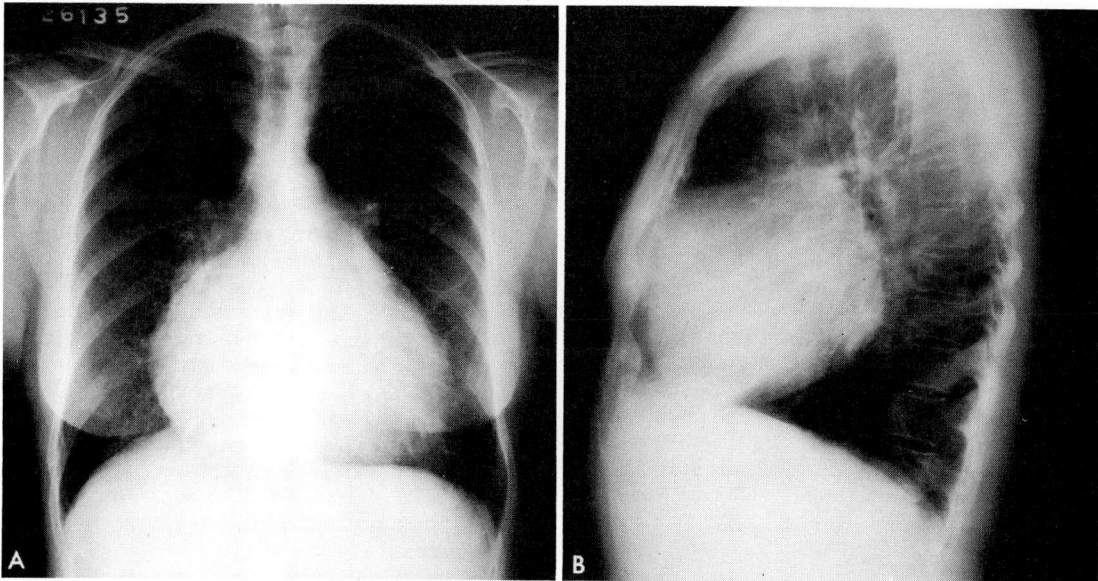

Figure 17. Classic roentgenograms of patient with tricuspid valvular disease. Right atrial enlargement is indicated by bulge of entire right heart contour extending to diaphragm on posteroanterior view (*A*). This finding superimposed on the changes of mitral stenosis, as indicated by evidence of pulmonary venous hypertension and left atrial enlargement (double contour on the right and elevation of left mainstem bronchus), indicates tricuspid valvular disease. Sharply angulated bulge into retrosternal space on lateral view (*B*) is probably large right atrial appendage.

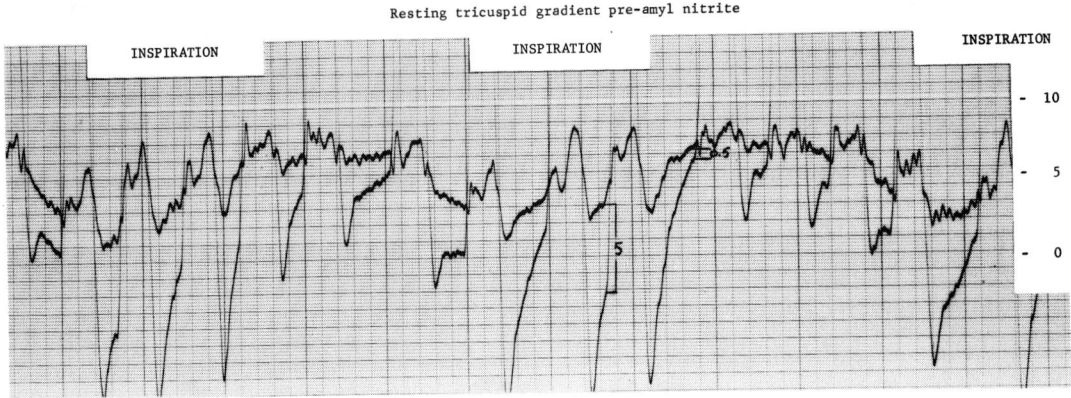

Resting tricuspid gradient pre-amyl nitrite

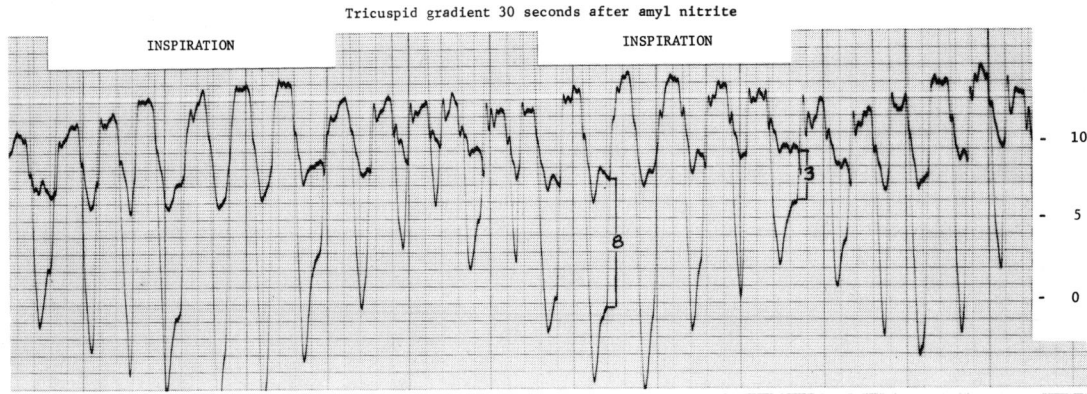

Tricuspid gradient 30 seconds after amyl nitrite

Figure 18. Typical cardiac catheterization findings in tricuspid stenosis: Simultaneous right atrial and right ventricular pressure tracings recorded through double-lumen catheter. Inspiration and amyl nitrite increase gradient by increasing venous return and hence flow across tricuspid valve. (From Sanders, C. A., Harthorne, J. W., DeSanctis, R. W., and Austen, W. G.: Circulation, 33:26, 1966. By permission of the American Heart Association, Inc.)

SURGICAL TREATMENT

Tricuspid valve surgery requires open techniques and cardiopulmonary bypass. Median sternotomy is usually employed because it allows the best exposure of the aortic, mitral, and tricuspid valves. If only the mitral and tricuspid valves are involved, a right anterolateral thoracotomy may occasionally be utilized. Cannulation and the other aspects of cardiopulmonary bypass have already been discussed. The tricuspid valve should be palpated through a right atrial purse-string suture before cardiopulmonary bypass is instituted to determine the degree of stenosis or regurgitation. If the tricuspid problem is functional regurgitation, the left-sided valvular lesions should first be corrected. Then cardiopulmonary bypass should usually be discontinued, and the surgeon should insert his finger again into the right atrium. If severe tricuspid regurgitation is still present, repair is required. Significant organic tricuspid stenosis or regurgitation is also an indication for tricuspid surgery.

Tricuspid Valve Replacement

In addition to the debate regarding the indications for corrective tricuspid valve surgery, there is argument concerning valve replacement versus annuloplasty or other valvuloplasty procedures. In general,

in patients with significant tricuspid malfunction, we believe that valve replacement is usually preferable. The right atrium is incised, and the tricuspid valve with its papillary muscle and chordae tendineae is removed. Because the bundle of His is in proximity to the septal leaflet, a rim of septal leaflet is preserved. Interrupted mattress or figure-of-eight sutures, with Teflon-felt buttressing if necessary, are placed around the circumference of the annulus and septal leaflet and then in the sewing ring of the valve substitute.

At present, we prefer the Starr-Edwards caged-ball prosthesis, but other types may be equally satisfactory. If a caged-ball valve is used, it is important to choose one that is not too large for the right ventricular cavity, since septal irritation and injury can occur if the prosthesis is too large. If a smaller valve is required, a low-profile caged-disc, eccentric-monocusp, or stented xenograft valve should be employed; some prefer these valves for all tricuspid valve replacements, partly because of the low pressures in the right side of the heart and the decreased force required for these valves to function.

Tricuspid Valvuloplasty

Various types of tricuspid valvuloplasty have been employed with different degrees of success. In the rare patient with relatively pure tricuspid stenosis, open valvuloplasty with incision of the fused commissures may be performed.[164] It is difficult to be sure of the exact location of all the commissures, and to avoid regurgitation it is usually best to incise just one or two of them. In the average-sized patient, an orifice size of more than 3 sq. cm. is probably satisfactory.

In patients with mixed organic disease or severe functional regurgitation, annuloplasty may be considered (in addition to incision of the commissures, if stenosis is also present). Traditionally, this procedure is difficult to perform, and enthusiasm for it is variable. Multiple mattress sutures are usually placed in the annulus at one or two commissures to decrease the annular size and to make the valve more competent. It is important that the annuloplasty not narrow the orifice too much, or significant stenosis may result. At the completion of the procedure, with cardiopulmonary bypass discontinued, the surgeon should palpate the valve with his finger through the right atrial wall. If there is significant tricuspid stenosis or regurgitation, valve replacement should be performed. Recent techniques of tricuspid annuloplasty, such as the methods of Carpentier and of De Vega, are enjoying early success.[74] It may well be that treatment with the Carpentier ring will represent a significant answer to this difficult problem.

EARLY POSTOPERATIVE COMPLICATIONS AND GENERAL POSTOPERATIVE CONSIDERATIONS

The postoperative complications and other considerations after tricuspid valve surgery are similar to those already discussed in association with mitral surgery. Patients with tricuspid valvular disease are usually sicker and undergo a more complicated operation involving repair of more than one valve. The most troublesome group are patients with pulmonary hypertension and severe functional tricuspid regurgitation. In addition to the complications already discussed in other sections of this chapter, patients undergoing tricuspid valve surgery may show evidence of postoperative hepatic failure because of long-standing high venous pressure secondary to the tricuspid valvular disease. Because of the high incidence of pulmonary hypertension and because most of these patients have severe, long-standing cardiac difficulties, prolonged respiratory support is usually necessary, and many patients require tracheostomy. Low cardiac output and cardiac failure are common, particularly if significant malfunction of the tricuspid valve is still present in the postoperative period, but also frequently when the tricuspid valve is functioning well. Cardiac arrhythmias and renal failure occur in a relatively high proportion of patients.

OPERATIVE RESULTS

Operative results depend on the other associated valvular lesions, the type of tricuspid valvular disease, and the degree of myocardial damage and secondary pulmonary effects. In patients with organic tricuspid valvular disease who undergo a satisfactory valvulo-plasty or valve replacement, the operative mortality is only slightly higher than that related to the operative procedure for the associated left-sided valvular problems, and is usually in the range of 5 to 15 per cent. In patients with significant functional tricuspid regurgitation, the long-standing severe cardiac disease and pulmonary hypertension result in a relatively higher operative mortality in the range of 20 to 25 per cent. Recurrence of tricuspid dysfunction may follow tricuspid valvuloplasty. Rarely, in patients with prosthetic valves, thrombosis of the prosthesis and pulmonary emboli may develop. In general, surviving patients do well, with considerable improvement in symptoms. Because of the multiple valve problems and secondary myocardial and pulmonary effects, the late mortality in this group of patients is somewhat higher than in patients with single mitral valve replacement.

ACKNOWLEDGMENT

The authors gratefully acknowledge the invaluable help and editorial advice of Catherine P. Fitzgerald.

REFERENCES

1. Akbarian, M., Austen, W. G., Yurchak, P. M., and Scannell, J. G.: Thromboembolic complications of prosthetic cardiac valves. Circulation, 37:826, 1968.
2. Amoury, R. A., Bowman, F. O., and Malm, J. R.: Endocarditis associated with intracardiac prostheses. Diagnosis, management and prophylaxis. J. Thorac. Cardiovasc. Surg., 51:36, 1966.
3. Amplatz, K.: The roentgenographic diagnosis of mitral and aortic valvular disease. Am. Heart J., 64:556, 1962.
4. Arbulu, A., Ganguly, S. N., and Robin, E.: Tricuspid valvulectomy without prosthetic replacement: Five years later. Surg. Forum, 26:244, 1975.
5. Aron, A. M., Freeman, J. M., and Carter, S.: The natural history of Sydenham's chorea: Review of the literature and long-term evaluation with emphasis on cardiac sequelae. Am. J. Med., 38:83, 1965.
6. Athanasuleas, C. L., Anagnostopoulos, C. E., and Kittle, C. F.: The autologous rectus sheath cardiac valve. III. Design and physical properties. J. Thorac. Cardiovasc. Surg., 65:118, 1973.
7. Auger, P., and Wigle, E. D.: Coarctation of the aorta associated with severe mitral insufficiency. Am. J. Cardiol., 21:190, 1968.
8. Austen, W. G., and Wooler, G. H.: The surgical treatment of mitral stenosis by the transventricular approach employing a mechanical dilator. N. Engl. J. Med., 263:661, 1960.
9. Bailey, C. P.: The surgical treatment of mitral stenosis (mitral commissurotomy). Dis. Chest, 15:377, 1949.
10. Bailey, C. P.: Surgery of the Heart. Philadelphia, Lea & Febiger, 1955.
11. Barlow, J. B., Bosman, C. K., Pocock, W. A., and Marchand, P.: Late systolic murmurs and non-ejection ("mid-late") systolic clicks: An analysis of 90 patients. Br. Heart J., 30:203, 1968.
12. Barnhorst, D. A., Oxman, H. A., Connolly, D. C., Pluth, J. R., Danielson, G. K., Wallace, R. B., and McGoon, D. C.: Long-term follow-up of isolated replacement of the aortic or mitral valve with the Starr-Edwards prosthesis. Am. J. Cardiol., 35:228, 1975.
13. Barratt-Boyes, B. G.: Homograft aortic valve replacement in aortic incompetence and stenosis. Thorax, 19:131, 1964.
14. Beall, A. C., Jr., Bloodwell, R. D., Liotta, D., Cooley, D. A., and DeBakey, M. E.: Clinical experience with Dacron velour covered Teflon disc mitral prostheses. Ann. Thorac. Surg., 5:402, 1968.
15. Beall, A. C., Jr., Morris, G. C., Jr., Howell, J. F., Jr., Guinn, G.

A., Noon, G. P., Reul, G. J., Jr., Greenberg, J. J., and Ankeney, J. L.: Clinical experience with an improved mitral valve prosthesis. Ann. Thorac. Surg., 15:601, 1973.

16. Beller, B. M., Frates, R. W. M., and Wulfsohn, N.: Cardiac pacemaking in the management of postoperative arrhythmias. Ann. Thorac. Surg., 6:68, 1968.

17. Bendixen, H. H., Egbert, L. D., Hedley-Whyte, J., Laver, M. B., and Pontoppidan, H.: Respiratory Care. St. Louis, The C. V. Mosby Co., 1965.

18. Biggers, J. T., Schmidt, D. H., and Kutt, H.: Relationship between the plasma level of diphenylhydantoin sodium and its cardiac antiarrhythmic effects. Circulation, 38:363, 1968.

19. Björk, V. O.: A new tilting disc valve prosthesis. Scand. J. Thorac. Cardiovasc. Surg., 3:1, 1969.

20. Björk, V. O., Böök, K., and Holmgren, A.: The Björk-Shiley mitral valve prosthesis: A comparative study with different prosthesis orientations. Ann. Thorac. Surg., 18:379, 1974.

21. Block, P. C., DeSanctis, R. W., Weinberg, A. N., and Austen, W. G.: Prosthetic valve endocarditis. J. Thorac. Cardiovasc. Surg., 60:540, 1970.

22. Bonchek, L. I., and Starr, A.: Ball valve prostheses: Current appraisal of late results. Am. J. Cardiol., 35:843, 1975.

23. BonTempo, C. P., Roman, J. A., Jr., deLeon, A. C., Jr., and Twigg, H. L.: Radiographic appearance of the thorax in systolic click–late systolic murmur syndrome. Am. J. Cardiol., 36:27, 1975.

24. Bousvaros, G. A., and Stubington, D.: Some auscultatory and phonocardiographic features of tricuspid stenosis. Circulation, 29:26, 1964.

25. Braunwald, E.: Mitral regurgitation: Physiologic, clinical and surgical considerations. N. Engl. J. Med., 281:425, 1969.

26. Braunwald, E., Braunwald, N., Ross, J., Jr., and Morrow, A. G.: Effects of mitral valve replacement on the pulmonary vascular dynamics of patients with pulmonary hypertension. N. Engl. J. Med., 273:509, 1965.

27. Braunwald, N. S., Ross, J., Jr., and Morrow, A. G.: Conservative management of tricuspid regurgitation in patients undergoing mitral valve replacement. Circulation (Suppl. 1), 35:63, 1967.

28. Brawley, R. K., Donahoo, J. S., and Gott, V. L.: Current status of the Beall, Björk-Shiley, Braunwald-Cutter, Lillehei-Kaster and Smeloff-Cutter cardiac valve prostheses. Am. J. Cardiol., 35:855, 1975.

29. Bristow, J. D., and Kremkau, E. L.: Hemodynamic changes after valve replacement with Starr-Edwards prostheses. Am. J. Cardiol., 35:716, 1975.

30. Brock, R. C., and Campbell, M.: Discussion on surgery of the heart and great vessels. Proc. R. Soc. Med., 44:995, 1951.

31. Brody, W., and Criley, J. M.: Intermittent severe mitral regurgitation. N. Engl. J. Med., 283:673, 1970.

32. Brunton, L.: Preliminary note on the possibility of treating mitral stenosis by surgical methods. Lancet, 1:352, 1902; Surgical operation for mitral stenosis. Lancet, 1:547, 1902.

33. Buch, W. S., Kosek, J. C., Angell, W. W., et al.: Deterioration of formalin-treated aortic valve heterografts. J. Thorac. Cardiovasc. Surg., 60:673, 1970.

34. Burch, G. E., DePasquale, N. P., and Phillips, J. H.: The syndrome of papillary muscle dysfunction. Am. Heart J., 75:399, 1968.

35. Burgess, J., Clark, R., Kamigaki, M., and Cohn, K.: Echocardiographic findings in different types of mitral regurgitation. Circulation, 48:97, 1973.

36. Carpentier, A., Deloche, A., Dauptain, J., Soyer, R., Blondeau, P., Piwnica, A., and Dubost, C.: A new reconstructive operation for correction of mitral and tricuspid insufficiency. J. Thorac. Cardiovasc. Surg., 61:1, 1971.

37. Carpentier, A., and Dubost, C.: From xenograft to bioprothesis: Evolution of concepts and techniques of valvular xenografts. In Ionescu, M. I., Ross, D. N., and Wooler, G. H. (Eds.): Biological Tissue in Heart Valve Replacement. London, Butterworths, 1972, p. 515.

38. Carpentier, A., Lemaigre, G., Robert, L., Carpentier, S., and Dubost, C.: Biological factors affecting long-term results of valvular heterografts. J. Thorac. Cardiovasc. Surg., 58:467, 1969.

39. Caulfield, J. B., Page, D. L., Kastor, J. A., and Sanders, C. A.: Dissolution of connective tissue in ruptured chordae tendineae. Circulation, 40(Suppl.):111, 1969.

40. Cheng, T. O.: Some new observations on the syndrome of papillary muscle dysfunction. Am. J. Med., 47:924, 1969.

41. Cohn, L. H., and Collins, J. J., Jr.: Life-table comparison of Han-

cock porcine and prosthetic disc valves for isolated mitral valve replacement. (Abstract) Circulation, 51 and 52 (Suppl. 2):30, 1975.

42. Cournand, A., and Ranges, H. A.: Catheterization of right auricle in man. Proc. Soc. Exp. Biol. Med., 46:462, 1941.

43. Cutler, E. C., and Levine, S. A.: Cardiotomy and valvulotomy for mitral stenosis. Boston Med. Surg. J., 188:1023, 1923.

44. Daley, R., Mattingly, T. W., Holt, C. L., Bland, E. F., and White, P. D.: Systemic arterial embolism in rheumatic heart disease. Am. Heart J., 42:566, 1951.

45. Dalichau, H., Gonzalez-Lavin, L., and Ross, D. N.: Autologous fascia lata transplantation for heart valve replacement: A two-year experience at the National Heart Hospital, London. Thorax, 27:18, 1972.

46. DeBusk, R. F., and Harrison, D. C.: The clinical spectrum of papillary muscle disease. N. Engl. J. Med., 281:1458, 1969.

47. Delman, A. J., Robinson, G., Stein, E., Yahr, W., and Lister, J. W.: Precise determination of cardiac arrhythmias during open heart surgery by monitoring of myocardial electrograms. Am. J. Cardiol., 21:714, 1968.

48. DeMaria, A. N., King, J. F., Bogren, H. G., Lies, J. F., and Maron, D. T.: The variable spectrum of echocardiographic manifestations of the mitral valve prolapse syndrome. Circulation, 50:33, 1974.

49. Dexter, C., Dow, J. W., Haynes, F. W., Whittenberger, J. L., Ferris, B. G., Goodale, W. T., and Hellems, H. K.: Studies of the pulmonary circulation at rest. Normal variations and the interrelations between increased pulmonary blood flow, elevated pulmonary arterial pressure and high pulmonary "capillary" pressure. J. Clin. Invest., 29:602, 1950.

50. Dietzman, R. H., Motsay, G. J., and Lillehei, R. C.: Drugs in the treatment of shock. Pharmacol. Physicians, 4:1, 1970.

51. Dinsmore, R. E., Sanders, C. A., and Harthorne, J. W.: Mitral regurgitation in idiopathic hypertrophic subaortic stenosis. N. Engl. J. Med., 275:1225, 1966.

52. Duchak, J. M., Jr., Chang, S., and Feigenbaum, H.: The posterior mitral valve echo and the echocardiographic diagnosis of mitral stenosis. Am. J. Cardiol., 29:628, 1972.

53. Duvoisin, G. E., Brandenburg, R. O., and Ellis, F. H., Jr.: Mitral valve replacement with a full-orifice ball valve: Experience with 108 operations. In Brewer, L. A., III (Ed.): Prosthetic Heart Valves. Springfield, Ill., Charles C Thomas, Publisher, 1969, p. 541.

54. Edwards, W. S.: Late results with autogenous tissue heart valves. J. Cardiovasc. Surg., 13:276, 1972.

55. Fadali, A. M., Ramos, M. D., Topaz, S. R., and Gott, V. L.: The use of autogenous peritoneum for heart valve replacement. J. Thorac. Cardiovasc. Surg., 60:188, 1970.

56. Feigenbaum, H.: Mitral valve. In Echocardiography. Philadelphia, Lea & Febiger, 1972, p. 43.

57. Fetterolf, G., and Norris, G. W.: The anatomical explanation of the paralysis of the left recurrent laryngeal nerve found in certain cases of mitral stenosis. Am. J. Med. Sci., 141:625, 1911.

58. Fishman, N. H., Hutchinson, J. C., and Roe, B. B.: Controlled atrial hypertension: A method for supporting cardiac output following open heart surgery. J. Thorac. Cardiovasc. Surg., 52:777, 1966.

59. Forssmann, W.: Ueber Kontrastdarstellung der Höhlen des labenden richten Herzens und der Lungen schlagader. Munch. Med. Wochenschr., 78:489, 1931.

60. Friedberg, C. K.: Acute pericarditis. In Diseases of the Heart, 3rd ed. Philadelphia, W. B. Saunders Company, 1966, p. 933.

61. Friedberg, C. K.: Tricuspid and pulmonic valvular disease. In Diseases of the Heart, 3rd ed. Philadelphia, W. B. Saunders Company, 1966, p. 1162.

62. Friedberg, C. K.: Surgical procedures in the cardiac patient. In Diseases of the Heart, 3rd ed. Philadelphia, W. B. Saunders Company, 1966, p. 1746.

63. Gans, H., and Krivit, W.: Problems in hemostasis during open heart surgery. III. Epsilon amino caproic acid as an inhibitor of plasminogen activator activity. Ann. Surg., 155:268, 1962.

64. Gerami, S., Messmer, B. J., Hallman, G. L., and Cooley, D. A.: Open mitral commissurotomy: Results of 100 consecutive cases. J. Thorac. Cardiovasc. Surg., 62:366, 1971.

65. Gerbode, F.: Transventricular mitral valvulotomy. Circulation, 21:563, 1960.

66. Gibbon, J. H., Jr.: Application of mechanical heart and lung apparatus to cardiac surgery. Minnesota Med., 37:171, 185, 1954.

67. Gibson, R., and Wood, P.: The diagnosis of tricuspid stenosis. Br. Heart J., 17:552, 1955.
68. Gold, H., and Hertz, L.: Death caused by fracture of Beall mitral prosthesis: Report of a case. Am. J. Cardiol., 34:371, 1974.
69. Goodwin, J. F.: Diagnosis of left atrial myxoma. Lancet, 1:464, 1963.
70. Goodwin, J. F., Hunter, J. D., Cleland, W. P., Davis, L. G., and Steiner, R. E.: Mitral valve disease and mitral valvotomy. Br. Med. J., 2:573, 1955.
71. Gorlin, R., and Gorlin, S. G.: Hydraulic formula for calculation of the area of the stenotic mitral valve, other cardiac valves, and central circulatory shunts. Am. Heart J., 41:1, 1951.
72. Gorlin, R., Lewis, B. M., Haynes, F. W., Spiegl, R. J., and Dexter, L.: Factors regulating pulmonary "capillary" pressure in mitral stenosis. Am. Heart J., 41:834, 1951.
73. Grismer, J. T., Levy, M. J., Lillehei, R. C., Indeglia, R., and Lillehei, C. W.: Renal function in acquired valvular heart disease and effects of extracorporeal circulation. Surgery, 55:24, 1964.
74. Grondin, P., Meere, C., Limet, R., Lopez-Bescos, L., Delcan, J.-L., and Rivera, R.: Carpentier's annulus and De Vega's annuloplasty: The end of the tricuspid challenge. J. Thorac. Cardiovasc. Surg., 70:852, 1975.
75. Hancock, E. W., and Cohn, K.: The syndrome associated with mid-systolic click and late systolic murmur. Am. J. Med., 41:183, 1966.
76. Harken, D. E., Ellis, L. B., Ware, P. F., and Norman, L. R.: The surgical treatment of mitral stenosis. N. Engl. J. Med., 239:802, 1948.
77. Harrison, D. C., Sprouse, J. H., and Morrow, A. G.: The antiarrhythmic properties of lidocaine and procaine amide. Circulation, 28:486, 1963.
78. Harthorne, J. W., Seltzer, R. A., and Austen, W. G.: Left atrial calcification: Review of the literature and proposed management. Circulation, 34:198, 1966.
79. Heikkila, J.: Mitral incompetence as a complication of acute myocardial infarction. Acta Med. Scand., Suppl., 475, 1967.
80. Heimbecker, R. O., Baird, R. J., Lajos, T. Z., Varga, A. T., and Greenwood, W. F.: Homograft replacement of the human mitral valve: A preliminary report. Can. Med. Assoc. J., 86:805, 1962.
81. Hildner, F. J., Javier, R. P., Cohen, L. S., Samet, P., Nathan, M. J., Yahr, W. Z., and Greenberg, J. J.: Myocardial dysfunction associated with valvular heart disease. Am. J. Cardiol., 30:319, 1972.
82. Hodam, R., Anderson, R., Starr, A., Wood, J., Dobbs, J., and Raible, D.: Further evaluation of the composite seat cloth-covered aortic prosthesis. Presented at the Society of Thoracic Surgeons, Dallas, Texas, 1971.
83. Hodam, R., Starr, A., Herr, R., et al.: Early clinical experience with cloth-covered valvular prostheses. Ann. Surg., 170:471, 1969.
84. Horowitz, M. S., Goodman, D. J., Fogarty, T. J., and Harrison, D. C.: Mitral valve replacement with the glutaraldehyde-preserved porcine heterograft: Clinical, hemodynamic, and pathological correlations. J. Thorac. Cardiovasc. Surg., 67:885, 1974.
85. Horsley, H. T., Jr., Rappoport, W. J., Vigoda, P. S., and Vogel, J. H. K.: Fatal malfunction of Edwards low-profile mitral valve. Circulation, Suppl., 40:111, 1969.
86. Hugenholtz, P. G., Ryan, T. H., Stein, S. W., and Abelman, W. H.: The spectrum of pure mitral stenosis: Hemodynamic studies in relation to clinical disability. Am. J. Cardiol., 10:773, 1962.
87. Hurst, J. W., and Logue, R. B.: Common diseases of the heart: Systemic tension in the heart. In The Heart, 2nd ed. New York, McGraw-Hill Book Company, 1970, p. 773.
88. Hurst, J. W., and Logue, R. B.: Less common diseases of the heart. In The Heart, 2nd ed. New York, McGraw-Hill Book Company, 1970, p. 863.
89. Hutter, A. M., Jr., Dinsmore, R. E., Willerson, J. T., and DeSanctis, R. W.: Early systolic clicks due to mitral valve prolapse. Circulation, 44:516, 1971.
90. Ionescu, M. I., Pakrashi, B. C., Mary, D. A. S., Bartek, I. T., and Wooler, G. H.: Long-term evaluation of tissue valves. J. Thorac. Cardiovasc. Surg., 68:361, 1974.
91. Ionescu, M. I., and Ross, D. N.: Heart-valve replacement with autologous fascia lata. Lancet, 1:355, 1969.
92. Ionescu, M. I., Wooler, G. H., Smith, D. R., and Grimshaw, V. A.: Mitral valve replacement with aortic heterografts in humans. Thorax, 22:305, 1967.
93. James, T. N.: Anatomy of coronary arteries in health and disease. Circulation, 32:1020, 1965.
94. Johnson, A. D., Daily, P. O., Peterson, K. L., LeWinter, M., DiDonna, G. J., Blair, G., and Niwayama, G.: Functional evaluation of the porcine heterograft in the mitral position. Circulation, 50 and 51 (Suppl. 1):40, 1975.
95. Jordan, S. C.: Development of pulmonary hypertension in mitral stenosis. Lancet, 2:322, 1965.
96. Karliner, J. S.: Intravenous diphenylhydantoin sodium (Dilantin) in cardiac arrhythmias. Dis. Chest, 51:256, 1967.
97. Kay, J. H., and Egerton, W. S.: The repair of mitral insufficiency associated with ruptured chordae tendineae. Ann. Surg., 157:351, 1963.
98. Kay, J. H., Tsuji, H. K., Redington, J. V., Mendes, A., Saji, K., Kamata, K., Yokoyama, T., Magidson, O., and Krohn, B.: Experiences with the Kay-Shiley disc valve. In Brewer, L. A., III (Ed.): Prosthetic Heart Valves. Springfield, Ill., Charles C Thomas, Publisher, 1969, p. 609.
99. Kiser, I. O., Hoeksema, T. D., Connolly, D. C., and Ellis, F. H., Jr.: Long-term results of closed mitral commissurotomy. J. Cardiovasc. Surg., 8:263, 1967.
100. Kitchin, A., and Turner, R.: Diagnosis and treatment of tricuspid stenosis. Br. Heart J., 26:354, 1964.
101. Kloster, F. E., Herr, R. H., Starr, A., et al.: Hemodynamic evaluation of a cloth-covered Starr-Edwards valve prosthesis. Circulation (Suppl. 1), 39:119, 1969.
102. Koch-Weser, J., Klein, S. W., Foo-Cantu, L., Kastor, J. A., and DeSanctis, R. W.: Antiarrhythmic prophylaxis with procainamide in acute myocardial infarction. N. Engl. J. Med., 281:1253, 1969.
103. Korn, D., DeSanctis, R. W., and Sell, S.: Massive calcification of the mitral annulus: A clinicopathological study of fourteen cases. N. Engl. J. Med., 267:900, 1962.
104. Kosek, J. C., Iben, A. B., Shumway, N. E., and Angell, W. W.: Morphology of fresh heart valve homografts. Surgery, 66:269, 1969.
105. Lang, D. L., Scolnick, E. M., and Willerson, J. T.: Association of cytomegalovirus infection with the postperfusion syndrome. N. Engl. J. Med., 278:1147, 1968.
106. Lavender, J. P., Doppman, J., Shawdon, H., and Steiner, R. E.: Pulmonary veins in left ventricular failure and mitral stenosis. Br. J. Radiol., 35:293, 1962.
107. Leatham, A.: Auscultation of the heart. Lancet, 2:703, 757, 1958.
108. Levinson, G. E., Schwartz, C. J., and Frank, M. J.: The effect of rest on the volume burden of mitral and aortic regurgitation. Clin. Res., 16:238, 1968.
109. Levisman, J. A., Abbasi, A. S., and Pearce, M. L.: Posterior mitral leaflet motion in mitral stenosis. Circulation, 51:511, 1975.
110. Levy, M., and Edwards, J.: Anatomy of mitral insufficiency. Progr. Cardiovasc. Dis., 5:119, 1962.
111. Lewis, B. M., Gorlin, R., Houssay, H. E. J., Haynes, F. W., and Dexter, L.: Clinical and physiological correlations in patients with mitral stenosis. Am. Heart J., 43:2, 1952.
112. Lillehei, C. W., Kaster, R. L., Starek, P. J., Block, J. H., and Rees, J. R.: A new central flow pivoting disc aortic and mitral prosthesis: Initial clinical experience. Am. J. Cardiol., 26:688, 1970.
113. Lillehei, C. W., Levy, M. J., and Bonnabeau, R. C., Jr.: Mitral valve replacement with preservation of papillary muscles and chordae tendineae. J. Thorac. Cardiovasc. Surg., 47:532, 1964.
114. Links, E., and Sysimetsa, E.: Clinical and radiological aspects of calcification of the mitral valve. Br. Heart J., 20:329, 1958.
115. Logan, A., and Turner, R.: Surgical treatment of mitral stenosis with particular reference to the transventricular approach with a mechanical dilator. Lancet, 2:874, 1959.
116. Lower, R. R.: Laboratory observations on homograft and autograft valve replacement. In Ionescu, M. I., Ross, D. N., and Wooler, G. H. (Eds.): Biological Tissue in Heart Valve Replacement. London, Butterworths, 1972, p. 125.
117. Lunger, M., Abelson, D. S., Elkind, A. H., and Kantrowitz, A.: Massive hemoptysis in mitral stenosis: Control by emergency commissurotomy. N. Engl. J. Med., 261:393, 1959.
118. MacLeon, L. D.: Venous pressure versus blood volume. Surg. Gynecol. Obstet., 118:594, 1964.
119. MacVaugh, H., III, Joyner, C. R., and Johnson, J.: Unusual complications during mitral valve replacement in presence of calcification of the annulus. Ann. Thorac. Surg., 11:336, 1971.

120. Malm, J. R., Bowman, F. O., Jr., Harris, P. D., and Kowalik, A. T. W.: Evaluation of aortic valve homografts sterilized by electron beam energy. J. Thorac. Cardiovasc. Surg., 54:471, 1967.

121. Manchester, G. H., Block, P., and Gorlin, R.: Misleading signs in mitral insufficiency. J.A.M.A., 191:87, 1965.

122. McEnany, M. T., Ross, D. N., and Yates, A. K.: Valve failure in seventy-two frame-supported autologous fascia lata mitral valves: Two-year follow-up. J. Thorac. Cardiovasc. Surg., 63:199, 1972.

123. McGoon, D. C.: Repair of mitral insufficiency due to ruptured chordae tendineae. J. Thorac. Surg., 39:357, 1960.

124. McIntosh, C. L., Michaelis, L. L., Morrow, A. G., Itscoitz, S. B., Redwood, D. R., and Epstein, S. E.: Atrioventricular valve replacement with the Hancock porcine xenograft: A five year clinical experience. Surgery, 78:768, 1975.

125. McLaughlin, J. S., Cowley, R. A., Smith, G., and Matheson, N. A.: Mitral valve disease from blunt trauma. J. Thorac. Cardiovasc. Surg., 48:261, 1964.

126. Morris, J. J., Jr., Estes, E. H., Whalen, R. E., Thompson, H. K., Jr., and McIntosh, H. D.: P-wave analysis in valvular heart disease. Circulation, 29:242, 1964.

127. Morrow, A. G., Oldham, H. N., Elkins, R. C., and Braunwald, E.: Prosthetic replacement of the mitral valve. Preoperative and postoperative clinical and hemodynamic assessments in 100 patients. Circulation, 35:962, 1967.

128. Mounsey, P.: Tricuspid incompetence following successful mitral valvulotomy. Br. Heart J., 21:123, 1959.

129. Murray, G.: Homologous aortic valve segment transplants as surgical treatment for aortic and mitral insufficiency. Angiology, 7:446, 1956.

130. Murray, G., Wilkinson, F. R., and MacKenzie, R.: Reconstruction of the valves of the heart. Can. Med. Assoc. J., 38:317, 1938.

131. Nanda, N. C., Gramiak, R., Shah, P. M., and DeWeese, J. A.: Mitral commissurotomy versus replacement: Preoperative evaluation by echocardiography. Circulation, 51:263, 1975.

132. Nathaniels, E. K., Moncure, A. C., and Scannell, J. G.: A fifteen-year follow-up study of closed mitral valvuloplasty. Ann. Thorac. Surg., 10:27, 1970.

133. Nelson, R. M., Jenson, C. B., Peterson, C. A., and Sanders, B. C.: Effective use of prophylactic antibiotics in open heart surgery. Arch. Surg., 90:731, 1965.

134. Nexlin, V. E., and Shamesova, L. C.: Infarction of papillary muscles: Clinical and anatomico-pathologic observations. (In Russian.) Klin. Med. (Moskva), 29:51, 1951.

135. Nichols, H. T., Blanco, G., Morse, D. P., Adam, A., and Baltazar, N.: Open mitral commissurotomy: Experience with 200 consecutive cases. J.A.M.A., 182:268, 1962.

136. Nixon, P. G. F., Wooler, G. H., and Radigan, L. R.: Mitral incompetence caused by lesions of the mural cusp. Circulation, 19:839, 1959.

137. Norman, J. C., McDonald, H. P., and Sloan, J.: The early and aggressive treatment of acute renal failure following cardiopulmonary bypass with continuous peritoneal dialysis. Surgery, 56:1, 1964.

138. O'Brien, M. F., and Clarebrough, J. K.: Heterograft aortic valves for human valve disease. Am. Heart J., 74:135, 1967.

139. O'Brien, M. F., Clarebrough, J. K., McDonald, I. G., Hale, G. S., Bray, H. S., and Cade, J. I.: Heterograft aortic valve replacement. Mitral follow-up studies. Thorax, 22:387, 1967.

140. Oh, W., Somerville, J., Ross, D. N., Ross, K. J., and Emanuel, R.: Mitral valve replacement with preserved cadaveric aortic homografts. J. Thorac. Cardiovasc. Surg., 65:712, 1973.

141. Olinger, G. N., Rio, F. W., and Maloney, J. V., Jr.: Closed valvulotomy for calcific mitral stenosis. J. Thorac. Cardiovasc. Surg., 62:357, 1971.

142. Osborn, J. R., Jones, R. C., and Jahnke, E. J., Jr.: Traumatic tricuspid insufficiency. Hemodynamic data and surgical treatment. Circulation, 30:217, 1964.

143. Oxman, H. A., Connolly, D. C., and Ellis, F. H., Jr.: Mitral valve replacement with the Smeloff-Cutter prosthesis: Experience with 154 patients and comparison with results of replacement with a Starr-Edwards prosthesis. J. Thorac. Cardiovasc. Surg., 69:247, 1975.

144. Perloff, J. K., and Harvey, W. P.: Clinical recognition of tricuspid stenosis. Circulation, 22:346, 1960.

145. Peter, R. H., Gracey, J. G., and Beach, T. B.: Significance of fibrillatory waves and the P terminal force in idiopathic atrial fibrillation. Ann. Intern. Med., 68:1296, 1968.

146. Phillips, J. H., Burch, G. E., and DePasquale, N. P.: The syndrome of papillary muscle dysfunction. Ann. Intern. Med., 59:508, 1963.

147. Pluth, J. R., Broadbent, J. C., Barnhorst, D. A., and Danielson, G. K.: Aortic and mitral valve replacement with cloth-covered Braunwald-Cutter prosthesis: A three-year follow-up. Ann. Thorac. Surg., 20:239, 1975.

148. Pocock, W. A., and Baslow, J. B.: Etiology and electrocardiographic features of the billowing posterior mitral leaflet syndrome. Am. J. Cardiol., 51:731, 1971.

149. Popp, R. L., Brown, O. R., Sliverman, J. F., and Harrison, D. C.: The echocardiographic abnormalities in the mitral valve prolapse syndrome. Circulation, 49:428, 1974.

150. Raftery, E. B., Oakley, C. M., and Goodwin, J. F.: Acute subvalvular mitral incompetence. Lancet, 2:360, 1966.

151. Reed, G. E., Clauss, R. H., and Spencer, F. C.: Controversy between replacement and repair of the mitral valve. In Brewer, L. A., III (Ed.): Prosthetic Heart Valves. Springfield, Ill., Charles C Thomas, Publisher, 1969, p. 458.

152. Roberts, W. C., Braunwald, E., and Morrow, A. G.: Acute severe mitral regurgitation secondary to ruptured chordae tendineae: Clinical, hemodynamic, and pathologic considerations. Circulation, 33:58, 1966.

153. Roberts, W. C., and Sjoersma, A.: The cardiac disease associated with the carcinoid syndrome (carcinoid heart disease). Am. J. Med., 36:5, 1964.

154. Robin, E., Thoms, N. W., Arbulu, A., Ganguly, S. N., and Magnisalis, K.: Hemodynamic consequences of total removal of the tricuspid valve without prosthetic replacement. Am. J. Cardiol., 35:481, 1975.

155. Ross, D. N.: Homotransplantation of the aortic valve in the subcoronary position. J. Thorac. Surg., 47:713, 1964.

156. Ross, J. K., and Johnson, D. C.: Mitral valve replacement with homograft, fascia lata and prosthetic valves: A long-term assessment of valve function. J. Cardiovasc. Surg., 15:242, 1974.

157. Rubin, J. W., Ellison, R. G., Moore, V., Harp, R. J., and Hitch, W. S.: Twelve-year experience with mitral valve replacement. Ann. Thorac. Surg., 19:659, 1975.

158. Salazar, E., and Levine, H. D.: Rheumatic tricuspid regurgitation. The clinical spectrum. Am. J. Med., 33:111, 1962.

159. Salomon, J., Shah, P. M., and Heinle, R. A.: Thoracic akeletal abnormalities in idiopathic mitral valve prolapse. Am. J. Cardiol., 36:32, 1975.

160. Salzman, E. W., and Britten, A.: Hemorrhage and Thrombosis. Boston, Little, Brown and Company, 1965.

161. Sanders, C. A., Armstrong, P. W., Willerson, J. T., and Dinsmore, R. E.: The etiology and differential diagnosis of acute mitral regurgitation. Progr. Cardiovasc. Dis., 14:129, 1971.

162. Sanders, C. A., Austen, W. G., Harthorne, J. W., Dinsmore, R. E., and Scannell, J. G.: Diagnosis and surgical treatment of mitral regurgitation secondary to ruptured chordae tendineae. N. Engl. J. Med., 276:943, 1967.

163. Sanders, C. A., Buckley, M. J., Leinbach, R. C., Mundth, E. D., and Austen, W. G.: Mechanical circulatory assistance: Current status and experience with combining circulatory assistance, emergency coronary angiography and acute myocardial revascularization. Circulation, 45:1292, 1972.

164. Sanders, C. A., Harthorne, J. W., DeSanctis, R. W., and Austen, W. G.: Tricuspid stenosis: A difficult diagnosis in the presence of atrial fibrillation. Circulation, 33:26, 1966.

165. Sanders, C. A., Scannell, J. G., Harthorne, J. W., and Austen, W. G.: Severe mitral regurgitation secondary to ruptured chordae tendineae. Circulation, 31:506, 1965.

166. Sanders, R. J., and Neubuerger, K. T.: Rupture of the papillary muscles. Occurrence of rupture of the posterior muscle in posterior myocardial infarction. Dis. Chest, 31:316, 1957.

167. Selzer, A., and Cohn, K. E.: Natural history of mitral stenosis: A review. Circulation, 45:878, 1972.

168. Selzer, A., Kelly, J. J., Jr., Vannitamby, M., Walker, P., Gerbode, F., and Kerth, W. J.: The syndrome of mitral insufficiency due to isolated rupture of the chordae tendineae. Am. J. Med., 43:822, 1967.

169. Semer, H., Hultgren, H., Kleiger, R., and Braniff, B.: Cardioversion following prosthetic mitral valve replacement. Circulation, 35:523, 1967.

170. Semler, H. J., and Pruett, R. D.: An electrocardiographic estimation of pulmonary vascular obstruction in 80 patients with mitral stenosis. Am. Heart J., 59:541, 1960.

171. Senning, A.: Fascia lata replacement of aortic valves. J. Thorac. Cardiovasc. Surg., 48:346, 1964.

172. Shanks, S. C., and Kerley, P.: A Text-book of X-ray Diagnosis, 3rd ed. Vol. 2. Philadelphia, W. B. Saunders Company, 1962.

173. Silver, M. D., Hudson, R. E. B., and Trimble, A. S.: Morphologic observations on heart valve prostheses made of fascia lata. J. Thorac. Cardiovasc. Surg., 70:360, 1975.

174. Souttar, H. S.: Surgical treatment of mitral stenosis. Br. Med. J., 2:603, 1925.

175. Starek, P. J. K., McLaurin, L. P., Wilcox, B. R., and Murray, G. F.: Clinical evaluation of the Lillehei-Kaster pivoting disc valve. (Abstract) Program of the 12th Annual Meeting of the Society of Thoracic Surgeons, 1976, p. 14.

176. Starek, P. J. K., Wilcox, B. R., and Murray, G. F.: Hemodynamic evaluation of the Lillehei-Kaster pivoting disc valve in patients. J. Thorac. Cardiovasc. Surg., 71:123, 1976.

177. Starr, A.: Mitral valve replacement with ball valve prostheses. Br. Heart J., Suppl. 33, 1971, p. 47.

178. Starr, A., and Edwards, M. L.: Mitral replacement: Clinical experience with a ball-valve prosthesis. Ann. Surg., 154:726, 1961.

179. Starr, A., Herr, R., and Wood, J.: Tricuspid valve replacement for acquired valve disease. Surg. Gynecol. Obstet., 122:1295, 1966.

180. Starr, A., Herr, R. W., and Wood, J. A.: Mitral replacement: Review of six years' experience. J. Thorac. Cardiovasc. Surg., 54:333, 1967.

181. Starr, A., Okies, E., Lambert, L., and Grunkemeier, G.: Mitral valve replacement: An appraisal at ten years of non-cloth covered vs. cloth-covered caged ball prostheses. (Abstract) Circulation, 51 and 52 (Suppl. 2):30, 1975.

182. Stinson, E. B., Griepp, R. B., Bieber, C. P., and Shumway, N. E.: Aortic valve allografts for mitral valve replacement. Surgery, 77:861, 1975.

183. Stinson, E. B., Griepp, R. B., and Shumway, N. E.: Clinical experience with a porcine aortic valve xenograft for mitral valve replacement. Ann. Thorac. Surg., 18:391, 1974.

184. Strober, W., Cohen, L. S., Waldman, T. A., and Braunwald, E.: Tricuspid regurgitation: A newly recognized cause of protein-losing enteropathy, lymphocytopenia, and immunologic deficiency. Am. J. Med., 44:842, 1968.

185. Sullivan, J. M., Harkins, D. E., and Gorlin, R.: Pharmacologic control of thrombo-embolic complications of cardiac valve replacement. N. Engl. J. Med., 284:1391, 1971.

186. Sweatman, T., Selzer, A., Kamagaki, M., and Cohn, K.: Echocardiographic diagnosis of mitral regurgitation due to ruptured chordae tendineae. Circulation, 46:580, 1972.

187. Wada, J.: Knotless suture method and Wada hingeless valve. Jap. J. Thorac. Surg., 15:88, 1966.

188. Watson, H. L.: Severe tricuspid stenosis revealed after aortic valvulotomy. Br. Heart J., 24:241, 1962.

189. Wellons, H. A., Jr., Strauch, R. S., Nolan, S. P., and Muller, W. H., Jr.: Isolated mitral valve replacement with the Kay-Shiley disc valve: Actuarial analysis of the long-term results. J. Thorac. Cardiovasc. Surg., 70:862, 1975.

190. West, J. B., Doller, C. T., and Heard, B. E.: Increased pulmonary vascular resistance in the dependent zone of isolated dog lung caused by perivascular edema. Circ. Res., 17:191, 1965.

191. Willerson, J. T., Kastor, J. A., Dinsmore, R. E., Mundth, E. D., Buckley, M. J., Austen, W. G., and Sanders, C. A.: Phonocardiographic and hemodynamic assessment of mitral paravalvular and intravalvular regurgitation. Br. Heart J., Suppl. 42, 1970, p. 32.

192. Wood, P.: An appreciation of mitral stenosis: I. Clinical features; II. Investigations and results. Br. Med. J., 1:1051, 1113, 1954.

193. Wood, P.: Systemic embolism. Br. Med. J., 1:1056, 1954.

194. Wukasch, D. C., Unger, F., Reul, G. J., Jr., Sandiford, F. M., Kyger, E. R., Hall, R. J., Norman, J. C., and Cooley, D. A.: Long-term results in cardiac valve replacements: Comparison of 6335 various type prostheses. 2nd Henry Ford Hospital International Symposium on Cardiac Surgery, in press.

195. Yeh, T. J., Brachney, E. L., Hall, D. P., and Ellison, R. G.: Renal complications of open heart surgery: Predisposing factors, prevention and management. J. Thorac. Cardiovasc. Surg., 47:79, 1964.

XVIII

EBSTEIN'S ANOMALY

Hassan Najafi, M.D.

The basic pathologic defect in Ebstein's malformation, a rare congenital cardiac anomaly, is the downward displacement of an abnormal tricuspid valve.[3] There is usually one functioning leaflet anteriorly, the others being rudimentary. The characteristic feature is that the single sail-like anterior leaflet extends from the anatomical annulus to the shortened chordae tendineae and partitions the right ventricular cavity into a proximal atrialized portion and a small, relatively inefficient distal pumping chamber. The atrialized portion varies in size and may be aneurysmal. The diminutive and misplaced posterior and septal leaflets inferior to the annulus often fuse to the interior of the ventricular wall and cause varying degrees of either tricuspid insufficiency or stenosis in different patients. Usually an associated veno-arterial shunt at the atrial level results in arterial desaturation and cyanosis.

CLINICAL MANIFESTATIONS

The severity of *symptoms* and *signs* and the incapacity caused by this disorder have been variable. Most of the reported patients, however, seem to have been limited in their activities from an early age, while a few have led almost normal lives until advanced ages. Congestive heart failure, arrhythmias, cyanosis, complications secondary to polycythemia, and paradoxical emboli are the cardinal clinical manifestations of this anomaly. In a collective review of 108 consecutive patients reported, the following observations were made: 55 were diagnosed clinically and the remainder at autopsy. Fifty-seven were male, 46 female, and in 5 patients the sex was not stated. The age ranged from 2 1/2 days to 79 years. The average age at the time of death in 60 patients not treated surgically was 23 years; sudden death was recorded in 16 patients.[18]

The *physical examination* invariably reveals a characteristic triple rhythm at the cardiac apex, a systolic murmur usually along the left sternal border, and in some patients a diastolic murmur may be audible in the same area. Clubbing of the fingers may be present in instances of longstanding severe cyanosis.

Roentgenogram of the chest in most instances shows increased cardiothoracic ratio, a large right atrium, and overall inverted funnel-shaped cardiac silhouette with narrowed pedicle and decreased pulmonary vascular markings. A convex and elevated left cardiac border constitutes a reliable diagnostic feature (Fig. 1). The typical electrocardiogram demonstrates a right bundle branch block with prolonged P-R interval. While large P waves are common, abnormalities of rate and rhythm and Wolff-Parkinson-White syndrome are uncommon. In recent years intracardiac electrocardiography has facilitated the diagnosis of Ebstein's anomaly. Echocardiography shows the characteristically abnormal pattern of movement of the anterior tricuspid leaflet with a late tricuspid valve closure not seen in other cardiac anomalies.

Angiocardiogram shows a greatly dilated right heart with marked delay in right ventricular emptying. The pulmonary vessels are poorly visualized and an atrial septal defect is often demonstrated by passage of contrast medium from the right into the left atrium. The characteristic finding is that of a curved linear protrusion into the right heart representing the abnormal tricuspid valve arising from the ventricular wall inferior to the annulus (Fig. 2).

In *cardiac catheterization* the catheter takes a characteristic course. As the tip of the catheter is maneuvered through the right atrium it passes toward the left heart border. At this point an atrial pressure is recorded rather than the usual right ventricular curve

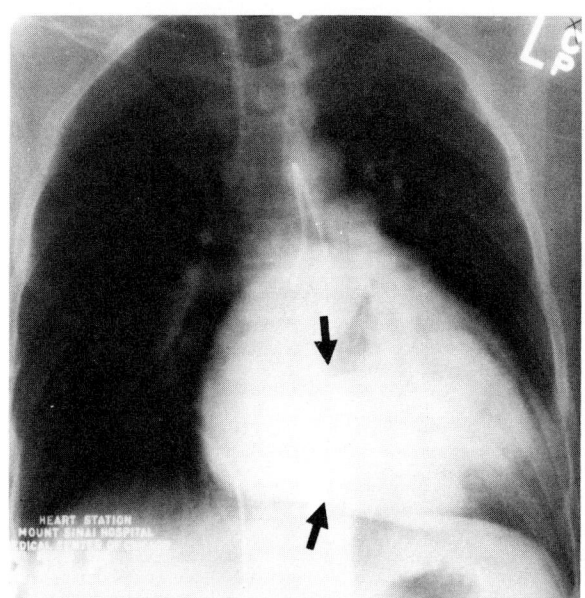

Figure 2. Right atrial injection of contrast medium shows enlargement of right heart chambers and partitioning of the right ventricle. Arrows point to the atrioventricular junction. Note the indentation produced by the displaced tricuspid valve.

due to the displaced valve leaflet and the tremendous size of the right atrium (Fig. 2). When the tip of the catheter does pass through the tricuspid valve, the ventricular outflow chamber appears to be extremely shortened. The catheter passes almost immediately into the pulmonary artery. Normal right ventricular and elevated right atrial pressures are the usual findings. The primary hemodynamic disturbance in Ebstein's anomaly is the decreased output of the right ventricle, causing low pulmonary blood flow. Because of the decreased volume and distensibility of the functioning ventricle (distal chamber), the receiving chamber, composed of the right atrium and the atrialized portion of the right ventricle, is unable to empty itself completely. This explains the right atrial hypertension, and in the presence of an atrial septal defect, a right-to-left shunt develops producing cyanosis.

SURGICAL MANAGEMENT

Progressive congestive heart failure, frequent arrhythmias, threatening sudden death, and symptomatic hypoxemia are the indications for surgery in the majority of these patients. Initially systemic pulmonary artery shunts were employed with uniformly poor results. Closure of the atrial septal defect was also associated with failure. Glenn in 1958 suggested partial circulatory bypass of the right side of the heart by superior vena cava–right pulmonary artery anastomosis.[5] In 1959 Gasul et al.[4] reported the first patient with Ebstein's disease in whom a successful superior vena cava–right pulmonary artery anastomosis was performed with improvement. Surgical efforts to completely correct this deformity were first directed

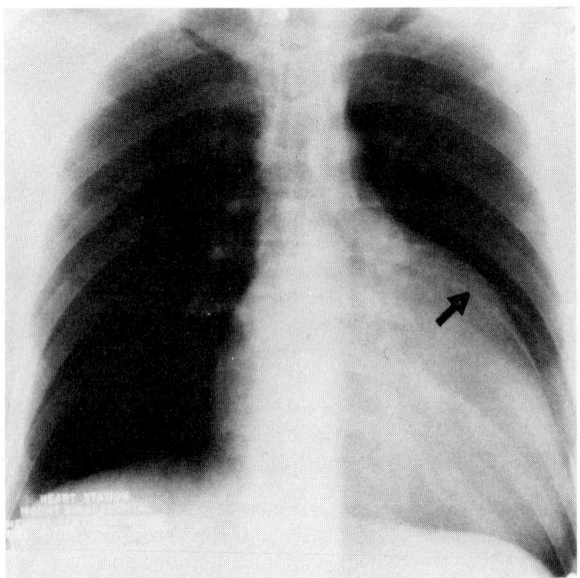

Figure 1. Chest roentgenogram in a patient with Ebstein's malformation. The arrow shows the characteristically elevated and convex left upper cardiac border representing the displaced and somewhat dilated distal right ventricular chamber or the infundibular outflow tract.

toward reconstructive procedures. In 1958 Hunter and Lillehei[9] suggested plication of the atrialized portion of the right ventricle by suturing the line of attachment of the septal and posterior tricuspid leaflets to the true annulus (Fig. 3). Subsequently this operation was successfully carried out by Hardy et al. in 1963 and reported in 1964.[7] Hardy and Roe[8] in 1969 reported the successful use of this definitive technique in a total of 6 consecutive patients with wide spectrum Ebstein's anomaly. Bahnson et al.[1] in 1965 reported three patients in whom correction of the downward displacement of the tricuspid valve was attempted, and this proved successful in two patients. They suggested that because of the degree of the deformity of the tricuspid valve in some patients this operation may not be feasible and valve replacement may be more appropriate.

In 1963 Barnard and Schrire[2] first reported on two patients with Ebstein's malformation in whom successful correction was achieved by excision of the anomalous anterior tricuspid leaflets together with replacement by valvular prosthesis. To avoid injury to the conduction system they sutured the prosthesis to the true annulus anteriorly but attached it to the right atrial wall several millimeters cephalad to the coronary sinus on the opposite side (Fig. 4). This displaced the coronary sinus into the right ventricle. Early attempts at valve replacement in five patients without such downward ventricular inclusion of the coronary sinus were not associated with satisfactory

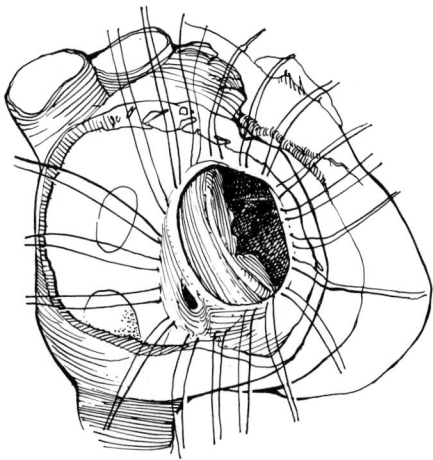

Figure 4. Diagram demonstrating placement of sutures for prosthetic valve insertion.

results. Surgically successful cases of prosthetic tricuspid valve replacement include two patients of Barnard and Schrire, three reported by Lillehei et al. in 1967,[12] two by Najafi et al. in 1967,[13] and a single instance by Gueron et al. in 1966,[6] Kay et al. in 1967,[10] Perez-Alvarez et al. in 1967,[14] Soulie et al. in 1967,[16] Timmis et al. in 1967,[17] Schumacker in 1969,[15] and Kittle and Balkoura-Christopoulos in 1973.[11] In addition to replacement of the valve, closure of the atrial septal defect or foramen ovale was carried out in the majority of these patients. A few patients had exclusion of the atrialized portion of the ventricle. The results have been encouraging, based on a high percentage of survivors and excellent postoperative achievements. Because of the possibility of chronic obliteration of the mechanical valve in the tricuspid position, recently consideration has been given to the use of a stented porcine heterograft valve. Even in children who require early surgery for relief of symptoms, valve replacement probably has a lower risk and results in better relief of symptoms than the palliative procedures that have been advocated. The dilated annulus invariably present in these patients makes it likely that a large-size valve can be utilized. The superior vena cava–right pulmonary artery anastomosis, however, remains as the operation of choice for infants and very small children who require surgery for relief of symptoms due to severe hypoxemia.

SURGICAL TECHNIQUE

A median sternotomy provides an excellent exposure. Both venae cavae are cannulated for gravity venous return, with arterial inflow achieved by cannulation of the distal ascending aorta. Cardiopulmonary bypass is established and systemic perfusion is maintained at close to normothermic levels. The right atrium is generously opened. The tricuspid valve and interior of the right heart chamber are carefully inspected and if primary repair is not feasible the valve is removed. Anteriorly sutures are placed in the annulus, while posteriorly and laterally sutures are

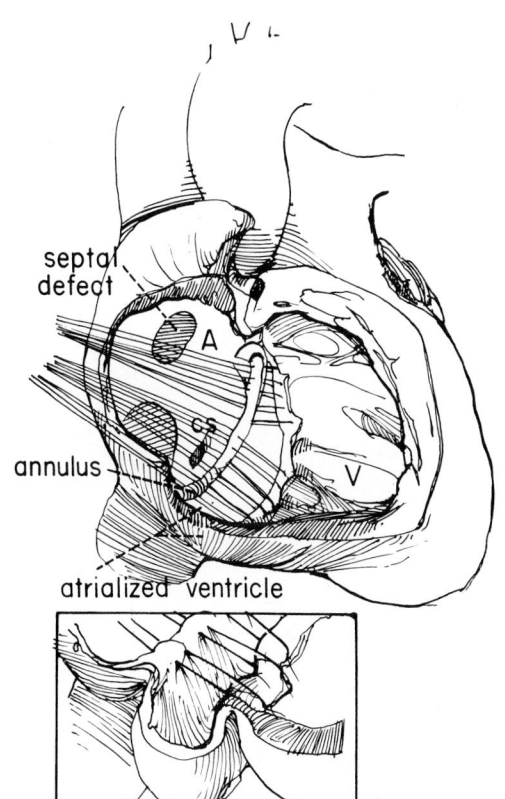

Figure 3. A diagram demonstrating placement of sutures for primary reconstruction of the tricuspid valve.

placed more superiorly so that in the region of the coronary sinus they are several millimeters on the atrial side of this orifice. This avoids injury to the conduction system (Fig. 4). These sutures are then passed through the sewing ring of the prosthesis. If the atrial portion is exceedingly large and had demonstrated paradoxical pulsation, it may be wise to exclude it to enhance right ventricular emptying. After replacement of the valve the atrial septal defect is closed. Since postoperative rhythm disturbances are common in these patients and intracavitary pacing is contraindicated in the presence of tricuspid valve prosthesis, permanent epicardial electrodes should be inserted and buried subcutaneously for possible permanent pacing after surgery. In addition, temporary pacemaker wires are used for management of immediate postoperative arrhythmias.

SELECTED REFERENCES

Hardy, K. L., and Roe, B. B.: Ebstein's anomaly: Further experience with definitive repair. J. Thorac. Cardiovasc. Surg., 58:553, 1969.
An exceptionally well-written article containing illustrations on primary reconstructive surgery for Ebstein's anomaly.

Lillehei, C. W., Kalke, B. R., and Carlson, R. G.: Evolution of corrective surgery for Ebstein's anomaly. Circulation, 35(Suppl. I):111, 1967.
A fine resume of surgical techniques for correction of Ebstein's anomaly, with emphasis on tricuspid valve replacement utilizing prosthetic devices.

Vacca, J. B., Bussmann, D. W., and Mudd, J. G.: Ebstein's anomaly: Complete review of 108 cases. Am. J. Cardiol., 2:210, 1958.
This is an excellent review of the literature carefully analyzing the clinical and pathophysiological features of Ebstein's anomaly in 108 patients.

REFERENCES

1. Bahnson, H. T., Bauersfeld, S. R., and Smith, J. W.: Pathological anatomy and surgical correction of Ebstein's anomaly. Circulation, 31(Suppl. I):3, 1965.
2. Barnard, C. N., and Schrire, V.: Surgical correction of Ebstein's malformation with prosthetic tricuspid valve. Surgery, 54:302, 1963.
3. Ebstein, W.: Ueber einem sehr seltenen. Fall von insufficiency der Valvular Tricuspidalis, bedengt durch eine angeborene hoch-gradige misserldung Derselbein. Arch. Anat. Physiol. Med., 1866, p. 236.
4. Gasul, B. M., et al.: Superior vena cava – right pulmonary artery anastomoses. J.A.M.A., 171:1797, 1959.
5. Glenn, W. W. L.: Circulatory bypass of the right side of the heart shunt between superior vena cava and right pulmonary artery: Report of clinical application. N. Engl. J. Med., 259:117, 1958.
6. Gueron, M., Hirsch, M., Stern, J., Cohen, W., and Levy, M. J.: Familial Ebstein's anomaly with emphasis on the surgical treatment. Am. J. Cardiol., 18:105, 1966.
7. Hardy, K. L., May, A. I., Webster, C. A., and Kimble, K. G.: Ebstein's anomaly: A functional concept and successful definitive repair. J. Thorac. Cardiovasc. Surg., 48:927, 1964.
8. Hardy, K. L., and Roe, B. B.: Ebstein's anomaly: Further experience with definitive repair. J. Thorac. Cardiovasc. Surg., 58:553, 1969.
9. Hunter, S. W., and Lillehei, C. W.: Ebstein's malformation of the tricuspid valve with suggestion of the new form of surgical therapy. Dis. Chest, 33:297, 1958.
10. Kay, J. H., Tsuji, H. K., Reddington, J. B., Yamada, T., Kaghwa, Y., and Kawashima, Y.: The surgical treatment of Ebstein's malformation with right ventricular aneurysmorrhaphy and replacement of the tricuspid valve with a disc valve. Dis. Chest., 51:537, 1967.
11. Kittle, C. F., and Balkoura-Christopoulos, M. H.: Post superior vena cava–right pulmonary artery shunt: Total surgical correction of Ebstein's anomaly with Starr-Edwards prosthesis. Chest, 63:120–123, 1975.
12. Lillehei, C. W., Kalke, B. R., and Carlson, R. G.: Evolution of corrective surgery for Ebstein's anomaly. Circulation, 35(Suppl. I):111, 1967.
13. Najafi, H., Hunter, J. A., Dye, W. S., Javid, H., and Julian, O. C.: Ebstein's malformation of the tricuspid valve: Surgical management. Ann. Thorac. Surg., 4:334, 1967.
14. Perez-Alvarez, J. J., Perez-Trevino, C., Gaxiola, A., and Reta-Villalobos, A.: Ebstein's anomaly with pulmonic stenosis. Am. J. Cardiol., 20:411, 1967.
15. Schumacker, H. B., Jr.: Miscellaneous congenital cardiac anomalies. In Gibbon, J. H., Jr., Sabiston, D. C., Jr., and Spencer, F. C.: Surgery of the Chest, 2nd ed. Philadelphia, W. B. Saunders Company, 1969, pp. 756–769.
16. Soulie, P., Vernant, P., Corone, P., and Baillot, F.: Traitement chirurgical de la maladie d'Ebstein. Acta Cardiol., 22:459, 1967.
17. Timmis, H. H., Hardy, J. D., and Watson, D. G.: The surgical management of Ebstein's anomaly: The combined use of tricuspid valve replacement, atrio-ventricular plication and atrioplasty. J. Thorac. Cardiovasc. Surg., 53:85, 1967.
18. Vacca, J. B., Bussman, B. W., and Mudd, J. G.: Ebstein's anomaly: Complete review of 108 cases. Am. J. Cardiol., 2:210, 1958.

XIX

SURGICAL TREATMENT OF SUPRAVENTRICULAR TACHYARRHYTHMIAS ASSOCIATED WITH THE WOLFF-PARKINSON-WHITE SYNDROME

Will C. Sealy, M.D.

In 1931, Wolff, Parkinson, and White[14] described a syndrome characterized by an electrocardiogram with a short PR interval, an abnormal QRS, and episodes of tachyarrhythmia as shown in Figure 1. The explanation of the mechanism in this disorder was unclear until 1932, when Holtzman[4] suggested that this could be related to the persistence of an anomalous pathway of conduction between the atrium and the ventricle,

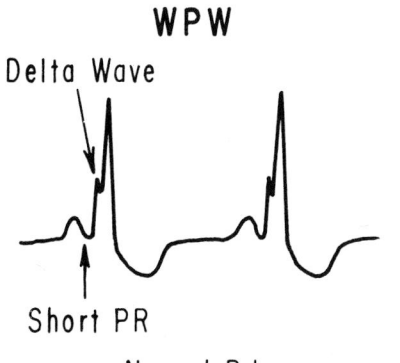

Figure 1. A copy of an electrocardiogram lead V_1 showing the pre-excitation of the ventricles.

such as described by Kent in 1914.[5] In 1942, Woods[15] had the opportunity to study the heart of a young boy who died suddenly and on whom a previous electrocardiogram showed changes typical of the Wolff-Parkinson-White (WPW) syndrome. Careful studies of the heart revealed an anomalous pathway on the right lateral wall of the ventricle similar to the one described by Kent. In 1969, Durrer and Roos[2] carried out epicardial mapping of the ventricular activation sequence in a patient who had the Wolff-Parkinson-White syndrome. This study proved that the ventricles did pre-excite. In 1969, the first patient at the Duke University Medical Center with Wolff-Parkinson-White syndrome was operated upon.[10] In this patient a Kent bundle was located by surface mapping and successfully divided at surgery. This operation corrected the pre-excitation and prevented further attacks of supraventricular tachycardia. This was the final evidence needed to prove that the Kent bundle was the cause of this syndrome.

ANATOMY AND PHYSIOLOGY

During embryologic development of man, there are numerous communications other than the His bundle that cross the annulus fibrosus connecting the atrial muscle to the ventricular muscle.[12] As the annulus fibrosus matures, these communications are obliterated. The persistence of one or more of them is the explanation for the origin of the anomalous pathways. Kent bundles are microscopic in size, composed of muscle, and course from the atrium to the ventricle either subendocardially or beneath the coronary fat pad.[6] Based on their embryologic development, it is obvious then that the pathways can be multiple and are located anywhere around the annulus fibrosus, as shown in Figure 1.

The physiologic properties of the Kent bundles have been studied in great detail.[3, 13] However, it is the observations of Durrer, Wellens, and their colleagues,[2, 13] using electrical stimulation and His bundle studies, that have been responsible for development of methods of study permitting the accumulation of in-

formation about these unusual cardiac anomalies. The effective refractory period of the pathway can be measured with these techniques. It has also been observed that the pathway's effectve refractory period is limited by the effective refractory period of either atrial or ventricular muscle. The pathways have been found to conduct differently from atrium to ventricle than from ventricle to atrium. In addition, anomalous pathways have been found that would conduct only from ventricle to atrium. With these methods it is possible to reproduce the patient's tachyarrhythmia and to determine the rapidity with which the ventricle will respond to atrial pacing. As shown in Figure 2, the supraventricular tachycardia is a re-entrant one which is caused by differences in the effective refractory periods of the Kent bundle and the AV node. This leaves a "window" and then an extra-atrial beat will be found to travel first down the AV node–His system and return retrograde over the Kent, for this "window" implies that one is excitable while the other one is refractory. Thus, when the impulse arrives at the ventricle, the Kent is now excitable and the circus movement is propagated. To break the circus movement, division of either Kent or His bundle will suffice. In some patients, the Kent bundle may have an effective refractory period that is quite short. If this occurs, then a fast atrial rate such as occurs in atrial fibrillation or flutter will be transmitted to the ventricle. Rates of over 400 beats per minute have been observed in some patients. This obviously would elicit an intolerable ventricular rate that can deteriorate into ventricular fibrillation. Only division of the Kent bundle would correct this.

There are other causes of pre-excitation of the ventricles and a short PR interval. Patients may have a direct connection, a Mahaim fiber, from the low AV node or His bundle to the ventricular muscle, thus bypassing the Purkinje system. Obviously, this would cause pre-excitation, although the PR interval would be only slightly shorter than normal or normal. The second anomaly may cause a short PR interval with a normal QRS. The fibers, described by James, may go directly from the atrium to the His bundle, bypassing the AV node. Once the impulse gets to the bundle of His, the QRS morphology is then normal. Both of these conditions can be the prerequisite for re-entry supraventricular tachycardia, and when associated with James fibers, it is called the Lown-Ganong-Levine syndrome.

CLINICAL PICTURE

This disorder is not a common one. It has been estimated that somewhere between 0.1 and 3.1 electrocardiograms per thousand examined show pre-excitation.[1] Perhaps 40 to 80 per cent of them have symptoms. The number who have serious symptoms is not known. At Duke University, we have examined more than 130 patients with this problem, and out of this group 50 were selected for surgery. Of this 50, 27 were thought to have a problem that was life-threatening in nature and, therefore, this served as an indication for surgery. A second group of 23 had disabling supraventricular tachycardia.

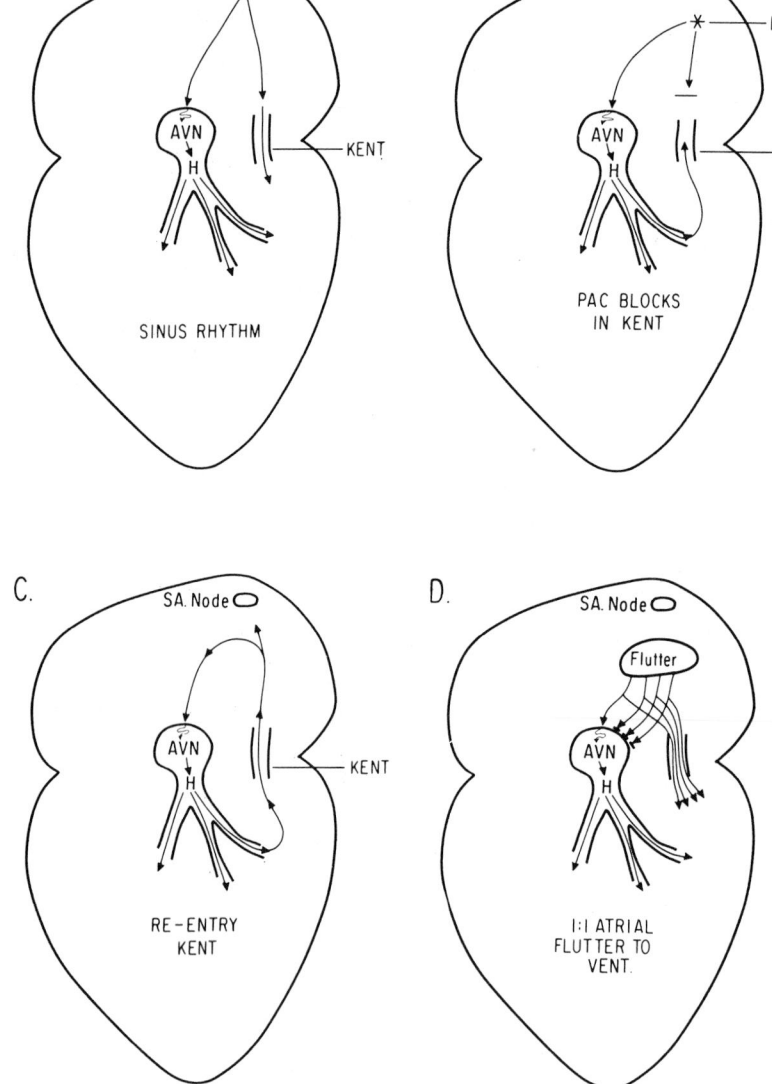

Figure 2. *A, B,* and *C* illustrate the mechanism for supraventricular tachycardia. A premature atrial contraction (PAC) is able to initiate the SVT because of electrophysiologic differences between the AV node and Kent. *D* shows how a fast atrial rate on a patient with a Kent bundle that has a short refractory period can be transmitted to the ventricle 1 to 1. (From Sealy, W. C., et al.: Ann. Thorac. Surg., in press.)

The patients in the Duke series who had a life-threatening problem are enumerated in Table 1. The age was lower, the pathways conducted rapidly, and many had ventricular fibrillation with terrifying episodes. One, a 14-year-old boy, was found by his father unconscious in the yard. He was given artificial respiration and cardiac massage for the 25 minutes required for him to be brought to a hospital where he was found to have ventricular fibrillation. Another, a 31-year-old woman, was found unconscious by her husband. He immediately carried her to the emergency room of a nearby hospital where she suddenly developed ventricular fibrillation and had to be resuscitated. This patient had a second similar episode a month later.

Those in the second group, with troublesome and poorly tolerated supraventricular tachycardia, were medical failures for various reasons. In some because of associated anomalies, such as cardiomyopathy, mi-

TABLE 1. Clinical Findings in 50 Patients with Kent Bundles Treated by Surgery*

	23 Pts. SVT		27 Pts. Lethal Potential
Above age 31 years	14		7
Syncope	4		20
Sick sinus syndrome	2		0
Cardiomyopathy	4		1
Ebstein's anomaly	4		0
Acquired heart disease	2		0
Ventricular fibrillation	0		12
Ventricular rate over 250 beats per min.	3/12		18/27
Effective refractory period of Kent over 250 msec.	10/12	0/8	0/8

*Sealy, W. C., et al.: Ann. Thorac. Surg., in press.

tral valve disease, and coronary artery disease, the tachycardias were poorly tolerated and were associated with symptoms of failure. Other patients could not tolerate the medication needed to control their tachyarrhythmia. Some had drug sensitivities. There was another group who, as they grew older, began to have more and more trouble with SVT.

Electrocardiogram in WPW shows a short PR interval and delta wave indicating pre-excitation of the ventricle. Rosenbaum was able to divide Wolff-Parkinson-White patients into Type A (left) and Type B (right) by an analysis of the vector of the delta wave. Usually Type A has a positive delta wave in V_1 and V_2, whereas a Type B has a negative one in these leads. Nearly half of the patients will exhibit a normal EKG at some time.

With the introduction of the His bundle studies and electrical stimulation studies of Durrer and Wellens, a precise preoperative clinical evaluation is possible in patients with WPW. The studies show the following: they confirm the presence of a Kent bundle. The role the Kent bundle plays in the tachyarrhythmia is determined. A judgment can be made of the potential of the Kent to cause a life-threatening tachyarrhythmia. The tachyarrhythmia can be induced and reversed. The presence of other Kent bundles as well as Mahaim and James pathways can be sought. The location of the pathway about the annulus fibrosus can be ascertained. The presence of a pathway that conducts only retrogradely can be detected. The effectiveness of various antiarrhythmic drugs can be tested.

With the preoperative electrophysiologic studies, and with mapping studies to be described below, we have separated our patients into free wall, anterior septal, and posterior septal problems, as shown in Figure 3. This classification is preferable to Type A and B.

Unusual variants of the Kent bundles have been noted. Among the most interesting are those that conduct only from the ventricle to the atrium, thus causing supraventricular tachycardia but not producing WPW syndrome. In six patients we found more than one Kent bundle. Mahaim and James fibers have been seen in combination with Kent bundles in others.

SURGICAL TREATMENT

The operation consists of two parts.[8] The first part is the mapping of the surface of the heart to detect the earliest area of ventricular and atrial activation which points to the Kent bundle. The surface of the heart is divided by an arbitrary grid. A pacing electrode is sutured to the atrium and a reference and pacing one to the ventricle as close to the suspected area of the Kent bundles as possible. Then the atrium is paced. The area on the ventricle that activates the earliest is the approximate site of the aberrant pathway. Supraventricular tachycardia affords an opportunity to map the atria. The ventricle can also be paced so as to find the earliest area of atrial activation. An example of a surface map is shown in Figure 4.

After the aberrant pathway has been located, the patient is put on cardiopulmonary bypass and the appropriate atrium is opened. In our earlier studies, we divided the aberrant pathway below the annulus just as it entered the ventricle. The incision is now made on the atrial side of the annulus. The coronary fat pad containing the coronary vessels is lifted up and the fibrous bands between the fat pad and the ventricle are carefully teased away and divided (Fig. 5).

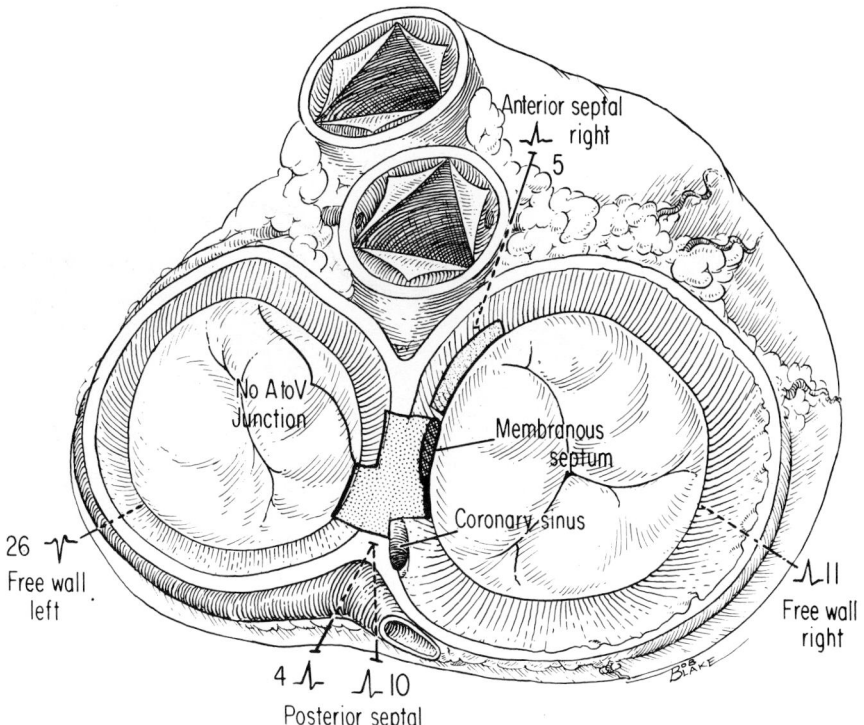

Figure 3. View of the heart looking down on the mitral and tricuspid valves. The classification of Type A and Type B, based entirely on electrocardiograms, is not always accurate. The numbers indicate the location of the Kent bundles in our 50 patients. Six patients had multiple pathways. We now use right and left free wall, postseptal, and right anterior septal. Note that there is no direct connection between atrium and ventricle where the mitral valve is attached to the aorta. The area with the stippling in the septal region indicates the possible points where the posterior septal Kent pathways enter the ventricle. In surface mapping, the activation in the anterior septal and posterior septal group shows a "loss of time" between this, the earliest area of ventricular activation, and the onset of the delta wave in the QRS. The activation point can be either to the right or left of the crux. (From Sealy, W. C., et al.: Ann. Thorac. Surg., in press.)

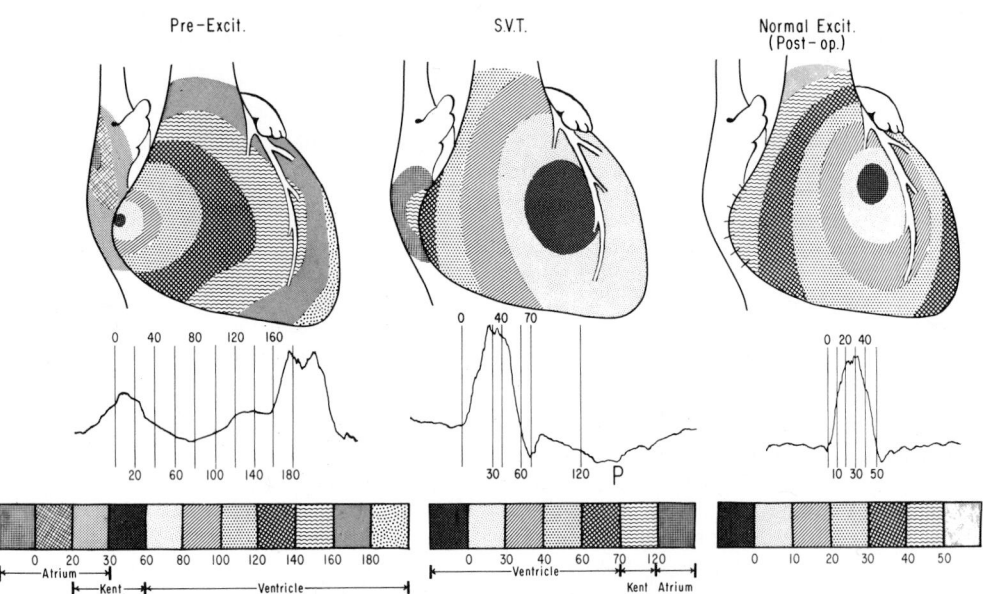

Figure 4. This is an isochronous map constructed from the epicardial mapping carried out at the time of surgery on a patient with a right lateral free wall Kent bundle. The earliest area of ventricular activation is shown with the time relationships between this point and the electrocardiogram. During SVT, activation occurs via the His-Purkinje route with the retrograde P shown. After surgery, the activation sequence is normal.

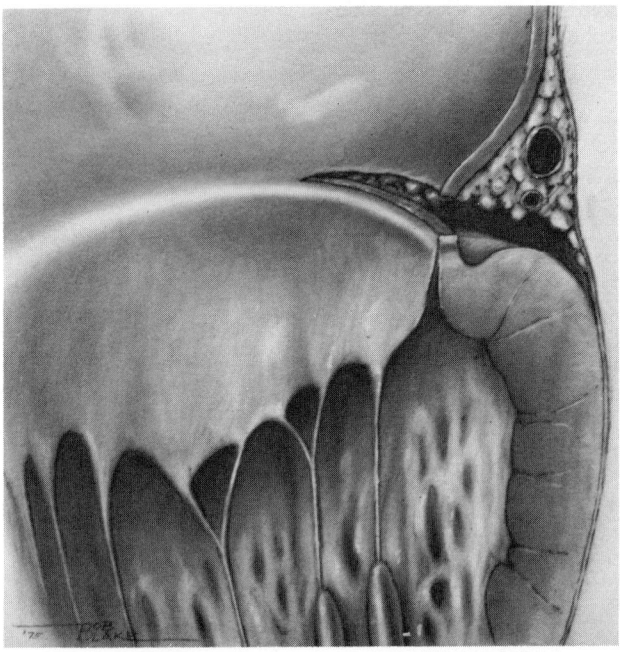

Figure 5. A drawing of the exposure of the coronary fat pad through an atrial incision just above the annulus fibrosus. The dissection is carried all the way to the epicardium. (From Sealy, W. C., et al.: Ann. Thorac. Surg., in press.)

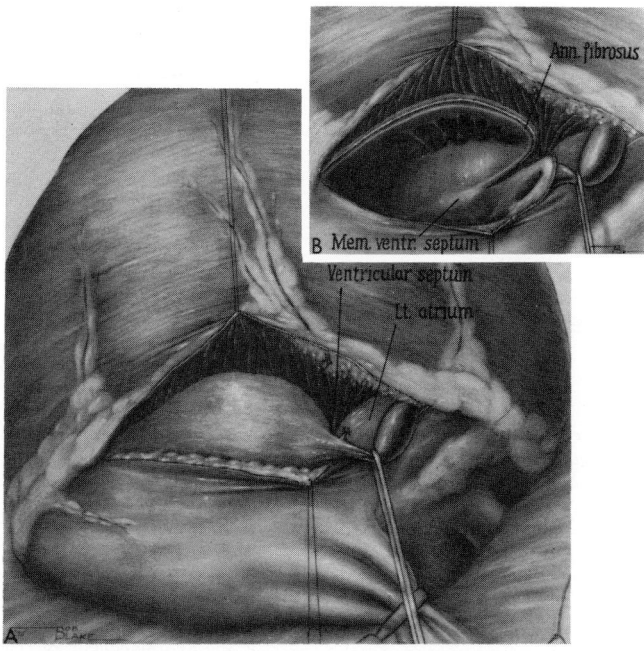

Figure 6. Drawing showing the approach to a right posterior septal pathway. The coronary sinus is dissected away from the ventricle, exposing the triangular space on top of the ventricular septum. The right atrium is then divided all the way to the central fibrous body. (From Sealy, W. C., et al.: Ann. Thorac. Surg., in press.)

On the left side, the incision, if necessary, can be started at the left trigone and carried around in a counterclockwise fashion all the way to the right trigone. On the right side, an incision can be made in the annulus fibrosus beginning just anterior to the point where the membranous ventricular septum protrudes into the right atrium. It can be carried around in a clockwise fashion, if needed, all the way to the posterior aspect of this structure.

The most difficult surgical problems in this disorder occur in those patients who have a pathway that emerges in the posterior septal area. This may either go to the right or to the left of the crux. The exposure we now use is shown in Figure 6. After interruption and while still on bypass, the patient is mapped again in order to be certain that the Kent pathway has been interrupted and that there are not other pathways present.

The His bundle may be divided as a means of breaking up the re-entry tachycardia. Obviously, this would have no effect on the patient whose problem is due to fast transmission of atrial impulses to the ventricle. After the operation, the patient requires a demand pacemaker even though the anomalous pathway may conduct the sinus impulse to the ventricle most of the time. Although easily injured during surgery for congenital heart disease, it may be difficult to interrupt electively. We have employed electrocauterization, freezing, and complete excision of the AV node.

In certain poor-risk patients, a pacemaker may be used to interrupt the supraventricular tachycardia but would be of little benefit for the ones with a life-threatening tachyarrhythmia. When an atrial pacemaker is used, it is activated by a radiofrequency unit. A random beat will interrupt the re-entry. The electrodes should be placed as close to the Kent bundle as possible. A ventricular demand one can be used in the same way, using the magnet to activate the pacing mechanism.

The results of treatment of the patients at Duke are shown in Table 2. In the last 20, all having free wall

TABLE 2. Summary of Results of Surgery in 50 Patients for Tachyarrhythmias Caused by a Kent Bundle*

	No. Pts.	Comments
Kent divided.		31	29 Asymptomatic
Death due to cardiomyopathy 2		
Delta absent. No arrhythmia.	3	1 Drug control
Antegrade conduction and		2 Asymptomatic, pacemaker
lethal rhythm abolished.		
His section 2		
Delta unchanged. No arrhythmia.	6	4 Asymptomatic, pacemaker
His section 4		2 Drug control
Delta changed. No arrhythmia.	6	4 Drug control
Kent damaged		2 With second Kent,
Second Kent present 2		asymptomatic
Mahaim pathway 2		
Elective His section.	1	Improved, pacemaker
Retrograde conduction only		Follow-up incomplete
Kent missed.	3	2 Status unchanged
Failure		1 Died 18 hours postop.,
		diagnosis questionable

*Sealy, W. C., et al.: Ann. Thorac. Surg., in press.

problems, we have been successful in dividing the Kent bundle. These operations represent the first surgical procedures for the cure of supraventricular tachyarrhythmia. As yet other re-entrant tachycardias, as well as tachyarrhythmias with fast conducting AV node–His system, can be treated only with His bundle interruption. It is hoped that as the electrophysiologic technique improves, surgical procedures can be devised that will correct the problem but preserve the supraventricular pacemaking function.

SELECTED REFERENCES

Boineau, J. P., and Moore, E. N.: Evidence for propagation across an accessory atrioventricular connection in types A and B pre-excitation. Circulation, *41*:375, 1970.
This is a description of a bundle of Kent that was studied very extensively in a dog, and this is correlated with the observations made on some of the early patients in the Duke series of WPW.

Durrer, D., and Roos, J. P.: Epicardial excitation of the ventricles in a patient with Wolff-Parkinson-White syndrome (Type B). Circulation, *35*:15, 1967.
This is the description of the epicardial mapping procedure used at the time of surgery.

Gallagher, J. J., Svenson, R. H., Sealy, W. C., and Wallace, A. G.: The Wolff-Parkinson-White syndrome and the pre-excitation dysrhythmias: Medical and surgical management. Med. Clin. North Am., *60*:101, 1976.
This is a review article and gives the reader a good insight into the mechanisms of pre-excitation as well as abnormalities other than the Kent bundle that cause this disorder.

Narula, O. S.: Wolff-Parkinson-White syndrome. A review. Circulation, *47*:872, 1973.
This is an excellent review of the whole subject of WPW.

Sealy, W. C., Gallagher, J. J., and Wallace, A. G.: The surgical treatment of the Wolff-Parkinson-White syndrome: Evolution of the improved methods of identification and interruption of the kent bundle. Ann. Thorac. Surg., *22*:(Nov.), 1976.
This is a publication of the details of the work from which this chapter was derived.

Wellens, H. J. J.: Electrical Stimulation of the Heart in the Study of Tachycardias. Baltimore, University Press, 1971.
This monograph describes the technique for programmed stimulation which defines the mechanisms in play that cause supraventricular tachycardia.

REFERENCES

1. Chung, K. Y., Walsh, T. J., and Massie, E.: Wolff-Parkinson-White syndrome. Am. Heart J., *69*:116, 1965.
2. Durrer, D., and Roos, J. P.: Epicardial excitation of the ventricles in a patient with Wolff-Parkinson-White syndrome (Type B). Circulation, *35*:15, 1967.
3. Gallagher, J. J., Svenson, R. H., Sealy, W. C., and Wallace, A. G.: The Wolff-Parkinson-White syndrome and the pre-excitation dysrhythmias: Medical and surgical management. Med. Clin. North Am., *60*:10, 1976.
4. Holzmann, M., and Scherf, D.: Über Elektrokardiogramme mit verkurzter Vorhof-Kammer-Distanz und positiven P. Zacken Z. Klin. Med., *121*:404, 1932.
5. Kent, A. F. S.: Illustrations of the right lateral auriculo-ventricular junction in the heart. J. Physiol., *48*:53, 1914.
6. Mann, R. B., Fisher, R. S., Scherlis, S., and Hutchins, G. M.: Accessory left atrioventricular connection in Type A Wolff-Parkinson-White syndrome. Johns Hopkins Med. J., *132*:242, 1973.
7. Rosenbaum, M. B., Hecht, H. H., Wilson, F. N., et al.: The potential variations of the thorax and the esophagus in anomalous atrioventricular excitation (Wolff-Parkinson-White syndrome). Am. Heart J., *29*:281, 1945.
8. Sealy, W. C., and Wallace, A. G.: Surgical treatment of Wolff-Parkinson-White syndrome. J. Thorac. Cardiovasc. Surg., *68*:757, 1974.
9. Sealy, W. C., Gallagher, J. J., and Wallace, A. G.: The surgical treatment of the Wolff-Parkinson-White syndrome: Evolution of the improved methods of identification and interruption of the Kent bundle. Ann. Thorac. Surg., *22*:(Nov), 1976.
10. Sealy, W. C., Hattler, B. C., Blumenschein, S. D., and Cobb, F. R.: Surgical treatment of Wolff-Parkinson-White syndrome. Ann. Thorac. Surg., *8*:1, 1969.
11. Sealy, W. C., Wallace, A. G., Ramming, K. P., Gallagher, J. J., and Svenson, R. H.: An improved operation for the definitive treatment of the Wolff-Parkinson-White syndrome. Ann. Thorac. Surg., *17*:107, 1974.
12. Truex, R. C., Bishof, J. K., and Hoffman, E. L.: Accessory atrioventricular bundles of the developing human heart. Anat. Rec., *131*:45, 1958.
13. Wellens, H. J. J.: Electrical stimulation of the heart in the study and treatment of tachycardia. Baltimore, University Press, 1971, p. 119.
14. Wolff, L., Parkinson, J., and White, P. D.: Bundle branch block with short PR interval in healthy young people prone to paroxysmal tachycardia. Am. Heart J., *5*:685, 1930.
15. Wood, F. C., Wolferth, C. C., and Geckeler, G. D.: Histologic demonstration of accessory muscular connections between auricle and ventricle in a case of short PR interval and prolonged QRS complex. Am. Heart J., *25*:454, 1943.

XX

CARDIAC NEOPLASMS

Brack G. Hattler, Jr., M.D.,
and David C. Sabiston, Jr., M.D.

Cardiac tumors have been recognized since the mid-sixteenth century. In 1559, Columbus[5] recorded the first known report of a cardiac neoplasm, and in the ensuing centuries these lesions continued to remain largely autopsy curiosities. Barnes[2] in 1934 reported the first clinical diagnosis of a cardiac tumor, in a patient who later died of a primary sarcoma of the heart. The true impetus to the premortem discovery of these tumors, however, came with the development of cardiac surgery and refinements in angiocardiographic techniques. Prior to the development of extracorporeal circulation in the performance of open-heart surgery, Steinberg[28] reported in 1953 an *unsuccessful* attempt to excise an atrial myxoma diagnosed by angiocardiography. The following year, Crafoord[6] performed the first successful removal of a cardiac neoplasm—an atrial myxoma—utilizing extracorporeal circulation. Since then cardiac tumors have been diagnosed and successfully excised from all chambers of the heart, a fact that is all the more important because of the frequently excellent prognosis with certain types of neoplasms. Of the cardiac tumors, metastatic lesions are most frequent, followed by primary benign lesions, and least common are primary malignant neoplasms.[24, 30]

Cardiac tumors, whether benign, malignant, or metastatic, produce clinical manifestations that vary with the location and size of the tumor and depend particularly upon whether or not cardiac function is compromised. In addition, intracavitary tumors produce bizarre symptoms mimicking a systemic illness. On occasion, these tumors are manifested initially by a peripheral arterial embolus or possibly an *immune reaction* to the tumor itself. Apart from this, cardiac tumors may continue to grow undetected, and it is interesting that more than 80 per cent of these neoplasms are first discovered at autopsy.[19] It is imperative, therefore, that the clinician be fully aware of the various presenting clinical manifestations.

METASTATIC NEOPLASMS

The most frequent cardiac tumors are of *metastatic* origin. Metastases to the heart may occur with all types of malignant diseases and spread is by direct extension or hematogenous or lymphatic routes.[11, 17] Melanomas have a definite propensity for vascular spread to the myocardium, where they may appear as tumor implants in as many as 50 per cent of cases.[19] In spite of limited cardiac lymphatic connections,[24] lymphatic spread of bronchogenic and mammary carcinoma to the heart has been reported in over 25 per cent of cases in which dissemination has occurred. The

spread within cardiac lymphatic channels is often retrograde. Metastatic infiltrates within the myocardium occur in over 15 per cent of cases of lymphoma and leukemia.[19] Direct cardiac extension of tumors from mediastinal structures or the surrounding lung also occurs. The pericardium is usually involved, and manifestations of acute pericarditis may appear. Associated pericardial friction rubs, hemorrhagic effusions with possible tamponade, and, on electrocardiogram, elevated ST segments and decreased voltage may be seen. Certain highly malignant tumors such as childhood rhabdomyosarcoma have a marked propensity to metastasize to the heart and have been found in as many as a third of the patients dying of this condition.[23]

Metastatic tumor to the heart should be suspected in any patient with a known malignant neoplasm in whom signs of cardiac arrhythmia, electrocardiographic changes, or heart failure develops. Lack of cardiac dysfunction does not exclude cardiac metastasis, however. Relatively small tumors may produce complete heart block if they involve the atrioventricular node, and yet metastatic tumors may become quite large without producing signs or symptoms. Thus, the heart may compensate for a purely space-occupying lesion if critical areas are not compromised. Bisel[3] has reported a 21 per cent incidence of cardiac metastasis in patients dying of malignant disease, but only approximately 10 per cent of affected patients have symptoms.[19] Diagnosis may be facilitated by careful examination of pericardial fluid, by pneumopericardiography following carbon dioxide injection into the pericardial space, or by direct biopsy of the lesion.

For metastatic tumors of the heart, treatment is palliative. Chemotherapy and irradiation have been tried with little benefit. Pericardicentesis for accumulated fluid provides temporary relief with improved cardiac filling. Rarely, pericardiectomy is indicated for treatment of metastatic pericarditis.

In addition to abnormalities due to direct involvement of the heart by metastasis, malignant carcinoids may affect the heart without actual mechanical invasion.[10] The overall manifestations of this endocrine-secreting tumor are discussed in detail elsewhere. Cardiac effects are of interest, however, because of their association with collections of fibrous tissue seen in the valvular cusps and endocardium, predominantly on the right side of the heart. Although the tumor actively produces serotonin (5-hydroxytryptophan), there is no evidence that the cardiac lesions are directly related to the production of this agent. Metastatic involvement of the liver is almost always encountered in patients with related cardiac abnormalities. Cardiac disturbances secondary to pulmonic stenosis or tricuspid insufficiency predispose to the development of right-sided heart failure. Because of the advanced state of the tumor when cardiac symptoms become manifest, chemotherapy directed at the carcinoid is of questionable benefit in alleviating the effects of the malignant neoplasm on the heart.

BENIGN NEOPLASMS

Benign tumors constitute 70 per cent of primary neoplasms of the heart; approximately half of them are myxomas. Lipomas, angiomas, teratomas, fibromas, hemartomas, and leiomyomas are rare benign cardiac neoplasms seen usually as incidental findings at autopsy.[16] Death from complete heart block or cardiac compression, however, has been reported with these tumors.[4, 15]

Rhabdomyoma is the most common cardiac tumor seen in infancy and childhood, with three fourths of the patients being under the age of one year.[9] In half the patients the tumor mass is intracavitary and obstructs one or more of the cardiac chambers or valve orifices. In 30 per cent, one or both atria are involved. More than 50 per cent of cases occur in association with tuberous sclerosis.[14] The tumor may be seen as single or multiple, ill-defined, grayish nodules within the myocardium. It is thought to be the result of a disturbance in glycogen metabolism leading to a glycogenic infiltration of the myofibrils. Characteristically, the nodules appear on histologic examination as areas of myofibril degeneration, with a prominent vacuolated cytoplasm surrounding the centrally placed nucleus. Rather than a true tumor of the heart, it is considered more a form of isolated glycogen storage disease. Death, frequently of undetermined cause, is seen in over 50 per cent of cases during the first year of life. The diagnosis of this histologically benign tumor should be suspected in infants with tuberous sclerosis in whom cardiac symptoms develop. With no specific therapy available, treatment in these cases is symptomatic.

Myxomas constitute the most significant of all cardiac neoplasms.[18] Not only are they the most common intracavitary tumor but also, once they are diagnosed, the probability of surgical cure is excellent. Although approximately 75 per cent originate in the left atrium and some 20 per cent in the right atrium, myxomas have been successfully removed from all chambers of the heart, Myxomas are more commonly found in females and have been diagnosed in all age groups. A familial tendency has recently been noted,[21] and a family has been described in which the mother and three of seven children had an atrial myxoma, and the mother's was biatrial.[27]

Myxomas characteristically arise from a portion of the interatrial septum on a rim of the fossa ovalis. The tumors are usually situated on a pedicle and may vary in size from less than 0.5 cm. to more than 10 cm. in diameter (Fig. 1). Rarely, these tumors are bilateral.[31] Although at one time thought to represent an organized atrial thrombus, myxomas are now considered to be true neoplasms. Grossly, they appear as a pale, gelatinous, extremely friable mass throughout which

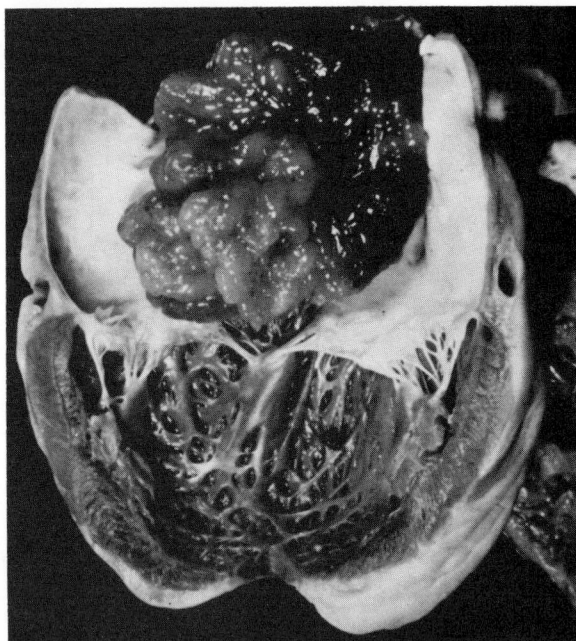

Figure 1.   A large left atrial myxoma in a patient who died from the condition. She presented with fever, petechiae, elevation of gamma globulin, and increased sedimentation rate. (From Cohen, A. I., McIntosh, H. D., and Orgain, E. S.: The mimetic nature of left atrial myxomas. Report of a case presenting as a severe systemic illness and simulating massive mitral insufficiency at cardiac catheterization. Am. J. Cardiol., *11*:802, 1963, with permission of authors and publisher.)

areas of calcification may be seen. Microscopically, the tumor is composed of fibroblasts scattered within a loose connective tissue stroma. Plasma cells and lymphocytes may be seen in all areas, and hemosiderin-laden macrophages are regularly found. Endothelium lines the outermost edges of the neoplasm. Glycoproteins and mucopolysaccharides form the main constituents of the tumor. It may grow slowly over a period of years without producing symptoms or may cause intermittent symptoms that are sometimes difficult to interpret. With left atrial tumors, especially the larger pedunculated ones, symptoms of left atrial obstruction may occur and may be erroneously attributed to mitral stenosis (Fig. 2). Recurrent pulmonary edema may be noted and is resistant to treatment. Murmurs of mitral stenosis or insufficiency may be heard, and a "tumor plop" sometimes confused with an opening snap has been described coinciding with movement of the pedunculated mass within the atrium or across the semilunar valves. These findings may vary with positional change. Right atrial myxomas producing atrioventricular valvular obstruction are most often confused with constrictive pericarditis, tricuspid stenosis, or Ebstein's anomaly. Hepatic enlargement, mild to severe peripheral edema, and varying tricuspid murmurs have been demonstrated in this setting. Acute circulatory failure may result from sudden blockage of the tricuspid or mitral valve.

Small tumors frequently remain asymptomatic unless they embolize or produce systemic symptoms.

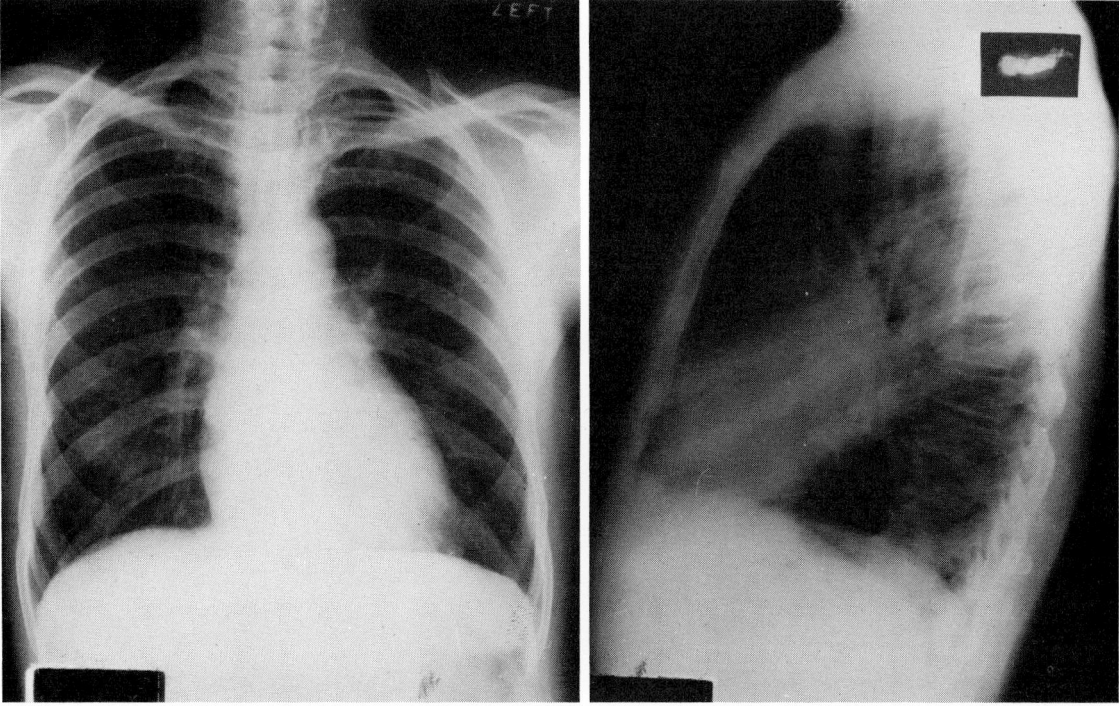

Figure 2. The calcified left atrial myxoma seen in the left lateral chest film was mistaken for the mitral valve. A roentgenogram of the removed myxoma is superimposed in the upper right corner. Although no calcium was present in the mitral valve, severe insufficiency was demonstrated. At the time of myxoma removal, the mitral valve was replaced with a ball valve prosthesis. The patient had had rheumatic fever as a young adult. (From Hattler, B. G., Jr., et al.: Ann. Thorac. Surg., *10*:65, 1970.)

In any large series of myxomas, a small percentage of patients present with initial symptoms of peripheral embolization. The diagnosis of myxoma is made on pathologic examination of the specimen at thrombectomy (Fig. 3). Systemic symptoms including recurrent fever, weight loss, arthralgia, and anemia may be encountered in these patients and suggest an inflammatory illness such as collagen-vascular disease, myocarditis, subacute bacterial endocarditis, or even acute rheumatic fever. Blood cultures, however, are usually negative, and the time course, intermittent symptomatology, and past history may help to differentiate the myxoma from a lesion of inflammatory etiology.

The *malignant potentiality* of atrial myxomas has been thoroughly established and although not well known is of considerable significance.[25] The first recurrence of a left atrial myxoma was reported in 1967,[12] and since then a number of recurrences have

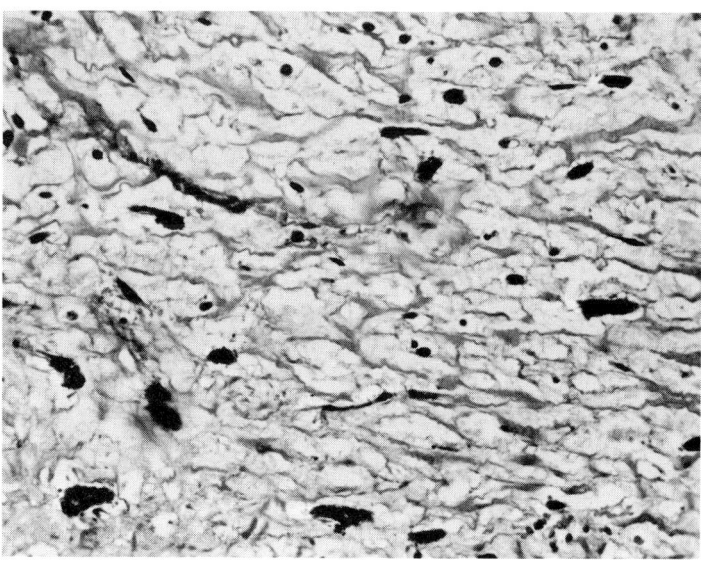

Figure 3. A section of myxomatous material from a saddle embolus. × 150. The patient presented with an acute obstruction of the right femoral artery. Histologic examination of the embolized material established the diagnosis. A left atrial myxoma was successfully removed. (From Hattler, B. G., Jr., et al.: Ann. Thorac. Surg., *10*:65, 1970.)

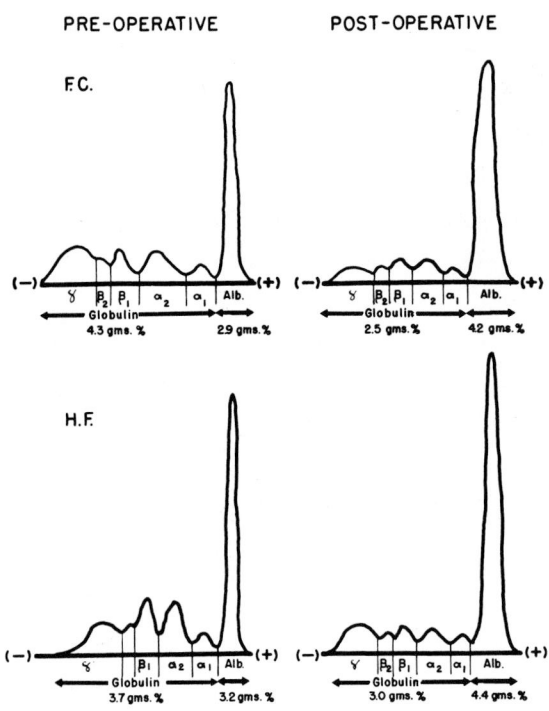

Figure 4. Serum protein electrophoresis demonstrating prominent alpha-2, beta-1, and heterogeneous gamma globulin peaks in the preoperative specimens. Reversion to normal is demonstrated postoperatively. Both patients presented initially with recurrent fever, weight loss, and arthralgias, which cleared following tumor removal. (From Hattler, B. G., Jr., et al.: Ann. Thorac. Surg., *10*:65, 1970.)

been described.[7] Metastases have been found in the mitral valve, left ventricle, atrial septum, sternum, chest wall, and pubis.

Patients with atrial myxomas may thus present with symptoms of peripheral embolization, atrioventricular valvular obstruction, or a systemic illness. In a consecutive series of 13 such patients, zone electrophoresis of serum proteins demonstrated elevated total globulin levels with prominent alpha-2, beta-1, or heterogeneous gamma globulin peaks. Immunoelectrophoresis localized the elevated globulins to either the IgM or IgA fractions. The levels return to normal with removal of the tumor (Fig. 4). Elevated erythrocyte sedimentation rates are usually seen. The electrocardiographic findings are usually nonspecific, although large right atrial P waves are sometimes seen in patients with right atrial tumors. Chest roentgenograms may be inconsistent, with a normal-sized heart evident in the presence of severe pulmonary venous and arterial congestion. *Echocardiography* is an excellent noninvasive method of making a definitive diagnosis of an intracardiac mass (Fig. 5). *Phonocardiography* may also be useful in demonstrating that the intensity of the first heart sound is almost uniformly increased, and in early diastole a low frequency sound or "plop" can be demonstrated in the majority of patients with left atrial myxomas. A diastolic murmur is also usually present. Hemodynamic findings on cardiac catheterization and the analysis of pressure tracings are best correlated with the degree of atrioventricular valvular obstruction. Their value lies mainly in localizing the site of the disorder. The definitive method of diagnosis is selective angiocardiography. In

the series of cases of atrial myxoma mentioned earlier, angiocardiograms were diagnostic in all patients on whom the study was performed (Fig. 6), while cardiac catheterization without angiography was unsuccessful in establishing a diagnosis in two patients. Radioactive precordial scans utilizing radioiodinated serum albumin may demonstrate defects in the area of the myxoma.

Management

Following diagnosis, all tumors should be surgically excised under direct vision with use of extracorporeal circulation. Operation should be performed promptly because of the constant threat of sudden death following any prolonged obstruction of the atrioventricular valve and the possibility of embolization. A right anterolateral incision provides ready access for incision into either the left or right atrium and it is often wise to open both atria so that they may be thoroughly inspected. During manipulation of these tumors, prophylaxis against embolization is accomplished by induction of ventricular fibrillation or temporary occlusion of the ascending aorta or both. Considerable care should be exercised in the removal of this very friable tumor, and a wide excision of the interatrial septum at its base is indicated to prevent local recurrence.[1, 12] The defect thus created in the atrial septum can be closed either directly or with a prosthesis.[22] Lavage of the atrium and ventricle aids in the removal of loose tumor fragments. Prognosis with surgery is excellent, and regression of all preoperative symptoms for follow-up periods of up to 10 years has been reported.

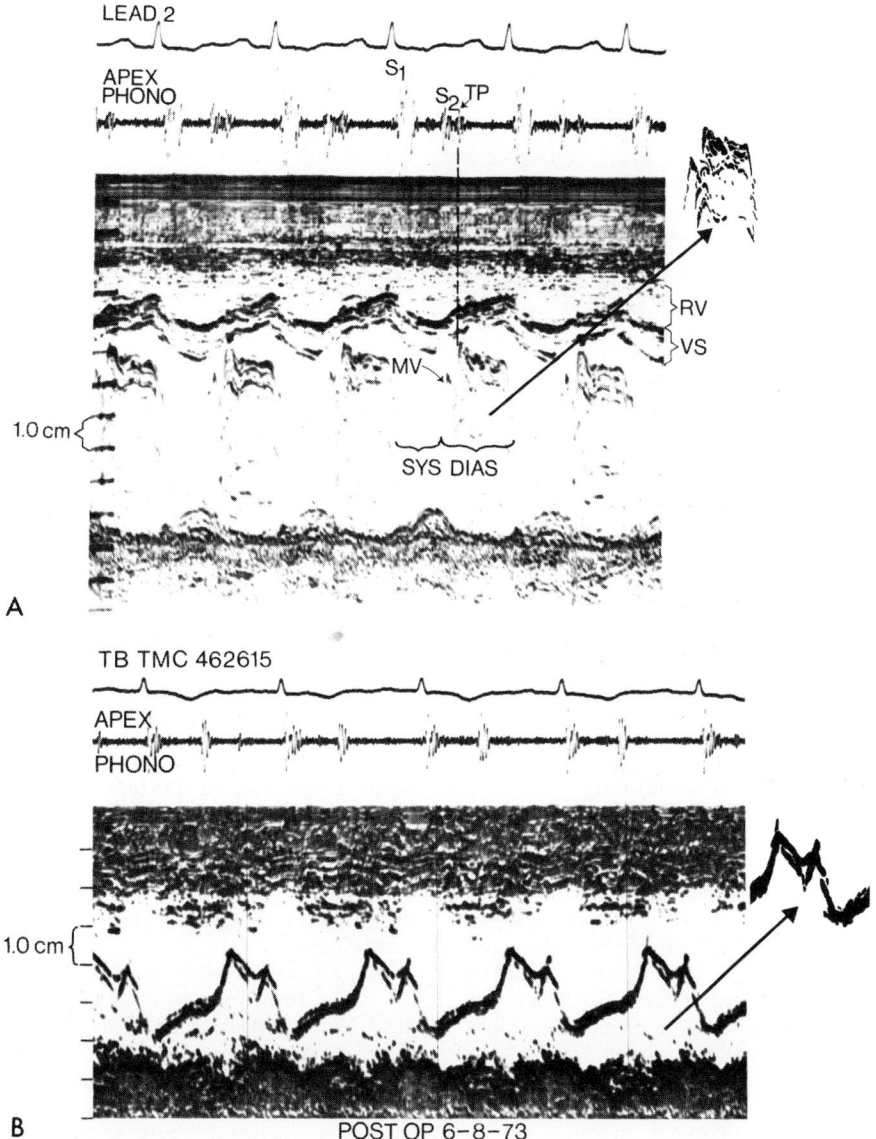

Figure 5. Mitral valve echocardiograms preoperative (*A*) and postoperative (*B*) from a patient with a pedunculated left atrial myxoma. A multitude of echoes is produced posterior to the anterior mitral valve echo during diastole. A simultaneous apex phonocardiogram demonstrates a "tumor plop" (TP) during this time interval. Both disappear after tumor removal. (Courtesy of Dr. Edward R. Byrne-Quinn. From Sabiston, D. C., Jr., and Spencer, F. C. (Eds.): Gibbon's Surgery of the Chest, 3rd ed. Philadelphia, W. B. Saunders Company, 1976.)

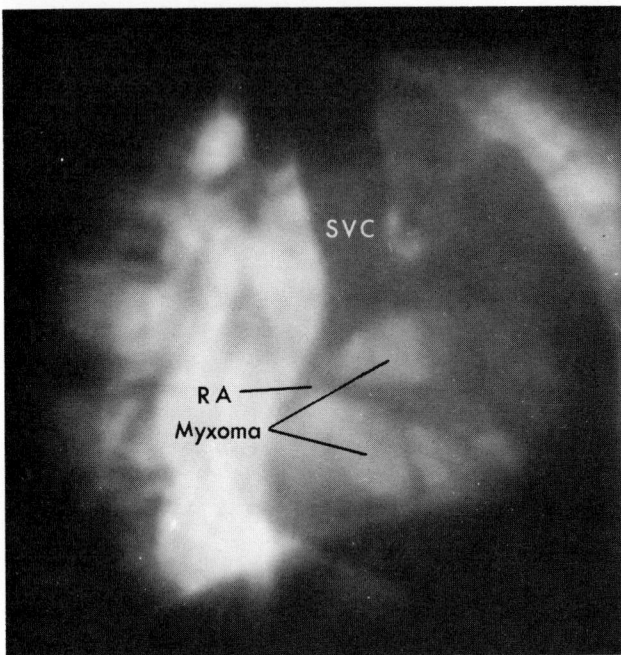

Figure 6. Angiocardiogram following injection of contrast medium into the superior vena cava (SVC). A large filling defect in the right atrium (RA) is demonstrated. A myxoma was removed the following day. (From Hattler, B. G., Jr., et al.: Ann. Thorac. Surg., *10*:65, 1970.)

MALIGNANT NEOPLASMS

The vast majority of primary malignant tumors of the heart are *sarcomas*.[29] With the exception of infants and children, in whom they are rarely found, these tumors are seen in persons of all ages and constitute approximately 20 per cent of primary cardiac neoplasms.[8] They originate most frequently from the endocardium or pericardium on the right side of the heart, occurring with equal frequency in the atrium and ventricle.[24] Grossly, neoplasms originating in the pericardium infiltrate diffusely, eventually obscuring the cardiac contour. Although an infiltrative lesion is commonly seen with tumors originating in the epicardium, intracavitary protrusions may also occur with more sessile forms of this neoplasm. Histologically, a wide range of sarcomatous tumors have been reported with round cell and spindle cell sarcomas and angiosarcomas being most frequent. Metastatic spread is encountered in over 25 per cent of cases, with involvement of the mediastinum, lung, and pleura. More rarely, hematogenous spread to abdominal organs including the liver, kidney, and adrenals has been noted.[24]

Clinically, patients with primary sarcomas of the heart have progressive heart failure that generally is unresponsive to medical therapy. Because of preponderant involvement of the right side of the heart, symptoms of tricuspid valve or superior vena caval obstruction may predominate. Invasion of the conduction system produces arrhythmias or may result in complete heart block. With epicardial and pericardial extensions, a picture of bizarre, irregular cardiac enlargement is seen on chest roentgenograms or by pneumopericardiography in association with hemopericardium. In contrast to benign myxomas, in which angiocardiograms are diagnostic, intracavitary sarcomas are only occasionally revealed by angiocardiog-

raphy. This may be attributed to the morphologic arrangement of the tumor, which is usually not pedunculated and has little or no free movement within the atrial or ventricular cavities.

A special malignant pericardial tumor is the *mesothelioma*.[26] It arises from the serous surface of the pericardium and is difficult to classify histologically. Both epithelial and connective tissue tumor components are seen microscopically with a frequently sarcomatous appearance intermingling in other areas with glandlike spaces or channels. Mesothelioma appears grossly as a flattened, nodular tumor mass spreading over the pericardium and resulting in voluminous hemorrhagic effusions. The clinical findings are those of pericarditis and tamponade. These highly malignant tumors grow rapidly and invade the surrounding myocardium. Distant metastases are commonly found.

Diagnosis of primary malignant cardiac tumors may be made from cytologic examination of pericardial fluid, but thoracotomy and direct biopsy may be required. With the exception of isolated reports, such as an instance of a right atrial rhabdomyoma in an infant, in which the entire right atrial wall was replaced with a pericardial graft with survival,[20] definitive therapy at the time of surgery is usually not possible. Symptomatic temporary relief can follow the removal of pericardial fluid or the excision of large space-occupying lesions. Further palliation may be obtained with drug and radiation therapy.[13] Death usually occurs within the first year following the onset of symptoms.

SELECTED REFERENCES

Freiman, A. H.: Cardiovascular disturbances associated with cancer. Med. Clin. North Am., *50*:733, 1966.
   This article considers in a concise fashion cardiac abnormalities that may arise as a result of either direct involvement of the heart by

metastatic tumor or secondary mechanisms associated with cancer that alter the function of the heart. It emphasizes the various clinical manifestations the clinician may encounter and the pitfalls to be avoided.

Gerbode, F., Keith, J. W., and Hill, J. D.: Surgical management of tumors of the heart. Surgery, *61*:94, 1967.

This concise, well-illustrated article describes the technical aspects and surgical management of 10 patients with tumors of the heart. Eight myxomas, one teratoma, and one fibroma were surgically excised. Recurrence of myxoma was noted in one case four years after simple excision. The recurrent tumor was removed along with a portion of atrial septum; the authors now recommend this procedure to insure against recurrence.

Gramiak, R., and Waag, R. C.: Cardiac Ultrasound. St. Louis, The C. V. Mosby Co., 1975.

This monograph includes selections by 18 contributors who are authorities in the field of the role of ultrasound in the diagnosis of cardiovascular disease. It provides excellent commentaries on basic features of ultrasound, recording methods, and specific disorders with their characteristic appearances. The illustrations are excellent and the text is highly recommended.

Hattler, B. G., Jr., Fuchs, J. C. A., Cosson, R., and Sabiston, D. C., Jr.: Atrial myxoma: An evaluation of clinical and laboratory manifestations. Ann. Thorac. Surg., *10*:65, 1970.

The diagnosis and management of 13 cases of atrial myxoma are reviewed. Emphasis is placed on the varied clinical manifestations these tumors may produce. Changes in the electrophoretic pattern of the serum proteins, with elevation in gamma globulins, are features of diagnostic importance that return to normal after excision of the myxoma. In 11 of the 13 patients the tumor was diagnosed correctly and managed by surgical excision.

Prichard, R. W.: Tumors of the heart: Review of the subject and report of one hundred and fifty cases. A.M.A. Arch. Pathol., *51*:98, 1951.

The article presents a general discussion of tumors of the heart, together with a report of 146 secondary and four primary cardiac neoplasms. Each type of tumor is reviewed at least briefly, and abundant gross and microscopic illustrations are included. The compilation of data and the references to works published up to that time make this paper a ready source of information.

Read, R. C., White, H. J., Murphy, M. L., Williams, D., Sun, C. N., and Flanagan, W. H.: The malignant potentiality of left atrial myxoma. J. Thorac. Cardiovasc. Surg., *68*:857, 1974.

In this review, the authors summarize the literature for patients with atrial myxomas, in whom spread to both local and distant sites has occurred. Metastases were demonstrated as far distant as the pubis.

Whorton, C. M.: Primary malignant tumors of the heart. Cancer, *2*:245, 1949.

The paper presents a review of 100 cases of primary sarcomatous tumors of the heart. Discussion of their localization, histology, and metastatic spread is amplified by a table concisely listing each case with its salient features and literature references.

REFERENCES

1. Bahl, O. P., Oliver, C. G., Ferguson, T. B., Schod, N., and Parker, B. M.: Recurrent left atrial myxoma: report of a case. Circulation, *40*:673, 1969.
2. Barnes, A. R., Beaver, D. C., and Snell, A. M.: Primary sarcoma of the heart: Report of a case with electrocardiographic and pathological studies. Am. Heart J., *9*:480, 1934.
3. Bisel, H. F., Wroblewski, F., and La Due, J. S.: Incidence and clinical manifestations of cardiac metastases. J.A.M.A., *153*:712, 1953.
4. Brandes, W. W., Gray, J. A. C., and MacLeod, N. W.: Leiomyoma of the pericardium: Report of a case. Am. Heart J., *23*:426, 1942.
5. Columbus, M. R.: De Re Anatomica. Paris, 1562, Libri XV, p. 482.
6. Crafoord, C.: Case report. In International Symposium Cardiovascular Surgery. Detroit, Henry Ford Hospital, 1955, p.202.
7. Dang, C. R., and Hurley, E. J.: Contralateral recurrent myxoma of the heart. Ann. Thorac. Surg., *21*:59, 1976.
8. Dong, E., Hurley, E. J., and Shumway, N. E.: Primary cardiac sarcoma. Am. J. Cardiol., *10*:871, 1962.
9. Fenoglio, J. J., Jr., McAllister, H. A., Jr., and Ferrans, V. J.: Cardiac rhabdomyoma: A clinicopathologic and electron microscopic study. Am. J. Cardiol., *38*:241, 1976.
10. Freiman, A. H.: Cardiovascular disturbances associated with cancer. Med. Clin. North Am., *50*:733, 1966.
11. Gassman, H. S., Meadows, R., Jr., and Baker, L. A.: Metastatic tumors of the heart. Am. J. Med., *19*:357, 1955.
12. Gerbode, F., Keith, J. W., and Hill, J. D.: Surgical management of tumors of the heart. Surgery, *61*:94, 1967.
13. Goldstein, S., and Mahoney, E. B.: Right ventricular fibrosarcoma causing pulmonic stenosis. Am. J. Cardiol., *17*:570, 1966.
14. Goyer, R. A., and Bowden, D. H.: Endocardial fibroelastosis associated with glycogen tumors of the heart and tuberous sclerosis. Am. Heart J., *64*:539, 1962.
15. Grant, R. T., and Camp, P. D.: A case of complete heart block due to an arterial angioma. Heart, *16*:137, 1932.
16. Griffiths, G. C.: Primary tumors of the heart. Clin. Radiol., *13*:183, 1962.
17. Hanbury, W. J.: Secondary tumors of the heart. Br. J. Cancer, *14*:23, 1960.
18. Hattler, B. G., Jr., Fuchs, J. C. A., Cosson, R., and Sabiston, D. C., Jr.: Atrial myxoma: An evaluation of clinical and laboratory manifestations. Ann. Thorac. Surg., *10*:65, 1970.
19. Hurst, J. W., and Cooper, H. R.: Neoplastic disease of the heart. Am. Heart J., *50*:782, 1955.
20. Kilman, J. W., Craenen, J., and Hosier, D. M.: Replacement of entire right atrial wall in an infant with a cardiac rhabdomyoma. J. Pediatr. Surg., *8*:317, 1973.
21. Magovern, G. J.: Discussion of Hattler, B. G., Jr., Fuchs, J. C. A., Cosson, R., and Sabiston, D. C., Jr.: Atrial myxoma: An evaluation of clinical and laboratory manifestations. Ann. Thorac. Surg., *10*:65, 1970.
22. Peters, M. N., Hall, R. J., Cooley, D. A., Leachman, R. D., and Garcia, E.: The clinical syndrome of atrial myxoma. J.A.M.A., *230*:695, 1974.
23. Pratt, C. B., Dugger, D. L., Johnson, W. W., and Ainger, L. E.: Metastatic involvement of the heart in childhood rhabdomyosarcoma. Cancer, *31*:1492, 1973.
24. Prichard, R. W.: Tumors of the heart: Review of the subject and report of one hundred and fifty cases. A.M.A. Arch. Pathol., *51*:98, 1951.
25. Read, R. C., White, H. J., Murphy, M. L., Williams, D., Sun, C. N., and Flanagan, W. H.: The malignant potentiality of left atrial myxoma. J. Thorac. Cardiovasc. Surg., *68*:857, 1974.
26. Reals, W. J., Russman, B. C., and Walsh, E. M.: Primary mesothelioma of the pericardium. A.M.A. Arch. Pathol., *44*:380, 1947.
27. Siltanen, P., Tuuteri, L., Norio, R., Tala, P., Ahrenberg, P., and Halonen, P. I: Atrial myxoma in a family. Am. J. Cardiol., *38*:252, 1976.
28. Steinberg, I., Dotter, C. T., and Glenn, F.: Myxoma of the heart: Roentgen diagnosis during life in three cases. Dis. Chest., *24*:509, 1953.
29. Whorton, C. M.: Primary malignant tumors of the heart. Cancer, *2*:245, 1949.
30. Yater, W. M.: Tumors of the heart and pericardium. Arch. Intern. Med., *48*:627, 1931.
31. Zajtchuk, R., Fitterer, J. D., Strevey, T. E., and Nelson, W. P.: Bilateral atrial myxomas. Preoperative diagnosis and successful removal. J. Thorac. Cardiovasc. Surg., *69*:291, 1975.

XXI

CARDIAC PACEMAKERS

William M. Chardack, M.D., Andrew A. Gage, M.D.,
and Anthony J. Federico, M.D.

Some accounts of the use of electrical currents to elicit contraction of the heart muscle date back to the eighteenth century, but the era of modern pacemaking began in 1932 when Hyman established the concept of pacing,[12] that is, the repetitive delivery of an electrical impulse that depolarizes only cardiac tissue adjacent to the electrode. The remainder of the myocardium is then activated by a propagated action potential. The pulse generator and needle electrode developed by him (Fig. 1) were cumbersome but adequate for clinical use, which he thought of as being in the domain of resuscitation from cardiac arrest. At that time, the serious nature of heart block complicated by asystole had been known for more than a century, but another 20 years elapsed before Zoll, in 1952, successfully treated the condition by repetitive electrical stimuli applied to the chest wall.[27] External pacemakers operating through surface electrodes gained immediate acceptance, but the painful side effects of the high voltages required by this technique made it difficult to use on a long-term basis.

With the development of open-heart surgery in the early 1950s, control of the heart rate became of great interest to surgeons because the inadvertent induction of heart block during the repair of intracardiac defects was then a not infrequent and often lethal complication; cardioaccelerating drugs were unsatisfactory, but the management of this complication was dramatically improved by the introduction of myocardial wires sutured to the myocardium and brought out through the chest wall at the time of operation.[26] The currents required to pacemake through such wires are below the threshold of sensation.

This approach stimulated the development of small battery-powered external pacemakers and of silicone rubber-insulated bipolar electrodes[11] and the application of pacing techniques to patients with other types of chronic heart block. About the same time, early clinical trials with pacing via transvenously placed endocardiac electrodes were reported.[8] However, long-term pacemaking with electrodes traversing the skin had limitations because of the risk of infection and accidental disconnection and the inconvenience of an externally worn apparatus. Two solutions to these problems were developed.

Partially implanted pacemaker systems were introduced in 1959, consisting of an externally worn pulse generator coupled by radio-frequency waves[1, 9] or by induction through the intact skin to an implanted receiver and electrode system. Other investigators pursued the concept of a completely implanted system, and the first successful long-term clinical use of a self-contained pacemaker carrying its own power supply was reported in 1960 (Fig. 2).[4] Since then, this approach has become the treatment of choice for chronic heart block.

In the ensuing decade, increasingly sophisticated instrumentation has been developed. Implanted pacemaker systems operating through transvenously placed endocardiac electrodes became popular in 1963,[24] and soon thereafter implantable devices were introduced, the output of which was programed from

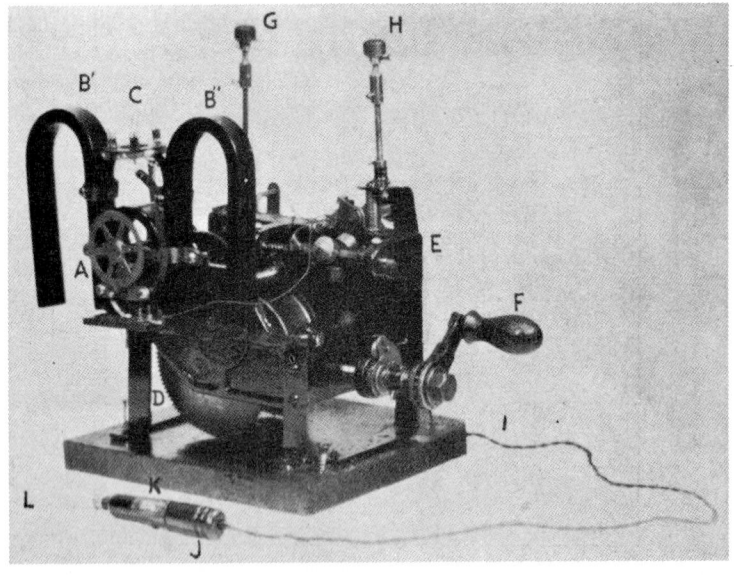

Figure 1. Artificial pacemaker consisting of a hand-operated magnetogenerator (A) and an electrode needle (L). (From Hyman, A. S.: Arch. Intern. Med., 50:289, 1932.)

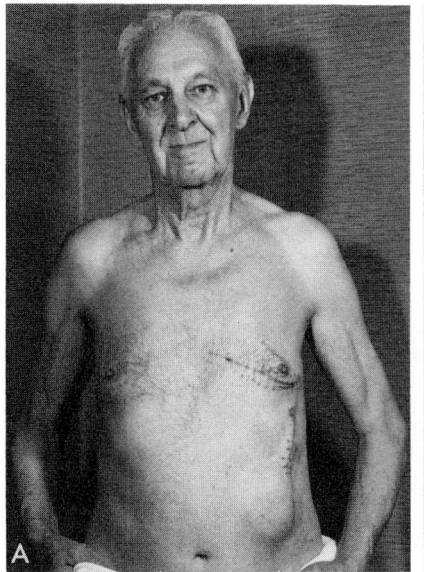
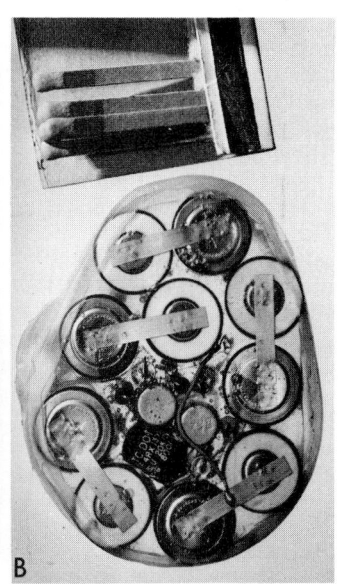

Figure 2. *A,* First patient treated successfully on a long-term basis with a self-contained, implantable pacemaker in 1960.[4] He was 77 years old, had sustained a skull fracture after innumerable Stokes-Adams attacks, and lived several years after receiving his pacemaker. *B,* Pacemaker similar to the one used in this patient, constructed by one of us (W. G.).[4] Note ten cells in series yielding a 14-volt pulse (very high by current standards). The long-term stimulation requirements were, of course, unknown and unforeseeable at that time. (From Chardack, W. M. *In* Sabiston, D. C., Jr., and Spencer, F. C. (Eds.): Gibbon's Surgery of the Chest, 3rd ed. Philadelphia, W. B. Saunders Company, 1976.)

spontaneous atrial[20] or ventricular electrical activity.[22] A recent report of the clinical use of a nuclear energy-powered pacemaker marked the introduction of an implantable power source with an extremely long life (Fig. 15).[15] Newly developed lithium batteries (and to some extent rechargeable batteries) have now been in use long enough to have established themselves as longer-lived power sources than the mercury cell used up to 1970. These new cells and the advent of integrated circuitry have culminated in hermetic sealing of the pulse generator, shielding it from body fluids and adding reliability to longer pacemaker life.

Temporary and permanent pacing techniques are now frequently used to treat arrhythmias other than block, and temporary pacing has become an important tool in the postoperative care of cardiac and other surgical patients.

The use of implantable pacemakers has grown rapidly and a survey in 1975* indicated that close to 60,000 new implantations were performed annually in the United States and that about one in 1300 persons was living with such a device, an increase in usage of about 100 per cent in a three-year period. Arrhythmias other than fixed complete heart block were the indication for implantation in 40 per cent of patients.

There has also occurred a change in the roles played by the cardiac surgeon and the cardiologist. The first pacemaker systems to be implanted used myocardial electrodes requiring thoracotomy and were in the surgical domain. Transvenously placed electrodes became popular in the mid 1960s and the cardiologist, conversant with cardiac catheterization, began to play an important role, especially in the development of pacing techniques for therapeutic and diagnostic purposes. The field of cardiac pacing is still changing and crosses the disciplines of surgery, cardiology, and bio-

medical and electronic engineering, and in the larger medical centers this has led to the development of specialized teams devoting full-time efforts to pacemaker therapy and the follow-up surveillance of the patients.

The surgeon is primarily concerned with the technique of installation of an implantable pacemaker system, and since patients with acquired chronic heart block still are the majority of those requiring this therapy, this entity will be dealt with first.

ETIOLOGY AND CLINICAL FEATURES OF ACQUIRED CHRONIC HEART BLOCK

Most patients are elderly; two thirds are over 70 years old and the ratio of males to females is 2:1.

The etiology of chronic heart block is still the subject of controversy. Histologic findings suggest that about 50 to 60 per cent of cases are caused by degenerative fibrous and calcific changes—probably related to the aging process—either of the conduction system itself or in the closely adjacent fibrous cardiac skeleton.[16, 17] There is convincing evidence linking the entity of chronic atrioventricular block in the elderly to bilateral bundle branch block, the so-called "hemiblocks," and "trifascicular blocks." Several of these entities, caused by various combinations of block in the distal branches of the bundle of His, are known to be precursors of complete block.[14] Recent techniques of recording an endocardiac electrogram (through a transvenously placed electrode) from various portions of the conduction system make it possible to localize accurately the site of the block (Fig. 3).[19] They may also lead to a more precise classification of block than that based on the conventional electrocardiogram, which distinguishes between (1) first degree block (prolongation of the atrioventricular conduction time); (2) second degree block (occasional dropped beats; higher grade block with 2:1, 3:1 atrioventricular conduction); and (3) complete block (atrial and ventricular activity are independent).

---

*Figures obtained in the State of New Jersey and extrapolated to the U.S.A. (Parsonnet, V. *In* Proceedings of Fifth International Symposium on Cardiac Pacing. See Selected References.)

The role of coronary artery disease in the genesis of heart block is changing. Autopsy data reported in the past have shown only inconspicuous involvement of the coronary arterial tree, but current clinical experience reveals an increase in the number of patients in whom permanent block is a direct sequela of an acute myocardial infarction. Heart block complicates about 8 per cent of acute infarctions, and in only a few of these does it become a permanent residual, but because of the high incidence of acute myocardial infarction, it may cause many thousands of cases of block per year in the United States.

Chronic block can also be caused by focal and diffuse lesions observed in a wide variety of diseases—rheumatic heart disease, myopathies, and bacterial and parasitic infections, to list but a few.

Atrioventricular block may be permanent or intermittent; episodes of complete or higher degrees of block can alternate with periods of normal conduction or lesser degrees of block. The features of the disease are caused by bradycardia (a slow subsidiary pacemaker substitutes for the sinus node), which is compensated for by an increase of the stroke volume, leading to dilatation and hypertrophy of the heart. When the rate falls to below 40 beats per minute, stroke volume approaches its maximum and cardiac output

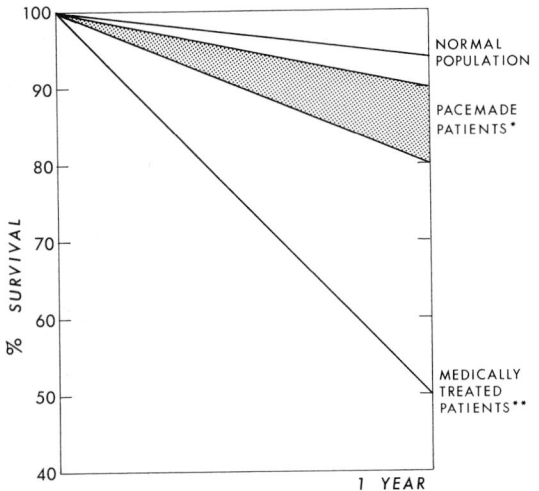

Figure 4. Comparison of per cent survival at the 1-year point in chronic acquired heart block. The asterisk indicates range of percentages from several large series. The double asterisk indicates average of percentages in several series of medically treated patients. (From Chardack, W. M. In Sabiston, D. C., Jr, and Spencer, F. C. (Eds.): Gibbon's Surgery of the Chest, 3rd ed. Philadelphia, W. B. Saunders Company, 1976.)

becomes entirely rate-dependent. Decompensation occurs, first under the stress of physical activity and then at rest. Cardiac output is then subnormal, the arterial pulse pressure and the arteriovenous oxygen difference are high, and secondary renal and cerebral manifestations make their appearance.

The occurrence of syncopal attacks (Adams-Stokes or Morgagni-Adams-Stokes syndrome) is the cardinal feature of the disease. Syncope is caused by the sudden reduction of cardiac output and cerebral blood flow. The underlying mechanism may be bradycardia, asystole, ventricular tachycardia, or ventricular fibrillation, and one or more of these may be observed in any one patient. Normal conduction may prevail between syncopal episodes. Tachyarrhythmias not caused by block also may produce syncope, and syncopal attacks unrelated to cardiac disease may occur in patients with low-degree block and erroneously be ascribed to the latter. Continuous recording of the electrocardiogram in combination with His bundle recording and temporary atrial pacing has become an essential diagnostic tool to recognize heretofore hidden conduction disorders (Fig. 3).

The natural course of chronic acquired heart block is unpredictable. Drug therapy has been unsatisfactory, and the ominous prognosis of the condition is well known. Without pacemaking, the mortality rate at the end of the first year following appearance of symptoms requiring treatment is between 50 and 60 per cent (Fig. 4).[3]

The indications for permanent pacemaking in heart block have been broadened in recent years based on the recognition of the underlying pathology in the branches. Therapy is indicated in the following:

Third degree block: symptomatic or not, fixed or intermittent.

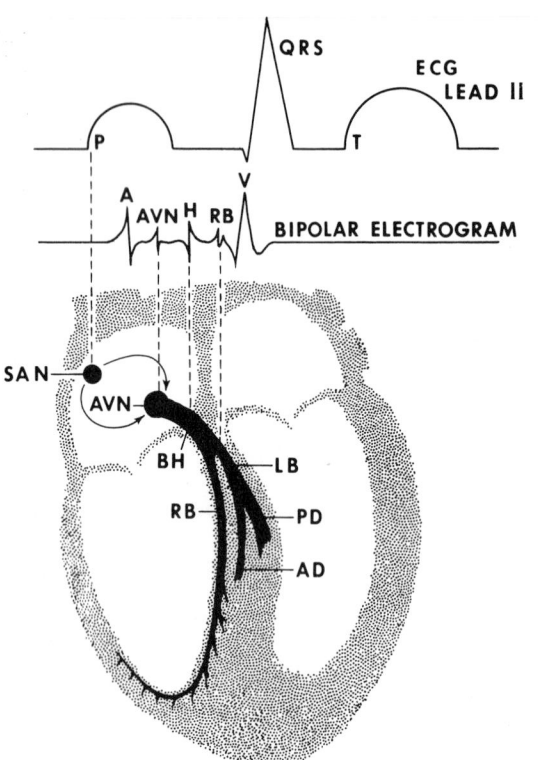

Figure 3. Diagram showing progression of conduction in the heart and the relationship between anatomic structures and the events observed in limb electrocardiogram and in an electrogram recorded from a transvenously inserted bipolar electrode positioned close to the conduction bundle (see text and references 14 and 19). SAN = Sinoatrial node, AVN = Atrioventricular node, BH = His bundle, RB = Right bundle branch, LB = Left bundle branch, (PD = posterior division; AD = anterior division).

Second degree block: symptomatic or not, fixed or intermittent.

Bilateral bundle branch block, right bundle branch block, and other partial blocks: symptomatic.

The discussion now revolves largely about patients with fascicular blocks who are asymptomatic. Prophylactic pacemaker therapy has been suggested for right bundle branch block and left axis deviation and trifascicular lesions. Definitive guidelines for therapy in these cases remain to be established by the cardiologists.

OPERATIVE INSTALLATION OF AN IMPLANTED PACEMAKER SYSTEM

Implantable pacemaker systems consist of a pulse generator and the electrode(s). Up to 1970, almost all implantable pulse generators were powered by zinc mercuric oxide batteries. Many patients still are wearers of such devices. Improved power sources are now coming rapidly into use. An electric circuit regulates the emission of an electrical impulse, ranging in amplitude from 4 to 7 volts and in duration from about 0.3 to 1 msec. The pulse is transmitted to the myocardium by either a myocardial or an endocardial electrode. This may be a single electrode structure (unipolar) which is used as the cathode (Fig. 5B) and the electrical circuit is completed by a metal plate or the metal housing of the pulse generator (anode) (see Fig. 10). It may be a bipolar electrode with both anode and cathode terminals on or in the heart (see Figs. 5A, 6, 9, and 15).

Implantation of systems operating through myocardial electrodes requires thoracotomy or an extra-pleural approach, usually under general anesthesia. Installation of a transvenously placed endocardiac electrode attached to a subcutaneously placed pulse generator can be carried out under local anesthesia. A wide variety of pulse generators are now available in combination with different electrode systems. The sophistication and complexity in terms of programing the output of the pulse generator has led to a three-letter identification code (Fig. 5, Tables 1 and 2).

At present there are about 50 pacemaker manufacturers in the world, each offering several models. A complete listing is beyond the purview of this review and only a few representative and innovative examples are described (see Figs. 9 to 16).

THORACOTOMY AND INSTALLATION OF A MYOCARDIAL-ELECTRODE PACEMAKER SYSTEM

Under general anesthesia, a left anterolateral thoracotomy is performed through the fifth intercostal space or through the bed of the resected fifth rib. The pericardium is incised anterior to the left phrenic nerve. The electrode(s) is affixed to a bare area of the left ventricular myocardium as shown in Figure 5. The pericardium is closed over the electrode leads with a small aperture left for drainage and with care to keep the phrenic nerve out of the immediate vicinity of the electrode. The pulse generator is then attached and placed subcutaneously either into a subcostal or more commonly now into a retropectoral position (Fig. 5). The chest is drained for 24 hours.

Important Considerations in the Management of Patients Treated by Thoracotomy

Preoperative pacing by a temporary endocardial electrode should always be used. It permits correction of congestive failure and electrolyte imbalance and an operation on a well-prepared patient. The temporary electrode also provides a high stimulation rate during certain phases of the operative procedure. Stimulation at a rate of about 100 beats per minute, suddenly interrupted, is followed by a controllable period of asystole which facilitates the installation of the electrode (Fig. 13G). This structure is subject to flex stresses at a rate of 80,000 to 100,000 duty cycles per 24 hours, and attention to details of placement and fixation is essential.

If a bipolar electrode system is used, the terminals are placed side by side on an avascular area of the left ventricle. The distance between the two electrode pins is not critical. An avascular area can usually be found near the apex of the left ventricle (Fig. 6).

The subcutaneous pocket for the pulse generator should be tight enough to avoid rotation of the apparatus and should be drained for 24 hours by a catheter brought out through a separate stab wound. Prophylactic antibiotic therapy is advisable to protect against infection, especially that caused by coagulase-positive staphylococci.

Several modifications of operative techniques have been devised to avoid entrance into the pleural cavity by either an upper abdominal or a subcostal trans-diaphragmatic approach (Fig. 8).

TABLE 1. Fully Implantable Pacemaker Systems*

ELECTRODES
Endocardiac ⎫
Myocardial ⎭ Unipolar or bipolar

PULSE GENERATORS
Asynchronous (Independent of intrinsic cardiac electrical activity)
  Fixed rate and output
  Programable rate and/or output
  Stimulus usually applied to ventricle but can be applied to atrium
  Atrioventricular sequential (stimulates both atrium and ventricle)

Synchronous (Programed from cardiac electrical activity)
  Programed from atrium (P wave synchrony)
  Programed from QRS
    QRS-suppressed-demand pacemaker (does not emit stimuli when patient is in NSR)

    QRS-triggered pacemaker (standby) (stimulus falls into absolute refractory during normal sinus rhythm)

    A-V bifocal, suppressed by QRS (may stimulate atrium and/or ventricle)

*From Sabiston, D. C., and Spencer, F. C.: Gibbon's Surgery of the Chest, 3rd ed. Philadelphia, W. B. Saunders Company, 1976.

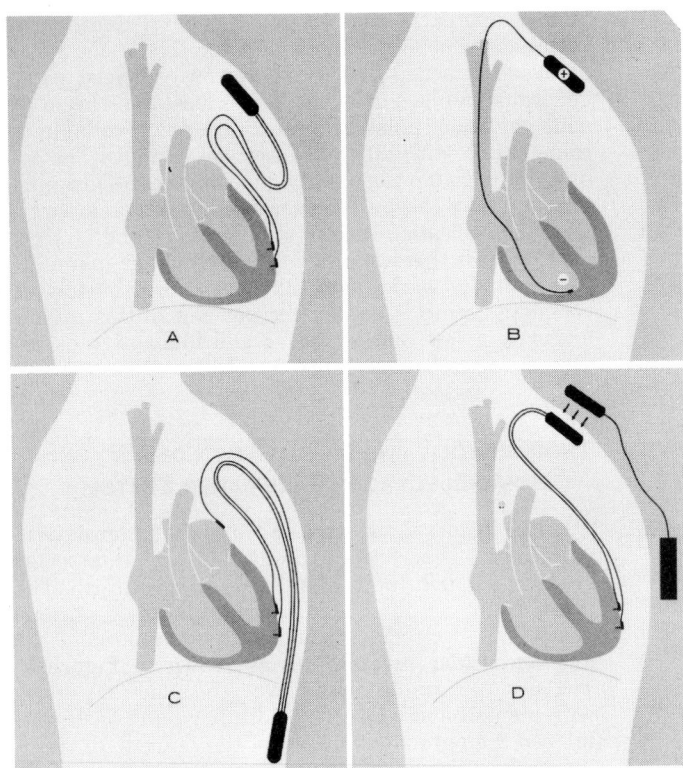

Figure 5. Diagram of pacemaker systems. *A*, Bipolar myocardial electrodes. Pulse generator in subcutaneous tissues of chest wall. *B*, Unipolar endocardiac electrode. Pulse generator in subcutaneous tissues of chest wall. *C*, Synchronous (atrial-programed) pulse generator. Note sensing electrode on left atrium. *D*, Partially implanted system. Note external transmitting coil placed over implanted receiver.

Management of Postoperative Complications

The pleural, pulmonary, and pericardial complications incident to a thoracotomy and pericardiotomy may have to be managed. Persistence of congestive failure may require drug therapy and a faster stimulation rate if the pulse generator allows adjustment of the rate. An important complication is the occurrence of runs of premature ventricular extrasystoles and multifocal ectopic activity (Fig. 14*A* and *B*). Myocardial injury and irritability, advanced dilatation and failure, and digitalis intoxication compounded by a low serum potassium concentration may play a part in the genesis of this complication. It should be treated immediately and aggressively by antiarrhythmic agents, restoration of a normal electrolyte pattern, and, if needed, an increase in the pacing rate (Fig. 14*C*).

Early infection around the implanted system is rare and usually caused by a coagulase-positive staphylococcus. It leads to an increase of the pacing threshold, often beyond the capabilities of the pulse generator. Aspiration and local and systemic administration of antibiotics are rarely successful. Exteriorization of the pulse generator is indicated, followed by implantation of a new permanent system at a different site.

Stimulation of the phrenic nerve(s), manifested by twitching of the upper abdomen and lower chest, is caused by too close proximity between the nerve and the electrode current field. It may subside but if persistent and symptomatic it can be corrected by crushing or transposition of the nerve.

In the past, the most common complication was breakage of the electrode. If only one lead of a bipolar system was affected, the complication could be corrected by transforming the broken lead into an indifferent subcutaneous electrode. Currently available electrodes have a flex resistance far in excess of requirements, and disruption of an electrode lead should be exceptional.

The pulse generator requires periodic replacement under local anesthesia when the batteries are near the end of their life. Infection may follow such secondary operation. The electrode leads are by then firmly encapsulated by a tight sleeve of fibrous tissue, and extension proximally of the infection and loss of pacing are infrequent. The pulse generator should be exteriorized and worn externally until a new system can be installed. The literature contains several reports of chronically infected systems that have been salvaged by antibiotics and relocation of the pulse generator. In the authors' experience, this appoach has always failed in the end and a new system has had to be installed.

TABLE 2.   Three-Letter Identification Code*

1st Letter *Chamber Paced*	2nd Letter *Chamber Sensed*	3rd Letter *Mode of Response*
V – Ventricle A – Atrium D – Both Chambers A and V		I – Inhibited T – Triggered O – Not applicable

*After Parsonnet et al.: Circulation, *50*:A21–A35, 1974.

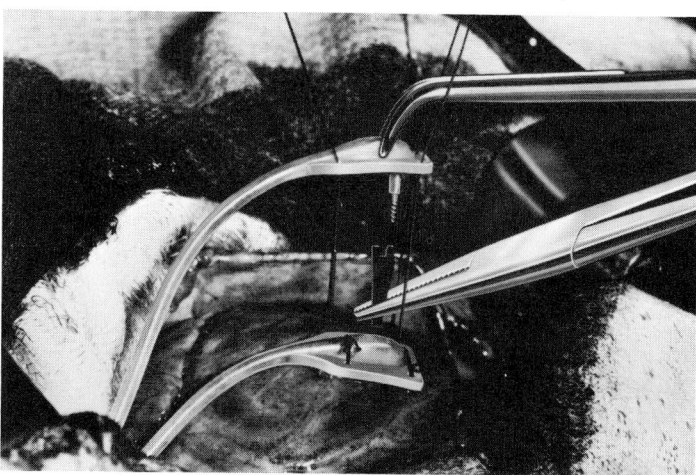

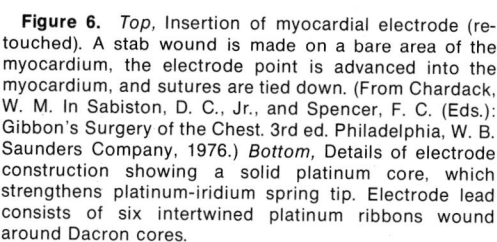

Figure 6. *Top,* Insertion of myocardial electrode (retouched). A stab wound is made on a bare area of the myocardium, the electrode point is advanced into the myocardium, and sutures are tied down. (From Chardack, W. M. In Sabiston, D. C., Jr., and Spencer, F. C. (Eds.): Gibbon's Surgery of the Chest. 3rd ed. Philadelphia, W. B. Saunders Company, 1976.) *Bottom,* Details of electrode construction showing a solid platinum core, which strengthens platinum-iridium spring tip. Electrode lead consists of six intertwined platinum ribbons wound around Dacron cores.

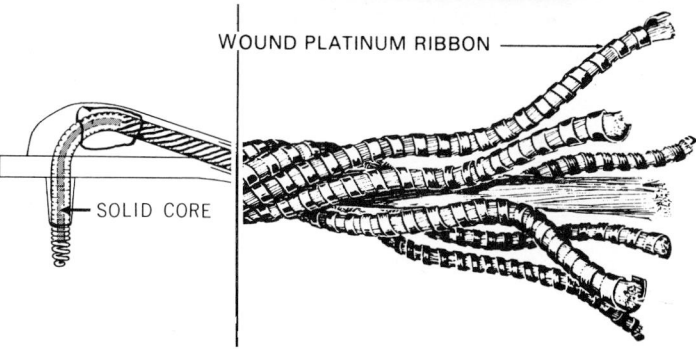

WOUND PLATINUM RIBBON

SOLID CORE

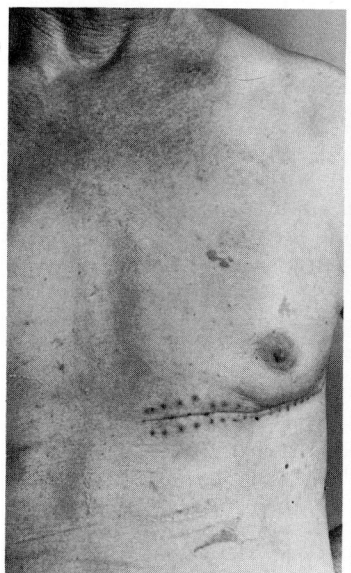
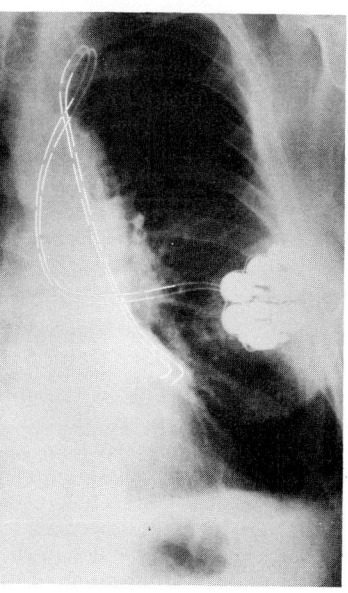

Figure 7. Patient with implanted myocardial-electrode pacemaker system. Pulse generator is in the subcutaneous tissues beneath the lateral margin of the pectoralis major muscle. (From Chardack, W. M. *In* Sabiston, D. C., Jr., and Spencer, F. C. (Eds.): Gibbon's Surgery of the Chest, 3rd ed. Philadelphia, W. B. Saunders Company, 1976.)

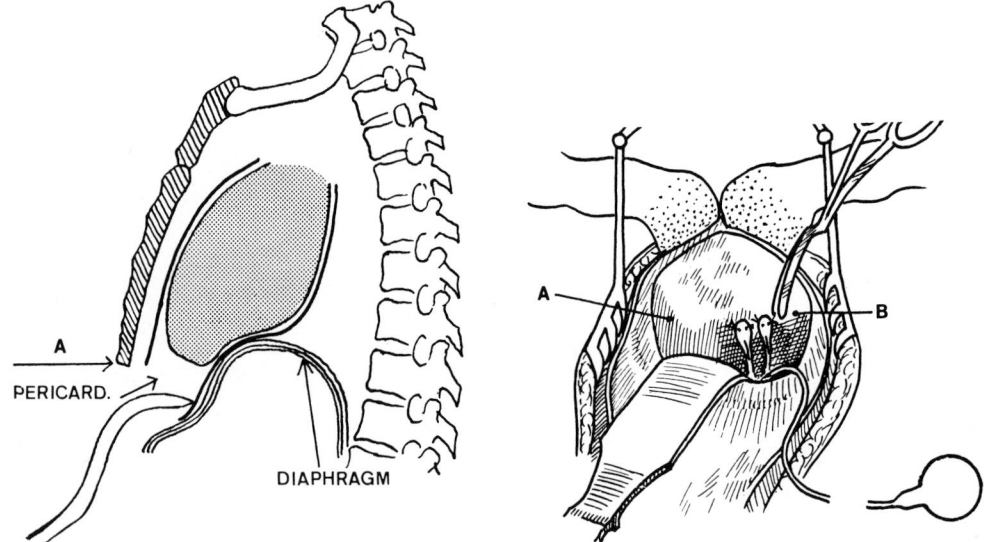

Figure 8. Drawing of epigastric midline approach. Larrey's space is enlarged (*A, left*) by blunt dissection and the pericardium is incised. The electrode(s) is affixed side by side on the bare inferior surface of the right ventricle. (After Castallani *et al.:* Ann. Chir. Thorac. Cardiovasc., 10(3):299–306, 1971.)

INSTALLATION OF AN IMPLANTED ENDOCARDIAC-ELECTRODE PACEMAKER SYSTEM

The technique and instrumentation for this approach are illustrated in Figures 9 and 10. Installation can be performed under local anesthesia. The electrical conductors of the electrode leads are one or two coils of a corrosion- and flex-resistant nickel or similar alloy. They terminate in a platinum ring and tip (bipolar) or in a tip only (unipolar). Stiffness and curvature required for insertion of the electrode are provided by removable stylets.

For patients with a clearly established indication, installation of a permanent endocardiac system can be the first therapeutic step, since it carries the same risk as the insertion of a temporary electrode. Support of the heart rate during insertion of the electrode is required rarely, usually only for a few minutes, and can be accomplished with an intravenous solution of isoproterenol (1 mg. in 500 ml. of 5 per cent dextrose). The rate of administration must be carefully titrated to avoid myocardial irritability. An intravenous solution of procaine amide (1 gm. in 250 to 500 ml. of normal saline) should be readily available. Positioning of the electrode requires an image intensifier, and in many centers the entire procedure is performed in the cardiac catheterization unit. Facilities must be available for monitoring the electrocardiogram and for defibrillation.

The right or left cephalic vein is now most commonly used, since this approach requires only one incision (Fig. 9). If this vein is inadequate in size, either the left or right external jugular vein can be used. If an internal jugular vein must be used, it should not be ligated, and the electrode entrance should be closed by a purse-string suture. The electrode with its stylets in place is guided into the right ventricle and advanced into the trabeculations of the apex. Accurate wedging of the electrode tip into the trabeculae of the right ventricular apex is essential (Fig. 9). Contact between the electrode terminals and the endocardium is critical and must be demonstrated not only by a satisfactory position of the electrode but also by the presence of appropriately low stimulation thresholds. An endocardiac electrogram recorded from the electrode may be helpful. A number of versatile battery-powered instruments are now available to ascertain stimulation thresholds as well as the QRS voltage to insure that they meet the requirements of programable pulse generators. Placement into the coronary sinus should be avoided unless specifically intended for atrial stimulation. To rule out a position in the coronary sinus, fluoroscopy in the lateral position and an endocardiac electrogram may be required. After placement of the electrode, the stylets are removed and the pulse generator is attached to the electrode terminal(s) and placed in a subcutaneous or retropectoral pocket. The pocket should be drained for 24 hours, and prophylactic antibiotics are recommended. Anticoagulants are not required.

Complications of the Endocardiac-Electrode Pulse-Generator System

Because of the elimination of thoracotomy and general anesthesia, the endocardiac technique has a low postoperative mortality rate; however, it has its own characteristic complications:

1. Only a few instances of septicemia and mycotic infections have been reported, even though part of the system resides in the bloodstream.

2. Disruption of the electrode leads is also rare. The flex stresses on the endocardiac electrode are less severe than those on a myocardial electrode.

3. Perforation of the right ventricular myocardium

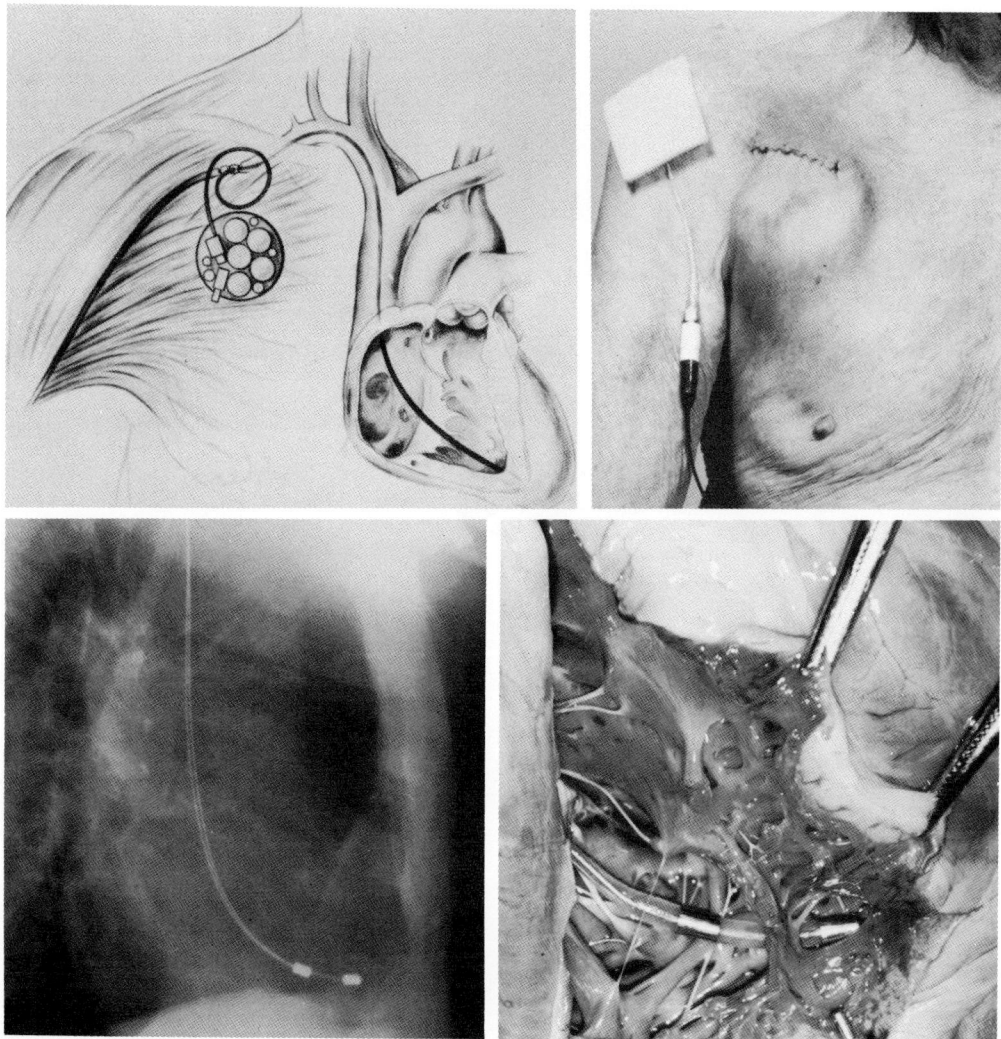

Figure 9. *Top left,* Schematic drawing of endocardiac approach. Electrode is inserted through right cephalic vein found in deltopectoral groove. (From Furman, S.: Ann. Surg., *164*:465, 1966.) *Top right,* Photograph of patient shortly after operation. Monitoring electrode is taped to right shoulder. *Bottom left,* X-ray showing anterior direction of endocardiac electrode. *Bottom right,* Interior of right ventricular cavity showing electrode wedged into trabeculations. Electrode was inserted for demonstration purposes only in the course of an autopsy on a patient who had no heart block. (From Chardack, W. M., et al.: Progr. Cardiovasc. Dis., 9:105, 1966. Reprinted by permission.)

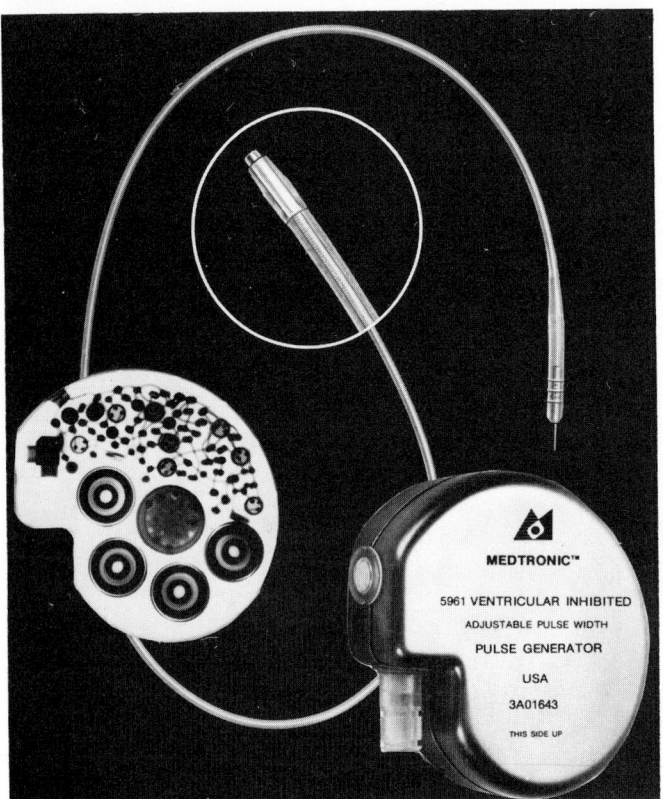

Figure 10. Demand pulse generator with adjustable pulse width and unipolar endocardiac small-tipped electrode (2 mm. diameter) (Manufactured by Medtronic, Inc., Minneapolis, Minnesota). This pulse generator was the first one with a noninvasively adjustable control of the output (1970). Impulse width rather than impulse amplitude was chosen because it provides an effective means of conserving battery capability and its absolute value can be detected from the electrical stimulus artifact appearing on the surface of the body. Note radiopaque circle on x-ray surrounded by four mercury cells (with translucent center). This is the gear train, actuated by a rotating magnet on the outside of the body regulating pulse width from 0.15 to 1.7 msec. Note the many small discrete components then in use. The pulse generator has a titanium housing as a shield against external electrical interference, but this is not a hermetic seal. The device is shown here (although of earlier technology) because of its programability, end of battery life characteristics (see following illustrations), and the excellent clinical results obtained by us and others.

or the interventricular septum can be caused by manipulation at insertion or later by erosion, resulting in one or more of the following: loss of pacing, pericardiac

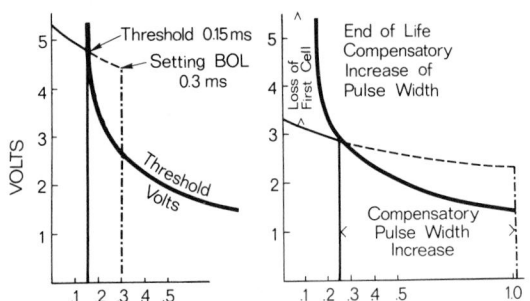

Figure 11. End of battery life characteristics in pulse generator shown in Figure 9 and of several other more current devices. The graph illustrates the basic "strength duration curve" showing the relationship between pulse duration and stimulus voltage (or current) required to depolarize the myocardium. This relationship is illustrated by the heavy line labeled "threshold volts" showing that threshold voltage decreases with pulse duration as an asymptote reaching the rheobase between 2 and 3 msec. In this patient, six weeks after implantation, the threshold was 0.15 msec. and was adjusted to 0.3 msec., about a 100 per cent margin. When battery voltage decreases (loss of one cell), the end of battery life pulse width increases to approximately 1 msec., maintaining an ample margin so that cardiac capture is maintained. In addition to a decrease in the rate, the increase in pulse width provides easily detectable end of battery life indicator by the physician, telephone transmission, or by patient self-check. (From Chardack, W. M.: *In* Sabiston, D. C., Jr., and Spencer, F. C. (Eds.): Gibbon's Surgery of the Chest, 3rd ed. Philadelphia, W. B. Saunders Company, 1976.)

rub, diaphragmatic contractions, and electrocardiographic patterns indicating left ventricular activation. None of these are pathognomonic, and their presence will depend upon the position of the electrode terminals in relation to myocardium. Tamponade following perforation has been exceptional, but it can be acute and require decompression by pericardiocentesis or thoracotomy. In most cases, the complication can be corrected by withdrawal of the electrode after its entrance site into the vein in the neck has been exposed.

4. Air embolism has occurred during insertion of an endocardiac electrode. In the reported cases, the complication remained harmless, but it should be kept in mind for prophylaxis and therapy.

5. Thromboembolic phenomena were conspicuously absent in early reports covering large series,[3] although prophylactic anticoagulants had not been used. More recently, thrombosis of the right atrium, the superior vena caval system, and the axillary and jugular veins and pulmonary embolizations have been observed. In some cases, congestive failure may have been a contributory cause. These complications have been rare, but they should be kept in mind because angiography can help with an early diagnosis, and surgical intervention may be warranted. Also, embolization may occur when an endocardiac electrode is withdrawn.

It is likely that thrombi form around most, if not all, endovascular and endocardiac electrodes, as can be demonstrated by venograms. As time goes by, organization of the thrombus occurs, resulting in a fibrous

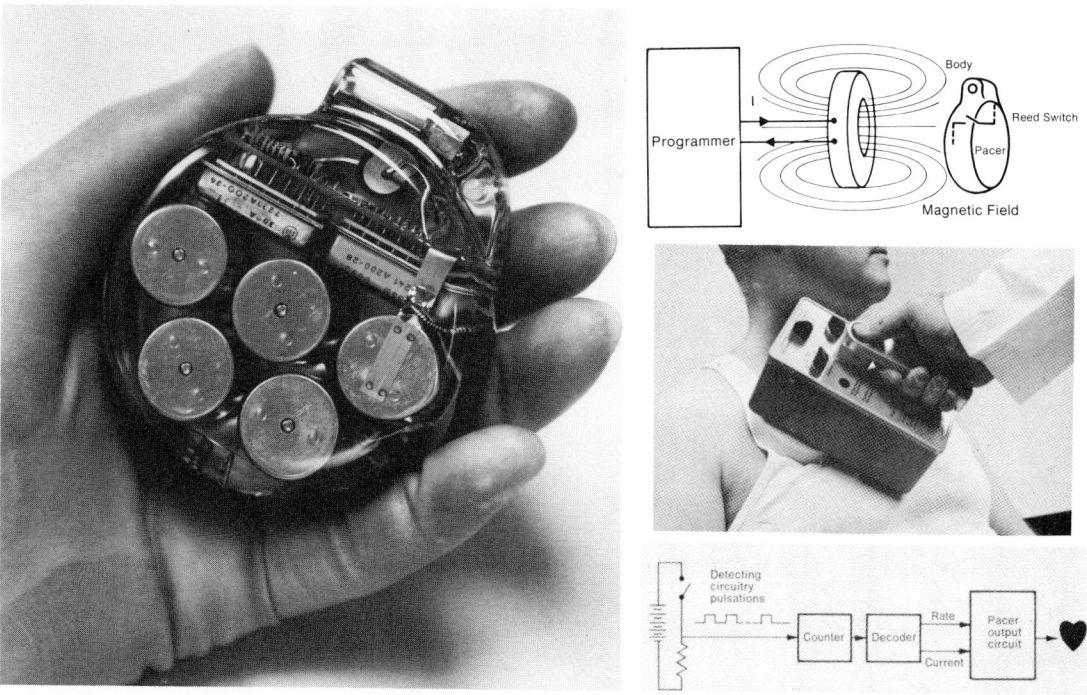

Figure 12. Programable pulse generator (Omnicor, manufactured by Cordis, Inc., Miami, Florida). Rate and current output can be programed noninvasively by a pulsating magnetic field which opens a reed switch in the implanted unit, which in turn provides a series of pulses transmitting a coded message. Note hybrid circuitry in sealed metallic containers. (Pulse generator may be of the fixed rate type, P-wave synchronous, or ventricular-suppressed demand.) (From Chardack, W. M. *In* Sabiston, D. C., Jr., and Spencer, F. C. (Eds.): Gibbon's Surgery of the Chest, 3rd ed. Philadelphia, W. B. Saunders Company, 1976.)

Figure 13. Commonly encountered electrocardiographic patterns in heart block and pacing. *A*, Complete heart block. *B*, Asynchronous pacing (stimulus has no relationship with P wave.) *C*, Competitive rhythm. Runs of conducted depolarizations (first five on left) alternate with runs of pacemade beats (last three on right). The arrow shows a pacemade beat interspersed between two conducted depolarizations, leading to a summation of rate. *D*, Competitive rhythm caused by extrasystoles. First three complexes on left are pacemade, the fourth is an extrasystole, and the next pacemaker stimulus (arrow) falls into the vulnerable period after extrasystole. In this particular patient, this phenomenon was innocuous for many years. Extrasystoles during the postoperative period should be suppressed. *E*, Intermittent pacing. Second stimulus from left fails to depolarize. In this case, intermittency was caused by perforation. *F*, Complete failure·to pace. None of the three stimuli depolarize. This may be because of inadequate pulse generator output, electrode displacement, or perforation. *G*, Long period of asystole during interruption of pacing. Note that this occurred even though the driving rate of the pacemaker was slightly below 60. *H*, Complete heart block corrected by synchronous pacemaking. Note constant time relationship between stimulus and preceding P wave. *I*, Resumption of normal conduction during synchronous pacemaking. Pacemaker stimulus (arrow) falls into absolute refractory period. (From Chardack, W. M. *In* Sabiston, D. C., Jr., and Spencer, F. C. (Eds.): Gibbon's Surgery of the Chest, 3rd ed. Philadelphia, W. B. Saunders Company, 1976.)

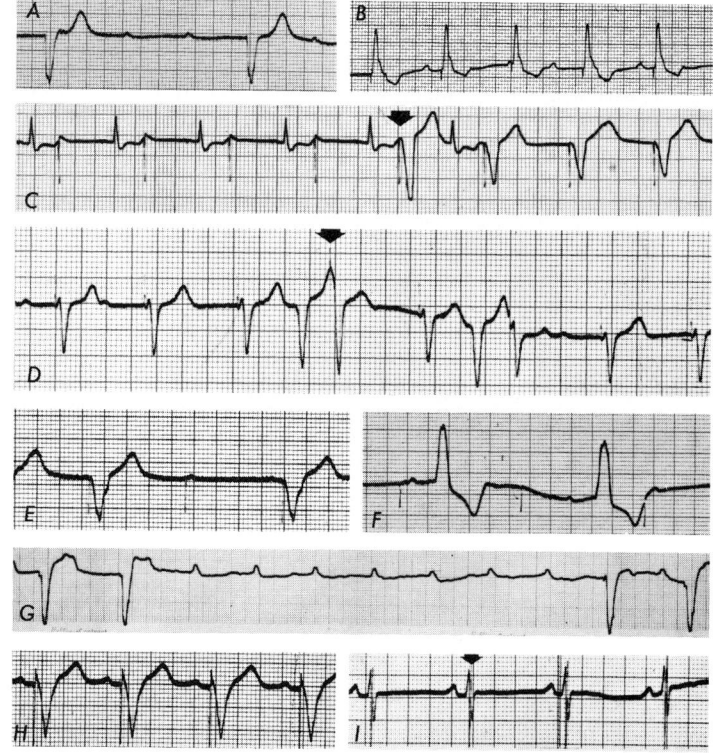

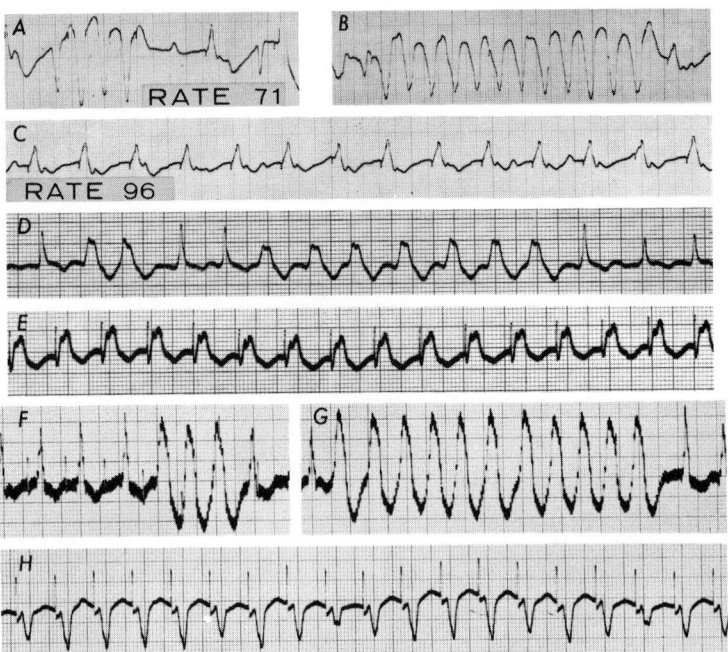

Figure 14. Important electrocardiographic patterns during pacing. *A* and *B*, Multifocal activity and repetitive ventricular tachycardia during postoperative period following implantation of an asynchronous pacemaker system. *C*, Correction of tachyarrhythmia following restoration of normal serum potassium level, administration of procainamide, and an increase of the pacemaker rate from 71 to 96 beats per minute. *D*, Repetitive tachycardia during postoperative period after myocardial revascularization; corrected by over driving (*E*). *F* and *G*, Repetitive episodes of ventricular tachycardia, many of which terminated in fibrillation, corrected by temporary overdriving (*H*). (From Chardack, W. M. *In* Sabiston, D. C., Jr., and Spencer, F. C. (Eds.): Gibbon's Surgery of the Chest, 3rd ed. Philadelphia, W. B. Saunders Company, 1976.)

sheath around the electrode and incorporation of the latter into the endothelium and endocardium. This sheath is covered by an outer endothelial layer, which may be important in preventing thrombosis and embolization in the majority of cases.[3]

6. The most common complication of the endocardiac approach is dislodgment of the electrode followed by loss of pacing. This has been reported in most series, with an incidence of 10 to 30 per cent. Usually dislodgment occurs in the early days or weeks following operation, and the electrocardiogram should be continuously monitored for a few days and longer if this can be done by telemetry techniques that do not interfere with mobilization of the patient. Displacement can often be corrected by repositioning of the electrode under local anesthesia. Late displacement of the electrode is uncommon, probably because of the firm attachment between the electrode and the endocardium.

It is held by some that the incidence of electrode dislocation can be decreased by increasing proficiency of the operator; others (including the authors) believe that these complications must be considered an inherent and, at least with currently available electrodes, unavoidable feature of the endocardiac approach.

INSTALLATION OF SYNCHRONOUS AND PARTIALLY IMPLANTED PACEMAKER SYSTEMS

A synchronous pacemaking system is programed from atrial activity and requires an additional electrode to sense the atrial potential (Fig. 5C). The most commonly practiced surgical approach consists of a left anterolateral thoracotomy and fixation of the sensing electrode to the atrium. Because of the popularity of the endocardiac electrode, synchronous pacemaking systems have also been installed by a transvenously placed atrial electrode and a second ventricular endocardiac electrode. Curved and hooked atrial electrodes have been devised for placement into the atrial appendage, and a sensing electrode placed close to the atrium by mediastinoscopy has also been used. The long-term reliability of these techniques remains to be demonstrated.

Partially implanted systems transmit electrical energy through the intact skin by radio-frequency waves or induction coupling.[1, 9] The receiver is implanted (Fig. 5D) and may be a myocardial electrode, an endocardiac electrode, or a miniaturized receiver with prongs directly attached to the myocardium. The advantage of a partially implanted system is that replacement of the pulse generator does not entail another operation, but the patient must wear an external appliance, the transmitting coil of which must remain secured to the skin in proximity to the implanted receiver. This requires constant watching, and rehabilitation is incomplete. For this reason, partially implanted systems have seen much less clinical application than fully implanted devices.

Pacemakers powered by rechargeable batteries can be considered partially implanted systems. The surgical techniques described above are applicable. Recharging is done by placing the transmitting part of the recharger over the pulse generator at specified intervals. Until recently this modality had not been given much consideration because the total life of the rechargeable cell did not exceed that available from mercury cells. In recent years, however, rechargeable cells have been developed for which a much greater life is claimed, and they are now under clinical trial.

TRANSVENOUS ENDOCARDIAC VERSUS MYOCARDIAC ELECTRODES (THORACOTOMY OR EPIGASTRIC APPROACH)

Most groups prefer the transvenous approach and some use it exclusively. Others favor myocardial electrodes inserted via thoracotomy or an upper epigastric approach. The literature begins to reflect a new interest in myocardiac electrodes. Our own position is eclectic, best summarized as follows:

The endocardiac system is ideally suited for the very elderly patient. The reported hospital mortality is about 1 per cent. Thoracotomy in the early years had an overall mortality rate of 7.5 per cent. The endocardiac approach is preferable when a thoracotomy would carry a high risk for reasons other than age or when it is impossible because of the presence of a previously installed myocardiac system that has become infected.

Most complications of the endocardiac approach can be corrected under local anesthesia, by repositioning of the electrode, or by replacement of the entire system. On the other hand, the potential risk associated with the long-term presence of an endovenous and endocardiac electrode structure still remains unknown. The presence of tricuspid valvular disease should be considered a contraindication. Major thromboembolism has seldom been a problem, but the presence of microembolism over long periods of time has not been excluded. The endocardiac approach should therefore be avoided in children and young adults. The most common complications of the endocardial system—albeit correctable under local anesthesia—are a potential hazard to life because of the associated cessation of pacing. Small as the risk may be, it should not be imposed upon patients in whom thoracotomy can be carried out with negligible risk. Where the line should be drawn in terms of chronologic or physiologic age is a matter of clinical judgment and cannot be covered by a rule of thumb. In considering this problem, one should keep in mind that the high mortality rate of 7.5 per cent ascribed to thoracotomy reflects the experience of an earlier period. The clinical material has changed over the years; the diagnosis is made earlier and the patient is better prepared. In our series, the hospital mortality of thoracotomy, epigastric, and endocardiac approaches has been about the same (1 per cent). In the early era of pacemaking, when myocardial electrode fractures were common, repeat thoracotomies were often required. This problem is now exceptional and one should not be deterred from thoracotomy by it. It is our feeling that with stable myocardial electrodes and the longer-lived pulse generators now available, thoracotomy or the epigastric approach should be given first consideration except in the old and debilitated.

PERMANENT PACING FOR CONGENITAL AND SURGICALLY INDUCED HEART BLOCK

Congenital block has been thought to occur mostly in association with congenital cardiac defects, but now it is known that it is an isolated entity more often than was suspected. In congenital block, the QRS is often narrow; this indicates a high location of the subsidiary pacemaker. The rate is relatively high (40 to 60 beats per minute) and increases during exercise. Physical work capacity can be close to normal, and the prognosis is said to be good. This classic picture does not always obtain, and congenital block can produce congestive failure, Stokes-Adams attacks, tachyarrhythmia, and death, particularly in the neonatal period or under the stress of exercise and intercurrent disease. A number of young children with congenital block, some in the neonatal period, have been treated with implanted pacemakers. This therapy should be considered if there is a history of syncope, especially in the very young child, if the QRS is wide (low idioventricular pacemaker), or if the block is diagnosed in utero.

With better knowledge of the anatomy of the conduction system, the incidence of block following repair of cardiac defects has been reduced (to about 1 per cent) but it remains high (about 13 per cent) following operations on the aortic valve. The immediate management of this complication is pacemaking through myocardial wires. In about two thirds of the cases, return of conduction can be expected to occur within several weeks because the block is caused by hemorrhage, edema, and ischemia rather than by severance of the conduction bundle.

The outlook for survival is poor when a surgically induced heart block remains a permanent sequela, and implantation of a pacemaker is indicated whether or not symptoms are present.

PERMANENT PACING FOR SINUS ARREST, SINOATRIAL BLOCK, AND SINUS DISEASE

These entities may produce symptoms because of slow or arrested impulse formation in the sinoatrial node, blocked conduction from the node to the atrium, or episodes of bradycardia alternating with tachycardia. Correction by an implanted pacemaker system is then indicated. In some patients, an atrial driving site has been used to preserve atrioventricular synchrony. Before selecting an atrial driving site, one must remember that sinus disease is frequently associated with or followed by atrioventricular conduction disturbances. These can be brought to light by preliminary atrial pacing[13] and by His bundle electrograms.[19] The use of ventricular-programed demand pacemakers is advantageous in such patients, since the pulse generator is suppressed during periods of adequate sinus impulse formation.

PERMANENT PACING FOR TACHYARRHYTHMIAS NOT ASSOCIATED WITH BLOCK

Temporary pacing alone or in combination with antiarrhythmic or beta-adrenergic blocking drugs has been shown to be effective in suppressing a variety of ventricular and supraventricular tachyarrhythmias not associated with block (Fig. 14D to G), and therefore implanted systems have been used in patients in

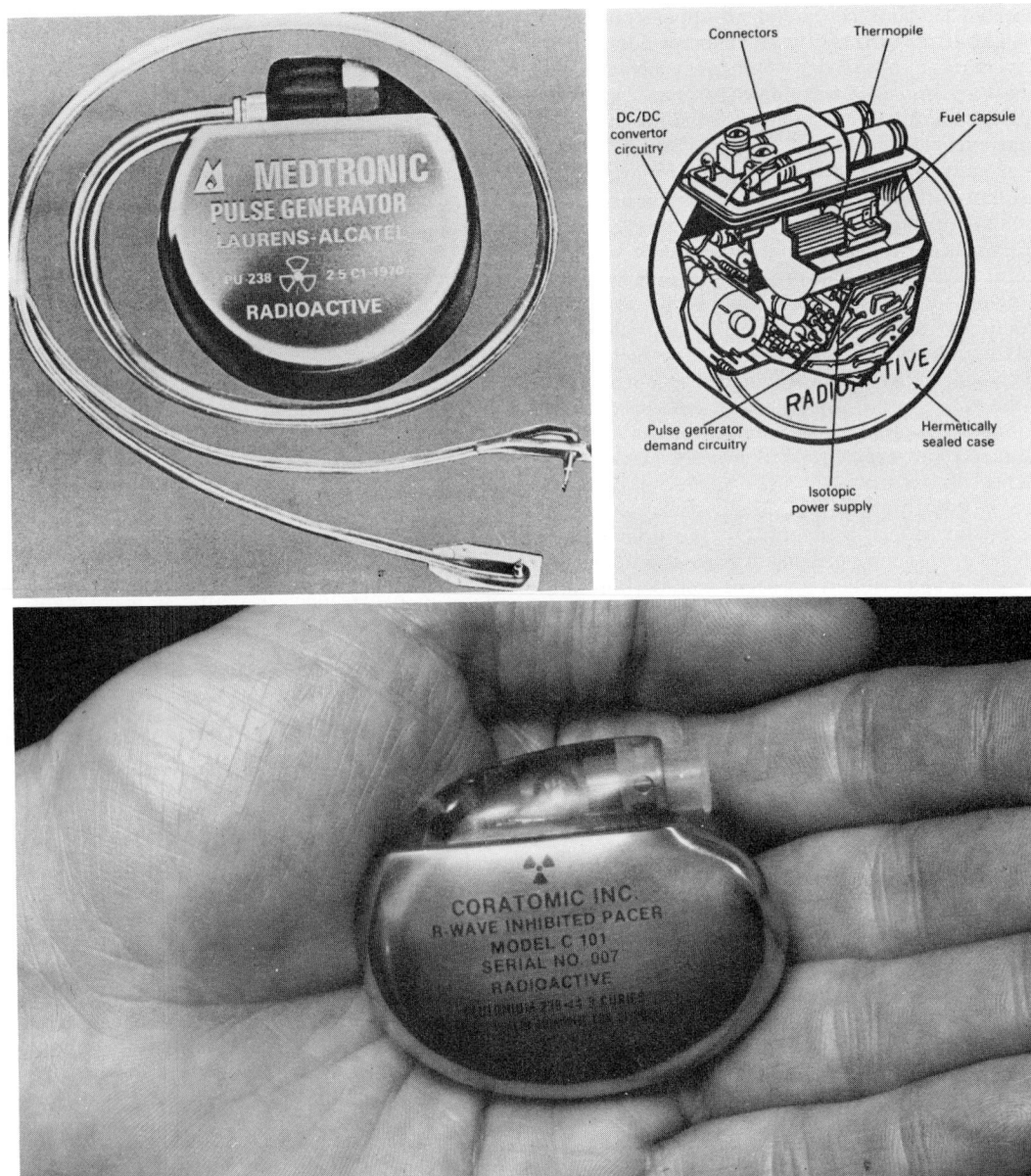

Figure 15. *Upper,* First (1970)[15] isotopic pulse generator (Medtronic-Laurens-Alcatel) (VVI) with myocardial helical spring electrodes (Medtronic Model 5814) (170 gm., 90 cc. volume). Radioactive fuel is plutonium-238, predominantly an alpha emitter with a half-life of 87.8 years. Heat from the fuel is transformed into electricity by a solid-state thermocouple. Appropriate multiple shielding and hermetic sealing is provided. The design life of this first unit was 10 years, with a potential of 20 years. Because of accountability to regulatory agencies, the follow-up of patients bearing this device has been complete and the device's performance in well over 1000 patients has been flawless. Power source failure has not been observed, and random component failures have been few. *Lower,* Second generation nuclear powered pulse generators that are lighter and smaller (61 gm., 33 cc., 6 cm. long) with a minimum design life of 45 years, have been in clinical use since 1974. (Courtesy of David Purdy, Coratomic, Inc., Indiana, Pennsylvania.) Radiation from these devices is negligible. For instance, the radiation dose to the patient's trunk is approximately 350 mrem per year as compared to an exposure of 5,000 to 30,000 mrem from a single GI series and fluoroscopy. (Upper photo from Chardack, W. M. *In* Sabiston, D. C., Jr., and Spencer, F. C. (Eds.) Gibbon's Surgery of the Chest, 3rd ed. Philadelphia, W. B. Saunders Company, 1976.)

whom such rhythm disturbances were uncontrollable by medication alone.[3, 7, 24] Maintenance of a moderately rapid rate ("overdriving"), faster than the normal sinus rate but slower than the rate during the episodes of tachycardia, suppresses the emergence of ectopic foci. In patients in whom atrioventricular conduction is normal, pacing from an atrial site is preferable. A few cases of uncontrollable supraventricular tachycardia have been managed by surgical division of the conduction bundle and installation of a pacemaking system.

CLINICAL RESULTS

There is agreement that long-term pacing prevents Stokes-Adams attacks regardless of the mechanism of their genesis. Pacing relieves, or palliates, congestive failure and the cerebral and renal symptoms induced by bradycardia. Opinion remains divided as to the degree of restoration of normal hemodynamics in these patients. Improvement is striking in most patients, but the gains are questionable in others, depending upon age and the degree of coexistent impairment of myocardial infarction. Data extending now over a period of more than a decade support the conclusion that, in addition to palliation, pacing increases survival in patients with heart block, which now parallels that of a normal population of comparable age and sex. This indicates that the mortality in most of these patients is determined by disease other than the cardiac lesion. The long-term prognosis is worse in patients paced for other arrhythmias or conduction disorders, suggesting that the mortality results from the different underlying cardiac pathology.

INSTRUMENTATION FOR LONG-TERM PACING

ELECTRODES FOR LONG-TERM PACING

A limited increase (after initial installation) in the threshold current required to initiate depolarization has been observed with every type of electrode. This is due to scar tissue around the electrode (and some degree of displacement in the case of an endocardiac electrode). The result is an increase in the distance between electrode and responsive myocardium and a corresponding decrease in current density at the latter. In the presence of infection, fluid accumulation around the electrode results in a greater separation between it and myocardium. A high current threshold is then observed. The absolute values of voltage or current required to set off a propagated action potential late in diastole (aside from the properties of myocardium) depend upon electrode surface, polarity, and metal and duration of the stimulus. Current practice favors smaller electrode surfaces (to minimize current drain). An optimal electrode surface has been calculated to be a hemisphere or short cylinder, the radius of which equals the diameter of the scar tissue which surrounds the electrode tip and constitutes the outer boundary of the interface where the stimulus is effective (about 0.7 to 1 mm.). This would indicate an electrode tip diameter of 2 mm. (Fig. 10).

The respective advantages of unipolar and bipolar electrode configurations have been the subject of much discussion. Unipolar cathodal threshold voltages are slightly lower than those of bipolar electrodes. The advantages of a bipolar configuration are redundancy, two opportunities instead of one to find a lower threshold (important mainly for endocardiac electrodes), and their lesser sensitivity to external electrical fields. Since pulse generators now are shielded against interference and electrode fracture is rare, there is little to choose between unipolar and bipolar electrode configurations.

Polarization and electrolyte corrosion effects on electrode metal are important considerations and support the choice of biphasic pulses and of platinum terminals for bipolar configurations. In unipolar configurations, the anodal surface should be large and the active cathode in the myocardium be made of platinum, since polarization is reduced (efficiency increased) and electrical thresholds with this material have been shown to be stable over periods in excess of 10 years.

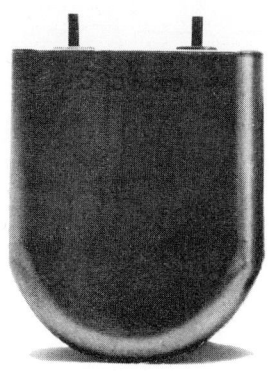
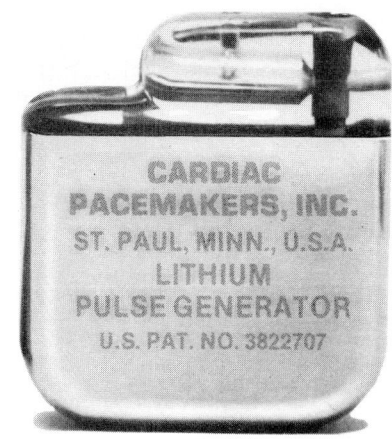

Figure 16. Photograph (actual size) of a second generation lithium pulse generator (manufactured by Cardiac Pacemakers, Inc., St. Paul, Minnesota). At left is solid state lithium battery modified and refined by W. Greatbatch. The battery is hermetically sealed. The electronic module is in a separate hermetic capsule and the entire assembly is contained by a third outer hermetic enclosure. The performance of the power source has been flawless in excess of five years in the laboratory and in excess of three years in clinical application. Its ultimate potential still remains to be verified. An 8- to 10-year capability is hoped for. This would cover the requirements of 80 to 90 per cent of patients requiring an implantable pacemaker system.

Pulse Generators

Asynchronous Pulse Generators (VOO)

Asynchronous pulse generators, the first to be developed, supply electrical stimuli at a fixed rate independent of the atrial and ventricular activity. Although the rate is fixed, in some pulse generators, it (as well as the output) is noninvasively adjustable (Figs. 10, 11, and 12). The ability to increase the pacing rate may be desirable in a few patients in whom one wishes to suppress ectopic activity or to increase cardiac output in the presence of myocardial failure.

Programmed Pulse Generators

Atrial-Programed Pulse Generators (VAT).* These require an additional electrode (Fig. 5C) to sense the atrial potential, which, amplified, triggers the pulse generator to deliver a stimulus to the ventricle after a set PR interval. To prevent tachycardia triggered from the atrium, a blocking circuit with a 2:1 reduction slows the rate of stimulation when the atrial signals occur at frequencies above 120 beats per minute. If the atrial potentials are inadequate, or if the atrial impulse formation is abnormally slow, the pulse generator reverts to a fixed rate of about 60 to 70 stimuli per minute.

Ventricular-Programed Pacemakers. Ventricular-programed pacemakers respond to any spontaneous QRS potential appearing at the electrode. The same

---

*Model Atricor, manufactured in the United States by Cordis, Inc., Miami, Florida.

electrode is used to carry the output stimulus from the pulse generator. Two types of ventricular-programed pulse generators are in clinical use.

Ventricular-Inhibited (VVI) Pulse Generators. Any spontaneous QRS potential appearing at the electrode resets the timing circuit of the pulse generator; for instance, if the device is set to a stimulation frequency of 60 pulses per minute, it will emit pulses at 1-second intervals as long as there is no spontaneous ventricular activity. However, if a depolarization, ectopic or conducted, occurs before the end of the 1-second escape interval, it recycles the pulse generator and suppresses the output for another cycle of 1-second's duration. Therefore, as long as spontaneous depolarizations occur at a beat-to-beat rate in excess of 60 per minute, the pulse generator remains quiescent. If none occur before the end of a 1-second cycle, the pulse generator will escape, emit a stimulus, and continue to do so in the absence of further spontaneous ventricular activity (Fig. 17A to C).

The purpose of ventricular-programed pacemaker systems is to preclude competitive rhythms from either conducted or ectopic depolarizations, a phenomenon that can occur with asynchronous pacemakers (Fig. 13C and D). The ventricular-suppressed pulse generator precludes delivery of a stimulus into the vulnerable period following a spontaneous depolarization and avoids the hemodynamic consequences of competitive rhythms. During periods of normal conduction, its output is suppressed; this reduces current drain. In order to demonstrate that the pulse generator is operational during these periods, an external

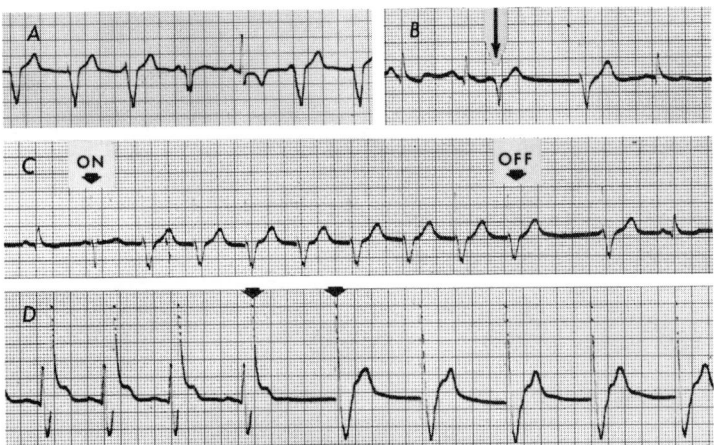

Figure 17. Electrocardiographic patterns with ventricular-programed pacemakers. *A,* Three pacemade beats on left followed by a fusion beat and a conducted depolarization. The latter suppresses output of pacemaker, which does not appear until preset interval has elapsed. *B,* Normal sinus rhythm—first two complexes on left. At the arrow, a ventricular extrasystole occurs and is followed by a pause that exceeds the programed cycle of the demand pulse generator. The next depolarization is pacemade, and the last (right) is again a normally conducted beat that suppresses pacemaker output. *C,* Normal sinus rhythm, pacemaker output suppressed, first complex on left. Between arrows, external magnet is applied and device functions as a fixed-rate pulse generator. All depolarizations are pacemade, and when the external control is turned off (arrow, right), a preautomatic pause follows, exceeding the standby interval. The next depolarization is therefore pacemade, and then the normal sinus rhythm (last complex on right) suppresses pacemaker output again. *D,* Ventricular-triggered standby pacemaker. First four depolarizations (left) are conducted, and a pacemaker pulse is directed into the absolute refractory period. Pressure is then applied to the carotid sinus, cardiac rate falls below the standby cycle, and the five depolarizations (beginning at second arrow) are pacemade. (From Chardack, W. M. *In* Sabiston, D. C., Jr., and Spencer, F. C. (Eds.): Gibbon's Surgery of the Chest, 3rd ed. Philadelphia, W. B. Saunders Company, 1976.)

magnet is applied that switches the device into fixed-rate operation (Fig. 17C).

VENTRICULAR-TRIGGERED PACEMAKERS (VTT). Ventricular-triggered pacemakers differ from true demand pacemakers in that the R wave triggers emission of a stimulus following a short delay so that it falls into the absolute refractory period. If there is no spontaneous ventricular activity within a preset interval, the pulse generator escapes and produces a stimulus. In ventricular-triggered pacemakers during normal sinus rhythm, the stimulus artifact can be seen in the absolute refractory period on the electrocardiogram (and makes interpretation difficult; Fig. 17D), but this does not insure that the stimulus is adequate to elicit depolarization were it needed. The current drain of ventricular-triggered pulse generators is high, since they emit a pulse even during periods of normal sinus rhythm, and they require protection against external electrical signals, which could accelerate the stimulation rate of these devices to a dangerous level.

A discussion of the respective merits of various types of pacemakers hinges upon the consideration of the hemodynamics during artificial pacing and the risks entailed by the pacing stimulus itself (see later).

RELIABILITY AND PERFORMANCE OF THE PULSE GENERATOR

Data on the long-term performance of pulse generators were slow to accumulate because in the early years electrode failure was the predominant cause of system malfunction. As the electrode problem abated, the performance of the pulse generator was recognized as the factor limiting the life of the system. The majority of failures either have been manifested by a limited increase or decrease of the stimulation rate or have led to intermittency or cessation of pacemaking and the resumption of an idioventricular rhythm. There have been rare instances in which the mode of failure was an inordinate increase of the rate, inducing a tachycardia that in some cases terminated in ventricular fibrillation. The "runaway" pacemaker failure has been rare but has been reported with many types and makes of pulse generators, even in recent years. This is difficult to understand, since protection against this failure mode is available. In some units this is achieved by letting the rate increase to approximately 120 beats per minute and holding it at that level. However, in elderly patients such a high rate may be poorly tolerated. A better approach would be to cut the rate to 60 when it reaches 120, which can be easily achieved. The "runaway" pacemaker constitutes an acute emergency that requires immediate disabling of the device and provision for prompt resumption of pacing by some other means.

The most important problem of implanted pacemakers has been their limited longevity (24 to 30 months), which was much below initial expectation. The responsibility for this discrepancy is often attributed to the manufacturers of the pulse generator. In fact, the initial estimate of a 5-year life was made by the authors[4] and was based on the then available ratings of the mercury zinc cell.* These ratings had been obtained at room temperature in an atmosphere with relatively low humidity. There had been no need at that time to test them under other conditions. However, at body temperature, at 100 per cent humidity, chemical losses within the battery reduced pulse generator life to an average of 2 years.

Because of the disappointing performance of the batteries, efforts have been made to predict impending failure of the pulse generator by oscillographic evaluation of the pacemaker stimulus potential as it appears on the surface of the body or by a measurement of the relative margin of pacemaker output over threshold requirement.[7, 21, 23-25] Specialized pacemaker clinics and the telephone transmission of the electrocardiogram or the pacemaker potential, or both, have been used to follow patients with implanted devices.[7, 21, 24, 25] Devices have been developed to permit a simple self-check of the pulse generator for integrity (rate and/or stimulus width) by the patient himself. Up to now the most important parameter in the follow-up has been the rate, since most pulse generators are programed for a decrease in the stimulation rate as the battery voltage drops. Recently, emphasis has been placed on an increase of pulse width as battery voltage drops. The purpose of this is to provide an additional end-of-battery-life indicator and to compensate for decreasing pulse amplitude by an increase in pulse duration, thus maintaining capture as the battery nears exhaustion (Fig. 11).

Pulse generator longevity and reliability have been improved. The main developments have been:

1. Improvements of the mercury cell itself and recognition that the threshold requirements were lower than originally thought.

2. Reduction of stimulus amplitude or duration and adjustment of these to each individual patient's threshold requirements, thus minimizing current drain.

3. Reduction of battery drain by the lower requirement of present-day circuit design (so-called "hybrids," making use of combinations of several integrated circuit chips) and the use of smaller electrodes.

4. Development of a nuclear power source (with a potential capability of several decades) for the small number of patients (about 5 to 7 per cent) who require a very long-lived pulse generator.

5. Development of the lithium iodine cell, which has been in clinical use now for over 3 years in more than 10,000 patients (and under laboratory evaluation for over 5 years). Battery depletion has not been observed with this cell and laboratory data project a pulse generator longevity of 6 to 10 years, depending upon the different battery models.

6. Nuclear and lithium power sources are hermetically sealed, and since the circuitry can also be sealed, the entire pulse generator becomes impervious to body fluids, eliminating an important cause of failure.

In the past, some deaths have been caused by pace-

---

*Mallory RM-1 cell, manufactured by Mallory Company, Tarrytown, New York.

maker failure. They have received disproportionate emphasis; the number has been quite small (26 in a recent 3-year period in the U.S.A., according to the Department of Health, Education, and Welfare) in comparison to the mortality from other devices such as heart valves or even from the side-effects of many drugs. No doubt, the developments cited above will further improve pulse generator performance in all respects.

TEMPORARY PACEMAKING SYSTEMS

Instrumentation and techniques for temporary pacemaking of the heart have been summarized in Table 3. Selection of a technique should be based on the circumstances in a given case. If ample time is available, introduction of an endocardiac electrode either under fluoroscopy or by monitoring its position by the intracardiac electrogram should be considered. In an acute emergency, repetitive blows on the chest may be effective, and the percutaneous insertion of myocardial wires should be considered. This requires only a few seconds and materials, suture wires and a spinal needle, that are readily available in a hospital environment.

Temporary pacing techniques are important in the preoperative and operative management of patients with block who require installation or repair of a permanent pacemaking system. They have also been applied to conduction and other rhythm disturbances complicating acute myocardial infarction.

Temporary pacing is also used either to increase an inadequate cardiac rate and output or to suppress tachyarrhythmias in postoperative states following cardiac and general surgery (Fig. 14D to H).[10] In patients with normal atrioventricular conduction, an atrial stimulation site should be used. Temporary ventricular and atrial pacing by single or repetitive stimuli (alone or in combination with drugs) has been employed to control a variety of ventricular and supraventricular tachycardias.[7, 24] Controlled hypotension during surgical procedures can be induced by rapid pacing, and atrial pacing at high rates has been used as a diagnostic procedure to bring to light latent disturbances of the atrioventricular conduction system.[13]

TABLE 3.   Instrumentation for Temporary Pacemaking*

EXTERNAL ELECTRODES (ZOLL, 1952)
ENDOCARDIAC ELECTRODES
   Positioned by fluoroscopy or by intracardiac electro-
      cardiographic monitoring
   Unipolar (Furman and Robinson, 1959), requiring
      indifferent subcutaneous electrode
   Bipolar (Parsonnet et al., 1962)
   Transvenously positioned (floated) endocardiac wire
      (Kimball and Killip, 1965)
ELECTRODE WIRES
   Installed at time of cardiac operation (Weirich et al.,
      1957)
   Introduced by cardiocentesis (Thevenet et al., 1958;
      Roe, 1965)

*From Sabiston, D. C., and Spencer, F. C.: Gibbon's Surgery of the Chest, 3rd ed. Philadelphia, W. B. Saunders Company, 1976.

Myocardial performance and the appearance of angina can be evaluated by electrically induced tachycardia.[24]

Pacing with paired electrical stimuli can slow the effective mechanical rate of the heart and induces postsystolic potentiation of cardiac contractility. The technique introduces a premature extrasystole into each cycle and creates a bigeminal rhythm in which mechanical ineffective beats alternate with potentiated effective contractions. The technique remains experimental, although the number of reported successful clinical trials is beginning to increase.[6]

ELECTRICAL HAZARDS OF PACEMAKING

The potential hazards of electrical stimulation of the heart involve three mechanisms: (1) leakage of 60 cycle current from line-powered instruments connected to pacing electrodes; (2) potential hazards of the pacemaker stimulus; and (3) the effects of external electromagnetic fields on implanted devices.

Leakage of Currents from Line-Powered Instruments

Pacing electrodes are low-resistant current pathways to the myocardium, and minute currents, of the order of 100 microamperes, can induce ventricular fibrillation. This danger is present when line-powered instruments are connected to an electrode, and if at the same time the patient is connected to a second line-powered instrument or in good contact with ground, such as through an x-ray table or an electrically powered bed. A case in point would be a patient paced with a line-powered pulse generator who then is connected to an electrocardiograph.

Only battery-driven devices should be connected to cardiac electrodes, and their terminals and connections to the electrodes should be protected against contact with potential sources of line current leakage. If a line-powered instrument must be used on a cardiac electrode (to obtain an endocardiac electrogram, for instance), it should be the only one in contact with the patient, and even then the hazard of ventricular fibrillation constantly must be kept in mind.

The dangers of line current leakage are always present with temporary electrodes traversing the skin and with permanent electrodes when they are being installed or exteriorized in the course of a pulse-generator exchange. With completely implanted devices, it is safe to use line-powered instruments, such as electrocardiographs and monitors, as well as X-radiation for diagnosis and therapy.

Hazards Arising from Pacemaker Stimulus

Ever since cardiac pacing was introduced, concern has been expressed about the risk of inducing ventricular fibrillation by the pacemaking stimulus itself. This possibility does not exist as long as the cardiac rhythm is dominated by the artificial pacemaker, because all stimuli are delivered in late diastole beyond the confines of the "vulnerable zone," which approximately coincides with the apex of the T wave. When there is competition between the artificial pacemaker and conducted or ectopic ventricular depolarizations, stimuli can fall into the vulnerable period following such an event (Fig. 13C and D). Extrasystoles and intermittent resumption of normal conduction commonly occur in pacemade patients.

Experimental data show that in the animal with a presumably normal myocardium, fibrillation can be initiated by brief pacing stimuli falling into the vulnerable period, but high currents are required to produce this effect. The threshold of fibrillation exceeds the threshold of stimulation (late in diastole) by a factor of about 20.[5] In general, the currents required for fibrillation are beyond the output capabilities of implantable pulse generators. However, physiologic and pharmacologic interventions can reduce the margin between fibrillatory and stimulating pulses. Fibrillation is facilitated by large electrode surfaces, stimuli of long duration, alterations in electrolyte composition, acidosis, hypoxia, and adrenergic and other agents commonly administered to cardiac patients, such as large doses of digitalis. The fibrillatory threshold also drops sharply following ligation of a coronary artery that supplies a myocardial electrode site. However, the threshold of stimulation also increases considerably in the ischemic area.[5]

The margin of safety between the amplitude of a pacemaker stimulus and that required to provoke ventricular fibrillation varies with the time that has lapsed since implantation of the electrode. At installation, the threshold for stimulation is low and then rises (over 2 to 3 weeks) as the electrode matures. The output of the pulse generator must be set to anticipate this increase as well as fluctuations of the stimulation threshold related to physiologic and pharmacologic causes.[23] Immediately after implantation, it exceeds the stimulation threshold by a considerable margin, which then decreases.

A review of the reported clinical experience[5] leads to the conclusion that electrical parasystole can be dangerous either during temporary pacing for block complicating an acute myocardial infarction or in the early postoperative period following installation of a permanent pacemaking system. Under the latter circumstances, a high ratio between stimulus and threshold is present, and myocardial irritability may be high, especially in the presence of digitalis intoxication and a low serum potassium concentration. In most observations (linking ventricular fibrillation to pacing), competition was the result of premature ventricular extrasystoles and multifocal ectopic activity. This type of arrhythmia (Fig. 14A and B) is intrinsically dangerous (whether electrical stimuli are administered or not) and must be treated aggressively even when a demand pacemaker is used. Furthermore, the insertion of an electrode causes some injury to myocardial fibers in its vicinity, and the risk may be compounded when the procedure is performed in the presence of an unsuspected infarction or when a coronary occlusion supervenes as a postoperative complication.

The danger of electrical parasystole is remote in patients in whom the electrode has matured and the stimulation threshold has increased. Temporary return to normal sinus rhythm has been observed in 20 to 50 per cent of patients with implanted pacemakers, and the real incidence may well be greater, since competitive rhythms are likely to escape documentation. Many thousands of patients with implanted fixed-rate pacemakers have now been observed for periods up to

a decade, and uncountable stimuli have been delivered into the vulnerable period. There is abundant evidence that such electrical parasystole is harmless in most cases. Pacemaker stimuli can be hazardous when the fibrillatory threshold decreases or the ratio between pacemaker stimulus and threshold is high. Because these circumstances are likely to be present in the postoperative period, ectopic ventricular activity and competitive rhythms should then be aggressively suppressed.

Pacemaker stimuli are also hazardous in the presence of an acute myocardial infarction when freshly placed electrodes are located in ischemic myocardium. Only demand pacemakers should be used in such patients, and excessive pulse amplitudes above threshold should be avoided.

Hazards Arising from External Electrical Fields

There is considerable electrical electromagnetic "noise" in the present day environment and the effects of these fields on implantable pulse generators have been studied extensively. They vary with the source of interference and the type of pulse generator. fields. Ventricular-programed pacemakers, since they must respond to QRS potentials of a few millivolts, are far more sensitive to external fields, and interference with their output has been observed when patients are exposed to radiated electromagnetic energy from sources such as radio and television transmitters, microwave ovens, diathermy, automobile ignitions, electric razors, and fluorescent lights. These fields penetrate the pulse generator itself, but they are also picked up by the electrode leads, which act as an antenna. Unipolar leads are more vulnerable than bipolar ones. Ventricular-programed pacemakers also can be interfered with by conducted electricity such as 60-cycle leakage currents (which may be below the level of sensory perception) from household appliances and machinery. The conducted currents are sensed principally through the electrodes. Magnetic fields are coupled to the circuitry mostly through the internal wiring of the pulse generator, with a modest contribution through the leads.

Protection of ventricular-programed pulse generators of current manufacture against radiated fields is obtained through shielding of a metal housing and by electrical filters.

In the presence of strong alternating conduction currents or magnetic fields, the demand pulse generator will revert to fixed-rate operation. However, extremely low conducted currents and magnetic fields have been observed to cause either reversion to a much lower than stimulation rate or, in some cases, to complete inhibition. Consequently, pacemaker wearers should be discouraged from operating appliances such as magnetic tape erasers, tool demagnetizers, large transformer-driven devices, and arc welding apparatus. If they must operate such devices, they should do so initially in the presence of another person capable of removing them to some distance from the device. These interferences affect the pulse generator only temporarily, while the patient is in close proximity or in direct contact with the source. Normal function of the pulse generator will resume as soon as contact with the source is broken or the patient withdraws from close proximity to the source. The reader should bear in mind that many of the reports dealing with electrical interference were made on devices manufactured many years ago and now obsolete. With appropriate shielding and filtering, electrical interference with implanted pulse generators is now viewed as a relatively minor clinical problem, although continued vigilance and further improvements are recommended.

Paradoxically, hazards to pacemaker patients exist in the medical environment. Notable examples are the use of 60-cycle devices on externalized electrodes or the use of electrosurgical and diathermy apparatus on patients with implanted pulse generators. Diathermy should never be used on body areas overlying an implanted pulse generator. If the latter is shielded by metal, severe localized heating of tissue adjacent to the metal capsule can occur. Unshielded pulse generators will not cause burns, but the device itself may be permanently damaged by the heating effects of diathermy. In regard to the use of electrosurgical apparatus, the administration of electroconvulsive therapy, and the use of certain dental instrumentation, interference with the pulse generator must be guarded against. Electrosurgical current should be applied in bursts separated by several seconds, and the pulse should be monitored manually. Many successful operations on pacemaker patients have been performed using these precautions. Cautery and cutting currents should not be used within two inches of implanted pulse generators. In summary, programed implantable devices are inherently sensitive to electrical signals, especially when they are modulated and resemble the QRS complex. With the patient's and the physician's awareness, these hazards can be minimized.

HEMODYNAMICS IN HEART BLOCK AND DURING ARTIFICIAL PACING

Oxygen demands of the body above the resting level are satisfied by an increase of cardiac output and of oxygen extraction from the blood. Cardiac output can be raised by an increase in the rate and the stroke volume. With maximal workloads, all three mechanisms—increasing rate, stroke, volume, and oxygen consumption—come into play. In untrained man, adjustment to mild to moderate exercise is mediated chiefly by an increase in heart rate, but in the presence of a heart rate that is fixed or held constant, cardiac output can increase solely by a higher stroke volume.

In the experimental animal in which heart block has been induced, pacing at increasing rates shows that cardiac output is relatively constant except at the very low and very high rates. While cardiac output remains relatively constant over this range of rates, myocardial oxygen consumption increases as the rate goes up and efficiency decreases.[3]

Many studies have dealt with the hemodynamics in patients with pacemakers. In evaluating the results, one should keep in mind that cardiac output decreases and arteriovenous difference increases in the aged, whose exercise performance is often limited before the cardiorespiratory system is maximally stressed, and one must differentiate between the response observed following an abrupt change of the rate or the mode of pacing (atrial to ventricular, for instance) and that seen if such interventions are permitted to reach a steady or chronic stage. In many patients, some myocardial insufficiency is present, and therefore the reported observations show some variations.

In many studies made at rest and during exercise, increases in cardiac output were observed as the rate

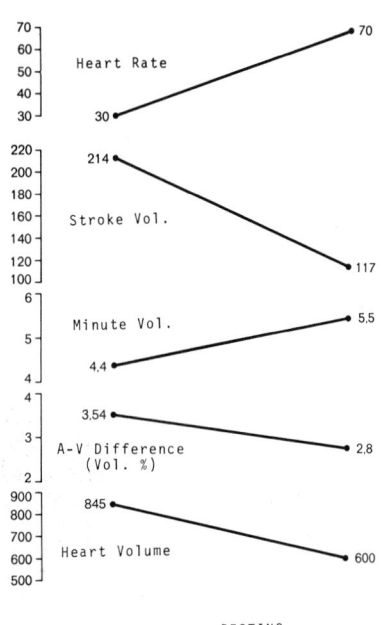

RESTING

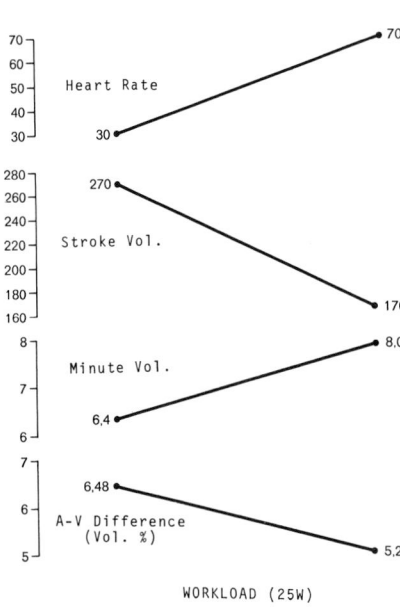

WORKLOAD (25W)

Figure 18. Hemodynamic changes (averages) in a series of patients at rest and after exercise. (After Büchner, C., Dragert, W., Schlosser, V., Arnold, T., and Nuber, B.: Schrittmacher Therapie des Herzens mit 123 Abbildungen. Forum Cardiol., *14*:1973 Boehringer-Mannheim, GmbH. Reproduced in Chardack, W. M. *In* Sabiston, D. C., Jr., and Spencer, F. C. (Eds.): Gibbon's Surgery of the Chest, 3rd ed. Philadelphia, W. B. Saunders Company, 1976.)

was raised by pacing (Fig. 18). This increase occurred as the rate was about 60 beats per minute, and, in general, cardiac output remained fairly constant from 60 to 110 beats, exhibiting a typical plateau type of curve. In other observations, cardiac output peaked between 70 and 90 beats and then decreased, and exercise produced only a negligible increment (Fig. 19).[3, 18, 24]

In regard to the energetics of the heart, an increase of cardiac output mediated by an increase in the stroke volume requires only a small increment of coronary blood flow and oxygen consumption, whereas increase of the output mediated by an increase of the rate requires large increments of these parameters. At slow rates, coronary arterial inflow is facilitated because of the long diastolic filling time. These considerations may be unimportant in regard to patients with block and relatively normal coronary arteries but they are quite relevant to patients who have coexisting coronary artery disease. Patients with angina are known to tolerate poorly the higher driving rates that are produced by atrial-triggered pulse generators.[7]

In general, fixed-rate pacemaking at about 70 beats per minute has been satisfactory and has produced a reasonable exercise tolerance. With pacing, cardiac size and volume decrease and cardiac reserve is restored, since now stroke volume can be increased again as a response to stress. A rate of 70 per minute is usually more than adequate to suppress multifocal ectopic activity and runs of ventricular tachycardia and fibrillation that are associated with very slow idioventricular rates. There are occasional patients in whom such tachyarrhythmias (similar to those observed in patients without block—Fig. 14D to H) require higher driving rates in combination with drugs, and in a few patients with refractory congestive failure a faster rate may be of help.

ASYNCHRONOUS VERSUS SYNCHRONOUS PACEMAKERS

With fixed-rate pacemakers, there is a limit to which cardiac output can increase in response to high workloads, but maximal performance is of little consequence in a group of patients of a mean age of 70 years. A fixed heart rate compels cardiac output to increase by augmenting stroke volume, which is less costly in energy than a rise in rate. Also, it has not been established that the rate response of the atrium by definition is an optimal response; in fact, it can be inappropriately high in many elderly patients and the "wisdom" of the node has been questioned.[7]

In most experimental and clinical studies made to assess the contribution of atrioventricular synchronization to cardiac output, the performance parameters of a single ventricular contraction preceded by an appropriately timed atrial contraction are compared with a ventricular contraction that is out of phase with the preceding atrial event. Under these circumstances, a contraction with a normal atrioventricular timing always produces a higher output, and if the driving rate is close to the atrial rate, cyclic variations occur in pressure and cardiac output (Fig. 20). When one compares mean cardiac output and pressure during synchronous driving and those obtained with asynchronous driving at a slightly lower rate, the fluctuations become negligible, especially if the experiment is carried out long enough to allow physiologic feedback mechanisms to come into play (Fig. 20).[4]

Most studies show a difference in cardiac output between synchronous and asynchronous pacemaking of the order of 10 to 20 per cent related to the loss of atrioventricular synchrony and the dyssynergia of abnormal ventricular activation. Even if synchronous pacing could produce a small increase of cardiac output of the order of 10 per cent, this would not matter except at the uppermost and lowermost limits of the range of cardiac outputs. In younger patients with good myocardial function, a fixed rate of 70 is well tolerated, and in many patients with congenital heart block, even rates around 50 are adequate for a normal work capacity. It seems fair to conclude that both the loss of atrioventricular synchrony and dyssynergia produce experimentally demonstrable but limited reductions in cardiac output, which, in most patients, are of little clinical significance. They may be of importance in the presence of myocardial insufficiency.[2] Synchronous pacing or sequential pacing (delivering appropriately timed stimuli to the atrium and ventricle) may also be of value when temporary stimulation is required in the treatment of acute myocardial infarction complicated by block or tachyarrhythmia or both, especially when high driving rates are used, since atrioventricular coordination becomes more significant as the rate increases.

Synchronous pulse generators require instrumentation of greater complexity and, in order to protect against atrial-triggered tachycardias, they must provide for an automatic cutoff of the rate once a preset atrial rate is reached. This cutoff point varies between 120 and 150 beats, and it is questionable whether a sudden decrease of the heart rate during physical or emotional stress is always well tolerated. Synchronous pacing is contraindicated when there is an increase or a decrease in frequency of atrial pulse formation and in the presence of angina.

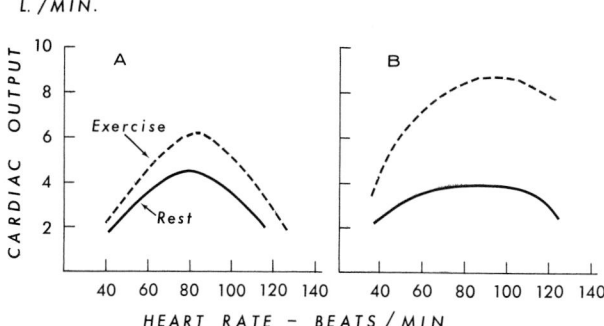

Figure 19. Cardiac output with increasing pacing rates. *A*, Peak response. *B*, Typical plateau (see text). (From McNally, E., and Benchimol, A.: Am. Heart J., 75:380, 679, 1968.)

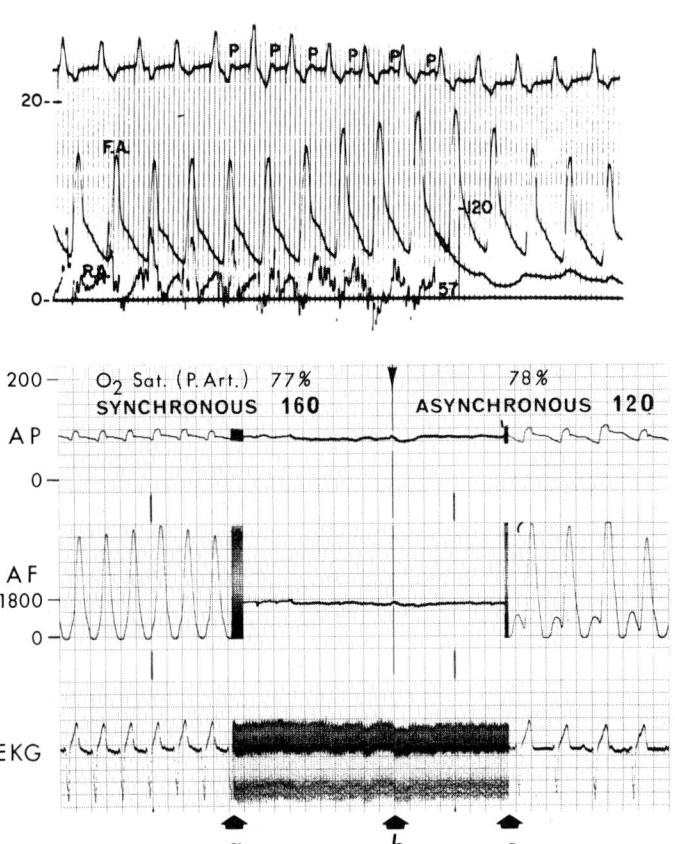

2/8/62

Figure 20. *Top,* Electrocardiogram and pressures of femoral artery and right auricle during asynchronous pacing. Note higher pressure during cycles in which the ventricular stimulus happens to follow a P wave with an appropriate delay (P). (From Samet, P., et al.: Am. J. Cardiol., *11*:594, 1963.) *Bottom,* Experimental comparison of synchronous pacing at rate of 160 beats per minute with asynchronous pacing at the slower rate of 120 beats per minute. Arterial pressure (AP), aortic flow (AF), and electrocardiogram recorded in an experimental animal with induced block. At *a,* slow paper speed is started and pressure and flow are recorded as mean values; at *b,* pacing is switched from synchronous to asynchronous mode. Paper speed increased again at *c.* Note that switch from synchronous to asynchronous mode has no significant influence on mean aortic pressure and flow.

It seems reasonable to conclude that although a pacemaker system programed from the atrium seems, at first glance, ideal because it accomplishes restoration of a normal physiologic state, in practice the gains have been more theoretical than practical, and for the majority of patients they do not warrant the increased complexity of the system and of its installation.

THE PLACE OF VENTRICULAR PROGRAMED PACEMAKERS

Pulse generators that are programed from ventricular activity are now used by many groups to the exclusion of other types. The purpose of ventricular-programed pacemaker systems is to preclude the delivery of a pacemaker stimulus into the vulnerable period as well as the hemodynamic consequences and the reduced efficiency inherent in a competitive rhythm. In regard to the risk of electrical parasystole, it is clear that external demand pacemaker systems should be the only ones used for temporary pacing for block complicating an acute myocardial infarction and in the suppression of various tachyarrhythmias when used in combination with otherwise dangerously high dosages of drugs.[5, 7] In regard to implanted pacemaker

systems, the available evidence indicates that there is no significant hazard associated with electrical parasystole in patients with fixed-rate pulse generators. Long-term follow-up studies show that the life expectancy of patients with pacemakers approaches that of a comparable normal population. Since competitive rhythms are common in these patients, a substantial unexplained mortality rate should now be clearly evident if electrical parasystole were a substantial hazard. In the experience of the authors and others, there has been no significant difference in the incidence of sudden or unexplained deaths (which conceivably could have been caused by ventricular fibrillation) in patients with implanted fixed-rate pacemakers and those with implanted demand pulse generators in whom electrical parasystole is precluded.

In the authors' experience, asynchronous pulse generators (less costly and less complex) have been satisfactory, especially as replacement units in patients with known fixed block (about 15 to 20 per cent of patients). On the other hand, however negligible the risk and loss of efficiency associated with electrical parasystole may be, the concept of eliminating electrical stimulation when it is not needed is obviously valid, provided the instrumentation required does not introduce new hazards and failure modes. The drawbacks formerly associated with demand systems, related to their sensitivity to external electrical interference, have been reduced with present-day devices. However, some problems remain, mostly related to proper sensing of the QRS complex. The ventricular-programed pulse generator must respond to a wide variety of QRS complexes and ignore other cardiac electrical signals. The demand pulse generator will be inhibited by an electrical signal that resembles the QRS complex. Two examples of such interference are muscle potentials in the vicinity of the pulse generator and potentials generated by respiratory muscular activity. Difficulties in sensing may also arise from inadequate QRS voltages such as those observed in infarcted areas and in Chagas' disease. In regard to higher current drain and greater complexity of components (liable to random failure), it is fair to state that these considerations are now less important because of the currently available power sources and hermetically sealed high-reliability devices.

In summary, the place of ventricular-programed devices is well established, certainly for all primary implantations, and their use is of particular importance in patients who most of the time are in normal sinus rhythm. Occasional sensing problems may occur, but they are the price that must be paid for this sophisticated therapy.

SUMMARY AND PERSPECTIVES

Implantable pacemakers have led to complete rehabilitation of patients with atrioventricular block, and their survival is very close to that of a normal comparable population, whereas before pacing the 1-year mortality was 50 per cent in this group. In addition, pacing is now applied to a wide variety of other rhythm disorders. It is true that these results have been achieved at the cost of many repeat operations (albeit minor ones and under local anesthesia) caused by failure of the electrode or the pulse generator and because the original estimates of battery life were not borne out.

Some components of the pacemaker system can be evaluated by accelerated testing, but the batteries cannot, at least not with acceptable confidence. To have delayed therapy until the "perfect" system had been designed and tested would have meant the loss of countless lives. To have taken such a course of "omission" would have gone unnoticed.

We now know that stimulation threshold levels are lower than was thought and that the efficiency of modern circuitry and of electrodes has improved to the point where current drains have been reduced by a factor of 3 to 4. Patients with devices (the output of which is programable) have been paced for 4 years, and a life of 5 years is attainable even with the mercury cell. Lithium batteries have operated for 4 years and promise to attain the 7- to 8-year range. Patients with radioisotope pulse generators have been paced since 1970, and safety and technical data indicate a potential pulse generator life of several decades.

The end-of-battery-life indicators now include a drop of the rate as well as a compensatory increase of the pulse width to keep the heart in capture. This will facilitate surveillance of the patient by self-check and by telephone transmission in addition to the direct contact between physician and patient.

Pulse generators are shielded against external electrical interference by their metallic housing and by metallic enclosures around the miniature circuitry now available. Electrical interference in the past has not been a danger to life but rather a nuisance. It should be greatly reduced in the future.

The indications for long-term pacing for rhythm disorders other than block may need further delineation by cardiologists.

ACKNOWLEDGMENT

We are grateful to Miss Lillian R. Klinko for the technical assistance in the preparation of this text and to the Medical Illustration Service, Veterans Administration Hospital, Buffalo, New York, for their assistance in the preparation of the illustrations.

SELECTED REFERENCES

Electrical control of cardiac activity is a recent and still ongoing development involving the disciplines of surgery, cardiology, electrophysiology, electronics, and bioengineering. A good overview can be gained from a review of the proceedings of the five international symposia on cardiac pacing which have been held every three years beginning in 1963. The proceedings of four of these symposia are in the English language and are the last four selected references. They contain contributions by numerous authors covering every technical and clinical aspect of cardiac pacing.

Chardack, W. M.: Cardiac pacemakers and heart block. *In* Sabiston, D. C., and Spencer, F. C. (Eds.): Gibbon's Surgery of the Chest, 3rd ed. Philadelphia, W. B. Saunders Company, 1976.
The bibliography in this chapter is up-to-date to 1975 and provides further documentation of the views of the author.

Parsonnet, V., Furman, S., and Smyth, N. P. D.: Report of the Intersociety Commission for Heart Disease Resources. Implantable Cardiac Pacemakers—Status Report and Resource Guidelines. Circulation, *50*:A21–A35, 1974.

Schechter, D. C.: Background of clinical cardiac stimulation. N. Y. State J. Med., *71–72*:2575, 1971–1972.
This article is a detailed account of the history of electrical stimulation of the heart.

Glenn, W. W. L. (Ed.): Cardiac pacemakers. Ann. N. Y. Acad. Sci., *111*:813–1122, 1964.

Furman, S. (Ed.): Advances in cardiac pacemakers. Ann. N. Y. Acad. Sci., *167*:515–1075, 1969.

Thalen, H. V. (Ed.): Cardiac Pacing. Proceedings Fourth International Symposium on Cardiac Pacing, Groningen, The Netherlands, April, 1973. The Netherlands, VanGorcum and Co., 1973.

Cardiac Pacing. Proceedings Fifth International Symposium on Cardiac Pacing, Tokyo, Japan, 1976. Amsterdam, Excerpta Medica, 1977.

REFERENCES

1. Abrams, L. D., Hudson, W. A., and Lightfoot, R.: A surgical approach to the management of heart block using an inductive coupled artificial cardiac pacemaker. Lancet, *1*:1372, 1960.
2. Braunwald, E.: Symposium on cardiac arrhythmias with comments on the hemodynamic significance of atrial systole. Am. J. Med., *37*:655, 1964.
3. Chardack, W. M.: Cardiac pacemakers and heart-block *In* Sabiston, D. C., Jr., and Spencer, F. C., (Eds): Gibbon's Surgery of the Chest, 3rd ed. Philadelphia, W. B. Saunders Company, 1976.
4. Chardack, W. M., Gage, A. A., and Greatbatch, W.: A transis-

torized, self-contained, implantable pacemaker for the long-term correction of complete heart block. Surgery, 48:643, 1960.

5. Chardack, W. M., Ishikawa, H., Fochler, F. J., Souther, S., and Gage, A. A.: Pacing and ventricular fibrillation. Ann. N. Y. Acad. Sci., 167:919, 1969.

6. Cranefield, P. F.: Paired pulse stimulation and postextrasystolic potentiation of the heart. Progr. Cardiovasc. Dis. 8:446, 1966.

7. Furman, S., and Escher, D. J. W.: Principles and Techniques of Cardiac Pacing. New York, Harper & Row, 1970.

8. Furman, S., and Robinson, G.: Stimulation of the ventricular endocardial surface in control of complete heart block. Ann. Surg., 159:841, 1959.

9. Glenn, W. W. L., Mauro, A., Longo, E., Lavietes, P. H., and Mackay, F.: Remote stimulation of the heart by radio-frequency transmission. N. Engl. J. Med., 261:948, 1959.

10. Hodam, R. P., and Starr, F.: Temporary postoperative epicardial pacing electrodes—their value and management after open heart surgery. Ann. Thorac. Surg., 8:506, 1969.

11. Hunter, S. W., Roth, N. A., Bernardez, D., and Noble, J. L.: A bipolar myocardial electrode for complete heart block. J. Lancet, 79:506, 1959.

12. Hyman, A. S.: Resuscitation of the stopped heart by intracardiac therapy. II. Experimental use of an artificial pacemaker. Arch. Intern. Med., 50:283, 1932.

13. Imparato, A., Reppert, E., and Spencer, F.: Rapid atrial pacing to produce transient heart block: A preliminary report. Surgery, 63:198, 1968.

14. Lasser, R. P., Haft, J. I., and Friedberg, C. K.: Relationship of right bundle branch block and marked left axis deviation to complete heart block and syncope. Circulation, 37:429, 1968.

15. Laurens, P., and Piwnica, A.: Stimulateur cardiaque isotopique, recherche sur la sécurité et la fiabilité à long terme. Communication à la Société Française de Cardiologie, May 10, 1970. Arch. Mal. Coeur, 63:906, 1970.

16. Lenegre, J.: Etiology and pathology of the bundle branch block in relation to complete heart block. Progr. Cardiovasc. Dis., 6:409, 1964.

17. Lev, M.: The pathology of complete atrioventricular block. Progr. Cardiovasc. Dis., 6:317, 1964.

18. McNally, E., and Benchimol, A.: Medical and physiological considerations in the use of artificial cardiac pacing. Am. Heart J., 75:380, 679, 1968.

19. Narula, O. S., Scherlag, B. J., Samet, P., and Javier, R. P.: Atrioventricular block—localization and classification by His bundle recordings. Am. J. Med., 50:146, 1970.

20. Nathan, D. A., Center, S., Wu, C-Y., and Keller, W.: An implantable synchronous pacemaker for the long-term correction of complete heart block. Am. J. Cardiol., 11:362, 1963.

21. Parsonnet, V., Myers, G. H., Gilbert, L., and Zucker, I. R.: Prediction of impending pacemaker failure in a pacemaker clinic. Am. J. Cardiol., 25:311, 1970.

22. Parsonnet, V., Zucker, I. R., Gilbert, L., and Myers, G. H.: Clinical use of an implantable standby pacemaker. J.A.M.A., 196:104, 1966.

23. Preston, T., Fletcher, R., Lucchesi, B., and Judge, R.: Changes in myocardial threshold. Physiologic and pharmacologic factors in patients with implanted pacemaker. Am. Heart J., 74:235, 1967.

24. Siddons, H., and Sowton, E.: Cardiac Pacemakers. Springfield, Ill., Charles C Thomas, Publisher, 1967.

25. Thalen, H. J., van den Berg, J. S., van der Heide, J. H. N., and Nieveen, J.: The Artificial Cardiac Pacemaker—Its History, Development and Clinical Application. Springfield, Ill., Charles C Thomas, Publisher, 1969.

26. Wierich, W. L., Gott, V. L., and Lillehei, C. W.: Treatment of complete heart block by combined use of myocardial electrode and artificial pacemaker. Surg. Forum, 8:360, 1957.

27. Zoll, P. M.: Resuscitation of the heart in ventricular standstill by external electric stimulation. N. Engl. J. Med., 274:768, 1952.

XXII

PHARMACOLOGY OF THE CARDIOVASCULAR SYSTEM IN THE SURGICAL PATIENT

Willard M. Daggett, M.D.,
Demetrios G. Lappas, M.D.,
and W. John Powell, Jr., M.D.

In this section, the pharmacology of low cardiac output states, cardiogenic shock, congestive heart failure, cardiac arrhythmias, hypertension, and protection of the myocardium against the effects of ischemia will be described. Discussions of the pharmacologic agents that act on the cardiovascular system can be found throughout other chapters within the context of the disease processes described. This section is not intended to cover all aspects of cardiovascular pharmacology pertinent to the surgeon, but rather emphasizes the treatment of pathophysiologic states commonly seen in patients with heart disease before, during, and after corrective cardiac surgical procedures.

LOW CARDIAC OUTPUT STATES

Inadequate cardiac output from a variety of causes may follow any cardiac surgical procedure. The first problem the surgeon faces in assessing this clinical situation is to determine the cause of inadequate peripheral perfusion. Measurement of cardiac performance is important in order to determine whether the low cardiac output has a myocardial basis or results from some other cause. In such patients with low cardiac output it is not uncommon to observe a discrepancy between left and right ventricular filling pressures, depending on which ventricle is more severely affected by the basic cardiac disorder. For example, in patients with coronary artery disease, left atrial pressure is frequently higher than right atrial pressure (Fig. 1). Conversely, in a patient with elevated pulmonary vascular resistance, right-sided filling pressure may exceed measured left atrial pressure. Thus, it is important to monitor filling pressures on both the left and right sides of the heart when assessing a patient with inadequate perfusion. This knowledge of intracardiac pressures is imperative to the selection of ap-

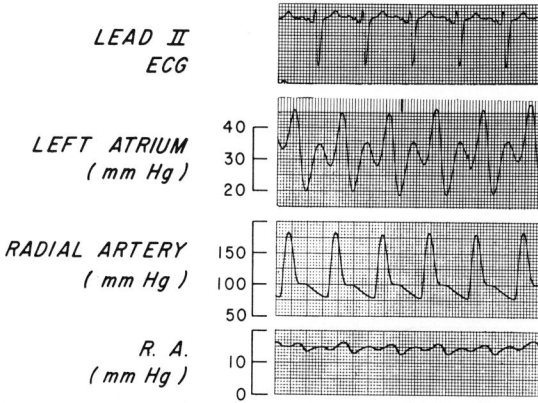

LEAD II
ECG

LEFT ATRIUM
(mm Hg)

RADIAL ARTERY
(mm Hg)

R. A.
(mm Hg)

Figure 1. Pressures recorded in a 52-year-old male under anesthesia immediately after coronary artery bypass grafting. Mean left atrial pressure exceeds 30 mm. Hg, while right atrial (R.A.) pressure has a mean value of approximately 15 mm. Hg. This type of discrepancy between right-sided and left-sided filling pressures, depending on the basic cardiac disorder, underscores the need for measuring left- and right-sided filling pressures in critically ill postoperative patients.

propriate pharmacologic therapy. The Swan-Ganz flow-directed balloon catheter[61] makes possible the continuous measurement of pulmonary capillary wedge pressure as an indirect index of left ventricular filling pressure. The measurement of central venous pressure as an index of right ventricular filling pressure is readily accomplished through an indwelling central venous cannula.

Careful assessment of the state of ventricular filling provides a rational basis for treatment of inadequate cardiac output. The baseline requirement for the treatment of the low cardiac output syndrome is adequate intravascular volume. Such patients may require higher ventricular filling pressures than would ordinarily be expected. It is not uncommon to observe improvement in cardiac output measured by the dye dilution technique in patients with chronic heart failure following elevation of left atrial pressure to 20 mm. Hg by expansion of intravascular volume.[36] Similarly, in those instances in which right ventricular failure is very prominent, a central venous pressure of 20 mm. Hg may be necessary for adequate cardiac output.

It is important to determine the arterial blood gas levels (pH, the Po_2, and the Pco_2) and to correct them if they are deranged. If the pH is low, this state should be corrected with the use of intravenous sodium bicarbonate even if the amount of sodium that must be administered causes a slight volume overload of the circulation. Both a low pH and a low Po_2 substantially depress left ventricular funtion.

It is also important to monitor cardiac rhythm and to maintain heart rate within an optimal range (approximately 80 to 120 beats per minute). If a sinus bradycardia or atrioventricular block exists and the ventricular rate is slow, it is advisable to increase the ventricular rate through the use of atrial and atrioventricular pacing, respectively. If there is a supraventricular tachyarrhythmia, it is advisable to convert the tachyarrhythmia to sinus rhythm or to slow the ventricular rate response by appropriate therapy. Whenever possible, the sequence of an atrial contraction followed closely by a ventricular contraction should be maintained. The hemodynamic importance of an appropriately placed atrial contraction in increasing cardiac output in the acutely ill patient has been well documented.[39]

Sepsis must always be considered in a patient with poor perfusion, since this is an important potential cause of low cardiac output.

In severe low cardiac output states, inotropic support of the circulation is usually required. Since the classification of catecholamine action by Ahlquist,[1] much insight has been gained into the mechanism of action of the various endogenous and synthetic symmines according to their ability to act on the cardiovascular system at hypothetical sites known as *beta-adrenergic receptors* and *alpha-adrenergic receptors*. This concept provides a convenient way of classifying catecholamines according to their biologic effects (Table 1). Agents that act on beta-adrenergic receptors increase heart rate, increase strength of myocardial contraction (increase contractility), and dilate arteries. Catecholamines that act solely upon alpha-adrenergic receptors do not influence directly either heart rate or strength of myocardial contraction. The primary action of such agents is constriction of peripheral arteries and veins. Thus, all naturally occurring and synthetic catecholamines can be classified according to beta- or alpha-adrenergic receptor stimulation or both. (See Table 2 for listing of catecholamines according to receptor site of action.)

In patients with the low cardiac output syndrome, peripheral vasoconstriction may be counteracted (and peripheral blood flow thereby improved) by the administration of isoproterenol (Isuprel) by intravenous drip. This synthetic catecholamine, an essentially pure beta-adrenergic receptor stimulator, causes active vasodilation of both systemic and pulmonary arterioles. In addition, the basic cause of peripheral vasoconstriction may be ameliorated by improvement in cardiac output secondary to enhancement of heart rate and myocardial contractile force by isoproterenol administration.[3] The reduction of preload and after-

TABLE 1. Cardiovascular Effects of Selective Adrenergic Receptor Stimulation

	Alpha	Beta
Cardiac:		↑ Heart rate
		↑ Contractility
		↑ Conduction velocity
		↑ Automaticity
		↑ Excitability
Vascular resistance:		
Coronary	↑	↓
Skeletal muscle	↑	↓
Abdominal viscera (excluding liver)	↑	↓

TABLE 2. Classification of Catecholamines According to Adrenergic Receptor Activity

Drug	Cardiac Effect	Peripheral Effect
Isoproterenol	Beta	Beta
Epinephrine	Beta ⎫	⎧ Beta — low dose
Dopamine	Beta ⎭	⎩ Alpha — high dose
Norepinephrine	Beta	Alpha
Metaraminol (Aramine)	Beta	Alpha
Phenylephrine (Neosynephrine)	Alpha	Alpha
Methoxamine (Vasoxyl)	Alpha	Alpha

load produced by this drug may result in a decreased diastolic arterial pressure.[7] Therefore, following initiation of treatment with isoproterenol it is often necessary to reassess the status of ventricular filling and to increase central blood volume with blood, plasma, or albumin.

Limitations to the amount of isoproterenol that can be delivered are related to its electrophysiologic effects. Isoproterenol increases rhythmicity, lowers threshold for pacemaker tissue, increases conduction velocity in Purkinje tissue,[18] and enhances excitability. Thus, marked increases in heart rate may attend higher doses of isoproterenol in association with either sinus tachycardia or a rapid ventricular response to atrial fibrillation owing to facilitation by this agent of atrioventricular conduction across the atrioventricular node. The enhancement of excitability may lead to ventricular irritability at the higher doses. In patients with regional myocardial ischemia, ventricular irritability may be manifest even at low doses. This effect is due both to lowering of diastolic arterial pressure by isoproterenol, which in turn lowers coronary perfusion pressure, and to an increase in myocardial oxygen consumption resulting from an increase in contractility. Because of these factors, isoproterenol is not ordinarily employed for treatment of low cardiac output on an ischemic basis. Therapy with isoproterenol should be initiated at a dose of 1 to 2 μg. per minute delivered intravenously (1 to 2 mg. of isoproterenol in 250 ml. of dextrose and water). Doses of isoproterenol in excess of 3 to 4 μg. per minute delivered intravenously are probably unwise owing to toxicity, which may cause subendocardial necrosis.[11]

Epinephrine is an endogenous catecholamine with mixed alpha- and beta-adrenergic stimulating effects.[56] This agent differs from isoproterenol in that, in addition to its capability for increasing strength of myocardial contraction and heart rate, it causes peripheral arterial and venous constriction at higher doses. Thus, arterial diastolic pressure is increased by high doses of epinephrine. The effect of epinephrine on heart rate is generally an increase, but it may vary as a result of reflex vagal enhancement secondary to an increase in arterial pressure. Epinephrine, like isoproterenol, increases rhythmicity, lowers threshold, and enhances excitability. This agent also facilitates atrioventricular conduction. Ventricular irritability may complicate high-dose therapy with epinephrine but usually in a lesser de-

gree than with isoproterenol. Therapy with epinephrine should be initiated at a dose of 1 to 2 μg. per minute delivered intravenously through a central venous cannula.

Dopamine, a precursor of norepinephrine, has in recent years found increasing clinical application to low cardiac output states because of three important effects of this agent: (1) it increases renal blood flow, (2) it enhances contractility, and (3) it has a lesser effect on heart rate and arrhythmia formation than isoproterenol.[32] For comparable increases in cardiac output, dopamine and isoproterenol cause comparable decreases in peripheral vascular resistance and, in the case of dopamine, only modest increases in heart rate.[32] The intravenous administration of 0.2 to 1.0 mg. per minute in patients with low cardiac output increases the cardiac output, stroke volume and, particularly at the higher doses, mean aortic pressure. At the higher delivery rates (above 0.6 mg. per minute) peripheral alpha-adrenergic receptor stimulation predominates, and an increase in peripheral vascular resistance occurs (see Table 2). This effect of dopamine is similar to the peripheral vascular effect of epinephrine in higher doses.

Recently a combination of norepinephrine and phentolamine has been advocated for support of the circulation in low cardiac output states.[2] The potentially adverse effects of peripheral vasoconstriction produced by norepinephrine are negated by the alpha blockade of phentolamine, while the beta-adrenergic stimulating effects of increased contractility and increased cardiac output are preserved. This combination of agents is reported to be superior to the administration of a pure beta agonist, such as isoproterenol. This superiority is probably related to the reversal by phentolamine of abnormal vasoconstriction which accompanies shock. Norepinephrine, after alpha blockade, does not produce the potentially harmful vasodilation associated with the administration of isoproterenol,[56] as the peripheral beta effect of norepinephrine is minimal (see Table 2). In patients with pulmonary artery hypertension and low cardiac output, the administration intravenously of required catecholamines for support of the circulation may actually aggravate the hemodynamic situation by increasing the afterload against which the right ventricle must pump. In addition to this adverse effect, significant clearing of norepinephrine from the pulmonary circulation has been documented,[28] making less of this catecholamine available for its beneficial effects on the coronary and systemic vascular beds. McEnany and co-workers[45] have described experimental results and clinical application of the administration of norepinephrine and epinephrine through a left atrial catheter inserted at the time of operation in patients undergoing corrective cardiac surgical procedures. The net effect of this maneuver was to markedly improve left heart performance and peripheral circulation without aggravating abnormal pulmonary arterial and right ventricular dynamics.

From the above discussion it is apparent that either dopamine or norepinephrine with phentolamine is currently thought to be most effective for treatment of low cardiac output. However, underlying disease states may modify catecholamine requirements both quantitatively and qualitatively. Thus, patients with chronic hypertension or arteriosclerosis may require higher perfusion pressures for adequate cerebral and renal blood flow and may, therefore, require a catecholamine with an alpha-adrenergic stimulating effect. In patients with low cardiac output, combinations of various catecholamines may be required for an optimal balance among cardiac output, peripheral blood flow, heart rate, perfusion pressure, and absence of arrhythmias.

Peripheral vasoconstriction in the presence of inadequate cardiac output may be so intense that additional specific pharmacologic agents are required. The catastrophic circle of events initiated by inadequate cardiac output and compounded by peripheral vasoconstriction often requires vigorous vasodilator therapy to break the chain of deterioration. Morphine given intravenously in increments of 5 to 10 mg.[40] may be of considerable aid in this regard, because of its relaxing effect on arterial smooth muscle.[41] Use of this agent in large doses will ordinarily require tracheal intubation and mechanical ventilation because of the resulting respiratory depression. Chlorpromazine and phentolamine, direct alpha-adrenergic receptor blocking agents, have also been found to be particularly effective when arterial constriction is most intense. In such patients, the administration of these agents should be initiated in small doses, since the effect of these agents is proportional to the degree of peripheral sympathetic activity present at the time the drug is administered. When sympathetic constriction is prominent, substantial decreases in arterial pressure may follow the administration of vasodilator agents in general, and alpha-adrenergic blocking agents in particular. Thus, the administration of these agents should be utilized cautiously, with plasma expanders readily available to counteract a sudden increase in vascular capacitance due to the action of the drug.

Recently another vasodilating agent, sodium nitroprusside, has been used effectively for treatment of acute heart failure (and also for acute myocardial ischemia)[14, 38] (Fig. 2). Like alpha-blocking agents described above, nitroprusside improves myocardial oxygen supply/demand ratios in the ischemic heart by coronary vasodilation and reduction of both afterload and preload (venodilation); nitroprusside, however, acts primarily on vascular smooth muscle and is independent of autonomic innervation.[34] Thus, nitroprusside, used in an intravenous drip, has a significant advantage over other vasodilator drugs. While alpha-adrenergic blocking agents, such as chlorpromazine and phentolamine, and ganglionic blocking agents, such as trimethophane, may be associated with significant "overshoot" or drift (i.e., arterial hypotension continuing for several minutes after administration of the agent has been discontinued), discontinuance of a nitroprusside intravenous drip results in almost immediate return of arterial pressure to previous levels.[52] Treatment of inadequate perfusion states with these potent vasodilators requires careful hemodynamic monitoring, usually through indwelling

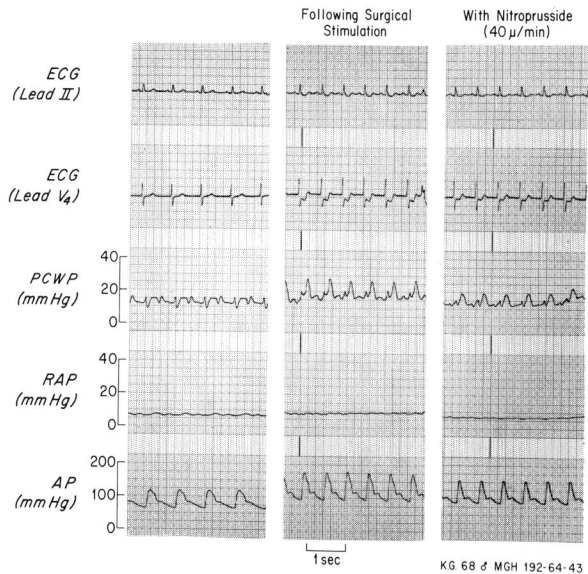

Figure 2. Hemodynamic data recorded intraoperatively in a patient with coronary artery disease prior to the institution of cardiopulmonary bypass. The left-hand panel shows data which were recorded after the induction of general anesthesia but prior to the start of the operation. The middle panel shows the hemodynamic response of the patient to the sternal incision. Abrupt arterial hypertension was associated with depressed ST segments particularly in lead V-4 and simultaneously acute left ventricular failure based on the elevation of pulmonary capillary wedge pressure. Of particular interest were the minimal effects of this important hemodynamic episode on central venous or right atrial pressure. The administration intravenously of sodium nitroprusside at 40 mcg. per min. resulted in a return of the arterial pressure toward control levels, a simultaneous fall in pulmonary capillary wedge pressure, and restoration of the ST segments back toward the isoelectric line. These data illustrate the importance of monitoring both left and right ventricular filling pressures during cardiac operations and also what can be accomplished with vasodilator therapy in the presence of abnormal intraoperative hemodynamics (PCWP = pulmonary capillary wedge pressure; RAP = right atrial pressure; AP = arterial pressure). Cardiac index was measured, using thermodilution technique and was, in the middle panel, 2.68 liters per minute per sq. meter. After the initiation of therapy with nitroprusside in the right-hand panel, the cardiac index increased to 3.55 liters per minute per sq. meter.

pulmonary arterial and systemic arterial catheters.[38]

Lillehei has presented data indicating that massive doses of corticosteroids (1 gm. methylprednisolone or its equivalent) may have a favorable effect in the low cardiac output syndrome,[21] but the use of corticosteroids in these doses must be considered developmental rather than established conventional therapy.

Mannitol, a hyperosmotic agent, may be particularly helpful, when given as a test bolus of 12.5 gm. intravenously, in assessing the underlying cause of oliguria in the patient with inadequate cardiac output. This agent increases intravascular volume almost immediately and thus may be used to determine whether hypovolemia is the cause of inadequate cardiac output from which oliguria results. For this type of situation, mannitol, given as a bolus, offers unique advantages as both a diagnostic and a therapeutic agent.[6]

CARDIOGENIC SHOCK

Cardiogenic shock may be defined as severe hypotension with inadequate perfusion of peripheral organs secondary to myocardial failure. It is accompanied by a vicious circle of ischemia or necrosis of the myocardium leading to a decrease in systemic arterial pressure, which leads to a decrease in coronary perfusion pressure and to a further reduction in myocardial oxygen delivery; this in turn results in further ischemia or necrosis of the myocardium.

Cardiogenic shock occurs in approximately 10 per cent of patients after acute myocardial infarction. Although the treatment of myocardial infarction was formerly the province of the internist or cardiologist, the advent of the surgical treatment of coronary artery disease makes adequate understanding of the treatment of acute myocardial infarction and its hemodynamic complications of the utmost importance to the surgeon. The therapy of cardiogenic shock is based on sound physiologic rationale.[31] First, as in all instances in which cardiac output is inadequate, it is necessary to be certain that there is adequate intravascular volume and oxygenation and to correct any disorder of acid-base balance. Cardiac rhythm must be closely monitored and arrhythmias treated appropriately.

Under conditions of severe hypotension, coronary blood flow varies directly with changes in systemic perfusion pressure. In these situations isoproterenol not only may increase the oxidative demands of the heart through its positive inotropic action, but also may lower systemic blood pressure through its peripheral vasodilatory effect. When this occurs, the demand for oxygen by the heart may outstrip the supply, and further ischemia and necrosis may ensue.[44] The importance of achieving an adequate systemic blood pressure in order to maintain coronary perfusion in severe hypotension bears emphasis. Norepinephrine, which increases peripheral vascular resistance through alpha receptor stimulation, may be very helpful. In addition, norepinephrine has a beta-adrenergic effect on the heart that is quantitatively equal to that of epinephrine and is the drug of choice for treatment of the uncommon patient in cardiogenic shock with low peripheral vascular resistance.

Calcium, delivered as a chloride or glucoheptonate salt, should be considered an important complementary agent for support of the injured or failing myocardium. The chloride delivers a much greater amount of ionized calcium. Confusion concerning which preparation is being used may lead to an overdose if the chloride is administered, or inadequate therapy may ensue if glucoheptonate is given. Calcium administered by intravenous drip is particularly helpful when large volumes of blood are being given rapidly to counteract loss of ionized calcium due to binding with citrate.[13] Intravenous calcium should be administered only when there is a firm cardiovascular indication for its use, such as hypotension in the presence of an elevated left atrial pressure or electrocardiographic evidence of hypocalcemia. As calcium augments the arrhythmogenic effects of digitalis glycosides, the two agents should be given together only with great caution, to avoid ventricular irritability.

When cardiogenic shock is refractory to these therapeutic measures, it is probable that severe injury to the left ventricle has occurred. Page, Caulfield, and their co-workers have shown that in death due to cardiogenic shock 40 per cent or more of the left ventricular myocardium has been lost.[51] If cardiogenic shock is refractory and resistant to pharmacologic therapy, mechanical circulatory assistance should be instituted in an attempt to stop the progression of extensive myocardial necrosis. Of the various means available, counterpulsation by means of intra-aortic balloon pumping[53] has yielded the greatest clinical success.[12] Patients who require mechanical circulatory assistance often, in addition, require emergency coronary revascularization[49] or infarct resection[17] or both for survival.

CONGESTIVE HEART FAILURE

The treatment of *congestive heart failure* in the surgical patient requires, in addition to the administration of cardiac glycosides and diuretic agents, treatment of the underlying cause. In patients undergoing cardiac surgical procedures, congestive heart failure may be temporarily aggravated by the stress of surgery and require vigorous treatment until the benefits of the operation are manifest. Since congestive heart failure in the surgical patient is often the result of fluid shifts that occur intraoperatively or postoperatively, the judicious use of diuretic agents assumes great importance. Because of the critical status of the patient, it is important to use a diuretic agent that is potent, rapid-acting, and parenterally administered.

Ethacrynic acid and *furosemide* are the two most potent diuretics available. Diuresis produced by these agents is associated with a urinary loss of sodium, chloride, potassium, and ammonium ions. This pattern is similar to that produced by the thiazide diuretics and must be kept in mind to ensure proper replacement of these electrolytes, particularly potassium and chloride. The indiscriminate use of these agents for the treatment of transient oliguria is to be discouraged, since large doses of either can produce irreversible auditory nerve damage. Rather, the cause of the oliguria should be sought and treated appropriately. If congestive heart failure is deemed the cause, then diuresis is appropriate. Since patients have been shown to tolerate sodium and water loading poorly after cardiac surgery, a central feature of prevention and treatment of congestive heart failure is stringent restriction of fluid and sodium intake.

Although the use of digitalis glycosides is important in the treatment of congestive heart failure in most clinical situations, the critically ill surgical patient presents special problems that dictate certain modifications in the use of glycosides. First, *long-acting* digitalis preparations are inappropriate for the treatment of the critically ill patient, since the usual signs of digitalis excess may be difficult to assess, and a rapid-acting and rapidly excreted preparation is required. Digoxin is generally the preparation of choice for treatment of the hospitalized patient. The onset of inotropy after the intravenous administration of 0.5 mg.

of digoxin occurs in approximately 30 to 60 minutes, and the half-life of this substance in the patient, assuming normal renal function, is 33 to 40 hours. Because of the arrhythmogenic effect of digitalis, significant impairment of renal function dictates a reduction of dosage. In the patient not treated with digitalis previously and with normal kidney function, 0.5 to 0.75 mg. intravenously can be given initially, followed by 0.25 mg. intravenously at 3- to 4-hour intervals over approximately 9 to 12 hours. During this time one should watch carefully for the onset of digitalis-induced arrhythmias, primarily *ventricular premature beats*. Other important signs of digitalis excess in the critically ill patient are the appearance of *paroxysmal atrial tachycardia with block* (see later discussion) and regularization of the ventricular response to *atrial fibrillation*. Gastrointestinal and visual signs are rarely of help in the severely ill patient. The recently developed technique of measuring glycoside blood levels by radioimmunoassay[59] adds significantly to the safe conduct of digitalis therapy.

The most important function of digitalis in the cardiac surgical patient is the control of the ventricular rate response to rapid atrial arrhythmias, such as atrial fibrillation and flutter, by induction of a graded degree of atrioventricular block. Although digitalis strengthens myocardial contraction significantly, it is no substitute for catecholamine pressor agents in the treatment of hypotension.

It is important to remember that the hypoxic or ischemic myocardium may be more susceptible to the arrhythmogenic effects of digitalis than the normal, well-oxygenated heart. Similarly, serum potassium must be monitored closely and deficits corrected, since hypokalemia significantly enhances the likelihood of a digitalis-induced arrhythmia for any given blood level of the glycoside.

Digitalis increases strength of contraction in the normal heart,[19] but it is of the greatest aid in situations in which severe congestive heart failure accompanies enlargement of the left ventricle. By improving contractility of the heart, digitalis may not only increase cardiac output but may also decrease the end-diastolic volume. Since lowering of the end-diastolic volume is associated with a decrease in wall tension, myocardial oxygen consumption should be reduced. Thus, an increase in myocardial efficiency may be achieved by use of the cardiac glycosides in congestive heart failure.

In treating the patient with ischemic heart disease the consideration of myocardial efficiency (or oxygen supply/demand) is of great importance. The relative balance between oxygen supply to the myocardium and the demand for oxygen by the myocardium may be favorably or adversely affected by the administration of a variety of cardiac active drugs.

Currently, extensive investigations are being pursued in relation to the effects of propranolol,[57] hyaluronidase,[43] nitroglycerine,[9, 15, 30] (Fig. 3) cobra venom,[43] hyperosmotic mannitol,[54] and corticosteroids[43] on acute myocardial ischemia and myocardial infarct size.[43]

PROTECTION OF THE MYOCARDIUM AGAINST THE EFFECTS OF ISCHEMIA

One of the unique features of cardiac surgical procedures on the ascending aorta, aortic valve, and coronary arteries is the finite time limit imposed upon the surgeon by the capability of the myocardium to withstand ischemia. Although successful results have been documented even with occasional lengthy periods of ischemia at normothermia,[8] approximate limits to this approach have been suggested.[22, 23] Methods of preventing the ischemic insult or protecting the myocardium against the effects of ischemia have been the subject of extensive investigation. Enright et al.[23] and

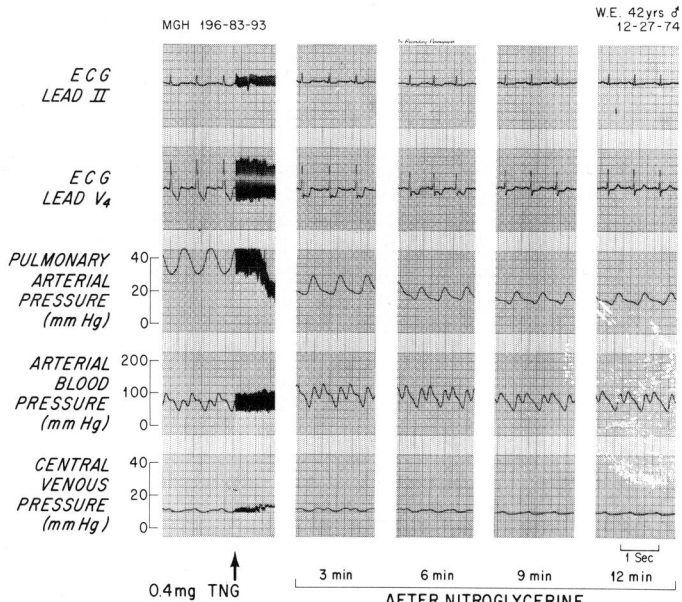

Figure 3. Hemodynamics recorded intraoperatively in a patient with both cardiogenic shock and recurrent angina pectoris four days following acute myocardial infarction. Because of this patient's hemodynamic instability and recurrent pain of myocardial ischemia, intra-aortic balloon counterpulsation had been initiated preoperatively as indicated by the deformation of the arterial blood pressure wherein a second peak is observed during diastole in the arterial blood pressure tracings. Under the influence of general anesthesia and after the surgical incision, the patient manifested acute left ventricular failure as evidenced by the exaggerated increase in pulmonary arterial pressure in the far left-hand panel. This episode was associated with relative arterial hypotension and acute ischemia as indicated in ECG lead V-4. Cardiac index at this time was 2.12 liters per minute per sq. meter. At the arrow 0.4 mg. of trinitroglycerin was administered sublingually with a prompt fall in pulmonary artery pressure and a concomitant increase in arterial blood pressure. The ST segments in ECG lead V-4 progressively returned toward the baseline in the panels recorded at 3, 6, 9, and 12 minutes after the administration of nitroglycerin. At nine minutes after nitroglycerin cardiac index was measured by the thermodilution technique and was 2.71 liters per minute per sq. meter. Note again the insensitivity of central venous pressure measurements to this dramatic series of hemodynamic events involving the pulmonary arterial, left ventricular, and systemic vascular systems.

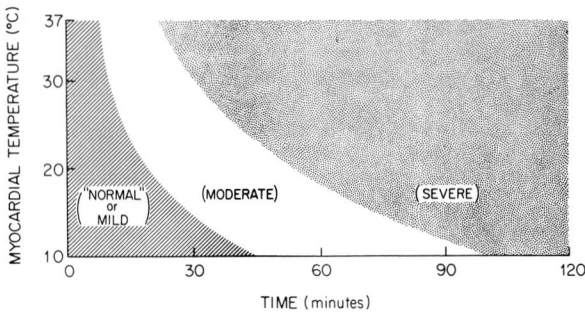

Figure 4. Myocardial depression following ischemic arrest relating time (horizontal axis) and myocardial temperature (vertical axis). The defined areas indicate the degree of myocardial injury resulting from various durations of ischemic arrest at different temperatures. The areas are approximations based on clinical and experimental data. (Reprinted from Maloney, J. V., Jr., and Nelson, R. L.: Myocardial preservation during cardiopulmonary bypass: An overview. J. Thorac. Cardiovasc. Surg., 70:1044, 1975.)

many other investigators have clearly documented the protective role of local cardiac hypothermia (Fig. 4). Topical cardiac hypothermia induced by bathing the heart in iced (4° C.) Ringer's solution with or without moderate systemic hypothermia (25 to 30° C.), appears to give good protection to the myocardium for periods of ischemic arrest up to 1 hour. While longer periods of ischemic arrest under local cardiac hypothermia have yielded successful results, the application of this approach to more lengthy ischemic periods is probably unwise. Coronary perfusion with blood has been shown to preserve myocardial function very satisfactorily,[4, 22, 23] but this method of preventing the ischemic insult presents its own technical problems, which include occasional episodes of subendocardial necrosis,[62] injury to the coronary ostia, and difficulties in exposing the small aortic root. Other investigators have emphasized the role of metabolic inhibitors such as magnesium sulfate in the protection of the myocardium against ischemic injury.[64] Pretreatment with steroids,[20] hypertonic glucose,[5] or propranolol[57] have also been shown to offer some degree of myocardial protection.

Iyengar and co-workers[33] have documented the protective effect of asanguineous coronary flushing with a heparinized dextran–multiple electrolyte solution. These investigators suggest that asanguineous coronary artery perfusion prevents the development of sludge formation within the coronary small circulation. Additional protective features of this method include prevention of vascular stasis and removal of acid metabolites by mechanical flushing; prevention of a fall in pH; maintenance of normal electrical charge; and glucose loading of the heart. Most recently, Gay and Ebert have investigated and advocated the use of potassium-induced cardioplegia to reduce the metabolic activity of the myocardium and therefore extend the time period that the heart will tolerate ischemia.[26, 27] Clinical trials of potassium-induced cardioplegia have been very promising. As Maloney and Nelson have pointed out,[42] the use of such metabolic inhibitors (Fig. 5) may significantly increase the time that the myocardium may be exposed to ischemia with-

out incurring significant damage. Conversely, factors such as hypertrophy, decreased perfusion pressure, ventricular fibrillation, and hemodilution may reduce that time interval within which the myocardium can escape ischemic damage.

The recent description of the "stone heart" in the absence of coronary artery disease presents an additional challenge to the cardiac biochemist in relation to ischemic injury.[16, 35] Ischemic contracture of the left ventricle (stone heart) is now a well-recognized complication of prolonged periods of interruption of coronary circulation during open-heart surgery. Hypothermia and metabolic inhibitors may significantly reduce the incidence of this infrequent but fatal manifestation of irreversible ischemic damage to the myocardium.

While aortic perfusion pressure has generally received less attention than some other factors which produce ischemic injury during cardiac surgery, this variable clearly may play a role, particularly when there is complicating coronary artery disease. Buckberg et al. have documented the occurrence of subendocardial ischemia in the presence of low diastolic pressure.[10] Increased resistance to myocardial perfusion during ventricular fibrillation has been thought by some to limit effective myocardial perfusion and has been shown to increase myocardial oxygen consumption.[46, 50]

The complexities of the problem of protecting the myocardium against ischemic injury are compounded by the profusion of methods currently in use and by

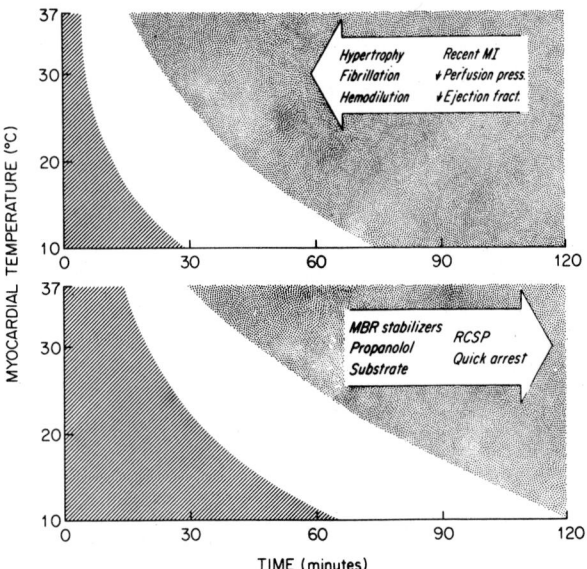

Figure 5. Increase or decrease of myocardial injury with ischemic arrest at different temperatures (vertical axis) and varying durations (horizontal axis) as influenced by a variety of factors both physical and pharmacologic. These curves are hypothetical representations of the effects of a variety of interventions (MI = myocardial infarction; MBR = membrane; RCSP = retrograde coronary sinus perfusion). (From Maloney, J. V., Jr., and Nelson, R. L.: Myocardial preservation during cardiopulmonary bypass: An overview. J. Thorac. Cardiovasc. Surg., 70:1046, 1975.)

the difficulties in obtaining statistical significance for any given method. At this time, however, certain principles or generalizations are probably applicable. (1) Total myocardial ischemia at normothermia for periods in excess of 30 minutes is probably unwise. (2) Topical cardiac hypothermia probably offers adequate myocardial protection for ischemic periods of 60 and possibly of 90 minutes. (3) Coronary perfusion should be employed, at least intermittently, for ischemic periods in excess of 90 minutes. (4) The use of metabolic inhibitors and asanguineous coronary flushing appear to be promising methods for protecting the myocardium against ischemic injury.

CARDIAC ARRHYTHMIAS

ATRIAL ARRHYTHMIAS

Of atrial arrhythmias, *atrial premature beats* are usually benign; however, if they are frequent and multifocal or if they are bigeminal in pattern, they may herald the onset of a more serious atrial tachyarrhythmia such as *atrial fibrillation*. Quinidine sulfate in a dose of 200 to 400 mg. every 4 to 6 hours orally (or quinidine lactate intramuscularly) is the drug of choice for treatment of atrial premature beats if it is deemed necessary to suppress them. If the patient cannot tolerate quinidine, procainamide (250 to 500 mg. every 3 hours)[38] may be used. The treatment of *sinus tachycardia*, during which the pulse rate is usually between 100 and 160 beats per minute, is usually directed at the underlying cause of the sinus tachycardia, which may be anxiety, congestive heart failure, hypovolemia, or a hypermetabolic state, such as hyperthyroidism or sepsis. Occasionally sinus tachycardia may, in and of itself, cause myocardial ischemia or impaired cardiac pumping capability. In such instances, by employing careful hemodynamic monitoring, one may control the tachycardia with increments (0.25 to 0.5 mg.) of propranolol administered intravenously.

Paroxysmal atrial tachycardia is an ectopic atrial arrhythmia with an atrial rate between 150 and 250 beats per minute. Usually each atrial complex is conducted to the ventricle. If atrioventricular block exists, underlying digitalis toxicity should be suspected. Carotid sinus pressure or the Valsalva maneuver will often abruptly convert the arrhythmia to normal sinus rhythm. The right carotid sinus should be massaged first for no longer than 5 to 10 seconds with continuous electrocardiographic monitoring. If this is ineffective, the left carotid sinus should be massaged. Simultaneous massage of both carotid sinuses should never be done, because of the possibility of resultant asystole or cerebral ischemia. If these maneuvers fail to convert the arrhythmia, edrophonium chloride (Tensilon) may be given intravenously in a dose of 5 to 10 mg. If the paroxysmal atrial tachycardia is well tolerated by the patient, as shown by a well-maintained systemic blood pressure, then rapid digitalization with intravenous digoxin is likely to convert the arrhythmia to sinus rhythm. Electrical cardioversion may be required

if these techniques fail to convert the arrhythmia, particularly in a patient who is hypotensive.

Atrial flutter is a rapid ectopic atrial tachyarrhythmia with an atrial rate between 250 and 350 beats per minute. The ventricular rate depends on the degree of atrioventricular block, which is usually either 2:1 or 3:1. In many patients, digitalization will convert this arrhythmia to sinus rhythm or, short of conversion, induce a stable degree of atrioventricular block leading to an acceptable ventricular rate. If this is not successful, cardioversion is the treatment of choice, particularly in a patient who is not tolerating the arrhythmia. If cardioversion is ineffective, digitalization followed by the administration of quinidine is the next treatment of choice. Prevention of recurrent attacks is best achieved by the oral administration of quinidine sulfate in a dose of 200 to 400 mg. every 4 to 6 hours. Atrial flutter is a common arrhythmia following cardiac surgery. If the patient has not had recent cardiac surgery or is not anticoagulated effectively, an underlying cause such as pulmonary embolism should be considered. A point of practical importance is the fact that atrial flutter can be resistant to digitalis therapy; larger than usual doses may be required either to convert flutter to sinus rhythm or to induce an acceptable, stable degree of atrioventricular block. Consideration must be given to the need for ultimate cardioversion in a given patient, lest the digoxin dose be pushed to toxicity level without success in treating the arrhythmia. The risk of ventricular fibrillation with cardioversion at this point is greater than it would have been had cardioversion been undertaken prior to the "digitalis push."

Atrial fibrillation is characterized by a rapid chaotic atrial rhythm at an atrial rate greater than 350 beats per minute. Digoxin is the drug of choice for controlling the ventricular rate. Digitalization should be continued until the ventricular rate is decreased to an acceptable range. In the acutely ill patient with chronic long-standing atrial fibrillation, attempts to convert the rhythm may not be successful or even hemodynamically useful. In such patients, satisfactory hemodynamics may be achieved merely by adequate ventricular rate control with digoxin. In the immediate postoperative period, attempts to reduce the ventricular rate below 100 with increments of digoxin should probably be avoided. Increased metabolic demands following surgery and augmented adrenergic activity, by facilitation of atrioventricular conduction, normally increase the heart rate. Thus, attempts to reduce the heart rate below this level with digoxin may lead to ventricular irritability without inducing block.

In a patient in whom digoxin therapy does not produce adequate rate control, propranolol in small doses (0.5 to 1.0 mg. intravenously as a single test dose, or 10 mg. orally 4 times a day) may be tried, assuming that the patient has basically good myocardial function. Use of this agent in this situation requires careful consideration, and the administration of propranolol to a patient with advanced myocardial disease is not recommended.

During digitalization, conversion to normal sinus rhythm may occur. If, however, neither conversion nor adequate rate control results from drug therapy, electrical cardioversion should be undertaken. Attempted conversion of atrial fibrillation with orally administered quinidine has little application in the acutely ill postoperative patient. If quinidine is given, full digitalization should be achieved prior to the administration of quinidine, because this drug is vagolytic and may increase the ventricular rate response to atrial fibrillation. Moreover, if atrial flutter develops, a 1:1 conduction to the ventricle with resultant hypotension or congestive heart failure or both may ensue.

As with atrial flutter, forethought is advisable concerning the need for cardioversion, which should be undertaken before digitalis therapy approaches toxicity level. When atrial fibrillation develops abruptly with a rapid ventricular rate response (160 to 170 beats per minute), increments of digoxin (and/or propranolol) are likely to be successful, particularly if administration of digoxin was discontinued for several days previously. However, when the onset of atrial fibrillation is accompanied by a lower ventricular rate (120 to 130 per minute) and the patient's response to the arrhythmia is poor, digoxin therapy is less likely to help, and immediate cardioversion is indicated.

Multifocal atrial tachycardia[58] is a rapid ectopic atrial rhythm involving at least several different atrial foci with a ventricular response of greater than 100 beats per minute. Patients with this arrhythmia frequently have accompanying lung disease (acute or chronic) with arterial hypoxia. Treatment is aimed primarily at correction of the arterial blood gas levels. In the patient not previously given digitalis therapy, digitalization may assist in slowing the ventricular response to the atrial tachycardia, but further increments of digitalis are not of benefit and may actually contribute to the patient's deterioration. This is a complex, life-threatening arrhythmia that is often resistant to pharmacologic therapy.

Nodal or Atrioventricular Junctional Rhythms

These arrhythmias may occur at any rate and are characterized electrocardiographically by relatively unchanged QRS complexes when compared to beats of supraventricular origin. However, an appropriately timed P wave does not appear before each QRS complex. From a hemodynamic standpoint, a nodal rhythm results in loss of an appropriately timed atrial systole prior to ventricular systole. This ectopic rhythm, if it occurs at a slow rate, as an "escape" rhythm, may be overcome by atrial pacing. Nodal tachycardia is a much more difficult problem, however, often indicating injury to or disease of the myocardium or digitalis excess. In the presence of nodal tachycardia, metabolic disorders such as acidosis, hypoxia, and hypokalemia must be corrected so that they can be excluded as possible etiologic factors. Phenytoin,* procainamide, lidocaine (Xylocaine), or propran-

olol may be used successfully on occasion, but nodal tachycardia is notoriously resistant to drug therapy. Resistant nodal tachycardia may respond to cardioversion, but if the arrhythmia is thought to be due to digitalis excess, cardioversion is most hazardous and drug treatment is far preferable. In the case of a refractory nodal tachycardia in a patient who cannot tolerate the arrhythmia hemodynamically, capture of the atrium by rapid atrial pacing and then gradual slowing of the atrial pacing rate to an acceptable level may suppress the nodal ectopic pacemaker.

Ventricular Arrhythmias

Ventricular premature beats are the most common ventricular arrhythmias. Indications for treatment include the following: the occurrence of more than three or four ventricular premature beats per minute, ventricular premature beats that are multifocal in origin, those that occur in salvos of two or three or more, and those that occur near the peak of the T waves of the preceding QRS complexes. The latter type is likely to initiate ventricular tachycardia. In the early postoperative period, ventricular premature beats should be suppressed vigorously with appropriate therapy, unless the patient has been known to have long-standing, singly occurring ventricular premature beats prior to operation.

There are many potential causes for ventricular irritability in the form of ventricular premature beats in the patient who has had cardiac surgery. Among these are digitalis excess, systemic hypoxia, regional myocardial injury or ischemia, acidosis, and hypokalemia. These defects, if present, must be quickly corrected when possible, and at the same time the ventricular irritability should be appropriately suppressed. It is helpful to recognize that although digitalis may aggravate ventricular irritability (particularly in the presence of hypokalemia), when ventricular premature beats occur in the presence of congestive heart failure, they may be eliminated by digitalis in a patient who has not received this agent previously. This latter effect of digitalis is probably due to a reduction in heart size by the drug which in turn reduces myocardial oxygen requirements secondary to the decrease in ventricular wall tension (La Place effect).

The usual treatment for ventricular premature beats after cardiac surgery is lidocaine delivered intravenously at a rate of 1 to 2 mg. per minute (1 gm. lidocaine in 250 ml. of 5 per cent dextrose in water). Continuing ventricular irritability may require additional intravenous boluses (50 mg.) of lidocaine. If lidocaine does not adequately suppress the ventricular premature beats, procainamide (250 to 500 mg. intramuscularly or orally every 3 hours) or quinidine (200 to 400 mg. of the sulfate orally or of the lactate intramuscularly) may be used to complement lidocaine therapy. In the patient with severe and threatening ventricular irritability but basically sound myocardial dynamics, propranolol (0.5 mg. to 1 mg. intravenously) may be used when other methods fail.

For ventricular irritability thought to be caused by digitalis excess, an intravenous potassium chloride in-

---

*New official name of diphenylhydantoin as of July 1, 1975.

fusion to replenish intracellular potassium losses may be effective. Phenytoin (100 mg. intravenously, intramuscularly, or orally every 6 to 8 hours) is particularly effective in the treatment of irritability due to digitalis excess.

Ventricular tachycardia should be treated immediately either with lidocaine by intravenous bolus (as described earlier) or, particularly if there is coexistent hypotension, with immediate electrical cardioversion. If immediate cardioversion is not successful with restoration of an acceptable systemic blood pressure (peak systolic pressure of 90 mm. Hg or greater), cardiopulmonary resuscitative efforts must be undertaken immediately. These include tracheal intubation, mechanical ventilation with 100 per cent oxygen, external cardiac massage, intravenous injection of sodium bicarbonate for acidosis, intravenous administration of 50 to 100 mg. lidocaine (once it has been established by electrocardiogram that the mode of the patient's cardiac arrest is not asystole), and repeated attempts at electrical defibrillation.[60] The intravenous administration of either norepinephrine or epinephrine may be indicated during and following the immediate period of cardiac "arrest" to effect an adequate coronary perfusion pressure initially.

The occurrence of *ventricular fibrillation* necessitates immediate electrical cardioversion. As with refractory ventricular tachycardia, failure to respond to electrical cardioversion should be treated with resuscitative maneuvers. If the condition is refractory to defibrillation, treatment should consist of intravenous administration of glucose (25 gm. in a 50 per cent solution) and crystalline zinc insulin (20 units), with or without 1 gm. of calcium chloride,[29] to correct probable hyperkalemia due to circulatory stasis.

Cardiac arrest in patients in whom the underlying rhythm disturbance is not readily discernible should be treated with electrical defibrillation immediately, since in the majority of these patients underlying *ventricular fibrillation* is the basis for cardiac arrest.

HYPERTENSION

Management of *hypertension* in the surgical patient is of importance in three distinct circumstances: (1) the routine management of the patient who is already hypertensive prior to surgery; (2) the antihypertensive treatment of the patient with an acute dissecting aneurysm of the aorta; and (3) severe paradoxical hypertension developing during or following surgery, as may occur in patients with ischemic heart disease (see Fig. 2), after repair of coarctation of the aorta, or during or immediately following surgery in a patient with pheochromocytoma.

For patients receiving antihypertensive medications preoperatively, it is appropriate to stop administration of these agents at least one day before surgery. Usually patients with even moderately severe hypertension prior to surgery will be normotensive during the administration of anesthesia. It is important that both the surgeon and the anesthesiologist know which antihypertensive agents were used. Although it was formerly thought that some drugs such as reserpine

should be withdrawn several weeks prior to surgery to allow repletion of cathecholamine stores, it has now become apparent that this agent may be given almost until the time of surgery and that depleted catecholamine stores may be replaced intraoperatively with intravenous norepinephrine if required.[25]

Although the majority of patients with dissecting aneurysm of the aorta are best managed by surgical repair, some very high-risk patients may be appropriately treated by means of a nonoperative antihypertensive program (see Chapter 54). Even the patient who has undergone operation will require pharmacologic control of blood pressure preoperatively and postoperatively to forestall further dissection. In addition to the usual antihypertensive agents, propranolol, a beta-adrenergic receptor blocking agent, may be of special benefit, since this drug lowers the rate of increase in pressure in the aorta with each ventricular systole and thereby decreases the tendency toward extension of the dissection.[65]

The third group of patients are those with severe paradoxical hypertension. Removal of pheochromocytomas is sometimes accompanied by a sharp increase in systemic blood pressure. This is particularly likely to occur at the time of manipulation of the tumor and is thought to represent a sudden release of catecholamines from the lesion. Prior treatment of these patients with phenoxybenzamine administered orally can substantially decrease the incidence of hypertension during and immediately following surgery (see Chapter 27).

Following surgical correction of coarctation of the aorta, paradoxical elevation of the blood pressure may occur. In some instances the extent of hypertension in this situation may be impressive. The exact mechanism of this change in blood pressure is not understood, but it is probably caused by neural release of catecholamines;[63] it can and should be treated, however, with the agents to be discussed in the succeeding paragraphs.

Diuretics such as chlorothiazide and spironolactone are mild antihypertensive agents that are commonly used, although their mechanism of action is not well understood. Either 500 mg. per day of chlorothiazide given orally or 100 mg. per day of spironolactone given orally (in four divided doses) or both, when not used in conjunction with other agents, may have a mild antihypertensive effect.[66] When used in conjunction with more potent antihypertensive agents, these drugs appear to potentiate the effect of the stronger medications. An advantage of using spironolactone, in contrast to other diuretics, is that potassium is conserved by this agent.

A second group of antihypertensive agents includes the rauwolfia alkaloids, of which reserpine is an example. These drugs act by inhibiting the binding of norepinephrine and epinephrine in the peripheral sympathetic nervous system. The usual oral dose of reserpine is in the range of 0.75 to 1 mg. per day in three or four equally divided doses. Reserpine can be administered intramuscularly to patients with severe hypertension in single injections of 0.5 to 1 mg., but there appears to be little added advantage to increasing the daily dose of parenteral reserpine above 8 mg.

Depression and peptic ulceration are important side effects of these agents.

Hydralazine, a drug that acts directly on vascular smooth muscle to promote arteriolar relaxation, is useful in patients whose hypertension is accompanied by renal failure. The drug does not adversely affect renal function and is not dependent upon the kidneys for inactivation. The usual dose is 75 to 100 mg. per day in three or four divided doses. Side effects include associated beta-adrenergic receptor stimulation with an increase in heart rate and in cardiac output. This effect may be detrimental to patients with angina or dissecting aneurysm. A collagen vascular disease resembling lupus erythematosus develops in a small percentage of patients receiving high doses of hydralazine over prolonged periods (usually longer than six months). The clinical manifestations of this disease appear to be reversible when the drug is discontinued.

Alpha-methyldopa (Aldomet) is metabolized into alpha-methylnorepinephrine, a less potent pressor agent than norepinephrine. This metabolite displaces stored norepinephrine at nerve endings. The usual dose of Aldomet is 1 to 2 gm. per day orally or intravenously in divided doses. Side effects include postural hypotension and somnolence; in 10 to 15 per cent of patients receiving Aldomet, a Coombs test produces positive results, which appear to be dose-related.

Guanethidine, a drug that is similar to Aldomet in its antihypertensive potential, probably acts by preventing the release of norepinephrine at myoneural junctions and by depleting peripheral stores of norepinephrine. Side effects include postural hypotension, which may become severe even when the drug is given in low therapeutic doses.

Diazoxide, a new agent that is structurally similar to chlorothiazide and is still under investigation, holds great promise as a therapeutic agent for the treatment of both malignant hypertension and chronic severe hypertension.[24, 48] Diazoxide appears to act directly on vascular smooth muscle to promote a lowering of vascular resistance.[55] The usual dose in acute severe or malignant hypertension is 300 mg. intravenously every 6 to 8 hours. Hypotension as a result of the use of this agent is unusual in a patient who is not being given other antihypertensive agents. Because of a lack of untoward side effects and because this agent increases renal blood flow, diazoxide may become an important agent in the treatment of hypertension.

Ganglionic blocking agents such as pentolinium tartrate (Ansolysen) and mecamylamine hydrochloride (Inversine) block both sympathetic and parasympathetic ganglia. These agents are indicated only for patients with severe hypertension. As might be anticipated, postural hypotension is a frequent complication of their use. Other side effects are attributable to blockade of the parasympathetic nervous system and include severe constipation and occasionally paralytic ileus.

All the antihypertensive drugs mentioned here, with the exception of diazoxide, can be administered orally. Trimethaphan camsylate (Arfonad) and nitroprusside are potent antihypertensive agents that are administered solely by the intravenous route. The delivery of both these agents must be titrated continuously with the patient's blood pressure. Failure to monitor continuously the rate of delivery of these drugs can result in severe hypotension and death. These drugs are indicated for treatment of severe hypertension refractory to other agents and for control of hypertension in situations in which the blood pressure must be rapidly controlled, as in acute dissecting aneurysm. The use of Arfonad or nitroprusside is best undertaken with continuous oscilloscopic display of the arterial blood pressure measured through an arterial catheter, since slight changes in rate of drug delivery may lead to precipitous changes in the blood pressure.

REFERENCES

1. Ahlquist, R. P.: Adrenergic drugs. In Drill, V. A. (Ed.): Pharmacology in Medicine, 2nd ed. New York, McGraw-Hill Book Company, 1958.
2. Argenta, L. C., Kirsh, M., Bove, E. L., Cimmino, V. M., and Sloan, H.: Comparison of the hemodynamic effects of inotropic agents. Presented at the 12th meeting of the Society of Thoracic Surgeons, Washington, D.C., January 19, 1976.
3. Armstrong, P. W., Gold, H. K., Buckley, M. J., Willerson, J. T., and Sanders, C. A.: Hemodynamic evaluation of rate augmentation produced by atrial pacing and isoproterenol in the early postoperative phase of cardiac valve surgery. Circulation, 44:649, 1971.
4. Austen, W. G.: Cardiac hypothermia versus coronary perfusion during aortic occlusion. Surg. Forum, 15:206, 1964.
5. Austen, W. G., Greenberg, J. J., and Piccinini, J. C.: Myocardial function and contractile force affected by glucose loading of the heart during anoxia. Surgery, 57:839, 1965.
6. Barry, K. G., and Berman, A. R.: Mannitol infusion: III. The acute effect of the intravenous infusion of mannitol on blood and plasma volumes. N. Engl. J. Med., 264:1085, 1961.
7. Bendixen, H. H., Osgood, P. F., Hall, K. V., and Laver, M. B.: Dose dependent differences in catecholamine action on heart and periphery. J. Pharmacol. Exp. Ther., 145:299, 1964.
8. Bloodwell, R. D., Hallman, G. L., Burdette, W. J., McMurtrey, M. J., and Cooley, D. A.: Cardiac valve replacement without coronary perfusion. In Brewer, L. A.: Prosthetic Heart Valves, 3rd ed. Springfield, Ill., Charles C Thomas, Publisher, 1969, pp. 397–418.
9. Borer, J. S., Redwood, D. R., Levitt, B., Cagin, N., Bianchi, C., Vallin, H., and Epstein, S. E.: Myocardial ischemia treated with nitroglycerin plus phenylephrine. N. Engl. J. Med., 293:1008, 1975.
10. Buckberg, G. D., Luck, J. C., and Hoffman, J. I. E.: Total and regional coronary blood flow after acute arteriovenous fistula. Surg. Forum, 21:171, 1970.
11. Buckberg, G. D., and Ross, G.: Effects of isoprenaline on coronary blood flow: Its distribution and myocardial performance. Cardiovasc. Res., 7:429, 1973.
12. Buckley, M. J., Mundth, E. D., Daggett, W. M., DeSanctis, R. W., Sanders, C. A., and Austen, W. G.: Surgical therapy for early complications of myocardial infarction. Surgery, 70:814, 1971.
13. Bunker, J. P.: Metabolic effects of blood transfusion. Anesthesiology, 27:446, 1966.
14. Cohn, J. N.: Vasodilator therapy for heart failure: The influence of impedance in left ventricular performance. Circulation, 48:5, 1973.
15. Come, P. C., Flaherty, J. T., Baird, M. G., Rouleau, J. R., Weisfeldt, M. L., Greene, H. L., Becker, L., and Pitt, B.: Intravenous nitroglycerin and phenylephrine in acute myocardial infarction. N. Engl. J. Med., 293:1003, 1975.
16. Cooley, D. A., Reul, G. J., and Wukasch, D. C.: Ischemic contracture of the heart: "Stone heart." Am. J. Cardiol., 29:575, 1972.
17. Daggett, W. M., Buckley, M. J., Mundth, E. D., Sanders, C. A., and Austen, W. G.: The role of infarctectomy in the surgical treatment of myocardial infarction. Am. Heart J., 84:723, 1972.
18. Daggett, W. M., and Wallace, A. G.: Vagal and sympathetic influences on ectopic impulse formation. In Dreifus, L., Likoff, W.,

and Moyer, J. H. (Eds.): Mechanisms and Therapy of Cardiac Arrhythmias. New York, Grune & Stratton, 1966, pp. 64–76.

19. Daggett, W. M., and Weisfeldt, M. L.: Influence of the sympathetic nervous system on the response of the normal heart to digitalis. Am. J. Cardiol., 16:394, 1965.

20. Davies, A. L., Juca, E. R., and Austen, W. G.: Left ventricular function in steroid pretreated dogs following total cardiopulmonary bypass. J. Cardiovasc. Surg., 9:273, 1968.

21. Dietzman, R. H., Castaneda, A. R., Lillehei, C. W., Ersek, R. A., Motsay, G. J., and Lillehei, R. C.: Corticosteroids as effective vasodilators in the treatment of low output syndrome. Chest, 57:440, 1970.

22. Ebert, P. A., Greenfield, L. J., Austen, W. G., and Morrow, A. G.: Experimental comparison of methods for protecting the heart during aortic occlusion. Ann. Surg., 155:25, 1962.

23. Enright, L. P., Staroscik, R. N., and Reis, R. L.: Left ventricular function after occlusion of the ascending aorta: Assessments of various methods for myocardial protection. J. Thorac. Cardiovasc. Surg., 60:737, 1970.

24. Finnerty, F. A., Jr., Davidov, M., and Kakaviatos, N.: Hypertensive vascular disease: The long term effect of rapid repeated reductions of arterial pressure with diazoxide. Am. J. Cardiol., 19:377, 1967.

25. Foëx, P., and Prys-Roberts, C.: Anaesthesia in the hypertensive patient. Br. J. Anaesth., 46:575, 1974.

26. Gay, W. A., Jr.: Postassium-induced cardioplegia. Ann. Thorac. Surg., 20:95, 1975.

27. Gay, W. A., Jr., and Ebert, P. A.: Functional, metabolic, and morphologic effects of potassium-induced cardioplegia. Surgery, 74:284, 1973.

28. Gillis, C. N., Greene, N. M., Cronau, L. H., and Hammond, G. L.: Pulmonary extraction of 5-hydroxytryptamine and norepinephrine before and after cardiopulmonary bypass in man. Circ. Res., 30:666, 1972.

29. Gilmore, J. P., Daggett, W. M., McDonald, R. H., and Sarnoff, S. J.: Influence of calcium on myocardial potassium balance, oxygen consumption, and performance. Am. Heart J., 75:215, 1968.

30. Gold, H. K., Leinbach, R. C., and Sanders, C. A.: Use of sublingual nitroglycerin in congestive failure following acute myocardial infarction. Circulation, 46:839, 1972.

31. Guyton, R. A., and Daggett, W. M.: The evolution of myocardial infarction: Physiologic basis for clinical intervention. Physiol. Rev., in press.

32. Holloway, E. L., Stinson, E. B., Derby, G. C., and Harrison, D. C.: Action of drugs in patients early after cardiac surgery: I. Comparison of isoproterenol and dopamine. Am. J. Cardiol., 35:656, 1975.

33. Iyengar, S. R. K., Ramchand, S., Charrette, E. J. P., and Lynn, R. B.: An experimental study of subendocardial hemorrhagic necrosis after anoxic cardiac arrest. Ann. Thorac. Surg., 13:214, 1972.

34. Johnson, C. C.: The actions and toxicity of sodium nitroprusside. Arch. Int. Pharmacodyn. Ther., 35:480, 1929.

35. Katz, A. M., and Tada, M.: The "stone heart": A challenge to the biochemist. Am. J. Cardiol., 29:578, 1972.

36. Kirklin, J. W.: Circulation and cardiac failure. In American College of Surgeons: Manual of Preoperative and Postoperative Care, 2nd ed. Philadelphia, W. B. Saunders Company, 1971, pp. 195–210.

37. Koch-Weser, J., Klein, S. W., Foo-Canto, L. L., Kastor, J. A., and DeSanctis, R. W.: Antiarrhythmic prophylaxis with procainamide in acute myocardial infarction. N. Engl. J. Med., 281:1253, 1969.

38. Lappas, D. G., Lowenstein, E., Waller, J., Fahmy, N. R., and Daggett, W. M.: Hemodynamic effects of nitroprusside infusion during coronary artery operation in man. Circulation, in press.

39. Leinbach, R. C., Chamberlain, D. A., Kastor, J. A., Harthorne, J. W., and Sanders, C. A.: A comparison of the hemodynamic effects of ventricular and sequential A-V pacing in patients with heart block. Am. Heart J., 78:502, 1969.

40. Lowenstein, E., Hallowell, P., Levine, F. H., Daggett, W. M., Austen, W. G., and Laver, M. B.: Cardiovascular response to large doses of intravenous morphine in man. N. Engl. J. Med., 281:1389, 1969.

41. Lowenstein, E., Whiting, R. B., Bittar, D. A., Sanders, C. A., and Powell, W. J., Jr.: Local and neurally mediated effects of morphine on skeletal muscle vascular resistance. J. Pharmacol. Exp. Ther., 180:359, 1972.

42. Maloney, J. V., Jr., and Nelson, R. L.: Myocardial preservation during cardiopulmonary bypass. J. Thorac. Cardiovasc. Surg., 70:1040, 1975.

43. Maroko, P. R., and Braunwald, E.: Effects of metabolic and pharmacologic interventions on myocardial infarct size following coronary occlusion. Circulation (Suppl. 1), 53:162, 1976.

44. Maroko, P. R., Kjekshus, J. K., Sobel, B. E., Watanabe, T., Covell, J. W., Ross, J., Jr., and Braunwald, E.: Factors influencing infarct size following experimental coronary artery occlusions. Circulation, 43:67, 1971.

45. McEnany, M. T., Morgan, R. J., Mundth, E. D., and Austen, W. G.: Circumvention of detrimental pulmonary vasoactivity of exogenous catecholamines in cardiac resuscitation. Surg. Forum, 26:98, 1975.

46. Moffitt, E. A., Rosevear, J. W., Townsend, C. H., and McGoon, D. C.: Myocardial metabolism in patients having aortic-valve replacement. Anesthesiology, 31:310, 1969.

47. Moran, N. C.: Adrenergic receptors within the cardiovascular system. Circulation, 28:987, 1963.

48. Mroczek, W. J., Leibel, B. A., Davidov, M., and Finnerty, F. A., Jr.: The importance of the rapid administration of diazoxide in accelerated hypertension. N. Engl. J. Med., 285:603, 1971.

49. Mundth, E. D., Buckley, M. J., Daggett, W. M., Sanders, C. A., and Austen, W. G.: Surgery for complications of acute myocardial infarction. Circulation, 45:1279, 1972.

50. Najafi, H., Henson, D., Dye, W. S., Javid, H., Hunter, J. A., Callaghan, R., Eisenstein, R., and Julian, O. C.: Left ventricular hemorrhagic necrosis. Ann. Thorac. Surg., 7:550, 1969.

51. Page, D. L., Caulfield, J. B., Kastor, J. A., DeSanctis, R. W., and Sanders, C. A.: Myocardial changes associated with cardiogenic shock. N. Engl. J. Med., 285:133, 1971.

52. Page, I. H., Corcoran, A. C., Dustan, H. P., and Koppanyi, T.: Cardiovascular actions of sodium nitroprusside in animals and hypertensive patients. Circulation, 11:188, 1955.

53. Powell, W. J., Jr., Daggett, W. M., Magro, A. E., Bianco, J. A., Buckley, M. J., Sanders, C. A., Kantrowitz, A. R., and Austen, W. G.: Effects of intra-aortic balloon counterpulsation on cardiac performance, oxygen consumption and coronary blood flow in dogs. Circ. Res., 26:753, 1970.

54. Powell, W. J., Jr., DiBona, D. R., Flores, J., Frega, N., and Leaf, A.: Effects of hyperosmotic mannitol in reducing ischemic cell swelling and minimizing myocardial necrosis. Circulation (Suppl. 1), 53:1–45, 1976.

55. Powell, W. J., Jr., Green, R. M., Whiting, R. B., and Sanders, C. A.: Action of diazoxide on skeletal muscle vascular resistance. Circ. Res., 28:167, 1971.

56. Powell, W. J., Jr., and Skinner, N. S., Jr.: Effect of the catecholamines on ionic balance and vascular resistance in skeletal muscle. Am. J. Cardiol., 18:73, 1966.

57. Reul, G. J., Jr., Romagnoli, A., Sandiford, F. M., Wukasch, D. C., Cooley, D. A., and Norman, J. C.: Protective effect of propranolol on the hypertrophied heart during cardiopulmonary bypass. J. Thorac. Cardiovasc. Surg., 68:283, 1974.

58. Shine, K. I., Kastor, J. A., and Yurchak, P. M.: Multifocal atrial tachycardia: Clinical and electrocardiographic features in 32 patients. N. Engl. J. Med., 279:344, 1968.

59. Smith, T. W., and Haber, E.: Digoxin intoxication: The relationship of clinical presentation to serum digoxin concentration. J. Clin. Invest., 49:2377, 1970.

60. Stephenson, H. E.: Cardiac Arrest and Resuscitation. St. Louis, The C. V. Mosby Co., 1969.

61. Swan, H. J. C., Ganz, W., Forrester, J., Marcus, H., Diamond, G., and Chonette, D.: Catheterization of the heart in man with use of a flow-directed balloon-tipped catheter. N. Engl. J. Med., 283:447, 1970.

62. Taber, R. E., Morales, A. R., and Fine, G.: Myocardial necrosis and the postoperative low-cardiac-output syndrome. Ann. Thorac. Surg., 4:12, 1967.

63. Verska, J. J., DeQuattro, V., and Woolley, M. M.: Coarctation of the aorta: The abdominal pain syndrome and paradoxical hypertension. J. Thorac. Cardiovasc. Surg., 58:746, 1969.

64. Webb, W. R., Dodds, R. P., Unal, M. O., Karow, A. M., Cook, W. A., and Daniel, C. R.: Suspended animation of the heart with metabolic inhibitors: Effect of magnesium sulfate or fluoride and adrenochrome in rats. Ann. Surg., 164:343, 1966.

65. Wheat, M. W., Jr., Palmer, R. F., Bartley, T. D., and Seelman, R. C.: Treatment of dissecting aneurysms of the aorta without surgery, J. Thorac. Cardiovasc. Surg., 50:364, 1965.

66. Wolf, R. L., Mendlowitz, M., Roboz, J., Styan, G. P. H., Kornfeld, P., and Weigl, A.: Treatment of hypertension with spironolactone. J.A.M.A., 198:1143, 1966.

XXIII _____

EXTRACORPOREAL CIRCULATION

Russell M. Nelson, M.D., Ph.D.

HISTORICAL ASPECTS

The idea of extracorporeal circulation was first recorded in 1812 by LeGallois,[41] who said, "If one could substitute for the heart a kind of injection of arterial blood, either natural or artificially made, one would succeed in maintaining alive indefinitely any part of the body whatsoever." The discovery of heparin by McLean[42] in 1916 became the enabling event. According to Edwards,[24] the first oxygenation of perfusion fluid may be credited to Charles A. Lindbergh. Working with Carrel in 1930, Lindbergh developed a system whereby perfusion fluid was oxygenated and driven by compressed oxygen gas. He also first demonstrated that bacterial contamination of gas could be prevented by filtering the gas through balls of cotton. Gibbon's report in 1937 of total pulmonary artery occlusion of cats supported successfully by cardiopulmonary bypass aroused the scientific community.[31] In Sweden, the filming disc oxygenator of Anderson, working with Crafoord, was used for perfusion of hearts of dogs by Björk,[9] who reported his work in 1948. In 1950, Clark et al.[12] first used a bubble oxygenator in a venovenous bypass and provided the important contribution of using silicone compounds as defoaming agents. The membrane oxygenator was discovered in Holland by Kolff and associates[39] in 1944 while they were developing an apparatus for renal dialysis.

The first complete cardiopulmonary bypass for open-heart surgery was performed in 1951 in Minneapolis by Dennis[16] and associates. The apparatus performed well, but the patient succumbed because of an imperfect repair of what was thought to be an atrial septal defect which turned out to be an endocardial cushion defect.

In 1952, Dodrill used selective left and right heart bypasses in humans with success.[20, 21] *In 1953, Gibbon[32] performed the first successful operation on a human utilizing total cardiopulmonary bypass for closure of an atrial septal defect.*

The fascinating history of the development of extracorporeal circulation is summarized in the reviews of Galletti and Brecher,[27] Bartlett and Gazzaniga,[7] Drinker,[22] Peirce,[52] Nelson,[47] Griffenhagen and Hughes,[34] and others.[1]

THE APPARATUS

The basic circuit employed is portrayed in Figure 1. The tasks of the extracorporeal circuit are simply to receive the venous blood from the body, to aerate it, and to pump it back to the arterial system. In addition to these basic requirements, provisions for intracardiac suction, filtration, sterility, and control of temperature and humidity add to the complexity of the apparatus, which consists of several components.

PUMPS

The majority of heart-lung machines utilize a simple roller pump, originally described by DeBakey in 1934.[15] This pump, as shown in Figure 2, uses a progression of rollers on adjustable heads to compress flexible tubing. The rotary movement of the rollers, which are adjusted to be almost or barely occlusive, propels the fluid within the tubing in a unidirectional, nearly nonpulsatile fashion. The volume of blood pumped per unit of time is dependent on the speed of rotation of the rollers, the degree of occlusion, and the diameter and compressibility of the tubing. The use of essentially nonpulsatile flow has the advantage of simplicity, accuracy, and reliability.

The prolonged use of nonpulsatile flow, however, may result in a gradual increase in vasomotor tone and peripheral resistance and may not be as physiologic as pulsatile flow.

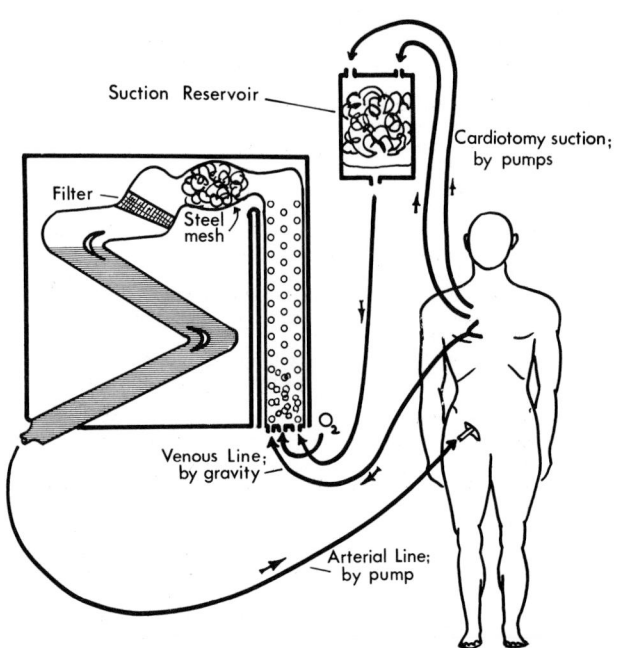

CIRCUIT FOR BAG OXYGENATOR

Figure 1. Diagrammatic illustration of an extracorporeal circuit. (From Paton, B. C.: J. R. Coll. Surg. Edinb., 8:301, 1963.)

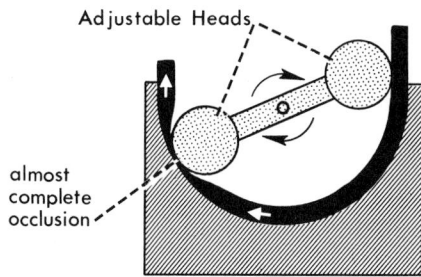

Figure 2. Diagrammatic illustration of a roller pump. (From Pomerantz, M.: Extracorporeal circulation. *In* Sabiston: Davis-Christopher Textbook of Surgery, 10th ed. Philadelphia, W. B. Saunders Company, 1972, p. 2108.)

OXYGENATORS

Although the term "oxygenator" is commonly used, the device must not only oxygenate, but allow for the elimination of carbon dioxide. Thus, the term "respirator" might be more accurate. However, this name is used for another device, so the term oxygenator is commonly employed despite the technical inaccuracy.

There are three types of oxygenators used clinically at present: (1) bubble oxygenators, (2) film oxygenators, and (3) membrane oxygenators.

BUBBLE OXYGENATORS

Blood may be oxygenated by introduction of bubbles of gas into it. Gas exchange occurs at the direct blood-gas interface. The bubbles then burst when coming in contact with silicone antifoaming compounds, thereby causing the gas to escape through portals for exhaust. The liquid blood is collected in a settling chamber to be filtered and reinfused into the arterial system of the patient.[17, 18] Usually the gas mixtures employed in bubble oxygenators utilize concentrations in the range of 97 per cent oxygen and 3 per cent carbon dioxide because of the respiratory alkalosis that ensues if no carbon dioxide is added. Gases are passed through microporous filters to eliminate bacterial contamination.[44] Most clinical perfusions at the present time are done with bubble units because they are compact, disposable, economical, well-standardized, easy to use, and safe for the time required for most human open-heart operations.

FILM OXYGENATORS

Bubbles are avoided in film oxygenators as the direct blood-gas interface is provided by filming blood in an oxygen-rich environment on rotating discs, cylinders, or stationary screens.[37] The use of film oxygenators has decreased from previous popularity because of the greater expense and labor associated with their preparation. In countries where labor is relatively less expensive than disposable materials, these oxygenators are often still preferred.

MEMBRANE OXYGENATORS

A direct blood-gas interface is avoided in these units, as a semipermeable membrane is partitioned between moving layers of blood and gas. The rate of gas transfer across the semipermeable membrane depends on the nature, thickness, surface, degree of hydration of the membrane, and formation of a boundary layer phenomenon, as well as the partial pressure differences of diffusing gases and other factors on opposite sides of the membrane.[6, 55] The advantages of a membrane oxygenator lie mainly in the avoidance of prolonged direct blood-gas interface with the resultant denaturation of proteins as shown by Lee and associates.[40] Thus, although used by some for cardiac surgery,[11, 25, 46] they are now more commonly used in perfusions of long duration such as prolonged cardiopulmonary assistance for patients with reversible pulmonary ventilatory insufficiency.[28, 35] Disadvantages are cost, limited capacity, complexity, reduced carbon dioxide exchange (related to thickness of boundary layers), and the possibility of increased resistance ratios should thrombus formation occur.

HEAT EXCHANGERS

Heat exchangers are incorporated into the extracorporeal circuit to control body temperature. Generally, it is lowered temporarily to reduce metabolic demand and returned to normal at the close of the procedure. The rewarming process is slower than cooling, as blood exposed to excessive heat is likely to be damaged. Most heat exchangers function by providing convection of heat or cold from water circulating in conduits in juxtaposition to blood conduits in the extracorporeal circuit. Heat exchangers may be used as separate components in the circuit or built in combination with disposable oxygenator units. A water dual cooler-heater may be used beside the heart-lung machine to insure adequate thermoregulation and control of the pressure of water to go into the heat exchanger.

FILTERS

Embolization of gas, platelet aggregates, fibrin, particles of calcium from diseased valves, and other detritus is an ever-present hazard in open-heart surgery.[23, 53] With addition of filters into the circuit, some protection from such embolization is afforded. They are generally included in the disposable bubble oxygenator unit, and others may be interposed between the reservoir from intracardiac suction, and occasionally used in the arterial line as well. Several types of filters of different porosity are available, but the characteristics of the ideal filter are as yet to be completely defined.[5]

TUBING

For most adult cardiac surgical operations, medical grade polyvinyl chloride (Tygon) tubing is employed. The venous line, generally draining by gravity siphonage, is 1/2 inch inside diameter, and the arterial line from the pump to the patient is generally 3/8 inch inside diameter. The tubing from the cardiotomy suction tips to the apparatus is usually 1/4 inch inside diameter. For pediatric surgery, the diameters may be reduced appropriately to keep the volume of priming fluid to a minimum. Care must be exercised in the sterilization and subsequent handling of the tubing to avoid crimping and kinking. Metal or rigid plastic connectors are employed. They must have highly polished and smooth interior surfaces tapered to ends free from heavy shoulders or rough edges which could cause damage to the blood moving rapidly through the tubing. Cannulae of plastic are generally employed in sizes as large as possible to allow adequate flow without the production of significant pressure gradients and turbulence.

PRIMING FLUIDS

Originally, extracorporeal circuits were usually primed with heparinized blood. The problems of blood procurement, storage, cross-matching, sludging of flow through the microcirculation, risk of hepatitis, and cost were reduced later by the introduction of 5 per cent dextrose in water as the priming fluid. This solution brought its own problems of rapid excretion, excessive urinary volumes, and potassium, sodium, and chloride depletion. However, the hemodilution was found to provide better flow through the microcirculation, decreased renal damage and acidosis, and less postoperative bleeding.

Currently, surgeons generally employ a solution of 5 per cent dextrose with a balanced electrolyte composition, often with the addition of salt-poor human serum albumin to prime the circuit. Whole blood is added in single-unit transfusions to the system to replace whole blood as it is lost during the operative procedure. In small children and infants, whole blood is added to the priming fluid to prevent excessive hemodilution. At the close of a hemodilution perfusion, the contents of the extracorporeal circuit are slowly reinfused into the patient to restore red cell mass. The water load is then excreted in the urine, aided by diuretics if needed, and the hematocrit is usually back nearly to normal at the close of the operation.

TECHNIQUE OF PERFUSION

After the preparatory surgical dissection has been completed and hemostasis is satisfactory, the patient is fully heparinized with a dose of 3000 units (approximately 3 mg.) per kilogram. Additional increments of 1000 units per kg. are added each hour, since the in vivo rate of disappearance is approximately 57 per cent per hour.[12] Arterial cannulation is first accomplished employing the aorta or any of its accessible branches, such as the common femoral artery, as preferred by the surgeon and as the individual circumstances may dictate. Coronary perfusion for operations on the aortic valve is provided by soft Silastic catheters connected to 1/4 inch tubing from side branches of the main arterial perfusion line. Retention of these catheters is simply and securely provided by U-shaped

sutures passed from the intima to the outside of the aorta, where they are retained by small Silastic catheter tourniquets.

Next, venous uptake catheters (3/8 inch) are inserted, usually into the inferior vena cava (via the right atrial appendage) and the superior vena cava (via the right atrium). Venous cannulation may be accomplished in certain operations by a single large (7/16 to 1/2 inch) catheter in the right atrium, right ventricle, or pulmonary artery. Bubble-free connections are then made to the previously primed tubing of the extracorporeal circuit. The left side of the heart is then vented, usually by insertion of a 3/16 inch catheter into the left ventricle via the apex. Venting through the left atrium or open aorta may also be employed, which is preferable in some instances. Mixing should be very gradual to allow accommodation to the hemodilution and filtration of any micro bubbles through the lower half of the body. A period of 5 minutes to allow for the transition to complete extracorporeal circulation has been found to be satisfactory.

Flow rates are generally determined by returning the blood to the patient at the same rate it flows to the oxygenator through catheters large enough to fill the venae cavae. These rates are usually in the range of 1.8 to 2.5 liters per minute per square meter. Flow rates may be augmented by elevating the height of the operating table and/or by adding fluid to the system. Flow rates of gas into the oxygenator are adjusted to maintain arterial oxygen tension near 100 mm. Hg and carbon dioxide tension near 40 mm. Hg. Generally, this requires one to two liters of gas flow per liter of blood flow in the commonly employed bubble oxygenators. Blood gases are determined periodically throughout the perfusion to ensure adequate and precise control.

The body temperature is then lowered to the desired range. For most adult intracardiac procedures, the temperature is reduced to the range of 30°C. This moderate hypothermia reduces the metabolic demand of each organ system.

Blood aspirated from the left ventricular sump and intracardiac sucker is returned to the oxygenator via a special intracardiac suction system. The source of this blood is the cardiac-thebesian system and bronchial flow, which can be voluminous in some cases. It is important not to aspirate blood which has pooled in the pericardial or pleural cavities, as that blood is rapidly lysed to yield free hemoglobin, fatty acids, and red cell ghosts. Such blood should be aspirated to the operating room suction system, and volumes of bank blood equivalent to that collected therein transfused into the circuit.

MONITORING OF PERFUSION

The adequacy of the extracorporeal perfusion must be assessed by adequate monitoring of various parameters. Central *arterial pressure* is monitored by an arterial catheter. The use of a plastic catheter introduced preoperatively via the radial artery has proved to be very satisfactory.[30] This catheter is connected to a closed strain-gauge system with manual flush control from a pressurized plastic container of saline.[29] Generally the mean arterial pressure gradually falls during the mixing phase at the onset of the perfusion. Once equilibration of flow has been achieved, the mean arterial pressure is maintained at or near the physiologic range by the speed of the arterial pump and the appropriate addition of blood and/or priming fluids as needed.

Central *venous pressure* is monitored by a previously placed catheter connected to a manometer and also by the anesthesiologist's watching the face of the patient to detect suffusion while also constantly watching for the possibility of kinking of the catheters or tubing.

The *electrocardiogram* is monitored throughout the procedure, being the first thing to be connected after the patient is positioned on the operating table and the last thing to be disconnected prior to moving the patient to the intensive care unit.

Electroencephalographic monitoring was originally done more than it is now and is generally not considered to be as essential as previously but continues to be used by some cardiac teams.

Blood is withdrawn from the oxygenator at regular and frequent intervals, usually every 15 to 30 minutes, for determination of *hematocrit, potassium, pH, Pco_2, Po_2, and derived data.* The assessment of venous Po_2 is used by many to monitor the adequacy of the perfusion.

Urinary volume is monitored continuously by measuring the flow from the bladder catheter into a calibrated container. This receptacle should be mounted in a location visible to the surgeons, anesthesiologist, and perfusionist.

Temperatures of the body (using rectal or esophageal probes), extracorporeal perfusate, and heat exchanger water should be monitored throughout the perfusion.

Body weights should have been determined on repeated occasions preoperatively for comparison with postoperative weights.

WITHDRAWAL FROM PERFUSION

The use of the monitoring systems just described becomes particularly important in the process of weaning the patient from extracorporeal circulation. In addition to the monitoring mentioned above, the left atrial pressure is monitored once the cardiac incisions are closed and additional volume loads are redirected to the patient's heart. After one of two venous uptake catheters is clamped, the left atrial pressure is monitored by inserting a 22-gauge needle into the left atrium or left atrial catheter. This is then connected to pressure tubing which goes to a separate strain-gauge. Experience has shown that one cannot infer from the pressure in one atrium what the pressure is in the other atrium.

The remaining venous drainage is gradually reduced by progressive occlusion of the tubing until adequate arterial pressures and left atrial pressures are maintained in the desired range (not to exceed 30 mm. Hg). Meanwhile, the right atrial pressure is monitored simply by holding the open end of one venous catheter which has been positioned into the mid right atrium. By this means, assisted circulation can be provided at a rate required to relieve any left atrial or right atrial hypertension and/or arterial hypotension. Such gradual withdrawal may be extended even to periods of two to three hours with success. It is imperative to avoid any period of left ventricular distention, as this is severely injurious to left ventricular function. The appearance of V waves in the left atrial pressure contour during the weaning phase usually indicates the presence of relative mitral regurgitation due to left ventricular dysfunction and calls for additional left ventricular support through either continued assisted circulation, digitalis, dopamine, diuretics, or other specific measures to enhance the force of the myocardial contractions.

Decannulation is accomplished in the reverse order of cannulation. To counteract the effects of heparin, it is advisable to begin the intravenous infusion of protamine sulfate (1.0 to 1.5 mg. per 100 units [1 mg.] of heparin given) slowly after the venous drainage has been stopped and before the arterial cannula has been removed. Protamine may cause a significant fall in cardiac output, stroke volume, and peripheral resistance.[53] The harmful consequences of these effects can be alleviated partially by concurrent reinfusion of the perfusate from the oxygenator as the dilute solution of protamine is being slowly administered. Once the protamine infusion has been completed and clot formation ensues, if the hemodynamics are stable, arterial decannulation and repair can then safely be accomplished.

METABOLIC CONSIDERATIONS

The requirements of the body for oxygen depend on the metabolic rate, the depth of anesthesia, body temperature, and other factors. Kirklin[38] has indicated that this value varies between 100 and 125 ml. per square meter per minute, while Clowes[14] estimated it to be between 120 and 150 ml. per square meter per minute. Lowering body temperature to 30°C decreases the oxygen requirement by approximately 50 per cent.[33] However, oxygen delivery during hemodilution or hypothermia may also be reduced by a shift of the oxyhemoglobin dissociation curve as blood is cooled. Low flow rates result in oxygen deficits producing lactic acidemia and metabolic acidosis. Accumulation of lactic acid is inversely proportional to the flow rate.[50] Hypocarbia and respiratory alkalosis may serve to decrease effective potassium levels.[2]

Increased urinary volume induced by hemodilution may also lower potassium levels. These factors must be borne in mind, and blood potassium values should be determined before using digitalis preparations in the immediate postperfusion period. It may be helpful to obtain urinary potassium concentrations as a guide to potassium replacement during the course of the perfusion.

COMPLICATIONS OF PERFUSION

All extracorporeal circulatory perfusions produce some damage to the blood and its constituents. Usually, the degree of damage is within limits of tolerance and, like starvation, can be endured if not carried out for too long a time. The risks of perfusion in the hands of experienced teams should be less than 1 per cent.[8]

AORTIC DISSECTION

Aortic dissection from the arterial cannulation requires immediate recognition and action. Once dissection has occurred, the extracorporeal perfusion is of no value. Venous and arterial tubing must be clamped immediately. Another arterial cannulation must be done quickly. If the initial cannula was in the aorta, the second cannulation may be done via the apex of the left ventricle by passing the catheter tip up through the aortic valve (if it is not an operation for aortic valve disease with an open aorta) or into the common femoral artery. If the primary cannulation was in the femoral artery, the second cannulation may be made into the aorta directly or indirectly via the apex of the left ventricle. Once the alternate arterial cannulation has been performed, the arterial line may be cut, filled, and connected to the newly placed cannula. Then the clamps may be removed and extracorporeal circulation resumed. Repair of the intimal tear in the femoral or iliac artery is not necessary, as simple withdrawal of the catheter and closure of the primary arteriotomy will suffice. A dissected aorta, previously thought to be fatal, is a salvageable situation, as heparinization and hypothermia prolong the tolerance of the brain to complete circulatory arrest long enough to permit recannulation and reconnection of the arterial line.

Prevention of this complication is uppermost in mind whenever an arterial cannula is inserted. The cannula must be inserted accurately and smoothly into the true lumen. If the adult femoral artery is used, the cannula should not be smaller than a 20F, because of the jet effect produced by high flows through a small aperture. If the femoral artery is not large enough to admit a 20F and preferably a 24F cannula, or if atherosclerotic plaques are extensive, the aorta should be used.

EMBOLIZATION

Air embolization is another complication of open-heart surgery much better prevented than treated. Most often, the source of the air is the open heart and not the open pump-oxygenators, owing to astute perfusionists, filters, and level controls. An open heart must not be pumping and/or the left ventricle must be thoroughly vented in order to keep the aortic valve closed. As the heart is being closed, there must be adequate evacuation of air from all chambers, and from the pulmonary veins as well, in addition to providing for release of any air from the aorta, before allowing the first effective beat of the heart to open the aortic valve. The patient should be positioned with the head down at this time of transition to prevent any retained air from entering the cerebral circulation. These precautionary measures become routine to the experienced cardiac surgeon and cannot be overemphasized.

Embolization of particulate matter is an especially important possibility in the presence of calcified aortic and mitral valves, thrombi in the left atrium or left ventricle, or tumors of the heart. If any of these possibilities exist, it is well to arrest the beating heart and/or cross clamp the aorta before manipulating or opening the heart. Meticulous removal of such material, if encountered in the open heart, is essential.

BLOOD DAMAGE

Extracorporeal circulation damages platelets and, to a lesser degree, red cells and white cells. Proteins may be denatured, which results in release of free lipids, an increase in blood viscosity, and hemagglutination. Experimental studies of the capillary microcirculation during perfusion have shown a progressive sludging of the blood elements, producing stasis and obstruction to blood flow through the capillaries.[55] The concentration of free hemoglobin in the plasma serves as an index to hemolysis, and the platelet count serves to quantitate the degree of damage to the platelets. This and other coagulation defects usually subside within one to seven days. Fat embolism has been observed, but this, as well as hemolysis, is not a serious problem if old changed blood from the pleural and pericardial cavities is not aspirated back into the oxygenator system.

FEVER

High fever, in the range of 40°C., was commonplace prior to the advent of completely disposable tubing and oxygenators. Now this problem has largely been eliminated, but not entirely so. It is common to see elevations to 38° or 39°C. in the first 48 hours, which gradually defervesce to normal by the fourth or fifth postoperative day.

POSTOPERATIVE CARE

Postoperative care and the management of complications following open-heart surgery with extracorporeal circulation involve problems unique to this field in addition to those common to other major surgical procedures. Some of these complications arise from the use of extracorporeal circulation itself. In general, perfusions with a bubble oxygenator up to four hours are well tolerated. Periods up to six hours may have moderate but reversible complications, while those beyond six hours approach the limits of tolerance of most patients to the effects of perfusion with present techniques. Moreover, the special circumstances requiring such prolonged support are usually a contributing factor to the increasingly higher mortality associated with prolonged perfusion.

GENERAL CONSIDERATIONS

In addition to the monitoring of vital signs as routinely done after other major operations, continuous monitoring of arterial pressure with an inlying arterial catheter and electrocardiogram is essential. Continuous surveillance and measurement of urinary output and thoracic drainage are likewise necessary. In patients with left ventricular dysfunction, it is well to leave a small catheter in the left atrium to sense pressures during the immediate postoperative period, or to use a Swan-Ganz catheter to assess changes in pulmonary artery diastolic pressure. The frequent determinations of hematocrit and arterial blood gases are necessary to guide blood replacement and respiratory control. Calculations of cardiac output are of great help if done serially to detect trends[57] but are of less value if done on a random basis, for the absolute values are less helpful than are the comparative values. The same might be said for estimation of total blood volume, which has been of very little help in the management of these critically ill patients.

Chest roentgenograms taken in the immediate postoperative period are helpful to confirm good expansion of the lungs and correct placement of endotracheal and thoracic tubes, and to rule out gastric distention, hemothorax, and pneumothorax. However, inferences regarding heart size cannot be interpreted well owing to edema, hematoma, parallax, and positioning factors.

Electrolyte studies for sodium, potassium, bicarbonate, and chloride are indispensable. Blood digoxin levels may be helpful but usually are not as definitive as are the biologic and electrocardiographic evidences of the effects of digoxin therapy.

The administration of prophylactic antibiotics has been very helpful in reducing the incidence of bacterial endocarditis.[45] The regimen currently preferred by many consists of cephalexin, 0.5 gm. orally four times daily starting the day before surgery, and cephalothin, 0.5 gm. four times daily intravenously and returning to cephalexin, 0.5 gm. orally four times daily once intravenous fluids are discontinued, up to seven days postoperatively.

Anticoagulant therapy is of two types. Patients with prosthetic valves are given warfarin to suppress the prothrombin time to the 25 to 35 per cent range. This level of anticoagulant therapy has proved to be adequate and avoids the risks of serious bleeding seen when the prothrombin time goes below 25 per cent. The prosthetic valves currently available have a relatively low risk of thromboembolic complication so that one should not burden the patient with the high risks of heavier anticoagulant therapy. The second type of anticoagulant therapy employed is with the hope of reducing the incidence of pulmonary embolism in patients undergoing coronary artery surgery. Heparin is administered subcutaneously in a dosage of 5000 units every 12 hours for about seven days postoperatively. There is no proof yet that this regimen is effective, but preliminary results suggest this may be the case.

SPECIFIC CONSIDERATIONS

Once these general postoperative management monitoring and precautionary measures have been instituted, concern may be directed to the management of specific complications of cardiac surgery and extracorporeal circulation. These complications, such as the low cardiac output syndrome, are ultimately manifest as multiple organ deterioration, and in the later stages, the causes may be difficult to differentiate. A system of thinking which has proved to be useful is to consider three categories of the patient's physiology as though they were separate, even though each is intimately associated with the function of the others. These three categories are circulatory, respiratory, and metabolic.

Circulatory

A normal circulation requires integrity of the heart as a pump, adequate blood volume, and an intact peripheral circulation. The low cardiac output syndrome can result from aberrations in any one or combination of these three factors.

Cardiac Factors. Rate disturbances can result in either bradycardia or tachycardia. Bradycardia from a junctional focus or complete atrioventricular block is best managed with a temporary pacemaker to control the rate at the desired range. The prophylactic placement of temporary wires is advisable whenever bradycardia may be anticipated. Sinus bradycardia may respond satisfactorily to infusions of isoproterenol and is often due to persistence of cardiac hypothermia.

Tachycardia may be sinus, supraventricular, or ventricular. Sinus tachycardia is usually secondary to some other cause such as hypovolemia, hypoxemia, fever, or pain. The primary cause must be determined and corrected. Tachycardias secondary to atrial fibrillation and flutter are common and generally respond to digitalization. Digoxin is the agent of choice. The dosage required to control the rate may be great, and one must be guided by the physiologic and electrocardiographic responses rather than by specific blood levels, which can only serve as a guide. Blockade of the beta-adrenergic receptors in the heart with propranolol may occasionally be employed but is generally not favored in the heart recently subjected to the trauma of surgery. Ventricular tachycardia is the forerunner of ventricular fibrillation and must be converted, usually with direct current shock. Rapid atrial fibrillation with bundle branch block is occasionally interpreted erroneously as ventricular tachycardia. With the former a satisfactory blood pressure is usually maintained, while with the latter it usually falls rapidly.

Rhythm disturbances, in addition to those mentioned above, frequently are premature atrial or ventricular depolarizations (PVDs), which are often associated with potassium depletion. Once a low blood potassium value is confirmed, these arrhythmias can be titrated away with the intravenous administration of solutions of potassium chloride (40 mEq. per 250 ml. of 5 per cent dextrose). If PVDs persist in spite of correction of potassium deficits, the use of an intravenous bolus of lidocaine may be required. Ventricular fibrillation is treated immediately with 400 watt-second direct current shock.

Cardiac power failure, as evidenced by rising atrial pressure and falling arterial pressure, is treated with positive inotropic agents. Digoxin is used commonly, even to the limit of tolerance. Isoproterenol is helpful in some cases, particularly if a more rapid rate is also needed, as it has positive chronotropic effects as well as positive inotropic effects. The use of a dopamine drip (200 mg. per 250 ml. of 5 per cent dextrose) has proved to be a great boon to those in need of increased stroke volume and cardiac output. It causes less irritability and rate increase than does isoproterenol and has now become the positive inotropic agent of choice for the short-term aid of the digitalized heart in failure. Some prefer mixtures of levarterenol and phentolamine (0.2 to 1.0 mg. per kg. per minute). Calcium is occasionally helpful, particularly in patients who have had massive bleeding and multiple transfusions of citrated bank blood.

Cardiac tamponade must be suspected in any patient failing to do well after open-heart surgery, particularly in those with larger than usual volumes of blood lost.[48] It is sometimes difficult to differentiate between tamponade and failure. Measurement of left atrial pressure may be helpful, for a low or normal value rules out congestive failure. Procedures used to diagnose tamponade in the nonoperative population, such as the chest roentgenogram, paradoxical pulse, and muffled heart tones, are of little value in this differential diagnosis postoperatively. Pericardiocentesis is of no value because clotted blood cannot be aspirated through a needle. If a reasonable doubt exists, it is safer to subject the patient to a second operation to make certain than to let an undiagnosed and otherwise fatal tamponade persist.

Failure of the operative procedure finally must be borne in mind. The clotting or malfunction of a prosthetic valve must be treated by reoperation, as must an acquired ventricular septal defect or other such complication inadvertently produced at the time of the operation.

Blood Volume Factors. The low cardiac output syndrome can result from either over- or undertransfusion. The key to distinguishing which of these mechanisms pertains is in knowing the left and right atrial pressures. The treatment of overload is digitalization, diuretics, and dopamine, as discussed previously.

Excessive bleeding in the postoperative period is generally due to mechanical problems with hemostasis rather than to coagulopathy. One can quickly determine if the blood from the chest tubes is clotting. The platelet count will help to assess the possible need for platelet transfusions, and the availability of fresh frozen plasma will provide clotting factors for those less common situations in which blood coagulation is a problem. It is well to anticipate those problems where excessive blood loss is likely to be encountered by having packs of platelets and fresh frozen plasma on hand for patients expected to have long pump runs, reoperations, or composite aortic valve replacement and aortic arch grafts.

If bleeding in excess of 300 ml. per hour persists after five hours or so, it is generally advisable to reoperate upon the patient to evacuate clots and control any bleeding points that may be found.

Peripheral Resistance Factors. Vasodilation associated with rewarming may produce a relative deficiency in blood, and arterial hypotension may become manifest. It is well, as a general principle, not to mask the effects of changes in the patient's peripheral resistance by the use of vasoconstrictor drugs. Physiologic rather than pharmacologic management is preferred. Occasionally, patients who have been on antihypertensive medication come to cardiac surgery with residual effects still evident, and they may require vasopressor therapy.

Respiratory

Pulmonary ventilatory insufficiency can come from central nervous system, major airway, alveolar, or pleural factors.

Central Nervous System Factors. Depression of the respiratory center from anesthetics or analgesics is well known and now is easily managed by continuous use of a mechanical ventilator and endotracheal intubation through the immediate postoperative period. Tracheal extubation is generally not done until the patient is fully awake and has an adequate tidal volume (greater than 5 ml. per kg.) and a vital capacity of approximately 10 ml. per kg. with satisfactory blood gases.

Major Airway Factors. Obstruction of the major airways by retained secretions is managed by endotracheal suction, liquefying agents, and vigorous physiotherapy. Emphasis to the patient about diligent coughing has been shown to be much more effective than intermittent positive pressure breathing therapy for most patients subjected to cardiac surgery, and use of the latter has largely disappeared. The use of incentive spirometry may also aid in encouraging the patient to breathe deeply and expand and deflate the lungs adequately.

A tracheostomy with a low-pressure, large-volume cuffed tube may be helpful for the patient who is either comatose or too weak to do the work of effective breathing, for the work of breathing can consume as much as 50 per cent of the oxygen derived by breathing. This may be the margin of success or failure in some cachetic individuals.

Alveolar Factors. Alveolar-capillary block and/or pulmonary shunting can be a problem in patients with ventilation-perfusion abnormalities or those in congestive failure. The maintenance of respiratory support until the blood gases are satisfactory may require days and weeks of care.

Pleural Factors. Mechanical interference with expansion of the lung results from significant hemothorax or pneumothorax. Adequate thoracic drainage usually allows re-expansion of the lung, but reoperation may be required to evacuate large collections of clotted blood. Small residual levels of retained blood and clot will generally be absorbed spontaneously and need not be aspirated by thoracentesis if the blood gases are satisfactory. Usually the chest roentgenogram taken six to eight weeks postoperatively will confirm the complete resolution of this problem.

Metabolic

Acid-base balance is crucial in the management of the postoperative patient, as acidosis per se causes a reduction in stroke volume and cardiac output. It also causes a relative increase in effective blood potassium concentrations. Correction by eliminating the cause of acidosis is preferable. The use of sodium bicarbonate or tris (hydroxymethyl) aminomethane (THAM), hydrogen ion acceptors, may be useful.[49] Alkalosis results in relative potassium shift downward and may contribute to cardiac irritability. Usually, this is a respiratory alkalosis and can be managed by altering the ventilation to allow for more retention of carbon dioxide.

Renal function is often measurably decreased. In addition, the use of significant fluid loads with hemodilution accounts for a relative oliguria seen commonly in the first four to five days after cardiac surgery. Treatment with fluid restriction to 750 ml. per square meter for that period is advisable. The use of intravenous ethacrynic acid or furosemide is very helpful in promoting rapid diuresis. These agents function as blockers of reabsorption of water in the proximal and distal tubules. The synergistic effects of chlorothiazide and triamterene are useful in promoting a slower, potassium-sparing diuresis for the patient with fluid retention in the mild range, as determined by a rise in body weight of 2 to 5 kg.

The degree of relative renal insufficiency, if progressive, can be assessed by performance of a urea clearance test comparing the simultaneous concentration of urea in the blood and the urine. Normally, urea should be concentrated at least fifteen times greater in the urine than in the blood. A urea concentration less than ten times greater in the urine than in the blood usually represents a severe degree of renal insufficiency. Progressive oliguria and anuria may require hemodialysis. This should be done frequently enough to control the potassium, creatinine, and urea nitrogen levels. Assuming adequate renal function preoperatively, recovery from the renal injury generally ensues in spite of prolonged renal insufficiency.

Other Factors

Less common but important problems are also considered as follows.

Postpericardiotomy Syndrome. This is characterized by fever, pericardial friction rub, and pericardial and/or pleural effusions. The leukocyte count is usually normal. Blood cultures are negative. The syndrome usually subsides with bed rest and aspirin. Steroid therapy is advisable in patients with coronary arterial bypass grafts or in other severe cases, utilizing 10 mg. prednisone four times daily with rapidly diminishing doses to wean off the steroid as quickly as possible.[26]

Urinary Infections. Because all of these patients have indwelling catheters in the urinary bladder, a small percentage may get urinary infections. The incidence is very low, possibly owing to the use of prophylactic antibiotics and the relatively early removal of the catheter, usually on the second postoperative day. Treatment of infection with the appropriate antimicrobial agent as determined by culture and sensitivities is indicated.

Gastrointestinal Complications. Acute abdominal complications have been observed relatively frequently. Acute appendicitis, acute cholecystitis, perforated cecum, perforated sigmoid colon, perforated duodenal ulcer, and ruptured spleen have been among the complications encountered. A high index of suspicion and a willingness to subject a critically ill postoperative patient with an acute abdomen to an abdominal exploration will be life-saving in certain circumstances. In patients who remain quite ill for prolonged periods, often on continuous respiratory support, erosive gastritis may occur. Therefore, appropriate prophylactic measures should be taken.

Anemia. As the donor red cells are rapidly destroyed, and as damaged autogenous red cells are more rapidly eliminated, an anemia generally ensues in the first week after operation. Mild degrees are managed with oral iron therapy. Symptomatic anemia is better managed with transfusions of packed erythrocytes to restore the hematocrit to safe levels. Anemia persisting after three months should be evaluated to determine cause.

Central Nervous System. Focal neurologic damage from embolization of intracardiac calcium or thrombi is a frequent and dreaded disaster encountered postoperatively. Although a carefully planned and executed procedure will prevent most emboli to the brain, there is no way adequately to ensure protection from this possibility for all, especially in those patients with unattached thrombi in the heart.

Postperfusion psychosis is very rare. In contrast, the emotional mood of these patients is generally one of encouragement and gratitude, as the relief of their preoperative distress is often rather dramatic and immediate.

PROFOUND HYPOTHERMIA AND TOTAL CIRCULATORY ARREST

Surgical access to the open heart may be achieved by this alternate or adjunctive technique. The rationale is based upon the fact that hypothermia reduces the metabolic requirements of the body. It has been found that total circulatory arrest in infants can be maintained at 20°C. for at least one hour without evidence of cerebral damage. Clinical use of profound hypothermia and total circulatory arrest, in conjunction with limited extracorporeal circulation, has improved the results of cardiac surgery in ill infants, especially in the correction of complicated congenital cardiac malformations.[3, 4, 10, 43, 56]

Several different techniques for the application of these principles have been devised. Special consideration must be given to the management of anesthesia, the induction of hypothermia, the evacuation of air from the heart, and the method of rewarming. Some surgeons have employed this technique by surface cooling and rewarming only, without the use of extracorporeal circulation.[19, 36] Others have added extracorporeal circulation of a limited degree to facilitate the process of cooling and rewarming and to aid the processes of resuscitation and evacuation of air.[4, 10] The various techniques and the results achieved with each have been summarized in a current review of this subject.[54]

The advantages of working in a bloodless field with complete relaxation of the heart unencumbered by the cannulations ordinarily employed for open-heart surgery with extracorporeal circulatory assistance have made it possible to correct complex congenital malformations in infancy. Anomalies currently being managed in this manner are transposition of the great arteries, total anomalous pulmonary venous connection, ventricular septal defect, and tetralogy of Fallot. Less encouraging results have been achieved in patients with infradiaphragmatic total anomalous pulmonary venous connection, complete atrioventricular canal, and pulmonary atresia.

SELECTED REFERENCES

Dennis, C., Spreng, D. S., Jr., Nelson, G. E., Karlson, K. E., Nelson, R. M., Thomas, J. V., Eder, W. P., and Varco, R. L.: Development of a pump oxygenator to replace the heart and lungs: An apparatus applicable to human patients and application to one case. Ann. Surg., 134:709, 1951.
   This is the report of the first application of extracorporeal circulation to permit open-heart surgery.

Drinker, A.: Progress in membrane oxygenator design. Anesthesiology, 37:242, 1972.
   This is a comprehensive review of the development of the artificial membrane oxygenator, as well as other aspects of extracorporeal circulation.

Galletti, P. M., and Brecher, G. A.: Heart-lung bypass — principle and techniques of extracorporeal circulation. New York, Grune & Stratton, 1962.
   This book represents an extensive review of the principles of extracorporeal circulation from its inception through 1961.

Gibbon, J. H., Jr.: Application of a mechanical heart and lung apparatus to cardiac surgery. Minn. Med., 37:171, 1954.
   This is Gibbon's report of the first successful use of extracorporeal circulation in man in an operation to correct an intracardiac defect.

Griffenhagen, G. B., and Hughes, C. H.: The history of the mechanical heart. Ann. Rep. Smithsonian Institution, 1955, p. 339.
   This historical review is written by two nonphysicians and published in a nonmedical journal. It is a scholarly review of this subject spanning the period from 1700 B.C. to 1955 A.D.

Hill, J. D., Ratliff, L., Fallat, J., Tucker, J., Lamy, M., Dietrich, H. P., and Gerbode, F.: Prognostic factors in the treatment of acute respiratory insufficiency with long-term extracorporeal oxygenation. J. Thorac. Cardiovasc. Surg., 68:905, 1974.
   This article reviews the unique and complex problems associated with the use of the extracorporeal membrane oxygenator for prolonged circulatory assistance for the patient with severe but reversible pulmonary insufficiency.

Nelson, R. M.: Era of extracorporeal respiration. Surgery, 78:685, 1975.
   This is a review of the development of the artificial lung from the first concept of extracorporeal oxygenation to the present time.

Peirce, E. C., II: Extracorporeal circulation for open-heart surgery. Springfield, Ill., Charles C Thomas, Publisher, 1969.
   This monograph provides much information necessary for those desiring a complete reference source in this field.

Rittenhouse, E. A., Mohri, H., Dillard, D. H., and Merendino, K. A.: Deep hypothermia in cardiovascular surgery. Ann. Thorac. Surg., 17:63, 1974.
   A comprehensive review of the various techniques of management of this adjunctive approach to open-heart surgery, this article summarizes the methods and results achieved in institutions throughout the world.

REFERENCES

1. Allen, J. G. (Ed.): Extracorporeal Circulation. Springfield, Ill., Charles C Thomas, Publisher, 1958.
2. Andersen, M. N., Mondelow, N., and William, O. G.: Relationship of respiratory alkalosis to metabolic acidosis during extracorporeal circulation. Surgery, 53:730, 1963.
3. Aoyagi, M., Flasterstein, A. H., Barnette, J., Von Koch, L., Ross, J. N., and Kennedy, J. H.: Cerebral effects of profound hypothermia (18°C) and circulatory arrest. Circulation (Suppl.), 51 and 52:52, 1975.
4. Barratt-Boyes, B. G., Simpson, M., and Neutze, J. M.: Intracardiac surgery in neonates and infants using deep hypothermia and surface cooling and limited cardiopulmonary bypass. In Mahoney, E. B. (Ed.): Cardiovascular Surgery 1970. Am. Heart Assoc. Monograph 34. Circulation, 43 and 44 (Suppl. 1):I-25, 1971.
5. Barrett, J., Dhurandhar, H. N., Miller, E., and Litwin, M. S.: A comparison in vivo of Dacron wool (Swank) and polyester mesh (Pall) micropore blood transfusion filters in the prevention of pulmonary microembolism associated with massive transfusion. Ann. Surg., 182:690, 1975.
6. Bartlett, R. H., Kittredge, D., Noyes, B. S., Willard, R. H., and Drinker, P. A.: Development of a membrane oxygenator: Overcoming blood diffusion limitation. J. Thorac. Cardiovasc. Surg., 58:795, 1969.
7. Bartlett, H., Gazzaniga, B., Fong, W., and Burns, E.: Prolonged extracorporeal cardiopulmonary support in man. J. Thorac. Cardiovasc. Surg., 68:917, 1974.
8. Bernstein, F., Castaneda, A., Blackshear, L., and Varco, R. L.: Prolonged mechanical circulatory support: Analysis of certain physical and physiologic considerations. Surgery, 57:103, 1965.
9. Björk, V. O.: Brain perfusions in dogs with artificially oxygenated blood. Acta Chir. Scand., 96:1, 1948.
10. Brunberg, J. A., Reilly, E. L., and Doty, D. B.: Central nervous system consequences in infants of cardiac surgery using deep hypothermia in circulatory arrest. In Kennedy, J. H. (Ed.): Cardiovascular Surgery 1973. Am. Heart Assoc. Monograph 42. Circulation, 49 and 50 (Suppl. II):II-60, 1974.
11. Carlson, R. G., Landé, A. J., Landis, B., Rogoz, B., Baxter, J., Patterson, R. H., Jr., Stenzel, K., and Lillehei, C. W.: The Landé-Edwards membrane oxygenator during heart surgery. J. Thorac. Cardiovasc. Surg., 66:894, 1973.
12. Clark, L. C., Gollan, F., and Gupta, V. B.: The oxygenation of blood by gas dispersion. Science, 111:85, 1950.
13. Clowes, G. H. A., Jr.: Bypass of the heart and lungs with an extracorporeal circulation. In Gibbon, J. H., Jr., Sabiston, D. C., Jr., and Spencer, F. C. (Eds.): Surgery of the Chest, 2nd ed. Philadelphia, W. B. Saunders Company, 1969, pp. 610.
14. Clowes, G. H. A., Jr., Hopkins, A. L., and Neville, W. E.: An artificial lung dependent upon diffusion of oxygen and carbon dioxide through plastic membranes. J. Thorac. Surg., 32:630, 1956.
15. DeBakey, M. E.: Simple continuous-flow blood transfusion instrument. New Orleans Med. Surg. J., 87:386, 1934.
16. Dennis, C., Spreng, D. S., Jr., Nelson, G. E., Karlson, K. E., Nelson, R. M., Thomas, J. V., Eder, W. P., and Varco, R. L.: Development of a pump oxygenator to replace the heart and lungs: An apparatus applicable to human patients and application to one case. Ann. Surg., 134:709, 1951.
17. DeWall, R. A., Warden, H. E., Gott, V. L., Read, R. C., Varco, R. L., and Lillehei, C. W.: Total body perfusion for open cardiotomy utilizing the bubble oxygenator. J. Thorac. Cardiovasc. Surg., 32:591, 1956.
18. DeWall, R. A., Bentley, D. J., Hirose, M., Battung, V., Najafi, H., and Roden, T.: A temperature controlling (omnithermic) disposable bubble oxygenator for total body perfusion. Chest, 49:207, 1966.
19. Dillard, D. H., Mohri, H., and Merendino, K. A.: Correction of heart disease in infancy utilizing deep hypothermia and total circulatory arrest. J. Thorac. Cardiovasc. Surg., 61:64, 1971.
20. Dodrill, F. D., Hill, E., and Gerisch, R. A.: Temporary mechanical substitution for the left ventricle in man. J.A.M.A., 150:642, 1952.
21. Dodrill, F. D., Hill, E., Gerisch, R. A., and Johnson, A.: Pulmonary valvuloplasty under direct vision using the mechanical heart for a complete bypass of the right heart in a patient with congenital pulmonary stenosis. J. Thorac. Surg., 25:584, 1953.

22. Drinker, A.: Progress in membrane oxygenator design. Anesthesiology, *37*:242, 1972.
23. Dutton, R. C., Edmunds, L. H., Jr., Hutchinson, J. C., and Roe, B. B.: Platelet aggregate emboli produced in patients during cardiopulmonary bypass with membrane and bubble oxygenators and blood filters. J. Thorac. Cardiovasc. Surg., *67*:258, 1973.
24. Edwards, W. S., and Edwards, P. D.: Alexis Carrel. Visionary Surgeon. Springfield, Ill., Charles C Thomas, Publisher, 1974, p. 91.
25. Eiseman, B., Birnbaum, D., Leonard, R., and Martinez, F. J.: A new gas permeable membrane for blood oxygenators. Surg. Gynecol. Obstet., *135*:732, 1972.
26. Engle, M. A., Zabriskie, J. B., Senterfit, L. B., and Ebert, P. A.: Post-pericardiotomy syndrome. Mod. Concepts Cardiovasc. Dis., *44*:59, 1975.
27. Galletti, P. M., and Brecher, G. A.: Heart-lung by-pass. New York, Grune and Stratton, Inc., 1962.
28. Galletti, P. M., Richardson, P. D., Snider, M. T., and Friedman, L. I.: A standardized method for defining the overall gas transfer performance of artificial lungs. Trans. Am. Soc. Artif. Intern. Organs, *18*:359, 1972.
29. Gardner, R. M., Warner, H. R., Toronto, A. F., and Gaisford, W. D.: Catheter-flush system for continuous monitoring of central arterial pulse waveform. J. Appl. Physiol., *29*:911, 1970.
30. Gardner, R. M., Schwartz, R., Wong, H. C., and Burke, J. P.: Percutaneous indwelling radial-artery catheters for monitoring cardiovascular function. N. Engl. J. Med., *290*:1227, 1974.
31. Gibbon, J. H., Jr.: Artificial maintenance of circulation during experimental occlusion of pulmonary artery. Arch. Surg., *34*:1105, 1937.
32. Gibbon, J. H., Jr.: Application of a mechanical heart and lung apparatus to cardiac surgery. Minn. Med., *37*:171, 1954.
33. Gordon, A. S.: Heat exchangers as hypothermia inducers in heart surgery. Ann. Rev. Med., *13*:75, 1962.
34. Griffenhagen, G. B., and Hughes, C. H.: The history of the mechanical heart. Ann. Rep. Smithsonian Institution, 1955, p. 339.
35. Hill, J. D., Ratliff, L., Fallat, J., Tucker, J., Lamy, M., Dietrich, H. P., and Gerbode, F.: Prognostic factors in the treatment of acute respiratory insufficiency with long-term extracorporeal oxygenation. J. Thorac. Cardiovasc. Surg., *68*:905, 1974.
36. Horiuchi, T., Koyamada, K., Matano, I., Mohri, H., Komatse, T., Honda, T., Abe, T., Ishitoya, T., Sagawa, Y., Matsuzawa, K., Matsumura, M., Tsuda, T., Ishizawa, E., Ishikawa, S., Suzuki, H., and Saite, Y.: Radical operation for ventricular septal defect in infancy. J. Thorac. Cardiovasc. Surg., *46*:80, 1963.
37. Kay, E. B., and Cross, F. S.: Direct vision repair of intracardiac defects utilizing a rotating disc reservoir oxygenator. Surg. Gynecol. Obstet., *104*:701, 1957.
38. Kirklin, J. W., and Theye, R.: Whole body perfusion from a pump oxygenator for open intracardiac surgery. *In* Gibbon, J. H., Jr. (Ed.): Surgery of the Chest. Philadelphia, W. B. Saunders Company, 1962, pp. 694–707.
39. Kolff, W. J., Effler, D. B., Groves, L. K., Peereboom, G., and Moraca, P. P.: Disposable membrane oxygenator (heart-lung) machine and its use in experimental surgery. Cleveland Clin. Q., *23*:69, 1956.
40. Lee, W. H., Jr., Krumhaar, D., Fonkalsrud, E. W., Schjeide, O. A., and Maloney, J. V.: Denaturation of plasma proteins as a cause of morbidity and death after intracardiac operations. Surgery, *50*:29, 1961.
41. LeGallois, J. J. C.: Experiences sur le principe de la vie. Notamment sur celui des movemens du coeur, et sur le siège de ce principe; suivies du rapport fait à la première classe de l'institute sur celles relatives aux movemens du coeur. Paris, D' Hautel, 1912.
42. McLean, J.: The discovery of heparin. Circulation, *19*:75, 1959.
43. Mori, A., Muraoka, R., Yokata, Y., Okamoto, Y., Ando, F., Fukumasu, H., Oku, H., Ideda, M., Shirotani, H., and Hikasa, Y.: Deep hypothermia with cardiopulmonary bypass for cardiac surgery in neonates and infants. J. Thorac. Cardiovasc. Surg., *64*:422, 1972.
44. Mortensen, J. D., Smith, S. M., and Hill, G.: Bacterial contamination of oxygen used in cardiopulmonary bypass. J. Thorac. Cardiovasc. Surg., *41*:675, 1961.
45. Nelson, R. M., Jenson, C. B., Peterson, C. A., and Sanders, B. C.: Effective use of prophylactic antibiotics in open-heart surgery. Arch. Surg., *90*:731, 1965.
46. Nelson, R. M., and Toronto, A. F.: Use of the hollow fiber membrane oxygenator in open heart surgery. Clinical experience. Bull. Soc. Intern. Chir., *4*:285, 1974.
47. Nelson, R. M.: Era of extracorporeal respiration. Surgery, *78*:685, 1975.
48. Nelson, R. M., Jenson, C. B., and Smoot, W. M., III: Pericardial tamponade following open-heart surgery. J. Thorac. Cardiovasc. Surg., *58*:510, 1969.
49. Nelson, R. M., Poulson, A. M., Lyman, J. H., and Henry, J. W.: Evaluation of Tris (hydroxymethyl) aminomethane (THAM) in experimental hemorrhagic shock. Surgery, *54*:86, 1963.
50. Neville, W. E.: Extracorporeal circulation. Curr. Probl. Surg., July, 1967.
51. Paton, B. C.: Cardiopulmonary bypass with diluted blood. J. R. Coll. Surg. Edinb., *8*:301, 1963.
52. Peirce, E. C.: Extracorporeal circulation for open-heart surgery. Springfield, Ill., Charles C Thomas, Publisher, 1969.
53. Pliam, M. B., and Nelson, R. M.: Unpublished data, 1975.
54. Reed, C., Romagnoli, A., Taylor, D. E., and Clark, D. K.: Particulate matter in bubble oxygenators. J. Thorac. Cardiovasc. Surg., *68*:971, 1974.
55. Rittenhouse, E. A., Mohri, H., Dillard, D. H., and Merendino, K. A.: Deep hypothermia in cardiovascular surgery. Ann. Thorac. Surg., *17*:63, 1974.
56. Varco, R. L. (Ed.): Conference on mechanical surface and layer effects on moving blood. Fed. Proc., *30*: 1971.
57. Venugopal, P., Alszowka, J., Wagner, H., Vlad, P., Lambert, E., and Subramanian, S.: Early correction of congenital heart disease with surface-induced deep hypothermia and circulatory arrest. J. Thorac. Cardiovasc. Surg., *66*:375, 1973.
58. Warner, H. R., and Gardner, R. M.: Computer-based monitoring of cardiovascular functions in postoperative patients. Circulation, *37* and *38* (Suppl. 2):68, 1968.

XXIV

ASSISTED CIRCULATION

John E. Connolly, M.D.

The explosive advances in cardiovascular surgery over the past two decades have clearly indicated both the feasibility of mechanical cardiopulmonary assistance for a few hours and the need for practical methods for mechanical assistance of the failing circulation for more prolonged periods. Many new diagnostic devices and methods for repair of cardiac dysfunction are now available if the patient can be kept alive long enough for these techniques to be put to use. Likewise, temporary mechanical support of some hearts that are successfully repaired may be necessary for some days until recovery from surgery is complete. Finally, in spite of the surgeon's ability to repair most varieties of cardiac disease, some patients with cardiomyopathy, advanced coronary artery disease, or irreparable congenital anomalies will be successfully treated only by a heart transplant or a totally implantable permanent artificial heart.

In the search for a simple, practical, and successful long-term method of mechanically assisting the failing circulation, three problems have been elucidated that are of minor importance during short periods of support for open-heart surgery but are major limiting factors for prolonged assistance. These are (1) control of clotting in the extracorporeal circuit without causing bleeding from the patient, (2) prevention of damage to blood cells and proteins associated with the prolonged use of currently available oxygenators, and (3) regulation of a physiologic pulse contour. Availability of durable materials that resist clotting and a self-contained power source are additional unsolved problems confronted in the development of a permanent implantable artificial heart.

The earliest accepted method of mechanical circulatory assistance has been partial vein-to-artery bypass using a nonblood-primed oxygenator and pump that can be preassembled and connected to a patient in a matter of minutes through the femoral vessels (Fig. 1). The power source may be a battery; this allows the system to be portable for emergency use. Such apparatus can maintain perfusion and oxygenation in a patient with massive pulmonary embolism until the diagnosis is confirmed and operative embolectomy performed. Patients suffering from cardiogenic shock secondary to myocardial infarction can be kept alive by such a portable pump-oxygenator until angiographic studies are performed which may delineate surgically correctable cardiac lesions and thus permit immediate operative correction. This method of mechanical circulatory assistance with a bubble-type disposable oxygenator poses problems if its use is required for more than six or seven hours. More prolonged pump-oxygenator assistance can be obtained by the use of a membrane oxygenator. Several centers have shown that two weeks of support is possible with the membrane oxygenator, but currently such prolonged extracorporeal oxygenation requires a massive effort with continuous sophisticated technical support.

Subsequent to the use of the pump-oxygenator for circulatory assistance, several simpler methods of mechanical support have been developed, which do not require oxygenation. One is counterpulsation by intra-aortic balloon pumping, which is currently being widely employed. The second technique is assistance by venoarterial bypass without oxygenation, employing the femoral vessels.

Other techniques of mechanical assistance to the failing circulation that should be noted are direct and indirect mechanical compression of the heart, counterpulsation by body compression, left heart bypass, and controlled ventilatory support.

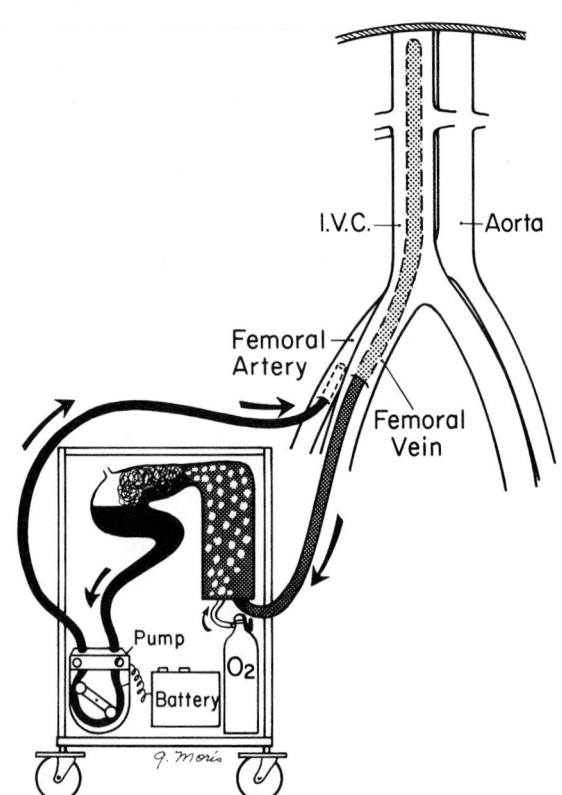

Figure 1. Diagram of venoarterial bypass with a disposable nonblood-primed pump-oxygenator connected to the patient through the femoral vessels.

EXTERNAL CARDIAC MASSAGE

Kouwenhoven and associates[26] in 1960 demonstrated that adequate systolic pressures of 60 to 100 mm. Hg could be obtained by repeated manual compression of the sternum toward the spine in patients with cardiac arrest. This technique of external cardiac massage has been widely applied and has saved many lives by maintaining the circulation until cardiac resuscitation could be performed. Harkins and Bramson[22] in 1961 described an ingenious mechanical device for providing prolonged external cardiac massage in patients who cannot be revived rapidly. They also speculated on the possibility of use of their mechanized unit to increase cardiac output in a failing but still beating heart. The apparatus consists of a cushioned piston rod that intermittently descends upon the sternum and compresses it toward the dorsal spine in a manner similar to external manual cardiac compression.

The compression is electronically synchronized with the electrocardiogram and occurs at the beginning of ventricular systole. This apparatus has subsequently been modified and simplified and is now widely used by rescue teams, in ambulances, and in hospitals. A commercially available external heart massager is shown in Figure 2. It is strapped about the patient's chest, and an oxygen mask is used to provide concomitant ventilatory support.

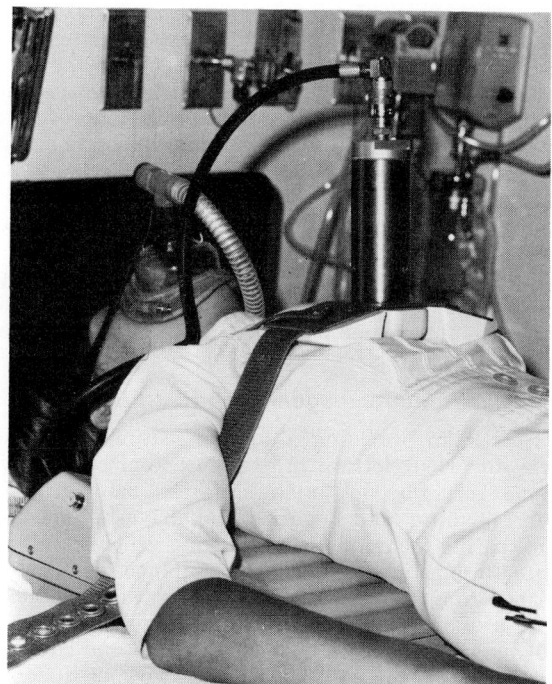

Figure 2. External mechanical heart massager. The mechanical pressure-driven pump is strapped to the chest. Note also the oxygen mask supplying positive-pressure breathing, which is part of the portable resuscitation apparatus.

COUNTERPULSATION

Clauss and associates in 1961 described another approach to mechanical assistance of the failing circulation called counterpulsation. This technique was based on observations of Sarnoff and Braunwald, who showed that myocardial oxygen consumption is related to ventricular pressure during systole and not to blood flow. If a quantity of blood is withdrawn from the arterial system immediately after the instant of isometric contraction, the pressure required during the phase of the maximal rate of ejection is reduced considerably. The same quantity of blood is then returned during diastole to enhance coronary artery perfusion in relation to the decreased myocardial work. Initial problems with counterpulsation or diastolic augmentation were related to inaccurate timing, with increased cardiac work resulting rather than assistance to the circulation.

Counterpulsation by Body Compression

A number of investigators (Birtwell et al.[6] and Osborn et al.[33]) have proposed and studied the effects of counterpulsation by encasing various portions of the body in alternating pressure suits to decrease peripheral resistance during systole and augment flow in diastole. The instant of compression is synchronized with the diastolic phase of the cardiac cycle. In most instances, the venous return, cardiac output, and systolic and diastolic pressures could be modified to reduce left ventricular work and at the same time increase cardiac output. From a practical standpoint, such pressure suit augmentation has lent itself most readily to the lower extremities. However, the amount of circulatory assistance provided by such devices is small and does not appear to be sufficient to answer the needs of most patients in cardiogenic shock.

An ingenious alternative to external pressure counterpulsation is the development by Arntzenius[2] of internal assistance or body acceleration synchronous with the heart (BASH). The entire patient in a BASH-bed is rapidly accelerated caudally during systole, and cranially during diastole; thus systolic resistance is reduced, and diastolic aortic root pressure is increased. Initial clinical trials in patients with cardiogenic shock were encouraging, but the technique has not gained wide acceptance.

Counterpulsation by Intra-aortic Balloon Pumping

A simplified approach to counterpulsation or diastolic augmentation has been provided by intra-aortic balloon pumping.[8, 9] A thin-walled polyurethane balloon is introduced retrograde from a femoral or subclavian artery into the descending thoracic aorta. The polyurethane helium-filled balloon is inflated during diastole and deflated at the beginning of systole, in electronic synchronization with the patient's electrocardiogram (Fig. 3). The theoretical physiologic benefits of this technique have been outlined earlier.

This technique has been used as supportive treatment in cardiogenic shock and as an adjunct to the preoperative and postoperative care of selected patients requiring open-heart surgery or myocardial

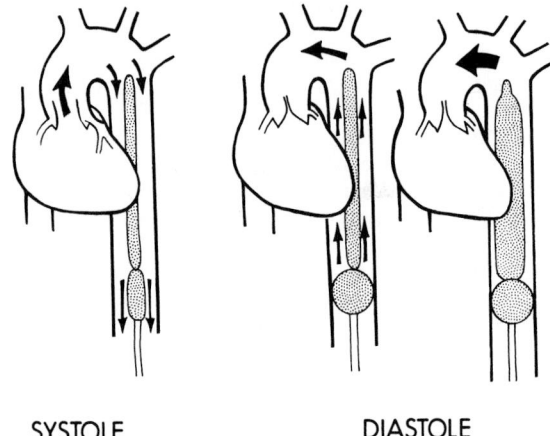

SYSTOLE   DIASTOLE

Figure 3. Intra-aortic balloon pumping. The double balloon deflates at the beginning of systole to decrease the work of ventricular ejection. The distal balloon, followed by the proximal balloon, inflates during diastole to increase the aortic root pressure and, in turn, the coronary blood flow.

revascularization. Laboratory investigation of this technique has shown its effectiveness in increasing coronary blood flow and decreasing left ventricular work. Improved survival in induced cardiogenic shock in animals after balloon pumping has been reported by some investigators. It would appear that diastolic augmentation by phasic balloon pumping may be helpful in sustaining circulation if the amount of infarcted or impaired ventricular muscle is not too great. Many centers have reported successful application of IABP, particularly after cardiac surgery. Although controls are not available, balloon pumping may also be helpful if applied within the first 20 hours of cardiogenic shock, and particularly if used in conjunction with surgical correction of ventricular aneurysm or myocardial revascularization or both. There is at present some disagreement about the design and number of balloons employed, but the major problems with this technique appear to be (1) difficulty in its introduction in patients with peripheral vascular occlusive disease, (2) problems with synchronization, (3) the possibility of balloon rupture, (4) trauma to the intima of the aorta, and (5) possible loss of extremity from arterial complications at the site of IAB.

LEFT HEART BYPASS

Another approach to mechanical support of the failing circulation is left heart bypass. Open-chest left heart bypass (left atrium to femoral artery shunting) has been a well-recognized adjunct to facilitate prolonged cross-clamping of the thoracic aorta since 1957.[15] However, few patients in cardiogenic shock can be expected to tolerate thoracotomy for institution of circulatory support. Closed chest left heart bypass for support of the failing circulation was first suggested by Dennis and associates in 1967.[17] Drainage of the left atrium was accomplished by passing a large metal cannula from a jugular vein through the right atrium, piercing the interatrial septum in the fashion of transseptal left heart catheterization, and entering the left

atrium. This ingenious form of support has many theoretical advantages. In addition to decreasing the work of the left ventricle, the use of the patient's own lungs for oxygenation eliminates a major source of difficulty in prolonged bypass.

Experiments have been performed to measure the oxygen consumption of the heart during left heart bypass. This was accomplished by determining arteriovenous oxygen differences between the root of the aorta and the coronary sinus and by measuring coronary blood flow during left heart bypass. Coronary blood flow was measured by placing a flowmeter directly on the coronary sinus. With these determinations, the oxygen consumption of the heart was calculated by means of the Fick principle and shown to be reduced 50 per cent or more with total or near-total left heart bypass.

Four hours of closed-chest left heart bypass significantly improved the survival of animals subjected to experimental cardiogenic shock.[10] It appears that even short periods of myocardial rest may reverse otherwise fatal cardiogenic shock. However, attempts to conduct closed-chest left heart bypass in animals for more than 12 hours were rarely successful. Both pulsatile flow for better organ perfusion and the elimination of anticoagulation appeared to be necessary to permit successful left heart bypass beyond 12 hours.

Pulsatile Versus Nonpulsatile Pumping

Several investigators have demonstrated that nonpulsatile flow for several hours provides inadequate perfusion for normal metabolism demands (Many,[30] Trinkle,[40] German[20]). In the study of German and associates,[20] the kidney was selected for assessment of the tissue effects of the two types of pumping. If renal oxygen flow (renal blood flow × oxygen content) was maintained at a constant level, oxygen uptake of the kidney was significantly higher with pulsatile than with nonpulsatile bypass; this indicated improved tissue perfusion with pulsatile pumping. Lactate production was significantly less in kidneys subjected to pulsatile as compared with nonpulsatile perfusion. One can conclude from these experiments that mechanical assistance to the circulation for prolonged periods of hours or days can be carried out with less physiologic derangement if a pulsatile pump rather than a nonpulsatile pump is employed, regardless of the variety of assistance employed.

Pulsatile Nonthrombogenic Left Heart Bypass

Success in providing a surface coating that would prevent blood clotting in extracorporeal circuits was first reported by Gott and associates,[21] using graphite, benzalkonium, and heparin. Wakabayashi[42] modified the coating technique by employing graphite impregnated in plastic. Wakabayashi combined his graphite-coated tubing with a pulsatile left ventricle pump coated with Dacron velour and employing tissue valves. He employed this type of pump and circuit to conduct prolonged left heart bypass without the use of heparin.[41] Bypass for 30 hours in dogs was successful. An endothelium-like membrane covered the velour lining and no clots were found in the pump or tubing after 30 hours of left heart bypass. These results were

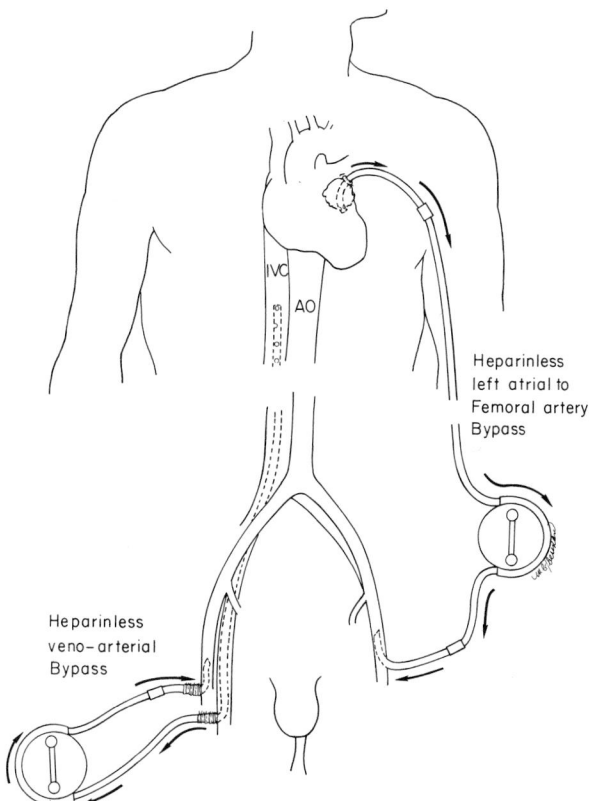

Figure 4. Diagram showing heparinless left atrial to femoral artery bypass for resection of descending thoracic aneurysms and venoarterial femorofemoral bypass without oxygenation for cardiac assistance.

significantly better than those in control animal experiments in which left heart bypass was performed with uncoated tubing, heparin, and conventional nonpulsatile pumping. A simplification of this athrombogenic left heart bypass circuit employing a roller pump[43] has been used to provide partial bypass for up to 4 hours in 25 patients undergoing thoracic aortic aneurysm resection and graft interposition (Fig. 4). No heparin was employed, and during these bypasses the mediastinum was noted to be remarkably free of bleeding. Postoperative bleeding was also significantly decreased as compared to that found when bypass techniques requiring heparin were used.

Transarterial Closed-Chest Left Ventricular Bypass

In 1969, Zwart[46] proposed bypass of the left ventricle by direct removal of left ventricular blood through a catheter introduced retrograde into the left ventricular cavity. The blood was then returned to a peripheral artery. Experience with this apparatus has demonstrated that a catheter of a size that can be introduced retrograde into the left ventricular chamber will permit total left heart bypass for several hours in sheep with a fibrillating heart. There is some question, however, whether a catheter of such a size can remove most of the left ventricular output in a

beating heart. Initial clinical trials have been technically successful but have not yet produced long-term survival or extensive application.

Direct Left Ventricle–Femoral Artery Bypass

For circulatory assistance at the completion of heart surgery, a coated athrombogenic cannula can be inserted through the apex of the left ventricle to aspirate blood which is then pumped through coated tubing to a femoral or axillary artery. The chest can be closed, with a stab wound for exit of the cannula. This technique has been employed in patients for periods of 6 to 9 hours, without the use of heparin, to decrease the work of the heart. None of the patients were long-term survivors, but all appeared to benefit during the bypass. The ultimate place for this type of bypass depends upon the ability of the heart to recover during the time of assistance.

Bernhard and associates[5] and Pierce and associates[35] have had considerable experimental success with the development of direct pumping of blood from the apex of the left ventricle to the descending thoracic aorta in calves using paracorporeal pumps. Calves have undergone synchronized assist pumping for over eight months with no evidence of thromboemboli. Infection and clotting in the pump continue to be problems requiring further investigation before such assist devices can be applied in the human. Lessons learned from these studies should lead to the successful replacement of the left heart and ultimately the total heart in man.

VENOARTERIAL BYPASS

Without Oxygenation

It is well known that phlebotomy can be life-saving in the treatment of cardiac failure and that intra-arterial transfusion can raise the aortic root pressure, increasing coronary perfusion, in patients with cardiogenic shock. Used separately, these techniques can be employed only briefly. However, in combination they can be maintained for hours or days. In experimental animals subjected to a fixed severe cardiac load, employment of partial venoarterial bypass has been shown to produce a remarkable restoration of myocardial strength.[13] The effectiveness of venoarterial bypass is directly related to its ability to raise the aortic root pressure and increase coronary blood flow.[14]

In 1958, emergency venoarterial bypass through the femoral vessels without oxygenation was performed at the bedside of four patients suffering from medically refractory cardiogenic shock due to myocardial infarction. The circulatory dynamics of all four patients improved during perfusions of up to 4 hours, but only one patient survived for any significant period beyond completion of the bypass.[3] Animal experiments were subsequently conducted to determine the length of time venoarterial bypass without oxygenation could be performed. With a roller nonpulsatile pump and total-body anticoagulation, 12 hours of bypass was tolerated with a high degree of success. However, significant mortality occurred with longer periods, and

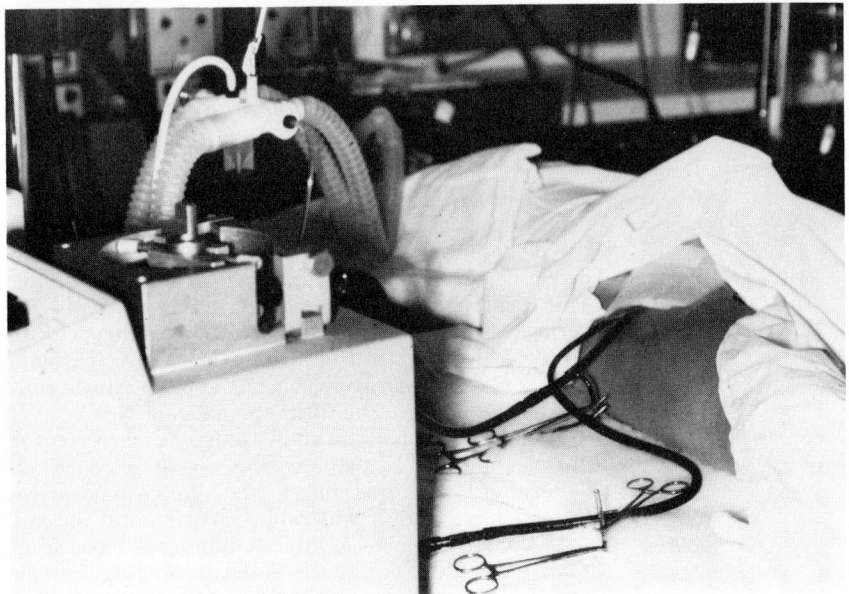

Figure 5. Femorofemoral venoarterial bypass employed at bedside for cardiac assistance in patient with cardiogenic shock. Note the athrombogenic coated tubing and roller pump.

there were few surviving animals bypassed for 24 hours. Postmortem examination showed gross and microscopic findings similar to those seen in hemorrhagic shock. These included loss of circulating blood volume and hemorrhage into the bowel. Bleeding associated with repeated heparin dosage, the adverse effects of prolonged nonpulsatile pumping, and effects of perfusing with hypoxic blood appeared to limit the feasibility of venoarterial bypass for longer than 12 hours.

However, the development of an athrombogenic surface by Wakabayashi and associates and the use of controlled ventilatory support to avoid potential desaturation from partial diversion of the pulmonary flow made the technique of venoarterial bypass without oxygenation feasible. Animal and human experience with the technique has shown that it can be conducted at the bedside via the femoral vessels for as long as six days without technical complication.[45] Figure 4 is a diagram of venoarterial bypass employed from femoral vein to artery for circulatory assistance and from left atrium to femoral artery to permit safe clamping of the descending thoracic aorta for surgery on that vessel. Note the cloth side-arms sewn to the femoral vessels to allow blood flow to and from the extremity during venoarterial bypass. Figure 5 shows the apparatus attached to a patient at the bedside. It was employed successfully in this patient for 80 hours, first to support the failing circulation following cardiogenic shock secondary to myocardial infarction and, subsequently, to permit coronary arteriography and corrective heart surgery, and thereafter to assist the heart in the postoperative period.

With Oxygenation

Total venoarterial bypass with oxygenation is routinely used for open-heart surgery, and partial venoarterial bypass with an oxygenator in circuit is an excellent method of assisting the circulation for a few hours. However, with conventional oxygenators, technical problems with the oxygenator, blood elements, and coagulation occur after 6 to 8 hours of oxygenation, and sometimes occur even sooner.

With a Membrane Oxygenator. It has been recognized that these adverse effects seen with bubble or film oxygenators are due to direct exposure of blood proteins to gas (Dobell[18] and Lee[29]) and can be alleviated by interposing a plastic film between gas and blood. Membrane oxygenators of this type were first described and used by Clowes in 1957.[11] However, the membrane lung was not a practical possibility until silicone polymer membranes with excellent gas-transfer properties were substituted for Teflon membranes in 1962. Bramson and colleagues[7] first demonstrated that an oxygenator employing such membranes could be successfully employed routinely for open-heart surgery in 1965. Subsequently, a number of investigators (Hill,[23] Kolobow,[25] Landé,[28] and Bartlett[4]) demonstrated that partial bypass can be carried out for periods up to two weeks without detrimental effects. The limiting factor is control of clotting and bleeding. Prolonged cardiopulmonary support using venoarterial bypass with a membrane oxygenator has been used clinically for three days with success (Hill and O'Brien[23]) and is undergoing clinical testing in many centers (Landé[28] and Peirce[34]).

CONTROLLED VENTILATORY SUPPORT

Controlled ventilatory support of patients following cardiac surgery reduces the work of breathing and, in turn, cardiac work and is thus an ancillary method of providing assistance to the circulation. Such ventilatory support is being increasingly employed after cardiac surgery and other types of surgery to maintain normal blood gases, but at the same time circulatory assistance is provided by relieving the work of breathing.

IMPLANTABLE ARTIFICIAL HEART

A considerable amount of laboratory investigation has been directed to the development of a permanent mechanical replacement for the heart. At present, a totally implantable power source capable of operating such a heart has not been developed. All such devices require external power sources with transmission lines penetrating the chest, and this leads to a high incidence of eventual infection. Likewise, all currently described artificial hearts continue to be complicated by problems of clotting and embolization.

Much progress has been made in solving some of the problems attendant upon use of artificial mechanical hearts by concentrating on implantable left heart bypass devices. In 1963 DeBakey and Liotta reported successful use of such a device in one of six patients.[16] However, this technique was subsequently discarded because of the problems previously mentioned. Bernhard and co-workers[5] have developed a pneumatically activated, double-valved pump that is interposed between the left ventricular apex and the descending thoracic aorta. The device accepts blood from the left ventricle during systole and ejects it into the descending thoracic aorta in diastole. Anticoagulant requirements are diminished by the culturing of a neo-intima of fibroblasts on the velour lining. Studies in calves have shown that this method of intermittent left heart bypass can be effective for several months.

Several groups (Akutsu,[39] Kolff,[27] Nosé,[32] Peirce[34]) have developed total artificial hearts of silicone or polyurethane and have employed them successfully for full support of the circulation in calves and sheep for longer than 100 hours. Multiple thromboses and infection continue to limit the long-term success of these experimental total replacement artificial hearts. These investigators, however, have shown that such devices can totally replace the heart and support life for short periods. They offer promise of success if the aforementioned problems can be solved.

FUTURE OF ASSISTED CIRCULATION

Although thousands of patients die each year of cardiogenic shock who might be kept alive with mechanical circulatory assistance, only those with borderline needs of assistance might be expected to recover after hours or days of assistance. In the majority of patients, the underlying cardiac lesion will remain and result in demise after termination of the bypass. Clearly, the place of assistance in patients with cardiogenic shock is to support the patient until diagnosis and surgical treatment of the underlying disease can be accomplished. In most patients, this will consist of cardiac catheterization and angiography followed by coronary artery bypass surgery or ventricular aneurysm resection or perhaps valve replacement.

An increasing number of patients are being supported by peripheral venoarterial cannulation and temporary pump-oxygenator bypass or by aortic balloon pumping while angiography is performed. Figure 6 shows a patient being transported to an angiography room while his circulation is supported by a portable pump-oxygenator. Following such definitive radiologic

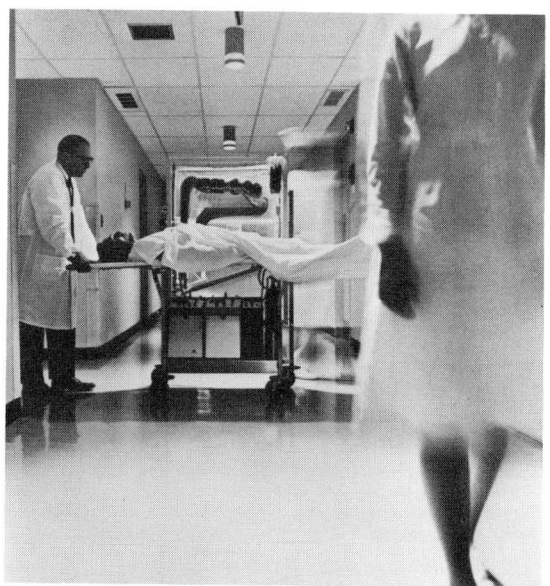

Figure 6. Emergency pump-oxygenator. Patient is being transferred to angiography room or operating room with circulatory support supplied by a portable pump-oxygenator.

examination, corrective surgery on the impaired ventricle or coronary vessels resulting in adequate myocardial function has been successfully performed (Mundth[31]). If left ventricular function is not adequate postoperatively, mechanical assistance may be required for several days or weeks until heart function improves or cardiac transplantation can be arranged. Either intra-aortic balloon augmentation or heparinless venoarterial bypass without oxygenation may be used as such a temporary assist device rather than a pump-oxygenator. Total left heart bypass without heparinization (extracorporeal or implanted) or the use of partial venoarterial bypass with a membrane oxygenator appears to provide the most promise in such situations requiring prolonged near-total assistance. Both intra-aortic balloon augmentation and athrombogenic venoarterial bypass without oxygenator appear to be practical techniques for prolonged partial assistance to the failing circulation. There is the possibility that mechanical assistance may one day be utilized to salvage ischemic myocardium not only in patients with established myocardial infarction and cardiogenic shock, but also in patients in the early stages of myocardial infarction to limit the extent of destroyed muscle.

While a totally implantable mechanical heart is not yet a reality, it is the author's belief that it will be in the next decade and that experience currently being gained with mechanical circulatory assistance for hours or days will contribute to the advances needed to solve the problems of a permanent artificial heart.

SELECTED REFERENCES

Clauss, R. H., Birtwell, W. C., Albertal, G., Lunzer, S., Taylor, W. J., Fosberg, A. M., and Harken, D. E.: Assisted circulation. I. The arterial counterpulsator. J. Thorac. Cardiovasc. Surg., 41:447, 1961.

This is the first paper to describe the technique of counterpulsation for mechanical assistance to the failing circulation. The technique has developed into the widely applied modality of intra-aortic balloon pumping.

Dennis, C., Carlens, E., Senning, A., Hall, D. P., Moreno, J. R., Capelletti, R. R., and Wesolowski, S. A.: Clinical use of a cannula for left heart bypass without thoracotomy. Ann. Surg., 156:623, 1962.
This paper describes an ingenious method of performing left heart bypass with a closed chest. A cannula is introduced through the jugular vein into the right atrium. It then pierces the atrial septum to enter the left atrium. Blood removed from the left atrium is pumped back to a peripheral artery.

Hill, J. D., Ratliff, J. L., Fallat, R. J., Tucker, H. J., Lamy, M., Dietrich, H., and Gerbode, F.: Prognostic factors in the treatment of acute respiratory insufficiency with long-term extracorporeal oxygenation. J. Thorac. Cardiovasc. Surg., 68:905, 1974.
This article reports 25 patients suffering from acute respiratory insufficiency, who were treated with extracorporeal membrane oxygenation when all other forms of conventional management had failed. With early recognition of favorable signs, ECMO offers the possibility of altering the course of acute respiratory insufficiency. In these patients, the reversal of pulmonary pathology was dramatic and beneficial.

Kolff, W. J., and Lawson, J.: Status of the artificial heart and cardiac assist devices in the United States. Trans. Am. Soc. Artif. Intern. Organs, 21:620, 1975.
Summary of present status of partial and total artificial heart development and the problems involved.

Mundth, E. D., Yurchak, P. M., Buckley, M. J., Leinbach, R. C., Kantrowitz, A., and Austen, W. G.: Circulatory assistance and emergency direct coronary-artery surgery for shock complicating acute myocardial infarction. N. Engl. J. Med., 283:1382, 1970.
This paper describes the successful use of intra-aortic balloon pumping to sustain the failing circulation while coronary arteriography and subsequently emergency coronary artery bypass surgery were performed in a patient suffering from an acute myocardial infarction and cardiogenic shock.

Wakabayashi, A., Connolly, J. E., Stemmer, E. A., and Nakamura, Y.: Clinical experience with heparinless venoarterial bypass without oxygenation for the treatment of acute cardiogenic shock. J. Thorac. Cardiovasc. Surg., 68:687, 1974.
This paper reports the successful clinical application of heparinless venoarterial bypass without oxygenation in six patients for the treatment of cardiogenic shock following acute myocardial infarction, open-heart surgery, and prophylactic circulatory support during the induction of anesthesia.

REFERENCES

1. Anstadt, G. L., Blakemore, W., and Baue, A.: A new instrument for prolonged mechanical cardiac massage. Circulation (Suppl.), 32:43, 1965.
2. Arntzenius, A. C.: Discussion of Ware, R. W., et al.: Inertial cardiac assistance. Trans. Am. Soc. Artif. Intern. Organs, 17:219, 1971.
3. Bacaner, M.: Human heart failure and shock treated by means of a mechanical veno-arterial bypass without oxygenation. Ann. Intern. Med., 55:837, 1961.
4. Bartlett, R. H., Gazzaniga, A. B., Fong, S. W., and Burns, N. E.: Prolonged extracorporeal cardiopulmonary support in man. J. Thorac. Cardiovasc. Surg., 68:918, 1974.
5. Bernhard, W. F., LaFarge, C. G., Husain, M., Yamamura, N., and Robinson, T. C.: Physiologic observations during partial and total left heart bypass. J. Thorac. Cardiovasc. Surg., 60:807, 1970.
6. Birtwell, W. C., Giron, F., Ruiz, U., Norton, R. L., and Soroff, H. S.: The regional hemodynamic response to synchronous external pressure assist. Trans. Am. Soc. Artif. Intern. Organs, 16:462, 1970.
7. Bramson, M. L., Osborn, J. J., Main, F. B., O'Brien, M. F., Wright, J. S., and Gerbode, F.: A new disposable membrane oxygenator with integral heat exchange. J. Thorac. Cardiovasc. Surg., 50:391, 1965.
8. Bregman, D., Goetz, R. H., and State, D.: Clinical experience with a new cardiac assist device: The dual-chambered intra-aortic balloon assist. J. Thorac. Cardiovasc. Surg., 62:577, 1971.
9. Buckley, M. J., Leinbach, R. C., Kastor, J. A., Laird, J. D., Phil, D., Kantrowitz, A. R., Madras, P. N., Sanders, C. A., and Austen, G. W.: Hemodynamic evaluation of intra-aortic balloon pumping in man. Circulation (Suppl. 2), 41:130, 1970.
10. Chapple, J. C., and Connolly, J. E.: Efficacy of left heart bypass in the treatment of acute heart failure. Surg. Forum, 15:262, 1964.
11. Clowes, G. H., and Neville, W. E.: Further development of a blood oxygenator dependent upon the diffusion of gases through plastic membranes. Trans. Am. Soc. Artif. Intern. Organs, 3:52, 1957.
12. Cohen, L. S.: Current status of circulatory assist devices. Am. J. Cardiol., 33:316, 1974.
13. Connolly, J. E., Bacaner, M. B., Bruns, D. L., Lowenstein, J. M., and Storli, E.: Mechanical support of the circulation in acute heart failure. Surgery, 44:255, 1958.
14. Connolly, J. E., Bacaner, M. B., Bruns, D. L., Lowenstein, J. M., and Storli, E.: The effect of venoarterial bypass on coronary blood flow. Arch. Surg., 81:58, 1960.
15. Connolly, J. E., Kountz, S. L., and Boyd, R. J.: Left heart bypass: Experimental and clinical observations on its regulation with particular reference to maintenance of maximal renal blood flow. J. Thorac. Cardiovasc. Surg., 44:577, 1962.
16. DeBakey, M. E.: Left ventricular bypass pump for cardiac assistance. Clinical experience. Am. J. Cardiol., 27:3, 1971.
17. Dennis, C., Carlens, E., Senning, A., Hall, D. P., Moreno, J. R., Cappelletti, R. R., and Wesolowski, S. A.: Clinical use of a cannula for left heart bypass without thoracotomy. Ann. Surg., 156:623, 1962.
18. Dobell, A. R. C., Mitri, M., Galva, R., Sarkosy, M., and Murphy, D. R.: Biologic evaluation of blood after prolonged recirculation through film and membrane oxygenators. Ann. Surg., 161:617, 1965.
19. Dunkman, W. B., Leinbach, R. C., Buckley, M. J., et al.: Clinical and hemodynamic results of intra-aortic balloon pumping and surgery for cardiogenic shock. Circulation, 46:465, 1972.
20. German, J. C., Chalmers, G. S., Hirai, J., Mukherjee, N. D., Wakabayashi, A., and Connolly, J. E.: Comparison of nonpulsatile and pulsatile extracorporeal circulation on renal tissue perfusion. Chest, 61:65, 1972.
21. Gott, V. L., Whiffen, J. D., Koepke, D. E., Daggett, R. L., Boake, W. C., and Young, W. P.: Techniques of applying a graphite-benzalkonium-heparin coating to various plastics and metals. Trans. Am. Soc. Artif. Intern. Organs, 10:213, 1964.
22. Harkins, G., and Bramson, M. L.: Mechanical external cardiac massage for cardiac arrest and for support of the failing heart. A preliminary communication. Surg. Res., 1:197, 1961.
23. Hill, J. D., Bramson, M. L., Osborne, J. J., and Gerbode, F.: Observations and management during clinical venovenous bypass for respiratory insufficiency. Adv. Cardiol., 6:133, 1971.
24. Hill, J. D., and O'Brien, T. G.: Personal communication.
25. Kolobow, T., and Zapol, W. M.: Partial and total extracorporeal respiratory gas exchange with the spiral membrane lung. Adv. Cardiol., 6:112, 1971.
26. Kouwenhoven, W. B., Jude, J. R., and Knickerbocker, G. G.: Closed-chest cardiac massage. J.A.M.A., 173:1064, 1960.
27. Kwan-Gett, C., Backman, D. K., Donovan, F. M., Jr., Eastwood, N., Foote, J. L., Kawai, J., Kessler, T. R., Kralios, A. C., Peters, J. L., Van Kampen, K. R., Wong, H. K., Zwart, H. H. J., and Kolff, W. J.: Artificial heart with hemispherical ventricles II and disseminated intravascular coagulation. Trans. Am. Soc. Artif. Intern. Organs, 17:474, 1971.
28. Landé, A. J., Edwards, L., Bloch, J. H., Carlson, R. G., Subramanian, V. A., Ascheim, R. S., Scheidt, S., Fillmore, S., Killip, T., and Lillehei, C. W.: Clinical experience with emergency use of prolonged cardiopulmonary bypass with a membrane pump-oxygenator. Ann. Thorac. Surg., 10:409, 1970.
29. Lee, W. H., Jr., Krumhaar, D., Fonkalsrud, E. W., Schjeide, O. A., and Maloney, J. V.: Denaturation of plasma proteins as a cause of morbidity and death after intracardiac operations. Surgery, 50:29, 1961.
30. Many, M., Giron, F., Birtwell, W. C., Deterling, R. A., and Soroff, H. S.: Effects of depulsation of renal blood flow upon renal function and renin secretion. Surgery, 66:242, 1969.
31. Mundth, E. D., Yurchak, P. M., Buckley, M. J., Leinbach, R. C., Kantrowitz, A., and Austen, W. G.: Circulatory assistance and emergency direct coronary-artery surgery for shock complicating acute myocardial infarction. N. Engl. J. Med., 283:1382, 1970.
32. Nosé, Y., Tajima, K., Imai, Y., Klain, M., Mrava, G., Schriber, K.,

Urbanek, K., and Ogawa, H.: Artificial heart constructed with biological material. Trans. Am. Soc. Artif. Intern. Organs, *17*:482, 1971.

33. Osborn, J. J., Russi, M., Salel, A., Bramson, M. L., and Gerbode, F.: Diastolic augmentation by external pulsed pressure. Fifteenth Conference on Engineering in Medicine and Biology. Chicago, November 4, 1962.

34. Peirce, E. C., II: A comparison of the Landé-Edwards, the Peirce, and the General Electric-Peirce membrane lungs. Trans. Am. Soc. Artif. Intern. Organs, *16*:358, 1970.

35. Pierce, W. S., Brighton, J. A., O'Bannon, W., Donachy, J. H., Phillips, W. M., Landis, D. L., White, W. J., and Waldhausen, J. A.: Complete left ventricular bypass with a paracorporeal pump. Ann. Surg., *180*:418, 1974.

36. Salisbury, P. F., Bor, N., Lewin, R. J., and Rieben, P. A.: Effects of partial and total heart-lung bypass on the heart. J. Appl. Physiol., *14*:458, 1959.

37. Salisbury, P., Cross, C. E., Rieben, P. A., and Lewin, R. J.: Comparison of two types of mechanical assistance in experimental heart failure. Circ. Res., *8*:431, 1960.

38. Sarnoff, S. J., Braunwald, E., Welch, G. H., Jr., Case, R. D., Stamsby, W. N., and Cruz, R.: Hemodynamic determinants of oxygen consumption of the heart with special reference to the time tension index. Am. J. Physiol., *192*:148, 1958.

39. Takano, H., Takagi, H., Turner, M. D., Henson, E. C., Crowell, J. W., and Akutsu, T.: Problems in total artificial heart. Trans. Am. Soc. Artif. Intern. Organs, *17*:449, 1971.

40. Trinkle, J. K., Helton, N. E., Bryant, L. R., and Griffen, W. O.: Pulsatile cardiopulmonary bypass: Clinical evaluation. Surgery, *68*:1074, 1970.

41. Wakabayashi, A., Dietrick, W., and Connolly, J. E.: Closed-chest left heart bypass without anticoagulation. J. Thorac. Cardiovasc. Surg., *58*:811, 1969.

42. Wakabayashi, A., Yim, D., Dietrick, W., Hirai, J., and Connolly, J. E.: Left heart bypass: A new nonthrombogenic device with homograft aortic valves. Am. J. Cardiol., *25*:540, 1970.

43. Wakabayashi, A., Connolly, J. E., Stemmer, E. A., and Nakamura, Y.: Clinical experience with heparinless venoarterial bypass without oxygenation for the treatment of acute cardiogenic shock. J. Thorac. Cardiovasc. Surg., *68*:687, 1974.

44. Wakabayashi, A., Connolly, J. E., Stemmer, E. A., Nakamura, Y., Kubo, T., and Ino, T.: Heparinless left heart bypass for resection of thoracic aortic aneurysms. Am. J. Surg., *130*:212, 1975.

45. Wakabayashi, A., Nakamura, Y., Woolley, T., Chen, C., Mullin, P. J. and Connolly, J. E. Successful prolonged heparinless venoarterial bypass in sheep. J. Thorac. Cardiovasc. Surg., *71*:648, 1976.

46. Zwart, H. H. J., Kralios, A. C., Kwan-Gett, C. S., Backman, D. K., Foote, J. L., Andrade, J. D., and Kolff, W. J.: Transarterial closed-chest left ventricular bypass for desperate heart failure. Adv. Cardiol., *6*:157, 1971.

59

THE RATIONALE AND SCIENTIFIC BASIS OF CURRENT EXAMINATIONS IN SURGERY

Arthur E. Baue, M.D.

The importance of examinations in the evaluation of an individual's capabilities in surgery make it appropriate that a textbook of surgery now include within its pages a discussion of the present state of the art and science of this process. Abraham Flexner emphasized that "professions are, as a matter of history — and very rightly — learned professions; there are no unlearned professions. Unlearned professions — a contradiction in terms — would be vocations, callings, or occupations."[5] Surgery, as a learned profession entrusted with the care of the sick, must be able to demonstrate that it is indeed learned, that it maintains the highest standards, and that it provides the best care possible for its patients. Care of the sick was once considered a sacred task. Now, society is requiring more rigorous review of those who are given the privilege of caring for the sick. Standards for professional care in surgery are being established and must be maintained and improved. Students of surgery in the mid-twentieth century are familiar with the series of evaluations which they must complete in order to be entrusted with these professional responsibilities. The MCAT, the NBE, FLEX, ECFMG, in-training examination, ABS, SESAP, and recertification examinations are examples of hurdles which must be overcome to demonstrate continued professional growth and development. The Medical College Admissions Test (MCAT) must be satisfactorily completed before entering medical school. The National Board Examination (NBE), or state board examinations, or FLEX examination must be satisfactorily completed for licensure. A foreign medical graduate must complete the ECFMG examination before entry into the graduate educational system of this country. An in-training examination has been developed for general surgical residents by the American Board of Surgery. Other surgical specialties also utilize this method to evaluate progress in graduate educational experience for a resident and to provide information about the educational program for the teaching staff.

The certifying examinations of the various specialty boards have been accepted as a standard of performance to be completed before beginning a career in an area. The recognition that a surgeon must continue educational endeavors throughout the career, as science and technology advance, has led to the development of a number of measuring devices which provide the opportunity for an individual in practice to assess capabilities. This is exemplified by the SESAP (Surgical Education and Self-Assessment Program) examinations prepared by the American College of Surgeons. Recently the need for some type of recertifying process has been recognized. A surgeon who has practiced a specialty for a period of years after completing the initial certifying process should be able to demonstrate, by some objective means, continued capability and competence.

The kinds of evaluations that are available to achieve the goal of providing excellent, safe surgeons and excellent, safe surgical care are (1) written examinations with multiple-choice questions and patient management problems using erasure techniques; (2) oral examinations; (3) careful observation of performance during the residency period; and (4) documentation of excellence in patient care during the surgeon's professional career.

The written examinations provide an objective evaluation of a number of characteristics required of a surgeon. These characteristics include a knowledge of the field and the ability to solve problems related to surgery. The oral examination is used to evaluate *clinical judgment* and to determine if it is *safe* and reasonable for the young surgeon to work independently in the care of the patients. Although the final certifying process is provided by a specialty board, it is the training program which must recommend the candidate for the certifying process. It is still necessary and even critical that the staff and program director of the teaching hospital testify from direct observation that the surgeon completing training has the maturity, judgment, morality, technical capability, and stamina to provide excellent patient care independently and without further supervision. Conscientious fulfillment of this responsibility must be a major consideration in determining which individuals and which hospitals should be responsible for educating surgeons. The final criterion must be the resultant product—the level of patient care provided. Methods to document that a surgeon is providing good care are being developed and must be utilized. Some of the early attempts to document the levels of patient care, such as through practice audits or by Professional Standards Review Organization (PSRO), have stressed length of hospitalization, laboratory studies, and other factors. The important measurements for an audit of surgical practice include: (1) Was an operation indicated, and if so, was the appropriate procedure done at the right time? (2) If an operation was not performed, should it have been? (3) What was the morbidity and mortality? and (4) What was the final outcome?

Historical Background

Just as the implementation of the Flexner report revolutionized and improved medical education, so the development of formal residency programs from previous informal preceptorships and apprenticeships has provided excellent surgical capability throughout the country. The first specialty board, the American Board of Ophthalmology, was founded in 1917. This board established requirements for training, required evidence of experience in the field, and developed an examination. Other specialties soon developed boards and their specific requirements for certification. The American Board of Surgery was organized in 1937 through the leadership of a committee of the American Surgical Assocation.

The development of present examinations in surgery can be seen in the evolution of the examination process of the National Board of Medical Examiners. The National Board was founded in 1915 with a single objective: "To provide examinations of high quality" for licensure in the several states. Through the years, the National Board has served as the epicenter for study and development of methods to measure clinical capability of physicians. Up until about 1950, all written examinations were of the essay type. The National Board examination consisted then of three parts: Part I (basic medical sciences), Part II (clinical sciences), and Part III (oral "practical" examination after the internship).

Meanwhile, the science of educational measurement was being developed and multiple-choice testing methods progressively came of age. These methods were called objective examinations because the answers could be scored as correct or incorrect by an impartial observer or machine. The American Board of Internal Medicine first introduced multiple-choice testing techniques into their board-certifying process and changed their examination from the previous essay test. Dr. Cecil Watson, the Chairman of the Board of Internal Medicine at that time, said, "I am satisfied that these examinations are superior to the essay type. They have permitted a much broader sampling of the candidate's general knowledge and the basic sciences pertaining thereto.... It has been argued that the multiple-choice examination does not probe the candidate's ability to reason as well as the essay type. This depends largely on the character of the questions, which may be devised to test nothing more than factual knowledge or experience, or to provide a situation which requires considerable analysis or reasoning."[9] This initial experience in medical testing led to a study of this type of approach by the National Board of Medical Examiners. As described by Dr. John Hubbard, "A study was undertaken with the cooperation of the Educational Testing Service to determine the applicability of multiple-choice testing methods to the field of medicine. After three years of deliberate, carefully designed experimentation, convincing evidence supported the conclusion that multiple-choice methods were superior to the time-honored essay methods for the purposes of the Board."[4, 6] The National Board of Medical Examiners then converted Parts I and II of their examination to the multiple-choice format. Subsequently, the specialty boards began to use this format for their written examinations. The National Board and the specialty boards, however, continued, as a predominant custom, a combination of a written and oral or practical examination. The written examination usually served as a screening procedure which the candidate was required to pass before being admitted to the oral examination.

For some years the National Board continued the Part III, or oral, examination as an oral bedside evaluation. The candidate completed a history and physical examination of an assigned patient, and was then questioned about the patient's diagnosis and the disease process. The Board found three variables in this process—the examiner, the patient, and the candidate—whereas the measurement of critical interest was the ability of the candidate. Therefore, in 1959 the National Board undertook a study to try to define clinical competence, which its Part III examination was intended to measure, and to develop testing methods which would permit a more objective, valid, and reliable assessment of such clinical competence. A two-year study was initiated in cooperation with the American Institute of Research, which had successfully developed objective methods for measuring the critical skills of airplane pilots. From this study came a new and different testing method which was called "Programmed Testing of Patient Management Problems," and more recently has simply been called the "PMP format." The candidate being evaluated is provided with a clinical situation and then is asked to solve the clinical problem by seeking more information from the history or physical examination or from the laboratory, and to accomplish a proper course of management for this patient. This type of evaluation was first used by the National Board in 1961 and has since been used by many of the specialty boards as part of their written examination.

Rationale

The purposes of examinations in surgery are fourfold: (1) to document clinical competence, (2) to serve as a guide to learning, (3) to guide continuing education, and (4) to recertify or demonstrate continuing competence.

A number of characteristics important for surgeons can be measured by objective means, and may generally be divided into two areas. One area is cognitive knowledge, the breadth of information which an individual has about a particular field of endeavor. This is important to measure, because no one can be an excellent practitioner without a basic fund of knowledge in his discipline which can be utilized on a moment's notice for the benefit of the patient. The fact that an individual is knowledgeable about the field of surgery does not, however, provide complete assurance that one is *clinically* capable. Secondly, problem-solving ability can certainly be measured by an objective examination. This is a necessary requirement for excellent patient care.

Test Preparation and Types of Questions

In preparing written or objective examinations, the committee method has been preferred by the specialty boards and by the National Board of Medical Examiners. This type of examination is developed by a committee composed of eight to ten specialists in the subject matter to be tested and several experts in test development. The criteria for selection of subject matter specialists to serve on such a committee are that they (a) be experts in their field, (b) be interested in participating in this type of educational and evaluating activity, and (c) have the willingness to subject themselves to the rigorous and exacting task of test preparation. Initially, such a committee must decide upon the purpose of the examination and what will be evaluated. From this initial plan, an outline or grid of material to be covered is prepared in which various categories or subjects are listed. This is necessary to ensure comprehensive coverage of the field or area, and to provide proper weighting for particularly important areas of subject matter. Following this, individual questions are written by each member of the committee according to the type of format decided upon. These are collated and prepared as a test draft and reviewed by each member of the committee, which then meets for several days in conference to review each question. Questions are approved, revised, or discarded. The important characteristics of an appropriate item or question are that it be accurate, concise, appropriate in content and difficulty for this particular examination, free from ambiguity, and representative of an important aspect of the subject. While an individual may feel competent as an expert in writing test material, it is the usual experience of everyone serving on such committees that what is unambiguous and appropriate to one expert may be confusing and too difficult to another expert in the same field. Thus, committee review is necessary to be certain that each question in the final draft of the test has been thoroughly evaluated and is as free of flaws as possible.

It has been customary in multiple-choice examinations to call a question an *item* and the format of a question an *item-type*, because a question may be in the form of a statement to be completed, rather than a query. The most common item-type used in multiple-choice examinations is the *one-best-response* format. This item-type consists of a stem, which is a statement or question, followed by four or five suggested answers or completions. One of the suggested answers is correct, and the other four are called distracters. Thus, the best or most appropriate choice of those given is correct. Such an item-type may be posed as a positive statement, such as:

A 32-year-old woman with recurrent hemoptysis and a 3 × 3 cm. mass in the hilum of the right lung, visible by chest x-ray, probably has:
1. tuberculosis
2. a squamous cell carcinoma of the lung
*3. a bronchial adenoma
4. an alveolar cell carcinoma
5. sarcoidosis

The asterisk indicates the correct response. This item-type may also be presented as a negative, using the word "except." Example:

All of the following are complications of regional enteritis (Crohn's disease) except:
1. obstruction
2. bleeding
3. perforation
4. fistula formation
*5. intussusception

These item-types may also be used with a case history as the stem. A patient and his problem are described, followed by three to five items which ask about the diagnosis, about therapy, or about other studies which might be carried out. Thus, following the previous stem about the 32-year-old woman, additional items could be included about diagnostic studies to be carried out and the treatment of this problem.

Another example of the multiple-choice item-type is the matching type, an example of which is:

Responses
A. left ventricular hypertrophy
B. cyanosis of the lower part of the body
C. notching of the ribs
D. right ventricular hypertrophy
E. clubbing of the fingers
Item Number
1. coarctation of the aorta (C)
2. mitral stenosis (D)
3. tetralogy of Fallot (E)
4. patent ductus arteriosis with reversal of shunt (B)
5. aortic stenosis (A)

The other type of multiple-choice item is the multiple true-false item. An example of this is:

Characteristics of early septic shock include:
1. increased cardiac output
2. decreased arteriovenous oxygen difference
3. decreased peripheral vascular resistance
4. hyperventilation
Select one:
A. 1, 2, 3 are correct
B. 1, 3 are correct
C. 2, 4 are correct
D. 4 only is correct
*E. all are correct

Another type of multiple true-false item is as follows:

Common complications of intravenous hyperalimentation are:
1. infection of the catheter (T)
2. hyperosmolality (T)
3. hyperphosphatemia (F)
4. inadequate caloric supply (T)
5. ketosis (F)

With these various item-types, pictorial, tabulated, or graphic material may be presented. The candidate is asked to interpret a photograph of a microscopic section of a surgical specimen, a photograph of a gross specimen, a chest x-ray or angiogram, or other types of pictorial material.

It is recognized that the standard multiple-choice items evaluate primarily cognitive knowledge—Can a candidate pick, from a list of possibilities, a correct response to a statement or question about a field? The use of pictorial or graphic material introduces another concept of evaluation, the ability to interpret a specimen, a set of laboratory values, or an x-ray.

In writing such items, a number of flaws or pitfalls may be introduced. Irrelevant clues to the correct response may be provided so that the candidate can answer the item correctly without having the appropriate knowledge which is sought. The correct response determined by the committee may not necessarily be the response utilized by all surgeons throughout the country. There may be honest disagreement about what is correct in that situation. There are situations where several approaches could be used but only one is listed. A candidate who would prefer another approach does not find it among the choices, and therefore must base his decision upon what is given. There are few absolutes in human biology, so that items which include *always* or *never* produce difficulty. It is easier to write an item which performs well about the unusual (bronchial adenoma) and more difficult to construct a test item about the commonplace (appendicitis).

The other examination format which is used by the National Board and many specialty boards at present is that called Programmed Testing of Patient Management Problems.[7] This testing method was introduced by the National Board in 1961 to test aspects of clinical competence that dealt with the ability to identify, to resolve, and to manage patient problems. This method simulates a clinical situation in which the candidate is presented a patient with an illness or injury. Limited information is provided in the case history or stem. Following this information, the candidate is asked what he would do next and is given a number of choices which may include further laboratory studies, other diagnostic procedures, therapeutic approaches, or further inquiries about history or past medical illness. The candidate is not told how many to select, but selects those which he feels are appropriate to a particular clinic situation. He is provided with a series of ink blocks in an answer book. He erases the blocks selected and beneath the block finds further information. This may reveal a value for a laboratory test, the findings of a diagnostic x-ray procedure, or the results of a therapeutic intervention. The information may lead him to make other choices in the same set. Following completion of one series of courses of action, he is given further information about the patient or a later time course in this patient's illness. There follows another list of courses of actions from which to select. Thus the candidate works his way through a patient's problem and may arrive eventually at a resolution of the problem or a correct diagnosis.

Example

A 29-year-old man strikes a bridge abutment while driving his car at a high rate of speed. On arrival at the emergency ward, he is semiconscious and has a dusky color. There are multiple lacerations about his face and neck. His respirations are 36/minute and shallow. Pulse is 130/minute and arterial blood pressure 80/60 mm. Hg. His right arm is deformed. There is a contusion of the anterior chest and this portion of his chest moves inward during inspiration. You would now:

Scoring	Item	Response Under Erasure Block
+1	Obtain a blood sample for typing and cross-matching	Obtained
+1	Insert endotracheal tube	Blood in larynx, tube doesn't pass
+1	Perform tracheostomy	Done
−1	Begin infusion of type specific uncross-matched blood	Done
−1	Determine passive range of motion of neck and all extremities	Patient becomes quadriplegic
−1	Begin assisted ventilation with 100% O_2	Done
+1	Obtain portable chest x-ray	Widened mediastinum, fluid in left pleural space
+1	Perform left tube thoracostomy	80 ml. blood removed
0	Obtain BUN determination	18 mg %

Scoring of patient management problems gives credit for correct decisions and a penalty for selecting inappropriate choices or omissions. Thus each course of action is classified as either (1) necessary for this patient, (2) should not be done because it may be harmful or is not needed, or (3) relatively unimportant and may or may not be done, depending upon local custom or conditions. In this third area the courses of action are scored as zero, whereas others are +1 or −1.

Analysis of Items and Scoring

In test development and review of performance, it is important to determine the accuracy of the measuring instrument. This can be done in three ways by statistical evaluation. The three areas of initial interest are the degree of difficulty of the examination, an index of discrimination or the extent to which the examination is successful in discriminating between the more knowledgeable and less knowledgeable candidates, and the relevance of the examination to the educational objectives or evaluation objectives of the examination. The difficulty of each item in an examination and for the total examination can be calculated and is called the P value. This is simply the per cent of candidates who have answered this item correctly. Thus a P value of 0.95 indicates that 95 per cent of the candidates answered this particular item correctly. From each individual item value, the degree of difficulty of the entire examination can be calculated. If an individual item or the entire examination has a very high P value (above 0.90), it contributes very little to evaluation because it does not discriminate between candidates. If, however, the P value is extremely low, the item may be too difficult or may be defective in construction. If the P value approaches 0.25 or 0.2, it suggests that the candidates are guessing without specific knowledge or understanding of that item. In examinations such as those for certification by a board, a satisfactory item should have a P value somewhere between 0.6 and 0.85.

If an objective of an examination is to discriminate between knowledgeable candidates and those with less than adequate knowledge of the field, the information about the ability of the various items to provide this discrimination is needed. This information can be provided by calculating the biserial correlation coefficient. This is done by calculating the relationship between how a number of individuals performed on a particular item and their total score for that portion of the test. The simple way to calculate this discrimination index is to select a random sample of candidates and obtain a frequency distribution of their scores. Those individuals whose scores fall in the upper 25 per cent or so of this distribution form a high group and those who fall in the lower 25 per cent or so form a low group and are used to determine how each group (high and low) performed on a particular item. A value is calculated for each item called an R value, or biserial R (r_{bis}). If all of the top candidates responded correctly to a particular item, and none of the bottom 25 per cent of candidates responded correctly, the r_{bis} would be 1.00. Obviously, no item performs in such a perfect way. If equal numbers of both groups responded correctly, the r_{bis} would be zero, indicating complete lack of discrimination. In the experience of test developers, an r_{bis} of 0.25 to 0.50 is quite satisfactory, indicating good discrimination.

The final area of evaluation, the relevance of test items to the real world of surgical competence, is more difficult to express in numerical terms. This requires an effort to correlate performance on the examinations with performance as a surgeon. Although this is never an exact determination, each group that develops such examinations must be sure the examination developed has been subjected to this scrutiny. Several approaches to validation may be used. Face or content validity means that the material tested is drawn from the real world of surgical care. The review of experts who prepare the test can best ascertain this. Predictive validity is harder to determine. This means that good performance on the test would predict good performance in practice. This, at present, cannot be measured.

Item analysis then consists of determining the P value or degree of difficulty, the r_{bis} or discrimination index, and a write-out of how high and low candidates answered each item, and particularly which of the various distracters were selected. An item which performs well is one which has a P value of 0.6 to 0.85 (fairly easy) and an r_{bis} of 0.4 to 0.5 (discriminates well).

Scoring of such an examination can be done rapidly with high-speed scoring equipment and computer hardware with the predetermined correct or incorrect responses. Since it is impossible for an examination committee to determine with complete accuracy how new test items will perform, it is possible that there will be flaws in various items. To eliminate such flaws it would be best to pretest such items. Since this is impossible, another approach is used which accomplishes this purpose and is called key validation. As the examination is being scored, a sample of candidates is selected and full item analyses of all their responses are obtained. This will indicate whether or not an item performed satisfactorily. If an item performed poorly with an extremely low P value and/or a negative discrimination index (r_{bis}), this item can be eliminated by the committee before the final scoring of the test is done.

After the final scores of all candidates are available, a decision must be made about who will pass and who will fail. The major purpose of any test of competence must be to distinguish between those individuals who have met some standard of achievement or excellence or knowledge or capability, and those who have not. The choice that must be made is between setting an absolute standard of capability and adopting a relative standard. An absolute standard for certification of physicians would seem in many ways to be preferable. One would like to believe that there is a minimal amount of knowledge and problem-solving ability which a candidate must have in order to pass this hurdle. Setting an absolute standard would be the determination that a percentage such as 75 per cent of the questions must be answered correctly for the candidate to pass. However, the use of an absolute standard for examination performance is a very difficult task. It requires that examination committees be able to determine fairly precisely what material a candidate should know in order to pass and examine him on that material in a clear, understandable way. This is hard to achieve. Some committees have tried to use certain key questions as critically important items that must be answered correctly to pass the examination. They have usually found that such an approach would yield an unacceptably high failure rate. Is this a fault of the committee, the candidate, the training program, or the item? Perhaps all are less than perfect.

Studies by the National Board of Medical Examiners[8] have indicated that absolute standards would have led to great variations in the pass-fail rate. Therefore, the National Board of Medical Examiners has decided that a relative standard is best. The examination is graded on a curve, with the failure rate established at a certain cut-off point. This course of action requires that a certain number of candidates fail the examination at any particular time. The arguments for and against these several approaches are beyond the scope of this presentation but have been thoroughly reviewed.[2]

Two other evaluations of a test are necessary: measurements of the *validity* and *reliability* of the examination. By validity is meant how well a scale or item or examination measures what it is intended to measure. The ultimate criterion for the validity of a board examination, for example, would be how the performance of a candidate in practice compares with his test score. Performance in practice, however, is far more complex and difficult to measure at the present time than are our capabilities of measurement. Thus, the ultimate criterion for validation of tests of competence for a physician is not available.[8] There are several intermediate criteria, however, which can be used as follows: (1) Does a specialty board examination or the National Board Examination measure what is being taught in the educational system? This seems to be true for present examinations. (2) Medical school grades can be compared with performance on the National Board Examination, and these seem to correlate fairly well. For specialty board examinations, performance of a candidate during residency as judged by his mentors can be compared with performance on the board examination. When this has been done, the correlation seems to be positive and fairly good. (3) Performance on an examination by several groups at different educational levels can be compared. In a study by the National Board of Medical Examiners, the Part III examination was given to third-year medical students and the results compared with those of a group completing an internship. The performance by those completing an internship was clearly superior to that of third-year students. This same comparison has been made at different levels of residency training.[1]

Another measure of an examination is its reliability. Does the examination instrument provide a measurement which is reproducible over time? If the same examination could be given again to the same group of candidates without their having learned anything from the prior administration, would their scores be the same? This cannot be done, but reliability can be measured by statistical means. Reliability means reproducibility but does not indicate that an examination is measuring that which it is designed to measure. Reliability of an examination may be determined by a procedure called the "split-half" technique. The examination can be divided into two parts so that odd-numbered questions are assigned to one half and even-numbered questions assigned to the other half. Scores are then obtained for each half of the test, and a correlation coefficient between the half tests is calculated. This approach has drawbacks, however, because splitting a test is always arbitrary. More satisfactory statistical measurements can be used in which each individual question serves as a subtest. One such method which is used by the National Board of Medical Examiners is called the Kuder-Richardson Formula 20. Reliability of an examination by such a calculation should have a coefficient of 0.9 or higher in order to distinguish adequately between individual candidates for certification. Thus, a high degree of reliability is necessary for a good examination, but it alone is not sufficient because validity must also be considered.

The Oral Examination

The oral examination has been the mainstay of professional qualifying examinations going back as far as the twelfth century, when members of the faculty of the University of Salerno met with representatives of the Emperor to determine the capabilities of a candidate. There are many features of an oral examination that cannot be included in a written measurement. The ease of communication, direct observation of the attitudes and train of thought of a candidate, the opportunity for a candidate to clarify or justify his position, the yes or no decision-making process of the surgeon ("I would operate," or "I would not operate"), all are unique to this type of evaluation.

Demonstration of competence by surgeons will always require direct observation of various behavioral aspects of learning, including technical skill, clinical judgment, assumption of responsibility, etc. In the early days of medical evaluation, and when the number of candidates was small, the oral examination included also an observation of the candidate's work. A surgical specialty board would visit a candidate and observe his performance during an operation which he performed on a patient. According to John Hubbard, the early examinations of the National Board required a candidate to demonstrate his surgical skill by performing a gastroenterostomy on postmortem specimens from a dog. Water from a faucet was then introduced into the esophagus, and if the anastomosis did not leak, the candidate passed this portion of the examination. Practical examinations or evaluations in the operating room or laboratory ceased when the number of candidates increased. In 1963, the National Board of Medical Examiners discontinued the bedside or practical oral examination, in part because of the large number of candidates and in part because their studies indicated that such an evaluation was not very objective. Recently, the American Board of Internal Medicine was faced with very large numbers of candidates to be examined. They concluded that the oral examination for certification in general internal medicine would be discontinued and objective measures as performed by the National Board would be used in its place. Most of the specialty boards in surgery and related disciplines continue to use the oral examination and find it essential for certain specific reasons. These reasons are that the multiple-choice examinations and patient management problem examination, although providing objective evaluation of cognitive knowledge and problem-solving ability, do not provide all of the information needed to determine that a surgeon is competent in his specialty. Surgical judgment, the type of operative procedure to be performed, when it is to be done, diagnostic criteria to be used, the ability of the young surgeon to work his way through a complex problem, all require at the present time an evaluation by a team of experts in the field. There certainly are legitimate criticisms of the oral examination, and subjective factors enter into this type of evaluation. Some feel that the oral examination is unreliable and invalid and should be discarded. Language problems for foreign medical graduates, personality clashes, nervousness, stress, and other factors all introduce subjectivity. However, a surgeon must make decisions rapidly on occasion and in stressing situations. The expertise of the examiner, not only in his specialty but in oral evaluation techniques, is an important factor in improving the objectivity of this process.

The Future of Evaluation of Clinical Competence

Part of the present research effort of the National Board of Medical Examiners is to develop a computer-based system for evaluation of clinical competence. This is an ongoing effort which will, in the future, probably provide even more precise evaluation of the capability of a physician. Special features of this approach are that it more closely simulates a patient and a clinical setting than is possible in a paper-and-pencil test. The candidate must initiate his own requests for information and develop his own decisions. The cues which are provided in a multiple-choice test are eliminated. It is one thing to select the best choice among five laboratory studies. It is another to ask for a specific, required laboratory study in a clinical setting. A primary problem in clinical judgment is to remember to consider all the diagnostic possibilities in a particular patient. If they are provided in a list in the examination, this departs from clinical reality where the surgeon must develop his own list. The candidate cannot look ahead to see what has happened later to the patient in a developing problem. The sequence of the candidate's decisions can be followed. Thus, a candidate would request data from the computer about a patient, and then could act upon that data and proceed further. At present, further research and development are needed to establish the reliability and validity of such an instrument, following which the logistics of hardware and software required for such an approach must be developed. It seems likely, however, in the future that more accurate evaluation can be done in this way. Whether this approach will eventually eliminate the need for oral examinations remains to be seen.

Summary

The *ideal* examination being sought is an exact, objective, fair, and easily administered instrument for evaluation of clinical competence. To say that such a goal is difficult to achieve is indeed an understatement. However, surgeons are known for their candor and honest assessment of capabilities and limitations. From this can only come good, as we work toward this goal. Our present evaluations may be disconcerting to those who think that human performance can be measured in exact terms.

Crawford Campbell, in his presidential address to the American Association for the Surgery of Trauma, stated, "There has been no written or oral examination or credentialing process so far that is known clearly to evaluate competency in surgery. Many problems related to attitude, judgment and technique do not lend themselves easily to ordinary examination techniques."[3] All realize that objective examinations cannot and will not measure various characteristics of human performance which are critical for the care of the sick. Honesty and integrity, decency and humaneness, industry and determination, kindness and consideration, persistence in adversity, and other characteristics required for excellent surgical care can be measured only by observation, by study of the health care provided, and by the results obtained, which in themselves introduce subjective evaluation. All recognize that observations on the battlefield or in the operating room or in the surgical intensive care unit introduce all of the subjective elements possible. Such observations must still be the mainstay in determining whether the surgeon, be he student or resident or practitioner, is capable of pursuing his appointed specialty. Such observations require an awesome responsibility on the part of those entrusted with leadership roles in the surgical community. It is the program director and associated colleagues who have observed the student of surgery and resident in the formative years of increasing responsibility and technical experience to the point of demonstrating independent capability. It is only the individual responsible for a program who can evaluate, on a day-to-day basis over the four to five years of a resident's experience, that he has indeed matured and developed the judgment, competence, and technical abilities to go out and care for patients independently. If a program director and teaching hospital staff feel that a resident is marginal, is not very good, or needs further training, they must make this decision. They are avoiding their responsibility if they recommend a candidate for examination by a surgical specialty board when they do not have complete confidence in that candidate. No examination will ever substitute for this detailed period of observation. An examination cannot determine that a surgeon will get out of bed in the middle of the night to evaluate a patient with abdominal pain or a postoperative complication. A written examination cannot evaluate whether or not a surgeon, in trying to extirpate a scarred and diseased gallbladder, will divide the common bile duct. A written and objective examination may have difficulty in determining whether a surgeon will recognize a patient with a ruptured aneurysm and take that patient immediately to the operating room for expeditious therapy.

Currently available examinations are necessary and extremely helpful in providing standards of capability. They can provide objective measurements of the adequate and the less-than-adequate. We must strive toward even better techniques of evaluation, as such instruments are used not only for the initial certifying process but also for continuing education and demonstration of continued competence as well. The final evaluation must always be the health and well-being of surgical patients.

REFERENCES

1. Baue, A. E., Saunders, R. H., Jr., Schumacher, C. F., Welch, J. S., and Hubbard, J. P.: In-training evaluation of surgical residents. J. Surg. Res., 8:341–344, 1968.
2. Cahn, S. M.: Philosophical reflections on evaluation. Am. J. Med., 57:152–156, 1974.
3. Campbell, C. J.: Continuing education for the trauma surgeon. J. Trauma, 14:97–101, 1974.
4. Cowles, J. T., and Hubbard, J. P.: Validity and reliability of the new objective tests. J. Med. Educ., 29:30, 1954.
5. Flexner, A.: Medical Education in the United States and Canada. New York, Carnegie Foundation for the Advancement of Teaching, 1910.
6. Hubbard, J. P.: Measuring Medical Education. Philadelphia, Lea & Febiger, 1971.
7. Hubbard, J. P., Levit, E. J., Schumacher, C. F., and Schnabel, T. G., Jr.: An objective evaluation of clinical competence. N. Engl. J. Med., 272:1321–1328, 1965.
8. Schumacher, C. F.: Scoring and analysis. In Hubbard, J. P.: Measuring Medical Education. Philadelphia, Lea & Febiger, 1971, pp. 51–65.
9. Watson, C. J.: Some activities and impacts of the American Board of Internal Medicine. J.A.M.A., 138:257, 1948.

NORMAL LABORATORY
VALUES

NORMAL LABORATORY VALUES

Prepared by REX B. CONN, M.D.,

NORMAL HEMATOLOGIC VALUES

Acid hemolysis test (Ham)	No hemolysis
Alkaline phosphatase, leukocyte	Total score 14–100
Bleeding time	
Ivy	Less than 5 min.
Duke	1–5 min.
Carboxyhemoglobin	Up to 5% of total
Cell counts	
Erythrocytes: Males	4.6–6.2 million/cu. mm.
Females	4.2–5.4 million/cu. mm.
Children (varies with age)	4.5–5.1 million/cu. mm.

Leukocytes			
Total		5000–10,000/cu. mm.	
Differential	*Percentage*	*Absolute*	
Myelocytes	0	0/cu. mm.	
Band neutrophils	3– 5	150– 400/cu. mm.	
Segmented neutrophils	54–62	3000–5800/cu. mm.	
Lymphocytes	25–33	1500–3000/cu. mm.	
Monocytes	3– 7	285– 500/cu. mm.	
Eosinophils	1– 3	50– 250/cu. mm.	
Basophils	0– 0.75	15– 50/cu. mm.	

(Infants and children have greater relative numbers of lymphocytes and monocytes)

Platelets	150,000–350,000/cu. mm.
Reticulocytes	25,000– 75,000/cu. mm.
	0.5–1.5% of erythrocytes
Clot retraction, qualitative	Begins in 30–60 min.
	Complete in 24 hrs.
Coagulation time (Lee-White)	5–15 min. (glass tubes)
	19–60 min. (siliconized tubes)
Cold hemolysin test (Donath-Landsteiner)	No hemolysis
Corpuscular values of erythrocytes	
(Values are for adults; in children, values vary with age)	
M.C.H. (mean corpuscular hemoglobin)	27–31 picogm.
M.C.V. (mean corpuscular volume)	80–105 cu. micra
M.C.H.C. (mean corpuscular hemoglobin concentration)	32–36%
Fibrinogen	200–400 mg./100 ml.
Fibrinolysins	0
Hematocrit	
Males	40–54 ml./100 ml.
Females	37–47 ml./100 ml.
Newborn	49–54 ml./100 ml.
Children (varies with age)	35–49 ml./100 ml.

Hemoglobin	
Males	14.0–18.0 grams/100 ml.
Females	12.0–16.0 grams/100 ml.
Newborn	16.5–19.5 grams/100 ml.
Children (varies with age)	11.2–16.5 grams/100 ml.
Hemoglobin, fetal	Less than 1% of total
Hemoglobin A_2	1.5–3.0% of total
Hemoglobin, plasma	0–5.0 mg./100 ml.
Methemoglobin	0.03–0.13 grams/100 ml.
Osmotic fragility of erythrocytes	Begins in 0.45–0.39% NaCl
	Complete in 0.33–0.30% NaCl
Activated partial thromboplastin time unactivated	35–45 sec.
	60–70 sec.
Prothrombin consumption	Over 80% consumed in 1 hr.
Prothrombin content	100% (calculated from prothrombin time)
Prothrombin time (one stage)	12.0–14.0 sec.
Sedimentation rate	
Wintrobe: Males	0–5 mm. in 1 hr.
Females	0–15 mm. in 1 hr.
Westergren: Males	0–15 mm. in 1 hr.
Females	0–20 mm. in 1 hr.
(May be slightly higher in children and during pregnancy)	
Thromboplastin generation test	Compared to normal control
Tourniquet test	Ten or fewer petechiae in a 2.5 cm. circle after 5 min. with cuff at 100 mm. Hg

Bone marrow, differential cell count	*Range*	*Average*
Myeloblasts	0.3– 5.0%	2.0%
Promyelocytes	1.0– 8.0%	5.0%
Myelocytes: Neutrophilic	5.0–19.0%	12.0%
Eosinophilic	0.5– 3.0%	1.5%
Basophilic	0.0– 0.5%	0.3%
Metamyelocytes	13.0–32.0%	22.0%
Polymorphonuclear neutrophils	7.0–30.0%	20.0%
Polymorphonuclear eosinophils	0.5– 4.0%	2.0%
Polymorphonuclear basophils	0.0– 0.7%	0.2%
Lymphocytes	3.0–17.0%	10.0%
Plasma cells	0.0– 2.0%	0.4%
Monocytes	0.5– 5.0%	2.0%
Reticulum cells	0.1– 2.0%	0.2%
Megakaryocytes	0.03– 3.0%	0.4%
Pronormoblasts	1.0– 8.0%	4.0%
Normoblasts	7.0–32.0%	18.0%

NORMAL BLOOD, PLASMA, AND SERUM VALUES

For some procedures the normal values may vary depending upon the methods used.

Acetone, serum	
Qualitative	Negative
Quantitative	0.3–2.0 mg./100 ml.
Aldolase, serum	0.8–3.0 mI.U./ml. (30°) (Sibley-Lehninger)
Amino acid nitrogen, serum	4–6 mg./100 ml.
Ammonia nitrogen, blood	75–196 mcg./100 ml.
plasma	56–122 mcg./100 ml.
Amylase, serum	80–160 Somogyi units/100 ml.
Ascorbic acid	See Vitamin C
Base, total, serum	145–160 mEq./liter
Bilirubin, serum	
Direct	0.1–0.4 mg./100 ml.
Indirect	0.2–0.7 mg./100 ml. (Total minus direct)
Total	0.3–1.1 mg./100 ml.
Calcium, serum	4.5–5.5 mEq./liter (9.0–11.0 mg./100 ml.) (Slightly higher in children) (Varies with protein concentration)
Calcium, serum, ionized	2.1–2.6 mEq./liter (4.25–5.25 mg./100 ml.)
Carbon dioxide content, serum	24–30 mEq./liter Infants: 20–28 mEq./liter
Carbon dioxide tension (Pco_2), blood	35–45 mm. Hg
Carotene, serum	50–300 mcg./100 ml.
Ceruloplasmin, serum	23–44 mg./100 ml.
Chloride, serum	96–106 mEq./liter
Cholesterol, serum	
Total	150–250 mg./100 ml.
Esters	68–76% of total cholesterol
Cholinesterase, serum	0.5–1.3 pH units
RBC	0.5–1.0 pH units
Copper, serum	
Male	70–140 mcg./100 ml.
Female	85–155 mcg./100 ml.
Cortisol, plasma	6–16 mcg./100 ml.
Creatine, serum	0.2–0.8 mg./100 ml.

Creatine phosphokinase, serum	
Male	0–50 mI.U./ml. (30°) (Oliver-Rosalki)
Female	0–30 mI.U./ml. (30°) (Oliver-Rosalki)
Creatinine, serum	0.7–1.5 mg./100 ml.
Cryoglobulins, serum	0
Fatty acids, total, serum	190–420 mg./100 ml.
Fibrinogen, plasma	200–400 mg./100 ml.
Folic acid, serum	7–16 nanogm./ml.
Glucose (fasting)	
blood	60–100 mg./100 ml.
plasma or serum	70–115 mg./100 ml.
Haptoglobin, serum	40–170 mg./100 ml.
Hydroxybutyric dehydrogenase, serum	0–180 mI.U./ml. (30°) (Rosalki-Wilkinson)
	114–290 units/ml. (Wroblewski)
17-Hydroxycorticosteroids, plasma	8–18 mcg./100 ml.
Immunoglobulins, serum	
IgG	800–1500 mg./100 ml.
IgA	50–200 mg./100 ml.
IgM	40–120 mg./100 ml.
Iodine, protein bound, serum	3.5–8.0 mcg./100 ml. (May be slightly higher in infants)
Iron, serum	75–175 mcg./100 ml.
Iron binding capacity, total, serum	250–410 mcg./100 ml.
% saturation	20–55%
17-Ketosteroids, plasma	25–125 mcg./100 ml.
Lactic acid, blood	6–16 mg./100 ml.
Lactic dehydrogenase, serum	0–300 mI.U./ml. (30°) (Wroblewski modified)
	150–450 units/ml. (Wroblewski)
	80–120 units/ml. (Wacker)
Lipase, serum	0–1.5 units (Cherry-Crandall)
Lipids, total, serum	450–850 mg./100 ml.

NORMAL BLOOD, PLASMA, AND SERUM VALUES (*Continued*)

Magnesium, serum	1.5–2.5 mEq./liter	
	(1.8–3.0 mg./100 ml.)	
Nitrogen, nonprotein, serum	15–35 mg./100 ml.	
Osmolality, serum	285–295 mOsm./liter	
Oxygen, blood		
Capacity	16–24 vol. % (varies with Hb)	
Content	Arterial	15–23 vol. %
	Venous	10–16 vol. %
Saturation	Arterial	94–100% of capacity
	Venous	60–85% of capacity
Tension, Po₂ Arterial	75–100 mm. Hg	
pH, arterial, blood	7.35–7.45	
Phenylalanine, serum	Less than 3 mg./100 ml.	
Phosphatase, acid, serum	1.0–5.0 units (King-Armstrong)	
	0.5–2.0 units (Bodansky)	
	0.5–2.0 units (Gutman)	
	0.0–1.1 units (Shinowara)	
	0.1–0.63 unit (Bessey-Lowry)	
Phosphatase, alkaline, serum	5.0–13.0 units (King-Armstrong)	
	2.0–4.5 units (Bodansky)	
	3.0–10.0 units (Gutman)	
	2.2–8.6 units (Shinowara)	
	0.8–2.3 units (Bassey-Lowry)	
	30–85 milliunits/ml. (I.U.)	
	(Values are higher in children)	
Phosphate, inorganic, serum	3.0–4.5 mg./100 ml.	
	(Children: 4.0–7.0 mg./100 ml.)	
Phospholipids, serum	6–12 mg./100 ml. as lipid phosphorus	
Potassium, serum	3.5–5.0 mEq./liter	
Proteins, serum		
Total	6.0–8.0 grams/100 ml.	
Albumin	3.5–5.5 grams/100 ml.	
Globulin	2.5–3.5 grams/100 ml.	
Electrophoresis		
Albumin	3.5–5.5 grams/100 ml.	
	52–68% of total	
Globulin		
Alpha₁	0.2–0.4 gram/100 ml.	
	2–5% of total	

Alpha₂	0.5–0.9 gram/100 ml.	
	7–14% of total	
Beta	0.6–1.1 grams/100 ml.	
	9–15% of total	
Gamma	0.7–1.7 grams/100 ml.	
	11–21% of total	
Pyruvic acid, plasma	1.0–2.0 mg./100 ml.	
Serotonin, platelet suspension	0.1–0.3 mcg./ml. blood	
serum	0.10–0.32 mcg./ml.	
Sodium, serum	136–145 mEq./liter	
Sulfates, inorganic, serum	0.8–1.2 mg./100 ml. (as S)	
Thyroxine, serum	4.6–11.2 mcg./100 ml.	
Thyroxine, free, serum	1.0–2.1 nanogm./100 ml.	
Thyroxine binding globulin		
(TBG), serum	16–26 mcg./100 ml.	
Thyroxine iodine (T₄), serum	2.9–6.4 mcg./100 ml.	
Transaminase, serum: SGOT	0–19 mI.U./ml. (30°)	
	(Karmen modified)	
	15–40 units/ml. (Karmen)	
	18–40 units/ml.	
	(Reitman-Frankel)	
SGPT	0.17 mI.U./ml. (30°)	
	(Karmen modified)	
	6–35 units/ml. (Karmen)	
	5–35 units/ml.	
	(Reitman-Frankel)	
Triglycerides, serum	0–150 mg./100 ml.	
Urea, blood	21–43 mg./100 ml.	
plasma or serum	24–49 mg./100 ml.	
Urea nitrogen, blood (BUN)	10–20 mg./100 ml.	
plasma or serum	11–23 mg./100 ml.	
Uric acid, serum		
Male	2.5–8.0 mg./100 ml.	
Female	1.5–6.0 mg./100 ml.	
Vitamin A, serum	20–80 mcg./100 ml.	
Vitamin B₁₂, serum	200–800 picogm./ml.	
Vitamin C, blood	0.4–1.5 mg./100 ml.	

NORMAL URINE VALUES

Acetone and acetoacetate	0		
Addis count			
Erythrocytes	0–130,000/24 hrs.		
Leukocytes	0–650,000/24 hrs.		
Casts (hyaline)	0–2000/24 hrs.		
Alcapton bodies	Negative		
Aldosterone	3–20 mcg./24 hrs.		
Amino acid nitrogen	50–200 mg./24 hrs.		
	(Not over 1.5% of total nitrogen)		
Ammonia nitrogen	20–70 mEq./24 hrs.		
Amylase	35–260 Somogyi units/hr.		
Bence Jones protein	Negative		
Bilirubin (bile)	Negative		
Calcium			
Low Ca diet (Bauer-Aub)	Less than 150 mg./24 hrs.		
Usual diet	Less than 250 mg./24 hrs.		
Catecholamines			
Epinephrine	Less than 10 mcg./24 hrs.		
Norepinephrine	Less than 100 mcg./24 hrs.		
Chloride	110–250 mEq./24 hrs.		
	(Varies with intake)		
Chorionic gonadotrophin	0		
Copper	0–30 mcg./24 hrs.		
Creatine			
Male	0–40 mg./24 hrs.		
Female	0–100 mg./24 hrs.		
	(Higher in children and during pregnancy)		
Creatinine	15–25 mg./kg. of body weight/24 hrs.		
Cystine or cysteine, qualitative	Negative		
Delta aminolevulinic acid	1.3–7.0 mg./24 hrs.		
Estrogens	Male	Female	
Estrone	3–8	4–31	
Estradiol	0–6	0–14	
Estriol	1–11	0–72	
Total	4–25	5–100	
	(Units above are mcg./24 hours.)		
	(Markedly increased during pregnancy)		
Glucose (reducing substances)	Less than 250 mg./24 hrs.		
Gonadotrophins, pituitary	5–10 rat units/24 hrs.		
	10–50 mouse units/24 hrs.		
	(Increased after menopause)		
Hemoglobin and myoglobin	Negative		
Homogentisic acid, qualitative	Negative		

17-Hydroxycorticosteroids		
Male	3–9 mg./24 hrs.	
Female	2–8 mg./24 hrs.	
	(Varies with method used)	
5-Hydroxyindole-acetic acid (5-HIAA)		
Qualitative	Negative	
Quantitative	Less than 16 mg./24 hrs.	
17-Ketosteroids		
Male	6–18 mg./24 hrs.	
Female	4–13 mg./24 hrs.	
Osmolality	38–1400 mOsm./kg. water	
pH	4.6–8.0, average 6.0	
	(Depends on diet)	
Phenylpyruvic acid, qualitative	Negative	
Phosphorus	0.9–1.3 gm./24 hrs.	
	(Varies with intake)	
Porphobilinogen		
Qualitative	Negative	
Quantitative	0–0.2 mg./100 ml.	
	Less than 2.0 mg./24 hrs.	
Porphyrins		
Coproporphyrin	50–250 mcg./24 hrs.	
Uroporphyrin	10–30 mcg./24 hrs.	
Potassium	25–100 mEq./24 hrs.	
	(Varies with intake)	
Pregnanetriol	Less than 2.5 mg./24 hrs. in adults	
Protein		
Qualitative	0	
Quantitative	10–150 mg./24 hrs.	
Sodium	130–260 mEq./24 hrs.	
	(Varies with intake)	
Solids, total	30–70 grams/liter, average	
	50 grams/liter	
	(To estimate total solids per liter, multiply last two figures of specific gravity by 2.66, Long's coefficient)	
Specific gravity	1.003–1.030	
Sugar	0	
Titratable acidity	20–40 mEq./24 hrs.	
Urobilinogen	Up to 1.0 Ehrlich unit/2 hrs. (1–3 P.M.)	
	0–4.0 mg./24 hrs.	
Vanillylmandelic acid (VMA)	1–8 mg./24 hrs.	

NORMAL LABORATORY VALUES

NORMAL VALUES FOR GASTRIC ANALYSIS

Basal gastric secretion (one hour)

	Concentration Mean ± 1 S.D.	Output Mean ± 1 S.D.
Male	25.8 ± 1.8 mEq./liter	2.57 ± 0.16 mEq./hr.
Female	20.3 ± 3.0 mEq./liter	1.61 ± 0.18 mEq./hr.

After histamine stimulation
Normal   Mean output = 11.8 mEq./hr.
Duodenal ulcer   Mean output = 15.2 mEq./hr.
After maximal histamine stimulation
Normal   Mean output   22.6 mEq./hr.
Duodenal ulcer   Mean output   44.6 mEq./hr.

Diagnex blue (Squibb):	Anacidity	0–0.3 mg. in 2 hrs.
	Doubtful	0.3–0.6 mg. in 2 hrs.
	Normal	Greater than 0.6 mg. in 2 hrs.
Volume, fasting stomach content		50–100 ml.
Emptying time		3–6 hrs.
Color		Opalescent or colorless
Specific gravity		1.006–1.009
pH (adults)		0.9–1.5

NORMAL VALUES FOR CEREBROSPINAL FLUID

Cells	Fewer than 5 cu. mm., all mononuclear
Chloride	120–130 mEq./liter
	(20 mEq./liter higher than serum)
Colloidal gold test	Not more than 1 in any tube
Glucose	50–75 mg./100 ml.
	(20 mg./100 ml. less than blood)
Pressure	70–180 mm. water

Protein, total	15–45 mg./100 ml.
Albumin	52%
Alpha$_1$ globulin	5%
Alpha$_2$ globulin	14%
Beta globulin	10%
Gamma globulin	19%

NORMAL VALUES FOR SEMEN

Volume	2–5 ml., usually 3–4 ml.
Liquefaction	Complete in 15 min.
pH	7.2–8.0; average 7.8
Leukocytes	Occasional or absent

Count	60–150 million/ml.
	Below 60 million/ml. is abnormal
Motility	80% or more motile
Morphology	80–90% normal forms

NORMAL VALUES FOR FECES

Bulk	100–200 grams/24 hrs.
Dry matter	23–32 grams/24 hrs.
Fat, total	Less than 6.0 grams/24 hrs.

Nitrogen, total	Less than 2.0 grams/24 hrs.
Urobilinogen	40–280 mg./24 hrs.
Water	Approximately 65%

NORMAL VALUES FOR SEROLOGIC PROCEDURES

Anti-hyaluronidase	Less than 1:200. Significant if rising titer can be demonstrated at weekly intervals.
Anti-streptolysin O titer	Normal up to 1:128. Single test usually has little significance. Rise in titer or persistently elevated titer is significant.
Bacterial agglutinins	Significant only if rise in titer is demonstrated or if antibodies are absent.
Complement fixation tests	Titers of 1:8 or less are usually not significant. Paired sera showing rise in titer of more than two tubes are usually considered significant.
C reactive protein (CRP)	Negative
Heterophile titer	Less than 1:56

Proteus OX-19 agglutinins	1:80	Negative
	1:160	Doubtful
	1:320	Positive
R. A. test (latex)	1:40	Negative
	1:80 –1:160	Doubtful
	1:320	Positive
Rose test	1:10	Negative
	1:20 –1:40	Doubtful
	1:80	Positive
Tularemia agglutinins	1:80	Negative
	1:160	Doubtful
	1:320	Positive

TOXICOLOGY

Arsenic, blood	3.5–7.2 mcg./100 ml.
Arsenic, urine	Less than 100 mcg./24 hrs.
Barbiturates, serum	0
	Coma level: Phenobarbital approximately 11 mg./100 ml.; most other barbiturates 1.5 mg./100 ml.
Bromides, serum	0
	Toxic levels above 17 mEq./liter
Carbon monoxide, blood	Up to 5% saturation
	Symptoms occur with 20% saturation
Dilantin, blood or serum	Therapeutic levels 1–11 mcg./ml.

Ethanol, blood	Less than 0.005%
Marked intoxication	0.3–0.4%
Alcoholic stupor	0.4–0.5%
Coma	Above 0.5%
Lead, blood	0–40 mcg./100 ml.
Lead, urine	Less than 100 mcg./24 hrs.
Lithium, serum	0
	Therapeutic levels 0.5–1.5 mEq./liter
	Toxic levels above 2 mEq./liter
Mercury, urine	Less than 10 mcg./24 hrs.
Salicylate, plasma	0
Therapeutic range	20–25 mg./100 ml.
Toxic range	Over 30 mg./100 ml.
Death	45–75 mg./100 ml.

OF CLINICAL IMPORTANCE (Continued)

LIVER FUNCTION TESTS

Bromsulphalein (B.S.P.)	Less than 5% remaining in serum 45 minutes after injection of 5 mg./kg. of body weight
Cephalin cholesterol flocculation	0–1 in 24 hours.
Galactose tolerance	Excretion of not more than 3.0 grams galactose in the urine 5 hours after ingestion of 40 grams of galactose.
Glycogen storage	Increase of blood glucose 45 mg./100 ml. over fasting level 45 minutes after subcutaneous injection of 0.01 mg./kg. body weight of epinephrine.

Hippuric acid	Excretion of 3.0–3.5 grams hippuric acid in urine within 4 hours after ingestion of 6.0 grams sodium benzoate,
	or
	Excretion of 0.7 gram hippuric acid in urine within 1 hour after intravenous injection of 1.77 grams sodium benzoate.
Thymol turbidity	0–5 units.
Zinc turbidity	2–12 units.

PANCREATIC (ISLET) FUNCTION TESTS

Glucose tolerance tests	Patient should be on a diet containing 300 grams of carbohydrate per day for 3 days prior to test.
Oral	After ingestion of 100 grams of glucose or 1.75 grams glucose/kg. body weight, blood glucose is not more than 160 mg./100 ml. after 60 minutes, 140 mg./100 ml. after 90 minutes, and 120 mg./100 ml. after 120 minutes. Values are for blood; serum measurements are approximately 15% higher.
Intravenous	Blood glucose does not exceed 200 mg./100 ml. after infusion of 0.5 gram of glucose/kg. body weight over 30 minutes. Glucose concentration falls below initial level at 2 hours and returns to preinfusion levels in 3 hours or 1 hour. Values are for blood; serum measurements are approximately 15% higher.

Cortisone-glucose tolerance test	The patient should be on a diet containing 300 grams of carbohydrate per day for 3 days prior to test. At 8½ and again 2 hours prior to glucose load patient is given cortisone acetate by mouth (50 mg. if patient's ideal weight is less than 160 lb., 62.5 mg. if ideal weight is greater than 160 lb.). An oral dose of glucose 1.75 grams/kg. body weight, is given and blood samples are taken at 0, 30, 60, 90, and 120 minutes. Test is considered positive if true blood glucose exceeds 160 mg./100 ml. at 60 minutes, 140 mg./100 ml. at 90 minutes, and 120 mg./100 ml. at 120 minutes. Values are for blood; serum measurements are approximately 15% higher.

RENAL FUNCTION TESTS

Clearance tests (corrected to 1.73 sq. meters body surface area)
Glomerular filtration rate (G.F.R.)

Inulin clearance, Mannitol clearance, or Endogenous creatinine clearance	Males	110–150 ml./min.
	Females	105–132 ml./min.

Renal plasma flow (R.P.F.)

p-Aminohippurate (P.A.H.), or Diodrast	Males	560–830 ml./min.
	Females	490–700 ml./min.

Filtration fraction (F.F.)

$$FF = \frac{G.F.R.}{R.P.F.}$$

	Males	17–21%
	Females	17–23%
Urea clearance (C_u)	Standard	40–65 ml./min.
	Maximal	60–100 ml./min.

Concentration and dilution	
Maximal Diodrast excretory capacity T_{M_D}	
Maximal glucose reabsorptive capacity T_{M_G}	
Maximal PAH excretory capacity $T_{M_{PAH}}$	
Phenolsulfonphthalein excretion (P.S.P.)	

	Specific gravity > 1.025 on dry day
	Specific gravity < 1.003 on water day
Males	43–59 mg./min.
Females	33–51 mg./min.
Males	300–450 mg./min.
Females	250–350 mg./min.
	80–90 mg./min.
	25% or more in 15 min.
	40% or more in 30 min.
	55% or more in 2 hrs.
	After injection of 1 ml. P.S.P. intravenously

THYROID FUNCTION TESTS

Protein bound iodine, serum (P.B.I.)	3.5–8.0 mcg./100 ml.
Thyroxine, serum	4.6–11.2 mcg./100 ml.
Thyroxine iodine, serum (T_4)	2.9–6.4 mcg./100 ml.
Free thyroxine	1.4–2.5 nanogram/100 ml.
T_3 (index of unsaturated T.B.G.)	10.0–14.6%
Thyroxine-binding globulin, serum (T.B.G.)	10–26 mcg. T_4/100 ml.
Thyroid-stimulating hormone, serum (T.S.H.)	0 up to 0.2 milliunits/ml.
Radioactive iodine (I^{131}) uptake (R.A.I.)	20–50% of administered dose in 24 hrs.

Radioactive iodine (I^{131}) excretion	30–70% of administered dose in 24 hrs.
Radioactive iodine (I^{131}), protein bound	Less than 0.3% of administered dose per liter of plasma at 72 hrs.

GASTROINTESTINAL ABSORPTION TESTS

d-Xylose absorption test	After an 8 hour fast 10 ml./kg. body weight of a 5% solution of d-xylose is given by mouth. Nothing further by mouth is given until the test has been completed. All urine voided during the following 5 hours is pooled, and blood samples are taken at 0, 60, and 120 minutes. Normally 26% (range 16–33%) of ingested xylose is excreted within 5 hours, and the serum xylose reaches a level between 25 and 40 mg./100 ml. after 1 hour and is maintained at this level for another 60 minutes.
Vitamin A absorption test	A fasting blood specimen is obtained and 200,000 units of vitamin A in oil is given by mouth. Serum vitamin A level should rise to twice fasting level in 3 to 5 hours.

REFERENCES

Castleman, B., and McNeeley, B. U.: N. Engl. J. Med., 290:39, 1974.
Davidsohn, I., and Henry, J. B.: Clinical Diagnosis by Laboratory Methods, 15th ed. Philadelphia, W. B. Saunders Company, 1974.
Department of Laboratory Medicine, The Johns Hopkins Hospital: Clinical Laboratory Handbook, Baltimore, July 1, 1975.
Henry, R. J., Cannon, D. C., and Winkleman, J. W.: Clinical Chemistry—Principles and Techniques, 2nd ed. New York, Harper & Row, 1974.
Long, C.: Biochemists' Handbook. Princeton, D. Van Nostrand Co., 1961.
Miale, J. B.: Laboratory Medicine—Hematology, 4th ed. St. Louis, The C. V. Mosby Co., 1972.
Miller, S. E., and Weller, J. M.: Textbook of Clinical Pathology, 8th ed. Baltimore, Williams & Wilkins Co., 1971.
Stewart, C. P., and Stolman, A.: Toxicology, Mechanisms and Analytic Methods. New York, Academic Press, 1960.
Sunderman, F. W., and Boerner, F.: Normal Values in Clinical Medicine. Philadelphia, W. B. Saunders Company, 1949.
Tietz, N. W.: Fundamentals of Clinical Chemistry, 2nd ed. Philadelphia, W. B. Saunders Co., 1976.
Wintrobe, M. M., Lee, G. R., Boggs, D. R., Bithell, T. C., Athens, J. W., and Foerster, J.: Clinical Hematology, 7th ed. Philadelphia, Lea & Febiger, 1974.

INDEX